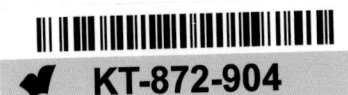

Oxford Textbook of
Medicine

VOLUME 1

Oxford Textbook of Medicine

FIFTH EDITION

Volume 1: Sections 1–12

Edited by

David A. Warrell

Emeritus Professor of Tropical Medicine, Nuffield Department of Clinical Medicine; Honorary Fellow, St Cross College, University of Oxford, Oxford, UK

Timothy M. Cox

Professor of Medicine, University of Cambridge; Honorary Consultant Physician, Addenbrooke's Hospital, Cambridge, UK

John D. Firth

Consultant Physician and Nephrologist, Addenbrooke's Hospital, Cambridge, UK

Sub-editor Immunological Mechanisms and Disorders of the Skin

Graham S. Ogg

Reader in Cutaneous Immunology, MRC Senior Clinical Fellow; Consultant in Dermatology, Churchill Hospital, Oxford, UK

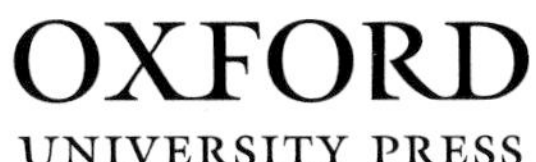

OXFORD
UNIVERSITY PRESS

Great Clarendon Street, Oxford OX2 6DP

Oxford University Press is a department of the University of Oxford.
It furthers the University's objective of excellence in research, scholarship,
and education by publishing worldwide in

Oxford New York

Auckland Cape Town Dar es Salaam Hong Kong Karachi
Kuala Lumpur Madrid Melbourne Mexico City Nairobi
New Delhi Shanghai Taipei Toronto

With offices in

Argentina Austria Brazil Chile Czech Republic France Greece
Guatemala Hungary Italy Japan Poland Portugal Singapore
South Korea Switzerland Thailand Turkey Ukraine Vietnam

Oxford is a registered trade mark of Oxford University Press
in the UK and in certain other countries

Published in the United States
by Oxford University Press Inc., New York

First edition published 1983
Second edition published 1987
Third edition published 1996
Fourth edition published 2003
Fifth edition published 2010

British Library Cataloguing in Publication Data
Data available

Library of Congress Cataloging in Publication Data
Data available

Typeset by Cepha Imaging Pvt. Ltd., Bangalore
Printed in Italy by LegoPrint s.p.A.

9780199204854 (three volume set)
volume 1: 9780199592852
volume 2: 9780199592869
volume 3: 9780199592876
Available as a three volume set only

1 3 5 7 9 10 8 6 4 2

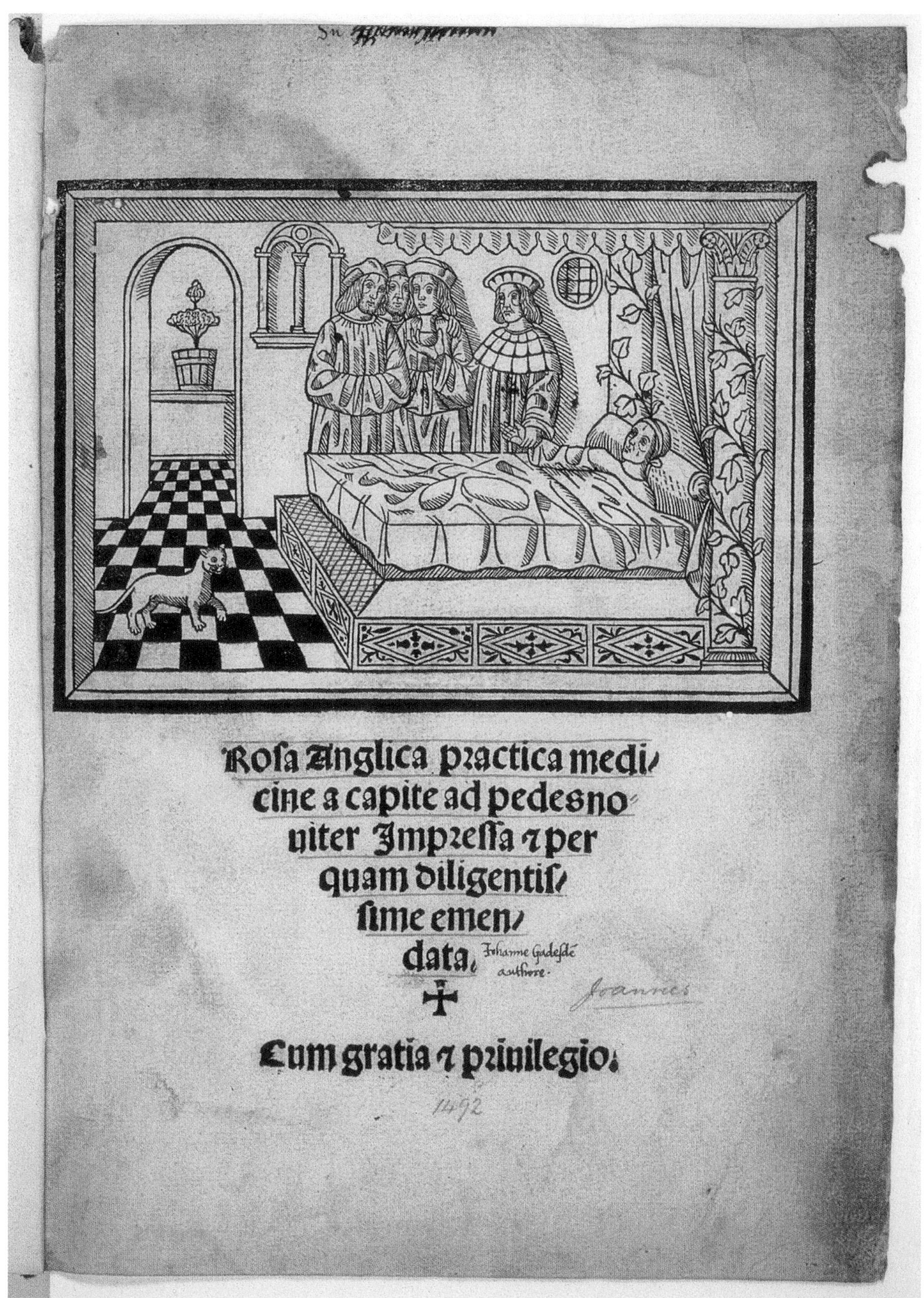

Rosa Anglica practica medicine a capite ad pedes no-
uiter Impressa ⁊ per
quam diligentis-
sime emen-
data.

Cum gratia ⁊ priuilegio.

The title page of the 1492 edition of *Rosa Anglica* by John of Gaddesden (1280–1361), which was probably written in 1314. The author was a well known physician attached to Merton College, Oxford in the early part of the 14th century. His famous book was probably the first 'Oxford Textbook of Medicine'. The author was the model for the unsavoury Doctor of Physick in Chaucer's *Canterbury Tales*.

Foreword

by Professor Sir Aaron Klug OM FRS

Since it first appeared 25 years ago, the *Oxford Textbook of Medicine* has established itself as an authoritative source for doctors to consult in everyday practice, particularly when questions arise outside their experience. The coverage is comprehensive and covers diseases and problems that occur anywhere in the world. It is very respected and has become a standard reference in the United Kingdom for journalists and for legal disputes in the courts.

In a book with such wide coverage, it is important for the practising physician to be able to find the topic of current interest speedily. The book seems to me to be less discursive than, say, *Harrison's Principles of Internal Medicine.* Indeed, the layout of the book is such that one can efficiently look up something specific. This is facilitated by a good index, with the right degree of cross-referencing.

The book begins with the basic biological science underlying medicine, cell and molecular biology, and the genomic basis of medicine. Despite these big issues, the text does not lose sight of the clinical implications of the science being presented, in keeping with the underlying philosophy of the book that the material must be of practical value to the physician. Thus the advances in understanding the modification of proteins by kinases, which add phosphate groups to selected amino acids, has led to the development of chemical inhibitors of the kinases. An example of such a successful designer drug is imatinib for chronic myologenous leukaemia.

A totally new modality for the treatment has appeared in recent years, namely monoclonal antibodies with high selectivity against protein targets. Originally developed in mice, they could not be used in patients because of the anaphylactic response to a foreign protein, but over the years they have been 'humanized', i.e. their relatively small, specific antigen- or immunogen-recognition regions have been fused to a human framework, which make up most of the antibody. Examples include palivizumab, against respiratory syncytial virus, and bevacizumab, against colorectal cancer, now in widespread use. Even more striking is the development of fully human antibodies, synthesized out of the cloned repertoire of the human genes making up the constituent antibody domains. The antibody adalimumab, released a few years ago, not only relieves the pain of rheumatoid arthritis, but also stops the progress of the disease.

These new modalities are of course costly, as are many of the new anticancer drugs such as Herceptin: their introduction is changing the setting in which medicine is practised, particularly in the United Kingdom where the National Health Service (NHS) is free at the point of delivery, and in the United States of America where the Health Maintenance Organizations (HMOs) are insurance based. As recognized by David Weatherall in his foreword to the fourth edition of this textbook, none of the richer countries has got to grips with the problem of financing the increasing number and costs of new treatments. In the United Kingdom where the decision to allow the use of a licensed drug is made by the local Health Authority, there is no uniformity of practice, so leading to the term 'postcode availability' of a drug. There is also the question of individuals receiving treatment under the NHS but wishing to top up privately with other or new drugs not available under the NHS. Despite much controversy, this practice has recently been allowed by the NHS.

Another issue likely to arise out of the sequencing of the human genome is the prospect of personalized and preventive medicine. This is fast becoming a potential reality with the decreasing cost of rapid DNA sequencing to determine an individual genome. The supporting clinical data to interpret individual susceptibility to disease is likely to come from 'genome-wide association' studies. These represent a powerful approach to the identification of genetic variations involved in common human diseases. In 2007, there appeared in the journal *Nature* a genomic study of seven common diseases, including coronary artery disease, type 1 and type 2 diabetes, hypertension, and bipolar disorders. This large study involved 14 000 cases and 3000 shared controls. Similar studies have been carried out in several forms of cancer. The association of a particular locus in the genome with a disease is still very modest. The overall increase in risk conferred by the genetic factors identified is of the order of 1.2- to 1.5-fold, and so thus far does not provide a clinically useful prediction of disease. But the work must be recognized as an important first step towards dissecting the genomic basis of common diseases. By the time of the next edition of the *Oxford Textbook of Medicine,* we may well see the results of these powerful genomic tools becoming available or already in use.

Preface

"Naught for your comfort"

Trevor Huddleston

The fruits of medical research

Publication of this new edition of the *Oxford Textbook of Medicine* prompts consideration of the precepts and practices of medicine in a world that faces unprecedented challenges. There is much to celebrate, and—with many new contributors—we have sought throughout the book to reflect the revolutionary effects of discovery in the medical sciences on clinical practice. Spectacular advances have been made at the most fundamental level and these continue to inspire our belief that improved prevention, diagnosis and treatment of disease will eventually relieve suffering. The popular term, 'translational medicine', reflects the shared optimism of many research agencies.

The Fifth edition has been rigorously revised and updated. It differs most blatantly from previous editions in having the gift of colour throughout and the inclusion of 'Essentials' (mostly written and all edited by John Firth) that summarize the main points of each chapter. The introductory Sections 2 and 3 include eight new chapters on topics ranging from the future of clinical trials, the evaluation and provision of effective medicines, to health promotion. This expansion reflects the ever burgeoning successes, constraints and frustrations of modern medicine. New sciences like stem cell biology, and emerging pathogens such as SARS, H1N1 and drug-resistant bacteria and malaria parasites, are well represented in our pages, and we have introduced some highly topical themes, notably Darwinian Medicine and the context of Human Disasters

Darwinian Medicine

Evolutionary medicine has a firm place in this book (Randolph Nesse and Richard Dawkins—Evolution: medicine's most basic science—Chapter 2.1.2), consistent with the 200th anniversary of Charles Darwin's birth and the 150th anniversary of the publication of *On the Origin of Species* in 2009. Darwin's remarkable synthesis (subtended in part by Gregor Mendel's later discoveries in heredity) has salient implications for understanding disease, rendering outmoded the crude analogy of the diseased body as a 'broken machine'. Much illness results from conflict between a person and the external influences to which he or she is uniquely maladapted at a particular time. Given that genetic and environmental variations are biological characteristics, the evolutionary concept has profound implications for any full description and understanding of disease. But while we have prodigious methods for determining genetic variation, our ability to measure environmental changes and interactions—or predict environmental disasters—is rudimentary.

Human disasters: political, sociological, and historical context

Human populations are dependent on the natural environment for food and water but exquisitely vulnerable to its storms, earthquakes and tsunamis. As demonstrated by one of our Nobel Laureate authors, Amartya Sen (Human disasters—Chapter 3.5), the effects of natural disasters are, irrespective of their origin, invariably magnified by dire socioeconomic circumstances resulting from human conquest. An agonising recent example was the seismic horror in Haiti, affecting a society dysfunctional and impoverished as an historical consequence of the European slave trade and more recent political interferences. Such disasters, including those attributable to wars, are also the province of medicine: in such catastrophes, doctors are needed to provide emergency treatment but, through proper involvement with governments, they are also critical for public health planning and the restoration of appropriate infrastructure and clinical services. In response to another human tragedy, the AIDS pandemic, and to mounting pressure on the industry, one of the world's largest pharmaceutical companies has recently agreed to cut the prices of its medicines in the poorest countries and to donate some of its profits to local hospitals and clinics. This initiative might be a bit late but is a significant first step taking other 'Big Pharmas' in a direction that improves access to treatments for stricken patients in poor countries.

The teaching and practice of medicine: a fine tradition betrayed

Irrespective of the political dimension of medicine, the care of patients and the prevention of disease depend on practising clinicians; the medicine of the future relies not only on scientific advances but on the education of doctors. Since the last edition, leaders of our profession in Britain have presided over, and in some cases acquiesced to the partial dismantling of arguably one of the finest systems of medical education. The implementation of a national process for the appointment of junior doctors has disaffected many trainees and their clinical mentors, who feel that they have become pawns in a bureaucratic political game. More important, if they understood the full implications, we believe that the British public and patients would be horrified. Within Europe, matters have been compounded by implementation of the European Working Time Directive, which threatens the professional apprenticeship and mentoring relationships between junior and senior doctors that best nurture young colleagues. The frequently heard mantra of the 'consultant-led service' is all very well, but the ideal will be short-lived if training is put in jeopardy.

We, the editors of this textbook, learnt how to practise as clinicians from such 'hands-on' apprenticeships and ask: how can young doctors accumulate adequate working knowledge and acquire essential skills if their clinical work is restricted to 48 hours each week? One might pose the question: would a patient prefer to be treated by a fully rested but inexperienced doctor whom they had never seen before, or a tired doctor with immense medical experience who knew them and their illness? We know whom we would prefer, as does Christopher Booth (On being a patient—Chapter 1.1). Short hours and other radical changes in the organization of clinical teams impair the continuity of medical care, an element of key importance for the patient but also critical for clinical education through time-honoured individual experience. Many countries are seeking to improve their systems of medical education, but for those who might consider adopting the current UK training timetables, we humbly offer advice—don't. It would be better to provide their medical students and young doctors with sufficient time and resources to acquaint themselves with the principles and practice of modern scientific medicine that are emphasized in this book.

Decline and fall of clinical trials evidence

How the profession responds to these old and new threats to the practice of medicine will influence the translation of new knowledge and scientific understanding into clinical benefit. Our contemporary environment is contaminated by countless man-made chemicals, including drugs and other medicinal products: many of the latter have untested effects on human health. One foundation of good practice is the evidence provided by clinical trials, but this is under threat from powerful self-interest groups. On one hand are those promoting alternative and so-called traditional treatments, which are ineffective and supported at best by what Robert Park has termed 'Voodoo Science', and who mount sustained attacks on anyone who might be brave enough to say so, including one of our authors, Edzard Ernst (Complementary and alternative medicine—Chapter 2.5). On the other hand are those who promote expensive health care, of which they take a financial cut: scaremongering occurs at every opportunity, and with the intensity that only billions of dollars can bring. Already most clinical trials are sponsored by pharmaceutical companies and instances where prompt release of all the results has been suppressed for commercial reasons continue to scandalize the profession.

Clinical trials require proper regulation, but burgeoning bureaucracy has become disproportionate; it is stifling the discipline and greatly discourages investigator-led clinical trials. Yet another vacuous meta-analysis, performed in the absence of sufficient data and therefore allowing of no conclusions, will be no substitute. We plead also for simplification of the legal and regulatory framework in which therapeutic trials and medical research can be conducted by individual doctors; for without the freedom ethically to test hypotheses prompted by the immediacy of clinical necessity, many imaginative advances will be thwarted.

Inalienable personal liberty versus the public good

The tension between the right to personal liberty and the desire for public good is ever more acute and is manifest in many ways. For the world as whole, population control (or lack thereof), is the most pressing issue. Even when we thought medicine might have solved a problem, the activities of the anti-vaccination lobby that resulted in the anti-MMR scandal reminded us that old battles sometimes need to be fought again. Many people in diverse populations are suffering because of this phenomenon and from the misguided public assessment of risk and disregard for specialist advice.

Bureaucratic targets

Well chosen targets are a good way of managing complex systems, but there is grave danger when those who set targets for clinical practice are intrinsically suspicious of doctors, take very selective advice, choose inappropriate limits, and compound the error by specifying crude and inappropriate mechanisms by which they should be achieved. What is being measured becomes of overwhelming importance, and the patient with the most pressing clinical need may not get the priority that he or she deserves. Many will suffer unless this state of affairs is remedied.

The future

Against a background of such uncertainty, we believe that sound clinical experience, combined with knowledge of the subject, based on authoritative books and peer-reviewed publications, remain the rocks upon which clinical management is based. The doctor whom doctors want to see, when they or their family are ill, is the one they recognize as having great knowledge, great experience, and good judgement, of patients and their disease. We have asked such doctors to write for this book, so that it will be of most value to those seeking a 'higher medicine'. Despite the many adverse factors detailed above, we are reassured that many bright young men and women training in medicine are motivated, hungry for knowledge, and prepared to challenge dogma in the struggle to provide the best care for their patients. We trust that this edition of the book hits the mark and will help those who use it to achieve this aim.

Our debts

This edition is a tribute to our long-suffering but ever-patient contributors who, faced by delays in publication, had to update their work or risk instant obsolescence.

We remember with gratitude seven authors who have died since publication of the 4th edition, but who contributed to the present edition, Richard S. Doll (Chapter 6.1), Ernest Beutler (Chapter 22.5.11), Philip A. Poole-Wilson (Chapter 16.1.2), Pauline de la Motte Hall (Chapter 15.22.7), Peter ('PK') Thomas (Chapter 24.16),

M. Monir Madkour (Chapter 7.6.21), and Richard Edwards (Chapter 24.24.4). Sir Richard S. Doll, who died in 2005, a giant of Oxford and World Medicine and a marvellous friend and inspiration to many, was a great supporter of this book. As a guest of the popular radio programme 'Desert Island Discs', he delighted us by choosing the *Oxford Textbook of Medicine* for his reading material.

Graham S. Ogg contributed his special skills and experience to the planning and editing of the sections on Immunological mechanisms and Disorders of the skin for which we are most grateful. We thank our wives, Mary, Sue, and Helen, and dedicated secretaries, Eunice Berry and Joan Grantham. In the publication team, we are particularly grateful to Helen Liepman, Anna Winstanley, Kate Wilson, Kathleen Lyle, and Aparna Shankar.

David A. Warrell
Timothy M. Cox
John D. Firth

Oxford and Cambridge
February 2010

Contents

Volume 1

Contributors *xxxi*

SECTION 1
On being a patient

1.1 **On being a patient** *3*
Christopher Booth

SECTION 2
Modern medicine: foundations, achievements, and limitations

2.1 **Scientific background to medicine** *9*
2.1.1 Science in medicine: when, how, and what *9*
W.F. Bynum
2.1.2 Evolution: medicine's most basic science *12*
Randolph M. Nesse and Richard Dawkins

2.2 **Medical ethics** *16*
Tony Hope

2.3 **Evidence-based medicine** *22*
2.3.1 Bringing the best evidence to the point of care *22*
Paul P. Glasziou
2.3.2 Evidence-based medicine—does it apply to my particular patient? *27*
Louis R. Caplan
2.3.3 Large-scale randomized evidence: trials and meta-analyses of trials *31*
C. Baigent, R. Peto, R. Gray, S. Parish, and R. Collins
2.3.4 The future of clinical trials *45*
Perry Nisen and Patrick Vallance

2.4 **Funding of health care** *48*
2.4.1 The evaluation and provision of effective medicines *48*
Michael D. Rawlins
2.4.2 Reasonableness and its definition in the provision of health care *54*
Norman Daniels
2.4.3 Priority setting in developed and developing countries *58*
Nigel Crisp
2.4.4 Sustaining innovation in an era of specialized medicine *60*
Henri A. Termeer

2.5 **Complementary and alternative medicine** *65*
E. Ernst

SECTION 3
Global patterns of disease and medical practice

3.1 **Global burden of disease: causes, levels, and intervention strategies** *73*
Ramanan Laxminarayan and Dean Jamison

3.2 **Human population size, environment, and health** *80*
A.J. McMichael and J.W. Powles

3.3 **Avoiding disease and promoting health** *86*
3.3.1 Preventive medicine *86*
David Mant
3.3.2 Medical screening *94*
Nicholas Wald and Malcolm Law

3.3.3 The importance of mass communication in promoting positive health *108*
Thomas Lom

3.4 Influence of wealth *112*

3.4.1 The cost of health care in Western countries *112*
Joseph White

3.4.2 A sinister pathogen corrupts two disciplines: the demographic entrapment of Middle Africa *116*
Maurice King

3.5 Human disasters *119*
Amartya Sen

SECTION 4
Cell biology

4.1 The cell *127*
George Banting

4.2 Molecular biology *135*

4.2.1 The human genome sequence *135*
Sydney Brenner

4.2.2 The genomic basis of medicine *136*
Paweł Stankiewicz and James R. Lupski

4.3 Cytokines *152*
Iain B. McInnes

4.4 Ion channels and disease *160*
Frances M. Ashcroft

4.5 Intracellular signalling *169*
R. Andres Floto

4.6 Apoptosis in health and disease *177*
Andrew H. Wyllie and Mark J. Arends

4.7 Discovery of embryonic stem cells and the concept of regenerative medicine *189*
Martin J. Evans

4.8 Stem cells and regenerative medicine *193*
Alexis J. Joannides, Roger Pedersen, and Siddharthan Chandran

SECTION 5
Immunological mechanisms
Editor: Graham S. Ogg

5.1 Structure and function *207*

5.1.1 The innate immune system *207*
Paul Bowness

5.1.2 The complement system *213*
Marina Botto and Mark J. Walport

5.1.3 Adaptive immunity *224*
Paul Klenerman

5.2 Immunodeficiency *235*
D. Kumararatne

5.3 Allergy *258*
Pamela Ewan

5.4 Autoimmunity *267*
Antony Rosen

5.5 Principles of transplantation immunology *280*
Ross S. Francis and Kathryn J. Wood

SECTION 6
Principles of clinical oncology

6.1 Epidemiology of cancer *299*
A.J. Swerdlow, R. Peto, and Richard S. Doll

6.2 The nature and development of cancer *333*
John R. Benson and Siong-Seng Liau

6.3 The genetics of inherited cancers *358*
Rosalind A. Eeles

6.4 Cancer immunity and clinical oncology *372*
Maries van den Broek, Lotta von Boehmer, Kunle Odunsi, and Alexander Knuth

6.5 Cancer: clinical features and management *380*
R.L. Souhami

6.6 Cancer chemotherapy and radiation therapy *396*
Bruce A. Chabner and Jay Loeffler

SECTION 7
Infection

7.1 Pathogenic microorganisms and the host *409*

7.1.1 Biology of pathogenic microorganisms *409*
Duncan J. Maskell

7.1.2 Physiological changes, clinical features, and general management of infected patients *413*
Todd W. Rice and Gordon R. Bernard

7.2 The patient with suspected infection *420*

7.2.1 Clinical approach *420*
Christopher J. Ellis

7.2.2 Fever of unknown origin *423*
Steven Vanderschueren and Daniël Knockaert

7.2.3 Nosocomial infections *428*
I.C.J.W. Bowler

7.2.4 Infection in the immunocompromised host *431*
J. Cohen

7.2.5 Antimicrobial chemotherapy *441*
R.G. Finch

7.3 Immunization *460*
D. Goldblatt and M. Ramsay

7.4 Travel and expedition medicine *465*
C.P. Conlon and David A. Warrell

7.5 Viruses *472*

7.5.1 Respiratory tract viruses *473*
Malik Peiris

7.5.2 Herpesviruses (excluding Epstein–Barr virus) *482*
J.G.P. Sissons

7.5.3 Epstein–Barr virus *501*
M.A. Epstein and A.B. Rickinson

7.5.4 Poxviruses *508*
Geoffrey L. Smith

7.5.5 Mumps: epidemic parotitis *513*
B.K. Rima

7.5.6 Measles *515*
H.C. Whittle and P. Aaby

7.5.7 Nipah and Hendra virus encephalitides *525*
C.T. Tan

7.5.8 Enterovirus infections *527*
Philip Minor and Ulrich Desselberger

7.5.9 Virus infections causing diarrhoea and vomiting *536*
Philip Dormitzer and Ulrich Desselberger

7.5.10 Rhabdoviruses: rabies and rabies-related lyssaviruses *541*
M. J. Warrell and David A. Warrell

7.5.11 Colorado tick fever and other arthropod-borne reoviruses *555*
M.J. Warrell and David A. Warrell

7.5.12 Alphaviruses *557*
L.R. Petersen and D.J. Gubler

7.5.13 Rubella *561*
P.A. Tookey and J.M. Best

7.5.14 Flaviviruses excluding dengue *564*
L.R. Petersen and D.J. Gubler

7.5.15 Dengue *575*
Bridget Wills and Jeremy Farrar

7.5.16 Bunyaviridae *579*
J.W. LeDuc and Summerpal S. Kahlon

7.5.17 Arenaviruses *588*
J. ter Meulen

7.5.18 Filoviruses *595*
J. ter Meulen

7.5.19 Papillomaviruses and polyomaviruses *600*
Raphael P. Viscidi and Keerti V. Shah

7.5.20 Parvovirus B19 *607*
Kevin E. Brown

7.5.21 Hepatitis viruses (excluding hepatitis C virus) *609*
N.V. Naoumov

7.5.22 Hepatitis C *615*
Paul Klenerman, K.J.M. Jeffery, and J. Collier

7.5.23 HIV/AIDS *620*
Graz A. Luzzi, T.E.A. Peto, P. Goulder, and C.P. Conlon

7.5.24 HIV in the developing world *644*
Alison D. Grant and Kevin M. De Cock

7.5.25 HTLV-1, HTLV-2, and associated diseases *650*
Kristien Verdonck and Eduardo Gotuzzo

7.5.26 Viruses and cancer *653*
R.A. Weiss

7.5.27 Orf *655*
David A. Warrell

7.5.28 Molluscum contagiosum *657*
David A. Warrell

7.5.29 Newly discovered viruses *659*
H.C. Hughes

7.6 Bacteria *663*

7.6.1 Diphtheria *664*
Delia B. Bethell and Tran Tinh Hien

7.6.2 Streptococci and enterococci *670*
Dennis L. Stevens

7.6.3 Pneumococcal infections *679*
Anthony Scott

7.6.4 Staphylococci *693*
Bala Hota and Robert A. Weinstein

7.6.5 Meningococcal infections *709*
P. Brandtzaeg

7.6.6 *Neisseria gonorrhoeae* *722*
D. Barlow, Jackie Sherrard, and C. Ison

7.6.7 Enterobacteria *727*

7.6.7.1 Enterobacteria and bacterial food poisoning 727
Hugh Pennington

7.6.7.2 *Pseudomonas aeruginosa* 735
G.C.K.W. Koh and S.J. Peacock

7.6.8 Typhoid and paratyphoid fevers *738*
C.M. Parry and Buddha Basnyat

7.6.9 Intracellular klebsiella infections (donovanosis and rhinoscleroma) *745*
J. Richens

7.6.10 Anaerobic bacteria *748*
Anilrudh A. Venugopal and David W. Hecht

7.6.11 Cholera *754*
Aldo A.M. Lima and Richard L. Guerrant

7.6.12 *Haemophilus influenzae* *759*
Derrick W. Crook

7.6.13 *Haemophilus ducreyi* and chancroid *763*
Nigel O'Farrell

7.6.14 Bordetella infection *764*
Cameron Grant

7.6.15 Melioidosis and glanders *768*
S.J. Peacock

7.6.16 Plague: *Yersinia pestis* *772*
Michael B. Prentice

7.6.17 Other *Yersinia* infections: yersiniosis *776*
Michael B. Prentice

7.6.18 Pasteurella *777*
Marina S. Morgan

7.6.19 *Francisella tularensis* infection *780*
Petra C.F. Oyston

7.6.20 Anthrax *783*
Arthur E. Brown and Thira Sirisanthana

7.6.21 Brucellosis *789*
M. Monir Madkour

7.6.22 Tetanus *795*
C.L. Thwaites and Lam Minh Yen

7.6.23 *Clostridium difficile* *800*
John G. Bartlett

7.6.24 Botulism, gas gangrene, and clostridial gastrointestinal infections *803*
Dennis L. Stevens, Michael J. Aldape, and Amy E. Bryant

7.6.25 Tuberculosis *810*
Richard E. Chaisson and Jean B. Nachega

7.6.26 Disease caused by environmental mycobacteria *831*
J.M. Grange and P.D.O. Davies

7.6.27 Leprosy (Hansen's disease) *836*
Diana N.J. Lockwood

7.6.28 Buruli ulcer: *Mycobacterium ulcerans* infection *848*
Wayne M. Meyers and Françoise Portaels

7.6.29 Actinomycoses *850*
K.P. Schaal

7.6.30 Nocardiosis *856*
Roderick J. Hay

7.6.31 Rat-bite fevers *857*
David A. Warrell

7.6.32 Lyme borreliosis *860*
Gary P. Wormser, John Nowakowski, and Robert B. Nadelman

7.6.33 Relapsing fevers *866*
David A. Warrell

7.6.34 Leptospirosis *874*
George Watt

7.6.35 Nonvenereal endemic treponematoses: yaws, endemic syphilis (bejel), and pinta *879*
David A. Warrell

7.6.36 Syphilis *885*
Basil Donovan and Linda Dayan

7.6.37 Listeriosis *896*
H. Hof

7.6.38 Legionellosis and legionnaires' disease *899*
J.T. Macfarlane and T.C. Boswell

7.6.39 Rickettsioses *903*
Philippe Parola and Didier Raoult

7.6.40 Scrub typhus *919*
George Watt

7.6.41 *Coxiella burnetii* infections (Q fever) *923*
T.J. Marrie

7.6.42 Bartonellas excluding *B. bacilliformis* *926*
Emmanouil Angelakis, Didier Raoult, and Jean-Marc Rolain

7.6.43 *Bartonella bacilliformis* infection *934*
A. Llanos-Cuentas and C. Maguiña-Vargas

7.6.44 Chlamydial infections *939*
David Taylor-Robinson and David Mabey

7.6.45 Mycoplasmas *950*
David Taylor-Robinson and Jørgen Skov Jensen

7.6.46 A check list of bacteria associated with infection in humans *961*
J. Paul

7.7 Fungi (mycoses) *998*

7.7.1 Fungal infections *998*
Roderick J. Hay

7.7.2 Cryptococcosis *1018*
William G. Powderly

7.7.3 Coccidioidomycosis *1020*
Gregory M. Anstead and John R. Graybill

7.7.4 Paracoccidioidomycosis *1023*
M.A. Shikanai-Yasuda

7.7.5 *Pneumocystis jirovecii* *1028*
Robert F. Miller and Laurence Huang

7.7.6 *Penicillium marneffei* infection *1032*
Thira Sirisanthana

7.8 Protozoa *1035*

7.8.1 Amoebic infections *1035*
Richard Knight

7.8.2 Malaria *1045*
David A. Warrell, Janet Hemingway, Kevin Marsh, Robert E. Sinden, Geoffrey A. Butcher, and Robert W. Snow

7.8.3 Babesiosis *1089*
Philippe Brasseur

7.8.4 Toxoplasmosis *1090*
Oliver Liesenfeld and Eskild Petersen

7.8.5 *Cryptosporidium* and cryptosporidiosis *1098*
S.M. Cacciò

7.8.6 *Cyclospora* and cyclosporiasis *1105*
R. Lainson

7.8.7 Sarcocystosis (sarcosporidiosis) *1109*
John E. Cooper

7.8.8 Giardiasis, balantidiasis, isosporiasis, and microsporidiosis *1111*
Martin F. Heyworth

7.8.9 *Blastocystis hominis* infection *1118*
Richard Knight

7.8.10 Human African trypanosomiasis *1119*
August Stich

7.8.11 Chagas disease *1127*
M.A. Miles

7.8.12 Leishmaniasis *1134*
A.D.M. Bryceson and Diana N.J. Lockwood

7.8.13 Trichomoniasis *1142*
Sharon Hillier

7.9 Nematodes (roundworms) *1145*

7.9.1 Cutaneous filariasis *1145*
Gilbert Burnham

7.9.2 Lymphatic filariasis *1153*
Richard Knight and D.H. Molyneux

7.9.3 Guinea worm disease (dracunculiasis) *1160*
Richard Knight

7.9.4 Strongyloidiasis, hookworm, and other gut strongyloid nematodes *1163*
Michael Brown

7.9.5 Gut and tissue nematode infections acquired by ingestion *1168*
David I. Grove

7.9.6 Parastrongyliasis (angiostrongyliasis) *1179*
Richard Knight

7.9.7 Gnathostomiasis *1182*
Valai Bussaratid and Pravan Suntharasamai

7.10 Cestodes (tapeworms) *1185*

7.10.1 Cystic hydatid disease (*Echinococcus granulosus*) *1185*
Armando E. Gonzalez, Pedro L. Moro, and Hector H. Garcia

7.10.2 Cyclophyllidian gut tapeworms *1188*
Richard Knight

7.10.3 Cysticercosis *1193*
Hector H. Garcia and Robert H. Gilman

7.10.4 Diphyllobothriasis and sparganosis *1199*
David I. Grove

7.11 Trematodes (flukes) *1202*

7.11.1 Schistosomiasis *1202*
D.W. Dunne and B.J. Vennervald

7.11.2 Liver fluke infections *1212*
David I. Grove

7.11.3 Lung flukes (paragonimiasis) *1216*
Udomsak Silachamroon and Sirivan Vanijanonta

7.11.4 Intestinal trematode infections *1219*
David I. Grove

7.12 Nonvenomous arthropods *1225*
J. Paul

7.13 Pentastomiasis (porocephalosis, linguatulosis/linguatuliasis) *1237*
David A. Warrell

SECTION 8
Sexually transmitted diseases and sexual health

8.1 Epidemiology of sexually transmitted infections *1243*
David Mabey

8.2 Sexual behaviour *1250*
Anne M. Johnson and Catherine H. Mercer

8.3 Sexual history and examination *1253*
Jackie Sherrard and Graz A. Luzzi

8.4 Vaginal discharge *1256*
Paul Nyirjesy

8.5 Pelvic inflammatory disease *1259*
David Eschenbach

8.6 Principles of contraception *1262*
John Guillebaud

SECTION 9
Chemical and physical injuries and environmental factors and disease

9.1 Poisoning by drugs and chemicals *1271*
J.A. Vale, S.M. Bradberry, and D.N. Bateman

9.2 Injuries, envenoming, poisoning, and allergic reactions caused by animals *1324*
David A. Warrell

9.3 Injuries, poisoning, and allergic reactions caused by plants *1361*

9.3.1 Poisonous plants and fungi *1361*
Hans Persson

9.3.2 Common Indian poisonous plants *1371*
V.V. Pillay

9.4 Occupational health and safety *1376*

9.4.1 Occupational and environmental health *1376*
J.M. Harrington and Raymond M. Agius

9.4.2 Occupational safety *1388*
Lawrence Waterman

9.5 Environmental diseases *1393*

9.5.1 Heat *1393*
M.A. Stroud

9.5.2 Cold *1395*
M.A. Stroud

9.5.3 Drowning *1397*
Peter J. Fenner

9.5.4 Diseases of high terrestrial altitudes *1402*
Andrew J. Pollard, Buddha Basnyat, and David R. Murdoch

9.5.5 Aerospace medicine *1408*
D.M. Denison and M. Bagshaw

9.5.6 Diving medicine *1416*
D.M. Denison and M.A. Glover

9.5.7 Lightning and electrical injuries *1422*
Chris Andrews

9.5.8 Podoconiosis (nonfilarial elephantiasis) *1426*
Gail Davey

9.5.9 Radiation *1429*
Jill Meara

9.5.10 Noise *1432*
Syed M. Ahmed and Tar-Ching Aw

9.5.11 Vibration *1434*
Tar-Ching Aw

9.5.12 Disasters: earthquakes, volcanic eruptions, hurricanes, and floods *1436*
Peter J. Baxter

9.5.13 Bioterrorism *1440*
Manfred S. Green

SECTION 10
Clinical pharmacology

10.1 Principles of clinical pharmacology and drug therapy *1449*
Kevin O'Shaughnessy

SECTION 11
Nutrition

11.1 Nutrition: macronutrient metabolism *1479*
Keith N. Frayn

11.2 Vitamins and trace elements *1487*
J. Powell-Tuck and M. Eastwood

11.3 Severe malnutrition *1505*
Alan A. Jackson

11.4 Diseases of overnourished societies and the need for dietary change *1515*
J.I. Mann and A.S. Truswell

11.5 Obesity *1527*
I. Sadaf Farooqi

11.6 Artificial nutrition support *1535*
Jeremy Woodward

SECTION 12
Metabolic disorders

12.1 The inborn errors of metabolism: general aspects *1549*
Richard W.E. Watts and Timothy M. Cox

12.2 Protein-dependent inborn errors of metabolism *1559*
Georg F. Hoffmann and Stefan Kölker

12.3 Disorders of carbohydrate metabolism *1596*

12.3.1 Glycogen storage diseases *1596*
Philip Lee and Kaustuv Bhattacharya

12.3.2 Inborn errors of fructose metabolism *1604*
Timothy M. Cox

12.3.3 Disorders of galactose, pentose, and pyruvate metabolism *1610*
Timothy M. Cox

12.4 Disorders of purine and pyrimidine metabolism *1619*
Richard W.E. Watts

12.5 The porphyrias *1636*
Timothy M. Cox

12.6 Lipid and lipoprotein disorders *1652*
P.N. Durrington

12.7 Trace metal disorders *1673*

12.7.1 Hereditary haemochromatosis *1673*
William J.H. Griffiths and Timothy M. Cox

12.7.2 Inherited diseases of copper metabolism: Wilson's disease and Menkes' disease *1688*
Michael L. Schilsky and Pramod K. Mistry

12.8 Lysosomal disease *1694*
P.B. Deegan and Timothy M. Cox

12.9 Disorders of peroxisomal metabolism in adults *1719*
Anthony S. Wierzbicki

12.10 Hereditary disorders of oxalate metabolism—the primary hyperoxalurias *1730*
Christopher J. Danpure and Dawn S. Milliner

12.11 Disturbances of acid–base homeostasis *1738*
R.D. Cohen and H.F. Woods

12.12 The acute phase response, amyloidoses and familial Mediterranean fever *1752*

12.12.1 The acute phase response and C-reactive protein *1752*
M.B. Pepys

12.12.2 Hereditary periodic fever syndromes *1760*
Helen J. Lachmann and Philip N. Hawkins

12.12.3 Amyloidosis *1766*
M.B. Pepys and Philip N. Hawkins

12.13 α_1-Antitrypsin deficiency and the serpinopathies *1780*
David A. Lomas

Index

Volume 2

Contributors *xxxi*

SECTION 13
Endocrine disorders

13.1 Principles of hormone action *1787*
Mark Gurnell, Jacky Burrin, and V. Krishna Chatterjee

13.2 Disorders of the anterior pituitary gland *1799*
Niki Karavitaki and John A.H. Wass

13.3 Disorders of the posterior pituitary gland *1819*
Aparna Pal, Niki Karavitaki, and John A.H. Wass

13.4 The thyroid gland and disorders of thyroid function *1826*
Anthony P. Weetman

13.5 Thyroid cancer *1845*
Anthony P. Weetman

13.6 Parathyroid disorders and diseases altering calcium metabolism *1851*
R.V. Thakker

13.7 Adrenal disorders *1869*

13.7.1 Disorders of the adrenal cortex *1869*
P.M. Stewart

13.7.2 Congenital adrenal hyperplasia *1891*
I.A. Hughes

13.8 The reproductive system *1901*

13.8.1 Ovarian disorders *1901*
Stephen Franks and Lisa J. Webber

13.8.2 Disorders of male reproduction *1913*
U. Srinivas-Shankar and F.C.W. Wu

13.8.3 Breast cancer *1928*
M. Cariati, L. Holmberg, J. Mansi, P. Parker, G. Pichert, S. Pinder, E. Sawyer, R. Wilson, and A. Purushotham

13.8.4 Benign breast disease *1940*
P. Jane Clarke

13.8.5 Sexual dysfunction *1942*
Ian Eardley

13.9 Disorders of growth and development *1948*

13.9.1 Normal growth and its disorders *1948*
Gary Butler

13.9.2 Puberty *1958*
I. Banerjee and P.E. Clayton

13.9.3 Normal and abnormal sexual differentiation *1963*
I.A. Hughes

13.10 Pancreatic endocrine disorders and multiple endocrine neoplasia *1976*
N.M. Martin and S.R. Bloom

13.11 Disorders of glucose homeostasis *1987*

13.11.1 Diabetes *1987*
Colin Dayan and Gareth Williams

13.11.2 Hypoglycaemia *2049*
Vincent Marks

13.12 Hormonal manifestations of nonendocrine disease *2059*
Timothy M. Barber and John A.H. Wass

13.13 The pineal gland and melatonin *2070*
J. Arendt and Timothy M. Cox

SECTION 14
Medical disorders in pregnancy

14.1 Physiological changes of normal pregnancy *2075*
David J. Williams

14.2 Nutrition in pregnancy *2079*
David J. Williams

14.3 Medical management of normal pregnancy *2085*
David J. Williams

14.4 Hypertension in pregnancy *2093*
C.W.G. Redman

14.5 Renal disease in pregnancy *2103*
John D. Firth

14.6 Heart disease in pregnancy *2108*
Catherine E.G. Head

14.7 Thrombosis in pregnancy *2116*
I.A. Greer

14.8 Chest diseases in pregnancy *2121*
Minerva Covarrubias and Tina Hartert

14.9 Liver and gastrointestinal diseases in pregnancy *2125*
Alexander Gimson

14.10 Diabetes in pregnancy *2133*
Moshe Hod and Yariv Yogev

14.11 Endocrine disease in pregnancy *2140*
John H. Lazarus

14.12 Neurological disease in pregnancy *2144*
G.G. Lennox and John D. Firth

14.13 The skin in pregnancy *2149*
Fenella Wojnarowska

14.14 Autoimmune rheumatic disorders and vasculitis in pregnancy *2154*
Sarah Germain and Catherine Nelson-Piercy

14.15 Infections in pregnancy *2165*
Lawrence Impey

14.16 Blood disorders specific to pregnancy *2173*
David J. Perry and Katharine Lowndes

14.17 Malignant disease in pregnancy *2181*
Robin A.F. Crawford

14.18 Prescribing in pregnancy *2186*
Peter Rubin

14.19 Benefits and risks of oral contraception *2191*
John Guillebaud

14.20 Benefits and risks of hormone replacement therapy *2196*
J.C. Stevenson

SECTION 15
Gastroenterological disorders

15.1 Structure and function of the gut *2201*
D.G. Thompson

15.2 Symptomatology of gastrointestinal disease *2205*
Graham Neale

15.3 Methods for investigation of gastrointestinal disease *2210*

15.3.1 Colonoscopy and flexible sigmoidoscopy *2210*
Christopher B. Williams and Brian P. Saunders

15.3.2 Upper gastrointestinal endoscopy *2214*
Adrian R.W. Hatfield

15.3.3 Radiology of the gastrointestinal tract *2219*
A.H. Freeman

15.3.4 Investigation of gastrointestinal function *2226*
Julian R.F. Walters

15.4 Common acute abdominal presentations *2232*

15.4.1 The acute abdomen *2232*
Chris Watson

15.4.2 Gastrointestinal bleeding *2237*
T.A. Rockall and H.M.P. Dowson

15.5 Immune disorders of the gastrointestinal tract *2244*
M.R. Haeney

15.6 The mouth and salivary glands *2257*
T. Lehner and S.J. Challacombe

15.7 Diseases of the oesophagus *2287*
Rebecca Fitzgerald

15.8 Peptic ulcer disease *2305*
Joseph Sung

15.9 Hormones and the gastrointestinal tract *2316*
A.E. Bishop, P.J. Hammond, J.M. Polak, and S.R. Bloom

15.10 Malabsorption *2326*

15.10.1 Differential diagnosis and investigation of malabsorption *2326*
Julian R.F. Walters

15.10.2 Small bowel bacterial overgrowth *2330*
P.P. Toskes

15.10.3 Coeliac disease *2335*
Patrick C.A. Dubois and David A. van Heel

15.10.4 Gastrointestinal lymphoma *2342*
P.G. Isaacson

15.10.5 Disaccharidase deficiency *2347*
Timothy M. Cox

15.10.6 Whipple's disease *2352*
H.J.F. Hodgson

15.10.7 Effects of massive small bowel resection *2354*
R.J. Playford

15.10.8 Malabsorption syndromes in the tropics *2357*
V.I. Mathan

15.11 Crohn's disease *2361*
Miles Parkes

15.12 Ulcerative colitis *2371*
D.P. Jewell

15.13 Irritable bowel syndrome and functional bowel disorders *2384*
D.G. Thompson

15.14 Colonic diverticular disease *2389*
S.Q. Ashraf, M.G.W. Kettlewell, and N.J. McC. Mortensen

15.15 Congenital abnormalities of the gastrointestinal tract *2395*
V.M. Wright and J.A. Walker-Smith

15.16 Cancers of the gastrointestinal tract *2405*
J.A. Bridgewater and S.P. Pereira

15.17 Vascular and collagen disorders *2417*
Graham Neale

15.18 Gastrointestinal infections *2424*
Davidson H. Hamer and Sherwood L. Gorbach

15.19 Structure and function of the liver, biliary tract, and pancreas *2435*
Alexander Gimson and Simon M. Rushbrook

15.20 Jaundice *2444*
R.P.H. Thompson

15.21 Hepatitis and autoimmune liver disease *2452*

15.21.1 Viral hepatitis—clinical aspects *2452*
H.J.F. Hodgson

15.21.2 Autoimmune hepatitis *2460*
H.J.F. Hodgson

15.21.3 Primary biliary cirrhosis *2464*
M.F. Bassendine

15.21.4 Primary sclerosing cholangitis *2468*
R.W. Chapman

15.22 Other disorders of the liver *2474*

15.22.1 Alcoholic liver disease *2474*
Stephen F. Stewart and Chris P. Day

15.22.2 Nonalcoholic steatohepatitis *2480*
Stephen F. Stewart and Chris P. Day

15.22.3 Cirrhosis and ascites *2482*
Kevin Moore

15.22.4 Hepatocellular failure *2493*
E. Anthony Jones

15.22.5 Liver transplantation *2505*
Gideon M. Hirschfield, Michael E.D. Allison, and Graeme J.M. Alexander

15.22.6 Liver tumours—primary and secondary *2512*
William J.H. Griffiths and Simon M. Rushbrook

15.22.7 Hepatic granulomas *2523*
C.W.N. Spearman, Pauline de la Motte Hall, M.W. Sonderup, and S.J. Saunders

15.22.8 Drugs and liver damage *2527*
J. Neuberger

15.22.9 The liver in systemic disease *2537*
J. Neuberger

15.23 Diseases of the gallbladder and biliary tree *2546*
J.A. Summerfield

15.24 Diseases of the pancreas *2557*

15.24.1 Acute pancreatitis *2557*
C.W. Imrie and R. Carter

15.24.2 Chronic pancreatitis *2567*
P.P. Toskes

15.24.3 Tumours of the pancreas *2574*
Martin Lombard and Ian Gilmore

15.25 Congenital disorders of the liver, biliary tract, and pancreas *2579*
J.A. Summerfield

15.26 Miscellaneous disorders of the bowel and liver *2584*
Alexander Gimson

SECTION 16
Cardiovascular disorders

16.1 Structure and function *2593*

16.1.1 Blood vessels and the endothelium *2593*
Patrick Vallance

16.1.2 Cardiac myocytes and the cardiac action potential *2603*
Kenneth T. MacLeod, Steven B. Marston, Philip A. Poole-Wilson, Nicholas J. Severs, and Peter H. Sugden

16.1.3 Clinical physiology of the normal heart *2618*
David E.L. Wilcken

16.2 Clinical presentation of heart disease *2628*

16.2.1 Chest pain, breathlessness, and fatigue *2628*
J. Dwight

16.2.2 Syncope and palpitations *2636*
A.C. Rankin, A.D. McGavigan, and S.M. Cobbe

16.3 Clinical investigation of cardiac disorders *2643*

16.3.1 Electrocardiography *2643*
Andrew R. Houghton and David Gray

16.3.2 Echocardiography *2662*
Adrian P. Banning and Andrew R.J. Mitchell

16.3.3 Cardiac investigation—nuclear and other imaging techniques *2671*
Nikant Sabharwal and Harald Becher

16.3.4 Cardiac catheterization and angiography *2678*
Edward D. Folland

16.4 Cardiac arrhythmias *2688*
S.M. Cobbe, A.D. McGavigan, and A.C. Rankin

16.5 Cardiac failure *2717*

16.5.1 Clinical features and medical treatments *2717*
Martin R. Cowie and Badrinath Chandrasekaran

16.5.2 Cardiac transplantation and mechanical circulatory support *2729*
Jayan Parameshwar

16.6 Heart valve disease *2736*
Michael Henein

16.7 Diseases of heart muscle *2758*

16.7.1 Myocarditis *2758*
Jay W. Mason

16.7.2 The cardiomyopathies: hypertrophic, dilated, restrictive, and right ventricular *2764*
William J. McKenna and Perry Elliott

16.7.3 Specific heart muscle disorders *2782*
William J. McKenna and Perry Elliott

16.8 Pericardial disease *2790*
Michael Henein

16.9 Cardiac involvement in infectious disease *2797*

16.9.1 Acute rheumatic fever *2797*
Jonathan R. Carapetis

16.9.2 Infective endocarditis *2806*
William A. Littler

16.9.3 Cardiac disease in HIV infection *2822*
Peter F. Currie

16.9.4 Cardiovascular syphilis *2826*
Krishna Somers

16.10 Tumours of the heart *2830*
Thomas A. Traill

16.11 Cardiac involvement in genetic disease *2834*
Thomas A. Traill

16.12 Congenital heart disease in the adult *2842*
S.A. Thorne

16.13 Coronary heart disease *2873*

16.13.1 Biology and pathology of atherosclerosis *2873*
Clare Dollery and Peter Libby

16.13.2 Coronary heart disease: epidemiology and prevention *2881*
Harry Hemingway and Michael Marmot

16.13.3 Influences acting *in utero* and in early childhood *2898*
D.J.P. Barker

16.13.4 Management of stable angina *2902*
Adam D. Timmis

16.13.5 Management of acute coronary syndrome *2911*
Keith A.A. Fox

16.13.6 Percutaneous interventional cardiac procedures *2935*
Edward D. Folland

16.13.7 Coronary artery bypass surgery *2942*
Graham Cooper

16.13.8 The impact of coronary heart disease on life and work *2946*
Michael C. Petch

16.14 Diseases of the arteries *2953*

16.14.1 Thoracic aortic dissection *2953*
Andrew R.J. Mitchell and Adrian P. Banning

16.14.2 Peripheral arterial disease *2959*
Janet Powell and Alun Davies

16.14.3 Cholesterol embolism *2966*
Christopher Dudley

16.14.4 Takayasu's arteritis *2968*
Yasushi Kobayashi

16.15 The pulmonary circulation *2974*

16.15.1 Structure and function *2974*
Nicholas W. Morrell

16.15.2 Pulmonary hypertension *2978*
Nicholas W. Morrell

16.15.3 Pulmonary oedema *2992*
Nicholas W. Morrell and John D. Firth

16.16 Venous thromboembolism *3002*

16.16.1 Deep venous thrombosis and pulmonary embolism *3002*
Paul D. Stein and John D. Firth

16.16.2 Therapeutic anticoagulation *3018*
David Keeling

16.17 Hypertension *3023*

16.17.1 Essential hypertension—definition, epidemiology, and pathophysiology *3023*
Bryan Williams

16.17.2 Diagnosis, assessment, and treatment of essential hypertension *3039*
Bryan Williams

16.17.3 Secondary hypertension *3057*
Morris J. Brown

16.17.4 Mendelian disorders causing hypertension *3071*
Nilesh J. Samani

16.17.5 Hypertensive urgencies and emergencies *3074*
Gregory Y.H. Lip and D. Gareth Beevers

16.18 Chronic peripheral oedema and lymphoedema *3083*
Peter S. Mortimer

16.19 Idiopathic oedema of women *3093*
John D. Firth

SECTION 17
Critical care medicine

17.1 Cardiac arrest *3097*
Jasmeet Soar, Jerry P. Nolan, and David A. Gabbott

17.2 Anaphylaxis *3106*
Anthony F.T. Brown

17.3 The clinical approach to the patient who is very ill *3115*
John D. Firth

17.4 Circulation and circulatory support in the critically ill *3122*
Michael R. Pinsky

17.5 Acute respiratory failure *3132*
Susannah Leaver and Timothy Evans

17.6 Management of raised intracranial pressure *3147*
David K. Menon

17.7 Sedation and analgesia in the critically ill *3153*
Gilbert Park and Maire P. Shelly

17.8 Discontinuing treatment of the critically ill patient *3158*
M.J. Lindop

17.9 Brainstem death and organ donation *3161*
M.J. Lindop

SECTION 18
Respiratory disorders

18.1 Structure and function *3169*

18.1.1 The upper respiratory tract *3169*
J.R. Stradling and S.E. Craig

18.1.2 Airways and alveoli *3173*
Peter D. Wagner

18.2 The clinical presentation of respiratory disease *3182*
Julian Hopkin

18.3 Clinical investigation of respiratory disorders *3189*

18.3.1 Respiratory function tests *3189*
G.J. Gibson

18.3.2 Thoracic imaging *3200*
Susan J. Copley and David M. Hansell

18.3.3 Bronchoscopy, thoracoscopy, and tissue biopsy *3216*
Pallav L. Shah

18.4 Respiratory infection *3227*

18.4.1 Upper respiratory tract infections *3227*
P. Little

18.4.2 Pneumonia in the normal host *3231*
John G. Bartlett

18.4.3 Nosocomial pneumonia *3243*
John G. Bartlett

18.4.4 Pulmonary complications of HIV infection *3246*
Mark J. Rosen

18.5 The upper respiratory tract *3254*

18.5.1 Upper airways obstruction *3254*
J.R. Stradling and S.E. Craig

18.5.2 Sleep-related disorders of breathing *3261*
J.R. Stradling and S.E. Craig

18.6 Allergic rhinitis *3277*
Stephen R. Durham and Hesham Saleh

18.7 Asthma *3283*
A.J. Newman Taylor and Paul Cullinan

18.8 Chronic obstructive pulmonary disease *3311*
William MacNee

18.9 Bronchiectasis *3345*
D. Bilton

18.10 Cystic fibrosis *3353*
Andrew Bush and Caroline Elston

18.11 Diffuse parenchymal lung diseases *3365*

18.11.1 Diffuse parenchymal lung disease: an introduction *3365*
A.U. Wells

18.11.2 Idiopathic pulmonary fibrosis *3375*
A.U. Wells, A.G. Nicholson, and N. Hirani

18.11.3 Bronchiolitis obliterans and cryptogenic organizing pneumonia *3382*
A.U. Wells and Nicholas K. Harrison

18.11.4 The lung in autoimmune rheumatic disorders *3387*
A.U. Wells and H.R. Branley

18.11.5 The lung in vasculitis *3395*
A.U. Wells and Roland M. du Bois

18.12 Sarcoidosis *3403*
Robert P. Baughman and Elyse E. Lower

18.13 Pneumoconioses *3414*
A. Seaton

18.14 Miscellaneous conditions *3425*

18.14.1 Pulmonary haemorrhagic disorders *3425*
D.J. Hendrick and G.P. Spickett

18.14.2 Eosinophilic pneumonia *3428*
D.J. Hendrick and G.P. Spickett

18.14.3 Lymphocytic infiltrations of the lung *3431*
D.J. Hendrick

18.14.4 Extrinsic allergic alveolitis *3434*
D.J. Hendrick and G.P. Spickett

18.14.5 Pulmonary Langerhans' cell histiocytosis *3446*
S.J. Bourke and D.J. Hendrick

18.14.6 Lymphangioleiomyomatosis *3447*
S.J. Bourke and D.J. Hendrick

18.14.7 Pulmonary alveolar proteinosis *3448*
D.J. Hendrick

18.14.8 Pulmonary amyloidosis *3451*
D.J. Hendrick

18.14.9 Lipoid (lipid) pneumonia *3452*
D.J. Hendrick

18.14.10 Pulmonary alveolar microlithiasis *3454*
D.J. Hendrick

18.14.11 Toxic gases and aerosols *3456*
D.J. Hendrick

18.14.12 Radiation pneumonitis *3458*
S.J. Bourke and D.J. Hendrick

18.14.13 Drug-induced lung disease *3460*
S.J. Bourke and D.J. Hendrick

18.15 Chronic respiratory failure *3467*
P.M.A. Calverley

18.16 Lung transplantation *3476*
K. McNeil

18.17 Pleural diseases *3486*
Robert J.O. Davies, Fergus V. Gleeson, and Y.C. Gary Lee

18.18 Disorders of the thoracic cage and diaphragm *3505*
John M. Shneerson

18.19 Malignant diseases *3514*

18.19.1 Lung cancer *3514*
S.G. Spiro

18.19.2 Pulmonary metastases *3533*
S.G. Spiro

18.19.3 Pleural tumours *3534*
Robert J.O. Davies and Y.C. Gary Lee

18.19.4 Mediastinal cysts and tumours *3539*
Malcolm K. Benson and Robert J.O. Davies

SECTION 19
Rheumatological disorders

19.1 Structure and function: joints and connective tissue *3547*
Tim E. Cawston

19.2 Clinical presentation and diagnosis of rheumatic disease *3554*
Anthony S. Russell and Robert Ferrari

19.3 Clinical investigation *3560*
Michael Doherty and Peter C. Lanyon

19.4 Back pain and regional disorders *3571*
Simon Carette

19.5 Rheumatoid arthritis *3579*
Ravinder Nath Maini

19.6 Ankylosing spondylitis, other spondyloarthritides, and related conditions *3603*
J. Braun and J. Sieper

19.7 Pyogenic arthritis *3617*
Anthony R. Berendt

19.8 Reactive arthritis *3622*
J.S. Hill Gaston

19.9 Osteoarthritis *3628*
Paul H. Brion and Kenneth C. Kalunian

19.10 Crystal-related arthropathies *3637*
Edward Roddy and Michael Doherty

19.11 Autoimmune rheumatic disorders and vasculitides *3649*

19.11.1 Introduction *3649*
I.P. Giles and David A. Isenberg

19.11.2 Systemic lupus erythematosus and related disorders *3652*
Anisur Rahman and David A. Isenberg

19.11.3 Systemic sclerosis *3665*
Christopher P. Denton and Carol M. Black

19.11.4 Polymyalgia rheumatica and temporal arteritis *3679*
Jan Tore Gran

19.11.5 Behçet's syndrome *3684*
Sebahattin Yurdakul, Izzet Fresko, and Hasan Yazici

19.11.6 Sjögren's syndrome *3688*
Patrick J.W. Venables

19.11.7 Polymyositis and dermatomyositis *3692*
John H. Stone

19.11.8 Kawasaki's disease *3698*
Brian W. McCrindle

19.12 Miscellaneous conditions presenting to the rheumatologist *3705*
Donncha O'Gradaigh

Index

Volume 3

Contributors *xxxi*

SECTION 20
Disorders of the skeleton

20.1 Skeletal disorders—general approach and clinical conditions *3719*
R. Smith and B.P. Wordsworth

20.2 Inherited defects of connective tissue: Ehlers–Danlos syndrome, Marfan's syndrome, and pseudoxanthoma elasticum *3771*
N.P. Burrows

20.3 Osteomyelitis *3788*
Anthony R. Berendt and Martin McNally

20.4 Osteoporosis *3796*
Juliet Compston

20.5 Osteonecrosis, osteochondrosis, and osteochondritis dissecans *3802*
Donncha O'Gradaigh and Adrian Crisp

SECTION 21
Disorders of the kidney and urinary tract

21.1 Structure and functions of the kidney *3809*
J. David Williams and A.O. Phillips

21.2 Electrolyte disorders *3817*

21.2.1 Disorders of water and sodium homeostasis *3817*
Steven G. Achinger and Juan Carlos Ayus

21.2.2 Disorders of potassium homeostasis *3831*
John D. Firth

21.3 Clinical presentation of renal disease *3846*
Richard E. Fielding and Ken Farrington

21.4 Clinical investigation of renal disease *3863*
A. Davenport

21.5 Acute kidney injury *3885*
John D. Firth

21.6 Chronic kidney disease *3904*
Eberhard Ritz, Tilman B. Drüeke, and John D. Firth

21.7 Renal replacement therapy *3930*

21.7.1 Haemodialysis *3930*
Ken Farrington and Roger Greenwood

21.7.2 Peritoneal dialysis *3943*
Simon Davies

21.7.3 Renal transplantation *3947*
P. Sweny

21.8 Glomerular diseases *3971*

21.8.1 Immunoglobulin A nephropathy and Henoch–Schönlein purpura *3971*
Jonathan Barratt and John Feehally

21.8.2 Thin membrane nephropathy *3977*
Peter Topham and John Feehally

21.8.3 Minimal-change nephropathy and focal segmental glomerulosclerosis *3979*
Dwomoa Adu

21.8.4 Membranous nephropathy *3985*
Dwomoa Adu

21.8.5 Proliferative glomerulonephritis *3988*
Peter W. Mathieson

21.8.6 Mesangiocapillary glomerulonephritis *3991*
Peter W. Mathieson

21.8.7 Antiglomerular basement membrane disease *3995*
Jeremy Levy and Charles Pusey

21.9 Tubulointerstitial diseases *4002*

21.9.1 Acute interstitial nephritis *4002*
Simon D. Roger

21.9.2 Chronic tubulointerstitial nephritis *4006*
Marc E. De Broe, Patrick C. D'Haese, and Monique M. Elseviers

21.10 The kidney in systemic disease *4021*

21.10.1 Diabetes mellitus and the kidney *4021*
Rudolf Bilous

21.10.2 The kidney in systemic vasculitis *4032*
David Jayne

21.10.3 The kidney in rheumatological disorders *4044*
Wai Y. Tse and Dwomoa Adu

21.10.4 Renal involvement in plasma cell dyscrasias, immunoglobulin-based amyloidoses, and fibrillary glomerulopathies, lymphomas, and leukaemias *4055*
P. Ronco, F. Bridoux, and G. Touchard

21.10.5 Haemolytic uraemic syndrome *4065*
Paul Warwicker and Timothy H.J. Goodship

21.10.6 Sickle-cell disease and the kidney *4069*
G.R. Serjeant

21.10.7 Infection-associated nephropathies *4071*
A. Neil Turner

21.10.8 Malignancy-associated renal disease *4076*
A. Neil Turner

21.10.9 Atherosclerotic renovascular disease *4078*
P.A. Kalra and John D. Firth

21.11 Renal diseases in the tropics *4082*
Vivekanand Jha

21.12 Renal involvement in genetic disease *4095*
D. Joly and J.P. Grünfeld

21.13 Urinary tract infection *4103*
Charles Tomson and Alison Armitage

21.14 Disorders of renal calcium handling, urinary stones, and nephrocalcinosis *4123*
Elaine M. Worcester, Andrew P. Evan, and Fredric L. Coe

21.15 The renal tubular acidoses *4133*
Fiona E. Karet

21.16 Disorders of tubular electrolyte handling *4140*
Nine V.A.M. Knoers and Elena N. Levtchenko

21.17 Urinary tract obstruction *4151*
Muhammad M. Yaqoob and Islam Junaid

21.18 Malignant diseases of the urinary tract *4162*
David Neal

21.19 Drugs and the kidney *4174*
Aine Burns and Caroline Ashley

SECTION 22
Disorders of the blood

22.1 Introduction *4191*
D.J. Weatherall

22.2 Haemopoietic stem cells *4199*

22.2.1 Stem cells and haemopoiesis *4199*
C.A. Sieff

22.2.2 Haemopoietic stem cell disorders *4208*
D.C. Linch

22.3 The leukaemias and other bone marrow disorders *4214*

22.3.1 Cell and molecular biology of human leukaemias *4214*
Alejandro Gutierrez and A. Thomas Look

22.3.2 The classification of leukaemia *4221*
Wendy N. Erber

22.3.3 Acute lymphoblastic leukaemia *4229*
Tim Eden

22.3.4 Acute myeloid leukaemia *4233*
Jonathan Kell, Steve Knapper, and Alan Burnett

22.3.5 Chronic lymphocytic leukaemia and other leukaemias of mature B and T cells *4240*
Clive S. Zent and Aaron Polliack

22.3.6 Chronic myeloid leukaemia *4247*
Tariq I. Mughal and John M. Goldman

22.3.7 Myelodysplasia *4256*
Lawrence B. Gardner and Chi V. Dang

22.3.8 The polycythaemias *4264*
Stefan O. Ciurea and Ronald Hoffman

22.3.9 Idiopathic myelofibrosis *4274*
Jerry L. Spivak

22.3.10 Thrombocytosis *4280*
Stefan O. Ciurea and Ronald Hoffman

22.3.11 Aplastic anaemia and other causes of bone marrow failure *4287*
Judith C.W. Marsh and E.C. Gordon-Smith

22.3.12 Paroxysmal nocturnal haemoglobinuria *4298*
Lucio Luzzatto

22.4 The white cells and lymphoproliferative disorders *4303*

22.4.1 Leucocytes in health and disease *4303*
Joseph Sinning and Nancy Berliner

22.4.2 Introduction to the lymphoproliferative disorders *4311*
Barbara A. Degar and Nancy Berliner

22.4.3 Lymphoma *4317*
James O. Armitage

22.4.4 The spleen and its disorders *4334*
D. Swirsky

22.4.5 Myeloma and paraproteinaemias *4342*
Robert A. Kyle and S. Vincent Rajkumar

22.4.6 Eosinophilia *4356*
Peter F. Weller

22.4.7 Histiocytoses *4361*
D.K.H. Webb

22.5 The red cell *4367*

22.5.1 Erythropoiesis and the normal red cell *4367*
Anna Rita Migliaccio and Thalia Papayannopoulou

22.5.2 Anaemia: pathophysiology, classification, and clinical features *4374*
D.J. Weatherall

22.5.3 Anaemia as a challenge to world health *4381*
D.J. Weatherall

22.5.4 Iron metabolism and its disorders *4386*
Timothy M. Cox

22.5.5 Normochromic, normocytic anaemia *4400*
D.J. Weatherall

22.5.6 Megaloblastic anaemia and miscellaneous deficiency anaemias *4402*
A.V. Hoffbrand

22.5.7 Disorders of the synthesis or function of haemoglobin *4420*
D.J. Weatherall

22.5.8 Anaemias resulting from defective maturation of red cells *4445*
James S. Wiley

22.5.9 Haemolytic anaemia—congenital and acquired *4450*
Amy Powers, Leslie Silberstein, and Frank J. Strobl

22.5.10 Disorders of the red cell membrane *4461*
Patrick G. Gallagher

22.5.11 Erythrocyte enzymopathies *4468*
Ernest Beutler

22.5.12 Glucose-6-phosphate dehydrogenase (G6PD) deficiency *4473*
Lucio Luzzatto

22.6 Haemostasis and thrombosis *4480*

22.6.1 The biology of haemostasis and thrombosis *4480*
Harold R. Roberts and Gilbert C. White

22.6.2 Evaluation of the patient with a bleeding tendency *4498*
Trevor Baglin

22.6.3 Disorders of platelet number and function *4507*
Kathryn E. Webert and John G. Kelton

22.6.4 Genetic disorders of coagulation *4518*
Eleanor S. Pollak and Katherine A. High

22.6.5 Acquired coagulation disorders *4531*
T.E. Warkentin

22.7 The blood in systemic disease *4547*
D.J. Weatherall

22.8 Blood replacement *4561*

22.8.1 Blood transfusion *4561*
P.L. Perrotta, Y. Han, and E.L. Snyder

22.8.2 Haemopoietic stem cell transplantation *4571*
E.C. Gordon-Smith and Emma Morris

SECTION 23
Disorders of the skin
Editor: Graham S. Ogg

23.1 Structure and function of skin *4583*
John A. McGrath

23.2 Clinical approach to the diagnosis of skin disease *4587*
Vanessa Venning

23.3 Inherited skin disease *4593*
Irene M. Leigh and David P. Kelsell

23.4 Vesiculobullous disease *4602*
Fenella Wojnarowska

23.5 Papulosquamous disease *4610*
Christopher Griffiths

23.6 Dermatitis/eczema *4618*
Peter S. Friedmann

23.7 Cutaneous vasculitis, connective tissue diseases, and urticaria *4626*
Susan Burge and Graham S. Ogg

23.8 Disorders of pigmentation *4656*
Eugene Healy

23.9 Photosensitivity *4665*
Jane McGregor

23.10 Infections and the skin *4672*
Roderick J. Hay

23.11 Sebaceous and sweat gland disorders *4676*
Alison Layton

23.12 Blood and lymphatic vessel disorders *4683*
Peter S. Mortimer

23.13 Hair and nail disorders *4698*
David de Berker

23.14 Tumours of the skin *4705*
Edel O'Toole

23.15 Skin and systemic diseases *4715*
Clive B. Archer

23.16 Cutaneous reactions to drugs *4724*
Peter S. Friedmann and Eugene Healy

23.17 Management of skin disease *4731*
Rod Sinclair

SECTION 24
Neurological disorders

24.1 Introduction and approach to the patient with neurological disease *4743*
Alastair Compston

24.2 Mind and brain: building bridges linking neurology, psychiatry, and psychology *4746*
A. Zeman

24.3 Clinical investigation of neurological disease *4749*

24.3.1 Lumbar puncture *4749*
Roger A. Barker, Wendy Phillips, and R. Rhys Davies

24.3.2 Electrophysiology of the central and peripheral nervous systems *4752*
Christian Krarup

24.3.3 Imaging in neurological diseases *4768*
Andrew J. Molyneux, Shelley Renowden, and Marcus Bradley

24.3.4 Investigation of central motor pathways: magnetic brain stimulation *4782*
K.R. Mills

24.4 Higher cerebral function *4786*

24.4.1 Disturbances of higher cerebral function *4786*
Peter J. Nestor and John R. Hodges

24.4.2 Alzheimer's disease and other dementias *4795*
John R. Hodges

24.5 Epilepsy and disorders of consciousness *4810*

24.5.1 Epilepsy in later childhood and adulthood *4810*
G.D. Perkin

24.5.2 Narcolepsy *4826*
David Parkes

24.5.3 Sleep disorders *4828*
Paul J. Reading

24.5.4 Syncope *4838*
A.J. Larner

24.5.5 The unconscious patient *4841*
David Bates

24.5.6 Brain death and the vegetative state *4847*
P.J. Hutchinson and J.D. Pickard

24.6 Disorders of the special senses *4851*

24.6.1 Visual pathways *4851*
Christopher Kennard

24.6.2 Eye movements and balance *4858*
Michael Strupp and Thomas Brandt

24.6.3 Hearing *4865*
Linda M. Luxon

24.7 Disorders of movement *4871*

24.7.1 Subcortical structures: the cerebellum, basal ganglia, and thalamus *4871*
Mark J. Edwards and Penelope Talelli

24.7.2 Parkinsonism and other extrapyramidal diseases *4879*
K. Ray Chaudhuri and Vinod K. Metta

24.7.3 Movement disorders other than Parkinson's disease *4889*
Roger A. Barker and David J. Burn

24.7.4 Ataxic disorders *4902*
Nicholas Wood

24.8 Headache *4911*
Peter J. Goadsby

24.9 Brainstem syndromes *4929*
David Bates

24.10 Specific conditions affecting the central nervous system *4933*

24.10.1 Stroke: cerebrovascular disease *4933*
J. van Gijn

24.10.2 Demyelinating disorders of the central nervous system *4948*
Siddharthan Chandran and Alastair Compston

24.10.3 Traumatic injuries to the head *4963*
Laurence Watkins and David G.T. Thomas

24.10.4 Intracranial tumours *4967*
Jeremy Rees

24.10.5 Idiopathic intracranial hypertension *4972*
N.F. Lawton

24.11 Infections of the central nervous system *4976*

24.11.1 Bacterial infections *4976*
Diederik van de Beek, Jeremy Farrar, and Guy E. Thwaites

24.11.2 Viral infections *4998*
Jeremy Farrar, Bridget Wills, Menno D. de Jong, and David A. Warrell

24.11.3 Intracranial abscesses *5013*
T.P. Lawrence and R.S.C. Kerr

24.11.4 Neurosyphilis and neuro-AIDS *5015*
Hadi Manji

24.11.5 Human prion diseases *5023*
R.G. Will

24.12 Disorders of cranial nerves *5033*
R.A.C. Hughes and P.K. Thomas

24.13 Disorders of the spinal cord *5039*

24.13.1 Diseases of the spinal cord *5039*
A.J. Larner

24.13.2 Spinal cord injury and its management *5045*
M.P. Barnes

24.14 Diseases of the autonomic nervous system *5055*
Christopher J. Mathias

24.15 The motor neuron diseases *5069*
Michael Donaghy

24.16 Diseases of the peripheral nerves *5076*
R.A.C. Hughes and P.K. Thomas

24.17 Inherited neurodegenerative diseases *5096*
Edwin H. Kolodny and Swati Sathe

24.18 Developmental abnormalities of the central nervous system *5134*
C.M. Verity, C. ffrench-Constant, and H.V. Firth

24.19 Acquired metabolic disorders and the nervous system *5150*
Neil Scolding and C.D. Marsden

24.20 Neurological complications of systemic disease *5158*
Neil Scolding

24.21 Paraneoplastic neurological syndromes *5166*
Jeremy Rees, Jerry Posner, and Angela Vincent

24.22 Autoimmune limbic encephalitis and Morvan's syndrome *5175*
Camilla Buckley and Angela Vincent

24.23 Disorders of the neuromuscular junction *5177*
David Hilton-Jones and Jacqueline Palace

24.24 Disorders of muscle *5185*

24.24.1 Structure and function of muscle *5185*
M.G. Hanna

24.24.2 Muscular dystrophy *5190*
K. Bushby

24.24.3 Myotonia *5207*
David Hilton-Jones

24.24.4 Metabolic and endocrine disorders *5212*
David Hilton-Jones and Richard Edwards

24.24.5 Mitochondrial encephalomyopathies *5221*
P.F. Chinnery and D.M. Turnbull

24.24.6 Primary (tropical) pyomyositis *5227*
David A. Warrell

SECTION 25
The eye

25.1 The eye in general medicine *5233*
Peggy Frith

SECTION 26
Psychiatry and drug related problems

26.1 General introduction *5257*
Michael Sharpe

26.2 Taking a psychiatric history from a medical patient *5259*
Eleanor Feldman

26.3 Acute behavioural emergencies *5263*
Eleanor Feldman

26.4 Neuropsychiatric disorders *5268*
Mervi L.S. Pitkanen, Tom Stevens, and Michael D. Kopelman

26.5 Psychiatric disorders as they concern the physician *5284*

26.5.1 Grief, stress, and post-traumatic stress disorder *5284*
Tim Dalgleish, Jenny Yiend, and Ann-Marie J. Golden

26.5.2 The patient who has attempted suicide *5292*
Keith Hawton

26.5.3 Medically unexplained symptoms in patients attending medical clinics *5296*
Michael Sharpe

26.5.4 Chronic fatigue syndrome (postviral fatigue syndrome, neurasthenia, and myalgic encephalomyelitis) *5304*
Michael Sharpe

26.5.5 Anxiety and depression *5308*
Lydia Chwastiak and Wayne J. Katon

26.5.6 Eating disorders *5317*
Christopher G. Fairburn

26.5.7 Schizophrenia, bipolar disorder, obsessive–compulsive disorder, and personality disorder *5324*
Stephen Lawrie

26.6 Psychiatric treatments *5329*

26.6.1 Psychopharmacology in medical practice *5329*
Philip J. Cowen

26.6.2 Psychological treatment in medical practice *5338*
Michael Sharpe and Simon Wessely

26.7 Alcohol and drug-related problems *5341*

26.7.1 Alcohol and drug dependence *5341*
Mary E. McCaul, Gary S. Wand, and Yngvild K. Olsen

26.7.2 Brief interventions against excessive alcohol consumption *5351*
Nick Heather and Eileen Kaner

SECTION 27
Forensic medicine

27.1 Forensic medicine and the practising doctor *5359*
Anthony Busuttil

SECTION 28
Sports medicine

28.1 Sports and exercise medicine *5375*
Roger L. Wolman

SECTION 29
Geratology

29.1 Medicine in old age *5389*
Gordon Wilcock and Kenneth Rockwood

29.2 Mental disorders of old age *5406*
Robin Jacoby

SECTION 30
Pain

30.1 Dealing with pain *5411*
Henry McQuay

SECTION 31
Palliative medicine

31.1 Palliative care *5419*
Bee Wee

SECTION 32
Biochemistry in medicine

32.1 Biochemistry in medicine—reference intervals: the use of biochemical analysis for diagnosis and management *5433*
P. Holloway and Heather Stoddart

SECTION 33
Acute medicine

33.1 Acute medical presentations *5453*
John D. Firth, David A. Warrell, and Timothy M. Cox

33.2 Practical procedures *5510*
John D. Firth, David A. Warrell, and Timothy M. Cox

Index

Contributors

P. Aaby Bandim Health Project, National Institute of Health, Guinea-Bissau
7.5.6: Measles

Steven G. Achinger Attending Nephrologist, Watson Clinic, Lakeland, Florida, USA
21.2.1: Disorders of water and sodium homeostasis

Dwomoa Adu Consultant Nephrologist, Department of Medicine, Korle Bu Hospital, Accra, Ghana
21.8.3: Minimal-change nephropathy and focal segmental glomerulosclerosis; 21.8.4: Membranous nephropathy; 21.10.3: The kidney in rheumatological disorders

Raymond M. Agius Professor of Occupational and Environmental Medicine and Honorary Consultant in Occupational Medicine, University of Manchester, Manchester, UK
9.4.1: Occupational and environmental health

Syed M. Ahmed Health Manager UK, Mediterranean & Shipping, Shell International, London, UK
9.5.10: Noise

Michael J. Aldape Assistant Research Scientist, Infectious Diseases Section, Veterans Affairs Medical Center, Boise, Idaho, USA
7.6.24: Botulism, gas gangrene, and clostridial gastrointestinal infections

Graeme J.M. Alexander Consultant Hepatologist, Cambridge University Hospitals, Cambridge, UK
15.22.5: Liver transplantation

Michael E.D. Allison Consultant Hepatologist, Cambridge University Hospitals, Cambridge, UK
15.22.5: Liver transplantation

Chris Andrews Mt Ommaney Family Clinic, Brisbane, Australia
9.5.7: Lightning and electrical injuries

Emmanouil Angelakis Faculté de Médecine et de Pharmacie, Université de la Méditerranée, Marseille Cedex, France
7.6.42: Bartonellas excluding B. bacilliformis

Gregory M. Anstead Associate Professor, Division of Infectious Diseases, Department of Medicine, University of Texas Health Science Center at San Antonio, and Medical Director, Immunosuppression and Infectious Diseases Clinics, South Texas Veterans Healthcare System, San Antonio, Texas, USA
7.7.3: Coccidioidomycosis

Clive B. Archer Consultant Dermatologist and Honorary Clinical Senior Lecturer, University Hospitals Bristol NHS Foundation Trust; The University of Bristol, UK
23.15: Skin and systemic diseases

Mark J. Arends University Reader and Honorary Consultant in Histopathology, Division of Histopathology, Department of Pathology, University of Cambridge, Addenbrooke's Hospital, Cambridge, UK
4.6: Apoptosis in health and disease

J. Arendt Professor Emeritus of Endocrinology, School of Biological Sciences, University of Surrey, Guildford, UK
13.13: The pineal gland and melatonin

Alison Armitage Consultant in Nephrology, The Richard Bright Renal Unit, Southmead Hospital, Bristol, UK
21.13: Urinary tract infection

James O. Armitage The Joe Shapiro Professor of Medicine, Section of Oncology/Hematology, University of Nebraska Medical Center, Nebraska Medical Center, Omaha, Nebraska, USA
22.4.3: Lymphoma

Frances M. Ashcroft Royal Society Research Professor, Department of Physiology, Anatomy and Genetics, University of Oxford, Oxford, UK
4.4: Ion channels and disease

Caroline Ashley Lead Specialist Pharmacist, Centre for Nephrology, Royal Free Hospital, London, UK
21.19: Drugs and the kidney

S.Q. Ashraf Academic Clinical Lecturer and Specialty Registrar, John Radcliffe Hospitals, Oxford UK
15.14: Colonic diverticular disease

Tar-Ching Aw Head of Department of Community Medicine, Faculty of Medicine & Health Sciences, United Arab Emirates University, Al-Ain, United Arab Emirates
9.5.10: Noise; 9.5.11: Vibration

Juan Carlos Ayus Director of Clinical Research, Renal Consultants of Houston, Texas, USA
21.2.1: Disorders of water and sodium homeostasis

Trevor Baglin Consultant in Haematology, Department of Haematology & Eastern Region Haemophilia Comprehensive Care Centre, Cambridge University Hospitals NHS Trust, Addenbrooke's Hospital, Cambridge, UK
22.6.2: Evaluation of the patient with a bleeding tendency

M. Bagshaw Director of Aviation Medicine, King's College, London, UK
9.5.5: Aerospace medicine

C. Baigent Clinical Trial Service Unit & Epidemiological Studies Unit (CTSU), University of Oxford, UK
2.3.3: Large-scale randomized evidence: trials and meta-analyses of trials

I. Banerjee Department of Paediatric Endocrinology, Royal Manchester Children's Hospital, UK
13.9.2: Puberty

Adrian P. Banning Consultant Cardiologist, John Radcliffe Hospital, Oxford, UK
16.3.2: Echocardiography; 16.14.1: Thoracic aortic dissection

George Banting Department of Biochemistry, University of Bristol, Bristol, UK
4.1: The cell

T.M. Barber Oxford Centre for Diabetes, Endocrinology and Metabolism, Churchill Hospital, Oxford, UK
13.12: Hormonal manifestations of nonendocrine disease

D.J.P. Barker Professor of Clinical Epidemiology, University of Southampton; Professor in Cardiovascular Medicine, Oregon Health & Science University
16.13.3: Influences acting in utero *and in early childhood*

Roger A. Barker University Reader in Clinical Neuroscience & Honorary Consultant, Cambridge Centre for Brain Repair and Department of Neurology, University Department of Clinical Neuroscience, Addenbrooke's Hospital, Cambridge, UK
24.3.1: Lumbar puncture; 24.7.3: Movement disorders other than Parkinson's disease

D. Barlow Consultant Physician, Department of Genitourinary Medicine, Guy's and St Thomas' Hospitals, London, UK
7.6.6: Neisseria gonorrhoeae

M.P. Barnes Professor of Neurological Rehabilitation, Hunters Moor Neurorehabilitation Ltd
24.13.2: Spinal cord injury and its management

Jonathan Barratt Senior Lecturer, University of Leicester; Honorary Consultant Nephrologist, University Hospitals of Leicester, UK
21.8.1: Immunoglobulin A nephropathy and Henoch–Schönlein purpura

John G. Bartlett Professor of Medicine, Johns Hopkins University School of Medicine, Baltimore, Maryland, USA
7.6.23: Clostridium difficile; 18.4.2: Pneumonia in the normal host; 18.4.3: Nosocomial pneumonia

Buddha Basnyat Oxford University Clinical Research Unit, Patan Hospital, Nepal
7.6.8: Typhoid and paratyphoid fevers; 9.5.4: Diseases of high terrestrial altitudes

M.F. Bassendine Professor of Hepatology, Institute of Cellular Medicine, Newcastle University, Newcastle upon Tyne, UK
15.21.3: Primary biliary cirrhosis

D.N. Bateman Professor in Clinical Toxicology, National Poisons Information, Edinburgh, UK
9.1: Poisoning by drugs and chemicals

David Bates Professor of Clinical Neurology, Newcastle University, UK
24.5.5: The unconscious patient; 24.9: Brainstem syndromes

Robert P. Baughman University of Cincinatti Medical Center, Cincinatti, Ohio, USA
18.12: Sarcoidosis

Peter J. Baxter Institute of Public Health, University of Cambridge, Cambridge, UK
9.5.12: Disasters: earthquakes, volcanic eruptions, hurricanes, and floods

Harald Becher Consultant Cardiologist and Honorary Senior Lecturer, Department of Cardiology, John Radcliffe Hospital, Oxford, UK
16.3.3: Cardiac investigation—nuclear and other imaging techniques

Diederik van de Beek Department of Neurology, Center of Infection and Immunity Amsterdam (CINIMA), University of Amsterdam, Amsterdam, The Netherlands
24.11.1: Bacterial infections

D. Gareth Beevers Professor of Medicine, University Department of Medicine, City Hospital, Birmingham, UK
16.17.5: Hypertensive urgencies and emergencies

John R. Benson Consultant Surgeon, Cambridge Breast Unit, Addenbrooke's Hospital, Cambridge, UK; Fellow and Director of Clinical Studies, Selwyn College, Cambridge, UK
6.2: The nature and development of cancer

Malcolm K. Benson Oxford Pleural Unit, Oxford Centre for Respiratory Medicine, John Radcliffe Hospital, Oxford, UK
18.19.4: Mediastinal cysts and tumours

Anthony R. Berendt Consultant Physician, Bone Infection Unit, Nuffield Orthopaedic Centre NHS Trust, Oxford, UK
19.7: Pyogenic arthritis; 20.3: Osteomyelitis

David de Berker Department of Dermatology, Bristol Royal Infirmary, Bristol, UK
23.13: Hair and nail disorders

Nancy Berliner Chief, Division of Hematology, Brigham and Women's Hospital, Professor of Medicine, Harvard Medical School, Baltimore, Maryland, USA
22.4.1: Leucocytes in health and disease; 22.4.2: Introduction to the lymphoproliferative disorders

Gordon R. Bernard Melinda Owen Bass Professor of Medicine, Division of Allergy, Pulmonary, and Critical Care Medicine; Associate Vice Chancellor for Research, Senior Associate Dean for Clinical Sciences, Vanderbilt University School of Medicine, Nashville, Tennessee, USA
7.1.2: Physiological changes, clinical features, and general management of infected patients

J.M. Best Emeritus Reader in Virology, King's College London, UK
7.5.13: Rubella

Delia B. Bethell Armed Forces Research Unit of Medical Sciences, Bangkok, Thailand (Clinical Trials Investigator); Oxford Radcliffe Hospital NHS Trust, Oxford, UK (Honorary Consultant Paediatrician)
7.6.1: Diphtheria

Ernest Beutler† Molecular and Experimental Medicine, The Scripps Research Institute, La Jolla, California, USA
22.5.11: Erythrocyte enzymopathies

Kaustuv Bhattacharya Staff Specialist, Metabolic Genetics Department, Western Sydney Genetics Program, The Children's Hospital at Westmead, Australia, NSW
12.3.1: Glycogen storage diseases

Rudolf Bilous Professor of Clinical Medicine, Newcastle University, Academic Centre, James Cook University Hospital, Middlesbrough, UK
21.10.1: Diabetes mellitus and the kidney

D. Bilton Consultant Physician, Royal Brompton Hospital and Honorary Senior Lecturer, Imperial College, London, UK
18.9: Bronchiectasis

A.E. Bishop Reader, Stem Cells & Regenerative Medicine, Department of Experimental Medicine & Toxicology, Imperial College Faculty of Medicine, Hammersmith Hospital, London, UK
15.9: Hormones and the gastrointestinal tract

Carol M. Black Professor of Rheumatology, Royal Free and University College Medical School, London, UK
19.11.3: Systemic sclerosis

S.R. Bloom Professor of Medicine, Imperial College, London, UK
13.10: Pancreatic endocrine disorders and multiple endocrine neoplasia; 15.9: Hormones and the gastrointestinal tract

Lotta von Boehmer Department of Oncology, University Hospital Zurich, Zurich, Switzerland
6.4: Cancer immunity and clinical oncology

Roland M. du Bois National Jewish Health, Denver, Colorado, USA
18.11.5: The lung in vasculitis

Christopher Booth Wellcome Centre for the History of Medicine, University College, London, UK
1.1: On being a patient

T.C. Boswell Consultant Medical Microbiologist, Nottingham University Hospitals, Nottingham, UK
7.6.38: Legionellosis and legionnaires' disease

Marina Botto Professor of Rheumatology, Rheumatology Section, Imperial College London, London, UK
5.1.2: The complement system

† It is with regret that we report the death of Professor Ernest Beutler during the preparation of this edition of the textbook.

S.J. Bourke Consultant Physician, Royal Victoria Infirmary, Newcastle upon Tyne, UK
18.14.5: Pulmonary Langerhans' cell histiocytosis; 18.14.6: Lymphangioleiomyomatosis; 18.14.12: Radiation pneumonitis; 18.14.13: Drug-induced lung disease

I.C.J.W. Bowler Consultant Microbiologist and Clinical Lead, Department of Medical Microbiology, Oxford Radcliffe Hospitals NHS Trust, Oxford, UK
7.2.3: Nosocomial infections

Paul Bowness Consultant Rheumatologist, Nuffield Orthopaedic Centre NHS Trust and Reader in Immunology, Nuffield Department of Medicine, Oxford University, UK
5.1.1: The innate immune system

S.M. Bradberry National Poisons Information Service and West Midlands Poisons Unit, City Hospital, Birmingham, UK
9.1: Poisoning by drugs and chemicals

Marcus Bradley Consultant in Radiology, Frenchay Hospital, Bristol, UK
24.3.3: Imaging in neurological diseases

Thomas Brandt Klinikum Groshadem, Neurologische Klinik, Munchen, Germany
24.6.2: Eye movements and balance

P. Brandtzaeg Department of Paediatrics, Oslo University Hospital, Oslo, Norway
7.6.5: Meningococcal infections

H.R. Branley Consultant in Respiratory Medicine, Whittington Hospital, London, UK
18.11.4: The lung in autoimmune rheumatic disorders

Philippe Brasseur Emeritus Professor of Parasitology, Faculty of Medicine of Rouen (France) and Research Unit (UMR 198), Institute of Research for Development, Dakar, Senegal
7.8.3: Babesiosis

J. Braun Rheumazentrum Ruhrgebiet, Herne, Germany; Ruhr University, Bochum, Germany
19.6: Ankylosing spondylitis, other spondyloarthritides, and related conditions

Sydney Brenner The Salk Institute, University of California, San Diego, California, USA
4.2.1: The human genome sequence

J.A. Bridgewater University College London Cancer Institute and UCLH/UCL Comprehensive Biomedical Centre, London, UK
15.16: Cancers of the gastrointestinal tract

F. Bridoux Department of Nephrology, Hopital Jean Bernard, Poitiers, France
21.10.4: Renal involvement in plasma cell dyscrasias, immunoglobulin-based amyloidoses, and fibrillary glomerulopathies, lymphomas, and leukaemias

Paul H. Brion Rheumatologist in Private Practice, Vista, California, USA
19.9: Osteoarthritis

Maries van den Broek Department of Oncology, University Hospital Zurich, Zurich, Switzerland
6.4: Cancer immunity and clinical oncology

Anthony F.T. Brown Professor of Emergency Medicine, Discipline of Anaesthesiology and Critical Care, School of Medicine, University of Queensland, Brisbane, Australia; Senior Staff Specialist, Department of Emergency Medicine, Royal Brisbane and Women's Hospital, Brisbane, Australia
17.2: Anaphylaxis

Arthur E. Brown Colonel, U.S. Army, Armed Forces Research Institute of Medical Sciences, Bangkok, Thailand
7.6.20: Anthrax

Kevin E. Brown Consultant Medical Virologist, Virus Reference Department, Centres for Infection, Health Protection Agency, London, UK
7.5.20: Parvovirus B19

Michael Brown Senior Lecturer, Department of Infectious & Tropical Diseases, London School of Hygiene & Tropical Medicine, London, UK
7.9.4: Strongyloidiasis, hookworm, and other gut strongyloid nematodes

Morris J. Brown Professor of Clinical Pharmacology, University of Cambridge, Addenbrookes Centre for Clinical Investigation (ACCI), Addenbrookes Hospital, Cambridge, UK
16.17.3: Secondary hypertension

Amy E. Bryant Research Scientist, Infectious Diseases Section, Veterans Affairs Medical Center, Boise, Idaho; Affiliate Assistant Professor, University of Washington School of Medicine, Seattle, Washington, USA
7.6.24: Botulism, gas gangrene, and clostridial gastrointestinal infections

A.D.M. Bryceson London School of Hygiene and Tropical Medicine, London, UK
7.8.12: Leishmaniasis

Camilla Buckley MRC Clinician Scientist and Honorary Consultant, Department of Clinical Neurology, University of Oxford, Oxford, UK
24.22: Autoimmune limbic encephalitis and Morvan's syndrome

Susan Burge Consultant Dermatologist, Oxford Radcliffe Hospitals NHS Trust, UK
23.7: Cutaneous vasculitis, connective tissue diseases, and urticaria

David J. Burn Professor in Movement Disorder & Neurology & Honorary Consultant, Institute for Ageing and Health, Newcastle University; Director, Clinical Ageing Research Unit, Campus for Ageing and Vitality, Newcastle upon Tyne, UK
24.7.3: Movement disorders other than Parkinson's disease

Alan Burnett Co-Director of the Center for Refugee and Disaster Response, Johns Hopkins, Department of Haematology, University of Wales College of Medicine, Cardiff, UK
22.3.4: Acute myeloid leukaemia

Gilbert Burnham Co-Director of the Center for Refugee and Disaster Response, Johns Hopkins, Department of International Health, Baltimore, Maryland, USA
7.9.1: Cutaneous filariasis

Aine Burns Consultant Nephrologist and Director of Postgraduate Medical Education, Centre for Nephrology, Royal Free NHS Trust and University College Medical School, London, UK
21.19: Drugs and the kidney

Jacky Burrin Department of Endocrinology, St Bartholomew's and the Royal London School of Medicine and Dentistry, London, UK
13.1: Principles of hormone action

N.P. Burrows Consultant Dermatologist and Associate Lecturer, Department of Dermatology, Addenbrooke's NHS Trust, Cambridge, UK
20.2: Inherited defects of connective tissue: Ehlers–Danlos syndrome, Marfan's syndrome, and pseudoxanthoma elasticum

Andrew Bush Consultant Physician, Royal Brompton and Harefield NHS Trust, London, UK
18.10: Cystic fibrosis

K. Bushby Professor of Neuromuscular Genetics, Institute of Human Genetics, International Centre for Life, Newcastle upon Tyne, UK
24.24.2: Muscular dystrophy

Valai Bussaratid Assistant Professor of Tropical Medicine, Department of Clinical Tropical Medicine, Mahidol University, Bangkok, Thailand
7.9.7: Gnathostomiasis

Anthony Busuttil Regius Professor of Forensic Medicine Emeritus, Forensic Medicine Section, University of Edinburgh, Edinburgh, UK
27.1: Forensic medicine and the practising doctor

Geoffrey A. Butcher The Malaria Centre, Department of Life Sciences, Imperial College London, London, UK
7.8.2: Malaria

Gary Butler Consultant in Paediatric and Adolescent Medicine and Endocrinology, University College London Hospital; Honorary Professor in Paediatric Endocrinology, UCL Institute of Child Health, Hospital for Children, London, UK
13.9.1: Normal growth and its disorders

W.F. Bynum Professor Emeritus of History of Medicine, Wellcome Trust Centre for the History of Medicine at University College London, UK
2.1.1: Science in medicine: when, how, and what

S.M. Cacciò Department of Infectious, Parasitic and Immunomediated Diseases, Istituto Superiore di Sanità, Viale Regina Elena, Rome, Italy
7.8.5: Cryptosporidium *and cryptosporidiosis*

P.M.A. Calverley Professor of Respiratory Medicine, School of Clinical Sciences, University of Liverpool, UK
18.15: Chronic respiratory failure

Louis R. Caplan Professor of Neurology, Harvard Medical School; Senior Neurologist, Beth Israel Deaconess Medical Center, Boston, Massachusetts, USA
2.3.2: Evidence-based medicine—does it apply to my particular patient?

Jonathan R. Carapetis Director, Menzies School of Health Research, Charles Darwin University, Darwin, Australia
16.9.1: Acute rheumatic fever

Simon Carette Professor of Medicine, University of Toronto; Deputy Physician-in-Chief, Education UHN/MSH; Head, Division of Rheumatology UHN/MSH, Toronto, Ontario, Canada
19.4: Back pain and regional disorders

M. Cariati Lecturer in Surgery, King's College London, UK
13.8.3: Breast cancer

R. Carter Consultant Surgeon, Lister Department of Surgery, Royal Infirmary, Glasgow, UK
15.24.1: Acute pancreatitis

Tim E. Cawston Professor of Rheumatology, Musculoskeletal Research Group, Institute of Cellular Medicine, The Medical School, Newcastle University, Newcastle upon Tyne, UK
19.1: Structure and function: joints and connective tissue

Bruce A. Chabner Clinical Director, Massachusetts General Hospital Cancer Center and Professor of Medicine, Harvard Medical School, Boston, Massachusetts, USA
6.6: Cancer chemotherapy and radiation therapy

Richard E. Chaisson Professor of Medicine, Epidemiology and International Health, Johns Hopkins University School of Medicine and Bloomberg School of Public Health, Baltimore, Maryland, USA
7.6.25: Tuberculosis

S.J. Challacombe Consultant in Oral Medicine, Guy's Hospital, London, UK
15.6: The mouth and salivary glands

Siddharthan Chandran MRC Centre for Regenerative Medicine, University of Edinburgh, UK
4.8: Stem cells and regenerative medicine; 24.10.2: Demyelinating disorders of the central nervous system

Badrinath Chandrasekaran Specialty Registrar in Cardiology, Wessex Cardiothoracic Unit, Southampton General Hospital, Southampton, UK
16.5.1: Clinical features and medical treatments

R.W. Chapman Consultant in Gastroenterology, Department of Gastrenterology, John Radcliffe Hospital, Oxford, UK
15.21.4: Primary sclerosing cholangitis

V. Krishna Chatterjee Professor of Endocrinology, Institute of Metabolic Science and Department of Medicine, University of Cambridge, Addenbrooke's Hospital, Cambridge, UK
13.1: Principles of hormone action

K. Ray Chaudhuri Co-director National Parkinson Foundation Centre of Excellence, Lead Neuroscience Research and Development Strategy, London South Representative, NIHR Nervous Systems Committee, Kings College/University Hospital Lewisham, Kings College and Institute of Psychiatry, London, UK
24.7.2: Parkinsonism and other extrapyramidal diseases

P.F. Chinnery Professor of Neurogenetics and Director of Newcastle, NIHR Biomedical Research Centre for Ageing and Age-related Disease, Institute for Ageing and Health, Newcastle University, Newcastle upon Tyne, UK
24.24.5: Mitochondrial encephalomyopathies

Lydia Chwastiak Assistant Professor, Department of Psychiatry, Yale University, Connecticut, USA
26.5.5: Anxiety and depression

Stefan O. Ciurea Assistant Professor, Department of Stem Cell Transplantation, Division of Cancer Medicine, The University of Texas MD Anderson Cancer Center, Houston, Texas, USA
22.3.8: The polycythaemias; 22.3.10: Thrombocytosis

P. Jane Clarke Consultant Breast Surgeon, Oxford Radcliffe Trust, Oxford, UK
13.8.4: Benign breast disease

P.E. Clayton Consultant in Paediatrics, Royal Manchester Children's Hospital, Manchester, UK
13.9.2: Puberty

S.M. Cobbe Consultant Cardiologist, Glasgow Royal Infirmary; former BHF Walton Professor of Medical Cardiology, University of Glasgow, Scotland
16.2.2: Syncope and palpitations; 16.4: Cardiac arrhythmias

Fredric L. Coe Professor of Medicine, Nephrology Section MC5100, University of Chicago, Chicago Illinois, USA
21.14: Disorders of renal calcium handling, urinary stones, and nephrocalcinosis

J. Cohen Dean of Medicine and Professor of Infectious Diseases, Brighton & Sussex Medical School, Brighton, UK
7.2.4: Infection in the immunocompromised host

R.D. Cohen Emeritus Professor of Medicine, University of London; Queen Mary University of London, Centre for Diabetes, Blizard Institute of Cell & Molecular Science, Bart's & The London School of Medicine & Dentistry, London, UK
12.11: Disturbances of acid–base homeostasis

J. Collier Consultant in General Medicine, John Radcliffe Hospital, Oxford, UK
7.5.22: Hepatitis C

R. Collins Clinical Trial Service Unit & Epidemiological Studies Unit (CTSU), University of Oxford, UK
2.3.3: Large-scale randomized evidence: trials and meta-analyses of trials

Alastair Compston Professor of Neurology, University of Cambridge, Cambridge, UK
24.1: Introduction and approach to the patient with neurological disease; 24.10.2: Demyelinating disorders of the central nervous system

Juliet Compston Professor of Bone Medicine, University of Cambridge School of Clinical Medicine, Cambridge, UK
20.4: Osteoporosis

C.P. Conlon Reader in Infectious Diseases and Tropical Medicine, University of Oxford; Consultant Physician, John Radcliffe Hospitals, Nuffield Department of Medicine, John Radcliffe Hospital, Oxford, UK
7.4: Travel and expedition medicine; 7.5.23: HIV/AIDS

Graham Cooper Consultant Cardiac Surgeon, Sheffield Teaching Hospitals NHS Foundation Trust, UK
16.13.7: Coronary artery bypass surgery

John E. Cooper The University of the West Indies, St Augustine, Trinidad & Tobago, West Indies; Department of Veterinary Medicine, University of Cambridge, Cambridge, UK
7.8.7: Sarcocystosis (sarcosporidiosis)

Susan J. Copley Consultant Radiologist and Reader in Thoracic Imaging, Imperial NHS Trust, London, UK
18.3.2: Thoracic imaging

Minerva Covarrubias Division of Allergy, Pulmonary and Critical Care Medicine, Vanderbilt University School of Medicine, Nashville, Tennessee, USA
14.8: Chest diseases in pregnancy

Philip J. Cowen Professor of Psychopharmacology, Warneford Hospital, Oxford, UK
26.6.1: Psychopharmacology in medical practice

Martin R. Cowie Professor of Cardiology, Imperial College London; Honorary Consultant Cardiologist, Royal Brompton Hospital, London, UK
16.5.1: Clinical features and medical treatments

Timothy M. Cox Professor of Medicine, University of Cambridge, Honorary Consultant Physician, Acting Head of Department, Addenbrooke's Hospital, Cambridge, UK
12.1: The inborn errors of metabolism: general aspects; 12.3.2: Inborn errors of fructose metabolism; 12.3.3: Disorders of galactose, pentose, and pyruvate metabolism; 12.5: The porphyrias; 12.7.1: Hereditary haemochromatosis; 12.8: Lysosomal diseases; 13.13: The pineal gland and melatonin; 15.10.5: Disaccharidase deficiency; 22.5.4: Iron metabolism and its disorders; 33.1: Acute medical presentations; 33.2: Practical procedures

S.E. Craig Research Fellow and Respiratory Medicine Specialty Registrar, Oxford Sleep Unit, Churchill Hospital, Oxford, UK
18.1.1: The upper respiratory tract; 18.5.1: Upper airways obstruction; 18.5.2: Sleep-related disorders of breathing

Robin A.F. Crawford Consultant Gynaecological Oncologist, Addenbrooke's Hospital, Cambridge, UK
14.17: Malignant disease in pregnancy

Adrian Crisp Consultant in Rheumatology and Metabolic Bone Diseases, Addenbrooke's Hospital, Cambridge, UK
20.5: Osteonecrosis, osteochondrosis, and osteochondritis dissecans

Nigel Crisp Independent Member of the House of Lords and London School of Hygiene and Tropical Medicine (formerly NHS Chief Executive and Permanent Secretary of Department of Health)
2.4.3: Priority setting in developed and developing countries

Derrick W. Crook Infectious Disease and Clinical Microbiology, Nuffield Department of Medicine, John Radcliffe Hospital, Oxford, UK
7.6.12: Haemophilus influenzae

Paul Cullinan Faculty of Medicine, Imperial College, London, UK
18.7: Asthma

Peter F. Currie Consultant Cardiologist & Clinical Lead for Cardiology, Perth Royal Infirmary & Ninewells Hospital, Perth, UK
16.9.3: Cardiac disease in HIV infection

Tim Dalgleish Senior Scientist, Medical Research Council, Cognition and Brain Sciences Unit, Cambridge, UK
26.5.1: Grief, stress, and post-traumatic stress disorder

Chi V. Dang Professor of Medicine, Cell Biology, Oncology & Pathology;Professor Vice Dean for Research, Johns Hopkins University School of Medicine, Baltimore, Maryland, USA
22.3.7: Myelodysplasia

Norman Daniels Mary B Saltonstall Professor and Professor of Ethics and Population Health in the Department of Global Health and Population at Harvard School of Public Health, Massachusetts, USA
2.4.2: Reasonableness and its definition in the provision of health care

Christopher J. Danpure Professor of Molecular Cell Biology, University College London, London, UK
12.10: Hereditary disorders of oxalate metabolism—the primary hyperoxalurias

A. Davenport Centre for Nephrology, University College London Medical School, London, UK
21.4: Clinical investigation of renal disease

Gail Davey Associate Professor, School of Public Health, Addis Ababa University, Ethiopia
9.5.8: Podoconiosis (nonfilarial elephantiasis)

Alun Davies Professor of Vascular Surgery, Imperial College School of Medicine, London, UK
16.14.2: Peripheral arterial disease

P.D.O. Davies Consultant Physician, Liverpool Heart and Chest Hospital and Aintree University Hospital, Liverpool, UK
7.6.26: Disease caused by environmental mycobacteria

R. Rhys Davies Consultant in Anaesthesia, Frenchay Hospital, Bristol, UK
24.3.1: Lumbar puncture

Robert J.O. Davies Professor of Respiratory Medicine, Oxford Centre for Respiratory Medicine, NIHR Oxford Biomedical Research Centre, University of Oxford and John Radcliffe Hospital, Oxford, UK
18.17: Pleural diseases; 18.19.3: Pleural tumours; 18.19.4: Mediastinal cysts and tumours

Simon Davies Professor of Nephrology and Dialysis Medicine, Institute of Science and Technology in Medicine, Keele University; Consultant Nephrologist, University Hospital of North Staffordshire, Stoke-on-Trent, UK
21.7.2: Peritoneal dialysis

Richard Dawkins Charles Simonyi Professor for the Understanding of Science, University of Oxford, Oxford, UK
2.1.2: Evolution: medicine's most basic science

Chris P. Day Institute of Cellular Medicine, Newcastle University, Newcastle upon Tyne, UK
15.22.1: Alcoholic liver disease; 15.22.2: Nonalcoholic steatohepatitis

Colin Dayan Head of Clinical Research and Reader in Medicine, Henry Wellcome Laboratories for Integrative Neuroscience and Endocrinology, University of Bristol, UK
13.11.1: Diabetes

Linda Dayan Senior Staff Specialist and Director of Sexual Health Services, Royal North Shore Hospital, Sydney; Clinical Lecturer, School of Public Health, University of Sydney, Sydney, Australia
7.6.36: Syphilis

Marc E. De Broe Professor of Medicine, Laboratory of Pathophysiology, University of Antwerp, Belgium
21.9.2: Chronic tubulointerstitial nephritis

Kevin M. De Cock Centers for Disease Control and Prevention, Nairobi, Kenya
7.5.24: HIV in the developing world

Menno D. De Jong Department of Medical Microbiology, Academic Medical Center, University of Amsterdam, Amsterdam, The Netherlands
24.11.2: Viral infections

Pauline de la Motte Hall† Late Professor, Division of Science, Murdoch University, Murdoch, Australia
15.22.7: Hepatic granulomas

P.B. Deegan Consultant in Metabolic Medicine, Department of Medicine, Addenbrooke's Hospital, Cambridge, UK
12.8: Lysosomal diseases

Barbara A. Degar Assistant Professor of Pediatrics, Dana-Farber Cancer Institute, Children's Hospital Boston, Harvard Medical School, Boston, Massachusetts, USA
22.4.2: Introduction to the lymphoproliferative disorders

D.M. Denison Emeritus Professor of Clinical Physiology, Royal Brompton Hospital and Imperial College London, London, UK
9.5.5: Aerospace medicine; 9.5.6: Diving medicine

Christopher P. Denton Professor of Experimental Rheumatology, Centre for Rheumatology, Division of Medicine, UCL Medical School, Royal Free Hospital, London, UK
19.11.3: Systemic sclerosis

Ulrich Desselberger Director of Research, Department of Medicine, Addenbrooke's Hospital, Cambridge, UK
7.5.8: Enterovirus infections; 7.5.9: Virus infections causing diarrhoea and vomiting

Michael Doherty Professor of Rheumatology, University of Nottingham, UK
19.3: Clinical investigation; 19.10: Crystal-related arthropathies

Richard S. Doll†† Emeritus Professor of Medicine and Honorary Member, Cancer Studies Unit, Nuffield Department of Medicine, Radcliffe Infirmary, Oxford, UK
6.1: Epidemiology of cancer

† It is with regret that we report the death of Professor Pauline de la Motte Hall during the preparation of this edition of the textbook; †† it is with regret that we report the death of Professor Richard S. Doll during the preparation of this edition of the textbook.

Clare Dollery Divisional Clinical Director, Consultant Cardiologist, The Heart Hospital, UCLH NHS Foundation Trust, London, UK
16.13.1: Biology and pathology of atherosclerosis

Michael Donaghy Department of Clinical Neurology, John Radcliffe Hospital, Oxford, UK
24.15: The motor neuron diseases

Basil Donovan Professor of Sexual Health, National Centre in HIV Epidemiology and Clinical Research, University of New South Wales; Senior Staff Specialist, Sydney Sexual Health Centre, Sydney Hospital, Sydney, Australia
7.6.36: Syphilis

Philip Dormitzer Senior Director, Senior Project Leader, Viral Vaccine Research, Novartis Vaccines and Diagnostics, Cambridge, Massachusetts, USA
7.5.9: Virus infections causing diarrhoea and vomiting

H.M.P. Dowson Consultant General and Laparoscopic Surgeon, Frimley Park Hospital, Surrey, UK
15.4.2: Gastrointestinal bleeding

Tilman B. Drüeke Division of Nephrology and Inserm U845, Necker Hospital, Paris, France
21.6: Chronic kidney disease

Patrick C.A. Dubois MRC Clinical Research Training Fellow, Specialty Registrar in Gastroenterology, Barts and The London School of Medicine and Dentistry, Queen Mary University of London, London, UK
15.10.3: Coeliac disease

Christopher Dudley Consultant Renal Physician. The Richard Bright Renal Unit, Southmead Hospital, North Bristol NHS Trust, Bristol, UK
16.14.3: Cholesterol embolism

D.W. Dunne Department of Pathology, University of Cambridge, Cambridge, UK
7.11.1: Schistosomiasis

Stephen R. Durham Professor of Allergy and Respiratory Medicine; Head, Section of Allergy and Clinical Immunology, National Heart and Lung Institute, Imperial College and Royal Brompton Hospital, London
18.6: Allergic rhinitis

P.N. Durrington Professor of Medicine, Cardiovascular Research Group Division of Clinical and Laboratory Sciences, University of Manchester Core Technology Facility, Manchester, UK
12.6: Lipid and lipoprotein disorders

J. Dwight Consultant Cardiologist, John Radcliffe Hospital, Oxford, UK
16.2.1: Chest pain, breathlessness, and fatigue

Patrick C. D'Haese Associate Professor, Laboratory of Pathophysiology, University of Antwerp, Belgium
21.9.2: Chronic tubulointerstitial nephritis

Ian Eardley Consultant Urologist, Leeds Teaching Hospital Trust, Leeds, UK
13.8.5: Sexual dysfunction

M. Eastwood Post-Retirement Honorary Fellow, Department of Medical Sciences, Western General Hospital, Edinburgh, UK
11.2: Vitamins and trace elements

Tim Eden Honorary Professor of Paediatric and Adolescent Oncology, University of Manchester, UK
22.3.3: Acute lymphoblastic leukaemia

Mark J. Edwards Sobell Department of Motor Neuroscience and Movement Disorders, Institute of Neurology, University College London; National Hospital for Neurology and Neurosurgery, London, UK
24.7.1: Subcortical structures: the cerebellum, basal ganglia, and thalamus

Richard Edwards† Late Emeritus Professor of Medicine, Liverpool University, UK
24.24.4: Metabolic and endocrine disorders

Rosalind A. Eeles Professor of Oncogenetics, The Institute of Cancer Research; Honorary Consultant in Cancer Genetics & Clinical Oncology, Royal Marsden NHS Foundation Trust, Sutton, UK
6.3: The genetics of inherited cancers

Perry Elliott The Heart Hospital, University College London, UK
16.7.2: The cardiomyopathies: hypertrophic, dilated, restrictive, and right ventricular; 16.7.3: Specific heart muscle disorders

Christopher J. Ellis Consultant Physician, Department of Infection and Tropical Medicine, Heartlands Hospital, Birmingham, UK
7.2.1: Clinical approach

Monique M. Elseviers Associate Professor, Department of Nursing Sciences, University of Antwerp, Belgium
21.9.2: Chronic tubulointerstitial nephritis

Caroline Elston Consultant Physician, Respiratory Medicine and Adult Cystic Fibrosis, King's College Hospital, London, UK
18.10: Cystic fibrosis

M.A. Epstein Nuffield Department of Clinical Medicine, John Radcliffe Hospital, Oxford, UK
7.5.3: Epstein–Barr virus

Wendy N. Erber Consultant Haematologist and Clinical Director of Haematology, Addenbrooke's Hospital, Cambridge, UK
22.3.2: The classification of leukaemia

E. Ernst Professor of Complementary Medicine, Peninsula Medical School, Universities of Exeter and Plymouth, Exeter, UK
2.5: Complementary and alternative medicine

David Eschenbach Professor and Chair, Department of Obstetrics and Gynecology, University of Washington, Seattle, Washington, USA
8.5: Pelvic inflammatory disease

Andrew P. Evan Chancellor's Professor, Department of Anatomy and Cell Biology, Indiana University School of Medicine, Indianapolis, Indiana, USA
21.14: Disorders of renal calcium handling, urinary stones, and nephrocalcinosis

Martin J. Evans School of Biosciences, Cardiff University, Cardiff, UK
4.7: Discovery of embryonic stem cells and the concept of regenerative medicine

Timothy Evans Professor of Intensive Care Medicine, Imperial College; Department of Anaesthesia and Intensive Care Medicine, Royal Brompton Hospital, UK
17.5: Acute respiratory failure

Pamela Ewan Consultant Allergist, Department of Medicine, Addenbrooke's Hospital, Cambridge, UK
5.3: Allergy

Christopher G. Fairburn Wellcome Principal Research Fellow and Professor of Psychiatry, Department of Psychiatry, University of Oxford, Oxford, UK
26.5.6: Eating disorders

Jeremy Farrar Oxford University Clinical Research Unit, Wellcome Trust Major Overseas Programme Vietnam; South East Asia Infectious Disease Clinical Research Network, Ho Chi Minh City, Vietnam
7.5.15: Dengue; 24.11.1: Bacterial infections; 24.11.2: Viral infections

Ken Farrington Consultant Nephrologist, Lister Hospital, Stevenage, UK
21.3: Clinical presentation of renal disease; 21.7.1: Haemodialysis

John Feehally Consultant Nephrologist, University Hospitals of Leicester; Honorary Professor of Renal Medicine, University of Leicester, UK
21.8.1: Immunoglobulin A nephropathy and Henoch–Schönlein purpura; 21.8.2: Thin membrane nephropathy

Eleanor Feldman Consultant Liaison Psychiatrist, John Radcliffe Hospital Oxford; Consultant in Eating Disorders, Warneford Hospital Oxford; Honorary Senior Clinical Lecturer in Psychiatry, University of Oxford, UK
26.2: Taking a psychiatric history from a medical patient; 26.3: Acute behavioural emergencies

Peter J. Fenner Associate Professor, School of Public Health, Tropical Medicine and Rehabilitation Sciences, James Cook University, Townsville, Australia
9.5.3: Drowning

† It is with regret that we report the death of Professor Richard Edwards during the preparation of this edition of the textbook.

Robert Ferrari Department of Medicine, University of Alberta, Edmonton, Alberta, Canada
19.2: Clinical presentation and diagnosis of rheumatic disease

C. ffrench-Constant Professor of Medical Neurology, MRC Centre for Regenerative Medicine, Centre for Multiple Sclerosis Research, The University of Edinburgh, Queen's Medical Research Institute, Edinburgh, UK
24.18: Developmental abnormalities of the central nervous system

Richard E. Fielding Locum Consultant Nephrologist, Brighton and Sussex University Hospital Trust, Brighton, UK
21.3: Clinical presentation of renal disease

R.G. Finch Professor of Infectious Diseases, Nottingham University Hospitals NHS Trust, Nottingham, UK
7.2.5: Antimicrobial chemotherapy

H.V. Firth Consultant Clinical Geneticist, Addenbrooke's Hospital, Cambridge, UK
24.18: Developmental abnormalities of the central nervous system

John D. Firth Consultant Physician and Nephrologist, Cambridge University Hospitals NHS Foundation Trust, Cambridge, UK
14.5: Renal disease in pregnancy; 14.12: Neurological disease in pregnancy; 16.15.3: Pulmonary oedema; 16.16.1: Deep venous thrombosis and pulmonary embolism; 16.19: Idiopathic oedema of women; 17.3: The clinical approach to the patient who is very ill; 21.2.2: Disorders of potassium homeostasis; 21.5: Acute kidney injury; 21.6: Chronic kidney disease; 21.10.9: Atherosclerotic renovascular disease; 33.1: Acute medical presentations; 33.2: Practical procedures

Rebecca Fitzgerald Honorary Consultant Gastroenterologist, Cambridge University Hospitals NHS Foundation Trust, Cambridge, UK
15.7: Diseases of the oesophagus

R. Andres Floto Wellcome Trust Senior Clinical Fellow, Cambridge Institute for Medical Research, University of Cambridge; Honorary Respiratory Consultant, Papworth & Addenbrooke's Hospitals, Cambridge, UK
4.5: Intracellular signalling

Edward D. Folland Chief of Clinical Cardiology, UMassMemorial Medical Center, Worcester, Massachusetts; Professor of Medicine, University of Massachusetts Medical School, Worcester, Massachusetts, USA
16.3.4: Cardiac catheterization and angiography; 16.13.6: Percutaneous interventional cardiac procedures

Keith A.A. Fox British Heart Foundation Professor of Cardiology, Centre for Cardiovascular Sciences, University of Edinburgh, Edinburgh, UK
16.13.5: Management of acute coronary syndrome

Ross S. Francis Transplantation Research Immunology Group, Nuffield Department of Surgery, University of Oxford, John Radcliffe Hospital, Oxford, UK
5.5: Principles of transplantation immunology

Stephen Franks Professor of Reproductive Endocrinology, Imperial College London, Hammersmith Hospital, London, UK
13.8.1: Ovarian disorders

Keith N. Frayn Professor of Human Metabolism, Oxford Centre for Diabetes, Endocrinology and Metabolism, University of Oxford, Oxford, UK
11.1: Nutrition: macronutrient metabolism

A.H. Freeman Consultant Radiologist, Addenbrooke's Hospital, Cambridge, UK.
15.3.3: Radiology of the gastrointestinal tract

Izzet Fresko Professor, Division of Rheumatology, Department of Medicine, Cerrahpasa Medical Faculty, University of Istanbul, Istanbul, Turkey
19.11.5: Behçet's syndrome

Peter S. Friedmann Emeritus Professor of Dermatology, University of Southampton, Southampton, UK
23.6: Dermatitis/eczema; 23.16: Cutaneous reactions to drugs

Peggy Frith Consultant Ophthalmic Physician, John Radcliffe Hospital, Oxford and University College Hospital London, UK
25.1: The eye in general medicine

David A. Gabbott Consultant Anaesthetist, Gloucestershire Hospitals NHS Foundation Trust UK; Chairman, Research subcommittee, Resuscitation Council (UK) Executive Committee Resuscitation Council (UK)
17.1: Cardiac arrest

Patrick G. Gallagher Professor of Pediatrics and Genetics, Yale University School of Medicine, New Haven, Connecticut, USA
22.5.10: Disorders of the red cell membrane

Hector H. Garcia Professor, Department of Microbiology, Universidad Peruana Cayetano Heredia, Lima, Peru; Head, Cysticercosis Unit, Instituto de Ciencias Neurológicas, Lima, Peru
7.10.1: Cystic hydatid disease (Echinococcus granulosus); 7.10.3: Cysticercosis

Lawrence B. Gardner Assistant Professor of Medicine and Pharmacology, Division of Hematology and the NYU Cancer Institute, New York University School of Medicine, New York, USA
22.3.7: Myelodysplasia

J.S. Hill Gaston Consultant in Rheumatology, Department of Rheumatology, University of Cambridge, Cambridge, UK
19.8: Reactive arthritis

Sarah Germain Senior Registrar in Obstetric Medicine, Guy's & St Thomas' Foundation Trust, London, UK
14.14: Autoimmune rheumatic disorders and vasculitis in pregnancy

G.J. Gibson Emeritus Professor of Respiratory Medicine, Newcastle University Newcastle upon Tyne, UK
18.3.1: Respiratory function tests

J. van Gijn Emeritus Professor of Neurology, University Medical Centre, Utrecht, The Netherlands
24.10.1: Stroke: cerebrovascular disease

I.P. Giles Centre for Rheumatology, Department of Medicine, University College London, London, UK
19.11.1: Introduction

Robert H. Gilman Professor, Department of International Health, Johns Hopkins Bloomberg School of Hygiene and Public Health, Baltimore, Maryland, USA
7.10.3: Cysticercosis

Ian Gilmore President, Royal College of Physicians, London, UK
15.24.3: Tumours of the pancreas

Alexander Gimson Consultant Physician and Hepatologist, Liver Transplantation Unit, Cambridge University Hospitals Foundation NHS Trust, Cambridge, UK
14.9: Liver and gastrointestinal diseases in pregnancy; 15.19: Structure and function of the liver, biliary tract, and pancreas; 15.26: Miscellaneous disorders of the bowel and liver

Paul P. Glasziou Department of Primary Health Care, University of Oxford, Oxford, UK
2.3.1: Bringing the best evidence to the point of care

Fergus V. Gleeson Oxford Pleural Unit, Oxford Centre for Respiratory Medicine, John Radcliffe Hospital, Oxford, UK
18.17: Pleural diseases

M.A. Glover Medical Director, Hyperbaric Medicine Unit, St Richard's Hospital, Chichester, UK
9.5.6: Diving medicine

Peter J. Goadsby Headache Group, Department of Neurology, University of California, San Francisco, California, USA
24.8: Headache

D. Goldblatt Professor of Vaccinology and Immunology, Consultant in Paediatric Immunology, Head, Immunobiology Unit, Director, Clinical Research and Development and, Director, NIHR Biomedical Research Centre, Great Ormond Street Hospital for Children NHS Trust and Institute of Child Health, University College London, UK
7.3: Immunization

Ann-Marie J. Golden Research Worker, Medical Research Council, Cognition and Brain Sciences Unit, Cambridge, UK
26.5.1: Grief, stress, and post-traumatic stress disorder

John M. Goldman Professor of Haematology (Emeritus), Imperial College, London, UK
22.3.6: Chronic myeloid leukaemia

Armando E. Gonzalez Dean, School of Veterinary Medicine, Universidad Nacional Mayor de San Marcos, Lima, Peru
*7.10.1: Cystic hydatid disease (*Echinococcus granulosus*)*

Timothy H.J. Goodship Professor of Renal Medicine, Newcastle University, UK
21.10.5: Haemolytic uraemic syndrome

Sherwood L. Gorbach Tufts University, Nutrition/infection Unit, Boston, Massachusetts, USA
15.18: Gastrointestinal infections

E.C. Gordon-Smith Emeritus Professor of Haematology, St George's, University of London, London, UK
22.3.11: Aplastic anaemia and other causes of bone marrow failure; 22.8.2: Haemopoietic stem cell transplantation

Eduardo Gotuzzo Instituto de Medicina Tropical Alexander von Humboldt Universidad Peruana Cayetano Heredia Av. Honorio Delgado, San Martín de Porres, Lima, Peru
7.5.25: HTLV-1, HTLV-2, and associated diseases

P. Goulder Wellcome Senior Clinical Fellow & Honorary Consultant Paediatrician, University of Oxford, Oxford, UK
7.5.23: HIV/AIDS

Jan Tore Gran Professor and Head, Department of Rheumatology, Oslo University Hospital, Rikshospitalet, Oslo, Norway
19.11.4; Polymyalgia rheumatica and temporal arteritis

J.M. Grange Visiting Professor, University College London, Centre for Infectious Diseases and International Health, London, UK
7.6.26: Disease caused by environmental mycobacteria

Alison D. Grant Department of Paediatrics, University of Auckland, Auckland, New Zealand
7.5.24: HIV in the developing world

Cameron Grant Department of Paediatrics, University of Auckland, Auckland, New Zealand
7.6.14: Bordetella infection

David Gray Reader in Medicine & Honorary Consultant Physician, Department of Cardiovascular Medicine, Nottingham University Hospitals NHS Trust, Nottingham, UK
16.3.1: Electrocardiography

R. Gray Clinical Trial Service Unit & Epidemiological Studies Unit (CTSU), University of Oxford, UK
2.3.3: Large-scale randomized evidence: trials and meta-analyses of trials

John R. Graybill Professor Emeritus, Division of Infectious Diseases, Department of Medicine, University of Texas Health Science Center at San Antonio, San Antonio, Texas, USA
7.7.3: Coccidioidomycosis

Manfred S. Green Professor and Head, School of Public Health, University of Haifa, Haifa, Israel
9.5.13: Bioterrorism

Roger Greenwood Consultant Nephrologist, Lister Hospital, Stevenage, UK
21.7.1: Haemodialysis

I.A. Greer Professor of Obstetric Medicine & Dean, Hull York Medical School, UK
14.7: Thrombosis in pregnancy

Christopher Griffiths Professor of Dermatology, Salford Royal NHS Foundation Trust, The University of Manchester, Manchester, UK
23.5: Papulosquamous disease

William J.H. Griffiths Consultant Hepatologist, Department of Hepatology, Addenbrooke's Hospital, Cambridge, UK
12.7.1: Hereditary haemochromatosis; 15.22.6: Liver tumours—primary and secondary

David I. Grove Formerly Director of Clinical Microbiology and Infectious Diseases, The Queen Elizabeth Hospital, Woodville and Clinical Professor, University of Adelaide, South Australia, Australia
7.9.5: Gut and tissue nematode infections acquired by ingestion; 7.10.4: Diphyllobothriasis and sparganosis; 7.11.2: Liver fluke infections; 7.11.4: Intestinal trematode infections

J.P. Grünfeld Université Paris Descartes, Department of Nephrology, Necker Hospital, Paris, France
21.12: Renal involvement in genetic disease

D.J. Gubler Director, Program on Emerging Infectious Disease, Duke-NUS Graduate Medical School, Singapore; Asian Pacific Institute of Tropical Medicine and Infectious Diseases, University of Hawaii, Honolulu
7.5.12: Alphaviruses; 7.5.14: Flaviviruses excluding dengue

Richard L. Guerrant Hunter Professor of International Medicine, Division of Infectious Diseases and International Health; Director, Center for Global Health, University of Virginia, Charlottesville, Virginia, USA
7.6.11: Cholera

John Guillebaud Emeritus Professor of Family Planning and Reproductive Health, University College, London, UK
8.6: Principles of contraception; 14.19: Benefits and risks of oral contraception

Mark Gurnell University Lecturer in Endocrinology, Institute of Metabolic Science and Department of Medicine, University of Cambridge, Addenbrooke's Hospital, Cambridge, UK
13.1: Principles of hormone action

Alejandro Gutierrez Instructor of Pediatrics, Harvard Medical School, Dana-Farber Cancer Institute and Children's Hospital Boston, Massachusetts, USA
22.3.1: Cell and molecular biology of human leukaemias

M.R. Haeney Consultant Immunologist, Salford Royal NHS Foundation Trust, Salford, UK
15.5: Immune disorders of the gastrointestinal tract

Davidson H. Hamer Associate Professor of International Health and Medicine, Boston University Schools of Public Health and Medicine; Director, Travel Clinic, Boston Medical Center, Adjunct Associate Professor of Nutrition, Tufts University Friedman School of Nutrition Science and Policy, Center for International Health and Development, Boston, Massachusetts, USA
15.18: Gastrointestinal infections

P.J. Hammond Consultant in Endocrinology, Harrogate District Hospital, Harrogate, UK
15.9: Hormones and the gastrointestinal tract

Y. Han Staff Physician, Transfusion Medicine, City of Hope Medical Center, Duarte, California, USA
22.8.1: Blood transfusion

M.G. Hanna Consultant Neurologist, National Hospital for Neurology and Institute of Neurology, London, UK
24.24.1: Structure and function of muscle

David M. Hansell Consultant Radiologist and Professor of Thoracic Imaging, Royal Brompton and Harefield NHS Trust, London, UK
18.3.2: Thoracic imaging

J.M. Harrington Emeritus Professor of Occupational Medicine, The University of Birmingham, Birmingham, UK
9.4.1: Occupational and environmental health

Nicholas K. Harrison Respiratory Unit, Morriston Hospital, Swansea, Wales, UK
18.11.3: Bronchiolitis obliterans and cryptogenic organizing pneumonia

Tina Hartert Associate Professor of Medicine, Vanderbilt University School of Medicine, Institute for Medicine and Public Health, Center for Health Services Research, Nashville, Tennessee, USA
14.8: Chest diseases in pregnancy

Adrian R.W. Hatfield Hepatobiliary Unit, The Middlesex Hospital, London, UK
15.3.2: Upper gastrointestinal endoscopy

Philip N. Hawkins Professor of Medicine, National Amyloidosis Centre and Centre for Acute Phase Proteins, UCL Medical School, London, UK
12.12.2: Hereditary periodic fever syndromes; 12.12.3: Amyloidosis

Keith Hawton Professor of Psychiatry, Centre for Suicide Research, Department of Psychiatry, University of Oxford, Oxford, UK
26.5.2: The patient who has attempted suicide

Roderick J. Hay Professor of Cutaneous Infection, Dermatology Department, King's College Hospital, London, UK
7.6.30: Nocardiosis; 7.7.1: Fungal infections; 23.10: Infections and the skin

Catherine E.G. Head Consultant Cardiologist, Guy's and St Thomas' NHS Foundation Trust, London, UK
14.6: Heart disease in pregnancy

Eugene Healy Professor of Dermatology, Dermatopharmacology, University of Southampton, Southampton General Hospital, UK
23.8: Disorders of pigmentation; 23.16: Cutaneous reactions to drugs

Nick Heather Emeritus Professor of Alcohol & Other Drug Studies, School of Psychology & Sport Sciences, Northumbria University, UK
26.7.2: Brief interventions against excessive alcohol consumption

David W. Hecht The John W. Clarke Professor and Chairman, Department of Medicine, Loyola University Medical Center, Maywood, Illinois, USA
7.6.10: Anaerobic bacteria

David A. van Heel Professor of Gastrointestinal Genetics, Honorary Consultant Gastroenterologist, Barts and The London School of Medicine and Dentistry, Queen Mary University of London, London, UK
15.10.3: Coeliac disease

Harry Hemingway Professor of Clinical Epidemiology, Department of Epidemiology and Public Health, University College London Medical School, London, UK
16.13.2: Coronary heart disease: epidemiology and prevention

Janet Hemingway Director, Liverpool School of Tropical Medicine, Liverpool, UK
7.8.2: Malaria

D.J. Hendrick Emeritus Professor, University of Newcastle upon Tyne, Consultant Physician Royal Victoria Infirmary, Newcastle upon Tyne, UK
18.14.1: Pulmonary haemorrhagic disorders; 18.14.2: Eosinophilic pneumonia; 18.14.3: Lymphocytic infiltrations of the lung; 18.14.4: Extrinsic allergic alveolitis; 18.14.5: Pulmonary Langerhans' cell histiocytosis; 18.14.6: Lymphangioleiomyomatosis; 18.14.7: Pulmonary alveolar proteinosis; 18.14.8: Pulmonary amyloidosis; 18.14.9: Lipoid (lipid) pneumonia; 18.14.10: Pulmonary alveolar microlithiasis; 18.14.11: Toxic gases and aerosols; 18.14.12: Radiation pneumonitis; 18.14.13: Drug-induced lung disease

Michael Henein Professor of Cardiology, Umea University, Sweden; Canterbury Christ Church University, UK
16.6: Heart valve disease; 16.8: Pericardial disease

Martin F. Heyworth Staff Physician and Adjunct Professor of Medicine, VA Medical Center and University of Pennsylvania, Philadelphia, Pennsylvania, USA
7.8.8: Giardiasis, balantidiasis, isosporiasis, and microsporidiosis

Tran Tinh Hien Vice Director, Centre for Tropical Diseases (Cho Quan Hospital), Ho Chi Minh City, Vietnam
7.6.1: Diphtheria

Katherine A. High Professor of Pediatrics, University of Pennsylvania School of Medicine, Children's Hospital of Philadelphia, Abramson Research Center, Philadelphia, Pennsylvania, USA
22.6.4: Genetic disorders of coagulation

Sharon Hillier Professor, Department of Obstetrics, Gynecology and Reproductive Sciences, University of Pittsburgh School of Medicine, Pittsburgh, Pennsylvania, USA
7.8.13: Trichomoniasis

David Hilton-Jones Clinical Director, Muscular Dystrophy Campaign, Muscle & Nerve Centre, Department of Clinical Neurology, John Radcliffe Hospital, Oxford, UK
24.23: Disorders of the neuromuscular junction; 24.24.3: Myotonia; 24.24.4: Metabolic and endocrine disorders

N. Hirani Consultant in Respiratory Medicine, Royal Infirmary, Edinburgh, UK
18.11.2: Idiopathic pulmonary fibrosis

Gideon M. Hirschfield Assistant Professor of Medicine, University of Toronto Liver Centre, Toronto Western Hospital, Toronto, Ontario, Canada
15.22.5: Liver transplantation

Moshe Hod Director, Division of Maternal Fetal Medicine, Helen Schneider Hospital for Women, Rabin Medical Center, Sackler Faculty of Medicine, Tel Aviv University, Petah-Tiqva, Israel
14.10: Diabetes in pregnancy

John R. Hodges Federation Fellow and Professor of Cognitive Neurology, Prince of Wales Medical Research Institute, Sydney, Australia
24.4.1: Disturbances of higher cerebral function; 24.4.2: Alzheimer's disease and other dementias

H.J.F. Hodgson Sheila Sherlock Chair of Medicine, University College London, London, UK
15.10.6: Whipple's disease; 15.21.1: Viral hepatitis—clinical aspects; 15.21.2: Autoimmune hepatitis

H. Hof Labor Limbach, Heidelberg, Germany
7.6.37: Listeriosis

A.V. Hoffbrand Consultant in Haematology. Department of Haematology, Royal Free Hospital, London, UK
22.5.6: Megaloblastic anaemia and miscellaneous deficiency anaemias

Ronald Hoffman Albert A. and Vera G. List, Professor of Medicine, Division of Hematology/Oncology, Director, Myeloproliferative Disorders Program, Tisch Cancer Institute, Departments of Medicine, Mount Sinai School of Medicine, New York, USA
22.3.8: The polycythaemias; 22.3.10: Thrombocytosis

Georg F. Hoffmann Chairman, University Children's Hospital, Department of General Pediatrics, Heidelberg, Germany
12.2: Protein-dependent inborn errors of metabolism

P. Holloway Consultant Chemical Pathologist and Honorary Senior Lecturer in Metabolic Medicine, Site Lead Clinician in Chemical Pathology and Immunology, St Mary's Hospital, Imperial College Healthcare NHS Trust, Medical School, London, UK
32.1: Biochemistry in medicine—reference intervals: the use of biochemical analysis for diagnosis and management

L. Holmberg Professor of Cancer Epidemiology, King's College London, UK
13.8.3: Breast cancer

Tony Hope Professor of Medical Ethics, University of Oxford; Fellow of St Cross College; and Honorary Consultant Psychiatrist
2.2: Medical ethics

Julian Hopkin Rector, Medicine & Health, School of Medicine, Swansea University, UK
18.2: The clinical presentation of respiratory disease

Bala Hota Division of Infectious Diseases, Department of Medicine, John H. Stroger Jr. Hospital of Cook County; Assistant Professor, Rush University Medical Center, Chicago, Illinois, USA
7.6.4: Staphylococci

Andrew R. Houghton Consultant Physician & Cardiologist, Grantham & District Hospital, Grantham, UK, and Visiting Fellow, University of Lincoln, Lincoln, UK
16.3.1: Electrocardiography

Laurence Huang Professor of Medicine, University of California San Francisco; Chief, AIDS Chest Clinic, HIV/AIDS Division, San Francisco General Hospital, San Francisco, California, USA
7.7.5: Pneumocystis jirovecii

H.C. Hughes Specialty Registrar (Infectious diseases/Microbiology), University Hospital of Wales, UK
7.5.29: Newly discovered viruses

I.A. Hughes Head of Department, Department of Paediatrics, Addenbrooke's Hospital, Cambridge, UK
13.7.2: Congenital adrenal hyperplasia; 13.9.3: Normal and abnormal sexual differentiation

R.A.C. Hughes Emeritus Professor of Neurology, King's College, London; Visiting Professor of Neurology, University College London; Cochrane Neuromuscular Disease Group, MRC Centre for Neuromuscular Disease
24.12: Disorders of cranial nerves; 24.16: Diseases of the peripheral nerves

P.J. Hutchinson Honorary Consultant Neurosurgeon and Senior Academy Fellow, Addenbrooke's Hospital, Cambridge, UK
24.5.6: Brain death and the vegetative state

Lawrence Impey Consultant in Obstetrics and Fetal Medicine, The John Radcliffe Hospital, Oxford, UK
14.15: Infections in pregnancy

C.W. Imrie Consultant Surgeon, Lister Department of Surgery, Royal Infirmary, Glasgow, UK
15.24.1: Acute pancreatitis

P.G. Isaacson Consultant in Histopathology, Department of Histopathology, Royal Free and University College Medical School, London, UK
15.10.4: Gastrointestinal lymphoma

David A. Isenberg Professor of Rheumatology, Centre for Rheumatology, Department of Medicine, University College London, London, UK
19.11.1: Introduction; 19.11.2: Systemic lupus erythematosus and related disorders

C. Ison Director, Sexually Transmitted Bacteria Reference Laboratory, Health Protection Agency Centre for Infections, London, UK
7.6.6: Neisseria gonorrhoeae

Alan A. Jackson Consultant in General Medicine, Southampton General Hospital, Southampton, UK
11.3: Severe malnutrition

Robin Jacoby Professor Emeritus of Old Age Psychiatry, University of Oxford; Department of Psychiatry, The Warneford Hospital, Oxford, UK
29.2: Mental disorders of old age

Dean Jamison Professor of Global Health, Department of Global Health, University of Washington, Seattle, Washington, USA
3.1: Global burden of disease: causes, levels, and intervention strategies

David Jayne Consultant in Nephrology and Vasculitis, Renal Unit, Department of Medicine, Addenbrooke's Hospital, Cambridge, UK
21.10.2: The kidney in systemic vasculitis

K.J.M. Jeffery Consultant Virologist, Oxford Radcliffe NHS Trust, John Radcliffe Hospital, Oxford, UK
7.5.22: Hepatitis C

Jørgen Skov Jensen Mycoplasma Laboratory, Copenhagen, Denmark
7.6.45: Mycoplasmas

D.P. Jewell Emeritus Professor of Gastroenterology, University of Oxford; Honorary Consultant Physician, John Radcliffe Hospital, Oxford, UK
15.12: Ulcerative colitis

Vivekanand Jha Additional Professor of Nephrology; Co-ordinator, Stem Cell Research Facility, Postgraduate Medical Institute, Chandigarh, India
21.11: Renal diseases in the tropics

Alexis J. Joannides Department of Clinical Neurosciences, University of Cambridge, UK
4.8: Stem cells and regenerative medicine

Anne M. Johnson Professor of Infectious Disease Epidemiology, Centre for Sexual Health and HIV Research, Research Department of Infection and Public Health, University College London, London, UK
8.2: Sexual behaviour

D. Joly Université Paris Descartes, Department of Nephrology, Necker Hospital, Paris, France
21.12: Renal involvement in genetic disease

E. Anthony Jones Former Chief of Hepatology, Academic Medical Center, Amsterdam, The Netherlands
15.22.4: Hepatocellular failure

Islam Junaid Consultant Urologist Barts and London NHS Trust Hospitals
21.17: Urinary tract obstruction

Summerpal S. Kahlon Melbourne Internal Medicine Associates, Melbourne, Florida, USA
7.5.16: Bunyaviridae

P.A. Kalra Consultant in Nephrology, Salford Royal NHS Foundation Trust, Salford, UK
21.10.9: Atherosclerotic renovascular disease

Kenneth C. Kalunian Professor of Medicine, Division of Rheumatology, Allergy and Immunology, University of California, San Diego School of Medicine, La Jolla, California, USA
19.9: Osteoarthritis

Eileen Kaner Institute of Health and Society, Newcastle University, UK
26.7.2: Brief interventions against excessive alcohol consumption

Niki Karavitaki Locum Consultant in Endocrinology, Department of Endocrinology, Oxford Centre for Diabetes, Endocrinology and Metabolism, Churchill Hospital, Oxford, UK
13.2: Disorders of the anterior pituitary gland; 13.3: Disorders of the posterior pituitary gland

Fiona E. Karet Professor of Nephrology, Honorary Consultant in Renal Medicine, University of Cambridge, UK
21.15: The renal tubular acidoses

Wayne J. Katon Professor and Vice-Chair, Department of Psychiatry & Behavioral Sciences, University of Washington, Washington, USA
26.5.5: Anxiety and depression

David Keeling Oxford Haemophilia & Thrombosis Centre, Churchill Hospital, Oxford, UK
16.16.2: Therapeutic anticoagulation

Jonathan Kell Department of Haematology, University Hospital of Wales and Cardiff University, Cardiff, UK
22.3.4: Acute myeloid leukaemia

David P. Kelsell Centre for Cutaneous Research, Blizard Institute of Cell and Molecular Science, Barts and the London School of Medicine and Dentistry, Queen Mary University of London, London, UK
23.3: Inherited skin disease

John G. Kelton McMaster University Medical Center, Hamilton, Ontario, Canada
22.6.3: Disorders of platelet number and function

Christopher Kennard Professor of Clinical Neurology, Head of Department, Department of Clinical Neurology, John Radcliffe Hospital, Oxford, UK
24.6.1: Visual pathways

R.S.C. Kerr Neurosurgery Consultant, John Radcliffe Hospital, Oxford, UK
24.11.3: Intracranial abscesses

M.G.W. Kettlewell Emeritus Consultant Colorectal Surgeon, John Radcliffe Hospital, Oxford, UK
15.14: Colonic diverticular disease

Maurice King Honorary Research Fellow, University of Leeds, Leeds, UK
3.4.2: A sinister pathogen corrupts two disciplines: the demographic entrapment of Middle Africa

Paul Klenerman Nuffield Department of Medicine, University of Oxford, Oxford, UK
5.1.3: Adaptive immunity; 7.5.22: Hepatitis C

Steve Knapper Department of Haematology, University Hospital of Wales and Cardiff University, Cardiff, UK
22.3.4: Acute myeloid leukaemia

Richard Knight Associate Professor of Parasitology (retired), Department of Microbiology, University of Nairobi, Kenya
7.8.1: Amoebic infections; 7.8.9: Blastocystis hominis *infection; 7.9.2: Lymphatic filariasis; 7.9.3: Guinea worm disease (dracunculiasis); 7.9.6: Parastrongyliasis (angiostrongyliasis); 7.10.2: Cyclophyllidian gut tapeworms*

Daniël Knockaert General Internal Medicine, University Hospital Gasthuisberg, Leuven, Belgium
7.2.2: Fever of unknown origin

Nine V.A.M. Knoers Professor in Clinical Genetics, Department of Human Genetics, Radboud University, Nijmegen Medical Centre, Nijmegen, The Netherlands
21.16: Disorders of tubular electrolyte handling

Alexander Knuth Department of Oncology, University Hospital Zurich, Zurich, Switzerland
6.4: Cancer immunity and clinical oncology

Yasushi Kobayashi Department of Immunobiology, Yale University School of Medicine, New Haven, Connecticut, USA
16.14.4: Takayasu's arteritis

G.C.K.W. Koh Honorary Specialist Registrar, Department of Medicine, University of Cambridge, Cambridge, UK
7.6.7.2: Pseudomonas aeruginosa

Stefan Kölker Consultant, Pediatric Metabolic Medicine, University Children's Hospital, Heidelberg, Department of General Pediatrics, Division of Inborn Metabolic Diseases, Heidelberg, Germany
12.2: Protein-dependent inborn errors of metabolism

Edwin H. Kolodny Bernard A. and Charlotte Marden Professor and Chairman, Department of Neurology, New York University School of Medicine, New York, USA
24.17: Inherited neurodegenerative diseases

Michael D. Kopelman Professor of Neuropsychiatry, Consultant Neuropsychiatrist, King's College London, St Thomas' Hospital, London, UK
26.4: Neuropsychiatric disorders

Christian Krarup Professor of Clinical Neurophysiology, Department of Clinical Neurophysiology, Rigshospitalet; Faculty of Health Science, University of Copenhagen, Copenhagen, Denmark
24.3.2: Electrophysiology of the central and peripheral nervous systems

D. Kumararatne Addenbrooke's Hospital, Cambridge, UK
5.2: Immunodeficiency

Robert A. Kyle Mayo Clinic, Rochester, Minnesota, USA
22.4.5: Myeloma and paraproteinaemias

Helen J. Lachmann Senior Lecturer, National Amyloidosis Centre and Centre for Acute Phase Proteins, University College London Medical School, London, UK
12.12.2: Hereditary periodic fever syndromes

R. Lainson Ex Director, The Wellcome Parasitology Unit, and research-worker, Department of Parasitology, Instituto Evandro Chagas, Rodovia, Bairro Levilândia, Ananindeua, Pará, Brazil
7.8.6: Cyclospora *and cyclosporiasis*

Peter C. Lanyon Consultant Rheumatologist, Nottingham University Hospitals Trust, UK
19.3: Clinical investigation

A.J. Larner Consultant Neurologist, Cognitive Function Clinic, Walton Centre for Neurology and Neurosurgery, Liverpool, UK
24.5.4: Syncope; 24.13.1: Diseases of the spinal cord

Malcolm Law Professor of Epidemiology and Preventive Medicine, Wolfson Institute of Preventive Medicine, St Bartholomews' and the Royal London School of Medicine and Dentistry, Queen Mary University of London, UK
3.3.2: Medical screening

T.P. Lawrence Neurosurgery Registrar, John Radcliffe Hospital, Oxford, UK
24.11.3: Intracranial abscesses

Stephen Lawrie Consultant in Psychiatry, Royal Edinburgh Hospital, Edinburgh, UK
26.5.7: Schizophrenia, bipolar disorder, obsessive–compulsive disorder, and personality disorder

N.F. Lawton Consultant Neurologist, Wessex Neurological Centre, Southampton General Hospital; Honorary Senior Lecturer, University of Southampton, UK
24.10.5: Idiopathic intracranial hypertension

Ramanan Laxminarayan Senior Fellow and Director, Center for Disease Dynamics, Economics, and Policy, Resources for the Future, Washington, DC, USA
3.1: Global burden of disease: causes, levels, and intervention strategies

Alison Layton Harrogate District Hospital, Harrogate, UK
23.11: Sebaceous and sweat gland disorders

John H. Lazarus Emeritus Professor of Clinical Endocrinology, Centre for Endocrine and Diabetes Sciences, School of Medicine, Cardiff University, Cardiff, UK
14.11: Endocrine disease in pregnancy

J.W. LeDuc Professor, Microbiology and Immunology, Robert E. Shope M.D. and John S. Dunn Distinguished Chair in Global Health, Deputy Director, Galveston National Laboratory, University of Texas Medical Branch, Galveston, USA
7.5.16: Bunyaviridae

Susannah Leaver Clinical Research Fellow/Specialty Registrar Respiratory and Intensive Care Medicine, Imperial College and Royal Brompton Hospital, London, UK
17.5: Acute respiratory failure

Philip Lee Lately Reader, Charles Dent Metabolic Unit, The National Hospital for Neurology and Neurosurgery, London, UK
12.3.1: Glycogen storage diseases

Y.C. Gary Lee Oxford Pleural Unit, Oxford Centre for Respiratory Medicine, John Radcliffe Hospital, Oxford, UK
18.17: Pleural diseases; 18.19.3: Pleural tumours

T. Lehner Professor of Basic & Applied Immunology, Kings College London at Guy's Hospital, London, UK
15.6: The mouth and salivary glands

Irene M. Leigh Vice Principal and Head of College, College of Medicine, Dentistry and Nursing, Ninewells Hospital and Medical School, Dundee, UK
23.3: Inherited skin disease

G.G. Lennox Consultant in Neurology, Addenbrooke's Hospital, Cambridge, UK
14.12: Neurological disease in pregnancy

Elena N. Levtchenko Pediatric Nephrologist, Radbound University Nijmegen Medical Centre, Nijmegen, The Netherlands
21.16: Disorders of tubular electrolyte handling

Jeremy Levy Imperial College Kidney and Transplant Institute, Imperial College Healthcare NHS Trust, London, UK
21.8.7: Antiglomerular basement membrane disease

Siong-Seng Liau Specialty Registrar in Hepatopancreatobiliary (HPB), Surgery, HPB Unit, Department of Surgery, Addenbrooke's Hospital Cambridge, UK
6.2: The nature and development of cancer

Peter Libby Chief, Cardiovascular Medicine, Brigham and Women's Hospital, Mallinckrodt Professor of Medicine, Harvard Medical School, Massachusetts, USA
16.13.1: Biology and pathology of atherosclerosis

Oliver Liesenfeld Professor of Medical Microbiology and Infection Institute for Microbiology and Hygiene, Charité Medical School Berlin, Berlin, Germany
7.8.4: Toxoplasmosis

Aldo A.M. Lima Professor of Medicine and Pharmacology, Faculty of Medicine, Federal University of Ceará, Fortaleza, CE, Brazil
7.6.11; Cholera

D.C. Linch Head of Department of Haematology, University College London, London, UK; Director of CRUK Cancer Centre at University College London, UK
22.2.2: Haemopoietic stem cell disorders

M.J. Lindop Consultant, John Farman Intensive Care Unit, Addenbrooke's Hospital, Cambridge, UK
17.8: Discontinuing treatment of the critically ill patient; 17.9: Brainstem death and organ donation

Gregory Y.H. Lip Consultant Cardiologist and Professor of Cardiovascular Medicine, Director, Haemostasis Thrombosis & Vascular Biology Unit, University of Birmingham Centre for Cardiovascular Sciences, City Hospital, Birmingham, UK
16.17.5: Hypertensive urgencies and emergencies

P. Little Professor of Primary Care Research, School of Medicine, University of Southampton, UK
18.4.1: Upper respiratory tract infections

William A. Littler Consultant Cardiologist, The Priory Hospital, Birmingham, UK
16.9.2: Infective endocarditis

A. Llanos-Cuentas School of Public Health & Administration and School of Medicine, Universidad Peruana Cayetano Heredia, Lima, Peru
7.6.43: Bartonella bacilliformis *infection*

Diana N.J. Lockwood Professor of Tropical Medicine, London School of Hygiene and Tropical Medicine, and Consultant Leprologist, Hospital for Tropical Diseases, London, UK
7.6.27: Leprosy (Hansen's disease); 7.8.12: Leishmaniasis

Jay Loeffler Herman and Joan Suit Professor, Harvard Medical School; Chair, Department of Radiation Oncology, Massachusetts General Hospital, Boston, Massachusetts, USA
6.6: Cancer chemotherapy and radiation therapy

Thomas Lom Senior Director, BBDO NY, New York, USA
3.3.3: The importance of mass communication in promoting positive health

David A. Lomas Department of Medicine, University of Cambridge; Cambridge Institute for Medical Research, Wellcome Trust, Cambridge, UK
12.13: α_1-Antitrypsin deficiency and the serpinopathies

Martin Lombard Liver and Pancreato-Biliary Unit, Royal Liverpool University Hospital, Liverpool, UK
15.24.3: Tumours of the pancreas

A. Thomas Look Professor of Pediatrics, Harvard Medical School; Vice Chair for Research, Department of Pediatric Oncology, Dana-Farber Cancer Institute, Boston, Massachusetts, USA
22.3.1: Cell and molecular biology of human leukaemias

Elyse E. Lower University of Cincinnati Medical Center, Ohio, USA
18.12: Sarcoidosis

Katharine Lowndes Specialty Registrar, Department of Haematology, Salisbury District Hospital, Wiltshire, UK
14.16: Blood disorders specific to pregnancy

James R. Lupski Baylor College of Medicine, Houston, Texas, USA
4.2.2: The genomic basis of medicine

Linda M. Luxon Professor of Audiovestibular Medicine, UCL Ear Institute and Consultant Neuro-otologist, National Hospital for Neurology and Neurosurgery, London, UK
24.6.3: Hearing

Lucio Luzzatto Chairman, Department of Human Genetics, Memorial Sloan-Kettering Cancer Center, New York, USA
22.3.12: Paroxysmal nocturnal haemoglobinuria;
22.5.12: Glucose-6-phosphate dehydrogenase (G6PD) deficiency

Graz A. Luzzi Consultant in Genitourinary Medicine and Honorary Senior Clinical Lecturer, University of Oxford, Wycombe Hospital, High Wycombe, UK
7.5.23: HIV/AIDS; 8.3: Sexual history and examination

David Mabey Professor of Communicable Diseases, Department of Infectious and Tropical Diseases, London School of Hygiene and Tropical Medicine, London, UK
7.6.44: Chlamydial infections; 8.1: Epidemiology of sexually transmitted infections

J.T. Macfarlane Lately Professor of Respiratory Medicine, University of Nottingham, and Consultant Respiratory Physician, Nottingham University Hospitals, Nottingham, UK
7.6.38: Legionellosis and legionnaires' disease

Kenneth T. MacLeod Reader in Cardiac Physiology, National Heart and Lung Institute (NHLI) Division, Faculty of Medicine, Imperial College London, London, UK
16.1.2: Cardiac myocytes and the cardiac action potential

William MacNee Professor of Respiratory and Environmental Medicine/Honorary Consultant ELEGI Colt Laboratories, MRC Centre for Inflammation Research, The Queen's Medical Research Institute, Edinburgh, UK
18.8: Chronic obstructive pulmonary disease

M. Monir Madkour‡ Consultant Physician, Military Hospital, Riyadh, Saudi Arabia
7.6.21: Brucellosis

C. Maguiña-Vargas Instituto de Medicina Tropical Alexander von Humboldt, Universidad Peruana Cayetano Heredia, Lima, Peru
7.6.43: Bartonella bacilliformis *infection*

Hadi Manji Consultant Neurologist and Honorary Senior Lecturer, National Hospital for Neurology and Neurosurgery, London, UK
24.11.4: Neurosyphilis and neuro-AIDS

J.I. Mann Professor of Human Nutrition and Medicine, University of Otago, Dunedin, New Zealand
11.4: Diseases of overnourished societies and the need for dietary change

J. Mansi Consultant Medical Oncologist, Guy's & St Thomas NHS Foundation Trust, London, UK
13.8.3: Breast cancer

David Mant Professor of General Practice, Department of Primary Health Care, University of Oxford, Oxford, UK
3.3.1: Preventive medicine

Vincent Marks Professor of Clinical Biochemistry Emeritus, Postgraduate Medical School, University of Surrey, Guildford, UK
13.11.2: Hypoglycaemia

Michael Marmot Professor of Epidemiology, Director of International Institute for Society and Health at University College London, Research Department of Epidemiology and Public Health, London, UK
16.13.2: Coronary heart disease: epidemiology and prevention

T.J. Marrie Dean, Faculty of Medicine, Dalhousie University, Clinical Research Centre, Halifax, Nova Scotia, Canada
7.6.41: Coxiella burnetii *infections (Q fever)*

C.D. Marsden* Late Professor of Neurology, National Hospital for Neurology and Neurosurgery, London, UK
24.19: Acquired metabolic disorders and the nervous system

Judith C.W. Marsh Professor of Clinical Haematology/Honorary Consultant Haematologist, Department of Haematology, St George's Hospital, St George's University of London, London, UK
22.3.11: Aplastic anaemia and other causes of bone marrow failure

Kevin Marsh Director, KEMRI Wellcome Research Programme, Kilifi, Kenya
7.8.2: Malaria

Steven B. Marston Professor of Cardiac Biochemistry, National Heart and Lung Institute (NHLI) Division, Faculty of Medicine, Imperial College London, London, UK
16.1.2: Cardiac myocytes and the cardiac action potential

N.M. Martin Consultant in Endocrinology, Hammersmith Hospital, London, UK
13.10: Pancreatic endocrine disorders and multiple endocrine neoplasia

Duncan J. Maskell Head of Department and Marks & Spencer Professor of Farm Animal Health, Food Science & Food Safety, Department of Veterinary Medicine, University of Cambridge, Cambridge, UK
7.1.1: Biology of pathogenic microorganisms

Jay W. Mason Professor of Medicine, Cardiology Division, University of Utah College of Medicine, Salt Lake City, Utah, USA
16.7.1: Myocarditis

‡ It is with regret that we report the death of Dr M. Monir Madkour during the preparation of this edition of the textbook.

*Deceased.

V.I. Mathan Vice-Dean and Campus Director, ICDDR.B, Dhaka, Bangladesh
15.10.8: Malabsorption syndromes in the tropics

Christopher J. Mathias Professor of Neurovascular Medicine and Consultant Physician, Imperial College at St Mary's and the National Hospital for Neurology and Neurosurgery, Institute of Neurology, University College London, UK
24.14: Diseases of the autonomic nervous system

Peter W. Mathieson Dean of the Faculty of Medicine & Dentistry, University of Bristol, Professor of Medicine and Honorary Consultant Nephrologist at North Bristol NHS Trust, UK
21.8.5: Proliferative glomerulonephritis; 21.8.6: Mesangiocapillary glomerulonephritis

Mary E. McCaul Professor, Department of Psychiatry & Behavioral Sciences, Johns Hopkins University School of Medicine, Baltimore, Maryland, USA
26.7.1: Alcohol and drug dependence

Brian W. McCrindle Professor of Pediatrics, University of Toronto, Staff Cardiologist, The Hospital for Sick Children, Toronto, Canada
19.11.8: Kawasaki's disease

A.D. McGavigan Associate Professor of Cardiovascular Medicine, Flinders University, South Australia, Australia
16.2.2: Syncope and palpitations; 16.4: Cardiac arrhythmias

John A. McGrath Professor of Molecular Dermatology, St John's Institute of Dermatology, King's College London (Guy's Campus), London, UK
23.1: Structure and function of skin

Jane McGregor Senior Lecturer and Honorary Consultant Dermatologist, Barts and the London NHS Trust, UK
23.9: Photosensitivity

Iain B. McInnes Professor of Experimental Medicine and Honorary Consultant Rheumatologist, Glasgow Biomedical Research Centre, University of Glasgow, Glasgow, UK
4.3: Cytokines

William J. McKenna The Heart Hospital, University College London, UK
16.7.2: The cardiomyopathies: hypertrophic, dilated, restrictive, and right ventricular; 16.7.3: Specific heart muscle disorders

A.J. McMichael Professor and NHMRC Australia Fellow, National Centre for Epidemiology and Population Health, ANU College of Medicine, Biology and Environment, Australian National University, Canberra, Australia
3.2: Human population size, environment, and health

Martin McNally Consultant Orthopaedic Surgeon, Nuffield Orthopaedic Centre NHS Trust, Oxford, UK
20.3: Osteomyelitis

K. McNeil Professor of Medicine, University of Queensland, CEO Metro North Health Service, Brisbane, Australia
18.16: Lung transplantation

Henry McQuay Nuffield Department of Anaesthetics, University of Oxford, Oxford, UK
30.1: Dealing with pain

Jill Meara Deputy Director/Public Health Consultant, Health Protection Agency Centre for Radiation, Chemical and Environmental Hazards, Chilton, UK
9.5.9: Radiation

David K. Menon Head, Division of Anaesthesia, University of Cambridge; Consultant, Neurosciences Critical Care Unit, BOC Professor, Royal College of Anaesthetists, Professorial Fellow, Queens' College, Cambridge, Senior Investigator, National Institute for Health Research
17.6: Management of raised intracranial pressure

Catherine H. Mercer Senior Lecturer in Sexual Health Research, Centre for Sexual Health and HIV Research, Research Department of Infection and Public Health, University College London, London, UK
8.2: Sexual behaviour

Vinod K. Metta Research and Clinical Registrar for Neurology and Movement Disorders, Kings College Hospital NHS Trust and University Hospital, London, UK
24.7.2: Parkinsonism and other extrapyramidal diseases

J. ter Meulen Executive Director Vaccine Basic Research, Merck Research Laboratories, West Point, Pennsylvania, USA
7.5.17: Arenaviruses; 7.5.18: Filoviruses

Wayne M. Meyers Visiting Scientist, Department of Environmental and Infectious Disease Sciences, Armed Forces Institute of Pathology, Washington DC, USA
7.6.28: Buruli ulcer: Mycobacterium ulcerans *infection*

Anna Rita Migliaccio Dirigente de Ricerca in Transfusion Medicine, Laboratory of Clinical Biochemistry, Istituto Superiore doi Sanità, Rome, Italy
22.5.1: Erythropoiesis and the normal red cell

M.A. Miles Professor of Medical Protozoology, Pathogen Molecular Biology Unit, Department of Infectious and Tropical Diseases, London School of Hygiene and Tropical Medicine, London, UK
7.8.11: Chagas disease

Robert F. Miller Professor, Reader in Clinical Infection, Centre for Sexual Health and HIV Research, University College London, London, UK
7.7.5: Pneumocystis jirovecii

Dawn S. Milliner Division of Nephrology, Departments of Pediatrics and Internal Medicine, Mayo Clinic, Rochester, Minnesota, USA
12.10: Hereditary disorders of oxalate metabolism—the primary hyperoxalurias

K.R. Mills Department of Clinical Neurophysiology, King's College Hospital, London, UK
24.3.4: Investigation of central motor pathways: magnetic brain stimulation

Philip Minor Division of Virology, National Institute for Biological Standards and Control, South Mimms, UK
7.5.8: Enterovirus infections

Pramod K. Mistry Department of Pediatrics, Yale School of Medicine, New Haven, Connecticut, USA
12.7.2: Inherited diseases of copper metabolism: Wilson's disease and Menkes' disease

Andrew R.J. Mitchell Consultant Cardiologist, Jersey General Hospital, Jersey, UK
16.3.2: Echocardiography; 16.14.1: Thoracic aortic dissection

Andrew J. Molyneux Consultant in Neuroradiology, The Manor Hospital, Oxford, UK
24.3.3: Imaging in neurological diseases

D.H. Molyneux Centre for Neglected Tropical Diseases, Liverpool School of Tropical Medicine, Pembroke Place, Liverpool, UK
7.9.2: Lymphatic filariasis

Kevin Moore Professor of Hepatology, Department of Medicine, University College London, London, UK
15.22.3: Cirrhosis and ascites

Marina S. Morgan Consultant Medical Microbiologist, Royal Devon & Exeter Foundation NHS Trust, UK
7.6.18: Pasteurella

Pedro L. Moro Immunization Safety Office, Centre for Disease Control and Prevention, Atlanta, Georgia, USA
*7.10.1: Cystic hydatid disease (*Echinococcus granulosus*)*

Nicholas W. Morrell British Heart Foundation Professor of Cardiopulmonary Medicine, University of Cambridge School of Clinical Medicine, Addenbrooke's and Papworth Hospitals, Cambridge, UK
16.15.1: Structure and function; 16.15.2: Pulmonary hypertension; 16.15.3: Pulmonary oedema

Emma Morris Senior Lecturer and Honorary Consultant, UCL Medical School, University College London, London, UK
22.8.2: Haemopoietic stem cell transplantation

N.J. McC. Mortensen Professor of Colorectal Surgery, University of Oxford and Consultant Colorectal Surgeon, John Radcliffe Hospitals, Oxford, UK
15.14: Colonic diverticular disease

Peter S. Mortimer Professor of Dermatological Medicine to the University of London, Consultant Skin Physician to St George's Hospital, London and the Royal Marsden Hospital, London, UK
16.18: Chronic peripheral oedema and lymphoedema; 23.12: Blood and lymphatic vessel disorders

Tariq I. Mughal Professor of Medicine and Hematology/Oncology, University of Texas Southwestern School of Medicine, Dallas, Texas, USA
22.3.6: Chronic myeloid leukaemia

David R. Murdoch Professor and Head of Pathology, University of Otago, Christchurch, New Zealand
9.5.4: Diseases of high terrestrial altitudes

Jean B. Nachega Associate Scientist, Department of International Health, Johns Hopkins University, Bloomberg School of Public Health, Baltimore, Maryland, USA; Extraordinary Professor, Department of Medicine, and Director, Centre for Infectious Diseases, Stellenbosch University, Tygerberg, Cape Town, South Africa
7.6.25: Tuberculosis

Robert B. Nadelman Division of Infectious Diseases, Department of Medicine, New York Medical College, Valhalla, New York, USA
7.6.32: Lyme borreliosis

N.V. Naoumov Immunology and Infectious Diseases, Novartis Pharma AG, Basel, Switzerland, and Honorary Professor of Hepatology, University College London, UK
7.5.21: Hepatitis viruses (excluding hepatitis C virus)

Ravinder Nath Maini Emeritus Professor of Rheumatology, The Kennedy Institute of Rheumatology Division, Imperial College London, UK
19.5: Rheumatoid arthritis

David Neal Professor of Surgical Oncology, Honorary Consultant Urological Surgeon, University of Cambridge; Department of Oncology, Addenbrooke's Hospital, Cambridge, UK
21.18: Malignant diseases of the urinary tract

Graham Neale Department of Surgery, Imperial College, London, UK
15.2: Symptomatology of gastrointestinal disease; 15.17: Vascular and collagen disorders

Catherine Nelson-Piercy Consultant Obstetric Physician, Guy's & St Thomas' Foundation Trust and Imperial College Healthcare Trust, UK
14.14: Autoimmune rheumatic disorders and vasculitis in pregnancy

Randolph M. Nesse Professor of Psychiatry and Psychology, Research Professor, Research Center for Group Dynamics, ISR, Director, Evolution and Human Adaptation Program, The University of Michigan, Ann Arbor, Michigan, USA
2.1.2: Evolution: medicine's most basic science

Peter J. Nestor University Lecturer in Cognitive Neurology, University of Cambridge, Department of Clinical Neurosciences, Cambridge, UK; Honorary Consultant Neurologist, Addenbrooke's Hospital, Cambridge, UK
24.4.1: Disturbances of higher cerebral function

J. Neuberger Honorary Consultant Physician, Liver Unit, Queen Elizabeth Hospital, Birmingham, UK; Honorary Professor of Medicine, University of Birmingham, UK; Associate Medical Director, Organ Donation and Transplantation, NHS Blood and Transplant, Bristol, UK
15.22.8: Drugs and liver damage; 15.22.9: The liver in systemic disease

A.J. Newman Taylor Consultant in Respiratory Medicine, Faculty of Medicine, Imperial College, London, UK
18.7: Asthma

A.G. Nicholson Consultant Histopathologist, Royal Brompton and Harefield NHS Trust; Professor of Respiratory Pathology, National Heart and Lung Institute, Imperial College School of Medicine, London, UK
18.11.2: Idiopathic pulmonary fibrosis

Perry Nisen Senior Vice President, Cancer Research, GlaxoSmithKline, Philadelphia, Pennsylvania, USA
2.3.4: The future of clinical trials

Jerry P. Nolan Consultant in Anaesthesia and Intensive Care Medicine, Royal United Hospital Bath, UK; Co-Chair International Liaison Committee on Resuscitation
17.1: Cardiac arrest

John Nowakowski Division of Infectious Diseases, Department of Medicine, New York Medical College, Valhalla, New York, USA
7.6.32: Lyme borreliosis

Paul Nyirjesy Professor of Obstetrics and Gynecology and of Medicine, Drexel University College of Medicine, Philadelphia, Pennsylvania, USA
8.4: Vaginal discharge

Kunle Odunsi Professor and Research Program Director, Roswell Park Cancer Institute, Buffalo, New York, USA
6.4: Cancer immunity and clinical oncology

Graham S. Ogg Reader in Cutaneous Immunology, MRC Senior Clinical Fellow; Consultant in Dermatology, Churchill Hospital, Oxford, UK
23.7: Cutaneous vasculitis, connective tissue diseases, and urticaria

Yngvild K. Olsen Assistant Professor, Department of Medicine, Johns Hopkins University School of Medicine, Baltimore, Maryland, USA
26.7.1: Alcohol and drug dependence

Petra C.F. Oyston Defence Science and Technology Laboratories in the Biomedical Sciences Department, Dstl Porton Down, Salisbury, UK; Chair at the University of Leicester in the Department of Infection, Immunity and Inflammation
7.6.19: Francisella tularensis *infection*

Nigel O'Farrell Consultant Physician, Ealing Hospital, London, UK
7.6.13: Haemophilus ducreyi *and chancroid*

Doncha O'Gradaigh Consultant Rheumatologist, Waterford Regional Hospital, Ireland
19.12: Miscellaneous conditions presenting to the rheumatologist;
20.5: Osteonecrosis, osteochondrosis, and osteochondritis dissecans

Kevin O'Shaughnessy Senior Lecturer/Consultant, Clinical Pharmacology Unit, Department of Medicine, Addenbrooke's Hospital, Cambridge, UK
10.1: Principles of clinical pharmacology and drug therapy

Edel O'Toole Centre for Cutaneous Research, Blizard Institute of Cell and Molecular Science, Barts and the London School of Medicine and Dentistry and Department of Dermatology, Barts and the London NHS Trust, London, UK
23.14: Tumours of the skin

Aparna Pal Centre for Diabetes, Oxford Endocrinology and Metabolism, Churchill Hospital, Oxford, UK
13.3: Disorders of the posterior pituitary gland

Jacqueline Palace Consultant in Neurology, The Horton Hospital, Banbury, UK
24.23: Disorders of the neuromuscular junction

Thalia Papayannopoulou Professor of Medicine (Hematology), University of Washington, Division of Hematology, Seattle, USA
22.5.1: Erythropoiesis and the normal red cell

Jayan Parameshwar Consultant Cardiologist, Transplant Unit, Papworth Hospital, Cambridge. UK
16.5.2: Cardiac transplantation and mechanical circulatory support

S. Parish Clinical Trial Service Unit, University of Oxford, Oxford, UK
2.3.3: Large-scale randomized evidence: trials and meta-analyses of trials

Gilbert Park Consultant in Anaesthesia and Intensive Care, Addenbrooke's Hospital, Cambridge, UK
17.7: Sedation and analgesia in the critically ill

P. Parker Head of Division of Cancer Studies, King's College London, UK
13.8.3: Breast cancer

David Parkes SGDP Research Centre, Institute of Psychiatry and Neurosciences Department, King's Healthcare, Denmark Hill, London, UK
24.5.2: Narcolepsy

Miles Parkes Consultant Gastroenterologist, Inflammatory Bowel Disease Genetics Research Unit, Addenbrooke's Hospital, Cambridge, UK
15.11: Crohn's disease

Philippe Parola Unité de Recherche en Maladies Infectieuses et Tropicales Emergentes, WHO Collaborative Centre for Rickettsioses and other Arthropod borne Bacteria, Faculté de Médecine, Université de la Mediterraníe, Marseilles, France
7.6.39: Rickettsioses

C.M. Parry Oxford University Clinical Research Unit, Hospital for Tropical Diseases, Ho Chi Minh City, Vietnam
7.6.8: Typhoid and paratyphoid fevers

J. Paul Regional Microbiologist, Health Protection Agency, South East Region, Regional Microbiologist's Office, Royal Sussex County Hospital, Brighton, UK
7.6.46: A check list of bacteria associated with infection in humans; 7.12: Nonvenomous arthropods

S.J. Peacock Professor of Clinical Microbiology, Department of Medicine, University of Cambridge Cambridge, UK
7.6.7.2: Pseudomonas aeruginosa*; 7.6.15: Melioidosis and glanders*

Roger Pedersen MRC Centre for Stem Cell Biology and Regenerative Medicine, University of Cambridge, UK
4.8: Stem cells and regenerative medicine

Malik Peiris Department of Microbiology, The University of Hong Kong, Queen Mary Hospital Pokfualm, Hong Kong SAR
7.5.1: Respiratory tract viruses

Hugh Pennington Emeritus Professor of Bacteriology, University of Aberdeen, UK
7.6.7.1: Enterobacteria and bacterial food poisoning

M.B. Pepys Head, Division of Medicine, Royal Free Campus, University College London; Director, UCL Centre for Amyloidosis & Acute Phase Proteins; UK NHS National Amyloidosis Centre, UK
12.12.1: The acute phase response and C-reactive protein; 12.12.3: Amyloidosis

S.P. Pereira Senior Lecturer in Gastroenterology, University College, London Medical School, London, UK
15.16: Cancers of the gastrointestinal tract

G.D. Perkin Emeritus Consultant Neurologist, Charing Cross Hospital, London, UK
24.5.1: Epilepsy in later childhood and adulthood

P.L. Perrotta Associate Professor of Pathology, Director of Clinical Laboratories, West Virginia School of Medicine, West Virginia, USA
22.8.1: Blood transfusion

David J. Perry Consultant Haematologist, Department of Haematology, Addenbrooke's Hospital, Cambridge, UK
14.16: Blood disorders specific to pregnancy

Hans Persson Senior Consultant Physician, Swedish Poisons Centre, Stockholm, Sweden
9.3.1: Poisonous plants and fungi

Michael C. Petch Consultant Cardiologist, Queen Elizabeth Hospital, Kings Lynn, UK
16.13.8: The impact of coronary heart disease on life and work

Eskild Petersen Department of Infectious Diseases, Aarhus University Hospital, Skejby, Aarhus, Denmark
7.8.4: Toxoplasmosis

L.R. Petersen Director, Division of Vector-borne Infectious Diseases, Centers for Disease Control and Prevention, Fort Collins, Colorado, USA
7.5.12: Alphaviruses; 7.5.14: Flaviviruses excluding dengue

R. Peto Clinical Trial Service Unit & Epidemiological Studies Unit (CTSU), University of Oxford, UK
2.3.3: Large-scale randomized evidence: trials and meta-analyses of trials; 6.1: Epidemiology of cancer

T.E.A. Peto Professor of Infectious Diseases, University of Oxford; Consultant Physician, Oxford Radcliffe Hospitals, Nuffield Department of Medicine, John Radcliffe Hospital, Oxford, UK
7.5.23: HIV/AIDS

A.O. Phillips Consultant in Nephrology, University Hospital of Wales, Cardiff, UK
21.1: Structure and functions of the kidney

Wendy Phillips Specialty Registrar in Neurology, Cambridge University Hospitals Foundation Trust, Cambridge, UK
24.3.1: Lumbar puncture

G. Pichert Consultant Clinical Geneticist, Guy's & St Thomas' NHS Foundation Trust, London, UK
13.8.3: Breast cancer

J.D. Pickard Professor of Neurosurgery, Academic Neurosurgery Unit, Department of Clinical Neurosciences, University of Cambridge, Addenbrooke's Hospital, Cambridge, UK
24.5.6: Brain death and the vegetative state

V.V. Pillay Chief, Poison Control Centre, Head, Analytical Toxicology, Amrita Institute of Medical Sciences, Cochin, Kerala, India
9.3.2: Common Indian poisonous plants

S. Pinder Professor of Breast Histopathology, King's College London, Consultant Histopathologist, Guy's & St Thomas NHS Foundation Trust, London, UK
13.8.3: Breast cancer

Michael R. Pinsky Professor of Critical Care Medicine, Pittsburgh, Pennsylvania, USA
17.4: Circulation and circulatory support in the critically ill

Mervi L.S. Pitkanen Consultant Neuropsychiatrist, Neuropsychiatry and Memory Disorders Clinic, Adamson Centre, London, UK
26.4: Neuropsychiatric disorders

R.J. Playford Professor of Medicine, Clinical Gastroenterologist, Vice Principal NHS Liaison and Deputy Warden, Barts and The London School of Medicine and Dentistry, UK
15.10.7: Effects of massive small bowel resection

J.M. Polak Emeritus Professor, Division of Investigative Science, Imperial Colllege London, London, UK
15.9: Hormones and the gastrointestinal tract

Eleanor S. Pollak Associate Professor, Hospital of the University of Pennsylvania, Children's Hospital of Philadelphia and the Philadelphia VA Medical Center, Abramson Research Center, Philadelphia, Pennsylvania, USA
22.6.4: Genetic disorders of coagulation

Andrew J. Pollard Professor of Paediatric Infection and Immunity, Department of Paediatrics, University of Oxford, Oxford, UK
9.5.4: Diseases of high terrestrial altitudes

Aaron Polliack Emeritus Professor of Hematology, and Head of Lymphoma, Leukemia Unit, Department of Hematology, Hadassah University Hospital and, Hebrew University Medical School Jerusalem, Israel; Senior Consultant, Emeritus Professor of Hematology, Department of Hematology and Bone Marrow Transplantation, Tel Aviv Sourasky Medical Center, Tel Aviv, Israel
22.3.5: Chronic lymphocytic leukaemia and other leukaemias of mature B and T cells

Philip A. Poole-Wilson† British Heart Foundation Simon Marks Professor of Cardiology, National Heart and Lung Institute (NHLI) Division, Faculty of Medicine, Imperial College London, London, UK
16.1.2: Cardiac myocytes and the cardiac action potential

Françoise Portaels Mycobacteriology Unit, Department of Microbiology, Institute of Tropical Medicine Nationalestraat, Antwerpen, Belgium
7.6.28: Buruli ulcer: Mycobacterium ulcerans *infection*

Jerry Posner Evelyn Frew American Cancer Society Clinical Research Professor—George C. Cotzias Chair of Neuro-oncology—Professor of Neurology and Neuroscience, Weil Medical School of Cornell University Department of Neuro-oncology, Memorial Sloan-Kettering Cancer Center, New York City, New York, USA
24.21: Paraneoplastic neurological syndromes

† It is with regret that we report the death of Professor Philip A. Poole-Wilson during the preparation of this edition of the textbook.

William G. Powderly Professor of Medicine and Therapeutics, Dean of Medicine, UCD School of Medicine and Medical Sciences, University College Dublin, Dublin, Ireland
7.7.2: Cryptococcosis

J. Powell-Tuck Emeritus Professor of Clinical Nutrition, Barts and the London School of Medicine and Dentistry, UK
11.2: Vitamins and trace elements

Janet Powell Department of Surgery & Cancer, Imperial College, London, UK
16.14.2: Peripheral arterial disease

Amy Powers Instructor, Harvard Medical School and Beth Israel Deaconess Medical Center, Boston, Massachusetts, USA
22.5.9: Haemolytic anaemia—congenital and acquired

J.W. Powles Department of Public Health and Primary Care, University of Cambridge, Cambridge, UK
3.2: Human population size, environment, and health

Michael B. Prentice Professor of Medical Microbiology, Department of Microbiology, University College Cork, Cork, Ireland
7.6.16: Plague: Yersinia pestis; *7.6.17: Other* yersinia *infections: yersiniosis*

A. Purushotham Professor of Breast Cancer, King's College London, Consultant Breast Surgeon, Guy's & St Thomas NHS Foundation Trust, London, UK
13.8.3: Breast cancer

Charles Pusey Imperial College Kidney and Transplant Institute, Imperial College London, UK
21.8.7: Antiglomerular basement membrane disease

Anisur Rahman Professor of Rheumatology, University College London, UK
19.11.2: Systemic lupus erythematosus and related disorders

S. Vincent Rajkumar Professor of Medicine, Division of Hematology, Mayo Clinic, Rochester, Minnesota, USA
22.4.5: Myeloma and paraproteinaemias

M. Ramsay Consultant Epidemiologist, Immunisation, Hepatitis and Blood Safety Department, HPA Centre for Infections, London, UK
7.3: Immunization

A.C. Rankin Professor of Medical Cardiology, BHF Glasgow Cardiovascular Research Centre, University of Glasgow, UK
16.2.2: Syncope and palpitations; 16.4: Cardiac arrhythmias

Didier Raoult Faculté de Médecine et de Pharmacie, Université de la Méditerranée, Marseille Cedex, France
7.6.39: Rickettsioses; 7.6.42: Bartonellas excluding B. bacilliformis

Michael D. Rawlins National Institute for Health and Clinical Excellence, London, UK
2.4.1: The evaluation and provision of effective medicines

Paul J. Reading Consultant in Neurology, Department of Neurology, The James Cook University Hospital, Middlesbrough, UK
24.5.3: Sleep disorders

C.W.G. Redman Emeritus Professor of Obstetric Medicine, University of Oxford; Honorary Research Fellow, Lady Margaret Hall, Oxford Nuffield Department of Obstetrics and Gynaecology, John Radcliffe Hospital Oxford, UK
14.4: Hypertension in pregnancy

Jeremy Rees Consultant Neurologist, National Hospital for Neurology and Neurosurgery, London, UK
24.10.4: Intracranial tumours; 24.21: Paraneoplastic neurological syndromes

Shelley Renowden Consultant in Neuroradiology, Frenchay Hospital, Bristol, UK
24.3.3: Imaging in neurological diseases

Todd W. Rice Assistant Professor of Medicine, Division of Allergy, Pulmonary, and Critical Care Medicine, Vanderbilt University School of Medicine, Nashville, Tennessee, USA
7.1.2: Physiological changes, clinical features, and general management of infected patients

J. Richens Centre for Sexual Health and HIV Research, Research Department of Infection & Population Health, University College London, London, UK
7.6.9: Intracellular klebsiella infections (donovanosis and rhinoscleroma)

A.B. Rickinson Institute for Cancer Studies, University of Birmingham, Birmingham, UK
7.5.3: Epstein–Barr virus

B.K. Rima Deputy Head of the School of Medicine, Dentistry and Biomedical Sciences, Belfast, Ireland
7.5.5: Mumps: epidemic parotitis

Eberhard Ritz Department of Internal Medicine, Division of Nephrology, Heidelberg, Germany
21.6: Chronic kidney disease

Harold R. Roberts Sarah Graham Kenan Distinguished Professor of Medicine, Department of Medicine; Division of Hematology/Oncology, University of North Carolina, Chapel Hill NC and Attending Physician, University of North Carolina Hospitals, North Carolina, USA
22.6.1: The biology of haemostasis and thrombosis

T.A. Rockall Director MATTU, University of Surrey, Guildford, UK
15.4.2: Gastrointestinal bleeding

Kenneth Rockwood Professor of Geriatric Medicine, Dalhousie University, Halifax, Nova Scotia, Canada
29.1: Medicine in old age

Edward Roddy Specialty Registrar in Rheumatology, Nottingham City Hospital, Nottingham, UK
19.10: Crystal-related arthropathies

Simon D. Roger Director of Renal Medicine, Gosford Hospital, Gosford, NSW, Australia; Clinical Associate Professor, Department of Medicine & Health Sciences, Newcastle University, Newcastle, NSW, Australia
21.9.1: Acute interstitial nephritis

Jean-Marc Rolain Faculté de Médecine et de Pharmacie, Université de la Méditerranée, Marseille Cedex, France
7.6.42: Bartonellas excluding B. bacilliformis

P. Ronco Professor of Renal Medicine, University Pierre et Marie Curie, Tenon Hospital, and Inserm Unit UMR_S702
21.10.4: Renal involvement in plasma cell dyscrasias, immunoglobulin-based amyloidoses, and fibrillary glomerulopathies, lymphomas, and leukaemias

Antony Rosen Mary Betty Stevens Professor of Medicine, Professor of Pathology, Director, Division of Rheumatology, Johns Hopkins University School of Medicine, Baltimore, Maryland, USA
5.4: Autoimmunity

Mark J. Rosen Chief, Division of Pulmonary, Critical Care and Sleep Medicine, North Shore University Hospital and Long Island Jewish Medical Center, Professor of Medicine, Hofstra University School of Medicine, New York, USA
18.4.4: Pulmonary complications of HIV infection

Peter Rubin Professor of Therapeutics, Division of Therapeutics & Molecular Medicine, University of Nottingham, Nottingham, UK
14.18: Prescribing in pregnancy

Simon M. Rushbrook Consultant Hepatologist, Department of Hepatology Norfolk and Norwich University Hospitals NHS Foundation Trust, Norfolk, UK
15.19: Structure and function of the liver, biliary tract, and pancreas; 15.22.6: Liver tumours—primary and secondary

Anthony S. Russell Professor Emeritus, Rheumatic Disease Unit, University of Alberta, Edmonton, Alberta, Canada
19.2: Clinical presentation and diagnosis of rheumatic disease

Nikant Sabharwal Consultant Cardiologist, Department of Cardiology, John Radcliffe Hospital, Oxford, UK
16.3.3: Cardiac investigation—nuclear and other imaging techniques

I. Sadaf Farooqi Metabolic Research Laboratories, Institute of Metabolic Science, Addenbrooke's Hospital, University of Cambridge, Cambridge, UK
11.5: Obesity

Hesham Saleh Consultant Rhiniologist/Facial Plastic Surgeon, Charing Cross Hospital and Royal Brompton Hospital, Honorary Senior Lecturer, Imperial College, London, UK
18.6: Allergic rhinitis

Nilesh J. Samani British Heart Foundation Professor of Cardiology, Department of Cardiovascular Sciences, University of Leicester, Leicester, UK
16.17.4: Mendelian disorders causing hypertension

Swati Sathe Assistant Professor of Neurology, New York University School of Medicine, New York, USA
24.17: Inherited neurodegenerative diseases

Brian P. Saunders Wolfson Unit for Endoscopy, St Mark's Hospital for Colorectal Disorders, Harrow, London, UK
15.3.1: Colonoscopy and flexible sigmoidoscopy

S.J. Saunders Division of Hepatology, University of Cape Town Medical School, University of Cape Town, South Africa
15.22.7: Hepatic granulomas

E. Sawyer Consultant Clinical Oncologist, Guy's & St Thomas NHS Foundation Trust, London, UK
13.8.3: Breast cancer

K.P. Schaal Emeritus Professor of Medical Microbiology; Member of the Expert Committee of the Federal Ministry of Labour and Social Affairs Institute for Medical Microbiology, Immunology and Parasitology, University Hospital, Bonn, Germany
7.6.29: Actinomycoses

Michael L. Schilsky Associate Professor of Medicine, Medical Director, Adult Liver Transplant, Yale-New Haven Transplantation Center, Department of Internal Medicine, Yale School of Medicine, New Haven, Connecticut, USA
12.7.2: Inherited diseases of copper metabolism: Wilson's disease and Menkes' disease

Neil Scolding University of Bristol Institute of Clinical Neurosciences, Department of Neurology, Frenchay Hospital, Bristol, UK
24.19: Acquired metabolic disorders and the nervous system; 24.20: Neurological complications of systemic disease

Anthony Scott Wellcome Trust Senior Research Fellow in Clinical Science, KEMRI Wellcome Trust Research Programme, Kilifi, Kenya; Nuffield Department of Clinical Medicine, University of Oxford, Oxford, UK
7.6.3: Pneumococcal infections

A. Seaton Honorary Senior Consultant, Institute of Occupational Medicine, Edinburgh, UK and Emeritus Professor of Environmental and Occupational Medicine, University of Aberdeen, Aberdeen, UK
18.13: Pneumoconioses

Amartya Sen Lamont University Professor and Professor of Economics and Philosophy, Harvard University, Cambridge, Massachusetts, USA
3.5: Human disasters

G.R. Serjeant University of West Indies, Kingston, Jamaica
21.10.6: Sickle-cell disease and the kidney

Nicholas J. Severs Professor of Cell Biology, National Heart and Lung Institute (NHLI) Division, Faculty of Medicine, Imperial College London, London, UK
16.1.2: Cardiac myocytes and the cardiac action potential

Keerti V. Shah Department of Molecular Microbiology and Immunology, Johns Hopkins Bloomberg School of Public Health, Baltimore, Maryland, USA
7.5.19: Papillomaviruses and polyomaviruses

Pallav L. Shah Consultant Physician, Royal Brompton Hospital, London, UK, Chelsea & Westminster Hospital, London, UK
18.3.3: Bronchoscopy, thoracoscopy, and tissue biopsy

Michael Sharpe Professor of Psychological Medicine, Psychological Medicine Research, School of Molecular and Clinical Medicine, University of Edinburgh, UK
26.1: General introduction; 26.5.3: Medically unexplained symptoms in patients attending medical clinics; 26.5.4: Chronic fatigue syndrome (postviral fatigue syndrome, neurasthenia, and myalgic encephalomyelitis); 26.6.2: Psychological treatment in medical practice

Maire P. Shelly Consultant in Intensive Care, Wythenshawe Hospital, Manchester, UK
17.7: Sedation and analgesia in the critically ill

Jackie Sherrard Consultant in Genitourinary Medicine, Churchill Hospital, Oxford, UK
7.6.6: Neisseria gonorrhoeae*; 8.3: Sexual history and examination*

M.A. Shikanai-Yasuda Professor of Department of Infectious and Parasitic Diseases, Endemic Diseases Group/Infections in Immunosupressed Host Programme, Faculdade de Medicina, University of São Paulo, Brazil
7.7.4: Paracoccidioidomycosis

John M. Shneerson Director, Respiratory Support & Sleep Centre, Papworth Hospital, Cambridge, UK
18.18: Disorders of the thoracic cage and diaphragm

C.A. Sieff Division of Hematology, Karp 080006C, Children's Hospital Boston, Boston, Massachusetts, USA
22.2.1: Stem cells and haemopoiesis

J. Sieper Free University, Berlin, Germany
19.6: Ankylosing spondylitis, other spondyloarthritides, and related conditions

Udomsak Silachamroon Assistant Professor of Tropical Medicine, Department of Clinical Tropical Medicine, Faculty of Tropical Medicine, Mahidol University, Bangkok, Thailand
7.11.3: Lung flukes (paragonimiasis)

Leslie Silberstein Professor, Harvard Medical School, Children's Hospital Boston, Dana-Farber Cancer Institute, Brigham and Women's Hospital, and Harvard Stem Cell Institute, Boston, Massachusetts, USA
22.5.9: Haemolytic anaemia—congenital and acquired

Rod Sinclair Professor of Dermatology, University of Melbourne, Director of Dermatology, St. Vincent's Hospital, Director of Research and Training, Skin and Cancer Foundation, Fitzroy, Australia
23.17: Management of skin disease

Robert E. Sinden The Malaria Centre, Department of Life Sciences, Imperial College London, London, UK
7.8.2: Malaria

Joseph Sinning Harold Leever Regional Cancer Center, Waterbury, Connecticut, USA
22.4.1: Leucocytes in health and disease

Thira Sirisanthana Professor of Medicine, Chiang Mai University, Thailand
7.6.20: Anthrax; 7.7.6: Penicillium marneffei *infection*

J.G.P. Sissons Regius Professor of Physic, Director, Cambridge University Health Partners, School of Clinical Medicine, University of Cambridge, Cambridge, UK
7.5.2: Herpesviruses (excluding Epstein–Barr virus)

Geoffrey L. Smith Wellcome Principal Research Fellow, Section of Virology, Faculty of Medicine, Imperial College London, London, UK
7.5.4: Poxviruses

R. Smith Emeritus Professor of Rheumatology, Nuffield Orthopaedic Centre NHS Trust, Oxford, UK
20.1: Skeletal disorders—general approach and clinical conditions

Robert W. Snow Head, Malaria Public Health Group, KEMRI/Wellcome Trust Programme and Advisor, National Malaria Control Programme, Ministry of Health, Nairobi, Kenya
7.8.2: Malaria

E.L. Snyder Professor, Laboratory Medicine, Yale University School of Medicine, New Haven, Connecticut, USA
22.8.1: Blood transfusion

Jasmeet Soar Consultant in Anaesthesia and Intensive Care Medicine, Southmead Hospital Bristol, UK; Chair, Resuscitation Council (UK)
17.1: Cardiac arrest

Krishna Somers Consultant Physician in Cardiovascular Medicine, Royal Perth Hospital, Perth, Australia
16.9.4: Cardiovascular syphilis

M.W. Sonderup Division of Hepatology, University of Cape Town Medical School, University of Cape Town, South Africa
15.22.7: Hepatic granulomas

R.L. Souhami Emeritus Professor of Medicine, University College London, London, UK
6.5: Cancer: clinical features and management

C.W.N. Spearman Division of Hepatology, University of Cape Town Medical School, University of Cape Town, South Africa.
15.22.7: Hepatic granulomas

G.P. Spickett Consultant Clinical Immunologist, Regional Department of Immunology, Royal Victoria Hospital, Newcastle upon Tyne, UK
18.14.1: Pulmonary haemorrhagic disorders; 18.14.2: Eosinophilic pneumonia; 18.14.4: Lymphocytic infiltrations of the lung

S.G. Spiro Professor of Respiratory Medicine and Honorary Consultant Physician Royal Brompton Hospital, London, UK
18.19.1: Lung cancer; 18.19.2: Pulmonary metastases

Jerry L. Spivak Division of Hematology. The Johns Hopkins University School of Medicine, Baltimore, Maryland, USA
22.3.9: Idiopathic myelofibrosis

U. Srinivas-Shankar Consultant Physician, Department of Diabetes & Endocrinology, St Helens & Knowsley Teaching Hospitals NHS Trust, St Helens, UK
13.8.2: Disorders of male reproduction

Paweł Stankiewicz Assistant Professor, Department of Molecular and Human Genetics, Baylor College of Medicine
4.2.2: The genomic basis of medicine

Paul D. Stein Visiting Professor, Department of Internal Medicine, Michigan State University, College of Osteopathic Medicine, East Lansing, Missouri, USA
16.16.1: Deep venous thrombosis and pulmonary embolism

Dennis L. Stevens Chief, Infectious Diseases Section, Veterans Affairs Medical Center, Boise, Professor of Medicine, University of Washington School of Medicine, Seattle, Washington, USA
7.6.2: Streptococci and enterococci; 7.6.24: Botulism, gas gangrene, and clostridial gastrointestinal infections

Tom Stevens Consultant Psychiatrist, Lambeth Hospital, South London and Maudsley NHS Foundation Trust, London, UK
26.4: Neuropsychiatric disorders

J.C. Stevenson Department of Metabolic Medicine, Imperial College London, Royal Brompton Hospital, London, UK
14.20: Benefits and risks of hormone replacement therapy

P.M. Stewart Professor of Medicine and Director of Research and Knowledge Transfer, University of Birmingham, Birmingham, UK
13.7.1: Disorders of the adrenal cortex

Stephen F. Stewart Institute of Cellular Medicine, Newcastle University, Newcastle upon Tyne, UK
15.22.1: Alcoholic liver disease; 15.22.2: Nonalcoholic steatohepatitis

August Stich Department of Tropical Medicine, Medical Mission Institute, Würzburg, Germany
7.8.10: Human African trypanosomiasis

Heather Stoddart Principal Clinical Scientist, Department of Chemical Pathology and Immunology, St Mary's Hospital, Imperial College Healthcare NHS Trust, London, UK
32.1: Biochemistry in medicine—reference intervals: the use of biochemical analysis for diagnosis and management

John H. Stone Associate Professor of Medicine, Harvard Medical School, Director, Clinical Rheumatology, Massachusetts General Hospital, Massachusetts, USA
19.11.7: Polymyositis and dermatomyositis

J.R. Stradling Professor of Respiratory Medicine & Consultant Respiratory Physician, Oxford Centre for Respiratory Medicine, John Radcliffe Hospitals, Oxford, UK
18.1.1: The upper respiratory tract; 18.5.1: Upper airways obstruction; 18.5.2: Sleep-related disorders of breathing

Frank J. Strobl Director of Scientific Affairs, Therakos, Inc. RandCD, Exton, Pennsylvania, USA
22.5.9: Haemolytic anaemia—congenital and acquired

M.A. Stroud Senior Lecturer in Medicine, University of Southampton, UK
9.5.1: Heat; 9.5.2: Cold

Michael Strupp Department of Neurology, Ludwig-Maximilians University, Munich, Germany
24.6.2: Eye movements and balance

Peter H. Sugden Professor of Cellular Biochemistry, National Heart and Lung Institute (NHLI) Division, Faculty of Medicine, Imperial College London, London, UK
16.1.2: Cardiac myocytes and the cardiac action potential

J.A. Summerfield St Mary's Hospital, London, UK
15.23: Diseases of the gallbladder and biliary tree; 15.25: Congenital disorders of the liver, biliary tract, and pancreas

Joseph Sung Professor of Medicine, Head, Shaw College, Associate Dean (General Affairs), Chairman, Department of Medicine & Therapeutics, Director, Institute of Digestive Disease, Faculty of Medicine, The Chinese University of Hong Kong
15.8: Peptic ulcer disease

Pravan Suntharasamai Mahidol University, Bangkok, Thailand
7.9.7: Gnathostomiasis

P. Sweny Emeritus Consultant Nephrologist, Royal Free NHS Trust, London, UK
21.7.3: Renal transplantation

A.J. Swerdlow Professor of Epidemiology, Institute of Cancer Research, University of London, UK
6.1: Epidemiology of cancer

D. Swirsky Consultant Haematologist, St James's University Hospital, Leeds, UK
22.4.4: The spleen and its disorders

Penelope Talelli Sobell Department of Motor Neuroscience and Movement Disorders, Institute of Neurology, University College London; National Hospital for Neurology and Neurosurgery, London, UK
24.7.1: Subcortical structures: the cerebellum, basal ganglia, and thalamus

C.T. Tan Professor, Department of Medicine, University of Malaya, Kuala Lumpur, Malaysia
7.5.7: Nipah and Hendra virus encephalitides

David Taylor-Robinson Emeritus Professor of Genito-Microbiology and Medicine, Imperial College London, Division of Medicine, London, UK
7.6.44: Chlamydial infections; 7.6.45: Mycoplasmas

Henri A. Termeer Chairman and Chief Executive Officer, Genzyme Corporation, Cambridge, Massachusetts, USA
2.4.4: Sustaining innovation in an era of specialized medicine

R.V. Thakker May Professor of Medicine, Academic Endocrine Unit, Nuffield Department of Clinical Medicine, University of Oxford; Oxford Centre for Diabetes, Endocrinology and Metabolism, Churchill Hospital, Oxford, UK
13.6: Parathyroid disorders and diseases altering calcium metabolism

David G.T. Thomas Department of Neurological Surgery, Institute of Neurology, London, UK
24.10.3: Traumatic injuries to the head

P.K. Thomas‡ Emeritus Professor of Neurology, Royal Free Hospital School of Medicine and Institute of Neurology, London, UK
24.12: Disorders of cranial nerves; 24.16: Diseases of the peripheral nerves

D.G. Thompson Professor of Gastroenterology, Epithelial Sciences Research Group, School of Translational Medicine, University of Manchester, Clinical Sciences Building, Salford Royal Hospitals Salford, UK
15.1: Structure and function of the gut; 15.13: Irritable bowel syndrome and functional bowel disorders

R.P.H. Thompson Gastrointestinal Laboratory, The Rayne Institute, St Thomas's Hospital, London, UK
15.20: Jaundice

S.A. Thorne Consultant Cardiologist, University Hospital, Birmingham, UK
16.12: Congenital heart disease in the adult

‡ It is with regret that we report the death of Professor P.K. Thomas during the preparation of this edition of the textbook.

C.L. Thwaites Oxford University Clinical Research Unit, Ho Chi Minh City, Vietnam
7.6.22: Tetanus

Guy E. Thwaites Department of Microbiology, Imperial College, London, UK
24.11.1: Bacterial infections

Adam D. Timmis Professor of Clinical Cardiology, London Chest Hospital, London, UK
16.13.4: Management of stable angina

Charles Tomson Consultant Nephrologist, Richard Bright Renal Unit, Southmead Hospital, Bristol, UK
21.13: Urinary tract infection

P.A. Tookey Senior Lecturer, MRC Centre of Epidemiology for Child Health, UCL Institute of Child Health, London, UK
7.5.13: Rubella

Peter Topham Consultant Nephrologist, John Walls Renal Unit, University Hospitals of Leicester NHS Trust Leicester, UK
21.8.2: Thin membrane nephropathy

P.P. Toskes Professor of Medicine, University of Florida College of Medicine, Gainesville, Florida, USA
15.10.2: Small-bowel bacterial overgrowth; 15.24.2: Chronic pancreatitis

G. Touchard Professor, Department of Nephrology, Poitiers University Hospital, Poitiers, France
21.10.4: Renal involvement in plasma cell dyscrasias, immunoglobulin-based amyloidoses, and fibrillary glomerulopathies, lymphomas, and leukaemias

Thomas A. Traill Adult Cardiology Faculty, Johns Hopkins, Hospital, Baltimore, Maryland, USA
16.10: Tumours of the heart; 16.11: Cardiac involvement in genetic disease

A.S. Truswell Emeritus Professor of Human Nutrition,University of Sydney, Australia
11.4: Diseases of overnourished societies and the need for dietary change

Wai Y. Tse Consultant Nephrologist and Senior Lecturer, Renal Unit, Derriford Hospital, Plymouth, UK
21.10.3: The kidney in rheumatological disorders

D.M. Turnbull Professor of Neurology and Director Newcastle Centre for Brain Ageing and Vitality, Institute for Ageing and Health, Newcastle University, Newcastle upon Tyne, UK.
24.24.5: Mitochondrial encephalomyopathies

A. Neil Turner Consultant in Nephrology, Royal Infirmary, Edinburgh, UK
21.10.7: Infection-associated nephropathies; 21.10.8: Malignancy-associated renal disease

J.A. Vale Director, National Poisons Information Service (Birmingham Unit) and West Midlands Poisons Unit; City Hospital, Birmingham, UK
9.1: Poisoning by drugs and chemicals

Patrick Vallance Senior Vice President Drug Discovery, GlaxoSmithKline, London, UK
2.3.4: The future of clinical trials; 16.1.1: Blood vessels and the endothelium

Steven Vanderschueren General Internal Medicine, University Hospital Gasthuisberg, Leuven, Belgium
7.2.2: Fever of unknown origin

Sirivan Vanijanonta Emeritus Professor of Tropical Medicine, Department of Clinical Tropical Medicine, Faculty of Tropical Medicine, Mahidol University, Bangkok, Thailand
7.11.3: Lung flukes (paragonimiasis)

Patrick J.W. Venables Professor of Viral Immunorheumatology, Kennedy Institute of Rheumatology. Imperial College, London, UK
19.11.6: Sjögren's syndrome

B.J. Vennervald DBL-Centre for Health Research and Development, Faculty of Life Sciences University of Copenhagen, Thorvaldsensvej, Denmark
7.11.1: Schistosomiasis

Vanessa Venning Consultant Dermatologist, Department of Dermatology, Churchill Hospital, Oxford, UK
23.2: Clinical approach to the diagnosis of skin disease

Anilrudh A. Venugopal Clinical Instructor, Division of Infectious Diseases, St. John Hospital and Medical Center, Detroit, Missouri, USA
7.6.10: Anaerobic bacteria

Kristien Verdonck Institute of Tropical Medicine Antwerp Nationalestraat, Antwerp, Belgium; Instituto de Medicina Tropical Alexander von Humboldt Universidad Peruana Cayetano Heredia Av. Honorio Delgado, San Martín de Porres Lima, Peru
7.5.25: HTLV-1, HTLV-2, and associated diseases

C.M. Verity Consultant Paediatric Neurologist, Child Development Centre, Addenbrooke's Hospital, Cambridge, UK
24.18: Developmental abnormalities of the central nervous system

Angela Vincent Consultant in Immunology, John Radcliffe Hospital, Oxford, UK
24.21: Paraneoplastic neurological syndromes; 24.22: Autoimmune limbic encephalitis and Morvan's syndrome

Raphael P. Viscidi Department of Pediatrics, Johns Hopkins University School of Medicine, Baltimore, Maryland, USA
7.5.19: Papillomaviruses and polyomaviruses

Peter D. Wagner Professor of Medicine & Bioengineering, Department of Medicine, University of California, San Diego, La Jolla, California, USA
18.1.2: Airways and alveoli

Nicholas Wald Professor of Environmental and Preventive Medicine, Wolfson Institute of Preventive Medicine, St Bartholomews' and the Royal London School of Medicine and Dentistry, Queen Mary University of London, UK
3.3.2: Medical screening

J.A. Walker-Smith Professor of Paediatric Gastroenterology, University Department of Paediatric Gastroenterology, Royal Free and University College Medical School, London, UK
15.15: Congenital abnormalities of the gastrointestinal tract

Mark J. Walport Director, The Wellcome Trust, London, UK
5.1.2: The complement system

Julian R.F. Walters Consultant Gastroenterologist and Reader, Imperial College, London UK
15.3.4: Investigation of gastrointestinal function; 15.10.1: Differential diagnosis and investigation of malabsorption

Gary S. Wand Professor, Department of Medicine Johns Hopkins University School of Medicine, Baltimore, Maryland, USA
26.7.1: Alcohol and drug dependence

T.E. Warkentin Professor, Department of Pathology and Molecular Medicine and Department of Medicine, Michael G. DeGroote School of Medicine, McMaster University, Hamilton, Ontario, Canada
22.6.5: Acquired coagulation disorders

David A. Warrell Emeritus Professor of Tropical Medicine, Nuffield Department of Clinical Medicine; Honorary Fellow, St Cross College, University of Oxford, Oxford, UK
7.4: Travel and expedition medicine; 7.5.10: Rhabdoviruses: rabies and rabies-related lyssaviruses; 7.5.11: Colorado tick fever and other arthropod-borne reoviruses; 7.5.27: Orf; 7.5.28: Molluscum contagiosum; 7.6.31: Rat-bite fevers; 7.6.33: Relapsing fevers; 7.6.35: Nonvenereal endemic treponematoses: yaws, endemic syphilis (bejel), and pinta; 7.8.2: Malaria; 7.13: Pentastomiasis (porocephalosis, linguatulosis/linguatuliasis); 9.2: Injuries, envenoming, poisoning, and allergic reactions caused by animals; 24.11.2: Viral infections; 24.24.6: Primary (tropical) pyomyositis; 33.1: Acute medical presentations; 33.2: Practical procedures

M. J. Warrell Oxford Vaccine Group, University of Oxford, Centre for Clinical Vaccinology & Tropical Medicine, Churchill Hospital, Oxford, UK
7.5.10: Rhabdoviruses: rabies and rabies-related lyssaviruses; 7.5.11: Colorado tick fever and other arthropod-borne reoviruses

Paul Warwicker Consultant in Nephrology, Lister Hospital, Stevenage, UK
21.10.5: Haemolytic uraemic syndrome

John A.H. Wass Professor of Endocrinology, University of Oxford Department of Endocrinology Oxford Centre for Diabetes, Endocrinology and Metabolism, Churchill Hospital, Oxford, UK
13.2: Disorders of the anterior pituitary gland; 13.3: Disorders of the posterior pituitary gland; 13.12: Hormonal manifestations of nonendocrine disease

Lawrence Waterman Director, Sypol Limited, Aylesbury; Head of Health and Safety, Olympic Delivery Authority, London
9.4.2: Occupational safety

Laurence Watkins Consultant in Neurosurgery, The National Hospital for Neurology and Neurosurgery, London, UK
24.10.3: Traumatic injuries to the head

Chris Watson Reader in Surgery and Honorary Consultant Surgeon, University of Cambridge Department of Surgery, Addenbrooke's Hospital, Cambridge, UK
15.4.1: The acute abdomen

George Watt Associate Professor of Medicine, University of Hawaii at Manoa, John A. Burns School of Medicine, Hawaii, USA
7.6.34: Leptospirosis; 7.6.40: Scrub typhus

Richard W.E. Watts Retired Professor & Honorary Consultant Physician, Imperial College School of Medicine, Hammersmith Hospital, London, UK
12.1: The inborn errors of metabolism: general aspects; 12.4: Disorders of purine and pyrimidine metabolism

D.J. Weatherall Regius Professor of Medicine Emeritus, University of Oxford; Weatherall Institute of Molecular Medicine, Oxford, UK
22.1: Introduction; 22.5.2: Anaemia: pathophysiology, classification, and clinical features; 22.5.3: Anaemia as a challenge to world health; 22.5.5: Normochromic, normocytic anaemia; 22.5.7: Disorders of the synthesis or function of haemoglobin; 22.7: The blood in systemic disease

D.K.H. Webb Consultant Paediatric Haematologist, Great Ormond Street Hospital for Children, London, UK
22.4.7: Histiocytoses

Lisa J. Webber Consultant in Reproductive Medicine, St Mary's Hospital, London, UK
13.8.1: Ovarian disorders

Kathryn E. Webert Assistant Professor, Haematology and Thromboembolism, McMaster University, Hamilton, Ontario, Canada
22.6.3: Disorders of platelet number and function

Bee Wee Consultant and Senior Clinical Lecturer in Palliative Medicine, Oxford Radcliffe Hospitals NHS Trust, and Fellow of Harris Manchester College, University of Oxford, UK
31.1: Palliative care

Anthony P. Weetman Professor of Medicine, Department of Human Metabolism, University of Sheffield, Sheffield, UK
13.4: The thyroid gland and disorders of thyroid function; 13.5: Thyroid cancer

Robert A. Weinstein The C. Anderson Hedberg Professor of Internal Medicine, Rush Medical College, Interim Chair, Department of Medicine, John H. Stroger Jr. Hospital of Cook County, Professor, Rush University Medical Center, Chicago, Illinois, USA
7.6.4: Staphylococci

R.A. Weiss Professor of Viral Oncology, Division of Infection and Immunity, University College London, London, UK
7.5.26: Viruses and cancer

Peter F. Weller Professor of Medicine, Harvard Medical School, Professor of Immunology and Infectious Diseases, Harvard School of Public Health, Chief, Infectious Disease and Allergy and Inflammation Divisions Beth Israel Deaconess Medical Center, Boston, Massachusetts, USA
22.4.6: Eosinophilia

A.U. Wells Interstitial Lung Disease Unit, Royal Brompton Hospital, London, UK
18.11.1: Diffuse parenchymal lung disease: an introduction; 18.11.2: Idiopathic pulmonary fibrosis; 18.11.3: Bronchiolitis obliterans and cryptogenic organizing pneumonia; 18.11.4: The lung in autoimmune rheumatic disorders; 18.11.5: The lung in vasculitis

Simon Wessely Professor, King's College, London, UK
26.6.2: Psychological treatment in medical practice

Gilbert C. White Executive Vice President for Research, Director, Blood Research Institute, Richard H. and Sara E. Aster Chair for Medical Research BloodCenter of Wisconsin; Associate Dean for Research, Professor of Medicine, Pharmacology, and Biochemistry Medical College of Wisconsin, USA
22.6.1: The biology of haemostasis and thrombosis

Joseph White Luxenberg Family Professor of Public Policy, Department of Political Science, Case Western Reserve University, Cleveland, Ohio, USA
3.4.1: The cost of health care in Western countries

H.C. Whittle Visiting Professor, London School of Hygiene and Tropical Medicine, MRC Laboratories, The Gambia, West Africa
7.5.6: Measles

Anthony S. Wierzbicki Department of Metabolic Medicine/Chemical Pathology Guy's & St Thomas Hospitals London, UK
12.9: Disorders of peroxisomal metabolism in adults

David E.L. Wilcken Emeritus Professor of Medicine, University of New South Wales, Prince of Wales Hospital, Sydney, Australia
16.1.3: Clinical physiology of the normal heart

Gordon Wilcock Professor of Clinical Geratology, University of Oxford, UK
29.1: Medicine in old age

James S. Wiley Professor of Haematology, Nepean Clinical School, University of Sydney, Penrith, Australia
22.5.8: Anaemias resulting from defective maturation of red cells

R.G. Will Professor of Clinical Neurology, Department of Clinical Neurosciences, University of Edinburgh, Edinburgh, UK
24.11.5: Human prion diseases

Bryan Williams Professor of Medicine, Department of Cardiovascular Sciences, University of Leicester School of Medicine, UK
16.17.1: Essential hypertension—definition, epidemiology, and pathophysiology; 16.17.2: Diagnosis, assessment, and treatment of essential hypertension

Christopher B. Williams Honorary Physician, Wolfson Unit for Endoscopy, St Mark's Hospital for Colorectal Disorders, London, UK
15.3.1: Colonoscopy and flexible sigmoidoscopy

David J. Williams Consultant Obstetric Physician, Institute for Women's Health, University College London Hospitals, London, UK
14.1: Physiological changes of normal pregnancy; 14.2: Nutrition in pregnancy; 14.3: Medical management of normal pregnancy

Gareth Williams Professor of Medicine, School of Clinical Science, University of Bristol, UK
13.11.1: Diabetes

J. David Williams Institute of Nephrology, University of Wales College of Medicine, Cardiff, UK
21.1: Structure and functions of the kidney

Bridget Wills Hospital for Tropical Diseases, Oxford University Clinical Research Unit, Wellcome Trust Major Overseas Programme, Vietnam, Ho Chi Minh City, Vietnam
7.5.15: Dengue; 24.11.2: Viral infections

R. Wilson Consultant Radiologist, Royal Marsden Hospital, London, UK
13.8.3: Breast cancer

Fenella Wojnarowska Professor Emeritus, University of Oxford, UK
14.13: The skin in pregnancy; 23.4: Vesiculobullous disease

Roger L. Wolman Consultant in Rheumatology and Sport and Exercise Medicine, Royal National Orthopaedic Hospital, Stanmore, UK
28.1: Sports and exercise medicine

Kathryn J. Wood Transplantation Research Immunology Group, Nuffield Department of Surgery, University of Oxford, John Radcliffe Hospital, Oxford, UK
5.5: Principles of transplantation immunology

Nicholas Wood Galton Professor of Genetics, Head of Department of Molecular Neuroscience, UCL Institute of Neurology, UK
24.7.4: Ataxic disorders

H.F. Woods Division of Molecular and Genetic Medicine, University of Sheffield School of Medicine, Sheffield, UK
12.11: Disturbances of acid–base homeostasis

Jeremy Woodward Consultant Gastroenterologist, Addenbrooke's Hospital, Cambridge, UK
11.6: Artificial nutrition support

Elaine M. Worcester Professor of Medicine, University of Chicago, Section of Nephrology, Chicago, Illinois, USA
21.14: Disorders of renal calcium handling, urinary stones, and nephrocalcinosis

B.P. Wordsworth Professor of Rheumatology, Nuffield Department of Orthopaedics, Rheumatology and Musculoskeletal Sciences, Nuffield Orthopaedic Centre, Oxford, UK
20.1: Skeletal disorders—general approach and clinical conditions

Gary P. Wormser Division of Infectious Diseases, Department of Medicine, New York Medical College, Valhalla, New York, USA
7.6.32: Lyme borreliosis

V.M. Wright Professor of Paediatric Gastroenterology, University Department of Paediatric Gastroenterology, Royal Free and University College Medical School, London, UK
15.15: Congenital abnormalities of the gastrointestinal tract

F.C.W. Wu Department of Endocrinology, Manchester Royal Infirmary, Manchester, UK
13.8.2: Disorders of male reproduction

Andrew H. Wyllie Head of Department, Department of Pathology, Cambridge, UK
4.6: Apoptosis in health and disease

Muhammad M. Yaqoob Professor of Nephrology, Barts and London NHS Trust Hospitals and School of Medicine and Dentistry, UK
21.17: Urinary tract obstruction

Hasan Yazici Professor and Chief, Department of Medicine and Division of Rheumatology, Cerrahpasa Medical Faculty, University of Istanbul, Istanbul, Turkey
19.11.5: Behçet's syndrome

Lam Minh Yen Hospital of Tropical Disease, Ho Chi Minh City, Vietnam
7.6.22: Tetanus

Jenny Yiend Research Scientist, Department of Psychiatry, University of Oxford, Oxford, UK
26.5.1: Grief, stress, and post-traumatic stress disorder

Yariv Yogev Director, Division of Maternal Fetal Medicine, Helen Schneider Hospital for Women, Rabin Medical Center, Sackler Faculty of Medicine, Tel - Aviv University, Petah-Tiqva, Israel
14.10: Diabetes in pregnancy

Sebahattin Yurdakul Professor, Division of Rheumatology, Department of Medicine, Cerrahpasa Medical Faculty, University of Istanbul, Istanbul, Turkey
19.11.5: Behçet's syndrome

A. Zeman Professor of Cognitive and Behavioural Neurology, Peninsula Medical School, Exeter, UK
24.2: Mind and brain: building bridges linking neurology, psychiatry, and psychology

Clive S. Zent Consultant Hematologist, Associate Professor of Medicine, Mayo Clinic, Rochester, Minnesota, USA
22.3.5: Chronic lymphocytic leukaemia and other leukaemias of mature B and T cells

SECTION 1

On being a patient

1.1 **On being a patient** *3*
Christopher Booth

1.1

On being a patient

Christopher Booth

Essentials

Those who practise medicine should remember that we are all patients at some time, but particularly at the beginning and end of our lives. Even distinguished professors and historians of medicine are not spared, as this account reveals. Doctors and those who manage and organize health services must recognize that patients may find it difficult to access care when they need it; that rapid relief of pain, by whatever means is appropriate, is absolutely crucial; that patients are often faced by a bewildering number of staff, who rotate on and off duty, and continuity of care is important—being looked after by a doctor or nurse whom you get to know and who understands your illness is essential for morale; that apparently simple procedures such as venesection or urinary catheterization require explanation, since they may cause great distress; that despondency mounts when there is unaccountable delay in carrying out scheduled procedures. Practical and important though many procedures are, requiring both skill and experience, for the patient, nothing can replace the compassion and sympathy that the caring professions owe the afflicted. So many aspects of excellent practice stem from these simple human qualities, which thankfully survive despite the strong business ethic that pervades medicine in many countries today. One other lesson remains. If you are a physician, no matter how important you may think you are, you should, so far as your own illnesses are concerned, consider yourself a layman.

We are all patients sooner or later, but particularly at the beginning and end of our lives. A general practitioner brought me into the world—a second twin—by manual removal when my mother was suffering from uterine inertia. Later, as a 4-year-old, I can recall being injected against an infectious disease and passing out cold on the floor. There were then many infections to which my generation was susceptible. Chickenpox, mumps, and measles were frequent. During the misery of measles, I remember seeing the flag on our nearby church flying at half-mast for the death of King George V. Our doctor, the one who had delivered me, was a tall, distinguished man, smelling—as they all did in those far-off days—of ether. Later, I contracted scarlet fever, a streptococcal illness of importance in those days before antibiotics. I was kept in strict isolation at home, with a resident nurse to care for me and daily visits from our general practitioner.

Between those childhood days and the years of maturity, I was but rarely a patient. There was a hazardous episode during training as a naval diver when I had an alarming allergic reaction to the sting of a jellyfish (a Portuguese man-of-war). The main symptoms were caused by severe oedema of the throat, and breathing became difficult. I had no idea then, long before I became a physician myself, that the large dose of morphine given by the naval doctor might well have exacerbated the respiratory distress. Beyond that, as a young man, I was a patient only for a brief period with glandular fever. I have been fortunate to escape those chronic conditions such as multiple sclerosis, Crohn's disease, or rheumatoid arthritis that blight young lives so terribly.

It was not until I was in my fifties that I developed any significant illnesses. I had intermittent atrial fibrillation, which usually subsided with antiarrhythmic drugs. My blood pressure was normal and has remained so. There were repeated electrocardiograms, but no attempts at cardioversion by direct current (DC) electric shock. For the first time, I began to make visits to hospital outpatient clinics or entered the sumptuous rooms of those who undertook private practice. This experience made me realize that the particular feature of 'being' a patient means 'having' patience. One came to accept that so much time is spent waiting—for an appointment, for a blood test or a radiograph, for a consultation, or for drugs from the hospital pharmacy.

As the years go by, you should realize that, like your patients, you become more liable to afflictions that may be truly frightening and threaten your life over prolonged periods. My next encounter with medicine in practice came about entirely by chance. I had been retired for some years when my partner encouraged me to have a 'check-up'. The excellent female general practitioner was not one of those many who spend more time staring at a computer screen than they do looking at you. She examined me carefully, found nothing amiss, but dispatched some blood tests. These too were normal, with one exception, a test with which I was then unfamiliar. The blood concentration of prostate-specific antigen

(PSA) was 15 μg/litre and thus above the healthy reference range. I was informed that this suggested the presence of a symptomless cancer of the prostate and, although I was reassured that the significance of the finding was uncertain, a subsequent prostate biopsy revealed that there was indeed cancer of the prostate, apparently localized to the gland. The question, therefore, arose as to what should be done.

Much today is made of choice; perhaps this has value when there can be a truly informed discussion, as subsequent events in my case show. So far as I was concerned, I had no interest in where I should be referred for treatment. My doctor could advise me about that. Nor had I much interest in choosing between the options available—surgery, radiotherapy, or hormonal treatment. It was for my advisers to recommend what they thought was best. It was only in later years that I realized that the choice of radiotherapy was unfortunate. At the time, daily treatment as an outpatient for more than 6 weeks was a tormenting experience since the resulting radiation cystitis caused excruciating pain. I was constantly reminded during those days of the urologist who prayed nightly to his maker, 'Lord, when thou takest me, take me not through my bladder'. In the end, the symptoms subsided. The PSA level returned to normal and has remained so. Mercifully, the cancer had been eradicated. I soon developed severe muscle pain—diagnosed by a rheumatologist as polymyalgia rheumatica, which required treatment with steroids. Nothing will ever convince me that these symptoms were not the result of the radiotherapy.

These events took place during my 70th year. A few years later, whilst in manifest good health, illness suddenly struck again. One evening, out of the blue, I developed severe upper abdominal pain. In the absence of an out-of-hours service from the local general practice, at midnight we attempted to obtain medical advice from 'NHS Direct' on the telephone. This was a fruitless task made very trying by 'language difficulties'. I finished up in the emergency department of our local hospital. There, a very competent doctor treated me with pethidine: and there too I first experienced lying on a trolley for the rest of the night. Lying on a trolley is no great problem for a patient blissfully enjoying the delight of repeated injections of pethidine, but it is extremely dispiriting for one's partner. Deeply troubled by my illness, seated in a small and uncomfortable plastic chair, my wife had nothing to do but watch and wait hopefully for the dawn. A week in the hospital taught me how to manage my life while attached to an intravenous drip, which had to accompany me at all times. It turned out that I had acute pancreatitis, possibly associated with a gallstone. The pain soon subsided and, apart from one other minor event, has not recurred.

All remained well for 4 or 5 months. Then, attending a clinic for a follow-up appointment, I found out why it was, I was thirsty and polyuric. My wife had noticed this and of course, had made the right diagnosis, which my medical adviser at once recognized when he smelt the acetone on my breath and found my blood sugar to be in excess of 30 mol/litre. I was immediately admitted, and the diabetes was brought under control. On this occasion, I was admitted to a geriatric ward where the noises at night generally made sleep no more than an aspiration. One particularly unfortunate man, suffering from expressive dysphasia caused by a stroke, kept shouting in frustrated attempts to make himself understood.

Becoming a diabetic changes your lifestyle at once. You find out how to control your blood sugar, initially on oral medication. But soon, as is so often the case, you require subcutaneous insulin, and you now have to learn how to inject yourself as well as keeping to a strict diet. You also have to ensure that you avoid the unpleasantness and fear of hypoglycaemic attacks. In addition, you may require visits to the foot clinic to ensure you develop neither ulcers nor infected toenails.

If, in the case of that illness, it was a matter of one thing following another, my next and most serious medical encounter was even more Odyssean. By my 82nd year, I had thought that the prostate cancer, 12 years after radiotherapy, could safely be forgotten. The PSA concentrations had remained within the normal range and I seemed in good health—but then haematuria developed. Cystoscopy as an outpatient failed to identify a source for the bleeding, and while waiting for an appointment for an in-patient cystoscopy I suddenly developed clot retention. It is no pleasant experience to drive through metropolitan rush-hour traffic with acute urinary retention. Nor was attention forthcoming in a hospital emergency department, dealing as usual with the overwhelming evening intake of drunks and dropouts. Finally, when I was installed once more on a trolley, a junior house officer attempted the necessary catheterization. Only after repeated and painful efforts was a more experienced registrar sent for; he, at last, blissfully relieved the obstruction. Then again, the long wait—and finally—admission to a high-dependency ward. I remained in hospital for treatment for the next 3 months.

The events of that first week in a high-dependency ward set the scene for what was to happen in the months to come. A regime of constant bladder washouts was instituted in the hope that the haematuria would subside. Several drugs were tried, all to no avail. There was obvious reluctance to undertake surgery in an elderly patient for a condition that showed no sign of being malignant. So, in due course, I was transferred to a single room in a urological ward where the haematuria persisted despite continuous bladder washouts. Maintaining the flow of fluid from two large containers hanging on a drip stand became one's constant concern, nurses not always leaving enough fluid supplies, particularly at night. If the flow ceased, clot retention would recur. For a brief period, I was sent home in the hope that the symptoms would subside. But it was to no avail—as was the search for the cause of the bleeding. Two careful cystoscopies under general anaesthesia failed to identify a bleeding point, another reason why there was reluctance to consider surgery at that time.

One soon became used to a ward routine that scarcely varied from day to day, with the exception that at weekends nothing ever seemed to happen. You might be gently woken by a kind nurse from the Philippines wanting to give you something, but whose command of English might not be fully up to the task. You would be increasingly less surprised to see the unfamiliar blank wall that had been there when you drifted off to sleep. You would at once be aware of noise, trolleys being pushed along corridors, the clatter of metal containers, and sometimes the cries of the afflicted. You have breakfast, the same cereal most days, sometimes porridge. You are given the morning's drugs. A phlebotomist takes your blood every day, the veins becoming progressively more difficult to find. Your blood pressure, oxygen saturation, and pulse rate are measured on a machine every 4 h or so and it may be necessary for a drip to be inserted, a task undertaken better by some than others. Your insulin dosage has to be adjusted, depending on the results of your blood glucose measurements repeatedly obtained by finger prick. Your bed is made, your body washed. You sometimes see the intern who has the responsibility for your care—but they change duties frequently. Then, there is the consultants' ward round. Instead of a single individual taking care of you, you find that up to five consultants, and their acolytes, visit together. They are invariably courteous and considerate, and you learn to hang on every word. There are those who find the recumbent position of the patient in bed, in the presence of massed ranks of consultants, to be demeaning. I have preferred not to acknowledge my obvious inferiority, but to imagine myself a medieval potentate receiving his courtiers.

Then, at last, another surgeon is brought to see me. The waiting is now over. Briskly and unhesitatingly, he decides to operate within 3 days. I am lucky—he is one of the best in the country. The operation is to be a total cystectomy and prostatectomy, the creation of an intestinal pouch to replace the bladder and transplantation of the ureters into this pouch. One can easily understand why my advisers had been so hesitant to inflict such a procedure on an individual in his 82nd year, irrespective of my status as a former professor of medicine. Fortunately, the surgery is brilliantly successful and we now have a diagnosis. The pathologist reports that there are no specific bleeding points in the bladder, but that there are signs of widespread radiation damage. As with my diabetes, one thing has again led to another: the diffuse pathological bleeding was caused by that course of radiotherapy given so long ago.

Surgical success depends on the support you receive before and after the operation. Languishing in hospital, I had lost a considerable amount of weight, and nutritional advice from a gastroenterologist was needed for recovery. There were other complications. My thumbs became septic because of a faulty technique in obtaining blood for sugar estimations and both were later shown to be infected with the near-ubiquitous methicillin-resistant *Staphylococcus aureus* (MRSA)—as was a small unhealed focus in my abdominal scar. More drugs—this time, antibiotics to treat the MRSA. Still feeling weak and scarcely able to walk the distance from the kerb to my front door, I was sent home.

I felt terrible that day and by evening had developed severe dysphagia. Back in hospital, I was soon drifting dreamingly in and out of consciousness; little did I know that my wife had been told by my advisers to expect the worst. By the next morning, however, the gastroenterologists had done an oesophagoscopy and identified oesophageal candidiasis. I was treated with nystatin and soon recovered. Although it took time to recover my appetite, I was able to eat again and returned home to convalesce. But it was to be a year or more before my strength fully recovered and my voice was weak and husky for some months.

Certain memories of life as a hospital patient persist. I encountered so many consultants during that time: seven urologists, a gastroenterologist, a cardiologist to check whether my heart would stand up to surgery, a diabetologist, a rheumatologist to check my steroid dosage and the status of my polymyalgia rheumatica, as well as a dermatologist when a presumed drug eruption occurred. There was also the infectious diseases expert who treated the MRSA infection. Throughout, the international nature of the team who contributed to my care was impressive. Among doctors, nurses, porters, radiographers, and other staff, I counted members of 38 nationalities, including many nurses from sub-Saharan Africa and the Philippines—clearly countries favoured for recruitment to the United Kingdom. One wonders about the loss of national skills.

Despite laudable attempts to make it tempting, hospital food was generally unappetizing and I depended largely on my wife for sustenance: she brought in dinner with a small bottle of red wine most evenings, and on this I survived. Yet above all, a patient depends on the support of friends and family, upon whom a greater burden lies than is often realized. My wife visited on every day of my incarceration—a task that she undertook despite her commitment to our household and her own affairs, when travel was not always easy, and when, on arrival at the hospital, parking might be difficult.

It is the doctors and nurses whom you meet every day who can do most to sustain your spirits. As a medical student in Scotland, I was taught to treat a duchess or a dustman just the same. The patient should, of course, always be treated with respect: I am convinced that this starts with their being addressed naturally using their surname rather than the all-too-prevalent belief that use of their first name would be preferred from the outset. Clearly, this familiarity may come later—by invitation—and when desired by the named individual! It is astonishing to see how frequently patients are offended by the presumption of first-name familiarity, at least in hospitals in the United Kingdom. It is a behaviour perceived as institutionally controlling by adults of all ages and status, not only by elderly professionals. But if the staff genuinely sympathize with your lot, spending time answering your questions and those of your family, you are greatly encouraged. It is so often the little things that count. I recall being much moved by a young Zimbabwean nurse who had cared for me during one of my hospital admissions and who later took the trouble to visit me in a far-off part of the hospital to see how I fared.

Continuity of care is also important. Being under the care of an intern or nurse whom you get to know and who understands your illness is essential for morale. Having to explain your problems to a stranger who drops in for a brief uncomprehending visit after normal working hours, or at a weekend, does nothing for confidence. There are also practical matters that may be overlooked. Whereas major interventions involving surgery, e.g. may be explained scrupulously, staff doing apparently simple procedures such as venesection, cannula insertion, arterial puncture for blood gas determination, or catheterization, often forget that these activities also require explanation since they may cause great distress to anxious or confused patients—to whom the slightest invasion of their person rapidly becomes anathema. Anxious despondency also mounts when there is unaccountable delay in carrying out procedures that have been arranged: timely explanation can often mollify this distress, but when it comes to the relief of pain, there is no excuse for delay—diagnostic or otherwise. The failure immediately to catheterize a patient with acute retention of urine is clearly unforgivable but, as I learnt, is still regrettably common.

Practical and important though many procedures are, requiring both skill and experience, for the patient, nothing can replace the compassion and sympathy that the caring professions owe the afflicted. So many aspects of excellent practice stem from these simple human qualities, which thankfully survive despite the strong business ethic that pervades medicine in many countries today.

Of the lessons that I have learnt, however, perhaps the most important is that to be a patient entails, as the *Oxford English Dictionary* puts it, 'enduring pain, affliction, inconvenience, etc., calmly, without discontent or complaint'. It is equally necessary to be 'able to wait calmly'. In our later years, it easier to agree with this advice. After all, as a man reaches his eighties he has little choice but to accept with equanimity the world of Shakespeare's sixth age, when he shifts

> Into the lean and slipper'd pantaloon,
> With spectacles on nose and pouch on side
> His youthful hose, well sav'd, a world too wide
> For his shrunk shank; and his big manly voice,
> Turning again towards childish treble....

That passage accurately describes me in the immediate postoperative period, even to the urostomy pouch—but my voice has now recovered. I do not, however, wish to survive into the last of Shakespeare's seven ages when we are doomed to 'mere oblivion; sans teeth, sans eyes, sans taste, sans everything'. While I have so far benefited from the courageous decisions of those who did not give up when the end looked inevitable, but who saw that there was a 'quality of life' worth striving for, I only hope that common sense, compassion, and proper conference with my nearest and dearest will be brought to bear when the seventh age draws nigh. One does wonder if such a perspective truly holds today—especially in wards for older people in modern Western hospitals.

One other lesson remains. If you are a physician, no matter how important you may think that you are, you should, so far as your own illnesses are concerned, consider yourself a layman.

SECTION 2

Modern medicine: foundations, achievements, and limitations

2.1 Scientific background to medicine *9*

2.1.1 Science in medicine: when, how, and what *9*
W.F. Bynum

2.1.2 Evolution: medicine's most basic science *12*
Randolph M. Nesse and Richard Dawkins

2.2 Medical ethics *16*
Tony Hope

2.3 Evidence-based medicine *22*

2.3.1 Bringing the best evidence to the point of care *22*
Paul P. Glasziou

2.3.2 Evidence-based medicine—does it apply to my particular patient? *27*
Louis R. Caplan

2.3.3 Large-scale randomized evidence: trials and meta-analyses of trials *31*
C. Baigent, R. Peto, R. Gray, S. Parish, and R. Collins

2.3.4 The future of clinical trials *45*
Perry Nisen and Patrick Vallance

2.4 Funding of health care *48*

2.4.1 The evaluation and provision of effective medicines *48*
Michael D. Rawlins

2.4.2 Reasonableness and its definition in the provision of health care *54*
Norman Daniels

2.4.3 Priority setting in developed and developing countries *58*
Nigel Crisp

2.4.4 Sustaining innovation in an era of specialized medicine *60*
Henri A. Termeer

2.5 Complementary and alternative medicine *65*
E. Ernst

2.1

Scientific background to medicine

Contents

2.1.1 Science in medicine: when, how, and what *9*
W.F. Bynum

2.1.2 Evolution: medicine's most basic science *12*
Randolph M. Nesse and Richard Dawkins

2.1.1 Science in medicine: when, how, and what

W.F. Bynum

Essentials

Science has always been part of Western medicine, although what counts as scientific has changed over the centuries, as have the content of medical knowledge, the tools of medical investigation, and the details of medical treatments. This brief overview develops a historical typology of medicine since antiquity. It divides the 'kinds' of medicine into five: bedside, library, hospital, social, and laboratory. These categories are still principal headings in modern health budgets, but they also have specific historical resonances. (1) Bedside medicine, developed by the Hippocratic doctors in classical times, has its modern counterpart in primary care. (2) Library medicine, associated with the scholastic mentality of the Middle Ages, still surfaces in the problems of information storage and retrieval in the computer age. (3) Hospital medicine, central to French medicine of the early 19th century, placed the diagnostic and therapeutic functions of the modern hospital centre stage in care and teaching. (4) Social medicine is about prevention, both communal and individual, and is especially visible in our notion of 'lifestyle' and its impact on health. (5) Laboratory medicine has its natural home in the research establishment and is a critical site for the creation of medical knowledge, setting the standards for both medical science and scientific medicine. François Magendie (1773–1855) was probably the first truly 'modern' medical scientist: he had little sense of medical tradition; instead, he sought to establish medicine on new, scientific foundations.

Introduction

At least since the Hippocratics, Western medicine has always aspired to be scientific. What has changed is not so much the aspirations but what it has meant to be 'scientific'.

'Science is the father of knowledge, but opinion breeds ignorance', opined the Hippocratic treatise *The Canon*, and Hippocratic practitioners developed an approach to health, disease, and its treatment based on systematic observation and cumulative experience. Even the word 'physic', whence physician as well as physicist, derives from the Greek for 'nature'. Further, Hippocratic medicine was experimental, that word stemming from the same classical roots which gave us 'experience'.

Words, however, can be slippery, as philosophers as divergent as Francis Bacon and Ludwig Wittgenstein have stressed. The science and experiment of the Hippocratics can still inspire, but they are not our science and experiment. During the past two or three centuries, an armoury of sciences and technologies has come to underpin medical practice. This essay attempts briefly to describe these, within the context of distinctive and perennial features of medical practice, i.e. suffering individuals whose problems and diseases demand attention.

A historical typology of Western medicine

The history of Western medicine can be divided into five 'kinds' of medicine: bedside, library, hospital, social, and laboratory. Each approach to medical care and knowledge emerged at a particular historical period, but each still has relevance to us today. Bedside medicine can be equated with the vision of the Hippocratics, with its emphasis on the individual patient, a tendency towards holism, and an abiding concern with the patient within his or her own unique environment. These are some of the reasons why Hippocrates (Fig. 2.1.1.1) is still claimed as the dominant father figure by both orthodox and alternative medical practitioners. What can be called 'library' medicine dominated in the Middle Ages, when learned medicine retreated into the universities and scholars sometimes assumed that everything worth discovering had been uncovered by the ancients, and everything worth being revealed could be found in the Bible. The millennium between the sacking of Rome and the discovery of the New World is often dismissed as a sterile period scientifically, but the physicians of the period, linguistically erudite and philosophically inclined, would

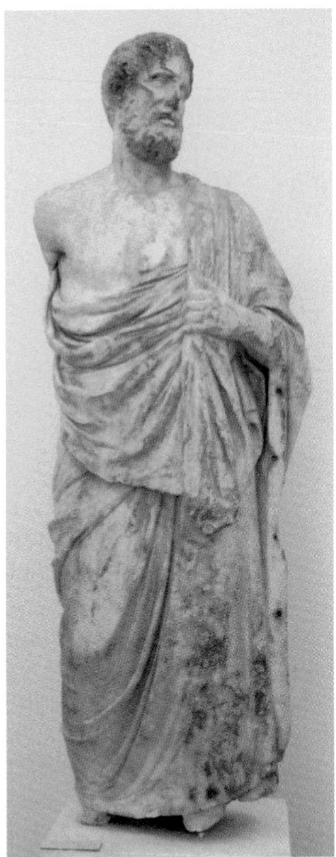

Fig. 2.1.1.1 Statue of Hippocrates, originally in Kos Odeion, now in the Archaeological Museum of Kos. Late Hellenistic Period copy of a classical prototype. No contemporary likeness of Hippocrates exists, but a number of busts and statues were created later in the classical period.
(Copyright © D A Warrell.)

have been surprised to be described as unscientific. They simply believed that the road to knowledge was through the book.

These medical men also sometimes engaged with nature, although it is undeniable that nature rather than words became an increasing source of truth and knowledge during the Scientific Revolution, a period stretching roughly from just before Andreas Vesalius (1514–1564) to Isaac Newton (1642–1727). Around 1600, it was becoming apparent to many that the Greeks had not left behind a complete and accurate account of the nature of the world, and that scientific knowledge was cumulative. This 'Battle of the Books', the debate over whether the ancients or the moderns knew more, was decided in favour of the moderns. Many of the outstanding scientific achievements of the era were in astronomy and physics, but medicine, both in its theory and its practice, was also affected. Theory has always been easier to change than practice, of course, and it was famously remarked that William Harvey's discovery of the circulation of the blood had no impact on therapeutics. Harvey (1578–1657) also notoriously lamented that his practice fell off mightily following the discovery, his patients fearing that he was 'crack-brained'. The fear that too close an identification with science was detrimental to patient confidence recurs in medical history, and is still part of the delicate negotiations between the profession and its public, and to the status of academic medicine.

Within the discipline of medicine itself there have always been individuals, some of them, like Thomas Sydenham (1624–1689), eminently successful, who believed that experimental science had little to offer to patient care. But these 'artists' of medicine could still invoke the authority of Hippocrates, with its older connotations of knowledge and experience. Sydenham himself did not demur from his being dubbed 'the English Hippocrates'. During the early modern period, the whole spectrum of the sciences—mathematics, physics, chemistry, the life sciences (not yet called biology)—made their ways into formulations of health and disease. Iatrophysics, iatromathematics, and iatrochemistry all had their advocates in the 17th and 18th centuries, as approaches to medical theory and practice.

That these systems tended to encourage speculation to run ahead of evidence was recognized at the time, and this was part of the reason why 'hospital medicine' had little recourse to those disciplines we now call 'basic medical sciences'. The founders of French hospital medicine, Xavier Bichat (1771–1802), J. N. Corvisart (1755–1821), R. T. H. Laennec (1781–1826), often referred to chemistry, physiology, and the like as sciences 'accessory' to medicine. The medicine that developed in the Paris hospitals, after the reopening in 1794 of the medical schools closed by the Revolution a couple of years earlier, emphasized above all the study of disease in the sick patient. In a sense, this was Hippocratic medicine writ large, but with some significant differences. First, the hospital offered the curious doctor a vast arena for observing disease. The equivalent of a lifetime's experience of a lone practitioner in the community could be experienced in a few months of hospital work. Hospitals offered the possibility of defining disease on the basis of hundreds of cases. Second, Hippocratic humoralism gradually disappeared as the dominant explanatory framework of health and disease, replaced by the primacy of the lesion, located in the solids: the organs and tissues, and by the mid 19th century, cells. In this new orientation, disease was literally palpable, its lesions to be discovered in life by the systematic use of physical examination—Corvisart rediscovered percussion, Laennec invented the stethoscope—and these findings to be correlated after death by routine autopsy. French high priests of hospital medicine brought diagnosis to a new stage and replaced the older symptom-based nosologies with a more objective, demonstrable one of lesions. The third feature of hospital medicine was what Pierre Louis (1787–1872) called the numerical method, the use of numbers to guide both disease classification and therapeutic evaluation.

The philosophy underlying early 19th century French medicine was most systematically expounded by one of the many American students who studied in Paris, Elisha Bartlett, in his *Philosophy of Medical Science* (1844). The medical science whose philosophy he chronicled was one of facts. Bartlett argued that all systems of medicine, past and present, were speculative, vague, and useless. Cullen, Brown, Broussais, and Hahnemann were all consigned to the historical dustbin. The new medicine was one of systematic observation and collection of facts, which, properly compared and organized, could provide an objective understanding of disease and a rational basis for its treatment. Bartlett's philosophy was essentially undiluted Baconian inductivism applied to medicine. Unsurprisingly, he counted Hippocrates as well as Pierre Louis among his heroes.

One consequence of the lesion-based medicine was the recognition that not much of what doctors did actually altered the natural history of disease. Therapeutic scepticism, or even nihilism, flourished among doctors whose lives were spent, as Laennec put it, 'among the dead and dying'. It was less likely to be expressed among doctors concerned with earning a living treating private, paying patients, but the concern with medicine's therapeutic impotency also fuelled the movement to prevent disease. The fourth kind of medicine, social, also flourished in the 18th century. Just as hospitals existed long before 'hospital medicine', so epidemics and preventive measures were not invented by the public health movement of the 1830s. Nevertheless, the preventive infrastructures developed partly in response to the cholera pandemics still exist, although of course much changed. The chief architect of the British public health movement, Edwin Chadwick (1800–1890), was a lawyer who thought that, on the whole, doctors were overrated. (He was neither the first nor the last lawyer to hold that opinion.) He held that filth spread via the foul smells (miasma) of rotting organic matter caused epidemic diseases. His solutions were engineering ones, clean water and efficient waste disposal, which he argued would leave the world an altogether more pleasant and healthier place. His ideas were formed during the 1830s and early 1840s, and they remained more or less fixed for the rest of his long life, which extended well into the bacteriological age. Nevertheless, Chadwick also invoked science in his public health reform programme, above all the science of statistical investigation. His use of statistics can easily be shown to have been naive, but it was ardent. In his own sphere of enquiry, Chadwick was as much in awe of the unadorned 'fact' as was his contemporary Bartlett. A later generation of Medical Officers of Health and others concerned with disease prevention (or containment) would develop new investigative techniques, more sophisticated statistics and, especially, new theories of disease causation and transmission. But the early public health movement was firmly based on the science of its time.

The final locus of medicine, the laboratory, was also largely a product of the 19th century, though of course laboratories (a place where one worked, especially to mutate gold from lead) had existed for much longer. A leading exponent of the laboratory, and one of its most thoughtful philosophers, had experienced Paris hospital medicine as a medical student. Claude Bernard's *Introduction to the Study of Experimental Medicine* (1865) is at once an intriguing account of his own brilliant career and a sophisticated analysis of the philosophy of experimentation within the life sciences. Hospitals, he argued, are merely the gateways to medical knowledge, and bedside clinicians can be no more than natural historians of disease. To understand the causes and mechanisms of disease, it is necessary to go into the sanctuary of the laboratory, where experimental conditions can be better controlled. There are in nature no uncaused causes: determinism is the iron law of the universe, extending equally to living systems and inorganic ones. However, organisms present special experimental problems, and it is only through isolating particular features, and holding other parameters as constant as possible, that reliability and reproducibility can be achieved.

Bernard identified three primary branches of experimental medicine: physiology, pathology, and therapeutics. His own research programme touched all three pillars: his research on the roles of the liver and pancreas in sugar metabolism contributed to understanding normal physiology as well as diseases such as diabetes; his investigations of the sites of action of agents such as curare and carbon monoxide foreshadowed structural pharmacology and drug receptor theory; his work on the functions of the sympathetic nerves buttressed his own more general notion of the constancy of *milieu interieur* as the precondition to vital action (and freedom), a precursor of Walter Cannon's concept of homeostasis. Bernard stands supreme as the quintessential advocate of the laboratory.

Who was the first modern medical experimentalist?

When Bernard wrote, experimental medical science was still a fledgling activity, best developed in the universities of the German states and principalities. The German university ideal of medical education was to be extolled by the American educational reformer Abraham Flexner (1866–1959) in the early 20th century. It was in the reformed and newly created German universities that the forms of modern scientific research were established. Research careers were created; copublication in specialist journals became common; scientific societies flourished. The microscope became the symbol of the medical scientist even as the stethoscope was becoming the hallmark of the forward-looking clinician. In the hands of scientists like Schwann, Virchow, and Weismann, the modern cell theory was developed and applied to medicine and biology more generally. These researchers established the drive to push units of analysis further and further. Eduard Buchner's identification of cell-free ferments in 1897 firmly established the importance of subcellular functions. Pasteur, Koch, Ehrlich, von Behring, and others advanced new notions of the causes of disease, the body's response to infection, and the possibilities of new drugs to combat disease. Any of these scientists might arguably be the answer to the parlour-game question: who was the first modern medical scientist?

The German-speaking lands perfected the modern forms of scientific research, but a good case can be made for a Frenchman to be crowned the first thoroughly modern experimentalist within medicine. François Magendie (1783–1855) (Fig. 2.2.1.2) was a child of the Enlightenment and product of the French Revolution. One of several eminent individuals (Thomas Malthus was another) raised according to the anarchic principles espoused by Jean-Jacques Rousseau, Magendie did not learn to read or write till he was 10. His subsequent precocity was such that he was ready for medical

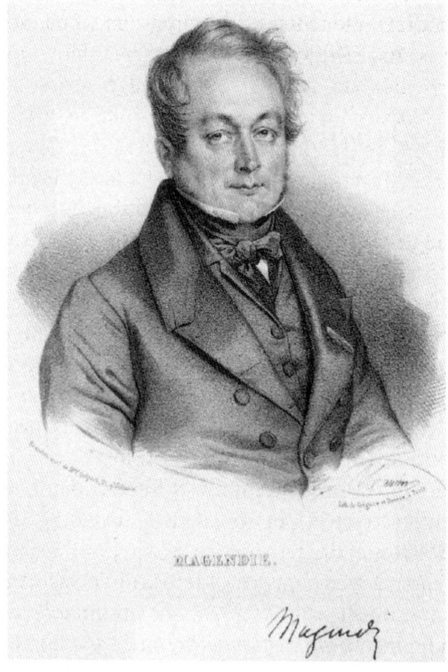

Fig. 2.1.1.2 François Magendie. Lithograph by N E Maurin.
(From Burgess R (1973). *Portraits of doctors and scientists in the Wellcome Institute, London*, no. 1870.2, by courtesy of the Wellcome Institute Library, London.)

studies by the age of 16, learned anatomy and surgery as an apprentice, and made his way through the Paris hospital system. Although he never lost interest in practical medical issues, his reputation was established primarily within the laboratory. His monographs on physiology and pharmacology marked new beginnings, and his life manifests three emblematic qualities which make him one of us. First, he valued facts above theories, evidence above rhetoric. But he went beyond Bartlett and the high priests of hospital medicine in insisting that in experiment, and not simply observation, lay the real future of medical knowledge. Like his pupil Claude Bernard, Magendie was a deft experimentalist. He used animals (and occasionally patients) to probe into a whole range of problems in physiology, pathology, and pharmacology: the functions of the spinal nerves, the physiology of vomiting, important facets of absorption, digestion, circulation, nutrition, and the actions of drugs and poisons. He described anaphylaxis a century before it was named. He was as philosophically naive as Bernard was sophisticated: of course he had theories, but his image of himself as a rag-picker with a spiked stick, gathering isolated experimental facts where he found them, is a telling one. Second, he was modern in sometimes backing the wrong horses. He judged cholera and yellow fever to be noncontagious, was suspicious of anaesthesia, and sometimes claimed more than we might for his newly introduced therapeutic substances, such as strychnine and veratrine. Magendie could often be mistaken in his beliefs; so can we. Finally, Magendie was the scientist who first expunged the double-faced Janus from the medical mentality. William Harvey worshipped Aristotle, Albrecht von Haller was steeped in history, and Isaac Newton popularized the pious conceit of pygmies standing on the shoulders of giants. Until the 19th century, doctors routinely looked to the past, not simply for inspiration but for useful information. Magendie looked only in one direction: the future. He had no sense of history and no use for it. He meant what he said when he insisted that most physiological 'facts' had to be verified by new experiments, and he undertook to provide a beginning. He made the laboratory the bedrock of medicine. With Magendie, the history of medicine became an antiquarian discipline.

What happened next?

Like everyone, Magendie was of his time. Nevertheless, his values were symptomatic of important themes within 19th century medicine and medical science. By the beginning of the First World War, most of the structures and the fundamental concepts of 'our' medicine were in place. Of course, both medical science and medical practice have been utterly transformed since. But the impulse of experimentation and its variable translation into practice were there. We have gone far beyond the cell in our analytical procedures, and our medical, surgical, and therapeutic armamentaria are vastly more sophisticated and powerful.

Our medicine is fundamentally different in one important respect, even if the trend was already evident in the 19th century: the fusion of science and technology. Science and technology have become so intertwined that the older distinctions between them are blurred. Technology made a real but minimal impact on 19th century medicine. Some instruments, such as Helmholtz's ophthalmoscope, came into clinical medicine through the laboratory; and German experimental scientists were eager to exploit the latest equipment such as kymographs, sphygmographs, and the profusion of artefacts (Petri dishes, autoclaves, etc.), which Koch and his colleagues devised for the bacteriological laboratory.

Most important of all was probably X-rays, discovered by Roentgen in late 1895. This made an immediate impact on medical diagnosis, and the associated science of radioactivity soon was felt within therapeutics. Significantly, perhaps, the pioneers of the radioactive phenomena—Roentgen, Becquerel, the Curies—got their Nobel Prizes in physics or chemistry. Hounsfield and Cormack got theirs for computer-assisted tomography in medicine or physiology. More recently, Kary Mullis's Nobel Prize was for a technological development within molecular biology.

Both medical science and medical practice are now inseparably rooted in technology. So is modern life, another reflection of a perennial historical truth: medical knowledge and medical practice are products of wider social forces with unique historical individualities.

Further reading

Ackerknecht EH (1967). *Medicine at the Paris Hospital, 1784–1848*. Johns Hopkins University Press, Baltimore, MD.

Bynum WF (1994). *Science and the practice of medicine in the nineteenth century*. Cambridge University Press, Cambridge.

Bynum WF (2008). *History of medicine: a very short introduction*. Oxford University Press, Oxford.

Bynum WF, Bynum H (eds.) (2007). *Dictionary of medical biography*. Greenwood, Westport, CT.

Bynum WF, Porter R (eds.) (1993). *Companion encyclopedia of the history of medicine*. 2 vols. Routledge, London.

Bynum WF, *et al.* (2006). *The Western medical tradition, 1800 to 2000*. Cambridge University Press, Cambridge.

Conrad LI, *et al.* (1995). *The Western medical tradition, 800 BC to AD 1800*. Cambridge University Press, Cambridge.

Cooter R, Pickstone J (eds.) (2000). *Medicine in the 20th century*. Harwood Academic Publishers, Amsterdam.

King LS (1982). *Medical thinking: a historical preface*. Princeton University Press, Princeton, NJ.

Reiser SJ (1978). *Medicine and the reign of technology*. Cambridge University Press, Cambridge.

Weatherall DJ (1995). *Science and the quiet art: medical research and patient care*. Oxford University Press, Oxford.

2.1.2 Evolution: medicine's most basic science

Randolph M. Nesse and Richard Dawkins

Essentials

The role of evolutionary biology as a basic science for medicine has been expanding rapidly. Some evolutionary methods are already widely applied in medicine, such as population genetics and methods for analysing phylogenetic trees. Newer applications come from seeking evolutionary as well as proximate explanations for disease.

Acknowledgement. Thanks to the Berlin Institute for Advanced Study for providing a fellowship to RMN that made preparation of this chapter possible.

Traditional medical research has been restricted to proximate studies of the body's mechanism. However, separate evolutionary explanations are also needed for why natural selection has left many aspects of the body vulnerable to disease. There are six main possibilities: mismatch, infection, constraints, trade-offs, reproduction at the cost of health, and adaptive defences. Like other basic sciences, evolutionary biology has limited direct clinical implications, but it provides essential research methods, it encourages asking new questions that foster a deeper understanding of disease, and it provides a framework that organizes the facts of medicine. Physicians who understand evolution recognize that bodies are not designed machines, but jury-rigged products of millions of years of natural selection that work remarkably well, given that no trait can be perfect, and that selection maximizes reproduction, not health.

Introduction

This medical textbook is, as far as we know, the first to offer a chapter on evolutionary biology. The occasion of the 150th anniversary of the publication of *The Origin of Species* makes it fitting, albeit somewhat delayed. Medical students are taught how the human body is (anatomy), and how it works (physiology), but seldom are they taught why it works (natural selection) or whence it comes (evolution). It is as though car mechanics were taught how a car works, and how to fix breakdowns, but never where it came from (factories and designers' drawing boards) nor the purpose for which it was designed (transport along roads).

Things are beginning to improve. The past 15 years have seen a series of books, articles, and meetings that report new applications of evolutionary biology to medicine. Evolution is as fundamental to medicine as physics or chemistry. This chapter cannot review its whole scope. We can only illustrate a few core principles in hopes of encouraging further reading.

Core evolutionary principles for medicine

Natural selection and adaptation

When individuals in a population vary in ways that influence their genetic contribution to future populations, the average characteristics of the population will change. This is not a theory; it is necessarily true. Natural selection involves no design, no planning, and no goal. The word 'evolution' refers more generally to any changes over time in a population, whether from selection, mutation, genetic drift, or migration.

Notwithstanding his most famous title, Darwin's greatest contribution was not his explanation of speciation, but his explanation of adaptation. Recent research on the Galapagos finches known as 'Darwin's finches' illustrates the point. During drought, only larger seeds are available, so individuals with larger beaks get more food and have more offspring. In just a few generations, the average beak in the population became significantly larger after a drought. When the rains came, and small seeds again became plentiful, selection switched to favouring smaller beaks. No trait is adaptive except in relation to a specific environment.

Levels of selection

Nonspecialists often assume that natural selection should shape traits to benefit groups. After all, if a species goes extinct, all the individuals and their genes are lost. This 'group selection' fallacy was unmasked over 40 years ago, but it continues to cause confusion in medicine.

For instance, one might expect pathogens to evolve low virulence: killing off the host is surely not good for the group! However, even long association of a host and pathogen does not necessarily decrease virulence. People who are out of bed transmit a rhinovirus faster; this selects for low virulence. The story is very different for insect-borne diseases. *Plasmodium* is transmitted faster from patients who are too sick to slap mosquitoes, so virulence is high for malaria in humans (infected mosquitoes feel just fine).

Ageing can be similarly misunderstood. One might think that senescence could speed the evolution of the species by making room for new individuals. The species, however, is not the level at which selection acts. Consider a lethal or deleterious gene that is expressed only late in life. Many carriers will have passed on the gene before it kills them. The same gene would be quickly selected out if it killed individuals before they reproduced. We are all descended from individuals who died after having children. Not one of our ancestors ever died in childhood! Moreover, a pleiotropic gene that gives a benefit early in life may be favoured, even if it causes deleterious effects later, when selection is weaker. This evolutionary explanation for senescence is now confronting remarkable new evidence that single-gene effects in the insulin signalling pathways can have huge effects. The reasons why selection has not incorporated such changes will prove most interesting.

Established applications

Some methods from evolutionary biology have long been applied to medicine. Population genetics describes how natural selection, mutation, migration, and drift account for shifting gene frequencies. This body of knowledge has been a foundation for medicine since the middle of the twentieth century, so we will only note a few new applications.

It is now clear that the ability to digest lactose as an adult is the exception, rather than the rule. In our ancestors, milk was a food for babies only. New analyses show that the ability to digest lactose as an adult has emerged on at least three separate occasions in human prehistory, always in dairying cultures. Remarkably, the selective advantage in these cultures has been huge, of the order of 5 to 15%. The exact benefits remain to be fully understood but calcium and vitamin D may be important, as well as getting more calories.

Another example is the prevalence of mutations influencing the alcohol dehydrogenase genes in some populations (especially in south-east Asia). Carriers get sick when they drink alcohol. Is the prevalence of this mutation a result of random genetic drift, or does it give some advantage, perhaps by decreasing the risk of alcoholism? New data show that it does protect against alcoholism and that strong selection has acted at this locus; it is at the centre of one of the largest haplotypes in some populations. This supports the role of alcohol, but the geographical distribution suggests that diet or other cultural variations may be responsible.

Genetic methods for tracing phylogenies of pathogens have long been available. Influenza strains are tracked so assiduously that it is possible now to predict some characteristics of likely future epidemic strains—invaluable information for vaccine design. Epidemics of pathogen-contaminated food are now routinely traced back to the source using genetic data. It has even been possible to trace specific cases of HIV back to a specific source, because rapid mutations leave a clear trail.

Evolutionary methods also can also be applied to somatic cell lines within a body, for instance to determine if the cells in a tumour are all identical or if subclones are competing in the tumour. The implications for customizing chemotherapy are substantial.

Evolutionary aetiology

Most medical research provides proximate explanations based on the anatomical and chemical details of the body's mechanisms. However, even knowing every detail about a trait offers only one half of a complete biological explanation. The other half is provided by an evolutionary explanation of how that trait came to exist in the first place. There are two kinds of evolutionary explanations. The first is a phylogenetic explanation based on the sequence of prior traits across evolutionary history. The other is an explanation of what evolutionary forces account for the changes across time. Most often, this requires understanding how the trait gives a selective advantage.

Explain vulnerabilities, not diseases

Evolution can explain why aspects of the body have been left vulnerable to disease. Why do we have wisdom teeth, and a small birth canal? Why do we so often develop lower back pain and hip problems? Why hasn't selection shaped our immune systems to better eliminate pathogens and cancer cells? Answering such questions in an evolutionary way is often challenging. A framework can help to organize the effort. There are six main reasons why bodies have vulnerabilities to disease despite the actions of natural selection (Box 2.1.2.1).

Mismatch

Chronic 'diseases of civilization' such as obesity, hypertension, and diabetes are now pandemic. The motivations that make us eat too much and exercise too little were shaped for an environment where sweet, fatty, or salty foods were good for us, and excess exercise could be fatal. Recognizing the origins of our unhealthy preferences does not change them, but it illuminates the source of the problem and possible solutions.

Similarly, allergies and autoimmune disorders are more common in developed societies. Our immune systems evolved when people were routinely exposed to intestinal parasites and pathogens. In their absence, inhibitory immune cells are not stimulated, leaving the system overactive and responsive to self. An attempt to recreate the original intestinal environment by administering whipworm ova has proved remarkably effective as a treatment for Crohn's disease.

Box 2.1.2.1 Six kinds of evolutionary explanations for vulnerability

- Mismatch between aspects of our bodies and novel environments
- Pathogens that evolve faster than we do, and resulting costly defences that cause harm themselves
- Constraints on what natural selection can do
- Trade-offs that keep any trait from being truly perfect
- Traits that increase reproduction at the cost of health
- Protective defences such as pain and fever

Coevolution

We remain vulnerable to infections because pathogens evolve faster than us. Just how fast is demonstrated by the rapid rise of resistance to every antibiotic. Evolutionary analysis of the phenomenon shows that initial intuitions may not be right. For instance, rotating the first-choice antibiotic in a hospital every few months does little to decrease multidrug resistance, and taking all of an antibiotic prescription may not prevent resistance. Most of our antibiotics are products of natural selection sifting through a vast range of molecules during a billion years of competition between microbes.

Pathogens also have strong selection effects on hosts, particularly in shaping defences such as fever, vomiting, diarrhoea, cough, and the many manifestations of inflammation. These adaptive responses often have harmful effects because they are products of an evolutionary arms race. Every defence creates selection for ways to escape it, and this shapes yet more expensive and dangerous defences. At equilibrium, we would expect the defences to become nearly as dangerous as the pathogens (natural selection would be expected to amplify them until they approach the danger level), a principle that should inform studies of anti-inflammatory agents in infection.

Constraints

Many of the body's limitations reflect the limits on what natural selection can do. It cannot maintain an information code without errors, nor can it start afresh to correct a poor 'design'. For instance, the eye's nerves and vessels are between the light and the retina, and their exit causes a blind spot. Such constraints can never be fixed, because intermediate stages don't work. Human engineers can, literally, go back to the drawing board, evolution cannot (imagine if the jet engine had had to 'evolve' from the propeller engine, step by step).

Trade-offs

Not only does selection result in many suboptimal 'designs', it cannot make any trait perfect. All traits involve trade-offs. Thicker wrist bones would break less easily, but they would inhibit free wrist rotation. Muscles fatigue, but careless use of a new drug that blocks fatigue may reveal just what damage fatigue prevents.

Bilirubin is, according to some medical teaching, a waste product from haem metabolism. However, an intermediate molecule, biliverdin, is relatively water soluble. Why not excrete biliverdin? Because bilirubin is an effective antioxidant.

If there are no such specific trade-offs to be seen, economics always furnishes an ultimate trade-off. Individuals could be built with thickened bones that never break, but they would spend extra energy moving those big bones while individuals with thinner bones would have more offspring because they divert the economic goods saved (e.g. calcium and energy) elsewhere in the economy of the body (e.g. milk) where they can do more good. Engineers know this as the principle of 'overdesign', in which risks of failure are minimized within available budgets. But whereas engineering budgets are arbitrary—civilian aviation standards are more risk averse than military, for example—evolutionary budgets are set by the competition. Individuals whose bones are 'too good' will end up having fewer children than rivals whose 'spending policy' accepts the increased risk of breakage.

Reproduction at the expense of health

A related point explains the differences in mortality between the sexes. A trait that increases reproduction will tend to spread, even if it harms health. Investments in competitive ability give greater reproductive pay-offs for males than for females, so men have been shaped to take more risks and to invest less in bodily repair. Data from developed societies shows that mortality rates for men at the age of sexual maturity are about three times higher than that for women.

Defences

The final explanation is not really a reason for vulnerability, but it is on the list because defences against disease are so often inadequately distinguished from direct manifestations of disease. Pain, fever, nausea, and vomiting are adaptations useful in certain situations. Unfortunately, they are often expressed as 'false alarms' when they are not essential. From a physician's point of view, it seems that selection has done a poor job. After all, much of general medicine involves of blocking normal defence reactions such as pain, fever, vomiting, and anxiety, and few patients expire as a result.

However, selection has not made a mistake. The costs of not expressing a response when it is needed are so huge relative to the costs of false alarms that the optimal threshold allows for many false alarms. This 'smoke detector principle' explains why blocking a defence is usually safe: the doctor can judge if the response is necessary. Nonetheless, we should expect that defences have been shaped to be expressed when they were needed on the average, in the long run.

Utility

In the clinic

Upon hearing about new evolutionary approaches to medicine, most journalists and many doctors ask how it can improve treatment in the clinic today. This is the wrong question. There are some direct clinical applications, such as hesitating before blocking a defensive response such as a raised temperature or vomiting. However, theory should not change practice directly. Instead, evolution offers established methods such as population genetics, new questions about why the body is vulnerable, strategies for answering them, and a scientific foundation for an integrative understanding of the body.

Research implications

Revisions and extensions of evolutionary methods will make them even more valuable. As extensions of the Human Genome Project move us towards individualized genetic medicine, an evolutionary view of genetic variations can get us beyond simply labelling some 'defective' and others 'normal'. There is, after all, no normal genome. There are just genes that construct phenotypes that result in more or fewer offspring in a given environment.

As outlined above, an evolutionary approach also suggests a new class of questions about the aetiology of disease. Research to answer these questions should eventually allow a book like this to provide an additional evolutionary section for each disease. The chapter on gout will describe comparative data that tests the hypothesis that uric acid's benefits as an antioxidant in a long-lived species justify its raised levels, despite the pain to some individuals. The chapter on jaundice will mention the costs, benefits, and evolution of bilirubin. The chapter on infectious disease will describe the arms races that shape pathogens and defences, and the costs and benefits of blocking defensive responses. The chapter on anxiety and depression will not treat them simply as pathological states, but as potentially useful responses, prone to dysregulation. So far, however, the benefits of seeking the evolutionary aetiology for every disease is only beginning to be recognized.

Teaching implications

There is more to teach than can be taught, so medical educators try to provide students with core facts, general understanding, and critical skills that allow them to learn more. Evolutionary knowledge is invaluable not only for itself, but because it offers a framework that can organize and relate the thousands of facts. It helps students realize why bodies fail, and therefore what disease really is. Evolution also offers opportunities for designing courses that provide deeper understanding. For example, a biochemistry course could emphasize the origins of certain pathways, and how adaptation is constrained by the limits of natural selection. Students in physiology would learn the evolutionary reason why the respiratory system relies on carbon dioxide, not oxygen, to regulate respiration.

A deeper understanding of the body

Physicians are increasingly being educated as if they are technicians, identifying problems and applying officially approved solutions. This makes very poor use of medicine's most valuable resource. We select medical students carefully because we want—or should want—doctors who think. Providing them with a deep evolutionary understanding of the body will foster clear thinking. Instead of viewing the body as a designed machine, they will see it as a product of natural selection with traits more exquisite than in any machine, some of which nonetheless leave us vulnerable to diseases. Doctors who understand the body in evolutionary terms will make better decisions for their patients because they will have a better sense of what it is that they are actually doing.

Further reading

Nesse RM, Stearns SC (2008). The great opportunity: Evolutionary applications to medicine and public health. *Evol Appl*, **1**, 28–48.

Nesse RM, Williams GC (1994). *Why we get sick: the new science of Darwinian medicine*. Vintage Books, New York.

Stearns SC, Koella JK (eds) (2007). *Evolution in health and disease*, 2nd edn. Oxford University Press, Oxford.

Trevathan WR, Mckkenna JJ, Smith EO (2007). *Evolutionary medicine*, 2nd edn. Oxford University Press, New York.

The Evolution and Medicine. Review http://evmedreview.com

2.2

Medical ethics

Tony Hope

Essentials

Medicine is a moral enterprise as well as a scientific one. It is as important to give reasons for the ethical aspects as it is for the scientific aspects of a decision. The corollary of evidence-based medicine is reason-based ethics.

Two concepts central to many ethical aspects of clinical practice are autonomy and best interests.

Mill argued that society has no right to exercise its power over individuals against their will purely for their own good. In the medical context a competent adult has the right to refuse any, even life-saving, treatment. Some conceptions of autonomy focus on competent choice, others emphasize the importance of reasons that relate to a person's long-term interests and goals. Respecting patient autonomy can be problematic when it either harms the patient, or others, or when a patient lacks capacity.

When patients lack capacity to make their own choices they should generally be treated in their own best interests. But what does this mean? Philosophers have given broadly three answers: maximizing positive states of mind, such as pleasure; maximizing the fulfilment of desires; and maximizing aspects of life that are objectively considered valuable. The legal concept of best interests is a composite of all these.

Three of the most common issues for which doctors seek ethics support are consent, end of life, and confidentiality.

A crucial issue if a patient is refusing beneficial treatment is whether he or she is competent to refuse. The assessment of competence involves three steps. First, identify the key information relevant to the decision. Second, assess the patient's cognitive ability: can the patient understand, retain, and weigh the key information to come to a decision? Third, assess other factors that may interfere with decision making, such as delusions. When patients lack capacity doctors must consider: patients' best interests; whether there is a proxy decision maker; and whether the patient has made any relevant advance directive.

Ethical principles may conflict in end-of life-decisions. Different ethical approaches disagree over the significance of two distinctions: that between acts and omissions; and that between intending and foreseeing an outcome. These distinctions are important in considerations of mercy killing; the moral difference between withholding life, extending treatment, and killing; and in giving treatments that relieve distress but might shorten life. The law varies on these issues in different countries.

When should doctors breach confidentiality either for the good of the patient or to prevent harm to someone else? There are differing accounts of the most important reason for medical confidentiality: respect for patient autonomy; keeping an implied promise; and bringing about the best consequences. These different accounts can have different implications for when it is right to breach confidentiality in problematic situations.

Introduction

Evidence-based medicine emphasizes the importance of critical assessment: an intervention should be evaluated on the basis of evidence not tradition. Critical skills are therefore crucial to modern scientific medicine. But medicine is a moral enterprise as well as a scientific one. Many clinical decisions involve a combination of factual concerns and ethical issues.

When making a clinical decision it is as important to be able to give the reasons for the ethical aspects of that decision as it is for the scientific aspects. Society increasingly expects this from doctors as part of transparent decision-making. Doctors' reasoning about ethical aspects of care will need to stand up to scrutiny—in a court if necessary—just as much as will the scientific aspects. The corollary of evidence-based medicine is reason-based ethics.

Acknowledgements. I would like to acknowledge with thanks the valuable discussions that I have had with Judith Hendrick and Julian Savulescu.

Two concepts: autonomy and best interests

Autonomy

John Stuart Mill's essay, *On Liberty*, is one of the great statements of liberal thinking that underpins much of the political philosophy of Western democracies. Mill wrote:

> ... the only purpose for which power can be rightfully exercised over any member of a civilised community, against his will, is to prevent harm to others. His own good, either physical or moral, is not a sufficient warrant. He cannot rightfully be compelled to do or forbear ... because, in the opinion of others, to do so would not be wise, or even right.
>
> (Mill, 1859, Chapter 1.)

This principle underpins the strict limits on the interference of the state into individual's lives. Mill articulates at its most general level a principle that in the medical setting is known as the principle of respect for (patient) autonomy. This principle has had an enormous effect in changing attitudes to the doctor–patient relationship over the last 30 years. It has been used to criticize medical paternalism, and has informed the development of 'patient-centred' medicine. It has led to ever-increasing standards in providing patients with information, and to the development of the concept of informed consent. It is one of the main grounds for the importance of patient confidentiality.

On those occasions when a competent adult patient is refusing treatment that is, objectively, good for him, a conflict arises between respecting the patient's wishes and doing what is best for him. This is widely seen as a conflict between the principle of respect for patient autonomy and the principle of acting in patients' best interests (often called the principle of beneficence). The concept of autonomy, however, is not straightforward, and respecting what a patient says (e.g. his refusal of treatment) and respecting his autonomy may, on some views of autonomy, be different.

Some aspects of autonomy

The term 'autonomy' has no clear single meaning.

> It is sometimes used as an equivalent of liberty ..., sometimes as equivalent to self-rule or sovereignty, sometimes as identical with freedom of the will. ... It is identified with qualities of self-assertion, with critical reflection, with freedom from obligation, with absence of external causation, with knowledge of one's own interests. ... It is related to actions, to beliefs, to reasons for acting, to rules, to the will of other persons, to thoughts and to principles.
>
> (Dworkin, 1988, p. 6.)

In the ideal of autonomy decisions should be rational, consistent with the person's life plans, and based on critical reflection. If a desire, or choice, is not based on a rational evaluation then, on some views, it is not autonomous. This is one reason why respecting a person's autonomy is not necessarily the same as respecting her choice.

Respecting patient autonomy can be problematic for doctors in at least three situations:

- when to do so harms the patient herself
- when to do so harms others, and
- when the patient lacks the capacity to make choices for herself

With regard to the first situation, patients sometimes refuse treatment that doctors believe is strongly in their best interests. This became a legal matter in England when an adult patient with motor neuron disease and who had capacity wanted to have her life support removed. Her doctors refused because they thought this was tantamount to killing her. The court, consistently with Mill's principle and English common law, said that her wishes must be complied with:

> The doctors must not allow their emotional reaction to or strong disagreement with the decision of the patient to cloud their judgment in answering the primary question whether the patient has mental capacity to make the decision.
>
> (Re B [2002].)

The conflict between respecting autonomy and harm to the patient or to others can also arise in the context of confidentiality (see below).

In the third situation, when a patient lacks capacity to make decisions for himself, is it possible to respect the patient's autonomy? Consider the following case.

> Mr D always valued academic and artistic pursuits. 'If I develop Alzheimer's disease allow me to die if given the chance', he says. Mr D subsequently develops Alzheimer's disease. He no longer recognizes his family, but he remains physically fit. He is looked after in a nursing home and appears to enjoy a simple life: flowers, food, TV. Mr D gets a chest infection. This could be treated with antibiotics. Without curative treatment he could be kept comfortable and would probably soon die.

On a straightforward view it would seem that we respect Mr D's autonomy by withholding antibiotic treatment and allowing him to die. This is consistent with the wishes that he expressed when he had the capacity to do so. But there are at least three concerns that we might have even if our only ethical value were to respect autonomy. First, do we know that when he expressed his view about being allowed to die he had taken into account all the relevant facts of his current situation? For example, at what stage in Alzheimer's disease did he want to be allowed to die; was he meaning to refuse even a simple treatment like giving antibiotics; and did he take into account the possibility that he would generally be enjoying life? Second, he might have changed his mind after he had made the statement about being allowed to die and before he lost capacity, but no one knows of this change of mind. Third, is it possible for a person when healthy to imagine sufficiently the state of having Alzheimer's? When we allow a person with capacity to refuse beneficial treatment we can take care to ensure that this is what the person really wants, and that he understands all the relevant issues.

Even if it is possible in this case to respect the patient's autonomy, in many (probably most) situations where a patient lacks capacity there will not be sufficient information about his previous views and values to make a decision about what to do based only, or even mainly, on this principle. The more useful principle in such situations is the principle of beneficence, that is treating people in their best interests.

Best interests

In many situations judging a patient's best interests is straightforward, but this is by no means always the case. Consider again Mr D. What is in his best interests? The answer may differ depending on your conception of best interests. The philosophical discussion relevant to best interests has been conducted mainly in terms of the concept of well-being. There are three main theoretical approaches to well-being.

Mental state theories

According to these theories well-being is defined in terms of mental states. At its simplest (hedonism) it is the view that happiness or pleasure is the only intrinsic good, and unhappiness or pain the only intrinsic bad. If Mr D with Alzheimer's disease is generally enjoying the 'simple' pleasures then, on this view, it will be in his best interests to continue to live by treating the infection. The fact that he might previously have despised enjoying the TV soaps he now enjoys is irrelevant.

Desire-fulfilment theories

According to desire-fulfilment theories, well-being consists in having one's desires fulfilled. If desire-fulfilment theories are to provide a plausible account of well-being it is necessary to restrict the relevant set of desires. On one view only those desires pertaining to life as a whole count as relevant in the analysis of well-being. These are desires that relate to a person's life plans. According to this view Mr D's prior intellectual values would be relevant. Withholding antibiotic treatment would be fulfilling his previous desires and these are the desires that fit with his long-term values. Desire-fulfilment theories of well-being have much in common with respecting autonomy but they are not the same. In the case of Mr D desire-fulfilment theories highlight the question of whether Mr D, at the time of deciding whether to give antibiotics, has relevant desires. From the perspective of autonomy the issue is whether he has capacity.

Objective list theories

According to objective list theories of well-being certain things can be good or bad for a person and can contribute to her well-being, whether or not they are desired and whether or not they lead to pleasurable mental states. Examples of the kind of thing that have been given as intrinsically good in this way are engaging in deep personal relationships, rational activity, and the development of one's abilities. Examples of things that are bad might include being betrayed or deceived, or gaining pleasure from cruelty.

An objective list theory does not give an unequivocal answer to what is in Mr D's best interests. On most lists—although not all—the pursuit of worthwhile life goals would normally take precedence over very simple pleasures. But that is not the choice that faces the carers of Mr D. The question is whether it is in Mr D's best interests to be dead, given that he can only enjoy these simple pleasures.

Composite theories

Each of the three theories of well-being outlined above identifies something of importance, but none seems adequate. Because of this, we might opt for a composite theory in which well-being is seen as requiring aspects of all the theories. A composite theory has some practical implications for medical practice. The main implication is that when considering what is in a patient's best interests, particularly when these are not clear, it may be relevant to consider the aspects of well-being that are highlighted by each of the three theories. This does not tell us how to balance these considerations but it does suggest that in coming to a decision about Mr D's best interests it is relevant to take into account all of the following factors: his previous values and wishes, his current experiences (e.g. of enjoyment), and any current desires.

Three issues in medical ethics

Doctors who seek help with ethical issues in their clinical practice often do so with regard to three types of issue: consent; end of life; and confidentiality. I will discuss each in turn.

Consent

The philosophical basis of informed consent rests on the principle of patient autonomy (see above). Valid consent is widely regarded as requiring three main criteria: that the patient be informed, and competent (or having capacity), and that the consent is voluntary (i.e. there is no external coercion).

In the legal and ethical analysis of treating people against their will, a great deal depends on whether the patient is competent (or has capacity) to make the relevant decision. The approach to competence endorsed by both law and most ethical analyses is what is known as the functional approach. This focuses on the process by which the person comes to the particular decision. One implication of this approach is that competence is specific to a particular decision. A person may, at one time, be competent to make one decision (e.g. whether to take a particular medication) but not a different decision (e.g. whether she is capable of living alone). When patients are making decisions (e.g. refusing treatment) that appear to be (significantly) contrary to their best interests, then doctors must carefully assess the capacity of that patient to make that decision. In broad terms, if patients have the capacity then their decision must be respected, although the doctor must make sure that the implications of the decision have been fully understood. The law in the United Kingdom and North America gives competent adult patients the right to refuse any, even life-saving, treatment. If, on the other hand, patients lack capacity to consent to (or refuse) treatment then they should be treated, generally, in their best interests (but see below).

Assessing competence

There are three main steps in assessing competence.

- Step 1: Identify the information relevant to the decision. The critically relevant information includes the likely consequences of different decisions (e.g. different possible treatments, or treatment vs no treatment) and including both wanted and unwanted effects; and understanding in broad terms what would be involved in carrying out a decision.
- Step 2: Assess cognitive ability. The Mental Capacity Act 2005, which is the key legislation in England and Wales, states that a person is unable to make a decision (i.e. lacks capacity) if he is unable:
    - to understand the information relevant to the decision
    - to retain that information
    - to use or weigh that information as part of the process of making the decision, or
    - to communicate his decision (whether by talking, using sign language or any other means)
- Step 3: Assess other factors that may interfere with competence. Cognitive impairment is only one factor that may interfere with the elements of information processing outlined above. It may also be important to assess whether there is such interference due to a mental illness. A delusion, for example, may interfere with believing the information. An affective illness (depression or mania) may interfere with the weighing-up of information and coming to a decision.

Making decisions for people who lack competence

There are four theoretically possible approaches to making decisions about the health care of incompetent patients.

Best interests

One approach for a doctor faced with an incompetent patient is to ask which plan of management serves the patient's best interests. I have outlined above some different approaches to the question of what is in a person's best interests (see case example of Alzheimer's disease above).

Proxy

An alternative approach is for a proxy to make decisions on behalf of an incompetent patient. Such an approach raises the question of why the proxy has such a right. The most obvious answer is that the patient had nominated the proxy at a time when she was competent to do so. The proxy of course is left with the question of the basis on which the decision should be made. English law, under the Mental Capacity Act 2005, allows a competent person to nominate someone else ('Lasting Power of Attorney') as proxy in the case of loss of capacity. The proxy (rather like a parent of a young child) must act in the person's best interests. If doctors believe a proxy is refusing highly beneficial treatment then they may need to seek a court ruling.

Substituted judgement

The criterion of substituted judgement asks the hypothetical question: suppose the patient were (magically) able to become competent, what treatment would he choose? In order to try to answer this question the doctor could use a range of evidence: reports of what the patient has said about this kind of situation in the past; the kind of general values the patient held; and experience with other patients. This criterion is problematic, not only in practice, but also theoretically since it is unclear precisely what are the person's abilities and beliefs in this magical state.

Advance directives

Advance directives (or 'advance decisions' as they are called in the English Mental Capacity Act 2005) are statements made by people at a time when they are competent, about how they want to be treated in the future were they to become ill and at the same time incompetent to give consent for treatment.

The central justification for advance directives is that they extend patient autonomy to include situations in which a person is no longer competent. One problem with advance directives is that they need to be interpreted when applied to the specific situation and this can be difficult. More fundamental is the concern that when completing the advance directive the person may not have been able to sufficiently imagine the situation at the time a decision needs to be made (see the discussion of Mr D above).

End of life

Killing someone is, of course, normally seriously immoral. Doctors often care for patients who are near the end of life and who are perhaps suffering. Modern medicine can in many circumstances prolong life through a variety of means. Paradoxically, it is the very fact that doctors care for patients that can make the general moral ban on killing ethically problematic. It is problematic in at least two ways. First, killing can, to some at least, appear merciful. Second, there is some ambiguity around what counts as killing.

Mercy killing

Lillian Boyes was an English patient with very severe rheumatoid arthritis, so severe that she was expected to die within a few weeks. She was in so much distress that she wanted to be killed, but she retained full decision-making capacity. Painkillers did not overcome her distress. Her caring relatives also wanted her to be killed. If the doctor caring for Mrs Boyes were to apply the principle of autonomy and respect her competent wishes, should he not kill her? And if every day of continued life was for her a burden, and there was no prospect of significant change until she died naturally, was it not in her best interests to be killed? The principles of autonomy and of beneficence point to the same action: to kill Lillian Boyes. In the United Kingdom or North America, however, a doctor who killed such a patient would commit murder. In some jurisdictions, e.g. the Netherlands, such a mercy killing (active voluntary euthanasia) can be legally carried out under carefully controlled conditions.

The principle of the sanctity of life

One reason why mercy killing might be wrong is because of an additional relevant principle: the principle of the sanctity of life.

There are differing versions of this principle. The most extreme form is called 'vitalism': human life is of absolute value. Whenever possible, human life should be maintained; and it is always wrong to take human life.

A less extreme form is one that sees life as a basic but not an absolute good. Preserving life on this view does not necessarily outweigh all other goods, but the value of life cannot be completely accounted for in terms of a person's experiences and beliefs.

In English law, and in that of many other countries, there are two components to the act of killing: first, the death results from a positive action on behalf of the killer, and second that the killer intends to cause the death. In a clinical setting this means that omitting to do something, such as withholding life-extending treatment (e.g. intravenous fluids or mechanical ventilation) on the grounds that it is kinder to the patient to 'let nature take its course' is not considered to be a positive action, and is not killing. Such withholding of treatment is not only perfectly legal but might be seen as good clinical practice, and morally required. Furthermore, in English law, withdrawing treatment (taking down the intravenous line or switching off the ventilator) is seen as equivalent to withholding treatment.

The intention too is crucial, at least legally. Sometimes a treatment for unpleasant symptoms can shorten life. This may be the case when large doses of morphine are given to very ill patients in order to control pain, because morphine may reduce respiratory drive. Giving morphine in such a situation is not killing and would normally be perfectly legal because the shortening of life is not intended, but is only foreseen.

If killing is wrong, but these two examples are not killing and not generally wrong, a lot of ethical weight rests on two distinctions: that between acts and omissions and that between intending and foreseeing.

Those who believe that what is of primary importance in judging the morality of an act is the foreseeable consequences will not find any significant moral difference in either of these distinctions. If we foresee, for example, that giving morphine will shorten life then this has the same moral weight as if we intend the shortening of life. We cannot close our eyes, on this view, to the foreseen consequences of our actions by claiming that although we foresaw them we did not intend them.

An alternative framework sees the nature of the choices and not only the foreseeable consequences as of moral significance. One idea within such a framework is known as the 'doctrine of double effect'.

At the core of this doctrine is the claim that there is a moral distinction between foreseeing a result and intending a result. Thus, it may be forbidden on moral grounds to bring about a bad result if that result is intended (even if as a means to a better overall outcome), but not forbidden to bring about the same result if the result is foreseen but not intended.

According to this doctrine, it may be right to give morphine, despite foreseeing an earlier death as a result, if four conditions hold:

1 The action (reducing pain) is good in itself.

2 The intention is solely to produce the good effect (i.e. to reduce pain and not to shorten life).

3 The good effect is not achieved through the bad effect (i.e. that reducing pain and distress is not brought about through the death of the patient).

4 There is sufficient reason to permit the bad effect, i.e. the good of reducing pain provides sufficient grounds to justify the earlier death (taking into account for example that the person is terminally ill).

Confidentiality

Much of the information that a doctor gains about a patient in her professional duties is confidential. By this it is meant that the doctor should not divulge that information to another person without the agreement (possibly implied) of the patient.

What is the basis for medical confidentiality? There are at least three different grounds. On all three approaches doctors should normally keep information about patients confidential. The ethically problematic situations are generally those in which breaching confidentiality will reduce a risk of harm either to the patient himself, or to someone else. The professional guidelines for doctors in the United Kingdom emphasize the importance of confidentiality but state that: 'Disclosure of personal information without consent may be justified where failure to do so may expose the patient or others to risk of death or serious harm' (General Medical Council 2000). Such guidelines need interpretation in applying to particular circumstances, and the interpretation will sometimes be affected by one's views about what underpins the importance of confidentiality. Three different answers to this question are: respect for patient autonomy; keeping an implied promise; and bringing about the best consequences.

Respect for patient autonomy

This principle implies that a person has the right, by and large, to decide who should have access to personal information about himself. If respect for patient autonomy is considered an important ethical principle then any breach of confidentiality is potentially serious and only the prevention of serious harm would justify it. Furthermore, on this approach, it might be argued that, *contra* to the GMC guidelines, if a competent patient refuses to give consent for a doctor to inform a third party, where failure to inform risks serious harm to that patient only, breaching confidentiality is wrong. After all, we allow a competent patient to refuse even life-saving treatment.

Can there be a serious breach of confidentiality if the patient never knows about the breach? On the view of confidentiality which considers that respect for patient autonomy is of key importance, the answer is yes.

Keeping an implied promise

Some views of the doctor–patient relationship see it as having elements of an implied contract. Such a contract may include an implied promise that doctors keep information about their patients confidential. Patients generally expect doctors to treat information confidentially, and professional guidelines emphasize the importance of high standards of confidentiality.

This view of confidentiality is different from that of patient autonomy. It does not ultimately depend on what the patient wants or believes. It depends on a concept of the doctor–patient relationship that is independent of what a specific patient believes. There are, however, two problems with this view: first, there has been no explicit promise, so the issue of an implied promise is to some extent a fiction; second, it raises the whole issue of why it is important to keep promises. The reason for the importance of keeping promises is likely to be grounded either in autonomy or consequences.

Bringing about the best consequences

From the perspective of a consequentialist ethical perspective it is the (foreseeable) consequences of the breach of confidentiality that determine the seriousness of the breach, and indeed that underlie whether breaching confidentiality is wrong in the first place. There are several different types of consequence that could be relevant, and the analysis of the situation depends in part on how these are viewed.

If respect for autonomy is the principal basis for confidentiality, then when maintaining confidentiality puts others at risk of harm there is a clash of two incommensurable values: respecting autonomy of the patient and preventing harm to others. From the consequentialist perspective the judgement is conceptually simpler. There is only one question: which action (breaching or maintaining confidentiality) has the better overall consequences? At first sight it might seem that on this consequentialist view the risk of even modest harm to others justifies a breach since we have to balance the harm to others against only the patient's emotional response to the breach. But this is too simplistic. Unless doctors are trusted to maintain high levels of confidentiality, patients in general may lose trust and not seek health care. The issue is not just about ill health: there are other consequences of untreated illness. For example, if people with uncontrolled epilepsy drive they may kill other road users. There is a public interest in ensuring that such people receive good health care in order to maximize control of the epilepsy. Even where the harm to others is potentially great, as in the example of epilepsy, it could be the case that more lives will be lost if doctors breach confidentiality because fewer people with fits will seek medical help. So although the consequentialist approach can deal with difficult cases in a conceptually clear way, in practice the lack of evidence and complexity can make judgements difficult.

From a consequentialist perspective, as opposed to the perspective of respect for patient autonomy, if a patient never finds out that a doctor has breached confidentiality and no harm comes to the patient as a result, that breach is trivial, even if it concerned something that the patient would strongly wish to keep confidential.

Conclusion

Ethics, like science, is at root a rational enterprise. For those of us who are concerned to do the right thing, and this includes most medical students and doctors, the questions arise: how can we examine our own moral standards and behaviour in specific situations; how can we develop these standards; and how can we ensure that our views stand up to scrutiny? I believe that rational enquiry is central to an answer to these questions. Such enquiry involves arguing with others, facing counter-arguments, and seeing how good are our own arguments. If the counter-arguments are stronger we need to change our views. If there is a contradiction between what we thought our principles were and what we think is right in a specific situation then we need to resolve that contradiction. There may be no final grounding of morality in nature but from that it does not follow that our personal moral system and our decisions in specific situations should be irrational or arbitrary.

Further reading

Ashcroft R, *et al.* (eds) (2007). *Principles of health care ethics*, 2nd edition. John Wiley & Sons, Chichester.

Battin M, Rhodes R, Silvers A (eds) (1998). *Physician assisted suicide: expanding the debate.* Routledge, New York.

Battin M, Rhodes R, Silvers A (eds) (2002). *Medicine and social justice.* Oxford University Press, New York.

Beauchamp TL, Childress JF (2008). *Principles of biomedical ethics*, 6th edition. Oxford University Press, New York.

Benn P (1997). *Ethics.* Taylor & Francis, London.

Blackburn S (2001). *Ethics: A very short introduction.* Oxford University Press, Oxford.

Buchanan A, *et al.* (2000). *From chance to choice: genetics and justice.* Cambridge University Press, Cambridge.

Campbell A, Gillett G, Jones G (2005). *Medical ethics*, 4th edition. Oxford University Press, Melbourne.

Doyal L, Tobias J S (eds) (2001). *Informed consent in medical research*, pp. 266–76. BMJ Books, London.

Dworkin G (1988). *The theory and practice of autonomy.* Cambridge University Press, Cambridge.

Fulford B, Thornton T, Graham G (2006). *Oxford textbook of philosophy and psychiatry.* Oxford University Press, Oxford.

Glover J (1977). *Causing death and saving lives.* Penguin, Harmondsworth.

Green S, Bloch S (2006). *An anthology of psychiatric ethics.* Oxford University Press, Oxford.

Harris J (1985). *The value of life: an introduction to medical ethics.* Taylor & Francis, London.

Hope T (2004). *Medical ethics: a very short introduction.* Oxford University Press, Oxford.

Hope T, Savulescu J, Hendrick J (2007). *Medical ethics: the core curriculum*, 2nd edition. Churchill Livingstone, Edinburgh.

Manson N, O'Neill O (2007). *Rethinking informed consent in bioethics.* Cambridge University Press, Cambridge.

Murray T (1996). *The worth of a child.* University of California Press, Berkeley, CA.

Nelson HL, Nelson JL (1995). *The patient in the family: an ethics of medicine and families.* Routledge, New York.

Parker M, Dickenson D (2001). *The Cambridge medical ethics workbook.* Cambridge University Press, Cambridge.

Radden J (2007). *The philosophy of psychiatry: a companion.* Oxford University Press, New York.

Shakespeare T (2006). *Disability rights and wrongs.* Routledge, London.

Singer PA (1991). *Companion to ethics.* Blackwell, Oxford.

Spriggs M (2005). *Autonomy and patients' decisions.* Rowan & Littlefield, Lanham, MD.

Steinbock, B. (2007). *The Oxford handbook of bioethics.* Oxford University Press, Oxford.

Young R (1986). *Personal autonomy: beyond negative and positive liberty.* Croom Helm, London.

2.3

Evidence-based medicine

Contents

2.3.1 Bringing the best evidence to the point of care *22*
Paul P. Glasziou

2.3.2 Evidence-based medicine—does it apply to my particular patient? *27*
Louis R. Caplan

2.3.3 Large-scale randomized evidence: trials and meta-analyses of trials *31*
C. Baigent, R. Peto, R. Gray, S. Parish, and R. Collins

2.3.4 The future of clinical trials *45*
Perry Nisen and Patrick Vallance

2.3.1 Bringing the best evidence to the point of care

Paul P. Glasziou

You must always be students, learning and unlearning till your life's end.

Joseph Lister

Essentials

Neither our memories nor our textbooks are complete and up to date with all the research relevant to the patients we will see today. The scattering of necessary research across a vast ocean of literature makes it inaccessible at the point of clinical decision. The consequences for patient care have given rise to the discipline of evidence-based medicine (EBM), whose two central concerns are with the quality of research evidence and with its appropriate usage in clinical care.

How can we keep abreast of new developments or fill gaps in our knowledge that we identify during our day-to-day clinical practices? Evidence suggests that the billions of pounds invested yearly in traditional continuing medical education does not change clinical behaviour. Part of the problem is due to not knowing, and part is due to not doing.

Not knowing

This arises from information overload, e.g. over 1500 studies and 55 randomized trials are added to Medline each day, hence filtering for the best research is a central concern of EBM. The key initial method is to employ a 'hierarchy of evidence' to identify the likely best research: e.g. if we are interested in the effects of a treatment, randomized controlled trials (RCTs) are usually the ideal study; but if no RCTs exist, we then go to the next level of evidence, and so on. This is a first step only: we then need to critically appraise any evidence found for its validity and the sizes of any effects.

Not doing

To use EBM in clinical practice we need to (1) keep abreast of major new studies that should alter our clinical practice; and (2) formulate and answer clinical questions as they arise with our patients—instead of trying to keep up to date with all areas of clinical practice, hoping that we have read and remembered the correct articles when we need to apply them, we shift focus to answering questions as they arise. The steps in answering clinical questions are: (1) formulating an answerable question; (2) formulating an information gathering strategy; (3) assessing the quality and relevance of the information retrieved; and (4) applying the results to our patient. Undergraduate and postgraduate students should be skilled in each of these steps, and use them in their ongoing medical practice.

Introduction

Neither our memories nor our textbooks are complete and up to date with all the research relevant to the patients we will see today. The scattering of necessary research across a vast ocean of literature makes it inaccessible at the point of clinical decision. The consequences for patient care have given rise to the discipline of evidence-based medicine (EBM), whose two central concerns are with the quality of research evidence and with its appropriate usage in clinical care.

One definition of EBM is:

> ... the conscientious, explicit and judicious use of current best evidence in making decisions about the care of individual patients. This practice involves integrating individual clinical experience with the best external clinical evidence from systematic research.
>
> (Sackett *et al.* 1996.)

Brief history

As our diagnostic and treatment modalities continue to expand, we would like to know which options have been demonstrated to be effective and which is best. These are not new questions. In 1536 Ambroise Paré, as a surgeon on campaign in Italy, followed the advice of the most authoritative texts and treated the French soldiers battle wounds with cautery using 'the oyle the hottest that was possible into the wounds'. However, when he ran out of oil he was 'constrained instead to apply a digestive'. After a troubled night, he awoke to find those he had cauterized in great pain, whereas those he had not were doing well. This accidental experiment changed Paré's and French treatment, but it was another 210 years before more deliberate experiments began. In 1747, James Lind examined alternative treatments for scurvy: he 'took 12 cases of scurvy on board the Salisbury at sea. The cases were as similar as I could have them'. Housing and diet were standardized. Of the six pairs of sailors, the two assigned oranges and lemons recovered within 3 weeks. However, unlike Paré's results, Lind's findings took several decades to be implemented. (See http://www.jameslindlibrary.org for more details on both examples.)

In 1948 Bradford Hill introduced the concept of the randomized trial to medicine in the Medical Research Council trial of streptomycin for pulmonary tuberculosis. Since then more than a quarter of a million such trials have been conducted. Almost simultaneously, Yerushalmy introduced greater rigour into the evaluation of diagnostic tests by quantifying the accuracy—the sensitivity and specificity—of chest radiograph screening for pulmonary tuberculosis.

The need for evidence-based medicine

Interest in improving clinical evaluation has grown in recent decades, giving rise to disciplines such as clinical epidemiology and EBM, and a flood of clinical research. This is welcome, but has also hampered the dissemination of research results. Medline started in 1966 and currently adds to its 15 million references over 1500 new articles per day (http://www.nlm.nih.gov/pubs/factsheets/medline.html). Though these are culled from over 5000 journals in 30 languages and 80 countries, it is only a modest portion of the estimated 13 000 to 15 000 biomedical journals currently being published. No clinician's reading time is sufficient to keep up with this flow directly, as many of the required articles are not in their speciality journal.

How can we cope with our information overload? Fortunately, most of the published information is insufficient to alter clinical practice: much is 'scientist to scientist' communication directed at unravelling mechanisms; and many of the clinically relevant studies are not of adequate quality. Thus filtering for quality and clinical relevance reduces the flow to a manageable trickle as illustrated in Fig. 2.3.1.1.

Filtering for the best research is a central concern of EBM. The key methods are to use initially a 'hierarchy of evidence' to identify the likely best research. For example, if we are interested in

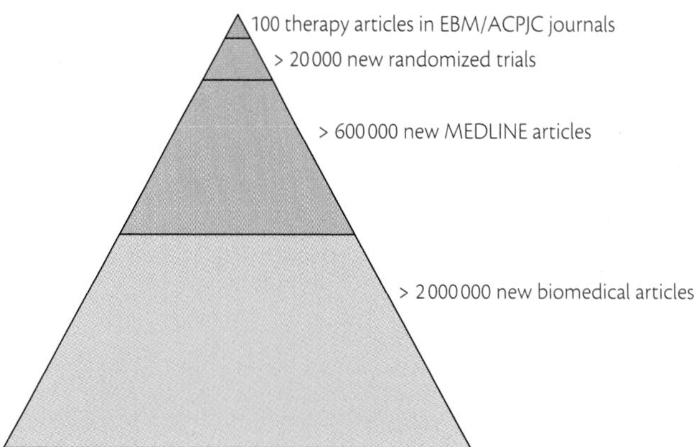

Fig. 2.3.1.1 The yearly flow of new biomedical publications.

the effects of a treatment, randomized controlled trials (RCTs) are usually the ideal study. But if no RCTs exist, we will go to the next level of evidence, and so on. This is a first step only. We then need critically to appraise the evidence found for its validity and the sizes of any effects. The key issues in the critical appraisal of different types of clinical questions are given in Table 2.3.1.1. There are usually three key issues: (1) the representativeness of the group studies, or the comparability of groups in experiments, i.e. random selection or randomization, respectively; (2) the need for good follow-up and ascertainment of a final outcome on most patients; and (3) a relevant outcome measure that is either objective or blinded to the factor being studied. (These issues can be remembered by the mnemonic RAMbo.)

Keeping up to date: 'push' or 'pull'

There are two complementary ways of obtaining filtered information. First we need to keep abreast of major new studies that should alter our clinical practice. However, rather than trying to scan hundreds of journals ourselves, it is wiser to enlist a group of our peers to do this. For example, journals such the *ACP Journal Club*, *Evidence-Based Medicine*, and *Evidence-Based Mental Health* review over 100 journals and appraise the articles for the quality of the research methods (fewer than 1 in 20 pass), relevance, and interest in order to identify new studies that could change the way we practice. The best systematic reviews and studies are reabstracted and an expert commentary helps place the new data in its current context.

The second, and complementary, process is to formulate and answer clinical questions as they arise with our patients. Instead of trying to keep up to date with all areas of clinical practice, hoping that we have read and remembered the correct articles when we need to apply them, we shift focus to answering questions as they arise. This implies being able to say 'I don't know' and adding 'but I will find out!' When a problem appears, we formulate an answerable question, devise an information gathering strategy, appraise the information achieved, and take it into account when deciding treatment with our patient. Learning becomes an active, integral and daily part of clinical practice.

Asking clinical questions

Answering patients' questions must be done rapidly: finding the information in about 30 s and assimilating it within a couple of minutes. This sounds formidable, but has been shown to

Table 2.3.1.1 Summary of types of clinical questions and the searching and appraising methods for each

Clinical question	Major appraisal issues	Possible sources	Best single Medline search term[a]
Pretest probabilities	Random or consecutive sample Ascertainment of final diagnosis (>80%) Measurement/classification adequate (adequate diagnostic workup)	PubMed	—
Diagnostic accuracy	Random or consecutive sample Adequate verification (>80% or adjustment for sampling) Measurement of an adequate reference standard, read blind to index test or objective	PubMed or EBM journal archives	(specificity[Title/Abstract])
Treatment effects	Randomized (concealed) allocation to groups Ascertainment of final outcome adequate (> 80%) Measurement of outcomes blind and/or objective	PubMed, Cochrane Library, Clinical Evidence	Clinical-trial (pt)
Prognosis	Random or consecutive sample of patients at first presentation (or other defined time-point) in disease Ascertainment of final outcome adequate (>80%) Measurement of outcomes blind and/or objective	EBM journal archives PubMed	Exp cohort studies
Multivariate prediction rules (prognostic or diagnostic)	As per diagnostic or prognostic question plus separate training and validation sets	PubMed, EBM journal archives	(validation[tiab] OR validate[tiab])

[a]See the PubMed: Clinical Queries filter table for a more complete listing of search strategies.

be feasible. In many ways it is similar to looking up drug doses: the information must be available in our consulting room, it must be well indexed, and the presentation must be readily usable. Currently none of the continually updated evidence-based resources is as comprehensive and rapid as a pharmacopoeia, and some skills are needed to navigate those available.

The steps in answering clinical questions are: (1) formulating an answerable question; (2) formulating an information gathering strategy; (3) assessing the quality and relevance of the information retrieved; (4) applying the results to our patient. To illustrate these steps, consider the following patient:

> Case 1. A 52-year-old woman presents with her second period of episodes of benign positional vertigo. She had previously been given stemetil, but says she had read about a nondrug treatment. You know about the Epley manoeuvre but are not sure of its efficacy or how to do it.

In answering questions, it is helpful to classify them into the types presented in Table 2.3.1.1: differential diagnosis, diagnostic accuracy, prediction/prognosis, and therapeutic effectiveness. For Case 1, the issue is therapy, and a useful breakdown of such questions is: the Patient, the Intervention, the Comparison, and the Outcome (remembered by the mnemonic 'PICO'). So with our patient this might be: 'In patients with BBPV, is the Epley manoeuvre effective in controlling symptoms?'

Finding answers

For treatment, we would generally first seek the results of RCTs (though there are some exceptional treatments whose effects are so clear that randomized trials are unnecessary). If there were several trials, we should seek existing systematic reviews. If we had answered this question previously, the stored result would provide the fastest answer. However, since we hadn't, the first try might be the archives of the *Evidence-Based Medicine* journal (or its sister journal the *ACP Journal Club*). Searching the term 'Epley' yields four abstracts within 10 s (but this will no doubt change by the time you read this textbook!).

The critical article of these four was a summary of a randomized trial of self-treatment with the Epley manoeuvre. The journal has appraised the critical features, so I do not need to repeat this: there was an unconcealed randomization procedure but with good balance between the groups, 99% follow-up, and both objective (Hallpike test) and subjective (symptoms) outcomes. The results showed that resolution at 1 week as judged by the Hallpike and cessation of symptoms was 88% in the self-treatment group compared to 69% in the Epley-only group. This is an absolute risk reduction (ARR) of 19% (88% –/+69%), or a number needed to treat of 6 (calculated as 1/ARR, i.e. 1/0.19 and rounded up). The patient handout can be found at: http://www.charite.de/ch/neuro/vertigo.html

The advantage of the self-Epley is that it not only treats the current episode, but can be used by patients to treat future episodes. In my own general practice, this has become standard practice for the clinicians and the handout is kept on an intranet for easy printing.

Another search alternative which would provide a more thorough review of trials, is to check the Cochrane Library (the Cochrane Database Systematic Reviews, CDSR), other systematic reviews (the Database of Abstracts of Reviews of Effectiveness, DARE), and a compendium of randomized trials (the Cochrane Controlled Trials Register, CCTR) identified in Medline, EMBASE, and the hand searching by contributors to the Cochrane Collaboration. This can be searched directly, but it is often more convenient to use PubMed Clinical Queries which will identify both the trials and the systematic reviews in the same search (using the 'Therapy' and 'Broad' filters in Clinical Queries). For the Epley this gives 37 hits, including a Cochrane review which identified 15 trials, only three of which were of sufficient quality to be included, and concludes 'Individual and pooled data showed a statistically significant effect in favour of the Epley manoeuvre over controls. There were no serious adverse effects of treatment'.

The application of results in Case 1 was straightforward, but this is not always so. The process varies depending on the type of question (Table 2.3.1.1) but there are some overall similarities.

First, is the study's illness group sufficiently similar (it need not be identical) to our patient to justify a judgement that the biological behaviour of the test or treatment would not be importantly different? Secondly, can we implement the test, measure, or treatment in a sufficiently similar manner? If these are fulfilled, then we need to consider how the individual features of our patient might influence the results. The next two sections look at the application of studies of diagnostic tests and of treatments.

Using the results of diagnostic test studies

Most clinical information is imperfect. This includes the history, signs, and laboratory tests. The simplest demonstration of this problem is the extensive data on the lack of agreement between experienced clinicians on the presence or absence of a clinical sign, and even between histopathologists looking at the same image. The sources of this variation and error may be in the patients, in the instruments, or in the observers. For example, true blood pressure varies considerably, but the measured blood pressure varies even more because of different calibration of instruments, cuff sizes, and clinical skill. While it is important to find ways to reduce this variation by standardization and training, some residual error is inevitable.

With experience we learn, implicitly or explicitly, some simple rules to minimize the problems of error. For example, we learn to repeat unexpected abnormal test results: the majority will have disappeared on a second reading, saving us and our patients much anxiety. Experience also teaches us that test results must be interpreted in the light of the clinical picture, or that we must combine our estimate of the chance that a patient has a disease (the pretest probability) with imperfect information from the test. A test's imperfection can be quantified by two measures: (1) the sensitivity, the probability of a positive test result in someone with the target disease, and (2) the specificity, the probability of a negative test result in someone without the target disease.

Case 2. A 70-year-old man being investigated for fatigue is found to have an iron deficiency anaemia. As part of the physical examination you do a faecal occult blood test which is negative. Does this obviate the need for a colonoscopy?

Colorectal cancer is clearly high in the differential diagnosis; investigations of consecutive cases of iron deficiency anaemia suggest a frequency of between 10% and 20%. Let us say our estimate is 16% for our case. To interpret the faecal occult blood test result we need to know its accuracy, that is, its sensitivity and specificity. A check of the *Best Evidence* CD provides the necessary information—Allison *et al.* (1996) followed over 8000 consecutive people screened with three different faecal occult blood tests. The gold standard was cancers detected immediately or within 2 years of follow-up (which was 96% complete). This study, which is acceptable according to the criteria in Table 2.3.1.1, tells us that the sensitivity is 69%, i.e. 69% of patients with cancer will have a positive faecal test, and the specificity is 94%, i.e. 94% of patients without cancer will have a negative faecal test.

The population of the study was quite different from our patient, who has a much higher chance of colorectal cancer. Hence, to apply this to our iron deficient patient we need to work backwards from his 16% chance of cancer before the test. We do this in Box 2.3.1.1 by beginning with a hypothetical cohort to construct a new 2 × 2 table as if the study had been done in group of patients identical to our case.

Box 2.3.1.1 Breakdown of HemeSelect results for a hypothetical 1000 patients

Using a hypothetical 1000 patients similar to our Case 2, we work through this probability in 3 steps:

Step 1. Of the 1000 similar patients, the 16% chance of cancer says we would expect 160 to have a colorectal cancer and 840 not (bottom row of table)

Step 2. Of these 160 with cancer, 69% (the sensitivity) will have a positive result, i.e. 0.69 × 160 = 110 and the remaining 50 will have a negative result (column 1)

Step 3. Of the 840 without cancer, 94% (the specificity) will have a negative result, i.e. 0.94 × 840 = 790 and the remaining 50 will have a positive result (column 2).

Thus our patient with the negative faecal test is among the 50 (false) + 790 (true) negatives, i.e. his chance of cancer is 50/(840) = 6% (the post-test probability after a negative test). With 6 chances in 100 of colorectal cancer, most people would probably still want to proceed with the colonscopy; i.e. the negative faecal test is insufficient to rule out cancer in the iron deficient 70-year old.

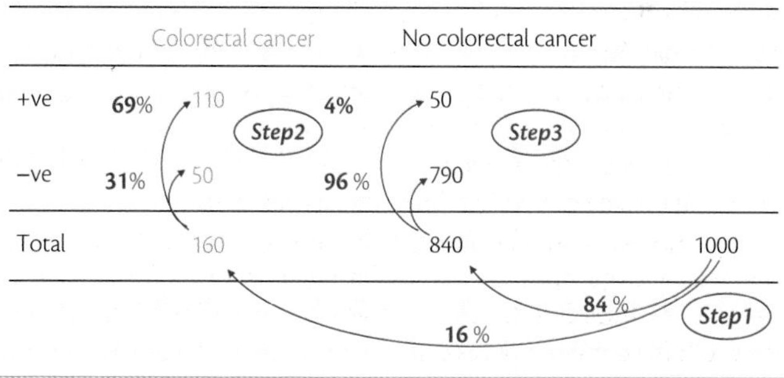

The process in Box 2.3.1.1 is clearly tedious. We do not want to repeat such calculations with every patient, but methods have been developed to simplify the process. However, the important principle illustrated here is the need to use both the clinical picture—quantified as the pretest probability—and the test accuracy. Harold Sox has expressed this succinctly: 'What you believe after the test depends on what you believed before the test.' In particular, it is important neither to be misled by false positives when screening, nor to be misled by false negatives when attempting to confirm the most likely diagnosis.

We could repeat the process of calculation in Box 2.3.1.1 for all possible pretest probabilities from 0 to 100%. Figure 2.3.1.2a illustrates this showing how the post-test probabilities vary with the pretest probabilities. For our Case 2, where even after a negative faecal test there is still substantial chance of colorectal cancer, whereas in the screening situation of Fig. 2.3.1.2b the positive faecal test is more likely to be a false than a true positive.

Using the results of treatment studies

The overall results of treatment trials apply to the 'average' patient and need to be individualized. If our patient is at a higher or lower

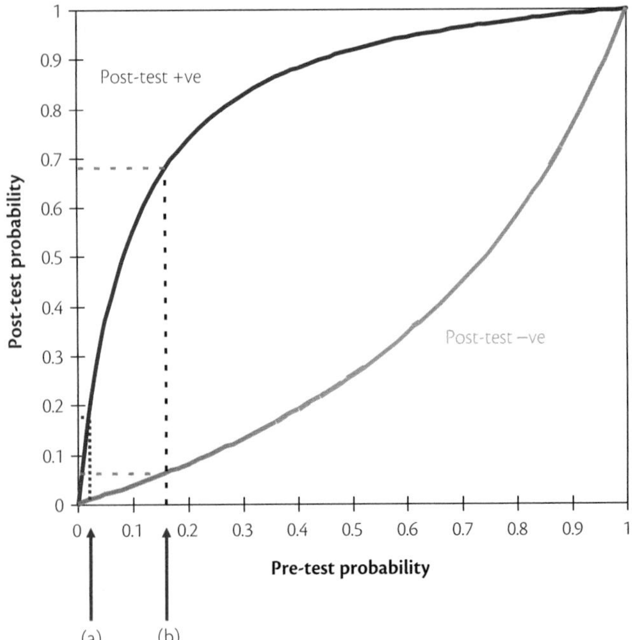

Fig. 2.3.1.2 Interpreting faecal occult blood results in different groups: 2 × 2 tables for (a) an asymptomatic 70-year-old being screened (2% chance of cancer), and (b) patient with iron deficiency anaemia (16% chance of cancer).

risk, then we need to adjust our estimate of the effects of treatment for this. Consider the following case:

> Case 3. During a routine check of his blood pressure, a 58-year-old man with stable angina and a history of hypertension was noted to have atrial fibrillation. A check of his chart showed this had been noted several months earlier. Routine investigations revealed no cause, and because of the duration, cardioversion was not warranted. But should he be taking aspirin or warfarin?

The Cochrane Library contains systematic reviews of the five relevant randomized trials: warfarin is extremely effective therapy, with a 68% reduction in the risks of ischaemic stroke. However, we must also be concerned about the dangers of anticoagulation, specifically the risks of bleeding, and most crucially the risks of intracranial haemorrhage. Should he be treated? Guidelines seem unhelpful here: a review by Thomson (1998) showed that the proportion of patients with atrial fibrillation recommended for anticoagulation by the 20 different guidelines ranged from 13 up to 100%!

So how do we apply the systematic review results? The following four questions have been suggested:

1 Is my patient so different from the study patients that the results cannot be applied?

The inclusion and exclusion criteria of clinical trials tell us about the broad category of patients tested in the trials, but are not necessarily a good guide to the applicability of the trials to individuals. A better approach is, first, to think about the potential modifiers of the therapeutic effect, and secondly, the benefits and harm in the individuals.

The biological effect of an intervention may be modified by several factors: patient characteristics, comorbidities, compliance, or cointerventions. To predict these may require pathophysiological knowledge and empirical data. For example, would a patient with Parkinson's disease having problems with dental hygiene be helped by an electric toothbrush? The randomized trials suggest that certain types of electric brush are clearly better than manual brushing, but did not include Parkinson's patients. However, our knowledge of Parkinson's does not suggest there would be any reduction in benefit, and it may be even greater given the effect of bradykinesia on manual brushing.

Treatment decisions must usually balance positive and negative effects of the intervention. For our patient on warfarin, the 68% relative reduction in the ischaemic stroke risk must be weighed against the inconvenience of therapeutic monitoring, and more serious, the risks of major bleeding, particularly the risks of intracranial haemorrhage: an excess of about 1% per year.

2 Is the treatment feasible in my setting?

Barriers to use include local organization of services, costs, and skills. Patients in remote settings may have difficulty with regular monitoring; service costs and hence access will vary across countries and settings; many new therapies or procedures may require skills or technology that are unavailable, e.g. cognitive behavioural therapy is helpful in many conditions but access to a skilled practitioner is often limited. These issues may make the treatment infeasible or threaten the balance of benefits and harms.

3 What are my patient's likely benefits and harm from the treatment?

Low-risk patients usually gain less absolute benefit and high-risk patients more than the 'average' patient in seen in the trials. Hence we need to predict the expected risk, based on the individual's clinical characteristics. By applying the relative risk reduction seen across the trials, this individualized prognosis can then be used to predict the gains of therapy. Figure 2.3.1.3 summarizes this process. The horizontal axis is the stroke rate per year; the vertical axis is the stroke equivalents prevented by anticoagulation using warfarin. This represents the 68% relative reduction seen across the trials.

Where does our patient lie in this spectrum? On the bottom and top axis are marked the clinical risk factors. Our 58-year-old male patient

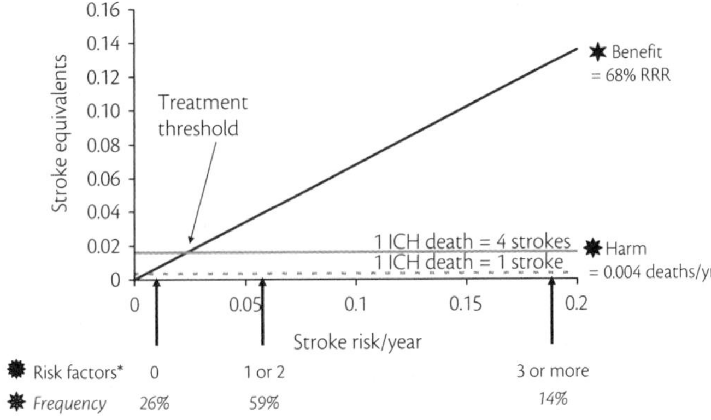

Fig. 2.3.1.3 Warfarin for atrial fibrillation, plotting how benefits and harm vary with stroke risk (horizontal axis): (1) expected benefit from a 68% relative reduction in risk of ischaemic stroke; (2) expected harms from intracranial haemorrhage: deaths (dashed line) or if one death is consider equal to four strokes (solid line); (3) predicted risk based on three clinical and two ECG risk factors; (4) the frequency of these risk categories in the Stroke Prevention in Atrial Fibrillation trial.

had a normal echocardiogram but ischaemic heart disease and a history of hypertension, and so fitted into the 1–2 risk factor category.

4 How will my patient's values influence the decision?

The essence of wise clinical management is to follow Hippocrates' aphorism, 'First do no harm'. We should now compare the absolute benefits and the absolute harm of therapy, then use the strength of the individual's preferences to weigh these. In large cohort studies of the use of warfarin in the community, the rates of excess intracranial haemorrhage deaths have been about 4/1000 per year. This rate is shown as the bottom line in Fig. 2.3.1.3. This line, however, would assume that one death was equivalent to one ischaemic stroke; the line above this values one death equivalent to four ischaemic strokes. The relative value is an individual judgement, but, measurements of quality of life in patients after stroke show an average quality of life of roughly 0.75 (on a scale of 0 for death to 1 for normal well health). Where the lines of benefit and harm cross one another, the expected benefit and harms are equal. It is only above this line that we begin to avoid our Hippocratic harm, and hence the treatment that could be considered worthwhile to the patient, as with Case 3 where the patient's risk factors put him clearly above the threshold.

Conclusions

If we are to advance the use of the best clinical research evidence in patient decision making, at least two things are required. First is the compilation of the necessary information so that it is quickly accessible by practitioners in the clinic and at the bedside. Answers are needed in minutes, not months. The Cochrane Collaboration has gone a long way towards achieving this for questions of therapeutic interventions, but similar efforts will be needed for prognosis, diagnosis, and other types of clinical questions. Second, we need to examine the several potential barriers to the application of research evidence. These include having the information and methods to decide for which patients benefits outweigh any harm of treatment, sufficient details and resources to carry out the treatment, and skills in communication and education of patients. At each stage we lose some of the impact of research, the net effect being that much of the potential benefit of good research is lost in the turbulence of everyday clinical practice.

Further reading

Allison JE, *et al.* (1996). A comparison of fecal occult-blood tests for colorectal-cancer screening. *N Engl J Med*, **334**, 155–9.

Antman EM, *et al.* (1992). A comparison of results of meta-analyses of randomized control trials and recommendations of clinical experts. Treatments for myocardial infarction. *JAMA*, **268**, 240–8.

Garg AX, *et al.* (2006). Lost in publication: Half of all renal practice evidence is published in non-renal journals. *Kidney Int*, **70**, 1995–2005.

Glasziou P, *et al.* (1998). Applying the results of trials and systematic reviews to individual patients. *ACP J Club*, **129**, A-15–16; *Evid Based Med*, **3**, 165–6.

Glasziou P, *et al.* (2007). When are randomised trials unnecessary? Picking signal from noise. *BMJ*, **334**, 349–51.

Glasziou P, *et al.* (1998). Applying the results of trials and systematic reviews to individual patients. *ACP J Club*, **129**, A-15–16; *Evid Based Med*, **3**, 165–6.

Glasziou P, Haynes B (2005). The paths from research to improved health outcomes. *ACP J Club*, **142**, A8–10.

Haynes RB (2006). Of studies, syntheses, synopses, summaries, and systems: the '5S' evolution of information services for evidence-based healthcare decisions. *Evid Based Med*, **11**, 162–4.

Hilton M, Pinder D (2004). The Epley (canalith repositioning) manoeuvre for benign paroxysmal positional vertigo. *Cochrane Database Syst Rev*, **2**, CD003162.

Jackson R, *et al.* (2006). The GATE frame: critical appraisal with pictures. *Evid Based Med*, **11**, 35–8.

Lind J (1753). *A treatise of the scurvy. In three parts. Containing an inquiry into the nature, causes and cure, of that disease.* Printed by Sands, Murray and Cochran for A Kincaid and A Donaldson, Edinburgh. (http://www.jameslindlibrary.org/)

McKibbon KA, Wilczynski NL, Haynes RB (2004). What do evidence-based secondary journals tell us about the publication of clinically important articles in primary healthcare journals? *BMC Med*, **6**, 33.

Medical Research Council (1948). Streptomycin treatment of pulmonary tuberculosis: a Medical Research Council investigation. *Br Med J*, **ii**, 769–82.

Sackett DL, Haynes RB (1997). 13 steps, 100 people, and 1,000,000 thanks. *ACP Journal Club*, **127**, A-14; *Evid Based Med*, **2**, 101.

Sackett DL, *et al.* (1995). Evidence-based medicine: what it is and what it isn't. *BMJ*, **312**, 71–2.

Straus S, *et al.* (2005). *Evidence-based medicine: how to practice and teach EBM*, 3rd edition, Churchill Livingstone, Edinburgh.

Stroke Prevention in Atrial Fibrillation Investigators (1996). Bleeding during, antithrombotic therapy in patients with atrial fibrillation. *Arch Intern Med*, **156**, 409–16.

Stroke Prevention in Atrial Fibrillation (SPAF) Investigators (1999). Factors associated with ischemic stroke during aspirin therapy in atrial fibrillation: analysis of 2012 participants in the SPAF I-III clinical trials. *Stroke*, **30**, 1223–9.

Tanimoto H, *et al.* (2005). Self-treatment for benign paroxysmal positional vertigo of the posterior semicircular canal. *Neurology*, **65**, 1299–300.

Thomson R (1998). Guidelines on anticoagulant treatment in atrial fibrillation in Great Britain: variation in content and implications for treatment. *BMJ*, **316**, 509–13.

Yerushalmy J (1947). Statistical problems in assessing methods of medical diagnosis, with special reference to X-ray techniques. *Public Health Rep*, **62**, 1432–49.

2.3.2 Evidence-based medicine—does it apply to my particular patient?

Louis R. Caplan

Essentials

Proponents of evidence-based medicine (EBM) have established a clear, unambiguous requirement for what they consider credible evidence, the randomized controlled trial (RCT), and especially the systematic review of several RCTs. They propose that clinical practice should be dominated by adherence to the 'evidence' as they define it.

It would be obtuse to argue that the doctor should ignore evidence from RCTs or aggregates thereof, but taking care of complex patients is very different from care during trials. Many conditions are unsuitable for trials, and many patients are not included in trials. Patients selected are often not representative of the conditions seen in the clinic by practitioners. Furthermore, there are important limitations in trial design and analysis that make the 'evidence' not very practically useful in everyday practice.

Instead of basing decisions largely on trial results of homogenized groups of patients, an alternative approach advocated in this chapter emphasizes spending more time at the bedside and in the clinic, finding out exactly what is wrong with each patient, and getting to know each patient and their circumstances, family situations, psychosocial and economic stresses, thoughts, fears, biases, and wishes. Therapeutic decisions are made with, by, and for complex individuals. Therapeutic decisions should be guided by detailed knowledge of the pathology, pathophysiology and circumstances in individual patients. One size does not fit all or most patients.

What is 'evidence-based medicine' and how is it new?

The latest medical crusade is to render the care of patients evidence-based. This term has become a shibboleth, a sacrosanct icon almost like motherhood. Who could possibly be against basing decisions on evidence? The *Oxford College Dictionary* defines evidence as 'something that furnishes proof; an outward sign; an indication, testimony'. Haven't doctors always prided themselves in having some evidence behind treatment selection? It is difficult to think of a polite term for actions and decisions not based on any evidence. The change from the past, however, is that advocates of evidence-based medicine have established a clear unambiguous requirement for what they consider credible evidence—the randomized controlled trial and especially the systematic review of several randomized controlled trials. But the almost religious zeal for cloaking all decisions about patient care under the banner of 'evidence-based' misses the real problem: that is, how well does the evidence from trials apply to the care of individual patients? Governmental organizations, insurance companies, and other funders embrace this new concept of evidence-based medicine since few treatments meet the strict criteria. They would prefer not to pay. He who pays the piper calls the tune.

In contrast to the situation envisioned by evidence-based medicine zealots, courts of law accept and evaluate many different types of 'evidence' and testimony. Judicial decisions depend on how the evidence applies to the individual case being considered.

How do trial data relate to treating individual patients?

Physicians in the free world are not compelled to give all patients with a condition the same defined treatment, as is the case in trials. Randomized trials mandate that numbers of patients with a general condition will be given treatment X and the results will be compared with patients given treatment Y or Z or placebo.

Doctors care for one patient at a time. Caring for individual patients is complicated. Care involves: (1) understanding what is wrong with the patient, and (2) understanding the patient's risks for disease, and (3) understanding the patient, their background, genetics, socioeconomic milieu, psychology, responsibilities, goals, etc., and (4) understanding the benefits and risks of potential therapeutic strategies to treat the patient's conditions (often multiple) and to prevent conditions that they are at risk for developing, and (5) communicating with the patient and sometimes family members and friends, listening and conveying information, and teaching. These functions are extensive and often difficult. They require much innate intelligence, experience, sensitivity, and training. They take time, a commodity now often jeopardized by large patient lists, managed care directives, and the need to support oneself and one's family. 'Evidence-based medicine' relates to only one of these doctor functions, number 4 above.

George Thibault said it very well:

> We then need to decide which approach in our large therapeutic armamentarium will be most appropriate in a particular patient, with a particular stage of disease and particular coexisting conditions, and at a particular age. Even when randomized clinical trials have been performed (which is true for only a small number of clinical problems), they will often not answer this question specifically for the patient sitting in front of us in the office or lying in the hospital bed.
>
> (Thibaud 1993).

Do randomized trials have theoretical and practical limitations?

Trials, the core of evidence-based medicine, have important theoretical and practical limitations. They are expensive, time consuming, and require enormous resources. To provide statistically valid results, randomized trials must contain large numbers of patients with enough end points for analysis. Sufficient endpoints must be obtained in a relatively short period. The condition studied must either be acute and cause adverse endpoints or rapid improvement within a short time. Chronic conditions must be severe enough to cause clear end points within 1 to 5 years of follow-up. Many medical conditions are unsuitable for study by trials. Less common, heterogeneous, and chronic conditions are difficult to study in trials. Patients who are too ill, too old, too young, female and 'of childbearing age', incapable of giving informed consent, too complex, or too full of coexisting illnesses are often not included in trials. But these are just the patients who visit doctors in their office and are under their care in the hospital.

The major theoretical limitation of trials is the issue of numbers vs specificity. For trials to yield statistically valid results, they must include many patients—numbers. For the results to be useful to practising physicians, the data must specifically apply to individual patients with the condition studied. To include enough patients, the condition to be studied must be common, and usually multiple physicians at multiple centres must be used. A single doctor or medical centre would have too few patients or would take an unacceptably long time to accrue the number of patients needed. To achieve numbers, a lumping strategy must predominate over splitting. For example, to study the effectiveness of a treatment to prevent embolism in patients with mitral valve prolapse, a study would not be able to obtain enough patients with mitral valve prolapse, mitral regurgitation, and mitral valve fibrinoid degeneration who had prior brain or systemic emboli and congestive heart failure even though this group is at highest risk and would be most likely to respond to prophylaxis. The study would have to include all patients with mitral valve prolapse to recruit enough patients.

The sample size of a trial will increase if: the projected effectiveness of the treatment (the percentage reduction in adverse outcomes) is low (10–15%); a number of treatments will be studied;

the follow-up period is short (otherwise many patients will be lost to follow-up, withdraw, or become noncompliant); the anticipated outcome event rate is low; and a high power of protection from type I and type II errors is desired. As an example of the extraordinary numbers of patients needed for some studies, the authors of a meta-analysis of randomized controlled trials of agents that decrease platelet aggregation for the secondary prevention of stroke calculated that 13 000 patients would be needed to detect, with 90% power, an observed reduction of 15% in endpoints with aspirin.

The greater the numbers of patients required, the more pressure there is to adopt a lumping strategy. The more a study lumps diverse subgroups, the more general are the results and their applicability to specific patients declines. For practising physicians, treatment must be very specific. Physicians are faced with individual patients for whom they must make therapeutic decisions. To be useful, trial results must help physicians treat individual patients in given situations. Subgroups can be managed either by prospective stratification, that is, by randomizing patients using predetermined criteria (e.g. sex, race, age) to ensure that subgroups will be relatively equally represented in the different treatment groups, or by analysing the treatment results by subgroup determinants that have been prospectively defined. But the subgroups must also be very large to satisfy statisticians.

A confounding issue is the number of treatments and agents that patients receive. For example, many trials consider secondary stroke prevention after an initial transient ischaemic attack or stroke. Patients are enrolled even 3 to 6 months after their initial cerebrovascular event. These trials have not taken into consideration the effect on the outcome of the initial treatment before randomization. Experience and outcome data show that treatments that are effective during the initial event (e.g. thrombolytics, mechanical clot extraction, anticoagulants, antiplatelets) often have durability and greatly influence the occurrence of later events. If initial treatments are taken into consideration, a much larger number of patients would be required to assess the results. Similarly, many patients with vascular disease are treated with polypharmacy prior to enrolment. It is difficult to balance the control and various treatment groups for all potential drugs and combinations of drugs.

There are also many practical problems confronting trialists. The logistics of performing randomized therapeutic trials can be problematical. Trials are big operations. Multiple centres require many physicians and clerical staff. Computer hardware and software and statistical skills are needed to record, manage, interpret, and analyse data. The personnel and equipment are very costly. Money for funding comes either from governmental, or private sources, most often pharmaceutical or device companies. Much time and effort is expended in writing grants and many pilot data are required. Government funding is becoming scarcer all over the world. Alternatively, private industry may be interested in funding grants if their products are being studied. Potential problems arise from involvement of private enterprises that have much to gain and much to lose, depending on trial results. Many companies strive to dictate trial methodology and/or play a role in analysis and publication of the results as a condition for funding studies. Companies have bailed out of studies depending on company finances and goals. Many worthwhile trials go unfunded.

Inclusion and exclusion criteria are designed so that patients entered will be 'pure breed' and can be followed until study completion. Most severe intercurrent diseases exclude patients, as do relative contraindications to treatments studied. Comorbid conditions such as alcoholism, cancer, liver, lung, blood, and renal disease are exclusions. The plethora of exclusions often make it difficult to recruit enough patients to meet sample size requirements. Estimates of the number of patients a centre predicts it will recruit are usually at least two or three times more than they actually manage to enter once the trial begins. In some trials, patients who are eligible under the inclusion/exclusion rules of a trial are not entered by physicians who feel that a particular patient needs the treatment and should not be randomized.

Eligible patients are not always easy to enrol in trials. Many patients decline because they don't want to be guinea-pigs and view trials as something others do, especially charity cases. Some patients are put off by the acknowledged lack of a scientific basis for treatment and cannot accept that a flip of the coin will decide treatment. Some are disturbed that neither they nor their physicians will know what treatment they receive. Especially disconcerting for many is the prospect that they may receive a placebo. They believe their problem is serious and warrants active treatment. With time and patience, some of these patients can be enrolled, but with much effort. Alas, some who have enrolled will be dissuaded later by their all-knowing friend or relative, and will drop out. To document that all procedures have been followed and all necessary examinations and evaluations have been performed, most studies require mountains of paper. Completion of forms takes time. Often, the filling out of forms is delegated to a clerk, a resident, or the most junior investigator. The validity of the data is thus jeopardized. The results are only valid if the data are reliable and accurate. Senior experienced clinicians should have seen all patients and personally reviewed the forms to ensure accuracy, but this is often not done.

To compare the effectiveness of different treatments, outcomes must be measured and quantified. Trials that study stroke prevention are an example. This is simple if large events such as death or new stroke are used, but are all strokes equal? In nonfatal diseases, other criteria, e.g. severity of deficits, disability, or other objective measures, must be used. Especially in neurology, severity and disability scores are problematic. How can aphasia be compared with diplopia, ataxia, facial numbness, and limb weakness? How are weights assigned to various abnormalities? For some patients, a hemianopia that makes reading difficult but does not effect daily living poses no major problem but to a physician, editor, or surveyor the same deficit is devastating.

Are some recommendations based on trial results useful?

Randomized trials that study common, relatively homogeneous, specific, acute conditions have been quite helpful to practising physicians. A randomized trial of high concentration oxygen therapy given to premature infants showed that blindness due to retrolental fibroplasia was an important complication of this treatment. The results prevented innumerable cases of blindness. Before this trial, renowned professors of paediatrics had embraced this treatment. Many trials and analyses have clarified the indications for carotid artery surgery in symptomatic patients with various severities of arterial narrowing. Many trials and analyses have shown that warfarin anticoagulation is superior in preventing strokes in patients with atrial fibrillation than aspirin and placebo treatment. Unfortunately, many doctors have not followed the recommendation to anticoagulate patients with atrial fibrillation unless there are important contraindications. Cardiac revascularization conveys more frequent and better survival from cardiac shock than medical stabilization. There are many such examples of very useful trials that have promoted changes in treatment of patients.

Are other trial-based guidelines and recommendations less useful?

Some other randomized trials are much less useful to practising physicians. In this category are the stroke prevention trials of drugs that decrease platelet aggregation. Some studies showed in full group analyses a benefit for aspirin, aspirin combined with sulfinpyrazone or dipyridamole, ticlopidine, and clopidogrel. Unfortunately, the mixture of patients treated with antiplatelet aggregants or placebo was probably not representative of patients in the community presenting with transient ischaemic attacks or minor strokes. In none of these studies was clarification of the nature and severity of the causative vascular and cardiac lesions required for entry. Patients with lesions thought favourable for carotid surgery were often operated on and were ineligible. Patients with 'surgical' lesions deemed unfit for surgery, and those unfit for angiography, were included in medical treatment groups. Some patients with detected cardiac sources of emboli were not entered. No systematic evaluation for carotid artery or cardiac disease was mandated. Subgroup analysis was only by sex and tempo of ischaemia (transient ischaemic attack, reversible ischaemic neurological deficits, minor stroke). The tempo of ischaemia does not predict the nature, severity, or location of causative vascular lesions. Since cardiac studies were not required, the groups must also have contained patients with cardiac-origin brain embolism as the cause of their brain ischaemia. A meta-analysis of randomized control trials of antiplatelet agents in the secondary prevention of stroke found that for aspirin compared with placebo there was a nonsignificant reduction in stroke of 15% and a trend in reduction of stroke for any regimen containing aspirin. The results of these studies are difficult for physicians to apply to individual stroke patients with identified stroke mechanisms, e.g stenosis of the vertebral artery, arterial dissection, fibromuscular dysplasia, cardiogenic embolism. In defence of the studies cited, the technology now available—high quality duplex ultrasound scans, pulsed and continuous wave Doppler ultrasound, transcranial Doppler ultrasound, CT angiography, brain MRI and MR angiography, and echocardiography—was not widely available when the studies were designed. To recruit enough patients, the decision was made not to require angiography for entry (the numbers vs specificity issue). The result is that, despite enormous expense, the data are not very useful for physicians treating patients with the conditions studied in the trials. Future trials of antiplatelet aggregants should be conceived differently and have sufficient subgroup data related to the presence and severity of vascular lesions to be meaningful to practising physicians.

Guidelines for thrombolysis in acute stroke patients are still based on a single study funded by the United States government, planned nearly two decades ago and published more than 10 years ago. Release of the results of the National Institute of Neurological Diseases and Stroke (NINDS) trial gave momentum to a movement to quickly introduce intravenous thrombolysis widely into the community. During the summer of 1996, about 6 months after the publication of the NINDS trial, the United States Food and Drug Administration approved the use of recombinant tissue plasminogen activator (rt-PA) for the treatment of stroke patients when the drug was given within the first 3 h. The NINDS trial did not include patients treated after 3 h. The American Heart Association and American Academy of Neurology published treatment guidelines that recommended intravenous administration of rt-PA according to the NINDS protocol. The recommendations suggested that a CT scan performed before thrombolysis should not show major infarction, mass effect, oedema, or haemorrhage. The guidelines did not require or suggest MRI or vascular tests before treatment, despite the fact that stroke is of course a vascular disease. The inclusions and exclusions of the NINDS trial were copied in the recommendation. Patients who had minor deficits, were improving, awakened with deficits, or had seizures were not recommended for intravenous thrombolysis. The recommendations have never been updated.

Before and since the NINDS trial, many thousands of patients have been given stroke thrombolyis throughout the world. Early studies involved angiography before and after intravenous or intra-arterial thrombolysis. These studies showed convincingly that outcome correlated highly and consistently with opening of arterial occlusions and reperfusion. Many patients treated after 3 h improved after thrombolysis, depending on the presence and amount of brain infarction and the nature and location of the arterial occlusion. These studies were only observational, since controls were seldom used and patients were not randomized, but successive patients meeting protocol requirements were treated. Unfortunately the results of these early studies were not included in the publications of the results of the NINDS and randomized European thrombolytic trials.

Many patients who awaken with deficits can be studied using modern brain and vascular imaging to determine the potential salvageability of brain tissue by thrombolysis. Patients with minor or improving deficits frequently worsen or crash in the ensuing 24 h after onset. Some patients with seizures have acute vascular occlusions as the cause. Modern brain and vascular imaging can be done safely and quickly and can yield the key information needed to logically choose those patients who are likely to benefit from thrombolysis, those who are likely to be harmed, and the best route of administration of the agent or the potential of device-engendered reperfusion.

The present thrombolytic recommendations are an embarrassment. They prevent many potentially eligible patients from being treated. They expose other patients who do not have occlusive arterial lesions to needless risks. Less than 5% of potentially eligible acute stroke patients are given thrombolysis. It should be obvious to even the most naive person that patients do not change from good candidates (queens) to no candidate (pumpkins) when the clock strikes four. Use of a clock and a plain CT scan to screen candidates in 2009 is archaic and is completely outmoded except in regions where skills and technological equipment are lacking. Organizations have failed to update the currently outmoded recommendations because the important information (evidence) gleaned from decades of experience is not 'evidence-based' according to their very strict criteria.

Conclusions

We need more and better randomized therapeutic trials designed by clinicians to answer clinically relevant specific therapeutic problems.

We need more critical reviews of trials and therapeutic dilemmas by experienced senior clinicians. Inexpert reviews by young academics often miss nuances and frequently lack clinical perspective and experience. All available information, not just that gleaned from randomized trials, should be included.

The panacea and saviour for medical therapeutics is not, and will not be, randomized trials or evidence-based reviews or meta-analyses. There are too many situations that cannot be clarified by trials. In other conditions general results are hard to apply to complex patients. Some envisage that the bulk of medical care will be delivered by primary care physicians who will spend much time at the computer reviewing evidence bases to guide therapeutic decisions. The role of specialists who have extensive experience and training in treating patients within their fields of expertise is minimized. After all, specialists are thought to be more expensive than primary care physicians (although no credible data proves this assumption). What a nightmare for present patients and for we doctors who ultimately will also become patients. Instead, I suggest that more time should be spent by general physicians and specialists at the bedside and in the clinic finding out exactly what is wrong with each patient, and getting to know each patient and their circumstances, family situations, psychosocial and economic stresses, thoughts, fears, biases, and wishes. Therapeutic decisions are made with, by, and for complex individuals. They cannot be readily homogenized without losing the essence of what being a doctor is all about.

Further reading

Antithrombotic Trialists' Collaboration (2002). Collaborative meta-analysis of randomised trials of antiplatelet therapy for prevention of death, myocardial infarction, and stroke in high-risk patients. *BMJ*, **324**, 71–86.

Biller J, *et al.* (1998). Guidelines for carotid endarterectomy. A statement of healthcare professionals from a special writing group of the Stroke Council, American Heart Association and the American Academy of Neurology. *Stroke*, **29**, 554–62.

Caplan LR (1988). TIAs—we need to return to the question, 'What is wrong with Mr Jones?' *Neurology*, **38**, 791–3. [Strongly advocates thorough diagnosis of the cause in each patient with brain ischaemia.]

Caplan LR (2000). *Caplan's Stroke, a clinical approach*, 3rd edition. Butterworth-Heinemann, Boston, MA. [Contains reviews of the results of trials and other data regarding treatment of patients with minor strokes and TIAs, carotid endarterectomy, atrial fibrillation, and stroke thrombolysis.]

Caplan LR (2001). Evidence-based medicine. Concerns of a clinical neurologist. *J Neurol Neurosurg Psych*, **71**, 569–76.

Chimowitz MI, *et al.* (2005). Comparison of warfarin and aspirin for symptomatic intracranial arterial stenosis. *N Engl J Med*, **352**, 1305–16.

Hochman JS, *et al.* (2006). Early revascularization and long-term survival in cardiogenic shock complicating acute myocardial infarction. *JAMA*, **295**, 2511–15.

Mohr JP, *et al.* for the Warfarin-Aspirin Recurrent Stroke Study Group (2001). A comparison of warfarin and aspirin for the prevention of recurrent ischemic stroke. *N Engl J Med*, **345**, 1444–51.

National Institute of Neurological Disorders and Stroke rt-PA Study Group (1995). Tissue plasminogen activator for acute ischemic stroke. *New Engl J Med*, **333**, 1581–7.

Quality Standards Subcommittee of the American Academy of Neurology (1996). Practice advisory: Thrombolytic therapy for acute ischemic stroke—summary statement. *Neurology*, **47**, 835–9.

Sackett DL, *et al.* (1996). *Evidence-based medicine. How to practice and teach EBM*. Churchill Livingstone, Edinburgh.

Stroke Prevention in Atrial Fibrillation Investigators (1991). The stroke prevention in atrial fibrillation study: final results. *Circulation*, **84**, 527–39.

Thibault GE (1993). Clinical problem solving: Too old for what? *N Engl J Med*, **328**, 946–50.

2.3.3 Large-scale randomized evidence: trials and meta-analyses of trials

C. Baigent, R. Peto, R. Gray, S. Parish, and R. Collins

Essentials

Reliable detection or refutation of realistically moderate effects on major outcomes often requires large-scale randomized evidence

As long as doctors start with a healthy scepticism about the many apparently striking claims and counter-claims that appear in the medical literature, trial results do make sense. The main enemy of common sense is over-optimism: there are a few striking exceptions where treatments for serious disease work extremely well, but many claims of vast improvements from new therapies turn out to be evanescent.

Clinical trials generally need to be able to detect or to refute realistically moderate (but still worthwhile) differences between treatments in long-term disease outcome. Large-scale randomized evidence should be able to detect such effects, but medium-sized trials or medium-sized meta-analyses can, and often do, yield false negative or exaggeratedly positive results. If the results of such studies seem too good to be true then they probably are; conversely, unpromising evidence can be misleading if it is from a study of inadequate size, or from one particular subgroup of a large study with a clearly favourable overall result. Realistically moderate expectations of what a treatment might achieve (or, if one treatment is to be compared with another, of how large any difference between the main effects of these two treatments is likely to be) should foster studies that can discriminate reliably between (1) a difference in outcome that is realistically moderate but still worthwhile, and (2) a difference in outcome that is too small to be of any material importance.

To assess moderate effects reliably, avoid both moderate biases and moderate random errors

To demonstrate or refute realistically moderate differences in outcome, studies must guarantee both (1) strict control of bias - which, in general, requires proper randomization and appropriate statistical analysis, with no unduly 'data-dependent' emphasis on specific parts of the overall evidence; and (2) strict control of the play of chance - which, in general, requires large numbers with the outcome of interest, rather than a lot of detail on each patient. The conclusion is obvious: moderate biases and moderate random errors must both be avoided if moderate benefits are to be assessed reliably. This leads to the need for large numbers of properly randomized patients with properly analysed data, which in turn should lead to some large but simple randomized trials (or 'mega-trials') and to large systematic overviews (or 'meta-analyses') of all related randomized trials.

Other forms of evidence may be untrustworthy

Non-randomized evidence, unduly small randomized trials, unduly small meta-analyses of trials and undue emphasis on particular subgroups (or on particular trials) are all much inferior as sources of evidence about current patient management or as foundations for future research strategies because they often cannot discriminate reliably between moderate (but worthwhile) differences and negligible differences in outcome, and the mistaken clinical conclusions that they engender could well result in the undertreatment, overtreatment, or other mismanagement of millions of future patients worldwide.

Benefits of large-scale randomized evidence

In contrast, many premature deaths each year could be avoided by seeking appropriately large-scale randomized evidence about various widely practicable treatments for the common causes of death, and by disseminating this evidence appropriately. The value of such large-scale randomized evidence is illustrated by the trials of fibrinolytic therapy for acute myocardial infarction; of anti-platelet therapy for a wide range of vascular conditions; of hormonal therapy for early breast cancer; and of drug therapy for lowering blood pressure. In these examples, proof of benefit that could not have been achieved by either small-scale randomized evidence or non-randomized evidence of benefit has led to widespread changes in practice that are now preventing hundreds of thousands of premature deaths each year, and appropriately large-scale randomized evidence could substantially improve the management of many important, but non-fatal, medical conditions.

Moderate (but worthwhile) effects on major outcomes are generally more plausible than large effects

Some treatments have large, and hence obvious, effects on survival: e.g. it was clear without the need for any randomized trials that prompt treatment of diabetic coma or cardiac arrest can save lives, and more recently the introduction of protease inhibitors for the treatment of HIV infection led to a reduction in AIDS-related morbidity and mortality that was large enough to be obvious even without randomized evidence; indeed, the remarkable effectiveness of antiretroviral drugs can be seen from the sudden reversal, after the mid 1990s, of the upward trend in mortality among men aged 30–34 in the United States of America (Fig. 2.3.3.1), the chief cause of which was HIV/AIDS.

However, over the past few decades the hopes of large treatment effects on mortality and major morbidity in many serious diseases have been unrealistically high. Of course, treatments do quite commonly have large effects on various less fundamental measures: certain drugs clearly reduce blood pressure, blood cholesterol, or blood glucose; many tumours or leukaemias in middle and old age can be controlled temporarily by radiotherapy or chemotherapy; and, in acute myocardial infarction, lidocaine (lignocaine) can prevent many arrhythmias and fibrinolytic therapy can dissolve many thrombi. However, although such effects on intermediate outcomes may be large, the net effects on mortality may be much more modest.

In general, if substantial uncertainty remains about the efficacy of a practicable treatment, its effects on major endpoints are probably either negligibly small, or only moderate, rather than large. Indirect support for this rather pessimistic conclusion comes from many sources, including: the previous few decades of disappointingly slow progress in the curative treatment of common chronic diseases of middle age; the heterogeneity of each single disease, as evidenced by the unpredictability of survival duration even when apparently similar patients are compared with each other; the variety of different mechanisms in certain diseases that can lead to death, only one of which may be appreciably influenced by any one particular therapy; the modest effects often suggested by meta-analyses (see later) of various therapies, and, in certain special cases, observational epidemiological studies of the strength of the

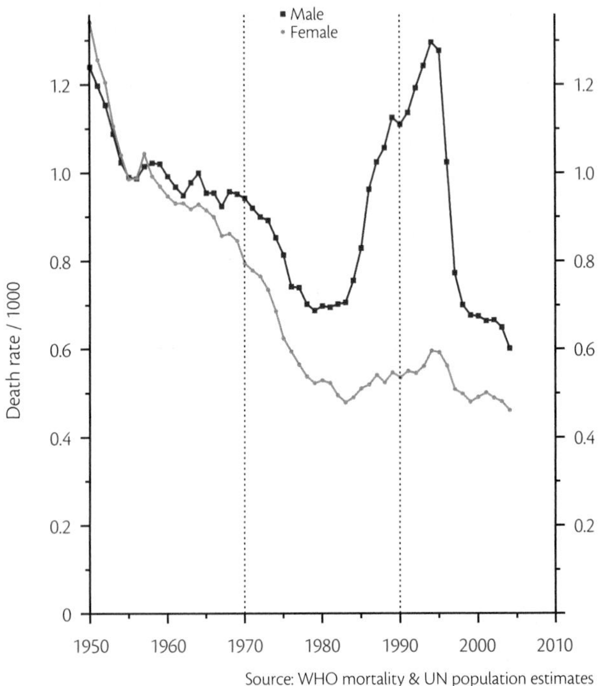

Fig. 2.3.3.1 Mortality trends in the United States of America among men and women aged 30–34 during the period 1950–2004. Antibacterial drugs caused a big decrease in mortality around the middle of the century in both sexes. The increase in AIDS-related mortality since the early 1980s caused a sharp increase in all-cause mortality, particularly in men, which continued until it was spectacularly reversed by effective antiretroviral drug combinations in the mid 1990s.

relationship between some disease and the factor that treatment will modify (e.g. blood pressure, blood cholesterol, or blood glucose: see later).

Having accepted that only moderate reductions in mortality are likely with many currently unevaluated interventions, how worthwhile might such effects be if they could be detected reliably? To some clinicians, reducing the risk of early death in patients with myocardial infarction from 10 per 100 patients down to 9 or 8 per 100 patients treated may not seem particularly worthwhile, and if such a reduction was only transient, or involved an extremely expensive or toxic treatment, this might well be an appropriate view. Worldwide, however, several million patients a year suffer an acute myocardial infarction, and if just one million were to be given a simple, nontoxic, and widely practicable treatment that reduced the risk of early death from 10% down to 9% or 8% (that is, a proportional reduction of 10 or 20%), this would avoid 10 000 or 20 000 deaths. (At least 1 million patients a year now receive fibrinolytic therapy for acute myocardial infarction, which is avoiding about 20 000 early deaths a year.) Such absolute gains are substantial, and might considerably exceed the number of lives that could be saved by a much more effective treatment of a much less common disease.

Reliable detection or refutation of moderate differences requires avoidance of both moderate biases and moderate random errors

If realistically moderate differences in outcome are to be reliably detected or reliably refuted, then errors in comparative assessments of the effects of treatment need to be much smaller than the difference between a moderate, but worthwhile, effect and an effect that is too small to be of any material importance. This in turn implies that moderate biases and moderate random errors cannot be tolerated. The only way to guarantee very small random errors is to study really large numbers, and this can be achieved in two main ways: by making individual studies large, and by combining information from as many relevant studies as possible in a systematic meta-analysis (Box 2.3.3.1). However, it is not much use having very small random errors if there may well be moderate biases, so even the large sizes of some nonrandomized analyses of computerized hospital records, where the complex factors involved in the decision to treat a person with a particular drug may not be recorded in sufficient detail, cannot guarantee medically reliable comparisons between the effects of different treatments (see later). For, the choice of treatment may be strongly affected by subtle patient characteristics that are correlated with the prognosis. (A crude illustration of such problems is provided by the old joke 'What's the most dangerous place in the world?' 'Bed—look at the number of people who die in bed!'.)

Box 2.3.3.1 Requirements for reliable assessment of moderate effects: negligible biases and small random errors

Negligible biases
(i.e. guaranteed avoidance of moderate biases)

Proper randomization

(nonrandomized methods might suffer moderate biases)

Analysis by allocated treatment

(including all randomized patients: 'intention to treat' analysis)

Chief emphasis on overall results

(no unduly data-dependent emphasis on particular subgroups)

Systematic overview of all relevant randomized trials

(no unduly data-dependent emphasis on particular studies)

Small random errors
(i.e. guaranteed avoidance of moderate chance fluctuations)

Large numbers in any new trials

(to be really large, trials should be 'streamlined')

Systematic overview of all relevant randomized trials

(which yields the largest possible total numbers)

Avoiding moderate biases

Proper randomization avoids systematic differences between the types of patient in different treatment groups. The fundamental reason for randomization is to avoid moderate bias, by ensuring that each type of patient can be expected (but for the play of chance) to have been allocated in similar proportions to the different treatment strategies that are to be compared. This means that only random differences should affect the final comparisons of outcome. Nonrandomized methods, in contrast, cannot generally guarantee that the types of patient given the new study treatment do not differ systematically in any important ways from the types of patient given any other treatment(s) with which the new study treatment is to be compared. For example, moderate biases may arise if the study treatment is novel and doctors are afraid to use it for the most seriously ill patients, or, conversely, if they are more ready to use it for those who are desperately ill. There may also be other ways in which the severity of the condition differentially affects the likelihood of being assigned to different treatments by the doctor's choice (or by the patient's choice, or by any other nonrandom procedure).

It might appear at first sight that by collecting enough information about various prognostic features it would be possible to make some mathematical adjustments that correct for any such differences between the types of patients who, in a nonrandomized study, receive the different treatments that are to be compared. The ill-conceived hope is that such methods, which are often carried out on routinely collected health care data, might achieve comparability between those entering the different treatment groups, but they cannot be guaranteed to do so, and often fail seriously. The difficulty is that some important prognostic factors may be unrecorded, while others may be difficult to assess exactly and hence difficult to adjust for reliably. Although there are examples of nonrandomized studies in which the estimated effects of treatment appear quantitatively close to those observed in analogous randomized trials, there are many examples where they do not, being either quantitatively incorrect—so that drugs appear either misleadingly promising or of misleadingly low efficacy—or even qualitatively incorrect, when a harmful drug might appear effective (or vice versa).

The machinery of a properly randomized trial

No foreknowledge of what the next treatment will be

In a properly randomized trial, the decision to enter a patient is made in ignorance of which of the trial treatments that patient will, once entered, be allocated. The treatment allocation is then made known after trial entry has been decided upon. (The purpose of this sequence is to ensure that foreknowledge of what the next treatment is going to be cannot affect the decision as to whether to enter the patient; if it did, those to be allocated one treatment might differ systematically from those to be allocated another.) Ideally, any major prognostic features should also be irreversibly recorded before the treatment is revealed, particularly if these are to be used in any treatment analyses. For, if the recorded value of some prognostic factor might be affected by knowledge of the trial treatment allocation, then treatment comparisons within subgroups defined by that factor might be moderately biased. In particular, treatment comparisons just among 'responders' or just among 'nonresponders' can be misleading unless the response is assessed before treatment allocation (which it can sometimes be, if all patients have a 'run-in' period on active treatment before randomization, partly to assess the response to treatment and partly to exclude those who seem during this prerandomization run-in unlikely to participate wholeheartedly in the main post-randomization study).

No bias in patient management or in outcome assessment

An additional difficulty, in both randomized and non-randomized comparisons of various treatments, is that there might be systematic differences in the use of other treatments (including general supportive care) or in the assessment of major outcomes. A non-randomized comparison may well suffer from moderate biases due to such systematic differences in ancillary care or assessment, particularly if it merely involves the retrospective review of medical records. In the context of a randomized comparison, however, it is generally possible to devise ways to keep any such biases small. For example, placebo tablets may be given to control-allocated patients and certain subjective assessments may be 'blinded' (although this may be less important in studies assessing mortality).

'Intention-to-treat' analyses with no post-randomization exclusions

Even in a properly randomized trial, unnecessary biases may be introduced by inappropriate statistical analysis. One of the most important sources of bias in the analysis is undue concentration on just part of the evidence; that is to say, on 'data-derived subgroup analyses' (see below). Another easily avoided bias is caused by the post-randomization exclusion of patients, particularly if the type (and hence prognosis) of those excluded differs from one treatment group to another. Therefore one of the fundamental statistical analyses of a trial that should be made available is an analysis that compares all those originally allocated one treatment (even though some of them may not have actually received it) with all those allocated the other treatment. This is sometimes referred to as an 'intention-to-treat' analysis. Additional analyses can also be reported: e.g. in describing the frequency of some very specific side effect it may well be preferable to record its incidence only among those who actually received the treatment. (This is because strictly randomized comparisons may not be needed to assess extreme relative risks.) However, in assessing moderate effects on the main outcome of interest such 'on-treatment' analyses can be misleading, and 'intention-to-treat' analyses are generally a more trustworthy guide as to whether there is any real difference between the trial treatments in their effects on long-term outcome.

Unduly data-dependent emphasis on results in particular subgroups

Treatment that is appropriate for one patient may be inappropriate for another. Ideally, therefore, what is wanted is not only an answer to the question, 'Is this treatment helpful on average for a wide range of patients?', but also an answer to the question, 'For which recognizable categories of patient is this treatment particularly helpful?' However, this ideal is difficult to attain directly because apparent differences between the *proportional* risk reductions in particular subgroups of patients are often surprisingly unreliable. Of course, patients who already have a very good prognosis anyway and are at low *absolute* risk cannot have a large absolute benefit (for even if a small risk is halved the absolute benefit is small). Classification of patients as being at low (or high) risk of an adverse disease outcome is often a useful guide as to which patients can expect little absolute gain even if the trial treatment works as expected (and as to which patients might expect a worthwhile gain). This low risk/high risk split may not require support from formal subgroup analyses—indeed, it could even be damaged by such analyses. For, even if the proportional effects of treatment in specific subgroups are importantly different, standard subgroup analyses are so insensitive that they may well fail to demonstrate these differences. Moreover, even if there are highly significant differences between the proportional risk reductions produced by the trial treatment in different subgroups, and the results seem to suggest that the treatment works in some subgroups but not in others (thereby giving the appearance of a 'qualitative interaction'), this may still not be good evidence for subgroup-specific treatment preferences. The play of chance often produces qualitatively wrong answers in particular subgroups in trials (or in meta-analyses of trials) that could, if interpreted incautiously, lead to millions of people being treated inappropriately, or untreated inappropriately.

Questions about such 'interactions' between patient characteristics and the effects of treatment are easy to ask, but are surprisingly difficult to answer reliably. Apparent interactions can often be produced by the play of chance and, in particular subgroups, can mimic or obscure some of the moderate treatment effects that might realistically be expected. To illustrate this, a subgroup analysis was performed based on the astrological birth signs of patients randomized in the very large Second International Study of Infarct Survival (ISIS-2) trial of aspirin for suspected acute myocardial infarction. Overall in this trial, the 1-month survival advantage produced by aspirin was conclusively demonstrated (804 vascular deaths among 8587 patients allocated aspirin vs 1016 among 8600 allocated no aspirin; 23% proportional reduction, two-sided p value $<0.000\,001$). However, when these analyses were subdivided into 12 subgroups by the patients' birth signs (in medieval Western astrology, the 'birth sign' is determined by the month of birth: e.g. 'Libra' means born 24 September to 23 October, and 'Gemini' means born 22 May to 21 June) to illustrate

Table 2.3.3.1 False-negative mortality effect in a subgroup defined only by the medieval astrological birth sign: the ISIS-2 (1988) trial of aspirin among over 17 000 patients with acute myocardial infarction

Astrological birth sign	No. of 1-month deaths (aspirin vs placebo)	Statistical significance
Libra or Gemini	150 vs 147	NS
All other signs	654 vs 869	$2p < 0.000001$
Any birth sign[a]	804 (9.4%) vs 1016 (11.8%)	$2p < 0.000001$

[a] Appropriate overall analysis for assessing the true effect in all subgroups. Medieval astrology divides birth dates into 12 'birth signs' (which depend only on the day and month of birth, not the year of birth). To demonstrate the potential unreliability of other subgroup analyses, the ISIS-2 patients were divided into 12 subgroups according to their astrological birth sign, and the apparent effects of aspirin were calculated separately in each of these 12 subgroups. Because of the play of chance the apparent effects differed from one subgroup to another, ranging from no apparent effect of aspirin in two subgroups (Libra and Gemini: see text for definition) to aspirin apparently halving mortality in another (Capricorn).

the unreliability of subgroup analyses, aspirin appeared totally ineffective for those born under Libra or Gemini (Table 2.3.3.1)! It would obviously be unwise to conclude from such a result that patients born under the astrological birth sign of Libra or Gemini should not be given aspirin if they have a heart attack. However, similar conclusions based on 'exploratory' data-derived subgroup analyses, which, from a purely statistical viewpoint, are no more reliable than these, are often reported and believed, with inappropriate effects on worldwide clinical practice.

There are three main remedies for this unavoidable conflict between the reliable subgroup-specific conclusions that doctors and patients want and need, and the statistically unreliable findings that direct subgroup analyses can usually offer. However, the extent to which these remedies are helpful in particular instances is one on which informed judgements differ.

First, where there are good *a priori* reasons for anticipating that the proportional effects of treatment might be very different in different circumstances then a limited number of subgroup analyses may be prespecified in the study protocol, along with a prediction of the direction of such proposed interactions. (For example, it was expected that the benefits of fibrinolytic therapy for acute myocardial infarction would be greater the earlier such patients were treated and so some studies prespecified that the analyses would be subdivided by the number of hours from the onset of symptoms to treatment: see later.) These prespecified subgroup-specific analyses can then be taken somewhat more seriously than other subgroup analyses, but they can still yield importantly wrong answers.

The second approach is to emphasize chiefly the overall results of a trial (or, better still, of all such trials) for the proportional reductions in particular outcomes, as a guide to—or at least a context for speculation about—the qualitative results in various specific subgroups of patients, and to give less weight to the actual results in each separate subgroup. This is clearly the right way to interpret the astrological 'findings' in Table 2.3.3.1, and if used sensibly, may also in many other circumstances provide the best assessment of whether one treatment is better than another in particular subgroups. The proportional effect of treatment as estimated from the overall results may well provide a useful approximation to the proportional effects of treatment in particular subgroups (and in future patients).

The third approach is to be influenced, in discussing the likely effects on mortality in specific subgroups, not only by the mortality analyses in these subgroups but also by the analyses of recurrence-free survival or some other major 'surrogate' outcome. For, if the overall results are similar but much more highly significant for recurrence-free survival than for mortality, subgroup analyses with respect to the former may be more stable and may provide a better guide as to whether there are any major differences between subgroups in the effects of treatment.

The appropriate interpretation of apparently different results in different subgroups of the randomized evidence is still one of the most difficult matters of judgement in the interpretation of randomized evidence; at present, many clinicians and regulatory agencies pay too much attention to irregularities in apparent effects that are consistent with chance.

Avoiding moderate random errors

The need for large-scale randomization

To distinguish reliably between the two alternatives that (1) there is no worthwhile difference in survival or that (2) treatment confers a moderate, but worthwhile, benefit (e.g. 10 or 20% fewer deaths), not only must systematic errors be guaranteed to be small (see above) compared with such a moderate risk reduction, but so too must any of the purely random errors that are produced just by chance. Random errors can be reliably avoided only by studying very large numbers of patients and hence large enough numbers of 'endpoints'. However, it is not sufficiently widely appreciated just how large clinical trials need to be in order to detect moderate differences reliably. This can be illustrated by a hypothetical trial that is actually quite inadequate—even though by some standards it is moderately large—in which a 20% reduction in mortality (from 10% to 8%) is supposed to be detected among 2000 heart attack patients (1000 treated and 1000 controls). In this case, one might predict about 100 deaths (10%) in the control group and 80 deaths (8%) in the treated group. However, if this difference were to be observed it would not be conventionally significant ($p = 0.1$); indicating that even if there is no real difference between the effects of the trial treatments, it would still be relatively easy for a result at least as extreme as this to arise by chance alone. Although the play of chance might well increase the difference enough to make it conventionally significant (e.g. 110 deaths vs 70 deaths, $2p < 0.001$), it might equally well dilute, obliterate (e.g. 90 deaths vs 90 deaths), or even reverse it. The situation in real life is often even worse, as the average trial size may include only a few dozen events rather than the several hundred (or few thousand) that would ideally be needed to guide the future treatment of millions.

Mega-trials: how to randomize large numbers

One of the chief techniques for obtaining appropriately large-scale randomized evidence is to make trials extremely simple, and then to invite hundreds of hospitals to collaborate. The first of these large streamlined trials (or mega-trials) were the ISIS and GISSI studies of heart attack treatment in the 1980s, and many other mega-trials have now been successfully undertaken, not only in the field of cardiology—where numerous large trials have already been performed—but also in other specialties where treatment might be expected to have only moderate effects on morbidity and mortality from a common disease or injury. Many such mega-trials have produced medically important results that would not otherwise have been reliably obtained. However, in terms of medically significant findings, what has been achieved so far is only a fraction of what would be possible if this research strategy could be more widely adopted. Any obstacle to simplicity is an obstacle to large size, and so it is worth making enormous efforts at the design stage to simplify and streamline the process of entering, treating, and assessing patients. Many trials would be of much greater scientific value if they collected 10 times less information, both at entry and during follow-up, on 10 times more patients. Since those responsible for entering patients into trials are generally busy people, it is particularly important to simplify the entry of patients, otherwise rapid recruitment may prove difficult (see later). Likewise, when allocating resources within large-scale trials, it is important to direct them to where it chiefly matters, namely the recruitment of large numbers of patients and counting how many suffer the main outcomes of interest, instead of wasting large sums of money on inappropriate audits or unnecessary or excessively frequent measurements, the analysis of which will contribute little to answering the main study question.

Simplification of entry procedures for trials: the 'uncertainty principle'

For ethical reasons, patients cannot have a commonly available treatment chosen at random for them if either they or their doctor are (for any reasons) already reasonably certain that another treatment is preferable. Hence, randomization can be offered only if both doctor and patient feel substantially uncertain as to which of the trial options is best. The question then arises, 'Which categories of patients about whose treatment there is such uncertainty should be offered randomization?' The obvious answer is all of them, welcoming the heterogeneity that this will produce. (For example, either the treatment of choice will turn out to be the same for men and women, in which case the trial might as well include both, or it will be different, in which case it is particularly important to study both.) In appropriately large trials, patient homogeneity is generally a defect while heterogeneity is generally a strength. Consider, for example, the trials of immediate fibrinolytic therapy for acute myocardial infarction. Some had restrictive entry criteria that allowed inclusion of only those patients who presented between 0 and 6 h after the onset of pain, and those trials contributed almost nothing to the key question of how late such treatment can still be useful. In contrast, the trials with wider and more heterogeneous entry criteria that included some patients with somewhat longer delays between pain onset and hospitalization were able to show that fibrinolytic therapy can have definite protective effects not only when given 0 to 6 h but also when given 7 to 12 h after the onset of pain (see later).

This approach of randomizing the full range of patients in whom there is substantial uncertainty as to which treatment option is best was used in the first Medical Research Council Asymptomatic Carotid Surgery Trial (ACST-1). Narrowing of the carotid artery (which is rapidly detectable by ultrasound) can eventually cause a stroke, or even a succession of strokes. It can be dealt with surgically by carotid endarterectomy, but in the 1990s there was much uncertainty as to whether such surgery, with its inherent perioperative risks, was appropriate for individuals with severe carotid artery narrowing who were currently asymptomatic (i.e. had not had a stroke in the past few months). The ACST was therefore designed to compare a policy of immediate carotid endarterectomy versus a policy of 'watchful waiting' in asymptomatic patients with substantial carotid artery narrowing. If a patient was prepared at least to consider surgery seriously, then the neurologist and surgeon responsible for that individual's care considered in their own undefined way whatever medical, personal, or other factors seemed to them to be relevant, including, of course, the patient's own preferences and values. Eligibility for randomization was defined by the 'uncertainty principle' (Fig. 2.3.3.2):

- If they or the patient were reasonably certain, for any reason, that they *did wish* to recommend immediate surgery for that particular patient, the patient was not eligible for entry into the ACST.
- Conversely, if they or the patient were reasonably certain, for any reason, that they *did not wish* to recommend immediate surgery, the patient was likewise not eligible for entry into the trial.
- If, but only if, the doctor(s) and patient were *substantially uncertain* what to recommend, the patient was automatically eligible for randomization between immediate vs no immediate surgery (with all patients receiving whatever their doctors judged to be the best available medical care, which generally included advice to stop smoking, low-dose aspirin, treatment of hypertension; and, in the latter years of the trial, a statin).

In ACST-1, there were substantial differences between individual doctors in the types of patient about whom they were uncertain (in terms of the severity of carotid stenosis [which was generally recorded on ultrasound as 70%, 80%, or 90% blockage], age, general health and various other characteristics). This guaranteed that no category of patient about which there was widespread uncertainty would be wholly excluded, and hence guaranteed that the trial would yield at least some direct evidence in a wide range of typical patients. As a result of the wide and simple entry criteria adopted by ACST-1, 3120 patients were randomized (which was more than in any previous vascular surgery trial), so the study was able to provide some clear answers about who needed carotid endarterectomy. In asymptomatic patients younger than 75 years of age, with carotid diameter about 70% or more on ultrasound, immediate carotid endarterectomy halved the net 5-year stroke risk from about 12% to 6% (even though this 6% included the 3% perioperative hazard). For patients with only moderate carotid artery stenosis on ultrasound, the 5-year risks of carotid stroke (excluding perioperative hazard) were 2% vs 9%, whilst among those with tighter stenosis the risks were 3% vs 10%, suggesting about as much benefit in moderate as in tight stenosis.

The 'uncertainty principle' simultaneously meets the requirements of ethicality, heterogeneity, simplicity and maximal trial size, and should be widely used. It states that the fundamental eligibility criterion is that both doctor and patient should be substantially uncertain about the appropriateness of each of the trial treatments for that particular patient. With such uncertainty as the fundamental criterion of eligibility, informed consent can often be simplified. For, the degree of 'informed consent' that is appropriate in a randomized comparison of two established treatments governed by the 'uncertainty principle' should probably not differ greatly from that which is applied in routine practice outside trials when treatment is being chosen haphazardly—or, to put it another way, 'double standards' between trial and non-trial situations are inappropriate. The haphazard nature of many

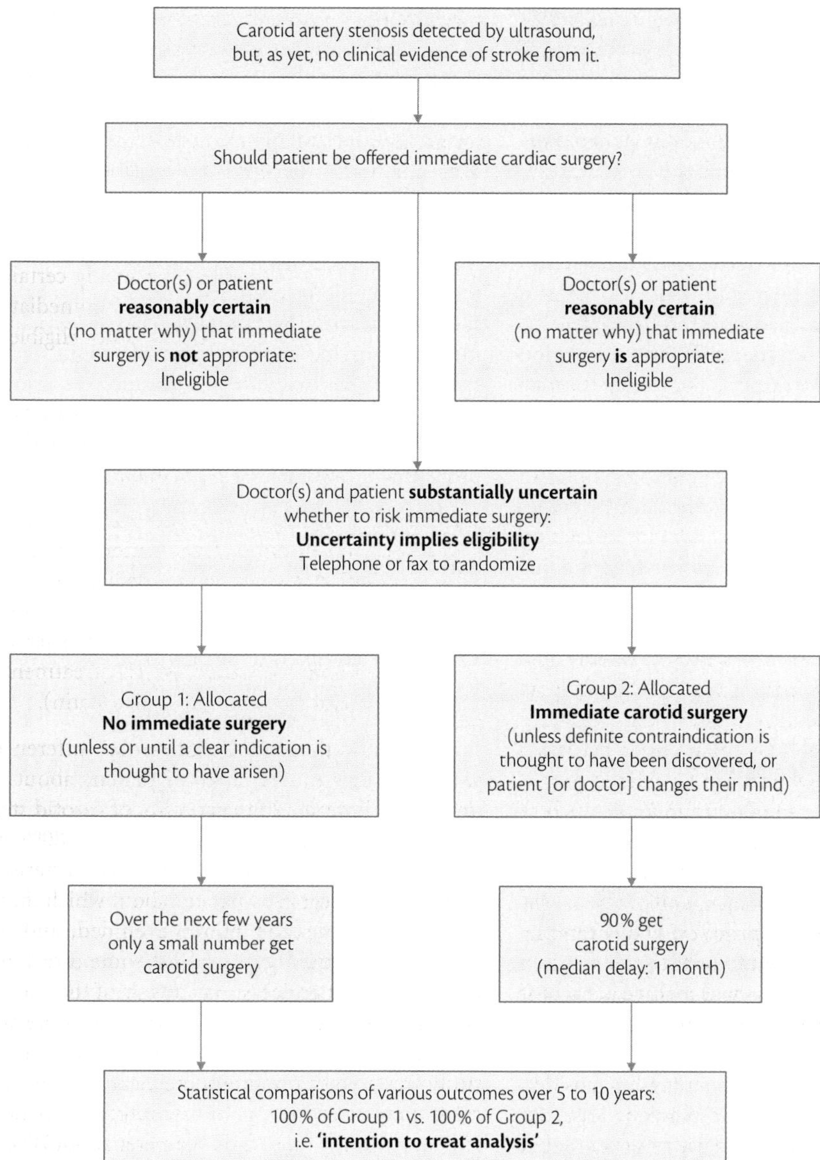

Fig. 2.3.3.2 Example of the 'uncertainty principle' to define eligibility for trial entry: the chief eligibility criterion for the Asymptomatic Carotid Surgery Trial (ACST) was that doctors and patients should be substantially uncertain whether to risk immediate carotid surgery. Partly because this criterion was appropriately flexible, ACST-1 became the largest-ever trial of vascular surgery, showing that the long-term benefits of carotid artery surgery could eventually outweigh the immediate hazards. ACST-2 (http://www.acst.org) is now randomizing surgery vs carotid stenting where the doctor(s) and patient are substantially uncertain which to prefer.

nonrandomized treatment choices is reflected in the wide variations in practice between and within countries. Even when a practice is similar, it may be similarly wrong: e.g. before the ISIS-2 results became available (see later), few doctors routinely used fibrinolytic therapy for acute myocardial infarction. Provided that trials are governed by the 'uncertainty principle', there is an approximate parallel between good science and good ethics. Indeed, in such circumstances, excessively detailed consent procedures (which can be distressing and inhumane, and so would not be considered appropriate in routine nontrial clinical practice) would not be humane or ethically appropriate in trials. Excessively detailed consent procedures are, unfortunately, quite common, but their chief purpose is to protect doctors against lawyers rather than to protect patients against anything.

This 'uncertainty principle' is just one of many ways of simplifying trials and thereby helping them to avoid becoming enmeshed in a mass of wholly unnecessary traditional complexity. If randomized trials can be substantially simplified (which, it must be admitted, requires a reversal of the current trend towards unnecessary complexity), as has already been achieved for a few major diseases, and hence made very much larger, then they will continue to play an appropriately central role in the development of rational criteria for planning treatment strategies and reducing death and disability.

Minimizing both bias and random error: meta-analyses of randomized trials

Archie Cochrane was one of the first people to emphasize the need to organize, by specialty, the results from all relevant randomized trials, and the Cochrane Library brings together in a single place a large number of systematic reviews (many of which include meta-analyses of randomized trials) summarizing the available evidence about a wide range of therapeutic questions. When several trials have all addressed much the same question, the traditional procedure of only a few of them becoming widely known may be a source of serious bias, since chance fluctuations for or against treatment may affect which trials become well known and widely cited.

To avoid this problem, it is appropriate to base inference chiefly on a meta-analysis of all the results from all of the trials that have addressed a particular type of question (or on an unbiased subset of such trials), and not on some potentially biased subset of these trials. Such meta-analyses will also minimize random errors in the assessment of treatment since, in general, far more patients are involved in a meta-analysis than in any contributory individual trial.

The separate trials may well be heterogeneous in their entry criteria, their treatment schedules, their follow-up procedures, their methods of treating relapse, etc. In view of this heterogeneity, at one extreme each trial might be considered in virtual isolation from all others, while at the opposite extreme the results from all trials could be combined, largely ignoring any heterogeneity. Both these extreme views have some merit, and the pursuit of each by different people may prove more illuminating than too definite an insistence on any one particular approach. However, the heterogeneity of the different trials merely argues for careful interpretation of any meta-analyses of different trial results, rather than arguing against meta-analyses. For, whatever the difficulties in interpreting meta-analyses may be, without them it is difficult to avoid moderate selective biases and substantial random errors, both of which could obscure any moderate treatment effects, or, conversely, imply an effect where none exists.

Which meta-analyses are trustworthy?

Since the 1970s, a rapidly increasing number of meta-analyses of the results of randomized trials have been reported, not all of which are trustworthy. When considering how reliable a given one might be there are two fundamental questions: what is the potential for bias, and what is the potential size of purely random errors? To answer the first question consideration must be given to whether biases might exist within individual trials (e.g. because of an unreliable method of randomization or because of postrandomization exclusions from the main analyses), and whether the subset of trials under consideration might be a biased subset of all relevant trials that have been performed (as might arise, for example, if certain trials were abandoned because of unpromising findings, or remained unpublished for this or any other reason).

The simplest approach to meta-analysis is merely to have collected and tabulated the published data from whatever randomized trial reports are easily accessible in the literature, and sometimes this may suffice. At the opposite extreme, extensive efforts may have been made by those organizing the meta-analysis to locate every potentially relevant randomized trial, including those never published, to collaborate closely with the trialists to seek individual data on each patient ever randomized into those trials, and then (after extensive checks and corrections of such data) to produce, in collaborative re-analyses with those trialists, agreed analyses and publications. The results of some of the largest such collaborative re-analyses will be described later: the Anti-Thrombotic Trialists' (ATT) Collaborative Group, the Fibrinolytic Therapy Trialists' (FTT) Collaborative Group, and the Early Breast Cancer Trialists' Collaborative Group (EBCTCG). Collaboration of the original trialists in the meta-analysis process, with collection of detailed data from each individual trial participant, can help to avoid or minimize the biases that could be produced by missing trials (e.g. owing to the greater likelihood of extremely good, or extremely bad, results being particularly widely known and published), by inappropriate post-randomization withdrawals, or by the failure to allocate treatment properly at random. If randomization was performed properly in the first place, the post-randomization withdrawals can often be followed up and restored to the study for an appropriate 'intention-to-treat' analysis. Knowledge of the exact methods of treatment allocation (backed up by checks on whether the main prognostic factors recorded are nonrandomly distributed between the treatment groups in a particular trial) may help to identify trials that were so improperly randomized that they should be excluded from a meta-analysis of the properly randomized trials. Meta-analyses based on individual patient data may also provide more information about treatment effects than the more usual overviews of grouped data, for they allow more detailed analyses—indeed, if they are really large then they may actually yield statistically reliable subgroup analyses of the effects of treatment in particular types of patient.

Conversely, even a perfectly conducted meta-analysis of an intervention with moderate effects on a major clinical outcome may not be reliable if the trials were all small. There are two reasons for this. First, when the true effect of an intervention is only moderate, most small trials will fail to reach statistical significance, and may be less likely to be published (or otherwise available) than the few with results that are misleadingly extreme. Hence, a meta-analysis consisting exclusively of small trials is particularly prone to bias. Secondly, the random errors may be too large to allow reliable interpretation. A meta-analysis that includes a total of only 100 deaths will have random errors about as great as a single trial with only 100 deaths. For these reasons small-scale evidence, whether from a meta-analysis or from one trial, is often unreliable and may well be found in retrospect to have yielded wrong answers. What is needed is large-scale randomized evidence; it does not matter much whether the totality of the evidence comes from a properly conducted meta-analysis of several trials or one properly conducted trial with such clear results that no further trials were done. The practical medical value of large-scale randomized evidence will be illustrated by a few examples.

Examples of important results in the treatment of vascular disease that could have been reliably established only by large-scale randomized evidence

Definite result from a single very large trial: benefit from medium-dose aspirin for patients with acute myocardial infarction (with benefits among other types of patient indicated by meta-analyses of smaller trials)

In the ISIS-2 trial, half of 17 000 patients with suspected acute myocardial infarction were allocated aspirin tablets (162 mg/day for 1 month, which virtually completely inhibits cyclooxygenase-dependent platelet activation) and half were allocated placebo tablets. Before 1988, when the ISIS-2 results were published, aspirin was not routinely used in the treatment of acute myocardial infarction, and no other major trial had (or has subsequently) compared aspirin with an untreated control group in cases of suspected acute myocardial infarction. However, the effects of 1 month of aspirin were so definite in ISIS-2 (804/8587 vascular deaths among those who were allocated aspirin vs 1016/8600 among those who

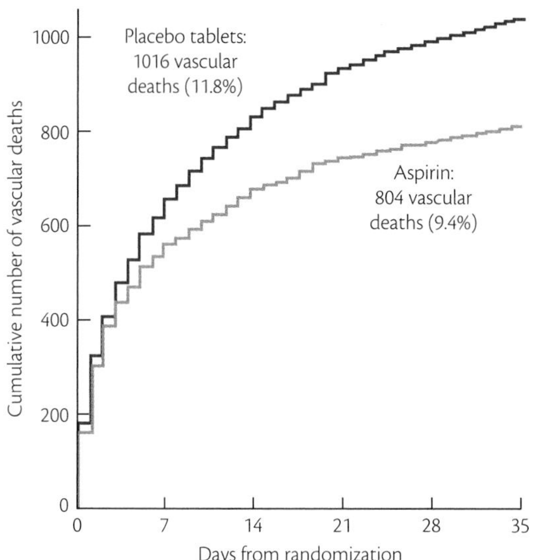

Fig. 2.3.3.3 Effect of administration of aspirin for 1 month on 35-day mortality in the 1988 ISIS-2 trial among 17 000 patients with acute myocardial infarction. (Absolute survival advantage: 24 SE 5 lives saved per 1000 patients allocated aspirin, 2*p*<0.00001. The COMMIT trial in 46 000 such patients has since shown aspirin plus clopidogrel to be slightly more effective than aspirin alone.)

were not) that even the lower 99% confidence limit would have represented a worthwhile benefit from this simple and inexpensive treatment (Fig. 2.3.3.3).

As a result, worldwide treatment patterns changed sharply when the ISIS-2 results emerged in 1988, and aspirin is now routinely used for the majority of emergency hospital admissions with suspected acute myocardial infarction not only in Europe and America but throughout Asia. In the United Kingdom, for example, two British Heart Foundation surveys found cardiologists reporting that routine aspirin use in acute coronary care had increased from under 10% in 1987 to over 90% in 1989. Worldwide, the annual number of patients with suspected myocardial infarction who would nowadays be given such treatment must be several million a year, suggesting that aspirin is already preventing several tens of thousands of premature deaths each year in this clinical context alone. However, if the ISIS-2 trial had been a factor of 10 smaller (i.e. 1700 instead of 17 000 patients), then exactly the same proportional reduction in mortality as shown in Fig. 2.3.3.3 would not have been conventionally significant and, therefore, would have been much less likely to influence medical practice—indeed, the result might by chance have appeared exactly flat, greatly damaging future research on aspirin in this context. (In fact, during the early interim monitoring of the ISIS-2 trial results by the independent Data Monitoring Committee there was no apparent difference in mortality on the basis of the first few hundred deaths.) Likewise, if the ISIS-2 trial had been nonrandomized, then it might well have produced the wrong answer since, in a nonrandomized study, doctors might tend to give active treatment to patients who are particularly ill, or who are rather different in various other ways from those not given active treatment. In addition, even if a nonrandomized study did happen to produce an unbiased answer, it would have been impossible to be sure that it had actually done so, so again a nonrandomized study might have had much less influence on medical practice than ISIS-2 did.

In the ISIS-2 trial, aspirin significantly reduced the 1-month mortality, but it also significantly reduced the number of nonfatal strokes and nonfatal reinfarctions that were recorded in hospital. Combining all these three outcomes into 'vascular events' (i.e. stroke, death, or reinfarction), 10% of those who were allocated aspirin vs 14% of the controls suffered a vascular event in the month after randomization (Table 2.3.3.2)—an absolute difference of 40 events per 1000 treated (or, perhaps more relevantly, 40 000 per million). The randomized trials of aspirin, or of other antiplatelet regimens, in other types of high-risk patients (e.g. a few years of aspirin for those who have survived a myocardial infarction or stroke) were not as large as ISIS-2, and so, taken separately, most yielded false-negative results. However, when the results from many such trials are combined, statistically definite reductions in 'vascular events' are seen (Table 2.3.3.2). Since such treatments do not appear to increase nonvascular mortality, all-cause mortality is also significantly reduced. More recently, a combination of aspirin and clopidogrel (which inhibits platelet activation through different pathways) has been shown to be slightly more effective than aspirin alone in acute myocardial infarction or acute coronary syndrome (Table 2.3.3.2).

The large-scale randomized evidence on anti-platelet drugs that is summarized in Table 2.3.3.2 has changed clinical practice worldwide, and may already have affected the treatment of hundreds of millions of patients in ways that, at low cost, have prevented millions of strokes, heart attacks, or vascular deaths. Small randomized trials and small meta-analyses of trials, or nonrandomized studies (however large), could not possibly have provided appropriately reliable evidence about such moderate risk reductions.

Definite result from a very large meta-analysis of trials: benefit from 'adjuvant' therapy with tamoxifen for patients with hormone-sensitive (ER-positive) 'early' breast cancer

By definition, in 'early' breast cancer all detectable deposits of disease are limited to the breast and the local or regional lymph nodes, and can be removed surgically. However, experience shows that undetectably small deposits of breast cancer cells may remain elsewhere that eventually cause clinical recurrence at a distant site, perhaps after a delay of several years, which is then usually followed by death from the disease. If the original tumour was 'ER-positive' (i.e. if the tumour cells were still expressing the oestrogen receptor protein) then the distant deposits of cancer cells that spread from it before it was removed may also be ER-positive, and may be continually stimulated by circulating hormones. Therefore, among women who have had breast cancer removed by surgery (or by surgery and radiotherapy), there have been many trials of 'adjuvant' daily treatment with tamoxifen, a drug that blocks the oestrogen receptor. Some involved only 1 to 2 years of treatment, some involved about 5 years, some compared 5 years vs 1 to 2 years and some that are still in progress compare 10 years vs 5 years of tamoxifen: in total, more than 100 000 women have been randomized in several dozen such trials.

Taken separately, most of these tamoxifen trials have been too small to provide reliable evidence about long-term survival. However, if the results of all of them are combined in various ways, some very definite differences emerge: 1 to 2 years of tamoxifen is better than nothing, 5 years is better than 1 to 2 years, and 10 years may be better still for delaying or avoiding the recurrence of

Table 2.3.3.2 Summary results of (a) trials of aspirin (or other antiplatelet drugs), and (b) trials of adding clopidogrel to aspirin

Type of patient	Study	Mean duration (total randomized)	Stroke, heart attack, or vascular death		
(a) Antiplatelet vs control			Antiplatelet (%)	Control (%)	Difference
Acute heart attack	ISIS-2	1 month (20 000)	10	14	40 per 1000 ($2p < 0.00001$)
Acute stroke	CAST and IST	1 month (40 000)	9	10	10 per 1000 ($2p = 0.001$)
Previous heart attack	ATT	2 years (20 000)	13	17	40 per 1000 ($2p < 0.00001$)
Previous stroke/TIA	ATT	2.5 years (23 000)	18	22	40 per 1000 ($2p < 0.00001$)
Other high risk (e.g. angina, peripheral vascular disease)	ATT	1 year (20 000)	8	10	20 per 1000 ($2p < 0.00001$)
(b) Aspirin plus clopidogrel vs aspirin alone			Aspirin + clopidogrel (%)	Aspirin alone (%)	
Acute coronary syndrome	CURE	9 months (13 000)	9	11	20 per 1000 ($2p < 0.001$)
Acute heart attack	CCS2-COMMIT	1 month (46 000)	9	10	10 per 1000 ($2p = 0.002$)

ER+ breast cancer (and, newer endocrine therapies may well have somewhat better effects than tamoxifen). Figure 2.3.3.4a shows the results from the trials of about 5 years of tamoxifen. Allocation to active treatment produces a 13% absolute difference in the 15-year risk of recurrence (34 vs 47%), and a 9% absolute difference in survival (25 vs 34%; both $2p < 0.00001$). Most of the effect on recurrence is seen during the first 5 years, while tamoxifen was still continuing to be given, but most of the effect on breast cancer mortality comes after this period (Fig. 2.3.3.4a). Indeed, the difference in the 15-year probability of death from breast cancer is about three times as great as that in the 5-year probability. Reliable assessment of the moderate improvements in long-term survival in early breast cancer that are produced by tamoxifen (and by radiotherapy and chemotherapy) would have been impossible without such a meta-analysis of all trials, with updated follow-up data provided periodically, because each of the trials was too small on its own to answer these questions convincingly.

Collaborative meta-analyses that involve hundreds of trialists from all around the world can also foster international acceptance of the totality of the randomized evidence. In the case of breast cancer this has, since the mid-1980s, helped lead to widespread adoption in many countries of a succession of improvements in treatment (earlier detection, better local control, progressively better chemotherapy and, in ER-positive disease, progressively better endocrine therapy). These have, in aggregate, resulted in a sustained fall in national mortality rates (Fig. 2.3.3.4b).

Promising meta-analysis of small trials confirmed by large trials: benefit from fibrinolytic therapy in acute myocardial infarction

If a recent thrombus has just blocked a coronary artery, thereby causing acute myocardial ischaemia or infarction, fibrinolytic drugs (such as streptokinase or tissue plasminogen activator) can sometimes rapidly dissolve the thrombus, restoring the flow of blood and reperfusing the heart muscle. These drugs were first introduced into clinical research in the late 1950s, but the trials of fibrinolytic therapy for suspected acute myocardial infarction in the 1960s and 1970s were too small to be statistically reliable (none involved even 1000 patients). So, by the early 1980s the haemorrhagic side effects were obvious, the benefits had not been convincingly demonstrated, and such treatments were generally considered to be definitely dangerous, probably fairly ineffective, and hence inappropriate for routine coronary care. Although meta-analyses published in the mid 1980s of the previous small trials (which had involved a total of only *c.*6000 patients in 24 trials) indicated a statistically definite benefit, they were not really believed by cardiologists and so such treatments were still not widely used. The situation was saved by two large randomized trials, GISSI-1 and ISIS-2, which together involved about 30 000 patients (and by their aggregation with the seven other randomized trials that each involved more than 1000 patients, yielding a total of 60 000; see below). In ISIS-2, not only were patients randomly allocated to receive aspirin or placebo tablets as described earlier (Fig. 2.3.3.3), but also they were separately allocated to receive intravenous streptokinase or a placebo infusion. In this 'factorial' design (which allows the separate assessment of more than one treatment without any material loss in the statistical reliability of each comparison), one-quarter of the patients were allocated aspirin alone, one-quarter were allocated streptokinase alone, one-quarter were allocated both streptokinase and aspirin, and one-quarter were allocated neither (i.e. they were given placebo tablets and a placebo infusion). Streptokinase, like aspirin, produced a highly significant reduction in mortality, and the combination of streptokinase and aspirin was highly significantly better than either aspirin alone or streptokinase alone (Fig. 2.3.3.5).

The results shown in Fig. 2.3.3.5 might suggest that there was no need to collect any more randomized evidence about fibrinolytic therapy, but this ignores the potential hazards of such treatment and the heterogeneity of patients. Taken separately, even ISIS-2 (the largest of these trials) was not large enough for statistically

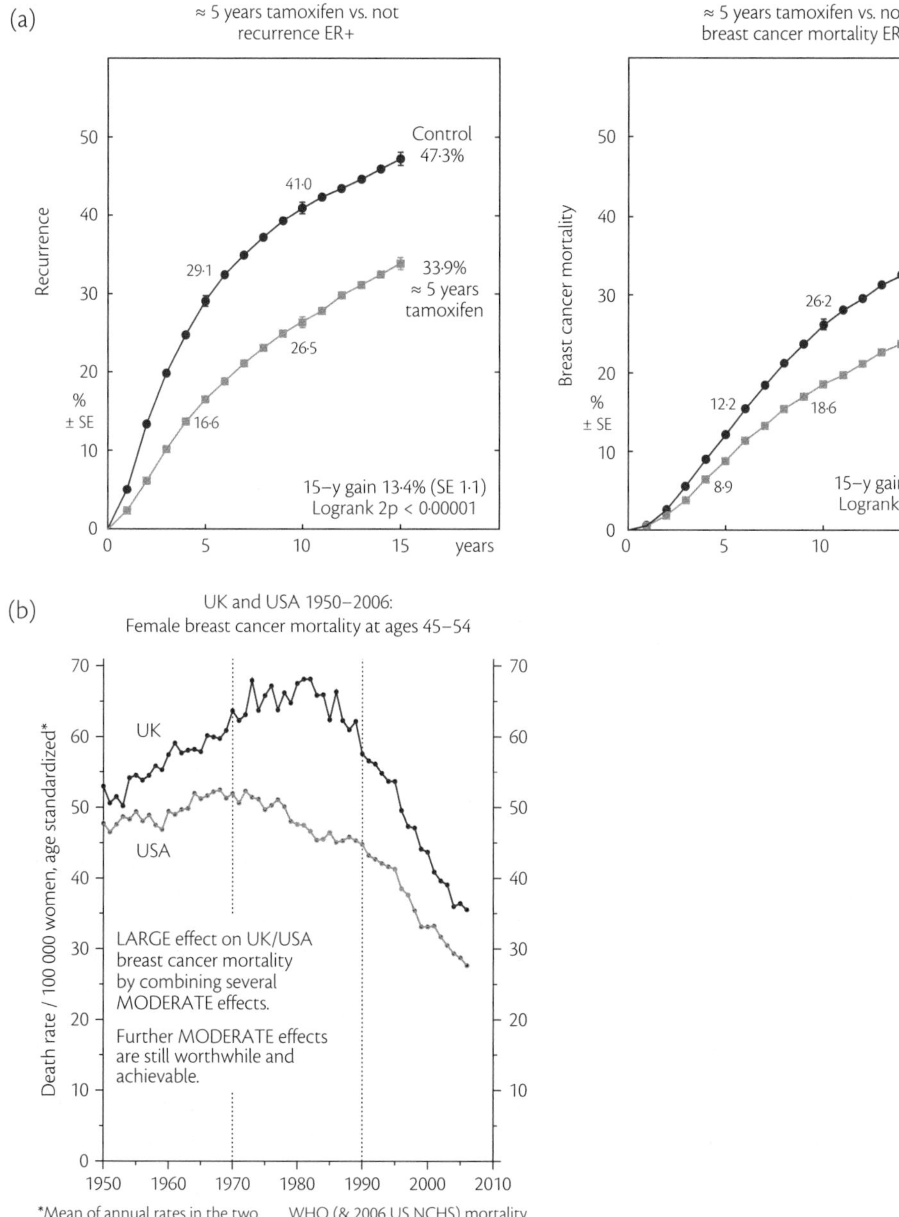

Fig. 2.3.3.4 (a) Effects of about 5 years of tamoxifen vs not in ER-positive disease: 15-year probabilities of recurrence and of breast cancer mortality (10 000 women in the 2005 worldwide EBCTCG meta-analysis). (b) Female breast cancer mortality in the United Kingdom and the United States of America at ages 45–54 during the period 1950–2006. (The United Kingdom breast screening programme has little effect on mortality at these ages.)

reliable subgroup analyses, but when the nine largest trials were all taken together they included a total of about 60 000 patients, half of whom had been randomly allocated fibrinolytic therapy. Those entering a coronary care unit with a diagnosis of suspected or definite acute myocardial infarction range from patients who are already in cardiogenic shock with low blood pressure and a fast pulse (half of whom will die rapidly) to those who have merely had a history of chest pain and no very definite changes on their ECG (of whom 'only' a small percentage will die before discharge). Fibrinolytic therapy often causes blood pressure to fall: should it be used in patients who are already dangerously hypotensive? It occasionally causes serious strokes: should it be used in patients who are elderly or hypertensive, and therefore already have an above-average risk of cerebral haemorrhage (or who have only slight changes on their ECG, and therefore have only a low risk of cardiac death)? Finally, if a coronary artery has been totally occluded for long enough, the heart muscle that it supplies will have been irreversibly destroyed: how many hours after the heart attack starts is fibrinolytic treatment still worth risking—3? 6? 12? 24?

These questions needed to be answered reliably before appropriate and generally accepted indications for and against such an immediately hazardous, but potentially effective, therapy could be devised. To address them, the main fibrinolytic therapy trialists collaborated in a systematic meta-analysis of the randomized evidence, based on individual patient data. On review of the 60 000 patients randomized between fibrinolytic therapy and control in trials of more than 1000 patients, some of the therapeutic questions were relatively easy to answer satisfactorily. For example, it appears that most of those whose ECG is still normal (or shows a pattern that indicates only a small immediate risk of death) can be left untreated, leaving open the option of starting fibrinolytic treatment urgently if their ECG changes suddenly for the worse over the

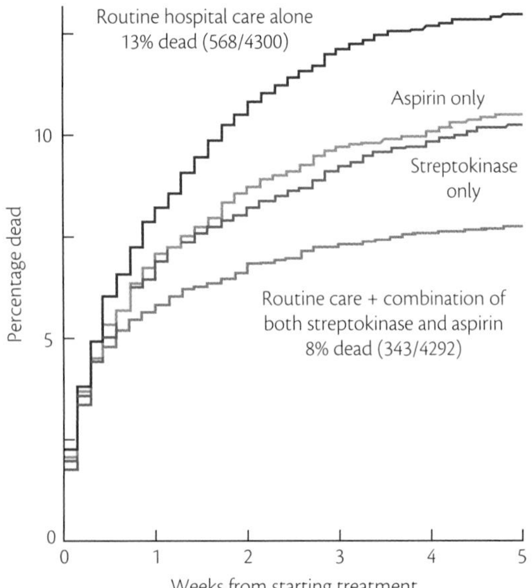

Fig. 2.3.3.5 Effects of a 1-h streptokinase infusion, and of aspirin for about 1 month, on 35-day mortality in the 1988 ISIS-2 trial among 17 000 patients with acute myocardial infarction who would not normally have received either treatment, divided at random into four similar groups to receive aspirin only, streptokinase only, both or neither.

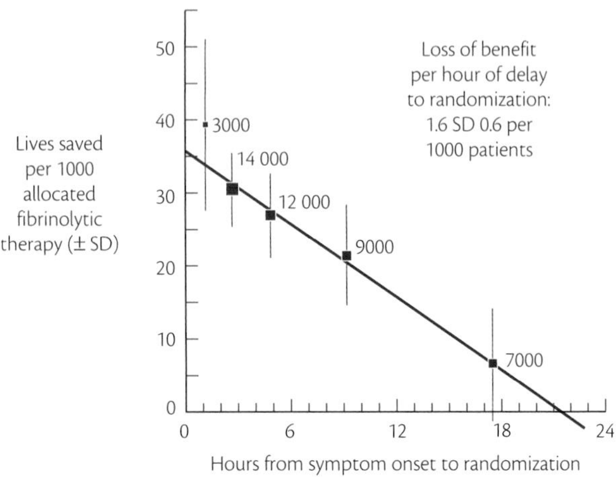

Fig. 2.3.3.6 Benefit vs delay (0–1, 2–3, 4–6, 7–12, or 13–24 h) in the nine largest randomized trials of fibrinolytic therapy vs control in patients with acute myocardial infarction. 1-month mortality results for 45 000 patients with ST elevation or bundle-branch block when randomized, showing the definite net benefit even for the 9000 randomized 7–12 h after the onset of pain.

next few hours or days. Conversely, among those who already had 'high-risk' ECG changes when they were randomized, the absolute benefit of immediate fibrinolytic therapy was, if anything, slightly greater than is indicated by Fig. 2.3.3.5. Age, sex, blood pressure, heart rate, diabetes, and a previous history of myocardial infarction could not identify reliably any subgroup that would not, on average, have their chances of survival appreciably increased by treatment.

By contrast, the longer that fibrinolytic treatment for such patients was delayed the less benefit it seemed to produce. Among the 45 000 whose ECG showed definite ST-segment elevation or bundle-branch block, the benefit was greatest (about 30 lives saved per 1000) among those randomized between 0 and 6 h after the onset of pain (Fig. 2.3.3.6).

However, the mortality reduction was still substantial and significant (about 20 per 1000; $2p$ <0.003) for the patients whose hospital admission had been delayed for some hours and who were therefore randomized 7 to 12 h after the onset of pain. Indeed, even if patients were randomized 13–18 h after the onset of pain, there still appeared to be some net reduction in mortality (about 10 per 1000, but not statistically definite). The regression line in Fig. 2.3.3.6 reinforces these separate subgroup analyses in a more reliable way. Yet, before these large trials it was forcefully, but mistakenly, argued that such treatments could not possibly be of any worthwhile benefit if given more than about 3 or 4 h after the onset of symptoms.

Such detailed inferences are difficult enough with large-scale properly randomized evidence, and would be impossible without it. Because of their unknowable biases (see above), nonrandomized database analyses are simply not a viable alternative to large-scale randomized evidence. Nor would randomization of 'only' several thousand patients have been sufficient. The availability of large-scale randomized evidence, in this case a meta-analysis involving about 6000 deaths among 60 000 patients, has been essential in determining which particular types of patient derive net benefit from fibrinolytic therapy.

Promising meta-analysis of small trials refuted by large trials: lack of significant benefit from magnesium infusion in acute myocardial infarction

In animal studies, infusion of a magnesium salt can limit the myocardial damage arising from sudden experimental blockage of a coronary artery. By the early 1990s, there was considerable optimism that a simple, inexpensive magnesium infusion might prove beneficial after acute myocardial infarction. Twelve small trials, involving between them a total of only about 2000 patients, had addressed this question, and their aggregated results indicated a highly statistically significant—but implausibly large—halving of risk (72/1199 deaths among those allocated magnesium vs 151/1191 among the controls, $2p$ <0.00001). At this time some argued that such results constituted proof beyond reasonable doubt that magnesium was of sufficient value to justify its widespread usage without seeking further randomized evidence, but others remained sceptical, arguing that the apparent results were far too good to be true.

Two trials, one (LIMIT-2) involving 2000 patients and one (ISIS-4) involving 58 000, were then set up to test the possible effects of magnesium more reliably. The first yielded a moderately promising result (Fig. 2.3.3.7), indicating avoidance of about one-quarter of the early deaths, but with its 99% confidence interval including the possibility that magnesium had no beneficial effect on early mortality. The second (which had continued in spite of intense lobbying of its data monitoring committee to stop the trial), however, yielded a completely unpromising result, so that the overall evidence, by that time based on over 60 000 randomized patients, indicated no net effect on mortality.

Nevertheless, some cardiologists remained hopeful that magnesium might prove to be effective among specific subgroups. Accordingly the MAGnesium In Coronaries (MAGIC) trial subsequently randomized 6000 patients, all of whom had received reperfusion therapy within the past few hours, to magnesium vs placebo, but this also found no evidence of any net benefit.

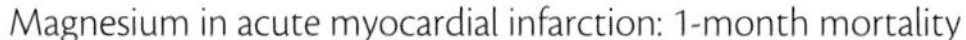

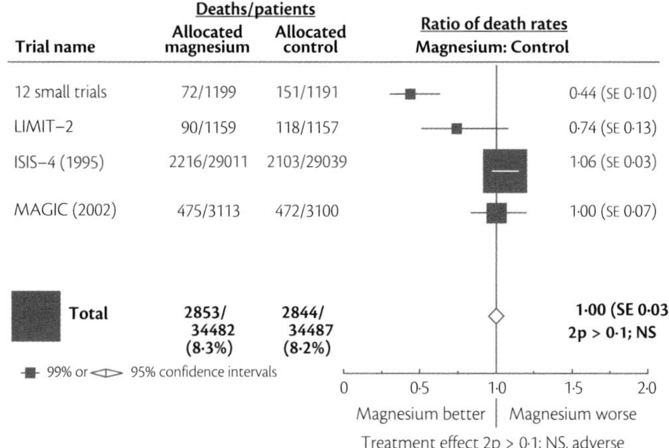

Fig. 2.3.3.7 Effect of a magnesium infusion on 1-month mortality among patients with acute myocardial infarction. Ratio of the death rate in the treatment group to that in the control group is plotted for each trial (as a black square with area proportional to the amount of statistical information) along with its 99% confidence interval (horizontal line). A stratified overview of the results of all these trials (and its 95% confidence interval) is represented by an open diamond.

It is interesting to consider what this sequence of magnesium trial results (Fig. 2.3.3.6) might mean for those wishing to interpret other randomized evidence. Our interpretation is that if something seems too good to be true then it probably is—or, more formally, that big benefits are often much less plausible than moderate benefits. None of the 12 small trials had sufficient power to detect a moderate effect on mortality, and although their aggregated results indicated that mortality could be reduced by more than half, such an effect is too extreme to be plausible, and could be misleading even though it is highly significant. The LIMIT-2 trial then suggested that magnesium might reduce mortality by about a quarter, a result that is somewhat more plausible but not clearly significant. The success of the ISIS-4 and MAGIC trials in refuting the implausibly large benefit suggested by the 13 smaller trials reinforces our point that often, when trying to distinguish between the two medically realistic possibilities of a moderate effect or no effect, only large-scale evidence suffices. Even the LIMIT-2 trial, which recruited 2000 patients, was in retrospect too small. (Another important methodological point is that 'random effects' methods for meta-analysis can produce importantly wrong answers: applied to the 15 separate trials in Fig. 2.3.3.7, a standard 'random effects' meta-analysis yields a summary odds ratio of 0.67 (95% CI 0.52–0.85; $2p < 0.001$), suggesting—clearly incorrectly—that magnesium reduces mortality by about one-third!)

Trials in their epidemiological context: blood pressure, stroke, and heart disease

Quantitative epidemiological evidence about the effects of long-term differences in risk factors such as blood pressure or blood cholesterol level can help in interpreting the results from trials of the effects of reducing these risk factors for only a few years. For example, appropriate meta-analyses of prospective observational epidemiological studies indicate that, throughout the range of usual systolic blood pressure in the populations studied (about 115–180 mmHg), a lower value is associated with a lower risk of ischaemic heart disease, with no apparent 'threshold' in this range below which the relationship reversed (Fig. 2.3.3.8). This analysis suggests that, in later middle age (60–69 years), 10 mmHg lower systolic blood pressure is associated with about 27% less mortality from ischaemic heart disease (and about 35% less stroke mortality: Prospective Studies Collaboration, data not shown).

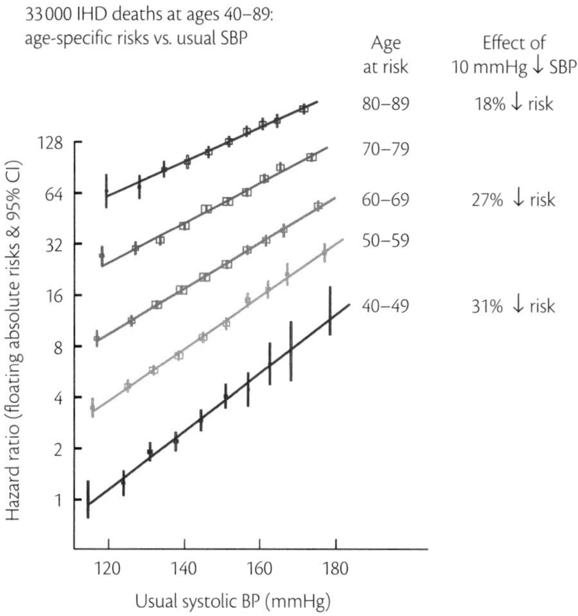

Fig. 2.3.3.8 Stroke and ischaemic heart disease mortality rate in each decade of age vs usual systolic blood pressure (SBP, mmHg) at the start of that decade, in a systematic overview of 61 prospective studies involving 1 million adults. Rates are plotted on a floating absolute scale, and each square has area inversely proportional to the effective variance of the log mortality rate.

By the mid 1990s, several trials had been conducted to determine whether a few years of blood pressure reduction in middle age reduces the risk of stroke and of coronary heart disease. Partly because of imperfect compliance, the mean difference in systolic blood pressure between the treatment and control groups in these trials was only about 10 mmHg. Even if such trial treatments would eventually produce about 27% less coronary heart disease after many years (as seen in observational studies), the effects seen within the 2 or 3 years that are available on average between randomization and death in a 5-year trial might well be somewhat smaller (perhaps only *c.*15%). But, considered separately, none of the trials recorded enough coronary heart disease events (or enough vascular deaths) for statistically reliable assessment of a 15% risk reduction.

For stroke, the trials provide direct and highly significant evidence that most, or all, of the risk reduction associated with 10 mmHg lower usual systolic blood pressure appears soon after the blood pressure is lowered (Fig. 2.3.3.9). In contrast, the significant reduction in coronary heart disease seen in the trials (16% SD 4, 95% CI 8–23%; $2p = 0.0001$) seems to fall somewhat short of the difference of about 27% suggested by the observational evidence. However, the coronary heart disease reduction in the trials is still substantial and real ($2p = 0.0001$).

Taken together, Figs. 2.3.3.8 and 2.3.3.9 suggest that antihypertensive regimens that produce differences of much more than 10 mmHg systolic blood pressure will eventually reduce stroke by more than half and heart disease by more than a quarter. They also

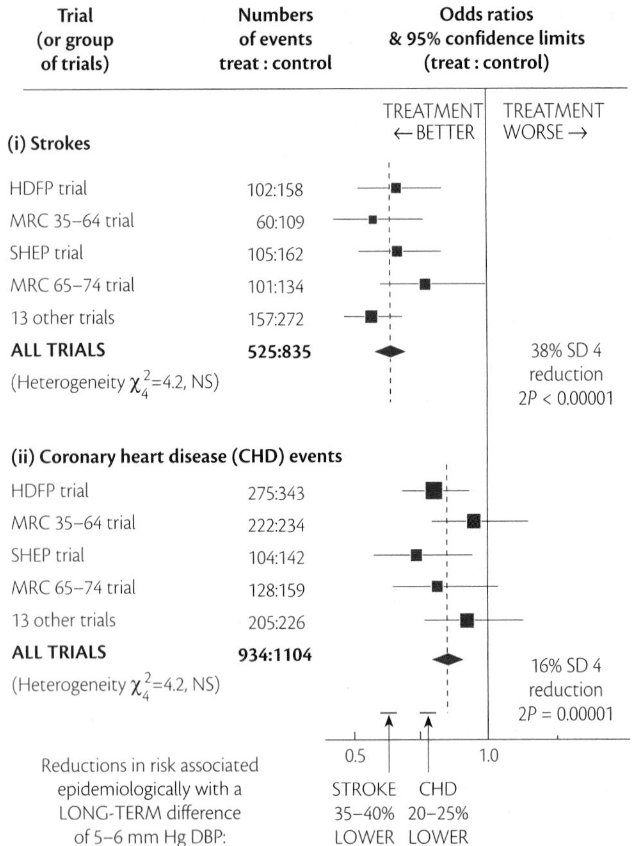

Fig. 2.3.3.9 Reduction in the odds of stroke and coronary heart disease in all unconfounded randomized trials of antihypertensive drug treatment (mean systolic blood pressure differences of *c.*10 mmHg for 5 years). Conventions are as for Fig. 2.3.3.7.

suggest that the proportional risk reduction produced by a given absolute reduction in systolic blood pressure will be approximately independent of the initial systolic blood pressure.

Results from large anonymous trials are relevant to real clinical practice

A clinician is used to dealing with individual patients, and may feel that the results of large trials somehow deny their individuality. This is almost the opposite of the truth, for one of the main reasons why trials have to be large is just because patients are so different from one another. Two apparently similar patients may run entirely different clinical courses, one remaining stable and the other progressing rapidly to severe disability or early death. Consequently, it is only when really large groups of patients are compared that the proportion of patients with truly good and bad prognosis in each can be relied on to be reasonably similar. One commonly hears statements such as: 'If the effect of a treatment isn't obvious in a few hundred patients then it isn't worth knowing about'. But, the accumulation since 1980 of large-scale randomized evidence of such moderate effects with treatments for heart disease, stroke, breast cancer, intestinal cancer, and various other conditions has transformed medical practice, and may already have avoided millions of deaths or recurrences.

It is also said that what is really wanted is not a blanket recommendation for everybody, but rather some means of identifying those few individuals who really stand to benefit from therapy. If any criteria (e.g. a short-term response to a non-placebo-controlled course of some disease-modifying agent) can be proposed that are likely to discriminate between people who will and will not benefit, then these can be recorded prospectively at entry and the eventual trial result subdivided with respect to them. However, there is a danger in too detailed an analysis of the apparent responses of small subgroups chosen for separate emphasis because of the apparently remarkable effects of treatment in these subgroups. Even if an agent brought no benefit, it would have to be acutely poisonous for it not to appear disproportionately beneficial in one or two such subgroups! Conversely, if an intervention really avoids an approximately *similar* proportion of the risk in each category of patient, it will, by chance alone, appear not to work in some category or categories of patient. The surprising extent to which this happens is evident from the example in Table 2.3.3.2. A large, anonymous trial will at least still help to answer the practical question of whether, on average, a policy of widespread treatment (except where clearly contraindicated) is preferable to a general policy of no immediate use of the treatment (except where clearly indicated). Moreover, without really large trials it is difficult to see how else many such questions relating to the effects of treatments on death or disability (or other major outcomes) are to be resolved reliably. Trials are at least a practical way of making some solid progress, and it would be unfortunate if desire for the perfect (that is, knowledge of exactly who will benefit from treatment) were to become the enemy of the possible (that is, knowledge of the average direction and approximate size of the effects of treatment in many large categories of patient).

Further reading

Antithrombotic Trialists' Collaboration (2002). Collaborative meta-analysis of randomised trials of antiplatelet therapy for prevention of death, myocardial infarction, and stroke in high-risk patients. *BMJ*, **324**, 71–86.

Chalmers I (1994). The Cochrane Collaboration: preparing, maintaining and disseminating systematic reviews of the effects of health care. *Ann N Y Acad Sci*, **703**, 156–63.

Chen ZM *et al.* for the COMMIT (ClOpidogrel and Metoprolol in Myocardial Infarction Trial) collaborative group (2005). Addition of clopidogrel to aspirin in 45, 852 patients with acute myocardial infarction: randomised placebo-controlled trial. *Lancet*, **366**, 1607–21.

Cochrane AL (1979). 1931–1971: a critical review, with particular reference to the medical profession. In: Teeling-Smith G, Wells N (eds) *Medicines for the year 2000*, pp. 1–11. Office of Health Economics, London.

Collins R, Peto R (1994). Antihypertensive drug therapy: effects on stroke and coronary heart disease. In: Swales JD (ed.) *Textbook of hypertension*, pp. 1156–64. Blackwell Science, Oxford.

Collins R, MacMahon S (2001). Reliable assessment of the effects of treatment on mortality and major morbidity I: clinical trials. *Lancet*, **357**, 373–80.

Collins R, Doll R, Peto R (1992). Ethics of clinical trials. In: Williams CJ (ed.) *Introducing new treatments for cancer: practical, ethical and legal problems*, pp. 49–65. John Wiley & Sons, Chichester.

Collins R, *et al.* (1987). Avoidance of large biases and large random errors in the assessment of moderate treatment effects: the need for systematic overviews. *Statist Med*, **6**, 245–50.

Early Breast Cancer Trialists' Collaborative Group (EBCTCG) (2005). Effects of chemotherapy and hormonal therapy for early breast cancer on recurrence and 15-year survival: an overview of the randomised trials. *Lancet*, **365**, 1687–717.

Fibrinolytic Therapy Trialists' Collaborative Group (1994). Indications for fibrinolytic therapy in suspected acute myocardial infarction: collaborative overview of early mortality and major morbidity results from all randomised trials of more than 1000 patients. *Lancet*, **343**, 311–22.

ISIS-2 (Second International Study of Infarct Survival) Collaborative Group (1988). Randomised trial of intravenous streptokinase, oral aspirin, both, or neither among 17,187 cases of suspected acute myocardial infarction: ISIS-2. *Lancet*, **332**, 349–60.

ISIS-4 (Fourth International Study of Infarct Survival) Collaborative Group (1995). ISIS-4: A randomised factorial trial assessing early oral captopril, oral mononitrate, and intravenous magnesium sulphate in 58050 patients with suspected acute myocardial infarction. *Lancet*, **345**, 669–85.

MacMahon S, Collins R (2001). Reliable assessment of the effects of treatment on mortality and major morbidity II: observational studies. *Lancet*, **357**, 455–62.

Magnesium In Coronaries (MAGIC) Trial Investigators (2002). Early administration of intravenous magnesium to high-risk patients with acute myocardial infarction in the Magnesium in Coronaries (MAGIC) Trial: a randomised controlled trial. *Lancet*, **360**, 1189–96.

MRC Asymptomatic Carotid Surgery Trial (ACST) Collaborative Group (2004). Prevention of disabling and fatal strokes by successful carotid endarterectomy in patients without recent neurological symptoms: randomised controlled trial. *Lancet*, **363**, 1491–502.

Prospective Studies Collaboration (2002). Age-specific relevance of usual blood pressure to vascular mortality: a meta-analysis of individual data for one million adults in 61 prospective studies. *Lancet*, **360**, 1903–13.

Prospective Studies Collaboration (2007). Blood cholesterol and vascular mortality by age, sex and blood pressure: meta-analysis of individual data from 61 prospective studies with 55,000 vascular deaths. *Lancet*, **370**, 1829–39.

Woods KL, *et al.* (1992). Intravenous magnesium sulphate in suspected acute myocardial infarction: results of the second Leicester Intravenous Magnesium Intervention Trial (LIMIT-2). *Lancet*, **339**, 1553–8.

Yusuf S, Collins R, Peto R (1984). Why do we need some large, simple randomized trials? *Statist Med*, **3**, 409–20.

2.3.4 The future of clinical trials

Perry Nisen and Patrick Vallance

Essentials

Clinical trials are the bedrock of evidence-based medicine. Introduced in the mid 20th century, they heralded a move away from opinion and anecdote to a more scientific evaluation of new treatments. Indeed, it could be argued that it is the clinical trial and the application of scientific method to determine which treatments work that distinguishes 'medicine' from 'alternative medicine'. The aim of this short section is to outline the way in which clinical trials are likely to evolve over the next few years.

Design of clinical trials

The gold standard for reliable and valid clinical trials is the frequentist statistical approach utilizing randomized, controlled, double-blinded studies that prespecify patient populations and the outcomes to be evaluated. These studies tend to be large, lengthy, expensive, and inflexible, but offer robust results that can directly influence clinical practice. However, Bayesian statistical designs are increasingly being utilized, particularly in early drug development, and this approach allows for the adaptation of information which accrues during a trial. An adaptive design means that trials may be smaller and more informative, and can limit exposure to inferior treatment. Information can be assessed at multiple time points (even continuously) and this can lead to the slowing, stopping or expansion of patient accrual, imbalance randomization to favour superior treatment, or focus on patient subsets that respond better. It also means that more dose levels can be tested. The challenge with these approaches is that the designs can be very complicated, implementation can be difficult, and analysis is often complex. There is also a perception that regulatory authorities will only accept frequentist designs.

There are additional examples of innovation in trial design that are increasingly being implemented. Positive results have been reported for oncology trials in which patients with progressive disease stop treatment, and those with stable disease or tumour shrinkage are randomized to either continue study drug or not (randomized discontinuation). Other trials enrich for subpopulations of patients most likely to benefit from a particular treatment. The targeted breast cancer therapy trastusimab was developed on the basis that only women whose tumours have *ERB2* gene amplification/over expression are likely to obtain benefit from this antibody therapy.

The 'n = 1' design is relatively underutilized but may have particular utility for chronic diseases in which there is a large placebo response rate and high levels of interindividual variability in treatment response rates. In this approach, each individual is randomized sequentially between placebo and active for several cycles. In this way, a statistically significant, reproducible, and robust response may be detected in individuals even if the overall patient cohort does not show significant benefit.

At a time when Bayesian design, composite endpoints, and new complex trial designs are to the fore, there is also a trend towards very large pragmatic trials undertaken in the real-life clinical setting with minimal exclusion criteria and simple monitoring such as 'all-cause mortality'. Such studies may make sense for definitive demonstration of efficacy in a large general population, but they may create challenges for safety assessment if extensive amounts of data are to be monitored.

Biomarkers and surrogate endpoints

For many diseases, the large size, length, and cost of conventional clinical trials creates an urgent need to find surrogate markers of efficacy including serum biomarkers and imaging. This approach has become mainstream in some therapeutic areas. For example, lipid profiles have become a routine proxy for antiatherosclerosis treatment to decrease cardiovascular risk. But the acceptance of LDL cholesterol as a surrogate for cardiovascular risk was preceded by many years of studies, ultimately culminating in validation of the endpoint with mortality outcomes studies. Other accepted surrogate endpoints include antibody titres as a measure of vaccine efficacy and viral load as markers of efficacy in trials for HIV or hepatitis C virus. In the coming years, it is likely that we will see the use of imaging as a surrogate for clinical benefit, for example MRI scans in multiple sclerosis, PET imaging for cancer, and possibly ultrasound detection of unstable atherosclerotic plaque.

Considerable challenges remain for many approaches, like chemoprevention of cancer, where extraordinarily long studies will be required to correlate changes in biomarkers with outcome. One path forwards may be to accept biomarkers for conditional approval of medicines for diseases with high unmet need and to withdraw marketing authority if subsequent studies fail to demonstrate benefit using hard clinical endpoints, such as survival.

Impact of advanced technology

Increased investment in electronic patient records (inpatient and outpatient) should provide an important opportunity to understand better the natural history of disease and the feasibility of conducting different types of clinical trials. For example, electronic patient records can be searched to determine very quickly how many subjects would be eligible for a particular study according to specific eligibility criteria. Electronic records may also allow the number of subjects amenable to participation in clinical trials to be increased by informing them of their eligibility and the opportunity to participate. These are becoming key issues for trialists as the number of centres recruited for multicentre studies expands and where the recruitment from individual centres may turn out to be very low.

Another important prospect would be to examine electronic patient records for the purposes of pharmacovigilance. At present, safety databases are largely dependent upon controlled clinical trials and spontaneous reporting of adverse events of marketed drugs. Further, electronic patient records should facilitate the conduct of large outcome studies and address the challenge of subjects dropping out from trials and being lost to follow-up.

Remote data entry, including the use of handheld devices, is also transforming the conduct of clinical trials. Remote data entry facilitates real-time monitoring and reconciliation of databases, allowing for more rapid closure or locking of databases. Technology also exists to record remotely clinical data in the outpatient or home setting, which would allow, for example, frequent assessment of vital signs and electrocardiograms. Such technologies also facilitate the assessment of adherence to treatments, an important factor in clinical trial outcomes, using medicine containers that record how often and when they are opened.

Finally, it is becoming possible to analyse data across multiple databases (e.g. sponsor-controlled studies, electronic patient records, and preclinical data). In addition to meta-analyses, this provides the opportunity to conduct more extensive modelling and simulation of clinical trial outcomes, which will facilitate optimal trial design with respect to dose selection, sample size and amount of required data collection. The ability to analyse across different databases will also enable regulatory authorities to evaluate class effects of medicines being developed by multiple sponsors.

Personalized medicine: the application of pharmacogenetics and pharmacogenomics

The notion that medicines should be personalized is hardly new. The mantra of 'the right drug at the right dose for the right patient' has been at the heart of rational therapeutics for many years. However, with advances in genetics there has been increasing interest in the idea that individual variation in the response to a medicine may, at least in part, be genetically determined. Even before the advent of easy genotyping there were examples of differences in responses to drugs based on simple mendelian patterns of inheritance. Examples include 'slow or fast acetylators' and the effects of glucose-6-phosphate dehydrogenase deficiency on susceptibility to adverse effects of drugs. Now of course it is possible to identify myriad genetic variations in coding and noncoding regions of every gene and the discipline of pharmacogenetics has emerged. How will this affect clinical trials? It is becoming routine in most major pharmaceutical clinical trials for blood to be collected for DNA. This is done largely for reasons of retrospective or 'post hoc' analysis, to explore potential mechanisms of unexpected unwanted effects or, less frequently, to search for reasons of nonresponse. Increasingly, however, patient stratification by genotype is used to enrich a population with potential responders, or to produce a group that will exhibit a more uniform pharmacokinetic response to the drug. Such approaches may be taken in the early phases of drug development to enable rapid decision making. It is less clear whether this approach will translate into meaningful differences in the clinic. The influence of common genetic variation on drug metabolism or effects tends to be relatively small and there is considerable overlap between groups. For example, although common variants in the gene for the p-glycoprotein drug transporter seem to predict poor response to certain antiepileptic drugs, the size of the effect is small and could not be used *a priori* to predict responders and nonresponders. It remains to be determined whether panels of gene variants can be clustered to establish a clinically meaningful marker profile of altered risk:benefit ratio for the individual who is the candidate to receive any particular drug.

The area in which genome-based stratification is a reality is in cancer. Here mutations within the tumour, or altered levels of expression of specific genes, can determine responses to treatment. As more specific molecularly targeted therapies for cancers are invented, the need to determine both genotype and gene or protein expression levels will become a routine part of oncology trials.

Presentation of results and comparison between treatment options

Increasingly, outcome studies use composite endpoints. Such endpoints assist in reducing the size of a trial and may facilitate the identification of clinically linked outcomes. In addition, outcomes may be presented in different ways. For example, the effects of a cancer drug may be presented in terms of absolute or relative changes in mortality, duration of survival, time to disease progression, or relapse-free interval. Although the endpoints may be comprehensible in terms of an individual study result, they may not translate easily between studies or allow prescribers and patients to make decisions between multiple treatment options. It seems likely that some sort of standardized form of outcome presentation will have to be agreed to allow informed assessment of treatment options. This will present a challenge for trialists, journals, and bodies such as the National Institute for Health and Clinical Excellence (NICE) in the United Kingdom.

A related question is the funding and organization of large comparative clinical trials. There have been several examples, particularly in cardiovascular and cancer trials, of partnerships between industry, charities, and governments. For trials designed to compare multiple treatment options in common conditions, this seems likely to be an increasing pattern of funding and organization.

Placebo controls and effects

Placebo responses are part of every trial and indeed every consultation. The randomized double-blind placebo-controlled trial was established to allow accurate assessment of the additional effect of the active ingredient. In some studies (e.g. in depression) the size of the placebo effect can be very large and make it difficult to separate active from placebo. Sceptics may argue that this reflects on the relative ineffectiveness of current antidepressants, but this interpretation is inconsistent with the positive effects seen in many large studies and in clinical practice. It is our opinion that advances in understanding of the biology of the placebo response will have a significant impact on trial design over the next decade.

Studies in the developing world

The demographics of clinical trials are subject to change. Growing demand for access to patients for clinical trials and skyrocketing costs are contributing to increased numbers of studies in the developing world. This phenomenon has created unique challenges to the safe, ethical execution of trials and the ability to generalize findings. The standards of medical care and comorbid conditions can vary and environmental factors can have an impact on clinical trial outcomes. For example, variation in diet can affect drug bioavailability, and the background incidence of smoking can shift clinical outcomes for certain diseases. Further, approaches to disease prevention differ; for example, treatment thresholds and medications for hypertension and dyslipaedemia vary around the world.

Ethical considerations permeate all aspects of the conduct of clinical trials in developing countries. If a new medicine is being tested in a developing world population, will it be marketed at an affordable price in that country? Is the informed consent understandable to the targeted population? Some clinical endpoints are descriptive and depend on language and culture. The Hamilton scale is used extensively in depression studies—do subtleties in the scale mean the same thing in Mandarin and Hindu? Will a strong treatment effect in a naive Chinese patient population translate into similar benefit for individuals who failed multiple prior courses of medication in the United States of America?

Ethnopharmacology is another complex issue. The frequency of functional polymorphisms for genes which influence drug metabolism varies greatly in different populations and the interactions of these multiple polymorphisms are highly complex. Nevertheless, these challenges are being addressed and medicines are increasingly being developed according to a common global standard. The imposition of agreed standards is itself creating a challenge for regulatory authorities as they struggle to understand the impact of these many variables on assessment of safety and efficacy in the populations they serve.

Further reading

Benedetti F, *et al.* (2005). Neurobiological mechanisms of the placebo effect. *J Neurosci*, **225**, 10390–402.

Berry DA (2006). A guide to drug discovery: Bayesian clinical trials. *Nat Rev Drug Discov*, **5**, 27–36.

Million RA (2006). Impact of genetic diagnostics on drug development strategy. *Nat Rev Drug Discov*, **5**, 459–62.

2.4

Funding of health care

Contents

2.4.1 The evaluation and provision of effective medicines *48*
Michael D. Rawlins

2.4.2 Reasonableness and its definition in the provision of health care *54*
Norman Daniels

2.4.3 Priority setting in developed and developing countries *58*
Nigel Crisp

2.4.4 Sustaining innovation in an era of specialized medicine *60*
Henri A. Termeer

2.4.1 The evaluation and provision of effective medicines

Michael D. Rawlins

Essentials

As more new medicines become available, often at a premium price, it has become imperative for individual practitioners, institutions, and health care systems to assess whether they represent good value for money. Are they an improvement on existing treatments (either in terms of improved efficacy or a better safety)? And, if so, do they represent a cost effective use of health care resources?

New medicines (and other treatments) are subject to evaluation on clinical evidence and on economic grounds. Several methods are used to evaluate medicines in terms of their efficacy and safety; these approaches seek also to determine whether a medicine has a safety and efficacy profile with advantages (or not) compared with existing treatments for the same condition. A further question relates to the practical utility of a new medicine in the context of current daily practice. The principal means of assessing clinical effectiveness use randomized controlled trials, controlled observational studies, and case-series together with expert opinion and systematic review.

Economic evaluation of medicines is more controversial and raises important philosophical societal (and political) questions. In practice, two main approaches are used to assess medicines—cost-effectiveness and cost–utility analyses.

Provision of medicines varies greatly between regions and individual nations. The issue is one of critical importance for sick persons and their families and arrangements can only be described as in a state of flux internationally—and highly influenced by economic factors as well as social structures and fiscal tradition. Nonetheless, the intrinsic conflict between the drive for demand for modern drugs as part of health care are an active focus of political discussion; the issues raised will continue to impinge on the practice of physicians worldwide, who, as a result, often face difficult ethical dilemmas.

Introduction

Over the past 50 years an extraordinary array of effective medicines has become available. Between 1960 and 1990, most new pharmacologically active compounds were discovered in the laboratories of commercial enterprises and almost none in academic or publicly funded research institutions. In recent years the balance has shifted somewhat and drug discovery has, once again, become an academic pursuit. The subsequent development of medicines, however, still depends on the resources and expertise of the pharmaceutical industry and this is unlikely to change.

Clinical evaluation

The clinical evaluation of a medicine seeks to answer four questions:

- Is it effective?
- Is it safe in relation to its efficacy?
- How does its efficacy and safety profiles compare with those of existing treatments?
- And how useful is it really likely to be in day-to-day clinical care?

Methodological approaches

A variety of methodological approaches are used to attempt to answer questions relating to the evaluation of clinical effectiveness:

- randomized controlled trials
- controlled observational studies
- case series
- expert opinion
- systematic reviews

Randomized controlled trials

Randomized controlled trials are generally regarded as the methodological 'gold standard' for evaluating clinical effectiveness. The technique, in principle, is straightforward. Patients with the condition to be studied are allocated, at random, to two or more treatments; and at the completion of the trial the fate of the two (or more) groups is compared.

The method is, unquestioningly, extremely powerful. Random allocation means that each patient in the trial has a known chance of being given each treatment(s); but the treatment to be given cannot be predicted. Provided that neither the patient nor the investigator is aware during the course of the study of which treatment has been given (i.e. a double-blind study), this design provides the best approach to minimizing bias. The principles underlying the design and analysis of randomized controlled trials are discussed in detail in Chapter 2.3.3.

Controlled observational studies

There are three types of nonrandomized, but otherwise controlled, study designs that are sometimes used to evaluate medicines.

- historical controlled trials
- case–control studies
- before-and-after designs

The application of these techniques, however, is controversial and careful consideration needs to be given before accepting any of them as providing reliable evidence of effectiveness.

Historical controlled trials

These involve comparing the health outcomes in a group of patients who have received a (usually) new treatment with outcomes in a 'historical' cohort of patients, collected previously, who did not receive the treatment but who were managed similarly in all other respects.

The traditional argument against the use of historical controlled trials is the difficulty in ensuring that comparisons are fair. Examples from the past have shown that they tend to exaggerate the value of new treatments. Nevertheless, a body of respectable opinion holds that under some circumstances historical controlled trials may provide a reasonably unbiased assessment of efficacy if all the following conditions are met:

- There is a biologically plausible basis for the particular treatment.
- The condition has a known and predictable natural history.
- The condition, untreated, is associate with a serious outcome.
- No other effective treatment is available.

Table 2.4.1.1 Some medicines for which the evidence for efficacy is based on (implicit or explicit) historical controlled trials

Treatment	Uses
Salicylate	Acute rheumatic fever
Insulin	Diabetic ketoacidosis
Thyroxine	Myxoedema
Sulphonamides	Puerperal sepsis
Neostigmine	Myasthenia gravis
Penicillin	Lobar pneumonia
Cortisone	Addison's disease
Streptomycin	Tuberculous meningitis
N-acetylcysteine	Paracetamol poisoning
Combination chemotherapy	Disseminated testicular cancer
Imatinib	Gastrointestinal stromal tumours

An additional approach to accepting the use of historical controls is in disorders where the signal-to-noise ratio—the magnitude of the effect in relation to the natural history of the condition—is more than 10-fold. Table 2.4.1.1 shows some common medicines whose efficacy is unquestioned but whose use is based on explicit (or more often implicit) historical controls. Historical controlled trials have been of special value in assessing the benefits of treatments for very rare diseases where assembling cohorts of patients for the purposes of a clinical trial sometimes poses almost insuperable obstacles.

Case–control studies

These involve comparisons of exposure to a particular agent in those with a condition of interest, compared to a control group without the condition in a 2 × 2 table (Table 2.4.1.2).

The odds ratio (and its 95% confidence interval) provides a measure of the strength of the association between exposure and the study condition:

$$\text{odds ratio} = a/b \div c/d$$

The odds ratio is greater than 1 if exposure to a drug (or some environmental factor) is harmful; and less than 1 if the association is beneficial. The relative risk is the ratio of the event rates in the exposed and unexposed groups:

$$\text{Relative risk} = [a/a + c] \div [b/b + d]$$

Again, a relative risk greater than 1 suggests that exposure is harmful and less than 1 that it is beneficial.

Case–control studies have been used primarily as an epidemiological tool to identify risk factors for specific conditions such as the association between smoking and lung cancer. In therapeutics they have been very important in the detection of less common adverse drug reactions: one important example is the association between

Table 2.4.1.2 A 2 × 2 table used in case–control studies

	Numbers with the study condition	Numbers (controls) without the study condition
Exposed	*a*	*c*
Unexposed	*b*	*d*

use of hormone replacement therapy (HRT) and the development of breast cancer.

Case–control studies appear, however, to have a limited role in demonstrating efficacy (and some would say none at all) because of the difficulties of avoiding bias. For example, during the 1980s and 1990s a series of case–control studies showed a consistent association between the use of HRT and reduction in coronary heart disease. This, together with HRT's effects on postmenopausal symptoms, resulted in it becoming the most frequently prescribed medicine in the United States of America. Since 1998, however, eight randomized controlled trials have shown that HRT certainly has no beneficial effect on coronary heart disease; and some trials have suggested its use might indeed increase the risk.

The explanation for these paradoxical findings remains unclear. It is likely to have been due, at least in part, to differences in baseline risk of coronary heart disease (including socioeconomic factors and lifestyle) which were not adequately controlled.

Before-and-after studies

As the name suggests, these compare patients' health status before treatment and after. In general this study design is unreliable, because of placebo effects as well as both allocation and ascertainment biases. Nevertheless there are some circumstances, similar to those used in validating historical controlled trials, where before-and-after designs can provide reasonably reliable evidence of clinical effectiveness particularly where change(s) in health can be measured objectively. Examples include the haematological response to vitamin B_{12} in pernicious anaemia, and the reduction of hepatomegaly and splenomegaly with enzyme replacement therapy in Gaucher's disease.

Case series

In the primary ascertainment of clinical effectiveness, observing the fate of a series of patients treated with a particular medicine is associated with the same problems as before-and-after designs. Nevertheless, case series can be useful in several ways. First, they may provide an indication of the generalizability (i.e. external validity or effectiveness in routine clinical practice) of the results of randomized clinical trials. Second, they may also be capable of detecting previously unrecognized adverse effects as well as providing an estimate of their incidence. Table 2.4.1.3 compares the fate of a group of patients with nonvalvular atrial fibrillation, undergoing routine anticoagulation with warfarin to prevent thrombotic stroke, with the pooled results from five independent randomized controlled trials. The case series indicates that, despite the difficulties in using warfarin in routine clinical practice, similar results can be achieved to those seen in formal studies. It provides a powerful message about generalizability (external validity).

Table 2.4.1.3 Annual events amongst patient on warfarin to prevent thrombotic stroke: a comparison between patients in routine practice and those in RCTs

Event	Annual event rate (95% CI)	
	Case-series (N = 167)	Pooled RCTs (95% CI)
Ischaemic stroke	2.0 (0.7–4.4)	1.4 (0.8–2.3)
Intracranial haemorrhage	0.3 (0.03–2.7)	0.3 (0.06–0.7)
Major bleeding	1.4 (0.2–4.6)	1.3 (0.7–2.1)
Minor bleeding	5.4 (2.4–10.2)	9.2 (3.7–12)

Kalra L, Yu G, Perez I, Lajhani A, Donaldson N. Prospective cohort study to determine if trial efficacy of anticoagulation for stroke prevention in atrial fibrillation translates into clinical effectiveness. *BMJ* 2000; **320**: 1236–9.

Expert opinion

The history of medicine is littered with the tombstones of patients who perished at the hands of their well-meaning, but unwise, physicians. In general even 'expert opinion', unsupported by reasonable evidence about the effectiveness of a particular medicine, has little place in therapeutics. Yet this, again, is not absolute.

In some instances expert judgement about the extrapolation of the results of one study from one clinical setting to another is both necessary and reasonable. This applies particularly to the use of a particular medicine in population subgroups which may have never been (and probably never will be) subjected to a randomized clinical trial. Where trials have been carried out in middle-aged men, can they reasonably be extrapolated to women? Or older men? Experience suggests that it is probably unusual for the efficacy (although not the risks) of treatments to vary with age and gender.

Systematic reviews

Reviews of the literature, about a particular topic, have an established place in assessing the clinical effectiveness of interventions. Conventional *ad hoc* approaches to reviewing, with an often incomplete scrutiny of the literature, have been superseded in favour of a formal, structured approach. This minimizes the possibility of bias and random error.

Systematic reviews (also sometimes known as research syntheses, secondary reviews, or overviews) have certain critical features:

1. A systematic review should always start with a clear definition of the question it seeks to address. It should also consider the type(s) of study design(s) that may be appropriate in answering the problem. In evaluating the effectiveness of new or established medicines, systematic reviews tend to consider only randomized controlled trials. A systematic reviewer also needs to decide whether the review will only consider comparisons with placebo or whether the review will encompass active comparators.

2. Ideally, the review will include all published and unpublished studies with no language limitation. Electronic searches of published studies, even using bibliographic databases, may exclude those indexed inappropriately. MEDLINE and EMBASE, the two most widely used databases for medical research, did not include the terms 'randomized trials' or 'controlled trials' until the mid-1990s. The Cochrane Collaboration has embarked on a project—the Cochrane Controlled Trials Register—to hand-search relevant journals and now contains 250 000 records. Additionally, the overlap between MEDLINE and EMBASE is only about 34% so any search strategy must include both. Conventional bibliographic literature searches will also fail to identify studies published in academic theses as well as those in the 'grey' literature (such as information placed in the public domain by drug regulatory authorities). They will also fail to identify unpublished studies undertaken by pharmaceutical companies. Unpublished studies, and those published in non English language journals, are important to identify because they are more likely to be negative. Their exclusion will overemphasize the benefits or, worse, result in false positive conclusions.

3 Abstraction of the relevant data from each of the studies that meet the predefined inclusion criteria is the next step. To avoid transcription errors this is often undertaken, independently, by two abstractors. The extracted data will include the methods used, the patient population, the nature of the interventions, the outcomes, and some assessment of the study quality. The extracted data is usually presented in the form of an evidence table from which the strengths, weaknesses, and conclusions of each study can be reviewed.

4 Where there are adequate data, and where the studies are broadly similar, the summary statistics from each trial can be pooled. The details of undertaking such a meta-analysis are beyond the scope of this chapter but there are well-developed methods for estimating the combined effects of treatments. These employ a weighted average so that larger trials have more influence on the pooled results than smaller ones. The results are commonly displayed, graphically, in the form of a 'forest plot' in which the means and 95% confidence intervals, for each study, are displayed horizontally. The size of the mean reflects the size of the contribution made by that study to the pooled results. An example of a forest plot, incorporating the results of five randomized controlled trials of the prevention of thrombotic stroke with anticoagulation in nonvalvular atrial fibrillation, is shown in Fig. 2.4.1.1.

Meta-analyses are not necessarily appropriate in a systematic review but, where they are, they can provide important information. First, they can provide a better estimate of the size of a treatment effect than can any study on its own. This is especially important where studies have yielded conflicting results; or where each, on its own, has not produced a statistically significant result (usually because of small sample sizes) but where the pooled data shows an overall beneficial (or adverse) effect. Second, they can be useful in subgroup analyses especially where subgroups in individual studies have included too few patients for significance to be achieved. Third, using special statistical techniques they can formally address the homogeneity of studies as well as provide strong hints of 'publication bias' (i.e. the possible/probable existence of unpublished negative studies). Finally, where there is a particular adverse event associated with the medicine (e.g. bleeding with anticoagulant therapy) this can be similarly be the subject of a meta-analysis to provide a better estimate of its incidence.

Clinical effectiveness

Clinical effectiveness is the term used to describe the extent to which an intervention (in this case a medicine) produces an overall health benefit in routine clinical practice. The methodological approaches described earlier (especially randomized controlled trials) are intended to provide solid evidence that, under the conditions of the study the results are free from bias and represent the 'truth' (i.e. internal validity). The results may not necessarily translate to the benefits accruing in practice (i.e. external validity). The issues include:

- the absolute magnitude of the benefits (effect size)
- the magnitude of the benefits in comparison with other available treatments
- use in heterogeneous patient populations (generalizability)

Absolute effect size

The results of a clinical trial may be expressed in several different ways:

1 The absolute risk reduction (also known as the absolute risk difference) is the event rate of interest in the control group less the event rate in the treated group. In the case of anticoagulation

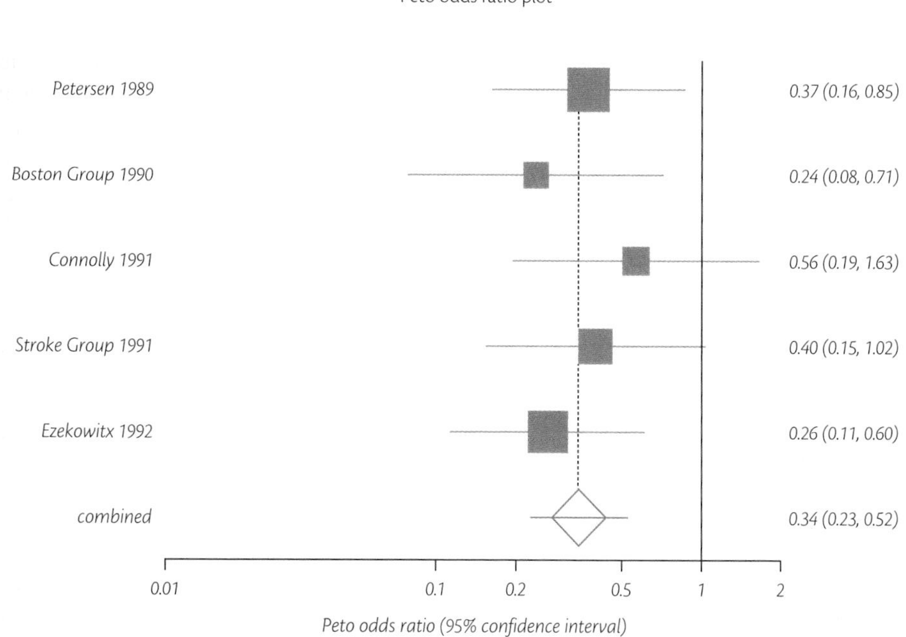

Fig. 2.4.1.1 Meta-analysis of the effectiveness of anticoagulant therapy vs placebo in the prevention of thrombotic stroke.
(From Aguilar MI, Hart R (2005). Oral anticoagulants for preventing stroke in patients with nonvalvular atrial fibrillation and no previous history of stroke or transient ischaemic attacks. *Cochrane Database of Systematic Reviews*, Issue 3, Art. No. CD001927.)

for nonvalvular atrial fibrillation, the absolute risk reduction in thrombotic stroke (Fig. 2.4.1.1) is 41 per 1000 (60/1000 less 19/1000). This represents a 68% decrease in the risk of thrombotic stroke, but such percentage changes should be regarded with caution because they ignore absolute risk.

2 The relative risk, like the hazard ratio and odds ratio, has important statistical properties and is widely (and rightly) used in the analysis of clinical trials. All of these suffer, though, from the same disadvantage of expressing change as a percentage.

3 The number needed to treat (NNT) is an estimate of the number of patients who would need to be treated for one patient to benefit. It is the reciprocal of the absolute risk reduction, expressed as a proportion, and in the anticoagulant example is 25 (1 divided by 0.04). In other words, to prevent 1 thrombotic stroke in patients with nonvalvular atrial fibrillation, 25 would need to be anticoagulated. NNTs for some other treatments are shown in Table 2.4.1.4.

4 There is an increasing interest in incorporating measures of health-related quality of life into the design and analysis of clinical trials. These measures fall into two distinct groups. Disease-specific quality of life questionnaires are designed to capture aspects as they apply to particular disorders; generic ones are designed to be used across all conditions. A variety of disease-specific measures have also been developed. They can be extremely useful in providing an assessment of the overall benefits of treatment as well as the frequency and severity of adverse effects. They are of varying quality, however, and none allows the improvement in health ('health gain') with a specific treatment for one condition to be compared with that for another. Generic instruments that attempt to capture global improvements in health gain are particularly important for economic evaluation in health care. The EurQol-5D (EQ-5D) was specifically designed for this purpose and is increasingly being used. The longer Medical Outcomes Study 36-Item Short Form questionnaire (SF-36), which primarily profiles various aspects of the quality of life, can also be used to a singly summary measure of health-related quality of life.

Table 2.4.1.4 Numbers needed to treat for a selection of common treatments

Treatment	Indication	NNT (95% CI)
Permethrin	Cure of head lice	1.1 (1.0–1.2)
Terbenafine	Cure of fungal nail infections	2.7 (1.9–4.5)
Isosorbide dintrate	Prevention of exercise-induced angina	5 (2.8–21)
Maternal antenatal steroids	Prevention respiratory distress syndrome in the baby	11 (8–16)
Statins	Secondary prevention of cardiovascular disease	11 (10–13)
Steroid and β-agonist (inhaled)	Prevention of severe exacerbations of asthma in children >1 year	11 (10–13)
Antimicrobials	Prevention of infection after dog bites	16 (9–92)
Statins	Primary prevention of cardiovascular disease	35 (24–63)
Finasteride	Prevention of benign prostatic hypertrophy (>2 years)	39 (23–111)

Comparative effectiveness

In evaluating the clinical effectiveness of a new treatment it is important to know whether it is an improvement on current practice and, if so, by how much. Where current practice comprises only 'supportive care', placebo-controlled trials provide a reasonably reliable approach to assessing a new medicine. Where alternative treatments exist, however, placebo-controlled trials cannot necessarily provide reliable answers. With the availability of more and more effective treatments the problem of comparators is becoming a major issue. Two approaches—direct and indirect comparisons—are available.

Direct comparisons

In this approach two or more treatments are compared in head-to-head trials. There are many instances, however, where such direct comparisons have not been undertaken. Comparative trials often require many more participants than placebo-controlled studies if they are to have the power to demonstrate the likely smaller differences. They are therefore much more costly to undertake. Moreover, national drug regulatory authorities do not generally require manufacturers of new medicines to undertake comparative trials, so there is a disincentive for them to do so. Although such trials would unquestionably be useful in evaluating new treatments, there are difficulties facing both regulatory authorities and manufacturers. International differences in clinical practice make it difficult—if not impossible—for manufacturers to identify comparator(s) that would meet the demands of all national drug regulatory authorities. Furthermore, the requirement to do so would escalate the cost of drug development (now claimed to be around US$1 billion per new medicine).

Indirect comparisons

These involve comparing the effectiveness of two (or more) medicines against their own, independent, placebo-controlled trials. Thus, if treatment A in a placebo-controlled study is associated with a relative risk of 0.8 (95% confidence interval 0.75–0.85), and treatment B (for the same indication) is associated with a relative risk of 0.6 (95% confidence interval 0.5–0.7), then it might be reasonably inferred that treatment B was superior. There are obvious pitfalls in this assumption but it often remains the only approach and, subject to certain caveats, it is often reasonably reliable.

Use in heterogeneous patient populations

Randomized controlled trials, especially those undertaken for regulatory purposes, are generally undertaken in homogeneous populations of patients. Manufacturers, not unreasonably, wish to ascertain whether their new medicine is both safe and effective in the particular condition for which they seek a licensed indication. Pregnant patients, children, the very old, and patients with comorbidities are therefore usually excluded. In routine clinical practice, however, such patient groups are very likely to be potential beneficiaries of the particular treatment.

There is no easy solution to this. In some instances so-called 'pragmatic trials', where exclusion criteria are kept to a minimum, are undertaken. Although valuable in themselves, they are not easy to undertake or evaluate. Even though it may be possible to conclude overall that efficacy is maintained in a mixed population, the study is unlikely to have been powered to encompass the full range of subgroups.

For the foreseeable future, decisions relating to the use of new (and existing) medicines in heterogeneous patient populations will often remain a matter of clinical judgement. The emergence of electronic patient records, and consequential developments in the analysis of case series, may allow us in the future to evaluate medicines in heterogeneous populations more adequately.

Economic evaluation

It is an uncomfortable but inescapable fact that—irrespective of their methods of financing—all health care systems have finite resources within which to deliver clinical services to the populations they serve. Moreover, no health care system meets all the demands of its patients. In general, the amount of money a country devotes to health care is a direct function of its wealth (as reflected by its gross domestic product).

The mismatch between resources and demand will only worsen in the future. The combination, in all developed countries, of an increasingly ageing population, the emergence of new innovative technologies, and heightened public expectations, are placing financial strains on every health care system. Part of the response to this emerging crisis, especially in countries where health care is largely provided from public funds, is the increasing recognition that new medicines should be subject to economic evaluation before being introduced into routine practice.

The economic evaluation of new and established medicines seeks to ensure they give reasonable value for money. This involves examining the benefits, and costs, accruing to the product, in comparison with current standard (or best) practice. Where two treatments are equally effective, it is obviously common sense to use the less costly one. This approach, known as cost minimization, depends on the demonstration of therapeutic equivalence. In many instances, however, one treatment is more costly but more effective than another. Deciding whether the increased cost appears to be worth the increased benefit is critically important because, if it is not, some other activity in the health care system will be displaced. This—the so-called 'opportunity cost'—means that the adoption of a more costly but more effective medicine may deprive other people, with other conditions, of more cost-effective treatment.

There are two approaches to examining the economic consequences of adopting more costly, but more effective, medicines (and other technologies) into a health care system. Both involve examining the costs (including not only the price of the product but also the costs of administration, monitoring, and treating adverse effects) and the benefits—in comparison to current standard practice—to derive the incremental cost-effectiveness ratio (ICER).

Cost-effectiveness analysis

In cost-effectiveness analysis benefits are expressed as natural units such as the magnitude of the reductions in blood pressure (for an antihypertensive agent) or serum cholesterol (for an antihyperlipidaemic product). The ICER for an antihypertensive agent (A), in comparison to the current standard (B), would be:

$$\text{cost per mmHg reduction with drug A} - \text{cost per mmHg reduction with drug B}$$

This approach is limited in its application because its use is confined to the circumstances of a single condition. An approach that has wider application is to express benefits in terms of the life-years gained (LYG) and hence the ICER as the cost per LYG. This has the obvious disadvantage, however, of limiting its use to treatments that prolong life rather than those that improve the health-related quality of life. What is important for a health care system is to know what economic impact the use of a particular treatment might have on its population as a whole—the opportunity cost.

Cost–utility analysis

Cost–utility analysis attempts to capture the benefits of a particular health technology (including medicines) using a metric that can be applied across all conditions and treatments. This approach involves assessing the 'utility' of a treatment taking account of improvements in both the increased longevity that it brings to patients and the enhanced health-related quality of life. Utility, in health care, is assessed on a scale of 0 (dead) to 1 (perfect health). The increase in utility that is brought about by a particular treatment is multiplied by the number of years for which it is enjoyed to provide the additional (incremental) quality-adjusted life year gained (QALY).

For example, if a new treatment for lung cancer costs an extra £5000 and confers an additional 6 months of life (over and above the current standard care), it will produce an ICER of £10 000 per LYG (cost-effectiveness analysis). If the utility during this period of prolonged life is 0.7, then the QALY gained over this time is 0.35 and the ICER will be £14 286 per QALY (£5000 divided by 0.35). ICERs for a selection of anticancer drugs appraised by the United Kingdom's National Institute for Health and Clinical Excellence (NICE) are shown in Table 2.4.1.5.

The application of cost–utility analysis in deciding how to allocate resources for health care requires a definition of the cut-off or threshold between cost-effective and cost-ineffective treatments.

Table 2.4.1.5 Incremental cost effectiveness ratios for some cancer drugs appraised by the National Institute for Health and Clinical Excellence (NICE)

Treatment	Condition	Incremental cost effectiveness ratio (£/QALY)
Rituximab	Aggressive nonHodgkin's lymphoma	6 100
Paclitaxel	Metastatic ovarian cancer	8 500
Gemcitabine	Metastatic pancreatic cancer	12 500
Vinorelbine	Metastatic breast cancer	14 500
Trastuzumab	Early breast cancer	18 000
Temozolomide	Recurrent glioma	25 300
Imatinib	Inoperable or metastatic gastrointestinal stromal tumour	32 000
Temozolomide	Newly diagnosed glioma	35 000
Bevacizumab	Metastatic colorectal cancer	62 857[a]
Cetuximab	Metastatic colorectal cancer	72 210[a]

[a] Considered by NICE to be a cost-ineffective use of resources in the UK NHS.

There is no empirical data that have reliably defined this, although it must bear some relation to a country's overall wealth and the amount (*per capita*) it is able to devote to health care. Indeed, the World Health Organization has suggested that ICERs (as cost per QALY) below a country's *per capita* gross domestic product should almost invariably be considered as cost effective; and those in excess of three times per the national *per capita* gross domestic product should be considered as cost ineffective.

In the United Kingdom, NICE usually regards ICERs below £20 000 per QALY as representing a cost-effective use of resources in the British National Health Service (NHS). As the ICER rises, there must be ever better reasons to recommend acceptance if other patients, with other conditions, are not to be denied cost-effective care. NICE therefore does not have a rigid threshold but makes decisions on a case-by-case basis, depending on various factors including confidence in the ICER, the seriousness of the condition, and the effectiveness of alternatives in relation to the particular product.

These case-by-case judgements require NICE to go beyond conventional scientific considerations of clinical and cost-effectiveness. Inevitably, this requires societal and ethical decisions about how the resources available in the United Kingdom health care system should be most appropriately be deployed. In its decision-making, NICE has therefore adopted principles and processes that are comparable (and compatible) with those enunciated by Norman Daniels in his approach to 'accountability for reasonableness' (see Chapter 2.4.2). The United Kingdom health care system, funded as it is from general taxation, is based on the principle of social solidarity. In attempting to resolve the problem of distributive justice, NICE therefore tries to balance the desire for efficiency (utilitarianism) with the need for fairness (egalitarianism).

Provision

National drug regulatory authorities (such as the Food and Drugs Administration in the United States of America and the European Medicines Agency in the European Union) permit new pharmaceutical products onto their markets, for specific (licensed) indications, provided they meet the requirements of quality, safety, and efficacy. Drug regulatory authorities do not expect manufacturers to show that their products are cost-effective. Nor, in general, do regulatory authorities expect manufacturers to demonstrate the superiority (or even equivalence) of a new product compared to existing ones used for the same indications.

Once a manufacturer has obtained a licence for a product, for a specific indication, it is available for prescription; and physicians may prescribe it for their patients in the private (independent) sector. The extent to which publicly funded health care systems are prepared to pay for, or reimburse the cost of, such prescriptions varies widely.

Historically, in the United Kingdom, the NHS allowed all new products to be available at a price set by the manufacturer. During the 1990s, however, local NHS organizations began to restrict access to some medicines. Because of a lack of consistency in decision-making, products could be available in some localities but not others (so-called 'postcode prescribing'). In 1999, the British government established NICE to examine the clinical and cost-effectiveness of selected new (and established) pharmaceutical products, and advise the NHS as to whether their use is appropriate. There is a legal obligation on local NHS organizations to provide those treatments that have been endorsed by NICE.

Arrangements in other countries differ. In the United States of America, most health care is provided through insurance arrangements. Insurers may restrict the availability of particular medicines but, more commonly, provide access to all licensed medicines and require patients to pay 'tiered' copayments. These are ones considered by the insurer to be less cost-effective than alternatives in the same therapeutic class. Medicare (the federally funded health care programme for older people) will provide any licensed medicine that is given to patients in hospital, or at a doctor's surgery, with no copayment required. Medicare recently also added coverage for outpatient medicines through federal subsidies of private drug insurance schemes. These schemes offer Medicare patients a choice from a wide variety of insurance packages with different monthly premiums and tiered copayment arrangements. In Europe arrangements vary between countries but, generally, prices are negotiated with companies before products are available under their national health care systems.

Provision, especially of new medicines, is in a state of flux in many countries because of the high price charged for many new products. Some countries have established health technology assessment centres to evaluate the clinical and cost-effectiveness of new pharmaceuticals (as well as devices, diagnostics, and procedures). The need to do so is predicated by the economic burdens that modern health care is placing on all countries. The inherent tensions between making medicines affordable, yet providing appropriate incentives for the development of new ones, remain to be resolved.

Further reading

Drummond MF, *et al.* (2005). *Methods for the economic evaluation of health care programmes.* Oxford University Press, Oxford.

Jadad AR, Enkin MW (2007). *Randomized controlled trials: questions, answers and musings.* BMJ Books, London.

Pocock SJ (1983). *Clinical trials: a practical approach.* John Wiley & Sons, Chichester.

Rawlins MD (2008). De Testimonio: on the evidence for decisions about the use of therapeutic interventions. *Lancet*, **372**, 2152–161.

2.4.2 Reasonableness and its definition in the provision of health care

Norman Daniels

Essentials

Two central goals of health policy are to improve population health as much as possible and to distribute the improvements fairly. These goals will often conflict. Reasonable people will disagree about how to resolve these conflicts, which take the form of various unsolved rationing problems. The conflict is also illustrated by the ethical controversy that surrounds the use of cost-effectiveness analysis. Because there is no consensus on principles to resolve these disputes, a fair process is needed to assure outcomes that are perceived to be fair and reasonable. One such process, accountability for reasonableness, assures transparency, involves stakeholders in deliberating about relevant rationales, and requires that decisions be revised in light of new evidence and arguments. It has been influential in various contexts including developed countries such as Canada, the United Kingdom, New Zealand, and Sweden, and developing countries, such as Mexico.

Introduction

Decisions about health-care provision are morally contentious because problems of distributive fairness are pervasive. We lack agreement on principles of distribution fine-grained enough to resolve the many disputes we have about how to balance maximization of aggregate measures of population health against the fair distribution of health benefits, yet both goals—improving population health and doing so fairly—are the primary goals of health policy. In the face of these pervasive and systematic controversies, a reasonable health policy will be one that emerges from a fair, deliberative process of the sort that holds decision-makers accountable for their reasonableness. Such a process must be based on reasons people can agree are relevant to the task, and on rationales that are fully transparent to those affected by the decisions and that allow for the revision of decisions in light of new evidence and arguments.

This process-based approach will leave some people unsatisfied: it does not tell us exactly how much a country should be spending on health care, for example, and it does not tell us exactly how what it does spend should be distributed. The answers to those questions must emerge from the fair process itself. What the process assures us of, however, is that the moral controversies about distribution—how to trade-off maximizing benefits against their equitable distribution—are thoroughly considered and that choices reflect careful consideration of the different values involved. That may be the best we can do in the pursuit of our two main goals, improving population health and distributing the improvements fairly.

Improving population health as much as we reasonably can is a requirement of justice because the departures from normal functioning that constitute ill health interfere with the satisfaction of various principles of justice. Thus ill health diminishes significantly the range of exercisable opportunities open to people, as I have argued elsewhere, or, as other philosophers have claimed, it diminishes their capabilities or their opportunity for welfare and advantage. Accordingly, different, prominent accounts of justice emphasize the importance of establishing institutions that protect or promote these goods (which is not to say that some theories deny any obligations to do so). Distributing those improvements fairly, however, is a further requirement of justice. A reasonable health policy must address and resolve the conflicts that may arise between these goals.

Since the conflict between these goals is so common, it may seem ironic that it ultimately disappears, at least if the goals are fully achieved. Health, conceived of as normal functioning, is a concept with a limit, unlike wealth or income. Consequently, the ultimate goal of maximizing population health is achieved if all people are made fully functional or healthy. But that outcome also fairly distributes the improvements, since all end up equally healthy. Ultimately, and surprisingly, the health maximizer and the health egalitarian (i.e. someone concerned about equity in health outcomes) aim for the same goal. In the real world where many are unhealthy, however, the goals rudely come apart. Health-maximizing strategies often ignore equity in health, and the pursuit of equity in health often requires foregoing some aggregate health benefits. It is in this uneven terrain that we must seek reasonable ways of balancing our two goals.

Reasonable people will, unfortunately, disagree about how to balance these objectives. In the absence of a prior, principled agreement that resolves these disputes, we require a form of procedural justice, a process accepted as fair by all. Then, outcomes of the fair process will be accepted as fair. A reasonable health policy will be what results from such a process, for the process holds decision-makers accountable for the reasonableness of their decisions. We illustrate more carefully in the next section why such a fair process is needed, but first one preliminary point needs to be addressed.

Some people might believe the problem of resolving these disagreements about priorities in health policy is artificially created by the presence of resource limits that are avoidable. They believe we should be able to do everything for everyone in need, and if we eliminated waste or arbitrary political constraints on funding, then we could meet all such needs. Some form of resource scarcity, however, is always going to be present: promoting health is not the only important good, for every society must meet other needs of its citizens. In addition, new technologies and ageing populations with more expensive health needs mean that we are always facing resource allocation problems with some novelty. Therefore, even very inefficient health delivery systems, such as the highly fragmented American system with its uniquely high unit costs and administrative costs, would face scarcity problems not due to waste were it to be dramatically reformed on the model of universal coverage systems elsewhere.

Health maximization vs health equity

To illustrate the types of conflict between health maximization and health equity that make health policy decisions difficult, consider one standard methodology for maximally improving population health; namely, cost-effectiveness analysis (CEA). The method permits us to compare the incremental health benefits of an intervention or policy with its incremental costs. The ratio of the two is the incremental cost-effectiveness ratio. Comparing the incremental cost-effectiveness ratios of two treatments for the same condition or two treatments for different conditions allows us to measure the marginal health benefit gained per unit of money spent.

Health benefits can be measured in various ways, but some way of combining the duration and the quality of changes in health states into health-adjusted life years (HALYs) is preferred so one can make comparisons across conditions with different kinds of outcomes. The most commonly used such unit in medicine is the quality-adjusted life year (QALY). Different health states are assigned a value on a scale from 0 (death) to 1 (perfect health), and this weighting function is then multiplied by the duration of live lived in that state to yield the number of QALYs gained. Thus, a year lived in perfect health is equivalent to 1 QALY, but if one is in a significantly compromised health state having a value of 0.6, then that same year is equivalent to 0.6 QALYs. The costs are similarly limited to treatment costs and do not include the indirect costs that result if people live longer and have to be assisted in other ways. If we select the most cost-effective intervention for treating a specific condition, we are getting the most health benefit per unit of money spent.

Although this method is often characterized as 'utilitarian' because it is a maximizing strategy, unlike utilitarianism, it ignores benefits other than the health benefit to the individual—for example the income stream generated by the extra life years the individual enjoys—and it ignores costs other than treatment costs. Arguably, some of these excluded benefits and costs are relevant to social policy, so cost-effectiveness analysis and full-blown utilitarianism will differ in some policy recommendations. Still, one ethical reason for avoiding some of these other benefits and costs is that it allows policy in the medical sector to avoid making social worth judgements about the consequences of treating some people rather than others. Arguably, this kind of respect for persons is owed to people in need of medical interventions and is part of the rationale for treating medicine as something of a 'separate sphere' from some other policy domains.

Despite this effort to keep CEA free from certain moral objections, it still faces other ethical criticisms. A key form of criticism is that the maximizing commitments of CEA mean it ignores important issues of distributive fairness. Consider three unsolved rationing problems in which CEA adopts an extreme position that puts it at odds with widely held concerns about equity.

- The priority problem. One widely held view is that we should give some priority in our thinking about whom to treat to those who are worse off. If, however, we give complete priority to those who are worse off, following a 'maximin' rule, then we may have to forego very significant benefits to others who have legitimate claims to them while we secure only minor benefits for the worst off. Maximin seems implausible. CEA, however, tells us to give no priority to those who are worse off. Rather, we are to distribute the chips—the QALYs—where they fall, aiming only to get the most chips. In effect, CEA denies or ignores the widely held view that it may be more morally important to give a QALY to someone who is worse off than another. But if both extreme views are implausible—no priority and maximal priority—then how much priority should we give those who are worse off? This is the priority problem, and reasonable people disagree about it.
- The aggregation problem. CEA tells us that all aggregations of benefit are permissible: we seek the maximum aggregate benefit regardless of whether it arises from significant benefits to a few or from very modest benefits to many. In contrast, most people think some trivial additional benefits should not count in deciding whom to save. At the other extreme, some people will rule out all forms of aggregation. Most people, however, believe that it is preferable to save more lives or life years or QALYS than fewer, even though they reject allowing every conceivable aggregation. Again, extreme positions seem implausible but reasonable people will disagree about which aggregations to allow in the middle range.
- The best outcomes/fair chances problem. As in the other problems, CEA takes an extreme view, always favouring best outcomes (greatest health benefit). But always favouring a group that would achieve best outcomes, say those who will gain the most life-years or QALYs from a transplant, means that others may have no chance at all at a significant benefit, say living more years but not as many as those in the 'best outcome' group. They would complain they ought to have a fair chance of some benefit and not be asked to sacrifice any chance of significant benefits just because others are lucky enough to have better outcomes. An extreme alternative to always favouring 'best outcomes' is to give everyone equal chances of a benefit. Many would think it implausible to give people equal chances of a benefit when that would mean foregoing much greater benefits for others. To find a middle ground, some theorists have therefore argued for a weighted or proportional lottery or chance. Reasonable people will disagree about how to set those weights or proportions.

Notice that standard policy choices about health interventions often face one or another of these problems. For example, in decisions to scale up antiretroviral treatments in high-prevalence, low-resource countries, it is often claimed that locating treatment sites in urban hospitals would lead more quickly to higher treatment rates. The decision means, however, that other populations fail to have any chance at significant benefit because 'best outcomes' favours another group. The problem of orphan drugs has the same form. Similarly, since CEA favours best outcomes, then wherever more QALYs are gained by treating people who are young than those who are old, the old lose any chance at a significant benefit while the young are favoured. (Some may want to give priority to the young for other reasons of fairness, such as Williams's 'fair innings argument', but always favouring best outcomes is not a fairness consideration.)

These distributive problems, and thus the conflict between health maximization and health equity, arise in two important and perhaps surprising contexts, efforts to reduce health inequities and human rights efforts to promote health. The distributive problems just reviewed are all presented with a morally unproblematic baseline. Some people are sicker than others, but we do not ask why. We only consider how much priority to give to them compared to others. Suppose, however, that some group is unjustly worse off with regard to health than another. Perhaps it is a traditionally excluded group, such as the indigenous population in some Latin American countries that has high maternal mortality rates, or African-Americans in the United States of America who have a higher prevalence of uncontrolled high blood pressure, or some ethnic minorities, like the Maori in New Zealand or Aboriginals in Australia, or the Roma in some European countries, all of whom have higher infant mortality rates than the dominant population, or young women in sub-Saharan Africa who have higher prevalence of HIV/AIDS than men. Because of the injustice of the baseline, we may have some good reason to want to give more priority to helping those who are worse off than we ordinarily might have, but how much more? Giving maximum priority ('maximin') means we forego all other benefits to others, whose illness gives them legitimate claims on assistance even it if is not the result of some broader social injustice. We may shift our priorities, but reasonable people will again disagree how much.

One promising movement in international health, the broad effort to improve population health and its distribution through the international legal framework of human rights, also encounters these controversial distributive problems. We might think this implausible because there is already agreement on general principles, the specific rights that are included in this framework. Nevertheless, we can often only improve realization of a specific right for some claimants and not others. For example, we may reach some young girls but not others in a programme to improve literacy among young women, a key determinant of maternal and child health. We can often improve population health in various ways that improve realization of some rights and not others, say by improving training of birth attendants or by changing the legal system to prevent young girls from being married and becoming pregnant too early. The choices among these alternatives raise the same priority, aggregation, and best outcomes/fair chances problems we already encountered, and the language of rights does not eliminate them. This means that different people affected by human rights efforts to improve population health will disagree about the fairness of one reform programme as opposed to another.

Accountability for reasonableness

When we lack prior agreement on principles fine-grained enough to resolve moral disagreements about fair distributions, we must rely on a form of procedural justice. For complex health policy choices, we need a process that is fair to all stakeholders, that is transparent to the broader public affected by these decisions, that permits appropriate deliberation about the reasons that are relevant to choices, and that allows decisions to be revisited in light of new evidence and arguments. One version of such a process is called 'accountability for reasonableness', and it requires compliance with the following conditions:

- Publicity. The rationales for all decisions must be publicly accessible so that people affected by them understand why choices that fundamentally affect their well-being were made.
- Relevant reasons. The rationales for decisions must be based on reasons that fair-minded people agree are relevant to making decisions of this sort. Fair-minded people are people interested in being able to justify their decisions to each other. Often, a mechanism for vetting such reasons is to involve a broad group of stakeholders in the decision, though the exact form for such involvement may vary considerably with the institutional level at which decisions are made. Stakeholder involvement should not be understood as 'democratic'; rather, it improves the deliberation and helps to assure a careful assessment of all relevant reasons, as well as adds transparency to the deliberation. (Stakeholder involvement may not be feasible in some private organizations, and then the publicity condition is the only assurance that broader critical discussion can take place.)
- Revisability and appeals. Decisions must be evidence and argument-based, and this means a fair process must allow for revisiting decisions as new considerations become available. Further, there are often specific groups or individuals who do not quite fit the rules or reasoning underlying some choices and who are unduly burdened by them. Such people need a fair hearing of their appeal against decisions that deny them fundamental goods.
- Enforcement. There needs to be assurance, often in the form of regulation, makes sure the procedures are ones that comply with the first three substantive conditions.

If these conditions are met, decision-makers are held accountable for the reasonableness of their decisions. Indeed, a kind of case law emerges that reveals the commitments underlying the decisions. In this way, the reasons underlying decisions are made explicit, even if all the grounds for them cannot all be articulated prior to considering specific cases, and they gradually accumulate as an explicit framework for priority setting. Since the public reporting of full rationales shows that deliberation about relevant reasons is at the core of the process, the public is assured that moral reasoning plays a role in what have historically been 'behind the scenes' decisions made by bureaucrats unaccountable for their reasons. The public reporting also means that morally controversial choices are exposed to broader public review and criticism. Ultimately, the fair process not only institutionalizes the importance of moral reasoning about these problems but contributes to a social learning process that can improve democratic regulation of the institutions over time.

Accountability for reasonableness is intended as a fair procedure for resolving disagreements about some problems of resource allocation problems, but it is constrained by some substantive moral commitments. For example, human rights considerations would restrict decisions about priorities to ones that are, among other things, nondiscriminatory. It is also assumed that there is a shared goal of meeting health needs fairly under resource constraints while promoting population health. More specifically, the shared goal might be characterized as a goal of protecting opportunity or capabilities by protecting health—and then more specific reasons for constraints must be the subject of deliberation in the fair process. Thus reasonable people may disagree about exactly what role to assign responsibility for healthy behaviours, especially given the difficulty of assigning responsibility, and this matter will have to be resolved along with others. A further issue that affects the legitimacy of outcomes of the fair process is specification of who should have the moral authority to make decisions. Much depends on the level within a health system at which decisions are made and the nature of the organization and funding of the system: it will be far more appropriate in publicly administered systems to be more inclusive about stakeholders involved in or consulted on decisions than it can be in systems that have private, indeed for-profit, components. In the latter, the publicity condition is an effort to include the broader public in the political oversight of the decisions as a whole.

A fair process such as this has broad appeal and broad application to many kinds of health care decisions at different institutional levels: international, national, and subnational. Internationally, the World Health Organization recently endorsed the value of such a process in its guidelines for assuring equity in patient selection for the scaling-up of antiretroviral treatments in its '3 by 5' programme. It also uses the features of that process as a framework for assessing decision-making in Tanzania about its AIDS treatment policy. At a national level, the Ministry of Health in Mexico recently embraced the features of accountability for reasonableness in constructing a fair, deliberative process for making decisions about incremental expansion of its catastrophic insurance plan. In the United States of America, an Institute of Medicine committee reporting on the use of CEA in regulatory settings insisted that the method, while valuable, cannot (by design and use) capture all value issues, so it should be one input among others into a fair deliberative process of the sort that meets the conditions of accountability for reasonableness. In the United Kingdom, Sir Michael Rawlins, director of the National Institute for Health and Clinical Excellence (NICE), affirms that the ideas underlying accountability for reasonableness should inform NICE's technology assessment recommendations. The Citizen's Council NICE established is one version of an appeal to a broader group of stakeholders and the commitment to full publicity for the grounds of decisions is similarly a positive feature of NICE's method of operation.

The process can be used to determine a reasonable health-care policy at subnational levels as well. Health authorities working at the regional and local levels face priority-setting decisions that encounter the same distributive problems noted earlier. Similarly, hospitals make priority and limit-setting decisions that inevitably encounter these distributive problems, and hospitals and their subdivisions could all comply with institutionally-appropriate versions of the conditions for accountability for reasonableness. Even general practitioners, acting as fundholders or commissioners of health services, would improve the legitimacy of their decisions were they to hold themselves accountable for their reasonableness.

Further reading

Brock D (2003). Ethical issues in the use of cost effectiveness analysis for the prioritization of health care resources. In: Khusfh G, Englehardt T (eds.) *Bioethics: a philosophical overview*. Kluwer, Dordrecht, pp. 203–19. [Explores a range of criticisms of cost-effectiveness analysis.]

Daniels N (2008). *Just health: meeting health needs fairly*. Cambridge University Press, New York. [Provides a comprehensive and integrated account of justice and health.]

Daniels N, Sabin JE (2002). *Setting limits fairly: can we learn to share medical resources?* Oxford University Press, New York. [Describes the theory underlying accountability for reasonableness and explains the need for it.]

Gold MR, *et al.* (1996). *Cost-effectiveness in health and medicine*. Oxford University Press, New York. [This Public Health Service report articulates a standard form of cost-effectiveness analysis.]

Ham C, Robert G (1999). *Reasonable rationing: international experience of priority setting in health care*. Open University Press, Maidenhead. [Evaluates the degree to which rationing conforms to conditions of reasonableness in five countries.]

Kamm F (1993). *Morality, mortality: death and whom to save from it*, vol. 1. Oxford University Press, Oxford. [Uses rigorous philosophical tools to explore problems of priority setting in health care.]

Miller W, Robinson LA, Lawrence RS (eds) (2006). *Valuing health for regulatory cost effectiveness analysis*. National Academies Press, Washington, DC. [This Institute of Medicine report supports the view that cost-effectiveness analysis should be seen as an input into a deliberative process.]

World Health Organization (2006). *Equity and fair process in scaling up antiretroviral treatments: potentials and challenges in the United Republic of Tanzania*. WHO, Geneva. [Evaluates the Tanzanian policy for scaling up antiretroviral treatments for AIDS in light of accountability for reasonableness.]

2.4.3 Priority setting in developed and developing countries

Nigel Crisp

Essentials

Priority setting is a normal and important task in any health system. The starting point is current knowledge and evidence, but priority setting is also about judgement, which goes beyond what can be based on evidence. Wherever possible, judgement needs to be based on transparent and systematic methods that are open to question and debate by others.

Public opinion and politics

Politics (in this context) embraces the activities of all those bodies—private, public, and professional alike—whose actions influence health care provision: these have a central place in priority setting, but also need to be transparent and accountable.

Leadership and management

It is essential to understand what leaders or managers are aiming to do in setting priorities at any time, whether this be responding to public pressure, dealing with a financial issue, setting a strategic direction, managing a transformation, or being opportunistic. Whatever is done, there are opportunity costs and there will be unexpected and negative consequences, which need to be anticipated and planned for, wherever possible, and responded to flexibly.

Introduction

This chapter offers a practical overview of priority setting. It is based on my own experience of running a large health system in a developed country (the National Health Service (NHS) in England, serving 51 million people and spending almost £100 billion a year) and my observation of systems in developing countries. There are many common threads. All systems prioritize through some means or other around key questions such as how much money should be spend on health, what are the most important needs to be addressed, what are the opportunity costs of using a particular therapy, judged by staff time and use of facilities as well as money spent, and what are the investments which need to be made in terms of buildings, research, and staff training? It is seen at its starkest in developing countries, where governments may have only \$10 or \$20 a head to spend each year on their populations. But it is also evident in the richest country in the world, the United States of America, where insurance systems put limits on coverage and politicians determine the budgets to be spent on disabled and older people. Only the limitlessly rich could have access to limitless health care!

Priority setting and the associated 'rationing of care', as it is sometimes referred to in more emotional terms, is a normal part of promoting health and providing health care in any system. It can, however, be done well or badly; it can be based on evidence or on popular perception or misconception. Equally, its unintended and detrimental consequences—because it will have some, even if the benefits outweigh them—can be well managed or simply ignored. Priority setting cannot be a purely rational and empirical process. A good starting point is, of course, the study of all the available evidence about the needs of a population and the clinical evidence about therapies and their relative benefits in cost and health terms.

There is now an increasing body of evidence and knowledge available to policy makers and clinicians. The number of documents, evidence-based protocols and systematic reviews is constantly increasing. The World Health Organization even has a listing of cost-effective interventions, which could be used to determine what are the most effective actions to take for any given amount of money. Why are they not widely used in developing and in developed countries? Why is it that Pang, Gray, and Evans needed to write in 2006 that:

> Applying what we know already will have a bigger impact on health and disease than any drug or technology likely to be introduced in the next decade.

It is tempting simply to blame ignorance, prejudice, poor systems, and raw politics. All apply, of course, in some cases, but the answers are more complex.

Judgement, politics, and management

First, there is judgement. This is about how people apply knowledge and goes far beyond what is based on evidence. In the United Kingdom, the National Institute for Health and Clinical Excellence (NICE) has developed a systematic approach to the judgement of which therapies to use. This involves clinical and financial assessments and, interestingly, taps into human judgements of value through a Citizens' Panel. Now there are also many sources of protocols and decision pathways to follow in looking after a patient. These are based on evidence and on consensus judgements of what are the most appropriate routes. Every clinician will also probably recognize the value of individual experience and wisdom in making judgements. The crucial point here is that these expert systems or the wise clinician are valuable, partly because they acknowledge the current state of knowledge in making their judgements.

The second key element is public opinion and politics. In the NHS Plan published in 2000, the United Kingdom government was explicit about targeting improvements in mortality from cancer and coronary heart disease and reductions in waiting times. Many other options were available, but they chose as priorities the issues that were seen as the public's greatest concerns. The dangers here are obvious. Once something is open to political decision making, there is the risk that lobbying, vested interests, and 'pork barrel' politics (spending for projects that are intended primarily to benefit particular constituents or campaign contributors) take over. In this sense of the word, politics covers all the manoeuvring of groups in society, not just the political parties. Doctors, with their powerful position that is often even more powerful in developing than developed countries, are particularly effective lobbyists and politicians in this sense.

In every health system there are examples of decisions that were clearly political: why was this hospital built here, not there? Why were investments made in these clinicians' services and not those? Why, in developing countries, were prestigious hospital projects funded at the expense of more effective community interventions? Why, in developed countries, is so little spent on public health? Public opinion and politics are, however, fickle. In the United Kingdom in 2000, there was great concern about deaths on the coronary heart disease waiting list. By 2005, when this had been largely solved, politicians received little if any credit. Public opinion had moved on. There were, and always will be, other pressing issues of the day.

While lobbying and politics can lead to some poor decisions, the interesting point is to identify where politics is appropriate. Priority setting is necessarily contextual and societal. The politicians in the United Kingdom were deliberately responding to public dissatisfaction. They recognized that the public were paying for the service and, crucially, that the public needed to see improvements if they were to keep faith with the NHS and continue to support it. In other words, they were making a decision not just about cancer or coronary heart disease but about who was paying for it and about how best to ensure the survival of the NHS. Politicians in other countries will consciously make decisions to demonstrate progress and point the direction for the future.

Priority setting is also about opportunity and sometimes needs to be opportunistic. There is sometimes a time and a place when something can be achieved that would not be possible at another.

Priority setting is also about will and determination. In the United Kingdom, we managers and politicians alike knew that we had to remain focused on a few priorities in order to make progress. We faced considerable opposition before there was visible progress. I recall well someone telling me that it was only after the second year of consistent focus that they knew we were serious about reducing waiting times. It was only in that second year that we saw change and began to generate momentum.

Priority setting is also about leadership and management. The decisions you make, although based on knowledge, need to take account of what you are trying to achieve and how you are planning to achieve it. Exercising judgement, responding to public opinion, and providing leadership and management are all necessary components of priority setting, but all need qualification and all have consequences.

Qualifications and consequences

The obvious question to ask at this point is what stops judgement, politics, and management riding roughshod over rational and empirically-based knowledge? Don't these arguments simply allow anything to be done under the heading of priority setting, and how can we make sure we don't end up with arbitrary and expedient priorities? I think that the best response to these questions is to consider how we can qualify judgement, politics, and management and how we can manage the consequences of decisions. Judgement, applied well, is largely but not entirely about balance. It is about taking into account all the relevant aspects of a situation. Arguably, we would not have achieved many of our targets in the NHS if they did not make any clinical sense or make sense to any clinicians. There needed to be some level of clinical support. Some targets were based purely on current medical knowledge, such as the targets to provide thrombolysis speedily after a myocardial infarct or to increase revascularization rates. Others, such as speeding up emergency treatment, were seen as appropriate for some but not all conditions. Peoples' beliefs and attitudes are also highly relevant, whether clinicians or members of the public. Examples from many countries show that the public often has clear views, e.g. in Oregon, where members of the public were asked to rate conditions in priority order for expenditure. The NICE example is perhaps the most sophisticated current example of a systematic way of bringing all these factors together to make a judgement. But such a system will not solve all our problems of judgement at the clinical or the societal level. Individuals and organizations still need to take responsibility for judgement and decisions. My experience does, however, lead me to believe that we need some systematic, consistent, and open way to bring together the various elements in a judgement about priority setting. NICE has taken a bold and important step in this direction.

This argument provides a good lead into the discussion about politics. NICE operates outside the political system and gains its legitimacy through a consistent and open methodology. Transparency and accountability play a similar role in a political system. Governments make decisions based on politics and public opinion and judgements about the needs of particular groups in society or of society as a whole. In health, as in other areas, such decisions and judgements are enhanced through consultation, communication, debate, transparency, and accountability. These considerations also apply to the other participants in the politics of health. Private and public organizations and professional groups all make decisions which affect the availability of treatments to patients.

Pharmaceutical companies—not surprisingly, given that they are business organizations—have concentrated on developing drugs they can sell in developed markets and have ignored the needs of the poor. Governments and donor organizations have had to step in to provide the incentives for investment in the diseases which primarily affect poor people and poor countries. In doing so they have changed the companies' priorities. These companies have enormous influence over many other aspects of health care and are also coming under increasing pressure to be transparent and accountable about the results of trials and about their decision-making processes. Professional organizations can also promote or block access to treatment. Sometimes this is about roles, standards and professional protectionism. In Brazil, for example, doctors have threatened strike action over the government's decision to allow nurses to prescribe certain drugs. Elsewhere nurses prescribe these drugs safely and effectively. In both cases, there is a strong argument that business and professional groups alike need to demonstrate transparency and accountability in the public realm to those, the general public, who will ultimately pay for and benefit, or not, from their decisions.

Decisions about priorities, however taken, will inevitably have some difficult consequences, some of which will be unforeseen. This could happen in a number of different ways. In the United Kingdom, some of the NHS Plan targets were resisted by clinicians because they were seen as 'distorting' priorities. For example, it was argued, rightly, that requiring all patients to be treated and out of hospital emergency departments in 4 hours ignored the fact that some patients needed a longer time there for tests and observation. We responded nationally by asking a senior clinician to identify to what proportion of patients this would apply and to exclude this percentage from the target. A more serious problem was that some managers and clinicians changed figures and reports to improve their performance against the targets. This may happen in any measurement system and needs to be anticipated, identified when it happens and dealt with very firmly. In the NHS, amongst other actions, we asked the independent Audit Commission to do spot checks on measurements.

Managing priorities has opportunity costs. In the NHS, we realized that for a relatively small amount of extra funding we could dramatically reduce waiting times for cataract surgery. However, at that time we wished to maintain our emphasis on existing priorities rather than add another, particularly one which seemed to favour a relatively less serious operation over other more serious ones. A year later, when waiting times were falling fast, we made the investment in cataract surgery, with dramatic results.

More serious is the current situation in developing countries. Tackling HIV/AIDS, tuberculosis, and malaria are priorities alongside maternal and child health in the Millennium Development Goals. The death and disability from these diseases, and the fact that so much can be done to ameliorate them, provides ample reason for this priority. However, this clear focus has consequences. In particular, the action of the 'vertical' funds set up to tackle these diseases is damaging broad based or 'horizontal' health systems in some countries. The projects funded by the vertical funds are well resourced and attract staff and attention away from basic services. In some countries the amount available to tackle these three diseases is greater than the expenditure on all other aspects of health, and inevitably has an unintended distorting effect. In the last year great efforts have been made to align these vertical programmes with other 'system strengthening' initiatives so as to gain the benefits of having priorities whilst not damaging other services.

The simple point here is that thought and planning needs to be given to identifying all the consequences of priority setting, good and bad, and there need to be ways to respond flexibly where problems arise.

Conclusion

Priority setting is both normal and important. Done badly, it can be arbitrary and expedient. Done well, it can bring together evidence, disciplined judgement, accountable politics and clear sighted leadership to improve health.

Further reading

Crisp N (2010). *Turning the world upside down: the search for global health in the 21st century*. RSM Press, London.

Pang T, Gray M, Evans T (2006). The 15th grand challenge for global public health. *Lancet*, **367**, 284–6.

2.4.4 Sustaining innovation in an era of specialized medicine

Henri A. Termeer

Essentials

We are living in an era of unprecedented biomedical innovation. In recent years, new therapies have improved the prognosis of numerous intractable disorders that were previously neglected—in some cases changing diseases from a death sentence to a manageable chronic condition.

Our increased understanding of the genetic basis of disease will continue to fuel the creation of innovative therapies for many decades. Many of even the most enterprising therapies being introduced today are only a bridge to the definitive cures that gene therapy, stem cells, and other advances may offer.

The current pace of innovation has spawned a public debate over the level of support that society should provide for access to progressive new medicines, particularly those designed for specialized patient populations. In this debate, the cost of these therapies is often highlighted while the specific and general benefits brought by providing access are often overlooked.

For individuals, access to innovative therapies has meant improved health, better quality of life and increased productivity—and often reduced spending on other medical interventions. For society more broadly, support for innovation allows the biopharmaceutical industry to continue with confidence in the creation of medicines for tomorrow; this investment supports the economic health of an industry that generates jobs favoured in developing and developed countries alike.

Here we examine the far-reaching impact of decisions by governments to support or deny access to biomedical innovation: we also outline the responsibility of all parties to address the issue of access to treatment in a global context.

Towards personalized medicine

This is a moment of transition at the world's biopharmaceutical companies. The ability of industry to create the largest-selling medicines upon which it has thrived for so long—so-called 'blockbuster' drugs—has diminished in part because advances in life sciences research have made drug development a more precise process. New therapies are increasingly refined, and as a result, the pool of patients who benefit from any one innovation has grown smaller. At the same time, the probability that any one individual patient within that pool will benefit from treatment has increased.

Some of the latest therapies are already fulfilling the promise of personalized medicine. In oncology, for example, targeted therapies have been developed not only for specific forms of cancer, but for patients with certain genetic mutations that make them most likely to respond to treatment or less likely to develop side effects. At the same time, a growing number of treatments for genetic diseases are being developed and prescribed only for those with a confirmed genetic diagnosis. Increasingly, genetics and therapeutics are being amalgamated, promising not only the development of highly effective and safe therapies, but also the efficient use of the resources spent to pay for them.

This transition—from the general to the specialized—has profound implications for drug makers and those who pay for innovation. Ultimately the degree of reimbursement support for these innovations, which may serve smaller patient populations and as a result cost more per patient, will dictate what treatments are available in the future. Owing to the large risk and substantial investment required to bring any new therapy to the market as a licensed agent, funding decisions made today will continue to reverberate for decades to come.

Innovation incentives

Strong financial incentives have long been the stimulus for biomedical innovation. Before 1983, when the United States Congress passed the first Orphan Drug Act, very few companies pursued treatments for rare diseases because the size of the market did not justify the risk and expense involved in their pharmaceutical development and marketing. The Orphan Drug Act, created in response to the will of society to address the needs of those with rare diseases, granted research and development tax credits and provided 7 years of market exclusivity to companies that successfully developed a therapy for a disease affecting fewer than 200 000 people in the United States of America.

The orphan drug legislation has been remarkably successful in the United States of America and other developed countries. Since 1983, more than 1600 product candidates have been designated for orphan disease status in the United States of America, and more than 290 of these have been successfully developed. Similar legislation was passed in Europe in 2000, leading to more than 390 designations and more than 30 approved therapies to date.

More important than the number of orphan drugs introduced is the nature of the benefits they provide. Many treatments supported by orphan drug legislation are first-ever, life-changing therapies for patients affected by chronic conditions. In some cases, they forestall or prevent the progressive deterioration that marks these chronic diseases, and allow patients who would otherwise be debilitated to enjoy a more normal productive life. In the most dramatic cases, these treatments not only alter patients' lives—they save them.

While tax credits and market protection have been valuable incentives, they are not enough by themselves to ensure that innovation reaches all who need it. Payment or 'reimbursement support' for treatments that can change lives is the engine that drives continued innovation and recovery. As discussed below, treatments for rare diseases will typically be more expensive on a per-patient basis because of the rarity of the condition. Long-term sustainability of this type of innovation depends on the ability of society to balance the needs of all citizens with the needs of a small number of severely affected individuals, and to make decisions that are equitable for all.

Societal investment

Health care is a basic human necessity. How individual countries seek to meet this need and the amount they are willing to spend on health care varies widely, yet greater spending does not necessarily buy better health outcomes—nor does it ensure that patients will have access to innovative treatment.

Spending on total health care in four major European countries (Germany, France, Spain, and Italy) ranged from 8% to 11% of gross domestic product in 2004, while the growth rate over that period ranged from 1% to 5%. In the United States of America, health care spending represented 15% of gross domestic product and grew at a rate of 4.6% over the same period. Pharmaceutical spending as a percentage of total health care costs in 2004 ranged from 14% to 23% in the four European countries and was 12% in the United States of America.

Spending on pharmaceutical and biological therapies is a visible, albeit relatively small, fraction of total health care costs. The increasing number of higher-priced, better-targeted specialty pharmaceuticals which treat smaller patient populations has led some to conclude that these therapies are driving a rise in health care costs. By restricting access to these new therapies, advocates believe they can control the growth of health care spending overall. There are several flaws in this argument.

1 Pharmaceutical spending is growing at, or only slightly above, the growth rate for total health care spending, and remains only a small fraction of total health care costs. The contribution made by therapies where the per-patient costs are the highest remains too small to be a driver.
2 By improving health, innovative new therapies can save society money in ways not easily captured by simple calculations related to direct costs.
3 A significant percentage of pharmaceutical spending is devoted to therapies destined to come off-patent in the next few years. As this occurs, the result will be increased competition and lower prices for consumers.
4 Restricting spending on innovative therapies will impede the very investment in research and development that is the central goal of the orphan drug legislation.

Despite advances in drug development, the process remains a very high-risk endeavour for pharmaceutical and biotechnology companies. Most treatments currently under development will fail. Indeed, most failures occur long before human clinical trials are undertaken—but even among those molecules which advance to human testing, only 20 to 30% of all product candidates will be approved. This failure rate has driven the cost of development for a new medicine from an estimated $154 million (in year 2000 dollars) to upwards of $1 billion today. In the 1980s it took less than 5 years to develop an average drug; today it takes an average of 8 to 10 years. This reality is reflected in the cost of new therapies.

Cost of therapy

Four main factors influence the price of any individual therapy: the cost of production, cost of development, size of the patient population, and the requirement of any commercial organization to make a profit.

The cost of production generally represents a small fraction of the overall drug cost in the case of small-molecule drugs, which can be chemically synthesized to exact specifications. Production of a biological therapy is more complicated, however, and therefore more costly. A biological therapy is produced in living systems with all of the inherent variability of those systems. Nevertheless, the final product must meet the same exacting standards as any medicine, to ensure that the individual patient can count on the expected level of safety and efficacy from that therapy.

Clinical development represents a major cost both before a therapy is approved for sale and after approval, when a manufacturer works to fulfil its post-approval regulatory commitments. In addition to investments in both manufacturing scale-up and preclinical development of the molecule, the bulk of the pre-market investment goes to demonstrate clinical safety and efficacy, which in the case of large-scale diseases may require clinical trials involving thousands of patients.

It is noteworthy that the cost of development of therapies for rare diseases is not necessarily less than for more common ones, despite much smaller-scale clinical trials. In the case of rare diseases, the major determinant of the ultimate cost of therapy is the size of the affected patient population. The costs associated with a therapy for a large indication can be spread over a much larger number of individuals, whereas the cost of therapy for a rare disease is borne by a much smaller number of people. As an example, consider Genzyme's enzyme replacement therapy for Gaucher's disease. Introduced in 1991, this treatment remains the standard of care, but is used by only 4900 people worldwide, including approximately 1500 in the United States of America—less than 1/100 of the patient population that may be considered as an orphan indication. If there were 100 000 individuals with Gaucher's disease on treatment in the United States of America—a total which would still qualify it as an orphan disease—the cost of enzyme replacement therapy would be proportionally less.

The revenues derived from marketed therapies like this one enable a company to cover the costs of other products that have failed in development, to invest in new therapies, and to create a sustainable business model with the necessary capital to invest in manufacturing and product support. By remaining profitable, companies are able to ensure that the enterprise is sustainable by rewarding the shareholders/owners who have borne the risk of funding the drug development process.

Special challenges with rare diseases

The approval in 2006 of Genzyme's treatment for Pompe's disease, a rare inherited genetic disease (see Chapter 12.8), demonstrates some of the special challenges posed when the drug development model is applied to an extremely rare disease. Pompe's disease affects fewer than 10 000 people worldwide. Before the development of a therapy, 9 in 10 infants born with the classic infantile form of Pompe's disease did not survive past their first birthday. The late-onset form of the disease progresses more slowly, but still results in substantial muscle deterioration and a vastly shortened life expectancy.

When Genzyme set out to develop enzyme replacement therapy for Pompe's disease in the late 1990s, they were building on a vast store of knowledge gained through the development of three similar treatments for other lysosomal storage disorders. Yet even with this considerable advantage, Pompe's disease would present one of the most vexing development challenges Genzyme had ever faced, one that would ultimately require 8 years of effort by hundreds of employees and outside collaborators, and an investment of more than $600 million by the end of 2006.

The impact of rarity on clinical trial design and patient recruitment is significant and proved particularly challenging in this case. For a condition like Pompe's disease, it is simply not possible to recruit patients for a large clinical trial, and small sample sizes can make it difficult to demonstrate the type of efficacy that regulatory agencies demand. The pivotal trial for Pompe's disease enrolled 18 infants. The primary end-point was ventilator-free survival after 18 months. Because of the rapidly fatal nature of this disease, the protocol called for initiation of treatment before 6 months of age.

Enrolling even this small number of patients required a massive international effort, first to educate physicians on the signs and symptoms of Pompe's disease, and then to ensure rapid diagnosis and enrolment for all eligible patients. For nearly all patients and their families, enrolment in the trial meant being relocated to one of four treatment centres around the world. Patients and their families were relocated for the duration of the trial from Japan,

Taiwan, Peru, Australia, South Africa, and the Middle East. An extraordinary partnership among academia, industry, and patient advocates helped us to fully enrol this trial as quickly as possible, mindful that every day there were families waiting and hoping for us to succeed.

The results were unequivocal. After 18 months of treatment, 83% of patients enrolled in the trial were alive and free of invasive ventilator support, compared with only 2% of patients in the historical comparator group. Within 6 months, the first treatment for Pompe's disease was made available to patients who need it. The ultimate success of this therapy underscores why it is so critical to support the availability of innovative therapies.

Global access

Ensuring global access is a critical issue facing society, as it acts on its collective responsibility to make innovative therapies available to all who need them.

Value is rewarded in a market-driven economy. The same should be true in health care. The health care system should not pay more for a second-generation therapy that offers no advantage over the first-generation option. Increasingly, governments are looking to agencies such as the National Institute of Health and Clinical Excellence (NICE) in the United Kingdom to assess the value of new therapies.

Using these analyses, society is beginning to apply cost-effectiveness measures to determine whether a therapy judged by regulatory agencies to be safe and effective should be reimbursed. This practice is being applied most broadly in assessing treatments for diseases affecting large patient populations. In these cases, much is often known about the natural history of the disease, and typically there have already been multiple therapies tested for use in this patient population, providing a solid benchmark against which new therapies can be compared.

Even in these cases, however, it is critical to assure that the procedure is used truly to clarify the incremental value of a new therapy, and not simply to control costs. The extremely rare 'ultra-orphan disease' patient population and the small fraction of severely affected patients with a more common disease—for example those with heart failure needing a transplant—are both particularly vulnerable in this process. In each instance, the cost of therapy for an individual patient is high, and even at the highest levels of efficacy, likely to exceed most cost-effectiveness thresholds by a significant amount.

To date, most private insurers and government payers have embraced their responsibility to provide patients access to innovative new therapies, even in countries where health budgets are limited. Most have recognized that the use of a highly effective and safe treatment by so few patients represents a prudent and compassionate use of resources, especially where it can help avert other health problems associated with progression of disease, and allow patients to live better, more productive lives. In a few countries such as Canada and Australia, however, the decision to fund treatment has come only after extensive and time-consuming negotiations with manufacturers regarding price. The protracted nature of these discussions has limited access, greatly disadvantaging waiting patients, particularly those with progressive diseases who will suffer irreversible damage or death.

The way pricing decisions are made on a global basis can also have an important impact on access. Genzyme has long approached pricing for its enzyme replacement therapies in a two-tiered way, which has allowed us to meet the obligation we feel to provide access to everyone who needs it, regardless of where they live or whether they are able to pay. In this scenario, all developed economies pay roughly the same price for treatment. And in those countries that are unable to pay, we provide the product for free. In addition, Genzyme has worked in developing economies to create sustainable health care systems capable of caring for patients with a rare disease. It is insufficient simply to ship product to an area lacking the required infrastructure to deliver the it, or the knowledge to ensure the patient can get appropriate long-term care. We partner with local physicians, patients, and responsible authorities to build the infrastructure that is required. Although the country may not have the resources to pay for the therapy, we work with them to make an initial commitment to the care of the patient with a rare disease. This major step moves them towards ultimately assuming full responsibility thereby creating a sustainable long-term outcome that is not totally dependent on the manufacturer. At present diseases are treated in countries as diverse as Algeria, Belarus, Chile, Cuba, Ecuador, Egypt, Haiti, India, Jamaica, Kenya, Malaysia, Pakistan, Palestine, Philippines, South Africa, Sri Lanka, Tanzania, Ukraine, Vietnam, and former Yugoslavia.

With increasingly free flow of products across borders and the use of reference pricing, it is becoming more difficult for manufacturers to preserve different pricing levels in different countries. Adopting uniform global pricing, with a strong parallel commitment to access in countries without the means to afford care, provides a solution that both supports innovation and enables more people globally to benefit from it.

Conclusions

The power of pharmaceutical innovation is twofold. In addition to improving the lives of patients today, these therapies are a bridge to the next generation of definitive treatments with the potential to provide greater health care benefits. For example, the enzyme replacement therapies that now provide the first specific treatments for a range of genetic diseases are life-changing—but they are not a cure.

Progress on gene therapy for even single-gene disorders has been made over the past decade, but this has been slower than anticipated. It is instructive to remember the advice that Genzyme's management was given by its board of scientific advisers when asked whether we should pursue development of an enzyme replacement therapy for Gaucher's disease. Their consensus—more than 20 years ago—was that it was foolish to pursue enzyme replacement therapy because it appeared gene therapy was 'just around the corner.' Fortunately for patients with Gaucher's disease, we decided to develop both approaches in parallel. The world now knows that these initial projections were wildly optimistic.

All potential breakthrough technologies—from stem cells to monoclonal antibodies to gene therapy—take decades of stops and starts before they begin to have a meaningful impact on human health. To continue to deliver on the potential of these innovations, the biopharmaceutical industry depends on society's continued willingness to reward value. The era of personalized medicine will force us to re-evaluate our current concepts of cost-effectiveness to accommodate targeted therapies for smaller patient populations that may carry a high per-patient price tag, but ultimately save money on an absolute basis by enabling more efficient use of society's investment.

Fully realizing society's hope for a healthier future will require a sustained and enlightened commitment on the part of companies, researchers, governments, and insurers. All will need to pursue the path that rewards and encourages innovation, and to bring the benefits of that innovation worldwide. The decisions we all make today will shape the health of generations to come.

Further reading

Danzon PM, Ketcham JD (2004). Reference pricing of pharmaceuticals for Medicare: evidence from Germany, The Netherlands, and New Zealand. *Front Health Policy Res*, **7**, 1–54.

Eng CM, *et al.* (2001). Safety and efficacy of recombinant human α-galactosidase: a replacement therapy in Fabry's disease. *N Engl J Med*, **345**, 9–16.

Feacham RG, Sabot OJ (2006). An examination of the Global Fund at 5 years. *Lancet*, **368**(9534), 537–40.

Gahl WA (2001). New therapies for Fabry's disease. *N Engl J Med*, **345**, 55–7.

Haffner ME (2006). Focus on research: adopting orphan drugs—two dozen years of treating rare diseases. *N Engl J Med*, **354**, 445–7.

Kakkis ED, *et al.* Enzyme-replacement therapy in mucopolysaccharidosis I. *N Engl J Med*, **344**, 182–8.

European Commission. *Register of Designated Orphan and Medicinal Products*. http://ec.europa.eu/enterprise/pharmaceuticals/register/orphreg.htm

Generic Pharmaceutical Association. *Upcoming Patent Expirations, 2005–2009*. http://www.gphaonline.org/AM/Template.cfm?Section=Resources&CONTENTID=1597&TEMPLATE=/CM/HTMLDisplay.cfm

Organisation for Economic Co-operation and Development. *Health Data 2006*. http://www.oecd.org/document/16/0,2340,en_2649_37407_2085200_1_1_1_37407,00.html.

Organisation for Economic Co-operation and Development. *Statistics Database*. http://stats.oecd.org/wbos/default.aspx

Ross JS, *et al.* (2004). Targeted therapies for cancer 2004. *Am J Clin Pathol*, **122**, 598–609.

Tufts Center for the Study of Drug Development (2005). *New drugs are taking longer to bring to market in the U.S.* http://csdd.tufts.edu/NewsEvents/NewsArticle.asp?newsid=58

Tufts Center for the Study of Drug Development (2006). *Average cost to develop a new biotechnology product is $1.2 billion*. http://csdd.tufts.edu/NewsEvents/NewsArticle.asp?newsid=69

US Food and Drug Administration. *List of Orphan Drugs and Approvals*. http://www.fda.gov/orphan/designat/list.htm

US Food and Drug Administration. *Text of Orphan Drug Act*. http://www.fda.gov/orphan/oda.htm

2.5

Complementary and alternative medicine

E. Ernst

Essentials

Complementary and alternative medicine (CAM) can be positively defined as diagnosis, treatment, and/or prevention which complements mainstream medicine by contributing to a common whole, by satisfying a demand not met by orthodoxy, or by diversifying the conceptual frameworks of medicine. It is popular, hence doctors should know about it.

Why is CAM popular?

The following motivations may be important: (1) to leave no therapeutic option untried; (2) to take control over one's own health; (3) to accord one's health care with one's global outlook; (4) to benefit from natural and, by implication, safe treatments; (5) to be given time, understanding, and empathy by a practitioner; (6) disenchantment with conventional medicine/science.

Types of CAM

The term covers a vast array of treatments and diagnostic techniques which have little in common except that they are not part of mainstream medicine. The most important modalities are (1) acupuncture—probably effective for some painful conditions and for nausea/vomiting; rarely causes severe adverse events. (2) Phytotherapy—treatment with herbal extracts; can be evaluated by assessing each of the many remedies separately; some phytomedicines are backed by sound evidence. (3) Homeopathy—based on irrational concepts of 'like cures like' and 'potentizing' (shaking and stepwise dilution of drugs); trial data fail to show efficacy for any condition. (4) Spinal manipulation—may be mildly effective for back pain as practised by chiropractors and other health care professionals; claims that it also works for many other conditions are not supported by sound evidence; can cause significant side effects, e.g. manipulation of the cervical spine causes transient adverse events in about half of all patients and has been associated with serious complications such as dissection of the vertebral artery.

Definition

Most health care professionals feel they know intuitively what is meant by complementary and alternative medicine (CAM). Yet an adequate definition is hard to find. Often CAM is described by characteristics that exclude it from mainstream medicine, e.g.

- not taught in medical school
- not scientifically proven
- not based on a scientific rationale
- not used in routine health care

CAM can be positively defined as 'diagnosis, treatment and/or prevention which complements mainstream medicine by contributing to a common whole, by satisfying a demand not met by orthodoxy or by diversifying the conceptual frameworks of medicine'.

CAM encompasses a large variety of techniques which have little in common except that they are not part of mainstream medicine, claim to offer help for most conditions, and pride themselves on a holistic approach to patient care (Table 2.5.1). Some relate to therapeutic modalities (e.g. herbalism), some to diagnostic techniques (e.g. iridology), and some include both diagnostic and therapeutic modalities (e.g. acupuncture).

There are considerable local differences in what are regarded as CAM or mainstream medicine. In Germany, massage therapy and herbalism are orthodox whereas in English-speaking countries they are usually regarded as CAM. Acupuncture is CAM in the West, while in China it is a widespread, traditional, and accepted form of treatment.

Since most CAM therapies are used as adjuncts to conventional treatments, 'complementary' is a more appropriate term than 'alternative'. When used as a true alternative to mainstream medicine, CAM can become a hazard to patients even if the treatment itself is without risks. In many countries including the United Kingdom, CAM is practised mostly by health care professionals who are not medically trained, often in the absence of stringent regulation.

Table 2.5.1 Various other forms of therapeutic and diagnostic methods

Name	Principle	Main indications/ reasons for use	Efficacy	Risks
Alexander technique	Training process of ideal body posture and movement; developed by F M Alexander	Musculoskeletal problems	Very few clinical trials	No serious adverse effects on record
Applied kinesiology	Diagnostic technique using muscle strength as an indicator; developed by G Goodheart	n.a.	Repeatedly shown to be not valid	Can delay reliable diagnoses
Aromatherapy	Application of essential oils usually through gentle massage techniques; developed by R M Gattefossé	Relaxation improvement of well-being	Systematic reviews are mostly inconclusive	Allergic reactions to oils
Autogenic training	Form of self-hypnosis for relaxation and stress reduction; developed by J Schultz	Stress management	Some evidence for effectiveness	No serious adverse effects on record
Chelation therapy	Intravenous infusion of EDTA used in CAM for 'deblocking' arteries from arteriosclerotic lesions	Circulatory disorders	Shown to be ineffective	Serious adverse effects, even deaths, reported
Chiropractic	Popular manual therapy based on the assumption that most health problems are due to misalignment of the spine and treatable through spinal manipulation; developed by D D Palmer; seen as mainstream by many proponents	Back pain, neck pain, and many others	Cochrane reviews of chiropractic for back pain show it is not superior to standard therapies, no good evidence for other indications	Serious adverse effects have been reported, their exact incidence is not known
Colonic irrigation (or colon therapy)	Cleansing of the colon through enemas with water or coffee for 'detoxication'	Various	No sound evidence for effectiveness	Serious adverse effects reported
Hypnotherapy	Induction of trance-like state to influence the unconscious mind	Various	Some evidence for effectiveness	Serious adverse effects probably infrequent
Iridology	Diagnostic technique using signs and impurities on the iris	n.a.	Repeatedly shown to be not valid	Can delay reliable diagnoses
Macrobiotic diet	Diet based on the yin/yang principle using whole grains and vegetables	Disease prevention	Positive effects on cardiovascular risk factors	Serious adverse effects reported
Massage	Various techniques of manual stimulation of cutaneous, subcutaneous or muscular structures (deemed mainstream on the European continent)	Musculoskeletal problems, anxiety, and many others	Some evidence for effectiveness in musculoskeletal and psychological problems	No serious adverse effects on record
Osteopathy	Health problems are thought to be due to misalignment of the spine and corrected through spinal mobilization; developed by T Still; seen as mainstream by many proponents	Back pain, neck pain, and many others	Systematic reviews of osteopathy for back pain are inconclusive	Adverse effects less than with chiropractic
Reflexology	Internal organs correspond to areas on the sole of the feet and can be influenced through massaging these	Relaxation	Systematic review was inconclusive	No serious adverse effects on record
Spiritual healing	Channelling of 'healing energy' through a healer into a patient	Re-establishing a wholesome balance	Best evidence fails to show effectiveness	No serious adverse effects on record
Yoga	Meditative, postural, and breathing techniques from ancient India	Various	Some evidence for effectiveness in asthma, or cardiovascalur risk factors for instance	No serious adverse effects on record

n.a., not applicable.

Prevalence

The 1-year prevalence of CAM usage by the general population ranges from 10% in the United Kingdom to 62% in Germany. In patient populations, these figures can be considerably higher. For instance, most cancer patients try one form of CAM or another. The annual expenditure for CAM exceeds US$20 billion in the United States of America and £1.6 billion in the United Kingdom.

In industrialized countries, typical users of CAM are middle-aged, female, well-educated members of a high socioeconomic class. Indications for CAM range from chronic benign conditions where mainstream medicine does not offer a cure (e.g. back pain) to life-threatening diseases like cancer and AIDS. Most patients try CAM in parallel with conventional treatment yet 30 to 50% do not tell their conventional health care providers that they do so. A medical history should include specific questions about CAM.

Reasons for CAM's popularity

The following motivations may be important:

- to leave no therapeutic option untried
- to take control over one's own health
- to align one's health care with one's global outlook
- to benefit from natural and, by implication, safe treatments
- to be given time, understanding, and empathy by a practitioner
- disenchantment with conventional medicine/science

Examples of CAM methods

Acupuncture

Description

Traditonally, the Chinese believed that the life energy (Qi or Chi) flowing in particular channels (meridians) governs human health. The energy is a balance of opposite characteristics: yin and yang. Illness is understood as an expression of an imbalance between yin and yang. One way of re-establishing the proper equilibrium would be to insert needles in acupuncture points located along the meridians. Instead of or in addition to needles, acupuncturists also use pressure (acupressure), laser light (laser acupuncture), electrical currents (electroacupuncture), heat (moxibustion), or other stimuli to stimulate acupuncture points. Neither the meridians nor the acupuncture points have a morphological basis and the theory of yin and yang is not supported by facts.

Mode of action

Neurophysiological research has created a (hypothetical) rationale for acupuncture: activation of brainstem nuclei, and the release of neural transmitters and endorphins in the brain and descending inhibitory control systems.

There are considerable differences between traditional Chinese and Western acupuncture. In traditional Chinese medicine, conventional diagnoses are not normally sought, treatment is highly individualized according to each patient's particular yin/yang imbalance, and acupuncture is employed as a 'cure all'. In contrast, Western acupuncturists tailor their treatment to the conventional diagnosis established beforehand and use acupuncture for indications for which it is demonstrably efficacious.

Efficacy

Many trials of acupuncture exist but are fraught with methodological problems, such as placebo and blinding patients or therapists. About 100 systematic reviews and meta-analyses of acupuncture trials for various conditions have been published. As they are often based on biased primary data, their conclusions are not always reliable. According to such reviews, acupuncture may be efficacious for the following conditions:

- chronic back pain
- dental pain
- gastrointestinal endoscopy
- idiopathic headache
- osteoarthritis of knee
- postoperative nausea and vomiting

In the following conditions, this evidence fails to support effectiveness:

- rheumatoid arthritis
- smoking cessation
- weight reduction

For all other indications, the data remain inconclusive, because of highly contradictory findings, insufficient primary data, or a total absence of studies. Recently, new nonpenetrating acupuncture devices have become available which can control adequately for placebo effects in clinical trials. The results of clinical trials employing such devices tend to suggest that most of the therapeutic response to acupuncture relies on placebo effects.

Safety

Serious complications of acupuncture include:

- trauma (e.g. cardiac tamponade, pneumothorax)
- infections (e.g. viral hepatitis)

With well-trained therapists, such complications are rare. However, mild adverse effects (e.g. pain or bleeding at the site of needling) occur in about 10% of all patients. In addition, there are indirect risks. For instance, some acupuncturists advise their patients about prescription drugs without having the medical competence to do so.

Phytotherapy

Description

Medical herbalism (phytotherapy) is treatment with whole plants, parts of plants, or plant extracts. The term does not cover treatment with single active constituents such as acetylsalicylic acid, originally derived from willow bark. Since all plants contain a multitude of chemicals, phytotherapy involves treatment with a mixture of potentially active compounds. In many cases, there is uncertainty about the most important active ingredients and their pharmacological actions. The claim of herbalists that the whole plant (extract) will yield more beneficial effects than any single isolated ingredient (synergy) is largely unproven.

Most medical cultures have their version of traditional herbalism. Traditional Chinese medicine has a long history of employing mixtures of herbs to prevent and treat disease. This tradition was modified by the Japanese and resulted in Kampo medicine. The Indian tradition has generated Ayurvedic medicine which relies heavily on plant-based remedies. Likewise, European herbalism has a tradition which is as old as European medicine itself. The scientific investigation of medicinal herbs is, however, a relatively recent innovation.

Mode of action

There are few differences in principle between pharmacotherapy and phytotherapy except that herbal remedies are multicomponent systems which render them pharmacologically more complex. There is no reason why the rules of pharmacokinetics and pharmacodynamics should not apply. Discernible modes of action exist for every plant-based medicine. In some cases these have been elucidated; in many other cases they remain hypothetical.

Efficacy

Based on authoritative systematic reviews and meta-analysis, good or at least encouraging evidence exists for the efficacy of the following herbal remedies:

- *Andographis paniculata* for upper respiratory tract infections
- black cohosh (*Actaea racemosa*) for alleviating menopausal symptoms
- cranberry (*Vaccinium macrocarpon*) for prevention of urinary tract infections
- devil's claw (*Harpagophytum procumbens*) for treating musculoskeletal pain
- garlic (*Allium sativum*) for hypercholesterolaemia
- *Ginkgo biloba* for intermittent claudication
- *Ginkgo biloba* to delay the clinical deterioration in dementias
- green tea (*Camellia sinensis*) for prevention of cancer and cardiovascular disease
- hawthorn (*Crataegus* spp.) for treatment of chronic heart failure
- horse chestnut (*Aesculus hippocastanum*) seed extract for primary venous insufficiency
- kava (*Piper methysticum*) as an anxiolytic drug
- nettle (*Urtica dioica*) for benign prostate hyperplasia
- red clover (*Trifolium pratense*) for hot flushes during menopause
- saw palmetto (*Serenoa repens*) for benign prostatic hyperplasia
- St John's wort (*Hypericum perforatum*) for mild to moderate depression
- valerian (*Valeriana officinalis*) for insomnia
- willow (*Salix* spp.) bark for pain

For many other popular medicinal herbs, too few clinical trials have been carried out, the studies are methodologically flawed, or their results are contradictory. No good evidence exists for the efficacy of traditional approaches to herbal medicine where plant mixtures with a multitude of ingredients are used depending not on a conventional diagnosis but on the individual patient's set of symptoms, constitution, or other circumstances. Yet these traditional approaches are the ones likely to be applied if a patient consults a medical herbalist.

Safety

Many medicinal herbs have been associated with serious adverse effects (see Chapters 9.3.1 and 9.3.2), e.g.

- aconite (*Aconitum*) cardiotoxic
- *Aristolochia* nephrotoxic
- black cohosh (*Actaea racemosa*) hepatotoxic
- broom (*Cytisus scoparius*) cardiotoxic
- chaparrall (*Larrea tridentate*) nephrotoxic
- comfrey (*Symphytum officinale*) hepatotoxic
- kava (*Piper methysticum*) hepatotoxic
- liquorice root (*Glycyrrhiza glaba)* induces hypokalaemia
- pennyroyal (*Mentha pulegium*) hepatotoxic
- skullcap (*Scutellaria lateriflora*) hepatotoxic

Herbal remedies can interact powerfully with synthetic drugs (Table 2.5.2), and Asian herbal medicines have been shown repeatedly to be adulterated with synthetic drugs or contaminated with heavy metals. In many countries (e.g. United Kingdom and the United States of America) herbal medicines are marketed as food (or dietary) supplements in the absence of stringent quality control.

Homeopathy

Description

Samuel Hahnemann, a German physician, believed in two major principles which formed the basis of an entirely new school of medicine: homeopathy. The 'like cures like' principle postulates that, if a given drug induces symptoms (e.g. a headache) in healthy individuals, it can be employed to treat headaches in patients who suffer from it. The second principle holds that 'potentizing' (i.e. shaking and stepwise diluting) drugs makes them more potent for the treatment of illness. Homeopathic dilutions prepared in this way are believed to be clinically effective even if not a single molecule of the original medicine is contained in the potentized remedy. For 200 years, scientists have pointed out that these principles fly in the face of science and that therefore homeopathy cannot possibly work beyond a placebo effect. Homeopaths, however, insist that their remedies act via 'energy' transfer from the original substance to the diluent (the theory of a 'memory of water').

Homeopaths do not treat diseases but claim to treat the whole individual. They take a detailed history with the aim to match the totality of the symptoms and characteristics of that patient with a 'drug picture' (the 'like cures like' principle). This homeopathic remedy, given in the correct potency, should then be the optimal treatment for that patient. Clinical improvement may, however, take weeks or months, and, in about 20% of all cases, symptoms may deteriorate before they become better, a phenomenon termed 'homeopathic aggravation'.

At the time of Hahnemann there were very few effective treatments and many that were overtly harmful. Homeopathic remedies had virtually no adverse effects. Hahnemann can therefore be credited with clinically exploiting the placebo effect to the best benefit of his patients. It is hardly surprising then that homoeopathy conquered many countries (e.g. France, the United States, India, South America) by storm. The advent of effective synthetic drugs lead to the sharp decline of homoeopathy; the recent boom of CAM, however, has brought about a revival.

Mode of action

Several hypotheses have been developed to explain the transfer of 'energy' from the mother tincture to the diluent. However, none has so far withstood the scrutiny of independent assessment. Neither has the 'energy' ever been defined in physical terms, nor are there rational explanations as to how this 'energy' (if it exists) might affect human health. Therefore homeopathy remains among the least plausible forms of CAM.

Efficacy

A meta-analysis of all 89 randomized and/or placebo-controlled clinical trials published by 1995 calculated an overall odds ratio of 2.45 in favour of homeopathy. When only the 26 most rigorous studies were meta-analysed, the odds ratio fell to 1.66 but remained statistically significant. This publication was criticized, e.g. for pooling data for all medical conditions and all homeopathic

Table 2.5.2 Possible interactions between some popular herbal remedies and synthetic drugs

Herbal remedy[a]	Usage or pharmacological effect[b]	Possible interaction
Aloe (*Aloe* spp.)	Various	With chronic use, potentiation of cardiac glycosides or antiarrhythmic drugs due to loss of potassium
Black cohosh (*Actaea racemosa*)	Oestrogenic	Increased effects of antihypertensives
Borage (*Borago officinalis*)	Anti-inflammatory	Interaction with antiepileptics, may increase risk of seizure
Broom (*Cytisus scoparius*)	Anti-arrhythmic, diuretic	Increased effects of antidepressants, β-blockers, and cardiac glycosides
Cascara (*Rhamus purshiana*)	Laxative, cathartic	Loss of potassium with chronic use, potentiation of cardiac glycosides or antiarrhythmic drugs
Chamomile (*Matricaria recutita*)	Spasmolytic, anti-inflammatory	May potentiate effects of anticoagulants through its coumarin content
Chasteberry (*Vitex agnus castus*)	Hormonal effects	Increased effects of other hormonal drugs
Cranberry (*Vaccinium macrocarpon*)	Urinary tract infections	May enhance elimination of drugs normally excreted in urine
Ephedra (*Ephedra sinica*)	CNS stimulant, sympathomimetic	Cardiac glycosides/halothane: arrhythmias, guanethidine: enhanced sympathomimetic effect, MAO inhibitors: enhanced sympathomimetic effect, secale alkaloids/oxytocin: hypertension
Garlic (*Allium sativum*)	Hypocholesterolaemic	Increased effects of anticoagulants and anti-platelet drugs
Ginger (*Zingiber officinale*)	Antiemetic	Increased effects of anticoagulants
Ginseng (*Panax ginseng*)	Various	Interaction with MAO inhibitors, interaction with stimulants and phenelzine, increased effect of hypoglycaemics
Hawthorne (*Crataegus* spp.)	Digitalis-like	Can increase hypotensive effects of nitrates, antihypotensives, cardiac glycosides, and CNS depressants
Hops (*Humulus lupulus*)	Hypnotic	Antagonism with antidepressants, can increase effects of CNS depressants and hypnotics, interference with hormonal drugs
Horse chestnut (*Aesculus hippocastanum*)	Anti-inflammatory	Increased effects of anticoagulants
Kava (*Piper methysticum*)	Anxiolytic	Potentiation with other axiolytics, can increase parkinsonian symptoms with levodopa
Lavender (*Lavandula angustifolia*)	Sedative	Increased effects of CNS depressants
Liquorice (*Glycyrrhiza glaba*)	Corticosteroid activity for gastric irritation	Potassium loss, e.g. with thiazide diuretics, water and sodium retention with corticosteroids, increased effects of digoxin, decreased effects of antihypertensives
Lily of the valley (*Convallaria majalis*)	Congestive heart failure	Increased (side) effects of quinodine, calcium, saluretics, laxatives, glucosteroids, β-blockers, calcium channel blockers, and digitalis
Mistletoe (*Viscum album*)	Anticancer drug	Increased effects of CNS depressants, antihypertensives, and cardiac drugs
Nettle (*Urtica dioica*)	Diuretic	May potentiate effects of other diuretics
Pumpkin seed (*Curcubita pepo*)	Anthelmintic, diuretic	Can increase effect of diuretics
Sage (*Salvia officinalis*)	Antispasmodic	Interaction with antiepileptics, may increase risk of seizure, decreased effect with antiglycaemics
St John's wort (*Hypericum perforatum*)	Antidepressant	Increased effects of digoxin MAO inhibitors or serotonin uptake inhibitors, decreased effect of drugs metabolized by the cytochrome P450 enzyme system

(*Continued*)

Table 2.5.2 (*Cont'd*) Possible interactions between some popular herbal remedies and synthetic drugs

Herbal remedy[a]	Usage or pharmacological effect[b]	Possible interaction
Valerian (*Valeriana officinalis*)	Hypnotic	Increased effects of CNS depressants and hypnotics
Yew (*Taxus* spp.)	Antirheumatic, anticancer	Chemotherapeutic agents may potentiate its effects

[a] Plant source in brackets.
[b] Not comprehensive.

remedies, and for including trials that were not randomized or placebo-controlled and studies of material (low dilution) remedies for which efficacy is not disputed. The results of about a dozen subsequent systematic reviews generally fail to demonstrate effects beyond placebo. Therefore the best evidence available to date fails to suggest efficacy.

Safety

Highly diluted homeopathic remedies cannot cause pharmacological adverse effects. Homeopaths claim that 'homeopathic aggravations'(an exacerbation of presenting symptoms after administration of the optimal remedy) occur in about 20% of cases; if that were true, they might represent a safety issue. 'Indirect' safety problems include the substitution of effective interventions by homeopathy. For instance, nonmedically qualified homeopaths tend to advise their clients against immunization and advocate homeopathic remedies instead. If this happens on a large scale, it jeopardizes herd immunity against serious infectious diseases.

Spinal manipulation

Description

In most cultures, spinal manipulation has been practised by bonesetters for centuries. Today this set of therapeutic techniques is practised by chiropractors, osteopaths, physiotherapists, doctors, and other health professionals. It is the hallmark therapy for chiropractors who use it to adjust 'subluxations', malalignments of the spine claimed to be at the root of all health problems. During spinal manipulation vertebrae are often manually moved beyond their physiological range of motion but not far enough to destroy joint structures. A typical technique is the short-lever, high-velocity thrust which is used by most chiropractors.

Mode of action

Chiropractors believe that vertebral 'subluxations' adversely affect human health and that consequent spinal manipulation will improve it. The mechanism of action is, however, unclear. Some theories hold that it breaks fibrous adhesions within joints, that it affects mechanoreceptors of the joint, or that it modulates central nervous system excitability.

Efficacy

Most of the trial data pertain to back pain. A Cochrane review of spinal manipulation found no evidence that it is superior to standard treatments for acute or chronic back pain but some evidence that is better than harmful interventions or sham treatments. For all other indications, e.g. neck pain, headache dysmenorrhoea, colic, asthma, the current best evidence fails to indicate effectiveness.

Safety

Several prospective studies have shown that spinal manipulation leads to transient, mild adverse effects such as local pain in about 50% of all patients. In addition, serious adverse effects such as arterial dissection, stroke, and death have been reported in about 700 cases. Chiropractors claim that the incidence of such complications is exceedingly low. Due to significant under-reporting, this may not be so. At present, the true incidence is not known.

Other forms of CAM

CAM is a highly diverse field comprising more than 150 different forms of therapeutic and diagnostic methods (see Table 2.5.1).

Further reading

Assendelft WJJ, *et al.* (2003). Spinal manipulative therapy for low back pain. A meta-analysis of effectiveness relative to other therapies. *Ann Intern Med*, **138**, 871–81.

Capasso F, *et al.* (2003). *Phytotherapy: a quick reference to herbal medicine.* Springer Verlag, Berlin.

Derry CJ, *et al.* (2006). Systematic review of systematic reviews of acupuncture published 1996–2005. *Clin Med*, **6**, 381–6.

Ernst E (2002). A systematic review of systematic reviews of homeopathy. *Br J Clin Pharmacol*, **54**, 577–82.

Ernst E (2006). Acupuncture—a critical analysis. *J Intern Med*, **259**, 125–37.

Ernst E (2008). Chiropractic: a critical evaluation. *J Pain Symptom Manage*, **35**, 544–62.

Ernst E, *et al.* (2008). *Oxford handbook of complementary medicine.* Oxford University Press, Oxford.

Singh S, Ernst E (2008). *Trick or treatment? Alternative medicine on trial.* Bantam, London.

SECTION 3

Global patterns of disease and medical practice

3.1 Global burden of disease: causes, levels, and intervention strategies *73*
Ramanan Laxminarayan and Dean Jamison

3.2 Human population size, environment, and health *80*
A.J. McMichael and J.W. Powles

3.3 Avoiding disease and promoting health *86*

3.3.1 Preventive medicine *86*
David Mant

3.3.2 Medical screening *94*
Nicholas Wald and Malcolm Law

3.3.3 The importance of mass communication in promoting positive health *108*
Thomas Lom

3.4 Influence of wealth *112*

3.4.1 The cost of health care in Western countries *112*
Joseph White

3.4.2 A sinister pathogen corrupts two disciplines: the demographic entrapment of Middle Africa *116*
Maurice King

3.5 Human disasters *119*
Amartya Sen

3.1

Global burden of disease: causes, levels, and intervention strategies

Ramanan Laxminarayan and Dean Jamison

Essentials

Recent decades have seen remarkable progress in quantifying the burden of disease in low- and middle-income countries and in gathering evidence on the effectiveness and cost-effectiveness of health interventions. This chapter reviews the major sources of death and disability in these countries and draws lessons from recent analytical work on the cost-effectiveness of interventions to address this disease burden. Four essential messages emerge:

1. Life expectancies worldwide improved dramatically from 1960 to 2002, with the largest increases being in low- and middle-income countries.
2. Improvements in immunization coverage, access to basic education, and spread of low-cost but powerful medical technologies—rather than income growth—appear to have been the primary causes of the gains in life expectancy.
3. The decline in childhood infectious disease burden has been partially offset by a dramatic, age-related increase in the incidence of HIV/AIDS and of chronic, noncommunicable diseases (cardiovascular disease, stroke, diabetes, cancer, psychiatric disorders), especially in low- and middle-income countries.
4. Cost-effective interventions can—if selected carefully and adopted widely—address the challenges of lowering under-5 and maternal mortality, and the burden of noncommunicable diseases.

Interventions that in appropriate circumstances can cost less (sometimes much less) than US$100 per disability-adjusted life year (DALY) include:

- improving care of children <28 days old
- expanded immunization coverage with standard child vaccines
- adding vaccines against additional diseases to the standard child immunization program (particularly *Haemophilus influenzae* B, hepatitis B)
- switching to use of combination drugs against malaria (when resistant to previous standard treatments)
- some measures to prevent and treat HIV/AIDS
- taxing tobacco products
- treating acute myocardial infarction with an inexpensive set of drugs
- detecting and treating cervical cancer
- operating a basic surgical ward at the district hospital level that focuses on trauma, high-risk pregnancy, and other common surgically treatable conditions

Introduction

For low- and middle-income countries, where nearly four in five people on the planet live, the latter half of the 20th century was characterized by two important changes. First, life expectancies increased rapidly, largely because of wider use of childhood immunization and access to basic education, and diffusion of medical technologies led to declines in the prevalence of infectious diseases. Second, the incidence of noncommunicable diseases, such as cardiovascular disease, diabetes, and cancer, also rose sharply. Although population ageing is the main reason for that increase, adverse changes in lifestyle and other risk factors are also occurring, and this new wave of diseases is poised to hit low- and middle-income countries especially hard.

This chapter describes the changes in life expectancy and disease burden during the past two decades, the major health challenges at the beginning of the 21st century, and the most promising interventions to address these challenges.

Changes in life expectancy: trends and causes

Increasing life expectancies during the latter half of the 20th century marked a significant improvement in living standards for populations around the world (Table 3.1.1). Life expectancies in low- and middle-income countries increased by an average of 6.3 years per decade between 1960 and 1990 and at a slower pace of

Table 3.1.1 Levels and changes in life expectancy by World Bank region, 1960–2002

Region	Life expectancy (years)			Rate of change (years per decade)	
	1960	1990	2002	1960–90	1990–2002
Low- and middle-income countries	44	63	65	6.3	1.7
East Asia and the Pacific	39	67	70	9.3	2.5
(China)	(36)	(69)	(71)	(11)	(1.7)
Europe and Central Asia	–	69	69	–	0.0
Latin America and the Caribbean	56	68	71	4.0	2.5
Middle East and North Africa	47	64	69	5.7	4.2
South Asia	44	58	63	4.7	4.2
(India)	(44)	(59)	(64)	(5)	(4.6)
Sub-Saharan Africa	40	50	46	3.3	−3.3
High-income countries	69	76	78	2.3	1.7
World	50	65	67	5.0	1.7

Reproduced from World Bank 2004 (CD ROM Version) World Bank (2004) World Development Indicators. With kind permission from The International Bank for Reconstruction and Development, The World Bank.
— = not available.
Note: Entries are the average of male and female life expectancies.

1.7 years in the century's final decade. Only in sub-Saharan Africa did life expectancy not increase at all, largely because of the HIV/AIDS epidemic.

Despite huge global improvements, many low- and middle-income countries have not shared in the gains, or have even fallen behind, and their citizens' poor health has impeded economic growth. Whereas income inequality between and within countries has increased, cross-country differences in life expectancy and overall welfare inequality have decreased markedly since 1950.

Income inequality explains the remaining health inequalities only partly. Dramatic improvements in health were achieved without significant income growth in Europe in the late 19th and early 20th centuries, and in Bangladesh, China, Costa Rica, Cuba, Sri Lanka, and the state of Kerala in India more recently. The rate of diffusion of knowledge about better interventions, and the willingness and ability to act on that new information, may determine the pace of a country's health improvement much more than its level of income.

Economic benefits of health

Better evidence is emerging on the economic consequences of good health, for both individuals and nations. Health has been found to be associated with greater individual productivity and living standards. Countries that have high levels of health but low levels of income tend to experience relatively faster economic growth. The initial health of a population has been identified as one of the most potent drivers of economic growth—among such well-established influences as the initial level of income per capita, geographical location, institutional environment, economic policy, initial level of education, and investments in education. An additional year of life expectancy has been associated with a roughly 4% increase in gross domestic product (GDP) per capita in the long run.

Conversely, health declines can precipitate downward spirals, setting off impoverishment and further ill health. For example, the effect of HIV/AIDS on per capita GDP could prove devastating. Human capital is wasted as prime-age workers die. A high-mortality environment deters the next generation from investing in education and creating human capital. Orphan children may be forced to work to survive and may not get the education they need. Savings rates are likely to fall, and retirement becomes less feasible. A foreign company is less likely to invest in a country with a high HIV prevalence rate because of the threat to the firm's own workers, the prospect of high labour turnover, and the potential loss of workers trained by the firm.

Major causes of death and disease

In this section, we discuss causes of death and disease burden measured in DALYs (see Box 3.1.1) in two age categories: children under the age of 5 who succumb to neonatal conditions, measles, malaria, diarrhoeal disease, HIV/AIDS, and respiratory infections; and adults whose deaths are due to chronic, noncommunicable conditions, including cardiovascular disease, stroke, diabetes, cancer, and psychiatric disorders.

Child mortality

From 1960 to 2002, the rate of under-5 mortality around the world steadily declined, largely because of expanded childhood immunization coverage, improved water and sanitation, and wider provision of medical treatment, such as antibiotics for respiratory infections. From 1990 to 2001, however, the under-5 mortality rate increased or remained stagnant in 23 countries. In another 53 countries (including China), the decline in under-5 mortality was less than half the 4.3% per year required to reach the fourth Millennium Development Goal of reducing under-5 mortality by two-thirds in the period 1990–2005. Progress has been slow in sub-Saharan Africa because of HIV/AIDS and, until very recently, the increasing prevalence of malaria, which is now widely resistant to the first-line drugs chloroquine and sulphadoxine–pyrimethamine.

Every year, an estimated 4 million babies die in their first month, accounting for 38% of all deaths among children under 5. Causes of death include infections (neonatal sepsis, pneumonia, diarrhoea, and tetanus, 36%), complications due to preterm birth (27%) and asphyxia (23%) (Table 3.1.2). Saving most of these babies does not require intensive care. Sri Lanka, to take one low-income country as an example, has lowered its neonatal mortality rate to 15 per 1000, less than one-third of the rates typical in sub-Saharan

Box 3.1.1 Measuring disease burden: DALYs

One challenge in measuring the burden of disease is aggregating disease morbidity and mortality in a single metric. Disability-adjusted life years (DALYs) have come into wide use by researchers and international organizations. One DALY represents a year of potential life lost to premature death or a year of less-than-full health. DALYs are the principal metrics used in the measurement of the global burden of disease; see 'Further reading' section.

Table 3.1.2 Estimated causes of under-5 mortality worldwide, 2001 (in thousands)

Cause	Total	0–4 years	Neonatal (0–27 days)	Stillbirths
HIV/AIDS	340	340		
Diarrhoeal disease	1600	1600	116	
Measles	557	557		
Tetanus	187	187	187	
Malaria	1087	1087		
Respiratory infection and sepsis	1945	1945	1013	
Low birth weight	1301	1301	1098	
Birth asphyxia and birth trauma	739	739	739	
Congenital anomalies	439	439	321	
Injuries	310	310		
Other	5375	2101	446	3274
Total	13874	10600	3900	3274

Notes: 1. Of the estimated 13.9 million under-5 deaths in 2001, only 0.9% occurred in high-income countries. Thus the cause distribution of deaths in this table is essentially that of low- and middle-income countries.

2. 'Stillbirths' are defined as fetal loss in the third trimester of pregnancy. The total column includes stillbirths among under-5 deaths. About 33% of stillbirths occur after labour has begun—so-called intrapartum stillbirths. No good estimates exist for stillbirths by cause, but since some of the cause categories (e.g. birth asphyxia, birth trauma, congenital anomalies) are the same as for ages 0–4, some deaths categorized as 'other' will be distributed among the existing categories when estimates become available.

Data from Bryce J, *et al.* (2005). WHO estimates of the causes of death in children. *Lancet*, **365**, 1147–52; Jamison DT, *et al.* (eds) (2006). *Priorities in health*. World Bank, Washington, DC; Mathers CD, Murray CJL, Lopez AD (2006). The burden of disease and mortality by condition: data, methods and results for the year 2001. In: Lopez AD, *et al.* (eds) *Global burden of disease and risk factors*. Oxford University Press, Oxford and New York.

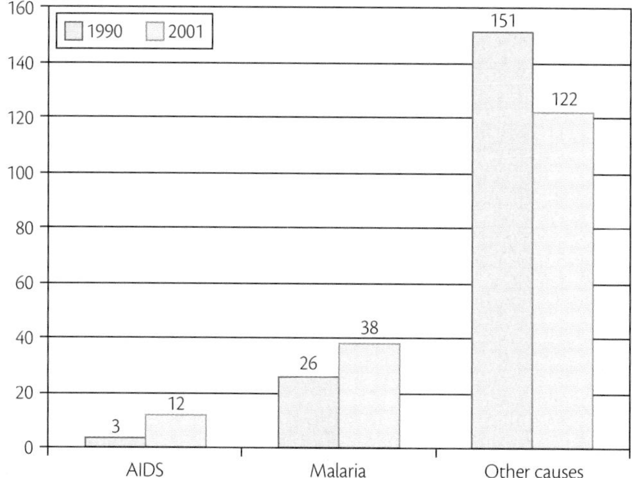

Fig. 3.1.1 Under-5 deaths from AIDS, malaria, and other causes per 1000 births in sub-Saharan Africa, 1990 and 2001.

Reproduced from *Disease Control Priorities in Developing Countries (2nd Edition)*, with kind permission from The International Bank for Reconstruction and Development, The World Bank.

Africa, without intensive care. Similar approaches would address the neglected global burden of over 3.2 million stillbirths each year.

Between 1990 and 2002, there were declining trends in deaths from acute respiratory infections (from 2.5 million to 1.9 million), diarrhoeal disease (from 2.4 million to 1.6 million), measles (from 0.8 million to 0.5 million), and injuries (from 0.6 million to 0.3 million). These improvements were partially offset by increases in under-5 mortality from malaria and HIV/AIDS (Fig. 3.1.1). From 1990 to 2001, child deaths due to malaria doubled from 5% to 10% worldwide and increased from 15% to 22% in sub-Saharan Africa, where few effective antimalarials are available.

Adult mortality

Ageing populations and changing lifestyles across the globe contribute to noncommunicable diseases that are imposing tremendous burdens. In 2001, cardiovascular disease, cancer, chronic respiratory illness, diabetes, and psychiatric conditions accounted for two-thirds of deaths in over-5 (see Table 3.1.3). Cardiovascular disease (including stroke) in low- and middle-income countries killed more than twice as many people in 2001 as did AIDS, malaria, and tuberculosis combined. In 2001, about 11.1 million people over the age of 5 in low and middle-income countries died of cardiovascular disease (including stroke), 4.9 million died of cancer, 2.4 million died of chronic respiratory disease, and 0.7 million died of diabetes—altogether, 25.2 million of the total 38 million deaths in over-5s in developing countries that year (Table 3.1.3). Deaths from ischaemic heart disease and stroke are expected to triple in sub-Saharan Africa, Latin America, the Middle East, and North Africa.

The largest increase in noncommunicable diseases is predicted to occur in low- and middle-income countries, which continue to suffer the burden of communicable diseases like malaria, tuberculosis, and HIV/AIDS. This 'double burden' is reversing many of the gains from expanded immunization and clean water and sanitation. Noncommunicable conditions, generally chronic, are overwhelming fragile health systems that are struggling with short-duration morbidities imposed by communicable diseases.

In high-income countries, the likelihood of dying from a chronic disease has declined dramatically. Among men over 30 in the developed world, for example, death rates from heart disease dropped by more than 50% between 1970 and 2005, from 600 to 800 per 100 000 to 200 to 300 per 100 000. The death rate for Brazilian men was 300 per 100 000 in 1980 (compared with 500–600 in high-income countries) but has remained unchanged since. The World Bank predicts that chronic conditions will be the leading cause of death in low-income countries by 2015.

Cardiovascular diseases are responsible for 17 million deaths worldwide each year. Of these, 13 million deaths are in low- and middle-income countries and represent more than a quarter of all deaths in these countries. Most cardiovascular deaths result from ischaemic heart disease (5.7 million) or cerebrovascular disease (4.6 million). Because such deaths occur at older ages, they are a smaller fraction of the total disease burden in DALYs—12.9%.

Tobacco use accounts for a substantial and avoidable fraction of cardiovascular disease and cancers. In 2000, the number of tobacco-related deaths in developing countries about equalled the number in high-income countries; by 2030, developing countries may have more than twice as many. Controlling smoking is a crucial element of any nation's strategy for preventing cardiovascular

Table 3.1.3 Causes of death in low- and middle-income countries, age 5 and older

	Deaths (in millions)	Percentage of total (%)
Communicable, maternal, perninatal, and nutritional conditions		
TB	1.5	4.0
AIDS	2.2	5.8
Respiratory infections	1.5	4.0
Maternal conditions	0.5	1.3
Other	2.5	6.6
Subtotal	8.2	21.7
Noncommunicable disease		
Cancers	4.9	13.0
Diabetes	0.7	1.9
Ischaemic and hypertensive heart disease	6.5	17.2
Stroke	4.6	12.2
Chronic obstructive pulmonary disease	2.4	6.3
Other	6.1	16.1
Subtotal	25.2	66.7
Injuries		
Road traffic accidents	1.0	2.6
Suicides	0.7	1.9
Other	2.7	7.1
Subtotal	4.4	11.6
Total	37.8	100

Data aggregated from Mathers CD, Murray CJL, Lopez AD (2006). The burden of disease and mortality by condition: data, methods and results for the year 2001. In: Lopez AD, *et al.* (eds) *Global burden of disease and risk factors*. Oxford University Press, Oxford and New York.

disease and promoting health more generally. Preventing the initiation of smoking is important because addiction to nicotine makes stopping smoking very difficult, even for those who want to quit. However, far more lives could be saved between now and 2050 by helping current smokers to quit. Reducing smoking levels is well within the control of public policy. Taxation is the principal proven instrument, but complementary measures such as bans on smoking in public places and tobacco advertising are also important.

The main risk factors for cardiovascular disease, such as high blood pressure, high cholesterol, smoking, obesity, excessive alcohol use, physical inactivity and poor diet account for very large fractions of the deaths (and even more of the burden) from ischaemic heart disease (collectively accounting for 78% of deaths in low- and middle-income countries) and stroke (61%). Measures to reduce the levels of those risk factors are the goals for prevention. Unlike the favourable experience with controlling tobacco use, attempts to change behaviour leading to obesity, hypertension, and high cholesterol appear to have had little success at a population level. However, many promising approaches remain to be tried. Common sense suggests that they should be initiated even while efforts to develop and evaluate behaviour-change packages are ramped up.

If sustained behaviour change proves difficult to achieve, medications have the potential to reduce cardiovascular disease risks by 50% or more. Pharmaceutical interventions to manage two major factors, hypertension and high cholesterol, are well established and are highly cost-effective for people at high risk of a stroke or heart attack. The low cost and high effectiveness of drugs to prevent the recurrence of a cardiovascular event have made their long-term use potentially cost-effective in low-income environments.

Lifelong medication for cardiovascular disease, however, like medication for psychiatric disorders, requires not only low-cost drugs but also health care personnel and systems that can perform reliably at all levels and be accessible to patients. Thus vertical programmes that sidestep the inherent weaknesses of health care systems are not really an option for dealing with chronic diseases. Since 1992, work by Feachem and others has indicated treatment and prevention approaches that could be adapted to developing countries with budget constraints.

From a patient's perspective, unfamiliarity with the risk factors for chronic diseases and lack of experience in dealing with heart disease or cancer are particularly important. The economic impact of chronic diseases is likely to be even more pronounced than that of communicable diseases, since they typically disable and kill adults of working age. Low-cost but effective approaches to long-term management of chronic conditions need to be developed and implemented.

Neurological and psychiatric disorders lead to only about 1.4% of deaths in low- and middle-income countries (1.8% in high-income countries), but they cause suffering and disability far beyond what the mortality numbers suggest. About 10% of the disease burden in DALYs in low- and middle-income countries results from these conditions, much of it attributable to three major psychiatric diseases: unipolar major depression (3.1% of DALYs), bipolar disorder (0.6%), and schizophrenia (0.8%).

Setting disease control priorities

Recent work in health has focused on identifying cost-effective interventions that policy makers are currently ignoring or underfunding, as well as investments that are now prevalent but not cost-effective. Setting priorities rationally makes limited resources go further. Without demonstrably improved efficiency in health spending, aid agencies and development partners may be less willing to pay for expansions of health programmes. Improving efficiency does not, however, reduce the importance of increasing resources for implementing these interventions and meeting broader objectives, such as the Millennium Development Goals. These objectives are complementary.

The Disease Control Priorities Project (DCPP), a joint effort of the Fogarty International Center of the United States National Institutes of Health, the World Health Organization, and the World Bank (and with substantial funding from the Bill & Melinda Gates Foundation) has analysed the cost-effectiveness of a wide range of population-based and personal health interventions. The project was launched in 2001 to identify policy changes and intervention strategies for the health problems of countries in need. It follows on from the first edition of *Disease Control Priorities in Developing Countries* (1993) and the World Bank's 1993 World Development Report, *Investing in Health*, which attempted to make global comparisons of interventions to improve health in developing countries.

Here we present results from the DCPP on the most cost-effective interventions to improve health in low- and middle-income countries. Cost-effectiveness is presented as US$/DALY averted, a metric that combines years of life lived with disability and years lost to premature death (see Box 3.1.1). Cost-effectiveness is only one consideration in allocating resources to specific diseases and interventions; epidemiological, medical, political, ethical, cultural, equity, and budgetary factors also matter. Interpreting the cost-effectiveness ratio as the 'price' of equivalent units of health using different interventions is a useful approach to deploying cost-effectiveness information alongside the other considerations in setting priorities. Cost-effectiveness information makes policy makers aware of differences in the price of improving health, using different interventions. All else being equal, those with a high price should be used less, whereas those with a low price should be used more.

Lowering under-5 mortality

Table 3.1.4 lists the most cost-effective interventions to reduce under-5 mortality and to prevent and treat HIV/AIDS and non-communicable diseases. Here we discuss interventions to lower under-5 mortality in detail.

Mortality of neonates and children under 5 can be greatly reduced with affordable interventions of proven effectiveness. Improvements can come from increasing coverage of preventive measures, such as breastfeeding, and expanding childhood vaccination programs beyond the traditional six antigens, in places where immunization coverage is already high and where new antigens, particularly pneumococcal and *Haemophilus influenzae* type B (Hib) vaccines, address diseases of significant burden. Implementation and increased coverage of interventions for acute respiratory infections, malaria, and diarrhoea should reduce the annual 6 million preventable deaths in this age group.

Adding essential care for newborn babies (warmth, cleanliness, and immediate breastfeeding), neonatal resuscitation, facility-based care of preterm babies and emergency care of ill neonates to the standard maternal and child health package has proved highly cost-effective in India ($11–265 per year of life saved, or $24–585 per DALY averted) and sub-Saharan Africa ($25–360 per year of life saved, or $46–657 per DALY averted); however, these interventions require a high initial investment. Addition of community-based interventions—promoting healthy behaviours, such as breastfeeding, providing extra care of moderately small babies at home through cleanliness, warmth, and exclusive breastfeeding, plus management of acute respiratory infections—to the maternal and child health package is likely to be highly cost-effective. A year of life saved could cost as little as $100 to $257 in India ($221–568 per DALY averted) and $100 to $270 in sub-Saharan Africa ($183–493).

Community-based approaches are now feasible in virtually all countries. If a midwife is available, resuscitation of newborns with a $5 self-inflating bag could save lives at low cost in low- and middle-income countries. Provision of two tetanus toxoid immunizations to all pregnant women could avert more than 150 000 neonatal deaths every year. Improvement of maternal- and child-health services delivered through a combination of family-level and community-level care, outreach, and clinical care would increase the survival rates of newborn and older children and reduce stillbirths and maternal deaths.

Childhood vaccinations, long recognized as among the most cost-effective uses of resources, prevented more than 3 million deaths worldwide in 2001. National immunization programs include vaccines against diphtheria, pertussis, and tetanus (DPT); tuberculosis; poliomyelitis; and measles at a cost of $13 to $24 per fully immunized child, depending on coverage levels and delivery strategy (health-facility based, special campaigns like national immunization days, or mobile team outreach). The estimated cost per death averted varies from less than $275 ($10 per DALY averted) in sub-Saharan Africa and South Asia to $1754 ($20 per DALY averted) in Europe and central Asia. The variation is largely attributable to differences in the underlying prevalence of disease. These same factors also affect the cost-effectiveness of scaling up coverage with the traditional Expanded Program on Immunization (EPI) vaccines. The cost per death averted varies by region, from $162 in sub-Saharan Africa to more than $1600 in Eastern Europe. Costs are less than $20 per DALY averted in all regions other than Europe and central Asia. Cost-effectiveness of the tetanus toxoid vaccine also varies widely, from less than $400 per death averted ($14 per DALY averted) in sub-Saharan Africa and South Asia to more than $190 000 ($15 000 per DALY averted) in Europe and central Asia.

Including a second measles vaccination through routine immunizations or special campaigns costs $23 to $228 per death averted and less than $4 per DALY averted in developing regions other than Europe and central Asia. New vaccines cost more per dose and are less cost-effective than the current EPI vaccines but might be worthwhile in regions of high disease prevalence. The pentavalent vaccine (DPT plus hepatitis B and Hib) has an estimated cost of $1433 to $40 000 per death averted and a cost-effectiveness of $42 per DALY averted in sub-Saharan Africa, and more than $245 elsewhere. Addition of a yellow fever vaccine costs between $834 per death averted ($26 per DALY averted) in sub-Saharan Africa and $2810 ($39) in Latin America and the Caribbean.

Multivalent pneumococcal conjugate vaccines could reduce the incidence of invasive pneumococcal disease while lowering antibiotic use and the likelihood of drug resistance. At $50 per dose, however, these vaccines are unaffordable to most people in low- and middle-income countries. After confirmation of efficacy and subsequent licensing, new vaccines that protect against rotavirus, malaria, human papillomavirus (associated with cervical cancer), and dengue could be included in the EPI schedule.

Although more demanding of health system capacity than vaccination, patient treatment is also an efficient use of resources. Management in the community and at a health care facility might be comparably cost-effective, but community-based strategies hold promise for more rapid coverage. Treatment of nonsevere pneumonia at facilities with oral antimicrobials and paracetamol ($24–424 per DALY averted) is slightly more cost-effective than similar treatment administered at home by a health care worker ($139–733). Treatment of severe pneumonia in a hospital is more expensive ($1486–14 719).

Of the interventions for diarrhoeal disease during the first year of life, breastfeeding promotion programmes ($527–2001 per DALY averted), measles immunization ($257–4565), and oral rehydration therapy (as low as $132, for a cost per child of $0.70) are more cost-effective than immunizations for rotavirus ($1402–8357) or cholera ($1658–8274). Lower prices and improved logistics for recently licensed rotavirus vaccines could make this intervention substantially more attractive. Because great reductions in mortality from this condition have already been achieved, the average case

Table 3.1.4 Cost-effectiveness of interventions to reduce under-5 mortality and to prevent and treat HIV/AIDS and noncommunicable diseases

Service or intervention	Cost per DALY (US$)	Estimated DALYs averted per million US$ spent
Reducing under-5 mortality		
Improving care of children under 28 days old (including resuscitation of newborns)	10–400	2500–100 000
Expanding immunization coverage with standard childhood vaccines	2–20	50 000–500 000
Adding vaccines against additional diseases to the standard child immunization programme (particularly Hib and HepB)	40–250	4000–24 000
Switching to the use of combination drugs (ACTs) against malaria where resistance exists to current inexpensive and previously highly effective drugs (sub-Saharan Africa)	8–20	50 000–125 000
Preventing and treating HIV/AIDS		
Preventing mother-to-child transmission (antiretroviral-nevirapine prophylaxis of the mother; breastfeeding substitutes)	50–200	5000–20 000
Treating STIs to interrupt HIV transmission	10–100	10 000–100 000
Using antiretroviral therapy that achieves high adherence for a large percentage of patients	350–500	2000–3000
Using antiretroviral therapy that achieves high adherence for only a small percentage of patients		Because of very limited gains by individual patients and the potential for adverse changes in population behaviour, it is possible that more life years would be lost than saved.
Preventing and treating noncommunicable disease		
Taxing tobacco products	3–50	24 000–330 000
Treating AMI (heart attacks) with an inexpensive set of drugs	10–25	40 000–100 000
Treating AMI with inexpensive drugs plus streptokinase (costs and DALYs for this intervention are in addition to what would have occurred with inexpensive drugs only)	600–750	1300–1600
Treating heart attack and stroke survivors for life with a daily polypill combining four or five off-patent preventive medications	700–1000	1000–1400
Performing coronary artery bypass grafting (bypass surgery) in specific identifiable high-risk cases—for example, disease of the left main coronary artery (incremental to treatment with polypill)	>25 000	<40
Using bypass surgery for less severe coronary artery disease (incremental to treatment with polypill)	Very high	Very small
Other		
Detecting and treating cervical cancer	15–50	20 000–60 000
Operating a basic surgical ward at the district hospital level that focuses on trauma, high-risk pregnancy, and other common surgically treatable conditions	70–250	4000–15 000

AMI; acute myocardial infarction.

Reproduced from *Global Burden of Disease and Risk Factors* with kind permission of the International Bank for Reconstruction and Development, The World Bank.

fatality rate from diarrhoea is now much lower than before oral rehydration therapy was introduced. Where none of these interventions has been adopted, diarrhoeal disease is still a major killer, and oral rehydration therapy and other measures are more cost-effective in preventing deaths even if diarrhoea incidence is unchanged. The situation is parallel with that for immunization: cost-effectiveness might look poor because of gains already achieved, but both continued and expanded coverage are needed. Similarly, improvements in water and sanitation ($1118–14 901 per DALY averted from diarrhoea) are less cost-effective where access to these amenities is adequate and other interventions against diarrhoea exist. In areas with little access to water and sanitation, however, improvements can be highly cost-effective because they reduce incidence of illness ($94 per DALY averted for installation of hand pumps and $270 per DALY averted for provision and promotion of basic sanitation facilities).

Conclusions

The 20th century has seen enormous gains in human health, but important challenges remain. The double epidemiological burden of communicable diseases (including HIV/AIDS) plus noncommunicable diseases is the most daunting. Existing cost-effective interventions need to be adopted on a wider scale. For communicable diseases, interventions that have been highly cost-effective in the past remain so despite emerging infections and drug resistance. Noncommunicable diseases, including ischaemic heart disease and stroke, can be prevented, importantly by comprehensive antismoking programmes, and managed effectively in low-income countries at a reasonable cost. Many interventions first developed in the industrialized world are now available in the developing world, but health care systems in low- and middle-income countries must first recognize the importance of the conditions. For health programmes to succeed, policy makers must have access to the best possible research and analysis to ensure that their investments in prevention and treatment save as many lives as possible.

Further reading

Adeyi O, *et al.* (2007). *Public policy and the challenge of chronic noncommunicable diseases.* World Bank, Washington, DC.

Becker G, *et al.* (2003). The quantity and quality of life and the evolution of world inequality. *Am Econ Rev*, **95**, 277–91.

Bloom DE, *et al.* (2004). The effect of health on economic growth: a production function approach. *World Dev*, **32**, 1–13.

Bourguignon F, Morrison C (2002). Inequality among world citizens: 1820–1992. *Am Econ Rev*, **92**, 727–44.

Bryce J, *et al.* (2005). WHO estimates of the causes of death in children. *Lancet*, **365**, 1147–52.

Deaton A (2004). *Health in an age of globalization.* Working paper 10669. National Bureau of Economic Research, Cambridge, MA.

Easterlin RA (1996). *Growth triumphant: The twenty-first century in historical perspective.* University of Michigan Press, Ann Arbor, MI.

Ezzati M, *et al.* (2006). Comparative quantification of mortality and burden of disease attributable to selected major risk factors. In: Lopez AD, *et al.* (eds) *Global burden of disease and risk factors*, Oxford University Press, Oxford and New York.

Feachem RGA, *et al.* (eds) (1992). *Health of adults in the developing world.* Oxford University Press, New York. [Initial work on approaches to treatment and prevention that could be adapted to developing countries.]

Haacker M (ed.) (2004). *The macroeconomics of HIV/AIDS.* International Monetary Fund, Washington, DC. [A collection of important studies of the multiple mechanisms through which an AIDS epidemic can be expected to affect national economies.]

Jamison DT, *et al.* (eds) (2006). *Disease control priorities in developing countries*, 2nd edition. Oxford University Press, New York. [With the next item, a new look at adapting health interventions to low-income countries.]

Jamison DT, *et al.* (eds) (2006). *Priorities in health.* World Bank, Washington, DC.

Jamison D, *et al.* (2004). *Why has infant mortality decreased at such different rates in different countries?* Working Paper 21, Disease Control Priorities Project, Bethesda, MD.

Laxminarayan R, *et al.* (2006). Advancement of global health: key messages from the Disease Control Priorities Project. *Lancet*, **367**, 1193–208.

Lopez AD, Begg S, Bos E (2006). Demographic and epidemiological characteristics of major regions of the world, 1990 and 2001. In: Lopez AD *et al.* (eds) *Global burden of disease and risk factors.* Oxford University Press, Oxford and New York.

Lopez AD, *et al.* (eds) (2006). *Global burden of disease and risk factors.* Oxford University Press, Oxford and New York. [Provides data sources, methods, and the current best estimates of disease and risk factor burden by age and sex for major regions of the world.]

Mathers CD, Murray CJL, Lopez AD (2006). The burden of disease and mortality by condition: data, methods and results for the year 2001. In: Lopez AD, *et al.* (eds) *Global burden of disease and risk factors.* Oxford University Press, Oxford and New York.

Murray C, Lopez A (1996). *The global burden of disease*, Volume 1. Harvard University Press, Cambridge, MA.

Murray CJ, *et al.* (1994). The global burden of disease in 1990: summary results, sensitivity analysis and future directions. *Bull World Health Organ*, **72**, 495–509.

Pearson TA, Jamison DT, Trejo-Gutierrez J (1993). Cardiovascular disease. In: Jamison DT, *et al.* (eds) *Disease control priorities in developing countries*, p. 746. Oxford University Press, New York.

Phillips M, *et al.* (1993). Adult health: a legitimate concern for developing countries. *Am J Public Health*, **83**, 1527–30. [How developing countries can adapt developed-world treatment despite budget constraints.]

Strong K, *et al.* (2005). Preventing chronic diseases: how many lives can we save? *Lancet*, **366**, 1578–82.

World Bank (1993). *World development report: Investing in health.* Oxford University Press, New York. [Global comparisons of interventions to improve health in developing countries.]

World Bank (2004). *World development indicators.* World Bank, Washington, DC. [Available annually.]

Yach D, *et al.* (2004). The global burden of chronic diseases: overcoming impediments to prevention and control. *JAMA*, **291**, 2616–22.

3.2

Human population size, environment, and health

A.J. McMichael and J.W. Powles

Essentials

The number of people has increased in a series of steps by around five orders of magnitude over the past 100 000 years as geographical dispersal and cultural changes expanded access to food and other resources. The last 10-fold increase has occurred in just over two centuries.

The main components of the complex relationship between environment and population size are: (1) the supply of environmental resources limits population size; (2) human societies typically extend that limit via cultural and technical developments; and (3) such extensions often cause depletion and degradation of the natural environment.

Historical perspective

Until the 19th century, all agrarian-based societies had both high death rates and high birth rates. Human populations have greatly increased pressures on the natural environment over the past two centuries by (1) expansion of numbers, and (2) increased material and energy intensities of productive activities. Initially, most environmental degradation was localized, such as urban-industrial air pollution, chemical pollution of waterways, and urban filth.

The situation today

Environmental damage is more extensive, systemic and cumulative—and the longer-term consequences for health are potentially much more serious. Global climate change is a prominent example of systemic overloading of the biosphere. Data on large-scale processes indicate that environmental resources and services are currently being used up at approximately 130% of the sustainable rate. This weakening of global life-supporting processes poses long-term risks to human health.

The future

Living within the environmental constraints will require radical changes in consciousness and institutional reconfigurations in both high- and low-income countries. A useful historical analogy lies in the radical and wide-ranging changes required between the mid 19th and early 20th centuries to render urban life in economically advanced countries compatible with child survival. High-income countries now generally enjoy high levels of health, but sustaining this historically remarkable level of population health will depend increasingly on achieving a secure world, and this in turn will require generalizing of health gains to the total human population. This will require the effective control of births, also a redefinition of 'progress' and the way we measure it, so that the interests of future generations are safeguarded. Physicians are well placed, individually and collectively, to foster public understanding of why large-scale environmental disruption jeopardizes the health of future generations and why it is in all our interests to avert this threat.

Introduction

Homo sapiens originated approximately 200 000 years ago from its archaic progenitor *Homo* lineage. Since then, this modern human species has undergone three population growth surges: (1) an estimated 50-fold increase as hunter–gatherer humans drifted out of north-eastern Africa and dispersed around the world over the course of 60 000 to 70 000 years; (2) a further 100-fold increase following the advent of agriculture, beginning from around 10 000 years ago; and then (3) another 10-fold increase from 0.5 billion to today's 6.7 billion since the beginning of the Industrial Revolution.

This third, incomplete, increase has occurred much faster than the previous two. Absolute annual additions to human numbers peaked during the past quarter-century, capping an almost-fourfold increase from 1.6 to 6 billion during the 20th century. The growth rate (percentage annual increase) has now been declining for several decades. Demographers expect that by the time the demographic transition is completed worldwide, and birth rates equilibrate with death rates (at historically low levels), world population will have reached between 7 and 11 billion, most probably between 8.5 and 9.5 billion. The United Nations medium variant projection for 2050 is approximately 9 billion.

Relationship between environment and population

All living things, including the human species, depend absolutely on access to environmental resources—the very resources and processes to which Darwinian evolution has attuned their biology. The relationship between the environment and population size is complex and multifaceted. The main components are (1) the supply of environmental resources (nature's 'goods and services') sets an upper limit on the size of the supportable population; (2) human societies typically extend that limit via cultural and technical developments; and (3) that extension process often results in the depletion and degradation of the natural environment, which can then pose detriment and risk to the dependent population.

Carrying capacity

In the natural world, the composition and assets of any particular species' niche determine the maximum number of individuals of that species that can be supported. That number defines the 'carrying capacity' of the species' local environment (habitat). Population size fluctuates around that number, as conditions vary over time. Uniquely, populations of the human species are not fully constrained by given environmental conditions. Through cultural and technical development, humans have been able to increase the carrying capacity of their local environments—at least temporarily. History is littered with examples of societies that overexploited and degraded their natural resource base, leading to decline or disappearance of that society.

From around 10 000 years ago, the domestication of plant species increased food yields and hence population carrying capacity. The subsequent domestication of wild animal species further increased carrying capacity. This advent of agriculture appears to have been associated with a substantial increase in fertility—from an average of 4 to 5 births per completed reproductive lifetime (as reported for traditional hunter–gatherers and, coincidentally, for great apes) to 5 to 7 births per reproductive lifetime in agrarian populations. This greater fecundity meant that the approximate balance between birth and death rates in slowly enlarging agrarian populations has long been attained at very high levels of both. This is well illustrated by India around 1900, when fertility was high (7 to 8 births per woman) and life expectancy was just 20 to 25 years with very high death rates throughout the lifespan.

Overloading the environment

Especially since the advent of agriculture, human communities have tended to overexploit the stocks of local natural resources—soil, water, and plants and animals—for food and materials. This has led, over time, to undernutrition and population decline.

The propensity to degrade the environment has accelerated over the past two centuries, as numbers have expanded and as the material and energy intensities of productive activities have increased. Over the past century or so, adverse environmental effects have mostly been of a localized kind, such as urban-industrial air pollution, chemical pollution of waterways, and urban filth. Today, damage to the natural environment is much more extensive, more systemic and cumulative. The longer-term consequences for health are likely to be commensurately more serious. Recent global assessments point to an increasing 'ecological deficit', with now-manifest decline in natural environmental and ecological resource stocks. Global climate change is perhaps the best known of these unprecedented environmental changes.

Environmental stresses also cause tensions and conflict between human communities. For example, Ethiopia and the Sudan, both upstream from Nile-dependent Egypt, increasingly need the Nile's water for their own crop irrigation. The disasters in Rwanda (1994) and Darfur, Sudan (this decade) are increasingly recognized as being grounded, respectively, in environmental overload due to excessive population size, and prolonged regional rainfall decline.

The sustained good health of any population, over time, requires a stable and productive natural environment that (1) yields adequate supplies of food and fresh water; (2) has a relatively constant climate in which climate-sensitive physical and biological systems are not adversely affected; and (3) retains biodiversity (a prerequisite for much ecosystem functioning and, more generally, a fundamental source of both present and future value). (For the human species, a 'social animal' in the extreme, the richness, texture, and stability of the social environment, i.e. 'social capital', is also important to population health, but this lies outside the scope of this chapter.)

Malthusian perspective on sustainability

Two hundred years ago, Thomas Malthus, responding to the utopian prospects held out by Godwin, de Condorcet, and others, foresaw instead a crisis arising from excessive human numbers within a food-limited environment. The exponential power of population growth would, he concluded, tend always to outstrip the (arithmetic) power of growth in food production. He grimly predicted that Europe faced famine, in order for nature's 'positive checks' to bring human numbers back in line with food supplies.

In fact, such a crisis did not materialize in Europe. Malthus could not have foreseen the remarkable increase in food-producing capacity that the second Agricultural Revolution, with mechanization and fossil-fuel energy, would bring during the 19th century, or the bonanza of imported grain and meat that Europe's newly established colonies would provide. Nor could he have foreseen the marked decline in fertility rates that emerged in European populations during the latter 19th century as social modernization occurred and the possibility of controlling fertility within marriage became widely understood.

There remains an important sense in which a 'malthusian' perspective remains relevant, albeit at another level of analysis. In the past several decades, we have begun to see evidence that there are limits to the carrying capacity of the globe as a whole. Human activities have damaged the stratosphere, induced climate change, begun to acidify the oceans, overloaded the environment with bioactive nitrogen compounds, degraded much land, and set in motion an accelerating loss of species. These are ominous signs that we are exceeding Earth's carrying capacity. What then might lie in store?

In the natural world, the tendency of plant and animal species to exponential population growth is generally constrained by predation, by limits to food supplies, by infectious disease, and, in many animals, by density-dependent changes in reproductive behaviour. As numbers increase, one of the following patterns comes into play:

1 logistic (asymptotic) growth, responding to immediate negative feedback as carrying capacity is approached

2 domed or capped growth, responding to deferred negative feedback, necessitating compensatory die-off following overshoot of carrying capacity

3 irruptive growth, with boom-and-bust and a chaotic post-crash pattern

While the first pattern might allow a sustainable outcome, the now palpable risks of overshoot and even catastrophic collapse (patterns 2 and 3) underlie the concern that, around the world, most human societies today are not on 'environmentally sustainable development' trajectories. Continuation of today's trends in excessive population size, globally and in many regions, and in escalating environmental pressures might therefore result in recurrent subsistence crises on a subnational or national level, or even more disastrous larger-scale environmental disruption.

Local subsistence crises

Much of the concern with 'overpopulation' in the latter half of the 20th century focused on the likelihood that local population growth would overload local environmental carrying capacities. Chronic food shortages would then ensue and undernutrition would force mortality rates up towards equilibrium with still-high fertility rates. The immiserating effects of population pressure would prevent economic development, prolong population growth, and leave such populations 'demographically entrapped' (see Chapter 3.4.2).

So far, however, there appear to have been few developments in this direction, other than in the several overt conflict situations that are deemed to be substantively due to environmental degradation and regional impacts of climate change. The famines that have occurred in recent times, the most serious being the Chinese famine of 1959 to 1961, which killed around 15 to 20 million people, have been attributable more to institutional disruption and failure than to the progressive reduction of food-producing resources per person. The recent generally favourable trends in per-person food supplies cannot be guaranteed to continue indefinitely; finite environmental resources always set limits. Indeed, the widespread crisis in food shortages and escalating prices in mid-2008 may foreshadow future difficulties in sustaining per capita production levels globally, especially in the face of rising consumer demands and the diversion of cereal grains into biofuels and livestock production. Meanwhile, populations in many poor countries are expected to double before stabilizing within the next half-century, inevitably amplifying the existing difficulties in overcoming food insecurity.

Planetary overload

While local subsistence pressures on the environment persist or increase in many parts of the world, a newer form of environmental pressure has recently emerged at the global level. Human population size and the material and energy intensity of most productive activities are now so great that the human population is beginning to disrupt some of the biosphere's life-support systems.

The best-documented early evidence of this human-induced 'global environmental change' has been the destruction of stratospheric ozone, particularly in polar and subpolar regions, over the past quarter-century, and, as an essentially separate problem in the lower atmosphere, the ongoing changes in world climate due to the increase in greenhouse gas emissions from human activities. The atmospheric concentration of heat-trapping ('greenhouse') gases, especially CO_2, is increasing at a rate of around 1% per year. This rate has itself increased over the past decade, and, probably in consequence, so has the documented rate of change in climatic variability around the world and in temperature-related physical, biotic and ecosystem changes. Recognition of this potentially disastrous climate change process has been slow on the part of most national governments, and the initial international remedial action (the Kyoto Protocol) is clearly inadequate. The Stern Report of 2006, commissioned by the United Kingdom government, argued strongly that, without immediate action by governments everywhere to substantially reduce emissions, the world's economy could experience up to a one-fifth slowing in the growth of gross global economic product by 2050. This report, with its great and immediate impact on policy discussion, focuses (as does conventional government policy nearly everywhere) on risks to the systems for commodity production. An even stronger motivation to pursue 'sustainable' policies may well emerge once it is better understood that the greater threat is to Earth's life-support systems.

It is important to note that climate change is one of a larger set of global environmental changes, part of a systemic overloading of the biosphere. Forests are in retreat in many tropical regions, especially in the Amazon as, now, the international demand for biofuels accelerates—largely as a way of reducing reliance on (increasingly costly) petroleum fuels. There is a continuing net loss of productive agricultural and pastoral soil on all continents. Most of the large ocean fisheries have been overexploited. Many of the great aquifers, upon which irrigated agriculture depends, are now seriously depleted. The widespread use of nitrogenous fertilizer, along with fossil fuel combustion, has approximately doubled the rate at which activated nitrogenous compounds are entering the global environment. Increasingly, persistent synthetic organic (especially chlorinated) chemicals are pervading the biosphere. And, most irreversible of all, human pressures are extinguishing species at a rising rate.

These various changes are disrupting the capacity of the natural world to stabilize, replenish, cleanse, and recycle; these were capacities that earlier generations were able to take for granted. Manifestly we no longer live in such a world. The currently foreseeable health risks from these environmental changes are diverse, and will impact very unevenly around the world. They include: (1) malnutrition and hunger in local populations whose agricultural productivity is adversely affected by changes in climate, soil fertility, freshwater supplies, and the ecology of pests and pathogens; (2) increased exposure, in some parts of the world, to weather extremes and disasters, consequent upon climate change; (3) changes in the geographical range and seasonality of vector-borne infectious diseases such as malaria and dengue fever because of climate change; (4) an anticipated increase in skin cancer rates (and perhaps in eye disorders and immune system suppression) due to the increase in ground-level ultraviolet radiation levels that, at least during the next decade or two, exists at middle-to-high latitudes; and (5) the many adverse health consequences from tensions, conflict, and displacement due to dwindling natural resources.

Contribution of population increase to environmental disruption

WWF, the global conservation organization, has analysed national trends over recent decades in the vitality and function of major categories of ecological systems, including freshwater, marine, and forest ecosystems. The WWF *Living Planet Report* (2006) highlights the 'ecological footprint' of humanity. This index is a composite measure of the area of Earth's surface environment required to supply and absorb in relation to the economic activities of a designated 'human' unit—a person, a community, or an entire population. This index tracks, over time, the area of biologically productive land and water needed to provide food, fibre, timber, and land on which to build, and sufficient land and ocean (vegetation, soil, water) to absorb CO_2 generated from fossil fuels. Freshwater consumption, a crucial human need, is not included in the WWF version of the ecological footprint; it is dealt with separately in their assessment.

Figure 3.2.1 shows the estimation by WWF for the period 1961–2003. The ecological footprint of the total human population is measured in the number of Planet Earths needed to meet the total environmental demands of our collective economic production, consumption, and waste generation. Overall, the Living Planet Index has declined by 30% since around 1980. Assessments by other international agencies and research teams approximately concur. (The figure also includes three scenario-based estimates of future aggregate demands, given certain policy and technological trajectories.)

The three main determinants of human disruption of the environment are: (1) the total number of humans, (2) the average wealth per human, and (3) the means by which that wealth is generated, sustained, and increased. The ongoing climate change debate illustrates well the relativities between the environmental effects of increases in population and production. During the 20th century, as population increased by just under fourfold, the annual emissions of CO_2 from fossil fuel combustion increased 12-fold. By the century's end, per capita emissions differed more than 20-fold between the richest and poorest nations. As economic development accelerates in many low- and middle-income countries, including the now rapidly growing economies of China, India, Brazil, and Mexico, and as population growth rates flatten gradually, economic intensification will become a relatively more important source of greenhouse gases and many other large-scale environmental pressures than will population growth.

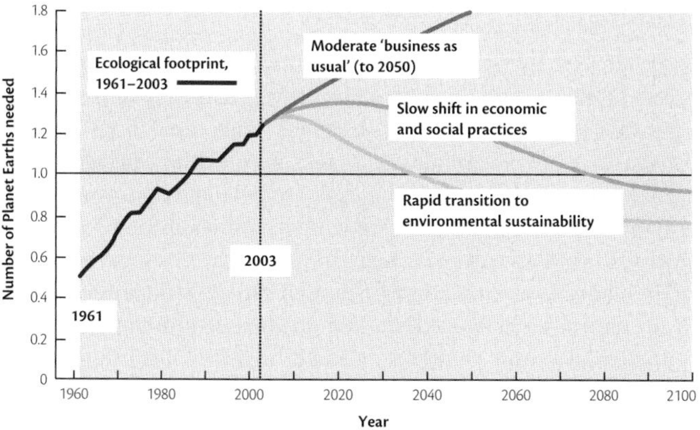

Fig. 3.2.1 Estimated recent time-trend and alternative future trajectories in the total human ecological footprint, expressed as 'number of Planet Earths needed', for 1963–2001 (data-based) and 2004–2100 (scenario-based).

Based on a figure from WWF International. Living Planet Report 2006. World Wildlife Fund International, Gland, Switzerland (http://assets.panda.org/downloads/living_planet_report.pdf). Figure 3.

Atmospheric concentrations of greenhouse gases are rising, with the dominant greenhouse gas, CO_2, having now reached 390 ppm, from a preindustrial level of 275ppm. The concentration of greenhouse gases is rising faster as more of the world industrializes and urbanizes. On current indications, it may not be feasible to limit this build-up of CO_2 to much less than a doubling of preindustrial concentrations. While some scientists think (or hope) that the resultant 550 ppm CO_2 would yield a climate that most ecosystems could tolerate, others point to increasing evidence that levels above 450 ppm CO_2 (currently likely to be reached by around 2025 to 2030) will involve a 'dangerous' climate with significant environmental and social disruption. Assuming the United Nations medium population projection of 9 to 10 billion by 2100, even limiting the rise to 550 ppm CO_2 would require (globally averaged) per capita CO_2 emissions no higher than those of the 1920s to 1930s, when world population was less than 2 billion. Re-attaining that level of emissions would require a 75 to 80% reduction below today's actual global rate of global emissions, around 30 Gt of CO_2 per year. (Note that CO_2 levels are being used here as proxy measures of the total greenhouse effect, from all greenhouse gases, to which CO_2 contributes about 75 to 80% of the warming effect. Important contributions also come from nonenergy sources, including methane and nitrous oxide from agricultural and livestock production.)

While achieving that level of reduction looms as an extraordinarily demanding task, we actually already have much of the necessary technology to reduce emissions greatly without decreasing our standards of living. Further, many of the necessary changes are identical or compatible with changes needed to achieve other health gains via the reduction of more familiar, localized risks to health (such as urban air pollution, labour-saving sedentarism, poorly insulated housing, and exposure to flood plains). The real and manifestly great challenge is political: to transform current economic priorities, technologies, institutions, and cultural practices (Fig. 3.2.2).

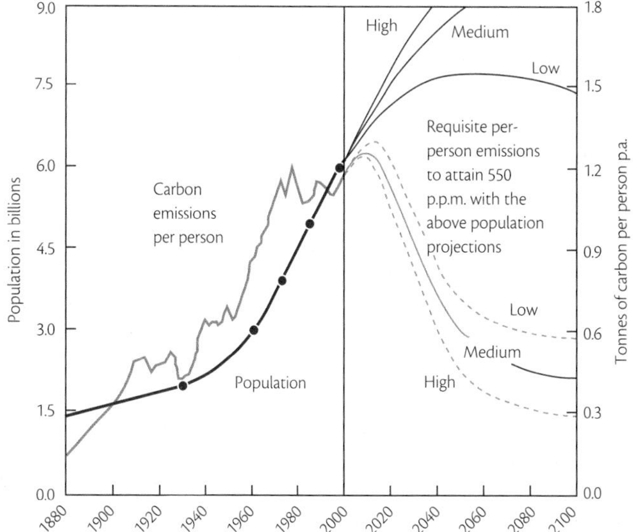

Fig. 3.2.2 Configuration of relationships between economic activity, wealth distribution (especially poverty), population size, environmental conditions, and human health. Note that poverty and the material (natural and social) environment are major determinants of health.

Overall, the larger potential threat comes less from an increase in the number of humans than from an increase in the average amount of environmental damage per human (due to a 'development' model that generalizes the patterns of production and consumption typical of today's rich countries). Current economic practices in rich countries cannot be applied to a total human population that is likely to stabilize at 8 to 10 billion. The Netherlands, for example, requires an estimated area ('ecological footprint') an order of magnitude times greater than its actual national size to support its population's way of life. The citizens of high-income countries today each require an estimated 4 to 9 ha of the Earth's surface to provide the materials for their lifestyle and to absorb their wastes, while India's population makes do with less than 1 ha per person. There is not enough Earth to provide more than about 1.5 ha of 'ecological footprint' per average person for a world population of 8 to 10 billion by 2050. The conclusion is unavoidable: living within the constraints now seen to be necessary will require radical changes in consciousness and institutional reconfigurations in rich and poor countries alike. The closest historical analogy may be the radical social, institutional, and infrastructural changes that were needed between the mid 19th and early 20th centuries in order to make urban life in economically advanced countries compatible with child survival.

To help political decision makers and the general public understand the choices to be made, various international scientific reviews and reports have postulated contrasting future scenarios, plausible storylines of economic, social, and political development, with their associated impacts on the environment. The United Nations Intergovernmental Panel on Climate Change (IPCC) has explored a basic set of four scenarios (also used in the Stern Report, which focused particularly on the more climate-disrupting of the scenarios). So, too, the comprehensive Millennium Ecosystem Assessment, conducted earlier this decade, used four contrasting scenarios with different estimated consequences for the future of major ecosystems around the world. WWF (see above) has developed three scenarios, with very different implications for the global ecological footprint over the course of this century.

Serious investment in the development and deployment of less environmentally disruptive technologies, and a much greater commitment to international equity, will be required if a smooth and timely transition to an ecologically sustainable world is to be achieved. Because rich countries remain the main source of new knowledge and new technologies, responsibility for finding paths to sustainability rests mainly with them. Minimizing the probabilities of long-term harm to health will be a major consideration—indeed, the protection and promotion of population well-being and health should, rationally, be the central criterion of sustainability. (Why else have an economy?) The need to achieve a sustainable path into the future is now the most crucial health-related aspect of the 'population debate'.

Green accounting

We cannot predict, with certainty, how the adverse health effects of ecological disruption will unfold. It therefore makes sense to concentrate, in the shorter term, on our society's direction of travel, on whether we are moving closer to, or further away from, sustainable paths of economic development. To this end we need to devise and implement new indicators of progress.

Sustainability has recently been defined by the Environment Department of the World Bank as leaving to future generations 'as many opportunities as we ourselves have had, if not more'. Sustainability can be more readily expressed in operational terms using measures of economic 'stock' (i.e. capital, including, critically, natural capital and human resources) than using measures of 'flow' (income). In this context, conventional national income accounts are both biased (they treat living off natural capital as income) and insensitive (they provide little indication of legacies for the future). A broad measure of wealth would combine the estimated values of natural and human resources with those of produced assets (capital as traditionally considered). Human resources include the 'human capital' embodied in individuals (augmented by health and education levels) and 'social capital' embodied in institutions, customs, and knowledge, though the latter cannot readily be quantified.

Employing these categories, a pattern of economically sustainable development can be envisaged as one that conserves natural capital while rebuilding (with 'green' technology) the stock of produced assets, and augmenting human and social capital. This shift of emphasis from flows to stocks accords with recent analyses of health trends. For example, in low- and middle-income countries, indicators of human capital such as school attendance rates for girls and literacy among adult women are correlated more strongly with the level of child mortality than is income. Countries at similar levels of income may have several-fold differences in child mortality, with the 'better performers' typically showing higher levels of relevant aspects of human and social capital.

For rich countries, this approach recognizes that health depends less on the consumption opportunities provided by gains in income than on personal and social capacities to protect and enhance health. Those capacities reflect, at the individual level, determinants such as schooling and, at the social level, determinants such as food cultures (e.g. the protection against cardiovascular mortality in Mediterranean populations) and elements of the built environment such as sewers, water supplies, and safe roads. Given that life expectancy differences among high-income countries are, at most, very weakly related to income, it makes little sense to see further increases in national income as an important contributor to sustainable improvements in population health.

Conclusion

Over the last two centuries, new knowledge of the nature and causes of disease and its control, improvements in material conditions, and the enhancement both of individual capabilities through education (human capital) and of social capacities through development of new institutional forms (social capital) have yielded previously unimaginable improvements in health and longevity. During the historical gap between the fall in the death rates and the fall in birth rates, populations increased rapidly, and are still doing so in many poorer countries. The citizens of most high-income countries have now generally attained high levels of health. Their future secure enjoyment of life will depend increasingly on achieving a secure world, an outcome that will require generalizing the advances in health that they have enjoyed to the total human population.

A first essential is to extend the effective control of births to all sections of the human population, for without it, death control will remain unsustainable. A second task is to redefine 'progress' and to reconstruct the milestones by which we measure it, so that the interests of future generations are safeguarded. Physicians are well placed, individually and collectively, to foster greater public understanding of why large-scale environmental disruption is likely to jeopardize the health of our grandchildren and why it is in all our interests to avert this threat.

Further reading

Intergovernmental Panel on Climate Change (2007). *Climate change 2001*, Vols. I, II, III. *IPCC Third Assessment Report*. IPCC, Geneva.

McMichael AJ (2001). *Human frontiers, environments and disease: Past patterns, uncertain futures*. Cambridge University Press, Cambridge.

Millennium Ecosystem Assessment. (2005). *Ecosystems and human well-being: synthesis*. Island Press, Washington. [Also related publications: http://www.maweb.org]

Stern N (2007). *The economics of climate change: The Stern review*. Cambridge University Press, Cambridge.

United Nations Department of Economic and Social Affairs, Population Division (2004). *World population prospects: The 2004 revision*. http://www.un.org/esa/population/publications/WPP2004/wpp2004.htm

WWF International. *Living Planet Report 2006*. http://assets.panda.org/downloads/living_planet_report.pdf

3.3

Avoiding disease and promoting health

Contents

3.3.1 Preventive medicine *86*
David Mant

3.3.2 Medical screening *94*
Nicholas Wald and Malcolm Law

3.3.3 The importance of mass communication in promoting positive health *108*
Thomas Lom

3.3.1 Preventive medicine

David Mant

Essentials

Most deaths before age 80 years are preventable.

Childhood and early adult life

Deaths from infectious diseases and trauma usually reflect poverty and political instability. Prevention requires political action to reduce the risk of war and improve the supply of food, clean water, sanitation, and shelter. Preventive medicine can augment, but not replace, this action by controlling spread of infection through vaccination, health education, control of insect vectors, and treatment of disease carriers to prevent onward transmission.

Middle age

The commonest cause of premature death is vascular disease—mainly heart attacks and stroke. The main causes are obesity, a high-fat diet, and tobacco smoking rather than starvation and lack of clean water. In this context political action is still very important to make it easy for people to take exercise and eat healthily, and to make it difficult for people to buy and smoke tobacco.

Preventive medicine

This can identify and treat people at increased risk of death from vascular disease (particularly those with diabetes, high blood pressure, and high blood lipids) and will save many lives by doing this effectively, but the need for medicines to treat vascular disease in individuals is a measure of public health failure. The coexistence of obesity and starvation as major causes of preventable mortality in many countries is a growing public health challenge. Many effective preventive interventions, such as legislation to make seatbelts compulsory or tax tobacco, should be targeted at the whole population, but preventive medicine provided by clinicians must target individuals. This often requires screening to detect early signs of disease (e.g. HIV infection, cancer) or markers of risk of disease (e.g. high blood pressure, intrauterine growth delay), but clinicians must be clear that something effective can be done to ameliorate the condition detected before any screening is undertaken (see Chapter 3.3.2).

Failure of evidence-based preventive interventions

The usual reason for failure is lack of effective implementation, with the three most important implementation failures being: (1) poor population coverage (only a small proportion of the at-risk population receiving the intervention); (2) inadequate staff training; and (3) inadequate quality control.

Preventive medicine and curative medicine

Preventive medicine is an important and integral part of good curative medicine. All doctors have a responsibility to think about why someone is ill. Whatever disease is diagnosed, the question of whether it could have been prevented, and whether the risk of progression can be reduced, must be addressed. For example, every clinician who diagnoses a stroke must ask themselves whether a previous clinical opportunity to measure and control blood pressure has been missed, and reflect on this in regard to their future practice relating to other patients.

Introduction

In his millennium address, Nelson Mandela reminded the world that 'we close the century with most people still languishing in poverty, subjected to hunger, preventable disease, illiteracy, and insufficient shelter'. The health gap between rich and poor nations is shameful. For example, life expectancy for men in Sierra Leone is 37 years compared to 79 years in Japan. But even in the economically developed world, many people still die prematurely. In England and Wales, almost 1.4 million years of working life are lost each year due to death before age 65 years. Again, there is a marked gap between rich and poor. Life expectancy at birth is 78 years in men from social class I compared to 68 years in social class V. It is naive to think that medicine will remedy this situation. The fundamental step in achieving good health remains the elimination of poverty, with consequent access to food, sanitation, education, and shelter. But the power of medicine lies in the scientific understanding it provides of the disease process. Preventive medicine uses this understanding both to try to reduce the risk of disease and to detect and treat appropriately emergent disease before it does damage.

What is the scope for prevention? Figure 3.3.1.1 shows the number of women expected to die at different ages if 10 000 were subject to the age-specific death rates in England and Wales of today compared to the 1870s (the pattern is similar for men). The dramatic fall in deaths during childhood and early adulthood demonstrates unequivocally that such deaths are preventable. However, the proportion of men or women who live to over 100 has changed little and remains low (no more than 1%). So there seems to be a reasonable expectation that effective preventive medicine might make death before age 80 years uncommon, but the achievable objective seems to be better quality of life before death, and avoidance of premature death, rather than extension of life beyond what appears to be a maximum span of about 100 years. What preventive medicine cannot offer is immortality.

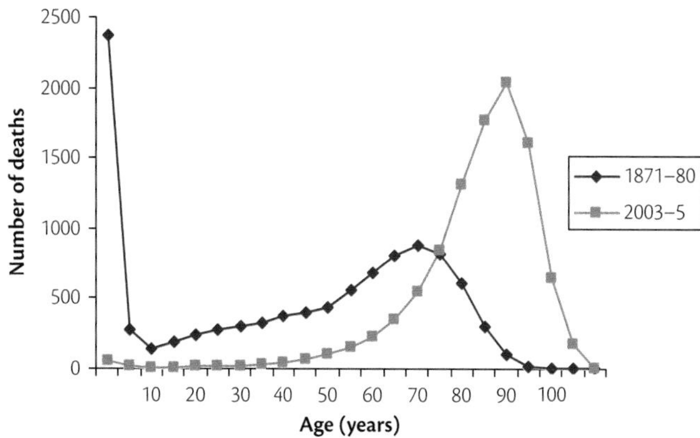

Fig. 3.3.1.1 Numbers of women dying in United Kingdom at different ages if 10 000 were subject from birth to the mortality rate current in 1871–1880 compared with that in 2003–2005.

Figure originally drawn by: Doll R. British Medical Journal 1982; 286: 445–53. Source of 2003–5 data: Office of National Statistics Interim Life Tables, United Kingdom.

Preventive strategies

Identifying and reducing risk

The main difference between preventive and curative medicine is the focus on risk. The World Health Organization's 2002 World Health Report focused on prevention and was entitled *Reducing Risks, Promoting Healthy Life*. The 10 leading global risk factors for ill health, estimated as together accounting for one-third of deaths worldwide, are shown in Table 3.3.1.1. The most disturbing fact for humanity is the occurrence of both starvation and obesity on the same list. While 170 million children are underweight because of hunger and 3 million each year die from starvation, 300 million adults are clinically obese. Figure 3.3.1.2 shows the impact of the

Table 3.3.1.1 Ten leading global risk factors causing a significant burden of disease

Risk factor	Attributable deaths/year (in millions)	Comment
Starvation and hunger	3.4	170 million children (27% of all children <5 years) are underweight
Unsafe sex	2.9	40 million people have HIV, 28 million (70%) in Africa; 99% of AIDS in Africa due to unsafe sex
Unsafe water Inadequate sanitation and hygiene	1.7	Most deaths from infectious diarrhoea, 9 out of 10 deaths are in children, virtually all (99.8%) in developing countries
Iron deficiency	1	2 billion people affected; pregnant women and children at highest risk
Indoor smoke from solid fuels	0.8	Half of world population exposed; causes 36% of all LRTI and 22% of all COPD cases
Tobacco consumption	4.9	1 million more deaths attributable to tobacco in 2000 than 1990, mostly due to increased smoking rates in developing countries
Alcohol consumption	1.8	Global alcohol consumption is increasing, most marked in developing countries; 60+ documented detrimental effects outweigh benefit of low to moderate consumption on vascular risk
Obesity	About 5	One billion overweight, 300 m clinically obese; causes 8–15% of life years lost in Europe and North America, less than 3% in Asia and Africa
High blood pressure	7.1	Main modifiable risk factors are diet (especially salt intake), obesity, and lack of exercise
High blood cholesterol	4.4	Mean cholesterol levels vary moderately between WHO regions but never more than 2.0 mmol/litre in any age group

Data from: World Health Report 2002, Reducing Risks, Promoting Healthy Life. World Health Organization, Geneva. www.who.int/whr/2002

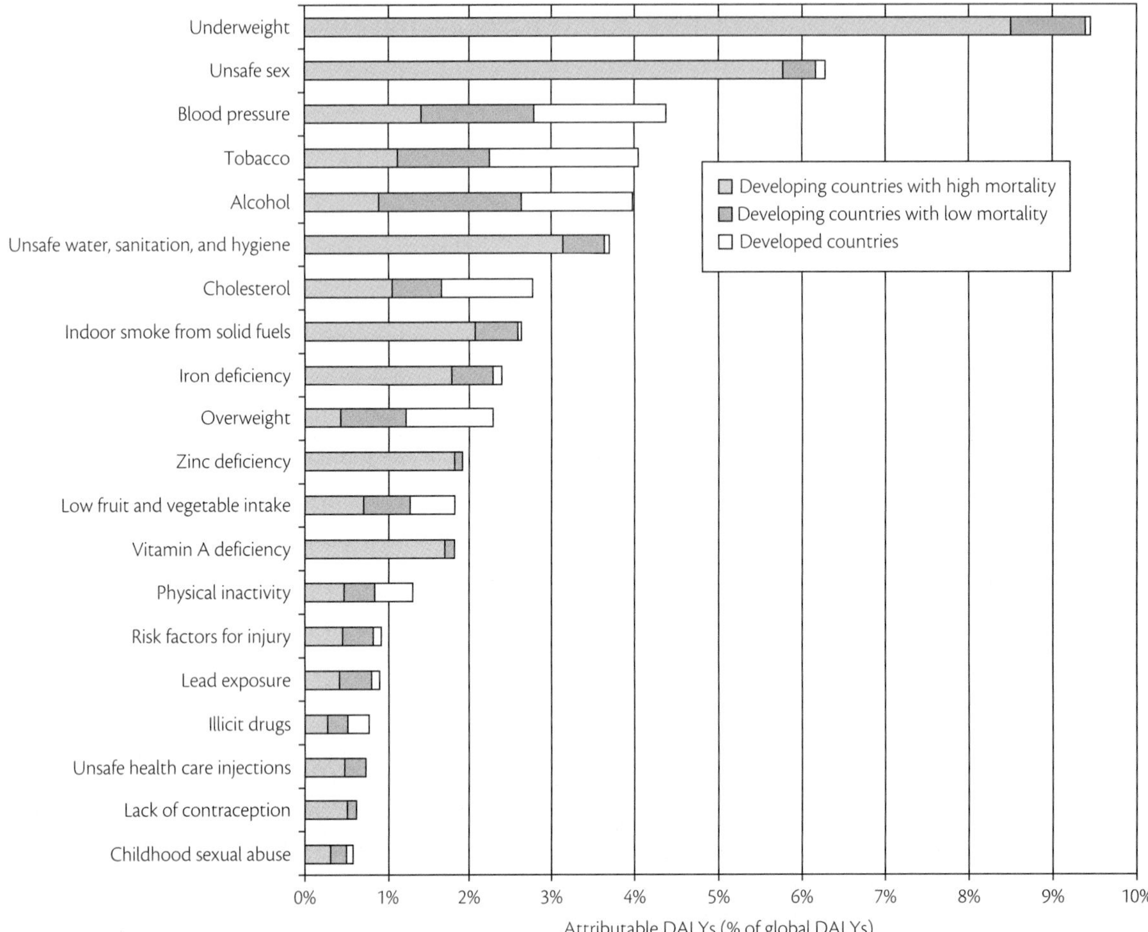

Fig. 3.3.1.2 Global burden of disease attributable to 20 leading risk factors in developed and developing countries.
Reproduced from The World Health Report 2002, with permission from The World Health Organization.

top 20 risk factors according to level of economic development. In developing countries with high mortality, the leading risk factors are hunger, unsafe sex, unsafe water, and nutritional deficiency of iron, vitamin A, iodine, and zinc. In developing countries with low mortality, they are alcohol, blood pressure, tobacco, and (paradoxically) both overweight and underweight. In developed countries they are tobacco, alcohol, blood pressure, cholesterol, and obesity. This overlap in health risk factors between developing and developed countries is a relatively recent phenomenon, creating a double burden of unconquered infection and increasingly unhealthy choices in individual consumption. This often reflects the unacceptable face of marketing in growing free-market economies.

The prevention paradox

Preventive medicine aims to reduce the risk of disease (or the risk of further morbidity and mortality in those who develop disease) so its benefit is the absence of disease in the future rather than the present. Absence of something is a difficult benefit to champion, particularly to the individual. As Geoffrey Rose pointed out many years ago, not only is the benefit intangible but many people must take precautions in order to prevent illness in only a few. Even in a country where diphtheria is common, several hundred children must be immunized to prevent one death. Rose called this the 'prevention paradox'—a preventive measure, which brings large benefits to the community may offer little to each participating individual.

The risk paradox

One of the three risk factors for cardiovascular disease identified by WHO is a high level of cholesterol in the blood. Figure 3.3.1.3 shows the prevalence of high blood cholesterol in the United Kingdom

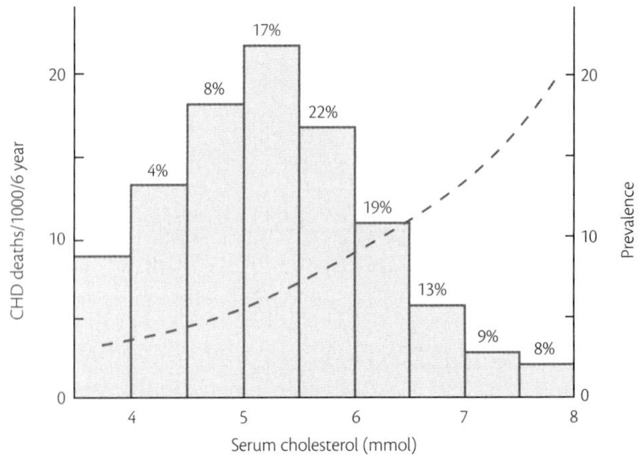

Fig. 3.3.1.3 Proportion of coronary heart disease deaths attributable to raised serum cholesterol (percentages above columns). Columns and left axis show population distribution of cholesterol levels. The broken line and left axis show the attributable mortality.
Reproduced from Rose G. Rose's Strategy of Preventive Medcine, 2008. With permission from Oxford University Press, Oxford.

population, the death rate associated with each cholesterol level, and the proportion of all deaths attributable to cholesterol occurring at each level. The risk paradox is that although those with a blood cholesterol >7.5 mmol/litre are at highest individual risk of disease they account for only 8% of total deaths. The group of people in whom most deaths occur (22%) is that with only a modestly increased cholesterol level of 5.5 to 6.0 mmol/litre. This is simply because of the number of people involved. There are far fewer in the high risk group than in the moderate risk group. Targeting preventive medicine at just the high risk group will often have relatively little impact on the total number of deaths in the population.

Primary and secondary prevention

Use of these terms has changed over time but commonly they can be interpreted as follows:

- Primary prevention—interventions to reduce the risk of disease in healthy people (e.g. use of seat belts to prevent injury in car accidents; tobacco control to prevent the occurrence of smoking-related disease; immunization against infectious disease)
- Secondary prevention—interventions to prevent avoidable morbidity in people with disease (e.g. treatment of vascular disease with aspirin; screening for early cancer)

It is immediately obvious that the distinction between primary and secondary prevention is sometimes difficult. Some interventions can fall into more than one category (e.g. stopping smoking reduces the progression as well as onset of many smoking-related diseases) and the definition of disease is not absolute (e.g. many apparently healthy people will have undetected disease). Nevertheless, the pragmatic categorization of preventive interventions into primary and secondary is often useful in practice.

Strategic choices

In choosing priority strategies for risk prevention, the WHO Report recommended that in general it is more effective:

- to focus on population-based rather than individual interventions
- to prioritize primary rather than secondary prevention
- to control distal before proximal risks to health

The recommendation to focus on population rather than individual interventions minimizes the importance of the risk paradox. Taking the cholesterol example, an effective intervention that focuses on reducing dietary fat intake in the whole population not only reduces the number of people at high risk but shifts the entire population distribution of risk to the left. In contrast, the recommendation to prioritize primary prevention aimed at distal risks (i.e. to provide clean water rather than focus on early recognition and treatment of dehydration from diarrhoea) exacerbates the prevention paradox. In public health practice, this may not matter if it is possible to convince the public to accept changes for the public good. However, in everyday clinical practice, individuals are concerned about their own health. It is often easier to persuade individuals to change their behaviour when they see early evidence of disease (e.g. to convince them to stop them smoking after they develop angina). In other words, secondary prevention may be easier to implement than primary prevention.

Defining and identifying the at-risk population

Public and individual interventions

Some public health interventions do not require anything other than a broad geographical definition of risk. Interventions are targeted at whole populations and do not require identification of individuals within that population—for example, road accidents can be reduced by seatbelt legislation and tobacco consumption by taxation without identifying the individual driver or smoker. However, some primary preventive strategies (e.g. vaccination) and most examples of secondary prevention (e.g. screening) have to be delivered to specific individuals at risk. You not only need to know that smokers are at risk, you need to know who smokes. These individuals can be defined in one of three ways: by demographic, phenotypic, or familial characteristics. Within each group of at-risk people so defined, further subpopulations may be identifiable as at particularly high risk.

Demographic risk

This is the most common way to define the target group for preventive-medicine services. For example, the United States Preventive Task Force defines the target group for most of the preventive services it recommends in terms of age. The other demographic risk characteristic used by the Task Force to define the target population is gender. It is obvious why it recommends that breast and cervical cancer screening should only be targeted at women, but gender-specific recommendations are also made for aortic aneurysm (based on differential risk) and gonorrhoea (based on the differential likelihood of asymptomatic infection). Some preventive programmes may target specific ethnic or racial groups—e.g. in Australia, interventions to reduce the risk of rheumatic fever associated with group A streptococcal infection of the throat have been restricted to the indigenous Aboriginal population who are at exceptionally high risk.

Phenotypic risk

A phenotype is a set of observable characteristics of an individual or group. Many epidemiological risk factors for disease are physical characteristics (e.g. obesity, hyperlipidaemia); other phenotypic categories often used to define at-risk target populations are behaviour (e.g. smoking, driving) and disease states (diabetes mellitus, angina). As some phenotypic risks interact (e.g. smoking and exposure to asbestos interactively increase risk of mesothelioma), multiple risk assessment is an increasingly common practice. A number of clinical tools have been developed to help estimate multifactorial risk in everyday practice, such as the New Zealand risk charts for cardiovascular disease.

Familial risk

Recent advances in genetic technology have increased our ability to characterize familial risk accurately, and further advance is likely in the next decade. At present, most preventive medicine programmes in this area use genetic assessment to refine assessment of individual risk in phenotypically identified high risk individuals or families (e.g. cystic fibrosis, neurofibromatosis) or demographically defined populations (e.g. pregnant women at risk of giving birth to a child with Down's syndrome). However, the characterization of risk based on population-based genetic screening is already technically feasible in the economically developed world, increasing the potential power of preventive medicine but also raising important ethical issues about how society deals with accurate predictions of high disease risk, particularly when evident at or before birth.

Registration, screening, and case-finding

It is much easier to identify specific individuals at risk when universal health registration is in place and its accuracy is systematically maintained. It not only allows efficient provision of primary prevention strategies, such as vaccination, but screening for disease risk is also much more efficient when based on an accurate population register. In the absence of a population health register, it is necessary to rely on case-finding. This requires identification of at-risk individuals during routine clinical work (normally in clinical consultations, but sometimes through contact or family tracing). It is less efficient than systematic population screening, but sometimes provides better access to socially disadvantaged groups who may respond poorly to screening invitations or have no registered address. It also allows some interventions to be given at a particularly appropriate moment (e.g. smoking cessation advice at a consultation for cough or contraceptive advice after termination of pregnancy).

Interventions to modify risk

The importance of public health

The marked improvements in health which have been achieved in economically developed countries over the past 150 years are not attributable to medicine. Life expectancy has doubled mainly because of environmental control of infectious pathogens (through sanitation and control of insect vectors) and a lifestyle that reduces individual susceptibility to infectious disease (better food, shelter, and education). So although medical science can play an important role in guiding public health policy by improving understanding of the mechanisms of disease, and specific medical interventions allow us to treat disease when it occurs, the role of preventive medicine should not be overestimated. In particular, the medical profession should not take upon itself responsibilities for public health, which are more appropriately assumed by governments and other social and environmental agencies.

The preventive responsibilities of all doctors

However, preventive medicine is an important and integral part of good curative medicine. All doctors have a responsibility to think about why someone is ill. Whatever cause is identified (physiological, social, or psychological), the question about whether the cause can be prevented (and the risk of future disease reduced) should be addressed. Clinicians should be held professionally accountable if they can be shown to have missed a previous clinical opportunity to measure blood pressure in an individual who subsequently develops a stroke. Doctors who work in a primary care role (particularly those with a registered population) have the added responsibility to ask themselves whether the risk should be addressed at a population rather than just an individual patient level.

Changing behaviour

Five of the ten leading risk factors for preventable mortality cited above are related to individual behaviour: smoking, diet, exercise, alcohol consumption, and unsafe sex. The most effective way to influence such behaviour is usually through public health policy (see below), but individual practitioners can play an important complementary role. People do listen to their doctors, and a number of clinical trials have shown advice on behaviour modification to be cost-effective, even though the impact may be small (e.g. in most studies only about 1 in 30 smokers given brief advice to stop smoking actually quit). Brief advice is most effective if practical in nature (giving guidance on how change can be achieved) and if backed up by written advice to take home. More intensive interventions may be even more effective but tend to be less cost-effective. In each case, it is important to take account of the scientific evidence about effectiveness and the local socioeconomic context.

Immunization

Vaccination is a very effective preventive strategy. Vaccination against smallpox has led to global eradication of the disease; eradication of polio seems a feasible global objective in the next decade. Vaccination against many diseases, particularly diseases of childhood such as measles, diphtheria, and polio, has led to rapid and dramatic falls in disease incidence. Figure 3.3.1.4 shows the impact of introduction of the Hib vaccine in 1992 on the incidence of *Haemophilus influenzae* infection in England and Wales. Table 3.3.1.2 shows the current routine vaccine schedule in the United Kingdom. Every individual in the population is vaccinated against 11 different organisms, 10 during childhood and 1 in old age. At-risk groups may be required to have specific vaccines to protect themselves (e.g. health workers against hepatitis B), and the general population and travellers to other countries can choose and pay for a range of vaccines for other diseases including hepatitis A, typhoid, and rabies. So the average person in the United Kingdom is now likely to receive vaccination against about 15 microorganisms during their lifetime.

A number of new and important vaccines are on the horizon, e.g. against malaria. But the existence of an effective vaccine does not guarantee the success of an immunization programme. This depends on the effective delivery of the vaccine to the at-risk population. Programmes are often limited in their effect by affordability (many vaccines are too expensive for developing countries), acceptability (parental anxiety about the adverse effects of pertussis vaccine has limited its uptake in many countries), and deliverability (vaccines may lose potency if stored outside a refrigerator). There are also potential problems with the antigenic variability of organisms (e.g. influenza) and the difficulty of immunizing at an age young enough to prevent morbidity but old enough to stimulate an immune response (e.g. measles). Nevertheless, immunization is probably the most important medical contribution to primary disease prevention.

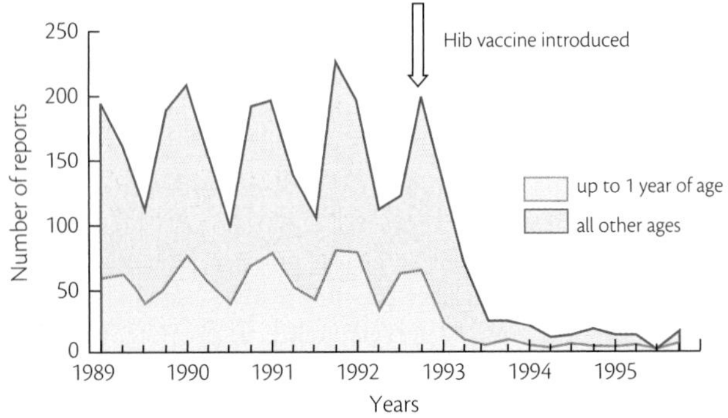

Fig. 3.3.1.4 Effect of introduction of *Haemophilus influenzae* type b (Hib) vaccination in the United Kingdom on laboratory reports of Hib infection. Reproduced by permission of the Controller, Her Majesty's Stationery Office.

Table 3.3.1.2 Routine immunization programme in the United Kingdom according to age

	2 months	3 months	4 months	12–13 months	3–5 years	13–18 years	65 years+	At-risk groups
Diphtheria	✓	✓	✓		✓	✓		
Tetanus	✓	✓	✓		✓	✓		
Polio	✓	✓	✓		✓	✓		
Pertussis	✓	✓	✓		✓			
Haemophilus influenzae B	✓	✓	✓	✓				
Meningococcus C		✓	✓	✓				
Measles				✓	✓			
Mumps				✓	✓			
Rubella				✓	✓			
Pneumococcus	✓		✓	✓			✓	✓
Influenza							✓	✓
TB								✓
Hepatitis B								✓

Data from: UK Joint Committee on Vaccination and Immunisation (2006). Immunisation against infectious disease. Report of UK Joint Committee on Vaccination and Immunisation. HMSO, London. www.dh.gov.uk/Policy and Guidance/HealthandSocialCareTopics/GreenBook/fs/en

Screening

The issue of screening is dealt with in Chapter 3.3.2. Three-quarters of the preventive services for adults recommended for implementation by the United States Preventive Services Task Force involve screening. The purpose of screening is to identify disease at an early and curable stage. The most important criterion that has to be met for screening to be ethical is that the condition identified can be ameliorated and cured. Good intention is not enough. Screening will do harm if it identifies conditions that cannot be ameliorated, either because of lack of effective interventions or lack of resources. It is particularly important to assess the effectiveness of screening interventions in randomized trials, as people whose disease was detected by screening will appear to clinicians to do well even if the screening is ineffective. This is because early diagnosis will lead to longer survival irrespective of treatment, and illness detected by screening will always tend to be more benign in its natural history than illness detected clinically.

Prophylactic treatment

Although most people think of medicines as cures for current illness, many medicines are prescribed with a view to preventing future illness. Antibiotics are given before surgery to prevent post-operative infection, antimalarials to prevent malaria in travellers, anticoagulants to prevent stroke in people with atrial fibrillation, and lipid-lowering agents to prevent heart attacks in people at high risk of cardiovascular disease. The duration of treatment may also be extended beyond the initial treatment phase to achieve a preventive effect. Antidepressants are continued after cure to prevent relapse, acetylcholinesterase inhibitors to prevent worsening of ventricular dysfunction, and uricosuric agents to prevent further episodes of gout.

It must be clear from these examples that many, perhaps most, drugs have the potential to be used for prevention as well as cure. In some cases (e.g. treatment of diabetes) the distinction between prevention and cure is unhelpful: treatment aims to prevent morbidity in both the short and long terms. However, in all the examples given, prescribing is limited to a defined high-risk group. Prophylactic treatment with drugs is less helpful when a high-risk population cannot be easily defined. It is almost always inappropriate to use prophylactic treatment to reduce population risk for three reasons: the strategy is seldom cost-effective, increasing the reliance of the population on medicine is an adverse social outcome, and uncommon adverse effects can easily outweigh any benefit.

Environmental change

Most environmental causes of disease are best modified on a public health rather than an individual basis. Such factors include the safety of the workplace, environmental pollution, transport safety, food hygiene, and provision of clean water. However, a number of diseases have environmental causes, which need to be recognized and avoided by the individual patient. On a global scale, avoidance of insect and other disease vectors (e.g. by netting) and attention to nutritional hygiene (e.g. by filtering water) are probably the most important. In economically developed countries, the most common diseases amenable to individual environmental intervention are those associated with atopy, such as asthma and eczema. Not all patients have an identifiable allergenic cause for their symptoms and, even if one is identified, avoidance (e.g. of house dust mite in asthma) may not be easy. But dramatic improvement can occur, and treating contact dermatitis without giving advice on contact avoidance, or treating louse bites without giving advice on how to rid clothes of lice, is bad medical practice.

What interventions work?

Public health interventions

It is impossible to list here all the public health initiatives that are known to be effective. There is no doubt that provision of clean

Table 3.3.1.3 Preventive interventions recommended for adults by the United States Preventive Services Task Force as providing important health benefit on the basis of research evidence rated as A (strong) or B (fair)

Medical problem	Men	Women	Target groups
Screening interventions			
Alcohol misuse	✓	✓	
Aortic aneurysm	✓		Once age 65–75 in ever smokers
Breast cancer	✓		Age 40+ (mammography); familial risk (genetic testing)
Cervical cancer	✓		Ever sexually active
Chlamydia infection	✓		Sexually active age <25 years or other at risk groups
Colorectal cancer	✓	✓	Age 50+
Depression	✓	✓	
Diabetes mellitus	✓	✓	Adults with hypertension or hyperlipidaemia
Gonorrhoea infection	✓		At risk groups
High blood pressure	✓	✓	
HIV infection	✓	✓	At risk groups
Lipid disorders	✓	✓	Men 35+, women 45+; younger if high CVD risk
Obesity	✓	✓	
Osteoporosis		✓	Women 60+
Syphilis infection	✓	✓	At risk groups
Other interventions			
Aspirin	✓	✓	Adults at increased CVD risk
Breastfeeding promotion		✓	Pregnant and recently delivered women
Breast cancer chemoprevention		✓	Women at high risk of breast cancer
Dietary counselling	✓	✓	Adults at high risk of CVD
Tobacco use counselling	✓	✓	All who use tobacco

Data from : The Guide to Clinical Preventive Services 2006, Recommendations of the U.S. Preventive Services Task Force. US Department of Health and Human Services, Washington, DC. www.ahrq.gov/clinic/pocketgd.pdf

water and sanitation; avoidance of war; progressive taxation; provision of education; fiscal policy to reduce tobacco and alcohol use; food policies to reduce community intake of salt, saturated fat, and excess calories; and education to promote safe sex, are all effective public health interventions. Their effective implementation depends on political will at a national and international level. In general, the effectiveness of public health interventions will reflect government attitude to regulation (e.g. whether the presumption of market-led development and free trade dominates individual and societal health concerns) and the understanding of health risk by the general public, politicians, and health practitioners. At an international level, the World Health Organization cites the Framework Convention for Tobacco Control as an exemplar of a very effective government-led international public health initiative. This covers advertising, regulation, taxation, and smoke-free zones as well as the individual treatment of addiction.

Individual interventions

As with public health interventions, it is impossible to list here all the preventive interventions targeted at individuals, which have been shown to be effective. Many are in any case better seen as part of good routine clinical care (and are included in the relevant chapters on specific diseases). Nevertheless, it is worth listing preventive interventions, which may not be included elsewhere, and for which there is very good evidence of effectiveness from clinical trials. One accessible source of regularly updated evidence on individual interventions is the United States Preventive Services Task Force and Table 3.3.1.3 lists the 20 conditions for which evidence of effectiveness is rated by them as A ('strong') or B ('at least fair'). The preventive interventions (other than vaccination) for two important at-risk groups—pregnant women and children—for which there is a similar level of evidence of effectiveness are listed separately in Table 3.3.1.4. Omission of interventions from these lists does not imply that they are unimportant or do not work, but it often implies lack of high-quality research evidence.

Implementation issues

Cultural constraints

Most behaviour aimed at preventing disease has a strong sociocultural component and reflects prevalent attitudes and norms in society. Preventive interventions are severely constrained by this social context. Convincing people to stop smoking, eat less salt, drink less beer, or drive more slowly is difficult if everyone else is doing the opposite. For example, Fig. 3.3.1.5 shows that the mean blood cholesterol level in Finland is almost twice that in Japan. Migrant studies show that this difference is dietary rather than genetic in origin and so medical advice to reduce fat consumption has the potential to reduce blood cholesterol level from

Table 3.3.1.4 Preventive interventions for pregnant women and children (other than vaccination) recommended by the US Preventive Services Task Force as providing important health benefit on the basis of research evidence rated as A (strong) or B (fair)

Recommendation	Children	Pregnant women
Alcohol misuse		✓
Asymptomatic bacteriuria screening		✓
Breast-feeding promotion		✓
Gonococcal ophthalmia neonatorum prophylaxis (antibiotic drops)	✓	
Infection screening (chlamydia, gonorrhoea, HepB, HIV, syphilis)		✓
Rhesus (D)-incompatibility screening		✓
Tobacco-use counselling		✓
Visual-impairment screening	✓	

Data from : The Guide to Clinical Preventive Services 2006, Recommendations of the U.S. Preventive Services Task Force. US Department of Health and Human Services, Washington, DC. www.ahrq.gov/clinic/pocketgd.pdf

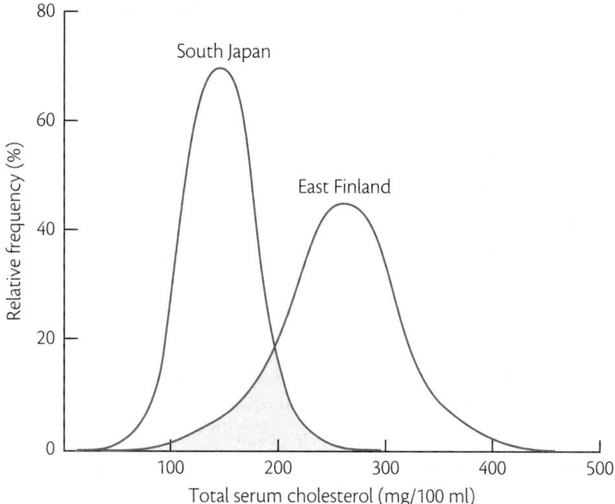

Fig. 3.3.1.5 Distribution of serum cholesterol in southern Japan and eastern Finland.
Reproduced from Rose G. Rose's Strategy of Preventive Medecine, 2008. With permission from Oxford University Press, Oxford.

the high level in Finland to the low level in Japan. However, even in clinical trials, dietary advice from health professionals in a community setting seldom achieves a reduction in blood cholesterol of more than 3 to 5%. Studies of salt restriction (to lower blood pressure) show a similar result. Intensive intervention and support is needed for an individual patient to achieve a physiologically significant reduction in intake and many find such a diet unpalatable. Countercultural change is difficult to achieve. The adverse consequence is the common use of medication (in this case statins) to treat what is effectively a sociocultural problem.

Time constraints

Things change over time. The North Karelia project was a large-scale, long-term programme to reduce mortality from cardiovascular disease in northern Finland, started in 1972, which involved both public health and individual intervention. Figure 3.3.1.6 compares mortality from cardiovascular disease in North Karelia with that in 10 other provinces in Finland before and during the intervention by plotting two regression lines. The difference in slopes of these two lines shows that the intervention was to some extent effective. However, far more impressive in magnitude is the absolute fall in mortality over time both in North Karelia and in the other provinces. The lessons for preventive medicine are two-fold: the effect of medical intervention may be small compared to the effect of other economic and social influences; and the change in baseline risk and social context over time may be so rapid that it will substantially influence the absolute benefit of any preventive intervention.

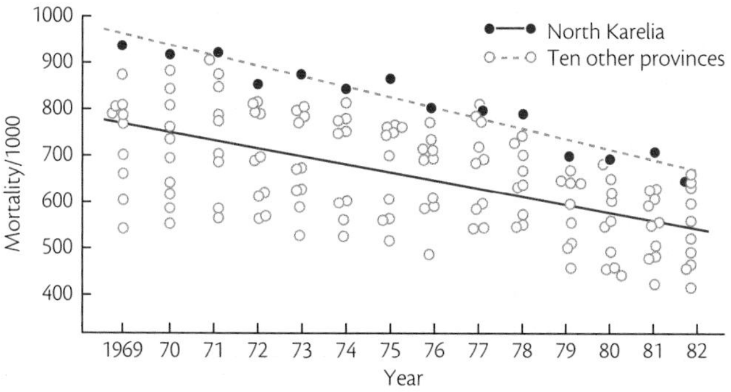

Fig. 3.3.1.6 The North Karelia project. Age-standardized annual mortality from cardiovascular disease in men aged 35–64 years in Finland, 1969–82.
Redrawn from original data published by Tuomilehto J et al, British Medical Journal 1986:293:1068–71.

Programme effectiveness

Many of the interventions cited earlier are known to work because they have been tested in clinical trials. However, clinical trials are often done in settings far removed from everyday life. Participants are compliant, those delivering the intervention are highly trained, the technology is of high specification, and quality control is rigorous. These conditions will not hold under ordinary working conditions. When recommended preventive interventions fail, the most common reason is lack of effective implementation of the programme, rather than lack of effectiveness of the intervention itself.

The importance of considering programme effectiveness is seen most vividly in immunization and screening programmes. The three most important issues that determine programme effectiveness are the following:

- Coverage—What proportion of the population at risk receives the intervention?
- Delivery—Are factors that affect the delivery of the intervention (like the maintenance of equipment, the training of staff, and the storage of biological materials) up to scratch?
- Quality control—Are standards set and monitored for key indicators of the intervention process (e.g. immune response or predictive value of screening)?

Failure in just one of these areas in the United Kingdom has damaged programmes promoting immunization (e.g. the resurgence of pertussis after media publicity about potential adverse effects of the vaccine led to a fall in uptake) and cervical screening (e.g. lack of quality control in cervical sampling and cytological assessment led to false negative results and avoidable mortality).

Conclusion

Preventive medicine is an integral part of clinical practice for all doctors. It is our responsibility as clinicians not only to cure the presenting illness but also to take action where possible to prevent future morbidity. However, we must display both humility and assertiveness in our approach. We need to be humble in our approach to patients and to recognize that medicine is not the main determinant of health. At the same time we must display assertiveness in our advocacy of prevention. In the United Kingdom, the Royal College of Physicians' reports, the campaigning of medical charities, and the decision by virtually all doctors to stop smoking have all played an important part in influencing both public and political opinion against tobacco use. As a profession, we can make a unique and powerful contribution to the prevention of premature death by identifying and publicizing the existence and causes of ill health. We also have a unique and powerful responsibility to act as advocates for our patients in ensuring that these causes are addressed and the risk to their health is ameliorated. Good clinical practice entails preventive medicine, but good preventive medicine is more than just good clinical practice.

Further reading

Rose G (1992). *The strategy of preventive medicine.* Oxford University Press, Oxford. [The definitive text on the theory of preventive medicine—short, readable, brilliant.]

UK Joint Committee on Vaccination and Immunisation (2006). *Immunisation against infectious disease.* Report of UK Joint Committee on Vaccination and Immunisation. HMSO, London. http://www.dh.gov.uk/en/Publichealth/Healthprotection/Immunisation/Greenbook/DH_4097254 [Annually updated short publication which provides a practical, but evidence based, summary of immunization recommendations in the United Kingdom.]

US Preventive Services Task Force (2006). *Guide to clinical preventive services—recommendations of the US Preventive Services Task Force.* US Department of Health and Human Services, Washington, DC. http://www.ahrq.gov/clinic/pocketgd.pdf [Summary of current evidence on the effectiveness of preventive health care.]

World Health Organization (2003). *World Health Report 2002. Reducing risks, promoting healthy life.* World Health Organization, Geneva. http://www.who.int/whr/2002 [Summary of the main global challenges to preventive health care; chapter 4 quantifies the major risk to health.]

3.3.2 Medical screening

Nicholas Wald and Malcolm Law

Essentials

Medical screening is the systematic application of a test or inquiry to identify individuals at sufficient risk of a specific disorder to benefit from further investigation or direct preventive action (these individuals not having sought medical attention on account of symptoms of that disorder). Key to this definition is that the early detection of disease is not an end in itself; bringing forward a diagnosis without altering the prognosis is useless and may be harmful.

Criteria for screening

Before a potential screening test is introduced into practice it must be shown to prevent death or serious disability from the disease to an extent sufficient to justify the human and financial costs. To this end, three screening parameters need to be determined: (1) the detection rate (sensitivity); (2) the false-positive rate (equivalent to the specificity); and (3) the odds of being affected given a positive screening result (equivalent to the positive predictive value). Where a detection rate cannot be directly determined, e.g. in cancer screening, or if the efficacy of the intervention is uncertain, a randomized trial is needed to show that screening and subsequent treatment reduce disease specific mortality.

Circumstances where screening is not appropriate

Screening tests should not be practised simply because they seem intuitively useful: chest radiography to screen for lung cancer and manual breast self-examination to screen for breast cancer were assumed to be worthwhile, but randomized trials showed they did not significantly reduce mortality from the cancer. Screening for prostate cancer is widely practised, yet it does harm (from hazardous treatment) with evidence of a relatively modest reduction in mortality from the disease. Causal risk factors, even important ones like serum cholesterol and blood pressure for cardiovascular disease, usually discriminate poorly between individuals who will and will not develop the disease they cause, because most of the population is 'exposed'.

Particular disorders where screening is justified

The number of disorders for which medical screening has been shown to be worthwhile is perhaps surprisingly small, but includes: (1) antenatal screening—e.g. various single gene disorders, Down's syndrome, neural tube defects, and some infections such as hepatitis B and HIV that may be asymptomatic in the mother but cause disease when transmitted to the fetus; (2) neonatal screening—e.g. congenital hypothyroidism, certain inborn errors of metabolism such as phenylketonuria, and congenital deafness; (3) adult screening—this has been shown to reduce mortality from only three cancers—breast, cervical, and colorectal; screening individuals with diabetes mellitus prevents blindness from retinopathy; screening men around the age of 65 prevents death from ruptured abdominal aortic aneurysm; and screening young women for chlamydia infection prevents pelvic inflammatory disease and its complications (including infertility).

Future prospects

Tests that arise out of technological development in the absence of a clear case of medical need, e.g. whole body scanning using MRI or CT scanning, should not be 'sold' to the public in the belief that they are helpful. As with all screening methods, their value needs to be shown before they are introduced into practice. Determining when medical screening is an effective method of preventing serious disease and disability is one of the most challenging areas in medical research.

Introduction

There is scarcely a medical discipline that does not include some aspect of screening. It has made significant inroads into the prevention of disease, but is often used inappropriately in circumstances where there is insufficient evidence that it benefits health. Determining when screening is an effective method of prevention is one of the most challenging areas in medical research today, requiring an understanding of the principles of screening, the pathology, natural history, and epidemiology of the diseases concerned, and quantitative information on the efficacy of the screening tests and the remedies available.

Medical screening contains three elements:

1 Identifying individuals at sufficiently high risk of having or developing a specific disorder to benefit from further investigation or direct preventive action.

2 It is systematically offered to a population that has not sought medical attention for symptoms of the relevant disease. It is usually initiated by medical authorities, not the patient.

3 Its purpose is to benefit screened individuals. On this basis, mass testing activities such as surveillance for HIV infection or

pre-employment examinations to test fitness for work are not classified as medical screening.

The following definition has been widely used and encapsulates these three elements:

> Medical screening is the systematic application of a test or inquiry, to identify individuals at sufficient risk of a specific disorder to benefit from further investigation or direct preventive action, among those who have not sought medical attention on account of symptoms of that disorder.

Worthwhile screening aims to prevent death or disability from specific disorders. Screening that simply brings forward a diagnosis without altering the prognosis is useless and may be harmful, prompting needless anxiety and possibly hazardous interventions. The early detection of disease is not an end in itself. As with any medical treatment, screening needs to be shown to offer medical benefit and to be acceptably safe. Many medical disorders are not candidates for screening, because they are too trivial or because treatment is no more effective following screening than following clinical presentation. The value of a screening test, in which the benefits are considered in the light of the human and financial costs, needs to be determined before it is introduced into practice.

Box 3.3.2.1 Requirements for a worthwhile screening test

1 Disorder: well defined

2 Prevalence/incidence: known

3 Natural history: medically important disorder

4 Remedy or treatment: more effective or acceptable than at clinical presentation

5 Screening test: simple and safe

6 Test performance:

(a) Detection rate can be determined: detection rate and false-positive rate known and acceptable. For a quantitative screening test, the distributions of test values in affected and unaffected individuals should be known, the extent of overlap sufficiently small, and a suitable cut off level defined

(b) Detection rate cannot be determined: randomized trial evidence shows that the combined effect of screening and treatment is sufficiently effective in preventing death and disability from the disease being screened for, with an acceptably low proportion of individuals requiring further investigation

7 Financial: overall cost acceptable to achieve the health benefit

8 Facilities: available or can easily be installed, including for diagnosis and treatment

9 Acceptability: procedures following a positive result are generally agreed and acceptable to the screening authorities and the screened individuals

Requirements for a worthwhile screening test (Box 3.3.2.1)

The disorder

The disorder needs to be clinically well defined and should, wherever possible, be specified independently of the screening test. The disorder should not be an 'abnormal' value of the screening test being offered, such as a value lying outside the 95% range. This creates a circularity ('tautological screening') that makes it impossible to determine whether screening is genuinely preventing disease or is just causing overdiagnosis. It is necessary to know the distribution of values of the screening test in individuals who have (or will develop) the clinical disease and in individuals who do not, in order to assess the value of the test.

An example is hypertension, or high blood pressure, an asymptomatic condition that increases risk of a heart attack or stroke. If hypertension were regarded as the medical disorder being screened for, then all the 'hypertensives' would have blood pressure above the cut-off and all the 'nonhypertensives' below it—i.e. a perfect test. The apparent screening perfection is a tautological misconception. A high blood pressure measurement is the result of a screening test (blood pressure measurement) for the clinical diseases (stroke and myocardial infarction) caused by high blood pressure. In fact, blood pressure measurement, although widely practised, is not a good screening test for stroke or myocardial infarction. Many people who will not have a stroke or myocardial infarction have high blood pressure, and many who do will not. This is considered in further detail below.

Prevalence or incidence

To derive an estimate of the odds of being affected among individuals with a positive screening result (see below), the prevalence, or incidence, of the disorder needs to be known. Prevalence is the number of cases of a disorder in a defined population at a given point in time, incidence is the number of new cases occurring in a defined population over a specified period. If the disorder is very rare screening may not be justifiable, unless it can easily be incorporated into an existing screening protocol. If the disorder is very common (e.g. heart attacks and strokes), screening may be pointless and a population-wide preventive strategy may be needed.

Natural history

Screening should be restricted to disorders that are medically important, i.e. associated with serious morbidity or premature mortality.

Remedy

A remedy or treatment must be available that is more effective or acceptable following screening than at clinical presentation. Offering an effective treatment is insufficient; the treatment must be more effective or acceptable if delivered early.

Screening test

The screening test should be simple and safe. Some screening tests are so simple or performed so routinely that they are not recognized as such. For example, asking a woman's age was once the antenatal screening test for Down's syndrome. A routine blood count includes the antenatal screening test for β-thalassaemia (mean corpuscular volume), so the issue is not one of introducing the test but of systematically interpreting a test already carried out.

The purpose of testing generally defines whether it is a screening or diagnostic test. If the aim is to identify a high-risk group for further investigation or preventive treatment, it is a screening test; if it is to make a diagnosis, it is a diagnostic test. Screening tests indicate a probability of having or developing a disorder, whereas diagnostic tests usually indicate whether an individual is affected or unaffected. The accuracy of each type of test does not itself define what type of test it is. Sometimes mass testing, perceived as screening, is in fact diagnosis, e.g. obstetric ultrasonography used routinely to diagnose anencephaly. Screening tests usually apply to healthy populations but this is not always the case, e.g. screening for retinopathy among people with diabetes.

Screening test performance

It is useful to separate screening tests for which detection rates can be determined from screening tests for which this is not possible.

Detection rate can be determined

The performance of screening and diagnostic tests is defined by three parameters: (1) the detection rate, (2) the false-positive rate, and (3) the odds of being affected given a positive result (OAPR).

Detection rate

The detection rate of a test (or test sensitivity) is the proportion of affected individuals with positive test results (Table 3.3.2.1).

An advantage of the term detection rate over sensitivity is that it avoids confusion with the usage of sensitivity in analytical biochemistry, where it means the minimum detectable amount in an assay. In cancer screening, 'detection rate' is often taken to mean the prevalence of detected cancers at a screening examination.

False-positive rate

The false-positive rate is the proportion of unaffected individuals with positive test results (Table 3.3.2.1).

The complement of the false-positive rate is the specificity, which is 100% minus the false-positive rate; e.g. a false-positive rate of 3% is the same as a specificity of 97%. Advantages of the term false positive rate over specificity are that (1) it is more easily understood and remembered; (2) it focuses attention on the group to be offered further medical intervention, and (3) a 10% false-positive rate is twice as 'bad' as one of 5%, whereas this is concealed within the corresponding specificity values of 90% and 95%.

Table 3.3.2.1 Algebraic summary of detection and false-positive rates of qualitative tests or quantitative tests using a specified cut-off

Test result	Affected	Unaffected
Positive	TRUE POSITIVES a	FALSE POSITIVES b
Negative	FALSE NEGATIVES c	TRUE NEGATIVES d
Total	$a + c$	$b + d$
Detection rate (sensitivity)	$\frac{a}{a+c}$	
False-positive rate (1 – specificity)		$\frac{b}{b+d}$

Odds of being affected given a positive result (OAPR)

The OAPR is the ratio of the number of affected to unaffected individuals among those with positive test results, i.e. true positives:false positives in the population in question.

The OAPR in Table 3.3.2.1 would be a:b if the numbers in Table 3.3.2.1 came directly from screening everyone in a study population. In practice this is uncommon because the disorder being screened for is rare and so it is sensible to estimate the detection rate on all the affected individuals but only a small sample of unaffected individuals. Because of this sampling difference, tables like Table 3.3.2.1 cannot be used to estimate the OAPR. It is best estimated indirectly using estimates of the prevalence of the disorder from one source and estimates of the detection rates and false-positive rates of the screening test from another source. This can be done using a flow diagram such as that in Fig. 3.3.2.1, in which the detection rate (80%) is applied to the number of affected individuals (prevalence 1%) and the false-positive rate (4%) to the number of unaffected. Then the ratio of true-positive to false-positive tests performed will be an unbiased estimate of the OAPR in a total population. The OAPR is 1:5 after the screening test, and 38:1 after the diagnostic test (detection rate 95%, false-positive rate 0.5%). If the prevalence of the disorder were halved (0.5%) the OAPRs would be halved to 1:10 and 19:1 respectively. Thus the less common the disorder, the less likely people with positive results will be affected.

The OAPR can be expressed as a probability ('true-positives/all positives') which is known as the positive predictive value (PPV). In the example in Fig. 3.3.2.1) the OAPR, 80:400 = 1:5, is equivalent to a predictive value of 1/(1+5) = 1/6 ≅ 17%. The OAPR is more useful than the PPV because it is numerically easier to compute when tests are performed in sequence (Fig. 3.3.2.1), and it provides a better impression of the relative performance of tests. In the example, the OAPR of 38:1 is equivalent to a PPV of 97% (38/39). If the detection rate of the screening test were halved (to 40%) the OAPR would also be halved (to 19:1) but the PPV, 95% (19/20), appears only a little lower.

A good screening test has a high detection rate, a low false-positive rate, and a high OAPR (e.g. 1:10 is better than 1:50).

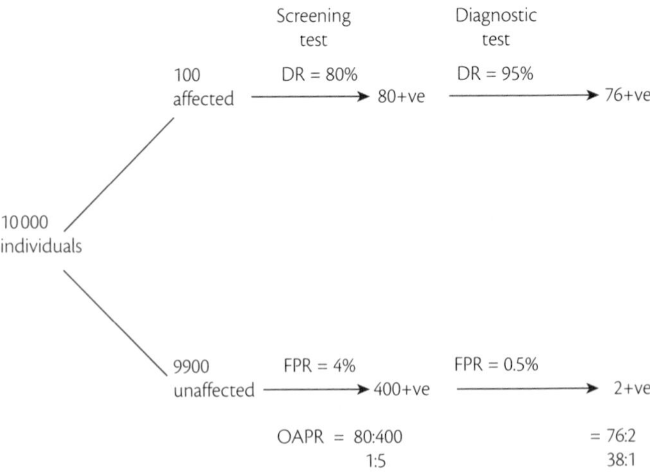

Fig. 3.3.2.1 Flowchart to show the performance of screening and diagnostic tests. The critical first step in constructing such a flowchart is to separate individuals into affected and unaffected, not into screen-positive and screen-negative.
Reproduced from Wald, N. An Introduction to Epidemiology in Medicine. London: Royal Society of Medicine Press, 2004.

Stating the detection rate for a test is uninformative unless a false-positive rate (or specificity) is also stated. Screening performance is assessed by specifying the detection rate for a given false-positive rate, or specifying the false-positive rate for a given detection rate.

The detection rates and false-positive rates are independent of the prevalence of the disease for tests that measure a consequence of the disease (e.g. the antenatal markers of Down's syndrome) but may not be independent for a screening test that is a measure of a cause of the relevant disease. For example when screening for an autosomal recessive disease such as cystic fibrosis by testing for a known DNA mutation in the gene for the disease, a higher gene prevalence will necessarily be linked to a higher disease prevalence.

The OAPR is always dependent on the prevalence. The higher the prevalence the higher the OAPR, even if the detection rate and false-positive rate are constant.

Estimates of the detection rate and false-positive rate can be applied from one population to others because they are generally independent of the prevalence of the disorder. This is not the case with the OAPR, which depends on the prevalence.

For a qualitative (or categorical) test, such as the presence or absence of a cystic fibrosis mutation among a given panel of mutations tested for, there is only one detection rate and false positive rate. This is not the case with quantitative (or noncategorical) tests, such as maternal serum α-fetoprotein (AFP) for open spina bifida screening, which yield numerical results. In such cases, the detection rate and false-positive rate depend on the screening cut-off level used to distinguish positive from negative results. No single pair of detection and false-positive rates summarizes the performance of tests; both will vary as the cut-off is changed. For example, at cut-off level A in the relative frequency distributions in Fig. 3.3.2.2 the test will have a detection rate given by the area under the curve for affected subjects to the right of cut-off level A (95%), and a false-positive rate given by the area under the curve for unaffected subjects to the right of the same cut-off level (10%). The higher the cut-off level (say, B or C) the lower the detection rate and false-positive rate.

It is common to summarize the performance of a test as a receiver–operator characteristic (ROC) curve. This is a plot of the detection rate against the false-positive rate, with both scales plotted from 0% to 100%. In such a graph a useless test is represented by the diagonal, indicating that the detection rate and the false-positive rate are always the same. As the screening test improves, the ROC curve bows out from the diagonal towards the axes. A perfect screening test clings to the detection rate axis up to 100% while the false-positive rate remains at zero. The area under a ROC curve is sometimes used to indicate the performance of a screening test, but it is not a satisfactory measure of this. It is better to state detection rate for specified false-positive rate or vice versa. A weakness of an ROC curve is that for screening tests that are potentially useful, the area of the graph that is informative is restricted to a small portion, namely the part covering false-positive rates up to about 10% and detection rates (from 40% to 100%) between about 50% and 100%. Figure 3.3.2.3 illustrates detection rates plotted against false-positive rates (from 0% to 10%) in multiple marker antenatal screening for Down's syndrome, showing the improvements in screening that have been made over the past 20 years.

Good screening tests are usually early manifestations of the disease being screened for, while causes of a disease that are highly prevalent in a community are usually poor screening tests.

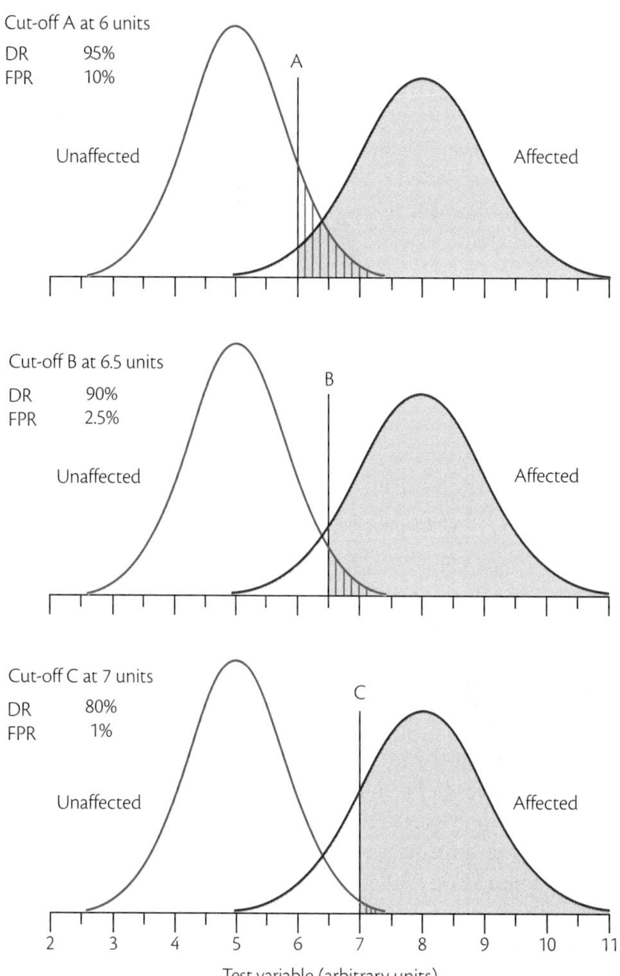

Fig. 3.3.2.2 Hypothetical example of the detection rate and false-positive rate of a screening test at three different cut-off levels. The implied vertical axis is the percentage of individuals at different levels of the screening test variables, considered separately for affected and unaffected individuals.

Reproduced from Wald, N. An Introduction to Epidemiology in Medicine. London: Royal Society of Medicine Press, 2004.

Causal risk factors such as blood pressure for stroke are important aetiologically and account for a large proportion of the disease they cause because they are usually common (e.g. most adults over 55 can be said to have a high blood pressure) yet many escape the consequences (e.g. a stroke). This means that causal risk factors usually do not discriminate well between individuals who will and who will not develop the disease.

Table 3.3.2.2 shows the detection rate for a 5% false-positive rate (DR_5) for various risk ratio estimates between the top and bottom fifths of the distribution of a risk factor. Even a 'strong' risk factor with a fivefold risk ratio between the top and bottom quintile groups (fifths) of the distribution (typical of LDL cholesterol and myocardial infarction) has only a 14% detection rate for a 5% false-positive rate. An interquintile risk ratio of around 1000 is necessary to achieve a detection rate of at least 75% for a 5% false-positive rate.

The OAPR can be determined by using the flowchart method illustrated in Fig. 3.3.2.1. It can also be determined using the likelihood ratio (LR) which is a measure of the 'concentrating' power of a test (Fig. 3.3.2.4). For a group of people with values of the

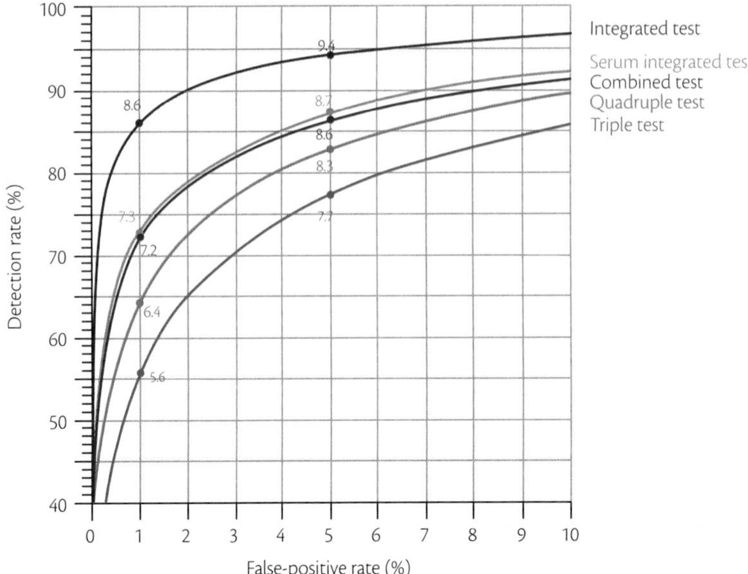

Fig. 3.3.2.3 Antenatal screening for Down's syndrome: detection rates and false-positive rates for specified screening tests.The Integrated test consists of the ultrasound marker nuchal translucency and pregnancy-associated plasma protein A (PAPP-A) measured in the first trimester, and AFP, unconjugated oestriol (uE3), human chorionic gonadotropin (hCG), and inhibin-A in the second trimester. The Serum Integrated test is the same as the Integrated test without nuchal translucency. The Combined test consists of nuchal translucency, PAPP-A, and hCG in the first trimester. The Quadruple test consists of AFP, uE3, hCG, and inhibin-A in the second trimester. The Triple test is the same as the Quadruple test without inhibin-A. All the tests include maternal age.

Reproduced from Wald NJ, *et al.* (2004). SURUSS in perspective. Br J Obstet Gynaecol, 111, 521–31, with permission from Wiley-Blackwell.

screening variable above a specified cut-off (i.e. all screen-positives), this is the proportion of the area for 'affecteds' to the right of the cut-off divided by the proportion of the area for 'unaffecteds' to the right of the cut-off. (Fig. 3.3.2.4a), which is equivalent to the detection rate divided by the false-positive rate (DR/FPR). It is the number of times individuals with positive results are more likely to have the disorder for which they are being tested compared with the general population (individuals who have not been tested).

That is, the OAPR is the likelihood ratio multiplied by the prevalence of the disorder (expressed as an odds):

$$\text{OAPR} = \text{LR} \times \text{prevalence as an odds}$$

Table 3.3.2.2 Detection rate for a 5% false-positive rate (DR_5) according to relative risk between top and bottom fifths of the distribution in unaffected individuals

Relative risk between top and bottom fifths of the distribution in unaffected individuals	DR_5 (%)
1	5
2	8
3	11
5	14
10	20
40	36
80	45
800	71
2000	79
10 000	89

Reproduced from Wald NJ, Hackshaw AK, Frost CD, *When can a risk factor be used as a worthwhile screening test?* BMJ 319,1562–65 © 1999 with permission from BMJ Publishing Group.

So (see Fig. 3.3.2.4a for example), if the detection rate is 80% and the false-positive rate is 1%, then the LR is 80%/1%, or 80. If the prevalence of the disorder were 1:1000 then

$$\text{OAPR} = 80 \times 1{:}1000 = 80{:}1000 = 1{:}1000/80 = 1{:}12.5$$

For an individual with the screening variable at some specific value, the likelihood ratio is the height of the relative distribution curve for 'affecteds' at the test value for that individual divided by the height of the curve for 'unaffecteds' at the same test value. So, for example, an individual with a test result of 7 (arbitrary units) in Fig. 3.3.2.4b has a likelihood ratio of 12, and so

$$\text{OAPR} = 12 \times 1{:}1000 = 12{:}1000 = 1{:}1000/12 = 1{:}83$$

In this way the likelihood ratio is used to estimate the risk for an individual.

Figure 3.3.2.5, showing the distribution of diastolic blood pressure in men who did and did not subsequently die of a stroke, illustrates how a particular blood pressure measurement of, say, 105 mmHg in a 70-year-old man, can be converted into a risk of developing a stroke. At a diastolic blood pressure of 105 mmHg the likelihood ratio is 3. The annual risk of a fatal stroke in all 70-year-old men regardless of blood pressure is 2:1000 (about 0.2%) so if his diastolic blood pressure is 105 mmHg the risk if 3 × 2:1000 or 6:1000 (about 0.6%).

To establish whether a quantitative screening test is worthwhile, the overlapping distributions of the values of the screening test in people with and without the disorder must be examined. If the two distributions are widely separated, as in the example in Fig. 3.3.2.6 (ultrasound measurement of the diameter of the abdominal aorta as a screening test for aneurysm likely to rupture), the test is good. If they substantially overlap, as in the example in Fig. 3.3.2.7 (serum cholesterol as a screening test for future death from ischaemic heart disease or blood pressure as a screening test for stroke, Fig. 3.3.2.5), it is not.

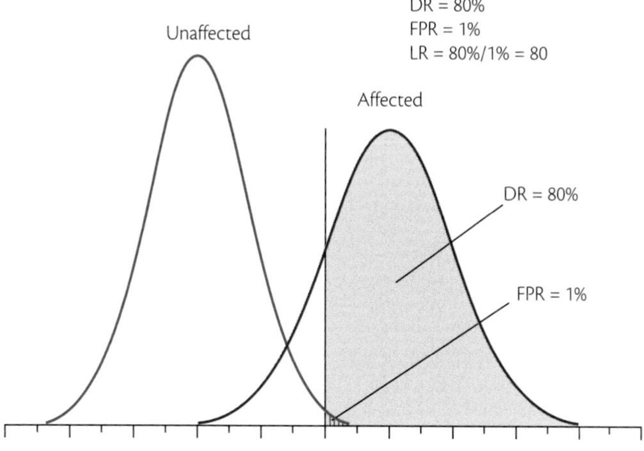

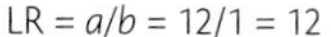

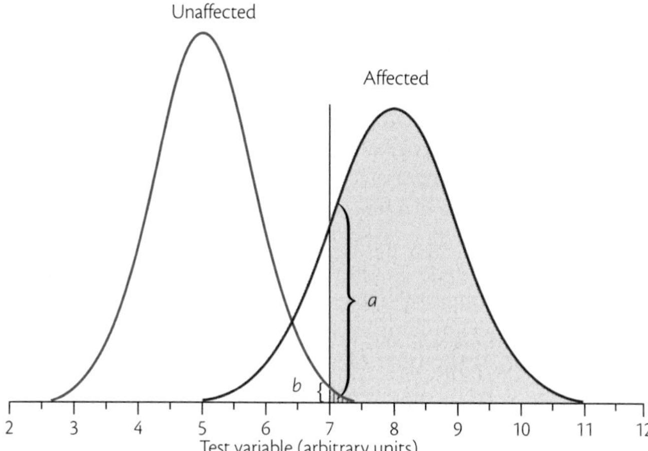

Fig. 3.3.2.4 Likelihood ratio for groups and for individuals.
Reproduced from Wald, N. An Introduction to Epidemiology in Medicine. London: Royal Society of Medicine Press, 2004.

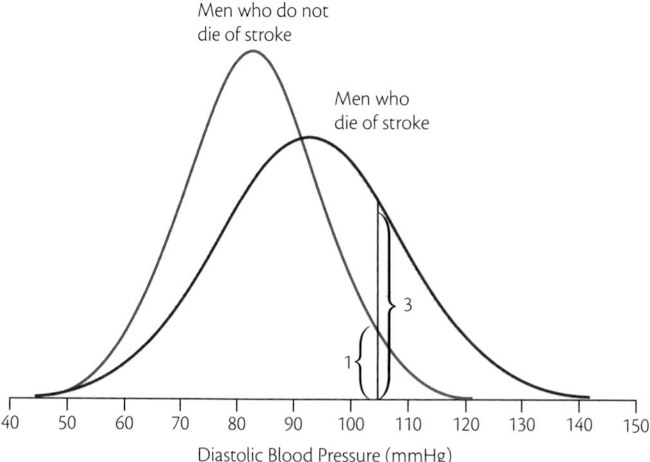

Fig. 3.3.2.5 Likelihood ratio of a fatal stroke in a man with a diastolic blood pressure of 105 mmHg.
Reproduced from Wald, N. An Introduction to Epidemiology in Medicine. London: Royal Society of Medicine Press, 2004.

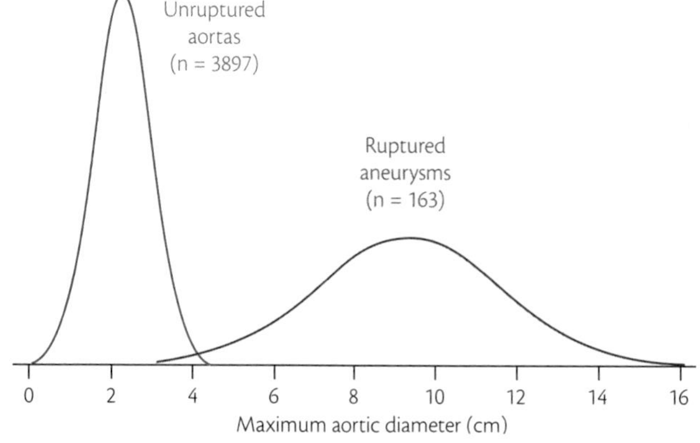

Fig. 3.3.2.6 Aortic diameter and ruptured aortic aneurysm. The distribution of less than 2 cm is not real but simply represents the lower half of the Gaussian distribution of more than 2 cm, which is based on data.
Data from Law MR, Morris J, Wald NJ (1994), Screening for abdominal aortic aneurysms. J Med Screen 1,110–116.

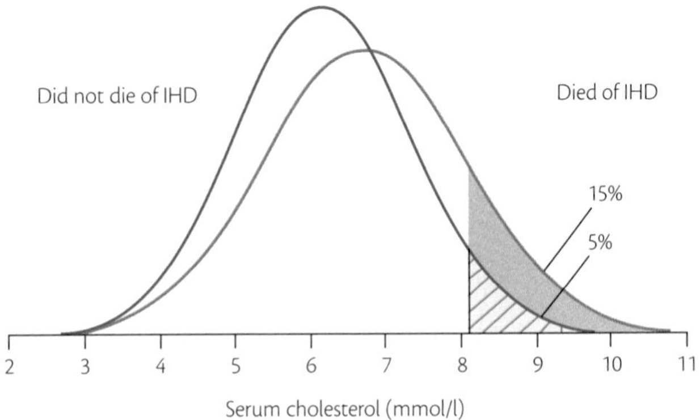

Fig. 3.3.2.7 Relative distributions of serum cholesterol in men who subsequently died of ischaemic heart disease (IHD) and in men who did not.

Reproduced from A strategy to reduce cardiovascular disease by more than 80%, NJ Wald & MR Law, British Medical Journal 2003, 326;7404 with permission from BMJ Publishing Group Ltd.

Detection rate cannot be determined

Determining the detection rate is straightforward when all individuals can be found to be either affected or unaffected. This is not always possible, notably in cancer screening, because if a lesion is found and a treatment carried out, one cannot know if that lesion would have become a clinical case had treatment not been given, or if it is 'overdiagnosis'. The problem arises for any progressive disorder in which the clinical outcome is not determined in a uniform way among all individuals, as would be the case if all screening research were initially observational without intervention dependent on the result of the screening test. Sometimes such an observational approach is possible, e.g. by storing serum samples in a population of adults (without testing them at the time of collection), and later identifying those who did and did not develop a cancer, retrieving the serum samples, and testing them on a case–control basis; this provides an unbiased estimate of the screening performance of the test. Such an approach is not practical with tests based on imaging, such as mammograms, which could not ethically be taken and stored without being examined at the time. In such circumstances, it may never be possible to know the screening performance of the test. The solution is to perform a randomized trial of screening (and treatment) vs no screening. If this shows that mortality from the disease is reduced, the combined effect of screening and treatment is known, though the relative contributions of the two in achieving the health benefit may not be.

Cancer screening must prolong survival (the time between diagnosis and death) to be effective, but because of two biases, prolonged survival alone is insufficient evidence that screening genuinely improves prognosis. The first bias, lead time bias, is the prolongation of survival from bringing forward the date of diagnosis, even though the date of death is unchanged. The second bias, length time bias, arises because cancer screening involves periodic examinations (say 3-yearly). So screening will detect slowly growing tumours more readily than rapidly growing ones because rapidly growing ones are more likely to develop and proceed to clinical presentation within the interval between two consecutive screening examinations, and thereby escape detection at screening. Survival with such rapidly growing screen-detected cancers will inevitably be shorter than average. This is biased sampling. Both biases can be avoided by comparing mortality from the specific cancer (the number of deaths divided by the number of people at risk) between screened and unscreened groups rather than comparing survival once a cancer is diagnosed. The biases are avoided because mortality measures deaths, whereas survival measures time.

Disease-specific mortality could be subject to bias if the screened and unscreened groups were at different risks of developing the disease. For example, women of higher socioeconomic status may be more likely to develop breast cancer and more likely to accept screening. So breast cancer mortality could still be higher in screened women even if screening were effective. The only way to reliably avoid such selection bias is to carry out a randomized controlled trial to be sure that like is compared with like.

Financial considerations

Having determined that the first six requirements for a worthwhile screening test are met (see Box 3.3.2.1), the financial considerations need to be assessed. Screening programmes should seek to minimize the cost for a given outcome, i.e. to maximize the cost-effectiveness. If the most medically effective form of screening is also the most cost-effective, it should be the programme of choice, provided it is affordable. If the best screening policy is not the most cost-effective, a judgement is needed on whether the extra health gain justifies the extra cost.

Facilities

Medical screening effectively 'creates' patients by identifying individuals at sufficient risk of a disorder to be offered further tests or treatment when they had no prior suggestion that they may have the disorder. This necessarily creates anxiety and a demand for medical attention, and an obligation to ensure that facilities exist for the necessary investigation, treatment and support. Screening should not be implemented until such arrangements have been made. Screening therefore needs to be offered in the context of programmes that are capable of meeting all the related needs of the people being screened.

Acceptability

Medical screening, including the treatment or remedy, must be acceptable to the population concerned and to the professional staff involved. The purpose, the benefits, and the limitations of screening need to be understood and regarded as important from the perspective of each individual who is offered screening. The decision not to be screened needs to be respected and programmes should not be driven by targets that set high uptake rates, though of course, if the rates are very low it would call into question the need for the screening programme. A key element in the acceptability of screening is individual choice set against a justifiable trust in the medical system that offers screening.

Requirements for a worthwhile public health screening programme (see Box 3.3.2.2)

Screening is a public health activity that should meet certain requirements that arise from a professional responsibility to achieve a collective health benefit. It is not the provision of a consumer commodity. Its purpose is to improve the health of individuals and thereby the health of the community.

Box 3.3.2.2 Requirements for a screening programme implemented as a public health service

1 Equitable: equal access to screening services
2 Organized: individuals are offered screening in an organized manner according to a specified protocol and with relevant information provided to permit an informed choice
3 Comprehensive: screening is the first step in a programme of service and care that includes counselling screen-positives, diagnosis, support, and treatment
4 Monitored and auditable: key aspects of the programme should be monitored so that remedial steps can be taken if they are below standard

Once the requirements for a worthwhile screening test shown in Box 3.3.2.1 are met, there are four additional requirements for a worthwhile screening programme implemented as a public health service. These are summarized in Box 3.3.2.2.

In public health terms, interventions that reduce exposure to the causes of disease should have priority over screening to detect early disease and offer treatment, but they are not mutually exclusive. A population approach correcting or reversing adverse risk factors is often more effective. For example, the human papillomavirus (HPV) vaccine is expected to steadily replace screening for cervical cancer after the next 40 years.

Screening for specific disorders

Antenatal screening (Table 3.3.2.3)

Much of antenatal care is screening—looking for problems before they arise clinically. Detecting rises in blood pressure to warn of the risk of pre-eclampsia (which may cause perinatal death and serious illness in the mother), and detecting maternal anti-D antibodies to warn of rhesus haemolytic disease of the newborn, are two examples. The purpose of such screening is usually the welfare of the mother and fetus, but in antenatal screening there is the unusual situation in which some fetal disorders are so severe or potentially disabling to justify screening and diagnosis, and the offer of a termination of pregnancy. Antenatal screening for open neural tube defects, Down's syndrome, severe congenital heart malformations, and severe, incurable single-gene disorders are examples.

Screening for four infections is worthwhile (syphilis, HIV, hepatitis B, and bacteruria) because they may not be clinically apparent in the mother but can cause serious preventable illness in the neonate (either immediately or in later life). Prognosis is substantially improved if the infection can be detected in the mother and appropriate treatment given to the mother before birth, the neonate at birth, or both. Routine screening for rubella syndrome in pregnancy is generally not worthwhile because it cannot prevent the disorder in the pregnancy screened; it can only lead to vaccination after birth in women without rubella antibodies. The preferred method of prevention is childhood vaccination.

In recent decades antenatal screening has taken on a scientific methodology and rigour that has permitted the development of screening programmes that are now standard throughout the world. The first such initiative arose with antenatal screening for open neural tube defects, first by measurement of maternal serum AFP and later by ultrasonography, which is used with AFP in many places and has replaced it in some. Screening now detects virtually all cases of anencephaly with scarcely any false-positives, and 87% of cases of open spina bifida with a false-positive rate of less than 1%. The birth prevalence of neural tube defects in Britain has declined by over 90% from 1 in 250 births in the early 1970s to less than 1 in 2500 now, due in part to screening, in part to an increase in folate intake through food and vitamin supplements.

Until the 1980s, antenatal screening for Down's syndrome was based on maternal age. In 1988 the triple test was described, based on combining second trimester serum markers with maternal age. Figure 3.3.2.3 shows the subsequent improvement in screening performance as the number of available markers increased over time. The Integrated test can detect about 85% of affected pregnancies for a false-positive rate of only 0.9%; the low false-positive rate is important because women with positive results usually have an amniocentesis, which may induce the miscarriage of a healthy fetus. Combining markers to obtain a single test result for an individual involves the multiplying of the likelihood ratios for each marker in that individual (as in Fig. 3.3.2.4a), allowing for any correlation between them (considered separately among affected and unaffected individuals). So, for example, in the simple situation of three independent screening markers that correspond to likelihood ratios of 3, 4, and 5, the combined likelihood ratio is 60 ($3 \times 4 \times 5$). To determine the screening performance of tests based on multiple markers, a hypothetical population of screened individuals is generated and the combined likelihood ratio for each individual calculated and converted to risk by multiplying it by prevalence expressed as an odds. The overlapping distributions of risk in affected and unaffected individuals are plotted, determining detection rates for specified false-positive rates in the same way as for a single screening marker. Then risk itself becomes the screening variable—which is convenient, because it is exactly what is needed in reporting results to screened individuals.

Most screening markers associated with Down's syndrome vary with gestational age, so a high level at one gestational age could be low at another. A widely used advance in screening is to express all values as 'multiples of the median' (MoM) for unaffected (or all) screened individuals at a specified gestational age, so that 1.0 MoM represents the median value ('normal'), 2.0 MoM is twice 'normal' and 0.5 MoM is half 'normal'. The MoM has the advantages that as a ratio it is unitless and so avoids the need to specify the original units of measurement (which vary from centre to centre), that it automatically adjusts for gestation, and that it indicates how high or low a particular value is.

Neonatal screening

Neonatal screening for phenylketonuria, one of the first population-wide screening programmes to be introduced, has proved to be effective and worthwhile in spite of the rarity of the disorder (about 1 per 10 000 births). A low-phenylalanine diet prevents severe mental retardation in affected infants. Neonatal screening has prevented cretinism, which is now extremely rare. Additional screening tests could be added to the blood already collected for phenylketonuria and hypothyroidism screening, e.g. MCADD (Table 3.3.2.4), and may be justified for other inborn errors of metabolism, given that much of the cost and effort is already spent.

Table 3.3.2.3 Summary of antenatal screening tests of proven value

Disorder	Approximate natural birth prevalence (per 10 000) in UK	Primary screening test	Secondary screening test(s) (if available)	Detection rate (%)	False-positive rate (%)	Odds of being affected given a positive result		Diagnostic test	Intervention
						1°ry screening test	2°ry screening test		
Autosomal or sex-linked recessive disorders									
Cystic fibrosis	4	Test for CF mutation in both parents ('couple screening')		72	0.09	1:3	–	CVS or amniocentesis	[a]
Sickle cell disease	3	Ethnic origin enquiry (black)	Sickling test; Hb electrophoresis in mother, and in father if positive in mother	99	3	1:100	1:3	CVS or amniocentesis	[a]
β-Thalassaemia	6	Red cell MCV or MCH in mother	Hb A_2 assay in mother, and in father if positive in mother	89	7	1:125	1:3	CVS or amniocentesis	[a]
Tay–Sachs disease	0.04	Ethnic origin enquiry (Ashkenazi Jew)	Hexoseaminidase assays in father, and mother if positive in father	50	1	1:3600	1:3	CVS or amniocentesis	[a]
Haemolytic disease of the newborn (D-antigen of Rh system)	40	Rh grouping and test for antibody in mother	Rh grouping of father; quantitation of maternal antibody	100	16	1:31	1:26	CVS or amniocentesis	Intrauterine transfusion, early delivery with exchange transfusion
Haemophilia	0.5	Recognition of affected male relative (carrier detection)	Test for mutation in mother	55	<0.01	1:35	1:3	CVS or amniocentesis	[a]
Chromosomal disorders									
Down's syndrome	18	Integrated 1st and 2nd trimester		86	1.0	1:5		CVS or amniocentesis	[a]
		1st trimester alone		72	1.0	1:22		CVS or amniocentesis	[a]
		2nd trimester alone		64	1.0	1:32		CVS or amniocentesis	[a]
Other congenital malformations									
Spina bifida (open)	8.5	Maternal serum AFP assay	Ultrasound	87	0.5	1:4		Amniotic fluid acetylcholinesterase + repeat ultrasound	[a]
Anencephaly	10	Ultrasound		100	0	1:0	–	Independent confirmation	[a]
Severe cardiac malformations	20	Ultrasound		46	≤0.6	≥1:6	–	Independent confirmation	[a]

Infections transmitted from mother to fetus									
Congenital rubella syndrome[b]	0.12	Absent antibodies in mother		>90	1.6	<1:1300	–	None	Vaccinate mother after delivery to protect subsequent pregnancies
Congenital syphilis	0.2	VDRL test or flocculation test in mother	Specific treponemal test in mother	>90	0.2	1:100	1:50	None	Penicillin
AIDS	1	ELISA test for IgG antibody in mother (repeated on same sample if positive)	ELISA test on repeat sample	99.9	0.13	1:13	1:<5	None	Antiretroviral drugs to mother and infant
Hepatitis B causing hepatoma and chronic liver disease	1.4	ELISA test for HBsAg in mother (repeated if positive)		≥98	0.14	1:10		None	Recombinant vaccine to neonate, hepatitis B immunoglobin at birth except when mother has antibodies to e antigen
Maternal bacteruria causing pyelonephritis[c]	200	Urine culture		76	4	1:4		None	Antibiotics to mother
Noninfectious maternal disease affecting fetus									
Maternal high blood pressure/pre-eclampsia causing perinatal death	93 (rate of all perinatal deaths)	Maternal blood pressure measurement	Test for proteinuria	38 (of all perinatal deaths)	30	1:77	1:41	None	Blood pressure lowering drugs

[a] Information on disorder and its prognosis, counselling, termination of pregnancy, or preparation for birth of affected child, advice on risk of recurrence.
[b] Worthwhile only with low uptake of childhood rubella vaccination in community.
[c] May cause low birthweight or fetal death.
AFP, α-fetoprotein; CVS, chorionic villus sampling.
Adapted from Wald NJ, Leck I, eds. Antenatal and Neonatal Screening (2nd ed). (2000) Oxford University Press, Oxford.

Table 3.3.2.4 Summary of neonatal screening tests of proven value

Disorder	Approximate natural prevalence (per 10 000 births) in UK	Primary screening test	Secondary screening test(s)	Detection rate (%)	False-positive rate (%)	Odds of being affected given a positive result		Diagnostic test	Intervention
						1°ry screening test	1°ry and 2°ry screening tests		
Congenital hypothyroidism	3	T_4 or TSH assay before hospital discharge	TSH and T_4 at 5–7 days	100	20	1:668	1:19	Clinical examination, T_4, free T_4, TSH, thyroid scan	Thyroxine
Phenylketonuria	1	Serum phenylalanine assay	Repeated serum phenylalanine assay	100	0.2	1:22	1:0.05	High plasma phenylalanine (>16.5 mg/dl) using quantitative technique; exclusion of biopterin defects	Diet low in phenylalanine
Medium chain acyl CoA dehydrogenase deficiency (MCADD)	1	Tandem mass spectrometry (together with PKU)		100	0	1:0		Repeat test	Avoidance of fasting, prompt treatment of minor illnesses
Deafness	14	Transient evoked otoacoustic emissions (TEORE)	Automated auditory brainstem response (AABR)	80	0.6%		1:5	Repeat test	Hearing aid or cochlear implant

Adapted from Wald NJ, Leck I, eds. Antenatal and Neonatal Screening (2nd ed). (2000) Oxford University Press, Oxford.

However, a line needs to be drawn; tandem mass spectrometry can identify over 40 disorders, but only a handful justify screening as defined. Neonatal screening for congenital deafness is worthwhile and has recently been introduced in the United Kingdom using technology that does not rely on voluntary subject response to noise, thus making it possible to test for hearing deficit in infancy.

Screening for congenital dislocation of the hip has been widely practised for many years, without good evidence of efficacy. Galactosaemia (an autosomal recessive inborn error of metabolism) may cause serious illness in the neonate, including septicaemia and encephalopathy, and cognitive impairment in later life, but it has not been shown that neonatal screening prevents these effects. Neonatal screening for cystic fibrosis has been introduced in some places without evidence that screening reduces the incidence or severity of the associated lung disease, the main cause of disability and death from cystic fibrosis.

Screening in childhood

Children are examined routinely to see if they are gaining weight and height as expected and to assess their hearing and vision. There is no evidence that systematic examination of children achieves greater health benefits than encouraging parents to take their child to a doctor if they are concerned, but nonetheless much such activity has taken place. In spite of the lack of formal evidence, it is probably sensible to check the visual acuity of children on starting school, as is current practice in many places. Unfortunately the lack of evidence to support screening in childhood is often camouflaged in the term 'childhood surveillance'. As with all screening, evidence of benefit should be sought before acceptance, even if this requires large-scale studies. One disorder that appears to merit screening, though still a subject for research, is screening for familial hypercholesterolaemia, an inherited disorder with a prevalence of 2 per 1000 that leads to early cardiovascular disease. Its detection is more effective in children over the age of 1 year than at birth or in adulthood.

Adult screening

Perhaps surprisingly, only a few disorders justify medical screening in adults. These are summarized in Table 3.3.2.5.

Cancers

Three cancers meet the screening requirements: breast, cervical, and colorectal. Cervical cancer screening illustrates the principle that effective adult screening programmes require a population age–sex register. Everyone in the appropriate age–sex group for screening can then be identified and sent written invitations at appropriate intervals. Formerly, cervical screening was carried out 'opportunistically' when women happened to consult doctors, and such screening failed because younger women, at lower risk, see doctors more frequently than older women, at higher risk, so cervical smears were carried out on the low-risk group, and at more frequent intervals than necessary for effective screening. It was only with the introduction of a systematic screening programme based on age–sex registers that the majority of older women were screened and cervical cancer mortality fell appreciably in the United Kingdom and other Western countries. Now women are invited 3-yearly between the ages of 25 and 49, and 5-yearly between the ages of 50 and 64. Screening in the United Kingdom is based on cytology, though combining cytology with HPV testing is more effective. The evidence on efficacy comes from nonrandomized studies: screening reduces mortality from cervical cancer by about 80%.

Mammographic breast cancer screening is offered in the United Kingdom at 3-yearly intervals to women aged 50 to 70 (though the age range may soon extend down to age 47 and up to 73). Randomized trials have shown that it reduces breast cancer mortality, by about a quarter in a population offered screening or a third in women who accept screening.

A colorectal cancer screening programme based on 2-yearly faecal occult blood testing in men and women aged 60 to 70 has been recently introduced in the United Kingdom. It reduces colorectal cancer mortality by about 15% in a population offered screening.

In systematic population-based cancer screening programmes, only people within a relatively narrow age range are invited for tests (effectively, age is used as the initial screening enquiry). Cancer screening tends to be most effective around the age of 60 in terms of cost per year of life saved; the lower incidence of cancer in younger people, and the shorter life expectancy in older people, mean that fewer years of life will be gained for the same number of people screened. The justification for a narrow age range is economic. Older women are not turned away, however, and the age range over which women are invited for mammographic screening has widened over time (it was originally 50–64). Usually it is not appropriate to stop inviting people for screening examinations above a certain age; if they are fit enough and willing to attend for screening examinations, they are suitable candidates for screening. Cancer screening is generally conducted at 2- to 3-yearly intervals; in principle more frequent screening would detect more cancers but the yield per 1000 screening examinations would be lower.

Screening for cancer and other diseases is sometimes widely practised simply because it seems intuitively useful. Chest radiography to screen for lung cancer, and manual breast self-examination by women to screen for breast cancer, are two examples of 'tests' that have been shown in randomized trials not to significantly reduce mortality from the cancer in question.

Screening for prostate cancer, mainly through measurement of serum prostate specific antigen (PSA) was introduced into medical practice with no evidence of reduction in mortality. PSA can distinguish between individuals who will and will not die of prostate cancer. However, discrimination weakens as the interval between the PSA test and clinical presentation or death from the cancer lengthens. By the time the PSA test is highly discriminatory, the disease may be too far advanced for treatment to be effective. The usual cut-off levels proposed for PSA screening (*c.*4 ng/ml) lead to a high proportion of older men being positive. A prostate biopsy in these individuals is often positive, because 25% of prostates in men aged 70 have histological evidence of cancer even though only a small minority of these men will suffer from or die of the disease. Such 'overdiagnosis' (the diagnosis of cancers that would otherwise never have come to clinical attention) is a potentially serious problem in cancer screening. These cancers are best never diagnosed; once diagnosed, anxiety and unnecessary hazardous investigation and treatment will ensue.

In 2009, two randomized trials of PSA screening for prostate cancer were reported, one showing a significant ($P = 0.01$) 20% reduction in prostate cancer mortality in men invited for screening (27% in those who were screened) and the other one showing a nonsignificant increase, but consistent with a 15% reduction. Both trials showed a high rate of overdiagnosis; in the larger of the two trials, for every one

Table 3.3.2.5 Summary of adult screening for selected disorders

Disorder	Prevalence	Screening procedure	Age range	Subsequent investigation	Detection rate	Positive rate	Odds of disorder in screen positives	Uptake of screening	Treatment	Reduction in disease
Breast cancer	4% of all deaths (women)	Mammography 2–3-yearly	50+	Further imaging; fine needle biopsy	Not applicable	8% first screen, 4% subsequent; biopsy rate 0.8%	1:6 (2:1 among women biopsied)	70–80%	Surgery (± chemotherapy, radiotherapy)	24% reduction in mortality at age 50–74; 16% at age 40–49 (from meta-analyses of randomized trials)
Colorectal cancer	3% of all deaths (men and women)	Faecal occult blood testing 2-yearly	60+	Colonoscopy ± barium enema	Not applicable	2–3%	1:10	50–60%	Surgery	15–18% reduction in mortality (from two randomized trials)
Cervical cancer	0.5% of all deaths (women)	Cervical smear ± HPV testing 3–5 yearly	25+	Repeat smear in 6 months (mild dyskaryosis); colposcopy (moderate/severe dyskaryosis)	Not applicable	5–10% (higher in younger than older women), lower with HPV test and smear	–	80%	Local ablation or excision (rarely hysterectomy)	90% reduction in mortality (from case-control studies)
Diabetic retinopathy	Proliferative retinopathy 50% IDDM 50% NIDDM Macular oedema 15% IDDM 10% NIDDM	Retinal photography with mydriatic yearly	All	Assessment by ophthalmologist	78%	0		50% if done in hospital clinics	Photocoagulation	Reduction in blindness >90% (proliferative retinopathy) 65% (macular oedema)
Abdominal aortic aneurysm rupture	Men aged 65+ 2% of all deaths 7% have aortic diameter ≥ 3.0 cm	Ultrasound scan	65 (men)	CT or MRI	86%	0.6%		75%	Open surgery	
Chlamydia trachomatis genital infection (subsequently causing PID)	Chlamydia: 5% among women under 25 PID 2%	Nucleic acid amplification test on urine sample	<25 (sexually active)	–	90–95%	<1%		64%	Doxycycline or azithromycin	56% reduction in PID

HPV, human papillomavirus; IDDM, type 1 diabetes; NIDDM, type 2 diabetes; PID, pelvic inflammatory disease.
Ashton *et al* 2002.

prostate cancer death prevented, 1410 men were screened, of whom 16% (230) had a biopsy, identifying 49 prostate cancers of which 48 were treated unnecessarily. Taking the two trials together, screening for prostate cancer by PSA testing probably does reduce prostate cancer mortality, but the reduction would generally be judged insufficient to warrant the level of overdiagnosis leading many men to receiving unnecessary hazardous treatment.

Three screening programmes that are currently under investigation are randomized trials of screening for lung cancer using spiral CT, ovarian cancer screening using a serum marker (CA125) and ultrasound examination of the ovaries, and screening for future stomach cancer by identifying people with *Helicobacter pylori* infection of the stomach.

Nonmalignant diseases

Screening for abdominal aortic aneurysms that, in the absence of surgery, are likely to rupture, by the ultrasound measurement of the aortic diameter, is worthwhile. The test is very discriminatory (see Fig. 3.3.2.6). Ruptured abdominal aortic aneurysms account for 2% of all deaths in men over 65, but are rare when the maximal aortic diameter is less than 5 cm. In the United Kingdom a screening programme based on aortic diameter using ultrasound is planned for men over 65 (rupture is rare in younger men). Over all ages ruptured abdominal aortic aneurysm is about twice as common in men as in women. Mortality rates for women for women are similar to those in men about 10 years younger.

Screening people with diabetes for retinopathy using retinal photography is very effective; it has been shown in randomized trials to reduce blindness by 90% with proliferative retinopathy and 65% with macular oedema. A national screening programme operates in the United Kingdom, based on inviting people from diabetic registers held in general practice.

Chlamydia infection in young women causes pelvic inflammatory disease (which may be complicated by chronic pelvic pain, ectopic pregnancy and tubal infertility and, when giving birth, causes neonatal eye and lung damage). Screening for chlamydia infection based on urine samples is followed by short term antibiotic treatment and is effective. Screening women under 25 has been recommended but no systematic screening programme has been introduced in the United Kingdom.

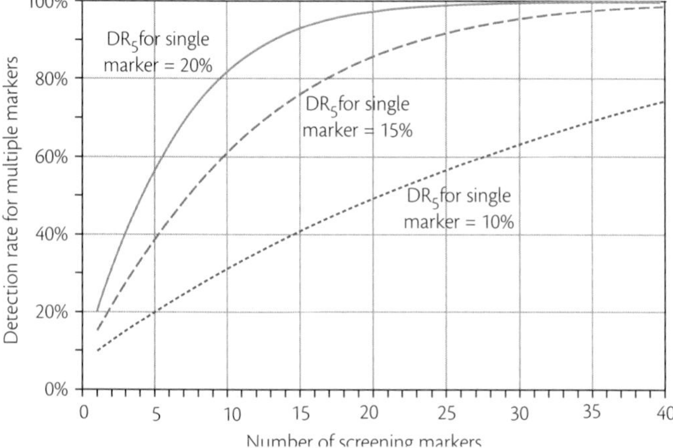

Fig. 3.3.2.8 Overall screening performance from combining individual screening markers: detection rate for a 5% false-positive rate (DR_5) according to the number of screening markers combined that individually have a DR_5 of 10% or 15% or 20%
Reproduced from Wald N, Morris J and Rish S, The efficacy of combining several risk factors as a screening test, J Med Screen 2005;12:197–201. London: Royal Society of Medicine Press, 2005.

Much screening activity falls under the category of 'risk factor screening' and such screening tends to be ineffective—e.g. cholesterol testing in screening for future ischaemic heart disease events (Fig. 3.3.2.7), blood pressure measurement in screening for future stroke, and bone density measurement as a screening test for future hip fractures. The problem arises because, for the reasons given above, risk factors that may be important causes of disease are usually poor screening tests. Most adults have high serum cholesterol and high blood pressure relative to levels in young adults (say at age 20), and all postmenopausal women have low bone density relative to premenopausal women, so nearly all older adults are 'exposed'.

Figure 3.3.2.8 shows the effect of combining different markers on the detection rate and false-positive rate where several markers that each have a detection rate for a 5% false-positive rate (DR_5) of 10%, 15%, or 20% and the standard deviation is the same in affected and unaffected individuals. Only when tests individually have a DR_5 of about 20% or greater will multiple marker screening become a realistic proposition. For example, combining five relatively weak independent markers, each with a DR_5 of 15%, yields only a 40% overall detection rate for a 5% false-positive rate, and combining ten yields a 60% detection rate for the same 5% false-positive rate. At present, screening for future coronary disease and most other diseases using causal risk factors is not effective because even in combination they are not sufficiently discriminatory.

Hypothyroidism in adults is widely regarded as a preventable cause of lethargy and depression. This has prompted attempts at screening for this disorder by measuring levels of thyroxine (T_4) or thyroid-stimulating hormone (TSH) and classifying individuals as positive if TSH is above or T_4 below the relevant reference range (which is usually the 95th centile range in the population). This is an example of the 'tautological screening' that arises from defining a disorder in terms of the test used to screen for it (see above). The solution to this circularity is to identify individuals from a population with TSH or T_4 outside specified TSH or T_4 limits and then offer each, in random order, thyroxine or placebo to determine whether thyroxine treatment relieves the symptoms more often than can be explained by chance. Each person is therefore their own control, and the response to treatment defines the clinical disorder. This approach can be used to see whether such screening is worthwhile, and if so to use it to identify which individuals will benefit from treatment.

Clarity of terminology and purpose

A number of terms used in screening are probably best avoided because they lack clarity. The term 'carrier screening' implies that carriers of autosomal recessive disorders (e.g. cystic fibrosis) themselves have a disease; they do not. The goal of such screening is to identify couples who are both carriers. 'Couple screening' involves collecting samples from both parents and reporting a positive result only when both are carriers. The term 'genetic screening' lacks clarity and tends to imply screening for inherited disorders even though some genetic disorders that are screened for (e.g. Down's syndrome) are usually not inherited. The term creates a false impression that something special is being offered that other forms of screening lack. For many people genes and consequently all things genetic are seen as highly determinant, even inevitable, influences, which is usually not the case. Genetic markers of a disease are in most instances too insensitive and too nonspecific for screening purposes. The term 'case finding' often implies the identification of cases of the disorder being screened for, while in fact it identifies individuals with a positive screening test for that disorder. For example, a case of 'hypertension' relates to the test result (high blood pressure), not the diseases it causes. The term 'opportunistic screening' is a euphemism for nonsystematic and nonorganized screening.

The purpose of medical screening is clear—to avoid disability and premature death at an acceptable level of safety. Determining efficacy is essential. Many screening tests are effective and should be part of public health practice. But particular care is needed in evaluating tests that arise out of technological development in the absence of a clear case of medical need. Whole-body scanning using MRI and fetal ultrasound examination are examples. Such screening, without defining the specific disorders being screened for, detects 'incidentalomas' (so-called 'abnormal' findings with little or no knowledge of their medical significance). There is no place for such screening in responsible medical practice. For example, total body MRI scanning is now advertised to the public as a screening test with little attention paid to whether it prevents serious disability or death, or meets the criteria set out in Box 3.3.2.1. A routine fetal anomalies scan at about 18 weeks of pregnancy has some proven specific applications (e.g. the detection of anencephaly, severe congenital heart disease, and placenta praevia extending to cover the internal cervical os), but the term 'fetal anomaly screening' lacks specificity. The challenge in performing a scan is to seek these specific anomalies but not to report other 'incidentalomas' which will undoubtedly lead to parental anxiety and further investigation but for which early detection has not been shown to be worthwhile. Under the ambiguous heading of genetic screening, so-called 'gene chips' have been developed, that can detect in one test many hundreds of genetic mutations with little or no evidence that knowledge of these will lead to useful medical intervention that will improve the health and quality of lives of the people being so tested. Medical screening needs to be driven by the medical need, not the technological capacity.

Doctors have a professional responsibility to discourage technologically driven screening and to ensure that all screening meets the requirements set out in Box 3.3.2.1. Screening promoted only in terms of the application of a particular technology should not be part of medical practice.

Further reading

Ashton HA, *et al.* (2002). The Multicentre Aneurysm Screening Study (MASS) into the effect of abdominal aortic aneurysm screening on mortality in men: a randomised controlled trial. *Lancet*, **360**, 1531–9.

Breslow N, *et al.* (1977). Latent carcinoma of prostate at autopsy in seven areas. *Int J Cancer*, **20**, 680–88.

Holland WW, Stewart S (2005). *Screening in disease prevention*. Nuffield Trust, Radcliffe Publishing, Oxford.

Journal of Medical Screening: screening briefs. (1994a, 1994b, 1995, 1996, 1997). *J Med Screen* **1**, 73; 1, 255; 2, 126; 3, 110; 4, 54.

Law MR, Morris J, Wald NJ (1994). Screening for abdominal aortic aneurysms. *J Med Screen*, **1**, 110–16.

McKeown T (1968). Validation of screening procedures. In: *Screening in medical care. Reviewing the evidence*. Nuffield Provincial Hospital Trust, Oxford University Press, Oxford.

Thorner RM, Remein QR (1961). *Principles and procedures in the evaluation of screening for disease*. Public Health Monograph No 67. Public Health Service Publication No 846. US Department of Health Education and Welfare, Washington, DC.

Wald NJ (1994). Guidance on terminology. *J Med Screen*, **1**, 76.

Wald NJ (2004). *The epidemiological approach: an introduction to epidemiology in medicine*, 4th edition. Wolfson Institute of Preventive Medicine/Royal Society of Medicine Press, London.

Wald NJ, Cuckle H. (1989). Reporting the assessment of screening and diagnostic tests. *Br J Obstet Gynecol*, **96**, 389–96.

Wald NJ, Law MR (2003). A strategy to reduce cardiovascular disease by more than 80%. *BMJ*, **326**, 1419–23.

Wald NJ, Leck I (eds) (2000). *Antenatal and neonatal screening*, 2nd edition. Oxford University Press, Oxford.

Wald NJ, Hackshaw AK, Frost CD (1999). When can a risk factor be used as a worthwhile screening test? *BMJ*, **319**, 1562–5.

Wald NJ, Morris JK, Rish S (2005). The efficacy of combining several risk factors as a screening test. *J Med Screen*, **12**, 197–201.

Wald NJ, *et al.* (2004). SURUSS in perspective. *Br J Obstet Gynaecol*, **111**, 521–31.

Wilson JMS, Jungner G (1968). *Principles and practice of screening for disease*. WHO Public Health Paper No. 34, World Health Organization, Geneva.

3.3.3 The importance of mass communication in promoting positive health

Thomas Lom

Essentials

Medical science is enabling an explosion of discovery in diagnostic tools and in the development of new treatments and products. But how do we take advantage if we are not aware? That is where the power of mass communication comes into play.

Stakeholders in communication about health

In a world with increasingly motivated and empowered patients, these go well beyond just the for-profit companies such as the pharmaceutical industry and include payers, governments, health care professionals, and institutions. The motivation for the dissemination of health information is a convergence of public health interest and public health policy with private sector commercial interests.

Communication technology

This is crucial to the dynamics of communication. The internet allows access to an enormous wealth of information that is not limited to the developed world alone, and this access fuels the interest in more and more education of both public and physicians, leading to a virtuous circle of communication with benefits including: (1) proper diagnosis of diseases previously undiagnosed or misdiagnosed and therefore untreated; (2) awareness of new and improved therapies that can save lives or improve the quality of life.

Introduction

Every day we seem to learn of another medical discovery, another medical breakthrough, another medical miracle. Medical science allows us to understand the human body as never before. We understand what makes our body tick and what makes it stop ticking. The science of medicine is discovering new therapies that can cure many diseases and slow the progression of others. Yet, amazing as the progress is, how do we get the word out? The challenge of making people aware of this innovation and turning that awareness into positive health behaviour is enormous.

Communication

To meet this challenge, many stakeholders develop all manners of communication in order to diffuse all of this innovation. It may take the form of journalism (broadcast, print, and internet) or advertising (paid and public service). In the United States of America, advertising spending on prescription medicines in 2006 reached $5.3 billion compared to $1.3 billion in 1998 and a mere $12 million in 1989. Consumer magazines and popular internet search engines devote any number of editorial pages to health care. The disease states covered by this explosion ranged from traditionally discussed ones such as arthritis pain, hypertension, and diabetes to newly discussed conditions such as osteoporosis, depression, and Alzheimer's disease.

Benefits of health information

The explosion of information has two benefits critical to our health. The first is that both the public and the physician are now aware of new and improved therapies that can save lives or improve the quality of life. People with HIV can have longer, better lives; people with poorly functioning joints can get new knees and hips; people with neurological disorders can cope more easily. The second benefit is that much of the information explosion has led to proper diagnosis of diseases previously undiagnosed or misdiagnosed and therefore untreated. We are now more aware of what distinguishes the symptoms of bipolar disorder from those of depression; we now know the benefits and risks of hormone replacement therapy; we now know that chemotherapy can cause anaemia that can be treated. As a result, we feel more empowered and better prepared to discuss our health with a physician.

Disease prevention

Not only does this process make people smarter about disease treatment, but communication also encourages disease prevention or, at the very least, early diagnosis. Journalistic coverage has especially increased awareness that certain kinds of cancers are far less deadly if caught early. Frequent and early screenings for breast, prostate, and colon cancer have led to a significantly improved prognosis for millions of men and women. The link between cholesterol and heart disease is well communicated and is leading to improved management of hypercholesterolaemia through lifestyle changes and drug therapy. The link between calcium and osteoporosis is also well communicated and has lead to much more proactive behaviour in the form of dietary changes and calcium supplementation. Importantly, these behaviours are happening at an earlier age.

Motives for advertising health

The motivation for the dissemination of all this information is driven by a convergence of public health interest and public health policy with private sector commercial interests. In fact, in a highly developed country such as the United States, it is the private sector that drives the process. The biggest private sector influence is the pharmaceutical industry. The industry is consistently investing in new drug development. In 2006 alone, the top 10 companies invested $17 billion in research and development. From 2002 to 2006, the United States Food and Drug Administration approved 172 new drugs. Is it any wonder, then, that this industry also invests heavily in educating people about these medicines?

Advertising to physicians

The first investment priority is in physicians. For years, drug company sales representatives have been calling on physicians to inform them of the clinical story behind a wide array of drugs. In fact, the number of such representatives continues to grow. Another trend is the increasing number of collaborative arrangements called 'co-promotes' in which the discovering company essentially rents sales force capacity from another company (often another company with which it competes in other areas). All of this has accelerated the process of diffusion of innovation. So, too, has the investment in industry-sponsored education for physicians. Be it in large medical conventions or smaller local meetings, physicians can review pharmaceutical science in more depth. Even if the science is commercially driven, good science is good science from any source.

As we moved into the new century, this science has been even more broadly and more quickly available via the internet. Medical journals that publish data from clinical studies can have that data posted in an instant for all to see. Company-sponsored websites also proliferate as a tool for physicians to gain access to clinical data. This is frequently accompanied by editorial comment from scientific opinion leaders. It can also be supplemented by commentary from practitioners as to their experience in clinical practice. Another trend that will accelerate is that information about experience with experimental drug trials will be shared over the internet. This is already happening in such areas as oncology and antiviral treatment, where specialists cannot wait to learn about promising new options.

Advertising to patients

The second investment priority is in patients. In the United States there is a broad trend in society toward self-reliance. We see it all around us. We do more of our own financial planning. We buy stocks online, not through a broker. Home improvement is driven by do-it-yourselfers. Health is no exception to this trend. Americans have become much more proactive about their health and their health care and are not shy about offering their opinions about diagnoses and helpful suggestions about treatment to their physicians.

Advertising by pharmaceutical companies

The pharmaceutical industry is only too happy to fuel this trend. Typically, when a new drug is introduced, a substantial patient-directed advertising programme almost always supports it within 6 to 12 months. There is no better or faster way for new therapies to work with their way into the public consciousness. It is especially valuable in encouraging patients to self-identify as having certain symptoms and to initiate a discussion with a physician. It also helps remove the stigma associated with certain diseases. Among the most notable of these is depression. Advertising has started many people on the road to a more normal life.

Advertising of medical devices

Other sectors of the health care industry have participated in these trends. Diagnostic devices, particularly for diabetes, are actively advertised to the growing number of diabetics. Orthopaedic devices, particularly for knees and hips, are being advertised as a major tool to help educate our ageing population about new ways to improve their mobility and quality of life. Similarly, cardiovascular device makers are educating people with angina or cardiac rhythm abnormalities on new and proven options for care.

Advertising by health care providers

Health care providers are another sector promoting themselves more and more to the general public. Leading hospitals, medical centres, and health systems with particularly strong reputations and capabilities in certain therapeutic areas are advertising aggressively, often beyond even their immediate geographical area. Providers of rehabilitation services are doing the same. So are other providers of health care services such as nursing homes, assisted-living communities, and providers of nursing care.

Advertising by the food industry

Yet another industry is joining the party of health education: the food industry. More and more is being learned about the positive health value of mainstream food, from calcium to oat bran, and new foods are being developed with clinically proven benefits derived from newly discovered natural ingredients (like plant sterols for cholesterol reduction). People are eager to learn about nature's solutions for more healthy living, and the food industry is providing that information. People are being educated about dietary supplements in much the same way.

Health education

In the 21st century, the consumer education process will only grow. Mass media like television, magazines, and newspapers will continue to be heavily used, and targeted media will become even more important. The 1990s saw major advances in sophistication of techniques that can get patients with specific diseases to identify themselves. Once that identification happens, targeted and specific educational material can be sent to that patient. The internet is also a tool of enormous value, as every health care product can have its own interactive website. Questions can be answered with an immediacy that used to require visiting a doctor. Professional experts can now be accessed easily via the internet.

Manufacturers are not alone in fuelling the public demand for health information. Books, newspapers, and magazines have also been major forces. Visit your local book store and notice the substantial health section filled with 'guides' of all sorts and notice that almost every newspaper has a weekly health section. Health sells. All of these media have websites to complement the printed word. Medical institutions also participate in this trend, whether nationally recognized names like the Mayo Clinic or local hospitals.

The public sector has also played an increasing role in the diffusion process by way of not-for-profit patient advocacy organizations. Although these have existed for many years, their number has grown. They have always been aggressive in 'spreading the word' on new treatments. However, today the internet gives enormous numbers of people immediate access to this information, not just in the United States but around the world. And with internet connectivity, these websites will increasingly steer people to a myriad of related sites on related topics. All of this fuels our tendency toward self-reliance.

The United States public sector also has a valuable tool in the Ad Council, which is a clearing house for public service messages of all kinds. They range from social issues to environmental issues to health issues. Perhaps the best-known health message is the anti-drug message sponsored by Partnership for a Drug Free America. In the fiscal year 2007, according to its website, Ad Council messages received \$2.0 billion worth of free media space and time. When the Ad Council puts its weight behind an issue, the message gets heard, and positive behaviour change usually follows. This is also the case when the federal government uses its 'public relations megaphone' to educate, e.g. on the perils of cigarette smoking.

In addition to physicians and patients, a third stakeholder has assumed increased prominence in the communication process—payers. Insurance companies, managed care organizations, and governments have an important stake in keeping people healthy in the most cost-effective way possible. Increasingly, they are using communications to encourage appropriate behaviour such as screening, early diagnosis, and proactive wellness activity. Payers recognize the financial cost of bad health and have a special incentive to promoting good health.

Health care advertising in the United States and the rest of the world

Health care communication abounds in the United States. To what extent can the United States communication paradigm be a constructive model elsewhere? That requires a review of participants and roles and depends on the state of economic development involved. In other developed countries, where the populace has the interest and means, the private sector is likely to take a dominant role. Just as in the United States, the pharmaceutical industry is well motivated commercially to invest in educating about new drugs. Companies will want physicians to be educated and patients to be aware in the same way. Similar dynamics will be at play ensuring that the diffusion of scientific innovation occurs.

Where Europe and Japan differ from the United States is in the regulatory environment. Regulations there do not allow for the kind of direct-to-consumer advertising permitted in recent years in the United States. However, since the internet is giving consumers access to the information anyway, governments are being forced to reconsider their regulations. Both directly and indirectly, the internet will accelerate globalization of the education process.

What about payers? Many developed countries have some form of nationalized health system. These systems place constraints on how much is spent on new and sometimes costly health care innovation. New diagnostic tools, new drugs, new treatments, and new surgical procedures all have a cost. How national health systems deal with that cost will have a substantial impact on how proactive the private sector will be. Private sector communication expenditure will be in proportion to the commercial incentive.

In less developed countries, the public sector will have to take more of the lead in health care communication. Where populations are poor and literacy rates are low, the dynamics are quite different. National governments must make communication a major part of public policy. However, health care needs and issues are more elementary. The media is more 'grass roots'. The workplace, schools, and clinics are more important media. Access to technology is as yet relatively limited, so the utility of the internet is less. Some physicians will benefit (more and more as the century progresses, I hope), as will the general public (libraries will provide access for the public). Unfortunately, public sector activity will not add much to the critical mass of educational activity, as it does, for example, in the United States.

Conclusions

Regardless of the differences, one central reality is common around the globe: public policy is focusing on health, individuals are focusing on health, and commercial enterprises are focusing on health. At the same time, there continues to be ever more progress in medical science. Communication will remain essential in ensuring that we fully take full advantage of that progress.

Further reading

Lom TP (2002). The role of communication and advertising. In: Koop CE, Pearson CE, Schwarz MR (eds) *Critical issues in global health*, 2nd edition. Jossey-Bass, San Francisco.

Wright KB, Sparks L, O'Hair HD (2008). *Health communication in the 21st Century*. Blackwell, Boston.

http://www.nche.org/index.htm [The website for the National Center for Health Education].

3.4

Influence of wealth

Contents

3.4.1 The cost of health care in Western countries *112*
Joseph White

3.4.2 A sinister pathogen corrupts two disciplines: the demographic entrapment of Middle Africa *116*
Maurice King

3.4.1 The cost of health care in Western countries

Joseph White

Essentials

All advanced industrial countries socialize most health care costs because their citizens view relatively equal access to such care as a mark of a decent society. This makes the costs of health care a policy issue, because governments need to relate costs to revenues, and there are limits to the willingness of citizens, especially wealthier citizens, to pay for others.

Why are health care costs rising?

Discussions about health policy often ascribe higher costs to technology, ageing, or 'moral hazard' (meaning the fact that people do not face price constraints when they consume care). None of these explanations gives useful guidance to policy makers. If technology were the dominant issue, then all systems would have the same costs; instead, policies affect both the adoption and price of technology. If ageing were crucial, costs across countries would be correlated with population age profiles; in fact there is little correlation. 'Moral hazard' is an inevitable consequence of the socialization of costs and does not prevent wide variation in costs across countries.

How can health care costs be controlled?

Cost control depends on policies that affect the price of care, volume of care, and system overhead costs. The most important direct measures are price regulation and measures to bundle services (meaning paying for a collection of services instead of for each individual service). The most important indirect approach is to limit system capacity. Measures to improve population health can be viewed as efforts indirectly to reduce volume, as can measures to make treatment more appropriate, such as 'managed care' (meaning mechanisms to regulate clinical decisions through some mix of guidelines, incentives, or governance arrangements). In practice, there is little evidence of success through such indirect methods. So far, much blunter measures such as price regulation and bundling have been more successful.

Reasons for interest

The countries conventionally called 'Western' (a term that refers to level of economic development, not geography) have the physical and financial resources needed to provide a high standard of health care to all citizens. Yet doing so at a socially acceptable cost is difficult. Policies to limit cost are controversial because they may also affect the quality of care, access to it, and the work and incomes of medical providers.

Why is cost a policy issue?

All societies view decent health care as a necessity, not a luxury. Yet need for care is distributed very unevenly, and the cost of serious illness may be unaffordable to many people. In order to protect themselves against the unpredictable risk of high costs, people either as citizens, employees, or consumers participate in systems of shared savings to pay for health care. Yet they have unequal ability to contribute to these systems, which means they must not only pool contributions but redistribute from those with higher income to subsidize those with lower incomes.

Except in the United States of America, rich democracies have created redistributive shared savings that pay for care for virtually all citizens. In most countries, most of the time, total spending on

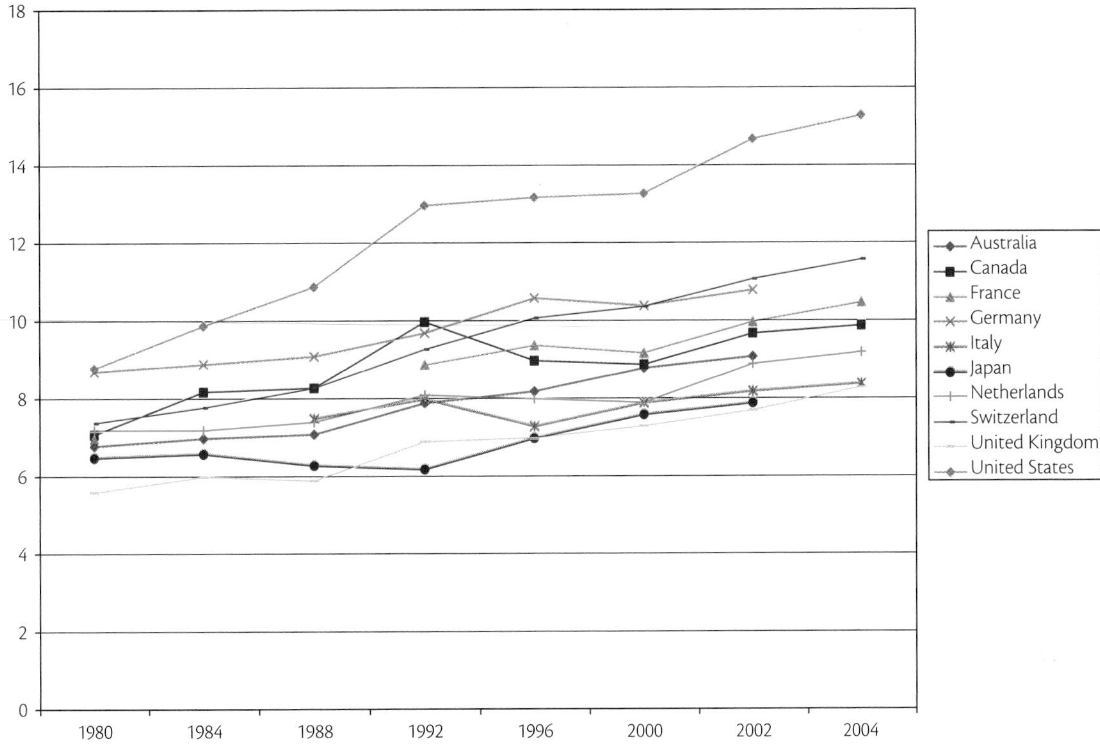

Fig. 3.4.1.1 Health care spending trends as a share of gross domestic product, 1980 to 2004.

health care rises more quickly than other economic production: Fig. 3.4.1.1 gives examples of the trend in 10 countries. So health care becomes a larger share of the national economy, and people have to contribute larger shares of their incomes. Richer people in particular may resent paying more and more for other peoples' care. Whether the fund is managed by a government whose leaders do not want to raise taxes, or by an employer whose shareholders do not want to reduce profits, the managers want to restrain the costs.

Medical providers will argue that higher costs are no problem, because medicine is continually offering new services that people value. But the usual test of what people value in a market is willingness to pay. Once medical care is funded by shared savings, the consumers (patients) do not have to pay out of pocket for new services, so willingness to consume only shows that the value to patients is greater than zero, not that it is close to the amount paid. Modern payers are aware that much medical care has not been scientifically demonstrated to be effective, never mind cost-effective. So payers do not assume that higher costs are justified, and seek ways to control them.

If there are multiple payers, any one payer will worry about the costs it incurs, not the total social costs. We therefore should distinguish cost control from cost shifting. If tight budgets for the United Kingdom's National Health Service cause many patients to 'go private', that is cost control from the government's perspective. From the vantage point of the patients, providers, and society, these costs have been shifted, but not reduced.

The basic issues are why societal costs rise so quickly and what can be done about it.

Three unhelpful explanations

The spending trends in Fig. 3.4.1.1 are often ascribed to three broad causes: population ageing, medical innovation ('technology'), or the fact that people do not face price constraints when they consume care ('moral hazard'). None of these explanations is helpful.

The varied trends among countries cannot be explained by patterns of ageing. Countries with more older citizens, like Japan, can have much lower costs than countries with fewer old people, such as the United States or Canada. Ageing has been only a modest cause of the increases experienced within countries.

To emphasize medical innovation can only beg the question of why countries vary at all. Innovation is, conceptually, international. Implementation can vary greatly—but if implementation varies, then whatever affects implementation, not the innovation itself, matters most.

Pooling resources to pay for health care makes it more affordable, and making it more affordable increases spending. The problem, however, is not how to do without pooled resources; it is how to control costs within a system that provides access to care, which must mean within a system that greatly reduces price constraints on consumption. There is no evident relationship between the level of price constraints in a system and its costs: the United States, with the least extensive insurance system, has the highest costs.

Controlling the components of cost

It is more useful to break costs down into components and then look at influences on those components. Figure 3.4.1.2 provides the simplest description. Costs of care depend on the costs of each service and how many services of each type are consumed. Some services (such as cardiac surgery) are bigger (more expensive) than others (such as an office visit for a bad cough). So costs depend on prices and volume, and volume on the quantity of each service and the mixture of services. Total costs rise because prices or volume increase.

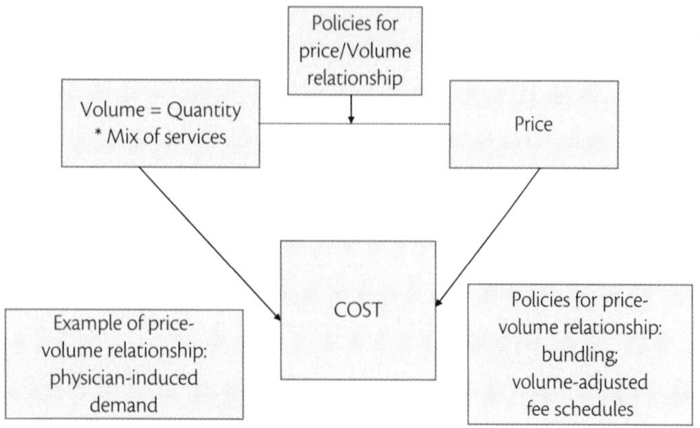

Fig. 3.4.1.2 Components of cost: simplest model.

The simplest way to control costs is to pay less per service, and any cost control methods must start with prices. Failure to limit prices makes all other methods irrelevant. The most expensive system, that of the United States, is characterized above all by higher prices per service, rather than greater volume of care. Most systems limit prices through some sort of collective contracting, in which payers combine to maximize their bargaining power with providers, or the government imposes prices that are distinctly lower than providers would like to charge. Some theories claim prices could be controlled by competing insurers that engage in selective contracting with some but not all providers. Proposals for reform of the health system in both Germany and the Netherlands have recently promoted that view. Yet savings from competition have only been observed for a short period of time, in the United States during the mid-1990s, and the country then returned to the normal pattern, in which selective contracting fails to sufficiently limit prices.

Controlling prices is necessary but may not be sufficient if volume rises quickly enough. The simplest way to slow volume increases is to create some price constraint on the consumers through cost sharing: limiting insurance either by having a deductible before insurance takes effect, requiring a flat fee for service (such as a $20 co-payment for an office visit), or that patients pay a portion of costs (co-insurance, such as 20% of the bill). Cost sharing, however, poses problems of finding the right balance. If the charge is too large, it will make insurance ineffective. If the charge is too small, the effects will be modest, and might not justify the administrative costs. Cost sharing also presumes consumption is in some sense voluntary. It therefore makes more sense as a way to encourage people to buy less expensive substitute drugs, for example, than for inpatient care (which is normally involuntary and always very expensive).

Most countries rely less on cost sharing than on methods to influence the relationship between prices and volume. In Germany, physicians' fees are reduced directly as their volume of billings increases. A more common approach is bundling: paying for a collection of services instead of for each individual service. The bigger the bundle, the harder it is to generate volume. For example, paying hospitals per hospitalization, according to the diagnosis (as in American Medicare), makes it much harder for hospital managers to generate extra fees than if the hospital were paid per service or per day of hospitalization. Paying a hospital with a budget bundles its entire set of services together, and so eliminates all volume effects. Similarly, paying physicians by capitation, a fixed amount per patient for which the doctor takes responsibility, is also a way to bundle services and protect the payer against volume increases. The main difficulty with bundling is that it gives providers an incentive to take the bundled payment and reduce services, thereby reducing quality.

Less direct cost-control policies

Both the theory and practice of cost control include many less direct methods. Figure 3.4.1.3 provides a way of reviewing those approaches.

The most important indirect approach, at 12:00 on the figure, consists of measures to limit system capacity. Constraining the number of physicians or hospital beds or MRI machines can limit volume. But limited capacity can also reduce prices, because if a piece of equipment has to be used more often, the cost per use declines. The absence of effective capacity limits is another major reason costs are higher in the United States than in other countries. If applied too stringently, however, capacity limits can contribute to waiting lists that create great public dissatisfaction.

At about 10:00 on Fig. 3.4.1.3 are measures to make treatments more appropriate. The literature that shows variation from community to community in service levels, without evident differences in health results, suggests to many observers that local medical communities cannot be trusted to decide what care is necessary. Thus, versions of 'managed care' seek to change medical decisions, or restructure medical delivery. One method is to require that the insurer pre-approve expensive treatments such as hospitalizations. Another is to have gatekeepers, usually primary care physicians, who have to approve referrals to specialists or hospitals. Sometimes, the gatekeepers will be placed at financial risk, so that if they refer 'too much', their own incomes are reduced. Another approach is to create an integrated network of providers and build a conservative practice culture ostensibly based on evidence about treatment effectiveness. This was the dominant dream of health policy analysts in the United States during the 1990s, who saw group-staff model Health Maintenance Organizations as the ideal.

What all of these measures have in common is that they seek to limit volume in the name of improving care. This presumes that patients are getting more inappropriate care than the amount of

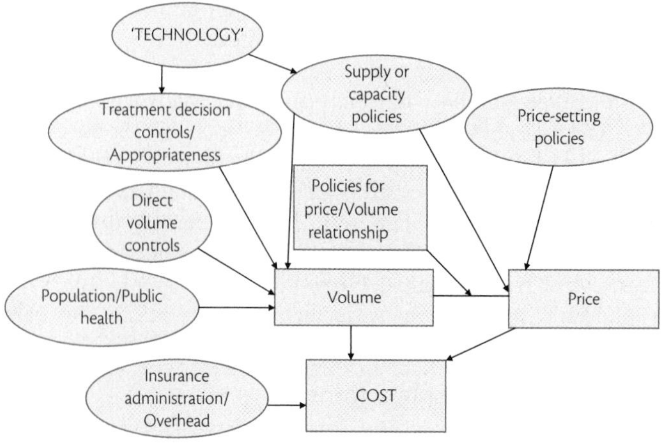

Fig. 3.4.1.3 Components of cost: multiple theories.

appropriate care that for some reason is not being provided. It also presumes that whoever manages the system can tell the difference; that the savings are worth the cost of management; and that the patients will trust the system rather than their physicians who might be recommending a treatment. Because there are few cases where all of these assumptions are true, measures to make care more appropriate have not generated substantial savings, and have had limited public legitimacy. The American experience with 'managed care' in the 1990s generated a backlash due to concern about legitimacy. Yet such savings as occurred were largely due to price restraint, and vanished when providers regained the upper hand in price bargaining. Since then, advocates for saving money by making care more appropriate have shifted to more modest, though still difficult, objectives such as better management of chronic disease. In that case, the argument is that changing the mix of care (e.g. better blood pressure control, thereby preventing strokes) can save money while not directly denying services to patients. Unfortunately, this requires difficult restructuring of both delivery and payment systems, so savings remain more theoretical than common.

The effects of new technology depend entirely on decisions about capacity and treatments. The technology has to be purchased and providers have to choose to use it. Conversely, policies that slow the purchase of equipment or training of providers, or that create impediments to a given service (such as gate-keeping) can limit volume of services. That is why the chart in Fig. 3.4.1.3 shows technology, at 11:00, only indirectly influencing costs. The effect of any technology also depends greatly on the price allowed for the service.

Another large set of cost-control arguments, though fewer effective policies, focuses on the level of disease that can result in medical expenses. Medical costs depend on the incidence of ill-health in the population. So costs could be reduced if pregnant women had better nutrition (leading to healthier babies); if the environment were cleaner; if there were less tobacco use; and even if a given society had less income and status inequality (inequality appears to be negatively correlated with population health statistics, though there is disagreement about the mechanism). Improving population health gets more attention in academic discussion than in cost-control politics in part because some of the desired changes (such as greater equality) are politically very difficult; in part because most countries have done most of the easier measures (such as systematic vaccinations and clean water); and in part because many of the good ideas (such as a cleaner environment) are things that neither medical providers nor those who pay for medical care can do much about.

A final major factor, at 7:00 on Fig. 3.4.1.3, is the overhead cost of the systems of medical care delivery and finance. Costs are higher if they must include profits for investors. They also increase as the insurance system includes more options, or if providers must face many different payment terms, or if insurers are allowed to underwrite (calculate premiums based on the likelihood any insured individual or group will incur costs), or if individuals get to choose among insurers or whether to insure at all (so insurers have to spend money on marketing). At the extreme, a system with one mandatory insurer with one set of payment rules, as for medical and hospital services in a Canadian province, will be much less expensive than a system with competing private insurers, as in the United States.

Consequences

Costs are much higher in the United States than in other countries because its payers pay more per service, there are few limits on capacity, administrative overhead is much higher and, perhaps, its inequalities lead to a modest amount of greater need (worse population health). The latter factor may not be significant because the victims of inequality could well be uninsured. Costs have been much lower in Japan mainly because of extremely stringent price regulation and restrictions on some forms of hospital capacity. Costs were much lower in the United Kingdom than in other major European countries for many years largely because of capacity controls and bundling. By the turn of the century, however, the perceived effects on volume had become so unpopular that the government felt compelled to increase spending, promising to spend up to the European norm as a share of the national economy.

The politics of health care costs are shaped by a simple equivalence: any cost is also an income. Cost controls require taking money from somebody, and whether they are physicians or nurses or insurance administrators or product manufacturers, they will resist. Drug companies will advertise to create demand for their products (manipulating volume); all providers will raise prices whenever they can. Providers always seek to enlist patients as allies, by claiming that any restrictions will worsen care. For instance, they will argue that high drug prices are needed to pay for the research that creates life-saving drugs, or that if physicians are not paid more they will simply cease practising. This is a basic reason why, in all countries, policy makers hope to save money by making care more appropriate, since, if care is more appropriate, nobody can legitimately complain about the savings. Unfortunately for payers, so far blunter methods of price regulation, bundling, and capacity control have been more successful.

Health care costs will probably continue to rise in Western countries because longer, less painful lives seem desirable to most people. In short, stringent control is not likely to seem optimal, even if there is no agreement on the proper level of cost. Some less useful innovation will be attractive just because it offers hope, and some innovation will actually reduce pain and extend life. Hence there are inherent pressures for greater volume. The trend will vary significantly across countries because they will have different policies about capacity, prices, cost sharing, and other options. The key question is whether countries will be able to maintain their systems of social sharing as costs rise. That will depend on whether political coalitions allow higher-income individuals to opt out of subsidizing their compatriates. The result, as in the United States, might not be lower overall costs. But it could make health care, also as in the United States, much less equal and, for many citizens, much less adequate. Whether health care costs are affordable is a political question, not an economic one.

Further reading

Barroa PP (1998). The black box of health care expenditure growth determinants. *Health Econ*, **7**, 533–44.

Dudley RA, *et al.* (1998). The impact of financial incentives on quality of health care. *Milbank Q*, **76**, 649–86.

Reinhardt U (1996). Our obsessive campaign to 'gut' the hospital. *Health Aff*, **15**, 145–54.

Reinhardt U, Hussey PS, Anderson GF (2004). U.S. health care spending in an international context. *Health Aff*, **23**, 10–25.

Rice T, Morrison KR (1994). Patient cost-sharing for medical services: a review of the literature and implications for health care reform. *Med Care*, **51**, 235–87.

White J (1999). Targets and systems of health care cost control. *J Health Polit Policy Law*, **24**, 653–96.

White J (2007). Markets and medical care: The United States, 1993–2005. *Milbank Q*, **85**, 395–448.

3.4.2 A sinister pathogen corrupts two disciplines: the demographic entrapment of Middle Africa

Maurice King

Essentials

Are starvation and violence 'diseases'? If they are, a textbook of medicine must be prepared to recognize some novel pathogens. The most sinister cause of these two diseases is 'demographic entrapment', which occurs when a subsistence community exceeds (1) the carrying capacity of its local ecosystem (too many people for the land to support), (2) its ability to migrate to new land, and (3) the ability of its economy to produce goods and services, which it can exchange for food and other essentials. The outcome of entrapment is severe poverty, starvation and violence, and the problem is at its worst in Middle Africa, where populations multiplied seven times during the 20th century, and are expected to triple again by 2050. Remedy will not be found unless fertility is reduced, if necessary to one child only per family, but discussion of this is prevented by the Hardinian taboo, named after Garrett Hardin.

Two kinds of corruption

Financial corruption is hugely important for the health of Africa, from the bribes that many health workers have come to expect to the misappropriation of funds by ministers. However, in the longer term, intellectual corruption is likely to be even more dangerous. This has nothing to do with money. It is the failure of both demography and development economics to tackle the distasteful problem of 'demographic entrapment', not because it is technically difficult, but because it presents such unwelcome ethical and political problems that they taboo it absolutely (Fig. 3.4.2.1).

Although the two disciplines of demography and development economics are indeed 'good in parts', it is their failure to confront the major problem facing both of them in Africa that merits the accusation 'corrupt'. The public, and indeed most of the practitioners in the two disciplines, are deluded into thinking that demographic entrapment does not exist, and therefore that these disciplines are sound, whereas in fact they are so gravely flawed as to be dangerous for the job in hand, in this case, improving the welfare of Middle Africa. The United Nations agencies, and the nongovernmental organizations, are also deluded into thinking that these disciplines are sound when they are not. They too have to be declared intellectually corrupt, but since they depend on what they imagine is the integrity of the two disciplines, their corruption is secondary, because they can rightly blame academia for the corruption.

If this corruption is the result of a powerful taboo, is the individual blameworthy? Or is it more charitable to assume that the corruption is corporate, so that there are no corrupt individuals, but only corrupt disciplines and institutions?

Two kinds of demographic entrapment

The ordinary person usually knows instinctively what is meant by 'demographic entrapment'. Technically, it has two equally valid and highly confusing meanings, which are conveniently distinguished by * and #. This paper is concerned with the * version, which is the only one that is taboo, and which is this:

> A subsistence community is *demographically trapped if it exceeds: (1) the carrying capacity of its local ecosystem (too many people for the land to support), AND (2) its ability to migrate to new land, AND (3) the ability of its economy to produce goods and services that it can exchange for food and other essentials. The outcome of *entrapment is the severest poverty, starvation, and violence.

*Entrapment has a definitive stage when there is starvation and/or violence already, and a warning stage when these can be confidently expected, because the population is increasing fast.

The two 'AND's are important, because a community is only *trapped if all three conditions are exceeded. If any one is not exceeded, it can be assumed to solve the problem.

The other version—#entrapment—is merely that the poor, being poor, have large families, and that this traps them in continuing high fertility, and thus in poverty. It is therefore only a particular aspect of the 'poverty trap'.

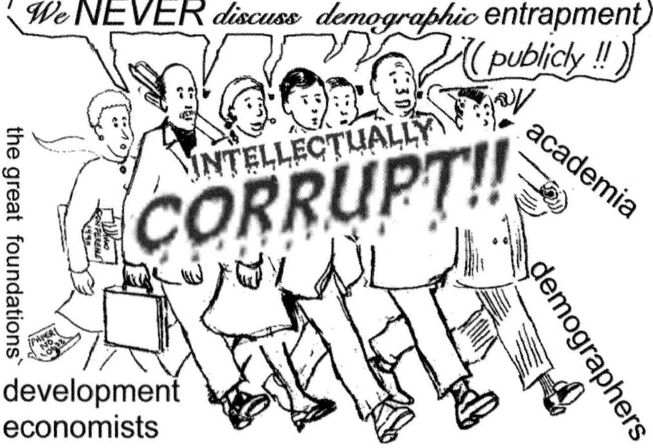
THE POPULATION POLICY LOCKSTEP
We NEVER discuss demographic entrapment
(publicly !!)
INTELLECTUALLY
CORRUPT!!
the great foundations
academia
demographers
development economists

Fig. 3.4.2.1 'Lockstep' is a way of marching very close together, with one's leg under the leg of the person in front. If anyone changes his step, the whole squad falls over. Nobody here ever discusses entrapment. Demography and development economics are therefore intellectually corrupt, as are the disciplines and agencies dependent upon them. If anyone here were to discuss demographic entrapment, everyone else would have to discuss it too, so that the squad would fall over and the lockstep would break up.

How widespread is *demographic entrapment?

*Entrapment would be less serious if it were only a local problem. Unfortunately, it appears to be widespread. I once asked Jack Caldwell, the most eminent demographer of Africa, how much of [Middle] Africa he thought was demographically trapped? His answer was that most of it is, except perhaps Ghana. Unfortunately, there are studies that already go a long way towards documenting entrapment for Niger, Ethiopia, Rwanda, North Kivu, Malawi, and other countries.

Jack Caldwell said I could quote him as having said that, for a long list of countries in Middle Africa, the chances of their economic and demographic transitions interacting are 'pretty bleak'. What he meant was that their fertility will not fall fast enough to allow them to develop, and they will not develop fast enough to allow their fertility to fall—before their rapidly increasing populations have exceeded the carrying capacities of their ecosystems (Fig. 3.4.2.2).

Sciences are not supposed to have taboos

Captain James Cook introduced the term 'taboo' in 1785, when he returned from the South Sea islands, as being something which is forbidden from discussion by general consent, without reasons being given. Although taboos appear to be largely nonrational, it must be assumed that there are partial reasons for them, even if they are not given. It is useful to call these reasons 'the Demons of the taboo', a Demon being anything that holds the taboo in place (see Box 3.4.2.1). For example, Demon 6 represents the many problems of one-child families, which may be necessary for disentrapment. Are they better or worse than starvation and violence, which is the likely alternative? The Chinese thought they were better.

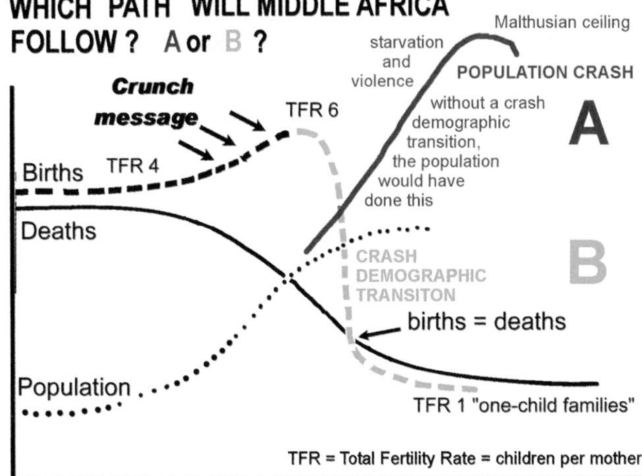

Fig. 3.4.2.2 Which path will Middle Africa follow? As things are at present, the population of many communities will continue to rise, so that they follow path A, with starvation and violence, until they reach their malthusian ceiling, followed by a population crash. The hope must be that some at least will follow path B and listen to the 'crunch message' delivered many times in many ways, and thus decide to reduce their fertility rapidly, if necessary to one child only, so that they can undergo a crash demographic transition.

Box 3.4.2.1 Some Demons

A Demon is anything that keeps a taboo in place. They are numbered arbitrarily; the list below is just a selection. Further discussion can be found on the internet, search for disentrapment.

1 Garrett Hardin's Demon—the inability of us humans to control our population numbers

6 The many problems of one-child families

7 Current notions of human rights, especially as they relate to human reproduction

9 The attitudes of many religious fundamentalists, Protestant, Catholic, and Muslim, to abortion

10 The Holy See's attitudes to most methods of family planning

11 The cultural attitudes of the South that favour high fertility

14 The metaphysical position of modern man: 'What are we here for anyway?'

16 Political correctness

17 Peer pressure

19 The accidie Demon: sloth, torpor, despair, cynicism, 'Why bother? What can we do about it anyway?'

40 The 'carrying capacity for man' Demon

'Disentrapment'—is demographic entrapment treatable?

If demographic entrapment is the result of an unfavorable state of all three factors in the earlier definition, a community could theoretically be 'disentrapped' by increasing carrying capacity (it is usually falling), increasing migration (difficult), increasing economic development (seldom possible fast enough), and reducing population growth.

The most hopeful option for trapped communities in Middle Africa is that, in addition to, what ever else might be done for them, there should be vigorous attempts to reduce fertility. Twenty times in the Democratic Republic of Congo recently, I have addressed communities with the following message in French. It forcefully breaks the taboo on telling African mothers that they have got to have fewer babies—or starve. It is called a 'crunch message', because messages of this kind need a generic title.

A CRUNCH MESSAGE

> Should I or should I not, say to you my friends in Africa, that if you don't reduce your fertility, if necessary to one child only, you can expect the direst poverty, starvation and violence, if indeed you are not experiencing it already. I argue that I have to, and that not to do so is gravest dereliction of duty in public health. If you want to lynch me, you are welcome, I trust that I will proceed to my martyrdom with a good courage.

I was not martyred. On one occasion I was even given a bunch of flowers. About one-third of the girls I spoke to in a slum in Kinshasa indicated that they were only going to have one child. Whether they actually will do so is another matter, but this was their stated intention. I was amazed! It does indicate that the dialogue on one-child families can at least be opened in Africa (Fig. 3.4.2.3). Where it will get to, is for

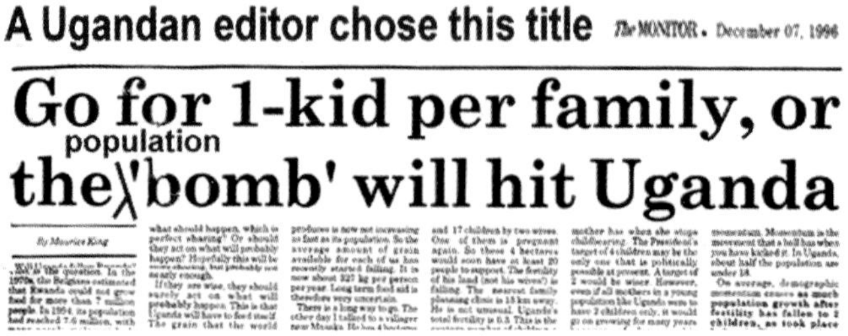

A Ugandan editor chose this title *The MONITOR*, December 07, 1996

Go for 1-kid per family, or the population 'bomb' will hit Uganda

Fig. 3.4.2.3 The dialogue on one-child families can open in Africa. Since Uganda's total fertility is 7.1, there is a long way to go.

the future to decide. What is certain is what will happen if the dialogue is not opened—ever-increasing starvation and violence. One-child families have problems, but they are soluble. If an only child dies, his parents should be using reversible methods of contraception so that they can have another one.

I sense that trapped communities know very well what is going to happen to them, and are happy to have somebody to discuss it with. Twice, after I had lectured in the Congo, members of the audience (a priest and a doctor) said: 'For Heaven's sake, do come and see us! Land is so scarce that our communities are killing one another.'

Lifting the Hardinian taboo and breaking up the population policy lockstep

Figure 3.4.2.1 suggests that there is a tight conformity in population policies, such that nobody dare change, but that if anybody ever did, everybody else will have to change also. The hope is that the editor of a high-profile journal can be found, who has sufficient courage to lift the Hardinian taboo, to denounce the two disciplines as being corrupt, and thus to break up the lockstep. Until this happens, the prospects for Middle Africa are bleak indeed—ever-increasing starvation and violence.

Further reading

Andre C, Platteau J-P (1998). Land relations under unbearable stress: Rwanda caught in a Malthusian trap. *J Econ Behav Organ*, **34**, 1–47.

Cleland J, Sinding S (2005). What would Malthus say about AIDS in Africa? *Lancet*, **366**, 1899–1901.

Cleland J, *et al.* (2006). Family planning: the unfinished agenda. *Lancet*, **368**, 1810–27.

Cook, J (1773). *Account of the voyages undertaken for making discoveries in the Southern Hemisphere in 1768–71.*

du Maurier G (1895). The curate's egg. *Punch*, 9 November.

Fisher NR (2006). *Food security in Malawi: A crisis waiting to happen.* Action against Hunger, Malawi.

King M (1997). To the point of farce: A Martian view of the Hardinian taboo—the silence that surrounds population control. *BMJ*, **315**, 1441–3.

May J, Guengant J-P (2007). Afrique: le grand rattrapage démographigue. *Le Monde*, 15 December.

Myers N, Kent J (2001). Food and hunger in Sub-Saharan Africa. *Environmentalist*, **21**, 41–69.

Wils W, Carael M, Tondeur G (1986). *Le Kivu montagneux: surpopulation—sous-nutrition—érosion du sol (étude prospective par simulations mathématiques)*. Royal Academy for Overseas Sciences, Brussels.

Yayé AD, Boureima AG (2007). *Histoire des crises alimentaires au Sahel: Cas du Niger*. University Abdou Moumouni de Niamey, Niger.

3.5

Human disasters

Amartya Sen

Essentials

Human disasters, as massive misfortunes long recorded over history, have great importance for medicine, rightly prompting the call for prevention, relief, and practical intervention by medical personnel. But why do human disasters happen? A sharp distinction is sometimes drawn between natural disasters, e.g. earthquakes, and social disasters, e.g. wars, but detailed knowledge often shows that this contrast is not always clear.

The example of famines

Take the example of famines. These are popularly understood in terms of food output decline caused by droughts, floods, or storms, but such explanations are contradicted by many famines that have occurred without any decline in food production. Such misunderstanding has been responsible for the loss of millions of lives, mainly by undermining the role of social intervention. Starvation is a characteristic of some people not having enough food to eat, not of there being not enough food in the economy. The critical connection of the command over food is with the purchasing power to buy it (in a market economy), linked to jobs and incomes and relative prices of what people have to sell (their labour and the commodities they can make) to buy staple food. A famine is in this sense an economic phenomenon—not just as an issue of agricultural production—and can be prevented by a willingness to start relief programmes, mainly in the form of emergency projects, which provide jobs and incomes to the afflicted population.

Disasters and policy interventions

Even when nature plays a part, society can make a huge difference. Interventions that can be effective include (1) environmental policies that can make floods and droughts less likely; (2) mitigation of effects of disasters on the economy—e.g. an earthquake may not lead to a famine, but can leave an economy unsettled, making lives precarious for those who are not killed in the physical event itself; these effects can be prevented or at least reduced in their impact through careful social intervention (as described above for famines); (3) health care actions—the morbidity and mortality associated with human disaster can be large and extend far beyond those who are directly hit. Taking note of the likely dangers from local contagions, the scale of both illness and death can be radically altered through preventive measures, such as immunization, ensuring safe water, influencing the routes of contact and spread, and by self education and prompt medical response.

Introduction

The term 'human disasters', has some plasticity of meaning. 'A sudden or great misfortune' is the way the *New Shorter Oxford English Dictionary* begins its definition of a disaster. This is a useful starting point for understanding the idea of 'human disasters'.

Human disaster is a common term in public discussion. The addition of the adjective 'human' to the word 'disaster' performs a double duty in narrowing the range of attention to a subset of disasters in general—a subset, though, that is still very large. The narrowing is done, first, by pointing specifically to the misfortunes of human beings (rather than those of animals or vegetables, except to the extent that these nonhuman plights may influence human mishaps), and second, by focusing particularly on the predicaments of groups of people with shared and interlinked predicaments, rather than on the personal tragedy or sadness of a particular individual. The term could be used differently, of course. There is nothing inherently odd in talking, for example, about the human disaster that befell King Lear—and Lear's gloomy problems can, of course, be of interest for a textbook of medicine. It would belong, however, to some other section of this book, linked with the psychological adversity of dejection and of betrayal of trust, with the need for clinical attention.

In contrast, the huge public interest in what are called 'human disasters' is linked with problems that are more mundane and also larger in the scale of tragedy. Furthermore—and this is where its social urgency lies—such disasters are seen to be more straightforwardly amenable to organizational remedy initiated by the state or society. Human disasters, in this sense, have come to be seen as sudden developments of huge misfortunes—in the form of death or debilitation or displacement or impoverishment—of substantial groups of people affected by such events as earthquakes, floods, epidemics, wars, or famines, which call for imperative social action for prevention or relief. That is the sense in which the idea of human disasters will be addressed in this chapter.

The natural–social distinction and its fragility

In the vast literature on the subject of human disasters, a sharp distinction is sometimes drawn between natural disasters, such as earthquakes, floods, or droughts, and social disasters, such as wars or genocide. There is some rudimentary logic in that distinction: political agitation can have more success in averting genocide or wars than in, say, preventing earthquakes. But probing investigation of the causation of disasters may often blur that contrast substantially. For example, though floods are natural phenomena in an obvious sense, their incidence is also influenced by social and economic operations, such as the making of canals or drainage systems, not to mention the climatic effects of global warming that may be significantly influenced by preventable human activities. Even though in understanding the immediate parameters of such events as floods or droughts or storms we can begin well enough by 'rounding up the usual suspects' in the natural world (such as rainfall, temperature, gales), it is important that the analysis does not insist on ending there.

Some other examples of human disaster are quintessentially mixed bags, such as epidemics, which depend on the working of nature (e.g. on the properties of viruses, bacteria, and other contagions), and yet are massively influenced by human behaviour (e.g. contacts and exposure) and social arrangements (e.g. immunization and medical care). In such cases, it would be very difficult even to begin the analysis of a disaster of this mixed type—epidemics and others—only as phenomena of nature, since the social–natural entanglement is rampant in every aspect of this type of human disaster.

As it happens, in some cases the inescapably mixed nature of the bag has tended to escape attention because of the popularity of allegedly 'obvious' causal explanations that fail to look far enough and are easily satisfied with finding a natural correlate. A good example of this kind of neglect can be seen in the popular understanding of the occurrence of famines in terms of food output decline, with much-repeated explanations that do not go beyond the proximate features of droughts, floods, or storms. This causal confusion, which is contradicted by the great many cases of famines that have occurred without any decline in food production, has been responsible for the loss of millions of lives, mainly through undermining the role of social intervention. The subject demands some discussion here, and to that I turn next. Indeed, by concentrating on famines, which have been much more extensively studied than other kinds of disasters, it is possible to illustrate the general points about the relationship between social and natural aspects of human disasters.

Famines: causes and prevention

Famines are gigantic events of carnage in which millions of people die from starvation and from diseases linked with debilitation, disruption, and movements of the destitute in search of something to eat, and the spread of communicable ailments associated with these phenomena. Even though a great many people die from a famine, the misfortune that a population experiences in a famine can go well beyond the mortality of those who succumb to hunger, since famines can leave an inheritance of huge disruption for many years to come.

The crude logic that if people are dying of starvation, there must be a shortage of food has had much influence in the world. That theory has had a particularly damaging effect in persuading governments to do nothing even when many people lose their livelihood (for one reason or another), which makes them unable to buy food. This hypothesis was relevant to the British Raj's strange inactivity as the Bengal famine of 1943 slowly gathered momentum—it would eventually kill more than 2 million people, indeed close to 3 million. The official statistics of food output in Bengal indicated that there had been no significant change in the availability of food there, and sticking to their theory, the government did little to relieve the relentless emergence of a large famine. Instead, it tried to deny the existence of the unfolding famine, sustained by the censorship of local press, and the complicity of silence of the British-owned newspapers. That gigantic cover-up ended when the British-owned leading English-language paper of India, *The Statesman*, broke rank, with the decision of the agonized editor (Ian Stephens) that he could no longer be a party to the concealment of a huge human disaster. Once the news went into the public domain, it received wide attention in the British press and in Parliament in London, making the government admit the existence of a famine and start relief work.

But, ever loyal to the theory that famines are caused only by a decline in food availability, the government would later revise the statistics downwards (to bring the revised 'facts' come in line with the government's deluded theory), even though the previous food statistics had been broadly right. What went wrong, of course, was not to see that starvation is a characteristic of some people not having enough food to eat—it is not a characteristic of there being not enough food in the economy. The critical connection of the command over food—what is sometimes called the 'entitlement' to food—is with the purchasing power to buy food (in a market economy), linked to jobs and incomes and relative prices of what people have to sell (their labour and the commodities they can make, such as services and crafts) in order to buy staple food. A famine is, in this sense, an economic phenomenon, not just as an issue of agricultural production.

However, going further, famines are not only an economic phenomenon, since they have both political aspects and medical ones as well. Famines are easy to prevent, since only a relatively tiny proportion of the population is affected, and it is easy to regenerate their purchasing power through emergency employment providing income in a region in which many people have lost their purchasing power, because of job loss or any other reason. Indeed, the fact that India, despite considerable regular undernutrition at a chronic level, has not had a famine since the end of the Raj in 1947, is only partly linked with the progress of food production and agriculture in the years since independence; it is also critically connected with the willingness to start relief programmes, mainly in the form of emergency projects, giving jobs and incomes to the afflicted population. But the urgency of that course of governmental intervention is largely governed by the imperatives of democratic governance. If a famine is allowed to develop, then no ruling party or coalition has a chance of being returned to office immediately thereafter (or even, before that, to survive blistering criticism in the media and in the parliaments). Indeed, in recent years, as in the past, famines have continued to occur only in countries without a regularly functioning democracy (e.g. military dictatorships, one-party states, or countries that do have elections but do not have other necessary features of a democracy such as a free media and room for public discussion and confrontation). Famines are, thus, political as well as economic phenomena.

Further, famines belong partly also to the domain of medicine and public health care. This is because most people who die from famines die from diseases of the region—occasional or endemic. While starvation is the prime mover of famine mortality, actual deaths very often come from people getting ill and succumbing to their illness. Debilitation due to severe undernourishment plays a part in this in making people vulnerable to fall ill and to die of disease. But no less importantly, hunger precipitates illness and death because of the propensity of hungry people to eat whatever scraps they can pick up from any source; because of vast population movements induced by search for jobs and food that spread contagions with great speed; and because of the breakdown of essential services including health care and medical attention. Famines typically kill not just directly as a result of starvation, but through intensifying and aggravating the forces of illness-based mortality common to the region.

Table 3.5.1 gives a breakdown of the causes of death in the excess mortality in the Bengal famine of 1943 from my 1981 book *Poverty and Famines*, looking over the period from 1943 to 1946 with elevated mortality, taking the average of the period between 1941 and 1942 as the standard for comparison.

More than four-fifths of the death toll resulting from the Bengal famine, in this estimate, was directly connected with diseases common to the region, with pure starvation death accounting for no more than only one-fifth of the total. A similar picture emerges from many other famines.

This aspect of famines has been taken as the centre of attention in Alex de Waal's important study of famines in Darfur in Sudan. This is certainly a rich and policy-relevant perspective on famines, particularly because even with the failure of food entitlements, the magnitude of deaths can be very substantially reduced through health interventions. If the emergence and survival of a famine is a largely economic and political issue, the mortality it generates is also very significantly an issue of health care and medical attention (including timely prevention, through immunization). The allegedly 'natural' phenomenon of famines may be intensely 'social' at many different levels.

Table 3.5.1 Proportionate breakdown of excess mortality in the Bengal famine: 1943–46 over 1941–42

Ailment types	Percentage contribution (%)
Malaria	36.7
Cholera	7.1
Smallpox	5.0
Dysentery, diarrhoea, and enteric group of fevers	5.0
Other fevers (often undiagnosed)	27.4
Respiratory diseases	0.4
Percentage share of ailment-related deaths	81.6

From Sen A (1981). *Poverty and famines: An essay on entitlement and deprivation*, Table D.3, p. 204. Oxford University Press, Oxford.

Before I move on from the subject of famines to other types of human disaster, let me briefly note the variety of circumstances in which famines have occurred and have killed with abandon across the world. It would be good to give firm mortality estimates with each famine, but this is a difficult exercise in many cases. Even though death tolls have been quite thoroughly studied for some famines, using reasonably good statistics, there is always an element of uncertainty in any such estimate, no matter how carefully it may have been prepared. Part of the difficulty lies in some conceptual issues. The death toll of a famine has to be calculated by contrasting the actual number of deaths in that period with the number of deaths that would have taken place in the absence of that famine (i.e. famine mortality is the difference between actual mortality in the famine period and the estimated number of people who would have died had the famine not occurred at all). Thus the uncertainties involved relate only partly to problems in getting good statistics of actual deaths—though that itself is not an easy task, especially at a time when many of the normal functioning of social institutions, including registration of deaths, are disrupted (sometimes because of death or migration of the staff involved in the social institution). But the uncertainty arises also from the ways and means of estimating—as a 'counterfactual'—what would have happened had the famine not occurred at all.

One can nevertheless get some general impression of the size and reach of a famine by looking at the estimates of death tolls that we have, along with reports of other events and predicaments connected with the respective famines. Table 3.5.2 gives data relating to a number of 'recent' famines that have occurred over the last couple of hundred years, beginning with the Irish famines of the period between 1845 and 1851 (drawing on a large number of sources).

The association of famines with political authoritarianism and civil disruption is well illustrated by the incidence of such events in countries with military governments (Ethiopia, Sahel countries), or one-party rule (Soviet Union, China, Cambodia, North Korea), or alien governance (India and Ireland before their independence), or civil disruption (Nigeria and to some extent Bangladesh, even though the death toll was kept in check).

Disasters and policy intervention

Human disasters can be of many types, varying from floods, droughts, wind storms, extreme temperatures, and earthquakes, where natural factors have some clear role, to wars and industrial accidents (like the Union Carbide disaster in Bhopal in 1984), where the story is almost entirely social in the broad sense. But the important point in the context of policy intervention is to recognize that even when nature plays a part, society can make a huge difference.

Consider floods and droughts, which have been associated with processes that have led to many more disaster deaths than other 'natural' causes. What can intervention achieve and how? There are three different types of influence.

- First, environmental policies can make floods and droughts less common. This is a subject that is being energetically discussed today—at long last—moved largely by the prospect of massive increases in their incidence related to global warming and other long-run environmental hazards.

Table 3.5.2 Some recent famines

1845–1951	Ireland	Recurrent famines linked with a blight in potato farming, with loss of jobs, incomes, and staple food; famine mortality around 1 million deaths (the largest proportionate mortality among all 'recent' famines)
1928–1929	China	Famines, particularly affecting farming population, especially in Shensi, Honan, and Kansu provinces, with mortality estimates >5 million deaths
1932–1934	Soviet Union	Connected with agricultural turmoil, at least partly linked with collectivization, especially severe in Ukraine, with mortality estimates >5 million deaths
1943	India	In the province of Bengal, during the Second World War, with a fairly normal food availability; mortality estimates now 2–3 million
1958–1961	China	Linked with the disastrous failure of the so-called Great Leap Forward, there was a sharp decline in food production, disruption of normal economic processes, and huge chaos; the famine was well hidden from those not directly exposed to it; the death toll was later estimated to be close to 30 million (making it the largest absolute size of famine mortality in the recorded history of famines in the world)
1967–1968	Nigeria	Connected with civil war and the blockade of Biafra; no reliable estimate of deaths has been made
1972–1974	Sahel region	Affecting a number of countries in the Sahel belt of Africa (Burkina Faso, Chad, Mali, Mauritania, Niger, Senegal), with some reduction in agricultural production, but also affecting pastoralists both through animal death and through a fall in the relative prices of animal products against staple food from agriculture; no reliable mortality estimates can be made
1973	Ethiopia	The drought in the Wollo province reduced the purchasing power of poor people, and even though there was no significant reduction in food output at all for Ethiopia as a whole (the reduction was confined mainly to Wollo), food did not move into Wollo, and some moved out of it, because of the relatively larger purchasing power of the rest of Ethiopia; no reliable mortality estimates can be made
1974	Bangladesh	This famine, which followed shortly after the disruption of civil strife that led to the break-up of Pakistan, occurred in a year of peak food availability; floods that would reduce food output the following year immediately affected employment and incomes of rural labourers, and also an exaggerated anticipation of a coming food crisis made food prices rise very steeply (followed by a price decline later on, after the famine); mortality estimates vary but it was kept very much in check by a huge food relief programme arranged by the government through which 4.35 million people (about 6% of the total population) were fed
1975–1979	Cambodia	Linked with the Khmer Rouge ravages of the rural economy, deportation of parts of the urban population, and systematic slaughter of unfavoured people; the death toll is estimated to be *c.*1 million
Since early 1990s	North Korea	Intermittent famines with economic disruption by an authoritarian regime with a strong ideological agenda; death estimates are increasingly put at *c.*1 million so far

- Second, any human disaster that kills directly will also tend to disrupt the economy through its effects on jobs and incomes and prices, thereby affecting the entitlement to food and other essentials that people need. The discussion on famines has already illustrated this general connection. That analysis can be extended: e.g. an earthquake may not lead to a famine, but can leave an economy unsettled, making lives precarious for those who are not killed in the physical event itself. These effects can be prevented or at least reduced in their impact through careful social intervention. The type of housing and the arrangements of city planning can also reduce the effects of earthquakes, floods, storms, and other hazards.
- Third, the morbidity and mortality associated with the human disaster can be large and even extend far beyond the immediately affected population who are directly hit by the physical events. However, taking note of the likely dangers from local contagions, the scale of both illness and death can be radically altered through a variety of preventive measures, such as immunization, ensuring safe water, influencing the routes of contact and spread, and also through health education and prompt medical response.

The divisiveness of disasters

The way so-called natural disasters kill depends greatly on social, economic, political, and medical arrangements that the afflicted population has. Indeed, the death toll from so-called natural disasters sharply goes down as we move to higher and higher income countries, even when they do not have any fewer natural events of that type. The contrast can be very sharp indeed, as Kofi Annan, the former Secretary General of the United Nations, has noted (*International Herald Tribune*, 19 September 1999):

> Ninety percent of the disaster victims worldwide live in developing countries where poverty and population pressures force growing numbers of poor people to live in harm's way on flood plains, in earthquake prone zones and on unstable hillsides. Unsafe buildings compound the risks. The vulnerability of those living in risk-prone areas is perhaps the single-most important cause of disaster casualty and damage.

A similar remark can be made about the role of medical services and epidemiology, which are often rudimentary in the poorer countries.

If low income is a predisposing condition for the penalty of disasters, the type of political rule can also be an important factor. The costs of insensitivity of ruling governments in authoritarian countries to the interests of vulnerable people have been illustrated in the specific context of famine prevention, but the problem of authoritarian insensitivity is a widespread phenomenon and goes well beyond the terrible record of authoritarian regimes with the incidence of famines. The neglect of medical services and health care that can be seen in many military dictatorships, for example, in sub-Saharan Africa, is itself a problem for disaster management. There are political parameters related to the medical, social, and economic interventions that can make disasters less likely, and less devastating when they do occur. The effects of the same types of natural phenomena can be widely different, depending on income levels, political voice, medical development, and other variable conditions.

Indeed, human disasters are very divisive events—not only between countries but also within them. Even in the same country, and within the same region of a country, a disaster can ruin some groups of people, while leaving others almost completely untouched. Famines, for example, tend to affect those who are already vulnerable because of poverty and the absence of safety nets on which they can rely—private or social. Policy intervention has to take note of the divisions along the lines of class and occupation group.

There are also differences related to age and gender. Children may be particularly vulnerable in some disasters, including in epidemics of some diseases. The need for immunization of children and arranging medical attention for children are important requirements in disaster management, and so is the institution of economic safety nets through state provision and other social arrangements for child support and income supplement at moments of dire need.

In some disasters (e.g. in the present phase of the AIDS epidemic), women are increasingly more affected. It is usually the case that the opposite is true in wars, which typically kill more men than women or children. But women may be particularly vulnerable when a civil war is targeted against a specific community where women are systematically raped, as has happened for example in Darfur in Sudan. Even though the mortality rate may be higher among men, leaving a lower ratio of men in the surviving population, the high incidents of rapes in the same brutal attacks amount to a gigantic vulnerability for women in particular. There are other kinds of special vulnerabilities in disasters, like breakdown of families in famines, from which women tend especially to suffer.

There is also a more subtle point that tends to be often neglected in journalistic reports. The life expectancy of women is typically longer than that of men for fairly well-established physiological reasons (the lower mortality rate applies even to female fetuses), unless this is reversed through gender bias in social care. There is some evidence that the life expectancy of women is comparatively more reduced by many types of so-called natural disasters than that of men. The greater vulnerability of women is sometimes hidden by the fact that even after the larger reduction, women may still have a higher life expectancy than men, but—as discussed in the context of famine analysis—the right comparison is between what actually happens with a disaster and what could have been expected to have happened in its absence. That distinction is as relevant for medical practitioners and public health experts as it is for social and economic investigators. So is the general need to see human disasters as highly divisive events.

Further reading

Depoortere E, *et al.* (2004). Violence and mortality in West Darfur, Sudan (2003–04): epidemiological evidence from four surveys. *Lancet*, **364**, 1315–20.

de Waal A (2005). *Famine that kills: Darfur, Sudan.* Oxford University Press, Oxford.

Dreze J, Sen A (1989). *Hunger and public action.* Oxford University Press, Oxford.

Guha-Sapir D, Hargitt D, Hoyois P (2004). *Thirty years of natural disasters 1974–2003: The numbers.* Centre for Research on the Epidemiology of Disasters, Presses Universitaires de Louvain.

International Federation of Red Cross and Red Crescent Societies (2006). *World Disasters Report 2005.* Eurospan, London; http://www.ifrc.org/publicat/wdr2005/index.asp

Kahn ME (2005). The death toll from natural disasters: the role of income, geography, and institutions. *Rev Econ Stat*, **87**, 271–84.

Neumayer E, Plumper T (2007). The gendered nature of natural disasters: the impact of catastrophe events on the gender gap in life expectancy, 1981–2002. *Ann Assoc Am Geogr*, **97**, 551–566.

Sen A (1981). *Poverty and famine: an essay on entitlement and deprivation.* Oxford University Press, Oxford.

Stern N (2007). *The economics of climate change.* Cambridge University Press, Cambridge.

Vaughan M (2007). *The story of an African famine.* Cambridge University Press, Cambridge.

SECTION 4

Cell biology

4.1 **The cell** *127*
George Banting

4.2 **Molecular biology** *135*

4.2.1 The human genome sequence *135*
Sydney Brenner

4.2.2 The genomic basis of medicine *136*
Paweł Stankiewicz and James R. Lupski

4.3 **Cytokines** *152*
Iain B. McInnes

4.4 **Ion channels and disease** *160*
Frances M. Ashcroft

4.5 **Intracellular signalling** *169*
R. Andres Floto

4.6 **Apoptosis in health and disease** *177*
Andrew H. Wyllie and Mark J. Arends

4.7 **Discovery of embryonic stem cells and the concept of regenerative medicine** *189*
Martin J. Evans

4.8 **Stem cells and regenerative medicine** *193*
Alexis J. Joannides, Roger Pedersen, and Siddharthan Chandran

4.1

The cell

George Banting

Essentials

This section emphasizes the cell as a dynamic entity. Cells are not simply building blocks that are linked together to create an organism: each cell comprises a dynamic network of interacting macromolecules. Just how dynamic has been brought home by recent advances in cell imaging technologies. A host of multisubunit molecular structures must assemble and disassemble in a highly coordinated, exquisitely regulated, and beautifully chöreographed manner in order to ensure the integrity of the cell and to provide its ability to function correctly as a single unit within a large multicellular organism.

Introduction

The cell is the fundamental unit of all forms of independent life on this planet, from the simplest single-celled prokaryote to the most complex multicellular eukaryote. A limiting membrane, the plasma membrane, encloses the contents of the cell and allows a host of enzymic reactions and intermolecular interactions to occur within a confined, and regulated, environment. This raises the question, 'What is the limiting membrane composed of and what are the contents of the cell?' The major component of the limiting membrane is a lipid bilayer and the major components of the lipid bilayer are amphipathic phospholipids. Amphipathic molecules have one part that is water soluble (hydrophilic) and one part that is water insoluble (hydrophobic). A property of amphipathic molecules is that, in an aqueous environment, they spontaneously organize themselves so that the hydrophobic regions face one another (shielding them from the surrounding water) leaving the hydrophilic regions (often referred to as 'head groups') exposed. In fact, an appropriate mixture of phospholipids in water will lead to the spontaneous formation of lipid vesicles, with water on the inside and water on the outside (Fig. 4.1.1). This gives us the basic template for the limiting membrane of the cell, but the contents of the cell, even though they are in an aqueous environment, are more than just water! The contents of the cell comprise, in fact, a vast range of biomolecules, from simple building blocks to large macromolecular complexes.

Prokaryotes compared with eukaryotes

Before going further it is probably best to clarify the difference between prokaryotes and eukaryotes. The defining difference between prokaryotes and eukaryotes is that prokaryotes have no nucleus whereas eukaryotes do. Prokaryotes can be divided into two major divisions, or domains, the eubacteria and the archaebacteria, which appear to have diverged from a common ancestor at around about the same time that ancestral eukaryotes evolved as the third domain of life on earth. All three domains use DNA as their hereditary material and information store. In prokaryotes this DNA resides within the cell alongside all the other cellular contents, in eukaryotes it is contained within the nucleus and thereby physically separated from the bulk of the contents of the cell. Just as the cell itself is a membrane-bound structure, so is the nucleus within each eukaryotic cell. In fact the membrane that surrounds the nucleus is a double lipid bilayer and is referred to as the nuclear envelope. The nucleus is just one of several membrane-bound structures within eukaryotic cells. The larger of these structures are referred to as organelles and they serve to compartmentalize the cell, allowing specific processes and reactions to occur within defined and controlled local environments. Smaller membrane-bound compartments are referred to as vesicles and tubules; these are generally involved in transport between organelles or between organelles and the plasma membrane. The contents of a eukaryotic cell are referred to as the cytoplasm; the aqueous part of the cytoplasm outside membrane-bound compartments is referred to as the cytosol and the inside of an organelle, vesicle, or tubule is termed the lumen of that compartment.

Transcription, translation, and macromolecular crowding

In all cells, DNA is transcribed into messenger RNA (mRNA) by RNA polymerase; the mRNA is, in turn, translated into protein by ribosomes. In prokaryotes this all occurs within the same space,

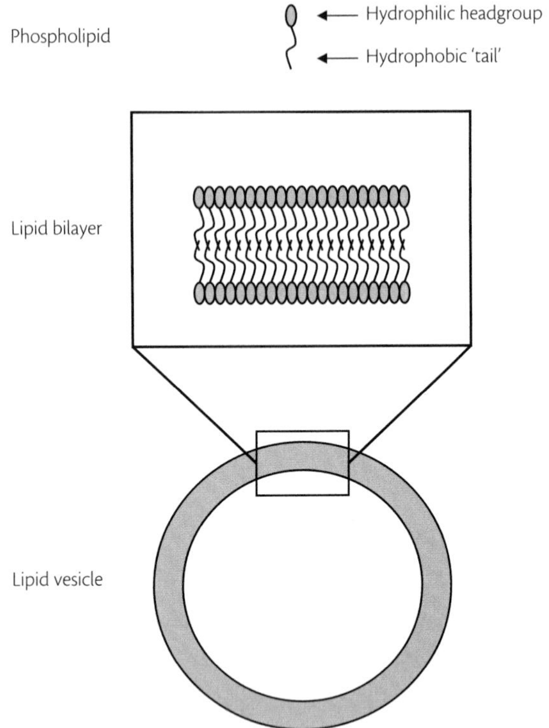

Fig. 4.1.1 Phospholipids spontaneously self-assemble in aqueous environments to form lipid vesicles.

since there are essentially no intracellular membrane-bound compartments and transcription and translation can be coupled, i.e. an mRNA can be being translated while still being transcribed. However, things are different in eukaryotes, since (in general) the transcribed mRNA leaves the nucleus (via protein-lined channels, nuclear pores, in the nuclear envelope) before being translated in the cytosol.

It has been estimated that, on average, each mammalian cell contains about 10^{10} protein molecules of about 10000 to 20000 different kinds. On top of this there are multiple copies of a range of other large macromolecules, notably nucleic acids and complex sugars. All of this within a cell that is around 20 μm in diameter (although there is massive variation here). It is, therefore, hardly surprising that there is a very high total concentration of macromolecules within mammalian cells—estimated to be up to 400 g/litre—meaning that anything up to 40% of the cell volume is physically occupied by these molecules. Thus, while the inside of the cell is clearly an aqueous environment, it is a very crowded and highly ordered aqueous environment, and probably has a consistency rather like that of thick soup or porridge.

Lipid bilayers and integral membrane proteins

A lipid bilayer, be it the plasma membrane at the cell surface or the defining membrane of an intracellular organelle, is, among other things, a permeability barrier. It is permeable to small lipophilic molecules, partially permeable to water, but impermeable to ions and large molecules. It therefore not only retains the contents of the cell or organelle, but also provides a physical barrier between the contents of the cell or organelle and the exterior environment. A cell, however, clearly has to interact with its exterior environment, whether it be a single-celled prokaryote (and most living organisms are single cells) or a complex multicellular organism such as a human being with an estimated 10^{13} cells assembled in such a way, and communicating with one another, so that they create a living being that is far more than the sum of the individual parts. This interaction with the exterior environment of the cell is dependent upon proteins that reside in the lipid bilayer. Many of these proteins actually span the lipid bilayer, with part of the protein residing outside the cell, part within the cell and part within the hydrophobic core of the lipid bilayer. In the case of eukaryotic cells, the vast majority of these membrane proteins have been post-translationally modified by the addition of specific sugar residues to create glycoproteins. In many cases the correct sugar modifications are critical for the correct function of the glycoprotein, particularly for those glycoproteins that are involved in cell–cell or cell–substrate interactions (NB: aberrant glycosylation is frequently observed on glycoproteins at the surface of cells present in tumours). Membrane proteins perform a multitude of roles, just about all of which can be considered to be involved, in some way, in communication between the inside and the outside of the cell. They act as transporters of ions, sugars, amino acids, peptides, hormones, and other molecules; they act as receptors for extracellular ligands such as hormones and neurotransmitters, and transmit signals to the inside of the cell; they act to link cells to one another or to the underlying substrate; in short they are the physical link between the inside of the cell and the outside world. It is not surprising, therefore, that it has been estimated that about a third of all the proteins encoded by the human genome are membrane proteins.

Organelles

What are the main organelles within eukaryotic cells? The major ones are the nucleus, the endoplasmic reticulum (ER), the Golgi apparatus, mitochondria, lysosomes, endosomes, and peroxisomes (and chloroplasts in plants), with a range of specialized organelles occurring in different cells of higher eukaryotes (see Fig. 4.1.2).

Nucleus

The nucleus can be considered to be at the heart of the eukaryotic cell. It harbours the vast majority of DNA within the cell, i.e. the nuclear genome. It is also, among other things, the site of gene transcription, the site of mRNA processing, and the site of ribosome assembly. The control of gene expression, which often occurs at the level of transcriptional regulation, is fundamental to the regulation of cell function and involves a complex interplay between the genomic DNA in the nucleus and a host of cellular proteins. Many of these proteins shuttle, in a controlled manner and in response to specific signals, between the nucleus and the cytosol. They are able to do so because there are gaps, termed nuclear pores, in the membrane that envelopes the nucleus. The nuclear membrane is, in fact not a single lipid bilayer, but a double lipid bilayer. Thus, there is an inner nuclear membrane in contact with the contents of the nucleus and an outer lipid bilayer in contact with the cytosol. The space between the two lipid bilayers is the lumen of the nuclear membrane and is a space that is contiguous with the lumen of the endoplasmic reticulum.

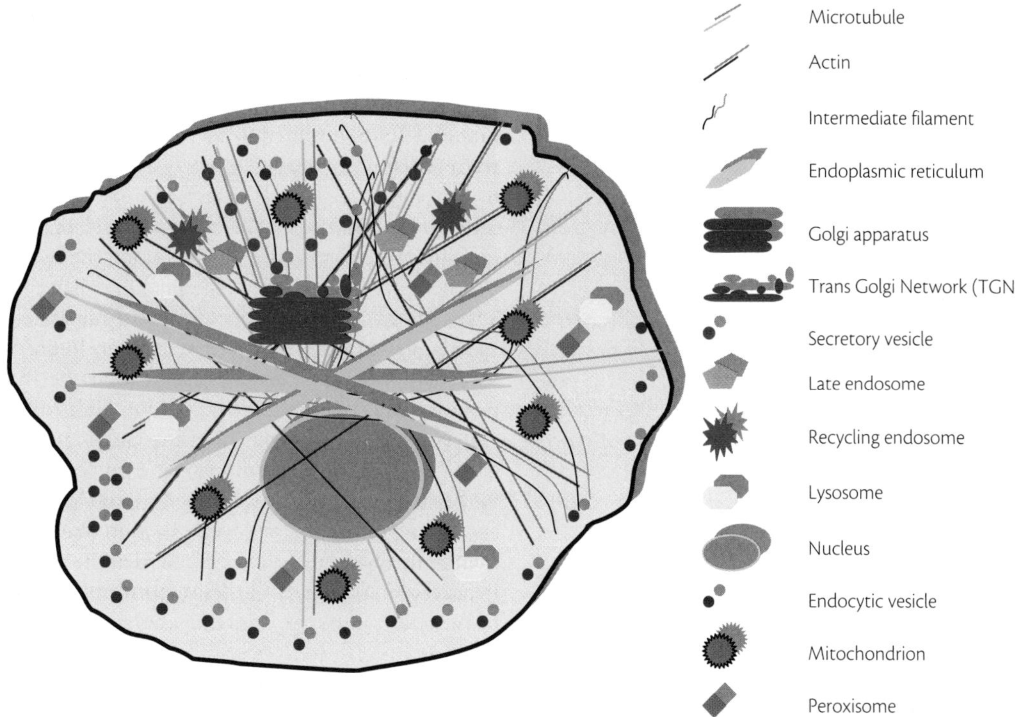

Fig. 4.1.2 Cartoon showing some of the main components of a higher eukaryotic cell.

Nuclear pores are complex multiprotein assemblies that allow certain proteins to pass in and out of the nucleus while excluding others. Fully processed mRNA also leaves the nucleus via nuclear pores before being translated in the cytosol by ribosomes. The dynamic traffic within, and in and out of, the nucleus is imperative for cell function.

Mitochondria

The mitochondria are also enveloped in two layers of membrane, an inner one and an outer one. They are involved in the oxidation of molecular fuels, including pyruvate derived form sugars and fatty acids, to generate the adenosine triphosphate (ATP) that is needed as an energy source for the reactions of the cell. They are thus fundamental to cell function. Other than chloroplasts, which are also enclosed in a double-layered membrane, mitochondria are the only nonnuclear organelles to contain DNA. It is likely that mitochondria arose by a process related to endosymbiosis (the process whereby certain bacteria enter eukaryotic cells and live within their cytoplasm) in which an aerobic eubacterium was engulfed by a eukaryotic cell—hence the double membrane, one from the engulfing eukaryotic cell and one from the engulfed prokaryote. The biogenesis of chloroplasts also probably occurred via a similar pathway. Mitochondrial disorders are an important cause of neurological diseases and disorders of muscle, including cardiac muscle. Mitochondrial abnormalities may be inherited or acquired. Those specifically affecting the intrinsic genome of this organelle are transmitted in a matrilinear fashion. Descriptions of important mitochondrial disorders are to be found in Chapter 24.24.5.

Peroxisomes

Peroxisomes are membrane-bound organelles that contain high concentrations of oxidative enzymes such as catalase and are therefore important for a range of oxidative processes necessary for the elimination of multiple substances (e.g. in the breakdown of very long chain fatty acids). Several diseases caused by defects in peroxisomal proteins are described in Chapter 12.9.

Endoplasmic reticulum (ER)

The membranes of the ER are contiguous with those of the nuclear membrane, thus the lumen of the ER is contiguous with the space between the two membranes of the nuclear envelope. The lumen of the ER serves as a calcium store for the cell, with concentrations of calcium in the ER lumen being around 10^{-3} M, compared with 10^{-8} M to 10^{-6} M in the cytosol. Regulated release of calcium from the ER, in response to extracellular signals detected by membrane proteins at the cell surface and transmitted via specific intracellular second-messenger molecules, leads to changes in the activity of a host of cellular processes. This is because many intracellular proteins bind calcium and their activities and/or interactions with other proteins are dependent upon whether or not they are calcium bound. In fact, the calcium concentration in the cytosol has to be very carefully controlled because it is an important regulator of many intracellular processes including muscle contraction and secretion. Excess calcium within the cytosol can rapidly lead to cell death. There is, therefore a complex array of transporters operating to ensure that calcium levels remain high in the lumen of the ER and are only transiently raised in the cytosol in response to specific stimuli. Some of these transporters are in the ER membrane, others in the plasma membrane, others in the mitochondria.

The ER is, however, not simply a calcium store. It is also a major site of lipid biosynthesis within the cell. Furthermore, it is also the site of synthesis for proteins that are destined to be secreted from the cell or to be membrane proteins. Such proteins are synthesized by ribosomes that become attached to the cytosolic face of the ER membrane soon after they have started to translate an mRNA encoding a secretory or integral membrane protein. Before folding up as a secretory protein in the lumen of the ER, or passing laterally from the translocation channel into the ER membrane if it is destined to be an integral membrane protein, the nascent protein is translocated through a protein-lined channel in the ER membrane. This channel opens only when a ribosome synthesizing a secretory or integral membrane protein is bound to its cytosolic face. The ER is thus the start of the secretory pathway in eukaryotic cells. The fact that the translocation channel opens only when a ribosome is bound to it preserves the integrity of the ER membrane as a permeability barrier and ensures no leakage of ions, such as calcium, from the ER lumen. Some of the most abundant proteins in eukaryotic cells reside in the lumen of the ER; these are proteins that are involved in assisting the correct folding of newly synthesized proteins in the secretory pathway and include proteins such as the enzyme protein disulphide isomerase (which ensures that the correct disulphide bonds are formed in proteins), calnexin, and calreticulin. The latter two are also calcium-binding proteins. Thus, although the majority of proteins that enter the secretory pathway at the ER are destined to be secreted or to become integral membrane proteins in the plasma membrane, certain proteins (both soluble proteins within the lumen of organelles along the secretory pathway and integral membrane proteins within the membranes of organelles along the secretory pathway) are primarily localized to specific compartments along the secretory pathway.

It has become increasingly clear over recent years that a combination of retention and retrieval signals within proteins serve to ensure these localizations, with retention signals serving to hold proteins in place and retrieval signals operating to bring proteins back to their steady-state localization from a point further along the secretory pathway.

Most diagrams of eukaryotic cells in textbooks, including Fig. 4.1.2 here, show the ER as a membranous organelle linked to the nucleus; this is correct, but it fails to illustrate the extent of the ER since, in most cells, it pervades much of the extranuclear space of the cell and is a highly dynamic organelle. More than half of the total membrane area of a mammalian cell can be ER.

Golgi apparatus

The step beyond the ER in the secretory pathway is the Golgi apparatus. The Golgi apparatus has been likened to a small stack of pitta bread, with each pitta corresponding to a cisterna (segment) of the Golgi. Vesicles, containing soluble and integral membrane protein cargo, bud off from the ER and are delivered to the cis face of the Golgi apparatus where they fuse with the Golgi membrane and deliver their contents. The recruitment of specific cargo into the vesicles, the budding of the vesicles and their fusion with the Golgi are all steps that involve discrete, and transient, assemblies of proteins. The different cisternae of the Golgi apparatus—known as cis, medial, and trans, although there may well be many more than three in certain cell types—represent the next steps along the secretory pathway. It now appears that passage through this part of the pathway can be quite complex, with both forward (anterograde) and backward (retrograde) vesicular traffic occurring. The anterograde traffic moves cargo towards the trans side of the Golgi apparatus and the retrograde traffic retrieves material that is required earlier in the secretory pathway, i.e. in the medial or cis cisternae of the Golgi apparatus or in the ER. Vesicular traffic within the Golgi apparatus also seems to be complemented by a process that has been termed cisternal maturation. This describes the maturation of a cis cisterna into a medial cisterna by the vesicular retrieval of material that should not be present in a medial cisterna. The retrieved vesicles fuse with newly arrived vesicles from the ER to form a new cis cisterna; meanwhile the medial cisterna matures into a trans cisterna via the same process. As all of this is happening, the proteins that are passing along the secretory pathway are being sequentially post-translationally modified, primarily by the addition of a series of sugar residues to generate glycoproteins, by specific enzymes with discrete steady-state localizations maintained by retention and retrieval signals, within specific cisternae of the Golgi apparatus.

Beyond the trans cisterna of the Golgi apparatus lies the trans Golgi network (TGN) from which a range of vesicles and tubules bud to deliver their cargo to its destination. This may be the cell surface, for proteins that are to be secreted or to become integral membrane proteins in the plasma membrane, but may also be an intracellular organelle. Thus, for example, lysosomal enzymes have to be delivered to the lysosome and this is done via the secretory pathway.

Lysosomes

Lysosomes can be considered as the recycling centres of the cell. Macromolecules are delivered to lysosomes to be broken down into their constituent building blocks (e.g. proteins to amino acids, polysaccharides to monosaccharides) by a host of acid hydrolases (proteases, glycosidases, nucleases, lipases, etc.). The building blocks are then exported from the lysosome and used by the cell to make new macromolecules. It is clearly important that the hydrolysis of macromolecules is strictly compartmentalized, otherwise the cell would destroy itself. In fact the cell not only compartmentalizes lysosomal enzymes within the lysosome, but also ensures that these enzymes only become fully active once they have been delivered into the lysosome. The lysosomal enzymes are acid hydrolases, that is to say that they function at low pH. The pH of the lumen of the lysosome is about 4.5. This is in contrast to the pH in the lumen of the Golgi and TGN (approximately 6.5 to 6.7) or the pH of the cytosol (approximately 7.4). Thus, as lysosomal enzymes are delivered from the TGN to the lysosome (by vesicular transport) they become activated because of the lower pH in the lysosome. In fact, lysosomal enzymes are not delivered directly from the TGN into the lysosome, but are delivered to an intermediate compartment, the late endosome. This is an interface between the secretory pathway and the endocytic pathway (a pathway carrying material that has been internalized from the cell surface). A late endosome fuses with a mature lysosome, delivering the contents of the late endosome into the lysosome. Membrane, and integral membrane proteins, that should be in the late endosome are then retrieved from the hybrid organelle to form a new late endosome and an immature lysosome. The lumenal pH of the late endosome is intermediate between that of the TGN and that of the lysosome (i.e. between 5 and 6). The reduced pH is generated by the action of a proton pump (a vacuolar ATPase) in the limiting membrane of the late endosome and lysosome. Many inherited disorders of lysosomal function have been identified. These diseases and their treatments are described in Chapter 12.8. The special capacity of the lysosomal compartment for complementation by internalizing proteins supplied externally has allowed several important therapeutic enzymes to be developed.

Endocytosis

The existence of late endosomes implies that there must also be early endosomes. There are. There is clearly a flow of membrane and protein along the secretory pathway culminating in the fusion of vesicles with the plasma membrane. In the absence of any compensatory membrane internalization, the surface area of the cell would therefore continually increase. Such internalization does occur, thereby ensuring that most cells remain relatively constant in size. The internalization of membrane from the cell surface (a process termed endocytosis) occurs via a variety of routes, the best characterized being clathrin-mediated endocytosis. The process involves the assembly of specific protein machinery at the cytosolic face of the plasma membrane, the invagination of the plasma membrane, and the pinching off of membrane-bound vesicles (or possibly tubules) from the plasma membrane. The protein coat that has been instrumental in the formation of these vesicles then generally disassembles and the uncoated vesicles fuse to form early endosomes; the vacuolar ATPase is already active in early endosomes and they have a lumenal pH of approximately 6.5 to 6.8. The endocytic process not only ensures that a balance is maintained between the amount of membrane inserted in the plasma membrane and the amount removed, but also allows the selective recruitment of specific integral membrane proteins (often with extracellularly bound ligand) into the endocytic pathway.

The different endocytic mechanisms selectively recruit different cargo and thereby serve as molecular filters, internalizing certain integral membrane proteins while leaving others at the cell surface. The complexity of the endomembrane system (i.e. the membranes of the endocytic compartments) in mammalian cells has become apparent in recent years. Thus, for example, in addition to early and late endosomes there are also recycling endosomes. These are compartments from which material that is to be returned to the plasma membrane is retrieved. Such material might be receptors that have been internalized along with their ligand, but which need to be returned to the cell surface having released their ligand at the lower pH of the early endosome/recycling endosome. An example of such a receptor would be the transferrin receptor which releases the iron that is bound to transferrin in the early endosome/recycling endosome, leaving the transferrin receptor and apotransferrin to be recycled to the cell surface for reuse. Other receptors that are internalized are destined for degradation in the lysosome and are delivered to the late endosome. An example of such a receptor is the epidermal growth factor receptor. When this receptor binds its ligand at the cell surface it transmits a cascade of signals across the cell which trigger cell growth and cell division. Such signals should only be transient, otherwise unregulated cell growth and cell division occur; the cell ensures that the signals transmitted by the receptor are transient by internalizing the receptor and sending it to the lysosome for degradation.

Cytoskeleton

All this movement of vesicles and tubules between compartments does not occur at random. It is dependent upon motor proteins and the cytoskeleton. The cytoskeleton is the name given to a framework within the cell which gives the cell its shape and which provides a structure to which organelles and proteins can be attached, thus providing an architecture that gives spatial organization to the cell. There are three main components of the cytoskeleton in mammalian cells: microtubules, actin filaments, and intermediate filaments (see Fig. 4.1.2). Each of these components is a polymer of protein subunits and all three are dynamic structures with the potential for assembly and disassembly according to the needs of the cell.

Microtubules are highly dynamic polymers of heterodimers of α- and β-tubulin which assemble to form long hollow tubes approximately 25 nm in diameter. Monomers of globular (G) actin polymerize to form filamentous (F) actin which is a double-stranded helical polymer with a diameter of 5 to 9 nm. Elongated and fibrous subunits assemble to form intermediate filaments with a diameter of approximately 10 nm (e.g. lamins A, B, and C assemble to form the nuclear lamina that provides the inner lining to the nuclear envelope).

The different components of the cytoskeleton provide complementary features of the cellular architecture. Microtubules serve to localize organelles within the cell and provide the tracks along which many classes of transport vesicles and tubules move, the movement being powered by motor proteins (notably kinesin and dynein) attached to the membranes of the vesicles or tubules. Microtubules also play a critical role during cell division, since they are pivotal in the physical separation of chromosomes during mitosis. Actin filaments can cross the cell and provide the structure that determines the shape of the cell's surface. These filaments play major roles in protrusions from the cell surface. For example, they run along the length of the microvilli that extend from the apical surface of polarized epithelial cells, and they are absolutely necessary for cell locomotion since concerted rearrangements of the actin cytoskeleton underlie cell movement. Myosin motor proteins also interact with actin, the best characterized such interaction being between actin and myosin II in skeletal muscle; this interaction is responsible for generating the force that is required for muscle contraction. Both microtubules and actin filaments are highly dynamic structures. Their assembly and disassembly is precisely and finely regulated by a host of cellular proteins in response to a range of extracellular signals. Intermediate filaments are relatively stable by comparison, and provide mechanical strength to the cell.

The dynamic cell

The preceding superficial overview of the secretory and endocytic pathways in mammalian cells highlights their dynamic nature. The elegant cartoons that grace most textbooks in this field indicate the subcellular organelles and other cellular components and their relative positions within the cell, but, because they are two-dimensional static images, they cannot give any indication of the complex dynamics that operate within cells. All the different vesicle budding, vesicle transport, vesicle targeting, and vesicle fusion steps involve the assembly and disassembly of specific and discrete macromolecular complexes. There is exquisite spatiotemporal control of each of these events. The dynamic nature of microtubules and actin filaments adds to the complexity of the interactions that occur within cells.

The dynamic nature of the eukaryotic cell has been made self-evident over the past 10 years or so following the increasingly widespread use of a range of tools and microscopy systems that allow the imaging of specific proteins within live cells. The real breakthrough came with the isolation of the DNA sequence encoding green fluorescent protein (GFP). GFP is encoded by the genome of the jellyfish *Aqueoria victoria*; it is a protein that is naturally fluorescent, emitting green light when it is illuminated with blue light. The now standard techniques of molecular genetics have allowed researchers to link the DNA sequence encoding GFP to the DNA sequences encoding a range of different proteins. These hybrid DNA sequences can be introduced into eukaryotic cells and the localizations, and intracellular movements, of the hybrid proteins they encode can be monitored by appropriate microscopy techniques. This has allowed us to see the dynamic instability of microtubules within living cells, the movement of proteins along the secretory pathway, the sorting of proteins in the endocytic pathway, and many other cellular processes. Genetic engineering has also provided us with a suite of spectral variants of GFP, each emitting light of a different wavelength (i.e. a different colour), thereby allowing the imaging of two or more different proteins in the same cell at the same time. It is remarkable that, in most cases, the presence of a fluorescent protein attached to a protein of interest has little if any effect on the function of that protein.

Biological membranes

It is over 30 years since Singer and Nicholson proposed the 'fluid mosaic' model for biological membranes. This proposed that integral membrane proteins could diffuse freely in the sea of the lipid bilayer. The imaging of populations of GFP-tagged proteins has confirmed earlier studies which show that this is essentially the case, but more sophisticated single-particle tracking studies have shown that the plasma membrane is partitioned with regard to molecular diffusion in the plane of the lipid bilayer. This is because of specific interactions with the underlying actin cytoskeleton. These interactions tend to be between actin and the cytosolic domain of specific integral membrane proteins (see Fig. 4.1.3). Such interactions are often indirect, i.e. via one or more intermediate proteins, thereby providing the opportunity for regulation of the interaction. For example the cytosolic domain of the cystic fibrosis transmembrane conductance regulator (CFTR) interacts with a cytosolic protein called EBP50 at the apical surface of polarized human airway epithelial cells. EBP50 in turn binds another protein, ezrin, and ezrin binds the actin cytoskeleton, thereby tethering CFTR to the actin cytoskeleton and keeping it in the right place in the plasma membrane. Similar interactions between the cytosolic domains of specific integral membrane proteins and the actin cytoskeleton most probably occur in the context of organellar membranes.

Differential gene expression

A human body clearly arises from a single cell, the fertilized egg. This single cell eventually gives rise to the multitude of different cell types within the body. For this to occur, cells must grow and divide (and sometimes die) in a highly regulated manner. Not only do the cells need to grow and divide, different populations of cells must differentiate along different lineages in order to generate the different cell types required to populate the different tissues and organs of the body.

Each of the 10^{13} or so cells in the human body is a phenomenally complex and dynamic entity. Furthermore, different subsets of the approximately 20 000 to 25 000 genes in the human genome are expressed in different cell types, with further variations in gene expression occurring during development and in response to external stimuli. This differential gene expression leads, at least in part, to the diversity of cell types found throughout the body. Thus, for example, a neuron is clearly very different from an epithelial cell lining the gut. However, both have the same fundamental organization described in the preceding paragraphs. They both express a core set of shared genes, providing the fundamental cellular organization, but each expresses a different set of specific genes. The specific genes expressed will help to define the phenotype of the cell. The differences between cells can often be quite subtle, e.g. different cell types have different protein subunits making up their intermediate filaments, different motor proteins are expressed in different cell types, and differential glycosylation of glycoproteins and glycolipids occurs in different cell types.

Alternative splicing and post-translational modifications

The fact that there appear to be only 20 000 to 25 000 genes in the human genome does not mean that only this number of proteins can be encoded by the genome. Many genes are subject to the process

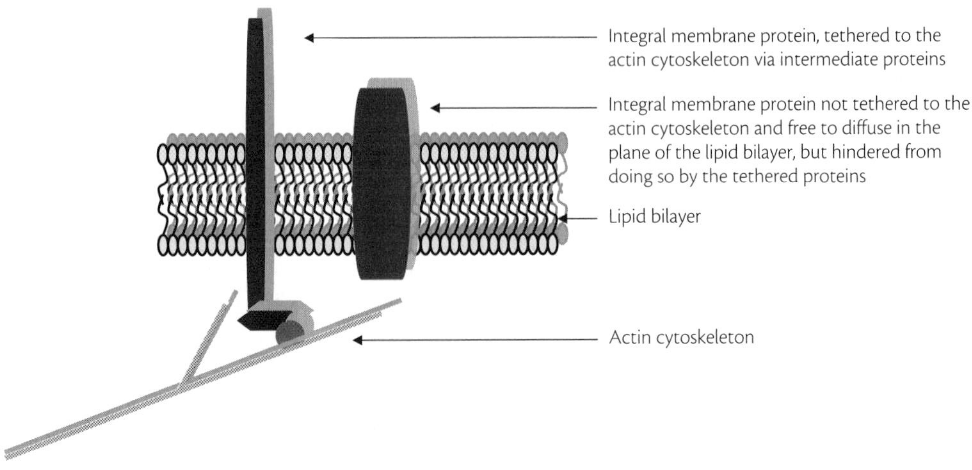

Fig. 4.1.3 Integral membrane proteins in the lipid bilayer. Some are tethered to the underlying actin cytoskeleton, keeping them in place and providing barriers to the free diffusion of those integral membrane proteins that are not so tethered.

of alternative splicing, whereby specific exons are included or excluded as the precursor mRNA is processed (spliced) in the nucleus to remove the noncoding intron sequences. Thus one gene can give rise to several related, but different, mRNA transcripts. Furthermore, differential processing and differential post-translational modification of proteins leads to further variety in the range of protein products produced from the genome.

The range of proteins in a cell (the proteome) is therefore potentially considerably larger than the number of genes in its genome. In the case of cytosolic proteins, and the cytosolic domains of integral membrane proteins, many of the post-translational modifications that occur are transient and reversible. Thus, many such proteins are subject to phosphorylation (the addition of a phosphate group to the side chain of a specific amino acid). This process is catalysed by specific enzymes (kinases) and occurs on specific serine, threonine, or tyrosine residues in target proteins. This modification is reversible by the action of members of another family of enzymes (phosphatases) that remove the phosphate. Phosphorylated proteins have different activities, and often interact with a different subset of proteins, from their nonphosphorylated counterparts; thus, reversible phosphorylation is a mechanism whereby the cell can regulate interactions, and thereby processes, occurring within it. It is not uncommon for a kinase to be activated by phosphorylation and it is not uncommon for one kinase to activate another by phosphorylation, thus establishing a signalling cascade that has built-in amplification of the initial signal—amplification because each kinase is an enzyme capable of acting upon multiple substrate molecules while it is in the active state. The initial signal might be the binding of a ligand to its receptor at the cell surface, e.g. the binding of epidermal growth factor to its receptor at the cell surface. As mentioned earlier, this initiates a cascade of signals across the cell which trigger cell growth and cell division; that cascade of signals is essentially a cascade of phosphorylation events. Such a process clearly needs to be transient or it would lead to unregulated cell growth and cell division. The initial signal is removed by the internalization and degradation of the epidermal growth factor receptor, as previously outlined, but this still leaves an activated kinase cascade perpetuating the 'grow and divide' message. It is the action of specific phosphatases removing the phosphate groups from the kinases in the cascade that turn off the signalling pathway. Thus, once again, we have a highly dynamic cellular system with exquisite spatio-temporal control.

Reversible phosphorylation is one example of several reversible post-translational modifications that serve to regulate cellular function. The principles relating to phosphorylation as a form of post-translational regulation, i.e. that phosphorylated proteins interact with different proteins compared to their nonphosphorylated counterparts, or that phosphorylated enzymes have different activities from their nonphosphorylated counterparts, and that this plays a role in the regulation of cell function, also applies to other forms of reversible post-translational modification.

Post-transcriptional gene silencing (miRNA)

The 20 000 to 25 000 genes in the human genome account for only about 2% of the total DNA in the genome. So, what is the role of all the other DNA? A significant amount of it serves structural purposes, e.g. the sequences at the centromeres (middles) and telomeres (ends) of chromosomes, but recent evidence shows that much of it plays crucial regulatory roles, working by the process of post-transcriptional gene silencing (PTGS).

The phenomenon of PTGS was first described in plants, but has subsequently been shown to be widespread in eukaryotes. In PTGS a short (19 to 23 nucleotides long) double-stranded RNA molecule associates with a target mRNA (the nucleotide sequence of one of the RNA strands in the double stranded molecule is complementary to the sequence of the target mRNA). This occurs in the context of a multiprotein complex and leads to either a block in translation or the degradation of the target mRNA. This mechanism therefore regulates protein expression post-transcriptionally, hence the designation PTGS. The short double-stranded RNA molecules are produced from slightly larger precursor RNA molecules known as micro RNAs (miRNAs) which are themselves produced by transcription of relevant DNA sequences by DNA polymerase in the cell's nucleus. The number of DNA sequences within the human genome that encode miRNAs has yet to be finalized, but there appear to be at least as many such sequences as there are protein-encoding DNA sequences (i.e. conventional genes). miRNA sequences have been shown to play critical regulatory roles in a range of processes, e.g. during development and in the immune response to pathogens. They have also been implicated as playing a role in several disease states, such as heart disease and cancer.

Future developments

The availability of the human genome sequence has given us access to information concerning the basic building blocks of the cell, but it is how those building blocks are modified and used in a multitude of different dynamic interactions that gives organization, function, and life to the cell. A major challenge of the next decade is to integrate the vast amounts of data that are now available, and will continue to become available, on the molecular mechanisms that underlie cellular organization, structure and function. Such a challenge will have to be met if we are to achieve a clearer, and more complete, understanding of the cell and are to develop the capacity to refine our means of modifying cellular functions that are disturbed in disease.

Further reading

Alberts B, *et al.* (2007). *Molecular biology of the cell*, 5th edition. Garland Science, New York. [Everyone should read this book. It is the best textbook on cell biology available.]

Ambros V, Chen X (2007). The regulation of genes and genomes by small RNAs. *Development*, **134**, 1635–41. [A thorough review of post-transcriptional gene silencing by miRNA.]

Berridge MJ (2006). *Cell signalling biology*. Portland Press, Colchester. http://www.cellsignallingbiology.org/ [This is a marvellous interactive resource covering signalling within cells.]

Brooks SA, *et al.* (2008). Altered glycosylation of proteins in cancer: what is the potential for new anti-tumour strategies. *Anticancer Agents Med Chem*, **8**, 2–21. [An overview of aberrant glycosylation of glycoproteins in cancer.]

Bushati N, Cohen SM (2007). microRNA functions. *Ann Rev Cell Dev Biol*, **23**, 175–205. [A thorough review of the roles of miRNA.]

Chalfie M, *et al.* (1994). Green fluorescent protein as a marker for gene expression. *Science*, **11**, 802–5. [The first description of the use of green fluorescent protein as a tool in cell biology.]

Clapham DE (2007). Calcium signaling. *Cell*, **131**, 1047–58. [A thorough review of calcium signalling.]

Derby MC, Gleeson PA (2007). New insights into membrane trafficking and protein sorting. *Int Rev Cytol*, **261**, 47–116. [A recent review of membrane trafficking and protein sorting in mammalian cells.]

Ellis RJ, Minton AP (2003). Join the crowd. *Nature*, **425**, 27–8. [A brief report on macromolecular crowding in cells.]

Giepmans BN, *et al.* (2006). The fluorescent toolbox for assessing protein location and function. *Science*, **14**, 217–24. [A review of the fluorescent tools available for live cell imaging.]

Goldman RD, *et al.* (2008). Intermediate filaments: versatile building blocks of cell structure. *Curr Opin Cell Biol*, **20**, 28–34. [A review of intermediate filament structure and function.]

Haggie PM, *et al.* (2006). Tracking of quantum dot-labeled CFTR shows near immobilization by C-terminal PDZ interactions. *Mol Biol Cell*, **17**, 4937–45. [A report of single particle tracking studies showing that CFTR is tethered to the underlying actin cytoskeleton via intermediate proteins.]

Kusumi A, *et al.* (2005). Paradigm shift of the plasma membrane concept from the two-dimensional continuum fluid to the partitioned fluid: high-speed single-molecule tracking of membrane molecules. *Annu. Rev. Biophys. Biomol Struct*, **34**, 351–78. [A thorough review of recent studies on the organisation of biological membranes.]

Lanzetti L (2007). Actin in membrane trafficking. *Curr Opin Cell Biol*, **19**, 453–8. [A review of the role of the actin cytoskeleton in membrane trafficking.]

Lewin B, *et al.* (2007). *Cells*. Jones and Bartlett, Sudbury, MA. [An excellent textbook on cell biology.]

Lippincott-Schwartz, J (2004). Dynamics of secretory membrane trafficking. *Ann N Y Acad Sci*, **1038**, 115–24. [A review highlighting the dynamic nature of membrane traffic.]

Luzio JP, Pryor PR, Bright NA (2007). Lysosomes: fusion and function. *Nat Rev Mol Cell Biol*, **8**, 622–32. [An authoritative review of lysosome biogenesis and function.]

Mellman I, Warren G (2000). The road taken: past and future foundations of membrane traffic. *Cell*, **100**, 99–112. [A thorough overview of membrane traffic in cells.]

Pelham H, Rothman J (2000). The debate about transport in the Golgi—two sides of the same coin? *Cell*, **102**, 713–19. [A review discussing vesicular transport and cisternal maturation as means of transport within the Golgi.]

Pfeffer SR (2007). Unsolved mysteries in membrane traffic. *Annu Rev Biochem*, **76**, 629–45. [A review highlighting questions still to be solved in membrane traffic.]

Ross JL, Ali MY, Warshaw DM (2008). Cargo transport: molecular motors navigate a complex cytoskeleton. *Curr Opin Cell Biol*, **20**, 41–7. [A review covering the roles of molecular motors and the cytoskeleton in intracellular transport.]

Stadler BM, Ruohola-Baker H (2008). Small RNAs: keeping stem cells in line. *Cell*, **132**, 563–6. [A review covering the role of miRNAs in the regulation of stem cells.]

Singer SJ, Nicolson GL (1972). The fluid mosaic model of the structure of cell membranes. *Science*, **18**, 720–31. [A classic paper presenting the fluid mosaic model for biological membranes.]

Stagg SM, LaPointe P, Balch WE (2007). Structural design of cage and coat scaffolds that direct membrane traffic. *Curr Opin Struct Biol*, **17**, 221–8. [A review discussing the macromolecular assemblies that are involved in sculpting vesicles involved in membrane traffic.]

Stefani G, Slack FJ (2008). Small non-coding RNAs in animal development. *Nat Rev Mol Cell Biol*, **9**, 219–30. [A review covering the role of miRNAs in development.]

Ungewickell EJ, Hinrichsen L (2007). Endocytosis: clathrin-mediated membrane budding. *Curr Opin Cell Biol*, **19**, 417–25. [A thorough review of the role played by clathrin in endocytosis.]

von Zastrow M, Sorkin, A (2007). Signaling on the endocytic pathway. *Curr Opin Cell Biol*, **19**, 436–45.

Zhang J, *et al.* (2002). Creating new fluorescent probes for cell biology. *Nat Rev Mol Cell Biol*, **3**, 906–18. [A review of fluorescent probes used for live cell imaging in cell biology.]

4.2

Molecular biology

Contents

4.2.1 The human genome sequence *135*
Sydney Brenner

4.2.2 The genomic basis of medicine *136*
Paweł Stankiewicz and James R. Lupski

4.2.1 The human genome sequence

Sydney Brenner

Essentials

The sequence of the entire human genome is now available. While it may be that ultimately this information will uncover numerous targets for therapeutic purposes, much additional biological and clinical research will be required on gene and protein function in living cells and in the context of the complete individual. Single mutations in human genes may be responsible for certain diseases and are thus informative about molecular pathogenesis. However, the genetic components of several much more common diseases are more difficult to unravel. This latter area is rapidly developing within medical science and there are early signs, for example in diabetes mellitus and Crohn's disease, that a molecular understanding of pathogenesis in terms of genetic and environmental factors will allow for predictive testing and improved treatments.

The modern period in biological research began in 1953 when JD Watson and FHC Crick discovered the double-helical structure of DNA. Within a very short period of time, about a decade, the new science of molecular biology uncovered the basic mechanisms of information transfer from genes to proteins in living cells. The nucleotide sequence of a gene was shown to be colinear with the amino acid sequence of the protein that it specified; the genetic code was found to be a triplet code; and the correspondences of the 3-base codons to each of the 20 amino acids was established. Although there were chemical methods for determining the amino acid sequences of proteins, the structure of the gene was accessible only through mutational changes as recorded by phenotypes. Such mutations defined genes, and these could be mapped by recombination. Research in molecular genetics proceeded most rapidly with bacteria and their viruses which could be handled easily in the laboratory. A beginning was also made to study more complex systems, such as *Drosophila* which had been long established as a laboratory organism for experimental genetics, and *Caenorhabditis elegans*, a small, free-living nematode worm.

In the mid 1970s there were two revolutionary, technical innovations which changed the entire course of genetics. The first was a method of cloning and propagating fragments of DNA in bacteria and yeasts and the second was the invention of methods for sequencing DNA. Thus the genome of any organism could be obtained as a library of fragments and the sequences of these fragments could be determined. In principle, therefore, the complete sequence of the genome could be obtained, and since it was possible to clone and sequence complementary DNA (cDNA) copies of messenger RNA, the expressed genes could be identified and the amino acid sequences of their proteins inferred from the nucleotide sequences. Characterization of cDNA became important when it was quickly discovered, by the new techniques, that the genes of higher organism were interrupted by intervening sequences called introns which were removed by splicing, leaving the coding exons to form a coherent sequence.

For some time the only complete genomes that were sequenced were small, of the order of 100 kb. In 1985, when it was suggested that the complete sequence of the human genome might be obtained, it was realized that not only would there have to be considerable technical improvements, but also the project would have to be on a large scale and require international cooperation. The technical improvements were the automation of many of the laborious steps of the sequencing process, and the availability of sequencing machines and their progressive enhancement in throughput. Larger genomes were tackled and an early accomplishment was the 14-Mb sequence of yeast. This was followed by the sequences of *C. elegans* and *Drosophila*, each of around 100 Mb.

In 2001, two groups announced that they had more or less completed the first draft of the human genome sequence, and this has since been subjected to much improvement.

The human genome sequence was seen by many to provide new approaches to human biology and, in particular, to medicine. For example, it was claimed that once all the genes were found, all the proteins specified by those genes would be known, and this would allow the uncovering of an enormous number of new targets for the development of new therapeutic agents. In the long run this may prove correct, but before we can use a protein as a drug target we have to know how it functions in the body, and whether any alteration of its activity will have the desired effects. Although the molecular function of a protein can often be specified by comparison of its sequence with proteins of known function, this is insufficient to decide how this activity is translated into a particular cellular process and how this is, in turn, integrated into the physiology of the whole human organism. Thus, for example, while we can readily identify domains with resemblances to proteases, we require additional information to decide what the proteolysis is doing; it may be involved in digestion, in gene regulation, in cell death, in blood coagulation, or in the complement pathway. For any protein to be a target we must have something much more than the protein sequence: we must have a therapeutic hypothesis, and this will be made possible only by the continuation of conventional biological and clinical research.

There can be no doubt, however, that knowing all or nearly all of the proteins made by cells will spur research on the biochemistry of cells. In particular, this has already had a profound effect on the development of knowledge about cell signalling pathways, DNA repair, protein traffic within cells, and ion channels, to name only a few. In addition, because many of these processes are common to other organisms such as *Drosophila*, nematodes, and even yeast and bacteria, we can draw on research in these organisms to illuminate function in mammalian cells. A whole area of research, called functional genomics by some, relies extensively on this comparative approach. Since mutations in genes are easily obtained in these model organisms, such mutant homologues can inform us about the cellular function of the gene, which can be carried over to the mammalian systems. The main experimental organism for functional analysis is the mouse, a mammalian model organism amenable to a special form of gene manipulation. A line of embryonic cells, ES cells, can be propagated in tissue culture, and when these are injected into a mouse blastula they become incorporated into the embryo and populate both the germline and somatic cells. In this way, as demonstrated by MJ Evans (see Chapter 4.7), transgenic mice can be constructed in which genes have been added or removed from the mouse genome. Mice in which genes have been deleted are called knockout transgenics and can reveal the contribution of the gene to the total phenotype. These methods were used to prove that prions cause the endogenous prion protein to adopt an incorrect form and so cause neurological disease. Complete removal of the prion gene has no effect of its own but the animals become resistant to infection.

The most significant contribution made by the new genetics has been the identification of the genes involved in single-gene mutations in humans. More than 1000 such monogenic inherited disorders have been identified; some rare, others, such as cystic fibrosis, quite common. These provide the direct test of function and they throw light on the pathogenesis of disease and the underlying molecular causes. In certain areas, such as cholesterol metabolism, the analysis of the changes in certain monogenic diseases has revealed the connections between cholesterol and the ensuing cardiovascular pathology. In addition, even very rare monogenic diseases which resemble the much more common diseases, such as the cases of breast cancer or Alzheimer's disease, can lead us to understand the pathogenic pathways involved.

There are, however, several very common diseases which can be shown to have a genetic component but are not due to single-gene mutations. Schizophrenia, diabetes, and Crohn's disease are common and are about 50% correlated in identical twins. There is, therefore, a large environmental component and the fact that the diseases are polygenic makes it difficult to discover the genes involved. However, the possibility that one might identify the genes with polymorphisms correlating with the disease state has led to the development of what is called predictive medicine or probabilistic medicine. We only have a few of these disease susceptibility markers, but the fact that genetic analysis may be predictive has raised many questions about the ethical, social, and legal consequences of genetic testing. There is very little established work in this field but already difficult issues have been raised, mostly created by health insurance.

It is clear that in the rush to obtain the sequence of the human genome, the understanding of the connections between genotype and phenotype has remained superficial. There is a tendency in popular media to talk about genes 'for' homosexuality, alcoholism, criminality, and so on. The unravelling of the complex skein of connections between the genes and the final phenotype has only just begun and it will occupy biomedical scientists for the next few decades, at least. DNA sequencing is a unique technology; one can feed a machine with DNA derived from anything—plants, bacteria, humans—and the linear sequence of bases which is the essential information in the DNA can be extracted. There has been an explosion in the amount of data available and there will be much more to come. However, data are not knowledge and only knowledge can lead to understanding the meaning of the sequence and enable us the better to diagnose and treat human disease.

4.2.2 The genomic basis of medicine

Paweł Stankiewicz and James R. Lupski

Essentials

During the last two decades it has become possible to determine the entire DNA content of living organisms—the genome. The completion of the human reference DNA sequence has provided an enormous amount of DNA sequence data and has extended our view of the genetic bases of disease.

Several structural variation studies (e.g. the HapMap and ENCODE projects) have revealed that human genetic variation is tremendous and consist of two major types: nucleotide sequence and genomic structural changes.

A first phase of the studies on genetic variation in humans has been focused on single nucleotide polymorphisms (SNPs). The large number of SNPs identified has enabled successful genome-wide association studies for disease risk of complex traits, e.g. diabetes and cancer.

Recent technology developments enabling a higher-resolution analysis of the human genome have uncovered extensive submicroscopic structural variation, copy-number variations (CNVs). CNVs involving dosage-sensitive genes result in several diseases and appear to contribute to human diversity and evolution.

An emerging group of genetic diseases have been described that result from DNA rearrangements rather than from single nucleotide changes. Such conditions have been referred to as genomic disorders.

Recurrent rearrangements, or those of common size and having clustered breakpoints, most frequently result from a mechanism of nonallelic homologous recombination (NAHR) between region-specific low-copy repeats, or segmental duplications. Nonrecurrent rearrangements, or those for which breakpoints do not cluster and that are generally different in size amongst families, can result from nonhomologous end-joining (NHEJ) recombination mechanism. Recently, a DNA replication mechanism has been shown to play an important role in the origin of nonrecurrent rearrangements.

The development of array-based comparative genomic hybridization (array CGH) has enabled high-resolution screening of genomic imbalances throughout the entire genome with the level of resolution depending only on the size and distance between the arrayed interrogating probes.

In the current postgenomic era both high-resolution genome analysis by array CGH and personalized diploid genomic sequencing applied to the study of inherited and complex traits promise a continued revolution in our understanding of normal physiology and the pathophysiology of disease heralding the genomic basis of medicine.

Introduction

The elucidation of the DNA double helix establishing the chemical basis of heredity in 1953 and the determination of the correct number of human chromosomes 3 years later laid the fundamentals for the development of two major fields in human and medical genetics: clinical molecular genetics and clinical cytogenetics. Although developing independently for the first four decades, molecular genetics and clinical cytogenetics have contributed enormously to provide a better understanding of the genetic bases of both human physiology and pathophysiology. In the last 10 to 15 years technological advances, mainly in fluorescence microscopy, have led to the development of molecular cytogenetics techniques that by enabling identification of submicroscopic chromosome rearrangements, bridged the 'resolution' gap between molecular genetics and clinical cytogenetics. As a consequence, since the early 1990s, the genomic aspects of inheritance have come to be recognized, as elucidated for example through studies of the submicroscopic CMT1A duplication causing Charcot–Marie–Tooth neuropathy.

The beginning of human genetics can be traced to the rediscovery of Gregor Mendel's observations on the inheritance of phenotypic traits in the garden pea *Pisum sativatum* and Archibald Garrod's elucidation of the genetics of biochemical traits such as alkaptonuria. Mendel found that during gamete formation, each member of the allelic pair separates from the other one to form the genetic constitution of the gamete. This phenomenon of independent segregation is now known as a Mendel's first law. Mendel's second law states that the segregation of two alleles (corresponding DNA loci on homologous chromosomes) during gamete formation is independent from the segregation of the alleles of other allelic pairs. We now know that linkage, the physical proximity of two genetic loci on a linear map, results in exceptions to Mendel's second law. Such linkage information has been used to map disease traits in humans. Mendel's 'inheritance factors' encoding the genetic information were further defined and termed 'genes' many years later.

During the last two decades it has become possible to determine the entire DNA content of the living organism—the genome. The first human reference genome sequence became available at the turn of this century. In the current postgenomic era both high-resolution genome analysis by array-based comparative genomic hybridization (array CGH) and personalized diploid genomic sequencing applied to the study of inherited and complex traits promise a continued revolution in our understanding of the genetic bases of normal physiology and the pathophysiology of disease.

Genes, chromosomes, and our genome

A gene is defined as a set of segments of DNA (desoxyribonucleic acid) or, that carries the information necessary to produce (transcribe) a functional RNA (ribonucleic acid). Despite the completion of the Human Genome Project (HGP), the exact number of genes in the human genome is still unknown; the current estimate is between 20 000 and 25 000.

The DNA double helix is a three-dimensional polymer composed of units called nucleotides. A combination of two purine bases, adenine (A) and guanine (G), and two pyrimidine bases, thymine (T) and cytosine (C), with desoxyribose sugars and linked by phosphodiester bonds (base + sugar + phosphate = nucleotide) constitute a single strand. The two strands are held together and stabilized by hydrogen bonds that enable Watson–Crick base pairs to form. The base A forms two hydrogen bonds with T while C forms three hydrogen bonds with G. A combination of three nucleotides constitutes a triplet codon that encodes an individual amino acid. Different triplets can encode the same amino acids or stop codons during translation (there are $4^3 = 64$ different codon combinations possible, but only 20 amino acids), making the genetic code degenerate.

Most genes consist of coding regions termed exons that are separated by intervening introns. The exonic and intronic portions of a gene are transcribed by ribonuclease II into messenger RNA, or mRNA, that usually begins with a cap on the 5′ end and terminates with a polyadenylated (polyA) tail on the 3′ end. The introns are deleted in a process called splicing and the resulting mature transcript, or spliced mRNA, is translated into a polypeptide chain starting with a methionine encoded by the AUG triplet (in RNA, thymine is replaced by uracil, U) at the 5′ end (N-terminal, NH_2, or amino end of polypeptide) and terminated by the stop codons: UAA (also known as ochre), UAG (amber), or UGA (opal) at the 3′ end (C-terminal, COOH, or carboxyl end of the polypeptide).

The normal flow of the genetic information is susceptible to perturbation at different levels. Changes in the base pairs are called mutations and can arise as a result of replication, recombination, and repair errors or by exposure to external factors (e.g. radiation or chemical mutagens). Structurally, small mutations can be divided into point mutations (substitutions), insertions, or deletions. The most common mutations involving exchange of pyrimidine for pyrimydine (e.g. C to T) or purine for purine (e.g. A to G) are called transitions. The rarer transversions substitute purine by pyrymidine (e.g. A to C) or the reciprocal (e.g. T to G). The CpG dinucleotide is particularly prone to transition mutations (about tenfold relative to other bases) because methylated C (after CpG island methylation) becomes T if deaminated, and now pairs with A.

DNA mutations that do not lead to a change in an amino acid, because of the degenerate code, are called silent mutations. These do not change an amino acid, but can have functional consequences if they create a cryptic splice site or affect an exon splice enhancer. Missense mutations result in an amino acid change and nonsense mutations introduce stop codons that truncate the protein prematurely. Small insertions and deletions called indels, which can shift a reading frame and thus alter the protein primary sequence structure, are called frameshift mutations. Abnormally truncated or erroneous transcripts with a premature termination codon (PTC) due to nonsense, frameshift, or splice mutations are eliminated from cells by a surveillance mechanism called nonsense mediated decay (NMD). NMD is usually triggered by a PTC in any exon except the last and a portion of the penultimate exon; PTCs in the last 50 to 55 bp of the penultimate exon or in the final exon escape NMD presumably because of the inability of the machinery to distinguish such a PTC from the normal stop codon. About one-third of all human disease-associated point mutations result from PTCs due to nonsense or frameshift alleles.

Mutations have been categorized also on the basis of their phenotypic outcomes. Loss-of-function mutations (hypomorphic if the loss is partial, amorphic if it is complete) manifest phenotypically when a decreased amount of protein is insufficient for the normal cell function (e.g. haploinsufficient genes). Gain-of-function mutations (neomorphic) enhance the normal or take on a new protein function, and dominant negative mutations (antimorphic) result in a protein that acts antagonistically with the normal product from the other allele or another subunit of a protein complex.

A genetic locus is said to be homozygous when two alleles have the same status (e.g. both alleles are mutated) and heterozygous when one allele is mutated and the second is normal (wild type). Compound heterozygotes have different mutations in both alleles of one gene. Double heterozygotes have two mutant alleles, but each is at a different locus. The status in which one of the alleles is absent, e.g. for most of the X chromosome genes in males, is described as hemizygous.

Typically, different mutations in a gene manifest with the same phenotype, a phenomenon described as allelic heterogeneity. However, different mutations in the same gene can sometimes lead to varied phenotypes. Such a situation is described as allelic affinity. Finally, if the same phenotype is caused by mutations in different genes, this is described as genetic or locus heterogeneity.

The human haploid genome consists of approximately 3×10^9 bp and the normal diploid human genome in each cell is approximately 6×10^9 bp. Most of the human genome is formed by repetitive DNA elements. They can be divided into tandem repeats represented by satellites (e.g. in centromeres), telomeric repeats, microsatellites and minisatellites, and interspersed repeats derived from transposable elements (e.g. *Alu* elements and L1 elements) and comprise up to 50% of the human genome. It has been estimated that about 4 to 5% of the haploid human genome is present in two or more copies, which have been termed low-copy repeats (LCRs) or segmental duplications.

The unique DNA sequence portion of the human genome includes genes, regulatory elements, and nongenic sequences. Recent data have shown that most of this DNA might be transcribed; however, the protein coding sequences occupy only about 1.5% of the human genome.

For every human, it is important to inherit the proper amount of genomic information with contributions from both parents and the correct copy-number of each genetic locus for proper function. The genes in a human genome are distributed along 46 chromosomes. There are 22 pairs of autosomal chromosomes and two sex chromosomes—X and Y in males and two X chromosomes in females. In a conventional clinical cytogenetic analysis using a light microscope, chromosomes can be recognized and distinguished from each other when their chromatin is condensed (arrested in metaphase of the cell cycle) and specifically stained, e.g. with Giemsa, revealing a characteristic G-banding pattern. Each human metaphase chromosome consists of two chromatids forming the chromosome arms connected by a centromere. Centromeres in the human genome consist of α-satellite DNA (arranged by monomers of approximately 171 bp) and occupy about 2 to 3% of the human genome. Depending on the relative location of the centromere, chromosomes have been divided into three types: metacentric (with similar-sized arms), submetacentric (with one arm significantly longer that the other, the shorter arm referred to as p and the longer as q), and acrocentric (with a centromere located very close to one end of a chromosome—chromosomes 13, 14, 15, 21, and 22). Human chromosome ends are capped by telomeres that contain thousands of copies of a telomeric repeat sequence TTAGGG. Based on the size and relative centromere position, human chromosome pairs have been enumerated and arranged in a karyogram that is routinely applied in clinical cytogenetics.

Patterns of inheritance

Mendelian inheritance

Genetic traits can show mendelian or nonmendelian inheritance patterns. Mendelian traits involve a single locus, are usually monogenic, and segregate in an autosomal dominant, autosomal recessive, or X-linked fashion.

In autosomal dominant inheritance, the mutated allele is transmitted to 50% of the gametes and thus is expected to be present in one-half of the progeny. However, if the trait is lethal, incompletely penetrant, age dependent, or results in variation in expressivity, this proportion may vary from 0 to 50%. In pedigree analysis, autosomal dominant inheritance is observed as a vertical transmission of the trait.

In an autosomal recessive trait the affected individuals carry two mutant alleles, each one usually inherited from both carrier parents, and represent one-fourth of the progeny. Of the remaining healthy sibs, two-thirds are carriers of the mutant allele and one-third (one-fourth of all progeny) have two wild-type alleles. When the mutated alleles in the affected subject are the same, the family is usually consanguineous. In pedigree analysis, autosomal recessive inheritance is revealed as horizontal transmission of the trait. Of note, for a few autosomal recessive genes it has been shown that the heterozygous carriers of the mutated allele may have an increased susceptibility to complex or multifactorial traits (Table 4.2.2.1).

In females, the vast majority of genes on the X chromosome undergo random inactivation and thus represent structural disomy but functional monosomy. If one of the X chromosomes harbours a mutated recessive allele, X inactivation is usually nonrandomly skewed with the X chromosome harbouring the mutant allele being preferentially inactivated. Therefore, X-linked recessive diseases are not present in females but affect all males since they have only one X chromosome. However, females with an incomplete X inactivation (e.g. the efficiency of X inactivation decreases significantly with age) or skewed X inactivation (e.g. 5–10% of females have a 80:20 ratio of X inactivation), females with Turner's syndrome and a 45,X karyotype, or females carrying a balanced translocation between the X chromosome and an autosome (X material on the derivative chromosomes is not inactivated) can manifest the X-linked recessive disease. In contrast, X-linked dominant diseases are present in both males and females and twice as many females as males are affected. However, the phenotype is usually milder in females than in males. Occasionally, if the disease is lethal in males, the trait can be visible only in females (e.g. Rett's syndrome). In the X-linked diseases, no male-to-male transmission is observed and all daughters of affected fathers are obligate carriers of the mutated allele.

Penetrance, expressivity, and age of onset

The determination of the mendelian segregation pattern can be challenged in pedigree analysis by incomplete penetrance, wherein a phenotypic feature can be present or absent (e.g. in Marfan's syndrome), variable expressivity, when the same mutation leads to different severity or pattern of the phenotype (e.g. in cystic fibrosis), or manifestations depending on age (e.g. in Huntington's disease).

Nonmendelian inheritance

There are many genetic abnormalities which show familial recurrence yet do not demonstrate mendelian segregation patterns. Such nonmendelian traits can be due to multiple aetiologies, including genomic imprinting, uniparental disomy, mosaicism, mitochondrial DNA mutations, digenic or triallelic inheritance.

Genomic imprinting

If a phenotypic trait is transmitted through only one gender (parent-of-origin effect), genomic imprinting should be considered. During the passage through meiosis, a number of genes are silenced (imprinted) in a sex-specific manner. For example, the paternal copy of the *UBE3A* gene on chromosome 15q11.2 is imprinted during spermatogenesis. In the progeny, only the allele inherited from the mother is expressed and is sufficient to produce enough RNA for normal cell function. When this single active allele is mutated or deleted, the individual is affected (in this case with Angelman's syndrome). The sex-specific imprint of *UBE3A* is erased upon the entrance of chromosome 15 into meiosis and, depending on the sex, a new imprint is established; again, only one allele is expressed.

Uniparental disomy

The active allele of the imprinted gene will not be transmitted to the progeny if both homologous chromosomes harbouring the imprinted allele are inherited from one parent. Such lack of normal biparental inheritance of homologous chromosomes has been defined as uniparental disomy. Two major types of uniparental disomy have been described, heterodisomy and isodisomy. In heterodisomy, two homologous chromosomes from one parent are transmitted to the child and in isodisomy, both homologous chromosomes in an offspring originate from only one of the parental homologues. If a recessive gene is present on the isodisomic chromosome, the disease will manifest even though only one parent is a carrier for the mutation. The most frequent mechanism responsible for uniparental disomy is chromosome nondisjunction in meiosis I followed by trisomy to disomy rescue in an early postzygotic stage of the embryo. In humans, among autosomes only trisomies 13, 18, and 21 are compatible with life. In certain tissues, the cells carrying an extra (trisomic) chromosome can survive only if one of the three copies of the homologous chromosomes (or a large portion thereof) is lost. This process of elimination of the extra chromosome is called trisomy rescue. Since this is a random event, in one third of cases the remaining chromosomes will be from the same parent, thus representing uniparental disomy. Because most cases result from an initial nondisjunction event, uniparental disomy is associated with advanced maternal age.

Table 4.2.2.1 Recessive disorders and heterozygous predisposition to multifactorial disease

Monogenic disease	OMIM	Gene	Multifactorial disease	OMIM
Familial hypercholesterolemia	143890	*LDLR*	Coronary artery disease	108725
Ataxia-telangiectasia	208900	*ATM*	Breast cancer	114480
α_1-Antitrypsin deficiency	107400	*AAT*	Chronic obstructive lung disease	606963
Hyperlipoproteinemia	238600	*LPL*	Ischaemic heart disease	612030
Cystic fibrosis	219700	*CFTR*	Pancreatic insufficiency, Chronic rhinosinusitis, Idiopathic bronchiectasis	167800, 211400
Progressive familial intrahepatic cholestasis	602347	*ABCB4*	Intrahepatic cholestasis of pregnancy	147480
Stargardt disease	248200	*ABCR* (*ABCA4*)	Age-related macular degeneration	153800

Mitochondrial inheritance

If a phenotypic trait is inherited only from mothers and never from fathers, then mitochondrial disease should be considered. Mitochondrial DNA (mtDNA) is present in multiple copies in the cell cytoplasm and is transmitted to progeny only through the oocytes; the sperm carries a negligible amount of mtDNA. Currently, at least 26 disease traits are known to be encoded by mitochondrial DNA. In some cases, both the mother and her child may present with various severity of the phenotype due to a different proportion of mutated mtDNA in the cytoplasm, a phenomenon called heteroplasmy. In mitochondrial disease, the most energy-dependent tissues (e.g. eyes, brain, heart) may be the first to reveal clinical signs and symptoms.

Digenic inheritance

A number of diseases that are not complex traits and are not inherited as simple single-gene mendelian disorders have been shown recently to be caused by mutations in two different genes, in which the other two alleles are normal. Such double heterozygotes that interact genetically to manifest the phenotype have been described for example in retinitis pigmentosa (*ROM1* and *RDS* encode interacting gene products) and deafness (*GJB6* and *GJB2*) (Table 4.2.2.2).

Triallelic inheritance

Bardet–Biedl syndrome, a pleiotropic mendelian recessive disorder characterized by postnatal obesity, postaxial polydactyly, and progressive retinal dystrophy, can be caused in some families by mutations in at least two genes. Mutation analyses in these genes have revealed that in some patients with Bardet–Biedl syndrome, three mutations in two different genes segregated with expression of the disease. This phenomenon has been described as triallelic inheritance and has been observed in other diseases also (e.g. familial hypercholesterolemia and cortisone reductase deficiency). Based on this observation, an oligogenic type of inheritance (i.e. mutations in a small number of genes combined rather than a single locus mutation) was proposed to explain some other phenotypes, such as Hirschsprung's disease (see Table 4.2.2.2).

Mosaicism

Another distortion of mendelian inheritance can be caused by mosaicism. Two or more cell lines can be present either in the gonads only (germline mosaicism) or in somatic cells. Mosaicism should be suspected when healthy parents have two or more children with a dominant disease.

Pleiotropy and epistasis

Pleiotropy occurs when a single gene has more than one distinguishable phenotypic effect. Epistasis refers to interaction between genes, in which a phenotypic effect is different from what would be expected if mutations of the genes were expressed independently.

Table 4.2.2.2 Models of disease allele transmission

Locus	Allele	Example (disease/gene)
Monogenic	Monoallelic	Angelman (*UBE3A*)
	Biallelic	Cystic fibrosis (*CFTR*)
	Triallelic	CMT1A (*PMP22*)
Digenic	Biallelic	RP (*ROM1-RDS*)
	Triallelic	BBS (*BBS1–8*)

In both situations, the inheritance pattern in pedigree analysis can appear as nonmendelian.

Genetic and genomic variation

Genetic variation

The Human Genome Project has provided an enormous amount of DNA sequence data; however, it did not assess the scale of genetic and genomic polymorphic variation between different individuals and among populations. The International HapMap Project (HapMap) was developed in 2002 to determine the common patterns of human DNA sequence variation and to generate a haplotype map (i.e. a linked set of genetic markers) of the human genome that in turn would help to identify genes affecting health, responsible for diseases and responses to drugs and environmental factors. Concurrently, the Human Genome Diversity Project (HGDP) was established to help to understand the diversity and unity of the entire human species, and the ENCODE (ENCyclopedia Of DNA Elements) Project was launched to help to interpret this information and to better understand the biology of human health and disease. By using high-throughput methods, the ENCODE Project has generated a comprehensive catalogue of the structural and functional components encoded in the human genome sequence, including protein-coding genes, nonprotein-coding genes, transcriptional regulatory elements, and sequences that mediate chromosome structure and dynamics. HGP, HapMap, HGDP, ENCODE, and several additional studies have revealed that human genetic variation is tremendous and consist of two major types: nucleotide sequence and genomic structural changes. Human genetic and genomic studies have resulted in the proliferation of several databases required to interpret the potential clinical significance or relevance of variation (Table 4.2.2.3).

Types of variations

Single nucleotide polymorphisms (SNPs)

A genetic polymorphism is defined as a heterozygous DNA variation found in more than 1% of the general population. A first phase of the studies on genetic variation in humans has focused on single-nucleotide polymorphisms (SNPs). A SNP is a nucleotide change that results from a base substitution during DNA replication. The frequency of such events has been estimated as 10^{-8} per base pair per generation. The vast majority of SNPs represent inherited changes that have accumulated over thousands of human generations. Depending on random genetic drift or natural selection models, the frequency of a particular SNP in the population can significantly change over generations.

Typically, there are two alleles for a SNP locus. SNPs are predominantly localized in the noncoding portion of the human genome; only 4 million out of over 27 million currently known SNPs map within genes. A SNP that does not change the polypeptide sequence is termed synonymous (or silent mutation) and if it leads to a polypeptide sequence change it is described as nonsynonymous. It has been shown that SNPs that are not in protein-coding regions may still have functional consequences; they can generate splicing mutations, modify transcription factor binding sites or gene regulatory elements, or change the sequence of noncoding RNAs.

A combination of closely linked SNPs is defined as a haplotype. Haplotypes result from reduced recombination (crossing-over) events between closely linked genetic markers during meiosis

Table 4.2.2.3 Summary of useful genomic websites

Name	URL	Description
DECIPHER, DatabasE of Chromosomal Imbalance and Phenotype in Humans	http://www.sanger.ac.uk/PostGenomics/decipher	Database of submicroscopic chromosomal imbalance describes clinical phenotype associated with submicroscopic rearrangements
Database of Genomic Variants	http://projects.tcag.ca/variation/	A curated catalogue of structural variation in the human genome
dbSNP	http://www.ncbi.nlm.nih.gov/projects/SNP/	A public-domain archive for a broad collection of simple genetic polymorphisms
ECARUCA	http://agserver01.azn.nl:8080/ecaruca/ecaruca.jsp	European Cytogeneticists Association Register of Unbalanced Chromosome Aberrations
Ensembl	http://www.ensembl.org/	Wellcome Trust funded software system which produces and maintains automatic annotation on selected eukaryotic genomes
GeneTests/GeneReview	http://www.genetests.org/	A publicly funded medical genetics information resource developed for physicians, other health care providers, and researchers
Human Gene Mutation Database	http://www.hgmd.cf.ac.uk/ac/index.php?	HGMD constitutes a comprehensive core collection of data on germ-line mutations in nuclear genes underlying or associated with human inherited disease
OMIM, Online Mendelian Inheritance in Man	http://www.ncbi.nlm.nih.gov/sites/entrez?db=OMIM	A catalogue of human genes and genetic disorders authored and edited by Dr Victor A. McKusick and his colleagues at Johns Hopkins and elsewhere
UCSC Genome Bioinformatics	http://genome.ucsc.edu/	This site contains the reference sequence and working draft assemblies for a large collection of genomes

and are generally shared between different populations; however, their frequency can differ widely. The nonrandom association of SNPs is described as linkage disequilibrium. The large number of SNPs identified has enabled successful genome-wide association studies (GWAS) for disease risk of complex traits, e.g. in diabetes and cancer (Table 4.2.2.4).

Repetitive DNA elements

Variable number of tandem repeats (VNTR); short tandem repeats (STRs)

Di-, tri-, and tetra-nucleotide repeats such as $(GT)_n$, $(CAA)_n$, or $(GATA)_n$ have been referred to as microsatellites. They are very unstable and polymorphic genomic loci, thus useful in population genetics, pedigree analysis, recombination and linkage studies, and in determining paternity or parental origin of chromosomes.

Minisatellites are DNA segments that consist of a short series (10–100 bp) of GC-rich tandem repeats and are present at more than 1000 locations in the human genome.

Retrotransposons

Alu elements are approximately 300 bp in size, present in approximately 1 million copies, and occupy approximately 10% of the human genome. The pathogenic function of *Alu* elements has been demonstrated to be exerted by two major mechanisms: insertional mutagenesis, utilizing an RNA intermediate to move or transpose *Alu* into exons or near spice junctions, and postinsertional 'activity', wherein *Alu* elements that share high sequence similarity serve as potential substrates for *Alu–Alu*-mediated nonallelic homologous recombination (NAHR) or Fork Stalling and Template Switching (FoSReS). Examples of diseases caused by *Alu* elements

Table 4.2.2.4 Whole genome association studies. SNPs and complex traits

Disease	Locus	Reference
Breast cancer	*FGFR2*	Easton *et al.* (2007), *Nature*, **447**, 1087–1093 Hunter *et al.* (2007), *Nat Genet*, **39**, 870–874
Coronary heart disease	SNP, rs1333049, 9p21.3	Samani *et al.* (2007), *N Engl J Med*, **357**, 443–453
Crohn's disease	*IRGM*	Parkes *et al.* (2007), *Nat Genet*, **39**, 830–832
Diabetes	12q24, 12q13, 16p13 and 18p11	Todd *et al.* (2007), *Nat Genet*, **39**, 857–864
Macular degeneration	*CFH*	Li *et al.* (2006), *Nat Genet*, **38**, 1049–1054 Maller *et al.* (2006), *Nat Genet*, **38**, 1055–1059
Obesity	*FTO*	Dina *et al.* (2007), *Nat Genet*, **39**, 724–726 Frayling *et al.* (2007), *Science*, **316**, 889–894
Prostate cancer	8q24	Gudmundsson *et al.* (2007), *Nat Genet*, **39**, 631–637 Yeager *et al.* (2007), *Nat Genet*, **39**, 645–649
Rheumatoid arthritis	SNP, rs10499194, 6q23	Plenge *et al.* (2007), *Nat Genet*, **39**, 1477–1482

insertion include haemophilia A and B and breast cancer due to disruption of the *BRCA1* gene and by *Alu–Alu* recombination in the *LDLR* gene and C1 inhibitor locus.

L1 elements are approximately 6 kb long, present in approximately 500 000 copies, and account for about 17% of the human genome. They are an important source of genomic variation. Like *Alu* repeats, using an RNA intermediate, L1 elements can be mutagenic by insertions into genes. Due to their abundance in the human genome, L1 elements that have high sequence identity can also stimulate and mediate NAHR. L1 elements have been shown to mutate the genes responsible, for example, for Alport's syndrome, colon cancer, and Duchenne muscular dystrophy. Both *Alu* and L1 elements can be responsible for structural variation, of approximately 300 bp or 6 kb, respectively, when heterozygous at a given locus.

Dynamic mutations

Unlike the aforementioned DNA changes, which are usually transmitted through many generations without any change, more than 20 diseases have been described to date that are caused by unstable dynamic mutations occurring during DNA replication, repair, or recombination. Most of these mutations are represented by an expansion of a simple triplet or trinucleotide repeat sequence (e.g. CAG, CGG, CTG, AAG) in either coding regions (e.g. in Huntington's disease) or noncoding regions such as introns (e.g. in Friedreich's ataxia), or either 5′ untranslated regions (e.g. in fragile X syndrome) or 3′ untranslated regions (e.g. in myotonic dystrophy). These triplet repeat diseases have been shown to be inherited as autosomal dominant (e.g. in myotonic dystrophy), autosomal recessive (e.g. in Friedreich's ataxia), or X-linked (e.g. in fragile X syndrome) traits due to gain- or loss-of-function mutations.

The minimal number of disease-causing triplet repeats varies among different disorders, with 36 in Huntington's disease and about 200 in fragile X syndrome. The intermediate number of repeats, lower than in affected individuals but greater than in normals, is called premutation. It has recently been shown that premutations can have phenotypic effects. An increased incidence of ovarian failure in females and a late-onset neurological disorder in males have been reported in individuals carrying premutations in the fragile X syndrome *FMR1* gene.

Premutations have a potential to expand during meiosis and thus manifest the disease in the next generation. The nucleotide expansion often occurs in a sex-specific manner and can be observed in a pedigree as a parent-of-origin effect. For example, expansions in fragile X syndrome arise during oogenesis and not in spermatogenesis. The number of the pathogenic repeats can correlate inversely with the onset and severity of the disease; this provides a molecular explanation for the clinical phenomenon referred to as anticipation. Anticipation is observed in pedigree analysis as reduced age of onset in successive generations.

In Huntington's disease, the expandable triplet repeat CAG encodes for the amino acid glutamine. Individuals with Huntington's disease have 36 or more CAG repeats, which leads to polyglutamine expansion with subsequent huntingtin protein misfolding, aggregation, and degradation that exert toxic effects upon neurons. Similar polyglutamine expansions have been reported in several other neurological diseases (e.g. in spinocerebellar ataxia type 1). Expansions of polyalanine tracts beyond a certain threshold have been described as pathogenic, for example in congenital malformations, skeletal dysplasia, and nervous system anomalies. Other pathogenic expansions have been shown to involve tetranucleotides (e.g. CCTG in myotonic dystrophy type 2) and pentanucleotides (e.g. ATTCT in spinocerebellar ataxia type 10).

Secondary DNA structures

Abnormal secondary DNA structures can also be mutagenic. A number of DNA conformations, different from the canonical right-handed *B*-form, have been described. The best known non-*B* DNA structures include triplexes, left-handed DNA, bent DNA, cruciforms, nodule DNA, flexible and writhed DNA, G4 tetrad (tetraplexes), slipped structures, and sticky DNA. Some of these structures have been described as pathogenic for more than 20 neurological and psychiatric diseases.

One of the best known examples of the pathogenic role of non-*B* DNA structures are AT-rich cruciforms in the proximal chromosome 22q11.2, responsible for the most common recurrent non-Robertsonian translocation t(11;22)(q11.2;q23.3) in humans.

Copy-number variation (CNV)

In contrast to the more than 400 000 insertion or deletion polymorphisms less than 1 kb in size that have been well studied and annotated, until recently little was known about the polymorphic changes larger than this. The application of array CGH to analyse the genomes of normal humans has led recently to the discovery of extensive genomic structural variation, ranging in size from thousands to millions of bases, that are not recognizable by chromosomal banding. These changes have been termed copy-number variations (CNVs).

Deletions, duplications, triplications, insertions, or translocations can all result in CNVs. The total number, position, size, gene content, and population distribution of CNVs remains elusive. Recent estimates have suggested approximate figures of 6000 CNVs in 4000 regions overlapping 1500 genes. CNVs may account for as much as 360 to 500 Mb and represent 12 to 20% of the human genome. These numbers can still represent a conservative estimate given that CNVs of 1 to 50 kb in size have not been ascertained well since there has not been an accurate molecular method available to study such smaller rearrangements on a genome-wide scale in different populations. It is anticipated that with the wider application of array CGH techniques, and next-generation sequencing to determine individual diploid genomes, the amount of structural variation identified will increase significantly. The genomic distribution of CNVs has been shown to be nonrandom and correlates with exons, segmental duplications, and the mobile elements such as *Alu* repeats, probably reflecting their ongoing evolutionary role.

Like many other genomic rearrangements, CNVs can be inherited or sporadic. A commonly used and useful standard is to assume that *de novo* CNVs in association with a sporadic clinical phenotype are more likely to be disease causative. However, the phenotypic effects of CNVs are unclear and depend mainly on whether dosage-sensitive genes are affected by the genomic rearrangement. Some CNVs have been shown to be responsible for mendelian diseases, nonmendelian traits such as complex diseases, and common traits (including behavioral traits), or to represent benign polymorphic variation (Fig. 4.2.2.1; Table 4.2.2.5).

Sporadic disease can also potentially result from a combination of two CNVs at a single locus (e.g. analogous to the autosomal recessive neuromuscular disease spinal muscular atrophy or the renal disease nephronophthisis type I) or theoretically from two or

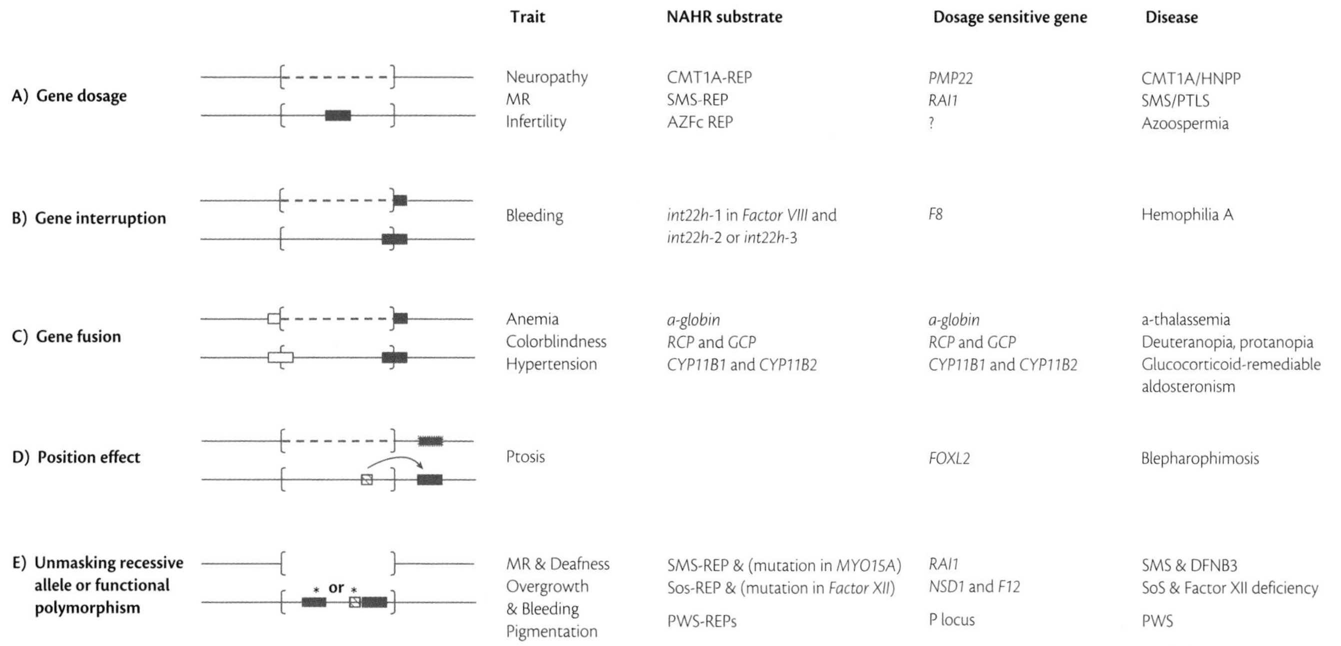

	Trait	NAHR substrate	Dosage sensitive gene	Disease
A) Gene dosage	Neuropathy MR Infertility	CMT1A-REP SMS-REP AZFc REP	*PMP22* *RAI1* ?	CMT1A/HNPP SMS/PTLS Azoospermia
B) Gene interruption	Bleeding	*int22h-1* in *Factor VIII* and *int22h-2* or *int22h-3*	*F8*	Hemophilia A
C) Gene fusion	Anemia Colorblindness Hypertension	*a-globin* *RCP* and *GCP* *CYP11B1* and *CYP11B2*	*a-globin* *RCP* and *GCP* *CYP11B1* and *CYP11B2*	a-thalassemia Deuteranopia, protanopia Glucocorticoid-remediable aldosteronism
D) Position effect	Ptosis		*FOXL2*	Blepharophimosis
E) Unmasking recessive allele or functional polymorphism	MR & Deafness Overgrowth & Bleeding Pigmentation	SMS-REP & (mutation in *MYO15A*) Sos-REP & (mutation in *Factor XII*) PWS-REPs	*RAI1* *NSD1* and *F12* P locus	SMS & DFNB3 SoS & Factor XII deficiency PWS

Fig. 4.2.2.1 Schematic models for molecular mechanisms of genomic disorders. For each model, examples of trait, NAHR substrate, and disease are shown. (A) gene dosage, where there is a dosage-sensitive gene within the rearrangement; (B) gene interruption, wherein the rearrangement breakpoint disrupts a gene; (C) gene fusion, whereby a fusion gene is created at the breakpoint that either fuses coding sequences or a novel regulatory sequence to the gene. For example, two genes encoding cytochrome P450 enzymes *CYP11B2* (aldosterone synthase) and ACTH-regulated *CYP11B1* (11-β-hydroxylase, cortysol biosynthesis) located on chromosome 8q21 are 45 kb apart and have 10 kb segments of 95% sequence identity. NAHR between these two genes results in a chromosome deletion, yielding a fusion hybrid *CYP11B1/CYP11B2* gene. *CYP11B1/CYP11B2* is under the regulation of ACTH and leads to glucocorticoid-remediable aldosteronism (GRA, MIM 103900). All symptoms of the disease can be normalized by the administration of glucocorticoid analogues and are exacerbated by administration of ACTH; (D) position effect, in which the rearrangement has effects on expression/regulation of a gene near the breakpoint, potentially by removing or altering a regulatory sequence; and (E) unmasking recessive allele, where a deletion results in hemizygous expression of a recessive mutation or further uncovers/exacerbates effects of a functional polymorphism. In each model, both chromosome homologues are depicted as horizontal lines. The rearranged genomic interval is enclosed by brackets. Dashed lines indicate genomic regions either deleted or duplicated, an absent line indicates deletion with phenotypic effects from the remaining allele unmasked because of the rearrangement, and a dotted line represents deletion but where phenotypic effects result from the absence of interactions between alleles. Gene is depicted by filled horizontal rectangle, while regulatory region is shown as a hatch-marked square. Asterisks denote point mutations.
CMT1A, Charcot–Marie–Tooth disease type 1A; DFNB3, deafness, neurosensory, autosomal recessive 3; HNPP, hereditary neuropathy with liability to pressure palsies; MR, mental retardation; PWS, Prader–Willi syndrome; SMS, Smith–Magenis syndrome; PMD, Pelizaeus–Merzbacher syndrome; PTLS, Potocki–Lupski syndrome; SoS, Sotos syndrome.
Adapted from Lupski JR, Stankiewicz P (2005). Genomic disorders: molecular mechanisms for rearrangements and conveyed phenotypes. *PLoS Genet*, **1**, e49.

more CNVs at different loci from two normal parents. CNVs have been proposed also to be a major factor responsible for human diversity and evolution.

CNVs have been catalogued in public databases such as the Toronto Database of Genomic Variants. Clinically relevant CNVs can be found in: DECIPHER and ECARUCA (see Table 4.2.2.3).

Genomic disorders

In the past 15 years, it has become evident that higher-order genomic architectural features can lead to a susceptibility to DNA rearrangements that are a frequent cause of diseases in humans. Such conditions that result from rearrangements of the human genome have been referred to as genomic disorders.

Table 4.2.2.5 CNVs and complex traits

Disease	Gene	Reference
Alzheimer's disease	*APP*	Rovelet-Lecrux *et al.* (2006), *Nat Genet*, **38**, 24–26
Chronic pancreatitis	*PRSS1*	Le Maréchal *et al.* (2006), *Nat Genet*, **38**, 1372–1374
Crohn's disease	*HBD-2*	Fellermann *et al.* (2006), *Am J Hum Genet*, **79**, 439–448
HIV	*CCL3L1*	Gonzalez *et al.* (2005), *Science*, **307**, 1434–1440
Lupus with glomerulonephritis	*FCGR3B*	Aitman *et al.* (2006), *Nature*, **439**, 851–855
Parkinson's disease	*SNCA*	Singleton *et al.* (2003), *Science*, **302**, 841
Systemic lupus erythematosus	*Complement C4 component*	Yang *et al.* (2007), *Am J Hum Genet*, **80**, 1037–1054

Table 4.2.2.6 New mutation rates for genomic rearrangements

Rearrangement hot spot	Mutation rate direct measure		Method	Mutation rate indirect estimate		Method
	Deletion	Duplication		Deletion	Duplication	
CMT1A-REP	4.2×10^{-5}	1.73×10^{-5}	Real-time PCR on sperm DNA		$1.7–2.6 \times 10^{-5}$	Prevalence + molecular
AZFa-HERV	2.16×10^{-5}	5.26×10^{-6}	Real-time PCR on sperm DNA			
LCR17p	1.87×10^{-6}	8.74×10^{-7}	Real-time PCR on sperm DNA			
WBS-LCR	9.55×10^{-6}	4.54×10^{-6}	Real-time PCR on sperm DNA	$2.0–12.5 \times 10^{-5}$		Prevalence
DGS/VCFS; SMS				$2.0–12.5 \times 10^{-5}$		Prevalence
DMD				1.0×10^{-4}	1.0×10^{-4}	Prevalence + molecular
α-Globin				4.2×10^{-5}		Sperm PCR
t(11;22)				$1.2–9.5 \times 10^{-5}$ (translocation)		Sperm PCR
Normal controls				1.7×10^{-6}	1.7×10^{-6}	Array CGH of trios

Adapted from Turner DJ, *et al.* (2008). Germline rates of *de novo* meiotic deletions and duplications causing several genomic disorders. *Nat Genet*, **40**, 90–5. and Lupski JR (2007). Genomic rearrangements and sporadic disease. *Nat Genet*, **39**, S43–7.

Many genomic disorders occur sporadically and these frequent events are often caused by *de novo* rearrangements. Different calculations have shown that the *de novo* locus-specific mutation rates for genomic rearrangements are between 10^{-4} and 10^{-5}, at least 100- to 10 000-fold more frequent than point mutations (Table 4.2.2.6).

Genomic rearrangements can cause mendelian diseases or complex traits such as behaviours, or may represent benign polymorphic changes. The major mechanism by which rearrangements convey phenotypes is gene dosage due to a variation in gene copy number. When the deleted or duplicated region harbours a dosage-sensitive gene, the rearrangement will lead to an abnormal phenotype. Other mechanisms include gene interruptions, gene fusions, position effects, and unmasking of mutations in coding region or other functional SNPs in the second allele (Fig. 4.2.2.1).

For a few genomic disorders, significant differences in incidences have been observed in different world populations. In some of them, structural variations of the genomic region in the patients' parents have been found, demonstrating that the variation of genomic architecture is a significant factor for disease susceptibility. For instance, submicroscopic genomic inversions can result in haplotype blocks (due to reduced recombination) and generate an architecture with directly oriented low-copy repeats that can act as NAHR substrates. This can lead to the susceptibility to deletion/duplication rearrangements only in the individuals within the population who harbour the inversion variant with the rearrangement-prone genome architecture (e.g. in Williams–Beuren syndrome or 17q21.31 microdeletion syndrome).

Low-copy repeats

DNA fragments larger than 1 kb in size and of more than 90% DNA sequence identity have been termed low-copy repeats or segmental duplications. Many low-copy repeats have a complex structure and have arisen during primate speciation over the last 25 to 40 million years as a result of serial segmental duplications.

Low-copy repeats longer than 10 kb and of more than about 97% sequence identity can lead to local genomic instability. Low-copy repeats have been shown to stimulate and/or mediate constitutional (both recurrent and nonrecurrent), evolutionary, and somatic genomic rearrangements.

Nonallelic homologous recombination (NAHR)

When located at a distance less than 5 to 10 Mb from each other, low-copy repeats can mediate NAHR, and potentially result in unequal crossing-over. NAHR between directly oriented low-copy repeats leads to deletions or reciprocal duplications of the genomic region located between them, and NAHR between the inverted low-copy repeats results in an inversion of the intervening genomic segment. In low-copy repeats of a more complex genomic structure consisting of both direct and inverted subunits, distinct portions can serve as NAHR substrates leading to deletions/duplications or inversions, respectively.

Recombination hot spots

Interestingly, the strand exchanges for NAHR sites are not scattered throughout the length of homology within low-copy repeats, but cluster in recombination hot spots. However, no specific primary or secondary DNA sequence motifs or features of DNA have been identified in these hot spots that may act in *cis* to stimulate recombination. Recent work demonstrates that normal allelic homologous recombination, like NAHR, is characterized by hot spots and cold spots throughout the genome.

Microdeletion and microduplication syndromes

Two common autosomal dominant peripheral neuropathies, CMT1A and hereditary neuropathy with liability to pressure palsies (HNPP) are amongst the first and best-characterized genomic disorders. CMT1A and HNPP are caused in over 99% of cases by copy-number change of a dosage-sensitive myelin gene *PMP22* as a result of reciprocal duplication and deletion, respectively, of an approximately 1.4-Mb genomic fragment within 17p12. This genomic segment is flanked by two low-copy repeats of about 24 kb, approximately 98.7% identical, termed the proximal CMT1A-REP and the distal CMT1A-REP, which serve as substrates for NAHR.

The proximal chromosome 17p also harbours another unstable genomic region with a haploinsufficient *RAI1* gene. Deletions and point mutations of *RAI1* result in Smith–Magenis syndrome (SMS), a disorder with multiple congenital anomalies and mental retardation characterized by minor craniofacial and skeletal anomalies such as brachycephaly, frontal bossing, synophrys, midfacial hypoplasia, short stature, and brachydactyly, neurobehavioral abnormalities such as aggressive and self-injurious behaviour and sleep disturbances, and ophthalmic, otolaryngological, cardiac, and renal anomalies. An genomic segment of approximately 4 Mb encompassing *RAI1* and flanked by large, complex, highly identical, and directly oriented, proximal (approximately 256 kb) and distal (approximately 176 kb) low-copy repeats termed SMS-REPs is deleted in 70 to 80% of patients with Smith–Magenis syndrome via the NAHR mechanism (i.e. common recurrent deletion).

The reciprocal duplication dup(17)(p11.2p11.2) of this region has been described in patients with Potocki–Lupski syndrome. Clinical features observed in patients with this syndrome are distinct from those seen with Smith–Magenis syndrome and include infantile hypotonia, failure to thrive, mental retardation, autistic features, sleep apnoea, and structural cardiovascular anomalies.

Other well-characterized microdeletion syndromes include Williams–Beuren syndrome (7q11.23), Prader–Willi and Angelman's syndromes (15q11.2q12), DiGeorge/velocariofacial syndrome (22q11.2), microdeletion 17q21.31 syndrome, and Sotos syndrome (5q35). For all these microdeletions, the reciprocal microduplications predicted by the NAHR model have been reported. The phenotypic manifestation of microduplication syndromes is milder than their reciprocal microdeletion counterpart. In chromosome duplications, the increase of 2 to 3 in gene copy number results in a 1.5-fold increase (50% change) of the protein amount, vs the 2 to 1 decrease in gene copy number leading to 2-fold reduction (100% change) of the protein amount in the reciprocal deletions.

With the exception of the X chromosome rearrangements, more pathogenic deletions than duplications have been identified in patients. This can be partially explained by the ascertainment bias due to the milder or even normal phenotype of patients with duplications vs deletions, and technical challenges with detecting duplications (3:2 vs 2:1 copies) as well as the fact that only deletion products of intrachromatid NAHR are transmitted to progeny (the reciprocal duplication product is acentric and thus lost in cell divisions).

Nonhomologous end joining (NHEJ) and fork stalling and template switching (FoSTeS)

The NAHR/low-copy repeat mechanism is most prevalent and responsible for the common recurrent deletions, duplications, or inversions. Nonrecurrent rearrangements have been shown in selected cases to arise by nonhomologous end joining (NHEJ) mechanism, where the low-copy repeats, if present, stimulate but do not mediate the recombination events.

Recently, DNA replication errors have been shown to play an important role in the origin of some genomic disorders due to nonrecurrent rearrangements. In some complex genomic rearrangements, consisting of deletions and/or duplications interrupted by either normal copy number or triplicated genomic segments, a replication-based mechanism called fork stalling and template switching (FoSTeS), similar to that described for *E. coli* genome amplifications induced under stress, has been proposed.

Chromosome aberrations

Variations of the human genome larger than about 5 Mb in size can be visible in the light microscope and are referred to as chromosome aberrations. Chromosome aberrations are frequent events, with the total incidence estimated as 1 in approximately 160 live births. They can be categorized as numerical or structural abnormalities. Numerical abnormalities (1 in approximately 250 newborns) are observed more frequently than structural ones (1 in approximately 375 newborns).

Numerical aberrations

Triploidies, tetraploidies

Deviations from the normal chromosome number are usually unbalanced and defined as aneuploidy. Triploid (3n) complements of chromosomes, 69,XXX, 69,XXY, or 69,XYY, typically result from an egg being fertilized by two sperms. Tetraploid (4n) sets, 92,XXYY or 92,XXXX, are caused by a failure in zygote division. Both triploidies and tetraploidies states are lethal.

Trisomies, monosomies

In contrast, the more common aneuploidies, trisomies and monosomies, result from chromosome nondisjunction in meiosis I, or sometimes in meiosis II, and in some cases (particularly those involving the sex chromosomes) are compatible with life. Although the most frequent aneuploidy in humans is trisomy 21 in patients with Down's syndrome (1 in 670 newborns), aneuploidies of sex chromosomes are more frequent (1 in 440 newborns) than those involving autosomes (1 in 700 newborns). This is due to the fact that, in addition to trisomy 21, only trisomies of chromosome 18 (Edwards' syndrome, 1 in 7500 newborns) and chromosome 13 (Patau's syndrome, 1 in 22 700 newborns) are compatible with life.

Although approximately 99% of fetuses with monosomy X are spontaneously aborted, patients with Turner's syndrome account for 1 in 4000 female newborns. Very often, however, the 45,X cell line is mosaic, accompanied by another cell line with either a normal cell chromosome complement or structural rearrangements of chromosome X (e.g. deletion of the short arm, ring chromosome, or isochromosome of the long or short arms). The most frequent aneuploidy during fetal life, trisomy 16 (one-third of all trisomies), leads to early miscarriages and is not identified in live newborns. The karyotype 47,XXY is found in patients with Klinefelter's syndrome (1 in 1000 male newborns).

Marker chromosomes

Marker chromosomes (SMCs) are small supernumerary chromosomes and are detected with a frequency of 0.24/1000 in newborns, 0.4 to 1.5/1000 in prenatal studies, 2 to 3/1000 among phenotypically abnormal individuals, and 0.5/1000 in the general population. Marker chromosomes are usually derived from acrocentric autosomes (*c.*85%), and particularly from chromosome 15 (some 40–50%). The risk of an abnormal phenotype in *de novo* cases has been estimated to be about 28%. The severity of the phenotype depends on the size of the marker chromosome and the extent of mosaicism.

Structural chromosome aberrations

Deletions and duplications

Chromosome deletions involving autosomes lead to structural and functional monosomies of the missing genomic material. In XY males, deletions of sex chromosomes result in structural and functional nullisomies. The phenotypic manifestation of a deletion is caused by the haploinsufficient gene(s) located in the deleted fragment or disrupted by the deletion breakpoint (Fig. 4.2.2.1).

If more than one haploinsufficent gene is present in the deleted region, the abnormality is referred to as a contiguous gene deletion syndrome, as in the Potocki–Shaffer syndrome (11p11.2) or Langer–Giedion syndrome (8q23q24). Many of the smaller deletions in the unstable genomic regions have been shown to have the same size and are recurrent. These microdeletion genomic disorders are usually caused by NAHR between directly oriented low-copy repeats and are frequent events (Table 4.2.2.6). For example, the deletions in chromosome 22q11.2 in patients with DiGeorge/velocardiofacial syndrome are found in 1 in 4000 newborns.

Reciprocal translocations

Reciprocal translocation is defined as an exchange of the chromosome segments between two chromosomes (homologous or nonhomologous). Balanced reciprocal translocations are found in approximately 1 in 600 individuals, so approximately 1 in 300 couples are at risk of unbalanced progeny. In most cases, balanced reciprocal translocations are not associated with an abnormal phenotype; however it has recently been shown that up to 40% of the apparently balanced reciprocal chromosome translocations in patients with abnormal phenotype are accompanied by a chromosome imbalance either at the translocation breakpoint or elsewhere in the genome. Balanced translocations can also have clinical consequences for normal individuals. Depending on the type of meiotic segregation and the size of the translocated chromosome material, the unbalanced meiotic products of the segregating translocation chromosomes can result in chromosome imbalance and be associated with either spontaneous abortions or births of affected children. The products of reciprocal chromosome translocation can be transmitted to progeny in a balanced or unbalanced form as a consequence of alternate or adjacent segregation.

In the vast majority of cases, reciprocal translocations appear to be random events. However, two of the most common constitutional non-Robertsonian translocations in humans have been shown to result from a specific genomic architectural features predisposing to recurrent events; the breakpoints of translocation t(11;22)(q11.2;q23.3) utilize AT-rich cruciforms whereas olfactory receptor gene clusters (constituting low-copy repeats on 4p and 8p) mediate the translocation t(4;8)(p16;p23). Genomic architecture involving low-copy repeats has also been shown to play a role in the formation of the most frequent somatic chromosome abnormality found in chronic myeloid leukaemia; translocation der(22) t(9;22)(q34;q11)—Philadelphia chromosome.

Robertsonian translocations

Translocation between two acrocentric chromosomes (13, 14, 15, 21, or 22), with breakpoints occurring in the short arms within or close to the centromere, is defined as Robertsonian translocation or centric fusion. Inverted repeats in acrocentric short arms have been proposed to mediate Robertsonian translocation.

One in approximately 900 newborns carry a Robertsonian translocation, making it the most common chromosome rearrangement in humans. In some cases, the rearrangement involving long arms of one chromosome is not a product of the centric fusion between two homologous chromosomes but a consequence of replication of one chromosome arm, and thus represents an isochromosome.

The karyotype of the carrier of Robertsonian translocation is balanced and consists of 45 chromosomes (the acentric heterochromatic short arms contain no genes and are lost during cell division). All combinations of acrocentric chromosomes have been found; however, translocations between chromosomes 13 and 14 or 14 and 21 are most prevalent, with the Robertsonian translocation 13;14 being the most common chromosome aberration in humans (1 in 1300). Carriers of Robertsonian translocation have a significantly increased risk of abnormal progeny; for example, carriers of translocation 21q21q have an almost 100% chance of having a child with Down's syndrome. The nonlethal trisomic products of Robertsonian translocation are those found in patients with Down's syndrome or Patau's syndrome (trisomy 13).

The carriers of Robertsonian translocation are also at increased risk of having offspring with uniparental disomy for the acrocentrics involved in the rearrangement due to the trisomy rescue mechanism (see above). Uniparental disomy has clinical consequences for carriers of Robertsonian translocations involving acrocentric chromosomes 14 and 15 that are known to contain imprinted genes.

Insertions

A nonreciprocal translocation of DNA material from one chromosome arm into another arm is described as an insertion or insertional translocation. The carrier of a balanced insertion has up to a 50% chance of an abnormal progeny.

Inversions

An inversion is defined as a double-break chromosome rearrangement, in which a segment of a chromosome is reversed and reinserted back into the chromosome. Some inversions (particularly those on chromosome 8p) have been shown to be mediated by a specific genomic architecture involving low-copy repeats in an inverted orientation.

When the inverted fragment contains the centromere, the inversion is described as pericentric. The recombination products of the pericentric inversion is a chromosome with a terminal deletion of one chromosome arm and a terminal duplication of the second arm. Paracentric inversions do not include the centromere; both breaks occur in one arm of the chromosome. The product of the paracentric inversion is either an acentric or dicentric chromosome; in both cases it is unstable and usually a lethal event. Typically, inversions are balanced; however, occasionally imbalances are found at their breakpoints. In addition, an inversion breakpoint can disrupt a dosage-sensitive gene (e.g. the most common cause of severe haemophilia A), resulting in an abnormal phenotype, or convey a phenotype because of a position effect.

Complex chromosome rearrangements

When more than two breakpoints involve two or more chromosomes the resulting aberration is referred to as complex chromosome rearrangement. These usually arise in spermatogenesis but are more often transmitted to subsequent generations through oogenesis.

Ring chromosomes

Ring chromosomes are usually formed when two chromosome arms break and fuse, thus forming a circular structure. Rings are often associated with abnormal phenotypes because of loss of genomic material at one or both chromosome ends. In rare cases, the breaks occur on one chromosome arm and the resulting ring chromosomes do not contain alphoid centromeres. Such acentric rings can generate neocentromeres from an euchromatic material and can be transmitted to the daughter cells. Rings are mitotically unstable, are often found in a mosaic state, and can form double ring structures as a result of crossing-over events.

Isochromosomes

When one chromosome arm is lost and the other is duplicated, the resulting mirror-image chromosome is called an isochromosome. When the breakpoint is within the centromere (centromere misdivision), the resulting isochromsome is monocentric and stable. If the original chromosome breaks outside the centromere, the derivative chromosome product is dicentric and thus unstable. To stabilize such a chromosome, one of the centromeres becomes inactive. Such chromosomes are then called pseudodicentric (pseudoisodicentric). The clinically relevant isochromosomes are, for example, isochromosomes of the long arms of chromosome X found in patients with Turner's syndrome. Moreover, an isodicentric chromosome idic(17)(p11.2) occurring as a somatic event is frequently found in chronic myeloid leukaemia and in childhood primitive neuroectodermal tumours. The idic(17)(p11.2) is recurrently formed utilizing large cruciform structures containing some 38 to 49 kb low-copy repeats of approximately 99.8% identity localized in the Smith–Magenis syndrome common deletion region in chromosome 17p11.2.

Centromere fission

Very rarely, as a result of centromere misdivision, the short arms of a chromosome are separated from its long arms and after replication form two isochromosomes, representing a balanced rearrangement. Such events are known as centromeric fission.

Heterochromatin variants

In addition to aberrations involving euchromatin, nonpathogenic variations of heterochromatin are often seen in karyotype analysis. The most common polymorphisms involve differences in size of satellite DNA of the short arm of acrocentric chromosomes and size or location of heterochromatin in 1qhet, 9qhet, 16qhet, and Yqhet.

Chromosome mosaicism

The presence of two or more different chromosome complements in one individual is defined as chromosomal mosaicism. Somatic chromosomal mosaicism is a well-known cause for birth defects, mental disability, and, in some instances, specific genetic syndromes such as hypomelanosis of Ito and Pallister–Killian syndrome (tetrasomy 12p). Chromosomal mosaicism is found in up to 50% of embryos at the eight-cell stage and up to 75% in blastocysts. The most common cause of chromosomal mosaicism is chromosome nondisjunction followed by trisomy rescue in a subpopulation of cells.

Routine clinical G-banded karyotype analysis is performed in a peripheral blood T lymphocytes stimulated to divide by phytohaemagglutinin. Thus, only a subpopulation of nucleated cells, and only those healthy enough to respond to stimulation, are expanded and examined. Recent applications of array CGH technology on genomic DNA extracted directly from uncultured peripheral blood has enabled the identification of mosaic chromosome abnormalities that were undetected by conventional karyotype analysis. Thus, array CGH has enabled better detection of mosaicism of unbalanced chromosome abnormalities than traditional cytogenetic techniques.

Genetic and genomic analyses

The pathogenic abnormalities in the human genome vary in size from single nucleotide changes (locus specific mutation rates approximately 10^{-6} to 10^{-8}) to copy number variation involving entire genes (mutation rate 10^{-4} to 10^{-5}) to microscopically visible chromosome aberrations (found in 1 in 160 newborns). Despite the broad spectrum of available techniques that have been developed recently to analyse the human genome, there is no single method that can identify all types of genetic and genomic variation. Thus, at different levels of resolution of human genome alterations, various techniques have to be used both in research and diagnostic applications (Fig. 4.2.2.2).

Single nucleotide changes

Point mutations are commonly analysed using conventional DNA sequencing with PCR amplification followed by chain termination with fluorescently labelled dideoxynucleotides. However, this method is low-throughput and relatively expensive. Novel 'next generation' DNA sequencing technologies have been developed recently for larger-scale genomic sequencing. The most promising technologies involve microarrays of amplified DNA or emulsion-based amplification of DNA fragments immobilized on beads. These technologies enable massive parallel sequencing that is robust, accurate, simple, fast, and cost effective. Tens of millions of high-quality bases per hour can be sequenced on a single instrument. Recently, the diploid genomes of two individuals have been sequenced: Craig Venter's personal genome was sequenced using conventional Sanger dideoxy technology and the diploid genome of James D. Watson was sequenced within a few weeks using the 454 Life Sciences technology.

A large number of SNPs analysed in genome-wide association studies are currently analysed using hybridization-based oligonucleotide microarrays (Table 4.2.2.4). The available technologies (Affymetrix, Illumina) enable analysis of more than 1 million SNPs in one experiment; however, they are still relatively expensive and in some cases require complicated equipment.

Small genomic rearrangements

Genomic rearrangements such as deletions, duplications, or inversions that are up to 30 kb in size can be detected using the polymerase chain reaction or Southern blot hybridization.

Genome structural changes

Large visible chromosome rearrangements can be analysed using the light microscope by conventional banding techniques (most often G-banding). The detection of genomic changes between 30 kb and 5 Mb in size had remained beyond the level of resolution of available methods until the development of the fluorescent *in situ* hybridization technique enabling identification and analysis of submicroscopic chromosome rearrangements. Likewise, pulsed-field gel electrophoresis enabled the resolution of genomic changes of such magnitude. However, both these technologies are still limited to the examination of specific genomic regions (i.e. they represent locus-specific tests).

The development of array CGH has enabled high-resolution screening of genomic imbalances throughout the entire genome simultaneously, with the level of resolution depending only on the size and distance between the arrayed interrogating probes. Initially, large genomic clones (bacterial or P1 artificial chromosomes) have

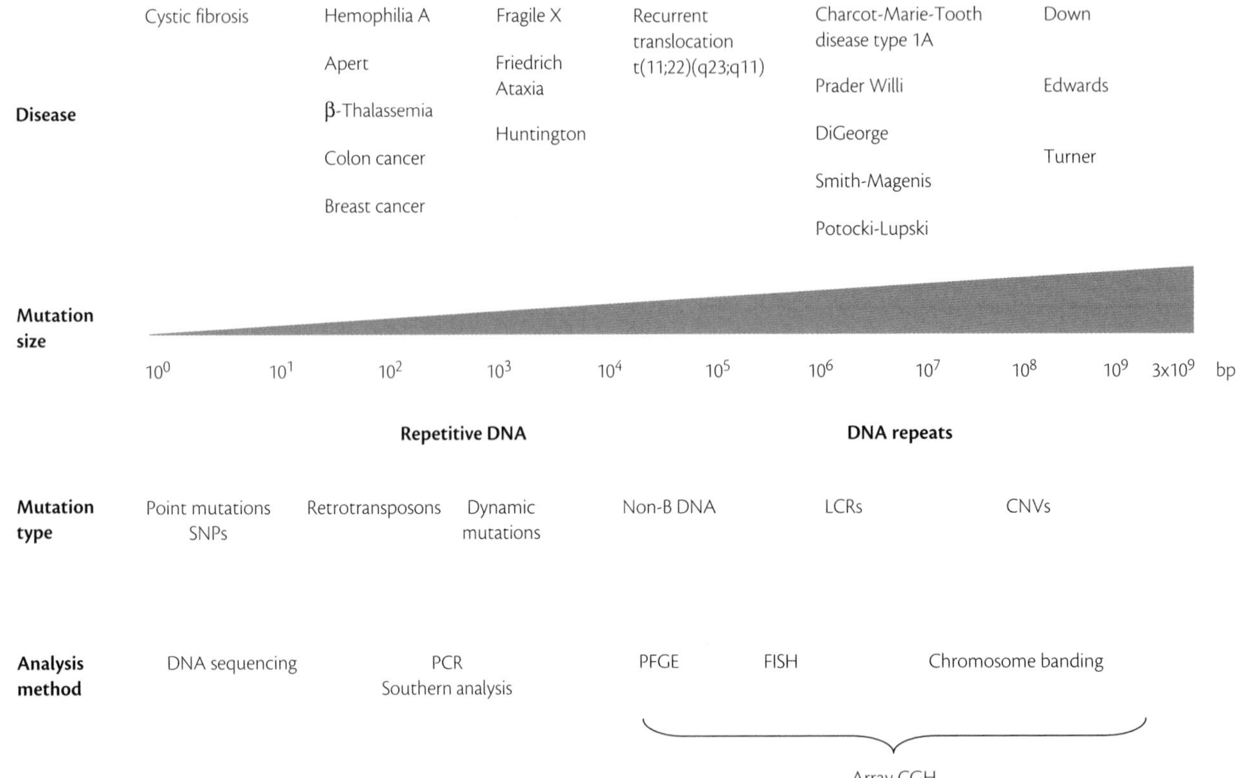

Fig. 4.2.2.2 Genomic rearrangements, phenotypic traits and methods used to assay. Above are shown the traits that can be due to DNA rearrangements. Below are ranges of DNA changes, descriptions of rearrangements, and the methods of assaying different sized changes.

been immobilized and arrayed on glass slides and used as interrogating probes. Such microarrays enabled detection of CNVs throughout the entire human genome with a resolution of approximately 100 kb, up to two orders of magnitude (i.e. 100-fold) greater genome resolving power than that afforded by the conventional CGH to the metaphase chromosomes in clinical cytogenetics laboratories.

Recently, the bacterial clones have been replaced by oligonucleotide probes. The currently commercially available arrays have several hundred thousand oligonucleotide probes and soon millions of probes will be offered. This technology has revolutionized clinical cytogenetics and may replace much of chromosome analysis with high-resolution genome analysis (Fig. 4.2.2.3).

As an alternative approach to genome-wide screening for the detection of specific large deletions or duplications in genomic DNA, a quantitative technique called multiplex ligation-dependent probe amplification (MLPA) based on the polymerase chain reaction, has been developed. This relies on sequence-specific probe hybridization to genomic DNA, followed by amplification of the hybridized probe and semi-quantitative analysis of the resulting polymerase chain reaction products. The relative peak heights or band intensities from each target indicate their initial concentration. This has proven to be an inexpensive, simple, rapid, and sensitive tool to detect dosage alterations in selected genomic regions.

Conclusions

Genetics of disease

In a classical mendelian monogenic model of a disease, Watson–Crick DNA base-pair changes in a single gene are recognized as a mechanism affecting the structure, function, or regulation of the encoded protein. Recent completion of the human reference DNA sequence and advances in novel technologies that enable us to study the entire human genome of a given patient have extended our view of the genetic bases of disease in humans. It has become apparent that many disease traits are caused by genomic alterations rather than by single nucleotide changes. The genetic heterogeneity of several complex traits has begun also to be resolved.

Studies of Bardet–Biedl syndrome, a genetically heterogeneous disorder, enabled identification of 12 causative genes. Mutation analysis of these genes has led to the discovery that a small number of them may interact genetically to manifest the disease phenotype. As a consequence, a triallelic and oligogenic model of inheritance has been proposed for Bardet–Biedl syndrome and other diseases (Table 4.2.2.2).

Charcot–Marie–Tooth disease is a very heterogenous peripheral neuropathy with mutations identified in more than 25 genes. Interestingly, the most common mutation, found in about 70% of all patients with CMT1, is a 1.4 Mb genomic duplication involving the dosage-sensitive *PMP22* gene. Thus, CMT1A represents a monogenic triallelic inheritance model (Table 4.2.2.2).

Recent genome-wide studies on genomic in copy number variation have led to important discoveries of large-scale CNVs in the human genome. The clinical consequences of the overwhelming majority of CNVs are not known. Many, if not most, CNVs are likely benign but some have been shown to be responsible for mendelian traits and others lead to increased susceptibility for complex traits such as Alzheimer's or Crohn's disease (Table 4.2.2.5).

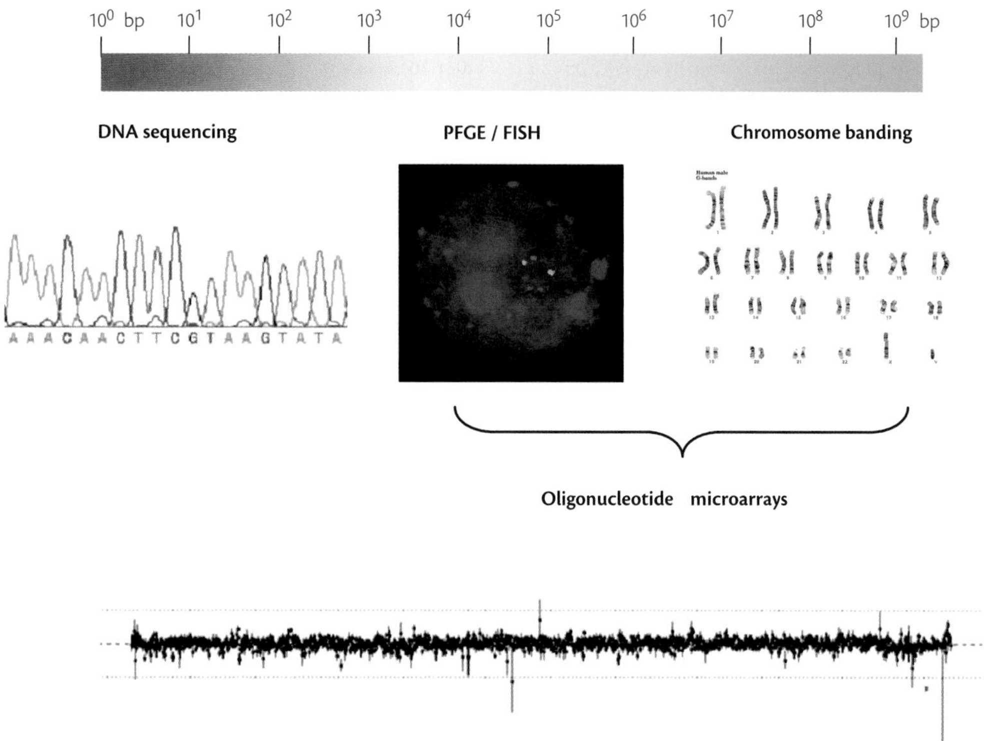

Fig. 4.2.2.3 Genome architecture and methods to resolve structure of varying DNA. Above is shown a scale of the human genome from 1(100) bp to 3×10^9 bp and the size ranges (colour coded) in which the different methods can physically resolve differences. Chromosomal banding (green) examines the whole genome at once, but cannot resolve changes of more than c.5 Mb (10^6–10^7 bp) in size. DNA sequencing (purple) can resolve single nucleotide changes and changes of several bases, but cannot identify CNVs. Pulsed-field gel electrophoresis (PFGE) and FISH (yellow) extend the reach of conventional karyotyping and resolve changes from 10^4 to 10^6 bp in size. Array CGH can resolve changes causing genomic imbalance from 10^3 to 10^8 bp (including aneuploidies), simultaneously performing thousands of locus-specific FISH procedures as well as detecting imbalances seen by chromosome analysis.

Adapted from Lupski (2003). 2002 Curt Stern Award Address. Genomic disorders recombination-based disease resulting from genomic architecture. *Am J Hum Genet*, **72**, 246–52; Lupski JR (2007). Genomic rearrangements and sporadic disease. *Nat Genet*, **39**, S43–7.

The pathogenic role of protein dosage can be illustrated by the β-amyloid encoded by the *APP* gene. Point mutations in *APP* localized on chromosome 21 have been described in patients with familial Alzheimer's disease. Recently, some patients with Alzheimer's disease have been found to have duplication of the entire *APP* gene, demonstrating that *APP* is a dosage-sensitive gene. Interestingly, mutations in the promoter region of *APP* have been reported as increasing *APP* expression leading to manifestation of Alzheimer's disease. Consistent with these findings is the well-known phenomenon that patients with Down's syndrome (carrying three copies of *APP*, since the gene maps to chromosome 21) are at risk of developing autosomal dominant early-onset Alzheimer's disease. Thus, trisomy 21 represents a model pathogenic role of CNV in a common trait.

Personalized genomic medicine

The concept of personalized medicine has been developed with the Human Genome Project. In contrast to conventional medicine, where the patients' diagnoses and treatments are based on disease signs and symptoms, personalized medicine refers to the genetic bases of the patient's traits and susceptibility to traits. The hypothesis underlying personalized genomic medicine is that personalized medical care can be guided by the unique genomic content of an individual patient. The aim of personal genomic medicine is the interpretation of unique information encoded in the individual patient's genome to be able to anticipate genetic risks and liability and adjust personal lifestyle changes, diet, medications, prevention, and therapy to mitigate the consequences of genetic risk.

The increasing ability to assay an individual's DNA polymorphisms (both SNPs and CNVs) will continue to further enable prediction of personal responses to different drugs depending on an individual's genetic background (i.e. pharmacogenomics). With the clinical implementation of new technologies, including massive parallel sequencing and high-resolution oligonucleotide array CGH that offer analysis of the individual diploid human genome (DNA sequence and CNVs) within a relatively short time, the information content of entire genomes of individuals is expected to become affordable. Recent whole-genome studies, however, suggest that interpretation of the complexity of the genetic load of an individual or selected patients will require better understanding of genotype/phenotype correlations to provide clinically relevant information in a format commensurate with clinical implementation. Such an approach will potentially revolutionize clinical diagnostics and therapy and may provide tremendous benefits for the patients' health.

Further reading

Badano JL, Katsanis N (2002). Beyond Mendel: an evolving view of human genetic disease transmission. *Nat Rev Genet*, **3**, 779–89.

Badano JL, *et al.* (2006). Dissection of epistasis in oligogenic Bardet-Biedl syndrome. *Nature*, **439**, 326–30.

Ballif BC, *et al.* (2006). Detection of low-level mosaicism by array CGH in routine diagnostic specimens. *Am J Med Genet A*, **140**, 2757–67.

Barbouti A, *et al.* (2004). The breakpoint region of the most common isochromosome, i(17q), in human neoplasia is characterized by a 220 kb region containing palindromic low-copy repeats. *Am J Hum Genet*, **74**, 1–10.

Bentley DR (2006). Whole-genome re-sequencing. *Curr Opin Genet Dev*, **16**, 545–52.

Chance PF, *et al.* (1994). Two autosomal dominant neuropathies result from reciprocal DNA duplication/deletion of a region on chromosome 17. *Hum Mol Genet*, **3**, 223–8.

Cheung SW, *et al.* (2007). Microarray-based CGH detects chromosomal mosaicism not revealed by conventional cytogenetics. *Am J Med Genet*, **143**, 1679–86.

Cooper DN, Youssoufian H (1998). The CpG dinucleotide and human genetic disease. *Hum Genet*, **78**, 151–155.

Coulondre C, *et al.* (1978). Molecular basis of base substitution hotspots in *Escherichia coli*. *Nature*, **274**, 775–780.

Dipple KM, McCabe ER (2000). Phenotypes of patients with 'simple' Mendelian disorders are complex traits: thresholds, modifiers, and systems dynamics. *Am J Hum Genet*, **66**, 1729–35.

Dumas L, *et al.* (2007). Gene copy-number variation spanning 60 million years of human and primate evolution. *Genome Res*, **17**, 1266–77.

Edelmann L, *et al.* (2001). AT-rich palindromes mediate the constitutional t(11;22) translocation. *Am J Hum Genet*, **68**, 1–13.

Eichers ER, *et al.* (2004). Triallelic inheritance: a bridge between Mendelian and multifactorial traits. *Ann Med*, **36**, 262–72.

ENCODE Project Consortium (2004). The ENCODE (ENCyclopedia Of DNA Elements) Project. *Science*, **306**, 636–40.

Giglio S, *et al.* (2002). Heterozygous submicroscopic inversions involving olfactory receptor-gene clusters mediate the recurrent t(4;8)(p16;p23) translocation. *Am J Hum Genet*, **71**, 276–85.

Hastings PJ, *et al.* (2009). Mechanisms of change in gene copy number. *Nat Rev Genet*, **10**, 551–64.

Iafrate AJ, *et al.* (2004). Detection of large-scale variation in the human genome. *Nat Genet*, **36**, 949–51.

Inoue K, *et al.* (2004). Molecular mechanism for distinct neurological phenotypes conveyed by allelic truncating mutations. *Nat Genet*, **36**, 361–369.

International Human Genome Sequencing Consortium (2004). Finishing the euchromatic sequence of the human genome. *Nature*, **431**, 931–45.

Kajiwara K, Berson EL, Dryja TP (1994). Digenic retinitis pigmentosa due to mutations at the unlinked peripherin/RDS and ROM1 loci. *Science*, **264**, 1604–8.

Kato T, *et al.* (2006). Genetic variation affects de novo translocation frequency. *Science*, **311**, 971.

Katsanis N, *et al.* (2001). Triallelic inheritance in Bardet-Biedl syndrome, a Mendelian recessive disorder. *Science*, **293**, 2256–9.

Kurahashi H, *et al.* (2000). Regions of genomic instability on 22q11 and 11q23 as the etiology for the recurrent constitutional t(11;22). *Hum Mol Genet*, **9**, 1665–70.

Lander ES, *et al.* (2001). International Human Genome Sequencing Consortium. Initial sequencing and analysis of the human genome. *Nature*, **409**, 860–921.

Lee JA, Carvalho CMB, Lupski JR (2007). A DNA replication mechanism for generating nonrecurrent rearrangements associated with genomic disorders. *Cell*, **131**, 1235–47.

Lee JA, Lupski JR (2006). Genomic rearrangements and gene copy-number alterations as a cause of nervous system disorders. *Neuron*, **52**, 103–21.

Levy S, *et al.* (2007). The diploid genome sequence of an individual human. *PLoS Biol*, **5**, e254.

Lifton RP, *et al.* (1992). A chimaeric 11-beta-hydroxylase/aldosterone synthase gene causes glucocorticoid-remediable aldosteronism and human hypertension. *Nature*, **355**, 262–5.

Lupski JR (1998). Genomic disorders: structural features of the genome can lead to DNA rearrangements and human disease traits. *Trends Genet*, **14**, 417–22.

Lupski JR (2006). Genome structural variation and sporadic disease traits. *Nat Genet*, **38**, 974–6.

Lupski JR (2007). Genomic rearrangements and sporadic disease. *Nat Genet*, **39**, S43–7.

Lupski JR (2007). Structural variation in the human genome. *N Engl J Med*, **356**, 1169–71.

Lupski JR, Stankiewicz P (2005). Genomic disorders: molecular mechanisms for rearrangements and conveyed phenotypes. *PLoS Genet*, **1**, e49.

Lupski JR, Stankiewicz P (eds) (2006). *Genomic disorders: the genomic basis of disease.* Humana Press, Totowa.

Lupski JR, *et al.* (1991). DNA duplication associated with Charcot-Marie-Tooth disease type 1A. *Cell*, **66**, 219–32.

Lupski JR, *et al.* (1992). Gene dosage is a mechanism for Charcot-Marie-Tooth disease type 1A. *Nat Genet*, **1**, 29–33.

Margulies M, Egholm M, Altman WE, *et al.* (2005). Genome sequencing in microfabricated high-density picolitre reactors. *Nature*, **437**, 376–380.

Pentao L, *et al.* (1992). Charcot-Marie-Tooth type 1A duplication appears to arise from recombination at repeat sequences flanking the 1.5 Mb monomer unit. *Nat Genet*, **2**, 292–300.

Redon R, *et al.* (2006). Global variation in copy-number in the human genome. *Nature*, **444**, 444–54.

Schmickel RD (1986). Contiguous gene syndromes: a component of recognizable syndromes. *J Pediatr*, **109**, 231–41.

Scriver CR, Waters PJ (1999). Monogenic traits are not simple: lessons from phenylketonuria. *Trends Genet*, **15**, 267–72.

Sebat J, *et al.* (2004). Large-scale copy-number polymorphism in the human genome. *Science*, **305**, 525–8.

Shaffer LG, Lupski JR (2000). Molecular mechanisms for constitutional chromosomal rearrangements in humans. *Annu Rev Genet*, **34**, 297–329.

Spence JE, *et al.* (1988). Uniparental disomy as a mechanism for human genetic disease. *Am J Hum Genet*, **42**, 217–26.

Stankiewicz P, Beaudet AL (2007). Use of array CGH in the evaluation of dysmorphology, malformations, developmental delay, and idiopathic mental retardation. *Curr Opin Genet Dev*, **17**, 182–92.

Stankiewicz P, Lupski JR (2002). Genome architecture, rearrangements and genomic disorders. *Trends Genet*, **18**, 74–82.

Stefansson H, *et al.* (2005). A common inversion under selection in Europeans. *Nat Genet*, **37**, 129–37.

The International HapMap Consortium (2003). The International HapMap Project. *Nature*, **426**, 789–796.

Tijo JH, Levan A (1956). The chromosome of man. *Hereditas*, **191**, 1268–70.

Todd JA, *et al.* (2007). Robust associations of four new chromosome regions from genome-wide analyses of type 1 diabetes. *Nat Genet*, **39**, 857–64.

Turner DJ, *et al.* (2008). Germline rates of *de novo* meiotic deletions and duplications causing several genomic disorders. *Nat Genet*, **40**, 90–5.

Watson JD, Crick FH (1953). Molecular structure of nucleic acids; a structure for deoxyribose nucleic acid. *Nature*, **171**, 737–8.

Wells RD (2007). Non-B DNA conformations, mutagenesis and disease. *Trends Biochem Sci*, **32**, 271–8.

Wheeler DA, *et al.* (2008). The complete genome of a single individual by massively parallel DNA sequencing. *Nature*, **452**, 872–6.

Willingham AT, Gingeras TR (2006). TUF love for 'junk' DNA. *Cell*, **125**, 1215–20.

Zhang F, Carvalho CM, Lupski JR (2009). Complex human chromosomal and genomic rearrangements. *Trends Genet*, **25**, 298–307.

Zhang F, *et al.* (2009). Copy number variation in human health, disease, and evolution. *Annu Rev Genomics Hum Genet*, **10**, 451–81.

4.3

Cytokines

Iain B. McInnes

Essentials

Cytokines are small glycoprotein mediators that are involved in every facet of immune effector function and regulation. More than 200 cytokines have been identified, which may usefully be classified in structurally related superfamilies. They can (1) function through binding to specific receptors that in turn signal via complex transduction pathways to regulate gene expression, thereby mediating positive and negative regulatory activities; (2) operate as soluble mediators in the extracellular domain or within cells, where they may also traffic to the nucleus and exhibit dual function as transcriptional regulators; (3) be expressed initially on the cell membrane, where they may exert effector function directly in cell–cell interactions, or from which they can be subsequently cleaved to yield bioactive soluble molecules, thereby mediating autocrine and paracrine activities around their cellular source.

The innate immune response—this is designed to offer immediate effector defence and comprises particular leucocyte lineages including neutrophils, eosinophils, monocytes/macrophages and natural killer cells. It is regulated by cytokines such as the type I interferons (IFN), tumour necrosis factor (TNF) α, and interleukin (IL) IL-1α, IL-6, IL-15, and IL-18. These are produced rapidly in large amounts, work along with pattern-recognition receptor families such as Toll-like receptors to coordinate local cellular activation, and are essential for the integrity of the innate immune response. Over time, additional cytokines such as IL-10 and tissue growth factor (TGF) β are synthesized, promoting resolution of immune responses and mediating healing of tissue damage. However, such responses are amnesic in that no specific molecular memory of the initiating stimulus is retained beyond pattern recognition.

Adaptive immune responses—these are an evolutionary refinement to facilitate recall responses to specific antigens derived from invading organisms or damaged self-tissue. Adaptive immunity to antigenic stimuli is initiated primarily via the activation of professional antigen-presenting cells, such as dendritic cells and macrophages, working in synergy with cytokines. Dendritic cells are activated by cytokines such as TNFα and IL-1α to increase antigen uptake, processing and presentation to naive T cells, and—critically—dendritic cells use cytokines to define the phenotype of subsequent T-cell responses: (1) production of IL-18 and IL-12 promotes a Th1 response (IFNγ predominant); (2) production of IL-1, IL-6, IL-21, and IL-23 favours the emergence of a Th17 response (IL-17A, IL-17F, IL-22 predominant); and (3) production of IL-4 and IL-33 favours Th2 cell differentiation (IL-4, IL-5, IL-13 predominant). Regulatory T-cell subsets may also be activated in this phase by cytokines such as IL-2, IL-10, IL-35 and TGFβ.

Activation of host-tissue cell types—cytokines mediate many effector functions in the immune system by action on host-tissue cell types, including (1) activation of endothelial and lymphendothelial cells to express adhesion molecules and to alter their permeabililty properties to facilitate induction and resolution of inflammation; (2) regulation of differentiated tissue specific cells, which can contribute indirectly to host tissue defence; (3) regulation of host tissue function in the context of inflammation, e.g. by facilitating metabolic responses to sustain energy requirements for host defence responses.

Clinical context—cytokines play a broad role in numerous biological systems. This renders them of basic scientific interest. Understanding of the cytokine network also has increasing importance in clinical practice with the advent of therapeutic strategies that target particular cytokines with exquisite specificity using biological agents, leading to remarkable advances in the treatment of inflammatory disorders, e.g. anti-TNF therapy in rheumatoid arthritis.

Introduction

In higher organisms, the immune system has evolved to provide flexible and comprehensive host defence against microbial organisms. It also plays a critical role in recognition of, and immediate response to, altered integrity of self-tissues, for example as occurs in trauma or neoplasia. The immune system itself comprises a complex interaction between cells of discrete lineage and function that must act in a cooperative manner to achieve satisfactory, long-lived protection with minimal damage to the host. Cytokines are small glycoprotein messengers (8–40 kDa) that facilitate regulation and effector function of cells in an autocrine or paracrine manner. Typically, cytokines exhibit functional activities that are of critical importance in the immune system, but also mediate wider effects across a range of tissues. Cytokines thus also play a role in a variety of normal physiological and metabolic processes. The field of cytokine biology has expanded considerably in the last decade with the recognition of large numbers of moieties and the advent of effective therapeutics based on cytokine targeting, particularly in inflammatory diseases.

Classification of cytokines

Cytokines were originally discovered and defined on the basis of their functional activities observed in bioassays e.g. macrophage activating factor, lymphocyte activating factor. Subsequent advances in molecular biology, bioinformatics, and recently the Human Genome Project have facilitated discovery of large numbers of cytokines, posing considerable challenges in resolving their individual and synergistic functions in complex tissues in health and disease. In the absence of a unified classification system, cytokines may be variously identified by:

- numerical order of discovery, e.g. the interleukins (IL): currently IL-1 to IL-35
- specific functional activity, e.g. tumour necrosis factor (TNF), granulocyte colony stimulating factor (G-CSF)—this is usually an underestimate of the potential activities of a given cytokine
- kinetic or functional role in inflammatory responses, e.g. early or late, innate or adaptive, pro-inflammatory or anti-inflammatory
- on the basis of predominant primary cell or tissue of origin (monokine = monocyte derived; lymphokine = lymphocyte derived; adipocytokine = adipose tissue derived)
- structural homologies shared with related molecules

The last represents a contemporary and logical approach. Cytokines should be considered in 'family groups' that share

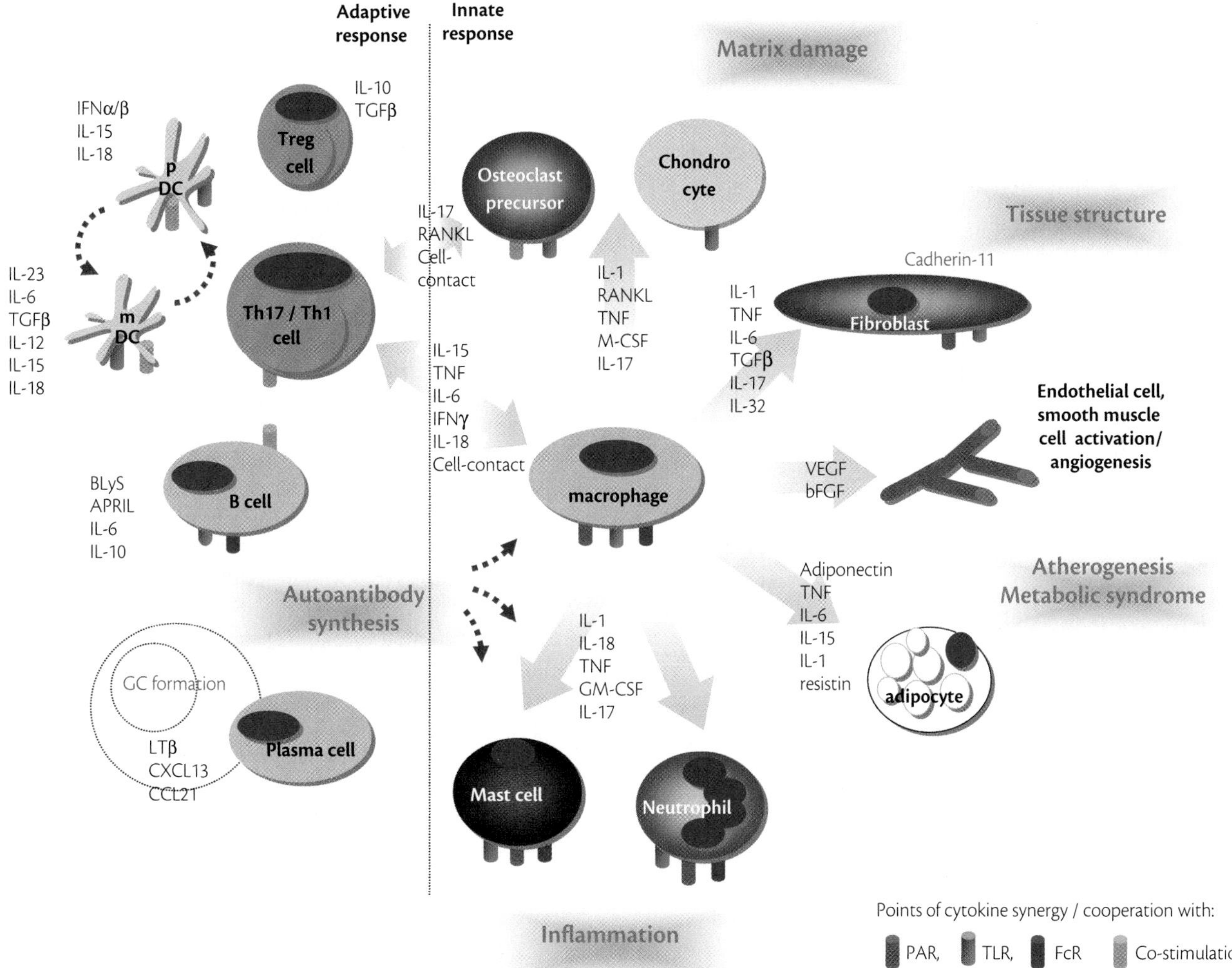

Fig. 4.3.1 Cytokines mediate pleiotropic activities within complex cellular systems. Cytokines form coordinated networks that regulate multiple cellular interactions locally and in turn promote systemic responses. This is particularly well defined in the pathogenesis of rheumatoid arthritis. The principle relationships existing between cellular lineages are consistent across a range of inflammatory disorders. The figure highlights the multifaceted roles played by cytokines in the range of manifestations of disease. The activities are broadly defined on the basis of their activities in promoting adaptive or innate immune function. In the novel immune response these will occur sequentially. In the context of chronic inflammation, or persistent recall responses, the two arms of the immune system will likely overlap allowing for considerable cross-talk and interlinked function for cellular components, but particularly in the cytokine network.

(Reprinted by permission from Macmillan Publishers Ltd: *Nat Rev Immunol*. Cytokines in the pathogenesis of rheumatoid arthritis. McInnes IB, Schett G. 2007 Jun; **7**(6):429–42, © 2007.)

sequence similarity and also exhibit homology and some promiscuity in their reciprocal receptor systems. Note that they need not exhibit functional similarity. These so called 'cytokine superfamilies' often contain regulatory cell membrane receptor–ligand pairs that use common structural motifs in diverse immune functions in higher mammals, reflecting evolutionary pressures. This is best exemplified in the IL-1/IL-1 receptor superfamily that contains cytokines such as IL-1β, IL-1α, IL-1 receptor antagonist, IL-1 F5–F10, IL-18, and IL-33, which mediate physiological and host-defence function. IL-1 receptor signalling cascades share remarkable similarities with the signalling pathways induced by toll-like receptors (TLR) and NOD-like receptors (NLR), a series of mammalian pattern-recognition molecules with a crucial role in recognition of microbial species early in innate responses. These common motifs allow integration of responses at the signal transduction level between cytokine and other immune receptor systems to allow fine tuning of responses over time.

Box 4.3.1 Factors that regulate cytokine production

- Cytokines (forming amplificatory and regulatory loops)
- Cell–cell contact (e.g. lectins, integrins, Ig superfamily members)
- Immune complexes/autoantibodies
- Complement activation products
- Microbial species and their soluble products (particularly via TLR/NLR pathways)
- Reactive oxygen and nitrogen intermediates
- Trauma
- Sheer stress and barotrauma
- Ischaemia
- Radiation
- Ultraviolet light
- Extracellular matrix components
- DNA (mammalian or microbial)
- Heat-shock proteins

Basic cytokine biology

Synthesis, expression, and regulation

Cytokines can be produced by almost every leucocyte and host tissue cell type (see below). They are synthesized in the Golgi apparatus and may traffic through the endoplasmic reticulum to be released as soluble mediators. Cytokines can also be expressed as cell membrane-bound proteins, or may be processed into cytosolic forms that can traffic intracellularly, even to the nucleus where they can act as transcriptional regulators. Thus, cytokines mediate autocrine function either through release or membrane expression and immediate receptor ligation on the source cell, or intracellularly within the source cell. Alternatively, cytokines operate in a paracrine manner, allowing cellular communication beyond that facilitated by local cell–cell contact.

The distance over which cytokines can mediate effects is unclear and probably depends on multiple factors—in tissues, *in silico* models predict meaningful bioactivity no further than a 40 µm diameter from the source cell due to physicochemical considerations of the peptide structure itself, extracellular matrix binding (e.g. to heparan sulphate), enzymatic degradation, or the presence of soluble receptors or cytokine-binding proteins. Nevertheless some cytokines clearly exhibit systemic activities, e.g. IL-6 induces the acute-phase response by circulating to the liver and IL-1β promotes pyrexia via either local expression or circulation to the central nervous system.

The triggers to cytokine release are diverse and depend upon the cell type and tissue concerned (Box 4.3.1). Many of these triggers can also be used *ex vivo* to study cytokine function, together with a variety of surrogate stimuli such as chemical entities, including phorbol esters, calcium ionophores, lectins and receptor-specific agonistic antibodies (e.g. anti-CD3/CD28 to mimic T-cell costimulatory activation). Detailed studies using such agents *in vitro* together with *in vivo* observations using gene knock-in and knockout mice have unravelled many layers of regulation for cytokine production. Since they exhibit such potent effects in immune function, it is unsurprising that these pathways are tightly regulated.

Transcriptional and post transcriptional regulation

Transcription of a cytokine gene depends upon the recruitment of usually multiple transcription factors (TFs) to the cytokine gene promoter region. TF binding allows numerous signal pathways to regulate cytokine expression. Some transcription factors, e.g. NF-κB, activator protein-1 (AP-1), nuclear factor of activated T cell (NF-AT), appear to have particular importance in cytokine regulation in disease states. For example inhibition of NF-κB activity using either chemical inhibitors or adenoviral delivery of regulatory proteins leads to amelioration of atherogenesis in *apoE–/–* mice, of inflammatory synovitis in murine arthritis models, or of colitis in inflammatory bowel disease models. However, many other TF binding sites exist in the majority of cytokine genes. Their recognition and manipulation represents both an area of enormous complexity at present but also great therapeutic opportunity to achieve context-specific inhibition of cytokine production e.g. inflammatory vs protective cytokine release.

Sequence polymorphism within cytokine promoters offers potential for differential cytokine expression between individuals that could confer selective advantage against infection, but could also increase susceptibility to, or progression of, autoimmunity or chronic inflammation. Thus, single nucleotide polymorphisms (SNP) in the TNFα promoter region (e.g. –308) are associated with altered TNFα release upon leucocyte stimulation *in vitro*. Similarly, homozygotes for the A2 allele at +3954 in the IL-1β gene produce more IL-1β to lipopolysaccharide (LPS) stimulation. In general, the net effect of haplotypes may be more important at the functional level, particularly when their relevance to disease entities is considered. Intronic SNPs elsewhere in the cytokine gene structure are also likely to be of importance although they are in general ill-clarified at present.

Post-transcriptional regulation is important in determining longevity of cytokine expression. This may operate by promoting translational initiation, mRNA stability, and polyadenylation. AU-rich elements (ARE) within the 5′ or 3′ untranslated regions (UTR) of cytokine mRNA are crucial for stability. For example 3′ UTR ARE down-regulate TNF expression—transgenic knock-in mice that lack TNF ARE develop spontaneous inflammatory arthritis and bowel disease. Regulatory proteins bind ARE to mediate such effects. Thus, HuR and AUF1 exert opposing effects, respectively stabilizing or destabilizing ARE-containing transcripts. TIA-1 and TIAR have been identified as RNA recognition motif family members that function as translational silencers. Alternatively, cytokines may generate stable mRNA *a priori* to facilitate subsequent rapid response in tissues. IL-15 mRNA 5′ UTR contains 12 AUG triplets that significantly reduce the efficiency of IL-15 translation but provides an intracellular pool of RNA. IL-15 forms generated by distinct processing of this mRNA can be rapidly synthesized and trafficked to cytosolic or extracellular domains as required.

Finally, the cytosolic activity of microRNA species provides a further level of cytokine regulation. These recently recognized small RNA sequences have the capacity to bind to mRNA and down-regulate translation to protein. Myriad microRNAs have now been identified, each considered capable of regulating up to 20 mRNAs, usually in a negative direction. Genetic targeting of such microRNAs *in vivo* has lead to remarkable effects on global immune function mediated through altered cellular differentiation and cytokine release.

Post-translational regulation

Cytokine production is also regulated by post-translational modifications. Patterns of glycosylation are important for cytokine function in the extra cellular domain and may also regulate intracellular trafficking. Modified leader sequences can alter intracellular trafficking of cytokines. Moreover, some cytokines are translated without functional leader sequences. Their secretion depends on nonconventional secretory pathways that are thus far poorly understood but may include ion channels, chaperone proteins or specific membrane pores. Enzymatic activation of preformed procytokines is common. Thus cleavage by caspase 1 of pro-IL-1β or IL-18 generates active cytokine species. Such enzymatic cleavage is often conducted within an assembly of proteins (e.g. inflamasome) designed to carefully coordinate and regulate the amount and duration of active cytokine release. A variety of other enzymes are implicated in similar processes including the serine proteases, proteinase 3, and elastase, and adamolysin family members. Enzyme cleavage pathways operate both within and outside cells, providing for extracellular cytokine activation. Thus, cell membrane enzymes serve to cleave membrane-expressed cytokine to generate soluble cytokines. In summary, extensive molecular machinery exists to tightly regulate not only the production and stability of cytokine mRNA, but also its translation and cellular expression and distribution.

How do cytokines mediate their effects?

Cytokines mediate their effects primarily via the binding of a cognate receptor(s). These are contained in structurally related superfamilies and comprise high-affinity molecular signalling complexes that facilitate cytokine-mediated communication. Such complexes often include heterodimeric or heterotrimeric structures that use unique, cytokine-specific recognition receptors together with common receptor chains shared across a cytokine superfamily. Thus, the common γ chain is used by receptor complexes of many α-helix cytokines (e.g. IL-2, IL-7, IL-15, IL-21) and the gp130 receptor is similarly utilized by IL-6 and many homologues. Similar promiscuity across cytokine receptors is shown by the intracellular molecules used to transduce the signal to the nucleus, e.g. JAK/STAT pathways. Distinct receptors may utilize shared signalling domains: homologous death domains are found in many TNF-receptor (TNF-R) family members and the TIR domain is common to IL-1R and TLR signalling. Single signal molecules in turn can function on behalf of many receptors although subtle differences may operate as to precise dimerization or phosphorylation events for any given receptor leading to specificity of the response.

Cytokines and their receptors can adopt a variety of orientations. Membrane receptors, with intracellular signalling domains intact, can transmit signals to the target cell nucleus following soluble cytokine binding and thereby promote effector function. Membrane receptors may bind cell membrane cytokines facilitating cross-talk between adjacent cells. Membrane-bound and soluble cytokines may promote distinct function. For example, TNFα binds TNF-RI and TNF-RII with similar affinity, but it has a slower rate of dissociation from TNF-RI. Soluble TNFα may rapidly dissociate from TNF-RII to bind TNF-RI, promoting preferential signalling by the latter (ligand passing). In contrast, during cell–cell contact, stable TNFα/TNF-RI and TNFα/TNF-RII complexes form, allowing for differential signalling contribution by TNF-RI and TNF-RII. Cytokine receptor–cytokine complexes may also operate in *trans*, whereby component parts of the ligand–receptor complex are derived from adjacent cells. Receptors also exist in soluble form, derived either from alternative mRNA processing to generate receptor-lacking transmembrane or intracellular domains, or by enzymatic cleavage of receptor from the cell surface. Soluble receptors can antagonize cytokine function, or preform complexes with cytokine to promote subsequent ligand–receptor assembly on the target cell membrane, and thereby enhance function. Furthermore, soluble receptors can deliver cytokine to the cell membrane via ligand passing. These details are crucially important in devising effective therapeutic inhibitors of cytokines. The homeostasis of cytokine release and function is maintained in this network. An inhibitor that blocks only part of the cytokine receptor interaction may be ineffective or, worse, paradoxically enhance effects.

Finally, although in general cytokines bind only their cognate receptor, there appears to be some plasticity in the system since close cross-communication on the cell membrane between seemingly unrelated cytokine receptor systems also occurs, thereby allowing a cell to integrate a variety of external stimuli to optimize signalling pathways. This allows cells to constantly sense and respond to complex changes in the local environment delivered by many cytokines either simultaneously or in sequence.

Principal cytokine activities

Members of the major cytokine superfamilies are listed in Table 4.3.1. Further hierarchical relationships exist within and between superfamilies, reflecting the ancestral genes from which cytokines have been derived. The diversity and density of data now available to describe the activities of individual cytokines are beyond the scope of this text, but the following paragraphs summarize the activities of selected cytokines implicated in inflammatory disorders.

TNF superfamily

Tumour necrosis factor (TNF) is the prototypic proinflammatory cytokine of this superfamily. It is produced by a wide variety of

Table 4.3.1 Members of the major cytokine superfamilies

Cytokine family/activity	Key members[a]
TNF-'like'	TNF, lymphotoxin, BLyS, APRIL, RANKL, TWEAK
IL-1-like	IL-1α, IL-1β, IL-1Ra, IL-18, IL-33, IL-1F5 to IL-1F10
IL-6-like	IL-6, oncostatin M, leukaemia inhibitory factor, IL-11, cardiotrophin-1, ciliary neurotrophic factor
IL-12-like	IL-12, IL-23, IL-27, IL-35
IL-10-like	IL-10, IL-19, IL-20, IL-22, IL-24
Growth factors	TGFβ, BMPs, PDGF
Angiogenesis	VEGF, bFGF, endostatin
Colony stimulating factors	G-CSF, M-CSF, GM-CSF
Adipocytokines	Adiponectin, resistin

[a] The cytokines shown for each family are examples, not an exhaustive list.

immune cell types, particularly macrophages, T and B lymphocytes, and neutrophils, but is also released by tissue cell types including keratinocytes, glial cells, and smooth muscle cells. It comprises a heterotrimer (each subunit of 26 kDa) that binds to either of two receptors TNF receptor I (p55) or TNF receptor II (p75). TNF and its receptors are synthesized as membrane proteins that can be cleaved to soluble form by the activity of members of the ADAMs family of enzymes. Downstream signalling is mediated via MAPK and NF-κB, and can if appropriate involve recruitment of death domains to facilitate apoptosis in target cells. TNF sits in a pivotal position in many inflammatory cytokine networks. Thus, inhibition of TNF in inflammatory tissues *in vitro*, such as those derived from inflammatory synovitis, psoriatic skin, or Crohn's mucosal biopsies leads to down-regulation of many other inflammatory cytokines such as IL-6 and IL-8. and of the production of many inflammatory chemokines. This 'cytokine hierarchy' is considered to explain in part the efficacy of single cytokine targeting in chronic disease states.

The precise effects of TNF receptor binding depend upon the lineage and activation status of the target cell. TNF induces monocyte activation and maturation and promotes chemokinesis, release of reactive oxygen and nitrogen intermediates (ROI/RNI), and prostaglandin/leukotriene production. Similarly, polymorphonuclear leucocytes are primed and induced to oxidative burst by TNF. Effects on T cells are predominantly regulatory such that long-standing exposure to TNF leads to relative hypofunction of T cells and impaired T-cell receptor signalling. Indeed, TNF blockade in humans leads to enhanced T-cell autoreactivity. TNF is a critical activator of tissue cells. Thus endothelial cells (vascular) and lymphendothelial cells (lymphatics) are induced to express high levels of adhesion molecules and chemokines upon TNF exposure. The net effect of this is to increase cellular trafficking into and out of inflammatory lesions. It further promotes vascular permeability and is directly implicated in the hypotension and oedema associated with septic shock. Local effects are also mediated upon nociception such that TNF increases pain sensation via modulated local neurotransmitter release. Systemic metabolic effects can promote cachexia and altered lipid metabolism in adipose tissues. Mice in which TNF is transgenically overexpressed develop spontaneous autoinflammatory diseases including inflammatory arthritis and inflammatory bowel disease. Targeting TNF is effective in numerous disease states, particularly rheumatoid arthritis, Crohn's disease, and psoriasis, providing formal proof of concept of a pivotal role for this cytokine in pathogenesis.

Lymphotoxin is a 22 to 26 kD cytokine that shares broad inflammatory properties with TNF but is particularly and additionally implicated in structural organization of the immune system. Thus formation of germinal centres in lymph nodes and spleen and the creation of 'ectopic' germinal centres (i.e. formed outwith lymphoid organs) in chronically inflamed tissues is particularly regulated by lymphotoxin, together with the chemokines CCL13 and CXCL21.

B lymphocyte stimulator protein (BLyS; also known as B cell activating factor, BAFF) and a proliferation inducing ligand (APRIL) are two recently described members of the TNF superfamily that regulate B-cell function. BLyS and APRIL can be synthesized by monocytes, T cells, dendritic cells, fibroblasts, and some tumour cells. Their primary activity lies in supporting B-cell maturation and activation transduced via BLyS receptor and TACI. Following antigen-driven B-cell activation, BLyS and APRIL promote isotype switching and immunoglobulin secretion and delay B-cell apoptosis. Effects beyond B cells have been observed including T-cell costimulation and tumour proliferation.

Receptor activator of NF-κB ligand (RANKL) was identified as a cytokine (35 kDa) promoting dendritic cell–T cell interactions but is now primarily recognized as a critical regulator of bone homeostasis. RANKL is produced by monocytes, T cells, osteoblasts, and stromal cells and binds to RANK, its cognate receptor. RANKL mediates effects in physiological bone remodelling by promoting maturation of osteoclast precursors to yield osteoclasts that are fully functional for resorption of calcified tissues. Production by osteoclasts facilitates integrated resorption and new bone formation to maintain structural integrity and morphology of bone. In inflammatory states, RANKL expression is increased leading to increased osteoclast maturation and effector function leading to net bone loss. RANKL exhibits synergistic effects with TNF, IL-1β, IL-17, and IL-6 in this regard. Osteoprotogerin (OPG) is a 55 kDa soluble decoy receptor for RANKL that acts as a competitive inhibitor to limit the activity of RANKL. OPG-deficient mice exhibit significant osteoporosis and transgenic mice are osteopetrotic, suggesting a critical role in physiologic bone remodelling. The balance between RANKL and OPG synthesis defines the net resorptive activity of bone and is dysregulated in inflammatory states leading to systemic bone loss, i.e. osteoporosis. An increased inflammatory milieu usually increases the RANKL/OPG ratio of expression leading to accelerated local bone loss, designated 'erosions'. These are particularly prevalent in rheumatoid arthritis and psoriatic arthritis, but also occur in septic arthritis.

IL-1 superfamily

The IL-1 superfamily contains a variety of moieties involved in local and systemic regulation of immune responses that share structural homology. IL-1α and IL-1β are synthesized as promolecules of approximately 35 kDa which are in turn cleaved by caspase 1 within the inflamasome to yield active 18 kDa cytokines. IL-1 receptor antagonist (IL-1Ra) is a homologue of IL-1α and IL-1β that competes with these agonists for receptor binding. The IL-1 cytokines effect function via binding to a heterodimeric receptor comprising IL-1 receptor I (IL-1RI) and IL-1 receptor accessory protein (IL-1RAcP). IL-1RII is a further receptor that has decoy function.

IL-1 cytokines signal through a canonical signal pathway that they share with the TLR superfamily. Via a series of protein interactions and kinase dependent events, this pathway leads to NF-κB activation and inflammation related gene activation.

IL-1α and IL-1β are differentiated by the primarily membrane expression of the former which also retains activity as a full-length promolecule. Their functions are, however, rather similar, reflecting the shared receptor components (and are designated 'IL-1' hereafter). Thus they promote monocyte activation, cytokine and ROI/RNI release, and prostaglandin production. They further drive fibroblast activation, collagen synthesis, prostaglandin release, and proliferation. IL-1 is a potent inducer of endothelial cell activation and adhesion molecule expression, osteoclast maturation and activation in synergy with RANKL, chondrocyte activation, catabolism, and matrix degradation via metallportinease production. IL-1 is a potent pyrogen commensurate with the fever syndromes that arise when genetic abnormalities occur in IL-1 regulation, e.g. Muckle Wells syndrome/cold autoinflammatory disorders. Such syndromes are accordingly amenable to therapeutic IL-1 blockade. IL-1 is implicated in the pathogenesis of a variety of common chronic inflammatory diseases including rheumatoid arthritis, ankylosing spondylitis, and psoriasis. Its hierarchical position in inflammation cascades relative to TNF is unclear since targeting with IL-1Ra in practice (anakinra) has proved disappointing in the majority of diseases in which TNF blockade is effective. There is interest in its metabolic activities in type II diabetes, however, in which therapeutic targeting may be beneficial. Finally, high levels of IL-1 expression within the central nervous system have been reported where it may regulate several central pathways implicated in cognition and mood state.

IL-18 is an innate response cytokine produced by monocytes, fibroblasts, neutrophils and dendritic cells as a 33 kDa promolecule that can be cleaved by the actions of caspase 1 in the NALP3 inflamasome to an 18 kDa active moiety. IL-18 activates a heterodimeric receptor (IL-18Rα/IL-18Rβ) and is antagonized *in vivo* by soluble IL-18Rα and by a distinct IL-18 binding protein family that contains several members generated by alternative mRNA splicing. IL-18 activates neutrophils to promote maturation, chemotaxis, ROI/RNI production and cytokine/chemokine release. It also drives NK-cell activation, and monocytes/macrophage maturation and activation. Its primary effects are likely mediated on driving T-cell differentiation towards a mainly Th1 phenotype in synergy with IL-12. IL-18 is expressed at high levels in rheumatoid arthritis, psoriasis and inflammatory bowel disease human tissues and rodent models and has net proinflammatory function therein. Very high systemic levels have been reported in Still's disease (juvenile and adult onset) and in systemic leukophagocytic syndromes. Recently effects on hepatocytes and adipocytes have been reported for IL-18. Their net effect on metabolism and accrued vascular risk is unclear since epidemiological and several *in vitro* studies suggest that IL-18 can promote atherogenic risk and metabolic syndrome whereas *in vivo* studies mainly in IL-18-deficient animals suggest that IL-18 may be protective in this regard. This may offer therapeutic opportunity in due course.

IL-33 is produced mainly by fibroblasts, and is synthesized as a 33 kDa protein that is cleaved by enzyme pathways as yet undefined. Its effects function via ST2L and IL-1RAcP binding and signals via the canonical IL-1 receptor pathway. It also acts within the nucleus of the synthesizing cell as a transcriptional repressor by virtue of a direct DNA binding domain. IL-33 activates Th2 cell differentiation and expansion. It directly activates mast cell and eosinophil activation and cytokine production. As such, the effects attributed to IL-33 are mainly in allergy and anaphylaxis.

Cytokines mediating and regulating T-cell function

T cells of CD4+ and CD8+ lineages are functionally defined on the basis of their release of effector cytokines. Th1 cells (defined by *t-bet* transcription factor expression) release IFNγ and TNFα and promote granuloma formation and host defence to intracellular organisms. Th1 cell formation is driven by IL-12 and IL-18 together with relative absence of TGFβ, IL-4, and IL-17. IFNγ is a 20 to 25 kDa molecule that has pleiotopic functions including priming and activation of neutrophils, activation of macrophages particularly to induce cytotoxic pathways, and activation of NK cells. However, IFNγ also promotes tissue repair and as such is an example of the multifunctional potential in cytokines that must be elucidated with care prior to therapeutic intervention. Inherited deficiencies in the IFNγ/IFNγR signalling pathway, or in the components of the IL-12 pathway, engenders susceptibility to intracellular infections, particularly tuberculosis, highlighting the critical role for this cytokine in host defence.

Th17 cells (RORγT) are a recently described subset implicated in autoimmunity and host defence. They release IL-17A, IL-17F, and IL-22 and when targeted in many rodent models of autoimmunity are found to be of profound pathologic importance. Their generation depends variously on the activities of IL-21, IL-1β, IL-6, IL-23, and TGFβ. IL-17A is a potent effector cytokine (20–30 kDa) that operates in synergy with IL-1 and TNF to promote leucocyte activation, bone marrow leucocyte maturation, haemopoiesis, and matrix degradation, the latter via direct effects on fibroblasts and chondrocytes. IL-22 similarly promotes autoimmune-mediated tissue damage by directly activating tissue cells such as keratinocytes and invading leucocytes.

Th2 cells (GATA3) are characterized by IL-4, IL-5, IL-13, and IL-25 release and have their primary role in driving humoral immunity and host defence to many parasites, particularly in mucosal/barrier defence. In disease states, Th2 cells promote especially allergy and anaphylaxis. Th2 differentiation is driven by IL-33 and IL-4. A further subset of regulatory T cells (Foxp3; T_r) is now described that comprises naturally occurring T cells that function in a predominantly suppressive manner via direct cell contact with adjacent leucocytes or via release of IL-10 and TGFβ. T_r differentiation is favoured by TGFβ and IL-35, although this is an area that is currently poorly understood.

Miscellaneous cytokine activities

IL-6 is a pleiotropic proinflammatory cytokine that mediates function via IL-6Rα and the common coreceptor, gp130. IL-6 also activates B cells, promoting isotype switching and immunoglobulin production and T cells promoting proliferation and differentiation. It has an important role in haemopoiesis and thrombopoiesis. IL-6 mediates intriguing systemic effects—it critically regulates the acute phase response via direct effects on hepatocytes. Moreover, it has a role in integrating inflammatory responses with function of the hypothalamic pituitary adrenal axis indicative of a role in the immediate stress response. High levels of IL-6 expression are described in rheumatoid arthritis and Crohn's disease and in juvenile inflammatory arthritis, particularly systemic variants thereof, and Still's disease. High levels of IL-6 are also detected in Castlemann's disease. IL-6 deficiency or blockade is anti-inflammatory in a number of *in vivo* and *in vitro* disease models, providing strong rationale for IL-6 blockade in the clinic.

In contrast, IL-10 exhibits predominantly anti-inflammatory effects. It is released by a variety of leukocytes including macrophages, and T and B lymphocytes. Acting via IL-10RI and IL-10RII, it inhibits macrophage cytokine and RNI/ROI production, T-cell activation, dendritic cell priming and maturation, and fibroblast activation. Note, however, that IL-10 promotes B-cell activation and immunoglobulin secretion. Several members of the IL-10 superfamily are now defined with effects often manifest in barrier defence. In particular, IL-20 and IL-22 are implicate in keratinocyte responses to cutaneous inflammation.

The range of known cytokine activities described is now substantial across a variety of tissue compartments and processes. Often their original designation belies pleiotropic effects across a range of physiology and pathologies. Colony stimulating factors such as GM-CSF, G-CSF, and M-CSF were originally defined on the basis of leucocyte precursor differentiation and maturation, but now are recognized to play a role in effector immune responses. TGFβ isoforms have broad effects in tissue maintenance and repair and enjoy broad expression and functional promiscuity. They initially promote inflammatory cell recruitment and activation together with a key role in fibroblast activation and matrix synthesis, but over time promote suppression of inflammation to permit efficient wound repair. The related cytokine family of bone morphogenetic proteins (BMP) exhibit similarly wide activities in tissue morphogenesis and repair. Comprising a large family of homo- and heterodimers, they regulate chemotaxis, mitosis, and differentiation during chondrogenesis, osteogenesis, and tissue morphogenesis in heart, skin, eye, and beyond, rendering them interesting moieties for therapeutic manipulation of tissue repair following injury, neoplasia, or inflammatory insult. Other fundamental processes in tissue repair also reside in cytokine regulation. Angiogenesis is critically regulated by VEGF and by basic FGF. Together with naturally occurring inhibitors of angiogenesis, such as endostatin, this pathway is permissive for tissue repair, but also for maintenance of inflammation, or metastasis. These angiogenins carefully orchestrate recruitment of endothelial precursors and their subsequent maturation and organization into vessel structure—relative deficiency or excess can have significant consequences for tissues.

Cytokines as therapeutic targets

General concepts in cytokine therapeutics

Cytokine immunology has provoked the creation of a dynamic new field in drug discovery. Cytokines represent therapeutic entities in themselves, best exemplified in their use to amplify cancer therapeutics via immune stimulation or to enhance immune competency in immunosuppressed patients. However, their short half-life and tendency to mediate systemic effects that are in general undesirable has limited their value in this respect. More success has been achieved in the treatment of chronic viral infection whereby treatment of hepatitis C infection with type I interferon as part of combination antiviral therapy leads to improved viral clearance.

Similarly, the utility of 'anti-inflammatory' cytokines as therapeutic entities *per se* in inflammatory diseases has been limited by their half-life and by toxicities arising from non-disease-related, but plausible, biological effector function. For example, IL-10, a cytokine with generally anti-inflammatory effects, exhibited some efficacy in patients with psoriasis and rheumatoid arthritis but offered an unacceptable toxicity/benefit ratio overall due in part to systemic adverse effects. Current efforts are focused upon delivering high local concentrations of cytokine, perhaps by gene delivery methodologies, often in structurally modified form (e.g. by addition of an Fc domain). Alternatively, tissue localizing molecules (e.g. monoclonal antibodies against tissue endothelium specific targets, or damaged tissue epitopes) may be engineered on to cytokines at the molecular level with the objective of providing high concentrations of local cytokine agonist activity in areas of maximal inflammatory insult. This remains an area under development.

The crucial advance in recent years, however, has been the recognition that specific cytokine inhibition can bring about remarkable changes in inflammatory disease expression. Cytokines can be inhibited by interruption of any part of their synthesis, secretion, and effector pathway (described in Chapters 4.2.1 and 4.2.2). Current therapeutics relies mainly on inhibition of cytokines in the extracellular or membrane compartment mediated by large biological drugs. Biological drugs generated thus far comprise antibodies and soluble cytokine receptor fusion proteins. Monoclonal antibodies specific for a given cytokine, which are either 'fully human' (human sequence, e.g. adalimumab, uzekinumab), 'humanized' (rodent sequence modified to resemble human structure) or chimaeric (part of the antibody is rodent derived and part of human structural origin, e.g. infliximab), offer effective high-affinity inhibition. Similarly, soluble cytokine receptors, fused with Fc domains of immunoglobulin to enhance their half-life and stability, similarly provide high-affinity therapeutic inhibitors, e.g. etanercept. Novel modifications to biologic agents, such as addition of polyethylene glycol residues (PEGylation), are in development to provide further refinement of their pharmacokinetic and pharmacodynamic properties.

Other approaches to cytokine inhibition include the generation of small-molecule inhibitors that may target several points in the synthesis and release pathway:

- enzymes that cleave cytokines intracellularly, or from the cell membrane, e.g. TACE, caspase 1
- signal transduction molecules that mediate receptor intracellular function, e.g. syk, JAK3, p38MAPK, JNK, NF-κB
- receptor antagonists selected for direct inhibition of cytokine–receptor protein interaction

An important corollary to small-molecule inhibition, at least for signal transduction inhibitors, is the loss of the exquisite specificity for a single cytokine contained in the biologicals. Thus, pathways such as the MAPK and JAK appear tractable to drug targeting, but since these molecules subserve several inflammatory cytokine receptor pathways, their inhibition is no longer specific to one pathway. The capacity to inhibit several cytokine effector pathways (and hence checkpoints) may be advantageous in bringing higher efficacy but must be carefully balanced with potential toxicity—predictable or idiosyncratic. Future approaches to cytokine inhibition will likely entail gene silencing via delivery of inhibitory RNA species, or gene therapeutic delivery of inhibitory biologic agents.

Cytokine targeting in inflammatory diseases

Cytokine inhibitors are now widely used in a number of chronic inflammatory diseases including rheumatoid arthritis, inflammatory bowel disease, sarcoidosis, psoriasis, psoriatic arthritis, uveitis, and vasculitis and are under investigation in many more conditions. They are dealt with in detail in disease related chapters. Whereas we have clearly used such therapeutics to inform the pathogenesis of diseases, we have also learned critical lessons from the use of these agents about the basic biology of cytokines:

- First, it appears that cytokines exist in highly regulated networks and that there are critical checkpoints in such networks at which inhibition leads to general suppression of the cascade.
- Second, there is redundancy in the cytokine system such that single cytokine blockade, although of therapeutic utility, does not lead to paralysis of the host defence capability. That said, there are some defence processes that may heavily rely on one cytokine—thus TNF appears critical for granuloma formation, hence susceptibility to tuberculosis and some fungal infections in TNF-blocked patients.
- Third, from pharmacokinetic (PK) studies we can deduce that cytokine effects in tissues are quantitatively regulated and thresholds may exist for some of their effector function.
- Fourth, we have not yet established sufficient rationale or understanding of cytokine networks to the level that we can formally combine targeting approaches. Combination targeting in rodent models is highly effective in many disease models, whereas in humans combined biological therapies have thus far led to increased toxicity with no yield in improved efficacy.

Measuring cytokines in biological fluids

There is increasing interest in measurement of cytokines in serum and plasma and *ex vivo* in cellular supernatants. This is in part driven by basic discovery research. However, there is intense interest in the potential for cytokines as biomarkers of disease activity and prognosis or for pharmacodynamic purposes to predict drug response or toxicities. Cytokines were originally measured and defined in bioassays using live cell assays *in vitro* that are impractical for such purposes. Thereafter, enzyme-linked immunosorbent assay (ELISA) or radioimmunoassay became the techniques of choice. Though these are validated and still widely used, the future analysis of cytokines will be facilitated by the use of multiplex technologies, based on laser analysis, which measure up to 30 cytokines in small ($<50\,\mu l$) volumes. Techniques based on protein chips offer further utility to measure the expression of wider ranges (up to 360 proteins per assay) of cytokines. The critical advance here will be to allow analysis of changes in patterns of cytokines as opposed to changes in single moieties that will in turn considerably increase the power of this approach. Moreover such techniques can be adapted to evaluate expression not only in fluid phase but also in tissue extracts to allow evaluation in biopsies.

Concluding remarks

The cytokine field has expanded considerably in recent years. The foregoing discussion highlights their broad functional profile and essential role in both physiologic and pathologic processes. The therapeutic potential in their manipulation has not yet been maximized and the future will hold remarkable advances as these molecular networks give up their secrets to provide for highly specific and well-tolerated interventions.

Further reading

Dayer JM (2004). The process of identifying and understanding cytokines: from basic studies to treating rheumatic diseases. *Best Pract Res Clin Rheumatol*, **18**, 31–45.

Dinarello CA (2005). Blocking IL-1 in systemic inflammation. *J Exp Med*, **201**, 1355–9.

Dong C (2008). TH17 cells in development: an updated view of their molecular identity and genetic programming. *Nat Rev Immunol*, **8**, 337–48.

Elliott MJ, *et al.* (1994). Randomised double-blind comparison of chimeric monoclonal antibody to tumour necrosis factor alpha (cA2) versus placebo in rheumatoid arthritis. *Lancet*, **344**, 1105–10.

Feldmann M, *et al.* (2004). The transfer of a laboratory based hypothesis to a clinically useful therapy: the development of anti-TNF therapy of rheumatoid arthritis. *Best Pract Res Clin Rheumatol*, **18**, 59–80.

McInnes IB, Schett G (2007). Cytokines in the pathogenesis of rheumatoid arthritis. *Nat Rev Immunol*, **7**, 429–42.

Moreland LW, *et al.* (1997). Treatment of rheumatoid arthritis with a recombinant human tumor necrosis factor receptor (p75)-Fc fusion protein. *N Engl J Med*, **337**, 141–7.

Ouyang W, Kolls JK, Zheng Y (2008). The biological functions of T helper 17 cell effector cytokines in inflammation. *Immunity*, **28**, 454–67.

4.4

Ion channels and disease

Frances M. Ashcroft

Essentials

Ion channels are membrane proteins that act as gated pathways for the movement of ions across cell membranes. They are found in both surface and intracellular membranes, and play essential roles in the physiology of all cell types. An ever-increasing number of human diseases are found to be caused by defects in ion channel function. Ion channel diseases may arise in a number of different ways:

- From mutations in the coding region of the gene, or its control elements, leading to the gain, or loss, of channel function. Diseases that result from ion-channel mutations are often known as channelopathies. As with all single-gene disorders, their frequency in the general population is usually very low. Many channelopathies are genetically heterogeneous and the same clinical phenotype may be caused by mutations in different genes, as is the case for long QT syndrome. Conversely, mutations in the same gene may produce different phenotypes. For example, gain-of-function mutations in the epithelial sodium channel produce Liddle's syndrome, whereas loss-of-function mutations cause pseudohypoaldosteronism type 1. Disease severity may also vary with different mutations in the same gene.
- From defective regulation of channel activity by intracellular or extracellular ligands, or by channel modulators, due to mutations in the genes encoding the regulatory molecules themselves, or defects in the pathways leading to their production. For instance, glucokinase mutations cause one type of maturity-onset diabetes of the young (MODY2), by impairing the metabolic regulation of ATP-sensitive potassium channels in pancreatic β cells.
- From autoantibodies to ion channel proteins, which may either down-regulate or enhance channel function. These diseases are discussed elsewhere.
- From ion channels that act as lethal agents. These are secreted by cells and insert into the membrane of the target cell to form large nonselective pores that cause cell lysis and death. Examples include bacterial toxins such as staphylococcal α-toxin and the amoebopore of *Entamoeba histolytica*. The membrane-attack complex of complement, perforin, and the defensins also acts in this way.

Properties of ion channels

To understand how ion channel defects give rise to disease, it is helpful to understand how these proteins work. This section therefore considers what is known of ion channel structure, explains the properties of the single ion channel, and shows how single-channel currents give rise to action potentials and synaptic potentials.

Ion channel structure

Some ion channels consist of a single subunit, as in the case of the calcium-release channel of the sarcoplasmic reticulum. In other cases, the channel pore is formed from a single (α) subunit but associated regulatory subunits may modify the ion channel properties, as in the case of voltage-gated sodium (Na^+) and calcium (Ca^{2+}) channels. Yet other ion channels are multimeric and several subunits are involved in pore formation—the nicotinic acetylcholine receptor comprises five subunits (2α, β, γ, δ, or ε), while the voltage-gated potassium (K^+) channels are composed of four subunits (which are sometimes, but not invariably, identical). Mutations in both pore-forming and regulatory subunits can cause disease.

The multimeric nature of an ion channel may influence whether a channelopathy is inherited in a dominant or recessive fashion. Individuals who are heterozygous for voltage-gated K^+ channel mutations will express both mutant and wild-type subunits in the same cell. If the mutant subunits co-assemble with wild-type subunits to form heteroligomeric channels that are nonfunctional, the resulting K^+ current will be much smaller than if heteromultimerization does not occur. This is known as the 'dominant negative' effect, and may give rise to a disease that is dominantly inherited.

Single-channel properties

An ion channel can either be open or closed. When it is open, permeant ions are able to move through the channel pore. The current flowing through the open pore is known as the single-channel current. Its magnitude is determined by the ion concentrations on either side of the membrane (the chemical gradient), by the membrane potential (the electrical gradient), and by the ease with which the ion can move through the channel pore (its permeability). At the equilibrium potential of an ion, the electrical and chemical gradients are equal in magnitude but opposite in direction, and thus there is no net ion flux. The single-channel conductance(γ) is a measure of the permeability of the ion and is given by the single-channel current (i) divided by the membrane potential ($\gamma = i/V$).

Ion channels are often highly selective in the ions they conduct. Potassium channels, for example, are about 100 times more permeable to K^+ than to Na^+, while Na^+ channels conduct Na^+ but discriminate against K^+. Ion selectivity takes place within a narrow region of the pore known as the selectivity filter. The basis of ion selectivity is only just beginning to be understood, but it is clear that while some ions are excluded on the basis of their size or their charge, hydrophobic interactions and the energy required to remove the waters of hydration are also important.

The fraction of time the channel spends in the open state is known as the open probability. Some channels open and close at random, but in other channels gating is regulated. In voltage-gated channels the open probability is determined by the membrane potential, whereas in ligand-gated channels it is regulated by the binding of extracellular or intracellular ligands. Gating may also be subject to modulation, a process in which channel opening or closing is modified, usually by one of a number of cytosolic substances (e.g. Ca^{2+} binding or phosphorylation). Gating is believed to involve conformational changes in the channel structure that result in the opening or closing of the pore.

At the resting potential of the cell, most voltage-gated channels are closed. In response to a membrane depolarization, the open probability of the channel is increased. This voltage-dependent activation may be followed by a further conformational transition (inactivation) to an inactivated state in which the channel no longer conducts ions. Recovery from inactivation occurs after a variable period following repolarization to the resting potential. Although most voltage-gated ion channels are opened by depolarization, a few types of voltage-gated channel are activated by hyperpolarization. Ligand-gated channels are opened (or more rarely closed) by binding of an appropriate ligand to a specific site on the channel protein, which induces a conformational change that allosterically opens the ion pore. The channel may open and close several times while the ligand remains bound to its receptor, but this intrinsic gating ceases on ligand dissociation.

There are numerous different types of channel. For example, even among the inwardly rectifying K^+ channels there are seven subfamilies, most of which have several members. In general, ion channels are named after their gating and/or selectivity properties.

Single-channel currents summate to produce macroscopic currents

The cell membrane contains many hundreds of ion channels. The macroscopic current (I) flowing through all ion channels of the same type is determined by the product of the number of channels in the membrane (N), the channel open probability (P), and the single-channel current (i); in other words $I = NPi$. Disease-causing mutations may affect any or all of these parameters and thereby influence the macroscopic current.

Cell membranes also contain several different types of channel. The total current that flows across the cell membrane (the membrane current) represents the sum of the ion fluxes through all the different kinds of ion channel open in the membrane. If it is sufficiently large, the membrane current may cause a change in membrane potential. The size of this voltage change is given by Ohm's law ($V = IR$) and is therefore influenced by both the current amplitude (I) and by the membrane resistance (R) (which in turn reflects the number of open channels). A change in the membrane potential to a more positive value is known as depolarization; hyperpolarization is a change to more negative potentials. The resting potential of most cells lies between –60 and –100 mV.

Action potentials

In excitable cells, a depolarizing stimulus may elicit an action potential. In nerve axons and skeletal muscle fibres, the action potential results from the initial activation of voltage-gated Na^+ channels followed shortly afterwards by activation of voltage-gated K^+ channels. Because Na^+ channels open rapidly on depolarization, there is an initial inward Na^+ current. If this is greater than the outward current flowing through (voltage-independent) K^+ channels which are open at the resting potential, it will produce a further depolarization. This activates more Na^+ channels and depolarizes the membrane even more. In this way, a regenerative increase in membrane potential (an action potential) is produced. The membrane is returned to its resting level by inactivation of the Na^+ channels (which reduces the inward current) and the opening of K^+ channels (which produces an outward, hyperpolarizing current).

The potential at which the inward Na^+ current exactly balances the outward current through resting K^+ channels is known as the threshold potential. It is a critical potential: any increase in the Na^+ current will elicit an action potential, while any reduction in the inward current (or increase in the outward current) will prevent action potential generation. Ion channel mutations may increase nerve or muscle excitability either by enhancing the inward current (as in hyperkalaemic periodic paralysis), or by reducing the outward current (as in some forms of long QT syndrome). This will produce a larger depolarization, so that the threshold potential is reached more easily and a subsequent action potential is initiated. Other mutations produce a depolarizing block of action potential activity. This results from a maintained membrane depolarization of sufficient amplitude to inactivate the voltage-dependent Na^+ channels.

In some cells, additional types of ion channel contribute to the action potential—the ventricular action potential is mediated by voltage-dependent Na^+ and Ca^{2+} channels, and at least four kinds of K^+ channel; several different kinds of K^+ channel contribute to the repolarization of action potentials in mammalian neurons; and chloride (Cl^-) channels play an important role in the electrical activity of skeletal muscle. The functional importance of these different ion channels is exemplified by the fact that mutations in the genes which encode them produce a range of nerve and muscle diseases.

Synaptic potentials

When a nerve impulse arrives in the presynaptic terminal it opens voltage-gated Ca^{2+} channels, producing a rise in the intracellular Ca^{2+} concentration ($[Ca^{2+}]_i$) that triggers the exocytosis of synaptic vesicles. The amount of transmitter released varies with $[Ca^{2+}]_i$ and thus with the magnitude of the presynaptic Ca^{2+} current. In turn, this is influenced by the duration of the membrane depolarization and thus by the amplitude of the voltage-gated K^+ current that underlies membrane repolarization. A reduction in the presynaptic K^+ current therefore leads to excess transmitter release and postsynaptic hyperexcitability, as in episodic ataxia type 1 and acquired neuromyotonia. Conversely, a reduction in the presynaptic Ca^{2+} current is associated with reduced transmitter release, as occurs in Lambert–Eaton myasthenic syndrome when the density of presynaptic Ca^{2+} channels is decreased by receptor internalization induced by the binding of autoantibodies.

Once released, the transmitter diffuses across the synaptic cleft and binds to receptors in the postsynaptic membrane. At the neuromuscular junction, for example, acetylcholine (ACh) binds to the nicotinic acetylcholine receptor (AChR), and opens an intrinsic ion channel. The resulting synaptic current produces a depolarization of the postsynaptic membrane (the endplate potential) which, if it is sufficiently large, triggers an action potential in the muscle fibre. A reduction in AChR density, as in myasthenia gravis, decreases effective transmission and leads to muscle weakness. Gain-of-function mutations in AChR may also induce myasthenia, by causing prolonged depolarization of the postsynaptic membrane and thereby Na^+ channel inactivation. This depolarizing block is the basis of the slow-channel syndromes. Mutations in the voltage-gated Na^+ channel of skeletal muscle may cause paralysis, or myotonia.

In skeletal muscle, the action potential is conducted into the interior of the fibre via invaginations of the surface membrane known as the transverse tubules (T-tubules). Depolarization of the T-tubule membrane stimulates the opening of Ca^{2+}-release channels (RyR) in the membrane of the sarcoplasmic reticulum (SR), the intracellular Ca^{2+} store. The T-tubule and SR membranes are not directly connected and the precise mechanism by which they interact is not fully understood. However, there is evidence that the α_1-subunit of the voltage-gated Ca^{2+} channel in the T-tubule membrane acts as the voltage sensor for the Ca^{2+}-release channels in the SR membrane. Mutations in the Ca^{2+}-release channel of skeletal muscles cause malignant hyperthermia and central core disease.

The channelopathies

This section provides brief descriptions of a selected range of channelopathies. Table 4.4.1 lists these diseases, the channels involved, their gene names and chromosomal locations. The list is far from exhaustive. Additional details may be found elsewhere in the *Oxford Textbook of Medicine* or in the books and Websites referenced.

Neuronal channelopathies

Epilepsy

Mutations in the α-subunit of the voltage-gated Na^+ channel *SCN1A* account for ~20% of cases of generalized epilepsy with febrile seizures plus (GEFS+). Affected individuals exhibit febrile seizures in childhood and afebrile generalized epilepsy in later life. GFES+ has also been linked to mutations in the β1-subunit of the voltage-gated Na^+ channel (*SCN1B*). The presence of the β-subunit accelerates both the rate of inactivation, and the rate of recovery from inactivation, of the voltage-gated Na^+ channel. Precisely how *SCN1A* and *SCN1B* mutations lead to GFES+ remains unclear.

De novo mutations in *SCN1A* also comprise 70% of cases of severe myoclonic epilepsy of infancy (SMEI). This severe childhood epilepsy is often associated with ataxia, motor developmental delay and cognitive impairments. Screening for *SCN1A* mutations is advised in children with early onset seizures as sodium channel blockers enhance their symptoms and should be avoided. Mutations in *SCNA2* and *SCNA3* channels have also been identified as the cause of epilepsy in some patients.

Benign familial neonatal convulsions

Benign familial neonatal convulsions (BFNC) is characterized by neonatal convulsions within the first 7 days after birth that normally show spontaneous remission by the third month of life. There is an increased risk of epilepsy in later life in 10 to 15% of individuals. Mutations in the voltage-gated K^+ channel genes *KCNQ2* and *KCNQ3* are associated with BFNC.

KCNQ2 and KCNQ3 associate in a heteromeric complex to form the M-channel. This channel plays a critical role in determining the electrical excitability of many neurons. It is slowly activated when the membrane is depolarized to around the threshold level for action potential firing, thereby hyperpolarizing the membrane back towards its resting level. This reduces neuronal excitability by limiting the spiking frequency and decreasing the responsiveness of the neuron to synaptic inputs. Some BNFC mutations result in reduced channel density. Others alter the channel kinetics. Both are expected to lead to neuronal hyperexcitability, accounting for the epileptic seizures. Because the M-channel is a heteromer of KCNQ2 or KCNQ3, mutations in either gene will disrupt channel function and cause BNFC.

Episodic ataxia type 1

Episodic ataxia type 1 (familial periodic cerebellar ataxia with myokymia) is an autosomal dominant disorder that causes ataxia accompanied by myokymia, nausea, vertigo, and headache. It results from mutations in the voltage-gated K^+ channel $K_V1.1$, which is expressed in the synaptic terminals and dendrites of many brain neurons. These mutations either prevent the formation of functional channels or result in a reduced K^+ current. This is expected to prolong the neuronal action potential, inducing repetitive firing and excessive and unregulated transmitter release, and thereby produce the clinical symptoms of ataxia and myokymia.

Familial hemiplegic migraine, episodic ataxia type 2, and spinocerebellar ataxia type 6

There are three human diseases with different phenotypes that are associated with mutations in the same Ca^{2+}-channel gene, *CACNA1A*. These are familial hemiplegic migraine (FHM), episodic ataxia type 2 (EA-2), and spinocerebellar ataxia type 6 (SCA-6). All three diseases result in progressive cerebellar atrophy, but they differ in the extent and rate of progression of neuronal degeneration, with SCA-6 showing the greatest atrophy, and FHM the least. Migraine-like symptoms also occur in all three diseases and are most severe in patients with FHM, who suffer transient hemiparesis. EA-2 and SCA-6 are also characterized by ataxia and nystagmus. FHM is associated with missense mutations. In mice, these lead to an increase in the P/Q type Ca^{2+} current of cerebellar and cortical neurons and an enhanced tendency to cortical spreading depression, which may underlie the migraine.

Startle disease (hyperekplexia)

Glycine is the major inhibitory transmitter in the brainstem and spinal cord. It binds to a ligand-gated Cl^- channel, producing an increase in Cl^- permeability that reduces the membrane depolarization and neuronal firing induced by excitatory neurotransmitters. The glycine receptor is a pentamer of three α-subunits, which contain the glycine-binding site, and two β-subunits. In humans, two types of the α-subunit have been identified. Mutations in the gene encoding the α_1-subunit of the glycine receptor give rise to startle disease (hyperekplexia). This is an autosomal dominant neurological disorder characterized by muscle spasm in response to an unexpected stimulus. It manifests as facial grimacing, hunching of the shoulders, clenching of the fists, exaggerated jerks of the limbs and sudden falls. Startle disease mutations produce a dramatic decrease in glycine-activated currents. Because glycinergic interneurons are important for normal spinal cord reflexes, muscle tone, and the pattern of motor neuron firing during movement, this leads to excessive and uncontrolled movements.

Charcot–Marie–Tooth disease

Charcot–Marie–Tooth disease type 1 (CMT1) causes progressive degeneration and demyelination of the peripheral nerves. It is genetically heterogeneous, but the X-linked form of the disease results from mutations in the gap junction channel connexin 32 (Cx32). It shows incomplete dominant inheritance, with heterozygous females being affected less severely than hemizygous males. The phenotype may vary from mild, in which the patient has a normal gait, to a severe form which may necessitate the use of a walking stick or wheelchair.

More than 100 mutations in *CX32* have been identified. They fall into two main groups—those in which the protein never reaches the plasma membrane, and those where the protein reaches the membrane but forms channels with altered functional properties. The former give rise to a severe phenotype, whereas the latter may be associated with either mild or severe phenotypes, according to whether they partially or completely disrupt channel function.

The Cx32 protein is primarily expressed in the Schwann cells of peripheral myelinated nerves, at the nodes of Ranvier and at Schmidt–Lanterman incisures. In these regions, the myelin is not complete and there is a thin layer of cytoplasm between each of the enveloping turns of the Schwann cell. This suggests that Cx32 may serve as a short-cut pathway for nutrients and other substances moving to the innermost layers of the Schwann cell, and perhaps also to the axon itself. This might explain why loss of Cx32 function causes axonal degeneration and demyelination.

Familial pain syndromes

Mutations in the peripheral nerve voltage-gated Na^+ channel Nav1.7 (*SCN9A*) cause familial pain disorders. Gain-of-function mutations produce erythermalgia and paroxysmal extreme pain disorder (PEPD). Conversely, loss-of-function mutations lead to a congenital inability to sense pain. Erythermalgia is characterized by episodes of erythema and burning pain of the lower legs and feet that usually are provoked by warmth or exercise. PEPD is associated with severe pain triggered by bowel movements: it may be accompanied by nonepileptic seizures and cardiac problems. These symptoms arise because Nav1.7 is expressed in nociceptive neurons and activating mutations enhance their excitability. Loss-of-function mutations lead to impaired action potential transmission and a reduced ability to sense pain: patients may not recognize they have hurt themselves as they feel no pain from bone fractures or walking on hot coals.

Cardiac muscle channelopathies

Long QT syndrome is a congenital cardiac disorder associated with an abrupt loss of consciousness and sudden death from ventricular arrhythmia in children and young adults. It is characterized by an abnormally long QT interval in the electrocardiogram, which reflects the delayed repolarization of the ventricular action potential. This predisposes to *torsade de pointes* and ventricular fibrillation. The duration of the cardiac action potential is determined by the balance between the inward and outward currents flowing during the plateau phase. Prolongation of the action potential can therefore be caused by a persistent inward current or by a reduction in outward K^+ currents.

Seven different cardiac ion channels are associated with long QT syndrome, the most common being *KCNQ1*, *KCNH2* (HERG), and *SCN5A* (Table 4.4.1). The I_{Ks} channel is a complex of two different proteins, KCNQ1 and minK. Likewise, I_{Kr} is a complex of HERG and Mirp1. Mutations in these four genes either abolish or markedly decrease the repolarizing K^+ currents I_{Ks} and I_{Kr}, and are therefore expected to prolong the cardiac action potential and increase the QT interval. Mutations in the cardiac muscle Na^+ channel gene (*SCN5A*) also cause LQT. These mutations affect Na^+ channel inactivation, producing a sustained inward current that results in an increased action potential duration. The larger the component of noninactivating current, the more severe the phenotype.

In many cases, long QT syndrome is not inherited but acquired. For example, drugs that block I_{Kr} or I_{Ks} currents prolong the cardiac action potential and induce long QT syndrome. Among these are the antibiotic erythromycin, the class III antiarrhythmic agents such as sotalol, dofetilide, and quinidine (which selectively block I_{Kr}) and the antihistamine H_1-receptor antagonists terfenidine and astemizole (which block HERG). In most people, terfenidine does not produce cardiac problems as it is rapidly broken down in the liver and its metabolite, terfenidine carboxylate, does not block I_{Kr}. However, if the activity of the P450 enzymes that break down terfenidine is impaired (due to liver disease or drugs such as ketoconazole and the macrolide antibiotics), there is a risk of *torsade de pointes.*

Skeletal muscle channelopathies

Myasthenia gravis, slow-channel, fast-channel, and AChR deficiency syndromes

Myasthenia gravis is usually produced by autoantibodies directed against the nicotinic acetylcholine receptor (nAChR), as discussed elsewhere. These antibodies lead to loss of nAChR due to internalization and thus to a smaller endplate potential that fails to reach the threshold for action potential initiation.

At least three different congenital myasthenic syndromes are produced by mutations in the muscle nAChR channel. Slow-channel syndrome (SCS) mutations are found in all four subunits of the adult channel (α, β, δ, ε) and result in protracted channel activation by acetylcholine. The increase in channel open probability produces a prolonged synaptic current and endplate potential. Impaired neuromuscular transmission is thought to result from a combination of three pathogenic mechanisms. First, temporal summation of endplate potentials can occur at physiological rates of stimulation, leading to prolonged depolarization of the muscle membrane, inactivation of voltage-gated Na^+ channels, and failure of muscle excitability. A similar 'depolarization block' is observed with acetylcholinesterase inhibitors or with nAChR agonists like suxamethonium. Second, the prolonged endplate potential causes excess Ca^{2+} entry and activation of proteolytic enzymes, which may account for the progressive destruction of the postsynaptic neuromuscular junction observed in SCS—loss of junctional nAChRs and destruction of the junctional folds has been reported. Abnormal channel openings in the absence of acetylcholine may also contribute to the 'endplate myopathy'. Third, the slow channel mutations give an increased propensity for the nAChR to enter a desensitized state in which it is unable to respond to acetylcholine.

Fast-channel syndrome (FCS) is the converse of SCS: nAChR mutations shorten channel openings thereby reducing the endplate potential amplitude below that required to trigger action potentials. nAChR deficiency, the most common congenital myasthenic syndrome, results from mutations (often in the ε subunit) that impair channel assembly and insertion into the plasma membrane.

Acetylcholinesterase inhibitors ameliorate the symptoms of nAChR deficiency and FCS but exacerbate those of SCS. However, SCS often benefits from treatment with open channel blockers of nAChR, such as fluoxetine or quinidine. All nAChR genetic disorders are unresponsive to immunotherapies.

The periodic paralyses

Hyperkalaemic periodic paralysis, paramyotonia congenita, and the potassium-aggravated myotonias result from mutations in the α-subunit of the human skeletal muscle Na^+ channel. All are inherited as dominant traits and usually present within the first or second decade of life.

Hyperkalaemic periodic paralysis (HyperPP) may occur spontaneously, but attacks are commonly precipitated by exercise, stress, fasting, or eating potassium-rich foods. Paralysis is often preceded by signs of muscle hyperexcitability such as myotonia or fasciculations. The duration is variable (minutes to hours) and may be so severe that the patient is unable to remain standing. It is associated with a raised blood K^+ concentration (5 to 7 mM). Paramyotonia congenita is precipitated by cold and (in contrast to most classical myotonias) aggravated by exercise. In some patients, the myotonia may be followed by prolonged paralysis. Potassium-aggravated myotonia is characterized by myotonia without muscle weakness or paralysis. It can be distinguished from classical myotonias by the fact that the myotonia is exacerbated by a mild elevation of the plasma K^+ concentration.

All three types of disorder result from mutations in the α-subunit of the skeletal muscle Na^+ channel (*SCN4A*), which disrupt Na^+ channel inactivation. As a consequence, they produce a persistent inward current that causes a tonic depolarization of the muscle membrane (the larger the current, the greater the depolarization). The magnitude of the depolarization determines whether myotonia or paralysis occurs. A small depolarization causes membrane hyperexcitability by lowering the action potential threshold, whereas a large depolarization can lead to Na^+ channel inactivation and thereby paralysis. It is still not understood how cold or an elevated plasma potassium level precipitate attacks.

Myotonia

Loss-of-function mutations in the gene *CLCN1* encoding the skeletal muscle Cl^- channel produce two forms of myotonia—the autosomal dominant myotonia congenita (Thomsen's disease) and the autosomal recessive generalized myotonia (Becker's disease). Clinical descriptions of the disease can be found in Chapter 24.24.4.

In normal skeletal muscle, the Cl^- conductance accounts for between 70 and 80% of the resting membrane conductance. Mutations in *CLCN1* that result in a loss of functional Cl^- channels will therefore produce a marked increase in the input resistance of the muscle fibre. Consequently, muscle excitability will be enhanced (because a smaller Na^+ current will be sufficient to trigger an action potential). The elevated input resistance also produces a reduced rate of action potential repolarization, which enhances muscle excitability. An important role of the muscle Cl^- conductance is to counteract the depolarizing effect of K^+ accumulation in the transverse tubular system that accompanies muscle activity. During an action potential, K^+ ions leave the muscle fibre. In normal muscle, the amount of K^+ entering the transverse tubular system during a single action potential is not sufficient to alter the membrane potential, because the tubular Cl^- conductance is very high. But in myotonic muscle, the Cl^- conductance is very low and a small rise in tubular K^+ produces a significant depolarization following an action potential. If several action potentials occur in rapid succession, summation of the after-depolarizations may be sufficient to trigger spontaneous action potentials and thereby myotonia.

Mutations in *CLCN1* give rise to both recessive and dominant forms of myotonia. This may be because the muscle Cl^- channel is a dimer. In heterozygotes, mutant subunits might combine with wild-type subunits to form heteromeric channels. The extent to which the mutant subunit reduced the function of the heteromeric channel would thus dictate the severity of myotonia. Total inactivation of the channel by a single mutant subunit (the dominant-negative effect) would produce dominant myotonia, whereas recessive myotonia might occur if the heteromeric channel was unaffected by the mutant subunit.

Malignant hypothermia and central core disease

Mutations in the ligand-gated Ca^{2+} channel of skeletal muscle cause malignant hyperthermia and central core disease. This channel mediates Ca^{2+} release from the sarcoplasmic reticulum (SR), allowing Ca^{2+} to enter the cytoplasm and activate the contractile proteins. It is also known as the ryanodine receptor (or RYR1) because it binds the alkaloid ryanodine with high affinity.

Malignant hyperthermia (MH) is one of the main causes of death due to anaesthesia. In susceptible individuals, common inhalation anaesthetics or depolarizing muscle relaxants trigger accelerated skeletal muscle metabolism, muscle contractures, hyperkalaemia, arrhythmias, respiratory and metabolic acidosis, and a rapid rise in body temperature (as much as 1 °C every 5 min). It is thought that this is due to stimulation of Ca^{2+} release from the SR, which produces a sustained increase in intracellular Ca^{2+}. This activates both metabolic and contractile activity; the former results in respiratory and metabolic acidosis and the latter produces the elevation in body temperature. The syndrome can be treated with dantrolene sodium, which blocks Ca^{2+} release from the SR. Malignant hyperthermia is genetically heterogeneous and is not linked to *RYR1* in all families.

Central core disease (CCD) is an autosomal dominant, non-progressive myopathy that presents in infancy as proximal muscle weakness and hypertonia. Diagnosis is by muscle biopsy, which reveals that regions of type 1 skeletal muscle fibres (known as 'central cores') are depleted of mitochondria and oxidative enzymes. The disease is often associated with a predisposition to malignant hyperthermia and results from mutations in *RYR1*. Thus CCD and MH are allelic disorders of the same gene. It is not clear how the different phenotypes arise, especially because the same mutation can give rise to MH in some individuals and CCD in others. Because all CCD patients are MH-susceptible, it is possible that additional factors are necessary for the development of central core disease.

Kidney channelopathies

Liddle's syndrome

Liddle's syndrome is a congenital form of salt-sensitive hypertension characterized by a very high rate of renal Na^+ uptake despite low levels of aldosterone, secondary hypokalaemia, and metabolic acidosis. It is caused by gain-of-function mutations in the epithelial sodium channel (ENaC). This channel consists of three subunits (α, β, γ), and disease-causing mutations have been identified in both the β- and γ-subunits. All are located in the C-terminus of the protein and result in constitutive channel hyperactivity.

The increase in ENaC current causes enhanced Na^+ uptake. This is accompanied by increased water uptake, thereby producing a chronic increase in blood volume and ultimately hypertension. An increased Na^+ uptake also has secondary consequences: in particular, K^+ secretion into the tubule lumen is stimulated because the apical membrane depolarizes and so increases the driving force for K^+ efflux. In addition, more K^+ enters the cell due to the enhanced activity of the Na^+/K^+-ATPase. This explains why excess ENaC activity in Liddle's syndrome is associated with hypokalaemia and, conversely, why reduced ENaC activity, as in pseudohypoaldosteronism type 1, is accompanied by hyperkalaemia. Treatment is a low salt diet and K-sparing diuretics like amiloride that directly block the ENaC channel.

Pseudohypoaldosteronism type 1

While gain-of-function mutations in ENaC cause enhanced Na^+ uptake and hypertension, loss-of-function mutations produce salt-wasting, hypotension, and dehydration in newborns and infants. Pseudohypoaldosteronism type 1 results from loss-of-function mutations in the α, β, or γ ENaC subunits. The marked reduction in ENaC activity leads to decreased Na^+ absorption by the kidney. This stimulates renin and aldosterone secretion, but salt reabsorption cannot be augmented as ENaC is not functional. The high Na^+ concentration in the tubular fluid causes water to be osmotically retained in the tubule lumen, leading to diuresis and dehydration.

Bartter's syndrome

Bartter's syndrome is characterized by severe salt-wasting, with elevated plasma renin and aldosterone levels. The syndrome is both phenotypically and genetically heterogeneous, and several subtypes have been distinguished. Antenatal Bartter's syndrome or hyperprostaglandin-E syndrome presents *in utero* with a marked fetal polyuria. Newborns fail to thrive and show polyuria, polydypsia, severe salt-wasting, moderate hypokalaemia, and metabolic acidosis, and elevated urinary excretion of prostaglandins. There is also marked calcinuria, osteopenia, and nephrocalcinosis.

Antenatal Bartter's syndrome results from loss-of-function mutations in the genes encoding proteins involved in salt transport in the cells of the distal kidney tubules. These include the inwardly rectifying K^+ channel Kir1.1 (*KCNJ1*; Bartter's syndrome type II), the NaK_2Cl cotransporter (*SLC12A1*, Bartter's syndrome type I), and the voltage-gated Cl^- channel CLC-Kb (*CLCNKB*, Bartter's syndrome type III). These variants may be distinguished clinically, because hypokalaemia is less pronounced (3.0 to 3.5 mM) in patients with mutations in *KCNJ1*, and the course of the disease is less severe. And in contrast to patients with Bartter's syndrome types I and II, patients with mutations in *CLCNKB* do not suffer from nephrocalcinosis, despite elevation of the urinary calcium concentration.

Disease-causing mutations in Kir1.1 or CLC-Kb impair NaCl uptake in the distal tubules by reducing channel function or decreasing protein expression. This leads to a high salt concentration in the urine and thus to an osmotic diuresis, which accounts for the salt-wasting, polyuria, and low plasma volume characteristic of Bartter's syndrome. A similar phenotype is observed with loop diuretics, such as frusemide (furosemide), which inhibit the NaK_2Cl cotransporter.

SeSAME syndrome

Loss-of-function mutations in the inwardly rectifying K^+ channel Kir4.1 (*KCNJ10*) give rise to SeSAME syndrome (also called EAST syndrome). This complex disorder is characterized by seizures, sensineural deafness, ataxia, mental retardation, and electrolyte imbalance (e.g. hypokalemia, hypomagnesemia, metabolic acidosis). Kir4.1 is expressed in the kidney, inner ear, and glial cells. It is postulated that K^+ recycling in the distal convoluted tubule is mediated by Kir4.1 and that in its absence the Na^+/K^+-ATPase is inhibited, reducing Na^+ uptake. This stimulates Na^+ uptake in other regions of the kidney tubule, which leads to increased K^+ and H^+ resorption and thereby hypokalemia and metabolic acidosis.

Dent's disease

Dent's disease describes a spectrum of related inherited disorders of renal function that result from mutations in the renal chloride channel gene, *CLCN5*. Different mutations can produce phenotypically distinct syndromes (Table 4.4.1), which may involve low molecular weight proteinuria, hypercalciuria, hyperphosphaturia, nephrocalcinosis and nephrolithiasis. ClC-5 is found in apical endosomes of kidney proximal tubule cells. Mouse models suggest that ClC-5 mutations result in reduced uptake of protein (including parathyroid hormone) by the proximal tubules. This leads to impaired metabolism of calciotropic hormones and ultimately to hyperphosphaturia and kidney stones.

Nephrogenic diabetes insipidus

Familial nephrogenic diabetes insipidus (NDI) results from impaired water uptake by the kidney tubules. The diseases manifests within the first few weeks of life and is characterized by the excretion of large amounts of hypotonic urine and excessive thirst. In early infancy these may not be noticed and the disease is often recognized by signs of dehydration, such as poor feeding, poor weight gain, irritability, and fever. In most cases, familial NDI is caused by a mutation in the vasopressin receptor, but in some families it results from loss-of-function mutations in the aquaporin 2 (*AQP2*) gene. AQP2 is expressed exclusively in the collecting duct of the kidney and plays a fundamental role in the production of a concentrated urine because it acts as a water channel. Vasopressin stimulates water uptake by causing the insertion of AQP2 channels into the apical membranes of the principal cells of the collecting duct, thereby enhancing water uptake. Loss-of-function mutations in *AQP2* result in a dramatic reduction in water channels, thereby accounting for the polyuria.

Table 4.4.1 Ion-channel genes associated with disease

Gene	Chromosome location	Protein	Disease
Neuronal diseases			
SCN1A	2q24	Voltage-gated Na^+ channel α-subunit, Nav1.1	Epilepsy (GEFS + type-2)
SCN2A	2q23–q24.3	Voltage-gated Na^+ channel α-subunit, Nav1.2	Benign familial infantile seizures
SCN9A	2q24	Voltage-gated Na^+ channel α-subunit, Nav1.7	Erythermalgia, Paroxysmal extreme pain disorder, Congenital indifference to pain
SCN1B	19q13.1	Voltage-gated Na^+ channel β-subunit	Epilepsy (GEFS + type-1)
KCNA1	12p13	Voltage-gated K^+ channel (Kv1.1)	Episodic ataxia type-1
KCNQ2	20q13.3	Voltage-gated K^+ channel	Epilepsy (BNFC)
KCNQ3	8q24	Voltage-gated K^+ channel	Epilepsy (BNFC)
CACNA1A	19p13.1	Voltage-gated Ca^{2+} channel (α-subunit P/Q type)	Episodic ataxia type-2, Familial hemiplegic migraine and Spinocerebellar ataxia type-6
CACNB4	2q22–q23	Voltage-gated Ca^{2+} channel β4-subunit	Juvenile myoclonic epilepsy Generalized epilepsy and praxis seizures
CHRNA4	20q13.2–13.3	nACh-receptor α_4-subunit	Epilepsy (nocturnal frontal lobe epilepsy type-1)
CHRNB2	1q21	nACh-receptor β-subunit	Epilepsy (nocturnal frontal lobe epilepsy type-3)
GLRA1	5p32	Glycine-receptor α_1-subunit	Hyperekplexia (startle disease)
GJB1	Xq13.1	Connexin 32	Charcot–Marie–Tooth disease
Cardiac muscle diseases			
SCN5A	3p21–24	Voltage-gated Na^+-channel α-subunit	Long-QT syndrome (LQT3), Brugada syndrome, Congenital conduction defects
KCNQ1	11p15.5	Voltage-gated K^+ channel α-subunit	Long-QT syndrome (LQT1) (Romano–Ward syndrome, Jervall–Lange–Nielsen syndrome)
KCNH2	7q35–36	Voltage-gated K^+ channel α-subunit (HERG)	Long-QT syndrome (LQT2), Short QT syndrome
KCNE1	21q22.1–q22.2	Voltage-gated K^+-channel β-subunit (MinK)	Long-QT syndrome (LQT5) Jervall–Lange–Nielsen syndrome
KCNE2	21q22.1	Voltage-gated K^+-channel β-subunit (MiRP1)	Long-QT syndrome (LQT6)
RYR2	1q42.1–q43	Ca^{2+}-release channel of cardiac SR	Ventricular tachycardia
Skeletal muscle diseases			
SCN4A	17q23–q25	Voltage-gated Na^+-channel α-subunit	HyperPP, PAM, paramyotonia congenita
CACNA1S	1q32	Voltage-gated Ca^{2+} channel α_{1S}-subunit (L-type)	Hypokalaemic periodic paralysis Malignant hyperthermia
KCNE3	11q13–14	Voltage-gated K^+-channel β-subunit (MiRP2)	Hypokalaemic periodic paralysis
KCNJ2	17q23	Inward rectifier K^+ channel Kir2.1	Andersen syndrome
CLCN1	7q35	Voltage-gated Cl^- channel, ClC-1	Myotonia congenita, generalized myotonia
RYR1	19q13.1	Ca^{2+}-release channel of SR	Malignant hyperthermia, central core disease
CHRNA1	2q24–q32	nACh-receptor α_1-subunit	Slow-channel syndrome (SCS), Fast-channel syndrome (FCS)
CHRNB1	17p12–p11	nACh-receptor β-subunit	SCS, nAChR deficiency syndrome
CHRND	2q33–q34	nACh-receptor δ-subunit	SCS, FCS
CHRNE	17p13.1	nACh-receptor ε-subunit	SCS, nAChR deficiency syndrome
Kidney diseases			
KCNJ1	11q24	Inward rectifier K^+ channel Kir1.1	Bartter's syndrome (type II)
KCNJ10	1q23.2	Inward rectifier K^+ channel, Kir4.1	SeSAME syndrome
CLCNKB	1p36	Voltage-gated Cl^- channel	Bartter's syndrome (type III)
CLCN5	Xp11.22	Voltage-gated Cl^- channel, ClC-5	Nephrolithiasis (Dent's disease*)
SCNN1A	12p13	Epithelial Na^+ channel α-subunit	Pseudohypoaldosteronism (PHA-1)
SCNN1B	16p13–p12	Epithelial Na^+ channel β-subunit	Liddle's syndrome, PHA-1, Bronchiectasis (BESC)

(Continued)

Table 4.4.1 *(Cont'd)* Ion-channel genes associated with disease

Gene	Chromosome location	Protein	Disease
SCNN1G	16p13–p12	Epithelial Na^+ channel γ-subunit	Liddle's syndrome, PHA-1, BESC
AQP2	12q13	Aquaporin 2 (water channel)	Nephrogenic diabetes insipidus
Other diseases			
KCNJ11	11p15.1	ATP-sensitive K^+ channel subunit, Kir6.2	Neonatal diabetes, Congenital hyperinsulinaemia of infancy
SUR1	11p15.1	ATP-sensitive K^+ channel subunit, SUR1	Neonatal diabetes, Congenital hyperinsulinaemia of infancy
CFTR	7q31	CFTR Cl^- channel	Cystic fibrosis
CLCN7	16p13	Voltage-gated Cl^- channel, ClC-7	Osteopetrosis
CNGA1	4p12–cen	Cyclic nucleotide-gated channel α-subunit	Retinitis pigmentosa
STIM1	11p15.5	CRAC channel subunit	Immunodeficiency and autoimmunity syndrome
ORAI1	12q24	CRAC channel subunit	Immunodeficiency and autoimmunity syndrome
GJB2	13q11–q12	Connexin 26	Deafness (DFNA3 and DFNB1) Vohwinkel's syndrome
GJB3	1p35.1	Connexin 31	Nonsyndromal sensineural deafness (DFNA2) Erythrokeratodermia variabilis
GJB6	13q12	Connexin 30	Deafness (DFNA3) Ectodermal dysplasia
GJA3	13q11	Connexin 46	Cataract (zonular pulverulent type-3)
GJA8	1q21.1	Connexin 50	Cataract (zonular pulverulent type-1)

BNFC, benign familial neonatal epilepsy; GEFS+, generalized epilepsy with febrile seizures plus; HyperPP, hyperkalaemic periodic paralysis; PAM, potassium-aggravated myotonia; PHA-1, pseudohypoaldosteronism type 1, BESC, Bronchiectasis with or without elevated sweat chloride

*Dent's disease is now recognized to include X-linked recessive nephrolithiasis, X-linked hypophosphataemic rickets, and a renal tubular defect in Japanese children

Other channelopathies

Cystic fibrosis

Of all the channelopathies, the best known is probably cystic fibrosis (CF). Its clinical features are described in Chapter 18.10. Cystic fibrosis results from mutations in an epithelial chloride channel known as the cystic fibrosis transmembrane conductance regulator (CFTR). Although its primary sequence is highly homologous to that of the ATP-binding cassette transporters, it is now well established that CFTR functions as a chloride channel. It also regulates the activity of the outwardly rectifying Cl^- channel and the epithelial Na^+ channel.

All disease-causing CF mutations result in the complete absence or a marked reduction in CFTR function. Those which result in the total loss of channel activity, either because the protein does not reach the plasma membrane or because it is present but completely inactive, give rise to a severe form of the disease. Mutations that result in a reduced Cl^- current are associated with a milder form of the disease. Compound heterozygotes carrying one allele with a severe mutation and another with a mild mutation will have significant residual channel activity and therefore a mild form of the disease.

Although a large number of mutations (more than 450) have been identified in CFTR, it is still far from certain how the loss of Cl^--channel function gives rise to the clinical features of the disease, especially in the lungs.

Insulin secretory disorders

The pancreatic β-cell ATP-sensitive K^+ (K_{ATP}) channel consists of two types of subunit: a pore-forming subunit Kir6.2 (*KCNJ11*), and a regulatory subunit SUR1 (*ABCC8*). Loss-of-function mutations in either subunit cause congenital hyperinsulinaemia (CHI) whereas gain-of-function mutations lead to neonatal diabetes. This is because the K_{ATP} channel plays a crucial role in glucose-stimulated insulin secretion. When the plasma glucose level is low (less than 3 mM), the channel is open and keeps the β-cell membrane potential at a hyperpolarized level. When plasma glucose levels rise, increasing glucose uptake and metabolism by the β-cell, K_{ATP} channels close. This produces a membrane depolarization that activates voltage-gated Ca^{2+} channels, increases Ca^{2+} influx, and so stimulates insulin release. Two classes of therapeutic drugs modulate insulin secretion by interacting with K_{ATP} channels. Sulphonylureas inhibit channel activity and are used to enhance insulin secretion in patients with type 2 diabetes mellitus, whereas K-channel openers (e.g. diazoxide) activate K_{ATP} channels, hyperpolarizing the β-cell and preventing insulin release.

CHI is characterized by unregulated insulin secretion and profound hypoglycaemia that presents at birth or within the first year of life. This is because CHI mutations result in loss of K_{ATP} channel activity, which causes continuous depolarization of the β-cell, persistent Ca^{2+} influx and thereby constitutive insulin secretion. Some patients respond to treatment with diazoxide, but in others the most effective treatment is resection of the pancreas (more than 90% is usual). Many patients develop diabetes in later life.

Mutations that increase K_{ATP} channel activity cause neonatal diabetes (ND), by holding the β-cell hyperpolarized and preventing Ca^{2+} influx and insulin secretion even when plasma glucose rises. Around 50% of ND patients have K_{ATP} channel mutations. All have diabetes, usually presenting within the first six months of life, which may be either permanent or exhibit a remitting-relapsing time course. These patients were once thought to have an unusually early form of type 1 diabetes and thus were treated with insulin. Recognition that they possess activating K_{ATP} channel mutations has enabled more than 90% of patients to switch to sulphonylurea therapy: these drugs close the open K_{ATP} channels so stimulating endogenous insulin secretion. In addition to diabetes, some mutations cause muscle weakness, motor and mental developmental delay and hyperactivity (iDEND syndrome), and occasionally also epilepsy (DEND syndrome). These symptoms are sometimes helped by sulphonylureas. Because of the marked clinical benefits of sulphonylurea therapy, it is advisable to test all patients with diabetes presenting before six months for K_{ATP} channel mutations.

Nonsyndromic deafness

About 70% of all cases of prelingual deafness are nonsyndromic. The disorder shows marked genetic heterogeneity, but in some families it results from loss-of-function mutations in the gene (*GJB2*) encoding the gap junction channel connexin 26. Both recessive and dominant mutations have been described. Connexin 26 is expressed in the cochlea, but the mechanism by which the lack of functional connexin 26 leads to hearing loss remains obscure. In some individuals, mutations in connexin 26 are associated with Vohwinkel's syndrome or other skin abnormalities. Many patients also suffer from deafness.

Further reading

Ashcroft FM (2000). *Ion channels and disease.* Academic Press, San Diego, CA.

Ashcroft FM (2006). From molecule to malady. *Nature,* **440**, 440.

Lehmann-Horn F, Jurkatt-Rott K (1999). Voltage-gated ion channel and hereditary disease. *Physiol Rev*, **79**, 1317–72.

National Center for Biotechnology Information, providing access to genetic sequence databases (e.g. GenBank) http://www.ncbi.nlm.nih.gov/

Online Mendelian Inheritance in Man (OMIM), a database of human genes and genetic disorders. http://www.ncbi.nlm.nih.gov/omim/

Washington University, Neuromuscular Disease Center. A website concerned with neurological and CNS disorders, including those associated with ion channel defects. http://www.neuro.wustl.edu/neuromuscular/mother/chan.html

4.5

Intracellular signalling

R. Andres Floto

Essentials

This section outlines the general principles of intracellular signalling. Focusing on cell surface receptors, the requirements for effective transmission of information across the plasma membrane are outlined. The principal mechanisms utilized in mammalian signal transduction are described. For each, the pathological consequences of aberrant signalling and means by which pathways can be pharmacologically targeted are described in molecular terms.

Intracellular signalling pathways permit the transmission and integration of information within cells. Mammalian receptor signalling relies on only a small number of distinct molecular processes which interact to determine cellular responses. Rapid advances in our knowledge of the mechanisms of intracellular signalling has greatly increased understanding of how cells function physiologically, how they malfunction pathologically and how their behaviour might be manipulated therapeutically.

Introduction

The evolution of cellular life was only possible through the development of an insulating barrier to the external world, the plasma membrane, allowing manipulation of the intracellular environment. However, to be able to respond to the extracellular milieu and to each other, primitive cells needed to transmit information across the plasma membrane, leading to the evolution of intracellular signalling processes. The progression to multicellularity appears to have depended on the development of robust and sophisticated signal transduction pathways. These evolved through episodes of gene duplication and subsequent protein sequence divergence which peaked at the time of animal–plant–fungi separation (1000 million years ago) and again after the Cambrian explosion (500 million years ago). Moreover, cooption of proteins originally involved in cell structure and metabolism further contributed to the diversification and development of signalling pathways. The resulting complex nomenclature, originating from diverse sources of biological research (especially the fruit fly, *Drosophila*), can be confusing and alienating for the non-specialist.

Transmitting information across the plasma membrane barrier is achieved in one of three ways:

1. *Nuclear receptor signalling* (utilized e.g. by steroid hormones) employs lipophilic, membrane-permeable ligands which diffuse through the plasma membrane and directly interact with intracellular receptors to alter gene expression and subsequently cell function. Nuclear receptor signalling is limited by the physical properties of the ligand, the absence of a signal amplification step (limiting sensitivity), and slow response times (since these depend on *de novo* protein synthesis).
2. *Ion channel activation* permits rapid changes in membrane voltage and intracellular ion concentrations. These processes, which underlie nerve conduction and muscle contraction, also mediate signalling events in nonexcitable cells and are discussed elsewhere.
3. *Cell surface receptors*, in contrast, detect extracellular ligand binding and transmit an intracellular signal to alter cell function. There are seven main solutions to the problem of transmembrane signal transduction that have evolved in mammalian cells. Heterotrimeric G-protein coupled-receptors (GPCRs), Wnt, and Hedgehog (Hh) signalling pathways all utilize cell surface molecules with seven transmembrane-spanning domains (7TM) which undergo conformational change on ligand binding triggering intracellular signalling cascades. Alternatively, ligand engagement can be sensed through activation (upon receptor aggregation) of intracellular enzyme cascades. This mechanism is utilized in tyrosine kinase (TK)-dependent receptor signalling and in the serine/threonine-dependent signalling of the transforming growth factor beta (TGFβ) receptor superfamily. Receptors have also evolved which, upon ligand-induced aggregation, recruit cytoplasmic molecules into large signalling complexes via homotypic protein domain interactions. These include the TNFα and Fas receptors as well as the Toll-like receptors (TLRs). Finally, Notch signalling employs ligand-dependent receptor cleavage and nuclear translocation of the receptor fragment to induce gene expression changes.

Principles of receptor signalling

Receptor signalling pathways, in transmitting an extracellular message to the cell interior, have to deal with the same fundamental problems of information transmission as other processes, such as electronic systems. These include signalling sensitivity, robustness, resolution, and integration.

Sensitivity

The sensitivity of signalling pathways varies enormously and is determined by both activation threshold and signal amplification.

The activation threshold for a pathway can be set by (1) the affinity, avidity and dissociation rates of receptor-ligand interaction and also (2) the amount of activated intermediary molecules required to propagate the signal. For example, activation of IgG receptors (FcγR) is determined by both the density and subclass of IgG coating an antigen (thereby affecting receptor engagement) but also by the level of receptor tyrosine phosphorylation achieved (which is influenced by the balance of receptor-associated tyrosine kinases and phosphatases).

Amplification is usually achieved through one or more enzymatic steps in the signalling pathway and permits extremely low levels of stimuli to trigger signal transduction. Examples include the ability of rod photoreceptors to respond to individual photons and the successful recognition of individual peptide-bound major histocompatibility complex (MHC) molecules by T-cell receptors. Very high amplification tends to lead to yes–no binary outputs (a pathway is either 'on' or 'off') as well as low signal-to-noise ratios. In contrast, nonamplified systems permit more fidelity of signal representation (with high signal-to-noise ratios), as illustrated by the response of TGFβ superfamily receptors to morphogenic gradients during development.

By altering sensitivity (through changes in threshold and amplification), signalling pathways can greatly extend the dynamic range of stimulus intensities they respond to without saturating. This process is known as adaptation.

Signal robustness

Robustness refers to the ability of systems to function correctly in the presence of invalid inputs or hostile environments. Robustness in cellular signalling can be enhanced by both positive and negative feedback loops. For example, a pathway which enhances the formation of its own ligand amplifies, stabilizes and prolongs signalling. Such events are commonly seen in development (where correct signal transmission is critical) but also occur aberrantly in cancer (through the establishment of autocrine signalling loops). Negative feedback cycles also stabilize fluctuations, rapidly returning signals to pre-excitation levels and thus minimize sub-threshold signalling. Another mechanism of increasing signal robustness is the use of parallel, redundant signalling cascades which ensure that interruption of one pathway does not disrupt signal transmission.

Signal resolution

Signalling pathways need to respond appropriately to temporal and spatial changes in stimulus.

- *Temporal resolution* is determined by the speed of initiation and termination of signalling and varies from milliseconds (e.g. ion channel activation and GPCR-like sensory transduction), seconds to minutes (as seen in TK-dependent signalling of immunoreceptors), or hours (such as Notch signalling in development). While fast temporal resolution permits rapid detection of changing external environments, slow receptor kinetics will, in effect, average extracellular signals over time, removing fluctuations in signal intensity and resulting in improved signal-to-noise ratios.
- *Spatial resolution* is the ability of cells to detect the localization of a stimulus. It is critical for many processes including cell migration during embryogenesis and inflammation, cell–cell interactions (e.g. immune synapse formation) and phagocytosis. Spatial resolution requires subcellular containment of activated signalling components which can be achieved by: (1) the restriction of lateral diffusion of activated membrane receptors by sphingolipid microdomains or cytoskeletal barriers; (2) the presence of a cordon of inhibitory molecules limiting signal spread (as observed at the leading edge of chemotactic cells where the phosphatase PTEN localizes phosphatidylinositol 3,4,5-triphosphate (PIP_3) production) and (3) the sequestration of active signalling proteins within a large multimolecular complex which localizes activity to a specific region of the cell.

Signal integration

As with complex neurological systems, individual cells can integrate multiple input signals (through interactions between different signalling pathways) to perform simple Boolean operations (combining 'signal 1 AND signal 2', 'signal 1 OR signal 2', and 'signal 1 NOT signal 2'). For example, to achieve full activation, T lymphocytes need to receive simultaneous signals from both the T cell receptor (TCR) and its coreceptor, CD28. They thus identify 'TCR signal AND CD28 signal'. However, if only TCR signalling is triggered (TCR signal NOT CD28 signal), cells respond by becoming unresponsive (anergic) to further stimulation. For certain aspects of T-cell function, however, another co-receptor, ICOS, may substitute for CD28 signalling and leads to full cellular activation (ICOS signal OR CD28 signal).

Cells also undertake more complex signal processing. The recent application of high-throughput genetic manipulation, the identification of protein–protein interactions by mass spectroscopy and the application of bioinformatic analysis has revealed that, far from being a series of linear processes, intracellular signalling is, in reality, a complex, integrated, and interdependent network of signalling pathways. However, within this web of multiple protein–protein interactions and enzymatic cascades, there are clear signalling 'nodes', important molecules where multiple signal inputs converge, which represent points of physiological, and potentially pharmacological, control of cellular responses.

Specific signalling pathways

The description of signalling pathways here is limited to the seven main types of receptor signal transduction mechanisms used by mammalian cells: GPCR, Wnt, Hh, tyrosine kinase-dependent signalling (using the B-cell receptor as an example), TGFβ superfamily receptors,Toll-like receptors (TLRs) (as an example of pathways utilizing homotypic protein domain interactions), and Notch signalling. For each pathway, the main physiological roles, the mechanism by which signalling is initiated and controlled, the pathological consequences of signalling dysfunction, and the potential for therapeutic manipulation are described.

G-protein-coupled receptors

The G-protein-coupled receptors (GPCRs) are a large family of approximately 800 7TM proteins which are involved in virtually all aspects of human biology including sensory transduction (of vision, olfaction, taste, and pain) and signalling by peptide hormones, glycoproteins, neurotransmitters and chemokines. More than 60% of all marketed drugs (and a large proportion of those in development) target GPCRs. The main signalling pathways are summarized in Fig. 4.5.1.

GPCRs constitutively associate with heterotrimeric G proteins which consist of a GDP-bound α subunit (of which there are 16 types) complexed to a βγ dimer. Ligand-induced GPCR conformational change permits the Gα subunit to bind GTP instead of GDP and allows Gα and βγ subunits to dissociate and interact with effector enzymes (such as adenylyl cyclase and phospholipase C) and small G proteins. Intrinsic hydrolysis of bound GTP to GDP inactivates Gα (thus acting as a molecular stopwatch to limit Gα activity) and permit binding to βγ subunits and re-association with receptors.

In parallel, GPCRs also interact, through c-terminal phosphorylation by G-protein-coupled receptor kinases (GRKs), with β-arrestins; molecules that mediate ubiquitination-dependent receptor endocytosis, recruitment of c-Src family tyrosine kinases (such as Hck and Yes) and activation of the ERK MAP kinase signalling pathway. Signalling by β-arrestins mediates receptor desensitization, cellular degranulation, chemotaxis, and cell survival.

As might be expected from their critical role in peptide hormone signal transduction, loss-of-function and gain-of-function mutations of multiple GPCRs and heterotrimeric G proteins have been implicated in both hereditary and sporadic endocrine diseases. Somatic Gsα mutations, which disrupt intrinsic GTPase function resulting in prolonged activation, are found in 40% of growth-hormone-secreting pituitary adenomas as well as McCune–Albright syndrome (bone fibrous dysplasia, endocrinopathy with hormone oversecretion). In contrast, heterozygous inactivating mutations of Gsα result in Albright's hereditary osteodystrophy.

GPCR signalling has also been exploited by pathogens. HIV binding to the chemokine receptor CCR5 mediates cellular invasion and alters immune cell function. *Vibrio cholerae* toxin A1 induces ADP-ribosylation of Gαs preventing GTP hydrolysis (resulting in persistent activation and leading to cyclic AMP-driven secretory diarrhoea). *Bordetella pertussis* toxin A freezes Gαi in an inactive GDP-bound conformation (through ADP-ribosylation) which prevents phagocyte chemotaxis, bacterial engulfment and intracellular killing.

Wnt signalling

Wnt signalling plays a major role in epidermal, haematopoetic, and neural stem cell development and has been implicated in oncogenesis (particularly of colonic, ovarian and hepatocellular carcinoma and melanoma) thought to arise through stem cell dysfunction. About 20 Wnt genes are defined in humans encoding secreted, palmitoylated proteins and their receptors (called Frizzled-class proteins). The name Wnt is derived from *Wingless*, a *Drosophila* gene and the molecule Int-1 (integration of mammary tumour virus).

Wnt signalling pathways are summarized in Fig. 4.5.2. In the absence of Wnt ligands, newly synthesized β-catenin is complexed within the cytoplasm to two scaffolding proteins, Axin and APC (adenomatous polyposis coli). Serine/threonine phosphorylation of β-catenin, by two proteins GSK3β and CK1, initiates its ubiquination and subsequent proteosomal degradation. In the absence of β-catenin, the transcriptional complex Tcf/Lef represses gene expression. Wnt ligands induce co-aggregation of LRP 5/6 (an LDL receptor family member) and the 7TM receptor, Frizzled, and results in phosphorylation of the scaffolding protein Dishevelled and sequestration of Axin. The resultant inhibition of the β-catenin destruction complex increases cytoplasmic levels of β-catenin and permits its nuclear translocation and binding to Tcf/Lef to form an activatory transcription complex which triggers gene expression. Although incompletely understood, noncanonical WNT signalling, involving engagement of β-arrestin, calcium signalling, and activation of heterotrimeric and Rho family G proteins, also occurs.

The critical role of Wnt signalling in stem cell regulation within intestinal villi underlies its association with colonic malignancies. Raised nuclear β-catenin levels (leading to persistent Wnt-dependent gene expression and eventually malignant transformation) occur in the presence of (1) mutations in either APC (found in most sporadic colorectal cancers as well as familial adenomatous polyposis) or

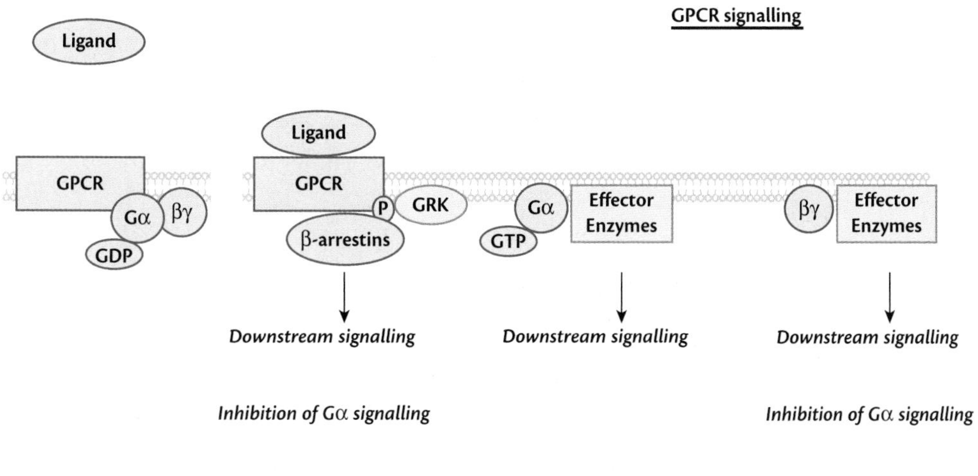

Fig. 4.5.1 G protein-coupled receptors (GPCRs). GPCRs constitutively associate with the guanosine diphosphate (GDP)-bound α (Gα) and βγ subunits of heterotrimeric G proteins. Ligand binding induces receptor conformational change allowing Gα to bind guanosine triphosphate (GTP) which permits the subunits to dissociate and interact with effector enzymes. GPCRs also interact with β-arrestins, following C terminal phosphorylation by GPCR kinases (GRK), which mediated receptor internalization and other signalling events.

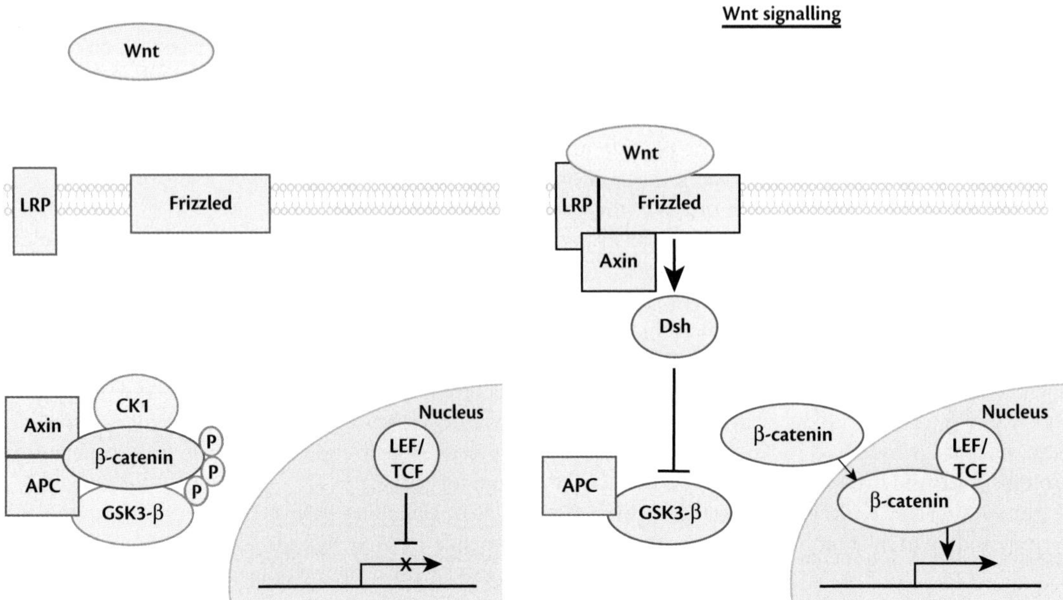

Fig. 4.5.2 Wnt signalling. In the absence of Wnt ligands, newly synthesized β-catenin is bound by Axin and APC (adenomatous polyposis coli), phosphorylated by GSK3β and CK1 and consequently degraded by the ubiquitin-proteosome system. Wnt ligands induce coaggregation of the surface receptors Frizzled and LRP, leading to phosphorylation of Dishevelled (Dsh), sequestration of Axin and inhibition of β-catenin degradation. β-catenin can then translocate to the nucleus, bind the transcription complex LEF/TCF and trigger gene expression.

Axin which impair β-catenin binding or (2) activating mutations of β-catenin, preventing its phosphorylation.

Therapeutic manipulation of Wnt pathway signalling is currently being investigated. Both small molecule agonists (to enhance tissue repair and wound healing) and inhibitors (as antitumour agents) are under development. Lithium, at least *in vitro*, enhances canonical Wnt signalling (through inhibition of GSK3β), which may underlie some of its effects in psychiatric disorders.

Hedgehog

Hedgehog (Hh) signalling has important roles in embryogenesis, tissue repair and tumorigenesis. During embryonic development, Hh proteins are named after the appearance of the embryo in classical *Drosophila* mutants and have been conserved as regulators of development in vertebrates. They act as short- and long-range morphogens (determining cell fate), mitogens (controlling cell proliferation) and as inducing factors (regulating the form of

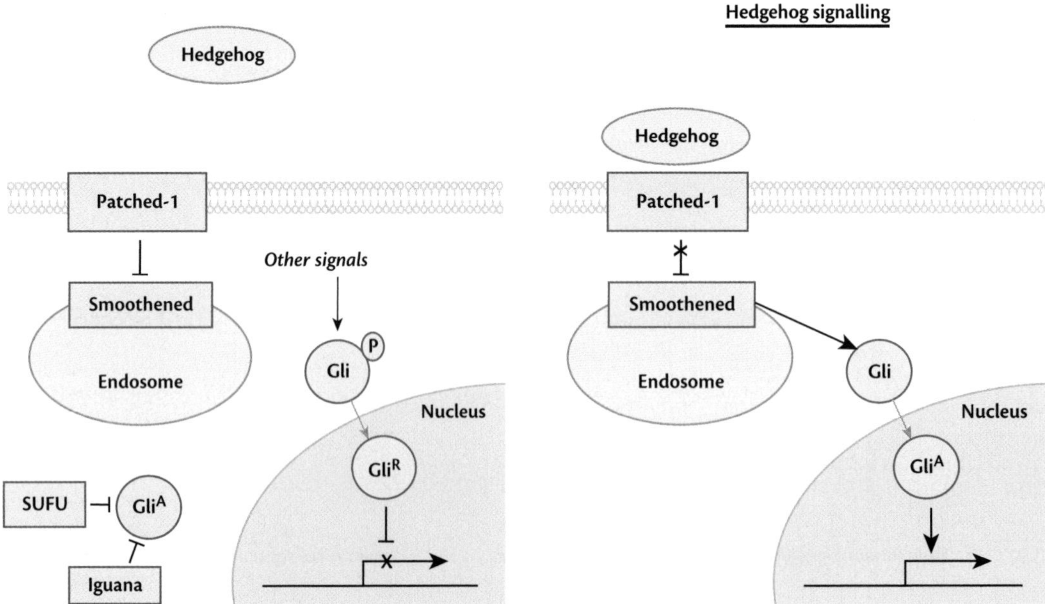

Fig. 4.5.3 Hedgehog signalling. Binding of the soluble ligand Hedgehog to its receptor, Patched-1, relieves constitutive repression of the protein Smoothened which now acts on the transcription factor complex Gli to increase the amount of activator form (Gli^A) relative to repressor form (Gli^R) and thus promote gene expression. Control of signalling is achieved by inhibition of nuclear translocation of Gli^A by two cytoplasmic proteins SUFU and Iguana, and phosphorylation of Gli (by a number of different signalling pathways including Notch) promoting Gli^R formation.

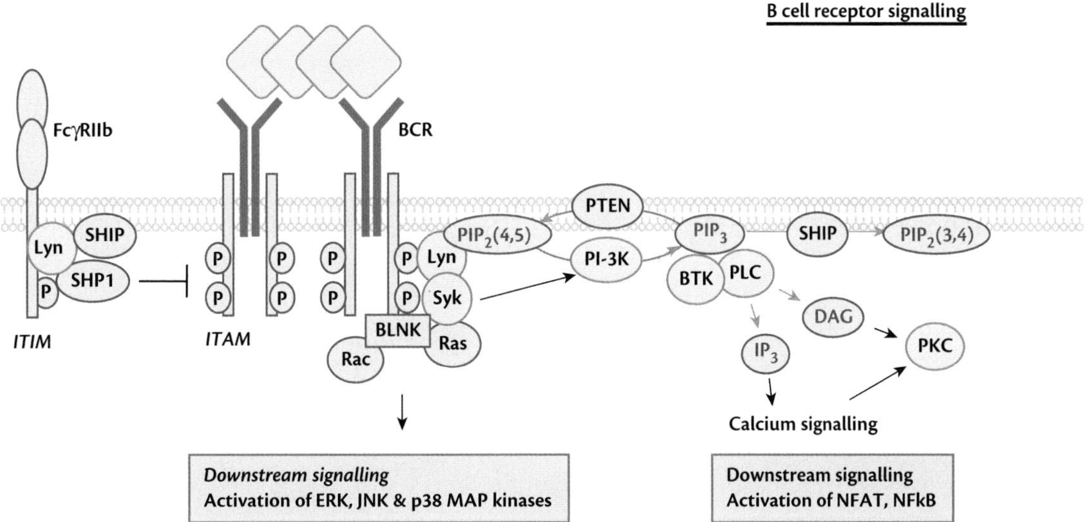

Fig. 4.5.4 B cell receptor (BCR) signalling. Antigen induces BCR aggregation leading to phosphorylation of cytoplasmic ITAMs (Immunoreceptor Tyrosine Activation Motifs) and subsequent binding and activation of soluble tyrosine kinases such as Lyn and Syk. A second wave of adaptor molecules (such as BLNK), small G proteins (such as Rac and Ras) and kinases, including phosphatidylinositol 3-kinase (PI-3K) are then recruited to the signalling complex. PI-3K generates phosphatidylinositol 3,4,5-triphosphate (PIP_3) from PIP_2(4,5) recruiting further molecules including Bruton's tyrosine kinase (BTK) and phospholipase C (PLC). The latter splits PIP_2(4,5) into inositol 1,4,5-trisphosphate (IP3) and diacylglycerol (DAG) leading to calcium signalling and protein kinase C activation. Signalling is controlled by co-aggregation of inhibitory receptors, such as FcγRIIb, which, through their ITIM (Immunoreceptor Tyrosine Inhibitory Motifs), recruit and activate tyrosine phosphatases (such as SHP1), limiting ITAM phosphorylation, and the inositol phosphatase SHIP, which together with the phosphatidylinositol phosphatase PTEN, reduce PIP_3 levels.

developing organs). There are three human homologues of Hh—Sonic Hh, Indian Hh, and Desert Hh—secreted as lipid-conjugated hydrophobic peptides with distinct patterns of spatial and temporal distribution.

Hedgehog binds to a cell surface receptor, Patched-1, relieving constitutive repression of a (predominantly endosomal) 7TM protein, Smoothened (Fig. 4.5.3). Active Smoothened increases the formation of the activator form of the transcription factor complex, *GLi* (*GLi*^{A}) which stimulates Hh target gene transcription. Control of Hh signalling occurs through (1) constitutive repression of *Smoothened*; (2) phosphorylation of GLi by other signalling pathways (such as Notch) which generates a repressor transcription complex GLi^R preventing gene expression, and (3) inhibition of nuclear translocation of GLI^A by two cytoplasmic proteins, *SUFU* and *Iguana*.

Mutations in human Sonic Hh, the best characterized member of these developmental regulatory proteins in mammals, result in developmental disorders such as holoprosencephaly which is

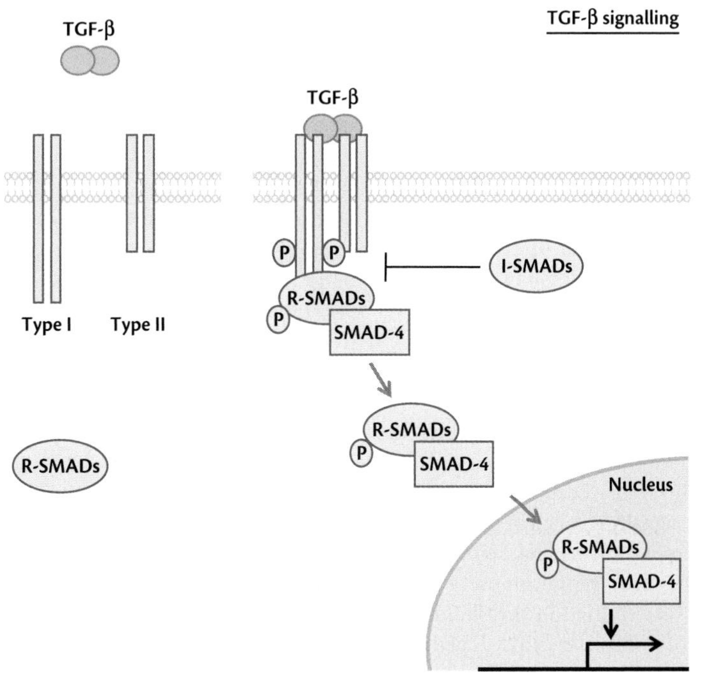

Fig. 4.5.5 TGF-β signalling. TGF-β binding induces heteromeric receptor complexes leading to phosphorylation of Type I receptor cytoplasmic tails permitting recruitment and activation of R-(receptor)SMADs which in turn bind SMAD-4. The R-SMAD/SMAD4 complex then translocates to the nucleus where it interacts with other co-factors to control gene expression. Inhibition of signalling is achieved by transcriptional induction of inhibitory SMADs (I-SMADs) which prevent R-SMAD/SMAD4 complex formation and target receptors for degradation.

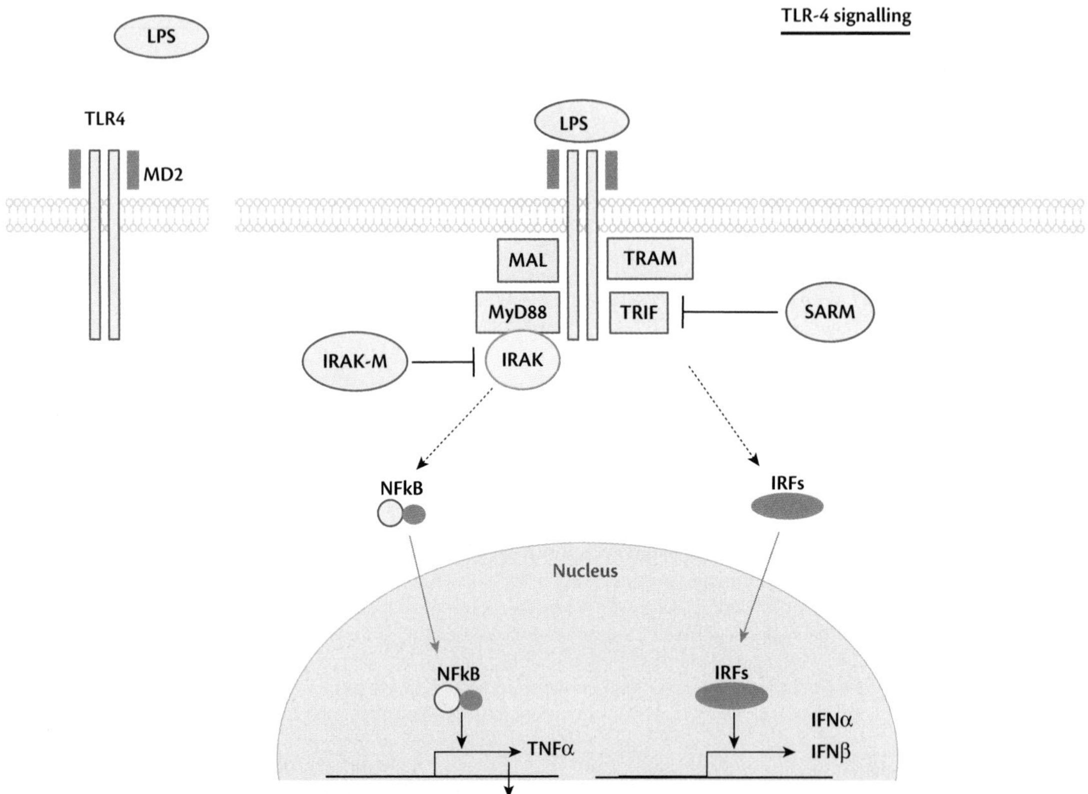

Fig. 4.5.6 Toll-like receptor signalling. Lipopolysaccharide (LPS) binding to TLR4 triggers receptor aggregation and conformational change recruiting cytoplasmin adaptor molecules (MyD88, MAL, TRIF and TRAM) through homotypic TIR (Toll/interleukin 1) domain interactions. MyD88 recruits and activates the serine/threonine kinases IRAKs (through Death domain interactions) which in turn activate the nuclear transcription factor NFkB and switch on transcription of pro-inflammatory cytokines such as TNF α. In contrast, TRIF activates interferon–regulatory factors (IRFs) which trigger generation of type 1 interferon (IFN α and β). Signal regulation is achieved at a number of levels including inhibition of signalling through IRAK and TRIF by IRAK-M and SARM respectively.

frequent in aborted fetuses and characterized by severe malfunctions including cyclopia. Drugs which interfere with sterol synthesis cause such malformations because they interfere with the addition of cholesterol to the N-terminal domain of the sonic hedgehog protein after processing, thereby preventing normal trafficking and secretion of the ligand. Uncontrolled Hh signalling appears to promote tumorigenesis. Gorlin syndrome, caused by an inactivating mutation of Patched-1, is characterized by the development of multiple basal cell carcinomas and medulloblastomas. Moreover, most sporadic basal cell carcinomas show evidence of inactivating mutations in Patched-1 or activating mutations in Smoothened, while a proportion of medulloblastomas demonstrate increased Hh signalling (due to inactivating mutations of Patched-1 or SUFU). Small-molecule antagonists to Hh signalling (inhibiting Smoothered function) have shown efficacy *in vitro* and *in vivo* as antitumour therapies.

Tyrosine kinase-dependent signalling

Tyrosine kinases (TK) mediate signalling by a number of different receptor families including those with receptor-associated TK activity (such as epidermal growth factor receptors) and those which recruit soluble TKs to initiate signalling (such as immunoreceptors, integrins, and cytokine receptors). In general, signal transmission is receptor aggregation-dependent, rapid in onset (of the order of seconds to minutes) and, once initiation thresholds are surpassed, greatly amplified (due to multiple enzyme-dependent steps). As expected, dysregulated TK signalling contributes to both oncogenesis and immunodeficiency.

The B cell receptor (BCR) serves as a useful example. The BCR complex consists of a surface immunoglobin noncovalently associated with Igα and Igβ subunits, each of which contains a cytoplasmic immunoreceptor tyrosine activation motif (ITAM). Antigen-induced receptor aggregation permits loosely associated c-Src family TKs (such as Lyn and Fyn) to phosphorylate subunit ITAMs which can then strongly bind c-Src family and Syk family tyrosine kinases. A second wave of adaptor molecules (such as BLNK), small G proteins (such as Ras and Rac), and kinases such as phosphatidylinositol-3-kinase (PI-3K) are recruited to the signalling complex. PI-3K generates phosphatidylinositol 3,4,5-triphosphate (PIP_3) from the plasma membrane lipid phosphatidylinositol 4,5-triphosphate (PIP_2(4,5)). PIP_3 recruits cytoplasmic molecules (through their Plextrin homology domains). These include: (1) Bruton's tyrosine kinase (BTK), mutation of which result in X-linked agammaglobulinaemia; (2) AKT, and (3) phospholipase C (PLC), which generates inositol 1,4,5-trisphophate (IP_3) and diacylglycerol (DAG) from PIP_2(4,5), leading to intracellular calcium signalling and protein kinase C (PKC) activation. The fully formed signalling complex can then activate downstream signalling pathways such as ERK, JNK and p38 MAP kinases, NFκB, and NFAT (Fig. 4.5.4).

Signal transduction is regulated at a number of steps including: (1) CD45-dependent dephosphorylation of src-family kinases which is necessary to permit ITAM engagement; (2) The activity

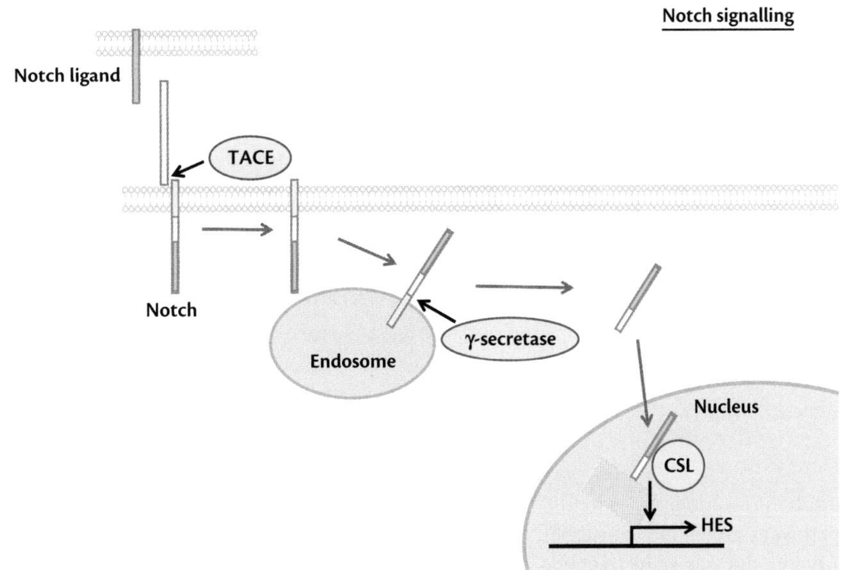

Fig. 4.5.7 Notch signalling. Ligand binding permits extracellular cleavage of surface Notch receptors (which form as heterodimers) by an ADAM protease TACE which allows ubiquitin-mediated internalization of membrane associated receptor fragment. Further cleavage by an endosomal γ secretase releases a cytoplasmic fragment which associates with the nuclear transcription factor CSL and drives gene expression.

of the phosphatidylinositol phosphatase, PTEN, which converts PIP_3 back to $PIP_2(4,5)$ thereby limiting signalling complex formation, and (3) the density of immunoreceptor tyrosine inhibitory motif (ITIM)-containing inhibitory receptors (such as FcγRIIb and CD22) associated with the signalling complex. *PTEN* (phosphotase and tensin homologue) is a human tumour suppressor gene; it is one of the most frequently lost tumour suppressors in cancer and is mutated in both Cowden's and Proteus syndromes. These inhibitory receptors recruit soluble tyrosine phosphatases (such as SHP1) which limit phospho-ITAM generation, inositol phosphatases (such as SHIP) which hydrolyse PIP_3 to $PIP_2(3,4)$ and inhibitors of small G-protein signalling (such as p62 DOK).

Small-molecule inhibitors of receptor tyrosine kinases are in clinical use in the treatment of chronic myeloid leukaemia (imatinib), renal cell carcinoma and gastrointestinal stromal tumours (sunitinib), and several PI-3K inhibitors are in development as anti-inflammatory and antitumour agents.

Transforming growth factor beta (TGFβ) superfamily

The TGFβ superfamily of about 20 ligands, including TGFβ, activin, nodal, endoglin, bone morphogenetic proteins (BMP), and growth and differentiation factors (GDFs), have important roles in embryogenesis (where they form morphogenic gradients), immunoregulation, and wound healing.

Receptors contain cysteine-rich extracellular domains, a single TM domain and an intracellular serine/threonine kinase domain. Ligands (all of which contain three intramolecular disulphide bonds termed a 'cysteine knot') are secreted as homodimers and trigger the aggregation of type I and type II receptor homodimers into heteromeric complexes (Fig. 4.5.5). Phosphorylation of type I receptors (by type II receptor serine/threonine kinases) permits recruitment and subsequent phosphorylation of intracellular signalling molecules called receptor (R-) SMADs. SMADs are homologues of the *Caenorhabditis elegans* protein SMA and the *Drosophila* protein Mothers against decapentaplegia. Phosphorylated R-SMADs, in turn, bind the key regulator, SMAD4. The R-SMAD/SMAD4 complex translocates to the nucleus where, after associating with other cofactors, it regulates gene transcription. Inhibition of signalling is achieved through transcriptional induction of inhibitory (I-) SMADs, which competitively bind type 1 receptors (preventing SMAD complex formation) and target receptors for ubiquitin-dependent degradation.

Defective signalling of TGFβ superfamily pathways has been implicated in Camurati–Engelmann disease (a progressive diaphyseal dysplasia affecting long bones), oncogenesis (particularly skin cancers), a number of fibrotic conditions (including systemic sclerosis), familial primary pulmonary hypertension (BMP receptor 2 mutations), and hereditary haemorrhagic telangectasia (endoglin mutations).

To date, preclinical studies have suggested antitumour and antifibrotic effects of small-molecule inhibitors of the kinase activity of TGFβ superfamily receptors.

Toll-like receptor signalling

A number of signalling pathways utilize protein-protein binding via homotypic domain interaction. These include TNFα receptor signalling, which uses death domains (DD), caspase signalling (utilizing CARD domains), and Toll-like receptor (TLR) signalling (which uses DD and Toll/interleukin 1 (TIR) domain interactions). I have focused on TLR signalling as an example.

The nine types of mammalian TLR are found on both the cell surface (TLR1,2,4,5,6,) and within endosomal compartments (TLR3,7,8,9) and recognize distinct microbial products (as well as some endogenous ligands). They direct the innate immune response against pathogens, triggering inflammatory and antiviral mediator release. In addition, TLR-induced maturation of dendritic cells permits processing and surface presentation of internalized antigen, resulting in stimulation of cognate T cells and induction of adaptive immunity.

In the case of TLR4 (summarized in Fig. 4.5.6), engagement of lipopolysaccharide (LPS) triggers receptor aggregation and conformational change which recruits cytoplasmic adaptor proteins (MyD88, MAL, TRIF, and TRAM) through TIR domain interactions. MyD88 in turn, through DD interactions, recruits and activates the serine/threonine kinases IRAKs which mediate ubiquitination-dependent activation of NFκB (generating production of pro-inflammatory cytokines such as TNFα). TRIF, in contrast, activates interferon-regulatory factors (IRFs) which trigger the generation of IFNα and β (which are crucial to antiviral host immunity). Regulation of signalling occurs at a number of levels including: (1) reduced membrane recruitment of MyD88; (2) disruption of IRAK signalling by the inhibitory molecule IRAK-M and (3) inhibition of TRIF signalling by the cytoplasmic protein SARM.

Polymorphisms in components of TLR signalling have been associated with increased susceptibility to Gram-negative infections (TLR4), Gram-positive infections (TLR2, IRAK4, MAL) and tuberculosis (TLR2, MAL). TLR polymorphisms have also been implicated in the development of atherosclerosis. Synthetic TLR agonists are in development as adjuvants for conventional and immunotherapy vaccines, and as antiviral therapies.

Notch

Named after a *Drosophila* protein mutation resulting in a 'notched' wing phenotype, Notch signalling pathways are widely conserved across species and have roles in embryonic development (particularly binary cell fate decisions and terminal differentiation), maintenance of stem cells, and lymphocyte differentiation and signalling. Four Notch receptors (Notch 1 to 4) and five canonical ligands (jagged1, jagged2, Delta-like 1, 3, and 4) have been identified (as well as several noncanonical ligands including contactin).

Although synthesized as a single polypeptide, surface Notch receptors are heterodimers consisting of an extracellular region noncovalently linked to a transmembrane/intracellular portion. As shown in Fig. 4.5.7, ligand binding permits extracellular cleavage of Notch heterodimers by TACE (TNFα converting enzyme), an ADAM protease. This allows ubiquitin-dependent endocytosis of Notch. Subsequent cleavage by an endosomal γ-secretase (presenilin) releases the intracellular fragment of Notch which can then associate with the nuclear transcription factor CSL, switching on gene expression (particularly of the HES family of transcription factors). In addition, Notch may also signal through CSL-independent nuclear and cytoplasmic pathways (although incompletely understood). Notch signalling can be modulated by alteration in receptor fucosylation (regulated by Fringe proteins) and re-routing of intracellular Notch fragments to lysosomes (leading to their degradation).

Mutations in Notch pathway proteins have been identified in developmental disorders such as congental aortic valve disease (Notch 1), neurovascular syndromes such as cerebral autosomal dominant arteriopathy with subcortical infarcts and leukoencephalopathy (CADASIL; Notch 3 mutations) and T-cell acute lymphocytic leukaemia (50% of which have activating mutations of Notch1 caused either by chromosomal translocation or viral promoter integration).

Therapeutic manipulation of Notch signalling has so far focused on γ-secretase inhibitors which have shown promise, in preclinical studies, as antitumour agents.

Conclusion

The transmission of information across the plasma membrane is achieved through a limited number of types of signalling pathway. Recent progress in defining the mechanisms of signal transduction ('learning the language of intracellular communication') has permitted huge advances in our understanding of disease pathophysiology and our ability to manipulate signalling therapeutically.

Further reading

Barolo S, Posakony JW (2007). Three habits of highly effective signaling pathways: principles of transcriptional control by developmental cell signaling. *Genes Dev*, **16**, 1167–81.

Call ME, Wucherpfennig KW (2007). Common themes in the assembly and architecture of activating immune receptors. *Nat Rev Immunol*, **7**, 841–50.

Clevers H (2006). Wnt/β-Catenin signaling in development and disease. *Cell*, **127**, 469–480.

Cook DN, Pisetsky DS, Schwartz DA (2004). Toll-like receptors in the pathogenesis of human disease. *Nat Immunol*, **5**, 975–9.

Fiúza U-M, Arias AM (2007). Cell and molecular biology of Notch. *J Endocrinol*, **194**, 459–74.

Ingham PW, McMahon AP (2007). Hedgehog signalling in animal development: paradigms and principles. *Genes Dev*, **15**, 3059–87.

Kanzler H, *et al.* (2007). Therapeutic targeting of innate immunity with Toll-like receptor agonist and antagonists. *Nat Med*, **13**, 552–9.

Lefkowitz RJ, Shenoy SK (2005). Transduction of receptor signals by β-Arrestins. *Science*, **308**, 512–17.

Milligan G, Kostenis E (2006). Heterotrimeric G-proteins: a short history. *Br J Pharmacol*, **147**, S46–55.

Nichols JT, Miyamoto A, Weinmaster G (2007). Notch signalling—constantly on the move. *Traffic*, **8**, 959–69.

Pires-daSilva A, Sommer RJ (2003). The evolution of signaling pathways in animal development. *Nat Rev Genet*, **4**, 39–48.

Rubin LL, de Sauvage FJ (2006). Targeting the Hedgehog pathway in cancer. *Nat Rev Drug Disc*, **5**, 1026–33.

Schmierer B, Hill CS (2007). TGFβ-SMAD signal transduction: molecular specificity and functional flexibility. *Nat Rev Mol Cell Biol*, **8**, 970–82.

Shi Y, Massagué J (2003). Mechanisms of TGF-β signalling from cell membrane to the nucleus. *Cell*, **113**, 685–700.

Takeda K, Akira S. (2003). TLR signalling pathways. *Seminars Immunol*, **16**, 3–9.

Weinstein LS, *et al.* (2006). Genetic diseases associated with heterotrimeric G proteins. *Trends Pharmacol Sci*, **27**, 260–6.

National Cancer Institute/Nature *Pathway Interaction Database*. http://pid.nci.nih.gov/browse_pathways.shtml#NCI-Nature

National Center for Biotechnology Information. *Online Mendelian Inheritance in Man (OMIN)*. http://www.ncbi.nlm.nih.gov/sites/entrez?db=omim

Science Signaling. *The signal transduction knowledge environment (STKE)*. http://stke.sciencemag.org/

UCSD Nature. *The signalling gateway*. http://www.signaling-gateway.org/

4.6

Apoptosis in health and disease

Andrew H. Wyllie and Mark J. Arends

Essentials

Apoptosis is the process by which single cells die in the midst of living tissues. It is responsible for most—perhaps all—of the cell-death events that occur during the formation of the early embryo and the sculpting and moulding of organs. Apoptotic cell death continues to play a critical role in the maintenance of cell numbers in those tissues in which cell turnover persists into adult life, such as the epithelium of the gastrointestinal tract, the bone marrow, and lymphoid system including both B- and T-cell lineages. Apoptosis is the usual mode of death in the targets of natural killer (NK) cells and cytotoxic T-cells, and in involution and atrophy induced by hormonal and other stimuli. It also appears in the reaction of many tissues to injury, including mild degrees of ischaemia, exposure to ionizing and ultraviolet radiation, or treatment with cancer chemotherapeutic drugs. Excessive or too little apoptosis play a significant part in the pathogenesis of autoimmunity, infectious disease, AIDS, stroke, myocardial disease, and cancer. When cancers regress, apoptosis is part of the mechanism involved. Here the cellular processes and molecular mechanisms of apoptosis are set out, together with a conspectus of its involvement in many diseases.

Structural changes in apoptosis

Apoptosis can be recognized because of its characteristic, stereotyped sequence of structural changes (Fig. 4.6.1). The dying cells lose contact with their neighbours and undergo a rapid loss of volume. There is explosive blebbing from the cell surface, followed by fragmentation of the cell into a cluster of subcellular bodies (apoptotic bodies), each membrane-bounded and containing a variety of compacted cytoplasmic organelles. The nucleus undergoes similar distortion and fragmentation. Chromatin condenses under the nuclear membrane in knob-like, hemilunar, or toroidal aggregates. Nuclear membranes overlying residual uncondensed chromatin are rich in pores but these are absent adjacent to condensed chromatin, suggesting that redistribution takes place. The nucleolus falls apart, its argyrophilic fibrillar centre remaining apparently tethered to the peripheral aggregates of chromatin, whilst the osmiophilic particles associated with transcription complexes disperse in the central nucleoplasm. Eventually the nuclear membrane disappears and the entire nuclear remnant becomes a mass of condensed chromatin.

Within the cytoplasm, the endoplasmic reticulum dilates. The cell surface loses any pre-existing microvilli or other indices of polarity. The shrunken cell and the apoptotic bodies into which it fragments tend to become spherical.

Isolated apoptotic cells lose the ability to maintain ionic homeostasis within an hour or so, lose density, swell in volume, and permit the entry of various dyes classically used to mark dead cells (such as Trypan Blue and propidium iodide). Within tissues, however, this phase is seldom seen, because the apoptotic cell and its fragments undergo phagocytosis. Often this is undertaken by 'professional' phagocytes—the resident tissue macrophages—but where unusually large numbers of apoptotic cells are generated, other cell types share in ingesting them, including their viable neighbours. Once within the phagosome of the ingesting cell, the apoptotic cell and its fragments rapidly become indistinguishable from the contents of any other large secondary lysosome.

For reasons to be expanded later, the process of apoptotic-cell phagocytosis inhibits the neutrophil-dominated inflammatory reaction that is often seen when macrophages are activated in other circumstances. Cell loss by apoptosis can therefore be effected with little disruption of the tissue concerned. Moreover, apoptosis, once initiated, is completed swiftly. Although the interval from the initial application of a lethal stimulus to the first manifestations of shrinkage and blebbing can vary from minutes to many hours, phagocytosis may be complete within an hour thereafter. Hence, the evidence for cell loss by apoptosis provided by the 'snapshot' of a histological section is often surprisingly scanty relative to the reduction in cell number that is being effected.

Apoptosis is not the only mode of cell death. Dying cells sometimes show a different pattern of change, dominated by volume overload and, eventually, plasma membrane breakdown and leakage of intracellular contents into the extracellular space. At first, the nucleus retains its general structure, although the chromatin

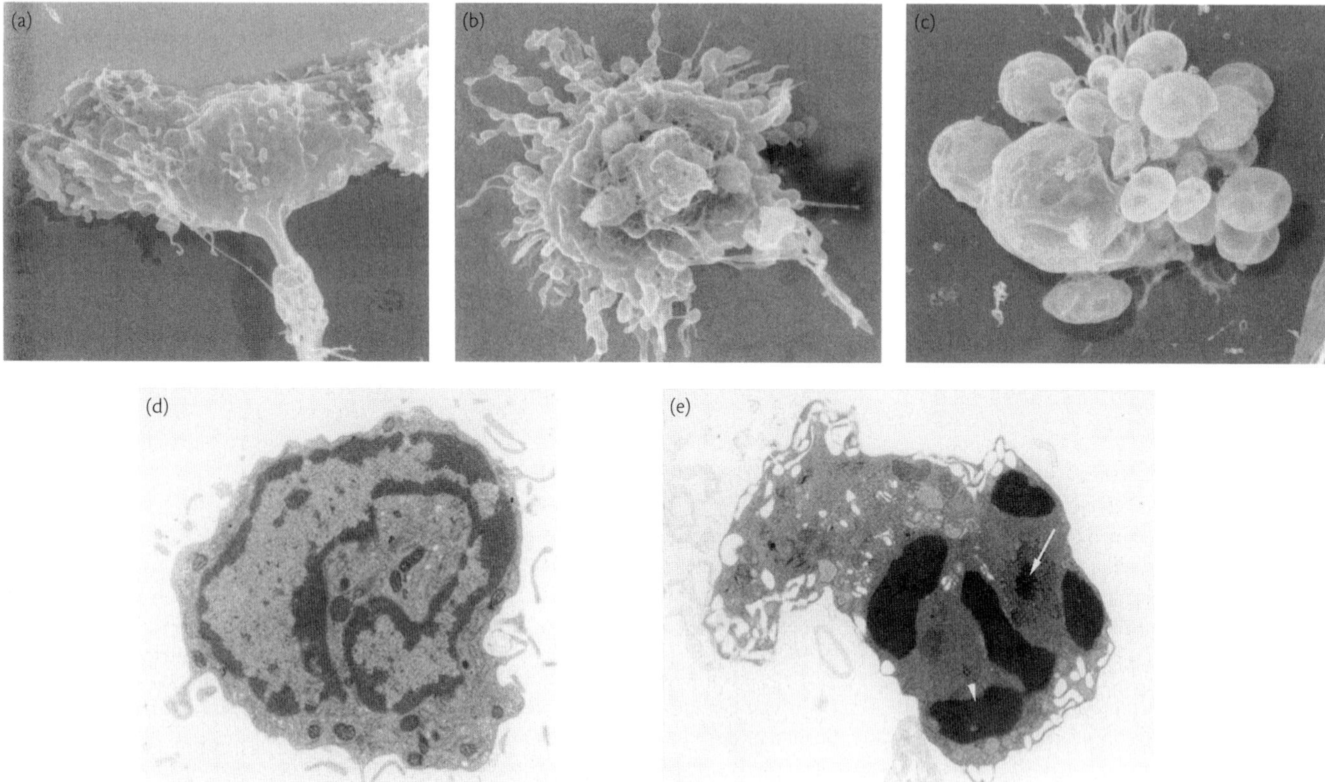

Fig. 4.6.1 The structure of apoptosis. (a) Scanning electron micrograph of a normal macrophage shows its surface sprouting many pseudopodia. In (b) the cell has been injured (in this case by oxidized lipid of the type often present in high concentration in atheromatous plaques) and is throwing out and retracting multiple surface blebs. In (c) the whole cell has fragmented into roughly spherical apoptotic bodies. Some of these are cratered by the orifices of the dilated endoplasmic reticulum. (d) Transmission electron micrograph of a thin section. (e) The condensed chromatin (arrowheads), nucleolar remnant (arrow), and highly convoluted surface are clearly visible. The scale bar is 1 μm.

(Micrographs by courtesy of Dr Jeremy Skepper and Dr Jing Xia, Cambridge School of Biology Multi-imaging Centre.)

patterns coarsen. Later, following equilibration of the cytosol with extracellular calcium, and the resultant widespread activation of degradative enzymes such as cathepsins, vestiges of nuclear structure fade away (karyolysis) and only ghost-like cellular outlines remain. Usually there is an associated acute inflammatory reaction. This pattern of death is frequently found when tissues are overwhelmed by high concentrations of toxic substances or in severe ischaemic damage, where vascular perfusion has been arrested. Classically, it is called necrosis.

Cells in tissues undergoing involution, or responding to exposure to toxins or other adverse environmental conditions often show a different set of structural changes, in which portions of cytoplasm including mitochondria and other organelles (but not the nucleus) become enveloped by their own cell's endosomal membranes and undergo destruction through fusion with lysosomes. This is the process of autophagy. It is one of the principal mechanisms responsible for cell atrophy (the organized reduction in volume and complexity of cytoplasm) but is probably not intrinsic to the process of death. Studies of gene expression show many differences between autophagy and apoptosis, and autophagy can occur without cell death. Although both may occur in parallel within involuting tissue, autophagy appears to be an adaptive response, effected by cells living through adverse conditions, but apoptosis always implies cell death.

Caspases: effectors of apoptosis

Many of the morphological features of apoptosis are attributable to activation of a family of proteases known as caspases (so called because of the presence of the amino acid *c*ysteine in their catalytic site, and their preferential cleavage of peptides immediately C-terminal to *asp*artate residues). There are at least 12 mammalian caspases. All are initially synthesized as inactive proenzymes and undergo proteolysis to generate two fragments of around 10- and 20-kDa molecular weight, together with a fragment of variable length from the original N-terminus (Fig. 4.6.2). These 10- and 20-kDa fragments oligomerize in pairs to form a tetramer, which is

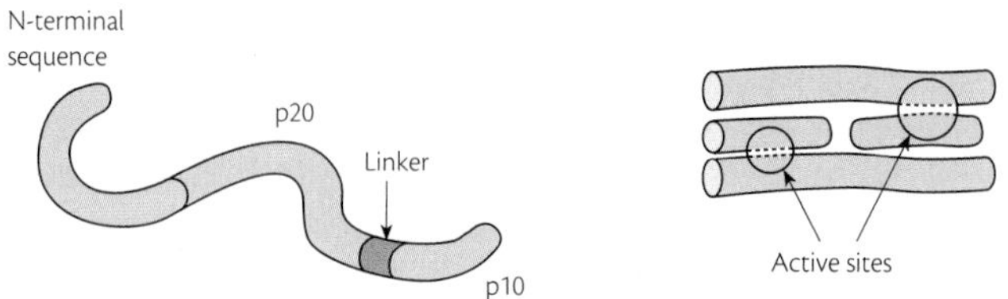

Fig. 4.6.2 Schematic diagram of caspase activation. The proenzyme is on the left. Following processing, as shown on the right, the N-terminal sequence and the linker are lost. The active sites of the enzyme each contain elements from both p10 and p20 subunits.

the active enzyme. Long N-terminal sequences provide the opportunity for regulation through interaction with various binding proteins.

Caspases recognize motifs of four amino acids that are present in many proteins. Significantly, such caspase target sites are often highly conserved between species, and frequently occur in strategic intramolecular locations, such that caspase cleavage would radically alter the function of the substrate protein. In particular, the cleavage of caspase substrates accounts for many of the structural changes of apoptosis already described. Particularly interesting substrates include proteases, kinases, cytoskeletal proteins, proteins involved in DNA damage and repair, and cell cycle regulatory proteins.

Caspases and proteases

The cleavage sites involved in the processing of caspases to their active form are themselves typical caspase target sequences. Hence, caspase activation can occur either by autocatalysis or through a sequential cascade-like process in which initiator caspases with long N-terminal sequences (caspases 8–12 and probably 2, 4, and 5) are activated first and then activate, by cleavage, the short effector caspases (3, 6, and 7). Caspases can also activate other proteases. Thus the calpain-inhibitor protein calpastatin is inactivated by caspase cleavage, so turning on calpain digestion within the dying cell.

Caspases and protein kinases

The small G-protein rho regulates the mobility of the cell surface. Two rho-dependent kinases, PAK2 and ROCK-1, are rendered constitutively active by caspase cleavage, through excision of their negative regulatory domains. PAK2 activity is a factor in the early retraction of the apoptotic cell from its neighbours or from substrate attachment, while ROCK-1 activity is responsible for the enhanced action of a myosin light-chain kinase that drives the cell-membrane blebbing immediately preceding fragmentation of the apoptotic cell.

FAK^{p125} is the kinase associated with focal adhesion plaques. It is a critical element in the signalling pathway that links cellular awareness of substrate attachment (through integrins) to other cellular functions, including movement, attachment, and new transcription. FAK^{p125} is cleaved and inactivated by caspases, hence isolating the cell from such signals, many of which would normally promote survival. Somewhat similarly, the adenomatous polyposis coli protein (APC) and β-catenin are cleaved by caspases, at molecular sites that ensure loss of their function. Both are members of the wnt-1 signalling pathway, connecting cell-to-cell signals with regulation of cell function.

Caspases and cytoskeletal proteins

Actin (the major protein of the cytoskeleton), fodrin (which provides the deformable shell underlying the plasma membrane), vimentin (an intermediate filament protein of the cytoskeleton), and the lamins (which form a major component of the nuclear envelope) are all caspase substrates. Caspase cleavage of these large polymeric proteins ensures they are rapidly disassembled to monomers. Gelsolin, a further caspase substrate, is an actin-binding protein that cleaves actin filaments in a calcium-dependent manner. Caspase cleavage of gelsolin separates the calcium-sensitive negative regulatory domain from the protease domain, and hence actin-filament cleavage is effected under normal intracellular calcium concentrations. These cytoskeletal proteolytic events probably contribute to the rounded shape of apoptotic bodies and to the eventual dissolution of the nuclear envelope.

Caspases and DNA damage and repair

ICAD (inhibitor of caspase-activated DNase) is a cytoplasmic chaperone that binds a double-strand DNase, CAD (caspase-activated DNase). The ICAD–CAD complex is normally cytoplasmic. ICAD, however, is a caspase substrate and once cleaved ceases to chaperone CAD, which unfolds, displaying a nuclear localizing signal. Once within the nucleus, CAD initiates the digestion of DNA, first to large fragments of around 50 kilobase pairs and eventually—through cleavage of chromatin at internucleosomal sites—to a series of fragments that are multiples of the 180- to 200-base pair unit wrapped around each nucleosome. The genesis of these DNA fragments is exploited in several cytological and electrophoretic methods for identifying apoptosis.

DNA-PK, ATM, PARP, and Rad51 are all DNA repair proteins concerned with the recognition and response to double-strand DNA breaks. Significantly, all are cleaved in apoptosis at sites that separate their DNA-binding and catalytic domains, thus removing their ability to repair DNA. This may be important in preventing re-ligation of the heavily digested DNA of the apoptotic nucleus, so avoiding the generation of large numbers of undesirable recombinant DNA molecules.

Caspases and cell-cycle proteins

Unexpectedly, several proteins that normally inhibit movement around the cell cycle are targets for caspase cleavage. These include p21WAF1 and p27KIP1(inhibitors of cyclin-dependent kinases that catalyse movement through the G_1 and S phases of the cell cycle), WEE-1 (which blocks movement from G_2 to mitosis), and CDC27 (which inhibits entry into mitosis). The purpose of this potential reactivation of cell cycle activity during the process of death is obscure. It occurs during the apoptosis of cells such as neurons that have long since ceased movement around the cycle.

The activation of apoptosis

Two well-documented pathways converge on and activate the effector caspases. One connects extracellular cytokine-based stimuli to the caspase cascade, through death-signalling receptors on the cell surface, and is often referred to as the extrinsic pathway. The other, termed the intrinsic pathway, links the caspase cascade to a great variety of signals from the cell interior, reflecting dysfunction in metabolism, genotoxic injury, hypoxia, and the status of the cytoskeleton. Both pathways may be triggered by physiological as well as pathological stimuli.

Death-signalling receptors coupled to apoptosis

The death-signalling receptors are all members of the tumour necrosis factor alpha (TNFα) receptor family. They are type 1 membrane receptors (that is, with the N-terminus on the external surface), containing a series of cysteine-rich incomplete repeats in the ligand-binding domain, a single transmembrane domain, and a cytoplasmic moiety with one or more signalling domains (Fig. 4.6.3). Their ligands are homologues of the cytokine TNFα. The prototype death-signalling receptor is fas (also called CD95

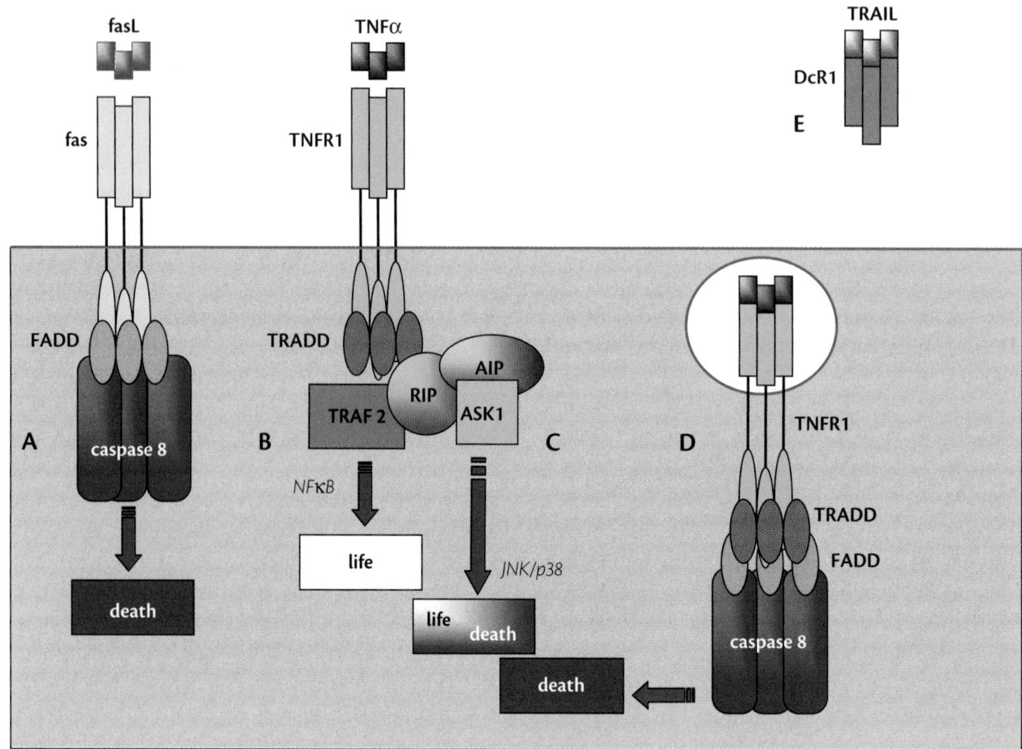

Fig. 4.6.3 Death-signalling receptors. The fas receptor, with its ligand and DISC, signalling exclusively to death, is shown in A. The more complex TNFα receptor 1 is shown in B, C, and D. One outcome of activation of this receptor (shown diagrammatically in B) signals for survival through the transcription factor NF-κB, by a RIP kinase dependent pathway. Another (C), dependent upon recruitment of ASK-1 to the DISC, activates the Jun Kinase/p38 pathway and can support either survival or apoptosis, depending on cell type and conditions. The third (D) requires internalization of the receptor, and activates caspase 8 through protein–protein interaction between TRADD and FADD. E shows DcR1, one of the decoy receptors for TRAIL (TNF-related apoptosis-inducing ligand). This receptor has no membrane anchor and so competes for TRAIL with the death-signalling membrane receptors, DR4 and DR5.

or Apo-1). On binding its ligand, FasL, this receptor trimerizes and immediately recruits to its cytoplasmic moiety a cluster of proteins collectively called the death-initiating signalling complex (DISC). The aggregation of DISC proteins is the result of protein–protein interaction at an α-helical region called the death domain (DD). Through their DDs, fas interacts with an adapter protein called FADD (fas-associated protein with death domain) that contains a further interactive region called DED (for death-effector domain). Through DED, FADD recruits procaspase 8 to the DISC, an initiator caspase with two DEDs in its N-terminal sequence. Because they are at high local concentration in the DISC, the procaspase 8 molecules can catalyse their own activation, and so initiate the proteolytic cascade that ultimately turns on the effector caspases. Whilst fas is widely expressed in many tissues, fasL expression is largely restricted to cytotoxic lymphocytes and to cells in immunologically privileged sites. In this way, the fasL/fas system plays a major role in cell killing by cytotoxic T-lymphocytes (CTLs) but can repulse CTLs at immunologically privileged sites.

TNFR1, the high-affinity TNFα receptor, also trimerizes on binding its ligand TNFα, but the downstream pathways are more diverse than those of fas. Three types of protein complex form around the cytoplasmic moiety of the activated TNF receptor. Each initially comprises a basic DISC that includes a DD-containing adapter protein called TRADD (for TNF receptor associated death domain protein), a threonine kinase called RIP (for receptor interacting protein), and a third protein, TRAF-2 (for TNF receptor associated factor). From this common origin, three types of protein complex develop, each responsible for a different pattern of signal transduction (Fig. 4.6.3 and Box 4.6.1).

DR3 is a receptor closely similar in structure to TNFR1 but with a narrower tissue distribution. Whereas TNFR1 is ubiquitous, DR3 is expressed predominantly in the lymphocytes of spleen, thymus, and peripheral blood. Interestingly, the expression of the ligands appears to adopt the opposite pattern, with TNFα being a product predominantly of activated macrophages and lymphocytes, whereas the DR3 ligand (variously also called Apo3L and TWEAK) is expressed in many tissue types.

DR4 and -5 are similar receptors that bind a ligand called TRAIL (TNF related apoptosis-inducing ligand). The downstream signalling appears to involve both FADD and caspase 8. Both TRAIL and its receptors are expressed in many tissue types. TRAIL has excited attention as a potential therapeutic agent because it is frequently cytotoxic to tumour cells under conditions in which normal cells are unharmed. Variant receptors that lack the cytoplasmic signalling moieties (e.g. DcR1, Fig. 4.6.3) are expressed in many normal tissues and appear to act as inhibitory decoys for TRAIL.

Mitochondrial signals coupled to apoptosis

The mitochondrial pathway depends upon the release of cytochrome *c*, together with deoxyATP (dATP), from the intermembranous space of mitochondria. Cytochrome *c* and dATP bind to and effect a conformational change in a protein of the outer

Box 4.6.1 TNFα signalling

When TNFα binds to its receptor, three pathways with different outcomes may be activated. First, the basic DISC—comprising TRADD, RIP, and TRAF2—may directly recruit regulatory elements of the MAP kinase pathway, leading to activation of the transcription factor NF-κB and a set of pro-survival, NF-κB dependent events. Second, and apparently following internalization of the receptor and its DISC, TRADD can recruit FADD and hence procaspase 8 or 10, so providing the means of activating apoptosis. Third, activation of the TNF receptor can lead to the dissociation from it of a protein called AIP (for ASK-interacting protein). While it is bound to the TNF receptor AIP is in an inactive, folded form, but on release it unfolds, becomes phosphorylated by RIP, and contributes to a new signaling complex comprising TRAF-2, RIP, AIP, and ASK-1. ASK-1 (for apoptosis signal-regulating kinase, also called MAP3K5) is an upstream kinase in the MAPKinase cascade and ultimately directs the activation of JNK and p38 kinase, as will be discussed later. Thus, activation of the TNF receptor may induce survival or apoptosis, depending on the cell type and local environmental conditions.

mitochondrial membrane, Apaf-1 (for apoptotic protease activating factor), so that it exposes a protein-binding domain (generically called a CARD, for caspase-activating recruitment domain) capable of recruiting and activating procaspase 9. This molecular assembly has been called the apoptosome. Caspase 9 then activates the effector caspases. Triggers for the release of cytochrome *c* include reactive oxygen species, cellular redox stress, and proteins of the BCL-2 family (Fig. 4.6.4).

BCL-2 is a protein with a C-terminal hydrophobic domain that allows it to anchor to the outer mitochondrial membrane. It was first identified because of its consistent activation (through a chromosome translocation) in follicular B-cell lymphoma. Its major physiological role, however, is that of a survival factor, and thus it can cooperate with other oncogenes during carcinogenesis to sustain the life of clones of cells that otherwise might be deleted by apoptosis. The mammalian Bcl-2 family contains at least 15 members in 3 major branches, distinguished on the basis of their function, which may facilitate either survival or apoptosis, and the presence or absence of certain conserved domains, called BH1 to BH4 (Fig. 4.6.5). Amongst the pro-survival molecules are BCL-2 itself, BCL-xL, BCL-w, MCL-1 and A1, all of which share all four BH homology domains. In contrast, bax and bak form a branch of the BCL-2 family that possesses BH3, BH2, and BH1 domains but exerts pro-death functions The third—and still expanding—family branch consists of pro-apoptotic proteins whose sole region of homology with the others is a single BH3 domain (amounting to no more than 9–16 amino acids): bid, bad, bim, bmf, bik, hrk, BNIP3, NOXA, PUMA, and Mule/ARF-BP1. Other more recently identified family members (Spike, BCL-rambo, BCL-B, BCL-G) are still being characterized.

The BH1, BH2, and BH3 domains of the pro-survival family members together form a hydrophobic groove into which BH3 domains of the BH3-only proteins and the multidomain pro-apoptotic proteins can fit, in much the same way as a ligand binds to its receptor. Such binding prevents the oligomerization of bak and bax and in so doing neutralizes their pro-apoptotic functions. However, in the presence of the 'BH3-only' family members, most of which bind to the hydrophobic cleft with high affinity, bax and bak are displaced from the groove to form homo-oligomeric structures that lodge in the outer mitochondrial membrane, creating there the conditions that permit efflux of cytochrome *c* and dATP (see Box 4.6.2) and hence procaspase 9 activation, as described above. An alternative scenario suggests that the

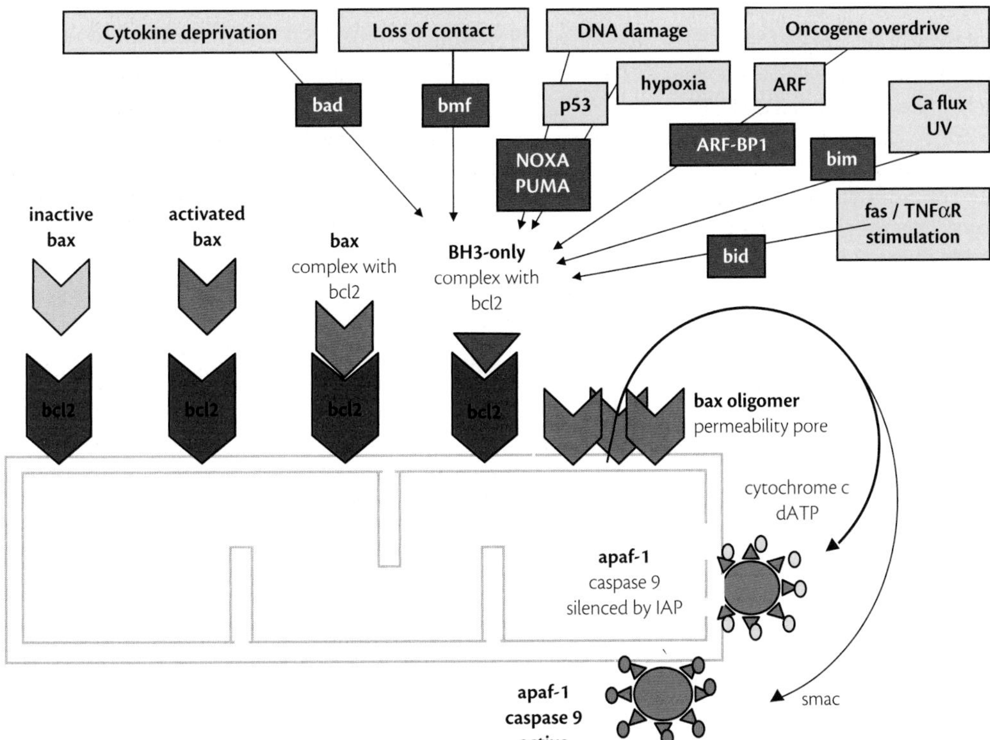

Fig. 4.6.4 A summary of the processes involved in activation of caspase 9, and the role of bcl-2 family proteins. Bax, activated in the cytoplasm, translocates to the surface of mitochondria where it initially binds to Bcl-2 (or combinations of bax or bak with bcl-2 or bcl-xL). Excess bax forms oligomers that are responsible for the permeability transition. Alternatively, bax may be displaced from bcl-2 by competition with the BH3-only proteins (and see Box 4.6.2). Caspase 9 complexed with apaf-1 is activated by cytochrome **c** and dATP from the intermembranous space, but this activation can be inhibited by IAPs. Release of smac from the intermembranous space releases this inhibition. The central role of several BH3-only proteins in connecting the apoptotic machinery to a variety of stimuli is also shown.

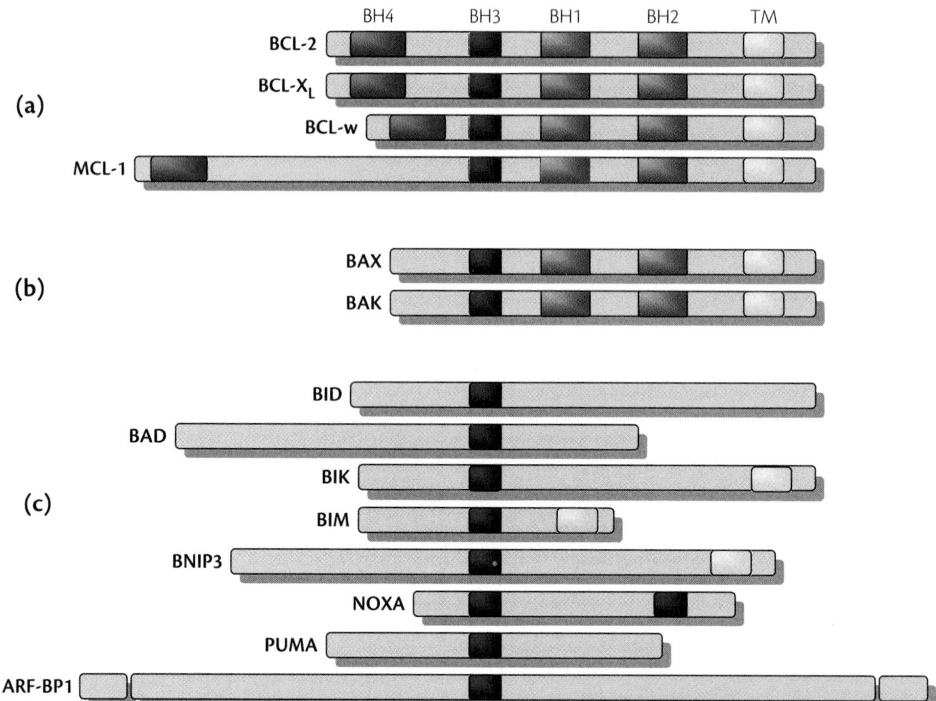

Fig. 4.6.5 Examples of the human Bcl-2 family, showing schematically the relative positions in the unfolded protein of the BCL-2 homology domains (BH1-4) domains, and the transmembrane domain (TM). (a) Four prosurvival members. The orientation of the BH domains in A1 is similar, but this protein lacks a transmembrane domain. (b) The two major multidomain pro-apoptotic proteins. (c) Some BH3-only proteins. Note that although some of these possess transmembrane domains, the great majority have only the BH3-homology domain in common, and they differ greatly in total size. Thus, PUMAα (the longest splice-variant isoform of the PUMA gene) has 193 amino acids, while ARF-BP1 has 4374, and hence is not drawn to scale relative to the others.

BH3-only proteins may bind to the hydrophobic groove of bax or bak, so catalysing their oligomerization directly.

The BH3-only, pro-apoptotic proteins play important roles in coupling the powerful mitochondrial pathway to a broad variety of stimuli—physiological and pathological—in the cellular environment (Fig. 4.6.4). Notably, bid is activated through cleavage by caspase 8 of a small peptide from its N terminus. The truncated, activated bid translocates from the cytosol to mitochondria and effects the mitochondrial release of cytochrome *c*. In this way, stimuli emanating from cytokine receptors but too small to activate the effector caspases directly can be amplified by recruitment of the mitochondrial pathway. Put another way, activation of bid lowers the threshold at which cytokines trigger apoptosis. Somewhat similarly, bad is involved in a mechanism to raise the threshold at which apoptosis is engaged, depending on the availability of cytokine growth factors. Bad is phosphorylated by the kinases Akt (protein kinase B) and Rsk, both in turn dependent on PI3 kinase and the growth factors responsible for its activation. Normally, phosphorylated bad is sequestered in the cytoplasm by the chaperone 14-3-3. In conditions of growth-factor deprivation, however, unphosphorylated bad becomes available, translocates to the mitochondria, and activates cytochrome *c* release. BNIP3 is a mitochondrial protein that accumulates under conditions of hypoxia. It may thus provide a trigger linking hypoxia to apoptosis. Normally, bim binds to the light chain of dynein and bmf to myosin V, cytoskeletal proteins that appear to generate signals relating to microtubule integrity and cell attachment respectively. The transcription of PUMA and NOXA is directly dependent on p53, hence providing a link between nuclear DNA damage and apoptosis. Mule/ARF BP1 is a ubiquitin ligase that targets for proteasomal destruction the cell cycle regulator cdc6. This has the effect of arresting the cell cycle, but as discussed below can also initiate apoptosis. There is also specificity as to which members of the pro-survival Bcl2 family proteins are targeted by individual BH3-only proteins: whereas t-bid, bim and PUMA bind to all five pro-survival Bcl-2 family proteins, the others have more limited affinities. In this way the BH3-only proteins provide a

Box 4.6.2 The mitochondrial permeability transition pore

There has been substantial controversy over the precise mode of action of bax and bak in effecting the release of cytochrome *c* and dATP from mitochondria. Under normal conditions, there is an electrical potential across the mitochondrial membrane ($\Delta\Psi m$) sustained by proton pumping through transmembrane protein complexes called permeability transition pores. In many circumstances, $\Delta\Psi m$ dissipates abruptly just prior to apoptosis, suggesting that the pores have become unselective ion channels. One consequence of this is osmotic expansion of the inner mitochondrial compartment, which could lead to rupture of the outer membrane and hence escape into the cytoplasm of cytochrome *c* and dATP. Direct experiments with artificial reconstructions of lipid bilayers, however, show that oligomers of bax can insert directly into such membranes, creating grommet-like channels through which large molecules can move. In this scenario, the collapse of $\Delta\Psi m$ would be secondary to the appearance of such channels.

summation of injury and physiological death signals from all over the cell, and translate that, in a cell-type-dependent manner, to the final decision between life and death.

Mitochondria are not unique amongst cellular organelles in providing the location for procaspase-containing protein complexes whose activation is affected by Bcl-2 family members. Procaspase 2 can be found in the nucleus and Golgi apparatus of some cells. Bcl-2 is present on nuclear and endoplasmic reticulum membranes. Activated bax locates to endoplasmic reticulum as well as to mitochondria. Hence, multiple organelles may contribute to the execution of apoptosis as well as the audit of its initiating stimuli.

Apoptosis and cell stress

The question arises how apoptosis relates to the other molecular mechanisms whereby cells respond to stresses of various kinds. Injured cells activate stereotyped reactions, of which the heat shock response, the unfolded protein response, the stress-activated kinase response and the DNA injury response are of particular relevance here.

The heat shock response

Heat shock proteins (HSPs) are molecular chaperones of diverse molecular weight that share the property of greatly enhanced transcription following cell stress. Thermal, osmotic, and redox stress, ultraviolet, and ionizing radiation all may induce HSP transcription. The heat shock response sustains cell survival under adverse circumstances and inhibits apoptosis in several different ways: Hsp27 inhibits caspase 8 cleavage of bid, and hence the release of cytochrome *c* from mitochondria; Hsp40 and Hsp70 inhibit bax translocation to mitochondrial membranes; Hsp70 and Hsp90 may dissociate the components of the apoptosome. Presumably each cell has a threshold at which full activation of caspases and the entry to apoptosis become inevitable. The HSPs raise that threshold, but little is known of how the threshold itself is defined in the first place.

The unfolded protein response (UPR)

This regulates the rate of protein synthesis so that correct folding and export from the endoplasmic reticulum occur. Without the UPR, insoluble aggregates of misfolded protein begin to accumulate in the ER, a manifestation of 'ER stress'. In summary, the UPR is initiated by three receptor proteins, PERK, ATF6 and IRE-1. PERK is a kinase, and responds to the presence of misfolded protein by inhibiting (by phosphorylation) the translation initiation function of eIF2. ATF6 is a transcription factor, and migrates to the nucleus where it stimulates the transcription of chaperone proteins, GRP78, GRP94, and XBP1. IRE is a dual function serine-threonine kinase and ribonuclease. It splices XBP1 mRNA to generate a further transcription factor for chaperones. However, the UPR has a clearly recognizable boundary at which its function changes from cytoprotective to pro-apoptotic. On prolonged stimulation, certain specific proteins are translated at high abundance, despite the general inhibition of eIF2. Amongst them is a protein called CHOP that lowers the cell's apoptosis threshold by inhibiting transcription of Bcl-2. Further, IRE-1 forms an activating complex with TRAF-2 and ASK-1, pro-apoptotic elements of the JNK/p38 kinase pathway to be described below.

The stress-activated kinase response

The MAP kinases are serine-threonine protein kinase cascades, described in detail elsewhere in this textbook (see Chapter 4.5). Activation of these cascades is initiated by phosphorylation of regulatory upstream members, MAP kinase kinase kinases (MAP3Ks), and leads ultimately to activation of transcription factors. Two of the three major sets of mammalian MAP kinase cascades are directly involved in transduction of stimuli that lead to apoptosis: the p38 kinases often being part of a stress-related pro-apoptotic process, the JNK kinases sometimes, depending on local circumstances. That these kinases have a role in the activation of apoptosis is clearly demonstrated by the attenuation of apoptosis in cells from appropriate knockout animals, but how and why these roles are played have proved more difficult to define. The stress kinase cascades appear to engage with the apoptosis effectors in several different ways. Thus, they activate (by phosphorylation) p53, CHOP, and several BH3-only pro-apoptotic BCL-2 family members, inactivate (again by phosphorylation) Bcl-2 and Bcl-XL, and activate the transcription of Fas ligand, all processes that lower the threshold for apoptosis. By stimulating cell cycle movement through transcriptional activation of c-myc, under conditions in which cycle movement is blocked (e.g. by p53) they also promote apoptosis, as described below. ASK-1 is a significant upstream MAP3K connecting the relevant environmental stimulus to the stress kinase cascades. ASK-1 is itself activated by reactive oxygen species, as it is normally bound in inactive conformation by the redox sensor thioredoxin. In the presence of a strong oxidative environment, thioredoxin dissociates, ASK-1 is activated, and the JNK/p38 cascades are stimulated. ASK-1 is also activated as part of a complex with TRAF-2 following TNF receptor stimulation and in the UPR, as described earlier.

The DNA damage response

Damage to nuclear DNA is a particularly important source of injury-related stimuli for caspase activation. Separate molecular mechanisms exist for responding to the presence of inappropriately inserted bases (base excision repair), nucleotides that have become modified through cross-linking or the formation of covalently bound adducts (nucleotide excision repair), nucleotide mismatch, insertion-deletion loops or abnormal methylation (mismatch repair), and double-strand breaks (homologous recombination or non-homologous end-joining). In mismatch repair, MSH-2 and MLH-1 are recruited sequentially into a molecular complex at the injury site, which activates p53, effects cell-cycle arrest, and, in the meantime, initiates repair at the site of damage. Similarly, amongst the first molecules to bind to DNA double-strand breaks in non-homologous end-joining are the DNA kinases ATM, ATR, and DNA-PK. In turn, these recruit and activate p53 and other molecules (e.g. CHK-1 and CHK-2). In surviving cells, these effect arrest at a variety of points around the cell cycle, so ensuring that there is opportunity to load the repair machinery on to the damaged DNA template before this is further altered by DNA replication (in S-phase) or chromatid separation (in mitosis).

A profoundly different means of limiting the effect of genome damage, however, is to commit the damaged cell to apoptosis. Elements such as p53 within the repair complex in both mismatch repair and non-homologous end-joining can also do this. The molecular basis for the decision between apoptosis or survival with repair is still largely unknown. Activation of p53 is common to both outcomes, and it is therefore reasonable to search in and around this molecule for clues to the nature of the life or death decision. Activated p53 alters the transcription of a large number of genes. Some are well-known inhibitors of cell-cycle progression, such as p21waf1/cip1, but others (e.g. bax, fas, a membrane protein called PERP, and the BH3-only pro-apoptotic molecules NOXA and PUMA) are associated almost exclusively with apoptosis. A further transcriptional target of p53 is the non-translated microRNA miR-34 (see Box 4.6.3), activation of which is associated with both cell-cycle arrest and apoptosis. The situation is further complicated by the fact that p53 also signals to the apoptosis effector process by non-transcriptional means, via an N-terminal sequence that does not appear to be instrumental in effecting cell-cycle arrest. Phosphorylation provides one of the critical signals for p53 activation, and there are several different phosphorylation sites that respond preferentially to the various kinases (including Jun kinase, as mentioned above). Thus the precise phosphorylation status of p53 could provide a molecular signature indicative of the nature, and perhaps the outcome, of the DNA damage.

Another potential factor in controlling the outcome of DNA injury is a kinase (called DAP kinase because it was originally discovered as a death-associated protein) that influences the selection of p14ARF rather than p16INK4A—alternative splice forms from the same gene. Whereas p16INK4A is a cell-cycle regulator, inhibiting the cyclin-dependent kinases, p14ARF displaces p53 from its inhibitor, MDM2, so generating a sustained p53 signal that may favour apoptosis.

Further evidence for integration of multiple factors in the response to double-strand DNA breaks comes from detailed study of the injured nucleus. Within an hour of DNA damage, large complexes of phosphorylated proteins form around the damaged site, including ATM, p53, many repair proteins and the phosphorylated histone γH2AX. Within a few hours, these foci come to lie in close juxtaposition with pre-existing intranuclear bodies called PML bodies, into which p53 and many other proteins in the DNA-injury response are recruited. Nuclei without PML mount only an attenuated version of the expected p53-dependent apoptotic response to DNA damage, even though p53 itself is available. One explanation for this is that the PML body is an intracellular location for the activation of p53 protein by acetylation. The PML body may thus form the local environment in which the state of the injured DNA is evaluated and final decisions made regarding the ultimate fate of the cell.

Box 4.6.3 MicroRNA

MicroRNAs are a family of short RNA species that are not translated, but exert profound influence over the patterns of transcription. They bind to regions of sequence homology in the 3′ untranslated regions of messenger RNA, inhibiting translation and creating double-stranded RNA that becomes a target for digestion by double-strand RNA specific ribonucleases called argonaute proteins. There appear to be only a few hundred distinct types of microRNA (miRNA), each capable of inhibiting its own spectrum of specific messenger RNA types. Hence altered patterns of miRNA transcription can swiftly alter the overall pattern of messenger RNA that is available for translation. Certain miRNA profiles are characteristic of some types of cancer.

The replicative status of the cell is a further important determinant of its sensitivity to apoptosis following DNA injury. The proto-oncogene c-*myc* is normally amongst the earliest gene products to be synthesized when cells are stimulated by growth factors to leave quiescence and enter their replicative cycle. Paradoxically, however, c-*myc* expression is also a powerful factor lowering the threshold for apoptosis. In particular, c-*myc* expression without concurrent molecular evidence of external growth-factor stimulation (such as phosphatidylinositol-3 (PI3) kinase and Akt activation) is interpreted as a death signal. Similarly, other early regulators of cell-cycle entry, including inhibition of function of the retinoblastoma protein and the release of the transcription factor E2F-1 from its binding pocket, also trigger apoptosis in the absence of concurrent evidence of external mitogenic stimulation. Perhaps this represents a means whereby tissues are protected from autonomous cell replication: survival of replicating cells is made conditional on the presence of appropriate stimuli in the cellular environment. The benefits of removing cells that show a tendency for such replicative autonomy are obvious, but the precise mechanism that couples replication to death except in acceptable circumstances is far less clear. It seems probable that the cell cycle itself includes checkpoints at which the decision to engage the apoptosis machinery can be taken should any of the appropriate conditions for replication be absent. Indeed, it is possible that injured cells may force the activation of such checkpoints as one way to access their apoptosis programme. This might explain the paradoxical activation of cyclin-dependent kinases by caspases in cells such as neurons that normally do not engage in replicative cycles at all, as mentioned earlier.

Inhibitors of caspase activation

The role of the BCL-2 family proteins in the activation and inhibition of apoptosis has been described, but there are other powerful endogenous inhibitors of caspase-associated cell death. One is FLIP, a DED-containing version of procaspase 8 that lacks caspase activity. High local concentrations of FLIP compete with procaspase 8 for recruitment into the DISC and so inhibit further propagation of death signals originating from the TNF family of receptors.

IAPs (inhibitors of apoptosis proteins) inhibit caspase activity after autocatalytic processing of the procaspase has begun. All contain an element called a BIR domain, which binds to the N-termini of the short fragment of partially processed caspases in such a way that adjacent elements of the IAP molecule drape across the caspase active site and sterically hinder substrate attachment. There are several such proteins—IAP1 and -2, ILP, the neuronal NAIP, and an X-linked family member X-IAP, all of which possess several BIR domains, and livin and survivin which contain a single BIR domain. One manifestation of the importance of IAPs is the presence of an IAP inhibitor, variously called smac or DIABLO, which is released from mitochondria along with cytochrome *c* during caspase activation by the mitochondrial pathway. The inhibitor smac has an N-terminal sequence that competes with partially processed caspase for the binding site in the BIR domain, and so allows the caspase to escape from the inhibitory embrace of the IAP.

The IAPs provide a further example of the interconnections between the cell cycle and cell death. Survivin, apparently associated with caspase 9, forms a complex with and is phosphorylated by active cdk1 (cyclin-dependent kinase-1) during mitosis. Loss of phosphorylation leads to dissociation of the survivin–caspase-9 heterodimer, activation of caspase 9, and apoptosis. As normal mitosis proceeds, survivin associates with kinetochore proteins, the spindle microtubules, and finally, at cytokinesis, with the midbody. Complexes of survivin with cyclin-dependent kinases active earlier in the cycle (e.g. cdk4) have also been identified and promote transit through G_1. Thus, survivin may form part of a regulatory network, providing a means whereby the threshold for apoptosis is varied through the cell cycle. Finally, IAPs are multifunctional proteins: they are themselves potential substrates of caspase attack, activators of the survival factor NF-κB, and downstream products of NFκB-directed transcription. They thus form part of positive-feedback systems for both survival and death.

Recognition of apoptotic cells

Macrophages recognize and bind to the surface of apoptotic cells by virtue of multiple molecular 'eat me' signals (Fig. 4.6.6). The disposition of phosphatidyl serine (PS) residues on the apoptotic cell surface is one of the most characteristic of these. Normally PS appears only on the inner leaflet of the cell membrane, but this strict polarity is lost very early in apoptosis: around the time of rounding up, substantially earlier than chromatin condensation and DNA cleavage, and probably prior to evidence of caspase activation. Macrophages possess a PS receptor that binds to the exposed PS residues. The exposed PS residues may also bind to molecules in the extracellular environment that then form linkers to receptors on macrophage surfaces. Thus thrombospondin helps bind PS on the apoptotic cell surface to β_1, β_3, and β_5 integrins on the macrophage surface. Similarly, the complement fragment iC3b links to macrophage β_2 integrins, whilst the near-ubiquitous extracellular molecule β_2 glycoprotein-1 links to a macrophage receptor specific for it. In the same way, extracellular complement component C1q links specific binding sites on the apoptotic cell surface to receptors on the macrophages. A group of scavenger receptors (SRA, CD36, CD68, LOX-1) may tether directly to poorly defined oxidized lipid groups (similar to those in oxidized low-density lipoproteins) exposed on the surfaces of apoptotic cells. CD14 on the macrophage binds to ICAM3, exposed on apoptotic cells. Endogenous macrophage surface lectins also bind to sugars (such as *N*-acetyl glucosamine) selectively exposed on apoptotic cell membranes. These multiple mechanisms that facilitate macrophage phagocytosis of apoptotic cells ensure that degradation of dying cells does not usually occur before they are securely engulfed within the phagosomes of the ingesting cells. Presumably this forestalls innate and acquired immune reactions to intracellular proteins, or the voiding into extracellular space of potentially recombinogenic fragments of genomic DNA.

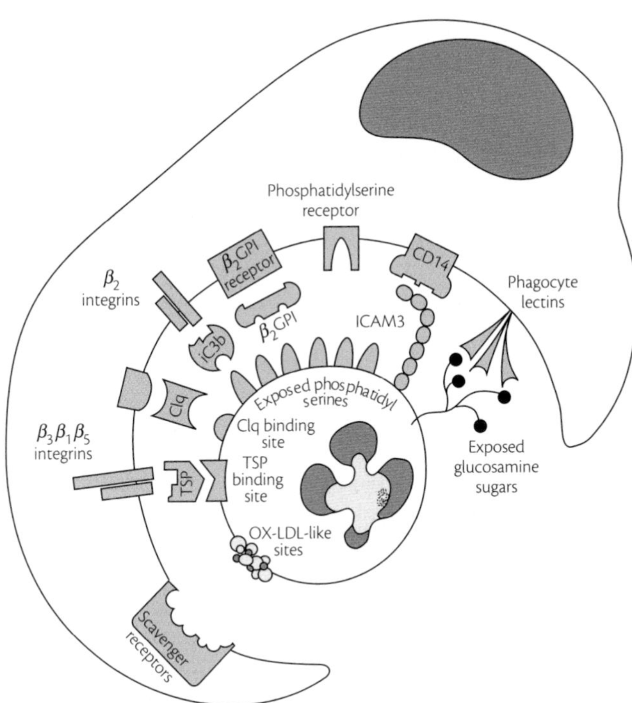

Fig. 4.6.6 Receptor–ligand interaction in the recognition of apoptotic cells by macrophages.

A distinctive feature of macrophage binding to apoptotic cells is the concurrent effect on macrophage function. Macrophages that phagocytose particles opsonized by immunoglobulin or complement component C3b effect a sharp increase in oxygen usage (the respiratory burst), generate reactive oxygen species and nitric oxide, and release of inflammatory cytokines such as TNFα. These recruit other acute inflammatory cells to the site. In contrast, macrophages that ingest apoptotic bodies show suppression of pro-inflammatory responses, mediated through the release of different cytokines, such as TGFβ. The basis of these contrasting effector responses appears to be the different signalling pathways that are activated by the macrophage receptors engaged by apoptotic bodies as opposed to opsonized particles.

Are caspases necessary and sufficient for cell death?

Although caspase activation plays a dominant role in the effector phase of apoptosis, it is not responsible for all the phenomena of apoptosis. One striking example is the surface exposure of 'eat me' signals described above: this is not affected by pharmacological blockade of caspases using inhibitors that competently block other aspects of apoptosis. Moreover, developmentally programmed cell death can sometimes occur on schedule in embryonic tissues in which caspases have been inhibited, or key members of the caspase activation system (such as Apaf-1) rendered deficient through germline gene knockout. In all these circumstances, the morphology of the caspase-free death is not that of apoptosis. The nuclei swell rather than undergoing chromatin condensation. The cytoplasm shows signs of fluid overload, sometimes with the formation of conspicuous fluid-filled vacuoles. Some of these changes are reminiscent of necrosis rather than apoptosis. Rather similar changes take place during the developmental death of phylogenetically ancient multicellular organisms that do not possess recognizable close homologues to the caspases, such as the slime mould *Dictyostelium discoides*.

These observations suggest that caspase activation, although intrinsic to the subtle and highly coordinated death process recognized as apoptosis, may not be the only event that commits cells to death. The existence of at least one caspase-independent death pathway is highlighted by a flavoprotein released from the mitochondria of injured cells called AIF (apoptosis-inducing factor). AIF translocates to the nucleus, where it can effect chromatin cleavage to large fragments, but not the extreme condensation observed in apoptosis. It also appears to reproduce the cellular volume overload described above, even in the presence of caspase inhibition. Phylogenetically close homologues of AIF are found in bacteria and plants as well as invertebrate and vertebrate animals.

Apoptosis and disease

There are few disease processes in which apoptosis does not feature, but the examples below are chosen because they exemplify how various steps in the apoptosis pathways may be critical for, or are subverted in, the course of disease pathogenesis.

Immunity and its disorders

Apoptosis is used extensively in the normal function of the immune system to facilitate the process of clonal selection. Antigen stimulation of T-cell proliferation is usually followed by expression of both fas and fasL, a recipe for apoptosis on a grand scale (called activation-induced cell death, AICD) unless there is rescue by a survival stimulus. This can be provided by co-stimulation from the immediate environment—adhesion molecules or cytokine receptors. A particularly important route for co-stimulation is through CD28, a receptor on T cells for signals transmitted from antigen-presenting cells, which increases the expression of several cytokines and their receptors. Similarly, clonally expanded populations of stimulated B cells in the bone marrow or those undergoing affinity maturation in lymph-node follicle centres are deleted by fas signalling, but can be selectively rescued by costimulation through CD40.

Cytotoxic T lymphocytes (CTLs) kill their targets by delivering to them the contents of their granules. Amongst these are perforin, which creates regions in the target-cell membrane of enhanced permeability at the points of contact with the CTL, and granzyme B, a protease that directly activates the caspases of the target cell. In this way, CTLs induce target-cell apoptosis.

The importance of apoptosis for the normal function of the immune system is underscored by the effects of genetic defects. Strains of mice with loss-of-function mutations in the genes encoding fas or fas ligand (called *lpr* and *gld*, respectively) show similar immunological phenotypes, characterized by massive lymphoproliferation and autoimmune disorders. The human homologue is the rare condition of Canale–Smith syndrome (childhood autoimmune lymphoproliferative syndrome or ALPS) in which there is a mutation in the DD of fas. Inherited deficiency in C1q also leads to an autoimmunity syndrome: affected individuals almost always develop systemic lupus erythematosus. The pathogenesis here appears to be ineffective recognition and phagocytosis of endogenous apoptotic cells, so that their intracellular antigens are inappropriately processed.

Infective disorders

Shigella dysentery is due to pathogenic strains of *Shigella flexneri*. Pathogenicity is conferred by plasmid-borne genes that neutralize the primary host defence: phagocytosis and destruction of the bacteria by macrophages in the intestinal lamina propria. The plasmid-encoded protein Ipa B activates macrophage caspase 1, so annihilating the defence by inducing macrophage apoptosis. This strategy appears to be successful, because the bacterium that would normally be destroyed if it persisted within the phagosome of the ingesting macrophage can escape from the cytoplasm of macrophages that undergo apoptosis.

The initial response to *Trypanosoma cruzi*, the parasite responsible for Chagas' disease, is dominated by T-lymphocyte activation. The resultant AICD generates a population of apoptotic lymphocytes. These impinge upon the macrophages that, suitably armed by pro-inflammatory cytokine stimulation, would be one of the most effective elements in the host defence against the parasite. As described earlier, sustained macrophage phagocytosis of these large numbers of apoptotic cells leads to suppression of pro-inflammatory cytokine release. The parasite subverts this aspect of the physiology of apoptosis into a source of protection from the host-defence reaction.

The intracellular parasite chlamydia makes a protein (CPAF) that comprehensively targets BH3-only pro-apoptotic molecules for proteasomal destruction. This illustrates the value to the organism of keeping a live cell environment around it, but also provides vivid affirmation of the key role played by BH3-only proteins in activating apoptosis.

Viruses engage with the machinery of apoptosis in many ways. Even lytic viruses have strategies designed to conserve the life of their host cells for some time. DNA viruses, in particular, require means to abort apoptosis, as they must activate the cellular DNA synthesis machinery in order to replicate their own genomes, yet must then avoid the apoptosis that would otherwise follow DNA synthesis unaccompanied by commensurate external stimuli. The *E6* gene of high-risk human papillomaviruses (HPV) 16 and 18 encodes a protein that targets p53 for ubiquitination and subsequent degradation, and so permits cellular survival as the viral E7 protein binds Rb and initiates entry into S-phase. The transforming genes of adenoviruses pair up to effect rather similar outcomes: E1A binds Rb and initiates DNA synthesis, the 55-kDa subunit of E1B binds and inhibits p53, and the 19-kDa subunit neutralizes proapoptotic members of the BCL-2 family. Human herpesviruses such as HHV8 encode their own version of FLIP (v-FLIP). They also have their own pro-survival BCL-2 family members, such as BHRF1 in the Epstein–Barr virus (EBV) and KS-BCL2 in HHV8. The HHV8 strategy is particularly subtle, because the virus also destroys the endogenous BCL-2. Unlike endogenous BCL-2, this viral surrogate lacks an internal caspase site, and cannot be converted into a killer peptide by caspase cleavage. Baculovirus encodes a 35-kDa protein with BIR domains that is a prototypical IAP.

Apoptosis plays a key role in the pathogenesis of AIDS. The progressive loss of circulating CD4+ T cells, by which the course of HIV-1 infection to clinical AIDS can be charted, involves numbers of cells that are several orders of magnitude greater than the numbers that ever carry the virus. It is therefore clear that the overwhelming majority of the dying cells must be bystanders, sensitized to apoptosis by the presence of infection but not infected themselves. Viral proteins released from infected cells effect this sensitization by several parallel routes. The HIV proteins Tat and Nef induce fas, fasL, and TRAIL. Tat alters the cellular redox equilibrium in a manner that may activate Ask-1. Vpr binds to the mitochondrial permeability transition pore. A type of AICD may be induced by stimulation of CD4 and the cytokine receptor CXCR4 (both of which bind HIV epitopes). In infected cells, however, Nef inhibits ASK-1, and so may selectively protect these from apoptosis. Rather similar mechanisms underlie the deletion of neurons in HIV-associated dementia.

Cardiovascular disease

Pathogenetic mechanisms that interface with apoptosis are relatively poorly understood in cardiovascular disease, but there are several observations of potential relevance. Laminar flow inhibits Ask-1 in endothelium, whilst the generation of reactive oxygen species induces the p38 and JNK stress kinase pathways. Thus, turbulence and the presence of generators of reactive oxygen species such as oxidized low-density lipoproteins—both known risk factors in the genesis of atheroma—are liable to promote apoptosis in endothelium. Other elements of the vascular wall are also abnormal in atheroma. Vascular smooth muscle cells from atheromatous vessels express p53, induce fas, and undergo apoptosis in increased numbers, particularly in the shoulders of the plaque, thus weakening attachment of the fibrous cap and rendering plaque rupture more probable. Macrophages also undergo apoptosis in response to the oxidized lipids that are present in atheromatous plaques. Death of the lipid-filled macrophages (foam cells) produces extracellular depots of oxidized lipid in the plaque core, a key step in plaque progression.

Although necrosis is the pattern of the cell death that immediately follows episodes of infarction, there is now substantial evidence that apoptosis occurs in the surrounding tissue over several hours thereafter, probably in response to relative ischaemia and the local generation of reactive oxygen species. In animal models of stroke, this apoptosis can be down-regulated by a variety of manoeuvres, including caspase inhibition, with objective evidence of improved cerebral function. These observations have generated enthusiasm for the development of antiapoptotic drugs for use following stroke and myocardial infarction. Another approach, potentially applicable to ischaemic myocardium, is to promote angiogenesis, perhaps by the use of angiogenic stem cells. Experimental models suggest that this improves the remodelling of the peri-infarct tissue, including decreased apoptosis of myocytes and improved cardiac function.

Degeneration of the central nervous system

Despite the importance of the subject, there is still much doubt over the role of apoptosis in the chronic degenerative disorders such as Alzheimer's and Parkinson's diseases. Much of the problem stems from the relative inaccessibility of the brain for sequential studies following injury. In both conditions there is clear evidence of a loss of neurons, and those that remain accumulate abnormal cytoplasmic material, such as presenilins 1 and 2, and amyloid protein Aβ in Alzheimer's disease. Cell culture and animal models suggest that the presence of these proteins may induce oxidative stress, which can lower the threshold for apoptosis. The protective effect of BCL-2 and caspase inhibition has also been recorded. The difficulties are compounded by the fact that neurons that undergo severe overstimulation (e.g. by local high concentrations of the neurotransmitter glutamate) can also be induced to die (a phenomenon called *excitotoxicity*), but it is not clear whether the pathways involved overlap with or are identical to those of apoptosis.

Tumour biology

Apoptosis is of significance in cancer biology for two major reasons. First, carcinogenesis is almost invariably associated with escape from mechanisms that normally activate apoptosis. Second, a large component of tumour regression following therapy is attributable to apoptosis.

Carcinogenesis involves inappropriate cell proliferation, driven by release from tumour suppressor gene inhibition or hyperactive oncogene expression. Under normal circumstances, however, the accelerated movement around the cell cycle renders the cells vulnerable to DNA damage, which activates p53 (the 'DNA damage checkpoint') and ensures either cessation of replication or apoptosis of the affected cells. For the inappropriately driven population to progress to tumour growth, the affected cells must silence this p53 response. This affords one reason for the frequent appearance of deletions and loss-of-function mutations of p53 in tumours, and the observation that the cells of many tumours and some premalignant (but progressing) hyperplasias appear to be in a perpetual state of uncompleted DNA repair. A more subtle mechanism couples inappropriate proliferation to activation of p14ARF. Uncoupling of this 'oncogene checkpoint' also permits the continuing replication of cells that would otherwise have been arrested in cell cycle or committed to apoptosis. The ARF and p53 pathways are not mutually exclusive, as ARF has the effect of increasing the half-life of p53. Suppression of these pathways in the early genesis of tumours has the effect of permitting repeated escape from the DNA damage or oncogene checkpoints and so giving cancer cells the opportunity to explore the consequences of further genomic rearrangements or mutations that are denied normal cells. Some of these prove incompatible with continuing life but others lead to selective, progressive growth advantage Fig. 4.6.7).

These considerations have an important bearing on therapeutically induced tumour regression. Many therapeutic agents are effective because they create DNA lesions that activate a DNA damage checkpoint. However, as discussed above, most if not all tumours will already be derived from clones of cells that have lost

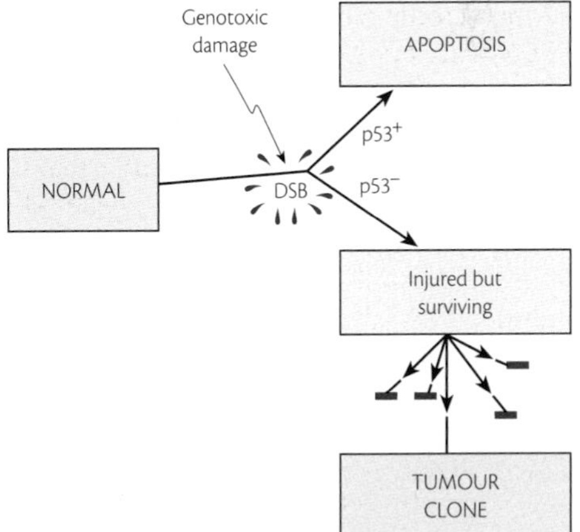

Fig. 4.6.7 Failure to activate apoptosis following damage by a genotoxic carcinogen, because of the absence of functional p53, leads to the inappropriate survival of clones of cells bearing double-strand breaks (DSB) and illegitimate recombination events. Although some of these clones may fail to proliferate further, others survive to become the founder clones of tumours. Constitutionally, these survivors have unstable genomes, as on further exposure to similar genotoxic stimuli they may again undergo genomic rearrangement or other forms of mutation yet fail to enact apoptosis. Although the example given is for cells lacking p53, and hence unable to respond appropriately to DNA DSBs, exactly the same argument applies to cells that fail to identify nucleotide mismatch through defective MSH-2 or MLH-1. Such cells sustain extremely high mutation rates, as mismatches occur (and are normally recognized and repaired) in the course of normal DNA replication, even in the absence of genotoxic carcinogens.

critical damage- or oncogene-activated checkpoints. If these happen to be the same as is targeted by the therapeutic agent, there is a high likelihood that the tumour will be resistant to the agent. Further, animal experiments have tested the effect on tumour behaviour of selective restoration of p53 function. Significantly, although regression was initiated almost immediately, tumour regrowth often occurred, accompanied by loss of function in the tumour cells of either ARF or the restored p53. The immediately effected regression of these tumours demonstrates that the downstream effectors of the p53 pathway are still intact in these tumours, and still capable of response to p53 when it is provided. However, the swift recurrence also shows that single-agent therapy has a high chance of failure: the tumour's genomic instability leads to rapid selection of alternative resistant clones.

Further reading

Adams J, Cory S (2007). The Bcl-2 apoptotic switch in cancer development and therapy. *Oncogene*, **26**, 1324–37.

Anwar S, Whyte MK (2007). Neutrophil apoptosis and infectious disease. *Exp Lung Res*, **33**, 519–28.

Danial NN, Korsmeyer SJ (2004). Cell death: critical control points. *Cell*, **116**, 205–19.

Feig C, Peter ME (2007). How apoptosis got the immune system in shape. *Eur J Immunol*, **37**, S61–S70.

LaCasse EC, Mahoney DJ, Cheung HH, *et al.* (2008). IAP-targeted therapies for cancer. *Oncogene*, **27**, 6252–75.

Levy OA (2009). Cell death pathways in Parkinson's Disease: proximal triggers, distal effectors, and final steps. Apoptosis, **14**, 478–500.

Lowe SW, Cepero E, Evan G (2004). Intrinsic tumour suppression. *Nature*, **432**, 307–15.

Li J and Yuan J (2008). Caspases in apoptosis and beyond. *Oncogene* **27**, 6194–6206.

Malhotra JD and Kaufman RJ (2007). The endoplasmic reticulum and the unfolded protein response. *Seminars in Cell and Developmental Biology* **18**, 716–731.

Merino D, Bouillet P (2009). The Bcl-2 family in autoimmune and degenerative disorders. *Apoptosis*, **14**, 570–83.

Serhan CN, Savill J (2005). Resolution of inflammation: the beginning programmes the end. *Nat Immunol*, **6**, 1191–97.

Takeda K, Noguchi T, Naguro I, *et al.* (2008). Apoptosis signal-regulating kinase-1 in stress and immune response. *Ann Rev Pharmacol Toxicol*, **48**, 8.1–8.27.

4.7

Discovery of embryonic stem cells and the concept of regenerative medicine

Martin J. Evans

In this chapter Sir Martin Evans, who was awarded the Nobel Prize for Physiology or Medicine in 2007, describes the identification of stem cells, initially from certain cultured tumour cells (teratocarcinoma cells) and latterly from early mammalian embryos.

Essentials

The differentiated cells of the adult vertebrate arise from a single fertilized egg and as development proceeds the commitment to differentiation becomes irreversible.

During early development a few cells give rise to all the differentiated tissues; these original cells are thus pluripotential.

In malignant tumours small populations of self-renewing cells may arise; these divide to generate rapidly differentiating cells and others, like themselves, which remain undifferentiated.

The original experimental observation that teratocarcinoma cells spontaneously differentiate into benign cell types, embryos, or primordial germ cells questioned the idea that the cellular differentiation was a spontaneous reversion from malignancy: perhaps stem cells within teratocarcinomas were essentially normal?

Discovery of embryonic stem cells made it possible to generate chimeras in the context of a carrier mouse embryo; the demonstration that these could contribute to the germline provided a route to genetic manipulation (transgenesis) from cells in culture to the intact adult mammal. This has been of critical importance for the generation of experimental animals that serve as authentic models of human inherited disease—with numerous technical refinements inducible and conditional models can be produced, almost at will, for study. It is moreover possible to disrupt any locus in the mouse (and now other mammalian) genome(s) in order to investigate the function of particular genes in the living animal.

Teratocarcinomas also occur in humans and their study has stimulated the developing concept of regenerative medicine—a concept further enriched by the isolation of human embryonic stem cells with differentiation properties similar to those of murine origin. In addition, knowledge about the factors that maintain pluripotency and suppress differentiation has allowed reprogramming of differentiated cells, such as skin fibroblasts, back into the embryonic stem-cell state. These scientific discoveries provide opportunities for using pluripotential cells in regenerative processes; those that are self-derived, would evade immune rejection.

Introduction

In this chapter I relate the history of isolation of mouse embryonic stem cells and their use as a vehicle for mammalian experimental genetic manipulation—and I will finish with some remarks on the possible future utility of the equivalent human embryonic stem cells as a vehicle for derivation of populations of tissue-specific precursor cells for cell transplantation, on which one form of regenerative medicine may be based.

Embryonic stem cells

During vertebrate development the entire organism with its panoply of diversely differentiated cells arises as the lineal descendant of the fertilized egg. Extensive studies in experimental embryology have demonstrated that commitment to differentiation becomes functionally essentially irreversible. At the earliest stages of development, when cell numbers are small, it is self-evident that there must be dividing cells, the descendants of which will give rise to a large range of differentiated tissues. Such cells would be termed pluripotential. It is not necessarily the case that there will be a self-renewing population of such cells in the normal embryo. Malignant transformation, on the other hand, can produce populations of self-perpetuating tumour cells and may provide a useful experimental source for cell types otherwise inaccessible.

Many tumours display a cell phenotype which is a caricature of their normal cell of origin. Teratocarcinomas are tumours which in addition to their malignancy and continued growth contain many patches of a wide variety of nearly normal tissues. In 1967, Leroy Stevens discovered and developed a strain of inbred mice which had a high spontaneous incidence of testicular teratocarcinomas. He was soon able to show that these arose by spontaneous overgrowth of primordial germ cells in the fetal testis. Stevens demonstrated that some of these tumours could be serially transplanted in the inbred strain of mouse and he said

> Following repeated serial transplantations, these tumours have retained their pleomorphic character. Pluripotent embryonic cells appear to give rise to both rapidly differentiating cells and others which like themselves, remain.

This is a definition of an embryonic stem cell.

In the course of this research, Leroy Stevens showed in 1970 that equivalent tumours could be formed by ectopic transplantation of preimplantation embryos. Dr Barry Pierce, as a human pathologist, was particularly interested in the observation that the differentiated cells appeared to be non-malignant whereas the stem cells provided the progressively growing malignant component of the tumours. Using the mouse model system, Pierce working with Kleinsmith in 1964 was able to transplant single cells and recover a fully differentiating tumour, thus proving that these tumours were indeed formed from a progressively growing population of pluripotential stem cells.

All these studies were carried out on tumours and cells derived from them, but increasingly there was evidence suggesting that the stem cells from these tumours were essentially behaving in a normal fashion. These cells, termed embryonal carcinoma cells, could be maintained in tissue culture and could be shown to differentiate *in vitro* in the tissue culture dish, *in vivo* in a tumour and *in vivo* in the context of a normal embryo to form a chimeric mouse. Moreover, by 1975 Gail Martin and I had shown that the differentiation observed *in vitro* followed a normal embryonic path. In discussion of this in 1981 I wrote

> Normal cells do not form tumours and conversely tumour cells are not normal. This concept lies at the heart of much of the study of tumour cell biology. Malignant teratocarcinoma stem cells spontaneously differentiate into benign cell types and normal embryos, or primordial germ cells, are able to initiate teratocarcinoma formation at a relatively high frequency. Is it reasonable to regard this process as a malignant transformation, and cellular differentiation as a spontaneous reversion from malignancy? One alternative ... [is that] the teratocarcinoma stem cell is essentially a cell showing a completely normal embryonic phenotype.

In the same year I also published a discussion of why, if these cells are indeed normal embryo cells, were we unable to derive them directly into tissue culture but it only through a tumour formed by ectopic transplantation of the embryo.

I surmised that there might be three explanations relating to number, timing, and rapidity of differentiation:

1 The number of pluripotential cells in the embryo at any one time might be very low; sufficient *in vivo* but insufficient *in vitro* where there is greater cell mortality.

2 There might be a short time window—*in vivo* this is extended by growth of the embryo up to this point or regression of some of the cells of a later embryo following damage of transplantation.

3 Embryonal carcinoma cells which differentiate readily are more difficult to maintain in tissue culture than those which are more culture adapted and differentiate less well; '... the genuine embryonic cell counterpart may differentiate and lose its pluripotency and rapid growth characteristics all too readily under culture conditions ...'

In retrospect we now know that it is possible to isolate these cells from mouse embryos between 1 and 4.5 days of normal development, so the second premise is unfounded, but the other two—cloning efficiency *in vitro* and use of culture conditions most conducive to maintenance of the undifferentiated state—are vital.

By that time I had, by using cloning efficiency assays, optimized all aspects of embryonal carcinoma cell culture; the media, serum, substrate, and feeder cells included. It was then that in 1981, in a collaboration with Matt Kaufman, we attempted to grow cells from implantationally delayed blastocysts and successfully isolated embryonic stem cell cultures. These diapause embryos have the advantage of a slight increase in cell number compared with the 3.5 day blastocyst. This technique was immediately effective in allowing pluripotential cell colonies to grow out directly from the inner cell mass. The use of delayed blastocysts was unnecessary but certainly improves efficiency of embryonic stem cell isolation. Much more is now known about the factors maintaining pluripotency and suppressing differentiation. Moreover, as shown by Takahashi and Yamanaka in 2006, by using conditions conducive to embryonic stem cell derivation and growth it has now proved possible to reprogram other differentiated cell types back to the embryonic stem cell state.

Because of all the antecedent work with culture of mouse embryonal carcinoma cells the expected properties for directly isolated mouse pluripotential stem cells were well understood and characterized. These were all rapidly verified, including—importantly—the ability to make chimeras in the context of a carrier mouse embryo. Andrew Bradley and other colleagues showed that these chimeras made with freshly isolated embryonic stem cell lines chimaerized not only the soma but also the germ line of the resulting mice, hence giving a route to genetic manipulation from culture to creature.

During normal early development there may be no more than a couple of dozen embryonic stem cells and they are constrained in the normal time course and present for only a short time. In contrast, many millions of embryonic stem cells may be maintained in tissue culture indefinitely and all of them retaining their pluripotentiality. This means that clones bearing a rare genetic change may be identified and used to pass that change into the mouse germ line and hence the breeding mouse genome. These cells are therefore a vector to an experimental mammalian genetics.

There are essentially two approaches: random mutagenesis and selection/screening, or targeted mutagenesis. Embryonic stem cells in culture are amenable to most forms of mutagenesis and it is therefore the screen that is pivotal. In the late 1980s, when we were first able to use embryonic stem cells to transfer mutation from culture to creature, sequence information for the mouse genome was very limited and many loci unidentified. When mutation is being induced randomly into as yet unidentified loci it is useful to ensure that these are marked and for this reason methods of insertion mutagenesis have tended to be favoured. With Andrew Bradley, I found that retroviral vectors were often the vehicle of choice because of their efficient transfection and clean integration leading to readily identifiable mutation.

With the notable exception of hypoxanthine-guanine phosphoribosyl transferase, informative mutations could not be readily selected *in vitro* and so screening of the resultant progeny after intercrossing was required—a lengthy process which did, however, result in the identification of some interesting loci. One of the more interesting was 413d/Nodal, found by Elizabeth Robertson and colleagues, which appeared as an organizational early embryonic lethal later identified by Zhou and colleagues as a factor resembling transforming growth factor beta (TGFβ). This was identified by the early death of homozygous mutant embryos.

The random mutagenesis approach was greatly strengthened by the introduction of the idea of gene trapping by transfection of embryonic stem cells using vectors with reporters which would be transcribed only when integrated into a suitable site in the genome. This allowed a screen not only of mutagenic effect (most usually in the homozygote) but of developmental and tissue-specific expression both *in vitro* and usefully in the immediate chimaera and the heterozygote offspring. Integration using a retroviral vector has the apparent disadvantage that the long terminal repeat sequences necessarily surround the trapping construct. But by using a splice acceptor as the trapping element and by having it in reverse orientation, thus avoiding interference with the transcription of retroviral vector itself, Friedrich and Soriano brought the advantages of retroviral transfection to gene trapping in the early 1990s. Intelligently constructed mutagenic reporters of gene function such as these have been used for extensive screens.

The alternative approach is directed mutagenesis. Two scientists who received the Nobel prize with me, Oliver Smithies and Mario Capecchi, both pioneered the method showing that a DNA construct with substantial homology with a chromosomal sequence could recombine into the endogenous sequence at relatively high efficiency when introduced into cells in tissue culture. With the advent of full knowledge of the genome, this method of gene targeting by homologous recombination has become the choice for gene inactivation. Even when a specific point mutagenesis or random point mutagenesis at a particular locus is desired it is more effective to recurrently target a marked locus with mutagenized vector rather than hitting the whole genome.

Homologous recombination works well with embryonic stem cells and is only limited by the need to keep the cells in conditions which retain their full pluripotentiality and germ line chimaerization ability. The design of the targeting vector and screening to find correctly targeted clones becomes the main consideration. In addition to simple mutation, methods have been developed which allow both spatial and temporal control of gene deletion or of function. All these studies are dependent upon the combination of *in vitro* cell genetic manipulation and selection coupled with true *in vivo* observation of the physiological consequences in the context of the whole animal. This has been made possible by tissue culture of embryonic stem cells. It is important to note that virtually any desired 'designer' change may be made by using the techniques of homologous recombination gene targeting ranging from single point mutation to large chromosomal alterations. All these techniques are applied to mice and this has provided the experimental genetic approach to mammalian genetics illuminating understanding of data emerging from the study of the human genome. Mouse embryonic stem cells have established at least two platforms for research: an *in vitro* system of cell differentiation equivalent to that in the early embryo and a vectorial system for experimental mammalian genetics *in vivo*.

Teratocarcinomas carcinomas occur not only in mice but also in humans. Thompson and colleagues showed in 1998 that embryonic stem cells isolated from human embryos have similar differentiation properties to those of mice. Clearly their use for genetical experiment would entirely unethical in addition to being impracticable, but their *in vitro* differentiation not only allows fundamental studies of human embryonic and cellular development but is also providing a possible platform for derivation of tissue-specific precursor cells *in vitro*. This concept of their utility to provide cells for tissue repair was clearly stated in the original publication by Jamie Thomson and the idea of both pluripotential and tissue-specific stem cells has been a very powerful stimulant for human regenerative medicine.

The beginnings of regenerative medicine

Regenerative medicine springs from the powerful idea of treatment of cellular insufficiency or tissue damage by replacement or supplementation with appropriately differentiated cells. Treatment with live cells is not a new concept; blood transfusion and bone marrow transplantation use cell suspensions and there are numerous transplantation therapies replacing whole organs. In some cases, such as liver transplantation, a regenerative tissue is introduced. Interestingly, skin grafting provides the example of transfer of organized tissue with the aim of transferring the regenerative skin stem cells and this therapy has advanced in some applications to the use of disaggregated cells either freshly isolated or from passaged tissue culture.

The question arises as to whether such treatments are medical or surgical. This is not just a question of professional demarcation: it affects which type of regulation is going to be applied. Will we see regenerative medicine and medical procedures regulated under rules designed for the safety of medicines, or under rules designed for the safety of tissue and organ transplantation? As presently framed, the two are very different. Regulations for drugs and other pharmacological formulations are framed both to ensure exact reproducibility and on the basis of large-scale clinical trials for efficacy. Regulations for organ and tissue transplantation focus upon the ethical source of the tissue and informed consent for its use and upon ensuring, as far as is practicable, that it does not transfer infection. The actual use is dependent upon professional judgement of its utility for the patient and good practice by the physician. It is much more a patient-specific approach than a specific formulation for use on many patients. Cell preparations, on the other hand, particularly when allogeneic, have been licensed by the United States Food and Drug Administration under conditions of good manufacturing practice and scrutiny not dissimilar to that of a drug. If the promise of widespread patient-specific treatment by autologously derived cells becomes a reality, then the personalized approach of the transplantation-based rules might be more appropriate.

There is another important practical question to be pondered; that is the cost of patient-specific treatment. Clearly, even when perfected and streamlined, preparing a specific precursor cell population autologous for each patient will be very expensive. On the other hand,successful treatment for what would otherwise be a chronic condition could be a one-off cure and the cost of this would have to be contrasted with the costs of long-term treatment and care, which might be only palliative. The current model of pharmaceutical intervention—using, in the main, small foreign molecules (drugs) to perturb and modulate the patient's physiology—should be contrasted with a future model of long-term regenerative repair by endogenous self-perpetuating natural effectors (cells). The cost-effectiveness of this approach may well eventually favour the cell model.

Further reading

Askew GR, Doetschman T, *et al.* (1993). Site-directed point mutations in embryonic stem cells: a gene-targeting tag-and-exchange strategy. *Mol Cell Biol*, **13**, 4115–24.

Bradley A, Evans M, *et al.* (1984). Formation of germ-line chimaeras from embryo-derived teratocarcinoma cell lines. *Nature*, **309**, 255–6.

Brennan J, Skarnes WC (2008). Gene trapping in mouse embryonic stem cells. *Methods Mol Biol*, **461**, 133–48.

Capecchi MR (2008). The making of a scientist II (Nobel Lecture). *ChemBioChem*, **9**(10), 1530–43.

Clarke AR (2000). Manipulating the germline: its impact on the study of carcinogenesis. *Carcinogenesis*, **21**, 435–41.

Evans M (1981). Origin of mouse embryonal carcinoma cells and the possibility of their direct isolation into tissue culture. *J Reprod Fertil*, **62**, 625–31.

Evans, M (2008). Embryonic stem cells: the mouse source—vehicle for mammalian genetics and beyond (Nobel lecture). *ChemBioChem*, **9**(11), 1690–6.

Evans MJ (1981). Are teratocarcinomas formed from normal cells? In: Anderson CJ, Jones WG, Milford-Ward A (eds) *Germ cell tumours*. Taylor & Francis, London.

Evans MJ, Bradley A, *et al.* (1985). The ability of EK cells to form chimeras after selection of clones in G418 and some observations in the integration of retroviral vector proviral DNA into EK cells. *Cold Spring Harbor Symp Quant Biol*, **50**.

Evans MJ, Bradley A, *et al.* (1983). EK cell contribution to chimeric mice: from tissue culture to sperm. *Genetic manipulation of the early mammalian embryo*. Banbury Report, Cold Spring Harbor Laboratory, **20**.

Evans MJ, Carlton MB, *et al.* (1997). Gene trapping and functional genomics. *Trends Genet*, **13**, 370–4.

Evans MJ, Kaufman MH (1981). Establishment in culture of pluripotential cells from mouse embryos. *Nature*, **292**, 154–6.

Evans MJ, Martin GR (1975). The differentiation of clonal teratocarcinoma cell culture *in vitro*. In Solter D, Sherman M (eds) *Roche symposium on teratomas and differentiation*. Academic Press, New York.

Friedrich G, Soriano P (1991). Promoter traps in embryonic stem cells: a genetic screen to identify and mutate developmental genes in mice. *Genes Dev*, **5**, 1513–23.

Joyner AL, Auerbach A, *et al.* (1992). The gene trap approach in embryonic stem cells: the potential for genetic screens in mice. *Ciba Found Symp*, **165**, 277–88. discussion 288–97.

Kleinsmith LJ, Pierce GB Jr. (1964). Multipotentiality of single embryonal carcinoma cells. *Cancer Res*, **24**, 1544–51.

Kuehn MR, Bradley A, *et al.* (1987). A potential animal model for Lesch-Nyhan syndrome through introduction of HPRT mutations into mice. *Nature*, **326**, 295–8.

Martin GR, Evans MJ (1975). Differentiation of clonal lines of teratocarcinoma cells: formation of embryoid bodies *in vitro*. *Proc Natl Acad Sci U S A*, **72**, 1441–5.

Martin GR, Evans MJ (1975). Multiple differentiation of clonal teratoma stem cells following embryoid body formation *in vitro*. *Cell*, **6**, 467–74.

Pierce GB (1967). Teratocarcinoma: model for a developmental concept of cancer. *Curr Top Dev Biol*, **2**, 223–46.

Robertson EJ, Conlon FL, *et al.* (1992). Use of embryonic stem cells to study mutations affecting postimplantation development in the mouse. *Ciba Found Symp*, **165**, 237–50. discussion 250–5.

Skarnes WC, Auerbach BA, *et al.* (1992). A gene trap approach in mouse embryonic stem cells: the lacZ reported is activated by splicing, reflects endogenous gene expression, and is mutagenic in mice. *Genes Dev*, **6**, 903–18.

Smithies O (2008). Turning pages (Nobel lecture). *ChemBioChem*, **9**, 1342–59.

Stevens LC (1967). Origin of testicular teratomas from primordial germ cells in mice. *J Natl Cancer Inst*, **38**, 549–52.

Stevens LC (1967). The biology of teratomas. *Adv Morphog*, **6**, 1–31.

Stevens LC (1970). The development of transplantable teratocarcinomas from intratesticular grafts of pre- and postimplantation mouse embryos. *Dev Biol*, **21**, 364–82.

Stevens LC, Little CC (1954). Spontaneous testicular teratomas in an inbred strain of mice. *Proc Natl Acad Sci U S A*, **40**, 1080–7.

Suh H (2000). Tissue restoration, tissue engineering and regenerative medicine. *Yonsei Med J*, **41**, 681–4.

Takahashi K, Yamanaka S (2006). Induction of pluripotent stem cells from mouse embryonic and adult fibroblast cultures by defined factors. *Cell*, **126**, 663–76.

Thomson JA, Itskovitz-Eldor J, *et al.* (1998). Embryonic stem cell lines derived from human blastocysts. *Science*, **282**, 1145–7.

Ying, QL, Wray J, *et al.* (2008). The ground state of embryonic stem cell self-renewal. *Nature*, **453**, 519–23.

Zhou X, Sasaki H, *et al.* (1993). Nodal is a novel TGF-beta-like gene expressed in the mouse node during gastrulation. *Nature*, **361**, 543–7.

4.8

Stem cells and regenerative medicine

Alexis J. Joannides, Roger Pedersen, and Siddharthan Chandran

Essentials

There is a great and unmet need for treatments that will deliver restorative solutions to patients with diseases hitherto considered irreparable. The twin properties of self-renewal and specialization common to stem cells offer unprecedented opportunities for regenerative medicine through the generation of unlimited numbers of defined human cells on the scale necessary for experimental study, drug discovery, and disease modelling. The field is fast developing, with the first wave of putative treatments necessarily drawn from autologous and adult stem cells, but the outstanding question remains whether these will lead to meaningful regenerative therapies.

Requirements for regenerative therapy

(1) A prerequisite for any regenerative therapy is the generation of scalable and enriched numbers of defined cell types appropriate to the target condition. The application of developmentally based insights offers the most rational route to generate functional cell types, and this approach is starting to yield success. (2) Preclinical work-up requires demonstration of sustained stem-cell mediated functional recovery in appropriate models of injury and this remains in its infancy, although for some diseases considerable progress and proof of concept has been achieved. (3) General principles include the need for ensuring appropriate distribution, connectivity, survival, and function of stem cells in the context of injury, without the hazards of tumour generation or immune rejection.

How might the promise of stem cells be realized?

(1) Consideration of three major target conditions for regenerative medicine—Parkinson's disease, heart failure, and diabetes—emphasize distinct and common challenges that must be overcome in order to realize the stem cell promise. (2) The emergence of novel approaches to induce pluripotency from differentiated somatic cells, along with insights based on human embryonic stem cells and increased recognition of endogenous stem cells, offers a range of mechanisms through which stem cells may be therapeutic. (3) In addition to classic cell/tissue replacement approaches, the ability of stem cells that include patient-specific material to model disease and enable drug discovery is likely to lead to significant therapeutic advances through the promotion of endogenous repair.

How long will it take before stem cell treatments are available?

The time it will take to deliver clinically useful stem cell treatments will vary from disease to disease and reflects the need for cell-based therapeutics to be competitive against established treatments. The history of haematological stem cell medicine, from which much of the template of regenerative medicine is borrowed, suggests an incremental and combinatorial approach to treatment, emphasizing the need for sophisticated clinical trial design to ensure correct clinical evaluation of putative regenerative stem cell based therapies.

Introduction

Regenerative medicine is not a new discipline. Indeed, the 1990 Nobel Prize in Physiology and Medicine to Joseph Murray and Donnall Thomas was in recognition of pioneering kidney and bone marrow transplantations undertaken in the 1950s. The current surge of renewed interest has been catalysed by recent and rapid advances in human stem cell biology and technology, which offer the prospect of the development of novel reparative strategies for a host of diseases hitherto considered irreparable. These include diabetes mellitus, neurodegenerative diseases, and heart failure.

The human body is organized into discrete but interrelated organs and tissues that each contain differentiated or specialized functional cells. Stem cells are defined as cells that possess three functional characteristics: an immature phenotype, self-renewal capacity, and the ability to differentiate into one or more functional or specialized derivatives (Fig. 4.8.1). The first or earliest stem cell is the embryonic stem cell (ESC) that arises from the epiblast (Fig. 4.8.2). Embryonic stem cells are pluripotent cells capable of generating all cell types in the body and can be considered as transient stem cells. During development and through adulthood other stem cells emerge that display progressively more restricted phenotypical range and can be considered tissue or organ specific. Endogenous tissue-specific stem cells are multipotent, with a differentiation repertoire normally confined to those cells of the tissue of origin.

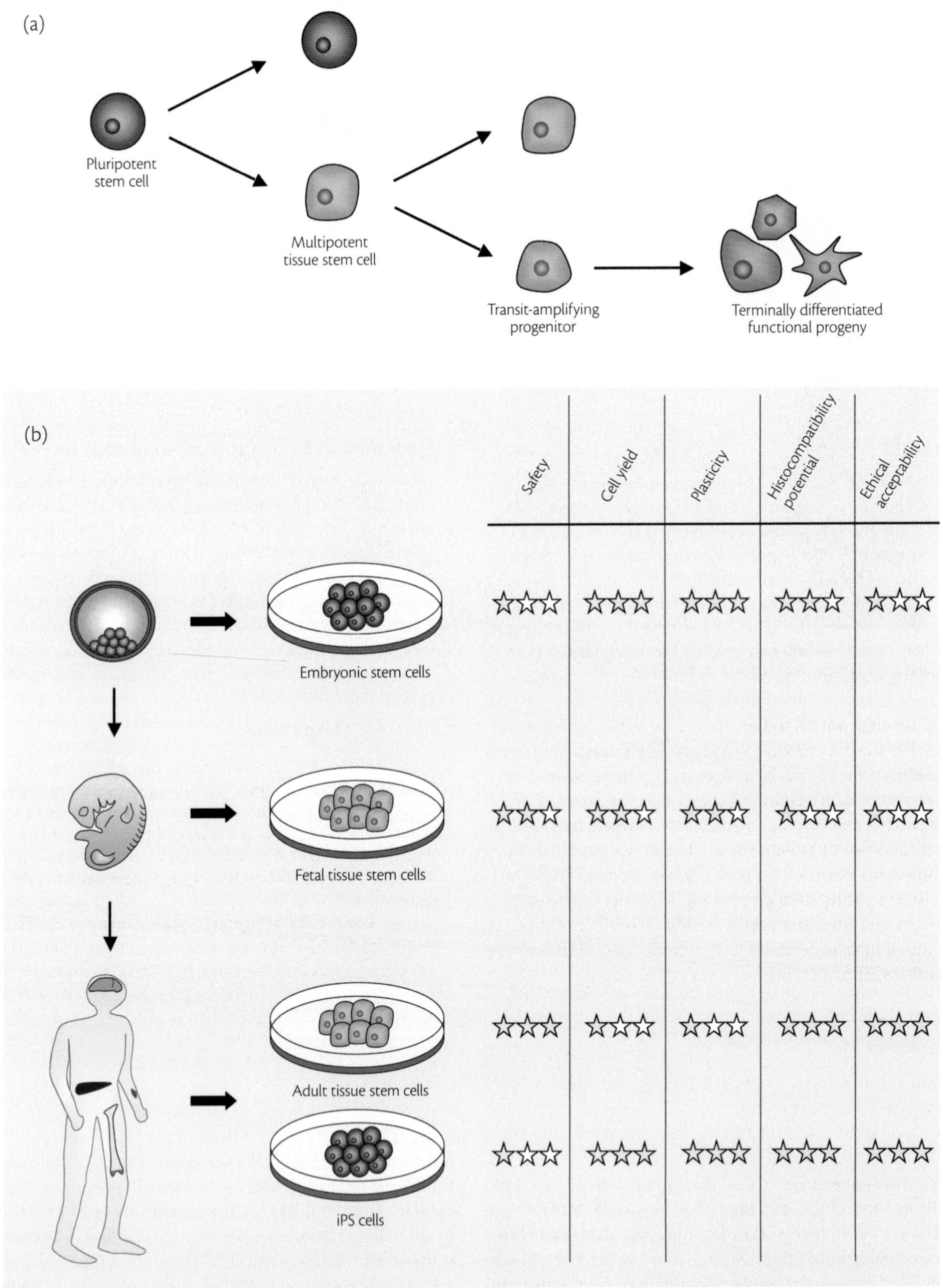

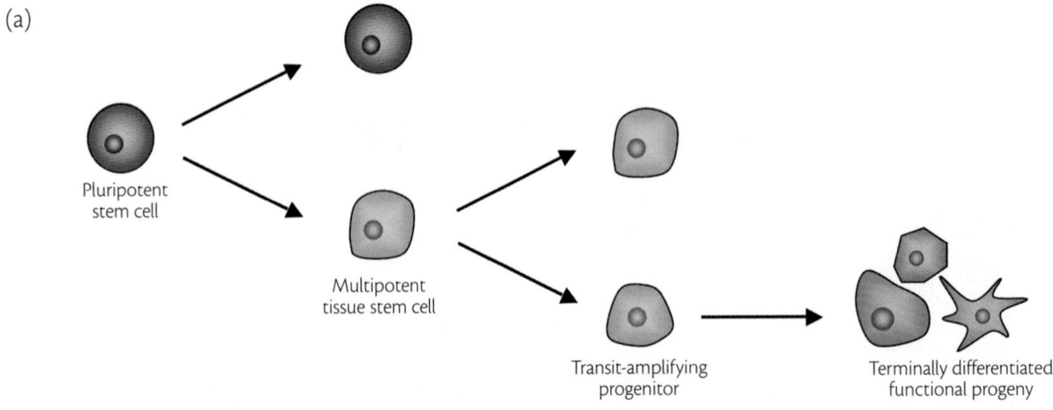

Fig. 4.8.1 Stem cells and their sources. (a) All stem cells, irrespective of developmental stage, share two fundamental properties: self-renewal and differentiation to progressively lineage-restricted cell types, ultimately generating terminally differentiated, functional progeny. (b) Human stem cells can be derived from embryonic, fetal, or adult tissue. Each has its relative merits and drawbacks, and choosing the most appropriate source largely depends on the requirements of each specific experimental or therapeutic context.

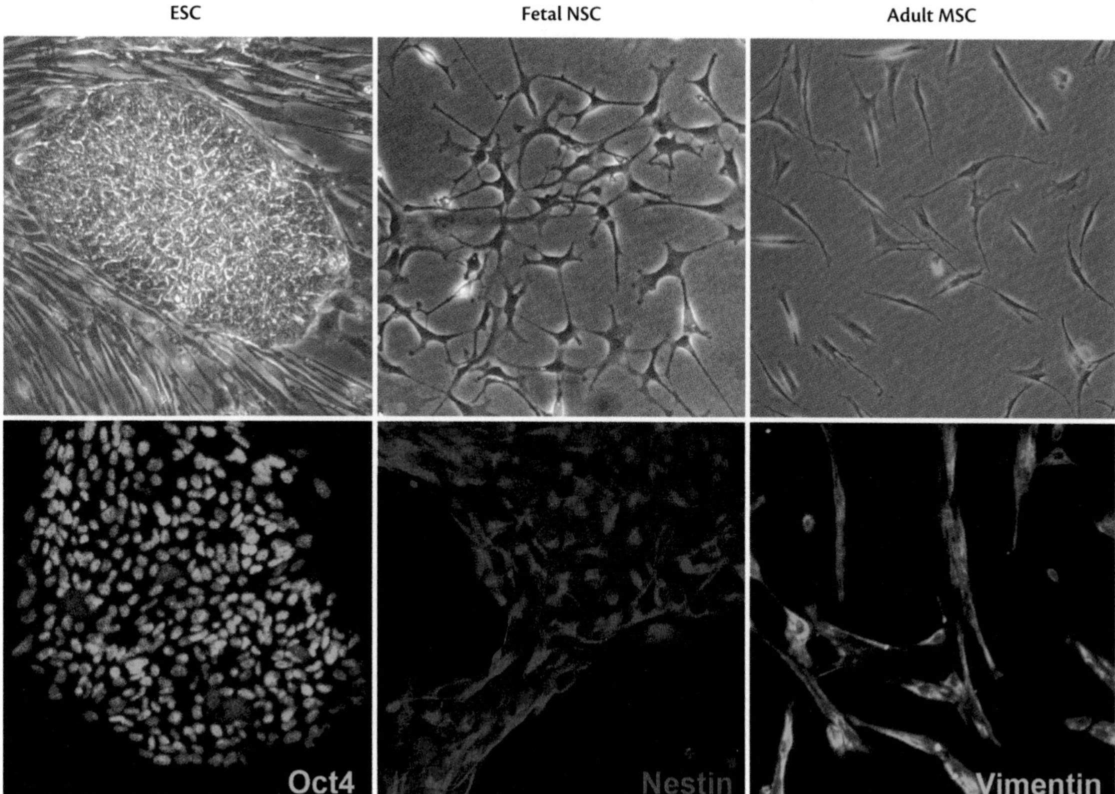

Fig. 4.8.2 Human stem cells *in vitro*. Representative light microscopy and immune micrograph pictures of embryonic stem cells (left panel), fetal-derived neural stem cells (centre), and adult skin-derived mesenchymal stem cells (right panel).

They persist through adulthood and are responsible for regenerating tissues with a rapid cell turnover, such as the gastrointestinal tract epithelium, skin epidermis, and haematopoietic system. Stem cells have also been identified in relatively quiescent tissues including the heart and central nervous system (CNS), where their precise functional role has yet to be determined. Recent technical advances enabling long-term *ex vivo* culture of human-derived embryonic and adult tissue-specific stem cells, along with increased recognition of endogenous adult stem cells and the possibility of directed reprogramming, have generated intense excitement in the experimental and therapeutic potential of stem cell biology.

What can human stem cells offer regenerative medicine?

Experimental and therapeutic opportunities are the short answer. Regenerative medicine can be summarized as treatments (cell and drug based) that seek to restore structure and function following injury (Fig. 4.8.3a). Stem cells can achieve this goal in a variety of ways, direct and indirect (Fig. 4.8.3b). Perhaps the simplest and most intuitive therapeutic contribution is through cell replacement of lost or damaged cells. Cultured autologous keratinocytes for skin loss is a well-established current example of cell-based therapy. Cell replacement therapy for Parkinson's disease and type 1 diabetes represents future therapeutic targets. Beyond stem cells as direct therapy, human stem cells offer complementary opportunities to study human development and model disease, as well as providing a unique resource for drug discovery and testing. Such insights are likely to lead to novel disease-modifying and regenerative therapies, and ultimately provide the largest clinical dividend.

Historical perspective

> Though it has long been known that the cells in certain tissues are constantly replaced, it is only recently that we have come to realise the number of these areas, the many ways by which a balance is achieved between cell production and loss, and particularly the speed of the renewal process ... such remarkable behaviour of many cell populations raises not only histological but biochemical questions which are yet unanswered.
>
> Leblond CP, Walker BE (1956). Renewal of cell populations. *Physiol Rev*, **36**, 255–76.

The concept of tissue stem cells emerged from the pioneering work of Charles Leblond, James Till, and Ernest McCullogh in the mid-20th century. Leblond developed the technique of autoradiography which led to the identification of continuous cellular self-renewal in a number of tissues and culminated in the description of what we now know as stem cell-mediated renewal in spermatogenesis. Till and McCullogh independently proposed a similar model for haematopoiesis. During the 1960s, they identified 'spleen colony-forming cells', which were able to reconstitute the haematopoietic system of a lethally irradiated animal host, and together with Louis Siminovitch went on to demonstrate their self-renewal capacity by serial transplantation.

Subsequent advances in stem cell biology have enabled identification, propagation and directed differentiation of stem cells from a variety of adult tissues, including bone marrow stroma, skin epidermis, and brain (Fig. 4.8.4). Parallel pioneering studies on embryonic carcinoma cells derived from teratocarcinomas led to the isolation of embryonic stem cells from mouse blastocysts in 1981. Recognition of the fundamental advance of this finding and

(a)

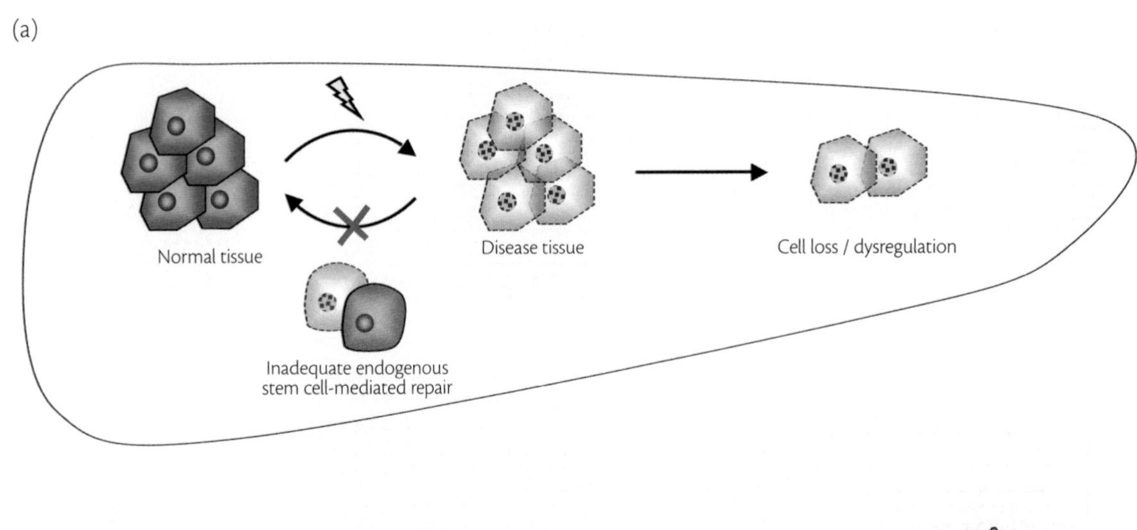

(b)

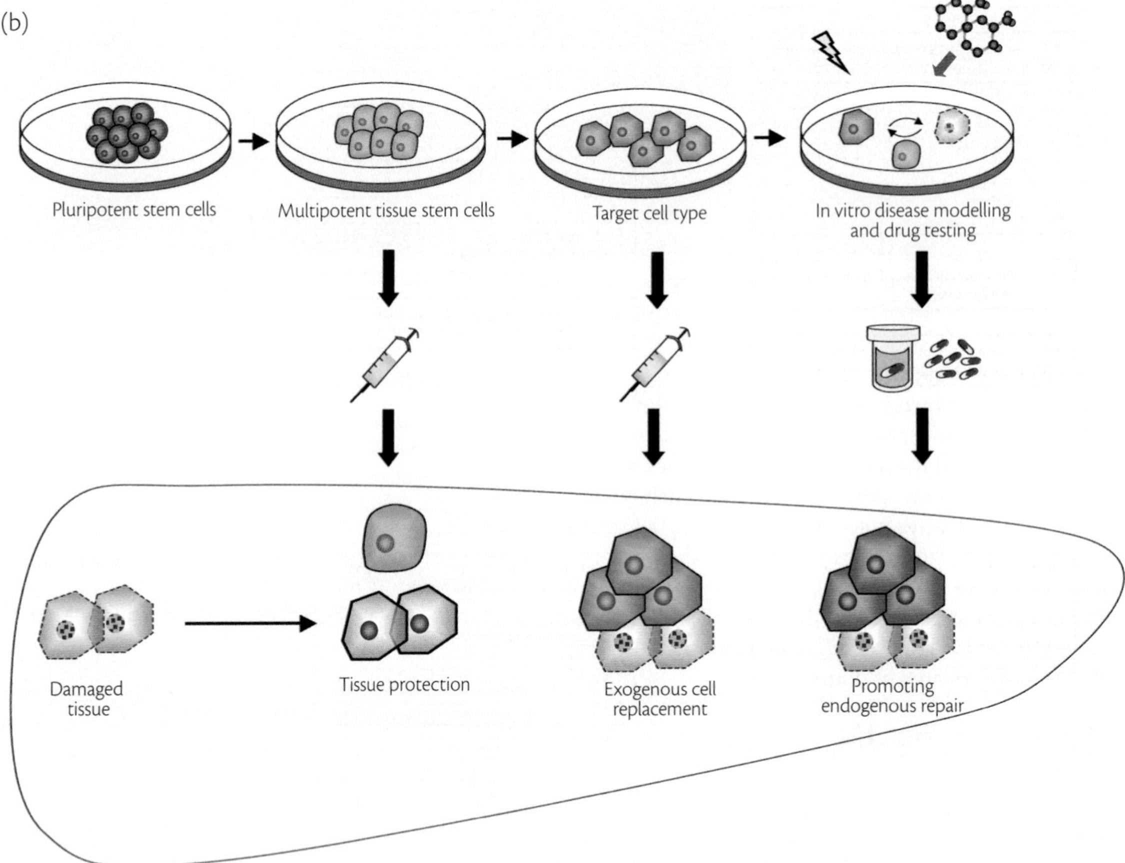

Fig. 4.8.3 Therapeutic principles of stem cell-based treatments. (a) Organ function is dependent on a dynamic equilibrium between the extent of pathological injury (from any cause) and the extent of self-repair from endogenous tissue stem cells (which is highly variable between organs). An imbalance leads to progressive tissue damage and/or loss, ultimately resulting in organ impairment and functional decompensation. (b) Stem cell-based interventions can be directed towards multiple points in disease progression. Stem cells and progenitors may have a disease-modifying effect independent of differentiation potential through trophic support or immunomodulatory properties, while differentiated progeny can be used to replace lost cells. In addition, *in vitro* stem cell-based studies can lead to the development of drug compounds for mobilizing endogenous stem cells and shifting the organ equilibrium towards self-repair.

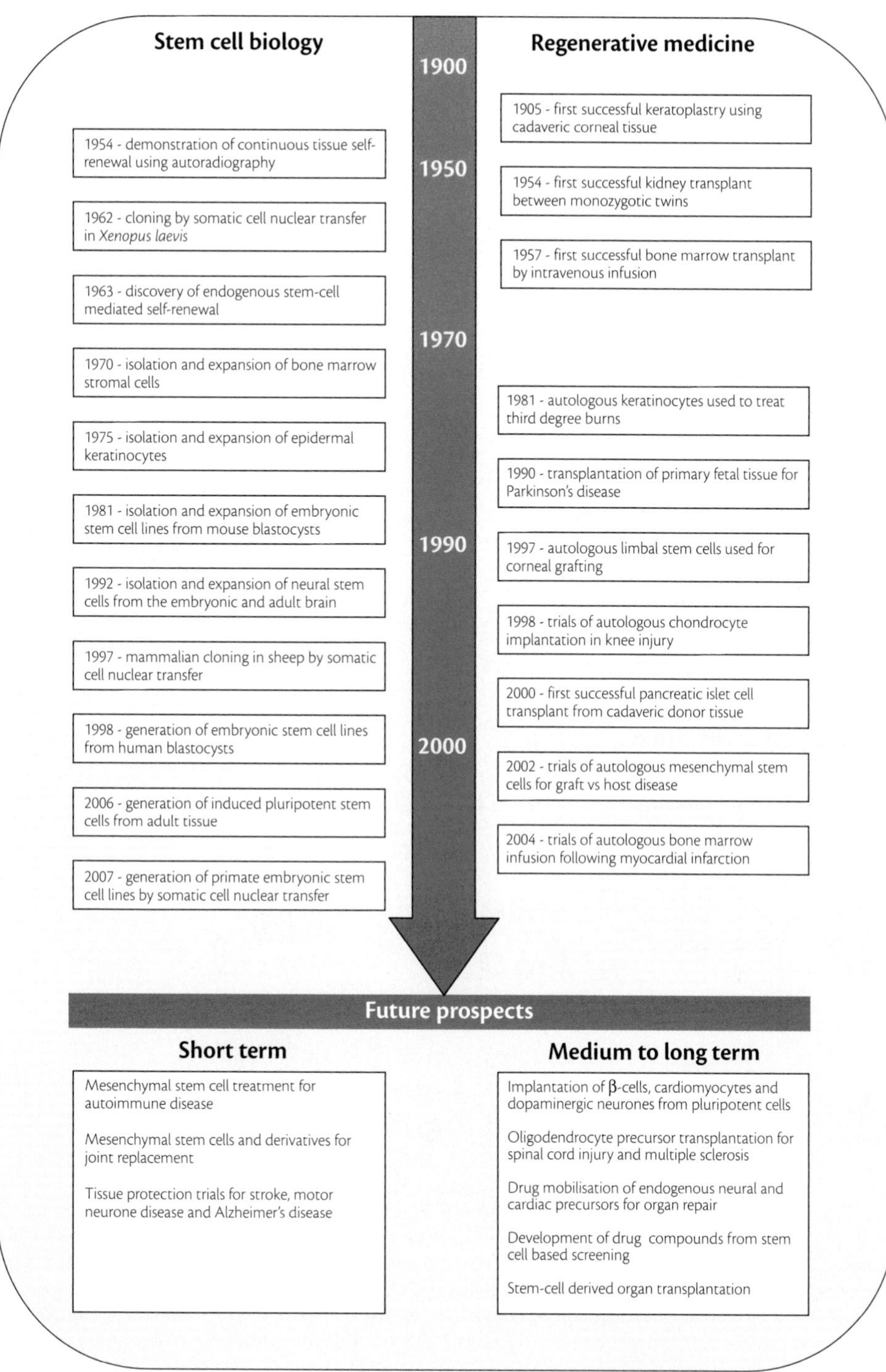

Stem cell biology
Regenerative medicine
1900
1950
1970
1990
2000
1954 - demonstration of continuous tissue self-renewal using autoradiography
1962 - cloning by somatic cell nuclear transfer in *Xenopus laevis*
1963 - discovery of endogenous stem-cell mediated self-renewal
1970 - isolation and expansion of bone marrow stromal cells
1975 - isolation and expansion of epidermal keratinocytes
1981 - isolation and expansion of embryonic stem cell lines from mouse blastocysts
1992 - isolation and expansion of neural stem cells from the embryonic and adult brain
1997 - mammalian cloning in sheep by somatic cell nuclear transfer
1998 - generation of embryonic stem cell lines from human blastocysts
2006 - generation of induced pluripotent stem cells from adult tissue
2007 - generation of primate embryonic stem cell lines by somatic cell nuclear transfer
1905 - first successful keratoplastry using cadaveric corneal tissue
1954 - first successful kidney transplant between monozygotic twins
1957 - first successful bone marrow transplant by intravenous infusion
1981 - autologous keratinocytes used to treat third degree burns
1990 - transplantation of primary fetal tissue for Parkinson's disease
1997 - autologous limbal stem cells used for corneal grafting
1998 - trials of autologous chondrocyte implantation in knee injury
2000 - first successful pancreatic islet cell transplant from cadaveric donor tissue
2002 - trials of autologous mesenchymal stem cells for graft vs host disease
2004 - trials of autologous bone marrow infusion following myocardial infarction
Future prospects
Short term
Mesenchymal stem cell treatment for autoimmune disease
Mesenchymal stem cells and derivatives for joint replacement
Tissue protection trials for stroke, motor neurone disease and Alzheimer's disease
Medium to long term
Implantation of β-cells, cardiomyocytes and dopaminergic neurones from pluripotent cells
Oligodendrocyte precursor transplantation for spinal cord injury and multiple sclerosis
Drug mobilisation of endogenous neural and cardiac precursors for organ repair
Development of drug compounds from stem cell based screening
Stem-cell derived organ transplantation

Fig. 4.8.4 Timeline of key advances and future prospects in stem cell biology and regenerative medicine.

the enabling of the gene modification era led to the Nobel Prize in Medicine 2007. Successful isolation of human ES cells, coupled with the discovery of a comparatively simple technique to induce pluripotency from adult differentiated cells, opened up the field of regenerative stem cell-applied biology to include the possibility of generating patient-specific cells or tissues.

Current therapeutic applications of stem cells

Not infrequently in medical discovery, application of scientific innovation precedes biological or mechanistic understanding. Stem cells are no exception. Within the translational arena, stem cell transplantation has been performed (even unknowingly) for over a century (Fig. 4.8.4). Eduard Zirm carried out the first successful keratoplasty in 1905, while E Donnall Thomas performed the first successful bone marrow transplantation by intravenous infusion in 1957. Haemopoietic stem cell transplantation for haematological disease is now routine procedure (see Chapter 22.8.2). Rheinwald and Green's success in using autologous, *ex vivo*, expanded human keratinocytes for treating patients with third-degree burns in 1981 established an important proof of concept for

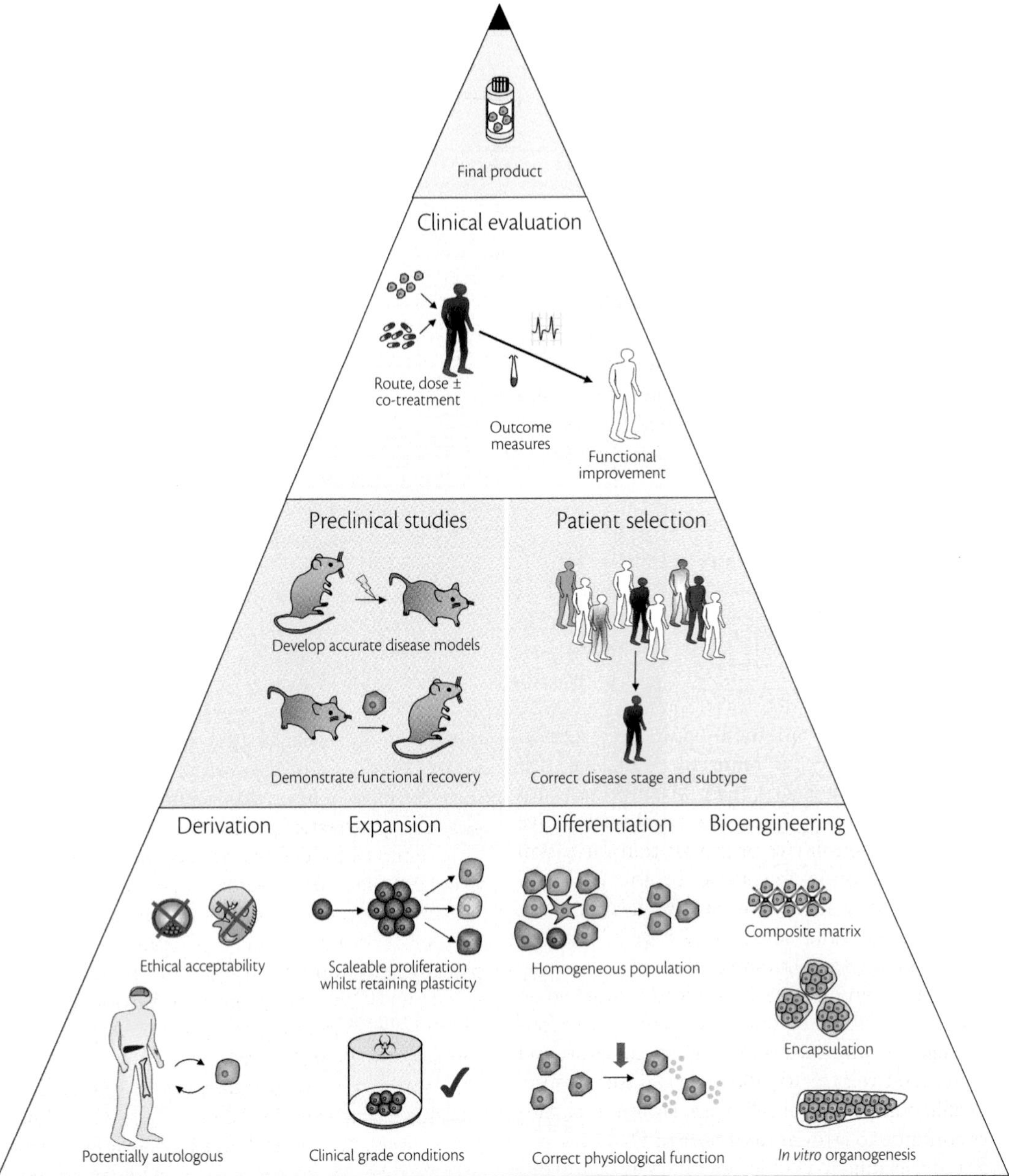

Fig. 4.8.5 Criteria for clinical implementation of cell-based therapy. The multiple challenges and requirements for cell-based strategies can be classified into three fundamental steps (see text for a detailed discussion). Initially, the right cell type needs to be generated in sufficient numbers, in high purity and in the right form for therapy (step 1). Subsequently, putative therapies need to be tested in accurate animal models of disease for both safety and efficacy, and criteria for patient phenotypes most likely to benefit from therapy should be established (step 2). Finally, clinical cell therapy needs to be evaluated in the context of other existing complementary therapies, and functional improvement should be monitored for a sufficient period to demonstrate benefits in disease morbidity and mortality (step 3).

stem cell-based therapy. The potential of regenerative therapy is apparent from the process of autologous epidermal grafting. Keratinocytes, although relatively quiescent *in vivo*, can be expanded exponentially in culture with a doubling time of 16 to 18 hours, achieving a 10 000-fold expansion over a 2- to 3-week period. Sufficient cell numbers can thus be obtained from very small full-thickness skin biopsies, thus making it possible to treat patients with large area skin loss, where split-thickness skin grafts are not feasible.

Together with autologous chondrocyte implantation for articular cartilage defects, this is a fast-growing area that is now mainstream. Use of limbal epithelial stem cells for corneal disease is a further example of an emerging clinical application of autologous adult stem cells. Finally, combination of autologous material with the disciplines of material science and biotissue engineering raises the imminent prospect of *ex vivo* tissue organogenesis. Use of tissue-engineered bladder augmentation for neurogenic bladders is an exciting advance and likely to herald wider application (see later).

Current barriers to clinical application

Clinical application of stem cells has now become routine practice in haematology, plastic surgery, orthopaedics, and ophthalmology. However, beyond these areas, the promise of using stem cells for therapy remains anticipated and unrealized, and raises multiple issues. Although comprehensive and detailed analysis of individual disease requirements is beyond the scope of this chapter, some general themes for clinical application of stem cell-based regenerative medicine emerge (Fig. 4.8.5). These include:

1 Identifying the correct stem cell source

2 Generating appropriate numbers of specialized cells and validating sustained *in vivo* function in injury models

3 Establishing the infrastructure to enable clinical evaluation of putative regenerative therapies

These separate areas are considered by way of illustration and in reference to three principal target medical conditions that could benefit from regenerative medicine: neurodegenerative diseases such as Parkinson's disease; cardiac failure; and type 1 diabetes mellitus.

Identifying the correct human stem cell source

Accepting the need for human material, this is in many ways an issue of determining the appropriate developmental stage of stem cells. Adult tissue-specific stem cells possess some advantage being potentially autologous, often readily accessible as well as being ethically less controversial (see Fig. 4.8.1b). However, their limited proliferative capacity and restricted differentiation potential place significant practical constraints on their widespread utility. Although a number of studies have reported adult stem cell 'transdifferentiation' to other lineages, these findings have not always been reproducible and remain controversial. Alternative explanations, such as cell fusion *in vivo* or genetic transformation *in vitro*, are likely to account for some of the findings. Notwithstanding their intuitive attraction, some populations (e.g. neural stem cells) are inaccessible and would require invasive methods, with attendant risks, for harvesting.

In contrast, embryonic stem cells are scientifically attractive on account of their unique ability to respond predictably to developmental cues, which together with their nontransformed nature and almost unlimited proliferative capacity, allow the realistic prospect of generating scaleable numbers of all cell types. However, significant ethical issues continue to swirl around human ES derivation, propagation, and study, leading to prohibition in many countries.

A stem cell source should thus ideally combine the practical and ethical acceptability of adult stem cells with the biological potential of embryonic stem cells. Successful somatic cell nuclear transfer (SCNT) in mammalian reproductive cloning demonstrated the conceptual feasibility of nuclear reprogramming to generate embryonic cells from an adult mammalian somatic cell source. Primate and human SCNT has since been demonstrated and independently confirmed. However, a significant practical hurdle of SCNT is the need for large numbers of oocytes. An alternative approach proposes fusion of existing embryonic stem cell lines and dermal fibroblasts. However, the most exciting development in this field has been the demonstration that somatic cell reprogramming can be induced by overexpression of a limited number of transcription factors in both adult mouse and human systems. The resulting induced pluripotent stem cells (iPS) show many of the characteristics of ES cells including pluripotency and germline transmission (in the mouse). This approach to 'reprogramming' is likely to mark an era of patient-specific stem cells.

Irrespective of source, stem cell culture and expansion need to fulfil a number of mandatory criteria for therapeutic application. Although clinical keratinocyte protocols presently use bovine serum and feeder cells, future stem cell therapies will need to conform to good manufacturing practice (GMP) conditions, which are most likely to stipulate exclusive use of chemically defined and human-derived components. Currently, most culture (and differentiation) protocols require animal products or unknown factors present in conditioned media or proprietary supplements. Regardless of the precise details, stem cell-based therapies will ultimately need to conform to internationally agreed guidelines laid down by regulatory bodies such as the United States Food and Drug Administration (FDA) and the European Medicines Evaluation Agency (EMEA).

Generating appropriate numbers of functional cell type(s)

GMP requirements for stem cell derivation and expansion also apply to differentiation protocols. There are two overriding requirements: generation of the correct functional cell type without any contaminant undifferentiated stem cell(s).

Although it is axiomatic that cells of appropriate regional identity and function are required for experimental or therapeutic application, directed differentiation has lagged behind advances in stem cell isolation and culture. Embryonic stem cells possess a clear advantage over (non-reprogrammed) adult stem cells, responding predictably to developmental signals and retaining imposed positional identity following transplantation. It is worth noting that most cell types in future regenerative therapies, including neuronal subtypes, pancreatic islet β cells, and cardiomyocytes, physiologically emerge at a defined developmental stage and are not normally generated from resident adult stem cell populations. Thus, it is unclear whether any other stem cell populations have the *in vitro* or *in vivo* potential to generate these functional cell types. Nevertheless applying insights borrowed from developmental principles of patterning and specification are likely to be critical of the generation of region-specific cell types regardless of age or source of origin of stem cell.

Minimizing the risk of tumorigenic 'rogue' cells is a major obstacle. Potential approaches include a combination of positive and negative *ex vivo* selection techniques, pre-differentiation, or insertion of inducible 'suicide' genes. Such methods will require customized developments particular to individual stem cells. Although standard practice in a laboratory setting, clinical application will require further refinement.

Donor cell developmental stage

The final stem cell-derived product can be either a progenitor population or *ex vivo* pre-differentiated cells. Pre-differentiation has the additional challenge of further controlled differentiation steps with complex protocols, and using specialized selection techniques to isolate a possibly rarer differentiated subtype (e.g. separating differentiating mature β cells from islet progenitors from other endocrine cell types). The increasingly evident role of the local cellular niche in cell fate subspecification also adds to the complexity of *ex vivo* differentiation. However, pre-differentiation may prove necessary particularly where the potential pathological host environment may otherwise impose inappropriate differentiation cues upon implanted progenitors. For example, the inflammatory environment in spinal cord demyelination models has been shown to promote astrocyte specification from neural precursors, while prior *ex vivo* oligodendrocyte lineage specification enables effective exogenous remyelination. Pre-differentiation is also a method to reduce the risk of uncontrolled *in vivo* proliferation.

Nervous tissue

The ability to program or direct neuroectodermal differentiation from human ESCs (hESCs) has progressed perhaps more rapidly compared with other lineages. This reflects in part the 'default' nature of neural induction from ES cells when grown in simplified conditions with limited extrinsic signalling. Several neural differentiation protocols exist, with the potential for scaleable derivation of neural stem cells under clinical grade conditions. Methods of derivation and/or enrichment include utilizing stage-specific cell surface markers (including CD133, Notch, and β_1-integrin) for neural progenitor selection. However, further differentiation from the neural stem cell platform to functional region-specific subtypes remains problematic. This is a major challenge for regenerative neurology given that regional identity subserves distinct physiological function(s), and thus absolute precision of spatial identity is a prerequisite for functional restitution. Midbrain dopaminergic and spinal cord motor neuron differentiation using developmental cues have been reproducibly reported, but derivation of other neuronal subtypes has been less successful. A combination of developmentally based approaches along with use of positive selection exploiting region-specific surface markers is likely to overcome this hurdle.

Cardiac tissue

The ability to reproducibly generate functional cardiomyocytes remains unresolved. Initial reports suggesting that bone marrow stromal cells and skeletal muscle satellite cells could 'transdifferentiate' into cardiomyocytes proved to be flawed. Embryonic stem cells or iPS cells are thus the most promising source for deriving cardiac tissue. This has been challenging due to the multiple stage-specific differentiation steps between hESCs and specified cardiac progenitors. Existing protocols depending on spontaneous differentiation or co-culture with visceral endoderm cells or conditioned medium have relatively low efficiency, highlighting the need for a more rational, developmentally rooted approach to differentiation. $Flk1^+CXCR4^+$ cells from differentiated mouse ESCs have been shown to retain cardiogenic capacity at the single cell level, raising the prospect of efficient selection of hESC-derived cardiac progenitors. Recently, $Flk1^+c\text{-}Kit^-$ cardiovascular progenitors have been generated from human ESCs using defined factors.

Pancreatic tissue

Cadaveric islet cell transplantation offers proof of concept of cell-based therapy for type 1 diabetes. The fundamental requirements are islet β-cell generation displaying physiological glucose-stimulated insulin secretion (GSIS). Earlier studies on hESCs demonstrated very low rates of differentiation to islet β cells, and several purported examples have since emerged as probable culture artefacts. A promising advance in this area has recently reported functional β-cell derivation from hES cells using a developmental approach via sequential differentiation to definitive endoderm, posterior foregut, pancreatic endoderm, islet precursors, and finally β cells over an 18-day period. However, although resulting β cells possessed a bona fide insulin biosynthetic pathway they coexpressed other islet hormones, and their insulin secretion was not responsive to glucose. These findings are consistent with an immature β-cell phenotype. Recently, implantation of hESC-derived pancreatic progenitors resulting in β-cell differentiation and correction of hyperglycaemia has been reported.

Validating stem cell-mediated functional recovery

Even when challenges in obtaining scaleable numbers of appropriate specialized cell type have been overcome, significant barriers to clinical application remain. Foremost is the need to demonstrate, in appropriate experimental systems, restoration of lost function. Notwithstanding the reasonable view that for certain diseases (untreatable and fatal, e.g. motor neuron disease) a lower burden of mechanistic proof is required before experimental clinical trials, it remains a fundamental tenet of drug or cell medicine development that prior demonstration of behavioural recovery is necessary. Although welcome evidence from animal studies of *in vivo* stem cell-mediated function is emerging, robust and sustained restoration of lost function remains elusive. This problem reflects in part the limitations of experimental systems in accurately modelling human disease.

The challenge of restoring lost function varies according to disease and organ involved, and is most severe in regenerative neurology where reconnection of circuitry is required over and above restoration of macroscopic structure. Due to the syncytial and pacing nature of myocardium, a prerequisite for regenerative cardiology is a method that ensures electrophysiological synchronization on cell implantation. In contrast, stem cell-based therapeutics for type 1 diabetes is comparatively straightforward; restoration of endocrine function does not require homotopic transplantation, and cadaver-derived transplantation of islet β cells into the hepatic portal vein has established proof of concept for a cell replacement strategy.

Survival, engraftment, and connectivity

Sustained functional integration represents the holy grail of regenerative medicine. It is largely unmet. Clinical context matters, but some general principles can be rehearsed. Donor cell survival, acute and chronic, requires a primed host environment as well as immunological mismatching to be overcome. Achieving long-term integration requires a permissive host environment. Combined approaches with, for example, immunomodulatory treatment are one way not just to manage ongoing disease activity but also to limit donor cell vulnerability to immune attack. For example, a common problem for treatment of autoimmune-mediated disease is to protect the implanted cell population, including autologous material, from the host immunological response.

Ensuring appropriate connectivity is likely to require supplementary approaches, e.g. brain and spinal cord injury is associated with an inhibitory glial scar that behaves as a physical and biochemical barrier to axonal growth. Co-treatment with enzymes targeting the inhibitory extracellular proteoglycan matrix is one approach, under clinical trial, to permit appropriate axonal regrowth. In cardiac repair, a functionally integrated cardiac syncytium with appropriate excitation–contraction coupling is a minimal requirement without the risk of potentially fatal arrhythmias. In contrast, studies reporting restoration of left ventricular function after human bone marrow cell infusion have failed to show histological integration or sustained improvement, with short-term benefits most likely due to trophic support.

Overcoming immune rejection

Stem cells allow the development of novel approaches, beyond classic immune suppression, to manage immune mismatch. Personalized cells, masking strategies, and derivation from predetermined tissue-matched banks of cell lines are all rational methods under study. Although a conceptually attractive method, generation of autologous stem cell lines for each patient would be impractical and cost prohibitive to implement for common conditions. However, a study focusing on the United Kingdom population has estimated that as few as 10 hESC lines homozygous for common HLA haplotypes (which could be derived by iPS, SCNT, or parthenogenetic ES cells) could achieve complete HLA matching for 38%, and a beneficial match for 67% of cases. Microencapsulation in a permeable substance such as alginate or poly-L-ornithine represents another option for creating an immunological protective barrier, with promising results in human islet transplantation trials. This approach is confined to grafts that do not require cell–cell contact for function.

Whether long-term immunotherapy is necessary is unknown in the context of some stem cell-based interventions, e.g. in the context of the relative immune privilege of the brain. Indirect evidence supporting such an idea comes from the demonstration of successful and early withdrawal of anti-rejection drugs after dopaminergic fetal neuroblast transplantation for Parkinson's disease.

Route and location of delivery

Distribution of cell therapy poses very different challenges compared with small molecules and macromolecules—again context matters. In some cases, such as β-cell replacement, donor cell function is largely independent of location. Conceptually there is no compelling reason for GSIS cells to be located within the pancreas. In contrast, precise focal targeting is required, in the meantime, for neurological disorders and cardiac failure. The problem is compounded in diseases characterized by nonfocal pathology. Stereotactic implantation is comparatively straightforward for site-specific disorders such as Parkinson's disease or spinal cord injury, but unfeasible for diffuse and multifocal disorders, such as Alzheimer's disease and multiple sclerosis, respectively.

However, recent studies that highlight the ability of some stem cells to 'home' in to sites of injury in response to cytokine/chemokine gradients offer a means to circumvent this long-standing conceptual obstacle to cell-based therapies for a range of disorders. Analysis by *in situ* hybridization of Y chromosomes of female heart transplants into male recipients provides some evidence for extracardiac origin of cardiac cells, although these were predominantly endothelial cells. In addition several experimental studies have shown homing of peripherally delivered cells to the injured heart and brain. However, the significance of limited homing is unclear. Estimates from experimental and clinical studies suggest that less than 5% cardiac retention 2 h after infusion of bone marrow-derived cells. This may, in part, also explain why clinical trials thus far in cellular cardiomyoplasty do not show long-term benefit.

Reproducibility and scale

Regardless of the precise method deployed to generate a functional cell type from stem cells, widespread clinical application requires scale and targeted delivery. In many ways this is essentially indistinguishable from standard pharmaceutical practice, which will require upscaling and automation. Ultimately, protocol effectiveness will need to be user independent with adoption of mass production techniques sufficient to generate scaleable production of cells. Aside from logistical and manufacturing issues, the variability of cell lines needs to be addressed. No two lines are the same with regard to epigenetic, molecular, or immunological factors, or indeed ease of differentiation to a given germ layer and its cellular derivatives. The potential for personalized cell lines both complicates and resolves these issues.

In summary, successful regeneration is an incremental process that begins with *in vitro* generation of uniform and scaleable numbers of correct cell type, followed by *in vitro* and ultimately *in vivo* demonstration of appropriate distribution, connectivity, survival, and function.

Translational considerations: testing novel regenerative therapeutics

An overlooked area in regenerative medicine is the critical importance of patient selection and optimal trial design to ensure correct evaluation of novel reparative therapies. This is more than identifying patients with the right disease, an obvious point but not as simple as it may appear. It is also essential that patients at the correct stage of disease appropriate for the proposed intervention be studied. To do otherwise is likely to introduce noise, account for type 2 errors, and contribute to inconsistent results from early phase clinical trials.

Furthermore, recognizing the limitations of preclinical animal studies, it is often necessary to enter the clinic in advance of understanding the mechanism of efficacy. Indeed creative trial design and outcome measures should be sought to allow early trials not only test efficacy but also to inform on putative mechanism of action. This is illustrated by the experience to date of cell replacement in Parkinson's disease, cellular cardiomyoplasty, and the use of adult mesenchymal stem cells in graft-versus-host disease (see below).

Neurological repair

Although more than 250 cell transplantations involving Parkinson's disease patients have been undertaken, it is only recently that the importance of patient selection has emerged. Historically, and not unexpectedly for a novel treatment, cell transplantation was undertaken in patients with comparatively advanced disease who had become refractory to conventional treatments. Unexpected results from a randomized study have since led to the revaluation of the role of cell implantation and an emerging consensus is that comparatively early onset Parkinson's disease is the ideal recipient of cell implantation therapy to minimize adverse events such as graft-induced dyskinesias. Disability scores, need for adjunctive pharmacological therapies and functional imaging together provide reasonable metrics of efficacy. The importance of identifying the right cohort for the proposed intervention can be further illustrated in neurological medicine with regard to multiple sclerosis. Patients with early active relapsing–remitting disease require disease-modifying therapy (immunomodulatory) whereas those with advanced progressive disease characterized by significant neurodegeneration require neuroprotection and repair.

Cardiac repair

Regardless of cell type, clinical indication and timing of intervention matter, e.g. the needs of acute versus chronic ischaemia differ from that of end-stage heart failure. Furthermore, in contrast to diabetes or Parkinson's disease, where the mechanism of efficacy is known, this is currently less understood in cardiomyoplasty. It follows therefore that standardization of endpoints should necessarily focus on functional (ventricular ejection fraction) and patient disability scores.

Diabetes

The Edmonton experience has been instrumental in providing proof of concept of islet transplantation and has also revealed that insulin independence, the ultimate goal, is short-lived. An understanding of the mechanisms of normal islet β-cell self-renewal and of the fate of transplanted islets is needed to take forward further transplantation studies. However, trials to date demonstrate that those with 'brittle' diabetes and recurrent hypoglycaemia appear to benefit the most regardless of insulin independence, illustrating the value of cohort subselection.

Future prospects

Solid organ transplantation

Using stem cells to generate solid organs is an important goal in regenerative medicine. *Ex vivo* organogenesis represents both an engineering and a biological challenge. The use of appropriate scaffolds for cells to grow and differentiate is one approach that has yielded some success. Tissue-engineered autologous bladders from urothelial and muscle cells seeded on a collagen–polyglycolic acid matrix have been successfully used in patients requiring cystoplasty. Use of a natural organ scaffold has been suggested as a potential solution for complex organs. Building on previous studies using decellularized heart valve grafts, a recent report has demonstrated successful recolonization of a completely decellularized heart (with an extracellular matrix and vascular structure) with cardiac and endothelial cells, with some demonstration of pump function.

A second challenge is achieving the right architecture when the organ is composed of multiple cell types, e.g. despite the success and life-saving nature of autologous keratinocyte grafts, reconstruction of sweat glands, hair follicles, and melanocytes has not been achieved. This challenge is particularly relevant to bioengineering an artificial kidney, arguably the organ with the highest demand. The kidney's characteristic anatomical and topographical nephron arrangement develops from a specific reciprocal induction process between the ureteric bud and the metanephrogenic mesenchyme—replicating this *in vitro* is still a long way from being achieved.

Stem cell repair independent of differentiation potential

Stem cells can be therapeutic by two mechanisms: (1) supplementing (exogenous) and (2) enhancing endogenous repair. Although exogenous repair through cell/tissue replacement is conceptually seductive, the promotion of endogenous repair and tissue protection is an area of active research that may ultimately deliver the larger clinical dividend. Using stem cells therapeutically for properties independent of their ability to be differentiated into a specific cell type is complementary to the classic view of stem cells as a means of replacing lost cells. This notion proposes that stem cells that display unexpected properties, including immunoregulation, pathotropism, and the ability to function as cellular 'mini-pumps', can be harnessed to promote tissue protection and endogenous repair.

Stem cells as cellular immunomodulators have already entered the clinic and are undergoing clinical trials in various disease contexts. In 2004, le Blanc and colleagues reported striking remission of severe treatment-refractory graft-versus-host disease following intravenous infusion of allogeneic mesenchymal stem cells. Interestingly, this innovative approach was undertaken in advance of definitive experimental proof of concept. Similar findings have since been reported in preclinical studies on animal models of autoimmune disease including multiple sclerosis, Crohn's disease, and rheumatoid arthritis. These studies highlight the potential value of stitching together two increasingly recognized properties of stem cells—ability to traffic to sites of injury and to recalibrate a dysregulated hostile immune system—in the context of inflammatory or immune-mediated disease.

Alternatively, stem cells can be used as cellular vehicles for the delivery of protective or reparative factors, which may be produced by default or by genetic overexpression. Growth factors have been shown to have a beneficial effect in a number of neurological diseases including Parkinson's disease and motor neuron disease. In this regard accumulating evidence suggests that some of the more promising results from stem cell trials in cardiac repair cannot be accounted for by graft-derived cell/tissue replacement but rather by graft-derived trophic-mediated support.

More recently, stem cells have also been used as a means of enzyme replacement in metabolic diseases. Implanted neural stem cells have been shown to prolong survival in an animal model of Sandhoff's disease through a variety of mechanisms, and display synergy with oral medication. This study further highlights the multifaceted action(s) of stem cells with cell replacement, anti-inflammatory, and enzyme replacement properties all implicated as contributory to efficacy.

Endogenous repair, disease modelling, and drug discovery

Endogenous repair

The promotion of endogenous repair is an intuitive and attractive long-term regenerative strategy. Recognition of adult stem cells in organs hitherto considered incapable of self-renewal—brain and heart—has only fuelled such a proposition. The evidence for endogenous niche-resident adult neural stem cells is irrefutable, notwithstanding the disputed 'multipotentiality' of widely distributed oligodendrocyte precursor cells. Increasingly persuasive studies also appear to confirm the presence of endogenous cardiac progenitor/stem cells. Indeed a recent mammalian report provides strong evidence for endogenous cardiac repair that occurs after injury but not age-related loss. Other findings that suggest endogenous replacement of islet β cells raise the prospect of parallel and complementary strategies to cell implantation in patients with diabetes with some intact β-cell tissue.

An outstanding question is whether limited numbers of stem cells in restricted niches are relevant to organ repair given that damage is often extensive and geographically distant. Furthermore, the physiological role of such cells as well as their response to injury is unknown. Nevertheless, these cells and their progeny provide a rational cellular target for pharmacological compounds to activate, mobilize, and thus promote cell-mediated repair (Fig. 4.8.6). A complementary cell-based approach could seek to isolate endogenous—typically slow cycling—stem cells and reimplant them to the injured organ after *ex vivo* expansion. Such a strategy is well established for haematological stem cell therapy in the context of malignancy.

Disease modelling and drug discovery

By virtue of their proliferation and differentiation, potential stem cells offer a unique experimental resource for drug discovery and

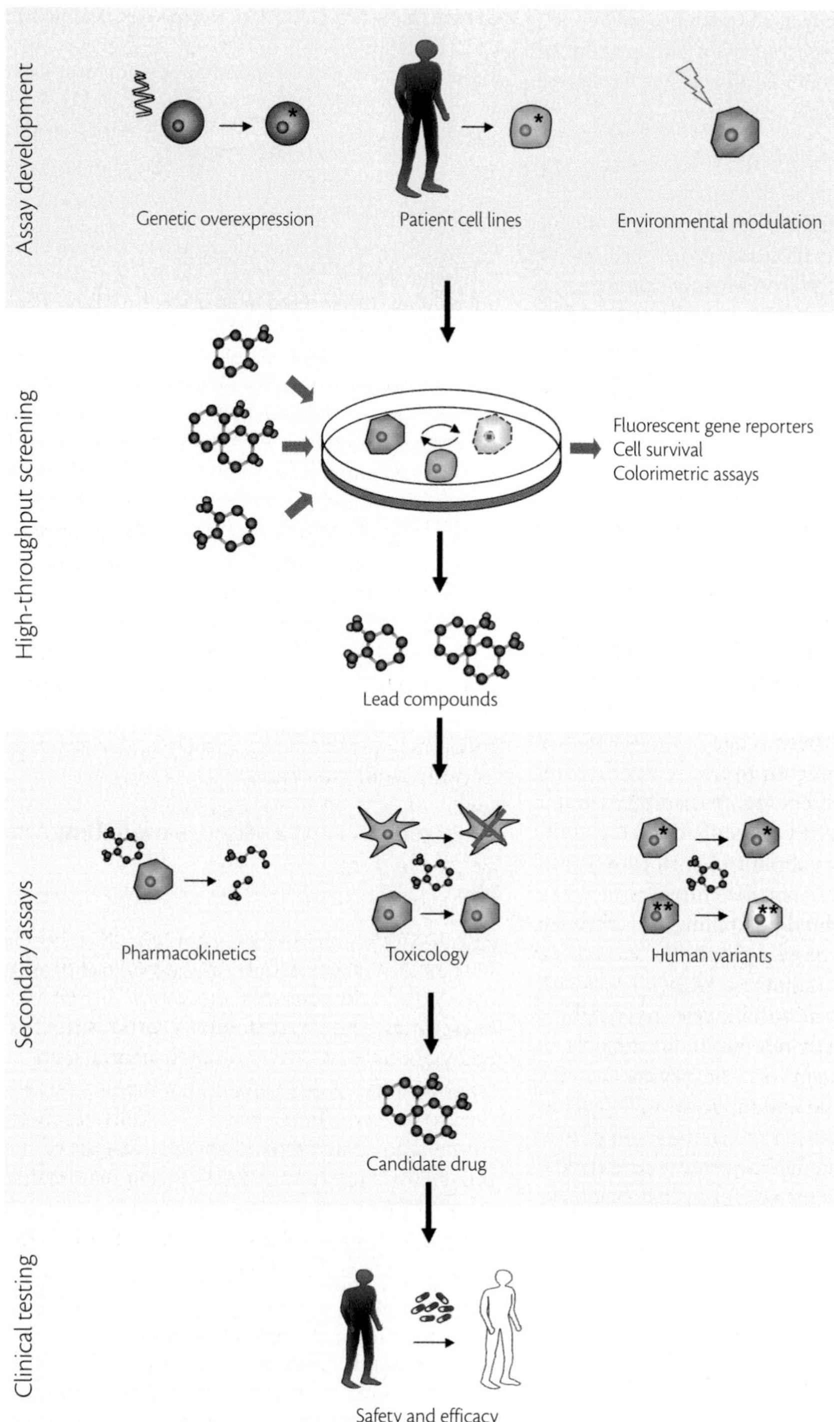

Fig. 4.8.6 Stem cells and drug discovery. A source of potentially unlimited numbers of nontransformed human cell types presents multiple opportunities in drug discovery and development. High-throughput stem cell-based screening can result in the identification of novel disease-modifying compounds. Their safety and differential efficacy can subsequently be determined in secondary assays utilizing stem cell-derived material, ultimately leading to the development of candidate drugs that can be evaluated through the conventional clinical trial route.

in vitro disease modelling. These opportunities converge on improved understanding of disease pathogenesis, endogenous repair, and failure to repair normally, and thus together they provide clues to novel regenerative approaches (Fig. 4.8.6). Human stem cells and their derivatives provide a unique opportunity for disease modelling and understanding genetic and/or environmental influences of many human disorders. This can be achieved by a number of complementary strategies: (1) generating iPS cells from patients with specific (or unknown) gene mutations or polymorphisms and differentiating these to lineages affected in the disease (e.g. cystic fibrosis); (2) modelling disease directly by genetic overexpression or gene inactivation or silencing; and (3) modulating environmental parameters to replicate disease conditions (e.g. hyperglycaemia in diabetes). Following on from an understanding of pathological mechanisms, *in vitro* disease models can be used for drug evaluation and testing. In this respect, stem cells offer distinct advantages over current human sources used in drug screening, which include primary tissue (capable of only limited proliferation) and tumour cell lines (which have a grossly aneuploid genome). Evaluation of drug targets can be approached through either a high-throughput screening approach (with subsequent deconvolution) or testing of candidate compounds with a disease-modifying rationale.

Simple and measurable outcomes, such as fluorescent gene reporters or cell survival over time, will be necessary for any drug-based assay in order to allow sufficient scalability. In addition to disease models, stem cell-derived lineages can be screened for potential drug toxicity.

Conclusion

Regenerative medicine, although in its infancy, will become of increasing importance in the face of the rising global challenge of diseases such as diabetes, neurodegeneration, and heart failure. Human stem cell biology is rapidly advancing. It is likely to lead to significant gains in understanding of disease mechanisms and thus open new therapeutic opportunities—cell and pharmacologically based—both to modify disease course and to promote repair of the injured organ.

Stem cells can be exploited directly and indirectly to promote repair. Specifically stem cell-based methods or insights seek to supplement and enhance, where appropriate, endogenous repair. Cell implantation strategies require the ability to generate large numbers of defined functional cell populations appropriate to clinical need, e.g. pancreatic islet cells for diabetes or midbrain dopaminergic neuroblasts for Parkinson's disease. In this regard human ESC- or iPS-derived populations offer significant advantages on account of their developmental competence. However, beyond generation of specific cell populations for replacement strategies, it is perhaps an oversimplification to view repair as simply recapitulation of development given the distinct cellular architecture of adulthood complicated by injury-related structural and biochemical changes. In addition to classic cell or tissue replacement, the evolving concept of 'therapeutic stem cell plasticity' offers additional methods through which stem cells may be useful for regenerative medicine. Outside of drug discovery, these include utilizing stem cells to limit damage and promote tissue repair by acting as cellular vehicles to deliver trophic/angiogenic factors or as cellular immunomodulators.

Time to clinic is less easily predicted. This will vary and, as with any innovative treatment, there will be a trade-off between justifiable risk and benefit. The ability of human stem cells to both inform on and potentially treat devastating and frequently untreatable disorders provides cautious grounds for optimism that stem cells will accelerate the emergence of novel therapeutics for regenerative medicine.

Further reading

Current cell-based clinical applications

Atala A, *et al.* (2006). Tissue-engineered autologous bladders for patients needing cystoplasty. *Lancet*, **367**, 1241–6.

O'Connor NE, *et al.* (1981). Grafting of burns with cultured epithelium prepared from autologous epidermal cells. *Lancet*, **i**, 75–78.

Pellegrini G, *et al.* (1997). Long-term restoration of damaged corneal surfaces with autologous cultivated corneal epithelium. *Lancet*, **349**, 990–3.

Wasiak J, *et al.* (2006). Autologous cartilage implantation for full thickness articular cartilage defects of the knee. *Cochrane Database Syst Rev*, **3**, CD003323.

Pluripotent stem cell derivation

Evans MJ, Kaufman MH (1981). Establishment in culture of pluripotential cells from mouse embryos. *Nature*, **292**, 154–6.

Gurdon JB, Melton DA (2009). Nuclear reprogramming in cells. *Science*, **322**, 1811–15.

Takahashi K, *et al.* (2007). Induction of pluripotent stem cells from adult human fibroblasts by defined factors. *Cell*, **131**, 861–72.

Thomson JA, *et al.* (1998). Embryonic stem cell lines derived from human blastocysts. *Science*, **282**, 1145–7.

Regenerative neurology

Eriksson PS, *et al.* (1998). Neurogenesis in the adult human hippocampus. *Nature Med*, **4**, 1313–17.

Gill SS, *et al.* (2003). Direct brain infusion of glial cell line-derived neurotrophic factor in Parkinson disease. *Nature Med*, **9**, 589–95.

Lee JP, *et al.* (2007). Stem cells act through multiple mechanisms to benefit mice with neurodegenerative metabolic disease. *Nature Med*, **13**, 439–47.

Lindvall O, *et al.* (1990). Grafts of fetal dopamine neurons survive and improve motor function in Parkinson's disease. *Science*, **247**, 574–7.

Suzuki M, *et al.* (2007). GDNF secreting human neural progenitor cells protect dying motor neurons, but not their projection to muscle, in a rat model of familial ALS. *PLoS ONE*, **2**(1): e689.

Cardiomyocytes and cardiac repair

Hsieh PC, *et al.* (2007). Evidence from a genetic fate-mapping study that stem cells refresh adult mammalian cardiomyocytes after injury. *Nature Med*, **13**, 970–4.

Laugwitz KL, *et al.* (2005). Postnatal isl1+ cardioblasts enter fully differentiated cardiomyocyte lineages. *Nature*, **433**, 647–53.

Ott HC, *et al.* (2008). Perfusion-decellularized matrix: using nature's platform to engineer a bioartificial heart. *Nature Med*, **14**, 213–21.

Schuldt AJ, *et al.* (2008). Repairing damaged myocardium: evaluating cells used for cardiac regeneration. *Curr Treat Options Cardiovasc Med*, **10**, 59–72.

Segers VFM, Lee RT (2008). Stem-cell therapy for cardiac disease. *Nature*, **451**, 937–42.

Yamashita, JK, *et al.* (2005). Prospective identification of cardiac progenitors by a novel single cell-based cardiomyocyte induction. *FASEB J*, **19**, 1534–6.

Pancreatic β cells and islet transplantation

Calafiore R, *et al.* (2006). Microencapsulated pancreatic islet allografts into nonimmunosuppressed patients with type 1 diabetes: first two cases. *Diabetes Care*, **29**, 137–8.

D'Armour KA, *et al.* (2006). Production of pancreatic hormone-expressing endocrine cells from human embryonic stem cells. *Nat Biotechnol*, **24**, 1392–401.

Dor Y, *et al.* (2004). Adult pancreatic beta-cells are formed by self-duplication rather than stem-cell differentiation. *Nature*, **429**, 41–46.

Kroon E, *et al.* (2008). Pancreatic endoderm derived from human embryonic stem cells generates glucose-responsive insulin-secreting cells in vivo. *Nat Biotechnol*, **26**, 443–52.

Shapiro AM, *et al.* (2006). International trial of the Edmonton protocol for islet transplantation. *N Engl J Med*, **355**, 1318–30.

Stem cell immunomodulation

Le Blanc K, Ringden O (2006). Mesenchymal stem cells: properties and role in clinical bone marrow transplantation. *Curr Opin Immunol*, **18**, 586–91.

Le Blanc K, *et al.* (2004). Treatment of severe acute graft-versus-host disease with third party haploidentical mesenchymal stem cells. *Lancet*, **363**, 1439–41.

Pluchino S, *et al.* (2005). Neurosphere-derived multipotent precursors promote neuroprotection by an immunomodulatory mechanism. *Nature*, **436**, 26671.

Zappia E, *et al.* (2005). Mesenchymal stem cells ameliorate experimental autoimmune encephalomyelitis inducing T-cell anergy. *Blood*, **106**, 1755–61.

SECTION 5

Immunological mechanisms

Editor: Graham S. Ogg

5.1 Structure and function *207*

5.1.1 The innate immune system *207*
Paul Bowness

5.1.2 The complement system *213*
Marina Botto and Mark J. Walport

5.1.3 Adaptive immunity *224*
Paul Klenerman

5.2 Immunodeficiency *235*
D. Kumararatne

5.3 Allergy *258*
Pamela Ewan

5.4 Autoimmunity *267*
Antony Rosen

5.5 Principles of transplantation immunology *280*
Ross S. Francis and Kathryn J. Wood

5.1

Structure and function

Contents

5.1.1 The innate immune system *207*
Paul Bowness

5.1.2 The complement system *213*
Marina Botto and Mark J. Walport

5.1.3 Adaptive immunity *224*
Paul Klenerman

5.1.1 The innate immune system

Paul Bowness

Essentials

The innate immune system comprises evolutionarily ancient mechanisms that mediate first-line responses against microbial pathogens, and are also important in priming and execution of adaptive immune responses, and in defence against tumours. These responses, which recognize microbial non-self, damaged self, and absent self, are characterized by rapidity of action and lack of plasticity, 'learning', or memory, and they involve various different cell types, cell-associated receptors, and soluble factors.

Cellular components—these are mainly derived from myeloid precursors in the bone marrow and include monocytes, macrophages, dendritic cells, and granulocytes (neutrophils, eosinophils, and basophils). Two small populations of lymphoid cells—NK and NKT cells—are also included because they lack the clonally rearranged receptors of B and T lymphocytes.

Receptors—the innate immune system uses a relatively small repertoire of germline-encoded largely non-rearranging receptors, including (1) Pattern recognition receptors (PRR)—these recognize invariant molecular signatures, usually microbial in origin, known as pathogen associated molecular patterns (PAMPs), Toll-like receptors and mannose receptors (2) Natural killer (NK) family of receptors—these largely have specificity for self or altered self molecules, e.g. recognizing conserved features of human leucocyte antigen (HLA) class molecules; can be either stimulatory or inhibitory. (3) Other pattern recognition receptors (PRRs).

Soluble mediators—these include (1) complement (see Chapter 5.1.2); (2) defensins—typically small microbicidal proteins, with other actions to stimulate both innate and adaptive immune responses; and (3) cytokines—frequently act over relatively short distances by binding to cell-surface receptors and initiating signalling via intracellular second messengers; play major roles in stimulating immune cell differentiation and proliferation.

Clinical features of dysregulation of the innate immune system—(1) hypofunction—can result in uncontrolled infections, e.g. in chronic granulomatous disease; (2) excess activity—can result in autoinflammatory disease, e.g. periodic fever syndromes; (3) dysfunction—may contribute to common conditions of multifactorial aetiology, e.g. Crohn's disease.

Introduction

The innate immune system is an evolutionary ancient defence system, with elements present in invertebrates, that mediates defence against microbial pathogens. It is also important in both the priming and the execution of adaptive immune responses. Although it is increasingly appreciated that the innate and adaptive responses are tightly interwoven, innate immune responses are characterized by rapidity of action and lack of plasticity, 'learning' or memory. The innate immune system frequently relies upon recognition of conserved molecular features of microbial pathogens—pathogen-associated molecular patterns (PAMPs). The innate immune system also recognizes damaged self and absent self, and hence also plays a role in rooting out malignant cells. It is useful to think of the components of the innate system separately. Most cells of the innate immune system are derived from the myeloid precursors in the bone marrow. These include monocytes and their derivatives—macrophages and dendritic cells, granulocytes (neutrophils, basophils, and eosinophils), and mast cells. Natural killer (NK) and natural killer T (NKT) cells,

Table 5.1.1.1 Cell types of the innate immune system

Myeloid lineage		
Monocyte/macrophage family	Monocytes (blood) Tissue macrophages including Kupffer cells (liver), mesangial cells (kidney), histiocytes (connective issue) and osteoclasts (bone) Dendritic cells including Langerhans cells (skin)	
Myelocytic family	Granulocytes Mast cells	Neutrophils Eosinophils Basophils
Lymphoid lineage	Natural killer (NK) cells Natural killer T (NKT) cells	

which are derived from the lymphoid cell lineage, are also included within the innate immune system as they lack the clonotypic receptors of lymphoid T and B cells characteristic of the adaptive immune system.

An increasing number of receptor recognition systems for nonself, damaged self, and missing self are being identified. The paradigm family of innate immune receptors are the Toll-like receptors (TLRs). These are present in *Drosophila melanogaster* (fruit flies), where for example the absence of Toll predisposes to overwhelming fungal infection. Important soluble factors include innate immune system cytokines, defensins, and pentraxins.

Dysregulation of the innate immune system is increasingly recognized as causing human disease. Hypofunction of the innate immune system can result in uncontrolled infections, as seen in chronic granulomatous disease. Excess innate immune activity can result in autoinflammatory disease; examples of this type of disease include the periodic fever syndromes. Innate immune dysfunction also contributes to common conditions of multifactorial aetiology such as Crohn's disease.

Cells of the innate immune system

Cells of the innate system are predominantly of the myeloid lineage, arising in the bone marrow (see Table 5.1.1.1 and Fig. 5.1.1.1), but do include two cell types of the lymphoid lineage, the NK and NKT cells.

Myeloid cell lineage

Monocytes/macrophages

Monocytes are derived from haematopoietic stem cell precursors in the bone marrow and make up 3 to 9% of circulating blood leucocytes in adults. Although lacking cytoplasmic granules, monocytes have lysosomes containing acid phosphatase and express the CD14 and CD68 markers. Monocytes themselves usually leave the blood within 48 h to further mature and reside in tissues as tissue-resident macrophages or dendritic cells. Different types of macrophage and dendritic cells are found in different anatomical locations.

Macrophages ('big eaters') are able to phagocytose (engulf) large particles including whole bacteria and apoptotic or necrotic dying cells. Phagocytosis is initiated following either recognition of antibody/complement coating (opsonization) or by PAMPs such as the mannose receptors. Phagoctosed microbes are usually killed, e.g. by production of reactive oxygen species (ROS). Organisms that are able to survive within macrophages, such as the mycobacterial species responsible for tuberculosis and leprosy, cause major disease.

Macrophages are also able to secrete and respond to cytokines (see below), and secrete proteases and growth factors important in tissue remodelling and repair. Uptake of modified low density lipoprotein (LDL) by macrophages in arterial vessel walls gives rise to foam cell formation and is thought to be critical in the pathogenesis of atherosclerosis. Excessive systemic macrophage

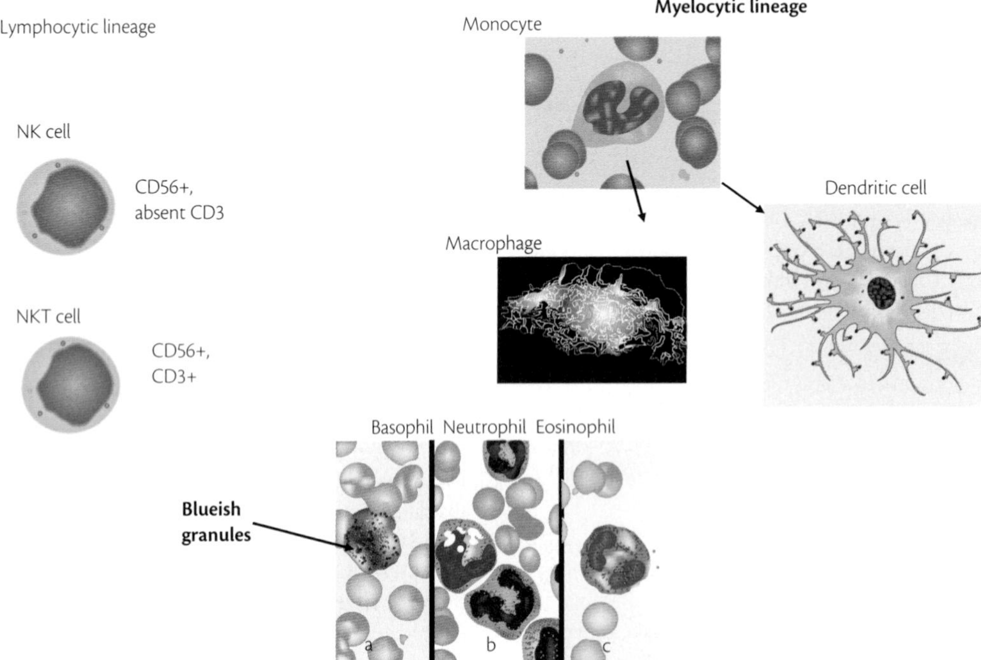

Fig. 5.1.1.1 Cell types of the innate immune system.

activation can result in the life-threatening haemophagocytic syndrome seen in children with viral infection and systemic juvenile idiopathic arthritis.

Dendritic cells

Dendritic cells are now recognized as vital players in the immune system. Although immature dendritic cells are largely tolerogenic, mature dendritic cells are the most potent known stimulators of immune responses. Dendritic cells are characterized by their ability to produce long cellular extensions known as dendrites (see Fig. 5.1.1.1). Dendrites are important both for sampling their environment for antigens and danger signals and for contacting other cell types. Immature dendritic cells patrol the tissues and transduce danger signals through recognition of PAMPs by PAMP receptors. These serve to drive both maturation of dendritic cells and their migration to adjacent lymphoid tissues, such as draining lymph nodes, where priming of adaptive immune responses occurs. A programme of cellular and molecular changes occurs, outlined in Table 5.1.1.2, which facilitate this migration and immune stimulation. Thus, for example, expression of the CCR7 receptor facilitates homing to lymph nodes or spleen. Mature dendritic cells show reduced antigen uptake but increased expression of HLA class II molecules, carrying antigen already taken up in the periphery for presentation to T cells. The HLA/antigen complex provides 'signal 1' and the costimulatory molecules CD80 and CD86 (formerly known as B7.1 and B7.2) give 'signal 2' to initiate T-cell adaptive immune responses.

It has recently become clear that a number of different types of dendritic cells exist, with differing functional properties, as shown in Table 5.1.1.2. The two principal types are myeloid and plasmacytoid dendritic cells. Myloid dendritic cells express CD11c and are now themselves recognized to include several different subpopulations, differing for example in their expression of other CD11 markers, and in their ability to preferentially stimulate CD4 and CD8 T-cell responses. Plasmacytoid dendritic cells probably have a different cellular origin and clearly have a different function. They are also known as interferon-producing dendritic cells, producing both α- and β-interferon, and may have an important role in response to viral infections, since they express the Toll-like receptor TLR9 (see below). α-Interferon production by plasmacytoid dendritic cells has been implicated in the pathogenesis of skin psoriasis and juvenile systemic lupus erythematosus.

Table 5.1.1.2 Human dendritic cell subtypes

Cell type	Example	Function	Phenotypic markers
Myeloid DC			
Immature	Skin Langerhans' cell	Antigen capture by endocytosis and phagocytosis	CD11c, CD1a
Mature	Lymph node	Stimulation of adaptive immune response	CD11c, CCR7 HLA class 2 CD40, CD80/86
Plasmacytoid pDC		Type 1 interferon production	CD123 hi lack CD11c

Granulocytes

Neutrophils, eosinophils, and basophils comprise the polymorphonuclear cells, all of which, together with monocytes, are capable of phagocytosis. Neutrophils are the most abundant white cells in the blood, and also the principle component of pus. They can rapidly leave the circulation to migrate to areas of inflammation. They are drawn down concentration gradients of cytokines such as interleukin (IL)-8 and γ-interferon (see below) in a process known as chemotaxis. Neutrophil granules contain abundant toxic defensins, cathepsins, and enzymes such as elastase. Deficiency of the NADPH oxidase enzyme (EC 1.6.3.1) in individuals (usually boys) with chronic granulomatous disease results in inability of phagocytes to generate superoxide and its bactericidal derivatives peroxinitrite, hydroxyl radicals, and hydrogen peroxide. As a result, bacterial and fungal infections are not cleared and large inflammatory granulomas form. By contrast, in familial Mediterranean fever (OMIM 240100), another genetic disorder (of the pyrin gene) primarily affecting neutrophils, results in excessive inflammatory activity causing peritonitis, arthritis, and amyloidosis. Eosinophils are short-lived granulocytes whose granules stain red on staining with eosin. IL-5 is a key mediator of neutrophil activation. Eosinophils are important in combating parasitic infections but are also implicated in asthma and allergy. Basophils are the least common form of granulocyte. Basophils are capable of releasing histamine and cytokines including IL-4 (see below).

Mast cells

Mast cells, also known as mastocytes, resemble granulocytes but almost certainly originate from a distinct lineage. They are found in the skin, lungs and gastrointestinal tract and express the high-affinity receptor for IgE (FcεRI). Mast cells play an important role in allergy, anaphylaxis, and immunity to parasites. Mast cells coated with antigen-specific IgE release granules containing histamine, cytokines, and eicosanoids upon antigen binding. The 'weal and flare' reaction is an example of such a response.

Lymphoid cells

NK cells

Natural killer or NK cells are a small but important blood lymphocyte population (*c.*2%), distinct from T cells and B cells. They do not express the T-cell receptor for antigen (or CD3), nor the surface immunoglobulin B-cell receptor, and in contrast to adaptive immune responses mediated by T cells, have the ability to kill target cells without prior sensitization. This is know as 'natural' killing. They therefore play a key early defence role against many infectious microbes. NK cells can be activated by NK receptors (see below), by the binding of antibody–antigen complexes to their Fc receptors, and by interferons and cytokines. Human NK cells are classified into two populations according to the intensity of CD56 (neural cell adhesion marker, NCAM) surface expression, as well as possession of CD16, the FcγIII receptor. $CD56^{dim}$ $CD16^{bright}$ make up approximately 90% of circulating NK cells and $CD56^{bright}$ $CD16^{negative/dim}$ comprises the remaining 10%. By contrast, $CD56^{bright}$ NK cells predominate in lymph nodes and sites of inflammation. $CD56^{bright}$ NK cells produce abundant cytokines (e.g. γ-interferon) and have immunoregulatory function, while $CD56^{dim}$ play a key role in natural and antibody-mediated cell cytotoxicity. They are capable of rapidly killing infected or malignant cells, sharing with cytotoxic (CD8) T cells the ability to induce apoptosis, and the cytolytic granules containing perforin and granzymes. The cytotoxic activity of NK cells is controlled by a balance of stimulatory and inhibitory receptors. Stimulatory receptors include the natural cytotoxicity receptors, some of which recognize microbial products, and some of the NK family of receptors (NKRs) including NKG2D, described below. Almost all NK cells also express inhibitory receptors for self HLA, which serve to limit killing of self cells under normal circumstances. Consequently NK cells have the ability to recognize absence of self or 'missing self'. NK cells have a major role in the early innate immune response to viruses, and can also kill antibody-coated cells through their FcγR3 receptors.

NKT cells

NKT cells are a minor population of lymphocytes (0.2% of peripheral blood lymphocytes) that coexpress both NK markers including CD56 and the T-cell receptor for antigen (TCR). They recognize foreign or self glycolipids presented by the nonpolymorphic MHC class 1-like molecule CD1. NKT cells can recognize relatively conserved glycolipids derived from bacteria and parasites, although the best-characterized ligand, α-galactosylceramide, is derived from a sponge. These glycolipids are bound and 'presented' by CD1 to the NKT cell TCR. Two types of human NKT cells are currently distinguished. Type 1 or iNKT express an invariant T-cell receptor (using the TCR α-chain AV24AJ18) and recognize α-galactosylceramide presented by CD1d. Type 2 NKT express variable TCRs and are CD1-restricted but do not respond to α-galactosylceramide, presumably recognizing distinct glycolipids. Upon activation NKT cells produce IL-4, γ-interferon and granulocyte colony-stimulating factor (G-CSF) (see below). The function of NKT cells is currently under intense investigation, with recent evidence in a murine model for a role in causing asthma. They may also play a role in immunity to tumours, and it is possibly relevant that the glycolipids lysosomal glycosphingolipid iGb3 and ganglioside GD3 are overexpressed by melanoma cells.

Receptors of the innate immune system

Unlike the adaptive immune system, the innate immune system uses a relatively small repertoire of germline-encoded largely nonrearranging receptors. Charles Janeway has suggested that conserved molecular patterns in microbes would be recognized by pattern recognition receptors (PRRs). These PAMPs would be both essential for the pathogen and distinct to host molecules. Recognition of such PAMPs is increasingly seen as a major function of the innate immune system. It is now recognized that innate immune receptor recognition systems can also have specificity for damaged self (e.g. necrotic cells) and missing self. Recognition of PAMPs or of damaged self by the innate immune system—the immunological 'danger' signals proposed by Matzinger—provides a key trigger in initiating both innate and adaptive immune responses. 'Missing self' is detected by loss of the inhibitory signals provided by receptors for self molecules including those for self HLA molecules. The TLRs principally recognize PAMPs; another very different grouping of receptors, the NKRs frequently recognize self and altered self.

Toll-like receptors

TLRs are transmembrane receptors, largely expressed at the cell surface, that recognize conserved microbial and, to a lesser extent, self molecules. These include conserved nucleic acids, lipoproteins, and lipopolyscaharrides. The principle TLRs and their ligands are shown in Fig. 5.1.1.2. One of the most important TLRs is TLR4,

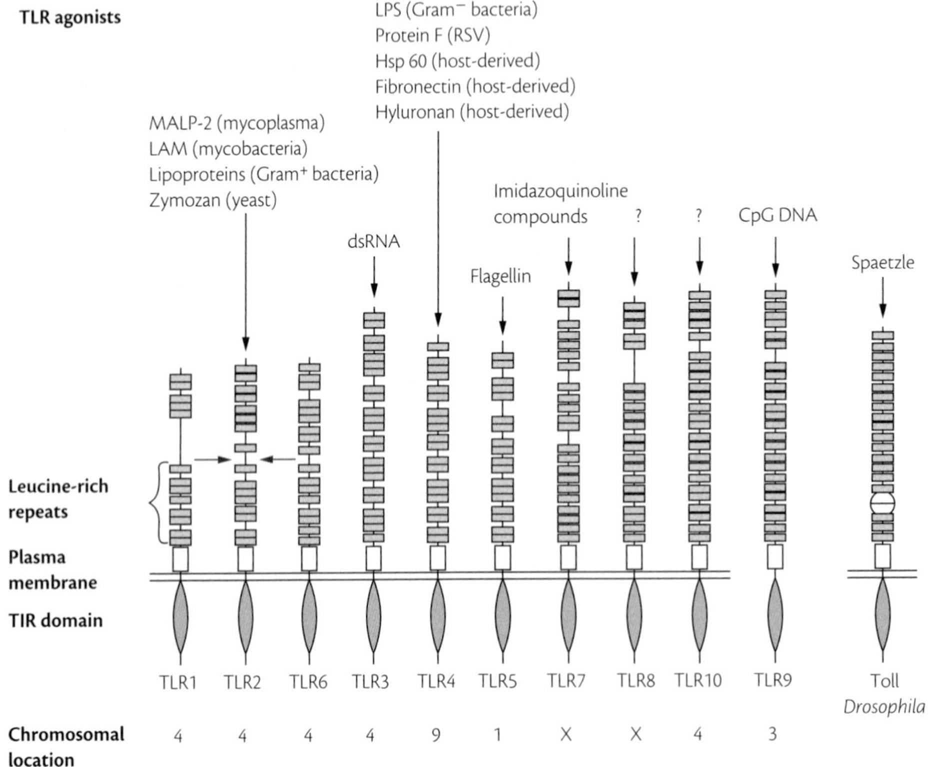

Fig. 5.1.1.2 Toll-like receptors and their ligands.

Table 5.1.1.3 Natural killer (NK) and related innate immune receptors

Receptor	Type	Cellular expression	Ligand
KIR	Ig	NK and T cells	HLA class 1, specific alleles e.g. KIR3DL1 recognizes HLA-B27 and related HLA-B alleles
LILR	Ig	Monocytes, DC, B	HLA class 1, general
NKG2D	Lectin activatory	All NK/some T	MICA/B
NKG2A/ CD94	Lectin	NK/T	HLA-E with HLA-derived peptide
Natural cytotoxicity receptors (NCR)			
NKp30, 46		NK	?Malignant cells
NKp44		Activated NK	?Malignant cells
NKp80		NK	AICL on monocytes

Ig denotes immunoglobulin family.

which was identified by Beutler and colleagues as a critical component of the receptor for bacterial lipopolysacharide (LPS). LPS is a major component of the outer cell wall of Gram-negative bacteria, (and hence known as an endotoxin), and is the principle cause of the fever associated with Gram-negative bacterial infection. Mice with a natural mutation in TLR4 exhibit both increased susceptibility to Gram-negative bacterial infection and resistance to LPS-induced fever. TLR4 is part of a cell-surface receptor complex, which includes CD14, the secreted helper molecule MD2, CCR5, and the intracellular signalling adaptor protein MyD88. In addition to bacterial LPS and certain viral proteins, some self molecules including heparan sulphate, fibrinogen, and hyaluran fragments can signal through TLR4. Other TLRs, illustrated in Fig. 5.1.1.2, include TLR3, which recognizes viral double-stranded RNAs. Another bacterial component, flagellin, is recognized by TLR5. TLR9 recognizes unmethylated CpG dinucleic acids, common in bacteria but very rare in mammalian DNA. Modulation of immune responses through therapeutic use of TLR ligands has huge potential for human therapy; e.g. the TLR7/8 ligand imiquimod is used in the treatment of skin malignancy.

Natural killer receptors (NKRs)

The term NKR loosely describes several groups of unrelated receptors that are frequently but not uniquely expressed on NK cells. These receptors can be either stimulatory or inhibitory and can recognize either self or foreign antigens. Killer-cell immunoglobulin-like receptors (KIR) recognize groups of HLA class 1 molecules, as illustrated in Table 5.1.1.3. KIRs can have either inhibitory functions, mediated through Immunoreceptor Tyrosine-based Inhibitory Motifs (ITIMs), or stimulatory functions mediated by adaptor proteins. Many KIRs have numerous different allelic variants. The KIR genes are located on chromosome 19q13.4 and are in linkage disequilibrium, thus a group of different variants are commonly inherited together, with 2 major haplotypes recently been recognized. Allelic forms have recently been implicated in progression to AIDS, and in susceptibility to autoimmune arthritis including psoriatic arthritis. In HIV progression and psoriatic arthritis it is the inheritance of a specific combination of KIR allele with HLA allele that determines disease progression/susceptibility. Leucocyte Immunoglobulin-like receptors (LILR), formally known as ILTs, are generally inhibitory, are expressed on a group of leucocytes and have broader specificity for most class 1 HLA molecules. NKG2D is important in cancer surveillance, at least in murine studies, and recognizes the MHC-like invariant molecules MICA and B. The natural cytotoxicity receptors are activatory molecules with poorly defined ligands that are also implicated in recognition of malignant cells. The outcome of an interaction of an NK cell with a potential target probably depends on the net balance of positive and negative signals.

Other cell-associated receptors

The discovery of new PRRs is occurring rapidly. Emerging cytoplasmic receptors of importance are the NLRs (nucleotide-binding domain, leucine-rich repeat) and the viral RNA sensors, retinoic acid-inducible gene I (RIG-I, and other RIG-1-like helicases) and melanoma differentiation-associated gene 5 (MDA5) which are important in responses to pathogens. The NLR family is large and increasing and includes the NOD, NALP, NAIP, and CIITA subfamilies. NOD2 variants are associated with Crohn's disease. Scavenger receptors (class A–H), sialic-acid-binding Ig-like lectins (Siglecs), and C-type lectins (e.g. DC-SIGN and mannose receptor) also have roles in recognition of pathogen determinants as well as some host molecules.

Soluble factors

Complement

The complement proteins comprise a vital arm of the innate immune response described in detail in Chapter 5.1.2. The classical, lectin, and alternative pathways comprise cascades that ultimately activate the membrane attack complex resulting in lysis of targeted cells. Covalent attachment of activated C3 to microorganisms is a key signal to the innate immune system to take up and destroy foreign material. The complement pathway is particularly important in immune responses to polysaccharide antigens and is discussed in detail in Chapter 5.1.2.

Defensins

These are small microbicidal proteins of usually 29 to 40 amino acids. α-Defensins are largely stored in the granules of neutrophils and, to a lesser degree, macrophages. Once released they exert direct antimicrobial (including anti-HIV) activity, and can also induce mast cell degranulation and attract both naive T cells and immature dendritic cells. β-Defensins are chemotactic for immature dendritic cells and memory T cells bearing CCR6. Other peptides with antiviral, antibacterial, or antifungal activity include cathelicidin, histatins, cathepsin G, azurocidin, chymase, eosinophil-derived neurotaxin, and lactoferrin.

Mannose-binding lectin (MBL)

MBL is a member of the collectin subfamily of C-type lectins. MBL and the related surfactant proteins A and D have an antimicrobial role in pulmonary defence against bacterial infections. MBL initiates the lectin pathway of complement activation following binding to mannose, *N*-acetylglucosamine, fucose, or glucose residues on microorganisms.

Table 5.1.1.4 Production and action of selected cytokines

Cytokine	Cell source	Target cell	Action
GM-CSF	Th cells	Myeloid progenitor cells	Growth and differentiation
		Monocytes	
Il-1α	Monocytes	T, B NK, other	Stimulation
IL-1β	Macrophages		Fever, inflammation
		Dendritic cells	
		B lymphocytes	
IL-2	Th1 CD4 T	T, B, NK	Activation, proliferation
IL-4	Th2 CD4 T	T, B, macrophages	Activation, proliferation, ? class switching
IL-6	Monocytes	B, plasma cells	Differentiation, antibody secretion
	Macrophages, etc.		
Il-8	Macrophages	Neutrophils	Chemotaxis
	Endothelial cells		
IL-12	Macrophages	e.g. NK cells	Activation
IFN-α	Leucocytes	Many	Inhibition of viral replication
			Increased HLA class 1 expression
IFN-β	Fibroblasts, pDCs	Many	Inhibition of viral replication
			Increased HLA class 1 expression
IFN-γ	Leucocytes	Many	Inhibition of viral replication
			Increased HLA class 1 expression
			T cell proliferation
			B cell class switching
MIP-1α	Macrophages	Monocytes, T cells	Chemotaxis
MIP-1β	Lymphocytes	Monocytes, T cells	Chemotaxis
TNFα	Macrophages	Macrophages	Cytokine production inc. IL-1
		NK, lymphocytes	Tumour killing
TGFβ	Monocytes, T lymphocytes	Monocytes, T cells	Chemotaxis, including IL-1 proliferation

GM-CSF. granulocyte macrophage colony stimulating factor; IFN, interferon; IL, interleukin; TGF, tissue growth factor.

Pentraxins

The pentraxins are a family of proteins with a ring structure made up of five monomers. They include C-reactive protein, a liver-derived acute-phase protein, induced by inflammatory cytokines such as IL-1 and IL-6, which protects against endotoxin-mediated mortality in animals.

Cytokines

Cytokines are a group of proteins important in host defence that are secreted by cells of the innate and adaptive immune systems. The first to be described was interferon, a compound produced by virally infected tissue that 'interfered' with subsequent viral infection of uninfected tissue. A number of overlapping terminologies are used to describe groups of cytokines, based upon their function. Thus monokines are made by monocytes, and lymphokines by lymphocytes; chemokines are cytokines with chemotactic activities; and interleukins are cytokines made by one leucocyte and acting on other leucocytes. Cytokines commonly have autocrine actions on the cells that secrete them, and paracrine actions on nearby cells. Cytokines are synthesized *de novo* in response to specific stimuli, frequently act over relatively short distances, and bring about their effects by binding to cell surface receptors and initiating signalling via intracellular second messengers. Cytokines frequently exhibit redundancy and pleiotropy (i.e. one cytokine can act on different cell types). Cytokine receptors fall into a number of categories: haematopoietin receptors such as the IL-2 receptor, TNF family receptors, interferon and chemokine receptors (see below). Many cytokines play major roles in stimulating immune cell differentiation and proliferation. The functions of some of the major cytokines are briefly summarized in Table 5.1.1.4. Cytokines are increasingly being targeted in human disease therapy, as their roles are elucidated. Thus tumour necrosis factor alpha (TNFα), also described as cachexin, is now known to play a central role in the joint pathology, malaise, and systemic eatures of rheumatoid arthritis as well as other inflammatory arthropathies including psoriatic arthritis, ankylosing spondylitis, and Crohn's disease. Treatment with monoclonal antiTNF antibodies or recombinant TNF receptors is highly effective in most patients. IL-1 has been shown to be important in the Muckle–Wells syndrome and treatment with interleukin receptor antagonists is effective.

Chemokines

These are small (*c.*8–10 kDa) glycoproteins, which are usually pro-inflammatory and result in cellular attraction along concentration gradient. Four major groups are recognized, C, CC, CxC, and CxxxC, based on the relative separation of their two N-terminal cysteines. CC and CxC are the major groups, C and CxxxC having only one member each, lymphotactin and fractalkine respectively. Most CxC chemokines are chemoattractants for neutrophils mediated by an ELR motif adjacent to the cysteines, e.g. IL-8, which induced migration from the bloodstream into tissues. By contrast, CC chemokines attract lymphocytes, monocytes, basophils, and/or eosinophils. Examples of CC chemokines are MCP-1, RANTES, and MIP-1α. Monocyte chemoattractant protein MCP-1 is a potent monocyte chemoattractant that induces monocyte migration from the bloodstream into tissues and subsequent maturation into macrophages. Chemokine receptors have seven transmembrane helices and signal through intracellular G proteins. CC chemokines bind to CC chemokine receptors, and CxC chemokines bind to CxC chemokine receptors, of which at least seven are described. The chemokine receptors CCR5 and CxCR4 are also coreceptors for HIV infection of macrophages and CD4 T-cells.

Interferons

The interferons are a group of cytokines with potent antimicrobial and antiproliferative effects that are produced in response to products of bacterial or viral infection, such as double-stranded RNAs, cytokines, or mitogens. They have multiple effects, characteristically mediated through JAK-Stat pathways, that include up-regulation of HLA class 1 and 2 expression, and generally have potent anti-viral activity. Type 1 interferons include α-interferons produced by lymphocytes (of which at least 13 are recognized), β-interferons produced by fibroblasts, and others. All type 1 interferons bind to a unique cell surface receptor, the interferon-α receptor. Only a single type 2 interferon is recognized, γ-interferon. This is produced by lymphocytes and activated NK cells, and binds to the type 2 interferon receptor. γ-interferon has a variety of activities including macrophage activation. Type 3 (λ) interferons have recently been recognized. Exogenously administered α-interferons 2a and 2b, which can be PEGylated to prolong their action, are effective in the treatment of hepatitis C infections, acting to greatly reduce viral replication. Interferons are also used in other viral infections, including hepatitis B.

Further reading

Banchereau J, Steinman RM (1998). Dendritic cells and the control of immunity. *Nature*, **392**, 255–62. [Review of function of dendritic cells.]

Beutler B, *et al.* (2006). Genetic analysis of host resistance: Toll-like receptor signalling and immunity at large. *Annu Rev Immunol*, **24**, 353–89. [Comprehensive review of TLRs.]

Farag SS, Caligiuri MA (2006). Human natural killer cell development and biology. *Blood Rev*, **20**, 123–37.

Feldmann M, Maini RN (2003). TNF defined as a therapeutic target for rheumatoid arthritis and other autoimmune diseases. *Nat Med*, **9**, 1245–50. [Overview of role of TNF and clinical use of anti-TNF monoclonal antibody therapy in rheumatoid arthritis.]

Hayakawa Y, Smyth MJ (2006). Innate immune recognition and suppression of tumours. *Adv Cancer Res*, **95**, 293–322. [Discussion of evidence of the role of innate immunity and the NKG2D receptor I tumour immunity.]

Janeway C, *et al.* (2005). *Immunobiology: the immune system in health and disease.* Churchill Livingstone, Edinburgh. [Excellent textbook; part I describes the innate immune system.]

Oppenheim J, *et al.* (2003). Roles of antimicrobial peptides such as defensins in innate and adaptive immunity. *Ann Rheum Dis*, **62** Suppl 2, ii17–ii21. [Review of roles of defensins.]

Orange JS, Ballas ZK (2006). Natural killer cells in human health and disease. *Clin Immunol*, **118**, 1–10. [Review of roles of NK cells in human disease.]

Plüddemann A, *et al.* (2006). The interaction of macrophage receptors with bacterial ligands. *Exp Rev Mol Med*, **8**, 1–25.

Pure E, Allison JP, Schreiber RD (2005). Breaking down the barriers to cancer immunotherapy. *Nat Immunol*, **12**, 1207–10. [Role of the immune system in cancer surveillance.]

Steinman R, Cohn Z (1973). Identification of a novel cell type in peripheral organs of mice. *J Exp Med*, **137**, 1142–62. [Discovery of the dendritic cell.]

Takeda K, Kaisho T, Akira S (2003). Toll-like receptors. *Ann Rev Immunol*, **21**, 335–76. [Comprehensive review of TLRs.]

Wantanabe, Y. (2004). Fifty years of interference. *Nat Immunol*, **5**, 1193. [Review of the discovery and functions of interferons.]

5.1.2 The complement system

Marina Botto and Mark J. Walport

Essentials

The complement system consists of over 20 distinct proteins and is an essential component of the innate immune system. It is a major effector mechanism of host defence against infection and inflammatory responses, has an important role in the physiological removal of immune complexes and dying cells, and plays an accessory role in the induction of antibody responses.

Complement activation and regulation

This occurs through three distinct pathways, each generating C3 convertases that cleave native C3 to form the active product C3b, which can deposit on foreign surfaces acting as opsonin or generate complexes capable of binding and cleaving C5. This culminates in the formation of the membrane attack complex, which disrupts target cell membrane integrity and can result in cell lysis.

Classical pathway of complement activation—plays a role in both innate and adaptive immunity; begins by the binding of C1q to (a) the Fc portion of antibodies complexed with antigens, or (b) directly to the surface of certain pathogens or host ligands such C-reactive protein complexed to its phospholipids; activated C1 complex then acts on the next two components of the classical pathway, cleaving C4 and then C2 to generate the classical pathway C3 convertase.

Alternative pathway of complement activation—is in a constant state of activation or 'tick-over'; activates through an amplification loop that can proceed efficiently on the surface of a pathogen or on abnormal host tissues (including virus-infected cells or tumour cells) but not on a host cell.

Lectin pathway of complement activation—mainly triggered following the binding of mannose-binding lectin (MBL) and ficolin proteins to carbohydrate residues on the surface of pathogens, leading to the activation of MBL associated serine protease (MASPs), one of which cleaves C4 and C2 sequentially to form C3 convertase.

Complement regulatory proteins—these tightly regulate complement activation, in the fluid-phase and on cell surfaces, preventing both depletion of complement proteins and limiting complement-mediated host cell damage.

Complement in disease

Hereditary or acquired abnormalities of complement activation components or of complement regulatory proteins can result in disease, including the following conditions.

Hereditary complement deficiency—(1) immunodeficiency—e.g. hereditary C3 deficiency leads to increased susceptibility to pyogenic infections; patients lacking one of the proteins of the membrane attach complex (MAC) display complex susceptibility to neisserial infection. (2) Autoimmune disease—e.g. homozygous hereditary deficiency of one of the early classical pathway components (C1q, C1r, C1s, C4, and C2) is associated with a markedly increased susceptibility to systemic lupus erythematosus (SLE). (3) Abnormalities of complement regulation—e.g. hereditary angio-oedema caused by deficiency of C1 inhibitor.

Acquired complement deficiency—(1) excessive classical pathway activation (C4 low, C3 normal or low)—e.g. SLE, mixed essential cryoglobulinaemia, rheumatoid vasculitis; (2) excessive alternative pathway activation (C3 low, normal C4)—e.g. caused by C3 nephritic factor (see below).

Abnormal complement regulation—(1) autoantibodies to complement proteins—e.g. C3 nephritic factor, an IgG autoantibody that binds to and stabilizes the fluid phase and cell-bound alternative pathway C3 convertase, is associated with partial lipodystrophy, membranoproliferative glomerulonephritis type 2, recurrent infections, and retinal abnormalities. (2) Paroxysmal nocturnal haemoglobinuria—caused by the loss through somatic mutation of expression of two membrane-bound regulators (CD59 and CD55) that prevent the formation and assembly of membrane attack complex in cell membranes and thereby inhibit the lysis by complement of autologous cells.

Measurement of complement in clinical practice

Diagnosis—measurement of complement activity in serum is required in the context of patients with possible (1) immunodeficiency—particularly recurrent pyogenic infections; (2) vasculitis and glomerulonephritis; (3) chronic infections—e.g. bacterial endocarditis, hepatitis C; or with (4) conditions specifically associated with abnormalities of the complement system.

Monitoring—there are very few diseases in which the repeated monitoring of complement levels is useful, but it may have a role in some patients with SLE.

Introduction

Complement was discovered by Jules Bordet as a heat-labile component of normal plasma that complemented the activity of antibody in the killing of bacteria—hence its name. Although complement was initially discovered as an effector arm of the adaptive immune system, it can be activated in the absence of antibodies and is also part of the innate immune system.

Complement consists of more than 20 plasma and cell-bound proteins that interact with each other in an enzymatic cascade. There are three distinct pathways through which complement can be activated: the classical pathway, the alternative pathway, and the lectin pathway (Fig. 5.1.2.1). The classical pathway is a predominantly antibody-dependent pathway, activated principally by aggregated IgG or IgM in immune complexes. The lectin pathway is antibody-independent and is initiated by the binding of mannose-binding lectin (MBL) or ficolin proteins to carbohydrates on bacteria or viruses. The third pathway, called the 'alternative pathway' because it was discovered as a second or alternative pathway for complement activation after the classical pathway had been identified, does not depend on a pathogen-binding protein for its initiation and is in a constant steady state of low-level activation, continuously generating fluid-phase C3b through a pathway termed the C3 'tick-over' pathway. After initiation, the activation of complement is amplified by the sequential activation of a series of enzymes, which lead to the cleavage of C3 and C5 and ultimately culminate in the formation of the membrane attack complex, which disrupts target cell-membrane integrity and can result in cell lysis. Thus a small initiating signal, e.g. from binding of a few MBL molecules to the surface of a bacterium, leads to cleavage of a large number of C3 and C5 molecules. These amplification steps in complement activation increase the effectiveness of complement as a host defence mechanism but also carry the risk to the host that inappropriate complement activation may cause bystander inflammatory injury to host tissues. To prevent this, there is a large array of regulatory mechanisms that avoid inappropriate complement activation and reduce the chance of complement injury to self tissues. Protein deficiency affecting either the complement activation pathways or the complement regulators can result in disease in humans.

A detailed description of the biochemistry of complement is beyond the scope of this chapter, which focuses on the diseases associated with abnormalities of the complement system. We first give a brief description of the pathways of complement activation and outline the different physiological activities of complement, which is necessary in order to understand the role of complement in disease. We then review the diseases associated with hereditary disorders of complement, followed by diseases in which there are acquired complement abnormalities. The chapter ends with a consideration of when and how assays of the complement system should be performed in the assessment and management of diseases.

Pathways of complement activation

Classical pathway

The classical pathway plays a role in both innate and adaptive immunity. The initial step in classical pathway activation is the binding of C1q, the first component of this pathway, to the Fc portion of antibodies complexed with antigens. The various IgG isotypes have different capacities to bind to and activate C1q. In humans, IgG3 is the most potent activator, followed by IgG1 and then IgG2. IgG4 does not bind C1q and thus cannot activate the classical pathway. C1q also binds to the CH3 domain of IgM that has adopted a stable configuration following binding of antigen. The classical pathway can also be triggered in an antibody-independent manner by the binding of C1q directly to the surface of certain pathogens or host ligands such C-reactive protein complexed to its phospholipids. C1q is part of a complex, the C1 complex, which consists of two serine proteases (C1s and C1r). Once activated, the C1 complex acts on the next two components of the classical pathway, cleaving C4 and then C2 to generate the classical pathway C3 convertase (C4b2a). This surface-bound convertase cleaves C3, resulting in the generation of large amounts of C3b, which coats the activating surface, a phenomenon termed opsonization. C4b2a is also able to bind C3b forming the classical pathway C5 convertase.

Alternative pathway

The main feature of the alternative pathway is that its activation can proceed on many microbial surfaces or on abnormal host tissues, including virus-infected cells or tumour cells, in the absence of antibody. The alternative pathway is in a constant state of

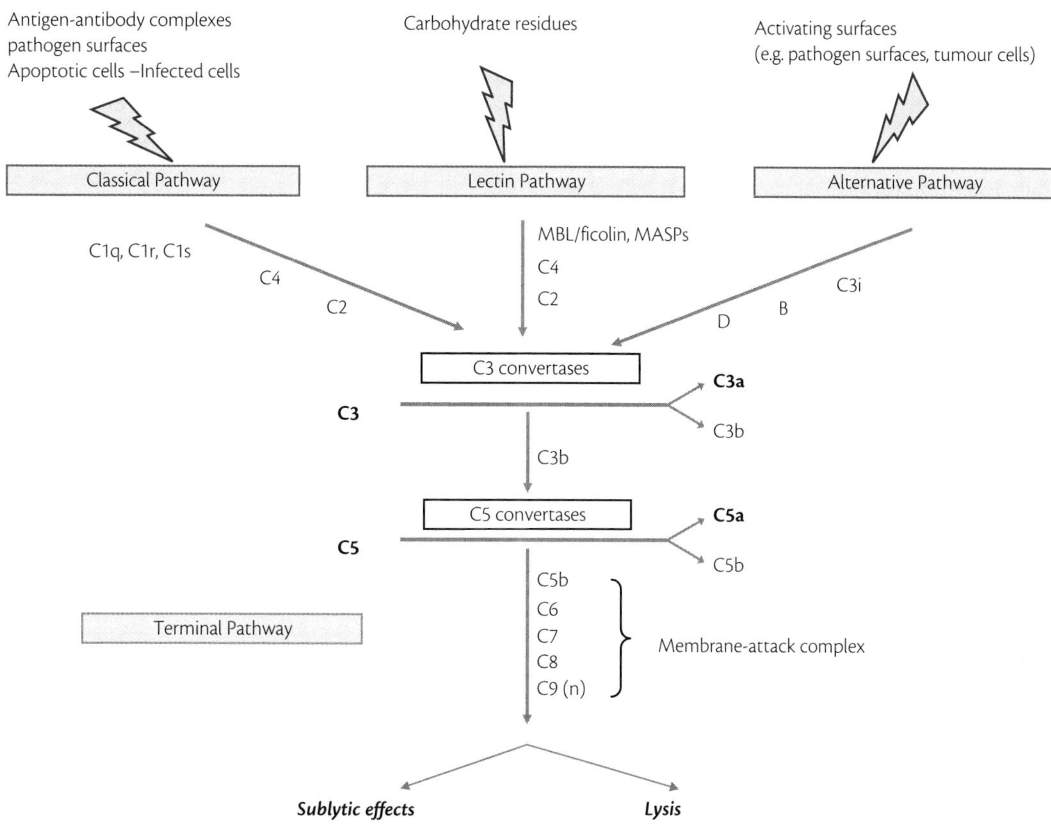

Fig. 5.1.2.1 Simplified overview of the complement system showing the three main activation pathways and the terminal pathway culminating in the formation of C5b–9.

activation or 'tick-over' that results in the generation of low levels of activated C3 fragment (C3b) in the fluid phase. Most of this fluid-phase C3b is inactivated by hydrolysis, but a small amount can bind to proteins and carbohydrates in the immediate vicinity of the C3 activation and act as acceptor site for factor B and initiate the amplification of the alternative pathway. Thus the fate of surface-bound C3b is critically dependent on the nature of the reactive surface and is controlled by two mechanisms. The first controlling mechanism is the presence of membrane-bound complement regulatory molecules which serve to protect host cells by inhibiting the formation of C3 convertases, promoting both their dissociation and the subsequent proteolytic inactivation of C3b. The second mechanism depends on the affinity of the surface-bound C3b for factor H. Factor H is the major fluid-phase regulator of C3 activation and binds preferentially to C3b bound to vertebrate cells, as it has a high affinity for the sialic acid residues present on these cells. In contrast, pathogen surfaces lack sialic acid residues and the affinity of factor H for surface C3b is low, rendering the bound C3b resistant to inactivation and allowing amplification to proceed. Thus the alternative pathway activates through an amplification loop that can proceed efficiently on the surface of a pathogen but not on a host cell. This same amplification loop enables the alternative pathway to amplify complement activation initially triggered through the classical or the lectin pathways.

Lectin pathway

The MBL pathway is the most recently described complement activation pathway. Activation of this pathway is mainly triggered following the binding of MBL to mannose residues, and to certain other sugars, on the surface of pathogens. However collagenous lectins, such as the ficolins, are also capable of activating this pathway. The lectin pathway proceeds in a closely similar way to the classical pathway. The binding of MBL or ficolin to carbohydrates on microorganisms leads to the activation of serine proteases, known as MASPs (mannose-binding lectin associated serine protease). The MASP system contains three different enzymes: MASP-1, MASP-2, and MASP-3 and a protein with no proteolytic activity named MAP19 or sMAP. The present consensus is that MASP-2, that is closely homologous to C1r and C1s of the C1 complex, cleaves C4 and C2 sequentially and thus is the main initiator of the lectin complement pathway. Although the functions of the other MASPs are poorly understood, MASP-1 appears to play a role as an amplifier of complement activation.

Terminal pathway

The final phase of complement activation is the assembly and formation of the membrane attack complex (MAC). The end result is a pore in the lipid bilayer membrane, firstly identified in electron micrographs as membrane 'pores' and 'hollow cylinders', that destroys the membrane integrity. The first step is the enzymatic cleavage of C5 to release C5a and a larger fragment, C5b, that binds sequentially and nonenzymatically to the plasma proteins C6, C7, C8, and C9. The polymerization of C9 produces a hydrophobic complex, commonly denoted as C5b-9_n, where n represents the number of polymerized C9 molecules, that forms 'pores' in lipid bilayers resulting in target lysis. Although the effect of MAC is very dramatic, particularly in experimental conditions in which antibodies against red cells are used to trigger complement activation, its role in host defence seems to be limited to the killing of a few pathogens such as neisseria, as described below.

Regulation of complement activation

Given the destructive effects of complement and the way in which its activation is rapidly amplified through a triggered-enzyme cascade, it is not surprising that its activation is tightly regulated both in the fluid phase and on cell surfaces, serving not only to prevent tissue damage from autologous complement activation but also to prevent the depletion of complement proteins. The evolution of the complement system has therefore been accompanied by the development of a sophisticated regulatory system consisting of fluid-phase and membrane-bound regulatory proteins summarized in Table 5.1.2.1. It is evident that many of these regulators inhibit both classical and alternative pathways of complement activation and there are also specific regulators of the terminal pathway. A detailed description of these molecules is beyond the scope of this chapter and here we review only the most important human conditions associated with abnormalities in complement regulatory molecules.

Table 5.1.2.1 Fluid-phase and membrane-bound complement regulatory molecules

Component	Function(s)
Fluid phase	
C1 inhibitor	Inhibits active C1r and C1s preventing uncontrolled fluid-phase C1 activation. inhibits other proteinases, e.g factor XIIa, kallikrein
C4-binding protein (C4bp)	Binds to C4b preventing binding of C2 Dissociates classical pathway C3 convertase: C4b2a Acts as cofactor for factor I-mediated inactivation of C4b
Factor I	Inactivates C3b and C4b with the aid of cofactors (e.g. factor H, MCP, CR1)
Factor H	Binds to C3b preventing binding of factor B Dissociates alternative pathway C3 convertase: C3bBb Cofactor for the factor I-mediated inactivation of C3b
Vitronectin (S protein)	Binds fluid-phase C5b-9 and prevents its insertion into cell surface
Clusterin	Binds fluid-phase C5b-9 preventing insertion into lipid membranes
Properdin	Positive regulator of the alternative pathway, stabilizes the C3/C5 convertases
Membrane bound	
DAF (CD55)	Accelerates the decay of the C3 and C5 convertases
MCP (CD46)	Cofactor for the factor I-mediated cleavage of C3b and C4b in C3/C5 convertases
CR1 (CD35)	Cofactor for factor I-mediated inactivation of C4b, C3b and iC3b Accelerates the decay of the C3/C5 convertases
CD59	Binds to C5b-8 preventing binding of C9 Binds to C5b-9 preventing polymerization of C9

C4bp, C4 binding protein; CR1, complement receptor 1; DAF, decay accelerating factor; MCP, membrane cofactor protein.

Table 5.1.2.2 Physiological activities of the complement system

Activity	Complement proteins responsible for activity
Opsonin	Covalently bound fragments of C3 and C4
Chemotaxis and activation of leucocytes	Anaphylatoxins C5a, C3a, and C4a
Lysis of bacteria and cells	Membrane attack complex: C5b-C9
Disposal of cellular debris	C1q, covalently-bound fragments of C3 and C4
Augmentation of antibody responses	C3b and C4b bound to immune complexes and antigen

Biology of complement

The physiological activities of complement are summarized in Table 5.1.2.2. The biological functions of complement can be divided into three activities. The first of these is the role of complement in host defence against infectious disease. Complement provides mechanisms for the killing and clearance of microorganisms; it does this by the covalent binding to their surface of C3 and C4 fragments that are ligands for receptors on phagocytic cells that ingest and kill the organism. The activation of complement also causes the generation of the anaphylatoxins C5a and C3a, which have chemotactic activity and recruit leucocytes to sites of infection and inflammation. These small complement fragments signal through transmembrane receptors (C5aR and C3aR) that activate G proteins and thus their action in attracting neutrophils and monocytes is analogous to that of chemokines. A further role of complement in host defence against infections is generation of the MAC. This may disrupt the cell membrane and kill the microorganism. The second activity of complement is as a bridge between the humoral adaptive immune system (antibody) and innate immunity. Activation of complement by immune complexes facilitates the clearance of antigen and thereby helps to prevent immune complexes from causing inflammatory damage to tissues, although, as we shall see, complement may contribute to inflammatory tissue injury in circumstances when immune complexes persist. Activation of complement also augments antibody responses and thereby enhances host defence against pathogens. The binding of complement to antigens reduces the threshold of B lymphocytes for activation. It enhances antigen presentation and B-cell memory by helping to localize antigen on antigen-presenting cells and on the follicular dendritic cells that are key to the maintenance of B cell memory for foreign antigens. The third activity of complement is in the resolution of inflammatory responses. It is in this role that complement may prevent the development of systemic lupus erythematosus (SLE) by promoting the clearance of tissue debris.

Complement in disease

Both inherited and acquired complement deficiencies are associated with disease. Studies of the inherited abnormalities of the complement system have illuminated our understanding of the major roles of the complement system *in vivo* (Table 5.1.2.3). In the following sections we will discuss inherited and acquired deficiencies and the significance of complement measurements in clinical practice.

Table 5.1.2.3 Examples of complete hereditary deficiency, disease association and typical complement profile

Component	Disease association	Complement profile
Early classical pathway components		
C1q, C1r, C1s, C4 and C2	SLE pyogenic infections including meningitis (many C2-deficient cases healthy)	C3 = normal or increased C4 = normal or increased (C4 = 0 in C4-deficient patients) CH50 = 0 AP50 = normal
Alternative pathway components		
Factor B[a] and factor D	*Neisserial* infections	C3 = normal C4 = normal CH50 = normal AP50 = 0
Properdin (X-linked)	Recurrent *Neisserial* infection; rarely pyogenic infection	C3 = normal C4 = normal CH50 = normal AP50 = low or normal
C3	Recurrent pyogenic infection MPGN	C3 = 0 C4 = normal CH50 = 0 AP50 = 0
Lectin pathway components		
MBL	Recurrent pyogenic infections particularly in childhood	C3 = normal C4 = normal CH50 = normal AP50 = normal
Terminal pathway components		
C5, C6, C7, C8, and C9	Neisserial infection many C9-deficient cases healthy	C3 = normal C4 = normal CH50 = 0 AP50 = 0
Deficiency of complement regulators		
Fluid phase		
C1 inhibitor	Angio-oedema	C3 = normal C4 = low CH50 = Low or normal AP50 = normal
Factor H	MPGN aHUS Recurrent pyogenic infection	C3 = low C4 = normal CH50 = very low or 0 AP50 = very low or 0
Factor I	Recurrent pyogenic infection Nephritis rare (MPGN not reported)	C3 = low C4 = normal CH50 = very low or 0 AP50 = very low or 0
Membrane-bound		
CD59*	Mild PNH-type anaemia	Normal complement profile
DAF	Healthy	Normal complement profile

aHUS, atypical haemolytic uraemic syndrome; MPGN, membranoproliferative glomerulonephritis; PNH, paroxysmal nocturnal haemoglobinuria; SLE, systemic lupus erythematosus.

[a] Single case reported.

Inherited complement deficiency and disease

There are three types of disease associated with hereditary complement deficiency. The first is immunodeficiency, which illustrates the role of complement in host defence against infection. The second is the association of SLE with deficiency of certain classical pathway proteins. This association has led to a greater understanding of the role of complement in the resolution of inflammation and in the clearance of immune complexes and tissue debris. The third category of disease is caused by deficiencies of proteins of the regulatory mechanisms of the complement system. This small group of disease illustrate the effects of unrestrained activation of the complement system. We consider each of these associations.

Complement deficiency and infection

Pyogenic infection and complement deficiency

Patients with hereditary C3 deficiency or with mutations in molecules leading to C3 consumption show increased susceptibility to pyogenic infections. They suffer from recurrent and severe bacterial infections, particularly those caused by encapsulated organisms such as *Streptococcus pneumoniae* and staphylococci. There is a similar susceptibility to infections in patients lacking antibodies or normal phagocytic function. This serves to illustrate that the normal pathway for host defence against such bacteria is binding of antibody, followed by complement, providing opsonins for uptake and bacterial killing by phagocytes. Disruption of any of the links in this chain causes increased susceptibility to infection by these pyogenic bacteria. In patients with C3 deficiency, major infections are most prominent in childhood and are less of a clinical problem in adults. This presumably reflects the lesser importance of complement in host defence to pyogenic bacteria as antibody responses mature in response to repeated infectious challenges.

Neisserial infection and complement deficiency

Humans who lack one of the proteins of the membrane attack complex (C5, C6, C7, C8, or C9) display a unique susceptibility to neisserial infection, especially by *Neisseria meningitidis*, which is frequently recurrent. This pattern of infection provides evidence that that extracellular lysis through formation of the MAC is critical in host defence against these organisms, which are capable of intracellular survival. C9 deficiency is rare in white individuals, but surprisingly frequent in Japanese, with an incidence of approximately 1 in 1000. These individuals are at an increased risk of neisserial infections, but otherwise healthy. Individuals lacking the earlier components of the complement system, which are the necessary precursors for the information of MAC, are also at increased risk of neisserial infection. Deficiency of properdin is also associated with neisserial infections. This protein stabilizes the alternative pathway C3 convertase enzyme and augments the cleavage of C3. It is encoded on the X chromosome and therefore properdin deficiency is found almost exclusively in males. Increased susceptibility to neisserial infections is also a feature of acquired complement deficiency, such as may be seen in patients with SLE or with C3 nephritic factor (see below).

MBL deficiency

MBL binds to terminal mannose groups in a spatial orientation that is present on many microorganisms, including certain Gram-positive and Gram-negative bacteria, mycobacteria, yeast, and parasites, but absent on mammalian cells. It is one of the 'pattern recognition' features of the innate immune system that binds molecules present on potential pathogens but not on the cells of the host. The physiological importance of the lectin pathway in humans can be appreciated from the phenotype described in individuals with MBL deficiency. MBL deficiency is associated with an opsonic defect and recurrent bacterial infections, particularly in childhood. The clinical effects of mannose-binding lectin deficiency are most apparent in childhood. At this stage of life the innate immune system is of particular importance in host defence against infection. Common causes of MBL deficiency are mutations of residues in the collagen domain of MBL, which cause misassembly of the multimer and thereby have a dominant effect suppressing mannose-binding lectin levels.

When should complement deficiency be suspected in a patient with infectious disease?

Immunodeficiency should be suspected in any individual who has recurrent or unexplained major infections. The type of the infection provides a clue to the relevant investigations of the immune system. Recurrent pyogenic infections imply a need to assay the activity of antibodies, the complement system, and phagocytic function. In the specific case of meningococcal sepsis, factors that point to complement deficiency are: (1) recurrent attacks; (2) a family history of meningococcal infection (especially if disseminated in time); (3) infection by unusual strains of *N. meningitidis;* (4) atypical clinical presentation; (5) consanguineous marriage. Individuals with complement deficiency remain susceptible to neisserial infection throughout life and may present at any age.

Complement deficiency and autoimmune disease

Homozygous hereditary deficiency of each of early classical pathway components (C1q, C1r, C1s, C4, and C2) is associated with a markedly increased susceptibility to SLE. There is a hierarchy of susceptibility and severity of SLE according to the position of the missing protein in the pathway of classical pathway activation with homozygous C1q deficiency showing the strongest association (approximately 93%). These cases of SLE associated with inherited complement deficiency are extremely rare and account for only a tiny minority of the population of patients with SLE. However, they provide an important clue to the aetiology of the disease. They illustrate that there is an important activity of the early classical pathway of complement that protects against the development of SLE. The source of the autoantigens that drive the autoimmune response in SLE is thought to be apoptotic cells. Apoptotic cells, unlike normal cells, have many of the lupus autoantigens (e.g. Ro) on the cell surface and thus in a position accessible to the immune system. There is a mounting body of evidence that suggests that the complement system, particularly C1q, is important in the physiological clearance of dying cells and in the processing of immune complexes. Loss of these activities might lead to abnormal processing of dying cells that, in the context of an inflammatory response, could initiate and drive an autoimmune response leading to the development of SLE. An *in vivo* defect in apoptotic cell clearance has been demonstrated in C1q-deficient mice that spontaneously develop a lupus-like disease on specific genetic backgrounds. Further support for the hypothesis that effective mechanisms of cellular waste disposal are essential to prevent the development of SLE is provided by a series of mice lacking molecules that have been implicated in the 'waste disposal' mechanisms of the body. These include mice lacking DNase 1 (which digests extracellular chromatin), IgM (which may augment the clearance of cellular debris), or membrane tyrosine kinase c-mer (thought to cause a loss of phosphatidylserine recognition by phagocytic cells). Each of these gene-targeted strains showed an impaired clearance of dying cells and developed a progressive SLE-like disease characterized by the presence of high levels of antinuclear antibodies.

Abnormalities of complement regulation

C1 inhibitor deficiency

The disease hereditary angio-oedema (OMIM 106100) is caused by deficiency of C1 inhibitor. This is inherited as an autosomal dominant disorder with partial penetrance. The disease is dominantly inherited because the production of C1 inhibitor from a single, normal allele is insufficient to maintain normal homeostasis of the complement and kinin pathways. The mutations may have two effects on protein production. In type I hereditary angio-oedema, which accounts for approximately 85% of cases of the disease, the mutant prevents any expression of protein from the mutant allele. This variety of disease is therefore associated with reduced levels of C1 inhibitor. Type II hereditary angio-oedema is caused by a series of point mutations in the C1 inhibitor gene that alter one of the amino acids at the active centre of the protein and abolish its activity as a serine proteinase inhibitor. These mutations allow expression of normal amount of protein, which is nonfunctional, or even abnormally high C1 inhibitor levels, because the mutant protein is not consumed by normal interaction with activated serine proteinases. It is easy to miss the diagnosis of this variant of hereditary angio-oedema, if it is not appreciated that levels of C1 inhibitor can be normal or high in patients with the disease. Functional C1 inhibitor assays are necessary to detect this particular deficiency. In normal circumstances, this inhibitor binds to and inactivates enzymatically active C1r and C1s. It also inhibits plasmin, kallikrein, and activated coagulation factors XIIa and XIa. Deficiency results in uncontrolled fluid-phase classical pathway activation and consequently reduced levels of both C4 and C2. Acute angio-oedema attacks are characterized by increased vascular permeability at the affected sites. The swellings are believed to be caused by the action of small peptides, called kinins, in particular bradykinin, that induce increased vascular permeability by their actions on vascular endothelium and smooth muscle. These kinins are produced by the action of serine proteinases that are ineffectively regulated in the presence of reduced activity of C1 inhibitor. Plasmin activation may be important in the precipitation of attacks, by consuming the reduced amounts of available C1 inhibitor in individuals with only half normal functional expression of the protein.

Individuals exhibiting clinical features of hereditary angio-oedema who have normal C1 inhibitor concentration and function have also been described. This new type of hereditary angio-oedema (OMIM 610618) has been termed hereditary angio-oedema type III or, more comprehensively, oestrogen-related hereditary angio-oedema or oestrogen-sensitive hereditary angio-oedema. In contrast to hereditary angio-oedema types I and II, hereditary angio-oedema type III has been observed exclusively in women, where it appears to be correlated with conditions of high oestrogen levels—e.g. pregnancy or the use of oral contraceptives. Recent reports have proposed mutations in *F12*, the gene encoding human coagulation factor XII (FXII, or Hageman factor) as a possible cause of hereditary angio-oedema type III.

Allergy is much more common than hereditary angio-oedema as a cause of angio-oedema. In hereditary angio-oedema, the swelling is not itchy and is not accompanied by other features of allergy such as asthma and urticaria. Oedema can affect any part of the integument, but is more common in the extremities. Classically, the oedema and swelling develop gradually over several hours and then subside over 2 to 3 days. In hereditary angio-oedema the involvement of the upper airways (including the tongue, pharynx, and larynx) may result in life-threatening airway obstruction. Swelling of the bowel mucosa may produce severe abdominal pain mimicking common surgical emergencies. On average, women have a more severe course of the disease than men. Patients with early onset of clinical symptoms are affected more severely than those with late onset.

Diagnosis of hereditary angio-oedema is made on the basis of the clinical findings described above, the presence of family history, and blood tests. A family history of angio-oedema makes diagnosis much easier but is not always present. This is because some cases of the disease are due to new mutations in the C1 inhibitor gene. In other families, other members with C1 inhibitor deficiency may have no clinical symptoms. All patients who are suspected of having hereditary angio-oedema should have a C4 level measured. Serum C4 level is a good screening test for hereditary angio-oedema as it is invariably low in untreated patients with hereditary angio-oedema. This is because the reduced C1 inhibitor activity allows C1s to cleave C4 and C2 in an unregulated fashion. In patients with type I hereditary angio-oedema C1 inhibitor protein levels are typically low (usually <30% of normal levels). However, in the 15% of patients with type II disease, protein levels may be normal or high. In these patients functional assays of C1 inhibitor are necessary. These are based on the ability of C1 inhibitor to block cleavage of a chromogenic substrate by activated C1s. Genetic tests are not indicated routinely and are usually not necessary to confirm the diagnosis of hereditary angio-oedema.

Treatment of the disease involves (1) the treatment of acute attacks and (2) prophylaxis to attempt to prevent their recurrence. Acute attacks of hereditary angio-oedema do not respond to adrenaline (epinephrine), though if there is any cause to suspect allergic rather than hereditary angio-oedema, then administration of epinephrine is unlikely to cause any harm and may be life saving. If attacks involve the airways, then respiratory support is the first priority. Acute attacks of angio-oedema may be arrested by infusion of purified C1 inhibitor concentrate. If this is not available, fresh frozen plasma may be infused. This is less satisfactory, as plasma not only contains C1 inhibitor but also kallikrein, C1r, and C1s, which may generate further kinin production. In patients with repeated attacks of angio-oedema or infrequent but life-threatening attack of disease, prophylactic treatment should be given. C1 inhibitor levels originating from the single normal allele increase in response to treatment with attenuated androgens, such as danazol, stanozolol, and oxandrolone. This is a moderately effective treatment, although these compounds still retain some virilizing activity. An alternative, though probably less effective therapy (there are no randomized trials), is the proteinase inhibitor tranexamic acid, which may reduce the consumption of C1 inhibitor by blocking the activity of the serine proteinases that interact with C1 inhibitor. New inhibitors of the fibrinolytic system, such as the kallikrein inhibitor DX88 and the bradykinin B2 receptor inhibitor icatibant have shown to be effective and safe for the treatment of C1 inhibitor deficiency in clinical trials. Advice on use of contraceptives and hormone replacement therapy should emphasize avoidance of oestrogen. Angiotensin-converting enzyme (ACE) inhibitors need to be avoided because of their effects on the kallikrein–bradykinin pathway. Angiotensin-II receptor antagonists may be used with caution in patients with hereditary angio-oedema.

Disease associated with unregulated C3 activation—factor I and factor H deficiency

A key step in the regulation of complement activation is control of the fate of the C3 fragment, C3b. This acts as the nucleus for formation of further C3 convertase enzyme, unless it is catabolized by the serine esterase enzyme, factor I, in conjunction with the cofactor protein, factor H. Complete deficiency of either of these proteins allows the unregulated formation of C3 convertase enzyme and continuing cleavage of C3 (Fig. 5.1.2.2). This results in secondary and severe C3 deficiency, together with depletion of the alternative pathway components (properdin and factor B). The typical associated complement profile is that of absent alternative pathway haemolytic activity (AP50) as well as absent total haemolytic activity (CH50), the latter a consequence of secondary C3 depletion. In some of the affected individuals terminal pathway components are low and most likely the result of uncontrolled C5 convertase formation. However the clinical manifestations associated with the complete deficiency of these fluid-phase regulators are different. Factor I is essential for the inactivation of C3b and C4b and cleaves the α-chain of C3b forming iC3b. Essential cofactors for this reaction include factor H in the fluid phase and membrane-bound regulators such as CD46 (MCP) and CR1 on cell surfaces. Patients with deficiency of factor I are susceptible to recurrent pyogenic infections, most likely a consequence of secondary C3 deficiency. Factor H inhibits alternative pathway activation by binding to C3b (thus preventing binding of factor B). It also has decay accelerating activity for both C3bBb and C3iBb and is an essential fluid-phase cofactor for the factor I-mediated proteolytic inactivation of C3b to iC3b.

In contrast to the phenotype associated with factor I deficiency, complete factor H deficiency in humans, pigs, and mice results in spontaneous membranoproliferative glomerulonephritis type II (MPGN2, also termed dense deposit disease; OMIM 609814). MPGN2 is characterized by the presence of C3 along the glomerular basement membrane (GBM) in the absence of immunoglobulin. The presence of C3 in tissue in the absence of immunoglobulin excludes classical pathway activation which is antibody-dependent. Hence, MPGN2 is considered to be a disorder of alternative pathway activation. This may arise as a consequence of genetic deficiency or abnormalities of factor H, a key alternative pathway regulator. The presence of C3 along the GBM results in a striking morphological change in the appearance of the GBM on electron microscopy. Thus the lamina densa of the GBM is replaced by intramembranous electron-dense material—hence the alternative name for MPGN2, dense deposit disease. The underlying mechanism of this form of nephritis is as yet not fully understood but recent studies in mice lacking factor H demonstrated that during uncontrolled alternative pathway activation, factor I-mediated cleavage of C3b is an absolute requirement for the development of C3 deposition on the glomerular basement membrane.

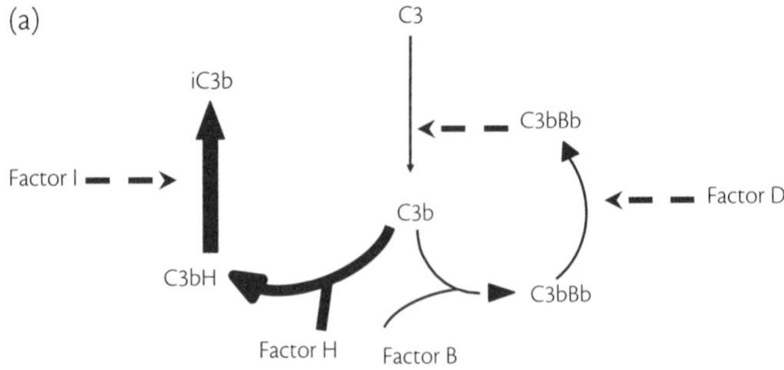

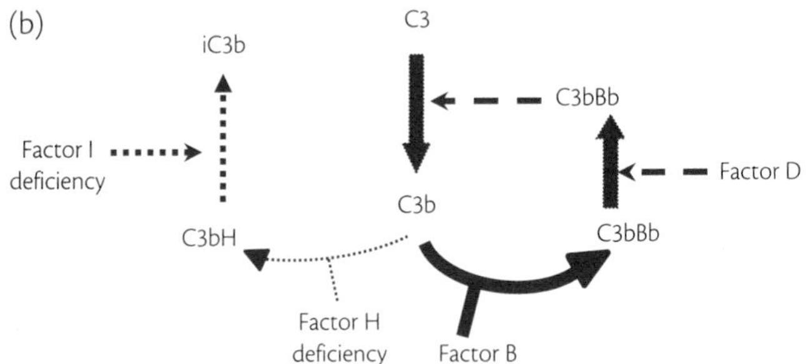

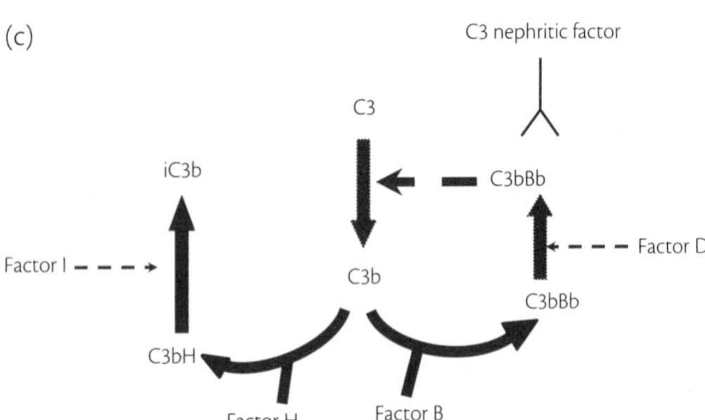

Fig. 5.1.2.2 Uncontrolled activation of C3 caused by Factor H or I deficiency, or by C3 nephritic factor. (a) Normal control of C3 cleavage. In plasma and tissues any C3b that is formed by the normal low-grade turnover of C3 is bound by factor H and catabolized by factor I to inactive products. (b) Effect of factor H or factor I deficiency. C3b cannot be catabolized to inactive products. Instead, there is increased formation of the alternative pathway, C3bBb C3 convertase, causing accelerated cleavage and depletion of C3. (c) Effects of C3 nephritic factor. This antibody stabilizes the C3bBb C3 convertase enzyme. This results in accelerated cleavage and depletion of C3.

In addition to the association of complete factor H deficiency with MPGN2, genetic studies have linked polymorphisms and mutations in the complement factor H gene with age-related macular degeneration (AMD), and atypical (non-Shiga toxin-associated) haemolytic uremic syndrome (aHUS). The underlying mechanism(s) of the genetic association between AMD and factor H polymorphisms are currently under investigation. aHUS is associated with particular factor H mutations (clustered in the C-terminal domains of the protein) that specifically impair complement surface regulation but do not alter plasma C3 regulation. Patients who present with aHUS should be tested first for serum C3 concentrations; however, normal C3 and factor H levels do not necessarily exclude a complement dysfunction. Measurement of factor H levels in serum is helpful to find out those few patients who carry factor H mutations that cause reduced factor H levels. Decreased CH50 values and factor B concentrations can be found in some but not all patients. aHUS is increasingly recognized to be a disease of defective complement regulation and genetic studies have documented that aHUS can be associated with partial genetic abnormalities of other complement regulatory proteins (e.g. factor I, factor B, MCP). A recent murine model of aHUS provided *in vivo* evidence that effective plasma C3 regulation accompanied by defective control of complement activation on renal endothelium, are the critical events in the molecular pathogenesis of factor H-associated aHUS. Interestingly, mutations in factor H, MCP, and factor I have recently been reported in C3 glomerulonephritis, a renal disease distinct from MPGN and aHUS and in the HELLP (haemolysis, elevated liver enzymes and low platelets) syndrome of pregnancy, suggesting that alternative pathway dysregulation is important in these conditions as well.

Acquired complement deficiency

Complement is activated *in vivo* by many stimuli, which include invading organisms, the formation of immune complexes, and tissue necrosis. When complement activation occurs on a substantial scale, this causes depletion of complement proteins, which may be measured as a reduction in their antigenic levels or as a reduction in the activity of the classical and/or alternative pathway (CH50 and AP50 respectively). The measurement of complement activation may be useful in both the diagnosis and monitoring of some diseases. In some conditions (e.g. SLE, mixed essential cryoglobulinaemia, rheumatoid vasculitis), there is excessive classical pathway activation (C4 low, C3 normal or low), whereas in others (e.g. partial lipodystrophy or MPGN with C3 nephritic factor), there is excessive alternative pathway activation (C3 low, normal C4).

In the case of sepsis associated with endotoxic shock, the large-scale systemic activation of the complement system may play an important part in the pathogenesis of this lethal condition. Activation of the classical and alternative pathways by bacterial endotoxin causes the generation of large amounts of the anaphylatoxins C3a and C5a, and of MAC which activate neutrophils and endothelial cells causing vascular and pulmonary injury, leading to death. Diagnosis of this condition is sadly all too easy and the measurement of complement in such patients does not play an important role in assessment or management.

Tissue necrosis is also an important cause of complement activation. Therapeutic studies of experimental models of myocardial infarction, and of ischaemia-reperfusion injury in other organs, including the brain, have shown that inhibition of complement causes a significant reduction in tissue injury and final infarct size.

The diseases associated with acquired complement activation may be divided into two categories. The first category comprises the diseases associated with abnormal regulation of complement, which is most commonly caused by certain autoantibodies to complement components. Paroxysmal nocturnal haemoglobinuria is a further example of an acquired disorder of regulation of the complement system. The second category is the diseases in which infection or autoimmunity cause clinically important activation of the complement system. Examples of diseases belonging to these categories will be presented below.

Diseases associated with acquired abnormal complement regulation

Here we review four diseases caused by acquired abnormalities of the regulation of complement. The first three of these are associated with the development of high-affinity autoantibodies to complement proteins, known as C3 nephritic factor, anti-C1q antibodies, and anti-C1 inhibitor antibodies. The fourth disease is paroxysmal nocturnal haemoglobinuria, in which a clone of haematopoietic cells loses expression of a family of cell surface molecules including regulatory proteins of the complement system.

Autoantibodies to complement proteins

C3 nephritic factor

C3 nephritic factor is an IgG autoantibody that binds to and stabilizes the fluid-phase and cell-bound alternative pathway C3 convertases (C3iBb and C3bBb respectively). The binding of C3 nephritic factor to the C3 convertase renders it resistant to inactivation by factor H. The consequent uncontrolled alternative pathway activation results in secondary C3 deficiency (Fig. 5.1.2.2). Patients with C3 nephritic factor have very low C3 levels in serum, accompanied by normal C4 levels. When serum from a patient with C3 nephritic factor is mixed with normal serum, the C3 in the normal serum is activated and converted to C3b, which forms the basis of an assay for C3 nephritic factor.

The presence of C3 nephritic factor is associated with four clinical manifestations. The first of these is partial lipodystrophy, in which there is disfiguring loss of fat from the face and upper part of the body. Adipocytes, or fat cells, produce several complement proteins including C3 and factor D, which was independently discovered in fat cells and named adipsin. It is thought that C3 nephritic factor stabilizes the assembly of a C3 convertase enzyme on adipocytes causing the activation of complement on these cells leading to their destruction. The second clinical feature is of MPGN2 (dense deposit disease). The pathogenic mechanism of this disease is similar to that for hereditary factor H deficiency, discussed above. MPGN2 has also been reported in an individual with an autoantibody to factor H and in families with inherited dysfunctional C3 molecules which form C3 convertases resistant to physiological inhibition by factor H. This form of nephritis may be severe, leading to renal failure, and there remains no definitive therapy for MPGN2. The third clinical feature is of recurrent infections, caused by the severe acquired deficiency of C3 associated with the presence of C3 nephritic factor. The fourth clinical manifestation is of retinal abnormalities (MPGN2 retinopathy) characterized by the presence of yellow, drusen-like lesions.

Anti-C1q antibodies

These IgG autoantibodies are directed against an epitope in the collagenous region of C1q, which becomes exposed when C1q is dissociated from the other proteins of the C1 complex, C1r and C1s. This type of epitope is known as neoepitope. Up to one-third of patients with SLE develop anti-C1q autoantibodies. These are associated with activation of the classical pathway, causing very low C4 levels and, to a lesser extent, reduced C3 levels. The mechanism of the hypocomplementemia associated with the presence of anti-C1q antibodies is not certain. Anti-C1q antibodies do not cause complement activation in the fluid-phase when added to fresh serum samples. The most likely mechanism is that they amplify complement activation by immune complexes in tissues, by binding to C1q fixed to immune complexes enlarging the complexes and promoting further complement activation. The presence of anti-C1q autoantibodies is a marker for severe SLE, especially for the presence of lupus nephritis. Increases in anti-C1q antibody titres have been shown to precede renal involvement in SLE and, in contrast to rises in anti-DNA antibody titres, appear to increase specifically prior to renal relapse.

Anti-C1q antibodies are also found as the sole autoantibody in the uncommon disease hypocomplementaemic urticarial vasculitis (HUVS). In this condition, very high titres of anti-C1q antibodies are typically found. Hypocomplementemia is characterized by reduction in both C4 and C3 levels, together with marked depression in C1q concentrations. Rarely, C3 levels may be normal, but a low C4 is invariably found. HUVS is clinically characterized by urticarial vasculitis, which, histologically, is usually a leukocytoclastic vasculitis. Other clinical features of HUVS include polyarthritis or polyarthralgia, glomerulonephritis (typically MPGN type 1), angio-oedema, neuropathy, and obstructive pulmonary disease. There is a considerable degree of overlap between the clinical manifestations of HUVS and SLE. This is analogous to the clinical relationship between SLE and the primary antiphospholipid syndrome.

Anti-C1 inhibitor antibodies

The third disease associated with an autoantibody to a complement protein is angio-oedema associated with autoantibodies to C1 inhibitor. The symptoms and signs of this are very similar to the disease of hereditary angio-oedema, though typically occur with a late onset. Measurement of complement proteins in the serum from patients with this disease show a similar abnormal profile to that seen in the blood of patients with hereditary angio-oedema, with low C1 inhibitor and low C4 levels. Additional abnormalities are low C1q levels and the presence of autoantibodies to C1 inhibitor. C1q antigenic protein levels are of value in diagnosing acquired angio-oedema because these are typically reduced in patients with acquired angio-oedema but normal in patients with hereditary angio-oedema. Acquired angio-oedema has an important association with lymphoproliferative disorders, particularly B-cell lymphoma.

Paroxysmal nocturnal haemoglobinuria (see Section 22.3.12)

Paroxysmal nocturnal haemoglobinuria (PNH; OMIM 311770) illustrates the role of membrane-bound complement regulatory proteins in protection against the activation of complement on normal cells. Haemolysis in the disease is caused by the loss of expression of two membrane-bound regulators named CD59 and CD55 (DAF). These molecules prevent the formation and assembly of MAC in cell membranes and thereby inhibit the lysis by complement of autologous cells. PNH is due to a somatic mutation in a clone of erythrocyte precursors which results in deficiency of phosphatidylinositol phospholipid glycan class A. This protein is required for synthesis of glycosylphosphatidylinositol phospholipid, which provides a 'lipid membrane anchor' for many proteins including both CD55 and CD59. As one might expect, the abnormal red cells in this condition are susceptible to lysis by autologous complement activation. It is notable that the few genetically DAF-deficient individuals described appear healthy with no evidence of significant red cell haemolysis *in vivo*. In contrast, the single reported case of CD59 deficiency was associated with a PNH-like phenotype indicating a key role for CD59 in protection of normal cells against homologous complement activation. The efficacy of eculizumab (a humanized monoclonal antibody against terminal complement protein C5 that inhibits terminal complement activation) in reducing transfusion requirements in patients with PNH provides further evidence for the central role of complement dysregulation in this condition.

Acquired hypocomplementemia in autoimmune disease

The measurement of complement is a useful diagnostic tool as part of the assessment of patients with vasculitis and glomerulonephritis (Table 5.1.2.4). Some of the causes of these conditions are associated with systemic activation of the complement system on a sufficient scale that plasma levels of C4 and C3 are significantly reduced below normal. In these diseases, it is the formation of immune complexes, either in the circulation or *in situ* in tissues, that is responsible for the activation of the complement system.

SLE

The relationship between the complement system and SLE are complex. As we have discussed, inherited deficiency of classical pathway complement proteins causes SLE. However, the vast majority of patients with SLE do not have homozygous deficiencies of complement proteins. Indeed, in these patients, SLE is associated with large-scale activation of the classical pathway of complement. The deposition of complement proteins in tissues, associated with the presence of immune complexes, has been thought to play a role in causing inflammatory lesions in tissues in SLE. Deficiency of C1q proteins is most strongly associated with the development of SLE, yet as we learnt above, approximately one-third of patients with SLE develop autoantibodies to C1q.

The explanation for these complex relationships between complement and SLE is partially understood. Studies in animal models of SLE show that the predominant manner in which immune complexes cause inflammation is by ligation of Fc receptors. Mice lacking Fc receptors were protected from glomerulonephritis caused by immune complexes, whereas mice lacking complement developed full-blown lupus glomerulonephritis. Fc receptors and complement mediate the normal processing of immune complexes. One important role of complement is to maintain immune complexes in solution. Complement is also important in enabling the recognition and capture of immune complexes by complement receptors on cells of the mononuclear phagocytic system. In the absence of complement, the clearance of immune complexes is abnormal, a phenomenon that has been demonstrated in many studies of patients with SLE. In the absence of efficient complement fixation, immune complexes may escape efficient clearance, deposit in tissues and cause tissue injury via ligation of Fc receptors on neutrophils and other leucocytes.

We have already discussed how C1q deficiency might cause the development of SLE. How might SLE cause the development of anti-C1q antibodies? The essential feature of SLE is the formation of autoantibodies to complexes of autoantigens, such as the spliceosome complex and chromatin. C1q binds to cellular debris that is thought to be the source of the autoantigens that drive the autoimmune response in SLE. As part of the debris, C1q may become antigenic and evoke an autoimmune response. This is a situation analogous to the association in SLE, and the primary antiphospholipid syndrome, of the presence of the anticardiolipin autoantibodies with anti-β_2 glycoprotein I antibodies. β_2-Glycoprotein I is a plasma protein that binds to negatively charged phospholipids that are exposed on the cell membranes of apoptotic cells and may thereby become part of the cellular debris that drives the autoimmune response in SLE.

The measurement of complement and of anti-C1q antibodies in SLE is of clinical value in both the diagnosis and management of patients. Serum from patients with active disease typically show evidence of classical pathway activation with reduced C4 and, to a lesser extent, reduced C3 levels. In patients with persistently very low C4 levels, there is a high likelihood that anti-C1q antibodies will be present and such patients are more likely to have, or to develop, glomerulonephritis.

There is one extremely important clinical association of both hereditary and acquired hypocomplementaemia from any cause in patients with SLE. Patients with chronic hypocomplementaemia are at particular risk of developing serious infection with encapsulated organisms such as *Streptococcus pneumoniae* and *Neisseria meningitidis*. These patients can be considered to be 'functionally asplenic' because the hypocomplementaemia, in addition to causing defective opsonization, also results in reduced splenic clearance of these organisms. There is a strong case that such patients, analogous to standard postsplenectomy prophylaxis, should receive prophylactic penicillin therapy and be considered for both pneumococcal and meningococcal vaccination.

Table 5.1.2.4 Levels of complement in patients with vasculitis and glomerulonephritis

Systemic vasculitis		**Glomerulonephritis**	
Normal complement	Reduced complement	Normal complement	Reduced complement
Polyarteritis nodosa	SLE	Minimal change GN	Poststreptococcal GN
Microscopic polyangiitis	Essential mixed cryoglobulinaemia	IgA nephropathy	MPGN associated with factor H deficiency or C3 nephritic factor
Wegener's granulomatosis	HCV-associated vasculitis		
Henoch-Schönlein purpura	SBE-associated vasculitis HUVS Waldenström's hypergammaglobulinaemic purpura		

GN, glomerulonephritis; HUVS, hypocomplementemic urticarial vasculitis syndrome; MPGN, membranoproliferative glomerulonephritis; SBE, subacute bacterial endocarditis. SLE, systemic lupus erythematosus.

Haemolytic anaemia

There is sometimes sufficient systemic complement activation associated with the haemolytic anaemias caused by autoantibodies to erythrocyte surface antigens to cause reduction in the levels of complement proteins measured in serum. This is most prominent in cold agglutinin disease in which IgM cold agglutinins, which bind to I antigen on red blood cells, cause the deposition of many thousands of C4 and C3 molecules per erythrocyte. The accelerated

Table 5.1.2.5 Viral subversion of the complement system

Activity	Virus	Host molecules	Viral molecule
Virus uses cell surface complement protein as receptor	Epstein–Barr virus Measles	CR2 (CD21) CD46 (MCP)	
Virus binds host complement protein to enter cell	HIV West Nile virus	C3b	
Virus expresses complement regulatory protein to avoid complement attack	Herpes simplex		Viral C3b receptor

CR2, complement receptor 2; MCP, membrane cofactor protein.

clearance of erythrocytes in autoimmune haemolytic anaemias is mainly caused by their ligation by mononuclear phagocytic cells bearing Fc receptors in the spleen, in the case of IgG autoantibodies. In the case of cold agglutinin disease, mediated by an IgM autoantibody which cannot bind to Fc receptors, there is typically low-grade intravascular haemolysis by complement.

Human red cells are well protected from complement-mediated lysis by complement regulatory proteins expressed on their cell membranes. As we have seen, the activity of these proteins is illustrated dramatically by PNH. Rarely, if there is extensive complement fixation, as in the case of a transfusion reaction caused by an ABO mismatch, then intravascular complement-mediated lysis of red cells may cause severe injury.

Complement and infectious disease

We have already discussed the role of complement in the innate immune system and as an effector arm of humoral adaptive immunity by illustration of the infections that accompany hereditary or acquired complement deficiency. Complement is also involved in the pathogenesis of infections in other ways. For example, several viral pathogens use the complement system in a subversive manner as part of their pathogenesis (Table 5.1.2.5). Several infections cause hypocomplementaemia through systemic activation of complement in a similar fashion to autoimmune disease and we shall consider some examples.

Complement activation is a feature of chronic bacterial sepsis, e.g. in subacute bacterial endocarditis or ventriculoatrial shunt infection. In both of these conditions there is chronic release of bacterial antigens in the presence of antibacterial antibody response that cannot eliminate the infection because of its relative inaccessibility to the immune system. This causes the chronic production of immune complexes with complement activation by the classical pathway, associated with low C4 and C2 levels and glomerulonephritis and small-vessel vasculitis.

Chronic viral infection by hepatitis C is a further important cause of acquired hypocomplementemia. This infection stimulates the production of large amounts of rheumatoid factor, which in some patients may lead to cryoglobulin production, causing complement consumption and vasculitis. Cryoglobulins should be tested in patients presenting with unexplained renal disease or peripheral neuropathy and low C4 (usually C3 concentration remain normal).

Another example of hypocomplementaemia associated with infection is the complement activation associated with poststreptococcal glomerulonephritis. In this disease, which is thought to be due to an immune response to a pathogen cross-reacting with host tissues, there is marked complement activation, which includes activation of the alternative pathway, associated with low C3 levels.

Measurement of complement in clinical practice

Throughout this chapter examples have been given of diseases which are associated with abnormal levels of complement proteins in the blood. Complement levels and activity can be assayed in clinical practice. It is useful to consider the value of measuring complement proteins in two categories: (1) in diagnosis of disease and (2) measurement repeatedly to monitor the activity of particular diseases.

When to measure complement

Complement in the diagnosis of disease

There are four groups of disease in which it is important to be able to measure complement activity in serum. The first is the immunodeficiencies—it is essential to measure complement in patients with recurrent pyogenic infections, particularly in the context of recurrent or familial meningococcal disease. In this group of diseases, simple antigenic measurement of C4 and C3 levels is insufficient—it is necessary to use tests that assay the activity of the whole complement system, preferably haemolytic assay of the classical and alternative pathways (CH50 and AP50 respectively). If absent or severely reduced activity is detected, then the sample should be referred to a specialist laboratory to try to identify the precise nature of the deficient component. Treatment should comprise counselling, prophylactic penicillin, and vaccination against meningococci.

The second group of diseases is vasculitis and glomerulonephritis. Table 5.1.2.4 shows how a very useful diagnostic subdivision of these diseases can be made on the basis of whether or not there is evidence of systemic complement activation. It is in these diseases that it can also be helpful to use assays of complement to monitor disease activity.

The third group are the chronic infections, which may masquerade as primary systemic vasculitis and, in this context, there should be a high index of suspicion for the presence of bacterial endocarditis or hepatitis C.

The fourth group of diseases are those specifically associated with abnormalities of the complement system, including hereditary and acquired angio-oedema, MPGN2 associated with factor H deficiency, and the syndrome of partial lipodystrophy with or without mesangiocapillary glomerulonephritis.

Complement in the monitoring of disease

There are very few diseases in which the repeated monitoring of complement levels is useful. In SLE, no single test acts as a reliable surrogate for the measurement of disease activity. However, there are some patients in whom fluctuation in complement levels correlates with the waxing and waning of disease activity and, in these individuals, it is useful to monitor regularly C4 and C3 levels. It should be kept in mind that SLE patients who have partial hereditary C4 deficiency (mainly C4A deficiency), C4 concentrations may remain low even during disease remission. Activation products of complement components such as C3degradation products (e.g. C3a, C3d) have been measured in an attempt to increase the correlation with disease activity. Although there is some evidence that measurements of these products correlate more strongly with disease activity, such assays are not routinely available and still provide only a crude marker of disease activity. It can also be useful to measure complement levels regularly in patients with autoantibodies to complement proteins; in these individuals the complement levels are a useful surrogate marker for the continuing presence of the autoantibody.

How to measure complement

Complement can be measured in a several ways. The simplest is antigenic measurement of the concentration of individual proteins, and measurement of levels of C3 and C4 are the most widespread assays in clinical use. The results of such assays need to be interpreted cautiously. The ranges of normality are wide, because there is substantial genetic variation in the levels of these proteins. Furthermore, proteins levels are a product of both synthetic and catabolic rates and both of these may vary in health and disease. Both C3 and C4 are acute phase reactants and concentrations of these proteins may rise, in the case of C3 by as much as 0.5 g/litre, in response to acute phase stimuli.

Measurement of C4 and C3 levels act as very crude surrogate markers of classical and alternative pathway activation respectively. However, further measurements are needed if there is any suspicion of the possibility of inherited complement deficiency or of an abnormality elsewhere in the complement system. Functional assays of complement are fairly straightforward and have the advantage that they measure the activity of all of the proteins in the complement system between activation and the end point, which is the lysis of target erythrocytes. The classical pathway is usually measured by assessment of the lysis by serum of sheep erythrocytes coated with antibody. The alternative pathway is measured by assay of the lysis of guinea pig erythrocytes, which directly activate the alternative pathway of complement in the absence of antibody, in the presence of a buffer that prevents classical pathway complement activity. Results of these assays are normally expressed as CH50 or AP50 units, which are measurement of the haemolysis of 50% of respective erythrocyte preparations.

Other approaches have been devised to assess the presence of complement activation *in vivo*. Many assays have been developed which identify the product of activation of the complement system. Although these assays are attractive in principle, the products of complement activation are only present in plasma very transiently and, in practice, assays of total C4 and C3 levels, together with measurement of CH50, have not been supplanted as the best 'rough and ready' estimates of complement activation in routine clinical practice.

Further reading

Botto M, *et al.* (2009). Complement in human diseases: Lessons from complement deficiencies. *Mol Immunol*, **46**, 2774–83.

Dommett RM, Klein N, Turner MW (2006). Mannose-binding lectin in innate immunity: past, present and future. *Tissue Antigens*, **68**, 193–209.

Janeway CA, *et al.* (2004). *Immunobiology: The immune system in health and disease*, 6th edition. Garland Publishing, New York.

Lambris JD, *et al.* (2008). Complement evasion by human pathogens. *Nat Rev Microbiol*, **6**, 132–142.

Liszewski MK, *et al.* (1996). Control of the complement system. *Adv Immunol*, **61**, 201–83.

Moffitt MC, Frank MM. (1994). Complement resistance in microbes. *Springer Semin Immunopathol*, **15**, 327–44.

Pickering MC, *et al.* (2000). Systemic lupus erythematosus, complement deficiency and apoptosis. *Adv Immunol*, **76**, 227–324.

Thiel S, Frederiksen PD, Jensenius JC (2006). Clinical manifestations of mannan-binding lectin deficiency. *Mol Immunol*, **43**, 86–96.

Walport MJ (2001). Complement. First part. *N Engl J Med*, **344**, 1058–66.

Walport MJ (2001). Complement. Second part. *N Engl J Med*, **344**, 1140–4.

5.1.3 Adaptive immunity

Paul Klenerman

Essentials

Following the innate immune response, which acts very rapidly, the adaptive immune response plays a critical role in host defence against infectious disease. Unlike the innate response, which is triggered by pattern recognition of pathogens, i.e. features that are common to many bacteria or viruses, the adaptive response is triggered by structural features—known as antigens or epitopes—that are typically unique to a single organism.

Cells involved in the adaptive immune response—these are B lymphocytes and T lymphocytes, the latter divided into CD4+ (helper) and CD8+ (cytotoxic) populations. All of these lymphocyte subsets can potentially respond to a huge variety of antigens through the generation of great diversity in their antigen receptors (T-cell receptors and B-cell receptors), some of which is genetically encoded, but much is created by recombination between gene segments as the receptors are expressed.

Recognition of antigens—(1) B cells—a membrane-bound form of the soluble antibody molecules that the cell is destined to secrete acts as the B-cell receptor, which can bind to a range of antigens, including nonprotein antigens such as carbohydrates. (2) T cells—these can only survey antigens that have been cleaved to short peptides and presented on surface of cells bound in the groove of the hugely diverse MHC class I and class II molecules. Dendritic cells have a central role since they can not only present the peptides efficiently, but also provide critical extra signalling in the form of specialized 'costimulatory' surface molecules and soluble cytokines.

Response to antigens—once T cell and B cells have been triggered by antigen, they proliferate rapidly and display a range of effector functions. (1) B cells—secrete antibodies, initially in the form of immunoglobulin M (IgM), but subsequently 'class switching' to IgG. (2) T cells—(a) CD8+ T cells—response includes migration to sites of infection, killing of infected cells, and secretion of soluble mediators; (b) CD4+ T cells—play a key role in providing 'help' for B cells, e.g. in class switching, 'help' for proliferation of CD8+ T cells, and also conditioning of dendritic cells. CD4+ T cells which secrete a panel of cytokines promoting cell mediated immunity (such as interferon-γ (IFNγ)) are described as Th1 (T helper 1), while others which secrete cytokines promoting B-cell functions (such as interleukin 4 (IL-4)) are Th2. and a third group which secrete IL-17 are termed Th17.

Immunological memory—once an infection is contained, the B- and T-cell populations contract and enter a phase of immunological 'memory'. These memory populations are found largely in lymph nodes, although some 'effector memory' T cells may be found in nonlymphoid organs (e.g. liver). They are retained long term at much higher cell frequencies than are found in an unexposed person, and can respond to re-encounter with antigen with very rapid proliferation and effector function.

Regulation of immune responses—the functions of the adaptive immune system are tightly regulated to limit immune-mediated pathology. T cells develop initially within the thymus, where those which recognize host ('self') antigens are eliminated ('central tolerance'). Self-reactive T cells may be further controlled in the periphery through a variety of mechanisms, including generation of a set of 'regulatory' T cells (Tregs). However, this multilayered control sometimes breaks down, thereby allowing pathological responses to harmless antigens (hypersensitivity) or self-antigens (autoreactivity), and pathogens such as HIV may exploit down-regulatory mechanisms to allow their long-term persistence in the body.

Clinical impact of understanding the adaptive immune system—this may be harnessed to generate novel diagnostics, therapies (e.g. monoclonal antibodies) and vaccines, but many challenges remain in translating our increasing knowledge about molecular control of adaptive immunity into protection against complex persistent infections.

Introduction

The adaptive immune response is distinguished from the innate immune response by two main features: its capacity to respond flexibly to new, previously unencountered antigens (antigenic specificity) and its enhanced capacity to respond to previously encountered antigens (immunological memory). These two features have provided the focus for much research attention, from the time of Jenner, through Pasteur onwards. In recent years, the molecular basis for these phenomena has become much better understood.

Historically, innate and adaptive immune responses have often been treated as separate, with the latter being considered more 'advanced', because of its flexibility. It is now clear this not the case. Innate immune responses provide the essential early controls and conditioning required for an adaptive immune response to function. This arises because of the differential speed of the two responses. Innate responses occur within minutes or hours of infection, whereas initiation of effective adaptive immunity may take days. Not only do mediators such as type I interferons have direct antiviral effects, but they also activate antigen presentation pathways and thus have a critical role in priming the adaptive immune response. Thus the adaptive immune response to a given antigen may be vigorous or absent depending on the quality of innate signalling that accompanies it.

The immune response evolved to deal with pathogens, of which viruses are the best examples. This is the focus of this chapter, but the same responses against self-, allo- or environmental antigens lead to auto-immunity (Chapter 5.4), transplant rejection (Chapter 5.5) and hypersensitivity/allergy (Chapter 5.3).

Antigen specificity of adaptive immune responses

Antigen is a word with a long history, originally associated with antibody binding, but currently used broadly to mean anything to which B or T cells can respond. An alternative description is 'immunogen'. Largely these are protein structures, and in the case of T cells short peptides, but for B cells the targets may be much more diverse. If a large molecule, such as influenza matrix protein, is defined as the antigen, the small regions within it which are recognized by the cells of the adaptive immune response are termed 'epitopes'.

Antigen recognition by T cells

T cells are divided simply into two lineages, CD4+ T cells (or T helper, Th cells), and CD8+ T cells (or cytotoxic T cells). These have distinct, if overlapping functions, but crucially they recognize antigen delivered through distinct pathways. Both sets of T cells can recognize antigen only if it is presented by specific host major histocompatibility (MHC) molecules at the cell surface. These molecules vary substantially between individuals, the basis of MHC restriction of the capacity of T cells to recognize a given antigen when presented by a specific MHC molecule.

Antigen presentation to CD8+ T cells

CD8+ T cells recognize antigen presented largely from intracellular compartments. In the case of a virus infection, this means newly synthesized viral proteins can be presented on the surface of an infected cell (Fig. 5.1.3.1).

The proteasome

Proteins destined for the antigen presentation pathway are tagged with ubiquitin and delivered to the cellular proteasome, a multi-component proteolytic complex present constitutively in all cells (although modified under inflammatory conditions to an immunoproteasome). The outputs from these proteasomes are sets of short peptides derived by specific cleavage of the larger input protein. Typically, these are 9 to 11 amino acids in length. Further peptide 'trimming' may occur at later stages.

Peptide transport

The next stage of antigen presentation is transport through an ATP-dependent peptide transporter (TAP, transporters associated with antigen processing) into the endoplasmic reticulum. Patients with genetically deficient TAP transporters have been described, which fail to present peptides at their cell surfaces bound to MHC class I molecules (see below). Their clinical presentation is with bacterial and vasculitic disease and they show overactivated natural killer (NK) cells.

Binding to MHC class I

The next step for antigenic peptides is loading on to an MHC class I molecule. These comprise a heavy chain with three major extracellular domains (α_{1-3}), which dimerizes with an invariant light chain β_2-microglobulin (β_2m). The α_3 domain acts as a membrane-proximal stalk, which provides the binding site for β_2m, and stability for the complex.

The α_1 and α_2 domains form a groove with closed ends lying above the stalk. Peptides lie stretched out lengthways in the groove, with two to four specific amino acid residues bound into 'pockets'

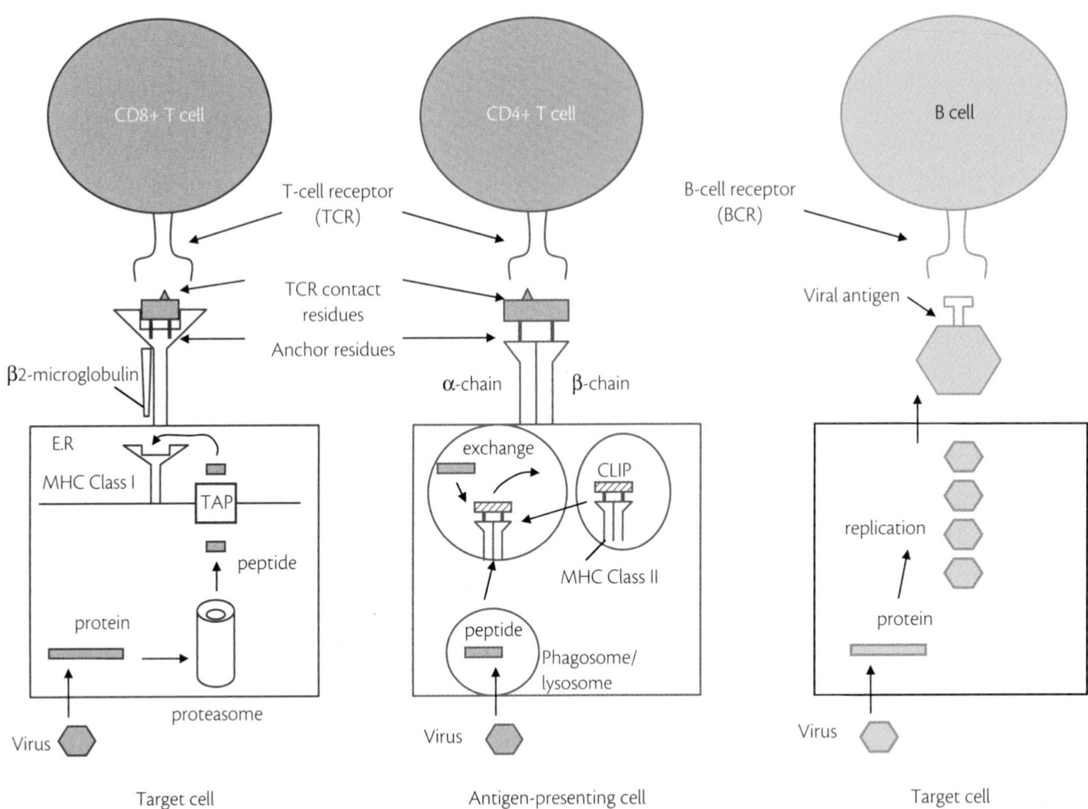

Fig. 5.1.3.1 Antigen presentation to T and B cells. A viral antigen is used as an example. Peptides are generated in infected (target) cells and in the case of class I transported to the endoplasmic reticulum (ER) via the TAP (transporters associated with antigen processing) complex. CD4+ T cells are triggered by professional antigen presenting cells, while B cells engage antigen directly.

in the floor. These act as 'anchors' and provide stability for the peptide–MHC interaction. Only specific amino acids can form anchor residues in any given MHC class I molecule. As a result, many peptides cleaved from a given protein will not be presented by host MHC molecules and the cellular immune system is essentially 'blind' to these. The other nonanchor amino acids within the peptide are displayed above the lips of the groove and are available for binding by the T-cell receptor.

Recognition by the T-cell receptor

The T-cell receptor (TCR) is the molecule responsible for sensitive and specific recognition of peptide–MHC complexes by T cells. TCRs are made up of pairs of chains—either α and β chains or γ and δ chains. TCRs comprising α and β chains (αβ T cells) are able to recognize MHC class I molecules through an interaction of low avidity but high specificity. Cocrystallization studies of a limited number of molecules have revealed that the tips of the TCR αβ complex interact in a diagonal fashion with the top surface of the MHC class I–peptide complex. Thus the strength of the interaction comes not only from binding of the TCR to the available peptide residues, but also from binding to the MHC class I molecule. This encapsulates the fundamental principle of the cellular immune response. The MHC molecule provides the central focus (restriction), but the peptide provides the essential specificity. Even subtle changes in the peptide sequence such as conservative amino acid exchanges (e.g. lysine to arginine) can substantially change the strength of the TCR interaction and radically affect the recognition by the T cell, a feature that has been fully exploited by variable viruses such as HIV (Chapter 7.5.25).

T-cells in which the TCR comprises γδ chain (γδ T cells) make up around 5% of the normal human T-cell pool in blood, although they may be concentrated in tissues. The molecular targets of such cells are, however, not fully established. These include relatively conserved molecules, and non-protein antigens and functionally γδ T cells are thought to play a role more aligned with innate immune responses.

Antigen presentation to CD4+ T-cells

Like CD8+ T cells, CD4+ T cells also survey antigens as peptides presented on the cell surface through MHC molecules. Unlike CD8+ T cells, these peptides are not principally derived from cytosolic antigens (Fig. 5.1.3.1). Two key points must be noted. First, while MHC class I molecules are present on virtually all cells, class II molecules are normally present on only a limited number of cell types. Secondly, the pathway requires specific machinery for soluble or particulate antigen outside the cell to be taken into the cellular endosome, which is notably greater in phagocytic cells. The recently discovered pathway of 'autophagy' may also provide a route into the class II pathway for intracellular proteins.

MHC class II molecules

Proteins within the endosome, after fusion with lysosomes, are degraded to peptides, which subsequently bind MHC class II molecules. These are polymorphic dimeric molecules, like class I, but differ in that both α and β chains are equal partners in peptide binding and presentation. An important difference from MHC class I is that the ends of the groove are open, allowing longer peptides to be bound (12–15 residues).

MHC class II molecules initially bind an 'invariant chain' (CLIP) in the endoplasmic reticulum which protects the binding groove. In the lysosome/endosome fusion compartment, the invariant chain is exchanged for peptides that can specifically bind into the groove if they possess the key anchor residues. Class II–peptide complexes are then presented at the surface of the cell, and can be recognized by specific CD4+ T cells.

Antigen recognition by B cells

Unlike T cells, which can only survey peptide antigens displayed on cells bound to MHC molecules, the range of antigens which can be bound by B cells and antibodies is much more diverse and includes non-protein antigens, such as carbohydrates. Recognition by B cells occurs through the B-cell receptor, a membrane-bound form of the soluble antibody molecules that the cell is destined to secrete (Fig. 5.1.3.1). The basic structure of an antibody (immunoglobulin G, IgG, in this case) is illustrated in Fig. 5.1.3.2. Essentially each antibody unit comprises one heavy (H) and one light (L) chain. Despite the functional differences from T cells, the basic structure of the TCR and the BCR/Ig is quite similar. The TCR resembles the key antigen-recognizing subunit of the Ig known as a Fab fragment.

Because B cells can react to intact antigen, no specific antigen presenting pathway is required (Fig. 5.1.3.1). However, there are similarities with T cell recognition of antigen, such as the size of the epitope recognized. Detailed mapping studies, using antigens such as influenza haemagglutinin, have revealed that the sites of B-cell recognition are discrete, each comprising less then 10 amino acids. Similar studies of carbohydrate antigens reveal a footprint of around seven sugars. Small synthetic molecules, typically described as haptens (haptenes), can also act as B cell targets but priming occurs only if they are linked to a conventional protein antigen.

One important difference from the peptide antigens recognized by T cells is that B cell epitopes may be conformational. This means that the amino acids which interact with the B-cell receptor need not be in a continuous sequence, but may come together as the protein folds. Other B cell responses may be directed against so-called 'linear' epitopes, in which case they can be mimicked by a shorter peptide. Perhaps more important functionally is the definition of epitopes that, when bound, lead to neutralization of a virus (i.e. loss of the capacity of the virion to enter a cell). Typically these epitopes occur on viral glycoproteins required for binding cellular entry receptors. The development of such neutralizing antibodies is the basis for many vaccines and for sterilizing immunity.

Generation of diversity within the immune system

The above discussion gives some indication of the nature of antigens and the common features of their presentation to T and B cells. However, the key feature of the system is its huge adaptability to diverse antigens. How is this diversity of antigen receptors generated?

Generation of diverse T-cell receptors

T-cell receptor diversity arises initially through genetically encoded variation, and is hugely expanded through combinatorial processes (Fig. 5.1.3.3). First, consider the β chain destined to become part of a TCR αβ complex. The genetic organization of this chain includes a variable (V), a diversity (D), and a joining (J) segment, which are spliced and recombined with a constant (C) chain to form the final sequence. The organization is similar for the α chain, but with the absence of the small D segment. The diversity arises first from

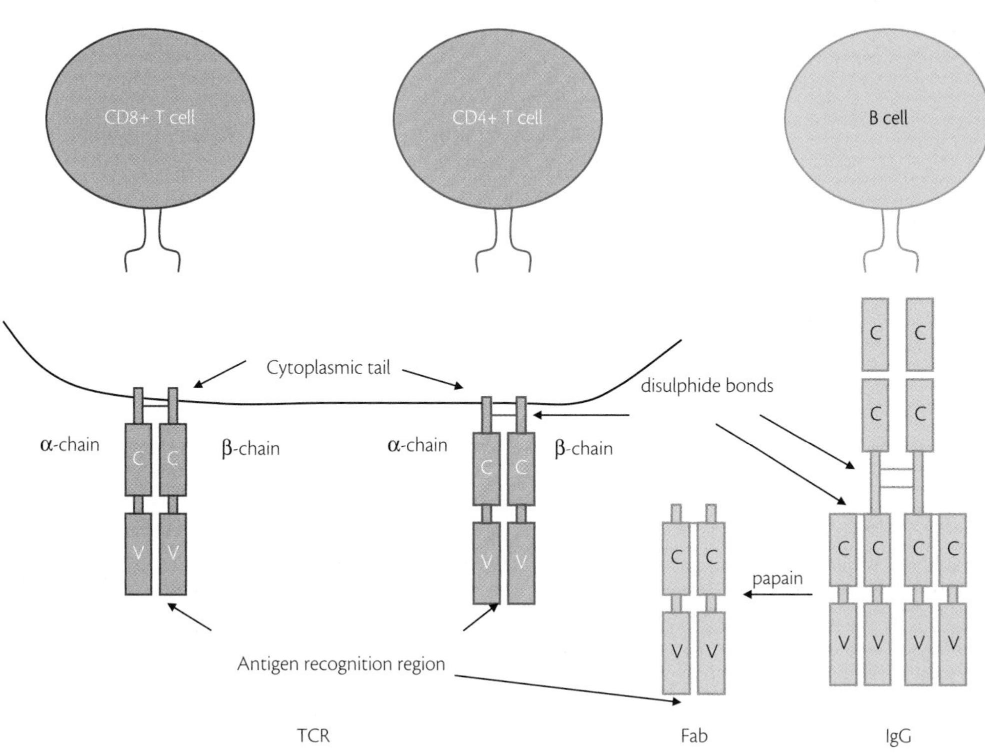

Fig. 5.1.3.2 Antigen binding by T and B cells. The T-cell receptor (TCR) is composed of two chains, bound by disulphide bonds, with antigen recognition occurring in a variable region. This is analogous to the variable region of an immunoglobulin molecule (IgG is illustrated here); the TCR-equivalent region (Fab fragment) may be cleaved from the full molecule using papain.

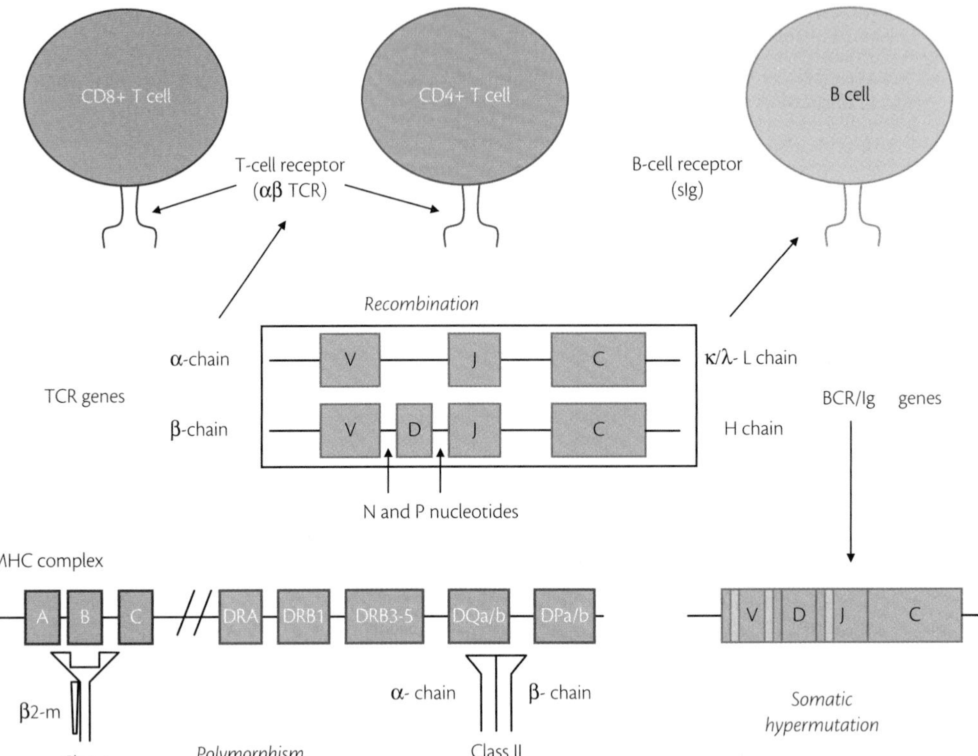

Fig. 5.1.3.3 Generation of diversity in the immune system. Both TCRs and BCRs are generated through recombination. For Ig H chains there are 65, 27, and 8, V, D, and J genes encoded in the germ line respectively. Somatic hypermutation occurs only in B cells. The MHC complex is highly polymorphic—the class II genes actually lie upstream of the class I genes on chromosome 6. DRA encodes the α chain which is conserved and pairs with polymorphic β chains from the DRB1 locus.

the fact that the V, D, and J regions exist in multiple copies, each distinct. It is expanded by the process of recombination whereby, in the process of generating a new T cell from a precursor, any combination of V, D, and J can be used to generate the new β chain. During this process, the action of the terminal deoxynucleotide transferase enzyme creates further diversity at junctions. Since α and β chains recombine independently, further diversity is generated as these form heterodimers. It has been estimated that this process could generate 10^{14} distinct T-cell receptors.

Table 5.1.3.1 Diversity of immunoglobulin types. The different immunoglobulins have different biological properties, some of which are illustrated here. There are further subtypes of the IgG classes

Isotype	H+L Chains	M_r (kDa)	Serum conc. (mg/ml)	$t_{1/2}$ (days)	C1q bound	Placental transport	Mast-cell binding
IgG1	2+2	146	9	21	+	+	±
IgG2	2+2	146	3	20	+	+	-
IgG3	2+2	165	1	7	+	+	±
IgG4	2+2	146	0.5	21	–	+	±
IgM	10+10	970	1.2	5	+	–	–
IgA1	2+2	160	2	6	–	–	–
IgA2	2+2	160	0.5	–	–	–	–
sIgA	4+4	405	0.5	–	–	–	–
IgD	2+2	170	0.06	3	–	–	–
IgE	2+2	190	0.0002	3	–	–	++

sIgA, secretory IgA; this also contains a J chain linking the multimeric structure.

Diversity of B-cell receptors and antibody

The generation of diversity is similar to that of the TCR α and β chains described above (Fig. 5.1.3.3). V, D, and J regions exist in multiple copies which, as the B cell develops, are recombined randomly (D regions are only present in the H chain), incorporating additional diversity as this occurs. Further variability is introduced as two loci for the generation of light chains exist, producing either κ or λ chains. However, in any given cell, only one heavy and one light chain is used, a process known as allelic exclusion.

The process above allows for a huge variability in the key regions which act as binding sites, within the 'variable' domain at the N-terminus. However, there is an additional biological variation between antibodies, not dependent on their specificity, which is provided by further recombination with a constant region (Table 5.1.3.1). In the heavy chain locus, nine potential C chains can be used to create a palette of diverse antibody types. For the heavy chains, the initial constant (C) chain used is μ, leading to the creation of an early IgM antibody in typical immune responses. Subsequent class switching, which is a one-way process through further recombination events, may lead to use of any of the other chains. This switching event is largely but not exclusively determined by T-cell help and cytokines. The constant regions determine critical factors in the distribution of the antibodies. Notably, only IgG can cross the placenta and protect the fetus, but IgA is secreted across epithelial membranes, including into breast milk, for protection of the newborn.

Finally, an important process which creates further diversity, and one which distinguishes B cells from T cells, is the emergence of somatic hypermutation. Once B cells have developed during an initial immune response, the action of the mutagenic enzyme AID within the hypervariable regions leads to the creation of somatic mutants. The B-cell receptors of some of these mutant clones may

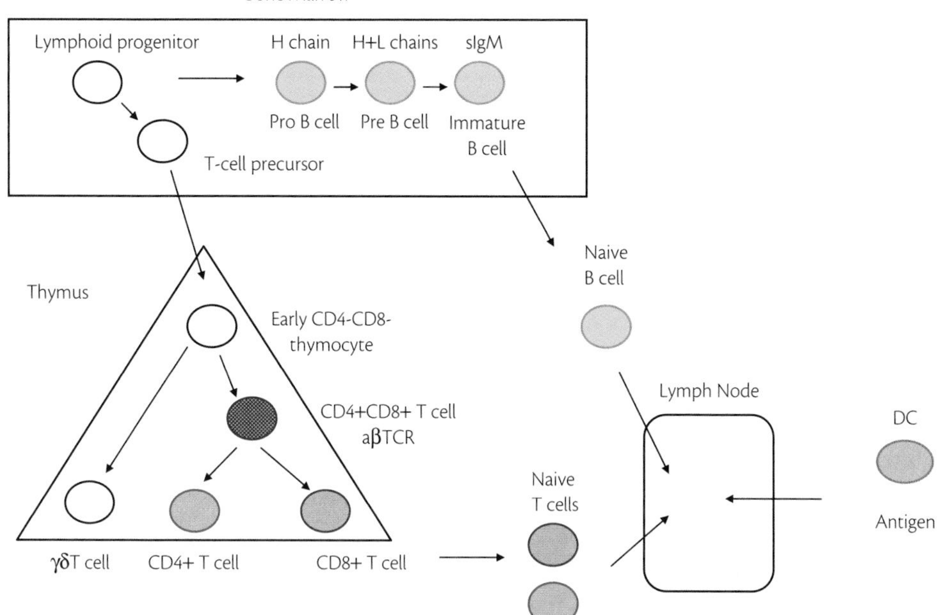

Fig. 5.1.3.4 Generation of a naive B- and T-cell repertoire. T- and B-cell precursors are generated in the bone marrow, but T-cell development occurs in the thymus. This includes negative selection and more than 90% of thymocytes die through apoptosis. Deletion and anergy of autoreactive immature B cells occur in the bone marrow.

have increased avidity for their original antigen, and are further selected. This molecular process is observed functionally by affinity maturation of the antibody response over time.

Diversity among MHC molecules

Class I molecules

These molecules provide the key platforms for antigen presentation, but only a small number of peptides can bind any given class I molecule, potentially limiting the T-cell response. This limitation has been solved for human MHC molecules (human leucocyte antigens, HLA) first by reduplication of these genes, such that for class I, there are three loci—A, B, and C (Fig. 5.1.3.2). However, more important, at each locus there exists a huge range of alleles or HLA types, which are represented at varying frequencies in different populations. In Western populations the commonest A allele is HLA A*0201, which occurs in up to 50% of individuals, but there are at least 20 other A types, and multiple subtypes, all of which are much less common. The B locus is even more diverse. Both A and B molecules play important roles in presenting antigens to T cells. HLA-C molecules are of more limited diversity, and play a role in signalling to NK cells.

Class II molecules

The principles are similar for HLA class II, although there are four loci, the most diverse of which is *DRB1*, encoding the β chain of a range of DR molecules (the α chain is invariant). The next locus encodes only three alleles, *DRB3*, *4* and *5* (previously *DR51*, *52*, and *53*). DR molecules are highly expressed on antigen-presenting cells and are restricting elements for important CD4+ T-cell epitopes. *DQ* and *DP* are also polymorphic loci, although the latter is less so, and is also expressed in lower amounts.

Thus an antigen-presenting cell will present potentially six different class I molecules and eight different HLA class II molecules, each binding distinct peptides from a given antigen. However, these molecules are not always inherited independently, since they are often in strong linkage disequilibrium.

Adaptive immune responses and the basis of immunological memory

The above discussion has outlined the molecular basis for antigen recognition, but how is this process coordinated in order to establish and maintain immune responses?

The naive state

Lymphocytes are generated from common lymphoid progenitors within the bone marrow and undergo a series of maturation steps to create naive B and T cells (Fig. 5.1.3.4). Naive in this context means ready to respond functionally to an as yet unencountered antigen. Reaching this stage requires education within the thymus (for T cells) and bone marrow (for B cells).

T-cell development

T-cell education occurs in the thymus, through interaction of thymocytes with specialized thymic cells (cortical epithelial cells and bone marrow derived cells). These present a range of self antigens, including nonthymic tissue-specific antigens (e.g. from pancreas), the expression of which is liberated by the *AIRE* gene.

The process of thymic development is initially similar for CD4+ and CD8+ thymocytes, which pass through a CD4+CD8+ phase, before down-regulating either receptor. Those that interact strongly with host MHC and self peptides receive signals which lead to elimination through a process termed negative selection. Thymocytes which fail to interact with host MHC molecules do not receive sufficient signals to survive and thus many thymocytes are eliminated at this stage. Positively selected CD8+ or CD4+ T cells are therefore those that interact weakly with MHC–self peptide complexes (class I or II respectively), providing a broad but non-self-reactive naive repertoire.

B-cell development

Early B-cell development within the bone marrow occurs through pro- and pre-B cell stages during which time immunoglobulin

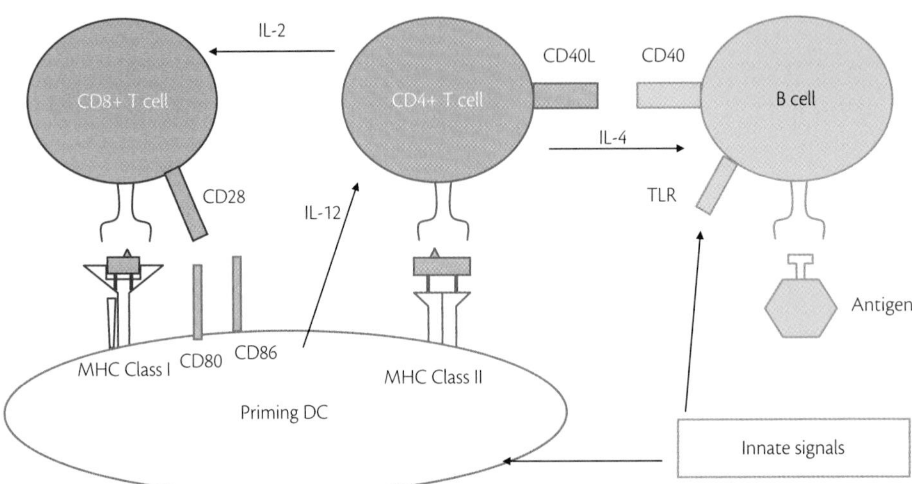

Fig. 5.1.3.5 Priming of naive B and T cells. Priming of T cells occurs through antigen presentation by a mature DC. Signals for maturation include innate signalling and also CD40L signals from primed T cells (not shown for the DC, but also occurring on B cells). A large number of other costimulatory molecules, and regulatory molecules are also expressed. Expression of these strongly modifies the quality of the T-cell response and thus the B-cell response.

genes are rearranged. Immature B cells possess rearranged surface IgM. Self-reactive B cells may be eliminated at this stage through clonal deletion, or induction of an anergic state. Further B cell maturation towards functional antibody-secreting cells occurs within lymphoid follicles.

Lymphocyte localization

Naive lymphocytes are found in blood and in lymphoid organs (spleen, lymph nodes, and the gut-associated lymphoid tissue or GALT). Within lymph nodes, the B and T cells segregate into the primary follicles and paracortex respectively (Fig. 5.1.3.4). The recirculation and organization of these cells is important in understanding the restrictions on priming of immune responses. Naive T cells do not home to tissues, even inflamed tissues. This is because their homing receptors and chemokine receptors (most importantly CD62L, or L-selectin, and CCR7) allow for entry through high endothelial venules into lymphoid organs. From there they can recirculate back into the blood via the efferent lymphatics. Since they cannot meet antigen at a peripheral site, it is therefore essential that antigen is delivered appropriately to the lymph node, and this is achieved by the dendritic cell (DC).

Priming of an immune response

DCs are the most important antigen-presenting cells as they possess not only the appropriate class I and class II molecules, but three further important biological features. First, within tissue, they are very efficient at taking up antigen and delivering this to the class II pathway. Some antigen may enter the cytosol and thus the class I pathway through a process known as cross-presentation. Secondly, they are mobile, and once antigen is taken up, they are able to migrate through chemokine signalling through afferent lymphatics to local lymph nodes. Thirdly, they possess an array of cell surface molecules and soluble mediators which allow for primary activation (priming) of naive T cells. All three of these functions are strongly influenced by local innate immune signalling including soluble factors such as interferon (IFN)-α, or direct signalling through TLRs that promote 'maturation' of the DC, improving its priming ability.

T-cell priming requires TCR interaction with cognate MHC–peptide. However, the TCR triggering requires support through signals from other cell surface molecules. A vast array of these is present, but some of the most important are shown in Fig. 5.1.3.5, including the interaction between CD28 on the T cell, with CD80/86 on the DC. Additionally soluble cytokines (e.g. interleukin (IL)-12) are secreted by the DC, which signal through cytokine receptors on the T cell to promote maturation to a full effector cell.

Triggering within the T cell requires the integration of all of these signals for full activation. Important signalling pathways within the cell include a cascade of tyrosine kinases starting at the TCR CD3 complex. Critical motifs on the cytoplasmic tails of signalling molecules (immunoreceptor tyrosine-based activatory motifs, ITAMs) initiate these cascades. Downstream, a number of cellular pathways are involved leading to a calcium flux and induction of key transcription factors such as NFAT, NF-κB, and AP-1. Similar intracellular pathways are involved in B-cell triggering.

T-cell effector functions

Proliferation

The most important consequence of T-cell priming is cellular proliferation. This is crucial because while there is huge diversity amongst the naive repertoire, the precursor frequency is extremely low, less than 1 in 10^6. Rapid clonal proliferation of responding CD4+ and CD8+ T cell may be observed, but particularly the latter. CD8+ T cell responses to specific epitopes may reach 20 to 50% of the CD8+ T cell pool within a few days of encounter with viruses such as Epstein–Barr virus (EBV).

Homing

A second key feature of T-cell activation is altered homing potential. Instead of homing to lymphoid tissue, these cells refocus their attention on peripheral organs (Fig. 5.1.3.6). They lose expression of CD62L and CCR7 and gain expression of chemokine receptors such as CCR5, which allow for distribution to inflamed sites (CCR5 is also the coreceptor for HIV entry). A diaspora of such cells therefore occurs to many organs, where innate mediators such as macrophages may secrete appropriate chemokines—a family of small molecules which play a crucial role in regulating cellular migration. A number of other cell surface receptors change in primed cells; one useful marker is CD45, which switches isoform from RA to RO.

CD8+ T-cell functions

These functions are broadly divided into killing and secretory. Killing of target cells occurs by two major means. (1) Lytic function

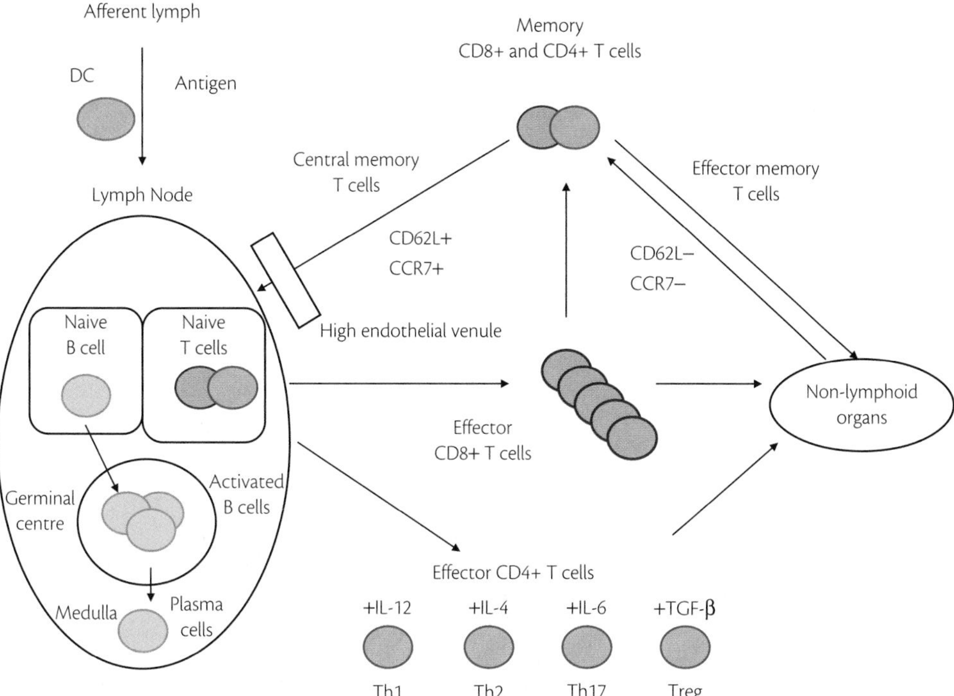

Fig. 5.1.3.6 Induction and maintenance of memory responses. Effector T-cell populations migrate from the lymph node and may enter nonlymphoid tissue. Subsequently they may revert to a central memory pool, in the absence of further antigenic encounter, or retain some effector functions and continue recirculating through nonlymphoid organs (effector memory).

is mediated through secretion of lytic granules, specialized secretory lysosomes which contain perforin, and a set of granzymes. When CD8+ T cells encounter a target cell, the molecules at the contact point reorganize to form an immunological synapse. Lytic granules are released across the synapse and lead to disruption of the target cell membrane and apoptosis. (2) Killing may also occur through interaction of Fas Ligand (FasL) on the CD8+ T cell with Fas on the appropriate target, leading to apoptosis.

CD8+ T cells also secrete a range of cytokines, the most important of which is IFN-γ, which has pro-inflammatory and antiviral effects. They may also secrete tumour necrosis factor (TNFα), interleukins, and chemokines. Some of the latter serve to attract further lymphocytes; they may also have important inhibitory effects on HIV entry, as they compete for binding to key entry receptors for the virus.

Overall these functions are critical in the control of intracellular pathogens such as viruses. Mice where CD8+ T cells are deficient (e.g. CD8 or perforin knockout) are susceptible to infection with lymphocytic choriomeningitis virus (LCMV). Similar inferences are made for human persistent virus infections. MHC class I genes such as HLA B27 and B57 are associated with protection against both HIV and HCV, probably through promoting efficient antiviral CD8+ T cell responses.

CD4+ T-cell functions

CD4+ T cells provide essential help for other cell types such as CD8+ T cells, B cells, DCs, and macrophages. This is largely through cytokine secretion, but one important interaction, through CD40L/CD40, serves as a further important maturation signal for DCs. The type of cytokines secreted by the priming DC, in turn influenced by the original innate signalling, has an important influence on the quality of the CD4+ T cell. Broadly, CD4+ T cells can mature in the direction of Th1 cells (which secrete IFN-γ and IL-2), or Th2 cells, which secrete IL-4, IL-5, IL-10, and IL-13. The former are critical in responses against intracellular pathogens such as viruses and mycobacteria, the latter are more involved in B-cell immunoglobulin switching, including IgE production and eosinophilia. A third effector subset, recently described, are cells secreting IL-17 (Th17 cells). Their evolution is driven by IL-6 and IL-23 and has been linked to autoimmunity and immunopathology. Still further subsets of CD4+ T cells with 'regulatory' roles can also emerge (see below).

Overall, CD4+ T cells play a central role in host defence, and, in their absence, there is failure of CD8+-mediated immunity, generation of new antibody responses, and macrophage-mediated immunity, creating susceptibility to viruses, mycobacteria, and tumours. This is most evident in the case of HIV, where CD4+ T-cell populations are depleted. Genetically determined variation in CD4+ T-cell responses plays a major role in host defence and also autoimmunity, e.g. the association of specific HLA class II alleles with protection and susceptibility to viral hepatitis.

Priming and functions of B cells

As with T cells, full activation of B cells requires encounter with antigen binding the B-cell receptor (BCR) on the lymphocyte surface, but also further signals. These can be provided through innate signalling via TLRs, but additionally signals from CD4+ T cells, both cell:cell (CD40L/CD40) and soluble (IL-4). Mutations in the gene for CD40L result in a failure of class switching and presents clinically as the hyper-IgM syndrome.

B cells also undergo clonal proliferation upon appropriate signalling, and move from the state of naive B cell, through lymphoblast and plasmablast to plasma cell (Fig. 5.1.3.6). Unlike T cells, a diaspora through the body is not seen, but reorganization within the lymph node occurs. Accumulation of B cells during an immune response leads to generation of a secondary follicle, containing additionally CD4+ T cells. Ultimately immunoglobulin secreting plasma cells migrate to cords within the medulla (and also bone marrow).

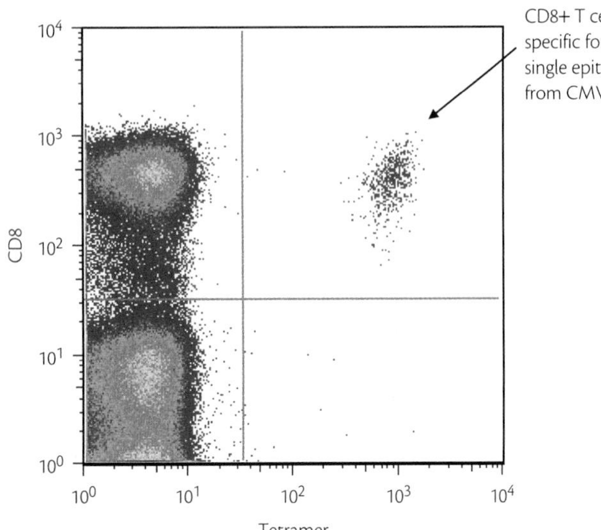

Fig. 5.1.3.7 Direct *ex vivo* evaluation of human antigen specific T cells using MHC class I peptide tetramers. The example is a healthy donor with a memory response to CMV. The peptide is derived from pp. 65 and the HLA restriction is A2. Approximately 1% of CD8+ T cells are visible after staining, using a flow cytometer.
Courtesy of Alison Turner.

As well as secreting antibody, B cells have roles as antigen presenting cells. They express MHC class II and can take up antigen, most efficiently cognate antigen via their BCR, for presentation to CD4+ T cells. They also secrete cytokines, including IL-10, which has an immunoregulatory role.

Generation and maintenance of memory

Once an immune response has been initiated, the first acute phase may last days to weeks, depending on the type of challenge, but typically the antigen is controlled through the effector mechanisms outlined above. Thus the expanded populations seen in the acute phase collapse down to smaller levels, although still much greater than seen previously. This elevated precursor frequency is the hallmark of immunological memory.

Central memory

For antigens that are not re-encountered or do not persist, memory T-cell pools over time lose their capacity for immediate effector functions (e.g. secretion of perforin), and their tendency to home to organs. They may regain expression of CD62L and CCR7 and home to lymph nodes (Fig. 5.1.3.6). These populations are termed *central memory*. They retain the capacity to respond very rapidly to antigen (within hours), proliferate, and regenerate effector populations. Similar features apply to memory B-cell populations.

Effector memory

For antigens which persist or are re-encountered, 'memory' populations exist which retain some features of effector cells (e.g. expression of perforin), and are found distributed throughout organs. These are termed effector memory cells and are thought to provide more immediate protective function. Within these pools, there is still further variation between cells which are considered more or less 'mature' as judged by a range of surface and intracellular markers which may be lost or gained over time. The net result of this is that such cells receive less costimulation (e.g via CD28) and more inhibitory signals (via NK-type receptors). The proportion of such cells varies in different infections, with CMV-specific memory CD8+ T cells showing the most mature phenotype, as well as the largest populations (often 1–10% of CD8+ T cells specific for a single epitope; Fig. 5.1.3.7).

Down-regulation of the immune responses

The focus so far has been on the initiation of responses against pathogens, but these responses must also be controlled to limit immune mediated pathology. Responses against self-antigens must also be minimized. The limitation of responses against self is termed tolerance, but many of the same mechanisms also limit responses against pathogens. These issues are briefly outlined below but also discussed further in Chapter 5.5 on transplantation and Chapter 5.4 on autoimmunity.

Mechanisms of T-cell tolerance

As discussed earlier, negative selection within the thymus serves to delete many autoreactive T cells. This process of central tolerance is, however, leaky and further peripheral tolerance mechanisms are required.

First, since naive T-cell priming occurs predominantly within lymphoid tissue, failure of antigen to reach this tissue provides an important checkpoint. This has been described as 'ignorance' and may be relevant so-called immune privileged sites, or rare antigens.

Secondly, anergy may occur through triggering of a T cell via its T-cell receptor, without costimulation (via cell surface signals and cytokines). Such anergic cells subsequently fail to respond to antigen. This may occur if the antigen is encountered on a non-professional antigen presenting cell that lacks costimulatory capacity. Another important contributor to anergy may be encounter of T cells with DCs which have not been fully activated. Antigens encountered without appropriate inflammatory or 'danger' signals (e.g. through TLRs) may lead to self-tolerance. The corollary of this is that self antigens encountered under conditions of 'danger' may prime autoreactive responses.

Thirdly, studies from the 1970s and 1980s had identified so-called suppressor T-cell activity, linked to the CD8+ T cell subset, but the failure to fully define these cells and their ligand brought this mechanism of regulation into disrepute. However, in the 1990s, the discovery of CD4+ T cell subsets with a regulatory role (Tregs) was made more robust by the linkage to expression of a specific gene, the forkhead transcription factor *FOXP3*. Such regulatory subsets may be generated in the thymus against self antigens (natural Tregs) or after antigen/cytokine stimulation (adaptive Tregs). The modes of action include secretion of TGFβ and IL-10, and also contact-dependent mechanisms.

Finally, downregulation may also be achieved through upregulation of inhibitory molecules on activated T cells. These include specific inhibitory molecules such as CTLA-4 and PD-1 (programmed death 1), which bind specific ligands on target cells or DCs, causing a down-regulation of T-cell triggering. Other direct cellular mechanisms include expression on NK inhibitory receptors (e.g. a range of killer inhibitory receptors, KIRs) on CD8+ T cells. Many such inhibitory molecules act through so-called immunoreceptor tyrosine-based inhibitory motifs (ITIMs) which recruit phosphatases and compete with ITAMs.

Mechanisms of B-cell tolerance

Since B cells do not receive education regarding self in the thymus, a potential self-reactive antibody repertoire is being generated continuously. One important mechanism for containing this is through the requirement for T-cell help for full maturation of antibody responses—in other words a crucial mechanism for B-cell tolerance is induction and maintenance of CD4+ T-cell tolerance.

The use of transgenic mouse models, where both a model antigen and antigen-specific antibody are expressed (classically hen egg lysozme, HEL) has shed important light on other mechanisms of B-cell tolerance. As they mature, B cells encountering self antigens may be controlled through deletion and anergy, as for T cells, or later suffer exclusion from germinal centres. Unlike T cells, autoreactive B cells get a second chance to rearrange their immunoglobulin genes through a process of receptor editing. This may rescue the B cell and allow further normal maturation.

Regulatory mechanisms and immune responses to pathogens

Induction of T-cell tolerance at high levels of viral replication has been observed in murine models and is probably occurring to some extent in chronic hepatitis B (HBV), hepatitis C (HCV), and HIV infection. Functional failure or anergy of T-cell responses under such conditions is termed T-cell exhaustion, and ultimately there may be deletion of such cells. It may be that such mechanisms have evolved to avoid potentially lethal immunopathology, e.g. in brain or liver, especially in noncytopathic virus infections.

Induction of Tregs may play an important role in persistent infection and such populations have been implicated in tuberculosis, leishmania, HCV, and HIV. To what extent they are a cause or consequence of persistent infection remains to be established. Up-regulation of PD-1 and IL-10 have been similarly implicated.

Failure of regulation of responses

The mechanisms of tolerance outlined above may limit self-reactivity, and also responses against pathogens. However, in all responses to pathogens, some immune-mediated pathology may occur as in acute hepatitis B or C. In most circumstances the benefit of the protective response outweighs the short-term cost of the tissue damage. However, immune mediated pathology can occur against harmless environmental antigens, where there is no net benefit and here it is termed hypersensitivity, or allergy (in the case of IgE-mediated responses; see Chapter 5.3). The underlying immunological mechanisms for this (and also for autoimmunity) are identical to those against pathogens. Classically they are divided into four forms, using the criteria of Coombs.

- Type I hypersensitivity describes immediate responses mediated by IgE and mast cells and is clinically the most critical (including anaphylactic responses to insect venom and asthma). Underlying this is a T-cell response predominated by Th2 cells.
- Type II responses are based on antibody binding antigen on the cell surface and fixation of complement, for example in red-cell or platelet sensitizing syndromes induced by drugs (e.g. penicillin).
- Type III responses involve antibody binding soluble antigen (e.g. drugs or therapeutic anserum) to form complexes. These may again fix complement in tissues leading to an Arthus reaction, or lead to a more generalized syndrome described as serum sickness. Both type II and III responses are mediated by IgG antibodies.
- Type IV responses are cell mediated, and thus delayed, requiring activation and migration of memory T cells. The best example of this is in the tuberculin test.

Harnessing adaptive immune responses

Diagnostics

B cells

The use of antibody induction to track exposure to specific pathogens relies on the specificity of responses. Early responses induce IgM, which is ultimately switched to IgG, except in the case of carbohydrate antigens. Direct detection of B cells may be performed using specific B cell ELISpot analysis, but these populations are very rare in blood. Affinity maturation of B-cell responses leads to increased antibody avidity over time, which may be used to date the onset of IgG responses.

T cells

Until recently, detection of antigen-specific T cells usually required culture *in vitro*, radioactive cytotoxicity assays (CD8+ T cells), or proliferation assays (CD4+ T cells) and was cumbersome and poorly quantitative. However techniques such as *ex vivo* ELISpot, intracellular cytokine staining, and MHC–peptide tetramer analysis have revolutionized the ability to measure T-cell responses in human disease.

ELISpot and intracellular cytokine staining rely on detection of cytokine (typically IFN-γ) after exposure to antigen, and subsequent capture of these single cell events on plates or using a flow cytometer. Direct *ex vivo* analysis of such populations has been used clinically to evaluate the T-cell response against tuberculosis, in a manner similar to the tuberculin skin test.

Tetramer analysis relies on *in vitro* synthesis of fluorescently labelled MHC–peptide complexes. These bind specifically to the T-cell populations of interest, which may be identified using a flow cytometer (Fig. 5.1.3.7). Such analyses may be of value in tracking the immune responses to infection or vaccines, or during immunosuppression.

Prophylaxis

Clearly the most successful clinical harnessing of the adaptive immune response is in the form of immunization, which relies on the antigen specificity and memory induction described above. This is dealt with in detail in Chapter 7.3. Overall, vaccines that induce neutralizing antibodies and provide sterilizing immunity have been the most successful. CD4+ T cell-based vaccines already exist for tuberculosis in the form of bacille Calmette–Guérin (BCG) and may be relevant in other settings. The ability to generate specific CD8+ T responses may be needed for complex infections such as HIV and HCV, where antibody responses are insufficient or are confounded by strain variation. Experimental vaccines based on recombinant virus and DNA technology to deliver antigen to the class I presentation pathway are in trial in such settings.

Therapy

B cells

Transfusion of serum enriched for particular antibodies has been used for many years, e.g in postexposure prophylaxis of herpes zoster, rabies, hepatitis B. Such antibodies are polyclonal (i.e. derived from a range of B cells). Fusion of antibody-secreting B cells with myeloma partners *in vitro*, followed by selection of specific hybridomas allows the generation of highly potent and specific monoclonal antibodies. This technology was first developed by Milstein and Kohler in 1975 and has in recent years led to the generation of a large range of antibodies with therapeutic potential, e.g. targeting cytokines/receptors, adhesion molecules, and tumour receptors. 'Humanization' of murine monoclonal antibodies by subsequent molecular modifications may be required for optimization.

T cells

In contrast with B-cell based interventions, transfusion of specific T cells has been limited by the ability to grow such cells *in vitro*, and problems of MHC restriction and rejection. However, the ability to detect and isolate specific T cells has allowed some intervention in specific cases, such as cytomegalovirus disease after bone marrow transplantation. *In vivo* expansion of donor-derived transfused T cells may be observed after bone marrow transplantation, and clinical effects even against established EBV-driven lymphomas have been reported.

Possible future developments

The molecular dissection of the adaptive immune response has recently allowed a clearer view of the basis for antigenic diversity and the mechanisms involved in induction and maintenance of functional responses. This has allowed improved diagnostics and targeted therapies to enhance or suppress specific responses. Further developments in this area leading to rationally designed immunosuppressant or adjuvant approaches are to be expected. The use of monoclonal antibodies to interrupt or target specific pathways has been greatly expanded recently, although there is caution since severe reactions can occur, as in the case of a trial antibody to CD28. Finally, viruses are by far the best immunologists. While their ability to manipulate host responses will remain a challenge to vaccine development, their ingenuity may be fruitfully harnessed further to provide novel immunization strategies.

Further reading

Ahern PP, *et al.* (2008). The interleukin-23 axis in intestinal inflammation. *Immunol Rev*, **226**, 147–59. [Review of the novel Th17 subset with special reference to inflammatory bowel disease.]

Antoniou AN, Powis SJ, Elliott T (2003). Assembly and export of MHC class I peptide ligands. *Curr Opin Immunol*, **15**, 75–81. [A description of the generation of MHC class I peptide complexes.]

Bromley SK, *et al.* (2001). The immunological synapse. *Annu Rev Immunol*, **19**, 375–96. [A review of studies of the interface between T cells and antigen-presenting cells, critical in T-cell activation and effector function.]

Cyster JG, Goodnow CC (1995). Antigen-induced exclusion from follicles and anergy are separate and complementary processes that influence peripheral B cell fate. *Immunity*, **3**, 691–701. [A classic paper using the HEL transgenic model to dissect diverse mechanisms of B cell tolerance.]

Davis SJ, van der Merwe PA (2006). The kinetic-segregation model: TCR triggering and beyond. *Nat Immunol*, **7**, 803–9. [A description of the molecular basis for T-cell activation, concentrating on the arrangement of molecules involved at the cell surface.]

Horton R *et al.* (2004). Gene map of the extended human MHC. *Nat Rev Genet*, **5**, 889–99. A description of the arrangement of genes within the MHC, the critical genetic region for the adaptive immune response.

Jung D, *et al.* (2006). Mechanism and control of V(D)J recombination at the immunoglobulin heavy chain locus. *Annu Rev Immunol*, **24**, 541–70. [A detailed review of the mechanism of B cell immunoglobulin gene rearrangement.]

Lanzavecchia A, Sallusto F (2001). The instructive role of dendritic cells on T cell responses: lineages, plasticity and kinetics. *Curr Opin Immunol*, **13**, 291–8. [Description of the role of dendritic cells in controlling T-cell quantity and quality.]

Marsh S, Parham P, Barber L (2000). *The HLA facts book*. Academic Press, London. [Comprehensive resource on HLA types.]

Rammensee H, *et al.* (1999). SYFPEITHI: database for MHC ligands and peptide motifs. *Immunogenetics*, **50**, 213–9. [Description of a very useful web resource for defining new peptide antigens.]

Sallusto F, Geginat J, Lanzavecchia A (2004). Central memory and effector memory T cell subsets: function, generation, and maintenance. *Annu Rev Immunol*, **22**, 745–63. [Description of the diverse qualities of immunological memory.]

Starr T, Jameson S, Hogquist K (2003). Positive and negative selection of T cells. *Annu Rev Immunol*, **21**, 139–76. [Review of thymic selection for T cells.]

Virgin HW, Wherry EJ, Ahmed R (2009). Redefining chronic viral infection. *Cell*, **138**, 30–50. [Review of the similarities and differences between distinct antiviral T-cell responses.]

Zinkernagel RM (1996). Immunology taught by viruses. *Science*, **271**, 173–8. [Classic paper describing evolution of the immune system in the context of virus infection.]

5.2

Immunodeficiency

D. Kumararatne

Essentials

Immunodeficiency is caused by failure of a component of the immune system and results in increased susceptibility to infections. The possibility that a patient has an underlying immunodeficiency should be considered in the following circumstances: (1) serious, persistent, unusual or recurrent infections; (2) failure to thrive in infancy; (3) known family history of immunodeficiency; (4) unexplained lymphopenia in infancy; (5) combination of clinical features characteristic of a particular immunodeficiency syndrome. The nature of the microbial infection in a particular patient provides a clue to the likely cause of immunodeficiency.

Primary immunodeficiency diseases are heritable disorders which result in defects in an intrinsic component of the immune system. Secondary immunodeficiencies are caused by conditions which impair the normal function of the immune system and include viral infections, myelomatosis, non-Hodgkin's lymphoma, severe renal or liver failure, and use of therapeutic agents which impair immunity.

Defects in anatomical and physiological barriers to infection

These are some the commonest predisposing causes of infection, e.g. obstruction of the biliary tract, urinary tract, or bronchi; presence of foreign bodies or avascular areas. Recurrent infections within the same anatomical locations are a characteristic feature, with typical organisms including pyogenic bacteria such as staphylococci, commensal organisms from the skin or intestinal tract, and fungi, especially candida.

Antibody deficiency

Clinical features—typical presentation is with recurrent infections by encapsulated bacteria, e.g. *Streptococcus pneumoniae*, *Haemophilus influenzae* type B; most patients suffer from repeated sinopulmonary infections, eventually resulting in structural lung damage; arthritis occurs in 20%; diarrhoea and malabsorption may occur due to chronic infection with intestinal pathogens or bacterial overgrowth in the small intestine.

Causes—major forms of antibody deficiency include (1) common variable immune deficiency—the commonest primary immunodeficiency disease; underlying molecular defect usually unknown; clinically defined by susceptibility to infection accompanied by low serum IgG and evidence of impaired specific antibody production in response to natural microbial exposure or vaccination. (2) X-linked agammaglobulinaemia—caused by a defect in a cytoplasmic tyrosine-kinase that results in the arrest of B-cell maturation; affected boys usually develop recurrent infections typical of antibody deficiency from around 6 months of age. (3) Other conditions—including (a) antibody deficiency associated with severe B lymphopenia; (b) hyper-IgM syndrome; (c) X-linked lymphoproliferative syndrome; (d) selective antibody deficiency with normal immunoglobulins; (e) antibody deficiency associated with thymoma; (f) IgA deficiency, (g) IgG subclass deficiency.

Treatment—immunoglobulin replacement therapy through the intravenous (IVIG) or subcutaneous (SCIG) routes is the mainstay of therapy.

Impaired T-cell-mediated immunity

Clinical features—these include increased susceptibility to infections caused by (1) viruses—e.g. children may develop fatal infection with common exanthematous viruses; adults may have considerable morbidity and mortality from reactivation of latent viruses, e.g. cytomegalovirus, herpes simplex, and varicella-zoster; (2) *Pneumocycstis jiroveci*—pulmonary infection is pathognomonic for T-cell deficiency; (3) fungal infections—e.g. mucocutaneous infection with candida; invasive infection caused by filamentous fungi like aspergillus and mucor; (4) intracellular bacteria—e.g. tuberculosis.

Causes—these may be inherited (rare) or acquired. Commonest causes of acquired T-cell deficiency include HIV infection or immunosuppressive therapy. Severe combined immunodeficiency, characterized by profound T- and B-cell failure, is caused by a variety of molecular defects. These patients present in early infancy with failure to thrive and recurrent, severe, potentially life-threatening bacterial, viral, and fungal infections, often including infections by organisms of low-grade virulence.

Treatment—(1) severe inherited T-cell disorders—invariably fatal unless treated with bone marrow stem cell transplantation or (in a very few instances) with gene therapy; (2) secondary T-cell deficiency—requires supportive therapy with antiviral and antibacterial chemotherapy agents.

Phagocyte deficiency

Clinical features—these typically include repeated visceral abscesses caused by *Staphylococcus aureus* or some species of Gram-negative bacteria, and invasive fungal infections are a particular risk.

Causes—these include (1) neutropenia—the commonest phagocyte deficiency seen in clinical practice; a neutrophil count <0.5 × 10^9/litre is associated with a high risk of life-threatening bacterial sepsis; (2) defects in bacterial killing—the best-characterized condition is chronic granulomatous disease, which is due to faulty post-phagocytic activation of the NADPH oxidase complex; (3) defects in leucocyte migration.

Treatment—this requires prophylactic antibacterial and antifungal agents, with the aggressive use of antibiotic chemotherapy of infections when they occur. Bone marrow transplantation is required for patients with defective leucocyte migration.

Other causes of immunodeficiency

These include (1) Mendelian susceptibility to mycobacterial disease; (2) Wiskott–Aldrich syndrome—characterized by eczema, thrombocytopenic purpura, with small, defective platelets and variable immunodeficiency; (3) DNA repair defects associated with immunodeficiency—e.g. ataxia telangiectasia; (4) defects in innate immunity—e.g. inherited deficiencies of components of complement system or impairment of the function of microbial pattern recognition receptors.

Introduction

The function of the immune system is to prevent infection. Immunodeficiency disorders are characterized by an increased susceptibility to infection. On a philosophical level, every infection results from a pathogen overcoming the immune defences of the body. However, most patients who suffer an infection do not have an underlying immunodeficiency, and the infectious episode is due to a shifting of the dynamic balance between the resistance of the host and the virulence of the pathogen.

The possibility of immunodeficiency should be considered under the following circumstances:

- Severe, potentially life-threatening infections. Immunodeficient patients may present for the first time with this type of infection
- Persistent infection, despite adequate and appropriate therapy
- Recurrent infection. Assessment of this criterion depends on age and clinical circumstances. For example, six to eight upper respiratory tract infections a year may not be unusual in young children, especially if they have recently joined a playgroup or started school. Such a pattern in adults would need investigation to exclude immunodeficiency
- Unusual infection. Infections caused by pathogens of low-grade virulence are pathognomonic of immunodeficiency. Examples are *Pneumocystis jiroveci* pneumonia, or persistent oral candiasis in an adult without a predisposing factor such as the use of inhaled steroids, dentures, or antibiotic therapy
- Failure to thrive in infancy. Immunodeficiency needs to be considered in the differential diagnosis, ideally as early as possible, since treatment of primary immunodeficiency is most successful if instituted before the onset of significant infections
- Known family history of immunodeficiency, especially if presenting with repeated or persistent infections
- Unexplained lymphopenia in infancy. Lymphocyte counts in infancy are higher than in adults (around 6 × 10^9/litre). Retrospective review of children with severe combined immunodeficiency (SCID) showed that most had absolute lymphocyte counts below the age-specific normal range
- Combination of clinical features characteristic of an immunodeficiency syndrome. For example, recurrent respiratory infections, eczema and thrombocytopenia associated with small sized platelets raise the possibility of Wiskott–Aldrich syndrome

The type of microbial pathogen causing infection in a particular patient is a clue to the likelihood of immunodeficiency (Tables 5.2.1) and will often indicate the category of immunodeficiency.

Classification of immunodeficiency disease

Primary immunodeficiency diseases are heritable disorders which result from defects in an intrinsic component of the immune system. Most primary immunodeficiency disorders are caused by single-gene defects. Others may represent the end result of an interaction between the genetic phenotype and environmental influences, including infections. Primary immunodeficiencies are rare, but it is difficult to give precise estimates due to the paucity of data, as well as variations between different ethnic groups. On the basis of data from national registries, these diseases are estimated to occur in 1 in 2000 to 1 in 10 000 live births.

The International Union of Immunological Societies (IUIS) convenes a committee which meets biannually to review the classification of primary immunodeficiency diseases. The main categories of primary immunodeficiency diseases are antibody deficiencies, where cell mediated immunity is substantially intact; T-cell deficiencies where T-cell mediated immunity is defective but antibody-mediated immunity is substantially intact; combined immunodeficiencies where both B- and T-cell function is defective; defects in phagocyte function; and complement deficiencies.

Each of these categories of immunodeficiency is characterized by a pattern of infection summarized in Table 5.2.1. The main primary immunodeficiency diseases currently identified are summarized in Table 5.2.2 and Fig. 5.2.1.

Secondary immunodeficiencies (Table 5.2.3) are caused by conditions which impair the normal functioning of the immune system. They are much more common than primary immunodeficiency diseases and result in a spectrum of infections, depending on which components of the immune system are deficient. Before investigating for a possible primary immunodeficiency disease it is essential to consider the history, examination and other investigations to exclude secondary immunodeficiency states.

Table 5.2.1 Immunodeficiency: usual patterns of associated infection and local pattern of associated infections

Physiological mechanism	Abnormality	Organisms[a]	Site: types of infection[b]
Nonimmune system			
Integumental barrier	Burns, eczema, skull fracture, sinus tract	Pyogenic and enteric bacteria occasionally fungi, especially candida	Recurrent in same location
Outflow	Obstruction of eustachian tube, urinary tract, or bronchi		
Vascular perfusion	Oedema, angiopathy, infarction		
Microbiological flora	Alteration by antibiotic therapy		
Phagocyte function			
Chemotaxis	Defects of neutrophil migration, e.g. leucocyte adhesin deficiency	Staphylococci, enteric bacteria	Skin, any site/localized and systemic
	Opsonin deficiency	(See 'Humoral systems')	Skin and respiratory tract
Phagocytosis	Neutropenia	Staphylococci, enteric bacteria pseudomonas species	Any site/localized and bactaeremic, stomatitis, perianal excoriation
	Asplenia	Pneumococcus, *Haemophilus influenzae* type b, (malaria, babesia)[c]	Septicaemia, meningitis, severe wound infection with *Capnocytophaga carnimorsus* following animal bites
Killing	Intrinsic cellular defects, e.g. chronic granulomatous disease	Staphylococci, enteric bacteria aspergillus, candida, BCG	Skin, lymph node and visceral[d] abscesses
Humoral systems			
Circulating antibody	Hypogammaglobulinaemia	Pyogenic bacteria, less commonly enteric bacteria, enteroviruses	Upper/lower respiratory tract; gastrointestinal, any site/localized and bacteraemic
Complement	Congenital deficiency C3, Factor I	Pyogenic bacteria, especially pneumococci	Bacteraemia, meningitis pyoderma
	Congenital deficiency C5,C6,C7,C8	*Neisseria meningitidis* or *N. gonorrhoeae*	Meningitis, pyogenic arthritis
	C1 inhibitor	No infections	Develop angio-oedema
	C2,C4	No infections or occasionally pneumococcal sepsis	
Cell-mediated immunity	Primary T-lymphocyte defects	Viruses, fungi, protozoa, intracellular bacteria	Any site/localized and systemic; mucocutaneous candida infections
	Th-1 cytokine/cytokine receptor defects e.g. IFNγ receptor, IL-12, IL-12 receptor	Poorly pathogenic mycobacteria e.g. *M. avium*, BCG; salmonella	Lymph node; disseminated

[a] Common infecting organisms are emphasized. 'Pyogenic bacteria' refers to pneumococci, *Streptococcus pyogenes*, *Haemophilus influenzae*, meningococci, and staphylococci. 'Enteric bacteria' refers to enterococci and the Gram-negative bacilli common to the intestinal tract, especially *Escherichia coli*, pseudomonas, klebsiella–enterobacter, and proteus species.
[b] Skin infections include furunculosis, subcutaneous abscesses, and cellulitis; respiratory-tract infections include recurrent pneumonia, otitis media, and sinusitis.
[c] Potentially fatal infections caused by blood-borne parasites if exposed by travel/residence in endemic area.
[d] Liver, lungs, lymph nodes, and spleen.
(Adapted from Johnston RB Jr. (1984) Recurrent bacterial infections in children. *N Engl J Med*, **310**, 1237–43, with permission.)

Defects in anatomical or physiological barriers to infection

One of the commonest predisposing causes of infection is a defect in the anatomical or physiological barriers to infection. Intact epithelial membranes, especially a stratified squamous epithelial surface such as the skin, constitutes an extremely effective barrier to infection.

The following defects predispose to infection:

- Integumentary damage caused by burns, eczema, or trauma (including surgery)
- Skull fracture, particularly damage of the cribiform plate, which may result in recurrent episodes of pyogenic meningitis
- Sinus tracts between deeper tissues and the skin surface
- Presence of foreign bodies or avascular areas (e.g. within bone)
- Obstruction to the drainage of hollow tubes and viscera (e.g. obstruction of the biliary tract, urinary tract, or bronchi)
- Impaired vascular perfusion of the tissues due to oedema, or angiopathy (including microvascular changes following diabetes mellitus)
- Alteration of the normal commensal flora by broad spectrum antibiotic therapy
- Damage from surgical instruments, perfusion lines, and catheters
- Damaged tissues such as damaged cardiac valves

Infections that recur in the same anatomical site are often due to defective anatomical or physiological barriers and hence should

Table 5.2.2 Classification of primary immunodeficiency states

Antibody deficiency diseases	Mutated gene/pathogenesis	Associated features
X-linked agammaglobulinaemia	*BTK*	Antibody deficiency and B lymphopenia
Autosomal recessive agammaglobulinaemia	Mutations in genes for μ, Igα, Igβ, λ5, or BLNK	Antibody deficiency and B lymphopenia
Thymoma with antibody deficiency	Unknown	Antibody deficiency and B lymphopenia
Hyper IgM syndome (autosomal recessive)	UNG or AICDA which encodes for AID or mutation in gene encoding the PMS2 component of the mismatch repair machinery	Low IgG and IgA, raised IgM
Common variable immunodeficiency	Unknown in most; *TACI* in *c.*10%, rarely *ICOS*, *CD19*, or *BAFFR*	Antibody deficiency; may have autoimmunity, lymphoproliferation, systemic granulomata
Selective IgA deficiency	Most unknown; few due to *TACI* mutations	Most remain healthy; increase in autommunity, atopy, coeliac disease
IgG subclass deficiency	Unknown	If associated with selective antibody deficiency may have recurrent sinopulmonary infections
Specific antibody deficiency with normal serum immunoglobulins	Unknown	Deficient antibody responses to some antigens. Anti-polysaccharide antibody deficiency may be associated with recurrent sinopulmonary infections
Transient antibody deficiency of infancy	Unknown	Reduced IgA and IgG; recovery by 3 years of age
Combined T-and B-cell deficiency		
Severe combined immunodeficiency (SCID)		Lymphopenia, low serum Igs, failure to thrive, severe recurrent infections by viruses, bacteria, and parasites; fatal without BMT
SCID due to failure of cytokine receptor signalling	*IL2RG* (common γ-chain), *IL2RA*, *IL7RA*, *JAK3*	T lymphopenia; B cell number normal (T−B+ SCID)
SCID due to defective VDJ gene recombination	*RAG 1*, *RAG2*, *DCLRE1C* (*Artemis*)	T-B-SCID
SCID due to defective nucleotide salvage	*ADA*, *PNP*	ADA deficiency gives rise to T-and B-cell lymphopenia (T-B-SCID); PNP deficiency give rise to T-lymphopenia and neurologic defects
SCID due to defective T-cell receptor function	*CD3D*, *ZAP70*, *CD45*	
SCID due to defective calcium entry into T-cells	Mutation in the *ORAI1* gene which encodes a subunit of the plasma membrane calcium channel CRAC. T-cell function is impaired	
SCID due to lack of T-cell egress from thymus	Mutation in *CORO1A* which encodes the actin regulator Coronin A, which is required for normal T-cell migration	Causes a T-B+NK+ SCID
SCID due to defective MHC class II transcription	*MHC2TA*, *RFXANK*, *RFX5*, *RFXAP*	Lack of MHC class II expression resulting in CD4 lymphopenia and severe failure of T-cell and B-cell function
Omenn's syndrome	hypomorphic mutation of *RAG1*, *RAG2*, DCLRE1C (*Artemis*), or IL7Ra	Variant of SCID. some T and B cells may develop but are oligoclonal. Features include erythroderma, lymphadenopathy, hepatosplenomegaly, eosinophilia. Outcome poor without BMT
MHC class I deficiency	*TAP1* or *TAP2*	Lack of MHC class I expression on cells; CD8 lymphopenia; present with bronchiectasis or vasculitis
X-linked hyper IgM syndrome	*CD40L*	Lack of CD40-ligand on activated T cells. Failure of Ig class- switching and affinity maturation; low IgG/IgA, raised or normal IgM; may develop neutropenia, autoimmune cytopenias, opportunistic infections and gastrointestinal and liver pathologies
CD40 deficiency (a type of autosomal recessive hyper IgM syndrome)	*CD40*	Lack of CD40 expression on B cells. Other features similar to CD40L deficiency

X-Linked lymphoproliferative disorder (XLP)	Mutation of *SAP* or *XIAP* genes. (see text for explanantion)	Clinical manifestations precipitated by EBV infection: hepaptitis, haemophagocytosis, aplastic anaemia, hypogammaglobulinaemia, Non-hodgkins lymphoma
DOCK 8 deficiency	Mutation in gene encoding dedicator of cytokinensis 8 (DOCK 8)	Recurrent sino-pulmonary infections and cutaneous viral infections (*Molluscum contagiosum* and HPV); low serum IgM and variable IgG responses
T cell deficiency		
MHC class I deficiency	*TAP1, TAP2 or TAPBP* (which encodes for the TAP binding protein Tapasin)	Lack of MHC class I expression on cells; CD8 Lymphopenia; present with bronchiectasis or vasculitis
Phagocyte deficiencies (excluding congenital neutropenias)		
Chronic granulomatous disease	Mutations in components of the phagocye oxidase (see text for details)	Pyogenic and fungal infections; lymph node and visceral abscesses; chronic granulomata (see text for details)
Leucocyte adhesin deficiency Type 1	Mutation of gene encoding CD18, which is a component of leucocyte adhesins (see text for details)	Delayed umbilical cord separating, omphalitis, pyoderma, periodontitis, leucocytosis
Leucocyte adhesin deficiency Type 2	Mutation of gene encoding GDP-fucose transporter (see text for details)	As above plus mental retardation
Leucocyte adhesin deficiency Type 3	Mutation in calcium and diacylglycerol-regulated guanine nucleotide exchange factor	Omphalitis, pyogenic infections, mulberry haematomas, bleeding tendency due to defective platelet activation, defect in leucocyte adhesion to endothelial surface due to defect in β1,2,3 integrin activation
Rac 2 deficiency	Mutation in RAC2 leading to impaired actin polymerization/ cytoskeletal function	Poor wound healing, leucocytosis, Clinical picture similar to Type1 Leucocyte Adhesin deficiency
Mendelian susceptibility to mycobacterial infection	Defects in the production or response to IFNγ. Mutated genes include *IL12B, IL12RB1, IFNGR1, IFNGR2, STAT 1, TYK2*. Intact response to IFNγ is essential for control of intracellular bacterial infection. Some *NEMO* mutations cause X-linked susceptibility to mycobacterial infection. See text for full explanation	Recurrent disseminated infections with poorly pathogenic mycobacteria (NTM or *BCG*) and systemic infections with non-typhi salmonella species
Miscellaneous well-characterized immunodeficiencies		
Wiskott–Aldrich syndrome	*WASP*: Lack or dysfunctional protein results in cytoskeletal defect affecting myeloid and lymphoid cells	Thrombocytopenia, small platelets, eczema, combined immunodeficiency, lymphomas, autoimmune disease
DNA repair defects		
Ataxia telangiectasia	*ATM*: Mutation causes dysfunction of cell cycle check point pathway leading to chromosomal instability	Ataxia, oculocutaneous telangiectasia, raised serum α-fetoprotein, increased malignancies (especially lymphoma), IgA/IgG subclass deficiencies with poor anti-polysaccharide responses, sino-pulmonary infections, Radiation sensitivity
Ataxia-like syndrome	*Mre 11*	
Nijmegen breakage syndrome	Mutation in NBS1: impaired DNA double strand break repair	Microcephaly, radiation sensitivity, lymphomas
DNA-ligase IV deficiency	Mutation in DNA ligase IV: defective DNA repair	Microcephaly, facial dysmorphism, radiation sensitivity
DiGeorge anomaly	Heterozygous deletion of 22q11 in 90%; mutation in *TBOX-1* gene in a few	Conotruncal defects, facial dysmorphism, hypoparathyroidism, velo-pharyngeal defects, thymic hypoplasia
Immunodeficiency with partial albinism		
Chediak–Higashi syndrome	Mutation in *LYST* gene. Impaired lysosomal function and defect in sorting cytolytic proteins into secretaory granules; poor NK-cell and T-cell mediated cytolysis	Partial albinism, giant lysosomes, recurrent pyogenic infections, mild mental retardation, peripheral neuropathy, eventually 85% develop accelerated phase with syndrome resembling haemophagocytic lymphohistiocytosis
Griscelli syndrome (type 2)	Deficiency of the RAB27A GTPase required for secretory vesicle function. Exocytosis of cytolytic granules deficient leading to poor NK-cell and T-cell mediated cytolysis	Partial albinism, giant lysosomes, recurrent pyogenic infections, encephalopathy, eventually 85% develop accelerated phase as in Chediak–Higashi syndrome

(Continued)

Table 5.2.2 (*cont'd*) Classification of primary immunodeficiency states

Antibody deficiency diseases	Mutated gene/pathogenesis	Associated features
Disorders of homeostasis of immune function		
Syndromes with autoimmunity		
Autoimmune lymphoproliferative syndrome (ALPS)	Defects of components in the apoptosis pathway in lymphocytes: mutations in genes encoding CD95 (*TNFRSF6*), CD95 ligand (*TNFSF6*), caspase 10 or caspase 8	Lymphadenopathy, hepatosplenomegaly, hypergammaglobulinaemia, deficient lymphocyte apoptosis, autoimmune diseases, increased CD4-CD8- T cells
Autoimmune polyendocrinopathy, candidiasis, ectodermal dysplasia syndrome (APCED)	Mutation in autoimmune regulator gene (*AIRE*) encoding protein required for expression of ectopic antigens in the thymic epithelial cells. This is required for induction of tolerance to autoantigens	Multiple endocrine autoimmunity; chronic mucocutaneous candidiasis
Immune dysregulation, polyendocrinopathy, enteropathy, X-linked (IPEX)	Mutation of *FOXP3* gene whose product is expressed by and is required for function of T-regulatory cells	Childhood onset autoimmune endocrinopathy, enteropathy, eczema
Familial haemophagocytic lymphohistiocytosis	Defective T-cell and NK-cell mediated cytotoxicity due to mutations in genes encoding perforin (PRF1), or MUNC protein (MUNK13-4) needed for fusion of intracellular vesicles	Viral infection triggers haemophagocytosis
X-linked lymphoproliferative syndrome	*SAP* (see text for explanation of function)	Clinical manifestations precipitated by EBV infection: hepatitis, haemophagocytosis, aplastic anaemia, hypogammaglobulinaemia, lymphomas
Disorders of homeostasis of inflammation (autoinflammatory syndromes)		
Familial Mediterranean fever	*MEFV*	Periodic fever, amyloidosis
Hyper-IgD syndrome	Partial mevalonate kinase deficiency; mechanism of disease uncertain	Periodic fever
TNF receptor associated periodic fever	*TNFRSF1*: results in decreased availability of soluble TNF receptor for mopping up TNF	Periodic fever, amyloidosis
Familial cold autoinflammatory syndrome	CIAS1: defect in cryopyrin required for leukocyte apoptosis NF-κB signalling and IL-1 processing	Cold induced urticaria, fever
Neonatal onset multisystem inflammatory disease (NOMID)	CIAS1: as above	Neonatal onset rash, fever, chronic meningitis, arthropathy
Muckle–Wells syndrome	CIAS1: as above	Urticaria, deafness, amyloidosis
Defects in innate immunity		
Anhydrotic ectodermal dysplasia with immunodeficiency	Hypomorphic mutation in *NEMO* which is a component in the NF-κB signalling pathway; results in defective NF-κB activation	Ectodermal dysplasia in some but not all patients, lack of anti-polysaccharide antibodies, failure to switch to IgG, pyogenic and mycobacterial infection; inheritance is X-linked recessive
Anhydrotic ectodermal dysplasia with immunodeficiency	Mutation in *IKBA* encoding a regulatory component of the NF-κB pathway	Ectodermal dysplasia and T-cell deficiency
IL-1 receptor associated kinase (IRAK4) deficiency	*IRAK4* encoding a component of the signalling pathway utilized by Toll-like receptors	Recurrent pyogenic infections especially with *S. pneumoniae*
WHIM syndrome	Gain of function mutation in gene encoding chemokine receptor CXCR4	Warts, hypogammaglobulinaemia, neutropenia with myelokathexis, bacterial infections

Severe herpes viral infections in childhood	Impaired production of IFNα and β in response to viral nucleic acids due to deficiency in UNC93B , a protein involved with Toll receptor activation. Similar syndrome produced by a mutation of gene encoding Toll Receptor 3 (TLR3)	Herpes simplex encephalitis in childhood
Severe herpes viral infections in childhood	Impaired response to IFNα and β due to lack of type-1 interferon receptor function. Caused by homozygous mutation of *STAT1*	Herpes simplex encephalitis in childhood; these patients also develop mycobacterial infections as STAT1 is required for signalling via IFNγ receptors
Hyper IgE syndrome	Heterozygous mutation in gene encoding signal transducing factor STAT 3	Recurrent bacterial and fungal infections, staphylococcal pneumonia with pneumatocoele formation, pyogenic infection causing cold abscess formation, poor acute phase responses, delayed shedding of primary dentition, facial dysmorphism, dermatitis, elevated serum IgE
CARD9 deficiency	Homozygous mutation in gene encoding Caspase recruitment domain containing protein 9 required for effective antifungal immune response (see text)	Recurrent mucocutaneous fungal infection and fatal invasive brain infection with Candida
Dectin-1 deficiency	Mutation in gene encoding Dectin-1, which is a pattern recognition receptor for fungal cell wall β glucan	Recurrent vulvo-vaginal candidiasis and fungal nail infection
Early onset Crohn's disease	Mutation in *IL10RA* and *IL10RB* genes encoding for the IL10R1 and IL10R2 components of the IL10-receptor. This abrogates responses to IL10, resulting in an increase in pro-inflammatory cytokine production, suggesting that IL10-dependent homesostasis of inflammatory pathways is abnormal in these patients.	Early onset severe , treatment refractory Crohn's disease. In one patient a cure was obtained by haemopietic stem cell transplantation.
Miscellaneous primary immunodeficiencies of unknown pathogenesis		
Idiopathic CD4 cell lymphopenia	CD4 lymphopenia of unknown cause	Infections typical of T-cell deficiency
Chronic mucocutaneous candidiasis without endocrinopathy	Unknown aetiology	Autosomal recessive and autosomal dominant cases of chronic mucocutaneous candida infection have been documented

JOHNSTON, R. B., JR. (1984) Recurrent bacterial infections in children. N Engl J Med, 310, 1237–43.)

(a)

Suspect immunodeficiency (see text for features raising suspicion)
The site and type of infection gives a clue to the category of immunodeficiency (see Table 5.2.1)
If infections recur in the same anatomical location: look for anatomical or physiological defect (see Table 5.2.1 and Text)
Exclude possibility of secondary immunodeficiency based on clinical features including drug history (see Table 5.2.3)
• Recurrent, severe or persistent sino-pulmonary infections
• Encapsulated bacterial infections
• Infants with failure to thrive
• Chronic diarrhoea, malabsorption, inflammatory bowel disease
Consider antibody deficiency
• Recurrent pyogenic skin sepsis (cellulitis, abscesses) without explanation (i.e. eczema, etc.) or visceral abscesses (lung, liver lymph nodes), often caused by *Staphylococcus aureus*
• Invasive fungal infection
• Recurrent or persistent oro/mucocutaneous ulceration
• Unexplained granulomatous inflammation
Consider phagocyte deficiency
• Failure to thrive from early infancy, especially if associated with infections
• Infants with features of graft versus host reaction: skin rash, diarrhoea, hepatosplenomegaly, lymphadenopathy
• Infants with lymphocyte count <2.5x10^9/litre
• Patients with one or more of the following infections or tumours:
Viruses, e.g. CMV
Intracellular bacteria, e.g. mycobacteria
Fungi, e.g. mucocutaneous candidiasis, *Pneumocystis*
Protozoa, e.g, *Toxoplasma, Cryptosporidium*
Certain malignancies, e.g. EBV-induced NHL, Kaposi's sarcoma
Consider defective cell-mediated immunity (If SCID is possible rapid diagnosis is essential)
• Encapsulated bacterial sepsis (*N. meningitidis, Pneumococcus, Hib*)
• Lupus-like syndrome/vasculitis
• Haemolytic uraemic syndrome
Consider complement deficiency
• Severe/recurrent encapsulated bacterial infection
• Severe malaria
• Babesia infection
• Cellulitis by *Capnocytophaga*
Consider hyposplenism

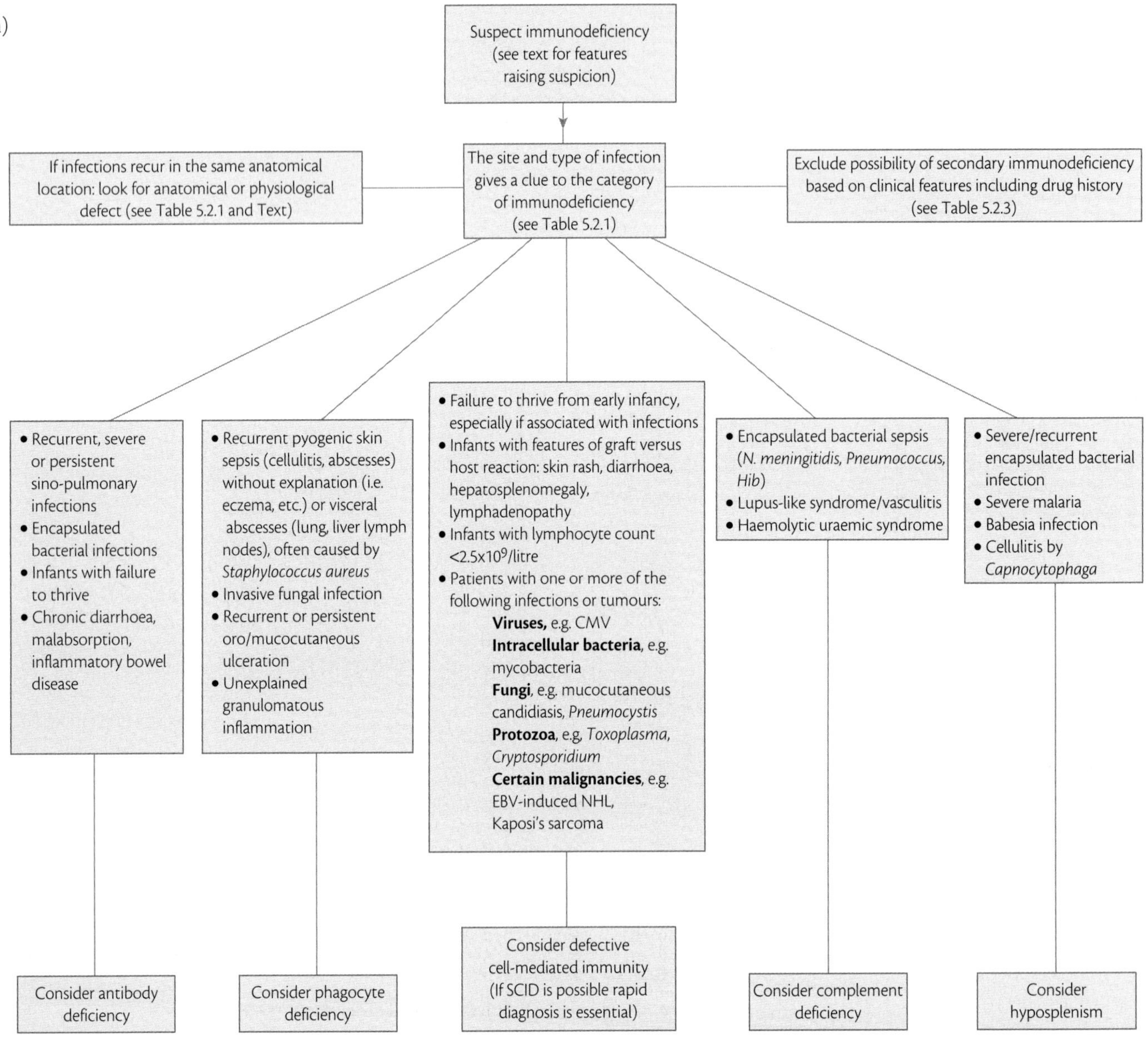

Fig. 5.2.1 Stepwise approach to the diagnosis of immunodeficiency.
Modified from The Lancet, 357, Alain Fischer, Primary immunodeficiency diseases: an experimental model for molecular medicine, 1863–1869, © 2001, with permission from Elsevier.

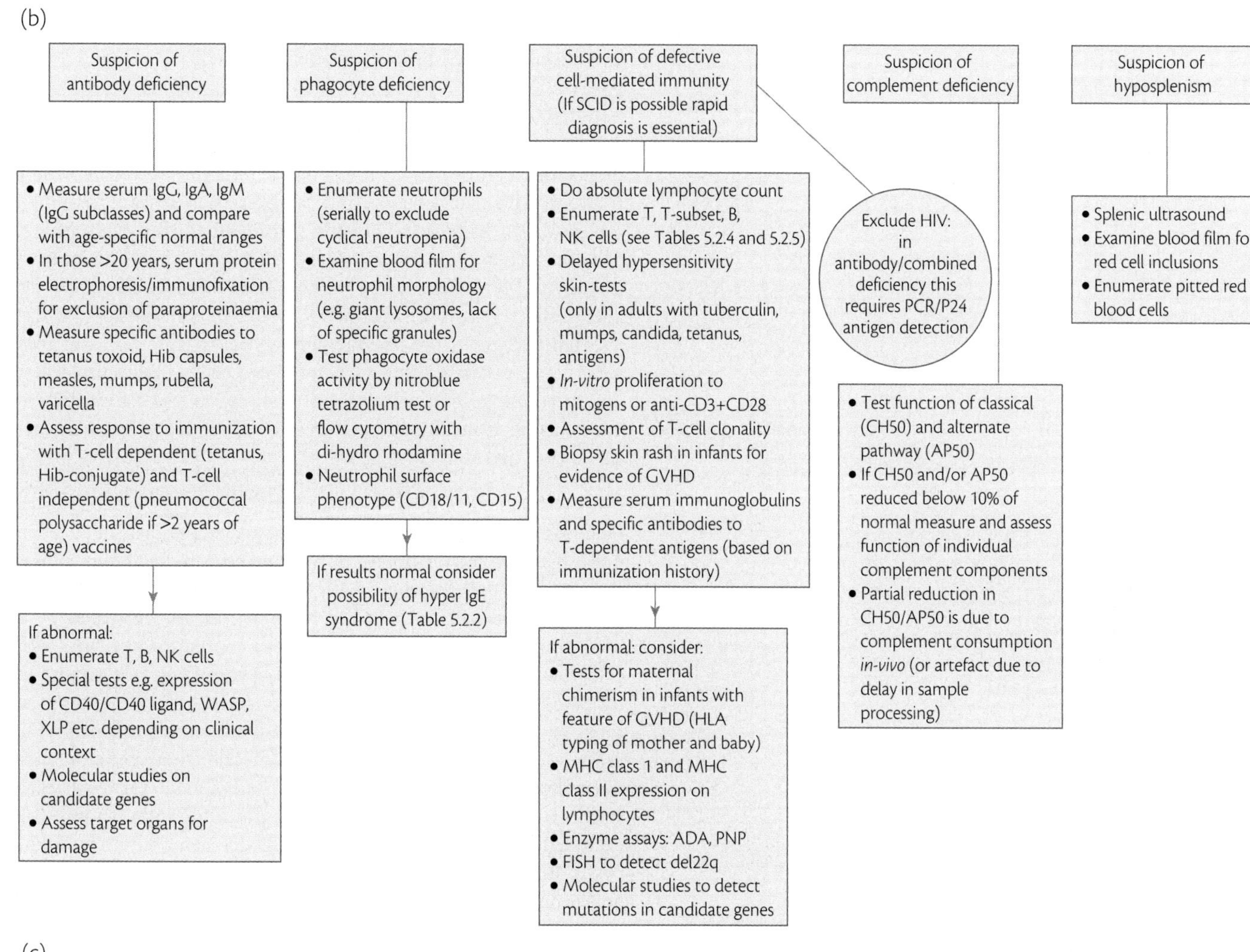

(c)

Possibilities to consider in patients with recurrent infections with same category of organism:	
Mycobacteria/Salmonella	Defects in IL-12/23-dependent IFNγ pathway; NEMO defect
S. pneumoniae	Antibody, complement, hyposplenism, defects in NEMO or IRAK4
N. meningitidis	Lack of terminal complement components (C5-9) or alternative pathway components (properdin)
S. aureus	Phagocyte deficiency, hyper IgE syndorme

Fig. 5.2.1 *(Cont'd)* Stepwise approach to the diagnosis of immunodeficiency.
(b) Modified from The Lancet, 357, Alain Fischer, Primary immunodeficiency diseases: an experimental model for molecular medicine, 1863–1869, © 2001, with permission from Elsevier.

Table 5.2.3 Causes of secondary immunodeficiency

	Defect
Defects in anatomical and physical barriers to infection	Various (see text for explanation)
Malignancies of the B-cell system	Antibody
Myelomatosis	
Non Hodgkin's lymphoma	
Chronic lymphocytic leukaemia	
Therapeutic agents	
Biological agents—	
Anti-B-cell antibodies (e.g. rituximab)	Antibody
Anti-TNF agents	Innate immunity and CMI
Cytotoxic drugs—alkylating agents, cytotoxic antibiotics, antimetabolites, vinca alkaloids, etoposide, etc.	Myelosupression and CMI
Immunosupressive drugs—corticosteroids, calcineurin inhibitors, antiproliferative immunosuppressants (azathioprine, mycophenelate)	CMI
Drugs causing antibody deficiency—gold, penicillamine, sulphasalazine, carbamazepine, valproate	Antibody
Radiotherapy	CMI
Metabolic/nutritional deficiencies	
Renal failure	CMI and innate immunity
Liver failure	CMI and innate immunity
Protein–calorie malnutrition	CMI
Vitamin A deficiency	CMI
Transcobolamine-II deficiency	Antibody
Increased loss of immunoglobulin	
Nephrotic syndrome	
Protein-losing enteropathy	
Dystrophia myotonica	
Virus infections	
HIV	CMI
Congenital rubella	Antibody
Congenital CMV	Antibody

CMI, cell-mediated immunity; CMV, cytomegalovirus;TNF, tumour necrosis factor.

induce a diligent search for such factors. Causative organisms are pyogenic bacteria such as staphylococci, commensal organisms from the skin or intestinal tract, and fungi, especially candida.

Primary antibody deficiencies

Antibody deficiency diseases (ADD) are characterized by a decrease in the levels of serum immunoglobulins below the fifth centile, for age. The reduction may be in all classes of immunoglobulins or a single isotype. Clinical features associated with antibody deficiency are summarized in Box 5.2.1 and Fig. 5.2.1.

Major forms of antibody deficiency

Common variable immune deficiency (CVID)

Patients with CVID are a heterogenous group, the diagnosis being based on the exclusion of other known causes of antibody deficiency. CVID is the commonest primary immunodeficiency disease with an estimated incidence of 1 in 10 000 to 1 in 50 000. It affects both sexes equally, and can present at any age, although the modal presentation is in the second or third decade of life. The underlying molecular defect in most CVID patients is unknown. Many cases are sporadic while others are familial, with autosomal recessive or dominant modes of inheritance. Within affected pedigrees, the phenotype may be variable ranging from selective IgA deficiency to CVID. In the last few years molecular defects resulting in impaired B-cell maturation and differentiation have been identified in about 10% of CVID patients. These defects are summarized in Table 5.2.3.

Diagnosis and differential diagnosis of CVID

Diagnostic criteria for major immunodeficiencies have been published by a consortium of European and American immunologists (see 'Further reading'). CVID is a clinically defined syndrome characterized by susceptibility to infection accompanied by a reduction of serum IgG below the fifth centile for age, and with evidence of impaired specific antibody production in response to natural microbial exposure or vaccination. Serum IgA is reduced in most patients with CVID, while IgM is often but not invariably reduced. Since CVID is a diagnosis of exclusion, patients with normal or elevated serum IgM should be evaluated for hyper-IgM syndromes and X-linked agammaglobulinaemia should be excluded in male patients with antibody deficiency and B lymphopenia. It is also essential to exclude secondary causes of antibody deficiency (see Table 5.2.3). The clinical features of antibody deficiency are summarized above.

X-linked agammaglobulinaemia

This is caused by a defect in a cytoplasmic tyrosine-kinase designated Bruton's aggammaglobulinaemia tyrosine kinase (BTK) which results in the arrest of B-cell maturation beyond pre-B-cell stage. As a consequence there is peripheral B lymphopenia associated with profound antibody deficiency. Affected males usually develop recurrent infections typical of antibody deficiency, commencing at around 6 months of age, when maternal immunoglobulin has been catabolized. Characteristic diagnostic features include profound reduction of all immunoglobulin isotypes (below the fifth centile for age), absent isohaemagglutins and responses to childhood vaccines. Numbers and function of T lymphocyte are normal. Demonstration of the absence of BTK protein in monocytes or platelets by flow cytometry or western blotting, or a demonstration of mutation in the BTK gene, confirm the diagnosis but are not essential. Patients with X-linked agammaglobulinaemia do not develop systemic granulomatous disease that is seen in CVID. In female carriers the chromosome carrying the BTK mutation is preferentially lyonized during B-cell development. During the characterization of the BTK gene defect, it has been recognized that the clinical phenotype may vary, even within the same family. Some affected males may therefore present at a later age and the condition should be considered in all males with antibody deficiency, especially in the presence of B lymphopenia.

Box 5.2.1 Clinical features associated with antibody deficiency

1 Recurrent infections caused by encapsulated bacteria, for example *Streptococcus pneumoniae* or *Haemophilus influenzae* type B (HIB). Sites involved are the upper and lower respiratory tract, middle ear, meninges, bones, and joints. The large majority of patients with antibody deficiency suffer from repeated sinopulmonary infections which eventually result in structural damage. Structural lung damage (bronchiectasis, pulmonary fibrosis) secondary to antibody deficiency is the most important cause of morbidity and mortality in these patients. Nontypable *Haemophilus influenzae* causes most exacerbations of sinopulmonary infections in these patients. Less common respiratory pathogens in patients with antibody deficiency include *Staphylococcus aureus* and Gram-negative bacteria such as *Pseudomonas* spp. Infections by fungi, intracellular bacteria (e.g. mycobacteria), or parasites are not usually a problem in these patients.

2 Viral infections are not a problem in antibody deficiency diseases except for the rare occurrence of enteroviral infections; ECHO viruses or coxsakieviruses can cause meningoencephalitis or dermatomyositis-like conditions. Poliomyelitis associated with oral polio vaccine has also been rarely reported, in patients with antibody deficiency.

3 Arthritis has been reported in about 20% of patients and may be septic caused by HIB, *S. pneumoniae* or mycoplasma/ureoplasma, or aseptic, resembling seronegative rheumatoid arthritis.

4 Diarrhoea and malabsorption may occur due to chronic infection with intestinal pathogens including giardia, campylobacter, salmonella, or cryptosporidium, or as a consequence of bacterial overgrowth in the small intestine. Chronic diarrhoea is often associated with a mild colitis and a minority may have Crohn's-like inflammatory bowel disease with iletis and occasional strictures. A few patients may have intestinal villous atrophy with a non-specific inflammatory infiltrate of the mucosa and submucosa. A minority of these will respond to a gluten-free diet, although antibody based screening tests for coeliac disease will be negative. Patients with antibody deficiency associated with common variable immune deficiency (CVID) (see below) may have nodular submucous lymphoid hyperplasia throughout the small intestine and occasionally the large intestine. This is usually clinically silent, although occasionally these lesions may bleed or cause obstruction.

5 Granulomatous lesions occurring in the lungs giving rise to sarcoid-like state with impaired gas transfer and secondary fibrosis. They may also affect other organs such as the liver, spleen, kidneys, or lymph nodes. The aetiology of this condition is unknown.

6 Autoimmune disorders are seen in approximately one-fifth of patients with CVID. These include autoimmune haematological disorders such as haemolytic anaemia, autoimmune thrombocytopenia, and pernicious anaemia, or neurological diseases such as Guillian–Barré syndrome, autoimmune endocrinopathies (e.g. thyroid disease), and, rarely, a lupus-like syndrome.

7 Splenomegaly can be seen in up to 30% of patients with CVID; in many this is due to infiltration with sarcoid-like granulomata.

8 Malignancies: there is an increased incidence of non-Hodgkin's lymphomas and gastric neoplasms in patients with CVID. The incidence of gastric carcinoma may be related to atrophic gastritis and *Helicobacter pylori* infection.

Provided X-linked agammaglobulinaemia is diagnosed early before organ damage is evident, and the patients are treated with optimum immunoglobulin replacement therapy, and antibiotics as required, the outlook is excellent.

Autosomal recessive antibody deficiencies with B lymphopenia

Five autosomal recessive gene defects have been identified as resulting in antibody deficiency associated with severe B lymphopenia. There are mutations in the μ heavy chain gene, the gene encoding the surrogate light chain which is utilized by the pre-B-cell receptors, a signalling component of the B-cell receptor complex, namely Igα and the signal transducing/scaffold protein called B-cell linker protein (BLNK). All these conditions are rare.

Hyper-IgM syndrome

During primary antibody responses, B cells initially produce IgM and later on in the response, they switch to the production and IgG, IgA and IgE. This process is called immunoglobulin class switching and is associated with somatic hypermutation of the immunoglobulin variable-region genes resulting in enhancement of antibody affinity for the stimulating antigens (affinity maturation). There are six known rare molecular defects which cause the failure of immunoglobulin class switching and affinity maturation, as well as the generation of B memory cells. A key requirement for this process is the interaction of CD40 on the surface of B cells with an activation-induced CD40 ligand (CD40L) protein on the surface of CD4 lymphocytes. Mutations in the CD40 ligand gene or the CD40 gene result in X-linked and autosomal recessive hyper-IgM syndrome syndrome respectively. Defects in the RNA editing enzymes activation-induced cytidine deaminase (AID) and uracil-DNA glycosylase (UNG) result in two further forms of hyper-IgM syndrome. Hypomorphic mutations of the gene encoding the NFκB essential modulator (NEMO), a component of the NFκB activation pathway which is required for the B-cell activation process (including signal transduction following CD40/CD40L interaction), causes a further rare form of X-linked hyper-IgM syndrome. Recently, homozygous mutations in the PMS2 component of the DNA mismatch repair machinery was identified to cause defective immunoglobulin class switching, resulting in low levels of serum IgG and IgA.

The commonest type of hyper-IgM syndrome is caused by CD40L deficiency. CD40L deficiency can be diagnosed by demonstrating the absence of this protein on the surface of *in vitro* activated T cells by flow cytometry, and confirmed by screening the CD40L gene for mutations. Patients with defects in CD40L suffer from recurrent bacterial infections typical of antibody deficiency. However, since CD40L function is required for optimum T-cell mediated immune responses, they also suffer from opportunistic infections characteristic of T-cell deficiency. About one-third have presented with *Pneumocystis jiroveci* pneumonia. Infections with

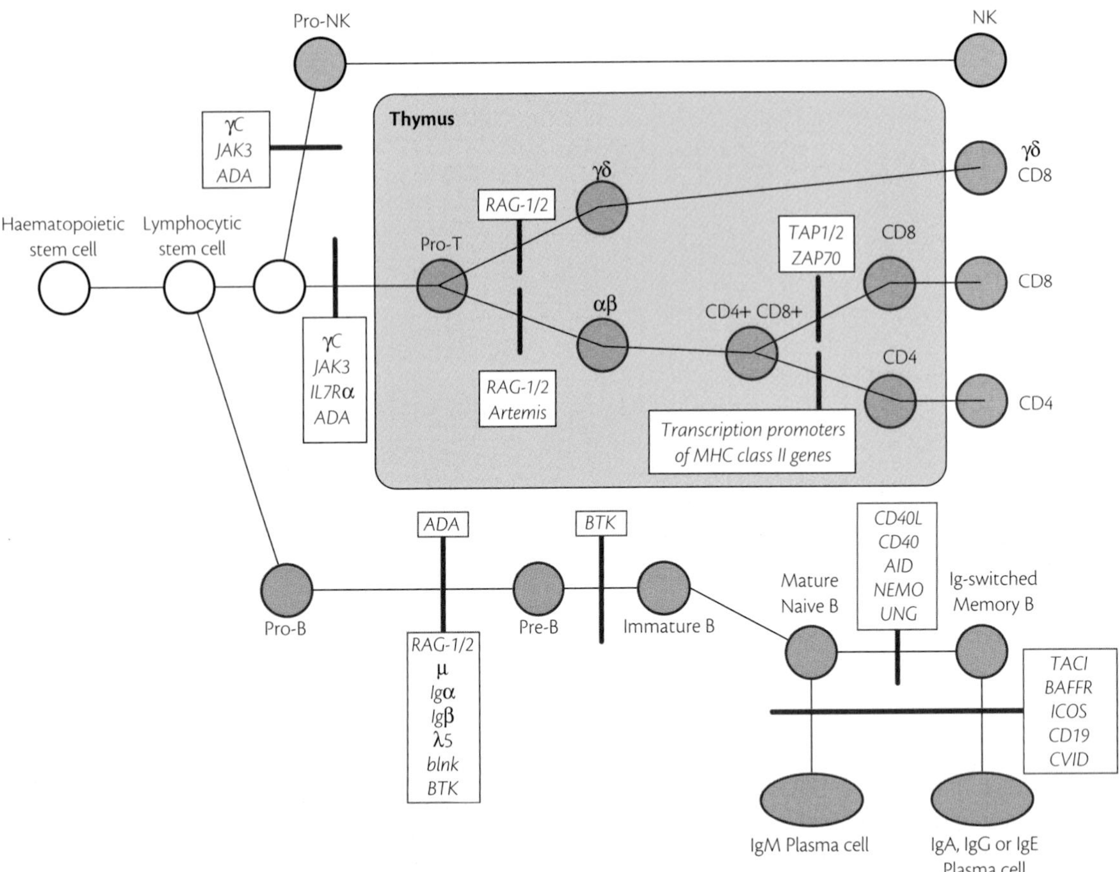

Fig. 5.2.2 Summary of immunodeficiencies resulting from a block in lymphocyte development. Haematopoietic stem cells differentiate in bone marrow into common lymphocyte precursors, from which NK, T, and B lymphocytes originate. γC, JAK-3, IL-7R deficiencies impair γC-dependent cytokine signalling necessary for T cell and NK lymphocyte development. *RAG1*, *RAG2*, and *DCLRE1C* (Artemis) gene mutations impair V(D)J recombination of T-cell receptor and immunoglobulin genes in pro-T and pro-B cells respectively. HLA class II deficiency prevents development of CD4 T-cells. ZAP70 kinase deficiency prevents CD8 T-cell development and leads to the development of non-functional CD4 T-cells. TAP 1/2 deficiencies impair positive selection of CD8 T-cells. μ heavy chain, Igα and β associated subunit, λ5, and BLNK deficiencies prevent the transition from pro-B to pre-B cells. BTK deficiency impairs B-cell development. CD40L,AID (activation induced cytidine deaminase), and uracil-DNA glycolase (UNG) deficiencies prevent immunoglobulin class switch recombination.

(Modified, with permission, from Fischer A (2001). Primary immunodeficiency diseases: an experimental model for molecular medicine. *Lancet*, **357**, 1863–9.)

cryptosporidium, toxoplasmosis and non-tuberculous mycobacteria may also occur. These opportunistic infections are explained on the basis that CD40L on activated T cells is involved in the activation of macrophages and dendritic cells which express CD40. A high proportion of patients with CD40L deficiency develop progressive liver damage (sclerosing cholangitis) probably as a result of cryptosporidial infection of the bile ducts. Recurrent or persistent neutropenia and thrombocytopenia occur in over one-half of patients with CD40L deficiency.

Immunoglobulin replacement therapy is required for patients with all forms of hyper-IgM syndrome. Patients with CD40L deficiency require prophylaxis for *Pneumocystis jiroveci* pneumonia and precautions to prevent cryptosporidial infection, including boiling drinking water. Because of the high risk of developing severe liver disease, haemopoietic stem cell transplantation has been used to treat CD40L deficiency diagnosed in infancy. However to date the mortality of this procedure is in excess of 30%.

X-linked lymphoproliferative syndrome

Affected males have a mutation in an adaptor protein called SAP (surface lymphocyte activation molecule associated protein), regulating the activation of T lymphocytes and NK cells. Patients with X-linked lymphoproliferative syndrome have defective regulation of CD8 T-cell responses to the Epstein–Barr virus. In these patients Epstein–Barr virus infection results in adverse consequences due to unregulated CD8 T-cell and NK-cell responses to the virus. Most patients present with severe infectious mononucleosis with a high mortality (80%), with death usually caused by a hepatic necrosis induced by activated cytotoxic (CD8) T-cells. Other consequences of Epstein–Barr virus infection in these patients include haemophagocytic lymphohistiocytosis, aplastic anaemia, the development of B-cell non-Hodgkin's lymphoma and/or hypogammaglobulinaemia. The outlook is poor, with most affected patients dying in childhood, unless treated with bone marrow transplantation.

Mutations in the gene *BIRC4* which encodes for the protein X-linked inhibitor of apoptosis (XIAP) also causes a form of X-linked lymphoproliferative syndrome. These patients too have reduced numbers of natural killer T cells.

Physiological antibody deficiencies

During the last trimester of pregnancy, maternal IgG is actively transported across the placenta to the fetus. At full term, neonates are born with IgG levels (including all four immunoglobulin subclasses) approximating to or even higher than the adult normal range.

Preterm babies are relatively IgG deficient at birth, to a degree that correlates with the degree of prematurity. Maternally derived immunoglobulins are metabolized after birth and the IgG levels reach a nadir around 4 to 6 months of age. Serum IgG levels begin to rise after this, due to increase in synthesis by the neonate, and reach approximately 70% of adult levels by 12 months. During the first 6 months of life, therefore, the neonate is protected by maternally transferred immunoglobulins. Children with inherited antibody deficiency do not usually develop infections until 5 to 6 months of age. Human infants, including preterm babies, have normal antibody responses to protein and protein-polysaccharide conjugate vaccines (e.g. *Haemophilus* B conjugate vaccine). Hence, primary immunization can start at 2 months of age. In contrast, children less than 2 years of age are unable to produce effective antibody responses to bacterial capsular polysaccharides. Antipolysaccharide antibody responses progressively mature after 2 years of age and it may take up to 5 to 7 years before the responses are quantitatively and qualitatively equivalent to those of adults.

Transient hypogammaglobulinaemia of infancy

In some infants there is a delay in the onset of *de novo* immunoglobulin synthesis and as a result serum IgG levels show a prolonged trough lasting up to 18 to 36 months of age. These infants can be differentiated from patients with primary antibody deficiency by their capacity to respond to immunization with T-cell dependent vaccines (tetanus, *Haemophilus* b conjugate vaccine) and their ability to produce blood-group isohaemagglutinins. If affected infants are asymptomatic, no treatment is required. However, if there are severe or recurrent bacterial infections, antibiotic prophylaxis is warranted. Replacement immunoglobulin is only very rarely required. Although this is a self-limiting disorder, the infants should be followed up until immunoglobulin levels are normal, to differentiate them from children with primary immunodeficiency disease. If immunoglobulin replacement therapy is used, it is important to stop this treatment after 3 to 6 months to allow re-evaluation of antibody responses.

Selective antibody deficiency with normal immunoglobulins

Some individuals with recurrent respiratory tract infections fail to respond to specific microbial antigens. The typical defect is an inability to respond to bacterial capsular polysaccharides, lasting beyond early childhood. Protein antibody responses are characteristically preserved. The prevalence of this condition is not known. Although most such individuals are asymptomatic, some develop recurrent sino-pulmonary infections.

The diagnosis is established by demonstrating normal IgG and IgM levels, accompanied by a failure to respond to immunization with some antigens, but with normal responses to others. Tetanus and the *Haemophilus* b (Hib) conjugate vaccine can be used to assess T-cell dependent responses. Measurement of serotype-specific responses to the pneumococcal polysaccharide vaccine (Pneumovax) is used to assess thymus-dependent antibody responses. Pneumococcal conjugate vaccine stimulates T-cell dependent antibody responses. In countries employing routine immunization of infants with the conjugate pneumococcal polysaccharide vaccine, therefore, antibody responses to five or more serotypes contained only within the polyvalent pneumococcal polysaccharide vaccine need to be assessed. Serotype-specific pneumococcal antibody assays need to be calibrated with an international reference standard (Food and Drug Administration SF 89) and the patient serum pre-absorbed with C-polysaccharide shared by all pneumococcal strains and 22F polysaccharide, which is cross reactive. Interpretation of pneumococcal antibody responses is difficult because of the lack of age-specific normal ranges. Furthermore, even healthy individuals may show reduced responses to individual serotypes. Pure polysaccharides are poor immunogens in infants less than 2 years of age. Between 2 and 5 years, response to at least 50% of the serotypes tested is the norm, while normal adults respond to about 70% of the capsular polysaccharides, when immunized with the pneumococcal polysaccharide vaccine. *Haemophilus* b and pneumococcal conjugate vaccines are powerful immunogens, and failure to respond to a full course of these vaccines should raise the suspicion of CVID. A consensus group in the United States of America has published provisional criteria for interpreting post-immunization responses to pneumococcal polysaccharide vaccines, as achieving an antibody level of at least 1.3 μg/ml against each serotype, or a greater than fourfold increase over baseline values.

Treatment of patients with selective antibody deficiency

Patients with selective antipolysaccharide antibody deficiency respond to and may benefit from conjugate vaccines. Antibiotic prophylaxis is sufficient for the management of most infection prone patients with selective antibody deficiency.

Antibody deficiency associated with thymoma

Patients with a thymoma may develop antibody deficiency with a clinical phenotype of CVID and presenting in the fourth decade or later. Such patients may exhibit features of T-cell deficiency and develop opportunistic infections including mucocutaneous candidiasis, *Pneumocystis jiroveci* pneumonia, cytomegalovirus, recurrent Herpes zoster and Herpes simplex infections. Autoimmune neutropenia, haemolytic anaemia, and red cell aplasia may occur. Laboratory findings are similar to those in CVID. Low serum IgM levels and B lymphopenia are seen in most. Plain radiographs may miss a thymoma and a CT scan of the chest may be required. These tumours can be locally invasive and a thymectomy is recommended, although the immunodeficiency is not reversed by this procedure. Due to the development of progressive T-cell deficiency, the condition has a worse prognosis than CVID.

IgA deficiency

This condition has an approximate incidence of 1 in 700 in white persons. It is rare in Africans and Japanese. Most individuals remain healthy, but long-term prospective studies indicate that a small proportion develop recurrent sino-pulmonary infections. Most infection-prone patients have concomitant IgG2 subclass deficiency and a selective inability to respond to pure capsular polysaccharides. IgA deficiency is associated with an increased incidence of atopy, coeliac disease, and a range of autoimmune diseases including arthritis, a lupus-like syndrome, autoimmune endocrinopathies, and autoimmune cytopenias. IgA-deficient patients with serum levels less than 0.07 g/litre are at risk of developing anti-IgA antibodies on receiving blood products. Such patients are at risk of anaphylactic reactions following the administration of blood or its fractions. IgA deficiency can coexist in families with other members affected by CVID. TACI mutations can cause IgA deficiency in some family members, while others develop CVID.

IgG subclass deficiency

Serum IgG is comprised of four subclasses, IgG1, -2, -3, and -4, in order of the relative abundance of these isotypes in the serum.

IgG subclass deficiency is diagnosed when there is a reduction in the serum IgG subclass concentration two standard deviations below the normal value for age, despite the total IgG level being normal. If the total IgG level is reduced, CVID is more likely. The lack of an internationally accepted reference preparation makes IgG subclass assays difficult to standardize. Furthermore, genetic variations influencing IgG subclass levels exist among different ethnic groups and age- and population-related normal bounds are not always available.

As with IgA deficiency, many individuals with IgG subclass deficiency are asymptomatic. Some individuals with IgG subclass deficiency are prone to recurrent sino-pulmonary and other infections. Most with sino-pulmonary infections exhibit impaired capacity to mount specific antipolysaccharide antibodies against antigens like the pneumococcal capsule. This is most often seen in individuals with IgG2 deficiency, with or without concomitant IgA deficiency. Most infection-prone patients with IgG subclass deficiency can be managed with antibiotic therapy or prophylaxis.

Immunoglobulin replacement should be limited to those with recurrent severe sino-pulmonary infections despite antibiotic prophylaxis. Such patients usually have specific antibody deficiency, especially to polysaccharides. Hence, in the United Kingdom there is a strong consensus that assessing specific antibodies is more useful than IgG subclass measurements for the assessment of infection-prone patients.

Treatment of antibody deficiency: immunoglobulin replacement therapy

Immunoglobulin replacement therapy through the intravenous (IVIG) or subcutaneous (SCIG) routes (Box 5.2.2), is the mainstay of therapy for antibody deficiency. Different products are licensed for IVIG and SCIG therapy, and are not interchangeable. IVIG and SCIG are equivalent in terms of safety and efficacy. All licensed immunoglobulin products have similar efficacy, safety, and tolerability, therefore product selection depends on availability. However, once patients are stabilized on one preparation, this should not be changed except for sound medical reasons.

Current practices of pre-screening donors and multiple antiviral steps employed by manufacturers have eliminated the risk of transmission of HIV and hepatitis B and C. Rare hepatitis C outbreaks occurred in the 1990s before the current multistage viral inactivation steps were introduced. Creutzfeldt–Jakob disease (classical and new variant) could theoretically by transmitted by immunoglobulin therapy, but the risk has been estimated to be exceedingly low. Plasma for manufacture of immunoglobulin products is not sourced in the United Kingdom, by government decree.

Adequacy of replacement therapy is judged by clinical well-being (freedom from infections and prevention of their complications) and preinfusion (trough) levels in the middle of the normal range (approximately 8 g/litre). Based on these criteria, replacement therapy needs to be individualized for each patient by altering the dose or frequency of administration. With adequate training and regular supervision, most patients can administer immunoglobulin replacement therapy at home.

Adverse effects of immunoglobulin replacement therapy

About 10% of patients experience mild reactions, including headaches, malaise, backache, nausea, and myalgia, during or immediately after IVIG therapy. This can usually be overcome by a combination of reducing the infusion rate, antihistamines, and antipyretics. Anaphylactic reactions, requiring cessation of therapy and adrenaline (epinephrine), are rare, and commoner during the first few infusions or the presence of intercurrent infections. These can be almost eliminated by administration of the initial infusion at a slow rate and postponing IVIG therapy until infections have resolved on antibiotic therapy. Rarely, anaphylactic reactions may be due to patients with severe IgA deficiency (serum levels less than 0.07 g/litre) producing anti-IgA antibodies. Premedication with paracetamol, antihistamines, and/or hydrocortisone, or changing the immunoglobulin product, often helps in patients who develop repeated adverse reactions. Apart from local pain and swelling, adverse reactions are rare with SCIG therapy. Switching to SCIG may be an option for patients who fail to tolerate IVIG.

Box 5.2.2 Dosage for immunoglobulin replacement therapy

- IVIG—from 400 to 800 mg/kg every 4 weeks
- SCIG—from 100 to 200 mg/kg once a week, or half the dose administered twice a week

Outcome of antibody deficiency

Prospective studies have shown that optimal immunoglobulin replacement therapy reduces the incidence of sepsis, especially by encapsulated bacteria. If this is instituted before structural lung damage is established, recipients are likely to have a normal lifespan. However, long-term studies in Italy have demonstrated that a proportion of patients with X-linked agammaglobulinaemia on optimum immunoglobulin replacement therapy may continue to develop lung damage. The cause for this is unclear, and this is a subject for future research. CVID patients with systemic granulomatous disease or interstitial lung disease exhibit reduced survival compared to those without these complications. The occurrence of non-Hodgkin's lymphoma (2–7%) and gastric carcinoma (approximately 1%) reduce survival.

Supplementary management of antibody deficiency

Even with optimum immunoglobulin replacement therapy, breakthrough infections can occur in these patients. There should be a low threshold for treating infections with antibiotics. Recurrent infections, especially when associated with structural lung damage, may require long-term prophylaxis. amoxicillin, co-amoxiclav, clarithromycin, doxicycline, and ciprofloxacin are useful agents for prophylaxis. Postural drainage of lung secretions and appropriate treatment of concomitant bronchial asthma is important.

Patients with serious lung disease, gastrointestinal disease, or impaired liver function should be managed with multidisciplinary input from relevant organ-based specialists. Patients should be encouraged to join support groups for education and counselling as well as practical help with social problems. Referral for genetic counselling should be considered in patients with a familial disorder or a known gene defect.

Defects in cell mediated immunity (T-cell dependent immunity)

These may be inherited (rare) or acquired (see Box 5.2.3 for classification of causes). Clearly, HIV infection is an important

Box 5.2.3 Cause of defective cell-mediated immunity (T-cell deficiency)

Congenital (primary)

See Table 5.2.2 for list of conditions.

Secondary

- Virally induced
  - HIV
  - Measles
- Iatrogenic
  - Irradiation
  - Bone marrow transplantation, until engraftment is complete
  - Chemotherapy for malignancy
  - Immunosuppressive therapy
- Loss of T cells from the gut (protein-losing enteropathy)
- Thymoma
- Lymphoma
- Severe renal failure or liver failure

cause of impaired cell mediated immunity and the incidence of this disorder varies with geographical location and the presence of risk factors for acquiring HIV infection (see Chapter 7.5.23).

Clinical phenotype of patients with impaired T-cell dependent immunity

Susceptibility to intracellular microbial pathogens including viruses, intracellular bacteria, and protozoans is increased. Infections caused by microbes of low-grade virulence (opportunistic infections) are common.

- Viral infections:
  - Children with T-cell deficiency may develop fatal infection with common exanthematous viruses (e.g. measles or chickenpox). These viruses are not a problem in adults, presumably because protective antibody responses following primary infection or immunization are robust, even when T-cell function is greatly diminished.
  - In children with SCID, chronic lung infection may be caused by respiratory syncytial virus, parainfluenza virus, cytomegalovirus, and adenovirus.
  - Adults with T-cell deficiency are often affected by reactivation of latent viruses which cause considerable morbidity and mortality. These include the cytomegalovirus, herpes simplex, and varicella-zoster. Epstein–Barr virus causes hairy leukoplakia of the tongue, seen in AIDS patients and may also cause a type of non-Hodgkin's lymphoma in these patients.
- Interstitial pneumonia caused by *Pneumocycstis jiroveci* is pathognomonic for T-cell deficiency
- Fungal infections:
  - T-cell deficient patients often develop mucocutaneous infection with *Candida* as well as invasive infection caused by filamentous fungi like *Aspergillus* and *Mucor*. Persistent oral candidiasis in an adult, without predisposing factors like broad-spectrum antibiotic therapy, the wearing of dentures, or the use of inhaled corticosteroids, and which recurs after antifungal treatment is highly suspicious of T-cell deficiency. In these patients *Candida* may affect the oesophagus and trachea as well. (Invasive candidasis, however, is not a feature of T-cell deficiency but is seen in patients with neutropenia or in intravenous drug users or those with intravenous lines or indwelling catheters.)
  - Cryptococcal infections involving the central nervous system or the lung, or in a disseminated form, may be seen.
- Intracellular bacterial infection:
  - T-cell deficient patients are highly susceptible to *de novo* infection or reactivation of tuberculosis, which may be disseminated, extra-thoracic or atypical in presentation.
  - Disseminated potentially fatal infections with poorly pathogenic mycobacteria including non-tuberculous mycobacteria and bacille Calmette-Guérin (BCG).
- Infants with T-cell deficiency usually exhibit failure to thrive.
- Infants with SCID may develop graft-vs-host disease due to maternal lymphocytes that have crossed the placenta, which may result in dermatitis and hepatosplenomegaly.
- Chronic diarrhoea caused by a variety of pathogens including *Cryptosporidium*, *Giardia*, and *Rotavirus*.
- Certain malignancies may develop where another infection is a cofactor, e.g. Epstein–Barr virus-induced non-Hodgkin's lymphoma and Kaposi's sarcoma where human herpesvirus 8 is the cofactor. There is an increased incidence of cutaneous malignancies in individuals who are exposed to significant amounts of ultraviolet light (e.g. basal cell carcinoma and squamous cell carcinoma of skin). Skin malignancies are not common in northern latitudes but are typically seen in sunny parts of the world.

The clinical phenotype of patients with impaired T-cell dependent immunity is summarized in Fig. 5.2.1.

Major categories of immunodeficiency exhibiting impaired T-cell function

Severe combined immunodeficiency (SCID)

This syndrome is characterized by severe failure of specific immune responses, dependent on lymphocyte function. Patients with SCID exhibit a clinical and immunological phenotype characterized by defects in both B and T cells. These are rare disorders, with an estimated incidence of 1 in 50 000 to 1 in 100 000 live births.

Clinical features of SCID

Most of these conditions present in early infancy, with failure to thrive and recurrent, severe, potentially life-threatening bacterial, viral, or fungal infections. These infections may be caused by a broad range of common pathogens, but often include persistent infections by organisms of low-grade virulence (e.g. *Candida*, *Pneumocystis*, cytomegalovirus). Diarrhoea, which is often due to viral infection, is common. Persistent respiratory infection may be caused by adenoviruses, respiratory syncytial virus or parainfluenza virus. Graft-vs-host disease, which is produced by transplacentally acquired maternal lymphocytes or the action of aberrant autoreactive T cells (Omenn's syndrome), manifests as skin rashes, or less commonly hepatosplenomegaly or lymphadenopathy.

Physical signs are chiefly those due to the presence of infection or complications of infection. The absence of tonsils or other lymph nodes may be noted, and radiographic studies may reveal the absence of a thymus. Immunologically, SCID is characterized by the presence of lymphopenia compared to age-related absolute lymphocyte counts, the severe reduction or absence of major lymphocyte subsets, deficient *in vitro* T-cell proliferation to mitogens, and markedly reduced total and specific antibody levels.

Immunological and molecular classification of SCID

Based on the blood lymphocyte phenotype, patients with SCID can be divided into two groups:

- T–B+ SCID—those who lack T cells but have normal or increased B cells
- T–B– SCID—those who lack both T and B cells

Defects in four functionally related genes cause T–B+ SCID. The commonest is X-linked SCID, due to a defective *IL2RG* gene that encodes the γ-chain common to the receptors for six cytokines (interleukins 2, 4, 7, 9, 15, and 21). The common γ-chain is the signal-transducing chain for all these receptors. The absence of response to these critically important cytokines explains the broad range of defects in specific B- and T-cell function in these patients. Interleukin 7 is required for early T-cell development and the lack of response to this cytokine results in the arrest of T-cell development at an early stage. Interaction of the common γ-chain with the JAK-3 tyrosine kinase is essential for signal transduction through the aforementioned cytokine receptors. Therefore JAK-3 gene mutations result in an autosomal recessive form of SCID with a similar phenotype. Mutations of the α-chains of the interleukin 7 and interleukin 2 receptors respectively are two further rare causes of T–B+ SCID.

About 50% of patients with T–B– SCID have a mutation in one of the recombinase activating genes (*RAG1* or *RAG2*). RAG1 and RAG2 recognize recombination signal sequences and introduce double-stranded DNA breaks, which initiates V, D, J gene rearrangements that are responsible for generating the normal repertoire of T- and B-cell antigen receptors. Without RAG1 and RAG2 function, T- and B-cell development fails, giving rise to T– B– SCID. Hypomorphic mutations of *RAG1* or *RAG2* cause a variant of SCID called Omenn's syndrome (OMIM 603554). In this condition a few T- and B-cell clones develop and undergo secondary expansion. Although patients with Omenn's syndrome may not be severely lymphopenic, their T-cells are oligoclonal and clinically the condition behaves like SCID.

A few patients with T–B– SCID who are also radiation sensitive have a mutation in a gene *DCLRE1C*, encoding for a protein (Artemis) required for DNA repair including the repair of strand breaks generated during VDJ recombinations.

About 15% of the cases of SCID are caused by adenosine deaminase deficiency, which has an autosomal recessive inheritance. This enzyme is essential for the salvage of nucleotides within lymphoid cells. The lack of adenosine deaminase results in the accumulation of toxic metabolites of purines within lymphocytes, which results in increased rates of death in T and B cells and their precursors, through mechanisms that are incompletely understood. Adenosine deaminase deficiency results in profound lymphopenia with reduced T, B, and NK cells. Rare mutations of adenosine deaminase which cause a milder defect may present with the milder immunodeficiency presenting in older patients.

Purine nucleoside phosphorylase is an enzyme which is also required for purine salvage within lymphocytes. Purine nucleoside phosphorylase deficiency causes a rare form of SCID which has a milder phenotype than seen in adenosine deaminase deficiency, but is nevertheless, fatal in childhood, without successful bone marrow transplantation.

A rare group of defects responsible for SCID impair signal transduction through the T-cell receptors. This includes a defect in the protein tyrosine phosphatase CD45 which is required for signalling through T- and B-cell receptors. Mutation of the δ-chain of the CD3 complex causes SCID but defects in the γ- and ε-chains of CD3 cause a milder, variable phenotype. A mutation of the gene encoding ZAP70 (zeta chain associated protein 70) which interacts with the ζ-chain of CD3 results in severe CD8 lymphopenia. In this condition, CD4 counts may be normal but their function is also reduced. A mutation of the *ORAI1* gene encoding a subunit of the plasma membrane calcium channel CRAC, causes a rare form of SCID due to defective calcium entry into T cells which impairs T-cell function.

The lack of expression of MHC class 2 on lymphocytes (MHC class 2 deficiency) leads to a severe form of SCID. Four gene defects encoding for components of a transcription complex promoting the transcription of MHC class 2 genes can lead to this condition. In the absence of MHC class 2, thymic CD4 T cell generation is abrogated, resulting in CD4 lymphopenia. CD4 cells recognize antigen in the context of MHC class 2 genes expressed by antigen-presenting cells. The absence of MHC class 2 therefore results in a profound failure of CD4 cell function. MHC class 2 deficiency therefore results in a severe failure of cell-mediated immunity and also defective generation of antibody responses. Recently, a T–B+ NK+ form of SCID due to lack of T-cell egress from the thymus, caused by a mutation of the gene *CORO1A*, encoding for the actin regulatory protein Coronin 1A, has been described.

Diagnosis of SCID

The diagnosis is readily suspected in most cases of infants who fail to thrive and suffer from recurrent severe infections from an early age. The clinical features raising the suspicion of SCID are summarized above. SCID is a medical emergency, as patients rapidly succumb to life-threatening infections. Untreated SCID is invariably fatal, with most dying in the first year of life, and the balance succumbing by the second year. Conversely, early bone marrow transplantation results in long-term survival in more than 95% of cases. The pretransplant occurrence of infections is associated with poorer outcome. For all these reasons, early diagnosis is essential (see Fig. 5.2.2).

HIV infection may present with a similar clinical picture and needs to be excluded by detection of the viral genome by the polymerase chain reaction. A detailed family history should enquire into consanguinity of parents, the occurrence of immunodeficiency in other family members, and deaths in early infancy within the pedigree.

The initial screening tests are:

- blood count and differential count
- enumeration of blood lymphocyte populations
- measurement of serum immunoglobulins.

Lymphopenia (absolute lymphocyte count $<3 \times 10^9$/litre in the first year of life) is a characteristic feature seen in over 80% of patients with SCID. Hence SCID needs to be excluded in all infants with a lymphocyte count below the age-related reference range. The second stage is to enumerate blood lymphocyte subsets (T cells, B cells, and NK cells) using flow cytometry. These results should be interpreted using age-matched reference ranges. The minimum panel of monoclonal antibodies recommended for lymphocyte phenotype determination are summarized in Table 5.2.4. The lymphocyte phenotypes typically associated with different molecular variants of SCID are summarized in Table 5.2.5.

Serum immunoglobulin levels are difficult to interpret in young infants. In SCID, IgM and IgA levels are usually low. The IgG level, which is maternally derived, may be normal in early infancy but progressively declines with time. In Omenn's syndrome, IgE levels may be elevated. The absence of lymphopenia does not completely rule out SCID. This can occur in SCID patients engrafted with transplacentally acquired maternal lymphocytes or in Omenn's syndrome. In these cases, the demonstration of oligoclonality of the T-cell repertoire (in contrast to the normal T-cell receptor repertoire) and poor *in vitro* T-cell proliferation to mitogens helps to confirm a diagnosis of SCID. These tests are only available in specialized centres. HLA typing of the mother and baby will help to identify maternal engraftment.

SCID is the probable diagnosis in infants who are less than 2 years of age and have (1) an absolute lymphocyte count $<3 \times 10^9$/litre, (2) CD3 cells <20% of the total lymphocyte count, and (3) proliferative responses to mitogens <10% of control values, in the absence of maternal engraftment.

Once the diagnosis of SCID is considered likely, additional investigations to identify the molecular phenotype of SCID are important, as these may guide the details of therapy, family counselling, and prenatal diagnosis. Such tests are available only in a few highly specialized centres. Specialist tests include metabolic studies (to identify adenosine deaminase or purine nucleoside phosphorylase deficiency), detection of proteins required for lymphocyte function by flow cytometry or western blotting (e.g. to identify common γ-chain defect), and mutation analysis of candidate genes.

Treatment and prognosis of SCID

Patients suspected of SCID should be transferred to expert paediatric centres as soon as possible. Immediate management of SCID includes protective isolation, prophylaxis for *Pneumocystis jiroveci* pneumonia infection, and a diligent search for existing infection and its treatment. If infection is suspected but the microbiological diagnosis is uncertain, empirical antibiotic therapy should be considered. Any blood transfusions should be irradiated and from cytomegalovirus-negative donors. Live vaccines are contraindicated. Once SCID is diagnosed, IVIG replacement should commence without delay. Untreated SCID has a fatality rate of 100%. Once a diagnosis of SCID is confirmed, irrespective of the molecular diagnosis, bone marrow haemopoietic stem cell transplantation from a HLA-identical or haplo-identical family donor is the treatment of choice. Treatment of SCID with bone marrow transplantation before 3.5 months of age has achieved good immune reconstitution and 95% long-term survival. In patients with SCID, bone marrow transplantation can be achieved with little or no immunosuppressive therapy. Delay in treatment or the occurrence of infection impairs outcome.

Infection and graft-vs-host disease are the main complications following bone marrow transplantation. European data indicate that long-term survival after transplants from HLA-matched unrelated donors was close to 60%. Review of European data between 1968 and 1999 indicates the progressive improvement of outcome, which is mainly due to better prevention of GVHD and the treatment of infection. Analysis of the outcome of European and American bone marrow transplant programmes for the treatment of SCID is ongoing and will be reported from time to time.

Gene therapy for SCID

Long-term immune reconstitution has been achieved in patients with SCID caused by the common γ-chain deficiency or ADA deficiency using gene therapy. This was achieved by *ex vivo* gene transfer to haemopoietic stem cells isolated from the patient's bone marrow. These gene-reconstituted stem cells were re-transfused into the patient. To date, gene therapy has been restricted to patients without an HLA-matched family donor.

Several cases of leukaemia have occurred among γ-chain deficient patients who received gene therapy. In these cases, the retroviral vector had integrated close to the *LMO2* proto-oncogene in the leukaemic clone leading to aberrant transcription and expression of *LMO2*. Because of this setback, clinical trials of gene therapy for SCID are being carefully evaluated and more experience is required before the exact role of gene therapy in SCID is established. Trials of gene therapy for SCID due to common γ-chain deficiency with improved vectors are underway.

Table 5.2.4 Blood lymphocyte profile in different molecular forms of SCID

SCID variant	CD3+	CD4+	CD8+	B cells	NK cells
IL2RG (common γ-chain), *IL2RA*, *JAK3*	Low	Low	Low	Normal	Low
IL7RA	Low	Low	Low	Normal or high	Normal or high
RAG 1, *RAG2*, *DCLRE1C* (*Artemis*)	Low	Low	Low	Low	Normal
ADA	Low	Low	Low	Low	Low
MHC class II deficiency	Normal	Low	Normal	Normal	Normal
ZAP-70	Normal	Normal	Low	Normal	Normal

Table 5.2.5 Designations of monoclonal antibody combinations recommended for lymphocyte phenotyping

Surface antigen recognized by antibody	Cells recognized
CD3	All T cells
CD3+CD4	T helper
CD3+CD8	T cytotoxic
CD16 and/or CD56	NK cells
CD19 or CD20	B cells
MHC class 11	B cells and monocytes
MHC class 1	All nucleated cells
CD3+TCR$\alpha\beta$	TCR$\alpha\beta$–bearing T cells
CD3+TCR$\gamma\delta$	TCR$\gamma\delta$-bearing T cells

MHC class 1 deficiency

Cell surface expression of MHC (major histocompatibility complex) class 1 molecules is deficient if one of the two transporters associated with antigen processing (TAP1 or 2) is absent. TAP1 and 2 transfer antigenic peptides from the cytosol across to the endoplasmic reticulum, to be loaded on to a newly synthesized MHC class 1 molecules. Subsequently the peptide-loaded MHC class 1 molecules are transported to the cell surface. In the absence of TAP1 or 2, cell surface expression of MHC class 1 molecules is deficient. CD8 T-cell receptors recognize only antigenic peptides that are bound to MHC class 1 molecules. In the absence of MHC class 1 molecules, CD8 cells are not generated in the thymus. The resultant immunodeficiency is milder than SCID and patients may present later in life. Paradoxically, viral infections are not a problem in these patients. Some patients develop a progressive bronchiectasis while others develop granulomatous destruction of the nose and face, resembling midline granuloma. The underlying pathology appears to be a vasculitis which is postulated to be due to self-destruction of endothelial cells by the unrestrained cytotoxicity of the NK cells.

DiGeorge syndrome (thymic aplasia)

Hemizygous deletion of chromosome 22q11 (del22q11.2) causes a complex syndrome including cardiac malformation, thymic hypoplasia, palatal abnormalities with associated velopharyngeal dysfunction, hypoparathyroidism, and facial dysmorphism, known as DiGeorge syndrome or thymic aplasia (OMIM 188400). 22q deletion has an incidence of about 1 in 2500 live births, but the clinical phenotype is highly variable. Some patients with 22q deletion have normal thymic development (and hence normal T-cell mediated immunity) but have cardiac, pharyngeal, and a wide range of other defects associated with the velocardiofacial (VCF) or Shprintzen syndrome (OMIM 192430). Cardiac, velopharyngeal, thymic, and parathyroid abnormalities arise from defective development of the third and fourth branchial arches during fetal development. Only about 20% of those with 22q deletion show evidence of reduced number and function of T cells. In most affected infants, the degree of T lymphopenia is modest, and a near normal repertoire and the function of T cells is acquired by 2 years of age. Infections characteristic of T-cell deficiency are therefore uncommon. A minority (<1%) exhibit profound T lymphopenia (CD3 count $<0.5 \times 10^9$/litre) and develop a SCID-like phenotype, with opportunistic infections (complete DiGeorge syndrome). Such patients have been successfully treated with HLA-matched bone marrow transplants or fetal thymic transplants.

The diagnosis of 22q deletion should be considered in any child with congenital heart disease, velopharyngeal abnormalities, or neonatal hypocalcaemia. The 22q deletion that is seen in 95% of patients with DiGeorge/velocardiofacial syndrome can be readily detected by cytogenic studies employing fluorescent *in-situ* hybridization. In the majority (96%) of affected individuals, the 22q deletion is *de novo* and in the remaining 4% it is inherited from a parent.

TBOX 1 (*TBX1*) is a gene which maps to the centre of the DiGeorge syndrome chromosomal region on 22q11.2. It is one member of the so-called TBOX genes, which are transcription factors involved in the regulation of developmental processes. *TBX1* mutations have been identified in patients with the clinical phenotypes that are seen in the del22q11.2 syndrome, including abnormal facies, cardiac defects, thymic hypoplasia, velopharyngeal defects, and hypoparathyroidism. This suggests that haploinsufficiency of the *TBX1* gene may be responsible for significant components of the phenotype of the 22q deletion syndrome.

Phagocyte deficiencies

Neutropenia

The commonest phagocyte deficiency seen in clinical practice is neutropenia, which results in increased susceptibility to a broad range of pyogenic organisms and fungi. In neutropenic patients commensal organisms including skin and intestinal bacteria often cause septicaemic illnesses. Invasive candidiasis and occasionally other fungal infections may also be seen in these patients. Neutrophils are particularly important for maintaining the integrity of mucous membranes. Hence, inflammation of mucous membranes, e.g. ulceration of mouth and perioral tissues and perianal inflammation and excoriation, can be features of neutropenia. A neutrophil count of less then 0.5×10^9/litre is associated with a high risk of life-threatening bacterial sepsis.

Defects in bacterial killing

Functional defects of neutrophils are rare. The best-characterized condition is chronic granulomatous disease, with an incidence of 1 in 20 000 births. Neutrophils and macrophages of these patients cannot kill ingested bacteria. This is due to a faulty post-phagocytic activation of the NADPH oxidase complex which produces superoxide (O_2^-) and generates a milieu within the phagosome that activates bactericidal enzymes cathespin and elastase. In the X-linked form (75% of total cases), this is due to a defect of the 91-kD chain of the cytochrome b ($gp91^{phox}$) whereas the rarer autosomal recessive form may be either due to deficiency of the 22-kD chain of cytochrome b ($p22^{phox}$) or cytosolic cofactors called $p47^{phox}$ and $p67^{phox}$ respectively.

Patients typically present in infancy with infections (see below) but initial presentation in adulthood is well documented. Chronic granulomatous disease patients develop infections with *Staphyloccocus aureus* or Gram-negative bacteria (*Burkholderia cepacia, Salmonella, Serratia*, enteric bacteria). Invasive fungal infections (*Aspergillus*) are life threatening. *Nocardia* is another pathogen seen in chronic granulomatous disease. Unusual environmental bacteria of low-grade virulence may be isolated from blood and lymph nodes. Characteristic sites of infection include skin, deep subcutaneous abscesses, or visceral abscesses involving lymph nodes, liver, spleen, or lung. Oral and perioral ulceration and gingivitis are common. These patients also develop granulomas in various tissues, giving rise to pathological problems. Granulomatous obstruction of the gastrointestinal tract or the urinary tract may occur and granulomatous infiltration of the lung may rarely be seen. Hepatosplenomegaly due to granulomatous involvement of these organs may also be a feature. Colitis resembling Crohn's disease is seen in approximately 15% of cases.

The diagnosis is based on the inability of neutrophils from these patients, when stimulated, to oxidize a dye called nitro blue tetrazolium and change it from yellow to a blue-black colour. Modifications of this principle using new methods such as the oxidation of the fluorescent dye dihydrorhodamine which can be detected by flow cytometry are reliable and sensitive for establishing the diagnosis.

Management consists of antimicrobal prophylaxis and prompt diagnosis and treatment of infections. Co-trimoxzaole at 5 mg/kg divided into two doses per day significantly reduces bacterial infections and daily itraconazole (100 mg for patients <50 kg body weight or 200 mg for, heavier individuals) reduces *Aspergillus* infections. A limited number of trials in the United States of America have shown reduced severe infections with prophylactic interferon at 50 μg/m^2, three times a week, via subcutaneous injection. Invasive fungal infections are difficult to treat and experience at major American centres suggests the need to use newer antifungal agents like voriconazole and pozaconazole. Granulocyte transfusions may be beneficial in those with severe, refractory infections. Bone marrow transplantation should be considered for patients with repeated severe infections with a matched sibling donor. Gene therapy has produced temporary physiological and clinical improvement for a few months in three patients, but has to be considered experimental at present.

Defects in leucocyte migration

Leucocyte adhesion deficiency type 1 is caused by deficiency of the CD18 which is the β-chain of three leucocyte surface receptors called CD11a/CD18 (leucocyte functional antigen), CD11b/CD18 (complement receptor 3), and CD11c/CD18 (complement receptor 4). The rarer form of leucocyte adhesion deficiency type 2 is due to a mutation of a GDP fucose transporter resulting in a failure of fucosylation of proteins within the Golgi apparatus.

To confer protection from infection, circulating phagocytes need to migrate along chemotactic gradients across capillary endothelium into sites of infection. Lymphocyte function-associated antigen 1 on leucocytes needs to bind tightly to the ligand intercellular adhesion molecule 1 (ICAM-1) on activated endothelial cells for emigration into tissues to occur. In leucocyte adhesion deficiency type 2, sialyl-lewis X, which is expressed on the surface of leucocytes and acts as the ligand for E selectin expressed on endothelial cells, cannot be synthesized. Without this interaction the initial adhesion of leucocytes to endothelial cells, a prelude to diapedesis, fails. Thus leucocyte adhesion deficiency types 1 and 2 exhibit impaired endothelial adherence, chemotaxis, and diapedesis of neutrophils and other leucocytes, which are held back in the circulation and cannot reach the sites of infection.

These patients characteristically develop delayed cord separation and periumbical sepsis during early infancy. Other features are recurrent pyogenic infections, persistent marked leucocytosis (>15 × 10^9/litre) due to the inability of leucocytes to migrate out into the tissues, and poor wound healing, with the development of pyoderma-like ulcers which may eventually heal, with paper-thin scars. Pus fails to form during infections. These inherited disorders of neutrophil function are characteristically associated with gingivitis and periodontal disease, again indicating the particular importance of normal neutrophil function for the maintenance of a healthy dental/gingival interface. Patients with leucocyte adhesion deficiency type 2 have facial dysmorphism, mental disability, and developmental delay.

Diagnosis of these conditions is by flow cytometry of blood leucocytes to detect CD18 or CD15 (sialyl-Lewis X) deficiency, respectively. In the complete form of leucocyte adhesion deficiency type 1 and in type 2, outcome is poor with early death from sepsis. Rare patients with a partial form of type 1, with a milder phenotype, may survive to adulthood. Bone marrow transplantation is curative in leucocyte adhesion deficiency type 1 and should be considered early. Oral fucose supplementation can result in clinical improvement in leucocyte adhesion deficiency type 2. For leucocyte adhesion deficiency type 3, see Table 5.2.3.

Leucocyte adhesion deficiency due to RAC 2 deficiency

Mutation of the gene encoding the Rac 2 GTPase causes impaired neutrophil motility and superoxide production in response to some stimuli. The clinical features in this case were similar to those seen in leucocyte adhesion deficiency.

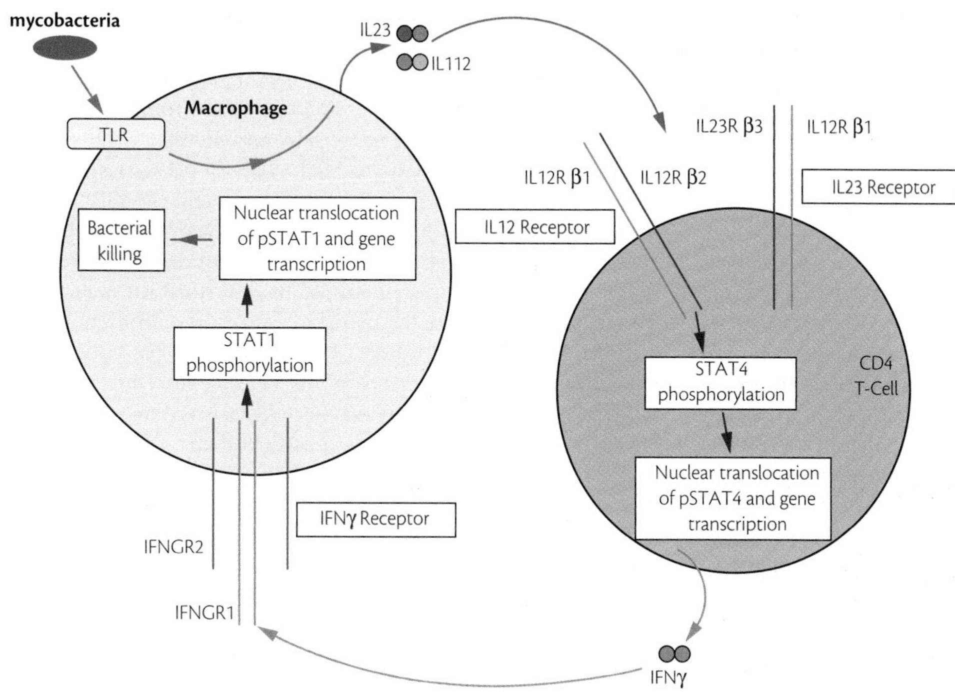

Fig. 5.2.3 A highly simplified diagrammatic representation of the key cytokine–receptor interactions relevant for immunity against intracellular bacteria, derived from observations in gene knock-out mice. Stimulation of macrophages/dendritic cells by mycobacteria by infection and via Toll receptors results in secretion of IL-12 which acts on antigen stimulated CD4 T cells (which express IL-12 receptors). IL-12 partitions responding CD4 T cells to develop along the Th1 pathway and secrete interferon-γ. Interferon-γ homodimers activate (a) macrophages enhancing their antimicrobial pathways and (b) T cells and NK cells in an autocrine fashion, via IFN-γR1/R2 dimers. Type I cytokine deficient patients indicate the relevance of these pathways for human immunity.

For information on rarer primary immunodeficiency diseases with impaired phagocyte function, see the sources listed in the 'Further reading' section.

Mendelian susceptibility to mycobacterial disease

Primary and secondary immunodeficiencies leading to severely impaired T-cell function result in increased susceptibility to mycobacterial infections, including those caused by poorly pathogenic mycobacteria (non-tuberculous mycobateria) and bacillus Calmette–Guérin (BCG). However, these infections may also occur in a disseminated, fatal form, sometimes with a familial distribution, in the absence of any recognized primary or secondary immunodeficiency. Genetic analysis of affected kindreds have, to date, defined mutations in six different genes participating in the interleukin 12 (IL-12)- and interleukin 23 (IL-23)-dependent, high-output interferon-γ pathway (see Fig. 5.2.3). This condition has been called mendelian susceptibility to mycobacterial disease (OMIM 209950).

Several gene defects responsible for mendelian susceptibility to mycobacterial disease have been documented:

- Recessive null mutations in the gene encoding the interferon-γ receptor (IFN-γR1) chain which either abolish receptor expression or their binding of interferon-γ. Dominant IFN-γR1 deficiency is due to the truncation of the intracellular domain of the receptor chain, resulting in the accumulation of non-functional receptors which interfere with the function of the residual normal receptors. Recessive mutations of the gene encoding the IFN-γR2 signalling chain are responsible for complete or partial IFN-γR2 deficiency.
- Null recessive mutations of the *IL-12RBI* gene encoding the IL-12 receptor chain, IL-12RβI, abrogate the cell surface expression of this chain which is shared by IL-12 and IL-23 receptors. This results in the inability to respond to IL-12 and IL-23. Mutation of the IL-12/23 receptor associated tyrosine kinase, Tyk 2, causes defective signal transduction via IL-12 receptors.
- Inability to produce IL-12 and IL-23, due to deletion within the gene encoding the inducible chain of IL-12 (*IL12B*) which is shared by IL-12 and IL-23.
- Partial or complete defects in the signal transduction molecule STATI, which is required for signalling via the interferon-γ receptor.

Recently, acquired interferon-γ deficiency due to the production of neutralizing autoantibodies to this cytokine has been identified in patients with disseminated mycobacterial infection.

The severity of the clinical phenotype depends on the genotype. Patients with complete IFN-γR1 or R2 deficiencies develop disseminated mycobacterial infections caused by BCG or non-tuberculous mycobateria, which present in early childhood and have a high mortality. The lesions in this patient cohort are characteristically multibacillary and are associated with impaired granuloma formation. In contrast, partial IFN-γR1 deficiency, complete IL-12B deficiency (resulting in IL-12 and IL-23 deficiency), and IL-12/IL-23 receptor deficiency predispose to curable mycobacterial infections, presenting at a later age. The dominant form of partial STAT1 deficiency, with impaired biological responses to interferon-γ, appears to primarily affect antimycobacterial defences. In contrast, recessive, complete STAT1 deficiency with impaired responses to interferon-γ and type 1 interferons leads to mycobacterial infections, and to fatal herpes simplex viral infections which present in infancy. In addition to this, extraintestinal or septicaemic relapsing infections caused by non-typhoid *Salmonella* species are the most common infections occurring in patients with defects in the IL-12/23 system.

Defective NFκB activation caused by X-linked hypomorphic mutations of the NFκB essential modulator gene (*NEMO*) which compromises the function of Toll-, IL-1, and tumour necrosis factor α (TNFα) receptors, also increases susceptibility to severe mycobacterial infections. Patients with inherited defects in the phagocyte NADPH-oxidase system are highly susceptible to *Salmonella* infections but exhibit only slightly increased susceptibility to mycobacteria.

Mycobacterial infections in patients with IL-12B, IL-12B1, and dominant partial IFN-γR deficiency that are refractory to chemotherapy respond to interferon-γ supplementation. Interferon-γ is of no use in complete IFNγ-R1 or -R2 deficiency, where the outcome is poor despite antimycobacterial chemotherapy, and bone marrow transplantation should be considered at an early age.

In conclusion, the above defects need to be sought by immunological and molecular methods in patients with refractory or disseminated mycobacterial infections in the absence of an underlying cause such as HIV infection, immunosuppressive therapy, or a recognized primary T-cell immunodeficiency.

Wiskott–Aldrich syndrome

This X-linked syndrome (OMIM 301000) is characterized by eczema and thrombocytopenic purpura with small, defective platelets and variable immunodeficiency. Patients usually present in infancy with a bleeding tendency, manifesting as petechiae, bruising, prolonged bleeding from wounds, or bloody diarrhoea. Eczema can vary in severity. Antibody production to bacterial capsular polysaccharides is deficient and protein antibodies often decline with time. Patients therefore commonly develop recurrent sino-pulmonary and middle ear infections. Progressive T lymphopenia develops with time, and T cells and NK cells display reduced functional capacity. Hence patients can develop opportunistic infections typical of T-cell deficiency. Autoimmune conditions, colitis, glomerulonephritis, vasculitis, and autoimmune cytopenias occur in these patients. The risk of malignancies in Wiskott–Aldrich syndrome patients has been estimated at 2% per year. Lymphomas are the most frequent tumours, most of which are induced by Epstein–Barr virus.

The gene defect responsible for Wiskott–Aldrich syndrome codes for the Wiskott–Aldrich syndrome protein (WASP). WASP is a cytoplasmic component which regulates actin polymerization and cytoskeletal reorganization, required for normal platelet and lymphocyte function. For example, WASP function is required for cytoskeletal changes required for formation of immunological synapses between cooperating T cells and antigen-presenting cells. Certain missense mutations of WASP cause X-linked thrombocytopenia or X-linked neutropenia. Rare female carriers with skewed X-chromosome inactivation can be symptomatic.

The diagnosis of Wiskott–Aldrich syndrome is suspected on identifying thrombocytopenia with small platelets and confirmed by demonstrating the absence of WASP by western blotting or flow cytometry. Some WASP mutations permit the prediction of the severity of disease. Mutations leading to absence of WASP result in a severe phenotype while the expression of a mutant protein results in X-linked thrombocytopenia. Hence a molecular diagnosis should be sought in every case.

Treatment and outcome of Wiskott–Aldrich syndrome

In the days before bone marrow transplantation, the outlook for these patients was poor, with a median survival of 5–7 years. HLA-identical sibling-derived bone marrow transplantation is curative and associated with an approximately 90% 5-year survival. HLA-matched unrelated transplants carried out before 5 years of age have a similar success rate. Above this age, individual risk assessment is needed. Splenectomy for thrombocytopenia, immunoglobulin replacement therapy, and antibiotics are supportive therapies.

DNA repair defects associated with immunodeficiency

Ataxia telangiectasia

Cerebellar ataxia, occulocutaneous telangestasia, growth retardation, variable immunodeficiency, and autosomal recessive inheritance are typical features of ataxia telangiestasia (OMIM 208900). Affected individuals exhibit increased sensitivity to ionized radiation and radiomimetic drugs and 80% of patients show increased susceptibility to malignancy, especially leukaemias and lymphomas. IgA deficiency, with or without IgG subclass deficiency, and defective responses to bacterial capsular polysaccharides are common. Patients therefore often develop recurrent sino-pulmonary infections. Lymphopenia and impaired T-cell function may also be detected. Chromosomal translocations corresponding to the locations of immunoglobulin heavy chain and T-cell receptor loci are commonly detected in T cells of ataxia telangiestasia patients.

The product of the affected gene, ATM, is required for detecting double-stranded breaks in DNA prior to their repair. Defective ATM results in defective control of checkpoints of the cell cycle. This explains the radiation sensitivity, abnormal immune cell development and function, and the cytogenic abnormalities that are frequently detected in ATM. Some 95% of affected individuals have elevations in serum α-fetoprotein, which is helpful for diagnosis.

There is no specific treatment, and most patients die by the third decade of lymphoreticular malignancy or complications of neurological disease. This complex condition should be managed with a multidisciplinary approach, with input from expert centres.

Other DNA repair defects associated with immunodeficiency

The Nijmegen breakage syndrome (OMIM 2551269), which is phenotypically similar to ataxia telangiestasia, is caused by mutation of the *MBSI* gene encoding for a protein acting as a substrate for ATM, and which is also critical for sensing damage to DNA. DNA-ligase 1 defect (OMIM 126391), which also causes defective DNA repair, results in growth retardation and immunodeficiency. Mutation of the *MRE11A* gene, which encodes for another component of the DNA damage-sensing machinery, causes a syndrome similar to ataxia telangiestasia (OMIM 604391), but without mutations in the ATM gene.

Other rare immunodeficiencies

Immunodeficiencies causing defective homeostasis of the immune system, rare defects in innate immunity and miscellaneous rare immunodeficiencies are summarized in Table 5.2.2.

Defects in innate immunity

Defects in the complement pathway resulting in immunodeficiency are described in Chapter 5.3 and summarized in Table 5.2.6.

Immune responses to pathogens are initiated by recognition of pathogen-associated molecular patterns by cell surface and intracellular pattern recognition receptors, e.g. Toll receptors. Defects in pathways involved in the recognition and response to pathogen-associated molecular patterns result in susceptibility to infection. Some of these recently described defects are outlined below.

Intracellular signalling downstream of Toll, IL-1 and IL-18 receptors, as well as CD40-ligand, utilize the NF-κB pathway. X-linked hypomorphic mutations of *NEMO* causes defective NF-κB activation resulting in defective responses to the engagement of Toll, IL-1, and TNFα receptors. These patients are susceptible to infections caused by a broad spectrum of microorganisms including mycobacteria, Gram-positive and Gram-negative bacteria, fungi, and viruses. Signalling via NF-κB is essential for ectodermal development and many (but not all) patients with *NEMO* defects have ectodermal dyplasia characterized by dental hypoplasia, reduced sweating, and hypoplastic hair. The CD40–CD40 ligand interaction is required for immunoglobulin class switching and some (but not all) patients with *NEMO* defects develop the hyper-IgM syndrome.

Table 5.2.6 Clinical consequences of complement deficiency

Deficient component	Clinical manifestations	Investigation
C3 deficiency; secondary C3 deficiency due to utilization (e.g. SLE; C3 nephritic factor; inherited factor I deficiency)	Recurrent pyogenic sepsis (especially by encapsulated bacteria)	Measure C3, C4 levels in serum. Test functional activity of classical and alternate complement pathway (CH50, AP50). Seek specialist advice
Deficiency of C1q, C1r, C1s, C4, or C2	SLE	Test functional activity of classical complement pathway (CH50). Seek specialist advice
Deficiency of properdin or factor D	Recurrent encapsulated bacterial sepsis	Test functional activity of alternate complement pathway (AP50). Seek specialist advice
Deficiency of C5, C6, C7, C8, or C9	Recurrent neisserial infection	Test functional activity of classical and alternate complement pathway (CH50, AP50). Seek specialist advice
Deficiency of factor H or factor I	Haemolytic uraemic syndrome, membrano-proliferative glomerulnephritis	Seek specialist advice
C1 inhibitor deficiency	Angio-oedema lasting more than 24 h; severe abdominal pain due to oedema of intestinal tissues	Measure C4 and C1 inhibitor levels in serum. 15% of patients have normal C1 inhibitor protein levels but absent functional activity
Inherited CD59 deficiency	Haemolysis	
Acquired CD59 deficiency	Paroxysmal nocturnal haemoglobinuria	

UNC93B is a protein of the endoplasmic reticulum involved in the activation of Toll receptors. Mutations in UNC93B results in defective interferon-α and -β production in response to herpes simplex and other viruses. These patients develop with herpes simplex encephalitis during childhood. Rarely heterozygous dominant negative mutations in the gene encoding Toll receptor 3 (*TLR3*) have been identified in patients with herpes simplex encephalitis. *TLR3* is expressed in the central nervous system where it helps to initiate interferon-α and -β responses toviral double-stranded DNA.

The interleukin receptor associated kinase-4 mediates signalling via Toll receptors and members of the IL-1 receptor superfamily. Individuals with homozygous mutations of the *IRAK-4* gene develop recurrent, life-threatening, pyogenic sepsis. They are especially susceptible to pneumococcal sepsis. The incidence of infections reduces by adolescence, with improvement in outcome. Mutation in the gene encoding the protein myeloid differentiation primary response gene 88 (MYD88), which is also required for signal transduction following Toll receptor engagement, causes a similar clinical syndrome.

Signal transduction via receptors to interferons -γ, -α, and -β involves the participation of the signal transducing molecule STAT-1. IFNγ-R-mediated signalling results in dimerization of phosphorylated STAT-1 molecules, which migrate to the nucleus and induce gene transcription. Signalling via interferon-α and -β receptors involves the formation of a complex between STAT-1, STAT-2, and a third protein called interferon stimulated gene factor 3-γ (ISGF3-γ). Complete (homozygous) defects of STAT-1 results in impaired responses to interferons- γ, -α, and -β, leading to the susceptibility to disseminated mycobacterial infections as well as fatal herpes simpex virus infection. Partial STAT-1 deficiency, which interferes with STAT-1 dimerization required for signal transduction via interferon-γ receptors, produces increased susceptibility to mycobacterial infections. In these patients, the cellular responses to interferon-α and -β are intact, thus preserving antiviral immunity.

The Warts hypogammaglobulinaemia infections myelokathexis (WHIM) syndrome (OMIM 193670) is characterized by severe warts, hypogammaglobulinaemia, and neutropenia due to retention of neutrophils in the bone marrow. This is an immunodeficiency caused by a gain of function mutation in the gene encoding the CXCR4 chemokine receptor. These mutant receptors show increased responsiveness to its ligands.

Hyper-IgE syndrome (OMIM 147060) is a condition characterized by recurrent bacterial (*S. aureus*, Gram-negative bacteria) and fungal infections of skin, lymph nodes, lungs, bones and joints; dermatitis; facial dysmorphic features; delayed shedding of primary dentition; and osteopenia. These patients have elevated serum IgE, levels, eosinophilia, and impaired acute-phase responses during infections. The majority have an autosomal dominant inheritance, but others are sporadic. Patients with hyper-IgE syndrome have heterozygous mutations in the gene encoding the signal transducing protein STAT3. These mutant proteins reduce the DNA binding of the phosphorylated STAT3 dimer, in response to interferon-α, IL-10, and IL-6. Reduced response to IL-6 would explain the defective acute-phase response and the defective response to IL-10 explains the overproduction of IgE. STAT3 is essential for the generation of T-helper 17 cells, which produce the cytokines IL-17 and IL-22 that are required for the secretion of the bactericidal peptides called β-defensins by epithelial cells of the skin and lungs, as well as for neutrophil mobilization and recruitment to the sites of infection. This may in part explain the increased incidence of severe bacterial and fungal sepsis, especially involving the lungs.

Dectin-1 is a pattern recognition receptor that recognizes β glucans found in the cell walls of candida. A recent study identified a family with four women who developed vulvo-vaginal candidiasis and onychomycosis who had the mutation Tyr238X in the gene encoding for Dectin-1. This defect was associated with impaired cytokine responses to candida by monocytes and macrophages. However this defect did not impair the ability of neutrophils to kill candida, explaining why these patients did not develop invasive candidiasis. Another study identified a family with four affected individuals who developed recurrent muco-cutaneous candidiasis as well as invasive candidiasis affecting the brain. These patients had an autosomal recessive defect due to a mutation in the gene encoding the caspase recruitment domain-containing protein CARD9. CARD9 is required for intracellular signalling downstream of Dectin-1. Operation of this signalling pathway results in the production of proinflammatory cytokines, including IL-1β, IL-6, and IL-23. CARD9-/- patients also had reduced IL-17 producing T cells that also contribute to mucosal immunity.

Mutations in the interleukin 10 receptor genes IL-10RA and IL-10RB, have been identified in a few children with severe progressive Crohn's disease commencing in early infancy. One of the patients was successfully treated with allogeneic haemopoietic stem cell transplantation.

Further reading

Antoine C, *et al.* (2003). Long term survival and transplantation of haemopoeitic stem cells for immunodeficiencies: report of the European experience 1968–99. *Lancet*, **361**, 553–60.

Bonilla FA, *et al.* (2005). practice parameter for the diagnosis and management of primary immunodeficiency. *Ann Allergy Asthma Immunol*, **94**, S1–63.

Buckley R, Fischer A (2007). Bone marrow transplantation for primary immunodeficiency diseases. In: Ochs HD, *et al.* (eds) *Primary immunodeficiency diseases: a molecular and genetic approach*, pp. 669–687. Oxford University Press, New York.

Bustamante J, *et al.* (2008). Novel primary immunodeficiencies revealed by the investigation of paediatric infectious diseases. *Curr Opin Immunol*, **20**, 39–48.

Dale DC, *et al.* (2008). The phagocytes: neutrophils and monocytes. *Blood*, **112**, 935–45.

Geha RS, *et al.* (2007). Primary immunodeficiency diseases: an update from the International Union of Immunological Societies Primary Immunodeficiency Diseases Classification Committee. *J Allergy Clin Immunol*, **120**, 776–94.

International Union of Immunological Societies (1999). Primary immunodeficiency diseases. Report of an IUIS Scientific Committee. *Clin Exp Immunol*, **118** Suppl 1, 1–28.

Jouanguy E, *et al.* (2007). Human primary immunodeficiencies of type I interferons. *Biochimie*, **89**, 878–83, T3.

Nortangelo L, *et al.* (2009). Primary immunodeficiencies: 2009 Update. *J Allergy Clin Immunol*, **124**, 1161–78.

Ochs HD, Smith CIE, Puck J (eds) (2007). *Primary immunodeficiency diseases: a molecular and genetic approach*. Oxford University Press, New York.

Orange JS, *et al.* (2006). Use of intravenous immunoglobulin in human disease: a review of evidence by members of the Primary Immunodeficiency Committee of the American Academy of Allergy, Asthma and Immunology. *J Allergy Clin Immunol*, **117**, S525–53.

Patel SY, *et al.* (2008). Genetically determined susceptibility to mycobacterial infection. *J Clin Pathol*, **61**, 1006–12.

Rosenzweig SD, Holland SM (2004). Phagocyte immunodeficiencies and their infections. *J Allergy Clin Immunol*, **113**, 620–6.

Wood P, *et al.* (2007). Recognition, clinical diagnosis and management of patients with primary antibody deficiencies: a systematic review. *Clin Exp Immunol*, **149**, 410–23.

Websites

European Society for Immunodeficiencies (2004). EBMT guidelines. http://www.esid.org/workingparty.php?party=1&sub=2&id=27

National Center for Biotechnology Information. *Online Mendelian Inheritance in Man (OMIM)*. http://www.ncbi.nlm.nih.gov/Database/index/html

5.3

Allergy

Pamela Ewan

Essentials

Allergy is common and becoming commoner: it now affects about one-third of the United Kingdom population. This is being driven by environmental changes, which are also leading to an increase in both the complexity and severity of the condition. In addition to the traditional allergic disorders—asthma, rhinitis, and eczema—multisystem allergic disease and reactivity to several allergens are now common; new allergies have appeared, including those due to foods, drugs, and diagnostic agents; and anaphylaxis is increasing.

Where possible, patients with significant allergy should be referred to an allergy specialist who can provide expertise not offered by- and complementary to—that of other specialties. Identifying allergic causes of disease leads to reduction or resolution of its manifestations.

Aetiology and pathogenesis

Mechanism—allergy in its classical form occurs following interaction of allergen with specific IgE antibody bound to high-affinity IgE receptors (FcεRI) on mast cells, which results in mast cell activation, degranulation, and mediator release, but the same clinical presentation can occur as a result of IgE independent mast cell degranulation e.g. idiopathic anaphylaxis. A normal subject has no specific IgE to common allergens and a low or normal total serum IgE level: production of specific IgE antibody requires a change in immunoregulation leading to sensitization (atopic state), with some sensitized subjects progressing to develop clinical allergy.

Allergens—common allergic triggers include (1) inhaled allergens—house dust mite, pollens, and animal danders are the commonest causes of allergic asthma, rhinitis and eczema; (2) foods—commonly egg, milk, peanuts, and tree nuts; mainly cause acute reactions of varying severity, e.g. urticaria, angio-oedema, or anaphylaxis; (3) drugs—particularly antibiotics, aspirin, NSAIDs, and drugs given during general anaesthesia; (4) bee and wasp stings; (5) latex rubber.

Clinical features and diagnosis

Clinical presentation—this can be in various guises acute or chronic, with common manifestations being (1) allergic rhinitis—timing of symptoms indicates the causative allergen; (2) nonallergic rhinitis—some have aspirin sensitivity, rhinosinusitis, nasal polyps, and asthma; (3) conjunctivitis; (4) asthma—timing of symptoms and exacerbations gives clues to aetiology; (5) eczema; (6) urticaria and angio-oedema—severe tongue swelling is a medical emergency and most often drug induced (especially ACE inhibitors) or idiopathic (non-IgE mediated); (7) anaphylaxis—presents with acute dyspnoea or hypotension/collapse, usually with cutaneous features such as erythema or urticaria (see Chapter 17.2).

History taking—a good history is the key to diagnosis: too often the underlying allergic trigger is not identified and disease which could be ameliorated by allergen avoidance continues unchecked; awareness of drug and latex allergy are essential.

Clinical investigation—(1) serum tryptase—may be transiently elevated for up to 4 h following an acute reaction; (2) skin prick tests or serum-specific IgE assays—many patients have positive tests without symptoms, hence performing them in the absence of appropriate clinical information is a common source of error; (3) intradermal and challenge tests—performed by allergy specialists, mainly for diagnosis of drug and food allergy.

Prevention and treatment

Prevention—there are no widely applicable proven methods for primary prevention of allergy.

Acute or chronic disease—management requires (1) allergen avoidance; and may also involve (2) pharmacotherapy—including nonsedative antihistamines and topical corticosteroids (nasal sprays, inhalers, and creams); and, less commonly, (3) immunotherapy (desensitization)—should be offered to patients with poorly controlled allergic rhinitis or venom anaphylaxis.

Anaphylaxis—first-line treatment is intramuscular adrenaline (epinephrine). All patients should subsequently be referred to an allergy specialist for diagnosis and management: allergen or trigger avoidance, e.g. food or drug, reduces further episodes and should be combined with an adrenaline autoinjector for early self-treatment. See Chapter 17.2 for further discussion.

Introduction

Allergic disorders are wide ranging, and include asthma, eczema, rhinitis, anaphylaxis, angio-oedema, and urticaria. Some disorders will always be allergy driven, e.g. food, venom, or latex allergy, whereas others, e.g. asthma or rhinitis, may be allergic or nonallergic, but the role of allergy is increasing. Allergy has increased in prevalence, severity, and complexity over the last three decades, with a resulting burden on patients and cost to health services. Failure to make an allergy diagnosis adversely affects management and outcome. Avoiding a food or a drug can completely ameliorate disease, yet many allergic disorders are treated with pharmacotherapy only.

Allergy practice involves both IgE-mediated (classical allergy) and non IgE-mediated disorders. In the latter group—which includes certain types of anaphylaxis, angio-oedema, and rhinitis—the signs and symptoms mimic IgE-mediated allergy because release of mast cell mediator occurs, but IgE is not involved.

Historical perspective

Early descriptions of allergy exist. Hay fever was described in 1873 by Charles Blackley, who demonstrated that pollen was the cause by applying pollen grains to his nose and eye in winter and reproducing the symptoms. Passive transfer of sensitivity to the skin by injecting serum from a fish allergic person to a nonallergic subject was demonstrated by Prausnitz and Kustner in 1921 but it was not until 1967 that the serum factor (reagin) was shown to be a new class of immunoglobulin, IgE, by the Ishizakas in the United States of America and then by Bennich and Johansson in Sweden in 1971.

Aetiology and pathogenesis

Type I hypersensitivity (allergic) reactions

The term 'allergy' is used variably. It is often used synonymously with the type I IgE-mediated reaction described by Gell and Coombs. Interaction of allergen with specific IgE antibody bound to high-affinity IgE receptors (FcεRI) on mast cells results in mast cell activation, degranulation, and mediator release (Fig. 5.3.1). Histamine and other mediators including leukotrienes and prostaglandins cause vasodilation, smooth muscle contraction, mucosal oedema, and secretions.

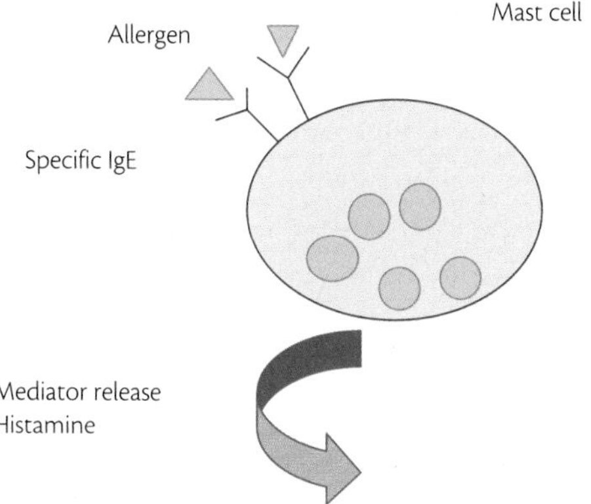

Fig. 5.3.1 The type I allergic reaction.
Reproduced from the BMJ, Pamela W Ewan, 316(7142):1442–5, © 1998, with permission from BMJ Publishing Group Ltd.

Non-IgE mediated reactions

Mast cell activation and mediator release may occur independent of IgE antibody. Certain drugs and physical stimuli (e.g. cold or exercise) do this in susceptible individuals. However, it can also occur without a recognized trigger. Mechanisms are poorly understood.

Steps in the development of allergy

A normal subject has no specific IgE to common allergens and a low or normal total serum IgE level—the nonatopic state. Production of specific IgE antibody requires a change in immunoregulation with a switch from the Th0/Th1 state to a Th2 dominant state. This may result from failure of function of T regulatory cells, which produce interleukin-10 (IL-10) and transforming growth factor β. Th2 cells secrete the cytokines IL-4 and IL-13 which result in B cell switching to IgE production (atopic) (Fig. 5.3.2). The atopic state often has no associated symptoms: this is known as sensitization. A proportion of sensitized subjects progress to develop clinical allergy (allergic).

Prevalence

Atopy

Atopy is defined as the presence of specific IgE to one or more common allergens. Specific IgE can be detected by skin prick testing. The incidence of atopy in the general population is high, many studies previously showing rates of about 40%, but this appears to be rising. In a study in the United States of America, the third National Health and Nutrition Examination Surveys conducted between 1988 and 1994, 54% of the population tested had positive skin prick tests to 1 or more of 10 common allergens, i.e. they were atopic. This was an increase compared to the findings in an earlier study (1970 to 1980), with prevalences 2 to 5 times higher for the 6 allergens common to both studies.

Sensitization as a predictor of allergy

Various studies suggest that sensitization is a predictor of later allergy. In some infants, sensitization to egg precedes and predicts the development of eczema. Early sensitization to food allergens in the first year of life is also a predictor of subsequent sensitization to inhalant allergens, which in turn predicts the incidence of asthma and hay fever in young adulthood.

Clinical allergy

It is not possible to provide precise prevalence data for allergy overall. There are incomplete or missing data for some allergic disorders, e.g. drug allergy and anaphylaxis; allergy is involved in a subset of certain diseases, e.g. eczema or asthma; and different manifestations of allergy occur in one individual (multisystem allergic disease).

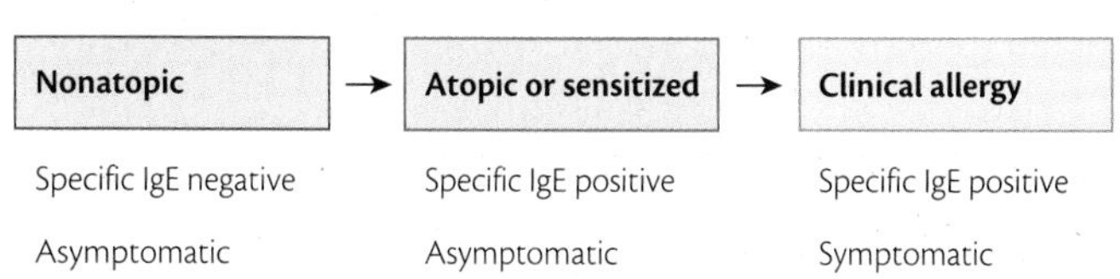

Fig. 5.3.2 Stages to the development of allergy.

A picture can be built up, however, with minimum estimates for number of people affected.

In the United Kingdom, about 18 million (39% of children and 30% of adults) have been diagnosed with one or more of asthma, eczema, and rhinitis. A considerable proportion of this is allergic in origin, e.g. 26% of the population has allergic rhinitis. Serial surveys show that the prevalence of asthma, rhinitis, and eczema has increased about threefold over the last three decades, and this is thought to be due to an increase in the prevalence of allergy. Comorbidity is common and increases the likelihood of allergy being involved.

Food allergy occurs in about 3% of adults and 4% of children—1.8 million people in the United Kingdom. Nut allergy, where there are more accurate data, occurs in more than 460 000 individuals in the United Kingdom. Venom allergy occurs in about 2% of the population.

There are no data for the prevalence of anaphylaxis overall (all causes). United Kingdom data shows that the number of hospital admissions for anaphylaxis has risen sevenfold over 10 years (Fig. 5.3.3). The absolute numbers do not reflect prevalence as only a minority is admitted, most being managed in emergency departments, however the trend is clear. A study was conducted in 1994, published in 1996 of Emergency Department attendances estimated that about 1 in 3500 of the catchment's population had an anaphylactic reaction in a 1-year period. A study of recorded diagnosis of anaphylaxis in primary care in England from 2001 to 2005 showed an increasing incidence and lifetime prevalence (75.5 per 100 000 in 2005) and that an estimated 1 in 1333 of the English population have at some point experienced anaphylaxis. Taking individual causes, food and venom allergy cause anaphylaxis in a few million people in the UK. Since 1990, hospital admissions for food allergy have increased fivefold; for urticaria they have doubled, and admissions for angio-oedema have risen by 40%.

Important areas where there are few data are drug allergy and angio-oedema. Even for penicillin allergy, where there are most data, prevalence data is incomplete. About 5.9 million people in the United Kingdom are labelled as penicillin allergic, yet only about of 10% of these are truly allergic. There are no data on prevalence of sensitivity to aspirin, non steroidal anti-inflammatory drugs (NSAIDs) or other analgesics—an increasing problem.

There are a number of new allergies, e.g. to fruits and vegetables and sesame, where again little information is available. Complex or multisystem allergic disease is now common. Allergic asthma, rhinitis, and eczema commonly coexist, and food and latex allergies occur mainly in patients with these disorders.

Aetiology: allergens

The allergic trigger varies with the disorder and to some extent with the age of the patient.

- Inhaled allergens are the commonest cause of allergic asthma, rhinitis, and eczema, especially house dust mite, pollens, and animal danders. These three allergens are the most common causes of allergy in the United Kingdom. Alternaria and cladosporium are important causes of acute seasonal severe asthma (and/or rhinitis) in late summer. Eczema in adults or older children may be driven by house dust mite allergy.
- Foods commonly responsible for allergy include egg, milk, peanuts, and tree nuts. Others are fish, shellfish, fruits, vegetables, sesame, seeds, and soya. These will mainly cause acute reactions of varying severity, e.g. urticaria, angiooedema, or anaphylaxis. In toddlers, foods, particularly egg or cow's milk, are important triggers for eczema.
- The important drugs are antibiotics, aspirin, nonsteroidal anti-inflammatory drugs, (NSAIDs) and drugs given during general anaesthesia, especially the neuromuscular blocking agents. Insulin, opiates, and vaccines are rarer causes of systemic allergic reactions. Local anaesthetic rarely causes allergy, although it is commonly perceived. Diagnostic dyes, chlorhexidine, and intravenous colloid occasionally cause anaphylaxis.
- Bee and wasp venoms cause systemic allergic reactions of varying severity including anaphylaxis.
- Latex rubber causes a variety of symptoms including urticaria, angio-oedema, asthma, rhinitis, and anaphylaxis.

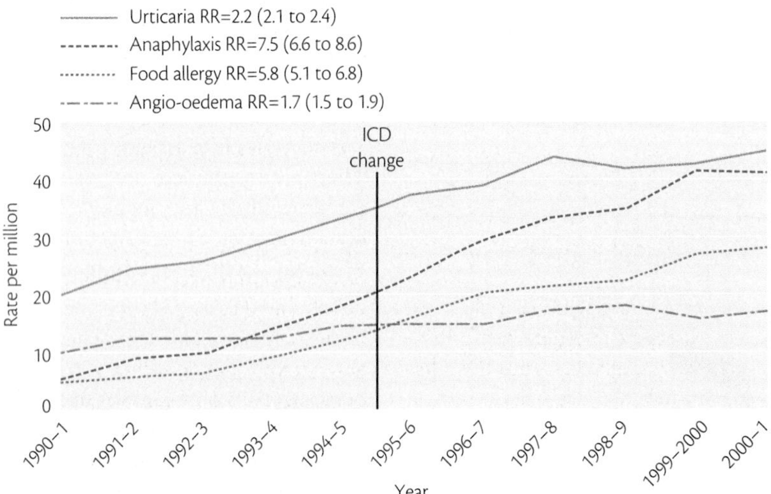

Fig. 5.3.3 Rising hospital admissions for anaphylaxis.
Reproduced from the BMJ, Gupta R. Sheikh A, Strachan D, Anderson HR, 327(7424):1142–3, © 2003, with permission from BMJ Publishing Group Ltd.

Prevention

Primary prevention

Environmental factors play an important role in the development of allergy. The hygiene hypothesis suggests that early exposure to microbial infection is protective, driving Th1 responses: e.g. children exposed to endotoxin from farm animals were less likely to develop allergic disease.

Avoiding exposure to food allergens in early life (maternal diet during pregnancy and lactation and the infant's diet), has been suggested as a means of preventing allergy, but the effect is not established. Advice from the Department of Health in relation to peanuts has been withdrawn. Another postulate is that early dietary exposure may induce tolerance.

Secondary prevention

Treatment with oral antihistamine has been shown to prevent or delay the development of asthma in infants with atopic dermatitis sensitized to grass pollen or house dust mite. Immunotherapy for rhinitis can prevent the development of asthma.

Clinical features

The history is the key to reaching an allergy diagnosis. This is supported by appropriate tests, particularly those for specific IgE. Knowledge of allergens, their seasons, sources, and disorders they may cause, as well as presentations and patterns of disease, is essential. Enquiry should be made into the timing of symptoms and the effect of allergen exposure (there may be multiple manifestations of allergy).

Some of the 'allergic' diseases, including asthma, rhinitis, eczema, and anaphylaxis, may be IgE-mediated or non IgE-mediated. This distinction needs to be drawn. In the allergic group, the allergic cause should be identified.

The likelihood of allergy is increased

- in children and young adults
- if multiple systems are involved, e.g. asthma, rhinitis, eczema, food allergy.

Allergic rhinitis

Symptoms include rhinorrhoea, nasal congestion or obstruction, and sneezing. The dominant symptom varies with the allergen. Pollen allergy (hay fever or seasonal allergic rhino-conjunctivitis) mainly causes sneezing, nasal itch, and profuse watery secretions as well as itchy watering eyes. The timing of the symptoms indicates the causative allergen, e.g. tree pollen allergy occurs in spring, grass pollen in early summer, and late summer and autumn symptoms are due to shrub or weed pollens or the moulds alternaria and cladosporium.

In perennial allergic rhinitis, nasal congestion and secretions are the main features. There may be a history of triggers responsible for exacerbations, as well as remissions when away from the allergen. House dust mite allergic patients are often worse on waking (following exposure from mattress and bedding overnight), or after cleaning, and better at altitude (dust mite does not survive above 1000 m). Animal allergy is usually evident from exacerbations on contact, or remissions away from home if a pet is kept there. Highly allergic subjects react to exposure to small amounts of hair on the clothing of others, without direct animal exposure. In horse allergy, a few hairs can cause severe periorbital oedema or asthma.

Nonallergic rhinitis

In non-IgE mediated rhinitis, symptoms are perennial but intermittent and variable. A subgroup have aspirin sensitivity, rhinosinusitis, nasal polyps, and asthma. This is often severe, with marked nasal obstruction, and difficult to control.

Conjunctivitis

This mainly occurs in association with rhinitis, especially due to pollen but also to animals and dust mites. In a small number of patients with hay fever, isolated conjunctivitis and periorbital oedema occurs. Severe disease can result in conjunctival oedema and impaired vision.

Asthma

Allergy plays an important role in most asthma in children and young adults. The importance of identifying the allergic trigger is that avoidance can significantly modify disease and reduce drug consumption. The timing of symptoms and exacerbations gives clues to aetiology. In pollen asthma, symptoms are seasonal. Alternaria allergy results in acute severe attacks of asthma at harvest time (July and August in the United Kingdom), when allergen is released resulting in sudden peak levels. Many patients have had hospital admissions with asthma at that time of the year. Accurate allergy diagnosis means that prevention measures can be put in place. Other causes are animals: exposure to cat, dog, or horse may induce acute wheeze. In a subset this can be life-threatening. House dust mite allergy is a major cause of perennial asthma.

Eczema

Atopic eczema in children most commonly affects the flexures and neck. In severe cases it may be widespread. It is more difficult in eczema to identify triggers from the history. Sometimes exacerbations are obvious, e.g. after contact with animals or if both eczema and rhinitis are exacerbated by dust exposure. House dust allergy is an important trigger. Scratching at night will rub allergen into the skin, driving the disease. Food allergy causes eczema in children. A problem is that many patients with eczema have specific IgE antibody to multiple allergens, many of which are not clinically relevant. If there is no clear history of flares with allergens, interpretation of allergy tests can be difficult. A trial of allergen exclusion over a few weeks is then required for diagnosis.

Urticaria and angiooedema

These may occur separately or together. Urticaria is common. Acute episodes may be allergic (see above) but chronic urticaria, defined as daily symptoms lasting for 6 weeks, is rarely allergic. Urticaria consists of itchy wheals, raised lesions with pale centres and surrounding erythema. Wheals are of varied size and usually occur in crops on the limbs or trunk but can be extensive. Lesions tend to be short lived, but as one crop fades another appears. In giant urticaria, lesions the size of the palm of the hand occur. These are more oedematous and take longer to resolve. When urticaria and angio-oedema coexist, urticaria is usually dominant with occasional episodes of angio-oedema.

It is important in chronic urticaria to determine aetiology. The usual assumption is that this is allergic, and foods are often implicated, leading to restricted diets, but most urticaria is non-IgE mediated (idiopathic). Ruling out allergy is important. Some is physical, triggered by heat, cold, exercise, pressure on the skin, or contact with water. In cold urticaria, chilling of the skin—e.g. by putting the hands in cool water or exposure to cold wind—causes erythema and pruritus. After more prolonged exposure, angio-oedema occurs. If a large surface area is involved, as in sea swimming, hypotension and loss of consciousness occur. Drugs, especially NSAIDs and aspirin, are an important cause. Infection can trigger urticaria, especially in children.

Angio-oedema

The commonest sites for angio-oedema are the lips and eyelids. This type of angio-oedema often occurs with urticaria but may occur alone. Angio-oedema may also involve the tongue and larynx, pharynx, or uvula. Swelling is often unilateral.

Tongue swelling usually occurs alone, without swelling at other sites or urticaria. Angio-oedema of the whole tongue can cause respiratory obstruction, cyanosis, or respiratory arrest. Severe tongue swelling is a medical emergency. Tongue swelling is mostly drug induced (especially acetylcholinesterase inhibitors) or idiopathic (non-IgE mediated). If the patient is taking an acetylcholinesterase inhibitor, the first step should be to stop the drug. Acetylcholinesterase inhibitor induced angio-oedema is thought to be due to bradykinin generation. Onset is either within weeks of starting medication or, confusingly, after an interval of many months or years. It is a class effect. Angiotensin II receptor antagonists are usually tolerated. Most isolated angio-oedema is non-allergic. There is no erythema or pruritus.

Allergic (IgE-mediated) angio-oedema

When angio-oedema is allergic, other features are usually present. Horse, other animal and pollen allergy cause periorbital oedema but usually with conjunctivitis and/or conjunctival oedema; there may also be rhinitis and asthma. Food allergy commonly causes perioral angio-oedema but there will also be perioral urticaria and oral pruritus. Systemic features may occur. In latex allergy the angio-oedema will be periorbital or perioral if there has been local rubber contact, e.g. rubber goggles, swimming cap, or blowing up a balloon. Pruritus, erythema, and urticaria will be present.

Hereditary angio-oedema (HAE)

This is a distinct disorder, due to the deficiency of the complement protein C1 inhibitor. The deficiency results in unopposed activation of the kallikrein system, leading to generation of bradykinin, which causes increased vascular permeability and oedema.

Angio-oedema occurs at one or more of three sites: cutaneous, intestinal, and laryngeal. Patients present with peripheral swellings, typically fleeting, involving different sites in different attacks—hence distinct from idiopathic or allergic angio-oedema which is restricted in site, usually lips or eyelids. The hand, limbs, and genitals are often affected. If the face is involved the swelling is more extensive and not limited to lip or eye. Intestinal mucosal oedema, which causes partial intestinal obstruction, presents with abdominal pain and vomiting. The least common but most severe manifestation is laryngeal oedema, which is life-threatening and can be fatal. Attacks are self-limiting, lasting 48 to 72 h, and of variable severity. They are intermittent, with many months between episodes when patients are well.

Treatment should be managed by a specialist. Prophylactic treatment is with danazol which increases the hepatic production (by the normal gene) of C1 inhibitor. Only a marginal increase in C1 inhibitor appears to be required. Other drugs that target the downstream pathways involved in HAE are being developed and include a bradykinin B2 receptor antagonist.

Anaphylaxis

Anaphylaxis is an acute severe systemic reaction of rapid onset. There is no universally agreed definition. There are many features, not all of which need be present (Box 5.3.1). One of the two severe features, respiratory difficulty or hypotension, should be present. Severe dyspnoea is due to laryngeal oedema, often described as a sensation of the throat closing up, or acute asthma. Hypotension presents as weakness, difficulty standing, collapse, or loss of consciousness. Cutaneous features are usually present.

The main causes of anaphylaxis are foods, drugs, venom, and latex allergy. In food-induced anaphylaxis, respiratory symptoms are the dominant severe feature. In contrast, in venom allergy or allergy to an intravenous drug, hypotension predominates. Thus the clinical picture varies with the cause of the anaphylaxis.

Non-IgE mediated (idiopathic) anaphylaxis is becoming more common. This usually presents in a different way and with a slower evolution over a few hours. It begins with pruritus of the palms and soles, then progresses to general pruritus, erythema, and urticaria, with diarrhoea, abdominal pain, and hypotension. Respiratory symptoms rarely occur.

Food allergy

Different foods cause different patterns of disease: with differences in severity, clinical features, comorbidities, and likelihood of resolution or persistence. Severity varies from mild, usually facial and oral urticaria/oedema, to anaphylaxis (Table 5.3.1). Egg and cow's milk are the commonest food allergies in infants and toddlers.

Box 5.3.1 Clinical features of anaphylaxis

- Erythema
- Pruritus
- Urticaria
- Angio-oedema
- Laryngeal oedema
- Asthma
- Nausea, vomiting, abdominal cramps
- Sense of impending doom
- Fainting, lightheadedness
- Collapse
- Loss of consciousness
- Fits (rare)
- Incontinence (rare)

Table 5.3.1 Varying presentations of acute allergic reactions to foods according to severity

Severity	Clinical features
Mild	Cutaneous features only: pruritus, erythema, urticaria or mild angio-oedema
Moderate	The above plus more severe angio-oedema and/or vomiting, abdominal pain and/or mild dyspnoea or tightening of throat
Severe	The above plus respiratory difficulty (laryngeal oedema or asthma) and/or hypotension (less common)

Egg allergy

Egg allergy is mostly mild or moderate. Symptoms include perioral or facial erythema, urticaria and angio-oedema often with vomiting. Diarrhoea is rare. In more severe egg allergy asthma and anaphylaxis occur. Egg allergy can be partial and at presentation the child may tolerate a low allergen dose, e.g. egg as an ingredient, but not whole cooked egg. Most egg allergy in infants and young children resolves by or before school age. Management includes exclusion of egg from the diet and review to decide on gradual egg reintroduction. In the minority where disease persists, this can be severe, as can adult-or teenage-onset egg allergy. Measles, mumps, and rubella (MMR) vaccine does not contain egg protein and can safely be given. Influenza vaccines contain egg protein, at very low levels, and are contraindicated in patients with egg anaphylaxis.

Cow's milk allergy

Mild to moderate cow's milk allergy causes similar symptoms to egg allergy, but gastrointestinal symptoms with vomiting, abdominal cramps, and diarrhoea are more common. Most milk allergy in infancy resolves early. Where disease persists it can be severe, tiny quantities of milk protein causing anaphylaxis. Nonimmunological reactions against cow's milk are described as cow's milk protein intolerance. Clinical presentation is similar to milk allergy and usually resolves by the age of 12 months.

Nut allergy

Nut allergy has the propensity to cause severe life-threatening reactions. In the mid 1990s, when this disorder first appeared in significant numbers, about two-thirds of cases were severe with airway involvement, either laryngeal oedema or asthma. Peanuts account for the majority of food-induced fatal and near-fatal reactions. In these airway obstruction and asphyxia occur. The diagnosis of peanut allergy therefore causes anxiety. However, about two-thirds of individuals now have mild disease.

Peanut is a legume, not a nut; it is thus botanically distinct from tree nuts—nonetheless, allergy to both in an individual is frequent. Peanut is the most common 'nut' to cause reactions. Of the tree nuts, Brazil nuts, almonds, and hazelnuts most frequently cause allergy. Brazil nuts and cashew nuts result in the highest proportion of severe reactions.

Nut allergy mostly begins in childhood. The average age of onset of peanut allergy is 2 years. Allergy to tree nuts then appears progressively during childhood, but some patients remain 'monoallergic'. Allergy presenting in older children or adults is more likely to be due to a tree nut. There is a strong association with atopy: 96% are atopic and about two-thirds have asthma, rhinitis or eczema.

Kiwi fruit allergy

This is one of a number of new food allergies. Kiwi allergy began to appear after the introduction of kiwi fruits to the United Kingdom food market, and the incidence gradually rose in parallel with consumption. The main symptoms are perioral urticaria and oral mucosal oedema, but anaphylaxis with laryngeal odema may occur.

Oral allergy syndrome

This is new disorder—allergy to fruits and vegetables in patients with tree or grass pollen allergy (spring or summer hay fever). Pollen IgE antibodies cross-react with allergens in the fruit. Stoned fruits, e.g. apple and peach, are the commonest cause. Symptoms are oral and palatal itch and mucosal oedema. The fruit can be tolerated when well cooked as the allergens are heat labile. This is thought to be a mild disorder.

Severe allergy to fruit are increasingly recognized. This appears to be a distinct disorder where the IgE is directed against different allergen components to those in oral allergy syndrome.

Fish and shellfish

These causes urticaria, angio-oedema, and vomiting. Severe anaphylactic reactions occur. Fish and shellfish allergy often occur separately.

Hymenoptera venom allergy (see Chapter 9.2)

Bee or wasp (yellow jacket) stings are an important cause of anaphylaxis but cause allergic reactions of varied severity, from urticaria through to anaphylaxis. Hypotension is common in severe venom reactions. Wasp sting allergy is more common in the UK. Bee sting allergy mainly occurs in beekeepers and their relatives, i.e. those frequently stung. The pattern of reactions varies but need not be progressively worse. A factor favouring a less severe reaction subsequently is a long interval between stings.

Drug allergy

Diagnosis can be difficult and many reactions are falsely labelled as drug allergy. Penicillin, muscle relaxants, insulin, and other hormones act via IgE-mediated mechanisms, whereas opiates, acetylcholinesterase inhibitors, NSAIDs, and radiocontrast media produce angio-oedema and anaphylaxis by non-IgE-mediated mechanisms. However this is a complex area and antibiotics including β lactams, may also cause reactions through other mechanisms e.g. T cell mediated. IgE-mediated reactions, e.g. to β-lactam antibiotics, result in rash, angio-oedema, or anaphylaxis. Less severe reactions involve rash which may be maculopapular or urticarial, and mainly follow oral administration. Reactions usually occur after one dose or 1 to 2 days into treatment. Anaphylaxis occurs after parenteral administration (within minutes of intravenous administration) but is described, rarely, after oral treatment. Always check for drug allergy before administering an intravenous drug.

Sensitivity to aspirin and NSAIDs presents with urticaria and angio-oedema or with asthma and laryngeal oedema. The time of onset in relation to drug administration depends on the route and formulation: 30 to 60 min after oral nonenteric coated preparations and several hours after slow-release preparations. Intravenous or rectal administration results in more rapid onset, often 15 to 30 min.

Anaphylaxis during anaesthesia may be due to the anaesthetic agent, usually a neuromuscular blocking agent. However, increasingly other drugs administered are responsible. These include antibiotics, NSAIDs, opiates, colloid, and diagnostic agents.

If a drug reaction is suspected, it is important to document the description, all drugs being taken at the time, and the time of onset in relation to these.

Latex allergy

Latex allergy causes reactions of varying severity. Most are mild to moderate, with contact erythema, urticaria, and angio-oedema. This can remain localized or become generalized as the allergen is absorbed. Most reactions occur in medical settings, from latex gloves or equipment. Thin, stretchy rubber products such as surgical gloves are most allergenic, whereas black solid rubber is inert and causes few reactions. Exposure through contact with dentists' gloves causes local symptoms in the mouth or face. Absorption from surgeons' gloves may occur through the peritoneum or mucosal surfaces, e.g. vaginal examinations during labour resulting in anaphylaxis. In daily life exposure may be from condoms, household gloves, swimming caps, etc. Blowing up balloons leads to perioral angio-oedema.

Inquiry into the effect of these exposures can elicit whether a patient has latex allergy. Almost all patients with latex allergy are atopic and have other allergies such as asthma, rhinitis, and eczema. There is a strong association with hand eczema, and broken skin increases absorption of latex. About 50% have food allergy due to cross-reacting allergens. This association was originally made for banana, avocado, and melon, but a wide range of foods may be involved. A latex allergic subject need only avoid foods to which allergy has been proved.

Many latex allergic subjects are health care workers—medical, nursing, dental, and ambulance staff—presumably sensitized through their increased exposure to latex. The commonest reaction is a local reaction on the hands with pruritus and urticaria. Longer exposure results in increased symptoms, including angio-oedema. In operating theatres where powdered latex gloves are used, repeated glove change leads to an aerosol of allergen in the powder, causing rhino-conjunctivitis. These symptoms can be linked to occupational exposure. Other groups at increased risk of developing latex allergy include children who have undergone repeated surgery, e.g. for spina bifida.

Until the 1980s latex allergy was rare, with only a few case reports. It then became common, especially in health care workers, probably because of the increased use of rubber gloves. There were deaths from anaphylaxis due to rectal absorption of allergen from latex rubber catheters for barium enemas.

Latex allergic patients require strict latex avoidance when undergoing medical procedures or surgery; latex-free equipment must be used. Most catheters and many other medical products are now non-latex, but the vaginal probe used in gynaecological ultrasonography is covered with a condom and reactions occur.

It is important to distinguish latex allergy from contact dermatitis due to a type IV reaction to chemicals used in rubber manufacture. This presents with hand eczema, and is diagnosed by a patch test to these chemicals. It is not dangerous and if the patient is admitted strict latex avoidance is not required.

Differential diagnosis

Anaphylaxis may present with collapse and loss of consciousness or severe dyspnoea and cyanosis. It is important to consider myocardial infarction, pulmonary embolus, diabetes, or severe asthma. The presence of urticaria or angio-oedema is helpful. Hypotension is usually accompanied by tachycardia.

It is usually straightforward to diagnose the disorder, e.g. asthma or anaphylaxis. The issue is to determine the cause: whether allergy is playing a role and if so which allergy(-ies).

Clinical investigation

Acute reactions

Tryptase

In acute severe reactions, including anaphylaxis, it is valuable to take a timed blood sample for serum tryptase. This is elevated transiently, so the sample should be taken within 1 to 2 h of onset. It may still be elevated up to 4 h, so if the 1–2 h time point is missed a later sample can still be useful. This confirms mast cell activation and degranulation. Tryptase is often but not always elevated in anaphylaxis.

Later investigation

A detailed allergy history is the key. Knowledge of allergens, the disorders, and symptomatology they cause is essential. Tests do not substitute for this; they can only be used as an adjunct to history, to confirm or refute suspected allergy.

Specific IgE: skin prick tests or serum specific IgE assays

Tests for specific IgE are best done by skin prick testing, but can also be measured in serum. The latter is commonly referred to as the radio-allergosorbent test (RAST) after the original test although this is now available as other assays including enzyme-linked immunosorbent assay (ELISA). Skin prick tests are superior, but mainly available in specialist settings.

The problem with these tests is interpretation, as many subjects have positive tests without symptoms. To aid interpretation, 95% predictive levels have been identified for some allergens, levels above which there is a high probability of clinical allergy. Although helpful, this does not resolve the problem, as for individual allergens, different predictive values are proposed depending on the cohort of patients (age, disease, etc.). In addition, there remains a grey area where the test is positive but below the predictive level, where some patients are allergic and others not. A simple rule of thumb is that about half of those with positive tests are sensitized but not allergic.

If the reaction is non-IgE mediated, tests for specific IgE are irrelevant. For most of these reactions there are no confirmatory laboratory tests. This applies to some drug allergies, e.g. NSAIDs and aspirin, where the reaction is a result of leukotriene generation.

Intradermal tests

There are performed by specialists, and can be useful in drug allergy to detect specific IgE when the skin prick test is negative.

Challenge tests

These are useful if the diagnosis cannot be reached from history and skin tests. They are used mainly for diagnosis of drug and food allergy, and to determine if resolution has occurred.

Challenge testing should only be undertaken in a specialist allergy unit because of the risk of anaphylaxis.

Criteria for diagnosis

For allergic disorders where there is a trigger, whether IgE-mediated or not, diagnosis is made by history ± confirmatory tests which may be skin prick tests (or serum specific IgE), intradermal test or challenge. For idiopathic anaphylaxis, angio-oedema, etc., diagnosis is made by exclusion of all other causes.

Treatment

Allergen avoidance

Treatment involves pharmacotherapy and avoidance of allergen or trigger. In the case of food or drug allergy, avoidance can completely stop further acute episodes or chronic disease, e.g. eczema. Avoidance of animals will significantly reduce or prevent allergic asthma and rhinitis. House dust mite avoidance measures can only reduce, not eliminate, exposure, but can impact on symptoms.

Drug avoidance is easier to achieve, but patients need education on over-the-counter medication and on drug groups to avoid. Alerts should be recorded in medical records. For some foods, avoidance is difficult to achieve because the food is an ingredient, often hidden, or listed under an obscure name. Patients therefore need detailed advice. However, data from large studies on nut allergy shows that if patients receive education on avoidance, significant reduction in further episodes with a 60-fold reduction in severe attacks can be achieved (Fig. 5.3.4). In contrast, if the advice is 'just avoid nuts', further reactions because of inadvertent ingestion are frequent.

Pharmacotherapy

Key drugs are nonsedative antihistamines (quick onset with once daily dosage) and topical corticosteroids, as nasal sprays, inhalers, and creams. Larger than standard doses of antihistamines may be required for difficult urticaria. For allergic rhinitis and conjunctivitis, step-up therapy tailored to severity is used, as for asthma. Mild disease can be controlled by oral antihistamines, and moderate by nasal corticosteroid ± oral antihistamines. Steroid nasules or nose drops alone or alternating with nasal steroid sprays are used in severe perennial rhinitis and nasal polyps. Cromoglycate eye drops are used long term, with steroid eye drops for short periods for more severe conjunctivitis.

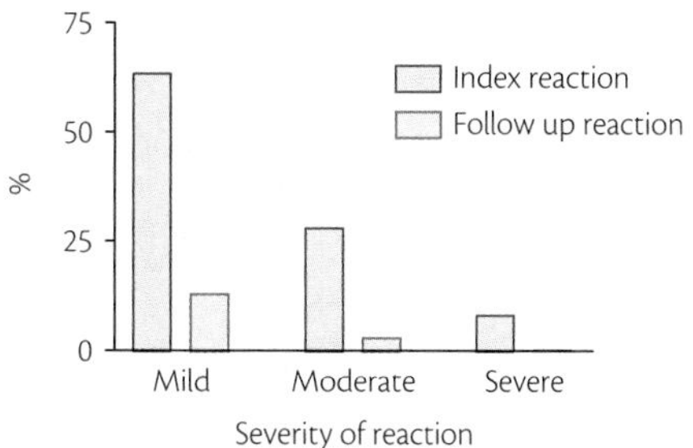

Fig. 5.3.4 Effect of a management plan in reducing subsequent reactions to nuts.

Reproduced from Ewan PW, Clark AT (2005). Efficacy of a management plan based on severity assessment in longitudinal and case-controlled studies of 747 children with nut allergy: proposal for good practice. *Clin Exp Allergy*, **35**, 751–6. With permission from Wiley-Blackwell.

Intramuscular adrenaline is the drug of choice for anaphylaxis, followed by intravenous chlorpheniramine and hydrocortisone. Further treatment with oxygen, nebulized salbutamol, and intravenous fluids may be required. If an acute reaction is evolving, with generalized urticaria and angio-oedema, but not clearly anaphylaxis, treatment can be begun with intravenous chlorpheniramine and hydrocortisone. Patients who have suffered anaphylaxis should carry an adrenaline auto-injector and be trained in its use, unless the allergen can be absolutely avoided.

Tongue swelling, depending on severity, requires oral antihistamine, adrenaline spray, soluble oral prednisolone or intramuscular adrenaline.

Montelukast is helpful as an adjunct to other therapy in certain subgroups with asthma, angio-oedema, urticaria (including exercise induced), and nasal polyps with rhino-sinusitis.

Immunotherapy

Allergen immunotherapy, or desensitization, is a different approach to treatment. It alters the immune response, 'switching off' the allergy. Conventionally it is given subcutaneously. Incremental doses of allergen are given at 1 to 2 weekly intervals until the top dose is reached, then maintenance therapy for 3 years. For pollen, shorter courses of preseasonal treatment are available. Recently sublingual immunotherapy has become available for pollen in the United Kingdom. A tablet is taken daily for 3 years and only the first dose has to be given in hospital, making it more accessible to patients. The safety profile remains to be fully determined.

Cochrane meta-analysis shows immunotherapy is effective for seasonal allergic rhinitis (subcutaneous) and allergic rhinitis due to pollen or other allergens (sublingual). Immunotherapy is highly effective for venom anaphylaxis. Issues are patient selection and safety. There is an incidence of severe allergic reactions to immunotherapy and deaths occurred in the 1980s. Immunotherapy should only be given by specialists with appropriate expertise.

Preliminary data has demonstrated it is possible to desensitise to foods, including peanut, using oral immunotherapy.

Anti-IgE

Monoclonal antibody therapy is available for severe asthma and has been shown to reduce repeated hospital admission. Expense and restrictive criteria limit its use.

Health economics

There is a significant burden of allergic disease, but much of this is not diagnosed or coded as allergy. The true size of this burden, the cost to the patient or to the health service, is unknown. In the United Kingdom direct health service costs for managing allergic problems are estimated at over £1 billion/year. However, the failure to diagnose allergy means disease is left unchecked, resulting in unnecessary cost to the National Health Service. Diagnosis of drug and food allergy stops further manifestation of the disease—anaphylaxis, acute allergic reactions, or eczema in a child. Other allergen avoidance leads to control of symptoms and lower drug consumption, again saving cost.

Incorrect labelling as allergy also has economic consequences. Only 10% of the 5.9 million people in the United Kingdom labelled as allergic to penicillin are in fact allergic. Costly alternative antibiotics are prescribed unnecessarily. Accurate diagnosis in the subset with high or specific antibiotic needs is cost effective.

Areas of uncertainty

- Requests for allergy tests, usually serum-specific IgE, without allergy knowledge to interpret the results is a common source of confusion and often results in the wrong diagnosis being made. This is because a 'positive' test does not necessarily correlate with disease. A common misconception is that the level of specific IgE correlates with severity.
- It is not known if sublingual immunotherapy is as effective as subcutaneous immunotherapy, and further studies are needed on its safety profile.
- Oral desensitisation for food allergy is a research area.
- The mechanism of idiopathic allergic-type reactions is not known. Better understanding of mast cell biology is needed.
- There are gaps in the epidemiology of allergy, especially for anaphylaxis and drug allergy.

Future developments

Research into new forms of allergen immunotherapy, including modified allergens and oral immunotherapy for food allergy, are likely to lead to changes in practice. Other types of immunotherapy, including monoclonal antibodies and drugs targeted against cytokines and other mediators, may become available.

Further reading

Calderon MA, *et al.* (2007). Allergen injection immunotherapy for seasonal allergic rhinitis. *Cochrane Database Syst Rev.*, **1**, CD001936.

Clark AT, Islam S, King Y, Deighton J, Anagnostou K, Ewan PW (2009). Successful oral tolerance induction in severe peanut allergy. *Allergy*, **64**, 1218–20.

Ewan PW, Clark AT (2005). Efficacy of a management plan based on severity assessment in longitudinal and case-controlled studies of 747 children with nut allergy: proposal for good practice. *Clin Exp Allergy*, **35**, 751–6.

Ewan PW (1998). ABC of allergies. Anaphylaxis. *BMJ*, **316**(7142), 1442–5.

Gupta R, *et al.* (2004). Burden of allergic disease in the United Kingdom: secondary analyses of national databases. *Clin Exp Allergy*, **34**, 520–6.

Gupta R, *et al.* (2007). Time trends in allergic disorders in the United Kingdom. *Thorax*, **62**, 91–6.

Sampson HA, *et al.* (2006). Second symposium on the definition and management of anaphylaxis: summary report—Second National Institute of Allergy and Infectious Disease/Food Allergy and Anaphylaxis Network symposium. *J Allergy Clin Immunol*, **117**, 391–7.

Soar J, *et al.* (2008). Working Group of the Resuscitation Council (United Kingdom). Emergency treatment of anaphylactic reactions—Guidelines for healthcare providers. *Resuscitation*, **77**, 157–69.

Wang J, Sampson HA (2007). Food anaphylaxis. *Clin Exp Allergy*, **37**, 651–60.

Wilson DR, Lima MT, Durham SR (2005). Sublingual immunotherapy for allergic rhinitis: systematic review and meta-analysis. *Allergy*, **60**, 4–12.

5.4

Autoimmunity

Antony Rosen

Essentials

Autoimmune diseases occur when a sustained, specific, adaptive immune response is generated against self-components, and results in tissue damage or dysfunction. They probably affect more than 3% of Western populations, more commonly women than men, and have peak incidence in the third to sixth decades.

Aetiology and pathogenesis

These can usefully be described in terms of (1) susceptibility—inherited or acquired defects in pathways required to maintain tolerance to self antigens render the individual susceptible to disease initiation; (2) initiation of autoimmunity—interaction between susceptibility genes and environmental events initiate an immune response directed at self antigens; (3) propagation—specific immune response to self antigens causes damage of tissues, with the release of more antigens that further drive the immune response; (4) transition—targets of immune response change and are amplified, with clinical symptoms assuming a recognizable phenotype.

Although a single immune effector pathway may predominate in generating tissue dysfunction and damage in some autoimmune diseases, it is much commoner for multiple effector pathways to participate in generating the final phenotype. Those pathways which generate tissue damage or dysfunction include autoantibody binding to target cells, immune complex-mediated activation of complement and Fc receptor (FcR) pathways, cytokine pathways, as well as lymphocyte-mediated cytotoxicity of target cells. The nature and sites of tissue damage determine the pathological and clinical features of specific diseases.

Tissue-specific autoimmune diseases

Immune-mediated damage is restricted to a particular tissue or organ that specifically expresses the targeted antigen, e.g. (1) Graves' disease—autoantibodies bind to and stimulate the TSH receptor, resulting in thyrotoxicosis; (2) myasthenia gravis—autoantibodies target the acetylcholine receptor at the neuromuscular junction, resulting in muscular weakness and fatigue due to the inefficient transmission of the acetylcholine signal; (3) type 1 diabetes—a cytotoxic T-cell response to the β cells of the pancreatic islets results in destruction of the insulin-producing cells.

Systemic autoimmune diseases

Typically characterized by simultaneous damage in multiple tissues, e.g. kidney, lung, skeletal muscle, nervous system, and skin. Unlike autoantibodies in tissue-specific autoimmune diseases, which target tissue-specific antigens, the autoantibodies in systemic autoimmune diseases are frequently directed against molecules expressed ubiquitously in multiple tissues, e.g. (1) aminoacyl-tRNA synthetases—targeted in autoimmune myositis and associated interstitial lung disease; (2) small nuclear ribonucleoproteins (snRNPs)—targeted in systemic lupus erythematosus (SLE); (3) toposiomerase-1—targeted in scleroderma. Each of these molecules is expressed in all cells, where they play critical roles in essential cellular processes, e.g. protein translation, mRNA splicing, and DNA replication and remodelling (respectively).

Nonsustained autoimmune diseases

Organ or tissue damage and dysfunction tend to be self-limited and resolve after the first attack, and are very unlikely to recur, e.g. epidemic Guillain–Barré syndrome. These diseases typically occur in the setting of infection, and are associated with cross-reactive antibody responses that recognize both components of the infecting organism as well as the target tissue.

Introduction

The effector mechanisms that the immune system utilizes to destroy extracellular pathogens, or host cells that harbour intracellular foreigners (e.g. mycobacteria or viruses) must be appropriately targeted if indiscriminate damage to normal host tissue is to be avoided. Under most inflammatory circumstances, some bystander tissue damage is unavoidable. In most situations, this damage is self-limited, due to efficient clearance of the exogenous antigen source and appropriate down-modulation of the immune response. Tissue damage in autoimmune diseases differs fundamentally from bystander damage, in that the host immune system is specifically activated and driven by self-components, focusing damaging immune effector pathways on host tissues expressing those components, in an autoamplifying and self-sustaining way. The danger inherent in initiating a self-sustaining, specific immune response directed against components of self-tissues is intuitively apparent, since antigen clearance under these circumstances is necessarily associated with complete tissue destruction.

It is now clear that an autoimmune component is a feature of many human diseases. Indeed, there are some estimates that autoimmune diseases afflict more than 3% of Western populations, and imposes a significant personal and economic burden on individuals and nations. This chapter will illustrate many of the principles unifying various autoimmune states, and will present a conceptual framework within which to understand their aetiology, pathogenesis, and pathology. The rapid advances in knowledge being made in this group of disorders predict that disease mechanisms will soon be more clearly understood, and will greatly impact therapeutics.

Epidemiology

Autoimmune diseases may affect individuals at all stages of life. In general, diseases have a predilection for beginning after the second decade, with peak incidence in the third to sixth decades. In many instances, there is a preference for the female gender, with the magnitude of this sex difference varying amongst the different diseases. Thus, for the systemic autoimmune diseases (e.g. systemic lupus eythematosus (SLE), rheumatoid arthritis, Sjögren's syndrome, scleroderma, and autoimmune myositis), and autoimmune thyroid disease, the female:male (F:M) ratio is approximately 4–9:1, while for type 1 diabetes, multiple sclerosis, and myasthenia gravis, the female predominance is much less prominent (F:M ratio <2:1). The exact mechanisms underlying this female predominance remain unknown, but this striking biological difference provides a major clue to pathways underlying susceptibility to autoimmunity. Recent studies describing possible gender-related differences in Toll-like receptor (TLR) expression may be relevant in this regard (see below).

Aetiology

An important theme related to the development of various autoimmune diseases has emerged in recent years. One of the most unexpected observations came from studies of patient populations in whom blood samples had been stored for a period of years prior to the onset of clinical disease (military cohorts or stored blood bank samples), allowing investigators to address whether autoantibodies are first generated coincident with clinical disease, or precede this. In a landmark study by Harley and colleagues in SLE, clear evidence was obtained showing that the relatively 'nonspecific' antinuclear autoantibodies and antiphospholipid antibodies generally precede the diagnosis of SLE, often by a period of several years. These investigators also showed that phenotype-specific autoantibodies in SLE (e.g. anti-Sm, anti-RNP) occurred around the time of onset of clinical disease, suggesting that different autoantibody specificities were marking different phases in the disease. Similar observations have been made in rheumatoid arthritis, where anti-cyclic citrullinated peptide antibodies predate clinical symptoms, whereas more specific antibodies (e.g. anti-vimentin) only occur when disease becomes established.

It is therefore operationally useful to divide autoimmune diseases into separate kinetic phases: (1) susceptibility—predisease, in which inherited or acquired defects in pathways required to maintain tolerance to self-antigens render the individual susceptible to disease initiation); (2) initiation of autoimmunity—the interface of susceptibility genes and unique environmental events, which initiate an immune response directed at self antigens—this phase may be prolonged, and is generally not accompanied by clinical symptoms; (3) propagation—a self-amplifying phase in which the specific immune response to self-antigens causes damage of tissues, with the release of more antigens, which further drive the immune response. It is important to note that this last, amplified phase does not manifest initially fully developed, but rather evolves over time towards the diagnostic phenotype. This generally occurs subacutely over weeks to months, and frequently begins with nonspecific symptoms and signs. Examples include the fatigue and constitutional symptoms that predate diagnosis of SLE and rheumatoid arthritis. This period—during which the targets of immune response change and are amplified, and during which clinical symptoms assume a recognizable phenotype—can be viewed as a transition phase, and its recognition is of importance in terms of diagnosis and early intervention.

Both genetic and environmental factors play important roles in initiation and propagation of autoimmune diseases. They probably play their central roles by regulating the activation, function, and targets of the host immune system. There is also evidence that stochastic processes play an important role in disease initiation, greatly complicating studies to define the causes and mechanisms of autoimmune disease (see below).

Genetic factors

Although autoimmune diseases in humans are genetically complex, significant advances in understanding have occurred over the past several years. In some cases, advances have come from the study of autoimmunity with mendelian patterns of inheritance (e.g. APECED, IPEX, C1q deficiency—see definitions below). Advances have also come from genetic association studies of various autoimmune phenotypes (e.g. rheumatoid arthritis, SLE, type 1 diabetes). Together, the studies stress that multiple genes interact in rendering an individual susceptible to autoimmunity, and highlight a critical role for pathways of tolerance induction, immunoregulation, and setpoints/thresholds for immune signalling in avoiding emergence of autoimmunity. A reciprocal role of target tissue pathways (e.g. antigen structure/expression) in regulating autoimmunity has also been recognized. The following are some general principles regarding the genetics of autoimmunity that have emerged in recent years.

Certain MHC class II alleles are associated with disease susceptibility

One of the most striking genetic associations with autoimmunity resides in the major histocompatibility complex (MHC), an area on chromosome 6 in humans which is highly enriched in genes that participate directly and indirectly in the immune response. The strength of association of different autoimmune phenotypes with MHC class II genes in this area is very robust (odds ratios in the 3–8 range). For example, patients with rheumatoid arthritis have an increased frequency of HLA DR4. HLA DR4 (initially defined serologically) encompasses numerous different alleles that have been defined by sequencing. Interestingly, not all subtypes of HLA DR4 are associated with an increased frequency of rheumatoid arthritis, but those alleles that are associated with rheumatoid arthritis share a short amino acid sequence (QKRAA) at positions 70 to 74 of the β chain of the HLA DR molecule. This sequence, termed the 'shared epitope' is located along the peptide-binding groove of HLA DR4 which presents peptides to the antigen receptor of T cells. Interestingly, this same 'shared epitope' is present in many HLA DR1-positive individuals with rheumatoid arthritis. A similar principle appears to hold for patients with type 1 diabetes, where there is a strong association of disease with specific DQβ genotype. Since MHC class II molecules function as a scaffold for presentation of specific peptides to CD4T cells (see below), it is possible that this MHC-encoded susceptibility to disease reflects the ability of these alleles to present unique self peptides to autoreactive T cells. The presence of significant linkage disequilibirum within the MHC region (i.e. large stretches of DNA do not undergo recombination, generating functional cassettes of associated genes) also creates the potential for the disease-association of particular MHC alleles to be influenced by additional genes on the extended haplotype in affected individuals. Studies to define these other genes, and the mechanisms whereby they influence development of autoimmunity, are challenging and are ongoing in many diseases.

Incomplete thymic tolerance induction predisposes to autoimmunity

Significant insights into basic mechanisms can derive from the study of rare human phenotypes. This has been true for autoimmunity, where several monogenic disorders have defined important pathogenic principles. Autoimmune polyendocrine syndrome type I (APS1; OMIM 240300), also called **a**utoimmune **p**olyendocrinopathy **c**andidiasis **e**ctodermal **d**ystrophy (APECED), is a rare disease in which patients develop multiple autoimmune diseases, often beginning in childhood. The syndrome is characterized by striking autoimmunity directed against multiple different target tissues, including parathyroids, adrenals, pancreatic β cells, parietal cells, thyroid, liver, and gonads. Numerous autoantigens have been defined as targets of autoimmunity in APS1, and include enzymes specifically expressed in various endocrine tissues (e.g. steroid 21-hydroxylase—specific for adrenal cortex; steroid 17a-hydroxylase—found in adrenal cortex and gonads, GAD65—found in pancreatic islets, and thyroid peroxidase). The genetic basis of APS1 was mapped to a gene on chromosome 21q22.3, subsequently termed *AIRE* (for autoimmune regulator). AIRE expression is highest in the thymus, where it is expressed in medullary thymic epithelial cells. Significant evidence has now been obtained that AIRE is a transcriptional regulator, which regulates expression in thymic epithelial cells of various peripheral autoantigens normally expressed exclusively in endocrine target tissues. Thus, AIRE appears to regulate the ectopic expression in the thymus of tissue-restricted autoantigens, and provide an antigen source against which to establish central tolerance. Several AIRE-deficient mouse models were subsequently generated; these animals developed various autoimmune endocrine phenotypes, resembling those found in human APS1.

Impaired clearance and tolerance induction by apoptotic cells: susceptibility defect in systemic autoimmunity

Although little is known in humans about the thymic pathways of tolerance induction to ubiquitously expressed autoantigens, there is accumulating evidence to suggest that in the periphery, apoptotic cells play an important role in providing a source of autoantigens against which the organism becomes tolerant. Apoptotic cells are generally very efficiently cleared by phagocytic cells; these events are normally associated with the production of anti-inflammatory cytokines and result in tolerance induction. Interestingly, early components of the classical complement pathway (e.g. C1q and C4) and C-reative protein (CRP) are required for efficient apoptotic cell clearance, with production of interleukin (IL)-10 and transforming growth factor β (TGFβ). It is of particular note, therefore, that homozygous C1q deficiency is associated with a striking susceptibility to SLE, suggesting that rapid, efficient, tolerance-inducing clearance of apoptotic cells may play a similar role to AIRE expression in the thymus in preventing subsequent emergence of autoimmunity to ubiquitously expressed autoantigens. Additional support for this model comes from recent studies of milk fat globule-EGF factor 8 (MFG-E8), a glycoprotein secreted from macrophages that is required for the efficient attachment and clearance of apoptotic cells by macrophages and immature dendritic cells. MFG-E8 is also expressed in tingible-body macrophages at the germinal centres of secondary lymphoid tissues. Interestingly, many unengulfed apoptotic cells are present in the germinal centres of the spleen in MFG-E8-deficient mice, which develop a striking lupus-like phenotype. Other examples exist in which defects in clearance of apoptotic cells are associated with development of systemic autoimmunity (e.g. Mer deficiency). Together, the data strongly suggest that efficient, anti-inflammatory clearance of apoptotic cells plays a central role in tolerance induction and prevention of autoimmunity.

Defective production of regulatory T cells

Although pathways exist that (1) regulate autoantigen expression at sites of tolerance induction, and (2) guide autoantigens towards tolerance-inducing outcomes, these pathways alone are clearly insufficient to prevent the emergence of autoimmune disease. This fact is highlighted by the emergence of autoimmunity when regulatory T-cell differentiation is abnormal in humans with IPEX syndrome (immune dysregulation, polyendocrinopathy, enteropathy, X-linked syndrome; OMIM 304790). IPEX is a rare X-linked recessive disorder, which is characterized by type 1 diabetes, thyroiditis, atopic dermatitis, and inflammatory bowel disease, and is caused by mutations in the *FOXP3* gene. FOXP3 is a member of the forkhead family of transcription factors, and is essential for the development of regulatory T cells (Tregs), which regulate the activation and differentiation of effector T cells at many different levels. It is therefore likely that induction of tolerance is incomplete under most circumstances, and that self-sustaining autoimmunity is normally limited by Treg function.

Signalling thresholds and susceptibility to autoimmunity

Several modulators of T-cell signalling have also been defined as important susceptibility determinants in autoimmunity. For example, CTLA4 polymorphisms are associated with increased risk of a variety of autoimmune diseases, including type 1 diabetes, Graves' disease, SLE, and rheumatoid arthritis. Similarly, a functional polymorphism in PTPN22 has been identified as a major risk factor for several human autoimmune diseases, including SLE, rheumatoid arthritis, and type 1 diabetes. Although the exact mechanisms underlying susceptibility to autoimmunity remain unclear, in both cases the polymorphisms appear to regulate the balance of stimulatory and inhibitory signalling in effector and regulatory T cells, favouring effector T-cell activation.

The genetic studies in autoiommunity therefore highlight that there are many barriers to the development of autoimmunity, including effective tolerance induction in the thymus and periphery, tightly regulated immune signalling, and homeostatic pathways of immunoregulation to limit self responses should these occur. There are also cassettes of immune response genes encoded in the MHC which appear to be more likely to capture specific self-antigens and generate a response to them. It is likely that the genetic susceptibility to autoimmunity in outbred humans represents an integrated threshold involving genes that regulate these various pathways, upon which environmental and stochastic events act to accomplish disease initiation and propagation.

Environmental factors

Twin studies in human autoimmune diseases showing that individuals with an identical genotype may be variably affected by disease (concordance rates vary widely, from 15 to 50%, in identical twins with SLE or rheumatoid arthritis) demonstrate that environmental insults and stochastic events likely play a significant role in the development of autoimmunity. Many potential environmental insults have been suggested to play a role in autoimmune diseases. These include infections, irradiation, and exposure to drugs and toxins. For example, exacerbations of SLE can follow sunlight exposure, and there are numerous reports that disease initiation may have a similar association with ultraviolet irradiation in rare patients. Numerous infections have been postulated to play a role in disease initiation across the spectrum of human autoimmune diseases. In rare cases, the association between antecedent infection and subsequent development of disease is evident (e.g. coxsackievirus infection-induced autoimmune myocarditis, acute rheumatic fever following streptococcal infection, Epstein–Barr virus infection and childhood SLE). In the majority of autoimmune diseases, however, it has not been possible to confirm this environmental connection with any certainty. This does not imply that a causal connection does not exist in these instances, but rather reflects several features of the diseases that greatly complicate the firm establishment of such a connection: (1) kinetic complexity of the autoimmune diseases—since development of autoimmunity occurs in several distinct phases, and once the propagation phase begins, establishment of a recognizable disease phenotype often takes months, evidence of the initiating insult may have disappeared by the time the environmental component is sought for the first time; (2) several different environmental insults may induce a similar response; (3) the environmental force may be extremely frequent in the population, but may only induce autoimmune disease in a unique subset of individuals with appropriate susceptibility genes.

How environmental forces influence initiation of autoimmune diseases is not yet known for most autoimmune diseases, but several plausible mechanisms have been advanced. These include (1) the disruption of cell and tissue barriers, allowing previously sequestered antigens access to a previously ignorant immune system (see below); (2) inducing novel pathways of antigen presentation, (3) alteration of the structure of self antigens, and (4) molecular mimicry. Some of these mechanisms are dealt with in more detail below.

Pathogenesis

Although extraordinarily complex in detail, the adaptive immune response operates by a set of relatively simple principles: (1) the immune system has the capacity to discern molecular structure in extremely fine detail; (2) it has a uniquely adapted set of signalling systems that computes the amount of antigen; (3) it responds in a binary way to contextual information, i.e. seeing an antigen in the setting of a dangerous context (e.g. infection) initiates an immune response, whereas seeing the antigen in the absence of such co-stimulatory signals leads to tolerance. Numerous studies over the past two decades have underscored that the sustained autoimmune response is extremely similar to adaptive immune responses directed against foreign pathogens, except that the driving antigens in autoimmune disease are self molecules. For example, autoantibodies in most autoimmune diseases display evidence of isotype switching (e.g. from IgM to IgG or IgA), and show features of having undergone affinity maturation through somatic hypermutation. These properties of autoantibodies require the activity of antigen-specific CD4+ T cells, and have therefore focused much attention on defining the mechanisms whereby self-reactive T cells are activated in autoimmunity. Since this is such a central issue in the understanding of autoimmunity, and since there are numerous mechanisms employed by the normal individual to prevent activation of autoreactive T cells, it is important to review briefly the mechanisms that the normal immune system uses to maintain tolerance against self proteins.

Central and peripheral tolerance

To prevent the survival of lymphocytes that will likely encounter their cognate antigens in healthy self tissues, with potential autoimmune destruction of tissues, the immune system spends significant energy on testing the specificity of all receptors generated during antigen-independent development of lymphocytes initially in the thymus, and subsequently in the periphery. When the T-cell receptor generated through somatic recombination recognizes a peptide–MHC complex in the thymus with high affinity/avidity, cells expressing this receptor are negatively selected (since they are likely self-reactive, and will recognize their cognate antigens at additional peripheral sites). These self-reactive cells undergo apoptosis in the thymus, and never make it into the periphery. In contrast, those T-cell receptors that have some affinity for the selecting MHC molecule, but not for the peptide contained in the groove, likely will recognize foreign peptides, and are positively selected. This process of establishing tolerance to self-proteins in the thymus is called 'central tolerance'. T cells exiting the thymus therefore include cells that can recognize peptides within the scaffold of the MHC molecule used to select that T cell, but have not encountered their specific peptide in the thymus. Since not all self-antigens are expressed in the thymus, there is still a chance that these T cells will encounter a self peptide–MHC complex in the periphery for which they have high affinity. Since cells that have left the thymus no longer have the developmental context that likely denotes a self peptide (i.e. recognition with high affinity of a peptide–MHC complex during development in the thymus), peripheral T cells utilize another binary system to define whether a high affinity interaction should lead to activation or inactivation. This binary system uses additional cell surface molecules (called costimulatory molecules) to denote context. Thus, when peripheral T cells recognize an MHC–peptide complex with high affinity in the absence of costimulation (through ligation of CD28 by surface CD80 or CD86 on the antigen-presenting cell), T cells are inactivated or tolerized. This is known as 'peripheral tolerance'. In contrast, when peripheral T cells recognize an MHC–peptide complex with high affinity in the presence of costimulation, these T cells are activated.

In addition to T-cell tolerance, B-cell tolerance to self components is also actively maintained. Thus, if B cells encounter either soluble or membrane-bound antigen during development in the bone-marrow, these cells are either deleted (tolerance) or inactivated such that they become refractory to specific stimulation by their antigen (anergy).

Mechanisms allowing an immune response to be directed against self antigens

Although tolerance to self molecules is stringently maintained at the T and B cell levels, reactivity against self molecules may still be possible for several reasons. These include:

Abnormal immunoregulation

There are numerous mechanisms used to establish and maintain T and B cell tolerance. There is accumulating evidence that defects in regulation of these pathways may result in the failure to eliminate autoreactive lymphocytes, or an altered activation threshold for lymphocytes. Examples include defects in the Fas/Fas-ligand system, a receptor–ligand pair which is required for removal of activated, self-reactive lymphocytes. Mice or humans with defects in this pathway manifest profound lymphadenopathy and a spectrum of autoimmunity. Similarly, defects in regulatory molecules which normally function to dampen the immune response (e.g. CTLA-4, the inhibitory T cell receptor for the costimulatory molecules B7-1 and B7-2) may result in profound autoimmune responses. Mice lacking CTLA-4 develop fatal autoimmunity, with widespread T-cell infiltrates, and CTLA-4 polymorphisms are associated with autoimmunity in humans. It should be remembered that the immune system is a highly complex system, with interdependent regulation present at numerous levels. It is likely that many of the other susceptibility genes in human autoimmunity impinge on these immunoregulatory pathways.

Existence of sites of immune privilege

Strict sequestration of tissue-specific antigens behind anatomical and immunological barriers prevents the development of tolerance to molecules expressed preferentially at these sites. Events (e.g. penetrating trauma) which breach this tight boundary may allow initiation of an immune response to these previously hidden self molecules. Relevant examples include antigens within the eye, testis, and central nervous system. In the eye, for instance, penetrating injury to one eye may be followed by development of inflammation in the contralateral eye (sympathetic ophthalmitis) approximately 1 to 2 weeks after injury. Several mechanisms have been proposed to be responsible for maintaining the immune-privileged status of these tissues. One powerful mechanism appears to involve the constitutive expression of Fas ligand in the relevant tissue (e.g. eye). When this molecule binds to and activates its receptor on lymphocytes, these cells undergo apoptotic death, and are prevented from entering the tissue.

Immunodominance and cryptic determinants

Not all regions of a molecule are equally immunogenic. Regions of the molecule that are well-captured by class II MHC molecules during natural processing of self-antigens are able to tolerize T cells (these determinants have been termed 'immunodominant' by Sercarz and colleagues). In contrast, regions of self molecules that are not generated in significant amount during natural antigen processing (so-called 'cryptic determinants') cannot effectively tolerize T cells, since they are never seen by these cells either in the thymus or peripherally. This immunodominance appears to be influenced by the intrinsic affinity of the peptide for MHC class II, as well as by neighbouring structural determinants on the antigen that may influence its binding to the peptide-binding groove. On self molecules, two sets of determinants can therefore be functionally defined (see Fig. 5.4.1):

- those that are easily processed and presented (comprising the dominant self), which readily tolerize developing T cells
- those that are not presented in appreciable amounts after natural processing (comprising the cryptic self), which do not tolerize

There are unusual circumstances in which natural processing of self-antigens is altered from the default pathway. Examples include novel proteolysis of autoantigen (which destroys the dominant epitope or generates a new dominant epitope) prior to entry into the processing pathway, as well as high-affinity binding to specific receptors or antibodies, which can hinder access of the dominant epitope to the antigen-binding groove of MHC class II molecules, or optimize the loading of a previously cryptic epitope. Since T cells recognizing these cryptic peptides have not previously been tolerized, such 'autoreactive' T cells can now be activated (see Fig. 5.4.2).

There are several clear demonstrations that autoreactive T cells recognizing cryptic epitopes can be activated *in vivo* through altered processing of self molecules to reveal these previously immunocryptic epitopes. For instance, high-affinity binding of the HIV surface protein gp120 to CD4 alters the processing of CD4, and activates T cells which recognize epitopes of CD4 not generated during normal antigen processing. This mechanism may account for the autoimmune response to CD4 seen during HIV infection. Similarly, although intact mouse cytochrome c is not immunogenic in mice, cleavage of the molecule into smaller peptides induces a robust T-cell response to cryptic areas of cytochrome *c*, which were never previously presented by the natural processing pathway, and therefore did not induce tolerance.

The revelation of cryptic epitopes in self-antigens is likely to be a highly relevant mechanism in many human autoimmune diseases, but the studies to demonstrate the importance of this mechanism have only recently begun in earnest. Since the structure of autoantigens influences the hierarchy of dominant and cryptic and determinants generated when the molecule is processed, unique processes which alter the structure of molecules may play critical roles in initiation of autoimmune diseases. These unique events likely do not occur during normal homeostasis, but may occur preferentially during infectious or other pro-immune events occurring at the host-environment interface. Relevant examples include:

- Activation of unique proteolytic pathways that specifically alter the structure of autoantigens during immune effector

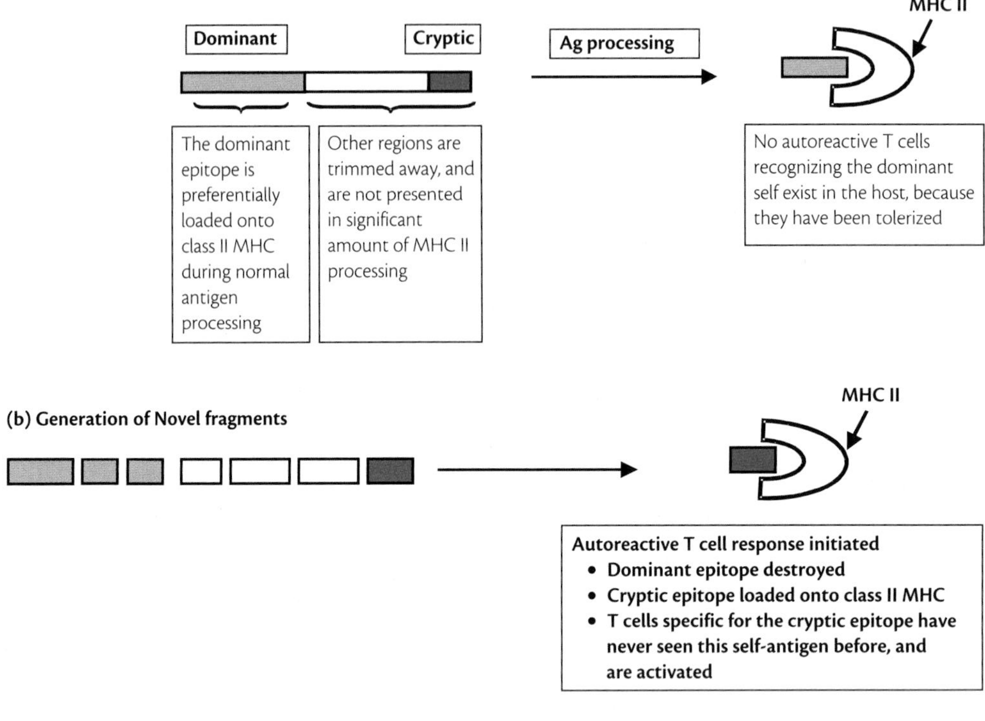

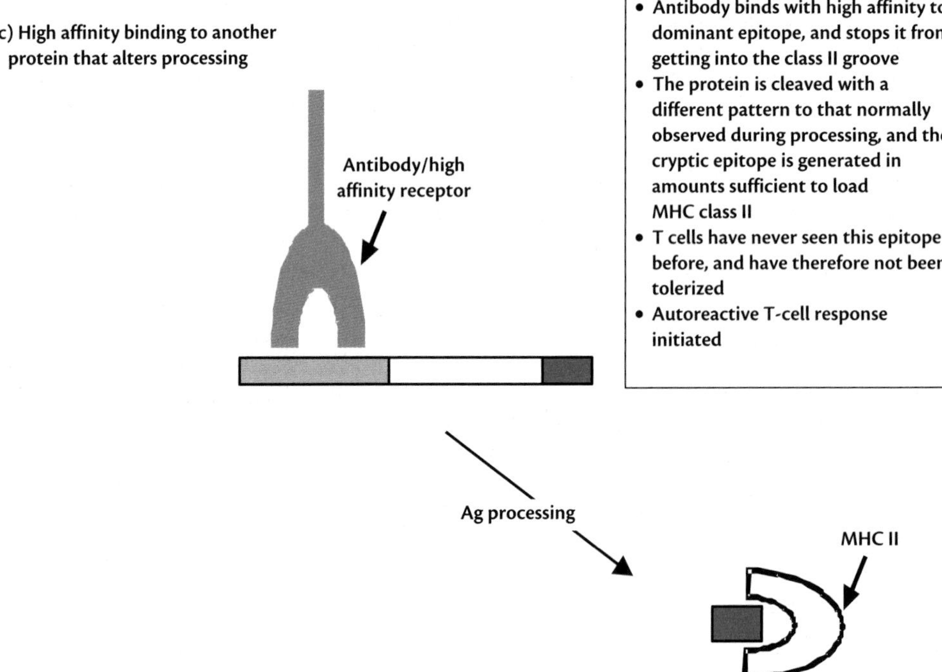

Fig. 5.4.1 Dominant and cryptic T-cell epitopes in autoimmune disease. (a) The default processing pathway for intact antigen results in the preferential and reproducible loading of the 'dominant' peptide determinant into the antigen-binding groove of MHC class II. During establishment of thymic and peripheral tolerance, T cells recognizing this dominant epitope are purged from the repertoire, but T cells recognizing cryptic epitopes do not encounter their antigens, and are not deleted or anergized. (b, c) When the processing of self antigens is altered (e.g. by novel proteolysis or through high-affinity binding to another molecule), a different hierarchy of epitopes is loaded on to class II MHC. If cryptic epitopes are loaded in sufficient amounts, these peptides can stimulate autoreactive T-cell responses directed against the cryptic self, and drive the autoimmune process.

pathways. It has recently been observed that the majority of autoantigens targeted across the spectrum of human autoimmune diseases are specifically cleaved by granzyme B during killing of infected target cells by cytotoxic lymphocytes. This cleavage generates unique molecular fragments never generated in the organism during development or homeostasis. Interestingly, this cleavage is a unique feature of autoantigens, and does not affect non-autoantigens. Although it has been proposed that these cleavage events allow the efficient presentation of previously cryptic epitopes, this remains to be formally demonstrated.

- Additional post-translational modifications that alter conformation of antigens, and modify their subsequent processing. It is noteworthy that numerous post-translational modifications of

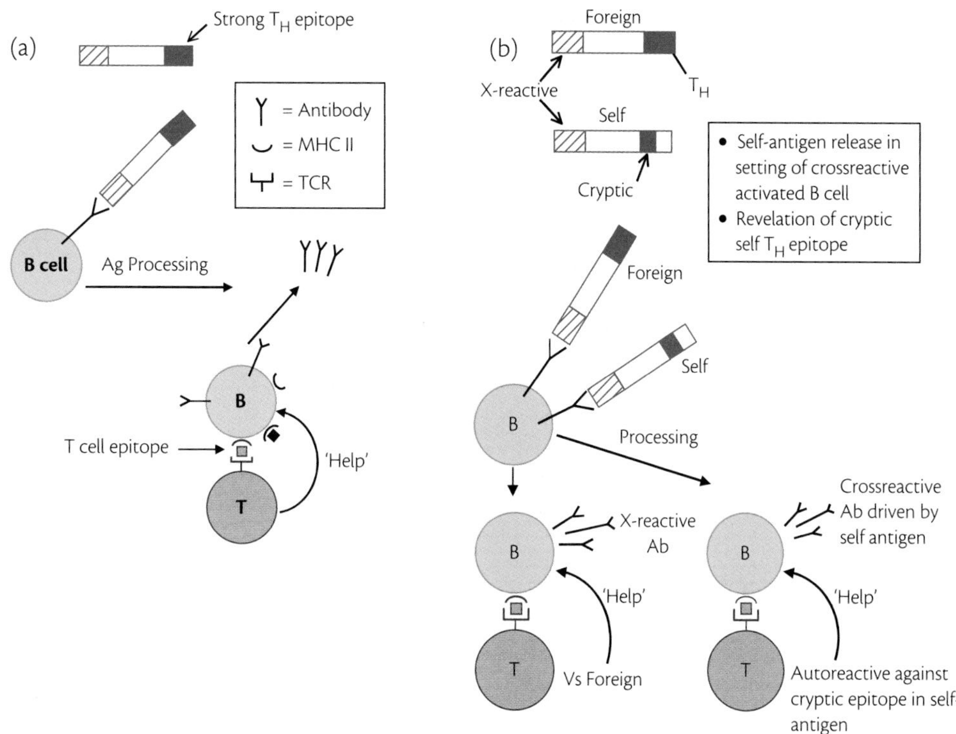

Fig. 5.4.2 Molecular mimicry. (a) Foreign antigens, which clearly differ from their homologous self antigens in some areas, may nevertheless bear significant structural similarity to self antigens in other regions. Initiation of an immune response to the foreign antigen may generate a cross-reactive antibody response that also recognizes the self protein. When the self antigen is a cell-surface molecule, antibody-mediated effector pathways can lead to host tissue damage. Although the antibody response is cross-reactive with self molecules, the T cells that drive this response are directed exclusively at the foreign antigen. (b) Under highly novel conditions, the simultaneous liberation of significant amounts of self antigen in the setting of a cross-reactive antibody response may allow effective presentation of cryptic epitopes in the self-antigen to autoreactive T cells by activated cross-reactive B cells. These autoreactive T cells can now continue to drive an autoantibody response to the self-antigen. If continued release of self antigen occurs as part of this process, a specific, adaptive immune response to self will be sustained.

autoantigens occur, and that in some cases the autoimmune response is strictly dependent on the occurrence of these modifications. Examples include phosphorylation, acetylation, deimination, and isoaspartyl formation, amongst others.

- Formation of high-affinity complexes between autoantigens and other viral or self-proteins.

In all these examples, it should be remembered that the initiating event in autoimmunity requires that, on the background of appropriate susceptibility genes, several stringent criteria needed to initiate a primary immune response must be simultaneously satisfied. These include the generation of suprathreshold concentrations of self molecules that have a structure not previously tolerized by the immune system, and the presentation of these unique molecular forms to T lymphocytes in the presence of costimulation (i.e. in a proimmune context).

Molecular mimicry

Foreign antigens, which clearly differ from their homologous self-antigens in some areas, may nevertheless bear significant structural similarity to self-antigens in other regions. Initiation of an immune response to the foreign antigen may generate a cross-reactive antibody response that also recognizes the self-protein (molecular mimicry). When the antigen is a cell-surface molecule, antibody-mediated effector pathways can lead to host tissue damage. Although the antibody response is cross-reactive with self molecules, the T cells that drive this response are directed at the foreign antigen (see below). Diseases involving this sort of antigen mimicry therefore tend to be self-limited. It is important to realize that molecular mimicry alone cannot explain self-sustaining autoimmune diseases, which are driven by self-antigens and autoreactive T cells. In these cases, there is a requirement for overcoming T cell tolerance to the self protein. The simultaneous liberation of self-antigen in the presence of the cross-reactive antibody response likely play critical roles in this regard (see below).

Mechanistic insights into molecular mimicry

Although a number of microbial and viral antigens have regions of high homology with various human autoantigens, a causal link between exposure to these foreign antigens and the onset or exacerbation of autoimmune disease has been extremely difficult to establish. There are, however, clear examples that suggest the existence of 'one-shot' autoimmune processes, in which cross-reactive antibodies directed against surface self-antigens are generated following infection, and result in tissue damage. This persists until infection is cleared, and the immune response wanes. Although the mechanistic details of this scheme are difficult to prove *in vivo*, several pertinent examples exist. One of these is a seasonal epidemic form of Guillain–Barré syndrome seen in northern China, which follows *Campylobacter jejuni* infection. Affected patients make antibodies recognizing gangliosides, and the disease has a self-limited course, which rarely recurs. The anti-ganglioside antibodies generated are likely responsible for the pathological findings of acute motor axonal neuropathy. Another plausible example of this mechanism (although with meager *in vivo* evidence) is immune thrombocytopenia (ITP) in children. This process characteristically (1) follows an infectious process; (2) demonstrates anti-platelet antibodies, and (3) frequently shows durable remissions. The mechanistic details of this process have been difficult to prove *in vivo*, and cross-reactive epitopes on potentially initiating pathogens have not yet been defined.

The single episodes of tissue damage in the setting of a cross-reactive immune response following infection must be contrasted to the sustained, autoamplifying disease frequently seen in other autoimmune syndromes. The central issues in this regard are (1) how T-cell tolerance to self antigens might initially be broken, and (2) once this has occurred, why these antigens continue to drive the immune response to self. Examination of tolerance to cytochrome *c*, a ubiquitous protein that has regions of homology and divergence across different species, has been very useful in understanding molecular mimicry of cross-reactive epitopes. Mouse cytochrome *c* shares significant homology with human cytochrome *c*, although the proteins are entirely different in other areas. When Mamula and colleagues used mouse cytochrome *c* to immunize mice, no T-cell or antibody response to the murine protein was observed. When human cytochrome *c* was similarly used to immunize mice, strong T-cell epitopes on the foreign cytochrome *c* were able to induce a strong antibody response to the foreign protein. The antibodies induced recognized both the murine and the human forms of cytochrome *c*, i.e. cross-reactive antibodies that recognize the self protein were produced. The T cell response to cytochrome *c* was, however, directed entirely against the foreign (human) form of the protein, and no T cells against the murine protein could be found. These cross-reactive antibodies disappear as the immune response to the foreign protein wanes.

Interestingly, when mouse cytochrome *c* was included with human cytochrome *c* during the immunization, a T-cell response to human cytochrome *c*, and a humoral response to the human protein that cross-reacts with the murine protein, was induced. Within a few days, a strong helper T-cell response specific for murine cytochrome *c* was detected. This breaking of T-cell tolerance to murine cytochrome *c* was dependent on activated B cells specific for cytochrome *c*, which likely exert their effect through altering the processing of mouse cytochrome *c*, potentially uncovering previously cryptic epitopes in the self-protein (see Fig. 5.4.2). In the presence of continued release of self antigen, this response may become self-sustaining—self-antigen driving autoreactive T cells, providing help to autoantibody-producing B cells (Fig. 5.4.2).

Molecular mimicry may therefore induce the production of cross-reactive antibodies, which, in the absence of liberation of significant amounts of self antigen, should disappear when the foreign pathogen is cleared. The form of epidemic motor axonopathy described above is likely representative of this scenario. Under highly novel conditions, the simultaneous liberation of significant amounts of self antigen in the setting of a cross-reactive antibody response may allow effective presentation of cryptic epitopes in the self-antigen to autoreactive T cells by activated cross-reactive B cells. If continued release of self antigen occurs, a specific, adaptive immune response to self will be sustained. Antigen release from tissues likely plays a critical role in driving this autoimmune process. Understanding the mechanisms of ongoing antigen release at sites of tissue damage in autoimmune disease (e.g. unique pathways of cell injury and death) is a high priority for future work, as it provides a novel target for therapy (see below).

It is clear from the above discussion that extraordinary complexity is operative in initiation of the human autoimmune diseases. The patient population is genetically heterogeneous, the human immune system is complex and extremely plastic, and it interacts with a plethora of environmental stimuli and stochastic events. The simultaneous confluence of susceptibility factors and initiation forces to

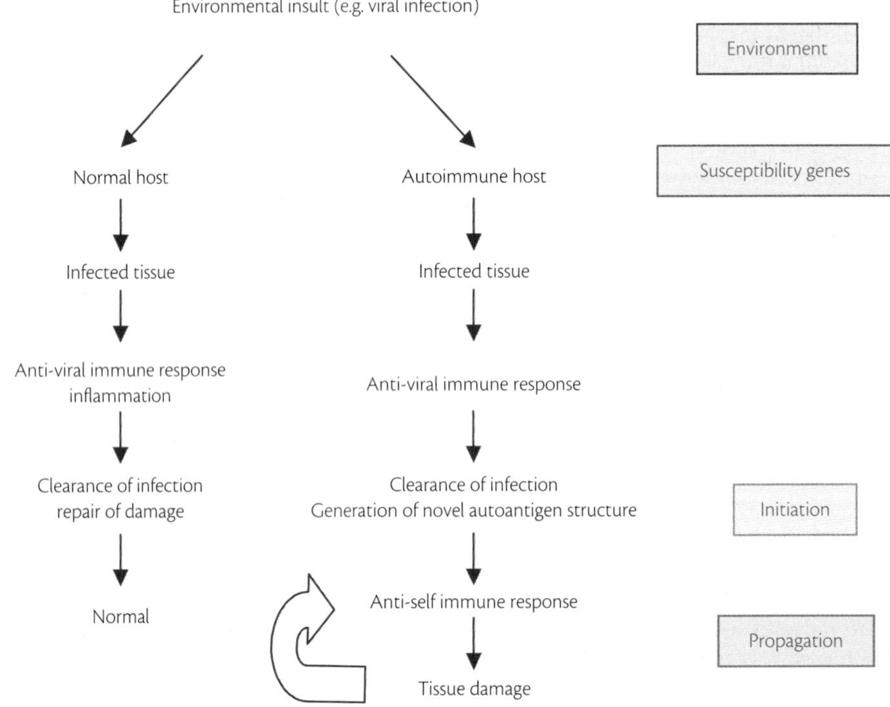

Fig. 5.4.3 Model of initiation and propagation of autoimmune disease. Autoimmune diseases are highly complex disorders, which require the simultaneous cooperation of multiple factors for their development. Numerous susceptibility genes (some of which regulate the immune response) appear to determine the threshold for disease initiation. In many diseases, a discrete, pro-immune environmental trigger likely plays a role in disease initiation, but is infrequently recognized. A critical requirement for disease initiation is the generation of suprathreshold concentrations of self-antigen with novel structure. Development of a recognizable disease phenotype generally requires marked antigen-driven amplification of the autoimmune response, in which immune effector pathways play a role in generating the ongoing supply of antigen to sustain the process.

set off the self-sustained and autoamplifying process is therefore an extremely rare occurrence. In contrast, once activation of autoreactive T cells has occurred, the ability of the immune system to vigorously respond to vanishingly low concentrations of antigen, to amplify the specific effector response to those antigens, and to spread the response to additional antigens in that tissue, greatly reduces the stringency that must be met to keep the process going (Fig. 5.4.3).

Effector mechanisms in autoimmune diseases

The initiation phase of autoimmunity requires cooperation between many different cell types, including antigen-presenting cells, T cells and B cells, as well as numerous soluble mediators including antibodies, chemokines, and cytokines. The effector phase of autoimmunity uses the same immune and inflammatory effector mechanisms that the immune system has evolved for removing and destroying pathogens. These include activation of the complement cascade, which generates signals that effect inflammatory cell recruitment and activation. Similarly, ligation of activating Fc receptors on inflammatory cells by immune complexes activates macrophage and neutrophil effector function. Autoantibodies directed against cell surface antigens initiate antigen-dependent cellular cytotoxicity (ADCC), likely mediated by macrophages and natural killer (NK) cells. Cytokines and chemokines play a central role in inflammatory cell recruitment and activation in the target tissue. Tissue damage can also be effected by cytolytic lymphocytes. The pathology characteristic of each autoimmune disease reflects both the particular antigens targeted, as well as the predominant effector mechanisms activated.

One principle of central importance in the effector phase of autoimmunity is autoamplification, which appears to play a central role in the self-sustaining nature of the autoimmune process. Thus, immune effector pathways cause damage of cells in the target tissue, liberating antigen which further stimulates the immune response and effector pathways, thus liberating more antigen. Although this is likely an oversimplification, the view that the immune system plays a role in generating an ongoing supply of autoantigen is useful therapeutically, since it focuses attention on controlling both the supply of antigen as well as immune effector pathways (see below).

Principles of amplification

One of the central features of human autoimmunity is the tendency of the process to amplify progressively with the accumulation of significant immune-mediated tissue damage. Furthermore, in the vast majority of cases, once such amplification begins, the process is very unlikely to resolve spontaneously. Properties of autoantigens themselves may be very important in this phase, in terms both of acquisition of adjuvant properties, and of regulation of expression. The essential features of amplification are a substrate cycle, in which antigen expression and adjuvant properties induce an immune response, which induces increased antigen expression and tissue damage—and further drive the immune response. The importance of tissue-specific autoantigen expression in focusing such immune responses is only beginning to be recognized.

Acquisition of adjuvant properties by disease-specific autoantigens

In recent years there have been dramatic advances in the understanding of the mechanisms whereby specific molecules are selected as antigens in the various autoimmune syndromes. In spite of the fact that tens of thousands of molecules could be targeted by the immune system in autoimmunity, the number of molecules that are frequently targeted in the different phenotypes are markedly restricted—limited perhaps to 100 or so molecules. This has led to the proposal that frequently targeted autoantigens may themselves have properties that make them proimmune. This was first suggested by Plotz and colleagues. who observed that the autoantigenic histidyl aminoacyl tRNA synthetase which is targeted in autoimmune myositis (but not non-auto-antigenic lysyl- and aspartyl-aminoacyl tRNA synthetases) is chemoattractant to immature dendritic cells and other leucocytes. The authors suggested that the selection of a self molecule as a target for an autoantibody response may be a consequence of proinflammatory properties of the molecule itself. They further suggested that modification of autoantigen structure during processes of cell damage or death may be critical in recruiting these additional functions of autoantigens.

Toll-like receptors (TLRs)

One of the most likely receptor systems to sense and transduce the pro-inflammatory properties of autoantigens is the Toll-like receptor (TLR) family, which is the primary innate immune system transducer of pathogen-associated molecular patterns. Ligands for TLRs include both microbial and endogenous molecules, the latter group being particularly relevant to autoimmunity (see below). Microbial ligands include components of Gram-positive bacteria, Gram-negative bacteria, yeast, and protozoans. Although viral and bacterial nucleic acids are the most likely ligands for TLRs, accumulating data demonstrates that complexes containing endogenous nucleic acids are also able to signal through TLRs. Although the exact nature and source of endogenous ligands for TLRs *in vivo* remains unclear, recent studies have demonstrated that components from stressed, injured and dying cells may play critical roles. Working in several models, numerous investigators have now provided evidence that the targeting of frequently targeted nucleoprotein autoantigens (which contain DNA or RNA) results from the ability of these nucleic acid components to ligate TLRs both *in vitro* and *in vivo*. For example, when TLR9-deficiency is bred on to MRL-lpr mice—which are an excellent model of SLE—animals no longer get autoantibody responses to chromatin. Similarly, when mice are rendered TLR7-deficient, the autoantibody response to Sm is markedly inhibited, and severity of the SLE phenotype is improved. These data confirm that autoantigens frequently selected in different autoimmune phenotypes likely have the dual property of being able to simultaneously activate the innate and adaptive immune systems, and that the ability to coligate TLRs plays a critical role. The likelihood that the TLR-autoantigen interface will be therapeutically relevant in autoimmune processes is very high.

One of the major pathways downstream of TLR ligation in autoimmunity appears to centre on a relatively rare class of immature dendritic cells (plasmacytoid dendritic cells or pDCs), which can secrete large amounts of type I interferons upon TLR ligation, and which express TLR7 and TLR9 at high levels. Ronnblom and colleagues have demonstrated that, when added to material from apoptotic or necrotic cells, autoantibodies from SLE and Sjögren's syndrome patients with specificity for DNA or RNA autoantigens induce striking interferon secretion. Type I interferons have a broad set of functions which likely contribute to the feed forward, propagation phase of systemic autoimmune diseases. For example,

Table 5.4.1 Autoantigens targeted in several tissue-specific autoimmune diseases

Disease	Tissue target	Prominent autoantigen(s)	Proposed disease mechanisms	Clinical features
Autoimmune haemolytic anaemia	Erythrocyte surface	Components of the Rh antigen, Band 3.1, glycophorin, and several unidentified molecules	Antibody-mediated destruction and clearance of erythrocytes	Anemia
Autoimmune hepatitis	Hepatocytes	Smooth muscle cell cytoskeletal components Cytochrome P450-2D6 ASGP-receptor	Multiple	Mild to severe chronic hepatic dysfunction in young women
Epidemic Guillain–Barré syndrome (N. China)	Motor axons	Axonal gangliosides	Infection with *Campylobacter jejuni* induces cross-reactive antibody, which mediates axonal damage	Acute autoimmune axonopathy Flaccid paralysis with areflexia Elevated cerebrospinal fluid protein
Grave's disease	Thyroid gland	TSH receptor	Antibody-mediated stimulation of TSH receptor, leading to excessive thyroid hormone secretion	Hyperthyroidism Goitere Grave's ophthalmopathy Localized dermopathy
Diabetes (type 1)	β cells of the islets of Langerhans	Glutamic acid decarboxylase (65-kDa form) Insulin Carboxypeptidase	Cytotoxic lymphocyte-mediated destruction of islet cells	Insulin deficiency and diabetes
Idiopathic thrombocytopenia	Platelet surface	Platelet integrins	Antibody-mediated platelet destruction and phagocytosis	Thrombocytopenia, bleeding
Inflammatory bowel disease	Gastrointestinal tract	Atypical p-ANCA ASCA	Cytokine and lymphocyte-mediated epithelial damage and dysfunction	Chronic intestinal inflammation marked by remission and relapse
Multiple sclerosis	Myelinated nerve fibers	Myelin basic protein PLP MOG Transaldolase	Activated cytokine pathways Activated effector lymphocytes Autoantibodies	Demyelinating disorder primarily affecting young adults: Protean clinical manifestations depending on location and size of classic plaques
Myasthenia gravis	Neuromuscular junction	Nicotinic AChR	Antibody-induced blockade and down-regulation of AChR	Striated muscle fatigue and weakness
Myocarditis	Myocardium	Cardiac myosin Adenine nucleotide transporter Branched-chain ketodehydrogenase	Infection with coxsackievirus induces myocardial damage and immunization with cardiac autoantigens	Subacute congestive heart failure
Pemphigus vulgaris	Hemidesmosome junctions	Desmoglein-3	Antibody-mediated disruption of epithelial cell junctions, with epidermal cell detachment	Blistering skin lesions
Rasmussen's encephalitis	Inhibitory neurons	Type 3 glutamate receptor	Antibody-mediated blockade of inhibitory neurotransmitter signalling	Severe epileptic seizures, progressive degeneration of a single cerebral hemisphere
Stiff man syndrome	GABA-ergic neurons modulating spinal cord reflexes	GAD67 Amphiphysin	Blockade of inhibitory neurotransmitter signalling, possible autoantibody-mediated	Rare disease characterized by severe, progressive stiffness with superimposed episodic muscle spasms, may be associated with autoimmune disease or malignancy
Vitiligo	Melanocytes	Tyrosinase, TRP-1	Cytotoxic lymphocyte-mediated damage of melanocytes	Skin depigmentation

AChR acetylcholine receptor; ASCA, anti-*Saccharomyces cerevisiae* antibodies; MOG, myelin/oligodendrocyte glycoprotein; PLP, proteolipid protein.

they (1) promote the differentiation of monocytes into mature DCs, which drive autoreactive T and B cell responses; (2) increase target cell sensitivity to killing pathways; (3) up-regulate cytotoxic effector pathways; and (4) up-regulate expression of autoantigens. Targeting interferon pathways in systemic autoimmunity may therefore have important therapeutic potential.

Table 5.4.2 Systemic autoimmune diseases

Disease	Prominent tissue target	Prominent autoantigen(s)	Proposed disease mechanisms	Clinical features
PM/DM	Skeletal muscle	Mi-2 helicase Aminoacyl-tRNA synthetases DNA repair machinery	Complement activation (DM) Activated effector lymphocytes (PM)	Proximal muscle weakness (PM/DM) Heliotrope/skin rash (DM) Interstitial lung disease
Rheumatoid arthritis	Synovial joints	IgG Fc Citrullinated peptides (CCP) Citrullinated vimentin, fibrin, calpastatin	Activated cytokine pathways (TNF) Activated effector lymphocytes Immune complex deposition	Symmetric, erosive polyarthritis
Scleroderma	Skin, lung, GI, kidney, heart	Topoisomerase-1 (diffuse form) RNA polymerases (diffuse) Centromere proteins (CREST form)	Blood vessel damage by activated effector lymphocytes and autoantibodies	Progressive fibrosis of skin, and multiple internal organs (including GI, lung, kidney and heart) Raynaud's phenomenon Vasculopathy
Sjögren's syndrome	Exocrine glandular epithelial tissue	Ro/SS-A; La/SS-B	Epithelial cell death induced by cytotoxic lymphocytes and other immune effector pathways	Keratoconjunctivitis sicca
Systemic lupus erythematosus	Numerous, including skin, kidney, joints, haematologic elements, nervous system	dsDNA/nucleosomes Splicing ribonucleoproteins (e.g. Sm, U1-RNP) Ro/SS-A; La/SS-B Ribosomal P proteins Phospholipid-protein complexes	Cell death/abnormal clearance of apoptotic cells Nucleoprotein complex ligation of TLRs inducing prominent interferon secretion Autoantibody-mediated pathology Immune complex deposition	Multisystem inflammatory disease Skin lesions Arthritis Renal disease Anemia, thrombocytopenia
Wegener's granulomatosis	Numerous, including upper airways, lungs, kidneys and skin	Neutrophil proteinase-3 (c-ANCA)	c-ANCA binding to neutrophil surface induces degranulation in the vessel wall with consequent damage	Multisystem inflammatory vascular disease with predominance of sinuses, middle ear, lung, and renal involvement

DM, dermatomyositis; PM, polymyositis.

Autoantigen expression in the target tissue in autoimmunity

Another important component of the amplification cycle is the target tissue itself, and particularly the amounts and forms of autoantigens expressed at these sites. Unfortunately, very little is currently known about such parameters *in vivo* in relevant target tissues, in either normal or pathological circumstances. Insights from studies on human autoimmune myopathies have begun to provide important insights into this problem. Thus, myositis-specific autoantigens are expressed at very low levels in normal muscle, but at high levels in myositis tissue, where antigen expression is at highest levels in regenerating muscle cells. These data suggest that enhanced autoantigen expression in the target tissue may be a feature of disease propagation, and that antigen expression during tissue repair may provide an ongoing antigen source to sustain and amplify tissue damage. In this regard, the regulation of antigen expression (rather than exclusively pathways of immune-mediated damage) may have important therapeutic potential.

Clinical features

The clinical features of the different autoimmune diseases are extremely diverse, and reflect the specific tissue dysfunction which results from activity of immune effector pathways. Almost all tissues may be affected, including prominent involvement of endocrine organs, nervous system, eye, bone marrow elements, kidney, muscle, skin, liver and gastrointestinal tract, blood vessels, lung, and joints. For tissue-specific autoimmune processes (e.g. type 1 diabetes, ITP, autoimmune haemolytic anaemia (AIHA)—see Table 5.4.1), symptoms may relate to tissue hypofunction resulting from (1) target cell destruction (for type 1 diabetes, destruction of the β cells of the pancreatic islets; for ITP and AIHA, destruction and phagocytosis of platelets and erythrocytes); (2) antibody-mediated interference with function or down-regulation of autoantigen expression (e.g. myasthenia gravis, bullous pemphigoid). In other cases, symptoms may arise from tissue hyperfunction (e.g. Graves' disease) due to activating effects of antibody binding (where antibodies to the TSH receptor induce nonphysiological secretion of thyroid hormone).

In the case of systemic autoimmune processes (Table 5.4.2), symptoms frequently result both from localized target tissue destruction (e.g. skeletal muscle in polymyositis, skin disease in SLE) as well as from the more general activities of inflammatory effector pathways. The latter result from (1) immune-complex deposition at multiple sensitive sites (e.g. joints, kidney, skin, and blood vessel walls) with activation of the complement cascade and recruitment and activation of myelomonocytic cells; (2) ongoing secretion of proinflammatory cytokines. In this regard, the profoundly positive effects of TNF inhibition recently observed on the inflammatory symptoms and joint destruction in rheumatoid arthritis underscore the central role of these general inflammatory mediators in generation and maintenance of the disease phenotype in systemic autoimmune diseases.

Prognosis

Although the barriers that need to be overcome in terms of initiating an autoimmune disease are stringent, and are difficult to satisfy even in the setting of appropriate susceptibility genes, the immune system is equipped with a powerful memory. The mechanisms of this memory are still incompletely defined, but include the generation of a population of memory cells specific for the antigen that initiated the response, which respond vigorously (both in terms of clonal expansion as well as effector function) to very low concentrations of antigen if they encounter it again. Since the autoimmune diseases are disorders driven by the ongoing release of self-antigen, this immunological memory constitutes a major barrier to complete cure. Autoimmune diseases therefore tend to be self-sustaining over long periods, and are often punctuated by clinical exacerbations (flares), which are likely due to re-exposure of the primed immune system to antigen (e.g. SLE, autoimmune myositis, rheumatoid arthritis). The possibility of disease recurring, even after long clinical remission, remains present in most of the autoimmune diseases. Tissue-specific autoimmune diseases may result in the complete destruction of the target tissue over time, with loss of function of that tissue accompanied by a waning immune response (e.g. type 1 diabetes). Interestingly, in cases where immune-mediated tissue pathology results from effector pathways being driven by a cross-reactive T-cell response to a foreign antigen (e.g. epidemic Guillain–Barré syndrome), disease has a finite duration, and generally does not recur.

Therapy

It is not possible to discuss the therapy of this broad group of disorders in any detail in this chapter, but a few principles that underlie current approaches to therapy are discussed. Autoimmune diseases cause significant tissue dysfunction through (1) inflammation, (2) tissue destruction with loss of functional units, (3) the consequences of healing, and (4) functional disturbances (e.g. interference with acetylcholine signalling by autoantibody to the acetylcholine receptor and inducing receptor down-modulation in myasthenia gravis). Therapeutic interventions in autoimmune diseases are generally focused on controlling immune and inflammatory pathways, and at replacing or accommodating lost function.

Control of immune and inflammatory pathways responsible for ongoing damage

Since in most instances the critical autoantigens and effector pathways responsible for unique diseases have not been defined, this goal is frequently extremely challenging. Thus, frequent use is made of anti-inflammatory and immunosuppressive therapies which broadly target many aspects of the immune response (e.g. steroids, azathioprine, cyclophosphamide, methotrexate, mycophenolate). Since a robust immune response is required to protect the host from a myriad of infectious threats, this nontargeted suppression of the immune system can have deleterious consequences in terms of increased susceptibility to infection, with its attendant high morbidity and mortality. In this regard, therapeutic targeting of specific inflammatory pathways is extremely attractive, and there are recent examples in which this approach has been highly successful. In rheumatoid arthritis, the maintenance of chronic inflammatory joint pathology appears to be dependent on the activity of tumour necrosis factor (TNF). Specific inhibition of TNF through the use of either soluble TNF receptors or humanized monoclonal antibodies has led to an astonishing effect on disease activity in rheumatoid arthritis, with abolition of systemic symptoms, and a striking decrease in the rate of joint destruction. These positive effects were associated with only a minimal increase in susceptibility to infection, although this risk is certainly present. This therapy also served as a model demonstrating that the use of injectable forms of biological therapies (monoclonal antibodies or receptors) as therapeutic agents in the general population was feasible. However, the significant expense associated with such therapies will be a major challenge to health care systems worldwide, particularly as additional effective and powerful agents have been discovered. Although the combinatorial use of agents targeting different pathways in autoimmune disease is attractive, the effects are unpredictable, and great caution will need to be exercised. As noted above, modulation of additional immune effector pathways, TLR signalling, or autoantigen expression in the target tissue are also important targets for novel therapy in the autoimmune diseases.

Another example of specific targeting of proinflammatory pathways is that of intravenous immunoglobulin (IVIG). This is prepared from pooled serum and its major component is immunoglobulin G (IgG). IVIG therapy has been used as a treatment of several autoimmune diseases, including ITP, autoimmune myositis, and acute demyelinating polyneuropathy, but is only available at prohibitive cost. Recent data from mice has demonstrated that IVIG induces surface expression of the inhibitory Fcγ receptor (Fcγ RII_B) on macrophages, and shifts the balance of signalling through Fc receptors towards inhibition, down regulating the pro-inflammatory response to immune complexes. It is likely that continued identification of additional agents that precisely modulate specific inflammatory pathways will have a major therapeutic impact on this group of diseases.

Interventions aimed at replacing or accommodating lost function

The majority of autoimmune diseases are associated with loss of function of organs and tissues, many of which perform essential physiological functions. Indeed, recognition of the autoimmune phenotype in many instances requires that tissue damage is sufficiently severe to have led to characteristic loss of function. For example, loss of insulin-secreting β cells of the pancreatic islets results in type 1 diabetes, and blockade and down-regulation of the nicotinic acetylcholine receptor causes striated muscle weakness and fatigue in myasthenia gravis. Similarly, chronic immune complex deposition in glomeruli causes renal inflammation and scarring in SLE. Where significant functional reserve is still present in a particular disease, a strong argument can be made for preventing further damage through specific or general immunosuppressive strategies described above. This is particularly relevant where the 'supply' of tissue that could be damaged is essentially inexhaustible (e.g. most instances of systemic autoimmune disease). Where functional impairment is already established, interventions aimed at replacing or accommodating lost function are indicated. For example, insulin replacement is required for type 1 diabetes, and treatment for hyperthyroidism is indicated in Graves' disease.

Further reading

Banchereau J, Pascual V (2006). Type I interferon in systemic lupus erythematosus and other autoimmune diseases. *Immunity*, **25**, 383–92. [A review of the critical roles of type I interferons in systemic autoimmunity.]

Casciola-Rosen L, *et al.* (2005). Enhanced autoantigen expression in regenerating muscle cells in idiopathic inflammatory myopathy. *J Exp Med*, **201**, 591–601. [Paper establishing tissue repair as a potential target of autoimmunity implicated in disease propagation.]

Diamond B, *et al.* (1992). The role of somatic mutation in the pathogenic anti-DNA response. *Annu Rev Immunol*, **10**, 731–57. [Comprehensive review of the evidence that autoantibodies are antigen-driven and T-cell dependent.]

Feldmann M, Maini RN (2001). Anti-TNF alpha therapy of rheumatoid arthritis: what have we learned? *Annu Rev Immunol*, **19**, 163–96. [A review of the discovery of anti-TNF agents as therapeutics in rheumatic disease.]

Filippi CM, von Herrath MG (2007). Islet beta-cell death—fuel to sustain autoimmunity? *Immunity*, **27**, 183–5. [Brief review highlighting the role of beta cell death in driving autoimmunity in diabetes.]

Gammon G, Sercarz EE, Benichou G (1991). The dominant self and the cryptic self: shaping the autoreactive T-cell repertoire. *Immunol Today*, **12**, 193–195. [Concise introduction to the concepts and consequences of immunodominance.]

Gregersen PK, Behrens TW (2006). Genetics of autoimmune diseases—disorders of immune homeostasis. *Nat Rev Genet*, **7**, 917–28. [Current and extensive review of the genetics of autoimmune diseases.]

Lanzavecchia A (1995). How can cryptic epitopes trigger autoimmunity? *J Exp Med*, **181**, 1945–8. [Important review of potential mechanisms of autoimmunity.]

Lin R-H, *et al.* (1991). Induction of autoreactive B cells allows priming of autoreactive T cells. *J Exp Med*, **173**, 1433–9. [Important demonstration that autoreactive B cells may alter the processing of self antigens to allow activation of autoreactive T cells.]

Marshak-Rothstein, A, Rifkin, IR (2007). Immunologically active autoantigens: the role of toll-like receptors in the development of chronic inflammatory disease. *Annu Rev Immunol*, **25**, 419–41. [Review of the pro-immune properties of autoantigens.]

Nimmerjahn F, Ravetch JV (2008). Fcgamma receptors as regulators of immune responses. *Nat Rev Immunol*, **8**, 34–47. [Extensive and current review of the signalling and functions of Fc receptors in inflammation.]

Plotz PH (2003). The autoantibody repertoire: searching for order. *Nat Rev Immunol*, **3**, 73–78. [Review of autoantibodies in systemic autoimmunity, introducing the concept that frequently targeted autoantigens have the capacity to directly activate the innate immune system.]

Radic MZ, Weigert M (1994). Genetic and structural evidence for antigen selection of anti-DNA antibodies. *Annu Rev Immunol*, **12**, 487–520. [Comprehensive review of evidence that autoimmunity is driven by self-antigen.]

Todd JA, *et al.* (2007). Robust associations of four new chromosome regions from genome-wide analyses of type 1 diabetes. *Nat Genet*, **39**, 857–864. [Paper using a genome-wide approach to confirm and extend previous genetic associations of type I diabetes.]

5.5

Principles of transplantation immunology

Ross S. Francis and Kathryn J. Wood

Essentials

Since the first successful transplant of a kidney between identical twins in 1955, transplantation has progressed from being an experimental procedure to a routine clinical therapy offering immense benefits for patients with organ failure, but the survival of transplanted organs remains limited by the body's immune responses, and many of the complications of transplantation result from the crude nature of our attempts to suppress these.

The immune system has evolved to protect the individual from invasion by pathogenic microorganisms as well as mutation of the individual's own cells that may be premalignant, hence stringent discrimination of 'self' from 'nonself' or 'altered self' is crucial.

The immune response to transplanted tissue

The immunological response that follows transplantation of tissue between genetically nonidentical individuals is complex. (1) Inflammatory signals generated at the site of transplantation as a result of local surgical trauma as well as injury from graft ischaemia and reperfusion activate cells of the innate immune system, promoting the presentation of alloantigens—particularly molecules of the major histocompatability complex (MHC)—to recipient T cells. (2) Activation and clonal expansion of alloreactive recipient T cells is a key event in allograft rejection, resulting in the production of populations of effector lymphocytes. (3) The resulting activated lymphocytes, together with other activated cells of the immune system such as macrophages and neutrophils, are able to migrate to the graft by following chemoattractant molecules that are also produced by the inflammatory response within the graft. (4) Many effector mechanisms contribute to graft destruction, including the delayed type hypersensitivity response, direct cytotoxicity and B cell alloantibody production.

Clinical features of allograft rejection

In clinical practice allograft rejection is frequently categorized depending on the timing in relation to the transplantation procedure, or the dominant arm of the immune system involved. (1) Hyperacute rejection—occurs if preformed complement-fixing antibodies against allogeneic MHC molecules or ABO antigens are present at the time of transplantation; modern crossmatch techniques have made this extremely rare, but in solid organ transplantation it is characterized by rapid widespread vascular thrombosis leading to infarction of the graft within minutes to hours. (2) Acute rejection—may be predominantly due to acute cellular rejection or acute antibody-mediated rejection; leads to a sudden deterioration in graft function over days to weeks; usually responds to treatment with intravenous corticosteroids, with or without increased baseline immunosuppression. (3) Chronic graft dysfunction ('chronic rejection')—may be partly due to chronic activation of the immune system; causes gradual deterioration in graft function occurring over weeks to months; there is no effective treatment.

Immunosuppressive therapy

Many different immunosuppressive regimens for solid organ transplantation are in clinical use. The agents employed include (1) glucocorticoids—act principally by binding to cytoplasmic glucocorticoid receptors, which then translocate to the nucleus and reduce the expression of many molecules important in the immune response; (2) antiproliferative agents—e.g. azathioprine, mycophenolate mofetil; interfere with DNA synthesis and prevent cell cycle progression, thus impairing the clonal expansion of alloreactive T cells; (3) calcineurin inhibitors—e.g. ciclosporin, tacrolimus; bind cytoplasmic immunophilins to form complexes that can inhibit the calcium-dependent phosphatase calcineurin, a rate-limiting enzyme in the T-cell receptor signal transduction pathway; (4) mammalian target of rapamycin (mTOR) inhibitors—e.g. sirolimus, everolimus; bind to the regulatory kinase mTOR, which has a critical role in cytokine receptor signal transduction; (5) depleting antibodies—e.g. anti-thymocyte globulin (ATG), alemtuzumab (a humanized monoclonal antibody directed against human CD52); cause profound lymphocyte depletion; (6) other biological agents—e.g. daclizumab, basiliximab, both of which are mouse–human chimeric monoclonal antibodies directed against CD25 (the high-affinity IL-2 receptor α-chain).

Clinical perspective and future prospects

Modern immunosuppressive therapy has improved 1-year graft survival to above 90%, but late graft loss and the adverse effects of chronic immunosuppression remain a significant problem. Challenges for the future include the development of better assays to monitor the immune response following transplantation and make it easier to individualize immunosuppressive therapy, improving the risk:benefit ratio, as well as facilitating trials of novel therapies that may lead to donor-specific hyporesponsiveness or even operational transplantation tolerance, which remains the holy grail of clinical transplantation and can be defined as the lack of a destructive immune response towards the graft without the requirement for indefinite nonspecific immunosuppressive therapy, while preserving immune responses to pathogens.

Introduction

The immune system has evolved to protect the individual from invasion by pathogenic microorganisms as well as mutation of the individual's own cells that may be premalignant. To achieve this, stringent discrimination of what has long been termed 'self' from 'nonself' or 'altered self' is crucial, both for avoiding autoimmunity and for limiting the immunological damage to self tissues that might occur during the response to a foreign pathogen. To complicate matters, the immune system is continually exposed to new antigens, and since many of these are harmless, or even beneficial (e.g. bacteria composing the intestinal flora), the immune response generated must be proportional to the threat that each new antigen poses.

The character of an immune response is determined partly by the particular antigens involved and partly by the context in which these antigens are encountered. In particular, priming of T cells with antigen from sites of inflammation is much more likely to produce an aggressive immune response aimed at clearing the antigen than priming with antigen in the absence of inflammatory signals.

Tissue transplanted between genetically disparate (allogeneic) individuals (see Table 5.5.1) contains many peptides (alloantigens) of donor origin that are recognized as foreign by the recipient immune system. Such foreign antigens are introduced in a highly inflammatory microenvironment and trigger a vigorous immune response that almost invariably results in destruction of the transplanted tissue unless active steps are taken to suppress the immune system.

Allograft rejection is a complex T-cell-dependent process, summarized in Fig. 5.5.1. Inflammation triggered by the retrieval of the donor organ or tissue and the transplant procedure itself generates so-called 'danger' signals that activate both the innate and adaptive immune systems. Triggering of the innate immune system creates an environment that promotes activation of the adaptive response that includes T cells and B cells. T-cell integration of signals delivered through recognition of alloantigen, costimulation, and inflammation leads to activation, clonal expansion, and differentiation of donor-reactive lymphocytes into effector cells. These events take place predominantly in the lymphoid tissue draining the transplant site and culminate in the migration of the mature effector lymphocytes generated to the graft, where they orchestrate the destruction of the transplant. The effector cells that have been shown to participate in rejection responses include cytotoxic T cells and activated helper T cells that act through delayed-type hypersensitivity mechanisms, as well as antibody-mediated destruction of the graft or so-called 'humoral immunity'. These elements of the adaptive immune system act in conjunction with activated components of the innate immune system, such as macrophages and natural killer (NK) cells, to destroy the allograft.

Table 5.5.1 Transplantation terminology

Autograft	Tissue transplanted from one part of an individual's body to another, e.g. skin grafts in patients with burns; vascular grafts for coronary or peripheral vascular disease
Isograft	Tissue transplanted between genetically identical (syngeneic) members of the same species, e.g. grafts between monozygotic twins; grafts between members of the same inbred strain of mouse or rat
Allograft	Tissue transplanted between genetically disparate (allogeneic) members of the same species, e.g. grafts between unrelated humans; grafts between different inbred strains of mice or rats
Xenograft	Tissue transplanted between individuals of different species, e.g. pig to human, rat to mouse

In clinical practice allograft rejection is frequently categorized depending on the timing in relation to the transplantation procedure or the dominant arm of the immune system involved (Table 5.5.2). For renal allografts, a classification system to define the severity of rejection observed in biopsy specimens has been developed, the Banff score, which has facilitated the decision-making process regarding the implementation of antirejection therapy.

This chapter will outline the cellular and molecular events involved in alloantigen recognition and subsequent allograft rejection, as well as the mechanism of action of the current pharmacological agents available in clinical practice to suppress graft rejection.

Role of the graft in initiating rejection

The physical process of removing and reimplanting tissue for transplantation initiates a sequence of changes in gene expression within the donor tissue that have a profound influence on the immunological response of the recipient. These changes are initiated in response to injury from the surgical procedures required to retrieve and reimplant the tissue, as well as injury from reactive oxygen species that are generated when the ischaemic tissue is reperfused. In the case of cadaveric donor transplantation, some of these changes are a direct consequence of brain death.

Cells of the innate immune system express invariant pattern-recognition receptors that enable them to recognize markers of tissue injury and to detect the presence of pathogens. The best characterized of these are the Toll-like receptors (TLRs), which bind to phylogenetically conserved molecular features unique to microorganisms, as well as endogenous molecules that are produced as a consequence of tissue injury, such as reactive oxygen species, activated complement components, and heat shock proteins.

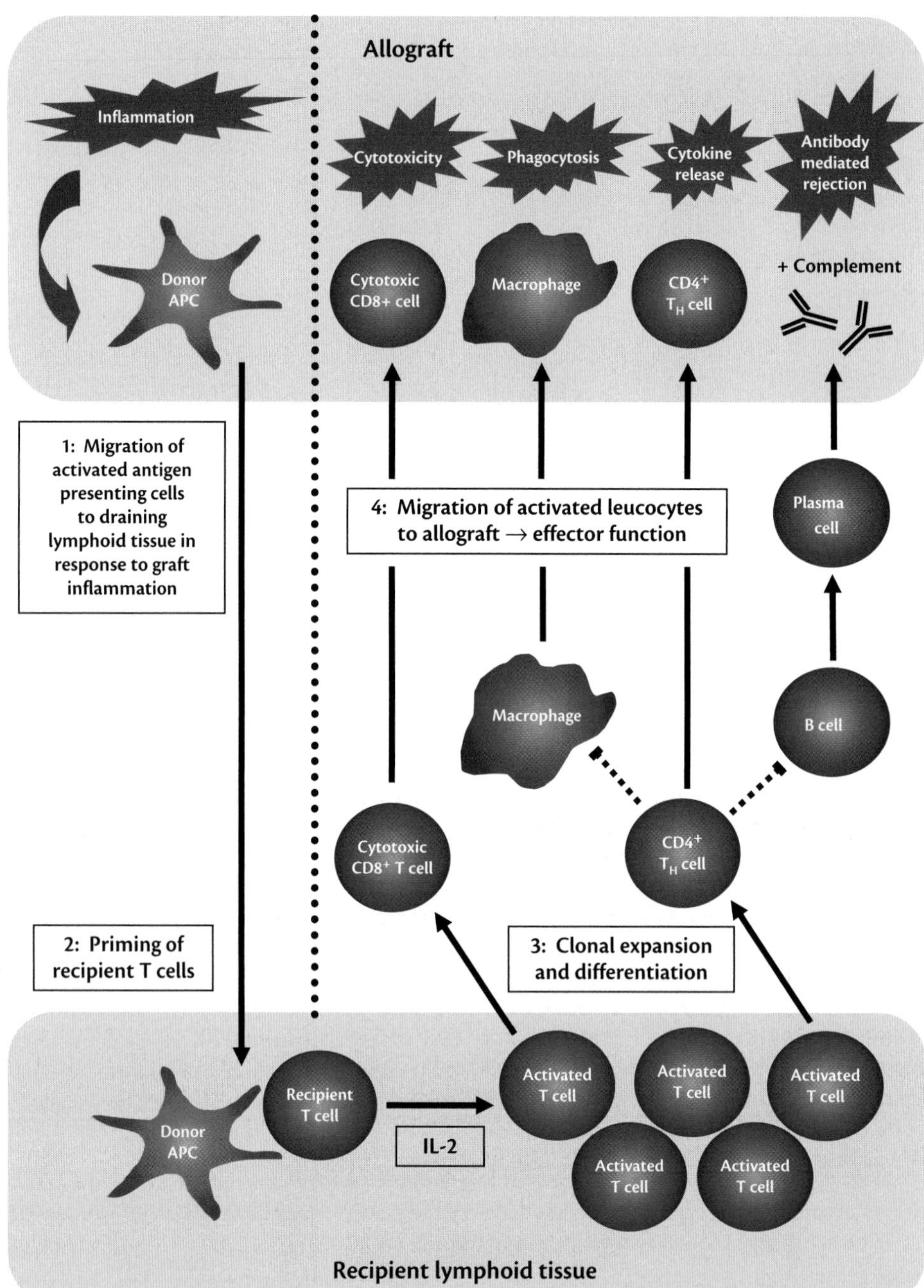

Fig. 5.5.1 Overview of allograft rejection. There are four phases in the immune response to an allogeneic transplant. Multiple cell types and effector mechanisms contribute to graft destruction, including cell mediated cytotoxicity (CD8+ T cells), delayed type hypersensitivity (CD4+ T cells), alloantibody production (B cells), and phagocytosis (macrophages and neutrophils).

Local tissue damage and ischaemia reperfusion injury that occur at the time of transplantation generates many potential TLR ligands, and result in the potent activation of innate immune system components that in turn contribute to activation of the adaptive alloimmune response (Fig. 5.5.2). The end result is the local production, i.e. within the transplanted tissue, of inflammatory mediators, chemokines (chemoattractant cytokines), and preformed P-selectin (CD62P), an adhesion molecule necessary for leucocyte transmigration into tissue. This identifies the transplanted tissue as a site of inflammation triggering the recruitment of inflammatory leucocytes into the graft, and stimulates the migration of donor-derived antigen-presenting cells contained within the transplant to recipient lymphoid tissue.

These events are a nonspecific response to tissue damage and happen irrespective of whether the transplantation procedure occurs between genetically identical or genetically disparate individuals. In transplantation procedures between genetically nonidentical individuals, the migration of donor-derived antigen-presenting cells to recipient lymphoid tissue allows priming of alloreactive recipient T cells and initiates an adaptive immune response against the allogeneic tissue. In this manner, implantation of the transplanted tissue initiates a series of events that contribute to its own destruction. In grafts between genetically identical individuals, an adaptive immune response is not generated as there are no allogeneic molecules, and the inflammatory processes subside with time, allowing repair of the graft and healing.

Table 5.5.2 Characterizing the immune response following transplantation

Hyperacute rejection	If preformed complement-fixing antibodies against allogeneic MHC molecules or ABO antigens are present at the time of transplantation, a particularly catastrophic form of rejection ensues. In solid organ transplantation this is characterized by rapid widespread vascular thrombosis leading to infarction of the graft within minutes to hours
Acute rejection	A sudden deterioration in graft function over days to weeks. This may be predominantly due to acute cellular rejection or acute antibody-mediated rejection. Most episodes of acute rejection respond to treatment with intravenous corticosteroids, with or without increased baseline immunosuppression
Chronic graft dysfunction	Gradual deterioration in graft function occurring over weeks to months. Histologically this is typically associated with fibrointimal proliferation in intragraft arteries and interstitial fibrosis. This term has replaced 'chronic rejection' since, although chronic graft dysfunction may be partly due to chronic activation of the immune system, other factors including toxicity from immunosuppressive medication contribute to the pathophysiology. Currently there are no therapies able to reverse chronic graft dysfunction

T-cell allorecognition and activation

Animals that lack T cells do not reject fully MHC-mismatched allografts or xenografts, but adoptive transfer of wild-type T cells to these animals is able to restore allograft rejection. In contrast, B cell deficient mice reject cardiac allografts at control rates. In clinical transplantation, therapies that deplete peripheral T cells are highly effective at reversing episodes of acute rejection. These observations highlight the non-redundant role of T cells in transplant rejection.

Several different approaches have been used to evaluate the relative contribution of $CD8^+$ and $CD4^+$ T cells to allograft rejection. The available data indicate that in general, $CD4^+$ cells are essential for allograft rejection. However, $CD8^+$ cells contribute to rejection, and in certain circumstances are capable of rejecting MHC class I mismatched allografts in the absence of $CD4^+$ cell help.

How T cells recognize alloantigens

There are many cell surface and intracellular molecules that are variant, or polymorphic, between different members of the same species, and recognition of this genetic variation by T cells is a crucial step in initiating transplant rejection. One of the reasons that transplantation induces such a dynamic immune response is the high precursor frequency of T cells able to respond to mismatched major histocompatibility complex (MHC) molecules, which can be as high as 1 in 10, orders of magnitude higher than the proportion of T cells that are able to react to a nominal peptide antigen–self MHC complex (1 in 20 000 to 1 in 100 000). However, although MHC molecules are the most important alloantigens, transplants between siblings with identical MHC molecules are still vulnerable to rejection, albeit at a slower tempo than MHC-mismatched transplants. Rejection in this setting is a result of T-cell recognition of other polymorphic non-MHC molecules called minor histocompatibility antigens (miH) that are derived from a wide variety of proteins and are not necessarily expressed by cells of the immune system. The genes encoding miH antigens are scattered throughout the genome.

Two pathways of allorecognition

Transplantation is a unique immunological situation in which priming of recipient T cells with antigen can occur via two distinct pathways. Direct allorecognition is the interaction of recipient T cells with intact allogeneic MHC–peptide complexes on the surface of donor-derived cells. Indirect allorecognition occurs when peptides derived from donor MHC or miH antigen are degraded and presented by recipient antigen-presenting cells (Fig. 5.5.3).

Direct allorecognition

Transplanted tissue contains bone marrow-derived haematopoietic cells of donor origin that have the characteristics of immature dendritic cells. In response to the inflammatory milieu that follows transplantation, the donor-derived passenger leucocytes rapidly leave the graft and migrate to the secondary lymphoid tissues of the recipient. During migration the passenger leucocytes acquire the phenotype and functional characteristics of mature dendritic cells, expressing high levels of MHC class I and II molecules as well as other cell surface costimulatory molecules necessary to fully activate naive CD4+ and CD8+ T cells. Once in the secondary lymphoid tissues they act as professional antigen-presenting cells, presenting any mismatched MHC molecules in the transplanted tissue to recipient T cells.

Antigen presentation via the direct pathway plays a dominant role in initiating the response to a transplant, and T cells that recognize alloantigen via the direct pathway constitute 90% of the total alloreactive T-cell repertoire. However, since there are a finite number of passenger leucocytes transferred within a transplanted organ, the role of the direct pathway in allograft rejection diminishes with time, as eventually only 'nonprofessional' antigen-presenting cells such as endothelial cells remain to stimulate direct-pathway T cells.

Indirect allorecognition

At the same time that donor-derived passenger leucocytes are leaving the graft, recipient leucocytes including antigen-presenting cells are attracted to the graft by the inflammatory mediators and chemokines released in the vicinity of the transplanted tissue. As these cells traffic through the graft, they phagocytose donor-derived debris arising from tissue damage at the time of transplantation before migrating to the draining lymphoid tissue. The ingested antigens are processed and presented on recipient MHC molecules to T cells in the recipient lymphoid tissue. In addition, soluble antigens released from the graft will also be transported in the blood to the draining lymphoid tissue, where they will be taken up and presented by resident antigen-presenting cells. In keeping with the direct pathway, the dominant antigenic peptides presented by the indirect pathway are the hypervariable peptide-binding regions of MHC molecules, but unlike direct pathway allorecognition, the indirect pathway is available for antigen presentation for as long as the graft remains *in situ* and therefore becomes the dominant mode of allorecognition in the long term.

Costimulation

Antigen-specific signals delivered via the TCR–CD3 complex (often described as 'signal 1') in isolation are insufficient to fully activate naive T cells (Fig. 5.5.4). The second essential signal ('signal 2') is provided by the interaction of pairs of cell-surface molecules present on T cells and antigen-presenting cells, called costimulatory molecules. Absence or blockade of costimulatory signals typically results

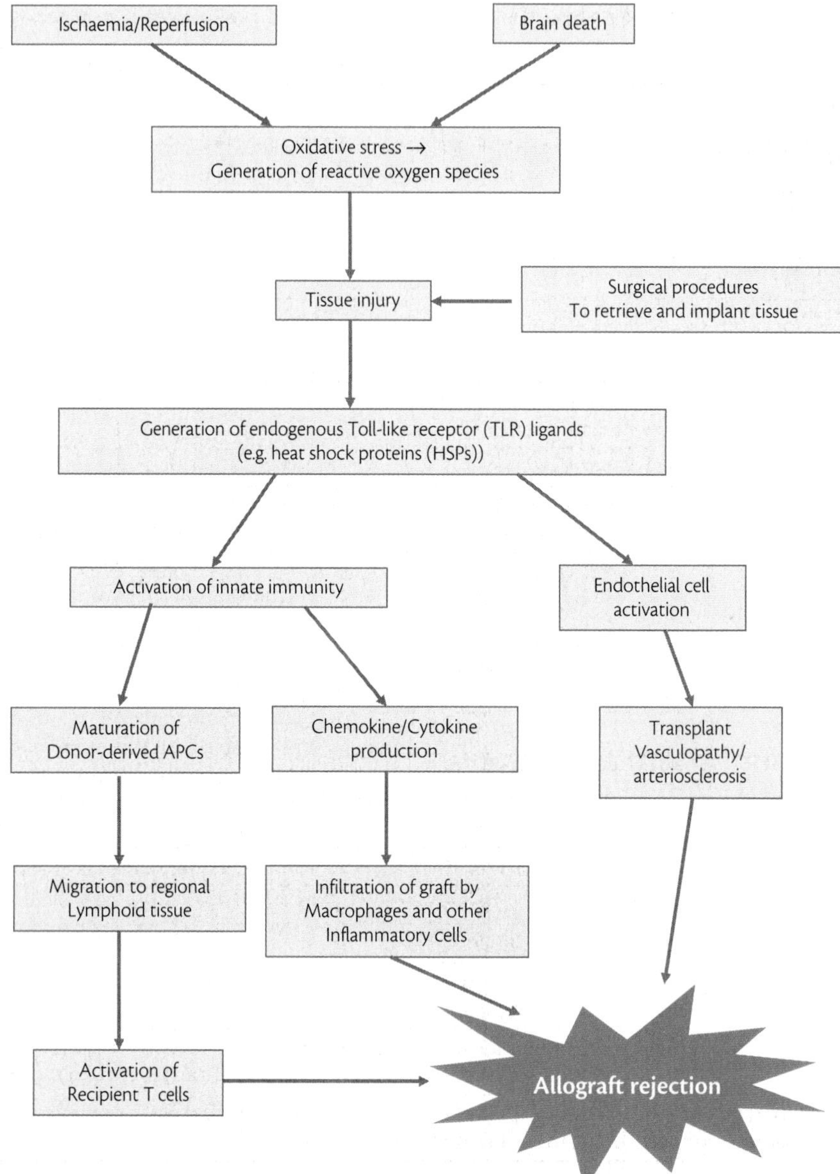

Fig. 5.5.2 The role of the graft in initiating rejection. The physiological stresses induced by the process of retrieving, storing, and reimplanting transplanted organs lead to graft damage and the generation of inflammatory compounds capable of activating cells of the innate immune system. This has a profound influence on the immunological response of the recipient. APC, antigen-presenting cell.

in T-cell unresponsiveness or 'anergy'. Many of these molecules are homologous and in general they can be divided into two families: the B7 family which is best characterized by the T-cell costimulatory molecules CD28 and CD152 (CTLA-4); and the tumour necrosis factor (TNF)/tumour necrosis factor receptor (TNFR) family of which the prototype receptor–ligand pair are CD40 and CD154 (CD40L) (Table 5.5.3).

T-cell costimnulatory molecules

CD28 is constitutively expressed by T cells and binds to the B7 family molecules CD80 and CD86 on antigen-presenting cells. Signalling via CD28 lowers the threshold for T-cell activation, increases the half life of mRNA for interleukin 2 (IL-2) and therefore expression of IL-2, and promotes T-cell proliferation and resistance to apoptosis.

During an immune response, activated T cells upregulate expression of CD152 (CTLA-4), a molecule that has close homology to CD28. CD152 also binds to CD80 and CD86, but it has an inhibitory effect on T-cell activation, and—because its binding affinity for CD80 and CD86 is 10–20 times greater than that of CD28—it is able to attenuate immune responses by competing with CD28 for ligation of these molecules. The importance of CD152 as a negative regulator of immune responses was demonstrated by the generation of CD152 knockout mice, which, when housed under normal conditions where they will be exposed to a wide range of environmental antigens, develop a fatal disorder characterized by massive proliferation of lymphocytes.

Another effect of CD28 signalling during T-cell activation is to up-regulate expression of other costimulatory molecules such as CD154 (CD40L). CD154 is the ligand for CD40 expressed by antigen-presenting cells, and as well as delivering a positive signal to the T cell, CD40–CD154 ligation activates antigen-presenting cells leading to increased expression of B7 family molecules and therefore a greater ability to activate further T cells.

As increasing numbers of novel costimulatory molecules are identified, it is becoming clear that the outcome of interaction

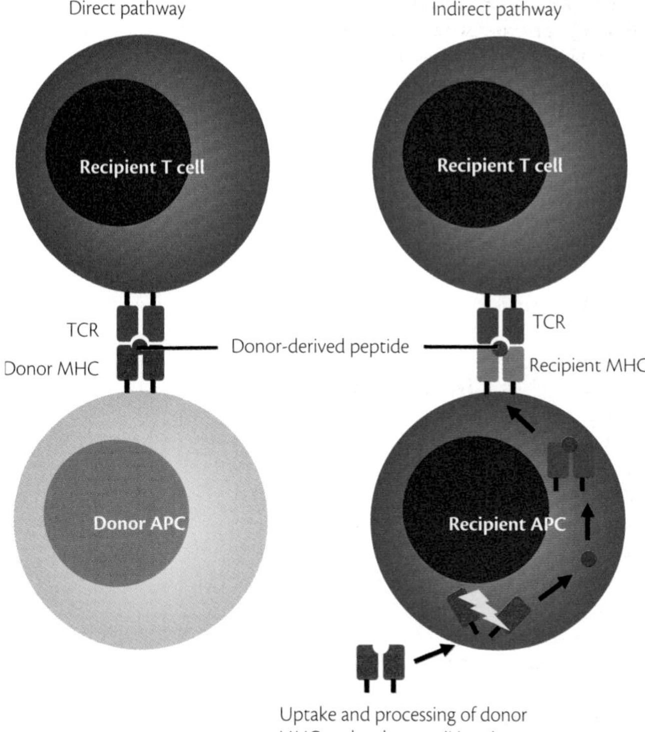

Fig. 5.5.3 Direct and indirect pathways of allorecognition. The dominant antigens that initiate an adaptive immune response following transplant procedures between nonidentical individuals are the highly polymorphic MHC molecules. There are two pathways through which the immune system is able to 'see' these antigens: (1) direct pathway—intact donor MHC–peptide complexes are presented to recipient T cells by donor-derived antigen-presenting cells; (2) indirect pathway—donor MHC and miH antigens are processed by recipient antigen-presenting cells and presented as peptides by recipient MHC molecules. TCR, T-cell receptor.

between T cells and antigen-presenting cells is determined both by the avidity of the cognate TCR–MHC–peptide interaction and the balance of positive and negative signals delivered by the costimulatory molecules present on the surface of the participating cells (see Table 5.5.3).

Transduction of costimulatory signals occurs in parallel to TCR–CD3 complex signalling and can be blocked independently, and the development of pharmaceutical agents able to interrupt costimulation has provided evidence of the importance of these pathways in transplant rejection. Administration of a fusion protein constructed from the extracellular domains of CD152 (CTLA-4Ig or CTLA-4Fc; see 'Immunosuppression in transplantation' below) or monoclonal antibodies directed against CD80 and CD86 are able to block costimulation via CD28, and this is sufficient to prevent allograft rejection. Monoclonal antibodies directed against CD154 are also able to prevent acute allograft rejection. In addition, both of these examples of costimulation blockade lead to long-term rejection-free survival of vascularized and nonvascularized allografts in experimental rodent models.

TCR signal transduction and 'signal 3'

Cell membranes are heterogeneous structures, and within the biphospholipid layer it is possible to identify cholesterol-rich regions that have been termed 'lipid rafts'. Some membrane-bound molecules are preferentially associated with lipid rafts, in particular those with lipophilic attachments to the cell membrane. In resting T cells the TCRs are usually not associated with lipid rafts, and as a result they are unable to interact with signal transduction molecules as these are usually found within lipid rafts. During the formation of an immunological synapse, clustering of signalling and adhesion molecules occurs as a result of multiple TCRs binding to the MHC–peptide complex on the surface of the antigen-presenting cell. The cell membrane reorganization that this produces allows TCR–CD3 complexes to integrate into lipid rafts, facilitating downstream signalling by placing them in close proximity to signal transduction molecules.

The intracellular signalling pathway downstream of the TCR is complex (Fig. 5.5.5). Briefly, TCR–MHC–peptide engagement results in the recruitment and phosphorylation of several signalling molecules. These phosphorylation events initiate a number of intracellular biochemical processes, resulting in activation of the Ras- and Rac- mitogen-activated protein (MAP) kinase pathways and hydrolysis of membrane phosphatidylinositol 4,5-biphosphate to generate the secondary messengers inositol triphosphate (IP_3) and diacylglycerol (DAG). IP_3 leads to the release of stored calcium from the endoplasmic reticulum and activation of the phosphatase calcineurin, which in turn dephosphorylates the transcription factor NFAT (nuclear factor of activated T cells), allowing it to translocate to the nucleus. Generation of DAG results in the activation of another transcription factor, NF-κB, and a third transcription factor, AP-1, is generated by the MAP kinase cascades. The action of these transcription factors alters expression of many genes, in particular leading to up-regulation of the T-cell growth factor IL-2 and the high-affinity IL-2 receptor α-chain (CD25).

Soon after activation the generation of large amounts of IL-2 and other pro-proliferative cytokines act in an autocrine and paracrine fashion to provide what has been described as 'signal 3' (see Fig. 5.5.4). Transduction of signals delivered by IL-2 promotes cell cycle progression and initiates the clonal expansion and differentiation of activated T cells.

Effector mechanisms

Although the initiation of allograft rejection is critically dependent on T-cell recognition of alloantigen, many components of the immune system subsequently contribute to the destruction of the transplanted tissue. Following activation, T cells play a key role in the recruitment of other cells of the immune response and also control their differentiation into effector cells. Additional factors modify the character of the immune response to an allograft, including the site of transplantation, the organ or tissue transplanted, the antigen-presenting cells involved in T-cell priming, and the immune status of the recipient at the time of transplantation.

Innate immune system in transplant rejection

The innate immune system comprises a group of cells and molecules (Table 5.5.4) that provide a first line of defence against pathogens, and which also play an important role in allograft rejection. Primary adaptive immune system responses that rely on the activation and expansion of antigen-specific lymphocytes take several days to reach maturity. In contrast, the innate immune system represents a 'pre-formed' defence that is immediately available to defend the host until either the dangerous stimulus is cleared or

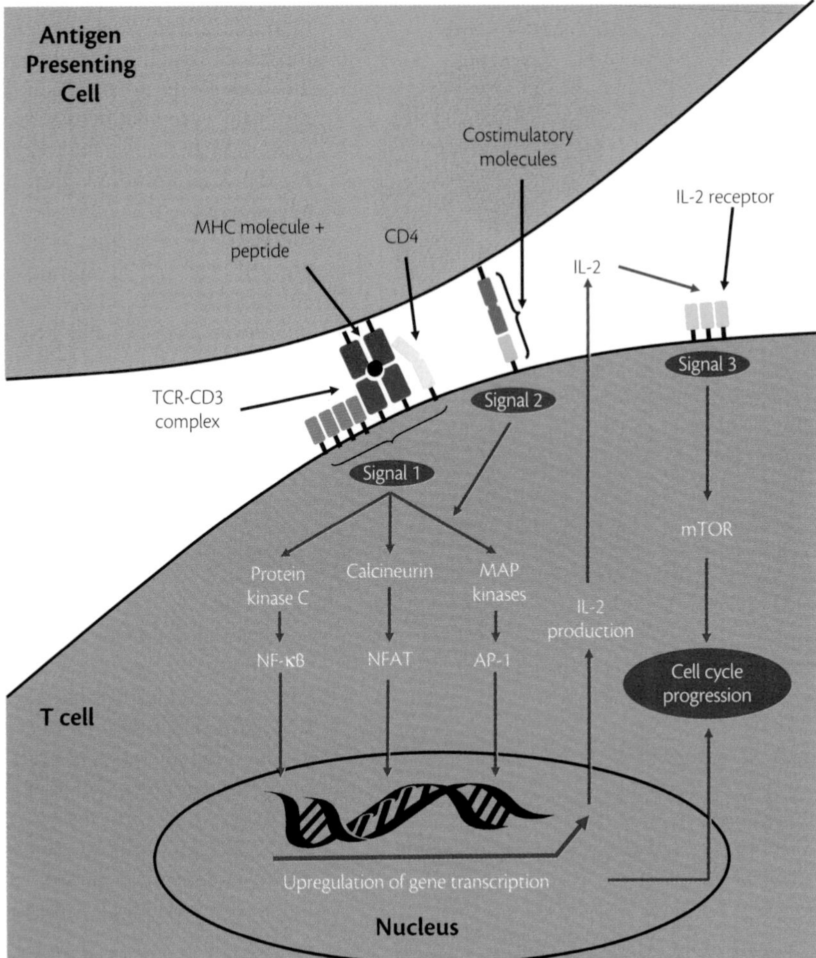

Fig. 5.5.4 Three-signal model of T-cell activation. The initiation of most adaptive immune responses is dependent on the activation and clonal expansion of T cells. Three types of signal are necessary for T-cell activation and proliferation: (1) Antigen specific signals delivered by the interaction between MHC–peptide complexes and the TCR–CD3 complex; (2) antigen-non-specific costimulatory signals; and (3) signals delivered by cytokines produced either by the T cell itself or by other inflammatory cells in the same microenvironment, in particular IL-2.

the adaptive immune system is able to mount an antigen-specific response.

As described above, the physical process of graft retrieval and implantation generates 'danger signals' in the form of heat shock proteins, complement breakdown products, and reactive oxygen species that activate cells of the innate immune system via TLR ligation. Macrophages and other phagocytic cells ingest necrotic tissue and when activated release cytokines such as tumour necrosis factor α (TNFα), interleukin 1 (IL-1), and interleukin 6 (IL-6) that contribute to the local inflammatory environment.

Activated complement components constitute a proteolytic cascade that generates a range of effector molecules. The anaphylatoxins C5a and C3a are chemoattractant molecules that assist leucocytes to home to the graft, while other soluble mediators are able to opsonize cells, targeting them for destruction by phagocytes. Recognition of C3b, C4b, or their fragments covalently bound to target cells by complement receptors on the surface of leucocytes facilitates antigen presentation and T-cell activation. Generation of the terminal components of the complement cascade (C5b-9) results in formation of the membrane attack complex within the target cell membrane and initiation of target cell lysis. This has been demonstrated to play an important role in ischaemia reperfusion injury.

NK cells are large granular lymphocytes that are able to kill virus-infected or mutated host cells in an identical manner to cytotoxic CD8+ lymphocytes. However unlike CD8+ cells they do not possess antigen-specific TCRs or require activation and expansion prior to effector function. Instead, NK cells express invariant cell-surface receptors including activating receptors that bind to widely expressed carbohydrate residues on self cells and inhibitory receptors that bind self MHC class I molecules. Some malignant or virally infected cells down-regulate MHC class I expression or express altered class I molecules as a strategy to evade CD8+ T-cell cytotoxicity. As a result they are unable to stimulate inhibitory receptors and are vulnerable to NK cell killing. Polymorphism of NK cell receptor targets should theoretically generate alloreactive NK cells that could contribute to tissue damage following transplantation. NK cells have been shown to be capable of rejecting bone marrow cells that express very low levels of MHC class I molecules, and NK cells with the ability to kill target cells *ex vivo* can be found in rejecting allografts, although to date there has been little evidence that they play an important role in solid organ allograft rejection.

Increasing evidence demonstrates the important role that components of the innate immune system play in activating the adaptive immune system. In particular, ligation of TLRs on dendritic cells induces maturation, as defined as up-regulation of costimulatory molecules and MHC class II, enhancing their ability to act as a bridge between the innate and adaptive immune systems.

Leucocyte recruitment

Traffic of naive lymphocytes is usually restricted to recirculation between the blood and lymphatic systems. However, once they have been primed in the secondary lymphoid tissues, activated

Table 5.5.3 T-cell costimulation molecules and their ligands

Expression	T cell	Antigen-presenting cell	Effect on T-cell activation
Constitutive	CD28	CD80 (B7–1) CD86 (B7–2)	Positive
	CD27	CD70	
Inducible	CD154 (CD40-L)	CD40	
	ICOS (inducible costimulator)	ICOS-L (ICOS ligand)	
	OX40 (CD134)	OX40-L (CD252)	
	4–1BB (CD137)	4–1BB-L (CD137L)	
	CD152 (CTLA-4—cytotoxic T lymphocyte antigen-4,)	CD80 (B7–1) CD86 (B7–2)	Negative
	CD279 (programmed death-1, PD-1)	CD274 (programmed death ligand 1, PD-L1, B7-H1) CD273 (programmed death ligand 2, PD-L2, B7-DC)	

lymphocytes as well as other activated leucocytes must be able to migrate into the graft in order to destroy the transplanted tissue, a process known as leucocyte recruitment.

The inflammatory processes at the site of transplantation generate chemotactic cytokines called chemokines, and up-regulation of chemokine receptor expression by activated leucocytes enables them to migrate along the chemoattractant gradient to reach the graft. Inflammatory signals also affect blood vessels in the vicinity of the transplant, causing vasodilation and endothelial activation. Activated endothelial cells rapidly externalize preformed granules called Weibel–Palade bodies that contain the adhesion molecule P-selectin. At the same time chemokines released from the graft become tethered to the endothelium, and these alterations in endothelial surface markers advertise to passing leucocytes that an inflammatory process is occurring in the neighbouring tissue.

Leucocytes are usually conveyed within the fast laminar flow at the centre of blood vessels, but once activated leucocytes reach postcapillary venules in proximity to the graft they are able to leave this rapid flow and move towards the edge of the vessel. This occurs in response to the local chemokine gradient and is assisted by the slower blood flow in the vasodilated blood vessels near the graft. Leucocyte extravasation is a multistep process (Fig. 5.5.6). Initially, low affinity interactions develop between endothelial P-selectin and sialyl-Lewis^X moieties that are present on the surface of activated leucocytes. These interactions continually form and break down, and the leucocyte 'rolls' along the endothelial surface. If chemokines are present on the endothelial surface, conformational changes in leucocyte integrin molecules occur that allow them to bind other endothelial adhesion molecules such as ICAM-1. These higher affinity interactions cause arrest of the leucocyte on the endothelial surface, allowing it to commence extravasation. Having entered the tissues, the activated leucocytes continue to migrate along chemokine gradients to invade the graft.

T cells

Cytotoxic T-cell response

Naive CD8+ cytotoxic T cells (CTLs) are activated either as a result of the formation of a three-cell cluster with the helper cell and the antigen-presenting cell, or as a result of an activated CD4+ T helper cell 'licensing' the antigen-presenting cell to activate CTLs. CD40/CD154 costimulatory signals play an important role in CTL activation.

Activated CTLs migrate to the graft site where they are able to identify their target cells by recognition of allogeneic class I MHC molecules. Once they have located their target cell they release granules containing cytotoxic molecules such as perforin and granzyme B, as well as up-regulating cell surface expression of Fas ligand (FasL) and secreting soluble mediators such as TNF. Target cell killing by CTLs is achieved by the induction of apoptosis. Perforins polymerize and insert into the target cell membrane, forming a pore that facilitates the entry of granzyme B and other compounds into the cell. Granzyme B is a protease that is able to initiate apoptosis by several mechanisms, including activation of caspase cascades. Binding of FasL to Fas on the target cell surface is also able to trigger apoptosis by activating caspases.

Delayed-type hypersensitivity

Alloantigen-specific CD4+ T cells (typically T helper 1 cells) contribute to the effector phase of allograft rejection via a nonspecific effector mechanism referred to as the delayed-type hypersensitivity (DTH) response. DTH reactions are characterized by the release of multiple soluble mediators including the proinflammatory cytokines IL-1, interferon-γ, and TNFα. Damage to the graft occurs as a result of the ensuing infiltration of activated leucocytes, including monocytes, macrophages and eosinophils, and the production of nonspecific mediators such as nitric oxide, reactive oxygen species, and inflammatory arachidonic acid derivatives (prostaglandin E_2, thromboxane, and leukotrienes). This activity is triggered in an antigen specific manner by the T helper cell, but the effector mechanisms that lead to the destruction of the graft are nonspecific. DTH reactions have been shown to directly affect graft physiology by altering cell permeability and vascular smooth muscle tone and play a role in both acute and chronic allograft rejection.

Activated CD4+ T cells also express cytokines and costimulatory molecules that allow them to provide help for B-cell proliferation, differentiation, antibody class switching, and affinity maturation.

Humoral immune response

The B-cell response to alloantigen following transplantation results in the generation of alloantigen-specific antibodies (alloantibodies) that play an important role in allograft rejection. B cells utilize surface immunoglobulin as an antigen receptor and are able to internalize antigens that are degraded and presented in conjunction with class II MHC molecules. For activation and differentiation into antibody-secreting plasma cells, B cells usually require both antigen-specific signals and costimulatory signals from activated CD4+ T helper cells.

As in the T-cell response to alloantigen, the predominant antigenic targets of alloantibodies are mismatched MHC molecules, but antibodies that recognize miH or blood group antigens also contribute to rejection.

The mechanism of antibody-mediated rejection is primarily via complement fixation and membrane attack complex formation

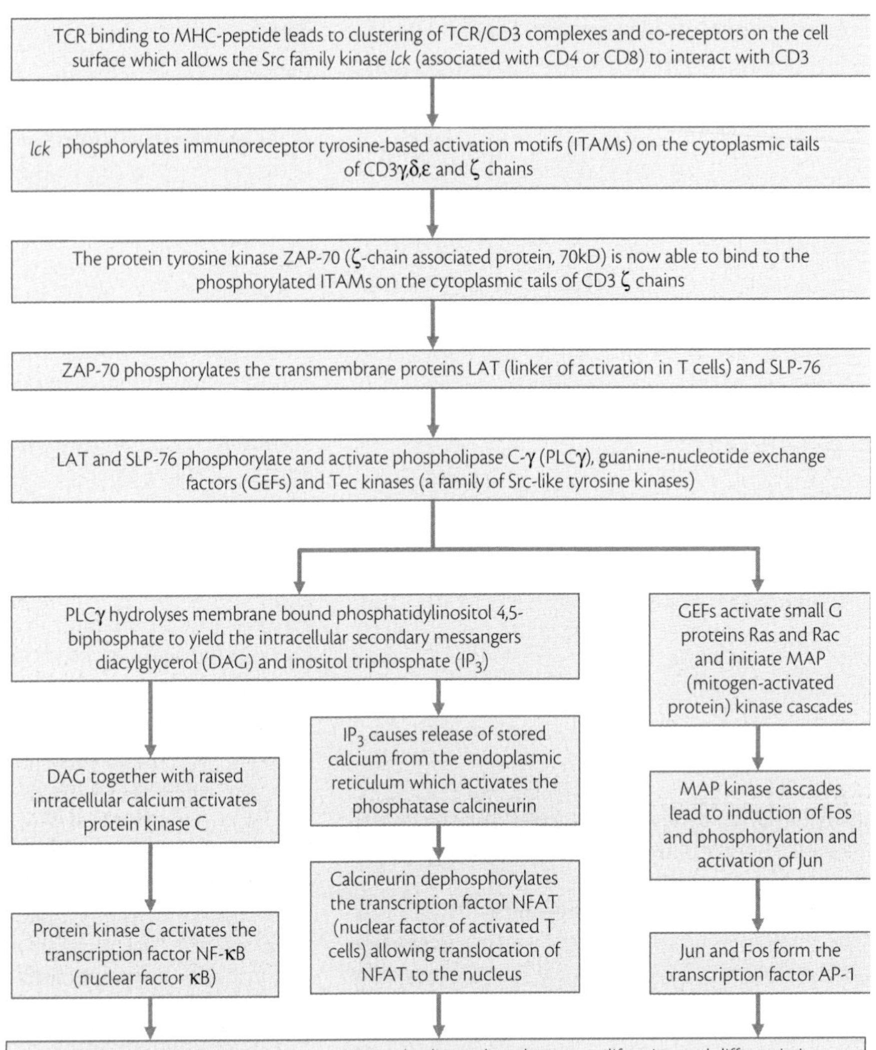

Fig. 5.5.5 T-cell receptor intracellular signalling pathway. The important intracellular molecular events that allow transduction of TCR-mediated signals into the T cell, ultimately leading to altered gene expression and T-cell activation.

leading to target cell lysis. NK cells and macrophages express receptors that bind to the non-antigen-specific (Fc) portion of antibodies, stimulating them to kill target cells that have antibody bound on the surface (a process called antibody-dependent cell-mediated cytotoxicity or ADCC), and this provides a second mechanism by which alloantibodies can induce donor cell death.

The humoral response to transplantation is demonstrated most dramatically if patients have preformed alloantibodies at the time of transplantation, where hyperacute rejection frequently results in graft destruction within minutes of organ reperfusion. In this situation the antibodies (which are usually directed at allogeneic MHC molecules or ABO blood group antigens expressed on graft endothelium) cause local activation of the coagulation and complement cascades, resulting in extensive thrombosis within the vascular supply to the graft culminating in infarction. Although modern cross-matching techniques have made hyperacute rejection extremely rare, the humoral arm of the immune system is increasingly being implicated in the pathogenesis of acute rejection episodes as well as chronic allograft damage.

Table 5.5.4 Components of the innate immune system

Cell	Primary function
Macrophage/ neutrophil	Phagocytosis; secretion of cytokines, enzymes and inflammatory mediators
Dendritic cell	Antigen uptake and presentation to lymphocytes
Natural killer (NK) cell	Cytotoxic to virally infected or mutated cells
Complement	Opsonisation, target cell lysis and chemoattraction
Eosinophil	Killing of antibody-coated parasites

Patients who have detectable anti-HLA antibodies at the time of transplantation have significantly poorer graft survival than those that are not sensitized, and the development of anti-HLA antibodies in previously unsensitized patients following transplantation is also highly predictive of early graft failure. The introduction of histological staining for complement 4d (C4d) in renal allograft biopsies allows indirect identification of antibody deposition and complement fixation, and peritubular C4d staining is strongly associated with early as well as late graft failure.

Immunological memory in transplantation

Following primary antigen exposure, long-lived antigen-specific memory T and B cells are generated that are able to deliver a

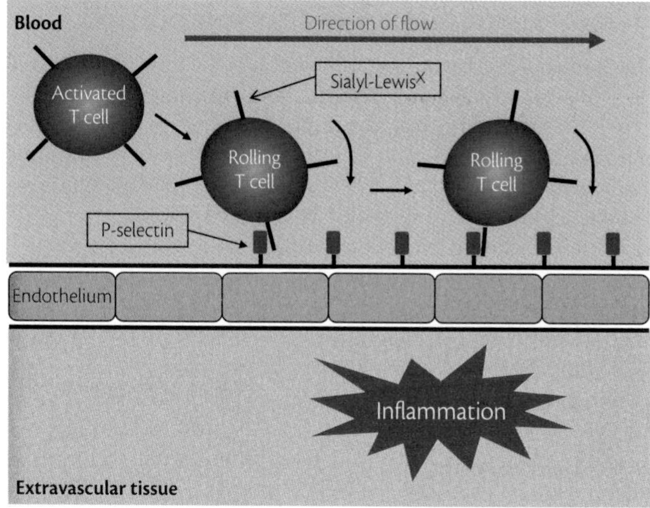

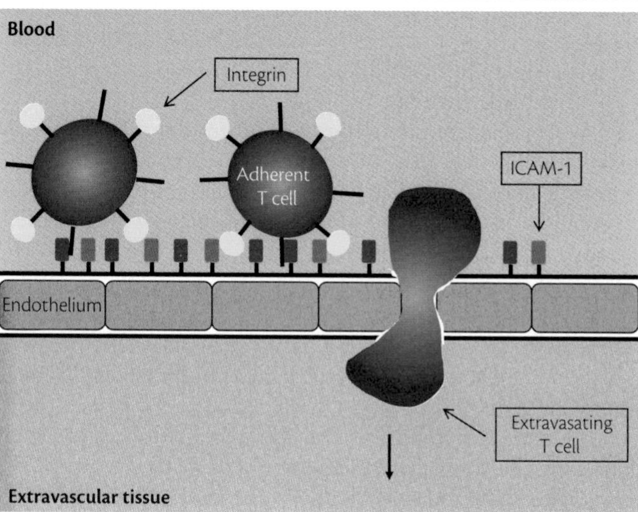

Fig. 5.5.6 Leucocyte extravasation. Activated effector lymphocytes are able to migrate to the graft along chemoattractant gradients generated by inflammation at the graft site. These inflammatory processes also affect the vascular bed within the graft, causing local vasodilation and endothelial activation. Leucocyte extravasation occurs in three steps. (1) Expression of sialyl-Lewis^X on activated leucocytes allows them to bind to P-selectin, an adhesion molecule that is released by endothelial cells following activation. The leucocytes are then able to 'roll' along the endothelium, constantly forming and breaking down bonds between sialyl-Lewis^X and P-selectin. (2) If chemokines and other inflammatory molecules are also present on the endothelium, conformational changes in other adhesion molecules (such as integrin and ICAM-1) allow higher-affinity binding and arrest of activated leucocytes on the endothelium. (3) Finally, the static leucocytes are able to migrate through the vessel wall and enter the graft tissue.

immune response that is more rapid and of higher magnitude if the same antigen is encountered on a subsequent occasion. Memory lymphocytes have a reduced activation threshold and are less dependent on costimulation. As a result they are able to up-regulate effector function and cytokine secretion more rapidly than naive lymphocytes. With increasing age the proportion of memory T cells within an individual's peripheral T-cell pool increases, reflecting cumulative antigen exposure, and can be as high as 50% in adult humans. While the generation of immunological memory is beneficial for protection against infectious pathogens, in transplantation the presence of allospecific memory produces an accelerated or 'second-set' rejection response. In clinical transplantation evidence of prior sensitization to donor antigens is associated with increased risk of acute rejection episodes and premature graft failure.

Memory-type responses towards alloantigens are frequently a result of exposure to alloantigens at the time of a previous blood transfusion, pregnancy, or transplantation. However, it is now recognized that memory-type responses may also be generated as a consequence of antigen receptor cross-reactivity (heterologous immunity) or by homeostatic proliferation of lymphocytes following an episode of lymphopenia.

Sensitization

Patients on transplant waiting lists are monitored for the development of anti-HLA antibodies as a marker of sensitization to potential donor antigens. The risk of sensitization from a single blood transfusion alone is highly variable, although overall sensitization rates are low. It was hoped that the introduction of routinely leucocyte-depleted blood products would reduce sensitization, although a randomized trial in patients undergoing cardiac surgery found no difference in rates of allosensitization after a single leucodepleted or whole blood transfusion. The prevalence of sensitization is much higher in multiparous women and patients with renal failure who have received a previous HLA-mismatched transplant.

Immediately before a transplantation procedure a final check is made to exclude the presence of complement-fixing and binding antibodies directed against donor HLA. The recipient's serum is incubated with donor splenocytes in the presence of exogenous complement and observed for donor cell lysis (the complement-dependent cytotoxicity assay or CDC). A positive CDC cross-match indicates the presence of complement-fixing IgG or IgM alloantibodies, and is an absolute contraindication to transplantation because it is associated with a greater than 90% risk of hyperacute rejection and graft loss. Increasingly, flow cytometry utilizing either donor cells or beads coated with recombinant HLA molecules is used to define the presence of anti-HLA antibodies prior to transplantation. These techniques are more sensitive than the CDC cross-match, and can also identify non-complement-fixing antibodies.

Patients who have become highly sensitized to HLA antigens have a reduced chance of transplantation and may remain on the transplant waiting list for extended periods, but patients with anti-HLA antibodies can be successfully transplanted following a program of 'desensitization'. Typically this involves a strategy of reducing alloantibody production by the administration of B-cell depleting agents (such as rituximab) in combination with other immunosuppressive agents (see 'Immunosuppression in transplantation', below), as well as removing existing alloantibodies by plasma exchange or immunoadsorption. Similar strategies have also been employed to allow transplantation between ABO-incompatible donor–recipient pairs (Table 5.5.5). However, in both situations the requirement for more powerful immunosuppression together with the higher rate of acute rejection observed compared to non-sensitized controls mean these therapies are currently appropriate only for selected patients.

Heterologous immunity

Experiments in mice demonstrated that viral infections could modulate the immune response to subsequent infection with a different virus. It is hypothesized that this phenomenon is due either

Table 5.5.5 ABO compatibility for transplantation

Blood group	Can receive transplant from:	Can donate transplant to:
O	O	O, A, B, AB
A	O, A	A, AB
B	O, B	B, AB
AB	O, A, B, AB	AB

to epitope sharing between different viruses or to TCR cross-reactivity within the population of memory T cells generated by the original virus. Other investigators found that sequential viral infections in mice also generated populations of alloreactive memory-phenotype T cells, and the presence of these cells prevented transplant tolerance induction by protocols that usually result in reliable long-term graft acceptance. It is therefore possible that memory lymphocytes generated by antecedent viral infections in humans may be able to cross-react with epitopes presented following transplantation, resulting in memory-phenotype responses towards the graft without prior sensitization to donor alloantigen.

Homeostatic proliferation

The size of the peripheral T-cell pool, as well as the relative ratios of CD4+ to CD8+ and naive to memory cells, are tightly regulated by homeostatic mechanisms. A consequence of this is that reduction of the overall T-cell population, either during illness or following medical intervention, strongly induces the residual T cells to proliferate, whether or not cognate antigen is present. A proportion of T cells undergoing homeostatic proliferation in response to lymphopenia differentiate into a phenotype that resembles that of antigen-experienced or memory T cells. These phenotypic changes typically include down-regulation of CD62L (L-selectin), an adhesion molecule that is highly expressed on naive T cells and is necessary for entry into lymph nodes via high endothelial venules, and up-regulation of CD44, an adhesion molecule that binds to hyaluronic acid and enables activated or memory-phenotype T cells to leave the vascular system and enter peripheral tissues. Other early markers of T-cell activation, including CD25 and CD69, do not appear to be up-regulated following homeostatic proliferation.

T cells that have undergone homeostatic proliferation not only have a phenotype that resembles memory T cells but also exhibit memory T-cell-like behaviour. They are less dependent on costimulation via CD28 and as a result have a reduced activation threshold. Moreover, following activation their capacity to secrete cytokines, proliferate, and manifest effector functions is enhanced compared to that of naive T cells. Homeostatic proliferation therefore presents a particular concern in transplantation for two reasons. Firstly, many patients receive monoclonal or polyclonal antibody therapy designed to deplete leucocytes and/or T cells either as part of induction immunosuppression or as therapy for an acute rejection episode. Since as many as 10% of naive T cells are able to respond to alloantigen, it is likely that homeostatic expansion in this setting could generate alloreactive memory-phenotype T cells. Secondly, T cells that have undergone homeostatic proliferation have also been shown to be resistant to tolerance induction in animal models.

Immunosuppression in transplantation

The dramatic improvements in allograft survival that have occurred since the first successful transplants were performed in the 1950s have been achieved by the development of potent immunosuppressant medications able to inhibit the aggressive immune response to the transplant. These agents work by depleting lymphocytes, interfering with lymphocyte signal transduction pathways, and/or altering lymphocyte trafficking.

The risk of acute graft rejection is greatest during the initial 3 months after transplantation, and therefore transplant recipients initially receive strong induction immunosuppression, often consisting of triple therapy with glucocorticoids, a calcineurin inhibitor, and an antiproliferative agent. Provided there are no episodes of acute rejection, the doses of these agents are gradually reduced and then maintenance immunosuppression is continued indefinitely.

Chronic immunosuppression is associated with several undesirable sequelae, in particular an increased relative risk of infections and malignancy. Recognized side effects of particular immunosuppressive agents are listed in Table 5.5.6.

Many different immunosuppressive regimens for solid organ transplantation are in clinical use, and a detailed discussion of these is beyond the scope of this chapter. What follows is an introduction to the immunosuppressive agents in widespread use currently (Fig. 5.5.7).

Glucocorticoids

Corticosteroids were developed in the 1950s and have complex immunosuppressive as well as anti-inflammatory effects. They act principally by binding to cytoplasmic glucocorticoid receptors, although at higher doses they can exhibit receptor-independent effects as well. The steroid–receptor complex translocates to the nucleus where it is able to alter the expression of multiple cytokines through DNA-binding and by targeting transcription factors such

Table 5.5.6 Principal side effects of immunosuppressive agents

Corticosteroids	Glucose intolerance, cosmetic changes, weight gain, hyperlipidaemia, osteoporosis
Ciclosporin	Nephrotoxicity, hypertension, glucose intolerance, gingival hyperplasia, hyperlipidaemia, hirsutism
Tacrolimus	Nephrotoxicity, hypertension, glucose intolerance, alopecia
Azathioprine	Bone marrow suppression, macrocytosis, hepatotoxicity
Mycophenolate	Diarrhoea, bone marrow suppression
Sirolimus	Hyperlipidaemia, thrombocytopenia, mouth ulcers, interstitial lung disease
Anti-CD25 (IL-2 receptor α-chain) antibodies	Occasional hypersensitivity reactions
ATG	Cytokine release syndrome (fever, influenza-like symptoms, hypotension), leukopenia, thrombocytopenia, serum sickness
OKT3	Cytokine release syndrome, pulmonary oedema, acute renal failure

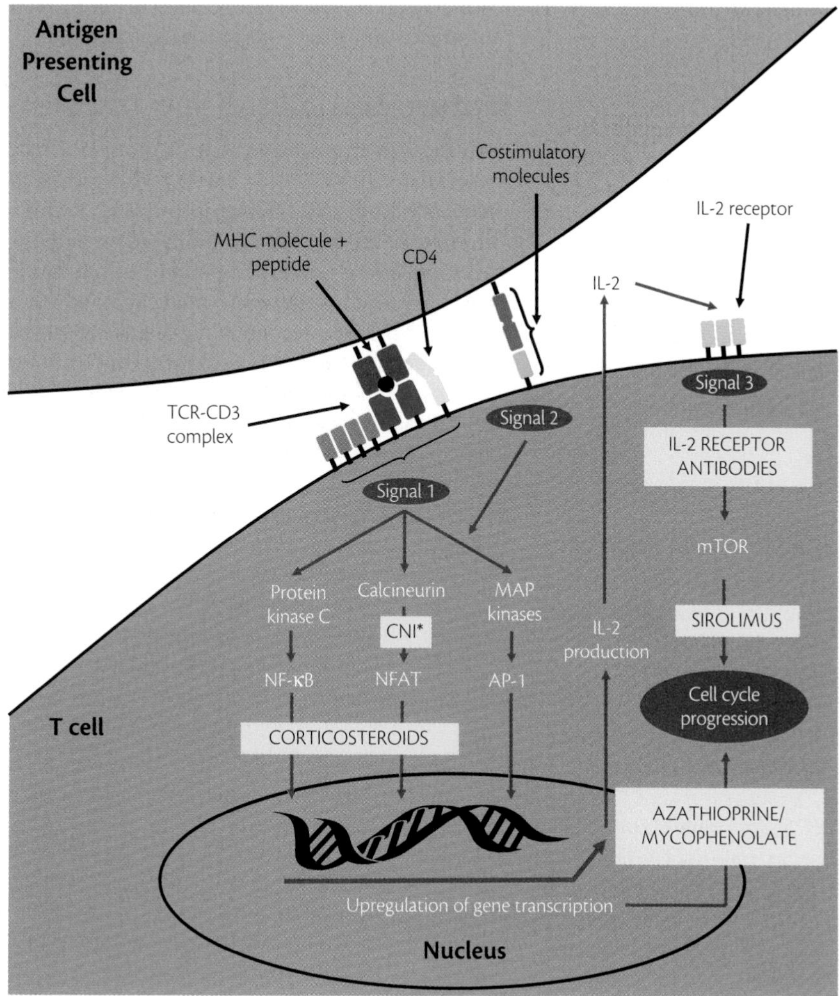

Fig. 5.5.7 Targets of immunosuppressive agents.

as AP-1 and NF-κB. Corticosteroids reduce the expression of many molecules important in the immune response, including interleukins 1, 2, 3, and 6, TNFα, interferon-γ and chemokines. By inhibiting cyclooxygenase, corticosteroids are also able to reduce the production of inflammatory mediators such as leukotrienes and prostaglandins.

Antiproliferative agents

Azathioprine and mycophenolate mofetil interfere with DNA synthesis and prevent cell-cycle progression. In the context of allograft rejection this impairs the clonal expansion of alloreactive T cells.

The introduction of azathioprine into clinical practice in the 1960s and its use in conjunction with corticosteroids allowed transplantation to progress from an experimental procedure into a practical therapy for patients with organ failure. It is metabolized in the liver to the purine analogue 6-mercaptopurine and incorporated into DNA. By inhibiting purine nucleotide synthesis (and therefore DNA and RNA synthesis), azathioprine reduces gene transcription and prevents cell cycle progression. The effects of azathioprine are not lymphocyte specific and patients must be monitored closely for bone marrow suppression.

Mycophenolate mofetil is metabolized in the liver to mycophenolic acid, which is a noncompetitive, reversible inhibitor of inosine monophosphate dehydrogenase (IMPDH). Cells are able to generate purines either *de novo* by converting inosine monophosphate to guanosine monophosphate (catalysed by IMPDH), or from guanine via the salvage pathway. The salvage pathway is less active in lymphocytes and therefore they are relatively dependent on the *de novo* pathway of purine synthesis compared to other cell types. As a result the effects of mycophenolate are more lymphocyte-specific than azathioprine, and it is less myelosuppressive.

Calcineurin inhibitors

The introduction of ciclosporin in the early 1980s presented a great step forward in transplant immunosuppression as this was the first drug able to selectively block T-cell activation. Subsequently a second calcineurin inhibitor, the macrolide antibiotic tacrolimus, has also been developed. Both drugs bind cytoplasmic immunophilins (cyclophilin in the case of ciclosporin and FK506-binding protein 12 (FKBP12) in the case of tacrolimus) to form complexes that can inhibit the calcium-dependent phosphatase calcineurin, a rate-limiting enzyme in the T-cell receptor signal transduction pathway. By preventing translocation of the transcription factor NFAT to the nucleus, calcineurin inhibition impairs up-regulation of many molecules important for T-cell proliferation and the generation of an effective immune response, including the cytokines IL-2, IL-4,

TNFα, and interferon-γ, and costimulatory molecules such as CD154 (CD40L).

mTOR inhibitors

Sirolimus and everolimus bind to the same immunophilin as tacrolimus (FKBP12), although the complexes they form are unable to interact with calcineurin. Instead they bind to the regulatory kinase mammalian target of rapamycin (mTOR), which has a critical role in cytokine receptor signal transduction. The usual actions of mTOR are to activate the ribosomal enzyme p70 S6 kinase and block an inhibitory protein 4E-BP1, both of which are required for translation of proteins necessary for progression from the G_1 (growth) phase to the S (DNA synthesis) phase of the cell cycle. Inhibition of this pathway ('signal 3') in T cells therefore blocks the action of cytokines such as IL-2, IL-4, and IL-15, preventing cell cycle progression and clonal expansion.

Depleting antibodies

Polyclonal antithymocyte globulin (ATG) is produced by immunizing either rabbits or horses with human lymphocytes. Immunoglobulins directed against lymphocyte epitopes can then be harvested from the animal's serum for clinical use. ATG causes profound lymphocyte depletion that does not fully recover for over several months, and is highly effective both as an induction agent and in the treatment of severe rejection episodes. OKT3 is a mouse monoclonal antibody against human CD3ε that is also able to effectively deplete T cells.

Administration of either ATG or OKT3 can result in the massive release of cytokines caused by the initial activation of lymphocytes prior to their depletion. Clinical manifestations of this range from fever and flu-like symptoms to a potentially fatal severe systemic inflammatory response syndrome characterized by hypotension, rigors, and pulmonary oedema.

CAMPATH-1H or alemtuzumab is a humanized monoclonal antibody directed against human CD52, which is a surface molecule that is expressed by most nucleated bone-marrow-derived cells, including T and B cells, monocytes, macrophages, and eosinophils, as well as Sertoli cells that line the male reproductive tract. Administration of alemtuzumab causes profound lymphopenia that can take months or years to recover from, and alemtuzumab has been used in a limited number of transplant recipients combined with conventional small-molecule immunosuppression since 1998.

Rituximab is a monoclonal antibody licensed for use in B-cell lymphoma and rheumatoid arthritis. It is directed against CD20, which is expressed on most B cells (except plasma cells), and there are reports of efficacy in patients with antibody-mediated rejection.

Other biological agents

Daclizumab and basiliximab are monoclonal antibodies directed against CD25 (the high-affinity IL-2 receptor α-chain). The addition of these agents to standard therapy reduces 6-month acute rejection rates by one-third, with minimal side effects, and they are now in widespread use as part of induction immunosuppression.

Another biological agent currently in clinical trials is belatacept (LEA29Y). This is a fusion protein consisting of the extracellular domain of CD152 (CTLA-4, cytotoxic-T-lymphocyte-associated antigen 4) combined with the Fc (non-antigen-binding) portion of IgG. As discussed earlier, CTLA-4 has a higher affinity for the costimulatory molecules CD80 and CD86 than does CD28, and belatacept is therefore able to block CD28:CD80/86 costimulation, thus increasing the T-cell activation threshold.

Future possibilities in transplantation

Advances in the management of transplant recipients have been accompanied by both improved 1-year graft survival and reduced acute rejection rates, offering many patients with organ failure great improvements in both morbidity and mortality. However, these advances still rely on the continuous administration of potent nonspecific immunosuppressive medication which is associated with increased risk of infection and malignancy as well as drug toxicity. The improvement in short- to medium-term outcomes has unfortunately not been followed by comparable reductions in long-term graft survival, with considerable late attrition of grafts resulting from the complex interaction of drug toxicity and chronic immune activation. A further major problem facing patients on transplant waiting lists is organ availability, with average waiting list time increasing for most organs in the United Kingdom at present, and rates of cadaveric donation falling. There is therefore considerable interest in strategies that might allow reduced exposure to immunosuppression medication with improved long-term outcomes (which in itself would decrease the pressure on scarce organ resources), as well as alternative sources of organs for transplantation.

Transplantation tolerance

In healthy individuals, autoimmunity is avoided by specific mechanisms that maintain immunological tolerance to self antigens (Table 5.5.7). The optimal outcome for patients after transplantation would be to harness these mechanisms to induce specific tolerance to the graft. Transplantation tolerance can be defined as the lack of a destructive immune response towards the graft without the requirement for indefinite nonspecific immunosuppressive therapy, while preserving immune responses to pathogens.

The science of immunological tolerance and the technology of transplantation have evolved hand in hand. The first description of acquired tolerance to foreign antigen in mice by Billingham, Brent and Medawar in 1953 (for which Medawar was awarded the Nobel Prize for medicine in 1960), actually preceded the first successful renal transplant (between syngeneic twins) by Murray and colleagues in 1955. Billingham, Brent and Medawar demonstrated that it was possible to acquire immunological tolerance to foreign antigen, and much effort has gone into defining strategies that would lead to tolerance to alloantigens in transplantation. Many successful experimental techniques can produce durable hyporesponsiveness to mismatched allografts in rodent models, but so far few of these have been successfully translated into large animal models or clinical trials. Progress in the field of transplantation tolerance is also hampered by the lack of definitive laboratory parameters able to give a clear indication of whether a particular recipient is tolerant of their graft.

Macrochimerism

The most robust experimental strategies for the induction of tolerance to foreign antigen utilize the mechanisms of central deletion to eliminate T-cell clones with specificity for the foreign antigens in question, thereby preventing them from entering the periphery. This can be reliably achieved by the establishment of haematopoietic chimerism through bone marrow transplantation.

Table 5.5.7 Mechanisms of immunological tolerance

Deletion	Deletion of autoreactive T cells occurs in the thymus during T-cell development (central deletion). Peripheral deletion of T cells can also occur if antigen is encountered under suboptimal condition (such as the absence or blockade of costimulatory signals)
Anergy	Anergy is the functional inactivation of T cells following antigen encounter and another possible outcome of antigen encounter under suboptimal conditions
Immunoregulation	Several populations of lymphocytes are able to suppress or regulate the ability of other lymphocytes to respond to a particular antigen
Ignorance	T cells do not have access to antigens present at certain sites of immune privilege (such as the anterior chamber of the eye)

Stable engraftment of donor haemopoietic stem cells results in repopulation of the recipient thymus with donor-type thymic dendritic cells, with the result that developing T cells with antidonor specificity are deleted by negative selection.

In experimental models, full donor chimerism induced by myeloablative therapy (frequently a combination of total body irradiation and cytotoxic medication) followed by donor bone marrow transplantation produces tolerance to a subsequent allograft from an identical donor. As proof of concept, there are a number of patients who have undergone successful bone marrow transplantation for haematological indications and have subsequently been successfully transplanted with a kidney from the same donor, without the requirement for increased immunosuppression. However, the establishment of full donor chimerism is not acceptable for most recipients on the transplant waiting list as the risk profile, i.e. the toxicity and mortality associated with myeloablative conditioning regimens and the high incidence of graft-vs-host disease in patients, is not acceptable when compared to the alternative, i.e. life-long immunosuppression with the agents described above.

A more promising approach is the induction of mixed haemopoietic chimerism, which can be achieved in experimental models with far less toxic induction therapy. Nonmyeloablative conditioning regimens have been applied in the clinical setting for patients who have developed renal failure as a consequence multiple myeloma. Further refinements of such protocols are being explored in experimental models. Examples of these include either a combination of depleting anti-CD4 and anti-CD8 antibodies, together with mild, nonmyeloablative total body irradiation or costimulatory blockade with anti-CD154 and/or CTLA-4-Ig. When these induction protocols are followed by bone marrow transplantation the result is mixed chimerism (the continued survival of both donor and recipient haematopoietic progenitor cells). Animals that have undergone these therapies demonstrate durable tolerance to donor type allografts, and have a much lower incidence of graft-vs-host disease compared to full chimeras.

Regulatory T cells

There is now abundant evidence for the existence of populations of regulatory lymphocytes with the ability to suppress immune responses by other leucocytes. The best studied regulatory or suppressor T cells (Treg) are a population of naturally occurring CD4+ cells that constitutively express the IL-2 receptor α-chain (CD25). These cells develop within the thymus under the direction of the transcription factor FOXP3 and have a critical role in limiting immune responses to self antigens, as demonstrated by experimental models where mice depleted of CD25+CD4+ cells subsequently develop inflammatory bowel disease and widespread autoimmune phenomena. Mutation of FOXP3 in humans is responsible for the IPEX syndrome (immune dysregulation, polyendocrinopathy, enteropathy, X-linked). There is evidence for the involvement of Treg in the down-regulation of immune responses to tumours, chronic infections, as well as allogeneic transplants.

A number of strategies in experimental models of transplantation result in the generation of Treg that are able to prevent rejection of a primary allograft. The best characterized of these involve either coreceptor (CD4 or CD8) blockade or costimulation blockade using monoclonal antibodies, administered either at the time of transplantation or prior to transplantation in conjunction with donor antigen (such as a donor specific blood transfusion). CD25+CD4+ Treg play a critical role in both the induction and maintenance of transplantation tolerance in these models. Depletion of CD25+CD4+ cells in tolerant animals results in allograft rejection. Alternatively, adoptive transfer of CD25+CD4+ cells from tolerant animals to naive animals induces tolerance in the recipient animal to grafts from the same donor strain as the original transplant, but not to grafts from third-party strains.

It is likely that the some of the nonspecific immunosuppressive agents in clinical use currently impair both effector T-cell function and the generation and function of Treg. As more is learned about the biology of Treg it will hopefully be possible to design protocols that enhance Treg function in clinical transplantation, either through the development of immunosuppressive agents that specifically target effector cells, or the expansion of alloreactive Treg *in vitro* for reinfusion after the initial alloresponse has been controlled by conventional immunosuppression or T-cell depletion.

Peripheral depletion

Therapies that deplete circulating leucocytes, and in particular T cells, have been used successfully both as induction immunosuppression and in the treatment of acute allograft rejection episodes for many years. The efficacy of this strategy in preventing allograft rejection led to the hypothesis that profound lymphocyte depletion at the time of transplantation may allow the development of donor-specific immunological hyporesponsiveness.

Initially, targeted irradiation of lymphoid tissue (by total lymphoid irradiation—TLI) was used alone or in combination with polyclonal antilymphocyte antibodies to induce lymphopenia at the time of transplantation. In experimental nonhuman primate models, therapy with TLI combined with anti-CD3 antibodies prolonged kidney or liver graft survival, with 50% of recipients demonstrating operational tolerance. Subsequently a series of human cadaveric renal transplant recipients who received TLI, ATG, and low-dose corticosteroids was reported. Only 9/28 patients had evidence of donor-specific hyporesponsiveness on mixed lymphocyte reaction (MLR), with 3/28 able to stop all immunosuppression.

An alternative approach used anti-CD3 immunotoxin (a monoclonal antibody to CD3 combined with a mutated diphtheria toxin) to induce T-cell depletion in rhesus monkeys. These animals received renal allografts which functioned for over 200 days, although biopsies taken beyond 100 days showed abnormalities consistent with chronic rejection.

Clinical trials have also been undertaken to evaluate leucocyte depletion using alemtuzumab (CAMPATH-IH) at the time of transplantation. The outcomes of 31 renal transplant recipients who received induction with alemtuzumab combined with low-dose monotherapy with ciclosporin were reported in 1999 and updated in 2005. Patients experienced a low incidence of acute rejection episodes in the early post-transplant period, prompting speculation that 'prope' or operational tolerance had been achieved, but as the trial progressed the alemtuzumab-treated patients experienced a relatively high incidence of late rejection, such that there was no significant difference in the overall incidence of acute rejection episodes compared with contemporaneous control patients at 5 years (30% vs 27% respectively). Overall graft and patient survival were not significantly different after 5 years. These findings were supported by a separate trial in which seven renal transplant recipients received induction immunotherapy with alemtuzumab followed by no maintenance immunosuppression. All seven patients experienced reversible acute rejection episodes within the first month requiring the introduction of immunosuppression. Further trials are in progress to investigate the effect of other immunosuppressive agents in combination with alemtuzumab induction.

Xenotransplantation

Since the 1960s attempts have been made to use animals as an alternative source of organs for transplantation. Initial attempts to transplant kidneys from nonhuman primates to humans resulted in renal function for weeks to months, although nonhuman primates are too scarce to be a realistic long-term source of organs. Instead, most research has focused on other mammals, and in particular pigs, which can be raised in sufficient numbers in pathogen-free facilities, can be genetically engineered, and have organs that are a suitable size. However, there remain significant practical as well as ethical hurdles to overcome before clinical xenotransplantation becomes a possibility.

The principal problem is the robust immune response induced by xenografts. Humans have naturally occurring xenoreactive antibodies that are thought to arise from interactions of the host immune system with gut bacteria early in life. The most important of these natural antibodies recognize Galα1, 3Gal, a carbohydrate determinant expressed by cells of pigs and other lower mammals but not humans or other primates. Antibody binding to Galα1, 3Gal and resultant complement activation invariably lead to hyperacute rejection following pig-to-primate organ transplantation. This process is exacerbated by porcine complement regulatory proteins (such as decay accelerating factor and CD59) which have reduced activity against human complement.

Some progress has been made in preventing hyperacute rejection, either by removal of preformed antibody before transplantation or the generation of genetically engineered pigs that lack Galα1, 3Gal or transgenically express human complement regulatory proteins. Unfortunately, where it has been possible to inhibit hyperacute rejection, downstream events involving the adaptive immune system have invariably resulted in acute vascular rejection over a period of days to weeks. The targets of the adaptive immune response to a xenograft include MHC molecules and a diverse range of other antigens expressed on foreign tissues.

Finally, although animals such as pigs can be raised in specific pathogen-free facilities, there remains a small risk of transmissible zoonoses. Some pig stocks carry the porcine endogenous retrovirus (PERV) which is able to infect human cells in culture. There is a theoretical risk that transmission of this virus to a xenotransplant recipient would allow the virus to spread more widely amongst humans, with unknown public health implications.

Further reading

Andrade CF, *et al.* (2005). Innate immunity and organ transplantation: the potential role of toll-like receptors. *Am J Transplant*, **5**, 969–75.

Barry M, Bleackley RC (2002). Cytotoxic T lymphocytes: all roads lead to death. *Nat Rev Immunol*, **2**, 401–9.

Becker YT, *et al.* (2004). Rituximab as treatment for refractory kidney transplant rejection. *Am J Transplant*, **4**, 996–1001.

Benichou G, *et al.* (1992). Donor major histocompatibility complex (MHC) peptides are presented by recipient MHC molecules during graft rejection. *J Exp Med*, **175**, 305–8.

Benichou G, Valujskikh A, Heeger PS (1999). Contributions of direct and indirect T cell alloreactivity during allograft rejection in mice. *J Immunol*, **162**, 352–8.

Billingham RE, Brent L, Medawar PB (1953). Actively acquired tolerance of foreign cells. *Nature*, **172**, 603–6.

Bingaman AW, Farber DL (2004). Memory T cells in transplantation: generation, function, and potential role in rejection. *Am J Transplant*, **4**, 846–52.

Brent L (1996). *A history of transplantation immunology*. Academic Press, London.

Bucher P, Morel P, Buhler LH (2005). Xenotransplantation: an update on recent progress and future perspectives. *Transpl Int*, **18**, 894–901.

Cascalho M, Platt JL (2001). The immunological barrier to xenotransplantation. *Immunity*, **14**, 437–46.

Clarkson MR, Sayegh MH (2005). T-cell costimulatory pathways in allograft rejection and tolerance. *Transplantation*, **80**, 555–63.

Colvin RB, Smith R N (2005). Antibody-mediated organ-allograft rejection. *Nat Rev Immunol*, **5**, 807–17.

Cosimi AB, Sachs D H (2004). Mixed chimerism and transplantation tolerance. *Transplantation*, **77**, 943–6.

Cosimi A *et al.* (eds) (1999). *Organ transplantation*. Blackwell Science, Oxford.

Fehr T, Sykes M (2004). Tolerance induction in clinical transplantation. *Transpl Immunol*, **13**, 117–30.

Feng G, *et al.* (2009). Donor reactive regulatory T cells. *Curr Opin Organ Transplant* doi: 10.1097/MOT.0b013e32832c58f1

Fuggle SV, Martin S (2004). Toward performing transplantation in highly sensitized patients. *Transplantation*, **78**, 186–9.

Gandhi AM, *et al.* (2008). Costimulation targeting therapies in organ transplantation. *Curr Opin Organ Transplant*, **13**, 622–6.

Grakoui A. *et al.* (1999). The immunological synapse: a molecular machine controlling T cell activation. *Science*, **285**, 221–7.

Halloran PF (2004). Immunosuppressive drugs for kidney transplantation. *N Engl J Med*, **351**, 2715–29.

Harder T (2004). Lipid raft domains and protein networks in T-cell receptor signal transduction. *Curr Opin Immunol*, **16**, 353–9.

Heeger PS (2003). T-cell allorecognition and transplant rejection: a summary and update. *Am J Transplant*, **3**, 525–33.

Janeway CA Jr, Medzhitov R (2002). Innate immune recognition. *Annu Rev Immunol*, **20**, 197–216.

Kissmeyer-Nielsen F, *et al.* (1966). Hyperacute rejection of kidney allografts, associated with pre-existing humoral antibodies against donor cells. *Lancet*, **ii**, 662–5.

Knechtle SJ (2005). Development of tolerogenic strategies in the clinic. *Phil Trans R Soc Lond B Biol Sci*, **360**, 1739–46.

Koo DD, *et al.* (2004). C4d deposition in early renal allograft protocol biopsies. *Transplantation*, **78**, 398–403.

Kroczek RA, Mages HW, Hutloff A (2004). Emerging paradigms of T-cell co-stimulation. *Curr Opin Immunol*, **16**, 321–7.

Krogsgaard M, Davis MM (2005). How T cells 'see' antigen. *Nat Immunol*, **6**, 239–45.

Land WG (2005). The role of postischemic reperfusion injury and other nonantigen-dependent inflammatory pathways in transplantation. *Transplantation*, **79**, 505–14.

Le Moine A, Goldman M, Abramowicz D (2002). Multiple pathways to allograft rejection. *Transplantation*, **73**, 1373–81.

Meier-Kriesche HU *et al.* (2004). Lack of improvement in renal allograft survival despite a marked decrease in acute rejection rates over the most recent era. *Am J Transplant*, **4**, 378–83.

Morris PJ, Russell NK (2006). Alemtuzumab (Campath-1H): a systematic review in organ transplantation. Transplantation, **81**, 1361–7.

Newell KA, Larsen CP (2006). Tolerance assays: measuring the unknown. *Transplantation*, **81**, 1503–9.

Obhrai J, Goldstein DR (2006). The role of toll-like receptors in solid organ transplantation. *Transplantation*, **81**, 497–502.

Patel R, Terasaki PI (1969). Significance of the positive crossmatch test in kidney transplantation. *N Engl J Med*, **280**, 735–9.

Quezada SA, *et al.* (2004). CD40/CD154 interactions at the interface of tolerance and immunity. *Annu Rev Immunol*, **22**, 307–28.

Racusen LC, Halloran PF, Solez K (2004). Banff 2003 meeting report: new diagnostic insights and standards. *Am J Transplant*, **4**, 1562–6.

Rocha PN, *et al.* (2003). Effector mechanisms in transplant rejection. *Immunol Rev*, **196**, 51–64.

Sacks SH, Chowdhury P, Zhou W (2003). Role of the complement system in rejection. *Curr Opin Immunol*, **15**, 487–92.

Sayegh MH, *et al.* (1991). Immunologic tolerance to renal allografts after bone marrow transplants from the same donors. *Ann Intern Med*, **114**, 954–5.

Schwartz RH (2003). T cell anergy. *Annu Rev Immunol*, **21**, 305–34.

Stegall MD, Dean PG, Gloor JM (2004). ABO-incompatible kidney transplantation. *Transplantation*, **78**, 635–40.

Stein JV, Nombela-Arrieta, C (2005). Chemokine control of lymphocyte trafficking: a general overview. *Immunology*, **116**, 1–12.

Stepkowski SM (2000). Molecular targets for existing and novel immunosuppressive drugs. *Expert Rev Mol Med*, **2**, 1–23.

Taylor DK, Neujahr D, Turka LA (2004). Heterologous immunity and homeostatic proliferation as barriers to tolerance. *Curr Opin Immunol*, **16**, 558–64.

Turka LA, Lechler RI (2009). Towards the identification of biomarkers of transplantation tolerance. *Nat Rev Immunol*, doi:10.1038/nri2568

Wekerle T, Sykes M (2001). Mixed chimerism and transplantation tolerance. *Annu Rev Med*, **52**, 353–70.

Whitelegg A, Barber LD (2004). The structural basis of T-cell allorecognition. *Tissue Antigens*, **63**, 101–8.

Wood KJ, Sakaguchi S (2003). Regulatory T cells in transplantation tolerance. *Nat Rev Immunol*, **3**, 199–210.

Worthington, J. E. *et al.* (2003). Posttransplantation production of donor HLA-specific antibodies as a predictor of renal transplant outcome. *Transplantation*, **75**, 1034–40.

Wu Z, *et al.* (2004). Homeostatic proliferation is a barrier to transplantation tolerance. *Nat Med*, **10**, 87–92.

Young NT (2004). Immunobiology of natural killer lymphocytes in transplantation. *Transplantation*, **78**, 1–6.

Websites

British Transplantation Society. http://www.bts.org.uk/

European Society for Organ Transplantation. http://www.esot.org/

Immune Tolerance Network. http://www.immunetolerance.org/

ImMunoGeneTics (IMGT) *Project HLA sequence database*. http://www.ebi.ac.uk/imgt/hla/

NHS UK Transplant. http://www.uktransplant.org.uk/ukt/default.jsp

Reprogramming the Immune System for Establishment of Tolerance. http://www.risetfp6.org/cgi-bin/WebObjects/Awo3.woa

Transplantation Society. http://www.transplantation-soc.org/

SECTION 6

Principles of clinical oncology

6.1 **Epidemiology of cancer** *299*
A.J. Swerdlow, R. Peto, and Richard S. Doll

6.2 **The nature and development of cancer** *333*
John R. Benson and Siong-Seng Liau

6.3 **The genetics of inherited cancers** *358*
Rosalind A. Eeles

6.4 **Cancer immunity and clinical oncology** *372*
Maries van den Broek, Lotta von Boehmer, Kunle Odunsi, and Alexander Knuth

6.5 **Cancer: clinical features and management** *380*
R.L. Souhami

6.6 **Cancer chemotherapy and radiation therapy** *396*
Bruce A. Chabner and Jay Loeffler

6.1

Epidemiology of cancer

A.J. Swerdlow, R. Peto, and Richard S. Doll[‡]

Essentials

The epidemiology of cancer is the investigation of the incidence and causes of the disease in people under different conditions of life. Such investigations have generally been the way in which reliable evidence about causal agents for cancer, and the magnitude of the risks from these agents, have been found. They have shown that any type of cancer that is common in one population is rare in some other, and that the differences between populations are mostly not genetic, but rather the consequences of behaviours and circumstances of life. In principle, cancers are therefore largely preventable.

The range of incidence rates between geographical and ethnic groups is more than 10-fold for each of the common cancers, and for some cancers is more than 100-fold. Large changes in rates of many tumours can occur in migrants compared with rates in their homeland, and large changes have occurred in rates within populations over time, indicating the scope for prevention.

The causes of cancer

These can be divided into nature (biological factors), nurture (environment and behaviours), and chance.

Biological factors—important biological factors are genetic susceptibility, age, and sex.

Tobacco smoking—this is the most important extrinsic factor causing cancer in developed countries, and is a major cause of cancers of the mouth, pharynx (other than nasopharynx), oesophagus, larynx, lung, pancreas, renal pelvis, and bladder (and it also causes a proportion of several other types of cancer). In 2005, smoking is estimated to have caused 28% of all fatal cancers in the United Kingdom.

Other extrinsic causes—there are many, including (1) alcohol—the cause of at least six types of cancer, including liver, various upper aerodigestive sites, and breast; (2) ionizing radiation—can cause cancer in most tissues; in the United Kingdom the main sources of exposure are natural sources including radon, and medical uses; (3) ultraviolet radiation—causes skin cancer; (4) infection, principally viral, but also bacterial and parasitic—a major cause of cancer of several sites, especially in developing countries; (5) immunosuppression—patients with persistent immunosuppression from therapeutic, infective, or genetic causes have raised risks of certain cancers, notably non-Hodgkin's lymphoma; (6) chemotherapeutic agents—about 20 of these, used for treatment of specific diseases and including several that are used to treat cancer, have been shown themselves to cause cancer, of different anatomical sites according to the agent; (7) other drugs—hormone replacement therapy and oral contraceptives, both widely used in the general population, affect the risk of certain female reproductive-related malignancies, increasing risk for some cancers but (for combined steroid contraceptives) decreasing it for others; (8) occupation—numerous occupational groups have been found to be at raised risk of cancer, mainly of the respiratory tract, especially the lung; (9) air, water, and food pollution—these are probably responsible for a small percentage of cancers in Western countries; (10) diet—this may well have an effect on the aetiology of a substantial proportion of cancers, but there is considerable uncertainty on the figure and specific dietary associations are largely unknown.

Other factors of particular note are (1) menstrual and reproductive history, also certain hormonal drugs—these affect the risks of breast, endometrial, and ovarian cancers in women; (2) obesity—relates to increased risks of breast, endometrial, colonic, kidney, and possibly other cancers; (3) physical inactivity—relates to increased risk of breast, endometrial, colonic, and possibly other cancers.

Epidemiology and aetiology of particular cancers

The most common cancers worldwide are those of the lung, breast, and colorectum, and the most common causes of cancer death are lung, stomach, and liver cancers. Descriptive and aetiological epidemiological information is given about 33 types of cancer in this chapter.

Lung cancer—the major cause is smoking tobacco, particularly cigarettes. Lung cancer became epidemic in men in Western countries during the mid 20th century, with rates rising later in women, and in Western countries there have been considerable decreases in men in recent years. In developing countries, however, the epidemic has arrived later, with rising rates to be expected in future years as a consequence of current smoking levels. Occupational causes of lung cancer include exposures to asbestos, polycyclic hydrocarbons,

[‡] It is with regret that we report the death of Professor Richard S. Doll during the preparation of this edition of the textbook.

and radon. Air pollution in towns may have been a factor, largely in smokers, and radon in indoor air contributes to a small percentage of cases.

Breast cancer—the most common cancer worldwide in women. It has greatest incidence in Western countries, where rates have tended to increase slowly over decades; rates have generally been much lower in Asia and Africa. Hormonal and reproductive factors are important to risk: early menopause, late menarche, nulliparity, and older age at first full-term pregnancy all increase risk, as do postmenopausal hormone replacement therapy and combined oral contraceptives, while tamoxifen treatment of unilateral breast cancer decreases risk in the unaffected breast. There is also raised risk of breast cancer in relation to a history of benign breast disease, alcohol consumption, lack of physical exercise, postmenopausal obesity, taller height, and ionizing radiation exposure at young ages, as well as genetic predisposition.

Introduction

All cancers have certain pathological and clinical characteristics in common, but those arising in different organs often have very different causes. The epidemiology of cancer, by which is meant the study of the incidence and causes of the disease in people under different conditions of life, is, therefore, the epidemiology of specific types of cancer, usually, but not always, defined as cancers of specific organs. In this sense, the subject has a history dating back nearly 300 years to Ramazzini's observation that cancer of the breast occurred more often in nuns than in other women of similar age and to Pott's observation, over 200 years ago, that scrotal cancer in young men occurred characteristically in chimney sweeps. The high risk in nuns (which largely reflected the protective effect of multiple pregnancies in the general population) helped the realization that hormonal factors can substantially affect the incidence of several types of cancer, while the latter led to the recognition that the combustion products of coal to which sweeps had been exposed could cause cancer on any part of the skin with which they came into repeated contact and to the isolation of the first specific chemical carcinogen. Many other similar observations were made over the next 150 years, mostly as a result of the acumen of individual doctors who noticed clusters of cases of a particular type of cancer occurring in patients with a similar occupational or cultural background. Lip and tongue cancers were found in pipe smokers, bladder cancer in certain aniline dye workers, buccal cancer in those who habitually chewed mixtures of tobacco and betel in India, lung cancer in miners of particular ores (who, it was subsequently realized, were heavily exposed to radon and its daughter products), and skin cancer in the early radiologists and radiographers who were heavily exposed to X-rays and in farmers and seamen heavily exposed to sunlight. Gradually, however, clinical anecdotes were replaced by statistics as the epidemiological methods that are described below began to be applied to the study of cancer and other noninfectious diseases. As a result, many other causes were identified with sufficient certainty to justify preventive action and data were obtained to suggest hypotheses that could be tested in the laboratory.

Preventability of cancer

Perhaps the most important result of such observations has been the realization that any type of cancer that is common in one population is rare in some other, and that the differences between populations are mostly not genetic. Hence, where they are common these cancers occur, in large part, as a result of the way people behave and the circumstances in which they live and they are, therefore, at least in principle, preventable. This does not mean that we can at present envisage a society in which any of the common cancers are completely eliminated (although this may prove to be possible when we understand more clearly the mechanisms by which they are produced). What it does mean is that we can envisage a society in which the age-specific risk of developing any type of cancer is low.

Differences in incidence between communities

Variation in incidence of cancer between different ethnic and geographical groups around the world can be ascertained from data provided by population-based cancer registries. Table 6.1.1 shows, for selected types of cancer, the range of variation recorded by cancer registries that have produced data sufficiently reliable for the purpose of international comparison, or, in one instance, the range determined by special surveys. The age ranges are constrained to exclude the oldest ages, at which the records of the incidence of the disease are least reliable. Types of cancer have been included if they are common enough somewhere to have a cumulative incidence among men or women of at least 2% by 75 years of age. The range of variation is never less than 13-fold and is sometimes more than 100-fold. Despite the selection of reasonably reliable registries, some of this tabulated variation may still be an artefact, due to different standards of medical service, case registration, and population enumeration. In many cases, however, the true ranges will be greater, because much of the world is not covered by reliable cancer registries, and because the data generally refer to cancers of whole organs and do not distinguish between different histological types or different locations within an organ, for which greater variation may apply.

The variation in incidence is not limited to the common cancers. Burkitt's lymphoma, for example, never affects more than 1 in 1000 of the population, but it is at least 100 times as common among children in parts of Uganda as it is in Europe and North America; while Kaposi's sarcoma, which was extremely rare in most of the world until the advent of AIDS, was so common in children and young adults in parts of Central Africa, even before 1970, that it accounted for 10% of all tumours seen in one of the African hospitals surveyed by Cook and Burkitt. Some few cancers occur with approximately the same frequency in all communities, but all are relatively uncommon. Acute myeloid leukaemia at 15 to 25 years of age is an example; nephroblastoma is another, except that it appears to be only half as common in Japan as elsewhere.

The figures above refer to cancer incidence in communities defined by geography, but substantial differences are found between communities defined in other ways such as by ethnic origin, religion, or socioeconomic status. Jewish women, for example, have a low incidence of cervical cancer irrespective of the country in which they live, and Mormons and Seventh Day Adventists living

Table 6.1.1 Range of incidence rates of common cancers (men, unless specified otherwise)

Site of origin of cancer[a]	High-incidence area[b,c]	Cumulative incidence (%) in high-incidence area[d]	Low-incidence area[c]	Ratio of cumulative rates in high- and low-incidence areas[e]
Nonmelanoma skin	Australia[f] (Queensland)	>20	Several nonwhite populations	>200
Prostate	US (Detroit, black)	28	China (Tianjin)	240
Oesophagus	China (Cixian)	23	Singapore, Malay	550
Stomach	China (Changle)	20	Thailand (Songkhla)	100
Lung	US (Detroit, black)	12	Mali (Bamako)	40
Breast[g]	Uruguay (Montevideo)	13	Gambia	18
Liver	Thailand (Khon Kaen)	11	Algeria (Algiers)	190
Colon	Japan (Hiroshima)	7	India (Karunagappally)	70
Uterine cervix[g]	Zimbabwe (Harare, black)	7	China (Tianjin)	40
Melanoma of skin	Australia (Queensland)	5	Mali (Bamako)	>300
Bladder	Italy (Genoa)	5	Uganda (Kyandondo)	24
Kaposi's sarcoma	Zimbabwe (Harare, black)	5	Several	>500
Rectum	Japan (Hiroshima)	3	Algeria (Algiers)	36
Corpus uteri[g]	US (Connecticut, white)	3	India (Karunagappally)	24
Non-Hodgkin's lymphoma	US (San Francisco, non-Hispanic white)	3	Mali (Bamako)	13
Kidney	Czech Republic	2	Vietnam (Hanoi)	40
Nasopharynx	Hong Kong	2	Mali (Bamako)	>200
Larynx	Spain (Zaragoza)	2	China (Qidong)	40

[a] Sites of cancer are shown if somewhere they reach a cumulative incidence by age 75 of at least 2% in either sex.
[b] The geographic area of highest recorded incidence by age 75.
[c] Excluding very small cancer registry populations, with unstable numbers.
[d] By age 75 years, in the absence of other causes of death.
[e] By age 65 years, in the absence of other causes of death.
[f] Special survey.
[g] Women.

in the United States of America have low incidence of cancers of the respiratory, gastrointestinal, and genital systems.

Few of the large differences between communities can be explained by genetic factors, apart from some of the differences in the incidence of cancer of the skin, the risk of which is much greater for whites than for blacks, and possibly also for some of those in the incidence of testis cancer, which rarely affects black populations, and in chronic lymphocytic leukaemia, which rarely affects people of Chinese or Japanese descent. Genetic factors cannot explain the differences observed on migration or with the passage of time, which are discussed below, nor can they explain the correlations observed between the national rates for particular types of cancer and aspects of the lifestyle in different countries.

Changes in incidence in migrant groups

That changes in the incidence of cancer occur on migration is certain. Numerous groups have been studied, particularly migrants from many countries to Australia, Israel, and the United States. These show, for example, that Afro-Americans experience incidence rates for internal cancers that are generally much more like those of white Americans than those of the black populations in West Africa from which most of their ancestors came, while Japanese in Hawaii have experienced rates that are much more like those of the white residents of Hawaii than those of Japanese living in Japan (Table 6.1.2). The ancestors of black Americans and Hawaiian Japanese will have come from many different parts of West Africa and Japan, some of which are likely to have cancer rates somewhat different from those cited in Table 6.1.2. Nevertheless, the contrasts are so great that there can be no serious doubt that new factors were introduced with migration.

Changes in incidence over time

Within one population there may be substantial changes in the incidence of a particular type of cancer over a period of a few decades that provide conclusive evidence of the existence of preventable factors. Changes in incidence over time may, however, be difficult to assess reliably, chiefly because it is difficult to compare the thoroughness of the selection and registration of particular types of cancer at different periods and partly because few incidence data have been collected for long enough, so we often have to fall back on changes in mortality rates even though these may be influenced by changes in treatment as well as by changes in incidence.

There are no simple rules for deciding which of the many changes in recorded cancer incidence and mortality rates are reliable indicators of real changes in incidence. Each set of data has to be assessed individually. It is relatively easy to be sure about changes in the incidence of cancer of the oesophagus, as the disease can be diagnosed without complex investigations and its occurrence is nearly always recorded, at least in middle age, because it is nearly always fatal. By contrast, it is much more difficult to be sure about changes in

Table 6.1.2 Comparisons of cancer incidence rates in migrants[a] and residents in homelands and adopted countries (men, unless otherwise specified), mid 1990s. Cumulative rate to age 65, per 1000 persons

		Hawaii		West Africa[b]	USA	
	Japan[b]	Japanese	Whites		Blacks	Whites
Oesophagus	6.5	3.0	1.7	1.9	7.4	2.6
Stomach	32.9	7.4	3.6	7.3	6.6	3.1
Colon	14.8	17.2	14.0	0.8	16.3	11.0
Rectum	10.0	11.6	6.6	0.9	6.8	6.4
Liver	17.3	3.5	2.6	32.1	4.9	1.9
Pancreas	4.4	4.0	3.9	1.3	7.0	3.4
Larynx	1.7	1.8	5.2	0.4	6.6	3.2
Lung	15.2	13.4	21.7	1.9	49.5	25.8
Breast[c]	24.2	61.7	72.2	10.5	59.8	65.1
Uterine cervix[c]	4.7	3.4	5.7	27.5	7.5	5.3
Corpus uteri[c]	3.0	13.1	9.9	1.9	7.6	12.4
Ovary[c]	4.7	7.4	10.2	1.4	5.5	9.1
Prostate	2.0	17.6	40.6	2.2	91.2	47.4
Testis	1.0	1.7	5.1	0.2	0.8	4.1
Non-Hodgkin's lymphoma	3.4	4.3	10.4	1.4	11.0	10.1

[a] 'Migrant' rates are based on ethnicity, and hence include all generations of migrant.
[b] Average of rates in two regions.
[c] Women.

the incidence of basal-cell carcinomas of the skin, which—although easy to diagnose—seldom cause death and can be treated effectively outside hospital, and so often escape registration. What appears to be a change in incidence may therefore be a change only in the completeness of registration. Cancers of the pancreas, liver, and brain, and myelomatosis, in contrast, usually cause death, but even when they do they may be misdiagnosed as another disease (e.g. brain tumours in old people could frequently in the past be misdiagnosed as other neurological conditions), so that an increased incidence or mortality rate may be wholly or partly due to improvements in diagnosis or in the availability of medical services. Such changes are particularly likely to affect the rates recorded for people over 65 years of age, as many old people who were terminally ill used not to be intensively investigated.

Despite these difficulties, some of the decreases and increases in the recorded rates of particular types of cancer have been so gross that there must have been real changes in their incidence. Examples include the increase in lung cancer throughout most of the world (and its recent large decrease in men in the United Kingdom), the increase in mesothelioma of the pleura in men in industrialized countries, the decrease in cancer of the tongue in the United Kingdom, and the decrease in cancers of the uterine cervix and stomach throughout western Europe, North America, and Australasia.

Identification of causes

More-specific evidence of the preventability of cancer, and of measures to enable this, has come from identification of agents and circumstances that cause the disease. In general, reliable evidence of causality (and particularly of the magnitude of any risks) has come from epidemiology and not from laboratory experiments, although the latter can often provide reinforcement of epidemiological findings and understanding of the mechanisms of cancer causation. Reliable epidemiological evidence does not require randomized trials within particular populations, but it does require the study of different individuals within populations and not just the comparison of incidence rates between populations. Nonrandomized epidemiological studies of individuals have often yielded proof of causation beyond reasonable doubt (like that required to convict in a court of law), and has been the decisive evidence of aetiology for almost all proven carcinogens. Action based on such evidence has, moreover, often been followed by the desired result—e.g. a reduction in the incidence of bladder cancer in the chemical industry on stopping the manufacture and use of 2-naphthylamine and, on a national scale, the reduction in the incidence of lung cancer in men in the United Kingdom following the decrease in smoking since the mid 20th century.

The causes of cancer can, briefly, be divided into nature (biological factors), nurture (behaviour and environment), and chance.

Biological factors

Genetic susceptibility

Various genetic factors are known that affect cancer risks to different extents. Very large risks are seen in patients with certain rare cancer-associated genetic syndromes in which bearers of one gene (if the condition is dominant) or two (if recessive) almost invariably develop a particular type of cancer. Examples include the dominant genes for polyposis coli that lead to cancer of the large bowel, and the recessive genes for retinoblastoma and xeroderma pigmentosum that lead (in the latter case) to squamous carcinoma and (less commonly) melanoma of the skin. Similar evidence has shown that other genetic syndromes frequently, but not invariably, lead to cancer, such as von Recklinghausen's neurofibromatosis leading to fibrosarcoma, the Peutz–Jeghers syndrome leading to carcinoma of the small bowel, the Wiskott–Aldrich syndrome leading to non-Hodgkin's lymphoma, and ataxia telangiectasia, Bloom's syndrome, and Fanconi's anaemia leading to leukaemia. Very high cancer risks are also present in individuals with various cancer susceptibility genes—e.g. raised risks of breast and ovarian cancers in patients with mutations in *BRCA1* and *BRCA2* genes. The recognition of these genes is important to the individual, as it may provide an opportunity for prophylactic surgery, or enable the diagnosis of malignancy to be made at an early stage when treatment is more likely to be effective, or (rarely) enable precautions to be taken to prevent exposure to the relevant carcinogens, as in the case of sufferers from xeroderma pigmentosum or albinism, who can be protected against sunshine. The proportion of all cancers that occur in people who are highly susceptible to cancer in this way is, however, very small, although substantially greater at young than at older ages.

Genes conveying less-raised risks of cancer are far more widespread in the population, and likely to be involved in the causation of a much larger proportion of cancers, but their discovery is only just beginning. It has been shown that many of the common types of cancer tend to cluster in families to some extent. Differences of this sort do not necessarily imply that the familial clusters are genetic in origin; they could be due to familial similarities of behaviour or environment. That socially important genetic variants exist is demonstrated by the greatly increased risk of developing basal-cell and squamous carcinomas of the sun-exposed skin in fair-skinned populations compared with dark-skinned, and there may be other genes associated with localized populations, which, for example, diminish the risk of chronic lymphatic leukaemia and myelomatosis in Chinese, Japanese, and Indians.

Discovery of genetic factors that affect particular types of cancer is unlikely to explain much of the social and geographical differences in the distribution of cancer other than skin cancer, but it should help to elucidate mechanisms and may help to focus health education and costly methods of early diagnosis on the sections of the populations that are most at risk.

Age

Some risk of cancer occurs at every age, but the risk of developing any particular type varies with age. The most common relationship with age is a progressive increase in incidence from near zero in childhood and adolescence to a high rate in old age. This type of relationship is shown by carcinomas of the skin, lung, and gastrointestinal and urinary tracts, and by myelomatosis and chronic lymphatic leukaemia. The rate of increase is rapid, being typically proportional to the fourth, fifth, or sixth power of age in years, so that the annual incidence may be 100 or 1000 times greater above age 75 than before age 25. It is probable that this reflects the cumulative effect of processes that operate steadily throughout life, starting at around the time of birth or at young ages (e.g. for lung cancer, in adolescence). With most of these cancers, the recorded incidence may stabilize, or even decrease, in the oldest age groups, but this is partly or wholly an artefact due to incomplete investigation of the terminal illnesses of old people.

A less common pattern is a peak incidence early in life, which may be followed either by a decline virtually to zero or by a slow rise in middle and old age. Retinoblastomas and nephroblastomas occur only in childhood, with peak incidences (respectively) in the first and second years of life. Teratomas and seminomas of the testis have peak incidence rates at about 25 and 35 years of age, respectively, and later almost cease to occur, while osteogenic sarcomas have a peak incidence in adolescence and then show a slow increase with age from a lower rate in young adult life.

The remaining cancers show a variety of patterns. Carcinomas of the breast and uterine cervix of women, for example, begin to appear in young adulthood and become rapidly more common up to the menopause. After the menopause the incidence of carcinoma of the breast may remain approximately constant, or may even become slightly reduced for a few years, before increasing again with age, though at a slower rate. Carcinoma of the cervix continues to increase fairly steeply for a few years after the menopause, before showing a stable or declining rate. Hodgkin's disease, on the other hand, appears in childhood but thereafter continues relatively evenly throughout life with only modest peaks in young adult life and at older ages, while connective tissue sarcomas become progressively more common from childhood on, but with a much slower rate of increase than is shown by the common carcinomas.

Some of these relationships with age, like that for retinoblastoma in early childhood, seem to be invariant everywhere and, as far as is known, at all times. Others vary from community to community, or from time to time. In postmenopausal women, for example, cancer of the breast becomes progressively less common with increasing age in parts of Asia, but more common in Europe, while carcinoma of the lung used to show a peak incidence at about 60 years of age in the United Kingdom, which gradually moved to older ages, as a generation that had not smoked substantial numbers of cigarettes throughout adult life was replaced by one that had, and the same process is now being repeated in many developing countries.

These various patterns provide information, either about the period of activity of the stem cells from which the cancers derive, or about the period when the main exposure to causative agents occurs and the duration of that exposure. Some of this variation has already helped to explain some of the causes of cancer, as was the case with the shift in the peak incidence of bronchial carcinoma, but much of it still awaits elucidation.

Sex

Cancer used to be more common in women than in men in many countries due to the great frequency of carcinoma of the breast and of the uterine cervix and to the rarity of bronchial carcinoma, and this is still the case in populations for which similar conditions persist, as in parts of Latin America. Elsewhere, cancer is now more common in men, among whom lung cancer often predominates. This overall male preponderance hides, however, a wide range of sex ratios for cancer of different organs. If the sites of cancer that are peculiar (or almost peculiar) to one sex are ignored, the sex ratio varies (in Britain) from a male excess of about 6 to 1 for pleural mesothelioma and carcinoma of the larynx, through many types of cancer with only a small male preponderance, to carcinoma of the thyroid, which is about twice as common in women.

For many types of cancer the sex ratio is much the same in different countries and at different times. For some, however, and particularly for cancers of the mouth, oesophagus, larynx, and bronchus, the sex ratio is extremely variable—not only between countries and at different times, but sometimes also between different ages at the same time and in the same country. The most marked variation is shown by cancer of the oesophagus, which may affect both sexes equally or be 20 times more common in men than in women. As with the various patterns of incidence with age, these different sex ratios and their variation can provide useful clues to the causation of the particular type of cancer, not all of which have yet been successfully followed up.

Delay between cause and effect

One reason why it has been difficult to recognize causes of cancer in humans is the long delay that characteristically occurs between the start of exposure to a carcinogen and the appearance of the clinical disease. This 'latent period', as it is commonly, but rather misleadingly, called is often several decades, although it may be as short as 1 year or as long as 60. The exact relation between the date of exposure and the date of the appearance of different cancers is still uncertain, partly because the interval is subject to random factors, partly because few cancers are induced by a single, brief exposure, and partly because there are still very few sets of quantitative data with detailed information about the dates when exposure began and ended.

When cancer is induced by short but intensive exposure to ionizing radiation, as following the explosions of the atomic bombs in Hiroshima and Nagasaki or in patients treated by radiotherapy, the excess incidence of solid tumours rises for 15 to 20 years and then may continue to rise, level off, or decline. In the case of acute leukaemia, however, a peak incidence occurs much earlier (*c*.5 years after irradiation) and relatively few cases appear after more than 30 years.

Short, intensive exposure to a carcinogen is, however, exceptional. The more usual situation is for sporadic or continuous exposure to a carcinogen to be prolonged for years—a decade or two in the case of occupational exposure, several decades in the case of tobacco smoking, and a lifetime in the case of ultraviolet radiation. In this situation the incidence of cancer increases progressively with the length of exposure. In the last two cases cited, the incidence appears to increase approximately in proportion to the fourth power of the duration of exposure, so that the effect after (say) 40 years is more than 10 times as great as that after 20 years, and more than 100 times as great as that after 10 years. Whether the same holds for occupational exposure is not known, but it has been shown to hold in some experiments in which chemicals were repeatedly applied to the skin of genetically similar mice and it may prove to be a general biological rule for many types of carcinoma and many carcinogens.

There is still less quantitative information about what usually happens when exposure ceases, but in the case of cigarette smoking the rapidly rising annual risk among those who continue to smoke stabilizes for one or two decades after smoking ceases before increasing again slowly. The ex-smoker consequently avoids the enormous progressive increase in risk suffered by the continuing smoker.

These delayed effects accord with the idea that the appearance of clinical cancer is the end result of a multistage process in which several mutations have to be produced in a single stem cell to turn it into the seed of a growing cancer. From the practical point of view, the important conclusions are that cancer may be very much more likely to occur after prolonged exposure to a carcinogen than after short exposure; that it is seldom likely to appear within a decade after first exposure (except in the case of leukaemia, certain hormone-related cancers, and the specific cancers of childhood); that it commonly occurs several decades after first exposure; and that some excess risk may continue to occur for decades after exposure has ceased. The exact relationship may, however, differ for different carcinogens and different types of tumour. Bladder tumours, for example, began to appear within 5 years of intensive exposure to 2-naphthylamine in the dye industry, while mesotheliomas of the pleura have seldom, if ever, appeared within 10 years of exposure to asbestos, but they continue to increase in incidence for up to 50 years after first exposure, even if the exposure was relatively brief.

Chance

There remains the influence of chance, which is commonly ignored; yet it is important for the individual as it is the reason why two animals of identical genetic constitution that have been treated in the same way do not, in general, develop cancer in the same place at precisely the same age. It reflects the element of chance that determines whether a particular series of events all occur in one particular stem cell out of the many thousands of stem cells that exist that do not give rise to a malignant clone. For any one individual the role of good or bad luck in determining the occurrence of cancer may be large (just as luck plays a substantial part in whether or not an individual driver has a traffic accident), but in a large population luck has little net effect on the incidence of cancer and only nature and nurture are important.

Avoidable factors

Tobacco

Tobacco is by far the most important single cause of cancer in developed countries. Chewed, it can cause cancers of the mouth and oesophagus; smoked, it is a major cause of cancers of the mouth, pharynx (other than nasopharynx), oesophagus, larynx, lung, pancreas, renal pelvis, and bladder. For these eight cancers, epidemiological evidence indicates that prolonged smoking of average numbers of cigarettes per day increases the risk 3 to 20 times. It is, however, now clear that cigarette smoking also causes a proportion of several other types of cancer, increasing the incidence up to twice that in nonsmokers: namely, cancers of the lip, nose, nasopharynx, stomach, liver, and renal body, and also myeloid leukaemia. Although the proportional increases are not large, the consistency of the findings in different countries, the evidence of dose–response relationships, the lower mortality in ex-smokers than in continuing smokers, the lack of evidence for important confounding, and the presence in the smoke of many different carcinogens provide strong grounds for believing that most or all of these observed associations are causal.

In sum, smoking is estimated to have caused 28% of all fatal cancers in the United Kingdom in 2005, down from 34% 30 years earlier. The reduction was substantial in men (down from 52% in 1975 to 39% in 1995 and 33% in 2005) but it was largely counteracted by the increase in women (from 12% in 1975 to 20% in 1995 and 22% in 2005). Comparable figures from the United States and from some other developed countries are shown in Table 6.1.3. In men, there have in the past decade been decreases in many developed countries, but in each the proportions remain substantial. In women, the proportion of cancer deaths attributed to smoking was generally low in 1975, but has subsequently increased in all developed countries and must be expected to increase further. It was, however, still small in countries such as France or Spain, where many young women now smoke but few middle-aged or elderly women have been smoking for long enough for any material effect to be produced.

Figure 6.1.1 shows the overall trends in UK cancer mortality at ages 35–69 since 1950 divided by whether or not they were attributable (in a statistical sense) to smoking; it can be seen how greatly the trends in men especially have been influenced by changes in smoking-attributed mortality.

Table 6.1.3 Per cent of cancer deaths attributed to smoking, 1955, 1975, 1995, and 2005, by sex: various countries

Country	Male				Female			
	1955	1975	1995	2005[a]	1955	1975	1995	2005[a]
Australia	20	40	33	29[a]	0	4	14	15[a]
Finland	38	46	37	31	1	1	5	8
France	17	34	37	35	0	0	3	7
Hungary	21	36	51	50	2	5	13	18
Spain	13	28	39	37	0	0	0	2
UK	41	52	39	33	3	12	20	22
USA	23	42	42	39	0	10	25	27

[a] 2005, except Australia for which the most recent year of data available from WHO was 2004.

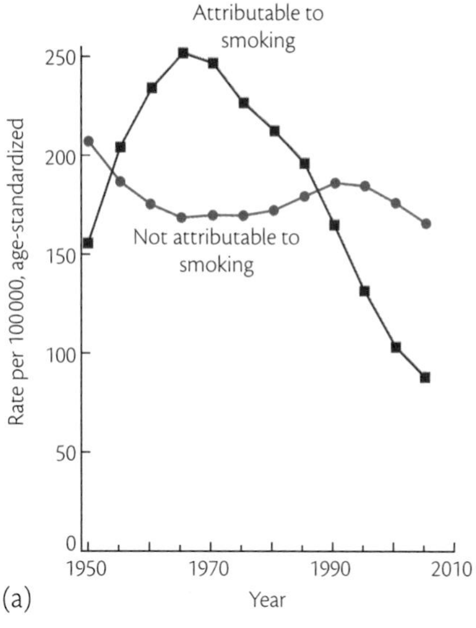

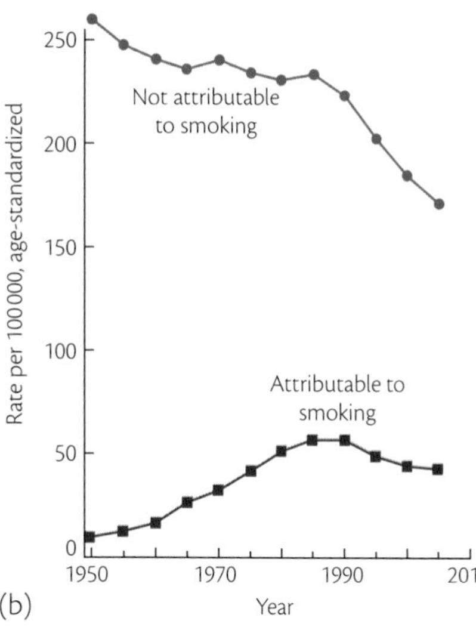

Fig. 6.1.1 United Kingdom cancer mortality at ages 35–69, 1950–2005, attributable to smoking and not attributable to smoking: (a) males (b) females.

In developing countries, the effects of smoking have only recently begun to be studied systematically and much remains unclear. Large, nationally representative studies of smoking and death have, however, been conducted in China and India. In general, women in developing countries do not smoke (although there are particular regions in China and India where they do so). In men, however, there has been a very large increase in worldwide cigarette consumption over the past few decades, the full effects of which have yet to materialize. China, with 20% of the world's population, smokes 30% of the world's cigarettes and by 1987 smoking was already responsible for about 20% of male cancer deaths (and 12% of all male deaths in China at ages 35–69), and this proportion is likely to at least double between the 1980s and the 2020s. In India, where many men have smoked 'bidis' (small, home-manufactured cigarettes) for decades, smoking now causes 32% of all male cancer deaths (and 20% of all male deaths in India at ages 35–69), partly because smoking can act as a cofactor for the production of cancers of the mouth, oesophagus, or stomach in those who habitually chew quids containing betel and tobacco. In some parts of South America and China the male lung cancer rates from smoking are already as high as in developed countries. Overall, tobacco may be causing about as many cancer deaths in developing as in developed countries, in which case it would be responsible for about 20% of cancer deaths throughout the world.

Alcohol

At least six types of cancer are caused in part by the consumption of alcohol. One, liver cancer, is produced mainly by the production of liver cirrhosis and is, consequently, caused mainly by heavy and prolonged consumption. Four are causally related to smoking as well as to alcohol: namely, cancers of the mouth, pharynx (other than nasopharynx), oesophagus, and larynx. The two agents act synergistically, increasing each other's effect, so that the risk from alcohol in nonsmokers or long-term ex-smokers is very small, while that in heavy smokers is disproportionately large. The remaining type, cancer of the breast, has been shown to be related to alcohol more recently. Epidemiological cohort studies show that the risk increases progressively with the amount drunk (at least up to moderately high levels) and laboratory studies that show that alcohol increases the level of oestrogen in the blood suggest a plausible mechanism.

Cancers of the large bowel have also been associated with alcohol in many studies, but the relationship is weak and its nature uncertain: it could be due to confounding by diet.

Ionizing radiation

Ionizing radiations, of whatever type, and whether from external sources or from inhaled or ingested radionuclides, share the characteristic of having sufficient energy to damage DNA through ionization when they pass through the tissues of the body. It is not surprising, therefore, that they have been found to increase the incidence of cancer in practically every organ. The radiosensitivity of different organs varies greatly, however, and particularly large risks, relative to background rates, occur for thyroid cancer in people exposed as children, for myeloid leukaemia, and for cancers of the breast and bladder. In contrast, there is no good evidence that exposure to ionizing radiation can increase the risk of chronic lymphocytic leukaemia, Hodgkin's disease, or testis cancer. Many exposures to ionizing radiation are specific to certain parts of the body or to certain organs or tissues, and this determines the site of the induced cancer. For example, the sites of cancers after radiotherapy depend on the sites exposed to radiation as a consequence of the treatment; Thorotrast (a radioactive contrast agent used in the mid 20th century) tends to be incorporated in the liver and bone marrow and hence to cause liver cancer and leukaemia; inhalation and ingestion of iodine-131 was the principal exposure from the Chernobyl accident to the general population in the surrounding areas, which led to an increase in thyroid cancer in children; and inhalation of the natural radioactive gas radon and its progeny gives rise to lung cancer.

Estimates of the carcinogenic effect of X-rays have been derived by following groups of people with unusual but well-documented exposures, including patients given radiotherapy, or repeatedly screened radiologically, and the survivors of the atomic bombings of Hiroshima and Nagasaki (in whom exposure was principally to γ-rays, which are high-energy X-rays). Estimates of the risk of lung cancer from the inhalation of radon and its progeny have been derived both from studies of uranium miners and from studies of indoor radon exposure carried out in the general population.

At low doses (<*c.*20 mGy) it seems probable that the carcinogenic effect of ionizing radiation is linearly proportional to the dose, while at higher doses the same is true for most cancers other than leukaemia, for which the risk is approximately proportional to the square of the dose. For most sites of cancer the risk is higher in people exposed in childhood than those exposed as adults, and it starts within the first 5 years and lasts for several decades. The International Commission on Radiological Protection (2007) has concluded that the lifetime risk of developing a fatal cancer is approximately 10%/Gy for X-rays (or per Sievert for other types of radiation) to the whole body if the radiation dose is moderate and given acutely, and about half that if the dose is low and spread out over time (that is 5 per 100 000 per mGy (or mSv)), with corresponding reductions if only part of the body is exposed.

It has not been possible to detect by direct observation the effect of very small exposures, including, for example, the effect of a single chest radiograph given to an adult. However, theoretical considerations and the dose–response relationship observed at larger doses both indicate that there is unlikely to be any threshold below which no effect is produced. This conclusion is reinforced by the observation that children who received doses of 10 to 20 mGy *in utero* (because their mothers were irradiated for diagnostic purposes while pregnant) were subject to an added risk of developing cancer in childhood of approximately 1 in 2000.

People are exposed to different amounts of radiation in different countries, depending principally on the concentration of radon in indoor air and the medical use of radiation for diagnosis. In the United Kingdom, the average indoor radon concentration is $20 Bq/m^3$ and this is estimated to give rise to about 1000 lung cancer deaths each year. In the United States the average radon concentration is about twice that for the United Kingdom and, within the United Kingdom, it varies from one part of the country to another. Most notably, Devon and Cornwall have average indoor radon concentrations three or four times greater than the national average and there are a few houses with concentrations that are 10 or even 100 times greater. Other sources of radiation are estimated to give rise to an average annual dose of about 1.4 mSv in the United Kingdom, which, on the basis of the risk estimate recommended by the International Commission on Radiological Protection, would lead to about 4200 deaths per year in the national population of about 60 million. This gives an estimated total of 5200 deaths per year from radiation-induced cancer, or just over 3% of total cancer deaths. The major contributors are radon (20%), other natural sources (55%), and medical uses (24%). In addition, there is a contribution from radiotherapy for cancer, but less than might at first sight be implied from the collective dose, because a substantial proportion is received by people who will not survive long enough for a radiation-induced cancer to appear. Less than 1% of all radiation-induced deaths in the United Kingdom can be attributed to occupational exposure, fallout from past nuclear weapons tests, manufactured products, or radioactive waste.

Ultraviolet radiation

Photon energies in the ultraviolet (UV) range are sufficient to damage DNA and hence to cause cancer mutations. UV does not penetrate much below the skin, so that it is chiefly within the skin that it is directly carcinogenic. Within the skin, however, it is the principal cause of all types of cancer, other than Kaposi's sarcoma. Whether it has any indirect carcinogenic effect on other tissues (notably the lymphopoietic tissue) remains uncertain. The main source of human exposure to UV radiation is sunshine.

Table 6.1.4 Viral causes of cancer

Virus	Cancer
Hepatitis B	Cancer of liver
Hepatitis C	Cancer of liver
HPV types 16, 18, and others	Cancers of cervix, vulva, vagina, penis, anus; some skin cancers
HHV type 4 (EBV)	Burkitt's lymphoma
	Post transplant lymphoproliferative disease
	Nasal T-cell lymphoma
	Other non-Hodgkin's lymphoma
	Hodgkin's disease[b]
	Nasopharyngeal cancer
HHV type 8 (Kaposi-associated herpesvirus)	Kaposi's sarcoma Primary effusion lymphoma
Human T-cell leukaemia type 1	Adult T-cell leukaemia/lymphoma
HIV[a]	Kaposi's sarcoma
	Non-Hodgkin's lymphoma
	Hodgkin's disease
	Conjunctival carcinoma

EBV, Epstein–Barr virus; HHV, human herpesvirus; HPV, human papillomavirus.

[a] In most cases, if not in all, by facilitating the effect of other viruses, probably via immunosuppression.

[b] Causal nature of observed association unproven.

Simian virus 40 (SV-40) has been suspected in the aetiology of mesothelioma and several other types of cancer, without clear proof.

Infection

Infection, principally viral, but also in some cases bacterial and parasitic, is a major cause of avoidable cancer, especially in developing countries: in sub-Saharan Africa about 40% of cancers in women and 30% in men, compared with about 10% in developed countries, are attributable to infections.

Viral infection

Viruses that are known to cause human cancers, or suspected of doing so, are listed in Table 6.1.4, along with the types of cancer with which they are associated. Not all infected people develop the disease. In some cases the proportion doing so is quite small, unless other factors are also present. Such cofactors include endemic malaria for Burkitt's lymphoma, the consumption of a type of salted fish for nasopharyngeal cancer, and the consumption of aflatoxin, a metabolic product of fungal infection with *Aspergillus flavus*, for liver cancer. What they are for the cancers produced by the human papillomavirus is not known.

Quantitatively, chronic infection with hepatitis B virus is one of the most important causes of cancer in many parts of the world. In China, for example, liver cancer accounts for about 18% of all cancer deaths, the large majority of which are due to chronic lifelong infection with the virus. Infant vaccination against the virus is now being introduced and will protect those born in the present century, but will not provide retrospective protection for those born in the 20th century.

Bacterial infection

Only one specific bacterial infection has been closely linked with the development of cancer: *Helicobacter pylori*. Persistent *H. pylori* infection acquired early in life leads to chronic gastritis in the antrum of the stomach and increases the risk of gastric cancer two- to three-fold. Nonspecific chronic infection in the bladder may increase the risk of bladder cancer.

Parasitic infection

In parts of Africa and Asia, parasitic infection is a major cause of cancer. Infection with *Schistosoma haematobium*, which excretes its eggs through the bladder wall, causes a high incidence of bladder cancer in Egypt and East Africa while infection with *S. japonicum*, which excretes its eggs through the wall of the large bowel, is responsible for a high incidence of intestinal cancer in parts of China. Liver flukes (*Clonorchis sinensis* and *Opisthorcis viverrini*) are similarly responsible for the high incidence of cholangiosarcoma of the bile ducts in parts of South East Asia. The parasites may not cause cancer directly, but chronic infection may start a chain of events that leads to cancer in other ways, such as chronic bacterial infection and the local formation of nitrites and nitrosamines.

Immunosuppression

Patients with persistent immunosuppression, either therapeutic (notably immunosuppressive drug treatment for organ transplant patients) or as a consequence of infection (e.g. HIV) or genetic (e.g. in ataxia telangiectasia and Wiskott–Aldrich syndrome) have greatly raised risks of non-Hodgkin's lymphoma, and often of other viral infection-related cancers including Kaposi's sarcoma, although the pattern of malignancy and scale of risk varies according to the type of immunosuppression—Kaposi's sarcoma, for instance, predominates after HIV, whereas non-Hodgkin's lymphoma is the most common consequence of genetic immunodeficiency and of transplantation.

Medical drugs

Apart from ionizing radiation, some 20 agents have been used therapeutically that are known to cause cancer in humans. These are listed in Table 6.1.5. That so many carcinogenic agents should have been prescribed medically is not surprising when it is borne in mind that treatment often requires modification of cellular metabolism and is sometimes intended to interfere with DNA. The hazard of cancer, however, need not necessarily be a bar to the use of a drug if this risk is outweighed by the therapeutic benefits, as is commonly the case with antineoplastic agents, immunosuppressive drugs, and radiotherapy.

Some of the chemotherapeutic agents listed in Table 6.1.5 were soon abandoned, while others have continued to be used for the treatment of uncommon conditions, and the sum of the cancers that these now produce cannot amount to more than 100 or so a year in the United Kingdom.

Two of the listed drugs are, however, used extensively in the general population: hormonal replacement therapy (HRT) for postmenopausal women, and selected steroids for contraception, which increase the risk of breast cancer. Both also increase the risk of endometrial cancer, but HRT does so substantially only when given in the form of oestrogen alone and steroid contraceptives do so only in the form (now abandoned) in which oestrogen and progestogen are given sequentially. The combined steroid contraceptives currently in use can also rarely cause liver cancer and they may possibly increase the risk of cervix cancer. Combined steroid contraceptives, however, also reduce the incidence of endometrial cancer and halve the risk of ovarian cancer for many years after they have been used, and HRT and combined steroid contraceptives are associated with a reduction of some 20% in the risk of colorectal cancer, although whether this is causally related to their use remains unknown.

Table 6.1.5 Carcinogenic agents used in medical practice (other than ionizing radiations)

Agent	Type of cancer
Antineoplastic agents including:	
Busulphan	Leukaemia[a]
Carmustine (BCNU)	Leukaemia
Chlorambucil	Leukaemia[a]
Chlornaphazine	Bladder
Cyclophosphamide	Bladder, leukaemia[a]
Lomustine (CCNU)	Leukaemia
Epipodophyllotoxins	Leukaemia
Melphalan	Leukaemia[a]
MOPP[b]	Leukaemia[a], probably lung[c]
Thiotepa	Leukaemia
Treosulfan	Leukaemia[a]
Arsenic	Skin, liver (angiosarcoma), lung
Immunosuppressive drugs:	
Azathioprine	Non-Hodgkin's lymphoma, Kaposi's sarcoma[d]
Ciclosporin	Non-Hodgkin's lymphoma, Kaposi's sarcoma[d]
Methoxypsoralen (plus UV radiation)	Skin
Phenacetin	Renal pelvis, bladder
Polycyclic hydrocarbons (coal-tar ointment)	Skin
Sex hormones:	
Unopposed oestrogens	Endometrium, breast
Transplacental diethylstilbestrol	Vagina and cervix (adenocarcinoma)
Oxymetholone (an anabolic steroid)	Liver (hepatoma)
Oral contraceptives (combined)[e]	Breast, liver (hepatoma)
Tamoxifen[e]	Endometrium

[a] Acute or nonlymphocytic.
[b] Combination of nitrogen mustard, vincristine, procarbazine, and prednisone.
[c] Lung cancer might also be caused by certain other alkylating agents or regimens.
[d] There have also been excesses of several other cancers in transplant patients treated with immunosuppressive drugs.
[e] Oral contraceptives also reduce the risk of ovarian and endometrial cancers and tamoxifen reduces the risk of contralateral breast cancer.

Other drugs that may inhibit cancer rather than cause it are the nonsteroidal analgesics, most notably aspirin, the prolonged use of which may somewhat reduce the risk of colorectal cancer and perhaps cancers of certain other sites.

Taken altogether, it seems unlikely that medically prescribed drugs can be responsible for more than 1% of all today's fatal cancers and may, in total, reduce the risk by somewhat more.

Occupation

In the years that followed Pott's observation that chimney sweeps tended to develop cancer of the scrotum, many other groups of workers were found to suffer from specific hazards of cancer; indeed, more substances that are known to be carcinogenic to humans have been unearthed by the search for occupational hazards than by any other means. Most of these occupational cancers are in the respiratory tract, especially the lung. The hazards are listed in Table 6.1.6. Many of the hazards that have been recognized caused large, or at least relatively large, risks, albeit for limited populations, and it may well be that other occupational causes exist that have not yet been detected, either because the added risk is small in comparison with that due to other causes, or because only a few workers have been persistently exposed, or simply because the hazards have not been suspected and so not looked for. It must also be borne in mind that cancer in humans seldom develops until one or more decades after exposure to the carcinogen first occurs and it is, therefore, too soon to be sure whether agents that have been introduced into industry only during the last 20 years are carcinogenic or not.

Many groups of workers not listed in Table 6.1.6 have been suspected of having a special risk, but it has not been possible to decide whether the risk is real and attributable to their work. Some of these excesses may have arisen by chance alone, especially if the excess has not been confirmed in other studies, and others may be due to confounding; i.e. they may have been produced by social factors or behaviours that are associated with the occupation in question rather than by the occupation itself.

Given sufficient details and the ability to repeat the observations, it is usually possible to obtain a fairly clear idea of whether an excess incidence in an occupational group reflects an occupational hazard e.g. by seeing whether the effect is related to the length of employment, the time after first exposure, and a specific type of work within the industry. Unfortunately these details are not always available and the reasons for many of the moderate excesses of cancer that have been reported in certain industries are still uncertain.

In addition to the directly occupational cancers discussed above, workers may be indirectly exposed to carcinogens while at work—e.g. tobacco smoke from clients or colleagues.

At present it seems likely that occupational hazards account for only a few per cent of all fatal cancers in developed countries such as the United Kingdom. The three principal causes are probably asbestos dust (lung and pleural cancer), the combustion products of fossil fuels (skin and lung cancer), and ionizing radiation (a wide range of cancers).

Table 6.1.6 Occupational causes of cancer

Agent	Type of cancer	Occupation[a]
Aromatic amines:	Bladder	Dye manufacturers
4-Aminodiphenyl		Rubber workers
Benzidine		Coal-gas manufacturers
2-Naphthylamine		Some chemical workers
Arsenic	Skin, lung	Copper and cobalt smelters
		Pesticide manufacturers
		Some gold miners
Asbestos (all forms)	Lung, pleura, peritoneum	Asbestos miners
		Asbestos textile manufacturers
		Carpenters and general builders
		Insulation workers
		Shipyard workers
Benzene	Leukaemia	Workers with glues and varnishes
Beryllium[b]	Lung	Beryllium refiners and machiners
Bis-chloromethyl ether and technical-grade chloromethyl methyl ether	Lung	Makers of ion-exchange resins
Cadmium[b]	Lung	Cadmium refiners
Chromium[b]	Lung[c]	Manufacturers of chromates from chrome ore; pigment manufacturers
Ionizing radiations	Lung	Uranium and some other miners
	Bone	Luminizers
	Leukaemia, skin	Radiologists, radiographers
Mustard gas	Larynx, lung	Poison-gas manufacturers
Nickel[b]	Nasal sinuses, lung	Nickel refiners
Polycyclic hydrocarbons in soot, tar, oil	Skin, scrotum, lung, and sometimes bladder	Coal-gas manufacturers, roofers, asphalters, aluminium refiners, and many groups exposed to tars and selected oils
Silica, when crystalline as quartz or cristobalite	Lung	Miners, stone workers, refractory brick workers
Sulphuric acid mists (strong acid)	Nasal sinuses, larynx	Many industries, isopropanol manufacture, 'steel pickling'
Ultraviolet radiation	Skin (melanoma and nonmelanoma)	Farmers, seamen
Vinyl chloride	Liver (angiosarcoma)	PVC manufacturers
?	Nasal sinuses	Hardwood furniture manufacturers
?	Nasal sinuses	Leather workers

[a] Typical occupations with proven hazards.
[b] Certain compounds or oxidation states.
[c] And possibly nasal sinuses.

Pollution

The idea that pollution might be an important cause of cancer has been in the forefront of the minds of cancer research workers since it was realized that the incidence of lung cancer tended to be higher in towns than in the countryside and that the combustion products of coal, which used to produce a pall of smoke over all large cities in Britain, contained carcinogenic hydrocarbons. Subsequently, with the rapid expansion of the chemical industry and the discovery that some of its products are mutagenic *in vitro* and carcinogenic in laboratory animals, anxiety increased about the possible effects of distributing such products ubiquitously in the air we breathe, the water we drink, and the food we eat.

The effects of pollution of this sort are, however, peculiarly difficult to assess directly by epidemiological methods, as pollutants are likely to be present in most areas, the absolute risk from each is likely to be small, and there may be little difference in the extent to which individuals are exposed over a wide area. Reliance is, therefore, often placed mainly on two indirect methods: extrapolation from the effects of chronic exposure to much larger amounts in an occupational setting, and prediction of the effects on humans from laboratory tests. Both, however, (but particularly the latter) involve substantial uncertainties.

So far as atmospheric pollution is concerned, the epidemiological picture is complicated by the personal pollution produced by tobacco smoke and the social distribution of smoking habits. Despite this complication, however, the various methods that have been discussed under lung cancer all lead to the conclusion that the pollution of the past may have contributed to the production of a few per cent of all lung cancers in Western countries, but that the levels over the last three decades (principally from the combustion of fossil fuels, but also from asbestos, dioxins, and various other materials) are unlikely to be responsible for more than a fraction of 1% of future cancers—although there may be exceptions awaiting discovery in the neighbourhood of particular factories. The greater effect of the modern type of pollution with ultra fine particles and of the intense indoor pollution with smoke that occurs in parts of China is examined later under lung cancer and of erionite in certain Turkish villages under pleural cancer.

The effect of polluted drinking water and food is more obscure. Modern analytical techniques permit the detection of chemicals at concentrations of less than 1 part per billion in both food and water and, in consequence, many have been detected that might arguably be carcinogenic, including pesticide residues and a variety of halogenated organic materials produced by the chlorination of water supplies. Relationships have been reported between the concentrations of some of these compounds in water and the mortality from cancers of the bladder and, possibly, the large intestine, in different localities, but it is extremely difficult to know what these relationships mean as there are many potentially confounding factors.

Mortality rates from cancers of the gastrointestinal and urinary tracts are, for the most part, stable or decreasing in early middle age, when the effects of new agents might be expected to show themselves first, and, in the absence of more specific evidence, it seems unlikely that chemical pollution of water and food could have a greater effect than the small effect already estimated for pollution of the air.

Diet

For many years there has been suggestive evidence that most of the cancers that are currently common could be made less so by modification of the diet, but, with few exceptions, there is still little reliable evidence as to the modifications that would be of major importance. If we define diet to include all materials that occur in natural foods, are produced during the processes of storage, cooking, and digestion, or are added as preservatives or to give food colour, flavour, and consistency, the ways in which diet could influence the development of cancer are legion.

Ingestion of preformed carcinogens

The most obvious is the ingestion of small amounts of powerful carcinogens or precarcinogens. Several have been identified in foodstuffs but only two have been related at all clearly to the production of cancer in humans. One is aflatoxin, a metabolic product of *Aspergillus flavus*, which contaminates stored or oily foods such as grains and peanuts in many countries, and is a major cause of liver cancer in the tropics among those individuals who are also chronic carriers of the hepatitis B (or less commonly hepatitis C) virus. Likewise, the salted fish eaten extensively in South China probably acts synergistically with Epstein–Barr virus to cause nasopharyngeal cancer. A third possible source is bracken fern, an extract of which is carcinogenic in animals. It is eaten extensively in Japan and has been tentatively linked with the development of oesophageal cancer. The polycyclic hydrocarbons and other mutagens that are produced in food by grilling or smoking have often been suspected of playing a role, but intensive investigation has failed to detect one.

It seems, therefore, that if diet does affect the incidence of cancer in the Western world in any material way, it is likely to do so by more indirect means, such as affecting the formation, transport, activation or deactivation of carcinogens in the body or affecting the secretion of hormones.

Overnutrition

That overnutrition could affect the incidence of cancer was first suggested by Tannenbaum's experiments on mice during the Second World War. These showed that the incidence of various spontaneous tumours and tumours produced experimentally could be halved by moderately restricting the intake of food without modifying the proportions of the individual constituents. This protective effect has subsequently been demonstrated repeatedly, but has attracted little attention. It is now clear, however, that what is considered normal nutrition in developed countries increases the risk of breast cancer (by bringing forward menarche and increasing body size). With greater consumption obesity (i.e. a body mass index $>25\,kg/m^2$) has been estimated to be responsible for 5% of all incident cancers in Europe and 10% of all cancer deaths in nonsmokers in the United States: most notably, cancer of the breast in women after the menopause and cancers of the endometrium, large bowel, and kidney, probably cancers of the oesophagus and gallbladder, and perhaps cancers of the prostate and thyroid. The increases in the two female cancers in postmenopausal women are probably attributable to the formation of oestrogen from androstenedione in adipose tissue, but for others the explanation is unclear.

Meat and fat

Figures for food consumption and cancer incidence and mortality rates in different countries show fairly close correlations between the consumption of fat, and to a lesser extent the consumption of meat, and the incidence of several types of cancer. The correlations are closest for breast cancer and cancer of the large bowel and are less strong for cancers of the endometrium, pancreas, and prostate. When, however, attempts are made to associate the consumption of either type of food with the disease in individuals within a country, the evidence is commonly conflicting. This could be because the international correlations are misleading, indicating only that the risks are correlated with something that is itself correlated with fat and meat consumption (e.g. some other aspect of a high gross national product), but it could be partly because of the inaccuracy of dietary histories and partly because people within developed countries eat such similar diets. Overviews of the published data, however, do suggest that a high consumption of fat is associated with a high risk of colorectal cancer, but the claim that a high consumption of fat (or of particular types of fat) is associated with high risks of breast and endometrial cancer after the menopause, other than by providing a high-calorie diet leading to obesity, is controversial.

Whether meat increases the risk of any type of cancer, apart from the contribution it makes through its calorie content, is also uncertain. The low incidence of several types of cancer that is commonly observed in vegetarian communities is not necessarily due to the absence of meat from the diet, as it can generally be explained by the increased consumption of protective foods (vegetables and fruits) and commonly by associated behavioural characteristics (below average use of tobacco and alcohol). Some studies that make allowance for these confounding factors have claimed that meat specifically increases the risk of large-bowel cancer, but the evidence is weak and the increase in risk, if any, is small.

Fibre

That fibre may play a part was suggested by Burkitt's observation that several intestinal diseases, including cancer of the colon, were common in countries in which cereals were processed to remove the fibre and rare in rural Africa and Asia where they were not. The idea was attractive, as 'fibre' passes through the small bowel unchanged and serves as pabulum for the colonic bacteria, thus increasing faecal bulk and possibly protecting mechanically against the development of cancer by diluting any carcinogens present and hastening their transit through the bowel. The idea was too simple, however, and has not been confirmed (using the original definition of fibre) by either epidemiological studies on individuals in developed countries or by experiments aimed at reducing the recurrence of colorectal adenomas. In fact, fibre is difficult to define and the term is better replaced by 'nonstarch polysaccharides' as there are many that share the characteristics of passing through the small bowel unchanged and being, for the most part, partially or wholly degraded by bacteria in the large bowel. Some starch, moreover, known as 'resistant starch' and found in green bananas and cold potatoes, has similar physiological characteristics. Further studies that take these complexities into account are, therefore, needed before 'fibre' in any of its manifestations can be considered as having any place in protecting against the development of cancer.

Retinoids and carotenoids

Experiments on animals and on cell cultures *in vitro* have suggested that vitamin A (retinol) and its esters and analogues (retinoids) may, in appropriate circumstances, reduce the risk of cancer by reducing the probability that partially transformed cells become fully transformed and proliferate into clinically detectable tumours, although in other circumstances they appear to have opposite effects. Human studies, however, did not support the idea that serum levels of retinol are related to the risk of any type of cancer, at least in countries in which clinical symptoms of vitamin A deficiency seldom or never occur. Such studies suggested that the risks were inversely related to the serum level of β-carotene, which acts as an antioxidant and is broken down to produce retinol. When β-carotene was put to the test of clinical trials, however, it provided no benefit and the inverse relationship commonly observed in epidemiological studies is presumably due to confounding with some other protective factors in vegetables.

Other components

Many other components of the diet, including lycopene in tomatoes, indoles in brassicas (e.g. cabbages and sprouts), phyto-oestrogens (plant chemicals structurally similar to oestradiol), fresh fruit and vegetables, vitamins C, D, and E, and calcium and selenium have also been proposed as protective agents. Conversely, nitrates, nitrites, secondary amines, and the preservation of food by salting, have been thought to increase the risk of cancer. For some the evidence is strongly suggestive: notably for vitamin C as protective against gastric cancer and for salt-preserved foods predisposing to it. In general, however, the evidence of benefit or harm is too weak to justify any firm conclusion.

Conclusion

Some of the uncertainties about the effect of diet could be resolved only by means of controlled trials in which volunteers are allocated at random to micronutrient supplements (such as vitamin C or lycopene) or a dietary schedule that requires a substantial reduction in the consumption of fat. Several such studies are under way, which may give answers within a few years. Practicable modifications of the diet may well provide the means for reducing cancer deaths in developed countries by one-third, but the range of uncertainty about this figure is large. Meanwhile the only dietary changes that can be recommended with confidence in developed countries are a general increase in the use of fresh fruit and vegetables and a sufficient limitation of calories to avoid obesity.

Reproduction, other factors affecting secretion of reproductive hormones, and other hormones

Epidemiological observations have shown clear relationships between a woman's menstrual and reproductive history and the risk of cancers of the breast, endometrium, and ovary, which are generally thought to reflect changes in hormonal secretions. Which hormones are concerned, however, and the mechanisms by which they act are, for the most part, still uncertain. An exception is endometrial cancer, the risk of which is directly related to the degree of exposure to oestrogen not followed after an appropriate interval by progestogen. Strong evidence that oestrogenic stimulation of the mammary tissues is a cause of most cases of breast cancer in developed countries has been provided by randomized trials of tamoxifen, an antioestrogenic drug that blocks the oestrogen receptors in the cells of the normal breast. The effect is large and rapid: 5 years of tamoxifen approximately halves the incidence of contralateral breast cancer in a woman who has had previous breast cancer, not only while the drug is being taken but also for some years afterwards. Exogenous oestrogen also increases the risk of breast cancer when given as hormonal replacement therapy and endogenous oestrogen accounts for the increased risk associated with adiposity after the menopause, as androstenedione, which continues to be produced by the adrenals, is converted to oestrogen in adipose tissue. It is presumably oestrogens, too, that cause a small increase in risk of breast cancer during and immediately after pregnancy and the oestrogen component of the steroid contraceptives that causes a similar small increase in risk during their use and for a few years after their use is stopped. It is, however, unclear which hormone-related processes are involved in reducing the long-term risk for the rest of a woman's life that occurs some years after the occurrence of each pregnancy and it is equally unclear why the use of oral contraception and the consequent suppression of ovulation reduces the long-term risk of ovarian cancer.

Sex hormones, it is thought, may also be involved in producing cancers of the testis and prostate in men. For testis cancer, the strongest evidence has been for an effect of maternal oestrogen levels on the developing testis *in utero*, whereas for prostate cancer the evidence relates to adult androgen levels, but for neither has causation been established. Randomized trials of the effects of physical or medical castration in men who already have prostate

cancer have shown that progression of the disease can be slowed substantially, presumably by the reduction of androgenic stimulation.

In recent years it has been found that prior raised endogenous levels of insulin-like growth factor-1 (IGF-1) are associated with raised risk of cancers of the breast, colon, and prostate, and there has also been evidence that endogenous and exogenous growth hormone affects the risk of colorectal cancer.

Physical inactivity

Physical inactivity contributes to the risk of cancer indirectly by increasing the risk of obesity but it may also contribute directly. Associations with colon, breast, and endometrial cancers have fairly consistently been reported, and an association with prostate cancer has been found in most studies. The mechanism of effect is uncertain, but possibilities include effects of exercise on hormone levels, on immune function, and on intestinal transit time and hence the duration of exposure of the colonic mucosa to faecal carcinogens.

Interaction of agents

Attribution of the risk of cancer to different causes is complicated by the fact that some agents interact with others to produce effects that are much greater than the sum of the separate effects of each on its own. An example is provided by smoking and asbestos, which multiply each other's effects so that, compared with non-smokers in general, the incidence of cancer of the lung was increased sixfold among a group of asbestos insulation workers in the United States of America who did not smoke, but were heavily exposed to asbestos dust in the 1940s, 10- to 20-fold among cigarette smokers in general who did not work with asbestos, and nearly 90-fold among the asbestos workers who also smoked cigarettes regularly. Other examples are provided by smoking and radon (which interact similarly, though somewhat less than multiplicatively, to produce cancer of the lung), by smoking and alcohol (which interact to produce cancers of the mouth, pharynx, larynx, and oesophagus), and by infection with the hepatitis B virus and aflatoxin (which interact to produce cancer of the liver).

Such interactions complicate the attribution of risk, as we may find ourselves appearing to claim that more cancer can be prevented than actually occurs by attributing, say, 80% of lung cancers in men heavily exposed to asbestos to their occupational exposure and 90% of the same cancers to cigarette smoking. Each, separately, is correct, but they cannot be added to show the combined effect.

Table 6.1.7 Estimated proportion of United Kingdom cancer deaths in the year 2005 attributed to previous exposure to different environmental and behavioural factors and proportion of future United Kingdom cancer deaths avoidable by known effects of practicable changes in current exposure levels

Factor or class of factors	Percentage of UK cancer deaths in 2005 attributed to previous exposure levels		Estimated percentage of future UK cancer deaths avoidable by known effects of practicable changes in current exposure levels
	Best estimate	Range of acceptable estimates	
Tobacco	28	25–30	<28[a]
Alcohol	6	4–8	<6[b]
Ionizing radiation	3[c]	2–4	<1
Ultraviolet radiation	1	1	<1
Infection (virus 3%, bacteria 2%)	5	4–15	<1[d]
Medical drugs	<1	0–1	<1
Occupation	4	3–5	<1[e]
Pollution	2	1–5	<1
Diet	25	15–35	<8[f]
Reproductive and hormonal[g]	15	10–20	<1
Other and unknown	?	?	?

[a] The proportion of UK cancer deaths attributed to smoking fell from 34% in 1985 to 28% in 2005 and is still decreasing (as current levels of smoking would cause less than 28% of future UK cancer deaths).

[b] Mostly cancer of the upper aerodigestive tract that could have been avoided by not smoking.

[c] 0.8% diagnostic x-rays, <0.1% all other manmade, 0.7% natural radon in houses, 1.8% other cosmic or terrestrial natural sources.

[d] Cervical cancer currently causes 1.4% of UK female cancer deaths. Without screening it would cause several per cent; with even better screening it would cause a fraction of 1%.

[e] Although asbestos exposure is now strictly controlled, the delayed effects of past exposure probably account for about 3% of current cancer mortality (including more than 1% from mesothelioma), and diesel, coal and other smoke must also have appreciable effects, especially if they potentiate tobacco smoke.

[f] In later middle age in the UK almost half are overweight (BMI 25–30 kg/m^2) and a quarter are obese (>30 kg/m^2); minimal cancer mortality is at c.25 kg/m^2, and about 8% of current cancer mortality would be avoided if the overweight and obese had a BMI of 25 kg/m^2. (Instead, BMI is increasing by about 1 kg/m^2 per decade.)

[g] Includes other factors affecting the secretion of reproductive hormones.

Conclusion

Estimates of the proportions of fatal cancers that can be attributed to environmental and behavioural factors, grouped into 11 main categories, are given in Table 6.1.7. The evidence on which these estimates are based is summarized in this chapter and in greater detail by Doll and Peto (1981), Tomatis *et al.* (1990), Stewart and Kleihues (2003), and Schottenfeld and Fraumeni (2006).

The sum of the best estimates in Table 6.1.7 amounts to less than 100%, despite the fact that some of the listed agents interact with one another to augment each other's effect and that some fatal cancers are consequently counted twice. The total would be somewhat more than 100%, however, if the true proportions attributable to some of the categories turn out to be nearer the upper end of the acceptable estimates.

The estimates in the second and third columns of Table 6.1.7 do not distinguish between factors (such as tobacco) that are sufficiently understood to enable specific action to be taken with a guarantee of success and those (such as diet) that are not. They should not, therefore, be taken as guides to the proportion of cancer deaths that can now be prevented by practicable means. This is illustrated by the fourth column in Table 6.1.7, which shows the proportions of United Kingdom cancer deaths in 2005 that are reliably known to be avoidable by practicable means. The percentage attributed to tobacco is more than the sum of the percentages reliably attributable to other specific factors for which practicable preventive measures are available: and tobacco causes about twice as many deaths from other diseases as it does from cancer. The position is different in countries such as China, where hepatitis B virus causes about as many cancer deaths as tobacco and the hazard for future generations can be avoided in a cost-effective way by infant vaccination.

Epidemiology of cancer by site of origin

In the following account of the epidemiology of cancers arising in specific organs, the description of each type is preceded by notes showing its importance in England. One figure gives the proportion of all cancers that arise at the site, from national cancer registrations for England in 2004 and another gives the proportion of all cancer deaths allocated to the site in the national mortality statistics for England and Wales for 2004. A third gives the ratio of the age-standardized incidence rates in England for each sex. The way in which the incidence of the disease varies with age is shown for males and females in a series of graphs, using data for England over a 5-year period (1993–7). Trends in incidence and mortality for each type, along with the trends in possible causative factors, are given by Swerdlow *et al.* (2001). Trends internationally are commented on in the text, and described more fully in Doll *et al.* (1994). Comments on the total worldwide frequency of different cancers are based on data from Parkin (2001); they disregard incidence of nonmelanoma skin cancers, for which reliable international statistics are not available.

Lip

- 0.1% of all cancers and 0.01% of cancer deaths
- Sex ratio of rates 2.0:1; age distribution like oesophageal cancer

Carcinoma of the lip was one of the first types of cancer to be related to an extrinsic cause when, more than 200 years ago, it was noted to occur characteristically in pipe smokers. Many years later it was realized that the disease could also be produced by smoking cigarettes, although much less readily, so that it must be produced by the chemicals in smoke rather than by the nonspecific effect of local heat. It is also much more common in outdoor than in indoor workers and is induced by ultraviolet radiation in the same way as other cancers of the exposed skin. Solar ultraviolet radiation and tobacco account, between them, for the great majority of all cases in the United Kingdom, probably multiplying each other's effects. The disease is much less common than it used to be, because of the decrease in both pipe smoking and outdoor work.

Oral cavity and pharynx (excluding salivary glands and nasopharynx)

- 1.2% of all cancers and 1.0% of cancer deaths
- Sex ratio of rates 2.2:1; age distribution like oesophageal cancer

Cancers of the tongue, mouth, and pharynx (other than nasopharynx) are all related to smoking (of pipes, cigars, and cigarettes) and to the consumption of alcohol. The two factors act synergistically and cancers in these sites are extremely rare in nonsmokers who do not drink alcohol. There is also fairly consistent evidence of an association of risk with low intake of fruit and vegetables.

Cancer of the tongue is much less common in Britain than it was 100 years ago, but the reason for this sharp decline is unknown. One explanation could be the decrease in syphilis, which was commonly believed to be a predisposing factor because of the clinical association with syphilitic leucoplakia. Recent increases in oral and pharyngeal cancer in men are partly due to increased consumption of alcohol and possibly, in the case of pharyngeal cancer, to human papillomavirus infection.

Cancers that occur low in the hypopharynx are distinguished by a tendency to affect women who have suffered from iron-deficiency anaemia and dysphagia.

Cancers of the mouth and pharynx (excluding nasopharynx) are particularly common in south east and central Asia where tobacco smoking is largely replaced by chewing tobacco, betel nut or leaf, and lime (calcium hydroxide). A close association with such chewing habits has been established by studies that have shown that the cancers tend to originate in the part of the mouth in which the quid is usually held—a characteristic that varies both between individuals and between areas. The materials chewed differ in different places and, although the disease is commonly described as 'betel chewer's cancer', betel is not invariably a component of the quid and the most characteristic constituent seems to be a small amount of lime and, in most cases, some form of tobacco. In parts of Asia, the disease is so common that it accounts for 20% of all cancers and in those populations the abandonment of chewing would be the single most effective means of reducing the total incidence of cancer—so long as the habit was not replaced by an increase in tobacco smoking. Among habitual quid chewers, the risks are particularly elevated in those who both chew and smoke—indeed, in parts of India the majority of deaths from betel chewer's cancer could have been avoided if those affected had not also smoked. The incidence might also be reduced by improved nutrition, as the disease in southern Asia tends to be associated with vitamin A deficiency.

In parts of India where women tend to smoke local cigars and cigarettes with the burning end inside the mouth to prevent them going out, the habit is associated with cancer of the palate.

Salivary glands

- 0.2% of all cancers and 0.1% of cancer deaths
- Sex ratio of rates 1.5:1; age distribution, see Fig. 6.1.2

The salivary glands are not common sites for cancer anywhere. They are, however, relatively more common in circumpolar Inuits than others. No causative factors are known other than ionizing radiation exposure, and no notable changes in incidence over time have been reported.

Nasopharynx

- 0.1% of all cancers and of cancer deaths
- Sex ratio of rates 2.5:1; age distribution, see Fig. 6.1.3

Cancers of the nasopharynx, unlike those in other parts of the pharynx, are not related to alcohol and are only weakly related to tobacco. They are rare in most populations but are common in southern China, especially so in Cantonese originating from parts of Guangdong, where the disease is the most common type of cancer. A weak relationship with HLA type has been reported. Moderately high rates have been observed in Eskimos, American Indians, Malays and Filipinos. Rates decrease over succeeding generations in Chinese migrants to (low-risk) Western countries.

DNA characteristic of the Epstein–Barr virus (EBV) has been detected in the nuclei of nasopharyngeal cancer cells and patients with the disease tend to have unusually high antibodies against EBV-related antigens. Among adults, sudden increases in certain EBV antigens in the blood often precede the appearance of a cancer by a few years. Infection with the EBV is, however, almost universal and can be only one of several agents that act in combination to produce the disease. One such agent in Southern China occurs in the 'salted fish' on which children are commonly weaned. This strongly flavoured delicacy bears little relation to the salted fish

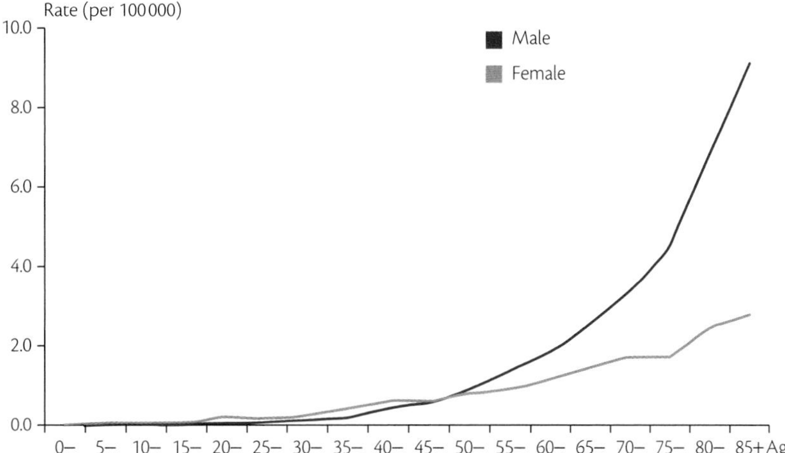

Fig. 6.1.2 Annual incidence of cancers of the salivary glands, by age and sex.

eaten elsewhere, and might better be described as decomposing fish: it contains various mutagens, and exposure to it in childhood when infection with EBV first occurs may alter the usual lifelong balance between host and virus in some hazardous way.

Oesophagus

- 2.1% of all cancers and 4.7% of cancer deaths.
- Sex ratio of rates 2.6:1; age distribution, see Fig. 6.1.4.

Cancer of the oesophagus is the eighth most common cancer in the world. It is exceptional among malignancies in the extent of geographical variation in incidence, both internationally and often also over relatively small distances. Like other cancers of the upper respiratory and digestive tracts, cancer of the oesophagus is closely related to prolonged smoking and the consumption of alcohol. All types of smoking have comparable effects and, so it appears, do all alcoholic drinks, although spirits may be slightly more effective per gram of ethyl alcohol than other alcoholic drinks. Alcohol and tobacco act synergistically and, in the absence of either, the incidence of the disease in Western countries would be greatly reduced. Smoking raises the risk of both squamous cell and adenocarcinoma of the oesophagus whereas alcohol affects largely or solely the former. A few cases originate from the scars produced by poisoning with corrosive substances and a very few in conjunction with a particular hereditary form of tylosis (presenting with keratoses of the palms and soles). The relatively small excess in men probably reflects the existence of other unknown causes in women, possibly nutritional in origin and similar to those responsible for cancers of the hypopharynx. Mortality (which, because of the high fatality rate, approaches incidence) fell progressively in men in Britain from the 1920s to the 1960s, in line with the fall in the consumption of alcohol, and rose again after 1960 when the trend in the consumption of alcohol reversed. Since pipe smoking affects oesophageal cancer risks at least as strongly as cigarette smoking, no large effects on male oesophageal cancer trends could be predicted from the male switch from pipes to cigarettes, although the switch by females from nonsmoking to cigarettes should, other things being equal, produce a large upward trend. It appears, however, that other things were not equal and some other, possibly nutritional, cause of oesophageal cancer seems to have decreased, for the upward trend in oesophageal cancer in women has been moderate. Oesophageal cancer is associated in several studies with low fruit and vegetable consumption. In men, in contrast, the rates have increased when based on smoking they might have been expected to decrease. To some extent this can be accounted for by the increased consumption of alcohol and possibly by an increase in the nitrosamine content of tobacco smoke, which has resulted from changes in the method of curing tobacco and which could have a specific effect on the oesophagus. A part of the increase is due to an increased risk of adenocarcinoma at the lower end of

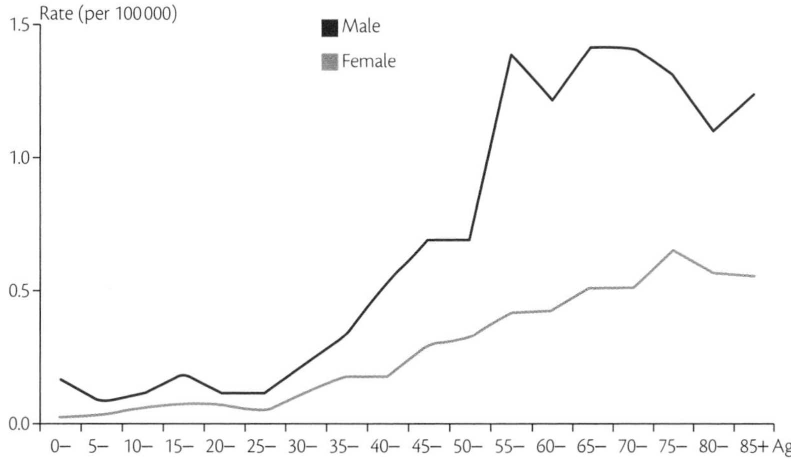

Fig. 6.1.3 Annual incidence of cancer of the nasopharynx by age and sex.

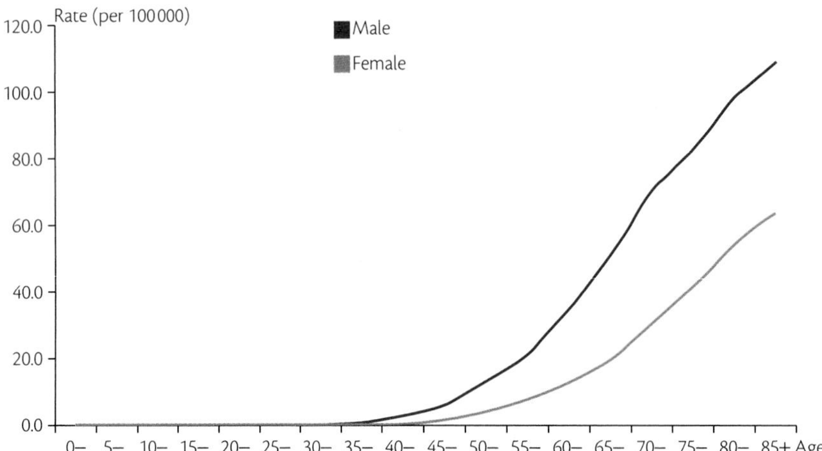

Fig. 6.1.4 Annual incidence of cancer of the oesophagus, by age and sex

the oesophagus, which may be associated with a decreased prevalence of *Helicobacter pylori* and gastritis, and an increase in gastro-oesophageal reflux and Barrett's oesophagus, which is a common precursor of the tumour. Obesity is associated with risk of adenocarcinoma of the oesophagus, perhaps via an effect on reflux. The balance of adenocarcinoma and squamous cell cancer of the oesophagus has altered greatly over time in Western countries, such that the former, which has been increasing, now generally predominates.

In Africa and Asia, the epidemiological features are quite different and present some of the most striking unsolved problems in the field of cancer epidemiology. In parts of China (particularly in north Henan but also elsewhere) and on the east coast of the Caspian Sea in Turkmenistan and Iran, oesophageal cancer is the most common type of cancer, with incidence rates in both sexes that are equal to the highest rates observed for lung cancer in men in European cities. Within China, the disease varies more than 10-fold from one county to another. In parts of Africa, particularly in the Transkei region of South Africa and on the east coast of Lake Victoria in Kenya, extremely high rates are also observed, sometimes equally in both sexes and sometimes only in men. In these and several other areas, the high incidence zones are strictly localized and the incidence falls off rapidly over distances of 200 or 300 miles (*c.*300–500 km).

When tobacco and alcohol are used they increase the hazard, but they are not the principal agents in these high-incidence areas. Many dietary causes have been proposed, including micronutrient deficiencies, contamination of food and pickled vegetables by fungi (particularly by species of fusaria) with the production of carcinogenic metabolites, an agent associated with the production of beer from maize, drinking very hot beverages, and the residues left behind in pipes from smoking opium (which are commonly swallowed). None, however, is supported by any impressive, consistent epidemiological data. The high-incidence area in Iran, which has been intensively investigated, is characterized by extreme poverty and a restricted diet consisting chiefly of home-made bread and tea, with some sheep's milk and milk products, and very little meat, vegetables, or fruit. In this area the disease has been common for centuries. In southern Africa, however, it seems to have become common only since the First World War. In China, where cancer of the oesophagus was the second most important neoplastic cause of death in the 1970s, the high incidence has persisted.

Stomach

- 2.3% of all cancers and 3.8% of cancer deaths
- Sex ratio of rates 2.4:1; age distribution like oesophageal cancer

Until about 1980, gastric cancer was responsible for more deaths from malignant disease worldwide than any other; it is now second to lung cancer, with over 600 000 deaths per year, mainly in developing countries. Over the last 50 years, the incidence has declined in Western countries (see Fig. 6.1.5), and recently it has begun to do so in South America and Japan.

The highest rates now are in parts of Japan and China, with high rates also in other parts of Eastern Asia, and countries in the ex-Soviet Union and Eastern Europe, while low rates are found both in North America and Australasia, and in some of the least

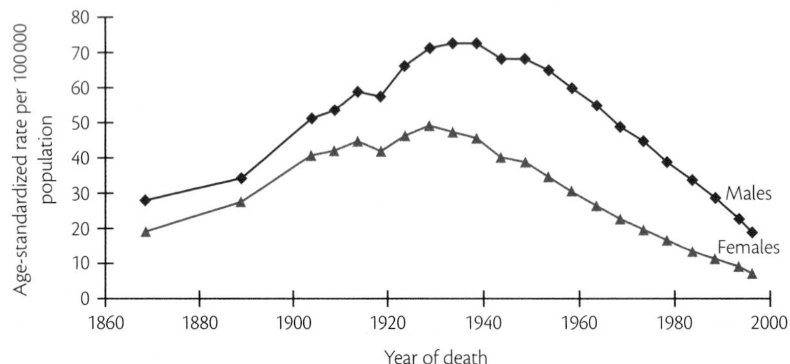

Fig. 6.1.5 Mortality from cancer of stomach, England and Wales, 1868–1997, ages 35 and older, by sex.

developed parts of Africa. This contrasts with the strong socioeconomic gradient in incidence of the tumour seen within Western countries. Irrespective of whether the incidence in a country is high or low, the sex ratio is generally between 1.5 and 3 to 1.

In migrants from high-risk to low-risk countries, for instance from Japan to the United States of America, risk decreases with longer time since migration, but can take two or more generations to reach local levels. Risk of gastric cancer is raised in relation to gastritis associated with chronic infection by *H. pylori* (sometimes leading to atrophic gastritis), a diet deficient in fruit and green and yellow vegetables, and a poor diet with large amounts of salt and salt-preserved food. Chronic infection with *H. pylori*, which is very common, is a major cause of peptic ulcer, a finding that is of considerable practical value in patients with ulcers, because the infection can generally be eliminated from the stomach by a short course of appropriate antibiotic therapy and this provides long-term protection against recurrence. Whether such treatments will have any material effect on the incidence of stomach cancer remains, however, to be shown. How these various factors influence the production of the disease is unclear. One possibility is that they encourage or discourage the formation of carcinogens *in vivo*, particularly perhaps the production of nitrosamines; but if they do, the intake of nitrates (which can be converted into nitrites by bacterial enzymes) is not a rate-limiting factor. Changes in the prevalence of the three factors above could have contributed to the decline in the incidence of the disease, but they could not have brought about such a large and widespread reduction in risk, and it seems probable that the better preservation of food, resulting from the extensive use of refrigeration, has played the major part.

No risk has been detected from the consumption of mutagens produced by the different methods of cooking meat and fish, nor from food additives or pesticide residues. Some food additives may, on the contrary, have served to reduce risk (by avoiding food spoilage and hence improving nutrition, by avoiding contamination by carcinogen-producing microorganisms, or by some antioxidant or other protective effect on the gastric epithelium).

Risk of gastric cancer is also raised, moderately, by smoking, and raised by exposure to ionizing radiation.

Large bowel

- 10.1% of all cancers and 10.5% of cancer deaths
- Sex ratio of rates 1.6:1; age distribution like oesophageal cancer

Cancers of the colon and rectum ought to be considered separately, as their causes are not identical. Cancer of the colon, for example, tends to occur more often in women than in men, particularly when it occurs on the right side, while cancer of the rectum is nearly twice as common in men. The geographical distribution also differs slightly, colonic cancer varying in incidence more than rectal cancer. Separate consideration may, however, sometimes be misleading as cancers commonly occur at the rectosigmoid junction and the site of origin of these cases is not recorded consistently. Moreover, there is a growing tendency to describe both diseases merely as 'cancers of the large bowel', which, according to the internationally agreed coding rules, are classed as cancers of the colon. The two diseases will, therefore, be considered together.

Cancers of the colon and rectum are the third most commonly incident cancer, and the fourth most common cause of cancer death, in the world. Almost a million cases occur per year worldwide, mainly in developed countries. The disease is most common in Western countries, but incidence has generally stabilized or decreased in these countries in recent years, especially at younger ages. In Japan, where incidence used to be very low, rates have risen to be similar to those in the United States of America and western Europe. Rates in migrants from low-risk to high-risk countries, for instance in previous times from Japan to the United States, tend to gain much or all of the host population risks within the first generation.

In most parts of Asia, and in Africa and eastern Europe, large-bowel cancer has been relatively uncommon (except in areas where chronic schistosomal infestation of the large intestine is prevalent; for example, high rectal cancer rates are found in Chinese counties in which *Schistosoma japonicum* was, until recently, a major cause of death). Rates tend to rise markedly, however, with the introduction of a Western lifestyle.

Incidence rates in different countries correlate closely with the *per caput* consumption of fat and meat and crudely with the consumption of processed foods from which the natural fibre has been removed. Ways in which these and other dietary constituents might influence the development of the disease have been discussed under diet. Other factors associated with increased risk are obesity and physical inactivity. A weak association with smoking has been observed in several cohort studies, which may be the result of confounding with the consumption of alcohol (which is associated with colorectal cancer risk in most studies) and a high-fat diet. It is possible, however, that smoking may cause a few cases indirectly by causing the diet to be modified in the direction of a higher fat content.

Cases in childhood or early adult life occur as a complication of familial adenomatous polyposis and of hereditary nonpolyposis colorectal cancer (HNPCC) syndrome. These conditions are determined by dominant genes, which increase the susceptibility to the disease so much that, unless prophylactic measures such as colectomy are undertaken, cancer is highly likely to develop at or before middle age. Many other cases develop from adenomatous polyps and a few occur as a complication of long-standing ulcerative colitis and Crohn's disease. There is substantial evidence of reduced colorectal cancer risk among long-term users of nonsteroidal anti-inflamatory drugs. There is also increasing evidence for an association of colorectal cancer risk with hormones of the growth hormone/IGF-1 axis: colorectal cancer risks are increased in patients with acromegaly; raised risks have been found in the general population in relation to prior greater levels of IGF-1; and raised risks have been found in patients treated with growth hormone.

Anal intercourse causing infection with types 16, 18 or some other specific types of the human papillomavirus is a probable cause of some anal carcinomas in both sexes, but patients who have sexually transmitted anal warts that are due to other types of human papillomavirus are not for this reason at special risk of anal cancer.

Liver

- 0.8% of all cancers and 1.7% of cancer deaths
- Sex ratio of rates 2.0:1; age distribution, see Fig. 6.1.6

Liver cancer is the third most common cause of cancer death in the world, with four-fifths of cases occurring in developing countries, and one-half occurring in China alone. Incidence is considerably

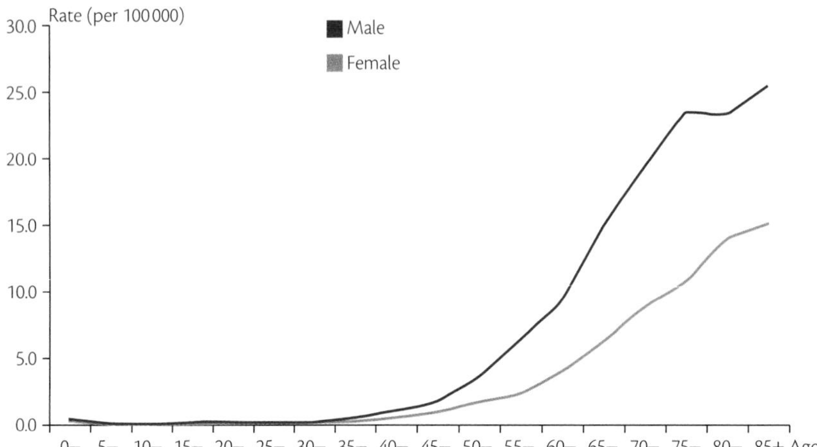

Fig. 6.1.6 Annual incidence of cancer of the liver by age and sex.

greater in men than women almost everywhere. Incidence rates have tended to be overestimated in developed countries because the primary condition is often confused with metastases to the liver from cancer in various other organs, particularly at older ages. Recently, however, there has been an increase in the United Kingdom and the United States from the very low level that existed previously, perhaps due in part to an increased prevalence of infection with hepatitis C.

The disease is common in South East Asia (the highest recorded rates are in parts of China and Thailand) and tropical Africa. In China it accounts for about 18% of all cancer deaths and in parts of Africa it is the most common cancer in men. Most cases derive from the main cells of the organ (hepatocellular carcinomas) and are attributable primarily to chronic active infection, established early in life, with the hepatitis B virus, exacerbated by consumption of some specific metabolite (e.g. aflatoxins) of particular types of fungi that contaminate stored foods. Neonatal vaccination against the virus produces a marked decrease in the proportion of children who become chronically infected. This has begun in many countries, now including the whole of China and parts of tropical Africa, and has already produced a decreased risk of hepatocarcinoma at young ages. Some cases, however, are caused by chronic infection with hepatitis C (a blood-borne RNA virus that cannot be avoided by immunization; see Chapter 7.5.22).

In developed countries, although some cases are also due to infection with hepatitis B and C viruses, more arise as complications of cirrhosis of the liver attributable to heavy and prolonged consumption of alcohol or, rarely, to haemochromatosis, certain types of porphyria, α_1-antitrypsin deficiency, and hereditary tyrosinaemia type 1. Occasionally, liver cancer is produced by drugs. A few cases have occurred in young men who have taken androgenic anabolic steroids to increase their muscular strength and a few from the use of steroid contraceptives, either arising *de novo* or from benign adenomas, which are themselves rare complications of the use of steroid contraceptives. Some can be attributed to smoking, for an association has been observed in parts of China where little alcohol is drunk and case–control studies in Europe have shown an association after alcohol consumption has been taken into account.

A second histological type (cholangiosarcoma) arises from the intrahepatic bile ducts, tends to occur at a somewhat later age than hepatocellular carcinoma, and, although generally less common than hepatocellular carcinoma, nevertheless accounts for an appreciable proportion of cases. In parts of China, Thailand, and elsewhere in south or east Asia it can be produced by chronic infection with liver flukes (*Clonorchis sinensis* or *Opisthorchis viverrini*). In north-eastern Thailand the latter fluke causes one of the highest rates of liver cancer in the world. In developed countries, primary sclerosing cholangitis is the main known risk factor for cholangiosarcoma.

A third histological type that is extremely uncommon everywhere has been variously described as reticuloendothelioma or angiosarcoma. It was first recognized as a complication of the use of Thorotrast as a contrast agent in neuroradiology, a long-abandoned practice that led to chronic retention of insoluble thorium radionuclides in the marrow, spleen, and liver. In 1973, the disease was found to be an occupational hazard for men exposed to vinyl chloride monomer. A few hundred cases have occurred throughout the world in men who were heavily exposed in the manufacture of vinyl chloride polymer, and linear extrapolation suggests that the minute amounts that have leached out of plastic consumer products might have caused only a dozen or so cases altogether in the general public, if indeed they have produced any. A third, and even rarer, cause is prolonged exposure to inorganic arsenic, such as used to result from the medical prescription of Fowler's solution. Despite these multiple causes only one case of hepatic angiosarcoma normally occurs annually per 10 million people, which is why the recognition of new causes has been easy.

The relative rarity of cancer of the liver in most developed countries is intriguing, since most of the carcinogens thus far discovered in experimental animals induce, perhaps with other cancers, tumours of the liver.

Gallbladder and extrahepatic bile ducts

- 0.4% of all cancers and 0.4% of cancer deaths
- Sex ratio of rates 0.9:1; age distribution like oesophageal cancer.

Cancers of the gallbladder and extrahepatic bile ducts are nearly always classed together, which is unfortunate as the causes differ. The former is more than twice as common in women as in men, is probably associated with obesity, and is usually preceded by (and probably caused by) cholelithiasis. The latter is slightly more common in men and is increased in incidence by liver fluke infection, primary sclerosing cholangitis and long-standing ulcerative colitis. Both types are uncommon, and their aggregate varies only moderately from one population to another. The highest rates are recorded among Japanese, Koreans, American Indians, and in women in Delhi (India) and parts of South America.

The incidence of cancer of the gallbladder has fallen sharply in the United States in the last 25 years, which may be partly due to the decreased consumption of animal fat and, perhaps more importantly, to an increase in the rate of cholecystectomy in people who, having gallstones, are at greatest risk of cancer of the gallbladder.

Pancreas

- 2.1% of all cancers and 4.7% of cancer deaths
- Sex ratio of rates 1.3:1; age distribution like oesophageal cancer

Cancer of the pancreas is two to three times more common in regular cigarette smokers than in lifelong nonsmokers. The chemicals in cigarette smoke that specifically cause pancreatic cancer have not been identified, but the volatile nitrosamines in smoke that are absorbed from the alveoli and carried to the pancreas in the bloodstream are likely candidates. The disease is twice as common in diabetics as in the population as a whole and risk is raised in patients with chronic pancreatitis.

Cancer of the pancreas is generally regarded as a disease of the developed world, but the diagnosis is difficult in the absence of a well-developed medical service and some of the relatively small geographical and temporal variations may be due to variation in diagnostic standards. The greatest reported rates are in African Americans. Mortality rates in Britain and the United States have begun to decrease under 65 years of age, and this is more likely to reflect a reduction in incidence from reduction in smoking than to any improvement in treatment, as the 5-year survival rate remains less than 5%.

Nose and nasal sinuses

- 0.1% of all cancers and of cancer deaths
- Sex ratio of rates 1.5:1; age distribution like oesophageal cancer

Surprisingly, in view of the widespread exposure of the human nose to tobacco smoke and other airborne toxins, cancers of the nasal cavity itself are extremely rare. Most arise from the paranasal sinuses. Several occupational hazards have been recognized, including the refining of nickel, processes giving rise to exposure to strong sulphuric acid mists, and the manufacture of hardwood furniture and leather goods. It would be wrong, however, to conclude that all contact with nickel, hardwood dust, and leather creates a hazard. The hazards have been observed in special occupational situations in which exposure has been intensive and prolonged. The nickel-refining hazard was first observed in South Wales where the nickel carbonyl process was used, but similar hazards were subsequently observed with other refining processes in Canada, Norway, and the Soviet Union. In the Welsh refinery the workplace exposures were much heavier before the Second World War, and (despite the continued use of the nickel carbonyl process in Wales) no hazard of nasal sinus cancer has been observed among men first employed there since 1950. The hazard in furniture workers was first observed in High Wycombe (southern England) and appears to have followed the introduction of high-speed woodworking machinery early in the 20th century. A hazard certainly affects some other groups of woodworkers, but should not be assumed to affect furniture workers in general.

Most nasal and nasal sinus cancers are squamous carcinomas, but the hazard from hardwood dust characteristically produced adenocarcinomas. In some of the groups exposed to this hazard, as many as 5% of the men developed the disease. This meant that the risk of adenocarcinoma was increased 1500 times (as this histological type of the disease is normally very rare) and the hazard was, in consequence, easy to confirm once suspicion had been aroused.

Chromate workers are sometimes said to experience a hazard of nasal cancer, but this may be an error due to confusion with the characteristic 'chrome ulcer' of the nasal septum. Such ulcers have not generally been found to become malignant. A causal excess of nasal sinus cancer has been seen, however, in women employed in the United States in the early 20th century to apply radium-containing luminescent paint to dials and clocks, who ingested the radium when they licked the brushes to shape their tips. Risk of nasal cancer is also modestly related to smoking.

Larynx

- 0.6% of all cancers and 0.5% of cancer deaths
- Sex ratio of rates 6.2:1; age distribution, see Fig. 6.1.7

Cancers of the larynx, like cancers of the oesophagus and buccal cavity, are closely associated with tobacco smoking and with the consumption of alcohol. The two agents act synergistically and in the absence of either the disease is rare. The different parts of this small organ are, however, related to the two agents differently. Cancers of the glottis are strongly related to smoking, particularly

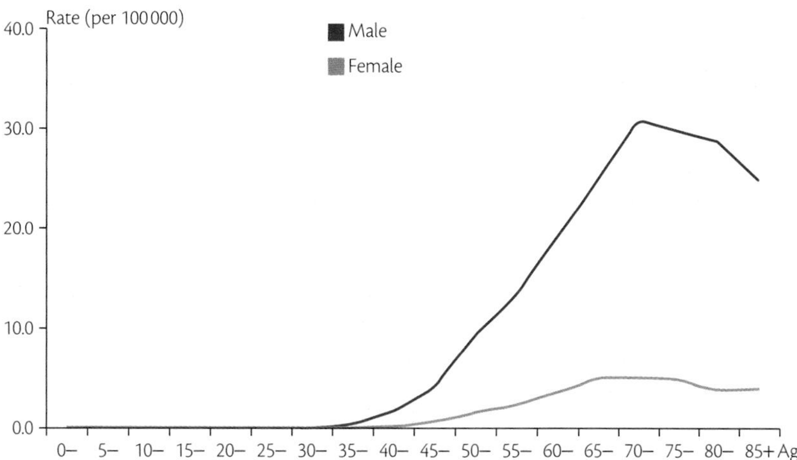

Fig. 6.1.7 Annual incidence of cancer of the larynx by age and sex.

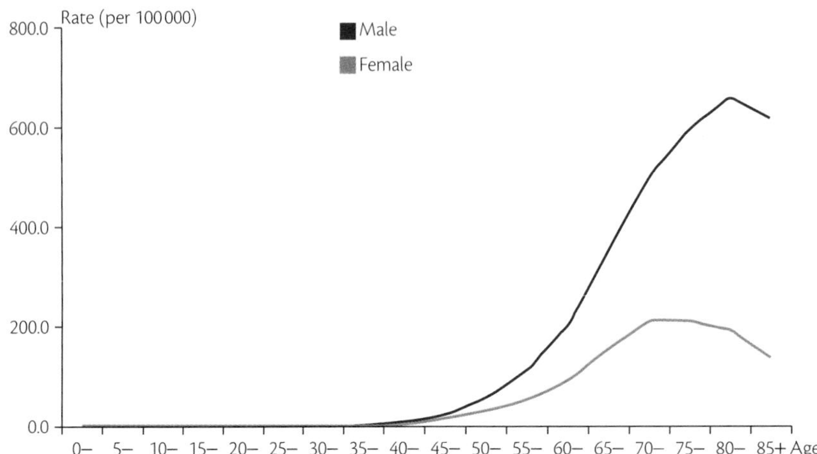

Fig. 6.1.8 Annual incidence of cancer of the lung by age and sex.

to cigarette smoking, and only weakly to alcohol, while cancers of the epilarynx resemble cancers of the neighbouring hypopharynx and are strongly related to both agents and to pipe and cigar smoking equally with cigarette smoking.

The highest reported incidence of laryngeal cancer in men is in African Americans in New Orleans (southern United States) and in parts of Spain. Rates in women are relatively low everywhere and generally a small proportion of those in men in the same place. Trends with time vary considerably between countries and between the sexes, reflecting trends in smoking and alcohol consumption, and probably some other aetiological factor, perhaps nutritional in character. There has been fairly consistent evidence for an inverse association of risk with fruit and vegetable consumption. That there are other causal factors is evident from the relatively high incidence rates in parts of India, Turkey, North Africa, and Brazil, which cannot be accounted for by tobacco and alcohol.

The disease has also occurred as an occupational risk in the manufacture of mustard gas and in processes that cause exposure to strong sulphuric acid mists.

Lung

- 10.4% of all cancers and 21.0% of cancer deaths
- Sex ratio of rates 1.8:1; age distribution, see Fig. 6.1.8

Nearly all lung cancers are bronchial carcinomas and should properly be so described. The term 'lung cancer' is, however, in such common use that it is used here as synonymous with bronchial carcinoma, although it actually includes a very small proportion of alveolar cell carcinomas and other rare types of cancer with different characteristics. Lung cancer is the most common cancer in the world, with over 1.2 million new cases per year, and the most common cause of cancer death.

Until the 1920s, lung cancer was uniformly rare (except in the Hartz mountains, see below). In the next two decades, German and then British pathologists began to comment on an apparent increase, but this tended to be dismissed as an artefact of the greatly improving methods of diagnosis and the establishment of special centres for thoracic disease. Gradually, however, the increase became so pronounced and the change in the sex ratio so marked that the increase could no longer be dismissed as wholly artefactual and by the late 1940s, when the age-standardized mortality rate in men in the United Kingdom had increased 20 times, it was clear that the developed world had begun to see an epidemic of lung cancer comparable in severity to the epidemics of infectious disease of the past, though with a longer time scale. Until the 1940s, the increase among British women was largely a diagnostic artefact. Since 1950, however, diagnostic standards in middle age have changed very little, the increase in British men has been replaced by a decrease, while the increase among middle-aged women has continued for longer, before also reversing (Fig. 6.1.9). As a result, the sex ratio (male rate divided by female rate), at e.g. 50 to 54 years of age, which rose from 1.8 after the First World War to 8.9 after the Second World War, was reduced to 1.3 in 2004. Changes in treatment have had little effect on the fatality rate, which remains extremely high, and real changes in mortality closely reflect real changes in incidence.

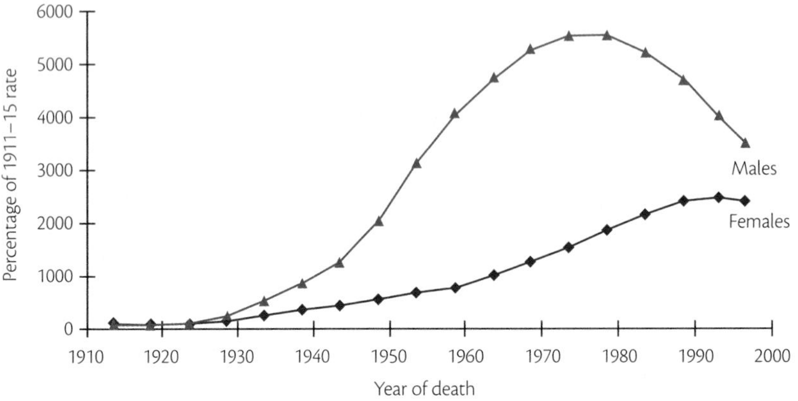

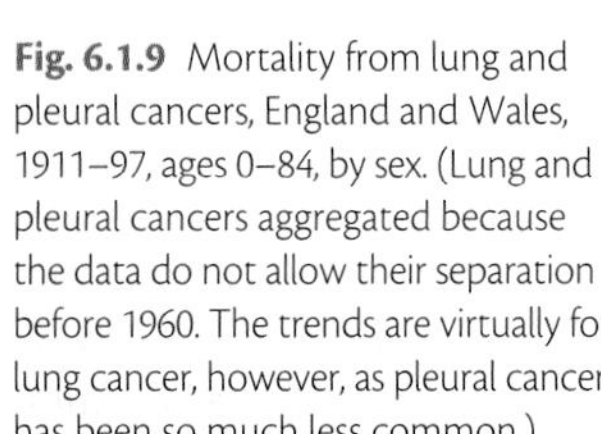
Fig. 6.1.9 Mortality from lung and pleural cancers, England and Wales, 1911–97, ages 0–84, by sex. (Lung and pleural cancers aggregated because the data do not allow their separation before 1960. The trends are virtually for lung cancer, however, as pleural cancer has been so much less common.)

Smoking

These time trends can be explained almost entirely by the effect of smoking tobacco, particularly in the form of cigarettes, which caused more than 90% of all lung cancers in the United Kingdom in the early 1990s. Evidence of this effect was first obtained in the middle of the last century by comparing the smoking histories of patients with different diseases (case–control studies). It was found that the proportion of patients who had never smoked was much smaller if they had lung cancer (the 'cases') than if they had some other disease (the 'controls'), and the proportion who had smoked heavily was correspondingly greater.

Further evidence was obtained by asking large numbers of apparently healthy men and women what they smoked and then following them up to determine the causes of death of those who had died. Cohort studies of this type, in the United States, in doctors in the United Kingdom, and in other groups, have all shown similar results, the risk increasing with the amount smoked, and varying with the length of time cigarettes had been smoked. If attention is restricted to populations in which most cigarette smokers had been smoking cigarettes regularly since early adult life, lung cancer is about 20 times more common in regular cigarette smokers than in lifelong nonsmokers and up to 40 times more common in very heavy smokers. At first the relationship was less marked in women than in men, but this was because female smokers who were old enough to have a high risk of cancer either had not begun smoking cigarettes so early in adult life or had smoked them less intensively when they began, and the sex differences in behaviour and risk have both been progressively eliminated with the passage of time.

Further studies have found that the relative risk of lung cancer has increased with decreasing age of starting to smoke and decreased with the number of years that smoking has been stopped (detectable at 5 years after stopping, but never reaching the risk of a lifelong nonsmoker); that the national increases in incidence have appeared at appropriate times after the increase in cigarette sales (after due allowance is made for a spurious increase due to improved diagnosis and appropriate differences in consumption by men and women); and that there is a general parallelism between the incidence of the disease in different countries and social and religious groups and the prolonged consumption of cigarettes. Finally, and most encouragingly, the trend in mortality has reversed following reduction in smoking. By 2004, the mortality from lung cancer among men in their thirties in Britain was only about one-fifth of that of men of the same ages some 50 years earlier, corresponding to the earlier changes in the prevalence of smoking. The reduction in tar delivery between 1939 and 1965 contributed to the reduction in lung cancer in young men after the war, but the later reduction had little effect because of changes in the way cigarettes were manufactured and in the way they were smoked to ensure an adequate intake of nicotine. At older ages the decreases are less striking, but they are now seen at all ages in British men, and up to 75 in British women.

In recent years, it has been shown that indoor air pollution with tobacco smoke—'passive smoking'—increases lung cancer risk, by about 20 to 30% from long-term adult exposure.

Occupation

Several other causes of lung cancer have been discovered as a result of observations in industry. Many thousands of men and women have experienced significant hazards from exposure to asbestos or to polycyclic hydrocarbons (from the combustion of fossil fuel). The former has given rise to hazards in asbestos mines, asbestos textile works, and insulation work in the shipbuilding and construction industries and the latter to specific hazards in the manufacture of coal gas in coking ovens, in steel works, in aluminium foundries, and wherever substantial amounts of incompletely combusted fumes were released into the working environment. Much smaller numbers of men have experienced substantial hazards from radon in the air of mines (not only when mining radioactive materials, but also when mining haematite and fluorspar under conditions in which radon seeped into the mine air from streams and the surrounding rock), from the manufacture of chromates and chrome pigments, from the refining of nickel, from arsenic (in the manufacture of arsenical pesticides and in the refining of copper, which is always contaminated with arsenic), from exposure to bischloromethyl ether in the chemical industry and exposure to vinyl chloride, from the manufacture of mustard gas, and, to a small extent, from exposure to silica if sufficient to cause silicosis. In one extreme situation (in the cobalt mines of the Hartz mountains in central Europe, which were subsequently mined for radium and uranium), the absolute risk of contracting lung cancer due to the occupational hazard of radon was so large that more than half the workers contracted the disease. In several other situations with heavy exposure to asbestos or the early stages of nickel refining, the occupational hazard has affected as many as 20 to 30% of the exposed men.

Atmospheric pollution

Some of the materials responsible for these occupational hazards—particularly the combustion products of fossil fuels—are or have been widely distributed in the air of towns and it is still uncertain how far they have, in this way, contributed to the production of the disease in the general population. That lung cancer was more common in big towns than in small towns and rural areas is certain, but this held as strongly for Oslo and Helsinki, two relatively unpolluted cities, as for more polluted ones. Differences between the largest towns and the least populated areas have seldom been more than threefold and much of the difference can be accounted for by past differences in cigarette smoking, a habit that has tended to spread outwards from the major cities. Attempts to 'allow for' cigarette smoking have usually been inadequate, as it is impossible to take full account of such factors as the age of starting to smoke cigarettes, the amount smoked daily at different periods, and the method of smoking (number of puffs, depth of inhaling, etc.). It is clear, however, that in the absence of cigarette smoking any effect of urban pollution in developed countries is relatively small. Estimates, based on extrapolation from the heavy pollution with coal smoke that used to occur in large towns, suggest that in such towns it may have contributed, in synergism with smoking, to as much as 10% of the risk of lung cancer, but would have caused very little risk in nonsmokers. On this basis, the present levels of pollution with benzo[*a*]pyrene and the other known lung carcinogens in town air can be only very small. Modern pollution with ultrafine particles ($<10\,\mu m$ diameter) may, however, be more hazardous. Study of residents in six contrasting cities in the United States in which information about personal smoking habits had been obtained suggests that the risk in the most polluted city compared with that in the least polluted could be increased by about one-quarter in both smokers and nonsmokers. The position in some developing countries is different: notably in parts of China, where intense indoor pollution with smoke and fumes from heating and cooking more than doubles the risk of lung cancer in nonsmokers.

Radon

The effect of another form of pollution—that of indoor air with radon arising from naturally occurring radium in rock and soil—has been estimated by extrapolation from the effects of the much larger doses to which some groups of underground miners have been exposed, and by direct observation in studies of people with and without lung cancer. These studies suggest that indoor radon may contribute to about 3% of lung cancers in the United Kingdom and about twice as much in the United States. The absolute effects are far greater in smokers than in lifelong nonsmokers, so that in the absence of smoking few cases would be produced.

Geographical differences

The development of the male lung cancer epidemic and the early signs of its departure have been most prominent in the United Kingdom and Finland, since the switch of young men to cigarettes was largely complete in these countries by the 1920s. In the United States, where cigarette consumption doubled during the Second World War, the peak of mortality occurred a little later. In some other developed countries, the development of the epidemic is still further behind and it is only just beginning to appear in many developing countries. For example, Chinese males, who now consume about 30% of the world's cigarettes, experienced a 10-fold increase in cigarette consumption per head between the 1950s and 1990s that may well eventually cause almost a million cancer deaths a year when the young men of today reach middle age.

In women, the development of the epidemic has generally been later than in men. (Only in the Maori population of New Zealand did it occur at the same time.) In the United Kingdom, the United States, and a few other developed countries, the female lung cancer rates from smoking are already substantial, but in others, such as France and Spain, the epidemic in women has scarcely begun. The greatest recorded incidence in men worldwide is in African Americans in New Orleans and Detroit, and the greatest in women is in the Canadian Northwest Territories. A relatively high risk has long been noted in Chinese women who are nonsmokers, irrespective of their country of residence, which is probably due to their exposure to mutagens in the fumes from oils used in cooking with a wok and from the coal smoke with which many Chinese homes have been heavily polluted.

Pleura and peritoneum

- 0.7% of all cancers and 1.3% of cancer deaths
- Sex ratio of rates approximately 3:1 (but 6.5:1 for mesothelioma); age distribution like laryngeal cancer.

The existence of a specific type of tumour arising from the pleura, or less commonly the peritoneum, was debated by pathologists until 1960 when Wagner and his colleagues reported that six African patients with a similar type of 'peripheral lung cancer' had all lived in villages that were heavily polluted with dust produced by the mining of blue asbestos (i.e. crocidolite). Since then, occupational asbestos exposure (in asbestos mines, shipyards, building construction, asbestos product manufacture, and other work) has been shown to be responsible for the great majority of mesotheliomas, which are the predominant cancers of the pleura and peritoneum. They are much less likely to be produced by white asbestos (chrysotile) than by brown asbestos (amosite) or blue, as the two last persist for longer in the lungs. A few cases arise from neighbourhood pollution with asbestos or secondary contamination (e.g. from household contact with asbestos workers) and some in Turkish villages are due to the weathering into the general atmosphere of erionite fibres in local rock and houses; these fibres are physically similar to asbestos although chemically different. A few cases have been caused by radiotherapy, and natural ionizing radiations may be responsible for most of those that are not associated with asbestos. An SV-40-like virus has been found in some tumours, but it is uncertain whether it plays a part in causing the disease.

Mesotheliomas seldom occur less than 15 years after first exposure to asbestos, commonly occur 25 to 30 years afterwards, and may be delayed for 50 years or more. Hence cessation of use of asbestos (peak imports to the United Kingdom, and peak production worldwide, were in the 1970s) will only lead to decreasing mesothelioma rates several decades later. In the last few years, the recorded mortality under age 70 in England and Wales has begun to decrease.

Almost all mesotheliomas are fatal. Due to confusion with lung or other types of cancer, it is still uncertain how many cases have occurred each year and some of the large increase in Western countries since 1960 may be artefactual. The highest recorded rates of mesothelioma incidence now are in men in Genoa, Italy and in Western Australia. Rates in women in Western countries tend to be much lower than in men.

Pleural mesothelioma is not related to cigarette smoking and the occupational hazard affects smokers and nonsmokers alike.

Bone

- 0.1% of all cancers and 0.2% of cancer deaths
- Sex ratio of rates 1.3:1; age distribution, see Fig. 6.1.10

Sarcomas can affect any bone, but characteristically affect the long bones in adolescence. After 45 years of age they occur most commonly in bones affected by Paget's disease (osteitis deformans), which predisposes to sarcoma so strongly that as many as 1% of all people affected by the disease eventually develop a bone tumour.

Many different histological varieties occur, some of which appear to have different causes. Osteogenic sarcomas and chondrosarcomas are the most common, the former accounting for nearly all the adolescent peak. One rare type (Ewing's tumour) occurs only in children and young adults and is almost unknown in black people, irrespective of the society in which they live.

Ionizing radiation is the main known extrinsic cause. Cases have been produced after high dose radiotherapy, especially such radiotherapy to childhood cancer patients, and after internal radiation from radionuclides including thorium in Thorotrast, an erstwhile contrast medium, radium in 'luminizers', once used to paint clocks and dials, and radium-224 therapy. Bone cancer risk has also been found raised after alkylating agent treatment of childhood cancers, and osteosarcoma risk is raised in several rare cancer syndromes, e.g. Li–Fraumeni syndrome (OMIM 151623), and in retinoblastoma patients.

National statistics in Britain record a reduction in mortality over the last 50 years, but are unreliable indicators of incidence as many

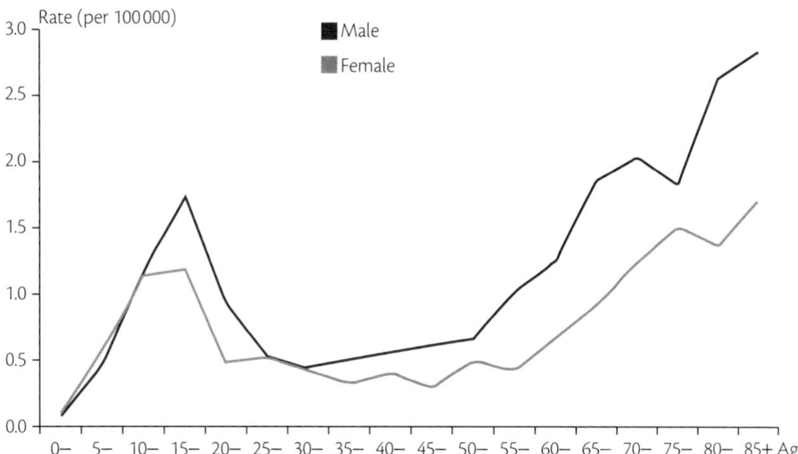

Fig. 6.1.10 Annual incidence of cancer of bone by age and sex.

deaths attributed to tumours of bone are due to cancers that have metastasized from other sites. The recorded decrease in mortality is, therefore, largely an artefact due to improved diagnosis (though it has been contributed to in recent years by higher survival rates in childhood) and the true incidence may have remained roughly constant. Internationally, bone cancer is relatively rare everywhere, with less geographical variation than for most cancers.

Connective and other soft tissue

- 0.4% of all cancers and of cancer deaths
- Sex ratio of rates 1.6:1; age distribution, see Fig. 6.1.11

Sarcomas of the soft tissues include a variety of different diseases, all of which are rare everywhere. Some occur in genetic syndromes, e.g. Li–Fraumeni syndrome and neurofibromatosis type 1 (OMIM 162200), and others are caused by ionizing radiation. A few might be caused by intensive immunosuppression or exposure to chlorophenols and related compounds, but the evidence is inconclusive.

Melanoma of the skin

- 2.5% of all cancers and 1.2% of cancer deaths
- Sex ratio of rates 0.9:1; age distribution, see Fig. 6.1.12.

Melanoma accounts for a small proportion of incident skin cancers but for most skin cancer deaths. Incidence, and to a lesser extent mortality, rates have been increasing in white populations as far back as data are available. In recently born generations in several populations, however, this trend has stabilized or reversed.

The incidence of the disease varies inversely with the amount of skin pigmentation, both comparing whites with nonwhites, and when comparing within whites, in whom skin sensitivity to sunshine (ease of burning and tanning) and fair or redhead complexion predict risk. Risk is also related strongly to numbers of benign moles and atypical moles on the skin, and less strongly to markers of cutaneous ultraviolet damage such as solar keratoses. There is a particularly great risk for patients with giant congenital naevi and those with xeroderma pigmentosum. In white people the tumour occurs most commonly on the legs in women and the trunk in men and is least common on the buttocks and soles of the feet (areas not exposed to the sun). In blacks, in whom melanoma is rare, a high proportion occur on the soles of the feet.

Incidence rates in white people vary roughly in proportion to the flux of sunshine (ultraviolet radiation) in the countries in which they live, although the reverse is true across Europe, probably reflecting darker complexions as one goes south. Risks rise in white migrants from countries with low insolation to those with higher insolation, especially if migration is at a young age. The greatest recorded incidence is in Queensland, Australia, where melanoma is the most common cancer (other than nonmelanoma skin cancer). For all skin sites combined, the incidence is not, however, greater in outdoor than indoor workers (rather the reverse, in fact, perhaps due to the protective effects of a semipermanent suntan).

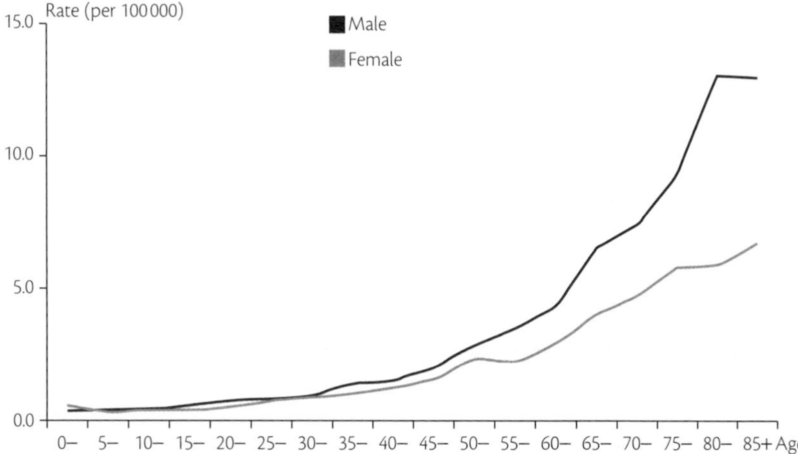

Fig. 6.1.11 Annual incidence of cancer of connective and other soft tissue by age and sex.

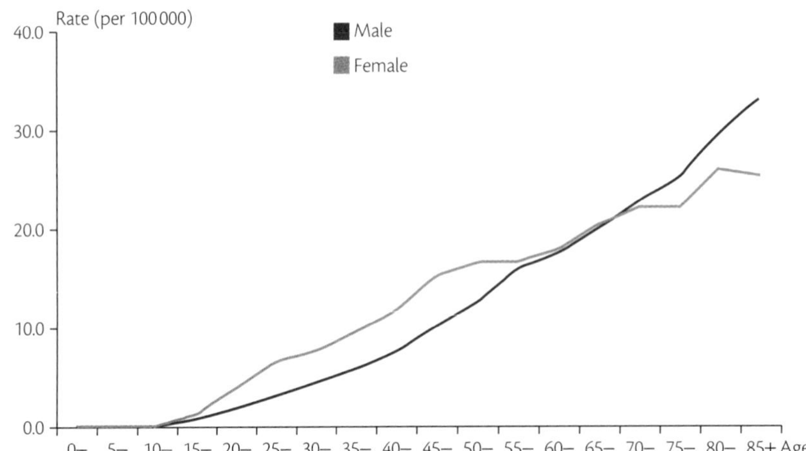

Fig. 6.1.12 Annual incidence of melanoma of the skin by age and sex.

The totality of the evidence suggests that recreational intermittent exposure of untanned skin to solar ultraviolet radiation, such as when sunbathing, is the principal cause of melanoma and the reason for the rising rates. The relationship is not simple, however, and indeed melanomas of the head and neck occur typically in elderly outdoor workers and appear to relate to chronic ultraviolet exposure. There is suggestive, but not decisive, evidence that use of sunbeds increases melanoma risk, and inconsistent evidence that PUVA (methoxypsoralen UVA) treatment can do so.

Skin (nonmelanoma)

- 20.4% of all cancers and 0.4% of cancer deaths
- Sex ratio of rates 1.5:1; age distribution like oesophageal cancer

Nonmelanoma skin cancers are the most common cancers in fair-skinned populations, although rarely fatal. The predominant cause is sunshine (ultraviolet) exposure, and correspondingly the highest reported rates of incidence are in Australia. Rates have been rising in white populations across the world for many years, and tend to be greater in men than in women. The tumours are of two main types, basal cell and squamous cell carcinomas. The former, also known as rodent ulcers, have a causation that appears to relate to both cumulative ultraviolet exposure and intermittent intense exposures such as sunbathing. They occur mainly on parts of the body that are regularly exposed to the sun and, in particular, on the face, head, and neck. They are more common in outdoor workers, such as seamen and farmers, than in indoor workers; more common in fair-skinned (and blond and red-haired) than in dark-skinned (and dark-haired) people; and are almost unknown in blacks (except those who suffer from albinism). Some few cases have been produced by exposure to X-rays, but the risk is very small unless the dose is very large and they seldom occur after normal courses of radiotherapy. People who suffer from xeroderma pigmentosum, a hereditary condition in which there is a defect in the enzyme responsible for the repair of the damage done to DNA by ultraviolet radiation, develop large numbers of skin tumours at an early age in response to even quite mild sun exposure (see Chapter 23.3).

Squamous cell carcinoma is also produced by ultraviolet radiation, risk being proportional to cumulative sun exposure, and in PUVA-treated patients proportional to cumulative PUVA dose. It accounts for about 20% of cancers on ultraviolet-exposed skin. It is, however, the principal type of skin cancer produced by various carcinogenic chemicals, and particularly by polycyclic hydrocarbons in the combustion products of coal. These chemicals have been responsible for the scrotal cancers of chimney sweeps, who accumulated soot in the folds of the scrotum; of mule spinners, whose clothes were saturated with carcinogenic oils; and of various other groups of workers whose clothes were contaminated with tar. They have caused (and still do cause) cancers of the forearm in industrial workers whose arms are regularly splashed with tar or carcinogenic oils, cancers of the groin in India, localized by the continued friction of the *dhoti* cloth, and cancers of the abdomen in Kashmir associated with the habit of carrying a *kangri*, or small stove, inside the clothes in winter to keep warm.

Squamous cell carcinoma has also been due to prolonged exposure to arsenic, which is excreted by the skin and in the hair, when it may be accompanied by arsenical pigmentation and keratoses. All these conditions have been produced by prolonged medical treatment with inorganic arsenic, which used to be prescribed for a variety of chronic conditions, by the consumption of well water from arsenic-rich soils, and by occupational exposure in the smelting of copper and cobalt (the ores of which often contain arsenic) and in the manufacture of arsenical pesticides.

How large a part human papillomaviruses play in the development of squamous carcinoma of the skin is unclear. The type 5 virus is responsible for the warty lesions of epidermodysplasia verruciformis, some of which progress to cancer, and other types of the virus may contribute to the greatly increased risk that follows the intensive immunosuppression given to permit the survival of organ transplants.

A third type is Kaposi's sarcoma, which is now classed as a skin cancer. It is associated with AIDS when AIDS results from homosexual intercourse, but probably only when this is accompanied by orofaecal contact. Frequent at first, particularly in the United States, the association has become progressively less common. Before the advent of AIDS, Kaposi's sarcoma was common in some parts of central Africa, where it occasionally affected children, progressed rapidly, and could account for as many as 10% of all hospital patients with cancer. Elsewhere it was rare, but indolent cases occurred occasionally in developed countries, principally on the legs of middle-aged and elderly men. The disease is initiated by infection with the human herpesvirus type 8, but cofactors are required for tumour development.

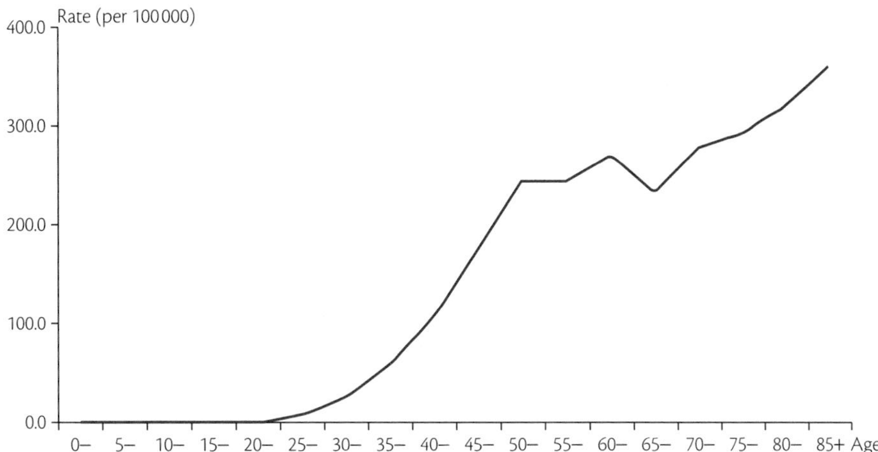

Fig. 6.1.13 Annual incidence of breast cancer in women by age.

Breast

- 12.7% of all cancers and 8.2% of cancer deaths
- Sex ratio of rates 0.01:1; age distribution, see Fig. 6.1.13

Cancer of the breast is the second most common cancer in the world and the most common in women, with a million cases occurring per year. Incidence rates are greatest in Western countries, somewhat lower in eastern Europe, and much lower in Asia and Africa. The geographical differences are unlikely to be chiefly due to genetic factors, as rates in migrants from low- to high-incidence countries rise considerably, to levels intermediate between the two, and there is a further rise in succeeding generations. In many countries incidence rates have tended to rise slowly over several decades, but mortality rates have started to decrease in recent years in Western countries because of more effective treatments and perhaps the effect of screening (Fig. 6.1.14).

Hormonal factors, particularly oestrogens, are important in the production of the disease. The duration of ovarian activity is relevant, as the disease is particularly common in women who have an early menarche and a late menopause (the former being more important than the latter). Pregnancy produces a short-term increase in risk, followed after a few years by a lifelong decrease, particularly after teenage or early adult pregnancies. The incidence in later life increases progressively with a woman's age at the time of her first full-term pregnancy, being about three times greater when the first birth occurs after 35 years of age than when it occurs before 18 years. Full-term pregnancies after the first have an additional protective effect. Pregnancies that end in abortion have little or no effect, however, suggesting that the effects of pregnancy depend on the induction of lactation. The duration of lactation has an additional protective effect but is not marked unless it continues for a year or more.

Risk of breast cancer is raised in women with benign breast disease, the degree of risk varying according to the type of disease. Risk is also raised by alcohol consumption, by lack of physical exercise, and by ionizing radiation exposure at young ages, with particularly high risks in women given high dose mantle radiation for Hodgkin's disease. There is not, however, good evidence for causation by any form of environmental pollution.

Parity and menstrual differences are insufficient to account for the large variations in the incidence of the disease between different countries, which seem to be correlated with a 'high' standard of living: i.e. with life in a developed country. Diet might play a part, but the evidence is complex and inconclusive. Obesity is associated with a reduced risk before the menopause, as it tends to be associated with ovarian dysfunction. After the menopause, obesity increases the incidence and probably the fatality of the disease. Height is associated with increased incidence both for pre- and postmenopausal women. Oestrogens prescribed medically, as hormone replacement therapy (HRT) after the menopause, increase the risk by about 2% for each year of use; combined with progestogens in the contraceptive pill they increase it by about 25% during use, but the increased risk gradually disappears over 10 years, when use is stopped, as it does after HRT is stopped. Tamoxifen, an antioestrogen prescribed

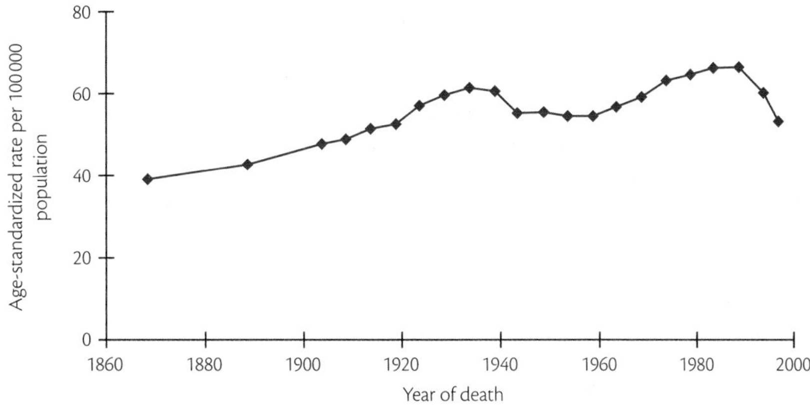

Fig. 6.1.14 Mortality from breast cancer in women, England and Wales, 1868–1997, ages 35 and older.

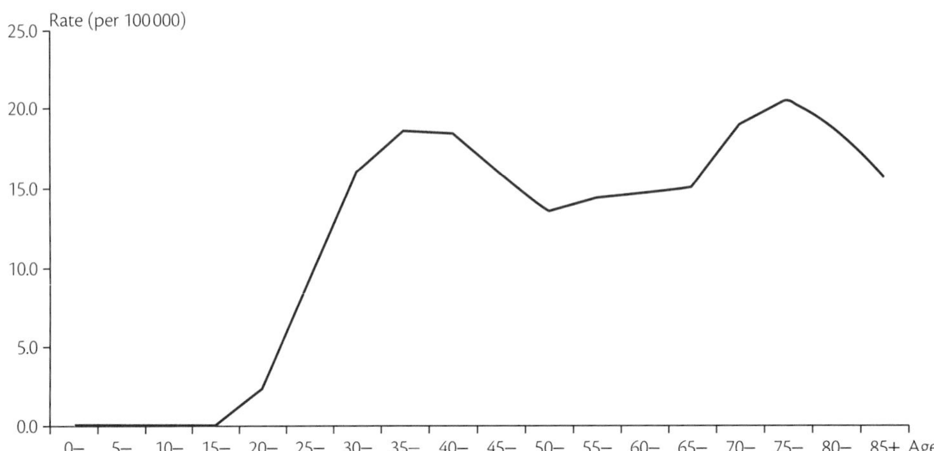

Fig. 6.1.15 Annual incidence of cancer of the uterine cervix by age.

for the treatment of breast cancer, reduces the subsequent incidence of the disease in the unaffected breast. As well as the relation to sex hormone levels, there is growing evidence that risk of premenopausal breast cancer relates to prior endogenous levels of IGF-1.

Breast cancer has been a particularly fertile area of genetic epidemiology in recent years, with the identification of several high risk genes, some related to clinical syndromes (e.g. Cowden's disease, and carriage of an ataxia telangiectasia mutation), but most related only to cancer risk, as described in Chapter 13.8.3.

Uterine cervix

- 0.8% of all cancers and 0.7% of cancer deaths
- Confined to women; age distribution, see Fig. 6.1.15

Carcinoma of the cervix is the second most common cancer in women worldwide, and the most common in parts of Africa and Asia; it used also to be common in Europe and North America. It has always been rare in Jewish women and has tended to be less common in Muslim women than in women of other faiths living in the same country (e.g. Hindus in India).

Changes in incidence over time have been difficult to assess, partly because mortality data have not always distinguished between deaths due to cancer of the cervix and those due to cancer of the corpus (or endometrium), partly because the introduction of screening programmes has made it possible to diagnose and treat premalignant lesions (see below), and partly because hysterectomy for benign conditions has become progressively more common, with a corresponding reduction in the number of uteri in which the disease could occur. Despite these complications there can be no doubt that the disease has become substantially less common in Europe and North America than it was before the Second World War.

The rarity of the disease in Jewish women and its relative rarity in Muslim women suggest that male circumcision may reduce the risk of its development, but this is unlikely as the state of circumcision of her husband has no substantial effect on a woman's risk of developing the disease in communities in which only some men are circumcised. Cleanliness is likely to be protective, as the disease is relatively uncommon in communities that practise ritual ablution before and after intercourse and, within each community, it becomes less common with rising socioeconomic status.

Squamous carcinoma, which constitutes the vast majority of all cases, is intimately connected with sexual activity. It almost never occurs in virgins and increases in frequency with the number of sexual partners that a woman or her partner has had and with younger age at first sexual intercourse. Almost all cases are attributable in part to infection with certain types of the human papillomavirus, most notably types 16 and 18. A vaccine effective against these two types has now been developed, and future vaccination should greatly reduce incidence.

The development of squamous carcinoma is preceded by pathological changes limited to the epithelium, known as cervical intraepithelial neoplasia (CIN) types I, II, and III. CIN III is associated with the same types of virus as squamous carcinoma, but CIN I and CIN II generally are not. The changes may progress from one to another, finally leading to carcinoma, but the early lesions (CIN I and II) commonly regress and even CIN III (previously known as carcinoma *in situ*) may do so occasionally. The lesions can be recognized in cervical smears and destroyed by lasers or extensive biopsy and the occurrence of clinical disease can be greatly reduced by the examination of all sexually active women every 2 or 3 years and the treatment of advanced CIN lesions.

Other factors associated with the production of the disease are high parity, the use of oral contraceptives, and cigarette smoking. Both of the latter tend to be associated with behaviour conducive to venereal infection, but it is uncertain whether this tendency can wholly account for their association with the disease. That smoking may be responsible for some cases is suggested by the presence of mutagens in the cervical mucus of smokers that are not present in the secretions of nonsmokers.

Adenocarcinoma of the uterine cervix is generally uncommon, but has become somewhat more common recently in several countries. It is related to human papillomavirus infection, but also appears to relate to factors similar to those for endometrial adenocarcinoma.

Endometrium (corpus uteri)

- 1.8% of all cancers and 1.1% of cancer deaths
- Confined to women; age distribution like cancer of ovary

The epidemiological features of endometrial cancer are in many respects the opposite of those of cervical cancer. Histologically, it is nearly always an adenocarcinoma. It is common in developed countries, especially parts of the United States of America, and rare in poor populations. It is inversely related to parity, but not otherwise related to coitus, and is unaffected by the number of

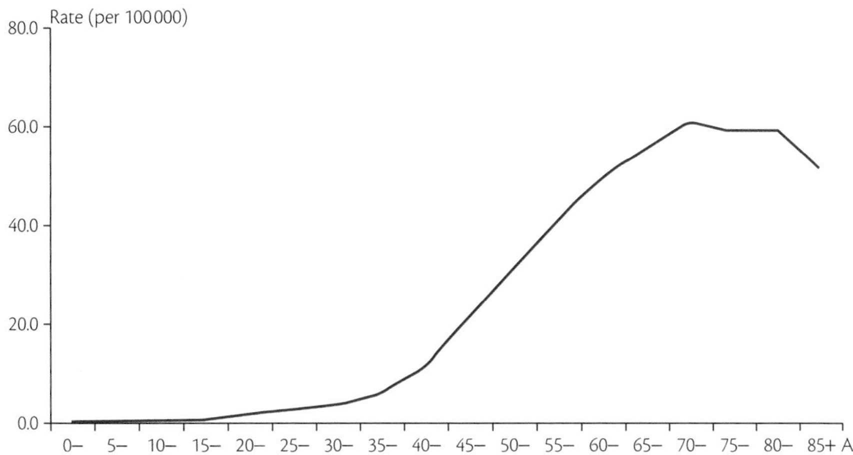

Fig. 6.1.16 Annual incidence of cancer of the ovary by age.

sexual partners. Like cancer of the breast, it is positively associated with late menopause, and perhaps with early menarche. Incidence in most Western countries has been fairly stable in recent decades, but in the United States there was a peak in the 1970s followed by a decline, as discussed below.

The one factor known to produce the disease is regular exposure to oestrogens, unopposed by progestogens. This leads to endometrial hyperplasia and eventually, in some cases, to cancer. Known causes include oestrogen-secreting tumours of the ovary, the use of oral contraceptives in which oestrogens and progestogens are prescribed sequentially (types that have now been abandoned), the use of unopposed oestrogens to relieve menopausal and postmenopausal symptoms, and adiposity. The last causes the disease because oestrogens are produced in the body after the menopause in adipose tissue from the adrenal hormone, androstenedione. Tamoxifen, an analogue of natural oestrogens, which blocks oestrogen receptors in the breast and hence acts as an antioestrogen, can, due to differences between the hormone receptors in different tissues, have a pro-oestrogenic effect in some other organs, and increases the incidence of endometrial cancer in proportion to the length of treatment. Endometrial cancer risks are reduced in users of combined (concurrent oestrogen and progestogen) oral contraceptives.

It is improbable that oestrogens are initiating agents. They are not mutagens *in vitro* and the changes that took place in the incidence of the disease in the United States following the increase and subsequent reduction in the use of unopposed premarin (a conjugated oestrogen) for the treatment of menopausal symptoms occurred so quickly that they make sense only if oestrogens act on some late stage(s) of the carcinogenic process. Endometrial cancer risk is raised in women who are physically inactive and in women with diabetes, in each instance with evidence that the relation may be more than just a consequence of obesity. Endometrial cancer risk, at least postmenopausally, appears to be reduced among smokers.

Ovary

- 1.8% of all cancers and 2.8% of cancer deaths
- Confined to women; age distribution, see Fig. 6.1.16.

About 90% of ovarian cancers are of the surface epithelium, and the causes of the tumour that have been recognized may refer only to these. Ovarian cancer incidence is greatest in countries with a high standard of living; the highest recorded rates are in part of Switzerland, in Iceland, and in Israeli Jews born in Europe or North America. Incidence decreases progressively with increasing number of children. There is no strong relation to age at menarche or age at menopause, however. Risk of the disease is reduced by the use of oral contraceptives, more greatly with longer use, and seems to depend on the lifetime number of ovulations. Risk is decreased by tubal ligation and perhaps by hysterectomy, and increased by mutations in the *BRCA1* and *BRCA2* genes.

Prostate

- 10.0% of all cancers and 6.8% of cancer deaths
- Confined to men; age distribution, see Fig. 6.1.17

Cancer of the prostate is the third most common cancer in men worldwide and is found mainly in Western countries. Rates are particularly low in Asia and some parts of Africa. It is more characteristically a disease of old age than any other cancer, so that it comes to play a much larger part in clinical experience as the proportion of old people in the population increases. It is unusual in that foci of cells resembling cancer can be found in a high proportion of clinically normal prostates, so that the recorded incidence is drastically increased by increasing the number of prostatic biopsies. Increases in incidence have been recorded in many Western countries. The introduction of prostate specific antigen (PSA) testing has given rise to considerable artefacts in recorded rates in the United States of America. Some increase in mortality had been recorded in Britain and the United States, but in the last 10 years there has been a modest decrease, and the weight of evidence suggests that the disease is principally due to factors that have affected society for many years. What these factors are remains obscure. Associations have been reported with both increased and decreased sexual activity and there is some evidence, not conclusive, for a reduced risk in men who eat more tomatoes and tomato products, the main source of lycopene. There is also some evidence for reduced risk in men who take considerable physical exercise. On general grounds it seems likely that the disease is dependent on sex hormone imbalance (particularly as castration or oestrogen administration slows the progression of clinical disease) but the nature of the imbalance is unknown. Decreased risks of prostate cancer have been found in patients with Klinefelter's syndrome and those with diabetes; the former, and there is some evidence

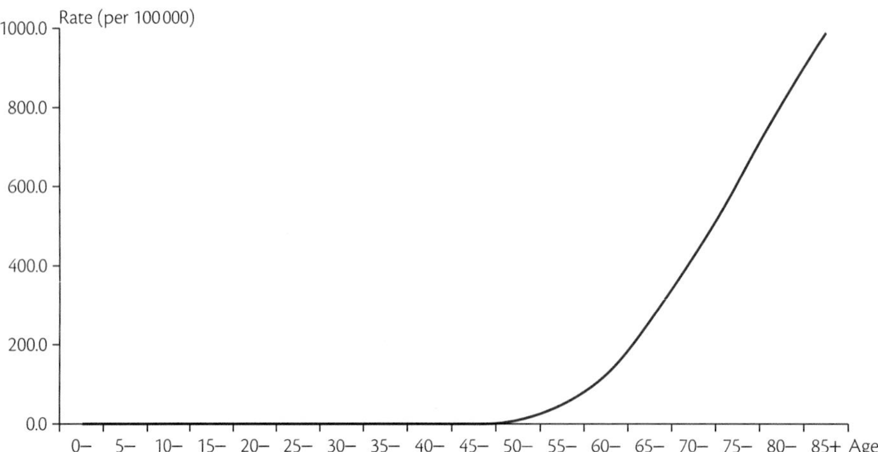

Fig. 6.1.17 Annual incidence of cancer of the prostate by age.

that also the latter, have reduced androgen levels. An association of prostate cancer risk has been found with prior raised circulating levels of IGF-1. Vasectomy was thought to increase the incidence of the disease, but probably does not.

Two epidemiological observations stand out: the exceptionally high incidence in African Americans (much the highest recorded), and the low incidence in Japan in contrast with other developed countries. Both may be partly due to genetic factors, but they are not wholly so, as Japanese and blacks have much higher rates in the United States than they have in Japan and Africa respectively.

Testis

- 0.6% of all cancers and 0.1% of cancer deaths
- Confined to men; age distribution, see Fig. 6.1.18

Testicular cancers are of two main types. Seminomas, which are the more common, have a peak incidence at about 35 years of age and teratomas, commonly called embryonal carcinomas in the United States, have a peak incidence about 10 years younger. Testicular cancer is the most common cancer in young white men in many countries, but much less common in nonwhite groups living in the same areas, except Polynesians. Tumours after 50 years of age are mostly lymphomas and are now classed as such. Both genetic and environmental factors are important. On the one hand, the disease is uniformly rare in black populations, whether in Africa or in the United States. On the other, it has increased in incidence over many decades in white populations around the world. In Britain, the increase began in the 1920s and affected first the higher socioeconomic groups. The increase trebled the mortality at 15 to 34 years of age and produced a sharp peak in young adult life that had not previously been present. Mortality has greatly decreased in recent decades, however, as treatment has improved (Fig. 6.1.19). The disease is more common in more prosperous populations, greatest in parts of Switzerland. Testicular cancer risk is greatly raised in men with XY gonadal dysgenesis, and in brothers, and to a lesser extent fathers, of cases. The cancer is much more likely to occur in an undescended than in a normal testis (*c.*10% of cases in whites are in men who have had maldescent), and in a testis opposite one that has been cancerous, and is also associated with prior inguinal hernia, but otherwise its causes are unknown. The leading hypothesis, in part because of the age distribution and association with cryptorchidism, has been that the aetiology is prenatal, due to exposure *in utero* to raised maternal oestrogen levels during the first trimester of pregnancy. Potential prenatal factors have been extensively investigated, with the strongest evidence for reduced risk with late birth order and raised risk for dizygous twins and boys born prematurely, but none are established.

Penis

- 0.1% of all cancers and of cancer deaths
- Confined to men; age distribution like cancer of the salivary glands

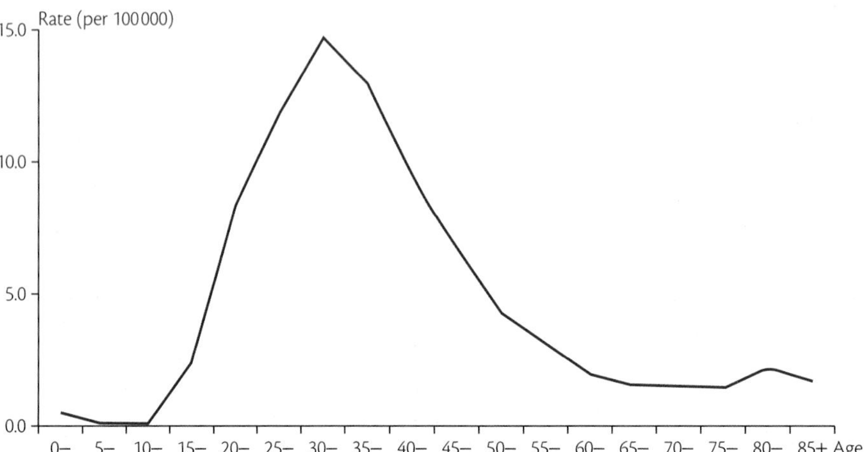

Fig. 6.1.18 Annual incidence of cancer of the testis by age.

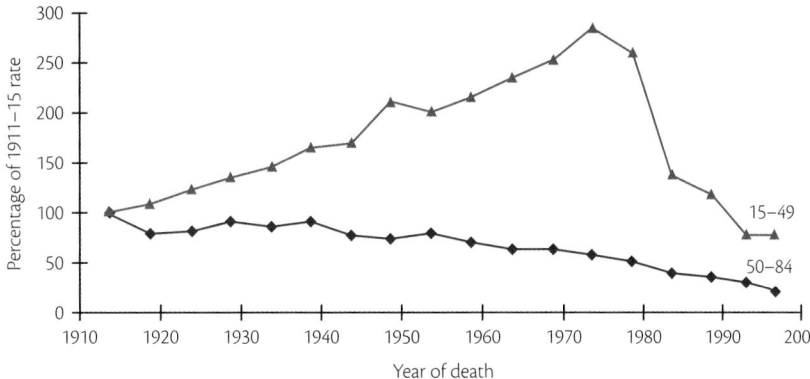

Fig. 6.1.19 Mortality from cancer of the testis, England and Wales, 1911–97, by age.

Carcinoma of the penis is at all common only in some parts of tropical Africa and Brazil, where it has accounted for 10% of all cancers in men. It is avoided almost entirely by circumcision at birth and is very rare if circumcision is carried out in boyhood. Phimosis is a risk factor. In developed countries penile cancer is rare even in the absence of circumcision if the glans, coronary sulcus, and foreskin are kept clean.

The oncogenic types of the human papillomavirus (principally types 16 and 18) can usually be identified in the malignant cells and are important causes of the disease.

Kidney

- 1.8% of all cancers and 2.2% of cancer deaths
- Sex ratio of rates 1.8:1; age distribution like liver cancer

Cancers of the kidney are of three main types: nephroblastomas (or Wilms' tumours), adenocarcinomas (or hypernephromas) of the renal parenchyma, and transitional- and squamous-cell carcinomas of the renal pelvis. The first are limited to childhood, occur with almost equal frequency everywhere, and apart from a few of genetic origin, are of unknown aetiology. The second constitute by far the majority of all cases, are more common in Europe (greatest in the Czech Republic) and North America than in Africa and Asia, and have been increasing in incidence in many Western countries. Cigarette smoking is one cause, but the association is weak and it does not account for more than about one-quarter of the cases. Obesity is also a risk factor, and phenacetin-containing analgesics may have been but the evidence is less clear than it is for renal pelvis cancers.

The third type of renal cancer (carcinoma of the pelvis) constitutes some 10% of all cases. Three established causes are occupational exposure to the chemicals that cause cancer of the bladder, cigarette smoking, and the consumption of phenacetin in large enough amounts to produce analgesic nephropathy. In all three cases the hazards are relatively small (two to three-fold). A fourth cause, Balkan nephropathy (Chapter 21.10.10), increases the risk several hundred-fold.

Bladder

- 2.8% of all cancers and 3.2% of cancer deaths
- Sex ratio of rates 3.4:1; age distribution like oesophageal cancer

Cancer of the bladder is almost universally several times more common in men than women. Greatest recorded incidence in men is in parts of Europe, with low rates in Africa, Asia and much of South America, and in nonwhites compared with whites in the United States of America. The tumour can be produced by cigarette smoking, occupational exposure to a group of chemicals classed together as aromatic amines, infection of the bladder with *Schistosoma haematobium*, the use of phenacetin-containing analgesics, and the medical prescription of chlornaphthazine (*N*,*N*′-bis(2-chloroethyl)-2-naphthylamine) and cyclophosphamide, and ionizing radiation. There has been evidence for a relation to chronic consumption of inorganic arsenic, a contaminant of the water supply in parts of Taiwan and other countries. There has also been some evidence for an association with urinary tract infection, supported by raised risks in paraplegics, who tend to have frequent urinary tract infections. Most bladder cancers are transitional cell carcinomas, but those associated with schistosomiasis are characteristically squamous carcinomas. It is not surprising that the bladder should be affected by many chemicals, as any noxious small molecules in the blood will tend to be found at greatly increased concentration in the urinary tract. Cigarette smoke contains several mutagenic chemicals that enter the bloodstream and thence the bladder, so that when tested *in vitro* on bacterial DNA the urine of cigarette smokers is found to be mutagenic, while that of nonsmokers is barely active.

Occupation

An occupational cause was first suspected in 1895 in Germany, when Rehn commented on a cluster of cases in men using aniline for the manufacture of dyes. Aniline, however, is not carcinogenic in experimental animals; more recent studies have failed to incriminate it epidemiologically, and it seems likely that other carcinogenic chemicals were present as impurities. Four aromatic amines that are carcinogenic in experimental animals have been shown to cause bladder cancer in humans: 2-naphthylamine, benzidine, 3,3′-dichlorobenzidine, and 4-aminobiphenyl. The first is one of the most powerful human carcinogens yet known and was responsible for the development of bladder cancer in all the 19 men who were employed in distilling it in a British factory. Its manufacture in Britain was stopped in 1949, but small amounts continued to be imported until the 1960s. Other aromatic amines that may cause bladder cancer include auramine, magenta, and, perhaps, 1-naphthylamine. The last is dubiously carcinogenic in experimental animals and it seems probable that the cases associated with its use have been due to a small proportion of 2-naphthylamine present as an impurity in the commercial material. These chemicals were used in the manufacture of dyes, in the rubber industry as antioxidants (1-naphthylamine and 4-aminobiphenyl) and

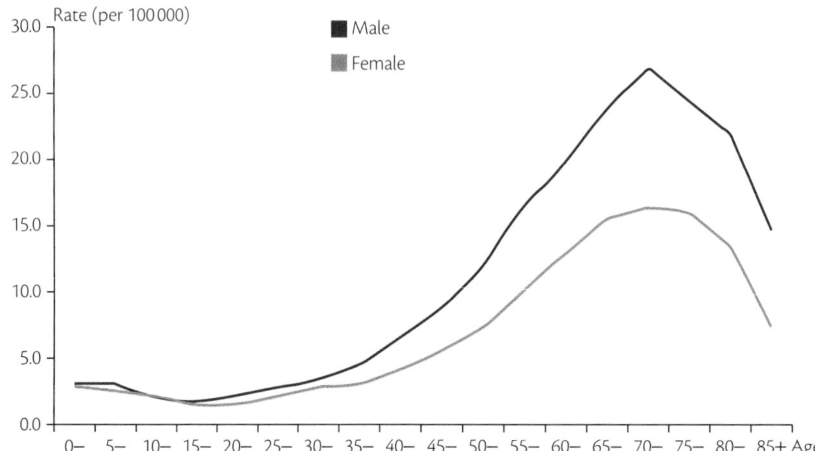

Fig. 6.1.20 Annual incidence of cancer of the brain and other CNS by age and sex.

hardeners (benzidine), and in laboratories as a reagent (benzidine). 2-Naphthylamine is also found in the combustion products of coal and may have been responsible for the hazard of bladder cancer in men who made coal gas. Various other occupational associations, including leatherworking and aluminium work, have been reported, but are less clearly aetiological. As many as 10% of cases were, at one time, attributable to occupational causes in Britain and North America; but the proportion should now be much less.

Smoking

The most important cause numerically is cigarette smoking, which probably accounts for about half the total number of cases in Britain and North America. 2-Naphthylamine and 4-aminobiphenyl are present in cigarette smoke, but whether the amounts are sufficient to account for the carcinogenic effect is uncertain.

Medicines

The medicinal causes have, by contrast, been responsible for relatively few cases. Chlornaphthazine was used briefly for the treatment of myelomatosis, until it was found to be metabolized into 2-naphthylamine. Cyclophosphamide is used primarily for the treatment of malignant disease, but it is also used as an immunosuppressant. In large doses it may cause sloughing of the bladder mucosa and, occasionally, cancer. High levels of consumption of phenacetin-containing analgesics led to bladder cancer as well as renal cancer risk, but these drugs have been banned in Western countries for the last 25 years.

Parasitic infection

Heavy infection of the bladder with *Schistosoma haematobium* has been found to be a cause of the disease, most notably in Egypt and Tanzania.

Artificial sweeteners

Artificial sweeteners came under suspicion as potential bladder carcinogens because of the results of animal experiments in which, first, mixtures of cyclamates and saccharin and then saccharin alone were shown to cause bladder cancer in rats. The human use of cyclamates was banned before saccharin came under suspicion and it now appears that the 'positive' results of animal experiments with cyclamates alone were due to impurities. Saccharin has been shown to cause bladder cancer in rats but the quantities that had to be given were large, constituting a few per cent of the feed. The human evidence is extensive and could hardly be more negative, except that it does not cover lifelong use.

Brain and other central nervous system

- 1.3% of all cancers and 2.3% of cancer deaths
- Sex ratio of rates 1.6:1; age distribution, see Fig. 6.1.20

Tumours of the brain and nervous system are of several different histological types, some of which may not be clearly either benign or malignant. One type occurs characteristically in childhood (medulloblastoma), another in adult life (glioblastoma), and a third (astrocytoma) at all ages. Despite the overall male excess, one type (meningioma) is more common in women. Recorded incidence of brain and other central nervous system tumours tends to be greatest in white populations in Western countries, but geographical variations are less marked than for most tumours.

A moderately large secular increase in incidence in old age has been recorded in many countries, which might be attributable to improved diagnosis with CT scans and MRI. Little or no increase in mortality has been reported in or before middle age and the recorded increases in incidence are certainly largely, and possibly wholly, artefactual. The only established external cause is ionizing radiation. No new environmental cause has been established, but many have been suspected without conclusive evidence, including electromagnetic fields associated with the use of electricity (50–60 Hz) and mobile telephones (cellphones). A small proportion of brain tumours are attributable to high-risk hereditary syndromes, most commonly neurofibromatosis. The presence of allergy is associated with reduced glioma risk, but the reason is unknown.

Thyroid

- 0.5% of all cancers and 0.2% of cancer deaths
- Sex ratio of rates 0.4:1; age distribution, see Fig. 6.1.21

The thyroid is particularly sensitive to ionizing radiation in childhood, but risks after adult exposures are relatively small. Substantial numbers of cases have occurred among the survivors of the atomic explosions in Hiroshima and Nagasaki, children who were exposed to large amounts of radioactive iodine following the Chernobyl accident, and young people whose necks were irradiated in infancy for the treatment of an enlarged thymus (a condition now considered to be perfectly normal, but at one time thought to be a cause

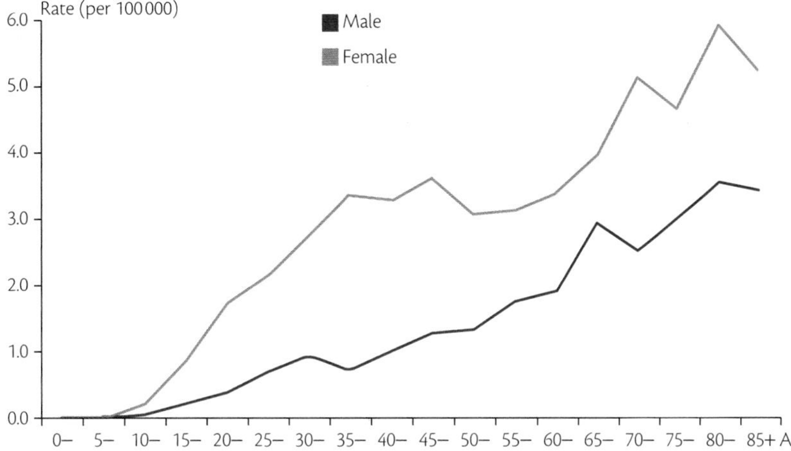

Fig. 6.1.21 Annual incidence of cancer of the thyroid by age and sex.

of sudden death). Fortunately, the thyroid tumours produced by ionizing radiation are nearly all of the papillary and follicular types, which respond well to treatment. No external causes are known of the medullary and anaplastic types, which have a high fatality and occur only in adult life. Many medullary thyroid cancers, however, are inherited as an autosomal dominant, alone or as part of the multiple endocrine neoplasia type 2 (MEN2) syndrome. Papillary and follicular thyroid cancers are less often genetic. Associations of thyroid cancer risk have been found with various benign thyroid conditions, but causality remains unclear.

The disease is most common in women in several Pacific islands and in Iceland. Increases in recorded incidence have been seen in recent decades in the United States of America and several other countries; it is unclear how much of this is due to changes in diagnostic completeness and criteria.

Hodgkin's disease (Hodgkin's lymphoma)

- 0.4% of all cancers and 0.2% of cancer deaths
- Sex ratio of rates 1.3:1; age distribution, see Fig. 6.1.22

Hodgkin's disease is best thought of as at least two diseases, one affecting primarily youths and young adults, the other primarily middle-aged and older people. This division is suggested partly by the existence of two peaks in the age-specific incidence rates, partly by the histological appearances (younger patients tending to have the nodular sclerotic form of the disease and older patients the mixed cellular form), and partly by the clinical distinction that young patients show mediastinal involvement in more than 50% of cases and infradiaphragmatic involvement in less than 5%, while the reverse tends to be true in older people.

There are several reasons for thinking that the characteristic type in young people is infective in origin. In developing countries, Hodgkin's disease occurs in childhood, but as the standard of living rises, the childhood cases disappear and are replaced by a larger number, and a peak of incidence, in young adults. This is reminiscent of what happened to poliomyelitis in the first half of the 20th century and suggests that the disease may be due to a ubiquitous infective agent that tends to be contracted at older ages as hygiene improves, rarely causes Hodgkin's disease, but is more likely to do so if infection is at an older age. Risk in young adults decreases with factors likely to facilitate early infection, e.g. late birth order. That the infectious agent is likely to be the Epstein–Barr virus (EBV or human herpesvirus type 4) is suggested by the findings that the incidence is increased 5 to 20 years after a clinical attack of infectious mononucleosis, that abnormal EBV antibody profiles can be present years before the disease, and that the virus is often present in the DNA of the malignant cells characteristic of the tumour (the Reed–Sternberg and tumour reticulum cells). As with other virus-induced cancers, there are likely to be cofactors (at present unknown) that determine whether cellular infection leads to the

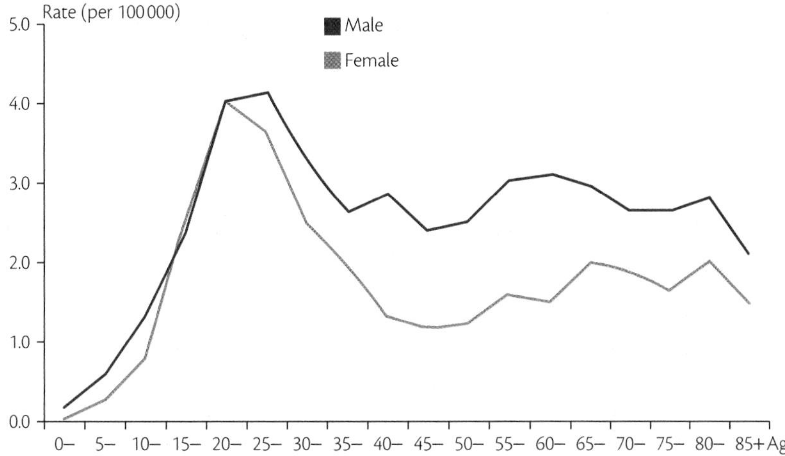

Fig. 6.1.22 Annual incidence of Hodgkin's lymphoma by age and sex.

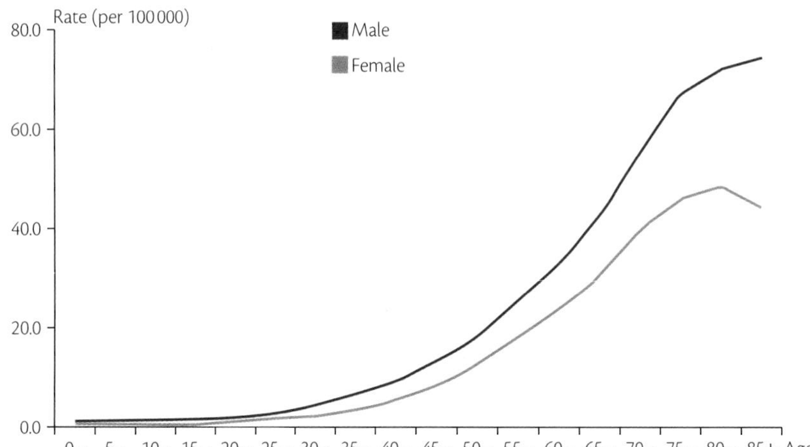

Fig. 6.1.23 Annual incidence of non-Hodgkin's lymphoma by age and sex.

production of a malignant clone. In recent years a raised risk has been noted in AIDS patients, with EBV genome detected in the tumour in most cases.

The principal trend in Hodgkin's disease in Western countries has been a dramatic decrease in mortality as modern radiotherapy and chemotherapy have transformed it from a disease that was largely incurable before the mid 20th century, to one with high survival.

Non-Hodgkin's lymphoma

- 2.8% of all cancers and 2.9% of cancer deaths
- Sex ratio of rates 1.4:1; age distribution, see Fig. 6.1.23

Non-Hodgkin's lymphoma embraces several diseases with different histological appearances. The histological classification has, however, varied from place to place and from time to time, and it has been difficult to collect epidemiological information about the individual types.

One type that has been clearly distinguished is Burkitt's lymphoma, derived from B lymphocytes. This affects children everywhere, but is common only in a few areas in which malarial infection is both heavy and widespread. In parts of Uganda, Tanzania, and Nigeria the disease is 100 times more common than in Europe and North America. In high-incidence areas, EBV can nearly always be recovered from the lymphomatous cells and part of its genome is identifiable in the cells' DNA. Infection with the virus is, however, not necessary for the development of the disease, as some cases occur in its absence; nor is it sufficient, as infection is almost universal and occurs at a very young age in high incidence areas. It seems, therefore, that EBV is a potential cause and that its carcinogenic effect is precipitated by the intense stimulation of the reticuloendothelial system that is characteristic of heavy and chronic malarial infection.

Another type occurs as part of the adult T-cell leukaemia–lymphoma syndrome that follows infection with the human T-cell lymphotropic virus-1 (HTLV-1), especially after infection in childhood. The disease is common in South Japan and the Caribbean, but may occur occasionally anywhere.

A third type, primary upper small-intestinal lymphoma (PUSIL), affects young people in many populations with a low standard of living, not only in North Africa and the Middle East (where its frequency gave it the earlier name of Mediterranean lymphoma) but also in South Africa and Central and South America. Malnutrition is not, however, a sufficient cause as it is uncommon in Bangladesh and several other malnourished populations.

A fourth type, the mucosa-associated lymphoid tissue tumour known as a maltoma, occurs in the stomach as a result of *H. pylori* infection and can be cured by aggressive treatment of the infection.

The remaining lymphomas, which constitute the majority in developed countries, should probably be divided further. Some in childhood might be better classed with acute lymphatic leukaemia, from which they are distinguished arbitrarily only by the number of lymphocytes in the blood. At present, however, they have to be considered as a group. As such they constitute one of the few types of cancer that have been increasing in incidence at all ages in Western countries for several decades. Internationally, recorded rates are greatest in these countries.

Two factors that have contributed to the increase, but which cannot account for it all, are the use of immunosuppressive drugs and the spread of AIDS. Intense immunosuppression for organ or bone marrow transplantation is followed within 1 or 2 years by an increase in the incidence of the disease of the order of 50- to 100-fold; most of the tumours are EBV-associated and are reversible by cessation of immunosuppression, but there is also an excess of non-EBV-related tumours. Smaller increases follow the less intensive use of immunosuppressive drugs for the medical treatment of patients with rheumatoid arthritis and other similar conditions. Raised risks have been see in patients with several immunological diseases including Sjögren's syndrome, systemic lupus erythematosus, coeliac disease, and dermatitis herpetiformis. AIDS leads to a 50 fold or greater risk in Western countries, with EBV often present in the tumour; a rare subtype is associated also with human herpesvirus type 8 infection. Greatly increased incidence rates, largely EBV-related, are also seen in a variety of rare hereditary disorders characterized by major immunological impairment, such as the Wiskott–Aldrich syndrome. There is also increased risk of non-Hodgkin's lymphoma in patients who have had Hodgkin's disease.

Multiple myeloma

- 1.0% of all cancers and 1.7% of cancer deaths
- Sex ratio of rates 1.5:1; age distribution like oesophageal cancer

Myelomatosis has been much easier to diagnose since marrow puncture and then serum electrophoresis became standard diagnostic tools and since the improvement in the management of renal failure, which is often the presenting symptom. As a result it is difficult to be sure whether the increase that was recorded until recently, in both incidence and mortality rates, was due solely to improved diagnosis, or whether it also reflects the introduction of major new causes into Europe and North America between the two World Wars. In southern Sweden, where there has been a long-standing interest in, and search for, cases of myelomatosis, no large increase was seen over the same period; the recorded rates were higher than in other developed populations, but in recent decades those in other populations have caught up.

The disease is uncommon in undeveloped areas, where it is almost certainly underdiagnosed. Genetic factors could be important, as in the United States it is twice as common in African Americans (who have the highest recorded incidence anywhere) as in whites, and is rare in Japanese and Chinese irrespective of where they live. Little is known about the causes of myeloma other than raised risk in patients with monoclonal gammopathy of undetermined significance (MGUS), some raised risk, although not entirely consistent, after ionizing radiation exposure, and probably raised risk in AIDS patients.

Leukaemia

- 2.0% of all cancers and 2.8% of cancer deaths
- Sex ratio of rates 1.7:1; age distribution, see Fig. 6.1.24

Leukaemia may be divided primarily into chronic lymphatic leukaemia (CLL), chronic myeloid leukaemia (CML), acute myeloid leukaemia (AML), and acute lymphatic leukaemia (ALL). CML, AML, and ALL are, in turn, amalgams of two or more different types, with different causes, different age distributions, and different prognoses, but the distinctions between them are still undergoing evolution and, with the exception referred to later, the epidemiological descriptions of each subtype are unclear.

CLL increases progressively with age in the same way as myelomatosis and most of the common epithelial cancers. It is extremely rare in Chinese, Japanese, and Indians, which is presumably due to genetic differences in susceptibility as it continues to be rare in these racial groups even when they migrate to other countries.

AML occurs at all ages. It becomes slowly, but progressively, more common from childhood on and is the most common type in young adult life. In this age group, its incidence is probably less variable throughout the world than that of any other reasonably common type of cancer. CML, by contrast, is very rare in youth, but becomes more common than AML in later middle age. The few cases that occur in childhood should perhaps be regarded as constituting a separate disease, as they lack the Philadelphia chromosome that normally characterizes CML in adult life.

ALL is the most common type of childhood cancer. Three main types can be distinguished. Common (c) ALL arises from B-lymphocyte precursors and is responsible for a peak incidence of the disease at 2 to 3 years of age. Null ALL also arises from B-cell precursors, but lacks the common antigen and accounts for most cases in the first year of life. T-cell ALL occurs more or less equally at all ages in childhood. ALL in adult life can be either B cell or T cell.

Many causes of leukaemia are known. The most important is ionizing radiation, which causes all types except CLL. The leukaemia risk appears, and peaks, sooner after exposure than the risk for solid cancers. The sparing of CLL may be because the relevant stem cells are so radiosensitive that they are killed by small doses that would otherwise be carcinogenic. The other main types are induced by ionizing radiation more easily than most other types of cancer and constitute about 10% of all fatal cancers from exposure of the whole body to moderate doses.

Whether extremely low-frequency nonionizing radiation can cause leukaemia, particularly ALL in childhood, is uncertain. There is evidence to suggest that the risk of ALL is approximately doubled in the small proportion of children who have exposure to power frequency magnetic fields in their homes of an intensity greater than 0.4 μT. The evidence for a causal relationship is, however, inconclusive.

One type of the disease (adult T-cell lymphoma/leukaemia) is caused by a virus (HTLV-1) and has been described under non-Hodgkin's lymphoma.

Other causes include smoking, which causes a small increase in myeloid leukaemia, several chemicals, and genetically determined diseases. The most important chemical is benzene, which is used widely in industry. Prolonged occupational exposure to large amounts has caused a substantial risk of AML (particularly one of its subtypes, erythroleukaemia) and, less commonly, acute lymphatic leukaemia. Many cases are preceded by periods of aplastic anaemia and there is still some doubt whether leukaemia can be caused by small doses.

Chemotherapy for malignancy can cause leukaemia, mainly AML but also ALL and CML. Several treatment agents are leukaemogenic.

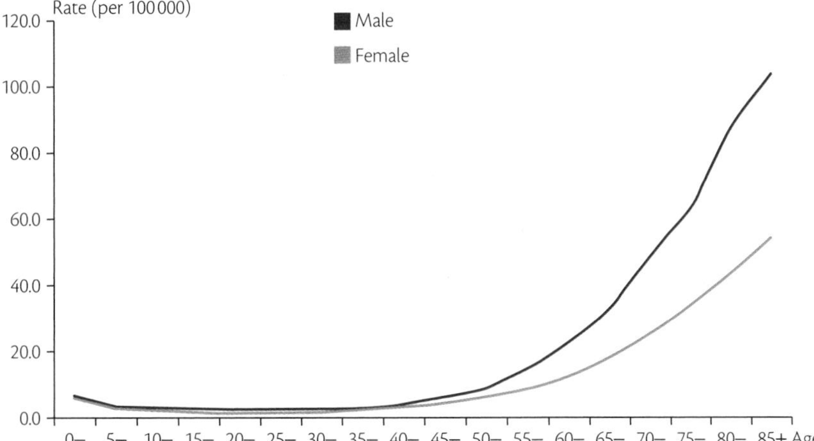

Fig. 6.1.24 Annual incidence of leukaemia by age and sex.

Treatment with alkylating agents, such as melphalan, lomustine, and mechlorethamine, greatly increases risk of AML, with a peak risk, as after radiotherapy, at about 5 to 9 years after treatment. Topoisomerase II inhibitors, particularly the epipodophyllotoxins, are leukaemogenic, with leukaemia often occurring within a year or two of treatment. There is evidence of raised risk after treatment with platinum compounds. Patients with chloramphenicol-induced aplastic anaemia may also be at raised leukaemia risk.

Of the hereditary causes, Down's syndrome is the most common and is probably responsible for the greatest number of cases, although the relative risk in some of the other rarer syndromes may be greater than the 20-fold increase in childhood leukaemia that occurs with Down's syndrome. Ataxia telangiectasia and Bloom's syndrome predispose to ALL, while Fanconi's anaemia predisposes to AML.

Further reading

Chen J, *et al.* (1990). *Diet, life-style, and mortality in China: a study of the characteristics of 65 Chinese counties.* Oxford University Press, Oxford.

Dockery DW, *et al.* (1993). An association between air pollution and mortality in six US cities. *N Engl J Med*, **329**, 1753–9.

Doll R, Peto R (1981). The causes of cancer: quantitative estimates of avoidable risks of cancer in the United States today. *J Natl Cancer Inst*, **66**, 1191–308.

Doll R, Fraumeni J, Muir C (eds) (1994). *Trends in cancer incidence and mortality. Cancer surveys*, Vol. 19 and 20. Cold Spring Harbor Laboratory Press, New York.

Doll R, *et al.* (2004). Mortality in relation to smoking: 50 years' observations on male British doctors. *BMJ*, **328**, 1519–33.

Hammond EC, Selikoff IJ, Seidman H (1979). Asbestos exposure, cigarette smoking, and death rates. *Ann N Y Acad Sci*, **330**, 473–90.

IARC Monograph on the Evaluation of Carcinogenic Risks to Humans (2004). *Tobacco smoke and involuntary smoking. Summary of data reported and evaluation.* Vol. 83. International Agency for Research on Cancer, Lyon.

International Commission on Radiological Protection (2007). Recommendations of the International Commission on Radiological Protection. Publication 60. *Ann ICRP*, **37**, nos. 2–4.

Jha P, *et al.* (2008). A nationally representative case-control study of smoking and death in India. *N Engl J Med*, **358**, 1137–47.

Office for National Statistics (2005). *Review of the Registrar General on deaths by cause, sex and age, in England and Wales, 2004* (Series DH2 no. 31). Office for National Statistics, London.

Office for National Statistics (2006). *Registrations of cancer diagnosed in 2004, England* (Series MBI no. 35). Office for National Statistics, London.

Parkin DM (2001). Global cancer statistics in the year 2000. *Lancet Oncol*, **2**, 533–43.

Parkin DM, *et al.* (eds) (2002). *Cancer incidence in five continents*, Vol. VIII. IARC Scientific Publications No. 155. International Agency for Research on Cancer, Lyon.

Peto J (2001). Cancer epidemiology in the last century and the next decade. *Nature*, **411**, 390–5.

Peto R, Chen ZM, Boreham J (1999). Tobacco—the growing epidemic. *Nat Med*, **5**, 15–17.

Peto R, *et al.* (1994) *Mortality from smoking in developed countries 1950–2000.* Oxford University Press, Oxford (2nd edition, 2006, available on http://www. deaths from smoking.net).

Peto R, *et al.* (2000). Smoking, smoking cessation, and lung cancer in the UK since 1950: combination of national statistics and two case-control studies. *BMJ*, **321**, 323–9.

Schottenfeld D, Fraumeni JF Jr (eds) (2006). *Cancer epidemiology and prevention*, 3rd Edition. Oxford University Press, New York.

Stewart BW, Kleihues P (eds) (2003). *World cancer report.* IARC Press, Lyon.

Swerdlow A, dos Santos Silva I, Doll R (2001). *Cancer incidence and mortality in England and Wales: trends and risk factors.* Oxford University Press, Oxford.

Tomatis L (ed.) (1990). *Cancer causes, occurrence and control.* IARC Scientific Publications No. 100. International Agency for Research on Cancer, Lyon.

6.2

The nature and development of cancer

John R. Benson and Siong-Seng Liau

Essentials

Contemporary ideas of carcinogenesis envisage a series of random genetic changes that confer a selective growth advantage over healthy cells. These changes collectively lead to the disruption of coordinated networks of intercellular communication and cause a fundamental change in cellular behaviour which affects processes such as proliferation, differentiation, and apoptosis. This progressive dysregulation of cellular function implies that cancer is not a morphological entity, but a process in which the malignant phenotype is gradually acquired.

Why are cells prone to become cancerous?

Cells have an inherent programme which influences rates of proliferation, differentiation, and cell death, but the rate of these processes is determined by the balance of positive and negative growth factors to which they are exposed. Whatever the mechanistic fault, aberrant function of these growth factor loops leads to excessive proliferation, promotes immortalization of cells, and in turn leads to neoplastic development.

Why do cells respond to multiple mitogenic growth factors? From a teleological perspective, these may guarantee a rapid growth phase during the early stages of embryogenesis, thereby maximizing the chances of sustained viability, and functional redundancy in the system may be an evolutionary safeguard to ensure an organism's survival in adverse circumstances where specific growth factor pathways are compromised and would otherwise threaten survival.

The process of carcinogenesis

Oncogenes and tumour suppressor genes—the malignant phenotype is thought to arise from an accumulation either randomly, or sequentially, of alterations within two operational classes of gene. (1) Oncogenes—these are derived from normal cellular counterparts termed proto-oncogenes, which code for a variety of proteins including polypeptide growth factors and their receptors, some key components of the signal transduction process, and nuclear regulators of the cell cycle. Activated oncogenes represent a positive or 'gain-of-function' change resulting in a growth advantage over normal cells. (2) Tumour suppressor genes—these are genes which exert a negative (suppressive) influence on cellular proliferation and promote pathways leading to programmed cell death. Mutations leading to loss of function remove a kind of 'brake' on the cell cycle or impair mechanisms involved in the maintenance of genomic integrity and fidelity of DNA replication.

The Knudson 'two-hit' hypothesis—this states that mutations in both alleles of a gene pair are a prerequisite for cancer development. Individuals with an inherited predisposition to cancer already possess a mutation in one allele (present in all cells) and thus require only one further somatic mutation for tumour formation, whereas sporadic forms of cancer are dependent upon two somatic mutations. This hypothesis is especially applicable to those tumours arising from loss of function in tumour suppressor genes, because inactivation of both alleles is usually essential before levels of the gene product fall sufficiently to induce malignant change; it is of less relevance to cancers produced by oncogenes.

The basis for malignant transformation—genetic alterations within a cell can be either inherited or acquired. Most human cancers are sporadic (meaning that there is no inherited risk) and these are dependent exclusively on somatic mutations, which result from one of two inter-related processes: (1) the intrinsic error rate for DNA synthesis and repair; and (2) augmentation of the spontaneous mutation rate by environmental factors interacting with cellular DNA either directly or indirectly, e.g. radiation and chemical carcinogens. These processes may (1) initiate tumour development—by producing a permanent change in cells, but insufficient to cause tumour development without other factors; and/or (2) promote tumour development—by inducing division of a cell that has been 'initiated'.

The origin of cancer cells—most human cancers are monoclonal, implying that a single cell undergoes malignant transformation and forms a primary clone from which further subclones are derived. It was previously believed that cancers arose from dedifferentiation of cells of mature phenotype, with reversion to a more primitive state to a greater (poorly differentiated) or lesser (well differentiated) degree. However, it is unlikely that mature somatic cells exist within tissues for a sufficiently long period to accumulate a mandatory number of mutations for malignant transformation. By contrast, stem cells have greater longevity and the capacity for self-renewal.

The cancer stem cell hypothesis proposes that the stem cell is the target for carcinogenesis and not mature somatic cells.

The malignant phenotype

Cancer cells possess the following *in vitro* characteristics: (1) reduced requirement for exogenous sources of polypeptide growth factors; (2) loss of contact inhibition once confluency is reached; (3) anchorage-independent growth; and (4) the ability to divide indefinitely after multiple passages in tissue culture (immortalization). Cells that have acquired these properties are referred to as 'transformed'.

Characteristics of malignant neoplasms—loss of responsiveness to normal growth control mechanisms is a hallmark of any tumour, but malignant neoplasms have three characteristic features: (1) growth is no longer subject to strict regulation by surrounding cells and tissues; (2) anaplasia or loss of cellular differentiation; and (3) the propensity to metastasize and form tumour foci at distant sites.

Clinical implications

Increasing understanding of the pathobiology of cancer has led to more targeted therapeutic approaches which focus on blocking, bypassing, or reregulating aberrant pathways, rather than nonspecific killing of cancer cells.

Introduction

Many biological processes including wound healing, development, and carcinogenesis involve well-defined patterns of cellular growth and differentiation. Rates of proliferation and differentiation are stringently regulated within normal tissues of a multicellular organism and ensure that organs do not exceed a specific size and that tissue renewal is proportionate and confined to replacement of damaged and/or effete cells only. Communication between cells is the essence of this 'cellular society' and may be based on several mechanisms. Direct cell-to-cell contact is restricted to cells in contiguous arrangement and involves specialized junctional elements permitting transfer of signals between cells. By contrast, indirect modes of communication allow interaction between neighbouring groups of cells which are not necessarily in direct contact. Thus cells may interact through the extracellular matrix which surrounds all cells *in vivo* and whose structure and composition is determined by tissue requirements. Alternatively, cells may communicate indirectly by means of soluble growth factors which are secreted by a particular cell type and diffuse through the extracellular matrix to reach target cells lying at variable distances from the source. An important mechanism for growth control in multicellular organisms is density-dependent growth inhibition which ensures that no single cell has unrestrained growth and competition for space and nutrients is 'fair'. This may be mediated by an increase in cellular requirements for macromolecular growth factors. As confluency is reached, with crowding of cells, their innate sensitivity to these growth factors decreases, perhaps as a result of a reduction in the density of cell surface receptors.

Polypeptide growth factors are a group of regulatory molecules which have been well characterized from serum and cell tissue extracts. There appears to be a close relationship between growth factor production and growth of many types of tumour. They are functionally divided into positive and negative growth factors depending upon whether epithelial proliferation is stimulated (mitogenic) or inhibited respectively. Polypeptide growth factors are produced and secreted locally by many cell types and interact with specific transmembrane receptors that are present on target cells. After the binding of growth factors to their cognate receptor, an intracellular signal is generated that translates an extracellular stimulus to an intracellular response. Growth factors are secreted into the intercellular space and have either an autocrine function acting on their cell of origin, or a paracrine action on adjacent cells of a similar or different type (Fig. 6.2.1).

Cells are exposed to a physiological cocktail of positive and negative growth factors in their microenvironment, and the balance of these determines the polarity and intensity of the overall signal delivered to epithelial cells. The excessive proliferation of cells that characterizes both preneoplastic lesions and established tumours could result from a breakdown of these autocrine and paracrine loops. The disturbance of cellular homeostasis might be associated with an excess of stimulatory growth factors derived from either epithelial cells or stromal elements. Conversely, there could be a deficiency of negative growth factors that normally serve to restrict proliferation of cells or induce nonproliferative states (e.g. differentiation or apoptosis). The breakdown of these loops could also be a result of an abnormal response from target cells. Failure of target cells to respond to negative growth factors could be secondary to defects in receptor function or signal transduction pathways, and constitutive activation of cognate receptors can increase sensitivity to normal amounts of growth factors.

Control of the cell cycle and hence rate of tumour growth is determined by the balance of growth factors acting upon a cell. Although cells have an inherent program which influences rates of proliferation, differentiation, and cell death, this 'sea' of soluble growth factors represents a principle mechanism for modulation

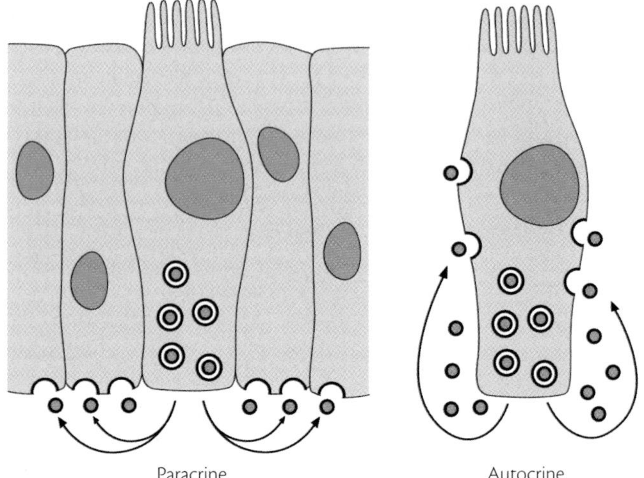

Fig. 6.2.1 Autocrine and paracrine modes of action for growth factors. Cells produce and secrete soluble growth factors which enter the extracellular space, from where they can act via cognate membrane receptors upon either the same (autocrine) or adjacent (paracrine) cells.

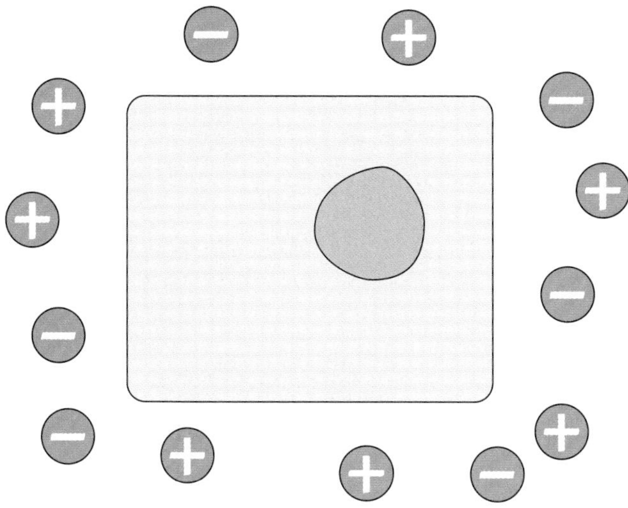

Fig. 6.2.2 Cellular growth factors. The local microenvironment of a tumour contains a pool of positive and negative growth factors, both autocrine and paracrine. The balance of these determines the polarity and intensity of the net signal delivered to epithelial cells.

and regulation of cellular activity by exogenous stimuli (Fig. 6.2.2). Whatever the mechanistic fault, aberrant function of these growth factor loops leads to excessive proliferation, promotes immortalization of cells, and in turn leads to neoplastic development.

From a teleological perspective, the existence of multiple mitogenic growth factors may guarantee a rapid growth phase during the early stages of embryogenesis thereby maximizing the chances of sustained viability. A degree of functional redundancy may be an evolutionary safeguard to ensure an organism's survival in adverse circumstances where specific growth factor pathways may be compromised and would otherwise result in an attenuated response and threaten survival.

Oncogenes and tumour suppressor genes

A consequence of this collective mitogenic potential of cells may be a lower threshold for development of hyperproliferative states which presage cancer. The sequence of events leading to formation of a tumour are ultimately attributable to genetic mutations and changes in gene expression, though the latter can be modified by host factors. Over the past 20 to 30 years, concepts of carcinogenesis have been dominated by the paradigm of oncogenes and more recently tumour suppressor genes. The malignant phenotype is considered to arise from an accumulation, either randomly or sequentially, of alterations within these two operational classes of gene. Oncogenes are derived from normal cellular counterparts termed proto-oncogenes which have some sequence homology with tumour-producing viruses. Activated oncogenes represent a positive or 'gain-of-function' change resulting in a growth advantage over normal cells in possession of the inactivated proto-oncogene. The latter code for a variety of proteins including polypeptide growth factors and their receptors together with several key components of the signal transduction process and nuclear regulators of the cell cycle. The term oncogene may be a misnomer as the 'normal' proto-oncogene product may simply be produced in excessive amounts rather than activation being associated with an abnormal gene product. In both scenarios, there are increased rates of cell proliferation and persistence of genetically aberrant cells. By contrast, tumour suppressor genes are characterized by mutations which lead to 'loss of function'. Tumour suppressor genes are natural elements of a cell's genetic code and products of these genes exert a negative (suppressive) influence on cellular proliferation but promote pathways leading to programmed cell death. In addition to acting as a kind of brake on the cell cycle, they have a crucial role in maintenance of genomic integrity and fidelity of DNA replication. Mutations within these tumour suppressor genes essentially produce tumours by default. Moreover, according to this paradigm, oncogenic events within a cell tend to be dominant and 'evil overrides good'.

The two-hit hypothesis

Epidemiological studies of inherited and sporadic forms of certain cancers have provided much insight into the genetic initiation process. Knudson proposed a 'two-hit' hypothesis in which mutations in both alleles of a gene pair were a prerequisite for cancer development. Individuals with an inherited predisposition already possessed a mutation in one allele (present in all cells) and thus required only one further somatic mutation for tumour formation. Sporadic forms of the cancer were dependent upon two somatic mutations, the chances of which were correspondingly smaller for any equivalent mutation rate. Knudson's hypothesis is especially applicable to those tumours arising from loss of function in tumour suppressor genes (see below); usually inactivation of both alleles is essential before levels of the gene product fall sufficiently to induce malignant change. By contrast, oncogenes behave in a dominant manner and mutation within a single allele may be sufficient for tumour development. Sometimes heterozygosity at an oncogene locus (e.g. 5q21) results in a premalignant phenotype such as colonic polyps (Fig. 6.2.3).

Increasing understanding of the pathobiology of cancer has led to more targeted therapeutic approaches which focus on blocking, bypassing, or reregulating aberrant pathways rather than non-specific killing of cancer cells. This accords with the concept that cancer cells are not 'foreign' and genetically disparate like endogenous

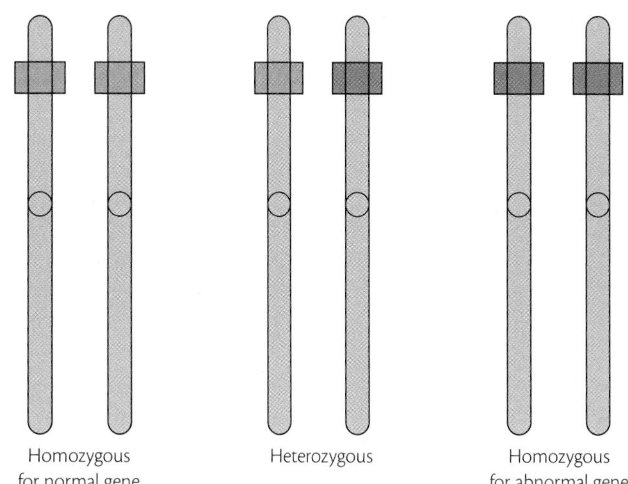

Fig. 6.2.3 According to Knudson's two-hit hypothesis, mutations in both alleles of a normal gene pair (shown in blue) are a prerequisite for cancer development (shown in orange). Individuals with an inherited predisposition already possess a mutation in one allele (heterozygous) and only one further mutation is necessary for tumour formation.

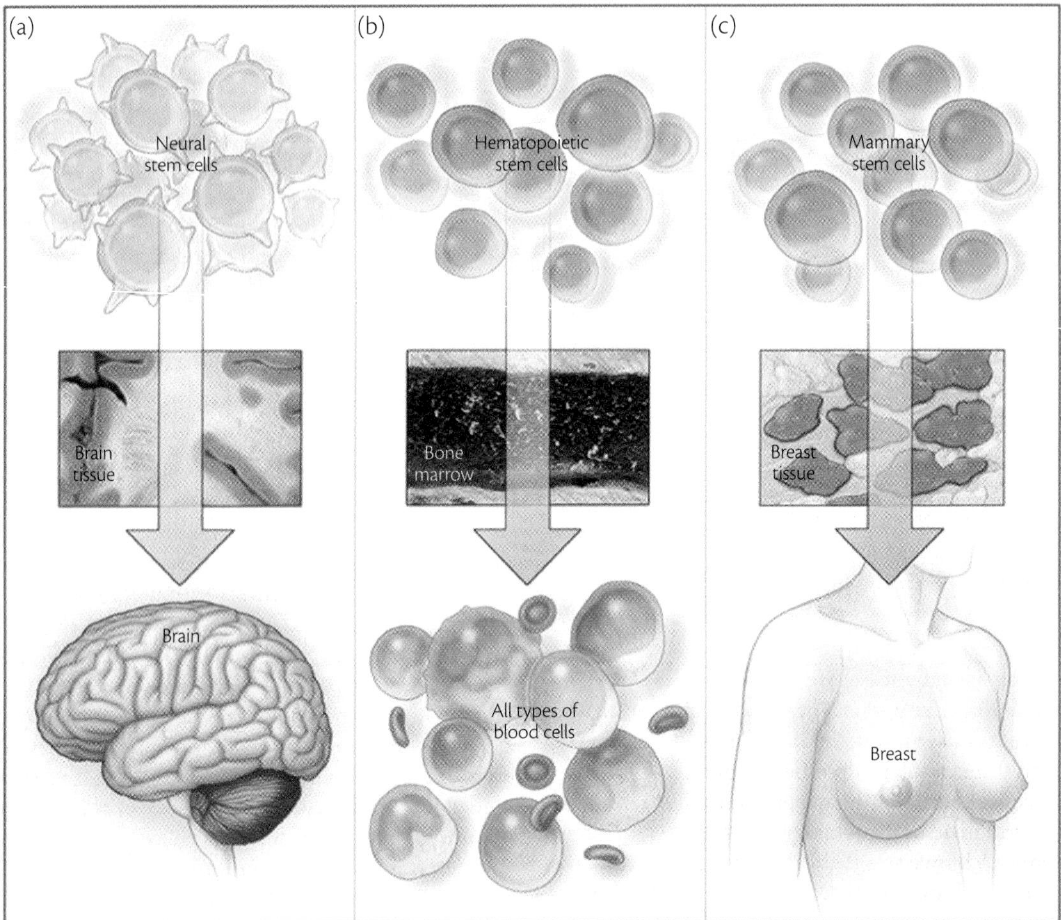

Fig. 6.2.4 Stem cells occur in many different somatic tissues and are responsible for phenotypic differentiation. Neural stem cells generate cells within the central nervous system (panel A), haemopoietic stem cells generate mature blood cells (panel B) and mammary stem cells generate breast tissue (panel C). Stem cells of one particular lineage cannot differentiate into another and are 'determined' once formed.

pathogens, but rogue cells with a finite number of genetic changes. Newer forms of biological therapies aim to control rather than kill cancer cells, with improvement of disease-free survival and quality of life.

Characteristics of the malignant phenotype

Growth and development of normal tissues proceeds to a point where the rate of cell proliferation is balanced by cell loss. Some tissues undergo hypertrophy or hyperplasia in response to normal physiological processes (e.g. breast and uterine tissues), but regress spontaneously upon withdrawal of an external stimulus. Furthermore, during the process of normal development and tissue renewal, the progeny of stem cells differentiate into mature cells which have characteristic biochemical and functional properties. Stem cells themselves originate from multipotential precursor cells which give rise to stem cells with a degree of genetic restriction and reduced potential. All stem cells have the capacity for self-renewal and can proliferate indefinitely. They undergo asymmetric cell divisions to produce a pool of identical progenitor cells or transit amplifying cells that differentiate into the cellular type appropriate for a particular location. Stem cells for one particular lineage cannot differentiate into cells of another lineage and are 'determined' once formed (Fig. 6.2.4). The phenotype of these stem cells is influenced by environmental factors which control replacement of senescent cells from undifferentiated stem cells (Fig. 6.2.5).

Loss of responsiveness to normal growth control mechanisms is a hallmark of any tumour, but malignant neoplasms have three characteristic features:

- Growth is no longer subject to strict regulation by surrounding cells and tissues. Cancers have achieved some degree of autonomy by dislocation of normal pathways of intercellular communication. However, a cancer cell is not completely autonomous and some channels of communication persist. In effect, a malignant tumour represents a state of regulatory imbalance in which cancer cells have attained various degrees of escape from the mechanisms that control rates of proliferation, cell death (apoptosis), and differentiation.
- Though many tumours are grossly similar to their parent tissue, all show degrees of anaplasia or loss of cellular differentiation. Cancers are a caricature of normal tissues and this is most evident for well differentiated tumours where there may be gross exaggeration of a normal characteristic. Poorly differentiated tumours appear disorganized with loss of normal tissue architecture and much variation in nuclear size and shape. Aneuploidy is also a prominent feature of less well differentiated tumours.

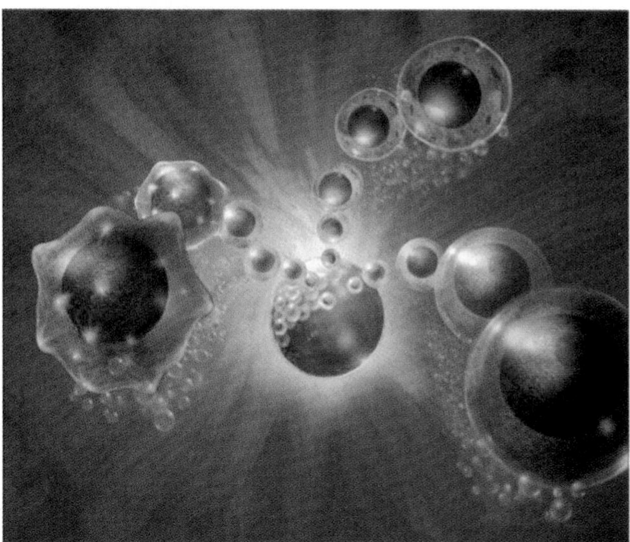

Fig. 6.2.5 Though stem cells of each tissue have particular features, all share the properties of self-renewal, multilineage potential, and high proliferative capacity. (From *The Lancet Oncology*, with permission. Copyright 2007 Elsevier Inc.)

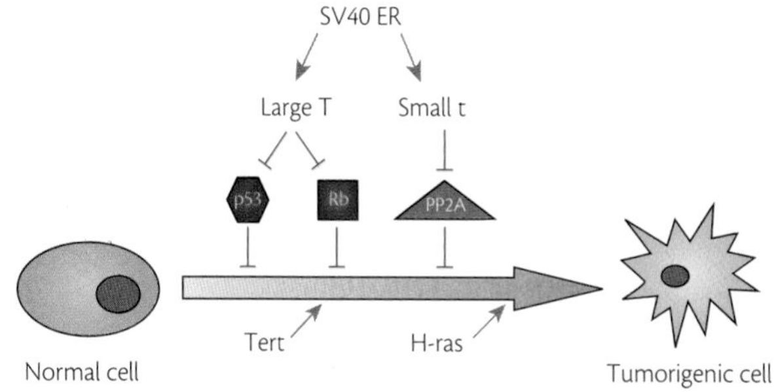

Fig. 6.2.6 At least four events are required to convert a normal human cell into a cancer cell *in vitro*. Introduction of clones specifying the SV40 large T antigen and small t antigens functionally disrupts the Rb and p53 protein pathways (events 1 and 2) while hTERT prevents telomere shortening (event 3). Finally, oncogenic H-ras results in malignant transformation (event 4).
(From the *Annual Review of Cell and Developmental Biology*, Volume 22, with permission. Copyright 2006 by Annual Reviews, http://www.annualreviews.org.)

- The fundamental feature of malignant neoplasms is the propensity to metastasize and form tumour foci at distant sites. Cancer cells within a tumour bolus have reduced cohesive properties and individual cells or tumour fragments can readily break away to enter either lymphatic or vascular channels within a nascent tumour. The endothelium lining these channels tends to be leaky and this facilitates entry of cancer cells. In the case of haematogenous spread, these cells must survive in the bloodstream and avoid immunological surveillance mechanisms (phagocytic cells and natural killer cells). There is evidence for some degree of organ specificity in terms of the capacity to invade and colonize distant sites with establishment of micrometastatic foci. The latter ultimately determine a patient's clinical fate and there is much heterogeneity between cells in the potential for metastatic spread, even within a single primary tumour.

Carcinogenesis

Carcinogenesis is a multistage process with the sequential acquisition of mutations within the genome. It remains unclear whether invasive malignancy develops once a critical number and type of mutations are present within a cell, or whether serial accumulation is mandatory whereby mutations are acquired in a particular order. Many genetic changes are already present in premalignant and *in situ* forms of cancer. The incidence of many common cancers (such as those of the breast, prostate, colon, or skin) increases with age with kinetics dependent on the fourth or fifth power of elapsed time. This observation suggests that a minimum of four or five events must occur before tumour development (Fig. 6.2.6). Moreover, the association of cancer with increasing age suggests that continuous exposure to low levels of environmental or endogenous carcinogens may have a cumulative effect and perhaps act upon tissues more susceptible to neoplastic change.

The genetic alterations within a cell which form the basis for malignant transformation can be either inherited or acquired. Germline mutations are present within all cells, whereas somatic mutations affect individual cells within a particular tissue. Approximately 1% of human cancers are attributable to inheritable (familial) forms of the disease whereby development of malignancy is almost inevitable. In such cases, either the homozygous (tumour suppressor genes) or heterozygous state (oncogenes) will confer a high level of genetic susceptibility and no further genetic mutation may be necessary for tumour initiation (e.g. retinoblastoma). In other circumstances, the chance of developing cancer will depend upon a balance of genetic predisposition and acquired mutations. For the majority of human cancers there is no inherited risk and these are termed sporadic tumours. They are dependent exclusively on somatic mutations. These latter genetic alterations result from one of two interrelated processes:

1. There is an intrinsic error rate for DNA synthesis and repair within normal tissues which results in acquired mutations that are passed on to the cell progeny during replication. This leads to a background rate of spontaneous mutation which has been estimated to be a one in a million chance for any particular gene each time a cell divides. This represents a very low baseline somatic mutation rate and the chance of a key cancer gene being mutated spontaneously must be extremely low. Moreover, the probability of serial mutations with functional impact occurring within a single cell must be a very rare event. However, carcinogenic mutations usually confer a growth advantage relative to neighbouring cells even before frank malignant transformation. A powerful positive selection pressure therefore operates from the outset for cancer-promoting mutations and this effectively magnifies the impact of low-frequency events. Once a mutation has occurred in a stem cell, a malignant clone of cells arises which will replicate the initial mutation thousands of times. As the clone size approaches about 100 cells, the chance of a second mutation within this primary clone increases significantly. This in turn will enhance any selective growth advantage and this new clone will outgrow the first one. This process is continued and leads to acquisition of a collection of cellular features typical of the malignant phenotype. Furthermore, this adaptive process can permit tumours to respond to treatment interventions with development of resistance (Fig. 6.2.7).
2. This baseline rate of spontaneous somatic mutation is augmented by environmental factors interacting with cellular DNA

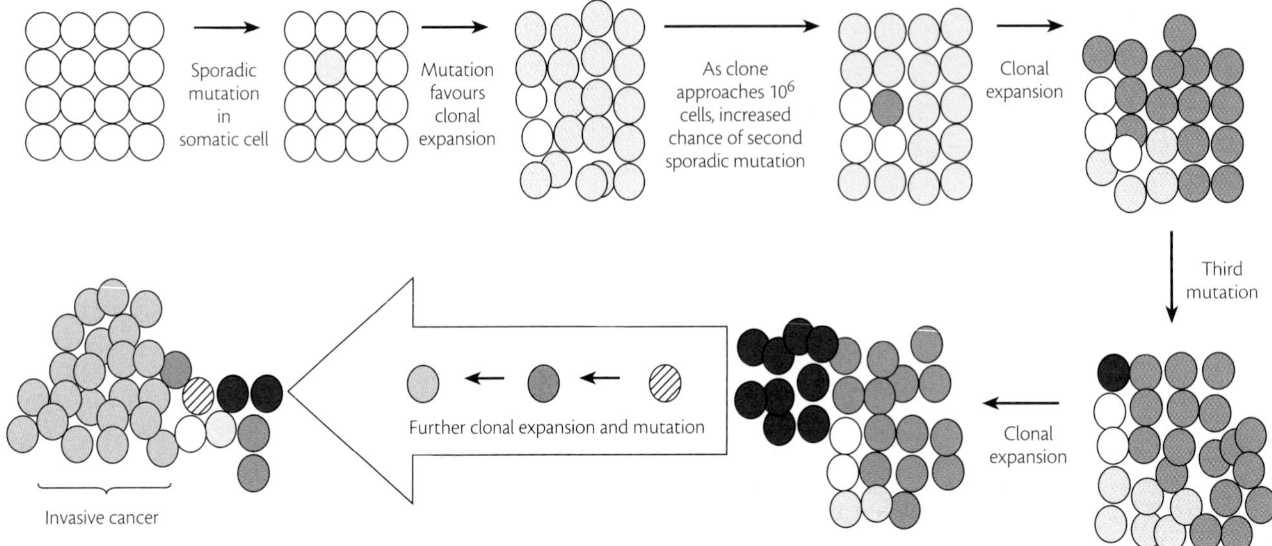

Fig. 6.2.7 Sporadic mutations which give a somatic cell a selective growth advantage encourage outgrowth of mutated clones. Successive clones continue to accumulate mutations and outgrow preceding clones. The process of clonal expansion and mutation eventually results in a clone of cells with a malignant phenotype. Established tumours continue to evolve by continuation of clonal expansion and acquisition of growth-promoting mutations.

either directly or indirectly. These include not only exposure to agents such as radiation and chemical carcinogens, but also the genotoxic effects of endogenous agents such as free radicals which induce oxidative stress. A variety of chemicals are known to be carcinogenic (Table 6.2.1) and some of the mechanisms for induction of tumours have been elucidated. For example, the carcinogenic potential of polycyclic hydrocarbons (coal tar) resides in the K-region of the molecule which is oxygenated by cellular enzymes to form an epoxide residue. This reacts directly with the genomic bases of DNA to effect mutagenesis. Aminophenols act in a similar manner after being released by the action of glucoronidase on β-naphthylamine and benzidine (aniline dyes).

Though many of the well documented industrial cancer risks have been minimized in recent years (coal mining; dye, rubber, and asbestos industries), several potential sources of carcinogens exist within the environment of contemporary Western society. Most of these involve low levels of exposure, including low-density ionizing radiation (X-rays, γ-rays) and ultraviolet irradiation. These will contribute to the background rate of somatic mutation and in some cases can greatly increase rates of malignancy (e.g. cigarette smoking, solar exposure).

Table 6.2.1 Chemical carcinogens

Category of carcinogen	Active constituent
Polycyclic hydrocarbons	3:4-Benzpyrene, 1:2, 5:6-dibenzpyrene
Nitrosamines	Dimethylnitrosamine
Aromatic amines/azo dyes	β-Naphthylamine, dimethylaminoazobenzene
Plant products	Aflatoxin, pyrrolozidium
Alkylating agents	Nitrogen mustard, melphalan, nitrosourea, etoposide
Inorganic chemicals	Arsenic, nickel, asbestos, cadmium

Initiators and promoters

Early studies on chemical carcinogenesis in animal models led to the conceptual division of tumour formation into separate phases of initiation and promotion. Agents classified as initiators produce a permanent change in cells but this is insufficient to cause complete tumour development. This initiating carcinogen most likely induces genetic damage within the stem cell population which involves segments of the genome containing cancer genes. Nongenetic changes may sometimes occur but genetic alterations will produce durable changes within cells which can last for a considerable time. Indeed, initiated cells will remain latent until acted upon by a promoter which yields transient changes in a repetitive manner over a prolonged period of time. These induce cell division and subsequent tumour development. Promoters are not usually carcinogenic, but some agents can act as both initiator and promoter. These are more likely to induce a widespread genetic insult which affects both the genes controlling malignant transformation as well as other sites. A breast cancer might be initiated during the early teenage years by a chemical carcinogen or radiation (e.g. radiation from the atomic bombs of Nagasaki and Hiroshima) and be promoted by oestrogens 20 to 30 years later. Promoters may encourage stem cells to remain undifferentiated and in a relatively hyperproliferative state. The rate of tumour development would depend on the balance of growth stimulatory and growth inhibitory influences converging upon cells.

Cellular transformation

The increased growth potential of cancer cells has been exploited empirically to study carcinogenesis in the laboratory setting. Most types of benign epithelial cells are difficult to grow in tissue culture, but their malignant counterparts more readily grow and survive *in vitro* and form tumour xenografts in animal models. Cancer cells possess the following *in vitro* characteristics:

- A reduced requirement for exogenous sources of polypeptide growth factors. This was originally observed for Rous sarcoma virus transformed chick fibroblasts and led to the 'autocrine hypothesis' by Sporn and Todaro in 1980.

- Loss of contact inhibition once confluency is reached. Instead of finite growth in two-dimensional systems, cells tend to pile up upon each other and form discrete tumour masses.
- Anchorage-independent growth in which cells can be propagated in suspension and grow in soft agar without the need for a solid, supporting substrate.
- The ability to divide indefinitely after multiple passages in tissue culture—a characteristic of immortalization.

Cells which have acquired the above properties are referred to as transformed cells. This term is also used to describe initiated cells which can potentially grow but cannot form tumours in the absence of a promoter. To some extent there are parallels between the concept of initiated cells and the *in vitro* correlate. The process of cellular transformation represents the first stage in a complex continuum of changes culminating in a cancer cell with full metastatic potential. Transformation at the molecular level has been defined in terms of disruption of four critical pathways (Fig. 6.2.6). Though these transformed cells all show anchorage-independent growth, not all of these transformed cells can form tumours in nude mice and even fewer yield metastatic foci at distant sites (e.g. lungs). Comprehensive expression of the malignant phenotype mandates further genetic changes specific to the processes of angiogenesis, invasion and metastasis. Furthermore, stromal–epithelial interactions are important for development of some tumours (e.g. breast, prostate) and monocultures of cancer cell lines do not fully simulate *in vivo* conditions.

A tumour is composed of several cell types in addition to neoplastic epithelium. These include various mesenchymal derivatives such as fibroblasts and endothelial cells, which *in vivo* have important interactions with epithelial cells in both topographical and functional contexts. The nature of these stromal–epithelial interactions remain ill defined and poorly understood, but mesenchymal elements are key determinants in fundamental mechanisms of cell proliferation and differentiation, even within the adult organism once morphological and functional maturity have occurred. Mesenchymal–epithelial interactions during embryogenesis and their continuance throughout an organism's lifespan raise questions about possible involvement in carcinogenesis:

- Does any derangement of epithelial proliferation and differentiation represent a regressive state in which features of the embryonal/fetal phenotype are re-expressed by transformed cells?
- If mesenchymal–epithelial interactions in the adult organism serve to keep in check any abnormal epithelial proliferation, then how are these interactions perturbed in cancer?
- Can therapies be directed at rectifying specific abnormalities in stromal–epithelial interaction?

Some of the genetic changes associated with invasion and metastases together with angiogenesis are discussed below.

The origin of cancer cells

One of the most challenging aspects in the research and treatment of cancer is tumour heterogeneity. Not only is there variation between individuals with respect to a designated tumour type, but cells composing a single tumour are far from homogeneous. Any theory for the origin of cancer cells must provide an explanation for cellular heterogeneity. Two questions are pertinent to this discussion:

- Is cancer monoclonal or polyclonal in origin?
- Do cancers originate from stem cells or from differentiated somatic cells?

Monoclonal theory

Much evidence has accrued supporting a monoclonal origin for most human cancers. This implies that a single cell undergoes malignant transformation and forms a primary clone from which further subclones are derived. This process of clonal evolution (Fig. 6.2.7) is predicated on a selective growth advantage for mutated cells which permits them to bridge 'bottlenecks' imposed by restrictions of space, nutrients, and oxygen (Fig. 6.2.8). Studies of enzyme expression in haematological malignancies arising in female heterozygotes for glucose-6-phosphate dehydrogenase have shown that cancers contain either the maternal or the paternal form of the enzyme. This suggests that the cancer is derived from a single cell containing one or other form of the enzyme. Similar evidence for the monoclonal nature of cancer comes from lymphomas and other cancers of the lymphoid system which invariably express a single class (monoclonal) of antibody with light chain restriction. A polyclonal origin for cancer might be feasible for some inherited forms of cancer where there are germ-line mutations in both alleles and genetic susceptibility operates as a 'field effect'. However, for most sporadic cancers and inherited forms that depend upon a further somatic mutation, polyclonality is highly improbable; multiple cells in close proximity would have to be transformed concurrently or within a relatively short time frame to form a single tumour.

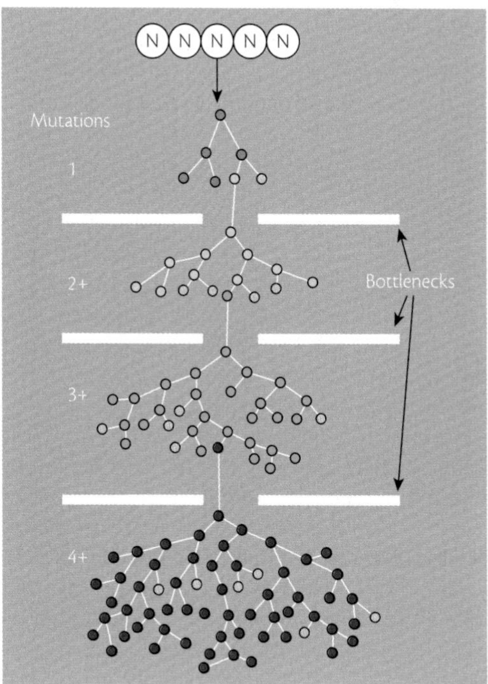

Fig. 6.2.8 Clonal evolution of a cancer. Sequential mutations result in successive descendent clones possessing a selective growth advantage which enables them to overcome 'bottlenecks' imposed by restrictions of space, nutrients and oxygen. First subclone shown in yellow, second in green, and third in red. Grey represents dying cells. N, normal stem cells.
(From *The Lancet Oncology*, with permission. Copyright 2002 Elsevier Inc.)

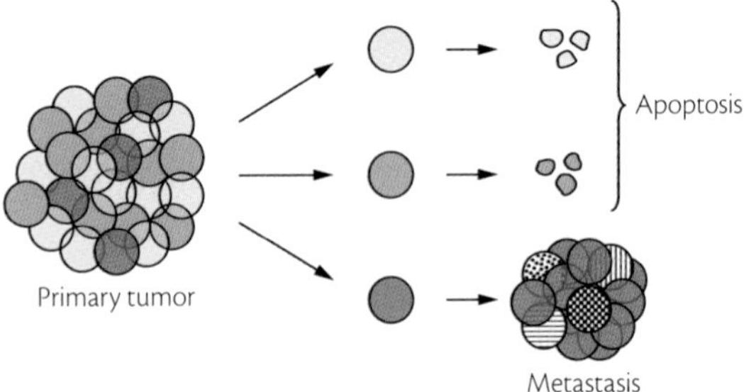

Fig. 6.2.9 The mature tumour contains cells of monoclonal origin but forming a heterogeneous mixture of independent subclones. These display phenotypic and genetic diversity and only a fraction of these will have the potential to migrate and form distant metastases (dark grey cells). Further mutations within this subclone will occur yielding metastases containing cells with diverse properties (striped and variously patterned cells).
(From *Annual Review of Medicine*, with permission. Copyright 2007 Annual Reviews.)

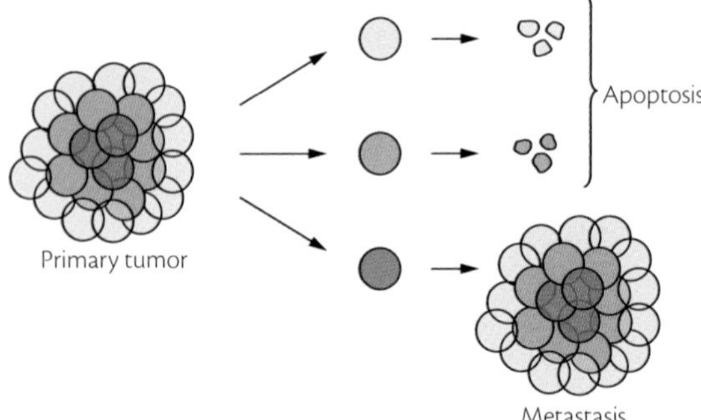

Fig. 6.2.10 According to the cancer stem cell hypothesis, intratumoral heterogeneity arises from cell differentiation and only cancer stem cells (dark grey cells) have the capacity to migrate and form distant metastases with differentiated cancer cells undergoing apoptosis. The proportion of differentiated/apoptotic malignant stem cells (light grey cells) relative to those which continue to proliferate determines tumour grade.
(From the *Annual Review of Medicine*, Volume 58, with permission. Copyright 2007 by Annual Reviews, http://www.annualreviews.org.)

So how might heterogeneity arise within the context of a monoclonal scenario? The sequential acquisition of mutations during clonal evolution not only provides a positive selection pressure, but also generates a degree of instability within the genome. This genetic instability favours further mutational change among individual cells of a clone. These additional and random mutations result in phenotypic differences between cells which will be manifest as variations in rates of proliferation, cell motility, and metastatic potential as well as sensitivity/resistance to therapeutic interventions. Thus the mature tumour contains cells of monoclonal origin but phenotypic and genetic diversity. This process generates subclones of cells with different functional properties, some of which will have the capacity to metastasize (Fig. 6.2.9).

Cancer stem cell hypothesis

Many tumours are grossly similar to their tissue of origin, which is most evident for well-differentiated lesions. It was previously believed that cancers arose from dedifferentiation of the mature phenotype with reversion to a more primitive state to a greater (poorly differentiated) or lesser (well differentiated) degree. It is rather unlikely that a mature somatic cell would exist within tissues for a sufficiently long period to accumulate a mandatory number of mutations for malignant transformation. By contrast, stem cells have greater longevity and have the capacity for self-renewal. The cancer stem cell hypothesis proposes that the stem cell, and not mature somatic cells, is the target for carcinogenesis (Fig. 6.2.10). A tumour would arise from differentiation of rapidly proliferating, undifferentiated stem cells and contain varying proportions of these two stem cell types (i.e. undifferentiated and differentiated malignant stem cells). Furthermore, the proportion of malignant stem cells which have undergone differentiation (and apoptosis) relative to those which continue to proliferate determines histological grade. Thus a cell may possess the typical features of a malignant phenotype yet still have gone through a sequential process of differentiation to a point comparable with the normal cell lineage. Studies with teratocarcinomas and haemapoietic malignancies support the cancer stem cell hypothesis and confirm that stem cells of individual lineages can be highly malignant. They have also been found to have the same immunophenotype as their healthy non-malignant counterparts.

In patients with acute myeloid leukaemia, a small fraction of undifferentiated cells were found to be the only cells isolated which had the capacity for reconstitution of tumours on implantation in NOD/SCID (nonobese diabetic/severe combined immunodeficient) mice. These undifferentiated cells resembled haemopoietic stem cells, suggesting that the latter are subject to carcinogenic processes. It is possible that partially committed progenitor cells which have acquired the capacity for self-renewal could be the origin of these malignant cells. Cancer stem cells have now been identified in tumours of the breast and nervous system and are the focus for novel and more targeted forms of treatment. Thus cancer stem cells form a functional group of cells which initiate tumour formation and can differentiate into a heterogeneous progeny that sustain tumour growth. A relatively small population of quiescent or slowly dividing cancer stem cells is responsible for the continued expansion of a tumour by spawning more differentiated cells. These latter cells constitute the bulk of the tumour (epithelial component) and have short-term proliferative capacity. The development of cancer therefore parallels normal tissue development with origin from an hierarchical lineage of cells (Fig. 6.2.11).

This cancer stem cell hypothesis is in accordance with the paradigm that cancer is an 'aberrancy in normal self'. Cancer cells resemble normal cells of their parent tissue and remain functionally part of a regulatory network which allows variable levels of intercellular communication.

Genetic alterations

The process of mitosis—division of a cell to produce progeny with identical genetic content—is extremely complex. Though cell division is well orchestrated with a high degree of fidelity, there is an innate fallibility which leads to errors in DNA replication. The cell possesses multiple mechanisms for ongoing repair of inappropriate alterations in base-pair sequences, and can activate programmed cell death when there is overwhelming DNA damage or gross chromosomal changes. Some of the enzymes involved in these repair processes can be susceptible to mutational events and will indirectly cause malignant transformation of cells by allowing persistence and propagation of gene alterations. Individuals with

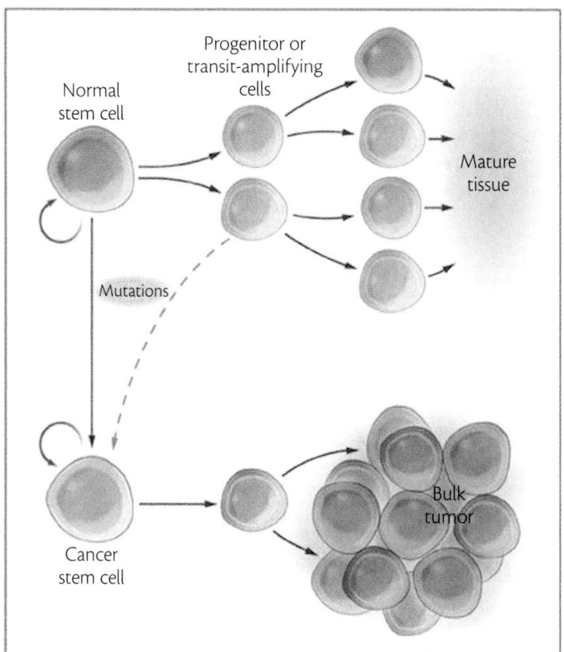

Fig. 6.2.11 Normal stem cells differentiate into mature tissue by generation of progenitor or transit-amplifying cells. Cancer stem cells arise from mutations in normal stem cells (or possibly progenitor cells) and subsequently undergo a sequential process of differentiation to form primary tumours. Cancer stem cells share the capacity to self-renew and can have high proliferative potential.
(From the *New England Journal of Medicine*, with permission. Copyright 2007, Massachusetts Medical Society.)

Bloom's syndrome have a deficiency of DNA ligase I and are highly susceptible to developing cancer.

Types of mutation

In recent years there has been major progress in understanding and unravelling the genetic alterations which lead to disruption and dislocation of molecular and biochemical pathways. Though no single genetic change has been identified which causes cancer, it is now appreciated that cancer cells display a finite number of aberrant pathways and the defective portion of the DNA is relatively small in proportion to overall genome size. Exogenous agents such as chemicals and irradiation induce direct DNA damage, but a background mutation rate occurs from the hydrolytic interaction of water itself with DNA. This results in the cleavage of glycosidic bonds which can depurinate or depyrimidate nucleotide bases or cause strand breaks. Genetic alterations associated with malignant change can be broadly divided into the following five categories:

- Changes in nucleotide sequence resulting from base-pair substitutions, deletions, or insertions. Deletions and insertions can lead to major problems with gene transcription and are sometimes referred to as 'missense' mutations. These often result in a truncated protein as the altered DNA sequence cannot be read. Up to 90% of pancreatic adenocarcinomas contain missense mutations. Tautomeric changes within individual nucleotides may have minimal impact and cause minor changes in protein structure and function. Indeed, a codon with a single base alteration could be 'silent' and not effect any change in amino acid sequence.
- Changes in the normal diploid number of chromosomes are common in cancer. Aneuploid cells usually have a reduced complement of chromosomal material (up to 50%), and result from inappropriate segregation of chromosomes during mitosis.
- Chromosomal translocations are the most common structural rearrangement in cancer cells and involve fusion of different chromosomes or segments of a single chromosome which are noncontiguous (Table 6.2.2). This interchange of chromosomal material can result in an oncogene being positioned next to transcription regulatory sequences, leading to overexpression. Alternatively, a fusion gene may be formed from combination of coding sequences on either side of the breakpoint (Table 6.2.2). A classic example of the latter is formation of the Philadelphia chromosome in chronic myelogenous leukaemia. This results from fusion of the C-terminus of the c-*abl* gene on chromosome 9 and the N-terminus of the *bcr* gene on chromosome 22 (*bcr-abl1* gene product) (Fig. 6.2.12).

Table 6.2.2 Translocations observed in specific malignancies. Gene fusion results in a chimeric protein which is under the influence of a cell-specific promoter and frequently affects regulation of cell cycle progression by modulation of transcription factors

Neoplasm	Description	Associated translocations	Genes disrupted in translocation
Lymphoma	Burkitt's lymphoma	t(8;14), t(2;8), t(8;22)	*myc* (TF) overexpression under control of immunoglobulin promoter sequences
	Follicular lymphoma	t(14;18)	BCL2 overexpression under control of immunoglobulin promoter sequences
AML*	Acute promyelocytic subtype	t(15;17)	Fusion of *PML* and *RARα* (TF)
CML†	90 percent of all CML	Philadelphia chromosome t(9;22)	Fusion of *BCR* and *ABL*
ALI‡	Pre-BALL	t(1;19)	Fusion of *PBX1* and *E2A* (TF)
Sarcoma	Ewing's sarcoma	t(11;22)	Fusion of *EWS* and *FLI1* (TF)
	Clear cell sarcoma	t(12;22)	Fusion of *EWS* and *ATF1* (TF)
	Alveolar rhabdomyosarcoma	t(2;13)	Fusion of *PAX3* (TF) and *FKHD* (TF)
	Synovial sarcoma	t(X;18)	Fusion of *SYT* (TF) and *SSX1* or *SSX2* (TFs)
	Myxoid liposarcoma	t(12;16)	Fusion *FUS* and *CHOP* (TF)

* Acute myeloid leukaemia.
† Chronic myeloid leukaemia.
‡ Acute lymphoid leukaemia.

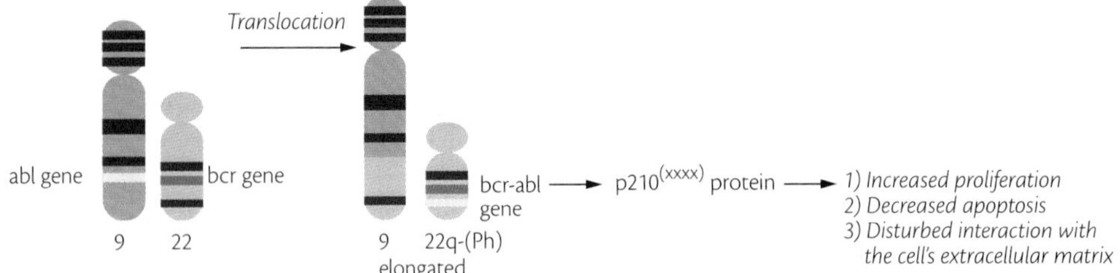

Fig. 6.2.12 Chronic myelogenous leukamia is characterized by a reciprocal translocation (t[9;22][q34;q11] which generates a small 22q chromosome referred to as the Philadelphia chromosome. This translocation results in the oncogene c-*abl* being transferred from chromosome 9 (band 9q34) to the *bcr* gene (band 22q11). Breakpoints can occur over variable distances on each chromosome to form the Philadelphia chromosome. This yields a fusion *bcr-abl1* gene product which is thought to lead to constitutive activation of a mitogenic growth factor receptor.

- Gene amplifications result from multiple copies of an 'amplicon' containing 0.5 to 10 Mb of DNA. This phenomenon occurs relatively late in the pathogenesis of cancer and probably reflects acquired genetic instability. When an amplicon encodes an oncoprotein, this will be overexpressed and promote tumorigenesis. Many oncogenes derive enhanced expression from this mechanism and are associated with particularly aggressive phenotypes. For example, the n-*myc* gene is frequently amplified in neuroblastomas which are highly lethal tumours (Fig. 6.2.13).
- Epigenetic changes represent a nonmutational pathway for modulation of gene expression. Instead of changes in nucleotide sequence, DNA methylation and histone modification are used to maintain a gene in a closed confirmation such that it cannot be accessed by DNA polymerase. Hypermethylation is a method for gene silencing and can prevent expression of tumour suppressor genes (e.g. *BRCA1*) even when the gene sequence is intact. Interestingly, tumorigenesis is generally associated with an overall reduction in levels of DNA methylation (up to 40%) but there is preferentially increased methylation of CpG islands associated with tumour suppressor genes (see below).

Genetic instability

As previously discussed, the process of clonal selection amplifies the rate of spontaneous mutation in somatic cells to permit emergence of tumours. The frequency of mutational events is further enhanced by the existence of genetic instability, which parallels clonal evolution. As cells progressively acquire cancer-related mutations, the genome becomes more unstable and prone to genetic alteration. This is a general property of the cellular DNA and not attributable to specific mutations. Genetic instability appears to be inherent in a large proportion of cancers and greatly increases the probability of further spontaneous mutations which contribute to neoplastic development.

Repair of genetic damage

Though cells are vulnerable to genetic damage, there are specific mechanisms which serve to maintain the integrity of the genome.

Caretaker genes

These are involved in recognition and repair of nucleotide base-pair abnormalities or DNA strand breaks. Two general mechanisms exist for repair of DNA:

- In base excision repair the abnormal sequence of nucleotides is removed enzymatically. Endonucleases initially cleave the DNA and the abnormal segment is removed by exonucleases. Polymerases subsequently resynthesize the missing segment which is united to the parent strand by action of a DNA ligase.
- Longer strands of DNA can be excised for repair of more extensive faults in a process termed nucleotide excision repair (see below).

These repair processes are fundamental to all living organisms including bacteria (*E. coli*). Importantly, should dividing cells contain any anomalous DNA, DNA is replicated as far as the damaged segment and the latter resynthesized using the other strand as a template.

Gatekeeper genes

These genes control entry of cells into the replicative cycle and activate cell cycle arrest in the presence of damaged DNA. This set of gatekeeper genes works in collaboration with caretaker genes so that sufficient time and opportunity exists for repair of damaged DNA prior to onset of cell division. If this gatekeeper function fails, there is a risk that damaged portions of DNA will be passed on to

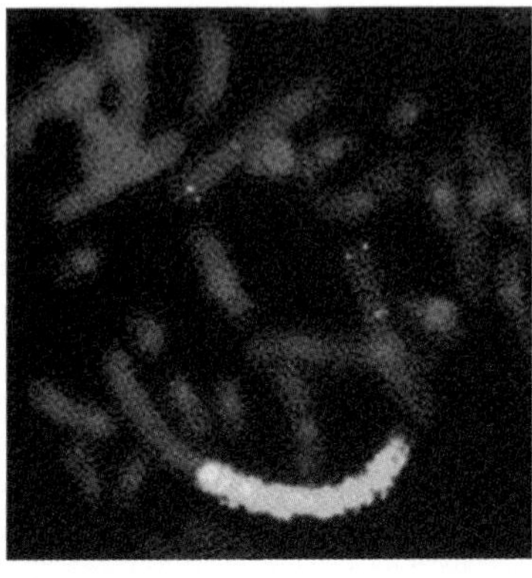

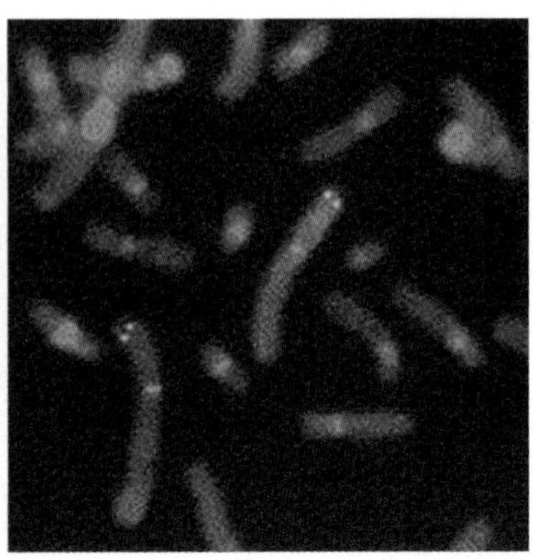

Fig. 6.2.13 Amplification is a principal mechanism for activation of oncogenes. Cytogenetic analysis reveals homogeneous staining of a chromosomal region in neuroblastoma indicates 150 fold amplification of the N-*myc* gene (right panel) compared with a normal cell (left panel)
(From *The Lancet Oncology*, with permission. Copyright 2003, Elsevier Inc.)

daughter cells as potential cancer-promoting mutations. There are two major control points in the cell cycle; the first is towards the end of G1 (G1/S) and the second at the initiation of mitosis (G2/M). Gatekeepers operate around these control checkpoints and interact with signal transduction pathways which are rapidly integrating stimulatory and inhibitory signals from within and outside the cell during the gap periods of the cell cycle (G1 and G2).

The cell will assess the final polarity of the net signalling and together with an analysis of DNA integrity will direct gatekeeper activities. Activation of gatekeeper pathways will influence one or other of these checkpoints and either prevent the onset of DNA synthesis (G1 checkpoint) or entry into mitosis (G2 checkpoint). Gatekeeper function also encompasses control of chromosomal segregation following alignment on the microtubular spindle (spindle checkpoint). In addition, these gatekeeper genes can trigger cell death in the face of extensive genetic damage or failure of basic DNA repair mechanisms of caretaker genes. This prevents propagation of potentially carcinogenic mutations and is an important mechanism for protecting a healthy genome. Specific defects in both caretaker and gatekeeper genes can lead to dramatic rates of genetic instability and rapid progression to a lethal phenotype.

Genetic instability can be manifest at one of two levels. Most instability is observed at the level of the chromosome, with large-scale deletions, duplication, or interchange of whole or large segments of chromosomes. Less commonly, nucleotide instability results from substitution, deletion, or insertion of nucleotides. Interestingly, there is an inverse relationship between instability at the chromosomal and nucleotide levels, suggesting that these pathways may be mutually exclusive.

Chromosomal instability

Karyotypic analyses indicate that most cancers of epithelial origin display aneuploidy. This suggests that several genes, when mutated, lead to this form of instability which is at least 10-fold higher in aneuploid compared with diploid tumours. Indeed, more than 100 genes may be predicted to result in chromosomal instability when aberrant; this includes those involved in chromosome condensation, sister chromatid cohesion, kinetochore assembly, and centrosome duplication. The molecular basis for this chromosomal instability is heterogeneous, with no obvious unifying theme. Moreover, defects in specific checkpoints discussed above will promote this form of genetic instability. 'Spindle checkpoint' genes ensure that segregation of chromosomes on the mitotic spindle proceeds without error, but mutations in these genes are commonly detected in human cancer. The genes involved in the spindle checkpoint response are *MAD1*, *MAD2*, *MAD3*, *BUBR1*, *BUB1*, *BUB3*, *MPS1*, and *CDC20*. Among these, somatic mutations in *BUB1* and *BUBR1* have been found in human cancers, the former being associated with massive chromosomal instability in colorectal cancers. Mutations in *BUB1* can act in a dominant negative manner by causing disruption of spindle checkpoint function in both mouse and human cells when expressed exogenously. Furthermore, *MAD2* expression appears to be repressed in several solid tumours, including breast cancers.

Defects in a second checkpoint, referred to as a 'DNA damage checkpoint', are probably a more frequent cause of chromosomal instability. This checkpoint prevents cells with damaged DNA from entering mitosis; replication of damaged DNA results in abnormalities of both chromosomal segregation and mitotic recombination. Gross structural alterations in chromosomes will occur if DNA replication goes ahead in the presence of either a single or double strand break. Some inherited forms of cancer predisposition are linked to these 'DNA strand break pathways' and genes such as *ATM* (ataxia telangiectasia mutated), *ATR* (ATM and RAD-3 related), *BRCA1*, *BRCA2*, and *TP53* are DNA damage checkpoint genes which have been implicated in human malignancy. Within normal cells, functional p53 will prompt cell cycle arrest in G1 in the presence of inappropriate chromosomal segregation. By contrast, a defective p53 protein allows cells to progress through the G1/S transition and eventually aneuploidy will occur in daughter cells.

A further mechanism for chromosomal instability is abnormal number and function of centrosomes. Centrosomes act to nucleate the ends of the mitotic microtubule spindle along which sister chromosomes separate during mitosis. Multiple (i.e. more than two) centrosomes have been noted in several common cancer types and result in multipolar spindles which cannot guide normal chromosomal segregation. Overexpression of centrosome-associated kinase genes induces formation of multiple centrosomes and abnormal karyotypes in human cancer cells. The Aurora kinases control duplication of centrosomes and transfection of the cognate gene for Aurora A kinase can transform cells in culture and promote tumour formation. Inactivating mutations of the gene abrogate this ability and therefore Aurora A has been classified as an oncogene. Another centrosome-associated kinase is PLK1 which is a homologue of *Drosophila* Polo. PLl1 is a serine/threonine kinase which has been found to be overexpressed in a subset of human cancers which display aneuploidy and chromosomal instability.

A final mechanism for chromosomal instability is via dysfunctional telomeres. The latter are ribonuclear protein complexes located at the ends of all functional eukaryotic chromosomes. They contain a high proportion of hexanucleotide repeat sequences TTAGGG spanning 4 to 15 kbp and are capped by associated proteins. Telomeric dysfunction promotes end-to-end fusions and fusion–bridge–breakage cycles which result in gross structural chromosomal abnormalities.

Therefore several mechanisms exist whereby cells may become aneuploid with chromosomal instability. Collectively, these are responsible for the relatively frequent occurrence of these complex lesions.

Nucleotide instability

Instability at the nucleotide level is relatively uncommon in cancers and probably reflects the impact of environmental carcinogens or the background rate of somatic mutation. However, defects in two main cellular DNA repair systems can lead to significant levels of genetic instability.

Nucleotide excision repair

This is a versatile DNA repair mechanism, alluded to above. It is responsible for detection and repair of bulky DNA lesions induced by exogenous mutagens, especially ultraviolet-induced lesions such as cyclobutane pyrimidine dimers and pyrimidine 6–4 photoproducts. The importance of nucleotide excision repair was first recognized in individuals with xeroderma pigmentosum who possess an inherited defect in this DNA repair system characterized by severe ultraviolet photosensitivity and susceptibility to skin cancers. The disease is autosomally recessive and heterozygotes are not at increased risk for malignancy. Thus the disease poses a significant clinical risk only in the context of an inherited predisposition.

DNA mismatch repair

This system is responsible for correction of DNA replication errors including base–base mismatches and abnormal nucleotide loops resulting from insertions/deletions of DNA and incorporated during the replicative process. Base–base mismatches typically affect nonrepetitive DNA sequences while insertional/deletion loops occur at sites of repetitive DNA sequences. These lesions lead to gains or losses of short mono- or dinucleotide repeat units (e.g. poly(A) or poly (CA) repeats) within sections of the genome, called microsatellite regions. The microsatellite sequences are characterized by identical nucleotide repeats and are frequently observed in the coding regions of genes. This type of nucleotide replication error is known as 'microsatellite instability' and has been identified in the majority of tumours developing in patients with hereditary non-polyposis coli (HNPCC), otherwise known as Lynch's syndrome. This disease is caused directly by mutations in genes required for DNA mismatch repair. However, mismatch repair defects accelerate the mutation rate for both hereditary and sporadic forms of colon cancer (cf. XP and NER mutations). Furthermore, mismatch repair defects can be detected in more than 10% of all colorectal, stomach, and endometrial cancers. Mismatch repair defects were first investigated in bacteria and yeast (*mutS* and *mutL*) and subsequently human homologues of these genes were identified. *MSH2*, the human homologue of *mut S*, has been located on chromosome 2 and is inactivated in kindreds of HNPCC patients with colon tumours. Moreover, *MLH1*, the human homologue of *mutL*, has been traced to chromosome 3 and is likewise mutated in HNPCC kindreds. It is now recognized that at least 95% of HNPCC cases are attributable to mutations in these two mismatch repair genes. A correspondingly lower proportion (15%) of sporadic colorectal cancers exhibit microsatellite instability and this often results from a nonmutational event (epigenetic inactivation of the *MLH1* gene). A total of seven human homologues of *mutS* (i.e. *MSH2*, *MSH3*, *MSH6*) and *mutL* (*MLH1*, *MLH3*, *PMS1*, *PMS2*) have thus far been identified. It is noteworthy that some genes involved in growth suppression have been found to be mutated at microsatellite sequences within their coding regions (Table 6.2.3).

Chromosomal translocations

Two principle forms of chromosomal translocations occur in human cancers: complex and simple.

Complex translocations

These are the more common type of translocation and probably represent a stochastic event with no predictable pattern of repetition within tumours of the same histopathological subtype. The molecular basis for these complex changes is unknown, but a fundamental fault involving caretaker and gatekeeper genes is likely responsible and translocations occur against a background of chromosomal instability. The complex type of translocation may result from cells entering mitosis before double strand breaks have been repaired. This will favour random union of free DNA ends through nonhomologous recombinations.

Table 6.2.3 Examples of genes containing microsatellite sequences and corresponding neoplastic tissues in which mutations within these microsatellite sequences have been demonstrated

Gene	Microsatellite sequence	Neoplasms
TGF-β1 type II receptor	AAAAAAAA	Gastrointestinal (HNPCC, colorectal, gastric and ampullary adenocarcinoma and Barrett's oesophagus). Glioma. Endometrial
IGFIIR	GGGGGGGG	Gastrointestinal (HNPCC and Barrett's oesophagus)
BAX	GGGGGGGG	Gastrointestinal (HNPCC and colorectal)

HPNCC: hereditary non-polyposis colon cancer.

Simple translocations

These appear to be nonstochastic events and are characterized by distinctive patterns of breakpoints and chromosomal rearrangements in specific cancers (namely leukaemias, lymphomas, and sarcomas). These simple types of translocation are most likely not due to any underlying genetic instability but instead may reflect low-frequency aberrations in normal physiological recombination events. This is most evident for lymphoid malignancies where DNA strand breaks are generated in lymphoid cells as part of the normal recombination process. This mechanism yields the potentially great diversity observed among genes encoding immunoglobulins and T-cell receptors. An alternative mechanism for existence of simple translocations in sarcomas is likely to appertain as gene rearrangements do not accompany physiological recombination. Translocations provide the opportunity for an oncogene to come under the influence of a strong promoter, either from repositioning next to regenerating sequences or fusion of two disparate coding regions.

Gene amplification

Gene amplification occurs towards the later stages of the neoplastic continuum and is a further manifestation of genetic instability. Gene amplification results in exaggerated expression of otherwise normal genes, though the term oncogene encompasses over-expression of a normal gene as well as an intrinsic gene abnormality which leads to enhanced functional activity of the gene (Fig. 6.2.13). Defects in the apoptotic pathway may permit cells with amplified chromosomal segments to survive (e.g. p53 abnormalities). A list of genes which are commonly amplified in human cancers is shown in Table 6.2.4.

Cell cycle checkpoints and cancer

The progression of cells through the normal cell cycle is closely regulated as part of the complex process of cell division. Specific cell cycle checkpoints exist which monitor the integrity and replication status of DNA. These checkpoints exert a restraining influence on cell cycle progression and help ensure fidelity of DNA replication and DNA repair processes are not compromised by time limitation. These control mechanisms minimize propagation of heritable mutations and reduce the risk of cancer development. Genes encoding proteins that promote cell cycling are frequently subject to activation in human cancers through gain of function mutation or gene amplification (see previous section). Oncogenes are discussed in more detail in the following sections, together with tumour suppressor genes which often encode components of cell cycle checkpoints. In contrast to oncogenes, these tumour suppressor genes are inactivated in malignant states and are among the most commonly documented mutations in human cancer.

The stimulus of DNA damage initiates a sequence of events which eventually halt cell cycle progression. Some of the molecular events involved have been elucidated, and activation of the genes for

Table 6.2.4 Examples of malignancies where gene amplification has been observed

Gene product	Description	Cancer type
Epidermal growth factor receptor	Receptor tyrosine kinase	Breast Head and neck Urogenital Glioblastoma multiforme
ErbB2/Her2	Related to epidermal growth factor receptor	Breast Ovarian Bladder Cervical Head and neck
Fibroblast growth factor 4	Growth factor	Oesophageal carcinoma
or Hst-1		Breast
Fibroblast growth factor 3 or Int-2	Growth factor	Breast Lung Gastric Oesophageal carcinoma Head and neck
Cyclin D1	Cell cycle regulation	Breast Oesophageal carcinoma Urogenital Head and neck
N-myc	Transcription factor	Neuroblastoma Small cell lung cancer Ovarian adenocarcinoma
Retinoic acid receptor	Transcription factor	Breast Prostate
Androgen receptor	Transcription factor	Breast
Topoisomerase IIa	Enzyme involved in DNA replication	

ATM and ATR kinases are key initial steps. ATM kinase is primarily activated in the context of double-stranded breaks while ATR kinase is a critical element in responses involving arrest of DNA replication forks (DNA structures formed during cellular replication). Both ATM and ATR are high molecular weight protein kinases (>300 kDa) that mediate phosphorylation of downstream substrates. In the presence of double strand breaks, ATM becomes activated by dissociation from a homodimeric to monomeric form. This is associated with autophosphorylation which triggers a rapid conformational change. Activated ATM coordinates the function of a series of proteins involved in DNA repair, cell cycle arrest and apoptosis. The phosphorylation targets for this kinase include p53, NBS1 (Nijmegan breakage syndrome), BRCA1, SMC1, and CHK2. By contrast, ATR is a constitutively active kinase whose function is regulated by subcellular localization. Thus when ATR is situated close to an abnormal stretch of single-stranded DNA such as occur at sites of replication fork arrest, it will phosphorylate critical substrates which include RAD17 and CHK1. The proximal checkpoint kinases ATM and ATR are themselves controlled by the effector kinases CHK2 and CHK1 respectively. In the following sections, the mechanisms through which ATM and ATR mediate cell cycle arrest will be discussed in more detail in the context of cell cycle regulation in general.

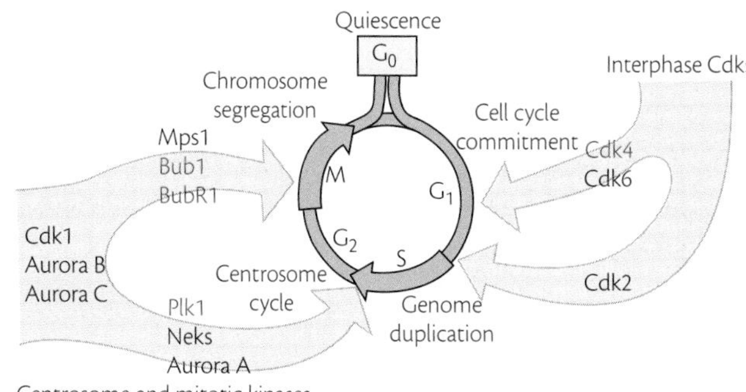

Fig. 6.2.14 A variety of cyclin-dependent kinases are involved in control of cell cycle progression (cdk1, cdk2, cdk3, cdk4, cdk6). Abnormal expression of *cdk4* and *cdk6* has been directly implicated in human malignancy and these are potential targets for therapeutic intervention.
(From *Current Opinion in Genetics and Development*, with permission. Copyright 2007 Elsevier Inc.)

G1/S checkpoint

The cyclin D family and their partner kinases (CDK4 and CDK6) are central players in cell cycle control mechanisms (Fig. 6.2.14). The activities of cyclins and cyclin-dependent kinases are closely regulated through specific cell cycle checkpoints. The retinoblastoma tumour suppressor gene product (pRb) is a 105-kDa protein which controls progression through the cell cycle and whose function is determined by its state of phosphorylation. pRb is phosphorylated by the cyclin D/cyclin-dependent protein kinase complex (Rb kinase) which itself is activated by a cyclin-dependent protein kinase–activating kinase (CAK). The unphosphorylated (active) form of pRb occurs in G1 (and G0) while phosphorylated forms dominate the S phase and G2/M. An increase in Rb phosphorylation releases a set of transcription factors termed E2F which collectively stimulate the expression of genes required for DNA synthesis (e.g. dihydrofolate reductase and thymidine kinase). E2F also coactivates cyclins A and B which further promotes cell cycle progression. The E2F proteins are regulated by a negative feedback loop involving a gene termed *CDKN2A*. This codes for a group of proteins ($p16^{CDKN2A}$) which inhibit Rb kinase by interfering with CAK activity and disrupting the cyclin-dependent protein kinase 4/Rb complex. These regulatory genes may be subject to either loss-of-function or gain-of-function mutations and are frequently found in cancer cells. Most of these mutations ultimately lead to deregulated E2F which favours the G1/S transition state. Gain-of-function mutations may occur in CDK 4 or cyclin D secondary to gene amplification. Both events will deregulate Rb kinase activity and increase E2F-dependent transcription. A similar outcome occurs when loss-of-function mutations affect the Rb protein directly or the negative feedback protein CDKN2A.

The G1/S checkpoint is the dominant pathway through which DNA strand breaks influence cell cycle progression. The molecular basis for this gatekeeper function has recently been clarified from studies on individuals with inherited cancer predisposition syndromes (Fig. 6.2.15). The kinases ATM and ATR can directly activate the tumour suppressor gene *TP53* by phosphorylation or indirectly modulate activity levels via phosphorylation of CHK2/CHK1. The p53 protein product is of paramount importance in DNA repair mechanisms throughout all cells and defective p53 function occurs in approximately half of all human cancers. Levels of this

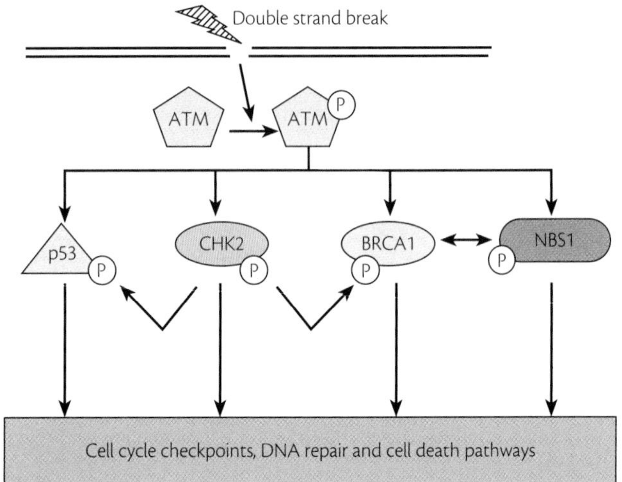

Fig. 6.2.15 Double-strand DNA breaks result in activation of ATM which in turn leads to phosphorylation of a variety of proteins including p53, CHK2, BRCA1, and NBS1. These collectively prevent propagation of DNA damage and interaction between BRCA1 (familial breast and ovarian cancer) and NBS1 (Nijmegen breakage syndrome) may coordinate DNA repair. p53 is also activated by the ATM-dependent kinase CHK2 and increases expression of genes such as *CDKN1A* and *BAX*.

nuclear phosphoprotein increase rapidly within cells in response to damage from ultraviolet light or cytotoxic drugs due to stabilization of the protein which can act in a dominant negative manner. It is indeed deserving of the title 'guardian of the genome' and appears to have a universal and over-arching role in maintenance of genomic integrity. Activation of *TP53* through any of the aforementioned pathways increases expression of p53-regulated genes which have critical caretaker and gatekeeper functions. One consequence of *TP53* activation is transcriptional activation of *TP21C1P1/WAF1* which inhibits another important cyclin-dependent kinase cyclin E/CDK2. The latter mediates arrest of cell growth in mink lung epithelial cells in response to negative growth factors. When cells are thus arrested in G1, DNA synthesis cannot be initiated. The p21 protein acts in a similar manner to p16 and inhibits Rb kinase. This maintains the Rb protein in an inactive, unphosphorylated state which prevents E2F activation (blockade of cells in G1).

In addition to repair of damaged cellular DNA, p53 can induce apoptosis in the presence of a severe genetic insult. This is partially accomplished by activation of the BAX protein which is a component of programmed cell death pathways. Thus mutations of p53 create a state of double jeopardy by allowing cells to continue replication with persistent strand breaks and failure of cell death in response to widespread irreparable DNA damage.

G2/M checkpoint

Cells will usually arrest in G2 in the presence of DNA damage. A specific checkpoint prevents the onset of mitosis and cells with mutant p53 can enter mitosis in the presence of DNA strand breaks and other forms of chromosomal abnormalities. This p53-dependent G2 arrest is mediated through upregulation of the CDK inhibitor p21, GADD45a, and 14-3-3 (sigma) proteins. The latter is an inhibitor of the cyclin B/cyclin-dependent protein kinase 2 complex required for initiation of mitosis. Perhaps the dominant pathway for halting all cell cycle progression does not directly involve p53; ATM and ATR can inhibit the cyclin B/cyclin-dependent kinase 1 through modulation of CDC25 phosphatases which normally activate CDK1 at the G2/M boundary. Drugs that selectively disrupt the G2/M checkpoint can potentially render cancer cells more susceptible to the genotoxic effects of chemotherapy and radiotherapy. This strategy would be especially pertinent to cancer cells containing abnormal p53 which will also have defective control of the G1/S checkpoint.

Oncogenes

The concept of the oncogene has been mentioned in the introductory section of this chapter in the context of paradigms for the pathobiology of cancer. It is now acknowledged that human cancer is a multifactorial process with several key steps being prerequisite for development of cancer. The term 'oncogene' originally implied that cancer might be caused by change in a single gene, but this is an oversimplified and outdated concept.

From an historical perspective, the revolution in understanding carcinogenesis at the molecular level originated from work on RNA tumour viruses which can rapidly induce tumours after inoculation into animal cells. These viruses contain reverse transcriptase and can synthesize DNA with a base pair sequence complementary to viral RNA. This DNA can then be incorporated into host DNA and cause malignant transformation. Both normal and malignant cells contain DNA sequences which are homologous or identical to the oncogenic segments of these so-called 'retroviruses'. These are termed cellular proto-oncogenes and correspond to viral (v-*onc*) oncogenes. These have probably arisen during evolution from incorporation of the cellular counterparts into viral structures. There is a remarkable level of conservation of these 'ancestral' oncogenes.

Seminal work by Peyton Rous on avian sarcomas led to isolation of the Rous sarcoma virus (RSV) which contains a gene (v-*src*) which, alone, is capable of transforming fibroblasts in cell culture and forming tumours (sarcomas) in chickens. RSV is one of several 'acutely transforming' retroviruses which can induce tumours in animal systems after a short latency period. Interestingly, RSV is the only retrovirus to contain both oncogenic and replicative sequences. Most of the RNA tumour viruses have lost some of the genetic information coding for replication as a consequence of incorporation of oncogenic sequences.

It was previously implied that the term 'oncogene' is a misnomer; the cellular homologue of viral oncogenes, the proto-oncogenes, are clearly not functioning in a tumorigenic capacity in most cells within animal tissues. These genetic sequences have oncogenic potential and this is expressed when the sequence is part of the viral genome—v-*onc* as opposed to c-*onc*. It may be surmised that cellular proto-oncogenes become activated either by overexpression of the normal gene product (quantitative change) or by alteration of the proto-oncogene to yield an abnormal product with oncogenic activity (qualitative change). The types of genetic alteration described earlier (point mutations, gene amplification, chromosomal translocation) can lead to either type of inappropriate expression of a proto-oncogene.

Not all cellular oncogenes have a viral homologue, and other methods have been employed to identify these oncogenes. These include gene transfer, insertional mutagenesis, and analysis of chromosomal translocation and sites of amplification. In the former process, viruses activate cellular oncogenes (for which

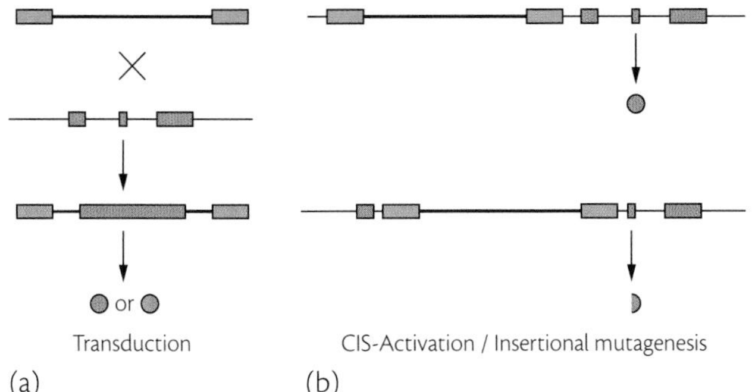

Fig. 6.2.16 Mechanisms of viral mutagenesis.

there is no viral counterpart, v-*onc*) by insertion of viral replicative sequences adjacent to the cellular DNA. These function as a promoter or enhancer and promote malignant transformation. An example of this process is the avian leukaemia virus which induces B-cell tumours in chickens. The virus does not contain a v-*onc* but insertional mutagenesis of a long terminal repeat unit (viral promoter sequence) activates the c-*myc* gene (Fig. 6.2.16).

The majority of oncogenes code for protein products which form components of mitogenic growth signalling pathways. Stimulation of these pathways leads to increased rates of proliferation and promotes tumour formation. One of the earliest oncogene products to be characterized was from the *src* gene. Antisera raised against the *src* gene product revealed a phosphorylated protein with a molecular weight of approximately 60 kDa (pp60 v-*src*). The protein product of the cellular homologue was similar (pp60 c-*src*) and located mainly on the cytoplasmic side of the plasma membrane. Furthermore, this protein was capable of autophosphorylation as well as phosphorylation of other proteins. Phosphorylation occurred on tyrosine residues and therefore the protein was known as a tyrosine protein kinase (as opposed to serine or threonine protein kinases). These tyrosine kinases can be divided into two main classes:

- Those forms which are membrane associated but without any obvious transmembrane or extracellular domains
- Those forms with a prominent extracellular domain constitute a potential site for ligand binding. These are members of the growth factor receptor family and play an important role in mediation of external growth stimulatory signals (e.g. erbB1, erbB2, PDGFR, IGFR1)

These two types of tyrosine kinases constitute distinct ways in which mutant forms of the protein can function as an oncogene. A third category of oncogene is represented by nuclear proteins which are more proximate effectors in cell cycle control.

Receptor protein tyrosine kinases as oncogenes

Receptor protein tyrosine kinases are growth factor receptors which have extracellular, transmembrane and intracellular domains. Binding of the cognate ligand to the extracellular binding site causes dimerization of receptors which leads to autophosphorylation of a tyrosine residue on the intracellular domain (which has intrinsic tyrosine kinase activity) (Fig. 6.2.17a). This in turn triggers a cascade of events which involves formation of a membrane complex with binding of cytoplasmic signalling proteins containing src homology-2 (SH-2) and protein tyrosine binding domains (PTB) (Fig. 6.2.17b). Amplification of the genes controlling receptor

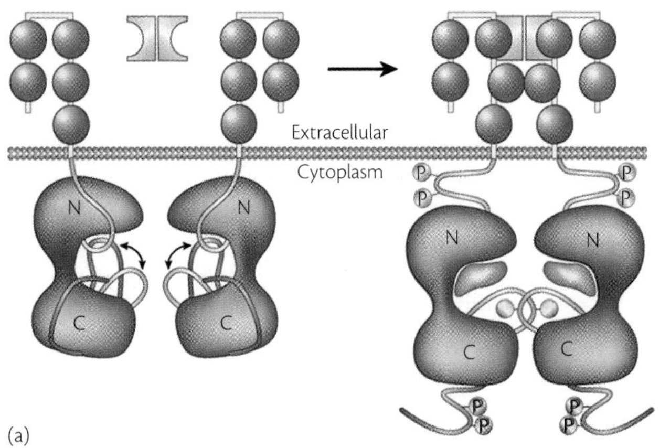

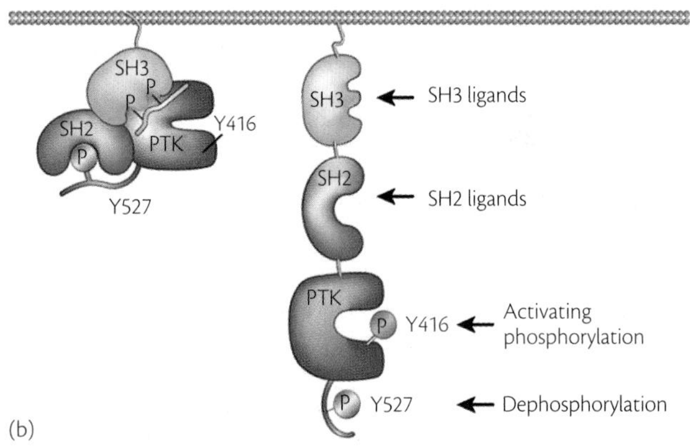

Fig. 6.2.17 A typical growth factor receptor is composed of extracellular, transmembrane, and intracellular domains. The latter may possess intrinsic tyrosine kinase activity which permits autophosphorylation. Some growth factor receptors do not have a cognate ligand.

protein tyrosine kinase is common in human cancers, resulting in overexpression and enhanced responsiveness to positive growth factor signals. This overexpression of receptors tends to promote ligand-independent dimerization with constitutive activation of the receptor which can lead to stimulation of downstream mitogenic pathways in the absence of any external stimulus. Epidermal growth factor receptor (EGFR) and HER2/neu are otherwise known as erbB1 and erbB2 respectively and belong to a family of receptor protein tyrosine kinases (erbB1–erbB4), so-called because of their homology to the erythroblastoma viral gene product v-erbB. Genes for both of these growth factor receptors are frequently amplified in breast, pancreas, and lung cancers. Furthermore, EGFR/erbB1 is overexpressed in up to 80% of head and neck cancers with levels of expression correlating inversely with survival (i.e. an adverse prognostic indicator).

Ligand binding to receptor protein tyrosine kinase usually leads to downstream activation of Ras and the mitogen-activated protein kinase (MAPK) cascades. The binding of epidermal growth factor (EGF) and similar ligands (e.g. tumour growth factor α, TGFα) to the EGFR is a classic example of this. Interestingly, HER2/neu (erbB2) has no natural ligand and functions as an amplifier by forming heterodimers with other members of the erbB family. Overexpression results in formation of homodimers of erbB2 which have constitutively active tyrosine kinase activity. In contrast to EGFR, this activated HER2/neu has a much broader range of potential downstream substrates which can transduce mitogenic, growth stimulatory signals.

Mutations in the c-*ret* and c-*met* receptor protein tyrosine kinase oncogenes are found in some familial cancer syndromes such as multiple endocrine neoplasia (MEN) 2A and 2B and familial forms of medullary thyroid cancer (c-*ret*). Papillary renal carcinoma can be associated with mutations of c-*met*. Both of these oncogenes are activated by missense mutations, leading to abnormal distribution of cysteine residues in the extracellular domain of the receptor. Inappropriate intermolecular disulphide bond formation encourages dimerization, constitutive tyrosine kinase activation, and enhanced mitogenic signalling.

Cytoplasmic protein tyrosine kinases as oncogenes

The existence of a cytoplasmic portion of the receptor tyrosine kinase molecule with intrinsic tyrosine kinase activity modifies the nature of the 'second messenger' system whereby an extracellular signal is translated into an internal cellular response. Receptor protein tyrosine kinase can directly phosphorylate a range of intracellular proteins leading to activation. Lay membrane bound receptors which do not possess tyrosine kinase activity must first bind a signal-transducing or G protein which then binds other molecules (guanine nucleotides) which will directly activate second messengers (Fig. 6.2.18).

The cytoplasmic portion of receptor protein tyrosine kinases converge upon a common second messenger system called ras proteins. The primary role of these proteins is to act as shuttling molecules that couple receptor activation to downstream effector pathways involved in regulation of cellular proliferation, differentiation and survival. Ras proteins are small GTPases which oscillate between inactive guanosine diphosphate (GDP)-bound and active guanosine triphosphate (GTP)-bound forms. Following ligand growth factor binding and dimerization, the receptor is autophosphorylated and forms an activated complex with recruitment of intracellular proteins to docking sites on the inner surface of the plasma membrane. The so-called 'docking proteins' form a scaffold structure which facilitates aggregation and interaction with downstream signalling components including the ras family of proteins. This complex also binds a series of adaptor molecules together with a protein termed SOS which catalyses the activation of ras proteins by exchange of GDP for GTP. This activated form of GTP-bound ras can interact with multiple downstream effectors to influence a spectrum of cellular processes varying from DNA synthesis to cell morphology and adhesion (Fig. 6.2.19). The system is switched off by GTPase activating proteins (GAPs) which hydrolyse GTP-bound ras to its GDP-bound form.

Activating mutations of ras are found in approximately 30% of human cancers and permit cells to partially bypass receptor protein tyrosine kinase signalling pathways. The *ras* oncogene was originally discovered in two retroviruses which gave rise to sarcomas in mice (Harvey and Kirsten murine sarcoma viruses). The two oncogenes *Hras* and *Kras* were found to yield almost identical gene products which resembled that of *Nras*, a further oncogene derived from neuroblastoma DNA. These three genes together with several other *ras*-related genes constitute the *ras* multigene family. Oncogenic sequences usually result from a missense point mutation and the Ras protein is maintained in the activated GTP-bound state. A single amino acid substitution can render the GTP-bound form resistant to hydrolysis by GAPs. Generation of a continuous mitogenic

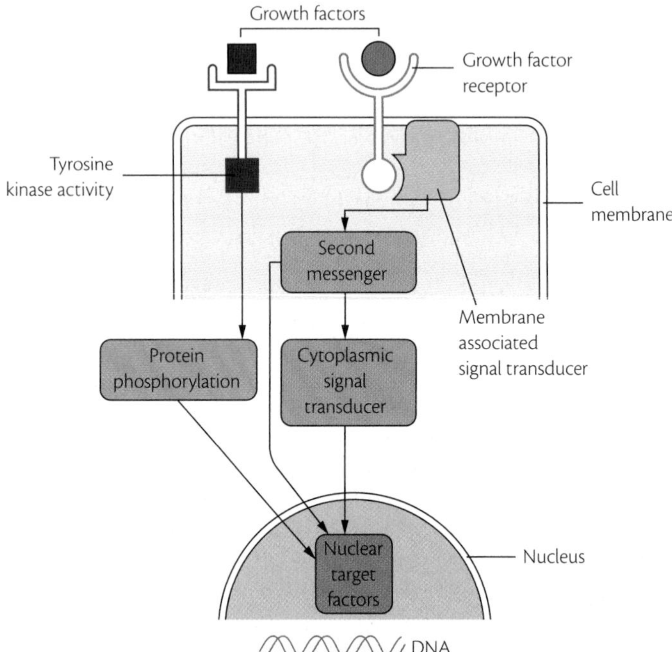

Fig. 6.2.18 Schematic diagram showing signal transduction via lay growth factor receptors (green) which are linked to membrane-associated signal transducer and interact with a second messenger. Growth factor receptors which have intrinsic tyrosine kinase activity (red) can interact directly with downstream effectors without the need for a second messenger.

signal provides a powerful driver for tumorigenesis. *KRAS* mutations are common in solid tumours; pancreatic (>90%), colorectal, endometrial, biliary tract, lung, and cervical. They occur together with *HRAS* mutations in about one-third of leukaemias and other myeloid malignancies, while *HRAS* mutations alone are found in bladder tumours.

Downstream targets regulated by Ras proteins include Raf which is a serine/threonine kinase that coordinates with Ras to phosphorylate the kinase MEK which in turn phosphorylates MAP kinase.

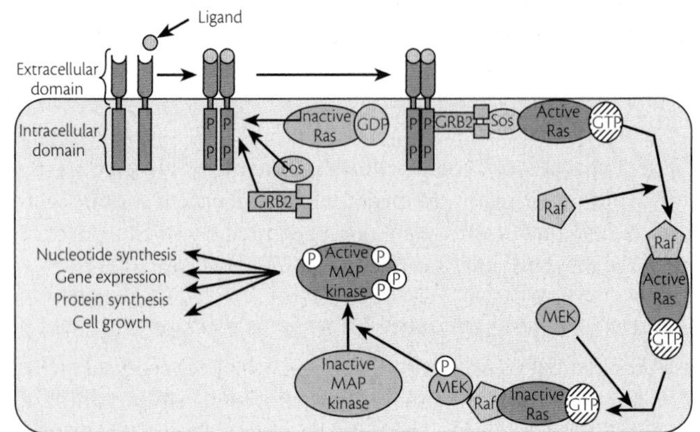

Fig. 6.2.19 Ligand binding to the extracellular domain of receptor tyrosine kinases triggers dimerization and receptor activation with autophosphorylation of specific tyrosine residues in the cytosolic domain. This leads to recruitment of intracellular proteins (GRB2) which bind to phosphotyrosine residues which constitute docking sites. This activated complex also binds a protein called SOS which catalyses activation of ras proteins by exchange of GDP for GTP. Active ras binds to Raf which in turn phosphorylates the kinase MEK. This phosphorylates MAP kinase which stimulates several potentially mitogenic pathways.

Ras also controls the rate of breakdown of inositol phospholipids (PI3-k/Akt/mTOR pathway).

Nuclear proteins as oncogenes

Oncogene products residing within the nucleus itself might be expected to have a more direct influence on gene expression then the aforementioned ones through binding to segments of DNA which contain gene regulatory elements. The *myc* oncogene is well characterized as a nuclear oncogene with growth stimulatory properties. The latter were first identified in avian retroviruses which transformed myeloid cell lines—hence the term myc (from myelomonocytic). These retroviruses also induced sarcomas and adenocarcinomas and were of interest because they lacked oncogenes. However, the *myc* gene is a member of a multigene family and a viral form v-*myc* corresponds to the cellular homologue. Distinct forms of the gene exist in neuroblastoma/retinoblastoma (N-*myc*) and small cell lung carcinomas (L-*myc*).

All three forms of the gene have been implicated in human malignancy. The *MYC* gene is universally expressed in cells and participates in a highly conserved pathway which is shared by most cells. Levels of the MYC product are generally increased in actively dividing cells and the *MYC* gene encodes transcriptional factors controlling proliferation, differentiation, and apoptosis. Abnormal expression within tumour cells may result from breakdown of a negative feedback loop whereby the MYC product fails to appropriately regulate activity of the gene. Oncogenic forms of *MYC* may result from a variety of changes including point mutation, amplification, and translocation. An example of the latter is Burkitt's lymphoma where translocation places the *MYC* gene in proximity to an immunoglobulin enhancer region. This results in augmented rates of transcription and overexpression of MYC protein.

Tumour suppressor genes

Though ultimately, oncogenic growth stimulatory activities may become dominant within malignant cells, defects in tumour suppressor genes may lead to excessive proliferation and neoplastic progression by default. Hence these genes are sometimes referred to as 'antioncogenes'; this term implies that mutations within these genes can be the primary driving force for malignant transformation, rather than representing a suppressor response to an established tumorigenic phenotype.

Tumour suppressor gene products are integral components of cell cycle regulatory pathways and have both gatekeeper and caretaker functions (see above). Some tumour suppressor genes possess functional duality and inactivation leads to major disruption of cell cycle regulation. Thus it is absence of a normal gene function rather than the presence of an abnormal gene as such which characterizes tumour suppressor gene disorders. A significant advance in the understanding of multistep carcinogenesis and in particular the concept of tumour suppressor genes came from studies into the genetic basis of retinoblastomas. Familial cases with bilateral tumours were noted to have loss of part of chromosome 13 (13q14). Sporadic cases with unilateral tumours also showed a similar chromosomal loss and Knudson proposed his famous 'two-hit' hypothesis (see Fig. 6.2.3); in familial cases of the disease, one hit is inherited as a germline mutation while the second is acquired early in life (perhaps *in utero*). It is now known that these two hits each correspond to allelic loss of a tumour suppressor gene—the retinoblastoma gene *RB1*. This gene was mapped to the chromosomal region 13q14 and its normal product is present in all cells except those of retinoblastoma tissue. Thus tumour formation is related to absence of the retinoblastoma gene product.

Transcriptional factors as tumour suppressor genes

The retinoblastoma gene

The Rb gene product is a universally expressed nuclear protein which has a fundamental role in controlling progression of cells through the G1 checkpoint at the transition from G1 to S-phase entry (see above). Levels of the Rb protein are critical determinants of overall functional status and when the amount of protein falls below a threshold value, 'suppressor' activity is lost and the cell acquires an oncogenic phenotype. Transfection of the retinoblastoma gene into tumour cells lacking retinoblastoma expression reasserts normal features and cell behaviour.

TP53 gene and p53 gene product

Like the retinoblastoma protein, the p53 gene product of the *TP53* gene is present in a wide variety of normal cells and levels of expression are increased in up to half of all cancers. Moreover, the protein product appears to be more stable with a longer half life in transformed cells. As previously discussed, p53 is often referred to as the guardian of the genome. It has an important cell cycle checkpoint function and protects cells from genotoxic damage. p53 causes cells to arrest in the G1 phase of the cell cycle and can act as a homotetrameric transcriptional factor which is activated in response to cellular insults such as irradiation, hypoxia, and drug-induced DNA damage. Though levels of *TP53* are increased in some tumours, the protein product is abnormal and p53 mutations are usually inactivating and associated with loss of gene function. Moreover, the *TP53* gene can act in a dominant negative manner whereby the presence of any abnormal protein product can impair function of normally expressed protein. Defective p53 introduced into the germline of transgenic mice leads to augmented tumorigenesis in the offspring of these p53 deficient mice. Therefore *TP53* functions as a tumour suppressor gene at the transcriptional level rather like the retinoblastoma gene. Indeed, the two proteins form part of a signalling network which regulates progression through the cell cycle and exerts a restraint on inappropriate growth promoting signals. Two further key components of this network include $p16^{ink4a}$ and $p14^{ARF}$. These are both encoded from a common locus on chromosome 9p21 called INK4a-ARF (alternate reading frame protein) which possesses two open reading frames. $p16^{ink4a}$ binds and inhibits the cyclin D-dependent kinases CDK4 and CDK6 and thereby induces Rb-dependent G1 arrest. Mutations of this gene are commonly found in familial and sporadic forms of melanoma, pancreatic, lung, and bladder cancers. $p14^{ARF}$ is also a potent tumour suppressor capable of activating p53 by binding directly to the p53 inhibitor MDM2. Mutations within this gene frequently occur in T-cell leukaemias (Fig. 6.2.20).

Cytoplasmic tumour suppressor genes

The development of colorectal cancers may be attributable to absence of a normal gene product. One form of colorectal cancer is associated with the hereditary condition familial adenomatous polyposis coli (FAP) which results in formation of hundreds of polyps within the colon and rectum. A proportion of these will become dysplastic and thereafter progress to carcinoma. An abnormality on chromosome 5 was originally identified in one of these patients and

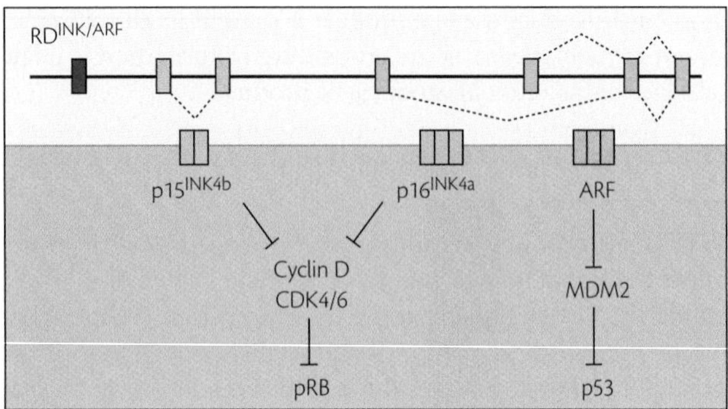

Fig. 6.2.20 The INK4a/ARF/INK4b locus encodes three genes: *ARF*, *CDKN2B* (p15^{INK4b}), and *CDKN2A* (p16^{INK4a}). Members of the INK4 family of cyclin-dependent kinase inhibitors bind to and inactivate CDK4/6. ARF inhibits MDM2 which results in stabilization of p53.
(From *Cell*, with permission. Copyright 2006 Elsevier Inc.)

the defective segment localized to 5q21. Furthermore, mutations at this site (the *APC* gene) can be found in more than three-quarters of cases of sporadic colorectal cancer. By analogy with retinoblastoma, a two-hit mechanism may apply; individuals with FAP will inherit a germline mutation of *APC* and require one further hit for development of cancer (heterozygosity predisposes to polyp formation alone). Sporadic forms of colorectal cancer require two somatic hits for tumour formation. Thus loss of function of tumour suppressor genes seems to be an important mechanism for carcinogenesis. The *APC* gene and its protein product have been characterized and the latter interacts with β-catenin which is a component of the Wnt/Wingless signalling pathway. Wild-type APC protein associates with β-catenin and targets it for proteosomal degradation. However, when APC is mutated, it is no longer able to negatively regulate β-catenin. Accumulated β-catenin translocates to the nucleus where it promotes cell cycle progression by interaction with transcriptional factors LEP/TCP (lymphoid enhancer factor/T-cell factor). Mutations in β-catenin have been identified in colorectal cancer and could be linked to abnormalities on chromosomes 17 and 18 which are frequently found in familial (nonpolyposis) and sporadic forms of the disease. Of note, chromosomal 17 mutations might lead directly to p53 dysfunction and impact on the (Rb/p53/p16/p14) signalling network discussed above (Fig. 6.2.21).

Receptor tumour suppressor genes

Transforming growth factor β (TGFβ)

This is a family of multifunctional regulatory peptides involved in a range of processes including development, wound healing, and carcinogenesis. It has three mammalian isoforms, each of which is a 25-kDa homodimeric peptide made from two identical peptide chains 112 amino acids in length. TGFβ is synthesized as part of a larger precursor molecule, with the mature moiety initially linked covalently to a precursor proregion from which it is proteolytically cleaved during synthesis. It remains loosely bound to the proregion which renders it functionally latent and is otherwise known as latency associated peptide (Fig. 6.2.22). TGFβ is generally secreted in an inactive form and the processes of sequestration and activation are potential checkpoints in controlling the biological activity of TGFβ. During activation, the mature moiety is dissociated from the proregion (and a specific TGFβ binding protein) and binds to cognate receptors with generation of an intracellular signal.

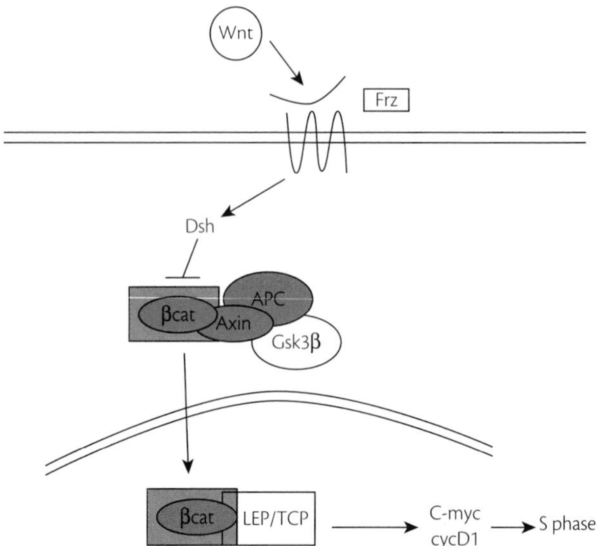

Fig. 6.2.21 Wnt signalling activates translocation of β-catenin to the nucleus where it acts as a transcription factor for specific target genes. Axin and APC modulate activity of β-catenin by regulating its degradation. Mutations involving β-catenin, APC, or Axin have been documented in human medulloblastomas and β-catenin abnormalities occur in both familial and sporadic forms of colorectal cancer where they may be linked to disorders of chromosomes 17 and 18.

Two forms of TGFβ receptor are recognized, type I and type II. These are transmembrane structures with an intracellular component that has intrinsic serine kinase or threonine kinase activity. TGFβ binds to the type II receptor which has a constitutively active kinase domain. After binding of the ligand, the phosphorylating activity of the type II receptor causes a conformational change leading to recruitment of the type I receptor into a heterodimeric complex. This complex formation leads to activation of the kinase domain of the type I receptor with signal propagation to downstream elements. Intracellular signal transduction is mediated by the Smad family of proteins; SMAD2 and SMAD3 are specific to TGFβ signalling and are recruited to the type I receptor where they subsequently form a heterooligomeric complex with SMAD4 which is a common mediator. This complex translocates to the nucleus, binds to DNA via a Smad-binding element and induces transcription of target genes. The latter inhibit phosphorylation of Rb protein and retention of E2F factors with cell cycle arrest or lengthening of G1 (Fig. 6.2.23). Smad4, also known as 'deleted in pancreatic cancer' (DPC4) is mutated in at least 50 to 90% of pancreatic cancers.

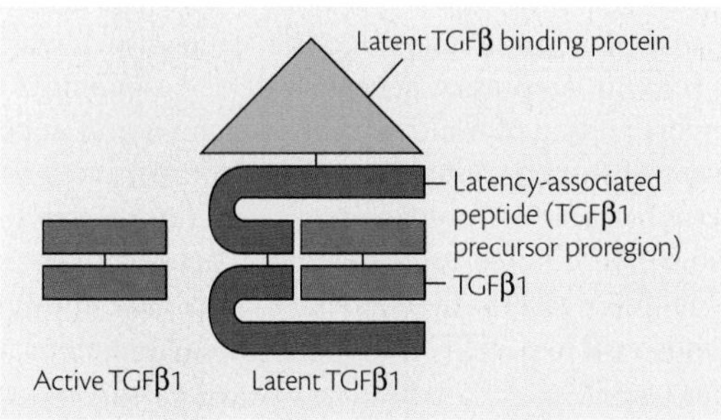

Fig. 6.2.22 TGFβ1 complex. Mature TGFβ is noncovalently bound to a precursor molecule called latency-associated peptide. This in turn is linked to the latent TGFβ binding protein which regulated activation and bioavailability of TGFβ1.
(From *The Lancet Oncology*, with permission. Copyright 2004 Elsevier Inc.)

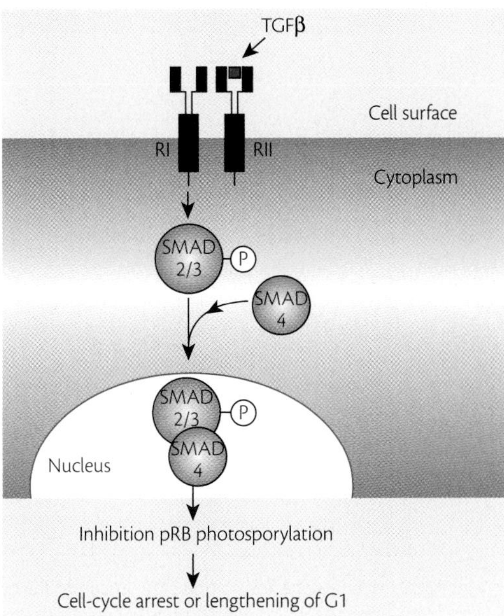

Fig. 6.2.23 After binding of TGFβ ligand to cognate receptors, signals are conveyed to the nuclear transcription site via intracellular proteins called smads. (From *The Lancet Oncology*, with permission. Copyright 2004 Elsevier Inc.)

TGFβ is a component of the complex language of intercellular communication and potentially acts as a switch that permits a biphasic functional profile. TGFβ is a pre-eminent inhibitory growth factor and in the premalignant and early stages of cancer this tumour suppressor activity is sustained. However, as cells pass along the neoplastic continuum, functional disruption occurs and malignant epithelial cells show a reduced or absent response to the growth inhibitory effects of TGFβ. Despite a dominance of growth inhibition in the early stages of carcinogenesis, during growth of a tumour there is a shift in the balance between tumour suppressor and potential prooncogenic activity. In the more advanced stages of malignant disease, TGFβ might promote tumour growth indirectly through the combined stimulation of stroma formation, angiogenesis, and immune suppression.

The tumour suppressor activity of TGFβ has generated much interest in the potential role of this growth factor in the process of carcinogenesis and the mediation of response to some therapies. The exact function of TGFβ depends upon both tumour stage and cellular context with relative amounts of ligand and receptor being a crucial determinant of response. TGFβ receptors jointly coordinate a cellular response and mutations in the type II receptor gene leads to loss of a growth inhibitory response in colon cancer cells lines which can be restored by transfection of the type II receptor subunit. The type II receptor is mutated in HNPCC through a mismatch repair error.

Hedgehog

The hedgehog (Hh) pathway is a signalling cascade with important roles in directing patterning and organ specificity during development and embryogenesis. Stimulation of this pathway can promote either proliferation or differentiation, depending on cell type and derangement of Hh signalling has provided valuable insight into mechanisms of cancer progression. The Hh pathway is activated by binding of ligand to a transmembrane receptor called patched-1 (ptch-1). Three mammalian Hh proteins have been identified, Sonic Hh, Indian Hh, and Desert Hh; these are secreted by cells following autoprocessing and can act in either an autocrine or paracrine manner upon adjacent cells. Unbound ptch-1 catalytically suppresses a transmembrane protein called Smoothened (Smo); ligand binding releases Smo from its repressed state where it can interact with downstream elements (Gli 1 and 2 factors) to upregulate Hh target genes.

Proliferation of tumour cells *in vitro* is increased by addition of Hh ligand and inhibited by neutralizing antibody. Moreover, constitutive activation of the Hh pathway by overexpression of Gli 1 leads to a metastatic phenotype in xenograft tumour models. Mutations in the PTCH gene have been found in Gorlin's syndrome where inactivation of this presumed tumour suppressor gene leads to basal cell carcinoma and medulloblastoma. The Hh pathway may be crucially involved in conversion of normal stem cells to cancer stem cells. One potential problem with inhibition of the Hh pathway as a therapeutic intervention in cancer is the adverse effects of Hh antagonists on normal stem cells of tissues such as bone marrow, gut, liver, and skin (Fig. 6.2.24).

Transgenic studies

The idea that epithelial proliferation is controlled by the net balance of positive and negative growth factors in the local microenvironment of tumours is supported by results of studies with transgenic models in which a selected protein is either not expressed (loss of function) or is overexpressed (gain of function) in target tissues. TGFβ can be overexpressed in the mammary gland of transgenic mice using a constitutively active construct of TGFβ linked to different promoters. Overexpression of TGFβ1 leads to apoptosis in the lobuloalveolar units with accelerated senescence of multipotent mammary stem cells. In the ductal compartment, proliferation is inhibited with impaired arborization and lateral branching. Furthermore, local overexpression of TGFβ1 in mammary tissues can suppress chemically induced carcinogenesis. These findings suggest that TGFβ1 can suppress events that initiate tumour formation and that it has an important role in the early phases of tumour development when changes in the amounts of growth factors in the local microenvironment might portend and encourage neoplastic progression.

By contrast with TGFβ1 transgenic mice, those which overexpress the mitogenic growth factor TGFα show mammary duct hyperplasia; and implantation of exogenous TGFα into regressed mammary glands reverses the changes of involution. Interestingly, cross-breeding experiments between MMTV-TGFβ1 and MMTV-TGFα transgenic mice hint at the interplay between positive and negative growth factors in determining overall proliferative activity of cells. Thus animals that have both transgenes do not develop carcinogen-induced tumours, suggesting that overexpression of a potent inhibitory growth factor can overcome the growth stimulatory capacity of oncogenic factors—'good overrides evil'.

Mutations in genes regulating apoptosis and cell death pathways

Programmed cell death or apoptosis is an essential feature of normal development and is an ongoing process throughout the life of a complex multicellular organism. For example, selective removal of cells during the phase of tissue remodelling in organogenesis is achieved by coordinated activation of cell death programmes. This leads to generation of digits and body cavities, for example. Apoptosis is also activated when cells are subjected to an insult, such

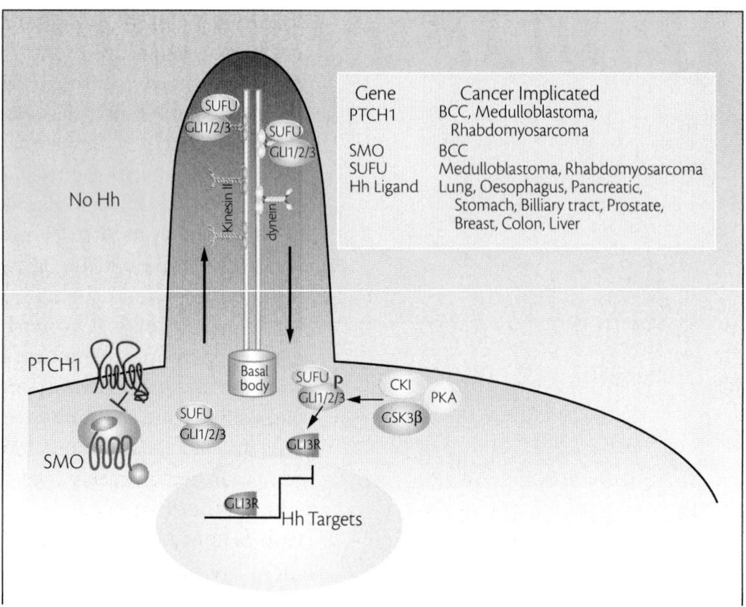

Fig. 6.2.24 Hh signalling in vertebrates. In the absence of Hh ligand, Ptch1 inhibits surface localization of Smo and protein kinases phosphorylate Gli proteins. N-terminal truncated forms of Gli (predominantly Gli3) act as repressors of Hh target gene expression. Sufu also regulates the pathway by binding to Gli within both cytoplasm and nucleus to prevent it from activating Hh target genes. The insert table lists genes which have been implicated in various human cancers where therapeutic approaches might include Hh antagonists or Hh antibodies (From *Clinical Cancer Research*, with permission. Copyright 2006 American Association for Cancer Research.)

as DNA damage. There are two distinct cellular programmes that trigger the 'intrinsic' and 'extrinsic' pathways. The intrinsic pathway is primarily responsible for apoptosis induced by cellular stress, external injury, and signals emanating from survival pathways. Any of these events will stimulate release of cytochrome *c* from mitochondria which subsequently activates a cascade of caspases that result in DNA fragmentation, plasma membrane destruction and the morphological features of apoptosis. The bcl-2 family of proteins determine the net cellular response through the balance of pro- (e.g. *bax* or *bad*) and anti- (*bcl-2, bcl-*X_L) apoptotic members. A dominance of proapoptotic bcl-2 proteins will permeabilize the mitochondrial membrane and permit egress of cytochrome c (Fig. 6.2.25). By contrast, the extrinsic pathway is activated by ligand binding to cell surface 'death' receptors which include Fas/CD95, TNFR (tumour necrosis factor receptor) and DF5. The respective cognate ligands are FasL, TNFα, and TRAIL. Each of these ligand/receptor complexes can activate the caspase cascade and trigger apoptosis.

Cancer cells possess the ability to evade mechanisms of programmed cell death. Overexpression of the antiapoptotic protein bcl-2 has been found in 85% of more aggressive lymphomas. The *BCL2* gene is up-regulated by a chromosomal translocation (14:18) and elevated levels of bcl-2 protein bind to *bad* and other proapoptotic factors (*bax, bid*). Bcl-2 is a potent cell survival factor and prevents cytochrome *c* release and in turn inhibits cell death. Inactivating mutations of *TP53* lead to impaired apoptotic pathways. Downstream effectors interact with proapoptotic members of the bcl-2 family. Functioning p53 protein increases transcription of the *BAX* gene which promotes release of cytochrome *c* from mitochondria.

Phosphatidylinositol-3-OH kinases (PI3-Ks) are a group of lipid kinases which can phosphorylate the 3′-OH group in the inositol ring of inositol phospholipids. A downstream mediator of PI3-K signalling is the serine/threonine kinase PKB/Akt, which is the cellular homologue of the acutely transforming retroviral oncogene v-*Akt*. Akt is another potent cell survival factor and protects cancer cells from apoptosis. It prevents mitochondrial release of cytochrome c by phosphorylation and inactivation of the proapoptotic protein *bad*. The tumour suppressor gene *PTEN* (phosphatase and tensin homologue deleted in chromosome 10) is mutated in human cancers at a frequency comparable to *TP53*. These mutations result in loss of function of the PTEN gene product (phosphatase) and have been identified in cancers of the breast, prostate, endometrium, and thyroid, together with melanomas and glioblastomas. However, haplodeficiency of *PTEN* may be sufficient to reduce phosphatase function and therefore *PTEN* does not conform to the classical two-hit paradigm. Germline mutations of *PTEN* have also been found in patients with Cowden's disease (characterized by development of multiple hamartomas and cancers of the breast and thyroid). The PTEN product normally antagonizes the action of PI3-K by neutralizing the active product of PI_3-K (phosphatidylinositol 3,4,5-triphosphate). PTEN negatively regulates Akt activity and loss of PTEN function effectively results in constitutive activation of Akt and shields cancer cells from apoptotic death. Interestingly, complete deficiency of PTEN is associated with embryonal lethality in mice but *pten* heterozygotes develop a variety of tumours.

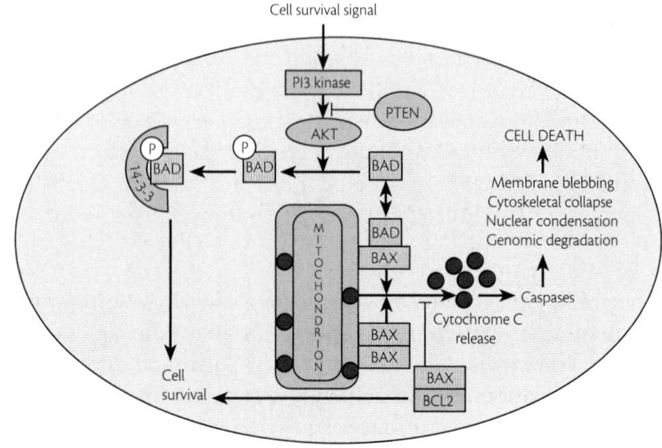

Fig. 6.2.25 Apoptosis is triggered by release of cytochrome *c* from mitochondria which activates the lytic enzymes caspase proteases. Cells possess highly regulated mechanisms to ensure that inappropriate cytochrome release does not occur. These operate through the Bcl2 family of cell death regulators.

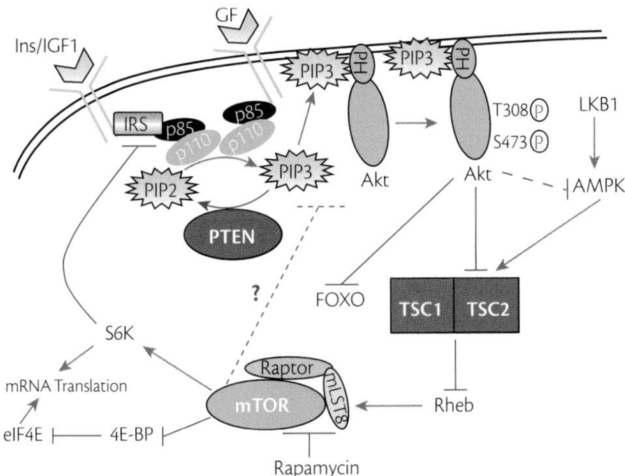

Fig. 6.2.26 In the PI13K/Akt/mTOR pathway, Akt is flanked by two tumour suppressor genes, *PTEN* and *TSC1/TSC2* heterodimer. PTEN antagonizes PI3K and thus inhibits Akt, while TSC1/TSC2 inhibits mTOR by suppressing activity of Rheb. (From *Cancer Cell*, with permission. Copyright 2005 Elsevier Inc.)

mTOR is an important downstream effector of Akt and a potential target for anti-cancer therapies. Akt activates mTOR via two pathways:

- Direct phosphorylation of TSC2 (tuberose sclerosis complex) within the TSC1/TSC2 heterodimer. This normally inhibits the activity of Rheb which is a small GTPase required for mTOR activation. Phosphorylation of TSC2 releases this inhibition and increases mTOR activity.
- Inhibition of AMPK which in turn can fully inhibit TSC2 and activate mTOR.

TSC1 and *TSC2* function as classic tumour suppressor genes with biallelic inactivation. Therefore Akt is essentially flanked by two tumour suppressor genes—*PTEN* and *TSC1/TSC2*. A feedback inhibition mechanism exists to negatively regulate activity of Akt. This involves multiple signal transduction factors including S6K and IRS-1 (insulin-receptor substrate-1) (Fig. 6.2.26).

MicroRNA as oncogenes and tumour suppressors

MicroRNAs are small, noncoding RNA molecules composed of short sequences of 20 to 22 nucleotides which exert a negative regulatory influence on gene expression in eukaryotic organisms. They generally reduce levels of both transcript and corresponding protein and have been shown to participate in several biological processes including cell proliferation (miR-125b; let-7) where microRNAs may enable stem cells to overcome the G1/S checkpoint of the cell cycle. These molecules are generated from hairpin-structured precursors by the action of members of the RNAase III group of enzymes (Dicer and Drosha). There are two proposed mechanisms by which microRNAs might silence genes following binding of microRNAs to complementary sequences located predominantly in the 3′ untranslated regions of genes. Firstly, such binding can result in decreased translation of specific mRNAs and reduced amounts of protein product. Secondly, binding of microRNA can divert mRNA to the RNA interference silencing complex (RISC) wherein mRNA transcripts are broken down and become void. Both of these mechanisms result in decreased expression of the corresponding gene.

Expression profiles of miRNAs differ between normal and malignant cells and cancer-specific microRNA fingerprints have been identified for many types of cancer, including leukaemias, lymphomas, breast, liver, gastric, colon, and pancreatic. Attention has recently focused on microRNA as a potential tumour suppressor. Abrogation of this negative gene regulation could promote cancer development. Indeed, microRNAs such as mi-R15 and mi-R16 appear to act in this capacity. Thus down-regulation of miR-15/16 results in overexpression of antiapoptotic bcl-2 and other genes which promote tumorigenesis. However, overexpression of other types of microRNA such as the polycistron miR-17–92 on chromosome 13q 32–33 can stimulate tumour growth suggesting that microRNA can have dual roles depending upon which particular genes are negatively regulated. In a mouse model of B-cell lymphoma, overexpression of the miR 17–92 cluster acts coordinately with c-*myc* upregulation to potentiate carcinogenesis.

It has been proposed that microRNAs act 'in cascade' over several cancer-specific protein coding regions which subsequently modulate transcriptional activity of other protein coding genes as well as noncoding RNAs. These mechanisms could be important in tumour initiation in somatic cells and genetic predisposition in germline cells (Fig. 6.2.27).

Epigenetics

The phenomenon of epigenetic change has previously been discussed in the context of genetic alterations and instability in cancer cells (see above). The majority of cancers display epigenetic changes which are reversible and heritable changes in gene expression without DNA sequence alterations. They act as 'translators' between the environment and the genome and represent an interface between genotype and phenotype.

Cancer cells have an imbalance of DNA methylation; though there is widespread loss of genomic DNA methylation with neoplastic progression, there is aberrant hypermethylation of cytosine residues in CpG islands in the promoter region of genes. These CpG islands are highly conserved segments of DNA with a GC content in excess of 50%. They are found in the promoter regions of almost one-half of mammalian genes. These CpG islands are normally protected from methylation, but aberrant methylation is widespread in human cancers and leads to selective gene silencing. Each tumour has its own pathways of methylation and hypermethylation profile. Epigenetic silencing tends to promote genetic instability with 5-methylcytosine being highly mutagenic and predisposing to C:G → A:T transitions. For example, in sporadic colon cancers there is evidence of hypermethylation and silencing of the DNA mismatch repair gene *MLH1* leading to microsatellite instability. Epigenetic silencing represents an important mechanism for inactivation of tumour suppressor genes. The *BRCA1* and *APC* genes can be inactivated by hypermethylation and in the case of the former this can act as a 'second hit' in hereditary forms of breast cancer. In sporadic cancers, there can be hypermethylation of one allele and genomic loss of the other allele. Targets for hypermethylation include the oestrogen, progesterone and prolactin receptors as well as the above genes. Hypermethylation of the tumour suppressor gene $p16^{INK4a}$ (*CDKN2A*) in lung cancer has been reported. A variety of novel genes which can be epigenetically silenced are likely to be discovered in the future. Furthermore, it may be possible to restore normal gene expression by pharmacological

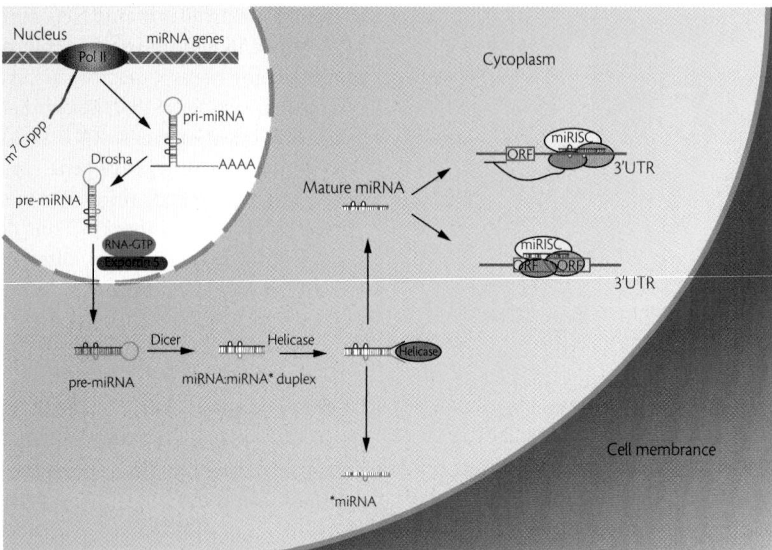

Fig. 6.2.27 MicroRNA genes are transcribed by RNA Pol II to form pre-microRNAs in the nucleus. These are then processed by RNase III, Drasha, and exported to the cytoplasm. The pre-microRNA is further processed by another RNase, Dicer, to generate a duplex form of microRNA and its complement microRNA* (microRNA:microRNA*). The enzyme helicase splits this duplex with release of mature microRNA which enters the microRNA-induced silence complex (miRISC). This blocks protein synthesis by one of two mechanisms: (a) imperfectly binding to the 3′ UTR of the mRNA; (b) base pairing to the target mRNA leading to endonucleolytic cleavage (microRNA* is degraded).
(From *World Journal of Gastroenterology*, with permission. Copyright 2007 WJG Press.)

manipulation of epigenetic changes without the need for genetic engineering.

Epigenetic therapy has focused on developing agents which can alter patterns of DNA methylation or histone modification. 5-Azocytidine is a protoype inhibitor of DNA methylation which inactivates DNA methyltransferases and can induce gene expression and differentiation *in vitro*. Like other cytotoxic agents, 5-azocytidine is effective in actively dividing S-phase cells and clinical trials are evaluating these agents in treatment of myeloid leukaemias. DNA methyltransferases can also be targeted with antisense molecules. Inhibitors of histone deacetylation can overcome epigenetic silencing and represent an alternative therapeutic strategy. Accumulation of acetylated proteins can switch on silenced genes and this approach may be appropriate if specific enzymes can be targeted (Fig. 6.2.28).

Cancer invasion and metastases

The properties of invasion and metastasis are essential for the malignant phenotype. These are complex and inter-related processes which are associated with multiple and sequential genetic changes. The transfer of cancer cells from a primary tumour focus to distant sites involves the following steps:

- invasion of normal surrounding tissues
- penetration of lymphatic and vascular channels with release of either single tumour cells or small cell clusters into these vessels
- survival within the lymphatic or circulatory systems
- arrest in the capillary beds of distant organs such as the lungs, bone, or liver (or the sinus of a lymph node)
- extravasation from the walls of these lymphovascular channels in distant organs and establishment of a viable metastatic focus

The initial stages of local tissue invasion involve cellular dissociation and migration. These two steps are dependent on changes in mechanical pressure within the tissues, together with release of proteolytic enzymes which reduce the adhesiveness and attachment between cancer cells and normal cells. Epithelial–mesenchymal transition (EMT) is characterized by loss of cell-to-cell contact with disruption of intercellular tight junctions. The latter maintain the orderly arrangement of cells in monolayers and loss of cohesion is accompanied by an increase in cell mobility. A group of enzymes called matrix metalloproteinases are key players in the process of tissue invasion; they include collagenases, gelatinases, and stromelysins. The genetic basis for invasion remains poorly understood, but so-called ‘invasion suppressor genes’ are being identified.

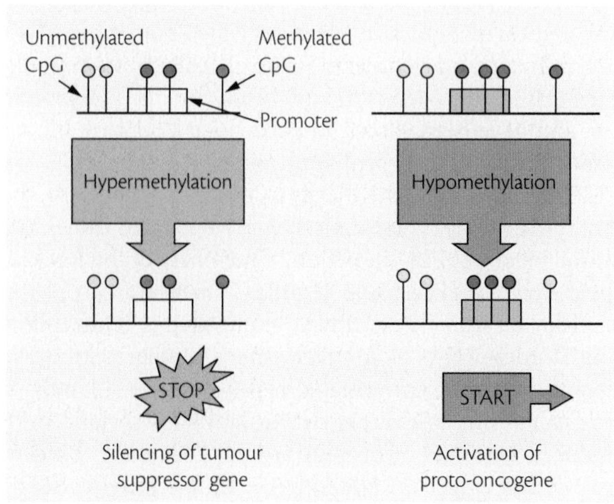

Fig. 6.2.28 Epigenetic regulation of gene expression by methylation. Methylation of CpG islands in cancer cells leads to silencing of suppressor genes.
(From *The Lancet Oncology*, with permission. Copyright 2002 Elsevier Inc.)

EMT is regulated by several growth factor pathways which link up with activation of metalloproteinases (via disruption of a sulphydryl group) and their tissue inhibitors (TIMPS). A checkpoint control for invasion has been proposed involving the ligand-receptor complex termed amphoterin/RAGE (receptor for advanced receptor glycation end products). This complex assists in generation of the enzyme plasmin which activates metalloproteinases. It is also involved in control of cell motility and modulation of adhesion receptors relating to the e-cadherin system. Mutations in the e-cadherin gene have been described for cancers of the breast, colon, and stomach. Collectively these mutations are associated with changes in cell morphology, enhanced motility and activation of the β-catenin/LEF pathway (see above).

Hepatocyte growth factor (HGF) or 'scatter factor' is produced by stromal cells and binds to the c-met receptor on cancer cells. Levels of this protein tyrosine kinase receptor can be elevated by either somatic or germline mutations in the c-*met* gene. Amplification of this gene has been found in liver metastases of colorectal carcinomas. Upregulation of the HGF/c-met signalling pathway activates an invasive programme which promotes invasion, migration, and cell survival—and in turn the metastatic phenotype.

Angiogenesis

Development of a tumour beyond the size of approximately 1 million cells is dependent upon an intact microvasculature. Blood vessels not only support further tumour growth by encouraging adequate supplies of oxygen and nutrients to cells deep within a tumour bolus, but also provide opportunity for metastasis, especially as newly formed blood vessels tend to be fragile and leaky.

Tumour angiogenesis factors stimulate capillary formation at an early stage of tumour development, leading to proliferation of endothelial cells which invade the stroma and produce capillary 'sprouts'. These become tubular structures which later canalize to form nascent capillary networks. One of the principle signalling pathways in tumour angiogenesis is the vascular endothelial growth factor (VEGF) receptor system. Endothelial cells possess two forms of the receptor, VEGFR1 and VEGFR2, which both bind the ligand VEGF-A. However, VEGFR1 is probably the dominant receptor for angiogenesis and ligand binding stimulates endothelial proliferation and formation of a neovasculature.

Normal cells respond to hypoxia by upregulation of a set of 'hypoxia-inducible' genes. VEGF-A represents one such gene and levels of VEGF-A are increased by cell hypoxia. This response is mediated by hypoxia-inducible factors, HIF1α and HIF2α, which function as transcription factors and are very sensitive to the ambient oxygen tension. In cancer cells, activity levels of HIF1α and HIF2α can remain high despite normoxic conditions. This generates a continuous and potent angiogenic signal which no longer represents a physiological response to hypoxia. This uncoupling of hypoxia-inducible gene expression from tissue oxygen tension can result from mutations in the von Hippel–Lindau (*VHL*) gene. The product of this gene normally targets HIF for proteosomal degradation via the ubiquitin pathway. Loss of this tumour suppressor gene activity leads to accumulation of excess HIF1α and HIF2α, which drives tumour angiogenesis. Inactivating mutations of the *VHL* gene are present in up to 50% of renal cell carcinomas which characteristically express high levels of VEGF-A. Of course, enhanced angiogenesis in most tumours is not linked to specific mutations of *VHL*; many other angiogenic factors exist (e.g. fibroblast growth factor) and levels of VEGF-A can be increased through other pathways which might involve activated EGFR, erbB2, and mutant ras signalling.

Inhibition of angiogenesis is a potential antitumour strategy and microvessel density is generally inversely correlated with tumour stage and clinical outcome (Fig. 6.2.29).

Viral causes of cancer

Both RNA and DNA viruses have been implicated as causative factors in a wide variety of animal tumours. Two patterns of carcinogenesis are recognized; the acutely transforming retroviruses rapidly transform cells in culture, while other viruses act more slowly and tumour induction occurs over a more prolonged period of time. The former group of viruses have provided much insight into mechanisms of oncogenesis and inspired the paradigm of the oncogene.

Despite the existence of proto-oncogenes in human tumours, viral oncogenesis is uncommon in humans. Human malignancy is very complex and there are potential problems with proof of causality; there may be an epidemiological association between a virus and a particular form of human cancer, but the former may not be a cause of the latter. Conclusions can be misleading when animal models are used to test the oncogenic potential of human viruses. Interestingly, recent data derived from polymerase chain reaction (PCR) studies suggests that human breast cancer is associated with human mammary tumour virus (HMTV) infection. The HMTV envelope can be detected in almost 40% of breast cancer patients, while expression is negligible in normal breast tissue.

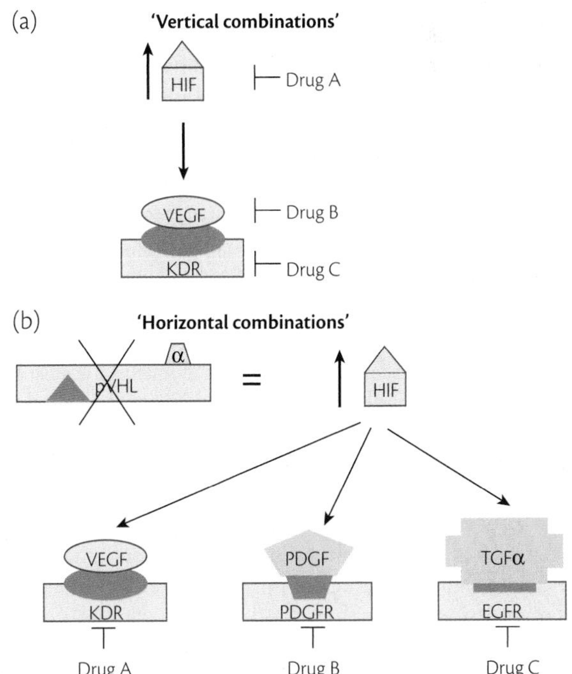

Fig. 6.2.29 Therapeutic strategies based on disruption of the HIF–VGEF pathway. (a) 'vertical' combination therapies in which multiple points are disrupted simultaneously in the HIF-VEGF pathway (b) 'horizontal' combinations in which multiple growth factors or their receptors are targeted. (KDR, kinase domain-related inhibitor; PDGFR, platelet-derived growth factor receptor). (From *Clinical Cancer Research*, with permission. Copyright 2004 American Association for Cancer Research.)

These observations imply that with HMTV infection is horizontally acquired and not vertically transmitted, but do not prove causation.

Notwithstanding these comments, up to one-fifth of cancer worldwide may be attributable to a viral aetiology. Invariably there is a relatively long latency period between infection and tumour development—no human malignancy is caused by an acutely transforming retrovirus. However, endemic retroviruses exist within the population and have been implicated in some forms of human cancer. Perhaps the most notable example is the HTLV-1 virus which is associated with T-cell leukaemia in Caribbean and Japanese populations. The prevalence of infection within these groups is much greater than the incidence of malignancy, with only 1 out of every 80 cases of HTLV-1 infection developing T-cell leukaemia. A viral protein (Tax) is required for T-cell transformation, but clearly other cofactors are essential for oncogenesis.

The host's immune system plays an important role at the initial stage of viral infection when the virus must penetrate the host's cells and proliferate. The immune response can also be critical at the second stage of neoplastic transformation when an infected cell is converted to a cancer cell. Only 'live' cells can form tumours and this will not occur if the host has mounted an immune response which is cytolytic and leads to the demise of infected cells (T-cell dependent). The immune system provides a degree of protection from the DNA tumour viruses which typically cause cancers in humans: Epstein–Barr virus (EBV), human herpes virus 8 (HHV-8), and human papilloma virus (HPV). These viruses are more likely to achieve both successful infection and induction of malignancy in an immunocompromised host. The human immunodeficiency virus-1 (HIV-1) indirectly causes a significant number of DNA viral tumours by weakening the immune surveillance mechanisms.

EBV infects more than 90% of the world's population and was the first virus to be directly implicated in development of human malignancy. It was present in cultured cells from a patient with Burkitt's lymphoma and virally encoded proteins were detected on the surface of these cells. Moreover, EBV will immortalize human B cells *in vitro* and levels of antibodies to viral antigens are much higher in affected individuals than in controls. In addition to Burkitt's lymphoma, EBV has a causative role in nasopharyngeal carcinoma and more aggressive forms of lymphoma. Often there is an impaired T-cell-dependent immune response due to either poor nutrition, malaria, or HIV infection. The genome of the EBV contains up to 100 gene sequences which code for a plethora of proteins that exhibit homology to various human cytokines, antiapoptotic factors, and signalling molecules. Several of these have potential oncogene-like properties such as the EBNA2 protein which acts as a transcriptional coactivator for the *myc* oncogene. The EBNA-LP protein cooperates with EBNA2 to inactivate the tumour suppressor genes *TP53* and *RB*. Though the exact mechanism for malignant transformation at the molecular level has yet to be elucidated, these viral gene products are likely involved in tumour initiation rather than continued growth and neoplastic evolution (Fig. 6.2.30).

It is estimated that up to 200 million individuals worldwide may be chronically infected with the hepatitis B or C virus. These are small DNA viruses and predispose to both cirrhosis and hepatocellular carcinoma, which is the commonest malignancy in some parts of the world. Nonetheless, this still represents a small proportion of those infected with the virus and other factors are necessary

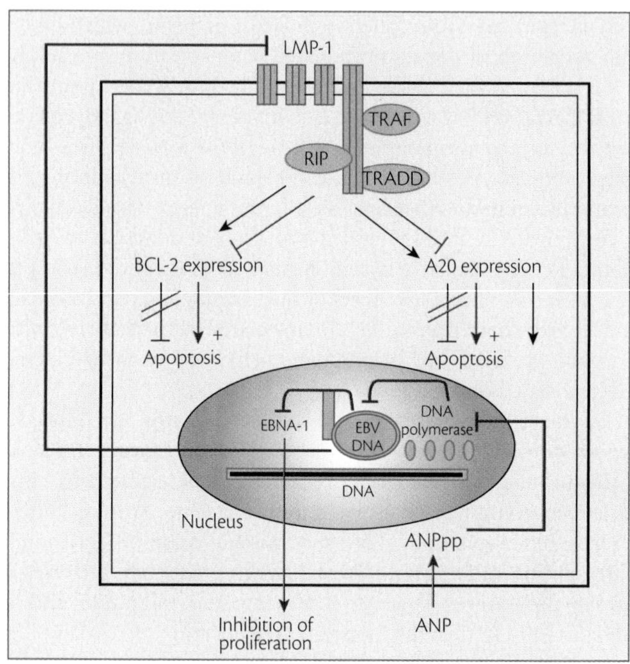

Fig. 6.2.30 The EBV oncoproteins LMP-1 and EBNA-1 are involved in cellular transformation and replication respectively. These proteins can be targeted using antisense strategies or diphosphonates which interfere with viral DNA synthesis. Down-regulation of these oncoproteins increases sensitivity to programmed cell death pathways in EBV-associated tumour cells. LMP-1 interacts with tumour necrosis factor receptor-associated factors (TRAF1 and TRAF2) together with tumour necrosis factor receptor-associated death domain which activates NF-κB. This is a key transcription factor involved in regulation of cell growth and apoptosis (increased levels of antiapoptotic proteins bcl2 and A20). ANP inhibits EBV gene expression and down-regulates both LMP-1 and EBNA-1 which promotes apoptosis and inhibits proliferation of EBV positive cells

(From *The Lancet Oncology*, with permission. Copyright 2001 Elsevier Inc.)

for tumour induction. The latter may be promoted by hepatocyte regeneration which occurs in response to chronic inflammatory changes caused by viruses, alcohol, or possibly aflotoxin B_1. The precise role of the hepatitis B virus in oncogenesis remains unclear, but HBV genes are integrated into the DNA of hepatocellular carcinomas. One of the sequences within the HBV genome is termed the 'x' gene and encodes a protein product of 154 amino acids which can complex with and inactivate p53. This x gene product can also transactivate oncogenes such as c-*fos*, c-*jun*, *myc*, and EGF.

There are more than 50 papilloma viruses which can infect humans, but the type that causes cervical carcinoma is best known and the molecular basis for oncogenesis has been characterized. Two viral genes, *E6* and *E7*, are responsible for HPV-induced cellular transformation, though other factors such as smoking and coinfection with the herpes simplex virus may contribute. The E6 protein mediates ubiquitination of p53 and subsequent proteosomal degradation. By contrast, the E7 protein binds to and abrogates the tumour suppressor function of the Rb protein by preventing association of Rb with E2F transcription factors. This interferes with the cell cycle checkpoint function of Rb and stimulates cell cycle progression and proliferation. This is also aided by an antiapoptotic function of E6. Therapeutic strategies include

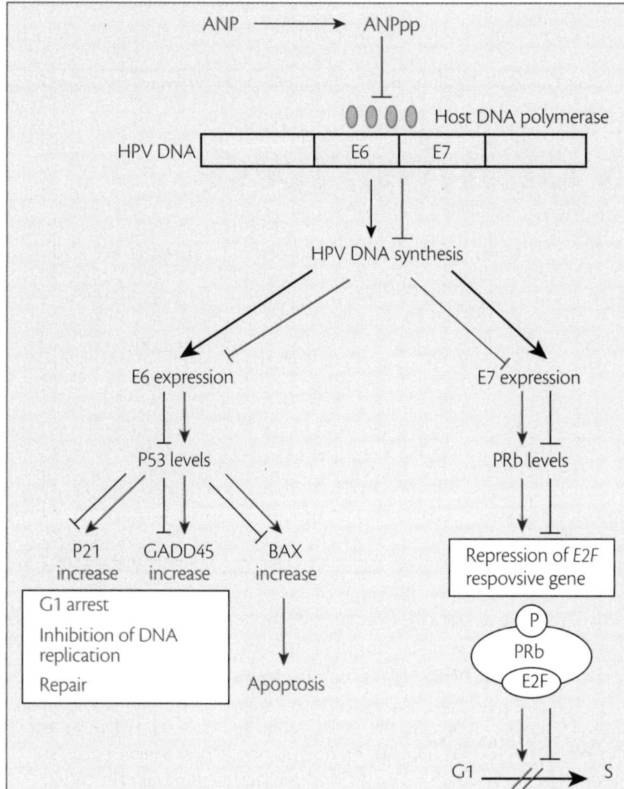

Fig. 6.2.31 HPV-induced cellular transformation results from enhanced activity of two viral genes, *E6* and *E7*. This results in loss of tumour suppressor activity by proteosome-mediated degradation of p53 and pRB which can be restored pharmacologically with agents such as acyclic nucleoside phosphonates (ANP) which interferes with viral DNA synthesis. The reduction in levels of *E6* and *E7* expression stabilizes p53 and pRb in HPV-infected cells and promotes cell cycle arrest and apoptosis.
(From *The Lancet Oncology*, with permission. Copyright 2001 Elsevier Inc.)

HPV vaccines which are currently being investigated in clinical trials with promising results. Other approaches target synthesis of the E6 and E7 proteins with antisense oligonucleotides or acyclic nucleoside phosphonates (ANP) (Fig. 6.2.31).

Conclusions

There have been great advances in our molecular understanding of carcinogenesis over the past two decades. The complete sequencing of the human genome has provided the impetus for translational research and novel therapeutic strategies which are underpinned by knowledge of pathobiological processes. The therapeutic goal has shifted from elimination of all cancer cells to re-regulation such that tumours can exist symbiotically and without detriment to the host for longer periods of time. By prolonging disease-free survival, it may be possible to achieve a 'personal' cure until patients succumb from causes unrelated to cancer. This may constitute a more realistic objective than striving for the elusive 'statistical' aim of clinical cure.

Cancer cells have great capacity to adapt and evolve in response to treatments. Targeting of specific growth factor pathways which drive tumour growth has become a clinical reality and this approach is consonant with the paradigm of control rather than cure. Chronic myeloid leukaemia is characterized by the fusion gene *bcr-abl1* which has enhanced tyrosine kinase activity. Selective tyrosine kinase inhibitors have been developed which can cure up to 90% of mice with chronic myeloid leukaemia and are highly effective in clinical trials. Likewise, a humanized monoclonal antibody directed against over-expressed HER2/neu receptor in breast cancer patients has dramatically improved short term clinical outcomes. This antibody (Herceptin) down-regulates tyrosine kinase activity by internalization of the receptor/antibody complex. Tyrosine kinases provide potent mitogenic signals and targeting of these pathways demonstrates the success of translational approaches.

The cellular heterogeneity of individual tumours presents a major therapeutic challenge. There is increasing recognition that phenotypic heterogeneity for some cancers may reflect an accumulation of mutations in a large number of less highly penetrant genes rather than being attributable to simple changes in one or two dominant genes. The sophisticated methods of genetic profiling with DNA microarrays and their integration with proteomics may ultimately allow treatments to be better tailored. If tumours arise from transformation of stem cells (or a closely related progenitor) into malignant stem cells, then the latter must be targeted therapeutically; these cells are either quiescent or cycle relatively slowly and are resistant to conventional chemotherapy. The ability of stem cells to self-renew provides the opportunity for 'regeneration' and clinical recurrence of cancer. Cancer stem cells retain programmes for invasion and metastases together with protective mechanisms which favour survival despite exposure to potentially noxious therapies. Future research will focus on identification of biochemical pathways which are unique to cancer stem cells and thereby permit selective targeting of this important subpopulation of tumour cells.

Further reading

Bishop JM (1987). The molecular genetics of cancer. *Science*, **235**, 305–11.

DeVita VT, Hellman S, Rosenberg SA (eds) (1995). *Biologic therapy of cancer*, 2nd edition. JB Lippincott, Philadephia, PA.

Franks LM, Teich NM (eds) (1995). *Introduction to the cellular and molecular biology of cancer*, 2nd edition. Oxford University Press, Oxford.

Hanahan D, Weinberg RA (2000). The hallmarks of cancer. *Cell*, **100**, 57–70.

Jordan CT, Guzman ML, Noble M (2006). Cancer stem cells. *N Engl J Med*, **355**, 1253–61.

Pierce GB, Speers WC (1988). Tumours as caricatures of the process of tissue renewal: prospects for therapy by directing differentiation. *Cancer Res*, **48**, 1996–2004.

Schipper H (1995). Shifting the cancer paradigm: must we kill to cure? (editorial). *J Clin Oncol*, **13**, 801–7.

6.3

The genetics of inherited cancers

Rosalind A. Eeles

Essentials

All cancer can be termed 'genetic' as cancer is caused by somatic cell mutations (alterations in the DNA code), which result in abnormal cellular growth and/or proliferation. Most of these mutations are sporadic (only occurring in the cancer cell), but some are due to the inheritance of a germ-line mutation in a cancer predisposition gene.

Cancer predisposition genes can be rare and confer a high cancer risk (about 10-fold lifetime relative risk), or common and confer a moderately increased risk (from just over onefold, up to two- to threefold). They have been shown to be involved in causing some of most common cancers as well as some rare cancers.

Mechanisms of inherited cancers

Cancer predisposition genes (see Chapter 6.2) are usually (1) tumour suppressor genes—e.g. retinoblastoma caused by mutations in *RB1*—when, although the mutations are recessively inherited at the cellular level, they tend to manifest with a dominant inheritance pattern because the chance of a mutation being inherited by the offspring is 50%, and a sporadic mutation of the remaining normal allele occurs in a somatic cell during the lifetime of the germ-line mutation carrier to lead to cancer development; (2) oncogenes—e.g. the *RET* oncogene in the multiple endocrine neoplasia (MEN) type 2A syndrome—when gain-of-function mutations act in a dominant manner; (3) mismatch repair genes—e.g. causing the hereditary nonpolyposis colorectal cancer (HNPCC, Lynch) syndrome.

Clinical features

Genetic predisposition to cancer should be suspected when cancers: (1) occur at a younger age than is seen in the general population; (2) occur in more than one site or at multiple times at the same site in an individual (multiple primary tumours); or when (3) rare cancers are seen in clusters in a family; or (4) common cancers are seen in clusters in a family, often at young age or with multiple primaries.

Genetic predisposition to common cancers—this includes (1) breast—*BRCA1* and *BRCA2* mutations confer 80 to 85% risk of breast cancer by 80 years (and also a significantly increased risk of ovarian cancer); *TP53* (Li–Fraumeni syndrome) mutations confer 90% risk of breast cancer by 60 years; (2) colon—mutations in the *APC* gene cause familial adenomatous polyposis (FAP) and a virtually 100% risk of colon cancer by the age of 40 years; HNPCC, which is also associated with other cancers in addition to colon cancer, particularly endometrial cancer (60% lifetime risk) and ovarian cancer (12% lifetime risk).

Rare inherited cancer syndromes—there are many of these, including hereditary retinoblastoma, neurofibromatosis type 1 (optic nerve glioma, sarcoma, phaeochromocytoma), neurofibromatosis type 2 (acoustic neuroma and other tumours of the central nervous system), MEN1 (parathyroid adenomas, pancreatic islet tumours and anterior pituitary tumours), MEN2A and 2B (medullary thyroid cancer, phaeochromocytoma, parathyroid adenomas), Cowden's syndrome (breast and other cancers), tuberous sclerosis (childhood brain tumours, cardiac rhabdomyomas), Gorlin's syndrome (multiple basal cell naevi/carcinomas), Von Hippel–Lindau syndrome (cerebellar and spinal hemangioblastomata, renal cell carcinoma, phaeochromocytoma, pancreatic tumours).

Clinical management

Patients and/or families known or suspected to carry cancer predisposition gene mutations require genetic counselling and risk assessment, which may lead on to (1) cancer screening—e.g. colonoscopy for some individuals at increased risk of colon cancer; (2) lifestyle changes—e.g. avoidance of known cancer-causing factors such as sunlight in Gorlin's syndrome; (3) prevention strategies—e.g. prophylactic total colectomy in the FAP syndrome; (4) cancer treatment considerations—e.g. tumours with a particular genetic abnormality may respond to particular treatments; and (5) genetic testing—which may either be diagnostic (the detection of a mutation in an individual affected by cancer) or predictive (the detection of a mutation in a clinically unaffected individual).

Future prospects—gene alterations that predispose to cancer affect prognosis and treatment, hence genetic information is increasingly recognized as important in oncological practice. Cancer genetics will become part of mainstream clinical pathways for cancer care in the next decade and is likely to contribute to health care that is tailored to individual patients.

Introduction

Cancer is a common disease; it affects up to one-third of the population during their lifetime. All cancer can be termed 'genetic' as cancer is caused by somatic cell mutations (alterations in the DNA code), which result in abnormal cellular growth and/or proliferation. Most of these mutations are sporadic (occurring only in the cancer cell) and only a proportion of these cases is due to the inheritance of a germ-line mutation in a cancer predisposition gene. In these latter cases, the genetic alteration is in all cells of the body with the exception of the gametes where, on average, the genetic alterations are in one-half of the gametes. It used to be thought that such alterations were rare, but each conferred a high cancer risk (about 10-fold lifetime). However, recent studies have shown that there are also more frequent alterations in cancer predisposition genes with each of such mutations conferring a slightly increased risk (with just over a onefold, up to a two- to threefold relative risk). This has implications for the role of genetic predisposition to cancer in general medical and oncological practice as a larger proportion of cases of cancer may harbour these latter alterations in the genetic code. Identification of such alterations will become important in the genetic profiling of the population to aid targeted cancer screening and prevention. There is emerging evidence that gene alterations that predispose to cancer affect prognosis and treatment and thus their significance is becoming incorporated into the clinical pathway for cancer care. Cancer genetics will become part of mainstream cancer care in the next decade and is likely to contribute to health care that is tailored to individual patients.

Historical perspective

Since Roman times, cancer has been known to run in families. In some families, the pattern of cancer incidence among family members is consistent with the inheritance of a mutated gene and carriers of this mutated gene have a high risk of cancer. The chance that cancer will develop if an individual has a mutation in a cancer predisposition gene is called the penetrance. Most cancer predisposition genes have incomplete penetrance (i.e. the cancer risk is <100%).

There are several types of evidence that inherited susceptibility plays a role in the development of cancer (also see Table 6.3.1):

- In some inherited syndromes, which are rare in the general population, there is an increased risk of cancer in carriers of genetic mutation(s) which give rise to the syndrome, e.g. neurofibromatosis type 1 (an autosomal dominant genetic syndrome—see later) which confers an increased risk (of a few %) of sarcoma and phaechromocytoma. Such syndromes can be accessed using the database initiated in the early 1960s by Dr Victor McKusick as a catalogue of mendelian traits and disorders, first entitled Mendelian Inheritance in Man (MIM), now the website Online Mendelian Inheritance in Man (OMIM).
- Some rare cancers cluster in families and form a 'cancer family syndrome', e.g. the association of tumours in multiple endocrine neoplasia type 2 (MEN2: the association of medullary thyroid cancer, phaeochromocytoma, and hyperparathyroidism). Such cancers are rare in the general population and so the occurrence of such rare cases either in relatives or in one individual is highly indicative of a genetic predisposition.
- The observation that families exist which have a number of cases of 'common' cancers. Even though these cancers are prevalent in the general population, the number of such cases in these families far exceeds the number predicted by population rates. Often these cancers occur at ages earlier than seen in the general population (see Fig. 6.3.1) and family members have an increased occurrence of synchronous and metachronous lesions.
- Epidemiological studies in the general population which show that there is an increased risk of cancer to relatives of cases and this risk markedly increases as the proband or index case with cancer is affected at a younger age or with bilateral cancers.
- Genes have now been identified which, when mutated, are associated with an increased risk of cancer. These may be rare mutations which confer a high (about tenfold) or moderate (just over two- to threefold) cancer risk, or common lower-penetrance genes (which confer an increased risk of just over onefold up to about twofold).

Historically, it was thought that genetic predisposition to cancer was a rare phenomenon and was predominantly observed in rare syndromes, such as multiple endocrine neoplasia, or was a rare component of other genetic diseases (such as neurofibromatosis). However, the advances in the Human Genome and HapMap projects (see below) have challenged this view and have shown that in fact genetic variants which are common in populations form an important contribution to cancer risk.

Inheritance, mechanisms of cancer predisposition, and the retinoblastoma story

Inheritance of germ-line mutations in cancer predisposition genes may be either dominant, recessive, or X-linked. We all carry two copies (alleles) of every gene, one copy from each parent, and as only one allele can be passed down to the next generation, there is a 50:50 chance as to which allele we inherit.

In dominant inheritance the presence of a single mutated allele is usually sufficient to cause the associated disease and approximately 50% of all offspring develop the disease. In recessive inheritance the presence of a single mutated allele is insufficient for disease expression and two mutated alleles are required. Usually both parents have to carry the mutated allele for the creation of an offspring affected by disease, but they themselves are unaffected, as their 'normal' allele overrides the effects of the mutated one. Two parents with a recessive mutated allele therefore have a 25% chance of having an affected child. An example of such a condition predisposing to colon cancer is the *MutYH* syndrome where adenomas occur in the colon. In such families colon cancer tends to cluster in siblings, as it is recessive (the colon cancer risk in mutation carrier parents is not thought to be raised above the general population). Most cancer predisposition genes are recessively inherited, at the cellular level, but dominantly inherited in families, i.e. there is a 50:50 chance that the mutated allele will be inherited, but in the cancer cell both copies of the allele have to be altered for cancer to occur.

In X-linked inheritance the mutated gene is carried on the X chromosome. Females have two X chromosomes, and can therefore be carriers of the condition but are not usually affected.

Table 6.3.1 Some of the 'rare' syndromes associated with an increased risk of malignancy and their mode of inheritance (for further details, see text)

Neoplasia or syndrome	Malignancy	Risk[a]	Mode[b]	Gene	Location
NF1	Plexiform Neurofibroma Optic glioma Sarcoma	 <4% <15% <5%	AD	*NF1*	17q11
NF2	Bilateral acoustic Neuroma Meningioma Spinal tumours Other brain tumours	 85% 45% 26% <10%	AD	*NF2*	22q12
Gorlin's syndrome	Basal cell carcinoma Medulloblastoma Meningioma	90% 5% 1%	AD	*PTCH*	9q22
Tuberous sclerosis	Renal cancer	<10%	AD	*TSC1* *TSC2*	9q34 16p13
Cowden's syndrome	Breast cancer Endometrial cancer Thyroid cancer	30% by age 50 <10% 15%	AD	*PTEN*	10q23
Li–Fraumeni syndrome	Brain tumours Breast cancer Sarcomas Leukaemia Adrenocortical cancer Other cancers Childhood cancer	All adult tumours: 90% by 60 in women, 74% in men 24% by 20	AD	*TP53*	17p13
MEN1	Pituitary tumour Pancreas Parathyroid Carcinoid	95%	AD	*MEN1*	11q13
MEN2A	Medullary carcinoma of thyroid Phaeochromocytoma	70% 50%	AD	*RET*	10q11
Retinoblastoma	Retinoblastoma Bladder/osteosarcoma	90% <10%	AD	*RB1*	13q14
Ataxia telangiectasia	Lymphoma Leukaemia	60% 27%	AR	*ATM*	11q22
Bloom's syndrome	Leukaemia Solid tumours	Rarely live to>40	AR	*BLM*	15q26
Werner's syndrome	Various		AR	*RECQL2*	8p12
Rothmund–Thomson syndrome	Various		AR	*RECQL4*	8q24
Fanconi anaemia	Leukaemia Head and neck cancer Oesophagus/cervix/anus		AR	*FANC* genes	
Xeroderma pigmentosum	Skin cancer	90% often <20 yrs	AR	*XP* genes	

NF, neurofibromatosis type; MEN, multiple endocrine neoplasia; NA, not available.
[a] Lifetime risk of cancer.
[b] Mode of inheritance is classified as autosomal dominant (AD) or autosomal recessive (AR).

Males have only one copy of the X chromosome, so if they inherit a mutated gene on the X from their mother, they will inherit the condition. A carrier female therefore has a 50% chance of passing the condition on to each of her sons, and a 50% chance that her daughters will be carriers. X-linked familial prostate cancer has been observed in a small number of families, although the causal locus has not yet been identified.

Mechanisms of action

Cancer predisposition genes are usually tumour suppressor genes, oncogenes, or mismatch repair genes. Recently, very rare instances have been described where alterations in the germ line have a down-stream effect which is called an 'epigenetic' effect; in most such cases the germ-line change results in alteration of methylation of genes, which alters their expression and this results in increased cancer risk.

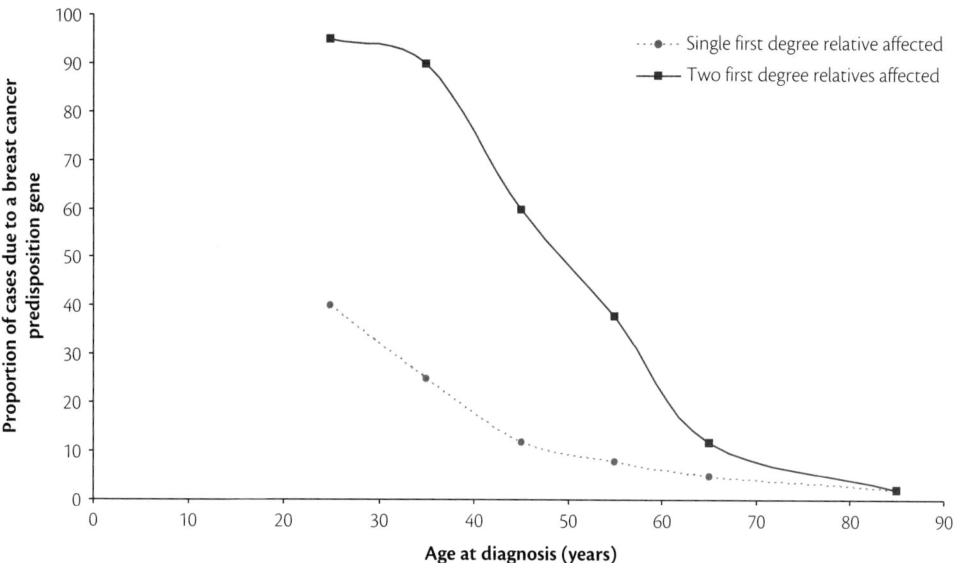

Fig. 6.3.1 Graph showing the probability that breast cancer is due to a predisposition gene by age at diagnosis of breast cancer (from Claus *et al.*, 1991). (Graph courtesy of Professor D T Bishop.)

Tumour suppressor genes are normal genes in which mutation tends to cause a 'loss of function' effect in the control mechanisms of growth and/or cellular proliferation pathways. The first example was retinoblastoma, a tumour of the eye, usually in children, caused by mutations in the tumour suppressor gene *RB1*. Most cancer predisposition genes are tumour suppressor genes and are recessively inherited at the cellular level. However, they tend to manifest dominant inheritance (the chance of a mutation being inherited by the offspring is 50%). A sporadic mutation of the remaining normal allele occurs in a somatic cell during the lifetime of the germ-line mutation carrier to lead to cancer development. This two-stage process in the development of cancers (where one stage is germ-line and the other is somatic) is known as Knudson's two-hit hypothesis (see Chapter 6.2).

Oncogenes or proto-oncogenes are mutated normal genes in which a mutation in only one allele tends to cause a 'gain of function' effect resulting in increased growth or proliferation of the affected cells. They act in a dominant manner. They rarely cause predisposition to cancer, but examples of those causing cancer include the *RET* oncogene in the multiple endocrine neoplasia 2A syndrome and the *MET* oncogene in familial papillary renal cancer.

Mismatch repair genes maintain the integrity of the genome and mutations in them allow acquired genetic damage to accumulate resulting in the creation of a cancer cell. They classically predispose to a colorectal cancer syndrome called Lynch syndrome (named after a famous cancer geneticist, Dr Henry Lynch, who was one of the first to recognize that predisposition to common cancers could be inherited), also known as HNPCC (hereditary nonpolyposis colorectal cancer; see below).

Hereditary cancer predisposition genes have also been classified into 'gatekeeper genes' and 'caretaker genes' (see Chapter 6.2). Gatekeeper genes are those that regulate progression through the cell cycle. Disturbance of their function leads to an imbalance of cell division over cell death. This cellular proliferation is followed by the accumulation of multiple somatic genetic events causing tumour development. Examples of gatekeeper genes include *TP53* and *RB1*. Caretaker genes maintain the integrity of the genome. Mutations occurring in these genes result in genetic instability, and it is this that results in mutation in other genes, including gatekeeper genes. The DNA mismatch repair genes in HNPCC are examples of caretaker genes.

The multistep pathway of carcinogenesis

The development of cancer is thought to be due to a multistep pathway involving several genetic changes. This is likely to be the explanation for incomplete penetrance, as not all genetic changes will occur in every individual who inherits the first genetic change. In inherited predisposition to cancer, the first change is inherited in most cases. Less commonly, the first change is still in the germ-line but the mutation has occurred *de novo* in the germ cells (i.e. the carrier of the germ-line genetic mutation is the first individual in the family to harbour the mutation; the rate at which this occurs is termed the 'new mutation rate'). This is more common in some types of inherited predisposition to cancer than others. For example, the new mutation rate in HNPCC is about 50%, but in familial breast/ovarian cancer due to *BRCA1* or *BRCA2* it is extremely rare. In the latter example, analyses of genetic variation flanking the region of the *BRCA1* gene and knowledge of the genetic recombination rate have enabled the occurrence of mutations in this gene in the Ashkenazi Jewish population to be dated to pre-Roman times.

The most classic multistep model which has been published is that of the progression from colorectal adenomatous polyp to invasive colorectal carcinoma; a multistep pathway which involves at least five genetic changes (the so-called colorectal adenoma–carcinoma sequence, proposed by Vogelstein). This is shown diagrammatically in Fig. 6.3.2.

Research approaches for the identification of cancer predisposition genes

There are several approaches to locate a cancer predisposition gene. Once it is located and characterized, genetic testing can then be offered in the clinical setting.

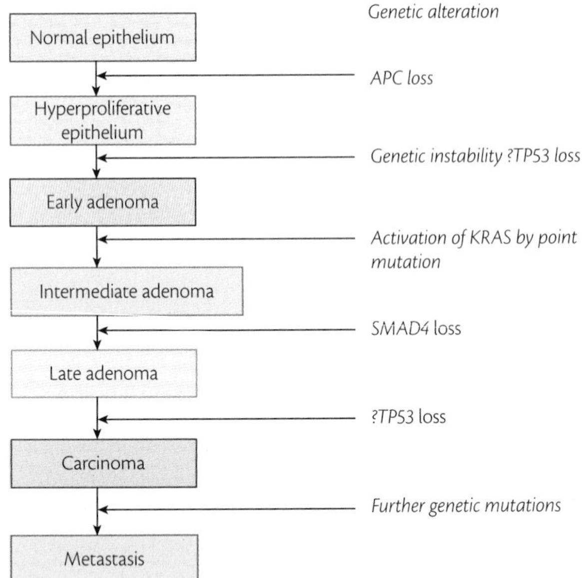

Fig. 6.3.2 The colorectal adenoma–carcinoma sequence.

Cytogenetic alterations

Gross chromosomal changes can be analysed by a karyotype or cytogenetic analysis from a blood sample. Rarely, karyotypic abnormalities in an individual who has an unusually early onset of cancer and other unusual phenotypic features have indicated the location of a cancer predisposition gene. The chromosomal study of a man with mental retardation and polyposis led to the finding of a loss of part of chromosome 5, subsequently found to be the location of the polyposis gene *APC* which predisposes to familial polyposis.

Linkage analysis

The concept of genetic linkage was first recognized by William Bateson, who noted that certain characteristics of his experimental plants tended to be coinherited, a phenomenon that had been described by the monk Gregor Mendel, 34 years previously. The explanation for this became clear once Morgan recognized that chromosomes contain the genetic material and two traits are coinherited (linked) only if the corresponding genes for them reside close together on the same chromosome. The search for cancer predisposition genes using linkage relies on collections of families with numerous cancer cases of the same cancer type. Coinheritance of specific genetic markers with the disease is said to show evidence of linkage if the coinheritance is greater than would be expected by chance. This is expressed as a 'LOD score' which is similar to a *P* value in clinical trials. A LOD score of >3 is considered statistically significant and equivalent to odds of linkage of 1000 to 1.

Phenotypic features

A physical characteristic associated with a cancer predisposition syndrome may give a clue as to its location. An example of this is the coexistence of aniridia and genitourinary abnormalities with Wilms' tumour in the WAGR syndrome. This is caused by a contiguous gene deletion on chromosome 11.

Association studies

A number of disease susceptibility loci have been identified using genome-wide association studies. In these case control studies, allele frequencies are compared between affected individuals and controls. It is important in such studies to have controls from the same ethnic/racial group to avoid false associations. Advances in the knowledge of the structure of the human genome have identified single nucleotide polymorphisms (SNPs or single base changes) throughout the genome (the HapMap project) and large-scale genomic analysis using chip array technology (e.g. the Illumina or Affymetrix systems) has enabled a million such SNPs to be analysed in each DNA sample at once. Such studies have identified common variants associated with disease risk which are present in at least 5% of the population: in some cases they are found in over one-half of the population. Although each SNP is associated with a small increased risk (usually less than twofold), the risks can be multiplicative and so a combination of SNPs can give different 'risk profiles' in different individuals. This therefore opens up the possibility of SNP profiling to determine the risk of cancer in defined populations.

Direct sequencing and the potential role of whole genome sequencing

As the Human Genome Project has identified a large proportion of the genetic code, parts or all of this can be subjected to direct analysis by sequencing of genes to look for base pair changes (point mutations or nonsense mutations), or insertions or deletions of bases (frameshift mutations). Most genetic tests for cancer predisposition now involve such sequencing technology of specific genes from blood DNA (e.g. the current breast cancer predisposition genetic tests sequence the *BRCA1* and *BRCA2* genes). One of the main current research activities is the sequencing of whole genomes (e.g. the '1000 genomes project' which aims to sequence 1000 human genomes to find genetic variation). Although at present a research tool, it is envisaged that this could become a routine investigation. The difficulty will arise in the interpretation of all the genetic variants, their potential interaction effects, and the accurate prediction of disease risk.

Detection of other mechanisms of gene alteration

Not all genetic changes involve alterations of DNA bases as above. Some mutations can be due to larger deletions or gene rearrangements and these can easily be overlooked by conventional sequencing methods. Most are detected by multiple probe ligation analysis (MLPA). For example the standard *BRCA1/2* genetic test for breast cancer predisposition also includes MLPA as well as sequencing, as up to 8% of *BRCA1/2* mutations in some populations can be caused by alterations which are only detected by MLPA. Epigenetic changes are often due to methylation of genes. Rarely, alterations in the germ line can cause downstream methylation of cancer predisposition genes; such changes have recently been described in Wilms tumour and some cases of HNPCC.

Cancer risks associated with cancer predisposition genes

Cancer risks depend on the presence of mutations in a cancer predisposition gene and its penetrance (Table 6.3.2). Penetrance may be affected by external factors, such as lifestyle, and other environmental effects; it may also depend on the ethnic origin of an individual due to population-specific mutation risks. For example, for *BRCA1* or *BRCA2*, which predispose to breast and ovarian cancer, using data from the Breast Cancer Linkage Consortium based on breast and ovarian cancer families identified from a worldwide

Table 6.3.2 Genes with high penetrance for the common cancers

Neoplasia or syndrome	Malignancies	Risk of cancer[a]	Location	Gene
Breast/ovary				
Breast/ovary cancer syndrome	Breast Ovary Other cancers, e.g. pancreas, young onset prostate, <65 years Breast Ovary Prostate, pancreas Other cancers, e.g. melanoma/bile duct/fallopian tube	80–85% 40–60% <10% 80–85% 27% <10% 10–14% by 74 years	17q21 13q12	*BRCA1* *BRCA2*
Colon				
Familial adenomatous polyposis	Bowel cancer Duodenum/periampullary Hepatoblastoma/ thyroid/brain Desmoid	*c.* 100% <5%	5q21	*APC*
HNPCC	Colon & endometrium Ovary Other cancers, e.g. renal tract	75–90% 12% <5%	2p22 3p21 2p16 2q31 7p22	*hMSH2* *hMLH1* *hMSH6* *PMS1* *PMS2*
Muir–Torre syndrome	As HNPCC (see above) with skin lesions		2p22	*hMSH2*
Peutz–Jeghers	Ovarian cancer (sex cord) Gastrointestinal	<10%	19p13	*STK11*
Juvenile polyposis	Colon	70%	18q21 10q23 10q22	*SMAD4* *PTEN* *BMPR1A*
MutYH	Colon	70%	1p34	*MUTYH*
Turcot's	Colon	70% can be <20		APC/HNPCC genes
Gastric cancer				
Diffuse gastric cancer	Stomach	90%	16q22	*CHD1*
Melanoma				
Melanoma	Melanoma	65%	9p21	*CDKN2A*
Renal				
Renal cancer (papillary)	Papillary renal	70%	7q31	*MET*
Von Hippel–Lindau	Cerebellar Haemangioblastoma Retinal angioma Renal cell carcinoma	 84% 70% 69%	3p25	*VHL*
WAGR	Wilms' tumour is part of syndrome		11p13	*WT1*
Birt–Hogg–Dube	Renal carcinoma	?	17p11	*FOLLICULIN*
Hereditary leiomyomatosis	Renal carcinoma	?	1q42	*FH*

[a] The risk is either the 'lifetime risk' quoted to age 80 years unless otherwise stated.

Note: The common cancers—colon, breast, prostate, lung, and lymphoma–have had numerous lower-risk variants identified by genome-wide association, and in breast cancer rare more moderately penetrant genes have been found by candidate genetic mutation analysis (see text).

population of high-risk families with breast cancer, the risk of breast cancer is estimated to be 85% by 80 years, but the risk associated with the Icelandic founder mutation in the *BRCA2* gene is estimated to be as low as 37% by this age. The ethnic population differences may be due to a founder mutation dependent risk, the effect of other modifying genes in a population, or the added effect of environmental influences, which may be shared within specific populations. Therfore it is important to ascertain the ancestry of the patient before genetic counselling is initiated. The estimate of penetrance can be confounded by the presence of phenocopies when research into the identification of a cancer predisposition gene is undertaken. Phenocopies are people who have developed the disease of interest but are found not to carry the disease predisposition gene, so that the disease has occurred by chance alone or may have been due to environmental influences. Phenocopies are a particular problem in the analysis of syndromes associated with common cancers such as breast or colon cancer.

When quoting cancer risks it is important to quote the risk by a specific age as the profile of risk may alter over time; for example the risk of breast cancer from a deleterious mutation in *BRCA1* is a sigmoid curve, starting to rise from the age of 30; the steepest part of the curve is in the 40s and there is still some risk until the age of 80 years. An unaffected woman with a *BRCA1* mutation will therefore have a lower residual cancer risk if she is aged 70 than she will at the age of 40 years.

Genetic predisposition to the common cancers

Breast cancer

Breast cancer is the most common noncutaneous cancer in women in the Western world. Several genes predispose to high risks of breast cancer, most notably *BRCA1* and *BRCA2* (breast cancer 1 and 2 genes) which were isolated in 1994 and 1995. These genes, when mutated, also predispose to ovarian cancer, and also have a small (<10%) risk of causing other cancers (e.g. pancreas, bile duct, melanoma, male breast cancer, prostate cancer). They are highly penetrant for female breast cancer (80–85% risk by 80 years) and ovarian cancer (40–60% risk for *BRCA1* and 27% risk for *BRCA2*). The profiles of the penetrance curves are slightly different (in general, those for *BRCA2* start to rise at an older age for both breast and ovarian cancer) and this is taken into consideration when considering the timing of preventative surgery (see below). A rarer breast cancer predisposition gene is *TP53* which usually predisposes to the Li–Fraumeni syndrome, the association of early onset sarcoma with cancer at <45 years in at least two close relatives. Often this syndrome is associated with childhood cancer. The penetrance of breast cancer is 90% by age 60 and this gene can cause breast cancer at particularly young ages (in the 20s). Other rarer cancer predisposition genes in the DNA repair pathway have been shown to be associated with increased breast cancer risk (*BRIP1*, *PALB2*, *ATM*, *CHEK2*), but these risks (about twofold) are not as high as those from mutations in *BRCA1/2* or *TP53*. Cowden's multiple hamartomatous syndrome has an increased risk of female and male breast cancer and also thyroid and uterine cancer. It is associated with gynaecological and brain abnormalities and bowel polyps, but there is debate as to whether there is also an increased risk of bowel cancer. The pathology of the breast cancer is characteristic in some of these conditions; in *BRCA1* mutation carriers, it is often hormone receptor and HER2 negative (so-called 'triple negative') and has cellular features of the basal type. There is an increased risk of lobular breast cancer in association with diffuse gastric cancer which is due to mutations in the *CDH1* E-Cadherin gene.

Colon cancer

It is thought that at least a proportion of colon cancers arises from polyps in the bowel. The colon cancer syndrome with the highest bowel cancer risk is associated with the presence of thousands of such polyps in the large bowel (familial adenomatous polyposis or FAP; Fig. 6.3.3). This is due to mutations in the *APC* gene. The APC protein is a negative regulator of β-catenin, a critical component of a signal transduction pathway that regulates cell–cell adhesion, cellular polarity, and tissue architecture. The penetrance is high, with a virtually 100% risk of colon cancer by the age of 40. There is also a risk of other cancers, such as hepatoblastoma, periampullary, thyroid and brain cancer, sarcoma, and desmoid tumours. Polyps can also occur in the upper gastrointestinal tract and pigment can be present in the retina. The polyps are so extensive that the mainstay of prevention is a colectomy once the polyps appear on sigmoidoscopic monitoring, of individuals who have *APC* mutations, from the age of 11 years.

Lynch's syndrome or HNPCC has fewer polyps (usually <100) and classical HNPCC conforms to a definition also known as the Amsterdam criteria, so-called because Vasen in Amsterdam found that if these criteria were used then over half of families had mutations in the mismatch repair genes *hMLH1* (chromosome 3p21), *hMSH2* (2p22), *hMSH6* (2p16), *PMS1* (2q31), and *PMS2* (7p22). These criteria are colon cancer in at least three individuals in two generations, at least two being first-degree relatives of each other and at least one of the colon cancers occurring at less than 50 years of age. Classically the cancers tend to occur more often in the right side of the colon whereas sporadic colon cancer is more often left sided. This condition is also associated with other cancers, particularly endometrial cancer (60% lifetime risk), ovarian cancer (12% lifetime risk), and smaller risks of biliary and pancreatic cancer, cancer of the renal tract (particularly transitional cell carcinoma), and upper gastrointestinal tract cancer.

Extracolonic cancers are more common in *hMSH2* mutation carriers, and *hMSH6* is particularly associated with uterine cancer. There are less stringent clusters which are also due to mutations in these genes and so more loose criteria have been developed (the so-called Bethesda criteria, but as the criteria get less stringent, the mutation frequency decreases). The mismatch repair genes are involved in DNA base excision repair and, if mutated, give rise to genetic instability, particularly of repeats in the DNA (microsatellite instability). This can be analysed in tumour specimens to determine if there is likely to be an underlying mismatch repair gene defect. Protein products of these genes can also be detected by immunohistochemical staining and so lack of staining in colonic tumours is used as a triage to determine which gene may be mutated. More rarely, brain tumours can occur in association with very early onset (often <20 years) colorectal cancer and these cases have been

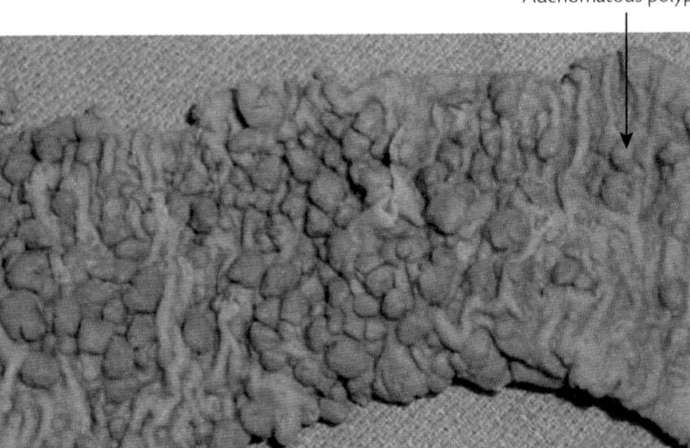

Fig. 6.3.3 Large bowel with numerous adenomatous polyps (arrowed) due to FAP. Google Images.

found to harbour homozygous (both gene copies are altered) mutations in mismatch repair genes (Turcot's syndrome). The presence of sebaceous adenomas or keratoacanthoma should raise the possibility of Muir–Torre syndrome which is HNPCC with these additional skin features and is also due to mutations in mismatch repair genes.

Genes predisposing to other rarer colorectal cancer syndromes have also been described. *STK11* predisposes to Peutz–Jeghers syndrome (autosomal dominant) where hamartomatous polyps are associated with pigmentation of the lips and buccal mucosa. This syndrome also has an increased risk of breast, ovarian, uterine, pancreatic, and testicular cancer. Juvenile polyposis is an autosomal dominant condition and causes diffuse hamartomatous polyps of the colon, small bowel, and stomach which develop at an early age (<10 years) or older (*c.*55 years). About half of patients have mutations in the *SMAD4* gene (which, interestingly, is mutated in the multistep pathway of colorectal cancer; see Fig. 6.3.2, within the cancer cells) or *PTEN* or *BMPR1A*. Rarely families with mutations in the *TGFBRII* gene have been described; this is in the *SMAD4* pathway.

If a family has a recessive pattern of inheritance (i.e. disease in siblings but not the parents) of multiple colonic polyps then *MutYH* should be considered. This gene usually has mutations at specific sites and so the genetic test can examine these regions specifically, at least in the first instance.

Upper gastrointestinal cancer and pancreatic cancer

There are rare reports of familial gastric cancer where the cancer can occur at a very young age (<20 years) and is of diffuse type. These are associated with mutations in the *CDH1* gene. The treatment is prophylactic gastrectomy. Duodenal cancers can occur as part of FAP. Familial pancreatic cancer is described but the genetic basis is still being researched; rare instances are due to mutations in the *BRCA2* gene.

Ovarian cancer

The main genes to consider are *BRCA1* (on chromosome 17q21) and *BRCA2* (on chromosome 13q12). These account for the majority of families with two or more cases of ovarian cancer and are predominantly associated with the serous type of ovarian adenocarcinoma. Peutz–Jeghers syndrome can cause unusual ovarian lesions such as mucinous tumours or sex cord tumour with annular tubules. Ovarian cancer can also be part of HNPCC but the penetrance is lower (about 12%) than with *BRCA1/2.*

Melanoma

Mutations in the multicancer tumour suppressor gene *CDKN2A* (*P16*) have been associated with melanoma. Mutations in this gene should only be considered if there are multiple melanomas in an individual, and/or at least three cases of melanoma in a family, often with early onset disease (≤40 years).

Prostate cancer

Prostate cancer is the most common noncutaneous cancer in men in the Western world. Over 80% of cases occur at more than 65 years of age. Rare cases (<5%), particularly at young age (<60 years), are due to mutations in the *BRCA* genes, particularly *BRCA2* which predisposes to more aggressive disease with a poorer prognosis. Most of the prostate cancer loci (>25) have been found by genome-wide association studies. Variation at these loci resulting in slightly increased risk is common. A man in the highest 1% of the risk profile from SNP combinations will have nearly three and a half times the average risk of the general population. As further SNPs are found, genetic profiling will be possible in the population. It is uncertain at present if these variants will help to identify more aggressive disease and further research is needed in this area.

Common lower-risk variants

Genome-wide association studies are revealing genetic changes (SNPs) associated with disease. These are more common than most of the genetic changes mentioned above, and often the SNPs are not in genes and so are presumably exerting their effect by altering gene function in another part of the genome. These types of alterations are currently the predominant types of variants predisposing to prostate and lung cancer. In the latter disease, one of the SNPs is on chromosome 15q25 which contains the nicotinic acetylcholine receptor subunit genes *CHRNA3* and *CHRNA5*, suggesting that susceptibility may be mediated through smoking behaviour.

Rare inherited cancer syndromes

Hereditary retinoblastoma: a classical example of a cancer predisposition syndrome

The first cancer predisposition genes were identified by studying rare but striking clusters of conditions that occur as part of recognized clinical syndromes (Box 6.3.1). Hereditary retinoblastoma is a classical example of this phenomenon. Retinoblastoma is a cancer of retinal cells and mainly occurs at in children less than 5 years of age (most occur at <2 years). One in 13 500 to 25 000 children are affected, with an equal sex distribution. About 10% of patients have a family history of the disease, with an autosomal dominant pattern of inheritance. Inherited forms of the disease are due to mutations in the *RB1* gene on chromosome 13q14; the new mutation rate is also high. The other cases are apparently sporadic but many of these have a germ-line mutation which has occurred *de novo* (see above). Knudson calculated that only one additional mutation is necessary for tumour development, leading to the two-hit hypothesis. All bilateral cases where retinoblastoma occurs in both eyes should therefore be considered to be gene mutation carriers. Eighty-five per cent of retinoblastomas presenting at less than 6 months of age affect both eyes and are likely to be the inherited form. The proportion of bilateral cases declines to 6% by 24 months, when most cases are of the sporadic type, with a much lower risk of genetic transmission (<5% of cases will be mutation carriers).

Box 6.3.1 Features of inherited cancer predisposition syndromes

- Earlier onset than sporadic cancer
- Bilateral or multifocal cancer
- Rare cancers either alone or more often in clusters in families than is expected by chance
- Phenotypic abnormalities indicating a disorder of tissue formation/regulation, e.g. overgrowth syndromes or skin manifestations
- New germ-line mutations may account for new cases where there is no family history

The penetrance of *RB1* mutations is 90%. Individuals with hereditary retinoblastoma are at an increased risk of developing a variety of other cancers (especially osteosarcoma and bladder cancer). Retinoblastoma illustrates the cardinal clinical features of inherited cancer predisposition syndromes: early onset, bilateral cancer, familial clustering, and predisposition to multiple tumours both within the eye and also at multiple sites. Many genetic alterations in *RB1* are gene deletions and insertions. Of interest, point mutations may be associated with a lower penetrance, suggesting a genotype–phenotype effect (the genetic and physical effects respectively).

Neurofibromatosis type 1

This is one of the most frequent single gene disorders with a frequency of 1 in 2500–3300 individuals. The diagnosis is clinical and the clinical features of neurofibromatosis type 1 (NF1, von Recklinghausen's disease) require at least two of the following:

- At least six café-au-lait spots larger than 5 mm (if prepubertal) or 15 mm (if postpubertal)
- At least two neurofibromas or one plexiform neurofibroma
- Axillary or inguinal freckling
- Optic nerve glioma
- At least two iris hamartomas (Lisch nodules)
- An osseous lesion such as sphenoid dysplasia or thickened long bone cortex ± pseudarthrosis
- A first-degree relative with NF1

Learning difficulties can also occur in about 30%. About 3 to 5% of cases have a malignancy which is usually an optic nerve glioma, sarcoma, or phaeochromocytoma. Recent analyses of other tumour risks have also reported a moderately increased breast cancer risk. The *NF1* gene (on chromosome 17q11) is very large (60 exons) and it encodes a guanosine triphosphatase activating protein known as the NF1-GAP-related protein, or neurofibromin. GAP proteins negatively regulate RAS to control cell proliferation. Mutations are numerous and varied in type, probably because the gene is so large. There is no genotype–phenotype correlation of the mutation with the NF1 features. Some patients have numerous neurofibromas while others have very few. The phenotype is thought to be controlled by other genes. The new germ-line mutation rate is high (30–50%), again probably because of the extremely large size of target locus.

Neurofibromatosis type 2

Neurofibromatosis type 2 (NF2) is less common than NF1 (1 in 33 000 births) and has an autosomal dominant pattern of inheritance. The neurological effects of neurofibromas predominate in NF2. There is a predisposition to development of tumours of the central nervous system, particularly schwannoma of the eighth cranial nerve ('acoustic neuroma', which occurs bilaterally in 85% of cases), meningioma, spinal cord schwannoma, and malignant gliomas. Deafness and tinnitus due to acoustic neuromas as well as muscle weakness and wasting due to spinal cord compression are not unusual. Criteria for diagnosis are bilateral acoustic neuromas or a family history of NF2 plus unilateral acoustic neuroma at <30 years or any two of the following: meningioma, glioma, schwannoma, and juvenile posterior subcapsular lenticular opacities. There is a milder and a more severe type with presentations at under and over 20 years of age respectively. The *NF2* gene, located at chromosome 22q12, encodes a protein named schwannomin (or Merlin, for Moesin Ezrin Radixin-like protein) which communicates between the extracellular matrix and cytoskeleton. About half the cases are *de novo*. There seems to be a genotype–phenotype correlation with milder phenotypes associated with point mutations and more severe phenotypes associated with nonsense and frameshift mutations. It is noteworthy that about 20% of apparently *de novo* cases will not have germ-line mutations, and the *NF2* mutation is only at the tumour site as a result of mosaicism (only some cells in the body have the mutation). Such patients have a lower risk of transmission to offspring as the chance of their gametes being involved in the mosaicism is less. Patients should be managed in specialist centres as complex screening and interdisciplinary management is needed.

Multiple endocrine neoplasia type 1

This syndrome (MEN1) is associated with parathyroid adenomas, pancreatic islet tumours, and anterior pituitary tumours (for ease of recall, the 3Ps) and is autosomal dominant. Carcinoid can also occur. The *MEN1* gene on 11q13 codes for menin which acts as a growth suppressor protein. Mutations can occur throughout the gene and there is no genotype–phenotype correlation. Only about 10% of cases are *de novo*. Multicentric pancreatic tumours and hyperparathyroidism at young age (<30 years), with or without pituitary tumour, should raise the possibility of MEN1 and genetic testing can be undertaken using gene sequencing, although in 20% of classical cases no mutation is found. The penetrance is high (95% by 70 years).

Multiple endocrine neoplasia types 2A and 2B and familial medullary thyroid cancer

Three disorders are due to activating mutations in the RET tyrosine kinase-linked cell surface receptor encoded by the *RET* gene at 10q11.2 which is an oncogene (only one mutated copy is necessary for disease development). Medullary thyroid cancer is common to all three conditions and is histologically associated with C cell hyperplasia which should be looked for in the pathology report. When no other features are present, the condition is termed familial medullary thyroid cancer. In multiple endocrine neoplasia (MEN) types 2A and 2B, additional unusual tumours arise including phaeochromocytoma (in 50%) and parathyroid adenomas in 20–30% (particularly in MEN2A). MEN2B is associated with marfanoid habitus, intestinal ganglioneuromas (causing Hirschsprung's disease), and mucosal neuromas, often in the lips, causing them to be prominent. Particularly in MEN2B, medullary thyroid cancer can occur at less than 10 years of age. In 95% of cases of MEN2A, mutations affect cysteine residues in the extracellular binding domain of RET, resulting in inappropriate disulphide bond formation, dimerization, and activation of the RET tyrosine kinase. Familial medullary thyroid cancer results from mutations which similarly involve cysteine residues in the majority of cases, but at different sites. The mutation found in MEN2B is distinct and involves a methionine to threonine substitution in the ATP binding site of the receptor tyrosine kinase, leading to excessive receptor activity. There is a strong genotype–phenotype correlation with certain mutations particularly associated with phaeochromocytoma.

Rarely other mutations may occur in other parts of *RET* and some of these are associated with a lower penetrance. As medullary thyroid cancer can occur in early childhood, current optimal management is genetic testing and prophylactic total thyroidectomy in gene mutation carriers. Many geneticists will undertake predictive tests from birth in families where there is a known *RET* mutation. Screening for phaeochromocytoma and monitoring of parathyroid hormone and calcium levels should be undertaken; the disease is penetrant by age 70. All cases of medullary thyroid cancer should be referred to a cancer geneticist to offer genetic testing for *RET* mutations; if no mutation is found in such a case then the chance that it is inherited is less than 5%.

Cowden's syndrome

This autosomal dominant condition is a multiple hamartomatous syndrome. It has characteristic skin and tongue hamartomatous lesions, gynaecological abnormalities, and intestinal hamartomas. Craniomegaly and mental subnormality occur in about 50% of affected individuals. The pathognomic mucocutaneous lesions include trichilemmomas, acral keratoses, papillomatous papules, hyperkeratoses, and oral fibromas. Breast cancer occurs in 30% of female gene carriers by age 50 and multiple painful fibroadenomas of the breast are common, often necessitating prophylactic mastectomy. Thyroid cancer, male breast cancer, and endometrial cancer can also occur. Glial masses may present as cerebellar ataxia and seizures (Lhermitte–Duclos disease). The gene concerned, 'phosphatase tensin homologue deleted in chromosome 10' or *PTEN*, is located on 10q23. The PTEN phosphatase, by operating in opposition to the phosphoinositol-3-kinase pathway, inhibits cell survival and growth.

Tuberous sclerosis

This is a disease of variable severity characterized by the development of multiple hamartomas involving many organs; it is autosomal dominant. Characteristic lesions—facial angiofibromas (adenoma sebaceum), shagreen patches, and ungual fibromas—along with epilepsy and learning difficulties often suggest the diagnosis. There is an association with cardiac rhabdomyomas. Often there is no family history since as many as 60% of cases are due to a *de novo* mutation. There is a 5 to 15% incidence of childhood brain tumours in affected individuals, mostly subependymal giant cell astrocytomas. In addition a weak association with renal cell cancer has been reported. A wide variety of benign tumours, including hamartomas, angiofibromas, and renal lesions occur. The renal tumours are characteristically angiomyolipomas which can cause renal haemorrhage or compress the normal kidney leading to renal failure. Linkage studies have identified two genes, *TSC1* at 9q34 and *TSC2* at 16p13. *TSC1* encodes a protein called hamartin. Most mutations described within this gene result in a truncated protein. *TSC2* encodes tuberin, a protein showing some homology to GTPase activating proteins.

Li–Fraumeni syndrome

This is a rare but important autosomal dominant syndrome. It is named after the two epidemiologists who noticed an increased cancer risk in first-degree relatives of patients with rhabdomyosarcoma. The key feature is sarcoma, particularly at young age (<45 years). The definition of classical Li–Fraumeni syndrome is sarcoma in the proband before age 45 years and cancer before age 45 years in two close relatives, one of whom is a first-degree relative. The tumour spectrum is wide and multiple tumours can occur in one individual; there is also a high (24% by age 20) risk of tumours in childhood. The lifetime penetrance by age 60 years is 90% in women and 74% in men; penetrance is increased by exposure to carcinogens, particularly smoking. The spectrum of early onset tumours particularly includes bone and soft tissue sarcoma (excluding Ewing's sarcoma), breast cancer, brain tumour, leukaemia, and adrenocortical carcinoma. Approximately 75% of Li–Fraumeni syndrome families have germ-line mutations within the *TP53* gene located at 17p13. *TP53* has been referred to as the 'guardian of the genome' because of a critical role in arresting the cell cycle in the presence of DNA damage (see Chapter 6.2). It can act as a tumour suppressor and also as a dominant oncogene. Radiation may increase the risk of second tumours (57% rate of second tumours over 30 years) and so should be avoided if possible.

Basal cell naevus syndrome (Gorlin's syndrome)

This condition should be considered in any patient presenting with a basal cell carcinoma before the age of 30 years, or with a personal or family history of multiple basal cell naevi/carcinomas. It is associated with abnormalities of skin, bone, and tooth formation, including polyostotic bone cysts, odontogenic keratocysts (jaw cysts), bifid ribs, ectopic calcification (lamellar calcification as seen on a posteroanterior skull radiograph is pathognomonic), and palmar or plantar pits. An increased incidence of other cancers, including medulloblastoma, ovarian carcinoma, and sarcomas, may also occur. The incidence has been estimated at 1 in 55 600. The gene responsible for the majority of cases, *PTCH* on 9q22.3, is a homologue of the *Drosophila patched* gene that encodes a transmembrane receptor for an extracellular ligand (Hedgehog). This pathway controls the fate of cells, body patterning, and growth by forming gradients in embryonic tissues. The most important management feature to note is that such patients should avoid therapeutic radiation as this induces further tumours.

Renal cancer and syndromes

Mutations in several genes have been demonstrated to predispose to renal cell carcinoma. These include the *VHL* gene (associated with von Hippel–Lindau syndrome), *FOLLICULIN* (associated with Birt–Hogg–Dubbe syndrome), *FH* (associated with leiomyomas), the succinate dehydrogenase genes, and rare reports of disruption of the *TRC8* gene (by a translocation).Translocations involving chromosome 3 have also been found constitutionally in renal cancer cases. Hereditary papillary renal cell carcinoma has been related to mutations in several genes, particularly the oncogene *MET*.

Von Hippel–Lindau disease

Von Hippel–Lindau syndrome (VHL) is a dominantly inherited familial cancer syndrome predisposing to a variety of malignant and benign neoplasms, most frequently retinal angioid streaks, cerebellar and spinal hemangioblastomas, renal cell carcinoma, phaeochromocytoma, and pancreatic tumours. There are numerous liver, pancreatic, and renal cysts which can be seen on imaging. The incidence in the United Kingdom is 1 in 36 000, with near complete penetrance by 70 years. There are two types, VHL type 1 and type 2 (without and with phaeochromocytoma respectively; type 2 is divided into three further types A–C depending on the combinations of associated features). The *VHL* gene at 3p25–p26 contains three exons that encode a 213-amino-acid protein. There is a genotype–phenotype correlation with missense mutations more often associated with phaeochromocytoma. The VHL protein plays a role in the transduction of growth signals generated by changes in oxygen tension, promoting the translation of target genes that include vascular endothelial growth factor. *VHL* is a classical tumour suppressor gene, with a second, somatic mutation required for the development of cancer. Mutations in *VHL* are common in sporadic renal clear cell carcinoma within the tumour cells only. Management of VHL patients should be in a multidisciplinary clinic as several systems need monitoring (eye, neurological, and urological). Specialist urological management is necessary as renal tumours are often multifocal, so nephron-sparing surgery is used.

Familial papillary renal cell carcinoma

Any case of the less common renal cancer type, papillary renal cell carcinoma, should be considered for genetic analysis of the *MET* oncogene (on chromosome 7q31) which predisposes to familial papillary renal cancer. It codes for a transmembrane tyrosine kinase receptor for hepatocyte growth factor or scatter factor, a peptide with essential roles in embryogenesis, cell motility, and tumour invasion. Germline *MET* missense mutations in cysteine residues, homologous to those involved in aberrant dimerization and activation of the RET receptor, are associated with familial papillary renal cell carcinoma. Monoallelic activating mutations in *MET* are also found in 15% of cases of the sporadic form of the disease. The spectrum of mutations found in sporadic papillary renal cell carcinoma is wider and includes activating mutations in the MET tyrosine kinase domain. Rarely other loci may be associated with papillary renal cancer, but *MET* is the gene to be most considered.

Birt–Hogg–Dubbe syndrome

This syndrome is a rare inherited genodermatosis characterized by hair follicle hamartomas, kidney tumours (usually a renal oncocytoma or chromophobe renal cancer), and spontaneous pneumothorax; fibrofolliculomas on the face are its hallmark and trichodiscomas (tumour of the hair disc) and acrochordons ('warts with a thin neck'; skin tags) are associated features. Onset is in adulthood. It is due to mutations in the *FOLLICULIN* gene on chromosome 17p11.

Hereditary leiomyomatosis and renal cell cancer

Multiple skin and uterine leiomyomas (fibroids) associated with renal cancer are associated with mutations in *FH* (on 1q42) causing fumarate hydratase deficiency.

Wilms tumour (nephroblastoma)

Wilms tumour is a poorly differentiated tumour of the kidney, usually in childhood. It occurs in 1 in 10 000 children and accounts for 8% of childhood cancers. It is associated with aniridia, hemihypertrophy, and developmental abnormalities of the genitourinary tract (the WAGR syndrome). Males and females are equally affected and usually present early in childhood, most often with an abdominal mass. Two sites of loss of heterozygosity have been identified in Wilms tumours, *WT1* at 11p13 and *WT2* at 11p15.5. There are also rare familial cases in which linkage to neither 11p locus has been established (referred to as the *WT3* group). In 10 to 30% of patients, the disease is bilateral or multifocal, but less than 1% of all cases are truly familial. Most cases of bilateral nephroblastoma are due to new germ-line mutations in *WT1*. The protein encoded by the *WT1* gene is a 'zinc finger' DNA-binding transcription factor. WT1 interacts with another tumour suppressor, TP53, to bind and suppress transcription from the epidermal growth factor receptor and insulin-like growth factor 2 gene promoters. When WT1 function is compromised, transcription from these growth- and survival-promoting proteins is increased, initiating tumour development. *WT1* is not, however, a strictly Knudson-type tumour suppressor. Statistical analysis of age at diagnosis and proportion of bilateral and unilateral tumours does not follow the pattern described for retinoblastoma. Furthermore, the children of patients who survive Wilms tumour are at lower risk of the disease than would be expected from a dominant-acting tumour suppressor gene. There is evidence that 'genomic imprinting' may explain some of these anomalies. Imprinting is a process of gene inactivation through DNA methylation that preferentially favours expression from genes inherited from one or other parental lineage. There is a recent report in some Wilms tumour cases of genetic alteration of a methylation centre in the genome, which is an example of a germ-line change that has epigenetic effects.

Chromosome fragility syndromes

All these syndromes are autosomal recessive and they cause other abnormalities of phenotype, such as short stature, autoimmune and immunodeficiency disease, and other features. Although they are very rare they are important as such patients are sensitive to DNA-damaging agents, which is an important consideration when treating the associated cancers with such agents.

Ataxia telangiectasia

This is a rare recessive condition (1 in 30 000–100 000). Ataxia telangiectasia patients who are homozygous for *ATM* mutations have telangiectases in the eye, progressive ataxia due to cerebellar degeneration, general neuromotor dysfunction, and immune defects. There is a 30 to 40% lifetime risk of malignancy including epithelial tumours, chronic T-cell leukaemia, and lymphoma. *ATM* heterozygotes do not exhibit any of these defects, but have a two- to threefold increase in the risk of cancer, particularly female breast cancer. The *ATM* gene (11q22) encodes a 350-kDa protein which contains a domain sharing homology with members of the phosphatidylinositol-3-kinase family and which is a signal transduction protein that regulates cell cycle checkpoints.

Bloom's syndrome

This a rare autosomal recessive disease of unknown incidence, more common in Ashkenazi Jews. Features include short stature, sensitivity to the sun, skeletal abnormalities (a bird-like face), and susceptibility to infection. An increased frequency of malignant neoplasms occurs throughout life, with dramatically reduced life expectancy; it is very rare to live into the 30s. Lymphoma and leukaemia predominate before the age of 25 years; those that survive into their 20s and 30s are prone to a variety of common solid tumours, particularly squamous cell carcinoma of the head and neck, breast cancer, and gastrointestinal tumours. The age at diagnosis for these carcinomas is usually 20 years earlier than in the general population. The gene responsible, *BLM* (15q26), is a RecQ DNA helicase, and mutations result in genetic instability with spontaneous chromosomal abnormalities and increased sensitivity to radio- and/or chemotherapeutic agents. Treatments therefore have to be appropriately tailored. Males are infertile because of a defect in meiosis.

Werner's syndrome

Werner syndrome is recessive and is characterized by a scleroderma-like, multisystem premature ageing phenotype which is also due to a RecQ helicase defect. It is associated with atherosclerosis and diabetes mellitus and short stature. The incidence is 1 in 50 000 to 100 000. Affected individuals have an excess of neoplasms (especially osteosarcoma, meningioma, and thyroid cancer). Mutation in the *RECQL2* gene (8p12) leads to genetic instability.

Rothmund–Thomson syndrome

This is a hereditary dermatosis characterized by atrophy, poikiloderma (marbleized pigmentation), and telangiectasia and frequently accompanied by juvenile cataract, saddle nose, congenital bone defects, disturbances of hair growth, short stature, and hypogonadism. Classical features are absent radii and a rudimentary/absent thumb. Survival is fairly good and can be into the 40s. This is a recessive cancer predisposition syndrome, due a defect in a different helicase (gene *RECQ4* at 8q24). There is a predisposition to malignancy, especially osteosarcomas and skin tumours.

Fanconi anaemia

Fanconi anaemia is a collection of recessive diseases characterized by a complex variety of developmental abnormalities, progressive marrow failure, and predisposition to acute myeloid leukaemia (15 000 times that of the general population). Fanconi anaemia commonly presents in early to middle childhood with anaemia and bruising. Progressive pancytopenia and chromosome breakage, worsened by exposure to alkylating agents, is characteristic. Fanconi anaemia homozygotes may develop a wide range of common cancers occurring at an early age. Squamous cell carcinomas, especially of the head and neck, oesophagus, cervix, vulva, and anus, occur with increased frequency, as do liver adenomas. Life expectancy is poor, around 12 years, with most deaths resulting from marrow failure and cancer. Approximately one-fifth of childhood aplastic anaemia is associated with Fanconi anaemia and treatment is bone marrow transplantation. Treatment using radiation and chemotherapy for the transplant has to be carefully given (reduced doses of conditioning are used as the cells are sensitive to DNA damaging agents). The heterozygote frequency is estimated to be 1 in 300 to 600; the frequency is greater in Ashkenazi Jews. Fanconi anaemia homozygous cells form abnormal chromosomes when exposed to cross-linking agents such as mitomycin C which is one of the diagnostic tests for the condition. Spontaneous chromosome aberrations are seen in a variety of cell types. There are several complementation groups and two of them are due to genes which also predispose to breast cancer in heterozygotes (*BRCA2* and *BRIP1*). The other groups do not appear to have an increased malignancy in heterozygotes.

Xeroderma pigmentosum

This is a group of rare autosomal recessive disorders, with an incidence of 1 in 1 000 000. The classical feature is photosensitivity, which starts in childhood, and freckling and telangiectasia leading to progressive degenerative skin changes and early development of cancers of the skin (squamous, basal cell, and melanoma) and eye. Fifty per cent of these children have a skin cancer by age 14 years. About 20% have concurrent neurological abnormalities and some have impaired immune systems. There is also an increased risk of solid and haematological tumours. Benign neoplasms include conjunctival papillomas, actinic keratoses, lid epitheliomas, keratoacanthomas, angiomas, and fibromas. Defects of several enzymes involved in excision repair of ultraviolet-induced pyrimidine dimers are responsible for this syndrome. There are several complementation groups which differ in their action in this process (damage recognition, nuclease function, DNA polymerase function).

Identification and management of known or suspected cancer predisposition gene mutation carriers

Cancer genetic counselling

This involves assessment of cancer risk, discussion of screening and management options, and the offer of genetic testing if appropriate.

Risk assessment

This can be complex; it involves a risk estimate and this information has to be communicated to the patient in the manner most appropriate to the individual concerned so that they can understand and retain the information but are not made inappropriately anxious about their risks.

The first risk estimation is the chance that a familial cluster is due to genetic predisposition (the 'prior probability' of a genetic predisposition gene being present in a family). An extensive family history is important to determine this, often out to third-degree relatives. Confirmation of diagnoses is important for some sites (e.g. abdominal tumours) as these can be misreported in families in about 17% of cases. The risk estimation is based upon published data or clinical experiences when published data are lacking, which unfortunately is often the case with rare genetic conditions. For example, for breast cancer clusters estimates can be made using data such as those shown in Fig. 6.3.1. There are also now computerized models for some common cancers which can aid prediction of the presence of a genetic mutation, such as the BOADICEA model for the chance of a *BRCA1/2* mutation.

The second risk estimation is the chance that the individual has inherited a particular gene based upon their cancer status (affected or unaffected), their position in the family tree, and their age. This is termed the 'posterior probability'.

The final calculation is the chance that cancer will develop, which is the posterior probability multiplied by the penetrance. The expression of this risk can be delivered in a number of formats: the optimal format is unknown. Currently, risk estimates tend to be given as a percentage risk or a '1 in X' value and followed up with a written summary, incorporating this risk estimate, to the individual attending the genetics consultation. There are data which suggest that individuals prefer not to have, or do not remember, numerical information, but are able to report the qualitative category of their risk (low, medium, high) with reasonable accuracy.

Identification of an at-risk family

A family at genetic risk of cancer must first be identified. This is usually via the general practitioner (family doctor) or a hospital oncology clinic; it is now becoming more common for family history to be requested by cancer geneticists working as part of the multidisciplinary team coordinating the patient's care. Because of the limited time available during most consultations, it is not appropriate to obtain a detailed family history from the patient. As a quick guideline, taking a history of all first-degree relatives only (parents, siblings, and children) and then asking if there are any other cancers in the family will detect 95% of familial syndromes. From this quick family history it should, however, be possible to make an assessment of whether the family history warrants further investigation. Referral guidelines have been developed; for example in the United Kingdom, there are national guidelines for familial breast cancer (http://www.nice.org.uk). These guidelines aim to delineate the management and referral pathway according to the Kenilworth model (http://www.macmillan.org.uk) whereby individuals whose risk does not exceed that of the general population are managed in the primary care setting, individuals at moderate risk are managed in secondary care, and individuals at high risk are managed in tertiary care in cancer genetics centres. In the cancer genetics clinic, after a full family history, initial clinical examination involves looking for any dysmorphic features and congenital anomalies. The skin should be carefully examined, as many cancer syndromes are associated with dermatological features, as noted above.

Throughout the consultation, it is important to be sensitive to any issues relating to bereavement due to the premature death of close relatives, particularly a parent or child. Unresolved bereavement may make it difficult for people to accept their own risks and make decisions about their own management. Some individuals are particularly worried when they are approaching the age at which their relatives were diagnosed. Others erroneously assume that they are more likely to have inherited the cancer predisposition gene because they resemble their affected relative, either physically or in temperament. Patients are sometimes unable to cope with their concerns, and referral for formal psychological counselling may be needed. Of particular concern are those individuals who have prophylactic surgery because of excess anxiety but who, while being temporarily relieved, could return at a later date with further cancer phobic symptoms. A psychological assessment and counselling should be part of the referral process before prophylactic mastectomy.

Clinical management

The subsequent management of an individual and their family will depend upon the final risk estimates regarding the inheritance of a cancer predisposition gene and the potential cancer risks. In general, management strategies fall into five categories, cancer screening, lifestyle changes, prevention strategies, cancer treatment considerations and genetic testing.

Cancer screening

Not all of the screening schedules have been proven to reduce mortality from the relevant cancer, but these schedules represent a pragmatic approach to the management of individuals at increased risk. There is, however, some evidence that screening individuals with HNPCC by colonoscopy reduces mortality due to colorectal cancer, as any suspicious polyps observed on colonoscopy may be removed at an early stage. The guidelines promulgated by the United Kingdom National Institute for Health and Clinical Excellence (NICE) mentioned above have made recommendations for mammographic and MRI screening in certain groups at risk of familial breast cancer. Prostate and ovarian cancer screening are contentious and are currently subjects of research.

Lifestyle changes

Lifestyle changes may involve avoidance of known cancer causing factors such as sunlight in Gorlin's syndrome and X-ray exposure in the Li–Fraumeni syndrome. Other lifestyle changes are less well established in the prevention of cancer and are being assessed in trials.

Prevention strategies

Primary prevention strategies include prophylactic surgery and chemoprevention. The evidence in support of the efficacy of these measures is variable, mainly due to the rarity of the genetic mutations making clinical trials difficult to perform. Established measures include total colectomy in the familial adenomatous polyposis syndrome, total thyroidectomy in the MEN2 syndrome, and bilateral salpingo-oophorectomy in women with *BRCA1/2* mutations. Limited retrospective data suggest that the risk of breast cancer is reduced by 90% following prophylactic mastectomy although there is still a small residual risk (about 1.5%) due to the inability to remove all breast epithelial tissues at mastectomy.

The role of chemoprevention is much less certain. In meta-analyses tamoxifen reduces breast cancer risk by at least 33%, but it should be noted that the type of tumour prevented is hormone receptor-positive, and this has a better prognosis. The oral contraceptive pill reduces ovarian cancer risk by about one-third in those on the pill for 2 years. Recent data report a reduction in colon cancer risk in HNPCC families in individuals who have taken aspirin after 5 years.

Cancer treatment

Data are emerging which report a difference in prognosis when certain genetic changes are present in the germ line; e.g. ovarian cancer due to mutations in *BRCA1/2* has a better prognosis and a higher response to platinum-based chemotherapeutic agents. Certain syndromes are associated with altered response to treatment, e.g. colonic tumours which have microsatellite instability are less responsive to 5-fluorouracil. Agents are now being developed which specifically target tumours with certain genetic defects, e.g. the PARP inhibitors, which enforce the cancer cell to use the homologous recombinant DNA repair pathway which is deficient in *BRCA1/2*-null cells, have resulted in promising early response rates in tumours in patients with germ-line *BRCA1/2* mutations.

Genetic testing

Genetic testing is possible for most cancer predisposition genes and is performed on DNA from venous blood after genetic counselling. Genetic testing may either be diagnostic (the detection of a mutation in an individual affected by cancer) or predictive (the detection of a mutation in a clinically unaffected individual). Mutations in cancer predisposition genes often occur throughout the gene and the vast majority of mutations so far have only been observed in limited numbers of families, except in specific ethnic groups with known founder mutations such as the Icelandic and Ashkenazi populations with *BRCA*1/2 mutations. Hence, unless an individual is a member of such a group, the specific mutation for that family must first be identified. An affected family member is tested first because they are the family member most likely to have the cancer-predisposing mutation. Once a mutation is identified, it is important to check that the 'mutation' is likely to be cancer causing and not a normal variant of the gene (polymorphism). When a pathogenic mutation is identified, predictive testing may be offered to unaffected family members for the identified mutation.

Misleading results may occur if an unaffected individual has a genetic test in order to identify a mutation without first identifying it in an affected relative. A negative result (i.e. no mutation is identified in the cancer predisposition gene tested) may not be a true negative for several reasons:

- The family history is caused by a gene other than the one being tested or may not be genetic at all.
- The alteration may be regulatory which means that it controls how the gene is expressed but the gene itself (and therefore the test which looks at the gene code) is normal.
- The genetic test sensitivity is not 100% for the genetic coding mutations and may therefore have missed mutations.

When the specific mutation has been identified in an affected individual, if it is not found in an unaffected relative, this is then a truly negative result. The personal and wider social implications of positive and negative results are issues discussed during genetic counselling sessions. A positive result could have psychological implications as well as widespread repercussions involving the rest of the family. A negative test result may have psychological consequences due to the recognized 'survivor guilt syndrome', which has been documented in the setting of Huntington's disease.

There is a moratorium on the use of some genetic information in the United Kingdom, as detailed on the Association of British Insurers' website http://www.abi.org.uk.

For genes predisposing to adult-onset cancers, testing of young children is not advised as the age of cancer onset permits the individual to make their own decision to have genetic testing once they have reached adulthood, following full genetic counselling. Children are offered genetic testing when it may alter management, for example, in the MEN2A syndrome when thyroidectomy is offered before age 5, in retinoblastoma to avoid unnecessary eye examinations, or in FAP where regular colonoscopies or colectomy may be avoided.

Recently genetic testing has been licensed for preimplantation genetic diagnosis for certain cases of hereditary cancer.

The future

Cancer is a common disease and only a proportion of cases will be due to the inheritance of mutations in specific genes that predispose to cancer. However, because cancer occurs with high frequency in the population, this represents a large number of individuals. The developments of more rapid genome sequencing will enable cancer genetics to become part of cancer care as more targeted treatments are developed for such individuals and targeted screening is undertaken in their relatives.

Further reading

Bodmer WF, *et al.* (1987). Localization of the gene for familial adenomatous polyposis on chromosome 5. *Nature*, **328**, 614–16.

Claus EB, Risch N, Thompson WD (1991). *Am J Hum Genet*, **48**, 232–42.

Easton DF, Peto J (1990). The contribution of inherited predisposition to cancer incidence. *Cancer Surv*, **9**, 395–416.

Easton DF, Eeles RA (2008). *Hum Mol Genet*, **17**(R2), R109–15.

Eeles RA, *et al.* (eds) (2004). *Genetic predisposition to cancer*. Arnold, London.

Ford D, *et al.* (1998). Genetic heterogeneity and penetrance analysis of the *BRCA1* and *BRCA2* genes in breast cancer families. The Breast Cancer Linkage Consortium. *Am J Hum Genet*, **62**, 676–89.

Foulkes WD (2008). Inherited susceptibility to common cancers. *N Engl J Med*, **359**, 2143–53.

Miki Y, *et al.* (1994). Isolation of *BRCA1*, the 17q-linked breast and ovarian cancer susceptibility gene. *Science*, **266**, 66–71.

Leach FS, *et al.* (1993). Mutations of a mutS homolog in hereditary nonpolyposis colorectal cancer. *Cell*, **75**, 1215–25.

Lynch HT, Lynch JF (1994). 25 years of HNPCC. *Anticancer Res*, **14**, 1617–24.

Nicolaides NC, *et al.* (1994). Mutations of two PMS homologues in herditary nonpolyposis colon cancer. *Nature*, **371**, 75–80.

Papadopoulos N, *et al.* (1994). Mutation of a mutL homolog in hereditary colon cancer. *Science*, **263**, 1625–9.

Wooster R, *et al.* (1995). Identification of the breast cancer susceptibility gene, *BRCA2*. *Nature*, **378**, 789–792.

Websites

Association of British Insurers. http://www.abi.org.uk

Genetic Interest Group. http://www.gig.org.uk

Online Mendelian Inheritance in Man (OMIM). http://www.ncbi.nlm.nih.gov/sites/OMIM

BOADICEA. http://www.srl.cam.ac.uk/genepi/boadicea/boadicea_home.html

6.4

Cancer immunity and clinical oncology

Maries van den Broek, Lotta von Boehmer, Kunle Odunsi, and Alexander Knuth

Essentials

Patients develop immune-mediated defence mechanisms against cancers, which are referred to as the 'three E's': (1) elimination—corresponding to immunological control of the tumour or immunosurveillance; (2) equilibrium—the process by which the immune response iteratively selects/promotes less immunogenic tumour variants; and (3) escape—when the immunologically sculptured tumour expands in an uncontrolled manner.

Human cancer antigens

These represent proteins that are uniquely (over)expressed in malignant tissues and function as target for immunotherapy. They can be divided in following categories: (1) cancer–testis (CT) antigens—silent in healthy tissues, except germ cells, but expressed in various cancer types (e.g. NY-ESO-1, which is probably the most immunogenic CT antigen known); (2) differentiation antigens of certain cell types, such as melanocytes or breast cell epithelia; (3) unique tumour-specific antigens that are the products of genetic alterations; (4) virus-encoded antigens in virus-associated cancers; (5) ubiquitous antigens that are overexpressed in tumours.

Cancer immunotherapy

Antigen-specific immunotherapy in cancer patients focuses either on (1) T-cell-mediated approaches or on (2) antibodies. T cells are generally directed against endogenous tumour-derived proteins that are processed and presented in the context of major histocompatibility complex molecules, whereas antibodies are directed at molecular targets expressed at the cancer cell surface.

Monoclonal antibodies—these are now established and integrated in many treatment regimens in cancer medicine, e.g. rituximab (targeting CD20) in non-Hodgkin's lymphoma and trastuzumab (targeting Erb2/HER2) in breast cancer).

Cancer vaccination—the keys to efficient vaccination are (1) availability of an immunogenic, tumour-associated antigen; (2) a route, schedule, and packaging of the antigen that will induce an optimal immune response *in vivo*; (3) the combination of antigen with an adjuvant to support the induction of a strong immune response *in vivo*; (4) sustained immunity; and (5) inhibition of regulatory pathways, such as CTLA-4, PD-1, and Tregs.

At this early stage of development, cancer immunotherapy should be offered only in the context of carefully monitored clinical trials conducted by experienced clinical research teams.

Introduction

The importance of the immune system in the control and defence of cancer is no longer in question. The origins of the field of cancer immunotherapy can be traced back to William Coley who, in the 1890s, observed that potentially fatal bacterial infections could induce an effective antitumour response in patients with partially resected tumours. Enthusiasm for this approach has waxed and waned over the last several decades. It is now well known that the immune system has the ability to recognize tumour-associated antigens (TAA) displayed on human malignancies and to direct cytotoxic responses to these targets. While the discovery of treatment modalities such as radiotherapy and chemotherapy focused the interest of the scientific community for decades, recent improved understanding of the molecular basis of immune recognition has revived the interest in cancer immunotherapy. In this chapter, we discuss the principles of tumour immunity, the tumour antigens that can be recognized by the immune system, cancer immunotherapy strategies, and selected clinical trials of immunotherapy.

The vertebrate immune system

The vertebrate immune system has evolved to combat pathogens that continuously threaten the integrity of the host. A wide variety of innate or natural resistance mechanisms have coevolved with adaptive immunity in vertebrates. The major function of these complex and efficient defence systems is to protect the host against deleterious infections with pathogens, such as bacteria, fungi, viruses, or parasites. This requires that the immune system discriminates between pathogens and self-antigens while precisely recognizing a vast array of antigens.

Within hours after an infection, the innate resistance system is activated. This evolutionary ancient defence system functions by pattern recognition, which is not target specific. It rapidly discriminates self and nonself, which leads to immediate inhibition of replication and spread of pathogens and gives the adaptive immune response time to develop. The innate response is composed of soluble and cellular effector mechanisms, such as the complement system, interferons, acute phase reactants, granulocytes, macrophages, and natural killer (NK) cells.

The adaptive immune response can be divided into either humoral (antibody) responses or cell-mediated (T-cell) responses. Antibodies recognize and bind to conformational determinants on soluble or cell surface proteins, and can kill the cell by either antibody-dependent cellular cytotoxicity (ADCC) or complement-mediated cell lysis. Antibodies alone, or in combination with chemotherapy, can be highly effective in mediating tumour regression in haematological malignancies, and have progressively also been introduced into clinical practice for the treatment of solid tumours. Conversely, T cells recognize antigenic peptides presented on the cell surface in the context of major histocompatibility (MHC) antigens with their T cell receptor (TCR). The TCR consists of an α and a β chain with constant and (hyper)variable regions, the latter interacting with the antigen MHC complex. Each T cell has only one type of antigen receptor, and is of single specificity. Theoretically, the T-cell repertoire can consist of more than 10^{10} different antigen receptors. However, the actual repertoire is considerably smaller, because most recombinations are not productive or because some will result in receptors that recognize self-antigens and are usually deleted. Interaction of thymocytes through their TCR with self-MHC molecules in the thymic medulla is a survival signal for these thymocytes: they will be positively selected and are MHC-restricted as a result. Most autoreactive T cells are deleted in the thymus by a process called negative selection, which takes place in the medulla and is thought to be mediated by macrophages and dendritic cells (DC) presenting self-antigens to immature thymocytes. However, some antigens may be absent from the thymus, especially those that are expressed only in peripheral tissues or those that are only present during certain periods of life (e.g. proteins involved in lactation). There is now evidence that many tissue-specific proteins are expressed ectopically in the thymus, and that AIRE, a thymus-specific transcription factor, may regulate this ectopic expression. However, as it is unlikely that all peripheral proteins are present in the thymus in sufficient quantities to mediate negative selection, there is an apparent need for induction and maintenance of peripheral T-cell tolerance in order to avoid autoimmunity (see below).

The activation of mature T cells is a complex process that requires a minimum of two signals. The first signal is mediated by the interaction of the TCR, expressed on T lymphocytes, with a specific antigenic peptide that has been processed by and presented on the surface of a professional antigen-presenting cell (APC) bound to an MHC molecule. Intracellular signalling, resulting in cellular proliferation, is then conveyed through an intracellular portion of the CD3 complex, which is associated with the TCR. The second costimulatory signal is also delivered by APCs through members of the B7 family of surface molecules that bind to their targets expressed on T cells. APCs also secrete critical cytokines such as interleukins IL-12 and IL-15 that contribute to T cell activation and memory. In the absence of costimulation, T cells may enter a state of nonresponsiveness or anergy.

Lafferty and coworkers first demonstrated the requirement for specialized stimulator cells for T-cell activation in a series of classical experiments, in which they observed that the rejection of histoincompatible organ grafts is dependent on donor leucocytes trapped in the graft. Based on their ability to express MHC class II and costimulatory molecules and to take up antigens, B cells, macrophages and dendritic cells are thought to have the capacity to stimulate naive T cells. During the past 10 years, however, a large body of evidence has accumulated suggesting that dendritic cells are the only cells fulfilling all criteria of an APC.

In the 1990s, Charles Janeway proposed that the induction of adaptive immunity depends on a distinct, innate recognition event involving primitive receptors, termed pathogen recognition receptors (PRRs). These receptors bind conserved microbial structures, the so-called pathogen-associated molecular patterns (PAMPs). Macrophages, dendritic cells, mast cells, neutrophils, eosinophils, and NK cells express different PRRs. A major class of PRRs consists of the Toll-like receptors (TLRs). In mammals at least 10 members of the TLR family have been described to date. TLRs specifically recognize microbial components, such as lipopolysaccharide (LPS), unmethylated CpG motifs, bacterial peptidoglycans, double-stranded (ds) RNA that naturally occurs during the replication of some viruses, flagellin, and many more. In addition to direct recognition of pathogens by receptors on the dendritic cell or inside the dendritic cell, indirect means of dendritic cell activation by pathogens have been described: dendritic cell maturation is induced in response to inflammatory mediators such as tumour necrosis factor α (TNFα), IL-1β, or prostaglandin E2 (PGE2) that are secreted in response to infections or by ligation of surface CD40 by activated CD4+ T cells (T-cell help).

The molecular understanding of PRRs has led to a better appreciation of adjuvants in cancer immunotherapy. A classic example is William B Coley's observation from the New York Hospital that some patients with sarcomas had spontaneous tumour regressions following a superficial streptococcal skin infection. Seeking to harness the power of the immune system, Coley deliberately infected some of his inoperable patients with erysipelas to stimulate tumour regression. He later refined this approach by using heat-killed *Streptococcus pyogenes* in combination with heat-killed *Serratia marcescens*—a mixture that is now commonly known as 'Coley's toxin'. Administration of Coley's toxin to patients with soft-tissue sarcomas resulted in response rates over 50%. Today, it is recognized that the induction of an efficient and protective immune response depends on the interaction between naive antigen-specific T cells and mature dendritic cells. Upon maturation dendritic cells have reduced capacity for antigen uptake, but change their pattern of homing receptors (e.g. up-regulation of CCR7), which allows them to migrate into the T cell areas of secondary lymphoid organs, and up-regulate costimulatory molecules. These changes are crucial for efficient priming of naive antigen-specific T cells.

Cancer immunosurveillance

During the last decade, there has been a re-emergence of interest in the concept of cancer immunosurveillance (Fig. 6.4.1). This concept,

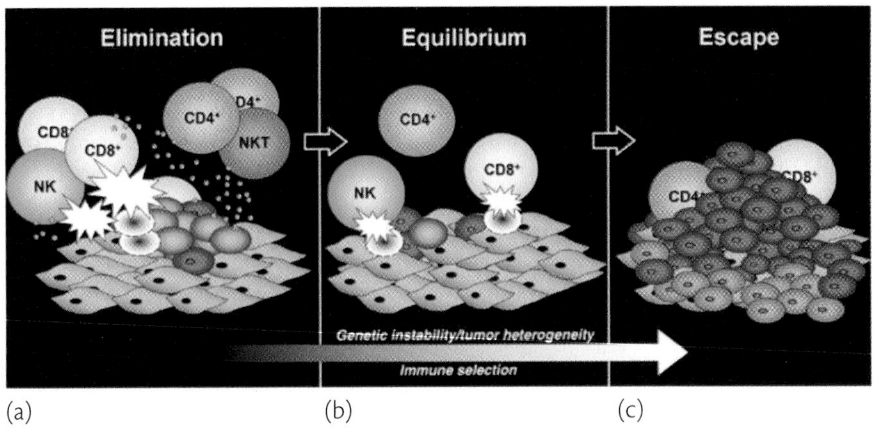

Fig. 6.4.1 The 'three Es'. Cancer immunoediting encompasses three processes. (a) Elimination corresponds to immunosurveillance. (b) Equilibrium represents the process by which the immune system iteratively selects and/or promotes the generation of tumour cell variants with increasing capacities to survive immune attack. (c) Escape is the process in which the immunologically sculpted tumour expands in an uncontrolled manner in the immunocompetent host. In a and b, developing tumour cells (blue), tumor cell variants (red) and underlying stroma and nontransformed cells (gray) are shown; in c, additional tumor variants (orange) that have formed as a result of the equilibrium process are shown. Different lymphocyte populations are as marked. The small orange circles represent cytokines and the white flashes represent cytotoxic activity of lymphocytes against tumour cells.

which was first put forward by Burnet, Thomas, and Medawar, is supported by several lines of evidence derived from murine tumour models as described by Schreiber, Smythe, and Old, and holds that the immune system not only protects the host against development of primary cancers but also sculpts tumour immunogenicity, a process referred to as immunoediting. Immunoediting is thought to consist of three phases: elimination, equilibrium, and escape. Elimination represents the classical concept of cancer immunosurveillance; equilibrium is the period of immune-mediated latency after incomplete tumour destruction in the elimination phase; and escape refers to the final outgrowth of tumours that have outstripped immunological restraints of the equilibrium phase. The elimination and equilibrium phases are accomplished via lymphocytes of both the adaptive and innate immune compartments including $\gamma\delta$T cells, $\alpha\beta$T cells, and natural killer T (NKT) cells. Tumours escape destruction by the immune system via a variety of active, regulatory mechanisms. These include down-regulation of MHC and tumour antigen loss, stimulation of the inhibitory receptor CTLA-4 on T-cells, tumour overproduction of indoleamine 2,3-dioxygenase (IDO), induction of increased tumour infiltration by regulatory CD4+CD25+ Fox P3+T cells (Tregs) and also certain types of NKT cells that inhibit tumour immune destruction.

Recent correlative human studies also support the concept of cancer immunoediting because of observations that tumour infiltration by lymphocytes is a reflection of a tumour-related immune response. Data from these studies indicate that the presence of tumour-infiltrating lymphocytes (TILs) may be associated with improved clinical outcome in several cancers including melanoma, colorectal, breast, prostate, renal cell, oesophageal, and ovarian carcinomas. In particular, recent data in epithelial ovarian cancer indicate significant differences in the distributions of progression-free survival and overall survival according to the presence or absence of intratumoral T cells. The 5-year overall survival rate was 38.0% among patients whose tumours contained T cells and 4.5% among patients whose tumours contained no T cells in islets. In addition, ovarian cancer patients whose tumours are infiltrated by CD4+CD25+FoxP3+ Tregs demonstrated reduced survival. In light of these considerations, clinical trials of cancer immunotherapy have attempted to activate the immune system in an effort to elicit effective antitumour responses.

The reasons why immune surveillance may fail in cancer patients are manifold. One possibility is escape, where the tumour down-regulates the presentation of target antigen/MHC or where antigen/MHC^{low} tumour cells preferentially grow out. A second possibility is inefficient migration of tumour-specific T cells into the tumour due to defective expression of lymphocyte homing receptors on the vascular endothelium of tumours. Finally, the tumour itself often provides an immunosuppressive environment such that effector cells become functionally impaired after tumour infiltration. The reason for this local unresponsiveness is not known at present and may be different in individual patients. These issues have been addressed in several studies. Some of the possibilities identified include production of cytokines by tumour cells or by the stroma that suppress dendritic cells through STAT3 signalling, or the conditioning of dendritic cells to support the development of FoxP3+ Tregs. There is evidence that Tregs mediate their suppressive activity by the production of TGFβ. Recently, tumour-infiltrating $\gamma\delta$ T cells were identified as a subset responsible for the suppressive environment within the tumour and their mode of action was found to be directed to T cells and to dendritic cells. It is clear that the major obstacles in developing effective cancer immunotherapies include: (1) the identification of targets with tissue-restricted expression and immunogenic potential, (2) development of strategies to induce an immune response sufficient to eradicate tumour or prevent relapse of disease, and (3) development of approaches to overcome the multiple mechanisms by which tumours evade the host immune response.

Tumour antigens

The era of modern cancer immunology started with observations made in two patients (SK-29 and MZ-2) with recurrent metastatic melanoma, who have been observed since 1978 and 1982 respectively. Both patients received intradermal immunizations with irradiated autologous tumour cells for an extended period of time, and complete regression of tumour manifestations in the presence of T-cell responses and strong, increasing T-cell responses under vaccination was documented. The patients have remained free of disease ever since, and are still alive after almost 30 years. On the basis of this favourable clinical effect, a systematic search was initiated to identify and characterize the cancer antigens and immune effector mechanisms that mediate tumour regression and tumour control *in vivo*. Thierry Boon and colleagues cloned the first T-cell defined human cancer antigens from these patients in 1991: MAGE-1, tyrosinase, and Melan-A. Since the initial reports by Boon *et al.*, a large number of tumour-associated antigens have been identified, many of which spontaneously induce humoral and/or cellular immune responses in cancer patients. Some antigens were identified by serological analysis of recombinant cDNA expression libraries (SEREX), others by differential gene expression analysis, T-cell epitope cloning (TEPIC), and bioinformatics. Nowadays, tumour-associated antigens are classified into one of the following categories:

- cancer–testis (CT) antigens, restricted expression in germ cells and cancer cells, e.g. MAGE, NY-ESO-1, and LAGE-1
- differentiation antigens, restricted to defined lineages like melanocytes, e.g. tyrosinase, Melan-A/MART-1, and gp 100
- mutated antigens, altered forms of constitutive proteins, e.g. CDK4, β-catenin, caspase-8, and p53
- amplification antigens, e.g. overexpressed Her2/neu and p53
- splice variant antigens, e.g. NY-CO-37/PDZ-45 and ING1
- glycolipid antigens
- viral antigens, e.g. HPV, EBV

Among the tumour antigens identified to date, the CT antigens are a distinct and unique class of differentiation antigens. The genes encoding CT antigens are frequently located on the X-chromosome and are often members of multigene families. CT antigens are not expressed in healthy tissues, except germ cells, but are expressed by a proportion of different tumour types in a lineage-nonspecific fashion. Often, a particular tumour expresses more than one CT antigen. The frequency of CT antigen expression in many cancer types ranges from 5 to 40%, with exceptionally high expression of individual CT antigens in certain cancers, e.g. MAGE-C1/CT7 in 70% of myeloma and NY-ESO-1 in 80% of synovial sarcoma. The function of CT antigens in germ cells and in malignant cells is unknown. How their expression is regulated is also unknown at present, but recent evidence suggests that epigenetic events including DNA demethylation and histone deacetylation play a role. Some well-characterized members of the CT antigen family include MAGE, GAGE/PAGE/XAGE, NY-ESO-1/LAGE-1, SSX, SPANX, TRAG-3, BAGE, SCP-1, OY-TES-1, and CT10.

The expression and immunogenicity of NY-ESO-1, a CT antigen initially defined by SEREX in oesophageal cancer, have been analysed extensively in various types of cancer and the findings illustrate several aspects of human tumour immunology. NY-ESO-1 is expressed at a variable frequency in several tumours (Fig. 6.4.2).

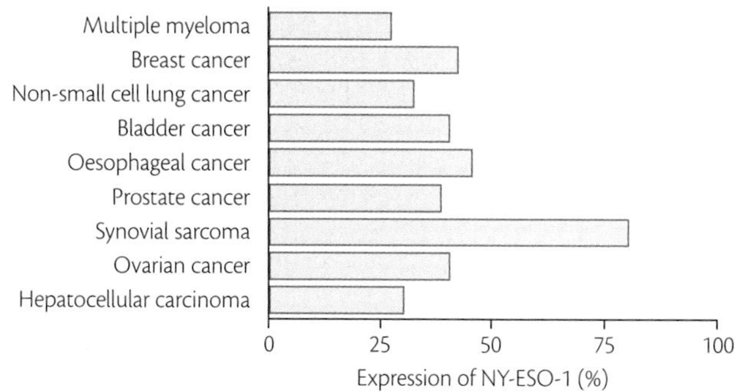

Fig. 6.4.2 Expression of NY-ESO-1 in different malignancies. NY-ESO-1 elicits both cellular and humoral immune responses in a high proportion of patients with advanced NY-ESO-1-expressing tumours. Several NY-ESO-1 MHC class I and II restricted epitopes (recognized by CD8+ cytotoxic and CD4+ helper and T cells, respectively) have been characterized, including those recognized in conjunction with HLA-A2, A24, B35, DR4, and DP4, and additional epitopes are still being characterized. These achievements are particularly important because they facilitate the monitoring of vaccine-induced immune responses in cancer patients. Correlating clinical evolution with immunomonitoring under cancer-specific vaccination strategies will eventually establish cancer immunotherapy as an additional treatment modality.

Cancer immunotherapy in clinical practice

Antigen-specific immunotherapy in cancer patients focuses either on antibodies or on T-cell mediated approaches. Targeting with antibodies generally requires the expression of molecular targets at the cancer cell surface, like peptides, proteins or lipids and glycosylated variants or sugar moieties. Since their development in the late 1970s, monoclonal antibodies have become established and integrated into many treatment regimens in cancer therapy (Table 6.4.1).

Crucial for an effective cancer vaccine is the use of an antigen that is immunogenic in cancer patients. This simple requirement, however, involves many issues that are still the subject of intense fundamental and clinical research. For instance, it is not known whether a monovalent (i.e. one antigen) or a polyvalent vaccine is better, or which form of antigen (peptide, protein, tumour lysate, recombinant attenuated pathogen that expresses tumour antigens) is most effective. Also, which adjuvants stimulate innate immunity such that a sustained and effective antitumour immune response is generated is largely unknown. The duration and frequency of vaccination, as well as the phase of disease in which the patient is vaccinated, may influence its efficacy. Importantly also, the choice of parameter to be monitored is not easy, because it is not really known which of many parameters actually correlates with clinical response. A number of current cancer vaccine strategies are summarized in Box 6.4.1, and some of the above-mentioned questions are considered in further detail below.

Adjuvants

An effective adjuvant treatment in bladder cancer is intravesical BCG (bacille Calmette–Guérin, heat-killed *Mycobacterium tuberculosis*). Multiple clinical trials have shown that BCG can give high response rates in recurrent superficial transitional cell carcinoma with significantly prolonged duration of remission. The mechanism of action of intravesical BCG is presumably the altered local cytokine production.

Unmethylated CpG (cytosine-phosphatidyl-guanosine) motifs are relatively common in bacterial genomic DNA, but not in human DNA. CpG interacts with TLR9 in the endosomal vesicles of APC, which licences the latter to activate T cells. Synthetic CpG has been used as a single agent in clinical trials in non-Hodgkin's lymphoma, non-small-cell lung cancer, melanoma, and renal cell

Table 6.4.1 Antibodies in cancer medicine

Drug	Target	Type	Type of cancer	Year of FDA Approval
Rituximab	CD20	Chimeric	Non-Hodgkin's lymphoma	1997
Trastuzumab	ErbB2/HER2	Humanized	Breast cancer	1998
Gemtuzumab ozogamicin	CD33	Humanized	Acute myeloid leukaemia	2000
Alemtuzumab	CD52	Humanized	Chronic lymphocytic leukaemia	2001
Ibritumomab tiuxetan	CD20	Murine, radiolabelled	Non-Hodgkin's lymphoma	2002
Tositumomab-131	CD20	Murine, radiolabelled	Non-Hodgkin's lymphoma	2003
Cetuximab	EGFR	Chimeric	Colorectal cancer	2004
			Head and neck cancer	2006
Bevacizumab	VEGF	Humanized	Colorectal cancer	2004
			Non-small-cell lung cancer	2006
			Advanced breast cancer	2008
Panitumumab	EGFR	Human	Colorectal cancer	2006

carcinoma with marginal success. The efficacy of the combination of tumour-associated antigen plus CpG as a strong adjuvant is further investigated in various types of cancer.

A variety of cytokines are or have been used alone or together with cancer vaccines in the clinic. Two examples are interferon-α (IFN-α) and the granulocyte–macrophage colony stimulating factor (GM-CSF). IFN-α has profound and diverse effects on gene expression: it up-regulates the MHC class I molecules, tumour antigens, and adhesion molecules. Most importantly, it promotes the activity of B cells, T cells, macrophages, and dendritic cells and increases the expression of Fcγ-receptors. INF-α is currently used for the treatment of malignant melanoma, follicular lymphoma, hairy-cell leukaemia, Philadelphia-positive chronic myelogenous leukaemia, condylomata acuminata, cutaneous T-cell lymphoma, and AIDS-related Kaposi's sarcoma. High-dose IFN-α has become a standard treatment option for adjuvant therapy in stage III melanoma patients. GM-CSF is used as an adjuvant because it may increase the number of APCs and thus enhances the ability to prime an immune response in the patient. A phase I trial comparing the cytotoxic T lymphocyte (CTL) reactivity after immunization with melanocyte differentiation antigen-derived peptides alone or with additional systemic GM-CSF as an adjuvant showed enhanced DTH reactions, CD8+ CTL responses and objective tumour regressions in patients that were treated with vaccine plus GM-CSF. The effects of GM-CSF were also tested with irradiated autologous melanoma cells engineered to secrete GM-CSF. Although only a few patients had major tumour-specific responses in classical terms, resected tumour nodules often demonstrated fibrosis and immune cell infiltrates attributed to the GM-CSF–transduced tumour cell therapy.

Box 6.4.1 Vaccine formulations

- Whole-cell or lysate cancer vaccines
- Gene-modified cancer cells
- *Ex vivo* activated lymphocytes
- Gene-modified lymphocytes
- Heat shock proteins
- Viral vectors
- Naked DNA
- Peptides
- Protein
- Dendritic cells—APCs

Peptide-based vaccines

The intracellular processing of proteins results in the generation of short peptide epitopes of 8 to 10 and 13 to 20 amino acids that bind MHC class I and class II respectively. The majority of peptides derived from tumour antigens are presented in association with MHC class I molecules and are recognized by CD8+ T cells. A smaller number of peptide epitopes have been defined for MHC class II molecules, and are recognized by CD4+ T cells. The major disadvantages of short peptides as a vaccine are the short *in vivo* half-life and the fact that they will be presented by other cells besides professional APCs, both of which result in limited immunogenicity. In addition, the use of peptides requires knowledge of the epitopes derived from the tumour-associated antigen and is often limited to patients with particular MHC alleles, such as HLA-A2. Nevertheless, phase I and II clinical studies in which melanoma patients were vaccinated with peptides plus different adjuvants showed the induction of peptide-specific CD8+ T cell responses. For example, in a recent phase I clinical trial, 12 HLA-A2+ patients with progressing NY-ESO-1-expressing metastatic tumours of different types were vaccinated intradermally with NY-ESO-1 peptides first alone and then in combination with GM-CSF as a systemic adjuvant. Five out of seven vaccinated patients, who were initially NY-ESO-1 antibody negative, developed stabilization or regression of individual metastases after induction of NY-ESO-1 specific CD8+ T-cell responses. In addition, there was disease stabilization following NY-ESO-1 immunization in three of five antibody-positive patients, indicating that vaccination may also result in clinical benefit in patients with baseline spontaneous immunity to NY-ESO-1.

Long peptides, recombinant proteins, tumour cell lysates, and DNA vaccines

In order to reduce the risk of immune escape, an immune response against a broad range of MHC class I and II epitopes is required. Vaccination with full-length antigens or (overlapping) long peptides has the potential to broaden the response and is not limited to patients with particular HLA alleles.

In a recent clinical trial evaluating the safety and immunogenicity of recombinant NY-ESO-1 protein with ISCOMATRIX adjuvant, 46 patients with resected NY-ESO-1-positive tumours received 3 doses of vaccine intramuscularly at monthly intervals. The majority of vaccinated patients demonstrated high-titre antibody responses, strong delayed-type hypersensitivity reactions, and circulating CD8+ and CD4+ T cells specific for a broad range of NY-ESO-1 epitopes, including known and previously unknown epitopes.

Autologous and allogeneic tumour cells have also been used as tumour vaccines, with mixed results. In theory, the main advantage of tumour cell vaccines is that they have all the relevant tumour antigens for the immune system to mount an effective antitumour response. In addition, tumour cell-based immunization allows the development of cancer vaccines without prior knowledge of specific antigens. However, the lack of knowledge of specific antigens responsible for anti-tumour immunity severely limits antigen-specific immunological monitoring.

Naked DNA vaccination introduces tumour antigens into dendritic cells for cross-presentation to cytotoxic T cells in draining lymph nodes. The advantages of this approach include simplicity, stability, and low cost. However, DNA vaccination has poorer efficacy than vaccination with recombinant viruses. In an attempt to improve the antitumour immune responses of DNA vaccines, several strategies have been employed including transdermal or mucosal delivery, gene-gun delivery of DNA-coated gold beads, DNA–liposome complexes, and the generation of chimeric recombinant constructs of antigen and IgG Fc, HSP 70, FLT3-L, and cholera toxin. Recombinant pathogens that express full-length tumour-associated antigens have the same advantage as recombinant proteins or long peptides, namely that they are exclusively presented by professional APCs. In addition, recombinant pathogens have natural adjuvant activity. Recombinant vaccinia virus, adenovirus, and fowlpox virus vaccines have been evaluated in preclinical models as cancer vaccines. Clinical trials with recombinant vaccinia virus vaccines expressing CEA, NY-ESO-1 or HPV E6 or E7 showed that such vaccines induce specific immune responses. Recent studies show that priming with one virus and boosting with another, the so-called prime–boost strategy, is well tolerated and is superior to priming and boosting with the same virus with respect to the induction of immune responses.

Dendritic-cell based vaccines

Dendritic cells are the most potent and efficient professional APCs and play a critical role in the initiation of the immune response through the uptake, processing, and presentation of antigens, including tumour antigens, to T cells. Dendritic cells pulsed with tumour lysates, tumour protein extracts, and synthetic peptide tumour antigen epitopes generate protective immunity to subsequent tumour challenge in mouse models. Studies of dendritic cell-based immunotherapy have been conducted in several tumour types including melanoma, colon cancer, prostate cancer, lymphoma, and multiple myeloma. All of these and other studies indeed suggest that monocyte-derived dendritic cells are capable of eliciting antigen-specific immune responses in humans, some of which have been associated with clinical responses. A major drawback of dendritic-cell based immunotherapy is the dependence on specialist preparation of cellular products, and this is likely to make the approach unavailable for widespread use.

Adoptive T-cell therapy

As cancer antigen specific T-lymphocyte expansion *ex vivo* under Good Manufacturing Practice conditions is feasible today, adoptive transfer of *in vitro* expanded effector lymphocyte populations may become an effective treatment modality. Positive results in infectious diseases have been published and early results in cancer point to a promising, yet challenging, modality in cancer therapy.

Immune intervention against virus-associated cancers

A number of human cancers are associated with viral infections. The best-characterized examples include primary hepatocellular carcinoma, which is linked to chronic infection with hepatitis B virus (HBV); anogenital carcinomas, which are associated with human papillomavirus (HPV); nasopharyngeal carcinoma, certain B-cell lymphomas and Hodgkin's disease, which are associated with the Epstein–Barr virus (EBV); and a form of adult T-cell leukaemia that is linked to human T-lymphotrophic virus (HTLV). Possible immune intervention strategies in these cancers include prevention of infection, thereby reducing the incidence of disease, or targeting the immune response against viral proteins expressed by tumour cells. Current vaccination approaches against these viruses include envelope glycoproteins, peptide epitopes, and the use of viral antigens. The use of these approaches in the context of HPV serves to illustrate advances in this field. Cervical cancer is the second most frequent cancer and the fifth most frequent cause of death from cancer among women in the world, with an estimated 471 000 new cases and 233 000 deaths in the year 2000. The relative importance of cervical cancer is even greater for women in developing countries, where more than 80% of cases occur, and where it comprises about 15% of cancers in women, with a lifetime risk of about 2%. In a recent report of a study involving 2392 young women, immunization with an HPV-16 virus-like particle (VLP) vaccine resulted in 0 per 100 woman-years at risk in the vaccine group while in the placebo group the incidence of persistent HPV-16 infection was 3.8 per 100 woman-years at risk (100% efficacy; 95% confidence interval, 90–100; $P < 0.001$). It is estimated that if women were vaccinated against all high-risk types of HPV before they become sexually active, there should be a reduction of at least 85% in the risk of cervical cancer, and a decline of 44 to 70% in the frequency of abnormal Pap smears attributable to HPV. Recently, programmes of prophylactic vaccination against oncogenic HPV types have been initiated in many countries. Unfortunately, even after vaccination is implemented, a reduction in the incidence of cervical cancer could not be expected to become apparent for at least a decade. Therefore, therapeutic vaccines are still very much needed to reduce the morbidity and mortality associated with cervical cancer.

The therapeutic approach to patients with preinvasive and invasive cervical cancers is to develop vaccine strategies that induce specific CD8+ CTL responses aimed at eliminating virus infected or transformed cells. The majority of cervical cancers express the HPV16-derived E6 and E7 oncoproteins, which are thus attractive targets for T cell-mediated immunotherapy. In a number of clinical trials, it was demonstrated that HPV 16 and 18 peptides can elicit CD8+ T-cell responses; however, tumour regression was minimal in most patients. In another recent clinical trial, 29 patients with clinical International Federation of Gynecologists and Obstetricians (FIGO) stage Ib or IIa cervical cancer were given 2 vaccinations with rVV-HPV (TA-HPV) at least 4 weeks apart, starting 2 weeks before radical hysterectomy. Vaccination with rVV was well tolerated in all patients with only mild to moderate local toxicity, and no serious adverse events were attributable to the vaccine. After a single vaccination, HPV-specific CTLs were found in four patients while eight patients developed HPV-specific serological responses. Other approaches currently undergoing preclinical development include the use of recombinant alphaviruses such as Venezuelan equine encephalitis virus (VEE), Semliki Forest virus (SFV), overlapping long peptides, and naked DNA vaccination.

Strategies to improve immunotherapy in cancer

Antigen

The ideal antigen for immunotherapy is exclusively expressed by tumour cells and is highly immunogenic, such as the CT-antigen NY-ESO-1. In addition, the majority, or even better, all cells of the tumour should express the antigen and present its epitopes on their surface in the context of MHC molecules in sufficient amounts.

Multiple injections of the entire antigenic protein in a free form, as long peptides, as mRNAs, or as cDNA encoding the antigen are considered a useful approach, as all forms will preferentially be taken up and presented by dendritic cells. More efficiently, the antigen can be coupled to substances targeting dendritic cells (e.g. anti-CD205 antibodies). Independent of the form of the antigen, it must be administered together with an appropriate signal to induce dendritic cell maturation. However, which signals are needed for appropriate dendritic cell maturation *in vivo* is not yet fully understood. Because the immune system developed to fight pathogens and is therefore efficiently activated by those, vaccination with recombinant (attenuated) pathogens that express tumour antigens may be superior to vaccination with recombinant protein, peptides, or tumour cell lysates. The amount and the biophysical nature of the antigen determine the duration of the antigenic stimulus and there is evidence that antigen persistence is required for the development and maintenance of effector function by responding T cells. This may require multiple injections in most cases, as most vaccines will be short lived *in vivo*. The relatively short half-life of endogenous dendritic cells (estimated to be <1 week) also argues for multiple vaccinations. If recombinant pathogens are used as a vaccine, it may be necessary to avoid neutralizing antibody activity to use another pathogen for each consecutive immunization (so-called prime–boost protocols), such as recombinant poxvirus, adenovirus, and herpesvirus or modified strains of salmonella or mycobacteria after cancer antigen encoding DNA transfection.

T cells and modulation of T cell function by antibodies

The activation of both naive and antigen-experienced T cells requires multiple signals and improving the quality of each of these signals may contribute to a more efficient response to persisting antigens such as tumours or some pathogens.

The quality of signal 1, the interaction between the TCR and the peptide/MHC complex, is determined by ligand density and TCR avidity. The current opinion is that this interaction must have a minimal duration and strength for adequate T-cell activation. As high-avidity T cells may have been purged from the repertoire of tumour-specific T cells, increasing the numbers of peptide/MHC complexes per APC may be considered during vaccine development. This may be achieved by targeting the relevant antigen to the compartments in which MHC class I- or class II-loading takes place. Signal 2 is delivered to the responding T cell as the net effect of costimulatory (CD80/CD28, CD86/CD28, CD70/CD27, B7RP1/ICOS, 4-1BBL/4-1BB, OX40L/OX40) and of coinhibitory (CD80/CTLA4, CD86/CTLA4, B7H1/PD-1, B7DC/PD-1) interactions that are mediated by surface molecules on the APC and T cell respectively. Costimulatory and coinhibitory molecules belong to the B7 or the TNF family and the number of known costimulatory and coinhibitory molecules is still increasing. Interference with these signals such that costimulation is increased and/or coinhibition is diminished is a promising approach for enhancing the magnitude and the quality of the tumour-specific T cell response. Diminishing coinhibition is presumably the better option, as mature dendritic cells usually express sufficient levels of costimulatory molecules. Nevertheless, positive effects of agonistic antibodies to 4-1BB and OX40 on tumour immunity were reported. PD-1 was shown to be important in peripheral tolerance induction and accordingly, PD-1-deficient mice spontaneously develop autoimmunity. In addition, it was shown that anergy of specific CD8+ T cells as a result of overwhelming antigen could be prevented by blocking PD-1/PD-1L interactions in mice and in humans. In cancer patients, the expression of PD-1L in the tumour or the expression of PD-1 by tumour-infiltrating lymphocytes was found to correlate with poor prognosis. The interaction of CD152 (CTLA4) with its ligands CD80 (B7.1) and CD86 (B7.2) has been studied more extensively in the context of tumour-specific immunity. CTLA4 is transiently expressed on T cells upon activation and plays a critical role in down-regulation of T cell responses as well as in peripheral T-cell tolerance, which is illustrated by the lethal generalized autoimmunity in CTLA4-deficient mice. Treatment with anti-CTLA4 antibodies resulted in rejection of established tumours in different mouse models, but in order to be effective in the poorly immunogenic B16 melanoma model it had to be combined with GM-CSF treatment. The beneficial effect in experimental systems encouraged the use of anti-CTLA4 treatment as a single agent or together with therapeutic vaccination in patients with melanoma. Major clinical responses were seen in these trials, also in patients with advanced disease. It has been suggested that anti-CTLA4 treatment acts through selective inhibition of Treg, which constitutively express CTLA4. This idea was challenged recently: First, it was shown that CTLA4 blockade had no impact on suppressive function *in vitro*. Second, Allison and co-workers used anti-CTLA4 and GM-CSF treatment in the B16 rejection model and elegantly showed that anti-CTLA4 had no effect on the number or function of tumour-infiltrating Tregs, but that instead the number of effectors in the tumour greatly increased resulting in an higher ratio of effector T cells to Tregs, which may explain the beneficial effect of anti-CTLA4/GM-CSF treatment.

Antigen-presenting cells (APCs)

Mature or activated dendritic cells have the unique capacity to activate naive CD4+ and CD8+ T cells and to reactivate memory CD8+ T cells *in vivo*. On the other hand, steady-state dendritic cells have been shown to induce peripheral tolerance in both CD4+ and CD8+ T cells. Thus, it is crucial that the vaccine is presented to T cells by mature, activated dendritic cells and that presentation by other cell types or by steady-state dendritic cells is avoided as much as possible. In addition and ideally, the vaccine should overcome peripheral tolerance that may have been induced by the tumour. In principle, two approaches may be considered: (1) loading of *in vitro* generated autologous dendritic cells with antigen (peptide, protein, tumour lysate, lentivirus, or nucleic acids encoding tumour antigens) followed by administration of dendritic cells to the patient; (2) *in vivo* targeting of the vaccine to dendritic cells with a simultaneous dendritic cell-maturation signal.

The major drawback for the therapeutic injection of antigen-presenting dendritic cells is their limited migration. Most dendritic cells were found to remain at the injection site and less than 1% were homing to draining lymphoid tissue. Nevertheless, many studies documented successful induction of immunity against viral and tumour antigens in healthy volunteers and in patients, respectively, although without significant clinical effects. A more promising alternative is targeting of antigen to dendritic cells *in vivo*, which circumvents problems of migration. Injection of proteins or long peptides together with adjuvants is presumably superior to the injection of short peptide epitopes, as dendritic cells are the only cells that efficiently take up and cross-present proteins or long peptides, and their *in vivo* half-life is probably longer. However, the process of cross-presentation is rather inefficient and may require the injection of relatively large amounts of antigen. Efficient targeting of antigen to dendritic cells can be achieved by coupling the antigen to an antibody specific to endocytic receptors on dendritic cells: It has been shown that antigens coupled to anti-DEC205 (CD205) potently induce CD4+ and CD8+ T cells in murine model systems and in humans when given together with a dendritic cell-maturation stimulus. The use of modified and attenuated pathogens as vectors may combine targeting to dendritic cells and delivery of correct maturation stimuli because many, if not all, pathogens infect dendritic cells or are efficiently taken up by them and because they provide 'danger' signals for dendritic cell maturation. Many vectors, including adenovirus, herpesvirus, and different poxviruses have been shown to efficiently induce the desired responses in patients. Pre-existing immunity to the vector due to previous immunization or infection, and safety issues especially in immunocompromised patients, limit the choice of viral vectors.

Concluding remarks

Significant advances have been made in the field of cancer immunotherapy over the last decade. The most important step forward has been the identification of tumour antigens with immunogenic potential. The utilization and improvement of cancer immunotherapy in the clinic demands carefully conducted and coordinated but discovery-oriented translational research in the form of clinical trials that include thorough monitoring of immune and clinical responses.

As selective outgrowth of antigen-loss variants due to immunoediting may occur during vaccination of cancer patients, antigen expression patterns of the tumour and metastases should be monitored during immunotherapy, if possible, followed by surgical resection of antigen-negative tumours. At this rather early stage of development cancer immunotherapy should be offered to cancer patients only within carefully monitored clinical trials of experienced clinical research teams. In addition, it may be rewarding to include patients with early-stage disease in immunotherapy trials, because immunoediting of the tumour and subversion of the immune response by the tumour is presumably less pronounced in those patients.

The keys to efficient cancer vaccination are: (1) availability of an antigen known to be a strong immunogen in cancer patients; (2) the route, schedule, and packaging of antigen to induce an optimal immune response *in vivo*; (3) combination of antigen with an adjuvant, to support the induction of a strong immune response *in vivo*; (4) long-term immunizations, and (5) inhibition of regulatory signals, such as CTLA-4, Tregs, and PD-1.

Further reading

Chen YT, *et al.* (1997). A testicular antigen aberrantly expressed in human cancers detected by autologous antibody screening. *Proc Natl Acad Sci U S A*, **94**, 1914–18.

Coley WB (1991). The treatment of malignant tumors by repeated inoculations of erysipelas. With a report of ten original cases. 1893. *Clin Orthop Relat Res*, **262**, 3–11.

Dunn GP, Old LJ, Schreiber RD (2004). The immunobiology of cancer immunosurveillance and immunoediting. *Immunity*, **21**, 137–48.

Dunn GP, *et al.* (2002). Cancer immunoediting: from immunosurveillance to tumor escape. *Nat Immunol*, **3**, 991–8.

Gnjatic S, *et al.* (2006). NY-ESO-1: review of an immunogenic tumor antigen. *Adv Cancer Res*, **95**, 1–30.

Ho W, *et al.* (2003). Adoptive immunotherapy: engineering T cell responses as biologic weapons for tumor mass destruction. *Cancer Cell*, **3**, 431–7.

Korman AJ, Peggs KS, Allison JP (2006). Checkpoint blockade in cancer immunotherapy. *Adv Immunol*, **90**, 297–339.

Krieg AM (2008). Toll-like receptor 9 (TLR9) agonists in the treatment of cancer. *Oncogene*, **27**, 161–7.

Maraskovsky E, *et al.* (2004). NY-ESO-1 protein formulated in ISCOMATRIX adjuvans is a potent anticancer vaccine inducing both humoral and CD8+ t-cell-mediated immunity and protection against NY-ESO-1+ tumors. *Clin Cancer Res*, **10**, 2879–90.

Marchand M, *et al.* (2003). Immunisation of metastatic cancer patients with MAGE-3 protein combined with adjuvant SBAS-2: a clinical report. *Eur J Cancer*, **39**, 70–77.

Sahin U, Türeci O, Pfreundschuh M (1997). Serological identification of human tumor antigens. *Curr Opin Immunol*, **9**, 709–16.

Steinman RM, Hawiger D, Nussenzweig MC (2003). Tolerogenic dendritic cells. *Annu Rev Immunol*, **21**, 685–711.

Stevenson BJ, *et al.* (2007). Rapid evolution of cancer/testis genes on the X chromosome. *BMC Genomics*, **8**, 129.

van der Bruggen P, *et al.* (1991). A gene encoding an antigen recognized by cytolytic T lymphocytes on a human melanoma. *Science*, **254**, 1643–7.

zur Hausen H (2002). Papillomaviruses and cancer: from basic studies to clinical application. *Nat Rev Cancer*, **2**, 342–50.

6.5

Cancer: clinical features and management

R.L. Souhami

Essentials

Cancer is common and will be the cause of death of about 20% of the population of developed countries. Every clinician should be aware of the many ways in which it presents. Delay in diagnosis may diminish the chances of successful treatment and always creates anxiety for the patient. Expert advice, immediate investigation, and definitive biopsy diagnosis should be obtained speedily.

Clinical features

Symptoms—common symptoms include (1) pain—a presenting feature of 30% of cases of cancer, with sites and distribution that may be characteristic of tumours in certain locations and indicators of a possible underlying malignancy; more likely to occur with rapidly growing tumours; when due to bone involvement is typically worse at night-time; (2) swelling—due to tumour mass; (3) weight loss—an invariable accompaniment of advanced cancer and also a frequent presenting symptom; may be due to direct interference with digestive function, production of factors leading to weight loss and anorexia by the tumour, and possible alteration in protein and energy metabolism.

Other clinical manifestations—these include (1) fever—particularly in lymphomas, renal carcinoma, and any cancer metastatic to the liver; (2) anaemia—usually normochromic; (3) hypercalcaemia—usually due to widespread skeletal metastases, but sometimes paraneoplastic and due to action of parathyroid hormone-related protein (PTH-rP); and (4) paraneoplastic manifestations—these may be endocrine, neurological, dermatological, musculoskeletal, or haematological; frequently present as puzzling medical problems at a time when the primary tumour may not be clinically apparent.

Emergency presentations—many presentations and complications of cancer are medical emergencies that require immediate treatment. These include spinal cord compression, raised intracranial pressure, pathological fractures, pleural and pericardial effusion, ascites, and metabolic disturbances such as hypercalcaemia.

General aspects of investigation and management

The diagnosis and immediate management of suspected cancer requires (1) a high index of clinical suspicion—cancer should be suspected with any unexplained illness, especially in older people; (2) obtaining a tissue diagnosis without undue delay—radiological imaging will often accelerate diagnosis but cannot provide a tissue diagnosis; every attempt should be made to make a histological or cytological diagnosis expeditiously; (3) initiation of treatment without undue delay—patients should start a planned programme of treatment within days, not weeks, of diagnosis.

The multidisciplinary approach—the management of a patient with cancer increasingly involves specialists in different disciplines who, at the outset, decide on the nature and sequence of treatment. These decisions are based on the stage of the tumour (local extent, presence of absence of lymph node spread, presence of absence of distant metastases) and other clinical and pathological determinants of prognosis, and on the likelihood of benefit from surgery, radiotherapy and chemotherapy.

Psychological and pastoral care, and management of pain—these are essential and rewarding aspects of cancer medicine. The attitudes of the medical team and the efficiency, openness, and responsiveness of the organization of care are of great importance in helping the patient cope with the stress of the diagnosis and its treatment.

Long-term consequences of cancer and its treatment—these are now occurring increasingly frequently as cure rates rise. They affect every aspect of general internal medicine and physicians in all specialties need to be aware of the nature of the problems that may occur, which include reduction in fertility, cognitive impairment, musculoskeletal problems, metabolic problems, and second cancers.

Introduction: cancer in general medical practice

Cancer is a common disease—approximately 20% of the population of the United Kingdom will die of cancer. It is a source of concern and perplexity to oncologists when patients are referred to them late in the disease. Symptoms may have been present for a long time, during which their significance has been overlooked, or multiple (and sometimes futile) investigations have been performed with a failure to appreciate the need for speed. To this delay can be added a frequent lack of understanding, on the part of the referring doctor, of the possibilities of treatment, and a failure to inform patients either of the nature of the diagnosis or of its implications and possibilities for therapy.

Yet almost every specialist sees patients with cancer affecting their particular field; unfortunately, these specialists may not be familiar with the principles of cancer medicine. General practitioners, seeing patients with diverse, and often minor, conditions, are in a vulnerable position when the early symptoms of a cancer first appear. Oncologists therefore frequently see patients with disease that has been present for a considerable time before diagnosis, or who have not had a proper explanation of their illness, and who have little idea of what treatment might involve. Every patient with cancer should be referred for expert advice as soon as the diagnosis is made. Delay in diagnosis and starting treatment is likely to worsen the outlook and may even deny the patient a chance of cure.

The complexity of modern cancer therapy, particularly the widening range of cellular targets for drug treatment, has led to the emergence of diverse short- and long-term consequences of treatment that involve every medical specialty.

The principles of cancer management are therefore important for every physician.

Diagnosis and immediate management of suspected cancer would be improved greatly if the following simple rules were adhered to:

- Cancer should be suspected with any unexplained illness, especially in older people.
- Imaging with CT, MRI, or isotopic methods (see Chapter 6.5), will often accelerate diagnosis. However, a tissue diagnosis cannot be made by these means and every attempt should be made to make a histological or cytological diagnosis expeditiously.
- Patients should start a planned programme of treatment within days, not weeks, of diagnosis. The need for speed in diagnosis and treatment is tacitly recognized in specialist centres for breast cancer where patients can, in well-regulated clinics, reasonably expect to have a diagnosis made within a few days of first consultation and to begin definitive treatment within 2 weeks. This admirable efficiency should be attainable for most cancers.

Common symptoms and signs of cancer

Many of the symptoms and signs of cancer are due to the local effects of the tumour infiltrating surrounding tissues and causing pressure and distortion of neighbouring structures. Tumours also produce symptoms that are, to some extent, common to all cancers. These are general symptoms due to the metabolic disturbances caused by the tumours and specific symptoms related to hormonal effects and immunological effects of the particular tumour—so-called paraneoplastic syndromes.

Pain

Most patients with cancer experience pain at some stage in their illness, as a direct result either of the tumour or of its treatment. Pain is a feature at presentation in about 30% of patients with cancer, but the incidence varies greatly with the site of the tumour. For example, over 90% of patients with primary bone tumours or with metastases to bone have pain, and this has the characteristic feature of being worse at night-time. In contrast, only 5% of patients with leukaemia develop pain. Pain also varies according to the rate of progression of the disease and is more likely to occur with rapidly growing tumours. No symptom of cancer causes greater demoralization than unremitting pain. Any patient with unexplained, persistent pain should be suspected of having malignant disease and appropriate investigations performed. In pain clinics, 80% of patients seen with cancer have pain due to direct tumour infiltration. If the pain is due to neurological infiltration it may be felt at the distribution of the nerve root. Certain pain syndromes are sufficiently common and misleading to warrant separate consideration.

Direct tumour infiltration of bone

The origin of the pain that occurs with tumour infiltration of bone is not fully understood. The periosteum is a pain-sensitive structure and may be the source in many patients. It is probable that osteolytic processes involving prostaglandins are also involved. Pain is a common feature of metastasis at the base of the skull. If the tumour is situated around the jugular foramen, pain is often referred to the vertex of the head and the ipsilateral shoulder and arm. Movement of the head may exacerbate the pain and, later, cranial nerve involvement may cause hoarseness, dysarthria, and dysphasia. Involvement of the 9th to the 12th cranial nerves and the development of ptosis and Horner's syndrome indicates involvement of the sympathetic nervous system extracranially adjacent to the jugular foramen. When metastases occur in the sphenoid sinus, severe headache, usually felt in both temples or retro-orbitally, is a common feature. There may be a full sensation in the head, nasal stuffiness, and a 6th nerve palsy.

When metastases occur in vertebral bodies the pain frequently precedes neurological signs and symptoms. Persistent thoracic vertebral pain and a positive bone scan is an indication for urgent investigation and treatment. In small-cell lung cancer, for example, a patient with thoracic vertebral pain and a positive bone scan has a 30% chance of developing a paraplegia. Ninety per cent of patients who have epidural spinal cord compression have vertebral body metastasis as the source of the epidural tumour (the management of spinal compression is described later). With metastasis to the odontoid process, patients complain of severe neck pain and stiffness radiating over the skull, up to the vertex. This is then followed by progressive neurological signs, often associated with autonomic dysfunction. In the lower cervical vertebrae pain is felt as an aching sensation, often radiating over both shoulders. If nerve root compression occurs at this site, there will be pain in the root distribution felt in the back of the arm, the elbow, and the ulnar aspect of the hand. The association with Horner's syndrome suggests involvement of the paravertebral sympathetic system. Lumbar metastases are associated with local pain, worse on lying or sitting and relieved by standing. In lesions in L1 the pain is often felt over the superior iliac crests. In the sacrum, pain may be accompanied by neurological signs with symptoms of bowel and bladder dysfunction and perianal sensory loss and impotence.

Nerve infiltration

When tumours infiltrate peripheral nerves they are often accompanied by an alteration in sensation, with hyperaesthesia, dysaesthesia, and sensory loss. This is a particularly common presentation when tumours invade the paravertebral or retroperitoneal region. Here the pain is often in a root distribution and is unilateral. Another common site is when a metastasis in a rib entraps the intercostal nerves. When tumour infiltrates the brachial plexus the pain is felt in the C7 or T1 distribution. Pain in this site is frequent with the Pancoast syndrome, where an apical lung cancer infiltrates the lower brachial plexus roots. Pain in the C5 distribution occurs with upper root infiltration.

Visceral pain

This is a frequent symptom of cancer; it can cause diagnostic confusion and be difficult to control when a tumour has already been diagnosed. Poorly localized abdominal pain is a frequent feature of ovarian and pancreatic cancer and of peritoneal carcinomatosis. Retroperitoneal pain may be particularly difficult to diagnose. It may vary greatly with position (being relieved on leaning forwards) and be felt variably in the back. Left upper quadrant pain may be a presenting feature of carcinoma of the tail of the pancreas involving the mesentery of the splenic flexure of the colon.

Weight loss

Weight loss is an invariable accompaniment of advanced cancer and also a frequent presenting symptom. Often it results from the physical presence of the tumour interfering with gastrointestinal function, such as in carcinoma of the stomach, pancreas, or colon, or with peritoneal carcinomatosis. Mechanical obstruction of the bowel and loss of appetite commonly accompany these tumours. Loss of appetite is a frequent symptom of any cancer that has metastasized to the liver and usually appears at a point when metastasis is replacing much of the normal liver tissue. The mechanism is not known. Pancreatic cancers, and cancers metastatic to the porta hepatis cause weight loss from a malabsorption syndrome due to obstructive jaundice or blockage of the pancreatic ducts.

Nevertheless, many tumours cause weight loss without direct involvement of digestive organs. It is well recognized that a weight loss of more than 5% is a very adverse prognostic feature in almost all cancers. Usually it indicates that the disease is more widespread than is apparent on clinical investigation, but the mechanisms of this symptom, which is often accompanied by alteration of taste, anorexia, and a general feeling of ill health, are obscure. Sometimes quite profound weight loss can accompany nonmetastatic tumours, which are relatively small. As with advanced cancer, the cachexia syndrome is then also accompanied by anorexia and altered taste. These tumours may produce circulating factors responsible for the weight loss and loss of appetite. Tumour necrosis factor α and interleukin-1β have both been shown to produce cachexic syndromes experimentally. Tumours may themselves contribute to weight loss by alteration in protein and energy metabolism. Negative nitrogen balance has been frequently documented in patients with cancer, particularly when advanced. An increase in whole-body glucose recycling via pyruvate and lactate has also been described in patients with cancer.

The loss of body weight is therefore due to an accumulation of events involving direct interference with digestive function, production of factors leading to weight loss and anorexia by the tumour, and possible alteration in protein and energy metabolism. Later in the course of the illness, antineoplastic treatment with chemotherapy, radiation, and surgery may exacerbate weight loss.

Tumour mass

It is astonishing that patients sometimes report the appearance of a swelling only to have the significance of the finding overlooked by their doctors. The appearance of any mass should lead to prompt investigation. Although imaging techniques can sometimes distinguish benign from malignant swellings, a biopsy will usually be necessary and should be taken without delay. Nowadays it is often unnecessary to undertake surgical excision biopsy. Indeed, doing so may sometimes make subsequent management very difficult. Where there is doubt about the nature of a swelling the correct procedure will usually be needle biopsy. Biopsy is in general preferable to aspiration cytological diagnosis because the precise diagnosis of many cancers depends on architecture as well as on cytology. The great advantage of early biopsy diagnosis is that a planned approach to treatment can then be undertaken by oncologists, radiotherapists, and surgeons together. Injudicious, and often marginal, surgical excision may lead to a greatly increased risk of local recurrence of the tumour. This is a frequent occurrence in sarcomas where an amputation that might have been avoided may then become necessary, or the local recurrence provoked by inadequate excision prove uncontrollable and fatal. Furthermore, for some tumours, chemotherapy may be the appropriate first line of treatment allowing assessment of the tumour response to drug treatment before surgery is undertaken: a good response may modify the need for surgery.

Fever

In cancer, fever is usually caused by infection. However, about 30% of patients with cancer develop fever at some stage in their illness and it may be the presenting feature of some tumours, particularly lymphomas, renal carcinoma, and any cancer metastatic to the liver. The fever may be accompanied by sweating, particularly at night. The characteristic feature of the sweats that accompany malignant lymphomas and other cancers is that the patients fall asleep and wake in the middle of the night to find themselves drenched with sweat. Rigors are very uncommon with febrile episodes in cancer, and should always lead to a suspicion that an infective complication is present. Characteristic patterns of fever are seldom observed; usually it is of a low-grade, remittent, type. The Pel–Ebstein fever of Hodgkin's disease, in which febrile periods are interspersed with several days of normal temperature, is well known but very uncommon.

The cause of the fever of malignant disease is unknown. Endogenous pyrogens may be liberated from mononuclear phagocytes in the liver or bone marrow. Tumour cells have also been shown to produce 'pyrogens'. The nature of the cytokines responsible is not clear. Exogenously administered tumour necrosis factor and interleukin 2 both produce fever and may be secreted in patients with cancer.

The fever of malignant disease may respond to simple antipyretics such as aspirin or paracetamol. In malignant lymphoma it will disappear with successful treatment of the tumour. In advanced cancer nonsteroidal anti-inflammatory agents may also help, but corticosteroids are more effective, at least for a short period.

Anaemia

The anaemia of malignant disease is multifactorial (see Section 22). Chronic blood loss may occur in cancer of the gastrointestinal tract, as a result of vaginal bleeding, or because of malabsorption of iron. Usually the anaemia is normochromic or slightly hypochromic in nature, and the plasma transferrin and serum iron are low. The iron stores are not reduced as judged by stainable iron in the bone marrow. The mechanism is discussed in Section 22.

Hypercalcaemia

Malignant disease is responsible for most of the very severe cases of hypercalcaemia seen in clinical practice. The patient will usually have widespread skeletal metastases, but occasionally the syndrome is paraneoplastic (see below). Parathyroid hormone-related protein (PTH-rP) may contribute to the pathogenesis of both paraneoplastic hypercalcaemia and that produced by bone metastases. For some cancers it appears that metastases in bone release PTH-rP locally and stimulate osteclastic resorption of bone. Resorption releases cytokines such as transforming growth factor-β and insulin-like growth factor 1 which, in turn, provokes more release of PTH-rP from the metastatic tumour. These cytokines may also cause proliferation of the tumour. Bisphosphonates may arrest the process by decreasing the activity of the osteoclasts. In the same way, bisphosphonates interrupt the activity of PTH-rP when this is liberated from a nonmetastatic tumour as a paraneoplastic phenomenon. Bisphosphonates are important both for the treatment of hypercalcaemia and containing growth of bone metastases.

Hypercalcaemic symptoms include anorexia, weight loss, and mental confusion, all of which may simulate metastatic disease. The symptoms and signs of hypercalcaemia and its management are discussed in Sections 13 and 22.

Paraneoplastic syndromes

Many patients with cancer have complications that are not due to direct invasion of adjacent tissues by the cancer or its metastases. The tumour produces hormones or cytokines, which are responsible for symptoms at a remote site. Alternatively, the tumour provokes an immune response to altered cellular constituents and the paraneoplastic syndrome arises from the resulting immunological reaction. Paraneoplastic syndromes are not rare but each syndrome only occurs in a minority of patients with cancer. Furthermore, although some syndromes, such as the production of parathyroid hormone-related peptide, are found in many cancers, others, such as Cushing's syndrome, are found in a few neuroendocrine tumours.

It is important to be aware of paraneoplastic syndromes because their appearance may be the first sign of malignant disease. Furthermore, they may lead the physician into believing that the patient has metastases and thus alter management inappropriately. The syndromes themselves may cause considerable disability, which is amenable to treatment. The diversity of paraneoplastic syndromes is such that only a brief description can be given in this chapter. A summary is shown in Table 6.5.1.

Cancer can cause almost any clinical syndrome, however bizarre, and should, therefore, enter the list of differential diagnosis in any unusual clinical disorder. There are, however, dangers in making a diagnosis of a paraneoplastic syndrome as a cause of symptoms. For example, most neurological problems in cancer are not due to paraneoplastic manifestations but to the local presence of the tumour. This means that spinal cord signs in a patient with cancer are much more likely to be due to direct compression of the cord than due to transverse myelitis as a paraneoplastic syndrome. Prompt treatment of the space-occupying lesion is essential and a mistaken diagnosis of paraneoplasia is potentially disastrous. Similarly, endocrine syndromes from cancer are often caused by resectable endocrine cancers themselves. Anaemia or thrombosis may be paraneoplastic in origin but more frequently a deep venous thrombosis is due to a direct compressive effect of cancer in the pelvis; and iron-deficiency anaemia should always raise the possibility of occult bleeding. Unless obviously paraneoplastic in nature, symptoms from cancer should, in the first instance, be regarded as likely to be produced by a direct effect of the tumour since this distinction has important therapeutic consequences. Some of these syndromes are described in detail in later sections: endocrine in Section 13, renal in Section 21, and neurological in Section 24.

Investigation and staging

Histopathological diagnosis

The foremost investigation of a cancer is to verify that the diagnosis is correct. Oncologists are completely dependent on the quality of the histopathological examination. Errors are not common but may be very serious, as they may lead to inappropriate investigation or the denial of curative treatment. The latter merits particular consideration of two cancer types.

Misdiagnosis of a lymphoma

Lymphomas may present with histological appearances that resemble anaplastic or undifferentiated carcinoma. The diagnosis should therefore always be considered when this is the pathology report on the biopsy. Nowadays diagnosis of lymphoma has been made much easier as a result of immunohistochemical techniques. An example is shown in Fig. 6.5.1. The use of antibodies to leucocyte common antigen, or a combination of B-cell and T-cell markers, is invaluable in diagnosis. If tumour cells do not stain, it makes lymphoma unlikely, but does not rule out the possibility. If positive, the diagnosis of lymphoma is virtually certain. Nevertheless, histologists may have difficulty either because the immunohistochemical technique is not sufficiently standardized in the laboratory, or because they mistake infiltrating lymphocytes for the tumour cells. Some undifferentiated pleomorphic lymphomas may be negative for leucocyte common antigen. These present considerable diagnostic difficulties, which may be resolved by examination of the tissue by molecular genetic techniques looking for rearrangement of the T-cell receptor genes or for immunoglobulin gene rearrangement. Other situations in which lymphoma may be overlooked, or a mistaken diagnosis made, are in the pulmonary lesions (or metastases) from small-cell carcinoma, which may be mistaken for lymphoma, or in biopsies from gastric ulcers where malignant lymphoma cells may wrongly be regarded as a chronic

Table 6.5.1 Paraneoplastic syndromes

Syndrome	Clinical features	Tumour	Comments
Endocrine syndromes[*]			
Cushing's syndrome	Metabolic features (BP ↑ K+↓ glucose ↑) are severe. Obesity, etc. occur in slower growing SCLC tumours	SCLC, carcinoid, other neuroendocrine tumours	Pro-opiocortin produced by tumour. Occurs in 0.5% of cases. Immunoreactive ACTH ↑ in many more. In SCLC, chemotherapy may help the syndrome. In other tumours resection is curative
Antidiuretic hormone excess	Low plasma sodium (less than 1 30 mmol/l with continued urine sodium excretion; below 120 mmol/l altered mental state, confusion, fits, coma, death)	SCLC	Tumour produces ADH. Slightly low plasma Na is common feature of all advanced cancer (due to pituitary ADH release). Treatment is by water restriction and demeclocycline. Hypertonic saline in emergency
Hypercalcaemia	Symptoms of hypercalcaemia often very severe	Squamous cancers	Immunoreactive PTH-related peptide. Possibly release of cytokines (IL-1 β, osteoclast activating factors) in some cases.Treatment described in Chapter 12.6
		T-cell leukaemia	
		Some lymphomas	
Gonadotrophin excess	Gynaecomastia in men, oligomenorrhoea, thyroid overactivity	Gestational trophoblastic tumours	β-hCG produced in excess. Clinical syndromes are uncommon. Mechanism of clinical syndrome is incompletely understood
		Germ cell tumours	
		Adenocarcinoma of the lung	
		Hepatoblastoma	
		Other adenocarcinomas	
Hypoglycaemia	Clinical features are of hypoglycaemia	Sarcoma	Major mechanism is non-suppressible insulin- like activity (NSILA, somatomedins) and insulin-like growth factors. Mesothelioma is usually abdominal
	Tumours are usually large	Mesothelioma	
		Hepatoma	
		Adrenal carcinoma	
Osteomalacia	Vitamin-D-resistant rickets with bone pain, phosphaturia	Benign mesenchyme tumours, fibromas, haemangiomas in soft tissue and bone	Low 1,25-OH vitamin D, low PTH. Treatment requires large doses of vitamin D and removal of tumour
Neurological syndromes			
Dementia	Variable-onset dementia	Lung cancer (SCLC)	May be due to vascular endothelial disorder induced by the tumour
Cerebellar degeneration	Subacute and progressive associated with dementia	Hodgkin's disease, uterine and ovarian cancer	CSF[1] protein raised and lymphocytosis
Limbic'encephalitis'	Dementia	SCLC	Pathologically there is hippocampal degeneration
		Hodgkin's disease	
Optic neuritis	Visual failure, papilloedema often bilateral	SCLC	Produced by antibodies (? to altered tumour- related proteins) which bind to retinal ganglion cell
Myelopathy	Rapid-onset cord degeneration often mid-thoracic. Usually quickly fatal	SCLC	CSF[1] protein elevated
Amyotrophic lateral sclerosis	Lower motor neurone weakness combined with spasticity fasciculation. Mostly in men. Slow course	Various	Cancer found in 5–10% of cases of ALS
Peripheral neuropathy	Either pure sensory neuropathy or a severe sensorimotor neuropathy	SCLC. Other intrathoracic tumours (thymoma, oesophageal cancer, lymphoma)	CSF1 protein may be elevated. May antedate tumour. Often does not improve if tumour removed. Sensory neuropathy is due to dorsal root ganglion degeneration and specific antibodies have been found
Guillain-Barré syndrome	Typical clinical features	Lymphomas	Association frequently noted but ? genuine

(Continued)

Table 6.5.1 (*Cont'd*) Paraneoplastic syndromes

Syndrome	Clinical features	Tumour	Comments
Dermatological syndromes			
Acanthosis nigricans	Hyperkeratosis and pigmentation in axillas, neck, and flexures	Gastric, other intra-abdominal	There is a congenital form which must be distinguished
Seborrhoeic keratoses	Sudden onset of keratoses (Leser–Tralat syndrome)	Gut, non-Hodgkin's lymphoma	Keratoses appear quickly in large numbers
Exfoliative dermatitis	Severe erythema and scaling	Lymphomas, especially T-cell type	Common cause of exfoliative dermatitis
			Responds to steroids and treatment of lymphoma
Migratory erythema	Blistering, necrotic erythema	Glucagonoma	
Panniculitis	Crops of tender, subcutaneous lesions which look like erythema nodosum	Pancreas	Probably due to fat inflammation caused by liberation of pancreatic lipases
Porphyria cutanea tarda	Nodular or erythematous skin lesions Photosensitive.	Hepatocellular carcinoma	Very uncommon
Ichthyosis	Dry scaly skin with hyperkeratosis of palms and soles	Lymphomas	Different from congenital form, which may be accompanied by carcinoma of oesophagus
Musculoskeletal syndromes			
Finger clubbing and hypertrophic pulmonary osteoarthropathy	Clubbing of finger nails.Tenderness over distal ends of radius and ulna, and tibia and fibula. Periosteal reaction on radiography	Bronchial carcinoma (not SCLC), benign mesothelioma, diaphragmatic Neurilemmoma	One of the great unsolved mysteries of medicine. Cause unknown
Dermatomyositis	Erythema of face—cheeks, eyelids—and over backs of hands	Wide variety of cancers, especially adenocarcinoma	May precede cancer by 6–24 months. In middle age approx. 30% of cases have underlying malignancy
Lambert–Eaton syndrome	A myasthenic syndrome with muscle weakness, especially in thighs and pelvis. Ptosis, dysarthria, double vision occur. EMG shows increase in action potential with repeated stimulation	SCLC	Syndrome often antedates cancer. Muscle strength does not deteriorate with exercise. An IgG autoantibody to voltage- gated calcium channels reduces acetylcholine release. Responds to treatment of tumour and to guanidine
Haematological syndromes			
Autoimmune haemolytic anaemia	Anaemia may be the presenting symptom. Splenomegaly may occur. Response to steroids is poor. May be associated with ITP	Non-Hodgkin's lymphoma (B-cell type), wide variety of epithelial cancers	Antibodies to red cell antigens.
			? cross-react with altered tumour surface antigens. Remits with successful treatment
Microangiopathic haemolytic anaemia	Mild forms are common, clinically apparent cases rare	Mucin-producing adenocarcinomas	May respond to anticancer treatment. Procoagulant appears to be produced by the tumour
Thrombocytosis	Usually asymptomatic. Mild elevation of platelet count is common. Thrombosis of haemorrhage is rare	Carcinoma, Hodgkin's disease	The tumour-associated cytokine has not yet been identified
Granulocytosis	Usually asymptomatic. Modest elevations frequently found with liver metastases	Adenocarcinomas, melanoma	Blood film does not show immature forms. CSFs[2] are assumed responsible, but IL-1 and IL-3 have been implicated in some tumours
Erythrocytosis	Elevated Hb with normal	PaO_2 and Hb electrophoresis	Renal carcinoma, Wilms' tumour, adrenal tumours, hepatomas
			Erythrocytosis resolves with removal of primary. Erythropoietin is made by the tumour or its release is stimulated

These are some of the most common paraneoplastic syndromes.

*The endocrine syndromes are those where the hormonal syndrome is produced by a non-endocrine cancer.

ACTH, adrenocorticotrophic hormone; ADH, antidiuretic hormone; ALS, amyotrophic lateral sclerosis; BP, blood pressure; CSF[1], cerebrospinal fluid; CSF[2], colony-stimulating factor; EMG, electromyography; Hb, haemoglobin; hCG, human chorionic gonadotrophin; IL, interleukin; ITP, idiopathic thrombocytopenia.

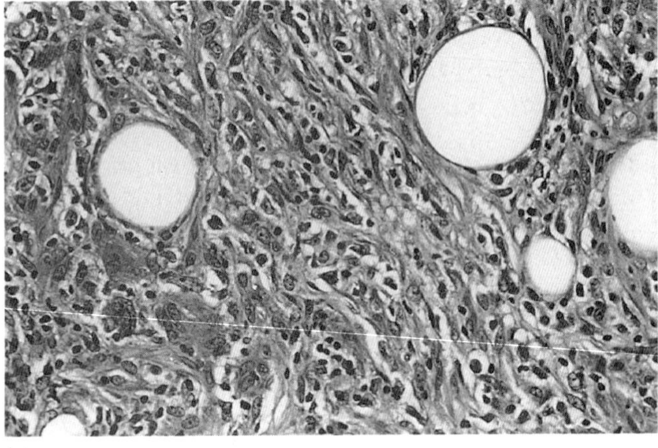

(a)

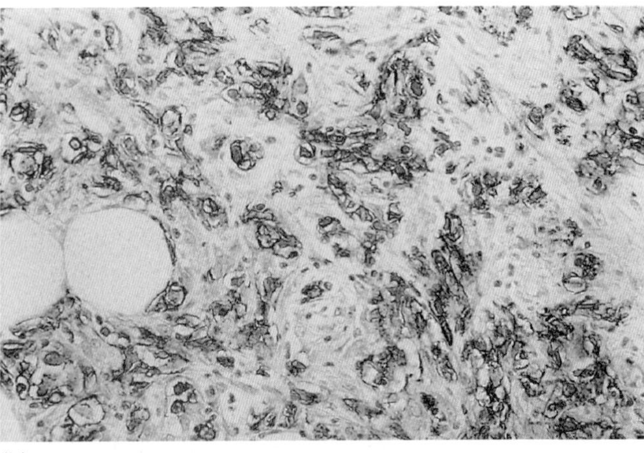

(b)

Fig. 6.5.1 (a) Section stained with haematoxylin and eosin of excision specimen of a retroperitoneal mass. The tumour is poorly differentiated, with fibrosis and infiltration of retroperitoneal fat. (b) Immunostaining with an antibody of CD20 (a B-lymphocyte marker) shows intense staining of tumour cells confirming that this is a B-cell non-Hodgkin's lymphoma.

inflammatory cellular infiltrate. As non-Hodgkin's lymphomas can present in many different sites, where the diagnosis is not clear a prudent physician will always ask the pathologist whether the diagnosis of lymphoma has been firmly excluded when a diagnosis of 'chronic inflammation' is made in an atypical clinical setting.

Mediastinal or metastatic germ cell tumours

These tumours may be mistaken for anaplastic carcinoma, but the recognition of a germ cell tumour is exceedingly important because many of them are curable. Mediastinal germ cell tumours typically present in young adults and with cervical node metastases. Special stains or serum tests for α-fetoprotein or β-human chorionic gonadotrophin may be very helpful, but if negative, do not exclude the diagnosis. Several studies have shown that the use of intensive combination chemotherapy, as for germ cell tumours at other sites, may result in lasting remissions of mediastinal poorly differentiated tumours in young adults, even when there were no other features of the germ cell nature of the neoplasm. In contrast, poorly differentiated adenocarcinoma in the mediastinum of young adults can seldom be ascribed to germ cell tumour, although occasional cases may respond dramatically to chemotherapy.

Investigation of local extent of a tumour

Following diagnosis, clinical staging is the most important first procedure. Clinical examination will often establish the likely extent of the tumour. This may require specialized techniques such as ear, nose, and throat examination and bronchoscopy. The extent of infiltration and fixation to surrounding structures is assessed. CT scanning and MRI have greatly improved the preoperative determination of tumour extent. They have largely replaced more invasive techniques such as angiography and lymphangiography. MRI is particularly valuable in the staging of sarcomas and central nervous system tumours. Both techniques show the extent of the tumour and infiltration of surrounding structures (Fig. 6.5.2). CT scanning is a valuable aid to needle biopsy diagnosis of deep-seated tumours.

Staging of lymph node spread

Spread to adjacent lymph nodes may be noted clinically or on straightforward investigations, such as chest radiography. Lymphangiography was used formerly to examine pelvic and lower para-aortic nodes but has largely been supplanted by CT. In fact the two techniques give slightly different information, as a CT scan will show enlarged lymph nodes (the assumption being that these are replaced by tumour when the lymph nodes become >2 cm in size), while lymphangiography may show abnormal appearances even when the nodes are not enlarged but contain foci of tumour cells within them.

An important development has been the introduction of so-called 'sentinel node' biopsy. In this technique a radioactive tracer, or a blue dye, is injected in the vicinity of the tumour, or into the tumour itself, and the lymph node at the first adjacent site of uptake is sampled, either by biopsy or surgical removal. In the case of breast cancer, the disease in which the technique is most widely used, the sampling may be at the time of operation. The presence or absence of tumour cells in the identified lymph node is taken as an indication of whether lymphatic spread has occurred. Surgery and subsequent treatment, can be modified accordingly. There are unresolved issues about accuracy and specificity of the technique in some tumours, and the confidence with which the results can be used to plan therapy.

Staging for distant metastases

Bone metastases are usually demonstrated by ^{99}Tcm-polyphosphate isotopic scanning. The sensitivity of the examination is high and abnormalities frequently precede detectable changes on plain radiography. However, the specificity is rather lower because any traumatic or inflammatory disorder in bone can give areas of increased uptake. When areas of increased uptake are seen on technetium scanning it is important to follow up with plain skeletal radiography, particularly in the long bones of the limbs. This is because isotope scanning gives no indication of the structural integrity of the bone and the risk of pathological fracture in a limb cannot be assessed on an isotope scan.

Liver metastases are detected by an increase in circulating enzyme levels, particularly alkaline phosphatase and serum glutamic oxaloacetic transaminase. Lactate dehydrogenase is also elevated in a somewhat greater frequency. Nevertheless, liver metastases can be present without alteration in serum enzyme levels and ultrasound scanning is an invaluable noninvasive method of detecting

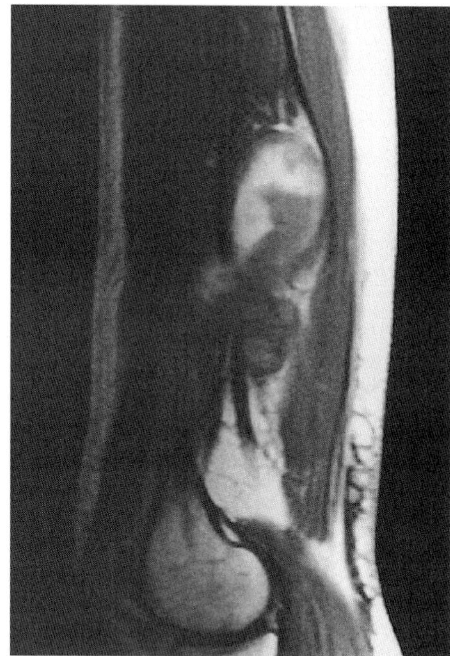

(a)

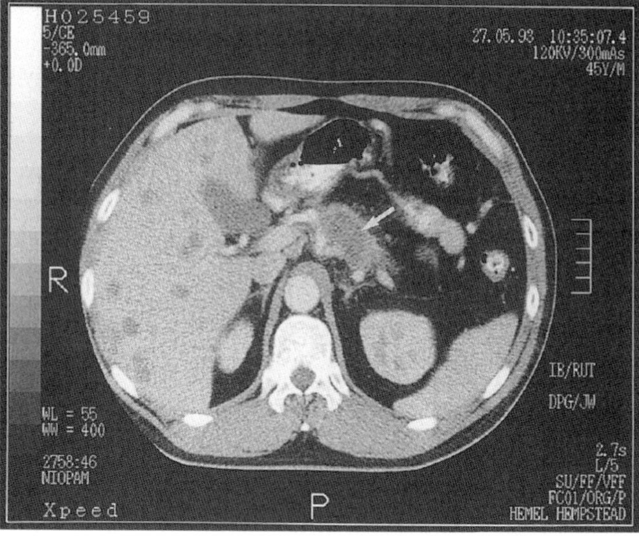

(b)

Fig. 6.5.2 (a) Longitudinal MRI of lower thigh. A large soft-tissue mass is seen displacing the muscle groups posteriorly. It lies behind the femur and the femoral artery is in close proximity to the mass, which at one point surrounds it. (b) CT scan of abdomen. A carcinoma of the body of the pancreas is shown (arrowed). The liver contains numerous small metastases.

liver metastases. CT and modern ultrasound scanning are approximately equal in sensitivity. Metastases down to 1 cm in size can be detected reliably.

Pulmonary metastases may be detected on the chest radiograph, but if they are less than 1.5 cm in size they may be present even when the radiograph appears normal. Metastases larger than this may also be overlooked if they are situated behind the heart or behind the diaphragm. CT scanning is the best method for demonstrating pulmonary metastases and lesions as small as 0.4 cm in diameter may be seen. CT scanning is therefore an essential investigation in patients who are to undergo extensive or mutilating surgery, such as for sarcomas where metastases to the lungs are particularly frequent, and the presence of metastases may influence the surgical decision.

Brain metastases are detected by CT scanning or, more reliably, by MRI. In a patient who is neurologically normal there is only a low chance of detecting asymptomatic cerebral metastasis by these methods (about 5%). For this reason the technique is not worthwhile as a routine investigation of most cancers.

Surgical staging of cancer

Surgery specifically for staging rather than for treatment is reserved for a few specific tumour sites. In lung cancer, investigation of the mediastinum is extremely important in deciding whether a tumour is operable. CT scanning may demonstrate inoperability either because the tumour is infiltrating the mediastinum or because there is lymph node spread to both ipsilateral and contralateral hilar nodes. However, in other patients, the mediastinum may appear normal and a mediastinoscopy may reveal tumour in mediastinal nodes implying the inoperability of the condition. Staging laparotomy used to be performed in localized Hodgkin's disease, but is now reserved for specific indications. In ovarian cancer thorough surgical staging is performed at the time of the initial resection, but surgical staging is in this case (as in many other tumour resections) part of the treatment.

The use of a staging notation

This has been valuable in the reporting of results of cancer treatment and is also helpful, in an individual patient, in focusing attention on the extent of the disease and the subsequent planning of treatment. The tumour–nodes–metastasis (TNM) system is widely used. This is particularly valuable for tumours that follow an orderly progression of spread from the primary site to adjacent lymph nodes and then to metastatic sites. Thus, tumours of the head and neck, breast, non-small-cell lung cancer, renal carcinoma, bladder carcinoma, and rectal carcinoma are all well defined by this means. In addition to the TNM system, many classifications contain a stage grouping, by which tumours with varying TNM assignments are grouped together because of equivalence of prognosis or similar approaches to management. An example of the TNM staging system and stage grouping for lung cancer is given in Table 6.5.2.

Not all tumours can be summarized by the TNM system. For example, small-cell lung cancer is usually widely metastatic at the time of presentation and a simpler classification into limited (confined to one side of the thorax with ipsilateral supraclavicular nodes) or extensive (disease that is bilateral within the chest or metastatic) is used. This simple classification serves to separate patients in whom radiation treatment may be worthwhile and those in whom it is unlikely to have any benefit. In leukaemia and myeloma, other staging criteria have been developed, which are based on prognostic factors and are not related to anatomical stage. In Hodgkin's disease and non-Hodgkin's lymphoma, the presence (B) or absence (A) of constitutional symptoms is added to the anatomical staging system, which is used to define the degree of lymph node spread. These additions were made because the presence of constitutional symptoms confers an adverse prognostic significance in addition to the prognosis related to the anatomical stage (see also Section 22).

Table 6.5.2 Staging of non-small cell lung cancer

T_1	<3 cm diameter		
T_2	>3 cm diameter but		
	>2 cm distal to carina, may be visceral pleural invasion		
T_3	Involves chest wall or mediastinum		
T_4	Invades heart, great vessels, trachea or oesophagus, malignant pleural effusion		
N_0	No involved nodes		
N_1	Ipsilateral peribronchial or hilar nodes		
N_2	Ipsilateral mediastinal or subcarinal		
N_3	Contralateral nodes or supraclavicular nodes		
M_0	No distant metastases		
M_1	Distant metastases		
Stage grouping			
Stage 1	$T_{1,2}$	N_0	M_0
Stage 2	$T_{1,2}$	N_1	M_0
Stage 3_a	$T_{1,2}$	N_2	M_0
	T_3	N_{0-2}	M_0
Stage 3_b	AnyT	N_3	M_0
	T_4	Any N	M_0
Stage 4	AnyT	Any N	M_1

Table 6.5.3 The management of tumours

Chemotherapy (including endocrine therapy)	Radiotherapy
May be curative in:	*May be curative in:*
Hodgkin's disease	Localized Hodgkin's disease
Non-Hodgkin's lymphoma	Non-Hodgkin's lymphoma
Germ cell tumours	Stage II seminoma
Wilm's tumour	Head and neck cancer
Ewing's sarcoma	
Osteosarcoma	
Rhabdomyosarcoma	
Leukaemia	
Adds to cure rate in:	*Adds to cure rate in:*
Stage II breast cancer	Ewing's sarcoma
? Colorectal cancer	Localized breast cancer
Ovarian cancer	Small-cell lung cancer
Small-cell lung cancer	Anal cancer
	Cervical cancer
	Skin cancer
	Rectal cancer
Produces remission and/or prolongs survival in:	*Produces remission and/or prolongs survival in:*
Small-cell lung cancer	Non-small cell lung cancer
Advanced breast cancer	Glioma
Prostate cancer	Prostate cancer
Ovarian cancer	Biliary tract cancer
Myeloma	
Palliates:	*Palliates:*
Non-Hodgkin's lymphoma (when incurable)	Small-cell lung cancer (extensive)
Bone metastases	Non-small-cell lung cancer
Brain metastases	Rectal cancer
	Oesophageal cancer

Principles of cancer management

The principles and details of cancer chemotherapy are discussed in Chapter 6.6. This section summarizes an integrated approach towards cancer management.

Nowadays the management of cancer will nearly always involve more than one specialist and more than one type of treatment. Increasingly, patients with cancer are seen in joint clinics where surgeons, medical oncologists, and radiotherapists plan treatment. Often there will be several possible approaches towards treatment, and these require discussion and assessment by the appropriate experts. It is of great value if a patient is referred for expert opinion before any definitive procedure is undertaken. For example, more information about gynaecological malignancy can often be obtained if a patient with abdominal swelling and ascites and an ultrasound-demonstrable mass in the pelvis is assessed preoperatively by a gynaecological oncologist. The subsequent laparotomy is likely to reveal much more information than if it is carried out as an emergency by an inexperienced surgeon. Similarly, a mass on a limb should be investigated thoroughly, including a biopsy diagnosis, before surgery is undertaken, because the nature of the histological diagnosis may profoundly alter management in the case of a sarcoma. Table 6.5.3 lists tumours in which radiotherapy and chemotherapy have an important part to play in management and where these modalities of treatment may sometimes be curative.

Surgery

Surgeons see more than 80% of patients presenting with cancer for the first time. Following diagnosis and staging to exclude metastases, curative surgery may be undertaken, e.g. in breast or colorectal cancer. The aim of the operation is complete excision of the tumour with a margin of normal, uninvolved tissue around the main tumour mass. The risk of local recurrence is very high with a marginal excision in which a tumour has been 'shelled out', because the pseudocapsule around the tumour is likely to be infiltrated with tumour cells. Removal or sampling of the draining lymph nodes will often be undertaken, e.g. in breast cancer, malignant melanoma, and other tumours where involvement of regional lymph nodes is likely (see the discussion of sentinel node biopsy above). In some cancers, such as breast cancer, it has become clear that extensive primary tumours are usually accompanied by distant metastasis. In this situation the role of surgery is mainly to prevent local recurrence and systemic treatment is essential. With other tumours, e.g. cancers of the head and neck, extensive surgery may be the only means of both gaining effective control and in obtaining a cure and in these cases a considerable degree of surgical expertise is necessary. In other situations the tumour may be approached either by surgery or by radical radiotherapy and there may be little to choose between the results. An example is in early prostate cancer where the results of radical radiation and surgery are probably equivalent, and in operable oesophageal cancer, particularly of squamous histology, where long-term results of radiation may be the same as those of surgery. In these situations the benefits of local control, survival, and long-term side-effects have to be judged together in making a decision.

Nowadays local treatment frequently involves surgery and radiation to maximize the chances of local control. Wide local excision is increasingly practised in carcinoma of the breast, and radiation to the breast and to axillary nodes is used as an adjunct. Radiation reduces the risk of local relapse, both in the breast and in the axilla. Local excision and radiotherapy have now replaced mastectomy for many patients with small primary breast cancers. Preoperative radiation of soft tissue sarcoma may sometimes increase the chance of successful compartmental excision of the tumour, and postoperative radiation decreases the risk of local recurrence in patients in whom the excision has been marginal. These are just two examples of the many ways in which the definitive local management of the primary tumour is a matter of discussion between surgical and radiation oncologists.

Optimum local management has become further complicated by the responsiveness of some tumours to modern chemotherapy. An example is the treatment of Ewing's tumour. In this highly malignant round-cell tumour of childhood, initial chemotherapy usually produces a prompt regression of the main tumour mass, both in the bone and in the surrounding soft tissues. However, the tumour permeates widely through the bone, and local irradiation, given after initial chemotherapy, is a standard means of maintaining local control. However, in large tumours, even with full-dose radiation, the risk of local relapse is still present. For this reason surgery is being used increasingly, provided that the cosmetic and functional results are reasonable. Surgical excision alone may be successful after chemotherapy, but frequently, because of the permeating nature of the tumour, viable tumour is present right up to the resection margins of the bone. In this situation radiation will be needed in addition to the chemotherapy and surgery. This is an example of how, in some tumours, very detailed planning of the approach to treatment by experienced specialists is essential for optimum results.

Specific management problems and medical emergencies

Spinal cord and cauda equina compression

Compression of the spinal cord and cauda equina are common and devastating complications of metastatic cancer. For successful management it is essential to remember one rule—every hour counts. Even if early treatment is not always successful, delay ensures that the patient will become permanently bed- or chair-bound, paralysed, and incontinent.

The metastasis often develops in a vertebra, from which it spreads directly or via the intervertebral foramina to compress the cord (or cauda equina below L1) from the extradural space (Fig. 6.5.3). Alternatively, the malignant mass may originate in a mass of retroperitoneal nodes, or the primary tumour (for example a bronchial carcinoma) may be in the posterior mediastinum or retroperitoneum (Fig. 6.5.3). Damage to the cord is by direct compression and by interruption of the arterial supply leading to infarction. It is uncommon for the tumour to be metastatic to the cord itself, although meningeal spread occurs and may cause compression (see carcinomatous meningitis, below). Cord compression may be the first manifestation of cancer but more commonly arises with metastases from a known primary.

Pain often precedes the onset of neurological symptoms. In the case of cord compression it is felt in the thoracic and cervical vertebrae. It is worse on coughing. An exceedingly sinister symptom is vertebral pain with a root distribution. A patient with this symptom needs urgent investigation, as cord compression may be imminent. The next symptom is usually weakness of the legs combined with sensory loss, of which loss of proprioception is especially characteristic. Loss of bladder and bowel sensation is late; once weakness and bladder disturbance begins, progression to irreversible paraplegia occurs in hours or a few days.

The patient often has a sensory level, motor weakness, brisk leg reflexes, and extensor plantar responses. The bladder may be palpable. Radiography of the spine often shows vertebral destruction—loss of a pedicle or compression of the body being typical. MRI (and, less reliably, CT scanning) is indispensible and has now largely replaced myelography. Treatment usually consists of surgical decompression, although for radiation-sensitive tumours such as lymphoma or Ewing's sarcoma, high-dose corticosteroids and radiation will produce quick relief of compression.

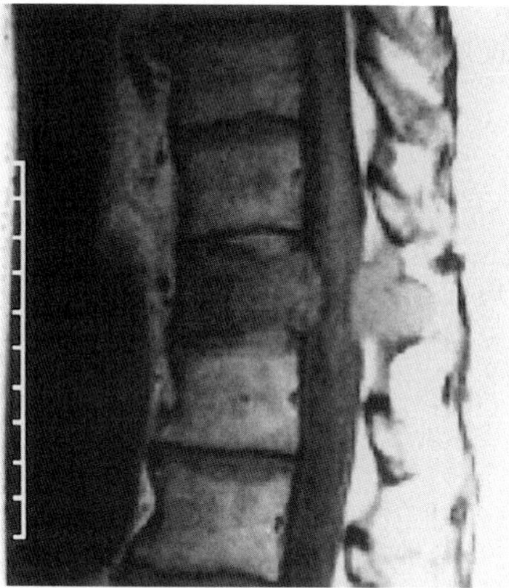

Fig. 6.5.3 MRI of thoracic vertebrae showing destruction of the body of T10 by a mass of Hodgkin's disease. The tumour extends posteriorly and compresses the spinal cord. The tumour mass has passed to the side of the vertebra (not shown), and is also compressing the cord posteriorly after infiltrating into the intervertebral foramen.

If there are multiple sites of block, radiation and steroids may be the only feasible option. The surgical approach to decompression varies according to the nature of the lesion—whether anterior or posterior, cervical or thoracic. Anterior decompression may involve removal of part of the vertebral body, but the risk of destabilization of the spine means that immediate stabilization may be necessary. It is not clear whether radiation is inferior to surgical decompression in patients with tumours that are sensitive to radiation. Radiation is, in any event, usually given after laminectomy.

Outcome is crucially dependent on the functional state of the patient before treatment. Less than 10% of those who are paraplegic before treatment will be able to walk later, 25% will do so if they have some motor function preserved, while almost all patients who can still walk on admission will continue to be able to do so.

Cerebral metastasis

Cerebral metastasis is clearly a serious complication of cancer, occurring in about 30% of all patients. Metastases are more than 10 times as common as primary brain tumours. About 15% of patients with cancer will develop symptomatic brain metastases during life. Thus, there will be approximately 15 000 deaths of patients with symptomatic cerebral metastasis each year in the United Kingdom. Metastasis at this site is life-threatening and disabling, causing severe deterioration in quality of life and great difficulty for patients and their carers.

Most cerebral metastases are intradural, usually in the substance of the brain extending to the meningeal surface. About 80% of these are situated in the cerebrum and the rest in the cerebellum and other regions. Lung cancer and breast cancer are the most common primary sites, and certain tumours are particularly associated with single metastases (cancer of the breast, ovary, and kidney). Although they may be the presenting symptom, cerebral metastases usually occur following diagnosis and treatment of a primary tumour.

In the brain substance, the metastases are vascularized from the cerebral circulation, but there is no evidence that a vascularized metastasis maintains a 'blood–brain' barrier—the vascularization is, after all, of nonnervous tissue without the tight endothelial junctions which characterize cerebral capillaries. Indeed, capillary leakiness appears to be a feature of cerebral metastasis and is responsible for the substantial amount of oedema of the brain that typically accompanies it. The blood–brain barrier may, however, be an important impediment to cytotoxic treatment when the metastasis is being established before it is vascularized and at the infiltrating periphery of an established metastasis. It will be a very significant factor in failure of treatment of leptomeningeal cancer.

Symptoms and signs

The typical signs of cerebral metastasis are headache, disturbance of cognitive function and affect, focal fits or grand mal convulsions, and limb paresis. Headache usually reflects a rise in intracranial pressure. It is typically present in the morning and increases in duration and frequency until other signs of raised intracranial pressure become apparent. Focal weakness is present in about half of all patients, and disturbance in higher cerebral function in about 60%.

Investigation

CT scanning or MRI is the essential diagnostic investigation. On a CT scan most metastases appear hypodense but enhance with contrast material. Typically there will be oedema around the metastases. Occasionally CT scans may be normal even in patients whose symptoms strongly suggest cerebral metastasis and where cerebral metastasis is sometimes proved by further scanning some weeks later or at autopsy. In these patients there may be multiple small metastases without oedema or leptomeningeal spread. MRI has a greater degree of sensitivity and is particularly valuable in detecting leptomeningeal spread of tumour. In the presence of a known primary it is not usually necessary to subject patients to histological confirmation of the tumour. However, after a very long disease-free interval, or where the primary is unknown, histological diagnosis will be essential.

Treatment

Dexamethasone is started as soon as the diagnosis is made. The usual dose is approximately 16 mg/day, although higher doses can be used if the patient does not respond. The clinical effects are rapid and usually noticeable within 24 h. The maximum effect is achieved in about 4 days. Approximately 80% of patients will respond. Phenytoin or carbamazepine are used to control focal fits.

The most useful nonsurgical treatment is radiation therapy. The therapeutic doses depend on the likely primary site, but usually consist of 30 Gy in 10 fractions in 2 weeks, or 40 Gy in 15 fractions in 3 weeks. The former is the most widely used schedule in the United Kingdom but no schedule has been proved to be superior over another. Solitary cerebral metastases may be removed if they are in an accessible site. The criteria for operation are usually that a solitary metastasis is present, that the diagnosis is uncertain, or that the response to radiation is unpredictable because of doubt about the nature of the primary tumour. The patient must be clinically fit in other respects to undergo surgery, and without life-threatening metastatic disease elsewhere.

There has been recent interest in the use of chemotherapy in the treatment of cerebral metastasis, as it is now clear, e.g. in small-cell lung cancer, that the response to chemotherapy in cerebral metastases is equal to that in metastases at other sites. Responses to chemotherapy in tumours such as small-cell lung cancer may be rapid and dramatic but cranial radiation will usually be necessary as an adjunct to chemotherapy.

Prognosis

The prognosis of cerebral metastasis depends on the clinical setting. If there is a solitary metastasis with no disease elsewhere then a long disease-free interval may result, particularly if the metastasis has occurred after a considerable interval following the primary treatment. In other tumours, where multiple metastases occur either synchronously with the primary tumour or after a short disease-free interval, and where the tumour is a particularly difficult type to treat (such as melanoma and non-small-cell lung cancer), the prognosis is very poor indeed. Overall, only 30% of patients will be alive at 1 year and the median survival is about 7 months. A small randomized trial has suggested that surgical resection of a solitary metastasis adds to survival when compared with radiation and steroids alone.

Carcinomatous 'meningitis'

Leptomeningeal spread of cancer seems to be increasing in frequency. In autopsy series about 4% of patients dying of advanced cancer have leptomeningeal spread. The frequency is higher in breast cancer (5–10%). This complication is increasing in lymphoma, small-cell lung cancer, ovarian cancer, and some sarcomas. Curiously, adenocarcinomas seem to have a greater propensity for this form of metastasis than other epithelial tumours. There may or may not be intracerebral metastasis at the same time. Malignant cells may enter the cerebrospinal fluid from intracerebral tumour via the arachnoid, or from vertebral deposits growing along nerve roots into the subarachnoid space. However, the most likely source of seeding appears to be directly from the bloodstream. Tumour is present as a thin covering of malignant cells, but the tumour cells may penetrate deeper into the substance of the brain along blood vessels. The tumour may also penetrate cranial and spinal cord nerves as they pass through the subarachnoid space.

Clinical features

The onset is usually over a few weeks and may be subtle at first. Headache is often severe and is due to raised intracranial pressure. Cranial nerve dysfunction is frequent, with diplopia, hearing loss, and facial numbness. There is often back pain and sometimes bladder and bowel dysfunction. A change in mental state may occur. Focal fits are uncommon. On examination there may be an abnormal mental state, signs of raised intracranial pressure, and extensor plantar responses. Focal neurological signs in the limbs are uncommon. Cranial nerve weaknesses are frequent, the most common being ocular muscle palsy, facial weakness, and hearing loss.

Diagnosis and treatment

The diagnosis is made by examining the cerebrospinal fluid. Typically, the opening pressure is high, the white count is raised, the cerebrospinal fluid sugar low, and the protein increased. Cytological confirmation on the first lumbar puncture is obtained in about 60% of patients, but a negative examination does not exclude the diagnosis. Myelography may show typical appearance of multiple small tumour seeds in the subarachnoid space, but MRI is proving invaluable and is now the preferred initial investigation if cerebrospinal fluid cytology is negative and the diagnosis strongly suspected.

Treatment is difficult and often unsuccessful. Temporary improvement can be obtained by the insertion of an intraventricular reservoir to deliver chemotherapy. Chemotherapy administered by lumbar puncture is uncomfortable and may not be effective if there is meningeal invasion supratentorially, since the drugs do not penetrate in high concentration beyond the foramen magnum. In breast cancer and lymphoma, intrathecal methotrexate is effective and may be administered in combination with thiotepa or, in the case of lymphoma, cytosine arabinoside. In addition, whole-brain irradiation is often given if the patient is improving and the clinical situation indicates that this treatment would produce further benefit. In general, however, the prognosis is poor when the meningeal infiltration is from an epithelial tumour, with a median survival of only 4 months.

Pleural effusion

Malignant pleural effusions occur either as a site of metastatic spread from outside the lung or due to direct invasion of the pleural space from an underlying primary bronchial carcinoma, or pulmonary metastasis. The effusions are typically exudates with a protein content of more than 3 g/dl. There is increased capillary permeability through inflammation and as a result of abnormal capillary endothelium in the tumour lining the pleural space. Typical primary sites are: breast and ovarian cancer, as common epithelial tumours metastasizing into the pleural space; lung cancer, as a cause of pleural effusion with underlying lung disease; and sarcomas, as a cause of pleural effusion due to invasion of the pleura by pulmonary metastasis.

Clinical features

The typical features are dyspnoea, which is directly related to the size of the effusion, dry cough, and chest wall discomfort. Even a small effusion may cause dyspnoea in a patient who has underlying lung disease such as chronic bronchitis and emphysema. Many patients have asymptomatic pleural effusions detectable on chest radiograph. The sequence of radiological appearances includes blunting of the costophrenic angle (occurring with volumes of more than 2–3 ml), increasing effusion, and, finally, mediastinal shift, which usually occurs when amounts in excess of 2 litres have accumulated. Ultrasound examination may assist in localizing the effusion and any loculi, which may influence the procedure for aspiration.

Diagnosis

The diagnosis, if the primary tumour is not known, is made by demonstrating malignant cells in the pleural fluid. The rate of positivity, in patients known to have an underlying cancer, is about 60% with a low false-positive rate. If pleural cytology is negative on the first aspiration it should be repeated using fresh aspirates. Occasionally, pleural biopsy will be necessary to make a diagnosis, and the combination of the two methods increase the diagnostic yield to about 90%. If both techniques fail, thoracoscopy is more successful, but is, of course, more invasive.

Treatment and prognosis

The primary tumour should be treated if possible. When a pleural effusion persists after treatment of the primary tumour, or if such treatment has been unsuccessful, treatment may need to be directed to the effusion itself. Frequently the effusion will need to be aspirated in order to make the patient comfortable, and pleural sclerotherapy considered. For best results of sclerotherapy it is important to drain the pleural cavity as completely as possible. A small flexible chest drain is ideal and is left in place for some time (12–24 h if possible) to allow the fluid to drain as far as possible. If there has been loculated effusion, the insertion of the drain is best done under ultrasound control. Sclerosis of the two pleural surfaces can be achieved by a variety of means; all give approximately equivalent results. The most favoured techniques are the instillation of talc, tetracycline, bleomycin, or *Corynebacterium parvum*. They all cause an inflammatory reaction in the pleural space and have an approximately 60% success rate in preventing immediate recurrence of the effusion. When pleural effusion complicates an underlying bronchial carcinoma it is more difficult to control than when it is a metastatic manifestation of a distant neoplasm, such as ovarian cancer. If the effusion is recurrent and is the major cause of morbidity, pleuroperitoneal shunting can be carried out, whereby the pleural fluid drains into the peritoneal cavity.

Pericardial effusion

The most common malignancies to cause pericardial effusion are breast, lung, ovary, and gastrointestinal cancers and non-Hodgkin's lymphomas. Pathologically, the pericardium may be infiltrated with tumour or diffusely nodular. The accumulation of fluid is due to obstruction of lymphatic and venous drainage of the pericardium.

Symptoms and signs

The symptoms are usually vague in onset, including orthopnoea, dyspnoea, and cough. Fatigue and dizziness also develop. If cardiac tamponade occurs it is associated with severe dyspnoea, vague central chest pain, and anxiety. The physical signs are usually minimal, although when tamponade occurs there will be jugular venous distension, pulses paradoxus, hypotension, and tachycardia.

Investigation

Investigations include a chest radiograph, which shows enlargement of the cardiac silhouette, and echocardiography, which is a rapid noninvasive technique for demonstrating pericardial effusion.

Diagnosis and management

The diagnosis is made by finding malignant cells in the pericardial fluid. False-negative results occur and the test may need to be repeated. Once the diagnosis has been established, the pericardial fluid may need drainage using a small rubber catheter. Installation of sclerosants can be carried out as for pleural effusions, but troublesome pericardial effusions can be controlled by the formation of a pericardial window through a small left anterior thoracotomy. Some patients, particularly those who have lymphoma, will respond to external-beam radiation with a dose of approximately 30 Gy given in 15 fractions over a 2- to 3-week period. Radiation is also considered for control of chronic pericardial effusion in breast cancer. The management of cardiac tamponade is discussed in Section 16.

Metastatic cancer from an unknown primary site

Approximately 3% of patients present with a metastasis from a cancer where the primary site is not known after full history, physical examination, blood count, and chest radiograph. This clinical situation requires considerable clinical expertise, as the diagnosis creates especial anxiety for the patient. The clinician has to decide on the most effective therapy and to sustain the patient without indulging in futile, invasive, and expensive investigations which will not alter management. The problem with extensive investigations is that they seldom alter management and the overall prognosis in this position is poor (4–6 months median survival). As one investigation after another fails to reveal the primary site, the patient and the doctor may come to consider this a failure and confidence can be badly shaken. Nevertheless, some tumours are potentially curable and, for these, investigation is justified. The common primary sites, when one is discovered, are cancers of the lung, pancreas, liver, gut, and stomach. The tumours for which therapy is possible, and which therefore must not be overlooked, are listed in Table 6.5.4.

Table 6.5.4 Metastasis from an unknown primary site. Possibilities for treatment

Potentially curable tumours
Germ cell tumours
Lymphomas
Trophoblastic tumours
Effective palliative chemotherapy
Breast cancer
Small-cell lung cancer
Ovarian cancer
Palliative hormonal therapy
Prostate cancer
Breast cancer
Endometrial cancer
Effective (potentially curative) local therapy
Head and neck cancer

Presentation

If the presentation is exclusively in cervical nodes, a full ear, nose, and throat examination is mandatory as local treatment with surgery and/or radiation may produce prolonged survival or even cure for primary cancers as this site. The higher the cervical node, the more likely it is that and ear, nose, and throat tumour is the primary source. Supraclavicular lymph nodes carry a worse prognosis because the likely primary site on the right-hand side is the lung or breast, and on the left-hand side intra-abdominal malignancy may have spread via the thoracic duct. Patients presenting with lymph node enlargement in the axilla are likely to have breast cancer as the primary site and this may not be excluded even with normal mammograms. Malignant melanoma is another possibility at this site and a careful examination for skin lesions should be made. Inguinal lymph nodes usually point to a primary site in the pelvis, vulva or rectum, or prostate. Malignant melanoma may also present with an inguinal mass. Cutaneous metastasis typically occurs from carcinomas of the lung, breast, and melanomas. A pulmonary metastasis may arise from a variety of different sites, of which breast, kidney, gut, melanoma, and sarcoma are the most common. In the liver, the likely source for the primary will be the gastrointestinal tract, although breast and lung primaries are other possibilities. A metastasis presenting in bone is particularly likely to occur from a cancer of the lung, breast, or prostate, the last being particularly likely if there is a mixed lytic and osteoblastic radiological appearance.

Investigation

The most important single investigation is a review of the histology. The clinician should discuss the diagnosis with the pathologist so that appropriate tests can be carried out. It is absolutely essential to distinguish between an epithelial tumour, a sarcoma, and a lymphoma. Immunohistochemistry may be invaluable in this respect. If there is any question of a germ cell tumour, the section should be stained for α-fetoprotein, β-human chorionic gonadotrophin, and placental alkaline phosphatase. If the histology is that of adenocarcinoma, the diagnosis will be more difficult and special stains may not serve to elucidate the diagnosis further. Where possible, the tissue should be examined for the presence of oestrogen or progesterone receptor, as this would make carcinoma of the breast or ovary more likely. The protein S100 is typically present in melanoma and may be invaluable in distinguishing this diagnosis from anaplastic carcinoma.

Further investigation and management

Investigation must be selective. Since there is specific treatment available for breast and prostate cancer, these diagnoses must always be considered when the histology is adenocarcinoma. Mammography is therefore justifiable, and measurement of serum acid phosphatase and prostatic specific antigen are simple and noninvasive. A pelvic ultrasound examination may show an ovarian mass, which may influence management as platinum-based combination chemotherapy might then be used, whereas it would not be contemplated in many patients with metastasis from an unknown primary site in view of its toxicity. The possibility of a germ cell tumour must always be considered in a young person, and in these circumstances full investigation is necessary if this diagnosis is possible.

Treatment follows pragmatic lines. Locally troublesome or painful metastases are treated with irradiation. If breast cancer seems a possible diagnosis a trial of hormone therapy is fully justified and, similarly, hormone treatment of prostatic cancer should be introduced if this seems a likely diagnosis. As mentioned above, radiation is frequently given to patients with enlarged cervical nodes when the diagnosis is poorly differentiated carcinoma, even if a head and neck primary has not been found.

The use of combination chemotherapy when the primary site is not known is more controversial. In general, responses are infrequent and are not long lasting. This drug treatment should be reserved for patients with more than one lesion and particularly when symptoms occur. It is important not to be dogmatic about this issue because many patients find it quite unacceptable to be told that no treatment of any kind is available to them, and are willing to accept the possible toxicities of chemotherapy in exchange for the chance of response. Most chemotherapy programmes will include an alkylating agent and some include doxorubicin or a taxane.

Supportive care of the patient with cancer (see also Section 31)

Psychological support

Nearly everyone will have had friends or relatives who have had cancer and who may have died of it, and they will have read articles and seen television programmes about cancer and its management. Many patients will have been worried about the possibility of cancer before they ever consult their general practitioner, or are subjected to a series of diagnostic tests, the effect of which may be to increase their anxiety. At each stage in the diagnostic process physicians should be aware of patients' feelings and be prepared to talk openly to them about why investigations are being performed. When the diagnosis is established it is essential for the physician to sit quietly with the patient, explaining the nature of the diagnosis and the broad principles that treatment will follow. Sometimes patients will like to have a member of the family with them during this conversation, in case they forget aspects of what is said. The conversation should take place quietly, not on a ward round, with both the patient and the physician seated and the physician calm and unhurried in approach. Avoidance of the word 'cancer', body language that indicates discomfiture or embarrassment, and evasion and vagueness are very likely to be interpreted by the patient as signs of a serious or hopeless outlook.

Many patients will be unable to take in all that is said in the first conversation, and physicians need to make it quite plain that they will be very pleased to talk again the next day, to go over points that need further clarification. There is much useful literature for patients to take home, there are professional and expert support groups that patients can contact and, in many hospitals, skilled counsellors who can provide follow-up support after the physician has outlined the basis of treatment. It is essential that all members of the medical team understand what was said and what words were used. The members of the family also need to understand exactly what information has been imparted. It may be necessary to hold back on a precise prognosis; first, because one may not be known until treatment starts, and second, because patients naturally tend to become fixated on the numerical prognosis, which is likely to be extremely inaccurate. If referral to an oncologist is to be made, it is critical to indicate exactly what has been said to the patient. Oncologists are put in an extremely difficult position when patients arrive with a diagnosis of cancer, without any indication at all of whether they know the diagnosis, or what words have been used.

A new difficulty in communication is now displacing the problems that formerly arose from concealment of the diagnosis. Modern cancer management is often complex, with equivalent results sometimes being obtained from approaches that have different early and late effects. A well-intentioned wish to 'share' the treatment decisions with the patient, and an increasing resort to litigation when events do not turn out well, has led doctors sometimes to present treatment options as a series of uncertainties in which the outcome will be strongly influenced by chance and fate. It is bad enough to be told you have cancer: worse still if your treatment seems mired in uncertainty. For some patients, treatment options will have been made even less clear by access to unfiltered advice on the internet, from reputable sources, charlatans, and cranks. There is nothing paternalistic in sensible advice from a well-informed, kind, sensitive, and experienced specialist. Questions which arise from complexity of choice and outcome in management increase the need for competent advice; they are not answered by passing the problem to the patient. Much distress, and a feeling of being abandoned, can come from lack of clear guidance.

Following treatment, patients frequently feel anxious and unsettled for many months or more. Even when unpleasant, treatment has the connotation of actively preventing recurrence of the disease. When this stops patients may need support, which they get most often from family and friends. Nevertheless minor symptoms are frequently the cause of anxiety for a year or two. A cancer service should offer all patients easy and informal access to advice that continues after treatment (a contact telephone number and an email address are what is needed). The simple fact of being available provides comfort and reassurance.

When treatment is to be palliative, after relapse or with widespread metastatic disease, it should none the less be made clear to the patient that it is 'treatment'. Patients dislike feeling that they are being abandoned. Indeed, many wise oncologists see their patients more frequently when they are having palliative treatment than they do during routine treatments or follow-up. They do this because palliative treatment requires great attention to detail, especially with respect to control of pain and other symptoms, and also to provide psychological support for the patient and the family. One of the most common reasons for patients seeking second opinions is that they have been given no feeling that there are possibilities for treatment in their case. Continuity in management is one of the most rewarding aspects of cancer medicine for the physician and for the patient. There is no place for impersonal clinics where patients see different doctors each time they attend, and where the emotional component of their illness cannot be properly explored.

Management of cancer pain

Pain is a common and distressing feature of cancer. A careful history is essential to determine the exact site and nature of the pain and to establish a close and trusting relationship with a patient who feels that the symptom is being taken seriously. Exacerbating factors should be noted and an anatomical diagnosis made as far as possible. If the pain is arising in a bone it may be quickly and effectively helped by radiation treatment. The primary tumour or metastasis may be responsive to treatment with irradiation or chemotherapy. If specific antitumour treatments of this kind are not appropriate, then the only approach is to control the pain with analgesics.

Nonnarcotic analgesics are used for mild or moderate pain. Useful agents include aspirin, paracetamol, and nonsteroidal anti-inflammatory drugs such as ketoprofen or naproxen. A combination may be useful. Combination drugs such as co-proxamol or co-dydramol are also helpful. Although prescribing each drug separately allows greater control over the constituents, in practice this may not be helpful, particularly for older patients who often find it difficult to take multiple medication. The aim of treatment should be to prevent pain as far as possible by taking regular analgesics, and to have additional analgesics on hand for an acute exacerbation. Side effects of nonopiate analgesics include gastric irritation (and they should therefore be used cautiously if steroids are being used at the same time), nausea, and constipation, particularly with codeine, oxycodone, or propoxyphene.

If these analgesics do not control the pain, opiate analgesics are essential. Two preparations have made an enormous contribution to pain relief. The first is long-acting morphine sulphate, which can be given twice daily, and the second is short-acting morphine sulphate. The former has a duration of action of 8 to 12 h and the latter of about 4 h. One curious feature of the use of morphine-like drugs is that the dose required to control pain varies greatly from person to person. It must therefore be found by trial and error, and the patient must be prepared to increase the dose under medical supervision. The aim is to produce background pain relief for most of the day and night. Short-acting morphine sulphate is particularly useful for dealing with acute exacerbations of pain.

If oral opiates are unable to control pain fully, continuous subcutaneous infusion is a useful alternative. This approach is particularly valuable in patients who cannot tolerate oral analgesics because of gastrointestinal symptoms, or where the tumour causes nausea or intestinal obstruction. Many pumps are now available, which are designed for continuous infusion through a small-gauge butterfly needle implanted subcutaneously. Patients can manage at home with these infusion pumps, with a nurse calling daily to change the infusion mixture.

Specialized forms of analgesia

A detailed discussion is beyond the scope of this chapter. Among the specialized techniques available are continuous epidural and intrathecal opiate infusion, nerve block procedures (including coeliac plexus block, peripheral nerve block, and epidural blocks), neurosurgical procedures, such as ablation of the peripheral nerve by neurectomy or, more radically, interruption of pain pathways by cordotomy. Each of these procedures has its value and limitations and the advice of specialists in the field of pain relief will be necessary.

Long-term consequences of successful cancer treatment

The welcome improvements in survival for many cancers has brought increasing realization that there are many subsequent medical and social problems that may affect patients, often several years after treatment has ended; their nature and frequency depending on the tumour and on the nature of the treatment. Medical personnel in almost every discipline will encounter these and they will continue to increase in frequency as cure rates improve and treatments are intensified. This is most apparent as a result of the increased cure rate of cancer in childhood and adolescence. This is one of the great triumphs of modern management but surveillance to detect long-term consequences, physical, psychological and metabolic, must extend for many years into adult life. Increasingly, this is true for adults as well. The following are some of the most important consequences.

- Fertility may be greatly reduced. In fertile boys and men, sperm storage is essential before cytotoxic chemotherapy begins. Cessation of spermatogenesis is almost immediate with many (but not all) chemotherapy agents. In a woman of child-bearing years chemotherapy, especially if it includes alkylating agents, will shorten the reproductive period of her life and may induce the menopause if she is in her mid-30s or later. Advice on this matter is essential if later regrets and unhappiness are to be avoided.
- Cognitive impairment is a serious consequence of tumours affecting the central nervous system. Children and young adults may suffer lifelong lost opportunity, both socially and occupationally. This may have a great impact on family life and require professional support.
- Musculoskeletal consequences are common. These are perhaps expected when the primary treatment has involved limb or trunk surgery, but bone rarefaction is a long term consequence of localized radiotherapy at any site when bone has been included within the field. Pathological fracture is more likely to occur in a weight-bearing bone. If the radiation field includes a growing epiphysisis, bone growth ceases with subsequent unilateral shortening. The use of aromatase inhibitors as adjuvant treatment for oestrogen receptor-positive breast cancer is associated with osteoporosis and risk of fracture.
- Metabolic problems are most frequently encountered when treatment has included drugs such as cisplatin and ifosfamide that frequently cause reduced glomerular filtration and tubular disorders (potassium and calcium loss, impaired acidification). Although these are monitored during treatment, these drugs are useful in the treatment of many tumours, especially in childhood, with long-lasting impairment.
- Second cancers are increasing in frequency. In adults these include radiation-induced cancers in bone, soft tissue and breast,

typically appearing within the radiation field 5–15 years after treatment. Secondary leukaemia is a well-recognized complication of chemotherapy, being particularly likely to occur when this has included etoposide or alkylating agents.

- Circulatory disorders mainly involve reduced cardiac output and arrythmias associated with anthracycline administration. With more complex regimens of treatment involving drugs that act on tumour vasculature, these complications may increase in frequency.

Further reading

Souhami R, Tobias J (2005). *Cancer and its management*, 5th edition. Blackwell, Oxford.

Tobias JS, Hochhauser D (2010). *Cancer and its management*. Blackwell, Oxford.

6.6

Cancer chemotherapy and radiation therapy

Bruce A. Chabner and Jay Loeffler

Essentials

The last two decades have brought significant improvements in cancer therapy: patients with previously fatal diseases, including acute leukaemia, non-Hodgkin's lymphoma, Hodgkin's disease, and germ cell tumours, now have a reasonable expectation of cure. For patients with the more common solid tumours, including lung, colon, and breast cancer, new chemotherapeutic and hormonal agents and monoclonal antibodies have improved treatment of both early and late stage disease and have extended survival. Nevertheless, cancer remains the second leading cause of death in the Western world, and nearly 40% of patients diagnosed with cancer will die of their disease.

Surgery, chemotherapy, and radiation therapy are the major modalities of cancer therapy, and are employed together in various sequences and combinations in most cancer patients.

Chemotherapy

Mechanism of action—most chemotherapy drugs block steps in the synthesis of DNA or its precursor nucleotides (purines and pyrimidines), or attack the integrity of DNA. These drugs are maximally effective if tumour cells are exposed during the S phase of the cell cycle, although some drugs (e.g. vinca alkaloids and taxanes) directly block cells during mitosis, and others (e.g. alkylating agents) act throughout the cell cycle.

Clinical use—chemotherapy can be applied as (1) combination chemotherapy with multiple drugs to cure some sensitive diseases, e.g. some types of leukaemia, or diminish tumour-related symptoms, improve the quality of life, and extend survival in less sensitive cancers, e.g. lung, colon; (2) palliative therapy for the treatment of advanced-stage or metastatic cancer; (3) adjuvant therapy, administered after the completion of definitive local surgery and/or radiation therapy to decrease the risk of recurrence of disease locally and at distant sites.

Complications—most of the commonly used chemotherapy agents cause acute myelosuppression; nausea and vomiting are frequent, but can often be helped by corticosteroids and serotonin uptake inhibitors (e.g. odansetron). Other problems specific to particular agents or classes of agent include (1) alopecia—doxorubicin and alkylating agents, (2) peripheral neuropathy—vinca alkaloids and platinum analogues, (3) left ventricular failure—doxorubicin, (4) pneumonitis—bleomycin, (5) infertility—alkylating agents. A very significant, delayed side effect of chemotherapy is the development of secondary leukaemias.

Radiation therapy

Mechanism of action—radiation therapy generates free radicals that damage DNA, producing breaks that must be repaired if the cell is to survive. Many tumours are less able than normal tissues to repair these breaks, providing a therapeutic window for successful treatment. Irradiation also inflicts potent damaging effects on tumour vasculature

Clinical use—radiation doses are usually delivered as an external beam from a source outside the body in a number of daily fractions, the total fractionated dose being determined by tumour sensitivity and normal tissue tolerance. Other methods of delivery include (1) brachytherapy—when the radiation source is implanted within the substance of the tumour, e.g. cervical cancer; (2) intraoperative radiation therapy—delivering a single, large fraction of radiation directly to the tumour bed; (3) radioisotopes—e.g. iodine-131 taken up by local and metastatic thyroid tissue; monoclonal antibodies coupled with radioisotopes to localize at tumour sites. For palliative irradiation of metastatic tumours, single large doses (radiosurgery) or abbreviated courses of irradiation (hypofractionated radiotherapy) may be administered to relieve symptoms.

Complications—toxicity to normal tissues within the field of radiation therapy or at its margins can be significant. Effects can be (1) acute—during the treatment course—particularly including damage to skin (erythema, desquamation, oedema), mucosal linings (diarrhoea, nausea, vomiting) and bone marrow (cytopenias); (2) subacute—after treatment but within a few months of therapy—e.g. radiation pneumonitis; and (3) late—permanent—including local tissue damage (e.g. transverse myelitis, bowel strictures, renal failure) and secondary tumours within radiation fields.

Chemotherapy

The rationale for cancer chemotherapy is based on principles of tumour biology. Cancer results from mutations in critical genes that control cell proliferation, DNA repair, and cell death. Tumours are usually clonal in origin, beginning with a single transformed cell that grows in an uncontrolled fashion, and invades and destroys normal neighbouring tissues (see Chapter 6.2). Tumour cells acquire the ability to secrete factors that promote the local growth of new blood vessels. This so-called 'angiogenic switch' represents a critical transition in their life history. Tumour cells may also acquire the capacity to migrate through the lymphatics and bloodstream to distant sites. Each of these important steps in the natural history of tumours requires the expression of specific proteins and pathways that have become the targets for new therapies.

The life cycle of a cancer cell is characterized by several phases: resting (G0), pre-DNA synthesis (G1), DNA synthesis (S), post-DNA synthesis (G2), and mitosis (M). Most chemotherapy drugs block steps in the synthesis of DNA or its precursor nucleotides (purines and pyrimidines), or attack the integrity of DNA. These drugs are maximally effective if tumour cells are exposed during the S phase of the cell cycle, although some drugs, such as the vinca alkaloids and taxanes, directly block cells during mitosis and others, such as the alkylating agents, act throughout the cell cycle.

Chemotherapy can be used in several different settings (Table 6.6.1). Foremost, chemotherapy is applied as primary therapy for the treatment of advanced-stage or metastatic cancer, when surgery or radiation therapy can no longer offer cure. Some diseases, including leukemias, lymphomas, and advanced-stage germ cell tumours are sensitive to multiple chemotherapy agents and can be cured with combination chemotherapy. In the less sensitive epithelial cancers, such as colon and lung cancer, combinations of agents are used to diminish tumour-related symptoms, improve the quality of life, and extend survival. For example, randomized clinical trials of chemotherapy vs best supportive care have demonstrated a survival advantage and quality of life improvement when patients with advanced-stage lung cancer receive multidrug chemotherapy.

Table 6.6.1 The role of chemotherapy in cancer management

Primary therapy (curative)
Acute lymphoblastic leukaemia, acute myeloblastic leukaemia
Hodgkin's disease
Non-Hodgkin's lymphoma
Germ cell tumours
Ewing's sarcoma
Small cell lung cancer (with radiation therapy)
Adjuvant therapy
Breast cancer
Colon cancer
Neoadjuvant therapy
Oesophageal cancer (with radiation)
Stage III non-small cell lung cancer
Head and neck cancer
Palliative therapy
Lung cancer
Breast cancer
Pancreatic cancer
Colorectal cancer

Secondly, chemotherapy is effective when given prior to radiation or surgery to cause shrinkage or disappearance of locally advanced disease. In this 'neoadjuvant' setting, the drugs, if effective, allow less extensive and less morbid surgery or irradiation, and make it possible to preserve organ function. Neoadjuvant chemotherapy is routinely given to patients with osteosarcoma, and to those with locally advanced lung, head and neck, breast, or oesophageal cancers, prior to surgery or radiation therapy. In the case of osteosarcomas, the response to neoadjuvant therapy can provide important information about tumour sensitivity, thereby permitting a more tailored approach to further management after surgery.

Finally, the drugs can be used as adjuvant therapy, administered after the completion of definitive local surgery and/or radiation therapy in order to decrease the risk of recurrence of disease locally and at distant sites. Adjuvant chemotherapy reduces the risk of tumour recurrence and improves survival in node-positive colon cancer, lung cancer, and breast cancer following surgical resection of the primary tumour. In the adjuvant setting and, more commonly, in the neoadjuvant setting, chemotherapy may be administered in sequence with, or simultaneously with, radiation therapy to optimize local effects of treatment.

Only in rare circumstances, such as methotrexate therapy for choriocarcinoma, can single agents cure advanced-stage cancer. Single agents tend to select for drug-resistant cells. Most often, therapy with multiple drugs has been required to effect cure. In combining drugs, it is imperative to employ agents that have independent activity and nonoverlapping toxicities so that the individual drugs can be used at their optimal dose and in their optimal schedule. Chemotherapy schedules are designed to permit marrow recovery before the next dose administration. Typically, peripheral blood counts will reach a nadir 5 to 10 days after therapy, with recovery by day 21. Hematopoietic growth factors such as granulocyte colony-stimulating factor (G-CSF) speed the recovery of neutrophils and allow regimens to be repeated every 2 weeks. Such 'dose dense' regimens may be more effective than the standard 3-week cycle in the adjuvant treatment of breast cancer.

Combinations of drugs circumvent tumour cell resistance, so treatments have been designed in which non-cross-resistant drugs are administered either together or in sequence. One of the earliest combination therapy programmes to cure a cancer was MOPP (mechlorethamine, vincristine, prednisone, and procarbazine), used for the treatment of Hodgkin's disease. Combination chemotherapy is now the mainstay for treating most acute leukemias, non-Hodgkin's lymphoma, testicular cancer, choriocarcinoma, and for most adjuvant and neoadjuvant regimens for epithelial cancers. Acute lymphoblastic leukaemia can now be cured in 90% of children using multidrug chemotherapy administered at frequent dosing intervals to avoid the development of resistant cells. Alternatively, extremely high doses of therapy can be used to overcome tumour resistance in patients with lymphoma who relapse after standard dose chemotherapy, but this may obligate the use of autologous haematopoietic stem cells harvested from peripheral blood or bone marrow to overcome the resulting profound bone marrow toxicity.

Chemotherapeutic drugs have both acute and late toxicities, and may affect virtually every organ system. The late toxicity may diminish organ function, causing congestive heart failure (after anthracyclines), pulmonary fibrosis (after alkylating agents or bleomycin), or kidney failure (after platinum-based therapies), or may damage reproductive tissues, brain, and other organs. In addition many drugs, particularly the alkylating agents, are leukaemogenic. Both the medical oncologist who manages the patient through the phase of active treatment, and the internist involved in later stages of follow-up must be alert to these toxicities and informed about their management.

Because of the serious toxicities of chemotherapy, physicians should administer regimens that have been carefully studied and reported in the peer-reviewed medical literature. New regimens tested in the context of well-designed clinical trials may offer the best alternatives to standard therapy. Clinicians should not routinely administer new drug combinations on the basis of anecdotal evidence.

Classes of chemotherapeutic agents

There are several distinct classes of chemotherapy agents (Table 6.6.2). In order to reduce interpatient variability in exposure to drugs, doses of most chemotherapy agents are calculated on the basis of body surface area, as determined by the patient's height and weight. In addition, doses of chemotherapy may need to be reduced in treating patients with renal dysfunction (methotrexate, bleomycin, hydroxyurea, fludarabine) or hepatic dysfunction (anthracyclines, vinca alkaloids, taxanes), depending on the primary route of drug clearance.

Adequate intravenous access, through an implanted central venous line, must be secured since many of the drugs are vesicants and extravasation can lead to tissue necrosis. Similarly, patients must be adequately hydrated before the administration of drugs such as high-dose methotrexate or routine doses of cisplatin, ifosfamide and cyclophosphamide, to prevent renal and/or bladder toxicity. Careful attention must be given to fluid and electrolyte balance with the administration of many agents. Cisplatin renal toxicity can cause profound hypomagnesaemia.

Table 6.6.2 Cancer therapy agents

Chemotherapy
Alkylating agents and platinating drugs
Anthracyclines
Antimetabolites
Topoisomerase inhibitors
Mitotic inhibitors
Hormone therapy
Biological therapy
Monoclonal antibodies
unconjugated antibodies
radioimmunoconjugates
immunotoxins
Cytokines
interferons
interleukin-2
Antisense oligonucleotides
Gene therapy
Targeted therapies

Antimetabolites

These exert their cytotoxicity by serving as inhibitors of pathways vital to cellular function and replication. Some are analogues of physiologic purines and pyrimidines, and are incorporated into DNA or RNA or alternatively inhibit enzymes involved in the synthesis of nucleic acids. Methotrexate inhibits the enzyme dihydrofolate reductase, which maintains intracellular pools of reduced tetrahydrofolates required for the synthesis of purine nucleotides and thymidylate. 5-Fluorouracil and the closely related prodrug capecitabine generate an active metabolite, fluorodeoxyuridine monophosphate, which inhibits thymidylate synthase, an enzyme required for the synthesis of deoxythymidine triphosphate, one of the precursors of DNA.

A third important antimetabolite is cytarabine (ara-C), which is converted to cytarabine triphosphate (ara-CTP) in the cell. Cytarabine triphosphate is incorporated into DNA and serves as a DNA chain terminator. A closely related deoxycytidine analogue, gemcitabine, is incorporated into DNA, but has the additional action of inhibiting the conversion of ribonucleotides to deoxyribonucleotides, which are DNA precursors. Prolonged exposure of tumour cells to some of the antimetabolites, such as 5-fluorouracil and cytosine arabinoside, through continuous intravenous infusion of drug, may be more effective than bolus injections alone. High dose ara-C is effective in remission consolidation for acute myelogenous leukaemia.

Purine analogues also have important roles as antimetabolites in the treatment of leukaemias and lymphomas; 6-mercaptopurinre (6-MP) is converted in the cell to a monophosphate, which inhibits the first step of purine synthesis. Moreover, the triphosphate nucleotides of 6-mercaptopurine and 6-thioguanine are incorporated into DNA resulting in an increase in strand breaks. Fludarabine, another purine analogue, serves as an adenosine mimic. Fludarabine is converted to 2-fluoro-ara-A in plasma and is then phosphorylated intracellularly. The resulting triphosphate inhibits DNA polymerase and ribonucleotide reductase. A closely related adenosine analogue, cladribine, has a similar mechanism of action and is highly effective in treating hairy cell leukemia.

As a group, the antimetabolites cause acute toxicity to bone marrow and are potent suppressors of the immune system. Methotrexate and azathioprine, a prodrug of 6-MP, have found important roles for suppressing graft rejection in organ transplantation and in treating autoimmune diseases.

Alkylating agents

These exert their cytotoxicity by binding to DNA and forming covalent bonds with electron-rich sites on DNA, blocking DNA replication and transcription. These drugs act throughout the cell cycle, but have their greatest effect on rapidly proliferating cells. Cyclophosphamide, melphalan, busulfan, and chlorambucil were among the first chemotherapy drugs and remain important agents in cancer therapy, with particular activity in haematological malignancies and breast cancer. Because there is a linear relationship between dose and cell kill, alkylating agents are commonly used in high dose regimens with bone marrow rescue. In a manner similar to alkylating agents, the platinum derivatives bind to, and cross-link DNA, leading to DNA breaks and apoptosis. Carboplatin is frequently included in high dose regimens.

Natural compounds

A variety of natural compounds, isolated as products of fungal fermentation, or from plants or marine organisms, possess antitumour activity. The anthracyclines, represented by doxorubicin and its analogues, bind to topoisomerase II, and thereby trigger double strand breaks in DNA. Etoposide, a semisynthetic compound derived from a plant source, also inhibits topoisomerase II. In a similar way, the camptothecins (irinotecan and topotecan) interfere with topoisomerase I, inducing single strand breaks in DNA. The anthracyclines are distinguished by their potent antileukaemic activity, as well as their activity against breast cancers, childhood sarcomas, and other solid tumours. Their primary disadvantage is their tendency to cause free radical damage to myocardial cells, with late-onset congestive heart failure.

Antimitotic compounds derived from plants have become increasingly important in the treatment of leukaemia and epithelial cancers. Vinca alkaloids (vincristine, vinorelbine, and vinblastine) interfere with microtubule formation and disrupt cell division. In contrast, the taxanes stabilize microtubule assembly, but they also arrest cells in mitosis. The taxanes are particularly valuable for breast and lung cancer treatment. As a group these drugs are hampered by neurotoxicity and myelosuppression.

Hormone-directed therapy

Along with the traditional cytotoxic agents, hormone-directed therapy can be critical in the treatment of breast and prostate cancers. Most breast cancers express receptors for oestrogen and progesterone, and most prostate cancers have androgen receptors. Depriving these tumours of the hormonal stimulus can exert cytostatic effects on the cell and induce apoptosis. Thus, more than 50% of breast cancers expressing the oestrogen receptor will respond to treatment with tamoxifen, an antioestrogen, or to aromatase inhibitors, which block the synthesis of oestrogen from adrenal androgens, an important source of oestrogen in postmenopausal women. The hormone antagonistics are included in regimens for adjuvant therapy of hormone-receptor positive breast cancer. Similarly, luteinizing hormone releasing hormone (LHRH) agonists (which reduce testosterone synthesis) and androgen receptor antagonists have inhibitory effects on most patients with metastatic prostate cancer, and are useful for decreasing tumour burden in locally advanced disease before radiation therapy. Side effects of hormonal agents result from deprivation of oestrogen or testosterone action, and include decreased libido, bone loss in both men and women, and profound metabolic effects such as an increased risk of endometrial cancer and thrombotic events in women on tamoxifen, and decreased muscle mass and an increased risk of myocardial infarction in men on anti-androgen treatment.

Chemotherapy resistance

Tumours may become resistant to the effects of cytotoxic chemotherapy by a number of different mechanisms (Table 6.6.3). Decreased accumulation of drug in the cell through loss of active membrane transport mediates resistance to methotrexate. Drug exporters, such as the *MDR* gene, may be overexpressed by drug resistant tumours, mediating resistance to natural products such as the anthracyclines, taxanes, and vinca alkaloids. Alternatively, the intracellular drug target may amplify in resistant cells, overwhelming the inhibitor and restoring pathway activity. Amplification of dihydrofolate reductase confers resistance to methotrexate. The target enzyme for 5-fluorouracil, thymidylate synthase, may be amplified and lead to resistance. Increased intratumoral drug metabolism, as occurs with ring reduction of 5-fluorouracil (by dihydropyrimidine dehydrogenase), also conveys drug resistance. In tumours resistant to alkylating agent and platinum analogues, the drugs may be inactivated through chemical reactions with thiol-containing compounds; resistance to DNA alkylators and platinum compounds is also mediated by up-regulation of DNA repair. It is now clear that even before therapy tumours harbour drug-resistant cells generated through spontaneous mutation, and these cells are selected for survival by exposure to chemotherapy. Thus, combinations of non-cross-resistant drugs are required for long-term effective treatment of most tumours.

Table 6.6.3 Mechanisms of chemotherapy resistance

Drug	Mechanism of resistance	Biological change
Methotrexate	Decreased drug uptake	Increased expression of folate transporter
	Decreased drug activation	Decreased folylpolyglutamyl synthetase
	Altered drug target	Altered dihydrofolate reductase
Doxorubicin	Altered drug target	Altered topoisomerase II
	Increased drug efflux	Increased MDR expression or MDR gene amplification
Alkylating agents	Increased detoxification	Increased glutathione or glutathione transferase
	Enhanced DNA repair	Increased nucleotide excision repair
Cisplatin	Defective recognition of DNA adducts	Mismatch repair defect
	Enhanced DNA repair	Increased nucleotide excision repair
Etoposide	Increased drug efflux	Increased MDR expression or gene amplification
	Altered drug target	Altered topoisomerase II
Most anticancer drugs	Defective checkpoint function and apoptosis	P53 mutations
5-Fluorouracil	Increased drug target	Amplified thymidylate synthase

MDR, multidrug resistance.

Side effects of chemotherapy

Most of the commonly used chemotherapy agents (Table 6.6.4) cause acute myelosuppression, although the timing of its onset and its duration differs with different groups of drugs. Most antitumour drugs cause an acute, 5- to 7-day depression in counts, affecting the white blood count more than platelets, allowing retreatment on 14- to 21-day cycles. By contrast, the nitrosoureas

Table 6.6.4 Side-effects of chemotherapy

Adverse effect	Representative agents
Nausea/vomiting	Cisplatin, doxorubicin
Alopecia	Cisplatin, adriamycin, taxol
Neuropathy	Taxol, cisplatin
Renal toxicity	Cisplatin, methotrexate
Pulmonary toxicity	Bleomycin, BCNU, methotrexate
Cardiotoxicity	Doxorubicin, daunorubicin
Bladder toxicity	Cyclophosphamide, ifosfamide
SIADH	Cyclophosphamide, vincristine
Mucositis	5-FU, Methotrexate, doxorubicin
Nail changes	Bleomycin, cyclophosphamide, 5-FU

lead to delayed-onset reductions in both neutrophils and platelet with nadir counts typically reached 4 to 6 weeks after therapy.

Nausea and vomiting remain significant side effects of chemotherapy, though corticosteroids and serotonin uptake inhibitors such as odansetron have diminished the incidence and severity of vomiting even with the most emetogenic agents, including cisplatin. Alopecia occurs in most patients receiving doxorubicin and the alkylating agents, but less commonly in patients treated with antimetabolites or antimitotic drugs. A peripheral neuropathy frequently results from treatment with vinca alkaloids and platinum analogues.

Many agents have unique side effects that are of concern to the practising internist. Doxorubicin causes a cumulative, dose-dependent decline in left ventricular ejection fraction, with a 7–20% incidence of congestive heart failure in patients receiving a cumulative dose of more than 550 mg/m^2. Bleomycin produces lung toxicity, including pneumonitis, which can progress to interstitial fibrosis. The carbon monoxide diffusing capacity of the lung diminishes with increasing cumulative bleomycin doses. Exposure to high concentrations of inhaled oxygen during surgery can precipitate acute respiratory failure in patients previously treated with bleomycin. Methotrexate in high doses can cause acute renal failure due to drug precipitation in the renal tubules, a complication that can prevented by intense hydration and urine alkalinization before and during drug infusion. The administration of paclitaxel can cause anaphylaxis due to Cremophor EL, the vehicle in which it is delivered. Hence, premedication with dexamethasone and antihistamines is required to reduce the risk of adverse reactions to paclitaxel. Cytarabine administered in high single doses (3 mg/m^2 or more) can cause irreversible cerebellar dysfunction. A careful neurological examination should be performed daily on patients receiving high-dose cytosine arabinoside so that it can be discontinued at the earliest sign of such toxicity.

Many of the chemotherapeutic drugs, particularly the alkylating agents, have profound effects on reproductive tissues. Men become azoospermic after receiving these drugs for lymphoma treatment, and the same drugs, with doxorubicin, may produce early menopause in women receiving adjuvant chemotherapy for breast cancer. These issues need to be discussed with young adults of childbearing age, as sperm banking is possible for men prior to lymphoma treatment, while egg harvesting and *in vitro* fertilization before treatment may allow conception after completion of adjuvant therapy in premenopausal women. Hormonal therapies, such as aromatase inhibitors and LHRH agonists, also have profound effects on oestrogen and testosterone levels, and thus can lead to changes in sexual function in patients with breast or prostate cancer, respectively.

A major, delayed side effect of cancer chemotherapy is the development of secondary leukaemias due to therapy. Leukaemia is most commonly seen in patients 2 to 4 years after receiving therapy with alkylating agents, as was the case for the treatment of Hodgkin's disease with MOPP chemotherapy. Newer regimens such as ABVD (adriamycin (doxorubicin), bleomycin, vinblastine, and dacarbazine) for Hodgkin's disease treatment avoid this devastating complication. More recently, topoisomerase II therapy (etoposide, anthracyclines) in high total doses has been associated with a risk of secondary leukaemias. High-dose therapy with alkylating agents such as cyclophosphamide, busulfan, or melphalan, followed by autologous stem cell infusion, confers a 10% risk of secondary myelodysplasia and leukaemia. As survival rates improve with intensive combination chemotherapy regimens, the long-term complications of cancer chemotherapy become more evident.

Targeted therapies

With advances in our understanding of cancer biology and the discovery of specific genetic changes that cause cancer, it has become possible to design therapies to block the master controls responsible for the proliferation, survival, and metastasis of tumour cells. These targeted drugs differ from cytotoxic chemotherapy, which block the synthesis of DNA or interfere with its function. Classic chemotherapy drugs have limited specificity for malignancy, and thus exert profound toxic effects on normal tissues. By contrast, the new targeted therapies attack features unique to the cancer cell or pathways upon which the cancer cell depends for survival. Examples of such pathways are activated growth factor receptors and their ligands, highly expressed signal transduction pathways, and tumour-induced angiogenesis. The first of these tumour-specific targets to be exploited was the bcr-abl1 kinase, created by the 9:22 translocation in chronic myelogenous leukaemia. Imatinib, an inhibitor of the ATP catalytic site of this enzyme, produces both haematological and cytogenetic remission in most patients with this disease. However, resistance to imatinib arises through the emergence of cells that carry mutations in the bcr-abl1 kinase. Dasatinib, an analogue of imatinib that binds to a slightly altered configuration of the enzyme, is highly effective in most patients who develop resistance to imatinib through kinase mutation.

Other targeted compounds block key growth factor receptors, such as the epidermal growth factor receptor (EGFR). Erlotinib and gefitinib proved highly effective in causing tumour regression in a subset of patients with non-small cell lung cancer whose tumours carry a constitutively activated mutant form of EGFR. Further mutations in EGFR lead to resistance to these drugs.

Tumours require new blood vessels to keep pace with their demands for oxygen and nutrients. They secrete potent angiogenic factors, including vascular endothelial growth factor (VEGF), which cause a proliferation of leaky vessels in the immediate environment of the tumour. Low molecular weight inhibitors of the VEGF receptor have proved effective in causing regression of renal cell cancers. The particular sensitivity of renal cell cancer to antiangiogenic agents is explained by their unique biology. These tumours are driven by loss of function of the Von Hippel–Lindau gene (*VHL*), which normally acts as an oxygen sensor for a highly angiogenic pathway. Loss of the *VHL* gene leads to high levels of expression of VEGF, cell transformation, and prominent angiogenesis. Sorafenib and sunitinib, both inhibitors of VEGFR, block angiogenesis and inhibit the growth of renal cell cancers, as does bevacizumab, a monoclonal antibody to VEGF. Bevacizumab partners effectively with chemotherapy in the treatment of many epithelial cancers, including tumours of the breast, lung, and colon.

Monoclonal antibodies have certain advantages over small molecules. They have long half-lives in plasma, and may, in addition to their own biological effect, recruit participation of the immune system in complement or cell-dependent cytotoxicity. Monoclonal antibodies that target receptors on the tumour cell membrane have become important components of regimens for treating lymphomas, breast and colorectal cancer. Rituximab binds to the CD20 antigen expressed on the surface of both normal and malignant B lymphocytes. Nearly 50% of patients with low-grade B-cell lymphoma respond to this targeted therapy. The most common side effects of Rituxan and other antibodies are infusion-related fevers, chills, and hypotension. Another biologically active antibody, herceptin, binds to the Her-2 receptor that is overexpressed in 25% of breast cancer cases. Herceptin is used exclusively for patients with breast tumours that have amplification of the Her-2 receptor. When given in conjunction with paclitaxel, herceptin prolongs survival for patients with metastatic breast cancer, and dramatically improves the effectiveness of adjuvant chemotherapy for the same disease. Antibodies to the EGFR receptor (cetuximab and panitumumab), and as mentioned previously, to VEGF (bevacizumab), are effective in a variety of epithelial tumours.

Naturally occurring cytokines, produced by the immune system, have found limited usefulness in cancer treatment. The interferons are a class of proteins produced by macrophages and lymphocytes in response to viral infections. α-Interferon has relatively modest antitumour activity, inducing responses in a minority of patients with melanoma and renal cancer. More consistent responses are seen in chronic myelogenous leukaemia and hairy cell leukemia. Except for its use in melanoma, it has been replaced by other, more effective drugs. Toxicities include fevers, chills, liver function test abnormalities, cytopenias, and depression. Activated T cells produce interleukin 2. It triggers proliferation of T-cells and produces long-term complete responses in a small fraction of patients with renal cell carcinoma and melanoma. However, its toxicities include fevers, renal dysfunction, and a capillary leak syndrome, with occasional severe pulmonary dysfunction.

Targeted therapies offer great promise for further contribution to cancer treatment. As the molecular pathways and specific mutations responsible for malignancy are elucidated by basic science, new targets will be exploited. The transition from laboratory to clinic is a complex process, in which information travels back and forth from clinician to scientist, informing the drug discovery and development process. Thus, it is becoming clear that current pathological classifications of disease inadequately describe the underlying heterogeneity of human tumours. This heterogeneity is most obvious in gene expression profiles of leukaemias, lymphomas, and many solid tumours, and in the variable expression of signalling pathways and receptor mutations. Further, there is a growing confidence that, with appropriate molecular and immunohistochemical tests, it will be possible to assign therapies to individual patients with a high chance of predicting response, as is now standard practice in hormonal therapy of oestrogen receptor-positive breast cancer and in the use of herceptin in Her-2 positive tumour treatment. An important study of EGFR receptor mutations has identified a subset of patients with non-small cell lung cancer who are uniquely responsible to EGFR inhibitors. Other molecular tests will likely be useful in identifying patients at risk for toxicity because of polymorphisms in enzymes responsible for drug metabolism or DNA repair. Most cancer researchers agree that cancer therapy will become increasingly individualized as molecular medicine helps identify the determinants of response and toxicity.

Radiation oncology

Since the earliest demonstration of the cytotoxic effects of high energy radioisotopes by Marie Curie more than 100 years ago, the use of ionizing radiation has become a critical component of the curative and palliative treatment options for patients with cancer. The field of radiation oncology has enjoyed a technical revolution that has provided more conformal and reproducible delivery capabilities. These improvements in radiation delivery have resulted because of the significant evolution of computer science, biomedical engineering, imaging, and robotics. High-energy (>4 MV) photons produced from linear accelerators coupled with three-dimensional image manipulation have allowed for intensity modulated radiation therapy (IMRT), robotic image-guided delivery (e.g. CyberKnife), and direct CT-guided radiation therapy (tomotherapy). High-energy electron beams carry no appreciable mass and are used to treat superficial structures such as skin cancer and tumours of the anterior eye. In the last 5 years (2004–09), the number of proton therapy centres has more than doubled around the world. Protons, unlike photons, have no exit dose beyond the treatment target and can reduce the integral dose by 50% or more. This is particularly important in the treatment of developing children with radiation as well as targeting tissues that are close to critical structures (e.g. spinal cord). Heavier charged particles (e.g. carbon, helium) have the same physical characteristics as protons, but have a greater biological effect. Two heavy-particle facilities are currently treating patients with resistant tumours.

The new technologies outlined above all provide much more conformal treatment delivery than was available a decade or so ago. A greater degree of conformality results in an improved therapeutic ratio. Highly conformal treatments can allow for dose escalation for resistant tumours while maintaining a fixed level of normal tissue complications and a resultant improvement in local tumour control. Improved treatment field planning is now possible with the help of advanced radiological techniques (MRI, functional MRI, PET). Treatment planning platforms can fuse or correlate images from a wide variety of radiographic studies to guide the selection of treatment volume and dose.

The principle mechanism for radiation-induced cytotoxicity appears to be damage to tumour DNA. Radiation therapy generates free radicals that damage DNA, producing breaks that must be repaired if the cell is to survive. Many tumours lack an effective capacity to repair DNA strand breaks, as compared to normal tissues. The difference in DNA repair between tumour and normal tissue provides a therapeutic window for successful treatment. Irradiation also inflicts potent damaging effects on tumour vasculature.

The dose of irradiation is defined as the unit of energy absorbed by each kilogram of tissue. The unit now used is the gray (Gy): 1 Gy (= 100 rad) is the absorption of 1 joule of energy by 1 kg of matter. Each normal tissue and each tumour type has a characteristic threshold of radiation dose above which the capacity to repair DNA damage is exceeded, and cell death occurs. As the dose of radiation is increased beyond the threshold, the percentage of cells killed increases. Simply stated, the higher the dose of radiation, the higher the probability of tumour control. Also, the higher the dose of radiation received by surrounding normal structures, the higher the probability of normal tissue injury.

Radiation doses are usually delivered in a number of daily fractions, the total fractionated dose being determined by tumour sensitivity and normal tissue tolerance. Seminoma is an exquisitely radiation controllable tumour and requires a low relative dose (30 Gy) for cure, while epithelial tumours such as lung cancer and melanoma, are relatively resistant to conventional doses (e.g. 60 Gy) of radiation.

Within 4–8 h after exposure to ionizing radiation, cells begin to recover from the effects of therapy. Thus, fractions administered too close together can offer increased toxicity to normal tissues, but those too far apart can permit repair of lethal or sublethal damage. Conventional therapy is usually given in daily radiation fractions of 1.8 to 2 Gy over 4–7 weeks, to total doses of 50 Gy or higher, but alternative schemes have been investigated. Hyperfractionated therapy, in which a smaller fraction sizes (<2 Gy) are used more than once daily, takes advantage of the more rapid repair of DNA by normal tissues as compared to tumour cells within the radiation treatment volume. This approach permits a higher total radiation dose to be administered over a shorter time interval, with tolerable late toxicity and slightly increased acute effects. This has been shown to be particularly helpful in the treatment of advanced epithelial tumours of the head and neck region.

The presence of oxygen is important in the generation of free radicals after exposure to ionizing radiation. Relatively hypoxic tissues are less sensitive to the toxic effects of radiation than those tissues that are well oxygenated. Attempts to overcome tumour hypoxia with biochemical manipulation or hyperbaric oxygen have failed. However, concurrent or neoadjuvant chemotherapy appears to improve the chances of curing a locally advanced head and neck cancer by reducing tumour bulk and restoring oxygenation prior to irradiation. Antiangiogenic drugs, such as bevacizumab may improve response to both chemotherapy and irradiation by reducing the tangled mass of leaky tumour vessels and partially re-establishing normal flow, thereby reducing intramural oncotic pressure and improving drug delivery and oxygenation.

Radiation used for the treatment of patients is generally delivered as an external beam from a source outside the body. In selected cases brachytherapy, in which the radiation source is implanted within the substance of the tumour, is effective in the treatment of cervical cancer and endometrial cancer, delivering high local doses and obviating the requirement for daily outpatient visits. For palliative irradiation of metastatic tumours, single large doses (radiosurgery) or abbreviated courses of irradiation (hypofractionated radiotherapy) may be administered to relieve symptoms, but this type of treatment offers limited expectation of long-term control except in the treatment of benign brain tumours (e.g. acoustic neuroma). At some centres, intraoperative radiation therapy can be used to deliver a single large fraction of radiation directly to the tumour bed. In some circumstances, radioisotopes themselves can be used for systemic treatment. For example, iodine-131 is taken up by thyroid tissue both locally and at sites of metastatic disease. Monoclonal antibodies such as tositumomab and ibritumomab tiuxetan, coupled with radioisotopes, may be administered intravenously, and localize at the tumour site. The radioisotope carried by the antibody emits β or γ particles that destroy malignant lymphomas.

Complications of radiation oncology

Radiation is highly effective in killing tumour cells, but toxicity to normal tissues within the field or at its margins can be significant. Effects of radiation can be acute (during the treatment course), subacute (after treatment but within a few months of therapy), and late (permanent). Tissues that proliferate rapidly, such as skin, mucosal linings, and bone marrow, are most susceptible to acute radiation injury. Thus, cutaneous erythema, desquamation, and oedema are important local effects of therapy. Oral and intestinal mucosae are particular susceptible to irradiation. Diarrhoea, nausea, and vomiting are common in patients receiving abdominal irradiation. If a significant radiation dose is delivered to the bone marrow, particularly the pelvis and spine, patients may develop cytopenias. In the case of whole-body irradiation, the lymphocyte count also falls and significant immune suppression may result. On occasion, these acute side effects are severe enough to require delays in treatment in order to allow recovery of the normal tissues and blood counts. When patients receive irradiation to a mass in the chest cavity, e.g. a lymphoma, the resultant radiation pneumonitis may cause fever, cough, dyspnoea, and pulmonary infiltrates. Relief from these pulmonary symptoms may require treatment with corticosteroids.

Long-term sequelae are tissue specific and occur most commonly if normal tissue tolerance is exceeded. Thus, careful radiation field planning and treatment delivery must be carried out to ensure that tissues do not receive treatment beyond their maximum predicted tolerated dose. For example radiation doses to the spinal cord in excess of 60 Gy can cause transverse myelitis, with paresthesias and neuropathies. Doses to large volumes of small bowel in excess of 45 Gy can cause strictures, and doses to an entire kidney above 25 Gy can cause irreversible renal damage. The whole liver tolerates radiation therapy up to doses of 40 Gy, above which hepatic necrosis and fibrosis result. However, partial liver irradiation to very high doses can be done safely as long as the volume of irradiation is restricted. Accelerated coronary artery disease was seen in patients with Hodgkin's disease years after they received mediastinal irradiation with the more primitive treatment techniques than are currently employed. Early results suggest that modern conformal radiation techniques can reduce both acute and late effects of treatment.

Perhaps the most distressing late effect of radiation therapy is the development of secondary tumours within radiation fields. Such radiation associated secondary neoplasms can occur 5 to 50 or more years after treatment. Ordinarily, this is not an issue for patients with metastatic cancer receiving radiation therapy for palliation of disease-related symptoms since the patients' survival will be limited. However, in treating paediatric tumours, and in patients with lymphomas, who will also be cured with radiation therapy, the development of solid tumours in the radiation field, including sarcomas and lung and breast cancers, represents a devastating complication. These secondary tumours can occur within the full-dose region as well as in the lower-dose regions of beam entrance and exit. Again, treatment techniques such as IMRT and proton therapy reduce the irradiated volume by 50% or more and will likely be associated with a reduced risk of secondary tumour formation.

Role of radiation therapy in cancer treatment

In the clinical management of patients, radiation therapy is used as the sole therapy for many localized tumours and as a component of primary therapy for many patients, either as an adjuvant after surgery to prevent local recurrence, or as neoadjuvant therapy to decrease tumour mass and thereby allow a less morbid procedure. It may be used alone or in conjunction with chemotherapy (which often acts as a radiation sensitizer). It is also valuable as palliative therapy for advanced stage treatment (Table 6.6.5).

Radiation therapy has a role in the management of several acute complications of cancer. Radiation can be valuable in the treatment of bone metastases, both to decrease painful lesions and to diminish the risk of pathological fractures. Radiation therapy can be delivered as an emergency procedure in patients with spinal cord compression to reduce the risk of permanent neurological toxicity. Likewise, radiation therapy has an important role in the management of brain metastases, either as primary therapy for patients with multiple lesions or as an adjuvant therapy for patients after excision of a solitary brain metastasis. In lung cancer, radiation can be used to palliate obstructive symptoms. In bleeding oesophageal or gastric tumours, radiation therapy can often assist in local control of haemorrhage.

In the management of many tumours, radiation therapy can serve as the sole modality or a component of definitive treatment.

Table 6.6.5 Role of radiation therapy in cancer treatment

Curative therapy alone
Hodgkin's disease
Non-Hodgkin's lymphoma (early stage, indolent histology)
Laryngeal carcinoma
Prostate cancer
Central nervous system tumours (e.g. medulloblastoma)
Cervical cancer
Breast cancer (postsurgery)
Curative in conjunction with chemotherapy
Small cell lung cancer (limited stage)
Non-Hodgkin's lymphoma (early stage aggressive histology)
Anal carcinoma
Adjuvant therapy
Rectal cancer (with 5-FU)
Gastric cancer (with 5-FU)
Neoadjuvant therapy
Oesophageal carcinoma
Lung cancer (stage III)

In early-stage Hodgkin's's disease, patients can be cured with either mantle radiation therapy alone or with mantle and para-aortic radiation. Similarly, 35 to 50-Gy doses of radiation therapy can cure 50 to 60% of patients with stage I/II non-Hodgkin's's lymphoma. Seminoma is exquisitely sensitive to irradiation and most patients with early stage disease can be cured with radiation therapy alone. Radiation therapy cures patients with early stage prostate cancer and laryngeal cancer, and causes less local morbidity than surgery. Finally, in early-stage breast cancer, lumpectomy and radiation therapy provides an equivalent survival outcome to a modified radical mastectomy.

In other diseases, combinations of radiotherapy and chemotherapy are highly effective. For example, in patients with squamous cell carcinoma of the anus, combined modality therapy using radiation therapy in conjunction with 5-fluorouracil and mitomycin C chemotherapy yields a high cure rate without surgery. Similarly, in patients with limited stage small-cell lung cancer, combined modality therapy using cisplatin-based chemotherapy and radiation therapy eradicates the primary tumour, and improves survival. Likewise, in cervical cancer, a combination of cisplatin and radiation after resection reduces tumour recurrence. It has been recently shown that radiation combined with concurrent and adjuvant temodar prolongs survival and disease-free progression in adults with malignant gliomas.

Radiation therapy also has an important role in adjuvant therapy. Prior to surgical resection of rectal cancer, radiation therapy administered in conjunction with 5-fluorouracil chemotherapy can reduce local, regional, and systemic recurrence and can improve both disease free and overall survival. In node-positive gastric cancer, a postoperative combination of 5- fluorouracil-based chemotherapy, with irradiation of the tumour bed, can reduce the risk of recurrence and improve survival. Recent studies have demonstrated that the administration of prophylactic cranial irradiation to patients with small-cell lung cancer who achieve a complete remission can reduce the risk of tumour recurrence in the central nervous system. In the neoadjuvant setting, radiation in combination with cisplatin-based chemotherapy improves survival and decreases recurrence in patients with stage IIIA lung cancer.

Conclusions

Advances in radiation therapy, chemotherapy, and biological therapy have revolutionized the care of cancer patients. Significant improvements in supportive care and the development of new, active anticancer agents have improved the prospects for long-term survival even for patients with metastatic disease. The internist has a pivotal role in coordinating care for such patients, recognizing the early and late consequences of treatment, and coordinating the long-term follow-up of such patients with the cancer specialists.

Further reading

Blaszkowsky LS, Erlichman C (2006). Carcinogenesis of anticancer drugs. In: Chabner BA, Longo D (eds) *Cancer chemotherapy & biotherapy principles and practice*, 4th edition, pp. 70–90. Lippincott Williams and Wilkins, Philadelphia, PA.

Chabner BA, Roberts TG Jr (2005). Timeline: Chemotherapy and the war on cancer. *Nat Rev Cancer*, **5**, 65–72.

Ferrara N, Kerbel RS (2005). Angiogenesis as a therapeutic target. *Nature*, **438**, 967–74.

Hahn WC, Weinberg RA (2002). Modelling the molecular circuitry of cancer. *Nat Rev Cancer*, **2**, 331–41.

Levin WP, *et al.* (2005). Proton beam therapy. *Br J Cancer*, **93**, 849–54.

Lynch TJ, *et al.* (2004). Activating mutations in the epidermal growth factor receptor underlying responsiveness of non-small-cell lung cancer to gefitinib. *N Engl J Med*, **350**, 2129–39.

Norton L (2006). Use of dose-dense chemotherapy in the management of breast cancer. *Clin Adv Hematol Oncol*, **4**, 36–7.

Roberts TG Jr, Chabner BA (2004). Beyond fast track for drug approvals. *N Engl J Med*, **351**, 501–5.

Sawyers C (2004). Targeted cancer therapy. *Nature*, **432**, 294–7.

SECTION 7

Infection

7.1 Pathogenic microorganisms and the host *409*

7.1.1 Biology of pathogenic microorganisms *409*
Duncan J. Maskell

7.1.2 Physiological changes, clinical features, and general management of infected patients *413*
Todd W. Rice and Gordon R. Bernard

7.2 The patient with suspected infection *420*

7.2.1 Clinical approach *420*
Christopher J. Ellis

7.2.2 Fever of unknown origin *423*
Steven Vanderschueren and Daniël Knockaert

7.2.3 Nosocomial infections *428*
I.C.J.W. Bowler

7.2.4 Infection in the immunocompromised host *431*
J. Cohen

7.2.5 Antimicrobial chemotherapy *441*
R.G. Finch

7.3 Immunization *460*
D. Goldblatt and M. Ramsay

7.4 Travel and expedition medicine *465*
C.P. Conlon and David A. Warrell

7.5 Viruses *472*

7.5.1 Respiratory tract viruses *473*
Malik Peiris

7.5.2 Herpesviruses (excluding Epstein–Barr virus) *482*
J.G.P. Sissons

7.5.3 Epstein–Barr virus *501*
M.A. Epstein and A.B. Rickinson

7.5.4 Poxviruses *508*
Geoffrey L. Smith

7.5.5 Mumps: epidemic parotitis *513*
B.K. Rima

7.5.6 Measles *515*
H.C. Whittle and P. Aaby

7.5.7 Nipah and Hendra virus encephalitides *525*
C.T. Tan

7.5.8 Enterovirus infections *527*
Philip Minor and Ulrich Desselberger

7.5.9 Virus infections causing diarrhoea and vomiting *536*
Philip Dormitzer and Ulrich Desselberger

7.5.10 Rhabdoviruses: rabies and rabies-related lyssaviruses *541*
M. J. Warrell and David A. Warrell

7.5.11 Colorado tick fever and other arthropod-borne reoviruses *555*
M.J. Warrell and David A. Warrell

7.5.12 Alphaviruses *557*
L.R. Petersen and D.J. Gubler

7.5.13 Rubella *561*
P.A. Tookey and J.M. Best

7.5.14 Flaviviruses excluding dengue *564*
L.R. Petersen and D.J. Gubler

7.5.15 Dengue *575*
Bridget Wills and Jeremy Farrar

7.5.16 Bunyaviridae *579*
J.W. LeDuc and Summerpal S. Kahlon

7.5.17 Arenaviruses *588*
J. ter Meulen

7.5.18 Filoviruses *595*
J. ter Meulen

7.5.19 Papillomaviruses and polyomaviruses *600*
Raphael P. Viscidi and Keerti V. Shah

7.5.20 Parvovirus B19 *607*
Kevin E. Brown

7.5.21 Hepatitis viruses (excluding hepatitis C virus) *609*
N.V. Naoumov

7.5.22 Hepatitis C *615*
Paul Klenerman, K.J.M. Jeffery, and J. Collier

7.5.23 HIV/AIDS *620*
Graz A. Luzzi, T.E.A. Peto, P. Goulder, and C.P. Conlon

7.5.24 HIV in the developing world *644*
Alison D. Grant and Kevin M. De Cock

7.5.25 HTLV-1, HTLV-2, and associated diseases *650*
Kristien Verdonck and Eduardo Gotuzzo

7.5.26 Viruses and cancer *653*
R.A. Weiss

7.5.27 Orf *655*
David A. Warrell

7.5.28 Molluscum contagiosum *657*
David A. Warrell

7.5.29 Newly discovered viruses *659*
H.C. Hughes

7.6 Bacteria *663*

7.6.1 Diphtheria *664*
Delia B. Bethell and Tran Tinh Hien

7.6.2 Streptococci and enterococci *670*
Dennis L. Stevens

7.6.3 Pneumococcal infections *679*
Anthony Scott

7.6.4 Staphylococci *693*
Bala Hota and Robert A. Weinstein

7.6.5 Meningococcal infections *709*
P. Brandtzaeg

7.6.6 *Neisseria gonorrhoeae* *722*
D. Barlow, Jackie Sherrard, and C. Ison

7.6.7 Enterobacteria *727*

7.6.7.1 Enterobacteria and bacterial food poisoning *727*
Hugh Pennington

7.6.7.2 *Pseudomonas aeruginosa* *735*
G.C.K.W. Koh and S.J. Peacock

7.6.8 Typhoid and paratyphoid fevers *738*
C.M. Parry and Buddha Basnyat

7.6.9 Intracellular klebsiella infections (donovanosis and rhinoscleroma) *745*
J. Richens

7.6.10 Anaerobic bacteria *748*
Anilrudh A. Venugopal and David W. Hecht

7.6.11 Cholera *754*
Aldo A.M. Lima and Richard L. Guerrant

7.6.12 *Haemophilus influenzae* *759*
Derrick W. Crook

7.6.13 *Haemophilus ducreyi* and chancroid *763*
Nigel O'Farrell

7.6.14 Bordetella infection *764*
Cameron Grant

7.6.15 Melioidosis and glanders *768*
S.J. Peacock

7.6.16 Plague: *Yersinia pestis* *772*
Michael B. Prentice

7.6.17 Other *Yersinia* infections: yersiniosis *776*
Michael B. Prentice

7.6.18 Pasteurella *777*
Marina S. Morgan

7.6.19 *Francisella tularensis* infection *780*
Petra C.F. Oyston

7.6.20 Anthrax *783*
Arthur E. Brown and Thira Sirisanthana

7.6.21 Brucellosis *789*
M. Monir Madkour

7.6.22 Tetanus *795*
C.L. Thwaites and Lam Minh Yen

7.6.23 *Clostridium difficile* *800*
John G. Bartlett

7.6.24 Botulism, gas gangrene, and clostridial gastrointestinal infections *803*
Dennis L. Stevens, Michael J. Aldape, and Amy E. Bryant

7.6.25 Tuberculosis *810*
Richard E. Chaisson and Jean B. Nachega

7.6.26 Disease caused by environmental mycobacteria *831*
J.M. Grange and P.D.O. Davies

7.6.27 Leprosy (Hansen's disease) *836*
Diana N.J. Lockwood

7.6.28 Buruli ulcer: *Mycobacterium ulcerans* infection *848*
Wayne M. Meyers and Françoise Portaels

7.6.29 Actinomycoses *850*
K.P. Schaal

7.6.30 Nocardiosis *856*
Roderick J. Hay

7.6.31 Rat-bite fevers *857*
David A. Warrell

7.6.32 Lyme borreliosis *860*
Gary P. Wormser, John Nowakowski, and Robert B. Nadelman

7.6.33 Relapsing fevers *866*
David A. Warrell

7.6.34 Leptospirosis *874*
George Watt

7.6.35 Nonvenereal endemic treponematoses: yaws, endemic syphilis (bejel), and pinta *879*
David A. Warrell

7.6.36 Syphilis *885*
Basil Donovan and Linda Dayan

7.6.37 Listeriosis *896*
H. Hof

7.6.38 Legionellosis and legionnaires' disease *899*
J.T. Macfarlane and T.C. Boswell

7.6.39 Rickettsioses *903*
Philippe Parola and Didier Raoult

7.6.40 Scrub typhus *919*
George Watt

7.6.41 *Coxiella burnetii* infections (Q fever) *923*
T.J. Marrie

7.6.42 Bartonellas excluding *B. bacilliformis* *926*
Emmanouil Angelakis, Didier Raoult, and Jean-Marc Rolain

7.6.43 *Bartonella bacilliformis* infection *934*
A. Llanos-Cuentas and C. Maguiña-Vargas

7.6.44 Chlamydial infections *939*
David Taylor-Robinson and David Mabey

7.6.45 Mycoplasmas *950*
David Taylor-Robinson and Jørgen Skov Jensen

7.6.46 A check list of bacteria associated with infection in humans *961*
J. Paul

7.7 Fungi (mycoses) *998*

7.7.1 Fungal infections *998*
Roderick J. Hay

7.7.2 Cryptococcosis *1018*
William G. Powderly

7.7.3 Coccidioidomycosis *1020*
Gregory M. Anstead and John R. Graybill

7.7.4 Paracoccidioidomycosis *1023*
M.A. Shikanai-Yasuda

7.7.5 *Pneumocystis jirovecii* *1028*
Robert F. Miller and Laurence Huang

7.7.6 *Penicillium marneffei* infection *1032*
Thira Sirisanthana

7.8 Protozoa *1035*

7.8.1 Amoebic infections *1035*
Richard Knight

7.8.2 Malaria *1045*
David A. Warrell, Janet Hemingway, Kevin Marsh, Robert E. Sinden, Geoffrey A. Butcher, and Robert W. Snow

7.8.3 Babesiosis *1089*
Philippe Brasseur

7.8.4 Toxoplasmosis *1090*
Oliver Liesenfeld and Eskild Petersen

7.8.5 *Cryptosporidium* and cryptosporidiosis *1098*
S.M. Cacciò

7.8.6 *Cyclospora* and cyclosporiasis *1105*
R. Lainson

7.8.7 Sarcocystosis (sarcosporidiosis) *1109*
John E. Cooper

7.8.8 Giardiasis, balantidiasis, isosporiasis, and microsporidiosis *1111*
Martin F. Heyworth

7.8.9 *Blastocystis hominis* infection *1118*
Richard Knight

7.8.10 Human African trypanosomiasis *1119*
August Stich

7.8.11 Chagas disease *1127*
M.A. Miles

7.8.12 Leishmaniasis *1134*
A.D.M. Bryceson and Diana N.J. Lockwood

7.8.13 Trichomoniasis *1142*
Sharon Hillier

7.9 Nematodes (roundworms) *1145*

7.9.1 Cutaneous filariasis *1145*
Gilbert Burnham

7.9.2 Lymphatic filariasis *1153*
Richard Knight and D.H. Molyneux

7.9.3 Guinea worm disease (dracunculiasis) *1160*
Richard Knight

7.9.4 Strongyloidiasis, hookworm, and other gut strongyloid nematodes *1163*
Michael Brown

7.9.5 Gut and tissue nematode infections acquired by ingestion *1168*
David I. Grove

7.9.6 Parastrongyliasis (angiostrongyliasis) *1179*
Richard Knight

7.9.7 Gnathostomiasis *1182*
Valai Bussaratid and Pravan Suntharasamai

7.10 Cestodes (tapeworms) *1185*

7.10.1 Cystic hydatid disease (*Echinococcus granulosus*) *1185*
Armando E. Gonzalez, Pedro L. Moro, and Hector H. Garcia

7.10.2 Cyclophyllidian gut tapeworms *1188*
Richard Knight

7.10.3 Cysticercosis *1193*
Hector H. Garcia and Robert H. Gilman

7.10.4 Diphyllobothriasis and sparganosis *1199*
David I. Grove

7.11 Trematodes (flukes) *1202*

7.11.1 Schistosomiasis *1202*
D.W. Dunne and B.J. Vennervald

7.11.2 Liver fluke infections *1212*
David I. Grove

7.11.3 Lung flukes (paragonimiasis) *1216*
Udomsak Silachamroon and Sirivan Vanijanonta

7.11.4 Intestinal trematode infections *1219*
David I. Grove

7.12 Nonvenomous arthropods *1225*
J. Paul

7.13 Pentastomiasis (porocephalosis, linguatulosis/linguatuliasis) *1237*
David A. Warrell

7.1

Pathogenic microorganisms and the host

Contents

7.1.1 Biology of pathogenic microorganisms *409*
Duncan J. Maskell

7.1.2 Physiological changes, clinical features, and general management of infected patients *413*
Todd W. Rice and Gordon R. Bernard

7.1.1 Biology of pathogenic microorganisms

Duncan J. Maskell

Essentials

Microorganisms are present at most imaginable sites on the planet, and have evolved to occupy these ecological niches successfully. A host animal is simply another ecological niche to be occupied.

The ability to cause disease may in some cases be an accidental bystander event, or it may be the result of evolutionary processes that have led to specific mechanisms allowing the pathogen to exploit the rich source of nutrients present in the host, before moving on to another fresh host.

Pathogenicity often relies on a series of steps, with specific and often distinct mechanisms operating at each of them. Some types of pathogen must adapt to the host environment by altering gene expression, and all must retain the ability to be transmitted readily between hosts. Specific mechanisms have evolved in microorganisms for the exploitation of the host and for evasion or avoidance of the innate and acquired immune systems.

The advent and application of hyper-rapid and ultra-high throughput whole-genome scale sequencing technologies is providing a mass of information, which—when sensibly and carefully gathered and used—will change fundamentally our way of looking at infectious diseases and our understanding of how pathogens work. This should enable the development of new intervention strategies, especially vaccines and antimicrobials, but the complexity of some of the biological mechanisms involved may make this a difficult exercise. Furthermore, pathogens may vary and evolve rapidly, and thus are likely to remain one step ahead of these strategies.

We live in a rapidly changing world. New pathogens will emerge to exploit new circumstances presented by changes in society, and ancient scourges will remain and re-emerge to plague us. Many of the new infectious disease challenges will arise from animals, and will be zoonoses, at least in the early stages of their emergence. It is therefore probably more important in this field than in any other to develop the vision of "One Medicine", with medical and veterinary clinicians and basic scientists working together, if we are to give ourselves the best chance of success in warding off threats of global infectious diseases.

Introduction

Microorganisms occupy almost all imaginable ecological niches. Microbes have been isolated from deep-sea sites, where they survive very high pressures, from extremely cold and extremely hot regions, where hyperthermophiles grow optimally at temperatures well in excess of 100°C, and even from rocks, where they can exploit chemical substrates for energy generation. It is no wonder, then, that microorganisms should also exploit other living organisms as potential habitats, from viruses that use other microorganisms as hosts through to microorganisms that occupy various ecological niches within and upon the mammalian body, sometimes to the benefit and sometimes to the severe detriment of the host. Microorganisms have been supremely successful in evolutionary terms and they contain enormous untapped reserves of biodiversity, much of which is to be found in those that we can neither isolate nor grow and which make up the vast majority of microbes on the planet. Since microorganisms reproduce much more rapidly than their mammalian hosts and have several specialized mechanisms for horizontal gene transfer, it is not surprising that they are often able to evolve quickly to stay one step ahead of any mechanisms that exist, or are invented by humans, to control them.

The control of infectious diseases over the last century or so has been a major achievement, relying mainly on improved public health systems and social conditions, as well as on technological advances such as antimicrobial drugs and vaccines. A wave of overconfidence led the United States Surgeon General, William H Stewart, to announce in the 1960s that the war against infectious diseases had been won. This optimistic proclamation was bolstered by the eradication of smallpox in 1977, achieved by a monumental worldwide public health and vaccination programme. But, as Aldous Huxley wrote, "Hubris against the … order of Nature would be followed by its appropriate Nemesis", and so it is was that very soon afterwards we had to learn to cope with the global catastrophe that is AIDS, along with the resurgence of ancient killers such as tuberculosis, and the emergence of apparently new threats such as bovine spongiform encephalopathy (BSE) and West Nile fever. In 2009, the world found itself dealing with the long-predicted global pandemic of influenza which is severely stretching and testing the ingenuity and organizational abilities of international human society in its attempts to control the spread and impact of the virus.

Pathogenicity in stages

It is important to break down pathogenesis into different steps and stages. Most viral and bacterial pathogens enter the host via the mucosa of the respiratory, gastrointestinal, or genitourinary tracts, although some important pathogens are introduced by injection from insect vectors or through abraded or wounded skin. Most pathogens then have to stick to a surface and have evolved structures to do so; these are usually constructed from proteins and many of them are complex and specialized. In bacteria, these protein molecules are known as adhesins and are often but not always delivered at the end of long proteinaceous organelles called pili or fimbriae. The precise amino acid sequence of the adhesin, and hence its structure, can dictate which host and even which tissues within the host the bacterium sticks to and can, therefore, play a major role in dictating host range and tissue tropism. For example, enterotoxigenic *Escherichia coli* (ETEC) expressing K88 fimbriae will stick to piglet intestine and cause disease, those expressing K99 will stick to calf and lamb intestine, and those expressing colonization factor antigen (CFA) I and CFAII will stick to human intestine. Similarly, *E. coli* expressing P fimbriae (otherwise known as PAP pili) will stick efficiently to the human urinary tract and cause infection at that site. After initial loose adherence, enteropathogenic *E. coli* (EPEC) will stick more firmly to the intestinal surface via the nonfimbrial adhesin, intimin. The receptor for intimin on the host cell surface is a protein called Tir, which is itself an *E. coli* protein that has been translocated into the host cell via a specialized needle-like structure, a type 3 secretory system (T3SS), which is itself closely related to bacterial flagella. This complex, coordinated series of events gives an insight into the extraordinary sequences of events that have evolved to enable bacteria to exploit their hosts as ecological niches.

Viruses also rely on surface structures for host specificity. An example of current interest is influenza virus. Among several other mechanisms, the host range and tissue tropism of influenza virus is dependent on the structure of its haemagglutinin molecule. On the respiratory epithelium, haemagglutinin binds to sialic acid which is linked to galactose on the host cell surface via either an α2,3 or an α2,6 linkage. Human influenza viruses bind preferentially to the α2,6-linked molecule, which is abundant on human tracheal epithelium, whereas avian influenza viruses bind preferentially to the α2,3-linked version, which is abundant in duck intestinal epithelium. The different binding capacities of the haemagglutinin molecules are also important in the transmissibility of the virus, which is clearly a major element in determining whether or not an epidemic will occur. Interestingly, pig trachea expresses plenty of both types of molecule, which may explain in part why pigs are susceptible to both avian and human influenza viruses, and why pigs may be a major source of reassorted virus that could jump species from avian to human. A caveat here is that a recent study suggests that the distribution of human and avian influenza viruses in the pig respiratory tract is such that they probably infect different cell types. For virus reassortment to occur, the same cell must be infected by both the avian and human types of virus, and therefore this observation may raise a serious problem for the dogma that the pig may be the 'mixing vessel'. A further recent observation indicates that the precise cell tropism in the human respiratory tract for viruses of different host origin may correlate with the type of disease caused, and maybe also the amount of virus that can be shed, leading to different disease severities and potentially different transmission dynamics.

Once established at a surface, pathogens have a wide array of possible strategies. They can stay at that surface and cause very little damage, and indeed be carried without causing any clinical signs. Bacteria such as *Haemophilus influenzae* and *Neisseria meningitidis* are good examples of this. Only as a result of some unknown and rare set of circumstances will these bacteria move into the bloodstream to cause septicaemia and sometimes meningitis. To survive and spread in the blood, bacteria have evolved a range of molecular strategies to inhibit the activation and activity of complement, and to avoid or resist phagocytosis. Alternatively, the bacteria can stay at the mucosal surface and cause considerable damage—by direct invasion and destruction of the tissue, by inducing a damaging inflammatory response, or by elaborating a toxin. The precise pathology caused, and consequently the clinical signs, depends on the precise nature of the toxin and the site at which it has its effects. Thus ETEC makes labile toxin (LT) and stable toxin (ST) which will usually result in watery diarrhoea, whereas enterohaemorrhagic *E. coli* (EHEC) can make Shiga toxin, which is spread systemically and acts at a distance from the gut with severe consequences such as thrombocytopenia and kidney damage, leading to haemolytic uraemic syndrome (HUS). Other bacteria invade and spread systemically, finally lodging in particular tissues and causing direct pathology or inducing inflammatory responses that result in immunopathology (e.g. the lesions associated with systemic salmonella infections such as typhoid fever). These pathologies often result from the binding of host receptors (pattern recognition receptors, PRRs) to relatively invariant structures on the invading organisms (pathogen-associated molecular patterns, PAMPs), such as endotoxin, peptidoglycan, flagella, or in viruses double-stranded RNA, leading to expression of a range of cytokines that mediate the inflammatory response. If this process gets out of control, or happens at the wrong time and in the wrong place, severe pathology can result. An example of this is the systemic inflammation that leads to sepsis, with attendant tissue damage, circulatory collapse, and often death.

Each of the different stages of infection relies on the bacterial pathogen being able to adapt physiologically and metabolically to the different niches in which it finds itself, and having the appropriate structures to survive the onslaught of innate and adaptive immune responses. It is becoming increasingly apparent that many bacteria can adapt gene expression profiles rapidly, and have sophisticated molecular mechanisms for rapid switching of many of the structures that are required for virulence or are recognized by the immune system.

Virulence factors versus fitness factors

Almost any gene product that has been identified as being required for infection has been called a 'virulence factor' in the literature. However, this is imprecise and can be misleading. For bacteria, many of the genes required for host exploitation might be better considered as 'fitness factors', but are no less important in the consideration of infectious diseases and how to combat them. Bacteria can often grow outside their hosts and so not all their genes are necessarily required for fitness inside the host. Those that are include classic virulence factors such as adhesins and toxins, and also various metabolic genes and pathways that enable the bacterium to survive for long enough and grow in the host causing damage.

Viruses on the other hand are obligate host parasites. They tend (with notable exceptions such as herpesviruses and poxviruses with genomes of 100–200 kb) to have rather small genomes with few genes. Therefore, in most viruses, each gene is required for exploitation of the host in some way and is highly likely to be a fitness factor in the sense of evolutionary fitness. It may well be appropriate to consider them as virulence factors in pathogenesis.

In considering virulence vs fitness in evolution, we might ask, 'Why do pathogens cause damage rather than simply existing in harmony with their host?' This question might be framed better as, 'What evolutionary pathway has resulted in pathogens that cause damage to their hosts?' There are many possible answers. The pathogen might have evolved to exploit a particular ecological niche rather than a particular host, but has found itself by accident in a host, which it then damages almost as a bystander event. Another answer might be that by inducing a certain pathology the pathogen liberates more nutrients for itself and/or facilitates its transmission to another host (preferably in most cases before it kills its original host). Whatever the truth is behind these evolutionary pathways, it is essential that people working with infectious diseases should recognize that there is more to the evolution of a pathogen than the acquisition of a toxin or two.

Adaptation to the environment

A major shift in the minds of infectious disease researchers in recent years has been the realization that pathogens are far from the relatively static entities they were once thought to be. It is now clear, from many different examples, that bacterial pathogens sense the environment in which they live, and alter gene expression profiles accordingly to enable exploitation of and survival in that environment. For example, a food-poisoning bacterium such as *Salmonella enterica* might be living on a nutrient-rich piece of meat, but at a cold temperature. The meat might then be cooked, providing the bacterium with heat stress. If the meat is undercooked the salmonellae will survive the heat stress by expression of different heat-shock operons, which incidentally might also lead to the expression of genes required to survive subsequent assaults in the host. On entry into the mouth, defences such as lysozyme and IgA must be overcome, and on entry into the stomach, a very low pH is encountered. Gene expression will again change in the salmonellae such that genes for acid tolerance and acid resistance are now to the fore. Once the bacteria exit the stomach, the pH will change again and they will be assaulted by bile salts and many other defence mechanisms until they arrive at their point of attachment to the small intestine. Although there are very few experimental data about these phenomena in actual host animals, experiments *in vitro* and a few experiments in cells or in animal models are beginning to reveal the complex changes that must take place in gene expression for a bacterium to establish itself in a host animal.

Many of these changes are orchestrated through well-understood environmental sensory and signal transduction systems. One of the most common is the two-component sensory system. One component is a membrane protein that senses external environmental cues and the second is an intracellular protein that binds to DNA and either activates or represses the transcription and expression of sets of genes, usually called regulons. A signal is transmitted from the sensor to the activator/repressor when the environment changes. Signal transduction is achieved via histidine protein kinases. These two-component systems are very common in bacteria. Those bacteria that can live in numerous environments tend to have many more of them (e.g. *c.*90 in *Pseudomonas*), whereas those bacteria that have become adapted to a lifestyle in a particular host have very few (e.g. 2 in *Chlamydia*, 0 in *Mycoplasma*) and there is often a concomitant loss of genomic size. A better understanding of how bacteria behave and of the genes that are actually expressed inside the host will very likely to lead to breakthroughs in the design of new antimicrobials and vaccines.

Interaction with the immune system: antigenic variation

The survival of pathogens in hosts is made particularly challenging by the existence of the immune system. Pathogens have responded to this challenge by evolving many specific mechanisms for the avoidance, evasion, or subversion of both innate and acquired host resistance mechanisms. For example, some viruses are inherently genetically unstable. The natures of the polymerases that replicate the RNA genomes of influenza virus and lentiviruses such as HIV result in errors being incorporated at a high rate. Many of these errors will be incompatible with the continued existence of the virus as an entity capable of self-reproduction. Consequently, many defective viruses can be isolated, but often the base pair changes do not effectively alter the functionality of the viral protein affected other than to alter its antigenicity. In this way, over time, these viruses evade the immunity that develops in response to infection. Viruses such as influenza have evolved segmented genomes. If two viruses happen to be occupying the same host cell, different segments can reassort and a new virus can be assembled. An intriguing question is how the proper segments are gathered together and packaged into the assembled virion, given that segments from different viruses can reassort. This type of large-scale reassortment leads to the antigenic shifts that overcome even solid levels of herd immunity and allow pandemics of influenza to occur. At a different level, within-host antigenic variation is thought to be one mechanism that allows HIV to continue to be carried chronically in the face of what might appear to be a strong immune response. Many other pathogens may also escape the immune response by antigenic variation within the host. Bacteria such as *Haemophilus influenzae, Neisseria meningitidis*, and *Campylobacter jejuni* have evolved tracts of repetitive DNA in single base pair repeats or repeats of four or more base pairs. The number of these repeats can change, apparently randomly. This is a powerful mechanism that allows the existence of a population of bacteria with a number of different antigens that may be 'randomly' expressed or not expressed in individuals within the population. This may be a kind of altruistic evasion strategy whereby some members of the population are lacking a particular structure which is itself a target for the immune system, such that they will survive and thus continue the existence of that bacterial population. Other mechanisms involving recombination and gene conversion exist in other pathogens, leading to the expression of alternative antigenic versions of the same protein and underlying the cycling of different forms of, e.g. variant surface glycoprotein in trypanosomes and the opportunistic fungal pathogen *Pneumocystis jirovecii* or pili in neisseriae.

Pathogens have also evolved mechanisms to subvert the immune system by mimicking elements of the innate response. Good examples are herpes and poxviruses that encode chemokine homologues and/or chemokine receptor homologues or analogues.

Genomes

Many bacterial, viral, fungal, and protozoal genome sequences are now complete. New genome sequencing technologies that are currently coming on stream are increasing massively our ability to generate raw sequence data. The availability of genome-scale sequence data for these pathogens has revolutionized our understanding of their biology and has opened up completely new methods of study and ways of thinking about how they interact with their hosts. Immediate benefits of having complete genome sequences include the obvious knowledge of the complete gene set. This means that we now 'know' every conceivable target for the immune system and every conceivable target for novel antimicrobial development. The real challenge for researchers and infectious disease physicians is to sift and unravel the whole mass of information and to select from it that which is genuinely useful. Once complete genome information is available, it will be interesting to see whether current vaccine target antigens, which have been derived empirically, really are the best targets. For example, *Bordetella pertussis* pertactin is one of a family of proteins called autotransporters. It is a very important component of the acellular whooping cough vaccine, and was discovered through much experimentation by several groups over many years. The genome sequence of *B. pertussis* contains a large number of other autotransporters, any one of which might be a vaccine candidate, and could conceivably be better than pertactin. Much research needs to be done to clarify these questions.

It might be better to invent strategies to let the host biology and the genome itself indicate which genes and antigens are likely to be useful as vaccine targets. Some of these methods are now being published and a good example is 'reverse vaccinology'. Here, genes for outer membrane proteins from a pathogen of interest are selected using computer algorithms, cloned by polymerase chain reaction (PCR) or synthesized, and the encoded protein expressed and purified. These proteins can then be used to interrogate sera from animals or humans that have been infected and are convalescent, to identify which of them is expressed as an antigen during infection, although this step is not essential. The proteins can subsequently be used to immunize animals with the intention of testing the resultant immune response for its ability to protect against virulent challenge in different infection models. The choice of read-out and model is of course crucial if an effective vaccine for humans is to be designed. Despite many possible pitfalls, reverse vaccinology is an exciting technology platform with great promise for the exploitation of genomes to generate completely new candidate vaccines against bacteria. Indeed a new vaccine against group B meningococcus has been developed using this strategy and was reported in 2008 as already having been through a successful phase II clinical trial.

Another fascinating story, emerging from the availability of many genome sequences and coupled with technology such as microarrays, has been the recognition of diversity within bacterial species and the evolutionary relationships between bacteria that this implies. It is clear that many bacterial species share their DNA promiscuously and that this can lead to rapid evolution of drug resistance and altered pathogenicity. Many tried and trusted schemes for classifying and typing bacteria need to be reassessed in the light of genomic information. Classic typing schemes, such as Kaufman–White for salmonellae, based on recognition of antigens on the bacteria by standardized antibodies, will be replaced by DNA-based methods such as multilocus sequence typing, analysis of single nucleotide polymorphisms (SNPs), and microarray-based approaches. The current advances in DNA sequencing technology and throughput are allowing rapid and routine acquisition of complete genome sequences of pathogen isolates in the laboratory and it is likely that in the relatively near future this will be a routine feature of the clinical laboratory. The high degree of diversity within certain bacterial species demands the use of many more than one genome sequence if approaches such as reverse vaccinology are to be exploited to their full extent.

Future challenges

Most infectious diseases are unlikely to be eradicated in the near future. Even if they were, new infectious agents would inevitably evolve to exploit the rich environments presented by host animals. It is probably fair to say that infectious disease biology and medicine are currently undergoing a renaissance, driven by the revolution in genome science, allied to the real and present dangers still presented by many pathogens. Infectious diseases still kill more people worldwide than any other class of disease. They have the capacity to deliver sudden severe global pandemics resulting in high global mortality. Emerging infections presenting acute public health problems are likely to be viral in nature, to have originated in an animal population and, therefore, at least initially, to be zoonoses, and to be spread quickly via air travel. Changing social conditions, e.g. increasing urbanization in certain parts of Africa, bring together animal and human populations that have rarely if ever been closely associated. This brings with it an increased chance for microorganisms to be shared between these species, with a resulting increased chance of new pathogens emerging. Even relatively minor changes in societal behaviour can lead to major disease problems. For example, changes to methods for preparing cattle feed led to the emergence of the BSE prion as a human disease problem in recent years in the United Kingdom and elsewhere.

This analysis does not take into account the added problem of possible biowarfare attacks, although the paranoia surrounding this subject is disproportionate to the threat.

To deal with these disease threats, the regulatory framework underlying the development and legal deployment of antimicrobials and vaccines will have to be adapted and evolved in step with the evolution of the diseases themselves. The pathogens are likely to win this race too! Artificial distinctions between 'human' and 'veterinary' medicine need to be removed. Most pathogens infect more than one species of host animal and certainly do not respect the anthropocentric division of research effort. The concept of 'One Medicine', introduced by Calvin Schwabe, is nowhere more pertinent than in consideration of infectious diseases and the biology of pathogens.

A concerted effort is needed to deal with pathogens in all parts of the world and not just in the developed world. Inexpensive but effective intervention strategies must be developed to defeat acute and chronic infectious diseases worldwide. The lives affected by pathogenic microorganisms in developing countries are just as valuable as those in more affluent areas, but are much more numerous. It is our task, whether from a medical, veterinary, or basic science background, to try to understand how pathogenic microorganisms work, and to harness that knowledge to defeat, wherever possible and by whatever means, these ever-adaptable scourges.

Further reading

Dean P, Maresca M, Kenny B (2005). EPEC's weapons of mass subversion. *Curr Opin Microbiol*, **8**, 28–34.

Galan JE, Wolf-Watz H (2006). Protein delivery into eukaryotic cells by type III secretion machines. *Nature*, **444**, 567–73.

Janeway CA, Medzhitov R (2002). Innate immune recognition. *Annu Rev Immunol*, **20**, 197–216.

Kuiken T, *et al.* (2006). Host species barriers to influenza virus infections. *Science*, **312**, 394–7.

Mora M, *et al.* (2006). Microbial genomes and vaccine design: refinements to the classical reverse vaccinology approach. *Curr Opin Microbiol*, **9**, 532–6.

Moxon R, Bayliss C, Hood D (2006). Bacterial contingency loci: the role of simple sequence DNA repeats in bacterial adaptation. *Annu Rev Genet*, **40**, 307–33.

Murphy PM (2001). Viral exploitation and subversion of the immune system through chemokine mimicry. *Nat Immunol*, **2**, 116–22.

Neumann G, Kawaoka Y (2006). Host range restriction and pathogenicity in the context of influenza pandemic. *Emerg Infect Dis*, **12**, 881–6.

Roumagnac P, *et al.* (2006). Evolutionary history of *Salmonella typhi*. *Science*, **314**, 1301–4.

van Riel D, *et al.* (2007). Human and avian influenza viruses target different cells in the lower respiratory tract of humans and other mammals. *Am J Pathol*, **171**, 1215–23.

7.1.2 Physiological changes, clinical features, and general management of infected patients

Todd W. Rice and Gordon R. Bernard

Essentials

Pathophysiological mechanisms

The host response to an infectious stimulus involves an intricate link between the inflammatory and coagulation systems, also mechanisms designed to limit damage to normal tissues. Key elements are: (1) the inflammatory cascade—antigens from infectious agents stimulate macrophages and monocytes (and other cells) via Toll-like receptors to release tumour necrosis factor α (TNFα), resulting in a cascade of pro-inflammatory cytokine release which is a vital component of the host's attempt to control and eradicate infection, but unfortunately can also result in damage to both infected and uninfected host tissues; inflammatory mediators with prolonged actions or appearing later in the course of sepsis are likely to play an important role in determining prognosis; (2) the anti-inflammatory cascade—a compensatory response involving anti-inflammatory cytokines, soluble receptors, and receptor antagonists directed against pro-inflammatory cytokines that is intended to localize and control the systemic proinflammatory response to the infection; (3) the coagulation cascade—activated in an attempt to contain infection locally and prevent spread to other parts of the body; platelets are activated, procoagulant pathways are initiated, and anticoagulant mediators are down-regulated; (4) the anticoagulation cascade—the coagulation response to sepsis is regulated via antithrombin, tissue factor pathway inhibitor (TFPI), activated protein C (APC), and fibrinolysis.

Clinical features

Definitions—(1) Systemic inflammatory response syndrome (SIRS)—which can occur as a result of an infectious or noninfectious insult—requires the presence of at least two of the following: (a) hyper- or hypothermia, (b) tachycardia, (c) tachypnoea or hyperventilation, (d) leucocytosis, leucopenia or left shift. (2) Sepsis—a suspected or confirmed infection plus criteria for SIRS. (3) Severe sepsis—sepsis resulting in the acute dysfunction of at least one organ system. (4) Septic shock—infection resulting in hypotension despite adequate fluid resuscitation.

Management—key elements are (1) antibiotics—often initiated empirically before culture results are available; (2) control of the source of infection—searching for the site of infection so that it can be eradicated should begin as soon as haemodynamic and respiratory status are stabilized; antibiotics without source control often fail; (3) early goal-directed resuscitation—requiring (a) crystalloid infusions to maintain central venous pressure, (b) vasopressors if arterial pressure remains low, and (c) transfusion of packed red blood cells and/or infusion of dobutamine if central venous oxygen saturation remains low; (4) consideration of other treatments—many specialists advocate recombinant APC for patients with severe sepsis who have a low risk of bleeding and a high risk of death.

Introduction

The term sepsis describes the physiological consequences of the activation of the systemic inflammatory cascade that occurs in infected patients. The cascade of events in response to infectious stimuli has been well characterized using both animal and human models. This response is the main focus of this chapter. Other aspects of sepsis, including epidemiology, clinical features, treatment, prognosis, and the controversial role of corticosteroids and tight glycaemic control will also be addressed.

Pathophysiology of infection

Initial investigations suggested that inflammatory cytokines mediated the physiological responses seen in patients with sepsis. However, information from studies of the coagulation system in sepsis and the subsequent examination of autopsy specimens demonstrated microthrombi in the arterioles and venules of various organs, suggesting that the coagulation system played at least some role in the pathophysiology. It is now clear that the inflammatory and coagulation systems are intricately linked and homeostasis of both is altered in infected patients.

Inflammatory cascade

Early phase

Sepsis syndrome describes the physiological effects of the systemic inflammatory cascade produced by the human body in response to any of a variety of infectious stimuli. Antigens from infectious agents stimulate macrophages and monocytes to release tumour necrosis factor-α (TNFα) resulting in a cascade of cytokine release. Numerous cell wall antigens are able to stimulate this response, including lipopolysaccharide (LPS) or endotoxin from Gram-negative bacteria, lipoteichoic acid from Gram-positive bacteria, peptidoglycan and flagellin from both Gram-negative and Gram-positive bacteria, and mannan from fungi. These antigens initiate an inflammatory response via type I transmembrane receptors called Toll-like receptors found on the surface of a variety of cell types including macrophages, neutrophils, fibroblasts, and some epithelial and endothelial cells. Numerous Toll-like receptors have been identified, but subtypes 2 (TLR2) and 4 (TLR4) appear to play a major role in mediating the inflammatory response to infectious stimuli. TLR2 binds both peptidoglycan and lipoteichoic acid from Gram-positive bacteria. On the other hand, TLR4 serves as the signal transduction component for LPS from Gram-negative bacteria. In macrophages and neutrophils, binding of LPS to TLR4 results in the release of TNFα via NF-κB, a eukaryotic transcription factor. Circulating TNFα stimulates the release of other proinflammatory cytokines from macrophages and neutrophils. These proinflammatory cytokines, especially interleukins 1 and 6 (IL-1, IL-6), trigger numerous additional proinflammatory events within endothelial cells and leucocytes (Fig. 7.1.2.1). TNFα acts in conjunction with IL-1 to produce the fever, tachycardia, and tachypnoea seen with systemic inflammation. In addition, their synergistic effects are probably responsible for the hypotension and resultant organ dysfunction seen early in the course of severe sepsis. The purpose of this proinflammatory response, which represents a vital component

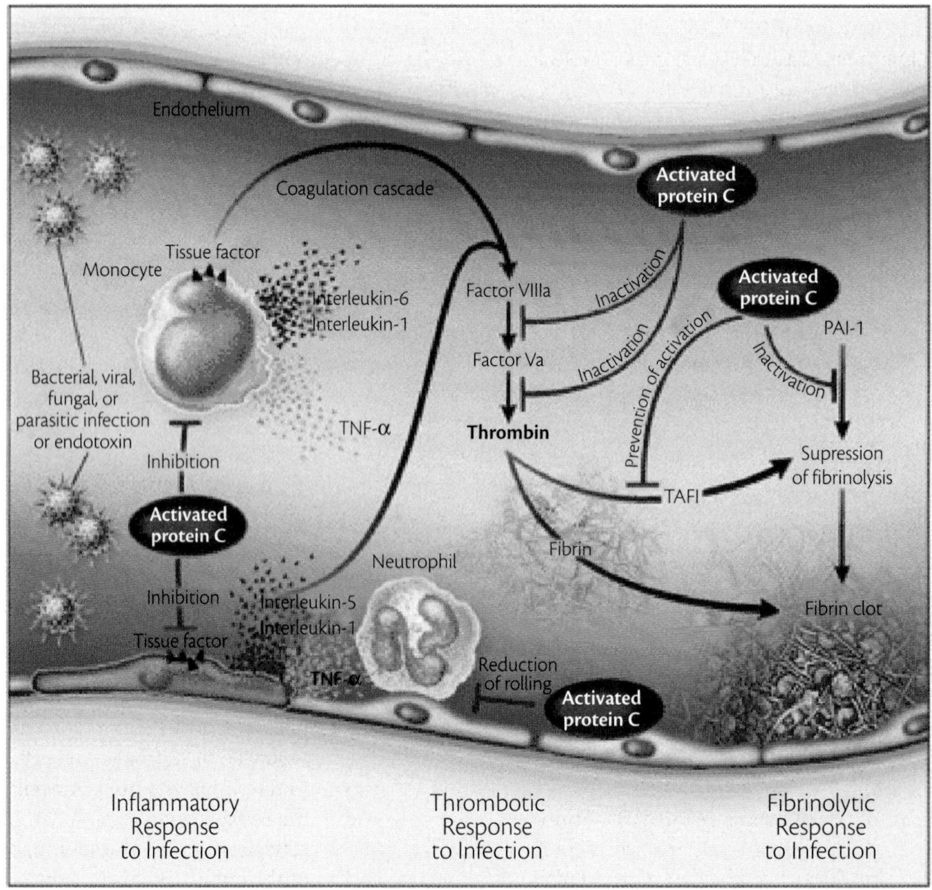

Fig. 7.1.2.1 The intricate link between the inflammatory and procoagulant response to infection with sites of action for activated protein C. PAI-1, plasminogen activator inhibitor type 1; TNF-α, tumour necrosis factor-α.
(From Bernard GR, *et al.* (2001). Efficacy and safety of recombinant human activated protein C for severe sepsis. *N Engl J Med*, **344**, 699–709. Copyright © 2001 Massachusetts Medical Society. All rights reserved.)

of the host defence, is to control and eradicate the infection. Unfortunately, the response is often so exuberant and poorly controlled that it results in damage to both infected and uninfected host tissues.

Late phase

The symptoms of sepsis, specifically tachypnoea, tachycardia, fever, or hypotension, are what prompt most patients to seek medical attention. Unfortunately, these result from the early inflammatory cascade which is already well into its course by the time patients present for medical care. Administration of endotoxin to humans demonstrates that TNF is the primary protagonist of the inflammatory response as serum levels rise almost immediately. However, the presence of TNF in the serum is short-lived and the majority of patients with sepsis have undetectable levels at the time of presentation, even the most critically ill with organ failure or shock.

Many sepsis deaths occur later in the course, at least 48 to 72 h after the onset of symptoms. This has prompted many to speculate that inflammatory mediators with more prolonged actions or appearing later in the course of sepsis are likely to play an important role in determining prognosis. High-mobility group box protein 1 (HMGB1) is one such late mediator; it is a 30-kDa protein, named for its rapid migration on electrophoretic gels, which was purified along with histones from nuclei in the 1970s and is now classified as a nonhistone chromatin-associated protein. The critical role played by HMGB1 in gene transcription and DNA repair and replication has been known since shortly after its discovery. However, recent data suggest that HMGB1 also possesses inflammatory properties. Using nuclear pores, HMGB1 is able to move from the nucleus to the cytosol, making it available for extracellular secretion from macrophages when stimulated with LPS or TNF. Cell necrosis, but not apoptosis, results in the passive release of HMGB1 from all nucleated cells. Once outside the cell, HMGB1 functions as an important mediator of both inflammation and coagulation, stimulating the release of proinflammatory cytokines, including TNFα, IL-1, and IL-6 from endothelial cells and monocytes. HMGB1 also helps regulate coagulation by inducing the expression of adhesion molecules on endothelial cells, resulting in the secretion of plasminogen activator inhibitor type 1 (PAI-1) and tissue plasminogen activator.

Animal models of sepsis demonstrate that serum levels of HMGB1 increase after LPS administration. However, unlike TNF and IL-1 which peak early in the course of sepsis and become undetectable within a few hours, serum levels of HMGB1 remain undetectable until 8 h after LPS administration and continue to increase until they plateau 24 to 32 h later. Similar elevations in levels of HMGB1 can be detected in the serum of humans with severe sepsis or septic shock and in plasma and bronchoalveolar lavage fluid of patients with sepsis and acute lung injury. Serum levels of HMGB1 may also have prognostic significance as higher levels are associated with mortality.

Mice treated with sublethal doses of HMGB1 develop signs of endotoxaemia within 2 h and higher doses result in death within 18 to 36 h, even in mice resistant to the effects of LPS. Numerous animal models have also demonstrated that antagonizing the effects of HMGB1 improves survival in sepsis, even when the antagonism is considerably delayed. Anti-HMGB1 antibodies, ethyl pyruvate (a nontoxic food derivative that inhibits the release of HMGB1 from LPS-stimulated and TNF-stimulated macrophages), and competitive inhibition of the HMGB1 binding site on macrophages all result in improved survival in animal models in which sepsis was induced with endotoxin and caecal ligation and puncture. However, treatment with these antagonists did not just extend the time to death, but allowed many of the animals to survive until necropsy and 'rescued' animals that already exhibited signs of severe sepsis.

Anti-inflammatory cascade

Although the initial inflammatory response in sepsis was originally believed to be largely uncontrolled, subsequent investigations have demonstrated that the body employs a compensatory anti-inflammatory response (CARS) in an attempt to maintain homeostasis. In addition to stimulating the release of other proinflammatory mediators, TNFα and IL-1 also stimulate leucocytes to release anti-inflammatory mediators, including IL-10, IL-13, and transforming growth factor β (TGFβ). These cytokines exert a direct anti-inflammatory effect on macrophages and endothelial cells and inhibit the synthesis of proinflammatory mediators. IL-10 and IL-13 also inhibit the ability of monocytes effectively to present antigens to other immune cells. The inflammatory response is further controlled by the release of soluble receptors and receptor antagonists directed against proinflammatory cytokines. This compensatory anti-inflammatory response is intended to localize and control the systemic proinflammatory response to the infection. Unfortunately, the anti-inflammatory response often exceeds the proinflammatory response in the later phases of sepsis, resulting in a hyporesponsiveness of immune cells and an inability to mount an effective immune response to additional infectious insults. This immunoparalysis late in the course of sepsis leads to delayed hypersensitivity, inability to clear infections, and an increased susceptibility to nosocomial infections, all of which contribute to the late morbidity and mortality in these patients.

Coagulation cascade

Earlier investigations implicated the inflammatory cascade in sepsis, but more recent work has demonstrated the involvement of the clotting and fibrinolytic systems which are intricately related to the inflammatory response (Fig. 7.1.2.1). As well as disrupting proinflammatory and anti-inflammatory homeostasis, sepsis also disturbs coagulation homeostasis. In response to infectious stimuli, the body rouses the coagulation cascade in an attempt to contain infection locally and prevent spread to other parts of the body. To accomplish this, platelets are activated, procoagulant pathways are initiated, and anticoagulant mediators are down-regulated. Unfortunately, this often results in a 'sepsis-associated coagulopathy', which may range from mild thrombocytopenia or increase in prothrombin time to overt disseminated intravascular coagulopathy. If the procoagulant response becomes too exuberant, microvascular thromboses can form resulting in local tissue hypoxia and subsequent organ dysfunction.

The activation of the coagulation response is intricately linked to the inflammatory response. TNFα and IL-1 both stimulate the release of tissue factor from monocytes and neutrophils and cause tissue factor normally present on endothelial cells, but not exposed to the circulation, to be 'unveiled' (Fig. 7.1.2.1). Tissue factor acts as the bridge between the inflammatory and coagulation pathways by activating the extrinsic clotting system and stimulating the formation of thrombin and fibrin clots. Specifically, the highly thrombogenic tissue factor (TF) combines with circulating factor VII to form a TF:VIIa complex. This complex activates factor X, which subsequently produces thrombin from prothrombin. Thrombin stimulates the formation of fibrin clots in the microcirculation with the aim of confining the infection to the local site. The disadvantage created by diffuse intravascular microthrombi is the creation of areas of regional hypoperfusion, resulting in tissue ischaemia, coagulation necrosis, and organ dysfunction.

Thrombin, TF:VIIa complex, and activated factor X also provide positive feedback to the inflammatory cascade. All three function as potent inflammatory mediators, stimulating neutrophil migration and release of additional proinflammatory cytokines. In turn, this positive feedback loop eventually fuels additional tissue factor release and more thrombin and fibrin clot formation.

Anticoagulation cascade

In similar fashion to its compensatory anti-inflammatory response, the body also regulates the coagulation response to sepsis. The anticoagulant response is mediated via four mechanisms: (1) antithrombin, (2) tissue factor pathway inhibitor (TFPI), (3) activated protein C (APC), and (4) fibrinolysis. Unfortunately, inflammation in sepsis suppresses many of these counter-regulatory measures, promoting a procoagulant environment.

Antithrombin

Antithrombin is synthesized in the liver and secreted into the circulation. It occurs free in the plasma and attached to platelets and endothelial cells, where it functions as an inhibitor of the coagulation system. Antithrombin directly suppresses thrombin-induced fibrin formation, inhibits factors IXa, XIa, and XIIa of the intrinsic coagulation pathway, and decreases the activation of factor Xa which is common to both the intrinsic and extrinsic coagulation pathways. The serum half-life of antithrombin, normally 36 to 48 h, is reduced to 8 h or less in sepsis-associated coagulopathy, resulting in a rapid depletion of antithrombin and a shift towards a procoagulant microvascular environment. Despite data showing that low or falling antithrombin levels were associated with a worse outcome in severe sepsis, administration of exogenous antithrombin failed to improve the prognosis in these patients.

TFPI

Endothelial cells synthesize and secrete TFPI, which inhibits the TF:VIIa complex and activated factor X. This results in suppression of the extrinsic pathway of coagulation and decreases the formation of thrombin and fibrin clots. Sepsis results in a truncated form of TFPI, with reduced anticoagulant properties. Although overall TFPI levels are elevated in septic patients, their reduced anticoagulant effect still favours thrombin formation and fibrin deposition at the endothelium. Unfortunately, administration of a recombinant TFPI also failed to produce clinical benefit in a large trial of patients with severe sepsis.

APC

Protein C is synthesized in the liver through a vitamin K-dependent pathway and is secreted into the blood as an inactive zymogen. In the presence of endothelial protein C receptor (EPCR) and a properly functioning endothelium, protein C is converted to its active form by complexing with thrombin and endothelial cell thrombomodulin. APC inhibits PAI-1 and inactivates clotting factors Va and VIIIa (Fig. 7.1.2.1). These profibrinolytic and antithrombotic properties restore and maintain, respectively, microcirculatory blood flow which help re-establish coagulation homeostasis and preserve the microcirculation. APC also has anti-inflammatory properties, such as limiting the inflammatory response induced by thrombin and inhibiting TNF production (Fig. 7.1.2.1). Unfortunately, severe sepsis down-regulates EPCR causing it to be sloughed from the cell surface, resulting in endothelial dysfunction. Sepsis also decreases plasma concentrations of thrombomodulin. These changes impair the conversion of protein C to its active form, resulting in a deficiency of APC. Most patients with severe sepsis have low levels of protein C and lower levels are associated with poorer outcomes.

Fibrinolysis

Under normal homeostatic circumstances, dissolution of fibrin clots (fibrinolysis) serves as an additional counter-regulatory measure to the coagulation cascade. Plasminogen activators convert plasminogen to active plasmin which then mediates clot lysis by degrading the cross-linked fibrin present in the clot. This fibrinolytic response is controlled primarily by plasminogen activator inhibitors, predominantly PAI-1. The production of PAI-1 is stimulated by proinflammatory cytokines, resulting in elevated levels which decrease plasminogen and plasmin levels over time (Fig. 7.1.2.1). Some plasmin-induced fibrinolysis still occurs in this environment, but is often insufficient to maintain coagulation homeostasis.

Epidemiology

The incidence of sepsis is about 240 cases per 100 000 people per year. It is the second most common cause of death in critically ill patients, after cardiovascular events, resulting in the deaths of 225 000 out of almost 750 000 patients with sepsis each year in the United States of America alone where the overall cost of caring for these patients exceeds $17 billion annually. In recent years, the incidence of sepsis has risen by almost 9% each year and will continue to increase with the ageing population, growing antibiotic resistance, increasing immunocompromised state of patients, and the expanding use of invasive procedures.

Although many patients afflicted with severe sepsis have obvious risk factors, the syndrome is not limited to the old, debilitated, or immunocompromised. Sepsis can affect anyone, including healthy young people, and often has devastating consequences. Men are more commonly affected than women and nonwhite people are affected almost twice as often as white people. Respiratory infections are the most common cause, but genitourinary sources predominate in women. Gram-positive bacteria account for over one-half of all infections, Gram-negative bacteria for about one-third, and fungi for 5%.

Clinical features and criteria for diagnosis

Definitions of systemic inflammatory response syndrome (SIRS), sepsis, and severe sepsis are frequently confused. SIRS, which can occur as a result of an infectious or noninfectious insult, is defined by demonstrating at least two of the following four criteria: (1) hyperthermia or hypothermia (temperature ≥38°C or ≤36°C), (2) tachycardia (heart rate >90 beats/min), (3) tachypnoea or hyperventilation (>30 respirations/min or $Paco_2$ <32 mmHg), and (4) leucocytosis, leucopenia, or left shift (≥12 or $\leq 4 \times 10^9$ white blood cells/litre or >10% immature neutrophils). Sepsis is defined as a suspected or confirmed infection plus at least two of the above

SIRS criteria. Severe sepsis is used to describe sepsis resulting in the acute dysfunction of at least one organ system. When the infection results in hypotension despite adequate fluid resuscitation, the patient has septic shock.

Tachypnoea is usually the first detectable clinical sign and is so common in severe sepsis that its absence should make the diagnosis suspect. The cause of the rapid breathing is often multifactorial. The lung is the most frequent site of infection and acute lung injury resulting from nonpulmonary sources of infection and respiratory compensation for metabolic acidosis also contribute. Tachycardia is virtually universal unless prevented by a cardiac conduction defect or pharmacotherapy (e.g. β-blockers). Increasing heart rate is an important compensatory mechanism to respond to the hypermetabolic state of sepsis as well as to maintain perfusion in response to intravascular volume deficits, reduced cardiac contractility, and vasodilation.

Differential diagnosis and clinical investigation

The diagnosis of sepsis may be obvious in some patients, but making the diagnosis in most requires a high level of suspicion and a fair amount of investigation. Noninfectious conditions such as pancreatitis, trauma, severe haemorrhage, myocardial infarction, drug overdose, and even heat stroke can mimic sepsis and often need to be ruled out before the diagnosis of sepsis syndrome can be established.

Laboratory abnormalities are often present, but are not specific for infection. Although suspicious, leucocytosis, bandaemia, and leucopenia are neither sensitive nor specific for the diagnosis. The hallmark of sepsis is a positive culture from a normally sterile body site, such as blood, urine, or cerebrospinal fluid, but culture results often take 24 to 48 h to return and are negative in up to one-third of cases. Clinical investigations, such as radiographs, urinalysis, or cerebrospinal fluid examination may demonstrate the site of infection. Other suggestive, but nonspecific laboratory results that may aid diagnosis include: elevated arterial lactate, metabolic acidosis with reduced serum bicarbonate, blood urea nitrogen, creatinine, glucose, bilirubin, alkaline phosphatase, and aminotransferase measurements. An elevated serum procalcitonin level may be a reasonable marker of sepsis in patients with SIRS, but is usually not readily available.

Treatment of sepsis

Antibiotics

Early administration of properly chosen antibiotics reduces morbidity and mortality in patients with sepsis. In clinical trials, an appropriate antibiotic regimen is begun in a timely fashion in 85 to 95% of occasions, but failure to do so is associated with a 25% higher overall case fatality. Since culture results are not immediately available for most septic patients, clinicians must use antibiotics empirically. When initiating therapy, the suspected site of infection, patient's immune status, recent antibiotic use, local resistance patterns, location in which the patient acquired the infection (i.e. nosocomial vs community), and Gram's stain and culture results should all be considered. Unless the causative organism and susceptibility are known, initial antibiotic therapy should cover a broader spectrum of possibilities when the patient is critically ill. Once microbiological data are available, therapy should be tailored promptly to the narrowest spectrum, least toxic, and least expensive agent.

Source control

Searching for the site of infection should begin as soon as haemodynamic and respiratory status are stabilized. Effective management relies on eradicating the source of infection, as antibiotics without source control often fail. Any devitalized tissue or sizeable collection of pus should be resected or drained, either surgically or using less invasive percutaneous drainage techniques. All foreign bodies, including intravascular catheters, should be carefully examined and removed promptly if there is any suspicion of infection.

Early goal-directed resuscitation

The inflammatory cytokines released in sepsis decrease systemic resistance, reduce filling pressure, and depress myocardial contractility. Increased venous pooling, greater insensible losses from anorexia, sweating, vomiting and diarrhoea, and worsening microvascular permeability all contribute to decreased intravascular volume. Consequently, many septic patients rapidly develop cardiovascular insufficiency manifested as hypotension. Aggressive resuscitation, aimed at restoring and maintaining an adequate blood pressure, should be initiated early in the course of treatment. In adults of normal size, this resuscitation often requires large amounts of colloid or 6 to 10 litres isotonic crystalloid. Although the endpoint for discontinuing aggressive resuscitation and the optimal measure of adequate perfusion pressure remains ill-defined, early goal-directed resuscitation (EGDT) during the first 6 h has been shown to lower mortality in one single-centre study of patients with severe sepsis and lactic acidosis or septic shock. The algorithm utilizes crystalloid infusions to maintain a central venous pressure of 8 to 12 mmHg. If mean arterial pressure remains below 65 mmHg, vasopressors are initiated. During resuscitation, central venous oxygen saturation ($Scvo_2$) is monitored continuously using a central venous catheter. If the patient has a central venous pressure and mean arterial pressure within the target ranges, but the $Scvo_2$ measurement remains below 70%, packed red blood cells are transfused to achieve a haematocrit of 30%. If the haematocrit is 30% or higher and the $Scvo_2$ is still below 70%, dobutamine is begun. Intention-to-treat analysis demonstrated that patients receiving EGDT during the first 6 h of care had a 33% relative reduction and 16% absolute reduction in hospital mortality (30.5% vs 46.5%; $P = 0.009$), with improvement in mortality persisting to at least 60 days. The reduction in mortality was largely attributable to a decrease in late, sudden cardiovascular collapse in patients treated with EGDT.

Drotrecogin alfa (activated) or recombinant human activated protein C

In late 2001, recombinant human activated protein C (rhAPC), or drotrecogin alfa (activated) (DAA), became the first drug approved for use in patients with a high risk of death from severe sepsis. A large phase III randomized blind placebo-controlled multinational trial was discontinued early, after 1690 of the planned 2280 patients were enrolled, because the predefined stopping boundary for efficacy was surpassed. rhAPC, administered as a continuous intravenous infusion of 24 μg/kg per h for 96 h, resulted in a 6% absolute and 19% relative reduction in 28-day all-cause mortality compared to placebo (24.7% vs 30.8%; $P = 0.005$). The survival difference became apparent shortly after initiation of the infusion, continued to increase for the duration of the study period, and persisted out to at least 1 year of long-term follow-up. Subsequent prospective data suggested that early treatment with rhAPC (i.e. within 24 h of organ dysfunction onset) resulted in better outcomes than delayed initiation. Although the criteria for high risk of death are hotly debated, patients with Acute Physiology and Chronic Health Evaluation II (APACHE II) scores of more than 25 or requiring vasopressors or mechanical ventilation are widely considered appropriate candidates for the drug.

Not unexpectedly given its anticoagulant properties, rhAPC increases the risk of bleeding. Although uncommon in both arms of the study, severe bleeding episodes were also almost twice as high in those receiving rhAPC compared to placebo (3.5% vs 2.0%; $P = 0.06$). These bleeding rates are similar to those seen with other forms of full systemic anticoagulation, such as full-dose heparin. Although patients at high risk of bleeding were excluded from the landmark study, those with either traumatic injury of a highly vascular organ or major blood vessel, ulcerations in the gastrointestinal system, meningitis, or markedly abnormal coagulation parameters (platelet counts <30 000/ml, INR >3, or activated partial thromboplastin time >120 s) had more bleeding.

Subsequent studies in adult patients with low risk of death (i.e. APACHE II <25, not on vasopressors, not in the intensive care unit) and children were stopped early because of inefficacy and side effects. Analysis of these data found that children with sepsis and postoperative patients with single-organ failure from sepsis did not derive benefit from administration of rhAPC, and both groups experienced higher bleeding rates. The drug is therefore not recommended for use in these populations.

Volume-limited and pressure-limited mechanical ventilation strategy

The vast majority of patients with severe sepsis require mechanical ventilation, many from sepsis-induced acute lung injury. Preventing undue distension of normally compliant segments of the injured lung, and subsequent release of inflammatory cytokines by using a volume-limited and pressure-limited ventilation strategy in patients with acute lung injury has been shown to decrease mortality and increase time alive and off the ventilator. To accomplish this, patients should be ventilated using volume-limited ventilation strategies with tidal volumes set at 6 ml/kg of predicted body weight. These tidal volumes should be titrated downwards as needed to maintain plateau pressure less than 30 cm H_2O. Ventilator weaning that is protocol-driven and employs daily spontaneous breathing trials results in earlier successful extubation.

Preventing complications and nosocomial infections

Since patients with severe sepsis possess multiple risk factors for deep venous thrombosis, prophylaxis for this complication should be nearly routine. Patients with low bleeding risk should receive a known effective dose of low molecular weight or unfractionated heparin, while intermittent compression devices should be used in patients at significant risk of bleeding. H_2-receptor antagonists have been shown to be superior to treatment with sucralfate in prevention of gastrointestinal bleeding for mechanically ventilated patients. Therefore, current therapy should almost always include an H_2-receptor blocker or a proton pump inhibitor.

The compensatory anti-inflammatory response and impaired host defence, along with numerous invasive procedures and broad-spectrum antibiotic exposure, predisposes patients with severe sepsis to nosocomial infections. Hand washing between patients and using barrier precautions (gloves and gowns) when examining patients colonized with resistant organisms should be universally employed. Likewise, inserting central lines using full barrier precautions, limiting the number of catheter manipulations, and utilizing closed infusion systems with minimal tubing changes can minimize vascular catheter infections. The risk of nosocomial pneumonia can be reduced by raising the head of the bed to 30 to 45 degrees in mechanically ventilated patients, especially those receiving enteral feedings. Draining the condensate from ventilator tubing and minimizing tubing changes also decreases the incidence of nosocomial pneumonia. If possible, all feeding and endotracheal tubes should be orally placed to reduce the incidence of sinusitis. If a tube must be placed through the nose, it should be small-bore and flexible to decrease the degree of sinus ostial obstruction.

Prognosis

Sepsis without organ dysfunction is a very serious condition, with in-hospital mortality rates ranging from 5 to 10%. However, once organ dysfunction is present, even with modern advances in the care of the critically ill, one-third to one-half of all patients with severe sepsis die before being discharged from hospital, and patients with septic shock have hospital mortality rates of 50 to 80%. Patients who survive their initial encounter with severe sepsis continue to have higher rates of death throughout the first year after hospital discharge for unknown reasons.

Areas of uncertainty

As with all diseases, areas of uncertainty exist in treating patients with severe sepsis. Corticosteroid treatment and tight glucose control with intensive insulin therapy represent two current areas of uncertainty. Although corticosteroids possess a variety of anti-inflammatory actions, numerous studies have demonstrated that high doses, aimed at suppressing the inflammatory response to infection, confer no benefit to patients with severe sepsis or septic shock. Meta-analyses of these studies confirm the lack of efficacy and even suggest a trend towards harm. More recent data suggest that lower, more physiological doses, administered over a longer period of time, may benefit a subset of patients with septic shock and relative adrenal insufficiency. Unfortunately, a multinational double-blind placebo-controlled study investigating this 'replacement dose' strategy found no difference in 28-day all-cause mortality or shock-free days. Given the numerous negative studies, the routine use of corticosteroids in patients with severe sepsis or septic shock cannot be recommended at this time.

The use of intensive insulin therapy, aimed at maintaining serum blood glucose levels between 80 and 110 mg/dl, also remains controversial. An initial study demonstrated that this tight glycaemic control improved survival, decreased bacteraemia, and reduced renal failure in cardiac surgery patients, regardless of a history of diabetes. A subsequent study in critically ill medical patients was unable to replicate the results, although some benefit was seen in patients requiring intensive care for longer than 72 h. Although hypoglycaemia is uncommon, patients who develop it have significantly higher mortality rates. Further research into this area will need to be undertaken to identify the optimal patient population and target glucose levels for intensive insulin treatment in patients with sepsis.

Further reading

Aird WC (2001). Vascular bed-specific hemostasis: role of endothelium in sepsis pathogenesis. *Crit Care Med*, **29** Suppl 7, 28–35.

Annane D, *et al.* (2002). Effect of treatment with low doses of hydrocortisone and fludrocortisone on mortality in patients with septic shock. *JAMA*, **288**, 862–71.

Bernard GR, *et al.* (2001). Efficacy and safety of recombinant human activated protein C for severe sepsis. *N Engl J Med*, **344**, 699–709.

Bone RC (1996). Sir Isaac Newton, sepsis, SIRS and CARS. *Crit Care Med*, **24**, 1125–8.

Cook DJ, *et al.* (1998). A comparison of sucralfate and ranitidine for the prevention of upper gastrointestinal bleeding in patients requiring mechanical ventilation. *N Engl J Med*, **338**, 791–7.

Dellinger RP, *et al.* (2004). Surviving Sepsis Campaign guidelines for management of severe sepsis and septic shock. *Crit Care Med*, **32**, 858–73.

Hotchkiss RS, Karl IE (2003). The pathophysiology and treatment of sepsis. *N Engl J Med*, **348**, 138–50.

Kollef MH, *et al.* (1999). Inadequate antimicrobial treatment of infections: a risk factor for hospital mortality among critically ill patients. *Chest*, **115**, 462–74.

Levi M, *et al.* (1993). Pathogenesis of disseminated intravascular coagulopathy in sepsis. *JAMA*, **270**, 975–9.

MacIntyre NR, *et al.* (2001). Evidence-based guidelines for weaning and discontinuing ventilatory support: a collective task force facilitated by the American College of Chest Physicians; the American Association for Respiratory Care; and the American College of Critical Care Medicine. *Chest*, **120** Suppl 6, S375–95.

Martin GS, *et al.* (2003). The epidemiology of sepsis in the United States from 1979 through 2000. *N Engl J Med*, **348**, 1546–54.

Rivers E, *et al.* (2001). Early goal-directed therapy in the treatment of severe sepsis and septic shock. *N Engl J Med*, **345**, 1368–77.

The Acute Respiratory Distress Syndrome Network (2000). Ventilation with lower tidal volumes as compared with traditional tidal volumes for acute lung injury and the acute respiratory distress syndrome. *N Engl J Med*, **342**, 1301–8.

Ulloa L, *et al.* (2002). Ethyl pyruvate prevents lethality in mice with established lethal sepsis and systemic inflammation. *Proc Natl Acad Sci U S A*, **99**, 12351–6.

van den Berghe G, *et al.* (2001). Intensive insulin therapy in critically ill patients. *N Engl J Med*, **345**, 1359–67.

van den Berghe G, *et al.* (2006). Intensive insulin therapy in the medical ICU. *N Engl J Med*, **354**, 449–61.

van Deventer SJH, *et al.* (1990). Experimental endotoxemia in humans: analysis of cytokine release and coagulation, fibrinolytic and complement pathways. *Blood*, **76**, 2520–6.

Wang H, *et al.* (1999). HMG-1 as a late mediator of endotoxin lethality in mice. *Science*, **285**, 248–51.

Yang H, *et al.* (2004). Reversing established sepsis with antagonists of endogenous HMGB1. *Proc Natl Acad Sci U S A*, **101**, 296–301.

7.2

The patient with suspected infection

Contents

7.2.1 Clinical approach *420*
Christopher J. Ellis

7.2.2 Fever of unknown origin *423*
Steven Vanderschueren and Daniël Knockaert

7.2.3 Nosocomial infections *428*
I.C.J.W. Bowler

7.2.4 Infection in the immunocompromised host *431*
J. Cohen

7.2.5 Antimicrobial chemotherapy *441*
R.G. Finch

7.2.1 Clinical approach

Christopher J. Ellis

Essentials

Infection is most often suspected when patients present with pyrexia and is certainly the most common cause of this presentation, whether in hospitalized patients or those in the community. The other principal causes of fever are primary inflammatory conditions and malignancy, but infections are likely to be most rapidly progressive and acutely life threatening and hence must be the physician's first concern.

The clinical approach to patients with likely infection begins with a focused history, leading on to a clinical examination which assesses the extent of the physiological derangement and looks for a focus of infection. Standard physiological measures define likely sepsis (see Chapter 7.1.2), which is the commonest reason for their sudden derangement in hospitalized patients. Investigations should be phased and must not delay the start of potentially life-saving treatment, the response to which must be carefully followed, especially when treatment has to be started before a complete or certain diagnosis is possible, and compared with the likely speed of response for the putative condition being treated. There is increasing evidence that delays in initiating appropriate therapy, especially antimicrobial medication and circulatory support, increase mortality.

Introduction

No diagnostic challenge better illustrates the power of traditional clinical methods than the patient with possible infection; clinicians rarely find themselves in a situation where there is potentially so much urgency in establishing a working hypothesis and management plan.

It is vital to keep in mind that previously healthy people with life-threatening infections may have few symptoms other than malaise, and little in the way of abnormality on examination other than an altered body temperature and tachycardia. However, at this point only decisive intervention will prevent a rapid decline into circulatory collapse, coagulopathy, and multiple organ failure with a high risk of death.

What suggests that the patient's life is in danger?

Standard observations (vital signs) are usually valuable pointers to life-threatening situations and have been combined to define sepsis syndromes (Box 7.2.1.1).

Observations made routinely on hospitalized patients are now codified to produce early-warning track and trigger systems, such as the modified early warning score (MEWS), which highlight developing sepsis. In general hospitals, the development of sepsis is currently the most common single reason for patients' scores reaching the trigger point.

Although these alarm calls are important, they will not identify all patients in whom urgent treatment is vital. Table 7.2.1.1 lists

Box 7.2.1.1 Sepsis syndromes

Sepsis (systemic inflammatory response syndrome, SIRS)

Defined by two or more of:

- Temperature >38 °C or <36 °C
- Pulse rate >90/min
- Respiratory rate >20/min
- Leucocyte count >12 or <4 × 10^9/litre

Severe sepsis

Sepsis with one or more of:

- Hypotension
- Confusion
- Oliguria
- Hypoxia
- Acidosis
- Disseminated intravascular coagulation (DIC)

Septic shock

- Severe sepsis with hypotension despite fluid resuscitation

some conditions that typically present in a bland and nonspecific manner although the patient may be only a day or two from death if not treated appropriately.

Infection may be mimicked by life-threatening noninfectious conditions. Primary vasculitic conditions commonly present with fever and skin infarcts identical to those seen in patients with endocarditis, while cerebral systemic lupus erythematosus (SLE) is clinically indistinguishable from an infective encephalitis.

Management before diagnosis

Acute medicine has been described as 'the art of making sufficient conclusions on insufficient information'. When confronted with a patient who fulfils the criteria for severe sepsis, attention must be paid to oxygenation, circulatory support, and intravenous antimicrobials, even if the clinician is still some way from a definitive diagnosis. In these fraught circumstances, organizational confusion can lead to vital actions being omitted or delayed. In particular, the prescriber should ensure the prompt administration of intravenous antimicrobials and deliver a fluid challenge to patients with hypovolaemia, bearing in mind that up to 40% of effective circulating volume can be lost, usually through vasodilatation, before vital signs register more than tachycardia. One litre of saline given over 30 min, and repeated if the pulse rate does not fall, is an appropriate prescription for an adult in this situation.

Table 7.2.1.1 Conditions presenting in a nonspecific manner

Condition	Key clue
Falciparum malaria	Travel history
Early meningococcaemia	Early purpura
Bacteraemia	Rigor, i.e. visible shivering for at least 10 s
Fasciitis	Tenderness to pressure beyond apparent bounds of cellulitis
Toxic shock syndrome	The patient has fainted on standing (because of incipient shock); erythematous rash

The history of the illness

Once immediate life-saving measures are in hand, if they are indicated, a thorough, focused history must include several questions that are not routinely asked (Table 7.2.1.2).

Clinical examination and chest radiograph

Examination of a patient with suspected infection can be both rapid and comprehensive. Having noted the vital signs, the clinician can proceed from head to toe. Temporal arteries should be examined in patients over the age of 50 with fever and headaches; the mouth should be examined for poor teeth and candidiasis (a pointer to possible HIV infection), and the heart for murmur(s). A chest radiograph may reveal areas of consolidation in patients without any respiratory symptoms and hilar lymphadenopathy in patients without palpably enlarged nodes elsewhere. Conversely, a normal chest radiograph does not exclude early pneumonia. Examination of the abdomen should pay particular attention to liver enlargement and/or tenderness and include several firm blows over the ribs overlying the posterior surface of the liver which may elicit tenderness in patients with posterior liver abscesses. Tenderness in the right iliac fossa might indicate bowel-related sepsis, such as an appendix mass, while bimanual examination may reveal an enlarged or tender kidney. The patient's posture should be noted; flexion of the hip points to a possible psoas abscess. Examination of the perineum is mandatory in febrile neutropenic patients; it may reveal septic necrosis spreading from the rectum.

Enlarged lymph nodes should be carefully sought in the neck and in the axilla, where they are easily overlooked. The entire skin should be inspected for rash or for areas of inflammation. The spine should be palpated and percussed looking for angulation or tenderness. The nervous system need not be examined unless symptoms suggest a pathological condition may be found there.

Investigations

These should be phased in the interests of both time and money and to avoid misleading false-positives. Initial blood tests must include a specific test for malaria, if indicated. Blood samples for culture should be taken before antibiotics are started. Patients who have been started on antibiotics before investigation should have them stopped, provided it is judged safe to do so, and blood taken for culture 24 h later. The chest radiograph should be inspected on the same day as the first consultation. All patients should have

Table 7.2.1.2 Questions that must be asked concerning the history of the illness

Open question	Possible significance
Have you travelled?	All cases of falciparum malaria imported into nonendemic areas are in people who have visited malarial areas in the preceding 3 months; most are within 1 month. In the UK, 90% of these infections will have been acquired in sub-Saharan Africa
	Approximately one-half of the cases of legionnaire's disease in the UK are in patients who have returned from Europe or Turkey in the preceding 2 weeks
Have you been sexually active?	Unprotected sex with a new partner (or a promiscuous regular partner) in the previous 2 months increases the probability of primary HIV and secondary syphilis
Have you been exposed to crowds of new social contacts (e.g. university freshers week, new military recruits, or large military deployments)?	Increased probability of meningococcal or pneumococcal infection
Have you been hospitalized or have you received medical attention recently?	Fever following the start of medication raises the possibility of drug fever (typically when a course of penicillin is extended beyond 1 week)
	Recent administration of antibacterial drugs predisposes to *Clostridium difficile* colitis
	Acquisition of a resistant strain of bacteria (e.g. extended-spectrum β-lactamase-producing bacteria)
	Dental work predisposes to endocarditis
	Previous splenectomy predisposes to fulminating pneumococcal septicaemia
	Infection of surgical wounds, retained surgical material, or prostheses
	Partial treatment of an abscess, most commonly intra-abdominal or retroperitoneal, including psoas abscess
Is the illness remittent?	Characteristically remittent conditions, including vivax malaria, systemic Still's disease, lymphoma
	Temporary improvement with antibacterial drugs suggests a possible 'collection', a concealed abscess

a properly taken midstream or clean-catch urine sample sent for analysis.

Liaison with the microbiology laboratory is essential, and prompt delivery of specimens is a priority. Investigations involving cell counts, i.e. cerebrospinal fluid and urine microscopy, must be carried out on the day they were obtained.

Initial investigations are therefore:

- Background—full blood count, urea and electrolytes, liver function tests, C-reactive protein (CRP)
- Specific—blood culture, malaria test if indicated, urine analysis, chest radiograph

In assessing the results of these tests, the clinician must be aware of the significance of collateral effects, such as thrombocytopenia in disseminated intravascular coagulation (DIC) and malaria, and moderate elevations of transaminases in bacteraemia from any focus. The nature of bacteria isolated from blood culture often indicates the need for attention to a likely source, e.g. *Streptococcus viridans* to endocarditis, *Streptococcus milleri* to endocarditis or liver abscess, *Streptococcus bovis* to both endocarditis and neoplasm of the colon, while a mixture of gram-negative rods and anaerobes points to liver abscess or gut-related sepsis.

Second phase investigations

If the first phase of test results do not point to a particular focus, imaging of the abdomen should be performed. Ultrasound examination is good for detecting fully liquefied liver abscesses and hydronephrosis and may point to focal sepsis or enlarged nodes. If negative, CT scanning should be considered.

Therapeutic trials

A therapeutic trial of an antibacterial may be indicated when, e.g. the patient reports temporary improvement following a previous course and the investigations outlined above have proved unhelpful. The spectrum covered by the previous antibiotic should be taken into consideration when selecting the trial agent. For example, a response to flucloxacillin suggests the need for a more protracted course of antistaphylococcal therapy. It is essential to compare the response to treatment with the response expected in the condition that has been provisionally diagnosed. In most bacterial infections pyrexia will settle within 48 h of starting appropriate antibacterial therapy, but there are notable exceptions, including typhoid fever, any abscess with a volume of more than about 10 ml, and conditions in which there is a significant host response to the infection, such as the development of pleural effusion in patients with pneumococcal pneumonia.

A trial of antituberculosis chemotherapy is routine in patients in whom this infection is likely on clinical grounds, while awaiting culture results. It should also be considered when a tissue biopsy reveals granulomata.

Finally, when the history suggests the possibility of systemic Still's disease with criteria either fulfilled or approximated, or when a patient over the age of 50 has intermittent fever and symptoms consistent with giant cell arteritis, a trial of corticosteroids should be considered. This should not be delayed, but if the patient does not show clear improvement within 5 days of starting prednisolone 60 mg daily, the trial should be stopped. Such a course carries only a small risk of significant adverse effects and the likelihood of infection 'lighting up' is, in practice, very small.

7.2.2 Fever of unknown origin

Steven Vanderschueren and Daniël Knockaert

Essentials

Fever of unknown origin (FUO) refers to a prolonged febrile illness that persists without diagnosis after careful initial assessment. Although over 200 causes have been described, including rare diseases, most cases are due to familiar entities presenting in an atypical fashion.

Causes of FUO—The 'big three' are (1) infections—including tuberculosis, endocarditis, abdominal and hepatobiliary infections and abscesses, complicated genitourinary tract infections, pleuropulmonary infections, bone and joint infections, salmonellosis, cytomegalovirus, Epstein–Barr virus and HIV; (2) tumours—including lymphoma; and (3) multisystem inflammatory conditions—including connective tissue diseases, vasculitic syndromes and granulomatous disorders. A miscellaneous category including factitious fever, habitual hyperthermia, and drug fever deserves consideration early in a patient's workup, since timely recognition may avert invasive and expensive procedures.

Clinical approach to the patient with FUO—The clinician must rely on a very careful and thorough clinical history and examination that does not neglect any part of the body, followed by appropriately targeted investigations directed by knowledge of the broad spectrum of diseases and local epidemiology. As advocated by Sutton's law—'go where the money is'—the approach should follow any possible diagnostic clues, which may sometimes be subtle. If clues are absent or prove misleading, then screening imaging techniques can focus further investigation, but a rigid algorithm and a blind pursuit of increasingly complex tests are ill-advised. Likewise, therapeutic trials without firm foundation are rarely diagnostically rewarding. If the diagnosis in a stable patient remains elusive despite vigorous effort, a watchful waiting approach is warranted as most patients with fever of persistently unknown origin do well.

Definition

Original definition

Most fevers are readily explained or resolve rapidly. Fever with unclear cause or source at first sight should not be labelled fever (or pyrexia) of unknown (or undetermined) origin (FUO). Defined properly, true FUO is uncommon and is encountered once or twice a month at most teaching hospitals. A strict definition, which should not be changed too rapidly, is necessary for comparison of literature data and to guide clinicians faced with this rather rare clinical problem. The three criteria initially proposed by Petersdorf and Beeson in 1961 are: (1) an illness of at least 3 weeks' duration, (2) a fever (temperature more than 38.3 °C on at least three occasions), and (3) no established diagnosis after 1 week of hospital investigation. The first criterion eliminates acute, self-limiting, frequently viral diseases and the second eliminates habitual hyperthermia, an entity commonly diagnosed at that time.

Update of the initial definition

In 1991, Durack and Street suggested modification of the third criterion to an uncertain diagnosis after at least three outpatient visits or at least 3 days in hospital. This revision reflected trends in medical practice, including a shift towards outpatient management, advances in diagnostic techniques, and an accelerated pace of investigation. They also divided FUO into four groups: classic FUO, nosocomial FUO, neutropenic FUO, and HIV-associated FUO. In the last three groups the case mixture differs from that of classic FUO, and the predominance of nosocomial and opportunistic infections in these often frail patients frequently justifies early empirical antimicrobial therapy. The present chapter focuses on classic FUO in adults.

Contemporary definition of classic fever of unknown origin

Recently, it has been suggested that the third criterion should be changed from a quantitative to a qualitative one, specifying which particular examinations are necessary before an unsolved prolonged febrile illness classifies as FUO, rather than an arbitrary number of hospital days or outpatient visits. These minimum requirements (Box 7.2.2.1) should be adapted to regional, mainly infectious, epidemiological factors. Finally, a protracted unexplained febrile illness with fever below 38.3 °C but with persistently raised inflammatory markers should probably be approached similarly. These proposed changes culminated in a modern definition of classic FUO (Box 7.2.2.2) which can be used for the next few decades.

Causes

Diagnostic spectrum

The list of differential diagnoses is among the longest and most challenging in internal medicine, encompassing more than 200 entities. Common and uncommon causes of FUO in adults are listed in Boxes 7.2.2.3 and 7.2.2.4. These causes are conveniently classified into five categories: (1) infections, (2) malignancies, (3) noninfectious inflammatory diseases, (4) miscellaneous causes, and (5) undiagnosed cases. Infections predominated in earlier case series, in paediatric series, and in series from developing countries and from secondary care hospitals. In recent series from western European and Japanese referral centres, noninfectious inflammatory disease (comprising connective tissue disorders, vasculitides, and granulomatous disorders) surpassed infections as the most prevalent category. In spite of innovative rapid microbiological techniques, old and emerging infectious diseases will remain an important source of FUO, due to increasing global travel, migration, implantation of devices, and resistance of microorganisms. Somewhat counterintuitively, the proportion of undiagnosed cases is highest in referral centres and has risen over recent decades, amounting to 25 to 50% of cases. This apparent loss of diagnostic yield is partially attributable to the improved diagnostic armamentarium that reveals the aetiology or source well before a febrile illness turns into FUO. Yet the cause of some prolonged fevers remains unknown despite vigorous clinical efforts. In larger series, even autopsy failed to unravel the cause of the FUO in a substantial minority.

Subpopulations

The cause of FUO differs among subpopulations. The importance of geographical origin and the immune status of the host have

Box 7.2.2.1 Minimum diagnostic evaluation to qualify as fever of unknown origin

- Comprehensive history (including accompanying symptoms, travel history, sexual risk behaviour, profession, hobbies, contact with animals (pets, birds, insects) and ill persons, family history, use of medications and illicit drugs, past medical and surgical history, presence of foreign material)
- Meticulous physical examination (eyes, mucosal surfaces, temporal arteries, skin, hands and nails, lymph nodes, thyroid, heart, lungs, abdomen, rectal examination, musculoskeletal system, neurological examination, vascular examination)
- ESR, C-reactive protein, protein electrophoresis
- Complete blood count, including differential and platelet count
- Routine blood chemistry, including creatinine, sodium, potassium, enzymes (lactate dehydrogenase, bilirubin, liver enzymes, creatine kinase)
- Antinuclear and antineutrophil cytoplasmic antibodies, angiotensin-converting enzyme
- Urinalysis, including microscopic examination
- Routine blood and urine cultures taken while not receiving antibiotics, cultures of other normally sterile fluids (e.g. from joints, pleura, or cerebrospinal space) whenever appropriate
- Tuberculin skin test
- Chest radiograph
- Abdominal ultrasonography (including pelvis)
- Further evaluation of any abnormalities detected by above tests (e.g. HIV testing in case of suspicious exposure, echocardiography in case of cardiac murmur, blood smear for malaria in the traveller, cytomegalovirus serology in case of reactive lymphocytosis)

already been alluded to, and age matters as well. In older people, giant cell arteritis, tuberculosis, malignancies, and drug fever are important considerations, while in younger adults, viral infections, particularly cytomegalovirus infection, adult-onset Still's disease, habitual hyperthermia, factitious fever, and undiagnosed cases are more prevalent. In recurrent or episodic FUO, defined as at least two episodes of fever with fever-free intervals of at least 2 weeks and seeming remission of the underlying illness, traditional causes

Box 7.2.2.2 Modern definition of classic fever of unknown origin

- Illness of more than 3 weeks duration
- Temperature of at least 38.3 °C, or lower temperature with laboratory signs of inflammation, on at least three occasions
- No diagnosis or reasonable (eventually confirmed) diagnostic hypothesis after an initial diagnostic investigation[a]
- Exclusion of nosocomial fevers and severe immunocompromise

[a] See Box 7.2.2.1

Box 7.2.2.3 Common causes of classic fever of unknown origin in adults

Infections

- Tuberculosis
- Endocarditis
- Abdominal and hepatobiliary infections and abscesses
- Complicated genitourinary tract infections
- Pleuropulmonary infections
- Bone and joint infections
- Salmonellosis (including typhoid fever)
- Cytomegalovirus, Epstein–Barr virus, HIV

Neoplasms

- Haematological
  - Non-Hodgkin's lymphoma
  - Hodgkin's disease
  - Leukaemia
- Solid
  - Adenocarcinoma (e.g. colon, kidney)

Noninfectious inflammatory diseases

- Connective tissue diseases
  - Adult-onset Still's disease
  - Polymyalgia rheumatica
  - Rheumatoid arthritis
  - Sjögren's syndrome
  - Systemic lupus erythematosus
- Vasculitis syndromes
  - Giant cell arteritis
  - Polyarteritis nodosa
  - Wegener's granulomatosis
- Granulomatous disorders
  - Inflammatory bowel disease
  - Sarcoidosis

Miscellaneous

- Drug fever
- Habitual hyperthermia
- Factitious fever
- Subacute thyroiditis
- Venous thromboembolism
- Haematoma

Box 7.2.2.4 Rare causes of fever of unknown origin in adults

Infections

- Bartonellosis (including *Bartonella henselae*, *B. quintana*), brucellosis, campylobacter, gonococcaemia, melioidosis, meningococcemia, listeriosis, tularaemia, yersiniosis
- Chlamydial infections (including psittacosis), ehrlichioses, rickettsioses (including Q fever)
- Atypical mycobacterioses, leprosy
- Febris recurrens, leptospirosis, Lyme disease, rat-bite fever, syphilis
- Actinomycosis, nocardiosis, Whipple's disease
- Human herpesvirus type 8, parvovirus B19
- Aspergillosis, blastomycosis, candidiasis, coccidioidomycosis, cryptococcosis, histoplasmosis, mucormycosis, pneumocystosis, sporotrichosis
- Amoebiasis, babesiosis, echinococcosis, fascioliasis, malaria, leishmaniasis, schistosomiasis, toxocariasis, toxoplasmosis, trichinosis, trypanosomiasis
- Malakoplakia, xanthogranulomatous pyelonephritis
- Central nervous system infection, dental infection, upper respiratory tract infection, wound infection
- Intravenous catheter infection, infected vascular graft, mycotic aneurysm

Neoplasms and related conditions

- Haematological
  - Angioimmunoblastic T-cell lymphoma
  - Intravascular lymphoma
  - Amyloidosis
  - Hypereosinophilic syndrome
  - Multiple myeloma
  - Myelodysplastic syndromes
  - Myelofibrosis
- Solid
  - Atrial myxoma
  - Hepatoma
  - Renal cell carcinoma
  - Other (more than 30 reported), with or without necrosis, with or without metastases

Noninfectious inflammatory diseases

- Connective tissue diseases
  - Acute rheumatic fever
  - Crystal-induced arthropathy
  - Eosinophilic fasciitis
  - Felty's syndrome
  - Mixed connective tissue disease
  - Polymyositis, dermatomyositis
  - Reactive arthritis, including Reiter's syndrome
  - Relapsing polychondritis
  - Seronegative spondylarthropathy
- Vasculitis syndromes
  - Behçet's disease
  - Henoch–Schönlein purpura
  - Mixed cryoglobulinaemia
  - Takayasu's arteritis
  - Urticarial vasculitis
- Granulomatous disorders
  - Granulomatous hepatitis

Miscellaneous

- Addison's disease, hyperparathyroidism, hyperthyroidism, hypothalamic hypopituitarism, phaeochromocytoma
- Erythema multiforme, erythema nodosum, linear IgA dermatosis, Sweet's disease
- Castleman's disease, inflammatory pseudotumour of lymph nodes, Kikuchi's disease
- Vogt–Koyanagi–Harada syndrome
- Giant haemangioma
- Dissecting aneurysm
- Retroperitoneal fibrosis
- Thrombophlebitis
- Cholesterol embolism, PTFE (Teflon) embolism, silicone embolism
- Antiphospholipid syndrome
- Cyclic neutropenia, haemolytic anaemia, haemoglobinopathies, macrophage activation (haemophagocytic) syndrome, vitamin B12 deficiency
- Schnitzler's syndrome
- Dressler's syndrome (postmyocardial infarction syndrome)
- Cerebrovascular accident, epilepsy
- Alcoholic hepatitis, autoimmune hepatitis, cirrhosis (with active necrosis), primary sclerosing cholangitis
- Extrinsic allergic alveolitis, hypersensitivity pneumonitis, interstitial pneumonia
- Hereditary periodic fever syndromes (familial Mediterranean fever, tumour necrosis factor receptor-1-associated periodic syndrome, hyper-IgD syndrome, Muckle–Wells syndrome, familial cold autoinflammatory syndrome)
- Gaucher's disease, Fabry's disease
- Hypertriglyceridaemia
- Erdheim–Chester disease

such as infections and malignancies are less frequently implicated. Recurrent FUO is especially challenging, as a final diagnosis is established in no more than one-half of the patients. As the duration of the fever increases, the likelihood of an infectious cause decreases.

Common diseases prevail

Although the possible aetiologies of FUO are myriad, a limited list of disorders (Box 7.2.2.3) accounted for the great majority of diagnoses in published series. Most patients do not have esoteric diseases, unfamiliar to the clinician, but rather are exhibiting atypical manifestations of common illnesses. A few examples may illustrate this point. The forms of tuberculosis that give rise to FUO are often disseminated disease, yet without the characteristic miliary pattern on chest radiograph, or extrapulmonary disease without clear localizing features; tuberculin skin tests and sputum smears are often negative. The forms of endocarditis that enter the FUO spectrum are frequently culture-negative or are caused by fastidious organisms; a new regurgitant murmur or signs of peripheral emboli are frequently absent. Leukaemia presents as an FUO characteristically in the aleukaemic phase. Giant cell arteritis may manifest with constitutional symptoms only (anorexia, weight loss, fever), without polymyalgia or arteritic signs and symptoms, and without a strikingly elevated ESR. Likewise, in subacute thyroiditis, localizing symptoms and signs may be subtle or nonexistent.

Approach to the adult with classic fever of unknown origin

Ruling out the 'little three'

For didactic and practical purposes, it is convenient to split the aetiologies into the 'big three' and the 'little three'. The 'big three' are infections, neoplasms, and noninfectious inflammatory diseases, which together represent the bulk of diagnoses. The 'little three' comprise factitious fever, habitual hyperthermia, and drug fever. While these three causes are numerically less important, considering them from the start may prevent painstaking and invasive investigations. For this reason, at an early stage, fever should be verified, temperature charts recorded, and an effort made to stop all nonessential medications and switch essential ones to unrelated alternatives.

Factitious fever

Due to either manipulation of the thermometer or self-induced disease (e.g. by self-injection of contaminated materials), this characteristically occurs in young women, often in the health professions. Discrepancy between symptoms and clinical and laboratory findings raises the suspicion of fraudulent fever. Unexplained polymicrobial bacteraemia, serial episodes of bacteraemia by different pathogens, or recurrent soft tissue infections suggest self-induced infection.

Habitual hyperthermia

This is also seen mainly in young women who complain of 'flu-like' and functional symptoms. In this syndrome, which overlaps with chronic fatigue syndrome and fibromyalgia, the diurnal variation in body temperature is maintained. Evening temperatures are on average 0.5 °C higher than morning temperatures, body temperature rises especially following physical and intellectual activity, the response to antipyretics is poor, and temperatures only occasionally exceed 38.3 °C. Laboratory evaluation, including acute-phase reactants, is entirely unremarkable.

Drug fever

Virtually any drug can cause fever, with the possible exceptions of digitalis and aminoglycosides. The mechanisms are multiple and often poorly understood, with hypersensitivity being most common. Examples of drugs causing FUO include anticonvulsants, antimicrobials (such as minocycline, β-lactams, sulphonamides, and nitrofurantoin), and allopurinol. Patients may have been on the offending drug for prolonged periods. Fever is rarely the sole manifestation but may be accompanied by rash, urticaria, mucosal ulceration, eosinophilia and other haematological abnormalities, hepatic or renal dysfunction, or pulmonary involvement. Phenytoin and carbamazepine are notorious for inducing a pseudolymphoma syndrome. Some patients with drug fever look severely ill and toxic, while others look and feel surprisingly well. Withdrawal of the offending drug usually results in defervescence within 72 to 96 h. Rechallenge is generally safe unless organ damage (e.g. hepatitis or interstitial nephritis) has occurred, but is rarely performed in clinical practice.

Fever characteristics

While recording and monitoring of body temperature are imperative, fever height and pattern do not contribute much to diagnosis. The few entities that have a distinctive fever pattern (e.g. nonfalciparum malaria or cyclic neutropenia) are rare, as are fever patterns thought to be characteristic of other diseases, such as Pel–Ebstein fever (a relapsing fever that disappears and reappears at intervals of several days) in Hodgkin's disease. Other features that lack diagnostic discrimination among the numerous sources of FUO are the presence of night sweats, weight loss, chills, and relative bradycardia (a heart rate lower than expected for the degree of fever). The naproxen test was proposed on the assumption of a selective antipyretic activity against neoplastic fever, but in clinical practice the accuracy of this test too is to low to be discriminative.

Go where the money is

The diagnostician confronted with FUO should keep in mind Sutton's law: 'go where the money is'. Possible diagnostic clues elicited from the history, physical examination, and the preliminary diagnostic evaluation (Box 7.2.2.1) should, of course, guide further investigation, but many cases become a FUO because these clues are misleading. Whenever possible, the clinician should strive to achieve microbiological or pathological confirmation. Any suspected focal abnormality that is accessible should be aspirated or biopsied. Close communication with the microbiologist and the pathologist will increase the diagnostic yield.

When diagnostic clues are either absent or misleading, an individualized approach is preferable. Indeed, there are no useful or evidence-based rigid algorithms.

Screening imaging techniques

Imaging is used primarily to localize abnormalities for further evaluation. Due to the higher spatial resolution compared with chest radiographs and ultrasound of the abdomen, CT scanning of thorax or abdomen is useful when looking for focal disease, mainly infectious or neoplastic. In the near future, the role of MRI in the work-up of FUO is anticipated to grow as its benefits relative to CT are demarcated. The choice between a whole variety of radiopharmaceuticals depends on local availability, cost, and skill. We do not advocate tracers that are more specific for infections, such as labelled leucocytes, because a wide range of inflammatory and neoplastic conditions enter the differential diagnosis, not just infections. In particular, ^{18}F-fluorodeoxyglucose positron emission tomography (FDG-PET) is a promising inflammation tracer technique in FUO, yielding the diagnosis in 25 to 40% of patients and performing at least as well as gallium scintigraphy. However, unlike gallium, fluorodeoxyglucose is taken up in vasculitic lesions in large blood vessels (giant cell arteritis and Takayasu's arteritis), which are classic causes of FUO.

Selective testing

The imaging studies may unmask hidden infectious, neoplastic, and inflammatory foci, but endoscopic techniques (e.g. gastrointestinal endoscopy, bronchoscopy), selective radiographs (e.g. of teeth, sinuses, sacroiliac joints), or contrast studies (e.g. gastrointestinal series, arteriography) should be ordered only when there is a well-founded and specific clinical suspicion. They should not be used as routine tests for FUO. This is even more the case for invasive procedures such as mediastinoscopy, thoracoscopy, or laparoscopy, techniques that are being replaced increasingly by less invasive ultrasound echoendoscopy, or CT-guided biopsy. Nowadays, exploratory laparoscopy is restricted to exceptional situations, e.g. when peritoneal carcinomatosis or tuberculosis are suspected and other tests have failed. Likewise, biopsies of lymph nodes, bone marrow, or liver, and lumbar puncture can be diagnostic, but should not be performed blindly, in the absence of firm suspicion of pathological involvement. The only biopsy that may be routinely performed is temporal artery biopsy in a patient over the age of 50 with a prolonged unexplained fever and vigorous acute-phase response, even in the absence of arteritic symptoms. Giant cell arteritis is one of the most frequent diagnoses in this age group and carries a serious risk of visual loss and other ischaemic complications.

Watchful waiting

An undirected pursuit of often increasingly costly and invasive tests is discouraged. Instead, when the diagnosis remains in doubt, all data including those from other hospitals should be critically reviewed and history taking, physical examination, and some basic tests (e.g. white blood cell count with differential, creatine kinase, urinalysis, chest radiograph) repeated in an effort to find clues that were previously overlooked or inapparent. There is no substitute for observing, talking to, and thinking about the patient. If the diagnosis can not be established after intelligent thorough investigation, an expectant approach is justified if the patient's condition is stable. In published series, most patients with FUO who left hospital without a diagnosis did remarkably well.

Therapeutic trials

Therapeutic trails are seldom diagnostically rewarding and tend to obscure rather than illuminate. In contrast to the approach to fever in immunocompromised patients (Chapter 7.2.4), the general goal when dealing with classic FUO is to ascertain the diagnosis before starting therapy. Antipyretics, mainly nonsteroidal anti-inflammatory drugs, may be symptomatically useful but rarely aid diagnosis. Blind administration of corticosteroids is discouraged. Infections such as tuberculosis may seemingly respond initially, only to deteriorate thereafter. Most patients have already had a failed trial of antibiotics before referral to secondary or tertiary care. Defervescence following administration of an antimicrobial agent is rarely diagnostic as the spectrum generally involves more than a single microorganism. Moreover, fevers caused by infections such as disseminated tuberculosis or culture-negative endocarditis may wane only several days after starting appropriate therapy. Spontaneous resolution of fever may coincide with a therapeutic trial, which is another argument against its routine use. The exception to the rule of withholding empirical therapy in classic FUO is the severely deteriorating patient. In such situations, antituberculosis chemotherapy is warranted, since tuberculosis is probably the most common cause of avoidable death in adults with classic FUO. Corticosteroid treatment is the next step in case of further deterioration of the clinical condition.

Prognosis

Not surprisingly, the outcome of classic FUO is highly variable and depends on the underlying disease. In the series of Larson *et al.* from the 1980s, for instance, only 9% of patients with malignancies were long-term survivors, while 78% of patients with infections and 88% of patients with FUO in other categories were alive after 1 year. Older age carries a worse prognosis. In a series from the 1990s, haematological malignancies (especially non-Hodgkin's lymphoma), while making up 12% of diagnoses, accounted for almost 60% of deaths. Treatable causes of death have included abdominal abscesses, endocarditis, vasculitis, pulmonary embolism, and especially tuberculosis.

Most patients who can not be diagnosed do well and over two-thirds have no recurrence of symptoms. Among the rest, a subgroup have clinical features suggesting protracted noninfectious inflammatory conditions, without meeting accepted diagnostic criteria for any particular disease. Most of these fevers respond to corticosteroid therapy.

Further reading

Arnow PM, Flaherty JP (1997). Fever of unknown origin. *Lancet*, **350**, 575–80.

Cunha BA (2007). Fever of unknown origin: Clinical overview of classical and current concepts. *Infect Dis Clin N Am*, **21**, 867–915.

Durack DT, Street AC (1991). Fever of unknown origin: reexamined and redefined. *Curr Clin Top Infect Dis*, **11**, 35–51.

Hirschmann JV (1997). Fever of unknown origin in adults. *Clin Infect Dis*, **24**, 291–302.

Knockaert DC, Vanderschueren S, Blockmans D (2003). Fever of unknown origin in adults: 40 years on. *J Intern Med*, **253**, 263–75.

Knockaert DC, *et al.* (1992). Fever of unknown origin in the 1980s. An update of the diagnostic spectrum. *Arch Intern Med*, **152**, 51–5.

Larson EB, Featherstone HJ, Petersdorf RG (1982). Fever of undetermined origin: diagnosis and follow-up of 105 cases, 1970–1980. *Medicine*, **61**, 269–92.

Petersdorf RB, Beeson PB (1961). Fever of unexplained origin: report on 100 cases. *Medicine*, **40**, 1–30.

Vanderschueren S, *et al.* (2003). From prolonged febrile illness to fever of unknown origin. The challenge continues. *Arch Intern Med*, **163**, 1033–41.

7.2.3 Nosocomial infections

I.C.J.W. Bowler

Essentials

Hospital-acquired or nosocomial infections—defined for epidemiological studies as infections manifesting more than 48 h after admission—are common. They affect 1.4 million people worldwide at any one time and involve between 5 and 25% of patients admitted to hospital, with considerable associated morbidity, mortality, and cost.

Clinical features—the commonest sites of nosocomial infection are the urinary tract, surgical wounds, and the lower respiratory tract. Bacteria are the most important causes, including *Escherichia coli*, *Staphylococcus aureus* (including MRSA), enterococcus, pseudomonas, and coagulase-negative staphylococci. The principal risk factors are extremes of age, the severity of underlying acute disease (e.g. neutropenia, organ system failure), and burden of chronic medical conditions (especially diabetes, renal failure, and alcohol abuse).

Prevention—between 15 and 30% of nosocomial infections are preventable, and hospital practitioners have a duty of care to minimize the risk of infection for their patients. Systematic surveillance to assess the incidence and prevalence of such infections, together with a regularly audited organized programme to prevent or minimize their impact, should be an important part of every hospital's quality assurance system. Hospital managers must ensure appropriate staffing and resources to provide (1) access to advice from well trained experts in infection control; (2) surveillance of infection with regular feedback of the data to staff; (3) isolation of patients with infections, with appropriate arrangements for their nursing and medical management; (4) appropriate arrangements for carrying out procedures likely to increase the risk of infection, e.g. insertion of central venous lines; and (5) policies for outbreak management. All staff should receive regular education to ensure that they recognize that infection control is 'everyone's business'.

Definitions

Nosocomial infections are distinct from community-acquired infections; they may affect patients and, less often, hospital staff. They can be usefully defined for epidemiological studies as infections manifesting more than 48 h after admission to hospital. However, some nosocomial infections may not be so easily identified as hospital acquired, e.g. hospital-acquired hepatitis B infection may not become clinically apparent until months after the patient has been discharged because of the prolonged incubation period. These are therefore called health care-associated infections. Iatrogenic infections are acquired as the direct consequence of a therapeutic intervention (e.g. insertion of a urinary catheter). Opportunistic infections are caused by organisms that do not ordinarily harm healthy people; they occur in people with impaired defences. Endogenous (autogenous) infections are produced by the patient's normal flora, while exogenous infections result from transmission of organisms to the patient from elsewhere. Although in practice it may not always be possible to distinguish endogenous from exogenous infections, this differentiation must be attempted because of important implications for control.

Scale and costs of nosocomial infections

Rates of nosocomial infections between 6.9 and 25 per 100 admissions have been reported. The urinary tract, surgical wounds, and the lower respiratory tract are the most common sites, in that order (Table 7.2.3.1). In the United States of America it is estimated that 80 000 deaths are directly attributable to nosocomial infection each year, and in 2005 costs were estimated at $4.5 to 5.7 billion. In England in 2000 the costs were estimated at £1 billion annually, and were mainly due to delayed discharge from hospital of infected patients. In Mexico an estimated 450 000 cases of nosocomial infection cause 32 deaths per 100 000 inhabitants each year at a cost of US$1.5 billion (World Health Organization 2005). Rapid changes in health care provision mean the frequency and nature of nosocomial infection are also changing. The increasing trend to early discharge, particularly for surgical patients, can lead to an underassessment of the disease burden. New interventions provide new opportunities for infection. For instance, flexible endoscopes, which have revolutionized the investigation and management of a wide variety of diseases, can transmit hepatitis B between patients if the endoscopes are not decontaminated between procedures.

Host factors

The principal risk factors are extremes of age and the severity of the underlying disease (e.g. neutropenia, organ system failure). The rapidly ageing population of the more developed world has had a major impact on the prevalence of hospital-acquired infection in these countries. In multivariate analysis, several medical diagnoses on admission, especially diabetes, renal failure, or alcohol abuse, are most strongly associated with risk. Treatment itself may lower host defences, e.g. surgical incisions, bladder catheterization, mechanical ventilation, and neutropenia following cancer chemotherapy. Pathogens are able to form biofilms on the increasingly used prosthetic devices (totally implantable, e.g. hip replacement, or transcutaneous, e.g. intravascular devices) subverting normal host clearance mechanisms.

Patients with similar clinical problems, who are likely to share similar risk factors for infection, tend to be nursed together for convenience, but the introduction of a microorganism into such a group can rapidly infect a number of patients. A good example

Table 7.2.3.1 Rates and sites of nosocomial infection in three countries

	USA (1996)	France (2001)	UK (2006)
Rates	9.8[a]	6.9[b]	7.6[b]
Sites (% of all infections)			
Urinary tract infection	34	40	20
Surgical wound infection	17	10	15
Lower respiratory tract infection	13	10	16
Other	36	40	49

[a] Cases/1000 patient days (incidence).
[b] Cases/100 admissions (prevalence).

is the rapid spread of norovirus gastroenteritis in geriatric wards. A poorly maintained hospital environment is a threat to vulnerable patients; for instance, in units caring for patients with solid organ transplants, outbreaks of legionellosis can result from defective air-conditioning and hot-water systems.

Microorganisms

Bacteria (*Escherichia coli, Staphylococcus aureus*, enterococcus, pseudomonas, and coagulase-negative staphylococci, in decreasing order of frequency) are the most important. Viruses, fungi, and protozoa play a minor part.

Whether endogenous or exogenous, the organisms causing nosocomial infection are usually part of a patient's colonizing flora. It may be difficult to distinguish infecting from colonizing organisms using bacteriological tests alone. The organisms are frequently multidrug resistant, since the widespread use of antibiotics in hospitals gives these strains a selective advantage. Empirical antibiotic therapy must accommodate the shift towards more resistant colonizing flora occurring in hospitals, particularly in burns and intensive care units. For example, *Pseudomonas aeruginosa*, methicillin-resistant *S. aureus* (MRSA), and enterococci exhibit multidrug resistance to antimicrobials, thus making them difficult and expensive to treat.

Principles of hospital infection control

The main aim of the hospital infection control programme is to prevent nosocomial infection. Infections must be identified as endemic or epidemic by clinical and epidemiological investigations. The identification and typing of isolates causing nosocomial infection allow recognition of organisms that are epidemiologically linked. Invasive multidrug-resistant organisms, such as MRSA, often require infection control measures to prevent their spread and so minimize the use of expensive, sometimes toxic, antibiotics required for their prophylaxis and treatment.

Epidemic infections account for less than 10% of the nosocomial disease burden but attract professional and media interest because they are unusual. They are amenable to measures that interrupt the spread of infection, such as the use of gowns and gloves, and careful hand washing by those attending patients. Transfer of colonized or infected patients to a single room or an isolation ward is a physical means of preventing spread. Patients infected with the same organism can be grouped together and attended to by a cohort of nurses not involved with uninfected patients. Identification of additional carriers and elimination of colonization may be necessary for some epidemic outbreaks. Controlled trials demonstrating the efficacy of such measures have not been made, but many observational studies support their use.

Endemic nosocomial infections are more difficult to control. The size of the problem may not be apparent because attack rates in individual units may be low or because some infection is seen as a normal consequence of certain interventions. It is important that information about endemic infections is collected systematically in a comprehensive surveillance programme, analysed, disseminated, and discussed so that preventive strategies can be improved. Control measures are applied to selected patients according to risk, e.g. correctly timed antimicrobial prophylaxis and meticulous sterile technique in prosthetic joint replacement surgery.

Site of nosocomial infections

Urinary tract

A bacterial count of at least 10^5 organisms/ml in freshly voided cultured urine indicates infection. However, counts as low as 10^2 organisms/ml are included by some and any organisms grown from a urine sample taken from a urinary catheter indicates infection. Most patients with catheter related urinary tract infection remain asymptomatic, but 20 to 30% develop the symptoms of urinary tract infection and about 1 in 100 of these develop bacteraemia.

Indwelling urinary catheters account for 80% of nosocomial urinary tract infections; 80% of patients catheterized for longer than 7 to 10 days develop bacteriuria. Most of the others result from instrumentation of the urinary tract. The main source of organisms is the periurethral flora, and *E. coli* is the dominant pathogen in all studies. Bacteria gain access to the bladder, usually by spreading up the outside of the lumen of the catheter. Occasionally, infection is acquired exogenously during an epidemic of nosocomial infection. Most symptomatic or bacteraemic infections occur within 24 h of the organisms gaining access to the bladder. Early recognition, by daily urine culture, of a urinary tract infection before it becomes symptomatic is not helpful. Treatment is with broad-spectrum antimicrobials administered empirically after obtaining appropriate cultures and later adjusted after receiving results of bacteriological studies. Asymptomatic patients need not be treated.

Since the important risk factor is the duration of catheterization, prevention is by avoiding catheterization or reducing the period of catheterization. Catheters should be inserted aseptically, and closed sterile drainage systems, uninterrupted gravity drainage, or intermittent or suprapubic catheterization employed. Some practitioners advocate a single prophylactic dose of antibiotic at the time of urinary catheter insertion or exchange in men to prevent bacteraemia. In other settings prophylactic antibiotics have not been shown to prevent infection for more than a few days. Catheters coated with antimicrobials such as silver have been shown to reduce infection rates in some patient groups, but their cost-effectiveness is disputed.

Surgical wound infection

One acceptable definition requires the presence of a purulent discharge in, or exuding from, a wound. Rates vary according to the definitions used. Internationally agreed definitions are used for high-quality epidemiological studies (Horan and Gaynes 2004).

Most wound infections follow direct inoculation of organisms into the wound at surgery or spread of bacteria to open wounds such as burns. The main risk factor is the degree of wound contamination at operation. Operations may be 'clean' (e.g. herniorrhaphy), 'clean–contaminated' (e.g. appendicectomy which requires incision of bowel), or 'contaminated' (e.g. gross spillage from the gastrointestinal tract during surgery). *S. aureus* causes most infections complicating clean surgery and rates below 2% are expected. 'Contaminated' surgery is associated with polymicrobial infections, especially with *E. coli* and mixed anaerobes originating from the patient's gut, and rates of infection are 5 to 15%. Other risk factors include age, underlying comorbidity including obesity, the length of the operation, and a remote infection.

Wound infections present with local symptoms and signs (pain, erythema, pus, dehiscence) and with general features of infection, such as fever. Appropriate cultures, including blood cultures, are taken, pus is drained, and broad-spectrum antimicrobials are given empirically, directed at the likely flora but later adjusted according to bacteriological results.

Prevention is by meticulous aseptic surgical techniques. Prophylactic antimicrobials, given no more than 2 h before the surgical incision, have been shown to reduce wound infection rates by between two- and fivefold for clean–contaminated and contaminated procedures, and in clean surgery when a prosthesis is inserted (e.g. vascular grafting).

Nosocomial pneumonia

Pneumonia is defined clinically by the production of purulent sputum, chest signs, a fall in arterial Po_2, and the appearance of new infiltrates on the chest radiograph not ascribable to pulmonary emboli, collapse, or pulmonary oedema. Between 0.55 and 1.5% of patients admitted to hospital develop lower respiratory tract infections. Crude case fatalities of between 20 and 30% are quoted, but death may be due to underlying disease. Intubated and ventilated patients have the highest risk of acquiring pneumonia. Bacteria colonizing the gastrointestinal and upper respiratory tracts are probably aspirated. This flora is often acquired after admission to hospital and the bacteria are often multidrug resistant. Organisms cultured from bronchoscopic samples are listed in Table 7.2.3.2.

Culture of expectorated sputum or tracheal aspirate is poorly predictive of the bacterial cause of nosocomial pneumonia, which is best determined by quantitative culture of specimens obtained by sampling the terminal airways (e.g. by bronchoalveolar lavage). Initially, broad-spectrum antimicrobials appropriate for likely infecting flora should be given empirically. Once the susceptibility of the causative pathogen has been determined, specific antimicrobial treatment can be instituted.

The risks of nosocomial pneumonia can be reduced by a variety of strategies, including avoidance of intubation and the use of noninvasive ventilation techniques. For those who are intubated, continuous aspiration of subglottic secretions and nursing in the semirecumbent position have been shown to be effective in good-quality studies. Selective decontamination of the digestive tract has reduced the occurrence of nosocomial pneumonia and mortality in ventilated patients, but has shown less benefit in units where there is a high prevalence of multidrug-resistant organisms. Short courses of antibiotics at the time of intubation have been shown to be effective in certain patient groups. Epidemic nosocomial pneumonia usually results from bacterial contamination of respiratory equipment, such as nebulizers, ventilators, or bronchoscopes, and can be prevented by ensuring that single-use respiratory devices are not reused, by cleaning and disinfecting equipment, and by hand washing after patient contact.

Table 7.2.3.2 Causative organisms identified in samples obtained at bronchoscopy by protected specimen brush (percentage of all pneumonias)

	France (2000)	Spain (2000)
Pseudomonas aeruginosa	22	33
Staphylococcus aureus including MRSA	17	26
Escherichia coli or 'coliform'	10	23
Streptococci	16	3
Haemophilus spp.	7	6
Acinetobacter spp.	5	0
Other species	23	9
Polymicrobial	12	0

MRSA, methicillin-resistant *Staphylococcus aureus*.

Intravascular device-associated infections

The most important intravascular device-associated infection is bacteraemia; it varies in prevalence from about 0.04% for subcutaneous central venous ports to about 0.2% for peripheral intravenous cannulae and approximately 10% for temporary nontunnelled central venous haemodialysis catheters.

Duration of intravascular cannulation is the greatest risk factor. Bacteria usually gain access to the blood by direct spread from the skin surface along the subcutaneous catheter tunnel to its tip in the blood vessel. Bacteraemia from intraluminal bacteria results from contamination of connecting devices. This is particularly important in catheters with subcutaneous cuffs, such as Hickman catheters, where the periluminal route of infection is less likely. The leading organisms causing intravenous device-related sepsis are *S. aureus*, pseudomonas, and candida. In patients with haematological malignancies, coagulase-negative staphylococci and enterococci are also frequently implicated.

Line-related sepsis presents with local inflammation or signs of thrombophlebitis often with features of bacteraemia and even thromboembolism. Blood cultures are obtained, the affected catheter is removed and cultures taken, and empirical antimicrobials are given. Sometimes, long-term intravenous catheters, such as Hickman lines, can be 'sterilized' by giving parenteral antibiotics down the line. Exit site infections involving these devices can usually be treated with antibiotics with the line *in situ*. Tunnel infections usually require line removal for resolution.

Prevention is by using aseptic techniques when inserting catheters, maintaining a high standard of line care, and removing catheters as soon as possible. Before insertion, the skin should be prepared with a reliable disinfectant such as an alcoholic solution of chlorhexidine. At insertion, the operators should wash their hands and, for long-line insertion, use a large sterile drape to isolate the insertion site and wear sterile gloves, gown, face mask, and hat. Central venous catheters are usually removed only if blocked or suspected as a source of sepsis. Removal of peripheral intravascular devices should be considered after 3 days. The skin at the exit site should be checked daily and the device removed if sepsis is suspected. Subcutaneous tunnelling, insertion of a subcutaneous cuff (Hickman line), burying them subcutaneously (e.g. portacaths), and incorporating antimicrobials onto the surface of the device can all reduce the infection rate significantly. Replacing the entire intravenous delivery set every 72 h is sufficient to reduce sepsis secondary to intraluminal contamination of 'giving' sets.

Prosthetic device-related infection

Infections of prosthetic devices such as heart valves, vascular grafts, cerebrospinal fluid shunts, artificial lenses, and joints are usually caused by the normal skin flora, e.g. coagulase-negative staphylococci. The devices become coated with a layer of host-derived macromolecules such as fibronectin and fibrin which have specific adhesion receptors for bacteria, particularly staphylococci. Once attached, these organisms multiply on the surface of the coated prosthesis forming a biofilm in a state physiologically different from rapidly dividing, 'free' microorganisms. They are inherently more resistant to antimicrobials, which explains the frequent failure of antimicrobial treatment. Bacteria gain access to prosthetic devices by direct inoculation, usually at surgery, or by settling on a prosthesis after bacteraemic spread. Direct inoculation at surgery is responsible for prosthetic-device infections occurring more than 1 year after insertion since the organisms involved are usually skin commensals of low virulence. Except for organisms that are exquisitely susceptible to antimicrobials, these infections are seldom cured with antimicrobial agents. Surgical removal of the device is frequently necessary. However, infections of artificial lenses in the eye are often cured by antimicrobial treatment.

Prevention is by avoiding contamination of the wound at surgery and by using strict aseptic surgical techniques. In orthopaedic implant surgery, a large randomized controlled trial showed that an ultraclean air supply to the operating theatre is of benefit. Prophylactic antimicrobials given at the time of surgery have also been shown to reduce the risk of prosthetic hip and knee device-related infection.

Antibiotic-associated diarrhoea

Up to 30% of patients treated with antibiotics will develop diarrhoea as a result of the disturbance of the complex gut flora. In a few, loss of 'colonization resistance' predisposes to acquisition of *Clostridium difficile*. Faecal colonization by this organism is usually harmless, but in about one-third of patients, particularly older patients, the organism may overgrow and produce a cytotoxin causing colitis.

The clinical picture varies from mild diarrhoea with fever to fulminating toxic megacolon requiring colectomy. More severe disease and a greater likelihood of relapse can be the result of infection with a quinolone-resistant clone of *C. difficile*, prevalent in North America, the United Kingdom, and the Netherlands, which produces large amounts of toxin due to the deletion of a regulator gene *tcdC*. *C. difficile*-associated diarrhoea delays discharge from hospital by about 3 weeks. Since attack rates in older patients are around 5% and relapse can occur in up to 30%, the disease can have a major impact on hospital resources. Diagnosis is by detection of the cytotoxin in a stool sample, but the test has poor specificity disease: toxin may be found in the stool of asymptomatic patients, and for many weeks after full recovery in those with symptoms. Patient management includes adequate rehydration, avoiding drugs which inhibit gut motility, and stopping the provoking antibiotics. More severe cases will require metronidazole or vancomycin, given by mouth, and surgical review.

Prevention is by restricting the use of antibiotics according to agreed and audited protocols. Hand washing after patient contact, isolation of patients with diarrhoea, and cleaning the ward environment are employed on microbiological grounds, despite a lack of prospective studies showing their efficacy.

Nosocomial bacteraemia

Bacteraemia may occur secondarily to the infections mentioned above. The incidence is approximately 3/1000 hospital discharges. The case fatality is about 40%, but varies with the severity of the underlying disease, being as low as about 2% in obstetric patients. Most cases are due to intravascular line or surgical space infection. The focus must be identified and, if possible, removed surgically. Appropriate antimicrobials are given after obtaining blood and other relevant cultures.

Future developments

The rapidly developing techniques of molecular biology are likely to reveal more clearly the relationship between hospital patients and the organisms which infect them, pointing the way to new risk-reducing strategies. The dissection of the genome of organisms causing outbreaks will reveal the basis for enhanced pathogenicity. Study of the human genome linked to carefully collected clinical data documenting infections in large populations will identify polymorphisms which predispose to infection, allowing prevention to be targeted to those patients most in need of it.

Further reading

Bennett JV, Brachman PS (eds) (1998). *Hospital infections*, 4th edition. Lippincott-Raven, Philadelphia.

Edgeworth JD, *et al.* (2007). An outbreak in an intensive care unit of a strain of methicillin-resistant *Staphylococcus aureus* sequence type 239 associated with an increased rate of vascular access device-related bacteraemia. *Clin Infect Dis*, **44**, 493–501.

Flores C, *et al.* (2006). A CXCL2 tandem repeat promoter polymorphism is associated with susceptibility to severe sepsis in the Spanish population. *Genes Immun*, **7**, 141–9.

Haley RN, *et al.* (1985). The efficacy of infection surveillance and control programs in preventing nosocomial infections in US hospitals. *Am J Epidemiol*, **121**, 182–205.

Horan TC, Gaynes RP (2004). Surveillance of nosocomial infections. In: Mayhall CG (ed) *Hospital epidemiology and infection control*, 3rd edition, pp. 1659–702. Lippincott Williams & Wilkins, Philadelphia.

National Nosocomial Infections Surveillance (NNIS) System Report, data summary from January 1992 through June 2004, issued October 2004. *Am J Infect Control*, **32**, 470–85.

World Health Organization (2005). *Global patient safety challenge: 2005-6/world alliance for patient safety*. World Health Organization, Geneva.

7.2.4 Infection in the immunocompromised host

J. Cohen

Essentials

The term 'immunocompromised host' embraces a group of overlapping conditions in which the ability to respond normally to an infective challenge is in some way impaired. This includes patients with underlying conditions such as protein–calorie malnutrition and diabetes, as well as organ transplant recipients, those with haematological malignancies and others receiving therapeutic immunosuppression, and patients with HIV. Many patients have multiple risk factors that increase the risk of opportunistic infection.

General clinical approach

A high level of awareness is essential to the management of patients who are immunocompromised; infections can progress with frightening rapidity, the early physical signs are often muted, and the microbiology can be confusing. Aside from a full history and detailed physical examination, assessment should take account of risk factors such as the depth and duration of neutropenia, or the dose and duration of steroid therapy. It is particularly helpful to try to form a judgement of how quickly the condition is progressing. Patients need to be reviewed frequently and will often need empirical therapy, but when possible it is better to try to establish the cause of the infection before starting treatment. This is partly because the differential diagnosis is wide and choosing the right treatment depends on knowing the causative organism, and partly because it is not uncommon for multiple organisms of different types to be involved.

Particular clinical syndromes

Fever of unknown origin—this is common in patients with neutropenia, with the risk of bacteraemia being most acute when the neutrophil count falls to less than 0.1×10^9/litre, but in 50% of cases an organism is never identified. Empirical antibiotic therapy is vital and needs to be directed against both Gram-negative and Gram-positive organisms. The risk of invasive fungal infection rises if fever persists, in which case empirical antifungal therapy is justified.

Fever and new pulmonary infiltrates—this is a challenging problem with a wide range of potential causes depending on the clinical setting, including conventional respiratory pathogens, nosocomial pathogens, 'atypical' organisms, mycobacteria and related organisms, viruses, fungi, parasites, and also noninfective causes such as pulmonary oedema, pulmonary haemorrhage, pulmonary emboli/infarction and drug toxicity. The clinical and radiological features are very rarely pathognomonic, hence a diagnostic procedure such as bronchoscopic lavage should be performed whenever possible.

Acute neurological syndromes—these include both (1) meningoencephalitis—associated with conventional bacterial infections, listeriosis and tuberculosis, as well as fungi such as cryptococcus and candida; and (2) space occupying lesions—caused by e.g. toxoplasma, aspergillus and nocardia. Once again there is a wide differential diagnosis and a low threshold of diagnostic suspicion is needed.

Gastrointestinal syndromes—these are frequent and include (1) stomatitis—the three commonest causes (candida, herpes simplex and chemotherapy-induced mucositis) are clinically indistinguishable and can coexist; (2) diarrhoea—graft-vs-host disease is very difficult to distinguish from infective causes in bone marrow transplant recipients; (3) abnormalities of liver function tests—mild derangements are a common accompaniment to many systemic infections, but hepatitis is a particular feature of both toxoplasmosis and cytomegalovirus infection.

Prevention

This is an integral part of the management of patients who are immunosuppressed and, depending on context, comprises interventions such as nursing them in single rooms and chemoprophylaxis, e.g. co-trimoxazole to prevent pneumocystis, but perhaps the single most important factor is being aware of the different and often subtle presentations of infection in this vulnerable group of patients.

Classification

The term 'immunocompromised host' has no formal definition but it embraces a group of overlapping conditions in which the ability to respond normally to an infective challenge is in some way impaired. It is helpful to think of such patients as falling into one of several distinct groups (Fig. 7.2.4.1).

Primary immunodeficiency syndromes

These are patients with congenital defects in immunity that render them more susceptible to infection. At the most extreme, children with severe combined immunodeficiency have virtually no functioning cellular or humoral immunity and, if unprotected, they will die from infection within a few months of birth. In contrast, some patients with chronic granulomatous disease, an inherited defect in neutrophil function, remain undiagnosed until early adult life. A complete description of the diagnosis and management of this group of disorders is given in Chapter 5.2.

AIDS

AIDS is a model for an acquired defect of cellular immunity leading to an increased risk of infection. Although there are inevitably parallels with other groups of immunocompromised patients, there are particular issues both in the diagnosis and management of infection in AIDS that warrant separate discussion (Chapters 7.5.23, 7.5.24).

Infection related to the underlying condition

The notion of opportunistic infection in the immunocompromised host is most familiar with haematological malignancy or organ transplantation, discussed in detail below. Less obvious, but probably more numerous, are the many physiological conditions and other diseases associated with an increased incidence of infection (Box 7.2.4.1). These immune defects are usually mixed and frequently poorly characterized. The susceptibility to infection varies considerably both in the pattern and severity of infection that occurs, but the clinical problem is real enough. For example, in malnutrition infection due to mycobacteria and salmonella is more common, and pneumocystis pneumonia was first described in children with protein-calorie malnutrition. There is extensive literature documenting multiple defects of host defence in association with alcohol abuse; clinically, this is reflected in an excess of lower respiratory tract infections with *Streptococcus pneumoniae*, *Mycobacterium tuberculosis*, and *Klebsiella pneumoniae*. In Cushing's disease, the excess endogenous steroid production can result in a pattern of opportunist infections that mirrors that seen in patients receiving steroid therapy (see below). Diabetes mellitus is a good example of a disease that is frequently complicated by infection, typically with staphylococcal skin abscesses.

Patients who have had their spleen removed or who have functional (or more rarely congenital) asplenia are at increased risk of certain infections caused by particular organisms, notably *S. pneumoniae* and *Haemophilus influenzae*. The degree of risk is related to the

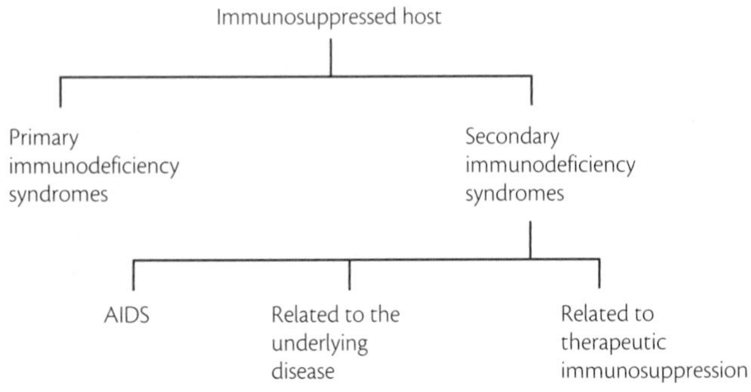

Fig. 7.2.4.1 A classification of the immunocompromised host.

Box 7.2.4.1 Examples of conditions associated with impaired immune responses and an increased risk/severity of infection

- Alcohol abuse
- Burns
- Cushing's disease
- Diabetes mellitus
- Down's syndrome
- Extremes of life
- Haemochromatosis
- Haemodialysis
- Intravenous drug abuse
- Malnutrition
- Pregnancy
- Severe liver disease
- Spinal cord injury
- Splenectomy
- Trauma/surgery
- Uraemia

underlying cause; overall, approximately 5% of patients will have a serious infection, but this varies from 1.5% following traumatic splenectomy to as high as 25% in patients with thalassaemia. Serious infections are most common during the first 5 years following splenectomy and particularly during the first year, but overwhelming postsplenectomy sepsis can occur decades after the surgery.

In myeloma and chronic lymphocytic leukaemia the primary defect is hypogammaglobulinaemia. This is manifested clinically by an excess of bacterial infections, typically those caused by encapsulated organisms such as *S. pneumoniae* and *H. influenzae*. These patients (and others, especially those with rheumatoid arthritis, systemic lupus erythematosus, or polyarteritis nodosa) all have impaired immunity as a consequence of their underlying disease, but because they also commonly receive treatment with immunosuppressive drugs it can be very difficult to attribute cause and effect.

Infection complicating therapeutic immunosuppression

In addition to the well-recognized risk groups, such as those with haematological malignancy or allograft recipients, infective complications of immunosuppression are now being recognized in a much broader range of patients. Conditions as diverse as severe skin disease, asthma, inflammatory bowel disease, and rheumatoid arthritis are routinely treated with immunosuppressive drugs such as prednisolone, azathioprine, ciclosporin, and cyclophosphamide. These patients are not so profoundly immunosuppressed as a bone marrow transplant recipient, but they are certainly at risk of opportunistic infections; a good example of this is the recent recognition of the increased risk of mycobacterial infections in patients with rheumatoid arthritis receiving the monoclonal antibody to tumour necrosis factor infliximab.

Immunosuppressed patients have multiple risk factors; a bone marrow transplant recipient may have been neutropenic, receiving corticosteroids and ciclosporin for management of graft-versus-host disease, and have an indwelling right atrial catheter for feeding purposes. Clearly each of these factors represents a substantial and very different type of risk factor for infection and it is important to remember that, in such patients, multiple pathogens can cause disease simultaneously.

Factors such as the precise nature and intensity of the immunosuppressive regimen, anatomical and/or surgical considerations, and the premorbid status of the patient will all have some influence on the pattern of opportunistic infections that occur. For instance, BK virus is a human polyoma virus that can cause renal allograft rejection but virtually never occurs in other organ recipients; liver transplantation is notable for the high incidence of invasive candida infections, and toxoplasmosis is recognized to be a particular problem following cardiac transplantation. The recent introduction of the anti-CD20 monoclonal antibody rituximab has led to an increase in the incidence of opportunistic viral infections such as cytomegalovirus and hepatitis C. A detailed consideration of these differences is beyond the scope of this chapter. The following sections describe the management of some of the common clinical syndromes that present as infection in immunosuppressed patients.

Common clinical syndromes

A general approach to management

Infections in immunosuppressed patients can progress with frightening rapidity; the early physical signs are often muted and the microbiology can be confusing. Patients need to be reviewed frequently and will often need empirical therapy, but this need not be totally 'blind'; a structured and informed assessment will generally allow a logical response to what are the most likely pathogens.

History

This may reveal exposure to community-acquired infections such as varicella zoster or tuberculosis, which can be particularly severe in the immunocompromised patient. Note should be made of any past history of infection; bronchiectasis, for instance, can be very troublesome in transplant recipients. A detailed travel history is important; patients who have visited certain parts of the United States of America may have been exposed to the systemic mycoses such as histoplasmosis or coccidioidomycosis, which are unfamiliar to many clinicians. Visitors to Central America or the Far East, even many years ago, may have acquired an asymptomatic infection with the helminth *Strongyloides stercoralis*; immunosuppression can lead to overt disease (the hyperinfection syndrome) with a high mortality (see below).

Physical examination

This may be unhelpful; immunosuppressed patients often do not mount a good inflammatory response. Thus there may be only a low-grade fever, a thin serous exudate may suffice for pus, and mild abdominal tenderness can be the only sign of peritonitis. Nevertheless, careful, and if necessary repeated clinical examination is worthwhile, as signs of inflammation may become apparent only when immune function returns. Particular attention should be paid to the presence of new skin lesions. In neutropenic patients, bacteraemias may be accompanied by striking embolic lesions (Fig. 7.2.4.2); pseudomonas infections (and less commonly klebsiella and aeromonas) can cause a focal necrotic cellulitis called ecthyma gangrenosum. Fungal infections present as indolent locally invasive

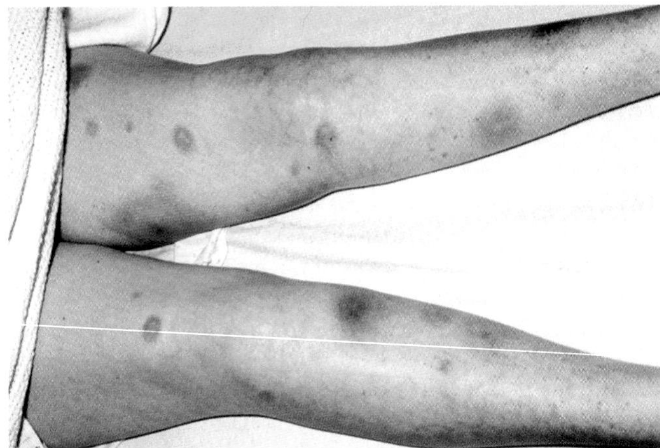

Fig. 7.2.4.2 Disseminated gram-negative sepsis in a neutropenic patient.

lesions (Fig. 7.2.4.3); aspergillus infections often have a black eschar. The perianal area and the insertion sites of indwelling right atrial catheters repay careful examination. Aspiration and/or biopsy of any new skin lesion in immunosuppressed patients are well worthwhile, since they may quickly point to an otherwise inapparent diagnosis. Lymphadenopathy is always important and will usually require aspiration or biopsy. It may be a manifestation of a lymphoproliferative condition, post-transplant lymphoproliferative disease (PTLD), arising as a consequence of the intense immunosuppressive regimens now in widespread use. Although the precise pathogenesis of PTLD is still unclear, it is generally accepted that Epstein–Barr virus (EBV) infection or reactivation and intensive anti-T-lymphocyte regimens play a major role. PTLD is emerging as one of the major causes of late death following renal transplantation.

Underlying disease

This can provide valuable clues. Neutropenia is a major risk factor for infection and renders the patient susceptible to bacteraemias, particularly with gram-negative organisms such as *Escherichia coli* and *Pseudomonas aeruginosa*. A patient with an obstructing bronchial neoplasm may develop a lung abscess due to inadequate drainage. Corticosteroids are used widely; when given in doses exceeding 15 to 20 mg daily for long periods they increase susceptibility to

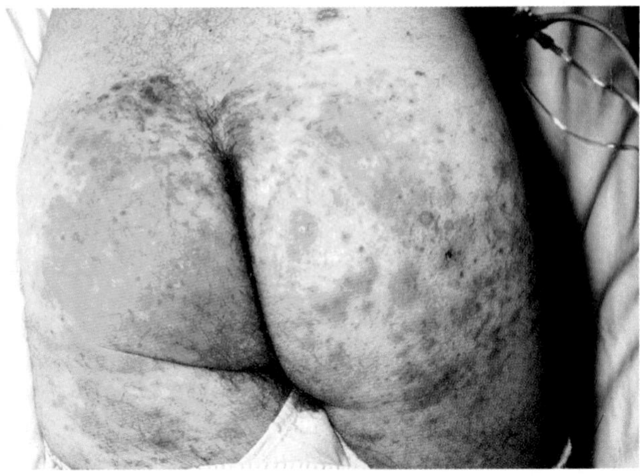

Fig. 7.2.4.3 Extensive dermatophyte infection in a bone marrow transplant recipient.

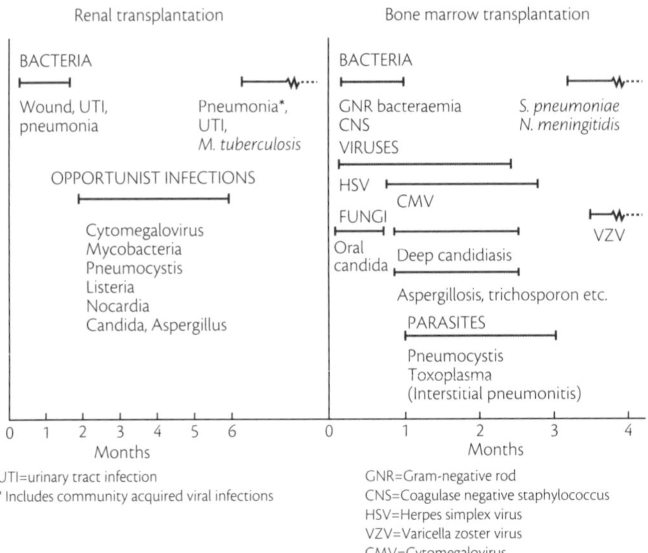

Fig. 7.2.4.4 Timetable for the development of infective complications in renal transplant and bone marrow transplant recipients.

infections with viruses, fungi, parasites, and bacteria such as *Mycobacterium tuberculosis*, all organisms normally associated with cellular immune defences.

Duration of immunosuppression

This often has a profound effect on the type of infection that occurs, and is well illustrated by comparing the 'timetables' of infections in renal transplant recipients with patients receiving bone marrow transplants (Fig. 7.2.4.4). In the first 6 weeks after renal transplantation bacterial infections predominate, typically surgical complications of the procedure or urinary infections. Between 6 weeks and 6 months post-transplantation the patient is most at risk from the 'classic' opportunistic infections; as time continues and the intensity of immunosuppression declines, typical community-acquired infections become more common. In bone marrow transplantation, the initial period of neutropenia is characterized by bacterial infections; later, when many patients receive high-dose steroids for graft-versus-host disease, cytomegalovirus and fungal infections (candida and aspergillus) develop.

Speed of progression

An assessment of this is helpful in both differential diagnosis and in deciding on empirical therapy. In neutropenic patients, the onset of fever is usually an indication for immediate empirical antibiotic therapy (see below). In contrast, the response to a fever and new pulmonary infiltrates in a patient who is 8 months post renal transplantation will depend on the pace of the illness. Rapid deterioration over the space of a few hours will suggest a bacterial infection or a noninfectious cause, and will need urgent therapy; a more indolent presentation would point to a fungal or mycobacterial aetiology, and treatment can be delayed for a short period to try and establish the diagnosis.

Investigations

It is important that the diagnostic laboratories be made aware of the clinical problem since handling of specimens from immunosuppressed patients—and interpretation of the results—will often differ substantially from routine procedures.

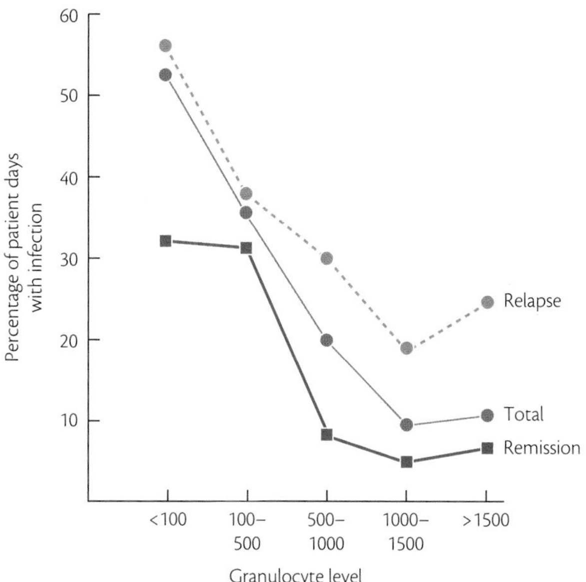

Fig. 7.2.4.5 Relationship between neutrophil count and the risk of invasive Gram-negative infection.
(From Bodey GP, *et al.* (1966). Quantitative relationships between circulating leukocytes and infection in patients with acute leukemia. *Ann Intern Med*, **64**, 328–40, with permission.)

Fever of unknown origin

In neutropenic patients, fever is often the first and only sign of bacteraemia, and prompt action is necessary. In this setting, a fever of unknown origin is defined as a fever of over 38 °C sustained for 2 h and not obviously due to an identifiable cause such as concomitant blood transfusion.

The risk of bacteraemia is directly related to the depth of the neutropenia; the incidence of infection rises when the neutrophil count falls to below 0.5×10^9/L, and is particularly severe when the count falls to less than 0.1×10^9/L (Fig. 7.2.4.5). Some years ago, the commonest bloodstream isolates were gram-negative bacteria such as *E. coli* and klebsiella, generally derived from the patient's gut flora, and *P. aeruginosa*, a common environmental pathogen. Gram-negative bacteraemia in neutropenic patients carried a very high mortality and led to the introduction of several preventative strategies such as the use of prophylactic antibiotics and colony-stimulating factors. Although these approaches have not been entirely successful, the incidence of gram-negative bacteraemias has declined substantially, and in most units gram-positive organisms, notably coagulase-negative staphylococci (*Staphylococcus epidermidis*) are now the commonest isolates. Importantly though, tissue-based infections such as pneumonia continue to be caused predominantly by gram-negative bacteria.

Clinical features are frequently unhelpful. Sometimes a focus will be suggested by erythema around the point of entry of an indwelling catheter, a finding often associated with staphylococcal infection. Septic shock is infrequent, although it can be associated with viridans streptococci; interestingly, endocarditis is rare.

Blood cultures should be drawn before treatment is begun. Ideally two sets should be obtained, at least one of which should be from a peripheral vein (rather than an indwelling catheter), although this is not always possible. Culturing larger volumes of blood (e.g. 30 ml compared to the more conventional 10 ml) will increase the yield. Appropriate samples must also be taken from other potential foci of infection. Nevertheless, it has been one of the enduring frustrations of this subject that even the most rigorous of microbiological investigations in the febrile neutropenic patient will yield only *c.*40 to 50% of positive cultures. The explanation for this is unknown; some studies have suggested that it is due to endotoxaemia in the absence of bacteraemia, but the data are inconclusive. What is clear, however, is that treatment must begin before the results of the cultures are available; delay will lead to unacceptable fatalities.

The choice of the initial empirical antibiotic regimen for the febrile neutropenic patient has been the subject of intense investigation. The ideal regimen will be safe and have good bactericidal activity against all the common pathogens. No single regimen is perfect; much will depend on the availability (and cost) of antibiotics in a given institution, and on local patterns of antibiotic susceptibility. The Infectious Diseases Society of America has published helpful guidelines on the management of these patients.

An important recent development in practice has been the risk assessment of febrile neutropenic patients. The goal is to distinguish those high-risk patients that need hospital admission and parenteral antibiotics, from a low-risk group (<5% risk of complications) who can be managed as outpatients with oral therapy. Well-validated hospital-based regimens include the combination of an antipseudomonal penicillin plus an aminoglycoside or the use of single agents such as a third- or fourth-generation cephalosporin (e.g. ceftazidime or cefepime), a penem such as meropenem, or a β-lactam/β-lactamase inhibitor combination (e.g. piperacillin–tazobactam). A recent meta-analysis concluded that monotherapy was on balance at least as effective as and probably safer than combination therapy.

All these regimens are very active against the common gram-negative organisms, but are relatively ineffective at treating gram-positive bacteria, such as coagulase-negative staphylococci or meticillin (methicillin)-resistant *Staphylococcus aureus* (MRSA), that are nowadays common problems in many units. Unfortunately, there are only a very limited number of drugs that are reliably active against these organisms, notably glycopeptides such as vancomycin and more recently linezolid. Some clinicians have advocated adding an anti-gram-positive agent to the initial empirical regimen; one disadvantage of this approach is the toxicity (and cost) of vancomycin which may not be justified, particularly because coagulase-negative staphylococci rarely cause death. Several prospective clinical trials have concluded that unless there are strong grounds for considering MRSA infection, vancomycin can usually be withheld until the results of blood cultures are known. A recent randomized controlled trial in febrile neutropenic patients concluded that linezolid was not inferior to vancomycin in either safety or efficacy.

Patients who are assessed as being in a low-risk group may be managed either with a brief period of inpatient parenteral therapy followed by rapid conversion to oral agents, or by oral therapy from the outset. A typical oral regimen is a combination of a quinolone plus amoxicillin/clavulanate.

In patients who respond to the initial regimen, the treatment should be continued for at least 7 days, and ideally until the neutrophil count has returned to over 0.5×10^9/L. Sometimes this is not possible; the patient may have a persistent or unresponsive neutropenia (e.g. aplastic anaemia, or following bone marrow transplantation). In these patients, treatment is usually cautiously stopped after an arbitrary period such as 14 days; rebound bacteraemias can occur and will need further treatment.

A common problem is the patient who continues to have high swinging fevers after 48 to 72 h of broad-spectrum antibacterial antibiotics. The patient must be carefully re-evaluated: Has some new clinical sign appeared? Could there be a resistant organism or an occult source of the sepsis? Simply changing the antibiotic regimen or adding vancomycin in the absence of any evidence to support these moves is not supported by clinical trial data. In this situation, deep fungal infection becomes more likely. Randomized clinical trials have demonstrated that empirical addition of an antifungal agent, either an amphotericin B formulation or an antifungal triazole such as voriconazole is associated with a response rate of approximately 30%.

Fever of unknown origin in the non-neutropenic immunosuppressed patient presents as a completely different problem. Fever in this setting is rarely immediately life-threatening, and the wide differential diagnosis means that it is generally better to pursue the cause rather than embark on empirical therapy.

Fever and new pulmonary infiltrates

The development of fever and new pulmonary infiltrates is one of the most challenging clinical problems in this group of patients. Pneumonia is the commonest infective cause of death in immunocompromised patients. In the presence of diffuse airspace disease, the mortality approaches 50% irrespective of the underlying defect in host defence, although the epidemiology varies both between different patient groups and at different times reflecting the intensity of the immunosuppression (Table 7.2.4.1).

Table 7.2.4.1 Aetiology of the 'febrile pneumonitis' syndrome in different patient groups

	Renal transplantation	Bone marrow transplantation
Less than 1 month	Aspiration Nosocomial LRTI	Aspiration Nosocomial LRTI Aspergillus
1–3 months[a]	Cytomegalovirus Pneumocystis Aspergillus Nocardia Mycobacteria Mucor	Cytomegalovirus Pneumocystis Aspergillus Respiratory syncytial virus Mycobacteria Mucor Noninfective causes[b]
More than 3 months[a]	Influenza Legionella Common respiratory bacteria	Varicella zoster GVHD Common respiratory bacteria and viruses

GVHD, graft-versus-host disease; LRTI, lower respiratory tract infection.

[a] Six months in renal transplant recipients.

[b] Includes idiopathic interstitial pneumonitis in bone marrow transplant recipients.

Modified from Wilson WR, Cockerill FR 3rd, Rosenow EC 3rd (1985). Pulmonary disease in the immunocompromised host (2). *Mayo Clin Proc*, **60**, 610–31.

The condition can progress extremely quickly, and conventional diagnostic procedures may be unhelpful. The list of possible causes is so daunting (Box 7.2.4.2) that clinicians may be tempted to use multiple empirical antimicrobial agents, sometimes to the patient's detriment. It is often not possible to 'guess' with any certainty the precise cause of the problem (indeed, it can be dangerous to do so, since it is not uncommon for multiple causes to be present simultaneously), but by considering the available information one can

Box 7.2.4.2 Causes of fever and new pulmonary infiltrates in the immunocompromised host

Infections

Bacterial

- Conventional respiratory pathogens
  - *S. pneumoniae*, *H. influenzae*, klebsiella
- Nosocomial pathogens
  - *E. coli*, *Pseudomonas* spp., *Legionella* spp
- 'Atypical' organisms
  - *Chlamydia psittaci*, *C. pneumoniae*, mycoplasma
- Mycobacteria and related organisms
  - *M. tuberculosis*, atypical mycobacteria, nocardia.

Viral

- Herpes viruses
  - Cytomegalovirus, herpes simplex, varicella zoster
- Respiratory viruses
  - Respiratory syncytial virus, (para)influenza, adenovirus, measles

Fungi

- Systemic mycoses
  - Blastomycosis, histoplasmosis, coccidioidomycosis
- Opportunist mycoses
  - Candida, aspergillus, mucor, cryptococcus
- Other rare fungi
  - Trichosporon, pseudallescheria/scedosporium

Parasites

- Pneumocystis, strongyloides, toxoplasma

Noninfective causes

Pulmonary pathology

- Pulmonary oedema, pulmonary infarction/emboli, pulmonary haemorrhage
- Primary or secondary malignancy

Other causes

- Drugs (e.g. busulfan)
- Activity of the underlying disease (e.g. systemic lupus erythematosus)
- Radiation pneumonitis

construct a 'short list' which will guide further investigation and treatment.

The initial evaluation should follow the approach outlined above, in particular making an assessment of the intensity of the immunosuppression and the speed of progression of the pulmonary disease. The main purpose of this is to determine the need for empirical therapy, either because the clinical picture is suggestive of a 'simple' bacterial pneumonia or because of a potentially more serious progressive cause of uncertain aetiology. Factors that would favour a bacterial aetiology include the presence of neutropenia, a rapidly developing clinical evolution (e.g. deterioration over a period of 12 h), progressive hypoxia, a sputum Gram stain showing a marked predominance of a single bacterial morphology (even in the absence of neutrophils), or a chest radiographic appearance that has worsened significantly over a short period. High fever is not necessarily a part of this syndrome; indeed, it is important to emphasize that this rapidly evolving clinical picture is not inevitably due to infection. Noninfective causes such as acute lung haemorrhage or pulmonary oedema can present in an identical fashion, and the most appropriate therapy may be diuretics rather than antimicrobials. However, antimicrobials will often need to be given as well because of what has been termed 'infection-provoked relapse'. In immunologically mediated diseases such as systemic lupus erythematosus or anti-glomerular basement membrane (GBM) disease (Goodpasture's syndrome) infection can precipitate a relapse of the underlying disease. Thus, the development of fever and new pulmonary shadows in a patient with anti-GBM disease may be primarily due to lung haemorrhage associated with a rise in anti-GBM antibodies, but this in turn can be precipitated by an infection that need not necessarily be in the lung. Treatment must be directed both towards improving oxygenation and the underlying infection.

Blood cultures should always be obtained, and sputum obtained if it is available. A chest radiograph and arterial blood gas analysis are essential. The initial treatment will be dictated by the clinical circumstances, but the temptation to use a complex regimen to provide very broad spectrum cover is best avoided. Rapid clinical deterioration is usually caused by bacterial infections; a combination of an extended-spectrum cephalosporin plus erythromycin will be appropriate. Where staphylococcal infection is suspected, flucloxacillin should normally be used, but vancomycin may be necessary if there are clinical or epidemiological grounds to be concerned about MRSA infection. Unusual ('opportunistic') organisms such as mycobacteria, nocardia, or cytomegalovirus rarely cause such a rapid clinical deterioration and it is extremely difficult to distinguish them on clinical grounds alone. For these reasons, the addition of further empirical agents is usually not warranted.

In patients in whom immediate empirical therapy is not necessary, additional diagnostic procedures can be done. These should include serological tests for atypical organisms (including histoplasma and coccidioides in patients who have been in endemic areas), and examination of blood and urine for cytomegalovirus. The chest radiograph should be repeated, but it is not as sensitive as arterial blood gas measurements, which should be done twice daily. The radiographic appearances are rarely sufficiently specific as to suggest a precise diagnosis, although they can provide helpful pointers. Thus a bilateral interstitial midzone infiltrate associated with marked hypoxia is typical of pneumonia due to *Pneumocystis jirovecii* (previously called *P. carinii*), and a pleura-based infarct is suggestive of aspergillus. However, there are pitfalls in relying on the radiographic appearance alone in guiding the choice of therapy. First, no radiographic appearance is pathognomonic of any single pathological process; e.g. cytomegalovirus or pulmonary oedema can mimic pneumocystis, and legionella pneumonia cannot be distinguished from aspergillus. Second, multiple agents can be present simultaneously, and each may require separate treatment. Other imaging techniques such as high-resolution CT can often provide useful additional information on the extent of the process, and will sometimes point to the cause (e.g. the 'halo sign' associated with invasive aspergillosis).

If the condition does not resolve and initial investigations are unhelpful it is often appropriate to try to make a specific diagnosis by obtaining material directly from the bronchial tree. In most cases the method of choice is bronchoscopy with bronchoalveolar lavage. This will provide adequate material without incurring a serious risk of bleeding (many such patients are thrombocytopenic). In most series, bronchial brush or transbronchial biopsy specimens produce only a marginal increase in the diagnostic yield, and are usually not done unless the clinical picture is suggestive of a noninfective process such as an infiltrating tumour. Close liaison with the microbiology laboratory is very important because additional diagnostic procedures will need to be performed.

Acute neurological syndromes

A large number of conventional and opportunistic pathogens can lead to neurological infection in immunocompromised patients. Although there is some degree of overlap, the underlying defect in host defence is often a good indicator of the likely cause (Table 7.2.4.2).

The clinical features may help suggest the diagnosis. Meningitic syndromes are more likely to be associated with conventional bacterial infections, listeriosis, and tuberculosis, as well as fungi such as cryptococcus and candida. In contrast, infections with toxoplasma, aspergillus, or nocardia more commonly present as space-occupying lesions. Pure encephalitic syndromes are less common, but can occur with herpes simplex. Rhinocerebral mucormycosis is a progressive, destructive infection caused by mucor and related moulds that

Table 7.2.4.2 Organisms causing neurological infections in different patient groups

	Bacteria	Fungi	Parasites	Viruses
Neutropenia	Enterics[a]	Candida		
		Aspergillus		
		Mucor		
T cell/ monocyte defect	Listeria	Cryptococcus	Toxoplasma	Varicella zoster
	Legionella	Aspergillus	Strongyloides	Herpes simplex
	Nocardia	Mucor		Polyomavirus
	Mycobacteria	Coccidioides		
Splenectomy	*S. pneumoniae*			
	H. influenzae			
	Neisseria			

[a] Gram-negative Enterobacteriaceae.

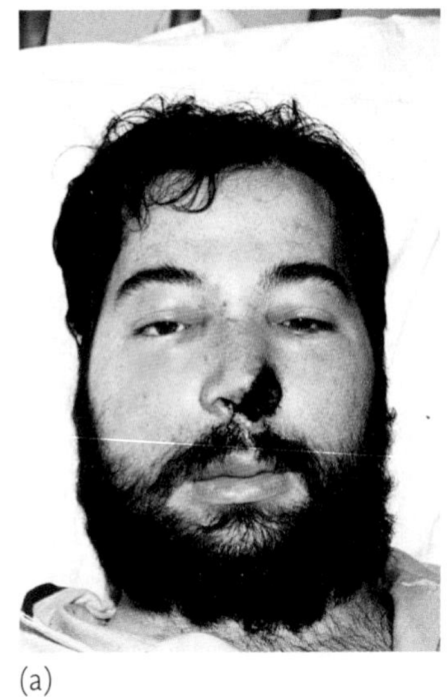

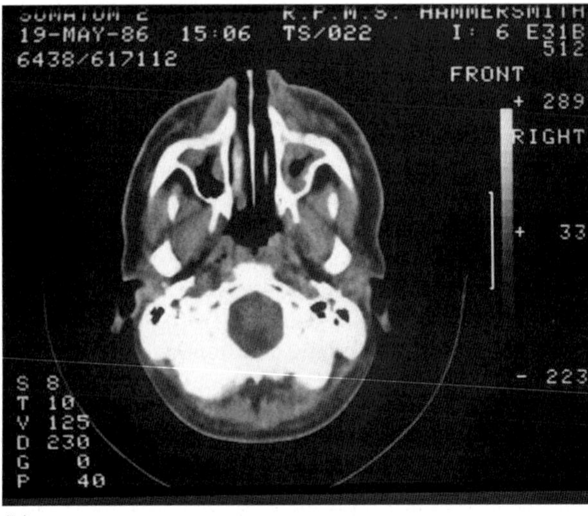

Fig. 7.2.4.6 Invasive mucormycosis. (a) Clinical appearances. (b) CT scan showing extensive sinus involvement.

usually begins in the paranasal sinuses and spreads caudally to involve the orbits or the frontal lobes of the brain (Fig. 7.2.4.6). It is seen particularly in patients with uncontrolled diabetes mellitus or as a complication of neutropenia. Progressive multifocal leukoencephalitis (PML) is a subacute neurological disease caused by the JC polyomavirus. PML presents with the insidious onset of impairment of speech, vision, and higher functions without evidence of raised intracranial pressure. The condition progresses inexorably, usually leading to death in about 6 months.

Bacterial infections generally proceed rapidly, while fungi and parasites pursue a more indolent course. However, exceptions to this are common and there is no substitute for obtaining a precise diagnosis. Examination of the skin (see below) and fundoscopy may be valuable. Retinitis is not usually a feature of systemic infection with toxoplasma or cytomegalovirus; in contrast, candida endophthalmitis may be the only manifestation of deep-seated infection (Fig. 7.2.4.7).

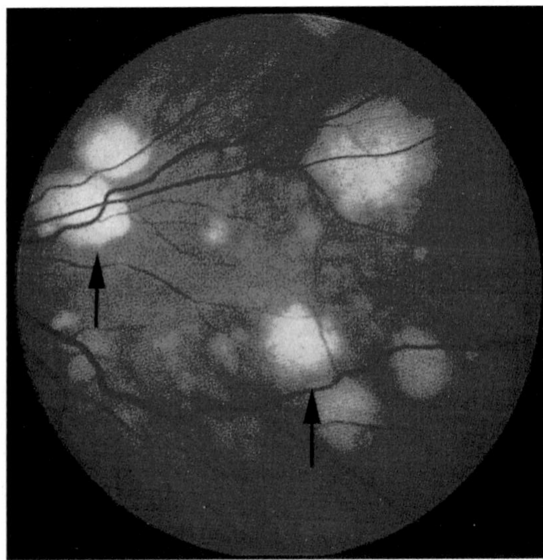

Fig. 7.2.4.7 Candida endophthalmitis.

Examination of the cerebrospinal fluid is mandatory. A high index of suspicion is necessary, since the clinical features of meningitis are often muted in these patients. An unexplained low-grade fever and mild headache may be the only clues; frank meningism, photophobia, or focal neurological signs occur late. Examination of the cerebrospinal fluid should include direct microscopy and culture for (myco)bacteria and fungi, a cryptococcal latex agglutination test, antigen tests for *S. pneumoniae*, and the demonstration of specific antibody production or DNA sequences by the polymerase chain reaction (e.g. for herpes simplex, polyomaviruses).

Certain organisms are notable for their absence on direct microscopy: mycobacteria are seen in less than 10% of cases, and nocardia and aspergillus only very rarely. A predominance of lymphocytes suggests partially treated bacterial infection, tuberculosis, or a viral aetiology, but not infection with listeria, despite its name. A low cerebrospinal fluid glucose points to tuberculosis but is not specific. Sometimes the only abnormality is a modest elevation of the cerebrospinal fluid protein; this should never be ignored, even in the seeming absence of other features of neurological infection. Where appropriate, cytological examination of the cerebrospinal fluid should be done to exclude carcinomatous or leukaemic meningitis, which can mimic an acute infective presentation.

Certain neurological infections are often associated with pulmonary disease; these include legionella, tuberculosis, aspergillus, mucor, and nocardia. A CT brain scan which should be contrast-enhanced is valuable. Focal, usually enhancing lesions are particularly associated with pyogenic abscesses and toxoplasmosis. Tuberculomas can appear as single lesions. MRI is better then CT scanning for abnormalities of the brain stem (e.g. the basal meningitis associated with cryptococcal infection), and frequently reveals lesions in toxoplasmosis that are not seen on CT scans. It may be particularly helpful in avoiding a brain biopsy when a diagnosis of PML is considered.

Any new skin lesions should be biopsied, and a nasal biopsy may reveal mucor. An electroencephalogram is rarely helpful. Brain biopsy is done very rarely; it should not be considered unless empirical therapy has failed and there is a real prospect of therapeutic benefit to the patient.

If the cerebrospinal fluid is nondiagnostic but bacterial infection cannot be excluded, empirical antibiotics should be given immediately. An extended-spectrum cephalosporin such as ceftriaxone is suitable. Serological tests for toxoplasmosis are not specific in this setting, and if the infection is suspected it is better to start empirical therapy with pyrimethamine and sulphadimidine. Cerebral aspergillosis and mucormycosis have a very poor prognosis; treatment should be begun with high-dose amphotericin B, and surgical debridement considered if possible. There is no effective treatment for PML.

Acute gastrointestinal syndromes

The organisms associated with specific gastrointestinal syndromes in immunocompromised patients are shown in Table 7.2.4.3.

Severe stomatitis is a common complaint in immunosuppressed patients. The three commonest causes candida, herpes simplex, and chemotherapy-induced mucositis are clinically indistinguishable and indeed can coexist and cause disease together. For these reasons, the diagnosis should always be confirmed by microscopy and culture. Herpetic stomatitis in particular can be atypical in these patients; the classic appearance of groups of small vesicles is unusual, and a more common presentation is ulceration, which can be extensive (Fig. 7.2.4.8). In profoundly immunosuppressed patients such as bone marrow transplant recipients oral candidiasis is very common, and in patients who are seropositive before transplantation, reactivation of herpes simplex is almost universal. For these reasons, prophylaxis is usually given. Both herpes simplex virus and candida can cause oesophagitis, generally (but not exclusively) as an extension of oral disease. If necessary, oesophagoscopy with brush cytology and/or biopsy is the investigation of choice. Proven oesophageal candidiasis should be regarded as 'invasive' disease and treated with systemic antifungals (amphotericin B or fluconazole).

A large number of organisms can cause acute diarrhoeal syndromes; in addition, noninfective conditions such as radiation enteritis, drugs, and graft-versus-host disease must be included in the differential diagnosis. There are no distinguishing clinical features of note, and diagnosis depends on microbiological examination of the faeces.

Table 7.2.4.3 Gastrointestinal syndromes in the immunocompromised host

	Bacteria	Fungi	Parasites	Viruses
Oral infection		Candida		Herpes simplex virus
Diarrhoeal syndromes	Neutropenic enterocolitis	Candida	Giardia	Enterovirus
	C. difficile		Isospora	Adenovirus
	Salmonella/shigella		Cryptosporidia	Cytomegalovirus
	Atypical mycobacteria		Microsporidia	Rotavirus
Hepatic syndromes		Candida	Toxoplasma	Cytomegalovirus
				Hepatitis B and C
				Herpes simplex
				Varicella zoster

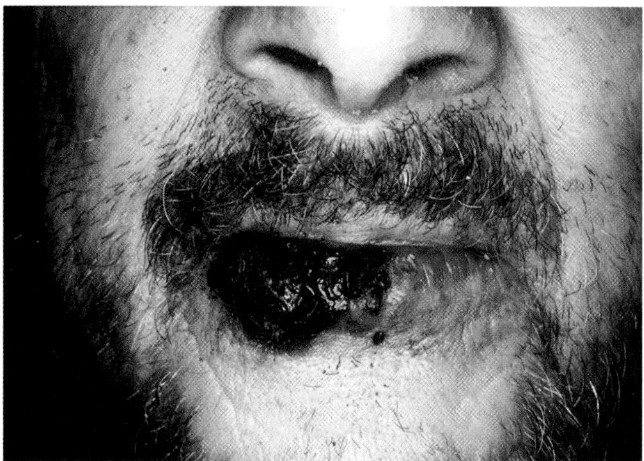
Fig. 7.2.4.8 Severe herpetic stomatitis in a patient with lymphoma.

The diarrhoea caused by *Clostridium difficile* is usually due to a pseudomembranous colitis. However, patients with leukaemia or aplastic anaemia may develop neutropenic enterocolitis (previously called typhlitis), a fulminating invasive colitis characterized by diffuse dilation and oedema of the bowel walls, haemorrhage, ulceration, and a high mortality. Classically this has been associated with clostridial bacteraemia, in particular *Clostridium septicum*, but other clostridia, including *C. difficile*, and even gram-negative bacteria can also be found.

Strongyloides stercoralis is a nematode that can be carried asymptomatically for many years after exposure. Strongyloidiasis has been recognized as a complication of human T-lymphotropic virus 1 (HTLV-1) infection, and also occurs secondary to immunosuppression (typically with high-dose steroids and in solid organ transplant recipients). A rise in the worm burden results in the hyperinfection syndrome, which may present as pneumonitis or intermittent intestinal obstruction. The movement of the worms through the gut wall can carry with them enteric bacteria, resulting in polymicrobial bacteraemias and gram-negative meningitis when the worms penetrate the cerebrospinal fluid.

Giardiasis is particularly associated with hypogammaglobulinaemia, and curiously is rarely seen in other groups. Cryptosporidium, microsporidia, and isospora are now well-recognized causes of severe and sometimes chronic diarrhoea in AIDS patients, but may also occur in other less severely immunocompromised patients. Among the viruses the most difficult problem is cytomegalovirus. Cytomegalovirus can cause a severe colitis, and in these cases ganciclovir is beneficial. Ideally the diagnosis should be confirmed by biopsy, but ultimately may depend on the result of a therapeutic trial since demonstration of the organism does not necessarily indicate that it is causing disease.

Mild abnormalities of liver function tests are a common accompaniment to many systemic infections, but hepatitis is a particular feature of both toxoplasmosis and cytomegalovirus infection. An increased prevalence of hepatitis B has been found in patients on chronic haemodialysis (10%) and those with Hodgkin's disease (8%) and lepromatous leprosy (20%). The acute hepatitic episode is mild, often anicteric, and may pass unnoticed. However, persistent viral replication and the development of complications

Table 7.2.4.4 Infection prevention strategies in organ transplant recipients and patients with neutropenia[a]

	Strategy	Comment
Bacterial infections		
Bacterial sepsis in neutropenia	Oral quinolones	Re-emerging following earlier concerns with efficacy and risk of resistance
	High-efficiency particulate air (HEPA)-filtered rooms	Very expensive and no clear advantage in survival
Overwhelming postsplenectomy sepsis	Oral penicillin and Pneumovax	
Tuberculosis	Isoniazid	In exposed or high-risk patients, especially if receiving prolonged high-dose corticosteroids
Viral infections		
Herpes simplex, cytomegalovirus	Aciclovir, ganciclovir	Dose and drug varies depending on specific indication
Influenza	Immunization	Not routine except in high-risk groups
Fungal infections		
Candida, aspergillus	Fluconazole, itraconazole	Amphotericin formulations and newer triazole drugs such as voriconazole may also have a role
Pneumocystis jirovecii	Co-trimoxazole	Used for both bone marrow transplantations and in some solid organ transplantations

[a] Excludes postexposure prophylaxis.

associated with chronic infection are more likely. Cirrhosis secondary to hepatitis C is currently the commonest indication for liver transplantation; recurrence of infection post-transplantation is almost inevitable and requires specific approaches to prevention and treatment. Other immunosuppressed patients are at risk of infection and nosocomial spread of hepatitis C among hospitalized patients being treated for cancer has been reported.

A particular form of systemic candidiasis has been called chronic hepatosplenic candidiasis, but the syndrome is better referred to as chronic disseminated candidiasis (CDC). Approximately 85% of the patients with CDC and underlying acute leukaemia are in remission at the time of diagnosis. The most common manifestation of CDC is persistent fever not responsive to conventional antibiotics. There is often abdominal pain; palpable hepatomegaly is unusual. The liver function tests show a markedly raised alkaline phosphatase and there may be hyperbilirubinaemia, but microbiological investigations (including fungal blood cultures) are frequently negative. Characteristic lesions are seen on MRI. Large doses of amphotericin B formulations are required to treat the infection and prevent further relapses.

Prevention of infection

Approaches designed to prevent infection in immunosuppressed patients have assumed increasing importance. For profoundly neutropenic patients, measures including nursing them in single rooms and taking great care to avoid nosocomial acquisition of infection from staff, visitors, or other patients is simple but effective. Chemoprophylaxis for a wide range of bacterial, viral, and fungal pathogens has had a major impact (Table 7.2.4.4). Immunization has only a limited role at present, although when feasible (e.g. providing pneumococcal vaccination before an elective splenectomy) it is worthwhile. In addition, routine screening of transplant recipients and donors should include serological tests for cytomegalovirus, hepatitis B, and HIV.

Further reading

Bucaneve G, *et al.* (2005). Levofloxacin to prevent bacterial infection in patients with cancer and neutropenia. *N Engl J Med*, **353**, 977–87.

Davies JM, Barnes R, Milligan D (2002). Update of guidelines for the prevention and treatment of infection in patients with an absent or dysfunctional spleen. *Clin Med*, **2**, 440–3.

Fischer SA (2006). Infections complicating solid organ transplantation. *Surg Clin North Am*, **86**, 1127–45.

Jaksic B, *et al.* (2006). Efficacy and safety of linezolid compared with vancomycin in a randomized, double-blind study of febrile neutropenic patients with cancer. *Clin Infect Dis*, **42**, 597–607.

Paul M, Soares-Weiser K, Leibovici L (2003). β lactam monotherapy versus β lactam-aminoglycoside combination therapy for fever with neutropenia: systematic review and meta-analysis. *BMJ*, **326**, 1111–19.

Pfaller MA, Pappas PG, Wingard JR (2006). Invasive fungal pathogens: current epidemiological trends. *Clin Infect Dis*, **43** Suppl 1, S3–14.

Richardson MD (2005). Changing patterns and trends in systemic fungal infections. *J Antimicrob Chemother*, **56** Suppl 1, i5–11.

Sipsas NV, Bodey GP, Kontoyiannis DP (2005). Perspectives for the management of febrile neutropenic patients with cancer in the 21st century. *Cancer*, **103**, 1103–13.

Viscoli C, Varnier O, Machetti M (2005). Infections in patients with febrile neutropenia: epidemiology, microbiology and risk stratification. *Clin Infect Dis*, **40** Suppl 4, S240–5.

Walsh TJ, *et al.* (2002). Voriconazole compared with liposomal amphotericin B for empirical antifungal therapy in patients with neutropenia and persistent fever. *N Engl J Med*, **346**, 225–34.

7.2.5 Antimicrobial chemotherapy

R.G. Finch

Essentials

The practice of medicine changed dramatically with the availability of effective antimicrobial agents. Fatal diseases such as bacterial meningitis and endocarditis became treatable; much minor community infectious morbidity became readily controlled; many surgical procedures became much safer, and developments in organ and bone marrow transplantation became possible. However, the very success of antimicrobial chemotherapy has led to overuse, misuse and inappropriate pressures from the public to prescribe. In many countries, antibiotics are freely available to the public for purchase 'over the counter', with few controls or guidance to ensure their safe and effective use.

Antimicrobial drugs

Pharmacological characteristics and antimicrobial spectrum—antibacterial drugs can be divided according to their mode of action into those that (1) inhibit cell wall synthesis—e.g. penicillins and cephalosporins; (2) interfere with protein synthesis—e.g. tetracyclines, aminoglycosides; (3) inhibit bacterial nucleic acid synthesis—e.g. fluoroquinolones; and (4) act on metabolic pathways—e.g. sulphonamides and trimethoprin. The antimicrobial spectrum of a drug is determined by the mode of action and ability to reach the relevant target site. Antibiotics active against a few particular bacteria are considered narrow spectrum (e.g. vancomycin), while others are active against many bacteria and are labelled broad spectrum (e.g. meropenem). Some antimicrobials are only active against anaerobically dividing bacteria (e.g. metronidazole).

Clinical effectiveness—to be effective clinically, sufficient drug must reach the infection site. The pharmacokokinetic characteristics of absorption, distribution, metabolism and excretion are critical to defining dose, efficacy and often safety. Poorly absorbed agents are often administered parenterally, some topically. Hydrophobicity and hydrophilicity are important in defining tissue and extracellular fluid concentrations, as are factors such as molecular size and pH. Highly protein-bound drugs such as flucloxacillin may achieve lower tissue concentrations in selected body sites.

Excretion, metabolism and drug monitoring—many drugs are metabolically degraded in the liver and/or excreted by the kidney via glomerular filtration or tubular secretion. It should therefore be anticipated that dose modification may be necessary to avoid toxicity in patients with compromised hepatic or renal function. Therapeutic drug monitoring is important in ensuring therapeutic and nontoxic concentrations of some drugs, e.g. gentamicin.

Antiviral, antifungal, and antiparasitic drugs—until recently, viral infections were largely without effective therapy, but this has changed with the availability of drugs to treat herpesvirus infections (herpes simplex, varicella–zoster and cytomegalovirus), and more recently the development of drugs active against HIV/AIDS. Advances in the management of invasive fungal disease have been slower: the reliance on polyenes, e.g. amphotericin, has only recently been eclipsed with the availability of potent azoles and triazoles and echinocandins. In the case of many parasitic diseases, advances have been extremely slow, but the importance of malaria has led to new compounds being discovered, also new ways of using established drugs in combination.

Resistance to antimicrobial drugs

Resistance mechanisms—loss of efficacy through resistance mechanisms is unique to antimicrobial drugs. There are four main types: (1) drug inactivation or destruction, (2) target site alteration, (3) reduced cell wall permeability (porin mutation) or increased removal from the cell (efflux resistance); and (4) inhibition as a result of metabolic bypass. Individual drugs can be subject to one or more mechanisms of resistance, which may vary by infecting microorganism.

Spread of resistance—genetic mutations that confer resistance do not just affect the target pathogen in the treated individual. They can disseminate both horizontally and vertically as a result of person to person or indirect spread of the pathogen. Spread through genetic mechanisms via plasmids, transposons, integrons, and phages between bacteria of the same and different species are common, as is spread between genera. Likewise, resistance mechanisms can spread to organisms making up the normal flora of the gut and skin.

Clinical impact—antibiotic resistance is of increasing medical and public concern, and affects all aspects of medicine. Infections become unresponsive to initial therapy, sometimes with fatal consequences in the seriously ill. In others, reassessment and alternative therapy with agents are often more toxic and more expensive are required, leading to increased morbidity and increased costs through prolonged hospitalization. The spread of resistant pathogens within hospitals, nursing homes and the community is a very significant concern. High rates of meticillin-resistant *Staphylococcus aureus* (MRSA) infections are present in many countries, including the United States of America, the United Kingdom, and Portugal. Public confidence in health care has been eroded, leading to major government initiatives in the European Union, North America, and Australia in efforts to contain these resistant pathogens.

Prescribing of antimicrobial drugs

A set of principles has emerged to support safe and effective prescribing, covering issues of choice of drug, dose and route of administration, duration of therapy, strategies to minimize adverse reactions, and what factors need to be considered should initial treatment fail. The complexity of modern therapeutics has led to the development of formularies and practice guidelines, the latter increasingly being evidence based, with the twin goals of supporting cost-effective safe prescribing whilst minimizing the risks of emergence of antibiotic resistance.

Introduction

The discovery and clinical application of antibiotics and antimicrobial chemotherapeutic agents is one of the major achievements in medicine. Life-threatening infections such as meningitis, endocarditis, and typhoid fever are now treatable, whereas before they were generally fatal. Likewise, the morbidity associated with many infectious diseases of a less life-threatening nature, such as urinary tract infections, skin and soft tissue infections, and bone and joint sepsis, has been substantially reduced. Major advances in medicine, such as organ and especially bone marrow transplantation, as well as the use of cancer chemotherapy, have become safer because of the availability of effective antimicrobial agents. In the field of surgery, perioperative prophylactic use of antibiotics has reduced the risk of infections complicating procedures such as large bowel and gall bladder surgery, vaginal hysterectomy, and implant surgery such as the insertion of prosthetic heart valves, joints, and neurosurgical shunting devices.

Antimicrobial chemotherapy is the use of antibiotics and chemotherapeutic substances to control infectious disease. The term 'antibiotic' was coined by Waksman to describe a substance derived from naturally occurring microorganisms and possessing antimicrobial activity in high dilution. The latter characteristic is essential in defining its selective toxicity to other microorganisms. True antibiotics include penicillin, derived from the mould *Penicillium notatum*, streptomycin from *Streptomyces griseus*, and the cephalosporins from *Cephalosporium* spp. Many chemotherapeutic substances with antimicrobial activity have been artificially synthesized, such as the sulphonamides, quinolones, and isoniazid. However, the term 'antibiotic' is loosely applied to both the true antibiotics and other antimicrobial agents.

Antibiotics are among the most widely prescribed drugs, accounting for an international expenditure of $33 billion. In the United Kingdom, around 80% of all prescribing is in the community where the emphasis is largely on oral agents; the remainder are used in hospitals where there is a greater emphasis on injectable drugs. More than 125 different antibiotics are available, but a relatively small number are necessary to deal with most prescribing needs. It is important that clinicians who prescribe these drugs are familiar with the principles of antimicrobial chemotherapy and that they adopt a continuous learning approach throughout their professional lives to ensure safe and effective prescribing. Table 7.2.5.1 summarizes the agents available for the treatment of bacterial, mycobacterial, fungal, viral, protozoal, and helminthic infections. More agents have been developed for the treatment of bacterial infections, but globally viral, fungal, and parasitic infections predominate. In recent years, there have been major advances in the availability of antiviral drugs particularly for the treatment of the herpesviruses and HIV. Likewise, safe and effective systemic antifungal agents have resulted from the discovery of azoles and triazoles.

The very success of antimicrobial chemotherapy has led to widespread and often excessive use, particularly in community practice where prescribing is largely empirical and clinical distinction between viral and bacterial infections is difficult. Antibiotics are used extensively in animal husbandry both for the treatment and prevention of infectious disease and, more controversially, in some countries as growth-enhancing agents among commercially raised poultry and swine. This has raised concerns about the emergence and spread of antibiotic resistance, which affects many classes of antibiotic, may be intrinsic to a particular pathogen, or may result from genetic mutation, and in 2006 led to the European Union banning the use of all such agents as growth promoters.

Table 7.2.5.1 Antimicrobial agents available by class or indication effective against bacterial, fungal, viral, protozoal, and helminthic infection (indicative number of agents available[a])

Antibacterial (68)	Antifungal (14)	Antiviral (37)	Antiprotozoal (9)	Anthelminthics (15)
Penicillins	Polyenes	Hepatitis B & C agents	Antimalarials	Anticutaneous larva migrans
Cephalosporins	Caspofungin	Herpesvirus agents	Amoebicides	Antihydatid agents
Carbapenems	Echinocandin	HIV nucleoside analogues	Trichomonacides	Antistrongyloidiasis
Tetracyclines	Flucytosine	HIV non-nucleoside agents	Antigiardials	Antithreadworm/hookworm
Aminoglycosides	Griseofulvin	HIV protease inhibitors	Leishmaniacides	Ascaricides
Macrolides	Azoles	HIV fusion inhibitor	Trypanocides	Filaricides
Clindamycin	Triazoles	Ribavirin	Antipneumocystis agents	Schistosomicides
Chloramphenicol	Terbinafine	Amantadine/rimantadine		Taeniacides
Sodium fusidate		Foscarnet		
Glycopeptides		Neuraminidase inhibitors		
Linezolid				
Quinupristin/dalfopristin				
Colistin				
Sulphonamides				
Trimethoprim				
Antituberculous				
Antileprotic				
Nitroimidazoles				
Quinolones				
Urinary antiseptics				

[a] Based on agents listed in the British National Formulary (www.bnf.org)

Resistance may be caused by enzymatic inactivation (β-lactamase), failure of drug penetration into the bacterial cell (porin mutation), alteration of the target binding site (e.g. penicillin-binding protein alteration in penicillin-resistant *Streptococcus pneumoniae*), or from efflux resistance whereby the drug is extruded from the bacterial cell (e.g. chloroquine-resistant *Plasmodium falciparum*). Organisms can also develop alternative metabolic pathways which bypass drug inactivation.

Resistance may be transferable between the same species or genera but may also spread between genera. Coding for multiple antibiotic resistance has been increasingly observed and results from several mechanisms, in particular plasmid transfer.

Despite the advances in antimicrobial chemotherapy, fresh challenges remain. These include the treatment of viral causes of enteric infection, hepatitis A and E, and viral meningitis, all of which are still without effective chemotherapy. Tuberculosis and malaria are among the world's major infectious disease killers and here problems of antibiotic resistance have escalated. In the case of tuberculosis, the continuing reliance on lengthy and complex regimens continue to frustrate disease management as a result of cost, toxicity, and patient compliance with these regimens.

Among the more worrying trends in antibiotic resistance is the emergence within hospitals of meticillin-resistant *Staphylococcus aureus* (MRSA) and vancomycin-resistant enterococci (VRE). Hospital-acquired MRSA has now spread into the community, largely among nursing home residents. Furthermore, more virulent strains of MRSA have recently arisen in the community in the United States of America and Australia. *Strep. pneumoniae* is another community pathogen which has rapidly become less sensitive to penicillin causing clinical failures when causing meningitis or otitis media. Internationally, multidrug-resistant tuberculosis and multidrug-resistant salmonellae, including *Salmonella typhi*, are of major concern.

Resistance is not confined to bacteria. Fungal resistance is increasing (e.g. *Candida albicans* and *C. krusei* to fluconazole). Resistance of the HIV to the nucleoside, non-nucleoside, and protease inhibitors is rapidly emerging with many treatment-naive patients acquiring virus resistant to one or more agents. Failure of chemotherapy is now a major factor responsible for progression of HIV disease.

Pharmacology

Mode of action

Knowledge of the pharmacological mode of action of an antimicrobial agents permits an understanding of the diverse mechanisms of microbial inhibition and the opportunities for drug resistance. This is best established for antibacterial and antiviral agents. In the case of antifungal and especially antiparasitic agents the modes of action are less well defined. This reflects the process of drug discovery whereby an understanding of the biochemical and molecular action of agents derived from natural or chemical sources has not always been a priority in establishing efficacy and safety, especially with regard to older agents.

Antibacterial drugs

Antibacterial agents may affect cell wall or protein synthesis, nucleic acid formation, or may act on critical metabolic pathways (Table 7.2.5.2).

The β-lactams (penicillins, cephalosporins, carbapenems, and monobactams (aztreonam)) and the glycopeptides (vancomycin and teicoplanin), inhibit cell wall synthesis. The β-lactams, which share the common β-lactam ring, act on cell wall transpeptidases to inhibit cross-linking of peptidoglycan. The glycopeptide antibiotics act at an earlier stage of cell wall synthesis by binding to acyl-D-alanyl-D-alanine. Despite their similar mode of action, the glycopeptides are less efficient bactericides than the β-lactams.

Table 7.2.5.2 Microbial site of action and targets for selected antibacterial drugs

Site of action	Drugs	Target
Cell wall peptidoglycan	Penicillins	Transpeptidase
	Cephalosporins	Transpeptidase
	Vancomycin	Acyl-D-alanyl-D-alanine
	Teicoplanin	Acyl-D-alanyl-D-alanine
	Daptomycin	Binds to bacterial membranes
Ribosome	Chloramphenicol	Peptidyl transferase of 50S subunit
	Clindamycin	50S ribosomal subunit transpeptidation
	Linezolid	Blocks initiation phase
	Macrolides	50S ribosomal subunit
	Tetracyclines	Ribosomal A site
	Aminoglycosides	Initiation complex and translation
	Fusidic acid	Elongation factor G
Nucleic acid	Quinolones	DNA gyrase
	Metronidazole	DNA strands
	Rifampicin	RNA polymerase
Folic acid synthesis	Sulphonamides	Pteroic acid synthetase
	Trimethoprim	Dihydrofolate reductase

Inhibitors of protein synthesis

Antibacterial agents that inhibit protein synthesis act on the 30S ribosomal subunit responsible for binding mRNA, or the 50S subunit which binds aminoacyl tRNA. The aminoglycosides, tetracyclines, and macrolide antibiotics are the most widely used inhibitors of protein synthesis. Chloramphenicol, clindamycin, and the recently introduced agent linezolid also act at this site.

Inhibitors of nucleic acid

Nucleic acid synthesis is targeted by quinolones, metronidazole, and rifampicin. The bacterial DNA gyrase is essential for the supercoiling of bacterial DNA. This, together with the enzyme topoisomerase IV, are the major targets for the quinolones. These enzymes are absent in humans, explaining the selective activity of these drugs. Rifampicin and other rifamycins interfere with DNA-dependent RNA polymerase, preventing chain initiation.

Metabolic inhibitors

The best known metabolic inhibitors are the sulphonamides and trimethoprim which interfere with folic acid synthesis by sequentially inhibiting the enzymes dihydropteroic acid synthetase (EC 2.5.1.15) and dihydrofolate reductase (EC 1.5.1.3). By acting sequentially, a combined bactericidal effect results. The selective activity of these compounds is dependent on the fact that humans are unable to synthesize folic acid and require preformed folic acid in their diet.

Table 7.2.5.3 Mode of action of selected antiviral drugs

Drug	Target virus	Antiviral activity
Aciclovir	HSV	Nucleoside analogue
Cidofovir	CMV	Nucleoside analogue
Famciclovir	HSV and VZV	Nucleoside analogue
Foscarnet	CMV	Inhibits DNA polymerase
Ganciclovir	CMV	Nucleoside analogue
Oseltamivir	Influenza A and B	Inhibits viral neuraminidase
Zanamivir	Influenza A and B	Inhibits viral neuraminidase
Amantadine	Influenza A	Uncoating and assembly
Rimantadine	Influenza A	Uncoating and assembly
Abacavir	HIV	Nucleoside reverse transcriptase inhibitor
Didanosine	HIV	Nucleoside reverse transcriptase inhibitor
Emtricitabine	HIV	Nucleoside reverse transcriptase inhibitor
Lamivudine	HIV	Nucleoside reverse transcriptase inhibitor
Stavudine	HIV	Nucleoside reverse transcriptase inhibitor
Tenofovir	HIV	Nucleoside reverse transcriptase inhibitor
Zidovudine	HIV	Nucleoside reverse transcriptase inhibitor
Delavirdine	HIV	Non-nucleoside reverse transcriptase inhibitor
Efavirenz	HIV	Non-nucleoside reverse transcriptase inhibitor
Etravine	HIV	Non-nucleoside reverse transcriptase inhibitor
Nevirapine	HIV	Non-nucleoside reverse transcriptase inhibitor
Atazanavir	HIV	Protease inhibitor
Indinavir	HIV	Protease inhibitor
Darunavir	HIV	Protease inhibitor
Fosamprenavir	HIV	Protease inhibitor
Nelfinavir	HIV	Protease inhibitor
Ritonavir	HIV	Protease inhibitor
Saquinavir	HIV	Protease inhibitor
Tipranavir	HIV	Protease inhibitor

CMV, cytomegalovirus; HSV, herpes simplex virus, VZV, varicella zoster virus

Antiviral agents

Viruses live and replicate within the host cell. Antiviral chemotherapy therefore presents a particular challenge if it is to be selectively toxic. The cycle of viral replication provides several opportunities for therapeutic intervention. Most available antiviral agents are nucleoside analogues, largely used in the treatment of HIV or herpesvirus infections (Table 7.2.5.3). The recent growth in numbers of antiviral agents has benefited greatly from HIV-related research through the identification of new drug targets (Fig. 7.2.5.1). Interference with cell surface attachment through ligand blockade of surface receptors provides a theoretical, but so far unfulfilled, target. Penetration into the host cell may be through a process of translocation or direct fusion between the outer lipid membrane of the virus and the cell membrane, before uncoating and release of viral nucleic acid. Replication differs among viruses, thereby providing several therapeutic options. Viral mRNA becomes translated into multiple copies of viral proteins encoded by the viral genome either as a result of virus-specific enzymes or by co-opting host-derived protein. For example, HIV employs its own reverse transcriptase to convert RNA to DNA before integration into the host cell chromosome. Transcription and translation follow. Before the virus can be released, new viral particles must be assembled for which host cell proteins and mechanisms of phosphorylation and glycosylation may be recruited. The protease inhibitors act at this stage and have been particularly successful. Virus release is the result of either transportation and budding or host cell lysis.

Antifungal agents

The polyene antifungals (amphotericin B and nystatin) act on ergosterol within the fungal cell membrane. Ergosterol is largely absent from bacteria and humans, explaining the selective toxicity of these agents. The azole antifungals include the imidazoles (e.g. clotrimazole, miconazole, and ketoconazole) and the triazoles (fluconazole, itraconazole, and voriconazole) which bind preferentially to fungal cytochrome P450 to inhibit 14-α-methylsterol demethylation to ergosterol. Caspofungin is a recently licensed agent which acts on fungal cell wall β(1-3)D-glycan to inhibit growth.

Antiparasitic agents

The mechanism of action of many antiparasitic drugs is only partially known. Among the antimalarials, chloroquine interferes with the digestion of haemoglobin taken up by plasmodia. Quinine is thought to act in a similar manner. Metronidazole is active against several protozoa such as *Entamoeba histolytica* as well as anaerobic bacteria. It acts as an electron sink, by reduction of its 5-nitro group activated by nitroreductase within the target pathogen, thus interrupting DNA synthesis.

Among the anthelmintic drugs, piperazine and praziquantel act by selectively inducing muscle paralysis in the target helminth. Others, such as thiabendazole, inhibit parasitic ATP synthesis and energy production.

Antimicrobial spectrum of activity

The antimicrobial spectrum of an agent is dependent on target site susceptibility among pathogenic organisms at clinically achievable drug concentrations. Some microorganisms are intrinsically resistant to certain antibiotics. For example, the aminoglycosides are inactive against anaerobic bacteria because cell entry is an energy-dependent process relying on respiratory quinones, which are absent in anaerobic bacteria. Certain strains of *Pseudomonas aeruginosa* are resistant to the aminoglycosides as a result of altered protein porin channels, which inhibit antibiotic penetration.

The antimicrobial spectrum of a drug in part dictates its clinical indications. While information on this spectrum is more easily determined *in vitro*, *in vivo* efficacy can only be confirmed through clinical use, which can be supported by animal model data during drug development. For example, *in vitro Salmonella typhi* is susceptible to gentamicin, but the drug is not effective clinically.

Narrow-spectrum and broad-spectrum agents

There are few truly narrow-spectrum agents. Fusidic acid, mupirocin, the glycopeptides (vancomycin and teicoplanin), and linezolid target specific pathogens and are mainly used to treat microbiologically confirmed infections.

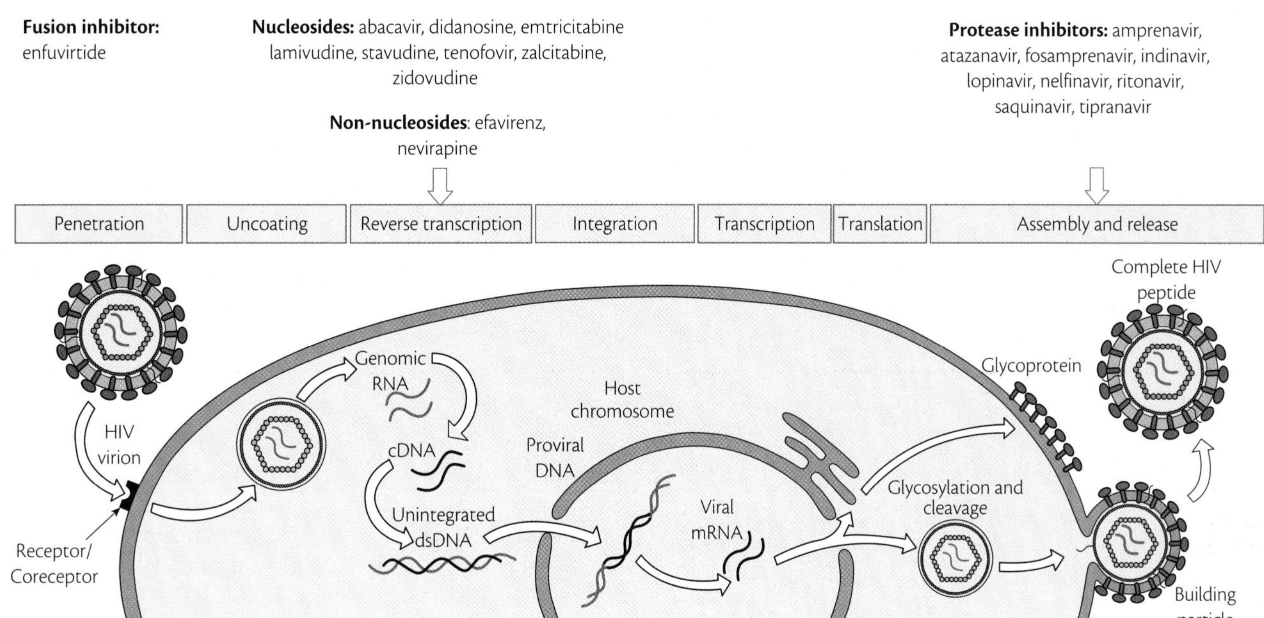

Fig. 7.2.5.1 Sites of inhibition of HIV replication by current antiretroviral drugs.

Broad-spectrum agents, such as the quinolone antibiotics and the parenteral cephalosporins such as cefotaxime and ceftriaxone, are active against many Gram-positive and Gram-negative pathogens. Metronidazole has activity against a large number of anaerobic bacteria and, because of this restricted activity, is considered to have a narrow spectrum. The aminoglycosides, although active against staphylococci and aerobic Gram-negative bacilli are inactive against streptococci and anaerobes and are, therefore, frequently prescribed in combination. The carbapenems (imipenem, meropenem, and ertapenem) possess the broadest spectrum of activity which includes most aerobic and anaerobic bacterial pathogens. Broad-spectrum agents are often used empirically in the initial management of severe infection. However, they frequently affect the normal flora so that superinfection with *Clostridium difficile* and yeasts are more likely to arise.

Susceptibility testing

Antibiotic susceptibility testing of clinical isolates is important for appropriate prescribing and for gathering epidemiological data. It is determined *in vitro* by using either broth-based or agar-based methods. Pathogens are exposed to known concentrations of an antibiotic and their degree of inhibition compared to a standard control. Disc susceptibility testing is the most widely used method. Zones of inhibition around the antibiotic-containing disc are measured, compared to a standard, and the pathogen designated sensitive, resistant, or of intermediate susceptibility to the drug. Currently, such methods require the isolate to be tested in pure culture. It is, therefore, difficult to obtain information on the susceptibility of a pathogen in less than 36 to 48 h from sample collection.

The minimum inhibitory concentration (MIC) in milligrams per litre provides more precise *in vitro* information on the activity of a drug against a bacterial pathogen. It is more time consuming and costly to determine, although automated systems and commercial strip tests are available (Fig. 7.2.5.2). Defining susceptibility by MIC determination permits greater predictive benefit in the treatment of certain infections such as gonorrhoea, bacterial endocarditis, and pneumococcal meningitis. Knowledge of the *in vitro* susceptibility of common pathogens to antimicrobial agents (Fig. 7.2.5.3) is helpful in selecting drug therapy but is only relevant to the achievable drug concentrations, which is important in predicting performance as discussed below.

Combined drug therapy

In hospital practice, it is common to combine agents when dealing with mixed infections or where initial broad-spectrum empirical therapy is required. Another important reason for combining drugs is to prevent the emergence of antibiotic resistance, such as in the treatment of tuberculosis and HIV infections. Antituberculosis regimens have been developed to ensure that naturally occurring minority populations of *Mycobacterium tuberculosis* resistant to isoniazid or rifampicin do not emerge during therapy. By combining isoniazid and rifampicin with pyrazinamide and ethambutol

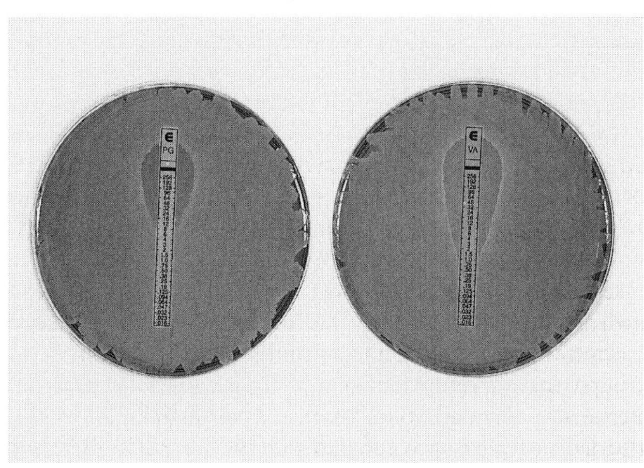

Fig. 7.2.5.2 *Staph. aureus* resistant to penicillin (MIC 8 mg/litre) on the left and sensitive to vancomycin (MIC 1.0 mg/litre) on the right, as demonstrated by a commercial strip test.

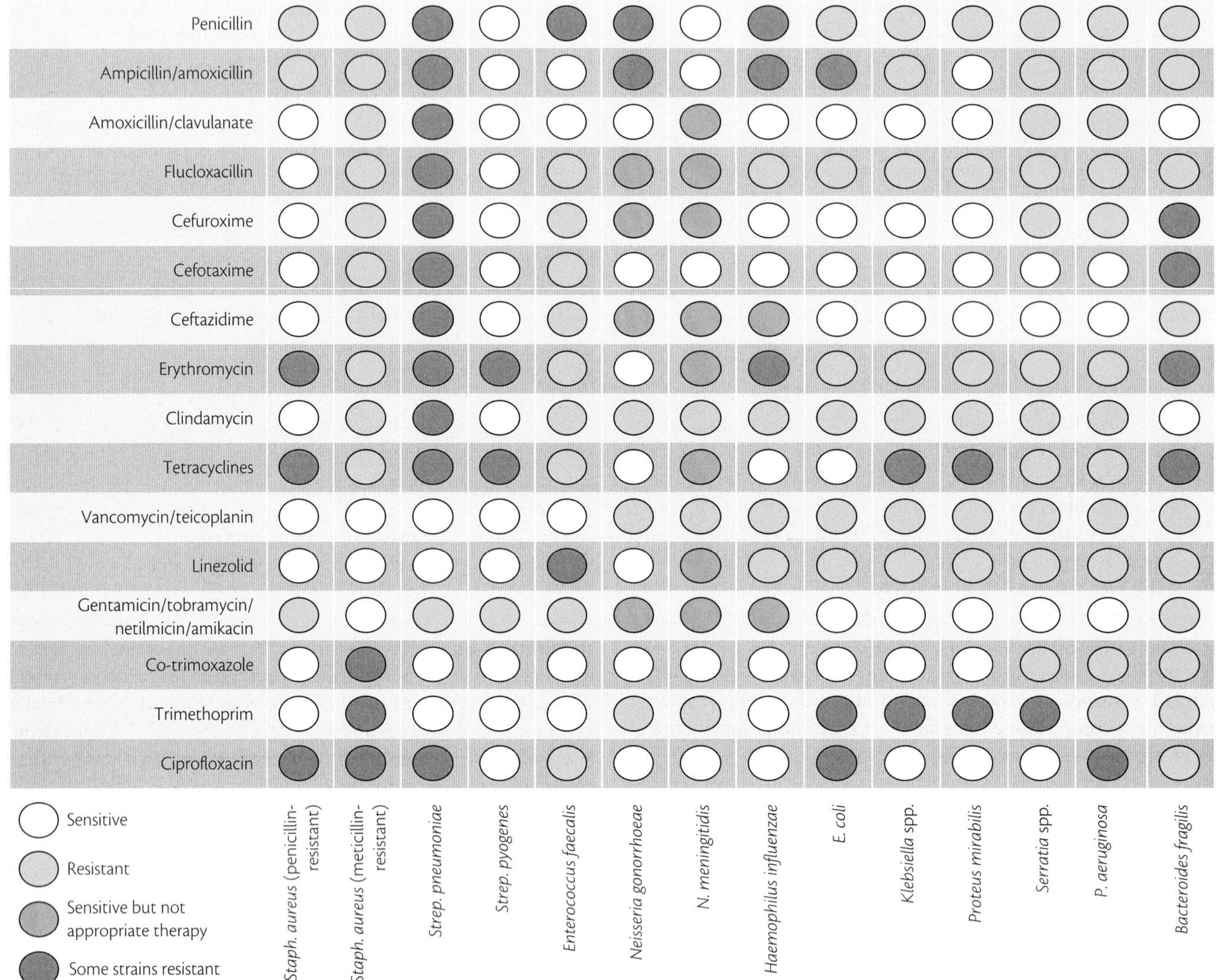

Fig. 7.2.5.3 Sensitivity of selected pathogenic bacteria to some common antibacterial agents.

for the initial phase of therapy (2 months), resistance is usually avoided. Therapy can be restricted to isoniazid and rifampicin for the continuation phase (4 months). The regimen is extended in those patients unable to tolerate pyrazinamide and in the treatment of tuberculous meningitis (Box 7.2.5.1).

HIV infection is treated with multidrug regimens. The success of highly active antiretroviral therapy, in which nucleoside analogues and protease inhibitors are combined in a three-drug regimen, is not only based on greater efficacy of the combined regimen but also on its ability to slow the emergence of drug-resistant mutants. The non-nucleoside reverse transcriptase inhibitors, such as efavirenz, appear to be equally effective in combination with nucleoside analogues and can delay the need for using protease inhibitors. This may increase the period of time in which an individual is responsive to antiretroviral therapy. The options for treating HIV infection are summarized in Box 7.2.5.2 (see also Chapter 7.5.23).

Occasionally, drugs are combined for the purpose of achieving a synergistic effect based on evidence that the *in vitro* activity of the combination is shown to be greater than the sum of the activity of the individual agents. Most drugs in combination will simply be

Box 7.2.5.1 Tuberculosis treatment regimens for pulmonary and nonpulmonary[a] tuberculous infection caused by *Mycobacterium tuberculosis*

Initial phase (2 months)

- Isoniazid
- Rifampicin
- Pyrazinamide[b]
- Ethambutol

Continuation phase (4 months)

- Isoniazid
- Rifampicin

[a] Central nervous system and tuberculous meningitis should be treated for 10 months after the initial phase of four drugs.

[b] If pyrazinamide is contraindicated or not given, the continuation phase is extended to 7 months.

Box 7.2.5.2 HIV infection: treatment regimens for drug-naive patients[a]

- Two nucleoside reverse transcriptase inhibitors + boosted protease inhibitor[b]
- Two nucleoside reverse transcriptase inhibitors + non-nucleoside reverse transcriptase inhibitor
- Three nucleoside reverse transcriptase inhibitors

[a] See Table 7.2.5.3 for agents available.

[b] Ritonavir + another agent.

additive in effect. One of the more frequently prescribed synergistic combinations is that of penicillin (or ampicillin) and streptomycin (or gentamicin) in the treatment of endocarditis caused by *Enterococcus* spp. The aminoglycoside alone is generally inactive against enterococci but in combination with ampicillin achieves synergistic killing (Fig. 7.2.5.4). A similar effect is employed in the treatment of viridans streptococcal endocarditis with this combination.

Another widely used example of synergistic inhibition is the combined effects of an antipseudomonal β-lactam, such as ceftazidime or piperacillin, and an aminoglycoside, such as gentamicin, tobramycin, or amikacin. This combination is used to treat documented or suspected *P. aeruginosa* infections occurring in neutropenic states complicating bone marrow transplantation, cytotoxic chemotherapy, and burn wound infections.

Antibiotic resistance

General considerations

Antibiotic resistance has been recognized since the introduction of effective antibiotics. For example, penicillin-resistant strains of *Staph. aureus* became widespread shortly after the introduction of this agent; penicillin-sensitive strains are now uncommon. Resistant strains of Gram-negative bacteria, such as *Klebsiella*, *Enterobacter*, *Acinetobacter*, and *Pseudomonas* spp. are commonly found in high-dependency units where they may cause epidemics. The international emergence of epidemic MRSA infections, primarily within hospitals and nursing homes, is very worrying. Conventional approaches to controlling these infections have been largely unsuccessful. The emergence of MRSA together with multiple-antibiotic-resistant coagulase-negative staphylococci has rapidly increased the use of vancomycin. Vancomycin-resistant enterococci have emerged in specialist hospital facilities such as dialysis and haematology units; therapeutic options are limited. Other problems include the emergence of penicillin-resistant pneumococci and β-lactamase-producing *Haemophilus influenzae*.

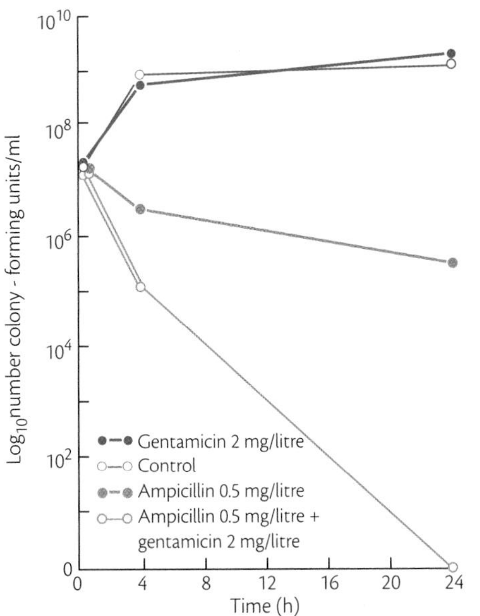

Fig. 7.2.5.4 Effects of ampicillin (0.5 mg/litre) and gentamicin (2 mg/litre) alone and in combination on a strain of *Enterococcus faecalis* from a patient with infective endocarditis. A synergistic effect is observed with the combined agents.

At present, there is great international concern among professionals, politicians, and, increasingly, the public about antibiotic resistance. In the United Kingdom, the House of Lords published an influential document in 1998 reviewing the issues surrounding this problem. This led to several initiatives including: (1) reducing the use of antibiotics, particularly in the treatment of minor upper respiratory tract infections in the community, (2) education strategies for prescribers and the public, and (3) better enforcement of infection control policies. Within the European Union, similar measures have been proposed together with a ban on the use of antibiotics as growth promoters in livestock animals. However, antibiotic resistance is a global problem. An increasing number of multidrug-resistant infections caused by *Salmonella* spp. and *Mycobacterium tuberculosis* are being imported from developing countries where the availability or prescribing of antibiotics is less controlled.

Antibiotic resistance drives changes in patterns of prescribing and is a major impetus to the pharmaceutical industry in its search for new therapies. Microorganisms differ in their ability to develop resistance, which may affect a particular drug, a class, or multiple classes of antibiotics. Genetic mutations select for antibiotic resistance, which frequently occurs under the influence of antibiotic pressure. The major mechanisms of resistance are summarized in Table 7.2.5.4. Resistance to single or multiple antibiotics may be either chromosomally or plasmid mediated, or both. In turn, genes may code for resistance to a single or multiple antibiotics. In addition to plasmid-mediated resistance, other transposable genetic elements (transposons) and insertion sequences (integrons) incapable of self-replication may exist within a chromosome, plasmid, or bacteriophage.

Resistance genes are most frequently transferred between organisms by conjugation. This occurs between the same or different species of bacteria and also between different genera. Other mechanisms of transferring resistance include transduction via a bacteriophage and, less commonly, transformation in which naked DNA released during cell lysis is taken up by other bacteria.

Transposon-mediated resistance reflects transfer of discreet sequences of DNA between chromosomes or plasmids whereby individual or groups of genes can be inserted into the host bacterial cell. Integrons may contain one or more gene cassettes which carry determinants of combinations of resistance genes within the bacterial chromosome, plasmid, or transposons. The antibiotic resistance genes are bound on each side by conserved segments of DNA. These individual resistance genes can be inserted or removed between the conserved structures and act as expression vectors for antibiotic resistance genes.

Table 7.2.5.4 Examples of resistance mechanisms for selected antibiotics

Enzymatic/inactivation	Altered target site	Altered permeability	Efflux	Metabolic bypass
Aminoglycosides	Erythromycin	β-Lactams	Tetracycline	Sulphonamides
β-Lactams	Chloramphenicol	Quinolones	Quinolones	Trimethoprim
Chloramphenicol	Fusidic acid		β-Lactams	
	Streptomycin			

While the molecular mechanisms of antibiotic resistance are legion, the ability of drug-resistant microorganisms to survive, disseminate, and cause disease varies widely. In many instances, antibiotic resistance may give a survival advantage only in the presence of continued antibiotic exposure to such agents. This is reflected in the occurrence of epidemic infections in high-dependency units such as intensive care facilities where antibiotic usage is often high. However, it is also clear that once the genetic mechanism for evading antimicrobial activity has been acquired, it is rarely lost and adds to the continuously expanding genetic memory that has steadily eroded the efficacy of many antimicrobial drugs.

Enzymatic inactivation

Aminoglycoside-modifying enzymes include adenylating, acetylating, and phosphorylating enzymes. Gentamicin is the most susceptible and amikacin the least susceptible to such inactivation. However, the largest group of inactivating enzymes are the β-lactamases (E.C. 3.5.2.6) which hydrolyse the β-lactam ring common to all penicillins and cephalosporins. Penicillinase was the first β-lactamase to be identified and is the reason why most strains of *Staph. aureus* are resistant to this drug. Another important β-lactamase is TEM-1, which is responsible for resistance to ampicillin by *Haemophilus influenzae*. The major impetus to the development of the broad-spectrum penicillins and cephalosporins was to extend their activity by resisting inactivation by β-lactamases present in many aerobic Gram-negative bacilli. However, new inactivating enzymes continue to emerge, including the extended-spectrum β-lactamases, which are now limiting the clinical utility of third-generation cephalosporins. A further example is the carbapenemase group of β-lactamases which hydrolyse imipenem, meropenem, and ertapenem.

Impermeability resistance

Drug uptake of antibiotics such as the penicillins, tetracyclines, and quinolone antibiotics by bacteria is through protein channels (porins) which cross the outer membrane. Alterations in the permeability of the outer membrane of Gram-negative bacteria is an increasingly important mechanism of drug resistance. Mutations in porin structure are responsible for resistance among pathogens such as *P. aeruginosa* and *Serratia marcescens.*

Alterations in target site

Another important mechanism of resistance is mutational modification of drug binding sites. This affects susceptibility to β-lactams, erythromycin, chloramphenicol, and rifampicin. Erythromycin and chloramphenicol bind to the bacterial 50S ribosomal subunit which is subject to genetic mutation. In contrast, the quinolones target DNA gyrase which is subject to subunit structure alteration resulting in one variety of resistance to drugs such as ciprofloxacin. The increasing resistance to penicillin among *Strep. pneumoniae* is the result of reduced binding of penicillin to several binding proteins (PBP2a and PBP2x). *Staph. aureus* resistance to meticillin is due to the presence of penicillin binding protein (PBP2a) which has reduced affinity for meticillin and other β-lactams and is encoded by the *mecA* gene.

The problem of vancomycin-resistant enterococci, which largely affects *Enterococcus faecium*, is the result of the production of enzymes (ligases) which permit continued cell wall synthesis despite the presence of vancomycin. To date, five different genes have been found responsible for this phenomenon (*vanA* to *vanE*) which result in different phenotypic patterns of resistance to the glycopeptides vancomycin and teicoplanin.

Metabolic bypass resistance

Bacteria must synthesize folic acid from the precursor *p*-aminobenzoic acid. The sulphonamide antibiotics competitively inhibit the enzyme dihydropteroate synthetase. Trimethoprim acts on the same metabolic pathway by inhibiting dihydrofolate reductase. The sequential inhibitory effects of trimethoprim and sulfamethoxazole (co-trimoxazole) result in synergistic bactericidal activity against many pathogens. Resistant organisms are able to synthesize their own enzymes thereby evading such competitive inhibition.

Surveillance of antibiotic resistance

Information on the susceptibility of pathogenic microorganisms is important. Such data can provide information on the relative frequency of pathogens and the pattern of susceptibility to prescribed agents. Surveillance, therefore, has a role in guiding prescribing, in developing prescribing policies, and in identifying and monitoring organisms that are subject to infection control measures. On a broader front, surveillance is also of value in alerting industry and health care planners to the need for new drug and vaccine strategies for disease control.

To be of maximum benefit, surveillance needs to be sensitive to a defined geographical base, which may simply reflect the catchment area of specimens submitted to a particular laboratory, providing information on the trends in community and hospital isolates. Within hospitals, more specific information can be provided about susceptibility patterns in high-dependency units, where antibiotic consumption is often greater, and more resistant pathogens such as *Klebsiella*, *Serratia*, *Enterobacter*, and *Acinetobacter* spp. and *P. aeruginosa* are found. Among Gram-positive pathogens, enterococci and, especially, *Staph. aureus* present an increasing challenge to prescribing and infection control practice.

National networks of surveillance often vary in their focus and include data on Gram-negative pathogens such as *Escherichia coli* and *P. aeruginosa*, *Staph. aureus*, penicillin resistance among pneumococci, and, more recently, vancomycin-resistant enterococci. There are important international networks which collect information on such pathogens as *Legionella pneumophila* and *Mycobacterium tuberculosis*. Drug-resistant tuberculosis is increasingly prevalent in the United Kingdom and elsewhere.

Surveillance of resistance to antiviral agents is largely confined to HIV in a few countries. Patient-specific data are increasingly sought in those with HIV infection to assess drug failure, guide change in management, and direct primary therapy in selected cases of person-to-person and mother-to-infant transmission. Determination of phenotypic resistance is still costly and time consuming, and most data relate to genotypic patterns of resistance to antiretroviral drugs among HIV isolates.

Pharmacokinetics

To be effective, antimicrobial agents must achieve therapeutic concentrations at the site of the target infection. This may be localized to a single anatomical site, such as the bladder or the cerebrospinal fluid, or involve major organs, such as the lung. Infections may also be generalized and affect many body sites. Drug selection must also take into consideration the fact that pathogens such as *Mycobacterium tuberculosis*, *Legionella pneumophila*, and *Salmonella typhi* replicate intracellularly. Antimicrobial drugs may be administered parenterally, orally, or topically to the skin, oral and genital mucosae, external auditory meatus, conjunctiva, and by intraocular application. In the case of systemically active agents, the effective drug concentrations are determined by the standard pharmacokinetic parameters of absorption, distribution, metabolism, and elimination. Since selective toxicity is crucial to safe prescribing, the dose regimen for each agent aims to avoid concentrations toxic to the host but inhibitory to the microorganism. This 'therapeutic window' varies by drug.

Table 7.2.5.5 Bioavailability and intestinal elimination of some commonly prescribed antibacterial drugs after oral administration

Drug	Bioavailability (%)	Intestinal elimination
Penicillins		
Amoxicillin	80–90	Concentrated up to 10-fold in bile
Ampicillin	50	Concentrated up to 10-fold in bile
Flucloxacillin	80–90	Negligible
Cephalosporins		
Cefalexin	80–100	Concentrated up to 3-fold in bile
Cefixime	40–50	Concentrated up to 50-fold in bile
Cefuroxime axetil	30–40	Bile concentrations of up to 80% of serum
Quinolones		
Ciprofloxacin	70–85	Concentrated up to 10-fold in bile
Nalidixic acid	90–100	Biliary concentrations similar to serum
Other antibacterials		
Erythromycin	18–45	Concentrated up to 300-fold in bile
Metronidazole	80–95	Concentrations in bile similar to serum
Rifampicin	90–100	Concentrated up to 1000-fold in bile
Sulfamethoxazole	70–90	Concentrations in bile 40–70% of serum
Tetracycline	75	Concentrated up to 10-fold in bile
Trimethoprim	80–90	Concentrated up to 2-fold in bile

Note that drugs which are well absorbed may still achieve high concentrations in the faeces because of secretion into bile or other enteral secretions.

Bioavailability

The rate and degree of absorption from the gastrointestinal tract is not only important for plasma concentrations reflected in the pharmacokinetic parameters of C_{max} and T_{max} of a drug, but also for potential adverse effects on the bowel (Table 7.2.5.5). For example, ampicillin, the first of the aminopenicillins, commonly caused gastrointestinal side effects, most notably diarrhoea. These effects have been reduced by increasing the bioavailability of the active drug through the introduction of hydroxyampicillin (amoxicillin) and various esters and prodrugs of ampicillin.

Some agents such as cefalexin, doxycycline, and several quinolone antibiotics are extremely well absorbed, achieving 80 to 100% bioavailability. In the case of some recent quinolones, the excellent bioavailability has raised the possibility of treating with oral antibiotics some severely ill patients who might normally require parenteral therapy. In contrast, drugs which are poorly bioavailable, such as cefixime and cefuroxime axetil, not only have a higher incidence of gastrointestinal side effects but also are more likely (although not uniquely) to select for *C. difficile*-associated large bowel disease.

Distribution

Most drugs are distributed in the blood via the plasma before gaining access to the extracellular fluid. Tissue concentrations of a particular agent are affected by pH, drug ionizability, lipid solubility, and the presence of an inflammatory reaction whereby the capillary fenestrations are increased in size. In the case of agents administered intravenously by infusion or by bolus injection, the distribution phase is rapid in comparison with orally, rectally, or intramuscularly administered drugs. Drugs which are poorly lipophilic, such as the β-lactams and aminoglycosides, achieve low concentrations in tissues such as the brain. However, the β-lactams achieve therapeutic concentrations in the cerebrospinal fluid as a result of the inflammatory reaction which accompanies meningitis.

Drugs may also be taken up intracellularly, as in the case of macrolides and quinolones, resulting in a large volume of distribution compared to drugs confined to the extracellular space, such as the β-lactams and aminoglycosides. This is important in relation to the treatment of intracellular pathogens such as *Mycoplasma pneumoniae*, *Legionella pneumophila*, and *Mycobacterium tuberculosis* which can only be effectively treated by drugs that are concentrated and remain biologically active within the cell.

The plasma half-life ($T_{½}$), which is the time required for the concentration of a drug in the plasma to fall by one-half, is affected by drug distribution and, in particular, its rate of elimination as a result of metabolism and excretion. This in turn affects the time taken to reach steady state. In the treatment of life-threatening infections, it is important that steady state kinetics are achieved

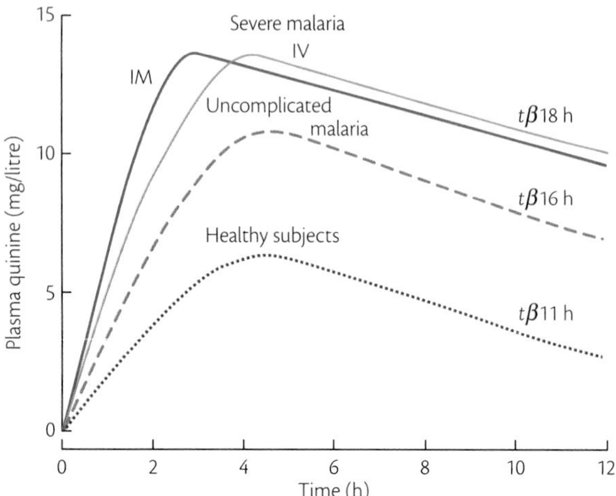

Fig. 7.2.5.5 Average plasma quinine concentrations following administration of a loading dose of 20 mg (salt)/kg to patients with severe and uncomplicated malaria, compared with those predicted to occur in normal subjects.
(From White NJ (1992). Antimalarial pharmacokinetics and treatment regimens. *Br J Clin Pharmacol*, **34**, 1–10, with permission.)

rapidly and the administration of a loading dose may be required. This applies to the use of agents such as intravenous quinine in the case of life-threatening malaria and gentamicin for the treatment of serious Gram-negative infections where the pharmacokinetic behaviour can be altered by the severity of the disease in comparison with healthy subjects (Fig. 7.2.5.5).

Drugs are commonly distributed in the blood and tissues bound to plasma proteins, mostly albumin, and they vary in their degree of protein binding. With agents such as flucloxacillin and ceftazidime it exceeds 95%. The importance of protein binding lies in the fact that the active moiety is the unbound drug. Dissociation from the bound to the unbound state is usually rapid, but this equilibrium may affect drug performance at certain sites such as the joints. The relationship between protein binding and drug performance has been emphasized from studies of the pharmacodynamics of drug activity (see below).

Metabolism

Antibiotics, like other drugs, are degraded at various sites in the body but predominantly within the liver. Degradation involves conjugation, hydrolysis, oxidation, glucuronidation, or dealkylation, according to the particular drug. Members of the hepatic cytochrome P450 group of enzymes play a dominant role in this process. Drug metabolites are usually but not always biologically inactive. For example, cefotaxime is degraded to desacetylcefotaxime and clarithromycin to hydroxyclarithromycin, both of which are biologically active and contribute to the overall antibacterial activity of these agents.

Excretion

Most drugs are excreted in the urine by glomerular filtration, tubular secretion, or a combination of these mechanisms. Thus high concentrations of drug will often be present in the urine; this has therapeutic importance in the treatment of urinary tract infections. Urinary pH affects the biological activity of many drugs; e.g. the activity of ciprofloxacin is markedly reduced at pH 5.5. Tubular excretion can be blocked by probenecid. This was formerly used to ensure higher plasma concentrations of penicillin and is still recommended in alternative treatment regimens for gonorrhoea when single doses of amoxicillin are prescribed. It is also important to note that any reduction in glomerular filtration rate will affect not only urinary concentrations of drug but also the plasma half-life and, in turn, serum concentrations of drugs which are primarily excreted by this route. In the case of antibiotics such as the aminoglycosides and vancomycin, the dose must be reduced in renal failure.

Biliary excretion is another important route for drug elimination either as the active compound or as a microbiologically active or inactive metabolite. Reabsorption from the gastrointestinal tract can result in enterohepatic recirculation, which in turn may affect plasma half-life. Drugs which achieve high concentrations in the bile are effective in the treatment of infections at this site such as cholecystitis. However, biliary obstruction or hepatic impairment may reduce therapeutic efficacy and require dose reduction to avoid toxic effects. Examples include clindamycin, efavirenz, mefloquine, and tetracyclines.

Therapeutic drug monitoring of some antibiotics is essential in order to ensure therapeutic yet nontoxic concentrations. This applies particularly to aminoglycosides which have a relatively narrow therapeutic index. Trough concentrations of gentamicin in excess of 2 mg/litre, if sustained, can result in nephrotoxicity and ototoxicity. The target cells for such toxicities are the renal tubular lining cells and the cochlear hair cells of the inner ear, respectively. Vancomycin is also frequently monitored, particularly in patients with impaired renal function.

Pharmacodynamics

The inter-relationship between drug, microorganism, and the infected host creates an important pharmacological dynamic. Antibiotics are unique in therapeutics in that they are targeted at an invading microorganism which may be present at a particular site or be more widely distributed in the body. The host's response to infection may modify the pharmacokinetic handling of a drug. Many antibiotics have a measurable effect on a variety of bacterial and host cell functions, even at subinhibitory concentrations. It is difficult to establish the exact role that these factors play clinically, but they are likely to contribute to the overall effect of an antibiotic. Macrolides such as erythromycin illustrate this point since they affect a variety of virulence characteristics (Table 7.2.5.6) as well as affecting the host's response to infection.

Table 7.2.5.6 Effect of macrolides on bacterial virulence at subinhibitory concentrations

Factor	Effect	Factor	Effect
Adhesins (pili, fimbriae)	↓	Exoenzyme production:	
Fibronectin binding	↓	Elastase	↓
Alginate production	↓	Protease	↓
Exotoxin A production	↓	DNAse	↓
β-Haemolysin activity	↓	Coagulase	↓
Serum susceptibility	↑	Leukocidin	↓
Flagellar function	↓		

From Shyrock TR, Mortensen JE, Baumholtz M (1998). The effects of macrolides on the expression of bacterial virulence mechanisms. *J Antimicrob Chemother*, **41**, 505–12.

Table 7.2.5.7 Postantibiotic effects (h) of selected drugs against *Staph. aureus*, *E. coli*, and *P. aeruginosa*

Drug	*Staph. aureus*	*E. coli*	*P. aeruginosa*
Ampicillin	1.7	0.1	NT
Cefotaxime	1.4	0.2	0.3
Ciprofloxacin	2.0	2.1	2.4
Erythromycin	3.1	NT	NT
Gentamicin	2.0	1.8	2.2
Imipenem	2.6	0.5	1.5
Rifampicin	2.8	4.2	NT
Vancomycin	2.2	NT	NT

NT, not tested.

Exposure of microorganisms to sublethal concentrations of an antibiotic may temporarily inhibit growth which recommences following removal of the drug. The time to recovery is known as the postantibiotic effect. This varies with the drug and the microorganism; e.g. the quinolones have a longer postantibiotic effect than β-lactams (Table 7.2.5.7). The relevance of this observation to the *in vivo* situation, where plasma drug concentrations are often well above the inhibitory concentration and are sustained through repeat doses, remains uncertain. It may have greater relevance to tissue concentrations, which tend to be lower than plasma concentrations. The postantibiotic effect certainly contributes to the effects of agents that are administered once daily, such as gentamicin.

The relationship between the pharmacokinetic characteristics of a drug and bacterial inhibition is critical to therapeutic outcome (Table 7.2.5.8). In the case of agents such as penicillins and cephalosporins, the time that drug concentrations are maintained above the MIC predicts the response. This contrasts with agents such as the quinolones and aminoglycosides, where it is more important to achieve high C_{max} to MIC ratios. Modelling the MIC of a particular organism against the dose response curve for a drug (Fig. 7.2.5.6) has established several important pharmacodynamic parameters, which have been supported by studies in animal models and man. For example, dosage regimens of quinolones such as ciprofloxacin and levofloxacin have been based on pharmacodynamic data. The ratio of C_{max} to MIC has been refined in the parameter area under the inhibitory concentration, which is the ratio of the area under the time curve (AUC) to MIC. This is more predictive of outcome. The importance of protein binding for drug performance has also emerged as an important modifying factor in this modelling. The AUC to MIC ratio of the free drug is the most sensitive predictor of response. The manner in which these ratios differ for selected quinolones is shown in Table 7.2.5.9.

Principles of use

In comparison with many other classes of drugs, antimicrobial agents are usually prescribed in short courses ranging from a single dose to a few days. Prolonged therapy is required for certain infections such as tuberculosis and bone and joint sepsis, and for HIV infection treatment is usually lifelong.

Most antibiotic prescribing, especially within community practice, is empirical. Even among patients in hospital, where there are greater opportunities for diagnostic precision based on laboratory investigations, the exact nature of the infection is established in only a minority of cases. Most therapeutic prescribing requires a presumptive clinical diagnosis that, in turn, is linked to a presumptive microbiological diagnosis based on knowledge of the usual microbial causes of such infections. Among the most widely treated infections are those affecting the upper and lower respiratory tracts, the urinary tract, and skin and soft tissues for which the likely microbial aetiology is restricted. For example, urinary tract infections arising in the community are usually caused by *E. coli* and other Gram-negative enteric pathogens and, less commonly, by enterococci or *Staphylococcus saprophyticus*. Local knowledge of the susceptibility of these pathogens to commonly used agents such as trimethoprim, ampicillin, and a quinolone such as ciprofloxacin is helpful in recommending initial empirical antibiotic management.

In more severe infections, such as community-acquired pneumonia, prompt empirical therapy is essential. Although the range of possible pathogens is more extensive (Table 7.2.5.10), *Strep. pneumoniae* predominates and must always be targeted. Assessment of severity, based on validated criteria, assists in defining the initial empirical antibiotic regimen. This is illustrated by the

Table 7.2.5.8 Summary of major pharmacodynamic differences between aminoglycosides and β-lactams

Pharmacodynamic measurement	Aminoglycosides	β-Lactam
Rate of bacterial killing	Rapid and dose related	Slower with little or no increase at higher doses
Number of bacteria killed per dose administered	Concentration-dependent over a wide concentration range	Little increase in degree or rate of killing at concentrations above minimum bactericidal concentration (MBC)
Postantibiotic effect	Concentration-dependent over a wide concentration range for Gram-positive and Gram-negative pathogens	Unpredictable in Gram-negative bacteria, always short with little or no increase related to concentration
Experimental models	Large, infrequent doses more effective than smaller, more frequent doses which supports once-daily dosing for Gram-negative infections	Frequent (hourly) injection or constant infusion most effective
Clinical trials	High peak serum concentration to *in vitro* minimum inhibitory concentration (MIC) ratio is strongly related to treatment outcome for Gram-negative bacteraemia or pneumonia	Limited supportive data in patients with neutropenia or nosocomial pneumonia with dosing regimens that keep serum concentrations above the MIC throughout therapy
	Clinical trials with amikacin, gentamicin, and netilmicin have shown single daily dosing to be effective	

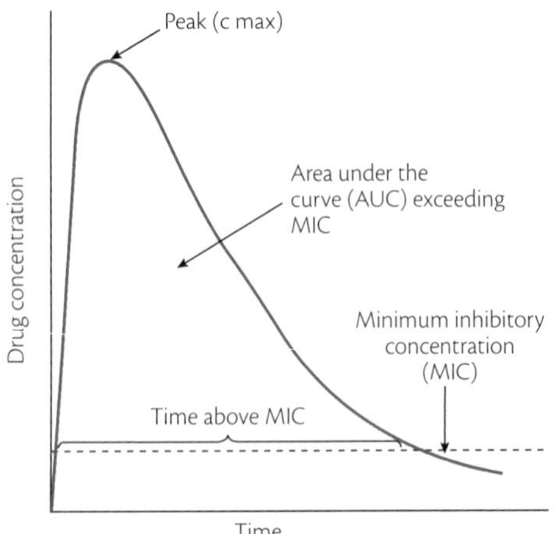

Fig. 7.2.5.6 Relationship between the minimum inhibitory concentration (MIC) of a drug and its pharmacokinetic profile.

British Thoracic Society's recommendations for the initial empirical antibiotic management of community-acquired pneumonia (Table 7.2.5.11).

The use of empirical therapy depends on the ease with which a clinical diagnosis can be made, as well as disease severity and drug toxicity. In the case of herpesvirus infections, the empirical use of aciclovir for the treatment of mucocutaneous herpes simplex infections or of shingles in older people is now common. However, it would be inappropriate to start treatment for HIV or cytomegalovirus infections without laboratory support for these diagnoses in view of the toxicity and cost of the antiviral agents used to treat these infections.

Antibiotic prophylaxis

Antibiotics are used widely in the prevention of infection, in association with surgery, and in a range of medical conditions (see above). Antibiotic prophylaxis is used for selected surgical procedures where the risk of infection, although relatively low, is of serious import should it occur. Examples include prosthetic joint implantation and cardiac surgery in which prosthetic valves and intracardiac patches are inserted. The principles of antibiotic prophylaxis are based on the selection of an agent active against the known potential target pathogen(s). The drug should be present in high concentrations at the site and time of surgery and be relatively free from adverse reactions. One or two doses are generally effective depending on the length of the procedure. No regimen can be effective against all potential pathogens, hence the importance of postoperative follow-up.

An important medical indication for the use of prophylactic antibiotics is the prevention of bacterial endocarditis in those with valve replacement, acquired valvular heart disease, structural congenital heart disease (including those structurally repaired or palliated) but excluding isolated atrial septal defect, surgically corrected ventricular septal defect and patent ductus arteriosus, hypertrophic cardiomyopathy or a previous episode of infective endocarditis, who are undergoing a gastrointestinal or genitor-urinary procedure at a site where infection is suspected, because of the risk of endocardial infection complicating an episode of transient bacteraemia. Here again, the principles governing the selection of the regimen are based on the recognition of the likely target pathogens, their pattern of susceptibility, and the necessity to ensure high bactericidal concentrations of drug at the time of the procedure. Another example of effective prophylaxis is the use of low-dose suppressive therapy to prevent *Pneumocystis jiroveci (carinii)* pneumonia in those with advanced HIV infection. Co-trimoxazole is the preferred agent; dapsone, atovaquone, or inhaled pentamidine are also used.

Anatomical or functional asplenia is associated with a 12.6-fold increased incidence of severe sepsis compared with the general population. This risk is related to the patient's age and, in those splenectomized, the reason for surgery and the period of time that has elapsed. Young children are particularly at risk, but this declines substantially after the age of 16 years. Hence the recommendation that immunization be supplemented with prophylactic oral penicillin (erythromycin for the intolerant) to prevent fulminant pneumococcal sepsis which predominates. Other recommended vaccines include *Haemophilus influenzae* type b and meningococcal group C conjugate. Apart from good evidence for the benefit of prophylaxis in children with sickle cell disease, there is poor support for efficacy in other populations of splenectomized patients. There remain, therefore, differences of opinion about the recommendation for the continued use of chemoprophylaxis in adults, although some recommend that a period of 2 years is appropriate. Issues of cost, compliance, and drug-resistant pathogens add further fuel to the debate. What is clear is that the patient or legal guardian(s) should be educated concerning this risk.

Dose selection

Few antibacterial drugs are specific to a single pathogen, hence the dosage regimen must capture a range of susceptibilities of the various target microorganisms to ensure a successful response. The dosage regimen is determined initially by pharmacokinetic studies in healthy volunteers. This is supplemented by information from standardized animal models that simulate infections such as peritonitis, endocarditis, meningitis, thigh abscess, otitis media, pneumonia, and sepsis complicating neutropenia. In man, information on drug penetration into the cerebrospinal fluid, bile, joint fluid,

Table 7.2.5.9 Pharmacokinetic and pharmacodynamic parameters of some recent quinolone antibacterial drugs

Drug (dose mg)	Protein binding (%)	MIC_{90} *Strep. pneumoniae*	AUC total (mg/h per litre)	AUC free (mg/h per litre)	AUIC (total drug)	AUIC (free drug)
Gatifloxacin (400)	20	0.5	51.3	41.0	102.6	82
Levofloxacin (500)	25	2.0	72.5	54.4	36.2	27.2
Moxifloxacin (400)	48	0.25	26.9	14.0	107.6	56.0

AUC, area under the concentration curve; AUIC, AUC to MIC ratio or area under the inhibitory concentration of total and free (unbound) drugs; MIC_{90}, minimum inhibitory concentration active against 90% of isolates tested.

Table 7.2.5.10 Microbiological aetiology (%) of adult community-acquired pneumonia in the United Kingdom

Pathogens	Community (n=236)	Hospital (n=1137)	ICU (n=185)
Strep. pneumoniae	36.0	39.0	21.6
Haemophilus influenzae	10.2	5.2	3.8
Legionella spp.	0.4	3.6	17.8
Staph. aureus	0.8	1.9	8.7
Moraxella catarrhalis	?	1.9	?
Enterobacteriaceae	1.3	1.0	1.6
Mycoplasma pneumoniae	1.3	10.8	2.7
Chlamydophila pneumoniae	?	13.1	?
Chlamydophila psittaci	1.3	2.6	2.2
Coxiella burnetii	0	1.2	0
Viruses	13.1	12.8	9.7
Influenza A and B	8.1	10.7	5.4
Mixed	11.0	14.2	6.0
Other	1.7	2.0	4.9
None	45.3	30.8	4.0

ICU, intensive care unit.
From Lim WS, *et al.* (2009). The British Thoracic Society guidelines for the management of community-acquired pneumonia in adults. *Thorax*, **64** Suppl III, 1–61.

and cutaneous blisters can be supplemented by data from biopsy specimens from sites such as tonsils, bronchus, and prostate. The role of pharmacodynamic assessment is of increasing importance in defining dose and predicting outcome as discussed earlier. Despite all this information, the definitive dosage regimen still requires support from large clinical trials in which the endpoints of response are precisely determined.

Bactericidal versus bacteriostatic agents

In the treatment of many common community infections which are usually of mild or moderate severity, the choice of either a bacteriostatic or a bactericidal antibiotic is of limited importance. However, in patients with severe infection, particularly when complicating an immunocompromised state, a bactericidal agent must be used. This applies particularly to those with severe granulocytopenia which is a common accompaniment of cytotoxic chemotherapy, especially in the treatment of haematological malignancies and following bone marrow transplantation. Another important indication for selecting a bactericidal regimen is in the treatment of infective endocarditis; although the infected vegetations are in the bloodstream, they are relatively protected from host phagocytic control. Effective penetration into the fibrin–platelet mass requires high concentrations of a bactericidal drug to sterilize the infected vegetations.

Duration of treatment

The duration of therapy for many common infections has not been rigorously determined. The treatment of many common conditions

Table 7.2.5.11 Preferred and alternative initial empirical treatment regimens for community-acquired pneumonia as recommended by the British Thoracic Society

Pneumonia severity (based on clinical judgement supported by CURB65 severity score)	Treatment site	Preferred treatment	Alternative treatment
Low severity (eg, CURB65 = 0–1 or CRB65 score = 0, < 3% mortality)	Home	Amoxicillin 500 mg tds orally	Doxycycline 200 mg loading dose then 100 mg orally *or* clarithromycin 500 mg bd orally
Low severity (eg, CURB65 = 0–1, < 3% mortality) but admission indicated for reasons other than pneumonia severity (eg, social reasons/unstable comorbid illness)	Hospital	Amoxicillin 500 mg tds orally If oral administration not possible: amoxicillin 500 mg tds IV	Doxycycline 200 mg loading dose then 100 mg od orally *or* clarithromycin 500 mg bd orally
Moderate severity (eg, CURB65 = 2, 9% mortality)	Hospital	Amoxicillin 500 mg–1.0 g tds orally *plus* clarithromycin 500 mg bd orally If oral administration not possible: amoxicillin 500 mg tds IV *or* benzylpenicillin 1.2 g qds IV *plus* clarithromycin 500 mg bd IV	Doxycycine 200 mg loading dose then 100 mg orally *or* levofloxacin 500 mg od orally *or* moxifloxacin 400 mg od orally*
High severity (eg, CURB65 = 3–5, 15–40% mortality)	Hospital (consider critical care review)	**Antibiotics given as soon as possible** Co-amoxiclav 1.2 g tds IV *plus* clarithromycin 500 mg bd IV (If legionella strongly suspected, consider adding levofloxacin†)	Benzylpenicillin 1.2 g qds IV *plus* either levofloxacin 500 mg bd IV *or* ciprofloxacin 400 mg bd IV **OR** Cefuroxime 1.5 g tds IV *or* cefotaxime 1 g tds IV *or* ceftriaxone 2 g od IV, *plus* clarithromycin 500 mg bd IV (If legionella strongly suspected, consider adding levofloxacin†)

bd, twice daily; IV, intravenous; od, once daily; qds, four times daily; tds, three times daily.
* Following reports of an increased risk of adverse hepatic reactions associated with oral moxifloxacin, in October 2008 the European Medicines Agency (EMEA) recommended that moxifloxacin "should be used only when it is considered inappropriate to use antibacterial agents that are commonly recommended for the initial treatment of this infection".
† Caution – risk of QT prolongation with macrolide-quinolone combination.
From Lim WS, *et al.* (2009). The British Thoracic Society guidelines for the management of community-acquired pneumonia in adults. *Thorax*, **64** Suppl III, 1–61.

is based on custom and practice and often varies internationally. The duration of treatment has been more thoroughly determined in the following cases:

- Gonococcal urethritis responds promptly to single-dose treatment with agents such as ceftriaxone, or a quinolone antibiotic such as ciprofloxacin or ofloxacin.
- Uncomplicated urinary tract infection, particularly when affecting women of child-bearing years, responds promptly to selected agents such as trimethoprim and norfloxacin. Although bacteriuria can be eliminated with a single dose, the symptoms of dysuria and frequency take longer to subside, hence a 3-day course is preferred.
- Pharyngitis caused by *Streptococcus pyogenes* improves symptomatically within a few days of antibiotics such as penicillin, but eradication of the infecting organism from the throat often takes up to 10 days. It is acknowledged that this presents major difficulties with regard to drug compliance.
- For pulmonary tuberculosis the current recommendation of an initial 2-month treatment with rifampicin, isoniazid, pyrazinamide, and ethambutol, reducing to isoniazid and rifampicin for a further 4 months provided the isolate is confirmed to be susceptible, is based on extensive clinical trials (Box 7.2.5.1).
- In cases of bacterial endocarditis, knowledge of the *in vitro* susceptibility of the infecting organism is crucial in determining dose, duration, and outcome of therapy. Highly penicillin-sensitive strains (MIC ≤0.1 mg/litre) of viridans streptococci are treated effectively with a 2-week regimen of parenteral penicillin and gentamicin or 4 weeks parenteral penicillin alone. Less sensitive strains should be treated with parenteral penicillin for a total of 4 weeks. If the infecting organism is an enterococcus, a minimum of 4 weeks' treatment with parenteral penicillin (or ampicillin) and aminoglycoside is essential.

Infections caused by *Staph. aureus* are a particular challenge since the severity is highly variable and yet the potential for metastatic infection and chronicity, as in the case of osteomyelitis, must be kept in mind. The isoxazolyl penicillins such as flucloxacillin are preferred with or without the addition of fusidic acid. Clindamycin and linezolid are useful alternative agents. Many *Staph. aureus* infections of the skin and soft tissues respond promptly to 7 to 14 days oral therapy. Where there is a severe systemic response to infection, parenteral therapy is appropriate initially. Where there is evidence of dissemination, treatment should be extended for periods of up to 4 weeks.

In the case of septic arthritis, antibiotics should be given promptly and joint aspiration carried out, sometimes repeatedly, to avoid damage to the articular cartilage. The duration of therapy has not been rigorously determined. Most infections will resolve in 2 to 3 weeks. One of the most challenging infections is staphylococcal osteomyelitis. To avoid chronicity, it is customary to treat for 4 to 6 weeks. Treatment is generally administered parenterally. In centres where skill, experience, and administrative support exist, patients are increasingly being managed in the community by parenteral administration through peripherally inserted venous catheters. Under these circumstances, a glycopeptide such as teicoplanin is convenient since it is administered once daily.

For most infections, the duration of therapy remains uncertain. However, many mild to moderate uncomplicated infections will defervesce within a 3- to 5-day period suggesting that 5 to 7 days of treatment is usually adequate. There is little evidence to suggest that treatment periods of 7 to 14 days, or longer, are any more effective. They are also likely to be associated with an increased risk of side effects, superinfection, and the selection of antibiotic-resistant organisms, as well as being more costly.

The parenteral administration of antibiotics is appropriate in the management of severe life-threatening infections and when oral therapy is contraindicated, such as in the postoperative period, if the patient is vomiting, or where gastrointestinal absorption cannot be relied on. However, the need for continued parenteral therapy should be reviewed regularly. In the treatment of many common infections, the acute features of infection such as temperature, tachycardia, and an elevated circulating neutrophil count usually improve within a period of 48 to 72 h. Provided there is no contraindication to oral therapy, this should be considered early in the course of patient management. The advantages are not just in the reduced cost of medication; the risk of intravenous line associated complications, such as infection, is also eliminated and discharge from hospital may be hastened.

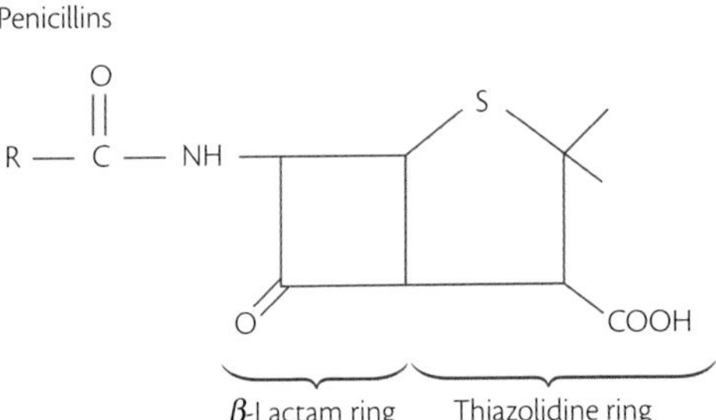

Fig. 7.2.5.7 Chemical structure of the β-lactam antibiotics (penicillins, cephalosporins, and monobactams) identifying the common β-lactam ring component which is subject to hydrolysis by β-lactamases.

Adverse drug reactions

Overall, antimicrobial agents have an outstanding record of safety. Nonetheless, no drug is without the potential for side effects. The risk varies by agent and sometimes by dose, while host genetic factors and pathophysiological status can also be important.

Oral antibiotics are largely used in the community where they are generally well tolerated and used in the treatment of minor infections in large populations. Injectable agents selected for short-course perioperative prophylaxis have a well-established safety record. However, agents such as the antiretroviral drugs and amphotericin B carry a higher risk of more serious adverse drug reactions, which must be balanced against the life-threatening nature of their target infections.

While drug safety is assessed during drug development, the full repertoire of adverse reactions becomes apparent only during widespread clinical use, hence, the importance of adverse drug reaction reporting systems. In the United Kingdom, the 'yellow card' system has been very successful and relies on voluntary reporting of possible adverse drug events to the Medicines & Healthcare products Regulatory Agency (MHRA, www.mhra.gov.uk) by doctors, dentists, coroners, pharmacists, nurses (including midwives and health visitors), radiographers, optometrists, and, most recently, patients. It is important to distinguish between adverse event reporting and adverse drug reaction reporting. The latter is more difficult to establish with certainty and may require rechallenge, which raises medical and ethical concerns.

It is essential to enquire about previous drug reactions as well as other forms of drug toxicities before prescribing. The relationship to a previously prescribed drug requires careful assessment. Hypersensitivity is among the more common of drug reactions and, in the case of β-lactam drugs, appears to be more a function of the five-membered thiazolidine ring (Fig. 7.2.5.7) of the penicillin molecule, since hypersensitivity reactions are less common with the cephalosporins which have a six-membered dihydrothiazine ring. The monobactam aztreonam has neither ring structure and hypersensitivity reactions appear to be rare. However, it is important to note that accelerated systemic hypersensitivity reactions (anaphylaxis) can be life-threatening such that any previous association with a β-lactam drug is an absolute contraindication to the use of all β-lactams.

Table 7.2.5.12 Dose-related adverse effects of selected antimicrobials

Drug	Adverse effect	Comment
Antibacterial drugs		
General	Superinfection by yeasts or *C. difficile*; selection of drug-resistant bacteria from the normal flora	These are universal adverse effects of antibacterial drugs and are generally related to the duration of exposure
β-Lactams	Myelosuppression	Neutropenia may occur after 1–2 weeks of high-dose IV therapy
	Drug fever	Occurs during prolonged (>1 week), high-dose IV therapy (e.g. endocarditis)
	Central nervous stimulation/convulsions	Can occur with overdose in renal failure
Aminoglycosides	Nephrotoxicity; ototoxicity	Monitoring of serum concentrations minimizes but does not avoid toxicity; risk of toxicity is related to the duration of the dose and concomitant therapy
Vancomycin	Nephrotoxicity; ototoxicity	May potentiate aminoglycoside nephrotoxicity
Macrolides (e.g. erythromycin)	Gastrointestinal stimulation	This is a prokinetic effect of erythromycin which does not occur with all macrolides
	Ototoxicity; cardiac arrhythmias	Only with high-dose IV therapy
	Drug interactions	Increased serum concentrations of theophylline and ciclosporin
Quinolones (e.g. ciprofloxacin)	Central nervous stimulation	Quinolones are weak GABA antagonists; this effect is potentiated by coadministration with NSAIDs, especially fenbufen
	Drug interactions	May inhibit metabolism of theophylline
Oxazolidinone (e.g. linezolid)	Anaemia, neutropenia, thrombocytopenia; neuropathy; lactic acidosis	Limit treatment to 28 days to reduce risk of haematological toxicity
Antifungal/antiprotozoal/ antiviral drugs		
Amphotericin B	Nephrotoxicity	Decreased creatinine clearance and renal potassium wasting are universal at clinically effective doses
	Rigors/hyperthermia/hypotension	Related to the rate of infusion
Ketoconazole	Inhibition of steroid synthesis	Occurs with prolonged (>1 week) high-dose therapy
Aciclovir	Central nervous adverse effects; crystalluria	Rare except with high-dose IV therapy
Quinine	Hypoglycaemia	

GABA, γ-aminobutyric acid; NSAID, nonsteroidal anti-inflammatory drug.

Some drug toxicities are genetically determined. For example, people who are genetically slow acetylators of isoniazid are more at risk of side effects such as peripheral neuropathy. Those genetically deficient in the enzyme glucose-6-phosphate dehydrogenase (EC 1.1.1.49) are at risk of drug-induced haemolysis. This risk is more common in those of African, Mediterranean, or Far Eastern descent. Hence, it is important to screen for this red cell enzyme deficiency before the administration of oxidant drugs such as primaquine.

Adverse drug reactions may not always be acute in their presentation but reveal themselves after prolonged drug exposure. Oral flucloxacillin and co-amoxiclav when administered for several weeks, particularly in older patients, are more likely to induce drug-associated hepatotoxicity. Likewise, parenteral formulations of selected drugs may be more toxic than their oral formulation, as is the case with fusidic acid where prolonged parenteral administration frequently gives rise to hepatotoxicity.

Concentration-dependent adverse reactions (Table 7.2.5.12) are more likely to occur in the presence of organ system failure. Aminoglycoside toxicity is more common in older people, in those with preexisting renal failure, and after repeated aminoglycoside doses or other nephrotoxic drugs. Concentration-dependent bone marrow suppression characterizes the use of chloramphenicol whereby pancytopenia arises when plasma concentrations are in excess of 25 mg/litre. This is to be distinguished from the idiopathic aplastic anaemia that is a rare accompaniment of chloramphenicol use, but unfortunately is rarely reversible.

Much has been learned about the structure–activity determinants of drug toxicity. For example, the quinolone antibiotics as a class have the potential to induce phototoxicity, arthrotoxicity, central nervous system (CNS) toxicity, cardiotoxicity, and interact with agents such as caffeine, theophylline, and nonsteroidal anti-inflammatory drugs (Fig. 7.2.5.8). Knowledge of such predictors has lead to the selection of agents with safer structural profiles. Despite this, adverse drug reactions have led to the withdrawal or modification of the licensed indications for several quinolones, notably temafloxacin, trovafloxacin and sparfloxacin, emphasizing the importance of clinical recognition and reporting of adverse events.

Few infectious conditions require lifelong therapy. The management of HIV infection has challenged this tenet. To date, drugs directed at the causative viruses or complicating opportunistic infections are suppressive rather than achieving eradication. It is also important to note that the drugs used in the treatment of HIV and AIDS are often licensed with limited information concerning their long-term safety. The potential for adverse reactions and especially interactions is considerable and requires careful attention to their detection and management. This has become an increasingly important challenge as life expectancy for those with HIV infection improves. It is important to balance drug safety while encouraging compliance and the maintenance of a reasonable state of health.

Failure of antibiotic therapy

Antimicrobial therapy may fail for several reasons. The agent selected may be inappropriate for the particular infection and fail to inhibit the target organism, or fail to reach the site of infection in sufficient concentration. For example, drugs such as nitrofurantoin and norfloxacin, while achieving high urinary concentrations, fail to deal adequately with parenchymatous infection of the kidney or bacteraemia which may complicate acute pyelonephritis.

The prostate also presents a chemotherapeutic challenge owing to the relatively low pH (*c*.6.4) in chronic bacterial prostatitis. Drugs which are weak bases, such as trimethoprim either alone or in combination with sulfamethoxazole (co-trimoxazole), are preferred, especially since they are also lipid soluble. Ciprofloxacin has similar characteristics and has also produced favourable results. However, treatment of acute bacterial prostatitis sometimes needs to be prolonged (4–6 weeks and occasionally longer), especially if there is a history of chronic relapsing infection.

The drug may be appropriate, but the dose selected may be inadequate. This may apply to such conditions as unsuspected bacterial endocarditis where high-dose parenteral antibiotic is required. Likewise, the concentration of penicillin required to deal with pneumococcal meningitis greatly exceeds that effective in the treatment of pneumococcal pneumonia; occasionally the two diseases may coexist. Infections caused by *Legionella pneumophila* and *Chlamydia* spp. require drugs that achieve high intracellular concentrations such as the macrolides, tetracyclines, or quinolones.

Resistance emerging during treatment is an uncommon cause of clinical failure but should be considered. Drug resistant *Mycobacterium tuberculosis* can develop on therapy as a result of the emergence of minority populations of organisms resistant to such first-line drugs as rifampicin and isoniazid. The current multidrug regimens are, in part, designed to avoid this occurrence. Likewise, in those with HIV infection, drug-resistant virus is an increasingly important cause of treatment failure and requires good compliance with multidrug regimens to slow its rate of emergence.

Mixed infections are commonly associated with intra-abdominal sepsis and occasionally with infections of the lung. They may fail to respond to treatment unless the regimen covers the full range of bacterial pathogens. In the case of intra-abdominal sepsis, the

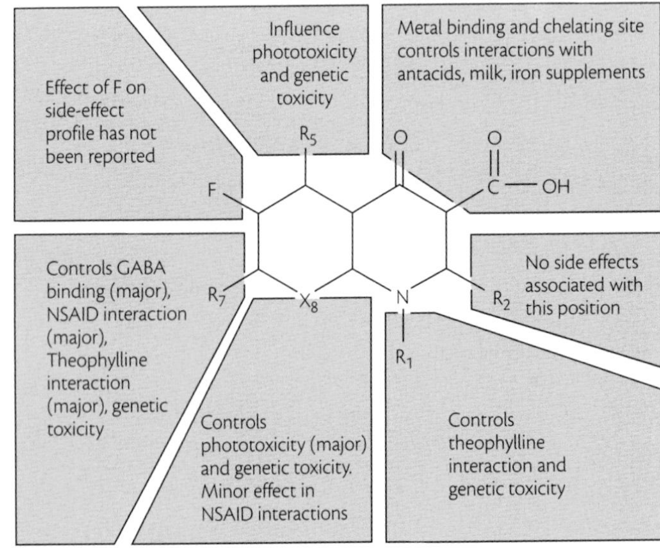

Fig. 7.2.5.8 Structure–activity side-effect relationships of the fluoroquinolone antibacterial drugs. GABA, γ-aminobutyric acid; NSAID, nonsteroidal anti-inflammatory drug.
(Redrawn from Domagala JM (1994). Structure–activity and structure–side-effect relationships for the quinolone antibacterials. *J Antimicrob Chemother*, **33**, 685–706.)

Table 7.2.5.13 The World Health Organization (2007) model list of essential drugs (anti-infectives)

Anthelmintics	Antibacterials	Antituberculosis medicines	Antifungals	Antivirals	Antiprotozoals
Albendazole	Amoxicillin	Ethambutol	Amphotericin B	Abacavir	Amodiaquine
Levamisole	Ampicillin	Isoniazid	Flucytosine	Aciclovir	Diloxanide
Mebendazole	Benzathine benzylpenicillin	Isoniazid + ethambutol	Potassium iodide	Didanosine	Metronidazole
Niclosamide	Benzylpenicillin	Pyrazinamide	Nystatin	Emtricitabine	Meglamine
Praziquantel	Cloxacillin	Rifampicin	Clotrimazole	Emtricitabine + Tenofovir	Pentamidine
Pyrantel	Phenoxymethylpenicillin	Rifampicin + isoniazid	Fluconazole	Lamivudine	Amphotericin B
Ivermectin	Procaine benzylpenicillin	Rifampicin + isoniazid + pyrazinamide	Griseofulvin	Stavudine	Amodiaquine
Praziquantel	Amoxicillin + clavulanic acid	Rifampicin + isoniazid + pyrazinamide + ethambutol		Stavudine + Lamivudine + Nevirapine	Artemether + Lumefantrin
Triclabendazole	Cefazolin	Streptomycin		Tenofovir	Chloroquine
Oxamniquine	Cefixime	Amikacin		Efavirenz	Primaquine
	Ceftazidime	*p*-Aminosalicylic acid		Efavirenz + Emtricitabine + Tenofovir	Doxycycline
	Ceftriaxone	Capreomycin		Nevirapine	Mefloquine
	Imipenem + cilastatin	Cycloserine		Ribavirin	Sulfadoxine + Pyrimethamine
	Azithromycin	Ethionamide		Ritonavir	Artemether
	Chloramphenicol	Kanamycin		Lopinavir + Ritonavir	Artesunate
	Ciprofloxacin tablet	Ofloxacin		Nelfinavir	Mefloquine
	Doxycycline			Saquinavir	Paromomycin
	Erithromycin			Zidovudine	Proguanil
	Gentamicin			Zidovudine + Lamivudine	Pentamidine
	Metronidazole			Zidovudine + Lamivudine + Nevirapine	Pyrimethamine
	Nitrofurantoin				Sulfamethoxazole + Trimethoprim
	Spectinomycin				Melarsoprol
	Sulfadiazine				Pentamidine
	Sulfamethoxazole + trimethoprim				Suramin sodium
	Trimethoprim				Eflornithine
	Clindamycin				Benznidazole
	Vancomycin				Nifurtimox
	Clofazimine				
	Dapsone				
	Rifampicin				

regimen should be active against anaerobic as well as aerobic bacterial pathogens.

Another important cause of antibiotic failure is the continued presence of a focus of infection. This may be an abscess that requires surgical drainage or the removal of an implanted medical device such as an intravascular catheter. Much more serious is infection of a prosthetic heart valve, hip joint, or CNS shunt where revision surgery carries significant risks. Many antibiotics fail to achieve therapeutic concentrations within abscess cavities, or are pH sensitive. Implant-associated infections present a similar challenge since bacteria often replicate slowly within a biofilm that is protective against normal host defences.

Finally, it should be remembered that a persistently elevated temperature in the presence of what appears to be adequate antibiotic treatment can reflect drug fever or indeed fever complicating a nonmicrobial diagnosis. This emphasizes the importance of monitoring the response to treatment and repeated patient assessment.

Practice guidelines and formularies

The plethora of therapeutic agents currently available presents a considerable challenge to the prescriber. Guidance on the choice of agent and the management of disease is becoming increasingly important. This is not only to ensure that the selection of treatment is appropriate for the target infection and consistent with current patterns of antimicrobial susceptibility but also that it reflects an acceptable safety profile as well as being sensitive to the appropriate use of health care resources. Such guidance is increasingly provided within formularies designed for local use, within either a hospital or a community practice. These frequently offer information on preferred and alternative regimens for particular infections. Formularies should include drugs currently tested by the diagnostic laboratory, since changing patterns of susceptibility may require modification of recommended drugs.

Within hospital practice, it is common for such formularies to identify drugs which may be prescribed freely according to specific indications and those for which expert advice from a clinical microbiologist or infectious disease specialist should be sought. The latter applies particularly to drugs that require specific skill and experience in their use, need drug levels to be monitored, or are expensive. For example, the treatment of deep-seated fungal infections with amphotericin B requires careful clinical assessment and guidance on dosage and monitoring. Likewise, the treatment of HIV infection is increasingly a specialist area. Antibiotics which are expensive to prescribe such as parenteral quinolones, third-generation cephalosporins, and the carbapenems may be restricted. The policy may also have recommendations for the timing of transfer from parenteral to oral therapy in order to minimize the use of injectable agents.

Formularies are educational and allow the prescriber to become familiar with indications and safety of the most commonly used agents. Their use should be supported by educational activities both at undergraduate and postgraduate level. Ideally, the selection of agents for inclusion in the formulary should be based on sound evidence of efficacy, safety, and economic benefit. However, such evidence-based medicine is often lacking or incomplete for commonly treated infections, since clinical trials of antibiotics, although increasingly robust in their design, are largely conducted to support licensing requirements rather than to address clinical use. They generally demonstrate the equivalence (or noninferiority) of a new agent in comparison with existing therapies. As a result, the recommendations of formularies and practice guidelines are based on a matrix of information derived from knowledge of the *in vitro* profile of an agent, its pharmacokinetic parameters, its clinical and microbiological efficacy, and its safety profile. This, in turn, is modified by custom and practice which explains why there is local and, sometimes, national and international variation in recommendations for some common indications such as community-acquired pneumonia and bacterial meningitis.

In developing countries, where medical resources are much more limited, greater reliance is placed on low-cost agents. The World Health Organization regularly updates its list of recommended essential drugs which includes anti-infective agents (Table 7.2.5.13). Despite the emphasis on low-cost agents, the drugs offered cover the majority of infections and prescribing needs of developing countries. The agents available in individual countries often vary according to local interpretation of the needs for these 'essential' drugs.

Recent developments in economically advanced countries have included an assessment of health care technologies for current management, national need, and the resources available. In the United Kingdom, the National Institute of Clinical Excellence (NICE, www.nice.org.uk) was established in 1999 to assess a variety of health care technologies including procedures as well as new therapies. Such assessments place greater emphasis on ensuring that new technologies are evaluated in a manner that more closely resembles clinical practice as well as demonstrating economic benefit, in contrast to drug licensing which addresses the quality, safety, and efficacy of new therapies. This new emphasis is likely to require a greater partnership between health care systems and pharmaceutical companies to ensure that the place of new technologies is rapidly assessed and that their use is consistent with health care strategies.

Further reading

American Thoracic Society, Centers for Disease Control and Infectious Diseases Society of America (2003). *Treatment of tuberculosis.* www.cdc.gov/mmwr/preview/mmwrhtml/rr5211a1.htm#top

Bennett WM, *et al.* (1994). *Drug prescribing in renal failure: Dosing guidelines for adults*, 3rd edition. American College of Physicians, Philadelphia.

Davies JM, Barnes R, Milligan D (2002). Update of guidelines for the prevention and treatment of infection in patients with an absent or dysfunctional spleen. *Clin Med*, **2**, 440–3.

Domagala JM (1994). Structure–activity and structure–side-effect relationships for the quinolone antibacterials. *J Antimicrob Chemother*, **33**, 685–706.

Elliott TSJ, Foweraker J, Gould FK (2004). Guidelines for the antibiotic treatment of endocarditis in adults: report of the Working Party of the British Society for Antimicrobial Chemotherapy. *J Antimicrob Chemother*, **54**, 971–81.

Finch RG, Williams RJ (1999). *Baillière's clinical infectious diseases: antibiotic resistance.* Baillière Tindall, London.

Finch RG, *et al.* (2003). *Antibiotic and chemotherapy*, 8th edition. Churchill Livingstone, Edinburgh.

Gould FK, Elliott TSJ, Foweraker J (2006). Guidelines for the prevention of endocarditis: report of the Working Party of the British Society for Antimicrobial Chemotherapy. *J Antimicrob Chemother*, **57**, 1035–42.

Hughes WT, *et al.* (2002). Infectious Diseases Society of America 2002 guidelines for the use of antimicrobial agents in neutropenic patients with cancer. *Clin Infect Dis*, **34**, 730–51.

Joint Tuberculosis Committee of the British Thoracic Society (1998). Chemotherapy and management of tuberculosis: recommendations. *Thorax*, **53**, 536–48.

Kerr KG (1999). The prophylaxis of bacterial infections in neutropenic patients. *J Antimicrob Chemother*, **44**, 587–91.

Kucers A, *et al.* (1997). *The use of antibiotics*, 5th edition. Butterworth Heinemann, Oxford.

Lim WS, *et al.* (2009). The British Thoracic Society guidelines for the management of community acquired pneumonia in adults. *Thorax*, **64** Suppl III, 1–61.

Russell AD, Chopra I (1996). *Understanding antibacterial action and resistance*, 2nd edition. Ellis Horwood, London.

Shyrock TR, Mortensen JE, Baumholtz M (1998). The effects of macrolides on the expression of bacterial virulence mechanisms. *J Antimicrob Chemother*, **41**, 505–12.

Standing Medical Advisory Committee Subgroup on Antimicrobial Resistance (1998). *The path of least resistance.* Department of Health, London.

Tuberculosis: clinical diagnosis and management of tuberculosis, and measures for its prevention and control. Clinical Guidelines 33 www.nice.org.uk/CG033 (accessed 22.10.09).

White NJ (1992). Antimalarial pharmacokinetics and treatment regimens. *Br J Clin Pharmacol*, **34**, 1–10.

Wise R, Honeybourne D (1999). Pharmacokinetics and pharmacodynamics of fluoroquinolones in the respiratory tract. *Eur Respir J*, **14**, 221–9.

World Health Organisation (2007) Model list of essential medicines (15th edition) http://www.who.int/medicines/publications/essentialmedicines/eu

7.3

Immunization

D. Goldblatt and M. Ramsay

Essentials

Immunization is one of the most successful medical interventions ever developed: it prevents infectious diseases worldwide.

Mechanism of effect—the basis for the success of immunization is that the human immune system is able to respond to vaccines by producing pathogen-specific antibody and memory cells (both B and T cells) which protect the body should the pathogen be encountered.

Clinical practicalities—most currently licensed vaccines contain live or killed bacterial or viral constituents, bacterial polysaccharides, or bacterial toxoids, while new types of vaccines are being developed that contain DNA. Most vaccines are delivered directly into skin or muscle via needles, or they are administered orally. New edible vaccines and vaccines delivered via the skin without the use of needles are being developed.

Who should be immunized?—vaccines can be used in a targeted way, i.e. only for those at high risk, or they can be recommended for mass immunization of whole populations. The latter approach may eventually lead to complete eradication of an infectious disease, as was the case with smallpox: polio eradication is the next global challenge. Vaccines that are able to interrupt the transmission of a pathogen between individuals are able to provide indirect protection, with the benefit of vaccination extending beyond the vaccinated population, e.g. infant immunization with pneumococcal vaccine has reduced the burden of disease in adults.

Global perspective—the Expanded Program on Immunization, set up by the World Health Organization to define which vaccines should be delivered in resource poor countries, has done much to increase coverage of vaccination amongst infants most at risk of infectious diseases. The evaluation of immunization programmes includes measurement of vaccine coverage, continuing surveillance for vaccine preventable infections, seroprevalence studies to assess population immunity, and systems for monitoring and reporting adverse events.

Introduction

Infectious diseases remain a major cause of mortality and morbidity worldwide. The prevention of certain infectious diseases by effective immunization programmes is one of the major triumphs of 20th century medicine. Most of this was achieved in the final third of that century, during which rapid strides in the understanding of the biology and pathogenicity of infectious agents or their components, and improved techniques for their purification, led to the development of safe and effective vaccines. The greatest triumph in the field of immunization was the eradication of smallpox. In 1959 the World Health Organization (WHO) declared its intention to eradicate smallpox, and in 1966 began to allocate sufficient resources to accomplish this ambitious goal. Thirteen years later, in 1979, the global eradication of smallpox was officially declared. Effective vaccines can eliminate infectious diseases, but to do this they must be implemented and used appropriately. Of the more than 12 million children under the age of 5 years who die annually, 2 million die of diseases that could be prevented by vaccines already available through the WHO's Expanded Program on Immunization (EPI). While rapid advances in vaccine science have introduced new techniques such as DNA vaccines, delivering vaccines to those most at risk must remain a priority.

Immunology of active immunization

Both nonspecific (innate) and specific (adaptive or acquired) immune systems are responsible for protecting humans against infectious diseases. The ability of the adaptive immune system to refine its antigen-recognition domains and establish immunological memory is the basis of successful active immunization. The specific immune system contains both cellular and humoral elements, whose relative importance differs depending on the nature of the infecting organism. The global eradication of type 2 poliovirus was achieved in 1999. In 2005, new monovalent vaccines targeting type-specific polio were developed and used for the first time. By 2008, however, poliovirus transmission continues in the four endemic countries, with importation into neighbouring countries and cases returning to 1999 levels. By 2009, polio eradication tools will be optimized with the availability of bivalent OPV against type 1 and type 3, as part of the framework for intensifying eradication efforts in 2010–2012.

Cellular responses are induced when antigen-presenting cells, such as dendritic cells, present antigens to T cells. T cells do not respond to soluble, unmodified antigens, and only recognize peptide antigens in association with major histocompatability complex (MHC) molecules. Two major forms of MHC molecules exist. Most nucleated cells produce MHC class I molecules, which stimulate a subset of T cells that produce the CD8 differentiation antigen. These T cells recognize and lyse infected target cells, hence their designation as cytotoxic T lymphocytes. By contrast, MHC class II molecules are produced by cells that participate in the immune response, and are recognized via a subset of T cells producing the CD4 differentiation antigen. A major role of such T cells is to augment the immune response, and so they are known as T helper cells. At least two subsets of T helper cells have been described: T helper 1 cells are involved in cytotoxic and delayed-type hypersensitivity responses, while T helper 2 cells support antibody production.

Immunoglobulin receptors on the surface of B cells are able to recognize soluble antigens, and so initiate the process of B-cell activation and differentiation. During differentiation, naive B cells become antibody-secreting plasma cells. In addition, B cells endocytose antigen bound to their surface immunoglobulins, and re-express it in the form of small peptides on the surface of the B cell in the context of MHC class II molecules. Thus B cells act as antigen-presenting cells and recruit T-cell help. The signals and soluble factors that result from such T-cell help drive the B-cell process of affinity maturation and memory formation. This takes place in the germinal centres of lymph nodes, where there is intimate contact between B cells, T cells, and dendritic cells. It is here that memory B cells are formed and then migrate to the bone marrow, spleen, and the submucosa of the respiratory tract and gut. On re-encountering the antigen, memory B cells undergo rapid activation and differentiation into plasma cells, and secrete large amounts of switched, high-affinity antibody.

Thus the ideal vaccine antigen will lead to the activation, replication, and differentiation of T and B lymphocytes. Ideally the antigen will persist in lymphoid tissue, conformationally intact, to allow the continuing production of cells that secrete high-affinity antibody, and the generation of memory cells.

Vaccine antigens

The ideal vaccine antigen is safe, with minimal side-effects, promotes effective resistance to the disease (although it does not necessarily prevent infection), and promotes lifelong immunity. It needs to be stable and remain potent during storage and shipping, and also has to be affordable to allow widespread use. Most currently licensed vaccines contain live or killed bacterial or viral constituents, bacterial polysaccharides, or bacterial toxoids (Table 7.3.1).

Live vaccines are ideal for certain diseases, as replication in the body mimics natural infection, thereby inducing appropriate and site-specific immunity. Live vaccines must be attenuated to remove the danger of clinical disease, but retain the beneficial effects of inducing immunity. Some live vaccines may be spread from person to person, and thus enhance herd immunity, although such spread may endanger immunocompromised individuals, in whom live vaccines should be avoided. Live vaccines are inherently less stable than killed vaccines, and the possibility of reversion of vaccine virus to the wild type exists (as in polio). Killed vaccines do not carry the risk associated with person-to-person spread, and are inherently more stable, but often require two or three doses to induce optimal immunity, especially when used in the first year of life.

Table 7.3.1 Currently licensed vaccines for use in humans

Vaccine type	Live vaccines	Killed/subunit vaccines
Viral	Rubella	Poliomyelitis (Salk)
	Measles	Influenza
	Poliomyelitis (Sabin)	Rabies (human diploid cell)
	Yellow fever	Hepatitis A
	Mumps	Hepatitis B
	Varicella zoster	Japanese encephalitis
	Rotavirus	Human papillomavirus
	Japanese encephalitis	
Bacterial	Bacillus Calmette–Guérin	Cholera
	Typhoid	Typhoid
	Cholera	Pertussis
		Borrelia burgdorferi
		Anthrax
		Plague
Bacterial polysaccharides		*Haemophilus influenzae* type b
		Neisseria meningitidis group A and C
		Streptococcus pneumoniae
Rickettsial		Typhus
Bacterial toxoid		Diphtheria
		Tetanus

New developments in vaccine antigens

Developments in molecular biology have begun to revolutionize the field of vaccine science, and provide a glimpse of the future, when the traditional reliance on live attenuated viral vaccines or purified bacterial or viral products as vaccine antigens may be reduced. The first licensed vaccine to contain recombinant genetic material was the hepatitis B vaccine. Despite the licensing of highly effective plasma-derived hepatitis B vaccines in the early 1980s, fears about safety, and their high cost, led to the search for other hepatitis B vaccines. Several vaccine manufacturers used recombinant DNA technology to express hepatitis B surface antigen in other organisms, which led to the development of new vaccines.

Recent developments have focused on the use of DNA as a vaccine antigen. The potential of naked DNA as a vaccine antigen was discovered by chance in 1989 during a gene therapy experiment, when it was shown that a gene inserted directly into a mammalian cell could induce the cell to manufacture the protein encoded by that gene. In early experiments, DNA was injected directly into muscle, and the resulting immune response was measured (Fig. 7.3.1).

DNA vaccines can induce protective immunity to a variety of pathogens in animals, but data in humans are limited. As DNA has the theoretical potential to be incorporated into the host genetic make-up and subvert the genetic working of cells, safety concerns have delayed studies in humans. Phase I studies, however, have assessed DNA vaccines designed to protect against hepatitis B,

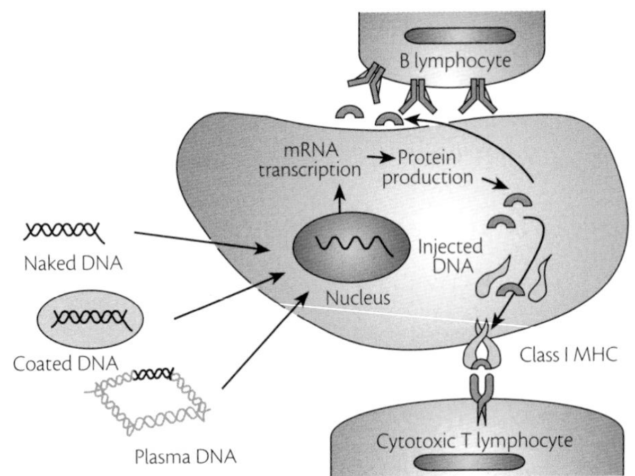

Fig. 7.3.1 Injection of DNA encoding a foreign protein can elicit antibodies and a cytotoxic T-lymphocyte response.

herpes simplex type 1 and 2, HIV, influenza, and malaria. So far clinical trials have proved disappointing, either because the level of the response was inadequate or because excessive doses of DNA were required to achieve an adequate response. To improve the response to DNA vaccines a number of newer techniques have been developed. These include:

- Incorporating DNA into microprojectiles that are shot into the target cell via the skin (the so-called gene gun technique)
- Coating DNA with cationic lipids or other materials that neutralize its charge; the lipids facilitate cellular uptake and membrane transfer
- Delivering DNA by incorporating it into a viral delivery system using disabled viruses
- Delivering DNA by incorporation into a bacterial delivery system such as attenuated *Salmonella typhimurium*
- Delivering DNA together with traditional adjuvants such as alum
- Improving immunogenicity by including a cytokine gene in the plasmid, adjacent to the gene encoding the protective antigen. Local expression of the appropriate cytokine (e.g. granulocyte–macrophage colony stimulating factor) may augment the immune response in a similar fashion to adjuvants.
- Combining priming immunization by a DNA vaccine with subsequent boost by a recombinant vaccine.

The huge potential of DNA vaccines, which offer the promise of cheap and stable vaccines that do not require a cold chain for distribution, will stimulate further development of these exciting products.

New developments in vaccine delivery

Research into different routes of vaccine delivery has been driven by the limitations of the parenteral route. These include the difficulty associated with the use of live viral vaccines in the first 6 to 9 months of life (because of the neutralizing effect of passively transferred maternal antibody) and the difficulty and expense of delivering mass immunization by injection. Mucosal delivery of vaccine via the intranasal route has been studied for a number of antigens, including measles, influenza, rubella, varicella, and *Streptococcus pneumoniae*. The induction of local immunity for pathogens that either enter the body via the nasopharynx (measles, influenza) or are commonly carried in the nasopharynx (*S. pneumoniae*) is attractive.

Edible vaccines are attracting increasing attention, providing as they do both a means of antigen production and delivery. Studies in animals, and phase I studies in humans, have demonstrated their potential. Mice fed with potatoes expressing a nontoxic fragment of the cholera toxin developed mucosal antibodies to the toxin, which reduced diarrhoea on challenge with whole cholera toxin. Humans fed raw potatoes expressing the B subunit of enterotoxigenic *Escherichia coli* also showed mucosal immune responses and an increase in neutralizing antibody levels. There are some problems with stability, but edible vaccines are a potentially simple and convenient method of vaccine delivery on a wide scale.

The aim of immunization programmes

Once a vaccine has been developed and shown to be effective it can be used in different ways. Many vaccines are used selectively in groups of the population who are at increased risk of infection (e.g. because of occupation or travel) or of severe consequences of the disease (e.g. because of an underlying medical condition). Other vaccines are employed for mass immunization targeting the whole population. Mass immunization can eradicate, eliminate, or control an infectious disease. Eradication, the state where a disease and its causal agent have been removed from the natural environment, has been achieved only for smallpox. Once eradication has been certified, mass immunization programmes can cease, and resources can be transferred to other programmes.

The next target for the WHO is the global eradication of poliomyelitis. Characteristics that favour eradication are the absence of an animal host, the absence of a carrier state, and lifelong protection given by vaccination. The polio eradication campaign has involved the use of National Immunization Days (NIDs), on which live attenuated polio vaccine is delivered to a high proportion of the childhood population on a single day. Millions of children have been immunized with trivalent oral polio vaccine (against types 1, 2, and 3) during NIDs. This had led to the successful interruption of poliovirus transmission in many previously endemic countries, and by 2005 only four countries remained where indigenous poliovirus transmission occurred (India, Pakistan, Nigeria, and Afghanistan). The global eradication of type 2 poliovirus was achieved in 1999, and type 3 is now largely confined to northern Nigeria. In 2005, new monovalent vaccines targeting type-specific polio were developed and used for the first time, and the Advisory Committee on Polio Eradication concluded that all polio-affected countries except Nigeria could stop poliovirus transmission by 2006. Preparations continue for the eventual cessation of routine polio vaccination.

For some infections, eradication by immunization is not possible. A good example is tetanus, where the agent is distributed widely in the environment. For these programmes the aim is to control infection to the point where it no longer constitutes a public health burden. To maintain control, immunization must be continued indefinitely.

For diseases that are transmitted from person to person, a good immunization programme provides protection by conferring both individual and herd immunity. For many vaccines, herd immunity can be achieved by vaccinating a high proportion of the childhood population; older individuals are generally immune as a result of previous natural infection. If such a situation can be sustained, transmission of the infection may be interrupted, and elimination or eradication becomes possible. If vaccine coverage or efficacy is suboptimal, however, then, in the absence of natural transmission, the number of susceptible people will gradually increase. Eventually, the proportion of susceptible people (those who did not receive vaccine or who failed to respond to it) may reach a level sufficient to support an epidemic. Although the size of these epidemics may be small by prevaccine standards, the average age of those infected will be higher than in the prevaccine era. For infections that have more severe consequences in older individuals the morbidity associated with such outbreaks can be substantial. A tragic example of this has recently been observed in Greece, where mass vaccination against rubella in childhood has been recommended since 1975. Implementation was poor, however, and during the 1980s coverage was below 50%. The low level of coverage was sufficient to interrupt transmission for several years, but by the time rubella infection recurred in 1993, a high proportion of pregnant women were susceptible to rubella and an epidemic of congenital rubella syndrome occurred.

The Expanded Program on Immunization

In 1974 the WHO launched the EPI, in recognition of the major contribution of vaccines to public health. At the start of the programme fewer than 5% of the world's infants were immunized against the six target diseases—diphtheria, tetanus, whooping cough, polio, measles, and tuberculosis. Between 1990 and 1997, around 80% of the 130 million children born each year were immunized by their first birthday, preventing around 3 million deaths each year. Each year, more than 500 million immunization contacts occur with children, and these have provided an opportunity for the delivery of other primary health care interventions.

During the 1990s the EPI added immunization against yellow fever and hepatitis B to its target diseases (Table 7.3.2). The introduction of these vaccines, however, has been less impressive, particularly in the poorest countries in greatest need. Of 33 African countries at risk of yellow fever, only 17 have included the vaccine in the childhood schedule. By 1998, hepatitis B vaccine had been incorporated into the national programmes of 90 countries, but it is estimated that 70% of the world's hepatitis B carriers live in countries without programmes. The major barrier to using new vaccines in the developing world is likely to be sustainable funding.

Table 7.3.2 Immunization schedule for infants, recommended by the WHO Expanded Program on Immunization

Age	Vaccines	Hepatitis B[a]	
		Scheme A	Scheme B
Birth	BCG, OPV	HB1	
6 weeks	DTP1, Hib1, OPV1	HB2	HB1
10 weeks	DTP2, Hib2, OPV2		HB2
14 weeks	DTP3, Hib3, OPV3	HB3	HB3
9 months	Measles		
	Yellow fever[b]		

BCG, Bacillus Calmette–Guérin; DTP, diphtheria, tetanus, pertussis; HB, hepatitis B; Hib, *Haemophilus influenza* type b; OPV, oral polio vaccine.

[a] Scheme A is recommended where perinatal transmission is frequent (e.g. in Southeast Asia); scheme B may be used where perinatal transmission is less frequent (e.g. in sub-Saharan Africa).

[b] In countries where yellow fever poses a risk.

Delivery of immunization programmes

For mass immunization to achieve its aims, high and uniform coverage of immunization must be reached and sustained. The level of coverage of immunization is associated with a variety of factors, including the sociodemographic characteristics of the population, the organization of health services, knowledge among health professionals, and parental attitudes.

Sociodemographic factors that may influence vaccine coverage include deprivation, maternal education, and family size. Centrally coordinated health services with few barriers to access, and standard record systems with facilities for call and recall are likely to achieve higher vaccine coverage. Health professionals with accurate knowledge of the indications and true contraindications to immunization are important. Excessive lists of contraindications for diphtheria–tetanus–pertussis immunization in the newly independent states of the former Soviet Union contributed to a massive resurgence of diphtheria in the early 1990s. The number of cases rose from 2000 in 1990 to over 47 000 in 1994; 2500 deaths from diphtheria occurred between 1990 and 1995.

Whether or not parents decide to have their children vaccinated depends on their perceptions of the severity of the disease and of the safety and effectiveness of the vaccine. Knowledge of parental perceptions can be used successfully to target health promotion campaigns. When coverage is high, the incidence of vaccine-preventable disease declines, and parental perception of the severity of that disease may decrease. In this situation, concerns about the safety of the vaccine become paramount and can lead to a decline in vaccine coverage. Such a situation arose in the United Kingdom in the early 1970s, when concern about the safety of pertussis vaccine led to a fall in coverage. This resulted in resurgence of the disease, with consequent mortality and morbidity (Fig. 7.3.2). Over the next decade vaccine coverage improved again, and the incidence of the disease fell to the lowest levels ever.

In 2003–4, concern about the safety of the polio vaccine led to the suspension of the programme in northern Nigeria. This led to an outbreak of polio in west and central Africa and the reintroduction of poliovirus into 22 previously polio-free countries. By 2005, after massive efforts from the international community, successful campaigns were launched to stop these outbreaks and transmission was contained in all but six of these countries. In 2008, a further polio outbreak occurred in Nigeria, leading to persistent importations into neighbouring countries and re-established transmission in Angola, Chad, the eastern part of Democratic Republic of Congo, and southern Sudan. This experience illustrates the major global implications of failure to sustain confidence in vaccination.

Evaluation of immunization programmes

Evaluation of an immunization programme may include the measurement of vaccine coverage, surveillance of disease incidence, assessment of prevalence of immunity, and the monitoring of adverse events.

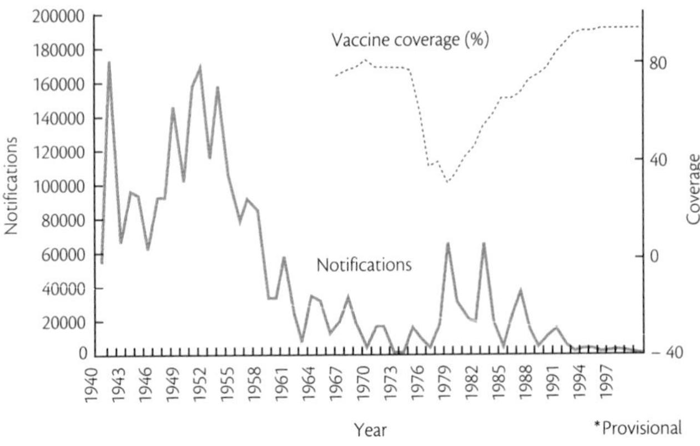

Fig. 7.3.2 Whooping cough cases and vaccine coverage in England and Wales between 1940 and 1998.

Vaccine coverage

Timely measurement is important for monitoring trends in vaccine coverage and identifying pockets of low coverage. Low coverage may be apparent before any increase in disease incidence is observed. Since the late 1970s, three outbreaks of poliomyelitis have been observed among groups in the Netherlands with religious objections to immunization. Despite national coverage of 96% for MMR vaccine, the same group has recently been the focus of a large epidemic of measles. Between April and December 1999, 1750 cases of measles occurred in the Netherlands, compared with only 9 in the whole of 1998.

Disease surveillance

Once an immunization programme has been implemented, disease incidence data can be used to monitor the effectiveness of the strategy. For example, the dramatic decline in the incidence of invasive *Haemophilus influenzae* infection described in both the Netherlands and the United Kingdom can be used to demonstrate the impact of conjugate vaccination. The age distribution of infection may change, as children above or below the target age form an increasing proportion of those infected. Various epidemiological methods, including case–control studies, cohort studies, and the screening method can be used to estimate the efficacy of the vaccine in the field. The introduction of a 7-valent pneumococcal conjugate vaccine into the routine infant immunization programme of the United States of America, and the associated surveillance for invasive pneumococcal disease, has revealed not only the direct impact of the vaccine in reducing disease in vaccinated children, but also a huge indirect effect, which has resulted in the reduction of invasive pneumococcal disease in unvaccinated adults.

Seroprevalence studies

Seroprevalence studies are used to assess population immunity to infection. Such immunity results either from immunization or from natural infection. This can detect groups that include a high proportion of susceptible individuals, who may be the focus of future outbreaks. In 1991, seroprevalence studies in the United Kingdom identified that a large proportion of school-age children was susceptible to measles, and therefore that an epidemic of measles was likely. A large campaign was mounted in November 1994 to immunize children from 5 to 16 years of age. The number of cases of measles fell rapidly and remained at low levels over the next 5 years.

Adverse events

The monitoring of adverse events is important for maintaining public confidence in an immunization programme and for detecting rare events that could not be identified before licensing the vaccine. The detection of such events may lead to the withdrawal of certain vaccines. In August 1998, a quadrivalent vaccine using reassortant rhesus rotavirus strains was licensed for use in the United States of America and recommended for the mass immunization of infants. During prelicensing studies, five cases of intussusception had been reported in around 10 000 recipients, compared with only 1 in almost 5000 controls; this difference was not statistically significant. During postlicensing surveillance, however, 15 cases were reported to the Vaccine Adverse Event Reporting System. On 22 October 1999, a review of scientific data concluded that there was an increased frequency of intussusception in the 1 to 2 weeks after vaccination, which led to withdrawal of the vaccine.

Further reading

Centers for Disease Control and Prevention (2005). Direct and indirect effects of routine vaccination of children with 7-valent pneumococcal conjugate vaccine on incidence of invasive pneumococcal disease—United States, 1998–2003. *MMWR Morb Mortal Wkly Rep*, **54**, 893–7.

Chen RT (1999). Vaccine risks: real, perceived and unknown. *Vaccine*, **17**, S41–46.

Czerkinsky C, *et al.* (1999). Mucosal immunity and tolerance: relevance to vaccine development. *Immunol Rev*, **170**, 197–222.

Leitner WW, Ying H, Restifo NP (1999). DNA and RNA-based vaccines: principles, progress and prospects. *Vaccine*, **18**, 765–77.

Orenstein WA, Bernier RH, Hinman AR (1988). Assessing vaccine efficacy in the field. Further observations. *Epidemiol Rev*, **10**, 212–41.

Tacket CO, *et al.* (1998). Immunogenicity in humans of a recombinant bacterial antigen delivered in a transgenic potato. *Nat Med*, **4**, 607–9.

Whitney CG, *et al.* (2006). Effectiveness of seven-valent pneumococcal conjugate vaccine against invasive pneumococcal disease: a matched case-control study. *Lancet*, **368**, 1495–502.

World Health Organization and the United Nations Children's Fund (1996). *State of the world's vaccines and immunization.* World Health Organization, Geneva.

World Health Organization (1997). *Polio: the beginning of the end.* World Health Organization, Geneva.

7.4

Travel and expedition medicine

C.P. Conlon and David A. Warrell

Essentials

Tourists, business people, pilgrims, and visitors to friends and relatives are making increasing numbers of trips to tropical and developing parts of the world, where the risk and range of infectious and environmental diseases and injuries may be much higher than in Western countries. The aim of travel and expedition medicine is to reduce risk through education, appropriate immunizations and other medical advice, hence enhancing the enjoyment and achievements of travelling abroad. Explorers, expeditioners, and wilderness travellers face the greatest health challenges, but risk can be minimized by technical competence, careful planning, training in practical medical skills, and rehearsing emergency evacuation.

Pretravel advice—this requires precise information about the mode of travel, geographical itinerary and the purpose of the visit, and must take into account the age, background health and immunocompetence of the traveller. Important provisions are (1) a first-aid kit, (2) sun-block, (3) insect repellent, (4) treatments for motion sickness, jet lag and high altitude sickness, (5) supplies of regular medications, and (6) generous, comprehensive travel insurance.

Pre-travel immunization – this involves (1) boosting childhood vaccinations - e.g. tetanus, poliomyelitis, and diphtheria; (2) adding protection against hepatitis A (and B in those at risk of parenteral or sexual exposure) and infections endemic in the areas to be visited, e.g. yellow fever in equatorial Africa and South America, Japanese encephalitis in South-East Asia, tick-borne encephalitis in northern Europe and Asia, *Neisseria meningitidis* in the meningitis belt of Africa, typhoid in South Asia, and rabies in most parts of the world. Pregnancy and immunocompromise present particular problems of vulnerability to infections and restrict the use of live vaccines.

Reducing the risk of infections—food and water hygiene are crucial for prevention of travellers' diarrhoea, the commonest medical problem likely to be encountered. Avoidance of bites by disease vectors such as mosquitoes and ticks and use of appropriate prophylactic drugs reduces the risk of malaria and many tropical other infections.

Other medical hazards of travel—long flights can lead to deep vein thrombosis and respiratory infection. Underestimated hazards of travel include sexually transmitted infections, schistosomiasis, drowning and road traffic accidents.

Introduction

International tourism has grown prodigiously over the last few years. From 2006 to 2007, the number of tourist trips worldwide increased by 4.1% to 880 million, 30% of which were to tropical or subtropical developing countries. United Kingdom citizens make 56 million visits abroad each year, 8% of these to developing countries, which carry a higher risk of illness (600-fold increased risk in Mexico, 1835-fold in the Indian subcontinent) than travel to European countries such as France. It has been estimated that 50 to 75% of short-term travellers to tropical or subtropical countries become unwell, usually because of an infection. Those travelling outside Europe need to be provided with adequate medical advice to minimize the risks of their journeys, while back at home, admitting physicians should consider a broader range of differential diagnoses, diagnostic tests, and specific treatments. Among the more common infectious disease health risks faced by travellers to developing countries are traveller's diarrhoea, malaria, dengue fever, acute lower respiratory tract infection, hepatitis A, gonorrhoea, and animal bites with rabies risk (Table 7.4.1).

Pretravel advice

This can be obtained from a variety of sources, but ideally should be sought from medical practitioners and clinics with a special interest in travel medicine. Other sources include the embassies of the countries to be visited, travel agencies, and, increasingly, the internet (see 'Further reading' below). People travel for a variety of reasons: business travel, pilgrimage, gap-year and educational travel, and tourism are all increasing. Many members of the immigrant

Table 7.4.1 Immunizations

Vaccine	Type	Route	Primary course	Booster
Routine				
Diphtheria	Adsorbed toxoid	IM/SC	Three doses at monthly intervals	Single low dose if under 10 years old
Polio (Sabin)	Live virus (attenuated)	PO	Three doses at monthly intervals	10 years
Polio (Salk)	Killed virus	IM/SC	Three doses at monthly intervals	10 years
Tetanus	Adsorbed toxoid	IM/SC	Three doses at monthly intervals	10 years (maximum 5 doses)
Combined tetanus, polio, diphtheria	–	IM/SC	Three doses at monthly intervals	10 years (maximum 5 total doses)
Haemophilus influenzae b	Conjugated polysaccharide	IM	Two to three doses, 2 months apart	Single dose
Influenza	Killed virus	IM	Single dose	Yearly
Pneumococcal	23-valent polysaccharide	IM/SC	Single dose	Repeat in those at high risk
Pneumococcal	7-valent conjugate polysaccharide	IM/SC	Three doses at 2, 4, and 13 months (not licensed for adults)	Repeat in those at high risk
Travel				
Hepatitis A[a]	Killed virus	IM	Two doses, 6–12 months apart	Probably not required
Hepatitis B	Adsorbed	IM[b]	Three doses at 0, 1, and 6 months	Single booster at 5 years (may not be required)
Japanese B encephalitis	Killed virus	SC	Three doses on days 0, 7, and 28	One year, then every 4 years
Meningococcal	Polysaccharide types A, C, W135, Y	IM/SC	Single dose	Every 3–5 years
Rabies	Killed virus	IM[b]/ID[b,c] 0.1 ml	Three doses on days 0, 7, and 28	Once, after 1–2 years
Tick-borne encephalitis	Killed virus	IM	Two doses 4 weeks apart, then at 9–12 months	Every 3 years
Tuberculosis: BCG	Attenuated	ID	Single dose	None
Cholera	Inactivated O1 strain plus recombinant B toxin subunit	PO	Two doses 1 week apart	6 months
Typhoid	Live Ty21a strain (attenuated)	PO	Three doses on alternate days	Every 5 years
Typhoid[a]	Capsular Vi polysaccharide	IM	Single dose	Every 3 years
Yellow fever	Live virus (attenuated)	SC	Single dose	Every 10 years

ID, intradermal; IM, intramuscular; PO, oral; SC, subcutaneous.

[a] Combined hepatitis A and typhoid vaccines are available.

[b] Should not be given into the buttock; deltoid or anterior thigh preferred. Double the dose for immunocompromised patients, or those on dialysis.

[c] Efficacy reduced if given with chloroquine antimalarial prophylaxis.

communities of Western countries travel to visit their friends and relatives abroad; such travellers are less likely to seek pretravel advice, and yet may be more vulnerable to endemic diseases in the tropics because of the living conditions at their destination.

At the pretravel clinic, the clinician elicits details about the proposed journey and the individual traveller's health and requirements. Such discussions allow a proper risk assessment to be made, so that advice and immunizations can be appropriately tailored. Issues that should be considered include general health advice, an assessment of the problems posed by different climates or environments, and the route, type, and duration of travel. Specific advice will include details of the necessary immunizations, and protection against malaria and other relevant diseases. It is important to discuss what might be done if the traveller were to fall ill while abroad or become unwell after their return. Travellers should be encouraged to take out generous and specific travel and health insurance including cost of repatriation in case of serious illness or accident.

General advice about health

First-aid kit

Travellers should carry a basic first-aid kit that should include a topical antiseptic solution; bandages; plasters; proprietary drugs for pain relief, diarrhoea, constipation, dyspepsia, allergy, and itch; sunscreen preparations; water purification tablets; and insect repellents.

Motion sickness

Antiemetic drugs such as cyclizine are effective, but they may cause sedation and a dry mouth. Long-acting transdermal skin patches containing scopolamine or antiemetics that can be absorbed through the buccal mucosa are preferable.

Air travel and jet lag

Long-haul air flights lead to jet lag: sleep disturbance, fatigue, a feeling of lightheadedness and unreality, and poor concentration. These symptoms may be attributable to a hangover if excessive alcohol has been drunk on the flight. A short-acting benzodiazepine such as temazepam, taken for the first couple of nights after flying, helps to re-establish a regular sleeping pattern. Some travellers have found that melatonin is helpful (Chapter 13.13), but obtaining products with the active ingredient can be a problem. The appropriate timing of exposure to daylight and meals can speed up the adjustment of circadian rhythms. People with diabetes may need advice on adjusting their insulin regimen or diet for changes in time zones, as may patients taking other regular medications. The closed recirculation of cabin air can spread respiratory pathogens. The risk of deep vein thrombosis from prolonged immobility and dehydration can be reduced by wearing tailored elastic stockings, moving about as much as possible, and frequently drinking water.

Regular medications

Patients with chronic illnesses such as diabetes or asthma should take plenty of their current medications, as these may not be available abroad. It is a good idea to divide the supplies among several bags in case one is lost or stolen. Patients should carry a letter from their physician outlining the condition and itemizing the medications to be carried.

Food and water hygiene

Strict food and water hygiene are important in countries with relatively poor sanitation. 'Boil it, peel it, or forget it' is a useful adage for the traveller, but is sometimes difficult to implement without causing offence when receiving hospitality. Water purification tablets and many types of portable water filters are available. Beverages made with boiled water are generally safe, whereas bottled water and especially ice cubes are unreliable. Treated water should always be used, even for tooth cleaning and washing fruit.

Climatic and environmental extremes

Sun and heat

Travellers should be reminded of the risks of sun exposure, and encouraged to dress and behave appropriately, and to use sunscreen. They must keep adequately hydrated and be aware of the risk of heatstroke. Several days of relative inactivity are needed to acclimatize safely to hot climates.

Swimming

Apart from the risk of drowning (Chapter 9.5.3), swimmers and bathers can be exposed to waterborne diseases such as schistosomiasis and leptospirosis in fresh water, together with the possibility of ingesting water and contracting gastrointestinal illnesses, even in swimming pools. Generally, swimming in chlorinated water is to be preferred. Schistosomiasis (bilharzia) occurs in Africa (including Madagascar), the Middle East, eastern South America, China and South-East Asia (Fig. 7.11.1). Infection is acquired by both bathing and washing with fresh water in lakes and sluggish rivers. Many United Kingdom cases are from scuba-diving schools in Lake Malawi, which has been declared 'bilharzia-free'. Travellers usually present weeks or months later with haematuria and, rarely, ascending flaccid paralysis.

Vector-borne diseases

Travellers should be warned about the risk of diseases transmitted by the bites of mosquitoes (e.g. malaria, dengue fever, chikungunya, Japanese encephalitis) and ticks (e.g. tick-borne encephalitis, Lyme disease, rickettsioses) and advised how to avoid bites.

High altitude

At high altitudes, snow blindness and severe sunburn can occur under clear skies, even at very low ambient temperatures. Those going to high altitudes should acclimatize slowly and build up their level of physical activity gradually (see Chapter 9.5.4). They should be aware of the symptoms and signs of altitude sickness. Acetazolamide in an adult dose of 250 mg twice a day, starting 12 h before starting the ascent, is effective prophylaxis for mild mountain sickness, especially if the traveller has to ascend rapidly (e.g. flying from sea level to more than 3 000 m). But gradual ascent allowing acclimatization is preferable, and if severe symptoms develop there is no substitute for rapid descent. In the tropics, heat, dehydration, and salt depletion may cause problems.

Blood-borne and parenteral infections

In many developing countries, blood-borne pathogens such as hepatitis B and C viruses, HIV, human T-cell leukaemia/lymphoma virus type 1, and, in some areas, malaria, trypanosomiasis, and other infections are prevalent. Screening of donated blood may not be rigorous, and needles are commonly reused, sometimes without adequate sterilization. As a result, travellers have been advised to take AIDS kits, usually containing needles, cannulas, intravenous giving sets, syringes, and artificial plasma expanders. These are too bulky and expensive for most travellers, but it is worth taking a few 21-gauge needles and 10-ml syringes in case blood must be taken for a laboratory test, or an injectable drug is needed. A covering letter from a doctor may allay the suspicion of customs officials that they are to be used for drug abuse.

Sexually transmitted infections

Surveys indicate that 4 to 19% of travellers have casual sex while abroad, and that these acts are unprotected on 50% of occasions. One result is about 7 new cases of HIV per 100 000 travellers per year. For United Kingdom residents, the risk of acquiring HIV is 300 times greater while travelling abroad than at home. Between 14 and 25% of cases of gonorrhoea and syphilis diagnosed in Europe are imported. Travellers are clearly more likely than usual to engage in unprotected sexual activity, especially when disinhibited by alcohol or other recreational drugs. Since sexually transmitted diseases, including HIV, are highly prevalent in many holiday resorts (not only in prostitutes), good-quality condoms, often not available when travelling, should be carried and used. Pretravel advice should include a discussion of the risks of unsafe sex.

Immunizations

Childhood vaccinations

The traveller's record of childhood immunizations should be reviewed (Chapter 7.3). Many adults will require booster doses for tetanus, polio, and diphtheria and may not have been adequately immunized against measles or mumps. Over the past few years, outbreaks of mumps and measles have occurred in many countries.

Since 1990 there has been an epidemic of diphtheria in the newly independent states of the former USSR. There were more than 150 000 cases and 5000 deaths reported from these states until 1998, but since then, widespread immunization campaigns have largely controlled the epidemic, although cases of diphtheria continue to be reported rarely in tourists and travellers to this region.

Previous travel immunizations should be noted, so that they are neither repeated unnecessarily nor allowed to lapse.

Hepatitis A

The incidence of hepatitis A in developing countries ranges from 300 to 2000 cases per 100 000 unprotected travellers per month of stay. Active immunization is safe, effective, and durable. Those who have received a full course of immunization will probably not need any further boosting doses (see Chapter 7.3).

Hepatitis B

This is a risk to medical or laboratory staff whose work involves contact with human blood and to those staying for prolonged periods, such that there is a possibility of receiving unscreened blood transfusions (see Chapter 15.21). It is also a risk of unprotected sexual activity. Vaccination in these circumstances is sensible.

Yellow fever

This is the only vaccination for which an internationally valid certificate is statutorily required for entry into countries where the disease is endemic, and for travellers returning from those places. Yellow fever is only endemic in tropical Africa and South America, not in Asia (see Fig. 7.5.14.4). Recently, there have been outbreaks of the disease in South America (Brazil, Ecuador, Peru, Bolivia, Argentina, Paraguay) and sub-Saharan Africa (Liberia, Togo, Cameroon, Central African Republic, Sudan). There have been worrying reports of adverse events associated with yellow fever vaccine, particularly in older people. Such reactions may be more common in those with thymic dysfunction or with other types of immune defect.

Cholera

Vaccination is no longer required by international regulations. Earlier vaccines were of little use, and although there is now a licensed oral vaccine, it is really only necessary for those, like aid workers in refugee camps, who have a high risk of exposure.

Typhoid

This potentially serious infection remains prevalent in Pakistan, India, Bangladesh, Indonesia, and Nepal, where the incidence of infection is approximately 1 in 3000 per month of stay. Those staying for long periods in rural areas, and especially those visiting friends and relatives abroad, are at greatest need of vaccination.

Meningococcal disease

In the meningitis belt of sub-Sahelian Africa (see Fig. 7.6.5.3), from Senegal to Sudan, and in some other areas, cool, dry-season meningococcal meningitis outbreaks are so predictable that immunization is recommended. The quadrivalent meningococcal vaccine (covering serogroups A, C, W135, and Y) is recommended. The new conjugate vaccine is very promising. Following outbreaks associated with the Hajj over the past few years, pilgrims to Mecca are required to be immunized and provide proof.

Rabies

Pre-exposure rabies vaccination is increasingly being used (see Chapter 7.5.10). Although the risk of transmission is fairly low, the lack of effective treatment for rabies encephalitis, and the fear engendered by a dog bite, and in many parts of the world, bat bites, justifies considering immunization.

Other encephalitides

Vaccination against Japanese encephalitis (see Fig. 7.5.14.2) and tick-borne encephalitis (see Fig. 7.5.14.5) may be considered after reviewing the travel itinerary and risk of exposure (Table 7.4.1).

Prevention of malaria

Both travellers and nonspecialist physicians must be educated about the prevention and recognition of malaria (see Chapter 7.8.2). It is important to be aware of the need to prevent mosquito bites by all possible means: wearing appropriate clothing, application of insect repellents to exposed skin and clothing, and the use of insecticide-impregnated bed nets and insecticide sprays or vaporizers in the sleeping quarters. Guidelines for antimalarial chemoprophylaxis are regularly updated (see 'Further reading: internet sites' below).

Prevention and management of travellers' diarrhoea

Box 7.4.1 Some causes of travellers' diarrhoea

Bacteria

Enterotoxigenic *Escherichia coli* (*c.*20–30%)

Aeromonas spp., *Plesiomonas* spp.

Campylobacter jejuni

Salmonella typhi

Other *Salmonella* spp.

Shigella spp.

Vibrio parahaemolyticus

Protozoa

Cryptosporidium parvum

Cyclospora cayetanensis

Entamoeba histolytica

Giardia lamblia

Plasmodium falciparum

Other

Rotavirus/norovirus

Schistosoma mansoni

Strongyloides stercoralis

Irritable and inflammatory bowel disease

Tropical sprue

Drug side effects,

Clostridium difficile toxin, fish/shellfish toxins

Diarrhoea is the most common health problem of travellers. Symptoms are usually mild, lasting only about 3 to 5 days, but holiday and business plans may be disrupted. The most common cause is enterotoxigenic *Escherichia coli* (ETEC). *Salmonella* spp., *Campylobacter* spp., *Shigella* spp., and other pathogenic *E. coli* are also common. Protozoan pathogens, such as *Giardia lamblia, Entamoeba histolytica, Cryptosporidium parvum, Cyclospora cayetanensis* and viruses are less common causes. Fish and shellfish poisoning cause similar symptoms, starting within minutes or hours of exposure (Chapter 9.2).

Strict food and water hygiene reduce the risk of gastroenteritis. Heating water to 100 °C will kill most pathogens, as will chemical treatment with chlorine or iodine (iodine is contraindicated in pregnant women and some patients with thyroid disease). Water filters are also effective. Antimicrobials such as trimethoprim–sulfamethoxazole, doxycycline, and the fluoroquinolones are protective to some extent, but are not cheap, may cause side effects, cannot be taken for prolonged periods, and may encourage antimicrobial resistance. Colloidal bismuth salts are cheaper, safer, and reasonably effective, but the large volumes are inconvenient. Vaccines against ETEC are in development.

Treatment involves maintaining an adequate fluid intake and using sachets of oral rehydration salts that can be made up with boiled water. Eating solid food may stimulate bowel action by the gastrocolic reflex. Antidiarrhoeal agents such as codeine phosphate and loperamide often relieve symptoms sufficiently to allow normal activities to continue. Short courses of empirical antimicrobials, e.g. ciprofloxacin (500 mg for 3 days, adults only), can be useful, particularly for patients with underlying diseases. Localized abdominal pain, high fever, and bloody diarrhoea are indications for seeking medical help immediately.

Special groups of travellers

Immunocompromised travellers

Except for asplenic patients, immunocompromised travellers—including those who have recently received chemotherapy or radiotherapy—should not be given live vaccines such as yellow fever, oral polio, and oral typhoid. Killed or synthetic vaccines are safe. Those patients with mild to moderate immune suppression will probably make a reasonable response to immunization; those with more severe immunosuppression may still make a useful, though less durable, response. Influenza, pneumococcal, and *Haemophilus influenzae* b conjugate vaccines are recommended, as these patients' risk of respiratory infection and bacteraemia is increased. Studies show that immunosuppressed patients can make a response to hepatitis A immunizations, although the durability of this response is again uncertain. People with HIV will often make a good response if they are on antiretroviral medication and have made a good CD4 response. Asplenic individuals should be on prophylactic antibiotics, such as amoxicillin, particularly if travelling, and should be dissuaded from travelling to areas with high rates of malaria transmission, as they are more likely to get severe disease if infected.

Immunocompromised patients should carry antimicrobials with them for treating respiratory or gastrointestinal infections, should seek medical help when abroad, and should carry a letter from their physician outlining their condition and medication.

Pregnant travellers

Commercial airlines will not normally convey a woman who is 36 weeks or more pregnant, without a covering letter from her physician. Insurance to cover the cost of delivery abroad should be considered. If possible, pregnant women should avoid travelling to areas where diseases are prevalent that pose a special risk in their condition, such as malaria and viral hepatitis E.

The risk–benefit assessment of immunizations and chemoprophylaxis is of particular importance for the pregnant woman and the fetus. Live vaccines should be avoided, but if there is a genuine risk of yellow fever the vaccine should be given, as there is no recognized associated teratogenicity. Inactivated polio vaccine may be given parenterally, and tetanus immunization is safe. Heat-killed typhoid vaccine is best avoided, as it might cause a febrile reaction and stimulate premature labour. However, the modern polysaccharide capsular Vi vaccine should be safe. Pneumococcal, meningococcal, and hepatitis B vaccines are safe in pregnancy, as is gamma globulin.

Malaria is especially dangerous in pregnant women (see Chapter 7.8.2). Chloroquine and proguanil are safe prophylactic drugs, and quinine in normal therapeutic doses is safe for treatment. Mefloquine is best avoided in the first trimester of pregnancy. Pregnant women should take special care with food and drink when abroad, as dehydration may threaten the fetus. There are concerns about congenital goitre when pregnant women use iodine to purify water; the maximum recommended daily intake is 175 µg. Loperamide as an antidiarrhoeal agent is safe, but antimicrobials such as tetracyclines and quinolones should be avoided.

Extremes of age

Young children should have completed their routine immunizations before travelling. Malaria chemoprophylaxis is recommended for all ages. Yellow fever vaccine should be given only to children older than 9 months, as a few cases of vaccine-associated encephalitis have occurred in younger children. Most other vaccines, including rabies, are safe. Hepatitis A is rarely symptomatic in children under 5 years old. Families planning to live in developing countries should be offered BCG vaccination for their children to reduce the risk of tuberculous meningitis.

Older people should have the same immunizations as younger adults, and should take antimalarial drugs. They are more prone to respiratory infection, and should therefore be given influenza, pneumococcal, and *Haemophilus influenzae* vaccines. Jet lag and changes in time zones may be very disturbing. Older people are more likely to have an underlying medical condition requiring medication; it is important that sufficient supplies of medicines are taken abroad and that the patient has a detailed list of these medicines and their dosages in case the tablets are lost or stolen. They should carry the name and contact address of their home physician, in case of emergency.

Explorers and expeditions

Because of their adventurous aims, expeditions are likely to involve exposure to greater environmental extremes and hazards than ordinary travel. Expeditions usually take place in areas remote from even rural health centres, and so a greater responsibility for dealing with medical problems will devolve to the expedition members. The explorer's greatest fear may be to fall victim to a lethal tropical disease or an attack by a wild animal, but the reality is much more mundane: road traffic accidents, mountaineering disasters, drowning, and attacks by humans claim most lives.

Table 7.4.2 Causes of fever in returned travellers

Tropical infections	Other infections	Noninfective causes
Short incubation; <3 weeks	Endocarditis	Connective tissue disease
African trypanosomiasis	Pneumonia	Drug reaction
Brucellosis	Prostatitis	Factitious inflammatory bowel disease
Dengue fever	Sexually transmitted disease	
Haemorrhagic fevers (e.g. Lassa)	Sinusitis	Malignancy
Hepatitis A	Urinary tract infection	
Malaria		
Relapsing fevers		
Tick/scrub typhus		
Typhoid		
Leptospirosis		
Malaria		
Long incubation; >3 weeks		
Amoebic abscess		
Brucellosis		
Coccidiomycosis		
Filariasis		
Hepatitis A, B, or C		
HIV (?incubation)		
Leishmaniasis		
Malaria		
Schistosomiasis (Katayama fever)		
Tuberculosis		
Typhoid		

The prevention and treatment of medical problems must be planned well in advance. Detailed advice and information can be obtained from a number of organizations, such as the Expedition Advisory Centre (Geography Outdoors) of the Royal Geographical Society in London, from clubs specializing in mountaineering, cave exploring, diving, and other activities, and from books, journals, and websites. All expeditions should have a designated medical officer, and all their members should receive first-aid training aimed at the particular needs of the expedition. The basics are clearing the airway, controlling bleeding, treating shock, relieving pain, and moving the injured person without causing further damage. Expedition medical kits should be more comprehensive than those carried by ordinary tourists and travellers. Lists of essential drugs are given in Johnson *et al.* (2008). Scissors, a generous supply of large triangular and crêpe bandages, adhesive plasters, and an AIDS kit (to reduce the risk of infection from dirty needles and intravenous fluids) are important. Lightweight emergency insulation must be taken if there is any risk of exposure in severe weather conditions; a lightweight collapsible stretcher should be taken for mountaineering, and an adequate water supply must be assured or taken if the expedition is into desert areas.

A covering letter on official notepaper, signed by a doctor, may be helpful in allowing drugs, even apparently innocuous ones such as codeine, through customs (e.g. the Russian Federation) and explaining the need for needles and syringes. The medical facilities nearest to the site of the expedition must be identified and contacted in advance. An emergency plan must be drawn up for the first-aid treatment and evacuation of severely ill or injured expedition members. In some areas, flying doctor and air evacuation services (such as AMREF in East Africa) are available. Medical insurance must be generous and comprehensive, and include repatriation of the injured. Before leaving their home country, expedition members should have a thorough dental check and treatment for any outstanding medical or surgical problems. Control of chronic medical problems such as diabetes mellitus, hypertension, and asthma should be stabilized. In selecting members for an expedition, the most important attributes are experience, possession of the necessary technical skills (e.g. diving and mountaineering), physical fitness, and proven psychological stability under stress. It is advisable always to appoint a reliable local agent in the country where the expedition will take place.

Illness in returning travellers

Details are needed about the countries visited, the activities undertaken while travelling, immunizations, and antimalarials taken. Common problems are fever, rash, diarrhoea, and eosinophilia (Tables 7.4.2 and 7.4.3, and Box 7.4.2).

The most important diagnosis to exclude in a traveller from the tropics with a fever is malaria. In travellers with acute diarrhoea, a dietary history, assessment of hydration state, stool microscopy and culture, abdominal films, and sigmoidoscopy may be needed. There are many possible causes (see Box 7.4.1). Patients with chronic diarrhoea may be infected with *Giardia* spp., *Cryptosporidium* spp., *Entamoeba histolytica*, shigellae, or salmonellae. Investigations should include a search for *Clostridium difficile* and its toxin, especially if the patient took antimicrobials while abroad. A minority of patients may develop postinfective enteropathy, the most common problem being

Table 7.4.3 Causes of rash in returning travellers

Infective	Non-infective
Cutaneous larva migrans; myiasis	Contact allergy
Cutaneous leishmaniasis	Drug reaction
Dengue fever	Erythema multiforme
Dermatophytes	Insect bites
Lyme disease	Sunburn
Meningococcal illness	
Mycobacteria	
Scabies/lice	
Sexually transmitted infections	
Tick/scrub typhus	
Tinea versicolor	
Typhoid/paratyphoid	

Box 7.4.2 Infective causes of eosinophilia in travellers

Angiostrongylus spp.
Ascaris spp.
Echinococcus spp.
Filariasis (onchocerciasis)
Gnathostoma spp.
Hookworm and other gut nematodes
Pulmonary eosinophilia
Schistosomiasis
Strongyloides spp.
Trichinosis
Trichuris spp.
Visceral larva migrans

secondary lactose intolerance. Rarely, bacterial overgrowth or tropical sprue develops.

The most common causes of eosinophilia are allergy, drug reactions, and helminths (Box 7.4.2).

Further reading

Auerbach PS (ed) (2007). *Wilderness medicine*, 5th edition. Mosby Elsevier, Philadelphia.

Backer HD, *et al.* (eds) (1998). *Wilderness first aid: emergency care for remote locations.* Jones and Barlett, Boston.

Barwick R (2004). History of thymoma and yellow fever vaccination. *Lancet*, **364**, 936.

Conlon CP (2001). The immunocompromised traveler. In: DuPont HL, Steffen R (eds) *Textbook of travel medicine and health*, 2nd edition. BC Becker, London.

Dawood R (2002). *Travellers' health: how to stay healthy abroad.* Oxford University Press, Oxford.

Forgey WW (2000). *Wilderness medicine: beyond first aid*, 5th edition. Globe Pequot Press, Guilford, Connecticut.

Hill DR, Ford L, Lalloo DG (2006). Oral cholera vaccines: use in clinical practice. *Lancet Infect Dis*, **6**, 361–72.

Johnson C, *et al.* (eds) (2008). *Oxford handbook of expedition and wilderness medicine.* Oxford University Press, Oxford.

Johnston V *et al.* (2009). Fever in returned travellers presenting in the United Kingdom: recommendations for investigation and initial management. *J Infect.* **59**, 1–18.

McMahon AW, *et al.* (2007). Neurologic disease associated with 17D-204 yellow fever vaccination: a report of 15 cases. *Vaccine*, **25**, 1727–34.

Martin M, *et al.* (2001). Fever and multisystem organ failure associated with 17D-204 yellow fever vaccination: a report of four cases. *Lancet*, **358**, 98–104.

Monath TP, Modlin JF (2002). Prevention of yellow fever in persons traveling to the tropics. *Clin Infect Dis*, **34**, 1369–78.

Potter SA (ed.) (1992). *ANARE Antarctic field manual*, 4th edition. Australian Antarctic Division, Kingston, Tasmania.

Steedman DJ (1994). *Environmental medical emergencies.* Oxford University Press, Oxford.

The Voluntary Aid Societies, St. John Ambulance, St. Andrew's Ambulance Associate and the British Red Cross (2006). *First aid manual.* Dorling Kindersley, London.

Ward MP, Milledge JS, West JB (2000). *High altitude medicine and physiology*, 3rd ed. Arnold, London.

Wilderness & Environmantal Medicine (formerly Journal of Wilderness Medicine) (1990–). Published for the Wilderness Medical Society by Chapman and Hall Medical, London.

Zuckerman JN, Connor BA, von Sonnenburg F (2005). *Hepatitis A and B booster recommendations: implications for travelers. Clin Infect Dis*, **41**, 1020–26.

Websites

General travel advice

Centers for Disease Control and Prevention. *Travelers' Health.* http://wwwn.cdc.gov/travel/

Health Protection Agency. http://www.hpa.org.uk/ http://www.hpa.org.uk/HPA/Topics/InfectiousDiseases/InfectionsAZ/1191942149486/

National Travel Health Network and Centre (NaTHNaC). *Protecting the Health of British Travellers.* http://www.nathnac.org

National Travel Health Network and Centre. *The Yellow Book.* http://www.nathnac.org/yellow_book/01.htm

Royal Geographical Society, Expedition Advisory Centre. http://www.rgs.org/OurWork/Fieldwork+and+Expeditions/Specialist+Advice/Medical+Cell/Expedition+Medical+Cell.htm

The International Society of Travel Medicine. http://www.istm.org

World Health Organization. *International Travel and Health.* http://www.who.int/ith/

Malaria

Centers for Disease Control and Prevention. *Malaria.* http://www.cdc.gov/malaria/index.htm

Health Protection Agency. *Malaria.* http://www.hpa.org.uk/webw/HPAweb&Page&HPAwebAutoListName/Page/1191942128239?p=1191942128239

World Health Organization (2006). *Guidelines for the treatment of malaria.* http://www.who.int/malaria/docs/TreatmentGuidelines2006.pdf

7.5

Viruses

Contents

7.5.1 **Respiratory tract viruses** *473*
Malik Peiris

7.5.2 **Herpesviruses (excluding Epstein–Barr virus)** *482*
J.G.P. Sissons

7.5.3 **Epstein–Barr virus** *501*
M.A. Epstein and A.B. Rickinson

7.5.4 **Poxviruses** *508*
Geoffrey L. Smith

7.5.5 **Mumps: epidemic parotitis** *513*
B.K. Rima

7.5.6 **Measles** *515*
H.C. Whittle and P. Aaby

7.5.7 **Nipah and Hendra virus encephalitides** *525*
C.T. Tan

7.5.8 **Enterovirus infections** *527*
Philip Minor and Ulrich Desselberger

7.5.9 **Virus infections causing diarrhoea and vomiting** *536*
Philip Dormitzer and Ulrich Desselberger

7.5.10 **Rhabdoviruses: rabies and rabies-related lyssaviruses** *541*
M.J. Warrell and David A. Warrell

7.5.11 **Colorado tick fever and other arthropod-borne reoviruses** *555*
M.J. Warrell and David A. Warrell

7.5.12 **Alphaviruses** *557*
L.R. Petersen and D.J. Gubler

7.5.13 **Rubella** *561*
P.A. Tookey and J.M. Best

7.5.14 **Flaviviruses excluding dengue** *564*
L.R. Petersen and D.J. Gubler

7.5.15 **Dengue** *575*
Bridget Wills and Jeremy Farrar

7.5.16 **Bunyaviridae** *579*
J.W. LeDuc and Summerpal S. Kahlon

7.5.17 **Arenaviruses** *588*
J. ter Meulen

7.5.18 **Filoviruses** *595*
J. ter Meulen

7.5.19 **Papillomaviruses and polyomaviruses** *600*
Raphael P. Viscidi and Keerti V. Shah

7.5.20 **Parvovirus B19** *607*
Kevin E. Brown

7.5.21 **Hepatitis viruses (excluding hepatitis C virus)** *609*
N.V. Naoumov

7.5.22 **Hepatitis C** *615*
Paul Klenerman, K.J.M. Jeffery, and J. Collier

7.5.23 **HIV/AIDS** *620*
Graz A. Luzzi, T.E.A. Peto, P. Goulder, and C.P. Conlon

7.5.24 **HIV in the developing world** *644*
Alison D. Grant and Kevin M. De Cock

7.5.25 **HTLV-1, HTLV-2, and associated diseases** *650*
Kristien Verdonck and Eduardo Gotuzzo

7.5.26 **Viruses and cancer** *653*
R.A. Weiss

7.5.27 **Orf** *655*
David A. Warrell

7.5.28 **Molluscum contagiosum** *657*
David A. Warrell

7.5.29 **Newly discovered viruses** *659*
H.C. Hughes

7.5.1 Respiratory tract viruses

Malik Peiris

Essentials

Viral respiratory infections, including rhinovirus, coronavirus, adenovirus, respiratory syncytial virus, human metapneumovirus, parainfluenza viruses, and influenza viruses, are a substantial cause of morbidity worldwide. Transmission occurs through direct contact, contaminated fomites, and large airborne droplets, with long-range transmission by small particle aerosols reported in at least some instances of influenza and severe acute respiratory syndrome (SARS).

Clinical syndromes affect the upper and/or lower respiratory tract, including coryza, pharyngitis, croup, bronchiolitis, and pneumonia. Each syndrome can potentially be caused by a number of viruses, and each respiratory virus can be associated with different clinical syndromes. Measles is a major cause of lower respiratory tract infections and fatality in tropical countries.

Diagnosis—nasopharyngeal aspirates, washes and swabs are superior to throat and nose swabs for diagnosis, with virus detected by culture or detection of antigen or nucleic acid (e.g. PCR-based methods). New respiratory viruses continue to be discovered, but some acute respiratory infections have no identifiable aetiology, and some patients have multiple respiratory viruses detectable in the respiratory tract in association with their disease—whether these have a synergistic role in pathogenesis remains unclear.

Particular respiratory tract viruses

Influenza—types A and B are clinically important causes of human disease; the viral envelope contains two glycoproteins, haemagglutinin (H) and neuraminidase (N), which are critical in host immunity and used to designate viral subtype, e.g. H1N1. Potential to cause pandemics makes influenza a unique challenge for global public health. Typically causes an illness associated with fever, chills, headache, sore throat, coryza, nonproductive cough, myalgia, and sometimes prostration. Can cause pneumonia directly or by secondary bacterial infections. Oseltamivir and zanamivir result in a reduction of 1 to 2 days in the time to alleviation of symptoms when administered within the first 48 h of illness, but recent emergence of resistance to antivirals is a cause for concern. Can be prevented by influenza vaccine, which contains antigens from the two subtypes of human influenza A (H3N2 and H1N1) and B viruses, but the composition of the vaccine must be updated on an annual basis to keep abreast of change in the surface antigens of the virus, and annual reimmunization is required. Synergic interaction with *Streptococcus pneumoniae* enhances pathogenesis, and pneumococcal conjugate vaccine reduces hospitalization associated with respiratory viruses.

Respiratory syncytial virus (RSV)—a major cause of bronchiolitis and pneumonia in infants. Infection in adults is often asymptomatic, but during the RSV season (winter months) it is an important cause of lower respiratory tract infection in adults, particularly elderly people. May be lethal (as can other respiratory viruses) in patients immunocompromised following organ or blood and marrow transplants (but is not a significant problem in patients with AIDS).

Severe acute respiratory syndrome (SARS)—this novel coronavirus of animals adapted to efficient human transmission and spread worldwide, causing a global outbreak in 2003 of an illness characterized by lower respiratory tract manifestations, severe respiratory failure, and death in about 10% of cases. Public health interventions interrupted viral transmission and it is no longer transmitting within humans, but the precursor virus remains in the animal reservoir (bats, *Rhinolophus* spp.) and may readapt to cause human disease in the future.

Introduction

Viral respiratory infections are one of the most common afflictions of humankind. They are the most frequent reasons for medical consultations, are believed to account for 30% of work absences and school absenteeism, and are a major reason for antibiotic prescriptions. Longitudinal family studies suggest that a person has on average 2.4 respiratory viral infections per year, a quarter of them leading to a medical consultation. The synergistic interaction between viruses and bacteria in pathogenesis are being increasingly recognized, for example that between influenza virus and *Streptococcus pneumoniae* and *Staphylococcus aureus*. With the exception of influenza in elderly people, these viral infections are not a major cause of mortality in otherwise healthy people in the developed world, but it is estimated that they contribute to over 1 million deaths annually in the developing world.

The term 'respiratory virus' is imprecise, but for the purpose of this discussion it will include those that have the respiratory tract as their primary site of clinically relevant pathology. Taxonomically, they belong to six virus families (Table 7.5.1.1) and are global in distribution. Other viruses cause systemic disease with respiratory tract involvement as part of an overall disseminated disease process in patients who are immunocompetent (e.g. measles, Hantavirus pulmonary syndrome) or immunocompromised (e.g. cytomegalovirus). These are dealt with elsewhere.

A respiratory virus may cause a range of clinical syndromes. Conversely, a respiratory syndrome may be caused by more than one virus. The major viral respiratory syndromes and their common aetiological agents are shown in Table 7.5.1.2. The pattern seen in tropical countries is similar, but a notable difference is the role of measles as a major cause of lower respiratory tract infections and fatality.

The anatomical demarcation between upper (URTI) and lower respiratory tract infections (LRTI) is the larynx. Influenza, respiratory syncytial virus, parainfluenza virus and adenoviruses are well-recognized causes of LRTI in adults as well as in children, although many other respiratory viruses may do so occasionally. Severe acute respiratory syndrome coronavirus (SARS CoV) and avian influenza H5N1 are unusual in that lower respiratory manifestations predominate over the involvement of the upper respiratory tract.

With newer molecular-based approaches to pathogen discovery, new respiratory viruses continue to be recognized. Some recently recognized viruses have been long endemic in humans (e.g. human metapneumovirus, coronavirus NL-63, HKU1, bocavirus) while others are novel pathogens, newly emergent as causes of human infections such as SARS and avian flu H5N1.

Table 7.5.1.1 Respiratory tract viruses: summary of classification, incubation period, duration of infectivity, and diagnostic options

Virus	Classification (virus family) and composition of virus	Subgroups, serotypes, and subtypes	Incubation period (days)	Duration of virus shedding in immunocompetent patients (days)	Options for laboratory diagnosis[a]
Rhinovirus	Picornaviridae Nonenveloped RNA viruses	>102 serotypes phylo-genetically divided into 3 groups A, B and C	1–2 days	5–6 days by culture; 50% remain positive by RT-PCR 2 weeks later	RT-PCR or viral culture (less sensitive)
Enterovirus	Picornaviridae Nonenveloped RNA viruses	65 serotypes	Few days	Up to 2 weeks from respiratory tract, much longer in faeces	RT-PCR. Viral culture less sensitive and not possible for some types unless animal inoculation is used.
Coronavirus	Coronaviridae. Enveloped RNA viruses	5 types (OC43, 229E, NL-63, HKU-1, SARS CoV	4–5 days	5–8 days	RT-PCR
Respiratory syncytial virus (RSV)	Paramyxoviridae Enveloped RNA virus	Subgroup A and B	5 days	6–7 days	Culture Rapid antigen detection,[a] RT-PCR Serology: useful in adults but less so in infants
Human metapneumovirus	Paramyxoviridae Enveloped RNA virus	Serotypes A and B	ND	ND	RT-PCR Viral antigen detection
Parainfluenza	Paramyxoviridae Enveloped RNA virus	Type 1, 2, 3, 4a, 4b	3–6 days	7 days	Culture Rapid antigen detection,[a] RT-PCR Serology: useful in adults but less so in infants
Influenza	Orthomyxoviridae Enveloped RNA virus	Types A, B, C Human influenza A subtypes currently in circulation are H1N1 and H3N2	Average 2–3 (range 1–7)	*c.*5 days in adults *c.*7 days in children	Culture Rapid antigen detection[2], RT-PCR Serology
Adenovirus	Adenoviridae Nonenveloped DNA virus	Subgroups A–F Types 1–51	Average 10 (range 2–15)	Days–weeks (from respiratory tract), weeks–months (in faeces)	Culture Rapid antigen detection,[a] RT-PCR, Serology
Bocavirus	Parvoviridae Nonenveloped DNA virus	One phylogenetic group	ND	ND	RT-PCR

ND, not defined.

[a] Best sensitivity from nasopharyngeal aspirates or nasopharyngeal swabs (in that order). Throat swabs give lower sensitivity.

Table 7.5.1.2 Viral aetiology of common respiratory syndromes

Virus	Coryza	Pharyngitis	Croup	Bronchiolitis	Pneumonia
Rhinovirus	+++[a]	++	+	+	Rare
Coronavirus	++	+	+ (NL-63)		SARS CoV, HKU-1
Adenoviruses	(+)	++	++	++	++ (all ages)
RSV	++	+	++	+++	+++ (children); + (elderly)
Human metapneumovirus	+	+	+	++	++ (children)
Parainfluenza 1	+	++	+++	+	
Parainfluenza 2	+	++	++	+	
Parainfluenza 3	+	++	++	++	++ (children)
Influenza A/B	+	++	++	+	++ (all ages)

[a] Frequency of cases caused by the virus: +++ the major cause (>25%); ++ a common cause (5–25%); + an occasional cause; blank, rare cause or not reported.

(Data adapted from Treanor 2009).

Transmission

The routes of respiratory virus transmission are through direct contact, contaminated fomites, and large airborne droplets (mean diameter >5 μm, range of transmission <1 m). There remains controversy over the potential for the spread of viruses such as influenza over longer distances by small particle aerosol (mean diameter <5 μm), but even here, large droplets, direct contact, and fomites are probably more important. Occasionally, SARS CoV appears to have spread by small particle aerosols, although droplets and fomites probably contributed to the major part of the transmission of this disease. Adenoviruses are transmitted by the faeco-oral route as well as by direct contact and large droplets.

Factors increasing transmission of respiratory viruses include the time of exposure, close contact (e.g. spouse, mother), crowding, family size, and lack of pre-existing immunity (including lack of breastfeeding). School-age children often introduce an infection into the family and the beginning of school term may affect transmission patterns in the community. Infected children shed higher titres of viruses than adults. The duration of virus excretion is shown in Table 7.5.1.1. Infectivity usually precedes the onset of clinical symptoms. Immunocompromised patients shed virus for a longer time.

Seasonality

Some respiratory viruses have a predictable seasonality, which varies regionally. For example, influenza A is a typically winter disease in temperate regions, a spring/summer disease in the subtropics (e.g. Hong Kong) and occurs all year round (e.g. Singapore) or predominantly in the rainy season (e.g. Thailand) in the tropics. The basis for such seasonality is unclear, but climatic factors such as high humidity and temperature may help virus survival in small particle aerosols or droplets, and on contaminated surfaces. Factors affecting population congregation such as commencement of school term and seasonal effects on social behaviour may also play a role.

Laboratory diagnosis

A well-collected specimen is the first and often most important determinant in successful laboratory diagnosis. Nasopharyngeal aspirates (secretions aspirated from the back of the nose into a mucus trap), nasopharyngeal washes, and nasopharyngeal swabs are superior to throat and nose swabs for the diagnosis of many respiratory viruses. They offer the advantage that rapid ('same day') diagnosis for a number of viruses is possible provided the appropriate methods are available. Swabs for viral culture are placed in viral transport medium immediately upon collection and kept cool (around 4°C) until processed. More invasive specimens such as endotracheal aspirates, bronchoalveolar lavage, or lung biopsy, when available, usually provide better information. However, the likely site of pathology must be kept in mind—the more invasive specimen is not always better.

Laboratory methods used for detecting a virus in clinical specimen/s are viral culture, antigen detection, and, more recently, nucleic acid detection (e.g. polymerase chain reaction (PCR)-based methods). The widespread use of molecular methods for viral detection has led to recognition that some viruses that are difficult to culture (e.g. coronaviruses and some rhinoviruses and enteroviruses) are found more often in patients with acute respiratory disease than previously recognized. Similarly, these methods have allowed the discovery of novel viruses associated with respiratory disease (e.g. coronaviruses NL-63, HKU1, bocavirus). They have also revealed that infection with multiple viruses is relatively common. These findings necessitate a reassessment of the clinical relevance of positive PCR results. Relevant questions include how commonly these viruses are detectable by these methods in age-matched healthy controls and how long viruses remain detectable after infection. It is important to understand the relevance of detection of multiple pathogens in a respiratory specimen. Are these viruses synergistic in pathogenesis or is one more important than another? Many of these questions remain to be resolved.

Demonstration of rising antibody titres in paired sera is used to diagnose some respiratory virus diseases, but serology is impracticable for others such as rhinoviruses where the large number of antigenically distinct serotypes have no common immunodominant antigen(s). However, adenoviruses and influenza viruses, though having many antigenic types or variants, have common antigen(s) and a single antigen can detect serological responses to many of them. IgM assays are not routinely available for diagnosis of respiratory viral diseases. Serology is also helpful in assessing the clinical relevance of a virus detected in a respiratory specimen (see above) by helping differentiating recent infection from more remote events.

'Near patient testing' is becoming a reality for some viruses (e.g. influenza, RSV) with availability of tests that can be performed in a general practice setting. These become more relevant with the greater availability of antiviral drugs.

Rhinoviruses

Rhinoviruses belong to the Picornavirus family and are adapted to replicate at temperatures of 33–35°C, as found in the external airways. Until recently, 102 serotypes of rhinoviruses were recognized phylogenetically clustered into two groups A and B. Recent studies have revealed at least one additional phylogenetic group (group C) and many more rhinovirus types. But only a few rhinovirus types will circulate in a region at any given time.

Epidemiology

Rhinoviruses remain one of the commonest infections of humans: 0.5 infections per person per year is a conservative estimate. Secondary attack rates in families may be around 50% overall and 70% in those who are antibody negative. They were thought to cause mainly mild community infections, but are being recognized increasingly as the commonest viral agent detected by RT-PCR in children hospitalized with acute respiratory illness. Many of these represent coinfections with other potential respiratory pathogens. As rhinoviruses are often detectable by RT-PCR for weeks after initial infection (50% remain positive at 2 weeks), the aetiological significance of this finding is unresolved and more studies with relevant control populations are needed.

Immunity

In experimental challenges, immunity is serotype specific. Homologous type specific protection lasts for at least 1 year and correlates with serum IgA, IgG, and secretory IgA antibody levels.

Pathogenesis

Viral replication occurs predominantly in the ciliated epithelial cells of the nasopharynx. The structure of the epithelium is preserved. Mucosal secretions associated with coryza appear to be due to the release of inflammatory mediators and neurogenic reflexes.

It was thought that the preference of the virus for a lower temperature for replication restricted it to the upper respiratory tract. However, this is not strictly true. The virus has been isolated from the lower respiratory tract (including bronchial brushings) and viral RNA has been demonstrated by *in situ* hybridization in bronchial epithelial cells. Rarely, the virus has been isolated post-mortem from lungs of immunocompromised patients.

Clinical manifestations

Rhinorrhoea, nasal obstruction, pharyngitis, and a cough are common features of rhinovirus infections. Fever and systemic symptoms are rare, but more common in the elderly in whom disease can be more severe. Rhinoviruses are a major cause of exacerbations of asthma and chronic obstructive respiratory disease in adults. Lower respiratory tract symptoms are uncommon in healthy young adults, but may occur in children (bronchiolitis), the immunocompromised, and the elderly. Rhinovirus infections associated with wheezing in the first 3 years of life is predictive of asthma in later childhood.

Treatment and prevention

There are no established antiviral drugs for treatment and management is symptomatic. Topical interferon-α prevents symptoms if given before onset of disease, but cannot be used for prophylaxis over prolonged periods because of side effects. Pleconaril is a viral capsid-binding agent that blocks viral attachment and uncoating and has had modest benefit in clinical trials, but concerns over side effects have prevented its licensing. Antibiotics are ineffective in preventing bacterial complications of the common cold. Mucopurulent discharges are part of the natural course of the common cold and are not an indication for antimicrobial treatment, unless it persists (e.g. >10 days). Given the large number of rhinovirus serotypes, vaccination is not an option.

Enteroviruses

Enteroviruses and rhinoviruses (see above) are genera within the family Picornaviridae. Enteroviruses have long been known as causes of central nervous system infections, myocarditis, or exanthema rather than as a respiratory pathogen, the latter role being assigned to rhinoviruses. As many enteroviruses fail to replicate in cell culture, the wider use of molecular diagnosis has revealed an increased role of enteroviruses in acute respiratory infections. Clinically, patients present with rhinitis, cough, fever, sore throat, or otitis media. There remains a need for studies of age-matched controls to better establish the clinical relevance of these molecular tests. In comparative studies done on the duration of shedding of enteroviruses and rhinoviruses, fewer enterovirus infected children continue to shed virus for longer than 2 weeks while 50% of rhinovirus infections do. This suggests that a positive enterovirus RT-PCR result in the respiratory tract is probably more likely to be clinically relevant than one for rhinovirus.

Coronaviruses

Five human coronaviruses are currently known, three of them being new viruses discovered since the SARS outbreak in 2003. Coronaviruses are taxonomically subdivided into three groups and the human coronaviruses 229E and NL-63 belong to group 1 while OC43, HKU1, and SARS CoV belong to group 2. There are no known human group 3 coronaviruses. Human coronaviruses OC43 and 229E have long been recognized as important causes of the common cold but coronaviruses cause a range of respiratory illnesses. SARS CoV is a newly emerged pathogen. Human coronaviruses are difficult to culture from clinical specimens and laboratory diagnosis largely relies on molecular methods.

Epidemiology

Infection with OC43 and 229E occur in early childhood and 85 to 100% of adults have antibody to both virus types. NL-63 has a similar epidemiology but less is presently known of HKU1. SARS CoV emerged from an animal reservoir, adapted to human transmission and caused a global outbreak in 2003 that affected 29 countries across 5 continents. However, determined public health interventions interrupted transmission of this virus and it is no longer transmitting within humans. However, the precursor virus remains in the animal reservoir (bats, *Rhinolophus* spp.) and these may at some future date, readapt to cause human disease.

Immunity

Volunteer reinfection studies with 229E show that 1 year after initial infection, protection from reinfection and illness following a challenge from the homologous virus is incomplete. Comparable data are not available for the newly recognized NL-63, HKU1, or SARS CoV.

Pathogenesis

In common with rhinoviruses, coronaviruses 229E induce little or no damage to the respiratory mucosa. The mucosal discharge is caused by the release of mediators from affected host cells. SARS CoV had a predilection to involve alveolar pneumocytes in the lower respiratory tract and consequently caused a severe viral pneumonia. Disease severity of SARS was markedly age related. Children had mild disease whereas those over 50 years had a poor prognosis. The basis for this age-related pathogenesis is unknown. The virus receptor for 229E is CD13, while both SARS CoV and NL-63 utilize the human ACE-2 molecule for virus entry.

Clinical findings

Coronaviruses 229E and OC43 typically cause URTI and the common cold but also cause a range of other respiratory manifestations and are significant pathogens in elderly people. NL-63 and HKU1 cause both upper and lower respiratory disease. NL-63 appears to be an important cause of croup, bronchiolitis, and pneumonia. HKU1 appears to be an important pathogen particularly in those with underlying respiratory complications.

SARS typically presented with lower respiratory tract manifestations and radiological changes with minimum involvement of the upper respiratory tract. Many patients had diarrhoea resulting from viral replication in the gastrointestinal tract. Overall case fatality was 9.6%. Terminal events were severe respiratory failure associated with acute respiratory distress syndrome (ARDS) and multiple organ failure. Autopsies showed diffuse alveolar damage corresponding to the clinical presentation of acute respiratory distress syndrome. Age, comorbidities, and viral load in the nasopharynx and serum during the first 5 days of illness correlated with an adverse prognosis.

Treatment and prevention

There are presently no clinically validated antiviral treatments for human coronaviruses disease, although a number of drugs have been documented to have *in vitro* activity against SARS CoV. A number of experimental vaccines were developed for SARS, but with its disappearance from the human population, the incentive to take these forward to human clinical trials and licensing has waned.

Adenoviruses

Currently there are 51 adenovirus types classified in six groups (A–F). Adenoviruses in subgroups A to D cause respiratory, ocular, hepatic, genitourinary, or gastrointestinal system disease in immunocompetent or immunocompromised individuals. Only respiratory diseases are considered here.

Productive replication and excretion of infectious virus can occur for a prolonged period (see below). In addition, adenoviruses can establish chronic persistence or 'latency', the virological basis and clinical significance of which is poorly understood.

Epidemiology

Adenovirus infections are common during childhood (usually serotypes 1, 2, 5 in early childhood, 3 and 7 during school years or later), but continue to occur throughout life. Reinfection with the same serotype occurs but is usually asymptomatic. Serotypes 1, 2, 5, and 6 are typically endemic, types 4 and 7 more typically associated with outbreaks, and type 3 can occur in either situation. Recently, adenovirus 14 has been spreading in the United States of America.

Clinical features

Adenovirus respiratory illness often leads to URTI with coryza and sore throat. Fever may last up to 2 weeks. The sore throat may be exudative and clinically difficult to differentiate from streptococcal infection. Adenoviral infection may present as pharyngoconjunctival fever. Otitis media is a complication in children. Unlike other respiratory viral infections, adenoviruses may be associated with elevated white blood cell counts (exceeding 15×10^9/litre), C-reactive protein, or ESR and thus more easily confused with bacterial diseases.

Though uncommon, pneumonia may occur sporadically or in epidemics (e.g. caused by serotypes 4 and 7), particularly in closed communities such as the military where stress and physical exertion may predispose to lower respiratory tract involvement. Community outbreaks of adenoviral pneumonia have been reported. Radiological appearance varies from diffuse to patchy interstitial infiltrates and pleural effusion may be present. Adenovirus type 7 pneumonia can lead to permanent lung damage, including bronchiectasis, bronchiolitis obliterans, and unilateral hyperlucent lung syndrome.

Adenoviral infection may disseminate and present as 'septic shock' in neonates. Manifestations in immunocompromised patients include hepatitis (especially in liver transplant recipients), colitis, and haemorrhagic cystitis (in renal and bone marrow transplant recipients) in addition to pneumonia. The serotypes associated with disease in these patients may differ from those typically found in the immunocompetent patient, and include the subgroup B2 serotypes 11, 34, and 35. With improving control of other common viral diseases of immunocompromised patients (e.g. cytomegalovirus), the role of adenovirus infections is being increasingly appreciated.

Isolation of an adenovirus from a clinical specimen presents a challenge in interpretation. Adenoviruses are excreted for a prolonged period after initial infection, especially, but not exclusively, from faeces. In children, one-third of patients shed viruses for longer than 1 month and 14% longer than 1 year. The clinical significance of a positive result depends on the specimen, the method, and the serotype. Isolation of viruses from the respiratory tract carries greater significance than that from faeces. Patients who have symptomatic adenoviral diseases have higher viral loads than those with asymptomatic carriage. Thus, a rapidly growing virus, a positive antigen detection test from a respiratory specimen (both reflecting higher virus load), or a detectable serological response all point to greater clinical significance.

Immunocompromised patients may be infected with unusual serotypes. The detection of the virus in the peripheral blood or in multiple body sites suggests greater clinical significance and is an indication that therapeutic intervention needs to be considered.

Treatment and prevention

Most adenoviral infections in immunocompetent patients are self-limited and require no specific therapy; however, some infections, especially but not exclusively in immunocompromised patients, are severe and life threatening. Ribavirin, vidarabine, cidofovir, and ganciclovir are active against adenoviruses *in vitro*. Although there are anecdotal reports of the therapeutic use of each of these drugs with variable success, on the basis of limited clinical studies cidofovir appears to be the antiviral of choice.

Live attenuated oral vaccines containing serotypes 4 and 7 (associated with outbreaks in military conscripts) are safe and effective, but not licensed for general use.

Respiratory syncytial virus

Respiratory syncytial virus (RSV) infects human and nonhuman primates and was first isolated from a chimpanzee with a 'cold'. The virus has two surface glycoproteins on its envelope (G and F) and the immune responses to them correlate with protection. Two subgroups (A and B) are recognized on the basis of antigenic differences of the G glycoprotein.

Epidemiology

Over two-thirds of infants acquire RSV infection during the first year of life. Of patients hospitalized with RSV disease, 75% are younger than 5 months. The peak of morbidity occurs around 2 to 4 months of age, a time when passive maternal antibodies protect against most other viral infections. Primary infection does not lead to solid immunity and reinfection is common. The first reinfection can still be associated with lower respiratory tract involvement. Subsequent reinfection occurs throughout life leading to asymptomatic or URTI. However, significant diseases may result in the immunocompromised or elderly.

Immunity

Both antibody and cell mediated immunity are important in protection. Antibody to the G protein prevents attachment of viruses to the cellular receptor, but immunity to the F protein is required to prevent cell to cell spread via fusion of virally infected cells. Cell mediated immunity is important in eliminating established viral infection.

Pathogenesis

The virus leads to a ballooning degeneration of the ciliated epithelial cells, lymphocytic infiltration, and necrosis of the epithelium. There is oedema and increased secretion from the mucous cells and the formation of plugs of mucous and cellular debris in the bronchioles. This results in obstruction and air trapping leading to collapse or over-distension of the distal alveoli. Cells throughout the respiratory tract are affected but the alveoli are spared unless there is RSV pneumonia. The pathogenesis of RSV bronchiolitis still remains controversial.

Severe RSV bronchiolitis is strongly associated with subsequent childhood asthma. RSV appears to promote type 1 hypersensitivity responses following subsequent exposure to unrelated antigens.

Clinical features

RSV infections of infants may lead to bronchiolitis and pneumonia. Bronchiolitis in infants is associated with expiratory wheeze, subcostal recession, hyperinflation of the chest, nasal flaring, and hypoxia with or without cyanosis. Fever is not prominent in one-half of the patients. Complete obstruction of a small airway leads to subsegmental atelectasis. Apnoea may occur (particularly in premature infants or in those <3 months of age) and may precede the development of bronchiolitis. Interstitial pneumonitis is uncommon but carries a bad prognosis. Otitis media is a common complication of RSV infection in children. Infants at highest risk from severe RSV disease are those <6 months, those with pre-existing congenital heart disease, chronic lung diseases (e.g. bronchopulmonary dysplasia), and those born premature.

Infection in adults is often asymptomatic or leads to URTI. However, during the RSV season, it is an important cause of LRTI in adults and elderly people and it is estimated to cause 2 to 9% of the hospitalizations and deaths associated with pneumonia in elderly individuals. Much of this morbidity is clinically indistinguishable from influenza.

RSV (as well as parainfluenza and influenza) infections in the immunocompromised patient can be life threatening. They usually occur during community outbreaks, but a significant proportion are nosocomially acquired. The disease typically commences as an URTI but may progress to involve the lower respiratory tract with more serious consequences. Factors that increase risk of disease progression appear to include bone marrow transplant recipients who acquire the infection in the period prior to engraftment and oncology patients with neutrophil counts less than 0.5×10^9/litre. Those immunocompromised by HIV appear to tolerate community acquired respiratory viruses better than oncology patients and transplant recipients.

Treatment and prevention

Ribavirin has activity against RSV *in vitro*. Administration of small particle aerosols via a mist tent, mask, oxygen hood, or ventilator has been recommended because it results in much higher concentrations in the respiratory tract than can be achieved by intravenous administration. There seems little therapeutic benefit of ribavirin therapy in RSV disease in immunocompetent children or adults. However, in patients at high risk for severe RSV disease such as adult bone marrow transplant recipients, an uncontrolled study of ribavirin together with intravenous immune globulin (selected batches with high neutralizing antibody titre) appeared to be beneficial when compared to historical controls. More information is required for deciding the best management strategy.

Monthly intravenous administration of a polyclonal immune globulin enriched in neutralizing antibodies to RSV (RespiGam) or a humanized monoclonal antibody to RSV (palivizumab) during the RSV season protects against disease of the lower respiratory tract and otitis media in children with pre-existing risk factors. Palivizumab appears to be more effective than RespiGam and there is less of a problem with fluid overload in children with chronic heart disease. High-titre RSV intravenous immunoglobulin by itself is ineffective in treatment of established RSV disease.

Candidate vaccines for RSV are undergoing clinical trials at present but none is yet available for routine use. Experience of early trials with inactivated RSV vaccines that led to enhanced RSV disease, rather than protection continues to haunt the field.

Parainfluenza virus

Parainfluenza viruses, despite their name, are not related to influenza viruses, and are more akin to respiratory syncytial virus with which they are classified (Table 7.5.1.1). They carry two envelope glycoproteins: HN containing both haemagglutinin and neuraminidase activity and F carrying fusion activity.

Epidemiology

The total impact on hospitalization of children by all four types of parainfluenza viruses taken together is similar to that of RSV but, in contrast to RSV, their impact is in later infancy and childhood. In temperate countries, parainfluenza virus type 3 occurs annually and infects two-thirds of all infants in their first year of life. Parainfluenza types 1 and 2 tend to occur in alternate years and infection is acquired more slowly over childhood. Reinfection with parainfluenza viruses occurs, but rarely leads to LRTI.

Pathogenesis

The virus is confined to the respiratory epithelial cells, macrophages, and dendritic cells within the respiratory tract. Dissemination is rarely documented even in immunocompromised patients.

Immunity

Reinfection with parainfluenza viruses continues throughout life. Presence of virus-specific IgE in nasopharyngeal secretions has been implicated in the development of parainfluenza croup or bronchiolitis.

Clinical features

Parainfluenza type 1 predominantly causes croup, while types 2 and 3 also cause bronchiolitis and pneumonia. Croup (or laryngotracheobronchitis) in children is associated with fever, hoarseness, and a barking cough and may progress to inspiratory stridor due to narrowing of the subglottic area of the trachea. The differential diagnosis is epiglottitis due to *Haemophilus influenzae* type b. Parainfluenza type 4 infection is less common, but causes bronchiolitis and pneumonia in children, often in those with underlying disease.

Reinfection in adults, when symptomatic, is a coryzal illness with hoarseness being prominent. Parainfluenza viruses (type 3 in particular) are significant causes of LRTI in adults when the virus is active in the community.

As with RSV, parainfluenza viruses cause problems in immunocompromised patients. Lower respiratory tract involvement is associated with wheezing, rales, dyspnoea, and diffuse interstitial infiltrates, and a fatal outcome in one-third of patients with allogenic bone marrow transplants. When pneumonia occurs, the histological appearance of the lung is that of a giant cell or an interstitial pneumonia.

Treatment and prevention

The need for specific antiviral therapy arises, particularly in the immunocompromised. Ribavirin is effective *in vitro* and was associated with a reduction of viral replication *in vivo* in anecdotal cases but there are no controlled trials documenting its clinical efficacy.

There are no options for prevention at present, either using vaccines or passive immunization. A live attenuated bovine-derived vaccine strain is currently undergoing clinical trials.

Human metapneumovirus

Human metapneumovirus (HMPV) belongs to the genus Metapneumovirus within the virus family Paramyxoviridae, subfamily Pneumovirinae. It closest known relative is the avian pneumovirus, an upper respiratory tract disease of turkeys and among human viruses is RSV which also belongs to the subfamily Pneumovirinae. It was first recognized in 2001 but is a virus that has circulated unrecognized in humans for many decades. There are at least two serotypes A and B which are antigenically distinct and appear to provide partial cross-protection.

Epidemiology

The virus is ubiquitous and most children have been infected with one or both serotypes by the age of 5 years. Symptomatic reinfection is common through life. Infection is commonest in the winter months in temperate regions and in late spring or summer in subtropical areas.

Clinical manifestations

HMPV is one of the common causes of hospitalization of children under 5 years of age and accounted for 12% of all LRTI hospitalization in one long-term study. However, the incidence in any given year may vary widely. The peak age for HMPV morbidity is between 6 and 12 months, which is later than that for RSV (2–4 months). Clinical features of HMPV are similar to that of RSV and range from URTI to bronchiolitis and pneumonia. In common with rhinovirus and RSV, HMPV appears to trigger exacerbations of asthma. Diarrhoea, vomiting, rash, febrile seizures, conjunctivitis, and otitis media have been reported. HMPV has on one occasion been isolated as the sole pathogen from the brain in a patient with encephalitis.

HMPV can cause respiratory disease in elderly or immunocompromised individuals, and those with underlying conditions at any age.

Since HMPV is difficult to grow *in vitro*, laboratory diagnosis is reliant on the detection of viral RNA in clinical specimens by molecular methods.

Treatment and prevention

There are currently no available vaccines. As with RSV, the F and G proteins are the main targets of the neutralizing antibody response and while the former is antigenically conserved, the latter is more variable. Thus the F protein has been the focus of vaccine development. Ribavirin has comparable *in vitro* activity against HMPV as against RSV but there is no clinical trial data that demonstrates therapeutic efficacy.

Influenza viruses

Influenza viruses contain a segmented RNA genome. Types A, B, and C are antigenically distinct; of these, types A and B are clinically important causes of human disease. The viral envelope contains two glycoproteins, the haemagglutinin (H) and neuraminidase (N) which are critical in host immunity. The M2 transmembrane protein is also found on the virion surface but does not appear to elicit a significantly protective host response following natural infection. Human influenza viruses are designated by the virus type, place of isolation, strain designation, year of isolation, and the H and N antigen subtype, e.g. A/Sydney/5/95 (H3N2).

Epidemiology

The H and N genes of influenza types A and B undergo mutational change resulting in the emergence of antigenic variants ('antigenic drift'). Every few years, a variant successful in evading the prior immunity of the human population emerges, to cause a global epidemic. Influenza viruses have a marked winter seasonality in temperate regions, making the disease burden of the virus more obvious. The more diffuse seasonality in tropical and subtropical regions leads to an obscuring of the clinical impact of the virus, leading to the illusion in some quarters that influenza is less significant in warmer climates. However, careful epidemiological studies demonstrate that the burden of mortality and morbidity in temperate and tropical regions are very similar. In those 65 years or older, influenza is associated with approximately 1 excess death per 1000 population annually in both the temperate and tropical regions.

In aquatic birds, the natural reservoir of the virus, 16 H and 9 N subtypes of influenza A are found. From 1918 till 1957, human influenza A viruses carried H1N1 surface antigens. In 1957, this virus acquired the novel H, N, and additional polymerase gene (PB1) from an avian influenza virus through genetic reassortment of its segmented genome giving rise to the H2N2 subtype virus ('antigenic shift'). As the human population lacked immunity to these novel viral antigens, this led to the 'Asian flu' pandemic. A similar reassortment event gave rise to the H3N2 virus and the 'Hong Kong influenza' pandemic of 1968. In contrast, the pandemic of 1918 is believed to have arisen by the direct adaptation of an avian influenza virus without reassortment with the pre-existing human influenza virus. Although all three influenza pandemics of the 20th century resulted in significant morbidity and mortality, the toll exacted by the 'Spanish flu' of 1918 was particularly horrendous—over 40 million deaths, greater than that of both World Wars combined. Since influenza B (and C) have no significant zoonotic reservoirs, antigenic shift and pandemics do not occur.

In early 2009, a novel H1N1 virus of swine-origin gave rise to the first pandemic of the 21st century. The pandemic arose in Mexico and rapidly spread worldwide along routes of air-travel. Unlike the two previous pandemics (1957, 1968) that arose through genetic reassortment of an avian virus with the prevailing human seasonal influenza virus, the pandemic virus of 2009 arose through reassortment between swine viruses previously documented in North America (so called 'triple reassortant' swine viruses that contained virus gene segments of swine, avian and human origin) and 'Eurasian-swine' viruses. Although the H1 haemagglutinin of both human and swine influenza viruses was originally derived from the 1918 'Spanish flu' H1N1 virus, they had antigenically diverged during their subsequent evolution in these two hosts so that the contemporary seasonal human H1N1 virus offered little cross-protection against the pandemic H1N1 virus of swine-origin. However, people born prior to the 1950s had substantial cross-protection against the novel pandemic virus, presumably derived by infection with H1N1 viruses circulating in the first half of the 20th century. Thus the pandemic was associated with explosive outbreaks in children and young adults while there was less infection in older adults. The disease was largely a mild-influenza-like illness comparable with seasonal influenza, sometimes associated with gastrointestinal symptoms of diarrhoea and vomiting. However, complications, severe illness, and fatalities did occur, especially in those who were pregnant or with underlying comorbidities including asthma and other lung disease, cardiovascular diseases, diabetes, neurological disorders, autoimmune disorders, and morbid obesity. While some of those with severe disease had secondary bacterial infections, others developed a primary viral pneumonia leading to acute respiratory distress syndrome.

Avian viruses (e.g. subtype H5N1, H9N2, H7N7) can zoonotically infect humans occasionally without undergoing prior reassortment with existing human strains. Currently, an H5N1 virus that is highly pathogenic for chickens has become entrenched in poultry flocks in a number of Asian and African countries and continues to zoonotically transmit to humans, often causing severe disease and pandemic concern. However, such transmission has so far not led to sustained human-to-human transmission that is the prerequisite for the generation of a new pandemic.

Pathogenesis

Viral replication occurs in the columnar epithelial cells leading to its desquamation down to the basal cell layer. The pathology typically involves the upper respiratory tract and the tracheobronchial tree. Infection results in decreased ciliary clearance, impaired phagocyte function, and increased adherence of bacteria to viral infected cells, all of which promote the occurrence of secondary bacterial infection.

While there may be differences in viral virulence, pre-existing cross-reactive immunity is a major determinant in reducing disease severity. Virus dissemination outside the respiratory tract is uncommon with human influenza viruses. However, zoonotic infections with the avian H5N1 virus may disseminate, and virus has been often detected in the gastrointestinal tract and occasionally in the central nervous system.

Immunity

Infection by an influenza virus results in long-lived immunity to homologous reinfection. However, the continued antigenic change in the virus allows it to keep ahead of the host immune response. Cross-immunity to 'drifted' strains within the same H or N subtype may provide partial protection, but there is believed to be little cross protection between different subtypes. Local and systemic antibody responses and cytotoxic T cells contribute to host protection.

Clinical features

The severity of influenzal disease ranges from asymptomatic infection, through the typical influenza syndrome, to the complications of influenza. Although it cannot always be distinguished from other viral infections on clinical grounds, the typical influenza syndrome is relatively characteristic in the adult. It is associated with fever, chills, headache, sore throat, coryza, nonproductive cough, myalgia, and sometimes prostration. The onset of illness is abrupt and the fever lasts 1 to 5 days. The pharynx is hyperaemic but has no exudate. Cervical lymphadenopathy is often present and crackles or wheezing are heard in around 10% of patients. While the acute illness usually resolves in 4 to 5 days, cough and fatigue may persist for weeks thereafter.

Common (>10% of symptomatic patients) complications of influenza include otitis media (in children) and exacerbation of asthma, chronic airways obstruction, and cystic fibrosis. Less common complications are acute bronchitis, primary (viral) and secondary (bacterial) pneumonia, myocarditis, febrile convulsions, encephalopathy, encephalitis, and myositis (especially in patients with influenza B infection). Age, prior immunity, virus strain, the presence of underlying diseases, pregnancy, and smoking all influence morbidity and severity.

Treatment and prevention

Antiviral therapy

Antiviral drugs with proven clinical efficacy for treatment of influenza A are the ion channel (M2) blockers that interfere with viral uncoating (amantadine, rimantadine) and the neuraminidase inhibitors (e.g. zanamivir, oseltamivir) which block virus release from infected cells. The neuraminidase inhibitors are also active against influenza B, while amantadine and rimantadine are only active against influenza A.

Since 2003, seasonal H3N2 and H1N1 viruses increasingly acquired resistance to amantadine and rimantadine and the 2009 pandemic H1N1 virus is also resistant to these drugs. Thus they are no longer drugs of choice in the treatment or prophylaxis of human influenza. Oseltamivir resistance to seasonal H1N1 viruses emerged in early 2008 and spread worldwide. The pandemic H1N1 virus (as well as seasonal H3N2 viruses) remains sensitive to oseltamivir although resistant pandemic H1N1 viruses have been occasionally reported. Zanamivir remains uniformly effective against seasonal and pandemic influenza viruses.

Zanamivir is administered by inhalation and oseltamivir orally. In patients infected with viruses sensitive to these drugs, zanamivir or oseltamivir treatment commenced within the first 48 h of disease onset leads to a 1 to 2 days reduction in the time to alleviation of clinical symptoms and also reduces incidence of influenza associated complications. Some studies have indicated benefit in reducing the complications of influenza even for patients in whom treatment commenced after the second day of clinical illness.

However, the sooner the drugs are used, the better the chance of clinical benefit. With a virus such as the highly pathogenic H5N1 virus which can disseminate beyond the respiratory tract, a systemically administered drug (oseltamivir) is likely to be superior to one administered by inhalation (zanamivir). However, oseltamivir has had variable success in the treatment of H5N1 influenza and although therapeutic failure may be partly due to late commencement of therapy, poor drug bioavailability in a severely ill patient and emergence of resistance may also contribute. Parenteral therapy is ideal for such patients and such options (e.g. peramivir) are currently undergoing clinical trials.

Aspirin should be avoided in children with influenza because of the increased risk of Reye's syndrome.

Vaccines

Influenza vaccine is a trivalent vaccine containing antigens from the two subtypes of human influenza A (H3N2 and N1N1) and B viruses. To keep abreast of change in the surface antigens of the virus, its composition must be modified on an annual basis and annual reimmunization is required. This updating of the vaccine is achieved through a collaborative effort of the global influenza virus surveillance network coordinated effort by the World Health Organization (WHO). As a result of this surveillance, the WHO makes recommendations of candidate vaccine viruses twice annually for vaccine production for the northern and southern hemispheres.

Vaccines currently in use are based on antigen derived from viruses grown in embryonated eggs or cell cultures and contain detergent-treated virus (split virus vaccines) or purified surface antigens (subunit of surface antigen vaccines). These vaccines have less side effects than killed vaccines containing the whole virus which were used in the past and are licensed for use in anyone 6 months of age or older. Previously unvaccinated children require two doses at least 1 month apart, whereas a single dose appears adequate for adults. These vaccines are generally safe, the most common side effect being soreness at the injection site lasting a few days. Vaccine efficacy is best when there is a good antigenic match between the vaccine and outbreak virus.

An intranasally administered, cold-adapted, live attenuated vaccine is now also licensed for use in those aged 5 to 49 years and offers the advantages of broader cross-protection across antigenic drifted viruses as well as easier administration and greater patient acceptability.

Inactivated and cold-adapted live attenuated monovalent vaccines containing the pandemic H1N1 were rapidly developed and used in 2009 in response to the pandemic. Some of these inactivated vaccines had adjuvents (MF59; AS03) added to enhance immune response. In 2010 and beyond, it is likely that the pandemic H1N1 virus will be included as one component of the seasonal influenza vaccine.

Immunogenicity and clinical protection are better in healthy young adults compared to patients with chronic renal failure and immunocompromised or elderly patients (all groups most at need of the vaccine). However, the vaccine is still effective in reducing influenza and pneumonia-related hospitalization and mortality in elderly people and is cost-saving. An additional option for protecting such high-risk individuals is the immunization of children and caregivers in contact with these individuals. In young adults, vaccination is associated with decreased absenteeism from work. The duration of protection is limited and therefore vaccine administration should be timed to precede the expected peak of influenza activity.

Influenza vaccine recommendations vary from country to country. In general, vaccine is recommended to those groups at highest risk of influenza related complications including (1) those aged 6 months to 5 years of age; (2) those aged 65 years or older (in the United States of America all those over 50 are recommended for vaccination); (3) pregnant women who will be in the second or third trimester during the influenza season; and (4) those with chronic medial conditions including persons with chronic disorders of pulmonary or cardiovascular systems (except hypertension), those with renal dysfunction, haemoglobinopathies, metabolic disorders, or immunodeficiency and those aged 6 months to 18 years who are on long-term aspirin therapy. Furthermore, vaccine is also recommended for health care workers and for persons living or caring for those at high risk, who may transmit influenza to such high-risk individuals.

Bocavirus and polyomavirus KI and WU

Human bocavirus is a member within a newly discovered genus Bocavirus within the family Parvoviridae. As with other parvoviruses, they are relatively resistant to inactivation by acid or alkaline pH or moderate heat (e.g. 56°C). Molecular detection by PCR in respiratory clinical specimens is the main option for diagnosis. The virus can also be sometimes detected in serum. Using these methods, it is one of the five most commonly detected viral agents in respiratory specimens from children with acute respiratory disease. However, relatively few studies have included age-matched healthy controls to assess the clinical relevance of the detection of these agents and the available data is at present contradictory. The peak age of detection is in children aged 6 months to 2 years and occasionally in adults. These patients presented with rhinitis, a cough that is often paroxysmal or 'pertussis-like', and wheezing and were categorized as bronchiolitis, pneumonia, or asthma. Some patients also had diarrhoea, vomiting, and a skin rash. The virus has been detected worldwide and is likely to have been long endemic in humans. Reliable tests to study the seroepidemiology of this infection are still awaited.

KI and WU are two novel polyomaviruses recently discovered in the respiratory tract of patients with acute respiratory infections. There are found in a proportion of children and adults with acute respiratory infection but often found as coinfections with other known respiratory pathogens. Their contribution to disease causation is still unclear.

Nosocomial infection

Respiratory viruses are efficient nosocomial pathogens. Though paediatric units face the brunt of the problem, adult wards are not exempt. Transmission may occur from patient to patient, patient to staff, and staff to patient, with visitors making their own contribution. Although influenza and RSV are the most notorious among the endemic respiratory viruses, even rhinoviruses cause problems when transmitted to immunocompromised patients. Once infected, immunocompromised patients have a prolonged period of viral shedding and pose a significant risk of transmission to other high-risk patients.

Transmission of many respiratory virus infections occurs by large respiratory droplets gaining access to the mucosa of a susceptible individual. Large respiratory droplets have a relatively short dispersal range (<1 m). On the other hand, direct hand contact is an important means of transmission within health care settings and adherence to strict hand-washing is the most critical preventive measure. Gloves are useful in reinforcing the 'hand-washing message', but will only be effective if they are changed between patients. Cohorting infected patients, either by symptoms (during the outbreak season) or by rapid viral diagnostic results, is useful. Influenza A vaccination of health care workers, especially those caring for high-risk children, is to be recommended. Staff education is vital, including awareness of the fact that some of these viruses manifest themselves as a mild 'cold' in adults, and that infected staff members can transmit to patients under their care.

The most dramatic example of the impact of nosocomial transmission with a respiratory virus occurred with SARS where health care facilities served as a major hub of virus transmission and health care workers accounted for one-fifth of all documented cases. Much of this transmission was preventable by basic (large) droplet and contact precautions, although protection from small particle aerosols was important when carrying out aerosol-generating procedures such as intubation.

Further reading

Abed Y, Boivin G (2006). Treatment of respiratory virus infections. *Antiviral Res*, **70**, 1–16. [Reviews role of antiviral therapy for respiratory virus infections.]

Centers for Disease Control and Prevention (2007). *Prevention and control of influenza: recommendations of the Advisory Committee on Immunisation Practices* (ACIP). *MMWR*, **56**, 1–54. Atlanta, GA. [Reviews the disease burden of influenza and the use of vaccines and antiviral therapy.]

Dolin R, Wright PF (eds) (1999). *Viral infections of the respiratory tract.* Marcel Dekker, Basel, pp. 1–432. [Comprehensive monograph with chapters on each of the respiratory viruses, antiviral therapy, and on infections in immunocompromised patients.]

Dowell SF (ed.) (1998). Principles of judicious use of antimicrobial agents for pediatric upper respiratory tract infections. *Pediatrics*, **101** Suppl, 163–84. [Journal supplement reviewing the use and abuse of antibiotics in upper respiratory tract infections.]

Falsey AR, Walsh EE (2006). Viral pneumonia in older adults. *Clin Infect Dis*, **42**, 518–24. [Reviews role of virus in lower respiratory tract disease of adults.]

Gern JE, Busse WW (1999). Association of rhinovirus infections with asthma. *Clin Microbiol Rev*, **12**, 9–18.

Kim YJ, Boeckh M, Englund JA (2007). Community respiratory virus infections in immunocompromised patients: hematopoietic stem cell and solid organ transplant recipients, and individuals with human immunodeficiency virus infection. *Semin Respir Crit Care Med*, **28**, 222–42. [Reviews the management of respiratory viral infections in the immunocompromised patient.]

Madeley CR, Peiris JSM, McQuillin J (1996). Adenoviruses. In: Myint S, Taylor-Robinson D (eds) *Viral and other infections of the human respiratory tract*, pp. 169–90. Chapman & Hall, London. [Reviews the adenoviral respiratory disease and laboratory diagnosis.]

Mallia P, Johnston SL (2006). How viral infections cause exacerbation of airway diseases. *Chest*, **130**, 1203–10.

Nicholson KG, Webster RG, Hay AJ (eds) (1998). *Textbook of influenza.* Blackwell Scientific, Oxford. [Comprehensive review of the ecology, clinical features, and control of influenza.]

Peiris JSM, De Jong MD, Guan Y (2007). Avian influenza virus (H5N1): a threat to human health. *Clin Microbiol Rev*, **20**, 243–67. [Reviews the threat from emerging zoonotic and potentially pandemic influenza viruses.]

Peiris JSM, *et al.* (2006). Severe acute respiratory syndrome (SARS). In Scheld WM, Hooper DC, Hughes JM (eds) *Emerging infections 7*, pp. 23–50. ASM Press, Washington DC. [Reviews the epidemiology, clinical features, pathogenesis and management of SARS.]

Siddell S, Myint S (1996). Coronaviruses. In: Myint S, Taylor-Robinson D (eds) *Viral and other infections of the human respiratory tract*, pp. 141–67. Chapman & Hall, London.

Treanor J (2009). Respiratory infections. In: Richmond DD, Whitley RJ, Hayden FG (eds) *Clinical Virology*, 3rd edition, pp. 7–27. ASM Press, Washington, DC. [Reviews viral respiratory infections.]

van den Hoogen BG, Osterhaus ADME, Fouchier RAM. (2006). Human metapneumovirus. In: Scheld WM, Hooper DC, Hughes JM (eds) *Emerging Infections 7*. pp. 51–68, ASM Press, Washington, DC.

7.5.2 Herpesviruses (excluding Epstein–Barr virus)

J.G.P. Sissons

Essentials

Eight human herpesviruses, all with a linear double-stranded DNA genome and divided into alpha-, beta-, and gamma-subfamilies on the basis of genomic and biological properties, share the capacity to produce latent infection. The diseases they cause may result from primary infection, or reactivation of the virus from latency, and tend to be more severe in immunosuppressed patients. Diagnosis of the various herpesvirus infections may be made on clinical grounds alone, by culture or demonstration of viral particles by electron microscopy of relevant samples, by serological testing, or (increasingly) by PCR-based tests.

Herpes simplex viruses (HSV)

These two alpha-herpesviruses infect epithelial cells and become latent in the central nervous system. (1) HSV-1—transmitted by direct contact with infected secretions from a carrier; predominantly causes orofacial infections; becomes latent in the trigeminal ganglion; reactivation may give rise to recurrent orolabial mucosal ulcers ('cold sores') on the lips or skin around the mouth; is the commonest identified cause of acute sporadic encephalitis occurring in immunocompetent subjects in Western countries. (2) HSV-2—usually acquired through sexual contact and is the predominant cause of genital HSV infection, which may also be recurrent.

Treatment of both HSV-1 and HSV-2 is with aciclovir, which is preferentially phosphorylated in HSV-infected cells, or other newer related drugs (famciclovir and valaciclovir). Oral treatment is used in immunocompetent patients, but intravenous therapy is indicated in severe infections, encephalitis and in immunosuppressed patients.

Varicella zoster virus (VZV)

This alpha-herpesvirus is presumed to spread by the respiratory route and after an incubation period of 10 to 20 days causes varicella (chickenpox), predominantly an exanthematous disease of childhood, but which may be complicated in adults by pneumonitis and encephalitis. The virus becomes latent in dorsal root ganglia after primary infection, whence it can reactivate to cause herpes zoster (shingles), with pain, erythema, and vesicular lesions occurring in a dermatomal distribution, particularly in elderly and immunosuppressed individuals. Treatment of severe varicella or herpes zoster is with aciclovir, with higher doses being required than for HSV. A live attenuated VZV vaccine is available: this induces 90% protection from natural varicella in children, and also diminishes the incidence of zoster and postherpetic neuralgia when given to older age groups.

Human cytomegalovirus (HCMV)

This beta-herpesvirus is the largest human herpesvirus. Infection is spread by close contact with body fluids of infected individuals: from 50 to 100% of adults are seropositive, depending on socioeconomic and sexual risk, with myeloid lineage cells being a principal site of HCMV latency. Primary infection in children and adults is usually asymptomatic, but infectious mononucleosis clinically indistinguishable from that caused by primary Epstein–Barr virus (EBV) infection can be produced (see Chapter 7.5.3), and HCMV can produce severe disease in two particular situations. (1) Fetal infection—congenital HCMV infection occurs in around 0.5 to 1% of live births in developed countries; most infected babies are asymptomatic, but classical 'cytomegalic inclusion disease' has a high mortality and surviving infants have mental, visual, and hearing impairment. (2) Infection in patients who are immunosuppressed patients—the most serious forms are pneumonitis in bone marrow transplant recipients and retinitis in HIV/AIDS patients. Specific treatment for HCMV is usually with ganciclovir, which requires intravenous administration and has limiting side effects including myelotoxicity; valganciclovir has higher oral bioavailability and is particularly used for prophylaxis.

Human herpesvirus 6 and 7 (HHV-6 and 7)

These are beta-herpesviruses, most probably transmitted via maternal saliva. Primary infection with HHV-6 in young children is associated with roseola infantum (exanthem subitum, sixth disease), and also with a febrile illness without rash. More than 90% of children are seropositive for HHV-6 by 2 years of age. HHV-6 reactivation may occur in immunosuppressed solid-organ and bone marrow transplant recipients, but it is not clear that HHV-6 causes disease in these patients. HHV-6 sensitivity to antiviral drugs corresponds with that of HCMV, but no treatment is usually required. HHV-7 has been associated with some cases of roseola, but there is no other evidence for its being pathogenic.

Human herpesvirus-8 (HHV-8)

This member of the rhadinovirus (gamma 2-herpesvirus) family is the most recently discovered human herpesviruses, having been isolated from Kaposi's sarcoma tissue in 1994. The mechanism of transmission is probably by saliva and sexual contact; reported seroprevalence is around 50% or more in many African adult populations, but 5% or less in blood donors in the United Kingdom and the United States of America, with intermediate rates in Italy and other Mediterranean countries.

HHV-8 (as other gamma-herpesviruses such as EBV) is potentially oncogenic: it is clearly associated with (1) Kaposi's sarcoma—HHV-8 can be detected by PCR in the blood of nearly all cases. Manifests clinically as purplish brown macules, papules and plaques, and is described in four clinical settings: (a) the classic form—typically presents in elderly Mediterranean or Jewish men with lesions on the extremities and an indolent course; (b) the endemic African form—accounts for 10% of cancer in equatorial Africa and is similar clinically to the classic form of the disease; (c) in patients with immunodeficiency states such as transplant recipients—lesions are more widespread and rapidly progressive, but visceral involvement is unusual; and (d) the AIDS-associated form—with widespread cutaneous lesions, involvement of the oral mucosa, visceral lesions in the lungs or gastrointestinal tract, and sometimes rapid progression. Kaposi's sarcoma lesions may regress with antiretroviral treatment, withdrawal of immunosuppression, and the disease can also be treated with radiation therapy and (for widespread cutaneous or visceral disease) with chemotherapy. (2) Primary effusion lymphoma—HHV-8 is present in the tumour cells of all cases of this rare and aggressive type of B cell lymphoma that presents in patients with AIDS. (3) Multicentric Castleman's disease (angiofollicular lymph node hyperplasia)—HHV-8 is present in most cases of this condition, especially those associated with HIV.

Cercopithecine herpesvirus 1

This alpha-herpesvirus (formerly named herpes B virus) is closely related to HSV found in Old World monkeys, its natural host. Transmission to humans from monkey bites results in a high incidence of severe disease, with progressive encephalitis. Treatment is with aciclovir or ganciclovir, but morbidity and mortality are high.

Human herpesviruses

The Herpesviridae family is widely distributed in the animal kingdom. More than 100 have been isolated from humans, primates, and other mammals, and from reptiles and fish. Comparative sequence analysis suggests they have been coevolving with their individual hosts for millions of years. Eight human herpesviruses have been identified to date (Table 7.5.2.1). Shared genomic and biological properties divide the herpesviruses into three subfamilies, the alpha-, beta-, and gammaherpesvirinae.

All the herpesviruses have a linear double-stranded DNA genome contained inside an icosahedral capsid that is surrounded by a protein tegument. The outer lipid envelope contains virus glycoprotein spikes. These large viruses have genomes consisting of unique segments of DNA flanked by inverted repeats, and encode most of the proteins needed for replication. All herpesviruses share an important biological feature, their capacity to produce latent infection in their natural host, during which the viral genome persists in cells, usually as a closed circle (episome), expressing only a limited subset of virus genes. This property results in their ability to produce lifelong infection in different types of cell, depending on the individual virus, and thus to persist in the population. Herpesvirus disease may result from primary infection, or reactivation of the virus from latency, and tends to be more severe in immunosuppressed patients. The gammaherpesviruses can induce cell transformation, and are associated with specific tumours.

Herpes simplex virus infections

Historical background

'Herpes' derives from the Greek, meaning to creep or crawl, apparently used since antiquity to describe the evolution of the skin lesions caused by herpes simplex virus (HSV) and varicella–zoster virus. HSV was the first of the herpesviruses to be isolated, in the

Table 7.5.2.1 The human herpesviruses

Common name	Designation	Subfamily	Genome size (kbp)	Site of latency and persistence
Herpes simplex virus 1	Human herpesvirus 1	α	152	Neurons (sensory ganglia)
Herpes simplex virus 2	Human herpesvirus 2	α	152	Neurons (sensory ganglia)
Varicella zoster virus	Human herpesvirus 3	α	125	Neurons (sensory ganglia)
Epstein–Barr virus	Human herpesvirus 4	γ	172	B lymphocytes (oropharyngeal epithelium)
Human cytomegalovirus	Human herpesvirus 5	β	235	Blood monocytes (probably epithelial cells)
HHV6	Human herpesvirus 6	β	170	Monocytes, T lymphocytes
HHV7	Human herpesvirus 7	β	145	–
Kaposi's sarcoma-associated herpesvirus	Human herpesvirus 8	γ	230	Uncertain

1930s, although the transmission of infection to animals had been demonstrated in 1919. The serological distinction between the two types, HSV-1 and HSV-2, and the association of HSV-2 with genital herpes, was made in the 1960s. HSVs are now some of the most intensively studied human viruses.

Aetiology

HSV has a genome size of 150 kbp, and codes for about 80 proteins. The genomes of HSV-1 and HSV-2 are largely colinear, but have different restriction endonuclease sites. Gene expression occurs in three temporally regulated phases: immediate early, early, and late. Immediate-early proteins are largely regulatory proteins that prepare the cell to produce further virus. The early genes code particularly for enzymes involved in the replication of virus DNA, and the late genes for the structural proteins of the virion. Antigenic differences in the surface glycoprotein G are used to distinguish between HSV-1 and HSV-2. The release of progeny virus is normally accompanied by cell death, i.e. the infection is lytic. The virus infects a relatively wide range of cells *in vitro*, and can also infect experimental animals, allowing studies of its pathogenesis.

Epidemiology

HSV is a ubiquitous virus, widely distributed in populations throughout the world. Although animals can be infected experimentally, there are no natural animal hosts, and humans are the only reservoir. Transmission occurs when a susceptible person has direct contact with infected secretions from an HSV carrier, usually from oral, genital, or skin lesions, to mucous membranes or abraded skin of the recipient. HSV carriers can excrete virus asymptomatically, and 1 to 15% of adult carriers excrete HSV at any one time. Conventionally, the prevalence of infection is assessed by demonstrating antibody to HSV-1 or HSV-2. The prevalence of HSV-1 increases with age, although the time of acquisition of HSV-1 antibody varies depending on socioeconomic factors. Seroprevalence in early life is higher among lower socioeconomic groups, 70 to 90% of children having antibodies by the age of 10, whereas only about 30% of children in higher socioeconomic groups have antibodies by this time. By mid life, 80 to 90% of people are HSV-1 seropositive.

HSV-2 infection is usually acquired through sexual contact; consequently, seroconversion correlates with the onset of sexual activity, and a progressive increase in seroprevalence to HSV-2 begins in adolescence. The number of sexual contacts is a major risk factor for the acquisition of HSV-2. Cumulative seroprevalence rates in adults vary from 10 to 80%, depending on the population and risk factors.

HSV can be transmitted to neonates by infection (usually HSV-2) from maternal genital secretions at the time of delivery. The mothers are most often asymptomatic excretors of the virus who have no history of genital herpes.

Pathogenesis

HSV infects and replicates in epithelial cells at the site of inoculation onto mucous membranes or abraded skin, with an incubation period of 4 to 6 days before clinical lesions appear. There is a marked local inflammatory response, but viraemia and dissemination may occur in the immunocompromised host. Following local epithelial replication, HSV enters the peripheral sensory nerves innervating the site of replication, and ascends the axons by retrograde transport to reach the dorsal root ganglia, or the trigeminal ganglion in the case of oral or conjunctival inoculation. The virus then becomes latent in the sensory ganglia, but despite extensive study, the mechanism of virus latency remains uncertain.

Latent HSV DNA is in an inactive state, with minimal gene expression. RNA species called latency-associated transcripts are the only detectable transcripts. These have no detectable protein product, and their deletion from the genome does not prevent the establishment of latency, although reactivation is impaired. Latent HSV is carried for the lifetime of the host, but may be reactivated in response to certain stimuli, including stress, menstruation, ultraviolet light, and immunosuppression. Upon reactivation, infectious virus is produced, travels down the peripheral nerves by anterograde axonal transport, and replicates in the epithelial cells at the nerve ending.

The neuronal latency of HSV and varicella–zoster virus is an extremely effective method of virus persistence. Latent virus in neuronal cells appears to be inaccessible to the immune response, and as it does not replicate is not susceptible to the action of antiviral drugs. In normal HSV carriers, reactivation at local sites is thought to be controlled by a specific effector T-lymphocyte response. However, HSV DNA encodes proteins that interfere with antigen processing by the class I MHC pathway, and are presumed to help the virus evade the T-cell immune response. There is no good evidence that the immune response to HSV of people who have symptomatic reactivation episodes differs from that of asymptomatic carriers.

Clinical features

Primary infection with HSV is often asymptomatic; among sexually active subjects, only 60% of primary infections with HSV-1, and 40% with HSV-2, are symptomatic. HSV-1 is the predominant

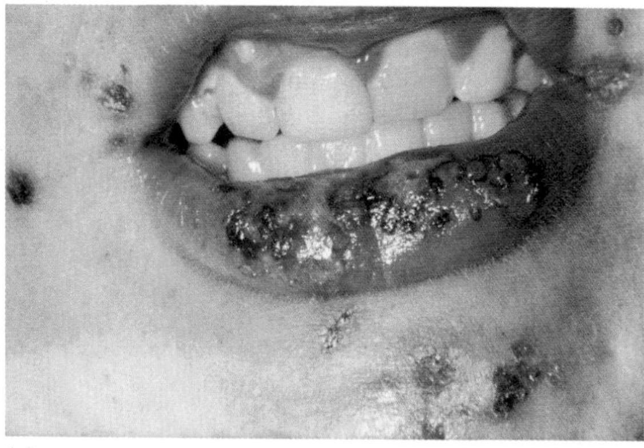
(a)

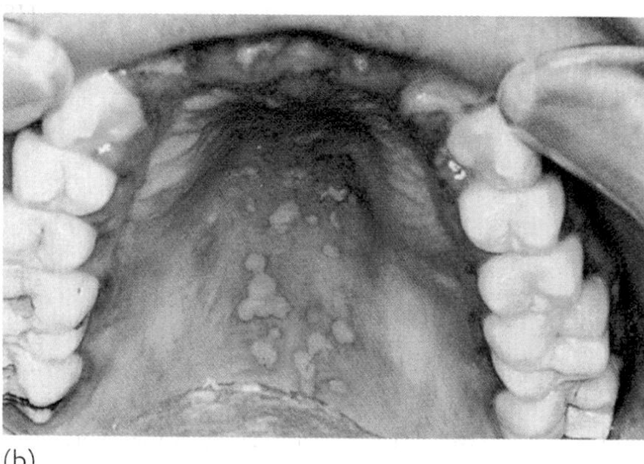
(b)

Fig. 7.5.2.1 Herpes simplex gingivostomatitis: (a) and (b).

cause of orofacial infections, whereas HSV-2 is the usual cause of genital HSV infection, but the clinical manifestations overlap.

Gingivostomatitis

This is the most common clinical form of primary infection with HSV-1. It is most often seen in children, following an incubation period of 2 to 12 days. Primary infection may be associated with a considerable systemic reaction, involving fever, sore throat, pharyngeal oedema, and redness. Painful vesicles appear a few days later on the pharynx and oral mucosa, the lips, and the skin around the mouth (Fig. 7.5.2.1). There may be cervical lymphadenopathy. Affected patients may have difficulty in eating, and the lesions last from 3 days to 2 weeks. The differential diagnosis includes other causes of pharyngitis, including bacterial pharyngitis and herpangina (from Coxsackie A virus infection) (Fig. 7.8.5 3). Anterior vesicles and ulceration affecting the lips and skin around the mouth are more suggestive of HSV infection. Stevens–Johnson syndrome and severe aphthous ulceration may appear similar, and staphylococcal impetigo affects the skin around the mouth, but is not associated with oral ulceration.

Reactivation of HSV may give rise to recurrent orolabial lesions, appearing as intraoral mucosal ulcers, but more frequently as the classical cold sore on the lips or skin around the mouth. A tingling sensation in the area of impending ulceration may precede the appearance of vesicles by 1 to 2 days. The lesions usually recur at the same site in individual patients. Around 25% of HSV-1 seropositive people develop recurrent orolabial lesions. The majority have only one or two reactivation episodes per year, although a minority (<10%) have more than one attack per month. The episodes are not associated with systemic symptoms, and diagnosis is usually straightforward.

Infection at other cutaneous sites

Herpetic whitlow

HSV infection of the finger, herpetic whitlow, may complicate primary oral or genital herpes by autoinoculation of virus, or may occur through occupational exposure (e.g. in nursing, medical, and dental staff). There is oedema, erythema, and local tenderness of the infected finger (Fig. 7.5.27.4). Lesions at the finger tip may be confused with pyogenic bacterial paronychias and incised, which is contraindicated for herpetic whitlow, and may even spread infection.

Herpes gladiatorum

This is mucocutaneous HSV infection occurring by transmission of virus via skin trauma resulting from wrestling or other contact sports.

Eczema herpeticum

HSV infections of the skin are more severe in patients with pre-existing skin disease. In patients with eczema, burns, or other blistering skin diseases, HSV infection may become disseminated.

Cutaneous HSV infection can be confused with herpes zoster, although the latter is usually easy to diagnose by its unilateral dermatomal distribution.

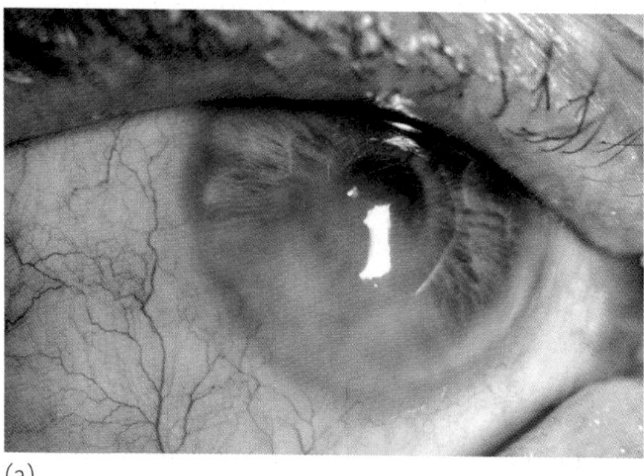
(a)

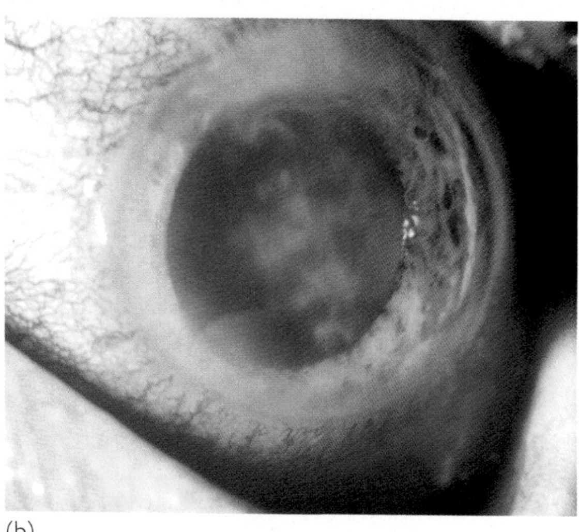
(b)

Fig. 7.5.2.2 Herpes simplex keratitis: (a) disciform, and (b) dendritic. (Courtesy of the late Dr B E Juel-Jensen.)

Herpes simplex and erythema multiforme

About 15% of all cases of erythema multiforme are preceded by a symptomatic attack of recurrent herpes simplex, and in susceptible people the characteristic rash can be induced by the intradermal inoculation of inactivated herpes simplex virus antigen. The rash of erythema multiforme starts several days after the onset of the herpetic vesicles, and in severe cases can involve the mucous membranes (Stevens–Johnson syndrome). The frequency of these attacks can be reduced by aciclovir prophylaxis.

Keratitis

HSV keratitis is characterized by the acute onset of pain, blurred vision, conjunctival injection, and dendritic ulceration of the cornea (Fig. 7.5.2.2). It can cause corneal blindness, and treatment is urgent. Topical aciclovir is the drug of choice; topical steroids may make the infection worse. HSV can also cause an acute necrotizing retinitis, usually only seen in immunosuppressed people, including those with HIV infection.

Genital herpes

Primary genital HSV infection is sexually transmitted, and may be associated with systemic symptoms such as fever, headache, and myalgias. Symptoms tend to be more severe in women than men. There is local pain and itching, dysuria, vaginal discharge, and inguinal lymphadenopathy, with vesicles and ulcers on the vulva, perineum, vagina, and cervix, and sometimes on the skin of the buttocks (Fig. 7.5.2.3). In males, primary HSV lesions are vesicles on the shaft or glans of the penis, and there may be associated urethritis. HSV-2 causes most genital infections, with a variable smaller proportion resulting from HSV-1. Only 40% of primary HSV-2 genital infections are symptomatic. In patients who have had prior HSV-1 infection, the symptoms of primary genital herpes tend to be less severe. HSV has been isolated from the urethra in 5% of women with urethral syndrome, in the absence of obvious genital lesions. Other manifestations of genital tract disease resulting from primary HSV infection are, rarely, endometritis and salpingitis in women, and prostatitis in men.

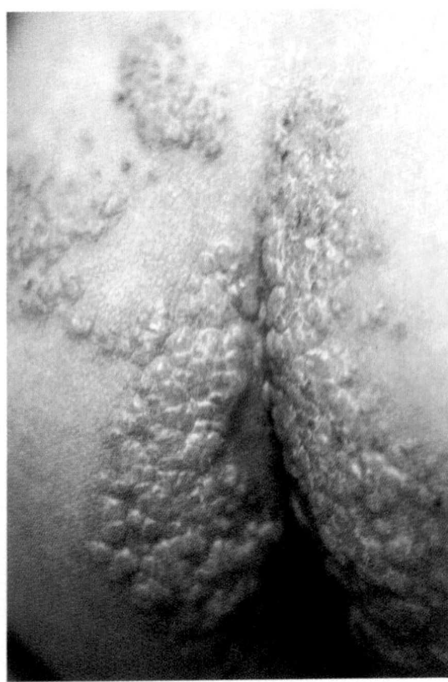

Fig. 7.5.2.3 Genital herpes in the natal cleft.
(Courtesy of the late Dr B E Juel-Jensen.)

HSV proctitis may follow rectal intercourse. There is anorectal pain and discharge, with ulcerative lesions visible on sigmoidoscopy. Perianal lesions are seen in immunosuppressed patients, and spreading perianal HSV infection and HSV proctitis occur in HIV-infected patients.

Recurrent genital herpes is frequent in the first year after primary genital disease (90% for HSV-2 and 55% for HSV-1). Thereafter, the recurrence rate tends to decrease with time, to around three to four attacks per year for HSV-2, but fewer for HSV-1. Severe recurrent genital herpes is particularly troublesome to women.

The complications of primary genital HSV infection include sacral radiculomyelitis, with urinary retention and hyperaesthesia of the perineal area, which usually resolves over several weeks. Aseptic meningitis requiring admission to hospital occurs in up to 7% of women and 2% of men, although suggestive symptoms are more common. Occasionally, and more seriously, transverse myelitis may occur.

HSV encephalitis (see also Chapter 24.11.2)

Encephalitis is the most serious type of disease produced by HSV in the immunocompetent host, and has an estimated annual incidence of two to three cases per million. It is the most commonly identified cause of acute sporadic encephalitis in Western countries. The great majority of cases are caused by HSV-1. A biphasic age incidence is reported, with higher rates between the ages of 5 and 30 years, and in those older than 50 years. The clinical features are of focal encephalitis, with acute onset of fever, confusion, and unusual behaviour, impaired consciousness, and possibly focal neurological abnormalities. However, there are no specific features, and the diagnosis of HSV should be considered in any patient with possible encephalitis.

The cerebrospinal fluid shows lymphocytic pleocytosis, although neutrophils and red cells may also be present, with a raised protein level. CT scans of the brain may show changes in the temporal lobe; MRI is a more sensitive method of detection. The electroencephalogram classically shows spike and slow-wave activity localized in the temporal lobes. The definitive way of establishing the diagnosis is brain biopsy. In the original trial of aciclovir for the treatment of HSV encephalitis, brain biopsy was an entry criterion, but confirmed the diagnosis in only 50% of clinically suspected cases. Since the advent of effective nontoxic chemotherapy for HSV, brain biopsy is very rarely used. There is good correlation between a positive polymerase chain reaction (PCR) test for HSV DNA in the cerebrospinal fluid, and a diagnosis of HSV encephalitis by brain biopsy and virus isolation. Evidence of intrathecal production of specific HSV antibody is also diagnostic, but as it usually not detectable until 1 week after onset, PCR-based diagnosis is more useful. Serum or cerebrospinal fluid titres of antibodies to HSV do not usually increase in the first week of the illness. In practice, the diagnosis is established by a compatible clinical picture, evidence of characteristic temporal lobe involvement on CT or MRI, and EEG, and by PCR-based detection of HSV DNA in the cerebrospinal fluid.

The pathogenesis of HSV encephalitis remains uncertain. Up to one-half of patients have primary infection, and in the rest the disease is presumed to result from reactivation. However, where HSV has been isolated from the brain and mouth simultaneously in the same patient, the two isolates differ by restriction endonuclease analysis in about 30% of cases, suggesting a new exogenous virus infection in an already seropositive patient. HSV DNA can be detected at autopsy in the brains of normal virus carriers, and the factors precipitating HSV encephalitis are not known. Immunosuppression is not usually associated with encephalitis, which predominantly affects normal immunocompetent adults, and very rarely patients with advanced HIV infection. The pathological features are of focal haemorrhagic necrotizing encephalitis affecting the temporal lobes.

Treatment with intravenous aciclovir should be started immediately if HSV encephalitis is clinically suspected, without waiting for confirmation of the diagnosis (in doses as below; see 'CNS infections'). The untreated mortality from HSV encephalitis is more than 70%, and very few survivors make a full neurological recovery. Intravenous aciclovir was established to be more effective than the previous best therapy of vidarabine in a randomized trial reported in 1986. Mortality in the aciclovir-treated group was 28%, although a lower Glasgow coma score on entry carried a higher risk of mortality. However, only 38% of those who received aciclovir had fully recovered at 6 months. There is still a high incidence of permanent neurological sequelae, particularly seizures, defects of memory, and personality changes, and the prognosis of HSV encephalitis remains poor.

Meningitis

HSV can cause aseptic meningitis, which is quite independent of, and not associated with progression to, HSV encephalitis. It is most commonly associated with primary genital HSV-2 infection, in which the incidence of proven HSV meningitis is 7% in women and 2% in men. There is pleocytosis, usually lymphocytic, but neutrophils may predominate in early meningitis. HSV may be isolated from the cerebrospinal fluid by culture, but is now more reliably detected by PCR for HSV DNA. In a high proportion of patients with Mollaret's meningitis (recurrent aseptic meningitis of unknown aetiology; Chapter 24.11.2), HSV DNA is reported to be detectable in the cerebrospinal fluid by PCR. The role of HSV in this syndrome remains uncertain.

Neonatal HSV infection and pregnancy

The incidence of neonatal HSV infection is approximately 1 in 3500 deliveries per annum in the United States of America, but appears to be lower in the United Kingdom, at 1 in 6600 live births. About 70% of cases are caused by HSV-2, and result from fetal acquisition of HSV-2 from maternal genital secretions during delivery. Most infants with neonatal HSV are born to mothers without clinically evident HSV infection. The risk of transmission from women with symptomatic primary HSV or clinically evident recurrent HSV-2 infection is about 50 and 20%, respectively. A small proportion (*c*.10%) of infections is acquired postnatally through contact with people with active lesions.

Neonatal HSV infection may appear as lesions on the skin, eye, and mouth, or as encephalitis or disseminated visceral infection. Although initial superficial infection may progress to visceral infection, visceral infection can present without cutaneous lesions, and the diagnosis should be considered in severely ill neonates. Untreated, visceral infection has a high mortality (around 60%). Primary infection in early pregnancy can lead to congenital HSV infection, which is rare, but can produce serious congenital abnormalities.

HSV in immunosuppressed patients

HSV infections in immunosuppressed people are usually because of reactivation, rather than primary infection. They tend to be more severe, are more likely to progress, and take longer to heal than in the immunocompetent host. Clinical manifestations in patients with HIV infection include severe perineal, orofacial, and oesophageal infection. HSV pneumonitis, hepatitis, and colitis are also described in immunosuppressed patients.

Pathology

The histological appearance of HSV infection remains the same, whether it is primary or recurrent. There is ballooning of infected cells, with condensed chromatin in the cell nuclei; intranuclear inclusion bodies (Cowdry type A bodies) may be seen; and multinucleated giant cells form. Varicella–zoster virus produces a similar appearance.

Laboratory diagnosis

Definitive diagnosis is made by virus isolation. Swabs from vesicular fluid or other body fluids in virus transport medium can be inoculated into tissue culture, producing typical cytopathic effects. Electron microscopy of negatively stained vesicle fluid is rapid, but will not differentiate HSV from varicella–zoster virus. The use of PCR-based techniques to detect viral DNA is becoming more widespread. It is particularly applicable to the detection of HSV DNA in cerebrospinal fluid.

Serological tests for antibody to HSV are useful only for making a retrospective diagnosis. Seroconversion provides proof of primary infection, and the absence of antibody to HSV-1 or HSV-2 rules out a diagnosis of recurrent HSV infection. However, making a diagnosis of reactivation by demonstrating rising antibody titres is of limited value.

Treatment

The introduction of aciclovir heralded a new era of specific antiviral drugs, and superseded the drugs previously used for the treatment of HSV infections, such as vidarabine and idoxuridine. Aciclovir is an acyclic nucleoside that is preferentially phosphorylated to the monophosphate in HSV-infected cells by the virus-encoded thymidine kinase. Cellular kinases then phosphorylate the monophosphate to the triphosphate, which is incorporated into nascent HSV DNA, where it acts as a chain terminator; aciclovir also directly inactivates the HSV DNA polymerase. Two newer, related drugs with the same mechanism of action are famciclovir, a prodrug of penciclovir, and valaciclovir, the valyl ester of aciclovir, which has greater bioavailability and less frequent dosage. All these drugs are relatively free of side effects, although intravenous aciclovir can crystallize in the renal parenchyma and produce renal impairment; it should be given by infusion over an hour, and patients should be adequately hydrated. The doses should be reduced in patients with renal impairment.

Primary mucocutaneous infection

In primary oral and genital infection, aciclovir 200 mg 5 times daily given orally for 10 to 14 days from the onset reduces the severity of infection, the duration of symptoms, and the duration of viral shedding. There is little evidence that the treatment of primary infection reduces the incidence of subsequent symptomatic reactivation episodes. If swallowing is difficult, intravenous aciclovir (5 mg/kg 8 hourly) may need to be given. Famciclovir 250 mg 3 times daily or valaciclovir 500 mg twice daily are alternatives.

Symptomatic reactivation of mucocutaneous infection

The treatment of recurrent infections in immunocompetent hosts is often unnecessary, as the symptoms are usually very mild. However, aciclovir can shorten the duration of symptoms if it is given very early in the course of the recurrence, preferably during the prodrome before vesicles appear. Oral aciclovir is effective, and anecdotal reports suggest that topical aciclovir is effective symptomatically. The same dosage as above for primary infection can be given for 5 days. Patient-initiated courses of single-day famciclovir (1 g twice daily) or 3-day valaciclovir (500 mg twice daily) have been shown to be effective for recurrent genital HSV.

Long-term suppressive therapy

This can be considered in immunocompetent patients with genital herpes who have frequent reactivation episodes. Trials of aciclovir in recurrent genital herpes have shown that a dose of 400 mg twice daily significantly reduces the frequency of attacks. However, patients may be able to find a lower effective dose, and in some, 200 mg daily prevents attacks. Because there is some evidence that resistant virus is a problem in this population, it is advisable to stop treatment for a month every 6 to 12 months. Valaciclovir 500 mg daily or famciclovir 250 mg twice daily are alternatives.

CNS infections

For HSV encephalitis, intravenous aciclovir (10 mg/kg 8 hourly for 10–14 days) should be given to any patient in whom the diagnosis is clinically suspected (see 'HSV encephalitis' above). For HSV meningitis, intravenous aciclovir 5 mg/kg 8 hourly can be used, with conversion to oral valaciclovir 1 g twice daily when improvement occurs, for a total of 10 days.

Systemic infection in the immunosuppressed

Oral treatment, as for primary HSV, can be used for mild mucocutaneous infection, but for more severe and for visceral involvement, intravenous aciclovir 5 mg/kg 8 hourly should be used. After resolution, continued prophylaxis is usually necessary until immunocompetence is restored, particularly in patients with HIV.

Aciclovir resistance

Resistance of HSV to aciclovir develops readily *in vitro*, but is clinically rare; it results from mutations in the HSV thymidine kinase or DNA polymerase genes. It is seen almost exclusively in immunocompromised patients who have received prolonged aciclovir prophylaxis, especially those with HIV infection, and is manifest as unresponsive or worsening HSV disease despite treatment with aciclovir. There is usually crossresistance to famciclovir and valaciclovir, and intravenous foscarnet is the most useful alternative drug in severe infection caused by resistant HSV, although it is more usually used for human cytomegalovirus (see 'Human cytomegalovirus' below).

Prevention and control

No vaccine is licenced for HSV, although a gD (glycoprotein D) based vaccine reduced new HSV2 infection in seronegative women, and other candidates are approaching phase III trials. There is particular interest in the use of vaccines for postinfective immunization to reduce the frequency of recurrent genital HSV attacks. This has proved possible in guinea pigs.

Special problems in pregnant women

Prevention of neonatal HSV infection is best achieved by preventing genital HSV infection late in pregnancy. There is no reason to give aciclovir prophylactically to women with a history of recurrent genital herpes who are asymptomatic, as the incidence of neonatal HSV infection is low in their children. However, women with clinically apparent genital herpes in the last trimester (and probably at any other time in pregnancy) can be treated with aciclovir, although the drug is not licensed for treatment in pregnancy. Women with no clinical lesions may have a vaginal delivery, but the presence of active lesions at the time of labour is an indication for Caesarean section. Babies born to mothers with clinically apparent genital HSV infection, or with a history of recurrent genital HSV infection, should be screened for HSV by cultures from the nasopharynx and eyes after birth.

Proven neonatal HSV infection should be treated with high-dose intravenous aciclovir (20 mg/kg per day every 8 h for 21 days).

Varicella–zoster virus infection

Historical background

There are clinical descriptions of varicella (chickenpox) and herpes zoster (shingles) in very early medical literature, although the skin lesions of herpes simplex and herpes zoster were grouped together under the term herpes. The similarities between the exanthematous rashes associated with smallpox and varicella meant they were not distinguished until the late 19th century. The characteristic clinical appearance of shingles, in a dermatomal distribution, was recognized as a discrete entity in the early Greek literature. The term zoster is derived from the Greek word for a girdle, and shingles from the Latin cingere meaning to encircle.

In 1892 von Bocquet observed that children developed varicella after contact with adults with herpes zoster, and in 1925 it was shown that vesicular fluid from patients with zoster, inoculated into susceptible people, produced chickenpox. The idea that zoster resulted from the reactivation of latent virus remaining in the tissues following childhood varicella was put forward by Garland in 1943, and strengthened by the work of Hope-Simpson, a British general practitioner. Varicella–zoster virus (VZV) was isolated in 1958, and Weller and colleagues showed the similarity between viral isolates from varicella and zoster patients. Restriction endonuclease analysis showed that the isolates from chickenpox and from later zoster in the same immunocompromised patient were identical. The long interval between the two illnesses has prevented such studies in immunocompetent people.

Aetiology

VZV is structurally similar to other members of the herpesvirus family. The genome is a linear double-stranded DNA of 125 kbp. VZV is an alphaherpesvirus, and encodes sets of genes that are largely colinear to those of HSV, and are also expressed in immediate-early, early, and late phases. The virus is closely cell associated, and spreads from cell to cell in tissue culture.

Epidemiology

VZV infects only humans, which are thus the only reservoir. The virus is presumed to spread by the respiratory route. Varicella is predominantly a disease of childhood, affecting both sexes. Ninety% of cases occur in children under the age of 13 years. The incubation period is about 2 weeks (with a range of 10–20 days); patients are infectious for about 48 h before the vesicles appear, and remain so for 4 to 5 days afterwards, until all the vesicles have crusted over.

The secondary attack rate in susceptible contacts with an index case in the household is 70 to 90%. The prevalence of VZV varies in different ethnic groups. In Europe, about 10% of the population over 15 years old is seronegative, and consequently susceptible to infection, although in tropical countries only 50% of young adults may be seropositive. Varicella in adults is uncommon in Europe, and less than 2% of all cases occur in patients older than 20 years. Subclinical infection is unusual, and accounts for less than 5% of all infections, but the disease may be mild, and in some surveys only 10% of people with a negative history were in fact seronegative for VZV. One attack of chickenpox usually confers lifelong immunity.

After primary infection, VZV becomes latent in dorsal root ganglia. Reactivation appears clinically as herpes zoster, which is a common disease affecting all age groups, but particularly older and immunosuppressed people; about 20% of the population will experience an attack. There is no evidence that exposure to people with active VZV infection predisposes to herpes zoster in their contacts, but a seronegative person may catch varicella from contact with the vesicles of a patient with shingles. Nosocomial varicella infection is well recognized, and the isolation of patients with varicella, and immunocompromised patients with herpes zoster, should be ensured in hospitals. Local unidermatomal zoster is less likely to cause infection, and consequently to need isolation.

Pathogenesis

During primary infection, initial virus replication probably occurs in the epithelial cells of the upper respiratory tract mucosa, followed by a phase of viraemia during which VZV can be isolated from leucocytes, and the disseminated rash appears. In the skin, the virus infects capillary endothelial cells, and adjacent fibroblasts and epithelial cells. During the viraemic phase, virus may spread to visceral organs, including alveolar epithelial cells, and transient subclinical hepatitis is probably a normal feature of varicella. VZV encephalitis may be a feature of primary infection, particularly affecting the cerebellum. Patients usually recover completely from encephalitis (unlike that associated with HSV), and it has been suggested its pathogenesis may be immune mediated. Following recovery from primary infection, the virus persists for life in a latent state in dorsal root ganglia. VZV reaches the ganglia by retrograde axonal transport from the skin lesions during primary infection, and all dorsal root ganglia and the trigeminal ganglion can potentially carry latent VZV in neurones and possibly in satellite cells.

As with other herpesviruses, the host response is critical in containing the initial infection. Cellular immunity is important, since varicella may be progressive in patients with severely impaired T-cell immunity. Both CD4 and CD8 cytotoxic T lymphocytes specific for VZV are present in normal people carrying latent VZV. The cellular immune response presumably plays a part in controlling reactivation, since impaired T-cell immunity increases the risk of developing zoster, and of having vesicles in multiple dermatomes, and cutaneous dissemination of reactivated virus. The increasing incidence of herpes zoster with age may reflect waning cellular immunity to VZV.

Clinical features

Primary infection and varicella

The most striking feature of varicella is the rash, which is centripetal (mainly on the trunk). The lesions are initially present on the face and scalp, before progressing to the trunk and later to the limbs (Fig. 7.5.2.4). A macular erythematous rash, papules, and vesicles may all be present together. Individual lesions progress from being papules to vesicles to pustules, and then crust over. The scabs normally separate after 10 days, without scarring. The systemic symptoms associated with varicella vary considerably. In most children there is a mild illness with fever. Adults characteristically have a more severe illness, with myalgia, headache, arthralgia, malaise, and higher fever, with the complications listed below. Symptoms may precede the rash by 1 to 2 days.

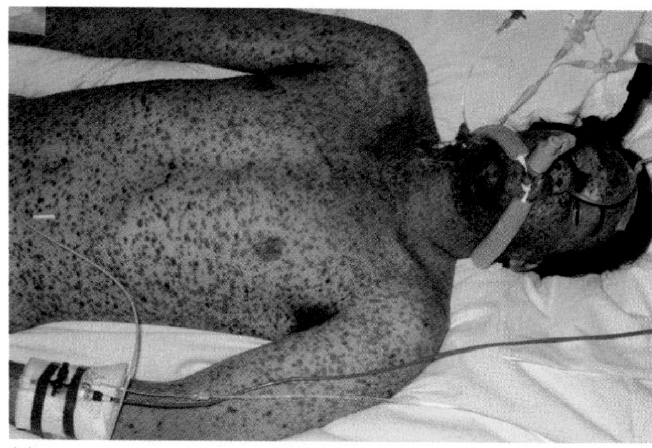

(a)

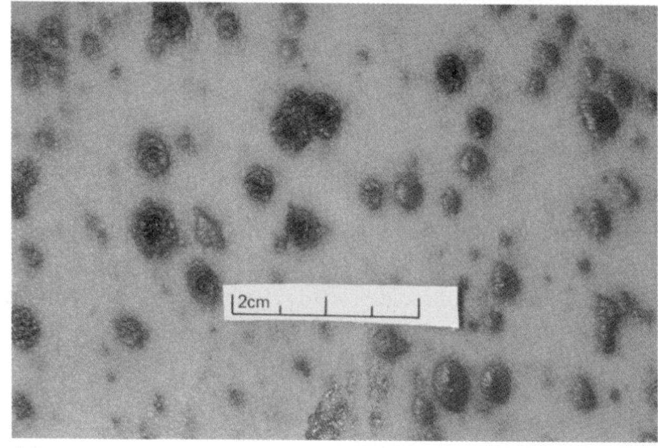

(b)

Fig. 7.5.2.4 Severe chickenpox: (a) and (b).
(Copyright D A Warrell.)

Complications of varicella

The principal complications of varicella in immunocompetent patients are pneumonitis and encephalitis.

Pneumonitis In a prospective study, 6% of young adults with chickenpox had respiratory symptoms, although 16% had changes on chest radiography, but the rate of admission to hospital for pneumonia in adults with varicella is only about 0.3%. Patients present with dyspnoea, cough, hypoxia, and bilateral infiltrates on the chest radiograph, occurring 1 to 6 days after the appearance of the rash. Hypoxia may be more severe than expected from the physical signs or the chest radiograph. The interstitial pneumonitis can progress to respiratory failure requiring artificial ventilation and intensive care (Fig. 7.5.2.4a), but it is more commonly transient, resolving completely within 2 to 3 days. Varicella pneumonia is said to be more common in smokers. Fatalities are rare, and VZV pneumonia

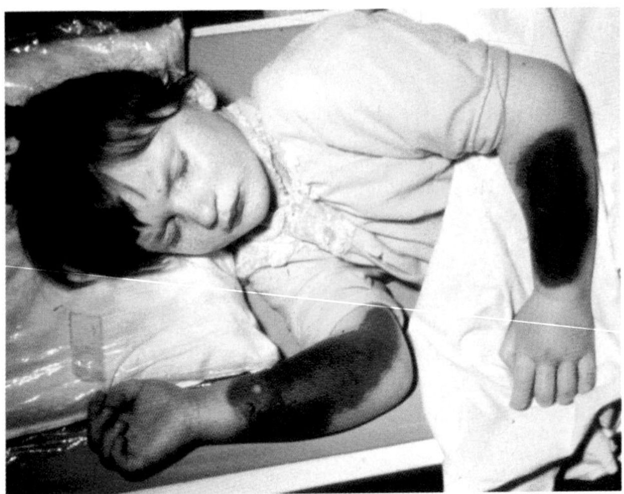

Fig. 7.5.2.5 Varicella purpura fulminans.
(Courtesy of the late Dr B E Juel-Jensen.)

is not associated with long-term respiratory problems. Benign nodular calcification throughout the lung occasionally follows.

Encephalitis Central nervous system involvement during varicella most commonly presents as acute cerebellar ataxia within 1 week of onset of the rash, although it may appear up to 21 days after the rash. It resolves completely over 2 to 4 weeks. A frequency of 1 in 4000 children aged less than 15 years has been quoted. The cerebrospinal fluid of these patients shows lymphocytosis and elevated protein concentration.

More serious encephalitis can occur in 0.1 to 0.2% of cases of varicella. This begins earlier in the course of infection than cerebellar ataxia, with headache, vomiting, confusion, and impaired consciousness. There is evidence of diffuse cerebral oedema, but no defined pattern of CT or MRI abnormality. The encephalitis may be progressive, and the mortality is between 5 and 20%, with neurological sequelae in up to 1% of survivors.

Varicella meningitis can occur. Other rarely reported neurological complications include optic neuritis, transverse myelitis, and Reye's syndrome.

Other complications Primary VZV infection may be complicated by acute thrombocytopenia, with petechiae, purpura, haemorrhage into vesicles, and other haemorrhagic manifestations. The platelet count can remain low for weeks after the illness has resolved. Secondary infection of the skin lesions with *Staphylococcus aureus* or *Streptococcus pyogenes* may occur. Purpura fulminans is a rare complication associated with arterial thrombosis and haemorrhagic gangrene (Fig. 7.5.2.5). Nephritis and arthritis have been reported as occasional complications, and myocarditis, pericarditis, pancreatitis, and orchitis are even more rare.

Special problems in pregnant women Varicella in pregnant women can be severe, with a maternal mortality of 1%. Varicella in the first trimester can cause varicella embryopathy. Affected infants may have a scarred, atrophic limb, microcephaly, cortical atrophy, and eye defects including chorioretinitis, microophthalmia, and cataracts. The autonomic nervous system may be damaged. Varicella embryopathy is rare; in recent reported series the risk was about 1 to 2% in mothers with varicella in the first 20 weeks of pregnancy. Varicella–zoster immunoglobulin should be considered for pregnant women in contact with varicella, and varicella in pregnancy should be treated with aciclovir on a named-patient basis. Neonatal varicella occurs in babies whose mothers contract varicella just before or after delivery, and is most severe when maternal disease appears from 2 to 7 days after delivery.

Herpes zoster

The clinical syndrome caused by the reactivation of VZV from sensory ganglia is herpes zoster. Typical prodromal localized pain or paraesthesia is followed by erythema and vesicular lesions occurring in a dermatomal distribution. The thoracic dermatomes, especially T4 to T12, are involved in about 50% of cases (Fig. 7.5.2.6); the lumbosacral dermatomes in about 16%; and the cranial nerves (mainly the Vth) in 14 to 20% of patients (Fig. 7.5.2.7a). The first symptoms are usually paraesthesia and shooting pains in the affected dermatome, which precede the eruption of vesicles by several days, occasionally 1 week or more. Erythematous maculopapular lesions then appear and quickly evolve into a vesicular rash, nearly always in a unilateral dermatome, with no vesicles beyond the midline. The vesicles usually form scabs after 3 to 7 days, and these separate after 2 weeks or so, but there is sometimes a more severe locally necrotic reaction (Fig. 7.5.2.8). There is a risk of secondary infection, particularly with *Staphylococcus aureus*. There may be malaise and low-grade fever, but laboratory investigations usually show no abnormalities, although up to 40% of patients with uncomplicated zoster may have lymphocytes and elevated protein in the cerebrospinal fluid. Involvement of the mandibular branch of the Vth cranial nerve can give intraoral lesions on the palate (Fig. 7.5.2.7b), floor of the mouth, and tongue. Involvement of the geniculate ganglion results in Ramsay Hunt syndrome, with pain and vesicles in the external auditory meatus, a loss of taste in the anterior two-thirds of the tongue, and a lower motor neurone VIIth cranial nerve palsy.

Complications of zoster

Ophthalmic zoster VZV reactivation from the trigeminal ganglion can affect the ophthalmic division of the trigeminal nerve, resulting in ophthalmic zoster (Fig. 7.5.2.7a). The features include conjunctivitis, anterior uveitis, keratitis, and sometimes iridocyclitis, with secondary glaucoma and panophthalmitis. However, these latter sight-threatening complications of ophthalmic zoster

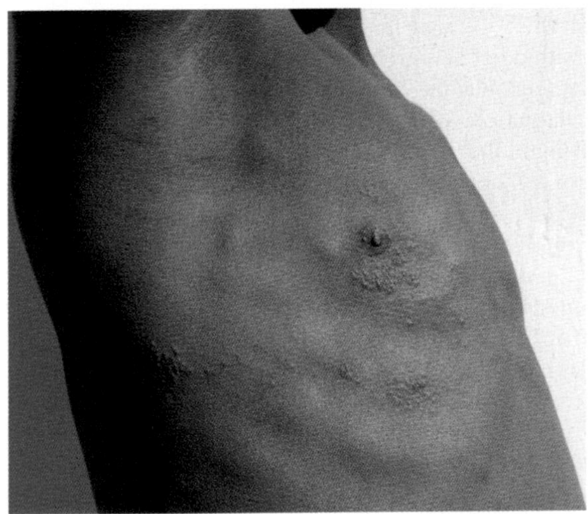

Fig. 7.5.2.6 Herpes zoster (shingles) of the T4 dermatome.
(Copyright D A Warrell.)

are unusual. A rare association with ophthalmic zoster is granulomatous cerebral angiitis, which can be associated with arterial thrombosis; cerebral angiography shows segmental narrowing in the cerebral arteries on the side of the ophthalmic zoster occurring weeks after the rash. CT may show cerebral infarcts, particularly in the middle cerebral artery territory, and contralateral hemiparesis can occur.

Motor zoster Weakness or paralysis can sometimes be associated with zoster, and results from the involvement of the anterior horn cells in the same segment of the spinal cord as the involved dorsal root ganglion. Depending on the segment involved, this can lead to a monoparesis affecting the upper or lower limb, or to diaphragmatic palsy (with the involvement of C5/6). Paralysis usually recovers completely, although the outlook for the recovery of facial nerve palsy is more variable. It is suggested VZV may be responsible for some cases of idiopathic VIIth nerve (Bell's) palsy.

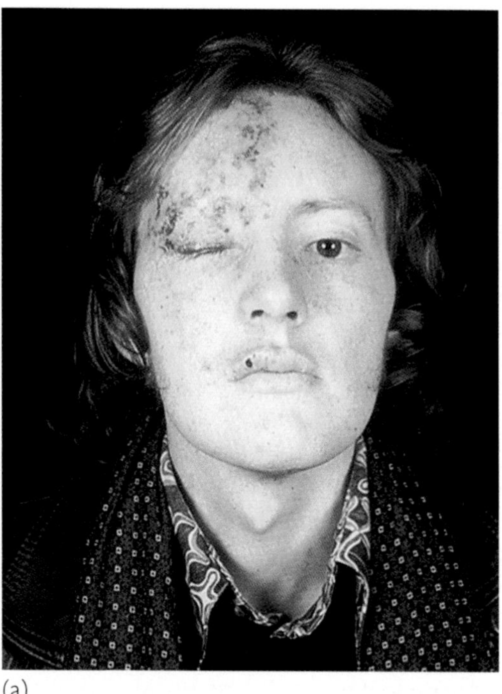

(a)

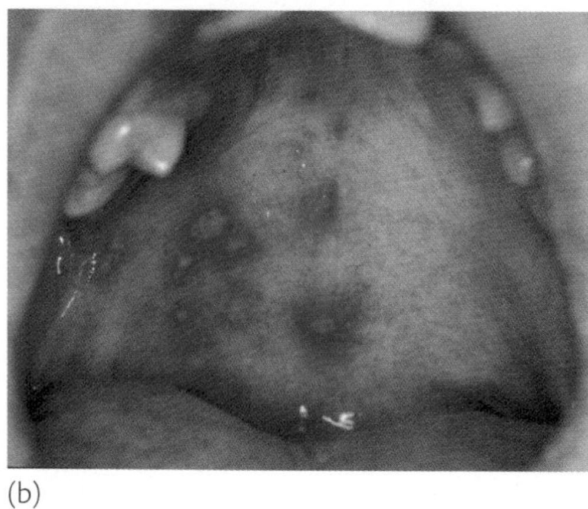

(b)

Fig. 7.5.2.7 Herpes zoster of the Vth cranial nerve: (a) ophthalmic division, and (b) lesions on the palate.
(Courtesy of the late Dr B E Juel-Jensen.)

Autonomic zoster Lumbosacral herpes zoster can be associated with neurogenic bladder, and acute retention of urine. This may be accompanied by haemorrhagic cystitis resulting from vesicles on the bladder wall. Intestinal ileus and obstruction may occur.

Zoster meningoencephalitis Meningoencephalitis may accompany zoster at any site, and is heralded by impaired consciousness, headache, photophobia, and meningism. The interval from the onset of skin lesions to symptoms is around 9 days, but may be as long as

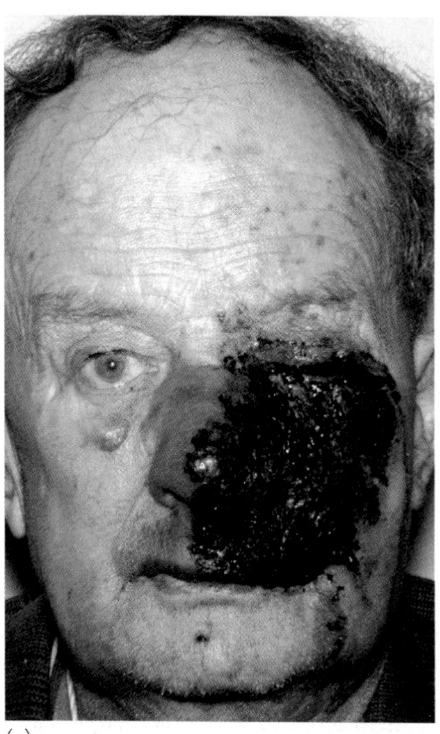

(a)

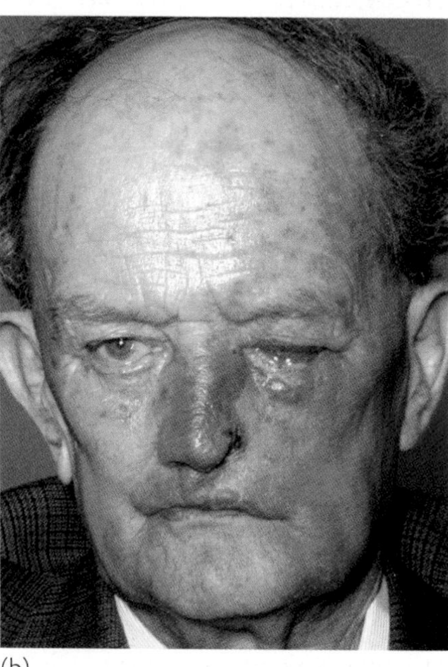

(b)

Fig. 7.5.2.8 Herpes zoster of the Vth cranial nerve, showing severe necrotic effects: (a) acutely, and (b) after recovery.
(Courtesy of the late Dr B.E Juel-Jensen.)

6 weeks. Symptomatic encephalitis usually lasts around 2 weeks, and is nearly always followed by full recovery without neurological sequelae.

Transverse myelitis, although rare, can occur at any level of the spinal cord.

Postherpetic neuralgia The incidence of postherpetic neuralgia rises with the increasing age of the patient. It is uncommon in young people, but can occur in 50% of patients older than 50 years. It is characterized by pain in the affected dermatome persisting for 1 month or more after the acute attack of zoster has resolved. The pain may be steady and burning, or paroxysmal and stabbing in nature; it may occur spontaneously, or be triggered by stimuli such as temperature or touch.

Zoster sine herpete This term refers to radicular pain similar to that experienced in zoster, but without the antecedent skin lesions of zoster. It was originally applied to patients who did have obvious zoster, but had dermatomal pain in areas distinct from those where there was rash. However, it is more commonly applied to patients with radicular pain and no rash at all. There have been reports describing the use of PCR testing for the detection of VZV DNA in the cerebrospinal fluid of patients with presumed zoster sine herpete. The literature is anecdotal, and it is difficult to regard zoster sine herpete as a diagnostic entity unless there is good evidence for VZV involvement, e.g. by the detection of VZV DNA in cerebrospinal fluid and/or blood mononuclear cells. It should be included in the differential diagnosis of radicular pain of unknown cause. Any possible mechanism is speculative.

VZV infection in immunosuppressed patients In patients with immunosuppression, particularly of cellular immunity, varicella can be much more severe. The skin lesions are more diffuse (Fig. 7.5.2.9), and can take up to 3 times as long to heal. There may be visceral dissemination to the lungs, liver and central nervous system. Patients with lymphoma undergoing chemotherapy are particularly susceptible.

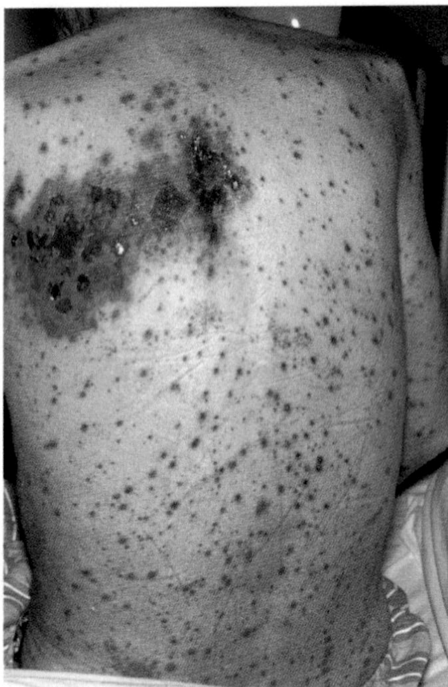

Fig. 7.5.2.9 Herpes zoster varicelliformis.
(Courtesy of the late Dr B E Juel-Jensen.)

Herpes zoster in immunosuppressed patients is also more severe than in healthy subjects. Before effective antiviral therapy was available, skin lesions were more extensive and could take several weeks longer to heal. Dissemination, presumably because of viraemic spread, with widespread skin lesions as in varicella, occurs in 10 to 40% of patients. Cutaneous dissemination is more likely to be associated with visceral dissemination to the same sites as those associated with varicella.

Patients with HIV infection or AIDS are prone to multidermatomal zoster, which can be one of the defining features of AIDS.

VZV retinitis This is a combination of pain and blurred vision in one eye, with progressive necrotizing retinitis seen on ophthalmoscopy. Adjacent cutaneous zoster indicates the diagnosis, but occasionally VZV retinitis occurs in immunocompetent patients as the sole manifestation of VZV reactivation. VZV retinitis may be difficult to distinguish from CMV retinitis. A severe form of the disease, seen particularly in patients with HIV infection, and named progressive outer retinal necrosis, is associated with a high incidence of retinal detachment, and may require treatment with ganciclovir, as aciclovir is often ineffective.

Differential diagnosis

Varicella is usually recognized relatively easily. Other causes of a vesicular rash are generalized herpes simplex in the immunosuppressed patient, and enteroviral disease, particularly hand, foot, and mouth disease caused by Coxsackie virus infection, but the rash on the hands and feet is unlike that of varicella, which has a centripetal distribution (Chapter 7.5.8). Human cases of infection with animal pox viruses (monkey pox and camel pox) have rarely been described (Chapter 7.5.4). Localized pain before the appearance of shingles or in zoster sine herpete may be severe enough to suggest myocardial ischaemia, or lung or intra-abdominal pathology if it involves the thoracic dermatomes.

Pathology

The histological appearance of VZV infection is similar or indistinguishable from that of HSV infection.

Laboratory diagnosis

The diagnosis of varicella and herpes zoster is usually made on clinical criteria alone. Virus can be seen in vesicular fluid by electron microscopy, or isolated in culture. A serological diagnosis of varicella can be made by demonstrating seroconversion or VZV IgM antibody. Urgent serology is needed to confirm the seronegative status of contacts at risk of severe VZV infection, to determine the need for VZV immunoglobulin (see 'Prevention and control' below). PCR-based tests for the detection of VZV DNA are available, and are of most use in testing cerebrospinal fluid in cases of suspected central nervous system disease.

Treatment

Pruritus may be alleviated by calamine lotion and antihistamines in patients with chickenpox. Fingernails should be closely cut to minimize scratching. Skin care is important to prevent secondary bacterial infection in patients with varicella and zoster. Aspirin should be avoided in children with chickenpox because of the risk

Box 7.5.2.1 The use of aciclovir in varicella–zoster infections

Indications for intravenous aciclovir (10 mg/kg 8 hourly)

Chickenpox:

- Immunocompromised patients
- Neonatal chickenpox
- Chickenpox with systemic complications
- Severe chickenpox in adults and in pregnancy (5 mg/kg 8 hourly)

Shingles:

- Severe shingles in immunocompromised patients
- Multidermatomal shingles
- Shingles complicated by ocular, motor, autonomic, or systemic involvement
- VZV retinitis (severe forms in AIDS may require foscarnet or ganciclovir)

Indications for oral aciclovir (800 mg 5 times daily)

- Uncomplicated chickenpox (except for mild chickenpox in children)
- Uncomplicated shingles in patients over 45 years
- Uncomplicated shingles in immunosuppressed patients
- Shingles presenting with severe pain

Infections not requiring active antiviral treatment

- Uncomplicated mild chickenpox in children
- Patients presenting more than 48 h after the appearance of the last lesion, or when all lesions have crusted
- Uncomplicated shingles in patients under 45 years
- Postherpetic neuralgia

of Reye's syndrome. Strong analgesia may be needed in patients with zoster.

VZV is sensitive to the nucleoside analogues aciclovir, famciclovir, and valaciclovir; as for HSV, VZV encodes a thymidine kinase that preferentially phosphorylates these drugs in infected cells. The median 50% inhibitory concentration of aciclovir against HSV is 0.1μM, but is 2.6μM against VZV, so 800 mg orally is necessary to achieve inhibitory concentrations.

The treatment recommendations for varicella and herpes zoster are summarized in Box 7.5.2.1.

Varicella

Whether to treat normal children with varicella (who are the great majority of patients) has been much debated; the argument can be made that the disease is not always mild and it is not possible to predict which child may have a severe case. Therapy with aciclovir is safe, and although it has been suggested that widespread treatment with antivirals might result in viral resistance, or failure to develop normal immune responses, there is no evidence of this in controlled trials. Treatment with aciclovir begun within 24 h of the onset of the rash leads to a 25% decrease in the duration and severity of chickenpox. The argument for treating all adolescents and adults is easier, as chickenpox is more severe for them than it is for young children. Chickenpox in neonates, children with leukaemia, and transplant recipients should always be treated with aciclovir. Intravenous aciclovir limits the visceral spread of the virus if given immediately on diagnosis. Treatment in these immunosuppressed patients can be changed from intravenous to oral aciclovir once the fever has settled, if there is no evidence of visceral varicella.

Herpes zoster

The major justification for the antiviral treatment of herpes zoster in immunocompetent patients has been to limit postherpetic neuralgia. Although there are difficulties in accurately and objectively quantifying the pain of postherpetic neuralgia, trial data indicate that aciclovir, valaciclovir, and famciclovir can limit the duration of zoster-associated pain, and that valaciclovir is slightly more effective. All three drugs accelerate the healing of cutaneous lesions by 2 days over placebo; valaciclovir and famciclovir have the advantage of more convenient dosage, as well as probably being slightly more effective.

Patients over the age of 50 years with zoster have the highest risk of postherpetic neuralgia, and so should be offered antiviral treatment. Younger patients may warrant treatment if they have marked pain. All patients with ophthalmic zoster should be treated urgently with antivirals, even if they present relatively late, as aciclovir reduces the incidence of keratitis. Immunosuppressed patients with herpes zoster should receive intravenous aciclovir to prevent cutaneous and visceral dissemination. Valaciclovir and famciclovir may be used if zoster presents in a localized form in less severely immunosuppressed patients.

Corticosteroids have been advocated in patients with herpes zoster, in order to reduce the severity of postherpetic neuralgia. However, the addition of oral prednisone to aciclovir slightly increases the rate of healing of skin lesions, but does not affect the incidence of postherpetic neuralgia; a role for corticosteroids thus remains unproven. Established postherpetic neuralgia can be managed with analgesics, tricyclic antidepressants, and other agents used for neuropathic pain, such as gabapentin and pregabalin, which were effective for the treatment of postherpetic neuralgia in large placebo-controlled trials. Although the use of opioids for the treatment of neuropathic pain is controversial, several studies support their efficacy and safety; oxycodone and tramadol have been shown to be superior to placebo for the treatment of postherpetic neuralgia. Topical agents such as lidocaine 5% patches and topical capsaicin have been useful in ameliorating postherpetic neuralgia, but are unsatisfactory for use as sole agents (see also Chapter 24.12).

Prevention and control

Varicella–zoster immune globulin, prepared from high-titre immune human serum, has been shown to prevent or ameliorate varicella in seronegative people at high risk, such as immunocompromised people and pregnant women. It should be given to seronegative immunodeficient patients (including those on high-dose corticosteroid treatment), and pregnant women with definite contact with varicella. It should be administered within 10 days (preferably 2–4 days) of exposure. Neonates whose mothers have had varicella less than 1 week before delivery, or within 28 days after delivery are also recommended to receive varicella–zoster immune globulin.

A VZV vaccine is available; a live attenuated Japanese vaccine containing the Oka strain of VZV. It confers 90% protection from natural varicella when administered to susceptible immunosuppressed people (such as patients with leukaemia and lymphoma receiving chemotherapy), but it produces rash in up to 40% of these recipients. In immunized healthy children the risk of subsequent varicella after community exposure is reduced to less than 5%, and the vaccine-induced rash is much less common (about 5% of recipients). This vaccine is licensed in Japan, some European countries, and the United States of America, where it is recommended for the routine immunization of children aged 12 to 18 months. However, in the United Kingdom it is recommended only for use in seronegative health care workers and children over 1 year in contact with individuals at high risk of severe varicella. Trials have shown that the postinfective immunization of subjects aged 60 years or over diminishes the incidence of zoster and postherpetic neuralgia, and the vaccine is now licensed in the United States of America for the prevention of herpes zoster in this age group.

The nosocomial transmission of VZV by patients with varicella requiring admission to hospital is a significant risk, as 10% of adults are seronegative. Nursing and managing patients with varicella in hospital should be restricted to those staff known to be seropositive for VZV. Patients with varicella in hospital should ideally be isolated in negative-pressure rooms to prevent airborne transmission.

Human cytomegalovirus infection

Historical background

The syndrome of congenital cytomegalovirus infection, cytomegalic inclusion disease, was described in children with fatal infection in 1904, but the intranuclear inclusions were attributed to a protozoan parasite. In 1921, the pathologist Goodpasture suggested that the inclusions in the parotid glands of infants were caused by a virus, because a filterable agent produced similar histology in guinea pig salivary glands, and the lesions were attributed in 1926 to 'salivary gland virus'. Human cytomegalovirus (HCMV) was finally isolated in 1956, and so named by Weller for the characteristic owl's-eye, or cytomegalic inclusions it produces in the nuclei of infected cells.

HCMV produces little morbidity in immunocompetent people, but can produce severe disease in the fetus if infection is acquired *in utero*, and in immunosuppressed patients.

Aetiology

HCMV is the largest human herpesvirus, with a linear double-stranded DNA genome of 250 kb encoding more than 200 proteins. Mammalian cytomegaloviruses are species specific, and so HCMV cannot be studied in animal models. The most widely studied laboratory strain, AD169, shows significant genomic variation from recent clinical isolates, which possess an additional 15 kb of DNA. HCMV replicates slowly compared with other herpesviruses, and gene expression occurs sequentially in immediate-early, early, and late phases.

Epidemiology

Following primary infection, HCMV persists for life as a latent infection, with periodic asymptomatic excretion of virus in saliva, breast milk, urine, semen, and cervical secretions. Infection is spread by close contact with these body fluids. In developing countries, HCMV is usually acquired in childhood, and nearly 100% of young adults are seropositive. In developed countries, seroconversion progresses with age, but seroprevalence is higher in lower socioeconomic groups. Overall, about 50% of adults are seropositive. In childhood, HCMV is acquired from breast milk or contact with infected children excreting virus in their saliva or urine. Children in day nurseries transmit the virus to each other, and to susceptible adult carers. Later, sexual transmission becomes a major route of infection, and seroprevalence approaches 100% in homosexual men, and sex workers.

Blood and blood products from normal seropositive donors can transmit HCMV. Transfusion recipients at risk of HCMV disease now usually receive screened seronegative blood; otherwise the risk of transfusion-related HCMV infection is 2.5% per unit of blood. The virus is carried in leucocytes, and leukodepletion of blood greatly reduces the risk of HCMV transmission. The technique is also being widely adopted as a preventive measure against transmissible spongiform encephalopathies. Finally, solid organ and bone marrow transplants from seropositive donors can transmit HCMV, producing particularly severe disease in seronegative recipients.

Pathogenesis

Current evidence suggests myeloid-lineage cells are a principal site of HCMV latency, and that virus may be reactivated from dendritic cells and monocytes as they differentiate. Endothelial cells, possibly epithelial and other cells, may also be sites of latency.

The immune response is critical for controlling infection in the normal host. Normal immunocompetent individuals infected with HCMV mount a strong T-cell response, with very high frequencies of cytotoxic (CD8+) T lymphocytes in the peripheral blood targeted particularly at the HCMV major tegument protein pp. 65, and the major immediate-early protein IE1. Impairment of this response is associated with the risk of disseminated infection. HCMV possesses multiple immune-evasion genes, whose products interfere with the class I MHC antigen-processing pathway, and recognition by natural killer (NK) cells, which may help the virus reactivate by delaying T- and NK-cell recognition of infected cells. Antibody probably limits blood-borne dissemination of HCMV, as maternal IgG appears to be especially important in preventing viral transmission to the fetus.

Subclinical reactivation occurs frequently in the normal host, but is controlled by the immune response. Immune deficiency, particularly of the T-cell response, such as iatrogenic or disease-induced immunosuppression, may allow uncontrolled replication and result in HCMV disease. Pathology is presumably produced by the direct cytopathic effects of the virus, although indirect effects produced by soluble virus-encoded proteins or the host response are also possible. The presence of HCMV in a diseased organ does not necessarily implicate the virus as a cause; reactivation of the virus can sometimes be nonpathogenic, and reflects its being a bystander, coexisting with another pathogenic process.

Clinical features of HCMV disease

Primary infection in immunocompetent subjects

Primary infection in children and adults is asymptomatic in most cases, but HCMV can produce an illness clinically indistinguishable from infectious mononucleosis caused by primary Epstein–Barr virus (EBV) infection, typically with fever, myalgia, cervical lymphadenopathy, and mild hepatitis. Tonsillopharyngitis is much less common than in primary EBV infection, and lymphadenopathy and splenic enlargement are less prominent features. The fever lasts 2 to 3 weeks, but can persist for up to 5 weeks. In developed countries an increasing proportion of HCMV seroconversion illness is seen in older adults, and the diagnosis should still be considered in patients aged over 50 years. Myocarditis, pneumonitis, and aseptic meningitis are rare complications. A proportion (5–10%) of patients with Guillain–Barré syndrome show serological evidence of primary HCMV infection; they are more likely to have antibodies to the GM2 ganglioside than other patients with Guillain–Barré syndrome, and a causal relationship has been postulated.

Primary HCMV infection acquired from blood transfusion results in a similar clinical picture occurring 3 to 6 weeks after transfusion, and is usually self limiting in the normal host. To distinguish between primary HCMV infection and other causes of mononucleosis syndromes, such as EBV and toxoplasmosis, requires serological testing (the Paul–Bunnell and monospot tests are negative in HCMV mononucleosis).

HCMV disease in immunosuppressed patients

HCMV infection is most severe in immunosuppressed patients, particularly solid organ and bone marrow transplant recipients, and those with AIDS, all of whom have impaired T-lymphocyte function. This strongly supports the importance of T cells in controlling infection.

Solid organ transplant recipients

The risk of HCMV disease is 3 to 5 times greater in a seronegative recipient receiving a graft from a seropositive donor, and it causes much more severe infection than in a seropositive recipient who has a reinfection or reactivation of latent virus. Many centres pair seronegative donors with seronegative recipients, although this is often thwarted by organ shortage. Clinically, there may be specific organ involvement, which is not seen in normal patients. Interstitial pneumonitis caused by HCMV is rare, except in bone marrow transplant recipients, and carries a poor prognosis; gastrointestinal disease includes oesophagitis, gastritis and peptic ulceration, and colitis; and HCMV retinitis may occur in severely immunosuppressed patients. HCMV has been reported to be associated with increased graft rejection and renal artery stenosis in renal transplant recipients; with accelerated coronary artery stenosis in heart transplant recipients; and with vanishing bile duct syndrome in liver transplant recipients. However, none of these associations is definitively established as causal.

Bone marrow transplant recipients

HCMV disease is a major problem in allogeneic bone marrow transplant recipients, with a 30 to 50% incidence of clinically significant infection. It is a lesser problem in autologous bone marrow transplant. If the donor and/or recipient is seropositive there is a risk of HCMV disease, but if both donor and recipient are seronegative, infection can be prevented if solely HCMV-seronegative blood products are used to support the patient. Pneumonitis is the most serious manifestation of HCMV infection after bone marrow transplant, occurring in 10 to 15% of allogeneic bone marrow transplant recipients, with a mortality of 80% without antiviral therapy. The clinical presentation is interstitial pneumonitis in the absence of any other identifiable pathogen, with increasing arterial hypoxaemia, and progression to respiratory failure. It is suggested that graft versus host disease may contribute to the lung injury in HCMV pneumonitis in bone marrow transplant recipients. The relationship between HCMV and graft versus host disease is controversial, with suggestions that HCMV may predispose to graft versus host disease, and vice versa.

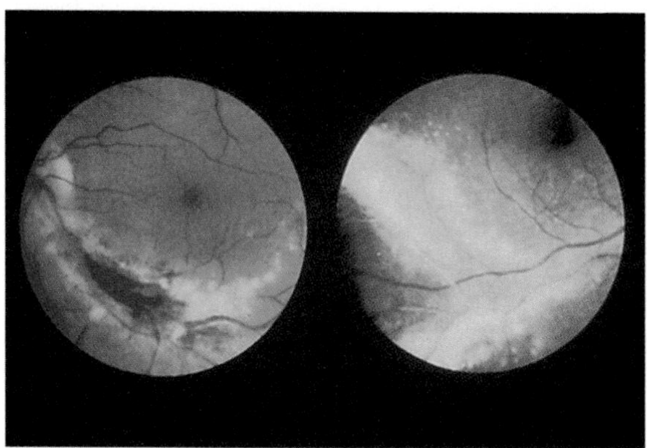

Fig. 7.5.2.10 CMV retinitis.

Patients with AIDS

HCMV disease is one of the most frequent opportunistic infections in patients with advanced HIV infection, of whom 40% develop sight- or life-threatening HCMV disease. A CD4 count of less than 50/μl carries a high risk of disease, although the widespread use of antiretroviral therapy in developed countries means that relatively few patients now have such low CD4 counts, and the incidence of HCMV disease in patients with AIDS has declined significantly.

HCMV retinitis has been seen in up to 25% of patients with AIDS not receiving effective antiretroviral therapy. Haemorrhagic retinal necrosis spreads along retinal vessels, and threatens sight when disease encroaches on the macula (Fig. 7.5.2.10). The clinical effect is visual impairment, and the risk of retinal detachment and haemorrhage is increased, hence those with low CD4 counts should have regular optic fundoscopy to detect retinitis before it becomes symptomatic. Diagnosis is made by the ophthalmological detection of typical retinal changes, preferably with accompanying evidence of HCMV viraemia. In the absence of treatment, HCMV retinitis almost invariably progresses to affect both eyes and destroy vision.

HCMV is reported to produce diffuse encephalitis in AIDS patients, but although the virus is sometimes seen in neuronal cells at autopsy, encephalitis attributable to HCMV is relatively rare in clinical practice by comparison with the other causes of encephalitis in AIDS. HCMV can also produce a progressive radiculopathy, causing low-back pain that radiates to the area supplied by the affected spinal nerve root, and the development of flaccid paraparesis.

In the gastrointestinal tract, HCMV is associated with oesophagitis, gastritis, and enterocolitis, and virus can be seen in biopsies from these sites, usually in shallow ulcers. HCMV pneumonitis is rare in patients with AIDS, suggesting that there must be additional factors to account for its frequency in bone marrow transplant recipients.

Congenital and neonatal HCMV infection

HCMV infection of the neonate may be congenital from intrauterine infection, perinatal from transmission during birth, or postnatal from breast milk. The frequency of congenital HCMV infection in developed countries is around 0.5 to 1% of live births, resulting from either primary maternal infection in pregnancy, or from reactivation of HCMV in a previously infected mother during pregnancy. The risk of primary maternal infection in pregnancy is about 1%, and it carries a 40% risk of congenital infection.

Fetal infection is more likely to be severe following primary infection in early pregnancy, whereas the risk of symptomatic congenital infection is much lower, although not absent, from reactivation of maternal HCMV. Pre-existing maternal immunity limits spread to the fetus.

Approximately 5 to 20% of congenitally infected babies are symptomatic at birth. In its most severe form, usually in babies of mothers with primary maternal infection, the clinical features of congenital HCMV are: microcephaly; chorioretinitis; nerve deafness; hepatitis with jaundice and hepatosplenomegaly; and thrombocytopenia with petechiae. This classical cytomegalic inclusion disease has a high mortality, and 80% of all infants symptomatic at birth who survive have serious sequelae, such as learning, visual, and hearing impairment. However, most congenitally infected babies are asymptomatic at birth, and only 5 to 15% of these subsequently develop sequelae on long-term follow up, the most common being sensorineural deafness, which also occurs in isolation in otherwise normal babies.

Perinatally or postnatally acquired HCMV infection is rarely symptomatic or associated with long-term sequelae, if the mother is seropositive.

Pathology

On light microscopy, typical HCMV-infected cells appear large, with a relative reduction in cytoplasm, and nuclei that contain prominent inclusions surrounded by a clear halo (described as owl's-eye inclusions). These cells contain replicating virus, and are associated with active infection and disease; they are diagnostic when seen in biopsies of affected organs. In patients dying of severe disease, histological evidence of HCMV involvement can be found in most organs, whereas it infects a restricted range of cells *in vitro*.

Malignancy

Although associations between HCMV and malignancy have been postulated in the past, there is currently no good evidence to associate the virus with any human malignancy.

Laboratory diagnosis

Primary infection is usually diagnosed by the detection of IgM antibody to HCMV in the absence of IgG antibody; there is a marked atypical lymphocytosis (mainly increased CD8+ T cells), but heterophile antibody (as detected in primary EBV infection by the monospot or Paul–Bunnell tests) is absent. IgG antibody is a useful marker of HCMV carriage, but titres do not rise reliably in disease; IgM antibody, a marker of primary infection, is also sometimes found with reactivation in immunosuppressed patients, and serology is of limited use in confirming HCMV disease in these patients. Culture of virus from urine may only indicate asymptomatic reactivation, but culture from the blood buffy coat suggests HCMV disease. The virus can never be cultured from the blood of normal HCMV carriers, and culture from an organ site (such as bronchoalveolar lavage fluid) may indicate locally active infection.

Rapid culture methods such as DEAFF (detection of early antigen fluorescent foci), which uses a monoclonal antibody against an immediate-early viral protein, or shell vial tests (centrifuging samples onto cell cultures) are now used less often. PCR techniques are increasingly used to detect and quantify the HCMV load in blood or plasma, and this is now the standard assay for detecting HCMV in many laboratories. As virus can never be detected in plasma (as opposed to leucocytes) in normal carriers, the presence of HCMV DNA in plasma indicates active viral replication. Detection of virus in biopsy specimens by histological and immunohistological techniques implies active HCMV infection in the relevant tissue.

In practice, HCMV disease is usually diagnosed by the combination of an appropriate clinical syndrome, and detection of HCMV DNA by quantitative PCR above a threshold level in blood or plasma, or in biopsies from involved organs, in the absence of any other likely causal microbial pathogen.

Treatment

Several drugs are now available for the treatment of HCMV disease. Aciclovir has little *in vitro* activity against HCMV, which does not possess a thymidine kinase (see 'Herpes simplex virus infections' above), and has no place in therapy (although valaciclovir is used in prophylaxis; see 'Antiviral prophylaxis' below).

Ganciclovir, another nucleoside analogue, is monophosphorylated in infected cells by the *UL97* gene product of HCMV, and is active against HCMV; its most limiting side effect is myelotoxicity, with leukopenia and thrombocytopenia, but it has many other potential side effects, including azoospermia, and intravenous administration is necessary. Valganciclovir, a valyl ester prodrug of ganciclovir, has much higher oral bioavailability, and produces equivalent plasma concentrations to intravenous ganciclovir; it is thus useful for prophylaxis. Resistance to ganciclovir results from a mutation in the HCMV DNA polymerase, or in the *UL97* gene, and is seen mainly in AIDS patients in whom prolonged use is necessary.

An alternative drug to ganciclovir is foscarnet, a competitive inhibitor of the viral DNA polymerase, which shows no crossresistance with ganciclovir. This also must be given intravenously, and its side effects include renal impairment and hypocalcaemia. Cidofovir, a nucleotide analogue acting on the viral DNA polymerase, is highly nephrotoxic (probenecid must be given concurrently to prevent irreversible renal damage), and therefore relatively rarely used. Another drug, maribavir, is not yet licenced.

Primary infection

In the immunocompetent host this usually requires no specific antiviral treatment, although occasionally, severe primary infection may lead to hospitalization and require treatment.

HCMV disease in immunosuppressed patients

Whether due to primary or secondary infection, or reactivation, this is usually treated with ganciclovir or foscarnet for 2 to 3 weeks, with full-dose induction intravenous therapy; for ganciclovir this is 5 mg/kg every 12 h and for foscarnet 60 mg/kg every 8 h. Oral valganciclovir 900 mg twice daily is an equivalent dose to intravenous ganciclovir. Secondary prophylaxis may well be needed if immunosuppression persists (see 'Prevention and control' below).

HCMV pneumonitis in bone marrow transplant recipients

This responds poorly to ganciclovir or foscarnet alone, but the combination of full-dose ganciclovir with intravenous immunoglobulin has been reported to reduce mortality. Specific anti-CMV immunoglobulin was initially used, then other trials suggest normal pooled intravenous immunoglobulin was equally effective, and recent reports question whether IVIg confers any additional benefit. Many centres monitor bone marrow transplant recipients, especially of allogeneic grafts, for CMV viraemia, and commence preemptive therapy with ganciclovir if viraemia is detected before the development of symptomatic or obvious organ disease.

HCMV retinitis in AIDS

This is treated with an induction course of ganciclovir or foscarnet (both drugs have also been used in combination) or valganciclovir 900 mg twice daily for 21 days. Continued prophylaxis is needed to prevent relapse until significant recovery of the CD4 count can be induced with antiretroviral therapy; valganciclovir 900 mg daily is most convenient. Implantable intraocular devices providing sustained release of ganciclovir into the vitreous humour have also been used. The use of combination antiretroviral therapy in HIV-infected patients is associated with much improved long-term control of HCMV infection. However, the syndrome of immune-recovery vitritis, characterized by posterior segment inflammation, can occur in patients with previously treated CMV retinitis when their CD4 count reconstitutes on antiretroviral therapy.

Congenital HCMV infection

Treating symptomatic congenital HCMV infection with ganciclovir (8 or 12 mg/kg daily for 6 weeks) reduces the excretion of CMV in the urine, but viruria returns to near pretreatment levels after cessation of therapy. Hearing improvement may occur, but the role of antiviral therapy in congenital HCMV infection remains to be established.

Prevention and control

The problem posed by HCMV in immunosuppressed patients has led to several approaches to prophylaxis.

Antiviral prophylaxis

There is a definite case for primary prophylaxis in solid organ and bone marrow transplant recipients at high risk of disease (seronegative recipients of a seropositive graft, or seropositive recipients), and in AIDS patients with fewer than 100 CD4 cells/µl. Ganciclovir has been widely used, and valganciclovir 900 mg daily is effective in many of these settings. Despite limited *in vitro* activity against HCMV, and lack of efficacy as therapy, oral valaciclovir has been shown to provide significant prophylaxis against HCMV disease in renal transplant recipients, and is licensed for this use.

Passive immunization

CMV hyperimmune globulin is reported to reduce the risk of HCMV disease in renal transplant recipients, but is expensive and little used in practice.

There are initial reports that HCMV-specific T-cell immunity can be reconstituted in bone marrow transplant recipients by the adoptive transfer of virus-specific T lymphocytes from the immune donor, but this is still being investigated.

Active immunization

A live laboratory strain (Towne) of HCMV has been tested as an experimental candidate vaccine in renal transplant recipients, with some evidence of protective immunity, perhaps equivalent to having previous natural HCMV infection. However, there is currently no available licensed vaccine.

Special problems in pregnant women

Pregnant women who are seronegative should avoid contact with possibly infected children in day-nursery settings, although this may be impractical. Ganciclovir must not be used in pregnancy.

Human herpesvirus 6 and 7

Human herpesvirus 6

Human herpesvirus 6 (HHV-6) was first isolated in 1986 from cultured human lymphocyte lines, and named human B lymphotropic virus, a misnomer since it is trophic principally for T cells, although replication also occurs in macrophages, glial cells, and EBV-transformed B cells. HHV-6 is widely distributed in humans. Primary infection causes roseola infantum (also known as exanthem subitum or sixth disease), an aetiological association first described in Japanese children in 1988.

Aetiology

HHV-6 has typical herpesvirus morphology, and is genetically classified in the betaherpesvirus subfamily. Two types of isolate, HHV-6A and HHV-6B, are now clearly distinguished by their genetic sequence, and some variation in biological properties. HHV-6B is associated with roseola, whereas HHV-6A has not been associated with disease.

Epidemiology

There is high seroprevalence of HHV-6 in all populations. More than 90% of children are seropositive at 2 years of age. The virus (usually the HHV-6B variant) can be detected in peripheral blood mononuclear cells by PCR-based tests in nearly all healthy people. It is most probably transmitted via maternal saliva, although intrauterine and perinatal transmission could occur. There is also evidence that chromosomally integrated maternal HHV6 can be transmitted in the germline, although the clinical significance is uncertain. The virus is not detectable in breast milk.

Pathogenesis

HHV-6 probably replicates in regional lymphoid tissue in the oropharynx during primary infection, and can be found in circulating lymphocytes. The virus replicates *in vitro* in CD4+ T-cell lines, but during persistent infection in the normal adult, virus can be detected by PCR in both CD4+ T cells and monocytes/macrophages in peripheral blood, which are probably the principal site of carriage during persistent infection. The mechanism of viral latency is uncertain.

Although HHV-6 cannot usually be isolated by culture from the peripheral blood of normal people, specific DNA is easily detected in blood during immunosuppression, indicating reactivation of HHV-6. The mechanism by which HHV6 produces its clinical manifestations remains unclear.

Clinical features

Primary infection with HHV-6 in young children is associated with roseola, and also with a febrile illness without rash.

Roseola infantum (exanthem subitum, sixth disease)

Roseola is an acute illness of infants and young children, typically 3 to 5 days of high fever with upper respiratory tract symptoms, and sometimes cervical lymphadenopathy. As the fever subsides, a rash appears and lasts for 1 to 3 days. The rash is diffuse, macular, or maculopapular, and appears similar to that of rubella. There is mild atypical lymphocytosis and maybe neutropenia. Infections may rarely be complicated by febrile convulsions, meningitis, encephalitis, and hepatitis, which is usually mild, but occasionally severe.

Roseola has been estimated to occur in only 10 to 20% of children, and primary HHV-6 infection is commonly subclinical.

Febrile Illness

Fever without rash is a more usual manifestation of primary HHV-6 infection than roseola. In a North American study, 10% of 1600 febrile children under the age of 3 years (including 20% of those aged 6–12 months) presenting with acute febrile illness were diagnosed as primary HHV-6 infection, but only 17% of them had clinical roseola.

Febrile convulsions

It is suggested HHV-6 may have a particular association with febrile convulsions in young children. Primary HHV-6 infection was reported to account for one-third of all the febrile seizures in children up to the age of 2 years; however, there were no seizures in 81 children with primary infection in a prospective cohort. HHV-6 DNA can be detected in the cerebrospinal fluid of children with primary infection, and any association may be because HHV-6 specifically infects the nervous system, rather than solely because of high fever.

HHV-6 infection in immunosuppressed patients

A number of studies have shown increases in antibody titres to HHV-6, and increased HHV-6 DNA levels in the peripheral blood of immunosuppressed solid organ and bone marrow transplant recipients. In bone marrow transplant recipients, HHV-6 has been associated with fever, skin rash, graft versus host disease, encephalitis, delayed engraftment, marrow suppression, and pneumonitis. It is not clear whether HHV-6 plays a specific aetiological role in all these syndromes; the evidence is perhaps stronger for a causal role in encephalitis. There is also good evidence that HHV-6 reactivates in patients with advanced HIV infection and AIDS, but again there is less firm evidence that this is associated with disease.

Other disease associations

Studies of chronic fatigue syndrome and multiple sclerosis have not provided convincing evidence of any significant aetiological association with HHV-6.

Differential diagnosis

Primary HHV-6 infection may be confused with many febrile childhood illnesses accompanied by a rash. Roseola may also be misdiagnosed as a sensitivity reaction to recent antibiotic treatment. Other virus infections (EBV, HCMV) may also be associated with atypical lymphocytes and a mononucleosis syndrome.

Pathology

HHV-6 replicates *in vitro* in cells originating from the central nervous system, particularly glial cell lines. HHV-6 DNA can be detected in the brains of apparently normal people, suggesting viral persistence in the central nervous system. No distinctive histopathology has yet been attributed to HHV-6.

Malignancy

HHV-6 DNA has been detected in the blood of patients with several lymphoproliferative disorders, but this probably reflects reactivation rather than any causal association with the tumour. HHV-6 DNA has been reported in some tumour tissues, including the nodular sclerosis variant of Hodgkin's disease, but without a convincing aetiological association between the virus and any tumour.

Laboratory diagnosis

Most assays for HHV-6 antibody do not distinguish between antibody to HHV-6A and HHV-6B, and may crossreact with antibodies to HHV-7. Seroconversion is evidence of primary infection. IgM assays for HHV-6 antibody are not reliable indicators of primary infection, as some HHV-6 carriers may periodically have IgM antibody.

Although HHV-6 can be cultured from peripheral blood mononuclear cells during acute primary infection, few laboratories will undertake this. PCR-based techniques for the detection of HHV-6 DNA in plasma and cerebrospinal fluid are the method of choice for clinical diagnosis, and are becoming more widely available.

Treatment

HHV-6 sensitivity to antiviral drugs corresponds with that of cytomegalovirus. Thus, HHV-6 replication is inhibited *in vitro* by ganciclovir and foscarnet, but not aciclovir; however, there are no controlled clinical trials of these drugs. Their use may be considered for immunosuppressed patients with suspected HHV-6-associated pneumonitis.

Prevention and control

There are no preventative measures for HHV-6 transmission. It seems unlikely that there will be a case for the development of a vaccine because infants may be infected so early in life, while they still have maternal antibody.

Special problems in pregnant women

Nearly all pregnant women will be carriers of HHV-6. There is no evidence that HHV-6 infection harms the fetus or the neonate.

Human herpesvirus 7

Human herpesvirus 7 (HHV-7) was isolated in 1990, and is a betaherpesvirus similar to, but distinct from, HHV-6. HHV-7 predominantly infects CD4+ T cells and can be reactivated from latency by T-cell activation.

Although there is serological crossreactivity between HHV-6 and HHV-7, data indicate that HHV-7 infects nearly all children, but later than HHV-6, with more than 90% being infected by the age of 5 years. The virus is excreted in saliva.

HHV-7 has been associated with some cases of roseola, which it was reported to cause in Japanese infants with a previous episode of roseola proven to be caused by HHV-6. There is no further evidence of pathogenicity.

The best method of diagnosis is PCR-based testing of serum or cerebrospinal fluid. Laboratory tests for HHV-6 often detect HHV-7 by multiplex PCR. There is no reason to consider any treatment for HHV-7.

Human herpesvirus 8

Human herpesvirus 8 (HHV-8) is the most recently isolated of the human herpesviruses; Chang and colleagues reported the detection of novel DNA sequences with homology to herpesviruses in Kaposi's sarcoma tissue in 1994. Initially named Kaposi's sarcoma-associated herpesvirus, it was subsequently designated HHV-8. It is genetically most closely related to a well characterized simian herpesvirus (herpesvirus saimiri), and less so to EBV; it has consequently been assigned to the rhadinovirus (γ2-herpesvirus) subfamily. Current culture techniques are unreliable, but the virus can be detected by PCR. Serological assays depend on the use of infected cell lines or synthetic antigens from predicted open reading frames. The seroepidemiology, biology, and disease associations of the virus are still being analysed, but HHV-8 is clearly associated with Kaposi's sarcoma, a tumour that has long been suspected of having a viral aetiology; with primary effusion lymphoma; and with multicentric Castleman's disease. Reported associations with multiple myeloma and other cancers are unconfirmed.

Aetiology

HHV-8 has the characteristic morphology of a herpesvirus. The viral genome is composed of a 141 kbp unique segment flanked by multiple 801 bp direct repeats. Sequence analysis suggests that HHV-8, like other herpesviruses, is an ancient human virus; comparative analysis of the variable genes *ORF-K1* and *K15* indicates there are at least four virus subtypes, A to D, reflecting the migrationary divergence of modern human populations. HHV-8 contains genes homologous to mammalian genes encoding cell-cycle regulatory proteins (the cyclins), chemokines, and inhibitors of apoptosis. On the evidence to date, the normal cellular site of latency of HHV-8 almost certainly includes the B cell.

Epidemiology

The emerging epidemiology of HHV-8 suggests it is less ubiquitous than other human herpesviruses. Initial serological assays detected antibodies to a latent nuclear antigen; assays using lytic-cycle antigens gave higher rates of seroprevalence, and newer assays using multiple HHV-8 antigens are currently being applied. Current data suggest a seroprevalence of 90% or more in patients with Kaposi's sarcoma, and 40% in HIV-positive homosexual men without Kaposi's sarcoma. Seroprevalence in normal adults is reported as being more than 50% in African adults in West Africa, 20% in black South African blood donors, and 53% in HIV-positive and -negative adults in Uganda. Seroprevalence is 5% or less in blood donors in the United Kingdom and the United States of America, with intermediate rates in Italy and other Mediterranean countries. HHV-8 can be detected by PCR in nearly all cases of Kaposi's sarcoma, but is less easy to detect in the blood of normal carriers.

The usual route of transmission is probably saliva and sexual contact, but intravenous drug use, blood transfusion, and organ transplantation also transmit the virus. A latent nuclear antigen-based assay detected seroconversion to HHV-8 in HIV-infected homosexual men at a median of 33 months before they subsequently developed Kaposi's sarcoma. HHV-8 infection in children correlates with seropositivity in their mothers, but whether this reflects vertical or horizontal transmission is uncertain.

Pathogenesis

There has been much uncertainty over the cell of origin of Kaposi's sarcoma, but the spindle cells of which the tumour is largely composed are thought to be of lymphatic endothelial origin. In Kaposi's sarcoma tumour tissue, HHV-8 DNA and latent nuclear antigen are present in every spindle cell, suggesting an aetiological role for the virus.

In HIV-associated Castleman's disease, the HHV-8 latent nuclear antigen is present in immunoblasts in the mantle zone of the tumour. HHV-8 is present in the tumour cells of all cases of primary effusion lymphoma so far studied (although so is EBV), and HHV-8 latently infected cell lines derived from these tumours can be induced to release infectious virus. These clear associations of virus DNA with tumour cells suggest a definite oncogenic role for HHV-8. The latent-cycle genes that maintain the virus DNA as an episome (latent nuclear antigen 1), and encode cyclin homologues and antiapoptotic proteins, are likely to be involved in cellular transformation and oncogenesis.

It has been suggested that HHV-8 may be involved in the pathogenesis of multiple myeloma, but this association is unproven, as is an association with primary pulmonary hypertension. The individual HHV-8 subtypes are not associated with any distinct pathology.

Clinical features

Apart from these malignancies, the only reported clinical syndrome accompanying primary or reactivated HHV-8 infection is fever and bone marrow graft failure in immunosuppressed transplant recipients.

Kaposi's sarcoma

Kaposi's sarcoma appears as purplish-brown macules, papules, or plaques. It is described in four characteristic clinical settings: the classical form in older Mediterranean or Jewish men, the endemic African form (accounting for 10% of cancer in equatorial Africa), in patients with immunodeficiency states, such as transplant recipients, and the AIDS-associated form. In the classical and African forms there are lesions on the extremities; systemic and mucosal involvement is rare, and the disease is indolent. In immunosuppressed patients (other than those with AIDS) the lesions are more widespread and more rapidly progressive, although visceral involvement is still unusual, and lesions may regress if immunosuppressive drugs are stopped. AIDS-associated Kaposi's sarcoma is seen predominantly in homosexual men in western countries, but is commonly associated with heterosexually acquired HIV infection in African countries. The clinical signs are widespread cutaneous lesions, with involvement of the oral mucosa (see Chapter 7.5.23, Figs. 7.5.23.12 and 7.5.23.13), and visceral lesions may occur in the lungs or gastrointestinal tract. Progression can be much more rapid than the other forms. HHV-8 has been isolated from all four types of Kaposi's sarcoma.

Primary effusion lymphomas

Previously known as body-cavity based lymphomas, these are a rare and aggressive type of B-cell lymphoma in patients with AIDS. They present as lymphomatous effusions of the peritoneal, pleural, or pericardial spaces, usually without any identifiable tumour mass. HHV-8 is present in the tumour cells of all cases so far studied, although so also is EBV.

Castleman's disease or angiofollicular lymph node hyperplasia

This can be localized, and is amenable to curative excision. However, a multicentric form is seen particularly in HIV-infected patients, and is more aggressive. HHV-8 is found in a high proportion of these multicentric cases, especially those associated with HIV.

Pathology

No distinctive histopathology has been identified for HHV-8 independent of the pathology of the tumours with which it is associated.

Laboratory diagnosis

HHV-8 can best be detected by PCR-based tests. The antibody assays described above may become commercially available in the near future.

Treatment

In vitro assays in HHV-8-infected lymphoma cell lines indicate that HHV-8 replication is moderately sensitive to foscarnet, ganciclovir, and cidofovir. AIDS patients treated with foscarnet and ganciclovir may be less likely to develop Kaposi's sarcoma. Antiviral drugs are not an established treatment for HHV-8 tumours.

Kaposi's sarcoma confined to the skin can be treated with radiotherapy or intralesional α-interferon. More widespread cutaneous or visceral disease can be treated with single-agent or combination chemotherapy. The treatment of Kaposi's sarcoma in AIDS patients is discussed in Chapters 7.5.23 and 7.5.24. Kaposi's sarcoma lesions may regress with antiretroviral treatment, possibly because of improved cellular immunity resulting from the reduction in HIV load.

Prevention and control

Given the uncertainty around the epidemiology and disease associations of HHV-8, prevention and control are not yet possible. No special problems of infection have been identified in pregnant women.

Cercopithecine herpesvirus 1 (herpes B virus)

Cercopithecine herpesvirus 1 is the formal name now given to herpes B virus (replacing the previous term, herpesvirus simiae), the natural hosts of which are members of the *Macaca* genus of Old World monkeys. It produces minimal disease in its natural hosts, but its transmission to humans results in a high incidence of severe disease. Although more than 30 other herpesviruses have been isolated from nonhuman primates, none of these has been unequivocally associated with a disease in humans. The virus was first isolated in 1932 from the brain of Dr W B, who died of encephalitis after a bite from a macaque (hence the name herpes B virus). There have since been about 45 cases of human infection resulting from accidental transmission from captive monkeys.

Aetiology

Herpes B virus is an alphaherpesvirus closely related to HSV, and appears to behave in an analogous manner to HSV in its natural primate host. Herpes B virus can also infect and produce disease in other nonhuman primates and small mammals.

Epidemiology

Herpes B virus is enzootic in Old World monkeys of the *Macaca* genus, principally rhesus (*M. mulatta*) and cynomolgus (*M. fascicularis*) macaques. The epidemiology in its primate host is similar to that of HSV in humans, with 80% or more of natural and captive adult monkeys being infected. Infected monkeys may develop vesicular oral lesions, and can shed virus intermittently from oral, conjunctival, and genital secretions.

Rhesus and cynomolgus macaques have been quite widely used in medical research, particularly for the development of polio vaccine in the mid 1950s, and in the late 1980s following the AIDS epidemic, for studies of retroviruses. Nearly all the reported human cases resulted from occupational exposure through bites and scratches in workers handling monkeys, but transmission from needlestick injuries and a splash in the eye have also been reported. One case of human-to-human transmission apparently occurred by inoculation onto inflamed skin.

Two clusters of infection have been described in the United States of America (in 1987, involving the case of human-to-human transmission, and 1989). A seroprevalence study of more than 300 monkey handlers showed that none was seropositive, and asymptomatic infection documented by seroconversion appears to be extremely uncommon.

Clinical features

The incubation period, from occupational exposure to the development of symptoms, has usually been 3 to 5 days, but can range from 3 to 30 days. Cutaneous vesicles may occur at or near the site of inoculation, accompanied by regional lymphadenitis. In the first 2 weeks, fever, malaise, headache, and abdominal pain are common, but the dominant and characteristic features are progressive multifocal haemorrhagic myelitis, and encephalitis. Visceral spread of herpes B virus is recorded in fatal cases. The untreated mortality is 80%. The history of monkey bite may lead to a suspicion of rabies (Chapter 7.5.10).

It is not clear whether herpes B virus in humans can become latent and then be reactivated. Viral shedding has recurred when antiviral treatment was stopped relatively early, so most patients have been maintained on antivirals for long periods.

Laboratory diagnosis

As herpes B virus is a category 4 pathogen, viral culture and isolation are only attempted in a few designated laboratories: in the United Kingdom at the Central Public Health Laboratory, Colindale, London; and in the United States of America at Georgia State University, Atlanta. Monkeys with suspected infection should have serum antibody tests. Serodiagnosis in humans is difficult because of antigenic crossreactivity between herpes B virus and HSV. The inoculation site should ideally be biopsied for culture and analysis. PCR-based methods are available in specialized centres, and are the standard for definitive diagnosis.

Treatment

Although injuries from macaques carry the risk of herpes B virus infection, most captive macaque colonies are now maintained free of the virus. A suspected contaminated wound should be debrided and cleaned with chlorhexidine or iodine soap. Postexposure prophylaxis may be initiated if the monkey is suspected to be positive for herpes B virus, and there is skin puncture or mucosal exposure. There may be a case for initiating immediate antiviral treatment if infection in the monkey is suspected, or for a deep wound.

Aciclovir and ganciclovir both inhibit herpes B virus replication *in vitro*. For postexposure prophylaxis, valaciclovir 1 g 8 hourly is recommended for at least 2 weeks. If symptomatic disease is suspected or proven, intravenous aciclovir is recommended if CNS symptoms are absent (15 mg/kg 8 hourly), and ganciclovir if CNS symptoms are present (5 mg/kg every 12 h). Treatment has been associated with the limitation of disease, and recovery, in some patients, but prolonged oral therapy with aciclovir or valaciclovir is advised to limit the risk of reactivation.

Prevention and control

Those working with macaques should follow standard procedures to avoid infection. The screening of newly imported monkeys, and the creation of colonies of macaques free of herpes B virus, are now becoming standard practice.

Further reading

Herpes simplex virus infections

Corey L, Wald A (2009). Current concepts: maternal and neonatal herpes simplex virus infections. *N Engl J Med*, **361**, 1376–85. [Useful review on this topic.]

Lakeman FD, Whitley RJ (1995). Diagnosis of herpes simplex encephalitis: application of polymerase chain reaction to cerebrospinal fluid from brain-biopsied patients and correlation with disease. NIAID collaborative antiviral study group. *J Infect Dis*, **171**, 857–63. [Study showing the detection of HSV DNA by PCR in 98% of 54 patients with brain biopsy-proven HSV encephalitis.]

Langenberg AGM, *et al.* (1999). A prospective study of new infections with herpes simplex virus type 1 and type 2. *N Engl J Med*, **341**, 1432–8. [Study of incident HSV-1/2 infections, reporting the proportion of symptomatic infections.]

Pellett PE, Roizman B (2007). The Herpesviridae: a brief introduction. In: Knipe DM, *et al.* (eds). *Fields virology*, 5th edition, vol. 2, pp. 2479–99. Lippincott, Williams and Wilkins, Philadelphia.

Roizman B, *et al.* (2007). Herpes simplex viruses. In: Knipe DM, *et al.* (eds). *Fields virology*, 5th edition, vol. 2, pp. 2501–601. Lippincott, Williams and Wilkins, Philadelphia.

Zhang SY, *et al.* (2007). Human toll-like receptor-dependent induction of interferons in protective immunity to viruses. *Immunol Rev*, **220**, 225–36. [Recent work on factors conferring susceptibility to HSV encephalitis.]

Varicella–zoster virus infection

Cohen JI, *et al.* (2007). Varicella–zoster virus. In: Knipe DM, *et al.* (eds). *Fields virology*, 5th edition, vol. 2, pp. 2773–818. Lippincott, Williams and Wilkins, Philadelphia.

Gilden DH, *et al.* (2000). Medical progress: neurologic complications of the reactivation of varicella–zoster virus. *N Engl J Med*, **342**, 635–46. [A good review of the subject, including postherpetic neuralgia.]

Gilden DH, *et al* (2002). The protean manifestations of varicella–zoster virus vasculopathy. *J Neurovirol*, **8** Suppl 2, 75–9. [A less well known aspect of VZV pathogenicity.]

Kimberlin DW, Whitley RJ (2007). Varicella–zoster vaccine for the prevention of herpes zoster. *N Engl J Med*, **356**, 1338–43. [Recent review of current status of the VZV vaccine.]

Wood MJ, *et al.* (1994). A randomised trial of acyclovir for 7 days or 21 days with and without prednisolone for treatment of acute herpes zoster. *N Engl J Med*, **330**, 901–5. [UK study showing that longer courses of aciclovir and prednisolone do not reduce the frequency of postherpetic neuralgia.]

Human cytomegalovirus infection

Boeckh M, Ljungman P (2009). How we treat cytomegalovirus in hematopoietic cell transplant recipients. *Blood*, **113**, 5711–9. [Useful discussion of treatment in this setting.]

Crumpacker CS, Wadhwa S (2005). Cytomegalovirus. In: Mandell GL, Bennett JE, Dolin R, (eds). *Principles and practice of infectious diseases*, pp. 1786–801. Elsevier Churchill Livingstone, Philadelphia.

Hodson EM, *et al.* (2008). Antiviral medications for preventing cytomegalovirus disease in solid organ transplant recipients. *Cochrane Database Syst Rev*, CD003774. [Systematic review of the evidence for the efficacy of primary prevention.]

Mocarski ES, *et al.* (2007). Cytomegaloviruses. In: Knipe DM, *et al.* (eds). *Fields virology*, 5th edition, vol. 2, pp. 2701–72. Lippincott, Williams and Wilkins, Philadelphia.

Sinclair J, Sissons JGP (2006). Latency and reactivation of human cytomegalovirus. *J Gen Virol*, **87**, 1763–79. [Review of mechanistic basis of latency and reactivation.]

Whitley RJ, *et al.* (1998). Guidelines for the treatment of CMV diseases in patients with AIDS in the era of potent antiretroviral therapy. *Arch Intern Med*, **158**, 957–69. [Recommendations of an international panel on the treatment of CMV disease in AIDS.]

Human herpesvirus 6 and 7

Hall CB, *et al.* (1994). Human herpesvirus-6 infection in children: a prospective study of complications and reactivation. *N Engl J Med*, **331**, 432–8. [A comprehensive study of primary HHV-6 infection in children presenting with febrile illness to a hospital emergency department.]

Yamanishi K, *et al.* (2007). Human herpesvirus-6 and 7. In: Knipe DM, *et al.* (eds). *Fields virology*, 5th edition, vol. 2, pp. 2819–45. Lippincott, Williams and Wilkins, Philadelphia.

Zerr DM, *et al.* (2005). A population-based study of primary human herpesvirus 6 infection. *N Engl J Med*, **352**, 768–76.

Zerr DM, *et al.* (2005). Clinical outcomes of human herpesvirus 6 reactivation after hematopoietic stem cell transplantation. *Clin Infect Dis*, **40**, 932–40.

Human herpesvirus 8

Antman K, Chang Y (2000). Medical progress: Kaposi's sarcoma. *N Engl J Med*, **342**, 1027–39. [Review of Kaposi's sarcoma and its association with HHV-8, including a review of therapy.]

Hayward GS (1999). Kaposi's sarcoma HV strains: the origins and global spread of the virus. Semin Cancer Biol, **9**, 187–99. [Summarizes the current molecular evidence for the evolution of the virus.]

Martin JN, *et al.* (1998). Sexual transmission and the natural history of human herpesvirus 8 infection. *N Engl J Med*, **338**, 948–54. [Provides evidence for the sexual transmission of HHV-8 and its association with Kaposi's sarcoma in homosexual men.]

Ganem D (2007). Kaposi's sarcoma-associated herpesvirus. In: Knipe DM, *et al.* (eds). *Fields virology*, 5th edition, vol. 2, pp. 2847–88. Lippincott, Williams and Wilkins, Philadelphia.

Cercopithecine herpesvirus 1

Cohen JI, *et al.* (2002). Recommendations for the prevention of and therapy for exposure to B virus. *Clin Infect Dis*, **35**, 1191–203. [Current US recommendations for the management of human herpes B virus infection.]

Sabin AB, Wright AM (1934). Acute ascending myelitis following a monkey bite, with the isolation of a virus capable of reproducing the disease. *J Exp Med*, **59**, 115–36. [The original description of herpes B virus and the case of Dr W B.]

Straus SE (2005). Herpes B virus. In: Mandell GL, Bennett JE, Dolin R, (eds). *Principles and practice of infectious diseases*, pp. 1832–5. Elsevier Churchill Livingstone, Philadelphia.

7.5.3 Epstein–Barr virus

M.A. Epstein and A.B. Rickinson

Essentials

Epstein–Barr virus (EBV) is a human herpesvirus with a linear double-stranded DNA genome that is carried asymptomatically by most people. Symptomless primary infection is usual in childhood, establishing a lifelong carrier state where the virus persists as a latent infection of circulating B cells. The virus replicates recurrently in oropharyngeal epithelial cells, with consequent shedding of virus in saliva transmitting infection.

Infectious mononucleosis

If delayed beyond childhood, primary infection causes infectious mononucleosis upto at least 50% of cases. This is typically characterized by sore throat, fever, anorexia, headache, fatigue, malaise (often disproportionately severe), generalized lymphadenopathy, splenomegaly (60%), hepatomegaly (10%), and jaundice (8%). Diagnosis can be confirmed by the Monospot test (which detects heterophil antibodies that are present in 85%) or the presence of IgM antibodies to virus capsid antigen. Treatment is supportive unless there are complications. Most cases resolve within 1 to 2 weeks; chronic or recurrent forms are described but are very rare. Primary infection in boys with the X-linked lymphoproliferative trait, a rare congenital immunodeficiency, gives severe or fatal disease. In other rare cases, most common in Asia, primary infection of immunocompetent people can lead to 'chronic active' EBV syndrome resembling persistent infectious mononucleosis but sometimes fatal.

B-cell tumours

Endemic Burkitt's lymphoma—all cells of this common malignancy of children in areas of Africa and New Guinea carry the EBV genome. A cofactor, hyperendemic malaria, explains the unusual geographical distribution of the high incidence disease. Presentation is with jaw and other tumours, peripheral lymph nodes and spleen are spared, and progression to death is rapid. Cyclophosphamide treatment is remarkably effective.

Other forms of Burkitt's lymphoma—a sporadic type occurs at low incidence worldwide. This is EBV-positive in only a few cases; jaw tumours are rare and lymph nodes are involved; response to treatment is poor—combination therapy is required, and survival after relapse is uncommon. Another form, EBV-positive in 30 to 40% of cases, occurs in AIDS patients.

Other lymphomas—where immune cell control over EBV is impaired in immunosuppressed transplant recipients or long-term AIDS patients, expansions of EBV-transformed B cells can occur as acute polyclonal lymphoproliferative lesions or later monoclonal large cell lymphomas. In transplant patients the first treatment is to reduce immunosuppressive therapy. EBV is also linked to Hodgkin's lymphoma, with the virus genome present in the Reed–Sternberg and mononuclear tumour cells in some 30 to 40% of cases.

Other malignancies and conditions associated with EBV

Undifferentiated nasopharyngeal carcinoma—this epithelial tumour is most common in southern Chinese and Inuit people, and is EBV genome-positive in all cases. Besides virus infection, dietary, genetic, and perhaps herbal remedy cofactors are involved. Radiotherapy is the treatment of choice.

EBV has more tenuous links with salivary gland tumours, some gastric carcinomas, rare smooth muscle tumours of the immunosuppressed, and certain nasal T and NK lymphomas. The nonmalignant lesions of oral hairy leukoplakia in HIV patients are interesting because the squamous epithelial cells forming them are driven by replicating EBV.

Background

The virus

Epstein–Barr virus (EBV) was discovered in 1964 during a sustained search for a viral cause of endemic Burkitt's lymphoma (see 'Endemic ('African') Burkitt's lymphoma' below). EBV is one of the eight human herpesviruses, and consists of an outer envelope, a protein capsid, and an inner double-stranded linear DNA genome. It is a very ancient parasite of humans, and related herpesviruses have been found in both Old World apes and monkeys and in New World monkeys. This indicates that the ancestor of such viruses infected early primates before the evolutionary split between Old World and New World primates occurred (about 35 million years ago based on palaeontology, or 45 million years ago based on DNA sequence analysis).

Viral infectious cycle

Natural infection is limited to humans, and the principal target cells of the virus are circulating B lymphocytes and squamous epithelial cells of the oropharynx. Lytic infection of these cells produces free viral progeny and cell death. The virus also causes latent infection of B cells *in vivo* and can transform normal B lymphocytes *in vitro* into continuously growing, latently infected lymphoblastoid cell lines.

Virus-coded proteins

Different sets of virus-coded proteins are expressed in lytic and latent infection. Lytic-cycle EBV-coded proteins are categorized as immediate early, early, or late antigens, according to when they appear. Many elicit cytotoxic T-cell and serum antibody responses, both of which are important in controlling the infection. Antibodies are used in diagnosis.

Epidemiology

The virus is widespread in all human populations. Primary infection usually occurs in early childhood, when it is almost always clinically silent. This leads to a lifelong carrier state, in which both humoral and cellular immune responses are maintained. The virus becomes latent in a few circulating memory B lymphocytes. There are also subclinical foci of lytically infected epithelial cells (and possibly intraepithelial B cells) in the mouth and pharynx, and perhaps also in the salivary glands and urogenital tract. Virus in the buccal fluid therefore provides the main source for transmission of the infection in the population. In developing countries, 99% of children are infected by the second to the fourth year of life. By contrast, in industrialized countries with higher standards of hygiene, as many as 50% of children, particularly those from high socioeconomic groups, enter adolescence uninfected (Fig. 7.5.3.1).

Infectious mononucleosis

Upto 50% of those who first acquire the virus in the second or third decade develop some clinical symptoms of infectious mononucleosis. Mononucleosis is therefore mainly a disease of upper socioeconomic groups in Western societies, and is exceptionally rare in developing countries (Fig. 7.5.3.1). Although most cases occur in adolescents and young adults, children and middle-aged people may sometimes develop the disease, and rarely also older people. Primary infection in adolescence or later is likely to be acquired by kissing a virus-shedding healthy carrier. This explains why case-to-case infection and epidemics are not seen, and why the incubation period, perhaps 30 to 50 days, is difficult to calculate. Symptomatic primary EBV infection may also be acquired through latently infected B lymphocytes present in blood transfusions or organ grafts.

Symptoms

Classical infectious mononucleosis may follow days of vague indisposition, or may start abruptly. It presents with sore throat, fever

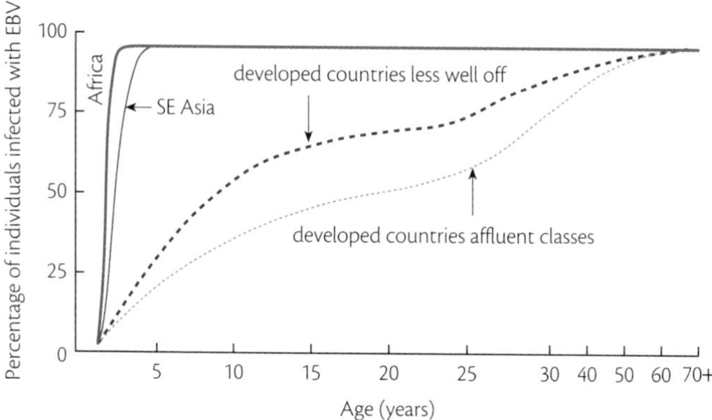

Fig. 7.5.3.1 Comparison of the ages at which people in different populations become infected with EBV. In developing countries, almost all children have acquired the virus by 2 to 4 years of age, depending on geographical region. In developed countries with high standards of living and hygiene, the time of infection is delayed for many, more markedly among the affluent than the less well off. Among the very rich, as many as 50% may reach adolescence or young adulthood without having encountered the virus, and will undergo delayed primary infection, with a high risk that this will be accompanied by the symptoms of infectious mononucleosis.
(Reprinted with permission from Epstein MA (2002). Infectious mononucleosis. In: *Encyclopedia of life sciences*, **10**, 211–16. Nature Publishing Group, London.)

with sweating, anorexia, headache, and fatigue, with malaise quite out of proportion to the other complaints. Dysphagia may be noticed, and also brief orbital oedema. Erythematous and maculopapular rashes occur in a small number of untreated patients, but much more frequently in those that have been taking ampicillin for sore throat before infectious mononucleosis has been diagnosed (Fig. 7.5.3.2). Tonsillar and pharyngeal oedema can rarely cause pharyngeal obstruction (Fig. 7.5.3.3).

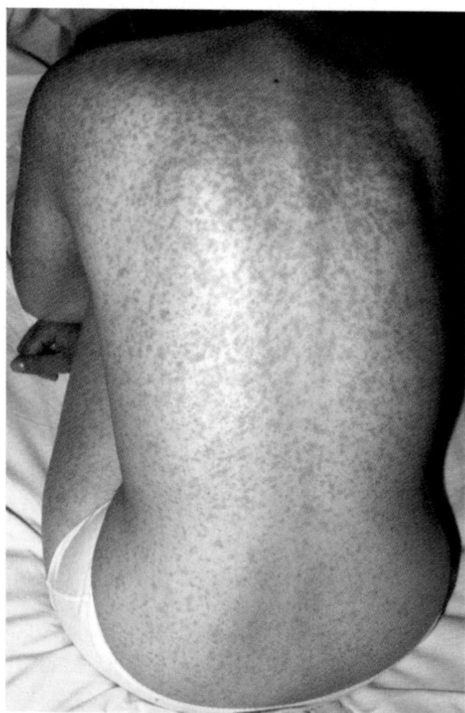

Fig. 7.5.3.2 Typical maculopapular erythematous rash in a patient with infectious mononucleosis who was treated with ampicillin.
(Copyright D A Warrell.)

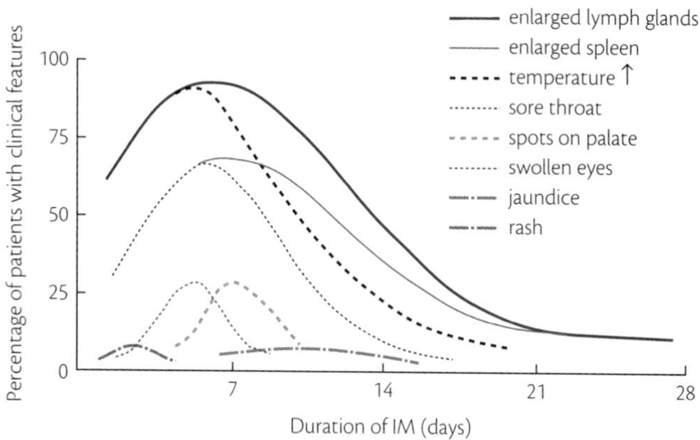

Fig. 7.5.3.3 Percentage of patients with infectious mononucleosis showing various clinical features during the course of the disease, and the timing and average duration of each.
(Reprinted with permission from Epstein MA (2002). Infectious mononucleosis. In: *Encyclopedia of life sciences*, **10**, 211–16. Nature Publishing Group, London.)

Signs

The fever may rise to 40°C, but swings are not seen. There is redness and oedema of the pharynx, fauces, soft palate, and uvula (Fig. 7.5.3.4a), and about half the patients develop greyish exudates on the tonsils (Fig. 7.5.3.4b). Generalized lymphadenopathy is almost always present, and is most marked in the cervical region; the glands are symmetrical, discrete, and slightly tender. Splenomegaly is seen in about 60% of cases and an enlarged liver in 10%. There is usually a moderate bradycardia. Besides the rash, characteristic palatal enanthematous crops of reddish petechiae (Fig. 7.5.3.4c) are found in about one-third of patients, and jaundice occurs in about 8%.

Clinical course

Mild cases may resolve in days, but 1 to 4 weeks is more usual, followed by a period of lethargy. The duration of this convalescence is influenced by psychological factors, particularly the speed with which patients are encouraged to resume full activity. About 1 case in 2000 may continue in a truly chronic or recurrent form for several months or years (see 'Chronic active EBV infection' below). Most other cases of so-called chronic infectious mononucleosis are manifestations of chronic fatigue syndrome (Chapter 26.5.4), but whether this is a true entity rather than a form of depression or a belief disorder is highly controversial. Credible connections with EBV have not been established.

Complications

Minor nonspecific complications may occur. Rare, more serious complications include secondary bacterial throat infections, traumatic rupture of the enlarged spleen, asphyxia from pharyngeal oedema, massive hepatic necrosis, Guillain–Barré syndrome, and autoimmune manifestations such as thrombocytopenia and haemolytic anaemia.

Differential diagnosis

Classical infectious mononucleosis is diagnosed by the clinical features, combined with serological and haematological laboratory investigations (see below). An infectious mononucleosis-like disease can occur in primary cytomegalovirus infection and in toxoplasmosis, but in both conditions the sore throat is much less severe,

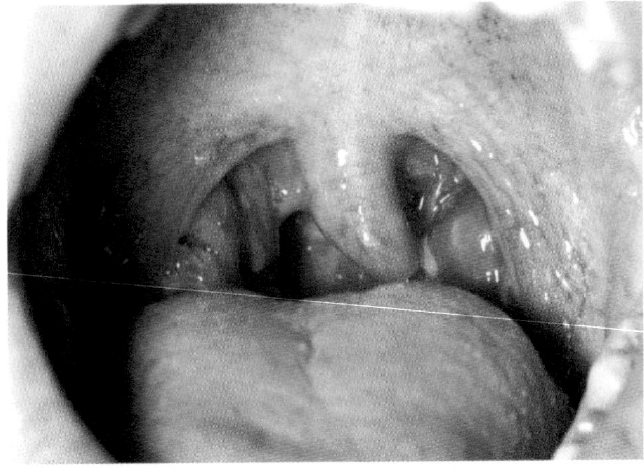
(a)

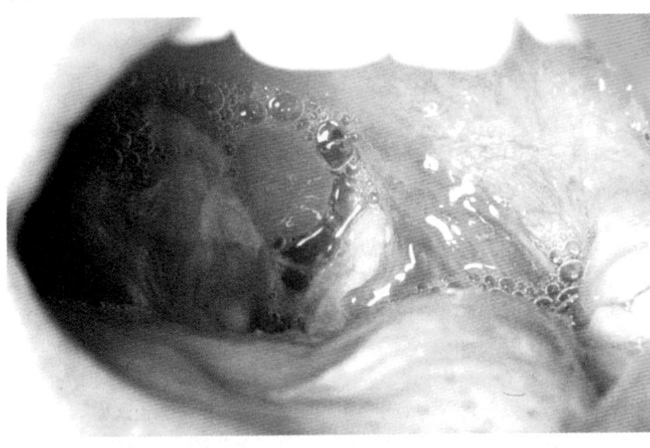
(b)

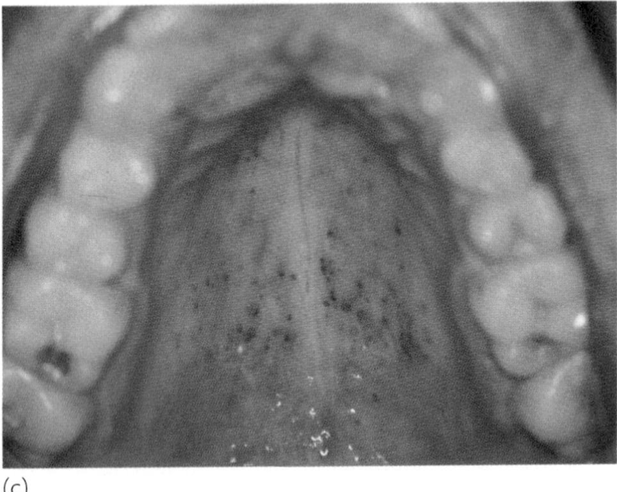
(c)

Fig. 7.5.3.4 Infectious mononucleosis: (a) Oedema of fauces, soft palate, uvula, and tonsils; (b) tonsillar exudates; and (c) palatal petechiae.
(Courtesy of the late Dr B E Juel-Jensen.)

and with cytomegalovirus the lymphadenopathy may be minimal or absent; an infectious mononucleosis-like syndrome is also sometimes seen during the acute phase of recent HIV infection.

Laboratory diagnosis

A rapid screening test (Monospot test) can be used to detect the presence of heterophile antibodies in the patient's serum. Although these heterophile antibodies are not directed against virally encoded proteins, they are present in up to 85% of acute infectious mononucleosis sera. Cases of Monospot-negative infectious mononucleosis tend to be outside the usual 15- to 25-year age range, and false-positive tests may occur in pregnancy and autoimmune disease. The diagnosis of infectious mononucleosis is confirmed by the presence of serum IgM antibodies to EBV capsid antigen (VCA), which can be detected for about 2 months. Another feature is the presence of lymphocytosis up to 15×10^9/litre, composed mainly of activated cytotoxic T cells with an atypical morphology.

Treatment

Bed rest and aspirin or paracetamol for headache and pharyngeal discomfort are the only treatments required. When the fever resolves the patient should be encouraged to get up and resume some activities as fast as is practicable, but violent exercise should be avoided for 3 weeks after an enlarged spleen ceases to be palpable. Only complications need active therapy; splenic rupture requires surgery, bacterial infections call for appropriate antibiotics, airway obstruction must be relieved by tracheostomy, and corticosteroids should be given for life-threatening pharyngeal oedema, and for neurological and haematological complications.

Pathogenesis

Why children are asymptomatic during primary EBV infection, whereas adolescents and young adults frequently develop infectious mononucleosis, is not fully understood. The higher virus dose likely to be acquired by kissing is one possible factor. In infectious mononucleosis patients, both epithelial and intraepithelial B cells in the oropharynx become productively infected, and infectious virus can easily be found in patients' saliva. The newly replicated virus initiates a latent growth-transforming infection of B cells, causing them to multiply and spread throughout the lymphoid system. These combined lytic and latent infections stimulate an exaggerated cytotoxic T-cell response in the circulation; in lymph nodes, tonsils, and other oropharyngeal lymphoid tissues; and in the spleen and the liver. This exaggerated response, and the cytokine storm that accompanies it, are thought to be responsible for the sore throat, fever, malaise, lymphadenopathy, and hepatosplenomegaly. Thus infectious mononucleosis is an immunopathological disease.

X-linked lymphoproliferative disease (fatal infectious mononucleosis) (OMIM 308 240)

An extremely rare genetically determined susceptibility to EBV occurs in young males of certain kindreds, who develop X-linked lymphoproliferative (XLP) disease following primary infection. This presents initially with acute mononucleosis-like symptoms, but progresses inexorably to haemophagocytosis, which culminates in the necrotic destruction of vital organs, leading to multisystem failure. The mutated X-chromosomal gene (*SAP; SH2D1A*) responsible for this defect is involved in the normal regulation of T cell and natural killer (NK) cell responses. In patients with XLP, the numbers of cytotoxic T and NK cells are amplified even more dramatically than in classical infectious mononucleosis, and the inflammatory cytokines released from these cells are probably responsible for initiating the haemophagocytosis.

Chronic active EBV infection

There are very rare cases of infectious mononucleosis that fail to resolve, and may continue for years, often developing serious complications leading to death. These cases of chronic active EBV infection can occur in both sexes, are not familially linked, and are more common in people of Asian than European descent.

Symptoms and signs

Persistent fever, lymphadenopathy, and hepatosplenomegaly are frequently accompanied or followed by anaemia, thrombocytopenia, and mononuclear cell haemophagocytosis. The disease can therefore lead to a clinical endpoint not unlike that seen in fatal XLP, but by a different pathogenetic route.

Pathogenesis and treatment

Chronic active EBV infection is unique, in that the virus infects T and/or NK cells, which appear to escape normal immune controls and so proliferate, infiltrating vital organs and releasing the cytokines that are thought to initiate haemophagocytosis. Later on, some of these patients develop monoclonal EBV-positive T- or NK-cell lymphomas.

There is no satisfactory treatment for this disease, but haematopoietic stem cell transplantation is being evaluated.

Endemic ('African') Burkitt's lymphoma

The classical form of this B-cell tumour, first described by Burkitt in 1958, is found in those parts of Africa and Papua New Guinea where the temperature does not fall below 16°C, and the annual rainfall does not fall below 55 cm. Endemic Burkitt's lymphoma is a disease of childhood, is extremely rare over the age of 14 years, and in endemic areas is more common than all other childhood tumours added together.

The association between latent EBV infection and the cells of endemic Burkitt's lymphoma is so close (virtually 100%) that it is generally accepted that the virus is essential, although it requires combination with cofactors in a complicated chain of events to lead to the malignancy. Hyperendemic malaria has been identified as an important cofactor, and its spread by anopheline mosquitoes requiring warmth and moisture explains the climate dependence.

A much rarer, sporadic form of Burkitt's lymphoma occurs worldwide, and there is a remarkably high incidence in AIDS patients (see 'Sporadic Burkitt's lymphoma' below).

Symptoms and signs

The endemic tumour is usually multifocal, and the symptoms depend entirely on the anatomical location. Jaw tumours are present in 70% of patients, are the usual presenting feature, may be multiple in all four quadrants, and are almost always accompanied by tumours elsewhere. The rapidly growing mass causes loosening of teeth, and exophthalmos from orbital spread. Abdominal tumours involve retroperitoneal nodes, liver, ovaries, intestines, and kidneys. Burkitt's lymphoma sometimes presents in the thyroid, the adolescent female breast, the testicles, and salivary glands; extradural tumours in the spine cause rapid paraplegia, and skeletal tumours also occur. Characteristically Burkitt's lymphoma does not involve the spleen or peripheral lymph nodes. The tumours are firm, very rapidly growing, painless, and cause minimal constitutional disturbance. Their site determines the clinical signs.

Differential diagnosis

In endemic areas, Burkitt's lymphoma can be diagnosed from the clinical picture. Unlike Burkitt's lymphoma, retinoblastoma is intraocular; rhabdomyosarcoma is extraorbital, and does not involve teeth; nephroblastoma is not multifocal; and neuroblastoma and ovarian tumours can be distinguished histologically. Paraplegia of tuberculous origin causes vertebral collapse, and acute transverse myelitis is preceded by pain and fever. The anatomical distribution of other lymphomas is quite different.

Laboratory diagnosis

Histological examination of a biopsy sample is clearly diagnostic. Antibodies to EBV antigens show a unique pattern, and titres rise or fall with disease progression or response to therapy. IgG anti-VCA titres are around 10-fold higher than in controls, and antibodies to EBV-restricted early antigens and membrane antigens are also detectable.

Clinical course and treatment

Tumour growth is relentless, and death ensues within a few months in the absence of treatment.

Surgery and radiotherapy are ineffective, but moderate courses of chemotherapy give excellent results. Cyclophosphamide, the drug of choice, remains effective after relapses.

Pathogenesis

EBV expresses a very limited range of latent gene products in Burkitt's tumour cells. When combined with a key cellular genetic change—a chromosomal translocation that causes hyperexpression of the *MYC* oncogene—these viral gene products appear to complete the malignant conversion of the target cell giving rise to Burkitt's lymphoma. Cofactors such as hyperendemic malaria may contribute, both by chronically stimulating cell—thought to be a germinal centre B cell—turnover in the B-cell system, thereby increasing the chances of rare chromosomal translocations occurring, and also by disturbing the normal virus–host balance, thereby enlarging the pool of EBV-infected cells in the body. It is clear that the virus is a necessary, but not sufficient element in the aetiology of endemic Burkitt's lymphoma.

Sporadic Burkitt's lymphoma

These tumours are seen in children worldwide, but generally at a much lower incidence than endemic Burkitt's lymphoma. The association of these tumours with EBV varies from 15 to 20% in the Western world, where the disease is quite rare, to more than 50% in other areas, where the incidence is intermediate between the two extremes. The role of EBV, when present, is unclear.

Symptoms and signs

Unlike endemic Burkitt's lymphoma, the sporadic form very rarely involves the jaws, and frequently presents in lymph nodes and within the abdomen. The clinical features depend on the location of the tumours.

Diagnosis

The tumour must be distinguished from large-cell and undifferentiated non-Hodgkin's lymphoma by histological examination of biopsies. The *MYC* translocation invariably found in endemic Burkitt's lymphoma is also present in sporadic tumours.

Treatment

The response to chemotherapy is not usually as good as in endemic Burkitt's lymphoma. Cyclophosphamide alone is inadequate; combination therapy is required, and survival after relapse is uncommon.

Lymphoproliferation in immunosuppressed states

T-cell impairment, whether congenital, or caused by immunosuppressive therapy or HIV infection, relaxes host control over persisting EBV infection, leading to increased virus replication in the oral cavity, and increased numbers of circulating virus-carrying B lymphocytes. The higher antigen load induces higher levels of serum antiviral antibodies. This reactivated infection is asymptomatic, but greater degrees of T-cell impairment can lead to the development of EBV-associated lymphoproliferative disease.

In transplant recipients

Transplant recipients who receive lifelong immunosuppressive drugs have up to 100-fold increase in their risk of developing lymphoproliferative disease and lymphoma, compared with normal immunocompetent individuals. Most of these tumours occur within the first year of transplantation, are frequently oligoclonal and consist of EBV-positive B cells expressing the same range of proteins as seen in EBV-transformed lymphoblastoid cell lines in culture. Such lesions arise through a failure of virus-specific immune T cell surveillance and, accordingly, occur with highest incidence in the most heavily immunosuppressed patients, particularly those (most often children) who were uninfected by the virus pretransplant and acquired it in the peritransplant period. The virus therefore appears to be both necessary and sufficient cause of such lymphoproliferative disease. Initial treatment is to reduce immunosuppressive drugs, with or without aciclovir therapy. Experimental treatments with EBV-specific cytotoxic T-cell infusions, or monoclonal antibody (rituximab) to the B-cell surface antigen CD20, have recently shown encouraging results. In addition, it is clear that transplant recipients receiving low but continual immunosuppression also have an increased longer term risk of lymphoma development. Some of these late tumours resemble the above lymphoproliferative lesions, whereas others are monoclonal B cell lymphomas of more varied type only some of which are EBV-positive; the role of the virus in this latter context is unclear.

In HIV/AIDS patients

Two types of lymphoma are seen in patients with HIV infection: large-cell lymphoma and Burkitt's lymphoma, both of which may be associated with EBV.

Large-cell lymphomas similar to those found in transplant recipients (see above) occur in severely immunocompromised patients with AIDS. Their distribution is extranodal, involving many unusual sites, most commonly the central nervous system. At least 50% of these tumours are EBV-positive, and this reaches 100% for cerebral tumours. The progress is rapid, with a mean survival time from diagnosis of 3 to 4 months. Radiotherapy is disappointing because patients with late-stage AIDS are in such poor general health.

Burkitt's lymphoma occurs earlier in the course of HIV disease, while the immune system is still relatively intact, and is therefore more amenable to treatment. Some 30 to 40% of these lymphomas contain EBV DNA.

Hodgkin's lymphoma

There has long been a suspicion that EBV is involved in the induction of Hodgkin's lymphoma, because of the similarity between the age and social class-dependence of this tumour's epidemiology and that of infectious mononucleosis. More recently it has become clear that infectious mononucleosis carries with it an increased risk of developing Hodgkin's lymphoma over the next 10 years. The overall risk is 4-fold but considerably higher within 2–3 years of the original attack of infectious mononucleosis; most of the resulting tumours are the EBV-positive form of Hodgkin's disease. The tumour is derived from post-germinal-centre B cells, and in virus-associated cases, EBV DNA is present and expressed as a monoclonal infection among the entire malignant population of Reed–Sternberg and mononuclear Hodgkin's cells.

In developed countries, up to 50% of Hodgkin's lymphomas are EBV-positive, and show an age-dependent distribution; EBV-positive cases occur relatively rarely in children (mainly boys), but more often in older adults, who characteristically develop the mixed cellularity type of disease. By contrast, nodular sclerosing type tumours, mainly occurring in young adults, are rarely EBV-associated.

In developing countries, the incidence of Hodgkin's lymphoma is high in young boys, and there is also an increased incidence in older people. Overall, 80% of these tumours are EBV positive.

Although the monoclonality of both the tumour cells and, where present, the virus suggest a causal relationship, there is insufficient evidence to be certain, indicating a pressing need for further investigations.

Nasopharyngeal carcinoma

This tumour is restricted to the postnasal space, where it arises from squamous epithelial cells. It is always heavily infiltrated by nonmalignant T cells, and is thus sometimes designated a lymphoepithelioma. The tumour is seen rarely throughout the world, but has a remarkably high incidence among the people of southern China, and the Inuit and related circumpolar peoples. In high-incidence areas, nasopharyngeal carcinoma is the most common cancer of men, and the second most common of women. The disease also occurs with intermediate incidence in Malays, Dyaks, Indonesians, Filipinos, and Vietnamese people, as well as in a belt stretching across North Africa, through Sudan, to the Kenyan highlands.

The tumour usually occurs in middle or old age, but in North Africa it has bimodal age peaks, one involving young people up to 20 years old and a second, much later in life. Irrespective of geographical region, nasopharyngeal carcinoma cells always carry the EBV genome and express viral latent proteins.

Symptoms and signs

Nasopharyngeal carcinoma causes nasal obstruction, discharge, or bleeding; deafness, tinnitus, or earache; and headache and ocular paresis from tumour spread to involve the cranial nerves. Patients may present with a single symptom caused locally by the tumour, or with several symptoms, and about one-third complain only of cervical lymph-node enlargement resulting from metastatic spread from an occult primary tumour.

Direct spread from the primary tumour may involve the soft tissues, bone, parotid gland, buccal cavity, and oropharynx. The neoplasm may extend into the nasal fossae, the paranasal sinuses, or the orbit, and can invade the eustachian tube or the parapharyngeal space, where cranial nerves IX, X, XI, and XII can be involved. Invasion of the skull or cranial foramina may damage cranial nerves II, IV, V, and VI. Lymphatic spread causes enlarged cervical lymph nodes, and subsequently extends to the supraclavicular glands. If bloodborne metastases occur, they are most frequent in the bones, liver, and lungs, but may be in any organ.

Differential diagnosis

Nasopharyngeal carcinoma must be distinguished from other tumours of the nasal cavities, namely adenocarcinomas, sarcomas, malignant lymphomas, and rare malignancies such as chordoma, teratoma, and melanoma.

Laboratory diagnosis

The diagnosis of nasopharyngeal carcinoma is made histologically on a biopsy sample of the primary tumour or an enlarged cervical lymph node. Serum antibody titres to EBV antigens show a characteristic reaction pattern—IgG and IgA antibodies to VCA and diffuse early antigen are raised, with the titre correlating with the tumour burden. Uniquely, IgA antibodies to VCA and early antigen are also found in patients' saliva. These antibody patterns often arise many months before the onset of tumour growth, and have been used in a high-incidence area of China to screen the population.

Treatment

Untreated nasopharyngeal carcinoma progresses inexorably to death, but it responds well to radiotherapy, which is the treatment of choice. In the earliest stages of the disease, radiotherapy gives 5-year survival rates of 50% or more, and of those surviving for 5 years, 70% remain permanently free of relapse. The more advanced stages of nasopharyngeal carcinoma have correspondingly worse prognoses.

Pathogenesis

EBV is now widely accepted as an essential element in the causation of nasopharyngeal carcinoma. Early studies showed that 100% of undifferentiated nasopharyngeal carcinomas are EBV positive, and recent studies have also detected viral DNA in some differentiated tumours. Thus all forms of nasopharyngeal carcinoma, irrespective of whether they originate in high- or low-incidence areas, may be associated with EBV. Both the tumour cells and the EBV genomes within them are clonal, indicating that the malignancy arises from a single malignantly transformed EBV-infected epithelial cell. Evidence from EBV latency genes expressed in nasopharyngeal carcinoma and premalignant lesions shows that viral gene products contribute to the abnormal proliferation.

Nonviral aetiological factors include racial and genetic predispositions; many cases among southern Chinese people show a clear familial link, and certain HLA haplotypes are associated with the disease. Epidemiological studies also suggest that environmental cofactors associated with the Chinese way of life play a role. Two likely candidates are (1) traditional herbal medicines containing tumour-promoting phorbol ester-type substances, taken as snuff, and (2) traditional salted fish, which has been shown to contain carcinogenic nitrosamines.

Salivary gland lymphoepithelioma

These relatively rare tumours resemble nasopharyngeal carcinoma, both histologically and in their prevalence in southern Chinese and circumpolar populations. Although some are in reality nasopharyngeal cancers that have spread to the parotid gland from occult primaries, others are clearly of salivary gland origin. The EBV genome, which is clonal in all the malignant epithelial cells, is not found in any other type of salivary gland tumour. The association with EBV has not been sufficiently explored to assess its significance.

Gastric carcinoma

About 10% of gastric carcinomas worldwide are EBV genome-positive, including all the rare gastric tumours of lymphoepithelioma type, and a minority of common adenocarcinomas. The viral genome is again found in every cell of the EBV-positive tumour, and is monoclonal, providing another example of a tumour arising from a single EBV-infected cell.

Although there is some evidence that EBV gene products contribute to the maintenance of the malignant condition, the role of the virus remains elusive.

Smooth-muscle tumours, T- and NK-cell lymphomas

Surprisingly, certain rare tumours of other cell lineages are consistently EBV positive. These include leiomyomas and leiomyosarcomas, whose incidence is raised in children immunosuppressed by AIDS or after organ transplantation, and those T- and NK-cell lymphomas of the nasal cavity that were previously categorized as lethal midline granulomas. The latter tumours are more common in men than women, and in Asian and South American populations than those of European descent. Presentation is usually in the midline of the face at the nose, or with destructive lesions of the soft palate, or multiple intranasal masses. Other rare forms of T- and NK-cell lymphoma are also associated with chronic active EBV infection (see 'Chronic active EBV infection' above).

Hairy leukoplakia

This nonmalignant lesion occurs in people with HIV, and in other immunosuppressed patients. It usually presents with painless white patches on the tongue or the lateral buccal mucosa. The lesions are usually multiple, up to 3 cm in diameter, slightly raised, poorly demarcated, and have a hairy or corrugated surface.

The differentiated squamous epithelial cells contain large amounts of actively replicating EBV, providing the only example of disease resulting from productive infection by the virus. Such exuberant production of EBV in epithelial cells is also exceptional. Aciclovir treatment arrests virus replication, and the lesions regress, but only for as long as the drug is continued.

Further reading

Bar RS, *et al.* (1974). Fatal infectious mononucleosis in a family. *N Engl J Med*, **290**, 363–7. [The first account of an XLP syndrome family.]

Burkitt D (1958). A sarcoma involving the jaws of African children. *Br J Surg*, **46**, 218–3. [The first description of Burkitt's lymphoma.]

Burkitt D (1963). A lymphoma syndrome in tropical Africa. *Int Rev Exp Pathol*, **2**, 67–138. [An early comprehensive review of Burkitt's lymphoma.]

de Thé, *et al.* (1978). Epidemiological evidence for a causal relationship between Epstein–Barr virus and Burkitt's lymphoma: results of the prospective Ugandan study. *Nature*, **274**, 756–61. [A massive investigation linking EBV to the causation of Burkitt's lymphoma.]

Dharnidkana VR, *et al.* (eds) (2010). Post-transplant lymphoproliferative disorders. Springer-Verlag, Berlin Heidelberg. [An up-to-date survey.]

Epstein A (1999). On the discovery of Epstein–Barr virus: a memoir. *Epstein–Barr Virus Report*, **6**, 58–63. [Details of how EBV was discovered.]

Epstein MA, Achong BG, Barr YM (1964). Virus particles in cultured lymphoblasts from Burkitt's lymphoma. *Lancet*, **i**, 702–3. [The first report of the discovery of EBV.]

Gottschalk S, Rooney CM, Heslop HE. Post-transplant lymphoproliferative disorders. *Annu Rev Med* 2005, **56**, 29–44. [A recent review of PTLD and its treatment.]

Greenspan JS, *et al.* (1985). Replication of Epstein–Barr virus within the epithelial cells of oral hairy leukoplakia, an AIDS-associated lesion. *N Engl J Med*, **313**, 1564–71. [The first description of the condition.]

Henle G, Henle W, Diehl V (1968). The relation of Burkitt's lymphoma tumor-associated herpesvirus to infectious mononucleosis. *Proc Natl Acad Sci (USA)*, **59**, 94–101. [The account of the original findings identifying EBV as the cause of infectious mononucleosis.]

Hjalgrim H *et al.* (2003). Characteristics of Hodgkin's lymphoma after infectious mononucleosis. *N Engl J Med*, **349**, 1324–32. [Describes associations between EBV and Hodgkin's lymphoma.]

Hislop AD, *et al.* (2007). Cellular responses to virus infection in humans: lessons from Epstein–Barr virus. *Annu Rev Immunol*, **25**, 587–617. [This review surveys current ideas on T-cell control of EBV infection.]

Hoagland RK (1955). Transmission of infectious mononucleosis. *Am J Med Sci*, **229**, 262–72. [The first recognition of infectious mononucleosis as the 'kissing disease'.]

Kuppers R (2003). B cells under influence: transformation of B cells by Epstein–Barr virus. *Nat Rev Immunol*, **3**, 801–12. [A good account of the pathogenesis of lymphomas.]

Rickinson AB, Kieff E (2007). Epstein–Barr virus. In: Knipe DM, *et al.* (eds). Fields Virology, 5th edition, vol. 2, pp. 2655–700. Lippincott, Williams and Wilkins, Philadelphia. [A comprehensive review of recent work on EBV.]

Robertson ES (ed) (2005). *The Epstein–Barr virus*. Caister Academic Press, Wymondham. [A multiauthor work covering all aspects of the virus and its associated diseases.]

Schlossberg D (ed) (1989). *Infectious mononucleosis*, 2nd edition. Springer Verlag, Berlin. [A multiauthor work covering many aspects of the disease.]

Sprunt TP, Evans FA (1920). Mononuclear leucocytosis in reaction to acute infections ('infectious mononucleosis'). *Bulletin of the Johns Hopkins Hosp*, **31**, 410–17. [The first description of infectious mononucleosis.]

Young LS, Rickinson AB (2004). Epstein–Barr virus: 40 years on. *Nat Rev Cancer*, **4**, 757–68. [A helpful discussion of the biology and oncogenicity of EBV.]

7.5.4 Poxviruses

Geoffrey L. Smith

Essentials

Poxviruses are large, complex DNA viruses that have played several seminal roles in medicine and biological science. Cowpox virus was introduced by Jenner as the first human vaccine in 1796; widespread vaccination with vaccinia virus led to the global eradication of smallpox in 1977, the only human disease to have been eradicated.

Smallpox—caused by variola virus, the most infamous poxvirus. A systemic infection, spread by the respiratory route, with characteristic skin blisters that had a centrifugal distribution on the body and, with variola major, produced mortality rates of 30 to 40% in unvaccinated populations.

Other poxviruses—molluscum contagiosum is the only other poxvirus that infects only humans, causing benign skin tumours that may be single or multiple, typically persisting for months before undergoing spontaneous regression (see Chapter 7.5.28). Several other poxviruses may cause zoonotic infections in humans, including cowpox virus, vaccinia virus, monkeypox virus, orf virus, psuedocowpox virus, tanapox virus and Yaba monkey tumour virus.

The development of vaccinia virus as an expression vector pioneered the concept of using genetically engineered viruses as live vaccines. Poxviruses remain excellent models for studying virus-host interactions and virus immune evasion strategies.

Introduction

Poxviruses are large DNA viruses that replicate in the cell cytoplasm. The most infamous was variola virus, which caused smallpox, a disease responsible for devastating epidemics with up to 40% mortality and which influenced human history. Smallpox was eradicated (in 1977) by immunoprophylaxis with vaccinia virus, a related orthopoxvirus. Since then, poxvirus infections in humans have been restricted to molluscum contagiosum (Chapter 7.5.28) and rare zoonoses such as monkeypox, cowpox, orf virus (Chapter 7.5.27), pseudocowpox, Yaba monkey tumour virus, and tanapox.

Classification

The *Poxviridae* is divided into the *Entomopoxvirinae* and *Chordopoxvirinae* subfamilies whose members infect insects and chordates, respectively. The *Chordopoxvirinae* is subdivided into eight genera (Table 7.5.4.1), although other genera are likely to be created based on the phylogenetic analysis of genome sequences of eclectic viruses such as deerpox virus and crocodilepox virus (see http://www.poxvirus.org). Viruses within different genera are antigenically distinct, while those within a genus are cross-reactive and cross-protective. Orthopoxviruses have been the most important for humans (Table 7.5.4.1), and four of the nine poxviruses that infect humans are orthopoxviruses: cowpox, variola, monkeypox, and vaccinia virus. Different orthopoxviruses are distinguishable by their biological properties such as pock type and ceiling temperature on the chorioallantoic membrane, or by the restriction pattern of genomic DNA and the genome sequences that have enabled development of species-specific polymerase chain reaction (PCR) detection methods. Vaccinia virus has no known natural animal reservoir and its origin remains a mystery. It caused human disease only as a rare complication after vaccination against smallpox. Cowpox and monkeypox viruses were named after the species from which they were isolated, but the natural reservoir of each virus is rodents. Infections in cows or monkeys, like the occasional transmission to humans, are zoonoses. Human monkeypox virus infections are often caused by handling or consumption of infected 'bush meat'. In 2003, there was an outbreak of monkeypox in the United States of America following the importation of Gambian rodents carrying the virus. Cowpox, monkeypox, and vaccinia viruses have a broad host range, while variola virus infected only humans and the lack of an animal reservoir aided the smallpox eradication campaign.

Poxvirus biology

Poxviruses replicate in the cytoplasm, encode enzymes for transcription and DNA replication, and have large, complex virions (Fig. 7.5.4.1) and double stranded DNA genomes of 134 to 360 kb. Vaccinia virus is the most intensively studied poxvirus. It encodes about 200 genes (the exact number varying with the strain of virus) of three classes (early, intermediate, and late) that are expressed in a strictly regulated manner. Transcription of each class is dependent upon the prior expression of the previous class.

Virus morphogenesis is complex (Fig. 7.5.4.2a) and produces two forms of infectious virion: intracellular mature virus (IMV) and extracellular enveloped virus (EEV). IMV remains within the cell until cell lysis and forms most of the progeny, whereas EEV is released by exocytosis (Fig. 7.5.4.2b) before cell death and represents a small fraction of total infectivity. EEV possesses an additional lipid envelope with which several virus proteins are associated, giving it distinct immunological and biological properties. EEV is necessary for efficient virus dissemination *in vitro* and within the infected host. Immunity to EEV-specific antigens, which are highly conserved among orthopoxviruses, is required for protection against disease and the B5 protein on the EEV surface is the only EEV-specific antigen against which neutralizing Abs are directed.

Pathogenesis

Poxvirus infections cause a local skin lesion or generalized pustular rash. Detailed experimental analysis of human smallpox was impossible, but generalized poxvirus infections have been studied in experimental models, namely monkeypox in monkeys, rabbitpox (a neurovirulent vaccinia virus) in rabbits, ectromelia virus in mice, and myxoma virus in European rabbits. The spread of variola virus in humans was probably similar to that of the ectromelia virus in mice and is characterized by sequential phases of virus infection, replication, and release accompanied by cell necrosis.

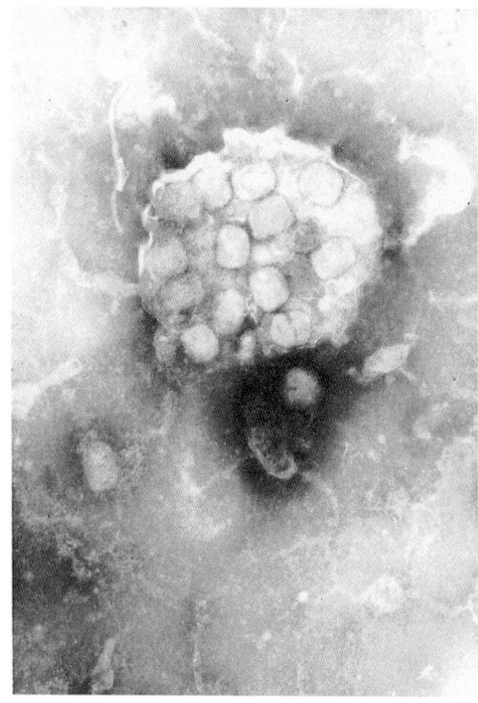

Fig. 7.5.4.1 Electron micrograph of material from smallpox lesion, viewed by negative contrast, showing a clump of poxvirus particles.
(Courtesy of the late Henry Bedson.)

Table 7.5.4.1 Poxvirus classification

Subfamily	Genus	Species
Entomopoxvirinae		
Chordopoxvirinae	*Orthopoxvirus*	*Variola virus
		*Vaccinia virus
		*Monkeypox virus
		*Cowpox virus
		Ectromelia virus
		Camelpox virus
		Taterapox virus
	Capripoxvirus	Sheeppox virus
		Goatpox virus
		Lumpy skin disease virus
	Parapoxvirus	*Orf virus
		*Pseudocowpox virus
	Avipoxvirus	Fowlpox virus
		Canarypox virus
	Suipoxvirus	Swinepox virus
	Leporipoxvirus	Myxoma virus
		Shope fibroma virus
	Molluscipoxvirus	*Molluscum contagiosum virus
	Yatapoxvirus	*Yaba monkey tumour virus
		*Tanapox virus

* Viruses that infect humans.

Virus enters through skin abrasions (ectromelia and cowpox) or inhalation of airborne virus and establishes a respiratory infection (ectromelia, rabbitpox, and variola). In smallpox, the respiratory route was the most important and sometimes the only possible route of transmission from index cases to contacts; also patients became infectious only after enanthem developed. A respiratory infection was established in the epithelial cells of the alveoli and small bronchioles. Here, alveolar macrophages became infected and transmitted the virus via lymphatics to the local lymph node, where further virus replication occurred. Virus released into the blood (primary viraemia) was mostly cell-associated and spread to other organs of the reticuloendothelial system, notably the liver, spleen, and lymph nodes.

Extensive replication here released larger amounts of virus into the blood (secondary viraemia) enabling the virus to infect other organs such as the kidneys, lungs, and intestines and to reach the skin and produce the skin lesions with the characteristic centrifugal distribution (Figs. 7.5.4.3–7.5.4.5). Lesions started with a papule that became pustular and then crusted. After 2 to 3 weeks the scab was shed leaving a scar. The incubation period of smallpox was approximately 12 days. Symptoms included headache, fever, malaise, vomiting, and, in severe cases, prostration, toxaemia, and hypotension. Delayed onset of the skin eruptions usually correlated with a grave prognosis. Haemorrhagic or flat confluent-type smallpox had very high mortality rates.

The outcome of infection depended upon the age and physiological and immunological status of the patient and the strain of virus.

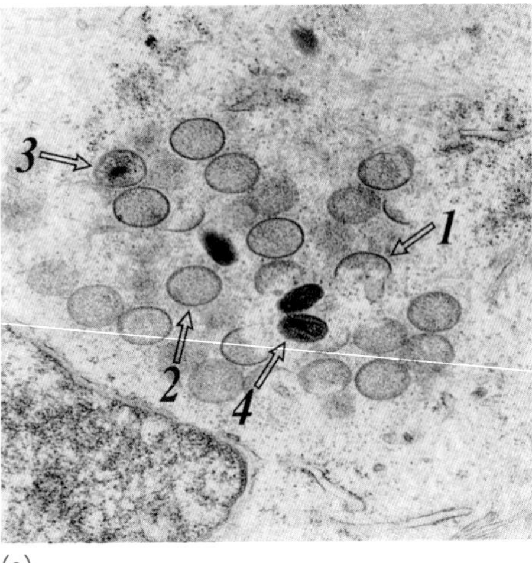

(a)

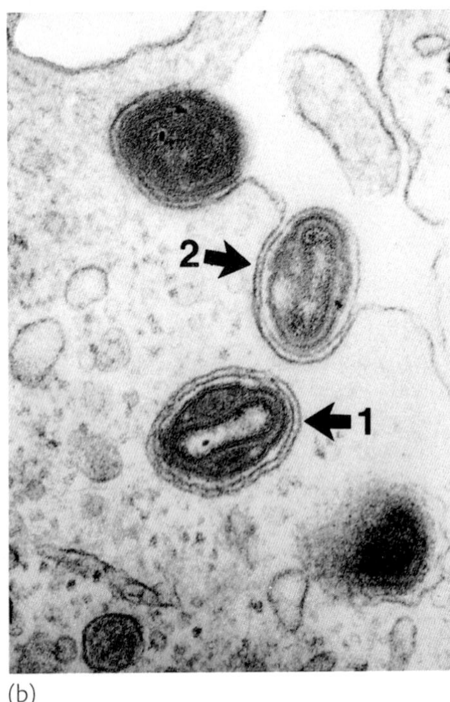

(b)

Fig. 7.5.4.2 Electron micrographs showing (a) a cytoplasmic vaccinia virus factory containing maturing virus particles with stages of morphogenesis numbered 1 to 4 and (b) fully enveloped virus particles, one of which is leaving the cell by exocytosis.

Variola major was more virulent and produced fatality ratesin unvaccinated patients of between 5 and 40%, while the milder variola minor, called alastrim in the Americas, caused only 0.1 to 2% mortality. Morphologically, the viruses were indistinguishable, and vaccination with vaccinia virus was equally effective against both. However, alastrim virus was consistently more thermolabile and had a lower ceiling temperature of 37.5 °C compared to 38.5 °C for variola major, 39 °C for monkeypox, 40 °C for cowpox, and 41 °C for vaccinia virus. The genomes of nearly 50 variola virus strains isolated from different places in the world at different times have been sequenced and compared, allowing the spread and evolution of variola virus in humans to be analysed. Comparisons of variola major and minor virus strains showed the genomes are very closely related, but there are too many minor differences to provide an understanding of why these viruses produced such different mortality rates in humans.

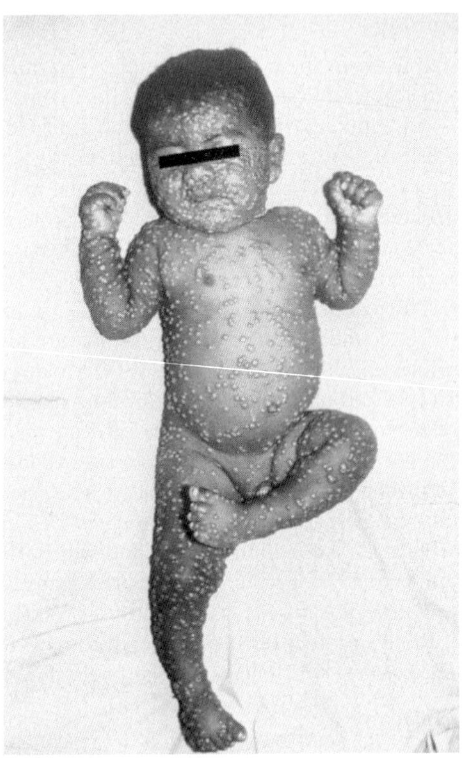

Fig. 7.5.4.3 Smallpox in a 9-month-old boy in Pakistan, photographed on the eighth day of the rash.
(Courtesy of the World Health Organization.)

Very young and old patients were most susceptible to smallpox, and those aged 5 to 20 years most resistant. Pregnancy and immunological deficiency, particularly in cell-mediated immunity, increased the severity of infection. Pregnant women were more likely than any other group to develop haemorrhagic-type smallpox, which was usually fatal. The greater importance of cell-mediated immunity rather than antibody in recovery from poxvirus infections was illustrated in several ways. Firstly, in children with severe defects in cell-mediated immunity there was a progressive and uncontrolled virus replication from the vaccination site that was usually fatal. In contrast, defects in antibody production were usually tolerated if the cell-mediated immune response was normal. Secondly, passive administration of antivaccinia virus serum had little effect on mice infected with ectromelia virus, whereas prior infection with vaccinia virus was protective. Thirdly, in mice infected with ectromelia virus, the effective mechanisms that combated infection in the liver and spleen were operative by 4 to 6 days postinfection and coincided with the maximum levels of cytolytic T cells, but preceded the development of systemic antibody.

The eradication of smallpox

Early attempts to control smallpox relied upon variolation or inoculation, in which material isolated from a mild case of smallpox was administered by sniffing or scratching. This was replaced by vaccination in 1798 after Jenner noticed that milkmaids, who often acquired cowpox infections on their hands from the teats of cows, were protected from smallpox. Jenner infected a boy (James Phipps) with poxvirus material (probably cowpox), derived from a cow via a milkmaid (Sarah Nelmes), and challenged him subsequently with smallpox. Protection was achieved and, due to the efficacy and greater safety of this procedure, it rapidly replaced

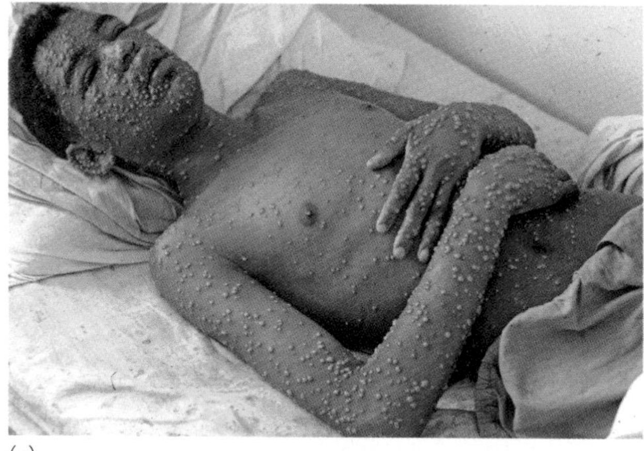

(a)

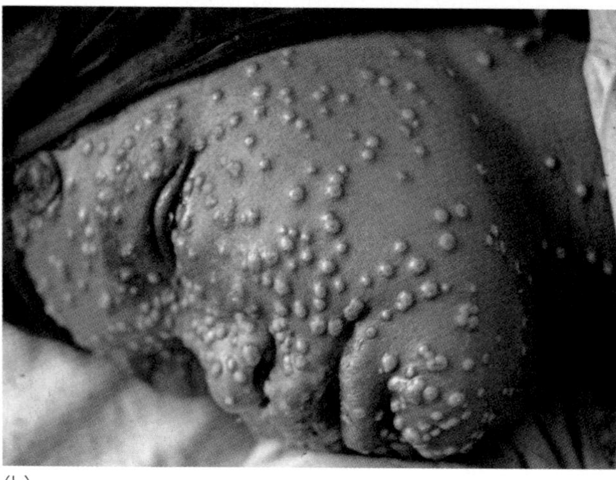

(b)

Fig. 7.5.4.4 Ethiopian patient, in 1968, showing classical centrifugal distribution of lesions with fewer on trunk (a) than on face (b).
(Copyright D A Warrell.)

variolation. Sometime between 1798 and the 20th century vaccinia virus replaced cowpox virus as the smallpox vaccine. In 1959, the World Health Organization (WHO) adopted a recommendation to achieve the global eradication of smallpox. With fresh funding and a plentiful supply of potent freeze-dried vaccine this goal was achieved in 1977. Two years later, the WHO certified that eradication was complete. This triumph of preventive medicine justifies the saying 'prevention is better than cure', but also demonstrates that prevention is best achieved by eradication.

Poxvirus genome sequences

The DNA sequence of about 80 orthopoxvirus genomes has been determined (see http://www.poxvirus.org), including 48 strains of variola virus, 14 vaccinia virus strains, nine strains of monkeypox virus, and at least one strain of most orthopoxviruses. The central region (about 100 kb) of these genomes is very highly conserved and 89 of the genes within this region are present in every sequenced chordopoxvirus. These genes probably represent the core genome of an ancestral poxvirus from which the current poxviruses evolved. During their evolution poxviruses acquired additional genes that became located in the more variable terminal regions of the genome and these give each virus its characteristic host range, virulence, and tropism. These genes vary in number and type between poxviruses, and encode nonessential proteins that affect virus virulence, host range, and immune modulation. A surprising feature of some orthopoxviruses is the fragmentation of several genes that are intact in other viruses, indicating that orthopoxvirus evolution has involved both gain and loss of gene function. The retention of these nonfunctional genes by some viruses, such as variola, suggests that they became nonfunctional in the relatively recent evolutionary past, and perhaps that variola virus is a 'recent' human pathogen that never became fully adapted to humans.

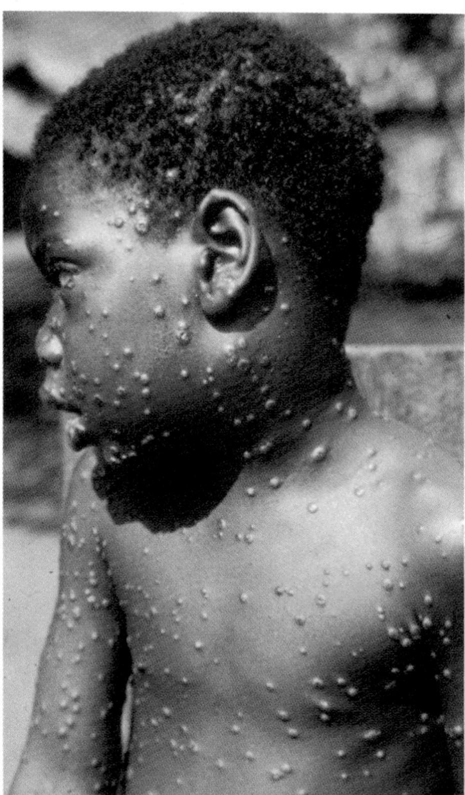

Fig. 7.5.4.5 Moderately severe monkeypox in a girl of 7 years from Équateur Province, Democratic Republic of the Congo.
(Courtesy of the World Health Organization.)

Poxvirus expression vectors

Vaccinia virus recombinants expressing foreign genes were developed in 1982 and have become a widely used laboratory tool; they are also being engineered as live vaccines for infectious disease and cancer. Infection with the recombinant virus allows expression and simultaneous delivery of the foreign antigen to the immune system. Moreover, the large capacity of vaccinia virus allows expression of multiple foreign genes from a single virus so creating polyvalent vaccines. Safer vaccinia virus strains that do not cause vaccination complications (eczema vaccinatum, generalized vaccinia, progressive vaccinia, encephalopathy (<2 years), or encephalitis (>2 years)) are being created by genetic engineering. An alternative strategy is to use poxviruses that establish only abortive infections in human cells, such as modified vaccinia Ankara (MVA) or the avipoxviruses fowlpox virus and canarypox virus.

Human monkeypox

Monkeypox was discovered in captive primates in 1958, but in 1970 was isolated in the tropical rainforests of West and Central Africa from humans who had suffered generalized poxvirus rashes visibly very similar to smallpox. The virus is quite distinct from variola in biological properties such as pock morphology, ceiling temperature, and lesion morphology on rabbit skin, and its genome sequence. Moreover, although monkeypox virus produced a very similar disease to smallpox in humans, person-to-person transmission was inefficient. Thus, human monkeypox virus infections are single or multiple sporadic cases restricted to dense tropical rainforests in Central and West Africa. Clinically, human monkeypox closely resembles ordinary, discrete-type smallpox except that there is a pronounced lymph node enlargement (Fig. 7.5.4.5). Two clades of monkeypox virus have been identified (from Central or West Africa) that differ in their virulence in humans. The Central African strains gave mortality rates in unvaccinated children (<8 years old) between 1970 and 1986 of 11.2%. In contrast, West African strains, such as the one that caused an epidemic in the United States of America in 2003, are milder and no mortalities were reported.

Cowpox virus and pseudocowpox virus

Cowpox virus has a broad host range including cattle, humans, large felines, and even elephants, but it is not enzootic in cattle and its natural hosts are rodents. It is distinguishable from vaccinia virus by the pock type, ceiling temperature, genome size and sequence, and the production of cytoplasmic type A inclusion bodies. Pseudocowpox is enzootic in cattle, unlike cowpox. Historically, pseudocowpox virus was important since it was sometimes used mistakenly for vaccination and, being a parapoxvirus, was ineffective in preventing smallpox. Its misuse compromised Jenner's correct assertion that cowpox virus was an effective smallpox vaccine.

In humans, cowpox virus produces an acutely inflamed, local lesion, similar to a primary smallpox vaccination. There is usually fever, enlargement of the local lymph nodes, and pain. Unlike vaccinia virus, which occasionally produced a generalized infection (Fig. 7.5.4.6), cowpox virus lesions are always local. Human lesions caused by pseudocowpox virus (milker's nodules) are extremely rare and are less painful than those caused by cowpox.

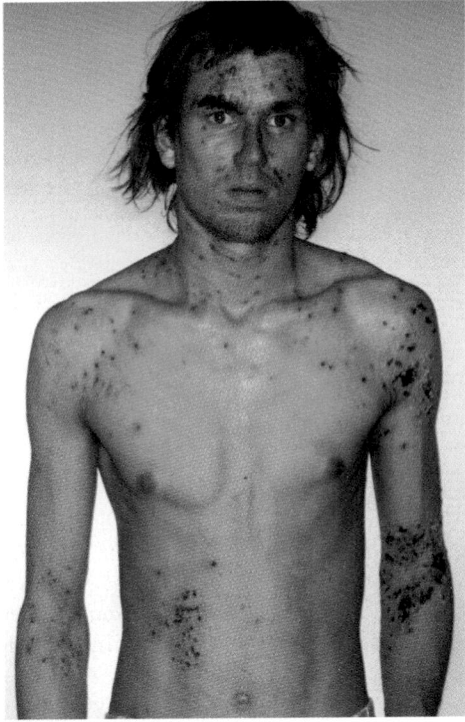

Fig. 7.5.4.6 Generalized vaccinia.
(Courtesy of the late Dr B E Juel-Jensen.)

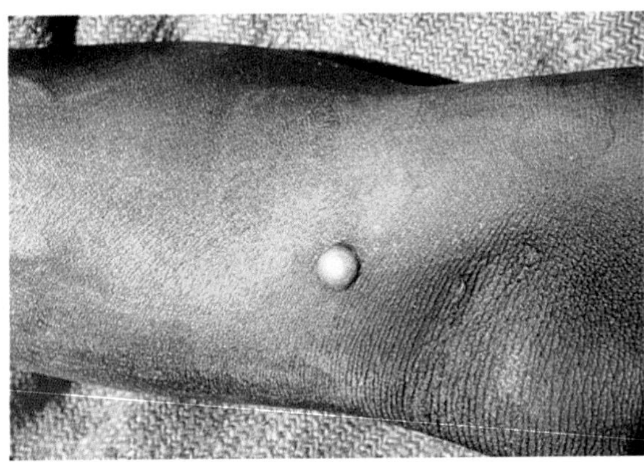

Fig. 7.5.4.7 Tanapox lesion on the leg of a Kenyan patient.
(Courtesy of the late P E C Manson-Bahr.)

Tanapox virus and Yaba monkey tumour virus

Tanapox virus and Yaba monkey tumour virus are the sole members of the *Yatapoxvirus* genus (another yatapoxvirus called Yaba-like disease virus, is considered a tanapox virus strain). These viruses are characterized by their slow replication rates in cell culture and can cause zoonotic infections in humans. Tanapox virus was isolated in the Tana valley in Kenya (1957–62) from humans suffering from localized skin lesions typical of poxviruses (Fig. 7.5.4.7). The virus is probably transmitted from infected monkeys by biting insects, particularly during wet weather conditions. It usually produces a solitary lesion that is preceded for a few days by a mild fever. The lesion takes 5 to 6 weeks to clear and is distinguished from other poxvirus lesions by its failure to become pustular. This virus cannot be cultured on the chorioallantoic membrane.

Yaba monkey tumour virus was discovered in Yaba, Lagos, Nigeria in 1957 as a virus causing cutaneous histiocytomas in rhesus monkeys and can infect humans if injected subcutaneously or intradermally. The lesions are not neoplastic and are cleared by the immune response.

Cutaneous poxviruses (orf virus and molluscum contagiosum virus)

See Chapters 7.5.27 and 7.5.28.

Further reading

Di Giulio DB, Eckburg PB (2004). Human monkeypox: an emerging zoonosis. *Lancet Infect Dis*, **4**, 15–25.

Fauquet CM, *et al.* (eds) (2005). *Virus taxonomy: Eighth Report of the International Committee on the Taxonomy of Viruses.* Elsevier, Amsterdam.

Fenner F, *et al.* (1988). *Smallpox and its eradication.* World Health Organization, Geneva.

Fenner F, Wittek R, Dumbell KR (1989). *The orthopoxviruses.* Academic Press Ltd, London.

Mercer AA, Schmidt A, Weber O (2007). *Poxviruses.* Berhäuser-Verlag, Berlin.

Moss B (2007). Poxviridae: the viruses and their replication. In: Knipe DM, *et al.* (eds) *Field's virology*, 5th edition, **2**, 2905–2946. Lippincott Williams & Wilkins, Philadelphia.

7.5.5 Mumps: epidemic parotitis

B.K. Rima

Essentials

Mumps is an acute, systemic, highly infectious, communicable infection of children and young adults, caused by a paramyxovirus (with an RNA genome). Transmission is by airborn droplet spread. After an incubation period of 14 to 18 days, typical presentation is with fever, pain near the angle of the jaw, and swelling of the parotid glands. Complications include orchitis, meningitis and encephalitis. Diagnosis is obvious clinically in cases with a contact history and parotitis, but serological (mumps-specific IgM and IgA) and RNA-based (RT-PCR) tests are used when this is not the case, e.g. the patient presenting with meningitis. Treatment is symptomatic. Prevention is by vaccination, often given as one component of a trivalent mumps/measles/rubella (MMR) vaccine at 14 to 16 months of age.

Introduction and historical perspective

The primary clinical manifestation in mumps, swelling of the salivary glands, is so characteristic that the disease was recognized very early as different from other childhood illnesses. Hippocrates described the disease in the 5th century bc and also noted swelling of the testes (orchitis) as a common complication of mumps. In 1790, Hamilton noted the infection in the central nervous system (CNS) and meninges. In 1934, mumps was shown to be a filterable virus by Johnson and Goodpasture, who also fulfilled Koch's postulates by infecting volunteers with virus propagated in monkeys. Since 1967, live attenuated vaccines have been licensed to control and prevent the infection.

Aetiology and genetics

Mumps virus (MuV) can be grown in tissue cultures of chick embryo, monkey kidney, and most human cells. The virus can also be cultured in the yolk sac or embryonic cavity of chick embryos. Cytopathic changes (syncytium formation and cell rounding) may be seen as early as 24 h postinfection and earlier if immunofluorescence is used. MuV is thermolabile. It can be stored for years at −70 °C, but infectivity is lost in a few days at room temperature. Treatment with ether or paraformaldehyde inactivates the virus rapidly, but does not destroy the antigens responsible for the complement fixation, haemagglutination, or reactivity in the skin test.

MuV is an enveloped RNA virus with a genome of 15 384 nucleotides. Its inner core is a ribonucleoprotein complex (the nucleocapsid) containing the nonsegmented, negative-strand, RNA molecule encapsidated by the nucleocapsid protein (N). The nucleocapsid has the herringbone structure characteristic of paramyxoviruses (Fig. 7.5.5.1a). Attached to this are two further proteins involved in transcription and replication of the RNA genome: the phosphoprotein (P) and the large replicase protein (L). The nucleocapsid is surrounded by a lipid bilayer (Fig. 7.5.5.1a, b). On the inner leaflet is a membrane or matrix protein (M) that plays an essential role in virus budding. On the outer surface are two glycoproteins, one carrying the haemagglutinin-neuraminidase activity (HN), the other responsible for fusion activity (F). The function of a nonstructural, small, hydrophobic protein (SH) is unknown; it is associated with the endoplasmic reticulum in MuV-infected cells. The SH protein sequence is hypervariable and this is used to assign MuV strains to one of 12 currently recognized genotypes. The nonstructural V protein functions in combating the host's innate immune response. The gene order (Fig. 7.5.5.1c) leads to an expression gradient in which the abundance of mRNAs decreases with increasing distance to the promoter at the 3'-terminal end of the genome, so that the N mRNA is more abundant than the L mRNA.

Epidemiology and pathogenesis

Mumps is highly infectious. Transmission depends on close personal contact with a patient who is excreting virus in the saliva and spreading it in droplets. In the prevaccine era, the peak incidence was in the late winter or early spring, in 3 to 7 year cycles. Most morbidity is associated with meningitis and orchitis. Case fatality is about 2 per 1000. The incubation period lies between 14 and 18 days. In any outbreak, 30 to 40% of those infected have subclinical illness.

MuV causes an infection of the upper respiratory tract that spreads to draining lymph nodes. The subsequent viraemia and infection of the lymphocytes and macrophages causes spread to many organs, but because mumps is so rarely lethal, details are scant. Lymphocytic infiltration and destruction of periductal cells lead to blockage of the ducts both in salivary glands and in the seminiferous tubules of the testes. The lymphatics in the tissues surrounding and overlying the parotid glands become obstructed, producing a gel-like oedema that may spread down over the chest wall, especially when the swelling of the salivary glands is severe.

Clinical features and diagnosis

Parotitis

A patient with mumps parotitis may have a fever without rigors (40–40.5 °C) as well as pain near the angle of the jaw. The face and neck become distorted with swelling. The skin over the gland is hot and flushed but there is no rash, unlike in the swelling of erysipelas. If the swelling is severe, the mouth cannot be opened for pain and tightness, and is dry because the flow of saliva is blocked. This discomfort lasts for 3 or 4 days. Sometimes, as one side clears, the parotid on the other side swells. When there is bilateral parotitis, clinical diagnosis is usually obvious. One condition that must be excluded is bull neck diphtheria (Chapter 7.6.1), which can look very like mumps.

Rarely, the submaxillary and sublingual salivary glands may also be affected. The symptoms are similar to those in parotitic mumps, but it is difficult or impossible to distinguish the swelling from other forms of submaxillary swellings, especially inflammation of various groups of lymph nodes and Ludwig's angina. In mumps, the neck swelling is ill-defined and the angle of the jaw is impalpable. To determine if cervical lymph nodes are swollen from some other cause, the pharynx must be examined carefully. The fauces must be examined for signs of tonsilitis that might cause cervical adenitis. The lymph nodes in contact with the submaxillary and sublingual salivary glands drain the corner of the eye, the side of the nose, the cheeks, the lips, and the floor of the mouth, all of which must be explored, before a diagnosis of submaxillary or

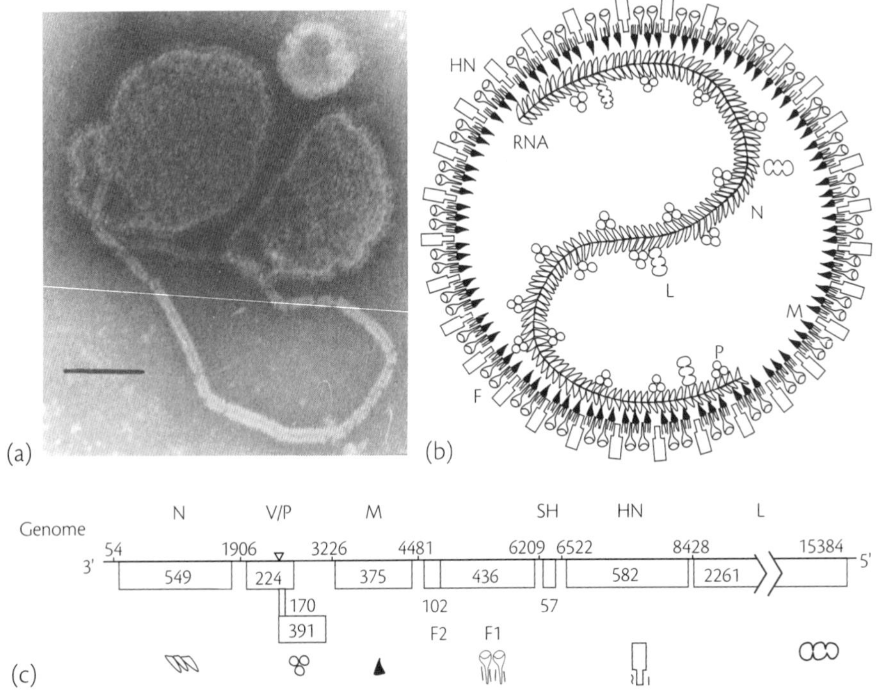

Fig. 7.5.5.1 Structure and genome organization of the mumps virus: (a) a disrupted, negatively stained, mumps virion. The viral nucleocapsid protrudes from the particle and the fringe of viral spikes is visible (bar = 100 nm); (b) diagram of the localization of the nucleocapsid (N), phospho- (P), large (L), matrix (M), haemagglutinin-neuraminidase (HN), and fusion (F) proteins in the mumps virion; and (c) structure of the genome of mumps virus indicating the localization of the genes, the nucleotide number of their starting and stopping position, and (in boxes) the number of amino acid residues in each of the viral proteins.

sublingual mumps can be made. Laboratory tests are needed to confirm the diagnosis.

In infectious mononucleosis, the glands stand out distinctly and the parotid is not affected. In septic parotitis there is more parotid tenderness; there may be fluctuation, and pus exudes from the orifice of Stensen's duct. Calculus causes spasmodic pain and swelling and may be detected radiographically. Recurrent parotitis and Mikulicz's syndrome are unlikely to be confused with mumps except in the earliest stages, nor are uveoparotid fever and tumours of the gland, as they are chronic conditions.

Orchitis

Orchitis may occur 4 or 5 days after the onset of parotitis. Quite often it occurs without preceding parotitis. It is an acute condition, with chills, sweats, headache, and backache, and a swinging temperature as well as severe local testicular pain and tenderness. The scrotum is swollen and oedematous, and the testicles are impalpable. Usually, only one testicle is affected but sometimes both: the second testicle may become affected just as the swelling of the first is subsiding. The illness lasts 3 or 4 days before the swelling begins to subside. Orchitis is unusual before the age of puberty, though it has occurred in young boys and even in infants. In adolescent and young males it develops in 1:5 cases. Some degree of atrophy of the testicle occurs in at least one-third of patients with orchitis. Azoospermia after mumps is rare and only temporary. The fear of sterility after mumps orchitis has been exaggerated and one can reassure the patient. Orchitis when it occurs without parotitis is difficult to distinguish from gonococcal epididymo-orchitis, unless there has been contact with mumps. The rare case of orchitis in infancy may resemble torsion of the testis and perhaps it is safer to operate than risk a serious misdiagnosis.

Meningitis and encephalitis

MuV frequently invades the nervous system: changes in the electroencephalogram and increased levels of protein and lymphocyte levels in the cerebrospinal fluid can be shown in at least half the patients. However, in most cases, neurological symptoms or signs are absent. Mumps virus was one of the most common known causes of lymphocytic meningitis. This may develop a few days after the start of parotitis, but almost as often it occurs in the absence of parotitis. Occasionally, the patient develops transient paralysis of limbs resulting in the occurrence of quadriplegia or single nerve paralysis in some patients. Polyneuritis, neuritis of the trigeminal or facial nerve, and retrobulbar optic neuritis have been described in mumps but all are rare. The meningitis is usually mild and self-limiting.

Mumps encephalitis is a different entity; cerebrospinal fluid is normal and contains no virus. The outlook is different. The patient is confused and may lapse into coma and remain comatose for days, weeks, or months. Almost 2% of the encephalitis cases are fatal. At autopsy there is perivascular demyelination as in other forms of postinfectious encephalitis (Chapter 24.11.2).

Other complications

Deafness is reported in up to 0.3% of the cases, but it is rarely permanent and often unilateral. Women sometimes complain of ovarian pain during an attack of mumps, but it is rarely as severe as in men with orchitis. There is no evidence that it affects fertility. Mastitis occurs in 15% of the cases, both in men and women, but it is usually mild and fleeting. Mild upper abdominal pain in about 50% of the cases may be related to viral changes in the pancreas. The amount of amylase in duodenal fluid may be less than normal. This is probably caused by a blockage of the ducts in the pancreas.

Although there are anecdotal reports of diabetes occurring after an attack of mumps, there is no virological or immunological evidence for a direct link though the virus is known to be able to infect the pancreatic islet B cells.

Mumps in the fetus and infant

Abortion may occur in women with mumps in the first trimester of pregnancy. It is not common and probably not caused by direct viral damage to the fetus. The connection between primary endocardial fibroelastosis and mumps remains vague. The disease's declining incidence has been attributed to mumps vaccination. Some studies using reverse transcription polymerase chain reaction (RT-PCR) indicate that viral RNA can be amplified from myocardial samples in a high percentage of cases. However, the latter technique is open to contamination problems and hence this link remains to be confirmed. Mumps virus has not been isolated from heart tissue at autopsy and these infants have no mumps antibody in their blood. They may show a delayed hypersensitivity response to the skin test. This has not been explained, but may reflect some immune defect in the fetus which could cause myocarditis and fibroelastosis.

In the normal infant, maternal IgG passes to the fetus and seems to protect the infant against mumps during the first year of life. The typical disease of mumps in infants is a rare clinical finding, even in populations with no previous experience of the disease. MuV may be isolated in vague respiratory infections in infants.

Laboratory diagnosis

In patients without parotitis, especially meningitis, and in the absence of contact history, serological tests and RT-PCR are the only means of reaching a firm diagnosis. MuV isolation is an insensitive method and now rarely used. MuV contains several different antigenic components, which provoke distinct antibodies that are useful for laboratory confirmation. Antibody to the N protein rises in the first 2 weeks of infection but then declines rapidly. Antibody to the HN protein appears at the end of the first week, usually in high titre: it may persist for years and indicates past infection. Neutralizing antibodies also develop, but titres are a poor correlate of protection. Nowadays, sensitive enzyme immunoassays allow early diagnosis by detection of mumps-specific IgM and IgA. In recent outbreaks in the United States of America and in the United Kingdom, IgM-negative cases have been identified. IgA can be detected in saliva or mouth washings on about the fourth day after infection, and in the serum early in the disease. Measurement of antibodies in acute and convalescent sera is a reliable method for diagnosis, especially in patients who have no parotitis.

Treatment

There is no specific antiviral treatment. Symptomatic treatment includes simple analgesics, but for the severe pain of orchitis, morphine (15–30 mg) may be required for a day or two. Corticosteroids are worth trying in severe cases of parotitis, more especially in orchitis. An adult dose of 60 mg prednisolone daily for 2 or 3 days sometimes gives dramatic relief from pain, though it may not reduce the swelling.

Prevention and control

The mainstay of prevention is vaccination of susceptible individuals. Isolation is not effective as the patient has been infectious for days before parotitis occurs and inapparent cases are frequent. Attenuated live vaccine gives 95% seroconversion, and protection lasts for at least 15 years. In developed countries, mumps vaccine is currently given between 14 and 16 months of age as one component of a live attenuated trivalent mumps/measles/rubella (MMR) vaccine. A two-dose schedule with follow-up at 4 to 5 years of age is now recommended. This has suppressed the incidence of mumps by more than 98% in the United States of America and in the United Kingdom. Nevertheless, both countries have had recent outbreaks of mumps in the college age population in both unvaccinated individuals as well as those with a documented vaccination history. It is not clear whether this is due to primary vaccine failure, waning immunity in the absence of frequent challenge, or the ability of new variant wild-type virus strains to break thought the protective immunity established by older vaccines. Mumps vaccination is contraindicated in pregnant women and patients with immunodeficiency due to immunosuppressive therapy or disease. However, HIV seropositive children should be vaccinated with the MMR vaccine.

Further reading

Carbone KM, Rubin S (2006). Mumps virus. In: Fields BN, *et al.* (eds) Fields Virology, 5th edition, pp. 1527–550. Lippincott Williams and Wilkins, Philadelphia.

Christie AB (1980). *Infectious diseases: epidemiology and clinical practice*, 3rd edition. Churchill Livingstone, Edinburgh.

Duprex WD, Rima BK (2006). Mumps virus. In: *Encyclopedia of the life sciences*. MacMillan Reference, Stockton Press, Basingstoke. Article number A4273 (CD ROM only).

Feldman HA (1989). Mumps. In: Evans AJ (ed). *Viral infections of humans*, 3rd edition, pp. 471–91. Plenum Medical, New York.

Rima BK (1999). Mumps virus. In: Granoff A, Webster RG (eds) *Encyclopedia of virology*, 2nd edition, pp. 988–994. Academic Press, London.

Wright KE (2006). Mumps. In: Newton VA, Vallely PJ (eds) *Infection And Hearing Loss*, pp. 109–126. John Wiley and Sons Ltd, Chichester.

7.5.6 Measles

H.C. Whittle and P. Aaby

Essentials

Measles is a single-stranded RNA virus that is spread by aerosolized droplets and is highly transmissible. It causes a spectrum of disease ranging from mild in the well nourished to severe in the malnourished or immunosuppressed: mortality is 3 to 10% in Africa.

Clinical features—10 to 14 days after infection the viral prodrome typically consists of runny nose and fever, sometimes also diarrhoea or convulsions; signs include mild conjunctivitis, red mucosae, and (on the buccal mucosa) Koplik's spots. After 14 to 18 days a morbilliform rash first appears on the forehead and neck, then spreads to involve the trunk and finally the limbs. Other manifestations include severe conjunctivitis (especially in those who are vitamin-A deficient), pneumonitis and enteritis (which may cause profuse diarrhoea). Early complications include (1) pneumonia—caused by secondary bacterial infection and responsible for most deaths; (2) stomatitis—caused by herpes simplex virus and/or candidal infection; (3) enteritis—due to candidal or bacterial superinfection; (4) eye infection—corneal ulceration may be caused by some combination of measles itself, herpes simplex infection, vitamin A deficiency, and use of traditional eye medicines; more than half of childhood blindness in Africa is related to measles; (5) skin and other infections, e.g. pyoderma; (6) encephalitis—occurs in 0.1 to 0.2% of cases; probably attributable to a neuroallergic process; mortality is 10 to 15%, and 25% of children are left with permanent neurological disability. Late complications include malnutrition, giant cell pneumonia and subacute sclerosing panencephalitis.

Diagnosis and treatment—diagnosis is primarily clinical, but signs may be less clear cut in vaccinated subjects. Detection of measles-specific IgM antibody or detection of measles antigen in saliva or urine may clinch the diagnosis if the rash is mild or atypical. Management is supportive, including administration of vitamin A, and with prompt treatment of secondary infections.

Prevention—(1) Passive immunization—human immunoglobulin is highly effective if given within 2 or 3 days of exposure and should be administered to those in whom vaccination is contraindicated. (2) Active immunization—live vaccine is often given in the developed world as one component of a trivalent mumps/measles/rubella (MMR) vaccine at 14 to 16 months of age. However, this is not appropriate for children in developing countries, who are infected by measles at a much earlier age, where substantial successes in controlling the disease has been obtained with a strategy combining (a) catch-up—a one-time mass campaign covering everybody aged 9 months to 14 years, regardless of previous measles or immunization; (2) keep-up—achieving a high coverage for each birth cohort; (3) follow-up—subsequent mass campaigns covering all children every 3 to 5 years; and (4) mop-up—campaigns that target children who are difficult to reach or during outbreaks.

Introduction

Measles is an acute, highly transmissible RNA viral infection of humans that is spread by aerosolized droplets. It causes much death and suffering, especially among poor children in developing countries. Its severity varies according to host and socioeconomic factors, not to antigenic variation or alteration in virulence of the virus. There is no reservoir of infection other than in humans and no evidence of a carrier state and as there is an effective vaccine, global eradication is possible but a dauntingly high vaccine coverage of more than 95% will be needed. The virus causes a generalized infection coupled with severe damage to the immune system due to destruction of T lymphocytes, disturbance of the Th1/Th2 cytokine balance, and impaired antigenic presentation. The chief clinical features result from infection of the skin, mucous membranes, and respiratory tract. Death, which occurs in up to 15% of hospitalized children in Africa, results from secondary infections and immunosuppression. Attack rates in home contacts are very high (of the order of 90%) and long-life immunity follows the disease but not vaccination. Supplemental immunization activities allowing repeated vaccination every 3 to 5 years in endemic countries have lowered measles deaths dramatically. However, although global coverage by measles immunization in 2005 was 77%, at least 20 million children are infected annually and 345 000 die, mainly in sub-Saharan Africa where immunization coverage is low.

Epidemiology

Measles has been the archetypical childhood infection, known and feared by all parents. Nearly everybody contracted this most infectious of childhood diseases. Measles was the single biggest cause of childhood deaths. In the prevaccination era, 6 million children may have died annually of measles. With advances in coverage during the last 25 years, the current estimate (2007) is 197,000 deaths, still the most important of the vaccine-preventable infections (Fig. 7.5.6.1). The severity and age of infection varies markedly between poor and rich countries. In the West, most children were infected between 3 and 6 years of age, when they attended nursery and primary schools. Mortality was low (<0.05%) and morbidity, although considerable when compared to many other common viral infections, was limited. Most cases occurred in the winter and spring, with a biannual epidemic pattern. Widespread immunization has dramatically reduced both the number of cases and complications in high income countries.

In low income countries, measles is still severe and behaves differently. It kills between 3 and 10% of children in the community and some 10 to 20% of those admitted to hospital. Mortality from measles is considerably higher in Africa (3–10%) than in Asia or South America (1%). West Africa has the highest case fatality rates.

There are many reasons for this increase in severity: children are infected at 1 to 2 years of age; severe malnutrition leads to prolonged, severe measles. Overcrowding is another strong determinant, for secondary and tertiary cases in large families are at great risk of death. Exposure to a large dose of the virus when in close contact with the index case may be the critical factor. The severity of measles depends on the severity of disease in the index case. The high mortality found in West Africa is due to this region having the largest polygamous and extended families, which increase the risk of intense exposure. When females stay at home and are constrained in their social contacts, mortality is higher in girls than boys. There is also a high case fatality in children with chronic disease, including kwashiorkor, tuberculosis, and HIV infection. Hospital wards and clinics in developing countries have been important centres of disease transmission.

Though measles may have permanent sequelae, recent research has provided limited support for the previous belief in long-term

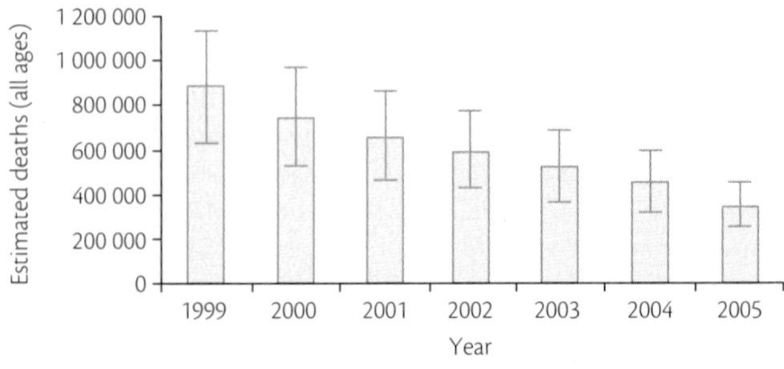

Fig. 7.5.6.1 Estimated worldwide mortality due to measles, 1999–2005. Bars are uncertainty bounds.
(Reproduced with permission from Wolfson L, *et al.* (2007). Has the 2005 measles mortality reduction goal been achieved? A natural history modelling study. *Lancet*, **369**,191–200.)

excess morbidity and mortality after the first 6 weeks of measles infection. Long-term consequences may also depend on intensity of exposure. Index cases apparently have better long-term survival than secondary cases, suggesting a beneficial effect of mild measles infection. Long-term morbidity is most likely to be experienced by young children who have severe measles following intensive exposure.

Measles immunization has dramatically decreased the number of cases, but measles deaths through vaccine failures are not infrequent. Immunized cases are characterized by a prolonged incubation period, a short prodrome, mild symptoms, and a favourable outcome. The mild measles of immunized cases leads to less risk of transmission or transmission of less severe disease. Immunization reduces the number of children being susceptible in the same household and hence reduces the risk of intensive exposure (Table 7.5.6.1).

However, immunization may have negative consequences on herd immunity for an increasing number of unvaccinated children, or children who have responded poorly to the vaccine will reach adulthood without having been exposed to measles. Thus, vaccinated people will have lower antibody levels than naturally infected people, which is particularly important because young immunized mothers will transfer lower antibody levels to their offspring. In West Africa, children of immunized mothers have only half the antibody levels of children of naturally infected mothers and they become susceptible as early as 3 to 5 months of age.

It has been argued that measles vaccines only saved 'weak' children who were likely to die anyway. However, many epidemiological studies, including small randomized trials, have shown remarkable reductions in all cause mortality after standard measles vaccine. In Bangladesh, measles vaccination was associated with a 49% reduction in all-cause mortality from the age of 9 months, even though acute measles accounted for only 10 to 12% of deaths. This unexpected benefit was not related to prevention of measles. In most studies, this nonspecific benefit is particularly marked for girls. More recent studies have shown that the combination of measles vaccine with other vaccines or vitamin A supplements may influence the nonspecific effects on child survival.

Popular beliefs

In most cultures, measles has a specific local name and is a much feared disease. Popular understanding is centred around the rash, which if it stays within the body will lead to severe disease. This belief has some basis in truth for the prodrome is prolonged in severe cases, and a proportion of deaths reportedly occur before the appearance of the rash during very severe epidemics. Therapeutic practices, such as rubbing the skin with palm oil or kerosene, are aimed at eliciting the rash quickly. In West Africa it is believed that cooling keeps the rash within the body, so the child may be bedded in warm sand or covered with blankets, and is not washed or given cold water to drink.

The virus and its antigens

Measles mainly infects humans, but like the other closely related morbilliviruses (such as rinderpest or canine distemper virus) it is able to cross species to infect other primates and, on occasions, dogs. It contains a single strand of RNA, is highly pleomorphic, and ranges from 100 to 300 nm in diameter. The virus propagates by budding from the cell membrane, from which it acquires an envelope. The membrane of infected cells and the virion envelope contain two surface glycoproteins, the haemagglutinin (H) and fusion (F) proteins, and a nonglycosylated matrix (M) protein, which forms the inner layer. The H protein, which allows attachment of the virus to cells, via the CD46 or CDw150 receptors, is the main target for neutralizing antibodies. The F protein is responsible for fusion and syncytium formation of infected cells. CD46 is a ubiquitous membrane cofactor protein, which together with five other proteins, protects cells from complement activation and lysis. Some wild-type viruses, but not all, bind to the receptor but do not down-regulate it, thus preventing lysis and allowing efficient viral replication. The CDw150 receptor (also known as signalling lymphocyte activation molecule, SLAM) is expressed on immature lymphocytes and on effector memory T cells, and is rapidly induced on T and B cells after activation. The internal components or nucleocapsid consist of RNA, the nucleoprotein (N), which is the major protein, the phosphoprotein (P), and the large protein (L). The F protein is remarkably stable, the H protein shows minor antigenic variation, but the N protein, which contains a variable region in the C-terminal, is highly divergent among different strains of virus. Genetic analysis of Haemagglutinin and Nucleoprotein genes allowed molecular surveillance of the measles virus to track the international spread of the virus. There is also variation in the M protein, which some claim is related to persistent infection. The virus and its antigens are shown in Fig. 7.5.6.2.

Pathogenesis and the immune response

The course of infection and the immune response to this invasion are shown in Fig. 7.5.6.3. The measles virus, which is thermolabile and survives best at low humidities, is spread to susceptible contacts in droplets during sneezing and coughing. First, it infects and multiplies in the epithelium of the upper respiratory tract or

Table 7.5.6.1 Impact of measles immunization on the transmission and severity of measles

Outcome measurements		Bissau 1980–1982	Senegal 1983–1990	Bissau 1991
Case fatality ratio: vaccinated / unvaccinated (95% CI)	Acute mortality within 1 month	0.39 (0.13–1.14)	0.0 (0–0.92)	0.30 (0.13–0.72)
	Delayed mortality from 1 month to 3 years			0.44 (0.22–0.90)
Secondary attack rate ratio according to vaccinated/ unvaccinated index cases		0.28 (0.10–0.79)	0.36 (0.15–0.87)	

Based on data from Aaby P, *et al.* (1986). Vaccinated children get milder measles infection: a community study from Guinea-Bissau. *J Infect Dis*, **154**, 858–63, and Samb B, *et al.* (1997). Decline in measles case fatality ratio after the introduction of measles immunization in rural Senegal. *Am J Epidemiol*, **145**, 51–7.

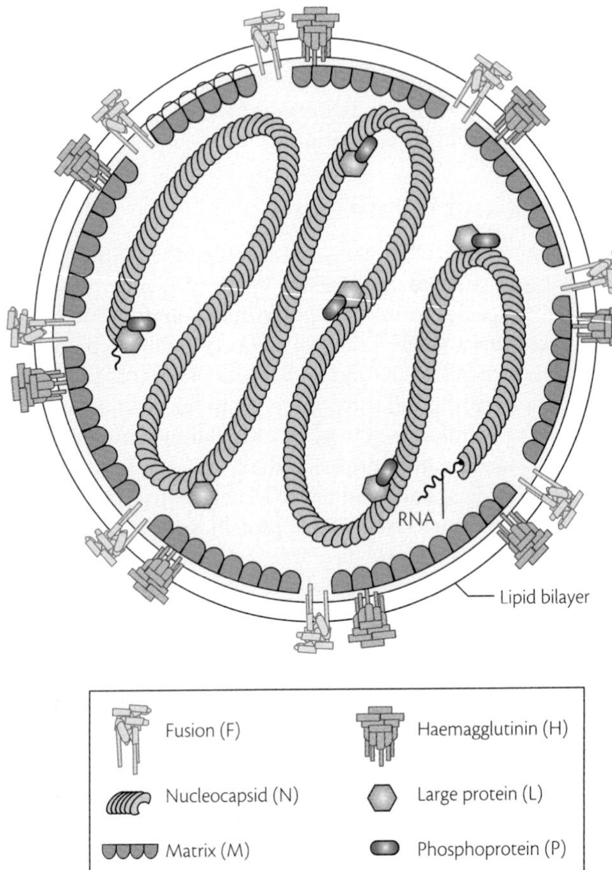

Fig. 7.5.6.2 The virus and its antigens.
(Reproduced with permission from Moss WJ, and Griffen D E (2006). Global measles elimination. *Nat Rev Microbiol*, **4**, 900–8.)

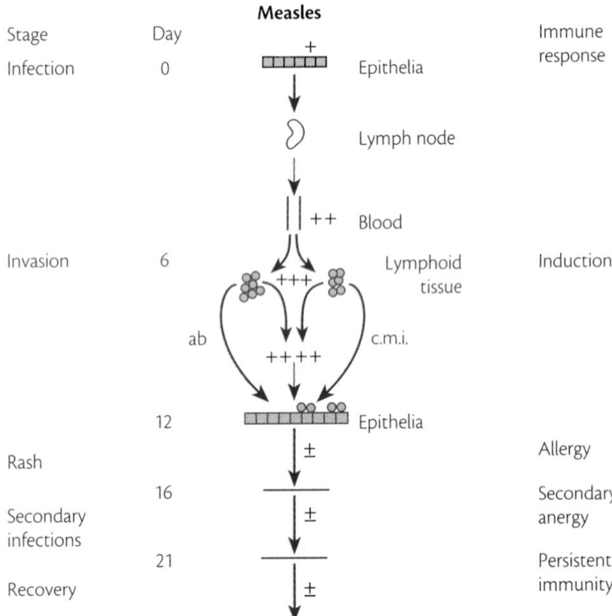

Fig. 7.5.6.3 Pathogenesis of measles. + Denotes, amount of virus; ab, antibody.
(Reproduced with permission from Parry EHOP (ed) (1984). *Principles of medicine in Africa*, 2nd edition. Oxford University Press, Oxford.)

the conjunctivae. Some 4 to 6 days later, the virus is found in the reticuloendothelial tissue of the liver and the spleen after passage through lymph nodes and spread via the blood. Here it multiplies, causing fusion of cells to form giant cells with many nuclei. Viral antigens, which can be found by immunofluorescent techniques in and on the surface of both these cells and lymphocytes, now induce the immune response. First, natural killer cells and cytotoxic T cells mount a cell-mediated reaction that contains the virus and limits its spread within cells. Later, B cells are primed to produce antibody. Defects in the cellular immune system, as in severe malnutrition, cancer, or primary and secondary immunodeficiencies, allow widespread multiplication of the virus to cause fatal giant cell pneumonia.

Around day 8, the measles virus is carried by the blood, either free or in mononuclear cells, to the target tissues, which are epithelia of the skin, eye, lung, and gut. Again, the agent multiplies to cause a bright erythema of the mucosae and Koplik's spots (see below), which are foci of viral multiplication. At this stage, measles virus may be cultured from nasopharyngeal secretions, and antigen can be detected by immunofluorescent techniques in the characteristic giant cells of the buccal mucosa, in epithelial cells, and in both B and T lymphocytes in the blood.

The rash, appearing around days 14 to 16, is the sign of a strong and complicated allergic reaction to the virus in epithelia. The extent and severity of the rash, which reflects the clinical severity of the disease, is determined by the number of target cells infected. Histological examination shows virus in the disrupted epidermis, in the corium, and in capillary endothelium. These tissues are infiltrated by mononuclear cells together with antibody, immune complexes, and complement. An intact cell-mediated immune response is essential to generate the rash and clear the virus, for if impaired, as in the case of children with leukaemia, or occasionally in severe kwashiorkor, the virus multiplies unchecked and no rash appears. Some 2 or 3 days after the start of the rash, around day 17 or 18, the virus can no longer be cultured from epithelia, for infected cells have been disrupted and the free virus neutralized by antibody. The first antibody to appear is to the nucleoprotein antigens. The second to appear, which is largely responsible for neutralization of the virus, is to the haemagglutinin. Finally, the antibody to the fusion glycoprotein appears in a low titre. This antibody stops cell-to-cell spread of the virus. At this stage the child is markedly immunosuppressed and thus susceptible to secondary infections of the eyes, mouth, gut, and lungs. Latent viruses, such as herpes simplex or cytomegalovirus, may be reactivated and in turn cause further damage to the immune system. The delayed hypersensitivity reaction, as measured by skin tests to old tuberculin or candida antigen, is absent or severely impaired.

By the third week, day 21, as the patient recovers, antibody is in full production. Levels remain elevated for the rest of the patient's life, either because of repeated subclinical infections or because the virus persists in latent form in the spleen and other organs, so stimulating antibody. Occasionally, the virus persists in the brain in a damaging form to cause subacute sclerosing panencephalitis (see below).

The mechanisms of immunosuppression are complex (Fig. 7.5.6.4). The CD4+ and CD8+ cytotoxic T-cell response, which is exuberant, may result in the destruction of infected T cells and dendritic cells thus leading to their depletion, deficient antigen processing, and generalized immunosuppression. Cross-binding of

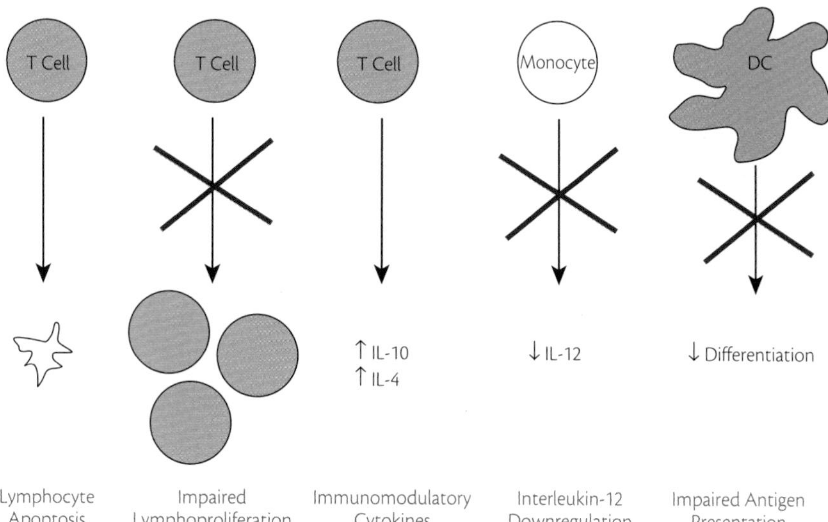

Fig. 7.5.6.4 Potential mechanisms of immune suppression following measles virus infection.
(Reproduced with permission from Moss WJ, Ota MO, and Griffen DE (2004). Measles: immune suppression and immune responses. *Int J Biochem Cell Biol*, **36**,1380–5.)

the CD46 cellular receptor down-regulates interleukin 12 (IL-12), a crucial cytokine in the development of Th1 and delayed hypersensitivity responses. Infection of CDw150+ lymphocytes, which are predominantly of the Th0/Th1 type, results in suppression of lymphoproliferation and cell death. Thus, measles ultimately dampens the Th1 response, resulting in a skewing towards a Th2 cytokine response and susceptibility to intracellular and other pathogens. However, this immunosuppression may be in the interest of the host by limiting further autoallergic damage of infected tissues.

Pathogenesis in the underprivileged, in the malnourished, and in the HIV-infected

Measles is severe, prolonged, and carries a high case fatality rate due to secondary infections in children of the developing world, as it was formerly in the underprivileged in Europe. Two explanations are offered. Crowding leads to a high dose of measles virus and also increases the chances of secondary infection. The period of incubation has been found to be short, around 10 to 12 days, in severe and fatal cases, consistent with the concept of infecting dose as a mechanism of severe disease. Alternatively, or in tandem, malnutrition diminishes the immune response to the virus, allowing great proliferation of virus and subsequent damage to the host. The immune response follows, which generates a severe and widespread rash followed by prolonged immunosuppression. Secondary bacterial infections with, e.g. *Streptococcus pneumoniae*, or latent infections such as herpes simplex or *Mycobacterium tuberculosis* occur in the wake of this intense damage to the immune system, often killing or maiming the child. Virus persists in lymphocytes and epithelial cells for up to 30 days after the start of the rash. Anorexia, increased catabolism, protein loss from the gut, and further malnutrition exaggerate the problem, which is worst in the weanling child (Fig. 7.5.6.5).

The death rate after measles in hospitalized infants is higher in HIV-infected children, and prolonged viral shedding occurs in these children. Thus, in regions of high prevalence, HIV-infected children may be important unrecognized transmitters of the virus. Asymptomatic HIV-infected children respond normally to vaccination, but those with AIDS are less likely to respond and may be threatened by persistent infection.

Clinical features

There is a spectrum of severity ranging from mild in the privileged and well nourished to severe in the blatantly malnourished or immunosuppressed. However, the rule is not inviolate and other factors such as the age and dose of infection are probably as important in determining the severity of disease. Measles, often severe, occasionally infects unvaccinated young adults or those who have lived in isolated communities. The clinical features of measles and some complications are shown in Fig. 7.5.6.6 and discussed below.

Prodrome (days 10–14)

A diagnosis of measles is often missed at this stage, when fever coupled with a runny nose, and sometimes complicated by convulsions, is the main feature. Other signs are mild conjunctivitis, red mucosa, Koplik's spots, and diarrhoea. Koplik's spots are found in the buccal mucosa (Fig. 7.5.6.7). They are small, irregular, bright-red spots with a minute bluish-white speck in the centre of each of them. The prodrome is prolonged in severe cases, and reduced in individuals with modified measles due to maternal antibodies or the prophylactic use of immunoglobulin.

Rash (days 14–18)

The morbilliform rash first appears on the forehead and neck and then spreads, over a period of 3 to 4 days, to involve the trunk and finally the limbs (Fig. 7.5.6.8).

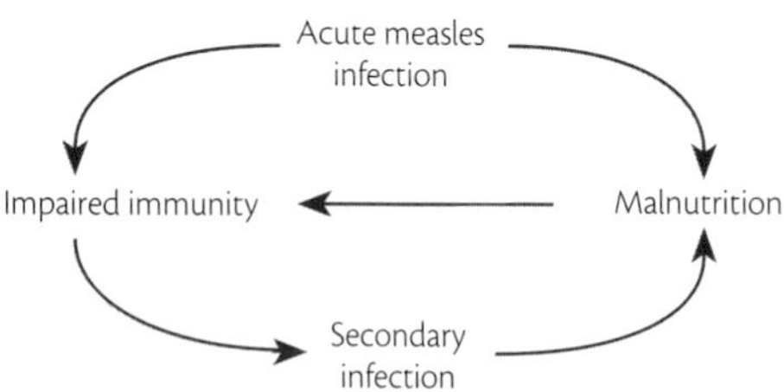

Fig. 7.5.6.5 The complex interaction between infection, nutrition, and impaired immunity seen in measles.
(Reproduced with permission from Greenwood BM (1996). The host's response to infection. In: Weatherall DJ, Ledingham JGGL, Warrell DA (eds) (1996). *Oxford textbook of medicine*, 3rd edition, p. 282. Oxford University Press, Oxford.)

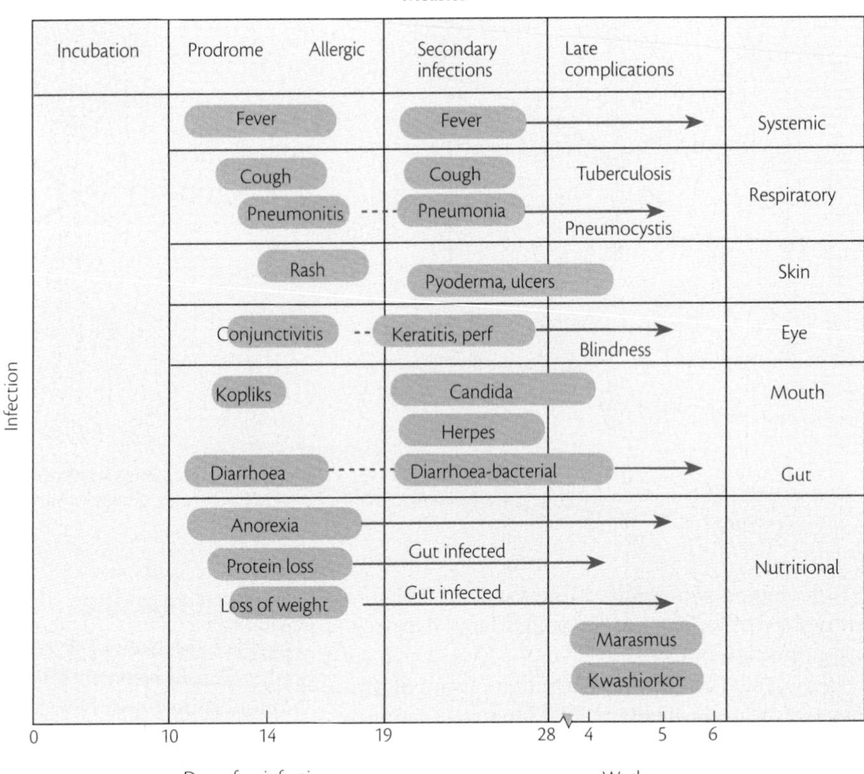

Fig. 7.5.6.6 Clinical features of measles and some of its complications. (Reproduced with permission from Parry EHOP (ed) (1984). *Principles of medicine in Africa*, 2nd edition, Oxford University Press, Oxford.)

In children in Africa and other parts of the developing world the rash is often red, confluent, raised (Fig. 7.5.6.9), very extensive, and sometimes accompanied by bleeding into the skin and gut. Later, the rash blackens (postmeasles 'staining', see Fig. 7.5.6.10), then the skin peels causing extensive desquamation (Fig. 7.5.6.11). Other epithelial surfaces are inflamed, the severity matching that of the rash. Cough may be hoarse and coupled with inspiration difficulty if the larynx and trachea are inflamed. Signs of pneumonitis are apparent, which in severe cases may cause cyanosis or be complicated by mediastinal and subcutaneous emphysema. Conjunctivitis, especially in those who are vitamin A deficient, can be severe. Enteritis may cause profuse diarrhoea with a resulting loss of protein, and malabsorption of food and water. The mouth is painful and red, which adds to the misery of the child, who becomes anorexic and may even refuse to suck the breast. In the uncomplicated case, as is usual in the West, the convalescent period is short, usually lasting less than a week. Complications should be suspected if fever persists while the rash is fading or desquamating.

Complications

Early complications (days 18–30)

As a result of the widespread, severe allergic reaction to the measles virus signified by the rash, the patient is left severely immunosuppressed and is susceptible to infection.

Pneumonia

This causes the most deaths (Table 7.5.6.2) and is heralded by a rise in fever, leucocytosis, and respiratory difficulties. Lobar pneumonia is usually caused by *S. pneumoniae*, but bronchopneumonia, which is more common, results from other bacteria, such as *Staphylococcus aureus*, or secondary viral infections with, e.g. herpes simplex or adenovirus. A variety of other organisms such as Gram-negative bacteria, cytomegalovirus, fungi, *M. tuberculosis*, and *Pneumocystis jirovecii* should be considered as potential lung pathogens in the malnourished or immunocompromised child.

Stomatitis and enteritis

Chronic diarrhoea and a sore mouth caused by candidal infection are common complications of measles in children in the developing world. The gut is often superinfected with bacteroides spp., *Escherichia coli*, pseudomonas spp., and *S. aureus*, which results in malabsorption and protein loss. Deep ulcers caused by herpes simplex virus erode the corners of the mouth, gums, and inner surface of the lips causing much misery, illness, and pain (Fig. 7.5.6.12).

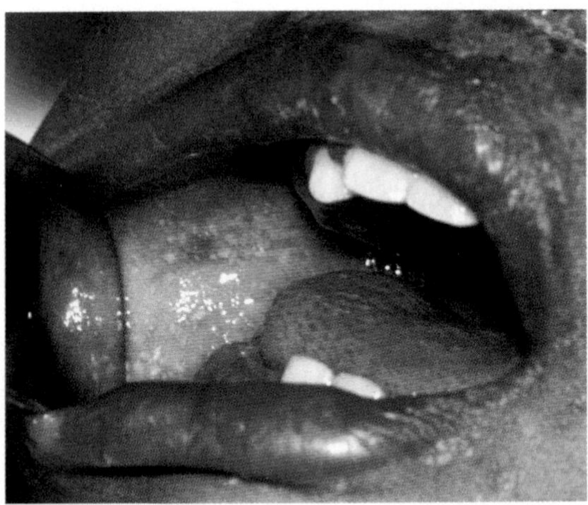

Fig. 7.5.6.7 Koplik's spots on the buccal mucosa. (Courtesy of the late Dr B.E. Juel-Jensen.)

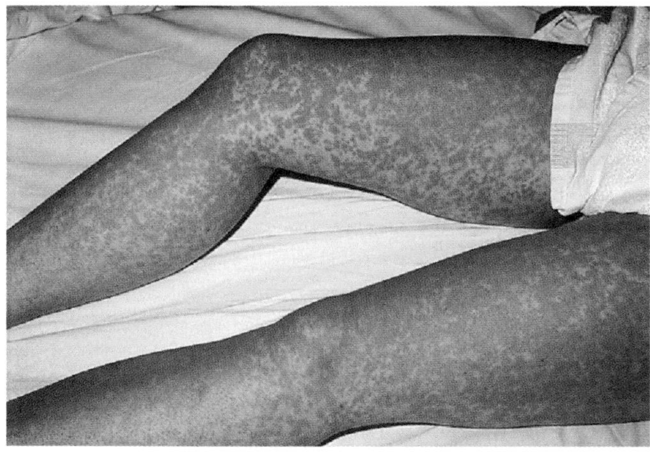

(a)

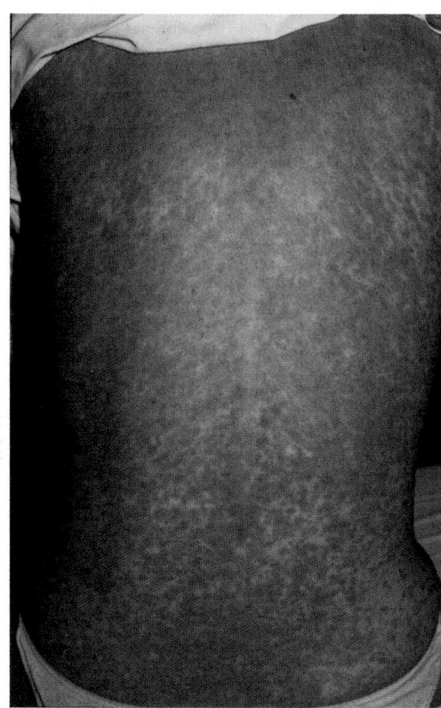

(b)

Fig. 7.5.6.8 (a, b) The morbilliform rash first appears on the forehead and neck and then spreads, over a period of 3 to 4 days, to involve the trunk and finally the limbs. (Copyright D A Warrell.)

Eye infections

Corneal ulceration leading to impaired vision or blindness is common after measles, especially in malnourished and vitamin A-deficient children (Fig. 7.5.6.13). Several studies from Africa have shown that more than half of childhood blindness is related to measles. The mechanisms are still under discussion. In northern Nigeria, herpes simplex was found in 47% of active corneal ulcers after measles, and measles virus in 12%: the children often had evidence of oral herpes. In a study in Tanzania, blindness precipitated by measles was associated with vitamin A deficiency (50%), herpes simplex infection (21%), and the use of traditional eye medicine (17%).

Skin and other infections

Pyoderma is common after measles. In the malnourished patient, deep eroding ulcers may bore through the skin even into bone.

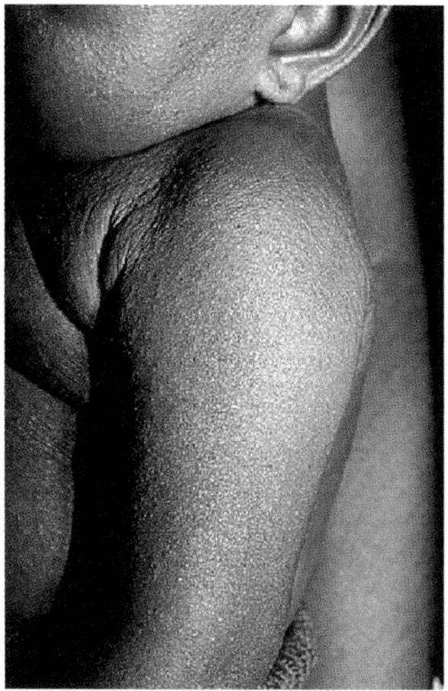

Fig. 7.5.6.9 Measles rash in an African child.

When originating in the mouth they are known as cancrum oris or noma (Fig. 7.5.6.14). Otitis media is also common.

Encephalitis

This is a rare, but much feared, complication found in approximately 1 to 2 per 1000 cases. The onset is usually between 4 and 7 days after the start of the rash, but, rarely, it may occur within 48 h or up to 2 weeks from the onset. In addition to seizures, there is often fever, irritability, headache, and a disturbance in consciousness that may progress to profound coma. The disorder is probably attributable to a neuroallergic process. Lymphocytes from the cerebrospinal fluid have been shown to respond to myelin basic protein, as in experimental allergic encephalomyelitis. The virus cannot be isolated from cerebrospinal fluid, which contains lymphocytes and raised levels of IgG but normal levels of measles antibody. Mortality and morbidity are high: 10 to 15% of patients die and 25% of children are left with permanent brain damage. Treatment is supportive; dexamethasone has no convincing beneficial effect.

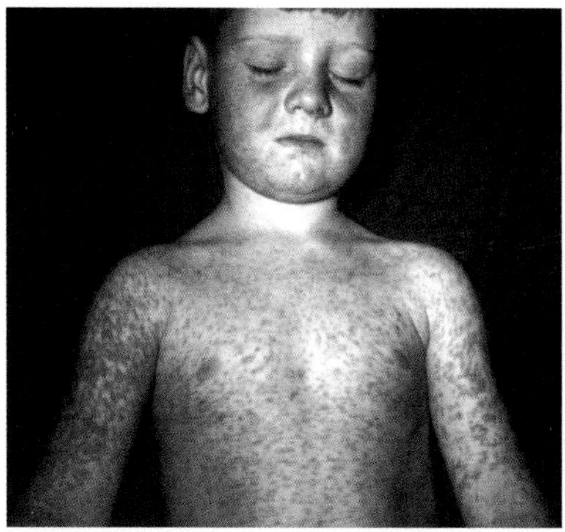

Fig. 7.5.6.10 Darkening measles rash after several days ('measles staining'). (Courtesy of the late Dr B.E. Juel-Jensen.)

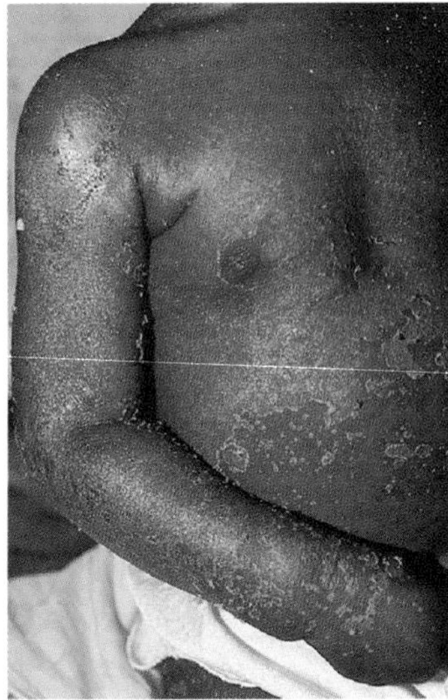

Fig. 7.5.6.11 Desquamating measles rash in an African child.

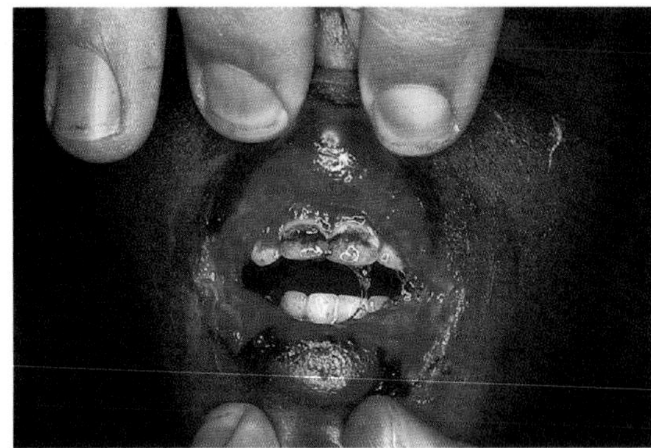

Fig. 7.5.6.12 Deep ulcers caused by herpes simplex virus.
(Copyright D A Warrell.)

Late complications

Malnutrition

This is the most frequent complication, for children of the developing world often lose a lot of weight during measles and may take many weeks to regain it. Those originally underweight, who have had severe measles, are at greatest risk, for anorexia in these children is prolonged, much protein is lost from the gut, and secondary infections, which lead to marasmus or marasmic kwashiorkor, are frequent. Measles has been shown to persist in the epithelia and lymphocytes of the severely malnourished for 30 or more days after the rash.

Persistent infection

Pneumonitis

Giant cell pneumonia is found in patients with defects in cell-mediated immunity. Children with leukaemia or kwashiorkor are particularly vulnerable, as are those with symptomatic HIV infection. The lung disease may develop weeks after measles, and in most cases the rash of measles has been absent and thus the diagnosis may not be suspected. The diagnosis is made by virological and/or histological examination of lung tissue. Most of these children die.

Subacute sclerosing panencephalitis (SSPE)

Persistent measles virus infection in the brain is responsible for this rare, progressive disease of the brain, which is found in 0.1 to 1.4 per million children after measles. The child with SSPE has usually experienced normal measles, albeit at a young age, 5 to 10 years earlier. The first indication is a disturbance in intellect and personality. Behavioural disorders and deterioration in school work are frequently mentioned. There then follows, over a period of weeks and months, myoclonus-like seizures, signs of extrapyramidal and pyramidal disease, and finally a state of decerebrate rigidity followed by death. The electroencephalogram shows a characteristic regular series of high-amplitude, spike-like waves. Very high titres of measles complement-fixing and haemagglutinin-inhibiting antibody are present both in serum and cerebrospinal fluid. Treatments for SSPE have included the use of transfer factor, plasmapheresis, and antiviral drugs, but to no avail.

Table 7.5.6.2 Complications and mortality in inpatients with measles, northern Nigeria, July–December 1978

	No.	Died	Percentage dead
Pneumonia	169	32	18.9
Gastroenteritis	65	9	13.8
Marasmic kwashiorkor	25	6	24.0
Laryngotracheobronchitis	21	4	19.0
Encephalitis	10	4	40.0

Reproduced with permission from Parry EHOP (ed) (1984). *Principles of medicine in Africa*, 2nd edition. Oxford University Press, Oxford.

Multiple sclerosis, autism, Crohn's disease

There is no convincing evidence that measles virus or immune responses to it have a causative role in these diseases. The alleged association between the measles, mumps, and rubella (MMR) vaccine, autism, and Crohn's disease was based on weak science and has now been convincingly refuted by larger and stronger epidemiological studies. Subsequent molecular studies have failed to

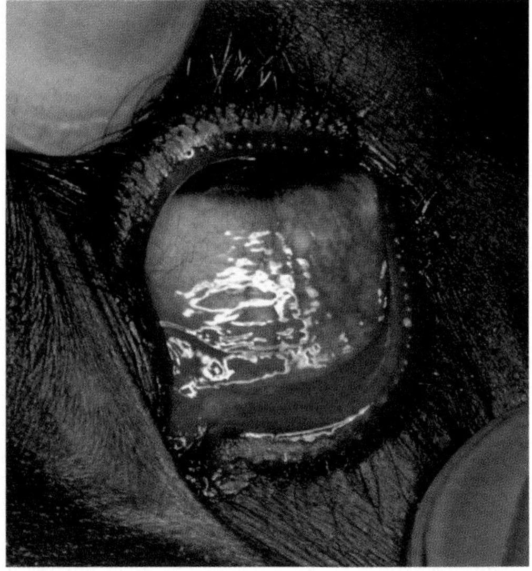

Fig. 7.5.6.13 Corneal ulceration leading to impaired vision or blindness after measles, especially in malnourished and vitamin A-deficient children.
(Copyright D A Warrell.)

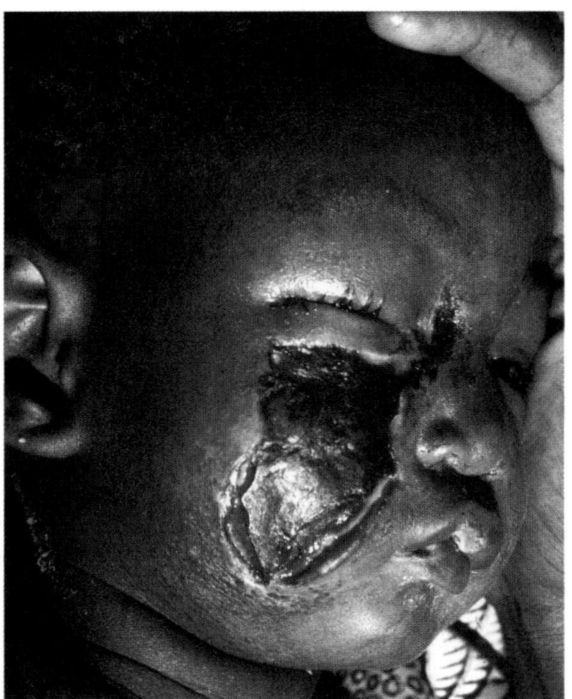

Fig. 7.5.6.14 Cancrum oris or noma following measles.

confirm the original finding of measles virus and genomic RNA in diseased bowel. The false alarm raised by this report caused a substantial reduction in the number of children vaccinated against measles in the United Kingdom.

Diagnosis

This is primarily clinical, although signs may be less clear-cut in vaccinated subjects. Thus, in areas of high vaccine coverage the detection of measles-specific IgM antibody by enzyme-linked immunoassay or, better still, the detection of measles antigen in saliva or urine may clinch the diagnosis if the rash is mild or atypical. Subclinical measles is common in vaccinated children after exposure to measles: the diagnosis is made by detecting a fourfold or greater rise in measles antibody within 2 to 6 weeks of exposure. It is not clear if such cases are infectious.

Treatment of measles and its complications

No effective antimeasles drug exists, yet some children do benefit from treatment in hospital. The following criteria indicate severe measles and a need for hospital admission: a widespread, confluent rash darkening to deep red or purple; signs of laryngeal obstruction; subcutaneous emphysema; marked dehydration; blood in the stool or more than five stools a day; convulsion or loss of consciousness; severe secondary pneumonia; corneal ulceration; severe ulceration of the mouth and skin. These signs should be taken particularly seriously when the child is underweight or frankly malnourished.

Hydrate the child orally or intravenously. Treat lobar pneumonia with benzylpenicillin, and bronchopneumonia with amoxicillin or, if severe, with combined antibiotics such as gentamicin and cloxacillin. Antibiotic eye ointments relieve discomfort and possibly prevent secondary infections of measles conjunctivitis. Antibiotics (topical and systemic) and vitamin A should be given routinely for the treatment of eye ulcers. If herpes simplex virus is the cause, use aciclovir topically or, when severe, systemically. Candida infections of the mouth or gut often respond dramatically to nystatin. Feeding, by tube if necessary, needs careful planning and presentation, for the anorexic infected child will be in severe negative energy balance due to a greatly increased catabolic rate. Case fatality rates are 30 to 50% lower in those children in hospital treated with vitamin A. This should be given orally at the time of diagnosis in a dose of 100 000 IU for children below 12 months of age and in a dose of 200 000 IU for older children. If eye signs of vitamin A deficiency are present, the initial dose should be repeated the next day and again 1 to 4 weeks later.

The prophylactic use of antibiotics such as amoxicillin or co-trimoxazole to prevent secondary infections after measles is a widespread practice based on slender evidence. The only community randomized placebo controlled trial was small: those children who received co-trimoxazole had less pneumonia and conjunctivitis and had a significantly higher weight gain (see Table 7.5.6.3).

Prevention

Passive immunization with human immunoglobulin is highly effective if given within 2 or 3 days of exposure, in a dose for children of 0.2 ml/kg. Immunoglobulin should be given to those in whom vaccination is contraindicated such as immunocompromised children with kwashiorkor, cancer, or AIDS or, if severe, combined antibiotics such as gentamycin and amoxicillin. If *S. aureus* is suspected, use gentamycin and cloxacillin.

The currently used vaccines are live strains, attenuated by culture in chick fibroblasts. The Edmonston–Zagreb strain, which has been cultured in human diploid cells, is also widely used. It is more effective than other vaccines in the presence of antibody, and should be used in a standard dose if vaccinating infants below 9 months of age, or if a booster dose is required. The complications of vaccination are few and generally mild. Fever of moderate severity is infrequent, and a mild rash with some signs of upper respiratory tract infection occurs rarely. Underweight children respond normally to the vaccine, as do ill children attending the outpatient department and those on the ward. As clinics and hospitals are major sites of transmission of the virus in the developing world, all susceptible children in these places should be vaccinated unless immunocompromised.

The measles vaccination policy for low income countries has seen major changes in the last 25 years. The optimal age for vaccination

Table 7.5.6.3 Prophylactic antibiotic to prevent complications after measles in Guinea-Bissau

Outcome	Co-trimoxazole (n = 46)	Placebo (n = 38)	Adjusted odds ratio (95% CI)
Pneumonia	1 (2%)	6 (16%)	0.14 (0.01–1.50)
Hospitalization	0	3	–
Diarrhoea	3 (7%)	5 (13%)	0.17 (0.01–1.55)
Severe fever	6 (13%)	11 (29%)	0.36 (0.09–1.43)
Stomatitis	4 (9%)	7 (18%)	0.43 (0.08–2.26)
Conjunctivitis	12 (26%)	17 (45%)	0.31 (0.10–1.03)
Weight gain (g/day)	32	15	–

(Adapted and reproduced with permission from Garly M-L, *et al.* (2006). Prophylactic antibiotics to prevent pneumonia and other complications after measles: community based randomised double blind placebo controlled trial in Guinea-Bissau. *BMJ*, **333**, 1245–50.)

in the developed world is between 14 and 16 months, when maternal antibody has disappeared. However, this recommendation could not be applied to children in developing countries, because there measles infects at a much earlier age. In 1982, the World Health Organization recommended vaccination at 9 months of age but, by then, 5 to 15% of children may have had measles. This policy was not based on good evidence; it is not known if vaccination at 9 months is better in saving children than vaccination at 7, 8, or 10 months of age, or a two dose regime in infancy.

Through the 1990s it became clear that several doses of measles vaccines were needed to improve measles control. The developed countries have used two-dose strategies with a second dose being given at school entry or to young teenagers. Latin America has obtained major successes with a combination of improved vaccination coverage and regular immunization campaigns providing a second opportunity for measles vaccination. The strategy has the following elements: (1) catch-up—a one-time mass campaign covering everybody between 9 months and 14 years of age regardless of previous measles or immunization; (2) keep-up—achieving a high coverage for each birth cohort; (3) follow-up—subsequent mass campaigns covering all children every 3 to 5 years; and (4) mop-up—campaigns that target children who are difficult to reach or during outbreaks. As a result of this strategy, Latin America has been declared free of internal measles transmission since 2002. Since there is no immediate risk of measles infection, the age of routine vaccination has been raised to 12 months as this is believed to be associated with better antibody responses.

The Latin American model has been transferred to other regions. Rebranded as SIA (supplementary immunization activities), it has assured a spectacular success in reducing measles mortality in Africa. The goal of reducing global measles deaths by 50% by 2005 compared to 1999 has been met. However, these campaigns which are donor driven are expensive and should not be seen as a substitute for an inadequate immunization service.

Elimination or eradication?

Global measles eradication has yet to be made official policy. However, the Americas have attained elimination (i.e. no internal transmission of the virus), and three other regions are pursuing such a policy. Measles satisfies the criteria for eradication for there is no animal reservoir, it is only transmitted between humans, it is easy to diagnose, and vaccines are available. Measles elimination can be accomplished for prolonged periods in defined geographical regions provided there is sufficient funding and political will. This was obtained for the first time in the Gambia in the mid 1960s as part of the smallpox eradication and measles vaccination campaigns.

However, eradicating measles will be a daunting task. First, it is the most infectious of diseases and will require vaccine coverage of greater than 95%. When there is no risk of infection, it will be increasingly difficult for parents to appreciate the necessity for vaccination especially as risk, although small, is perceived. Secondly, herd immunity will become a problem as with less exposure to the virus vaccine induced immunity will wane more rapidly. Thirdly, Africa will be a stern test for due to political instability, wars, and natural disasters it will be difficult to maintain sufficiently high coverage. Fourthly, with the growing HIV epidemic, there is a risk that the vaccine may be less effective and that infected individuals will be difficult to diagnose and excrete virus for long periods. Fifthly, with the growing fear of bioterrorism, it is unlikely that all immunization can be stopped in the posteradication era. Lastly, but most difficult, will be to assure long-term funding as donors have a tradition of changing priorities.

The international health community is split over whether eradication can be attained with the Latin American strategy using existing vaccines or whether new vaccines and delivery systems such as aerosolization are needed. New vaccines, which can be given in early infancy, or two-dose strategies using the standard vaccine at 4 and 9 months of age, might be necessary to contain measles in the developing world. Coverage of at least 95% of all susceptible children, including those between 3 and 9 months of age, with a vaccine that is at least 95% effective is assumed to be necessary if the virus is to be eradicated. Current vaccines do not meet these standards except when two doses have been given in national campaigns. New vaccines such as the modified vaccinia Ankara (MVA) recombinant virus, a nonreplicating mutant of horsepox made to express the F and H proteins, or a DNA vaccine expressing these proteins may possibly fulfill such exacting requirements, for they have been shown to protect macaques from measles. High titre vaccines were used to vaccinate young infants, but were discontinued when an unexplained increase in mortality in girls was found 1 to 3 years after vaccination. Thus, new vaccines need long-term monitoring in order to fully understand the potential nonspecific immunological interactions that may occur between the many vaccines in use and with infections that are common in infants.

Further reading

Aaby P, *et al.* (1983). Measles mortality, state of nutrition, and family structure. A community study from Guinea-Bissau. *J Infect Dis*, **147**, 693–701. [Groundbreaking paper showing measles mortality depends on family structure and intensity of exposure but not nutrition.]

Aaby P, *et al.* (1986). Vaccinated children get milder measles infection: a community study from Guinea Bissau. *J Infect Dis*, **154**, 858–63.

Aaby P, *et al.* (1995). Non-specific beneficial effects of measles immunization: analysis of mortality studies from developing countries. *BMJ*, **311**, 481–5.

Aaby P, *et al.* (2003). Differences in female-male mortality after high-titre measles vaccine and association with subsequent vaccination with diphtheria—tetanus-pertussis and inactivated poliovirus: re-analysis of West African studies. *Lancet*, **361**, 2183–88. [An interesting theory invoking nonspecific effects of vaccines.]

Aaby P, *et al.* (2003). The survival benefit of measles immunisation may not be explained entirely by the prevention of measles disease. *Int J Epidemiol*, **32**, 106–115.

de Quadros CA, *et al.* (1996). Measles elimination in the Americas. Evolving strategies. *JAMA*, **275**, 224–229.

Duke T, *et al.* (2003). Measles: not just another viral exanthema. *Lancet*, **361**, 763–73. [An excellent review.]

Fenner F (1948). The pathogenesis of the acute exanthems. An interpretation based on experimental investigations with mouse-pox (infectious ectromelia of mice). *Lancet*, **2**, 915–20.

Garly ML, *et al.* (2006). Prophylactic antibiotics to prevent pneumonia and other complications after measles: community based randomized double blind placebo controlled trial in Guinea Bissau. *BMJ*, **333**, 1245–1250. [The only randomized controlled trial of prophylactic antibiotics for measles in Africa.]

Jaye A, *et al.* (1998). Ex vivo analysis of cytotoxic T lymphocytes to measles antigens during infection and after vaccination in Gambian children. *J Clin Invest*, **102**, 1969–77. [The largest and most complete study of cytotoxic T-cell responses in natural measles.]

Morley D (1969). Severe measles in the tropics. *Br Med J*, **1**, 363–5. [Classic clinical studies.]

Moss WJ, Ota MO, Griffen DE (2004). Measles: immune suppression and immune responses. *Int J Biochem Cell Biol*, **36**, 1380–84. [A succinct review of an important aspect of measles.]

Moss WJ, *et al.* (2006). Global measles elimination. *Nat Rev Microbiol*, **4**, 900–908.

Samb B, *et al.* (1997). Decline in measles case fatality ratio after introduction of measles immunization in rural Senegal. *Am J Epidemiol*, **145**, 51–57.

Whittle HC, *et al.* (1979). Severe ulcerative herpes of mouth and eye following measles. *Trans R Soc Trop Med Hyg*, **73**, 66–9.

Whittle HC, *et al.* (1999). Effect of sub-clinical infection on maintaining immunity against measles in vaccinated children in West Africa. *Lancet*, **353**, 98–101.

Wolfson LJ, *et al.* (2007). Has the 2005 measles mortality reduction goal been achieved? A natural history modelling study. *Lancet*, **369**, 191–200.

7.5.7 Nipah and Hendra virus encephalitides

C.T. Tan

Essentials

Nipah and Hendra are two related viruses of the Paramyxoviridae family that have their reservoir in large *Pteropus* fruit bats. Human disease manifests most often as acute encephalitis, which may be late-onset or relapsing, or pneumonia, with high mortality. Transmission from bats to human includes direct spread from consumption of food contaminated by infected bats' secretions, and contact with infected animals: human-to-human spread can also occur.

Introduction

Nipah and Hendra viruses are two new zoonotic viruses that have emerged in recent years. Both are paramyxoviridae family sharing many similar characteristics. Because of their homology, a new genus called Henipavirus (Hendra + Nipah) was created for these two viruses.

Hendra virus infection

Hendra virus was first isolated in an outbreak of acute respiratory illness involving horses in Australia in 1994. A horse trainer and stable hand were also infected, manifesting with respiratory illness from which the horse trainer died. A second human death occurred in 1995, where a farmer who had contact with ill horses about a year earlier died from encephalitis. Another death involving a veterinary surgeon occurred in the Hendra virus outbreak in July 2008, also in Australia. Thus, till 2008, there have been 11 spillover events of Hendra virus to horses, 4 of these involving subsequent horse-to-human transmission.

Thus, Hendra virus is able to cause respiratory and encephalitic illness in humans who have close contact with infected horses. There could be considerable delay before the manifestations of the encephalitic illness. The reservoir of Hendra virus is the *Pteropus* genus of fruit bats (see Chapter 7.5.10, Fig. 7.5.10.18) which also harbour Nipah, Menangle, Tioman, and Australian bat lyssaviruses.

Nipah virus infection

In late 1998 to early 1999, there was an outbreak of viral encephalitis in several pig-farming villages in peninsular Malaysia which subsequently involved abattoir workers in Singapore. More than 300 patients were affected. Isolation of virus from cerebrospinal fluid specimens of several patients indicated that this was due to previous unknown Napah virus.

Epidemiology

Human Nipah virus infection was transmitted by close contact with infected pigs. Human-to-human transmission was thought to be rare, although the virus could be readily isolated from patients' respiratory secretions and urine.

Clinical manifestations

During the outbreak, more than half of the patients had affected family members, suggesting a high infection rate. Some of the household members had seroconversion without clinical disease, indicating subclinical infection at a ratio of asymptomatic vs symptomatic infection of 1 to 3. The infection involved all age groups.

The incubation period was less than 2 weeks in most patients. The clinical manifestations were those of an acute encephalitis with fever, headache, vomiting, and reduced level of consciousness. Distinctive clinical features were areflexia, hypotonia, and prominent autonomic changes such as tachycardia and hypertension. Segmental myoclonus found in about one-third of patients was characterized by focal, rhythmic jerking of muscles, commonly involving the diaphragm and anterior muscles of the neck. Respiratory tract involvement with cough was seen at presentation in 14% of patients. There were some patients who had nonencephalitic infection with seroconversion and systemic symptoms but no evidence of encephalitis.

The overall mortality of acute Nipah encephalitis was 40%. Severe brainstem involvement was associated with poor prognosis.

Laboratory investigations

Cerebrospinal fluid examination was abnormal in 75% of patients with elevated protein levels or elevated white cell counts. Glucose levels were within normal limits. These features are nonspecific. IgM and IgG antibody detection in serum and cerebrospinal fluid were critical to the diagnosis of Nipah virus infection. The antibody test utilized an enzyme-linked immunosorbent assay (ELISA) test. The rate of positive IgM was 100% by day 12 of illness. For IgG, it was 100% by 4 weeks of illness.

Brain MRI in acute encephalitis showed multiple, disseminated, small discrete hyperintense lesions best seen in the FLAIR sequence particularly in the subcortical and deep white matter (Fig. 7.5.7.1). The lesions were likely to correspond to the microinfarctions noted in postmortem tissues. Similar changes were also seen in asymptomatic patients with Nipah virus infection.

Treatment

Treatment is mainly supportive with mechanical ventilatory support for seriously ill patients. Ribavirin, a broad-spectrum antiviral agent, appeared to reduce the mortality rate.

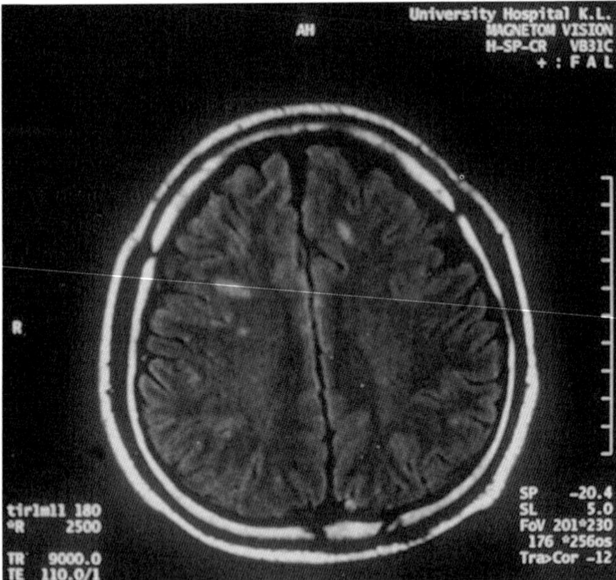

Fig. 7.5.7.1 Nipah virus encepahalitis: MRI FLAIR showing disseminated, small discrete hyperintense lesions.

Pathology and pathogenesis

Vasculitis of the medium-sized to small blood vessels in brain, causing thrombosis, and vascular occlusion with areas of necrosis and ischaemia, were the major findings (Fig. 7.5.7.2). There were also viral inclusions indicating direct viral involvement of the neurons. Vasculitis was also seen in lung and kidney.

Relapse and late-onset Nipah encephalitis

Close to 10% of patients suffered a second or even a third neurological episode months or years following recovery from acute encephalitis. About 5% who were either asymptomatic or only had mild nonencephalitic illness initially, also developed similar neurologic episodes (late-onset Nipah encephalitis) for the first time after a delayed period. Clinical, radiologic and pathologic findings indicate that relapse and late-onset Nipah encephalitis was the same disease process,which was distinct from acute Nipah virus encephalitis. The common clinical features were fever, headache, seizures, and focal neurological signs. There was an18% mortality. MRI showed patchy areas of confluent cortical lesions. Necropsy showed focal confluent encephalitis due to a recurrent infection.

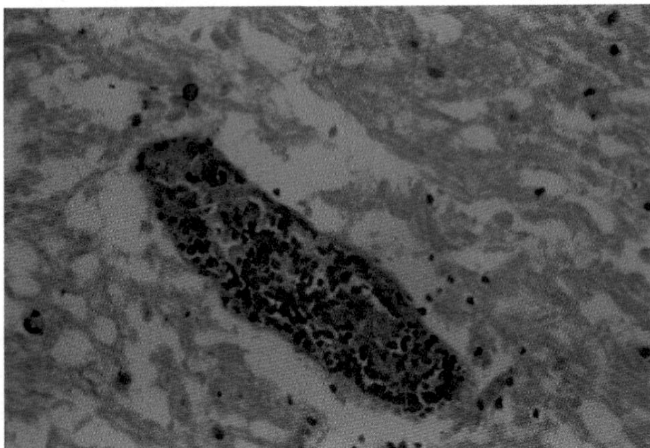

Fig. 7.5.7.2 Nipah virus encepahalitis: vasculitis of a medium-sized cerebral blood vessel, showing thrombosis and vascular occlusion with areas of necrosis and ischaemia.

The bat as reservoir host

As for Hendra virus, the reservoir of Nipah virus is fruit bats of the *Pteropus* species. Half-eaten fruits dropped by bats near pig farms may have infected an animal that subsequently ingested them. Pigs were the amplifying hosts for the virus. There was pig-to-pig transmission which subsequently spread to human.

Nipah encephalitis in Bangladesh and India

Nine outbreaks of Nipah encephalitis has been reported in Bangladesh from 2001 to 2008 and in Siliguri district, north-eastern India, in 2001.

As in Malaysia, Nipah virus caused a fatal encephalitic illness in humans in Bangladesh and India. However, the Bangladeshi and Indian outbreaks showed prominent human-to-human spread of infection, with florid pulmonary involvement in some patients. Brain MRI in some patients showed confluent high signal lesions involving both grey and white matter, which is unlike the acute Nipah encephalitis in the Malaysian outbreak, suggesting some differences in the pathology from the Malaysian patients. The RNA of Nipah virus in Bangladesh and India was close to but not identical with that causing the outbreak in Malaysia. *Pteropus* bats were also the reservoir of Nipah virus in Bangladesh. There may be a variety of mode of transmission from bats to humans in the Bangladesh and Indian outbreaks. Consumption of raw date-palm juice contaminated by secretions from bats is a suggested mode of transmission.

Pteropus bats are widespread in large parts of Asia, Africa, and Australia. Nipah virus has been isolated in urine of *Pteropus* bats in Cambodia, and Nipah viral antigen has been found in saliva of *Pteropus* bats in Thailand. Serological evidence of *Henipavirus* infection has been reported in fruit bats from Papua New Guinea to Ghana, Africa from East to West, and Yunnan, China to Australia from North to South, indicating potential human Nipah virus infection elsewhere.

Menangle and Tioman viruses

These are two other newly identified paramyxoviruses harboured by *Pteropis* fruit bats. Menangle causes disease in pigs but neither has been implicated in human infections.

Further reading

Chadha MS, *et al.* (2006). Nipah virus-associated encephalitis outbreak, Siliguri, India. *Emerg Infect Dis*, **12**, 235–40.

Chong HT, Jahangir Hossain M, Tan CT (2008). Differences in epidemiologic and clinical features of Nipah virus encephalitis between the Malaysian and Bangladesh outbreaks. *Neurol Asia*, **13**, 23–6.

Chua KB, *et al.* (1999). Fatal encephalitis due to Nipah virus among pig-farmers in Malaysia. *Lancet*, **354**, 1257–9.

Goh KJ, *et al.* (2000). Clinical features of Nipah virus encephalitis among pig farmers in Malaysia. *N Engl J Med*, **342**, 1229–35.

Hsu VP, *et al.* (2004). Nipah virus encephalitis reemergence, Bangladesh. *Emerg Infect Dis*, **10**, 2082–7.

Tan CT, *et al.* (2002). Relapse and late-onset Nipah encephalitis. *Ann Neurol*, **51**, 703–8.

7.5.8 Enterovirus infections

Philip Minor and Ulrich Desselberger

Essentials

Enteroviruses are single-stranded RNA viruses comprising poliomyelitis viruses (3 types), Coxsackie A viruses (23 types), Coxsackie B viruses (6 types), and echoviruses (28 types). They have recently been reclassified into 4 human enterovirus species (A–D) on the basis of sequence comparisons. Transmission is by the faeco-oral route, with seasonal peaks of infection in areas of temperate climate, but infections occurring all year round in tropical regions.

Pathogenesis—following transmission, enteroviruses undergo a first round of replication in cells of the mucosal surfaces of the gastrointestinal tract and in gut-associated lymphoid cells, followed by viraemia, which leads to infection of distant organs (brain, spinal cord, meninges, myocardium, muscle, skin, etc.), where lesions may be produced. Shedding of virus occurs from throat and faeces for many weeks.

Clinical manifestations and diagnosis

Most enterovirus infections are silent or only produce minor illness, but severe major illness can develop in a few of the infected.

Poliomyelitis—infection with poliovirus is normally inapparent, but a few of the infected (1% or less) develop neurological symptoms comprising (1) aseptic meningitis, or (2) paralytic poliomyelitis—5 to 10 days after a mild upper respiratory tract infection presentation is with flaccid paralysis resulting from motor neuron destruction; this may affect the limbs (spinal form) or muscles supplied by the medulla oblongata or bulb (bulbar form), with potentially life-threatening respiratory muscle involvement. Treatment is supportive; mortality is 2 to 5% in children and 15 to 30% in adults, and there is residual paralysis in 90% of survivors.

Other clinical syndromes include: (1) aseptic meningitis, the most frequent clinical presentation of enterovirus infection, caused by Coxsackie viruses and echoviruses; (2) encephalitis, a rare event, possibly following aseptic meningitis; (3) pleurodynia (Bornholm disease), presenting abruptly with fever and chest pain and usually caused by Coxsackie B viruses; (4) myopericarditis; (5) herpangina; (6) exanthema, rubella-like or hand-foot-and-mouth disease; and (7) conjunctivitis.

Diagnosis is by virus isolation in cell culture or by viral genome detection using RT-PCR.

Prevention

Paralytic poliomyelitis has been eradicated in most countries of the world following universal mass vaccination with formaldehyde-inactivated poliovirus (Salk vaccine) and/or live-attenuated viral vaccine (Sabin vaccine). However, it persists in a few countries (e.g. India, Pakistan, Afghanistan, Nigeria). As long as there are pockets of infection, the world remains at risk of re-emergence of the disease.

Introduction

Enteroviruses are a major group of viruses causing systemic infection in humans. They form two genera of the *Picornaviridae* family (the *Enterovirus* and *Parechovirus* genera) and occur in at least 66 serotypes in humans. They infect via the gastrointestinal tract and are mostly clinically inapparent. However, viraemia can be followed by infection of organs distant from the site of entry with often devastating effects in the form of meningitis, encephalitis, paralysis, myopericarditis, and also rashes and conjunctivitis.

The viruses

Viruses of the *Picornaviridae* are nonenveloped icosahedral particles of 27 to 30 nm in diameter and contain single-stranded RNA of positive polarity and 7.2- to 8.4-kb size as their genome. The nucleic acid is polyadenylated at the 3′ end and carries a small protein, VPg, covalently linked at its 5′ end. The enteroviruses and parechoviruses form two of the nine current genera of the Picornaviridae family, the others being the genera of *Rhinovirus*, *Cardiovirus*, *Aphthovirus*, *Hepatovirus*, *Erbovirus*, *Kobuvirus*, and *Teschovirus*. Three serotypes of poliomyelitis virus (poliovirus), 23 types of Coxsackie A virus, 6 types of Coxsackie B virus, and 28 types of enteric cytopathic human orphan (echo) viruses are recognized within the *Enterovirus* genus. The parechoviruses comprise echoviruses 22 and 23 and were established as a separate genus on the basis of highly divergent sequence of their genomes. Other classic features of the enteroviruses, such as their stability at acid pH (in contrast to rhinoviruses or aphthoviruses), their buoyant density in caesium chloride gradients, and the nature of their broad clinical effects and persistence in the environment are also shared by the parechoviruses.

The three-dimensional structure of the poliovirus particle has been elucidated by crystallographic analysis (Fig. 7.5.8.1). The viral capsid consists of 60 protein subunits, each containing the four unglycosylated viral proteins VP1 to VP4. The capsid proteins are arranged in such a way that VP1 molecules form the apices at the fivefold symmetry axis of the icosahedron, whereas two other proteins VP2 and VP3 are arranged in the centre of the triangular face near the threefold axis of symmetry; VP4 is an internal protein. All proteins interact with each other. The N-terminus of VP4 is myristoylated.

Viruses initiate replication by attaching to their cellular receptors, and some of these have been characterized. The poliovirus receptor (PVR) is a member of the immunoglobulin superfamily. Transgenic mice expressing the human PVR become susceptible to poliovirus infection with a pathology similar to that of infected primates. Tests using these animals have been incorporated into regulatory requirements as supplements and eventual replacements for primates for vaccine testing (see below). Other enterovirus receptors are the decay accelerating factors (DAF; receptor for various echovirus types, Coxsackie B virus types, and coxsackievirus A21), implicated in the complement pathway, and the integrin VLA-2 (receptor for echovirus types 1 and 8). Other cell surface molecules may be involved as coreceptors in the virus–cell receptor interactions of many enteroviruses, as the expression of a single identified receptor is not always sufficient to make a previously resistant cell line susceptible to productive infection. It is also of interest that some strains of poliovirus, mainly of serotype 2, are able to paralyse mice if injected. The receptor involved in mice has not been identified.

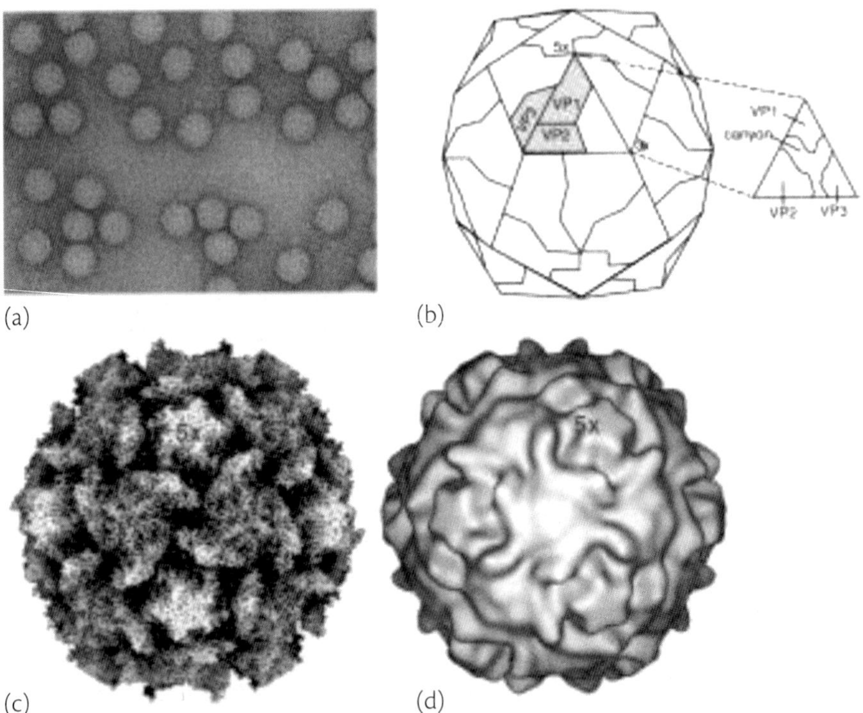

Fig. 7.5.8.1 Structural features of picornaviruses. (a) Electron micrograph of negatively stained poliovirus. Magnification ×270 000. (b) Diagram of the picornavirus capsid, showing the packing arrangements of VP1, VP2, and VP3, and the interspersed canyon. VP4 is located on the interior of the capsid. The biological protomer (grey) is different from the icosahedral subunit (triangle shown at right). (c) Model of poliovirus type 1, Mahoney, based on X-ray crystallographic structure determined at 2.9 Å. The fivefold axis of symmetry is marked (5×). Surrounding the fivefold axis are canyons, the receptor-binding site. (d) Model of poliovirus type 1, Mahoney, produced by image reconstruction from cryoelectron microscopy data obtained at 20 Å resolution.

From Racaniello VR (2007). Picornaviridae: the viruses and their replication. In: Knipe DM, *et al.* (eds) *Fields virology*, 5th edition, pp. 795–838. Wolters Kluwer Health/Lippincott Williams & Wilkins, Philadelphia. With permission of author and publisher.

The positive-sense RNA genome acts as a messenger molecule. All enterovirus RNAs have a long 5′ end untranslated region (UTR) of approximately 750 nucleotides in length, which is highly structured and contains an internal ribosomal entry site (IRES). The IRES is important for binding of the RNA to ribosomes and subsequent translation of the RNA into protein. Downstream of the 5′ UTR is a large single open reading frame containing three parts: P1, coding for structural proteins VP1 to VP4; P2, coding for proteins 2A, 2B, and 2C; and P3, coding for proteins 3A to 3D. Proteins 2A and 3C are viral proteases and protein 3D is the RNA-dependent RNA polymerase (RdRp). P2 and P3 proteins (with the exception of VPg = 3B) are only found in infected cells. The P1 to P3 proteins are synthesized as one large precursor from which the individual proteins are produced by complex autocleavage and cleavage cascades. RNA replicates via double-stranded replicative intermediates. The ratio of positive-stranded to negative-stranded RNA molecules in infected cells is approximately 100:1. During replication, RNA recombination does not infrequently occur. Replication of and translation from the same RNA cannot occur at the same time. Poliovirus-infected cells undergo a shut off of cellular mRNA synthesis and cellular protein translation. Naked enterovirus RNA is infectious on transfection (poliovirus was the first RNA virus rescued this way) and can be transcribed from full-length cDNA clones permitting biochemical manipulation and structure–function studies at the molecular level (reverse genetics).

The extensive antigenic variation of enterovirus capsid proteins allows typing into polioviruses, coxsackieviruses, and echoviruses using type-specific neutralizing antisera, but there is some cross-reactivity. The main antigenic sites are located on all three major virion proteins (VP1–VP3), and some involve sequences from more than one protein. The molecular mechanisms for the high genomic diversity of picornaviruses are thought to be based on misincorporations of nucleotides during chain elongation (due to the high error rate of the viral RdRp) and to frequent RNA recombination events, which also occur in natural infections.

Comparison of complete RNA genome sequences of many enteroviruses shows a very close relationship between some enterovirus and rhinovirus sequences. Within the echoviruses, however, there is great diversity, e.g. echovirus 22 shows a very low degree of homology with any other enteroviruses.

A subdivision of human enteroviruses into four species according to genomic relatedness has been proposed:

1 Human enterovirus A: coxsackieviruses A2 to A8, A10, A12, A14, and A16, human enterovirus 71, and human enterovirus 76

2 Human enterovirus B: coxsackieviruses B1 to B6, A9, all echoviruses except types 22 and 23, and human enteroviruses 69, 73 to 75, 77, and 78

3 Human enterovirus C: poliovirus types 1 to 3, coxsackieviruses A1, A11, A13, A17, A19 to A22, and A24

4 Human enterovirus Group D: human enterovirus enteroviruses 68 and 70

Hepatitis A virus has previously been designated enterovirus 72, but is now in its own genus *Hepatovirus*. Echoviruses types 22 and 23 form the *Parechovirus* genus.

Pathogenesis

The most widely accepted model of the pathogenesis of enterovirus infection is based on that developed by Bodian for poliovirus, in which the virus infects the host via the gastrointestinal tract and undergoes primary replication in lymphoid cells lining the alimentary tract (oropharyngeal, intestinal). A viraemic phase follows, allowing infection of distant target organs: spinal cord and brain, meninges, myocardium, skeletal muscles, skin, and mucous membranes. Other tissues, e.g. lymph nodes and brown fat tissue, can also become infected. Intensive multiplication in the central nervous system (CNS) leads to the destruction of motor neurons and results in paralysis.

A slightly different and more subtle model of poliovirus pathogenesis was proposed by Sabin, in which the virus infects the mucosal surface, thus accounting for the fact that virus can be shed in faeces long after it has become undetectable in lymphoid tissues and when neutralizing antibody is detectable in the blood. The primary replication creates a viraemia which seeds distant, still unknown, sites and virus replication there results in a second viraemia, which may be detected about 1 week postinfection and can lead to systemic infection including CNS involvement.

Shedding of virus occurs from the throat and faeces for many weeks and even months after infection and thus ensures transmission (see below). Virus replication in sites distant from the port of entry normally terminates with the appearance of neutralizing antibody, first IgM at 1 to 2 weeks after infection and then IgG and secretory IgA. Children with B-cell immunodeficiencies may develop persistent infections.

Most enterovirus infections are silent or produce a 'minor illness' with the symptoms of a mild upper respiratory tract infection with or without fever. In a minority of infections (1% or less) one of the following systemic 'major diseases' may develop:

- Paralytic poliomyelitis, aseptic meningitis (polioviruses)
- Aseptic meningitis, herpangina, conjunctivitis, hand-foot-and-mouth disease (Coxsackie A viruses)
- Aseptic meningitis, myopericarditis, encephalitis, pleurodynia (Coxsackie B viruses; enterovirus 71)
- Aseptic meningitis, rashes, conjunctivitis (echoviruses)
- Polio-like illness, aseptic meningitis, hand-foot-and-mouth disease, epidemic conjunctivitis (enterovirus types 68–71)

Symptoms of clinical illness caused by enteroviruses are summarized in Table 7.5.8.1 and are discussed in more detail below.

Clinical symptoms

Central nervous system infections (Chapter 24.11.2)

Poliomyelitis

Evidence of poliomyelitis as an ancient human disease is revealed on a funerary stele from Middle Kingdom Egypt, about 1300 bc, but there is little documentation of its occurrence until nearly the end of the 19th century when it appeared in epidemics in children (hence the alternative name 'infantile paralysis'). The appearance of poliomyelitis coincided with the improvement in standards of public hygiene and is explained by the consequent exposure of infants to infection at a later age. Maternal antibody is capable of confining infection to the gut, where the virus can persist until the immune response develops to eliminate it. In contrast, when maternal antibody has declined in older infants, the virus can spread to sites outside the intestine, causing paralysis.

Even under modern conditions of hygiene, infection with all three poliovirus types is normally inapparent, but illness with neurological symptoms results in about 1% of infections or less. This can present as aseptic meningitis with neck stiffness, usually recovering after 10 days (abortive or nonparalytic poliomyelitis). Meningitis is also caused by several other enteroviruses (see below). The more serious presentation is paralytic poliomyelitis, appearing 5 to 10 days after a mild upper respiratory tract infection ('minor illness') and progressing to flaccid paralysis resulting from motor neuron destruction ('major illness'). This may be accompanied by spasms and lack of coordination of nonparalysed muscles. Various forms of the 'major illness' reflect infection of different parts of the CNS. Paralysis of limbs (Fig. 7.5.8.2) results from destruction of motor neurons in the lower part of the spinal cord ('spinal form'), while the more life threatening bulbar poliomyelitis ('bulbar form') involves infections of the medulla oblongata or bulb. Respiratory functions can be affected in both the spinal and bulbar forms of the disease; encephalitis is rare. In children under 5 years old, paralysis of one leg is most common; in children 5 to 15 years of age, weakness of

Table 7.5.8.1 Clinical symptoms and their possible enteroviral causes

Clinical symptom (phenotype)	Poliovirus			Coxsackievirus															Echovirus									Enterovirus	
	Type			Group A type										Group B type					Type									Type	
	1	2	3	2	4	5	6	7	9	10	16	21	24	1	2	3	4	5	1	2	4	6	9	11	16	19	30	70	71
Aseptic meningitis (rarely encephalitis)	✓	✓	✓	✓	✓			✓	✓	✓				✓	✓	✓	✓	✓			✓	✓	✓	✓	✓		✓	✓	✓
Paralysis	✓	✓	✓					✓	✓						✓	✓	✓	✓		✓	✓	✓	✓	✓			✓		✓
Severe systemic infection (neonates)														✓	✓	✓	✓	✓				✓	✓	✓	✓				✓
Myo(peri)carditis					✓						✓				✓	✓	✓	✓	✓			✓	✓			✓			
Epidemic pleurodynia									✓					✓	✓	✓	✓	✓	✓			✓	✓						
Exanthemata, enanthema					✓	✓	✓		✓	✓	✓				✓	✓	✓	✓	✓			✓	✓			✓			✓
Conjunctivitis													✓	✓				✓										✓	
Respiratory symptoms (herpangina)									✓		✓	✓	✓	✓		✓	✓	✓			✓		✓	✓					
Diarrhoea																								✓					

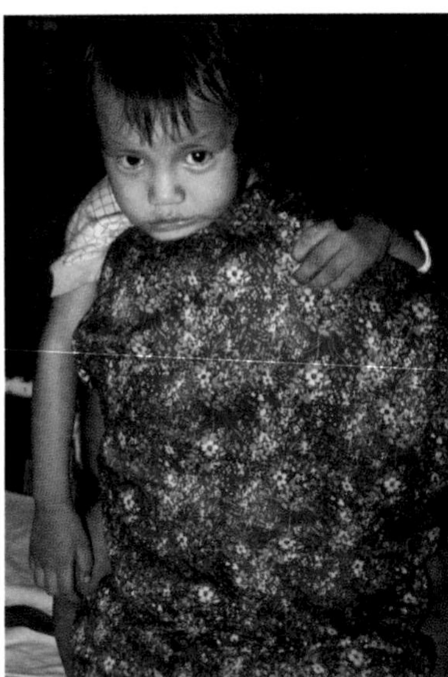

Fig. 7.5.8.2 Acute monoplegia in a Thai child in 1979 caused by poliomyelitis. Copyright D.A. Warrell.

one limb or paraplegia are frequent; quadriplegia is most common in adults and is often accompanied by urinary bladder and respiratory muscle dysfunction. Muscular function in limbs may return slowly, but there is residual paralysis in 90% of survivors. Of paralytic cases, 10 to 25% have bulbar symptoms with hypertension, shock, and dysphonia. Complications are nosocomial pneumonias (by staphylococci or gram-negative bacteria), urinary tract infections, and emotional problems. The mortality from paralytic polio is 2 to 5% among children and 15 to 30% among adults. Muscle weakness may develop many years after the initial polio disease (postpolio syndrome or postpolio neuromuscular atrophy). A persistent poliovirus infection as cause of this has been assumed, based on the presence of viral RNA in cerebrospinal fluid and neural tissue. However, such RNA has also been found in patients with other neurological and non-neurological diseases and is, therefore, less likely to be related to the postpolio syndrome. The alternative view is that the postpolio syndrome is anatomical in origin, such that the initial attack of polio destroys motor neurons and reduces the backup available as the patient ages.

Aseptic meningitis

Aseptic meningitis is the most frequent clinical presentation of enterovirus infection and can be caused by coxsackieviruses of both groups A and B, and echoviruses, mainly types 4, 6, 11, 14, 16, 25, 30, and 31 (see Table 7.5.8.1). The disease starts with fever, headache, neck stiffness, and photophobia. Sensory or motor deficits are unusual, but confusion is common. The symptoms may persist for 4 to 7 days. The cerebrospinal fluid usually shows pleocytosis consisting of 10 to 500 leucocytes/μl, mainly lymphocytes. Polymorphonuclear cells may predominate at the onset, but bacterial infection and possibly abscesses should be considered if they persist. The protein concentration in cerebrospinal fluid may be normal or slightly increased; the glucose level is normal. Complete recovery is the usual outcome of aseptic meningitis.

Encephalitis

Enterovirus encephalitis is rare but may follow aseptic meningitis. Enterovirus infection in patients with hypogammaglobulinaemia or agammaglobulinaemia may persist for years with chronic meningitis or encephalitis and a high mortality rate as sequelae.

Enterovirus 71 infection, which is normally associated with hand-foot-and-mouth disease, has been found to cause severe meningoencephalitis (with brain stem involvement), polio-like acute flaccid paralysis, and a high case fatality rate in children during several recent outbreaks in Bulgaria, Taiwan, and Malaysia. In some of the fatal cases there may have been coinfections with a species B adenovirus. Enterovirus 71 occurs in three genotypes and is rapidly evolving; it is most closely related to coxsackievirus A16.

Neonatal infections

Neonatal infection followed by severe generalized disease may be caused by Coxsackie B viruses and echoviruses, mainly of types 6, 7, and 11. These viruses seem to be transmitted late in pregnancy, perinatally, or postnatally by the mother or other virus-infected infants in neonatal wards or special care baby units. The infants develop either heart failure due to a severe myocarditis or a meningoencephalitis; hepatitis and adrenalitis may also occur. The mortality is high. Viruses may be recovered from brain, spinal cord, myocardium, and liver at autopsy.

Bornholm disease (epidemic pleurodynia)

This is usually caused by Coxsackie B viruses but can also be caused by echoviruses of types 1, 6, 9, 16, and 19 and by Coxsackie A viruses of types 4, 6, 9, and 10. The disease can strike families in small outbreaks. It typically starts abruptly with fever and chest pain due to the involvement of the intercostal muscles or abdominal pain resulting from involvement of muscles of the abdomen. There may be severe frontal headache. The symptoms last 3 to 14 days and are followed by complete recovery.

Myopericarditis

Enterovirus-induced myocarditis is mostly due to infection with Coxsackie B viruses in the young. The onset of disease is usually acute, very severe, and may be fatal in neonates; however, in adolescents and adults it is normally mild. The virus may persist after the initial infection and cause dilated cardiomyopathy. In fatal cases (usually neonates 2–11 days after onset of disease) there is cardiac dilatation, myocyte necrosis, and an inflammatory reaction. The diagnosis is often difficult, particularly in older patients, as pericarditis, coronary artery occlusion, or heart failure may have been diagnosed initially. Typical clinical findings are often tachycardia, arrhythmias, murmurs, rubs, and cardiomegaly.

Besides causing acute myocarditis, chronic enterovirus infection may lead to chronic myocarditis and dilated cardiomyopathy, possibly due to immunopathological mechanisms. In chronic disease, neither infectious virus nor viral antigens are normally detected in heart biopsies; however, viral RNA is regularly found in cardiac muscle suggesting that the viral genome persists. The true significance of the presence of the viral genome in such cases is still under discussion.

The disease can be produced with Coxsackie B viruses in mice. In this animal model there is also initial viraemia and replication in myocytes, but this is followed by disappearance of infectious virus and destruction of myocytes, possibly by autoimmune mechanisms.

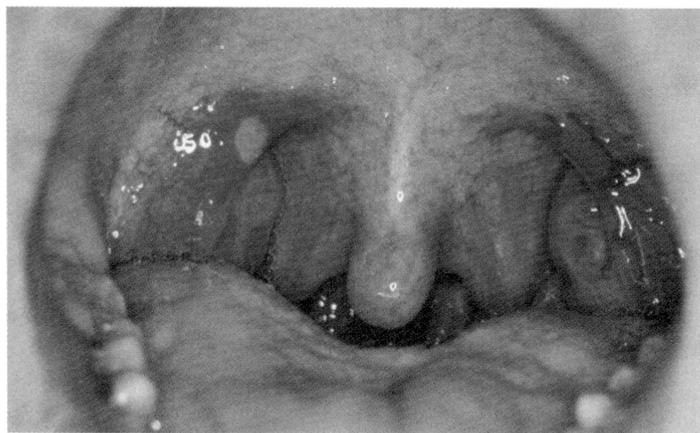

Fig. 7.5.8.3 Herpangina due to coxsackievirus A6 infection.
Courtesy of the late Dr B.E. Juel-Jensen.

Herpangina

This is caused by coxsackieviruses of types A1 to A6, A8, A10, and A22. Children and young adults between 2 and 20 years of age are mainly affected. The disease presents with acute onset of fever, sore throat, and pain on swallowing, as well as vomiting and abdominal symptoms. Small vesicular lesions or white papules surrounded by a red halo can be seen on the fauces, pharynx, palate, uvula, and tonsils (Fig. 7.5.8.3). The disease is mild and self-limiting.

Exanthemas

Rubella-like rashes can be produced by echoviruses of types 4, 9, and 16, but also coxsackieviruses A9, A16, and B5 (Fig. 7.5.8.4). They usually occur in the summer and may be accompanied by fever, malaise, cervical lymphadenopathy, and aseptic meningitis.

Hand-foot-and-mouth disease

A typical distribution of vesicular lesions in hands, feet, and mouth (but also buttocks and genitalia) is produced by infection with coxsackievirus type A16 and enterovirus 71, and less frequently with coxsackieviruses A4, A5, A9 and A10, B2, and B5 (Fig. 7.5.8.5a,b). Enterovirus 71 may produce more severe clinical symptoms (see above).

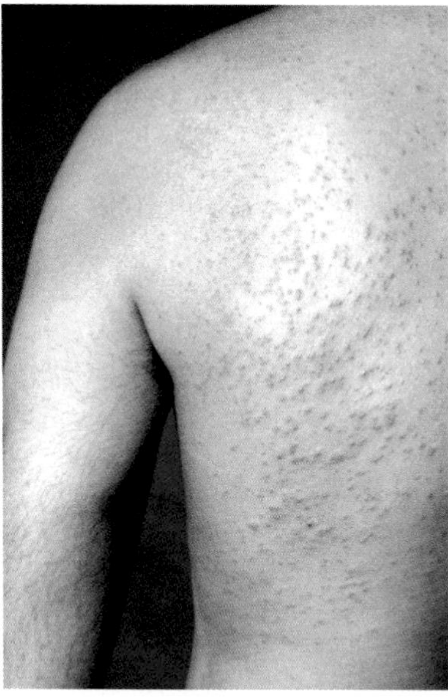

Fig. 7.5.8.4 Exanthema due to coxsackievirus infection.
Courtesy of the late Dr B.E. Juel-Jensen.

Foot-and-mouth disease

The aphthovirus causing foot-and-mouth disease in cloven-hoofed animals is endemic in Africa, Asia, and South America. Virus is secreted before blisters on the mouth and feet appear in animals. The zoonosis in humans is very rare, with about 37 recorded cases. Human infection occurs from virus entering through broken skin, drinking unpasteurized milk, or by inhalation of droplets. A 2- to 6-day incubation period is followed by blisters of hands, feet, and mouth, fever, and sore throat; complete recovery ensues. No person-to-person spread is recorded.

Conjunctivitis

Several enterovirus types cause conjunctivitis, often affecting large numbers of people epidemically. Most notable causes are echovirus types 7 and 11, coxsackievirus A24 and B2, and enterovirus 70 that often produces a haemorrhagic conjunctivitis.

Diabetes and pancreatitis

Insulin-dependent diabetes mellitus (IDDM, or type 1 diabetes) is likely to be an autoimmune disorder in which the insulin-secreting pancreatic islet cells (β cells) are destroyed. The human disease has long been thought to be caused by infectious agents, particularly since association between enterovirus infection and the development

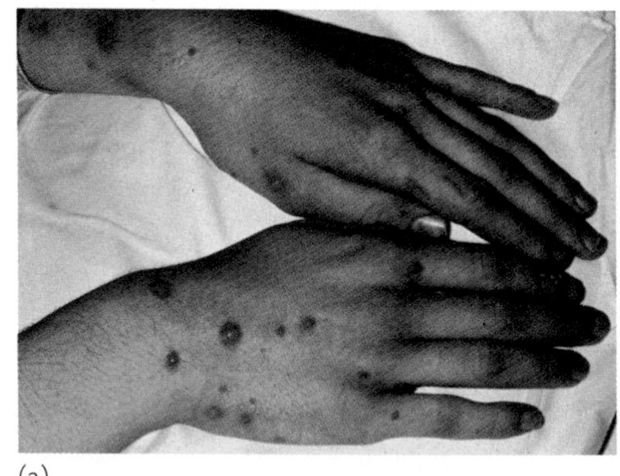

(a)

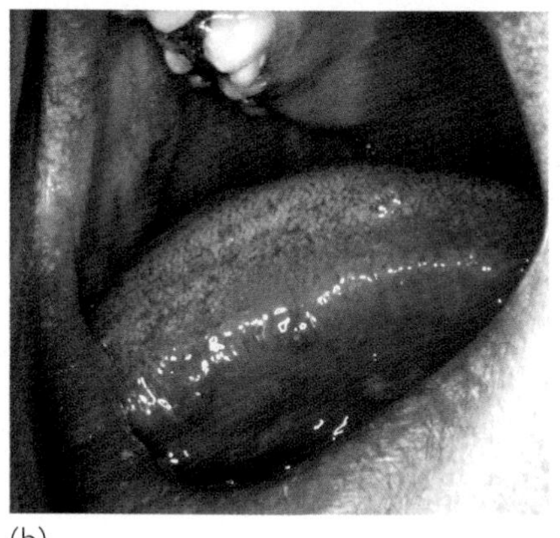

(b)

Fig. 7.5.8.5 (a, b) Hand-foot-and-mouth disease due to coxsackievirus infection.
Courtesy of the late Dr B.E. Juel-Jensen.

of IDDM has been shown in animal model studies (infection of mice with Coxsackie B3–B5 viruses). However, there is also a strong genetic component in the development of IDDM.

Chronic fatigue syndrome (Chapter 26.5.4)

Chronic fatigue syndrome (CFS), also known under the names of myalgic encephalomyelitis (ME), Royal Free disease, Iceland disease, postviral fatigue syndrome, and neuromyasthenia, can occur both sporadically and epidemically. The main clinical feature is excess fatigability of skeletal muscle, accompanied by pain. Other symptoms include headaches, inability to concentrate, paraesthesia, and impairment of short-term memory. A major problem in diagnosis is a clear definition of the clinical entity. Several virus infections have seemed to precede the development of CFS; they are mainly enterovirus infections, chronic Epstein–Barr virus (EBV) infection, and also infections with *Toxoplasma* and *Leptospira* spp. The stringency of the association of chronic enterovirus infection with the appearance of CFS is controversial. A report of a joint working group of the Royal Colleges of Physicians, Psychiatrists, and General Practitioners has concluded that persistence of enteroviruses is unlikely to play a role in the development of CFS. Similar conclusions have been drawn for the possibility of a causal link between chronic EBV infection and CFS (see Chapter 7.5.3).

Gastroenteritis

Although enteroviruses infect via the gastrointestinal tract and readily replicate there, they very rarely cause diarrhoea. Outbreaks of diarrhoea with echovirus type 11 have been reported. In Japan, an enterovirus termed Aichi virus, which is proposed as the type species of the new genus *Kobuvirus* of the Picornaviridae family, has been identified as the cause of multiple outbreaks of gastroenteritis in humans, mostly associated with the consumption of raw oysters. This virus seems to circulate widely in populations of Japan and other south-east Asian countries, with subclinical infections likely to be common (see Chapter 7.5.9).

Laboratory diagnosis of enterovirus infections

Virus isolation

Virus isolation is an excellent procedure to diagnose enterovirus infections. Virus is shed for weeks, and sometimes months, from the primary infection sites (cells lining the gut, see above). Starting from a few days after infection, virus can be found in concentrations of 10^5 to 10^6 tissue culture infectious doses 50%/g ($TCID_{50}$/g) of faeces. Throat swabs are also a good source for virus, particularly early in infection and when there are respiratory symptoms. In cases of meningitis, enteroviruses can be propagated in cell culture from the cerebrospinal fluid, but the method is much less sensitive than genome detection (see below). Viruses are readily isolated in secondary cultures of monkey kidney cells, or in cultures of permanent cell lines derived from human embryonic kidney, human amnion, or human fetal lung. The cytopathic effect (CPE) produced by enteroviruses is nonspecific. Typing of a cytopathic agent is carried out using antiserum pools (see below) or in multistep procedures. Most Coxsackie A viruses (with the exception of coxsackievirus A9) do not grow well in cell culture but can be readily isolated by intracerebral, intraperitoneal, or subcutaneous infection of mice, causing flaccid paralysis and death. In contrast, Coxsackie B viruses cause spastic paralysis. Polioviruses or echoviruses do not usually grow in mice although polioviruses will replicate in transgenic animals that have appropriate receptors (see above).

Serology

Neutralization assays are the method of choice for typing enteroviruses. Due to the large number of enterovirus types, these tests are labour intensive and not apt for rapid diagnosis. Pools of type-specific antisera (prepared by Drs Lim, Benyesch, Melnick, and LMB pools) have greatly helped to establish the epidemiology of enterovirus infections worldwide. Recurrent enterovirus infections during a lifetime often result in elevated serum antibody titres which obscure diagnostic changes. Significant antibody rises are, therefore, rarely observed in paired sera (taken at the onset of and during convalescence from disease).

A Coxsackie B virus-specific IgM test (using an IgM antibody capture technique) has been developed for rapid diagnosis. However, there is cross-reactivity between the IgM responses to different enteroviruses, including different genera of the picornaviruses, and so this test is not very specific. Prolonged presence of enterovirus-specific IgM has also been observed. In summary, the usefulness of serology for the diagnosis of enterovirus infection is limited.

Genome detection

Hybridization procedures and, more recently, reverse transcription–polymerase chain reaction (RT-PCR) techniques have been applied to test for the presence of enterovirus genomes. This approach has been very productive, particularly in diagnosing CNS infections from cerebrospinal fluid specimens, and has become the 'gold standard' of diagnosis, surpassing viral culture. Enterovirus RNAs have also been detected in myocardial biopsies from patients with myocarditis and dilated cardiomyopathy, in muscle of people with inflammatory muscle disease and chronic fatigue syndrome, and in brain biopsies. The significance of these findings is not clear, as infectious virus can rarely be isolated and viral antigen cannot be detected. Highly conserved sequences in the 5′ end of enterovirus genomes have allowed the design of PCR primers detecting most enterovirus RNAs. As the echovirus 22 genome is very different from that of the other enteroviruses (see above), tailor-made primers have to be added in a multiplex RT-PCR to include these viruses, which cause infections particularly in neonates and infants. A modified RT-PCR procedure can differentiate between wild-type and vaccine-derived poliovirus infections.

Epidemiology of enterovirus infections

Enteroviruses are mainly transmitted by the faeco-oral route, due to the fact that viruses are shed in faeces for weeks or months after infection. Spread is particularly intense within families, usually starting from the primary infection of young children. In temperate climates, there are seasonal peaks (July–September in the northern hemisphere and December–February in the southern hemisphere), whereas in subtropical and tropical climates enterovirus infections occur all the year round. The vast majority of primary human enterovirus infections occur during the first decade of life. Type-specific surveillance in several geographical regions has shown that coxsackieviruses A9, A16, and B4 and echovirus types 6, 9, 11, 19, 22, and 30 are most frequently found.

Prevention of enterovirus infections

As there are only three poliovirus types and no significant animal reservoir, it has been possible to develop very successful poliovirus vaccines. In 1954, a formalin-inactivated poliovirus vaccine (IPV) was introduced by Dr Jonas Salk in the United States of America, and in 1962 Dr Albert Sabin introduced a vaccine consisting of live attenuated strains of the three poliovirus types which could be given orally (OPV). Protection by the live attenuated vaccine is effected mainly at the site of entry by eliciting locally virus-specific IgAs and IgGs. Inactivated vaccine mainly elicits serum IgGs which prevent infection of the CNS and other sites distant of the port of entry by neutralization of viraemic virus. The main characteristics of IPV and OPV are summarized in Table 7.5.8.2.

Inactivated poliovirus vaccine

The early IPVs developed by Salk were of relatively low potency. High potency vaccines, based on large-scale cell culture systems but the same inactivation procedures, were developed in the Netherlands in the 1980s and form the basis of IPVs used today. Much of the developed world including Europe and the United States of America now uses only IPVs, having previously used the live attenuated vaccines which were thought to be better able to eradicate poliomyelitis and were proven to be able to break epidemic transmission. However, Scandinavian countries and the Netherlands had eliminated the disease with IPVs. IPV is given by injection and is more expensive per dose than the oral vaccine, but has advantages as outlined below, mainly the avoidance of vaccine-associated paralysis. IPV is the vaccine of choice in cases of immunodeficiency.

Live attenuated poliovirus vaccine

This vaccine has several advantages compared to the inactivated vaccine (Table 7.5.8.2) as it:

- parallels the natural infection;
- stimulates both local secretory IgA in the pharynx and alimentary tract, and systemic circulating virus-specific IgG antibody;
- is easy to administer as an oral vaccine;
- is more cost effective; and
- is proven to be capable of interrupting virus circulation and epidemics.

The disadvantage is that in a few cases the attenuated vaccine strains have reverted to virulence in vaccine recipients or their contacts. Since the early 1980s, all cases of polio in the United States of America and Europe were found to be vaccine-related, due to infection with reverted poliovirus, or were imported from endemic countries and were not indigenous original wild-type strains. The risk of vaccine-associated poliomyelitis is between 0.5 and 3.4 cases/million of susceptible children immunized. Vaccine-related polio is mostly caused by type 2 or type 3 viruses, probably due to the fact that the number of point mutations in type 1 vaccine virus compared to wild-type virus is much higher than in type 2 and type 3 vaccine viruses. However, as the disease becomes increasingly rare in the countries concerned and the world at large, indigenous cases or importation of virus are increasingly rare, and the risks of oral vaccination begin to outweigh its benefits. The reintroduction of polio by the use of oral vaccine has been documented as described below, and poses a risk to the eradication programme. These risks are not associated with the use of IPV, which has become the vaccine of choice in many countries.

Table 7.5.8.2 Characteristics of poliovirus vaccines

Characteristic	Live attenuated poliovirus vaccine (OPV)	Inactivated poliovirus vaccine (IPV)
Virus source	Attenuated virus (Sabin strains)	Virulent virus strains
Primary course	3 doses at monthly intervals starting at age of 2 months (temperate climates; more doses in tropics)	Three doses at 2-month intervals
Administration route	Oral	Parenteral (injection)
Immunity produced—systemic	IgA, IgM, IgG	IgM, IgG, (IgA)
—local	IgA	(IgA, minimal)
Booster doses required	1. at school entry 2. between 15 and 19 years 3. in adult life when exposed (last dose 10 years or more ago)	Yes (every 3–5 years or when exposed)
Efficacy	Good in temperate climates, variable in tropics	Good
Spread to contacts	Yes	No
Vaccine-associated paralysis	0.5–3.4 cases/million first doses in susceptible children	No
Production cost per dose	$0.07	$0.7
Requirement on personnel	Not highly trained	Trained and skilled
Requirement of 'cold chain'	Yes	Less than OPV
Combination with other vaccines	No	Possible
Use in immunodeficient children	No	Possible

Polio eradication and surveillance

For many years it was thought that the Sabin oral poliovirus vaccines were ineffective in tropical countries. While many reasons were put forward, the lack of impact of polio vaccination programmes was probably due to loss of vaccine potency through failure to maintain storage at cool temperatures ('cold chain'), and also the epidemiology of poliovirus infection. In temperate countries, poliomyelitis is seasonal with infections peaking in the summer months. A strategy of vaccination based on immunization of young children at a set age (usually a few months) is, therefore, able to build up a highly immune population in the winter so that transmission of the wild-type virus becomes more difficult. In tropical countries, where exposure is year round. It is a matter of chance whether a child will first be naturally infected or immunized. This was recognized by Sabin in 1960, but not acted upon until some 20 years later when the strategy of National Immunization Days was developed in South America. This approach involves immunizing all children below a certain age in a country within a very short period, so that all susceptible children's intestinal tracts are occupied by vaccine virus and are, therefore, resistant to infection by the wild-type virus. Transmission of wild-type virus is therefore broken, and the virus dies out.

The World Health Organization has pronounced the intention of eliminating poliomyelitis due to wild-type virus. The Americas have been free of polio since 1992. The last case of polio in South East Asia occurred in March 1997. In 2000, the Western Pacific Region was declared polio-free by the World Health Organization, and the European region in 2002. The enormous achievement between 1988 and 2004 is shown in Fig. 7.5.8.6. The scale of the undertaking is colossal, and the progress towards eradication is extraordinary. For example, in 1992 in China, all children aged 5 or less were immunized over a 1-week period. This amounts to one-quarter of the world's children. At the time of writing, virus is still known to be endemic in only a few countries: India, Pakistan, Afghanistan, Nigeria, and a few Central African countries (Fig. 7.5.8.7). Eradication before long is a real possibility although it is not a trivial matter. In 2004, immunization stopped in Nigeria when it was suggested that the vaccine contained oestrogens to render recipients sterile. The result was the re-emergence and reintroduction of polio into much of Central Africa, where it had been previously considered eradicated, and the situation was only brought under control by massive coordinated immunization activities throughout the region. However, polio remains in northern Nigeria, which was recently the source of outbreaks in Yemen and Indonesia; it is surmised pilgrims returning from Mecca were infected by coreligionists from Nigeria and reintroduced the virus. Finally, in 2006, polio was reintroduced into Angola from northern India, and spread from Angola to Namibia. So long as pockets of infection persist the world remains at risk of the re-emergence of polio. Thus part of the challenge is to demonstrate that the virus has in fact been eliminated, and this depends on rigorous effective surveillance. One approach is to obtain data on cases of acute flaccid paralysis of whatever cause, including the Guillain–Barré syndrome. All cases should be investigated to see whether they are due to poliovirus infection or not, and it is considered that the background rate in the absence of poliomyelitis should be one case per 100 000 members of the population, providing a control for the adequacy of the surveillance scheme. Alternative approaches include the investigation of poliovirus isolates to establish whether they are derived from vaccine or represent wild-type strains. There are possible concerns over the adequacy of either approach.

Once wild-type poliovirus has been eradicated, the only sources of the virus will be manufacturers of vaccines, laboratories holding stocks, and recipients of live attenuated vaccine. While manufacturers and laboratory workers can be required to work under high containment level conditions to avoid escape of virulent virus, vaccinees pose a particular problem. The vaccine works by establishing an infection in the recipient, but the virus may adapt to the gut and eventually undergo major molecular changes to improve its fitness. In principle, such viruses could spread to others forming a focus for a return of poliovirus infections and poliomyelitis. In practice, the vaccine virus seems to be poorly transmissible compared to the wild type. In countries such as Cuba where it has been given only in the early part of the year as a matter of policy, virus is not detectable after 6 months. Thus, it might be possible to stop vaccinating with no further precautions, as the vaccine strain of poliovirus will die out more rapidly than susceptible individuals will accumulate to provide a population to maintain its circulation.

However, in recent years there have been outbreaks of polio attributable to the vaccine strains that had regained the ability to spread efficiently from person to person. This has been observed in Haiti, Egypt, the Philippines, and Madagascar and may be

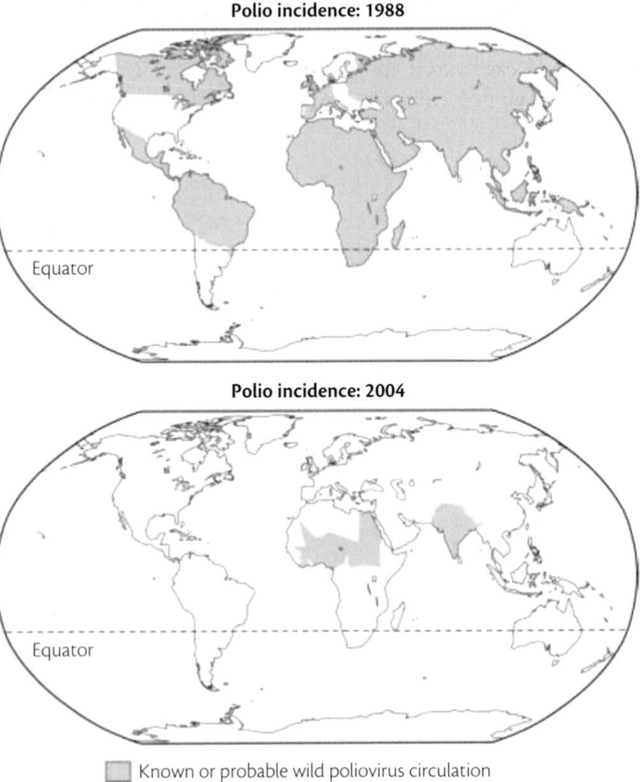

Fig. 7.5.8.6 World maps depicting the circulation of wild-type poliomyelitis virus for 1988 and 2004, as reported by the World Health Organization.
From Pallansch M, Roos R (2007) Enteroviruses: polioviruses, coxsackieviruses, echoviruses, and newer enteroviruses. In: Knipe DM, *et al.* (eds) *Fields virology*, 5th edition, pp. 839–93. Wolters Kluwer Health/Lippincott Williams & Wilkins, Philadelphia. With permission of author and publisher.

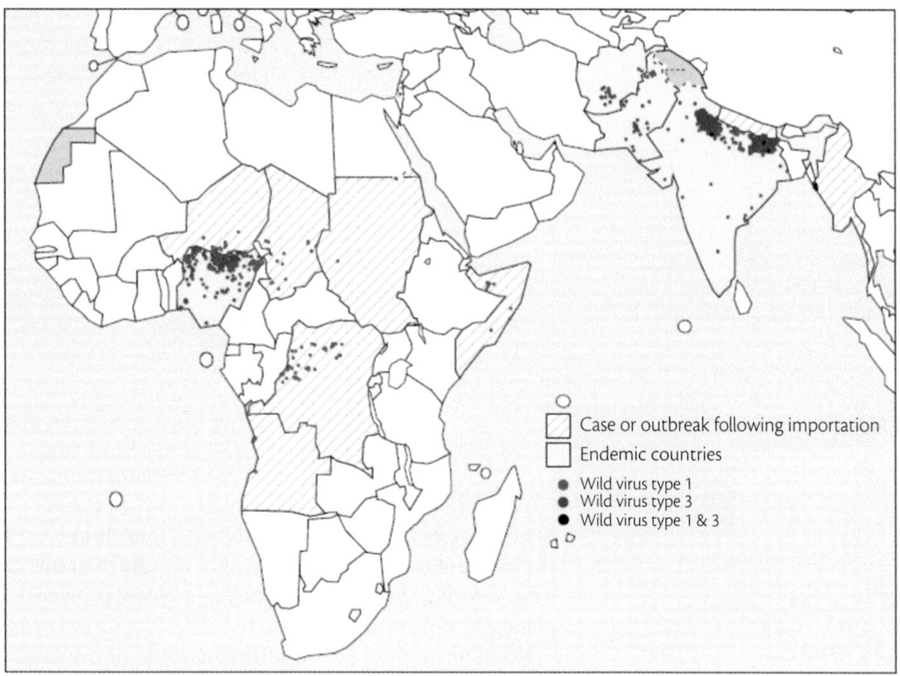

Excludes viruses detected from environmental surveillance and vaccine derived polioviruses.
Data in WHO/HQ as of 22 Apr 2008

Fig. 7.5.8.7 Wild-type poliovirus cases in 2007.
From World Health Organization (2008). *Global polio eradication initiative. Annual report 2007. Impact of the intensified eradication effort.* WHO, Geneva. www.polioeradication.org/content/publications/AnnualReport2007_English.pdf. With permission of the publisher.

relatively common, particularly where vaccination continues with the live vaccine for a long time with poor coverage so that vaccinated and unvaccinated individuals mix, providing the ideal conditions for the selection of transmissible virus. The solution may be to cease vaccination abruptly, or, as is increasingly the case in developed countries, use IPV which does not pose this risk.

A further concern comes from people with B-cell immunodeficiency who can become chronically infected but be apparently healthy for up to 15 years. During this time the virus may adapt to an extent that neurotropism is regained, and an unvaccinated population will again be highly susceptible. The numbers and geographical distribution of such long-term excretors are unknown but most exposed individuals do not excrete virus for very long periods, and even those that do usually cease excreting virus spontaneously, albeit after a period of a few years.

The fact that serious consideration has to be given to how to deal with the cessation of vaccination is a tribute to the extraordinary progress which has been made towards polio eradication.

The *de novo* synthesis of infectious particles from poliovirus RNA transcribed from synthetic cDNA in a cell-free HeLa cell extract has created a huge debate on the scientific value of such an experiment, concerns about poliovirus eradication, issues of national security and freedom of virological/biological research. Since then, other viruses (ΦX174, the 1918 H1N1 influenza virus a.o.) have been synthesized *de novo*, allowing the effect of more drastic changes in viral sequence on viral properties to be examined than is possible by established methods of genetic manipulation. The usefulness of the method to carry out broad-based research into questions of viral pathogenesis and attenuation for vaccine production (e.g. by changing codon usage) is becoming appreciated but it has also led to considerable efforts by the scientific community and industry to define and assess possible misuse of this technology.

Further reading

Cello J, Paul AV, Wimmer E. (2002). Chemical synthesis of poliovirus cDNA: generation of infectious virus in the absence of natural template. *Science*, **297**, 1016–18.

Joint Working Group of the Royal Colleges of Physicians, Psychiatrists, and General Practitioners (1997). *Chronic fatigue syndrome*, pp. 58. Royal College of Physicians Publication Unit, London.

Kew OM, *et al.* (2002). Outbreak of poliomyelitis in Hispaniola associated with circulating type 1 vaccine-derived poliovirus. *Science*, **296**, 356–9.

Martin J, *et al.* (2000). Evolution of the Sabin strain of type 3 poliovirus in an immunodeficient patient during the entire 637-day period of virus excretion. *J Virol*, **74**, 3001–10.

Melnick JL (1996). Enteroviruses: polioviruses, coxsackieviruses, echoviruses, and newer enteroviruses. In: Fields BN, *et al.* (eds) *Fields virology*, 3rd edition, pp. 655–712. Lippincott-Raven, Philadelphia.

Mendelsohn C, Wimmer R, Racaniello VR (1989). Cellular receptor for poliovirus: molecular cloning, nucleotide sequence and expression of a new member of the immunoglobulin superfamily. *Cell*, **56**, 855–65.

Minor PD (1990). Antigenic structure of picornaviruses. *Curr Top Microbiol Immunol*, **161**, 122–54.

Minor PD (1996). Poliovirus. In: Nathanson N, *et al.* (eds) *Viral pathogenesis*, pp. 555–74. Lippincott-Raven, Philadelphia.

Minor P (2005). Picornaviruses. In: Mahy BW, ter Meulen V (eds) *Topley and Wilson's microbiology and microbial infections. Virology*, 10th edition, pp. 857–87. Hodder Arnold, London.

Offit PA (2005). The Cutter Incident, pp. 256. Yale University Press, New Haven.

Pallnsch M, Roos R (2007) Enteroviruses: polioviruses, coxsackieviruses, echoviruses, and newer enteroviruses. In: Knipe DM, *et al.* (eds) *Fields virology*, 5th edition, pp. 839–93. Wolters Kluwer Health/Lippincott Williams & Wilkins, Philadelphia.

Racaniello VR (2007). Picornaviridae: the viruses and their replication. In: Knipe DM, *et al.* (eds) *Fields virology*, 5th edition, pp. 795–838. Wolters Kluwer Health/Lippincott Williams & Wilkins, Philadelphia.

Racaniello VR, Baltimore D (1981). Cloned poliovirus complementary DNA is infectious in mammalian cells. *Science*, **214**, 916–19.

Stanway G, *et al.* (2005). Picornaviridae. In: Fauquet CM, *et al.* (eds) *Virus taxonomy. Classification and nomenclature of viruses. Eighth Report of the International Committee on Taxonomy of Viruses*, pp. 757–78. Elsevier Academic Press, London.

Wimmer E. (2006). The test-tube synthesis of a chemical called poliovirus. The simple synthesis of a virus has far-reaching societal implications. *EMBO Rep*, **7 Spec No**, S3–S9.

Wimmer E, *et al.* (2009). Synthetic viruses: a new opportunity to understand and prevent viral disease. *Nat Biotechnol*, **27**, 1163–72.

World Health Organization (2008). *Global polio eradication initiative. Annual report 2007. Impact of the intensified eradication effort.* WHO, Geneva. www.polioeradication.org/content/publications/AnnualReport2007_English.pdf

Yamashita T, *et al.* (2000). Application of a reverse transcription-PCR for identification and differentiation of Aichi virus, a new member of the picornavirus family associated with gastroenteritis in humans. *J Clin Microbiol*, **38**, 2955–61.

7.5.9 Virus infections causing diarrhoea and vomiting

Philip Dormitzer and Ulrich Desselberger

Essentials

Gastroenteritis is frequently caused by rotaviruses, enteric adenoviruses (group F), human caliciviruses (noroviruses, sapoviruses), and astroviruses: these cause much disease worldwide and considerable mortality, mainly in developing countries. Other viruses found in the human gastrointestinal tract are not regularly associated with diarrhoeal disease, except in patients who are immunosuppressed and in whom herpes simplex virus, cytomegalovirus, and picobirnaviruses can cause diarrhoea, as can HIV itself.

Epidemiology—(1) Rotaviruses—the major cause of endemic infantile gastroenteritis worldwide; transmission is by the faeco-oral route; there is a strict winter peak of infections in temperate climates, but these occur year round in tropical and subtropical regions; many animals and birds harbour a large diversity of rotaviruses and may act as a reservoir for human infections. (2) Human caliciviruses—the most important cause of nonbacterial gastroenteritis outbreaks worldwide—frequently spread by contamination of food (oysters, green salads, fresh fruit, cold foods, and sandwiches) and water.

Clinical features and management—following an incubation period of 1 to 2 days, there is sudden onset of watery diarrhoea lasting between 4 and 7 days, vomiting, and varying degrees of dehydration. Other features include abdominal cramps, headache, myalgia and fever. Treatment is supportive, mainly with oral rehydration solutions or—in more severe cases—intravenous rehydration.

Diagnosis—viral infection can be demonstrated by passive particle agglutination tests, virus-specific enzyme-linked immunosorbent assays, and by viral genome detection using the polymerase chain reaction (PCR) (for adenoviruses) or reverse transcription-PCR (RT-PCR) (for rotaviruses, caliciviruses, and astroviruses).

Prevention and control: two live attenuated oral rotavirus vaccines have recently been licensed in numerous countries, in some of which universal mass vaccination of children as part of childhood vaccination schemes has been accepted. There are no vaccines against other viruses causing gastroenteritis in humans. Outbreak control measures relate mainly to calicivirus-associated gastroenteritis and focus on the interruption of person-to-person transmission and the removal of common sources of infection (food, water, etc).

Introduction

Acute gastroenteritis and vomiting in humans is a well-characterized clinical entity caused by various different agents (viruses, bacteria, parasites, etc.). Viral gastroenteritis is a global problem, particularly in infants and young children.

Many viruses are found in the human gut but not all of them produce acute gastroenteritis (Table 7.5.9.1). Viral infections normally associated with gastroenteritis are caused by rotaviruses, human caliciviruses (noroviruses, sapoviruses), enteric adenoviruses (group F), and astroviruses. Other viruses found in the human gastrointestinal tract (enteroviruses, reoviruses, non-group F adenoviruses, toroviruses, coronaviruses, parvoviruses) are not regularly associated with diarrhoeal disease. Finally, there are viruses found in the gut of immunosuppressed patients (most commonly those infected with HIV), including herpes simplex virus (HSV), cytomegalovirus (CMV), and picobirnaviruses. HIV itself can also infect the gut directly.

Only the major virus groups regularly causing gastroenteritis in humans are described here in separate sections. Clinical symptoms, diagnosis, treatment, epidemiology, and vaccine development are reviewed under common headings.

Rotaviruses

Structure

Rotaviruses are the major cause of infantile gastroenteritis worldwide and also of acute diarrhoea in the young of many mammalian species. They are members of the *Reoviridae* family, with a genome of 11 segments of double-stranded RNA encoding six structural viral proteins (VP1–VP4, VP6, VP7) and six nonstructural proteins (NSP1–NSP6). The icosahedral virion has three concentric protein layers and no lipid envelope (Fig. 7.5.9.1).

The inner layer (consisting of VP2) encloses the genome segments, the polymerase VP1, and the capping enzyme VP3. The addition of a middle layer consisting of VP6 leads to the formation of a transcriptionally active subviral particle, referred to as the double-layered particle (DLP). VP6 is the most immunogenic rotavirus protein. Infectious virions have an additional layer, which mediates the translocation of the DLP into the cytoplasm during cell entry. This outermost layer consists of two proteins VP4 and VP7, both of which elicit and are the targets of neutralizing antibodies. VP7 forms a shell, which is shed in the low calcium environment of the cytoplasm. VP4 forms spikes, which are important

Table 7.5.9.1 Virus infections of the human gut

Viruses found as	Genus (Family)
Regular cause of diarrhoea and vomiting	Rotaviruses (*Reoviridae*)[a]
	Human caliciviruses (*Caliciviridae*)[a]
	Group F adenoviruses (*Adenoviridae*)
	Astroviruses (*Astroviridae*)
Occasional cause of diarrhoea and vomiting	Enteroviruses (*Picornaviridae*)[b]
	Reoviruses (*Reoviridae*)
	Adenoviruses other than Group F (*Adenoviridae*)
	Toroviruses (*Coronaviridae*)
	Coronaviruses (*Coronaviridae*)
	Parvoviruses (*Parvoviridae*)
Cause of diarrhoea in immunodeficient patients	Human immunodeficiency virus (*Retroviridae*)
	Herpes simplex virus (*Herpesviridae*)
	Cytomegalovirus (*Herpesviridae*)
	Picobirnaviruses (*Birnaviridae*)

[a] Not all infections cause disease (see text).

[b] Outbreaks of diarrhoea caused by echovirus type 11 infections have been reported (see Chapter 7.11.8).

for attachment and membrane penetration. To achieve maximal infectivity of the virion, the VP4 spike must be cleaved by intestinal trypsin. In electron micrographs of negatively stained specimens, virions have a characteristic appearance as 75-nm wheel-like particles (Fig. 7.5.9.2), the name of the virus being derived from Latin *rota* = wheel.

Classification

Rotaviruses are classified according to the immunological reactivities and genomic sequences of three of their structural components. Specific epitopes on the inner-shell protein VP6 allow five groups (A–E) to be distinguished, and two more groups (F, G) probably exist. Group A rotaviruses cause the vast majority of human gastroenteritis infections and have been divided into subgroups on the basis of additional determinants on VP6. Group B rotaviruses have caused epidemics of diarrhoea affecting adults and children. Group C rotaviruses generally cause more mild diarrhoeal disease. The remaining groups are only known to infect nonhuman hosts.

Both surface proteins VP4 and VP7 elicit neutralizing antibodies and thus confer type specificity. A dual-type classification system has been devised for group A rotaviruses, which differentiates glycoprotein (G) types (VP7-specific) and protease-sensitive protein (P) types (VP4-specific). For example, G1P1A[8] is G serotype and genotype 1, P serotype 1A, P genotype 8. At present, rotaviruses carrying a relatively restricted number of G types (G1–G4 and G9) and P types (P[4] and P[8]) cause most human disease in temperate climates. However, at least 11 G types and 11 P types have been found in humans. Zoonotic rotovirus infections of humans are well documented, and previously rare serotypic variants have become established among strains pathogenic to humans (mainly in tropical and subtropical regions). In addition, rotaviruses can exchange genome segments (reassort) during mixed infections, providing an additional mechanism to introduce genetic diversity. Hence, rotavirus epidemiology continues to evolve, and eradication of rotaviruses is not feasible.

Replication

The primary targets of rotavirus infection are the mature epithelial cells at the tips of the villi of the small intestine. Viral entry requires penetration of a membrane to deliver an intact DLP to the cytoplasm. It is not known whether the plasma membrane or an endosomal membrane is the primary site of entry. In the cytoplasm of an infected cell, the DLP extrudes 11 different newly synthesized

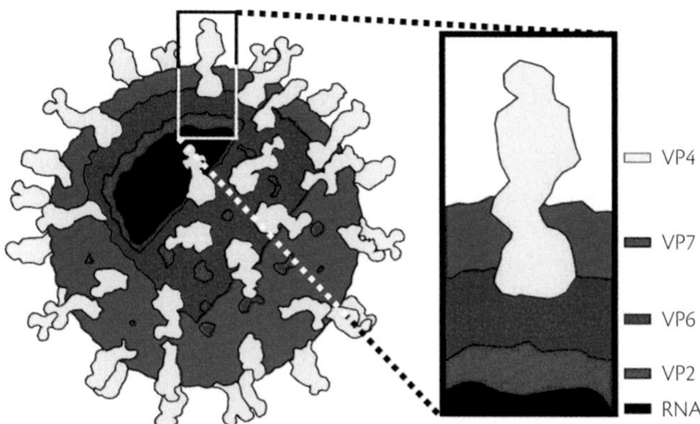

Fig. 7.5.9.1 The icosahedral rotavirus virion has three layers: (1) an inner VP2 layer that contains the genome, polymerase, and capping enzyme; (2) a middle VP6 layer; and (3) an outer VP7 layer. The VP4 spike is anchored in the VP6 layer and protrudes through the VP7 layer.

(Based on Dormitzer P, *et al.* (2004). Structural rearrangements in the membrane penetration protein of a non-enveloped virus. *Nature*, **430**, 1053–58; Yeager M, *et al.* (1990). Three-dimensional structure of rhesus rotavirus by cryoelectron microscopy and image reconstruction. *J Cell Biol*, **110**, 2133–44.)

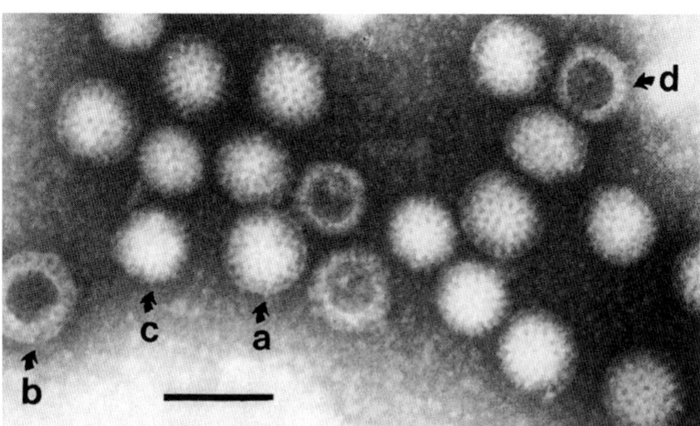

Fig. 7.5.9.2 Rotavirus particles in the faeces of a child admitted to hospital with acute gastroenteritis. Negative staining with aqueous 2% potassium phosphotungstate, pH 7.0. Scale bar represents 100 nm. Four different morphologies of particles are shown: (a) triple-layered particle containing RNA; (b) triple-layered particle without RNA (empty, core penetrated with stain); (c) double-layered particle containing RNA; and (d) double-layered empty particle.

Courtesy of M. Jenkins, Regional Virus Laboratory, East Birmingham Hospital.
From Desselberger U (1992). Reoviruses. In: Greenwood D, Slack R, Peutherer J (eds) *Medical microbiology*, 14th edition, p. 620. Churchill Livingstone, Edinburgh, with permission of the publisher.)

mRNAs without releasing the genome segments. One viral nonstructural protein, NSP3, binds to the nonpolyadenylated 3′ ends of viral mRNAs, substituting for host poly(A) binding protein in circularizing mRNA, and shutting off host translation by depleting pools of the translation initiation factor eIF4G. New DLPs assemble in the cytoplasmic inclusion bodies, termed viroplasms. Because each infectious unit corresponds to a small number of virus particles, it is likely that one of each of the 11 genome segments is packaged into each new DLP. The mechanism of this specific and highly selective packaging remains a puzzle. Nascent particles bind a virally encoded integral endoplasmic reticulum membrane glycoprotein, NSP4, and bud into the endoplasmic reticulum lumen, acquiring a transient envelope. This envelope is lost as the outermost protein layer is added to complete the virions. Virions are released from infected enterocytes after transport to the cell surface by a vesicular transport pathway that bypasses the Golgi apparatus. Replication in the gut results in very high concentrations of viral particles (up to 10^{11}/ml) in faeces at the peak of the acute diarrhoea. The physical hardiness of the shed particles ensures their efficient transmission to new hosts.

Pathogenesis

The pathogenesis of rotavirus diarrhoea is complex. Viral infection causes direct damage to the enteric epithelium, resulting in the blunting and denudation of villi. The villous damage is repaired by cells emerging and differentiating from the crypts of the gut epithelium, which show a reactive hyperplasia. Loss of functioning absorptive cells leads to a degree of malabsorption and osmotic fluid loss. However, there also appears to be a secretory component to rotavirus diarrhoea. By raising intracellular calcium concentrations in infected cells, NSP4 activates a plasma membrane anion channel causing fluid secretion. There is evidence that a fragment of NSP4 is released from infected cells, acting as a viral enterotoxin to induce a secretory state of uninfected cells. The cellular receptor for the NSP4 fragment has recently been identified. The enteric nervous system also plays a role in pathogenesis. Enteric nervous system inhibitors diminish fluid secretion in the gut of rotavirus-infected animals.

Immune response

A primarily serotype-specific humoral immune response is elicited after neonatal or primary rotavirus infection. However, during the first 2 years of life children are repeatedly infected with rotaviruses leading to multiple serotype-specific, and also partially heterotypic, protection. The presence of rotavirus-specific secretory IgA coproantibodies seems to correlate best with protection against disease, although the exact correlates remain to be determined. Rotavirus-specific cytotoxic T-cell responses are capable of clearing infections, but appear to be less important than humoral immune responses in protecting against repeated infections. The abundant antibody that is produced against VP6 during infection does not neutralize extracellular virus. However, anti-VP6 IgA, which is transported across enterocytes for secretion into the gut lumen, can inhibit viral replication by binding DLPs in the cytoplasm ('intracellular neutralization'). The role of this phenomenon in protection against human infection is not yet known.

Enteric adenoviruses

Structure and classification

Adenoviruses are nonenveloped icosahedral viruses possessing a genome of linear double-stranded DNA approximately 35 000 bp in size. Their capsid is between 70 and 80 nm in diameter and consists of 240 hexons and 12 pentons that stand out as projecting fibres at the corners of the icosahedral virus particle. Human adenoviruses occur in 51 distinct serotypes, ordered in six different subgroups (A–F). Those adenoviruses regularly associated with gastroenteritis are classified as subgroup F, consisting of serotypes 40 and 41. Adenoviruses of different groups (causing respiratory tract infections) are also found frequently in the human gut, but are not regularly associated with diarrhoea.

Replication

Adenoviruses attach to susceptible cells via the fibre proteins, and enter via receptor-mediated endocytosis. Phased early and late gene transcription of the viral DNA in the cellular nucleus is followed by translation and morphogenesis in the cytoplasm, and numerous particles are released after cell death. The virally encoded early proteins E1A and E1B induce host cells to enter the S phase, prevent apoptosis, and inhibit antiviral responses. Late adenovirus gene expression blocks cellular DNA expression. Some adenoviruses seem to decrease the expression of major histocompatibility complex class 1 antigens on the surface of infected cells, thus reducing susceptibility to adenovirus-specific cytotoxic T cells. There is a serotype-specific humoral immune response providing homotypic protection.

Human caliciviruses

Structure and classification

These viruses were first recognized as the cause of gastroenteritis during outbreaks in Norwalk, Ohio, in the late 1960s. Norwalk virus (NV) particles are spherical and measure 27 to 35 nm in diameter. Norwalk virus and Norwalk-like viruses (NLVs) are all members of the *Caliciviridae* family. Their 7.7-kb genome consists of single-stranded RNA of positive polarity. Cup-shaped depressions on the surface of virions have given the name to this viral family (Latin *calix* = goblet, cup) (Fig. 7.5.9.3c,d). Phylogenetic trees of full-length sequences of caliciviral cDNAs have led to their classification into four genera: viruses of the genera *Norovirus* and *Sapovirus* infect humans, and viruses of the genera *Vesivirus* and *Lagovirus* only infect animals. Until recently viruses of the *Norovirus* genus were often termed 'small round structured viruses' and those of the *Sapovirus* genus 'classical caliciviruses'.

Replication

Details of the replication of human caliciviruses can only be deduced from those of animal caliciviruses, as there is no reproducible *in vitro* cell culture system for the human caliciviruses. The viruses seem to interact with species-specific receptors and a single protein precursor is cotranslationally and post-translationally cleaved in a way similar to that observed in picornaviruses.

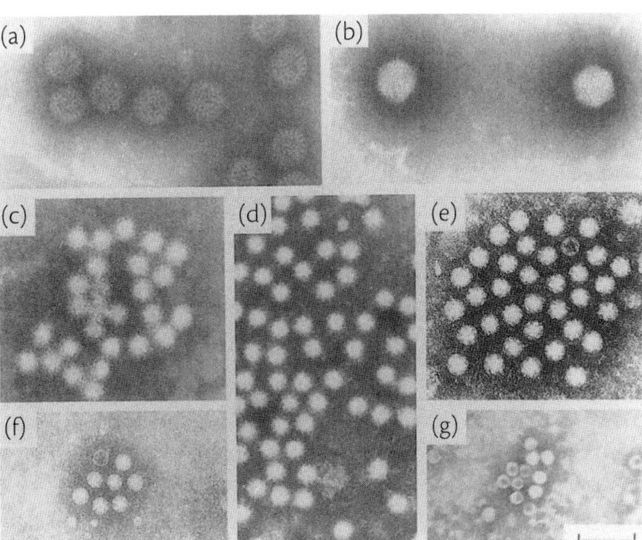

Fig. 7.5.9.3 Electron micrographs of (a) rotavirus, (b) enteric adenovirus, (c) Norwalk-like virus, (d) sapovirus, (e) astrovirus, (f) enterovirus, and (g) parvovirus. Negative staining with 3% phosphotungstate, pH 6.3; bar represents 100 nm. (Courtesy of Dr J. Kurtz, Oxford Public Health Laboratory (astroviruses) and Dr J. Gray, Clinical Microbiology and Public Health Laboratory, Cambridge (all other viruses). Reproduced from Zuckerman A, Banatvala J, Pattison J (eds) (2000). *Principles and practice of clinical virology*, 4th edition, p. 236. Wiley & Sons, Chichester, with permission of the publisher.)

Immune response

Although calicivirus infections elicit human immune responses, they do not seem to give full protection against subsequent infection. Higher pre-existing antibody levels may be associated with more severe illness on reinfection. Certain histo-blood group antigens can act as receptors for noroviruses, and secretors of such antigens have been found to be more susceptible to norovirus infections than nonsecretors. Due to the genetic variability in human susceptibility to some norovirus strains, pre-existing antibody may not necessarily correlate with protection from re-infection.

Astroviruses

Structure and classification

Astroviruses are members of the family Astroviridae. They possess a 6.8-kb genome of single-stranded RNA of positive polarity. So far, eight different serotypes have been distinguished that correlate well with major differences in genome sequences (i.e. genotypes).

Replication

Human astroviruses grow well in particular cell cultures. After viral absorption to unidentified cellular receptors and uncoating in the cytoplasm, full-length and subgenomic RNAs are made. These direct the production of protein precursors, which are post-translationally cleaved. Replication takes place purely in the cytoplasm.

Viral gastroenteritis

Clinical features

The onset of acute viral gastroenteritis follows a short incubation period of 1 to 2 days. It is sudden, with watery diarrhoea lasting between 4 and 7 days, vomiting, and varying degrees of dehydration. Over one-third of children with rotavirus infection have a fever of more than 39°C. Fewer children have a high fever after infection with caliciviruses, and the duration of diarrhoea after infection with caliciviruses is, as a rule, shorter (1–2 days) than after infection with rotaviruses or enteric adenoviruses (4–7 days). Disease due to calicivirus infection may be accompanied by abdominal cramps, headache, and myalgia. In rotavirus infection all degrees of severity are seen. Inapparent infections are not infrequent, particularly in neonates, in whom the infection is caused by so-called nursery strains. It is not known whether the asymptomatic nature of rotavirus infection in neonates is due to infection with particular strains or depends on the presence of maternal antibodies that provide partial protection. Rotavirus infections are frequently accompanied by respiratory symptoms, but there is no strong evidence that rotavirus replicates in the respiratory tract. Viraemia commonly accompanies rotavirus infection; however, the clinical significance of this finding in immunocompetent hosts is not yet established. In immunodeficient children, rotavirus may replicate at extraintestinal sites, and chronic gut infections with rotaviruses, adenoviruses, and astroviruses have been observed, accompanied by virus shedding over weeks and even months.

Diagnosis

The diagnosis of rotavirus, astrovirus, and enteric adenovirus infections is relatively easy as large numbers of particles are shed during the acute phase of the illness. In contrast, human caliciviruses replicate for a shorter period and are shed at lower concentrations. Diagnosis is commonly carried out by passive particle agglutination tests (PPATs), virus-specific enzyme-linked immunosorbent assays (ELISAs), and more recently by viral genome detection using the polymerase chain reaction (PCR) (for adenoviruses) and reverse transcription–PCR (RT-PCR) (for rotaviruses, caliciviruses, and astroviruses). PCRs are extremely sensitive diagnostic tools, allowing both viral detection and typing. Aliquots of PCR amplicons can also be sequenced and the information used to establish phylogenetic trees. Such trees are becoming increasingly important not only for virus classification but also for epidemiological studies and surveillance (see below). Electron microscopy of negatively stained specimen suspensions is a 'catch all' method that can diagnose less common viral enteric pathogens that are not detected by standard assays, such as nongroup A rotaviruses. The morphological appearances of the main viruses pathogenic for humans are shown in Fig. 7.5.9.3.

Treatment

Treatment is mainly with oral rehydration solutions or, in more severe cases, intravenous rehydration. The enkephalinase inhibitor racecadotril, used as a supplement to oral rehydration, has been shown to significantly decrease the duration and total fluid loss in rotavirus-infected children. In severe rotavirus infections, treatment with oral immunoglobulins can decrease the duration of diarrhoea and virus shedding; however, this is not a routine treatment. Otherwise treatment is symptomatic, but the use of antimobility drugs (codeine phosphate, diphenoxylate, loperamide) in children is not advised. Specific antiviral agents have been tested in animal models of rotavirus infections but are not used for human treatment.

Epidemiology

Rotaviruses

Rotavirus infections occur endemically worldwide and cause over 600 000 deaths annually in children below the age of 2 years, mainly in developing countries. Therefore, development of vaccine candidates has been a major goal since the early 1980s (see below).

The epidemiology of rotaviruses is complex. Besides children, elderly patients and patients with immunodeficiencies can be affected. There is a strict winter peak of rotavirus infections in temperate climates, but infections occur year round in tropical and subtropical regions. Transmission is by the faeco-oral route. Nosocomial infections on infant hospital wards occur and are difficult to eliminate. Group A rotaviruses of different G and P types are found to cocirculate in various populations within the same geographical location, and the relative incidence of different types changes over time. Various surveys have shown that usually more than 90% of cocirculating strains in temperate climates are types G1 to G4 and occur in combination with different P types as types G1P1A[8], G2P1B[4], G3P1A[8], and G4P1A[8]. Other G types may also be represented, particularly in tropical and subtropical areas but increasingly in temperate climates as well. For instance, G9 strains have recently been found to cause outbreaks of acute gastroenteritis in the United States of America and in many European countries. Most mammalian as well as avian species harbour a large diversity of rotaviruses and may act as a reservoir for human infections. An animal source is suspected for many of the more unusual human group A rotavirus isolates and possibly for group B rotavirus isolates. The latter caused outbreaks in children and adults in China during the 1980s and have also been isolated from patients with diarrhoea in different regions of India and Bangladesh. Group C rotaviruses are associated with small outbreaks in humans.

Human caliciviruses

Age-related seroprevalence studies of human caliciviruses have shown that infection is much more frequent and occurs from younger ages onwards than previously thought. Approximately 50% of children have been infected by the age of 2 years. The rate of inapparent infection is high, particularly in the young. In contrast to rotavirus infections, human caliciviruses cause outbreaks of acute gastroenteritis, mostly due to contamination of food or water, and are now recognized as the most important cause of non-bacterial gastroenteritis outbreaks worldwide. Contaminated oysters, green salads, fresh fruit, cold foods, and sandwiches are often implicated as sources of infection. Outbreaks occur in older children and adults in recreational camps, hospitals, nursing homes, schools, cafeterias, hotels, cruise ships, at banquets, etc. Human calicivirus outbreaks occur worldwide throughout the year, in contrast to the regular winter peaks of rotavirus infections in temperate climates. The viruses are highly infectious (i.e. a few virus particles constitute an infectious dose) and spread rapidly. Transmission is by the faeco-oral route and also by projectile vomiting, which scatters viruses into the environment by aerosol. There is cocirculation of different genotypes.

Astroviruses

Endemic infections with astroviruses occur in infants and elderly people, but they can also cause food-borne outbreaks of diarrhoea. There are at least eight genotypes, correlating well with known serotypes, which cocirculate. Serotype 1 is most frequently found, followed by serotypes 2 to 4 at intermediate frequencies and serotypes 5 to 8 at low frequencies. Seroprevalence studies have indicated that infection by more than one serotype is not unusual.

Vaccine development

Vaccines have been confirmed as the best individual and also population-based tools to restrict infection with epidemic viruses. Of the gastroenteritis-inducing viruses, vaccine development has only been intensively directed towards rotaviruses. After many trials with variable success, a live attenuated rhesus rotavirus (RRV)-based human reassortant vaccine eliciting immunity to human rotavirus strains G1 to G4 was found to confer significant protection (70–80%) from severe disease including dehydration. Protection from infection alone was only moderate (40–50%). This vaccine was recommended by the Advisory Committee on Immunization Practices (ACIP) in the United States of America in 1998. However, after 1.5 million doses had been used, the rare complication of gut intussusception was found to be temporally associated with vaccination. In 1999 the ACIP withdrew the recommendation, and the vaccine has been taken off the market by the manufacturer. Studies of the epidemiological findings and possible mechanisms of pathogenesis have not explained the association definitively.

In the search for alternative vaccines, two further live attenuated oral rotavirus vaccines have been developed (Rotarix and Rotateq). The underlying concepts of the vaccines are different. The pentavalent vaccine, containing the human antigens G1 to G4 and P[8] in monoreassortant viruses on a bovine rotavirus (WC3 strain) genetic backbone, is aimed at eliciting type-specific antibodies against all the rotavirus types that are recognized to circulate most frequently. The monovalent vaccine, an attenuated human G1P[8] strain, is based on two clinical observations: (1) cross-protection is accumulated through successive natural infections and rotavirus disease can be prevented by repeated natural infection and (2) vaccination with one rotavirus type can provide protection, even if subsequent infections are by rotaviruses of a different type. Both vaccines have recently been licensed in numerous countries, and in some of them universal mass vaccination of children as part of childhood vaccination schemes has been accepted. The introduction of rotavirus immunization in Australia, the United States of America, and other countries has been associated with substantial reductions in rotavirus disease and some evidence of herd immunity. There will be ongoing postmarketing surveillance in order to estimate the global impact of the vaccine and also to monitor whether or not novel rotavirus strains may emerge. It also remains to be seen to what extent the new vaccines will have an effect in developing countries where they are most needed.

Next generation approaches to immunization against rotavirus infection are under investigation, such as the use of virus-like particles obtained from baculovirus-recombinant coexpressed rotavirus proteins, enhancement of rotavirus immunogenicity by microencapsidation, DNA-based candidate vaccines, and possibly 'edible vaccines'.

No vaccines against other viruses causing gastroenteritis in humans have been developed so far. For human caliciviruses, vaccine development will be a challenge due to antigenic variation and uncertainty about the duration of acquired immunity.

Outbreak control

Nosocomial rotavirus outbreaks among paediatric populations (on hospital wards and in day-care centres) are common. There have been numerous reports of outbreaks of diarrhoea and vomiting occurring in adults and children due to infections with caliciviruses acquired from banquets, travel on cruise ships, cafeterias, schools, hotels, fast-food restaurants, etc.

Outbreak control measures should focus on the interruption of person-to-person transmission and the removal of common sources of infection (food, water, etc.) in conjunction with measures to improve environmental hygiene (by food-handlers, etc.).

Further reading

Ball JM, *et al.* (1996). Age-dependent diarrhoea induced by a rotaviral nonstructural glycoprotein. *Science*, **272**, 101–4.

Carter MJ, Willcocks MM (2005). Human enteric RNA viruses: astroviruses. In: Mahy BWJ, ter Meulen V (eds) *Topley and Wilson's microbiology and microbial infections*, 10th edition, pp. 888–910. Hodder Arnold, London.

Clarke IN, Lambden PR (2005). Human enteric RNA viruses: noroviruses and sapoviruses. In: Mahy BWJ, ter Meulen V (eds) *Topley and Wilson's microbiology and microbial infections*, 10th edition, pp. 911–31. Hodder Arnold, London.

Cortese MM, Parashar UD (2009). Prevention of rotavirus gastroenteritis among infants and children. Recommendations of the Advisory Committee on Immunization Practices (ACIP). *Morb Mort Wkly Rec MMWR*, **58**, 1–25.

Desselberger U (2000). Viruses causing gastroenteritis. In: Zuckerman A, Banatvala J, Pattison J (eds) *Principles and practice of clinical virology*, 4th edition, pp. 235–52. Wiley, Chichester.

Desselberger U, Gray J, Estes MK (2005). Rotaviruses. In: Mahy BWJ, ter Meulen V (eds) *Topley and Wilson's microbiology and microbial infections*, 10th edition, pp. 946–58. Hodder Arnold, London.

Dormitzer PR (2010). Rotaviruses. In: Mandell GL, Bennett JE, Dolin R (eds) *Principles and practice of infectious diseases*, 7th edition, pp. 2105–15.Churchill Livingston Elsevier, Philadelphia.

Estes MK, Kapikian AZ (2007). Rotaviruses. In: Knipe: DM, Howley PM, *et al.* (eds) *Fields Virology*, 5th edition, pp. 1917–74. Lippincott Williams & Wilkins, Philadelphia.

Green KY (2007). Caliciviridae: The noroviruses. In: Knipe DM, Howley PM, *et al.* (eds) Fields Virology, 5th edition, pp. 949–80. Lippincott Williams & Wilkins, Philadelphia.

King CK, *et al.* (2003). Managing acute gastroenteritis among children: oral rehydration, maintenance, and nutritional therapy. *Morb Mort Wkly Rec MMWR*, **52**, 1–16.

Mendez E, Arias CF (2007). Astroviruses. In: Knipe DM, Howley PM, *et al.* (eds) *Fields Virology*, 5th edition, pp. 981–1000. Lippincott Williams & Wilkins, Philadelphia.

Offit PA (1994). Rotaviruses. Immunological determinants of protection against infection and disease. *Adv Virus Res*, **44**, 161–202.

Pesavento JB, *et al.* (2006). Rotavirus proteins: structure and assembly. *Curr Top Microbiol Immunol*, **309**, 189–219.

Vesikari T, *et al.* (2008). European Society for Paediatric Infectious Diseases/European Society for Paediatric Gastroenterology, Hepatology, and Nutrition evidence-based recommendations for rotavirus vaccination in Europe. *J Pediatr Gastroenterol Nutr*, **46**, S38–S48.

Wold WSM, Horowitz MS (2007). Adenoviruses. In: Knipe DM, Howley PM *et al.* (eds) *Fields Virology*, 5th edition, pp. 2395–436. Lippincott Williams & Wilkins, Philadelphia.

7.5.10 Rhabdoviruses: rabies and rabies-related lyssaviruses

M.J. Warrell and David A. Warrell

Essentials

The *Rhabdoviridae* are a large family of RNA viruses, two genera of which infect animals: the genus *Lyssavirus* contains rabies and rabies-related viruses that cause at least 55 000 deaths annually in Asia and Africa.

Transmission and epidemiology

The risks and problems posed by rabies and other lyssaviruses vary across the world. Virus can penetrate broken skin and intact mucosae. Humans are usually infected when virus-laden saliva is inoculated through the skin by the bite of a rabid animal, usually a dog. Although the greatest threat to man is the persistent cycle of infection in stray dogs, several other terrestrial mammal species are reservoirs of infection. In the Americas, bat viruses are also classic genotype 1 rabies and insectivorous bats have become the principal vectors of infection to humans in the United States of America. Elsewhere in the world, there is increasing evidence of widespread rabies-related lyssavirus infection of bats. Unrecognized infection of organ donors has proved fatal to transplant recipients.

Clinical features

After a highly variable incubation period (usually 20 to 90 days), prodromal symptoms include itching at the site of the healed bite wound. These are followed by symptoms of either furious or paralytic rabies, reflecting whether infection of the brain or spinal cord predominates.

Furious rabies—the diagnostic symptom is hydrophobia, a combination of inspiratory muscle spasms, with or without painful laryngopharyngeal spasms, associated with terror, initially provoked by attempts to drink water. Patients may suffer generalized arousal, during which they become wild, hallucinated, fugitive, and rarely aggressive.

Paralytic rabies—flaccid ascending paralysis develops, starting in the bitten limb.

Diagnosis

The diagnosis can be made during life using rapid laboratory methods such as immunofluorescence of brain or punch biopsy specimens of skin taken from a hairy area. The polymerase chain reaction is used increasingly to detect rabies in saliva and skin biopsy material. However, lack of facilities hampers the confirmation of disease in developing countries where the diagnosis usually relies on recognition of hydrophobic spasms and other clinical features of furious rabies. Paralytic disease is rarely identified. Rabies has been misdiagnosed as cerebral malaria, or even drug abuse.

Management and prognosis

The few human survivors of rabies encephalomyelitis had received vaccine and, with one exception were left with severe neurological sequelae. Recently an unvaccinated patient bitten by a bat in North America made a good recovery. However, dog rabies virus infection remains universally fatal in man. Patients with furious rabies rarely live more than one week without intensive care but survival can be up to one month with paralytic disease. The mechanism of neuronal dysfunction remains elusive, and no treatment has proved effective experimentally.

Management—intensive care treatment may be appropriate for patients infected by a bat in the Americas if they present early and are already seropositive. Other patients with rabies should be sedated heavily and given adequate analgesia to relieve their pain and terror.

Prevention

Highly effective methods for control and prevention of rabies are available.

Control of rabies in domestic dogs—95% of human rabies deaths could be prevented by controlling the transmission of dog rabies, but education and resources are lacking.

Pre-exposure prophylaxis—a three-dose course of rabies vaccine is recommended for travellers and indigenous people in dog-rabies endemic areas, but the cost is often prohibitive.

Postexposure prophylaxis—at the time of a bite, correct cleaning of the wound and optimum postexposure immunization virtually eliminate the risk of rabies (compared to c. 45% in untreated cases). Effective prophylaxis demands urgent wound cleaning with copious amounts of soap and water, followed by vaccine and rabies immunoglobulin. A new improved economical 4-site intradermal postexposure vaccine regimen could increase the availability of affordable treatment in developing countries.

Epidemiology

Rabies is a zoonosis of mammals that remains endemic in most parts of the world (Fig. 7.5.10.1). A cycle of infection is maintained in several reservoir species, of which the domestic dog is by far the most important. Many wild mammals including bats are also independent rabies reservoirs (sylvatic infection) with identifiable strains of virus. Any mammalian species is potentially susceptible to rabies and may be a vector, e.g. a cat infected by a dog may then bite and infect a person. However, there is no persistent virus transmission between cats. The vector origin of human disease depends on the likelihood of contact with an infected animal. Hence domestic dogs and cats are the source of more than 95% of human cases worldwide, mainly in Africa, Asia, and parts of South America. Rabies control programmes can reduce the risk of rabies in domestic animals to such an extent that wild animals, e.g. insectivorous bats in the United States of America, become the principal vectors of infection to humans. Rabies in wild mammals is usually spread by bites or by ingestion of infected prey.

Rabies and rabies-related viruses

The *Lyssavirus* genus currently includes classic rabies virus, genotype 1, and six rabies-related genotypes that are continent-specific in Europe, Australasia, and Africa, and are, with one exception, zoonoses of bats (Fig. 7.5.10.2) (see also 'Rabies-related viruses known to infect humans'). All but Lagos bat virus have caused fatal human disease. New unclassified lyssaviruses are now emerging. No rabies-related viruses have been found in the Americas. All terrestrial rabies reservoir mammal species (dogs and wildlife) carry genotype 1 rabies, except for the rare Mokola virus in Africa.

Countries currently reported as rabies free include Iceland, Norway, Sweden, Finland, Portugal, Greece, Cyprus and most other Mediterranean islands, Singapore, Sabah, Sarawak, Antarctica, Oceania (including New Guinea and New Zealand), Hong Kong islands (but not the New Territories), Japan, South Korea, Taiwan, and Caribbean islands with the notable exceptions of Cuba, the Dominican Republic, Grenada, Haiti, and Trinidad and Tobago. The British Isles, together with other Western European countries, and Australia have no rabies in terrestrial species, but do harbour rabies-related lyssaviruses in bats (Fig. 7.5.10.1). Inadvertent importation of infected animals is a global risk.

Cyclical epizootics of rabies may result from an uncontrolled increase in the population of the key reservoir species, such as the fox epizootic in Europe in the late 20th century. This started in Poland and spread across France, but it has now been eliminated from Western Europe. The AIDS pandemic has increased indirectly the risk of rabies infection in South Africa because many dogs abandoned by people who are sick or dying from AIDS have become feral and rove in packs. Outbreaks in dogs have also followed the movement of refugees.

Although the fox is one of the species most susceptible to rabies, about 3% of animals survive the infection and become immune. Seropositive bats are not uncommon, and rabies antibody has been found in several other species, exceptionally even in dogs. There is no evidence that animals can become chronically infected or be infectious carriers, although an apparently healthy animal may be infectious during the prodromal stage of infection.

Wild mammal reservoir species

Wild mammal reservoir species vary in different areas.

North America

Reservoir species in the central United States of America and California are striped skunks *Mephitis mephitis* and, to a lesser extent, spotted skunks *Spilogale putorius*; in Arizona and Texas grey foxes *Urocyon cinereoargenteus* and red foxes *Vulpes vulpes*; and in Alaska arctic foxes *Alopex lagopus*. However, in the east, rabies is most commonly found in raccoons *Procyon lotor* that transmit it to skunks and foxes. In North America many insectivorous bats are reservoirs, including big brown bats *Eptesicus fuscus*, Mexican free-tailed bats *Tadarida brasiliensis mexicana*, little brown bats *Myotis lucifugus*, and silver-haired bats *Lasionycteris noctivagans* whose virus is the main cause of human rabies infections in the United States of America (see below) where bat infection has been found in every state except Hawaii. All bat rabies in the Americas is due to genotype 1 virus.

Latin America and the Caribbean

Dog rabies persists in some urban areas of South America despite successful control programmes. The three species of true vampire bats *Desmodus rotundus*, *Diaemus youngi*, and *Diphylla ecaudata* (Desmodontinae) occur from sea level to over 3500 m but usually

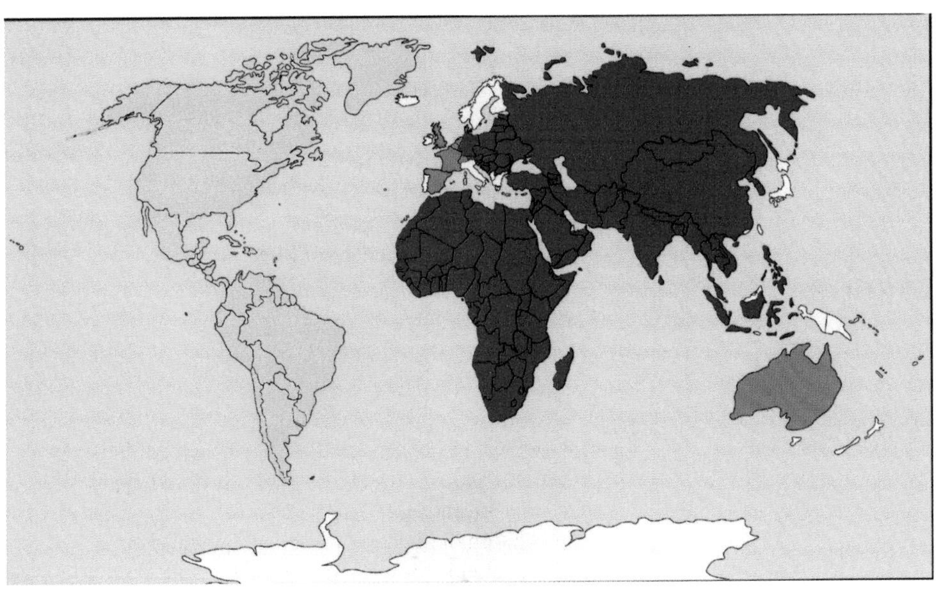

Fig. 7.5.10.1 Global distribution of rabies.

below 1500 m only in Mexico, Central and South America, and some Caribbean Islands (Fig. 7.5.10.3). The common vampire bat *D. rotundus* (Fig. 7.5.10.4) is the main reservoir of vampire bat rabies in Trinidad, Mexico, and Central and South America, where humans are occasionally bitten (Fig. 7.5.10.5). Carnivorous bats of the family Megadermatidae, such as the Indian 'vampire' *Megaderma lyra*, have given rise to the myth that vampires occur elsewhere. In Latin America, thousands of head of cattle are lost each year from vampire bat-transmitted paralytic rabies (derriengue) with locally serious economic consequences. Mongooses *Herpestes auropunctatus* are reservoirs of sylvatic rabies in Central America, Grenada, Puerto Rico, Cuba, Haiti, and the Dominican Republic.

Africa and Asia

Dog rabies predominates but there is sylvatic rabies in Africa in foxes, wolves, jackals, and small carnivores of the families Mustelidae and Viverridae (e.g. the yellow mongoose *Cynictis penicillata* in South Africa), and in Asia in wolves, jackals, ferret-badgers *Melogale moschata* in China, and palm civets *Paradoxurus hermaphroditus* in Indonesia.

Europe

Foxes, wolves, raccoon dogs *Nyctereutes procyonoides*, and insectivorous bats are infected (see also 'Rabies-related viruses known to infect humans').

Rodents

There are reports of rabies virus being isolated from wild rodents in many countries but there is no evidence that they are a reservoir species or that rodent bites, which are very common in some places, pose a threat of rabies.

Incidence of human rabies

The true incidence of human rabies throughout the world is not reflected in official figures; 55 000 deaths annually have been estimated to occur in Asia and Africa, including about 20 000 in India alone. However, it is suggested that only 3% of cases are recorded. High mortalities also occur in Bangladesh and Pakistan, and recently the incidence has been rising in China. There are very few data from Africa. In Latin America, mortality from canine rabies persists in Brazil, El Salvador, Mexico, Bolivia, Colombia, Venezuela, and Haiti. There have been recent outbreaks due to vampire bat rabies in Peru, Ecuador, and Brazil. In the United States of America there are on average two human deaths annually. Among 37 indigenous infections occurring in the last 40 years, 92% were caused by insectivorous bats. Europe reported 45 deaths in the last 5 years, mainly from the Russian Federation and the Ukraine. Rabies was apparently eliminated from the United Kingdom by 1903, but, since 1980, there have been nine imported cases and one indigenous European bat lyssavirus infection.

Virology

The Rhabdoviridae are a family of more than 100 rod-shaped or bullet-shaped RNA viruses found in vertebrates, insects, and plants (Fig. 7.5.10.6). Two genera infect animals, *Vesiculovirus* and

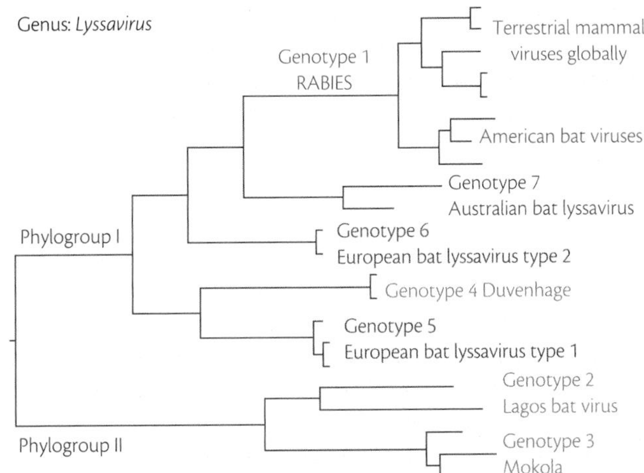

Fig. 7.5.10.2 Phylogenetic relationships between whole genomes of the lyssaviruses. Viruses in green type are confined to Africa.
(From Delmas O, *et al.* (2008). Genomic diversity and evolution of the lyssaviruses. *PLoS One*, **3**, e2057, with permission.)

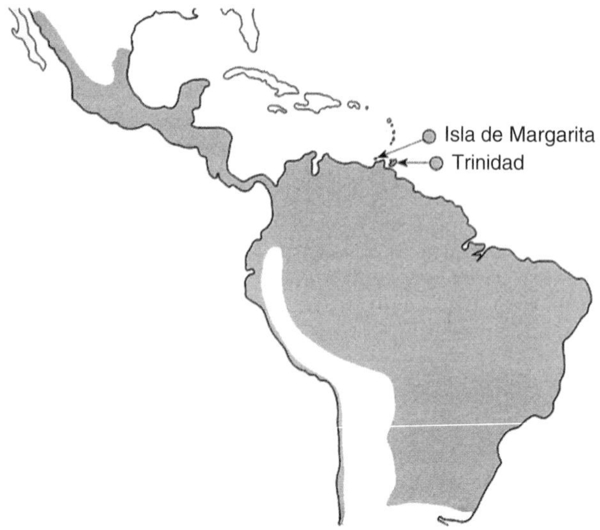

Fig. 7.5.10.3 Distribution of the three species of true vampire bats (Desmodontinae).

Lyssavirus. Vesicular stomatitis virus is a vesiculovirus of cattle and horses, which occasionally causes an influenza-like illness in farmers or laboratory workers. The genus *Lyssavirus* contains rabies and rabies-related viruses.

The rabies virion is approximately 180 × 75 nm. Its core is a single spiral strand of negative nonsegmented RNA associated with a nucleoprotein, a phosphoprotein, and an RNA polymerase to form a helical ribonucleoprotein (RNP) complex. This is enveloped in a matrix protein, host cell-derived lipid, and a coat of protruding glycoprotein (G) molecules bearing spikes or knobs 10 nm long. The composition of the glycoprotein determines viral virulence.

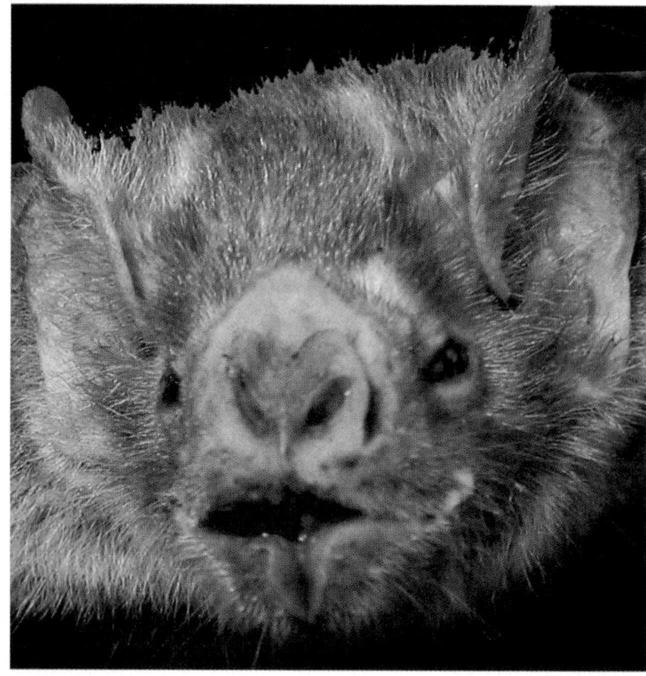

Fig. 7.5.10.4 *Desmodus rotundus* (Peru).
(Courtesy of Dr Vargas Meneses, Lima, Peru.)

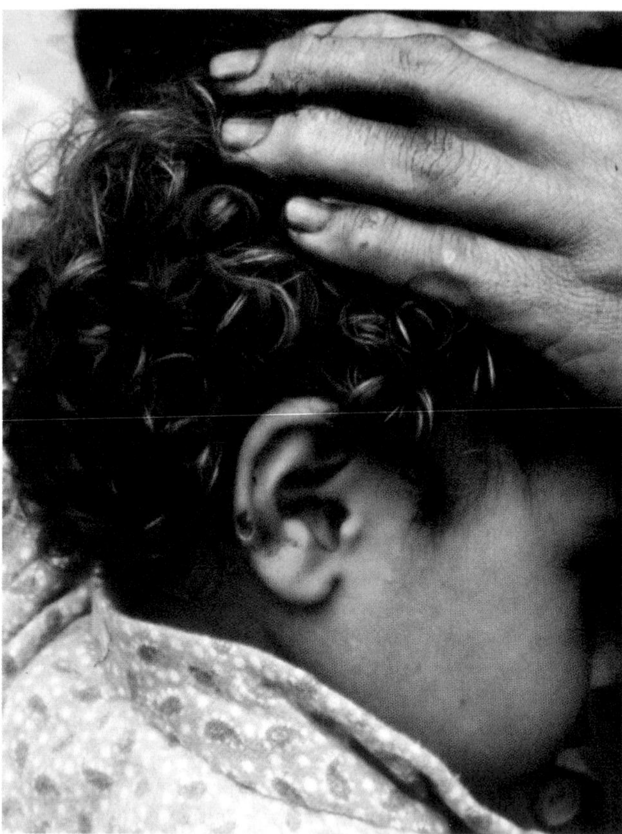

Fig. 7.5.10.5 Vampire bat bite inflicted on the ear of a sleeping child in Tapirái, São Paulo, Brazil.
(Courtesy of Dr João Luiz Costa Cardoso, São Paulo, Brazil.)

The virus is readily inactivated by ultraviolet light, drying, boiling, most organic lipid solvents including at least 45% ethanol, soap solution, detergents, hypochlorite, and glutaraldehyde solutions.

Typing by means of monoclonal antibodies or genetic sequencing techniques allows the identification of diverse strains of rabies and rabies-related viruses from different geographical areas and vector species.

Transmission

Virus can penetrate broken skin and intact mucosae. Humans are usually infected when virus-laden saliva is inoculated through the skin by the bite of a rabid dog or other mammal (Fig. 7.5.10.7). Saliva from a rabid animal can infect if the skin is already broken, e.g. by the animal's claws. In North America, contact with bats leading to rabies has passed unnoticed; only 39% of patients reported a bat bite and 34% had no history of exposure to bats. Animals can be infected through the gastrointestinal tract, but there is no evidence that this happens in humans.

Inhalation of aerosolized virus created by infected nasal secretions of bats may be an important method of transmission among cave-dwelling bats. In Texas, two men died of rabies after visiting caves inhabited by millions of Mexican free-tailed bats *Tadarida brasiliensis mexicana*, some of which were rabid, however fleeting bat contact may have caused the infection. Two laboratory workers in the United States of America developed rabies after inhaling

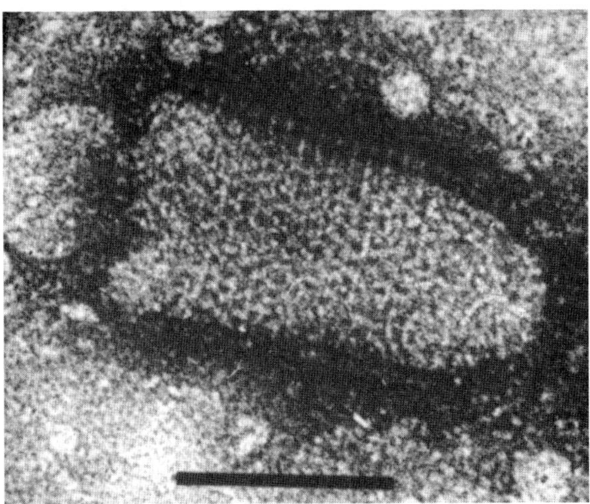

Fig. 7.5.10.6 Rhabdoviruses. Virion of rabies virus.
(Note the surface projections composed glycoprotein (G). The marker line is 100 nanometres long)

aerosolized fixed strains of rabies virus during the preparation of vaccines. The accidental use of vaccine in which the virus was not inactivated has led to fixed virus rabies (rage de laboratoire), e.g. in Fortaleza, Brazil in 1960.

Transmission of rabies between people has been proved in 13 cases of tissue transplantation from donors who had died of undiagnosed neurological diseases. Six recipients of infected corneal grafts developed retro-orbital headache on the side of the graft 22 to 39 days after transplantation and died soon afterwards (other infections spread by corneal grafts include Creutzfeldt–Jakob disease and cryptococcosis). In Texas and Germany, seven recipients of kidney, liver, lung, pancreas, or even just a segment of iliac artery developed rabies encephalitis. Rabies was not suspected in the two young donors despite a history of recent rough travel in India in one and later discovery of a bat bite in the other. Recreational drug abuse was detected in both. One surviving liver transplant patient had had rabies vaccine previously. Postexposure prophylaxis following corneal transplants from infected donors has been successful.

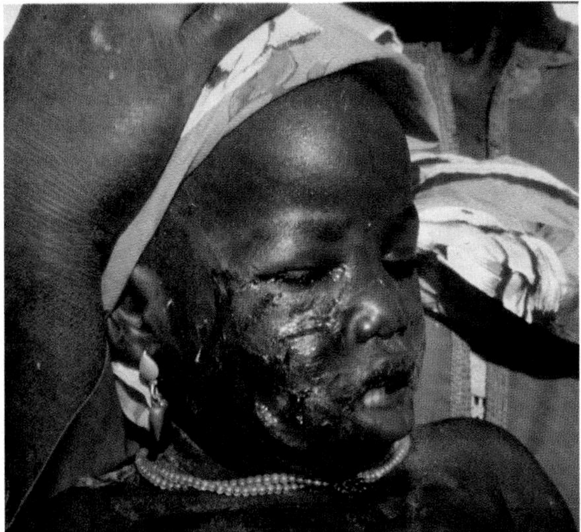

Fig. 7.5.10.7 Child bitten on the face by a rabid dog. This wound carries a high risk of rabies with a short incubation period.
(Copyright D A Warrell.)

Considering that the saliva, respiratory secretions, and tears of rabies patients contain virus, it is surprising that the disease has not been spread to intimate relatives and nurses.

Transplacental infection has been observed in animals but has only been reported once in humans. Several women with rabies encephalitis have given birth to healthy babies. The transmission of rabies from mother to suckling infant via the breast milk has been suspected in at least one human case and is well known in animals.

Pathogenesis

The mechanism by which the highly neurotropic rabies virus enters the nervous system and travels into the brain and out again to many organs is intriguing. The virus may replicate locally in muscle cells or attach directly to nerve endings. It can bind to many types of receptors including the neural cell adhesion molecule and the nicotinic acetylcholine receptors at motor endplates, which are blocked by α-bungarotoxin. Several other neuronal binding mechanisms may be involved. Once inside peripheral nerves, virus travels in a strictly retrograde direction within the axoplasm. This progression can be blocked experimentally by local anaesthetics, metabolic inhibitors, and nerve section. The axonal dynein molecular motor is assumed to be the vehicle of transport but the attachment mechanism is elusive. Viral binding might be directly via the naked ribonucleoprotein complex or indirectly as a vesicle containing a whole virion. Rabies virus is experimentally inaccessible to antibodies while concealed in the peripheral nerves.

On reaching the central nervous system, the virus replicates massively within neurons and is transmitted directly from cell to cell across synaptic junctions. Dramatic symptoms can appear before histopathological changes are apparent. Viral virulence is inversely related to neuronal apoptosis. Rabies alters host cell gene expression, but the mechanisms of gross neuronal dysfunction are speculative. Centrifugal spread of virus from the central nervous system, apparently in the axoplasm of somatic and autonomic efferent nerves, deposits virus in many tissues including skeletal and cardiac muscle, adrenal medulla where infection may be clinically significant, and also in kidney, retina, cornea, pancreas, taste buds, respiratory tract, and the skin in nerve twiglets around hair follicles (see below 'Laboratory diagnosis'). At this stage, productive viral replication occurs, with budding from outer cell membranes in the salivary and lacrimal glands. This is how rabies is transmitted by bites to other mammals. Viraemia has been detected very rarely, only in animals, and is not thought to be involved in pathogenesis or spread.

Immunology

Immunological response to rabies infection in humans

Some patients die without any detectable immune response, suggesting that rabies virus evades or suppresses the immune system. Rabies antibody might become detectable in serum 7 days or more after the onset of illness and in cerebrospinal fluid a little later. It may rise to high levels in patients whose lives are prolonged by intensive care. A small amount of rabies-specific IgM is sometimes detectable, but is not useful as a means of diagnosis.

There is little evidence of a lymphocyte-mediated immune response to rabies encephalitis. A pleocytosis appears in only 60% of patients, with a mean leucocyte count of 75×10^3/mm. Peripheral blood lymphocyte transformation has been shown in a few patients with furious rabies, but not in those with paralytic disease. Experimentally, in fatal rabies there is suppression of the cytotoxic T-lymphocyte response to unrelated viral antigens and a T-cell response is associated with survival in mice.

Interferon is induced by rabies infection, but appears to be at a very low level in human patients. In animals, latent infections can be reactivated by corticosteroids and stress. This provides a possible explanation for occasional reports of long incubation periods.

Immunological response to rabies vaccination

The viral glycoprotein induces neutralizing antibody, which is detectable by 2 weeks after the start of primary immunization. In animal studies, the neutralizing antibody titre is the best available measure of protection against death. The nucleoprotein antigens also stimulate antibody that is more cross-reactive between lyssaviruses than the more strain-specific glycoprotein. Although peripheral blood lymphocyte transformation occurs following human vaccination, the role of T lymphocytes in protection remains to be demonstrated.

Although neutralizing antibody is undoubtedly protective in the early stages after inoculation of virus, it may be deleterious once central nervous system infection is established. In animals, acceleration of the terminal phase of the encephalitis ('early death phenomenon') is associated with the presence of low titres of rabies antibody.

Transient low levels of interferon may be induced after the first dose of tissue culture rabies vaccines. Interferon is effective postexposure prophylaxis against experimental rabies.

Rabies in animals

All warm-blooded animals can be infected with rabies but their susceptibility varies. However, only mammals are infected naturally.

In dogs, the incubation period ranges from 5 days to 14 months, but is usually between 3 and 12 weeks. The first symptom, as in many humans, is intense irritation at the site of the infection. Despite the popular idea of the 'mad' rabid dog, probably only a minority develop furious rabies. There is an early and striking change in the dog's behaviour with dysphagia, ptosis, altered bark, paralysis of the jaw, neck, and hind limbs (Fig. 7.5.10.8), hypersalivation, congested conjunctivae, pruritus, shivering, trembling, snapping at imaginary objects, pica, and extreme restlessness causing the animal to wander miles from home. Dogs with furious rabies attack inanimate objects, often seriously injuring their mouths in the process. Virus has been found in the saliva 3 days before symptoms appear, and the animal usually dies within the next 7 days.

This is the basis for the traditional 10-day observation period for dogs that have bitten humans. Very rare old reports from India, Ethiopia, and Nigeria of persistent or intermittent excretion of virus in the saliva of apparently healthy dogs have not been confirmed by subsequent thorough searches. 'Oulou fato', a clinical variant of canine rabies with reduced virulence, was seen in West Africa 50 years ago. In Tanzania, a rabies virus of apparently low virulence has been identified in hyenas.

Rabid foxes lose their fear of humans and the majority develop paralytic rabies. An extreme degree of furious rabies is seen in 75% of infected cats. Cattle usually develop paralytic symptoms with dysphagia, hypersalivation, groaning, trembling, colic, diarrhoea, tenesmus, and rectal prolapse. Most other domestic ungulates develop paralytic symptoms. Horses often show furious features with sexual excitement. Most wild animals, like foxes, lose their fear of humans and may appear tame. Rabid skunks, raccoons, badgers, martens, and mongooses may become very aggressive. Dysphagia and inability to drink is common in rabid animals, but they do not exhibit hydrophobia.

Clinical features in humans

The incubation period ranges from 4 days to many years, but it is between 20 and 90 days in three-quarters of cases. It tends to be shorter after bites on the face (average 35 days) than after those on the limbs (average 52 days).

Prodromal symptoms

Often, the first symptom is itching, pain, or paraesthesia at the site of the healed bite wound (Fig. 7.5.10.9). Nonspecific prodromal symptoms include fever, chills, malaise, weakness, tiredness, headache, photophobia, myalgia, anxiety, depression, irritability, and symptoms of upper respiratory tract and gastrointestinal infections. Subsequently, symptoms of either furious or paralytic rabies will develop, depending on whether the spinal cord or brain are predominantly infected.

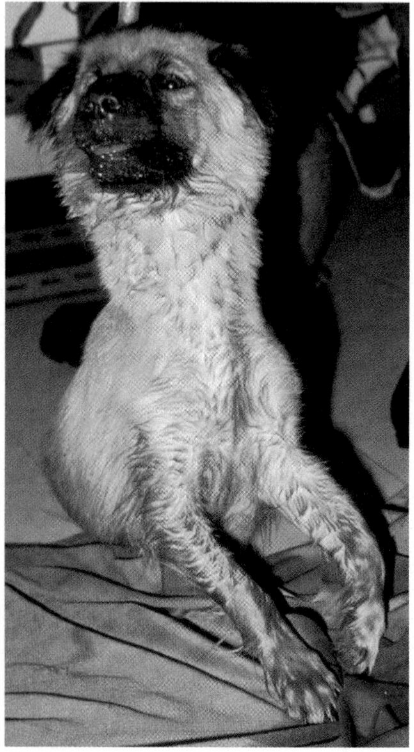

Fig. 7.5.10.8 Dog with paralytic rabies showing paralysis of the limbs and hypersalivation.
(Copyright D A Warrell.)

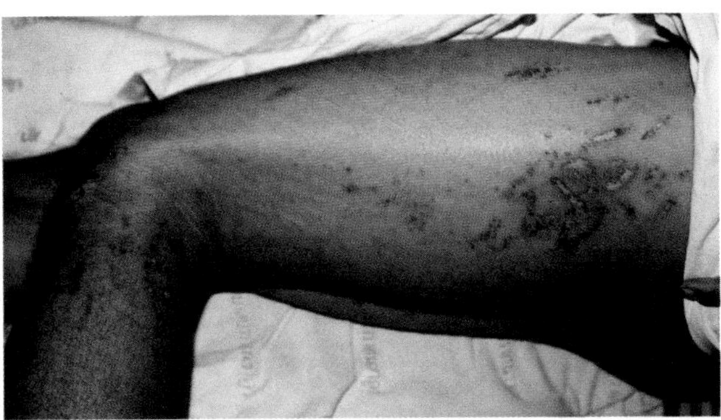

Fig. 7.5.10.9 This man developed intense itching in the left leg, provoking scratching and excoriation, 6 weeks after being bitten in that limb by a rabid dog. He died with furious rabies a few days later.
(Courtesy of the late Professor Sornchai Looaresuwan.)

Furious rabies

Furious rabies is the more common presentation. Most patients have the diagnostic symptom of hydrophobia, which is a combination of inspiratory muscle spasm, with or without painful laryngopharyngeal spasm, associated with terror (Fig. 7.5.10.10a–e). Initially provoked by attempts to drink water, this reflex can be excited by a variety of stimuli including a draught of air ('aerophobia'), water splashed on the skin, irritation of the respiratory tract or, ultimately, by the sight, sound, or even mention of water. The inspiratory spasm is violent and jerky. The neck and back are extended, the arms thrown up, and the episode may end with a generalized convulsion complicated by cardiac or respiratory arrest.

Patients experience hyperaesthesia and, at times, generalized arousal during which they become wild, hallucinated, fugitive, and sometimes aggressive (Fig. 7.5.10.11). This behaviour alternates with periods of mental lucidity during which patients may become distressingly aware of their predicament. Despite these dramatic symptoms, attributable to brainstem encephalitis, conventional neurological examination may prove surprisingly normal, leading to the false assumption of hysteria. Reported abnormalities include meningism, cranial nerve lesions (especially III, VI, VII, IX–XII), upper motor neuron lesions, fasciculation, and involuntary movements. Disturbances of the hypothalamus or autonomic nervous system are reflected by hypersalivation (Fig. 7.5.10.12), sweating, lacrimation, hypertension or hypotension, hyperthermia or hypothermia, inappropriate secretion of antidiuretic hormone or diabetes insipidus, and, rarely, priapism with spontaneous orgasms, satyriasis, or nymphomania. Hypersexuality suggests similar aetiology to the Klüver–Bucy syndrome created in rhesus monkeys by bilateral ablation of the hippocampus.

Without supportive treatment, about one-third of the patients will die during a hydrophobic spasm during the first few days. The rest lapse into coma and generalized flaccid paralysis, and rarely survive for more than a week without intensive care.

Paralytic or dumb rabies

This is the clinical pattern in less than one-fifth of human cases except in the case of bat-transmitted rabies, especially vampire bat infection, which is usually paralytic. Patients may become literally dumb ('rage muette') because their laryngeal muscles are paralysed, but symptoms are quieter ('rage tranquille') than in furious rabies. The largest reported outbreak was in Trinidad between 1925 and 1935 when there were 89 human cases, initially misattributed to poliomyelitis or botulism; others have been described from Mexico, Guyana, Brazil, Peru, Ecuador, Bolivia, and Argentina. The paralytic form of rabies was also seen in patients with post-vaccinal rabies, in the two patients who inhaled fixed virus, and is said to be more likely to develop in patients who have received antirabies vaccine. After the usual prodromal symptoms, especially fever, headache, and local paraesthesias, flaccid paralysis develops, usually in the bitten limb, and ascends symmetrically or asymmetrically with pain and fasciculation in the affected muscles and mild sensory disturbances. Paraplegia and sphincter involvement then develop, and finally fatal paralysis of deglutitive and respiratory muscles (Fig. 7.5.10.13). Hydrophobia is unusual, but may be represented by a few pharyngeal spasms in the terminal phase of the illness. Even without intensive care, patients with paralytic rabies have survived for up to 30 days.

Other manifestations and complications

Respiratory system

Asphyxiation and respiratory arrest may complicate the hydrophobic spasms or generalized convulsions of furious rabies and the bulbar and respiratory paralysis of dumb rabies. Bronchopneumonia is a predictable complication if life is prolonged by intensive care, but a primary rabies pneumonitis may occur. Various abnormal patterns of respiration have been described, including cluster and apneustic breathing. There are some similarities to respiratory myoclonus. Pneumothorax may complicate inspiratory spasms.

Cardiovascular system

A variety of dangerous cardiac arrhythmias have been reported, including supraventricular tachycardias, sinus bradycardia, atrioventricular block, and sinus arrest, together with T wave and ST segment changes (Fig. 7.5.10.14). Hypotension, pulmonary oedema, and congestive cardiac failure are attributable to myocarditis.

Nervous system

Raised intracranial pressure resulting from cerebral oedema or internal hydrocephalus has been reported in a few cases, but spinal fluid opening pressure is usually normal and papilloedema is rarely seen. There is clinical and electrophysiological evidence of diffuse axonal neuropathy, consistent with histological appearances of degeneration of peripheral nerve ganglia and axons.

Gastrointestinal system

'Stress' ulcers and the Mallory–Weiss syndrome are possible explanations for the haematemesis often reported in rabies.

Clinical and differential diagnosis

Rabies should be suspected in any patient who develops neurological symptoms after being bitten by a mammal in a rabies endemic area. However, some patients fail to remember that they have been bitten and others may be infected while they are asleep possibly by contact with lip mucosae (North American insectivorous bats) or near-painless bites by vampire bats in parts of Latin America.

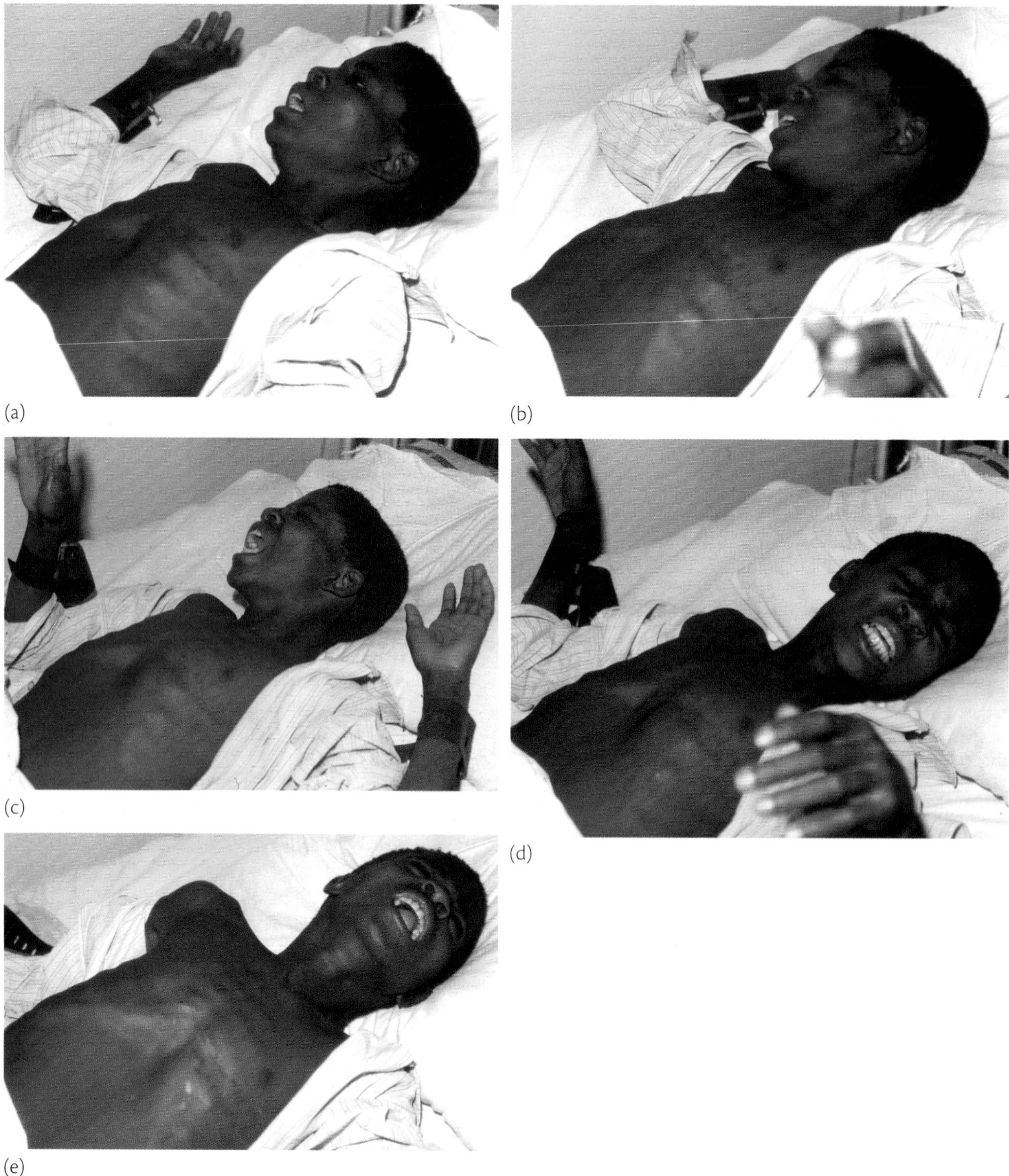

Fig. 7.5.10.10 (a–e) Hydrophobic spasm in a 14-year-old Nigerian boy with furious rabies. Note the violent contraction of inspiratory muscles, sternomastoids and diaphragm, depressing xiphisternum.
(Copyright D A Warrell.)

Furious rabies

Pathognomonic inspiratory spasms with associated emotional response are provoked by asking the patient to swallow accumulated saliva or by directing a draught of air on to the face.

- Psychiatric conditions: Rabies encephalitis has been misdiagnosed as a variety of psychiatric conditions, including hysteria and behavioural disturbances attributed to recreational drugs. Conversely, patients with a morbid fear of rabies (rabies phobia, lyssaphobia, pseudohydrophobia) may simulate the more melodramatic features of the disease but hydrophobia is unlikely to be mimicked accurately, the incubation period after the bite (hours or a few days) is usually much too short for rabies encephalitis, and the prognosis is, of course, excellent.

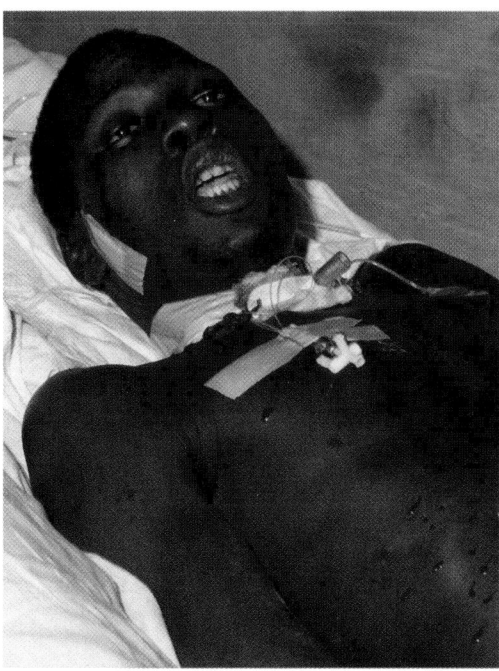

Fig. 7.5.10.11 Episode of intense arousal in a Nigerian patient with furious rabies.
(Copyright D A Warrell.)

- Otolaryngological conditions: Pharyngeal and upper airway symptoms of hydrophobia may be misinterpreted as pharyngitis or laryngitis so that the patient is referred to an otolaryngologist.
- Tetanus: This can also follow an animal bite and is similar to rabies in some respects, especially the pharyngeal form of cephalic tetanus ('hydrophobic tetanus'). It is distinguished by its shorter incubation period (usually less than 15 days in severe tetanus), the presence of trismus, the persistence of muscle rigidity between spasms, the absence of meningoencephalitis (cerebrospinal fluid is universally normal), and the better prognosis.
- Other encephalopathies/encephalitides: The typical encephalitic progression from severe headache to continuous coma is unusual in furious rabies. Hydrophobia with intermittent excitation and lucid intervals of full consciousness does not occur in other encephalitides. Among children with suspected cerebral malaria in Malawi, some were proved at biopsy to have died of rabies.
- Toxic encephalopathies: Delirium tremens, some drugs (phenothiazines, amphetamines, modafinil, cocaine, and other recreational drugs), and plant poisonings (e.g. *Datura fastuosa*) can cause excitable and aggressive behaviour that might be confused with rabies.

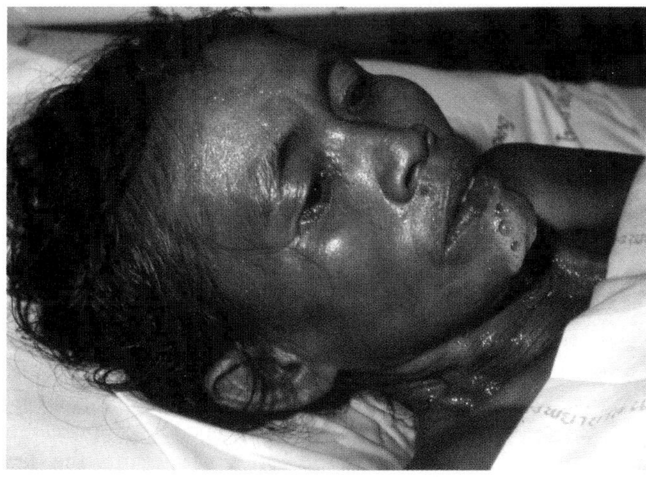

Fig. 7.5.10.12 Hypersalivation in a Thai woman with furious rabies.
(Copyright D A Warrell.)

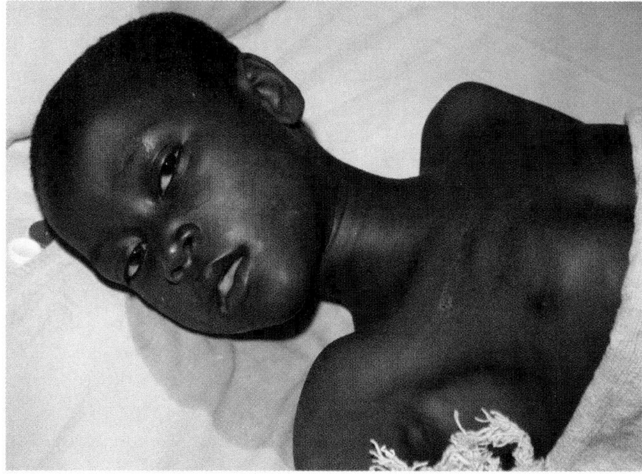

Fig. 7.5.10.13 Paralytic rabies.
(Copyright D A Warrell.)

Paralytic rabies

Other causes of ascending (Landry-type) paralysis may enter the differential diagnosis.

- Postvaccinal encephalomyelitis (see below): This usually develops within 2 weeks of the first dose of the now rarely used nervous tissue rabies vaccines.
- Poliomyelitis: Objective sensory disturbances are absent and fever rarely persists after paralysis has developed.
- Acute inflammatory polyneuropathy (Guillain–Barré syndrome): Cerebrospinal fluid examination will help to distinguish this condition.
- *Cercopithecine herpesvirus* (B virus) encephalomyelitis: Bites and other types of contact with Asian macaque monkeys (genus *Macaca*), especially rhesus (*M. mulatta*) and cynomolgus (*M. fascicularis*) transmit this dangerous infection. The incubation

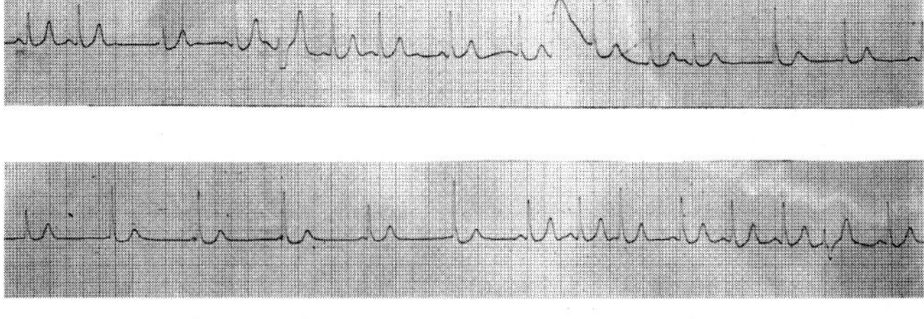

Fig. 7.5.10.14 Electrocardiogram in a Nigerian patient with furious rabies showing sinus tachycardia, atrial and ventricular premature beats, and a wandering atrial pacemaker.
(Copyright D A Warrell.)

period (3–4 days) is usually shorter than in rabies and symptoms develop within 1 month of contact. Vesicles may be found in the monkey's mouth and at the site of the bite, and the diagnosis can be confirmed virologically.

Pathology

The brain, spinal cord, and peripheral nerves show ganglion cell degeneration, perineural and perivascular mononuclear cell infiltration, neuronophagia, and glial nodules. Inflammatory changes are most marked in the midbrain and medulla (Fig. 7.5.10.15) in furious rabies and in the spinal cord in paralytic rabies.

Negri bodies (Fig. 7.5.10.16) are eosinophilic intracytoplasmic inclusions predominantly consisting of masses of viral ribonucleoprotein, with a basophilic inner body containing fragments of cellular organelles including ribosomes and occasional virions. They can be demonstrated by haematoxylin and eosin stains in histological sections of grey matter in up to 75% of human cases, especially in hippocampal pyramidal cells and cerebellar Purkinje cells.

In view of the appalling prognosis of rabies encephalitis, neuronolysis is often surprisingly mild and patchy, and death can occur without any inflammatory response. Vascular lesions such as thrombosis and haemorrhage have also been described. The brainstem, limbic system, and hypothalamus appear to be most severely affected and, in paralytic disease, the spinal cord and medulla. Outside the nervous system, there is focal degeneration of salivary and lacrimal glands, pancreas, adrenal medulla, and lymph nodes. An interstitial myocarditis with round cell infiltration is found in about 25% of cases.

Laboratory diagnosis

If a mammal suspected of being rabid has bitten, scratched, or otherwise risked infecting a person, it should be killed and its brain examined without delay. The best way to detect rabies antigen in acetone-fixed brain impression smears is by the direct immunofluorescent antibody (IFA) test. Alternatively, if no fluorescent microscope is available, rapid enzyme immunodiagnosis can be used. Sellers' stain is insensitive and rarely used. Virus isolation takes up to 3 weeks by intracerebral inoculation of mice, or about 4 days in murine neuroblastoma cell culture.

In humans, rabies can be confirmed early in the illness by demonstration of viral antigen by the direct IFA test in frozen sections of full-thickness skin biopsies taken from a hairy area, usually the nape of the neck. Specific diagnostic staining is seen in nerve twiglets around the base of hair follicles (Fig. 7.5.10.17). This rapid method is positive in 60 to 100% of cases, and no false-positive results have been reported. Antigen can also be found in brain biopsies, but tests on corneal impression smears are usually falsely negative. The polymerase chain reaction is being used increasingly to detect rabies in saliva, and occasionally cerebrospinal fluid, and also skin biopsy material.

During the first week of illness, virus may be detected in saliva, brain, cerebrospinal fluid, and very rarely urine. Rabies antibodies are not usually detectable in serum or cerebrospinal fluid before the eighth day of illness in unvaccinated patients. Serum antibody may leak into the cerebrospinal fluid in patients with postvaccinal encephalomyelitis, but a very high titre suggests a diagnosis of rabies. A specific IgM test has not proved useful diagnostically.

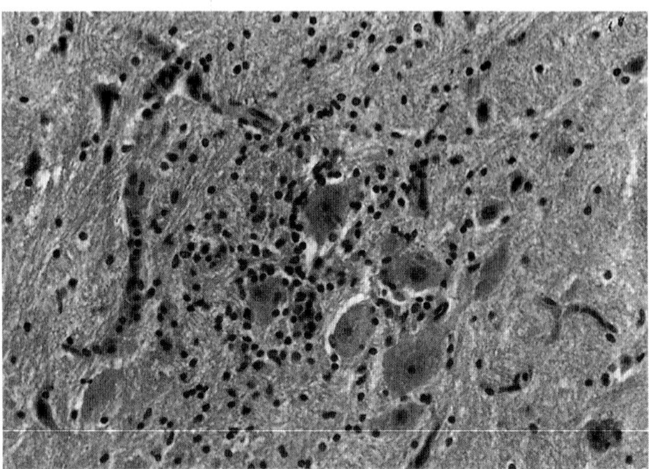

Fig. 7.5.10.15 Inflammatory cells around neurons in the central medulla (para-ambigualis region) of a patient who died of rabies encephalitis. Magnification × 400.
(Courtesy of Dr P Lewis, London.)

Treatment

Patients with rabies must be sedated heavily and given adequate analgesia to relieve their pain and terror. If intensive care is undertaken, the aim is to prevent complications such as cardiac arrhythmias, cardiac and respiratory failure, raised intracranial pressure, convulsions, fluid and electrolyte disturbances including diabetes insipidus and inappropriate secretion of antidiuretic hormone, and hyperpyrexia. Antiserum, antiviral agents, interferon-α, corticosteroid, and other immunosuppressants have proved useless.

Prognosis

Rabies was formerly regarded as a universally fatal disease, but there are reports of seven cases of recovery or prolonged survival following intensive care. All the diagnoses were made serologically and no virus or antigen was identified. Two patients had been given postexposure prophylaxis with nervous tissue vaccines and then intensive care. Four further patients, a microbiologist who inhaled

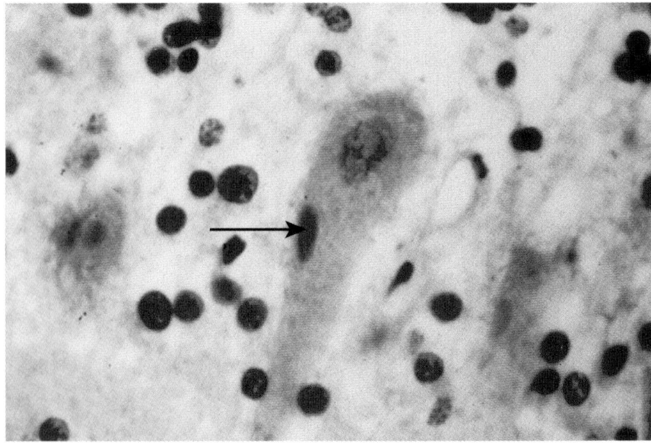

Fig. 7.5.10.16 Street virus in human cerebellar Purkinje cells as seen with the light microscope. Several Negri bodies can be seen (one is arrowed). Magnification × 615.
(Courtesy of Armed Forces Institute of Pathology 73–12 330.)

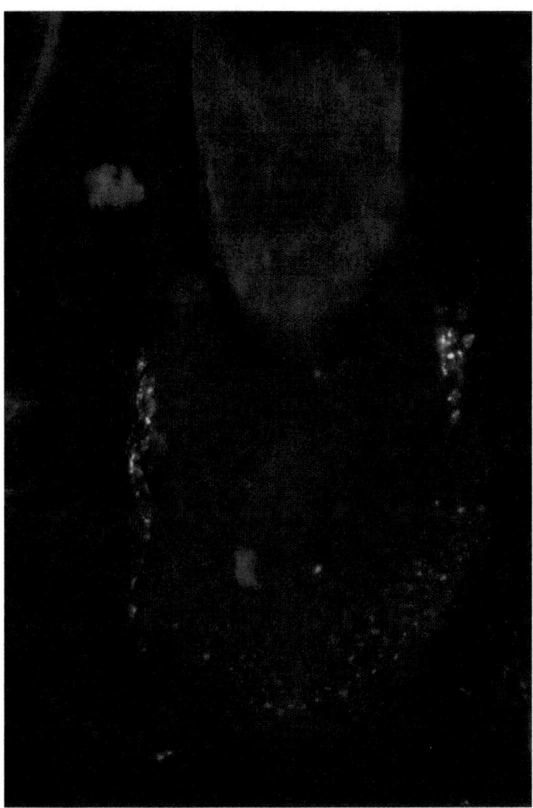

Fig. 7.5.10.17 Diagnosis of human rabies during life. Vertical section through a hair follicle and shaft showing fluorescence of nerve cells around the follicle indicating the presence of rabies antigen. Magnification × 250.
(Copyright M J Warrell.)

fixed rabies virus, two boys in Mexico, and a girl in India, were given pre-exposure or postexposure tissue culture vaccines, and survived months or years with profound neurological impairment.

The first unvaccinated patient to survive rabies has returned to near normal life following intensive care and antiviral therapy. She was bitten by a bat in Wisconsin in 2004, had no rabies prophylaxis, and developed typical encephalitis without hydrophobia. Rabies neutralizing antibody was detected on the sixth day of illness. Treatment comprised coma induction and antiviral drugs. She made a slow recovery over 5 years and has returned to normal life, although with minor neurological deficits. The antiviral treatments have not proved effective against rabies experimentally; however, she developed antibody at an early stage of the disease. Her treatment possibly maintained her vital functions until the spontaneous specific immunity immune response eliminated the virus, probably with loss of infected neurons. In animal experiments, American bat rabies virus infection differs from that of canine virus in that it is slower to evolve and progress, virus replication is not restricted to neurons, and histopathological changes are milder with less apoptosis. This suggests that the virus maybe less pathogenic and may also explain the complete recovery of a boy infected by a similar virus in 1970 who had delayed treatment with a nervous tissue vaccine. It is likely that he too had rabies antibody present at an early stage of illness.

The treatment protocol used in Wisconsin has since been used unsuccessfully in several other patients with rabies encephalitis who were infected by bats or dogs. Recently, however, a vaccinated Brazilian boy bitten by a bat survived symptomatic rabies, but the residual neurological deficits are unknown.

No treatment has proved effective in animal models. Human rabies of canine origin remains 100% fatal. Until a new treatment is proved effective experimentally, palliation of the patient and immunization of contacts is recommended. Intensive treatment may be appropriate for patients infected by an American bat, who present early, and are already seropositive. Intensive care treatment is inappropriate for canine virus infection, especially in developing countries, and the cost is prohibitive.

Control of rabies in animals

The elimination of dog rabies would reduce the human mortality by over 95% and drastically reduce the need for human vaccination. Rabies control has been achieved most effectively where the principal reservoir is the domestic dog, as in 19th-century United Kingdom, Malaysia, and Japan, and since then in other areas including Western Europe, Taiwan, North America, and parts of urban Latin America.

In countries where rabies is endemic

The control strategy depends on the local pattern of rabies occurrence in wild and domestic animals. Education and publicity about rabies is always needed. Domestic animals can be protected by regular vaccination. Owned dogs can be muzzled or kept off the streets. People should be discouraged from keeping wild carnivores such as skunks, raccoons, coatis, and mongooses as pets. Unnecessary contact with mammals should be avoided (e.g. stroking stray dogs or apparently friendly wild animals, exploring bat-infested caves). Culling reservoir species has proved an unpopular and ineffective method of long-term control. Impressive reduction of urban rabies in stray dogs has proved possible in India by vaccination, population control, and reducing available food and shelter by removing refuse. Effective oral vaccination of dogs is not yet practicable.

Control of sylvatic rabies has been achieved by vaccination of key wild animal reservoir populations with live oral vaccines distributed in bait. Repeated campaigns distributing attenuated rabies or vaccinia-recombinant rabies glycoprotein vaccines have eliminated fox rabies in Western Europe, and the latter has been used in North American coyotes, foxes, and raccoons. New vaccines are being developed for other species. Vaccination of bats is unlikely to be feasible. Vampire bat rabies is controlled by destroying roosts and poisoning the bats with anticoagulants.

In countries where rabies is not endemic

The inadvertent importation of a mammal incubating rabies is a universal risk. The movement of potential vectors, especially domestic dogs and cats, wild carnivores, and bats, should be strictly controlled. Serological evidence of successful vaccination should be provided for imported mammals, or they should be vaccinated on arrival and quarantined.

Prevention of human infection

Pre-exposure prophylaxis

Pre-exposure vaccination is the most effective form of rabies prevention. No rabies deaths have been reported in anyone who had pre-exposure vaccine followed by postexposure booster doses. It is recommended for people who handle imported animals, workers in zoos and rabies laboratories, and those who are resident in or intend to travel to dog rabies-endemic areas, especially children. Others particularly at risk in certain areas include veterinarians, dog catchers, farm workers, cave explorers, naturalists, and animal collectors. In dog rabies-endemic areas, pre-exposure prophylaxis is advisable but is rarely used. Travellers should be educated to seek immediate local medical help if they are bitten, scratched, or licked by animals. However, recommendations vary in different areas and local advice may be unreliable. Tissue culture vaccine and especially rabies immune globulin may not be readily available.

Primary pre-exposure vaccine course

A course of three doses of tissue culture rabies vaccine (see below) is given intramuscularly into the deltoid, or the anterolateral thigh in children, on days 0, 7, and 28. The last dose may be advanced towards day 21 if time is short. An effective economical alternative is intradermal injections of 0.1 ml at the same intervals. If the injection is too deep to produce a papule, withdraw the needle and repeat the procedure. The whole vaccine ampoule should be used within a day or discarded. If chloroquine is being taken for malaria prophylaxis (unlikely today), or in other cases of suspected immunosuppression, the intramuscular route must be used. Many travellers cannot afford three doses of an expensive vaccine, so the economical intradermal route is ideal for family, student, or other groups who can be vaccinated on the same day.

Booster doses

A booster dose 1 to 2 years after the primary course enhances and prolongs the presence of antibody. Although the titre falls more rapidly after intradermal than intramuscular inoculation, the response to a booster dose is equally prompt. Confirmation of seroconversion is recommended only if immunosuppression is suspected. Further booster doses may be given intradermally or intramuscularly at intervals of 2 to 10 years depending on the risk of exposure. If the rabies neutralizing antibody level is at least 0.5 IU/ml, boosters are not necessary. Laboratory staff at high risk should have more frequent serology tests. Travellers who will have rapid access to vaccine if exposed need not have further immunization, but, if medical resources will be unreliable, a booster vaccination should be given before departure if 3 to 5 years have elapsed since the previous dose. A personal record of immunization must be kept, and urgent treatment is essential after possible exposure. Lyophilized rabies vaccine is relatively stable even at tropical ambient temperatures. It is sensible to take a dose on expeditions to remote rabies endemic areas. An extra emergency injection can then be given immediately after a risky encounter with an animal. If more than one person is exposed, the ampoule can be shared by giving multiple intradermal doses to each, using the whole dose (see postexposure regimens). This does not replace the normal postexposure treatment, which must still be given as soon as possible.

Postexposure prophylaxis

Despite intensive care, rabies encephalomyelitis of canine origin remains 100% fatal. At the time of the bite, however, correct cleaning of the wound (see below) and optimum postexposure immunization reduce the risk of rabies to nearly zero compared to about 35 to 57% in untreated cases. The risk varies with the biting species and the site and severity of the bites. It is highest following bites to the head by proved rabid wolves, which carries a case fatality exceeding 80% in unvaccinated people. The decision to give postexposure treatment depends on an assessment of the risk of infection by asking about the precise geographical location of the exposure; its severity, whether it was a bite or lick on broken skin; the site of the lesion; and the nature, appearance, behaviour, and fate of the biting animal, and, whether it had been recently vaccinated against rabies. The animal's brain must be tested for rabies if possible. If there is any doubt, the patient should be given full postexposure prophylaxis, even if the bite is several months old.

The aim of prophylaxis is to neutralize inoculated virus before it can enter the nervous system. Wound cleaning and active and passive immunization must be implemented as soon as possible.

Wound cleaning

This is effective in killing virus in superficial wounds, but is often neglected. First aid includes vigorous cleaning of the wound with soap or detergent and water under a running tap for at least 5 min. Foreign material should be removed and a viricidal agent such as povidone iodine, or 40 to 70% alcohol, should be applied liberally. Quaternary ammonium compounds such as benzalkonium chloride are inactivated by soap and so are not recommended. Hospital treatment of wounds involves thorough exploration, debridement, and irrigation of deep wounds, if necessary under local or general anaesthetic. Suturing should be avoided or delayed and the wound left without occlusive dressings. Attention should be given to tetanus prophylaxis (Chapter 7.6.22) and the large range of viral, bacterial, and fungal pathogens particularly associated with mammal bites. These include *Cercopithecine herpesvirus* (B virus) from Asian macaques (Chapter 7.5.2); *Pasteurella multocida* (Chapter 7.6.18), *Francisella tularensis* (Chapter 7.6.19), *Streptobacillus moniliformis*, and *Spirillum minus* (Chapter 7.6.13) from rodents; and *Pasteurella multocida, Capnocytophaga canimorsus*, and *Bartonella henselae* (Chapter 7.6.42) from dogs and/or cats. Most of the bacteria are sensitive to amoxicillin/clavulanic acid, cefoxitin, or tetracycline.

Active immunization

Rabies vaccines

Three highly immunogenic tissue culture vaccines that meet the World Health Organization (WHO) recommended standards are human diploid cell vaccine (HDCV), purified chick embryo cell (PCEC) vaccine, and purified VeRO cell rabies vaccine (PVRV).

Several tissue culture vaccines are produced, mainly for national use, in China, India, Japan, Russia, and other Asian and South American countries.

Obsolete nervous tissue rabies vaccines, no longer sanctioned by the WHO, are still produced in a few countries. Semple vaccine, a sheep or goat brain suspension, or suckling mouse brain (Fuenzalida) vaccine is used in a few countries in Asia, Africa, and South America. Daily subcutaneous doses for 7 to 21 days, followed by booster doses, are usually given over the abdomen. Neurological reactions including postvaccinal encephalomyelitis still occur.

Postexposure tissue culture vaccine regimens

The standard intramuscular five-dose (Essen) regimen is 5 × 1-ml (PVRV 0.5 ml) doses injected into the deltoid (or anterolateral thigh in children) on days 0, 3, 7, 14, and 28.

The alternative 2-1-1 intramuscular regimen is two full doses (1.0 ml or for PVRV 0.5 ml), injected into the deltoids on day 0, and one dose on days 7 and 21. A total of four full doses are given, but the antibody level may fall more rapidly.

The intramuscular regimens are unaffordable in many countries. However, two economical multisite intradermal methods are available, each requiring only 40% of the vaccine used in the standard intramuscular method. Each of the intradermal injection sites drains to a different group of lymph nodes, intended to stimulate more lymphoid tissue to produce antibody.

The new simplified four-site intradermal regimen consists of a whole ampoule of vaccine divided between four intradermal injections over the deltoid and the thigh or suprascapular areas. The volume per site is about 0.1 ml for PVRV and the equivalent dose for vaccines containing 1 ml per ampoule is 0.2 ml. On day 7, two intradermal injections of 0.1/0.2 ml in the deltoid and thigh areas are followed by a single intradermal dose on day 28. If PCECV (1 ml/ampoule) is used, a reduced ID dose of 0.1 ml/ID site was found to be immunogenic. If resources are limited and more than one patient is treated on the same day, ampoules of vaccine can be shared, and an alternative dose is 4 x 0.1 ml ID on day 0, and thereafter 0.1 ml per ID site x 2 on day 7 and one on day 28. The 4-site regimen has several advantages as it requires only three clinic visits on days 0, 7, and 28 and is economical even without sharing any ampoules, using a maximum of 3 doses instead of 5 for the IM regimen. However this involves some vaccine wastage.

The two-site intradermal regimen was designed for use with PVRV. A dose of 0.1 ml for PVRV, or 0.2 ml for vaccines formulated in ampoules containing 1 ml, is given intradermally at two sites in the deltoid area on days 0, 3, and 7 and at two sites on day 28. An intradermal dose of 0.1 ml per site has also been used with PCEC 1 ml vaccine.

For all other vaccines, the manufacturer's instructions should be followed.

Postexposure vaccine regimen for people who have already received vaccination

If a complete pre-exposure or postexposure course of a potent tissue culture vaccine has been given in the past, or if the neutralizing antibody level has been over 0.5 IU/ml, only two doses of tissue culture vaccine should be given on days 0 and 3. The first dose can be divided between four intradermal sites on day 0. Rabies immune globulin is not required, but otherwise full postexposure treatment must be given.

Side effects of tissue culture vaccines

Mild and transient local redness, itching (especially after intradermal injection), or pain at the site of injection are not uncommon. Influenza-like symptoms and rashes are infrequent. Type I immediate hypersensitivity occurs rarely during primary courses. Type III immune-complex hypersensitivity was reported in 6% of those receiving booster doses of HDCV in the United States of America. This consisted of urticaria, rash, angio-oedema, and arthralgia 3 to 13 days after injection. No fatal reactions have been reported. Very rarely polyneuritis, Guillain–Barré syndrome, or local limb weakness have been reported in patients receiving tissue culture vaccines but no more frequently than for other commonly used virus vaccines.

Neurological reactions to nervous tissue vaccines

These occur in up to 1 in 220 courses of Semple vaccine, with a 3% mortality, and are an allergic response to myelin and related neural proteins in the vaccine. Reactions to suckling mouse brain vaccine are rare. The incubation period ranges from 3 to 35 days after the first vaccine injection. Clinical forms include localized neuropathy, transverse myelitis, paralysis with sensory loss or pain (a Landry-type ascending paralysis), meningoencephalitis, and meningoencephalomyelitis. These can be clinically indistinguishable from paralytic rabies, but recovery is usually complete. Permanent neurological sequelae are rare. Corticosteroids are thought to be helpful, and cyclophosphamide therapy has been suggested. Vaccination should be stopped as soon as symptoms appear and the course continued with a tissue culture vaccine.

Passive immunization: rabies immune globulin

Rabies immune globulin (RIG) has proved valuable in providing protection before neutralizing antibody has been actively generated, presumably by neutralizing rabies virus during the first week after initial vaccination. It is recommended as part of primary postexposure treatment, but it is vital following severe bites (on the head, neck, hands, and multiple or deep bites) (see Box 7.5.10.1).

The dose of human RIG is 20 IU/kg body weight and for equine RIG is 40 IU/kg. Reactions to equine and human RIG have been observed in 1.8% and 0.09% of recipients, respectively, and serum sickness in 0.72% and 0.007%, respectively. These are not predicted by a previous intradermal hypersensitivity test and, since RIG must be given even if the test is positive, skin tests are time-wasting and unnecessary. Adrenaline (epinephrine) should always be available in case of reactions.

All the RIG is infiltrated into and around the bite wound if anatomically possible, but any remaining is injected intramuscularly preferably into the thigh, not the buttock, at a site distant from the vaccine. If RIG is given hours or days before the first dose of vaccine, the active immune response will be impaired. RIG is prohibitively expensive and is neither available nor affordable for 99% of people in developing countries for whom postexposure treatment is indicated.

Failures of postexposure prophylaxis

Deaths from rabies have occurred despite prophylaxis. Failures are attributable to delay in starting vaccination, incomplete vaccine course, use of a substandard (nervous tissue) vaccine, and omission of RIG. Failure to infiltrate RIG around the wound, injection of vaccine into the buttock, or impaired immune responsiveness of the patient may also contribute. Low vaccine potency has been held responsible only with nervous tissue vaccines. Vaccine protection against rabies-related lyssaviruses may be less efficient than against genotype 1 rabies viruses (see below), but no case of vaccine failure has been attributed to this phenomenon.

A reduced or delayed immune response to vaccine can sometimes be predicted. If treatment is started late (e.g. more than 2 days after exposure), no RIG is available for severe bites, the patient is immunocompromised, or a rabies-related virus infection is suspected, the immune stimulus might be enhanced by dividing the first dose of tissue culture vaccine between four sites intradermally, as for the economical four-site regimen (see above).

Rabies-related virus infections of humans

The genus *Lyssavirus* contains seven genotypes: genotype 1, classic rabies, and six rabies-related genotypes (Fig. 7.5.10.2). Continent-specific rabies-related viruses occur in Africa, Europe, and Australia, and there is serological evidence of lyssavirus infection

Box 7.5.10.1 Specific postexposure prophylaxis for use in a rabies endemic area[a] following contact with a domestic or wild rabies vector species, whether or not the animal is available for observation or diagnostic tests

Minor exposure (including licks of broken skin, scratches, or abrasions without bleeding)

- Start vaccine immediately
- Stop treatment if animal remains healthy for 10 days
- Stop treatment if animal's brain proves negative for rabies by appropriate laboratory tests

Major exposure (including licks of mucosa, minor bites on arms, trunk or legs, or major bites i.e. multiple or on face, head, fingers, or neck)

- Immediate rabies immune globulin and vaccine
- Stop treatment if domestic cat or dog remains healthy for 10 days
- Stop treatment if animal's brain proves negative for rabies by appropriate laboratory tests

[a] This scheme is a simplification of the recommendations of the World Health Organization Expert Committee on Rabies (1997).

across Asia. With the exception of Mokola virus, all are viruses of bats. All are known to be capable of infecting humans except Lagos bat virus. They are occasionally detected in other species, but diagnostic tests are available only in highly specialized laboratories, infection is rarely suspected, and the routine tests for genotype 1 rabies virus may be weakly positive or negative. Their true prevalence is, therefore, unknown. Only 13 human cases of rabies-related virus infections have been reported, and disease is likely to remain unrecognized and misdiagnosed.

African lyssaviruses

- Lagos bat virus (genotype 2) has not been implicated in any human case.
- Mokola virus (genotype 3) has been isolated from shrews (*Crocidura* spp.) and rodents, as well as cats and dogs which are presumably vectors. It was isolated from a child with meningitis who recovered, and from another with fatal encephalitis. Mokola virus also caused mild disease in a rabies-vaccinated laboratory worker.
- Duvenhage virus (genotype 4) has been identified in three people, all of whom had had skin lesions inflicted by bats and had developed a fatal illness with clinical features identical to rabies encephalitis.

European bat lyssaviruses

Infected insectivorous bats have been found in Europe since 1954. The European bat lyssavirus (EBLV) group comprises genotype 5 (also known as EBLV 1) and genotype 6 (EBLV 2), both of which have subgroups a and b. EBLV type 1a is found across Northern and Eastern Europe from the Netherlands to Russia; EBLV type 1b in the Netherlands, France, and Spain; EBLV type 2a in the Netherlands and the United Kingdom; EBLV type 2b very rarely in Switzerland and an untyped EBLV 2 in Finland. Five unvaccinated people with bat bites died of encephalitis indistinguishable from rabies: two in Russia, one in the Ukraine, one in Scotland, and a Swiss zoologist visiting Finland was infected with EBLV 2b. Four new, so far unclassified, lyssaviruses have been found in bats in Eastern Europe.

Australian bat lyssavirus

Australian bat lyssavirus (ABL) (genotype 7) has been found in fruit bats (genus *Pteropus*) (Fig. 7.5.10.18) and insectivorous bats in Eastern Australia since 1996. It caused a fatal rabies-like encephalitis in two women who had handled bats.

The lyssavirus genotypes have been classified into two phylogroups. Mokola and Lagos bat viruses form phylogroup II and the other lyssaviruses are in phylogroup I. All phylogroup I genotypes have caused fatal rabies-like encephalitis in humans, but experimentally phylogroup II viruses are less pathogenic. This is in keeping with the clinical cases reported. The genetic relationships between the whole genome of the genotypes (Fig. 7.5.10.2) correlates with the degree of serological cross-protection. Since all rabies vaccines are prepared from genotype 1 rabies virus, protection against ABL, which is closely related to genotype 1, should be undiminished. Protection is less efficient against phylogenetically more distant EBLVs and there is little if any protection against Mokola virus. However, there have been no failures of prophylaxis after exposures to bats, and no other treatment is available. Pre-exposure and postexposure immunization

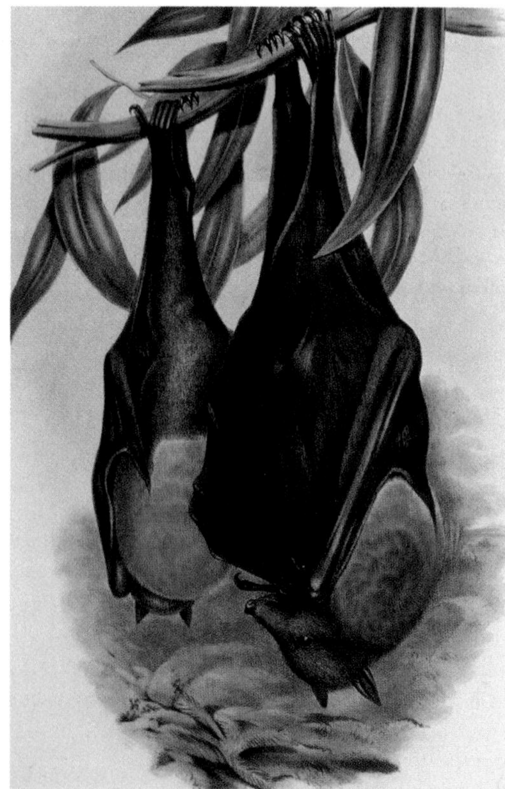

Fig. 7.5.10.18 Pteropid fruit bat (flying fox) (*Pteropis poliocephalus*), the natural reservoir of Nipah, Hendra, and Menangle paramyxoviruses and of Australian bat lyssavirus.
(From a painting by John Gould.)

is, therefore, more urgent if exposure to a rabies-related virus infection is suspected.

Further reading

Delmas O, *et al.* (2008). Genomic diversity and evolution of the lyssaviruses. *PLoS One*, **3**, e2057.

Helmick CG, Tauxe RV, Vernon AA (1987). Is there a risk to contacts of patients with rabies? *Rev Infect Dis*, **9**, 511–18.

Jackson AC (2007). Pathogenesis. In: Jackson AC, Wunner AH (eds) *Rabies*, 2nd edition, pp. 341–81. Elsevier, Academic Press, London.

Kaplan C, Turner GS, Warrell DA (eds) (1986). *Rabies the facts*, revised edition. Oxford University Press, Oxford. [Detailed review of clinical features with illustrative case histories.]

Nel LH, Markotter W (2007). Lyssaviruses. *Crit Rev Microbiol*, **33**, 301–24. [A comprehensive compilation of the lyssaviruses from all continents and their distribution.]

Nel LH, Rupprecht CE (2007). Emergence of lyssaviruses in the Old World: the case of Africa. *Curr Top Microbiol Immunol*, **315**, 161–93. [Epidemiological, historical, and genetic details of lyssaviruses in Africa.]

Schnell MJ, *et al.* (2010). The cell biology of rabies virus: using stealth to reach the brain. *Nat Rev Microbiol*, **8**, 51–61.

Warrell MJ, Warrell DA (2004). Rabies and other lyssavirus diseases. *Lancet*, **363**, 959–69. [Erratum: *Lancet*, **364**, 2096.]

Warrell DA, *et al.* (1976). Pathophysiologic studies in human rabies. *Am J Med*, **60**, 180–90. [Physiological and histopathological investigations of the mechanism of hydrophobia and brain damage in human rabies encephalitis.]

Warrell MJ, *et al.* (1985). Economical multiple-site intradermal immunisation with human diploid-cell-strain vaccine is effective for post-exposure rabies prophylaxis. *Lancet*, **i**, 1059–62. [A randomized controlled trial of intradermal treatment with Semple vaccine in patients bitten by proven rabid animals. Rabies immune globulin was only given if severe exposure.]

Warrell MJ, *et al.* (2008). A simplified 4-site economical intradermal post-exposure rabies vaccine regimen: a randomised controlled comparison with standard methods. *PLoS Negl Trop Dis*, **2**, e224. [Demonstration of the immunogenicity of a new regimen that has advantages over both the previous intradermal methods.]

World Health Organization (2007). Rabies vaccines. WHO position paper. *Wkly Epidemiol Rec*, **82**, 425–35. Available from: www.who.int/wer/2007/wer8249_50.pdf

7.5.11 Colorado tick fever and other arthropod-borne reoviruses

M.J. Warrell and David A. Warrell

Essentials

Human pathogens are found in six genera of *Reoviridae*: *Reovirus*, *Rotavirus*, *Orthoreovirus*, and three arthropod-borne genera—*Coltivirus* (Colorado tick fever, Salmon River virus, and Eyach viruses), *Orbivirus* (Kemerovo, Changuinola, Orungo, and Lebombo) and *Seadornavirus* (Banna virus).

Colorado tick fever—common in parts of north-western North America; acquired from tick (ixodid) bites, most often by hikers and campers, presenting 3 to 6 days later with sudden fever, rigors, generalized aches, myalgia, headache and backache, rashes (12%) and gastrointestinal symptoms (20%). Diagnosis confirmed by detection of viral antigen in erythrocytes or serum, or by serodiagnosis. Management is symptomatic. Illness usually resolves in 10 to 14 days, but convalescence may be prolonged. Prevention is by avoiding, repelling, and rapidly removing ticks; no vaccines are available.

Coltiviruses

Colorado tick fever

The virus responsible for Colorado tick fever or 'mountain fever' is an 80-nm double-shelled particle covered with capsomeres. The icosahedral core contains 12 segments of double-stranded negative-sense RNA. The virus can infect human erythrocytes and this may also occur with the other coltiviruses and orbiviruses.

Colorado tick fever is a zoonosis involving hard (ixodid) ticks (principally *Dermacentor andersoni*, but also *D. occidentalis*, *D. parumapertus*, *D. albipictus*, etc.) and wild mammals, including porcupines, deer, coyotes, squirrels, chipmunks, deer mice, and other rodents. Ticks pass Colorado tick fever virus trans-stadially and transovarially.

Epidemiology

Colorado tick fever is acquired from tick bites in western and north-western parts of the United States of America (including California) and Canada (British Columbia and Alberta). Very rarely, it has been caused by an infected blood transfusion. Several hundred cases are reported each year in the United States of America, but the true incidence is thought to be at least 10 times higher than that. It is the second most commonly diagnosed arboviral infection in the United States of America, after West Nile virus. Hikers and campers are at special risk in rodent- and tick-infested terrain. The prevalence of antibody to Colorado tick fever among shepherds is 32%. The highest incidence is from May to July when ticks are most active. Infection usually confers lasting immunity.

Clinical features

In adults, the infection is nearly always mild, but in children it is occasionally severe but rarely fatal. Three to 6 days after the tick bite (extreme range 1–19 days) there is a sudden fever for about 3 days, with rigors, generalized aches, myalgia, headache, and backache. In one-half of the patients there is a biphasic fever. Rashes then appear in up to 12% of patients, usually a transient peripheral maculopapular rash or petechiae on flexor surfaces of arms or perhaps widespread and it may be hyperaesthetic. Gastrointestinal symptoms occur in 20% of patients. Laboratory findings include leukopenia with relative lymphocytosis, occasional thrombocytopenia, and mild lymphocyte pleocytosis.

The illness usually resolves in about 10 to 14 days, but convalescence may be prolonged. Severe manifestations include meningism and drowsiness, sometimes associated with gastrointestinal symptoms, spontaneous bleeding, thrombocytopenia, and disseminated intravascular coagulation. Late, possibly immunological effects, include myocarditis, pericarditis, pleurisy, arthritis, and epididymitis. Colorado tick fever infection may precipitate abortion, or transplacental infection but the teratogenic effects reported in mice have not been observed in humans.

Diagnosis

Viral antigen may be detected in erythrocytes by immunofluorescence 1 to 120 days after the start of symptoms. Erythrocyte precursors are infected in the marrow, but their survival is apparently not affected. Virus can be isolated from the blood and, if there is central nervous system involvement, the cerebrospinal fluid. Colorado tick fever virus produces a cytopathic effect on several cell lines, but intracerebral injection of ground blood clot or preferably washed erythrocytes into suckling mice is more sensitive for diagnostic isolation. Antigen can be detected in serum during acute infections by polymerase chain reaction (PCR) or Western blot, but enzyme-linked immunosorbent assay (ELISA) techniques have been less sensitive. An indirect fluorescent antibody test can provide early serodiagnosis. Neutralizing antibody and specific IgM enzyme immunoassays become positive after 14 to 21 days and the IgM disappears after 45 days.

Differential diagnosis

Many other tick-borne acute febrile illnesses, some with rashes and nervous system involvement, can be acquired in the area endemic for Colorado tick fever. These include Rocky Mountain spotted fever, tularaemia, Lyme disease, and relapsing fever. Tick paralysis caused by *D. andersoni* and other ixodid ticks presents as a poliomyelitis-like, ascending, flaccid paralysis that is unlikely to be mistaken for the meningitic or encephalitic syndromes of Colorado tick fever.

Treatment

The symptomatic treatment of fever and pain should exclude salicylates in case of thrombocytopenia. Tribavirin (ribavirin) inhibits the replication of Colorado tick fever virus experimentally, but its use in humans has not been reported. Immunity is long lasting.

Salmon River virus

This virus is closely related to Colorado tick fever virus. It was isolated from a patient with similar symptoms in Idaho.

Eyach

This European coltivirus has been found in Germany and France. There is serological evidence of human infection in Czechoslovakia causing meningoencephalitis or neuropathies.

Orbiviruses

Although antibody to the tick-borne Great Island virus and insect-borne Corripata orbiviruses have been found in humans, there is no evidence of their pathogenicity.

Kemerovo

Three serotypes of Kemerovo virus have been isolated from ixodid and hyalomma ticks in Russia and Central Europe. They cause benign febrile illnesses and, occasionally, meningitis or encephalitis in spring and early summer when ticks are active. Rodents and birds are involved in the zoonotic cycle.

Oklahoma tick fever is another Kemerovo virus rarely causing febrile illness in the United States of America.

Changuinola

There is a single report of human febrile illness with the orbivirus Changuinola in Panama. The virus has been isolated from phlebotomine flies and mammals in that area.

Orungo

Orungo virus is found mainly in West Africa but also in Uganda and the Central African Republic. Up to 75% of some human populations are seropositive. The clinical effects are unknown, but fever and diarrhoea occur in some people, perhaps with encephalitis as in experimental mice. There is no rash or jaundice. It is transmitted by anopheles, aedes, and other mosquitoes. Monkeys, sheep, and cattle may be infected.

Lebombo

This orbivirus was isolated from one febrile child in Nigeria. Lebombo is also found in mosquitoes and rodents.

Seadornaviruses

These viruses from south-east Asia and Indonesia include Banna virus from China, which has been isolated from patients with encephalitis. It is likely to be misdiagnosed as Japanese encephalitis.

Prevention

Tick-borne infections are prevented by avoiding, repelling, and rapidly removing ticks. No vaccines are available.

Further reading

Attoui H, *et al.* (2005). Coltiviruses and seadornaviruses in North America, Europe, and Asia. *Emerg Infect Dis*, **11**, 1673–9.

Brown SE, Knudson DL (1995). Coltivirus infections. In: Porterfield JS (ed.) *Exotic viral infections*, pp. 329–42. Chapman & Hall, London.

Labuda M, Nuttall PA (2008). Viruses transmitted by ticks. In: Bowman AS, Nuttall PA (eds) *Ticks: biology, disease and control*, pp. 989–92. Cambridge University Press, Cambridge.

Libikova H, *et al.* (1978). Orbiviruses of the Kemerovo complex and neurological diseases. *Med Microbiol Immunol*, **166**, 255–63.

McGinley-Smith DE, Tsao SS (2003). Dermatoses from ticks. *J Am Acad Dermatol*, **49**, 363–92.

Romero JR, Simonsen KA (2008). Powassan encephalitis and Colorado tick fever. *Infect Dis Clin North Am*, **22**, 545–59.

7.5.12 Alphaviruses

L.R. Petersen and D.J. Gubler

Essentials

There are 29 registered alphaviruses belonging to the family Togaviridae, 16 of which are known to cause human infection. They are RNA viruses with global geographical distribution and complex transmission cycles between wild or domestic animals or birds and one or more mosquito species; humans are infected by mosquito bites. They cause a spectrum of clinical manifestations ranging from nonspecific febrile illness to acute encephalitis and death. Diagnosis of infection is made serologically by detection of IgM and IgG antibody responses, virus isolation, or by polymerase chain reaction and immunohistochemistry on tissue samples.

Old World alphaviruses, including Chikungunya, Ross River, Sindbis, Barmah Forest, Mayaro and O'nyong-nyong, generally have mammals as their natural vertebrate host and, cause acute febrile illness characterized by rash and arthritis. Management is symptomatic; prevention and control is by reducing vector mosquito populations and by avoiding mosquito bites.

New World alphaviruses, including Eastern, Western and Venezuelan Equine Encephalitides, generally have birds as their natural vertebrate hosts; about 2% of adults infected with Eastern Equine Encephalitis virus (less for other types) develop encephalitis, which can be fatal, with permanent neurological sequelae in many survivors; management is symptomatic; prevention and control is by reducing vector mosquito populations and by avoiding mosquito bites. Various vaccines have been used in laboratory workers and others at high risk of exposure. New generation vaccines are in clinical trials.

Introduction

The genus *Alphavirus* of the family Togaviridae comprises 29 registered viruses, 16 of which are known to cause human infection (Table 7.5.12.1). Alphaviruses are lipid-enveloped virions with a diameter of 60 to 70 nm whose genome is a molecule of single-stranded, positive-sense RNA approximately 12 000 nucleotides in length. Most alphaviruses are maintained in nature in complex transmission cycles between wild or domestic animals and one or more mosquito species. Humans are infected when the infective mosquito takes a blood meal. Patients develop high viraemias with some alphaviruses and this may contribute to the transmission cycle by infecting mosquitoes. The epidemiology and geographical distribution of the alphaviruses depend on several factors including the presence of suitable amplifying hosts, the presence and feeding behaviour of a suitable arthropod vector, and the frequency of exposure of nonimmune reservoir hosts and humans to infected vectors. Alphavirus infections are not directly communicable between humans.

Most infections in humans are asymptomatic, but alphaviruses can cause a spectrum of clinical illness ranging from nonspecific febrile illness, often with rash, myalgia, or arthralgia, to frank encephalitis and death. They cause two main clinical syndromes: Old World alphaviruses generally cause illness characterized by rash and arthritis while New World alphaviruses are generally associated with neuroinvasive disease. No specific therapy is available. Vaccines for some alphaviruses are used in animals, although none have been licensed for humans.

Laboratory diagnosis

Alphavirus infections are diagnosed serologically by detection of IgM and IgG responses. All alphaviruses have common antigenic determinants that result in cross-reactions in immunodiagnostic tests. Neutralization tests may be necessary for serological confirmation in areas where multiple alphaviruses are endemic/enzootic. Isolation of virus from acute-phase serum is possible with some alphaviruses, but they are seldom recovered from the central nervous system, including cerebrospinal fluid, except from fatal cases. Virological diagnosis may also be made using polymerase chain reaction and immunohistochemistry on tissue samples.

Alphaviruses associated with arthritis and rash

Chikungunya

Aetiology and epidemiology

Chikungunya virus is found in Africa and Asia and is transmitted primarily by day-biting aedes mosquitoes. Nonhuman primates such as monkeys and baboons may be the primary maintenance hosts in sylvatic environments in Africa. In urban surroundings in Africa and Asia, the virus is transmitted between humans by *Aedes aegypti* mosquitoes, although *Ae albopictus* mosquitoes have been implicated in some outbreaks. Explosive urban epidemics occur during the rainy season. Since 2004, a major epidemic has occurred in India (more than 1.3 million cases), adjacent Asian countries, Kenya, and Indian Ocean islands (Comoros, Mauritius, Seychelles, Madagascar, Mayotte, and Réunion where 34% of the population was infected), and in 2007 it reached Gabon in Central Africa and Italy. This epidemic was exacerbated by a new variant virus. A single mutation in the envelope protein increased infectivity to *Ae albopictus*, a mosquito that has spread throughout the tropics and subtropics and has a wider distribution in urban, semiurban, and rural habitats than *Ae aegypti*, which favours urban environments. Serosurveys following outbreaks have shown antibody prevalences generally ranging from 30 to 70%. Infections in travellers returning to Europe and the United States of America from areas experiencing outbreaks have been frequently reported. More than 800 cases were imported into France and 100 into the United Kingdom from Réunion and the other islands popular with tourists. In August 2007, local transmission of chikungunya by *Ae albopictus* mosquitoes was confirmed around Ravenna in Italy, resulting in 205 cases and one death. Neonatal infection has occurred from mothers ill shortly before or at the time of delivery.

Clinical characteristics

'Chikungunya' means 'that which bends up' in Makonde, an East African language, and refers to the crippling arthralgia that characterizes the disease. After an incubation period of 2 to 3 days (range 1–12 days), there is sudden fever and severe arthralgia. In some patients, the fever may remit for 1 to 2 days and then recur ('saddleback'

Table 7.5.12.1 Known disease associations of alphaviruses [a]

Virus	Geographical distribution	Disease in humans	Outbreaks	Other features
Aura	South America		No	
Barmah Forest	Australia	SFI, arthropathy	Yes	Clinically similar to Ross River virus infection
Bebaru	Malaysia		No	Laboratory infection only
Cabassou	French Guiana		No	
Chikungunya	Tropical Africa, India, Southeast Asia, Philippines	SFI, arthropathy	Yes	Large outbreaks in urban settings
Eastern equine encephalitis	North and South America on Atlantic and Gulf Coasts, Caribbean	SFI, encephalitis	Yes	Isolated cases or small outbreaks occur mainly in North America
Everglades	Florida	SFI, encephalitis	No	Variant of Venezuelan equine encephalitis
Fort Morgan	Colorado		No	
Getah	Asia	SFI	No	
Highlands J	North America		No	
Mayaro	Trinidad, Brazil, Bolivia, Surinam, French Guiana, Peru, Venezuela	SFI, arthropathy	Yes	
Middleburg	South, West, and Central Africa	Not described	No	
Mosso das Pedras	Brazil		No	Venezuelan equine encephalitis complex
Mucambo	Trinidad, Brazil, Surinam, French Guiana, Colombia, Venezuela	SFI	No	Proposed species in the Venezuelan equine encephalitis antigenic complex
Ndumu	Africa		No	
O'nyong-nyong	East and West Africa, Zimbabwe	SFI, arthropathy	Yes	Igbo-ora virus is a subtype of o'nyong-nyong
Pixuna	Brazil	SFI	No	Laboratory infection only
Rio Negro	Argentina		No	
Ross River	Australia, South Pacific	SFI, arthropathy	Yes	Periodic epidemics in South Pacific
Salmon Pancreas disease	North Atlantic		No	
Semliki Forest	Sub-Saharan Africa	SFI, encephalitis	No	
Sindbis	Africa, East Mediterranean, South and Southeast Asia, Borneo, Philippines, Australia, Sicily, Scandinavia	SFI, arthropathy	Yes	
Babanki	West and Central Africa	SFI, arthropathy	Yes	Subtype of Sindbis
Kyzylagach	Azerbaijan	SFI, arthropathy	Yes	Subtype of Sindbis
Southern elephant seal	Antarctica		No	
Tonate	French Guiana	SFI, encephalitis	No	Venezuelan equine encephalitis complex
Trocara	South America		No	Proposed species in the Venezuelan equine encephalitis antigenic complex; fatal encephalitis in one infant
Una	South America, Trinidad		No	
Venezuelan equine encephalitis	Northern South America, Central America, Mexico	SFI, encephalitis	Yes	
Western equine encephalitis	North and South America	SFI, encephalitis	Yes	Human disease rare outside of North America and Brazil
Whataroa	New Zealand, Australia		No	

SFI, systemic febrile illness.

Adapted from Griffin D (2007). Alphaviruses. In: Knipe DM, Howley PM (eds) *Fields virology*, 5th edition, vol. 1, pp. 1023–67. Lippincott Williams & Wilkins, Philadelphia.

fever). Arthralgias are polyarticular, with the knees, ankles, elbows, and small joints of the hands and feet most commonly affected. They are often associated with low back pain. A useful sign is pain on squeezing the wrists (tenosynovitis). Headache, injected pharynx, gastrointestinal symptoms, and myalgias are frequent during the acute illness. Rashes, typically on the trunk and limbs, occur in about one-half of the patients usually during the second to fifth day of illness. They are very variable in appearance: papular or maculopapular erythemas (blanching as in dengue), vesicular, bullous, dyshidrotic, keratolytic, purpuric and hyperpigmented associated with facial oedema, erythema nodosum, and aphthous ulcers. Arthralgia may last several months and is associated with effusions and bursitis; a few patients may have symptoms 5 years after infection. Haemorrhage, meningoencephalitis, Guillain–Barré polyradiculopathy, myocarditis, and hepatic and renal complications are uncommon but may be fatal. Rheumatological manifestations are less frequent in children. Conjunctival suffusion and cervical or generalized lymphadenopathy are common. Serological surveys suggest that asymptomatic infections may occur.

Diagnosis

Leukopenia and elevation of liver and muscle enzymes are common early in infection. Detection of viral RNA by reverse transcription–polymerase chain reaction (RT-PCR) is useful for diagnosis during the first week of illness. Haemagglutinin inhibition and IgM antibodies will be present in nearly all patients by the seventh day of illness. IgM antibodies detectable in serum by IgM antibody capture enzyme-linked immunosorbent assay (MAC-ELISA) may persist for 6 months after infection. Virus isolation is confirmatory.

Prevention, control, and treatment

Prevention and control can only be achieved by reducing vector mosquito populations in the large urban centres of the tropics and by avoiding mosquito bites. The American military has an effective vaccine, but it is not licensed for general use. Several new vaccines are all in late stage development. There is no specific treatment. Anti-inflammatory drugs may relieve arthralgia. An uncontrolled study suggested that chloroquine phosphate may be helpful for refractory arthralgias.

Ross River virus

Aetiology and epidemiology

This virus causes 'epidemic polyarthritis' in Australia, south-western Pacific islands, and Fiji. *Aedes vigilax* is an important vector in Australia and *Ae scutellaris* complex mosquitoes in some south Pacific islands, although the virus has been isolated from more than 30 mosquito species. An epidemic in various Pacific islands in 1979 to 1980 affected more than 50 000 people. An average of 4800 cases is reported annually from Australia. Explosive outbreaks and viraemias in humans implicate virus transmission from human to human by certain mosquitoes. Outbreaks tend to be associated with periods of increased rainfall. Camping is a significant risk factor in tropical Australia.

Clinical characteristics

The incubation period ranges from 2 to 21 days (7–9 days on average). The illness begins suddenly with fever and arthralgias predominantly in the ankles, wrists, knees, fingers, and feet. A maculopapular rash occurs in about one-half of patients within 2 days of onset and is most prominent on the trunk and limbs, but can cover the entire body; the rash may progress to small vesicles. Myalgias, headache, anorexia, nausea, and tenosynovitis are common, but the temperature is only slightly elevated. Arthralgia generally resolves within 3 to 6 months. Symptomatic infection is rare in children.

Diagnosis

Isolation of virus from serum is possible for the first few days of illness. IgM antibodies will be detected by MAC-ELISA within 5 to 10 days of onset. Complement fixation, haemagglutinin inhibition, and neutralization tests may be useful, particularly when paired serum samples are available. Virus isolation and PCR are confirmatory.

Prevention, control, and treatment

Avoidance of mosquito bites and peridomestic mosquito control can effectively reduce the risk of infection. No specific treatment is available. Nonsteroidal anti-inflammatory drugs may relieve symptoms. One study suggested that corticosteroids might hasten recovery.

Sindbis

Aetiology and epidemiology

Sindbis virus is widely distributed in Africa, India, tropical Asia, Australia, and Europe. However, clinical disease is common only in geographically restricted areas. In Europe, the main vectors to humans are late summer, ornithophilic mosquitoes of the genera *Culex* and *Culiseta*. High antibody prevalences in Africa suggest that human exposure is common. Several outbreaks have been noted.

Clinical characteristics

In northern Europe, symptomatic disease is recognized from Sweden (Ockelbo disease), through Finland (Pogosta disease), to the former Karelian Soviet Socialist Republic (Karelian fever). The clinical features include mild fever, rash, arthralgia, myalgia, malaise, headache, and pruritus. The maculopapular rash progresses from trunk to extremities and vesicles can occur on the palms and soles. Ankle, finger, wrist, and knee joints are most commonly affected. Prominent rheumatic symptoms, sometimes persisting for several years, have been noted in Europe and South Africa.

Diagnosis

Haemagglutinin inhibition and IgM antibodies will be present in nearly all patients by the eighth day of illness. IgM antibodies detectable in serum by MAC-ELISA may persist for 6 months after infection. Virus can be infrequently detected by culture or RT-PCR from blood or skin lesions.

Prevention, control, and treatment

Avoidance of mosquito bites can reduce the risk of infection. No specific treatment is available.

Barmah Forest virus

Since its first recognition as a cause of human disease in 1988, the geographical distribution of Barmah Forest virus has expanded recently in Australia. It causes sporadic disease and epidemics, with up to 300 serologically confirmed cases. The disease resembles that of Ross River virus infection, although the rash tends to be more florid and true arthritis is less common. The illness is prolonged in some patients. Little is known about the ecology of Barmah Forest virus, although outbreaks have coincided with Ross River virus outbreaks and the virus has been identified in the same mosquito species.

Mayaro virus

Mayaro virus has been isolated from humans and various mosquito species (mostly *Haemagogus* ssp.) in Trinidad, Brazil, Bolivia, French Guiana, Surinam, Peru, and Venezuela. Serosurveys suggest the virus is widespread in South America. Several outbreaks have been identified, most recently in Venezuela in 2000. Following an incubation period of approximately 1 week, illness onset is abrupt with fever, chills, headache, retro-orbital pain, myalgia, gastrointestinal symptoms, and arthralgia mostly in the small joints of the extremities. A maculopapular rash may occur 2 to 5 days after defervescence. Arthralgia may persist for several months.

O'nyong-nyong virus

From 1959 to 1962, this virus caused epidemics in Uganda, Kenya, Tanzania, and Malawi involving approximately 2 million people. The virus was isolated in 1978 from *Anopheles funestus* mosquitoes in Kenya after a long period of no apparent o'nyong-nyong virus activity. In 1996 to 1997, an outbreak occurred in Uganda. In 2003, an outbreak occurred among refugees in the Côte d'Ivoire and a human infection was confirmed in Chad in 2004. O'nyong-nyong is closely related to chikungunya and produces a similar illness, although fever is less pronounced and lymphadenopathy is more common. *An funestus* and *An gambiae* transmit the virus.

Alphaviruses associated with neuroinvasive disease

Eastern equine encephalitis

Aetiology and epidemiology

The virus is widely distributed throughout North, Central, and South America and the Caribbean. However, little is known about the epidemiology of eastern equine encephalitis outside North America, where it is maintained in a bird–mosquito cycle in hardwood swamps in coastal areas from the Great Lakes to the Gulf Coast. In the United States of America human infections are usually sporadic, and small outbreaks occur each summer mostly along the Atlantic and Gulf Coasts. In recent years, 1 to 21 cases have been reported annually. In North America, wild birds and *Culiseta melanura* mosquitoes maintain the virus.

Clinical characteristics

Most infections are inapparent. The incubation period exceeds 1 week and the onset is abrupt with high fever. About 2% of infected adults and 6% of children develop encephalitis. Eastern equine encephalitis is the most severe of the arboviral encephalitides, with a mortality of 35 to 75%. Symptoms and signs include dizziness, decreasing level of consciousness, tremors, seizures, and focal neurological signs. Death can occur within 3 to 5 days of onset. Sequelae are common in nonfatal encephalitis and include convulsions, paralysis, and mental retardation. Illness due to eastern equine encephalitis in South America appears to be less severe.

Diagnosis

Cerebrospinal fluid pressure may be raised, with slightly increased protein, normal sugar, and up to 2000 cells/mm^3. IgM antibodies are readily detected in serum or cerebrospinal fluid by ELISA. Paired serum samples can be tested by haemagglutinin inhibition, ELISA, or neutralization tests. Horse or pheasant deaths and the proximity to swamps provide clues to the diagnosis.

Prevention, control, and treatment

Prevention depends on the avoidance of mosquito bites and mosquito control in suburban areas. Inactivated vaccines have been used successfully in horses, and an inactivated vaccine has been used experimentally in laboratory workers and others at high risk of exposure. No specific treatment is available.

Venezuelan equine encephalitis complex

Aetiology and epidemiology

Six subtypes (I–VI) within the Venezuelan equine encephalitis virus complex have been identified. Five antigenic variants exist within subtype I (IAB, IC, ID, IE, IF). These subtypes and variants are classified as epizootic or enzootic, based on their apparent virulence and epidemiology. Epizootic variants of subtype I (IAB and IC) cause equine epizootics and are associated with more severe human disease. Enzootic strains (ID–F, II (Everglades), III (Mucambo [A,B,D], Tonate [B]), IV (Pixuna), V (Cabassou), VI (Rio Negro)) do not cause epizootics in horses, but may produce sporadic disease in humans. Large epizootics (IAB and IC) have occurred in equines in northern countries of South America and Central America, sometimes reaching the United States of America. In 1969 to 1972, a massive epizootic extending from Ecuador to Texas killed more than 200 000 horses and caused several thousand human infections. In 1995, a large epizootic, which began in Venezuela and spread to Colombia, affected thousands of horses and caused approximately 90 000 human infections. Epizootic strains are carried by a wide variety of mosquitoes including *Aedes*, *Mansonia*, and *Psorophora* spp. Horses are the principal amplifying hosts during epizootics but are not amplifying hosts for enzootic transmission. Enzootic strains are maintained in a cycle involving *Culex* (*Melanoconion*) mosquitoes and rodents.

Clinical characteristics (epizootic virus infections)

After an incubation period of 1 to 6 days, there is a brief febrile illness of sudden onset characterized by malaise, nausea or vomiting, headache, and myalgia. Acute symptoms last 2 to 5 days, and generalized asthenia up to 3 weeks. Among those with clinical illness, less than 0.5% of adults and less than 4% of children develop encephalitis. Nausea and vomiting, nuchal rigidity, ataxia, convulsions, paralysis, and death may occur. Long-term sequelae following encephalitis are uncommon.

Diagnosis (epizootic virus infections)

A marked leukopenia is universal, often accompanied by neutropenia and thrombocytopenia, with moderate lymphocytosis in the cerebrospinal fluid. Virus can be detected by isolation or by PCR from serum or throat swab is possible within the first few days of illness. Paired sera can be tested by haemagglutinin inhibition and neutralizing tests. Specific IgM can be detected by MAC-ELISA in the second week of illness.

Prevention, control, and treatment

Equine immunization is effective in controlling epizootic disease. Venezuelan equine encephalitis is highly infectious by the aerosol route; many laboratory infections have occurred. Live attenuated and inactivated vaccines have been used in laboratory workers. People in affected areas should avoid mosquito bites. No specific treatment is available.

Western equine encephalitis

Aetiology and epidemiology

This is a complex of closely related viruses found in North and South America, but human disease is rare outside North America and Brazil. Summer outbreaks may be precipitated by flooding, which increases breeding of *Culex* mosquitoes (particularly *Culex tarsalis* in the western United States of America). Large outbreaks of western equine encephalitis in humans and horses occurred in the western United States of America in the 1950s and 1960s; however, a declining horse population, equine vaccination, and improved vector control have reduced the reported number of human cases to zero in most recent years.

Clinical characteristics

The ratio of apparent to inapparent infection in adults is less than 1 in 1000; however, this ratio increases to 1:1 in infants under 1 year of age. Following an incubation period of about 7 days, headache, vomiting, stiff neck, and backache are typical; restlessness and irritability are seen in children. Weakness and hyporeflexia are common. Convulsions occur in 90% of affected infants and 40% of affected children between 1 and 4 years, but are rare in adults. Recovery in 5 to 10 days is common, but convalescence may be protracted. Although rare in adults and older children, sequelae are common in infants, with one-half of those with encephalitis being left with convulsions and/or severe motor or intellectual deficits. The case fatality rate is 3 to 7%.

Diagnosis

Clinical laboratory findings in western equine encephalitis are often unremarkable. IgM antibodies are readily detected in serum by ELISA. Paired sera can be tested by haemagglutinin inhibition, IgG ELISA, or neutralization tests. Virus can occasionally be isolated from serum or cerebrospinal fluid.

Prevention, control, and treatment

Prevention of western equine encephalitis relies on mosquito control and the avoidance of mosquito bites. Vaccine is available for horses. An inactivated vaccine has been used for laboratory staff and others at high risk of exposure. No specific treatment is available.

Further reading

Centers for Disease Control and Prevention (2006). Eastern equine encephalitis: New Hampshire and Massachusetts, August–September 2005 *MMWR Morb Mortal Wkly Rep*, **55**, 697–700.

Griffin D (2007). Alphaviruses. In: Knipe DM, Howley PM (eds) *Fields virology*, 5th edition, vol. 1, pp. 1023–67. Lippincott Williams & Wilkins, Philadelphia.

Harley D, *et al.* (2001). Ross River virus transmission, infection, and diseases: a cross-disciplinary review. *Clin Microbiol Rev*, **14**, 909–32.

Kiwanuka N, *et al.* (1999). O'nyong-nyong fever in South-Central Uganda, 1996–1997: clinical features and validation of a clinical case definition for surveillance purposes. *Clin Infect Dis*, **29**, 1243–50.

Laine M, *et al.* (2004). Sindbis virus and other alphaviruses as cause of human arthritic disease. *J Int Med*, **256**, 457–71.

Pialoux G, *et al.* (2007). Chikungunya, an epidemic arbovirosis. *Lancet Infect Dis*, **7**, 319–27.

Weaver SC, Frolov IV (2005). Togaviruses. In: Mahy BWJ, ter Meulen V (eds) *Topley and Wilson's microbiology and microbial infections*, 10th edition, vol. 2, pp. 1010–24. Hodder Arnold, London.

Weaver SC, *et al.* (2004). Venezuelan equine encephalitis. *Annu Rev Entomol*, **49**, 141–74.

7.5.13 Rubella

P.A. Tookey and J.M. Best

Essentials

Rubella is caused by an enveloped RNA virus, for which humans are the only known host. Transmission is by airborne droplet spread, with infection seen predominantly in spring and early summer in temperate zones.

Postnatally acquired infection—presents after incubation of 14 to 21 days with rash (maculopapular, usually beginning on the face before spreading to the trunk and extremeties), lymphadenopathy (suboccipital and posterior cervical), and mild fever. Sore throat, coryza, cough, conjunctivitis, and arthralgia may be seen. The illness is usually mild. Management is symptomatic.

Rubella in pregnancy—in the first 10 weeks of gestation this is associated with a 90% risk of congenital fetal abnormalities, most typically comprising sensorineural hearing loss, alone or combined with cataracts and/or cardiac anomalies. Clinical diagnosis is unreliable, hence rapid investigation is essential when a woman develops a rubella-like illness in the first 16 weeks of pregnancy, comprising (1) testing of maternal serum for rubella IgG and IgM antibodies; and sometimes (2) amniotic fluid and/or fetal blood testing; and (3) ultrasonography to detect fetal defects. If a fetus is infected, termination of pregnancy is considered.

Prevention—live attenuated rubella vaccines provide protection to about 95% vaccinees and are usually given in combination with measles (MR) or measles and mumps (MMR) vaccines. Vaccination of >80% of children is required to prevent circulation of rubella virus. Health care workers and women of childbearing age whose rubella status is unknown (including recent immigrants) should also be targeted for MMR vaccination. Immunization of pregnant women is contraindicated, but women found to be susceptible at antenatal testing should be offered MMR vaccination after delivery.

Introduction

Rubella is a mild exanthematous disease of little clinical significance. However, infection in early pregnancy may result in multiple congenital abnormalities, often referred to as 'congenital rubella syndrome'. As a result of the widespread use of rubella vaccine, congenital rubella syndrome is now rare in many countries.

Aetiology

Rubella is caused by rubella virus, an enveloped RNA virus, which is classified in its own genus *Rubivirus* within the family Togaviridae. There are no major antigenic differences among rubella virus isolates, although at least seven genotypes have been described.

Epidemiology

Humans are the only known host for rubella virus. In temperate zones the infection is seen predominantly in spring and early summer. Before the introduction of rubella vaccine, rubella was endemic in virtually all countries. Epidemics were superimposed on the endemic infection every 4 to 9 years and pandemics every 10 to 30 years. In most populations, in the absence of a mass immunization programme, 10 to 20% of women are still susceptible to rubella infection when they reach child-bearing age. A review by the World Health Organization in 2000 estimated that more than 100 000 infants were born with congenital rubella syndrome each year in developing countries.

Postnatally acquired infection

The rash usually begins on the face and spreads to the trunk and then the extremities; the pink maculopapular lesions are initially discrete but later tend to coalesce. The suboccipital and posterior cervical lymph nodes are characteristically enlarged. Mild fever, sore throat, coryza, cough, and conjunctivitis may be present; symptoms are usually mild and last 3 to 7 days. There may be a prodrome with malaise and fever, especially in adults. There is no specific treatment.

Transient arthralgia with or without arthritis occurs in up to 70% of postpubertal women, but is less common in men and children. Less common complications include thrombocytopenia with or without purpura, postinfectious encephalitis, transverse myelitis, and rarely the Guillain–Barré syndrome. When rubella is acquired in early pregnancy congenital infection may occur (see below).

Rubella is clinically indistinguishable from several other infections and 20 to 50% of infections are subclinical. Therefore, a history of clinically diagnosed rubella infection is unreliable.

The incubation period is 14 to 21 days. The exact mode of transmission is uncertain but airborne spread by the respiratory route is likely and close contact is usually necessary for transmission. Individuals are most infectious just before the onset of symptoms, and the infectious period lasts from about a week before to a week after the rash appears. Infection usually produces lifelong immunity; however, when rubella is circulating reinfection may occur and is usually asymptomatic.

Congenital infection

Risk to the fetus

The possible consequences of rubella in pregnancy are the birth of an infant with congenital rubella infection with or without congenital defects, the birth of a normal infant, or spontaneous abortion. Infection before conception is not a risk to the fetus. Spontaneous abortion may occur when rubella is acquired early in pregnancy. When maternal infection occurs during the first 10 weeks of pregnancy the rate of fetal infection is about 90%; it then declines until the last few weeks of pregnancy when the rate rises again. Virtually all of those infected during the first 10 weeks of pregnancy are likely to have congenital defects, but the risk declines over the next 6 weeks. After 16 weeks' gestation even sensorineural hearing loss and growth retardation are rare, and no abnormalities have been demonstrated following serologically confirmed maternal infection after 18 weeks' gestation. Most prospective studies of the risk to the fetus have been carried out on women with symptoms, but asymptomatic primary infection is thought to carry a similar risk.

Following maternal reinfection in pregnancy the risk of transmission to the fetus is probably less than 10% and the risk of damage less than 5%, although it may be higher following symptomatic reinfection.

Clinical features

Congenital rubella is typically associated with cataracts, cardiac anomalies, and sensorineural hearing loss, and the term congenital rubella syndrome (CRS) refers to this classic triad of defects. The teratogenic effects may result in a wide range of defects (Box 7.5.13.1), but sensorineural hearing loss alone or combined with other abnormalities is most common. Severe multiple problems are more likely when infection occurs early in pregnancy.

Some defects, particularly sensorineural hearing loss, may not develop or become apparent until late infancy or childhood. Other reported late-onset problems include diabetes mellitus, thyroid dysfunction, autism, and other behavioural and psychiatric disorders. A rare progressive rubella panencephalitis has also been reported.

Laboratory diagnosis

The diagnosis of congenital rubella infection is relatively easy if suspected early, but more difficult to confirm after 3 months of age. The presence of rubella IgM antibody in early infancy is virtually diagnostic of congenital infection because acquired infection is rare at this age. Using sensitive assays, rubella IgM may be detected in 85% of infected infants at 3 to 6 months and about 30% at 6 to 12 months of age. The presence of IgG antibody alone is not diagnostic since it is likely to indicate passively transferred maternal antibody, but persistence of IgG between 6 and 12 months is strongly suggestive of congenital infection. When abnormalities present late, a presumptive diagnosis can be made based on a compatible clinical picture and the presence or persistence of rubella IgG antibodies in a young child who has not yet been vaccinated.

Congenital infection can also be diagnosed by detection of virus during the first months of life when it can be isolated or detected by polymerase chain reaction from a variety of specimens including nasopharyngeal swabs, urine, oral fluid, and conjunctival fluid. Congenitally infected infants shed large amounts of virus from the oropharynx and may be a source of infection for many months; viral shedding occasionally persists for more than a year.

Management of rubella-like illness during pregnancy

Appropriate management of a rash illness in pregnancy will depend on the local epidemiology of rubella. Routine antenatal rubella testing is not designed to identify rubella infection in pregnancy, and specific diagnostic investigations are needed. Pregnant women with a rubella-like rash should be investigated simultaneously for rubella and parvovirus B19, since they are clinically indistinguishable,

Box 7.5.13.1 Most common defects associated with congenital rubella

Classic triad

- Deafness
  - Sensorineural
  - Central auditory
- Abnormalities of the cardiovascular system
  - Patent ductus arteriosus
  - Pulmonary stenosis
  - Pulmonary arterial hypoplasia
- Abnormalities of the eye
  - Retinopathy
  - Cataracts
  - Microphthalmos
  - Iris hypoplasia

Other defects

- Growth retardation
- Microcephaly
- Mental retardation
- Speech defects

Other signs in the neonatal period and infancy

- Low birthweight
- Hepatosplenomegaly
- Jaundice
- Meningoencephalitis
- Rash
- Thrombocytopenia with or without purpura
- Adenopathies
- Bony radiolucencies
- Hypogammaglobulinaemia
- Pneumonitis

and even women previously reported to be immune should be investigated in case of laboratory error. Blood should be tested for rubella IgG and IgM antibodies. Rising IgG or detectable IgM antibody indicates recent infection; a positive IgM result alone should be confirmed with a second serum sample. Pregnant women who are susceptible or of unknown rubella antibody status and are in contact with a rubella-like illness should also be investigated as rapidly as possible. The detection of rubella IgM in a woman without a rash or history of contact should be interpreted with caution as rubella IgM may persist for some months or even years after infection or vaccination, or the IgM may be due to cross-reaction with autoantibodies or other viral IgM antibodies. Investigations must be done in consultation with a virologist who should be aware of the date and type of contact, stage of pregnancy, and history of previous immunization and testing. Prenatal diagnosis of congenital infection using amniotic fluid and/or fetal blood may sometimes be indicated. Ultrasound examination may detect such defects as microcephaly, dystrophic calcification, cataracts, microphthalmos, hepatosplenomegaly, and intrauterine growth restriction.

Prevention

Rubella can be prevented by live attenuated rubella vaccines. The RA27/3 strain is commonly used and this produces antibodies in about 95% of recipients; protection is probably lifelong in most vaccinees. Rubella vaccine is usually combined with measles (MR) or measles and mumps (MMR) vaccines.

In children, rubella vaccine causes few side effects. Low-grade fever and rash are occasionally reported, and transient arthralgia has been seen in about 3% of vaccinees; there have also been rare reports of myositis and vasculitis. Joint symptoms are more common in adult women, affecting up to 60% of vaccinees, but are transient and less severe than following naturally acquired rubella.

When rubella vaccines were first licensed in the late 1960s, universal childhood vaccination was implemented in the United States of America with the aim of eliminating rubella. A different strategy was pursued elsewhere, and the selective programmes established in Australia and some European countries targeted prepubertal girls and women of child-bearing age. This provided individual protection while allowing the continued circulation of wild virus and the acquisition of natural immunity by the majority of individuals. When the combined MMR vaccine became available, many countries with high vaccine uptake moved to a universal offer of MMR vaccine for children in the second year of life, usually with a second dose offered preschool or later.

The MMR vaccine was introduced into the United Kingdom schedule in 1988, and uptake by the age of 24 months reached 92% between 1992 and 1996. The schoolgirl programme was discontinued in 1996 and replaced by the offer of a second MMR for four-year-olds. Uptake of MMR subsequently declined to a low point of 80% in 2003, because of unfounded concerns about safety; however, by 2005 there were signs of recovery and uptake increased to over 85% by 2008. Antenatal screening continues. Although the circulation of rubella virus has dropped to very low levels since the introduction of MMR, prolonged periods of low vaccine uptake may lead to outbreaks of rubella in the future, putting susceptible pregnant women at risk.

Use of rubella-containing vaccines has led to the elimination of rubella in the United States of America and Scandinavian countries, although outbreaks have occurred in the United States of America due to importations of rubella virus. Similarly, in the United Kingdom there have been dramatic declines in the numbers of susceptible pregnant women, rubella-associated terminations, and children born with congenital rubella syndrome. Less than five congenitally infected infants were reported on average each year between 1990 and 1999, compared with about 50 per year in the 1970s. Between 2000 and 2008 fewer than 15 cases were identified, and in about half of these the infant's mother acquired infection abroad. Termination of pregnancy associated with rubella disease or contact is also now a rare occurrence.

The World Health Organization has recommended that all countries undertaking measles elimination should consider the introduction of MR or MMR vaccine in order to eliminate rubella as well. By 2005, rubella vaccine was used by 117 of 214 countries, with particularly good progress seen in the Americas. In 1997 the Pan American Health Organization recommended a regional initiative to eliminate rubella and congenital rubella syndrome, and by 2004 all countries in the region, except Haiti, had incorporated rubella vaccine into their routine vaccination programmes leading to a significant fall in cases of rubella and congenital rubella syndrome. The World Health Organization European Region established a goal of reducing congenital rubella syndrome cases to less than 1 per 100 000 births by 2010. The strategy to be adopted in any country seeking to control congenital rubella by vaccination must depend on the projected uptake of vaccination and the long-term prospects for continuing the programme. An important element should be the immunization of susceptible health personnel, particularly those in contact with pregnant women. It is also important to target women who have emigrated from countries without rubella vaccination programmes, as they are more likely to be susceptible than women born in countries with well-established vaccination programmes.

Vaccination in pregnancy

There have been persistent concerns that the vaccine virus might be teratogenic if given during pregnancy. Although vaccinees cannot infect other susceptible individuals, the virus can cross the placenta. Data from studies of children born to several hundred women inadvertently vaccinated up to 3 months before conception or during pregnancy show less than 3% with serological evidence of congenital infection, and no reported case of abnormalities attributable to congenital rubella. At least 80 of these infants were born to women vaccinated in the month of conception, probably the period of greatest vulnerability. These data suggest that the likely maximum theoretical risk of rubella-associated abnormalities is less than 5%.

Likely developments

- Elimination of rubella by further countries
- Introduction of rubella vaccine in additional countries worldwide
- Use of mathematical models to guide rubella vaccination strategies in different countries
- Use of genotyping to track the source of rubella outbreaks as countries approach elimination of rubella virus
- Development of techniques for the diagnosis of congenital rubella syndrome after the age of 3 months

Further reading

Banatvala JE, Brown DWG (2004). Rubella. *Lancet*, **363**, 1127–37.

Banatvala JE, Peckham C (eds) (2007). *Rubella viruses. Perspectives in medical virology*, vol. 15. Elsevier, London.

Best JM, Cooray S, Banatvala JE (2005). Rubella. In: Mahy BWJ, ter Meulen V (eds) *Topley and Wilson's microbiology and microbial infections*, 10th edition, pp. 959–92. Hodder Arnold, London.

Cooper LZ, Alford CA (2006). Rubella. In: Remington JS, *et al.* (eds) *Infectious diseases of the fetus and newborn infant*, 6th edition, pp. 894–926. Elsevier, Saunders, Philadelphia.

Department of Health (2006). Rubella. In: *Immunisation against Infectious Disease—'The Green Book'*. Available from: www.dh.gov.uk/assetRoot/04/13/79/28/04137928.pdf

Morgan-Capner P, Crowcroft NS; PHLS Joint Working Party of the Advisory Committees of Virology and Vaccines and Immunisation (2002). Guidelines on the management of, and exposure to, rash illness in pregnancy (including consideration of relevant antibody screening programmes in pregnancy). *Commun Dis Public Health*, **5**, 59–71. Available from: www.hpa.org.uk/infections/topics_az/pregnancy/rashes/default.htm

Robertson SE, *et al.* (2003). Rubella and congenital rubella syndrome: global update. *Pan Am J Public Health*, **14**, 306–15.

7.5.14 Flaviviruses excluding dengue

L.R. Petersen and D.J. Gubler

Essentials

Flaviviruses, family *Flaviviridae*, are small single-stranded, positive sense RNA viruses. They comprise 53 species (40 of which can cause human infection), divided into three major groups based on epidemiology and phylogenetics. They are maintained in nature in complex transmission cycles involving a variety of animals and hematophagous arthropods, which transmit infection to humans. IgM antibody capture enzyme-linked immunosorbent assay (MAC-ELISA) is widely used for diagnosis, with confirmation requiring isolation of the virus, or detection of specific antigen or of viral RNA by nucleic acid amplification from a tissue sample.

Mosquito-borne flaviviruses

Dengue and dengue haemorrhagic fever—see Chapter 7.5.15.

Japanese encephalitis virus—widespread distribution throughout Asia; the most important cause of arboviral encephalitis; maintained in a cycle involving *Culex* mosquitoes and water birds; about 1/250 infections are symptomatic, with manifestations ranging from a febrile illness with headache, through aseptic meningitis, to encephalitis, and death. Many survivors have residual neurological abnormalities. There is no specific treatment. Vaccination should generally be offered to people spending a month or more in endemic areas, especially if travel includes rural areas.

St Louis encephalitis virus—prevalent throughout the western hemisphere from southern Canada to Argentina; maintained in a cycle involving *Culex* mosquitoes and water birds; 1/16 to 1/425 infections are symptomatic, with manifestations ranging from fever with headache, to aseptic meningitis, to encephalitis, and death. There is no specific treatment. No vaccine is available.

West Nile virus—found in Africa, the Middle East, western Asia, parts of Europe and the Americas; maintained in a cycle involving *Culex* mosquitoes and water birds; most infections are asymptomatic, but 30% develop a febrile illness, and 1% neuroinvasive disease including meningitis, encephalitis and acute flaccid paralysis.

There is no specific treatment. Several equine vaccines are available, and human vaccines are in clinical trials.

Yellow fever virus—found in tropical America and Africa; forest/jungle transmission cycle involves canopy-dwelling mosquitoes and monkeys, urban cycle involves humans as the vertebrate host and *Aedes aegypti* as the principal vector; 5% of infections present clinically with a viraemic illness, which may be followed after a transient period of remission by relapse with shock, neurological deterioration, jaundice, haemorrhagic manifestations and renal failure. Treatment is symptomatic. A live, attenuated, single-dose vaccine is highly effective.

Other mosquito-borne flaviruses—these include Kunjin, Murray Valley, and Rocio encephalitides and Zika virus.

Tick-transmitted flaviviruses

Tick-borne encephalitis, louping ill, Powassan encephalitis—geographical distribution determined by that of relevant hard tick vectors; rodents are the principal vertebrate hosts, with occupational and vocational pursuits favouring tick exposure risk factors for human disease; most infections are subclinical, but a nonspecific influenza-like febrile illness may be followed after a few days of apparent recovery by aseptic meningitis or meningoencephalitis that may lead to permanent paralysis in some cases. Treatment is supportive. Effective inactivated vaccines are available.

Tick-borne haemorrhagic fevers—these include Kayasanur Forest disease and Al Khumra and Omsk haemorrhagic fevers.

Introduction

The genus *Flavivirus* of the family *Flaviviridae* comprises 53 virus species, 40 of which can cause human infection (Table 7.5.14.1). Flaviviruses are small (37–50 nm), spherical particles whose genome is a molecule of single-stranded, positive-sense RNA approximately 11 000 nucleotides in length. Based on epidemiological and phylogenetic characteristics, the flaviviruses are classified into three groups: (1) those that are mosquito-borne, (2) those that are tick-borne, and (3) those for which no arthropod vector has been demonstrated. All flaviviruses of human importance belong to the first two groups; the last group contains a few viruses found in vertebrates.

Most flaviviruses are maintained in nature in complex transmission cycles between wild or domestic animals and one or more haematophagous arthropod vectors. Humans become infected from infected arthropod vectors that take a blood meal, but for most of the flaviviruses humans do not usually develop high viraemias and are not thought to contribute to the transmission cycle. However, some flaviviruses such as dengue and yellow fever viruses do produce high-level viraemias in humans and can be maintained in urban surroundings through a mosquito–human–mosquito transmission cycle.

The epidemiology and geographical distribution of the flaviviruses depend on several factors including the presence of suitable amplifying hosts, the presence and feeding behaviour of a suitable arthropod vector, and the frequency of exposure of nonimmune reservoir hosts and humans to infected vectors. Globalization of trade and travel, human population growth, urbanization, and neglect of mosquito control programmes have produced conditions conducive to increasing incidence and geographical expansion of the flaviviruses. A recent dramatic example is the introduction and subsequent spread of the West Nile virus in the western hemisphere. Flavivirus infections are not directly communicable between humans.

Flavivirus infection in humans can result in asymptomatic infection or a spectrum of clinical illness ranging from nonspecific febrile illness, fever with rash or arthralgia or both, haemorrhagic fever, hepatitis, encephalitis, and death. The same virus can cause a variety of syndromes, and often the majority of those infected are asymptomatic. Although no specific therapy is available, prompt supportive treatment and proper management may substantially reduce mortality from some flavivirus infections.

Laboratory diagnosis

All flaviviruses have common group epitopes on the envelope protein that result in extensive cross-reactions in serological tests. The specificity of antibody should, therefore, be confirmed by cross-neutralization tests in areas where multiple flaviviruses are endemic/enzootic.

The IgM antibody capture enzyme-linked immunosorbent assay (MAC-ELISA) is widely used for diagnosis of flaviviruses. IgM antibody is usually detectable 5 to 8 days after onset of symptoms. Because detectable IgM antibody persists for one or more months after infection with most flaviviruses, its presence does not confirm current infection; people with detectable IgM antibody are considered recent or presumptive cases. Confirmatory laboratory diagnosis of most flaviviruses requires isolation of the virus, detection of specific viral RNA by nucleic acid amplification (NAA) or specific antigen in a clinical sample, or virus-positive immunohistochemistry in autopsy tissues. A fourfold or greater rise in specific neutralizing antibody is confirmation in some infections.

Important mosquito-borne flavivirus infections

For dengue and dengue haemorrhagic fever, see Chapter 7.5.15.

Japanese encephalitis

Aetiology and epidemiology

Japanese encephalitis virus is the type species of the Japanese encephalitis antigenic group of flaviviruses that includes several antigenically related viruses, including St Louis encephalitis, West Nile, Koutango, Usutu, Murray Valley encephalitis, Kunjin (a subtype of West Nile), Alfuy, Cacipacore and Yaounde viruses. Sequence analysis of the structural proteins suggests there are several genotypes of Japanese encephalitis in distinct geographical areas.

Japanese encephalitis has a widespread distribution throughout Asia, and its distribution has expanded in recent years with outbreaks in the Pacific, Australia, Nepal, and western India (Fig. 7.5.14.1). It is the most important cause of arboviral encephalitis and about 50 000 cases are reported annually. The highest incidence is in temperate and subtropical countries where epidemics may occur. The virus is maintained in a cycle involving *Culex* mosquitoes and water birds and is transmitted to humans by *Culex*

Table 7.5.14.1 Taxonomy of flaviviruses

Group	Species name[a]	Strain name, synonyms, and tentative species names	Abbreviation
Mosquito-borne viruses			
Aroa virus group	*Aroa virus*	Aroa virus	AROAV
		Bussuquara virus	BSQV
		Iguape virus	IGUV
		Naranjal virus	NJLV
Dengue virus group	***Dengue viruses***	**Dengue virus 1**	**DENV-1**
		Dengue virus 2	**DENV-2**
		Dengue virus 3	**DENV-3**
		Dengue virus 4	**DENV-4**
	Kedougou virus	Kedougou virus	KEDV
Japanese encephalitis virus group	*Cacipacore virus*	Cacipacore virus	CPCV
	Japanese encephalitis virus	**Japanese encephalitis virus**	**JEV**
	Koutango virus	Koutango virus	KOUV
	Murray Valley encephalitis virus	**Alfuy virus**	**ALFV**
		Murray Valley encephalitis virus	**MVEV**
	St Louis encephalitis virus	**St Louis encephalitis virus**	**SLEV**
	Usutu virus	Usutu virus	USUV
	West Nile virus	**Kunjin virus**	**KUNV**
		West Nile virus	**WNV**
	Yaounde virus	Yaounde virus	YAOV
Kokobera virus group	*Kokobera virus*	Kokobera virus	KOKV
		Stratford virus	STRV
Ntaya virus group	*Bagaza virus*	Bagaza virus	BAGV
	Ilheus virus	Ilheus virus	ILHV
		Rocio virus	**ROCV**
	Israel Turkey meningoencephalitis virus	Israel Turkey meningoencephalitis virus	ITV
	Ntaya virus	Ntaya virus	NTAV
	Tembusu virus	Tembusu virus	TMUV
Spondweni virus group	***Zika virus***	**Spondweni virus**	**SPOV**
		Zika virus	**ZIKV**
Yellow fever virus group	*Banzi virus*	Banzi virus	BANV
	Bouboui virus	Bouboui virus	BOUV
	Edge Hill virus	Edge Hill virus	EHV
	Jugra virus	Jugra virus	JUGV
	Saboya virus	Potiskum virus	POTV
		Saboya virus	SABV
	Sepik virus	Sepik virus	SEPV
	Uganda S virus	Uganda S virus	UGSV
	Wesselsbron virus	Wesselsbron virus	WESSV
	Yellow fever virus	**Yellow fever virus**	**YFV**

(Continued)

Table 7.5.14.1 *(Cont'd)* Taxonomy of flaviviruses

Group	Species name[a]	Strain name, synonyms, and tentative species names	Abbreviation
Tick-borne viruses			
Mammalian tick-borne virus group	*Gadgets Gully virus*	Gadgets Gully virus	GGYV
	Kyasanur Forest disease virus	**Kyasanur Forest disease virus**	**KFDV**
		Al Khumra haemorrhagic fever virus	**AKHFV**
	Langat virus	Langat virus	LGTV
	Louping ill virus	**Louping ill virus**	**LIV**
		British subtype	**LIV-Brit**
		Irish subtype	**LIV-Ir**
		Spanish subtype	**LIV-Span**
		Turkish subtype	**LIV-Turk**
	Omsk haemorrhagic fever virus	**Omsk haemorrhagic fever virus**	**OHFV**
	Powassan virus	**Powassan virus**	**POWV**
	Royal Farm virus	Karshi virus	KSIV
		Royal Farm virus	RFV
	Tick-borne encephalitis virus	**Tick-borne encephalitis virus**	**TBEV**
		European subtype	**TBEV-Eu**
		Far Eastern subtype	**TBEV-FE**
		Siberian subtype	**TBEV-Sib**
Seabird tick-borne virus group	*Kadam virus*	Kadam virus	KADV
	Meaban virus	Meaban virus	MEAV
	Saumarez Reef virus	Saumarez Reef virus	SREV
	Tyuleniy virus	Tyuleniy virus	TYUV
Viruses with no known arthropod vector			
Entebbe bat virus group	*Entebbe bat virus*	Entebbe bat virus	ENTV
		Sokoluk virus	SOKV
	Yokose virus	Yokose virus	YOKV
Modoc virus group	*Apoi virus*	Apoi virus	APOIV
	Cowbone Ridge virus	Cowbone Ridge virus	CRV
	Jutiapa virus	Jutiapa virus	JUTV
	Modoc virus	Modoc virus	MODV
	Sal Vieja virus	Sal Vieja virus	SVV
	San Perlita virus	San Perlita virus	SPV
Rio Bravo virus group	*Bukalasa bat virus*	Bukalasa bat virus	BBV
	Carey Island virus	Carey Island virus	CIV
	Dakar bat virus	Dakar bat virus	DBV
	Montana myotis leukoencephalitis virus	Montana myotis leukoencephalitis virus	MMLV
	Phnom Penh bat virus	Batu cave virus	BCV
		Phnom Penh bat virus	PPBV
	Rio Bravo virus	Rio Bravo virus	RBV
Viruses tentatively placed in the genus Flavivirus			
	Cell fusing agent virus		CFAV
	Tamana bat virus		TABV

[a] Species in bold are discussed in the text.

Adapted with permission from Fauquet C, Fauquet CM, Mayo MA (eds) (2005). *Virus taxonomy: classification and nomenclature of viruses; eighth report of the International Committee on the Taxonomy of Viruses*, pp. 986–8. Academic Press, New York.

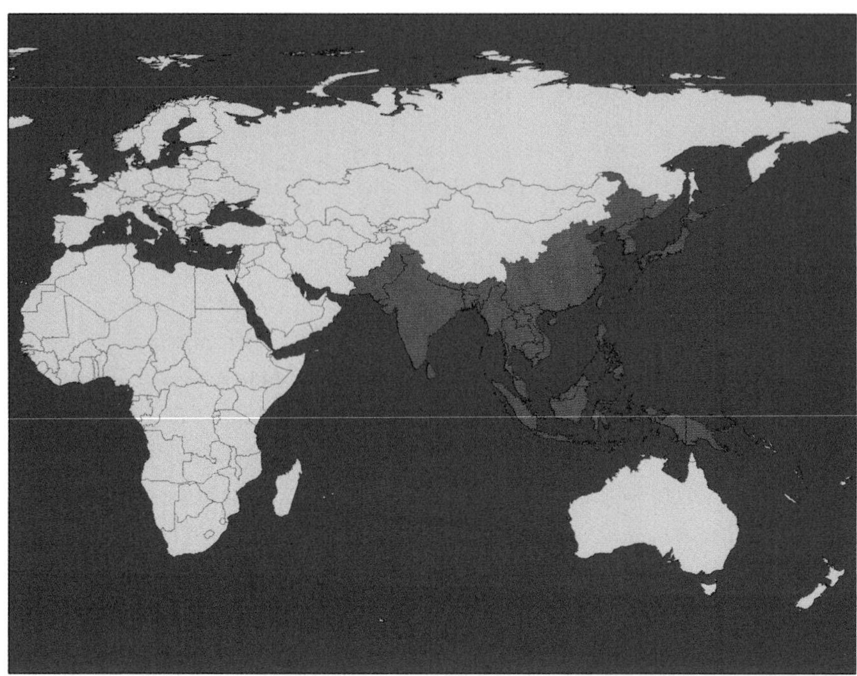

Fig. 7.5.14.1 Approximate geographical distribution of Japanese encephalitis virus.

mosquitoes, primarily species of the *Culex tritaeniorhynchus* complex which breed in rice fields. Pigs are the primary amplifying host in the peridomestic environment. Epidemics occur in late summer in temperate regions and throughout the year in some tropical areas of Asia. Children have the highest attack rates because of cumulative herd immunity with age.

Clinical characteristics (see also Chapter 24.11.2)

Only about 1 in 250 infections results in symptomatic infection, which ranges from a febrile illness with headache, through aseptic meningitis, to encephalitis, and death. After an incubation period of 6 to 16 days, illness usually begins with a prodrome lasting several days followed by abrupt high fever, change in mental status, nausea and vomiting, and headache. Early onset seizures occur in at least one-half of hospitalized children and one-quarter of adults. They are usually generalized tonic–clonic, but may also be partial motor or with more subtle clinical manifestations, such as twitching of a digit or eyebrow, or nystagmus. Patients with subtle seizures are usually in status epilepticus. Extrapyramidal features include dull, expressionless facies, generalized hypertonia, and cogwheel rigidity. Focal motor deficits, including cranial nerve palsies and acute flaccid paralysis resulting from anterior horn cell destruction may also occur. This poliomyelitis-like illness may be the only neurological manifestation of the illness or may proceed or accompany encephalitis. Respiratory dysregulation, coma, abnormal plantar reflexes, and prolonged convulsions are associated with a poor prognosis.

Laboratory examination often reveals a moderate peripheral leukocytosis and mild anaemia. Hyponatraemia, reflecting inappropriate antidiuretic hormone secretion, is common. Cerebrospinal fluid pressure is usually normal, pleocytosis ranges from a few to several hundred cells/mm^3, and cerebrospinal fluid protein is moderately elevated in about one-half the cases.

Five to 40% of cases are fatal; young children are more likely to die, and if they survive are more likely to have residual neurological defects. Overall, up to 70% of survivors have residual neurological abnormalities including parkinsonism, paralysis, behavioural changes, and psychological deficits. Evidence suggests that infection fails to clear in some patients, with clinical relapse several months after resolution of the acute illness. The clinical effects of congenital infection are unknown. Spontaneous abortions of women infected in the first and second trimesters have been reported.

Diagnosis

The differential diagnosis includes other viral encephalitides including arboviruses, herpes, and enteroviral infections, cerebral malaria, and bacterial infections. Epidemiological features such as place of residence or travel, season, and occurrence of other cases in the community provide clues to the diagnosis. Patients with encephalitis are rarely viraemic, although they may be so during the early acute stage of illness. Specific IgM can be detected in cerebrospinal fluid, serum, or both in nearly all patients by the seventh day after onset. Confirmation can be obtained by demonstrating fourfold or greater changes in specific IgM or neutralizing antibody titre.

Prevention and control

A formalin-inactivated mouse brain vaccine has been used widely in Japan, Korea, Taiwan, Thailand, and other countries in Asia for childhood immunization and is licensed in the United Kingdom, the United States of America, and other developed countries to protect travellers. Hypersensitivity reactions to this vaccine, including generalized urticaria, angio-oedema, and even anaphylaxis, have occurred within minutes to as long as 2 weeks following vaccination at a rate of 1 to 104 per 10 000. An inactivated tissue culture-based vaccine has been used in China and inactivated tissue culture-based vaccine is replacing the mouse brain vaccine in many countries, including for adults in the United States of America. A tissue culture-based live attenuated vaccine (SA 14-14-2) used extensively in China appears to have a remarkably good safety profile and currently is being introduced elsewhere in Asia. The risk to travellers in endemic areas during the transmission season can reach 1 in 5000 per month of exposure. The risk for most short-term travellers may be less than 1 in a million. In general, vaccine should be offered to people spending a month or more in endemic areas during the transmission season, especially if travel includes rural areas. However, there is perennial transmission in both urban and rural areas in Vietnam. Water and crop management and animal husbandry have been used to decrease human exposure to mosquito bites in the peridomestic environment.

Treatment

No specific therapy is available, but supportive treatment can reduce morbidity and mortality. Interferon-α2a failed to improve clinical outcome in a double-blind placebo-controlled trial. Dexamethasone did not prevent death caused by oedema-induced increases in intracranial pressure in patients with severe encephalitis.

St Louis encephalitis

Aetiology and epidemiology

St Louis encephalitis virus is prevalent throughout the western hemisphere from southern Canada to Argentina. The natural transmission cycle involves wild birds and *Culex* mosquitoes. Although clinical illness has been sporadically reported throughout much of the western hemisphere, the highest incidence occurs in North America during epidemics. Fewer than 100 human cases are generally reported annually; epidemics with hundreds to thousands of cases have occurred in North America every 10 to 20 years.

Clinical characteristics

The ratio of infection to clinical illness is high, ranging from 425:1 in children to 16:1 in elderly persons. Illness ranges from fever with headache, to aseptic meningitis, to encephalitis, and death. Advanced age is the principal risk factor for both symptomatic disease and severity of encephalitis. After an incubation period of 4 to 21 days, the typical presentation of encephalitis is fever, headache, chills, nausea, and dysuria. Within 1 to 4 days, central nervous system signs appear and may include meningism, tremor, abnormal reflexes, ataxia, cranial nerve palsies, convulsions (especially in children), stupor, and coma. Recovery is usually complete, except that 10 to 25% of very young infants have residual mental deficits, personality changes, muscle weakness, and paralysis. Underlying diseases such as hypertension, diabetes, and alcoholism affect the outcome. The case fatality rate is about 7% overall, but is only 1% of those under 5 years of age as the disease is generally milder in children. Short-lived sequelae of nervousness, memory impairment, and headache occur uncommonly in older children and adults.

The peripheral leucocyte count, serum transaminases, and creatine phosphokinase may be elevated. Hyponatraemia due to the syndrome of inappropriate antidiuretic hormone secretion may be noted in up to one-third of patients. The cerebrospinal fluid contains fewer than 500 cells/mm^3, principally leucocytes.

Diagnosis

The differential diagnosis includes other viral encephalitides such as West Nile virus and other arboviruses, herpes, and enterovirus, as well as other bacterial and fungal infections of the central nervous system. Epidemiological features (residence, season of the year, and occurrence of other cases in the community) provide diagnostic clues. Because of serological cross-reactivity with other flaviviruses, positive serum samples should be subjected to cross-neutralization tests. From fatal cases, virus may be isolated from brain tissue or demonstrated by immunohistochemistry. Virus has not been isolated from the blood during the acute phase of illness.

Prevention and control

No vaccine is available. Prevention is aimed at personal protection from mosquito bites and mosquito abatement.

Treatment

Treatment is supportive; no specific therapy is available.

West Nile encephalitis (see also Chapter 24.11.2)

Aetiology and epidemiology

West Nile virus is maintained in a cycle involving *Culex* mosquitoes and wild birds and is enzootic in Africa, the Middle East, western Asia, parts of Europe, and the Americas (Fig. 7.5.14.2). From the 1950s to the 1970s, sporadic epidemics, rarely associated with severe neurological disease and death, occurred in Israel, France, and Africa. No epidemic activity was then reported until the mid-1990s when epidemics associated with severe neurological disease and death in humans and/or equines and birds were recorded in Algeria, Morocco, Tunisia, Italy, Romania, Israel, southern Russia, and France. The virus was first detected in the New World during an outbreak in New York City in 1999; subsequently, the virus has become enzootic throughout most of the United States of America and southern Canada and has been detected as far south as Argentina. While large outbreaks have occurred annually in the United States of America, human or equine cases have been uncommonly reported in the tropical regions of the Caribbean and Latin America despite serological evidence of widespread enzootic transmission.

In temperate regions, outbreaks typically occur in late summer and early autumn, times when sufficient viral amplification in the bird–mosquito cycle has occurred to produce high mosquito infection rates. Although mosquito transmission accounts for nearly all human infections, infection resulting from receipt of contaminated blood transfusions and transplanted organs, transplacental transmission, needlestick exposure, aerosol exposure in the laboratory, mucous membrane splashes of infected fluids, and possibly ingestion of breast milk from an infected mother have been documented.

Phylogenetic studies indicate five and possibly as many as seven viral lineages: lineage one includes most strains isolated in recent outbreaks in Europe, the Middle East, and North America; lineage two includes many of the strains enzootic in Africa. Kunjin virus (see below) is a variant of West Nile virus and fits within lineage one. The strain introduced into North America was genetically identical to a strain circulating in the Middle East.

Clinical characteristics

Most infections are asymptomatic. Approximately 30% of those infected develop a systemic febrile illness, while less than 1% develop neuroinvasive disease including meningitis, encephalitis, and acute flaccid paralysis. Advanced age is the most important risk factor for developing both encephalitis and death. Certain immunosuppressed persons, such as organ transplant patients, are at extremely high risk of developing neuroinvasive disease after infection. The incubation period is usually 2 to 15 days, but may be longer in the immunosuppressed.

West Nile fever presents as a dengue-like illness with fever, headache, backache, myalgia, muscle weakness, anorexia, nausea, and vomiting that lasts 3 to 6 days. Roseola or a maculopapular rash on

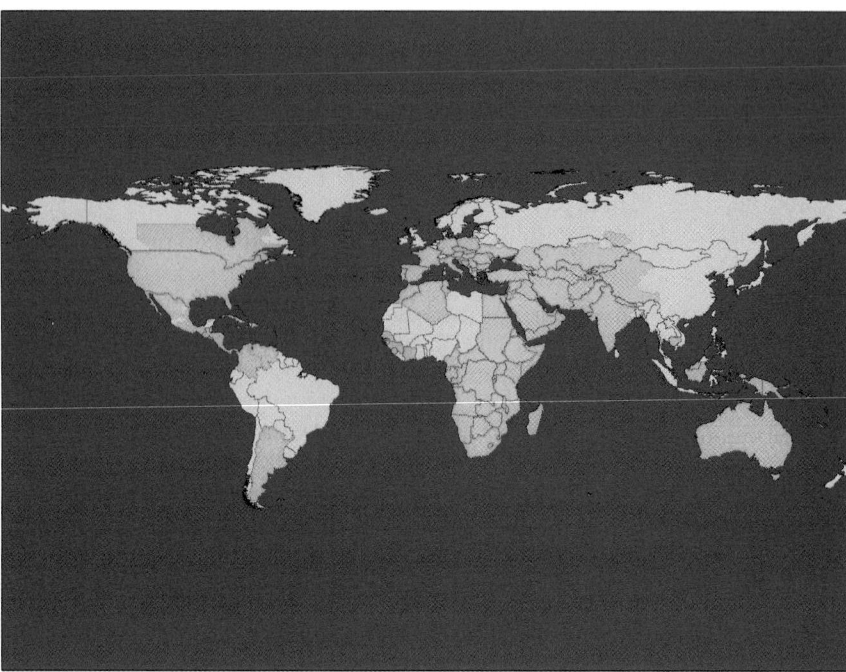

Fig. 7.5.14.2 Approximate geographical distribution of West Nile virus.

the trunk and extremities occurs in about one-half the patients with West Nile fever and generally arises during convalescence. The rash is present in about 20% of neuroinvasive disease patients. Fatigue lasting longer than a month after acute infection is common.

Among patients developing meningitis or encephalitis, fever is present in at least 90%, with weakness, nausea, vomiting, and headache in approximately one-half of patients. Other neurological manifestations include tremor, myoclonus, and parkinsonian features such as rigidity, postural instability, and bradykinesia. West Nile virus infection can cause an acute flaccid paralysis syndrome, even without concurrent meningitis or encephalitis; the paralysis usually results from involvement of the anterior horn cell process. Cranial nerve abnormalities may produce facial paralysis, which has a favourable prognosis. Dysarthria and dysphagia accompanied by acute flaccid paralysis indicate a high risk of impending respiratory failure. West Nile virus infection infrequently causes other forms of weakness, including brachial plexopathy, radiculopathy, and a predominantly demyelinating peripheral neuropathy similar to Guillain–Barré syndrome. Other neurological complications include seizures, cerebellar ataxia, and optic neuritis.

Numerous other manifestations of West Nile virus infection have been reported. Chorioretinitis and vitritis appear commonly, but are usually of minor clinical significance. Other reported ocular findings include iridocyclitis, occlusive vasculitis, and uveitis. Rhabdomyolysis, myocarditis, hepatitis, pancreatitis, central diabetes insipidus, and haemorrhagic manifestations have been documented.

Recovery from West Nile fever and meningitis is usually complete. Among those with encephalitis, approximately one-half of survivors have residual neurological deficits and initial disease severity may not predict eventual clinical outcome. Case fatality rates among those with encephalitis are approximately 10%. Most patients with acute flaccid paralysis have incomplete recovery of limb strength, often resulting in profound residual deficits. Quadriplegia and respiratory failure are associated with high morbidity and mortality, and recovery is slow and typically incomplete.

Diagnosis

Epidemiological features (residence, season of the year, and occurrence of other cases in the community) provide diagnostic clues. The differential diagnosis includes other causes of acute febrile illness; other viral encephalitides including arboviruses, herpes, and enterovirus, as well as other bacterial and fungal infections of the central nervous system; and other causes of acute flaccid paralysis. West Nile virus should strongly be considered when myoclonic jerking, parkinsonian features, or acute flaccid paralysis occur with encephalitis during peak transmission times. In patients with acute flaccid paralysis, neurological examination should differentiate anterior horn cell dysfunction from Guillain–Barré syndrome.

The cerebrospinal fluid usually contains moderately elevated protein and up to 2000 cells/mm^3, with neutrophils predominating early in infection followed by lymphocytic predominance. IgM ELISA of serum or cerebrospinal fluid samples is positive in nearly all patients by the eighth day after clinical onset, although some immunocompromised patients may either fail to develop or have delayed onset of demonstrable IgM antibodies. Nucleic acid amplification testing (NAT) of serum or cerebrospinal fluid may aid in the diagnosis of these patients. In patients with West Nile fever, NAT may increase the yield of testing of early acute-phase samples. In areas endemic for other flaviviruses, serological cross-reactivity may complicate diagnosis and positive samples should be tested by cross-neutralization.

Prevention and control

Several equine vaccines are available. Human vaccines are in clinical trials. Mosquito repellents containing *N,N*-diethyl-3-methylbenzamide (DEET), picaridin, or oil of lemon eucalyptus are recommended. Community prevention is aimed at surveillance and mosquito abatement. Universal blood donor screening using NAT has markedly reduced the risk of transfusion-related transmission in the United States of America and Canada.

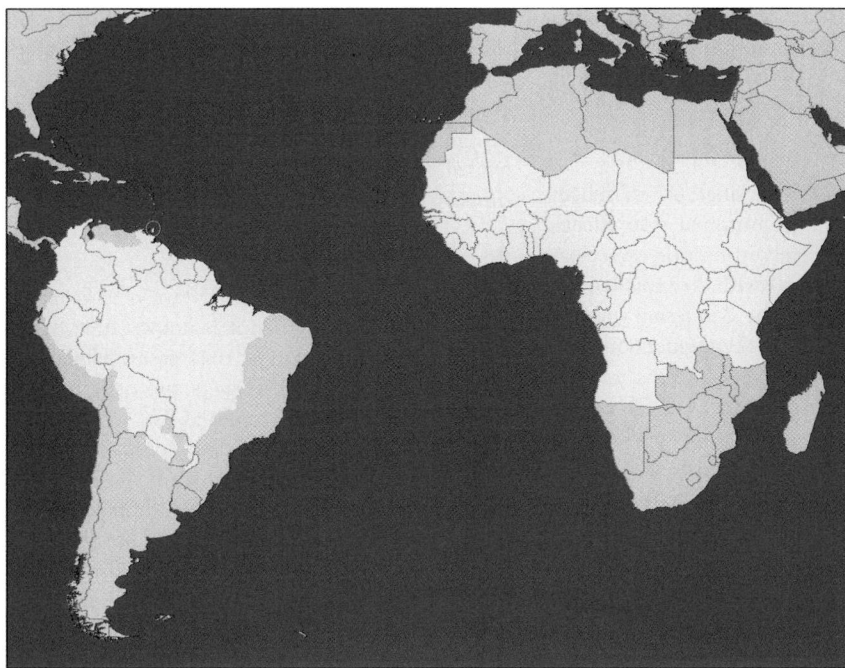

Fig. 7.5.14.3 Approximate geographical distribution of yellow fever virus.

Treatment

Treatment is supportive; no specific therapy is available. It is imperative that appropriate diagnostic testing including lumbar puncture, electromyography, and nerve conduction studies be obtained before initiating therapies for Guillain–Barré syndrome or other inflammatory neuropathies.

Yellow fever

Aetiology and epidemiology

Yellow fever was first described in the 17th century and was one of the great plagues of humans for over 400 years. In 1900, mosquito transmission and the viral aetiology were proved. The virus was isolated in 1927 and a vaccine developed in 1937. The virus is present in tropical America and Africa, but does not occur in Asia (Fig. 7.5.14.3). Epidemics still occur, especially in West Africa. Between 1986 and 1991, a series of outbreaks in Nigeria caused an estimated 100 000 cases (although only about 5000 were officially reported), with attack rates in affected areas of 30/1000 and case fatality rates exceeding 20%. In South America, the disease affects up to 300 people annually, principally young men working in forest areas exposed to haemagogus mosquitoes breeding in tree holes (jungle yellow fever). Disease in unvaccinated travellers is rare; however, at least six have died in the United States of America and Europe of infection acquired in South America and Africa in recent years. In 2008, yellow fever was reported from the Democratic Republic of the Congo, Côte d'Ivoire, Central African Republic, Liberia, Peru, Brazil, Argentina, and Paraguay.

Yellow fever virus has two cycles of transmission, jungle (sylvatic) yellow fever and urban yellow fever. The forest or jungle transmission cycle involves canopy-dwelling mosquitoes and monkeys. The urban cycle involves humans as the vertebrate host and *Aedes aegypti* as the principal vector. In the past 30 years, *Ae aegypti* has reinvaded Central and South America and a small outbreak of urban yellow fever occurred in Bolivia in 1998. Sporadic urban transmission has occurred in other South American countries in recent years, including Brazil and Paraguay. Epidemics in Africa often occur in moist savannah regions, involving forest (sylvatic) or peridomestic *Aedes* mosquitoes and humans as viraemic hosts. In dry areas and urban centres, epidemic transmission occurs where water-storage practices breed domestic *Ae aegypti*. Several hundred thousand people are infected annually and outbreaks are frequent.

Clinical characteristics

Approximately 1 in 20 infections results in clinical disease with jaundice. In its classic form, disease occurs abruptly after an incubation period of 3 to 6 days. The initial phase ('period of infection') is characterized by viraemia, fever, chills, headache, photophobia, lumbosacral pain, myalgia, nausea, and prostration. On examination, the patient may have a relative bradycardia and conjunctival injection. Within several days, the patient may recover transiently ('period of remission') only to relapse ('period of intoxication') with jaundice, albuminuria, oliguria, haemorrhagic manifestations (especially 'black vomit' haematemesis), delirium, stupor, metabolic acidosis, and shock. The prognosis in such cases is poor; 20 to 50% die during the second week of illness.

Clinical laboratory tests reveal leukopenia, thrombocytopenia, hepatic dysfunction, and renal failure. The bleeding diathesis is caused by decreased synthesis of clotting factors and may be complicated by disseminated intravascular coagulation. Pathological findings include midzonal hepatic necrosis and eosinophilic degeneration of hepatocytes (Councilman bodies), possibly representing apoptosis, and acute renal tubular necrosis. Focal myocarditis, brain swelling, and petechial haemorrhages contribute to pathogenesis. Recovery is complete, without postnecrotic hepatic cirrhosis.

Diagnosis

Exposure and travel history provide important clues to aetiology. The differential diagnosis includes viral hepatitis, leptospirosis, rickettsial infections, dengue haemorrhagic fever, Rift Valley fever, Ebola, and Crimean–Congo haemorrhagic fever. Serological cross-reactions with other flaviviruses may complicate serology.

Postmortem histopathological examination of the liver is diagnostic, with or without immunocytochemical staining for viral antigen. Liver biopsy should never be performed on living patients as it may precipitate haemorrhage.

Prevention and control

The live attenuated 17D vaccine, delivered as a single 0.5-ml subcutaneous dose, is highly effective and has minimal side effects. Immunity is probably lifelong, but for travel certification revaccination is recommended every 10 years. People with documented egg allergy should not be immunized or should be skin tested with the vaccine. The vaccine must not be given to children under 6 months of age, in whom there is a risk of postvaccinal encephalitis, and it is best to delay vaccination until 9 months of age. On theoretical grounds, immunosuppressed patients (including those with clinical AIDS) should not be immunized. The immune response in HIV-infected persons is impaired. Evidence suggests that vaccine-associated viscerotropic disease is much more common in patients with a history of thymic tumour and thymectomy is contraindicated. No evidence of clinical congenital infection has been found. Immunization during pregnancy is contraindicated, but, if inadvertently performed, recipients should be reassured and followed. The immune response in pregnancy was found to be impaired. Fatal infection following vaccination with the 17D strain has been rarely reported, although postvaccination encephalitis and Guillain–Barré syndrome in adults (incidence 0.4 and 1.9 cases per million doses of vaccine, respectively) and viscerotropic disease (incidence 0.1–2.5 per million vaccinees) may be increasing. Both of these conditions are more frequent among older vaccinees. Other control measures include reducing the principal urban mosquito vector *Ae aegypti* in tropical urban centres.

Treatment

Treatment is symptomatic. Intensive care requires prompt awareness and treatment of acidosis, shock, and metabolic imbalance. Patients with renal failure may require dialysis.

Other mosquito-borne infections

Kunjin

Genomic sequencing indicates that Kunjin virus is a variant of West Nile virus. It is found over most of tropical Australia and Queensland and has a similar transmission cycle involving birds and *Culex* mosquitoes. Infection is usually asymptomatic, but occasional cases of encephalitis have been reported. Infections are generally milder than with Murray Valley encephalitis and are not life threatening. Kunjin virus infections that are nonencephalopathic usually present with fever, often with polyarthralgia. Cases occur sporadically with only 43 reported from 1998 to 2005. Treatment is supportive; there is no vaccine.

Murray Valley encephalitis

Murray Valley encephalitis is enzootic in New Guinea, north Western Australia, and the Northern Territory, and possibly in northern Queensland. The virus has a transmission cycle involving birds and *Culex* mosquitoes and is transmitted to humans by *Culex annulirostris* mosquitoes from the end of March to early June. Only 1 in 1000 to 2000 infections results in clinical illness; of those that have neurological disease, approximately one-third are fatal and one-quarter have residual neurological deficits. Clinical illness resembles Japanese encephalitis. Children and elderly people are at the highest risk. In 1974, the largest recorded epidemic involved 58 cases and 10 deaths; since then, sporadic cases have been identified. Serological diagnosis is complicated by the presence of the closely related Kunjin virus, which also causes encephalitis. Treatment is supportive; there is no vaccine.

Rocio encephalitis

Rocio virus is a member of the Ntaya virus group and is considered a subtype of Ilheus virus; it is known only in Brazil. Epidemics from 1973 to 1980 caused 1021 cases, principally among young adult male agricultural workers and fisherman. Since then, only sporadic illness has been reported. The virus has been isolated from *Psorophora ferox* mosquitoes and *Aedes scapularis* mosquitoes may be involved in Rocio virus transmission. Wild birds are the likely amplifying hosts. Symptoms include fever, headache, anorexia, nausea, vomiting, myalgia, and malaise followed by confusion, reflex disturbance, motor impairment, and cerebellar dysfunction. The mortality rate is approximately 10%, and 20% of patients have neurological sequelae. Virus is not recoverable from blood, but postmortem diagnosis may be made by virus isolation from brain tissue. Treatment is supportive; there is no vaccine.

Zika virus infection

This flavivirus was first identified in 1947 in rhesus monkey serum in Uganda. It has been responsible for small epidemics in Uganda, Nigeria, Malaysia, and Indonesia. It causes a mild dengue-like illness (fever, conjunctival injection, rash, and arthralgia). A total of 120 confirmed and probable cases occurred in Yap, Micronesia, and possibly Guam, from March to May 2007. Mosquitoes (*Aedes aegypti, Ae africanus*) are known vectors.

Tick-borne infections of the central nervous system

Tick-borne encephalitis

Aetiology and epidemiology

There are three subtypes of tick-borne encephalitis virus defined phylogenetically, European, Far Eastern, and Siberian, which differ only slightly in viral protein structure. These viruses, along with the louping ill, Powassan, Kyasanur Forest disease, and Omsk haemorrhagic fever viruses, belong to the tick-borne encephalitis antigenic complex. The disease caused by the Far Eastern subtype is also known as Russian spring/summer encephalitis and Russian epidemic encephalitis; the European subtype as also known as FSME (Frühsommer-Meningoenzephalitis), early-summer encephalitis, and Kumlinge's disease. The geographical distribution of disease is determined by that of their hard tick vectors: *Ixodes persulcatus* for the Far Eastern subtype causing human disease principally from the Baltic countries to north-eastern China and northern Japan, and *Ixodes ricinus* for the European subtype which occurs from the Urals in Russia to the Alsace region of France, Scandinavia to the north, and parts of the Mediterranean areas along the Adriatic coast to the south (Fig. 7.5.14.4). Several other tick species play a role as minor vectors. Switzerland reports more than 100 cases each year, while 3000 clinical cases are reported in Europe. The incidence is increasing in all countries except

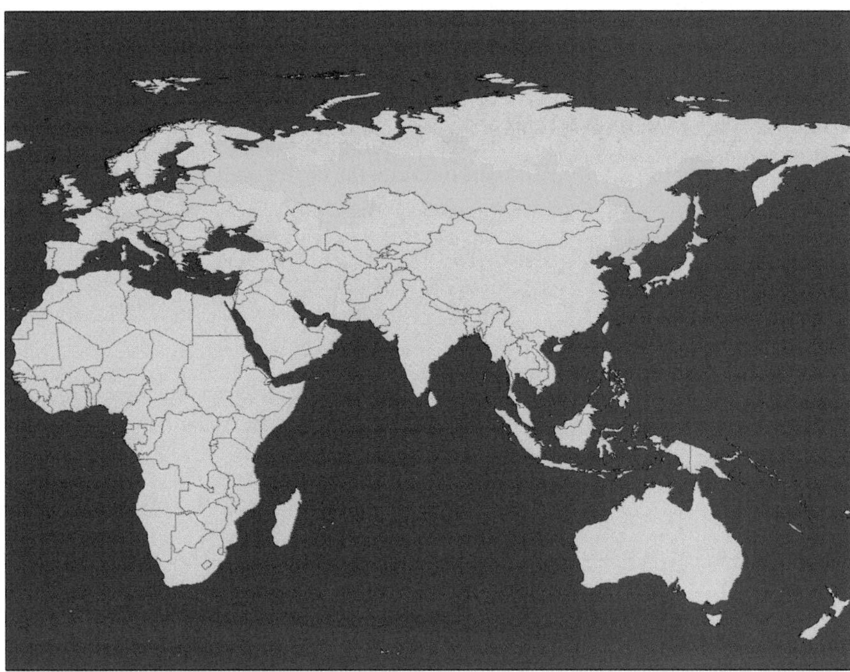

Fig. 7.5.14.4 Approximate geographical distribution of tick-borne encephalitis virus.

Austria where an aggressive vaccination policy has proved effective. The Siberian subtype is found in Siberia and the Baltic states. In Russia more than 10 000 cases of tick-borne encephalitis are reported each year.

Infections occur during the period of tick activity from April to November. In Novosibirsk, south-west Siberia, more than 20 000 tick bites are reported annually. Tick-borne encephalitis is largely a rural infection; occupational and vocational pursuits favouring tick exposure are risk factors. Human infection and outbreaks following consumption of raw milk or cheese from asymptomatic goats or, more rarely, sheep or cows have been described. Hundreds to thousands of cases occur annually, with reported attack rates up to 200/100 000 residents in Latvia, the Urals, and western Siberia. Aerosolized virus has caused laboratory infections.

Clinical characteristics

Most human infections are subclinical. The illness produced by each subtype is generally similar but that produced by the Far Eastern subtype carries a worse prognosis. The incubation period is 7 to 14 days (range 2–28 days); incubation periods of 3 to 4 days follow milk-borne exposure. The European subtype typically produces a biphasic illness. The first phase is a nonspecific, influenza-like, febrile illness lasting 2 to 7 days followed by an afebrile and relatively asymptomatic period lasting 2 to 10 days. Flushing, conjunctival haemorrhage, nausea, vomiting, dizziness, and myalgia are common findings. Approximately one-third of patients then develop higher fevers with aseptic meningitis or meningoencephalitis. The Far Eastern subtype usually progresses without an asymptomatic phase. Signs and symptoms of meningitis, meningoencephalitis, meningoencephalomyelitis, myelitis, or meningoradiculitis include somnolence, coma, asymmetrical paresis of the cranial nerves, tremors of the extremities, nystagmus, severe pain in the extremities, and flaccid paralysis of the neck and upper extremities.

Permanent paralysis develops in 2 to 10% of patients with the European subtype and 10 to 25% with the Far Eastern subtype. Corresponding case fatality rates are 0.5 to 2.0% and 5 to 20% for the European and Far Eastern subtypes, respectively. Severity of illness with the Siberian subtype is intermediate between the European and Far Eastern subtypes, with a case fatality rate of 1 to 3%.

Laboratory findings include neutrophilia, although neutropenia, thrombocytopenia, and elevated liver enzyme levels may occur early. The cerebrospinal fluid white blood cell count is usually below 500 cells/mm^3, primarily of mononuclear cells.

Diagnosis

The differential diagnosis is similar to Japanese encephalitis; the pattern of flaccid paralysis may be confused with poliomyelitis. A history of bite by small ixodid ticks is elicited in fewer than one-half of patients. Specific diagnosis is made by virus isolation from blood or cerebrospinal fluid during the first week of illness, or by serological tests including IgM enzyme immunoassay and a neutralization test.

Prevention and control

Effective inactivated vaccines are available in Europe in formulations for adults and children. Two doses 4 to 6 weeks apart followed by a booster at 1 year are recommended for those walking and camping in tick-infested coniferous forests of endemic areas, especially during the tick season (May–October). Mass vaccination in Austria produced a dramatic decline in disease incidence. Vaccines appear to produce equal protection against the eastern and western strains. Rapid immunization schedules are available for those with impending travel to endemic areas during the tick season. Tick bites should be prevented by the use of repellents containing DEET and use of permethrin on clothing and camping gear, and attached ticks should be discovered and removed as soon as possible. Unpasteurized goats' milk products should be avoided.

Treatment

Treatment is supportive.

Louping ill

This is a disease of veterinary importance causing neurological illness in sheep and to a lesser extent in cows, horses, farmed deer, sheepdogs, and pigs. The virus, isolated in 1931, is a member of the tick-borne encephalitis complex and is transmitted by *Ixodes ricinus*. Louping ill occurs in the hill country along the western coast of Scotland and northern England, Ireland, and Norway. Natural infections resulting in human disease have been rare, but laboratory infections are not uncommon. Naturally acquired human infections have mainly occurred in persons with occupational exposure to animals. Some of these cases were attributable to contact with sheep blood. Infection from tick bite is rare. The human disease is typically aseptic meningitis or encephalitis; no fatal infections have occurred. Avoidance of tick bites in enzootic areas is recommended. The licensed tick-borne encephalitis vaccine may be protective.

Powassan encephalitis

The virus was first isolated from the brain of a patient who died in Powassan, Ontario in 1958. Since then, more than 30 human cases have been recognized in eastern Canada and the eastern United States of America, primarily in children, with a case fatality rate of 10% and a high incidence of residual neurological dysfunction. Serological surveys indicate an antibody prevalence of 1 to 4%. The distribution of the virus in North America is considerably wider than indicated by human cases, and the diagnosis should be suspected in any case of summer–autumn encephalitis. The virus is transmitted between *Ixodes Cookei* (ricinus complex) ticks and rodents. Cases have also occurred in Russia where the primary vector is *IX. persulcatus*. The clinical features are those of viral encephalitis, with localizing neurological signs and convulsions. There is no specific treatment or vaccine.

Tick-borne haemorrhagic fever

Kyasanur Forest disease

Aetiology and epidemiology

This virus is a member of the tick-borne encephalitis antigenic complex. The virus has been isolated from humans, monkeys, and ticks since it was first recognized in 1957 during an outbreak of haemorrhagic fever affecting wild monkeys in Karnataka (then Mysore) State, India. Several hundred cases are reported annually, principally among people working in the forest in Karnataka State. In 1983, 1555 cases, including 150 deaths, occurred. The peak seasonal incidence is from January/February to May. The virus is transmitted by *Haemaphysalis spinigera* ticks in a life cycle that involves small mammals, monkeys, birds, cattle, and large mammals at various stages. Humans are incidental hosts and are primarily infected by nymphs. Al Khurma virus, a subtype of Kyasanur Forest virus, causes haemorrhagic fever in Saudi Arabia (see below).

Clinical characteristics

After an incubation period of 3 to 8 days, fever starts abruptly with chills, headache, myalgia, abdominal pain, nausea, vomiting, and diarrhoea. Physical signs include bradycardia, lymphadenopathy, and haemorrhagic manifestations. Hypotension is frequently noted during the end of the acute stage. Fatal cases develop shock and pulmonary oedema. A biphasic illness is not uncommon, with resolution of the first phase in 5 to 12 days and return of the fever and signs of meningoencephalitis after an interval of 1 to 3 weeks. Localizing neurological signs are infrequent, and residual defects are rare; convalescence is prolonged. Laboratory abnormalities include leukopenia, thrombocytopenia, and elevated serum transaminases during the acute phase. Fatality rates are 2 to 10%.

Diagnosis

Diagnosis is by virus isolation from blood collected during the first week after onset or by serological tests. Virus isolation should be conducted under biosafety level 4 conditions.

Prevention and control

Tick bites should be avoided in endemic areas. A formalin-inactivated vaccine is available in India.

Treatment

Treatment is supportive; specific therapy is not available.

Al Khumra ('Alkhurma') haemorrhagic fever

In 1995, a subtype of Kyasanur Forest disease virus was isolated from patients from Al Khumra, south of Jeddah, Saudi Arabia, with clinical symptoms ranging from febrile illness with headache, malaise, myalgia, nausea, and vomiting to fatal haemorrhagic disease. It has been referred to incorrectly as 'Alkhurma haemorrhagic fever'. From 2001 to 2003, 20 cases were identified by national surveillance in Saudi Arabia. Human infections are associated with handling meat or drinking unpasteurized camels' milk. The virus seems to be associated with sheep, goats, and camels, which do not manifest disease themselves, and to be transmitted by ticks. Its natural reservoir is unknown but the camel tick *Hyalomma dromedarii* is a prime suspect. Fever, headache, malaise, and myalgia are common. About one-half of patients exhibit haemorrhagic manifestations ranging from mild bleeding (epistaxis) to haemorrhagic shock and disseminated intravascular coagulation with thrombocytopenia. Most have elevated serum concentrations of liver transaminases, lactate dehydrogenase, creatine kinase, and bilirubin, and some develop renal failure. About 35% of patients develop encephalitis and the case fatality rate is 25%. Important differential diagnoses include Crimea–Congo haemorrhagic fever and Rift Valley fever which share its epidemiological features. Compared to Rift Valley fever, there is no visual loss, scotomas, or haemolysis in Al Khumra haemorrhagic fever, but haemorrhage is more common and the case fatality rate is higher.

Omsk haemorrhagic fever

This disease was first recognized in 1945 in western Siberia. Cases were frequent between 1945 and 1949, with morbidity rates of 500 to 1400/100 000, but subsequently have been rare, mainly occurring among residents of rural areas working in the fields. Human infections are acquired by dermacentor tick bite or contact with infected muskrats. After an incubation period typically of 3 to 7 days, the disease begins with the abrupt onset of fever, headache, myalgia, facial flushing, conjunctival suffusion, minor haemorrhagic manifestations, and leukopenia. Recovery occurs in the second week, and the case fatality rate is low (0.5–3%). The differential diagnosis includes tularaemia, rickettsial infection, and leptospirosis. Specific diagnosis is made by virus isolation from blood during the acute phase or by serological tests. Only a few laboratories outside Russia with biocontainment level 4 facilities are capable of providing laboratory assistance. Tick-borne encephalitis vaccines may cross-protect against Omsk haemorrhagic fever.

Further reading

Gould EA, *et al.* (2006). Potential arbovirus emergence and implications for the United Kingdom. *Emerg Infect Dis*, **12**, 549–54.

Gritsun TS, Lashkevich VA, Gould EA (2003). Tick-borne encephalitis. *Antiviral Res*, **57**, 129–46.

Gubler DF, Kuno G, Markoff L (2007). Flaviviruses. In: Knipe DM, Howley PM (eds) *Fields virology*, 5th edition. Lippincott Williams & Wilkins, Philadelphia.

Günther G, Haglund M (2005). Tick-borne encephalopathies. Epidemiology, diagnosis, treatment and prevention. *CNS Drugs*, **19**, 1009–32.

Hayes EB, Gubler DJ (2006). West Nile virus: epidemiology and clinical features of an emerging epidemic in the United States. *Annu Rev Med*, **57**, 181–94.

Hayes EB, *et al.* (2005). Virology, pathology, and clinical manifestations of West Nile virus disease. *Emerg Infect Dis*, **11**, 1174–9.

Mackenzie JS, Gubler DJ, Petersen LR (2004). Emerging flaviviruses: the spread and resurgence of Japanese encephalitis, West Nile and dengue viruses. *Nat Med Suppl*, **10**, S98–109.

Madani TA (2005). Alkhumra virus infection, a new viral hemorrhagic fever in Saudi Arabia. *J Infect*, **51**, 91–7.

Marfin AA, *et al.* (2005). Yellow fever and Japanese encephalitis vaccines: indications and complications. *Infect Dis Clin North Am*, **19**, 151–68.

Pattnaik P (2006). Kyasanur forest disease: an epidemiological view in India. *Rev Med Microbiol*, **16**, 151–65.

Solomon T (2003). Recent advances in Japanese encephalitis. *J Neurovirol*, **9**, 274–83.

7.5.15 **Dengue**

Bridget Wills and Jeremy Farrar

Essentials

Dengue is caused by a flavivirus and is the most important mosquito-borne viral infection of humans. Some 40 million symptomatic infections are estimated to occur annually. The disease is hyper-endemic in many large Asian cities, and is also a significant problem in the Pacific region and in the Americas. The primary mosquito vector is *Aedes aegypti*. Infection can be caused by any one of four closely related but serologically distinct dengue viral serotypes. Following infection with a single serotype there is life-long immunity to that serotype but the possibility of more severe disease during a subsequent infection with a different serotype.

Clinical features and diagnosis—symptomatic disease ranges from a nonspecific febrile illness through to a syndrome characterized by plasma leakage that may, if severe, result in the development of potentially fatal dengue shock syndrome. Thrombocytopenia and deranged haemostasis also occur, but clinically significant bleeding is unusual except it patients with profound shock. Severe hepatic and neurological complications are also seen in some patients. Diagnosis depends on viral isolation, detection of viral antigen or viral RNA, or serological testing.

Management and prevention—treatment is supportive, with particular emphasis on careful fluid management. Prompt volume resuscitation is essential for patients with shock, with regular monitoring of the pulse rate, blood pressure, and haematocrit to minimize the risk of fluid overload. No vaccine is available as yet but a number of candidates are entering clinical trials. Currently prevention relies on elimination of potential vector breeding sites, biological and chemical vector control strategies, and avoidance of mosquito bites.

Introduction and aetiology

Dengue is the most important mosquito-borne viral infection of humans. 'Dengue' is a West Indian Spanish word derived from Ki Swahili 'ka dinga pepo' ('a kind of cramping plague') that was brought from Africa to the Caribbean. In the British West Indies it was called 'dandy fever' because of the stiff posture of its victims, and in Cuba dengue was later termed 'quebranta huesos' or 'breakbone fever' because of the severe myalgias and arthralgias. Infection can be caused by any one of the four closely related but serologically distinct dengue viral serotypes (DEN-1, -2, -3, and -4) that together constitute one subgroup of the genus *Flavivirus*, family Flaviviridae. Since there is only transient cross-protective immunity between the four serotypes, people living in a dengue-endemic area can be infected up to four times during their lifetime.

Epidemiology

Humans are infected with dengue viruses by the bite of a mosquito. *Aedes aegypti*, the principal vector, is a highly domesticated tropical mosquito that lays its eggs in artificial water containers commonly found in and around homes. The adult mosquitoes rest indoors and prefer to feed on humans during daylight hours, with peak biting activity in the early morning and late afternoon. The adult female mosquitoes are nervous feeders and, if their feeding is interrupted, will return to the same person or different persons to continue feeding. Thus, during a single blood meal several persons may become infected, making *Ae aegypti* a highly efficient epidemic vector. The transmission cycle of most importance is *Ae aegypti*–human–*Ae aegypti* in large urban centres of the tropics. Multiple virus serotypes often cocirculate within the same city causing periodic epidemics. Epidemics of febrile illness attributed to dengue have been reported at intervals over the last 200 years across Asia, Africa, and North America, likely reflecting progressive expansion in the global distribution of the *Aedes* mosquito vectors. However, from the 1950s onwards a new clinical syndrome, characterized by vascular leakage and bleeding and given the name dengue haemorrhagic fever (DHF), began to emerge in south-east Asia. The first epidemic of DHF in the Americas appeared in 1981 in Cuba, associated with the arrival of a new Asian strain of DEN-2 virus of different genotype from the American strain.

Dengue is now hyperendemic in most Asian cities, with epidemics occurring every 3 to 5 years superimposed on background endemic transmission. It has also become established as a significant problem in the Pacific region and in the Americas. More than 3 billion people live in areas of risk and approximately 40 million symptomatic infections are estimated to occur each year,

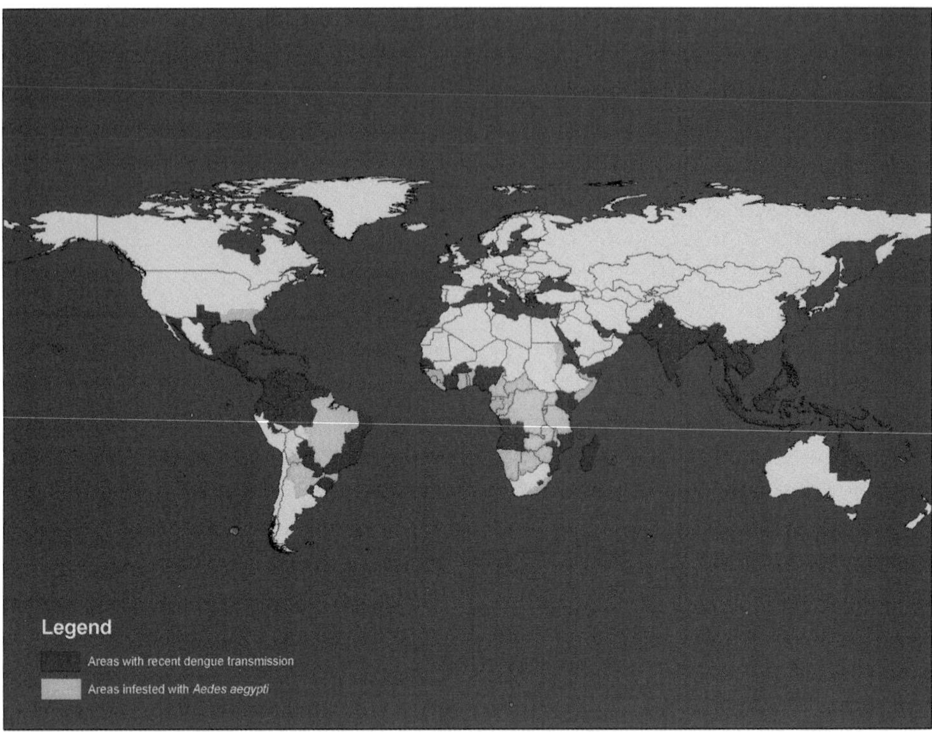

Fig. 7.5.15.1 Global distribution of dengue.

with some two million severe enough to require hospitalization. Although low mortality rates (0.1–0.2% for severe disease) are usual in experienced hands, much higher rates are still reported from some regions.

Pathogenesis

All four serotypes can cause disease. Infection with one serotype elicits immunity to that serotype but does not provide long-term cross-protective immunity to the remaining serotypes. Severe disease occurs predominantly in patients experiencing a second or subsequent infection with a dengue serotype different from their first infection, or else in infants with transmitted maternal antibody experiencing their first infection. The generally accepted antibody-dependent enhancement (ADE) hypothesis suggests that residual heterotypic non-neutralizing antibodies bind to the new virus enhancing its infectivity by increasing the efficiency of binding and uptake of virus–antibody complexes through Fc receptors on blood monocyte or tissue macrophage cells, thus amplifying viral replication. The resulting increase in viral load drives an immunopathogenic cascade that alters microvascular function in some way, resulting in capillary leakage and coagulopathy. Rapid mobilization of serotype cross-reactive memory T cells has been suggested as an alternative mechanism to trigger the inflammatory cascade. Other factors considered to influence disease severity include differences in viral virulence, molecular mimicry, and immune complex and/or complement-mediated dysregulation, as well as age and genetic predisposition. However, the pathogenesis of the vascular leakage and coagulopathy associated with severe infections remains poorly understood and, so far, no mechanism has been identified that links the established immunological derangements with a definitive effect on microvascular structure or function.

Clinical manifestations

Dengue virus infection in humans causes a wide variety of illnesses ranging from inapparent infection to mild febrile illness to severe and fatal disease. Most infections are asymptomatic. In the past, symptomatic disease was conventionally separated into two major clinical syndromes, dengue fever (DF) and dengue haemorrhagic fever (DHF), with case definitions and management guidelines for these entities published by the World Health Organization (WHO). The pathognomonic feature of DHF is increased vascular permeability, which may be severe enough to result in hypovolaemic shock; in addition, to qualify for a diagnosis of DHF, a patient must have some evidence of bleeding and a platelet count below 100 x 10^9/litre. Due to practical difficulties in using the old WHO scheme a revised classification system has recently been developed, based on prospective data collected from over 2000 children and adults with dengue from endemic areas around the world, and this has now been adopted in the latest WHO guidelines for dengue published in 2009. The new scheme classifies the disease into dengue and severe dengue, in line with several other complex diseases such as malaria and pneumonia. It is hoped that in the future this will prove to be a simpler system that will be useful for triage, aid clinical management, and improve the quality of surveillance and epidemiological data.

Symptomatic dengue is primarily a disease of older children and adults. After an incubation period of c.4 to 7 days symptoms start suddenly and typically follow three phases—an initial febrile phase, a critical phase around the time of defervescence, and a spontaneous recovery phase.

Febrile phase

There is sudden onset of high fever often accompanied by facial flushing, headache, retro-orbital pain, lumbosacral pain, severe malaise, myalgias, bone pain, anorexia, altered sense of taste, mild

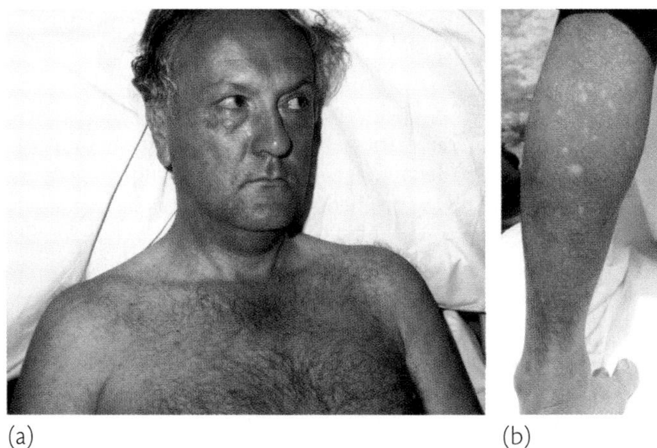

(a) (b)

Fig. 7.5.15.2 (a) Early macular rash on the shoulders and conjunctival injection in a European traveller with primary dengue.
(Copyright D A Warrell.)
(b) Convalescent rash in a Vietnamese adult with dengue.
(Copyright OUCRU-VN.)

sore throat, nausea, and vomiting. Younger children experience high fever, but are generally much less symptomatic. Some patients may have a transient rash or skin mottling in early illness (Fig. 7.5.15.2a). Other findings associated with infection may include generalized lymphadenopathy, mild haemorrhagic manifestations (e.g. petechiae or easy bruising, Fig. 7.5.15.3a,b), and palpable hepatomegaly but rarely splenomegaly. Haematuria is uncommon and jaundice is rare. Clinical laboratory findings during the first week include thrombocytopenia and leukopenia, often with moderate elevation of hepatic transaminases.

Critical phase

Most patients recover around the time of defervescence, usually between days 3–7 of illness, but in a small proportion an increase in capillary permeability becomes apparent at this time, marking the onset of the critical phase for complications. A capillary leak syndrome manifests with increasing haemoconcentration, hypoproteinaemia, pleural effusions and ascites, and, if severe, may compromise the circulating plasma volume so that the patient develops the potentially life-threatening dengue shock syndrome (DSS) (Fig. 7.5.15.4a,b). When the pulse pressure narrows to less than 20 mmHg with a rapid weak pulse and impaired peripheral perfusion, or if hypotension develops, the patient is defined as having DSS. If fluid resuscitation is not instituted promptly the ongoing depletion of plasma becomes critical, the systolic pressure falls rapidly, and irreversible shock and death may follow. However, with judicious fluid management the majority of patients make a full recovery. Warning signs that the patient may be at risk for severe disease include severe vomiting, intense abdominal pain, and increasing tender hepatomegaly.

Haemorrhagic manifestations are common during this period but often limited to the presence of skin petechiae or bruising, or a positive tourniquet test. Mucosal bleeding (e.g. epistaxis, gastrointestinal bleeding, haematuria, menorrhagia) may occur, but is rarely clinically significant in children except in association with profound or prolonged shock. However, adults tend to experience more severe bleeding problems than children (Fig. 7.5.15.5a,b);

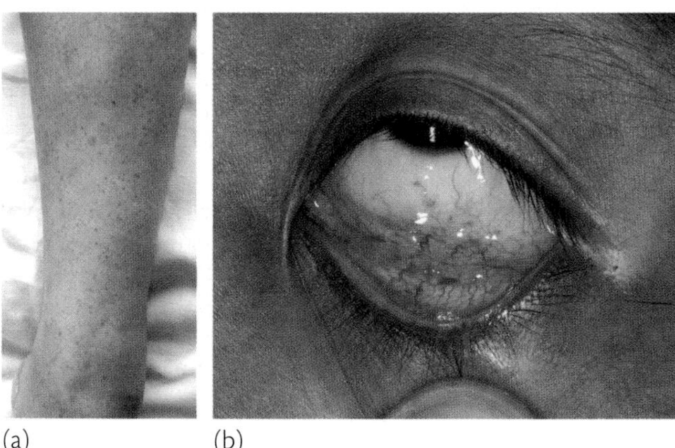

(a) (b)

Fig. 7.5.15.3 (a) Petechial rash on the leg of a Vietnamese child with dengue.
(Copyright Dinh The Trung.)
(b) Conjunctival petechiae in a Vietnamese adult with dengue.
(Copyright D A Warrell.)

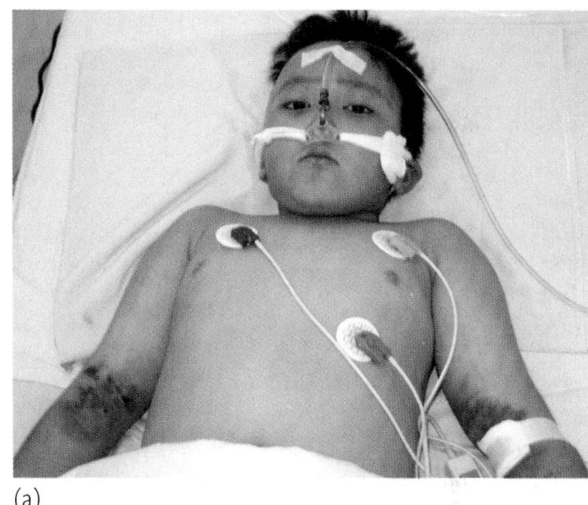

(a)

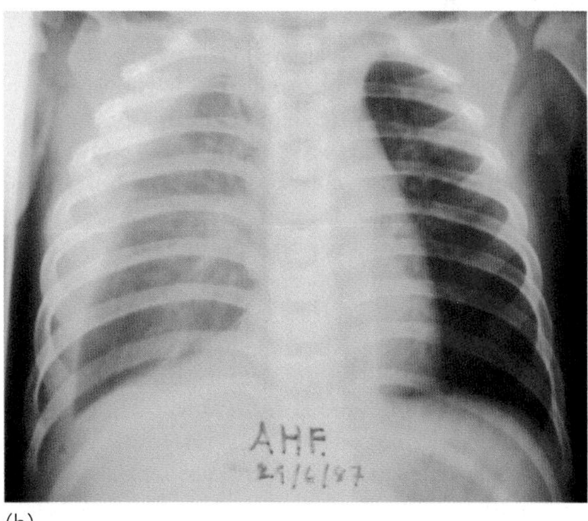

(b)

Fig. 7.5.15.4 (a) Vietnamese child with severe DSS, pleural effusions, ascites, oedema, and bruising at venepuncture sites. He required crystalloid and colloid infusions, inotropic support, and nasal continuous positive airway pressure (CPAP) but made a good recovery.
(Copyright B A Wills.)
(b) Pleural effusion in a 14-month-old Thai child with DHF and DSS.
(Courtesy of the late Professor Sornchai Looareesuwan.)

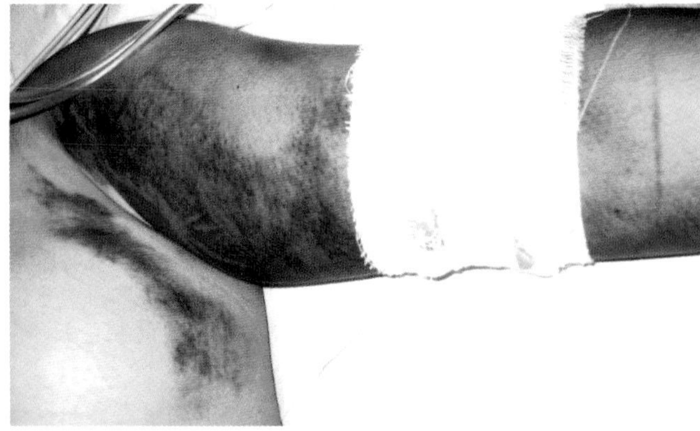
(a)

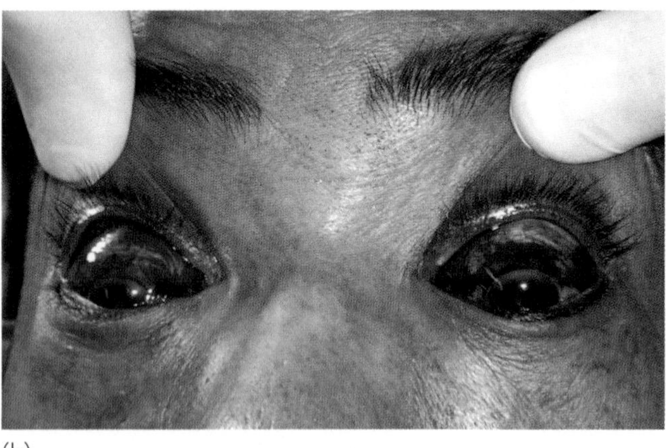
(b)

Fig. 7.5.15.5 (a) Major bleeding at a venepuncture site in a Vietnamese teenager with severe DSS. (b) Extensive subconjunctival haemorrhages and severe epistaxis requiring nasal packing in a Vietnamese adult with dengue.
(Copyright Dinh The Trung.)

gastrointestinal bleeding and menorrhagia may be significant even in patients with little evidence of vascular leakage. Moderate to severe thrombocytopenia is usual, with nadirs below 20×10^9 /litre often observed during the critical period followed by rapid improvement during the recovery phase. An increase in the activated partial thromboplastin time and a reduction in fibrinogen levels are also frequently noted. However, these findings are not indicative of classic disseminated intravascular coagulation and the true nature of the coagulopathy remains unknown. Other laboratory investigations show similar but usually more profound abnormalities to those seen in uncomplicated cases.

Recovery phase

The increase in permeability is transient and reverts to normal after approximately 24–48 h. Fluid is reabsorbed quite rapidly, often with an obvious diuresis, and the patient improves. A second rash, varying in form from scarlatiniform to maculopapular, may appear around day 6 to 7 of illness, typically on the extremities although sometimes involving the trunk and face (Fig. 7.5.15.2b). The rash blanches on pressure, may be accompanied by intense pruritus, and often resolves with desquamation.

Other syndromes

Unusual manifestations, including acute liver failure and encephalopathy/encephalitis, may be noted, even in the absence of severe plasma leakage or shock. Myocarditis has also been reported in a few cases.

Severe dengue

Under the new scheme, patients who recover without complications are classified as having dengue, while those who experience any one of the following problems are classified as having severe dengue: plasma leakage resulting in shock and/or fluid accumulation sufficient to cause respiratory distress; severe bleeding; severe organ impairment, e.g. liver failure, myocarditis etc. However, most deaths from dengue occur in patients with profound shock, particularly if the situation is complicated by fluid overload.

Differential diagnosis

The differential diagnosis during the acute phase of illness includes influenza, Epstein–Barr virus, measles, rubella, typhoid, leptospirosis, rickettsial infection, malaria, other arboviral infections with rash, other viral haemorrhagic fevers, and meningococcaemia.

Laboratory diagnosis

During the early febrile stage (up to about day 5 of illness) laboratory confirmation of dengue infection relies on viral isolation or detection of viral antigen or viral RNA by reverse transcription–polymerase chain reaction (RT-PCR) in blood. After this time IgM antibody capture enzyme-linked immunosorbent assay (MAC-ELISA) is the most widely used serological test for dengue diagnosis; seroconversion or a rising titre of dengue-specific IgM or IgG in paired samples indicates acute infection. Patients with secondary infection (either dengue or another flavivirus infection) often develop high levels of IgG antibodies in the acute phase and the IgM response may be less intense. Serological diagnosis is also complicated by the existence of flavivirus cross-reactivity, making it necessary to perform tests for other locally prevalent flaviviruses in parallel with dengue serology. Because antidengue antibodies persist for several months, diagnosis based on a single positive MAC-ELISA result should be considered provisional. Bedside rapid serological tests are now available but, in common with conventional serological tests, may not become positive until the end of the first week of illness. ELISA tests to detect circulating dengue nonstructural protein 1 during the first few days of fever may be a promising tool for early diagnosis.

Management

Good supportive care, with a particular focus on careful fluid management, remains critical for a favourable outcome. For patients with mild disease, oral rehydration is usually sufficient. No antimicrobial therapy is yet available for the treatment of dengue, although several viral inhibitors are in preclinical trials. No ancillary drugs have been shown to be beneficial. Corticosteroid therapy showed no convincing benefit on mortality from shock in several small clinical trials, but whether deployment before the development of shock influences outcome remains unknown. Fever should be controlled with tepid sponging and paracetamol. Aspirin and nonsteroidal anti-inflammatory drugs are contraindicated.

Persistent vomiting, severe abdominal pain, mucosal bleeding or severe skin bleeding, a rapidly rising haematocrit, or a marked drop in the platelet count indicate the need for close observation and frequent monitoring of vital signs and haematocrit. Judicious parenteral fluid therapy is indicated for those with a rapidly rising haematocrit. For patients with established DSS, prompt but careful restoration of circulating plasma volume is crucial, followed by maintenance fluids to support the circulation at a level just sufficient to maintain critical organ perfusion until vascular permeability reverts to normal. However, fluid overload with respiratory compromise is a common complication and one of the major contributors to mortality. Thus the volume of parenteral fluid given must be kept to the minimum required to maintain cardiovascular stability and adequate urine output during the phase of active leakage, and as soon as reabsorption begins, usually about 1 to 2 days later, intravenous fluids should be stopped. Isotonic crystalloid solutions should be used initially. Colloid solutions should be reserved for patients presenting with severe DSS and those who fail to improve with crystalloid therapy. Correction of metabolic acidosis, electrolyte imbalance, and hypoglycaemia are also essential. Platelet concentrates are not indicated, even for profound thrombocytopenia unless there is overt bleeding, as the thrombocytopenia improves rapidly during the recovery phase without intervention. However, in the event of significant bleeding transfusion of fresh blood, platelets, and other blood products may be indicated, but should be undertaken with great care because of the risk of fluid overload.

Outcome

The majority of patients with dengue make a full recovery. Those with DSS and/or significant bleeding usually do well provided they receive appropriate supportive care from experienced health care personnel during the critical phase of the illness. Adults may go on to experience several weeks of extreme tiredness, weakness, skin desquamation, pruritus, and depression during convalescence after infection, but there are no permanent sequelae. In general, children recover more rapidly and do not experience such problems.

Prevention

Although major efforts are being directed towards development of safe and effective dengue vaccines, it seems unlikely that a suitable candidate will be available for large-scale deployment for some years. Until then prevention of epidemics will continue to rely on elimination of potential vector breeding sites together with biological and chemical vector control strategies. Community control of *Ae aegypti* by eradication of mosquito larvae from stagnant water sources is recommended but has been difficult to achieve in contemporary tropical urban settings. Insecticide-treated bednets have limited use since *Ae aegypti* mosquitoes are primarily daytime feeders. Avoidance of mosquito bites in areas infested with *Ae aegypti* by using repellents containing *N*,*N*-diethyl-3-methylbenzamide (DEET) or picaridin and protective clothing are the most effective preventive measures for the traveller.

Further reading

Deen JL, *et al.* (2006). The WHO dengue classification and case definitions: time for a reassessment. *Lancet*, **368**, 170–3.

Halstead SB (1965). Dengue and hemorrhagic fevers of Southeast Asia. *Yale J Biol Med*, **37**, 434–54.

Halstead SB, Nimmannitya S, Cohen SN (1970). Observations related to pathogenesis of dengue hemorrhagic fever. IV. Relation of disease severity to antibody response and virus recovered. *Yale J Biol Med*, **42**, 311–28.

Kay B, Vu SN (2005). New strategy against *Aedes aegypti* in Vietnam. *Lancet*, **365**, 613–7.

Mackenzie JS, Gubler DJ, Petersen LR (2004). Emerging flaviviruses: the spread and resurgence of Japanese encephalitis, West Nile and dengue viruses. *Nat Med*, **10** Suppl, S98–109.

Mongkolsapaya J, *et al.* (2003). Original antigenic sin and apoptosis in the pathogenesis of dengue hemorrhagic fever. *Nat Med*, **9**, 921–7.

Screaton G, Mongkolsapaya J (2006). T cell responses and dengue haemorrhagic fever. *Novartis Found Symp*, **277**, 164–71.

Wilder-Smith A, Schwartz E (2005). Dengue in travelers. *N Engl J Med*, **353**, 924–32.

Wills BA, *et al.* (2005). Comparison of three fluid solutions for resuscitation in dengue shock syndrome. *N Engl J Med*, **353**, 877–89.

World Health Organisation (1997). *Dengue haemorrhagic fever: diagnosis, treatment, prevention and control.* World Health Organisation, Geneva.

World Health Organisation (2009). Dengue: Guidelines for diagnosis, treatment, prevention and control. World Health Organisation, Geneva.

7.5.16 Bunyaviridae

J.W. LeDuc and Summerpal S. Kahlon

Essentials

Viruses of the family Bunyaviridae contain a 3-segmented, single-stranded, negative-sense RNA genome. They are divided into five genera, of which four are known to include human pathogens—*Orthobunyavirus*, *Phlebovirus*, *Hantavirus*, and *Nairovirus*. These viruses are found throughout the world and are transmitted between vertebrate hosts and to humans through the bite of infected arthropod vectors (mosquitoes, ticks, others), or from infectious excreta of rodents and other small mammals, and rarely person to person. Many of viruses are transmitted from infected arthropod vector females to the next generation by transovarial transmission, thereby surviving adverse environmental conditions and leading to marked seasonal distribution of disease. There are few vaccines available to protect against infection. Prevention is by avoidance of exposure to potentially infected arthropod and small-mammal vectors.

Clinical features

Bunyaviridae cause a wide range of clinical illnesses, ranging from self-limited febrile disease to severe, life-threatening haemorrhagic fever, acute respiratory distress, or encephalitis. The most important human diseases include those caused by:

La Crosse virus—the commonest cause of 'California encephalitis', most cases of which are relatively mild and with good prognosis; treatment is supportive.

Oropouche fever—causes epidemics of febrile illness, sometimes with meningitis, throughout the Amazon basin; prognosis is good; treatment is supportive.

Haemorrhagic fever with renal syndrome—caused by four distinct viruses (Hantaan, Dobrava, Puumala, Seoul); Hantaan and Dobrava cause the most severe disease, characterized sequentially by (1) febrile phase with features including headache, myalgias, petechiae and conjunctival haemorrhage, (2) hypotensive phase with shock, (3) oliguric phase, when one-third of cases have severe haemorrhage,

(4) diuretic phase, (5) convalescent phase, which may be prolonged; ribavirin is effective if started early in disease. Inactivated vaccines against Hantaviruses are available for use in Asia.

Hantavirus pulmonary syndrome – most commonly reported from the western United States, Canada, Central and South America; symptoms are primarily those of acute unexplained adult respiratory distress syndrome; treatment is supportive; mortality is 20-40%.

Other diseases caused by Bunyaviridae—these include sandfly fever, Rift Valley fever and Crimean-Congo haemorrhagic fever. Some viruses of the family, e.g. Rift Valley fever virus and Nairobi sheep disease virus, are important pathogens of domestic animals.

Viral taxonomy and vectors

The family Bunyaviridae currently contains around 300 viruses, and is divided into five genera (Table 7.5.16.1). The family name, and that of the genus *Orthobunyavirus*, is derived from the type species Bunyamwera virus, which was isolated in Uganda from *Aedes* mosquitoes. The other genera are *Hantavirus* named after Hantaan virus (the cause of Korean haemorrhagic fever), *Nairovirus* after Nairobi sheep disease virus, *Phlebovirus* after phlebotomus or sandfly fever virus, and *Tospovirus* after tomato spotted wilt virus. All members of the family share structural, biochemical, and genetic properties, such as a spherical enveloped virion 80 to 120 nm in diameter (Fig. 7.5.16.1) and a genome of single-stranded negative-sense RNA divided into three segments (L, M, S). Members of different genera vary substantially in their biological and biochemical properties and in their mechanisms of replication. Orthobunyaviruses, nairoviruses, and phleboviruses, which together make up most of the family, are all arthropod-borne animal viruses (arboviruses). These circulate in a wide variety of different vertebrate hosts and are transmitted between vertebrates, including humans, by the bites of blood-sucking arthropods, principally mosquitoes for orthobunyaviruses, sandflies for phleboviruses, and ticks for nairoviruses. Hantaviruses are zoonotic agents infecting rodents and other small mammals. They may spread to humans who are in close contact with infected excreta. Tospoviruses are arthropod-transmitted plant viruses of no known medical importance.

Viruses within the larger genera are further subdivided into serogroups; orthobunyaviruses have at least 18 serogroups and nairoviruses have 7 (Table 7.5.16.1). Of over 60 Bunyaviridae that are known to infect humans, the type species and those causing major human diseases are shown in bold type in Table 7.5.16.1 and are described in more detail. Table 7.5.16.2 lists the distribution of the remaining viruses that cause minor human infections with their principal arthropod vectors. The habitats of the different viruses and their vectors range from arctic to tropical. The enzootic cycles of arboviruses are poorly understood. Most viruses undergo alternate cycles of replication in vertebrate and invertebrate hosts, but transovarial and trans-stadial transmission within some mosquitoes, ticks, and phlebotomine flies, and venereal transmission from vertically infected male mosquitoes to uninfected females is also known to occur. Most arboviruses have a narrow host range, occur within a limited area, and are transmitted by specific vectors to a limited number of vertebrate hosts, but some viruses infect a wider host range, are transmitted by more than one type of vector, and may occur in more than a single continent. Tick transmission predominates in Asia, but is unknown in South or Central America, and although some Bunyaviridae have been isolated in Australia, none is known to infect humans in that continent. Viruses of this family are among the most common apparently emerging diseases. Following viral entry, whether through the skin after the bite of an infected arthropod or by another route, there is replication in draining lymph nodes, which may be enlarged, and then viraemia. Symptoms develop when virus is deposited and replicates in other sites. The viruses are killed by bleach, phenolic disinfectants and detergents, autoclaving, boiling, and γ-irradiation. Enzymes such as nucleases also inactivate these viruses. Biosafety level 3 is recommended for handling most human pathogens with the ability to spread by aerosol (e.g. hantaviruses and Oropouche virus), but level 4 is required for Crimean–Congo haemorrhagic fever virus. Added precautions are necessary when handling hantavirus-infected animals and virus concentrates.

Genus *Orthobunyavirus*

Studies with Bunyamwera and similar viruses show reassortment within the three-segmented genome when two closely related viruses infect the same cell, either in nature or in the laboratory. Such studies have been used to analyse the molecular basis of virulence for vertebrate and invertebrate hosts. Two orthobunyaviruses, Akabane and Aino viruses in the Simbu serogroup, produce congenital deformities in sheep, goats, and cattle in Japan, Australia, Africa, and the Middle East. However, there is no evidence that any member of the genus or family produces teratogenic effects in humans, but there is concern that Oropouche virus, a Simbu serogroup pathogen of Central and South America, may be a threat to pregnant women.

Bunyamwera virus

Symptoms

A mild febrile illness, usually with headache, joint and back pains, sometimes with a rash, and occasionally with mild involvement of the central nervous system. Serological surveys indicate widespread human infection in sub-Saharan Africa but it is rarely recognized. Laboratory infections have been recorded. Garissa virus, isolated from haemorrhagic fever patients during outbreak investigations in Kenya and Somalia, has genome segments virtually identical to both Bunyamwera and Cache Valley viruses, but neither of these is known to cause haemorrhagic disease in humans.

Treatment and prognosis

No treatment is necessary and the prognosis is excellent.

California encephalitis, Inkoo, Jamestown Canyon, La Crosse, Tahyna, and snowshoe hare viruses

The viruses named above, and perhaps others currently unrecognized, are responsible for the clinical condition known as California encephalitis. The viruses are widely distributed throughout many parts of North America, Europe, and Eurasia. In the United States of America most reported human infections are due to La Crosse virus in Ohio, Wisconsin, West Virginia, and Minnesota. From 1995 to 2005, 70 to 167 cases were reported annually. Most occurred in children, usually in boys, although Jamestown Canyon virus is found more often in adults. There is nearly always a history of outdoor exposure during warmer months in areas where woodland mosquitoes are prevalent. The incubation period is 5 to 10

Table 7.5.16.1 The family *Bunyaviridae*: its genera, serogroups, vectors, and viruses infecting humans

Genus	Serogroup	Vector	Viruses infecting humans
***Orthobunyavirus* (over 150)**	Anopheles A (12)	Mosquito	Tacaiuma
	Anopheles B (2)	Mosquito	
	Bakau (5)	Mosquito	
	Bunyamwera (33)	Mosquito	**Bunyamwera**, Calovo, **Garissa**, Germiston, Ilesha, Maguari, Shokwe, Tensaw, Wyeomyia
	Bwamba (2)	Mosquito	**Bwamba**, Pongola
	C group (14)	Mosquito	Apeu, Caraparu, Itaqui, Madrid, Marituba, Murutucu, Nepuyo, Oriboca, Ossa, Restan
	California (14)	Mosquito	**California encephalitis,** Guaroa, **Inkoo, Jamestown Canyon, Keystone La Crosse,** snowshoe hare, **Tahyna**, trivittatus
	Capim (10)	Mosquito	
	Gamboa (8)	Mosquito	
	Guama (12)	Mosquito	Catu, Guama
	Koongol (2)	Mosquito	
	Minatitlan (2)	Mosquito	
	Nyando (2)	Mosquito	Nyando
	Olifantsvlei (5)	Mosquito	
	Patois (7)	Mosquito	
	Simbu (24)	Mosquito	**Oropouche**, Shuni
	Tete (5)	Mosquito	
	Turlock (5)	Mosquito	
	Unassigned (3)	Mosquito	
***Hantavirus* (8)**	Hantaan (26)	None	**Andes, Bayou, Black Creek Canal, Dobrava, Hantaan, Juquitiba, Laguna Negra, Lechiguanas, Monongahela, Oran,** Prospect Hill, **Puumala, Seoul, Sin Nombre**
***Nairovirus* (32)**	Crimean–Congo (3)	Tick	**Crimean–Congo haemorrhagic fever**, Hazara
	Dera Ghazi Khan (6)	Tick	
	Hughes (10)	Tick	Soldado
	Nairobi sheep disease (3)	Tick	Dugbe, Ganjam, Nairobi sheep disease
	Qalyub (3)	Tick	
	Sakhalin (7)	Tick	Avalon
	Thiafora (2)	Tick	
***Phlebovirus* (57)**	Phlebotomus (44)	Sandfly[a]	Alenquer, Candiru, **Chagres,** Corfou, **Punta Toro, Rift Valley fever**[a], **Naples, sandfly fever, Sicilian, Toscana**
	Uukuniemi (13)	Tick	Uukuniemi, Zaliv-Terpeniya
***Tospovirus* (1)**		Thrips	
Unassigned (53)		Mosquito	Bangui, Kasokero, Tataguine
		Tick	Bhanja, Issyk-kul Keterah, Tamdy, Wanowrie

Numbers in parentheses indicate the approximate number of viruses in the genus or serogroup.
Bold type indicates the type species and viruses causing major disease in humans.
[a] Mosquito vector for Rift Valley fever virus.

days. Most cases of La Crosse encephalitis are relatively mild with headache, fever, and vomiting, progressing to lethargy, behavioural changes, and occasional brief seizures, followed by improvement. Severe cases (10–20%) develop sudden fever and headache, disorientation, and seizures during the first 24 h of illness, sometimes progressing to coma and requiring intensive supportive care. Overall, about 50% of symptomatic children have seizures with status epilepticus in 10 to 15%. The case fatality rate approaches 1%. Residual seizures occur in 6 to 13%, persistent hemiparesis in about 1%, and cognitive dysfunction in a few. In appropriate epidemiological settings, the disease should be considered in children presenting with aseptic meningitis or encephalitis.

In Europe, Tahyna virus is widely distributed in Austria, former Czechoslovakia, France, Germany, Italy, Norway, Romania, former Yugoslavia, and the former Soviet Union. Seroprevalence exceeds 95% in parts of former Czechoslovakia, and is about 50% in the Rhone valley in France and the Danube basin near Vienna, but overt disease is seldom recognized. Inkoo virus is prevalent in Finland

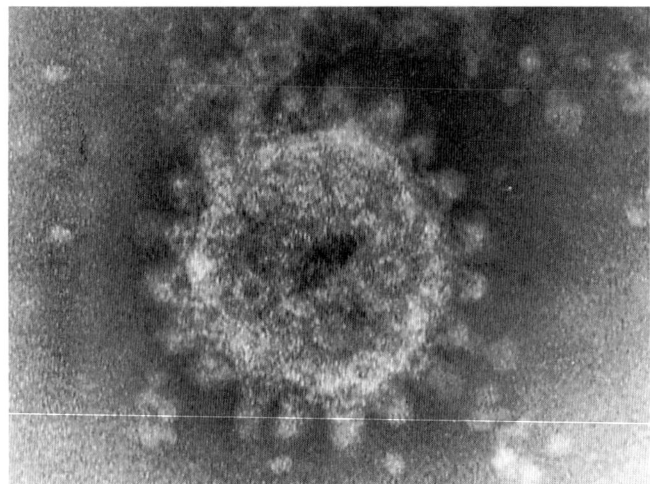

Fig. 7.5.16.1 Electron micrograph of Crimean–Congo haemorrhagic fever virus. Magnification × 400 000.
(Courtesy of Dr D S Ellis.)

and also in neighbouring regions of Russia. Most adult Lapps have antibodies. Small children may have signs of central nervous system involvement during acute infection. Antibodies reactive with California serogroup viruses have also been found in human sera collected in Sri Lanka, China, and in the far northern latitudes of Eurasia where several California serogroup viruses have been isolated from mosquitoes, some related to Inkoo and Tahyna viruses, but others to snowshoe hare virus. In another Russian study of *c.*50 people, mainly 14 to 30 years old, with infections caused by California serogroup viruses, about two-thirds had influenza-like illnesses without central nervous system involvement, while the remaining one-third had aseptic meningitis.

Control, treatment, and prognosis

Measures to limit mosquito breeding, particularly of *Aedes triseriatus*, are useful in endemic regions. No vaccines are available, and there is no specific treatment. Fluid and electrolyte balance must be maintained, and anticonvulsive drugs may be required to control seizures. Intravenous ribavirin has been used to treat severe La Crosse encephalitis.

Oropouche virus

Symptoms

Before 1961, Oropouche virus was known to have caused only a mild fever in a single forest worker in Trinidad, but that year it was responsible for a substantial epidemic in the Belém area of northern Brazil, where *c.*7000 people were affected. Over the ensuing 50 years, massive epidemics of febrile illness have been recorded throughout the Amazon Basin and beyond, with many thousands infected. Symptoms include headache, generalized pain including back pain, prostration, and fever (40°C). Rash, meningitis, or meningism occasionally accompany infection (Fig. 7.5.16.2). Illness lasts from 2 to 5 days, occasionally with protracted convalescence. No fatalities have been reported.

Control, treatment, and prognosis

No vaccine is available. Transmission is probably by the biting midge *Culicoides paraensis* and outbreaks appear to be a consequence of agricultural development of the Amazon Basin. Accumulated organic waste from cacao and banana production provides ideal breeding sites for *Culicoides*, leading to massive populations and subsequent epidemic Oropouche disease. Measures to reduce *Culicoides* breeding may be beneficial. Treatment is supportive and the prognosis is good, although convalescence may be protracted.

Genus *Hantavirus*

Haemorrhagic fever with renal syndrome

Hantaan virus of the genus *Hantavirus* is the cause of Korean haemorrhagic fever in Korea. The Hantaan River is near the

Table 7.5.16.2 *Bunyaviridae* causing only mild or trivial infections in humans, arranged on a geographical basis

Africa	North America	Central America	South America	Europe	Asia
Bangui (M)	Avalon (T)	Fort Sherman	Alenquer (P)	Bhanja (T)	Batai (M)
Bhanja (T)	Keystone (M)	Madrid (M)	Apeu (M)	Calovo (M)	Bhanja (T)
Dugbe (T)	Prospect Hill	Nepuyo	Candiru (P)	Corfou (P)	Issyk-Kul (T)
Germiston (M)	Tensaw (M)	Ossa (M)	Caraparu (M)	Tamdy (T)	Ganjam (T)
Ilesha (M)	Trivittatus (M)	Restan (M)	Catu (M)	Uukuniemi (T)	Hazara (T)
Kasokero (M)		Soldado	Guama (M, P)		Keterah (T)
Nairobi sheep disease		Trivittatus (M)	Guaroa (M)		Wanowrie (T)
Nyando (M)			Itaqui		Zaliv-Terpeniya (M, T)
Pongola (M)			Maguari (M)		
Shokwe (M)			Marituba (M)		
Shuni (M)			Murutucu (M)		
Tataguine (M)			Oriboca		
Thiafora			Restan (M)		
Wanowrie (T)			Tacaiuma (M)		
			Wyeomyia (M)		

M, virus transmitted by mosquitoes; P, virus transmitted by phlebotomine flies; T, virus transmitted by ticks.

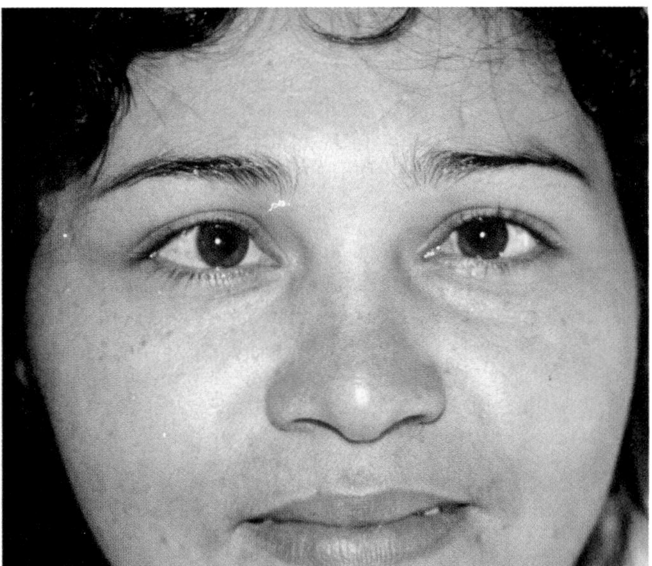

Fig. 7.5.16.2 Patient convalescent after Oropouche virus encephalitis in Belém, Para, Brazil, showing a left VIIth cranial nerve palsy.
(Courtesy of Dr Pedro Pardal, Hospital Universitário João de Barros Barreto, Brazil.)

demilitarized zone between North and South Korea where the virus was first recovered in 1976 from its rodent host *Apodemus agrarius*. The clinical diseases caused by Hantaan and related viruses in the Eurasian continent have long been known by different synonyms: epidemic haemorrhagic fever, Korean haemorrhagic fever, or nephropathia epidemica, but haemorrhagic fever with renal syndrome (HFRS) is preferred. Four distinct viruses are responsible for most recognized cases of HFRS: Hantaan virus, found primarily in Asia; Dobrava virus in an enclave of disease in the Balkan region and sparsely elsewhere in Europe; Puumala virus in Scandinavia, western Russia, and much of Europe; and Seoul virus is probably global wherever uncontrolled populations of *Rattus norvegicus* exist. Hantaan and Dobrava viruses cause severe life-threatening disease with mortality of about 5%, reaching up to 30% in select populations. Puumala virus infections are less severe, although patients still require admission to hospital, but fewer than 1% of admitted patients die. Seoul virus is thought to be the least severe of the pathogenic strains of Old World hantaviruses, although it has been associated with human deaths.

Each hantavirus is associated with a particular rodent host: Hantaan virus with the striped field mouse *Apodemus agrarius*; Dobrava virus with the yellow-necked mouse *Apodemus flavicollis*; Puumala virus with the bank vole *Myodes*; and Seoul virus with the Norway rat *Rattus norvegicus*. Humans are infected by aerosols of rodent excreta, or rarely by rodent bites. It is seen among adult men in rural environments and may be an occupational disease. Those at greatest risk include farmers, woodcutters, shepherds, and, especially, soldiers in the field. Most hantavirus disease is seasonal, with a peak incidence in late autumn and early winter, although the Balkan form is found most often during summer months in Greece and adjacent countries.

Symptoms

The incubation period for hantaviruses is variable; it is usually 12 to 16 days but it can be up to 2 months. Severe disease, typically associated with Hantaan or Dobrava virus infections in Asia or the Balkans, is characterized by five phases:

1 Febrile: 3- to 7-day duration

2 Hypotensive: lasting from a few hours to 3 days

3 Oliguric: from 3 to 7 days

4 Diuretic: from a few days to weeks

5 Convalescent: prolonged

Signs and symptoms of the febrile phase include fever, malaise, headache, myalgia, back pain, abdominal pain, nausea and vomiting, facial flushing, petechiae, and conjunctival haemorrhage (Fig. 7.5.16.3). In the hypotensive phase, patients have nausea, vomiting, tachycardia, hypotension, blurred vision, haemorrhagic signs, and shock. About one-third of fatalities occur during this phase. In the

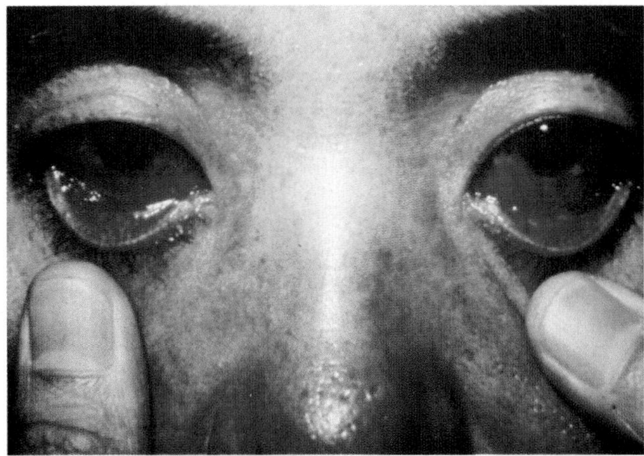

(a)

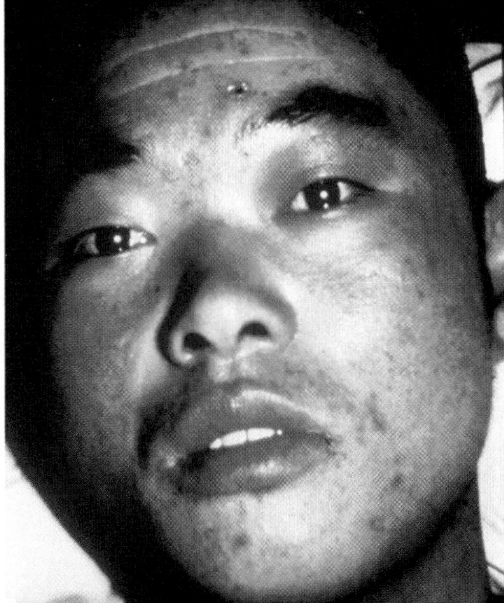

(b)

Fig. 7.5.16.3 Patient with acute Korean haemorrhagic fever, showing extensive conjunctival haemorrhages (a) and facial swelling (b).
(Courtesy of Professor H W Lee.)

oliguric phase, nausea and vomiting may persist and blood pressure may rise. Renal failure develops with anuria, and about one-third of cases have severe haemorrhage (epistaxis, gastrointestinal, cutaneous, or bleeding at other sites). Nearly one-half of the deaths occur during the oliguric phase. In the diuretic phase, urine output increases to several litres per day. Convalescence is protracted and it maybe months before full strength and function are regained.

Not all the phases are seen in the less severe forms of the disease. The milder forms of HFRS, such as nephropathia epidemica due to Puumala virus, follow a similar but less severe course, with abrupt onset of fever of 38 to 40°C, headache, malaise, backache, and generalized abdominal pain. Back or loin pain is especially common. Signs of renal failure are usually not as pronounced, and the need for renal dialysis varies. Transient blurred vision occurs in about 10% of cases. Infection due to Seoul virus follows a similar course, but may present with more evidence of liver involvement. There is no evidence of person-to-person transmission.

Treatment and prognosis

Admission to hospital, avoidance of trauma and unnecessary movement, close observation, and careful supportive care are essential for patient survival. Treatment is phase specific, with special attention to fluid balance and volume, and control of hypotension and shock. Renal dialysis may be required. Antiviral therapy using ribavirin has been shown to be effective if started early in disease. Recovery is protracted but complete, with the exception of Seoul virus infection which carries the risk of chronic renal disease, hypertension, or stroke.

Hantavirus pulmonary syndrome

Hantavirus pulmonary syndrome, first reported from the United States of America in 1993, also occurs in Canada, Central and South America. The initial cases had a mortality of more than 50%, but rates have declined to 20 to 40% as clinical experience has increased. Most disease was reported from the western United States of America and Canada, and more recently from Argentina, Chile, Brazil, and other Central and South American countries. Sin Nombre virus was first associated with HPS, but many additional hantaviruses have now been recognized as likely causes of this syndrome (Table 7.5.16.1). As Old World hantaviruses are generally associated with specific microtine rodents (Microtinae: voles, lemmings, muskrats, and their allies, distributed worldwide), so each American hantavirus appears to be associated with a specific sigmodontine host (Sigmodontinae: cotton rats and their allies found in the western hemisphere). Apparent human-to-human transmission of Andes virus occurred during an outbreak in southern Argentina, including transmission to medical staff. Protective precautions are recommended when treating suspected cases of HPS.

Symptoms

Symptoms are primarily those of acute unexplained adult respiratory distress syndrome, rather than the expected renal disease. Nonspecific prodromal features of fever, myalgia, and malaise may last 4 to 6 days, with nausea, vomiting, and abdominal pain, often accompanied by dizziness. On admission, physical examination of patients with confirmed infection reveals fever (more than 38°C), tachycardia (more than 100 beats/min), tachypnoea (more than 20 breaths/min), and often hypotension (systolic pressure less than 100 mmHg), with audible rales in the chest. Laboratory findings include hypoxia, leukocytosis, haemoconcentration, thrombocytopenia, atypical lymphocytosis, elevated transaminases, and prolonged prothrombin time. Chest radiography shows progression from subtle interstitial findings to bilateral frank pulmonary oedema; pleural effusions are usually present (Fig. 7.5.16.4). Thrombocytopenia and haemoconcentration are independent statistical predictors of HPS, although not infallible. In a patient with rapidly progressive pulmonary oedema, a blood smear showing four of the following five characteristics is a highly sensitive and specific means of establishing the diagnosis of HPS: (1) thrombocytopenia, (2) haemoconcentration, (3) lack of toxic granulation in neutrophils, (4) more than 10% immunoblasts, and (5) myelocytosis. Disease progresses rapidly once the lungs begin to fill, and death is commonly seen 24 to 48 h after admission, or sooner if there is hypoxia or circulatory failure. The severity of disease correlates with the degree of pulmonary oedema on chest radiography. Hypotension and shock may occur independently in patients whose hypoxaemia is medically controlled.

Treatment and prognosis

Treatment is supportive, ideally in a modern intensive care unit, with careful management of hypoxia, fluid balance, and shock. About two-thirds of patients require intubation and mechanical ventilation. Fluid loss into the lungs leads to haemoconcentration, but infusion of fluids exacerbates pulmonary oedema; therefore

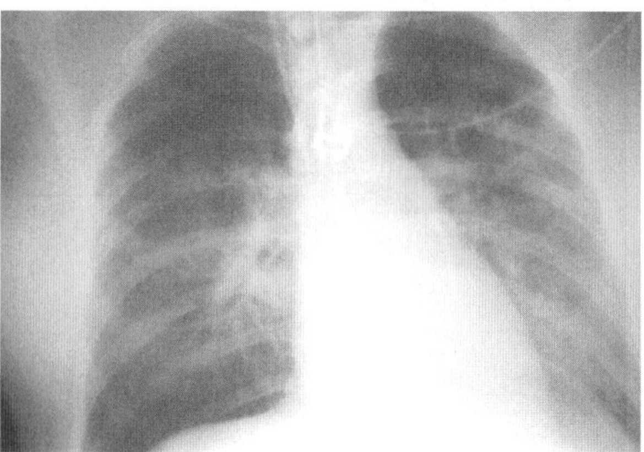

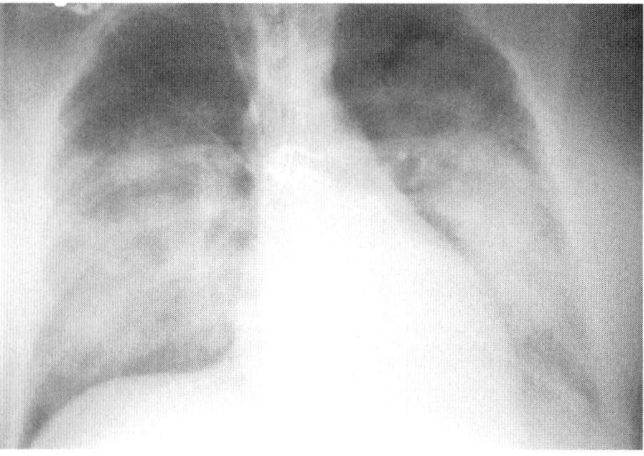

Fig. 7.5.16.4 Chest radiograph of a patient with early hantavirus pulmonary syndrome (left), and the same patient 24 h later (right) showing development of bilateral perihilar alveolar oedema.
(Courtesy of Dr Loren Ketai.)

fluids should be administered cautiously with careful monitoring. Limited experience suggests that intravenous ribavirin has little effect on the course of HPS, perhaps because of the speed with which the disease progresses.

Control

Prevention involves avoidance of infected rodents either through efficient rodent control programmes in cities, for Seoul virus, or maintenance of clean campsites so that waste food is not allowed to accumulate and attract rodents. Nationally approved inactivated vaccines, reported to be safe and effective against hantaviruses, are available for use in Asia.

Genus *Nairovirus*

The genus *Nairovirus*, named after Nairobi sheep disease, is an acute haemorrhagic gastroenteritis affecting sheep and goats in East Africa, with transmission by the sheep tick *Rhipicephalus appendiculatus*. It has caused laboratory infections, but the genus includes Crimean–Congo haemorrhagic fever virus and several other viruses known to infect humans, e.g. Ganjam virus, almost indistinguishable from Nairobi sheep disease virus but first isolated in India from *Haemaphysalis intermedia* ticks collected from healthy goats; Hazara virus, recovered from *Ixodes redkorzevi* ticks collected from the vole *Alticola roylei* in a subarctic habitat at an altitude of 3660 m in the Kaghan valley of Hazara district, Pakistan; Dugbe virus, isolated in Nigeria from *Amblyomma variegatum* ticks collected from healthy cattle; and Soldado virus, repeatedly isolated from a variety of bird ticks but recently linked to a mild illness in humans.

Crimean–Congo haemorrhagic fever virus

This was first recognized as a cause of an acute febrile haemorrhagic disease affecting humans in the Crimean region of the former Union of Soviet Socialist Republics, transmitted by ticks and carrying a mortality of 5 to 30%. In Africa, Congo virus was first isolated in the then Belgian Congo (now Democratic Republic of the Congo) from the blood of a local 13-year-old boy, and it caused a moderately severe laboratory infection. Related viruses were isolated in Uganda where more laboratory infections occurred, one of which ended fatally after a severe haematemesis. In Asia, a virus indistinguishable from Congo virus was isolated from pools of ticks collected from a variety of wild and domestic animals in western Pakistan. Crimean haemorrhagic fever virus was later proved to be serologically indistinguishable from Congo virus, hence the use of the term Crimean–Congo haemorrhagic fever virus. Different strains of this virus have been associated with outbreaks of severe and sometimes fatal disease in the Crimea, Rostov, and Astrakhan regions of Russia, in Albania, Bulgaria, and the Balkans, in East, West, and South Africa, in Iran, Iraq, and western Pakistan, and in China. From 2002 to 2008, ~2500 cases were reported in Turkey, although it was virtually unknown there previously. Most infections are seen among farmers or abattoir workers and acquired by tick bites or exposure to viraemic animal blood, but infections have occurred in both hospitals and laboratories.

Symptoms

The incubation period is 3 to 7 days. Fever usually starts suddenly and is normally continuous, although occasionally it is remittent or biphasic. Other clinical features are headache, nausea, vomiting, joint pains, backache, photophobia, circulatory disorders, thrombocytopenia, and leukopenia. Haemorrhagic manifestations are common. Patients show cutaneous petechiae and extensive ecchymoses, and bleed from nasal, gastric, intestinal, uterine, and urinary tract mucosae (Fig. 7.5.16.5). Patients may present with acute abdominal pain, mimicking an acute surgical emergency, and operating-theatre staff have become infected and died through exposure to infected blood or secretions at operation. The mortality is about 5 to 30%, but may be up to 40% or higher in hospital or nosocomial outbreaks. Transient hair loss has been reported.

Control, treatment, and prognosis

No vaccine is available. Avoidance of tick bites may reduce the risk of infection. In hospital outbreaks, meticulous attention to the containment of infected secretions is essential and barrier nursing should be used. Overt disseminated intravascular coagulation usually indicates a poor prognosis, and haematemesis, melaena, and somnolence are significantly more common in fatal cases. Supportive therapy is essential, with monitoring of fluid and electrolyte balance. The antiviral ribavirin is recommended for severe cases based on observational studies. Limiting injections and avoidance of aspirin or other drugs affecting coagulation

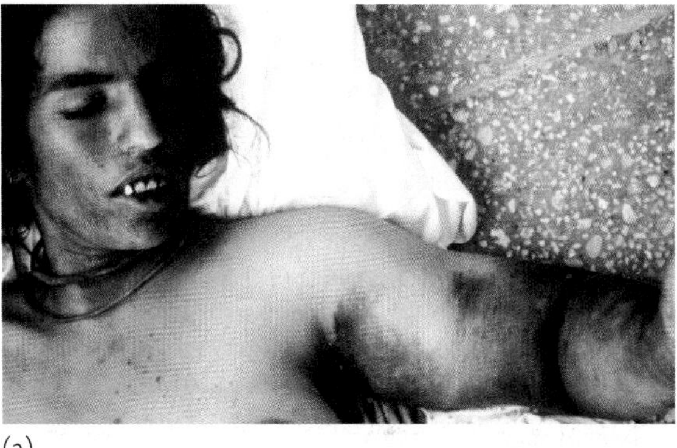
(a)

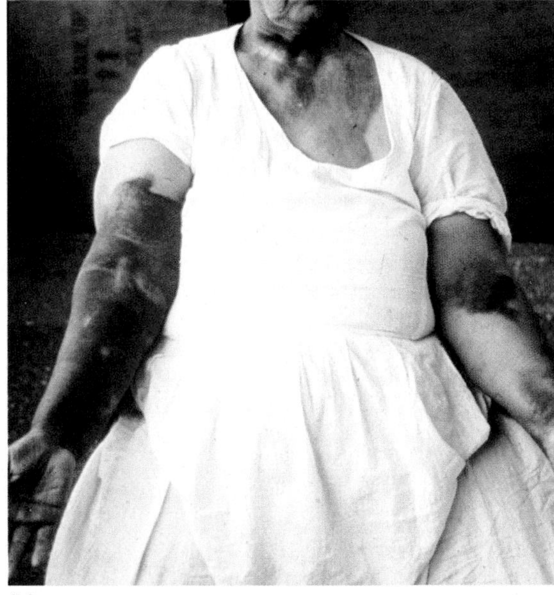
(b)

Fig. 7.5.16.5 Turkish patients with Crimean–Congo haemorrhagic fever showing petechiae (a) and extensive ecchymoses (a,b) on the arms and thorax. (Courtesy of Professor D I H Simpson.)

may reduce bleeding. Patients who recover may have residual polyneuritis persisting for months, but eventual recovery is to be expected. Laboratory investigations with live virus require biological safety level 4 containment.

Genus *Phlebovirus*

At least nine different phleboviruses are known to infect humans (see Table 7.5.16.1). Pappataci fever, sandfly fever, or phlebotomus fever was recognized as a clinical entity in the Mediterranean area during the 19th century, and the association with *Phlebotomus papatasi* sandflies was demonstrated by showing that filtrates of human blood reproduced the disease in human volunteers. It was thought that humans were the only vertebrate host, but antibody studies indicate that gerbils, cattle, and sheep may also be infected. Naples virus was isolated from human serum collected during an outbreak of sandfly fever in Naples, and the Sicilian virus was isolated from American troops with a similar disease in Palermo, Sicily. The two viruses have many common properties, but are serologically quite distinct. Sandfly fever is widespread throughout the Mediterranean area, and also occurs in Egypt, Greece, Iran, Turkey, the former Yugoslavia, Bangladesh, India, Pakistan, and the southern states of Russia. Toscana virus, serologically related to the Naples virus, is found in countries bordering the Mediterranean; it is notable for its ability to infect the central nervous system, especially in central Italy where it is thought to be responsible for at least 80% of acute summertime infections of the central nervous system in children. The viruses that cause sandfly fever do not occur in the New World, but in South and Central America a similar clinical condition follows infection with Alenquer, Candiru, Chagres, and Punta Toro viruses.

Rift Valley fever has long been known as a disease of domestic animals, mainly sheep, in East Africa, which occasionally spreads to farm workers and others handling infected animals. The infection is endemic, but seldom recognized, in many wild game animals in Africa. Rift Valley fever virus differs from the sandfly fever viruses, Punta Toro virus, and most other members of the genus in being normally transmitted by mosquitoes rather than sandflies. Uukuniemi and Zaliv-Terpeniya viruses are tick-transmitted; the only evidence that Uukuniemi virus can infect humans is the finding of specific antibodies in some human sera collected in Estonia and in former Czechoslovakia. Zaliv-Terpeniya virus was isolated from bird ticks collected on an island in the Sea of Okhotsk, Sakhalin region, and there is some evidence that it may be pathogenic to humans.

Sandfly fever, Naples, and Sicilian viruses

Symptoms

After an incubation period of 2 to 6 days, fever starts abruptly with chills, nausea and vomiting, epigastric pain, and often severe generalized headache leading to incapacitating prostration. Fever of 38 to 40°C usually resolves after 2 to 3 days, but may be biphasic and persist for a week. There is no rash, but small haemorrhages into the skin and mucous membranes may be seen. Photophobia and eye pain occur, lymphadenopathy is often seen, and the liver may be tender although jaundice is rare. The disease is self-limiting, with complete recovery. No deaths have been attributed to either sandfly fever, Naples, or Sicilian viruses.

Rift Valley fever virus

Following its initial isolation in 1930 as the agent of enzootic hepatitis of domestic animals in Kenya, Rift Valley fever virus was recognized as the cause of sporadic human infections in East, Central, and West Africa, with a particular tendency to infect laboratory workers handling the virus. In East and Central Africa the virus has been isolated from a variety of mosquito species and it is capable of persisting in mosquito eggs during the dry season, emerging when larvae hatch in the rainy season. From 1951 to 1956 there were severe epizootics in lambs in southern Africa, and many human cases occurred. Further human cases with several deaths were seen in South Africa in 1975, and a major outbreak occurred in East Africa following El Niño flooding in 1997 to 1998, apparently seeding a 'virgin soil' outbreak in Saudi Arabia and Yemen in 2000. In 1997–8 and 2006–7 there were epizootics in Kenya, Tanzania, Burundi, and Somalia. In the recent epidemic, 684 cases with 155 deaths were reported in Kenya (case fatality 23%), 264 cases with 109 deaths in Tanzania (case fatality 41%), and 114 cases with 51 deaths in Somalia (case fatality 45%). Heavy rains in East Africa during 2006–7 triggered another outbreak with many human and animal cases.

In the Central African Republic in 1969, a virus isolated from *Mansonia africana* mosquitoes and named Zinga virus was associated with several cases of haemorrhagic fever; Zinga virus was later shown to be a strain of Rift Valley fever virus. In West Africa, Rift Valley fever virus was isolated from mosquitoes in Nigeria and from bats in Guinea, but despite the presence of antibodies in human sera collected in Nigeria and Senegal, human disease was unrecognized until 1987 when a substantial epidemic occurred in Mauritania, with further epidemics in following years. In 1977 the virus spread, apparently for the first time, into Egypt, producing a major epizootic in domestic animals, principally sheep and goats but also cattle, and causing about 600 human deaths within 3 months. The virus has been detected intermittently since then in Egypt. The principal known vector is the mosquito *Culex pipiens*. Both the Egyptian and the Mauritanian epidemics appeared to be linked to major ecological changes following the construction of the Aswan Dam on the Nile and dams on the Senegal River.

Symptoms

After an incubation period of 3 to 6 days, fever starts abruptly with shivering, nausea and vomiting, epigastric pain, arthralgia, and often severe generalized headache. The fever may be biphasic, with temperatures between 38 and 40°C, and may remain elevated for at least a week. There is no rash, but small haemorrhages appear on mucous membranes. Photophobia and eye pains occur. There may be conjunctival inflammation, and a central serous retinitis leading to central scotoma and sometimes to retinal detachment can occur late in disease. The fundus may show macular exudates that are slow to disappear. There is often a lymphadenopathy and although the liver is frequently involved and may be tender, jaundice is rare. Convalescence may be protracted but is usually uncomplicated.

A few patients develop severe disease with haemorrhage, encephalitis, or eye lesions. Haemorrhagic disease presents as above but progresses with cutaneous and mucous membrane petechiae, ecchymoses (Fig. 7.5.16.6a), gastrointestinal haemorrhage, and jaundice with severe liver and renal dysfunction often progressing to disseminated intravascular coagulation, hepatorenal syndrome,

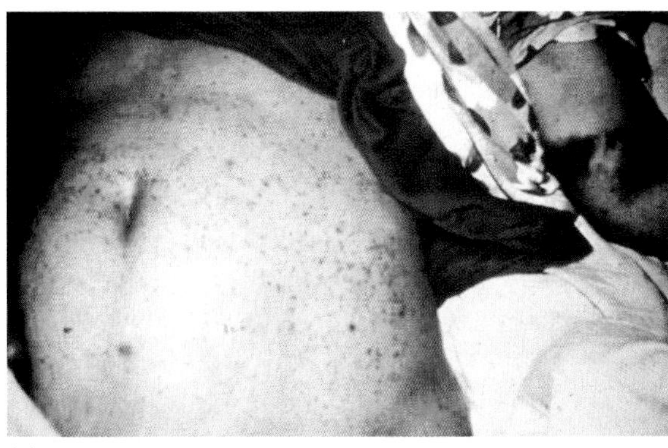
(a)

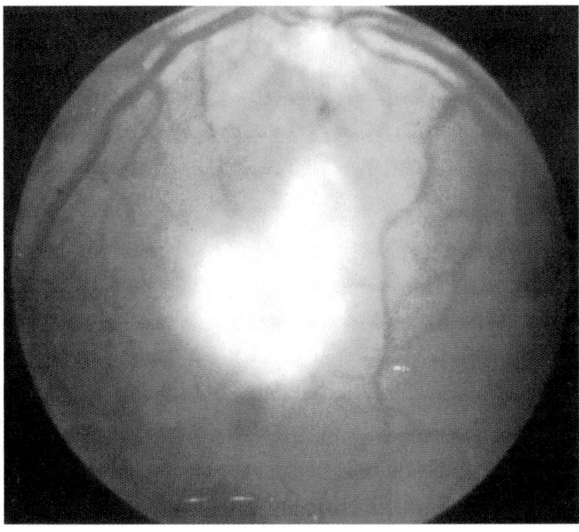
(b)

Fig. 7.5.16.6 Severe Rift Valley fever. (a) Cutaneous petechiae and ecchymosis. (b) Severe central retinal lesion.
(Courtesy of Professor D I H Simpson.)

and death. Patients with encephalitis usually recover from acute febrile disease only to present within a few days to 2 weeks later with headache, meningism, confusion, and fever, often leading to residual defects or ending in death. Ocular complications are characterized by rapid onset of decreased visual acuity with scotomas due to retinal haemorrhage, exudates, and macular oedema (Fig. 7.5.16.6b). These are also seen after apparent recovery from the initial disease. About one-half of these patients have some degree of permanent visual loss. Death from Rift Valley fever was rarely recognized before the 1977 outbreak in Egypt, but the Mauritanian epidemics with mortality due to jaundice and haemorrhagic manifestations, and the recent East African and Arabian Peninsula outbreaks with several hundred suspect fatalities establish it as a life-threatening infection.

Control, treatment, and prognosis

Veterinary vaccines have been used for some years, and formalin-inactivated vaccines have also had limited use for the prevention of disease in laboratory workers and others exposed to high risk of infection. Improved vaccines based on molecular techniques are under development. Treatment is supportive. Although there are no reports of nosocomial transmission, barrier nursing would be a sensible precaution.

Unassigned viruses and viruses causing only minor disease in humans

The great majority of the viruses listed in Table 7.5.16.2 cause only a mild febrile illness, but the following show certain additional features.

Bhanja virus (unassigned)

This virus was first isolated from *Haemaphysalis intermedia* ticks collected from healthy goats in India, but has since been isolated in Sri Lanka, Africa, and Europe. Infection of goats is widespread in Italy and the Balkans where there have been several reported human cases, including some with severe neurological disease and at least two deaths. Laboratory infections have also occurred.

Bwamba virus (*Orthobunyavirus*)

This was first isolated in Uganda in 1941 and is very widespread throughout sub-Saharan Africa. More than 75% of adult human sera collected in Nigeria and over 95% of human sera collected in Uganda and Tanzania have antibodies against Bwamba virus. The original cases showed fever, headache, generalized pain, and conjunctivitis but no rash, although a rash has been described in the Central African Republic. No fatalities have been reported.

Nyando virus (*Orthobunyavirus*)

This virus was first isolated from mosquitoes in Kenya. It has since been isolated from humans in the Central African Republic where it caused fever, myalgia, and encephalitis.

Tataguine virus (unassigned)

This causes fever, rash, and joint pains in at least five African countries (Cameroon, Central African Republic, Ethiopia, Nigeria, and Senegal).

Wanowrie virus (unassigned)

This virus was first isolated in India from *Hyalomma marginatum* ticks collected from sheep. It has also been isolated in Egypt and Iran, and in Sri Lanka where it was recovered from the brain of a 17-year-old girl who died following a 2-day fever with abdominal pain and vomiting.

Further reading

Bartelloni PJ, Tesh RB (1976). Clinical and serologic responses of volunteers infected with phlebotomus fever virus (Sicilian type). *Am J Trop Med Hyg*, **25**, 456–62.

Calisher CH, Thompson WH (eds) (1983). *California serogroup viruses. Progress in clinical and biological research*, vol. 123. Liss, New York.

Ergonul O (2006). Crimean-Congo haemorrhagic fever. *Lancet Infect Dis*, **6**, 203–14.

Koster F, *et al.* (2001). Rapid presumptive diagnosis of hantavirus cardiopulmonary syndrome by peripheral blood smear review. *Am J Clin Pathol*, **116**, 665–72.

LeDuc JW (1995). Hantavirus infections. In: Porterfield JS (ed) *Exotic viral infections*, pp. 261–84. Chapman & Hall, London.

LeDuc JW, Pinheiro FP (1989). Oropouche fever. In: Monath TP (ed) *The arboviruses: epidemiology and ecology*, vol. 4, pp. 1–14. CRC Press, Boca Raton.

Lee HW, Calisher C, Schmaljohn CS (1999). *Manual of hemorrhagic fever with renal syndrome and hantavirus pulmonary syndrome.*

WHO Collaborating Center for Virus Reference and Research (Hantaviruses), Seoul.
Madani TA, *et al.* (2003). Rift Valley fever epidemic in Saudi Arabia: epidemiology, clinical and laboratory characteristics. *Clin Infect Dis*, **37**, 1084–92.
Monath TP (ed) (1989). *The arboviruses: epidemiology and ecology*. CRC Press, Boca Raton.
Peters CJ (1997). Emergence of Rift Valley fever. In: Saluzzo JF, Dodet B (eds) *Factors in the emergence of arbovirus diseases*, pp. 253–64. Elsevier, Paris.
Peters CJ (1998). Hantavirus pulmonary syndrome in the Americas. *Emerg Infections*, **2**, 17–64.
Peters CJ, LeDuc JW (1991). Bunyaviridae: bunyaviruses, phleboviruses, and related viruses. In: Belshe RB (ed) *Textbook of human virology*, 2nd edition, pp. 571–614. Mosby Year Book, St. Louis.
Peters CJ, Simpson GL, Levy H (1999). Spectrum of hantavirus infection: hemorrhagic fever with renal syndrome and hantavirus pulmonary syndrome. *Annu Rev Med*, **50**, 531–45.
Saluzzo JF, Dodet B (eds) (1999). Factors in the emergence and control of rodent-borne viral disease (hantaviral and arenal diseases). Elsevier, Paris.
Swanepoel R (1995). Nairovirus infections. In: Porterfield JS (ed) *Exotic viral infections*, pp. 285–93. Chapman & Hall, London.

7.5.17 Arenaviruses

J. ter Meulen

Essentials

Arenaviruses are zoonotic RNA viruses that are distributed worldwide and are adapted to various rodent genera. Some are highly pathogenic and cause haemorrhagic fevers that are endemic in restricted regions of a few countries. Humans are thought to become infected mainly through inhalation of aerosolized rodent urine or dust particles to which infectious urine has dried, or by ingestion of contaminated foodstuff: prevention therefore depends on rodent control and avoidance of contact with rodents, their excreta, and nesting materials.

Clinical approach—because arenaviruses cause diseases that start insidiously and therapy is life-saving, they should be considered in all patients with fever of unknown origin and a history of possible exposure in the well-known endemic areas.

Specific infections

Lassa fever—reservoir is a small rodent (*Mastomys natalensis*); occurs regularly in rural areas of Nigeria, Liberia, Sierra Leone and the Republic of Guinea, but may occur also in other West African countries. Clinical picture is highly variable and can be difficult to distinguish from other febrile infections, but may include chest pain, nausea/vomiting/diarrhoea/abdominal pain, facial swelling, pulmonary oedema, and bleeding. Case-fatality is 15 to 30%, but may be reduced by up to 90% through prompt administration of ribavirin. Irreversible sensorineural deafness is a frequent complication. Body fluids of patients are highly infectious and Lassa virus has been transmitted directly from person-to-person, hence strict 'barrier nursing' measures are required and (if possible) patients with severe disease and bleeding should be managed in a negative-pressure room by personnel wearing appropriate protective gear, including respiratory filters; postexposure prophylaxis with ribavirin should be considered. No vaccine is available.

Lymphocytic choriomeningitis virus infection—reservoir is the house mouse. Most commonly causes an influenza-like illness, sometimes with subsequent aseptic meningitis or encephalomyelitis. Intrauterine infection has resulted in nonobstructive hydrocephalus with periventricular calcifications, chorioretinitis, and psychomotor retardation. Use of ribavirin has not been systematically evaluated.

South American haemorrhagic fevers—the reservoir(s) for Argentinian haemorrhagic fever is the vesper mouse, for Bolivian haemorrhagic fever *Calomys callosus*, and for Venezuelan haemorrhagic fever the cotton rat and the cane mouse. These cause an influenza-like illness with marked skin erythema and (in almost half of cases) haemorrhagic manifestations; a late neurological cerebellar syndrome occurs in about 10%. Treatment with convalescent-phase plasma is very effective in Argentinian haemorrhagic fever, and ribavirin may be effective. A live attenuated vaccine for Argentinian haemorrhagic fever is licensed in Argentina.

Introduction

Arenaviruses are pleomorphic enveloped negative-stranded segmented RNA viruses with a characteristic internal granular structure, hence their family name Arenaviridae (Latin *arenosus* = sandy). Several arenaviruses are known to be responsible for severe diseases in humans. Lymphocytic choriomeningitis virus (LCMV) is distributed worldwide and occasionally causes acute central nervous system (CNS) disease and congenital malformations and has been transmitted through solid organ transplantation. Lassa virus in West Africa, and Junin, Machupo, Guanarito, and Sabia viruses in South America cause viral haemorrhagic fevers (VHF). Certain rodent species are the principal hosts of arenaviruses and shed them lifelong in high titres in their urine. Humans are thought to become infected mainly through inhalation of aerosolized rodent urine or dust particles to which infectious urine has dried, or by ingestion of contaminated foodstuff. Human-to-human transmission occurs with some of the viruses. In geographically confined endemic rural areas, sporadic infections with these viruses occur regularly and are often linked to seasonal agricultural activities. Novel related viruses are emerging from time to time in previously unaffected areas. In 2000, three patients from California were fatally infected with a novel arenavirus related to Whitewater Arroyo virus, originally isolated from rodents in New Mexico.

Aetiology, genetics, pathogenesis, and pathology

Common to all arenavirus haemorrhagic fevers is disruption of vascular endothelial integrity, originating most likely from the release of endogenous mediators from infected macrophages or endothelial cells, and resulting in extravasations of fluid into extravascular spaces ('capillary leakage syndrome'). Coagulation disorders are subtler than in filovirus infections and disseminated intravascular coagulopathy is not observed. Platelets are dysfunctional despite their adequate or only mildly depressed numbers, and evidence for a soluble protein inhibitor of platelet function, presumably of host origin, has been described in Lassa virus (LASV) and Junin virus (JUNV) infections. Experimentally, LASV-infected nonhuman primates also showed a marked decrease in endothelial prostacyclin production.

Arenaviruses initially infect macrophages and immature dendritic cells, compromising the ability of the latter to mature and stimulate T-cell responses. Infected dendritic cells seem to be eliminated by immunopathological mechanisms, correlating with a decline in the number of lymphocytes and destruction of the architecture of lymphatic organs. In LCMV and LASV infections, this suppression of the innate immune responses is shown by the absence or delayed appearance of a neutralizing antibody response. In contrast, infection with JUNV induces neutralizing antibodies. Hence, immune plasma is used for passive immune therapy.

Arenaviruses replicate in many epithelial cell types with only modest cytopathic effect and there is ominous absence of an inflammatory response in infected organs. Autopsy of LASV-infected nonhuman primates shows pulmonary congestion, pleural effusion, and pericardial oedema and effusion. Major microscopic lesions are necrotizing hepatitis and interstitial pneumonia. The degree of hepatic damage is not sufficient to implicate hepatic failure as the cause of death. In JUNV infection, there are large areas of intra-alveolar or bronchial haemorrhage, petechiae on organ surfaces, and ulcerations of the digestive tract, although bleeding is not massive. Pneumonia with necrotizing bronchitis or pulmonary emboli is observed in one-half of cases. Haemorrhage and a lymphocytic infiltrate have been observed in the pericardium, and splenic haemorrhage is common. Renal damage occurs in about one-half of the fatal cases and consists of severe structural damage in the distal tubular cells and collecting ducts with relative sparing of the glomeruli and proximal tubules.

Neurological involvement during the acute phase of the disease is common in the South American haemorrhagic fevers, but there is no evidence of direct viral infection of the CNS. In Lassa fever, neurological complications, mainly sensorineural deafness, are very common during convalescence and are thought to be due to immunopathology. There is evidence that LASV persists at least for some time because it has been isolated in human urine for up to 60 days.

In one report of a fatal human LCMV infection there was perivascular macrophage infiltration in multiple areas of the brain and antigen was observed in the meninges and cortical cells. LCMV has been recovered from the CNS of newborn children with malformations.

Epidemiology

Lassa fever

Clinical cases of Lassa fever are reported regularly in rural areas of Nigeria, Liberia, Sierra Leone, and the Republic of Guinea, but may occur also in other West African countries. The reservoir of LASV is a small rodent (*Mastomys natalensis*) that lives in and around human dwellings. In West Africa, 300 000 to 500 000 LASV infections are estimated to occur annually, resulting in approximately 150 000 clinical cases, ranging in severity from flu-like illness to haemorrhagic fever, and approximately 5000 deaths. In endemic areas, 75% of all LASV infections are probably asymptomatic, with an overall mortality of 1 to 5%. Lassa fever patients are not infectious during the incubation period and quite close contact with body fluids is required for person-to-person spread of the virus. However, airborne transmission, probably through direct contact with droplets produced during heavy coughing and presumably originating from Lassa pneumonitis, has been reported in a few instances.

Presumed nonpathogenic arenaviruses have been isolated from *Mastomys* spp. and other rodents throughout Africa, and serological evidence of human infection has been detected. Recently, a novel, highly pathogenetic arenavirus (named Lujo virus) was isolated from a Zambian patient hospitalized with a fatal Lassa fever-like illness in South Africa, who transmitted the infection to several care givers.

Expatriates working in endemic areas have repeatedly imported Lassa fever into Europe and North America.

Lymphocytic choriomeningitis virus infection

The distribution of LCMV is highly variable within populations of its natural host *Mus musculus*. From infected mouse colonies, LCMV spreads to humans in rural settings or when human habitats are substandard in urban areas. Infected laboratory and pet rodents have also been associated with disease in humans, and aerosol transmission may have occurred. Clinical cases of LCMV infection seem to be rare in the United States of America, even though 9.0% of house mice and 4.7% of residents had measurable antibodies in the Baltimore area in the 1990s. Person-to-person spread has not been demonstrated. Intrauterine LCMV infection has resulted in fetal or neonatal death, as well as hydrocephalus and chorioretinitis in infants, and the virus may be a more frequent cause of CNS disease in newborns than previously recognized. Two clusters of transplantation-associated transmission of LCMV have been reported.

Argentine haemorrhagic fever

The endemic area of Argentine haemorrhagic fever (caused by JUNV) comprises the provinces of Buenos Aires, Córdoba, Santa Fe, and La Pampa. The major rodent hosts of JUNV are the agrarian rodents (vesper mice) *Calomys musculinus* and *C. laucha*. Most human cases are male agricultural workers. About 21 000 cases have been reported since the early 1960s, averaging about 360 a year with wide annual fluctuations. Peak incidence is during summer and early autumn. Overall human antibody prevalence is about 12% and about 30% had no history of typical illness. Occasional hospital or family epidemics have occurred, but cases have not been observed outside of Argentina. Recent introduction of a live attenuated vaccine has reduced the incidence of the disease dramatically.

Bolivian haemorrhagic fever

Bolivian haemorrhagic fever (caused by Machupo virus) is limited to rural areas of Beni department in Bolivia. The only known reservoir is *Calomys callosus*. The largest known epidemic of Bolivian haemorrhagic fever, involving several hundred cases, followed a marked and unusual increase in the *Calomys* population in homes in the town of San Joaquin in 1963 and 1964. This seems to have been a unique event, and there were almost no further cases until 1994, when there was an outbreak in north-eastern Bolivia. Since all ages and both sexes are affected, it can be assumed that most patients were infected in their homes. Person-to-person spread is rarely reported.

Venezuelan haemorrhagic fever

Venezuelan haemorrhagic fever (caused by Guanarito virus) is endemic to the southern and south-western parts of Portuguesa state and adjacent regions of Barinas state in Venezuela. From 1989 to 1995, a total of 105 confirmed or probable cases of Venezuelan haemorrhagic fever were reported, of which 34% were fatal. All ages and sexes were infected suggesting that transmission had occurred in and around houses. The incidence peaked each year between November and January, during the period of major agricultural activity. In addition, epidemic activity of the illness appears cyclically every 4 to 5 years. The cotton rat *Sigmodon alstoni* and the cane mouse *Zygodontomys brevicauda* are the rodent reservoirs. Seroprevalence in humans living in the state of Portuguesa is below 2%. Human-to-human transmission has not been reported.

Other arenavirus infections

Sabia virus was isolated in 1990 from a fatal case in São Paulo, Brazil. Its natural distribution and host are still unknown. One patient who acquired the infection in the laboratory treated himself immediately with ribavirin, and made a rapid and full recovery.

Whitewater Arroyo virus was isolated in 1996 from white-throated wood rats or pack rats (*Neotoma albigula* and *Neotoma* spp.) collected in McKinley county, New Mexico. A related virus has caused three fatal human infections in California in 1999 and 2000; they are believed to be rare events because the abundance and habits of wood rats suggest that potential contact with humans is limited. One patient reportedly cleaned rodent droppings in her home during the 2 weeks before illness onset; no history of rodent contact was solicited for the other two patients. Several other arenaviruses isolated from North American rodents have not yet been shown to cause human infections.

Prevention

Rodent control

In endemic areas, rodent control is essential and direct contact with rodents, their excreta, and their nesting materials should be avoided.

Management of infected patients

Safe and orderly care of the ill and adequate disinfection procedures should be instituted early (barrier nursing, guidelines from Centres for Disease Control and World Health Organization, see Box 7.5.17.1), with effective surveillance of high-risk contacts and prompt isolation of further cases. Direct person-to-person transmission occurs in Lassa fever and, although rare, has been documented for some New World viruses. Nosocomial transmission can occur through direct contact with an infected patient's blood, urine, or pharyngeal secretions. If possible, patients with severe disease and bleeding should be placed in a negative-pressure room and all personnel should wear protective gear with P3 filters for respiratory protection. High-risk contacts are associated with percutaneous or mucosal contact with blood or body fluids. Medium-risk contacts (unprotected contact with blood or body fluids) may safely be observed for development of persistent high fever for 3 weeks from the last date of contact by daily temperature measurement and telephone reporting.

Box 7.5.17.1 Principles of barrier nursing in resource-poor settings (World Health Organization)

Protective clothing

- Double gloves
- (Single-use) gown
- Plastic apron
- Mask (P3 protection)
- Goggles
- Disinfect within isolation area or destroy (single-use) material.

Hand washing

- After each patient contact or contact with infected material
- Rinse in disinfectant, then wash with soap and water
- Disinfectant/washing facilities must be located just outside isolation rooms.

Instruments

- Individual thermometer for each patient, keep in receptacle with disinfectant
- Disinfect stethoscope and sleeve of sphygmomanometer between each use
- Place all reusable instruments in disinfecting fluid after use

Bed covering and linen

- Use of plastic sheet to cover and protect entire mattress is essential
- Disinfect after discharge or death of the patient
- Place bedding and linen in plastic bag for sterilization (soak in disinfectant, boil, or autoclave)

Food

- Food should be supplied by hospital, not relatives
- Each patient must have own eating utensils
- Wash and disinfect in isolation area
- Dispose of uneaten food

Charts/records

- Keep outside isolation area

Disinfection methods

- Household bleach—viruses causing viral haemorrhagic fevers are killed by exposure to a 1:10 solution for 1 min, or to a 1:100 solution for 10 min
- Heat sterilization—if autoclave not available, boil at 100°C for 20 min

Ribavirin postexposure prophylaxis

There are no evidence-based data to support oral ribavirin as postexposure prophylaxis, but, anecdotally, a German physician seroconverted asymptomatically under ribavirin prophylaxis after examining a coughing Lassa fever patient without respiratory protection and gloves (medium-risk contact). Prophylaxis should be given to high-risk contacts of Lassa fever and South American haemorrhagic fever patients, and offered to medium-risk contacts of Lassa fever patients on an individual basis. One recommended dosage is 600 mg orally four times a day for 10 days. Temporary side effects of this regimen were skin rash, tachycardia, myalgia, diarrhoea, and abdominal pain. In one case, there may have been an association between ribavirin and worsening of a pre-existing tachyarrhythmia. Among 16 people there were reversible increases in plasma bilirubin concentrations in 11 and a decrease in haemoglobin concentration in 9. One person stopped prophylaxis after 4 days because of jaundice, and in another the serum lipase concentration increased.

Vaccines

Experimental vaccines based on different viral vector systems have protected against lethal challenge with LASV in animal models, but are far from licensure. A live attenuated vaccine (candid No. 1) against JUNV is licensed in Argentina and produced by the Maiztegui Institute, Pergamino. It was tested in over 200 000 volunteers, showed an estimated effectiveness of 95.5%, and may be cross-protective against Machupo virus only. The Salk Institute, Swiftwater, PA, also produced some quantities of the vaccine, which has an investigational new drug (IND) status from the United States Food and Drug Administration for high-risk populations.

Clinical features

Lassa fever

The clinical picture of Lassa fever is highly variable and may be very difficult to distinguish from other febrile infections. Following an incubation period of 7 to 21 days, Lassa fever begins insidiously with fever, weakness, malaise, severe usually frontal headache, and a painful sore throat. One-half of patients develop joint and lumbar pain and a nonproductive cough. Severe retrosternal chest pain, nausea with vomiting or diarrhoea, and abdominal pain are also common. Respiration rate, pulse rate, and temperature are elevated and blood pressure may be low. There is no characteristic rash; petechiae and ecchymoses are not seen. About one-third of patients will have conjunctivitis. More than two-thirds of patients have pharyngitis, one-half with exudates; the posterior pharynx and tonsils are diffusely inflamed and swollen, but there are few ulcers or petechiae (Fig. 7.5.17.1). The abdomen is tender in one-half of the patients. Neurological signs in the early stages are limited to a fine tremor, most marked in the lips and tongue. Thirty per cent of patients progress to a prostrating illness 6 to 8 days after onset of fever, usually with persistent vomiting and diarrhoea. Patients are often dehydrated with elevated haematocrit. Proteinuria occurs in two-thirds of patients, with moderately elevated blood urea nitrogen. About one-half of Lassa fever patients have diffuse abdominal tenderness without localizing signs or loss of bowel sounds. The severe retrosternal or epigastric pain seen in many patients may be due to pleural or pericardial involvement. Facial and conjunctival swelling develop, and severe pulmonary oedema and adult respiratory distress syndrome are common in fatal cases, with gross head and neck oedema, stridor, and hypovolaemic shock (Fig. 7.5.17.2a,b). Renal and hepatic failure are not seen. Bleeding is seen in only 15 to 20% of patients and is restricted to mucosal surfaces, conjunctiva, and gastrointestinal and/or genital tracts. Over 70% of patients have abnormal electrocardiograms (nonspecific ST-segment and T-wave abnormalities, ST-segment elevation, generalized low voltage complexes, and changes reflecting electrolyte disturbance), but none correlate with disease severity or outcome. There is no clinical evidence of myocarditis. Neurological signs are infrequent but carry a poor prognosis; they progress from confusion to severe encephalopathy with or without general seizures and without focal signs (Fig. 7.5.17.3). There has been a report of an imported fatal Lassa fever case presenting with only neurological symptoms. Cerebrospinal fluid is usually normal, apart from a few lymphocytes. Pneumonitis and pleural and pericardial rubs develop in early convalescence in about 20% of hospitalized patients, sometimes associated with congestive cardiac failure.

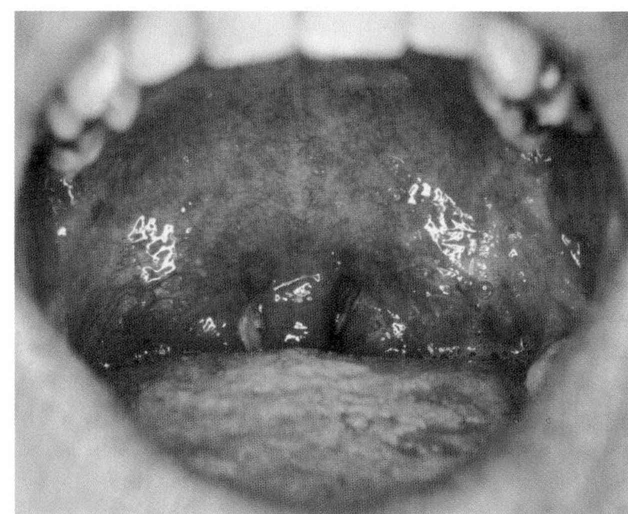

Fig. 7.5.17.1 Lassa fever: pharyngitis. (Copyright D A Warrell.)

Lassa virus is present in the breast milk of infected mothers, and neonates are therefore at risk of congenital, intrapartum, and puerperal infection. Lassa fever may be difficult to diagnose in children. In very young babies marked oedema has been reported.

Laboratory findings

A normal mean white blood cell count on admission to hospital (6×10^9/litre) may mask early lymphopenia with later relative or absolute neutrophilia as high as 30×10^9/litre. Thrombocytopenia is moderate, even in severely ill patients, but platelet function is markedly depressed. The ratio of aspartate aminotransferase (AST, SGOT) to alanine aminotransferase (ALT, SGPT) is as high as 11:1. Prothrombin times, glucose, and bilirubin levels are nearly normal, excluding biochemical hepatic failure. Platelet and fibrinogen turnover are normal and there is no indication of disseminated intravascular coagulopathy.

Complications and sequelae

Nearly 30% of patients develop unilateral or bilateral deafness beginning during convalescence. About one-half show a near or complete recovery after 3 to 4 months, but the other one-half remain permanently deaf. Many patients also show transient cerebellar signs during convalescence, particularly tremors and ataxia.

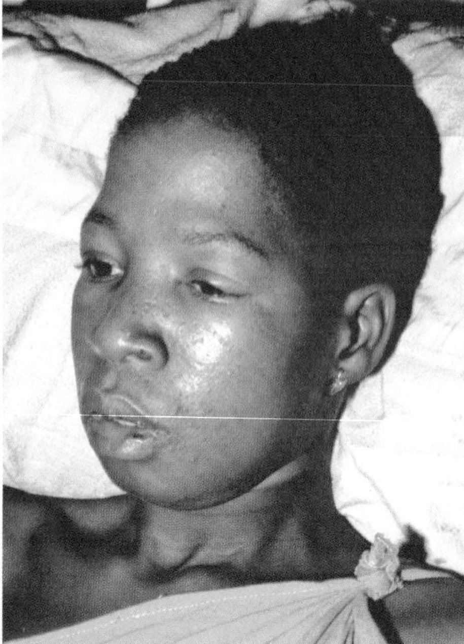

(a)

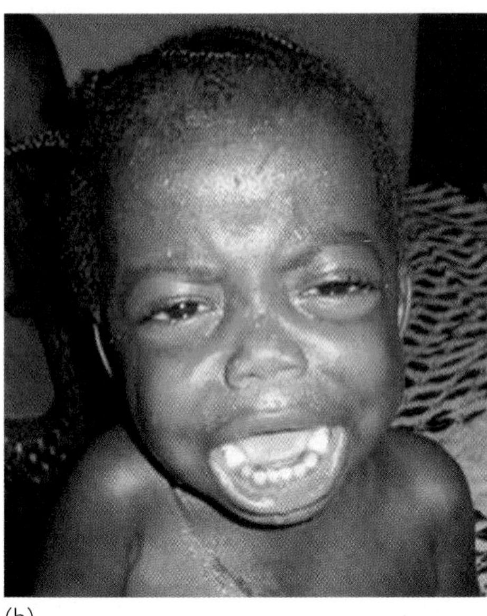

(b)

Fig. 7.5.17.2 (a) Lassa fever: facial and generalized oedema and hypovolaemic shock in a pregnant woman in Sierra Leone.
(Copyright D A Warrell.)
(b) Lassa fever: facial oedema in a child.
(Courtesy of Dr S. Mardel.)

Other complications include uveitis, pericarditis, orchitis, pleural effusion, ascites, and acute adrenal insufficiency.

Prognosis

The case fatality rate of hospitalized patients in West Africa is approximately 15%, but it exceeds 50% in patients with haemorrhage. CNS manifestations carry a poor prognosis. Lassa fever is a common cause of maternal mortality in parts of West Africa. Mortality is 20% in the first trimester and 30% in the second trimester of pregnancy, with fetal loss occurring in 87%, apparently not varying with the trimester. Mortality was reduced fourfold in women who spontaneously or were therapeutically aborted.

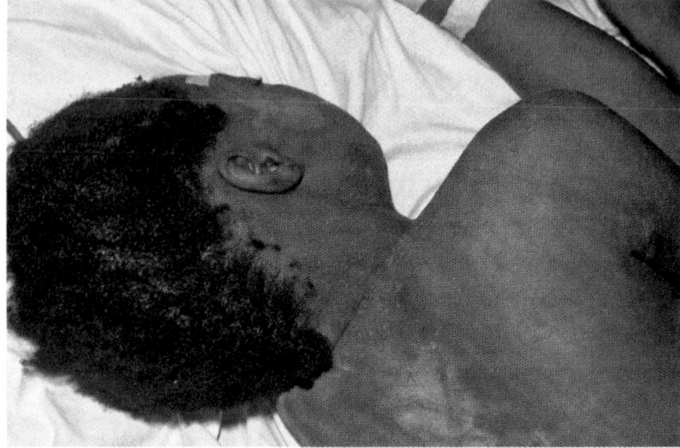

Fig. 7.5.17.3 Lassa fever: generalized oedema and encephalopathy in a pregnant woman in Sierra Leone.
(Copyright D A Warrell.)

High viral titre in serum (exceeding 10^4 $TCID_{50}$/ml), AST (SGOT) raised above 150 U/litre, and bleeding, each worsen the prognosis, with the combination of high viral titres and high AST (SGOT) carrying a risk of death of approximately 80%. High neutrophil counts (more than 30×10^9/litre) may be observed in these patients.

In most patients with imported Lassa fever treated in developed countries, diagnosis and ribavirin therapy have often been delayed, and the patients have died despite full supportive care.

Lymphocytic choriomeningitis virus infection

An influenza-like illness is the most common clinical presentation of LCMV. Fever (up to 40°C) with rigors is always present. Frequently noted are malaise, retro-orbital headache, photophobia, lumbar myalgias, anorexia, nausea, bradycardia, and pharyngeal injection without exudate. Mild nontender cervical or axillary lymphadenopathy may occur. Up to 50% of patients have vomiting, sore throat, and dysaesthesias, and one-quarter of patients complain of chest pains and cough, associated with pneumonitis. Arthritis, parotitis, orchitis, myocarditis, rash, and alopecia have also been noted. In some patients, the disease is biphasic with subsequent aseptic meningitis of about 1 week's duration or encephalomyelitis in a smaller number of cases. Other neurological manifestations such as myelitis, Guillain–Barré syndrome, and sensorineural deafness have been reported. The onset of CNS disease may also occur without any prodrome.

Intrauterine infection

This has resulted in nonobstructive hydrocephalus with periventricular calcifications, chorioretinitis, and psychomotor retardation. No cardiac abnormalities were observed. Some mothers had a history of febrile illness during pregnancy.

Transplantation-associated lymphocytic choriomeningitis virus infection

In two clusters of cases, the solid organ transplant recipients had abdominal pain, altered mental status, thrombocytopenia, elevated aminotransferase levels, coagulopathy, graft dysfunction, and either fever or leukocytosis within 3 weeks after transplantation. Diarrhoea, peri-incisional rash, renal failure, and seizures were variably present. Seven of the eight recipients died 9 to 76 days after transplantation.

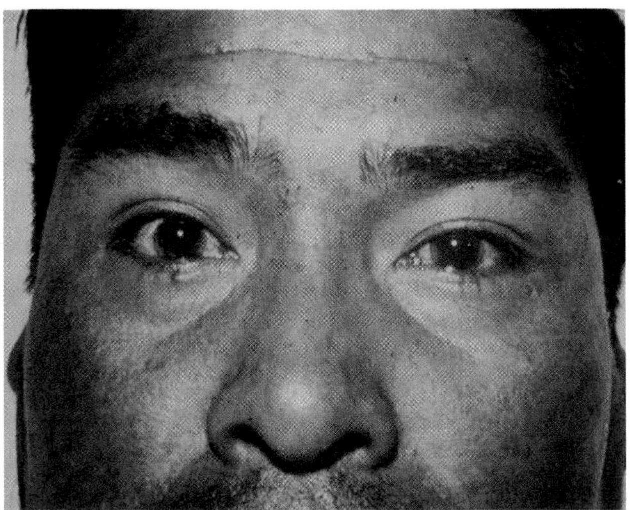

Fig. 7.5.17.4 Argentine haemorrhagic fever: facial swelling and erythema. (Courtesy of Professor D.I.H. Simpson.)

Prognosis

Patients with aseptic meningitis almost always recover without sequelae, but 25 to 30% of patients with encephalitis have neurological residua.

South American haemorrhagic fevers

In Argentine and Bolivian haemorrhagic fevers, after an incubation period of 7 to 16 days, there is insidious development of malaise, chills, fever, severe myalgia, anorexia, lumbar pain, epigastric pain, abdominal tenderness, conjunctivitis, retro-orbital pain often with photophobia, and constipation. Nausea and vomiting occur frequently after 2 or 3 days of illness. There is no lymphadenopathy, splenomegaly, sore throat, or cough, but there is high fever (up to 40°C), marked erythema of the face, neck, and thorax, and conjunctivitis (Fig. 7.5.17.4). Respiratory symptoms are uncommon. Petechiae appear by the fourth or fifth day of the illness. There may be a pharyngeal enanthema, but pharyngitis is uncommon. The infection either resolves after about 6 days or progresses to severe disease.

South American haemorrhagic fevers are associated with haemorrhagic manifestations in nearly one-half of patients: gingival haemorrhages (Fig. 7.5.17.5), epistaxis, metrorrhagia, petechiae (Fig. 7.5.17.6), ecchymoses, purpura, melaena, and haematuria.

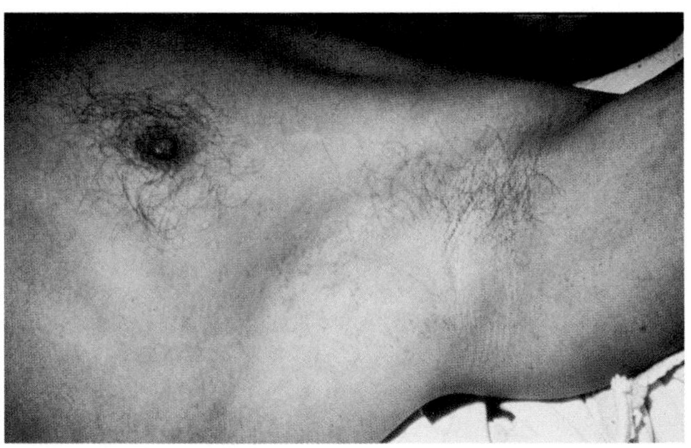

Fig. 7.5.17.5 Argentine haemorrhagic fever: petechial haemorrhages. (Courtesy of Professor D I H Simpson.)

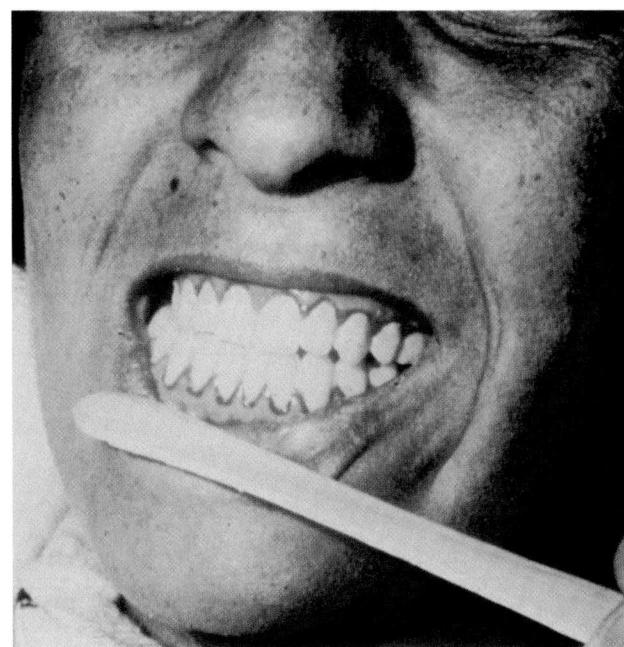

Fig. 7.5.17.6 Argentine haemorrhagic fever: gingival bleeding. (Courtesy of Professor D I H Simpson.)

Severe cases have nausea, vomiting, intense proteinuria, microscopic haematuria, oliguria, and uraemia. Fatal cases develop hypotensive shock, hypothermia, and pulmonary oedema. Renal failure has been reported but glomerular filtration rates, renal plasma flow, and creatinine clearance are usually normal. There is some electrocardiographic evidence of myocarditis. Fifty per cent of patients have neurological symptoms during the second stage of illness, such as tremors of the hands and tongue, progressing in some patients to delirium, oculogyration, and strabismus. Meningeal signs and cerebrospinal fluid abnormalities are rare.

The clinical presentation of Venezuelan haemorrhagic fever is similar. Patients are toxic and usually dehydrated, with pharyngitis, conjunctivitis, cervical lymphadenopathy, facial oedema, or petechiae.

Laboratory findings

Thrombocytopenia (below 150×10^9/litre) and neutropenia (range 0.8–6.6×10^9/litre) are almost invariable. Bleeding and clot retraction times are concomitantly prolonged. Although reductions of levels of factors II, V, VII, VIII, and X and of fibrinogen are observed, alterations in clotting functions are usually minor and full-blown disseminated intravascular coagulopathy is not a feature.

Complications and sequelae

A late neurological syndrome in about 10% of cases, consisting mainly of cerebellar signs, is associated with treatment using high titre antiserum. Among survivors of South American haemorrhagic fevers, convalescence typically takes 1 to 3 months, with weight loss, fatigue, autonomic instability, and occasional hair loss. Mild permanent damage to acoustic centres has been detected in a small group of patients.

Prognosis

In endemic areas, the case fatality rate of Argentine haemorrhagic fever is 15 to 30% for untreated hospitalized patients and 1% for patients who received plasma therapy. CNS manifestations carry a poor prognosis. The case fatality rate of Bolivian haemorrhagic fever is higher. In one series of hospitalized patients with Venezuelan haemorrhagic fever, the case fatality rate was reported to be 33% despite vigorous supportive care. Argentine haemorrhagic fever is reported to be severe in pregnancy.

Whitewater Arroyo-like virus

Illnesses were associated with nonspecific febrile symptoms including fever, headache, and myalgias. Within the first week of hospitalization, lymphopenia was observed in all three patients, and thrombocytopenia (30–40×10⁹/litre) was seen in two. All three patients had acute respiratory distress syndrome and two developed liver failure and haemorrhagic manifestations. All patients died 1 to 8 weeks after becoming unwell.

Criteria for diagnosis and differential diagnosis

Due to the variable clinical presentation of arenavirus infections, the diseases should be suspected in any patient presenting with a severe febrile illness and evidence of vascular involvement (low blood pressure, postural hypotension, petechiae, haemorrhagic diathesis, flushing of face and chest, nondependent oedema). Sore throat, abdominal symptoms, and CNS symptoms are likewise important. For many regions in the world, the major differential diagnose is malaria.

Lassa fever

Lassa fever should be suspected in a patient living in or coming within the incubation period (7–21 days) from rural areas in Sierra Leone, Liberia, Nigeria, the Republic of Guinea, and adjacent territories, and presenting with otherwise unexplained high fever (above 38.5°C), pharyngitis with dry cough and chest pain or abdominal pain and diarrhoea, facial oedema, mucosal bleeding, or CNS symptoms. In West Africa, fever with pharyngitis, proteinuria, and retrosternal chest pain had a predictive value for Lassa fever of 81% and a specificity of 89%. Due to the variable clinical picture of Lassa fever, there are many differential diagnoses including severe malaria, typhoid fever, rickettsial diseases, relapsing fevers, shigellosis, leptospirosis, meningococcaemia, and gram-negative sepsis. Viral haemorrhagic fevers such as yellow fever, Rift Valley fever, and Marburg and Ebola virus infections are much more likely to cause haemorrhage, disseminated intravascular coagulopathy, and severe liver dysfunction than Lassa fever.

South American haemorrhagic fevers

These should be considered in patients coming from endemic areas of Argentina (particularly male agricultural workers), Bolivia, Venezuela, and Brazil who present with unexplained fever and a bleeding diathesis. Differential diagnoses are similar to those for Lassa fever and, in addition, yellow fever and dengue fever must be considered. Appearance of the blanching maculopapular rash and a shorter duration of fever differentiate dengue from the early stages of arenavirus infections.

The combination of a platelet count of less than 100×10⁹/litre and a white blood cell count of less than 2.5×10⁹/litre has a sensitivity of 87% and a specificity of 88% for Argentine haemorrhagic fever. These criteria are recommended when screening Argentine haemorrhagic fever patients for treatment with immune plasma or ribavirin in endemic areas.

LCMV infection should be considered in patients presenting in autumn or winter with a biphasic disease characterized by fever and persistent meningeal signs, particularly if there is a history of rodent contact. Other rat bite fevers (Chapter 7.6.31) enter the differential diagnosis.

Laboratory diagnosis

Laboratory diagnosis of arenavirus infection is by isolation of virus from serum, demonstration of a fourfold rise in antibody titre, or high-titre IgG antibody with virus-specific IgM antibody in association with compatible clinical disease. More recently, detection of viral sequences by reverse transcriptase–polymerase chain reaction (RT-PCR), or by detection of viral proteins using an enzyme-linked immunosorbent assay (ELISA) system have been introduced.

For handling of clinical specimens from suspected cases, see Table 7.5.17.1.

Treatment

Lassa fever

Ribavirin is effective but must be given as early as possible while laboratory confirmation of the diagnosis is pending. It is administered by intravenous infusion as a 2-g loading dose followed by 1 g every 6 h for 4 days then 0.5 g every 8 h for 6 more days. Another recommended intravenous regimen is an initial dose of 30 mg/kg followed by 15 mg/kg every 6 h for 4 days, followed by 7.5 mg/kg every 8 h for 6 days. Rigors may occur if the drug is infused too rapidly. Oral ribavirin doses are a 2-g loading dose followed

Table 7.5.17.1 Inactivation of blood/serum from viral haemorrhagic fever patients for laboratory analysis

Material	Examination	Inactivation
Blood	Thick film	Add formalin to a final concentration of 1% to solution used for lysis of erythrocytes
Blood	Thin film	Methanol fixation
Blood	Leucocyte count	1:100 in 3% acetic acid, 15 min room temperature
Serum/plasma	Serological tests	Heat for 60 min at 60°C[a]
		0.25% β-propiolactone (final concentration), 30 min 37°C
Serum/plasma	Clinical chemistry	Heat for 60 min at 60°C[b]
		0.25% β-propiolactone (final concentration), 30 min 37°C[c]
		0.1% Triton X-100 (final concentration), 60 min room temperature[d]

[a] Loss of reactivity. Heating at 56°C for 1 h preserves antibody reactivity better but leaves sample with residual infectivity. Only recommended if sample can be safely handled in biological safety level 2 cabinet (laminar air flow).

[b] No influence on sodium, potassium, magnesium, urea, creatinine, urate, bilirubin, glucose, C-reactive protein. Reduced levels of bicarbonate, aspartate aminotransferase, calcium, phosphate, albumin, total protein. Measurement not possible for alkaline phosphatase, alanine aminotransferase, γ-glutamyl transpeptidase, creatine kinase.

[c] Liver enzyme values reduced by 20%. pH and bicarbonate not useful.

[d] Influence on clinical chemistry not evaluated.

by 4 g/day in four divided doses for 4 days followed by 2 g/day for six doses. Oral ribavirin is believed to be only half as effective as intravenous therapy. A five- to tenfold decrease in the case–fatality ratio was demonstrated in patients treated with ribavirin compared to untreated patients when therapy was given within the first 6 days of illness. Patients with high AST (SGOT) and viraemia, who were treated within the first 6 days of illness, had a 5 to 9% case fatality, and a 26 to 47% fatality when treated after 6 days, compared with 52 to 78% when untreated. Ribavirin is contraindicated in early pregnancy because of potential teratogenicity, but the fetus rarely survives the infection. Fluid, electrolyte, respiratory, and osmotic imbalances should be corrected, and full intensive care support, including mechanical ventilation, offered as required. However, even vigorous support may be insufficient to prevent fatal progression of advanced disease.

Interferon-α has shown efficacy against arenaviruses in animal models but only if given within a couple of days of challenge. A synergistic effect with suboptimal doses of ribavirin was observed.

Lymphocytic choriomeningitis virus infection

Ribavirin treatment has not been evaluated in human CNS disease caused by LCMV. In a cluster of transplantation-associated systemic LCMV infections, one recipient, who received ribavirin and reduced levels of immunosuppressive therapy, survived.

South American haemorrhagic fevers

Convalescent-phase plasma has been shown to be highly successful in Argentine haemorrhagic fever, reducing the mortality from 15 to 30% to 1% in patients treated in the first 8 days of illness. Efficacy is directly related to the concentration of neutralizing antibodies, and delayed treatment is less successful. Availability of appropriately screened plasma may, however, be a problem. Ribavirin is effective against the causative JUNV in experimentally infected primates, but does not prevent CNS involvement. In one small double-blind trial with 18 patients, mortality was 12.5% in those treated compared to 40% in the placebo group. One human case of Bolivian haemorrhagic fever has been successfully treated with ribavirin and Venezuelan haemorrhagic fever is also likely to respond.

Other issues

Lassa fever is a truly neglected re-emerging disease that has a considerable impact on West African health care systems and the economy of affected rural areas. The absence of local diagnostic capacity and the high price of intravenous ribavirin preparations are the main barriers to the introduction of specific therapy to endemic areas.

Areas of uncertainty or controversy

The pathogenic events leading to plasma leakage, bleeding, and shock are not well understood in arenavirus infections, compared to filoviruses. A lack of understanding of the inhibition of neutralizing antibody responses is the main hurdle to the development of a Lassa fever vaccine.

Likely developments in the near future

Candid No. 1 is likely to be licensed in the United States of America. Several experimental antiviral drugs with efficacy against arenaviruses and other haemorrhagic fever viruses relevant to biodefence will enter clinical development.

Further reading

Bonthius DJ, *et al.* (2007). Congenital lymphocytic choriomeningitis virus infection: spectrum of disease. *Ann Neurol*, **62**, 347–55.

Fischer SA, *et al.* (2006). LCMV in transplant recipients. Transmission of lymphocytic choriomeningitis virus by organ transplantation. *N Engl J Med*, **354**, 2235–49.

Geisbert TW, *et al.* (2005). Development of a new vaccine for the prevention of Lassa fever. *PLoS Med*, **2**, e183.

Günther S, Lenz O (2004). Lassa virus. *Crit Rev Clin Lab Sci*, **41**, 339–90.

McCormick JB, *et al.* (1986). Lassa fever. Effective therapy with ribavirin. *N Engl J Med*, **314**, 20–6.

McCormick JB, *et al.* (1987). A case-control study of the clinical diagnosis and course of Lassa fever. *J Infect Dis*, **155**, 445–55.

7.5.18 Filoviruses

J. ter Meulen

Essentials

Filoviruses are large RNA viruses, of which Ebola virus and Marburg virus cause the most severe forms of viral haemorrhagic fever and have been best-studied because of fear of their misuse as bioterrorism agents. These are zoonotic viruses with reservoirs, most likely fruit-eating bats, in the rainforests of tropical Africa, where they cause sporadic infections and outbreaks among great apes and humans.

Epidemiology—the primary mode of transmission of Ebola virus to humans often involves contact of hunters with dead animals, especially chimpanzees, whose meat is consumed as 'bush meat'; contact with bats has been implicated for Marburg virus. However, the viruses are highly infectious and are transmitted from the index case and subsequently from person to person by all body fluids, including sweat and respiratory droplets.

Clinical features—Ebola haemorrhagic fever is clinically indistinguishable from Marburg haemorrhagic fever. Presentation is with an influenza-like illness, often with gastrointestinal symptoms, followed by development of a maculopapular rash and haemorrhagic manifestations including epistaxis, gum bleeding, haematemesis, melaena, petechiae, and ecchymoses. There is no specific treatment, although recombinant activated protein C (Drotrecogin α) and the investigational anticoagulant rNAPc2 have reduced mortality by 20 to 30% in animal models. Mortality is 50 to 90%.

Diagnosis and prevention—viral haemorrhagic fever is a clinical diagnosis which requires the immediate instalment of the strictest barrier nursing procedures and notification of public health authorities. Care must be taken in both drawing and handling blood specimens, which must be inactivated before performing routine laboratory tests, and samples must be shipped immediately to a reference laboratory for diagnosis by detection of virus by cell culture, viral antigen by ELISA, and viral RNA by PCR. A prophylactic vaccine based on a replication-deficient adenoviral vector is in clinical development.

Introduction

Filoviruses are large, enveloped, negative-stranded, nonsegmented RNA viruses with a characteristic thread-like morphology, hence the family name *Filoviridae* (Latin *filum* = thread). Ebola viruses (EBOV), comprising three genetically distinct species from Côte d'Ivoire, the Democratic Republic of the Congo (DRC, formerly Zaire), and Sudan, and Marburg virus (MARV), cause the most severe forms of viral haemorrhagic fever (VHF). They are now among the best-studied agents of these diseases, mainly because of fear of their misuse as bioterrorism agents (Chapter 9.5.13). The first appearance of these viruses was in Marburg in 1967, when laboratory, medical, and animal care personnel exposed to tissues and blood from African Green monkeys (*Cercopithecus aethiops*) were infected. In 1976 and 1979, epidemics of a haemorrhagic disease with very high mortality in northern DRC (then Zaire) and in southern Sudan were found to be due to two strains of a related filoviruses, named Ebola virus. Over the next 10 years, rare, sporadic cases of filovirus infections in Africa were the only continuing evidence of the existence of these viruses. Another species of the virus, Ebola virus Reston (EBOv-R), was imported on four occasions between 1989 and 1996 with wild-caught monkeys (*Macaca fascicularis*) from Mindanao, Republic of the Philippines, to animal facilities in the United States of America and Italy. This virus, which is highly lethal for monkeys, has caused asymptomatic infections in animal keepers. Since 1990, both Ebola and Marburg viruses have re-emerged across tropical Africa between latitudes 5° north and 5° south, causing several devastating epidemics.

In total, 18 instances of human Ebola haemorrhagic fever (EHF) have been recorded in Côte d'Ivoire, in the DRC, Gabon, Sudan, and northern Uganda. The outbreaks varied in size from 17 to 425 cases totalling 1880 cases, of which 1302 were fatal. The largest outbreak of Ebola virus disease so far (caused by EBOV Sudan) occurred in 2000 in Gulu, Uganda. There were 425 cases with a case fatality of 53%. Until 2007, Marburg virus cases totalled 567 with 467 fatalities. Outbreaks varied in size from 3 to 374, the largest in Uige, Angola where MARV appeared for the first time in 2005.

Aetiology, genetics, pathogenesis, and pathology

Filovirus infections are characterized by massive, unchecked, and destructive replication of virus in several organs, profound immunosuppression due to infection of immune cells and apoptosis of infected and noninfected cells, and triggering of a cascade of immune-mediated mechanisms resulting in a cytokine storm, endothelial damage, and coagulopathy culminating in shock and organ failure. The immunological and pathological aspects in end-stage filoviral disease resemble, in several aspects, those of bacterial sepsis.

Through minute lesions in the skin and mucosa, the pantropic filoviruses infect initially dendritic cells, monocytes, and macrophages. Lymphocytes are spared from the infection. EBOV and MARV infected dendritic cells fail to mature to the antigen-presenting stage and do not produce proinflammatory cytokines required for activation of natural killer cells and T cells. At the molecular level, the expression of viral proteins interferes with the production of interferon-α (IFN-α) and β, and with the ability of these and IFN-γ to induce an antiviral state in cells. Dendritic cells show no increase in costimulatory molecules such as CD40, CD86, and interleukin 12 (IL-12). The early immune response dysfunction originating in dendritic cells is aggravated by continued replication of filoviruses in monocytes and macrophages, accompanied by the secretion of noninhibited proinflammatory cytokines and activation of polymorphonuclear leucocytes. This accumulated release of proinflammatory mediators culminates in a 'cytokine storm', causing thrombocytopenia and endothelial injury, e.g. through the action of tumor necrosis factor-α (TNFα). Fatal human Ebola cases showed a marked elevation of serum levels of IFN-γ, IL-2, and IL-10, whereas elevated IFN-α, TNFα, and IL-6 were associated with fatalities in some, but not all, studies. Increased blood levels of nitric oxide, which has been shown to contribute to hypotension, cardiodepression, and vascular hyporeactivity in sepsis, were also found to be associated with mortality. The likely reason for the variations of cytokine and chemokine release observed *in vivo*, as well as in experimentally infected primary human cells, is currently unknown genetic differences of the host. Both humans and experimentally infected nonhuman primates show massive apoptotic death of noninfected CD4+, CD8+, and NK cells in the blood and peripheral lymph nodes, a phenomenon which has been termed 'bystander apoptosis', that appears to play a pivotal role in pathogenesis. In addition, there appears to be also massive apoptotic death of infected macrophages.

The expression of tissue factor is up-regulated in infected monocytes and triggers the extrinsic pathway of coagulation. The procoagulant state amplifies the production of proinflammatory cytokines and the development of vascular leakage, which further provokes activation of coagulopathy. The terminal stage of the disease is therefore characterized by plasma leakage, disseminated intravascular coagulopathy, and bleeding. It is thought that triggering the above outlined cascade of events is more critical to the development of the observed pathology than direct organ damage due to cytopathic virus replication. However, infection of the liver and adrenal glands impairs the synthesis of clotting factors and steroids, thus aggravating hemorrhage and shock. Whether infection of endothelial cells contributes to the overall pathology remains controversial.

At autopsy, both Marburg and Ebola infected humans and primates show widespread haemorrhagic diathesis of skin, membranes, and soft tissue. Extensive necrosis with little infiltration is seen in parenchymal cells of many organs, including liver, spleen, kidneys, and gonads. The most characteristic histopathological features are seen in the liver. Large disseminated deposits of viral antigen can be found in different organs, including the sweat glands and the skin. Virus is also detectable in pneumocytes and as cell-free virions in the alveoli.

Spleen and lymph nodes show various degrees of lymphoid depletion with extensive vascular follicular necrosis. Fatal infection is marked by absence of specific IgG and presence of low levels of specific IgM in only 30% of cases, whereas in human survivors early and increasing levels of Ebola-specific IgM and IgG is followed by activation of cytotoxic T cells. During two outbreaks in Gabon, asymptomatic seroconversion with PCR-proven infection occurred in several people who mounted an early, strong inflammatory response, with high levels of proinflammatory cytokines. This unexpected observation suggests that the early inflammatory response is able, on occasions, to control viral replication and disease.

The recent successful immunization against EHF in animal models revealed that protection is clearly mediated by cellular immunity, because CD8+ T-cell depletion abrogated vaccine protection in nonhuman primates. Neutralizing antibodies are found neither in natural infection nor after immunization. However, antibodies may contribute to protection by non-neutralizing mechanisms.

Epidemiology

Central African nonhuman primates and monkeys are victims of EBOV, as are other animals such as bushpigs, porcupines, and antelopes living in the tropical rainforest. Data from wildlife surveillance show that epizootics occur more often than previously thought and that EBOV has caused massive die-offs of gorillas and chimpanzees. Phylogenetic analysis of the viruses further suggests that the outbreaks are epidemiologically linked and that EBOV, strain Zaire (EBOV-Z), has spread south-westward since 1976 in a wave-like manner from Yambuku, its site of appearance in the DRC, to the Republic of the Congo and to Gabon at a speed of approximately 50 km per year. This argues against the hypothesis that EBOV-Z was resident, but undetected, in the central African forest block before the mid 1970s. Evidence has now accumulated that fruit-eating bats (*Hypsignathus monstrosus, Epomops franqueti, Myonycteris torquata* and others) are one, but possibly not the primary, natural reservoir of EBOV, and hunting of bats for human consumption has been linked to an EBOV outbreak in DRC in 2007. Recently, EBOV Reston was detected in domestic swine in the Philippines and a few asymtomatic human infections were reported. The pathogenicity of the virus for these animals and their possible role in a transmission cycle are currently not known.

The primary mode of transmission of EBOV to humans often involves contact of hunters with dead animals, especially chimpanzees, whose meat is consumed as 'bush meat'. In several outbreaks, however, the mode of infection of the index case could not be elucidated. The index cases usually transmit the virus to caring family members, often women, who come into contact with blood and body fluids. These are highly infectious, so that the average rate of secondary cases generated from the index case is around 10 to 20%, but may be considerably higher. Occasionally, the virus has been spread through sexual contact. Nosocomial spread through improperly sterilized reusable syringes or other medical equipment has caused explosive Ebola epidemics in Sudan and the Democratic Republic of the Congo. The mortality among surgical staff operating on EHF patients misdiagnosed as having acute abdominal conditions was also extremely high. Nursing activities and preparing the corpse for burial carry a high risk of infection, as do burial practices which include touching of the corpse and collectively washing hands in a common bowel thereafter. There is no epidemiological evidence that Ebola or Marburg viruses are transmitted as true, small particle aerosols between humans. However, direct mucosal exposure to droplets generated by a patient during coughing poses a considerable risk of infection.

MARV epidemiology is similar to that of EBOV. Evidence of infection has been detected in fruit-eating bats (*Rousettus aegyptiacus*) from Uganda and Kenya, and in insectivorous bats in DRC (*Miniopterus inflatus, Rhinolophus elocuens*). However, epizootics have not been observed in mammals. Contact with bats during mining activities was reported for several index cases of Marburg haemorrhagic fever (MHF), in accordance with cave roosting of *R. aegyptiacus*, a habit that is not observed in the bat species implicated in EBOV transmission. Until 2000, the viral origins of cases could be traced to eastern Africa. However, in 2005 the largest outbreak of MHF occurred in Uige, Angola, expanding the known range of the disease to the far western edge of the Congo basin. Continuing population movements in central Africa, destruction of the rainforest, and increased consumption of 'bush meat' increase the likelihood of future filovirus outbreaks. In 2008 a fatal and a nonfatal case of Marburg haemorrhagic fever occurred in the Netherlands and the United States of America, respectively, imported by tourists who had visited a bat-roosting cave in Uganda (Python cave, Queen Elisabeth park). Touching bat excrements or being hit by low flying bats were identified as possible risk factors for acquisition of the infection.

Prevention

In endemic areas, avoidance of contact with bats and their excrements, with dead and diseased monkeys, and control of monkey sellers are currently the only feasible options for prevention. In case of outbreaks, interruption of person-to-person spread of the virus is essential for control. Early institution of safe and orderly care of the ill, using barrier nursing and disinfection procedures, should be set up with effective surveillance of high-risk contacts and prompt isolation of further cases (barrier nursing, guidelines from the CDC and WHO, see Chapter 7.5.17, Box 7.5.17.1). In fully equipped hospitals, patients must be placed in negative-pressure rooms and all personnel must wear protective gear with P3 filters for respiratory protection. Cutaneous or mucosal contact with blood or body fluids from an Ebola patient poses a high risk. Contacts must be followed up for development of persistent high fever for 3 weeks from the last date of contact by daily temperature measurement.

Development of vaccines against filoviruses has recently made astonishing progress, after decades of futile efforts. The first effective vaccine protocol against EBOV in nonhuman primates was based on a prime/boost regimen, expressing the viral nucleoprotein (NP) and glycoprotein (GP) from a plasmid (DNA immunization) and a recombinant, replication-deficient adenovirus, serotype 5 (Ad5). This vector has the advantage of having been tested extensively in humans and found to be safe. Subsequently, a protocol was developed in which a single shot of Ad5-GP given 4 weeks before challenge with 1000 infectious EBOV particles conferred 100% protection in nonhuman primates. This vaccine is currently in clinical trials performed by the National Institutes of Health, United States of America, and may be licensable within a few years. However, Ad5 vectors have the drawback of facing a high level of pre-existing neutralizing antibodies in the general population, which may impede the induction of anti-EBOV immunity. Prime/boost schemes will be required to overcome this problem. The latest amazing finding was that replication-competent vesicular stomatitis virus expressing the EBOV-GP could protect 50% of nonhuman primates when given 30 min after a lethal challenge, making it an ideal postexposure vaccine for health care workers. However, clinical development of this viral vector system faces higher regulatory hurdles, because it has so far not been evaluated in humans. Recently, an experimental preparation of the vaccine was given as a postexposure prophylaxis to a German researcher after a possibly EBOV contaminated needle-stick injury. No severe systemic side effects of the vaccination were reported.

Protection against MARV infection in animal models has been much easier to achieve using a variety of vaccines, including recombinant proteins, than against EBOV. This is probably due to the slightly slower replication of the virus in these models. A vaccine is likely to enter clinical trials soon.

Fig. 7.5.18.1 Rash of Ebola haemorrhagic fever acquired through a laboratory accident.
(Courtesy of Professor D I H Simpson.)

Clinical features

MARV and EBOV cause identical clinical diseases. After an incubation period of 5 to 12 days, the disease starts suddenly with fever, headache, myalgia, and extreme fatigue. Early signs also include conjunctivitis, bradycardia, and sore throat, often associated with severe swelling and dysphagia, but no exudative pharyngitis. Severe nausea, vomiting, abdominal pain, and profuse watery diarrhoea are common. Around the fifth day, a perifollicular, nonitching, maculopapular rash frequently appears on the trunk, back, and shoulders, spreading to the face and limbs and becoming confluent (Fig. 7.5.18.1). It may be difficult to see and has a measles-like appearance on dark skin. The rash fades in 3 to 10 days and is followed by a desquamation in survivors. In about half of the patients, haemorrhagic manifestations occur between the 5th and 7th day, including epistaxis, gum-bleeding, haematemesis (Fig. 7.5.18.2), melaena, petechiae, ecchymoses (Fig. 7.5.18.3), haemorrhages from needlesticks and post-mortem evidence of visceral haemorrhagic effusions. Dehydration and prostration are frequent; patients show the ghost-like facial expression typical of the disease. During the first week, the temperature remains high around 40°C, falling by lysis during the second week, to rise again between days 12 and 14. Other clinical signs during the second week include hepatosplenomegaly, oedema, orchitis, scrotal or labial reddening, myocarditis, and pancreatitis. Jaundice is not a feature. A poor prognosis is marked by haemorrhagic signs, oliguria or anuria, chest pain, shock, tachypnoea, and neurological symptoms (sudden hearing loss, blindness, painful paresthesia, intractable hiccups). Death in shock usually occurs 6 to 9 days after onset of clinical disease. Infection in pregnancy results in high maternal mortality and virtually 100% fetal death. Central nervous system involvement has led to hemiplegia and disorientation, and sometimes frank psychosis.

The recovery of Marburg and Ebola disease is prolonged with arthralgia or persistent arthritis, ocular disease (ocular pain, photophobia, hyperlacrimation, loss of visual acuity, uveitis), hearing loss and orchitis occurring as late manifestations. Serious but reversible personality changes have been recorded in a few survivors, namely confusion, anxiety, and aggressive behaviour. Blindness has been reported as a sequel.

Marburg virus has been isolated from the anterior chamber of the eye and from seminal fluid 7 weeks after the onset of clinical disease and there has been a documented case of sexual transmission. The shedding of EBOV RNA has been detectable in semen and vaginal fluid by polymerase chain reaction (PCR) for months, but not by virus isolation. Patients should therefore refrain from sexual activities during early reconvalescence.

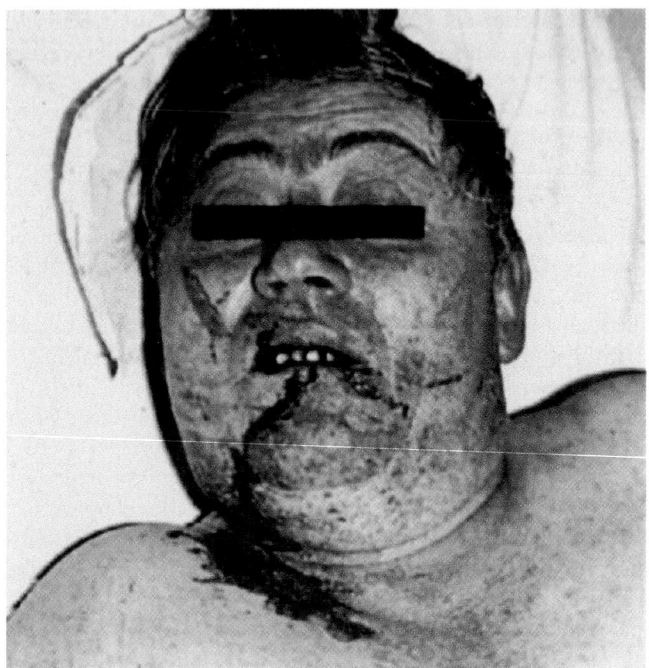

Fig. 7.5.18.2 Hemorrhage and oedema of face and neck in Marburg haemorrhagic fever.
(Courtesy: Professor S Stille.)

Haematological studies reveal early leucopenia, thrombocytopenia accompanied by abnormal platelet aggregation, subsequent relative neutrophilia, and the appearance of atypical lymphocytes. Liver enzymes are elevated (AST/SGOT >ALT/SGPT) consistent with histopathological evidence of hepatitis (Fig. 7.5.18.4), but alkaline phosphatase and bilirubin levels are usually normal or only slightly elevated. Although disseminated intravascular coagulation (DIC) is a prominent manifestation of EBOV infection in primates (prolonged prothrombin (PT) and partial thromboplastin time (PTT), D-dimers, fibrin split products), the presence of DIC in

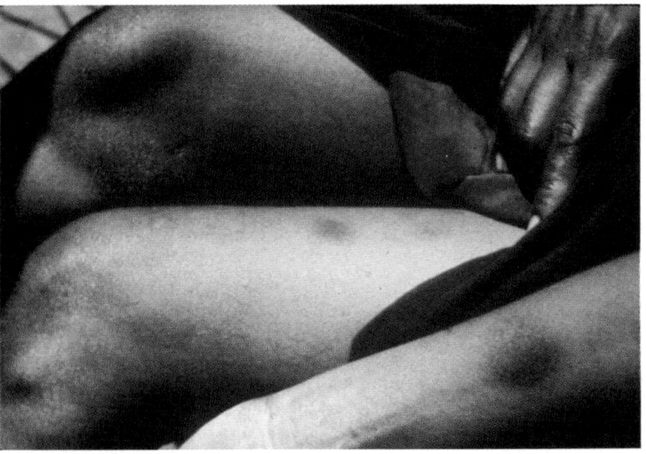

Fig. 7.5.18.3 Ecchymoses in a patient with Ebola haemorrhagic fever.
(Courtesy of Professor D I H Simpson.)

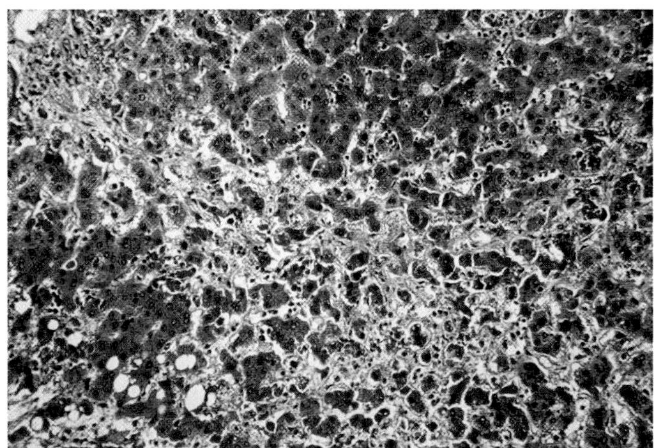

Fig. 7.5.18.4 Hepatic histology in Ebola haemorrhagic fever. (Courtesy of Professor D I H Simpson.)

human filoviral infections has been a controversial topic, because logistical problems have hampered systematic studies in the past. However, fibrin deposition has been documented at autopsy, and clinical laboratory data suggest that DIC is likely to be also a prominent feature of human disease. In nonhuman primates, a rapid decline in plasma protein C levels was observed in EBOV infection, preceding clinical symptoms.

Differential diagnosis and criteria for diagnosis

Clinically, filovirus infections can be confused with nonviral infections such as severe malaria, typhoid fever, shigellosis ('diarrhée rouge' in francophone Africa), leptospirosis, rickettsial diseases, meningococcaemia, Gram-negative sepsis, and other conditions resulting in DIC. There is overlap of clinical presentation with other VHFs. Filovirus HF should be suspected in a patient living in or coming from, within the incubation period, a known endemic area (currently Angola, Côte d'Ivoire, the DRC, Gabon, Sudan, Kenya, and Uganda) and presenting with otherwise unexplained high fever (above 38.5°C) and vascular involvement (subnormal blood pressure, postural hypotension, petechiae, haemorrhagic diathesis, flushing of face and chest, nondependent oedema). Reported contact with another VHF patient or a known VHF vector is obviously a very important risk factor.

Because VHF is a purely clinical diagnosis which requires the immediate instalment of barrier nursing procedures and notification of public health authorities, rapid laboratory confirmation is mandatory. Care must be taken in both drawing and handling blood specimens since virus titre may be extremely high, and the virus is stable for long periods, even at room temperature. During the first week of clinical illness, virus is easily detected by cell culture, viral antigen by enzyme-linked immunoabsorbent assay (ELISA), and viral RNA by PCR, but all methods require specialized equipment. Blood samples have to be handled and shipped to a reference laboratory using special precautions (triple packaging: primary, secondary, and outer container with absorbent material in between) and have to be inactivated for performing routine laboratory tests (Chapter 7.5.17, Table 7.5.17.1). If the patient dies in the second week, antiviral antibodies remain undetectable or very low in the majority of cases. Otherwise the appearance of IgM and IgG antibodies can be detected by ELISA or immunofluorescence, preferably in paired serum samples. A diagnostic test has been developed based on immunohistochemical detection of abundant filovirus antigen in biopsies. Skin snips taken from the axilla or nape of the neck are fixed with formalin and can be shipped without further safety requirements to reference laboratories.

For handling of clinical specimens from suspected cases, see Chapter 7.5.17, Table 7.5.17.1.

Treatment

Conceptually, therapy of EHF and MHF consists of specific antiviral approaches, modulation of the host immune response, and symptomatic treatment. Currently, no specific antiviral therapy is available. The guanosin analogue ribavirin is not effective against filoviruses. Prophylactic treatment of EBOV infection in nonhuman primates with high doses of either polyclonal immune serum, a potent neutralizing human monoclonal antibody (50 mg/kg), or IFN-α2b (2×10^7 IU/kg per day) delayed time to death but did not reduce mortality. In contrast, modulation of the coagulation/inflammation cascade showed some promising results. Treatment with recombinant human activated protein C (continuous perfusion of 48 µg/kg per h drotrecogin-α, on days 0–7) resulted in 18.2% survival and a prolonged time-to-death. Similarly, treatment of nonhuman primates with the recombinant nematode anticoagulant protein c2 (rNAPc2), a potent inhibitor of FVIIa/tissue factor-initiated blood coagulation, by subcutaneous injections of 30 µg/kg bodyweight, administered once daily for up to 14 days after a high-dose lethal injection of Ebola virus, resulted in a 33% survival rate and prolonged survival time. The molecule is being developed as an anticoagulant by ARCA Biopharma, Colorado, United States of America.

Fluid, electrolyte, respiratory, and osmotic imbalances should be managed carefully. Patients may require full intensive care support, including mechanical ventilation, along with blood, plasma, or platelet replacement. The maintenance of intravascular volume is a particular challenge, but every effort is justified since the crisis is short lived, and complete recovery can be expected in survivors. Treatment of all concurrent (tropical) infections is important.

Management of an imported EHF or MHF case will therefore require, to a certain degree, experimental therapy, such as the use of investigational drugs for modulation of immune responses and coagulation cascades, which are being evaluated in bacterial sepsis.

Prognosis

The case fatality of filovirus infections is extremely high and possibly dependent on the infecting species, with up to 90% for EBOV Zaire and MARV Angola. Because the lesions in filovirus infections are so widespread and the immune response is so ineffective, it is uncertain whether good supportive care alone has a major effect on the clinical outcome. Despite good clinical care being delivered to the majority of patients during the Ebola outbreak in Uganda in 2000, the overall mortality was not significantly lower than the 50% which would be expected for the Sudan strain of Ebola, which caused the epidemic. Common denominators of survival in filovirus-infected macaques are maintenance of D-dimer levels, maintenance of protein C activity (>50%), maintenance of levels of proinflammatory/procoagulant cytokines, and low viral load.

Areas of uncertainty/controversy

Despite concerted international actions, it has so far neither been possible to implement true standard of care patient treatment during filovirus outbreaks in Africa nor to conduct clinical trials. Therefore, most of the knowledge of the pathogenesis of these diseases and the few available therapeutic data come from experimental infection of nonhuman primates and uncontrolled clinical studies.

Likely developments over next 5 to 10 years

The licensing of a recombinant, adenovirus-based EBOV and possibly MARV vaccine is to be expected in the United States of America within 5 years. Combined therapies using antiviral drugs, immune modulators, and anticoagulants will most likely improve survival rates in nonhuman primate models beyond the currently reported 20 to 30%.

Further reading

Feldmann H, *et al.* (2007). Effective post-exposure treatment of Ebola infection. *PLoS Pathog*, **3**, e2.

Geisbert TW, *et al.* (2003). Treatment of Ebola virus infection with a recombinant inhibitor of factor VIIa/tissue factor: a study in rhesus monkeys. *Lancet*, **362**, 1953–8.

Hensley LE, *et al.* (2007). Recombinant Human Activated Protein C for the Postexposure Treatment of Ebola Hemorrhagic Fever. *J Infect Dis*, **196** Suppl 2, S390–9.

Marty AM, Jahrling PB, Geisbert TW. (2006). Viral hemorrhagic fevers. *Clin Lab Med*, **26**, 345–86.

Mohamadzadeh M, Chen L, Schmaljohn AL. (2007). How Ebola and Marburg viruses battle the immune system. *Nat Rev Immunol*, **7**, 556–67.

Rollin PE, Bausch DG, Sanchez A. (2007). Blood chemistry measurements and D-Dimer levels associated with fatal and nonfatal outcomes in humans infected with Sudan Ebola virus. *J Infect Dis*, **196** Suppl 2, S364–71.

World Health Organization. *Infection control for viral haemorrhagic fevers in the African health care setting* (WHO/EMC/ESR/98.2.). http://www.who.int/csr/resources/publications/ebola/WHO_EMC_ESR_98_2_EN/en/

Zaki SR, *et al.* (1999). A novel immunohistochemical assay for the detection of Ebola virus in skin: implications for diagnosis, spread, and surveillance of Ebola hemorrhagic fever. *J Infect Dis*, **179** Suppl 1, S36–47.

7.5.19 Papillomaviruses and polyomaviruses

Raphael P. Viscidi and Keerti V. Shah

Essentials

Papillomaviruses and polyomaviruses are small, nonenveloped, double-stranded DNA viruses.

Human papillomavirus

There are over 100 human papillomavirus (HPV) types that infect epithelia of skin and mucous membranes. They infect only humans, and cause conditions including the following:

Skin warts and verrucas—caused by types 1 and 2; infection initiated when, after e.g. minor skin abrasions, the basal cells of the epithelium come in contact with infectious virus.

Anogenital warts—caused by types 6 and 11; transmitted by direct sexual contact, these are the most common sexually transmitted infection; present clinically as multiple exophytic lesions or as subclinical flat lesions. Can be treated topically with podophyllin or imiquimod, or by ablative surgical methods. Recurrences are common. A highly efficacious prophylactic vaccine is available.

Cervical cancer—the second most common tumour in women worldwide; most often caused by types 16 and 18, whose DNA can be recovered from nearly all cases of invasive disease and squamous intraepithelial lesions of the cervix, which precede invasive cancer. Prevention is by cervical screening and vaccination (two highly effective vaccines are available).

Other cancers—HPVs can cause cancers at other lower anogenital tract sites and in the oropharynx. HPV DNA is often detected in nonmelanoma skin cancers, but it is not known whether this is pathogenic.

Respiratory papillomatosis—caused by types 6 and 11; usually involves the vocal cords, leading to presentation with hoarseness or voice change; may rarely cause life-threatening airway obstruction; mainstay of treatment is surgical removal of papillomas, which commonly recur.

Human polyomaviruses

Exposure to polyomaviruses is nearly universal: they cause asymptomatic infection in childhood and then persist as latent infections, primarily in the kidney, producing disease in the context of immunosuppression.

BK virus—can cause (1) nephropathy and renal failure in renal transplant patients; management is by gradual reduction in immunosuppression, but more than 50% of patients lose their allograft; (2) haemorrhagic cystitis in bone marrow transplant patients.

JC virus—causes progressive multifocal leucoencephalopathy, a demyelinating disease of the central nervous system that is usually relentlessly progressive and fatal. Most often seen in patients with HIV/AIDS, but recently reported as a rare complication of treatment with natalizumab in patients with multiple sclerosis or Crohn's disease.

Introduction

Papillomaviruses and polyomaviruses are small, spherical, nonenveloped, doubled-stranded DNA viruses that multiply in the nucleus. The two virus groups are unrelated. Papillomaviruses infect surface epithelia and produce disease at these sites. Polyomaviruses are carried by viraemia, after initial multiplication at the site of entry, to affect internal organs such as the kidney and the brain. Viruses of both families produce experimental tumours in laboratory animals, but only papillomaviruses are related to naturally occurring cancers. Within each family the viruses are immunologically related and share nucleotide similarity.

More than 120 human papillomaviruses have been recognized, about 35 of which infect mucous membranes (genital and respiratory tracts, and the oral cavity) and the remainder infect skin. Human papillomaviruses cause skin warts, genital warts, respiratory papillomas, and papillomas at other mucosal sites (e.g. mouth, eye). In addition, infection with some genital tract human papillomaviruses causes cervical cancer, one of the most common

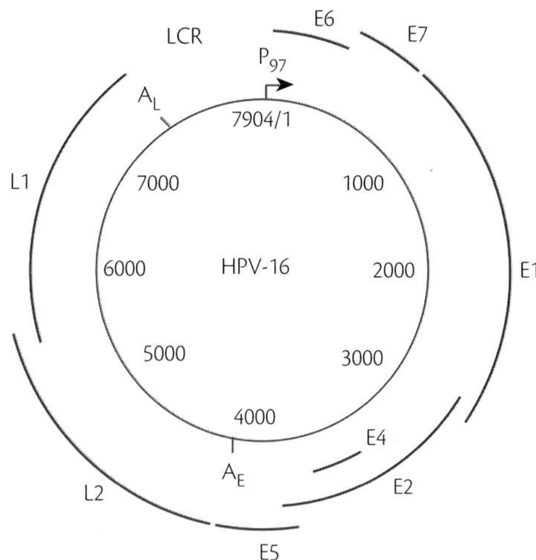

Fig. 7.5.19.1 Genomic map of HPV-16. On the inner circle, P97 represents the transcriptional promoter and A_E and A_L designate early and late polyadenylation sites. The location of the early region open reading frames (E1–E8), the late region open reading frames (L1, L2), and of the long control or regulatory region (LCR) are shown.

(Reproduced from Shah KV, Howley PM (1996). Papillomaviruses. In: Fields BN, *et al.* (eds) *Fields Virology*, vol. 2, pp. 2077–109. Lippincott-Raven, Philadelphia., with permission.)

female malignancies in the world, as well as a proportion of cancers at other genital tract sites and the oropharynx.

Two polyomaviruses, BK virus and JC virus, infect humans. JC virus is the aetiological agent of progressive multifocal leukoencephalopathy, a fatal demyelinating disease occurring in immunodeficient people. BK virus is associated with haemorrhagic cystitis in bone marrow transplant recipients, and with nephropathy and renal failure in renal transplant recipients.

Human papillomaviruses (HPVs)

Human papillomaviruses cannot be propagated in tissue culture and require nucleic acid hybridization assays for their identification. Their double-stranded circular genome contains about 8000 bp, divided into an early region, necessary for transformation, a late region, encoding for capsid proteins, and a regulatory region, containing control elements (Fig. 7.5.19.1). Open reading frames of the viral genome are located on one strand: E1 to E8 in the early region and L1 and L2 in the late region. The functions assigned to the different open reading frames are listed in Table 7.5.19.1.

Table 7.5.19.1 Functions of human papillomavirus open reading frames

Function	ORF
Replication of viral DNA	E1, E2
Regulation of transcription	E2
Coding for late cytoplasmic protein	E4
Cellular proliferation	E5[a]
Transformation	E6, E7
Not known	E3, E8

Abbreviations: ORF, open reading frame.

[a] In bovine papillomavirus, the major transforming activity is in E5.

(Modified from Shah KV, Howley PM (1996). Papillomaviruses. In: Fields BN, *et al.* (eds) *Fields Virology*, vol. 2, pp. 2077–109. Lippincott-Raven, Philadelphia.)

Table 7.5.19.2 Mucosal human papillomaviruses: chief clinical associations

Clinical association	Viral type(s)
Exophytic condyloma; respiratory papillomas; oral and conjunctival papillomas	HPV-6, -11
Cervical cancer:	
High-risk infections	HPV-16, -18, -31, -45, -33, -35, -39, -51, -52, -56, -58, -59
Low-risk infections	HPV-6, -11, -40, -42, -43, -44, -54, -61, -70, -72, -81
Vulval, vaginal, penile, anal, and oropharyngeal cancers	HPV-16
Focal epithelial hyperplasia of the oral cavity	HPV-13, -32

(Modified from Shah KV, Howley PM (1996). Papillomaviruses. In: Fields BN, *et al.* (eds) *Fields Virology*, vol. 2, pp. 2077–109. Lippincott-Raven, Philadelphia. Includes material from *The Oxford textbook of medicine*, 3rd edition, pp. 3366–9.)

Human papillomaviruses infect only humans. They show a marked degree of cellular tropism. Mucosal human papillomaviruses do not readily infect cutaneous epithelia and cutaneous human papillomaviruses are rarely present on mucous membranes. Infection is initiated when, after minor trauma (e.g. during sexual intercourse or after minor skin abrasions), the basal cells of the epithelium come in contact with infectious virus. The virus stimulates the proliferation of basal cells. The early region open reading frames are expressed in all layers of the infected epithelium, but expression of the late region open reading frames and synthesis of viral particles occur only in the upper differentiating and keratinizing layers.

Important disease associations and characteristics of mucosal HPVs are listed in Table 7.5.19.2. The burden of human cancers attributable to HPVs is shown in Table 7.5.19.3. The genital tract is the reservoir for all but a few mucosal human papillomaviruses and genital human papillomavirus infections constitute the most common viral sexually transmitted infections. Genital human papillomaviruses may sometimes infect nonanogenital mucosal sites, e.g. the respiratory tract, the mouth, and the conjunctiva. Transmission of genital tract HPV types 6 and 11 from an infected mother to the baby at birth results in juvenile onset recurrent respiratory papillomatosis. Infection with two types, HPV-13 and HPV-32, appears to be confined to the oral cavity.

Table 7.5.19.4 lists disease associations of cutaneous HPVs, which are transmitted by direct contact with infected tissue or by contact with a contaminated object.

Table 7.5.19.3 Cancers attributable to HPV infection in 2002

Site	Attributable to HPV (%)	Total cancers	Attributable to HPV	% of all cancers
Cervix	100	492 800	492 800	4.54
Penis	40	26 300	10 500	0.10
Vulva, vagina	40	40 000	16 000	0.15
Anus	90	30 400	27 300	0.25
Oropharynx	12	52 100	6200	0.06
All sites	~5	10 862 500	552 800	5.1

(Modified from Parkin DM and Bray F (2006). The burden of HPV-related cancers. *Vaccine* **24**, Suppl 3, S11–S25).

Table 7.5.19.4 Cutaneous human papillomaviruses: chief clinical associations

Clinical association	Viral type
Deep plantar wart	HPV-1
Common wart	HPV-2, -4
Mosaic wart (superficial spreading wart)	HPV-2
Flat warts	HPV-3, -10, -28, -41
Macular plaques of epidermodysplasia verruciformis	HPV-5, -8, -9, -12, -14, -15, -17, -19, -20, -21, -22, -23, -24, -25, -36, -47, -50
Squamous cell carcinoma	HPV-5,-8, -20, -36, -38

Modified from Shah KV, Howley PM (1996). Papillomaviruses. In: Fields BN, *et al.* (eds) *Fields Virology*, vol. 2, pp. 2077–2109. Lippincott-Raven, Philadelphia.)

Anogenital warts

Anogenital warts (condylomas) are the most commonly recognized clinical manifestations of genital HPV infections. More than 90% of condylomas result from infections with HPV-6 and HPV-11. In the United States of America, there are more than a million annual consultations for anogenital warts.

Epidemiology

Genital and anal warts are most common between the ages of 16 and 24 years. They are transmitted by direct sexual contact. Anogenital warts in children can also be due to close but nonsexual contact within a family but, in many cases, sexual abuse by an infected adult is responsible.

Clinical features

The incubation period is between 3 weeks and 8 months (mean=2.8 months). In men, condylomata acuminata (exophytic condylomas) most often appear on areas exposed to coital trauma, the glans penis, coronal sulcus, prepuce, and terminal urethra. The soft fleshy vascular tumours are usually multiple and may coalesce into large masses (Fig. 7.5.19.2). Sessile or papular warts are more likely to occur on dry areas such as the shaft of the penis (Fig. 7.5.19.3). The raised pink or grey lesions, 0.5 to 3 mm in diameter, may occur alone or with exophytic condylomas. Subclinical HPV lesions (flat condylomas) are identified by examining the genitalia with magnification after the application of 5% aqueous acetic acid solution. The affected areas are slightly raised and shiny white (acetowhite), with a rough surface. Flat condylomas affect the same areas as exophytic condylomas.

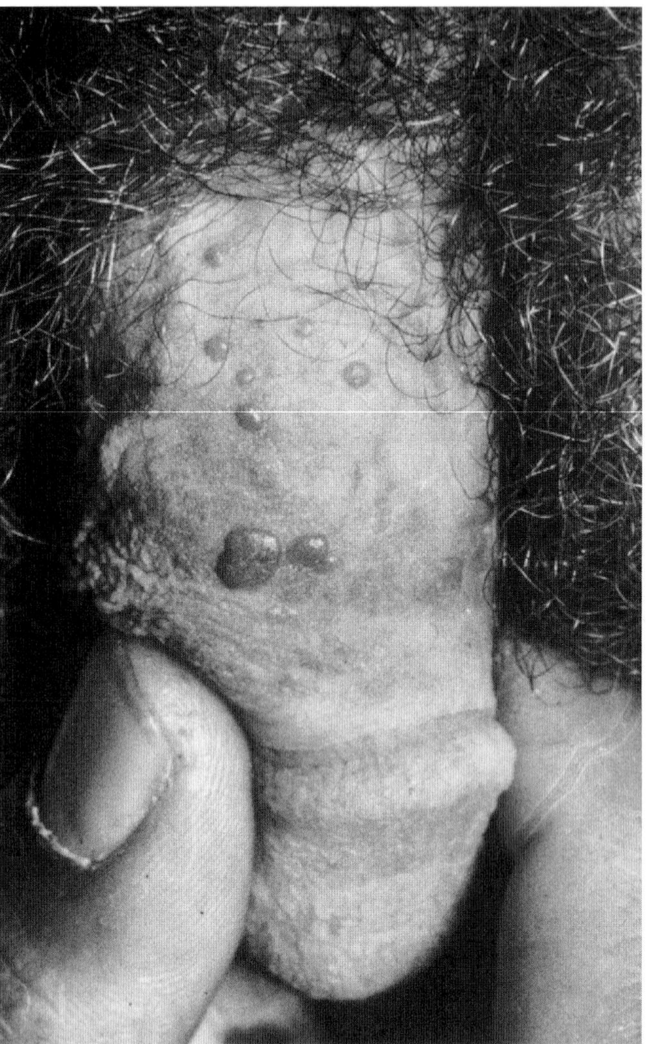

Fig. 7.5.19.3 Sessile (papular) warts of the penis.

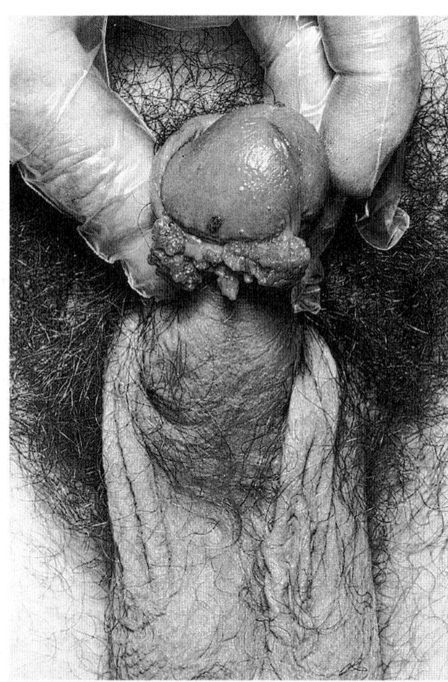

Fig. 7.5.19.2 Condylomata acuminata (exophytic condylomas) of the penis.

Perianal warts are usually exophytic and in moist conditions around the anus may reach a large size. In 50% of cases, condylomas also appear in the anal canal. Areas of acetowhite epithelium indicative of subclinical HPV infection may be associated with perianal warts or occur alone.

In women, exophytic condylomas (Fig. 7.5.19.4) appear at the fourchette and adjacent areas, and may spread to the rest of the vulva, the perineum, anus, vagina, and cervix. Multiple sessile warts may affect the labia and perineum. Subclinical HPV infection presents as slightly raised acetowhite lesions: the fissuring of these may cause dyspareunia. About 15% of women with vulval

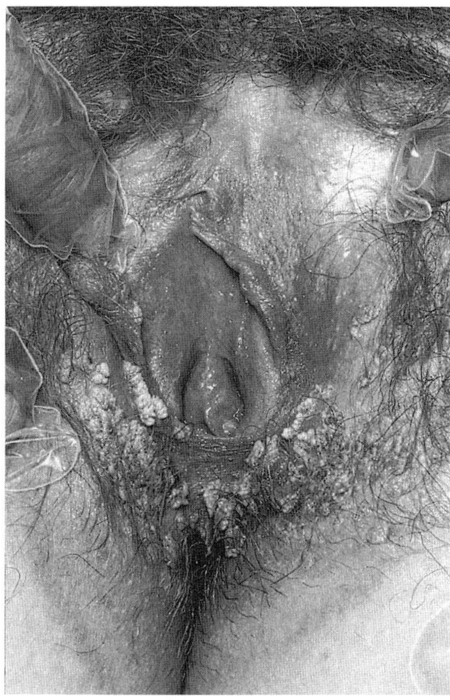

Fig. 7.5.19.4 Condylomata acuminata of the vulva.

warts have exophytic condylomas on the cervix. Subclinical infection is more common, and consists of acetowhite lesions with punctation due to capillary loops, which can be identified by colposcopy. Large, exophytic vulval condylomas may develop during pregnancy and may become so large that they compromise delivery. Most regress post-partum.

Even with therapy (see below), recurrence of genital warts occurs within 3 months in 25 to 67% of cases. Recurrences are often at sites of previous genital warts and are attributed to persistent infection that then reactivates.

Diagnosis and management

Genital warts must be distinguished from Fordyce's spots, fibroepithelial polyps, molluscum contagiosum, and the papillar lesions of secondary syphilis. Lesions that appear atypical or respond poorly to treatment must be biopsied early.

Associated sexually transmitted diseases must be excluded. Sexual partners should be examined. Intraepithelial neoplasia must be excluded. Cervical cytological examination should always be done on women with vulval warts and on female partners of men with penile warts.

Treatments for genital warts can be classified as topical, immunomodulatory, or surgical. Podophyllin and podophyllotoxin, which are derived from the root of the mayapple plant, are antimitotic agents that disrupt viral activity by inducing local tissue necrosis. Patient-applied topical podophyllotoxin, 0.5%, has a clinical cure rate of 56%; however, recurrence rates range from 23 to 65%. Disadvantages of podophyllin compounds include local adverse reactions, risk of systemic absorption, and teratogenicity. Imiquimod, a topical treatment for genital warts, induces macrophages to secrete cytokines, principally interferon-α, and is thought to work by stimulation of a cell-mediated immune response against HPV. Imiquimod is as effective as podophyllin for initial clearance of genital warts and results in a lower recurrence rate. The side effect profile of imiquimod is benign. Warts may be destroyed by cryotherapy with liquid nitrogen, electrocautery, electrodessication, scissor excision, or carbon dioxide laser therapy. Although these ablative therapies are successful in initially removing genital warts, recurrences are common. In a comparative trial, imiquimod 5% cream alone or in combination with ablative treatments was superior to ablation alone in reducing the recurrence rate of successfully treated anogenital warts. A prophylactic vaccine that prevents 100% of genital warts due to HPV-6 and HPV-11, if administered prior to exposure to HPV, is now commercially available in many countries (see below).

Respiratory papillomatosis

This rare disease may have onset in childhood or in adult life. It is most common in children under the age of 5 years. It may become life-threatening if it obstructs the airways. Papillomatosis usually involves the vocal cords and the patient presents with hoarseness or voice change. Papillomas may recur after surgical removal.

HPV-6 and HPV-11, genital tract HPVs that are responsible for most of the exophytic genital warts, also cause respiratory papillomatosis. Patients with juvenile-onset disease are infected at birth during passage through an infected birth canal. In adult-onset disease, transmission may occur by sexual contact. Respiratory papillomas rarely progress to invasive cancer. Irradiation of papillomas with X-rays (a practice now discontinued) increases the risk of malignancy.

Caesarean delivery for mothers who are found to have genital warts or are infected with HPV-6 or HPV-11 would reduce the risk of juvenile-onset respiratory papillomatosis, but it is not generally recommended because of the small risk of disease following perinatal infection. The mainstay of treatment is surgical removal of papillomas; however, recurrence of lesions is common. Various adjunct therapies have been tried, including interferon-α, indole-3-carbinol, cidofovir, and photodynamic treatment. These therapies have had only modest success in reducing the need for surgery. It is anticipated that a child born to a mother who has received the HPV Gardasil vaccine, will have a markedly reduced risk of developing respiratory papillomatosis.

Cervical cancer (Chapter 6.1)

Human papillomavirus DNA is recovered from nearly 100% of cases of invasive cervical cancer and squamous intraepithelial lesions of the cervix, which precede invasive cancer. The viral genome is present in the tumour cells of primary as well as metastatic cervical cancer. The progression from low grade squamous intraepithelial lesions to invasive cancer may take more than 10 years; human papillomaviruses are found throughout this disease process. The viruses are recovered much less frequently from cytologically normal women of comparable age. In prospective studies of women with normal cervical cytology, the presence of HPV is a strong risk factor for the subsequent development of squamous intraepithelial lesions.

Certain HPV types are preferentially associated with invasive cancers. From their distribution in normal individuals and in preinvasive and invasive cervical disease, genital tract HPVs have been categorized as high-risk, or low-risk types (Fig. 7.5.19.5; Table 7.5.19.2). HPV-16 and HPV-18 are the predominant viruses in invasive cancers and account for 40 to 60% and 5 to 20%, respectively, of HPV-positive cancers in different studies. About a dozen additional types of HPV are found in small proportions of

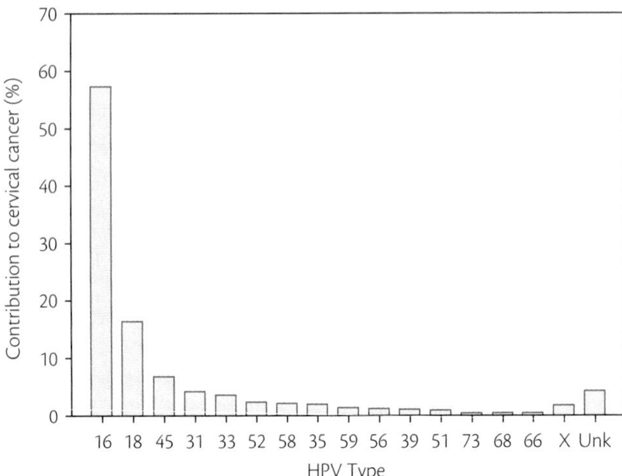

Fig. 7.5.19.5 Percentages of cervical cancer cases attributed to the most frequent HPV types in all world regions combined. X includes the rare types 40, 42, 53, 54, 55, 83, and 84. 'Unk' includes specimens that were positive for HPV DNA but could not be genotyped by current methods.
(Data from Munoz N, *et al.* (2004). Against which human papillomavirus types shall we vaccinate and screen? The international perspective. *Int J Cancer*, **111**, 278–85.)

invasive cancers. The low-risk HPVs are almost never detected in invasive cervical cancers.

Comparisons of different HPV types for their ability to transform human keratinocytes *in vitro* show that HPV-16 and HPV-18, types most clearly associated with naturally occurring cervical cancers, also have the greatest oncogenic potential in laboratory studies. The transforming functions of HPVs are localized to open reading frames E6 and E7; these are the viral genes consistently expressed in naturally occurring HPV-positive cancers. The viral genome is integrated into the cellular DNA in most cervical cancers. The break in the circular viral genome that is required for integration occurs most frequently in the E1/E2 region and results in an enhanced expression of the transforming E6 and E7 open reading frames. The transforming HPV proteins E6 and E7 interact with cellular tumour suppressor proteins p53 and Rb, respectively. The oncogenic effect of HPVs is mediated largely by their ability to inactivate the tumour suppressor proteins which normally regulate the cell cycle.

Epidemiology

Human papillomavirus infections of the genital tract are extremely common in sexually active populations. In young sexually active women, point prevalence (single sampling) of HPV infection as measured by the detection of HPV DNA in genital tract specimens by the sensitive polymerase chain reaction (PCR) may be as high as 40%, and the cumulative prevalence (multiple sampling of women over time) may be as high as 80 to 90%. The prevalence decreases with increasing age. Most of these infections are found in women with normal cervical cytology and undoubtedly resolve without leaving a trace. Only a small proportion of infections persists and progresses to squamous intraepithelial lesions and then to invasive cancer. The cofactors that might be associated with progression to cancer include smoking, use of oral contraceptives, parity, and presence of other sexually transmitted diseases. Human immunodeficiency virus (HIV) infection and associated immunosuppression, leads to a much higher prevalence, and longer persistence, of HPV infections and to greater incidence of squamous intraepithelial lesions.

Prevention and control

Screening for cervical cytological abnormalities by cervical smear and treatment of preinvasive and invasive cancers identified by screening, have been credited with the decrease in incidence of cervical cancer and mortality due to the disease that has been observed in many developed countries over the last 40 to 50 years. Women who have cytological abnormalities which are low grade or of uncertain significance may benefit from an HPV diagnosis. The presence of cancer-associated HPVs would indicate a need for closer monitoring and colposcopy; HPV-negative women would be monitored routinely. Tests for the presence of high risk HPVs may replace cervical smears as cervical cancer screening strategy.

Prophylactic vaccines

The discovery that the L1 coat protein of papillomaviruses could assemble into a virus-like particle (VLP), when expressed as a recombinant protein, and the demonstration that immunization of rabbits, cattle, and dogs with VLPs of their respective papillomaviruses protected against papillomavirus-induced disease, stimulated the development of vaccines for human papillomaviruses. L1 VLPs appear to induce very limited cross-neutralization against other genotypes necessitating a multicomponent vaccine to provide coverage against disease caused by more than one type. Two HPV L1 VLP vaccines have been developed commercially; Cervarix is a bivalent HPV-16/18 L1 VLP vaccine and Gardasil is a quadrivalent HPV16/18/6/11 L1 VLP vaccine. Both vaccines are generally safe and well tolerated and are highly immunogenic. Both vaccines have demonstrated truly remarkable efficacy, preventing nearly 100% of incident infections and preinvasive cervical cancers due to the HPV types in the vaccines. Gardasil is also 100% effective in preventing genital warts associated with HPV 6/11. Since genital HPV infection is sexually transmitted, the vaccines ideally should target prepubertal and young adolescent girls. The vaccines are also recommended for young women 13 to 26 years of age, because many of them may not yet have been exposed to the HPV types in the vaccines. If HPV vaccines are proven to be safe and efficacious in males, future recommendations will likely include immunization of boys and young men in order to reduce the risk of genital warts, protect against penile and oropharyngeal cancer, and provide herd immunity. The durability of the immune response engendered by HPV vaccines and thus the possible need for a booster in vaccinated individuals is unknown. Because protection may wane over time and because vaccination does not protect against the HPV types not included in the vaccines, screening programmes will need to be maintained, but the strategy may change with longer intervals between screening and a greater emphasis on HPV DNA testing as a screening method.

Therapeutic vaccines

Human papillomavirus-associated cancers express HPV E6 and E7 proteins in their tumour cells. Candidate therapeutic vaccines targeted to these proteins are being developed for the treatment of high grade squamous intraepithelial lesions and invasive cancer.

Cancers at other lower anogenital tract sites

Human papillomavirus infections are very common on the vulva, vagina, penis, perineum, and anus. Synchronous neoplasia at multiple sites in the female lower genital tract is almost always associated with HPVs, especially HPV-16. Carcinoma of the vulva is aetiologically heterogeneous. Vulval cancers occurring in younger women are associated with HPVs, but the typical squamous cell carcinoma of the vulva in older women is not. Neoplasia of the anal canal, seen frequently in HIV-seropositive homosexual men, is strongly associated with HPVs.

Cancer of the oropharynx

A subset of oropharyngeal cancers, especially tonsillar cancers, is aetiologically linked to high-risk HPVs, most often HPV-16. Patients with HPV-associated cancers have risk factors related to their sexual history rather than to alcohol and tobacco use. As compared to HPV-negative cancers, the HPV-positive cancers are characterized by more frequent basaloid pathology, less frequent p53 and Rb mutations, and better prognosis.

Skin warts (Chapter 23.10)

Skin warts and verrucas may occur anywhere on the skin and are morphologically diverse. They are most common in older children and young adults. Except in the rare condition known as epidermodysplasia verruciformis (see below), they almost never become malignant. Most regress within 2 years. Specific HPV types are strongly associated with specific types of warts (Table 7.5.19.4).

Epidermodysplasia verruciformis

This is a rare, lifelong disease in which a patient has extensive warty involvement of the skin that cannot be resolved. It generally begins in infancy or childhood with multiple, disseminated polymorphic wart-like lesions on the face, trunk, and extremities that tend to become confluent. The warts are either flat or reddish-brown macular plaques that resemble pityriasis versicolor. In about a third of the cases, foci of malignant transformation occur in macular plaques in areas of the skin exposed to sunlight. The tumours are slow growing and rarely metastasize.

Epidermodysplasia verruciformis (EV) is often a familial disease. Patients sometimes have a history of parental consanguinity. A susceptibility locus has been mapped to chromosome 17q25 and truncating mutations in either of two novel adjacent genes, *TMC6* and *TMC8*, are associated with the disease in different pedigrees. The function of the gene products of TMC6 and TMC8 and how they confer increased risk for EV are unknown. A second putative susceptibility locus is located on chromosome 2p21-p24. The flat warts yield the same HPV types as those of normal individuals, but a very large number of HPVs that are seldom encountered in normal individuals are recovered from the macular plaques (Table 7.5.19.3). It is unclear how patients with epidermodysplasia verruciformis become infected with these particular papillomaviruses. The factors that contribute to the occurrence of carcinoma in these patients therefore include a genetic defect, infection with specific HPVs, e.g. HPV-5 and HPV-8, and exposure of the affected area to sunlight.

Nonmelanoma skin cancers

HPV DNA has been detected in 30 to 50% of nonmelanoma skin cancers (NMSC) in immunocompetent populations and in up to 90% of NMSC from immunocompromised populations, in particular organ transplant recipients. The HPV prevalence is generally higher in squamous cell carcinoma than in basal cell carcinoma. The sequences represent cutaneous HPV types, EV-associated HPVs, and many novel HPV sequences. No single HPV type predominates and there is no evidence of high-risk types analogous to those seen in cervical cancer. The amount of HPV DNA in skin tumours is very low, indicating that not every tumour cell harbours an HPV genome. Because HPV DNA is frequently detected in normal skin samples, it is not clear to what extent HPVs contribute to the development of NMSC. Ultraviolet (UV) light is considered the most significant risk factor for NMSCs. Cutaneous HPVs through the antiapoptotic activity of their E6 gene may act as cocarcinogens by preventing elimination of cells with UV-induced DNA damage.

Human polyomaviruses

In 1971, BK virus was isolated from the urine of a renal transplant recipient and JC virus was recovered from the brain of a patient with progressive multifocal leukoencephalopathy. Recently, two new human polyomaviruses, KI virus and WU virus, were detected in respiratory tract secretions of children by using molecular techniques. The viruses were detected in upper respiratory tract specimens in the presence of other recognized respiratory tract pathogens and thus their role in disease is unclear. In 2008, another new human polyomavirus, Merkel cell virus, was identified in tumour cells from patients with Merkel cell carcinoma, a rare aggressive skin cancer. Polyomaviruses have a double-stranded DNA genome of about 5000 bp, which is divided into an early region encoding viral T proteins, a late region encoding viral capsid proteins, and a noncoding regulatory region. The T proteins regulate viral transcription, initiate viral DNA replication, and mediate inactivation of host cell tumour suppressor proteins, which contribute to the oncogenic potential of polyomaviruses. The viral regulatory region contains elements for viral DNA replication and promoters for transcription of early and late genes, as well as binding sites for cellular transcription factors, which determine the host and tissue tropism of polyomaviruses.

The early and late regions are transcribed from different strands of the viral DNA. Although BK and JC viruses are homologous for 75% of their nucleotide sequence, the infections are readily distinguishable by conventional tests.

Infection occurs in childhood and is largely subclinical. Most children acquire antibodies to BK virus by the age of 10; infection with JC virus occurs at a later age. Infection occurs by the respiratory route and possibly by ingestion. Both viruses establish latent, often lifelong, infection in the kidney and are often shed in the urine of normal people. Reactivation in immunodeficient people is responsible for most associated illnesses. The viruses are reactivated in pregnancy, but without any apparent harm to the mother or the newborn.

Polyomavirus-associated illnesses

Nephropathy in renal transplant recipients

This condition is associated most often with BK virus and rarely with JC virus. It occurs in 3 to 10% of renal transplant recipients and results in a loss of the allograft in 50 to 80% of the affected patients. The recent increase in the incidence of this complication is related to the introduction of new and intensive immunosuppressive therapies. Pathologically, the disease is characterized by inclusion-bearing enlarged nuclei in renal tubular and glomerular epithelial cells which are readily detected by microscopy (Fig. 7.5.19.6). Monitoring of the patients for BK virus viraemia has predictive value for the incidence of the disease.

Haemorrhagic cystitis in bone marrow transplant recipients

Late-onset haemorrhagic cystitis in bone marrow transplant recipients is associated with BK virus infection. Large amounts of BK virus are shed in urine during the haemorrhagic episodes.

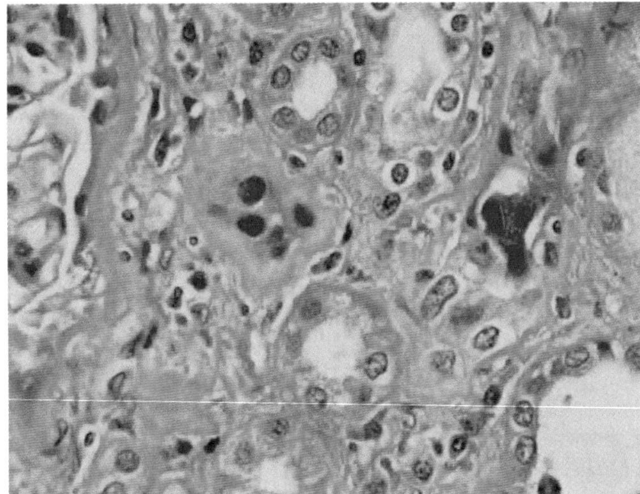

Fig. 7.5.19.6 BK virus infected cells (dark and hyperchromatic) in renal parenchyma, with some cells shed in the tubular lumen.

Progressive multifocal leucoencephalopathy (PML) (Chapters 7.5.23 and 24.11.2)

JC virus causes progressive multifocal leucoencephalopathy, a subacute demyelinating disease of the central nervous system occurring in individuals with impaired cell-mediated immunity. Until the advent of AIDS, it was a rare disease found mainly in older patients with lymphoproliferative disorders or chronic diseases. Because PML is a complication in 1 to 2% of AIDS cases, it is a more common disease and is seen much more frequently in younger patients. It has also been recognized in children who have inherited immunodeficiency diseases or have AIDS. Recently, PML has been recognized as a complication in patients with Crohn's disease or multiple sclerosis participating in clinical trials of natalizumab monoclonal antibody, which inhibits migration of cells across the blood–brain barrier.

The key pathogenetic event in PML is the cytocidal JC virus infection of oligodendrocytes, which are responsible for the production and maintenance of myelin. This leads to foci of demyelination that tend to coalesce and eventually involve large areas of the brain. Infected oligodendrocytes, containing large inclusion-bearing nuclei filled with abundant virus particles, surround the foci of demyelination (Fig. 7.5.19.7). Enlarged astrocytes often show bizarre nuclear changes but are mostly virus negative. They are found within the foci of demyelination. JC virus is disseminated haematogenously to the central nervous system, probably through virus-infected B lymphocytes.

PML starts insidiously. Early signs and symptoms indicate the presence of multifocal asymmetrical lesions in the brain and involve impairment of vision and speech, and mental deterioration. The disease is usually relentlessly progressive and fatal within 3 to 6 months, but rarely it can become stabilized with survival for many years. CT and MRI have been successfully used for

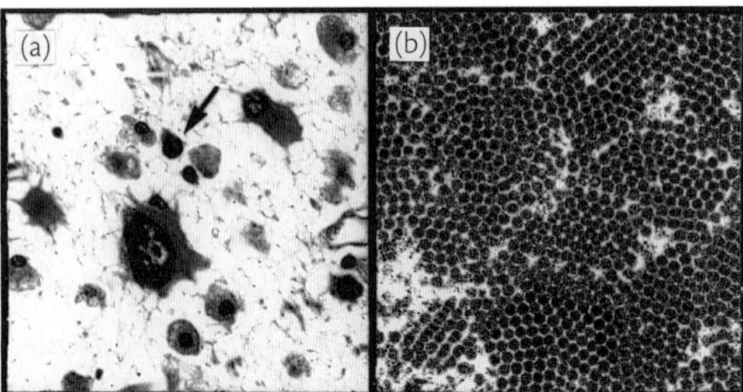

Fig. 7.5.19.7 A lesion of progressive multifocal leukoencephalopathy showing oligodendrocytes with enlarged, deeply staining nuclei (arrow) and giant astrocytes (left), and a crystalloid array of JC virus particles in an infected oligodendrocyte nucleus (right).

(Reproduced, with permission, from Shah KV (1992). Polyomavirus, infection and immunity. In: Roitt IM (ed) *Encyclopedia of Immunology*, pp. 1256–8. Academic Press, New York.)

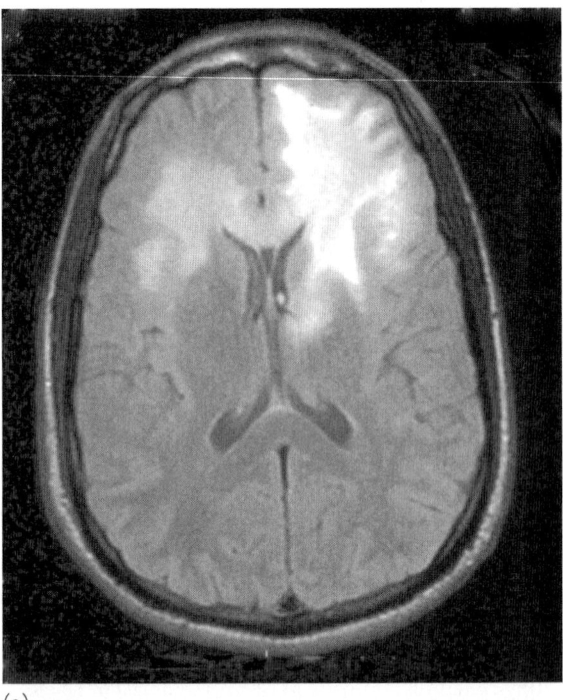

(a)

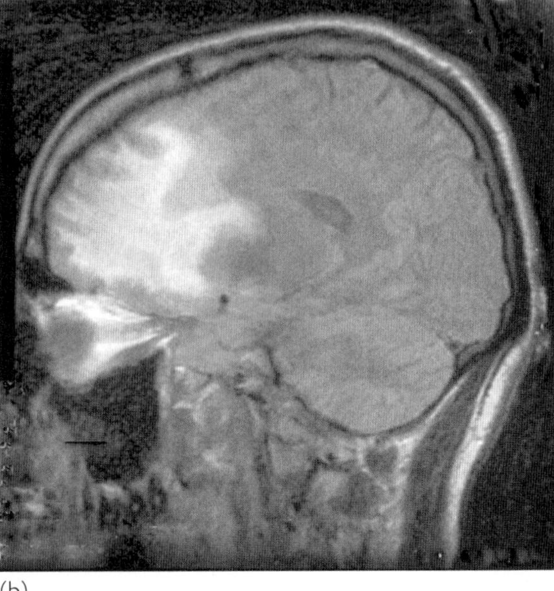

(b)

Fig. 7.5.19.8 Brain fluid attenuation inversion recovery (FLAIR) MRIs in axial (a) and sagittal (b) planes of a 36-year-old man with AIDS and progressive multifocal leukoencephalopathy proven by detection of JC virus DNA in cerebrospinal fluid by PCR.

diagnosis (Fig. 7.5.19.8). Treatment with cytosine arabinoside and the presence of an inflammatory response in the brain have been associated with the few relatively successful outcomes.

Role of polyomaviruses in human tumours

The role of polyomaviruses in human tumours is the subject of debate. JC virus and BK virus are oncogenic for laboratory animals and they transform cultured cells. There are reports of finding JC virus DNA in brain and colon tumours and BK virus DNA in prostate, bladder, and brain tumours, as well as neuroblastomas and insulinomas. However, a reproducible and consistent aetiological association of either virus with any human tumour has not been demonstrated. The Merkel cell virus provides a more convincing example of a polyomavirus-induced human tumour, since the viral genome was found to be integrated into tumour cell DNA, a key event in experimental polyomavirus-induced animal tumours. However, the prevalence of the Merkel cell virus in human populations is unknown and the precise role of the virus in the aetiology of Merkel cell carcinoma remains to be established.

Further reading

Berger JR, *et al.* (1998). Progressive multifocal leukoencephalopathy in patients with HIV infection. *J Neurovirol*, **4**, 59–68.

Bosch FX, *et al.* (2002). The causal relation between human papillomavirus and cervical cancer. *J Clin Pathol*, **55**, 244–265.

D'Souza G, *et al.* (2007). Epidemiological evidence that human papillomavirus is a cause of oropharyngeal squamous cell carcinomas. *N Engl J Med*, **356**, 1944–56.

Koutsky LA, *et al.* (2002). A controlled trial of a human papillomavirus type 16 vaccine. *N Engl J Med*, **347**, 1645–51.

Munoz N, *et al.* (2004). Against which human papillomavirus types shall we vaccinate and screen? The international perspective. *Int J Cancer*, **111**, 278–85.

Randhawa P, Brennan DC. (2006). BK virus infection in transplant recipients: an overview and update. *Am J Transplant*, **6**, 2000–5.

Shah KV. (1992). Polyomavirus, infection and immunity. In: Roitt IM (ed) *Encyclopedia of immunology*, pp. 1256–8. Academic Press, New York.

Shah KV, Howley PM. (1996). Papillomaviruses. In: Fields BN, *et al.* (eds) *Fields virology*, vol. 2, pp. 2077–109. Lippincott-Raven, Philadelphia.

Yousry TA, *et al.* (2006). Evaluation of patients treated with natalizumab for progressive multifocal leukoencephalopathy. *N Engl J Med*, **354**, 924–33.

7.5.20 Parvovirus B19

Kevin E. Brown

Essentials

Parvovirus B19 (B19V) is a small DNA virus that replicates in erythroid progenitor cells, with virus-induced cytotoxicity stopping red cell production. It only infects humans, is endemic in most places, and is transmitted predominantly by the respiratory route. In healthy people it causes erythema infectiosum, also known as 'fifth disease' or 'slapped cheek disease', associated with minimal drop in haemoglobin, but in patients with increased red cell turnover, e.g. haemolytic anaemia or haemoglobinopathy, it causes transient aplastic crisis; in immunocompromised patients it causes chronic anaemia; and following maternal infection it leads to hydrops fetalis or fetal loss. Treatment is supportive in most instances, but reduction in iatrogenic immunosuppression and/or intravenous immunoglobulin may be appropriate in some cases. No vaccine is available.

Introduction

Parvovirus B19 (B19V) is a member of the Parvoviridae, small (*c.*22 nm), nonenveloped, icosahedral-shaped viruses (Fig. 7.5.20.1), with a linear single-stranded DNA genome of about 5000 nucleotides. At least four types of parvovirus infect humans: B19V; adeno-associated viruses (AAVs); the recently described Parv4/5, and human bocavirus. To date, only B19V has definitively been shown to be a human pathogen.

Aetiology, pathogenesis, and pathology

Based on viral sequence, B19V can be divided into three distinct genotypes (1, 2, and 3). Genotypes 2 and 3 are infrequently detected in Europe or the United States of America. No differences in pathogenicity are observed between the different genotypes, and they are all a single B19V serotype.

B19V replication occurs primarily in erythroid progenitors, with the specificity in part due to the limited tissue distribution of the B19V receptor, blood group P antigen (globoside). Infection leads to high titre viraemia (>10^{12} virus particles/ml or IV/ml) (Fig. 7.5.20.2), and the virus-induced cytotoxicity stops red cell production.

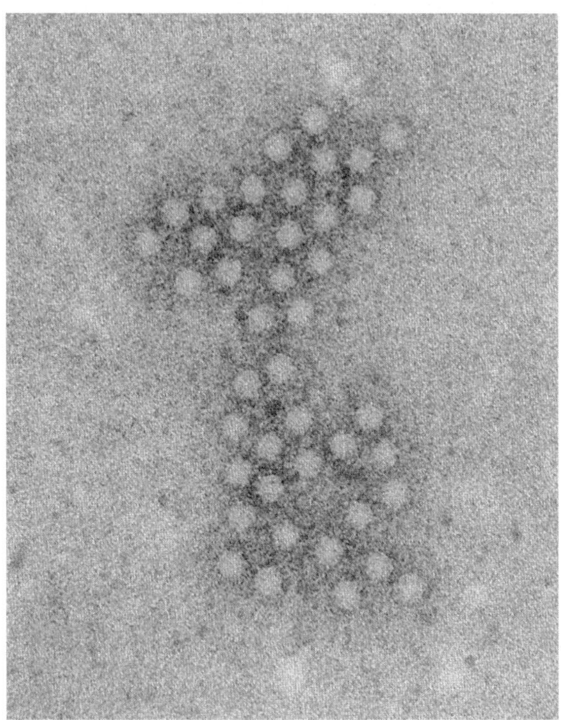

Fig. 7.5.20.1 Typical appearance of parvovirus B19, with characteristic 22 nm icosahedral particles.
(Courtesy of Dr Hazel Appleton, Virus Reference Department, Health Protection Agency.)

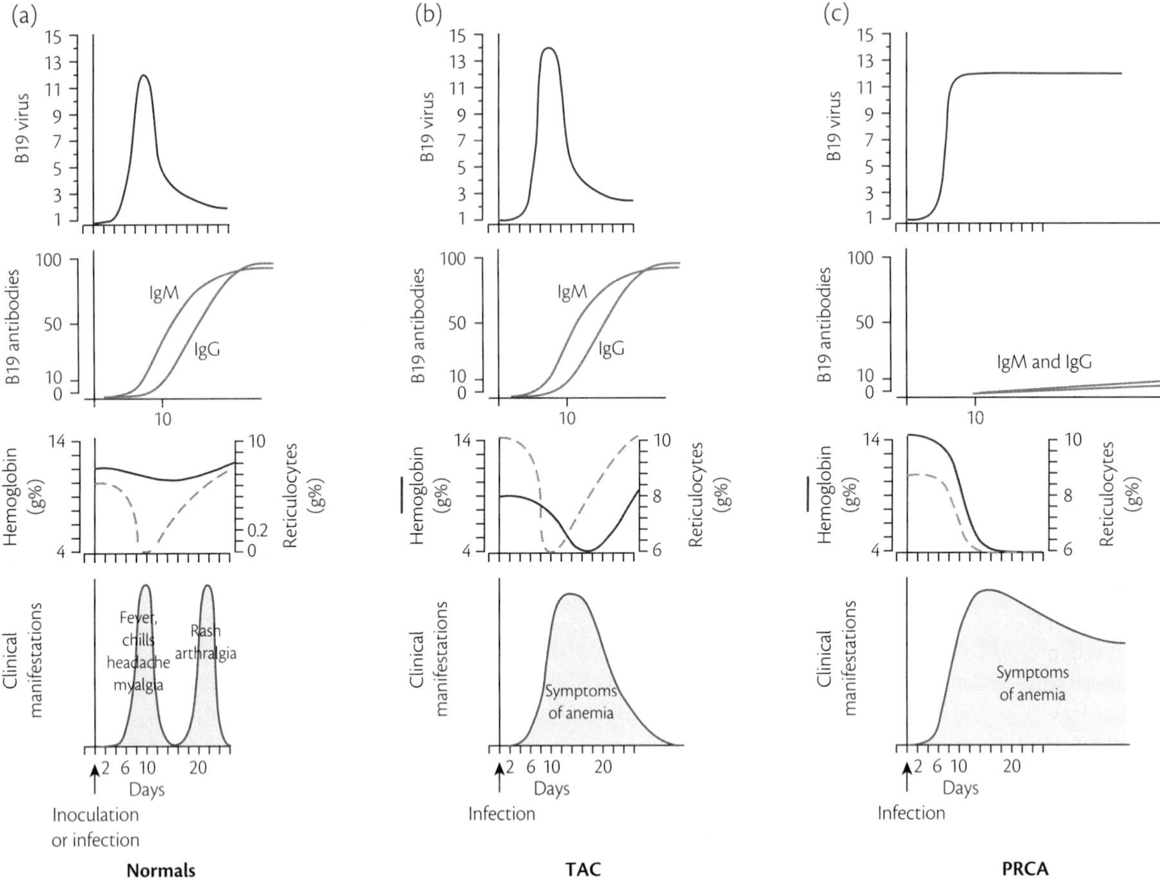

Fig. 7.5.20.2 Schematic of the time course of B19 infection in (a) erythema infectiosum (EI), (b) transient aplastic crisis (TAC), and (c) pure red cell aplasia (PRCA) or chronic anaemia. The B19 virus titres are given in log 10 IU/ml.
(From Young NS, Brown KE (2004). Parvovirus B19. *N Engl J Med*, **350**, 586–97.)

In immunocompetent people, viraemia and arrest of erythropoiesis is transient, and resolves as the antibody response is mounted. In those with normal erythropoiesis the drop in haemoglobin is minimal, but in patients with increased red cell turnover, infection induces a transient crisis with severe anaemia (Fig. 7.5.20.2b). Similarly, in the fetus or anyone who does not mount a neutralizing antibody response which halts the lytic infection, erythroid production is compromised and patients develop chronic anaemia (Fig. 7.5.20.2c).

The immune-mediated phase of illness begins 2 to 3 weeks postinfection as the IgM response peaks, and the rash of fifth disease, arthralgia, and/or frank arthritis appear.

The B19 receptor is found on other cell types, including megakaryocytes, endothelial cells, placenta, myocardium, and liver. B19 infection at these sites may be responsible for some of the more unusual presentations. Rare people who lack P antigen are naturally resistant to B19V.

Epidemiology

B19V exclusively infects humans, and the virus is endemic in virtually all parts of the world. Transmission is predominantly via the respiratory route, prior to the onset of the rash or arthralgia. About 50% of 15-year-old children have detectable IgG, increasing to more than 90% of older people. In pregnant women there is an estimated annual seroconversion rate of approximately 1%. The secondary infection rate within households approaches 50%.

Prevention

High titre B19V is not unusual in blood, and transmission occurs via transfusion, particularly of pooled components. B19V is resistant to heat and solvent/detergent inactivation. Plasma pools are currently screened by nucleic acid testing (NAT) and high titre pools are discarded.

Clinical features

The clinical manifestation of B19V infection varies widely, depending on the host (Table 7.5.20.1). The majority of infections are asymptomatic. In healthy, immunocompetent people, B19 infections causes erythema infectiosum (EI), also known as 'fifth disease' or 'slapped cheek disease' due to the characteristic facial rash which appears several days after a minor febrile prodrome. The rash may spread and develop a lacy reticular appearance, but the intensity and distribution of the rash varies and is difficult to distinguish from other viral exanthems. In adults, the 'slapped cheek' may not be apparent. Although uncommon in children, a symmetrical polyarthropathy, affecting the small joints of the hands and occasionally the ankles, knees, and wrists occurs in *c*.50% of adults, more often in women than men. Resolution usually occurs within a few weeks, but recurring symptoms can continue for months.

Patients with increased erythropoiesis (i.e. those with haemolytic anaemia or haemoglobinopathy) develop transient aplastic crisis

Table 7.5.20.1 Diseases associated with parvovirus B19 infection and methods of diagnosis

Disease	Host(s)	Pathogenesis	IgM	IgG	Quantitative PCR
Fifth disease	Healthy children	Immune-mediated	Positive	Positive	(Low positive)
Polyarthropathy syndrome	Healthy adults (especially women)	Immune-mediated	Positive within 3 months of onset	Positive	(Low positive)
Transient aplastic crisis (TAC)	Patients with increased erythropoiesis	Erythroid cytotoxicity			Often $>10^{12}$ IU/ml, but rapidly decreases
Persistent anaemia/ pure red cell aplasia	Immunocompromised patients	Impaired neutralizing antibody	Negative/weak positive	Negative/ weak positive	Often $>10^{12}$ IU/ml, but should be $>10^{6}$ IU/ml in the absence of treatment
Hydrops fetalis	Fetus	Erythroid cytotoxicity and impaired neutralizing antibody			Positive amniotic fluid or tissue

(TAC), with symptoms of acute anaemia. Bone marrow examination reveals an absence of erythroid precursors and the presence of characteristic giant pronormoblasts.

In the immunocompromised (i.e. patients with AIDS, leukaemia, and following transplantation), B19 infection may lead to chronic anaemia or pure red cell aplasia. Patients have persistent anaemia with reticulocytopenia, absent or low levels of B19 IgG, high levels of B19 DNA in serum, and often scattered giant pronormoblasts in the bone marrow. Transient neutropenia, lymphopenia, and thrombocytopenia, may be seen and B19V occasionally causes a haemophagocytic syndrome.

Infection with B19V during pregnancy can lead to hydrops fetalis and fetal loss. The risk of transplacental fetal infection is about 30%, and the risk of fetal loss, predominantly in the second trimester, 9%. The risk of congenital infection is less than 1%. Although B19V does not appear to be teratogenic, there are anecdotal reports of eye damage and CNS abnormalities. Cases of congenital anaemia have also been described. B19V probably causes 10 to 20% of all cases of nonimmune hydrops.

B19V infection is rarely associated with hepatitis, vasculitis, myocarditis, glomerulosclerosis, and CNS disease.

Diagnosis

In immunocompetent people, B19V infection is usually diagnosed by the detection of B19 IgM antibodies (Table 7.5.20.1). IgM can be found at the time of rash in EI and by the third day of TAC in patients with haematological disorders. IgM remains detectable for about 3 months. B19 IgG appears by the seventh day of illness and remains for life. Detection of B19 DNA should be used for the diagnosis of early TAC or chronic anaemia. Although levels fall rapidly with the development of the immune response, low levels of DNA can be detectable by polymerase chain reaction (PCR) for months and even years after infection, even in healthy people, so a quantitative PCR should be used for diagnosis. At the height of viraemia, more than 10^{12} B19 DNA IU/ml of serum can be detected, but titres fall rapidly within 2 days. Patients with aplastic crisis or B19-induced chronic anaemia generally have more than 10^{5} IU/ml B19 DNA.

Treatment

No antiviral drug is available, and treatment is often only symptomatic. B19-induced TAC may require blood transfusions, and intrauterine blood transfusion can prevent fetal loss in some cases of fetal hydrops. In patients on chemotherapy, stopping treatment temporarily may result in an immune response and resolution, but if unsuccessful or inapplicable, intravenous human normal immunoglobulin (HNIG) may cure or improve persistent B19 infection. These patients and those with TAC should be considered infectious. Administration of immunoglobulin is not beneficial for EI or B19-associated polyarthropathy.

Prevention in the future

No vaccine is currently approved for parvovirus B19. A vaccine based on viral-like particles expressed in insect cells is under development and results of phase 1 trials were promising.

Further reading

Brown KE, Young NS (2006). Parvovirus B19. In: Young NS, Gerson SL, High KA (eds) *Clinical Hematology*, pp. 981–991. Mosby Elsevier, Philadelphia.

Brown KE, *et al.* (1994). Resistance to parvovirus B19 infection due to lack of virus receptor (erythrocyte P antigen). *N Engl J Med*, **330**, 1192–96.

Kerr JR, *et al.* (eds) (2006). *Parvoviruses.* Hodder Arnold, London.

Kurtzman GJ, *et al.* (1987). Chronic bone marrow failure due to persistent B19 parvovirus infection. *N Engl J Med*, **317**, 287–94.

Young NS, Brown KE (2004). Parvovirus B19. *N Engl J Med*, **350**, 586–97.

7.5.21 Hepatitis viruses (excluding hepatitis C virus)

N.V. Naoumov

Essentials

The group of hepatitis viruses includes five unrelated human viruses (A to E), which differ in their genome organization, biology, and epidemiology, while being united by their hepatotropism. About 10 to 15% of cases of viral hepatitis are considered as non-A to E hepatitis, whose aetiology is still unknown, but the search for which has led to the identification of several new viruses (e.g. HGV or GB virus-C, TT, and SEN viruses) of uncertain pathogenic significance.

Clinical aspects of viral hepatitis are discussed in Chapter 15.21.1.

Hepatitis A virus (HAV)

Single-stranded RNA genome. Replicates primarily in hepatocytes and excreted via the biliary system into the faeces, where it can be found in high concentrations prior to clinical symptoms. Does not cause chronic infection. Anti-HAV IgG remains detectable after acute infection and provides protective immunity.

Hepatitis B virus (HBV)

The smallest human DNA virus. Eight genotypes, designated A to H, have been determined, each having a distinct geographical distribution. The virus is noncytopathic, with virus-specific cellular immunity being the main determinant for the outcome of infection. Eradication of HBV is rare, but in cases with resolution of HBV infection an effective immune response controls HBV replication and there is no liver disease. The natural evolution of chronic infection includes four consecutive phases: (1) early 'immunotolerant' phase—high levels of virus replication and minimal liver inflammation; (2) immune reactive phase—significant hepatic inflammation and elevated serum aminotransferases; with some patients progressing to (3) 'non-replicative' phase—seroconversion to anti-HBe; undetectable or low level of viraemia (below 2000 IU/ml by polymerase chain reaction-based assays); resolution of hepatic inflammation; and (4) HBeAg-negative chronic hepatitis B—due to the emergence of viral mutations; characterized by fluctuating serum HBV DNA and serum ALT levels, and progressive liver disease.

Hepatitis C virus (HCV)

See Chapter 7.5.22.

Hepatitis delta virus (HDV)

A defective virus with a single-stranded circular RNA genome, causing acute or chronic liver diseases only in association with hepatitis B virus. Can infect a person either simultaneously with HBV (coinfection) or subsequently, with duration of infection determined by that of HBsAg positivity.

Hepatitis E virus (HEV)

An RNA virus. May be zoonotic, with evidence of infection in pigs, cattle and sheep in endemic regions. No chronic infection. Immunity can be transient and may wane if acquired in childhood.

Introduction

Viral hepatitis (Fig. 7.5.21.1) is an ancient disease which remains a major health problem worldwide. Five viruses have been identified as aetiological agents and named A, B, C, D, and E (Table 7.5.21.1). These unrelated human viruses differ in their genome organization, biology, and epidemiology, while being united by their hepatotropism. Approximately 10 to 15% of cases with viral hepatitis are considered as non-A to E hepatitis and the aetiology is still unknown. The search for additional hepatitis agents led to the identification of several new viruses, named hepatitis G virus (HGV or GB virus-C), TT, and SEN viruses. These viruses have been detected in high proportions of the general population and their pathogenic role, if any, remains uncertain. Thus, the search for new hepatitis agents responsible for the small proportion of cases with cryptogenic hepatitis continues. Clinical aspects of viral hepatitis are discussed in Chapter 15.21.1.

Hepatitis A virus (HAV)

HAV particles were first discovered by immune electron microscopy in 1973 in stool samples of patients with hepatitis A. The virus is classified in the genus *Hepatovirus* of the family Picornaviridae. The genome of HAV is a single-stranded, linear RNA of approximately 7500 nucleotides (Table 7.5.21.1). This includes a 5′ nontranslated region (5′ NTR) of approximately 740 nucleotides, followed by a single, long, open reading frame (ORF), which encodes a polyprotein of 2200 amino acids and a short 3′ nontranslated segment. After translation, HAV polyprotein undergoes multiple cleavages by a virally-encoded enzyme, 3C protease. The polyprotein contains three functionally separate domains. At the N-terminal end is domain P1 which includes the major structural polypeptides of HAV in the following sequence—VP2, VP3, and VP1. A fourth very small polypeptide, VP4, which is presumed to be involved in HAV capsid formation, is located at the extreme N-terminal end of the polyprotein. These four structural polypeptides assemble into a viral capsid containing 60 copies of each. It is not known how the viral RNA is incorporated into the virion, but both empty and RNA-containing capsids have been observed in most virus preparations. The other P2 and P3 domains of the viral polyprotein include at least six separate proteins which are involved in viral replication. These include 2B and 2C helicase, 3A and 3B proteins, 3C (the viral protease), and 3D (an RNA-dependent RNA polymerase).

Hepatocytes are the predominant site of HAV replication *in vivo*. Recent data indicate that HAV may also replicate within the epithelial cells of the gastrointestinal tract. However, the mechanism by which HAV reaches the liver remains unknown. The maximal HAV replication in hepatocytes occurs before serum aminotransferases rise. The virus is excreted via the biliary system into the faeces where it can be found in high concentrations around 1 to 2 weeks prior to the onset of clinical symptoms. Viraemia is present from the earliest phase of infection and is due to HAV replication within hepatocytes. HAV differs from other picornaviruses because of its noncytolytic replication. Liver injury is immune mediated by natural killer cells, virus-specific CD8+ cytotoxic T lymphocytes, and nonspecific inflammatory cells recruited to the liver. At the onset of clinical symptoms there is a humoral immune response

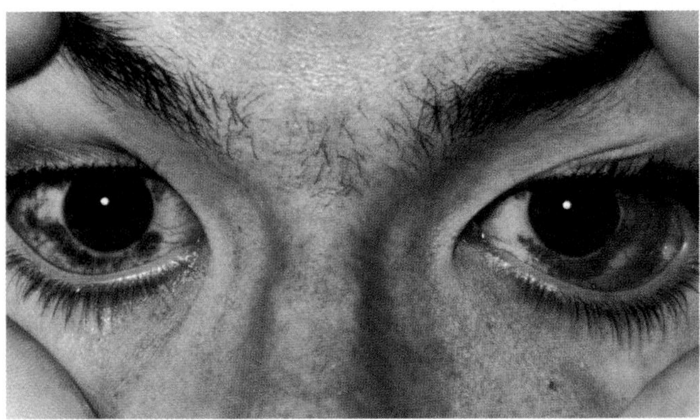

Fig. 7.5.21.1 Acute viral hepatitis (HBV) with jaundice and subconjunctival haemorrhages.
(Copyright D A Warrell.)

Table 7.5.21.1 Main characteristics of hepatitis viruses

Virus	Family	Morphology	Genome	Proteins	Antibodies	Pathogenesis	Specific features
HAV	*Picornaviridae*	27–28 nm nonenveloped spherical particles	Single-stranded linear RNA, 7500 nt	Four capsid proteins, viral polymerase, and proteases	Anti-HAV	Noncytopathic virus Immune-mediated acute hepatitis	No chronic infection Effective vaccines available
HBV	*Hepadnaviridae*	42 nm particle with nucleocapsid (core) and outer envelope (surface)	Partially double-stranded, circularDNA, 3200 nt	*Envelope* Major protein (HBsAg) Middle protein (PreS2+S) Large protein (PreS1+S2+S) *Nucleocapsid* (HBcAg) HBeAg nonstructural, soluble protein	Anti-HBs Anti-HBc Anti-HBe	Noncytopathic virus Immune-mediated acute and chronic hepatitis Weak T-cell reactivity—a dominant cause for persistent viral replication	In chronic infection spontaneous evolution from HBeAg(+) to anti-HBe(+) phase Mutant strains (surface, precore, polymerase) evolve under selection pressure DNA integration into host genome Transactivation of cellular genes Effective vaccines available
		22 nm spherical and filamentous subviral particles		Envelope proteins only	Anti-HBs		
HCV	*Flaviviridae*	50–60 nm enveloped spherical particles	Single-stranded linear RNA, approx. 9500 nt	*Structural* Envelope 1 (E1) Envelope 2 (E2) Nucleocapsid (core)	Anti-E1 Anti-E2 Anti-core	Usually noncytopathic virus Neutralizing antibodies (?)	High degree of virus heterogeneity (genotypes and quasi species) High propensity to chronic infection No integration in host genome
			Six major genotypes	*Nonstructural* NS2 NS3 NS4 NS5	Anti-NS3 Anti-NS4 Anti-NS5	T-cell reactivity—major role for resolution of acute infection	
HDV	Resembles viroids and plant viruses	35–37 nm enveloped particles	Single-stranded circular RNA, 1700 nt	HD-Ag (nucleocapsid) HBsAg (envelope)	Anti-HD Anti-HBs	Direct cytopathic and/or immune-mediated liver injury	Defective RNA virus Requires help from HBV for providing the envelope HBsAg
HEV	*Caliciviridae*	32–34 nm nonenveloped spherical particles	Single-stranded linear RNA, 7500 nt	ORF1—nonstructural proteins ORF2—structural proteins ORF3—unknown function	Anti-HEV	Probably immune mediated (?)	Enterically transmitted hepatitis mainly in Asia, Middle East, and Central America No chronic infection
HGV/ GBV-C	*Flaviviridae*	?	Single-stranded linear RNA, 9400 nt	Conserved E2 No core protein	Anti-E2	Primary site of replication unknown Does not cause hepatitis	Can establish chronic infection No clear pathogenic role
TTV	*Circinoviridae* (?)	?	Single-stranded, circular DNA, approx. 3850 nt	?	?	Does not cause hepatitis	Can establish chronic infection High degree of virus heterogeneity No clear pathogenic role

NS, nonstructural; nt, nucleotides; ORF, open reading frame.

and antibodies to structural HAV proteins (anti-HAV) are detectable in patients' serum. Initially, these are mainly IgM antibodies (IgM anti-HAV) which usually persist for approximately 6 months. During convalescence, anti-HAV of IgG class become the predominant antibodies, which remain detectable indefinitely and represent protective immunity to HAV.

Hepatitis B virus (HBV)

Two discoveries related to HBV mark the beginning of the understanding of hepatitis viruses. In 1965, Baruch Blumberg identified the surface antigen (HBsAg) of HBV, initially termed 'Australia antigen', and in 1970 the complete virion (a 42 nm particle) was identified by Dane and colleagues using electron microscopy. HBV belongs to a virus family named Hepadnaviridae, which includes similar hepatotropic DNA viruses specific for woodchucks, ground squirrels, and Pekin ducks.

Genome organization

The HBV genome contains only 3200 nucleotides and is the smallest DNA virus (Table 7.5.21.1). One of the DNA strands, known as the 'minus' strand, is almost a complete circle and contains four overlapping reading frames: precore/core, polymerase, envelope, and *X* genes (Fig. 7.5.21.2). The other ('plus') strand is shorter and varies in length.

The envelope ORF contains 3 start codons which separate the pre-S1, pre-S2, and S sequences. The surface gene encodes the major envelope protein (HBsAg), which has 226 amino acids. The translation product of the pre-S2 and S gene is the middle envelope protein and the product of pre-S1, pre-S2, and S gene is the large envelope protein. In addition to the complete virion, a much greater amount of noninfectious, 22 nm in diameter, spherical, and filamentous subviral particles are produced in infected hepatocytes. HBsAg and the middle envelope protein are present in all viral and subviral particles, while the large protein is present in the virions and in some subviral filaments. The domain which binds to a specific HBV receptor (still not defined) on the plasma membrane of hepatocytes resides within the pre-S1 region.

The precore/core ORF has two start codons which encode two closely related proteins. Translation from the preC start codon produces a precursor molecule, designated precore protein. In the endoplasmic reticulum this protein undergoes two proteolytic steps at the N- and at the C-terminal ends, and the resultant polypeptide is secreted from hepatocytes as hepatitis B e-antigen (HBeAg). This is a nonstructural protein, which is not essential for viral replication. Translation from the C start codon results in the nucleocapsid protein (HBcAg), which has 183 amino acids. In the cytoplasm of hepatocytes HBcAg assembles spontaneously into nucleocapsid particles. HBeAg and HBcAg share about 90% of the amino acids but differ substantially in their conformation.

The polymerase ORF encodes the HBV polymerase protein with 832 amino acids. It has three functional domains—terminal protein, reverse transcriptase, and RNAse H activity. The X ORF encodes a protein with 154 amino acids. Its role is not fully understood, but it functions as a transactivator of cellular and other viral genes. The X protein is not essential for the replication of hepadnaviruses, but is believed to contribute to HBV-related hepatocarcinogenesis.

Eight genotypes of HBV (designated with the letters A to H) have been determined. The variations involve approximately 10% of the genome. Data on the geographical distribution indicate that genotype A is predominant in central and northern Europe, genotypes B and C in Asia, genotype D in the Mediterranean basin, and genotype E in Africa.

Viral replication

Following HBV entry into hepatocytes, the nucleocapsid is transported to the nucleus (Fig. 7.5.21.3). Cellular enzymes repair the open circular HBV DNA into covalently closed circular DNA

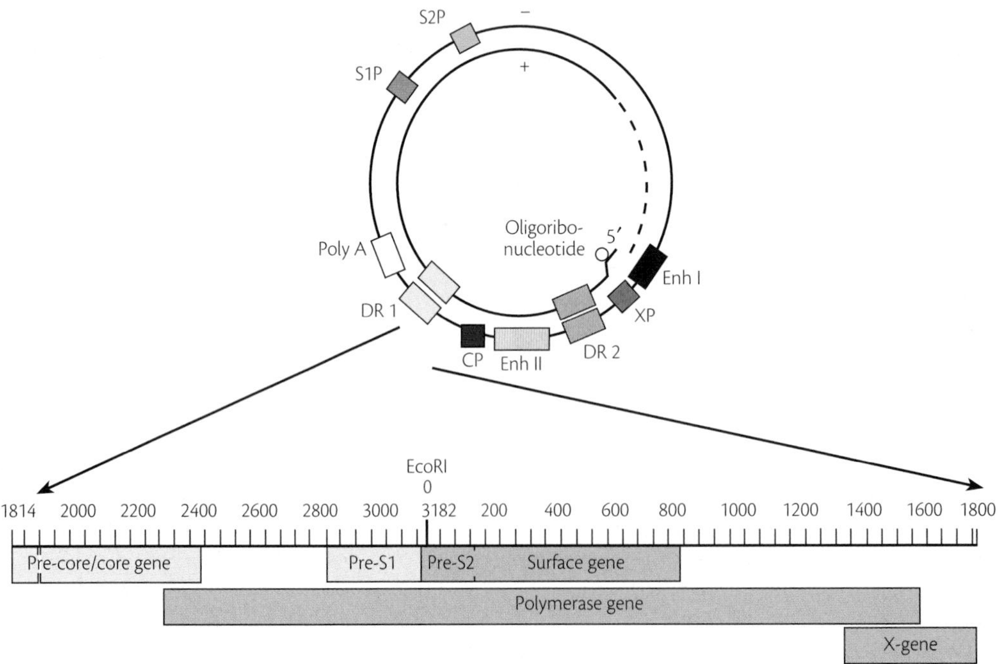

Fig. 7.5.21.2 Schematic representation of hepatitis B virus genome. CP, core promoter; DR1, direct repeat 1; DR2, direct repeat 2; EcoRI, restriction site for EcoRI enzyme used as a starting point for numbering; EnhI, enhancer I; EnhII, enhancer II; S1P, pre-S1 promoter; S2P, pre-S2 promoter; XP, X gene promoter.

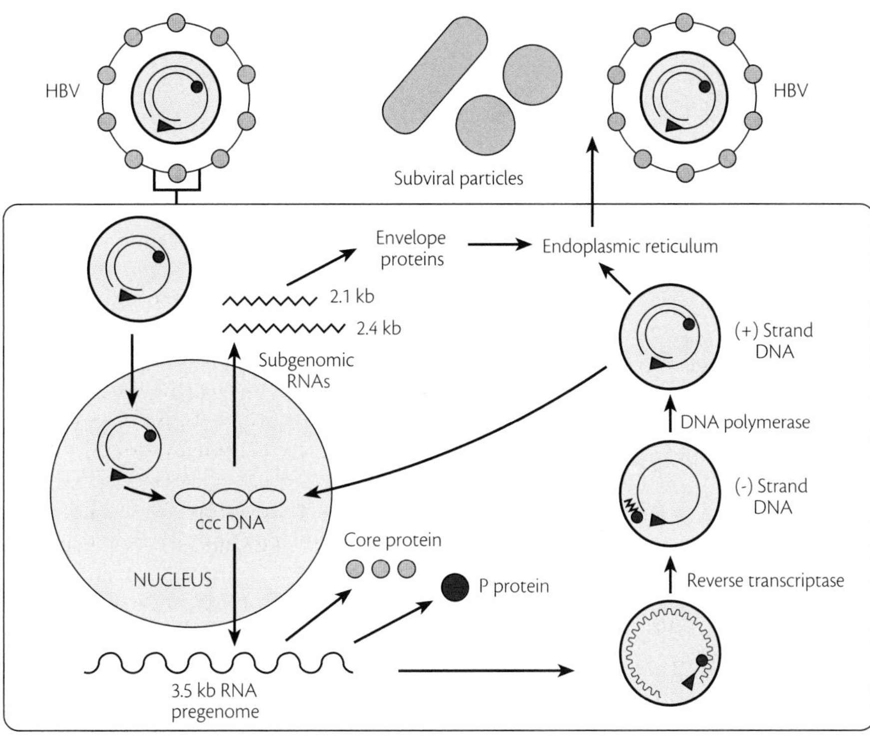

Fig. 7.5.21.3 Replicative cycle of hepatitis B virus.

(cccDNA), which serves as a template for the synthesis of pregenomic and messenger RNAs. Viral DNA does not integrate into the host genome as part of the normal replication cycle. The pregenomic RNA is transported to the cytoplasm and serves as mRNA for translation of new core and polymerase proteins. When these three components (pregenomic RNA, core, and polymerase proteins) reach sufficient quantities, they assemble into nucleocapsid particles, with the polymerase protein being directly involved in the pregenomic RNA encapsidation. Inside the particles the pregenomic RNA is reverse transcribed into DNA 'minus' strand, while the RNA template is simultaneously degraded by RNAse H. Finally, the 'plus' strand is produced which completes a new, partially double-stranded, HBV DNA. Some of the newly synthesized nucleocapsids with HBV DNA are transported back to the nucleus, which maintains a stable pool of cccDNA. Others are enveloped and leave the cell as new virions. The replication strategy used by hepadnaviruses differs from that of retroviruses in two main aspects: 1) integration into the host genome is not obligatory during replication; 2) functional mRNAs are produced from several internal promoters of the circular DNA genome.

Host immune response and pathogenesis

HBV is a noncytopathic virus. The virus-specific cellular immune response mainly determines the outcome of infection. Both HLA class I and class II-restricted T-cell responses are strong and directed to multiple viral antigens in patients with acute self-limited hepatitis B. Despite clearance of serum HBsAg, HBV DNA remains detectable by polymerase chain reaction (PCR) in most cases, and HBV-specific CD4+ and CD8+ T-cell reactivity has been demonstrated 10 to 20 years after the time of acute infection. Cytokines released from these cells, especially interferon-γ, have been shown to exert a noncytolytic inhibition on HBV replication without causing cell death. Thus, eradication of HBV may be rare, but an effective immune response controls HBV DNA expression and there is no liver disease. Patients with chronic HBV infection (defined by detection of HBsAg in serum for longer than 6 months) show weak virus-specific T-cell reactivity, which is the dominant cause for HBV persistence. This ineffective response, together with antigen nonspecific inflammatory cells recruited at the site of inflammation, is responsible for the progression of liver damage.

The humoral immune response involves antibodies directed at different HBV antigens (Table 7.5.21.1). The clinical significance is based on several aspects: 1) diagnosis—the antibody profile in the serum, together with the result of HBsAg and HBeAg, is used to define different phases of HBV infection; 2) prophylaxis—the development and the level of the protective antibody (anti-HBs) is used to monitor the response to vaccination; 3) pathogenesis—the humoral immune response contributes to viral elimination from the circulation by forming immune complexes. In some cases, the tissue deposition of antigen-antibody complexes is responsible for extrahepatic pathology such as glomerulonephritis, polyarteritis nodosa, arthritis, and skin changes.

Evolution of chronic HBV infection

HBV-host interactions change over time, typically in four consecutive phases, which are characterized by different levels of HBV replication and associated liver disease. The early 'immunotolerant' phase is associated with high levels of virus replication. HBeAg and HBV DNA are readily detectable in serum, while there is minimal liver inflammation. Over the years this is followed by a phase with enhanced immune reactivity to the virus, as reflected by significant hepatic inflammation and elevated serum aminotransferases. Serum HBeAg is still positive and serum HBV DNA level is usually lower. Some patients will progress spontaneously to the next 'non-replicative' or low-replicative phase, manifested by seroconversion to anti-HBe, undetectable or less than 2000 IU/ml viraemia (by polymerase chain reaction-based assays), and resolution of hepatic inflammation. In a proportion of patients, HBeAg loss may be due to the emergence of mutations in the core promoter and/or in the precore region (usually the $G_{1896}A$ stop codon), which prevent the translation of HBeAg. These HBe-minus mutants are replication competent and when viraemia levels are high, they cause HBe-negative chronic hepatitis B. The latter is characterized by fluctuating serum HBV DNA levels, mirrored by serum alanine aminotransferase (ALT) fluctuations, and progressive liver disease.

Hepatitis C virus (HCV) (Chapter 7.5.22)

Hepatitis D virus (HDV)

HDV is a defective virus that causes acute and chronic liver disease only in association with hepatitis B virus. This unique pathogen was discovered in 1977 by Mario Rizzetto in liver biopsies from patients with hepatitis B. HDV particles contain the viral RNA nucleocapsid, which is hepatitis delta antigen (HDAg), and an outer envelope (HBsAg), which is provided by the helper virus HBV. The HDV genome is a single-stranded, circular RNA (Table 7.5.21.1), and is the smallest known animal virus genome. Because of a high degree of internal complementarity, 70% of the nucleotides are base-paired. This gives an unusual, rod-like structure of the HDV genome. HDV RNA replicates via RNA-directed RNA synthesis by transcription of genomic RNA to a complementary antigenomic delta RNA. The latter serves as a template for subsequent genomic RNA synthesis. HDV produces a single protein, hepatitis delta antigen (HDAg), which is encoded by the antigenomic RNA. RNA editing of the antigenomic RNA allows the virus to make two forms of HDAg—small (HDAg-S, 195 amino acids) and large (HDAg-L, 214 amino acids). Both forms are present in the virions and have different functions in the HDV replicative cycle. HDAg-S facilitates HDV RNA replication, while HDAg-L inhibits replication and is required for assembly of the virion. Although the formation of delta virions requires the helper function of HBV, the replication of HDV RNA within the cell can occur without HBV.

Three phylogenetically distinct HDV genotypes have been identified. The most widespread is genotype 1, identified in Africa, Asia, Europe, and North America, which is associated with a broad spectrum of chronic liver disease. Genotype 2 is found only in East Asia and seems to cause mild hepatitis delta. Genotype 3 is found exclusively in northern parts of South America and is associated with particularly severe hepatitis.

Host immune response and pathogenesis

HDV can infect a person either simultaneously with HBV (coinfection) or as superinfection of a person with chronic HBV infection. Because HDV requires the helper function of HBV, the duration of delta infection is determined by the duration of HBsAg positivity. Analogous to the antibodies to HBV nucleocapsid (anti-HBc), antibodies to HDAg are not protective. Chronic HDV infection is accompanied by high titres of IgG anti-HD. A high serum level of IgM anti-HD indicates acute delta infection or exacerbation of chronic hepatitis D. The relative role of cellular immune reactions to HDAg, HBV antigens, or both in the immunopathogenesis of hepatitis D is not fully understood. The lack of liver pathology in transgenic mice expressing HDV and data from experimental infections suggest that HDV is not cytopathic. This is supported by the experience with patients undergoing liver transplantation for HDV cirrhosis. Although HDV recurs universally in the graft, necroinflammation is absent unless HBV recurs as well. The presence of microvesicular steatosis in severe hepatitis D indicates a possible direct cytopathic effect in some circumstances.

Hepatitis E virus (HEV)

HEV was first identified in 1983 by immune electron microscopy in the faeces of patients and classified in the family Caliciviridae. The HEV genome is a single-stranded, polyadenylated RNA of approximately 7500 nucleotides and contains three open reading frames (Table 7.5.21.1). ORF1 encodes nonstructural proteins involved in virus replication—helicase and RNA-dependent RNA polymerase. ORF2, comprising approximately 2000 nucleotides, codes for the major structural proteins. ORF3 has 328 nucleotides and also appears to code for a structural protein. The genomic organization of HEV is different from HAV and HCV because the structural and nonstructural proteins are coded by discontinuous, partially overlapping ORFs. Unlike HAV, HEV infection may be zoonotic. HEV RNA has been found in the faeces of wild pigs and serological evidence of infection was found in pigs, cattle, and sheep in endemic regions.

Four genotypes of HEV have been identified, which show 25% nucleotide variability. Geographically, genotype 1 has been isolated from tropical countries in Asia and Africa; genotype 2 was found in Mexico, whereas genotype 3 has worldwide distribution, including America, Asia, and Europe. Genotype 4 in contrast has been found only in Asia. Non-travel-associated hepatitis E has been diagnosed in indigenous patients in England and Wales. In the majority of cases it was caused by HEV genotype 3. For vaccine development, it is important that all HEV strains share at least one major, serogically cross-reactive, epitope.

The primary site of HEV replication is not fully understood. Following intravenous HEV inoculation in experimental models, serum aminotransferases levels rise after 24 to 38 days. Expression of HEV antigens has been detected in the cytoplasm of hepatocytes as early as 7 to 10 days after inoculation. Experimental data indicate that during an initial phase with high HEV replication the virus may be released from hepatocytes into bile, which occurs before the elevation of liver enzymes and morphological changes in the liver. The virus shedding appears to end with the normalization of serum aminotransferases. HEV RNA is detectable by reverse transcriptase polymerase chain reaction (RT-PCR) in the serum of virtually all patients within 2 weeks after the onset of hepatitis. Prolonged periods of viraemia, between 4 to 16 weeks, have also been reported. The detection of anti-HEV by enzyme immunoassays, involving recombinant HEV antigens or synthetic peptides, is the most frequently used method for diagnostic purposes and for epidemiological studies.

In most outbreaks, the route of transmission is water contaminated with faeces. Food-borne transmission has been suggested in some outbreaks. Person-to-person transmission of HEV appears to be less common than for HAV. During acute infection, the humoral immune response gradually develops in parallel with the ALT rise. The serum level of anti-HEV IgM reaches a maximal titre around the time of peak ALT levels and is detectable for 5 to 6 months. Although the IgG anti-HEV response persists for several years after the acute phase, the natural history of protective immunity to HEV is not fully established. In contrast to HAV, hepatitis E shows an unusually high attack rate amongst adults, suggesting that immunity to HEV, if acquired in childhood, may wane. Pregnant women show increased susceptibility to severe disease with increased case fatality.

New hepatitis-associated viruses

GB virus C (GBV-C) or hepatitis G virus (HGV)

The genome of GBV-C was identified in 1995 by molecular hybridization techniques in the serum of a patient with the initials GB. In parallel, another group of investigators identified the genome of a new RNA virus, named hepatitis G virus. The comparison of HGV and GBV-C genomes revealed very high homology, both at nucleotide (86%) and amino acid level (100%). It is now accepted that they represent two isolates of the same virus. GBV-C/HGV is an RNA virus with a single ORF encoding a polyprotein of approximately 3000 amino acids (Table 7.5.21.1). Together with another two RNA viruses, GBV-A and GBV-B, it belongs to the Flaviviridae and these three viruses show various similarities with HCV. Specific features of the GBV-C/HGV genome include absence of core gene (nucleocapsid); long 5′ and 3′ NTR and lack of poly A tail. Unlike HCV, this virus has a very conserved E2 region. Longitudinal studies have shown that GBV-C/HGV can establish chronic infection with RNA persistence in serum for up to 15 years. A proportion of patients clear the virus spontaneously and develop anti-E2 reactivity, which is used as a marker of past infection. Anti-E2 also seems to confer protective immunity. A large body of evidence suggests that GBV-C/HGV does not cause liver disease.

TT virus (TTV)

TTV was identified in 1997 by investigators in Japan. By applying the methodology used for the identification of GBV-C, they detected the genome of a new DNA virus in the serum of a patient with cryptogenic post-transfusion hepatitis. The patient's initials (TT) prompted the name of this new virus and a causative role for acute and chronic hepatitis was suggested. TTV and its smaller variant are now spelt as Torque teno virus (TTV) and Torque teno mini virus (TTMV), after the Latin for 'thin necklace'.

The TTV genome is circular, single-stranded DNA of approximately 3850 nucleotides (Table 7.5.21.1). Three partially open reading frames have been predicted, but TTV proteins have not been expressed, so far. It is suggested that TTV belongs to a new family—Circinoviridae. TTV DNA has been detected in nonhuman primates and in farm animals. The primary site of TTV replication and the biological nature of TTV are still unknown.

Unlike other DNA viruses, TTV shows remarkable genomic variability. Phylogenetic analyses of TTV isolates have identified at least 20 genotypes, which differ between each other by more than 40% of the DNA sequences. As recombinant viral proteins are not available, the diagnosis of TTV infection is based on the detection of TTV DNA by PCR. TT virus population is very heterogeneous, and frequently a mixed infection with 3 to 5 TTV genotypes is present in one patient.

TTV infection is ubiquitous in more than 90% of adults worldwide. The virus was initially thought to have mainly a parenteral route of transmission, although the high prevalence of TTV infection in the general population indicates the importance of nonparenteral routes as well. The prevalence of TTV infection was shown to increase with age in paediatric and adult groups.

The pathogenic role of TTV, if any, is unknown. Analysis of liver histology in patients with TTV infection, longitudinal studies, as well as experimental TTV inoculation in chimpanzees all demonstrate that this virus does not cause hepatitis. Possible associations with other diseases, such as severe idiopathic inflammatory myopathies, lupus, and acute respiratory diseases in infants, have been suggested. However, TTV remains an example of a human virus with no clear disease association.

SEN virus (SEN-V)

SEN-V is a recently discovered single-stranded DNA virus, distantly related to TTV, with a worldwide distribution. Eight genotypes of SEN-V, designated A to H, have been identified. SEN-V is transmitted via transfusion of blood products and parenteral contact. Interest in SEN-V was triggered by the initial reports that two SEN-V genotypes, SEN-V-D and H, were associated with post-transfusion non-A, non-E hepatitis. No causative agent and no evidence of hepatitis due to SEN-V infection have yet been established.

Further reading

Hino S, Miyata H (2007). Torque teno virus (TTV): current status. *Rev Med Virol*, **17**, 45–57.

Hoofnagle JH, *et al.* (2007). Management of hepatitis B: summary of a clinical research workshop. *Hepatology*, **45**, 1056–75.

Naoumov NV (2006). Hepatitis A and E. *Medicine*, **35**, 35–38.

Rehermann B, Nascimbeni M (2005). Immunology of hepatitis B virus and hepatitis C virus infection. *Nat Rev Immunol*, **5**, 215–29.

Taylor JM (2006). Structure and replication of hepatitis delta virus RNA. *Curr Top Microbiol Immunol*, **307**, 1–23.

Tellinghuisen TL, *et al.* (2007). Studying hepatitis C virus: making the best of a bad virus. *J Virol*, **81**, 8853–67.

7.5.22 Hepatitis C

Paul Klenerman, K.J.M. Jeffery, and J. Collier

Essentials

Hepatitis C virus (HCV) is an RNA virus that has evolved into multiple genotypes (1–6) and subtypes. Humans are the only known natural host. HCV replication is highly error-prone, hence within any one person the virus exists as a swarm of closely related variants, known as 'quasispecies'.

Epidemiology—HCV is a major cause of liver disease worldwide, with 170 million people probably infected. Spread is parenteral and usually associated with needle use, most commonly by intravenous drug users in the West; mother to child infection does occur but is infrequent, as is sexual spread. Before the screening of blood products was introduced, blood recipients and patients with haemophilia were also at risk, and outbreaks in some countries (e.g. Egypt) have been associated with mass parenteral therapy programmes.

Clinical aspects—these are discussed in detail in Chapter 15.21.1, but HCV tends to become persistent in most of those infected, although around 25% clear the virus as a result of effective innate and adaptive immune responses at the time of acute infection.

The clinical course is variable in those with persistent infection: most develop some degree of hepatic inflammation and fibrotic liver disease, with a fraction going on to develop cirrhosis, with an increased risk of hepatocellular carcinoma. Cofactors which predispose to progression include simultaneous HIV infection and drinking alcohol.

Treatment: now and in the future—treatment is currently a combination of pegylated interferon-α and ribavirin, with outcome dependent on viral genotype. In future, therapies directed against specific viral gene products such as protease and polymerase may be useful, but the capacity of the virus to mutate and thus evade both drug therapy and immune responses is a major barrier to progress.

Introduction

Hepatitis C virus (HCV) is a major global pathogen. Humans are the only known natural hosts, although chimpanzees have been infected experimentally. The origin of the virus in humans is not well established, but the huge genetic diversity and global distribution, together with analyses of the viral molecular clock, suggest that it has coevolved with human populations for centuries. In the 1990s, spread through changes in medical practice and intravenous drug use was recognized to have created an emerging problem. The capacity of the virus to persist despite host innate and adaptive immune responses makes it extremely hard to develop vaccines. Although there have been major improvements in the efficacy of treatment regimens, they are still expensive, hard to deliver, and associated with serious side effects. Therefore, it is important to identify those who are most likely to benefit from the available therapies, based on the observed progression and likely response to treatment. Improved understanding of the viral replication cycle and the most effective immune responses is leading to more selective drugs and vaccines.

Historical perspective

Previously known as non-A, non-B hepatitis, HCV was recognized for many years before its discovery by Kuo and Houghton in 1988. It was soon identified as a major infectious agent and the development of antibody-based assays revealed its prevalence, and allowed the development of screening tools for blood products. The majority of chronic viral carriers were identified by detection of viral RNA in blood, while sequencing and bioinformatics approaches led to the description of diverse viral genotypes. Inability to culture the virus proved a major obstacle, but the development of a replicon system by Bartenschlager in 1999 was a major breakthrough, allowing a dissection of viral replication *in vitro*. However, no infectious virus system was available until 2005, when several groups used an unusual Japanese strain (JFH-1) to develop cell culture infectious systems.

Aetiology, genetics, pathogenesis, and pathology

HCV is a positive-sense single-stranded RNA virus. It is classed individually as an hepacivirus and is genetically closely related to flaviviruses, such as dengue. The viral RNA genome is approximately 10 kb in length and comprises a long, single open reading frame. The genome is typically divided into structural and nonstructural proteins. The structural proteins, contained within virions, comprise core and envelope (E1 and E2). The latter are glycosylated, form a heterodimer, and are important targets for antibodies. They are also highly variable and contain hypervariable regions (HVR1 and HVR2), which evolve rapidly under antibody selection pressure. The nonstructural proteins include enzymes with defined protease and helicase activity, and a viral polymerase.

Viral replication is initiated using an internal ribosomal entry site (IRES) in the 5′ untranslated region (5′ UTR). The latter is highly conserved, varying only slightly between genotypes and so is an important target for molecular diagnosis. The polymerase replicates the virus through a double-stranded intermediate, which is a substantial trigger for host innate responses. However, the virus can disable triggering of one of these pathways (RIG-I; retinoic acid inducible gene I) through the action of the protease, which cleaves a cellular target (Cardif; CARD adapter inducing interferon (IFN)-β). Another important feature is that replication is highly error-prone. Thus, within any one person, the virus exists as a swarm of closely related variants, known as 'quasispecies'.

HCV usually replicates in hepatocytes. Virus has been observed in other cell types, including lymphocytes and dendritic cells, and within the central nervous system, but it is uncertain how this contributes to disease pathogenesis. A number of cellular receptors for HCV have been described including: CD81 (a member of the tetraspanin family with signalling properties on lymphocytes); the LDL (low-density lipoprotein) receptor; DC-SIGN (dendritic cell-specific ICAM3-grabbing nonintegrin); a macrophage scavenger receptor class B1 (SR B1); and Claudin-1, a component of tight junctions. None of these fully explains the hepatotropism of the virus.

After natural or experimental infection, virus may be detectable for weeks or months without any apparent clinical, biochemical, or immunological disturbance. During this time, virus may replicate to high levels in blood and within the liver, indicating the minimal direct cytopathic effects of the virus in the absence of host immune responses. This silent phase is followed by the onset of acute hepatitis, which is not always clinically apparent. Detailed intrahepatic studies in animal models (not possible in man) reveal that the first responses at this stage of infection are production of innate immune mediators (IFNs, NK cells), followed by an influx of T cells (both CD4+ and CD8+). In studies of human acute hepatitis C, the emergence of highly activated, virus-specific CD8+ T cells correlates quantitatively and temporally with the peak of the alanine aminotransferase (ALT), suggesting that tissue damage at this stage is a result largely of the host T-cell response.

The subsequent events vary substantially between different patients, but three clinical patterns are observed: clearance of virus below the level of detection in blood; persistence of virus without host control; or an intermediate state, where the virus is transiently controlled, but relapses. The immunological differences determining these outcomes are not clear, but the association of specific HLA genes, both class II (such as *HLA DR11/DQ3*) and class I (such as *HLA B27* and *B57*), with spontaneous resolution point to the importance of T-cell responses. The broader and more sustained in number and function the responses are, the more likely they are to be successful in viral control. B-Cell responses are also likely to be involved. However, the rapid emergence of viral escape mutants in the hypervariable envelope regions may limit the efficacy of neutralizing antibody responses in containing viral replication. Viral mutation within T-cell epitopes is also a major cause of persistence despite T-cell responses, although other phenomena such as T-cell exhaustion and the emergence of regulatory T-cell subsets also contribute to T-cell failure.

In the 25% in whom virus is cleared below the level of detection long term, antibody and T-cell responses may be detected for many years. In most people, virus persists after the acute hepatitis, despite the presence of antibody. T-Cell responses in blood at this stage are weak, but infiltrates of T cells may be found within the liver.

Liver histopathology due to HCV infection can vary greatly, and there is no diagnostic staining pattern. Portal tract infiltrates of T and B cells are typical, sometimes with the emergence of lymphoid follicles within liver tissue. Histological scores (Ishak's, Metavir) have been developed to quantify the degree of liver damage. These assess the degree of hepatic inflammation (typically portal tract infiltration, 'interface' hepatitis, lobular infiltration and necrosis), and the degree of hepatic fibrosis.

The viral genotype is not thought to have a major effect on pathogenesis, although genotype 3 has been associated with the development of hepatic steatosis, which might contribute to increased inflammation and fibrosis.

Epidemiology

HCV is estimated to infect around 170 million people worldwide. Spread is parenteral, and usually associated with needle use (intravenous drug users, patients in parenteral therapy programmes, nosocomial spread) and exposure to infected blood products (recipients of unscreened blood or plasma fractions, haemophiliacs). Mother to child infection does occur, but at relatively low rates (around 3–5%), and sexual spread is also infrequent.

In the West, intravenous drug users have particularly high rates of acquisition and now represent the main focus of the infection. In some countries, notably Egypt, medical programmes have resulted in the spread of HCV in specific groups, and the 20 to 30% prevalence of HCV in some communities in Egypt is the highest worldwide.

HCV has evolved into multiple genotypes (1–6) and subtypes. Molecular typing techniques can trace the spread of individual strains within populations (including those from a single source). The Egyptian outbreak is genotype 4a, the older circulating western strains were typically genotype 1a and 1b, and the more recent strains acquired by western drug users are 3a. Genotype 3 viruses were originally found in Asia, where genotype 6 is still prevalent. Genotypes 2 and 5 have remained mainly localized to West and South Africa respectively, but all strains are tending to spread worldwide.

Prevention

Primary prevention

There are no licensed HCV vaccines. Primary prevention of HCV worldwide depends on ensuring a safe blood supply and sterile injection devices for all health care applications. Provision of sterile equipment to intravenous drug users has been shown to reduce the prevalence of HCV. Infection is not transmitted by normal household exposure, but household contacts of HCV positive people should avoid sharing razors and toothbrushes. Sexual transmission of HCV is inefficient and studies show a low prevalence (average: 1.5%) of HCV infection in long-term partners of patients with chronic HCV infection who had no other risk factors. Multiple published studies have demonstrated that the prevalence of HCV infection among homosexual men who were not injecting drugs, was similar to that in heterosexuals, although there has been recent spread within HIV-positive communities.

No intervention has been shown clearly to decrease the risk of mother to child transmission of HCV, and breastfeeding is not discouraged. The risk of mother to child transmission is increased two to threefold if there is HIV/HCV coinfection. Medical workers should ensure aseptic techniques and appropriate equipment and facilities to reduce the risk of percutaneous injury.

Postexposure prophylaxis

Immune globulin is not effective in preventing HCV infection postexposure. Anyone exposed to the virus, e.g. via an injury or perinatally, should be offered follow-up testing for HCV. The average risk of infection following a percutaneous injury is 1.8% (range 0–7%) and those who become infected should be offered early antiviral therapy.

Clinical features

Acute hepatitis C

Acute HCV infection is usually asymptomatic, but is otherwise clinically indistinguishable from other causes of acute viral hepatitis. There is prodromal fever, myalgia, and malaise. Compared with hepatitis A or B, classical symptoms of jaundice, pruritus, pale stools, and dark urine are unusual. Serum transaminase levels can be markedly elevated, although values of up to 10 times the upper limit of normal would be more usual. Fulminant hepatic failure is rare in acute HCV. There is evidence that patients with symptomatic acute HCV have a higher rate of spontaneous viral clearance than those with asymptomatic infection. Overall, approximately one in four patients will clear the virus spontaneously. In those with persistent virus, serum transaminases may return to normal, but they usually remain elevated at about twice the upper limit of normal (Fig. 7.5.22.1).

Chronic infection

Chronic infection with HCV is defined as the persistence of HCV RNA in blood for more than 6 months. Most patients with chronic HCV are unaware of their diagnosis, and many will have been tested following an incidental finding of abnormal liver function tests or on routine screening, e.g. for blood donation, or having given a history of potential HCV exposure, such as intravenous drug use. Such patients may be asymptomatic or have nonspecific symptoms such as fatigue. Clinical features of liver disease are unlikely to be present unless cirrhosis has developed. Hypoalbuminaemia, thrombocytopenia, and coagulopathy suggest cirrhosis, although this can only be diagnosed definitively by liver biopsy.

HCV is associated with several extrahepatic manifestations, the best documented of which are HCV-related lymphoproliferative disorders, characteristically with mixed cryoglobulinaemia. Although studies suggest a high prevalence of serum cryoglobulins in HCV-positive patients, they are generally present at low levels with few, if any, symptoms. Occasionally, patients will present with neuropathies, arthralgias, and purpura. In more severe cases, there may be kidney involvement. In some studies, B-cell non-Hodgkin's lymphomas, porphyria cutanea tarda, Sjögren's syndrome, lichen

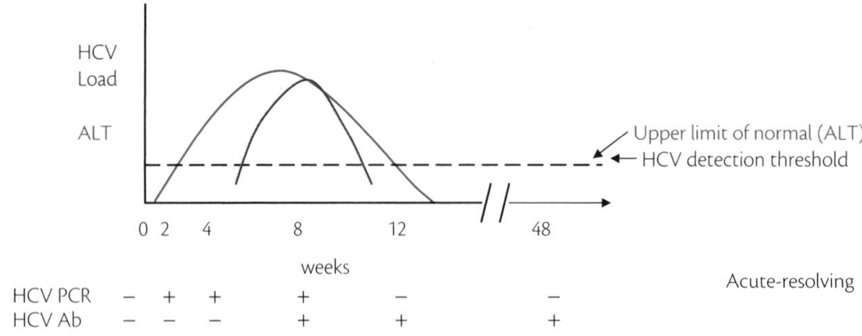

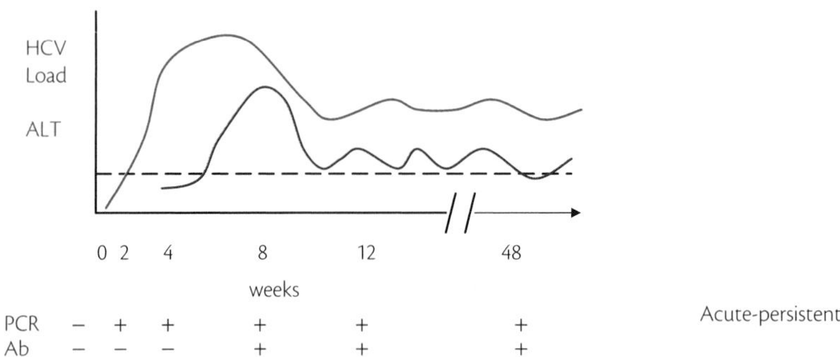

Fig. 7.5.22.1 Typical virological and biochemical test results following infection with hepatitis C in (a) patients who clear the virus (acute resolving) and (b) those that go on to get persistent infection (acute persistent). The time lines vary between patients and these are approximations based on human and chimpanzee model infections. Some patients, such as those with HIV, may never develop an antibody response. ALT, alanine aminotransferase.

planus, autoimmune thyroiditis, and type 2 diabetes mellitus have been found more commonly in association with HCV infection than in control groups.

Prognosis

The rate of progression of HCV is highly variable. Risk factors for progression include: older age at acquisition of infection; male gender; immunosuppression including coinfection with HIV; and concurrent heavy alcohol consumption. It is estimated that 7 to 20% will develop cirrhosis within 20 years of infection. Progression rates are highest in those with transfusion-associated hepatitis. However, some groups, such as a cohort of Irish women infected in 1977 through contaminated blood products, show very low rates, with only 3% developing cirrhosis within 20 years of infection.

Once cirrhosis has developed, 80% will have complications such as ascites and variceal bleeding within 10 years. Fifty per cent of these patients will develop liver failure within a further 5 years. Hepatocellular carcinoma occurs only in the presence of cirrhosis, with an incidence of 1 to 5% per year. HIV coinfected patients progress more rapidly to liver failure once complications of cirrhosis have occurred.

Liver transplantation is indicated for decompensated HCV cirrhosis and for cirrhotics who develop a small hepatocellular carcinoma despite good liver function. The infection always recurs in the transplanted liver and progression to cirrhosis occurs in about 10% of transplant recipients within 5 years. Only about 20% of patients with recurrent HCV post-transplantation can be cured with pegylated IFN and ribavirin, which is often poorly tolerated.

Diagnosis

Serology

Initial diagnosis of HCV infection is usually made by detecting HCV antibody to recombinant HCV proteins in sensitive screening immunoassays. In low prevalence populations, the probability of a false positive antibody result is high, and supplementary confirmatory tests should be performed, such as immunoassays using different antigens. Alternatively, highly specific line or strip immunoblots (which have individual synthetic or recombinant antigens applied as separate lines to a solid phase) can distinguish different antigens to which the serum is reacting, and confirm the presence of HCV antibody.

Recent developments include assays which combine tests for antibody and HCV core antigen. These are more useful for the diagnosis of acute infection (Fig. 7.5.22.1). These assays are likely to be particularly useful for screening blood donations in developing countries. The appearance of HCV antibody after infection can take up to 2 months in immunocompetent people, and may be delayed or even absent in immunocompromised patients, such as those with HIV infection or those who are on haemodialysis. By 6 months, 97% of those infected will have developed an antibody response. It is good practice to confirm the presence of HCV antibody with a second sample.

HCV RNA testing

Nucleic acid tests are essential for the diagnosis of acute and chronic HCV infection, and are increasingly being used as supplementary tests for confirmation of HCV antibody tests. HCV RNA can be detected by polymerase chain reaction (PCR) as early as 2 weeks postinfection, before the appearance of antibody. Several amplification techniques, including reverse transcriptase PCR (RT-PCR), transcription-mediated amplification (TMA), and branched DNA (bDNA) are available. Most commercial assays now produce quantitative results with increasingly sensitive limits of detection. Although quantitative tests (i.e. a measure of viral load, which may vary across several logs between individuals) may be important to predict the response to IFN therapy (see below), in contrast to HIV infection they are not useful in predicting disease severity or long-term progression. Some countries have successfully introduced nucleic acid screening of pools of samples for blood donation.

Pretreatment evaluation

HCV virus genotyping is essential before treatment as it determines the duration of treatment and the response (see below). Most genotyping methods are based on viral sequencing and subsequent phylogenetic analysis, or on the detection of nucleic acid mutations specific for individual genotypes. A pretreatment liver biopsy is frequently, but not always, performed to assess the degree of fibrosis. Noninvasive methods of assessing the degree of liver fibrosis using serum markers, and assessment of liver stiffness using an ultrasound probe (e.g. Fibroscan, FibroSure/FibroTest) are being evaluated.

Treatment

The aim of HCV therapy is to eradicate HCV RNA from serum. Although loss of viraemia is associated with improvement in liver histology, the risk of hepatocellular carcinoma remains if cirrhosis is present. Tumours have been detected up to 5 years after successful treatment with antiviral therapy. Screening of cirrhotic patients for hepatocellular carcinoma should therefore be continued.

HCV viraemia may re-emerge within 6 months of stopping treatment (relapse), but those who remain HCV RNA negative for 6 months are considered to be cured (sustained response) and viraemia will not recur.

Chronic hepatitis C

Interferon-α and ribavirin are the treatments for chronic infection. Interferon-α induces the expression of multiple genes with antiviral and antiproliferative actions, including those encoding RNAses, 2′,5′-oligoadenylate synthetase, and protein kinase R. It is administered subcutaneously three times a week. It has been largely superseded by pegylated IFNs which have the advantages that they need only be given once weekly and are more effective when used with ribavirin. The two types of pegylated IFN-α, 2a and 2b, are IFN-α molecules with modified side chains that prolong their half-lives.

Ribavirin is a guanosine analogue which does not reduce HCV RNA levels when used alone but sustains virological suppression when combined with IFN-α. Combination treatment with ribavirin (800–1000 mg/day orally) and pegylated IFN-α180 μg/kg subcutaneously weekly for IFN-α2a, or 1.5 μg/kg subcutaneously weekly for IFN-α2b) is successful in 56% of all patients. It is less effective against genotype 1 than genotype 3, which in turn is less effective than genotype 2. Up to 12 months of therapy is required for genotype 1 patients to give a sustained virological response in 42 to 46%. A shorter duration of therapy, 6 months, and lower doses of ribavirin can be given for genotypes 2 and 3, which achieve a cure in 76 to 82%. Twelve months therapy is needed for the rarer genotype 4 infection, with slightly better outcome than for genotype 1.

For genotype 1 infections, treatment is usually stopped after 3 months of therapy if HCV RNA is detected in serum, because continuing for 12 months is only curative in 6%. Coinfection with HIV is not a contraindication to therapy, although the efficacy of treatment is reduced. Twelve months of ribavirin and pegylated IFN-ααresults in a sustained viral response in 29% of genotype 1 HCV/HIV coinfected patients and 62% in those with genotype 2 or 3.

Side effects of treatment are common and the quality of life is universally affected, although many patients are able to continue work during therapy. Treatment with IFN-α is associated with fatigue, depression, and mood swings. Other side effects include rashes and thyroid abnormalities. Flu-like symptoms are frequent within 6 h of the first dose, but often improve over the first few weeks. Bone marrow suppression is common and may warrant dose reductions, a particular problem in cirrhotic patients who are pancytopenic before starting treatment. IFN-α is contraindicated in renal and cardiac transplant recipients for fear of inducing acute cellular rejection. Ribavirin causes haemolysis and frequently leads to a 2 to 3 g/dl drop in haemoglobin during treatment. As it is excreted by the kidney, it is contraindicated in renal failure.

Acute hepatitis C

The results of treating acute HCV are much better than in chronic infection. Up to 50% of patients with acute symptomatic HCV may clear the virus spontaneously within the first 3 months. Treatment should be started between 12 and 24 weeks of infection, allowing time to assess whether spontaneous resolution has occurred, without losing the clinical benefit of early treatment. Genotype does not substantially affect response and cure rates of 80 to 95% can be achieved with 6 months of monotherapy using pegylated IFN.

The optimal regimen for treatment of acute hepatitis C remains to be determined. Guidelines suggest that pegylated IFN should be used in equivalent doses to those in chronic infection, and that ribavirin may be added (800 mg daily), although success may be achieved with monotherapy. At least 24 weeks of therapy is recommended.

Areas of uncertainty or controversy

The significance of finding residual viral RNA in lymphocytes and liver tissue after successful treatment with HCV or spontaneous resolution of acute infection is unclear. The mechanism of action of ribavirin, including its effect on the immune response, is not understood. The role of immunity in the pathogenesis of HCV and the response to treatment in acute and chronic infection is debated.

Likely future developments

Treatment is likely to become tailored according to the dynamics of the initial response to therapy. Patients with genotype 2 and 3 virus who become nonviraemic within a month of starting combination therapy (a rapid virological response (RVR), defined as an undetectable serum HCV RNA at week 4 of treatment) may be treated with a shorter 12 to 16 week course of therapy. Similarly, genotype 1 patients with a low baseline viral load (e.g. below 200 000 IU/ml) who have an RVR at 4 weeks may have their treatment shortened to 6 months, as studies show that the sustained virological response rates are comparable with treatment for 12 months in this group.

New drugs have been developed which interfere with viral proteases, RNA polymerase, as well as Toll-like receptor agonists and caspase inhibitors. Recent Phase II studies of the protease inhibitor Telapravir in combination with standard of care medication show an 80% sustained response rate in treatment naive genoytpe 1 patients; other agents show similar promise. Treatment regimes in the future are likely to include these drugs in combination with pegylated IFN-α and ribavirin; the addition of such novel drugs has been shown to shorten treatment times and increase response rates.

Accessibility of current and newer HCV treatments on a global scale is essential if cirrhosis and hepatocellular carcinoma are to be prevented in most of the world's HCV-infected population.

Further reading

Benvegnu L, *et al.* (2004). Natural history of compensated viral cirrhosis: a prospective study on the incidence and hierarchy of major complications. *Gut*, **53**, 744–49. [Important study showing the risk of complications of cirrhosis occurring over a 10 year period of follow-up.]

Dienstag JL, McHutchison JG (2006). American Gastroenterological Association technical review on the management of hepatitis C. *Gastroenterology*, **130**, 231–64. [Comprehensive review of the management of HCV.]

Feld JJ, Hoofnagle JH (2005). Mechanism of action of interferon and ribavirin in treatment of hepatitis C. *Nature*, **436**, 967–72. [A review of how interferon and ribavirin act to eliminate HCV, with data on viral kinetics during treatment.]

Gee I, Alexander G (2005). Liver transplantation for hepatitis C virus related liver disease. *Postgrad Med J*, **81**, 765–71. [Comprehensive review of management of recurrent HCV following liver transplantation and natural history.]

Hadziyannis SJ, *et al.* (2004). Peginterferon –alpha 2a and ribavirin combination therapy in chronic hepatitis C: a randomized study of treatment duration ribavirin dose. *Ann Intern Med*, **140**, 346–55. [A study showing that it is possible to treat genotypes 2 and 3 HCV with lower doses of ribavirin and shorter courses of pegylated interferon-α.]

Pépin J, Labbé AC (2008). Noble goals, unforeseen consequences: control of tropical diseases in colonial Central Africa and the iatrogenic transmission of blood-borne viruses. *Trop Med Int Health*, **13**, 744–53.

Levine RA, *et al.* (2006). Assessment of fibrosis progression in untreated Irish women with chronic hepatitis C contracted from immunoglobulin anti-D. *Clin-Gastroenterol Hepatol*, **4**, 1271–7. [Study of young women infected with hepatitis C showing that the risk of progression to cirrhosis 20 years following infection is much lower than 20% in some cohorts.]

Johnson RJ, *et al.* (1993). Membranoproliferative glomerulonephritis associated with hepatitis C virus infection. *N Engl J Med*, **328**, 465–70. [One of the earliest papers to make a clear association between hepatitis C infection and an extrahepatic disorder.]

Maheshwari A, Ray S, Thuluvath PJ (2008). Acute hepatitis C. *Lancet*, **372**, 321–32. [A comprehensive review of the presentation and treatment of acute hepatitis C.]

Manns MP, *et al.* (2001). Peginterferon alfa -2b plus ribavirin compared with interferon alfa-2b plus ribavirin for initial treatment of chronic HCV: a randomised trial. *Lancet*, **358**, 958–65. [One of two large studies showing the improved efficacy of pegylated interferon in combination with ribavirin over standard interferon-α.]

McHutchison JG, *et al.* (2009). Telaprevir with peginterferon and ribavirin for chronic HCV genotype 1 infection. *N Engl J Med*, **360**, 1827–38. [Shows the added benefit of a novel targeted protease inhibitor in improved SVR and reduced treatment times for genotype 1.]

Micallef JM, Kaldor JM, Dore GJ (2006). Spontaneous viral clearance following acute hepatitis C infection: a systematic review of longitudinal studies. *J Viral Hepat*, **13**, 34–41. [Although clearance rates in the 19 studies (682 individuals) reviewed in this paper range from 0–80%, the overall clearance rate was 26%, with the largest study (67 individuals) having a clearance rate close to this. Women appeared to have a higher clearance rate than men.]

Poynard T, Bedossa P, Opolon P (1997). Natural history of liver fibrosis progression in patients with chronic hepatitis C. The OBSVIRC, METAVIR, CLINIVIR, and DOSVIRC groups. *Lancet*, **349**, 825–32. [The first large retrospective cross-sectional study showing the wide variation in progression of hepatitis C fibrosis with cirrhosis occurring in around 20% within 20 years of infection.]

Thursz M, *et al.* (1999). Influence of MHC class II genotype on outcome of infection with hepatitis C virus. The HENCORE group. Hepatitis C European Network for Cooperative Research. *Lancet*, **354**, 2119–24. [A host genetics study confirming the importance of specific HLA Class II genes (and CD4+ T cells) in determining the outcome of HCV.]

Walker C, Bowen, D (2005). Adaptive immune responses in acute and chronic hepatitis C virus infection. *Nature*, **436**, 946–52. [A comprehensive account of the immunological responses against hepatitis C virus in human and model studies, including a discussion of the importance of immune escape through mutation.]

Wakita T, *et al.* (2005). Production of infectious hepatitis C virus in tissue culture from a cloned viral genome. *Nat Med*, **11**, 791–6. [A description of tissue culture replication competent virus—one of the studies opening the way to address fundamental aspects of HCV biology *in vitro*.]

Zignego AL, *et al.* (2006). Extrahepatic manifestations of Hepatitis C Virus infection: A general overview and guidelines for a clinical approach. *Dig Liver Dis*, **39**, 2–17. [A review outlining recent evidence for extrahepatic disorders possibly associated with hepatitis C.]

7.5.23 HIV/AIDS

Graz A. Luzzi, T.E.A. Peto, P. Goulder, and C.P. Conlon

Essentials

Since its discovery in 1983, the human immunodeficiency virus (HIV) has been associated with a global pandemic that has affected more than 50 million people and caused many millions of deaths. The highest prevalence rates are in sub-Saharan Africa and other parts of the developing world. The impact of HIV in some African countries has been sufficient to reverse population growth and reduce life expectancy into the mid thirties, although HIV incidence has recently declined in some of these high-prevalence countries. However, there are large-scale epidemics of HIV elsewhere, e.g. India, the Russian Federation, and eastern Europe.

Transmission

Worldwide, the principal mode of transmission is heterosexual intercourse. Other risk factors for acquisition of HIV include unprotected sex between men, injecting drug use, blood or blood products, and mother to child transmission.

Cellular biology

HIV-1 (derived from a simian immunodeficiency virus in the chimpanzee) and HIV-2 (animal reservoir the sooty mangabey monkey) belong to the lentivirus subfamily of retroviruses. The viral genes in infectious particles are carried as RNA, but upon infection of the host cell, reverse transcriptase catalyses the synthesis of a double-stranded DNA viral genome that is inserted into the chromosomal DNA of the infected cell by viral integrase.

Genomic structure—HIV has only nine genes: (1) *gag*—encoding the core proteins p17, p24, and p15; (2) *pol*—encoding the enzymes protease, reverse transcriptase, and integrase; (3) *env*—encoding envelope glycoproteins (gp120 and gp41); (4) two major regulatory genes—*tat* and *rev*—encoding proteins that are not assembled into the virus but are essential for replication in the cell; (5) four accessory genes, whose functions are not clearly understood.

HIV receptors and cellular tropism—CD4 is the cell surface receptor for HIV, which binds to it via gp120; gp41 is then thought to effect membrane fusion. However, another cellular component or coreceptor is required, and different substrains of HIV (even those isolated from the same patient) exhibit specific tropisms for different cell types in culture, dependent on the ability of each particular substrain to bind to particular chemokine receptor family coreceptors.

Knowledge of the cell biology of HIV has facilitated the development of pharmacological agents that have transformed the disease from a uniformly fatal illness to a chronic condition in those countries able to provide antiretroviral treatment.

Diagnostic tests and screening

Reliable tests that detect HIV antibodies are used for diagnosis and screening. In all countries, many HIV-infected people are unaware of the fact, increasing the risk of sexual and perinatal transmission and requiring the development of targeted screening programmes.

Clinical features

Primary HIV infection—a few weeks after acquisition of HIV, many people develop a nonspecific influenza-like illness (seroconversion illness/acute retroviral syndrome), with a transient macular or maculopapular rash affecting the upper body. Rarely, there are neurological complications and severe immunodeficiency with secondary opportunistic infections. Most do not seek medical help, and whether treatment of primary HIV infection with antiretroviral drugs would improve long term prognosis is not known.

Clinical latency—following primary infection (symptomatic or asymptomatic) a period of clinical latency follows, typically lasting 8 to 10 years before development of further illness. The infected person is asymptomatic, but some have persistent generalized lymphadenopathy, and they may develop minor opportunistic conditions affecting the skin and mucous membranes, e.g. viral warts, oropharyngeal candidiasis, oral hairy leucoplakia.

Progression to symptomatic HIV disease (AIDS)—the value of making a distinction between AIDS and HIV infection at other stages is questionable, especially in industrialized countries: it is more useful to consider progressive HIV disease as a continuous spectrum. Complications of late-stage HIV disease include (1) opportunistic infections—e.g. pneumocystis pneumonia, oesophageal candidiasis, cerebral toxoplasmosis, and cytomegalovirus retinitis; (2) opportunistic tumours—e.g. Kaposi's sarcoma and non-Hodgkin's lymphoma; and (3) direct HIV effects—e.g. HIV encephalopathy/dementia.

Clinical management and prognosis

CD4 lymphocyte count and HIV viral load are the two laboratory markers with the best prognostic value. (1) CD4 count—this is an indicator of HIV-related immune impairment, with decline to below 200/mm^3 associated with the risk of life-threatening opportunistic infection; antiretroviral treatment is currently considered when it has fallen to around 350/mm^3. (2) Viral load—quantitative estimation of HIV RNA in the blood plasma adds additional prognostic information before starting antiretroviral treatment, and is useful in monitoring the effectiveness of therapy, which aims to maintain suppression of viral RNA at undetectable levels (<20 copies/ml). The choice of initial antiretroviral regimen should take into account the results of baseline genotypic resistance testing.

Prognosis—the outlook for people with HIV infection in well-resourced countries was transformed in the late 1990s by the advent of highly active antiretroviral therapy (HAART), but access to antiretroviral drugs continues to be difficult in less-developed countries (see Chapter 7.5.24).

Drug regimen—more than 20 agents are now available: a minimum of 3, drawn from at least 2 drug classes, is required for effective treatment. Initial regimens usually include (1) a backbone of two nucleoside analogues (inhibitors of HIV reverse transcriptase), e.g. lamivudine, emtricitabine, abacavir, or zidovudine, with either (2) a non-nucleoside reverse transcriptase inhibitor (NNRTI), e.g. efavirenz or nevirapine, or (3) a protease inhibitor, e.g. lopinavir, atazanavir, fosamprenavir. or saquinavir (usually ritonavir-boosted). Factors considered when selecting the initial antiretroviral combination include potential drug interactions with other medications, presence of renal or hepatic dysfunction, likelihood of pregnancy, and the presence of cardiovascular risk factors. An important development has been the availability of simplified regimens involving small numbers of tablets taken once or twice daily. Adherence to treatment and avoidance of suboptimal therapy (such as regimens involving fewer than three active agents, or use of agents in the presence of HIV mutations conferring resistance) are important in avoiding treatment failure.

Other drugs for HIV—(1) Nucleotide agent—tenofovir, which acts on the same target as the nucleoside analogues, has been a useful addition. (2) New agents in established drug classes—these have activity against HIV despite mutations conferring resistance to other drugs in the class, e.g. etravirine (a NNRTI), and tipranavir and darunavir (two relatively new protease inhibitors). (3) New drug classes—(a) entry inhibitors, including two subgroups, the fusion inhibitors (e.g. enfuvirtide), and the CCR5 co-receptor antagonists (e.g. maraviroc); (b) integrase inhibitors (e.g. raltegravir). The place of these newer agents in HIV therapy has not yet been clearly determined.

Adverse reactions to antiretroviral drugs—these are relatively common and include. (1) Short-term reactions—gastrointestinal disturbances, rashes, and neuropsychiatric reactions may require early adjustments to the treatment regimen. (2) Longer-term reactions—metabolic complications include (a) mitochondrial toxicity; and (b) disturbances of lipid and glucose metabolism associated with a risk of cardiovascular disease including myocardial infarction—the absolute risk is small but requires consideration in patients with pre-existing cardiovascular risk factors. (3) Paradoxical reactions—called immune reconstitution syndromes, these occur in up to 20% of patients starting treatment and include new or worsening inflammatory symptoms, especially in patients who have tuberculosis, *Mycobacterium avium* infection, cryptococcal meningitis, and cytomegalovirus retinitis.

Co-infections involving HIV and tuberculosis, hepatitis B or hepatitis C are common and require specialized treatment.

Prevention

Strategies to raise awareness and provide education, and promote risk reduction, underpin HIV control programmes worldwide. Control of coexistent sexually transmitted genital ulcers and other genital infections reduces HIV transmission. Mother to child transmission can be reduced to below 1% if antiretroviral treatment is administered to the mother during pregnancy, delivery is by planned caesarean section, and breastfeeding is avoided. No vaccine is available.

Introduction

Acquired immunodeficiency syndrome (AIDS) was first recognized in 1981 in the United States of America, when outbreaks of pneumocystis pneumonia and Kaposi's sarcoma were reported in homosexual men in New York and California. The variety of unusual infections and other conditions declared a new form of cellular immunodeficiency. In 1983, the causative retrovirus was isolated and subsequently named human immunodeficiency virus (HIV). At the time of its discovery, HIV was already widespread, the earliest infections probably having occurred before the 1950s.

In 1986, a second retrovirus causing AIDS, HIV-2, was identified in West Africa. It remains largely confined to this region, while HIV-1 is the cause of the world pandemic of AIDS. HIV infection may be regarded as a zoonosis: HIV-1 is derived from a simian immunodeficiency virus in the chimpanzee (*Pan troglodytes troglodytes*), and the animal reservoir for HIV-2 is the sooty mangabey monkey (*Cercocebus atys*).

Epidemiology

The global HIV-1 pandemic has had the greatest impact in developing countries (see Chapter 7.5.24). The World Health Organization (WHO) estimated that in 2006, 40 million people were living with HIV worldwide, of whom two-thirds were in sub-Saharan Africa (Fig. 7.5.23.1). Worldwide, the WHO estimated there were over 4 million new infections in 2006, 400 000 more than in 2004. Globally, AIDS caused 2.9 million deaths in 2006, almost three-quarters of which were in sub-Saharan Africa.

In North America, western Europe, and Australasia the epidemic began among homosexual men and injecting drug users. However, in these regions the proportion attributable to heterosexual transmission subsequently increased. In 2006, over 70 000 people were living with HIV in the United Kingdom, a third of whom were unaware of their diagnosis. The proportion of newly diagnosed cases in the United Kingdom attributed to heterosexual transmission rose steadily from 1999 onwards, largely due to increased numbers arriving from countries with high prevalence, and increased HIV detection through routine antenatal testing. However, injecting drug use, unprotected sex between men, and unprotected paid sex remain important modes of transmission in Europe, as well as in Asia and Latin America.

In contrast, HIV transmission in regions with the highest prevalence rates, such as sub-Saharan Africa, is predominantly heterosexual and perinatal. The estimated overall adult prevalence there is 6%, rising to between 20 and 30% in some countries such as Botswana and Zimbabwe, where AIDS has curtailed population growth and life expectancy has fallen into the mid 30's. Swaziland (population 1 million) is the country with the highest adult seroprevalence, of 33%. The country with more infected people than any other is believed to be South Africa (5.5 million adults living with HIV, adult seroprevalence 20%), although in India, where prevalence data are less easily accessible, the overall numbers may be similar (despite adult seroprevalence below 1%).

The overall prevalence of HIV has risen worldwide in recent years because new transmissions exceed AIDS-related deaths, and because antiretroviral treatment has reduced mortality. However, there have been notable declines in some high prevalence countries such as Kenya, Zimbabwe, and parts of India, and a levelling off in other parts of sub-Saharan Africa, attributable to prevention efforts. Uganda is seen as one of the best examples of

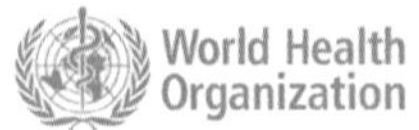

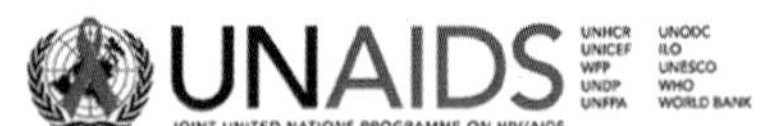

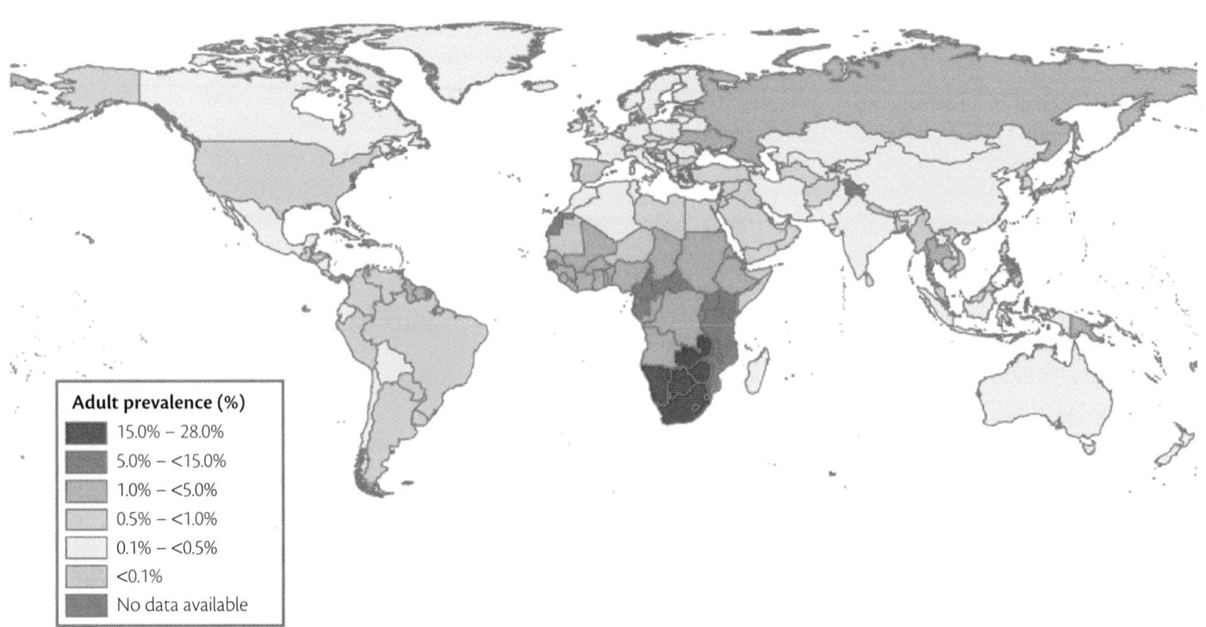

Fig. 7.5.23.1 World distribution of HIV, 2007.
(Reproduced with permission from: UNAIDS. *2008 Report on the global AIDS epidemic*, http://www.unaids.org/en/KnowledgeCentre/HIVData/GlobalReport/2008/2008_Global_report.asp)

a country where prevalence has declined significantly, believed to be, at least in part, due to the timely government campaign of public education.

The global distribution of HIV is currently characterized by very variable rates of prevalence and scattered areas of very high transmission in epidemics. Consequently, the risk of acquisition of HIV is also highly variable from region to region. In some countries, such as Russia and Ukraine, HIV has caused large scale epidemics and transmission rates remain high. The risk of onward transmission is especially high soon after sexual acquisition of HIV, when plasma viral load is high, and the virus is present in genital secretions in sexually active people. Therefore, it is particularly important to detect primary HIV infection in population screening programmes. HIV transmission continues at a high level in many countries because of poverty, low condom usage, high rates of other sexually transmitted infections, and higher risk behaviour such as unprotected paid sex and use of nonsterile injecting drug equipment.

HIV-2 is endemic in parts of West Africa and is also prevalent in Angola, Mozambique, France, and Portugal. In other parts of the world, the prevalence is very low, although it is present in India. The clinical features of HIV-2 are similar to those of HIV-1, but some patients with HIV-2 appear to progress much more slowly than those with HIV-1 for unknown reasons.

Variation of HIV-1 RNA sequences has been identified, leading to a classification of 11 sequence subtypes (or clades), A to K, of the main group M, and N (new) and O (outlier) as two quite distinct groups in west central Africa. The subtypes have varying geographical distributions. For instance, subtypes A and D are found in central Africa, B in North America and Europe, and E in Thailand. More people are infected with clade C virus than any other, being the predominant clade of virus in southern Africa as well as India. Study of the genetic and geographical divergence of subtypes has shed light on the emergence and global spread of HIV.

Cellular biology of HIV

The viral replication cycle

HIV-1 (Fig. 7.5.23.2) and HIV-2 belong to the lentivirus subfamily of retroviruses. Retrovirus implies a 'backwards' step in biological information during viral replication attributable to its enzyme, reverse transcriptase. As with all retroviruses, the viral genes in infectious particles are carried as RNA, but upon infection of the host cell, reverse transcriptase catalyses the synthesis of a double-stranded DNA viral genome (Fig. 7.5.23.3). Insertion of the DNA genome into the chromosomal DNA of the infected cell is effected by viral integrase. The integrated provirus may remain latent, particularly in resting lymphocytes. In actively infected cells, however, RNA transcripts and proteins are synthesized, leading to the formation of new virus particles.

The core proteins derived from the *gag* and *pol* genes are made as large polypeptides that are then cleaved into smaller components representing the enzymes and building blocks of the virus. This cleavage is achieved by the viral protease. The unique reverse transcriptase and protease are targets of antiretroviral therapy (see below). Reverse transcriptase inhibitors such as zidovudine and lamivudine affect an early step in HIV replication, whereas the protease inhibitors, such as saquinavir or lopinavir, block a late stage of virus assembly (Fig. 7.5.23.3). Compounds that inhibit any stage of HIV replication, without being too toxic to the infected person,

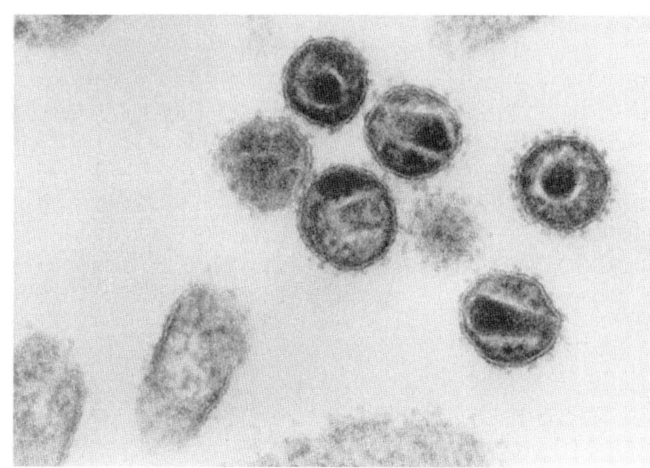

Fig. 7.5.23.2 Electron micrograph of HIV-1.
(Reproduced by courtesy of H Gelderblom.)

are potential antiviral drugs. Agents have recently been developed to block viral entry (e.g. fusion inhibitors) and integration into the host cell DNA (integrase inhibitors).

Although regarded as a complex retrovirus, HIV has only nine genes (Fig. 7.5.23.4). The three structural genes are *gag*, *pol*, and *env*, encoding the core proteins p17, p24, and p15, the enzymes (protease, reverse transcriptase, and integrase), and the envelope glycoproteins (gp120 and gp41), respectively. The major regulatory genes *tat* and *rev* encode proteins that are not assembled into the virus but are essential for replication in the cell. The Tat protein acts in positive feedback to enhance transcription of viral RNA from the DNA provirus, while the Rev protein helps the efficient transport of viral RNA from the nucleus to the cytoplasm. Either of these proteins could be a suitable target for antiviral therapy, particularly Tat, because the synthesis of all the other viral proteins depends on its activity.

The functions of the four accessory genes of HIV are less well understood. *Vif* encodes a protein assembled in virus particles that appears necessary for the infectivity ('viral infectivity factor') at a stage soon after entry. Vif binds and hastens the degradation of the cellular protein APOBEC which, in the absence of Vif, hypermutates HIV, thereby disabling it. *Nef* also affects an early postentry function; it is not needed by laboratory-adapted HIV strains or

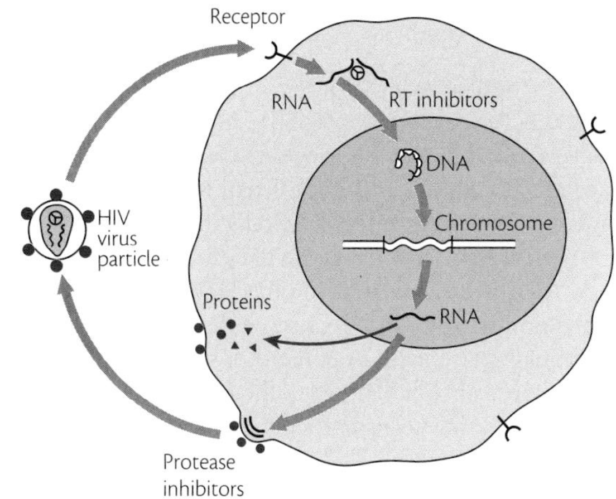

Fig. 7.5.23.3 Replicative cycle of HIV.

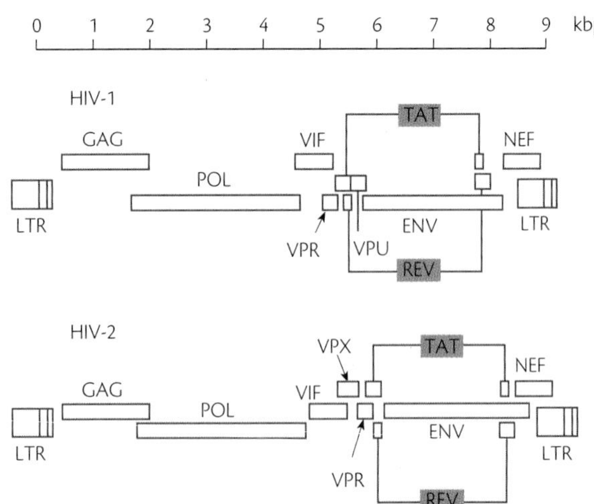

Fig. 7.5.23.4 HIV genome map.

if virus enters via endosomal vesicles rather than fusing with the outer cell membrane. It also down-regulates surface expression of the primary cell-surface receptor for HIV, the CD4 antigen, by drawing CD4 into clathrin-coated pits. *Vpu* similarly interacts with CD4, promoting its degradation by directing it to the ubiquitin–proteasome pathway. *Vpr* has dual functions; first, it directs the preintegration complex of the virus, containing the newly synthesized DNA, into the nucleus so that it can integrate into chromosomal DNA; second, it blocks cell proliferation in the G2 phase of the cell cycle, thereby enhancing the amount of viral progeny released per cell.

Unlike HIV-1, HIV-2 and the simian immunodeficiency viruses (SIV) lack *vpu*, but have an alternative gene, *vpx*. HIV-2 Vpr leads the viral genome into the cell nucleus, but does not arrest the cell cycle. These proteins presumably recognize cellular proteins and some of these interactions are species-specific. Thus the Vpr and Vif proteins in SIV of African green monkeys do not function in human cells, while the equivalent proteins of SIV from sooty mangabey monkeys work well in human cells. This could explain why sooty mangabey SIV was able to infect humans and become HIV-2, whereas the more widespread African green monkey SIV has not led to a zoonosis. Another difference is that HIV-1 incorporates the cellular protein cyclophilin A (the target of the drug ciclosporin A) into virus particles, where it may cooperate with Vif and is required for steps early in the infection. In contrast, HIV-2 does not contain cyclophylin A and replicates well without it.

HIV receptors and cellular tropism

CD4 is the cell-surface receptor for HIV; it is expressed on T-helper lymphocytes, the cells that become depleted in AIDS. CD4 is also expressed (to a lesser extent but sufficient to permit infection) on macrophages, Langerhans dendritic cells in mucous membranes, and brain microglial cells. These are the other target cells for HIV infection. CD4 is necessary to initiate HIV infection but is not sufficient to allow the virus to fuse with host-cell membranes: another cellular component or coreceptor is required.

Different substrains of HIV, even those isolated from the same patient, exhibit specific tropisms for different cell types in culture. All isolates can infect primary CD4 lymphocytes, but only some infect macrophages while others can infect cell lines established from CD4+ leukaemic cells. Macrophage-tropic strains predominate early in the course of HIV infection, and may be more transmissible from person to person. They do not cause CD4 lymphocytes to fuse together in culture and hence are referred to as non-syncytium-inducing (NSI) strains. In contrast, many HIV isolates established from late-stage infection rapidly adapt in culture to infect T-cell lines and are syncytium-inducing (SI). Approximately 50% of patients with AIDS develop SI strains in addition to NSI strains. The differences in cellular tropism and SI/NSI phenotype occur in all HIV subtypes or clades, which appear to reflect geographical variation of HIV rather than specific biological properties of the virus.

The complex cellular tropism of HIV has been explained by the discovery that different members of the chemokine receptor family act as coreceptors to CD4 for HIV entry into cells. Chemokines are chemoattractant, locally acting hormones or cytokines that bind to one or more receptors which are structurally related to olfactory and neurotransmitter receptors. Following binding to the CD4 receptor, primary NSI strains use CCR5, the chemokine receptor for macrophage-inhibitory proteins (MIP-1α, MIP-1β) and RANTES. In contrast, the SI strains of HIV use the CXCR4 coreceptor, the receptor for another chemokine, stromal-derived factor-1 (SDF-1). Other receptors such as CCR3 (the receptor of eotaxin) can be used by some NSI strains.

High levels of MIP-1α or -β in the blood correlate with relative resistance to HIV infection. Some exposed yet uninfected individuals are homozygous for an inherited defect of the CCR5 receptor involving a 32 bp deletion in the *CCR5* gene. This mutation is present in approximately 20% of white people (approximately 1% of white people are homozygous), but is not found in African and Asian populations. Individuals who are homozygous for the deletion are healthy, indicating that the CCR5 receptor is not essential for the development of immune competence, probably because MIP-1 and RANTES can also bind to alternative receptors. However, homozygotes are genetically resistant to infection by NSI strains of HIV, and the few homozygotes with Δ32 deletions who are HIV-positive appear to have been infected with SI strains that utilize CXCR4 instead. Other, more subtle, mutations in the promoter region of the *CCR5* gene allowing only low levels of coreceptor expression may confer relative resistance to HIV infection and also, if infection occurs, slower the progression to AIDS.

Recently, a blood group antigen on red blood cells, the Duffy antigen receptor for chemokines (DARC), was shown to be another non-HLA genetic factor influencing HIV transmission and disease progression. In addition to forming a receptor for certain HIV-suppressive and proinflammatory chemokines such as RANTES, DARC serves as the red cell receptor for *Plasmodium vivax* malaria and consequently nonexpression of DARC on red cells (Duffy negative phenotype) confers complete resistance to *P. vivax.* As a result of selection pressure from malaria, most West Africans and two-thirds of African Americans do not express DARC on red cells (although expression is preserved on endothelial cells). The DARC-negative red cell phenotype is associated with an increased risk of acquisition of HIV-1; however, it is also associated with slower HIV-related disease progression.

The outer envelope glycoprotein, gp120, is the molecule on HIV that binds to CD4 and subsequently to the coreceptor. Gp120 is anchored to the viral envelope via gp41, the viral protein that is thought to effect membrane fusion. The gp120–gp41 is present in the viral envelope as a trimeric complex. SI strains have a gp120–gp41 structure that is less stable than NSI strains, readily undergoing conformational change on binding to CD4. This property makes SI strains more sensitive to neutralization by gp120 antibodies and also to inactivation by soluble forms of recombinant CD4, which were once seen as promising therapeutic agents. NSI strains, however, are more resistant. Mutations in the V3 loop of gp120 can convert NSI strains to SI strains. These mutations arise naturally during progression to AIDS and may allow HIV to switch to infect different cell types via new coreceptors.

The natural chemokines act as competitive inhibitors of HIV entry; certain chemically modified chemokines and chemical analogues act as strong HIV inhibitors without triggering the downstream signalling of the receptor. This has led to a new class of potential anti-HIV drugs, called coreceptor antagonists.

Diagnosis of HIV infection

Following seroconversion, antibody to envelope protein persists indefinitely in the serum and forms a highly specific test for HIV infection. Most laboratories use one or more sensitive enzyme immunoassay tests that detect HIV-1 and HIV-2 antibodies and p24 antigen as the initial screening test. Positive screening tests are usually referred to a specialist laboratory for additional tests to confirm the presence of HIV antibodies. Most seroconversions occur within 3 months of infection, and very rarely up to 6 months. Routine diagnostic tests, if negative, should be repeated 3 months after the last possible exposure. If primary infection is suspected, or after high risk exposure, additional tests may be indicated (see Primary HIV infection, below). Near patient testing for HIV, e.g. using saliva, is available, but the place for such testing is not well defined. Easy availability of near patient testing or home testing could potentially increase higher risk behaviour.

Many people are unaware of their HIV infection. Detection of HIV is important for timely intervention with antiretroviral treatment, reduction of risk of perinatal transmission, and behavioural change to protect sexual partners. However, early diagnosis may cause distress and disruption of domestic, social, and professional lives, although the infected person may not need antiretroviral treatment for many years. Psychological support and counselling may be needed, especially soon after the diagnosis.

Many industrialized countries are developing strategies to increase HIV detection. In the United Kingdom, it is policy that all patients attending sexual health clinics for screening or treatment for sexual infections are offered HIV testing. In the United States of America, where more than 25% of those infected are unaware of their HIV infection, the Centers for Disease Control and Prevention (CDC) has recommended that HIV testing should be routinely offered in all health care settings. In patients with unexplained symptoms that could be caused by HIV, testing is essential for diagnosis so that appropriate treatment can be provided. If the patient is too ill to give consent, testing is justified on these grounds as being in the patient's best interest. A high level of confidentiality must be maintained; disclosure of HIV-positive status is acceptable only in the medical interests of the patient and in general with their knowledge and consent. Patients unwilling to inform their sexual partners should be advised of the possible legal implications of nondisclosure, if transmission occurs. In the United Kingdom, there have been successful prosecutions of individuals knowingly exposing their partners to HIV.

Clinical presentation and features

Primary HIV infection

Between 2 and 6 weeks after exposure to HIV, 50 to 70% of those infected develop a transient, often mild, nonspecific illness (sometimes called seroconversion illness or acute retroviral syndrome) similar to infectious mononucleosis, with fever, malaise, myalgia, lymphadenopathy, and pharyngitis. However, unlike infectious mononucleosis, over 50% of people develop a rash, typically erythematous, maculopapular, and affecting the face and trunk. Other rashes and patterns of distribution, and oral and genital ulcers have also been reported. The illness begins abruptly and usually lasts for 1 to 2 weeks, but may be more protracted. Neurological complications include acute encephalitis, lymphocytic meningitis, and peripheral neuropathy. Severe or long-lasting illness and neurological involvement are associated with accelerated progression to AIDS and a bad prognosis, which may be influenced by early antiretroviral therapy. A transient decrease in CD4 lymphocytes is usual during primary illness. Occasionally, this may be substantial and associated with opportunistic infections such as oral or oesophageal candidiasis, and rarely pneumocystis pneumonia (PCP).

Diagnosis requires a high index of suspicion. Primary HIV infection is a time of high viraemia (typically 10^5–10^6 viral particles/ml) during which antibodies to HIV may initially be absent (Fig. 7.5.23.5). Serum antibodies to the core and surface proteins of the virus usually appear within 2 to 6 weeks. Therefore, if primary infection is suspected additional tests may be required; rapid diagnosis may be provided by detecting HIV viraemia using tests for HIV RNA or proviral cDNA (by polymerase chain reaction, PCR), which may confirm HIV infection before antibodies become detectable.

Aggressive therapy of primary HIV infection with antiretroviral drugs does not eradicate the infection but, on theoretical grounds, might alter the natural history. After primary infection, the viral load becomes relatively stable after 6 to 9 months at an average level of 30 000 HIV RNA copies/ml plasma (Fig. 7.5.23.5). The plasma HIV RNA level at this virological steady state or 'set point' is of prognostic importance; therefore, treatment of the initial

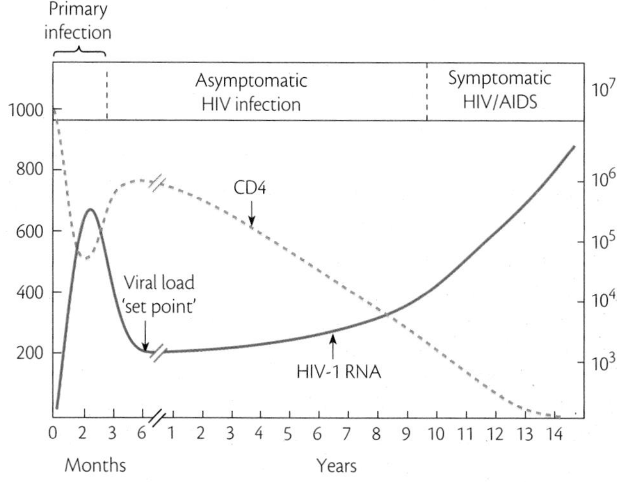

Fig. 7.5.23.5 Schematic representation of typical changes in CD4 lymphocyte count (left axis, per mm^3) and plasma HIV-1 RNA (right axis, copies/ml) with time, during the natural history of HIV infection.

viraemic illness may lower the risk of progression if viral set point off therapy is lowered. A placebo-controlled trial of zidovudine monotherapy during primary HIV infection showed a short-term benefit, but it is not known whether the rate of progression is affected by early treatment. There are also concerns about the long-term toxicity of antiretroviral drugs. A major trial currently underway (Short Pulse Anti Retroviral Therapy at HIV Seroconversion, SPARTAC) aims to determine whether early treatment for a limited period, early treatment that is continued indefinitely, or no treatment for primary infection, will affect virological and immunological set points and which strategy will lead to better clinical outcomes.

Early HIV infection

Following the primary illness or subclinical seroconversion, there usually follows an asymptomatic period lasting an average of 10 years without antiretroviral therapy. Although a time of clinical latency, there is intense viral turnover: 10^9 to 10^{10} viral particles are replaced daily and the half-life of circulating CD4 lymphocytes is substantially reduced.

During the asymptomatic period, physical examination may be normal, but about one-third of patients have persistent generalized lymphadenopathy. The enlarged nodes, caused by a reactive follicular hyperplasia, are usually symmetrical, mobile, and nontender. The cervical and axillary nodes are most commonly affected. Nodes that are markedly asymmetrical, painful, or rapidly enlarging should be biopsied to exclude tumours such as lymphoma and opportunistic infections such as tuberculosis.

Symptoms of progressive HIV infection can be prevented by antiretroviral treatment. In the absence of treatment, patients often develop minor opportunistic conditions affecting the skin and mucous membranes. These are also common throughout the later stages of HIV disease. They include a range of infections: fungal (e.g. tinea, pityrosporum), viral (e.g. warts, molluscum contagiosum, herpes simplex, herpes zoster), and bacterial (e.g. folliculitis, impetigo); and also eczema, seborrhoeic dermatitis, and psoriasis.

Oral hairy leucoplakia usually appears as corrugated greyish-white lesions on the lateral borders of the tongue in homosexual men. The condition is symptomless and nonprogressive, but may be a clue to HIV seropositivity. Epstein–Barr virus DNA has been demonstrated in these lesions.

One of the characteristic clinical presentations of HIV disease is a sore mouth and throat due to oropharyngeal candidiasis (oral thrush) (Fig. 7.5.23.6). This is a sign of worsening immunodeficiency and may be recurrent. *Candida albicans* is usually responsible, but other species (e.g. *Candida glabrata*) may be implicated.

There is an increased incidence of periodontal disease in those with untreated HIV, including inflammation of the gums (gingivitis) and the more serious and extensive periodontitis that can lead to loss of teeth. Two distinctive forms are associated with HIV: a linear gingival erythema that causes a typical red band along the gum line, and in advanced immunosuppression, necrotizing ulcerative periodontitis which may require extensive debridement and antimicrobials. Recurrent oropharyngeal aphthous ulceration is common and may be painful. Recurrent ulcers may occur in the oesophagus and other parts of the gastrointestinal tract. They usually respond to local or systemic corticosteroid therapy. Resistant cases may respond to thalidomide. The availability of antiretroviral therapy has reduced the need for specific treatment.

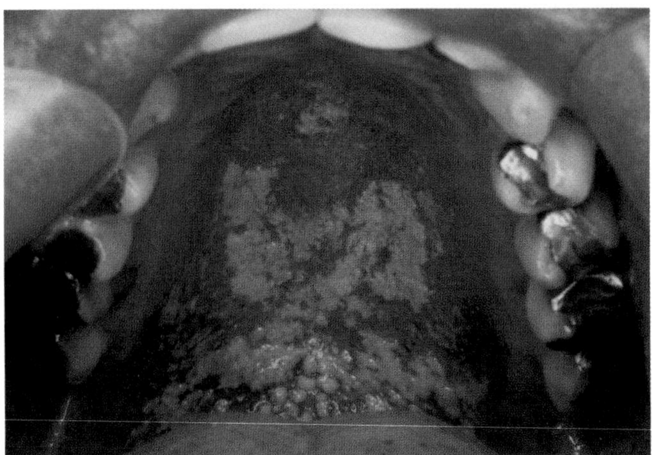

Fig. 7.5.23.6 Oral candidiasis.
(By courtesy of the late Dr B E Juel-Jensen)

Later in the course of untreated HIV infection, intermittent or persistent nonspecific constitutional symptoms may develop, which include lethargy, anorexia, diarrhoea, weight loss, fever, and night sweats. These symptoms may presage severe opportunistic infections or tumours.

Progression to symptomatic HIV disease (AIDS)

Various staging systems for HIV infection and case definitions of AIDS were developed and modified as understanding of the pathogenesis and natural history increased (Fig. 7.5.23.7). The CDC in the United States of America listed a range of specific diseases and other criteria, such as a CD4 lymphocyte count of less than 200/mm^3 (0.2×10^9/litre), as indicative of AIDS. AIDS-defining illnesses were essential for surveillance when HIV status was frequently unknown, the natural history of HIV infection was poorly understood (the proportion developing opportunistic complications was uncertain), and disease-modifying drugs were not available.

Effective prevention of many of the opportunistic infections has led to an increase in the proportion of symptomatic patients who

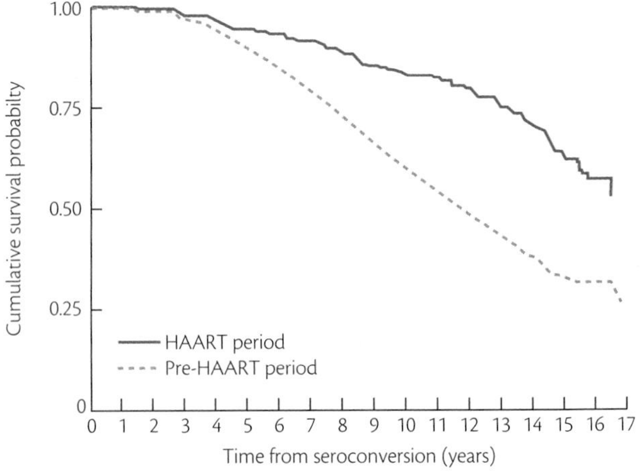

Fig. 7.5.23.7 Natural history of HIV. Estimated proportions of individuals surviving from HIV-1 seroconversion in the pre-HAART era. HAART, highly active antiretroviral therapy.
(From CASCADE collaboration (2000). Survival after introduction of HAART in people with known duration of HIV-1 infection. The CASCADE Collaboration. Concerted Action on SeroConversion to AIDS and Death in Europe. *Lancet*, **355**, 1158–59.)

do not fulfil the criteria for AIDS. Antiretroviral therapy usually improves the clinical condition and survival, even when started after progression to AIDS. These factors have undermined the epidemiological value and prognostic importance of a strict AIDS case definition. Therefore, the current value of making a distinction between AIDS and HIV infection at other stages is questionable, especially in industrialized countries. It is more useful to consider progressive HIV disease as a continuous spectrum.

However, clinical criteria to identify symptomatic HIV disease and AIDS were needed in resource-poor countries, if laboratory confirmation of HIV was not possible. The WHO therefore adopted clinical case definitions for AIDS surveillance in resource-limited countries, based on clinical manifestations with or without laboratory confirmation of HIV infection. This approach has been superseded by the WHO clinical staging system, which assumes that an HIV test has been done. Rapid HIV tests can now be done even in field conditions. For surveillance, it is suggested that HIV case reporting should supersede AIDS case reporting, though that may not yet be possible everywhere (Chapter 7.5.24).

Nonprogression

While the average time between infection with HIV and the development of AIDS is about 10 years, approximately 20% of patients progress rapidly to AIDS within 5 years and 10 to 15% remain clinically well for 15 to 20 years. Age is an independent risk factor for progression; acquisition of HIV in later life is associated with a less favourable prognosis. Long-term healthy survivors are often called nonprogressors, and this subgroup generally represents the tail end of a normal distribution of progression rates. Cohort studies have demonstrated that most apparent nonprogressors are actually slow progressors, in whom a gradual decline in the CD4 lymphocyte count and increments in HIV viral load can be demonstrated. Although several investigators have reported virological, genetic, and cellular and humoral immunological factors that may be associated with nonprogression, limitations in study design have made it difficult to identify what was responsible.

In white cohorts of antiretroviral treatment-naïve, HIV-infected persons who show unusually successful control of HIV to levels of below 50 copies/ml plasma, more than 50 to 90% express one or both of the HLA class I alleles HLA-B*5701 and HLA-B*2705. The protective value of these HLA class I alleles is related to the importance of the CD8+ T-cell response in successful immune control of HIV, and in particular where the CD8+ T-cell response includes broad targeting of epitopes in the conserved internal Gag protein. Infected persons expressing the HLA class I alleles HLA-B*3502 or B*5802 tend not to make Gag-specific CD8+ T-cell responses, and progress to AIDS significantly more rapidly. In addition to defining the nature of the CD8+ T-cell response, the particular HLA alleles expressed have important influences on the natural killer cell response against HIV, also affecting rates of progression to HIV disease. Non-HLA genes that affect rates of progression include the macrophage chemokine receptor CCR5 gene mutation (see Cellular biology of HIV, above) associated with nonprogression in the heterozygous state.

Late complications and their management

Pneumocystis jiroveci pneumonia (Chapter 7.7.6)

P. jiroveci (previously *Pneumocystis carinii*) pneumonia, one of the hallmarks of AIDS, is now less common because of primary prophylaxis and antiretroviral therapy. Some 85% of cases occur in patients with CD4 lymphocyte counts below 200/mm^3, and mostly at counts below 100/mm^3. Symptoms typically include increasing shortness of breath, dry cough, and fever, usually developing subacutely over a few weeks. Malaise, fatigue, weight loss, and chest pains or tightness may occur. Chest signs are usually minor (crackles) or absent. The characteristic chest radiograph shows bilateral mid zone interstitial shadowing (Fig. 7.5.23.8), but can be normal. Other appearances include localized infiltrates or consolidation, upper lobe shadows resembling tuberculosis, nodular lesions, and pneumothorax; effusions are very rare. The arterial oxygen saturation is usually less than 95% at rest or falls after exercise.

Infection with *P. jiroveci* is associated with an interstitial inflammatory infiltrate and progressive impairment of lung function. The diagnosis can sometimes be confirmed by microscopy of sputum, which is induced by nebulized saline in properly ventilated isolation rooms to reduce the risk of tuberculosis transmission (see Multidrug-resistant tuberculosis, below). *P. jiroveci* cysts and trophozoites are visualized by the use of special stains. If the result is negative, fibreoptic bronchoscopy with bronchial lavage is indicated (Fig. 7.5.23.9); other causes of lung disease or coexistent infection may also be diagnosed by this technique, including tuberculosis, fungal infections, and Kaposi's sarcoma. Immunofluorescence using monoclonal antibodies, or DNA amplification by PCR, may improve diagnostic sensitivity when compared with conventional staining techniques, but these methods are not yet used routinely. In a minority of patients with *P. jiroveci* pneumonia the diagnosis is not confirmed but treatment is given empirically.

High-dose co-trimoxazole (120 mg/kg daily in divided doses) for 3 weeks is the first-line treatment for pneumocystis pneumonia. Oral therapy is often adequate, but in moderate and severe cases the drug should be given intravenously. The drug can be given orally if fever, symptoms, and oxygenation have improved after 10 days. Adverse reactions to co-trimoxazole—especially neutropenia, anaemia, rash, and fever—occur in up to 40% of patients, usually after 6 to 14 days. Intravenous pentamidine (4 mg/kg per day) is the second-line choice for patients who do not tolerate co-trimoxazole.

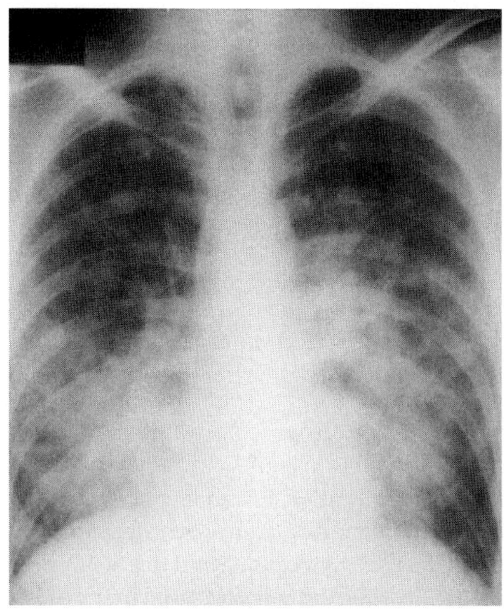

Fig. 7.5.23.8 Chest radiograph: *Pneumocystis jiroveci* pneumonia.

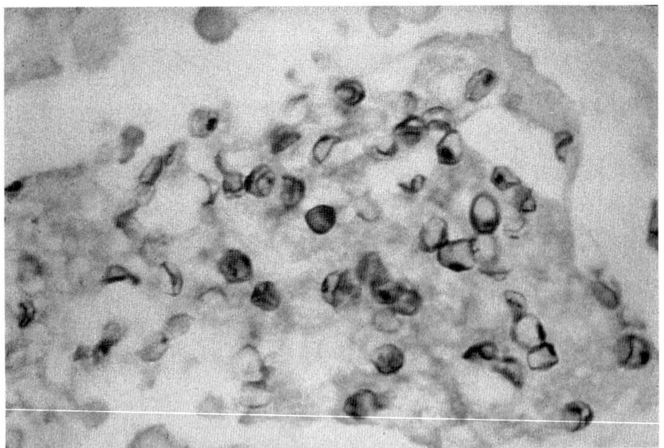

Fig. 7.5.23.9 *Pneumocystis jiroveci* cysts in bronchoalveolar lavage aspirate.

Patients intolerant of co-trimoxazole and pentamidine may be treated with clindamycin plus primaquine or dapsone plus trimethoprim. These regimens have only been evaluated in patients with mild to moderate pneumocystis pneumonia, as has atovaquone, an antiprotozoal drug that is active against *P. jiroveci.* Although slightly less effective than co-trimoxazole, atovaquone causes fewer adverse effects.

In patients with moderate or severe pneumocystis pneumonia, high-dose corticosteroids reduce morbidity and mortality. If the arterial partial pressure of oxygen (Pao_2) is less than 9.3 kPa or the alveolar–arterial oxygen gradient is greater than 4.7 kPa, oxygen and intravenous methylprednisolone or oral prednisolone should be given for 5 to 10 days. Patients who develop respiratory failure may require ventilatory support. After treatment for pneumocystis pneumonia has been completed, secondary prophylaxis should be given to prevent recurrence. This can be discontinued if there is a good response to antiretroviral treatment, with a rise in the CD4 count sustained above 200/mm^3.

Bacterial pneumonia

The risk of bacterial pneumonia is increased in HIV, especially if the CD4 lymphocyte count is below 200/mm^3. The most common cause is *Streptococcus pneumoniae*, although *Haemophilus influenzae* and *Moraxella catarrhalis* are also relatively common, and *Staphylococcus aureus*, klebsiella spp., and other Gram-negative rods are important causes in advanced HIV disease. Rare causes include nocardia spp. and *Rhodococcus equi.* The presentation may be atypical, and radiological appearances frequently include diffuse infiltrates that resemble pneumocystis pneumonia, as well as more typical segmental or lobar patterns. Cavitation with abscess formation, pleural effusion, and empyema may occur. HIV predisposes to recurrent invasive pneumococcal infections with bacteraemia; recurrent bacterial pneumonia in a 12-month period is an AIDS-defining condition. Chronic lung damage with bronchiectasis and colonization by *Pseudomonas aeruginosa* have been reported.

Other pulmonary complications

Disseminated fungal infections, including cryptococcus spp., may involve the lungs (Chapter 7.2.4, Section 7.7). In endemic areas, histoplasmosis, coccidioidomycosis, and disseminated *Penicillium marneffei* infection need to be considered (see below). Invasive *Aspergillus fumigatus* infections may occur in patients with advanced HIV disease who have additional risk factors such as severe neutropenia. Patients usually have severe systemic illness. The radiographic appearances in all these fungal infections are usually nonspecific. Bronchoalveolar lavage may be needed for diagnosis. HIV-associated lymphocytic interstitial pneumonitis causes diffuse abnormalities, usually in children but occasionally in adults. Bronchiolitis obliterans-organizing pneumonia (BOOP) is a steroid-responsive cause of lung infiltrates, probably a tissue response to various underlying conditions, which has also been reported in HIV and may be confused with pneumocystis pneumonia.

Tuberculosis (Chapter 7.6.25)

The interaction between HIV and tuberculosis (TB) was recognized early in the HIV epidemic. Studies in central Africa in the mid 1980s showed that more than 60% of newly diagnosed tuberculosis patients were HIV-positive at a time when the background seroprevalence of HIV in the population was much lower. Intravenous drug users were shown to have an increased risk of developing active tuberculosis if they were HIV-positive. After decades of progressive decline in the incidence of tuberculosis in the United States of America, notifications increased during the mid-1980s, soon after the emergence of the HIV epidemic. A similar trend was subsequently observed in western Europe. Globally, tuberculosis remains the most frequent life-threatening opportunistic infection in AIDS.

Most cases of tuberculosis in HIV-positive individuals represent reactivation of dormant bacilli. However, molecular typing of isolates of *Mycobacterium tuberculosis* by restriction fragment length polymorphism (RFLP) analysis suggests that up to 40% are new infections. The WHO estimates that one-third of the world's HIV-positive population is coinfected with tuberculosis. In communities where *M. tuberculosis* is a common endemic organism, those who are immunosuppressed by HIV have an increased risk of relapsing or contracting new infections. Where the background prevalence of tuberculosis is low, the disease is uncommon in HIV-positive patients unless they become exposed, e.g. through travel. Testing for HIV should be done in all patients presenting with active tuberculosis, and tuberculosis should be considered as a cause of unexplained symptoms in patients with HIV.

Active tuberculosis may occur at any time during the course of HIV infection. In early-stage HIV, it is more likely to present with the typical clinical features: subacute history of cough, fever, and weight loss, upper lobe cavitary disease and/or pleural disease on chest radiographs, and a positive skin test to tuberculin. In late-stage HIV, infected patients are more likely to present atypically with unusual chest findings, extrapulmonary involvement, and cutaneous anergy. The chest radiograph may be normal in up to 40% of cases and, when abnormal, upper lobe involvement is less common. Sputum smears should be examined for acid-fast bacilli, but are less likely to be positive in HIV. Blood cultures may be positive for *M. tuberculosis.*

Patients with HIV and TB are more likely to relapse after completion of therapy and to die prematurely if their HIV disease is not treated. Patients with advanced HIV infection are more likely to develop extrapulmonary tuberculosis involving lymph nodes, pericardium, liver, bone marrow, or meninges. Diagnosis can be difficult and frequently relies on invasive procedures to obtain appropriate specimens. The role of interferon-γ tests in HIV is uncertain.

The standard 6-month regimen of three or four antituberculosis drugs (isoniazid, rifampicin, pyrazinamide, and ethambutol) is generally effective in patients with HIV, unless there is resistance to one or more of these first-line drugs. The drug regimen may need to be adjusted when *in vitro* sensitivity results are known. For fully sensitive organisms, after 2 months on three or four drugs, isoniazid and rifampicin should be continued for a further 4 months. It should be noted that rifampicin interacts with many of the antiretroviral drugs, particularly protease inhibitors, and these interactions need to be considered in deciding on drug regimens. Patients with pulmonary tuberculosis should be isolated initially. Contact tracing is important; HIV-positive contacts of a smear-positive TB case are at particular risk and should be offered isoniazid preventive therapy (unless known multidrug-resistant TB). The tuberculin skin test may be negative, especially if the CD4 count is low.

Up to 20% of patients with HIV experience adverse reactions to antituberculosis drugs. In HIV-positive patients with tuberculosis in Africa, the sulpha-based drug thiacetazone has been associated with serious skin reactions, including toxic epidermal necrolysis and fatal cases of Stevens–Johnson syndrome. Whereas response rates for conventional short-course tuberculosis treatment in industrialized countries are similar to those achieved in HIV-negative patients, in resource-limited countries and where compliance is less easily achieved, cure rates are lower and there is a risk that resistance will develop. Several countries have adopted a 'directly observed therapy' strategy (DOTS) to address this problem. Supervised swallowing is a component of this strategy but political commitment, secure drug supply, and good organization are needed for this to be effective.

Multidrug-resistant tuberculosis

Over 15 outbreaks of multidrug-resistant tuberculosis (MDR-TB) have been reported since the late 1980s. MDR-TB isolates are resistant to at least two first-line antituberculosis drugs, most commonly isoniazid and rifampicin, and are often resistant to several agents. Most have occurred in HIV units in hospitals, but there have been outbreaks in prisons, drug treatment centres, and nursing homes. Most documented outbreaks have been in the United States of America. Elsewhere, over 200 people were involved in Buenos Aires, Argentina, and another outbreak affected over 100 people in Lisbon, Portugal. In MDR-TB outbreaks, health care workers may become infected. Initially, the mortality among HIV-positive patients was very high (up to 93%), but the outcome has subsequently improved because of more rapid diagnosis and treatment with at least four drugs to which the *M. tuberculosis* isolate is sensitive *in vitro*. More recently, extensively drug-resistant TB (XDR TB) in HIV infected patients in South Africa has caused outbreaks, with 100% mortality.

To prevent outbreaks of MDR-TB, special precautions are required when HIV-positive patients with possible tuberculosis are admitted to hospitals. Diagnosis must not be delayed, appropriate treatment must be started as soon as possible, and drug resistance identified. Precautions include the isolation of patients in negative-pressure rooms, use of respiratory protection for staff, and special care during certain procedures such as bronchoscopy or nebulized pentamidine administration. With effective treatment, patients rapidly become noninfectious, but precautions need to be continued until the sputum is repeatedly culture-negative.

Mycobacterium avium complex

In the absence of antiretroviral treatment, patients with advanced HIV infection and CD4 lymphocyte counts below 50/mm^3 are at high risk of disseminated *Mycobacterium avium* complex (MAC) infection, particularly in industrialized countries where historically it was reported to develop in up to 40% of patients with AIDS. *M. avium* is a ubiquitous environmental organism of low pathogenicity that can be isolated from domestic water supplies. Infection is likely to be through the gastrointestinal tract. MAC infection becomes widely disseminated in those with advanced HIV and causes fever, night sweats, weight loss, diarrhoea, abdominal pain, anaemia, disturbed liver function, and reduced overall survival. The organism can usually be cultured from blood or bone marrow, or may be recognized as acid-fast bacilli in tissue biopsies (e.g. from lymph node, small bowel, or liver). It is unclear why the diagnosis is uncommon in underdeveloped countries; high mortality from other opportunistic infections at earlier stages of immunosuppression may be partly responsible.

MAC infection is intrinsically resistant to most first-line antituberculosis drugs. Comparative trials suggest that initial therapy should be with two or three drugs: clarithromycin or azithromycin and ethambutol should be used, and additional rifabutin or a quinolone (e.g. ciprofloxacin) considered. In severely ill patients, intravenous amikacin may be useful as the third agent. In the absence of antiretroviral treatment, lifelong treatment may be required to prevent relapse; but if immunity is restored by highly active antiretroviral therapy, such maintenance therapy can be discontinued.

Other nontuberculosis mycobacteria

Other mycobacteria, notably *Mycobacterium kansasii*, *Mycobacterium genavense*, and *Mycobacterium celatum*, may cause opportunistic infections in those with HIV. *M. genavense*, which colonizes pet birds, was discovered in European patients with HIV and causes fever, diarrhoea, and severe weight loss. HIV does not seem to affect the incidence or natural history of leprosy (*Mycobacterium leprae*).

Gastrointestinal disease

Oesophageal candidiasis

Oesophagitis presents with retrosternal pain on swallowing, and in patients with HIV is most commonly caused by *C. albicans*. Oesophageal candidiasis indicates advanced immunosuppression and is an AIDS-defining condition. The diagnosis should be suspected in a patient with oral candida and dysphagia, and may be supported by barium swallow or confirmed by endoscopy and biopsy. Treatment is with oral azole antifungal agents such as fluconazole. It may recur and in patients with severe immunosuppression, and in the absence of antiretroviral treatment, candida may become resistant to prolonged azole treatment. Resistance tends to develop gradually and can be monitored by *in vitro* testing. Such patients require treatment or continuous suppression with high doses of fluconazole (which is better tolerated than high doses of ketoconazole or itraconazole) or intermittent treatment with intravenous amphotericin. Azole-resistant oro-oesophageal candidiasis has become rare since the advent of highly active antiretroviral therapy.

The differential diagnosis of oesophageal candidiasis includes oesophagitis caused by cytomegalovirus (CMV) or herpes simplex virus (HSV), which require specific antiviral therapy, and aphthous ulceration, which may respond to oral prednisolone or thalidomide.

Intestinal infections

Some infections are much more common in HIV disease than in other settings. *Cryptosporidium parvum* can lead to cholera-like diarrhoea. An ascending cholangitis may occur with fever, pain, and jaundice and have the imaging appearance of sclerosing cholangitis. Other protozoan parasites, such as *Cystoisospora (Isospora) belli* and *Cyclospora cayetanensis* may also cause diarrhoea, as can microsporidia. Cytomegalovirus can cause an acute colitis with pain and bloody diarrhoea. Sigmoidoscopy shows ulceration and biopsies show characteristic CMV inclusions. Tuberculosis may also present as intestinal disease.

HIV enteropathy

Many patients with HIV, especially in the tropics, present with diarrhoea and malnutrition leading to wasting in the absence of detectable gastrointestinal opportunist infections. Biopsies often show villous blunting and increased inflammatory cells in the lamina propria of the small bowel and functional tests suggest increased bowel permeability. The pathogenesis of this enteropathy is poorly understood, but may involve cytokine activation secondary to HIV infection.

HIV and the nervous system (Chapter 24.11.4)

The nervous system is a major site of involvement for direct and indirect complications of HIV at all stages of infection. All parts of the nervous system may be affected. In advanced HIV, opportunistic infections and tumours (lymphoma), and tissue damage caused by HIV replication in the brain and spinal cord, are important and relatively common during progressive HIV disease.

Cerebral toxoplasmosis (Chapter 7.8.4)

Cerebral infection with the intracellular protozoan *Toxoplasma gondii* is the most frequent infection of the central nervous system in AIDS, occurring when the CD4 lymphocyte count is below 200/mm^3. It usually results from reactivation of toxoplasma cysts in the brain, leading to the formation of focal lesions that are typically multiple but may be single. Symptoms develop subacutely and include focal neurological disturbance, headache, confusion, fever, and convulsions. On CT the lesions appear as ring-enhancing masses with surrounding oedema (Fig. 7.5.23.10). MRI is more sensitive and frequently detects lesions not visible on CT. Serum antibodies to toxoplasma spp. are usually detectable; their absence makes the diagnosis unlikely but does not exclude it. Detection of toxoplasma DNA in cerebrospinal fluid by PCR is being evaluated as a diagnostic test. The principal differential diagnosis is cerebral lymphoma; other causes of focal brain lesions in AIDS include cryptococcoma, cerebral abscess (including infection with nocardia spp.), tuberculoma, progressive multifocal leukoencephalopathy, and neurosyphilis. Brain biopsy is required for a definitive diagnosis, but is rarely performed. As toxoplasmosis is by far the most common treatable cause of focal cerebral lesions in HIV, it is standard practice to treat for this and only consider biopsy if there is no clinical improvement in 7 to 10 days.

The condition responds well if treatment is started early; a combination of sulfadiazine at 4 to 6 g/day and pyrimethamine at 50 to 75 mg/day is the treatment of choice. More than 40% of patients experience adverse effects, especially rash and nephrotoxicity caused by sulfadiazine. The haematological toxicity of pyrimethamine may be reduced by adding folinic acid (10 mg/day). If sulpha drugs are not tolerated, clindamycin with pyrimethamine is an effective alternative. Corticosteroids can be used to reduce cerebral oedema in patients with large lesions and serious mass effects, but this is controversial.

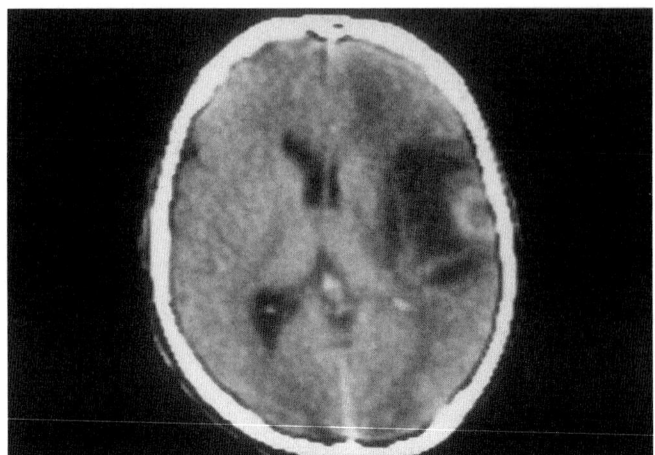

Fig. 7.5.23.10 Cerebral toxoplasmosis: ring enhancement and surrounding cerebral oedema (CT with contrast).

Treatment is usually given for 3 to 6 weeks, and in the absence of effective antiretroviral treatment relapse is common after stopping. In these circumstances, lifelong maintenance treatment is usually required using pyrimethamine (25–50 mg/day) with a sulpha drug or clindamycin. However, these can be discontinued if antiretroviral treatment leads to sustained immunological recovery. The use of primary prophylaxis against PCP also reduces the risk of toxoplasmosis.

Cryptococcal meningitis (Chapter 7.7.2)

Although infection of the central nervous system with *Cryptococcus neoformans* can occur in the absence of immunodeficiency, it most commonly arises in association with HIV infection. Before the widespread use of azole antifungals for mucosal candidiasis, it accounted for 5 to 10% of opportunistic infections in patients with AIDS. The presentation is usually subacute and may be subtle and nonspecific with headache, vomiting, and mild fever, and few neurological signs. Less frequently, psychiatric disturbance, convulsions, cranial nerve palsies, truncal ataxia, or focal intracerebral lesions may occur. Neck stiffness is unusual. The diagnosis is made by identifying cryptococci in the cerebrospinal fluid by India ink staining, detection of cryptococcal antigen in the cerebrospinal fluid (uniformly positive), and culture. Cryptococcal antigen is also usually detectable in serum. *C. neoformans* in patients with AIDS causes minimal inflammation, so the white cell count of the cerebrospinal fluid is often only mildly raised and the protein and glucose levels of the cerebrospinal fluid may be normal.

A randomized, controlled trial showed that the combination of amphotericin B and flucytosine was superior to amphotericin B alone or fluconazole alone for the treatment of cryptococcal meningitis. Amphotericin B and flucytosine together lead to more rapid sterilization of the cerebrospinal fluid, but are not as well tolerated as fluconazole. Resistance of cryptococci to fluconazole is very rare. Itraconazole can be effective, but is not generally recommended. Adverse reactions to amphotericin are frequent, especially fever, myalgia, renal impairment, and electrolyte disturbances. Close monitoring is required. Lipid formulations of amphotericin are increasingly used and likely to become the standard of care; otherwise they are used for patients intolerant of the conventional formulation. Raised intracranial pressure is associated with clinical deterioration and the risk of blindness: repeated lumbar punctures and, sometimes, ventricular shunting are needed in these circumstances.

Without secondary prophylaxis, cryptococcal meningitis relapses in 50 to 80% of patients with HIV in the absence of antiretroviral treatment. Oral fluconazole (200 mg/day) is effective for maintenance, and can be discontinued if antiretroviral treatment leads to sustained immunological recovery.

Progressive multifocal leukoencephalopathy

Progressive multifocal leukoencephalopathy is a progressive demyelinating condition of advanced HIV disease caused by JC virus, a polyomavirus cytopathic for oligodendroglia. It presents with focal neurological deficits, personality changes, or ataxia; headache and mass effects are absent. Brain MRI, the investigation of choice, usually shows multiple white matter lesions. JC virus is detectable in cerebrospinal fluid by PCR, but this is not usually necessary for diagnosis. There is no specific treatment. Survival of less than 6 months is usual, but progression may sometimes be halted or reversed by highly active antiretroviral therapy. Cidofovir is active against JC virus and is being evaluated. The other human polyomavirus, BK virus, is a very rare cause of encephalitis and interstitial nephropathy in AIDS.

Cerebral lymphoma

These are B-cell lymphomas that arise, usually, due to EBV infection and the cerebrospinal fluid may be positive for EBV with PCR. Lymphoma of the central nervous system may present in a manner similar to toxoplasmosis, with focal signs or seizures. CT or MRI of the brain reveal a single space-occupying lesion. Treatment has little impact on the course of the disease and the prognosis is very poor; death usually occurs within 3 months of diagnosis.

HIV encephalopathy

HIV can infect the nervous system directly, leading to a variety of clinical problems. Most patients dying of AIDS show histological evidence of brain involvement including neuron loss. A smaller number (up to 10%) develop the cognitive, behavioural, and motor abnormalities of dementia. In the early stages, there is impairment of concentration and memory and mood changes mimicking depression; gradual progression leads to intellectual incapacity and motor disability so that patients cannot care for themselves. Neurological signs include slow movement, incoordination, motor weakness, hyperreflexia, and extensor plantar responses; brain imaging shows reduced grey matter volume in the cortex and basal ganglia. Ultimately, a nearly vegetative condition develops with virtual mutism, inability to walk, and incontinence. These patients die within 2 years. Antiretroviral treatment prevents, and in the earlier stages reverses, AIDS dementia.

Other psychological/psychiatric problems include anxiety, panic attacks, and depression. Psychotherapy may be helpful. Antidepressants may be needed in severe cases. Acute psychosis is rare. Dystonic reactions to various drugs, such as metoclopramide, are more common in patients with HIV.

In the late stages of HIV disease, the differential diagnosis of HIV dementia includes cytomegalovirus (CMV) encephalitis. This usually presents with rapidly progressive confusion and dementia, impaired consciousness, fever, cranial nerve lesions, and convulsions. MRI shows necrotizing periventriculitis; protein levels in cerebrospinal fluid may be elevated and CMV DNA is detectable in the cerebrospinal fluid by PCR. Ganciclovir and other anti-CMV agents may reduce progression.

Peripheral neuropathy and myelopathy

Peripheral neuropathy can occur at any stage of HIV infection, even at seroconversion, but is most common in advanced disease, when 10 to 15% of patients have a distal symmetrical sensorimotor neuropathy of axonal type causing pain and paraesthesias that may limit walking and, less often, distal weakness and atrophy. Mononeuritis multiplex and acute inflammatory demyelinating polyneuropathy resembling the Guillain–Barré syndrome are also described, generally at an earlier stage. Drugs used in patients with HIV, including stavudine, didanosine, and vincristine, may cause or exacerbate peripheral neuropathy. HIV-related autonomic neuropathy may cause postural hypotension, diarrhoea, impotence, impaired sweating, and bladder symptoms. CMV infection in patients with AIDS presents with a lumbosacral polyradiculopathy causing sacral paraesthesiae and numbness, lower limb weakness, and urinary retention that may progress to flaccid paraparesis if untreated.

HIV may involve the spinal cord directly, causing a vacuolar myelopathy. This usually presents with bilateral leg weakness and sensory symptoms, usually paraesthesias, and may progress to spastic paraparesis, ataxia, and incontinence. Rarely, a myopathy can occur.

Ocular disease

Cytomegalovirus retinitis

Without antiretroviral therapy, up to 30% of patients with AIDS (and a CD4 lymphocyte count below 50/mm^3) develop reactivation of CMV in the form of a destructive and blinding retinitis. This is rare in other types of immunosuppression. It usually presents with blurring of vision, scotomas, floaters, or flashing lights. The characteristic retinal changes are patches of irregular retinal pallor, caused by oedema and necrosis, and haemorrhages in a perivascular distribution (Fig. 7.5.23.11). The retinitis usually starts peripherally and progresses rapidly to involve the macula and whole retina, leading to blindness. Complications include retinal detachment, branch retinal artery occlusion, persistent iritis, and cataract. CMV retinitis should not be confused with cotton wool spots (HIV retinopathy)—small, pale retinal lesions without haemorrhages that commonly occur in patients with HIV. These are benign and often come and go.

The diagnosis of CMV retinitis is clinical, based on the characteristic retinal appearance (see Chapter 25.1). CMV viraemia may be detectable by PCR, and high or rising CMV viral load is associated with an increased risk of developing retinitis and other CMV disease. Anti-CMV drugs (ganciclovir, foscarnet, cidofovir) are viristatic; before the availability of highly active antiretroviral drug combinations, the aim of treatment was to stop progression rather than to cure disease. First-line treatment is with intravenous ganciclovir, which may cause severe neutropenia and thrombocytopenia that are dose-limiting in about 10% of patients. Foscarnet (phosphonoformate) is a relatively toxic second-line agent that causes dose-limiting reversible renal impairment and symptoms of hypocalcaemia in about 20% of patients. Ganciclovir can also

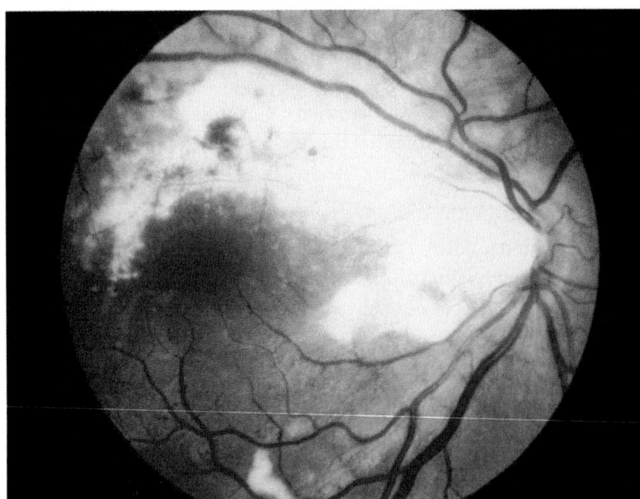

Fig. 7.5.23.11 CMV retinitis.

be given as a slow-release intraocular implant, but this may allow CMV to develop at other sites including the other eye.

For maintenance therapy, oral valganciclovir may be adequate, convenient, and well tolerated, although there is a greater risk of disease progression than with daily intravenous infusions of ganciclovir or foscarnet, and the eyes must be examined frequently. Cidofovir is more active against CMV than the other anti-CMV drugs. It can be given by intermittent intravenous infusion, initially weekly and then every 2 weeks. Whereas ganciclovir and foscarnet require a central venous catheter, cidofovir may be given in short infusions through a peripheral vein because of its prolonged antiviral effect. However, cidofovir is relatively toxic, causing irreversible nephrotoxicity, neutropenia, and peripheral neuropathy in over one-third of patients.

With the advent of highly active antiretroviral therapy, CMV retinitis is much less common in developed countries. Sustained suppression of HIV viral load and improvement in immune status can allow discontinuation of maintenance treatment. New manifestations of ocular CMV, such as vitritis, have been reported in patients treated with highly active antiretroviral therapy (see Immune reconstitution syndromes, below).

Other ocular syndromes

Acute retinal necrosis is a rare condition originally reported in reactivation of varicella zoster virus in otherwise healthy adults. In patients with advanced HIV infection, it is usually preceded by dermatomal herpes zoster and typically presents with blurring of vision and pain in the affected eye. Progressive necrotizing retinitis leads to visual deterioration that may be associated with uveitis. An outer retinal necrosis syndrome with little ocular inflammation also occurs in patients with AIDS. There is a high risk of visual loss and retinal detachment. Both eyes may be affected. Suspected acute retinal necrosis should be treated with intravenous aciclovir.

Acute toxoplasma choroidoretinitis may resemble CMV retinitis, but the retinal scarring that follows treatment is distinctive. The disease is more common in countries such as Brazil and France where the background prevalence of toxoplasmosis is much higher than in the United Kingdom. Choroidoretinitis is also a rare complication of histoplasmosis and cryptococcosis, and uveitis may occur in syphilis.

HIV-related tumours

Kaposi's sarcoma

Kaposi's sarcoma characteristically presents as multiple, purplish, nodular skin lesions (Fig. 7.5.23.12). Lesions start as small, pink, deep purple, or brown macules, and develop into nodules or plaques that may ulcerate. They also occur on mucosal surfaces, most commonly on the hard palate. Local or regional oedema and lymph node enlargement may occur. Mucocutaneous lesions are cosmetically and psychologically important but are rarely of clinical importance (Fig. 7.5.23.13). However, visceral disease, which most commonly affects the lungs and gastrointestinal tract, is an important cause of morbidity and even mortality. Lung lesions cause dyspnoea, cough, or haemoptysis, and gut involvement may cause abdominal pain, bleeding, or a rare protein-losing enteropathy. Extensive visceral involvement can cause constitutional symptoms such as fevers, night sweats, and weight loss. Kaposi's sarcoma rarely affects the central nervous system.

In industrialized countries, Kaposi's sarcoma is over 2000 times more common in HIV-infected individuals than in the general population. Classic Kaposi's sarcoma in HIV-negative individuals occurs in middle-aged and older men of Eastern European or Mediterranean origin. Endemic Kaposi's sarcoma in Africa has been known for decades. It is predominantly a disease of older men that has a fairly indolent course. HIV-related Kaposi's sarcoma, on the other hand, is a more aggressive disease and occurs mostly in those people who have acquired HIV via a sexual route, namely homosexual and bisexual men and in younger African men and women. The epidemic of Kaposi's sarcoma in central and East Africa exactly mirrors the HIV epidemic in these regions. Kaposi's sarcoma is rare in intravenous drug users and very rare in recipients of blood products, including those with haemophilia. These epidemiological features suggested a sexually transmissible aetiological agent.

In 1994, a new herpesvirus, human herpesvirus 8 (HHV-8), was found in HIV-related Kaposi's sarcoma and was soon detected in the lesions of all forms of Kaposi's sarcoma. Seroepidemiological studies show that HHV-8 is common only in certain geographical regions, corresponding to where Kaposi's sarcoma was endemic before the era of HIV. HHV-8 is detectable in saliva but less often in semen. This may explain why both sexual and other routes of transmission occur. In Africa, where HHV-8 infection is common, it is transmitted perinatally from mother to child.

Kaposi's sarcoma lesions are characterized by proliferating spindle cells, possibly of endothelial origin, thin-walled slit-like vascular spaces, infiltration by lymphocytes and plasma cells, and extravasated red cells. Multiple lesions appear synchronously in widely dispersed areas. The clonality of Kaposi's sarcoma lesions has not been fully resolved. Although some studies have suggested a monoclonal origin, others have shown a mixed picture and the lesions may be reactive proliferative rather than truly cancerous. HHV-8 is detectable in spindle cells and flat endothelial cells lining the vascular spaces of Kaposi's sarcoma lesions. It is likely that the virus triggers the release of cellular and virus-encoded cytokines that promote the proliferation of spindle cells.

Highly active antiretroviral therapy has led to a dramatic reduction in the frequency and mortality of Kaposi's sarcoma in developed countries. In early Kaposi's sarcoma, the progression is often halted or reversed by starting antiretroviral treatment alone. Otherwise, cutaneous lesions may be left untreated or treated with local radiotherapy, cryotherapy, or intralesional vinblastine.

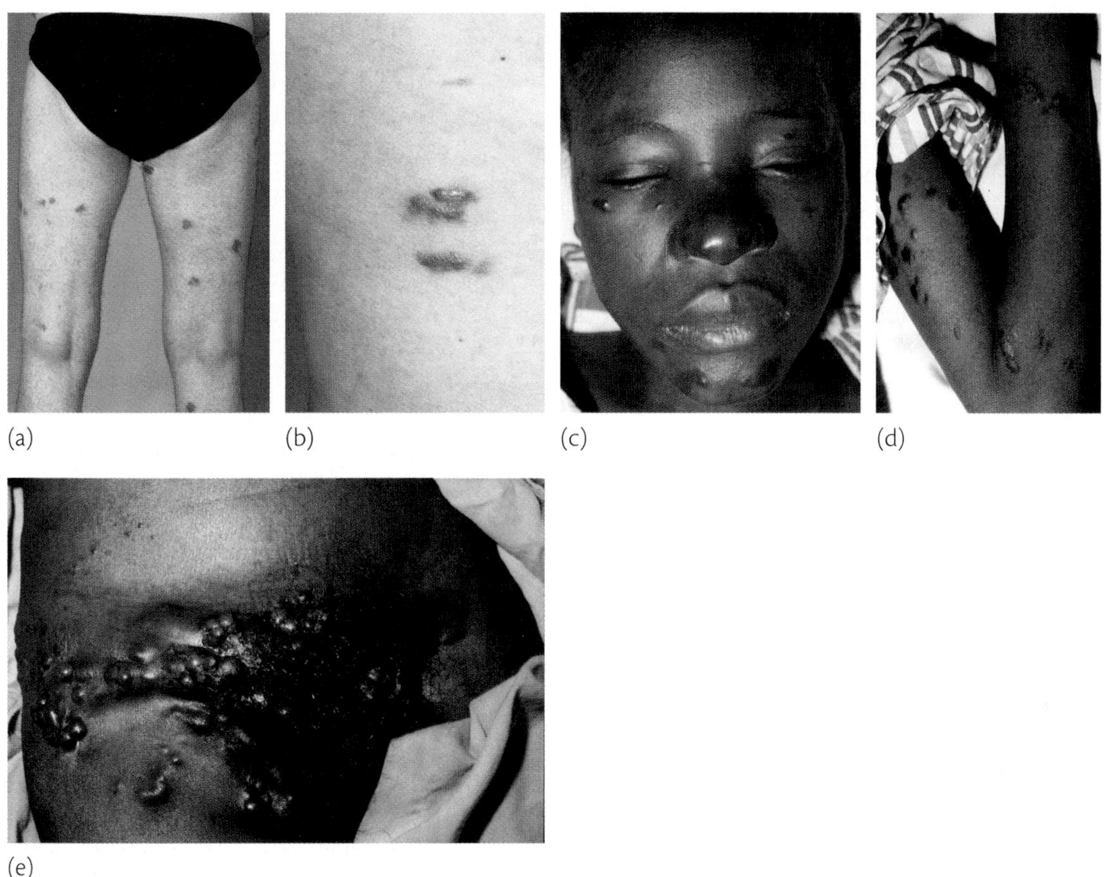

Fig. 7.5.23.12 Kaposi's sarcoma. (a, b) cutaneous Kaposi's sarcoma in a white man; (c, d), cutaneous Kaposi's sarcoma in a Zimbabwean; (e) invasive Kaposi's sarcoma in a Kenyan.
(Copyright D A Warrell)

Widespread skin or visceral disease is usually treated by systemic chemotherapy, usually with a liposomal anthracycline such as daunorubicin or doxorubicin, which are more effective than the previously used combination of vincristine and bleomycin. Paclitaxel, a taxane, is potentially more toxic than liposomal anthracyclines, but may be useful as a second line agent after treatment failure. Treatment of disseminated Kaposi's sarcoma has not been considered to be curative, but remissions may be induced by a combination of highly active antiretroviral treatment and systemic chemotherapy.

Non-Hodgkin's lymphoma

Non-Hodgkin's lymphoma develops in 3 to 10% of HIV-positive patients, an incidence 60 to 100 times higher than in the general population. Most tumours are extranodal and, histologically, 60% are large cell B-cell lymphomas; 30% are Burkitt's type and the rest are of T-cell or non-B-, non-T-cell origin. Some 50% are associated with Epstein–Barr virus (EBV) infection and are more aggressive with a shorter survival. A minority of HIV-related lymphomas are associated with HHV-8. They present as body cavity lymphomas, causing pleural or peritoneal effusions (primary effusion lymphoma). Patients on highly active antiretroviral therapy have a reduced risk of developing non-Hodgkin's lymphoma, and consequently the incidence of HIV-related lymphomas in developed countries has declined in recent years.

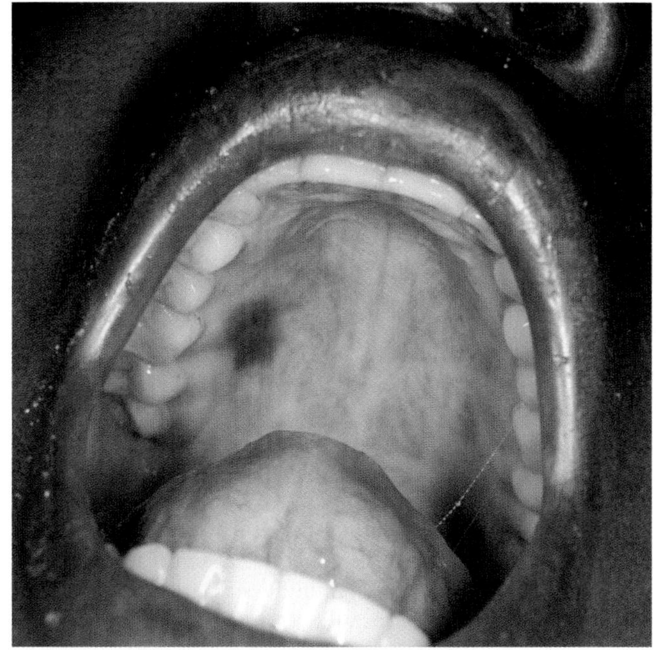

Fig. 7.5.23.13 Palatal Kaposi's sarcoma.
(Copyright D A Warrell.)

HIV-associated lymphoma outside the central nervous system may respond well to standard lymphoma chemotherapy regimens, in addition to highly active antiretroviral treatment. Response is better in those who are less immunosuppressed (CD4 above 200/mm^3 and no previous AIDS diagnosis). Opportunistic infections cause many deaths during chemotherapy. Lower dose or less toxic chemotherapy protocols are sometimes advocated for patients with more advanced HIV disease.

Other tumours in AIDS

Some studies have reported an increased frequency of Hodgkin's disease in patients with HIV, particularly of the mixed cellularity type. Disseminated disease with a poor prognosis seems to be more frequent than for HIV-negative Hodgkin's disease. Castleman's disease (angiofollicular lymph node hyperplasia) is a lymphoproliferative condition that can be HHV-8 related and, in the multicentric form, is associated with HIV. There is an increased incidence of squamous cell carcinoma of the conjunctiva in patients with HIV infection, especially in Africa. HIV-infected women suffer a higher incidence of cervical intraepithelial neoplasia (CIN) and predisposition to cervical carcinoma; cervical cancer has been designated an AIDS-defining condition. The incidence of vulvar intraepithelial neoplasia (VIN) is also increased by HIV infection. The incidence of squamous cell anal carcinoma is increased in homosexual men, but the risk does not seem to be greatly magnified by HIV while the risk of anal intraepithelial neoplasia (AIN), a precursor of anal carcinoma, is significantly increased. The development of CIN, VIN, and AIN may be related to coinfection with oncogenic types of human papillomavirus, especially type 16.

Miscellaneous conditions

Bacillary angiomatosis

Disseminated infection with *Bartonella henselae*, the principal agent of cat-scratch disease, is the cause of bacillary angiomatosis, an HIV-associated condition that typically causes multiple subcutaneous vascular lesions, fever, liver lesions (bacillary peliosis hepatis), and osteolytic bone lesions. The skin lesions are usually purplish nodules that may be mistaken for Kaposi's sarcoma, but the histology is distinct—acute neutrophilic inflammation and capillary proliferation, and clusters of bacilli revealed by modified silver staining. The organism may be cultured from blood. A similar syndrome in HIV-positive patients can be caused by the agent of trench fever, *Bartonella quintana.* Bacillary angiomatosis usually responds to treatment with a macrolide antibiotic. Cats and cat fleas form a reservoir for *B. henselae*, and patients who develop bacillary angiomatosis frequently have a history of contact with cats.

Disseminated fungal infections

In regions where invasive fungal infections are endemic (such as *Histoplasma capsulatum* in the Mississippi river region, *Coccidioides immitis* in the southern United States of America, and *Penicillium marneffei* in South East Asia) or where there is a relevant travel history, disseminated fungal infection should be considered in HIV-positive patients presenting with fever, weight loss, anaemia, pulmonary infiltrates, lymphadenopathy, and hepatosplenomegaly. Papular skin lesions may be seen in disseminated histoplasmosis and *P. marneffei* infection. Similar lesions resembling giant molluscum (see below) may occur with disseminated cryptococcosis. Blood or bone marrow cultures or direct identification by the use of special stains on tissue obtained from skin lesions, bone marrow, or liver are required for diagnosis. Initial therapy is generally with intravenous amphotericin; itraconazole (for histoplasmosis and *P. marneffei*) or fluconazole (for coccidioidomycosis) may be adequate for subsequent maintenance treatment.

Leishmaniasis

HIV-associated disseminated leishmaniasis is mostly reported from the Mediterranean littoral, South America, and Africa. It is caused by dissemination of leishmania spp., protozoan parasites transmitted by sandflies. A high index of clinical suspicion is required, because although the classic features are fever, weight loss, anaemia, and hepatosplenomegaly, a high proportion of patients have fever alone. The disease may present months or years after exposure in an endemic country. Leishmania may be transmitted by shared needles in injecting drug users. Most cases can be diagnosed by bone marrow examination or splenic aspirate; serology may be helpful. Treatment is with lipid formulations of amphotericin B.

Haematological conditions

Thrombocytopenia is relatively common (5–15%) in HIV infection and may be how the disease first presents. It is associated with antiplatelet antibodies. Symptomatic thrombocytopenia is uncommon but more likely in the later stages of HIV infection. Life-threatening bleeding is rare. Thrombocytopenia is not a marker for HIV progression and spontaneous remissions are frequent. Antiretroviral treatment is first-line when the CD4 count is low; zidovudine is known to increase platelet production. When specific treatment for thrombocytopenia is required, the principles and response are similar to those that apply in the treatment of HIV-negative immune thrombocytopenia, and include the use of prednisolone, intravenous immunoglobulin, and splenectomy.

Anaemia is common in patients with advanced HIV infection, and is frequently related to medications (such as zidovudine). Human (B19) parvovirus infection is a reversible cause of chronic anaemia in HIV infection. Bone marrow biopsy typically shows an absence of erythroid development with occasional giant pronormoblasts, and B19 parvovirus is detected by PCR. The anaemia may respond to treatment with intravenous immunoglobulin.

Mild neutropenia is common in HIV-positive patients at all stages of infection, and may be partly responsible for the increased risk of pyogenic bacterial infections; however, profound neutropenia (below 0.5×10^9/litre) is rare. Antineutrophil antibodies may be present. Drugs (such as co-trimoxazole, ganciclovir, and antiretrovirals) may increase the incidence and severity of neutropenia. In selected HIV-positive patients with refractory or life-threatening bacterial or fungal infection and severe neutropenia, the addition of recombinant human granulocyte colony-stimulating factor to the treatment regimen may improve the outcome.

Skin conditions in advanced HIV

In the later stages of HIV infection, a number of infections have atypical cutaneous manifestations. All have become rare in settings where antiretroviral treatment is available to prevent advanced immunosuppression. These conditions include giant molluscum contagiosum, characterized by large, flesh-coloured, nontender umbilicated lesions often affecting the face in homosexual men. In advanced HIV disease, genital herpes simplex infection may cause painful chronic genital or anal ulcers that can become resistant to aciclovir and related compounds; intravenous foscarnet or cidofovir are effective. Aciclovir-resistant varicella zoster virus also occurs in AIDS; and reactivation of varicella zoster virus can take an unusual form, with a subacute course and dissemination causing scattered vesicular lesions in the absence of dermatomal zoster. CMV is a cause of chronic perianal ulceration that can be treated with ganciclovir. Atypical cutaneous presentations of syphilis may occur at any stage of HIV infection. In Asia, the varied skin manifestations of *P. marneffei* infection are familiar.

HIV-associated nephropathy (HIVAN)

HIV infection may be complicated by renal impairment and often presents as nephritic syndrome, but with minimal oedema. This condition appears to be more common in Africans and African Americans than in the white population. There is evidence that HIV directly infects glomerular and tubular epithelial cells. Renal biopsy reveals a collapsing focal glomerulosclerosis and there may be tubular dilatation. Renal function usually improves with the use of antiretroviral medication, but some patients progress to chronic renal failure and require renal replacement therapy or transplantation.

HIV and hepatitis virus coinfections

Because of common risk factors for blood-borne virus infections, there are increasing numbers of individuals with HIV who are coinfected with either hepatitis C (HCV) or hepatitis B (HBV) virus, or both. Over the past few years, new data have become available on the size of this problem and some management strategies have emerged.

HIV/HCV coinfection

Hepatitis C coinfection occurs in up to a third of those with HIV. The group with the highest prevalence is the haemophiliac population, but the group most at risk now is injecting drug users (IDU). Anywhere between 50 and 75% of IDU with HIV are coinfected. More recently, there is an awareness that growing numbers of men who have sex with men (MSM) are acquiring HCV sexually.

HCV/HIV coinfection increases the risk of liver disease progression compared to HCV infection by itself. In addition, the treatment of HIV with antiretrovirals may carry an increased risk of hepatotoxicity in those with coinfection. There is little evidence to suggest that HCV worsens HIV disease.

Treatment aimed at clearing HCV in those with coinfection can be successful, but is less likely to lead to a sustained virological response compared to HCV infection alone. Trials in HIV coinfected patients show that pegylated interferon-α 2a with ribavirin is the treatment of choice and, as in those without coinfection, HCV genotypes 2 and 3 respond better than genotypes 1 and 4. Treatment in those with coinfection is more likely to lead to anaemia and may cause transient drops in CD4 count.

HIV/HBV coinfection

The scale of the HIV epidemic in Africa and, now, in Asia means that up to 90% of those with HIV will have evidence of past or current HBV infection. Estimates vary, but up to 10% of those with HIV may be HBV carriers.

Unlike with HCV, there is no evidence that liver disease due to HBV is worse in HIV coinfected individuals. Although HBV DNA levels are higher in HIV coinfection, there is evidence that there is less liver injury. New HBV infections in HIV positive individuals are less likely to cause acute hepatitis and jaundice, but are more likely to result in chronic HBV carriage. HBV infection does not seem to affect the progression of HIV disease.

Treatment of HBV coinfection is less well defined than treatment of HCV coinfection. Although pegylated interferon may be useful, there are no large trials of its efficacy in HIV. Lamivudine monotherapy is more likely to lead to resistant HBV with the 'YMDD' mutant in the presence of HIV. Drugs currently used to treat HBV in the absence of HIV coinfection also have anti-HIV activity, particularly lamivudine, emtricitabine, and tenofovir. Caution must be used in treating HBV with these agents in coinfected patients as monotherapy with these drugs will lead to resistant HIV. A recently introduced drug to treat HBV, entecavir, was thought not to have activity against HIV but had now been shown to have an anti-HIV effect and this can also lead to HIV resistance. By contrast, if HBV coinfected patients require antiretroviral therapy, a combination of lamivudine and tenofovir, or emtricitabine and tenofovir, is recommended as part of the antiretroviral regimen to decrease HBV replication.

Management of HIV infection

The advent of highly active antiretroviral therapy (HAART) in the mid 1990s led to marked reductions in morbidity and mortality attributable to HIV and its complications—although not in resource-limited countries, where the epidemic is concentrated and access to antiretroviral treatment remains limited. A decline in the incidence of opportunistic infections, notably pneumocystis pneumonia, disseminated *M. avium* complex (MAC) infection, CMV retinitis, cerebral toxoplasmosis and cryptococcal meningitis, and associated mortality was reported from the United States of America and Europe after the introduction of treatment based on a minimum of three antiretroviral drugs. HIV infection in adults in resource-rich countries is now almost exclusively managed on an outpatient basis.

There is no evidence that HAART can ever achieve eradication or 'cure' of HIV. Although HIV may be undetectable in plasma for many months, a long-lived reservoir of infectious virus can be recovered from latently infected (resting) memory CD4 lymphocytes. The half-life of this cell population is long, about 6 months, and it is not known whether HIV can ever be eradicated from this infected cell line. Other compartments exist that are relatively inaccessible to drugs—e.g. in the central nervous system, retina, and testes—and unless viral replication can be successfully prevented at such sites there is also the risk of reinfection of compartments previously cleared by therapy.

Initial assessment and management

Ideally, HIV infection should be identified at the asymptomatic stage. At the time of diagnosis, patients should undergo a baseline assessment that includes taking a detailed history, including a sexual history, and determination of risk factors for HIV infection. An assessment of cardiovascular risk factors should be made, including smoking and family history. A detailed physical examination should be performed with attention to the skin and mucous membranes, blood pressure, and body mass index (BMI), fundoscopy, and should include a search for lymphadenopathy and signs of liver disease. Initial investigations include full blood count, biochemical screen including liver profile and estimated GFR, fasting lipids, chest radiography, and serological screening for infections that may require additional treatment (hepatitis B and C, syphilis) or which can reactivate during immunosuppression (CMV and toxoplasma). Baseline investigations include CD4 lymphocyte (T-helper cell) count (lymphocyte subsets profile), quantitative estimation of HIV RNA in the blood plasma (viral load), and HIV genotypic resistance testing; and should include tissue typing for HLA-B*5701, a marker for abacavir hypersensitivity. In women, cervical cytology screening is indicated at annual intervals.

Following initial assessment, hepatitis B immunization may be provided to susceptible individuals, and pneumococcal vaccine may be offered. Psychological support and counselling are often needed. There should be a discussion on who should be informed about their HIV status, including the primary care physician, and family members and friends for support. The issue of disclosure to sexual partners should also be raised, with advice on reducing risk of transmission (including the importance of barrier methods such as condoms).

The CD4 lymphocyte count and HIV viral load are the two laboratory markers that have the best prognostic value. The CD4 count is a reliable indicator of HIV-related immune impairment. CD4 counts, normal at or above 600/mm^3, vary considerably, even in the absence of HIV infection. A fall in the CD4 lymphocyte count to below 200/mm^3 is associated with a risk of opportunistic infections of about 80% over 3 years without antiretroviral treatment. However, progression is variable and a minority remain well for several years with stable low CD4 counts. This variability is explained partly by differences in HIV viral load. The level of CD4 lymphopenia generally determines the spectrum of potential infections (Table 7.5.23.1). For instance, whereas oral and oesophageal candidiasis and pneumocystis pneumonia are frequent at CD4 counts of 100 to 200/mm^3, disseminated MAC infection and CMV retinitis are rarely seen until the CD4 count is below 50/mm^3.

The prognostic value of measuring HIV RNA in plasma was reported from the United States of America in 1996. In HIV-positive men, in a subgroup of the Multicenter AIDS Cohort Study, only 8% with less than 5000 copies of HIV RNA/ml progressed to AIDS over 5 years, whereas 62% with viral loads above 35 000 developed AIDS. For a given level of CD4 lymphocytes, variations in viral load broadly predict the risk of progression. The most useful prognostic information is therefore derived from the CD4 count and viral load taken together (Fig. 7.5.23.14).

In industrialized countries, HIV viral load measurements are widely available. Techniques include reverse transcription followed by amplification by the polymerase chain reaction (RT-PCR), branched DNA (bDNA) signal amplification, and nucleic acid sequence-based amplification (NASBA). Highly sensitive tests with very low detection limits (50 copies/ml) are generally used.

Antiretroviral therapy

Nucleoside analogues

Knowledge of the viral lifecycle (Fig. 7.5.23.3) led to the development of a number of antiretroviral compounds with clinically useful activity against HIV (Table 7.5.23.2). The forerunner of these was zidovudine (AZT or ZDV), first shown to be active against HIV *in vitro* in 1985. Zidovudine, a nucleoside analogue that inhibits HIV reverse transcriptase, slowed down the rate of disease progression over a 12-month period in patients with AIDS and improved short-term survival, well-being, body weight, and neurological features. However, clinical progression associated with viral resistance to the drug was observed after a year or two of therapy. When early treatment with zidovudine was compared to deferred zidovudine, there was no difference in survival or disease progression after 3 years.

The clinical failure of monotherapy prompted combination therapy in an attempt to reduce the development of drug resistance. Double nucleoside combinations proved superior to zidovudine monotherapy, especially in patients without prior exposure to zidovudine. Treatment with at least three drugs is more effective and has become the standard of care. In general, two nucleoside drugs are used with either a non-nucleoside reverse transcriptase inhibitor or a protease inhibitor. A combination of three nucleoside analogues (zidovudine, lamivudine, and abacavir) can also be used in a single tablet taken twice daily, but is less effective than other combinations and is not routinely recommended (Table 7.5.23.3). A nucleotide agent, tenofovir, has similar properties and is usually grouped in the same category as the nucleoside analogues.

Non-nucleoside reverse transcriptase inhibitors

The prototype of the class is nevirapine, a potent and selective inhibitor of HIV reverse transcriptase. When nevirapine is given alone, resistance develops rapidly; this drug is of limited effectiveness in double therapy or when added to failing regimens. However, in antiretroviral-naive patients without AIDS (CD4 200–600/mm^3), over 50% of patients treated with nevirapine plus two nucleosides (zidovudine and didanosine) had undetectable plasma HIV RNA after 1 year of therapy, compared with 12% for zidovudine/didanosine only. Efavirenz and delavirdine (which is not licensed for use in the United Kingdom) are other non-nucleoside reverse transcriptase inhibitors (NNRTIs) with similar properties to nevirapine. More recently, a new NNRTI, etravirine, has been licensed and has activity against viral isolates resistant to the older NNRTIs. None of these drugs is active against HIV-2.

Protease inhibitors

The HIV-encoded protease (or proteinase) is required for the production of mature infectious viral particles. This enzyme cleaves a number of structural proteins and enzymes from the polyprotein precursors produced by translation of the *gag* and *gag–pol* genes. Inhibitors of HIV protease act synergistically with nucleoside drugs and are potent inhibitors of HIV replication.

In early studies, indinavir, in combination with two nucleoside analogues (zidovudine/lamivudine or stavudine/lamivudine) produced good results in a large controlled trial with clinical endpoints (ACTG 320 clinical trial). Similar results were subsequently reported for combination therapy with other protease inhibitors (PIs). The PIs in current use are generally 'ritonavir-boosted', i.e. they are used in combination with low dose ritonavir to improve pharmacokinetics (via cytochrome P450 interactions) of the principal PIs (especially saquinavir, lopinavir, atazanvir, and fosamprenavir).

PIs have a higher threshold for development of resistance mutations compared to NNRTIs, so that when resistance does occur it is more likely to be due to poor absorption and suboptimal blood levels. Nevertheless, PI mutations do occur and can be a problem in drug-experienced patients. Newer PIs, such as tipranavir and darunavir, are active against some of the PI-resistant isolates and have an increasing role in salvage therapy.

Entry inhibitors

HIV entry inhibitors are a new class of antiretroviral drugs that target viral entry into cells. This class contains two subgroups, fusion inhibitors and coreceptor antagonists. The fusion inhibitor enfuvirtide (T-20) stops the HIV glycoprotein gp41 from effecting

Table 7.5.23.1 Principal complications of HIV infection

Infections	Neoplasms	Direct HIV effects
Early/intermediate HIV infection (CD4 >200/mm^3)		
Herpes zoster	Non-Hodgkin's lymphoma[a]	Persistent generalized lymphadenopathy
Oral hairy leucoplakia	Cervical intraepithelial neoplasia	Atopy; eczema
Oral candidiasis; candidal vaginitis	Anal intraepithelial neoplasia	Recurrent aphthous ulcers (oral and gastrointestinal tract)
Pulmonary tuberculosis[a]		Immune thrombocytopenia
Bacterial pneumonia, especially pneumococcal		Neutropenia
Bacteraemia, especially pneumococcal and salmonella		Neuropathy (mononeuritis multiplex; Guillian–Barré syndrome)
Bacillary angiomatosis		HIV-associated nephropathy (HIVAN)
		Lymphocytic interstitial pneumonitis (LIP)
Late HIV infection (CD4 <200/mm^3)		
Pneumocystis pneumonia[a]	Kaposi's sarcoma[a]	HIV enteropathy
Candidal oesophagitis[a]	Primary cerebral lymphoma[a]	Peripheral neuropathy (distal, axonal)
Cerebral toxoplasmosis[a]	Hodgkin's lymphoma	Autonomic neuropathy
Cryptococcal meningitis[a]	Conjunctival carcinoma	Myelopathy
Chronic cryptosporidial diarrhoea[a]	? Cervical carcinoma[a]	HIV dementia[a]
Chronic isosporiasis[a], microsporidiosis	? Anal carcinoma	Wasting syndrome[a]
Chronic HSV[a] ulceration		Cardiomyopathy
Extrapulmonary tuberculosis[a]		
Disseminated *M. avium* complex (MAC)[a]		
CMV (retinitis and disseminated)[a]		
Progressive multifocal leucoencephalopathy[a]		
Recurrent bacterial pneumonia[a]		
Recurrent bacteraemia, especially salmonella[a]		
Disseminated histoplasmosis[a], and *P. marneffei*		

[a] AIDS-defining conditions; incomplete list.

? Signifies suspected but unproven association. Many of the early/intermediate manifestations also occur in late-stage HIV disease; non-Hodgkin's lymphoma is more common during the later stages.

fusion of the viral and cellular membranes, and thereby prevents HIV entry into host cells. This drug is licensed for use in treatment-experienced patients in combination with other drugs. It must be given by subcutaneous injection and is associated with a high rate of injection site reactions.

Coreceptor antagonists act as functional antagonists of the chemokine receptor CCR5 and are active against the R5-tropic subgroup of HIV-1 viruses. Maraviroc is the first to be licensed from this subgroup, but others, such as vicriviroc, are in clinical trials. These drugs are not effective against strains of virus using CXCR4 (more common in late disease), so assays to determine the type of coreceptor usage of a patient's virus are needed before these drugs are used. The place of these agents in HIV therapy is yet to be determined.

Integrase inhibitors

This new class of drugs inhibits an essential enzyme that catalyses the integration of HIV proviral DNA into the host cell genome. The enzyme, integrase, is also involved in viral assembly and is not a feature of host cells. The first drug to be licensed in this group, raltegravir, is a potent inhibitor of HIV replication which currently should

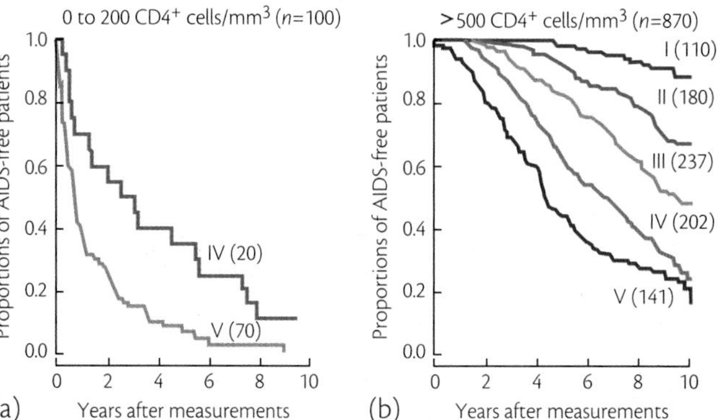

Fig. 7.5.23.14 Curves showing AIDS-free survival with time among groups with different baseline CD4 lymphocyte counts, according to HIV-1 RNA category. The five categories were (copies/ml): I, 500 or less; II, 501–3000; III, 3001–10 000; IV, 10 001–30 000; and V, above 30 000. (Sample sizes are shown in brackets).

Table 7.5.23.2 Principal antiretroviral agents

Nucleoside reverse transcriptase inhibitors	Non-nucleoside reverse transcriptase inhibitors	Protease inhibitors	Entry inhibitors
Zidovudine (AZT/ZDV)	Nevirapine	Lopinavir[a]	*Fusion inhibitor*
Lamivudine (3TC)	Efavirenz	Ritonavir	Enfuvirtide
Emtricitabine (FTC)	Etravirine	Atazanavir[a]	
Abacavir (ABC)		Saquinavir[a]	*CCR5 antagonists*[b]
Didanosine (ddI)		Fosamprenavir[a]	Maraviroc
Stavudine (d4T)		Indinavir[a]	Vicriviroc[b]
		Nelfinavir	
Nucleotide reverse transcriptase inhibitor		Tipranavir[a]	*Integrase inhibitors*
Tenofovir (TDF)		Darunavir[a]	Raltegravir
			Elvitegravir[b]

Other compounds (not shown) are at earlier phases of development and evaluation.

[a] Given with low-dose ritonavir for pharmacokinetic enhancement.

[b] Experimental, in advanced clinical trials.

only be used in combination with other active antiretrovirals in patients with high exposure to all three major drug classes. Another drug in this class, elvitegravir, is at an advanced stage of development.

Other drugs

There is a need for new drug classes for use after development of drug resistance, allowing additional options for switching after treatment failure or drug intolerance, and also to provide compounds that avoid the long-term toxicities associated with current antiretrovirals. Immunotherapy with interleukin-2 (IL-2), which raises CD4 lymphocyte counts and is given by subcutaneous injection, has been shown to be clinically ineffective in recent studies.

Table 7.5.23.3 Initial antiretroviral regimens

Regimen	Examples	Comment
2 NRTIs + NNRTI	3TC/ABC + efavirenz OR nevirapine	Preferred initial regimens[a]; avoid efavirenz if risk of pregnancy
	TDF/FTC + efavirenz OR nevirapine	
	AZT/3TC + efavirenz OR nevirapine	Alternative regimen; avoid efavirenz if risk of pregnancy
2 NRTI + 2PIs[b]	AZT/3TC + ritonavir/other PI[b]	Alternative initial regimen; caution about drug interactions with ritonavir
	3TC/ABC + ritonavir/other PI[b]	
	TDF/FTC + ritonavir/other PI[b]	

3TC, lamivudine; ABC, abacavir; AZT, zidovudine; FTC, emtricitabine; NNRTI, non-nucleoside reverse transcriptase inhibitor; NRTI, nucleoside reverse transcriptase inhibitor; PI, protease inhibitor; TDF, tenofovir.

[a] If HLA-B*5701 -ve

[b] Low-dose ritonavir (to improve pharmacokinetics) plus usually lopinavir, atazanavir or fosamprenavir.

When to start antiretroviral treatment

The optimum time to start antiretroviral therapy is not known, and no trials have adequately addressed this question; large scale, long-term clinical trials are needed. Data from several clinical cohorts suggest that patients who start treatment when the CD4 count is below 200/mm^3 have an increased mortality when compared with those starting at higher CD4 levels. Therefore, treatment should be started before the CD4 count drops to 200/mm^3 or if the patient develops symptoms related to HIV. In asymptomatic patients, current guidelines recommend that antiretroviral treatment should be considered when the CD4 count falls to around 350/mm^3. The decision to start treatment should take into account other factors of prognostic importance, including the rate of CD4 decline, the viral load, age, and presence of coinfection with hepatitis B or C. Patients who are clinically well and have high CD4 counts at presentation should be seen for follow-up at intervals of 3 to 6 months for CD4 and viral load measurements.

What to start with

Highly active antiretroviral therapy consists of at least three drugs from two different drug classes, usually a backbone of two nucleosides with either a non-nucleoside reverse transcriptase inhibitor or a protease inhibitor (see Table 7.5.23.3). For improved pharmacokinetics, the protease inhibitor is usually combined ('boosted') with a second protease inhibitor, i.e. low-dose ritonavir. A triple nucleoside regimen is also available, but is not suitable for initial therapy because of lower potency. A number of initial regimens have equivalent efficacy.

The most important cause of treatment failure is inadequate treatment, which may relate to failure to take the drugs regularly, i.e. nonadherence, lack of availability of drugs, or poor absorption. Before starting treatment it is therefore important to discuss the patient's views about taking medication regularly. Simplified regimens have helped with adherence (see below). A number of other factors also influence the selection of the initial regimen, including potential drug interactions (e.g. with antituberculosis treatment), toxicity (e.g. avoidance of stavudine in initial regimens), ease of administration (didanosine is taken on an empty stomach), presence of renal or hepatic dysfunction, female gender (avoidance of efavirenz in women who may be at risk of pregnancy). HIV viral load and CD4 count should be checked within 2 months. The aim of initial treatment is to achieve a sustained reduction in viral load to undetectable levels (<40 copies/ml) within 2 to 3 months of starting treatment.

Patient adherence

A substantial proportion of HIV patients do not follow treatment recommendations. Reasons for nonadherence include poor communication, the complexity of drug regimens and number of tablets, disruption of life (including timing and food restrictions), side effects, concerns about long-term effects, and lack of confidence in noncurative treatments of indefinite duration. Adherence to treatment requires a high level of understanding and motivation in the patient. This is of particular concern in HIV therapy because of the risk of developing drug resistance mutations during suboptimal therapy. The recent development of simplified regimens (one or two tablets taken once or twice daily) has helped. Patients may be helped to be adherent by skilled support from trained professionals such as counsellors or pharmacists.

Changing therapy

The principal reasons for changing antiretroviral treatment are treatment failure, toxicity, and poor adherence. There is no agreed definition for treatment failure. Patients whose viral load is not suppressed to less than 40 copies/ml within 3 months, or was initially suppressed and subsequently rises, should be considered for changing to a completely new regimen of at least three drugs. This should be guided by a resistance test (see below). Continuing viral replication in the presence of antiretroviral treatment should be avoided because of progressive accumulation of resistance mutations which can compromise future treatment options. However, the optimal point at which the switch should be made has not been clearly defined. If adherence is poor or likely to be the cause of treatment failure, changing to a combination that is simpler to take should be considered, e.g. based on once or twice daily dosage and low pill burden.

Poor absorption of protease inhibitors may sometimes cause treatment failure related to low blood levels, without development of resistance; measurement of blood levels may be useful in this context. If treatment needs to be changed because of drug toxicity (e.g. a severe rash), a single drug substitution can be made if the responsible agent is identified.

'Salvage' therapy

Salvage therapy is generally defined as treatment following exposure to multiple antiretroviral drugs. In this situation, numerous drug resistance mutations are usually present and the likelihood of achieving sustained viral suppression below the detection level is much lower than for patients who have limited or no previous antiretroviral exposure. This is especially true if drugs from all three major classes have previously been used. Studies using clinical endpoints suggest that declines in viral load correlate with improvements in clinical outcome, even if suppression to below the detection limit is not achieved. Several factors may be considered when selecting a treatment regimen in these circumstances, including the history of drug classes to which the patient has not been exposed and the results of tests for viral resistance. It may be possible to recycle some drugs with less likelihood of resistance, or to include new drugs active against resistant isolates (e.g. darunavir) or new classes of drugs (e.g. raltegravir). When initiating salvage therapy it is important to use at least two new drugs to which the patient has not been exposed in order to reduce the risk of further resistance developing.

Drug resistance

Viral resistance is a major factor in treatment failure. Resistant mutants can arise spontaneously even in the absence of antiretroviral therapy; however, the selection of drug-resistance mutants occurs rapidly when HIV replicates in the presence of subtherapeutic levels of antiretroviral drugs, and is eliminated when HIV replication is completely suppressed by a potent drug combination.

Extensive genotypic variation of HIV occurs because of very high viral turnover and transcription errors by the reverse transcriptase enzyme, so that all possible single point mutations are likely to occur over time. Although mutations causing resistance to single agents may arise before antiretroviral treatment is started, on statistical grounds it is unlikely that specific combinations of multiple mutations will be present. Control of viral replication with a highly potent treatment regimen limits the appearance of resistant HIV mutants.

Genotypic and phenotypic assays have been developed to test for drug resistance in HIV isolates. Genotypic assays that identify codon mutations correlating with *in vivo* resistance to antiretrovirals are relatively easy to perform, inexpensive, and most widely used. Phenotypic assays that measure the ability of the virus to grow in increasing concentrations of drugs are time-consuming and expensive, but provide more direct evidence of resistance to a particular drug. Resistance assays are widely used in the selection of drug regimens and investigation of treatment failure. Interpretation of resistance patterns is increasingly difficult as the number of drugs and mutations involved increases.

Resistance mutations to antiretroviral agents in newly acquired HIV, indicating transmitted drug resistance, are identified in approximately 10% of recent seroconverters in Europe and may be increasing. However, the presence of a mutation does not necessarily denote clinical resistance. In the absence of therapy, wild-type virus predominates and resistance mutations may be undetectable though present in small copy numbers. This can lead to treatment failures with the resistant mutants increasing as wild-type virus is eradicated by drugs. For this reason, baseline resistance testing at diagnosis is now advocated in an attempt to identify resistance mutations at the outset.

Drug toxicity and interactions

Adverse reactions to antiretroviral agents are relatively common and may lead to the patient stopping their therapy (Table 7.5.23.4). Minor gastrointestinal disturbances (nausea, vomiting, and diarrhoea), rashes, and headache are common, but some adverse reactions are serious. Drug interactions must be considered when prescribing antiretroviral drugs, especially in advanced HIV disease. Antiretroviral agents may interact with each other and with other drugs. For example, phenytoin drastically reduces plasma levels of efavirenz. Ritonavir, a potent inhibitor of cytochrome P450, is especially prone to raising blood levels of other drugs and should not be given with most antiarrhythmics, anxiolytics, and antihistamines. Caution is required with several analgesics, anticonvulsants, and other categories of medication.

Metabolic complications, especially mitochondrial toxicity and disturbances of lipid and glucose metabolism, have emerged as important adverse effects of antiretroviral therapy. Mitochondrial toxicity is associated with nucleoside drugs (especially didanosine and stavudine) and may result in neuropathy, myopathy, pancreatitis, hepatic steatosis, hyperlactataemia, and lactic acidosis. Lactic acidosis causes nonspecific symptoms, including malaise, gastrointestinal disturbance, and liver function abnormalities, and can progress to death, particularly if antiretrovirals are not stopped. There is no evidence that routine monitoring of lactate levels is helpful. Nucleoside drugs are thought to cause mitochondrial dysfunction by inhibiting mitochondrial DNA polymerase-γ.

A syndrome of lipodystrophy (progressive loss of fat from face and limbs) and hyperlipidaemia is associated with thymidine analogue nucleoside drugs, especially stavudine, and to a lesser extent zidovudine. Truncal fat accumulation, hyperlipidaemia, and insulin resistance have been associated with protease inhibitors.

After the introduction of antiretroviral treatment, early reports suggested a possible increase in cardiovascular disease. Several variables potentially affect the risk of myocardial infarction and other cardiovascular events in patients with HIV. Uncontrolled viraemia may cause endovascular inflammation. The Data Collection on

Table 7.5.23.4 Principal toxicities of antiretroviral drugs

Nucleoside reverse transcriptase inhibitors (NRTI)	
Class effects	GI disturbances, raised liver enzymes, hepatic steatosis, lactic acidosis
AZT	Headache, nausea (usually resolve within 2–4 weeks)
	Anaemia (avoid if anaemic at baseline)
	Macrocytosis (benign)
	Nail pigmentation
	Myopathy (rare on lower dosages 500–600 mg/day)
	Lipodystrophy with facial wasting (long-term effect, unknown incidence)
ABC	Hypersensitivity 5%; may be fatal if rechallenged (closely associated with HLA B*5701)
ddI	Pancreatitis, peripheral neuropathy
d4T	Lipodystrophy with facial wasting; peripheral neuropathy
3TC, FTC	No major toxicities
Nucleotide RTI	
Tenofovir	Renal failure (case reports, rare, incidence unknown)
Non-nucleoside RTI (NNRTI)	
Efavirenz	Neuropsychiatric disturbances (8%) – vivid dreams, impaired concentration, mood changes (usually transient, <4 weeks duration); rash
Nevirapine	Rash (20%, severe 6%); rarely Stevens–Johnson syndrome; hepatitis (esp. in women with CD4 >250/mm^3 or men with CD4 >400 / mm^3—avoid)
Protease inhibitors (PI)	
Class effects	GI disturbances; hyperlipidaemia, truncal fat accumulation, diabetes, bleeding in haemophiliacs, raised liver enzymes
Lopinavir	Diarrhoea
Ritonavir	Circumoral and peripheral parasthesiae (unusual in low dosage)
Saquinavir	Rash, peripheral neuropathy
Nelfinavir	Diarrhoea
Indinavir	Renal calculi, haemolysis
Atazanavir	Hyperbilirubinaemia, jaundice
Tipranavir	Rash (caution in sulphonamide allergy), liver dysfunction
Darunavir	Diarrhoea, rash (caution in sulphonamide allergy)
Entry inhibitors	
Fusion inhibitors	
Enfuvirtide	Injection site reactions (painful, erythematous nodules); headache, dizziness, nausea, eosinophilia
CCR5 antagonists	
Maraviroc	Cough, muscle and joint pain, diarrhoea, sleep disturbance, raised liver enzymes (and possibly hepatitis)
Integrase inhibitors	
Raltegravir	Nausea, diarrhoea, headache; raised CPK in some patients

Adverse Events of Anti-HIV Drugs (DAD) study group has shown an association with antiretrovirals and cardiovascular events. The relative risk of myocardial infarction may be increased by about 10% when other factors, such as lipid levels, are taken into account. The INITIO trial has shown an increased incidence of the metabolic syndrome with antiretroviral treatment, with an associated increased risk of cardiovascular disease. The absolute risk is very small when compared to the risks associated with smoking and diabetes mellitus. Nevertheless, increasing attention is being paid to modifying cardiovascular risk factors in those on HIV therapy, such as smoking cessation programmes, treatment of hypertension, and managing hyperlipidaemia.

More recently, attention has also focused on changes in bone metabolism. Patients on HIV therapy may have an increased risk of osteoporosis and there is an increased incidence of avascular necrosis of the femoral head. The latter may be a consequence of vascular disease, but the mechanism involved in the development of osteoporosis is not clear.

Treatment interruptions

In general, once treatment is started it is continued indefinitely. There has been recent interest in whether interrupting treatment (in supervised or structured treatment interruptions) can be beneficial. In theory, such interruptions might enhance immune responses, reduce long-term toxicity, or reduce resistant virus by allowing repopulation with wild-type virus. A recent large trial (SMART) was stopped early because of a paradoxical result. The study randomized patients with stable disease on therapy to continuing therapy or to stopping (and restarting if the CD4 count fell below 250). Not only were there more HIV complications in the stopping group, but this group, surprisingly, also had a higher incidence of cardiovascular disease. It is postulated that the increased cardiovascular risk is related to endothelial inflammation secondary to uncontrolled viraemia. It is thus unlikely that treatment interruption will be a sensible management strategy and patients should be counselled about the need for long-term treatment.

Immune reconstitution inflammatory syndrome (IRIS)

Since the introduction of highly active antiretroviral therapy (HAART), there have been reports of unusual symptoms and signs appearing in patients some time after starting therapy. Because these clinical problems arise in the face of increasing CD4 counts, the syndrome has been called the immune reconstitution inflammatory syndrome (IRIS) or immune reconstitution disease (IRD). In the absence of HIV, paradoxical clinical responses have been described in tuberculosis and in leprosy. In the setting of HIV, IRIS often takes the form of an exacerbation of a previously treated opportunist infection or an unusual clinical presentation of an opportunist infection that was subclinical at the time HAART was started.

The incidence of IRIS is difficult to determine, particularly as there is no currently agreed definition, but it may occur in up to 20% of patients starting HAART. Usually, IRIS starts within a few months of starting HAART and is temporally related to a rise in CD4 count. A proposed definition includes (1) new or worsening symptoms of an infection or inflammation after starting antiretrovirals, (2) symptoms not explained by a new infection or the expected course of an infection previously diagnosed, and (3) a decrease in viral load by at least 1 log10. The pathogenesis of IRIS is poorly understood, but many patients have been found to have raised IL-6 levels, possibly related to a brisk Th-1 lymphocyte response.

The most common opportunist infections complicated by IRIS are tuberculosis, *M. avium* (MAC) infections, cryptococcal meningitis, and cytomegalovirus. IRIS complicating tuberculosis is probably the most common problem. Patients may develop fever or lymphadenopathy or may present with pleural effusions. Bone and joint involvement also occurs. IRIS is possibly more common in those presenting with extrapulmonary tuberculosis.

IRIS may occur in those receiving treatment for MAC and in one series complicated 30% of cases. The usual problem is lymph node enlargement, which may be massive and can mimic lymphoma. Some cases are complicated by hypercalcaemia.

Cryptococcal meningitis, when complicated by IRIS, may present as an apparent relapse with fever, headache, and signs of meningeal irritation. Rapidly expanding cerebral cryptococcomas may lead to fatal increases in intracranial pressure. Cytomegalovirus infections may also be complicated by IRIS with a worsening of signs of retinitis or a more benign vitritis. Rarely, patients have presented with a uveitis some years after starting HAART.

Some of the common features in the above conditions are that affected patients often started HAART at very low CD4 counts and with very high HIV viral loads. There is no consensus on the best management of IRIS, but there is no rationale for stopping HAART and most cases are self-limiting. Steroids and nonsteroidal anti-inflammatory drugs are frequently used, but there are no trial data to provide guidance.

Children and HIV

Most paediatric infections result from the mother-to-child transmission (MTCT) of HIV, although some children may be infected by blood products or sexual abuse. The risk of MTCT is increased during advanced maternal HIV disease, by vaginal delivery, and by breastfeeding (see Mother-to-child transmission, below). Diagnosis is important during the first year of life because about 20% of HIV-infected children progress rapidly to AIDS during that time; however, a special diagnostic approach is needed before 18 months of age, because over this period uninfected children may have maternal HIV antibody. Techniques for virus detection (e.g. HIV DNA by PCR) allow confirmation of HIV infection in 95% of nonbreastfed perinatally infected infants by 1 month of age.

The natural history is very different in resource-rich versus resource-limited countries. In the latter, HIV-infected children without antiretroviral therapy have a mortality rate of 45 to 59% at 2 years. In Europe and the United States of America, about 20% of untreated children would develop AIDS or die in infancy; by 5 years, 40% of children would have developed AIDS and 25% would have died. The most common AIDS diagnosis in infancy is pneumocystis pneumonia, typically presenting at 10 to 14 weeks of age. HIV encephalopathy is also common in untreated HIV-infected infants, with severe developmental delay occurring in about 10% and more subtle delays in an additional 40%.

In older children, clinical conditions suggestive of HIV infection include persistent oral candida, parotid swelling, and recurrent or frequent serious bacterial infections including pneumonia, meningitis, and sepsis. Failure to thrive, diarrhoea, fever, lymphadenopathy, and hepatosplenomegaly are more common in HIV-infected infants but are nonspecific and less predictive. HIV dementia and other neurological and developmental problems are associated with a poor prognosis. HIV-related lymphocytic interstitial pneumonitis (LIP) typically occurs in children and is characterized by progressive, widespread, reticulonodular shadowing on chest radiography. LIP develops insidiously and may initially be asymptomatic; chronic lung disease develops with cough, breathlessness, hypoxia, clubbing, and secondary bacterial infections, and bronchiectasis occurring in severe cases. LIP is often associated with other lymphoproliferative manifestations (such as parotitis) and relatively well-preserved immune function, and may be treated with oral prednisolone.

HIV-infected children should be managed by paediatricians with experience in HIV care, usually in specialized units. The absolute CD4 lymphocyte count is less valuable for monitoring than in adults, particularly in very young children; consequently, prophylaxis against pneumocystis is usually given regardless of the CD4 count during the first year. In older children, the principles of monitoring are similar to those in adults, using clinical status, CD4 counts, and viral load estimation by plasma HIV-1 RNA measurement. The CD4 percentage (percentage of total lymphocytes) varies less with age and is more useful than absolute CD4 counts in children under the age of 5 years.

Principles of antiretroviral treatment are similar in children and adults. Particular challenges to the effective use of HAART that are specific to children include the need to adjust drug dose as the child grows (to avoid underdosing and drug resistance), the lack of paediatric formulations suitable for infants, fewer drug choices, limited paediatric toxicity data and nonspecific presentation of drug toxicity in children, reliance of children on caregivers who themselves may have HIV and be ill, and, in adolescents, problems of adherence and coming to terms with an HIV diagnosis. An additional problem in the use of HAART in infants, where infected mothers have received single-dose nevirapine (or other antiretroviral therapy during pregnancy to reduce MTCT), is that the transmitted virus in such a setting is usually drug resistant. Clinical trials are used to determine optimal antiretroviral combinations, when to start treatment, and the tolerability of the newer drugs in all the major categories. Triple and even quadruple therapy regimens are well tolerated in infants and older children and may produce sustained elevations in CD4 lymphocyte counts, but adherence is particularly difficult. As HIV-infected children grow older, the number of adolescents with perinatally acquired HIV is increasing, raising the need for advice on reducing the risk of sexual transmission.

Prevention of opportunistic infections (see Table 7.5.23.5)

The risk of developing an opportunistic infection rises greatly once the peripheral CD4 lymphocyte count falls consistently below 200/mm^3. It is standard practice to introduce low-dose co-trimoxazole prophylaxis for pneumocystis pneumonia at this stage. This also reduces the risk of cerebral toxoplasmosis and may prevent bacterial pneumonia. Studies in Africa, in both children and adults, have shown that co-trimoxazole prophylaxis is associated with decreased mortality.

The risk of developing active tuberculosis in HIV-positive American intravenous drug users with positive tuberculin skin tests has been shown to be about 8% per year and can be reduced by taking isoniazid for a year. In developing countries, in particular, the risk of active tuberculosis in HIV-positive individuals is high

Table 7.5.23.5 Prophylaxis of major opportunistic infections in HIV

Infection	Indications	Regimens		Comments
		First line	Alternatives	
Pneumococcal pneumonia	All HIV-positive patients	Pneumococcal vaccine	None	Clinical effectiveness unproved; antibody response greater if CD4 >350/mm^3
P. jiroveci pneumonia	CD4 <200/mm^3; or symptomatic HIV; or following PCP	Co-trimoxazole 480–960 mg daily (or 960 mg, 3 times per week)	Dapsone; dapsone with pyrimethamine; monthly nebulized pentamidine; atovaquone	May be stopped if CD4 is sustained >200/mm^3 on anti-HIV treatment
Cerebral toxoplasmosis	CD4 <100/mm^3 plus toxoplasma IgG-positive following treatment of cerebral toxoplasmosis	As above	Dapsone with pyrimethamine	Primary prophylaxis usually incidental to that for PCP prophylaxis; pentamidine not protective
		Sulfadiazine 0.5–1 g, 4 times daily with pyrimethamine 25–75 mg/day, and folinic acid; protects against *P. carinii* as well	Clindamycin with pyrimethamine, and folinic acid;	May be stopped if CD4 is sustained >200/mm^3 on anti-HIV treatment
Tuberculosis[a]	Tuberculin reaction >5 mm induration with no previous BCG; or high-risk exposure to tuberculosis[a]	Isoniazid 300 mg/day with pyridoxine 50 mg/day for 6–12 months	Rifampicin with isoniazid for 3 months	Rifampicin should not be given with protease inhibitors or nevirapine
M. avium complex (MAC)	CD4 <50/mm^3 following treatment of disseminated MAC	Clarithromycin 500 mg, twice daily, or azithromycin 1200 mg/week	Rifabutin; rifabutin with azithromycin	Primary prophylaxis usually unnecessary
		Clarithromycin 500 mg, twice daily, with ethambutol 15 mg/kg per day with or without rifabutin 300 mg/day	Azithromycin with ethambutol, with or without rifabutin	May be stopped if CD4 is sustained >200/mm^3 on anti-HIV treatment
Cytomegalovirus (CMV)	CD4 <50/mm^3 and CMV antibody-positive	Valganciclovir 900 mg daily	None	Primary prophylaxis usually unnecessary
	Following CMV retinitis or other CMV disease	Valganciclovir 900 mg daily; or ganciclovir 5–6 mg/kg IV on 5–7 days/week	Foscarnet IV; cidofovir IV; ganciclovir intraocular implant	May be stopped if CD4 is sustained >200/mm^3 on anti-HIV treatment
Cryptococcal meningitis	CD4 <50/mm^3 following treatment of cryptococcal meningitis	Fluconazole 100–200 mg/day orally	Itraconazole orally	Primary prophylaxis usually unnecessary
		Fluconazole 200 mg/day orally	Amphotericin B IV weekly or 3 times/week; itraconazole orally	Fluconazole superior to itraconazole for secondary prophylaxis May be stopped if CD4 is sustained >200/mm^3 on anti-HIV treatment

IV, intravenous; PCP, pneumocystis pneumonia.

[a] In circumstances of contact with MDR-TB, specialist advice about prophylaxis should be sought.

and isoniazid alone or in combination with rifampicin can reduce the risk, but there is a challenge in implementation, which includes addressing the need to exclude active TB. BCG vaccination does not appear to be protective in HIV.

Primary prophylaxis may prevent other conditions, such as CMV retinitis, cryptococcal meningitis, and histoplasmosis, but because of the relatively low incidence and lack of predictors of risk for these conditions, it is not cost-effective. Before the advent of highly active antiretroviral therapy, after treatment of an opportunistic infection the predisposition to the infection usually remained. Thus, in early studies, following an episode of pneumocystis pneumonia, patients had a 50% chance of a further episode within a year. Secondary prophylaxis with co-trimoxazole proved effective. Secondary prophylaxis for pneumocystis and other opportunistic infections, including MAC and CMV, is now discontinued if there is a good response to antiretroviral treatment, with CD4 counts sustained above 200/mm^3 and low plasma levels of HIV RNA.

Simple measures, other than drugs, may reduce the risk of some infections. Avoiding undercooked eggs and poultry may reduce the risk of disseminated salmonella infection and adequate boiling of drinking water can prevent cryptosporidiosis. Stopping cigarette smoking reduces the risk of bacterial chest infections.

Prevention of HIV transmission

Sexual transmission

Sexual transmission accounts for most new cases of HIV infection. Education to alter behaviour and reduce the risk of HIV infection is a key component of HIV control programmes. Condom promotion in Thailand has made an impact on HIV transmission rates.

The presence of other sexually transmitted infections, especially those causing genital ulcers, facilitates HIV transmission. Accordingly, studies in Tanzania and elsewhere have demonstrated that programmes to prevent and treat sexually transmitted infections reduce the incidence of new HIV infections. Herpes simplex virus type 2 (HSV-2) is of particular importance in facilitating HIV-1 transmission, because of its high prevalence worldwide, including developing countries. Aciclovir suppression of HSV-2 infection has been shown to reduce genital shedding of HIV-1 and plasma HIV viral load, but field studies have not demonstrated a consequent reduction in risk of HIV acquisition.

The foreskin in males, rich in Langerhans cells, is an important portal of entry for HIV infection. Randomized trials in Africa have confirmed that the risk of acquiring HIV is reduced by half in circumcised men compared to uncircumcised men. Adult male circumcision, although not fully protective, may therefore be a valuable addition to HIV prevention programmes in resource-limited countries.

There are large studies underway to assess the efficacy of vaginal microbicides in the prevention of sexually transmitted infections (STIs) and HIV and these will report in the near future. In addition, there are pilot studies to assess the feasibility of using antiretroviral drugs for pre-exposure prophylaxis (PrEP) of sexually acquired HIV. Studies of tenofovir with and without emtricitabine are in progress.

Mother-to-child transmission

As the number of women infected with HIV increases, the problem of mother-to-child transmission (MTCT) of the virus assumes greater importance. Currently, an estimated 1500 infants are infected by MTCT daily worldwide. In developed countries, the risk of MTCT without interventions is 15 to 30%, but 25 to 40% in sub-Saharan Africa because of population differences and breastfeeding. Without interventions, approximately one-third of peripartum MTCT occurs in late pregnancy, the remaining two-thirds during labour. Post-partum transmission through breastfeeding can double the risk of MTCT. However, in resource-limited settings where the vast majority of infected mothers live, breastfeeding for 6 months is still recommended because of the substantial nutritional and immunological benefits that accrue, and these outweigh even the increased risk of HIV infection in the infants. In resource-rich settings, the risk of MTCT is below 1% as a result of HAART administered to the mother during pregnancy and delivery by elective Caesarean section. Vaginal delivery is a safe option if the viral load is fully suppressed by HAART. Simpler, cheaper regimens have been employed widely in resource-limited settings, such as single-dose nevirapine given to the mother during labour and to the infant within the first 72 h of life. These have also been shown to be effective (50% reduction in MTCT); but not as effective as highly active antiretroviral treatment. The routine offer of HIV testing is incorporated into antenatal care in developed countries where antiretroviral treatment is available.

Blood products

Screening of blood products began as soon as testing for HIV became available, and heat treatment for factor VIII concentrate was also introduced. These measures dramatically reduced the risk of virus transmission by blood and blood products in industrialized countries. However, there may still be a problem in resource-limited countries where screening is not efficient, or where the background seroprevalence of potential donors is so high that HIV-infected blood may be screened as negative when donated by an individual in the 'window period' immediately after initial infection (see Diagnosis of HIV infection, above).

Injecting drug use

Needle exchange programmes and the prescription of controlled drugs to registered addicts may reduce the incidence of new HIV infections in injecting drug users. Major problems still exist in countries such as India and Russia, where injecting drug use is more common and education about the risk and the availability of clean needles is very limited.

Occupational exposure and postexposure prophylaxis

Based on data from more than 3000 occupational exposures to HIV, the average risk of HIV infection after needlestick injury or other percutaneous exposure was calculated to be 0.3% (about 1 in 325). The risk following mucous membrane exposure has been estimated to be around 0.1%. The risk of transmission is greatest for deep injuries; if there is visible blood on the device; during procedures involving direct cannulation of blood vessels; or if the source patient has advanced HIV disease. A small retrospective case-control study demonstrated an 80% reduction in the likelihood of seroconversion in health care workers who took zidovudine soon after percutaneous exposure to HIV. In view of the greater activity of antiretroviral drug combinations but without direct evidence, it is currently recommended that high-risk occupational exposures to HIV are treated as soon as possible with two nucleoside inhibitors and a protease inhibitor (such as zidovudine, lamivudine, and lopinavir/ritonavir) for 1 month. Nevirapine is not currently recommended in postexposure prophylaxis regimens because of a relatively high rate of adverse reactions. A careful risk assessment should be done, and if a significant risk of HIV transmission is identified antiretroviral therapy should be offered and started promptly to maximize the chance of success.

Following possible sexual exposure to HIV, antiretroviral therapy may reduce the risk of seroconversion, but there are no randomized studies to confirm this. A comparative study in men who have sex with men in Brazil reported that individuals who took antiretroviral therapy after sexual intercourse were less likely to acquire HIV infection (0.6% vs 4.2%). Unprotected receptive anal intercourse (including sexual assault) is associated with the greatest risk (estimated up to 3%). After possible sexual exposure to HIV, a risk assessment is recommended and antiretroviral therapy should be offered if a significant risk is identified. Treatment should be started as soon as possible and is unlikely to be effective if started more than 72 h after exposure.

Vaccine development

The high degree of viral variation and immune escape present difficulties for the development of an effective preventive HIV vaccine. Nonetheless, group-specific neutralizing antibodies have been identified. In particular, there is evidence that broad CD8+ T-cell responses directed against the relatively invariant, internal p24 Gag 'capsid' protein can be successful in achieving durable immune control of HIV at very low or undetectable (below 50 HIV RNA copies/ml plasma) levels. Current vaccine efforts are therefore focused principally on inducing broad CD4+ and CD8+ T-cell responses against HIV. These responses, however, would be expected to control rather than eliminate the virus altogether, and may lead to disease modification rather than complete prevention. Although a vaccine capable of inducing broadly neutralizing antibodies against the range of HIV variants would eliminate the virus, no antigen capable of doing so has been identified to date.

So far, noninfectious killed whole virus or recombinant subunit vaccines have not been successful in protecting chimpanzees from HIV infection, or macaques from SIV infection and disease. Certain live attenuated strains of SIV, with deletion mutations in *nef* and other regulatory genes, initially appeared to protect adult monkeys from challenge with virulent SIV strains, but subsequently were reported to cause AIDS in neonatal macaques.

Human testing of candidate HIV vaccines, including a vaccine made from tiny recombinant fragments of gp120, the surface glycoprotein of HIV that binds to host cell CD4 receptors, has so far not been successful. Large phase III trials in Thailand and the United States of America involving over 5000 uninfected high risk volunteers showed no protection by a vaccine using recombinant gp120 (VaxGen) that had produced good neutralizing antibodies in pilot studies.

Several new approaches are being examined, which may prove more effective in inducing protective humoral and killer T-cell-mediated immunity. These include DNA vaccines, consisting of pieces of HIV DNA incorporated into harmless plasmid DNA from bacteria, and the use of live vectors (e.g. poxviruses such as canarypox and modified vaccinia) to deliver portions of the HIV envelope. A common approach now is to use a 'prime-boost' strategy whereby a DNA vaccine dose is given, followed by a boosting with the DNA incorporated in a vector, such as modified vaccinia. One of the most potent vaccines uses a replication-incompetent adenovirus type 5 as the vector. However, a phase IIb efficacy trial (STEP/HVTN 502) using the adenovirus type 5 vector with *gag*, *pol*, and *nef* genes was stopped prematurely. Not only was no efficacy shown, but there was evidence that those already immune to human adenovirus from natural infection were more likely to become infected by HIV. The reasons for this are not clear, but the National Institutes of Health (NIH) has stopped or paused other trials using adenovirus vectors as a result. Trials with canarypox and other vectors continue.

This approach, using DNA vaccines to stimulate CD8+ responses, is also being evaluated for therapeutic vaccination in HIV-positive patients with suppressed viraemia who are being treated with antiretroviral agents, to determine if vaccination will allow interruption of treatment without loss of virological control. Effective vaccination is likely to hold the greatest promise for controlling HIV infection in the future, but experience to date would indicate that researchers face a formidable challenge.

Further reading

Abdool Karim SS, Naidoo K, Grobler A, *et al.* (2010). Timing of initiation of antiretroviral drugs during tuberculosis therapy. *N Engl J Med*, **362**, 697–706.

Altfeld M, Goulder P (2007). 'Unleashed' natural killers hinder HIV. *Nat Genet*, **39**, 708–10.

Bartlett JG, Gallant JE (2006). *Medical Management of HIV infection*. Johns Hopkins Medicine, Health Publishing Business Group, Baltimore.

Fisher M, *et al.* (2006). UK guideline for the use of post-exposure prophylaxis for HIV following sexual exposure. *Int J STD AIDS*, **17**, 81–92.

Friis-Møller N, *et al.* (2003). Cardiovascular disease risk factors for HIV patients—association with antiretroviral therapy. Results from the Data Collection on Adverse Events of Anti-HIV Drugs (DAD) study. *AIDS*, **17**, 1179–93.

Goulder P, Watkins D (2004). HIV and SIV CTL escape: implications for vaccine design. *Nat Rev Immunol*, **4**, 630–40.

He W, *et al.* (2008). Duffy antigen receptor for chemokines mediates trans-infection of HIV-1 from red blood cells to target cells and affects HIV-AIDS susceptibility. *Cell Host Microbe*, **4**, 52–62.

Johnston MI, Fauci AS (2008). An HIV vaccine—challenges and prospects. *N Eng J Med*, **359**, 888–890.

McMichael AJ (2006). HIV vaccines. *Ann Rev Immunol*, **24**, 227–255.

Prendergast A, *et al.* (2007). International perspectives, progress, and future challenges of paediatric HIV infection. *Lancet*, **370**, 68–80.

Robertson J, *et al.* (2006). Immune reconstitution syndrome in HIV: validating a case definition and identifying clinical predictors in persons initiating antiretroviral therapy. *Clin Infect Dis*, **42**, 1639–46.

The Strategies for Management of Antiretroviral Therapy (SMART) Study Group. (2006). CD4+ count-guided interruption of antiretroviral treatment. *N Eng J Med*, **355**, 2283–96.

Online resources

Joint United Nations Programme on HIV/AIDS. *2008 Report on the Global AIDS Epidemic*. http://www.unaids.org/en/KnowledgeCentre/HIVData/GlobalReport/2008/2008_Global_Report.asp

Joint United Nations Programme on HIV/AIDS. *UNAIDS, Uniting the world against AIDS*. http://www.unaids.org

NAM. *Aidsmap*. http://www.aidsmap.com [UK national guidelines (British HIV Association, regularly updated).]

University of California (San Francisco). *HIV InSite Gateway*. http://hivinsite.ucsf.edu/ [University of California Center for HIV Information.]

US Department of Health and Human Services (DHHS). *AIDSinfo*. http://www.hivatis.org [United States of America HIV Treatment Guidelines Library; regularly updated.]

7.5.24 HIV in the developing world

Alison D. Grant and Kevin M. De Cock

Essentials

The developing world is disproportionately affected by the HIV pandemic. In many countries in sub-Saharan Africa, HIV infection is established in the general population: in southern Africa, which is particularly severely affected, HIV prevalence among pregnant women reached around 40% by 2003 in some areas. Local epidemiology depends on the relative contribution of the three major routes of HIV transmission: sexual contact (heterosexual and homosexual); mother to child; and exposure to blood or blood products. The main route of transmission is sex between men and women.

Clinical features—these vary by geographical region, reflecting increased exposure in developing countries to common pathogens such as tuberculosis, nontyphoid salmonellae, and *Streptococcus pneumoniae* throughout the course of HIV infection. People with advanced immunosuppression are also at risk of disease due to geographically-restricted opportunistic pathogens, e.g. leishmania and *Penicillium marneffei*.

Diagnosis and management—diagnosis of HIV-related disease may be difficult where there is limited access to laboratory diagnostics, and presumptive therapy based on the most likely aetiologies is often necessary. Antiretroviral therapy is increasingly available using clinical eligibility criteria, standardized drug regimens, and simpler monitoring.

Prognosis—the underlying natural history of HIV infection in the developing world is little different from that in industrialized nations, but survival with advanced HIV disease is short if there is no access to antiretroviral therapy or interventions to prevent and treat HIV-related infections.

Prevention—this requires political commitment to creating an environment that supports education about HIV, and prevents stigma and discrimination. Some countries have implemented successful control programmes and have seen declining HIV prevalence, but the goal of preventing HIV transmission remains elusive in many settings. Prevention interventions for general populations should include information and education; promotion of partner reduction and of condoms, which are highly protective against sexual transmission if used correctly and consistently; and encouragement of universal knowledge of HIV serostatus. Targeted interventions should be focused on groups and situations in which HIV transmission is most intense, guided by local epidemiology. Male circumcision has a protective efficacy of almost 60% against heterosexual acquisition of HIV infection in men, but other methods of prevention must still be promoted among circumcised men. No vaccine is available.

Epidemiology

At the end of 2008, the Joint United Nations Programme on HIV/AIDS (UNAIDS) and the World Health Organization (WHO) estimated that 33.4 million people were living with HIV infection worldwide (Chapter 7.5.23.1). This global pandemic comprises a mosaic of local epidemics, each with its own characteristics. Variation, both between regions and between groups of individuals affected within one region, is one of the pandemic's striking features. Broadly, there are two patterns: generalized epidemics, established in the general population in most countries in sub-Saharan Africa; and concentrated epidemics, in specific populations in most other regions.

Local epidemiology depends on the relative contribution of the three major routes of HIV transmission: sexual contact (heterosexual and homosexual); mother-to-child; and exposure to blood or blood products. Within sub-Saharan Africa, there have been substantial regional differences in the evolution of the epidemic. The main route of transmission is sex between men and women, although recent studies have shown that in some cities, sex between men is more important than had been realized. In West Africa, where the HIV epidemic was recognized from the mid 1980s, the highest prevalence among women attending antenatal clinics was in Abidjan, Côte d'Ivoire, peaking at around 14% in 1999 and subsequently falling to around 10% in 2002. By contrast, in southern Africa, where HIV prevalence was very low until the 1990s, HIV prevalence among pregnant women in some areas reached around 40% by 2003.

The reasons for these regional differences are not clearly understood. In a study comparing countries with high (Zambia and Kenya) and lower (Benin and Cameroon) prevalences, the main behavioural differences in cities with high prevalence were young age of sexual debut in women, young age at first marriage, and a large age difference between spouses. The main biological risk factors were herpes simplex virus type 2 (HSV-2) infection, trichomoniasis in women, and lack of male circumcision.

Global HIV incidence probably peaked in the late 1990s, and in 2008 was estimated at 2.7 million new cases (1.9 million in sub-Saharan Africa). In South Africa, the country with the highest number of HIV-infected people, the national prevalence of HIV infection among women aged 20 to 24 in 2008 was 21.1% compared with 5.1% among men of the same age, implying very high HIV incidence among young women. Since the turn of the 21st century, the global prevalence of HIV has stabilized. In many places, stable prevalence reflects high incidence balanced by high mortality. In 2008, global deaths due to HIV were estimated at 2.0 million, and in sub-Saharan Africa at about 1.4 million. Some countries have seen falls in prevalence, attributable both to a reduction in HIV-related deaths, partly due to improved access to treatment, and to a reduction in the number of new HIV infections, in some countries resulting from successful prevention campaigns. However, as antiretroviral therapy (ART) becomes more widely used, the prevalence of HIV infection will rise as treatment prolongs survival. Prevention of new infections remains the key to controlling the epidemic. Understanding the local epidemiology is essential to guide prevention and control efforts.

Prevention

Prevention of HIV infection requires political commitment to creating an environment that supports education about HIV, and prevents stigma and discrimination. Everyone should know about prevention, but efforts must be focused on groups and situations in which HIV transmission is most intense, guided by local epidemiology. Involvement of civil society and those living with HIV is especially important, as is emphasis on 'positive prevention' to ensure that people with HIV benefit from interventions and support to prevent transmission to others.

Sexual transmission

A traditional approach has been that of 'ABC', standing for Abstinence, Being faithful, and using Condoms if neither abstinent nor monogamous. While abstinence is an appropriate strategy for the youngest age group, there is no evidence that promoting abstinence is effective as a broader strategy. Reduction in the number of sexual partners, and avoidance of concordant different partnerships and intergenerational sex are important. Correct and consistent use of condoms is highly protective against acquiring HIV infection, but is difficult to sustain in long-term relationships. HIV-infected people who are aware of their HIV status tend to alter their behaviour to prevent transmission to others. Voluntary counselling and testing can help prevent transmission within discordant relationships.

Male circumcision appears to have a protective efficacy of almost 60% against heterosexual acquisition of HIV infection in men, but it affords only partial protection and other methods of prevention must still be promoted among circumcised men. Male circumcision could have considerable public health impact in southern and, to a lesser extent, East Africa, but cultural difficulties, logistical challenges, and health system weaknesses pose practical obstacles to its implementation.

For commercial sex workers and their clients, correct and consistent condom use and prompt diagnosis and treatment of other sexually transmitted infections must be promoted. Important interventions for men who have sex with men include voluntary HIV counselling and testing, correct and consistent condom use, and addressing drug abuse that may lead to unsafe behaviour. The quests continue for an effective HIV vaccine and microbicide. Clinical trials of herpes suppressive therapy have failed to show reductions in HIV acquisition. Results are awaited of trials assessing the use of ART taken as pre-exposure prophylaxis or to prevent HIV transmission in discordant couples.

Transmission by injecting drug use

The public health approach emphasizes harm reduction. Essentials include information and education, access to HIV testing and counselling, sterile needle and syringe programmes, interventions to assure safe disposal of contaminated injection equipment, treatment for drug dependence including opioid substitution, and interventions to prevent sexual transmission of HIV.

Blood transfusion and nosocomial transmission

Although eliminated in the industrialized world, transmission of HIV by blood transfusion remains a possibility in many countries. Basic measures to prevent transfusion-transmitted HIV include appropriate management of conditions predisposing to the need for transfusion (such as childbirth and malaria), and avoidance of all but essential transfusions. Family and paid donors should be avoided in favour of regular, low risk donors. All blood destined for transfusion should be screened for HIV, and, as far as possible, obtained from centralized services that can assure safe blood.

Preventive measures against nosocomial transmission include universal precautions, which treat all body fluids as potentially infectious, not to be handled without gloves. Infection-prone procedures may require other protection such as masks, gowns, and goggles. Injection safety requires absolute avoidance of re-use of needles and syringes, and assurance of their safe use and disposal. Health care institutions require policies and availability of postexposure antiretroviral prophylaxis following occupational exposure.

Mother to child transmission

In industrialized countries, combination antiretroviral therapy for pregnant women, elective caesarean section, and avoidance of breastfeeding have rendered perinatal HIV transmission rare. An integrated approach in developing countries requires primary prevention of HIV infection in girls and young women, prevention of unintended pregnancy in HIV-infected women, interventions to prevent transmission of HIV from infected women to their offspring, and diagnosis and care of infants and their mothers.

Health care workers should recommend HIV testing and counselling to all pregnant women. Pregnant women requiring antiretroviral therapy for their own health should receive standard therapy, but avoid starting efavirenz during the first trimester because of possible teratogenicity. WHO recommendations for pregnant women in low and middle income countries are shown in Table 7.5.24.1.

All women should receive information and support about infant feeding. Exclusive breastfeeding is recommended for HIV-infected women for the first 6 months of life unless replacement feeding is acceptable, feasible, affordable, sustainable, and safe, when avoidance of all breastfeeding is recommended.

Table 7.5.24.1 WHO recommendations for antiretroviral therapy for pregnant women

Women needing antiretroviral treatment for their own health	
Mother	
Preferred	Zidovudine plus lamivudine plus nevirapine or efavirenz[a]
Alternative	Tenofovir plus lamivudine (or emtricitabine) plus nevirapine or efavirenz[a]
Infant	
Breastfeeding	Nevirapine daily until 6 weeks of age
Nonbreastfeeding	Zidovudine or nevirapine daily until 6 weeks of age
Women who do not yet require antiretroviral therapy for their own health	
Option A: maternal AZT	
Mother	
Antepartum	Zidovudine daily starting from 14 weeks of pregnancy, or as soon as possible when women present late in pregnancy, in labour or at delivery
Onset of labour	Single-dose nevirapine[b]
During labour and delivery	Zidovudine plus lamivudine[b]
Postpartum	Zidovudine/lamivudine x 7 days[b]
Infant	
Breastfeeding	Nevirapine daily until one week after all exposure to breast milk has ended
Nonbreastfeeding	Zidovudine or nevirapine for 6 weeks
Option B: maternal triple antiretroviral therapy prophylaxis	
Mother	From 14 weeks gestation until one week after all exposure to breast milk has ended: ◆ Zidovudine plus lamivudine plus lopinavir/ritonavir OR ◆ Zidovudine plus lamivudine plus abacavir OR ◆ Zidovudine plus lamivudine plus efavirenz[a] OR ◆ Tenofovir plus emtricitabine plus efavirenz[a]
Infant	
Breastfeeding	Nevirapine daily from birth to 6 weeks
Nonbreastfeeding	Zidovudine or nevirapine for 6 weeks

[a] Avoid starting efavirenz in the first trimester of pregnancy.
[b] Single dose nevirapine and zidovudine/lamivudine intrapartum and postpartum may be omitted if mother receives more than 4 weeks of zidovudine during pregnancy.

Clinical features

Acute HIV disease

Symptoms associated with seroconversion, which is rarely specifically diagnosed, are described in Chapter 7.5.23. In a study of women in Kenya, the most common symptoms reported by seroconverters were fever, headache, fatigue, and arthralgia, whereas the clinical features most strongly associated with seroconversion were lymphadenopathy, vomiting, diarrhoea, fever, and myalgia.

Progression from HIV infection to symptomatic disease

Contrary to early assumptions, recent data from representative cohorts with well-defined dates of seroconversion show that the progression of HIV disease from seroconversion to the stage of advanced immunosuppression in developing countries is little different from that observed in the pre-ART era in industrialized countries. Once people reach the stage of advanced immunosuppression, survival is likely to be shorter than in industrialized countries if they do not have access to ART and interventions to prevent and treat opportunistic infections.

People with early HIV disease in developing countries frequently experience symptoms suggestive of more advanced immunosuppression such as weight loss, chronic fever or diarrhoea, and severe bacterial infections, which may give the impression of rapid HIV disease progression. However, such symptoms are also common among individuals without HIV infection, and thus are more likely to be explained by a high background morbidity in the community.

Symptomatic HIV disease

HIV-infected people suffer much higher incidence of diseases caused by pathogens common in developing countries, such as tuberculosis, pneumococcal disease, and nontyphoid salmonella, than those uninfected with HIV. Tuberculosis is often the first manifestation of HIV disease, although by the time they present with tuberculosis about half the patients will already have a CD4 count below 200/mm^3. Other early presenting symptoms of HIV disease are skin conditions such as generalized pruriginous dermatitis and herpes zoster, both of which have a high positive predictive value for underlying HIV infection among populations with high HIV prevalence.

Advanced HIV disease

When HIV-infected people reach the stage of advanced immunosuppression, the spectrum of disease varies by geographical region. Tuberculosis, bacterial infections due to pathogens such as *Streptococcus pneumoniae* and nontyphoid salmonella sp., and cryptococcal disease are common worldwide, whereas the risk of some other opportunistic infections depends on the risk of exposure, which differs by geographical region. Penicilliosis, caused by *Penicillium marneffei*, is largely confined to South-East Asia and southern China (Chapter 7.7.7). Pneumocystis pneumonia is relatively common in Asia and South Africa, but in many countries in sub-Saharan Africa, it is less common as a cause of severe respiratory symptoms than bacterial infections and tuberculosis. Diseases characteristic of very advanced immunosuppression such as those due to cytomegalovirus and *Mycobacterium avium intracellulare* have been rare in many developing countries, probably because survival with advanced disease in the absence of ART is short. This could change as ART becomes more widely available, particularly if ART prevents death but does not fully restore immunocompetence.

Tuberculosis (Chapter 7.6.25)

Tuberculosis is the most important cause of HIV-related severe morbidity and mortality in developing countries. It results both from reactivation of latent infection as well as rapid progression following new or re-infection. Molecular epidemiological studies show that new infections are an important mechanism of recurrence, which is common in HIV-infected people.

The diagnosis of tuberculosis is more challenging in developing countries. The changing clinical presentation of tuberculosis with advancing immunosuppression is described in Chapter 7.5.23. HIV-infected people are more likely to have atypical clinical presentations and to have smear-negative tuberculosis, making the diagnosis harder to confirm, particularly where the main diagnostic test is sputum microscopy. This is a particular problem for those with advanced immunosuppression, among whom a delay in initiating tuberculosis treatment may be fatal. Sputum culture has higher sensitivity than microscopy, particularly if liquid culture media are used, but in many developing countries facilities for mycobacterial culture are very limited. Current initiatives are improving microscopy-based tuberculosis diagnosis and are making culture-based diagnosis more widely available.

A particular challenge is posed by drug-resistant tuberculosis. Extensively drug-resistant tuberculosis (XDR-TB) (defined as resistance to at least rifampicin, isoniazid, any quinolone, and one of the injectable agents amikacin, capreomycin, or kanamycin) has been identified in every world region. The susceptibility of HIV-infected people to drug-resistant tuberculosis was highlighted by a survey in rural South Africa in 2005 to 2006. All those with XDR-TB who were tested had HIV infection, and almost all died rapidly after diagnosis. The victims included health care workers, raising concerns about nosocomial transmission. This problem is made worse by the paucity of facilities for drug susceptibility testing in most countries that carry the highest burden of tuberculosis, making interruption of transmission or rapid appropriate treatment challenging. This emphasizes the urgent need for stronger tuberculosis programmes, improved detection and treatment of people with resistant tuberculosis, and better infection control in health facilities to prevent nosocomial transmission to both patients and staff.

Everyone with newly diagnosed HIV infection should be screened for tuberculosis. Those who do not have active tuberculosis may benefit from isoniazid preventive therapy. Those with newly diagnosed tuberculosis should be recommended testing for HIV infection because in some places more than 70% will also have HIV infection. Patients with HIV-associated tuberculosis should receive co-trimoxazole prophylaxis. In patients whose HIV infection is diagnosed at the time of a tuberculosis episode, early data from a randomized controlled trial in South Africa suggest that mortality is higher if ART is deferred until the end of tuberculosis treatment. WHO guidelines from 2009, therefore, recommend that tuberculosis treatment should be started first, followed by ART as soon as possible afterwards, regardless of the CD4 count.

Interaction between HIV infection and 'tropical' diseases

Malaria (Chapter 7.8.2)

In areas of year-round (stable or holoendemic) malarial transmission, studies from Uganda and Malawi suggest that HIV infection impairs acquired immunity to falciparum malaria, resulting in increased frequency of malarial parasitaemia and clinical malaria among adults and older children proportional to the degree of immunosuppression, but no increase in severe or complicated malaria. However, HIV-infected infants in a holoendemic area of Kenya were at increased risk of severe anaemia and hospitalization for malaria. In studies from South Africa of nonimmune adults and older children resident in areas of intermittent (low or unstable) malaria transmission, HIV was associated with an increased risk of severe and fatal falciparum malaria, inversely proportional to their CD4 counts. In HIV-infected pregnant women, the beneficial effects of parity on severity of malaria are attenuated, and their peripheral and placental parasitaemia, and risk of suffering an episode of malaria or anaemia during pregnancy are increased. Malaria-HIV coinfection is associated with an increased risk of low birth weight, preterm birth, intrauterine growth retardation, and postnatal infant mortality. Malaria transiently increases peripheral blood and placental HIV viral load, but whether this affects the risk of vertical transmission of HIV infection or accelerates HIV disease progression is unknown. ART and co-trimoxazole reduce the risk of febrile malarial episodes; HIV-infected patients in malaria endemic areas should sleep under insecticide-treated bed nets; and nonimmune people travelling to malarial areas should use bednets and antimalarial chemoprophylaxis. Pregnant women who are not taking continuous co-trimoxazole should receive at least three doses of intermittent preventive therapy. In malaria-endemic areas, those on co-trimoxazole prophylaxis who develop fever should be investigated for causes other than malaria rather than being treated presumptively for malaria. They should not be given pyrimethamine with sulfadoxine as malaria treatment. ART may interact with antimalarial drugs (see http://www.hiv-druginteractions.org).

Leishmaniasis (Chapter 7.8.12)

The HIV epidemic has led to localized increases in visceral leishmaniasis, predominantly in people with CD4 counts below 200/mm^3, particularly among injecting drug users around the Mediterranean; in the north-east of Africa (Ethiopia and Sudan); Brazil; and India. In those with HIV infection, visceral leishmaniasis most often presents classically with fever, hepatosplenomegaly, and pancytopenia, although presentations range from asymptomatic to multi-organ involvement. The treatment of choice is liposomal amphotericin B. Amphotericin B deoxycholate or sodium stibogluconate are less satisfactory. Without secondary prophylaxis, relapse after treatment is almost inevitable until the CD4 count has risen on ART.

Cutaneous leishmaniasis may present with atypical skin lesions, which may be disseminated and may recur after treatment.

Trypanosomiasis (Chapters 7.8.10–7.8.11)

Asymptomatic infection with Chagas' disease (*Trypanosoma cruzi*) may be reactivated by HIV-related immunosuppression, most often resulting in meningoencephalitis or cerebral mass lesions. Myocarditis is common at autopsy, although rarely apparent clinically. There is no evidence of an interaction between human African trypanosomiasis and HIV infection, although reports suggest high mortality among HIV-infected patients treated for central nervous system disease.

Helminths

There is little evidence of interaction between intestinal nematodes and HIV infection; the expected association with *Strongyloides stercoralis* hyperinfection has not been observed, although it is common with another retroviral infection, human T-lymphotropic virus (HTLV-1) (Chapter 7.9.4). HIV infection does not affect the management of onchocerciasis, although skin disease may be more severe. Higher prevalence of *Wuchereria bancrofti* infection in HIV-infected than uninfected people has been reported. Schistosomiasis does not appear to be more common or more severe in HIV-infected people, although genital schistosomiasis in women is associated with HIV infection and could be a risk factor for HIV transmission. Atypical forms of neurocysticercosis, such as giant brain cyst and spinal epidural lesions, are reported.

Fungi

Penicilliosis (Chapter 7.7.7) is a common opportunistic infection among those with advanced immunosuppression in South East Asia and China. Paracoccidioidomycosis (*Paracoccidioides brasiliensis* infection—Chapter 7.7.4) is the most common invasive fungal infection in South America, but reports of coinfection with HIV are uncommon.

There is no evidence of important interactions between HIV infection and typhoid fever, melioidosis, amoebiasis, or giardiasis. Leprosy may be unmasked by ART as an immune reconstitution phenomenon.

Clinical staging of HIV disease

Given limited laboratory facilities in many developing countries, HIV viral load estimation and CD4 counts are often not available. A system designed to estimate HIV disease stage based on clinical symptoms, modified by absolute lymphocyte count or CD4 count if available, was published by WHO in 1990 and revised in 2006 (Table 7.5.24.2). This has become widely used in developing country settings to guide when to start interventions such as preventive therapy with co-trimoxazole and ART.

Diagnosis and testing

Serological tests for HIV infection first became available in 1985, the driving force for their development being concern to assure the safety of blood for transfusion. From early on, because of concerns about discrimination, there was a strong commitment to ensure HIV testing was only conducted with informed consent after pre- and post-test counselling and with assured confidentiality (voluntary counselling and testing, VCT), unlike the approach to diagnostic testing for other communicable diseases. Compulsory testing was not thought to bring public health benefit and was strongly discouraged. VCT emphasized discussion with a counsellor about the desirability of being tested, the implications of positive or negative results, advice about disclosure, etc. An important

Table 7.5.24.2 WHO clinical staging system

WHO clinical stage	HIV-associated symptoms	Examples of defining conditions
1	Asymptomatic	Asymptomatic Persistent generalized lymphadenopathy
2	Mild symptoms	Recurrent respiratory tract infections Herpes zoster Seborrhoeic dermatitis
3	Advanced symptoms	Unexplained severe (>10%) weight loss Persistent oral candidiasis Pulmonary tuberculosis Severe bacterial infections
4	Severe symptoms	HIV wasting syndrome Extrapulmonary tuberculosis Recurrent severe bacterial pneumonia Kaposi's sarcoma

Table 7.5.24.3 WHO recommendations for provider-initiated counselling and testing

Type of HIV epidemic	HIV testing and counselling recommended to:
All	All patients with signs, symptoms, or conditions which could indicate HIV infection, including tuberculosis Children born to HIV-infected women Men seeking male circumcision for HIV prevention
Generalized	All patients presenting to health facilities, regardless of the reason for presentation. Priorities may include: medical wards and outpatient facilities, antenatal, childbirth, and postpartum health services, sexually transmitted infection services
Low level or concentrated	Prioritize symptomatic and perinatally-exposed people, as above. Consider for: Sexually transmitted infection services Most-at-risk populations Maternal health services

incentive for VCT was to avoid people at risk donating blood primarily to discover their HIV serostatus. As HIV treatment has improved, VCT has become more popular and services, especially in Africa, have increased substantially, facilitated by the advent of simple rapid tests. If the initial test is positive, confirmatory testing using a test based on a different antigen and/or platform is important to minimize false positive results.

As HIV treatment programmes began to be introduced, VCT was recognized to be poorly adapted to the needs of clinical medicine, and patients were going undiagnosed. WHO and UNAIDS introduced the concept of provider-initiated HIV testing and counselling, where health care providers recommend HIV testing to patients. Pretest information is provided and patients have the right to decline, ensuring that the test is voluntary. Results must be returned with post-test counselling, and patients must be linked to appropriate services. To distinguish it from provider-initiated testing, VCT is now also referred to as client-initiated HIV testing and counselling. Table 7.5.24.3 shows the indications for provider-initiated HIV testing and counselling according to different epidemic situations.

HIV testing is also conducted for surveillance. In low and middle income countries, blood collected for syphilis testing from pregnant women attending antenatal services is most often used. To ensure completeness of testing, identifiers from the specimens are removed and the blood is tested for HIV anonymously (unlinked anonymous testing).

Treatment, care, and prevention of HIV-related disease

Since 2000, there has been a radical change in policies for providing ART in developing countries. Previously, it was considered too expensive and too complex to be made widely available in developing countries, but the number of people receiving ART in low and middle income countries has increased dramatically from around 240 000 in 2001 to over 4 million by the end of 2008. Unprecedented funding has been made available from initiatives such as the Global Fund to Fight AIDS, Tuberculosis and Malaria, and the United States President's Emergency Plan for AIDS Relief.

Table 7.5.24.4 WHO guidelines on when to start antiretroviral therapy in adults and adolescents

WHO clinical stage	Action
1 or 2	Treat if CD4 350/mm^3 or below
3 or 4	Treat irrespective of CD4 count

Discussion has moved from whether expanded access is feasible to how it can be achieved. Despite this success, more needs to be done to make ART available to all of the estimated 9.5 million people in need of it.

The approach to ART delivery in developing countries takes a public health rather than an individualized approach. The aim is to maximize the survival of all HIV-infected people in the population by using ART regimens which are standardized rather than tailored to the individual; by simplifying management so that HIV care can be undertaken by health care workers where there are few doctors; and using clinical and basic laboratory monitoring so that ART can be delivered even if CD4 counts and HIV viral load measurements cannot be done. The current WHO guidelines for adults and adolescents (2009) for starting ART are summarized in Table 7.5.24.4.

The recommended first line regimen for HIV-1 infections comprises two nucleoside reverse transcriptase inhibitors (NRTIs) and one non-nucleoside reverse transcriptase inhibitor (NNRTI). For HIV-2 infections, NNRTIs are ineffective, and a boosted protease inhibitor-based regimen would be the preferred first line regimen. Second line therapy is based on a boosted protease inhibitor in combination with two previously unused NRTIs.

Aside from the provision of ART, much can be done to prevent illness among HIV-infected people. Co-trimoxazole prophylaxis reduces morbidity and mortality among HIV-infected children and symptomatic adults. WHO guidelines recommend, in the absence of CD4 counts, starting co-trimoxazole prophylaxis for those with symptomatic HIV disease (WHO stage 2, 3, or 4), or, if CD4 counts are available, at any WHO stage if the CD4 count is below 350/mm^3, or for WHO stage 3 or 4, irrespective of the CD4 count. Where health infrastructure is limited, co-trimoxazole may be offered to everyone with HIV infection, regardless of their CD4 count or clinical disease stage. People with HIV should be screened for symptoms of active tuberculosis at each clinical encounter, and those who do not have active tuberculosis should be offered a course of isoniazid preventive therapy. Where cryptococcal disease is common, antifungal prophylaxis may be considered for severely immunosuppressed people after exclusion of active disease. Interventions to prevent malaria should be offered. Appropriate vaccines may include those against hepatitis B, pneumococcal disease, and influenza. Nutritional support should be provided for the malnourished. To reduce infective diarrhoea, household-based water treatment methods are recommended, along with proper disposal of faeces and hand washing with soap.

The WHO document 'Priority interventions: HIV/AIDS prevention, treatment and care in the health sector' brings together recommendations relevant to HIV care in resource limited settings and is available on the WHO website (details in the reading list).

Further reading

Corbett EL, *et al.* (2006). Tuberculosis in sub-Saharan Africa: opportunities, challenges, and change in the era of antiretroviral treatment. *Lancet*, **367**, 926–37.

Friedland G, Churchyard GJ, Nardell E (2007). Tuberculosis and HIV infection: current state of knowledge and research priorities. *J Infect Dis*, **196** Suppl 1, S1–S3.

Joint United Nations Programme on HIV/AIDS. *UNAIDS epidemic update.* http://data.unaids.org/pub/Report/2009/JC1700_Epi_Update_2009_en.pdf

Karp LC, Auwaerter PG (2007). Coinfection with HIV and tropical infectious diseases. I. Protozoal pathogens. *Clin Infect Dis*, **45**, 1208–13.

Karp CL, Auwaerter PG. (2007). Coinfection with HIV and tropical infectious diseases. II. Helminthic, fungal, bacterial, and viral pathogens. *Clin Infect Dis*, **45**, 1214–20.

Mermin J, *et al.* (2005). Developing an evidence-based, preventive care package for persons with HIV in Africa. *Trop Med Int Health*, **10**, 961–970.

Sanders EJ, *et al.* (2007). HIV-1 infection in high risk men who have sex with men in Mombasa, Kenya. *AIDS*, **21**, 2513–20.

Slutsker L, Marston BJ (2007). HIV and malaria: interactions and implications. *Curr Opin Infect Dis*, **20**, 3–10.

Todd J, *et al.* (2007). Time from HIV seroconversion to death: a collaborative analysis of eight studies in six low and middle-income countries before highly active antiretroviral therapy. *AIDS*, **21** Suppl 6, S55–S63.

World Health Organization. *Rapid advice: Antiretroviral therapy for HIV infection in adults and adolescents. November 2009.* http://www.who.int/hiv/pub/arv/rapid_advice_art.pdf

World Health Organization. *Essential prevention and care interventions for adults and adolescents living with HIV in resource-limited settings.* http://www.who.int/hiv/pub/prev_care/OMS_EPP_AFF_en.pdf

World Health Organization. *Priority interventions: HIV/AIDS prevention, treatment and care in the health sector.* http://www.who.int/hiv/pub/priority_interventions_web.pdf

7.5.25 HTLV-1, HTLV-2, and associated diseases

Kristien Verdonck and Eduardo Gotuzzo

Essentials

Human T-lymphotropic virus (HTLV)-1 and HTLV-2 belong to the genus *Deltaretrovirus* of the family *Retroviridae*. They only infect humans, produce a lifelong infection, and can be transmitted from mother to child, through sexual intercourse, and via cellular blood components. Both viruses are present in all continents. The highest HTLV-1 prevalence in the general population (10%) has been found in southern Japan: there are endemic foci of HTLV-2 among native Amerindians and Central African pygmy tribes. It is unclear why some infected people develop associated diseases while others remain asymptomatic.

Clinical features—(1) HTLV-1—up to 10% of carriers develop clinical manifestations, of which adult T-cell leukaemia/lymphoma and HTLV-associated myelopathy/tropical spastic paraparesis are the most severe; treatment options are limited. (2) HTLV-2—causes a milder form of HTLV-associated myelopathy/tropical spastic paraparesis and pulmonary disorders.

Diagnosis and prevention—HTLV enzyme immunosorbent assays and particle agglutination tests are used for screening, followed by confirmatory testing of positive results. Mother-to-child transmission of HTLV-1 can be reduced by avoiding breastfeeding; condom use protects against sexually transmitted infection; screening of blood donors is performed in many countries. No vaccine is available and there are no effective antiviral drugs.

Historical perspective

In 1979, human T-lymphotropic virus 1 (HTLV-1) was isolated from a patient with a T-cell malignancy. In the years that followed, several syndromes, previously considered idiopathic, were linked to this virus: adult T-cell leukaemia/lymphoma (ATL), tropical spastic paraparesis, and infective dermatitis. Originally, tropical spastic paraparesis had been attributed to malaria by Strachan in Jamaica in 1897, but was named Jamaican neuropathy by Cruickshank in the 1950s. HTLV-2 was discovered in 1982, and HTLV-3 and HTLV-4 in 2005. It is not yet known whether HTLV-3 and -4 cause human disease.

Pathogenesis

The genomes of HTLV-1 and HTLV-2 consist of RNA, which, during infection, is transcribed to DNA and inserted into the DNA of human lymphocytes. HTLV-1 shows tropism for CD4 and HTLV-2 for CD8 lymphocytes. During chronic infection there is little production of mature virions, and the viruses propagate via mitosis of infected lymphocytes (clonal expansion). A viral protein, Tax, regulates the expression of viral genes and interferes with host cell gene expression, resulting in spontaneous proliferation of infected lymphocytes among other phenomena. In HTLV-1 infection, the effects of Tax can lead to ATL. There are no vaccines and no effective antiviral drugs against HTLV-1 and HTLV-2.

The proviral load (the proportion of peripheral blood mononuclear cells carrying integrated HTLV provirus) remains relatively stable in any given subject, but varies between subjects. A high HTLV-1 proviral load is related to the risk of human T-lymphotropic virus associated myelopathy (HAM)/tropical spastic paraparesis (TSP), and perhaps also of ATL.

HTLV infection is a necessary but insufficient condition for the development of associated diseases. Other viral, host genetic and environmental factors contribute to the risk of disease. The risk of HAM/TSP in HTLV-1 carriers is influenced by the viral subgroup, the rate of HTLV-1 expression, and the efficiency of the cytotoxic lymphocyte response against the virus, which in turn depends on human leucocyte antigen (HLA) type, cytokine, and cytokine receptor genes.

Epidemiology

The origin of HTLV is in Africa. Several HTLV-1 and HTLV-2 subtypes have spread to the rest of the world, in ancient and more recent times. Nowadays, about 20 million people are infected with HTLV-1 worldwide. The number of HTLV-2-infected people may also amount to several millions.

The highest HTLV-1 prevalence (>10% of the general population) is found in southern Japan. Countries with a moderate prevalence (1–10%) include Papua New Guinea and the Solomon Islands in

Oceania; Guinea-Bissau, Togo, and Cameroon in Central Africa; Jamaica and Martinique in the Caribbean; and Guyana, French Guyana, and Peru in South America. In Brazil, Iran, Romania, and Taiwan, the prevalence is 0.1 to 1%. The infection is uncommon in Western Europe and the United States of America.

For HTLV-2, there are two endemic foci: among native Americans (prevalence 1–58%) and Central African pygmy tribes (prevalence up to 14%). The virus is also frequent among injecting drug users (IDU) in all continents (prevalence up to 20%).

In endemic populations, the prevalence of HTLV-1 and HTLV-2 increases with age and is higher in women than in men. Other risk factors include prolonged breastfeeding, unsafe sexual practice, blood transfusion, and drug abuse.

There are six molecular subtypes of HTLV-1 and four of HTLV-2 connected with specific populations and geographical locations, but they have little or no influence on disease outcome.

Diagnosis of infection

HTLV enzyme immunosorbent assays and particle agglutination tests are available for screening. In samples with a positive result, confirmatory testing with western blot, line immunoassay, immunofluorescence, and/or polymerase chain reaction (PCR) is recommended to eliminate false-positive reactions and to discriminate between HTLV-1 and HTLV-2.

Prevention

HTLV-1 mother-to-child transmission can be reduced from 15 to 25% to less than 5% by avoiding breastfeeding.

The incidence of sexual transmission among stable partners is about 1 per 100 person-years for HTLV-1 and -2. Condom use protects against infection.

Transfusion of HTLV-1-contaminated cellular blood components leads to infection in more than 40% of recipients. In many countries, candidate blood donors are screened for HTLV.

HTLV-1 disease outcomes (see Table 7.5.25.1)

The lifetime risk for HTLV-1 carriers to develop ATL is 1 to 5%. HAM/TSP occurs in 0.3 to 4%, and for HTLV-1-associated diseases in general, the risk is estimated in 10%.

Adult T-cell leukaemia/lymphoma (ATL)

ATL is an aggressive malignancy of HTLV-1-infected CD4 lymphocytes. Clinical features include lymphadenopathy, hepatosplenomegaly, skin lesions, and opportunistic infections. Hypercalcaemia and lytic bone lesions are found in up to 70% of patients. Peripheral blood smears may show lymphoid cells with basophilic cytoplasm and convoluted nuclei ('flower cells').

HTLV-1-induced ATL is classified as acute, lymphoma-type, chronic, and smouldering, based on total lymphocyte count, presence of abnormal lymphocytes in peripheral blood, calcium and lactate dehydrogenase levels, and lymphadenopathy. Recently, a fifth category, cutaneous T-cell lymphoma, was proposed.

The median survival time after diagnosis of acute ATL is 6 months. Chronic and smouldering forms have a better prognosis, but can evolve to acute ATL.

Table 7.5.25.1 HTLV-1 and HTLV-2 disease outcomes and main clinical features

HTLV-1	
Malignant disease	
ATL	Lymphadenopathy, hepatosplenomegaly, skin lesions, opportunistic infections, hypercalcaemia. Poor prognosis. Affects more men than women, mostly adults.
Inflammatory syndromes	
HAM/TSP	Weakness of the legs with signs of pyramidal tract involvement (hyperreflexia, clonus, spasticity, Babinski's sign), loss of vibration sense, back pain, urinary problems, constipation, and sexual disorders. Progressive disease. Affects more women than men; mostly adults.
Uveitis	Blurred vision with floaters, iritis, vitreous opacities, retinal vasculitis, uni- or bilateral. Intermediate uveitis in >50% of cases. Sometimes preceded by an episode of thyroiditis. Resolves spontaneously, but more rapidly with corticosteroids. Relapse is frequent. Affects more women than men; mostly adults, sometimes children.
Arthritis	Resembles rheumatoid arthritis.
Infectious complications	
Strongyloidiasis	Disseminated, life-threatening strongyloidiasis can develop. Relapse after treatment is common.
Infective dermatitis	Generalized papular rash, with exudates and crusting on scalp, ear, eyelid margins, paranasal skin, neck, axilla, and groin. Watery nasal discharge, lymphadenopathy. Chronic syndrome; good response to antibiotics but frequent relapse. The syndrome has an inflammatory as well as an infectious component. Affects usually young children.
Scabies	Severe forms can occur, with extensive, crusted lesions, located mainly in pressure areas.
Tuberculosis	Increased risk of active tuberculosis. Specific clinical features remain to be clarified.
HTLV-2	
HAM/TSP	Similar symptoms as in HTLV-1, but milder and more slowly progressive disease.
Acute bronchitis and pneumonia	Specific clinical features remain to be clarified.
Arthritis	

ATL, adult T-cell leukaemia/lymphoma; HAM/TSP, HTLV-associated myelopathy/tropical spastic paraparesis.

Allogenic haematopoietic stem cell transplantation, intensive chemotherapy, and the combination of interferon-α with zidovudine have been evaluated for the treatment of ATL. In most reports, the median survival remained less than one year despite treatment.

HTLV-associated myelopathy/tropical spastic paraparesis (HAM/TSP)

HAM/TSP is characterized clinically by spastic weakness of the legs (Fig. 7.5.25.1), back pain, bladder problems, sensory signs and symptoms, constipation, and/or sexual dysfunction. The main pathological feature is an inflammation of the white and grey matter of the spinal cord. Cerebrospinal fluid examination may show mild lymphocytosis and protein increase.

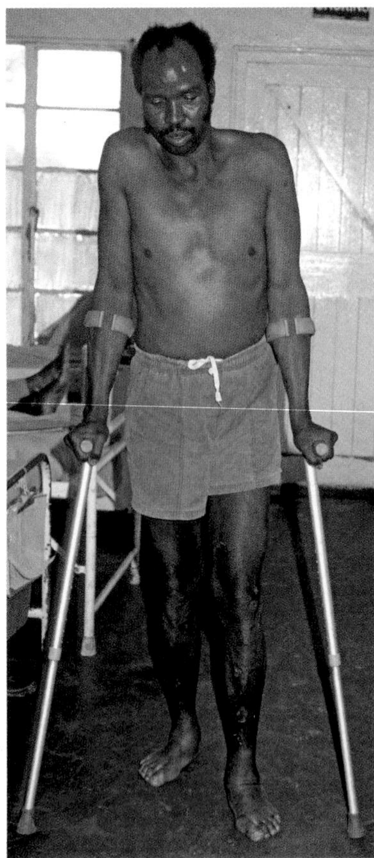

Fig. 7.5.25.1 Spastic paraplegia in a South African patient with HTLV-1 infection. (Copyright D A Warrell.)

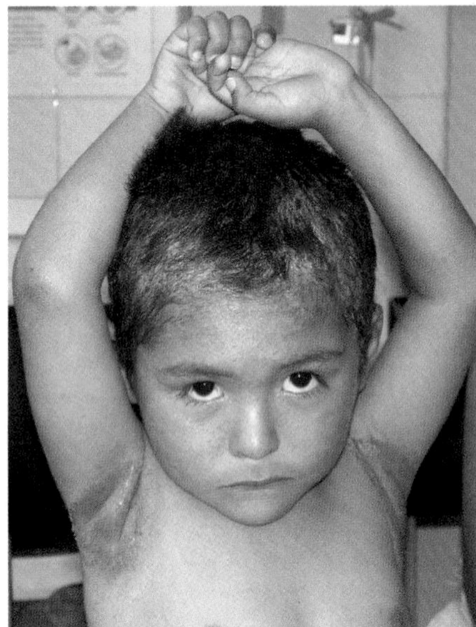

Fig. 7.5.25.2 Patients with HTLV-1-associated infective dermatitis.
The child has a papular rash on the forehead, crusting on the scalp, and lesions in the armpits.
(Courtesy of Dr Francisco Bravo, Institute of Tropical Medicine Alexander von Humboldt, Lima, Peru.)

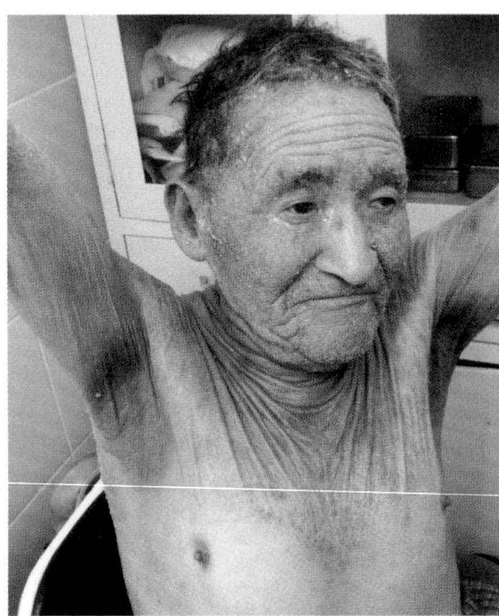

Fig. 7.5.25.3 Patient with HTLV-1-associated infective dermatitis. This disease can affect adults, although it mostly occurs in children. Typical characteristics are crusting on the scalp and lesions on the eyelid margins, in the neck and in the armpits.
(Courtesy of Dr. Francisco Bravo, Institute of Tropical Medicine Alexander von Humboldt, Lima, Peru.)

The diagnosis of HAM/TSP requires demonstration of HTLV-1 and exclusion of other causes of myelopathy, such as spinal cord compression, vitamin B_{12} and folate deficiency, multiple sclerosis, amyotrophic lateral sclerosis, and lathyrism.

Several treatment strategies have been proposed, including corticosteroids, interferon-α, interferon-ß-1a, and the combination of two nucleoside analogues (zidovudine + lamivudine). There are reports of good response to zidovudine + lamivudine in combination with corticosteroids in patients with rapidly progressive disease. However, all regimens evaluated in clinical trials so far, showed no satisfactory effect on symptoms or proviral load.

Infective dermatitis

Infective dermatitis is a chronic, relapsing disease that affects mostly children. Clinical characteristics include a papular rash, with exudates and crusting, mainly on the scalp, but also on the ears, eyelid margins, paranasal skin, neck, axilla, and groin (Figs. 7.5.25.2, 7.5.25.3). Watery nasal discharge and crusting of the nostrils are frequent. Clinical and histopathological images may resemble atopic dermatitis. The response to corticosteroids and antibiotics is generally good, but relapses are frequent after withdrawal of treatment. Case reports suggest that HTLV-1-infected children with infective dermatitis have an increased risk to develop HAM/TSP and ATL.

Other diseases

Arthropathy, uveitis, and thyroiditis are other inflammatory conditions linked to HTLV-1. Carriers of HTLV-1 are also at increased risk of infectious complications, notably invasive strongyloidiasis (superinfection) (Chapter 7.9.4), scabies, and perhaps also tuberculosis. Other diseases have been reported in association with HTLV-1 infection, but because the aetiological role of HTLV-1 is uncertain, they are not mentioned here.

HTLV-2 disease outcomes (see Table 7.5.25.1)

HTLV-2 is less pathogenic than HTLV-1, but has been linked with HAM/TSP, arthritis, and pulmonary problems. A prospective study of blood donors in the United States of America found an increase in mortality compared to uninfected control subjects.

Likely future developments

Developments in the near future will probably include the following:

- Treatment trials for HAM/TSP and ATL
- Clear picture of HTLV-1, -2, -3, and -4 disease outcomes
- Better understanding of pathogenesis of associated diseases (role of viral, genetic, and environmental factors)
- Availability of surrogate markers (e.g. proviral load)
- Better understanding of interaction with HIV
- Research into vaccines and antiretroviral therapy

Further reading

De Castro-Costa CM, *et al.* (2006). Proposal for diagnostic criteria of tropical spastic paraparesis/HTLV-I-associated myelopathy (TSP/HAM). *AIDS Res Hum Retroviruses*, **22**, 931–5.

Mosley AJ, Asquith B, Bangham CR (2005). Cell-mediated immune response to human T-lymphotropic virus type I. *Viral Immunol*, **18**, 293–305.

Proietti FA, *et al.* (2005). Global epidemiology of HTLV-I infection and associated diseases. *Oncogene*, **24**, 6058–68.

Roucoux DF, Murphy EL (2004). The epidemiology and disease outcomes of human T-lymphotropic virus type II. *AIDS Rev*, **6**, 144–54.

Taylor GP, Matsuoka M (2005). Natural history of adult T-cell leukemia/lymphoma and approaches to therapy. *Oncogene*, **24**, 6047–57.

Verdonck K, *et al.* (2007). Human T-lymphotropic virus 1: recent knowledge about an ancient infection. *Lancet Infect Dis*, **7**, 266–81.

7.5.26 Viruses and cancer

R.A. Weiss

Essentials

Viruses are important in cancer for three main reasons: (1) As a cause of cancer—about 15% of the worldwide cancer burden is due to viruses: retroviruses can activate cellular oncogenes; Tax, a viral protein encoded by HTLV-1, contributes to malignancy by transcriptional activation, up-regulation of cellular genes, and 'immortalizing' CD4+ T lymphocytes; polyomaviruses (HPV), adenoviruses, and HHV-8 interfere with tumour suppression. Viral cancers are prevented by early screening for tumours, screening for the virus to prevent transmission, and immunization as in the cases of hepatitis B virus and HPV. (2) In understanding of the biology of cancer—the discovery and characterization of oncogenes and tumour-suppressor genes. (3) In the treatment of cancer—parvoviruses and mutant adenoviruses replicate in and destroy proliferating cells; viruses as foreign antigens may aid the recognition of cancer cells by the host's immune system ('xenogenization'); viruses are also used as vectors for immunization and for gene therapy.

Viruses as aetiological agents of cancer

Oncogenic viruses establish persistent infections, which usually occur decades before malignancy. Table 7.5.26.1 lists the viruses implicated in human cancer. In most but not all cases, the viral genome is present in the malignant cells; the exceptions appear to be those that promote cancer indirectly, such as HIV and hepatitis C virus (HCV). Table 7.5.26.1 also lists the diseases associated with oncogenic viruses that are not malignancies.

Cancer is usually a rare outcome of virus infection, and other cofactors play a part in viral carcinogenesis. For example, Epstein–Barr virus (EBV) is a ubiquitous infection, yet childhood Burkitt's lymphoma occurs only in areas of holoendemic malarial infection, whereas undifferentiated nasopharyngeal carcinoma occurs mainly in southern Chinese populations. Aflatoxin acts synergistically with hepatitis B virus (HBV) to induce liver cancer, and in hereditary epidermodysplasia verruciformis the ultraviolet radiation acts with human papilloma virus strains (HPV-5 and HPV-8) to cause skin cancer. The underlying cause of all forms of Kaposi's

Table 7.5.26.1 Viruses implicated in human cancer

Virus	Malignancy	Nonmalignant disease
DNA viruses		
HPV-16, 18	Cervical cancer	
HPV-5, -8	Skin cancer	Warts
HBV	Primary liver cancer	Hepatitis
MCPyV	Merkel cell skin cancer	
	Burkitt's lymphoma	
	Immunoblastic lymphoma	
	Hodgkin's disease	
	Leiomyosarcoma	
EBV	Nasopharyngeal carcinoma	Infectious mononucleosis
KSHV	Kaposi's sarcoma	
	Primary effusion lymphoma	
	Castleman's disease	
Retroviruses		
HTLV-1	Adult T-cell leukaemia	Tropical spastic paraparesis
HIV-1	Non-Hodgkin's lymphoma	AIDS
	Kaposi's sarcoma	
XMRV	Prostate cancer?	
RNA virus		
HCV	Primary liver cancer	Hepatitis

EBV, Epstein–Barr virus; HBV, hepatitis B virus; HCV, hepatitis C virus; HPV, human papillomavirus; HTLV, human T-lymphotropic virus; MCPyV, Merkel cell polyomavirus; XMRV, xenotropic murine leukaemia virus-related virus.

sarcoma (KS) is human herpes virus 8 (HHV-8 or KSHV), which also causes primary effusion lymphoma and plasmablastic multicentric Castleman's disease. KS occurs much more frequently in immunodeficient patients. Its relative risk in recipients of organ transplants is about 400, and in persons with AIDS about 20 000.

Oncogenic viruses belong to many virus families with different routes of transmission. HBV is frequently acquired perinatally or through subsequent exposure to blood. Human T-cell lymphotropic virus type 1 (HTLV-1) is transmitted vertically through infected cells in breast milk. Sexual transmission is common to HIV, HTLV-1 (with a male to female bias), HBV, and HPV. Oncogenic viruses do not appear to be transmitted by the respiratory route or via arthropod vectors, except for some veterinary cases, e.g. bovine leucosis virus. Whereas EBV (transmitted through saliva) occurs worldwide, HBV, HTLV-1, and HHV-8 have a higher prevalence in those population groups in which the associated cancers occur.

Certain common human viruses are highly oncogenic in experimental animals but are not linked epidemiologically to human cancer, namely the polyomaviruses BK and JC, and the adenoviruses types 2 and 12. There are claims that a simian relative of BK virus, simian vacuolating virus 40 (SV40), is linked with mesothelioma, osteosarcoma, and ependymoma in humans, but these findings remain controversial. In 2008, a novel human polyomavirus, MCPyV, was linked to Merkel skin cell cancer. A retrovirus related to murine leukaemia virus (XMRV), has been clearly detected in the certain human prostate cancers, but there is also a large literature on 'false alarms' of human retroviruses.

Mechanisms of viral carcinogenesis

Physical and chemical carcinogens are usually mutagens. They cause DNA mutations in specific genes that contribute to the eventual malignant phenotype of the cancer. Oncogenes were first discovered in animal retroviruses, such as the Rous sarcoma virus of chickens, and are now known to originate from cellular genes. Most retroviruses do not carry oncogenes, but the DNA provirus integrates into chromosomal DNA and can activate adjacent cellular oncogenes. Oncogene activation by retroviruses is comparable to activation by chromosomal translocation.

The mechanism of cell transformation by HTLV-1 is different from that of the majority of animal retroviruses. HTLV-1 encodes a viral protein, Tax, which is essential to promote full viral gene transcription. Tax acts as a transcriptional activator, by associating with host nuclear proteins which activate expression of the viral genome. However, Tax also up-regulates certain cellular genes such as the interleukin-2 receptor. HTLV-1 'immortalizes' CD4+ T lymphocytes in culture, rather as EBV 'immortalizes' B lymphocytes, but this is only one step in the pathway to malignancy.

Cell transformation by DNA viruses is best understood for polyomaviruses and adenoviruses. The transforming genes of these viruses are expressed early in the infection cycle and prevent tumour suppressor protein function. Adenovirus proteins E1A and E1B and BK T antigen bind to p53 and retinoblastoma (Rb) proteins and block their normal interaction in the cell cycle. Thus, instead of mutating these cellular tumour suppressor genes, DNA tumour viruses block the normal function of their proteins, which similarly results in unregulated cell proliferation. The KSHV genome carries several oncogenes, including a homologue of *cyclin D2* (*CCND2*), which inactivates Rb by a different mechanism, phosphorylation.

Most oncogenic viruses persist in the tumour cells, often by integrating into chromosomal DNA. Oncogenic herpesviruses do not integrate but are maintained episomally. Epstein–Barr virus-associated nuclear antigen 1 (EBNA-1) is required for episomal replication of EBV (and latency-associated nuclear antigen (LANA) for KSHV), while other nuclear and latent membrane proteins are responsible for the transformed cell phenotype. With HBV, integrated copies are found in many liver carcinoma lines, but a requirement for integration has not been unequivocally shown. HBV expresses transactivating functions from the *X* gene, so its transformation may resemble that of HTLV-1.

Indirect carcinogenic effects are those in which damage to tissues by viruses may allow clones of premalignant cells to proliferate that would not otherwise do so. HCV and possibly HBV do this by destroying normal liver cells, resulting in a much greater rate of liver cell regeneration. HIV promotes tumour development by destroying helper T-cell immunity to other oncogenic viruses. The cancers elevated in AIDS are also seen in immunosuppressed transplant patients, e.g. non-Hodgkin's lymphoma and Kaposi's sarcoma, and themselves have a viral aetiology.

Treatment and prevention

Oncogenesis is multifactorial, requiring several sequential events before a patient presents with a fully malignant tumour. Yet, if a virus plays a crucial role in oncogenesis, its elimination should prevent that type of cancer. Currently, there is no special approach to the treatment of cancers that have a viral aetiology. Among the lymphoid malignancies, some respond well to radiotherapy or chemotherapy, such as Hodgkin's disease, whereas others seldom show remission, such as adult T-cell leukaemia (ATL). Cancers that express viral antigens should be responsive to immunotherapy. For tumours in which viral proteins are required for the maintenance of the malignant state, those proteins are potential molecular targets, as drugs that block them might spare normal cellular functions.

Prevention is preferable to cure, and offers the greatest promise of reducing cancer mortality due to viruses. Prevention can be accomplished by three strategies: (1) early screening for tumours, (2) screening for the virus with prevention of transmission, and (3) immunization. Early screening is exemplified by cervical smears. Screening to prevent iatrogenic transmission via blood and blood products is routinely employed in many countries for potentially oncogenic viruses such as HBV, HCV, HIV, and HTLV-1. In Kyushu, Japan, where infection was endemic, HTLV-1 is being steadily eradicated through a policy of antenatal screening to prevent milk transmission.

Prevention of cancer by immunization against infection by oncogenic viruses is likely to have a major impact on world cancer mortality in the 21st century. The HBV vaccine is based on surface antigen and two HPV vaccines protective against cervical cancer were licensed in 2006. Intensive research is also being undertaken on vaccines for HIV and HCV, but there are immense obstacles to successful immunization against HIV as the virus is extraordinarily variable. Nevertheless, immunization against oncogenic viruses is becoming a most effective cancer prevention strategy.

Viruses as therapeutic agents

Viruses may be put to use in the fight against cancer. First, some cytopathic viruses preferentially replicate in proliferating cells and destroy them, such as parvoviruses and mutant adenoviruses. Second, viruses as foreign antigens may aid the recognition of cancer cells by the host's immune system. Although the mechanism is ill understood, 'xenogenization' of tumour cells by virus infection can, in some cases, enhance immune attack against noninfected cells in the same tumour. Third, viruses are used as vectors for immunization and for gene therapy, by restoring tumour suppressor functions, by enhancing immune responses through the expression of antigens or cytokines, and by locally delivering genes for enzymes that convert inert prodrugs into active, chemotherapeutic agents.

Further reading

Astbury K, Turner MJ (2009). Human papillomavirus vaccination in the prevention of cervical neoplasia. *Int J Gynecol Cancer*, **19**, 1610–13.

Boshoff CH, Weiss RA (2002). AIDS-related malignancies. *Nature Cancer Rev*, **2**, 373–82.

Feng H, *et al.* (2008). Clonal integration of a polyomavirus in human Merkel cell carcinoma. *Science*, **319**, 1096–100.

Plymoth A, Viviani S, Hainaut P (2009). Control of hepatocellular carcinoma through hepatitis B vaccination in areas of high endemicity: perspectives for global liver cancer prevention. *Cancer Letters*, **286**, 15–21.

Voisset C, Weiss RA, Griffiths D (2008). Human RNA rumor viruses: the search for novel human retroviruses in chronic disease. *Microbiol Mol Biol Rev*, **72**, 157–96.

Zur Hausen H (2009). Papillomaviruses in the causation of human cancers. *Virology*, **384**, 260–65.

7.5.27 Orf

David A. Warrell

Essentials

Orf ('ecthyma contagiosum') is caused by an epitheliotropic parapox DNA virus of sheep and goats that is able to subdue the host's immune response. It is an occupational zoonosis of people working with these animals. A painful papule/pustule develops, usually on a finger, the site of contact with lesions on the animal's muzzle. Systemic effects are unusual, but include local lymphadenopathy, fever, erythema multiforme, and other generalized rashes. Spontaneous resolution within 6 weeks is usual. Multiple, giant lesions may develop in the immunosuppressed. Topical cidofovir is effective in severe cases.

Aetiology

Orf virus, a member of the *Parapox* genus of the Chordopoxvirinae subfamily, causes 'scabby mouth' (ecthyma contagiosum, contagious pustular dermatitis), a debilitating disease of sheep and goats. Orf virions are ovoid (approximately 260 × 160 nm), with a characteristic basketweave pattern visible by negatively stained and transmission electron microscopy. Other parapoxviruses infect cattle (pseudocowpox; bovine papular stomatitis virus, BPSV), camels, seals, and reindeer. Full genome sequences of orf and BPSV have been published. The orf virus genome is double-stranded DNA of 135 kbp, encoding a polypeptide homologous to interleukin 10 (IL-10), inhibitors of interferon, interleukin 2 (IL-2), and granulocyte-macrophage colony-stimulating factor (GM-CSF), and a vascular endothelial growth factor. These contribute to the dermal lesions characterized by capillary proliferation and dilatation.

Epidemiology

Orf has been recognized for more than 200 years as a disease of mainly young lambs and kids, which contract the infection from one another, or possibly from persistence of the virus in the pastures where the virus can remain viable for long periods in dried scabs from lesions. Human disease is an occupational zoonosis, following contact with infected sheep. Since orf is familiar to veterinarians, shepherds, farmers, abattoir workers, and butchers and is generally self-limiting, it often goes unreported. In the United Kingdom it is known to be prevalent in sheep farming communities in Wales. Outbreaks are associated with the end of the lambing season and with Islamic religious festivals associated with animal sacrifice. Transmission is by direct contact with the animals' lesions and possibly with fomites. Human to human spread has not been recorded. Infection confers only partial immunity, so that repeated milder attacks are possible.

Immunopathology

Orf virus infects skin keratinocytes and excites a brisk immune response locally and in lymphoid tissue, involving CD4+ and CD8+ cells, interferon, and antibody. However, orf virus genome encodes a variety of virulence and immunomodulatory factors that subvert or suppress the host's immune response, allowing viral replication. These include viral IL-10, interferon resistance protein, chemokine binding protein, GM-CSF, vascular endothelial growth factor, and heparin binding protein. In vaccinology, orf is proving a promising viral vector for delivering pathogen antigens to the immune system, and inactivated virus is immunoenhancing.

Clinical features

In sheep and goats, papules and vesicles appear on the muzzle or nostrils (Fig. 7.5.27.1) and gradually heal without scarring over 4 to 8 weeks, although more persistent infections may occur. In humans, after an incubation period of 2 to 6 days, a painful, small, red, firm papule enlarges to form a flat-topped haemorrhagic pustule or bulla with prominent margin and an eroded, crusted centre, sometimes surrounded by pustular satellite lesions (Fig. 7.5.27.2). The lesion is usually 1 to 3 cm in diameter, but may be as large as 5 cm. They are usually solitary or few in number and commonly occur on the extensor surface of a finger or hand, but also on the palm, forearm, and occasionally the face or scalp. The surrounding skin may be reddened, sometimes diffusely, and erysipelas-like lesions have been described. Lymphangitis or regional lymphadenopathy is not uncommon. Giant, multiple, fungating granulomatous or tumour-like lesions have been reported, usually in immunocompromised patients with haematological malignancies. Slight fever and malaise can occur. Complications include secondary infection, generalized vesicular rashes, usually classified as erythema multiforme, in as many as one-third of cases (Fig. 7.5.27.3), which develop typically

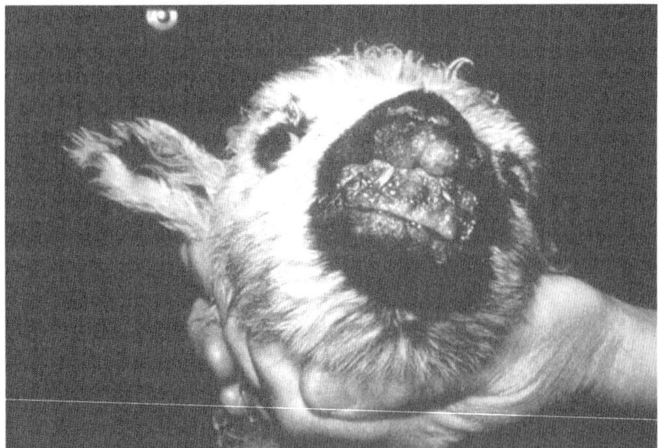

Fig. 7.5.27.1 Contagious pustular dermatitis ('orf') in a lamb.

10 to 14 days after the initial lesion, and other generalized rashes. An autoimmune bullous disease, previously designated as bullous pemphigoid, has been reported. A lesion on the precanthal skin resulted in follicular conjunctivitis. Spontaneous recovery without residual scarring is usually complete within 6 weeks.

Diagnosis

The characteristic lesion in someone exposed to sheep or goats, especially to lambs or kids, allows a clinical diagnosis. This can be confirmed in the laboratory by electron microscopy of a biopsy of the orf lesion, by polymerase chain reaction (PCR), viral culture, and fluorescent antibody staining.

Skin biopsy specimens show distinctive histopathological changes. There is hyperkeratosis with cellular swelling, balloon degeneration and vacuolation in the upper epidermis, and the presence of eosinophilic B type intracytoplasmic inclusion bodies.

Differential diagnosis

In those at occupational risk of orf, differential diagnoses include milkers' nodules, caused by another parapox virus, and cowpox (Chapter 7.5.4), an orthopoxvirus. Whitlows (felons), including herpetic whitlow (Fig. 7.5.27.4), impetigo, pyogenic granuloma, cutaneous anthrax, and tumours might also cause confusion.

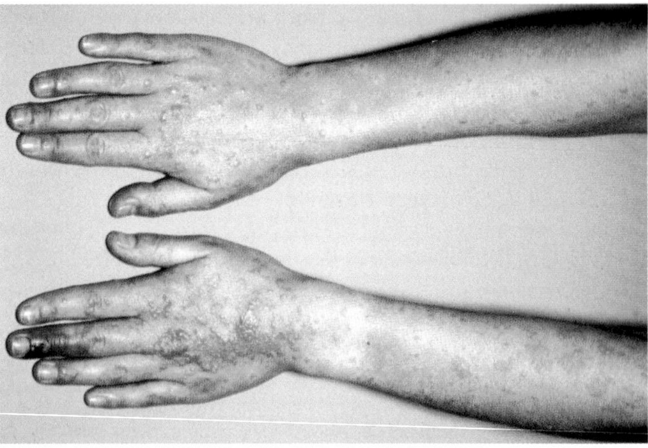

(a)

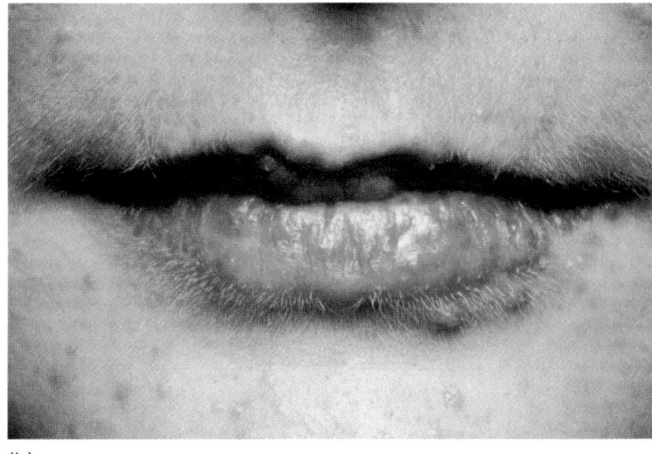

(b)

Fig. 7.5.27.3 Generalized vesicular eruption 'erythema multiforme' complicating orf of the left middle finger in a veterinary student: (a) arms, (b) mouth.

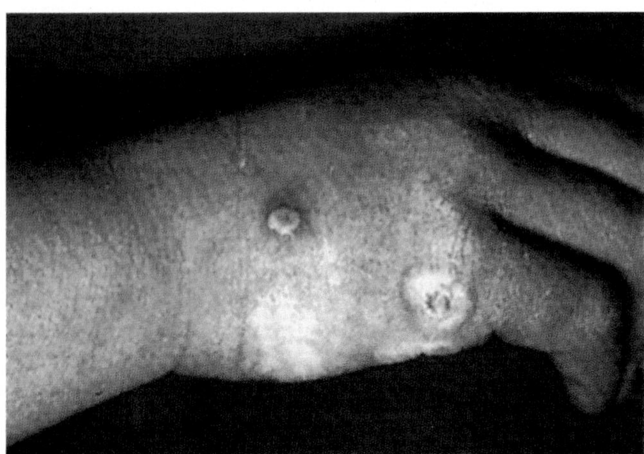

Fig. 7.5.27.2 Typical lesions of orf on a farmer's hand.

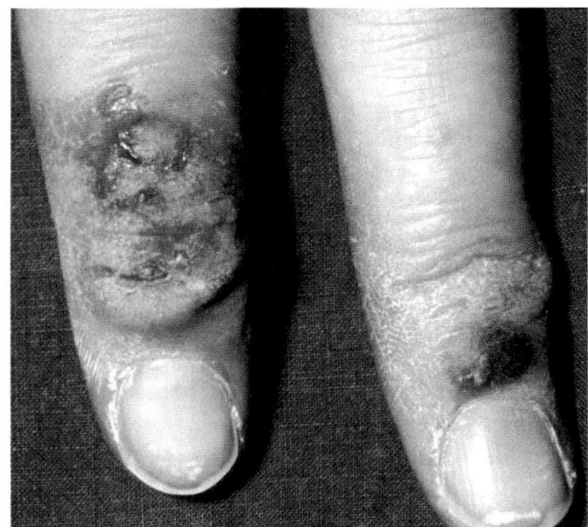

Fig. 7.5.27.4 Herpetic whitlows on adjacent fingers.
(Courtesy of the late Dr B E Juel-Jensen.)

Treatment

Secondary infection should be treated if it occurs. Large lesions can be removed surgically, but recurrence can occur in the immunocompromised. Cidofovir (topically or intravenously) and imiquimod (topically) have been used successfully to treat giant or persistent lesions, especially in immunosuppressed patients.

Further reading

Al-Salam S, *et al.* (2008). Ecthyma contagiosum (orf)—report of a human case from the United Arab Emirates and review of the literature. *J Cutan Pathol*, **35**, 603–7.

Gill MJ, *et al.* (1990). Human orf. *Arch Dermatol*, **126**, 356–8.

Groves RW, Wilson-Jones E, MacDonald DM (1991). Human orf and milkers' nodule: a clinicopathologic study. *J Am Acad Dermatol*, **25**, 706–11.

Haig DM (2006). Orf virus infection and host immunity. *Curr Opin Infect Dis*, **19**, 127–31.

Torfason EG, Gunadóttir S (2002). Polymerase chain reaction for laboratory diagnosis of orf virus infections. *J Clin Virol*, **24**, 79–84.

7.5.28 Molluscum contagiosum

David A. Warrell

Essentials

Molluscum contagiosum is caused by a Molluscipox DNA virus which infects keratinocytes of the epidermal stratum spinosum, producing distinctive small umbilicated papules on the skin. Its genome encodes a variety of proteins that suppress the host's immune response. In children it is spread by skin contact, producing few or many lesions, while in sexually active adults it causes anogenital lesions. Molluscum is self-limiting within a few years in the immunocompetent, but those with preexisting atopic eczema and immunosuppression, notably AIDS, commonly develop persistent diffuse eruptions with larger papules. Lesions can be removed mechanically or chemically. More severe infections can be treated with imiquimod or cidofovir.

Aetiology

Molluscum contagiosum (MCV), first described clinically in the early 19th century, is caused by a virus of the genus Molluscipox. This enormous (200–300 nm long), brick-shaped, double-stranded DNA virus, is a member of the Chordopoxvirinae subfamily of the Poxviridae. It multiplies in the cytoplasm of keratinocytes of the deep epidermal stratum spinosum. MCV shares unique genomic features with parapoxviruses such as orf (Chapter 7.5.27), including a GC-rich nucleotide composition, three orthologous genes, and a paucity of nucleotide metabolism genes. Restriction endonuclease analysis of the genome has identified four types, MCV-1, MCV-1a, MCV-2, and MCV-3. MCV-1 causes most childhood infections while MCV-2 is transmitted sexually in older people.

Like orf virus, MCV encodes several proteins that suppress host immunity. MC54L is a human (IL-18) binding protein homologue. MC148 antagonizes CC chemokine receptor 8. MC013L promotes viral replication by inhibiting the differentiation of infected keratinocytes. MC159L causes abnormal proliferation of epithelium by inhibiting tumour necrosis factor (TNF) and apoptosis-inducing factors. MC80R, an MHC class I homologue, interferes with the presentation of MCV peptides. Glutathione peroxidase protects infected cells from oxidative damage by peroxides.

MCV has not been transmitted to laboratory animals and no *in vitro* cultivation system is available. It has been grown in human prepuce grafted to athymic mice.

Epidemiology

Molluscum contagiosum has a worldwide incidence of 2 to 8%. It also affects animals: chimpanzees, kangaroos, dogs, horses, and birds. In tropical climates, it is more common in younger children (1–4 years), and in temperate climates, in older school-age children (10–12 years). The prevalence in American children is less than 5%. It is highly contagious by skin-to-skin contact, especially in humid and unhygienic conditions. Fomites such as shared towels, the use of communal bathtubs and swimming pools, and contact sports such as wrestling, all promote infection. Lesions are spread over the body by autoinoculation. Sexual transmission accounts for a second peak of incidence in young adults. The risk and extent of infection is increased in those with generalized skin diseases such as atopic eczema and in those with congenital or acquired immunodeficiency, caused by HIV, lymphomas, sarcoidosis, organ transplantation, and immunosuppressive therapy. In HIV seropositive people, the prevalence of molluscum contagiosum is 5 to 20%, but in those with CD4 cell counts below 100/ml it increases to 30%.

Clinical features

The incubation period varies from 7 days (in newborns) to 50 days or even up to 6 months. The classic lesion is a painless, discrete, shiny, pearly, hemispherical, firm papule with a central umbilication (depression).

In immunocompetent children, lesions can occur singly but are commonly multiple, fewer than 30 to several hundred (Figs. 7.5.28.1, 7.5.28.2). They grow gradually to a diameter of 5 to 10 mm over 6 to 12 weeks. Occasionally, a single lesion may grow to 1.5 cm in diameter, or a plaque of very small lesions develops (agminate form). New lesions may continue to appear for 6 to 8 months, but spontaneous clearance is complete without scarring within 2 to 4 years. In about 10% of cases, especially where there is a history of atopy, a patchy erythema or dermatitis develops around the lesions, causing itching which encourages scratching and autoinoculation. Lesions are most commonly seen on the axilla and other flexures, trunk, neck, or face, but any part of the skin can be affected. Conjunctival inoculation may result in unilateral conjunctivitis or corneal or conjunctival nodules. Lesions are rare on the palms, soles, and buccal mucous membrane. In immunocompetent sexually active teenagers and adults, infections usually result in anogenital lesions.

In patients with HIV and other types of immunosuppression, molluscum can be widespread, but particularly involves the face

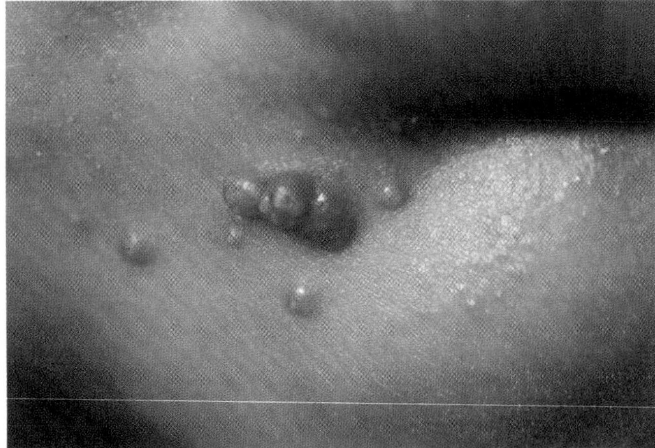

Fig. 7.5.28.1 Molluscum contagiosum: cluster of lesions in an immunocompetent child.
(Courtesy of Dr Susan M Burge.)

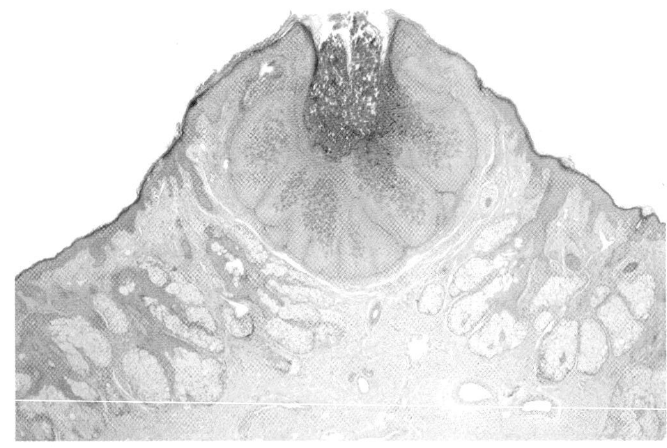

Fig. 7.5.28.3 Molluscum contagiosum showing the characteristic demarcated lesion.
(Courtesy of K Hollowood.)

(eyelids), neck, trunk, and around and inside the mouth in homosexual men. Lesions often lack the classic umbilication and may become so large, atypical, and even necrotic that they are mistaken for basal cell carcinomas or other skin tumours. The disease persists and spreads, especially when HIV is advanced.

Diagnosis

The diagnosis is usually clinical, but histological and electron microscopic examination of a curetted papule establishes the diagnosis. The demarcated lesion shows lobules of epidermis, depleted of Langerhans cells, penetrating down to the dermis with a central crater opening onto the surface through a narrow pore (Fig. 7.5.28.3). It contains keratinocyte debris with numerous Henderson–Paterson molluscum bodies. These are 35 μm in diameter, ovoid, eosinophilic, intracytoplasmic inclusion bodies within keratinocytes (Fig. 7.5.28.4). They stain purple with Tzanck reagent in scrapings from the lesions. In HIV patients, histological appearances may different.

Differential diagnosis

The differential diagnosis includes lepromatous leprosy, Darier's disease (keratosis follicularis), epithelial naevi, and skin tumours such as basal cell epithelioma or trichoepithelioma. Giant lesions might be confused with keratoacanthoma, common warts, or warty dyskeratoma. In the genital area, genital warts (condylomata acuminata) may look similar. In immunosuppressed people, cutaneous lesions of disseminated *Penicillium marneffei* infection, histoplasmosis, paracoccidioidomycosis, or cryptococcosis may appear identical to molluscum.

Treatment (see also Section 23)

Treatment may not be necessary, depending on the site and number of lesions and the age of the patient. An enormous number of local treatments are claimed to be effective, but evidence is lacking. Mechanical methods include picking out lesions on the tip of a needle or with adhesive tape, curettage, cryotherapy with liquid

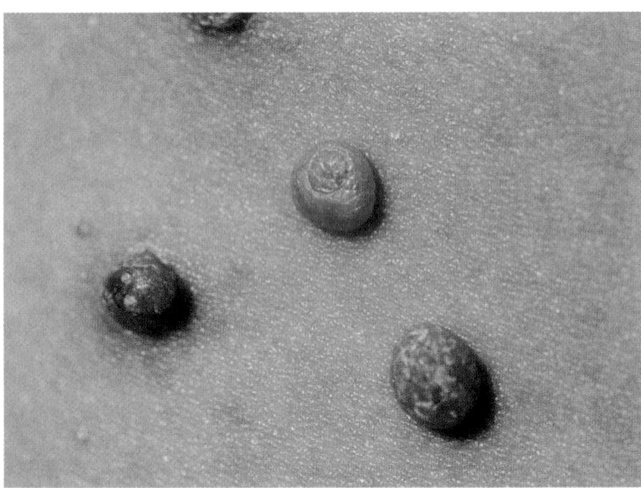

Fig. 7.5.28.2 Molluscum contagiosum: characteristic papules with central punctum.
(Courtesy of Dr Susan M Burge.)

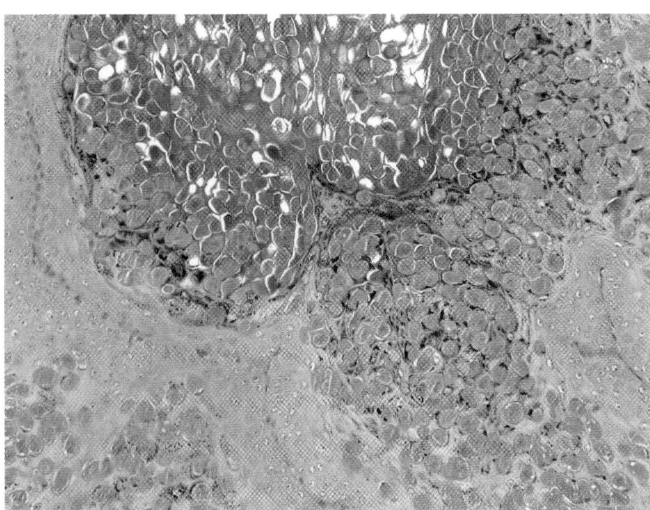

Fig. 7.5.28.4 Molluscum contagiosum showing keratinocyte debris with Henderson–Paterson molluscum bodies.
(Courtesy of K Hollowood.)

nitrogen, and diathermy. Topical chemicals include tretinoin, podofilox, cantharidin, acetic acid, phenol, salicylic acid, silver nitrate, trichloroacetic acid, lactic acid, and benzoin. Agents can be delivered to the inside of the lesion using the sharpened end of a wooden applicator stick. In children, local anaesthetic cream should be applied beforehand.

In patients with HIV, molluscum usually responds dramatically to highly active antiretroviral therapy (HAART). In severe cases, 5% imiquimod cream or cidofovir (intravenously or topically) have proved effective.

Prevention

In schoolchildren, spread can be prevented by avoiding swimming pools, contact sports, and shared towels, until the lesions have resolved.

Further reading

Brown J, *et al.* (2006). Childhood molluscum contagiosum. *Int J Dermatol*, **45**, 93–9.

De Clercq E (2003). Clinical potential of the acyclic nucleoside phosphonates cidofovir, adefovir, and tenofovir in treatment of DNA virus and retrovirus infections. *Clin Microbiol Rev*, **16**, 569–96.

Schwartz JJ, Myskowski PL (1992). Molluscum contagiosum in patients with human immunodeficiency virus infection. A review of twenty-seven patients. *J Am Acad Dermatol*, **27**, 583–8.

Smith KJ, Skelton H (2002). Molluscum contagiosum: recent advances in pathogenic mechanisms, and new therapies. *Am J Clin Dermatol*, **3**, 535–45.

Smith KJ, Yeager J, Skelton H (1999). Molluscum contagiosum: its clinical, histopathologic, and immunohistochemical spectrum. *Int J Dermatol*, **38**, 664–72.

van der Wouden JC, *et al.* (2006). Interventions for cutaneous molluscum contagiosum. Cochrane Database Syst Rev, **2**, CD004767.

7.5.29 Newly discovered viruses

H.C. Hughes

Essentials

Although humans are affected by an enormous range of micro-organisms, almost all newly discovered emerging pathogens are viruses that are often zoonotic or vector-borne. These emerging viruses often have high baseline mutation rates, allowing them to adapt relatively easily to new hosts and enabling them to take advantage of new epidemiological opportunities provided by the changing environment. A range of apparently new human viral pathogens has been reported increasingly in international outbreak information over the last few years. How they will influence global public health remains to be seen.

Emerging viruses that may be of particular public health importance include (1) respiratory SARS-like coronaviruses; (2) Garissa and Ngari viruses, Alkhurma virus and Lujo virus—discovered during investigations of haemorrhagic fever; (3) KI and WU human polyomaviruses, new human coronaviruses, human bocavirus, human parechovirus and mimivirus—causing predominantly respiratory disease; (4) Toscana and, Usutu, viruses—causing viral meningitis and encephalitis. (5) Merkel cell polyomavirus—with oncogenic potential. The human pathogenicity of other emerging viruses, e.g. vesivirus, Ljungan virus, gamma-retrovirus and Saffold virus is less certain.

SARS-like coronaviruses (Chapter 7.5.1)

Coronaviruses (CoV) are single-stranded RNA viruses commonly associated with respiratory illness and less often with gastrointestinal and neurological disease in a wide variety of mammals and birds. The severe acute respiratory syndrome (SARS) outbreak of a new human coronavirus, SARS-associated coronavirus (SARS-CoV), between November 2002 and July 2003 spread across 5 continents and caused over 700 human deaths. This pandemic triggered renewed interest in this area, leading to increased understanding of the origin of SARS-CoV, as well as the discovery of two previously unknown human coronaviruses.

In the early phase of the outbreak, the infecting SARS viruses showed closer similarities to animal viruses than later on in the pandemic. Virological studies suggest that the animal viruses crossed over to humans on more than one separate occasion, so repeated similar events should be expected in the future. Bats are increasingly recognized as reservoirs of emerging viruses. The discovery of species-specific, SARS-like coronaviruses in horseshoe bats with the same genome organization as human SARS coronaviruses indicates that a human SARS virus originated in one or more bat species. It is likely that an intermediate animal host is also required to allow modification of the mutating progenitor virus before transmission to humans is possible. Understanding this reservoir might help to prevent future human outbreaks of SARS-CoV.

New human coronaviruses

Two new human coronaviruses have been discovered since the SARS epidemic: HCoV-NL63 and HCoV-HK. HCoV-NL63 was first identified in a child with bronchiolitis in the Netherlands. Studies published in 2004 and 2005 found 8 to 9% of children under 5 years old with known respiratory illness were positive for HCoV-NL63 by polymerase chain reaction (PCR), while tests for common respiratory viruses were negative. Longitudinal studies showed that seroconversion usually occurred by the age of 3.5 years. Significant sequence heterogeneity exists and it is likely therefore that there are two closely related genotypic subgroups.

In 2005, another human coronavirus was discovered, HCoV-HKU1. It was first described in Hong Kong in a 71-year-old man with pneumonia who had recently returned from China. It has since been reported in patients in Australia and the United States of America. Common clinical findings in young children included rhinorrhoea, cough, fever, and abnormal breath sounds on auscultation. The possibility of central nervous system infection and hepatitis (in a liver transplant recipient) were suggested in two separate patients in one study. Genomic and phylogenetic analysis suggests that this virus is most closely related to the mouse hepatitis virus, a coronavirus studied since the 1930s.

New human polyomaviruses: KI, WU, and Merkel cell polyomavirus

The double-stranded DNA human polyomaviruses, JC virus and BK virus, are ubiquitous worldwide and are pathogenic in immunocompromised hosts. In 2007, two new human polyomaviruses were described, KI virus and WU virus. They share a phylogenetic relationship and together may form a new subclass. They have been isolated primarily from respiratory secretions. KI was discovered after molecular screening of respiratory samples. WU was first detected by high-throughput sequencing of respiratory secretions from a patient with an acute respiratory disease of unknown aetiology. Analysis of two more cohorts in different continents revealed that the majority of patients positive for WU were under 3 years old, and that all infected adults were immunocompromised. The clinical spectrum of the disease included upper and lower respiratory tract infection, bronchiolitis, croup, and, rarely, gastroenteritis. However, the role of these viruses as respiratory pathogens has since been questioned after further studies detected them both in asymptomatic children and those concurrently infected with other respiratory viruses. Studies to establish the role of WU and KI in immunocompromised adults have also been inconclusive.

In 2008, another novel polyomavirus termed 'Merkel Cell polyomavirus' was found to be integrated within the cellular genome of cells of the rare skin cancer Merkel cell carcinoma. This is consistent with the oncogenic potential of other polyomaviruses. Merkel cell polyomavirus has also been isolated in respiratory samples from symptomatic adult and paediatric patients though its precise role as a pathogen in this context is yet to be confirmed.

Human bocavirus

Human bocavirus (HBoV) is a nonenveloped, single-stranded DNA virus in the family Parvoviridae, first described in September 2005 following isolation by random PCR in pooled respiratory samples from hospitalized children in Sweden. HBoV is closely related to canine minute virus and bovine parvovirus. The only other parvovirus known to be pathogenic in humans is parvovirus B19, the cause of fifth disease in children (Chapter 7.5.20).

Although Koch's postulates have not yet been fulfilled, supportive molecular evidence demonstrated this virus in respiratory samples from children with lower respiratory tract disease who tested negative for common respiratory viruses. It has been found most commonly in children under 3 years old, particularly in preterm infants with mild to severe respiratory symptoms. A more recent study conducted in the Netherlands showed no difference between the detection of HBoV in children with or without LRTI in paediatric intensive care. However, higher levels of HBoV were seen in the symptomatic patients compared to asymptomatic controls which may reflect differences in viral load of acute infection versus asymptomatic shedding.

Related viruses HBoV2 and a recombinant HBoV-1/-2 have more recently been identified in faecal samples of children in several countries including the United Kingdom, Pakistan, and Thailand. An association with acute gastroenteritis has been described: in one study, HBoV2 was the third most prevalent virus seen in children with AGE after rotavirus and astrovirus. Absence of HBoV2 in >6500 paediatric respiratory samples in one study suggests a very different tissue tropism to HBoV despite its close phylogenetic lineage. HBoV-3 has also been described though a clinical association is yet to be shown.

Further quantitative studies are needed before the precise role of these viruses in human disease is reliably established.

Vesivirus

Single-stranded RNA vesiviruses of the Calciviridae family are common marine microorganisms, but are also known to infect land mammals. They cause a broad spectrum of disease in animals including vesicular rash, encephalitis, haemorrhagic disease, spontaneous abortion, and hepatitis. Their effect on humans is not well established, but a recent seroprevalence study has shown that 12% of tested successful blood donors had evidence of past exposure to vesivirus. This was significantly higher (29%) in patients with hepatitis of unknown but suspected infectious cause, and even higher (47%) in patients with hepatitis of unknown cause associated with blood transfusion or dialysis. Vesivirus viraemia was also shown to be present in some of those tested.

New parechoviruses: Human parechovirus and Ljungan virus

Human parechovirus and Ljungan virus are the two species of the genus parechovirus of the family *Picornaviridae*. Human parechoviruses are single-stranded RNA viruses which differ from other family members in having only three, rather than four, capsid proteins, and in exerting atypical cytopathic effects. HPeV-1 and HPeV-2 were previously designated Enterovirus 22 and 23 but were reclassified in 1999. At the start of 2010, 14 human parechoviruses had been described (HPeV-1 to HPeV-14).

HPeV infections are common with at least 95% of the adult population positive for HPeV-specific antibodies. Most infections are thought to predominantly affect neonates and young children and the clinical spectrum of disease differs between the viruses. Earlier studies of HPeV-1 suggested infection resulted in more gastrointestinal and respiratory illness which was often severe, and was occasionally found as a copathogen with other respiratory viruses such as respiratory syncytial virus (RSV). The role of HPeV-1 as a respiratory pathogen has since been challenged. HPeV-2 and HPeV-3 have been shown to present as sepsis-like syndromes, predominantly affecting neonates. More recently described HPeV-8 (Brazil, 2009) and HPeV-10 (Sri Lanka, 2010) were both found in stool specimens of children with acute gastroenteritis. It is also likely that further novel human parechoviruses will be discovered and their contribution as human pathogens investigated.

Another parechovirus, Ljungan virus (LV) has recently been postulated as a major aetiological agent in sudden infant death syndrome (SIDS). LV mainly affects rodents and is known to be associated with perinatal rodent death both in the wild and in laboratory mice. Interestingly, a strong epidemiological link between small rodent numbers and human intrauterine fetal death has been described in Sweden. In addition, LV has been detected in brain, heart and lung tissue in cases of SIDS. Whether true causation can be proven is yet to be established.

Human cardiovirus: Saffold virus

Investigation of an 8 month old girl with pyrexia of unknown origin, led to the discovery of a novel cardiovirus of the family

Picornaviradae, provisionally named Saffold virus (SAFV). Several strains of SAFV have since been described and have been detected in faecal and respiratory specimens of children worldwide. Although this may be the first human cardiovirus, a specific clinical association is yet to be found.

Usutu virus

Usutu virus, named after a river in Swaziland, was first isolated from mosquitoes in South Africa in 1959. It is a mosquito-borne flavivirus of the Japanese encephalitis group and was isolated once from a man with fever and rash. Although a virus of tropical or subtropical Africa, the epidemiology might be changing, following its isolation from several bird species during a die-off in Austria in 2001. This reflects the pattern of the emergence of West Nile virus in the United States of America in 1999, which first affected birds and subsequently humans. Neuroinvasive infection secondary to Usutu virus was reported for the first time worldwide in 2009 when USUV was detected by RT-PCR in CSF and serum samples in two immunocompromised patients. The extent of the human pathogenic potential of USUV remains to be seen, but there is concern that it may follow a recurrent theme of flavivirus emergence in previously cooler climates following climate change.

Garissa and Ngari virus

Genetic reassortment of segmented RNA viruses such as influenza is well known to have an important role in the emergence of viruses with new disease potential and host range. There is less genetic information on bunyaviruses, but there is increasing evidence that this mechanism could account for their evolution and increase their potential to cause disease in humans.

The first association of Ngari virus with human haemorrhagic fever (HF) was discovered during an extensive investigation of a large outbreak in Kenya, Tanzania, and Somalia in 1997 to 1998. A previously unidentified member of the orthobunyavirus genus (family Bunyaviridae) was found in two cases. The virus was initially named Garissa virus, but subsequent genetic analysis showed that it was not a separate orthobunyavirus but had arisen by genetic segment reassortment between two known orthobunyaviruses, Bunyamwera virus and Ngari virus. Further sequence analysis of multiple orthobunyaviruses revealed that Ngari virus is a reassortment Bunyamwera virus.

Alkurma virus

Alkhurma virus, a re-emerging tick-borne flavivirus, is related to Kysanur Forest disease and shares clinical features with Dengue Fever. It was first described in a butcher in Saudi Arabia in the 1990s, and over the next 10 years, had a case fatality rate of around 25%. In 2009, 4 further sporadic cases were described in Jeddah in the post Hajj period and all may be linked to the slaughtering/processing of sheep. The cases have highlighted the need to further understand the epidemiology of this re-emerging disease.

Lujo virus

Lujo virus is the proposed name for a novel genetically distinct arena virus associated with haemorrhagic fever with an exceptionally high case fatality rate of 80%. It was first isolated in South Africa in 2008 during a nosocomial outbreak of 5 cases following the transfer of the index case from Zambia. The technique of unbiased pyrosequencing used during the investigation of this outbreak may well be useful in identifying other novel pathogens in the future.

Toscana virus

Toscana virus (TOSV) is an arthropod-borne bunyavirus transmitted by sandflies. Though it was first identified in Italy in 1971, epidemiological studies and clinical research over the last three decades has shown that it is an increasingly important cause of seasonal aseptic meningitis and encephalitis across the Mediterranean. It is the most common cause of this disease in Italy from May to October and has also been associated with human infection in France. The RNA of TOSV has been isolated in a different species of sandfly in France from that in Italy, although there is no confirmation that human disease is arthropod-borne.

Mimivirus

With a diameter of 600 nm and with a dsDNA genome of 1.2 Mb, mimivirus is the largest virus so far discovered. It was initially thought to be a Gram-positive coccoid bacterium and is visible with the light microscope.

The virus species *Acanthamoeba polyphaga mimivirus* is within a family of its own, the Mimiviridae. Phylogenetic analysis has shown its relationship to other large DNA viruses including the Iridoviridae and Poxviridae, though its precise position in the phylogenetic tree remains under debate. Discovered during the investigation of respiratory pathogens using an amoeba coculture system, it may have originated in marine environments. Although it replicates within amoebae, it is yet to be shown to multiply effectively in mammalian cells. Mimivirus may have a role in respiratory disease. A pneumonic illness can be produced in mice and a laboratory technician occupationally exposed to high concentrations of mimivirus antigens developed a subacute, spontaneously resolving pneumonia with seroconversion to Mimivirus. The prevalence of antibodies to mimivirus was 9.66% in 376 Canadian patients with community acquired pneumonia compared to 2.3% of healthy controls. Two studies of pneumonia in intensive care units have shown seroconversion to the virus in more patients with ventilator-associated pneumonia than in controls. Seropositivity to mimivirus in ventilated patients in a prospective matched cohort study was associated with longer duration of ventilation and longer ICU stay. There was no mortality difference between seropositive patients and matched seronegative controls. Mimivirus antibodies have been found to be more prevalent in populations admitted from nursing homes and in those rehospitalized after discharge. These seroprevalence studies must be interpreted cautiously because of possible cross-reactivity with other pathogens. However, mimivirus DNA was recovered from a bronchoalveolar lavage of a patient with relapsing pneumonia in the absence of other causative pathogens.

Gamma-retrovirus: xenotropic murine leukaemia virus-related virus

A novel retrovirus termed xenotropic murine leukaemia virus-related virus (XMRV) was linked previously to prostate cancer in the USA but no in Europe. In 2009, it was reported that 68 of 101 patients with chronic fatigue syndrome in the USA were infected with the virus though this finding has not been replicated in a similar UK cohort. It may be that these findings reflect differences in the prevalence of this virus in North America and Europe rather than a specific association with CFS per se.

Further reading

Abed Y, *et al.* (2006). Human parechovirus types 1, 2 and 3 infections in Canada. *Emerg Infect Dis*, **12**, 969–75.

Allander T, *et al.* (2005). Cloning of a human parvovirus by molecular screening of respiratory tract samples. *Proc Natl Acad Sci U S A*, **102**, 12891–96.

Allander T, *et al.* (2007). Identification of a third human polyomavirus. *J Virol*, **81**, 4130–36.

Arthur JL, *et al.* (2009). A novel bocavirus associated with acute gastroenteritis in Australian children. *PLoS Pathog*, **5**, e1000391.

Charrel RN, *et al.* (2005). Emergence of Toscana virus in Europe. *Emerg Infect Dis*, **11**, 1657–63.

Charrel RN, *et al.* (2005). Low diversity of Alkhurma hemorrhagic fever virus, Saudi Arabia, 1994–1999. *Emerg Infect Dis*, **11**, 683–88.

Drexler JF, *et al.* (2009). Novel human parechovirus from Brazil. *Emerg Infect Dis*, **15**, 310–13.

Erlwein O, *et al.* (2010). Failure to detect the novel retrovirus XMRV in chronic fatigue syndrome. *PLoS One*, **5**, e8519.

Esper F, *et al.* (2006). Coronavirus HKU1 infection in the United States. *Emerg Infect Dis*, **12**, 775–79.

Gaynor AM, *et al.* (2007). Identification of a novel polyomavirus from patients with acute respiratory tract infections. *PLoS Pathog*, **3**, e64.

Gerrard SR, *et al.* (2004). Ngari virus is a Bunyamwera virus reassortant that can be associated with large outbreaks of hemorrhagic fever in Africa. *J Virol*, **78**, 8922–26.

Harvala H, *et al.* (2008). Epidemiology and clinical associations of human parechovirus respiratory infections. J Clin Microbiol, **46**, 3446–53.

Kim Pham NT, *et al.* (2010). Novel human parechovirus, Sri Lanka. *Emerg Infect Dis*, **16**, 130–32.

Nguyen NL, *et al.* (2009). Serologic evidence of frequent human infection with WU and KI polyomaviruses. *Emerg Infect Dis*, **15**, 1199–1205.

Pyrc, K *et al.* (2007). The novel human coronaviruses NL63 and HKU1. *J Virol*, **81**, 3051–57.

Raoult D, *et al.* (2007). The discovery and characterization of Mimivirus, the largest known virus and putative pneumonia agent. *Clin Infect Dis*, **45**, 95–102.

Ren, L *et al.* (2009). Saffold cardiovirus in children with acute gastroenteritis, Beijing, China. *Emerg Infect Dis*, **15**, 1509–11.

Smith AW, *et al.* (2006). Vesivirus viremia and seroprevalence in humans. *J Med Virol*, **78**, 693–701.

Vabret A, *et al.* (2005). Human coronavirus NL63, France. *Emerg Infect Dis*, **11**, 1225–29.

van de Pol AC, *et al.* (2009). Human bocavirus and KI/WU polyomaviruses in pediatric intensive care patients. *Emerg Infect Dis*, **15**, 454–57.

Vincent A, *et al.* (2009). Clinical significance of a positive serology for mimivirus in patients presenting a suspicion of ventilator-associated pneumonia. *Crit Care Med*, **37**, 111–8.

Wang LF, *et al.* (2006). Review of bats and SARS. *Emerg Infect Dis*, **12**, 1834–40.

Wattier RL, *et al.* (2008). Role of human polyomaviruses in respiratory tract disease in young children. *Emerg Infect Dis*, **14**, 1766–68.

Weissenbock H, *et al.* (2002). Emergence of Usutu virus, an African mosquito-borne flavivirus of the Japanese encephalitis virus group, central Europe. *Emerg Infect Dis*, **8**, 652–56.

7.6

Bacteria

Contents

7.6.1 Diphtheria *664*
Delia B. Bethell and Tran Tinh Hien

7.6.2 Streptococci and enterococci *670*
Dennis L. Stevens

7.6.3 Pneumococcal infections *679*
Anthony Scott

7.6.4 Staphylococci *693*
Bala Hota and Robert A. Weinstein

7.6.5 Meningococcal infections *709*
P. Brandtzaeg

7.6.6 *Neisseria gonorrhoeae* *722*
D. Barlow, Jackie Sherrard, and C. Ison

7.6.7 Enterobacteria *727*

7.6.7.1 Enterobacteria and bacterial food poisoning *727*
Hugh Pennington

7.6.7.2 *Pseudomonas aeruginosa* *735*
G.C.K.W. Koh and S.J. Peacock

7.6.8 Typhoid and paratyphoid fevers *738*
C.M. Parry and Buddha Basnyat

7.6.9 Intracellular klebsiella infections (donovanosis and rhinoscleroma) *745*
J. Richens

7.6.10 Anaerobic bacteria *748*
Anilrudh A. Venugopal and David W. Hecht

7.6.11 Cholera *754*
Aldo A.M. Lima and Richard L. Guerrant

7.6.12 *Haemophilus influenzae* *759*
Derrick W. Crook

7.6.13 *Haemophilus ducreyi* and chancroid *763*
Nigel O'Farrell

7.6.14 Bordetella infection *764*
Cameron Grant

7.6.15 Melioidosis and glanders *768*
S.J. Peacock

7.6.16 Plague: *Yersinia pestis* *772*
Michael B. Prentice

7.6.17 Other *Yersinia* infections: yersiniosis *776*
Michael B. Prentice

7.6.18 Pasteurella *777*
Marina S. Morgan

7.6.19 *Francisella tularensis* infection *780*
Petra C.F. Oyston

7.6.20 Anthrax *783*
Arthur E. Brown and Thira Sirisanthana

7.6.21 Brucellosis *789*
M. Monir Madkour

7.6.22 Tetanus *795*
C.L. Thwaites and Lam Minh Yen

7.6.23 *Clostridium difficile* *800*
John G. Bartlett

7.6.24 Botulism, gas gangrene, and clostridial gastrointestinal infections *803*
Dennis L. Stevens, Michael J. Aldape, and Amy E. Bryant

7.6.25 Tuberculosis *810*
Richard E. Chaisson and Jean B. Nachega

7.6.26 Disease caused by environmental mycobacteria *831*
J.M. Grange and P.D.O. Davies

7.6.27 Leprosy (Hansen's disease) *836*
Diana N.J. Lockwood

7.6.28 Buruli ulcer: *Mycobacterium ulcerans* infection *848*
Wayne M. Meyers and Françoise Portaels

7.6.29 Actinomycoses *850*
K.P. Schaal

7.6.30 Nocardiosis *856*
Roderick J. Hay

7.6.31 Rat-bite fevers *857*
David A. Warrell

7.6.32 Lyme borreliosis *860*
Gary P. Wormser, John Nowakowski, and Robert B. Nadelman

7.6.33 Relapsing fevers *866*
David A. Warrell

7.6.34 Leptospirosis *874*
George Watt

7.6.35 Nonvenereal endemic treponematoses: yaws, endemic syphilis (bejel), and pinta *879*
David A. Warrell

7.6.36 Syphilis *885*
Basil Donovan and Linda Dayan

7.6.37 Listeriosis *896*
H. Hof

7.6.38 Legionellosis and legionnaires' disease *899*
J.T. Macfarlane and T.C. Boswell

7.6.39 Rickettsioses *903*
Philippe Parola and Didier Raoult

7.6.40 Scrub typhus *919*
George Watt

7.6.41 *Coxiella burnetii* infections (Q fever) *923*
T.J. Marrie

7.6.42 Bartonellas excluding *B. bacilliformis* *926*
Emmanouil Angelakis, Didier Raoult, and Jean-Marc Rolain

7.6.43 *Bartonella bacilliformis* infection *934*
A. Llanos-Cuentas and C. Maguiña-Vargas

7.6.44 Chlamydial infections *939*
David Taylor-Robinson and David Mabey

7.6.45 Mycoplasmas *950*
David Taylor-Robinson and Jørgen Skov Jensen

7.6.46 A check list of bacteria associated with infection in humans *961*
J. Paul

7.6.1 Diphtheria

Delia B. Bethell and Tran Tinh Hien

Essentials

Diphtheria is a potentially lethal infection caused by toxin-producing strains of *Corynebacterium diphtheria*, a Gram-positive bacillus. Humans are the only known reservoir, with spread via respiratory droplets or direct contact with skin lesions. Although now rare in developed countries, this vaccine-preventable disease remains an important problem in countries with poor or failing health systems, and is estimated to cause about 5000 deaths per year worldwide, most in children under 5 years of age.

Pathogenesis—diphtheria develops when toxigenic bacteria lodge in the upper airway or on the skin of a susceptible individual. An intense inflammatory reaction develops, leading to a characteristic greyish-coloured pseudomembrane that is adherent to underlying tissues. Systemic effects are caused by release of diphtheria toxin, carried by a lysogenic corynebacteriophage, a single molecule of factor A of which can kill a eukaryotic cell.

Clinical features—after an incubation period of 2 to 6 days the disease presents acutely in a number of ways, classified by the location of the pseudomembrane: (1) anterior nasal—usually relatively mild; (2) tonsillar (faucial)—the commonest form, with malaise, fever, sore throat, painful dysphagia and tender cervical lymphadenopathy; (3) tracheolaryngeal—with particular risk of airway obstruction; (4) malignant—with rapid onset, circulatory shock, cyanosis, gross cervical lymphadenopathy ('bull neck'), and very poor prognosis; (5) cutaneous—usually mild but chronic; morphological features can be extremely variable. Later complications include (1) myocarditis—seen in 10% of cases; and (2) segmental demyelinative neuropathy—most often palatal paralysis, and more sinister paralyses of pharyngeal, laryngeal, respiratory and limb muscles.

Diagnosis—infection may be confirmed by bacterial culture, with detection of toxin production by one of several laboratory techniques, or of the toxin-producing gene by PCR.

Treatment and prognosis—aside from supportive care, this involves (1) antitoxin—20 000 to 100 000 units, depending on disease severity; preferably given within 48 h of the onset of symptoms; (2) antibiotics—benzylpenicillin (or penicillin V), or erythromycin in those allergic to penicillin; (3) maintaining the airway—life-saving procedures such as tracheostomy may be required. Recovery is usually complete if the patient survives.

Prevention—diphtheria is completely preventable by vaccination, but immunity is not life-long and may wane in adult life if booster doses are not given regularly. Similarly, infection does not necessarily confer complete protection and the disease may recur in previously infected individuals.

Introduction

Diphtheria is an acute and potentially highly lethal infection of the upper respiratory tract caused by toxigenic strains of *Corynebacterium diphtheriae* and *C. ulcerans*. Today diphtheria has been virtually eliminated from most developed countries by mass immunization, yet it remains a threat in countries with poor vaccine coverage. During the 1990s there was a huge epidemic in parts of the former Soviet Union. Smaller outbreaks have been reported in several other countries.

Historical perspective

Since ancient times diphtheria has been one of the most feared childhood diseases, characterized by devastating outbreaks. Diphtheria was recognized as an infectious disease by Brentonneau in 1819. The causative bacillus was described by Löffler in 1884 and a soluble toxin was identified by Roux and Yersin in 1889. In 1890, Fränkel developed an attenuated vaccine and von Behring produced an antitoxin, the first therapeutic antiserum that was first used clinically by Roux in 1894. Before the introduction of antitoxin, mortality in some epidemics had exceeded 50%. In 1913, von Behring produced a successful vaccine and the Schick (skin) test was used to detect immunity. In the United Kingdom there was an average of 50 000 cases and 4000 deaths each year from 1915 to 1942 and it was the leading cause of death among children aged 4 to 10 years. During the Second World War, more than a million cases were reported, including 50 000 deaths. In the United States of America, W. Barry Woods Jr declared in 1961 that: "Were it possible merely to apply what is now known about diphtheria to every part of the world, this devastating malady could be wiped from the face of the earth". However, even in that country, epidemic outbreaks continued in major cities, e.g. the 1970 San Antonio epidemic involving 201 cases with 3 deaths mainly in the unimmunized poor nonwhite population aged less than 15 years. In the United Kingdom, mass vaccination had reduced diphtheria to approximately 8–10 notified cases each year. In 2002 there were still an estimated 5000 deaths from diphtheria worldwide, of which 4000 were in children under 5 years of age.

Pathogenesis

C. diphtheriae are slender pleomorphic Gram-positive rods or clubs. There are four biotypes: *gravis*, *intermedius*, *belfanti*, and *mitis*, any of which can cause diphtheria if they produce exotoxin. Early manifestations of diphtheria, including pseudomembrane formation, result from an inflammatory reaction to the multiplying toxigenic *C. diphtheriae*. Fluid and leucocytes move from dilated blood vessels to surround necrotic epithelial cells. The fluid clots to enmesh dead cells, leucocytes, diphtheria bacilli, cellular debris, and occasionally small blood vessels. The resulting pseudomembrane is therefore adherent to underlying tissues and bleeds when pulled away.

C. diphtheriae does not usually pass beyond the pseudomembrane site; it is the toxin that causes the later complications of diphtheria. Diphtheria toxin is a 535-amino acid residue 62-kDa exotoxin consisting of three domains, A (enzymatic), B (binding), and T (translocation). Domain B binds on the cell surface to heparin-binding epidermal growth factor (EGF)-like growth factor precursor and CD9 complex, allowing the lethal factor A to pass through the endosome membrane into the cytosol where it catalyses the NAD^+-dependent ADP-ribosylation of eukaryotic elongation factor 2 preventing protein synthesis leading to cell death, facilitated by apoptosis. Delivery of a single molecule of factor A to the cytosol of a eukaryotic cell will kill it. Employing this mechanism, recombinant diphtheria toxin with its B domain truncated and fused with the human interleukin (IL)-2 receptor is marketed as denileukin diftitox (DT388-IL2) for the treatment of cutaneous T-cell lymphoma, chronic lymphocytic leukaemia, and non-Hodgkin's lymphoma.

The structural gene of the toxin (*TOX*) is carried by a lysogenic corynebacteriophage. However, *TOX* gene expression is regulated by the bacterial chromosome and requires low extracellular iron concentrations. Locally the toxin causes tissue necrosis and, when absorbed into the bloodstream, systemic complications. In addition to bacterial exotoxin, cell wall components such as the O- and K-antigens are important in disease pathogenesis.

Pathological changes may be seen in all human cells, but the most profound changes are seen in the myocardium, peripheral nerves, and kidneys. Common cardiac changes include fatty degeneration of cardiac muscle (myocarditis) and infiltration of the interstitium with leucocytes, which may involve the conduction fibres. Although the heart can recover completely from these effects, severe fibrosis and scarring may lead to death in late convalescence. Mural endocarditis may cause embolism leading to cerebral infarction and hemiplegia. Valvular endocarditis is extremely uncommon. Neuritic changes may be seen in the nerves to the heart during the late paralytic stage of the disease. Diphtheria toxin also causes demyelination and degeneration of both sensory and motor nerves. It affects the nerves to the eye, palate, pharynx, larynx, heart, and limb muscles. It is unclear whether the toxin crosses the blood–brain barrier to cause central lesions.

Epidemiology

Humans are the only known reservoir for *C. diphtheriae*. In most cases transmission to susceptible individuals results in transient pharyngeal carriage rather than disease. Spread is via respiratory droplets or direct contact with skin lesions. Cutaneous diphtheria is more contagious than respiratory diphtheria and chronic skin infections are the main reservoir in environments of poverty and overcrowding. Patients may become carriers of the infection and continue to harbour the organism for weeks or months. The organism can survive for up to 5 weeks in dust or on fomites.

Today diphtheria remains an important health problem in countries with poor vaccine coverage. In these areas, children generally meet *C. diphtheriae* early, sometimes becoming a carrier, and young children may have severe or fatal attacks of diphtheria. *C. diphtheriae* tends to die out in highly immunized populations, and children may grow to adult life without encountering the bacillus. Recent serological studies in several countries indicate that up to 50% of adults are susceptible to diphtheria, and their immunity decreases significantly with increasing age. This potential risk is becoming increasingly important with the growth in international travel.

Immunity to systemic disease depends on the presence of IgG antitoxin antibodies. Type-specific protection against carriage and mild forms of local disease is induced by antibodies to the variable K antigens of the bacterial cell wall. Infection does not always confer protective immunity and outbreaks of mild disease have been reported even in highly vaccinated populations. In endemic countries protective immunity is boosted naturally through circulating strains of toxigenic *C. diphtheriae*.

Diphtheria is a devastating but preventable disease. Experience suggests that declining immunity in adults poses the risk of outbreaks, but is probably not sufficient in itself to sustain a large diphtheria epidemic unless there are large numbers of susceptible children and adolescents. In the newly independent states of the former Soviet Union (NIS), economic hardship, large urban migration, and low vaccination coverage due to failing health systems probably contributed to the massive outbreak of the 1990s. This started in Russia but spread to all the NIS, leading to more than 150 000 cases and 5000 deaths between 1990 and 1998 and more than 2700 cases subsequently. Widespread immunization campaigns have largely controlled the epidemic but the risk of diphtheria remains in all countries of the former Soviet Union (e.g. there were outbreaks in Western Siberia in 2003 and the southern Urals in 2004) and rare cases of diphtheria continue to be reported in tourists and travellers to the NIS.

Clinical features

Early features

Diphtheria has an incubation period of 2 to 6 days and presents acutely in a variety of forms, classified according to the location of the pseudomembrane:

Anterior nasal

This is usually unilateral and relatively mild unless it coexists with other forms. It is relatively common in infancy. There is a nasal discharge, initially watery, then purulent and blood-stained. The nostril may be sore or crusted and a thin pseudomembrane can sometimes be seen within the nostril itself.

Tonsillar (faucial)

This is the commonest form of diphtheria. Malaise, sore throat, and moderate fever develop gradually. At the onset of symptoms only a small, yellow-grey spot of pseudomembrane may be present on one or both tonsils and is easily mistaken for other types of tonsillitis; it is associated with marked fetor. The surrounding areas are dull and inflamed. Over the next few days the pseudomembrane enlarges and may extend to cover the uvula, soft palate, oropharynx, nasopharynx, or larynx (Fig. 7.6.1.1). There is tender cervical lymphadenopathy, nausea, vomiting, and painful dysphagia. The pseudomembrane becomes greenish-black and eventually sloughs off.

Tracheolaryngeal

Some 85% of tracheolaryngeal presentations are secondary to faucial diphtheria, but occasionally there may be no pharyngeal pseudomembrane. Initial symptoms include moderate fever, hoarseness, and a nonproductive cough. Over the next day or two, as the pseudomembrane and associated oedema spread, the patient becomes increasingly dyspnoeic with severe chest recession, cyanosis, and eventual asphyxiation unless the obstruction is relieved. Tracheostomy brings instant relief if the obstruction is confined to the larynx and upper trachea. In a minority of cases the pseudomembrane also involves the bronchi and bronchioles and tracheostomy has little effect.

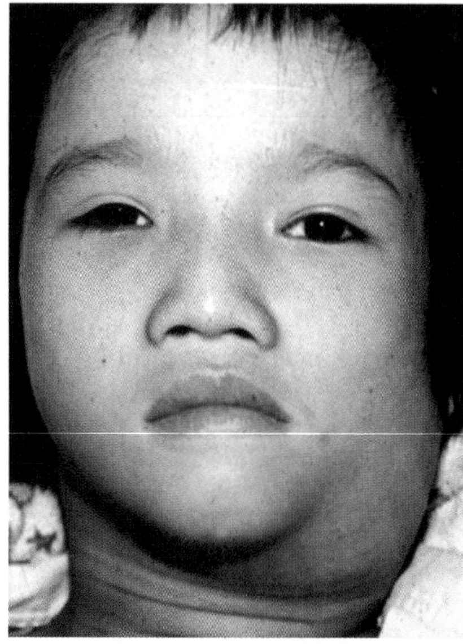

Fig. 7.6.1.2 Malignant diphtheria with typical bull neck.
(Copyright Rachel Kneen.)

Malignant

The onset is rapid, with high fever, tachycardia, hypotension, and cyanosis. Pseudomembrane spreads from the tonsils to cover much of the nasopharynx. It has a thick edge and as this advances the earlier parts become necrotic and foul-smelling. There is gross cervical lymphadenopathy. Individual lymph nodes are difficult to feel because of surrounding oedema; this is the characteristic 'bull neck' of malignant diphtheria (Fig. 7.6.1.2). The patient may bleed from the mouth, nose, or skin (Figs. 7.6.1.3, 7.6.1.4). Cardiac involvement with heart block occurs within a few days. Acute renal failure may ensue. Survival is unlikely.

Cutaneous

In contrast to respiratory forms, cutaneous diphtheria is usually chronic but mild. The morphological features of individual

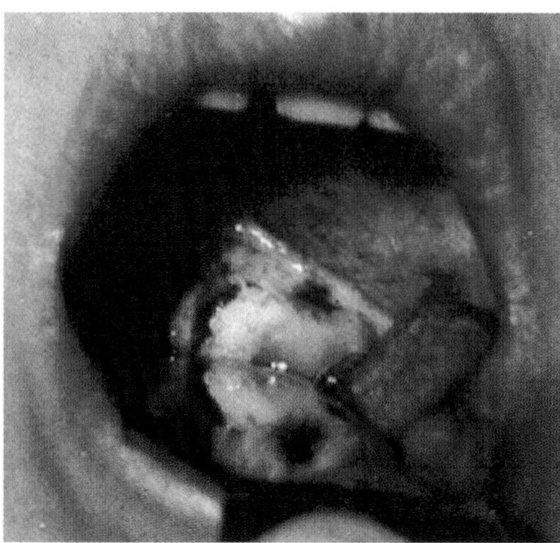

Fig. 7.6.1.1 Severe diphtheria in Vietnamese children. Typical faucial pharyngeal pseudomembrane.
(Copyright Bridget Wills.)

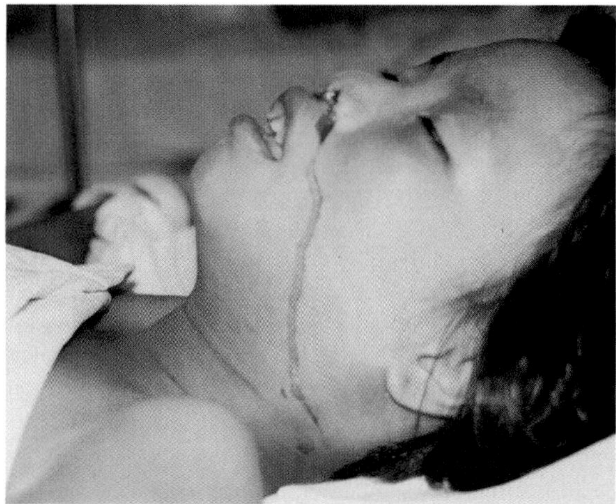

Fig. 7.6.1.3 Malignant diphtheria with serosanguinous nasal discharge.
(Copyright Rachel Kneen.)

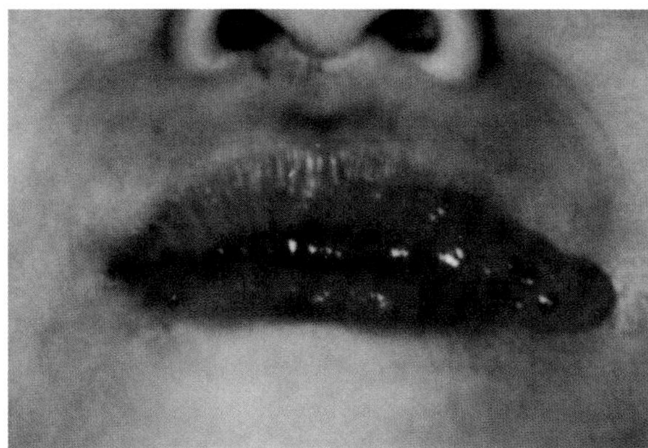

Fig. 7.6.1.4 Malignant diphtheria with serosanguinous oral discharge. (Copyright Tran Tinh Hien.)

lesions can be extremely variable as *C. diphtheriae* can colonize any pre-existing skin lesion (such as impetigo, scabies, surgical wounds, or insect bites) without altering their picture. However, the ulcerative form is the most frequent and typical (Fig. 7.6.1.5). Initially vesicular or pustular, and filled with straw-coloured fluid, it soon breaks down to leave a punched-out ulcer several millimetres to a few centimetres across. Common sites are the lower legs, feet, and hands. During the first 1 to 2 weeks it is painful and may be covered with a dark pseudomembrane which separates, revealing a haemorrhagic base, sometimes with a serous or serosanguinous exudate. The surrounding tissue is oedematous and pink or purple in colour. Spontaneous healing to leave a depressed scar usually takes 2 to 3 months, and sometimes much longer. Systemic complications such as myocarditis are rare. Occasionally, the affected limb becomes paralysed.

Other sites

A mild conjunctivitis may accompany faucial diphtheria. Occasionally, pseudomembrane forms in the lower conjunctiva and spreads over the cornea causing considerable damage. Dysphagia may indicate that pseudomembrane has spread from the tonsils to the oesophagus. Other parts of the gastrointestinal tract are not usually affected, but melaena with colicky abdominal pain is described. Diphtheria may spread by fingers from the throat to vulva or penis causing localized sores. *C. diphtheriae* occasionally invades the vagina and cervix, allowing the absorption of toxin. Endocarditis is rare, but at least one reported case recovered following antimicrobial treatment.

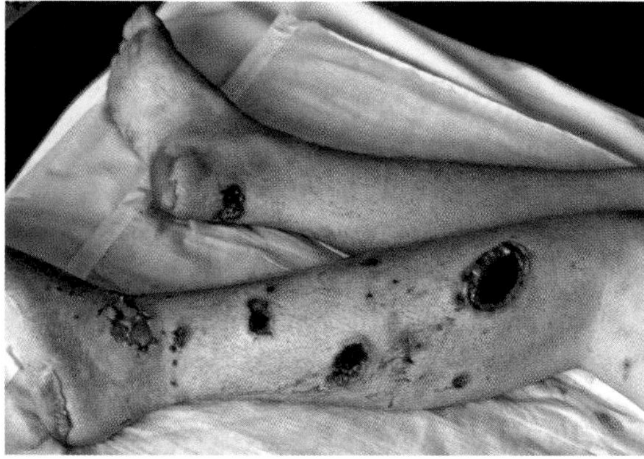

Fig. 7.6.1.5 Cutaneous diphtheria. (Courtesy of the late Dr B.E. Juel-Jensen.)

Diphtheria caused by other corynebacteria

C. ulcerans produces two toxins, one of which seems to be the same as diphtheria toxin. It may cause membranous tonsillitis but toxic manifestations are rare. *C. ulcerans* has been spread to humans in cows' milk.

C. pseudodiphtheriticum is commonly present in the flora of the upper respiratory tract. It is nontoxigenic, but can cause exudative pharyngitis with a pseudomembrane identical to that produced by *C. diphtheriae*. More commonly it causes endocarditis in patients with anatomical abnormalities or infections of the lungs, trachea, or bronchi in immunosuppressed patients or those with pre-existing respiratory disease.

Later complications

Patients surviving acute diphtheria may develop one or more later complications. These result from delayed effects of the toxin following haematogenous spread. The risk and severity of complications correlates directly with the extent of the pseudomembrane and the delay in administration of antitoxin.

Cardiovascular

Approximately 10% of patients with diphtheria will develop myocarditis, usually those with clinically severe infection. There is a much greater frequency of cardiac involvement in laryngeal and malignant diphtheria than in faucial diphtheria, and where antitoxin administration was delayed more than 48 h after onset of symptoms.

Cardiac toxicity usually appears after the first week of illness, but in malignant diphtheria can occur after just a few days. Patients complain of upper abdominal pain and may vomit. They become very lethargic and tired. Examination reveals a rapid, thready pulse with hypotension. At this stage profound shock may lead to death. In less severe cases, congestive cardiac failure may develop with a displaced apex beat, gallop rhythm, and murmurs audible over all areas of the heart. Profound bradycardia may result from heart block. There is hepatomegaly and oliguria.

Electrocardiography (ECG) is the best way to demonstrate cardiac involvement (Fig. 7.6.1.6). The most common abnormalities are T-wave inversion with ST-segment changes in one or more chest leads and prolonged QTc and PR intervals. There may be right or left axis deviation, bundle branch block, or heart block. Very occasionally, atrial fibrillation or tachyarrhythmias are seen. Many more bursts of arrhythmias can be demonstrated if 24-h ECG monitoring is performed. Numerous ectopic beats have been recorded in patients who lacked other manifestations of cardiac involvement. Although most patients surviving myocarditis recover completely, the presence of left bundle branch block at discharge is associated with poor long-term outcome.

Neurological

Diphtheria toxin causes a segmental demyelinative neuropathy. Neurological complications usually appear weeks after the onset of the disease, when the patient appears to be recovering, and may show a temporal progression. Palatal paralysis is relatively common and may be seen from the third week onwards. The patient develops a nasal voice and regurgitates fluids through the nose. This usually resolves within a week or so. From the third to the fifth week there may be blurred vision from paralysis of accommodation, or a transient squint from external rectus paralysis. About the sixth or seventh week more sinister paralyses may develop

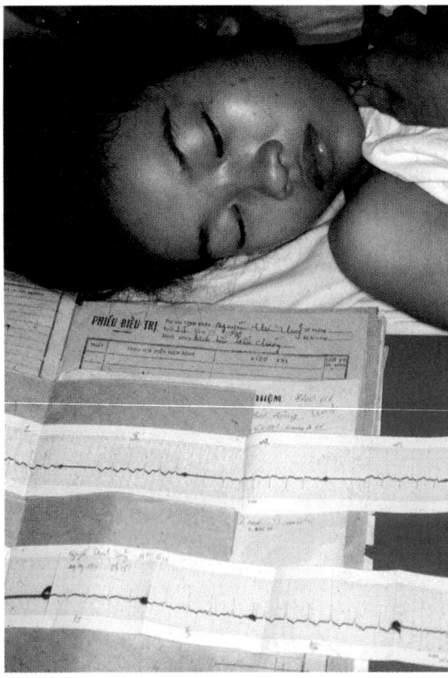

Fig. 7.6.1.6 Fifteen-year-old girl with cardiac and neurological complications (paralysis of muscles innervated by cranial nerves IX, X and XII). (Copyright D.A. Warrell.)

involving pharyngeal, laryngeal, respiratory, and limb muscles (Fig. 7.6.1.7). The nerves to the heart may be affected causing tachycardia and dysrhythmias. In severe cases patients may become profoundly hypotonic over a few hours and can die from respiratory arrest. However, if intensive care facilities and skilled staff are available, complete recovery over the following weeks or months should ensue.

Differential diagnosis

Clinical diagnosis is difficult where diphtheria is rare. The differential diagnosis includes infectious mononucleosis, streptococcal or viral tonsillitis, peritonsillar abscess, Vincent's angina, oral thrush, anthrax (Chapter 7.6.20, Fig. 7.6.20.2), Lassa fever (Chapter 7.5.17), and leukaemia and other blood dyscrasias. The bull neck of malignant diphtheria may be mistaken for mumps. In adults, secondary syphilis can sometimes cause a glairy (resembling egg white) exudate on the tonsils, and may be accompanied by rash and laryngitis.

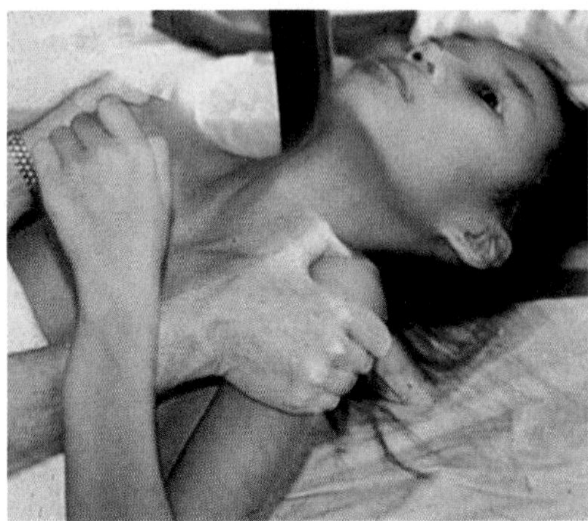

Fig. 7.6.1.7 Generalized muscle weakness. (Copyright Rachel Kneen.)

Clinical investigation

Bacterial culture of *C. diphtheriae* is the mainstay of investigation. Material for culture should be obtained preferably from the edges of the mucosal lesions and inoculated onto appropriate selective media. Suspected colonies may be tested for toxin production by gel precipitation (Elek's test), guinea pig inoculation, or enzyme immunoassay. Direct smears of infected areas of the throat are often used for diagnostic purposes, but are only of value in experienced hands. More reliably the diphtheria toxin gene may be detected directly in clinical specimens using polymerase chain reaction techniques.

Criteria for diagnosis

In areas where diphtheria is relatively common and during outbreaks, the disease should be suspected in any patient with exudate in the throat. Treatment must not be delayed until the disease is confirmed, except in cases of suspected cutaneous diphtheria without associated respiratory symptoms.

Other corynebacterial skin infections

C. diphtheriae and some other corynebacteria are associated with cutaneous 'desert sores'. Erythrasma is caused by *C. minutissimum* and, in HIV-immunosuppressed patients, *C. striatum* can cause exuberant ulceration (Fig. 7.6.1.8).

Treatment

Antitoxin is the mainstay of treatment, but to be maximally effective it must be given before the toxin has reached tissues such as the heart and kidneys, preferably within 48 h of the onset of symptoms, implying that it must be given empirically before bacteriological confirmation. Dosage depends on the site of primary infection, the extent of pseudomembrane, and the delay between the onset of symptoms and antitoxin administration. Between 20 000 and 40 000 units are given for faucial diphtheria of less than 48 h duration or for cutaneous infection, 40 000 to 80 000 units for faucial diphtheria in excess of 48 h duration or for laryngeal infection, and 80 000 to 100 000 units for malignant diphtheria. For doses over 40 000 units a portion is given intramuscularly followed by the bulk of the dose intravenously after an interval of 30 min to 2 h. Anaphylaxis can occur following antitoxin administration, and adrenaline (epinephrine) should always be available.

Antibiotics are given to eradicate the organism and prevent further toxin production. Benzylpenicillin 150 000 to 250 000 units/kg per day (90–150 mg/kg per day) is given intravenously in four to six divided doses in children aged 1 month to 12 years. In adults the dosage is 12 million to 20 million units/day (7.2–12 g/day) in four to six divided doses. Oral penicillin V is substituted when the patient is able to swallow. Erythromycin may be used for penicillin-sensitive individuals, but it may not be as effective in eradicating carriage. Antibiotic therapy should continue for 10 to 14 days.

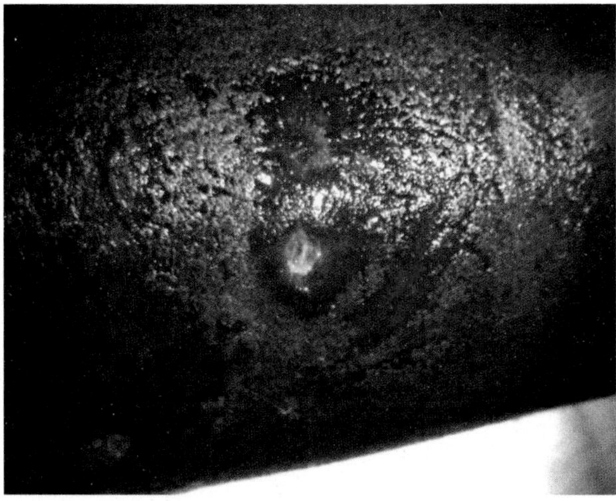

(a)

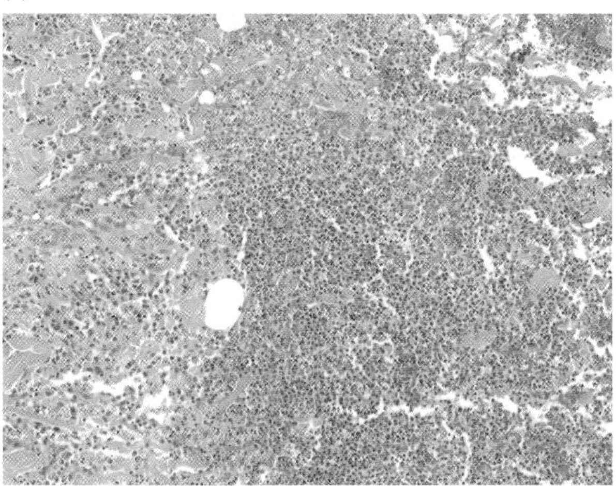

(b)

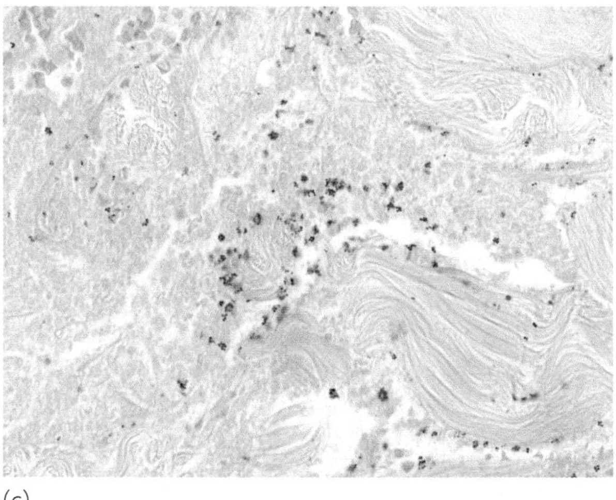

(c)

Fig. 7.6.1.8 *Corynebacterium striatum* infection on the thigh of an African patient with HIV-immunosuppression (a) clinical appearance of exuberant ulcerative lesion, (b) and (c) histopathological appearances of a biopsy of the lesion showing Corynebacteria (Gram-positive short rods, banded forms that look like diplococci and clubbed forms).
(a) (Courtesy of Dr C.P. Conlon, Oxford.) (b) and (c) (Courtesy of Kevin Hollowood, Oxford.)

Facilities for urgent tracheostomy should always be available in case of respiratory obstruction. Indications include increasingly laboured breathing and agitation. This procedure will be lifesaving in many cases. Most tracheostomies can be closed after just a few days. Steroids may be used in conjunction with tracheostomy to reduce airway swelling, but there have been no controlled trials to support their use. Steroids are of no benefit in preventing myocarditis or neuritis.

Patients with signs or symptoms of cardiac involvement need to be managed in intensive care units. Oxygen should be given. Temporary cardiac pacing is useful in patients with heart block, but is of doubtful value in cases of malignant diphtheria. An isoprenaline infusion may buy valuable time while the patient is transferred to a centre with facilities for pacing. Digoxin has been used in congestive cardiac failure. It has been suggested that carnitine may prevent some cases of myocarditis.

There is no specific treatment for neuritis. The severest cases will need mechanical ventilation and intragastric or intravenous feeding. With skilled nursing care full recovery can be expected. Patients recovering from clinical disease should complete active immunization during convalescence.

Prevention

Diphtheria toxoid is highly effective in conferring protection against clinical disease. Circulating antitoxin levels of less than 0.01 IU/ml are considered nonprotective, while levels of 0.01 IU/ml may confer some protection. Levels of 0.1 IU/ml or more are considered fully protective, and levels above 1.0 IU/ml are associated with long-term protective immunity. The potency of diphtheria vaccine is reduced in children aged 7 years and older so that reactogenicity is minimized.

The recommended schedule for vaccination against diphtheria varies between countries. In the United Kingdom three primary doses of adsorbed diphtheria–tetanus–pertussis–haemophilus influenzae type b vaccine (DTP-Hib) are given at 2, 3, and 4 months; a first booster dose with DTP at age 3 to 5 years, and a second booster dose with DT at school leaving. The primary course does not need to be repeated if boosters are delayed. People living in low-endemic or nonendemic countries should receive booster doses of DT approximately every 10 years. It is now recommended by the World Health Organization that DT rather than T (tetanus toxoid alone) should be used when tetanus prophylaxis is needed following injury.

Where diphtheria is endemic the primary course alone should be sufficient to prevent an epidemic of diphtheria, as natural mechanisms such as frequent skin infections caused by *C. diphtheriae* probably contribute to maintaining immunity. One or two DT or DTP booster doses may need to be added to the routine schedule in areas at increased risk of diphtheria. Adults in developing countries do not require routine immunization.

Aggressive action is needed in the event of a diphtheria outbreak. Groups at risk should be immunized, there should be prompt diagnosis and management of cases, and identification of close contacts should be made so that the spread of infection can be halted. A single dose of DTP should be used for children under 3 years of age, and DT for children aged over 3 years and adults. Additional doses of vaccine will be needed in nonimmunized (Schick test positive) people.

Susceptibility to diphtheria may be assessed using the Schick test: 0.1 ml of toxin is injected into the skin of one forearm (test site) and the same quantity of a heat-inactivated toxin injected into the other forearm (control site). A positive reaction occurs in individuals without toxin-neutralizing antibodies and consists of an area of redness appearing after 24 to 36 h at the test site only and persisting for 4 to 5 days. If no toxin-neutralizing antibodies are present there will be either no reaction at either site (negative test) or a pseudoreaction at either site due to antibodies to substances other than diphtheria toxin in the test materials. This test is no longer commonly performed due to limited availability of the test materials.

Further reading

Celik T, *et al.* (2006). Prognostic significance of electrocardiographic abnormalities in diphtheritic myocarditis after hospital discharge: a long-term follow-up study. *Ann Noninvasive Electrocardiol*, **11**, 28–33. [Thirty-two patients surviving diphtheritic myocarditis were followed after discharge. All seven with left bundle branch block at discharge eventually died.]

Christie AB (ed) (1987). Diphtheria. In: *Infectious diseases: epidemiology and clinical practice*, 4th edition, pp. 898–928. Churchill Livingstone, New York. [Still the best clinical account.]

Crowcroft NS, *et al.* (2006). Screening and toxigenic corynebacteria spread. *Emerg Infect Dis*, **12**, 520–1. [A brief discussion of the factors influencing diphtheria surveillance in the United Kingdom.]

Health Protection Agency (n.d.). *Diphtheria.* http://www.hpa.org.uk/HPA/Topics/InfectiousDiseases/InfectionsAZ/1191942152928 [Includes information on United Kingdom notifications and vaccine uptake.]

Hofler W (1991). Cutaneous diphtheria. *Int J Dermatol*, **30**, 845–7. [A useful review of cutaneous diphtheria.]

Jayashree M, Shruthi N, Singi S (2006). Predictors of outcome in patients with diphtheria receiving intensive care. *Indian Pediatr*, **43**, 155–60. [Myocarditis was found to be the only independent predictor of death in 48 children admitted to a paediatric intensive care unit.]

Mikhailovich VM, *et al.* (1995). Application of PCR for detection of toxigenic *C. diphtheriae* strains isolated during the Russian diphtheria epidemic, 1990 through 1994. *J Clin Microbiol*, **33**, 3061–3. [A comparison of PCR with Elek's plate method.]

Rakhmanova G, *et al.* (1996). Diphtheria outbreak in St. Petersburg: clinical characteristics of 1,860 adult patients. *Scand J Infect Dis*, **28**, 37–40.

Statutory notifications of infectious diseases 1994–2008—England and Wales.

Vitek CR (2006). Diphtheria. *Curr Top Microbiol Immunol*, **304**, 71–94. [A comprehensive review of the disease and its epidemiology.]

World Health Organization (2006). Diphtheria vaccine: WHO position paper. *Weekly Epidemiol Rec*, **81**, 24–32. [A detailed yet concise summary of the disease and its prevention.]

World Health Organization (2009). *Diphtheria.* www.who.int/topics/diphtheria/en [Up-to-date information on global and regional figures for diphtheria.]

Wren MW, Shetty N (2005). Infections with *Corynebacterium diphtheriae*: six years' experience at an inner London teaching hospital. *Br J Biomed Sci*, **62**, 1–4. [Suggests C. diphtheriae infections are underdiagnosed in the United Kingdom.]

7.6.2 Streptococci and enterococci

Dennis L. Stevens

Essentials

The streptococci are a diverse group of Gram-positive pathogenic cocci that cause clinical disease in humans and domestic animals. They are traditionally classified on the basis of serological reactions, particularly Lancefield grouping based on cell-wall carbohydrates, and haemolytic activity on blood agar. Six groups can be defined by genetic analysis: pyogenic streptococci, milleri or anginosus group, mitis group, salivarius group, mutans group, and bovis group.

Group A streptococci (*S. pyogenes*)

Carried, usually in the nose or throat, by 5 to 20% of children and 0.5% of adults. More than any other human pathogen, group A streptococci cause a wide variety of infections ranging from pharyngitis, erysipelas, cellulitis, and necrotizing fasciitis to the postinfectious sequelae—rheumatic fever and poststreptococcal glomerulonephritis. These microbes continue to evolve, as evidenced by over 150 different genetic types and the emergence of novel infections such as streptococcal toxic shock syndrome.

Group A streptococci are easy to culture in the laboratory from appropriate samples; diagnosis can also be made by detection of the group A antigen or confirmed serologically. All strains remain sensitive to penicillin, which is the antibiotic of choice, with erythromycin usually given to those who are penicillin allergic, although epidemics of pharyngitis caused by erythromycin resistant strains have been widely reported. Genetic differences and the presence of multiple virulence factors have frustrated efforts to develop effective vaccines.

Group B streptococci (*S. agalactiae*)

Carried in the throat by 5 to 10% of adults, also in the urethra, vagina, perineum, and anorectum. Cause (1) neonatal infection—including bacteraemia and meningitis; screening for vaginal carriage during the third trimester of pregnancy and intrapartum treatment with intravenous penicillin has reduced the incidence of early onset neonatal disease; (2) postpartum infection—puerperal infection usually manifests as endometritis with fever and uterine tenderness, occurring within 24 to 48 h of delivery or abortion; also (3) skin and soft tissue infections (especially in patients with diabetes), urinary tract infections, and bacteraemias.

Group B streptococci are readily isolated from any clinical specimen in the laboratory, and detection of group B antigen in body fluids by latex particle agglutination enables rapid diagnosis. They are sensitive to penicillin (the antibiotic of choice), erythromycin and cephalosporins. The polysaccharide capsule of group B streptococcus is a major virulence factor, with at least six different serotypes identified: experimental immunization using the polysaccharide provides type specific protection, but no such vaccine has yet been developed for human use.

Acknowledgement: The author of the present chapter and the editors acknowledge the inclusion of much material from the chapter in the previous edition by Professor S K Eykyn.

Other groups of streptococci

Groups C and G—produce infections that are similar to those caused by *S. pyogenes*, but tend to be less virulent. Are important causes of cellulitis, particularly recurrent cellulitis associated with saphenous vein donor site infections in patients with coronary artery by-pass surgery.

Milleri or anginosus group—includes *S. constellatus*, *S. intermedius*, and *S. anginosus*. Found in the normal flora of the upper respiratory tract, gastrointestinal tract and genital tract; commonly isolated from a range of pyogenic infections (e.g. dental or other abscesses), sometimes in pure culture, but often with other organisms, particularly anaerobes.

Mitis, salivarius, and mutans groups of streptococci (oral/viridans streptococci)—these include *S. pneumoniae* (see Chapter 7.6.3) and those oral streptococci that are the commonest causes of infective endocarditis of oral or dental origin. Occasionally cause bacteraemia in neutropenic patients, particularly those who have received prophylaxis with fluoquinolones such as ciprofloxacin.

Bovis group of streptococci—a gastrointestinal commensal; most patients with *S. bovis* bacteraemia will have endocarditis in association with colonic pathology.

Streptococcus suis—an occupational cause of septicaemia, meningitis, septic arthritis, pneumonia, and endophthalmitis among those working with pigs and pork in South-East Asia.

Enterococci

Part of the normal gut flora of humans and animals, these are an increasingly important cause of nosocomial infection and colonization, possibly the result of the large-scale use of antibiotics such as cephalosporins and quinolones to which they are inherently resistant. *Enterococcus faecium* and *E. faecalis* have also become vancomycin resistant, a characteristic dramatically increasing treatment failures, although they remain sensitive (at the time of writing) to linezolid, an oxyzolidinone antimicrobial.

Introduction

The term streptococcus was first used by Billroth in 1874 to describe chain-forming cocci found in infected wounds. In 1879, Pasteur also found them in the blood of women with puerperal sepsis. In 1884, Rosenbach defined these streptococci as *Streptococcus pyogenes*. This organism remains one of the most important human pathogens. The genus *Streptococcus* contains many other species of varying degrees of pathogenicity for humans and animals. *S. faecalis* and *S. faecium* were split from the genus *Streptococcus* in 1984 and became *Enterococcus* spp. and numerous other species have since been included in this genus. The nutritionally exacting streptococci *S. adjacens* and *S. defectivus* have also been assigned to a new genus *Abiotrophia* to which the newly described species *A. elegans* has been added.

Classification

Traditionally, classification of streptococci has relied on serological reactions, particularly the Lancefield grouping based on cell wall carbohydrates, and haemolytic activity on blood agar, which has led to rather unsatisfactory streptococcal taxonomy. Genetic analysis has now enabled the subdivision of the species of *Streptococcus* into six clusters or groups as follows: pyogenic streptococci, milleri or anginosus group, mitis group, salivarius group, mutans group, and bovis group. Since the medically important members of the mitis, salivarius, and mutans groups are all oral streptococci and are of clinical relevance predominantly in endocarditis, they will be considered together.

Pyogenic streptococci

The pyogenic streptococci include the major human pathogen *S. pyogenes* (Lancefield group A), group B streptococci (*S. agalactiae*), and groups C and G streptococci. These organisms are β-haemolytic on blood agar.

S. pyogenes (β-haemolytic group A)

The prevalence and severity of streptococcal pharyngitis has remained constant over the centuries of recorded history, although the incidence of complications such as peritonsillar abscess and mastoiditis have declined with the advent of antibiotics. However, since the beginning of the last century, and long before the introduction of antibiotics, the prevalence and severity of scarlet fever and rheumatic fever following infections with *S. pyogenes* declined until the 1980s. In the mid-1980s, highly virulent streptococci appeared causing very severe infections such as streptococcal toxic shock syndrome and necrotizing fasciitis, often in otherwise healthy people. Such cases occurred not only in the United Kingdom but also in most of the developed world. *S. pyogenes* infection is usually community-acquired but may be acquired in hospital where the most serious infections are postoperative.

Carriage

Although *S. pyogenes* is an invasive organism, it survives on epithelial surfaces (asymptomatic carriage) usually in the nose and throat. Carriage can also be anal, vaginal, and on the scalp. Pharyngeal carriage rates are usually much higher in children (5–20%) than in adults (0.5%) and also vary with season, year, and geographical location. They are higher in crowded living conditions. *S. pyogenes* can persist for months after acute pharyngitis, though in decreased numbers. Survival in the environment is poor and *S. pyogenes* can only survive on skin and inanimate objects for a limited period of time.

Pathogenicity, virulence, and typing

S. pyogenes is an extracellular pathogen and produces virulence factors that enable it to avoid host defences and spread in tissues. An important virulence factor is the M protein and streptococci rich in M protein resist phagocytosis by granulocytes. Immunity to *S. pyogenes* infection is associated with the development of opsonic antibodies to antiphagocytic epitopes of M protein; the immunity is usually type specific and lasts for many years. M protein was first described in the 1920s by Rebecca Lancefield; over 100 M types have now been differentiated. Lancefield also developed the supplementary T typing system which distinguishes 26 serotypes of a trypsin-resistant surface protein (T antigen), most of which can be expressed by several different M types. Certain M types also produce a serum opacity factor (OF+). These typing systems are still widely used in epidemiological studies to distinguish between strains of *S. pyogenes*. However, more modern methods utilize procedures to sequence the M protein gene. Recent studies have shown considerable genetic diversity in *S. pyogenes*, and horizontal transfer and recombination of virulent genes have played a major role.

This finding is likely relevant to the emergence of new unusually virulent clones of the organism.

In addition to M protein, lipoteichoic acid, important in the host–bacterial interaction, is expressed on the surface of the organism and is the adhesin that binds the organism to fibronectin on the surface of the oral epithelial cell membranes and initiates the colonization that precedes infection. *S. pyogenes* has a hyaluronate capsule which, like M protein, is also antiphagocytic, and is an additional virulence factor. The extent of encapsulation varies, and colonies with prominent capsules are very mucoid on blood agar. Strains of *S. pyogenes* that are both rich in M protein and heavily encapsulated are readily transmitted from person to person and have been associated with epidemics of acute rheumatic fever.

S. pyogenes produces many extracellular substances, several of which are important in the pathogenesis of infection. The most familiar are streptolysin O, deoxyribonuclease (DNase) B, and hyaluronidase, as serum antibodies to these provide retrospective confirmation of recent streptococcal infection. Other extracellular products include DNases A, C, and D, streptolysin S, proteinase, streptokinase, and the substances previously known as erythrogenic toxins. These toxins have now been designated streptococcal pyrogenic exotoxins (SPE)-A, -B, -C, and more recently several others. SPE-A and SPE-C are coded by a phage gene and readily transmitted to susceptible strains. These toxins, known as superantigens, have diverse effects on the host. In addition to the rash of scarlet fever, they cause fever and induce lethal shock in animals. They have profound effects on the immune system including increasing susceptibility to endotoxic shock, induction of cytokine production, and cause clonal proliferation of T lymphocytes.

Recently, nicotine adenine dinucleotidase (NADase) has been found in 100% of strains of group A streptococci (GAS) associated with invasive GAS infections such as toxic shock syndrome and necrotizing fasciitis. There is evidence that the gene for NADase is found in all strains of GAS but only produced extracellularly in these invasive strains. In addition, production of NADase by M1 strains, the most common strain associated with invasive types of infections, began around 1985, just before the recognition of severe invasive GAS infections.

S. pyogenes may penetrate the upper respiratory tract mucosa or a break in the skin causing local infection or may spread along tissue planes or lymphatics. The M protein is not toxic in itself but protects the streptococcus from phagocytosis, and antibodies to the M protein are opsonic. In about two-thirds of patients with serious invasive disease, who may present with fever, shock, and renal impairment, the portal of entry is the skin and infection of soft tissue is apparent, but in others the site of infection may be deep in the fascia or muscle.

Infections caused by *S. pyogenes*

S. pyogenes causes a variety of illnesses ranging from very common infections such as pharyngitis, impetigo, and cellulitis to less common more severe infections such as puerperal sepsis, necrotizing fasciitis, bacteraemia, and toxic shock. *S. pyogenes* is also associated with the nonsuppurative sequelae of acute rheumatic fever and acute glomerulonephritis.

Streptococcal pharyngitis

Streptococcal pharyngitis or tonsillitis is one of the commonest bacterial infections in children from 5 to 15 years, but all ages are susceptible. The incubation period, at least in outbreaks, is short (1–3 days) and the onset of the infection is marked by the abrupt onset of sore throat and pain on swallowing with malaise, fever, and headache. The signs are redness and oedema of the pharynx, enlarged red tonsils (Fig. 7.6.2.1) with spots of white exudate, fever, and enlarged tender anterior cervical lymph glands. Nausea, vomiting, and abdominal pain are common in children, and in infants and preschool children there may be few definite signs of pharyngitis but fever, nasal discharge, enlarged cervical lymph glands, and otitis media occur.

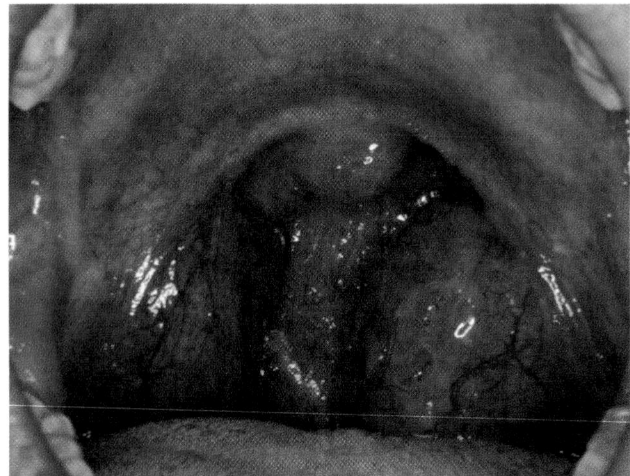

Fig. 7.6.2.1 Streptococcal tonsillitis: suppurative complications. (Copyright D A Warrell.)

Direct extension of streptococcal pharyngitis can give rise to acute sinusitis or otitis media, and other suppurative complications include peritonsillar abscess (quinsy), mastoiditis, retropharyngeal abscess, and suppurative cervical lymphadenitis.

Scarlet fever

Scarlet fever results from infection with a strain of *S. pyogenes* that produces SPE (erythrogenic toxin). It is usually associated with streptococcal pharyngitis but may follow streptococcal infections at other sites including surgical site infections. Scarlet fever rarely follows streptococcal pyoderma. Most cases occur in school-age children and the rash must be distinguished from viral exanthems, Kawasaki's disease, and staphylococcal toxic shock syndrome. The rash, which generally appears on the second day of clinical illness, is usually a diffuse erythema, symmetrical, and blanches on pressure. It is seen most often on the neck, chest, folds of the axilla, and groin. Occlusion of sweat glands gives the skin a 'sandpaper' texture, a useful sign in dark-skinned patients. The face appears flushed with circumoral pallor. There are small red haemorrhagic spots on the palate, and the tongue is initially covered with a white fur through which red papillae appear ('strawberry tongue'); after the rash develops, the white fur peels off leaving a raw red papillate surface ('raspberry tongue'). The rash persists for several days and later (up to 3 weeks) peeling (desquamation) may occur, usually on the tips of the fingers, toes, or ears and less often over the trunk and limbs. A similar rash may develop as a reaction to streptokinase thrombolytic therapy.

Streptococcal perianal infection (cellulitis)

This is a superficial well-demarcated rash spreading out from the anus in young children, usually boys, associated with itching, rectal pain on defaecation, and blood-stained stools. *S. pyogenes* is isolated from perianal cultures and usually also from pretreatment throat swabs.

Streptococcal vulvovaginitis

Vulvovaginitis in prepubertal girls is often caused by *S. pyogenes* and presents with serosanguinous discharge and erythema of the labia and vaginal orifice. As with perianal infections, *S. pyogenes* is usually also found in the throat. In both streptococcal perianal infection and vulvovaginitis, more than one child in the family may be affected and nasopharyngeal carriage is likely in both infected and uninfected children.

Streptococcal skin and soft tissue infections

Pyoderma/impetigo Almost any purulent lesion of the skin can yield *S. pyogenes*, sometimes with *Staphylococcus aureus*. Such lesions include impetigo, infected cuts and lacerations, insect bites, scabies, intertrigo, and ecthyma. *S. pyogenes* often causes secondary infection in varicella, occasionally with resultant bacteraemia. The term pyoderma is used synonymously with impetigo for discrete purulent apparently primary infections of the skin that are prevalent in many parts of the world, especially in children. These lesions are initially papules, then vesicular with surrounding erythema, and finally pustules with crusting exudate; they may be localized to one part of the body or generalized. Outbreaks of impetigo can occur among adults subject to skin trauma, such as rugby football players (scrumpox), and streptococcal infection of cuts on the hands and forearms are an occupational hazard for workers in the meat trade. Epidemics of impetigo can occur in day care centres, prisons, and schools. Ecthyma is an ulcerated form of impetigo in which ulceration extends into the dermis. In recent times, approximately 50% of cases of impetigo are caused by *Staphylococcus aureus*.

Invasive streptococcal infections of skin and soft tissues

Erysipelas This is an acute inflammation of the skin with lymphatic involvement. The streptococci are localized in the dermis and hypodermis. It usually affects the face, particularly in elderly people, but may occur elsewhere. It may be bilateral (Fig. 7.6.2.2) and is sometimes recurrent. There is generally a history of sore throat, but the mode of spread to the skin is unknown. It is usually accompanied by fever, rigors, and toxicity. The cutaneous lesion begins as a localized area of brilliant erythema and swelling and then spreads with rapidly advancing raised red margins that are well demarcated from adjacent normal tissue. Facial erysipelas begins over the bridge of the nose and spreads over the cheeks. Vesicles and bullae appear, which become crusted when they rupture. There is marked oedema and the eyes are often closed. When the infection resolves it is often followed by desquamation. Intense local allergic reactions to topical agents, such as cosmetics, may cause confusion.

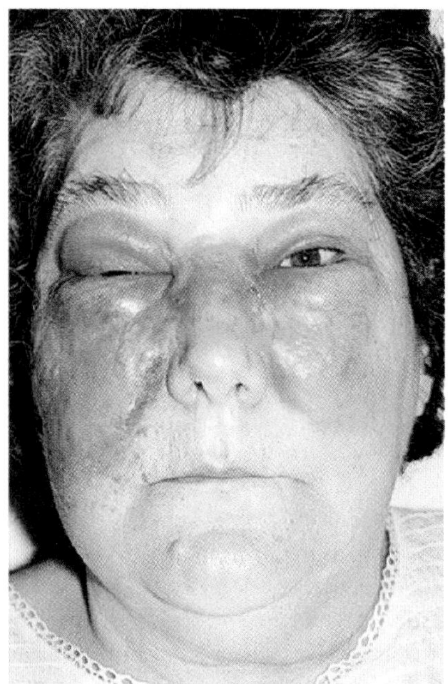

Fig. 7.6.2.2 Bilateral facial erysipelas.
(Copyright S J Eykyn.)

Cellulitis Cellulitis (Fig. 7.6.2.3) is commonly caused by streptococci and *Staphylococcus aureus*. This is an acute spreading inflammation of the skin and subcutaneous tissues with local pain swelling and erythema. Fever, rigors, and malaise may precede by a few hours the appearance of the skin lesion and associated lymphangitis and tender lymphadenopathy. Streptococcal cellulitis differs from erysipelas in that the lesion is not raised and the demarcation between affected and unaffected skin is indistinct. It may result from infection of burns, mild trauma, or surgical wounds. When this involves the leg, fungal infection of the feet is often present and predisposes to streptococcal invasion. After the first episode, there is a tendency for recurrence in the same area. Recurrences are more common in patients with chronic venous insufficiency, lymphatic obstruction, and at the saphenous vein donor site in patients following coronary bypass surgery. These latter infections are most commonly caused by group C or G streptococci. Intravenous drug users are also at risk of streptococcal cellulitis associated with skin and tissue infection and septic thrombophlebitis.

(Type II) necrotizing fasciitis (streptococcal gangrene) This infection, described by Meleney in 1924, involves the deep subcutaneous tissues and fascia (and occasionally muscle as well) with extensive necrosis and gangrene of the skin and underlying structures. It is generally community-acquired, usually involving the arm or leg, but may also occur after surgery, which can sometimes be quite minor. Some people with this infection are diabetic, but the majority are previously healthy. Risk factors providing a portal of entry include surgery, trauma, childbirth, intravenous drug abuse, and chickenpox. Blunt trauma and muscle strain and the use of nonsteroidal anti-inflammatory agents are also risk factors. The infection begins at the site of trivial or even inapparent trauma with

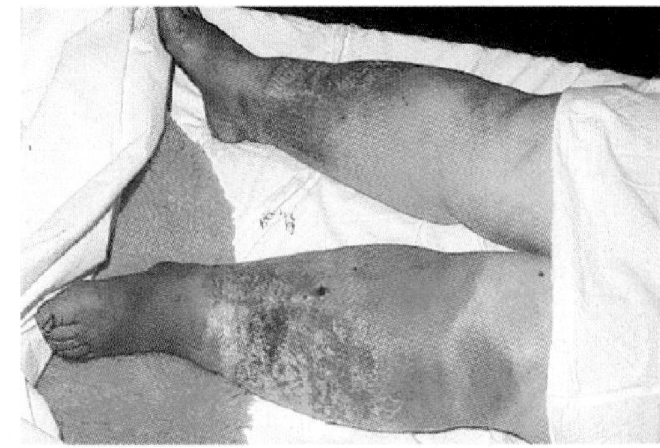

Fig. 7.6.2.3 Cellulitis.
(Copyright S J Eykyn.)

redness, swelling, fever, and rapidly escalating focal pain followed by purple discoloration and the development of bullae, which are often haemorrhagic. In patients who develop infection deeply in traumatized tissue such as muscle, fever and severe pain may be the only initial signs and symptoms of infection. Bacteraemia is often present and within days skin necrosis occurs followed by extensive sloughing. The patient is profoundly ill and the disease has a high case fatality rate of 30 to 70%. Features of streptococcal toxic shock syndrome are associated in many cases. The United Kingdom media memorably dubbed *S. pyogenes* the 'flesh-eater' in reports of a cluster of cases of necrotizing fasciitis in 1994. Treatment involves early intravenous antibiotics. The organisms are sensitive to penicillin but, paradoxically, the drug may not be effective in high concentrations (the 'Eagle effect'). Clindamycin has advantages over penicillin, based on animal studies and one retrospective study in humans. The efficacy of clindamycin is likely due to its ability rapidly to inhibit toxin production by Gram-positive pathogens. Urgent surgical debridement of necrotic tissue and intensive care to support failing organs and systems (e.g. cardiovascular and renal) are extremely important. Benefits of immunoglobulin are suggestive but inconclusive.

Streptococcal toxic shock syndrome

This syndrome was described in 1989 in patients with severe *S. pyogenes* infection and clinical features remarkably similar to those of the staphylococcal toxic shock syndrome described a decade earlier. Streptococcal toxic shock syndrome is defined as any acute *S. pyogenes* infection associated with the sudden onset of shock and multiorgan failure. Streptococcal toxic shock syndrome may be associated with necrotizing fasciitis, myositis, pneumonia, peritonitis, or postpartum sepsis. It can occur at all ages and many of those affected are young and previously healthy. Most cases have been community-acquired, though it can be acquired in hospital. M1 has been the predominant serotype in many countries, though others, especially 3, 4, 6, 11, 12, and 28, have also been implicated. Most strains produce SPE-A. Interestingly there is an amino acid homology of 50% and immunological cross-reactivity between SPE-A and staphylococcal enterotoxins B and C, which together with staphylococcal toxic shock syndrome toxin-1 are relevant in nonmenstrual staphylococcal toxic shock syndrome. Diffuse scarlatina type rash is present in only 5 to 10% of cases (Fig. 7.6.2.4).

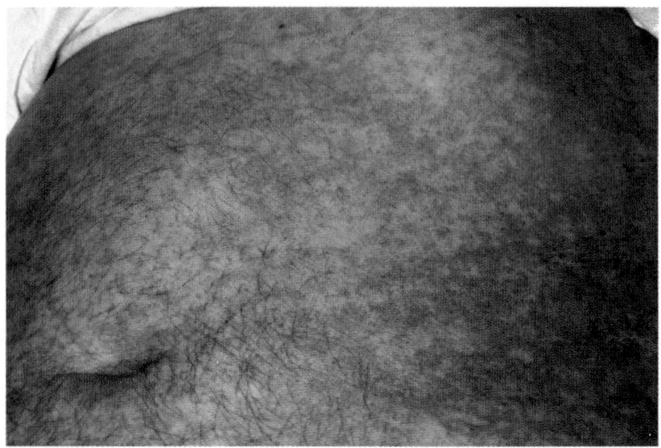

Fig. 7.6.2.4 Scarlatina-like rash of streptococcal toxic shock syndrome.
(Copyright D A Warrell.)

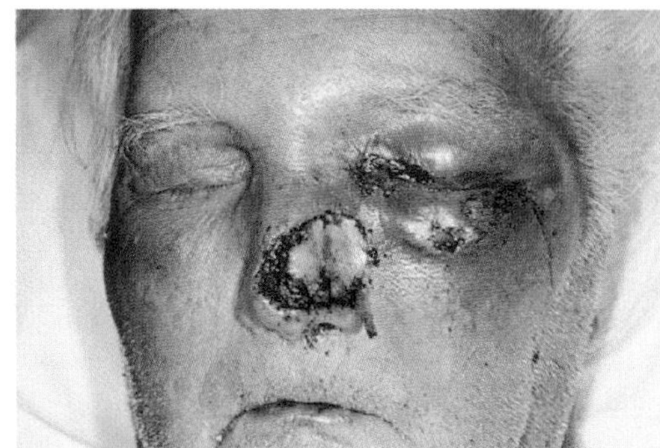

Fig. 7.6.2.5 *S. pyogenes* bacteraemia 3 days after a skin graft.
(Copyright S J Eykyn.)

Streptococcal bacteraemia

In parallel with the increase in serious *S. pyogenes* infections, there has been an increase in bacteraemic infections, both community- and hospital-acquired (usually postoperative) (Fig. 7.6.2.5). While many patients have an underlying disease, generally malignancy, immunosuppression, or diabetes, others are previously healthy adults between 20 and 50 years old. The portal of entry is usually the skin. The mortality is higher in patients with underlying disease, those with necrotizing fasciitis, myositis, pneumonia, or postpartum sepsis, and the very young or old.

Puerperal and neonatal infection

Historically *S. pyogenes* has always been an important cause of puerperal sepsis ('childbed fever'). However, in the postantibiotic era, it was rarely encountered in obstetric practice until the 1980s when sporadic cases occurred, some with streptococcal toxic shock syndrome, and some women have died. These infections follow abortion or delivery when streptococci (usually colonizing the patient herself) invade the endometrium, lymphatics, and bloodstream. They can be devastatingly severe and present with nonspecific signs such as restlessness and gastrointestinal upset that may not immediately suggest sepsis. Fever may be absent resulting in further diagnostic confusion. The streptococcal infection involves the uterus and adnexa and sometimes distant sites such as joints as well. It can also affect the baby, causing serious neonatal infection including meningitis. Instrumentation in the presence of asymptomatic vaginal or anorectal carriage of *S. pyogenes* can result in severe infection. Small epidemics of puerperal sepsis have been reported where a health care provider has been a carrier that caused infection.

Other infections

S. pyogenes can cause pneumonia (usually associated with viral infection or pulmonary disease), osteomyelitis, septic arthritis, meningitis, pericarditis (Fig. 7.6.2.6), endophthalmitis, and endocarditis.

Laboratory diagnosis of *S. pyogenes* infection

S. pyogenes is easy to culture in the laboratory and usually grows on blood agar in 24 h in atmospheres containing 10% CO_2. Throat swabs must be taken before antibiotics are given or the chance of recovery is greatly reduced. Kits for the detection of the group A antigen directly from throat swabs are available and give few false-positive reactions; they are seldom used in the United Kingdom but are commonly used in the United States of America. Ideally, two swabs are obtained. One is used for the rapid test and, if negative, the other is cultured appropriately. Even trivial

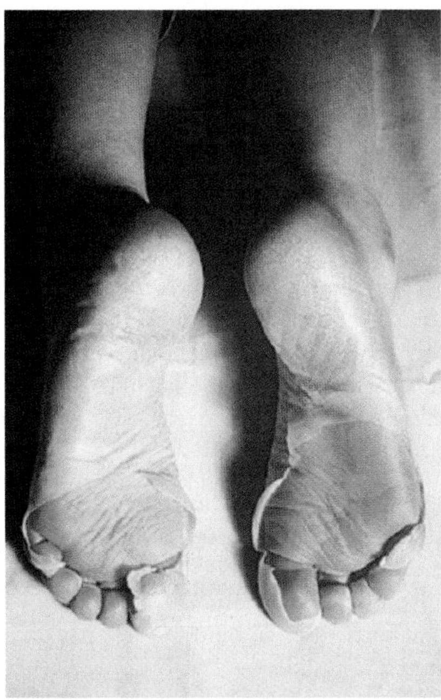

Fig. 7.6.2.6 Peeling of the skin of the soles of the feet in a patient with *S. pyogenes* pericarditis.
(Copyright S J Eykyn.)

skin lesions such as impetigo or surgical site infection are worth swabbing (if necessary with a moistened swab). Swabs from the surface of cellulitis and erysipelas rarely yield streptococci, although they may be recovered from specimens obtained by aspiration approximately 20% of the time. In practice this is seldom carried out. Blood cultures should be done in any patient who is ill whether febrile or not. Serological confirmation of infection with *S. pyogenes* when the organism has not been isolated can be obtained by the detection of raised antibodies to its extracellular products. Most laboratories tend to use two or more tests. Interpretation requires knowledge of the level of titres in the community for those without a history of recent streptococcal infection. In the United Kingdom the upper limit of titres in teenagers and young adults without such a history is antistreptolysin O (ASO) 200, antideoxyribonuclease B (ADB) 240, and antihyaluronidase (AHT) 128.

Management and antibiotic treatment of *S. pyogenes* infection

Remarkably, *S. pyogenes* remains exquisitely sensitive to penicillin and this is the antibiotic of choice for treatment, parenterally for severe infections and orally otherwise. Conventionally, 10 days treatment is recommended for pharyngeal infections to eradicate the organism and prevent acute rheumatic fever. In practice, compliance with this regimen is poor as once the symptoms abate there is a natural reluctance to continue the antibiotic. Treatment of patients allergic to penicillin is usually with erythromycin or the newer macrolides (azithromycin and clarithromycin), but some 3 to 5% of strains are erythromycin resistant in most of the western world. Epidemics caused by erythromycin-resistant strains have been described in Japan, Finland, Sweden, and the United States of America. *S. pyogenes* is also sensitive to cephalosporins. Topical agents such as mupirocin and fusidic acid are useful in addition to systemic antibiotic treatment in impetigo and other skin lesions. Patients with streptococcal toxic shock syndrome require intensive care and many require inotropic support, ventilation, and haemodialysis. Urgent surgical intervention is needed for necrotizing fasciitis and myositis. Clindamycin (in addition to penicillin) has been recommended for patients with established invasive streptococcal infections since this drug stops the metabolic activity of the streptococci and thus halts further production of toxin. This is especially relevant in type II necrotizing fasciitis/myositis and streptococcal toxic shock syndrome. Intravenous immunoglobulin has also been used in an attempt to neutralize the streptococcal toxins, but reports of its effects are inconclusive. Prevention of recurrent cellulitis of the lower legs involves meticulous foot hygiene with treatment of 'athlete's foot' fungi and reduction in skin carriage using topical mupirocin. Oedematous limbs can benefit from elastic stockings. Antibiotic prophylaxis may be required in cases of frequent recurrence refractory to these measures. Lastly it should be remembered that *S. pyogenes* is readily transmitted from person to person and thus appropriate infection control precautions should be taken until swabs show that the organism has been eradicated.

β-Haemolytic group B streptococci (*S. agalactiae*)

The group B streptococcus has been known for over a century as a cause of bovine mastitis, and in the 1930s it was recognized as a vaginal commensal, an occasional cause of puerperal fever, and an uncommon cause of invasive disease in adults. Not until the 1960s was it realized that the group B streptococcus was an important neonatal pathogen, and some 20 years later it had replaced *Escherichia coli* as the predominant neonatal pathogen. Group B streptococcus can also cause septic arthritis, osteomyelitis, and cellulitis in adult patients with diabetes or peripheral vascular disease.

Carriage

Group B streptococci can be recovered from various sites in healthy adults but vaginal carriage has been most extensively investigated. Swabs from the lower vagina are more often positive than cervical swabs and carriage rates of 3% to over 40% have been reported. Higher rates have been obtained with selective media and enrichment techniques. Carriage also increases with sexual activity and is highest in women attending genitourinary clinics. The urethra, vagina, perineum, and anorectal region have all been suggested as the prime site of carriage. Approximately 5 to 10% of healthy adults carry group B streptococci in the throat, independent of urogenital and anorectal carriage.

Pathogenicity, virulence, and typing

The chief determinant of virulence appears to be the capsular polysaccharide, and most human strains carry one of six sialic acid-containing polysaccharides that surround the cell wall. In addition, a protein antigen (c, X, or R) may be carried. Certain combinations are common; serotypes III or III/R form one-quarter of all isolates from superficial sites on women, but three-quarters of all group B streptococci causing meningitis in infants. They are also the commonest serotypes found in adult (nonpregnant) infections. The type polysaccharide, like the M protein of *S. pyogenes*, inhibits phagocytosis. Colonization of the mucous membranes of the neonate results from vertical transmission of the organism from the mother either *in utero* by the ascending route or at delivery. The rate of vertical transmission in neonates born to mothers colonized with group B streptococci is about 50%, but the incidence of symptomatic infection in neonates born to colonized mothers is only about 1 to 2%. It is much higher in preterm infants. Nosocomial colonization of neonates can also occur. In most cases of adult infections (other than in pregnant women) the source of the infection is unknown.

Infections caused by group B streptococci

These are commonly neonatal or puerperal infections, but group B streptococci also cause infection in nonpregnant adults.

Neonatal infection

The frequency of neonatal infection (bacteraemia, meningitis, or both) has been variously quoted as between 0.3 and 5.4 cases/1000 live births, but these figures have wide confidence limits. Two fairly distinct clinical patterns of disease predominate, but the spectrum is wide and includes impetigo neonatorum, septic arthritis, osteomyelitis, pneumonitis, peritonitis, pyelonephritis, facial cellulitis, conjunctivitis, and endophthalmitis.

Early-onset disease Symptoms develop within the first 5 days of life with a mean of 20 h, although they can present at birth suggesting an intrauterine onset of infection. Early-onset disease is usually a bacteraemia with no identifiable focus of infection, but can also be pneumonia or, infrequently, meningitis. The presenting signs include lethargy, poor feeding, jaundice, grunting respirations, pallor, and hypotension and they are common to all types of disease. Respiratory symptoms are nearly always present. The only reliable way of detecting meningitis is by lumbar puncture. Mortality rates are high in low birth weight babies. In addition to positive blood cultures, the infecting strain can be found in the mother's vagina and cultured from 'screening' sites on the baby; these include ear, throat, and nasogastric aspirate.

Late-onset disease This usually presents between 7 days and 3 months after birth, often in previously healthy babies born after a normal labour who are admitted unwell from home. The pathogenesis is less clear than in cases of early-onset disease and only about one-half of these cases are associated with mucosal colonization during delivery. Most babies have meningitis and concomitant bacteraemia and present with nonspecific symptoms such as lethargy, poor feeding, irritability, and fever. Neurological sequelae are common among survivors.

Puerperal infection

Puerperal infection with group B streptococci usually occurs within 24 to 48 h of delivery or abortion. The source of the organism is always the vagina and infection is more likely when there has been premature rupture of the membranes and chorioamnionitis. Most infections are endometritis with fever and uterine tenderness sometimes associated with retained products of conception, but group B streptococci can also cause wound infection after caesarean section. Bacteraemia is common. Other bacteria, both aerobes and anaerobes, are sometimes isolated from the genital tract and wounds in addition to the group B streptococcus. Very rarely the streptococcus may spread to other sites in puerperal women.

Infection in nonpregnant adults

The prominence given to group B streptococci as neonatal and puerperal pathogens has tended to overshadow their importance in men and nonpregnant women in whom they cause significant morbidity and mortality. Most infections are community-acquired, occur in middle-aged and elderly people, and are as common in men as women. Many, though by no means all, patients with group B streptococcal infection have underlying diseases, particularly diabetes, peripheral vascular disease, and myeloma. Skin and soft tissue infections are especially common in patients with diabetes. Occasional urinary tract infections occur, in men as well as women. Bacteraemic infections serve to emphasize the virulence of group B streptococci, and they have increased in incidence, or perhaps have been increasingly recognized, since the early 1990s. Community-acquired group B streptococcal bacteraemia is similar in many respects to that caused by *Staphylococcus aureus* since common clinical manifestations include endocarditis, vertebral osteomyelitis, septic arthritis, endophthalmitis, and meningitis. As with staphylococcal infections, some bacteraemic patients have more than one metastatic focus of infection, which can lead to diagnostic confusion.

Laboratory diagnosis of group B streptococcal infection

Group B streptococci are readily isolated from any clinical specimen in the laboratory and easily identified by Lancefield grouping. The group B antigen is not shared by any other streptococcus. Importantly the antigen can be reliably detected in fluids such as blood, urine, or cerebrospinal fluid by latex particle agglutination enabling a rapid diagnosis.

Treatment of group B streptococcal infection

Group B streptococci are sensitive to penicillin and this is the antibiotic of choice for treatment. They are rather less sensitive to penicillin than *S. pyogenes* with minimum inhibitory concentrations some fourfold to tenfold higher. For this reason penicillin is sometimes combined with gentamicin for meningitis and other serious infections, though this is not of proven benefit. Certainly, the maximum recommended dose of parenteral penicillin should be given whether combined with gentamicin or not. Penicillin allergy is not likely to be an issue in neonates; adults with meningitis can be treated with chloramphenicol. Most group B streptococci are sensitive to erythromycin and they are sensitive to cephalosporins.

Prevention of neonatal infection with group B streptococci

During the 1990s, the incidence of disease caused by mother-to-child transmission of group B streptococci in the United States of America fell by two-thirds as a result of the increased use of intrapartum penicillin in women at high risk of transmitting the infection, an intervention largely brought about by parental pressure. The American authorities recommend either prenatal screening or a risk-based strategy to identify women to receive intrapartum antibiotics. Similar recommendations are to be introduced in the United Kingdom. Any protocol for prophylactic penicillin based on the isolation of group B streptococci in late pregnancy would present difficulties in a busy obstetric unit, and culture methods may also fail to detect the organism unless vaginal and rectal swabs are cultured in selective broth media. Maternal colonization with group B streptococci can be identified rapidly and reliably by polymerase chain reaction assay, but this is unlikely to be adopted as a routine round-the-clock service. An effective vaccine is an alternative approach, but is so far unavailable. In any event pregnant women should have vaginal cultures during the third trimester of pregnancy.

β-Haemolytic groups C and G streptococci

These streptococci are sometimes referred to as 'large colony-forming group C and G streptococci' to distinguish them from the small colony-forming strains of streptococci with the same Lancefield antigens that belong to the anginosus or milleri group (see below). Groups C and G streptococci are closely related genetically. They are most conveniently regarded as 'pyogenes-like' as the infections they cause are similar to those caused by *S. pyogenes* though these streptococci tend to be less virulent than *S. pyogenes*. Infections with these streptococci are less common than *S. pyogenes* infections. Although poststreptococcal glomerulonephritis has been associated with pharyngitis caused by both groups C and G streptococci, acute rheumatic fever has not. Group C streptococci are less frequently encountered in human infections than group G and most group C infections are caused by *S. equisimilis*; those caused by *S. zooepidemicus* have an animal source. Group G streptococci are frequently isolated from leg ulcers and pressure sores, usually with other bacteria. In such patients cellulitis and systemic toxicity are rare and the organisms may merely be colonizing the lesions. They, like *S. pyogenes*, can cause cellulitis in lymphoedematous limbs. Recurrent cellulitis caused by group C and G streptococci has been described at the site of saphenous vein excision in patients following coronary artery bypass surgery.

Streptococci of the anginosus or milleri group

This group of streptococci has been a source of considerable taxonomic confusion, partly as a result of a lack of international consensus on nomenclature but also because of a lack of reliable phenotypic differences between taxa within the group. Most clinicians are familiar with the organism they know as '*Streptococcus milleri*'. There are three species of milleri streptococci, *S. anginosus*, *S. constellatus*, and *S. intermedius*, but despite increasing awareness of the clinical significance of the milleri group little is known about the association between individual species and specific sites of isolation and diseases. These streptococci are found in large numbers in the normal flora of the upper respiratory tract, gastrointestinal tract, and genital tract, and are commonly isolated from a range of pyogenic infections, sometimes in pure culture but often with other organisms, particularly anaerobes. These infections include dental abscesses, intra-abdominal abscesses (especially of the liver), subphrenic abscesses, lung abscesses and empyema, and brain abscesses. Such is the propensity of these organisms to cause deep-seated abscesses that isolation of a milleri streptococcus from a blood culture should prompt investigations to detect such a focus. Milleri streptococci are also commonly isolated from inflamed appendices and postappendicectomy wound infection. Unlike other viridans and nonhaemolytic streptococci, milleri streptococci seldom cause endocarditis. They form minute colonies on blood agar and are preferentially anaerobic on primary isolation. They may be α-, β-, or nonhaemolytic. Some have the Lancefield antigens A, C, G, or F. All group F streptococci are milleri group whereas not all milleri streptococci are group F. Another useful clue to their identity in the laboratory is the distinct caramel smell of many strains on blood agar, the result of the diacetyl metabolite. Most strains are very sensitive to penicillin; however, routine susceptibility assays are not readily available.

Streptococci of the mitis, salivarius, and mutans groups (oral/viridans streptococci)

This group of usually α-haemolytic (viridans) streptococci includes *S. pneumoniae* and those oral streptococci (*S. mitis*, *S. oralis*, *S. sanguis*, *S. gordonii*, and, rarely, *S. salivarius*) that are the commonest cause of infective endocarditis of oral or dental origin. These streptococci occasionally cause bacteraemia in neutropenic patients, who sometimes have detectable mouth lesions, and neonatal infection, as they are found as part of the normal vaginal flora. These infections should be suspected in neutropenic patients who have received prophylaxis with fluoroquinolones such as ciprofloxacin.

Streptococci of the bovis group

Although this group comprises at least three species, *S. bovis* is the main species of medical importance. *S. bovis* is similar to the enterococci in that it bears the Lancefield group D antigen and is a gastrointestinal commensal, but, unlike the enterococci, it is sensitive to penicillin. It can be misidentified in the laboratory either as an oral streptococcus or as an enterococcus. Most patients with *S. bovis* bacteraemia will have endocarditis and it is seldom isolated from other sites. It is important to recognize *S. bovis* in a blood culture as the organism is associated with colonic pathology, and patients should be specifically investigated for this.

Nutritionally variant organisms previously classified as streptococci, now *Abiotrophia* spp.

These organisms, which occasionally cause endocarditis, require pyridoxal or thiol group supplementation for growth in the laboratory and tend to form satellite colonies surrounding colonies of *Staphylococcus aureus*. Although most blood culture media will support their growth, successful subculture requires supplementation or cross-streaking of the plates with *Staphylococcus aureus* to provide the necessary growth factors. The *Abiotrophia* include three species, *S. adjacens*, *S. defectivus*, and the recently described *A. elegans*. They are less susceptible to penicillin than other streptococci.

S. suis

This streptococcus, which can be misidentified in the laboratory as *S. bovis* or an enterococcus as it reacts with group D antiserum, is an important pathogen of young pigs causing meningitis, septicaemia, arthritis, pneumonia, and endocarditis and is also carried in the pharynx of healthy pigs. *S. suis* type II (also referred to as group R streptococci) is not only the most invasive type in pigs, it can cause serious infection—mainly septicaemia and meningitis, but also septic arthritis, pneumonia, and endophthalmitis—in humans, in whom it is an occupational disease of pig farmers, abattoir workers, and factory workers handling pig meat (Fig. 7.6.2.7) (see Chapter 24.11.1). The streptococcus probably enters the bloodstream via skin abrasions that are common in the above

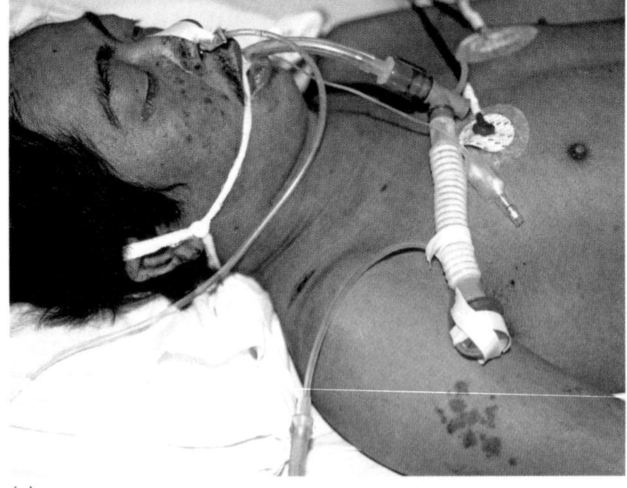

(a)

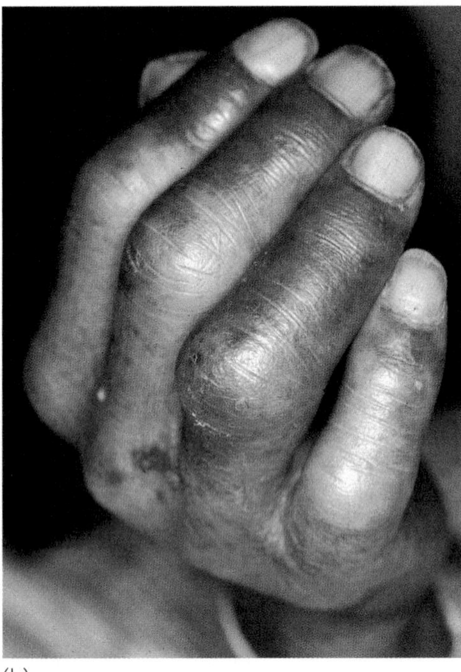

(b)

Fig. 7.6.2.7 (a) *S. suis* septicaemia with meningitis in a Vietnamese pig farmer. (b) *S. suis* pyogenic arthritis in a Thai abattoir worker.
(a) (Copyright D A Warrell.) (b) (Courtesy of the late Professor Prida Phuapradit.)

occupations. *S. suis* type II meningitis results in deafness in about one-half of those affected.

Enterococci

Enterococci are Lancefield group D, Gram-positive cocci that can grow and survive in extreme cultural conditions, and are also more resistant to antibiotics than streptococci. They form part of the normal gut flora of humans and animals. Overall, the commonest clinical isolates of enterococci are *Enterococcus faecalis*, but the more antibiotic-resistant species *E. faecium* is increasingly encountered in hospitals. Nosocomial isolates of enterococci have dramatically increased in the 1990s. Other species, including *E. casseliflavus*, *E. durans*, and *E. avium*, are occasionally isolated. In most cases it is unnecessary to determine the species of enterococci in a clinical laboratory but sometimes differentiation between *E. faecalis* and *E. faecium* is helpful, e.g. in epidemiological studies and in endocarditis because of their different antibiotic susceptibilities.

Infections caused by enterococci

Enterococci are an increasingly important cause of nosocomial infection and colonization, possibly as a result of the large-scale use of antibiotics such as cephalosporins and quinolones to which they are inherently resistant. They occasionally cause community-acquired urinary tract infections but the most important community-acquired infection is endocarditis, which is increasing in incidence. This infection is almost always caused by *E. faecalis*. Any patient admitted from the community with *E. faecalis* in blood cultures should be assumed to have endocarditis until proved otherwise. Enterococci are predominantly hospital pathogens and cause urinary infection, particularly after instrumentation, intra-abdominal infections, wound infections (usually with other organisms), infections associated with intravascular devices and dialysis, and occasionally endocarditis.

Antibiotic sensitivity and treatment

Enterococci are not only intrinsically resistant to many antibiotics, they show a remarkable ability to acquire new mechanisms of resistance. This allows them to survive in environments in which large quantities of antibiotics are used and also has important therapeutic consequences, particularly for the treatment of endocarditis and other serious infections. Fortunately many patients from whom enterococci are isolated do not require antibiotic treatment. Sensitive enterococci cannot be killed by ampicillin/amoxicillin alone, although combination with an aminoglycoside is bactericidal (synergy); but many strains now exhibit high-level gentamicin resistance and for them the combination is not bactericidal. *E. faecium* is almost always resistant to ampicillin/amoxicillin and *E. faecalis* is occasionally. The first published report of vancomycin-resistant enterococci (VRE) was in 1988 from a London hospital outbreak, though such strains had been recognized a year before in Paris. Most strains of VRE in the London outbreak were *E. faecium* and overall most VRE are *E. faecium*. There are four recognized phenotypes of vancomycin resistance; the first isolates of VRE were highly resistant to vancomycin and teicoplanin and exhibit what is known as the VanA resistance phenotype. Since then, levels of resistance to teicoplanin in this phenotype have been more varied. Most VanA enterococci are *E. faecium*, but this phenotype also occurs in *E. faecalis* and occasionally in other species. The VanB phenotype is associated with low-level vancomycin resistance and sensitivity to teicoplanin and is found in both *E. faecalis* and *E. faecium*. Both VanA and VanB are acquired traits. The VanC phenotype is an intrinsic property of *E. casseliflavus* and *E. gallinarum* and these species have low-level resistance to vancomycin but are sensitive to teicoplanin. A fourth phenotype, VanD, has been described in a single strain of *E. faecium*. Vancomycin-resistant *E. faecium*, though not vancomycin-resistant *E. faecalis*, is sensitive to quinupristin/dalfopristin and all VRE are sensitive to the oxazolidinone linezolid.

The antibiotic susceptibilities of the enterococci outlined above serve to emphasize that these bacteria are the most antibiotic-resistant Gram-positive bacteria now encountered in hospital practice. Fortunately many, perhaps most, of the patients from whom they are isolated do not require antibiotic treatment at all, but for those who do, the effective treatment of serious infection caused by enterococci and particularly antibiotic-resistant strains requires microbiological expertise.

Further reading

Bisno AL, Stevens DL (2000). *Streptococcus pyogenes* (including streptococcal toxic shock syndrome and necrotizing fasciitis). In: Mandell GL, Bennett JE, Dolin R (eds) *Principles and practice of infectious diseases*, pp. 2101–17. Churchill Livingstone, New York.

Bisno AL, Brito MO, Collins CM (2003). Molecular basis of group A streptococcal virulence. *Lancet*, **3**, 191–200.

Colman G, *et al.* (1993). The serotypes of *Streptococcus pyogenes* present in Britain during 1980 to 1990 and their association with disease. *J Med Microbiol*, **39**, 165–78.

Edwards MS, Baker CJ (2000). *Streptococcus agalactiae* (group B streptococcus). In: Mandell GL, Bennett JE, Dolin R (eds) *Principles and practice of infectious diseases*, pp. 2156–67. Churchill Livingstone, New York.

Jacobs JA (1997). The 'streptococcus milleri' group: *Streptococcus anginosus*, *Streptococcus constellatus* and *Streptococcus intermedius*. *Rev Med Microbiol*, **8**, 73–80.

Katz AR, Morens D (1992). Severe streptococcal infections in historical perspective. *Clin Infect Dis*, **14**, 298–307.

Murray BE (1990). The life and times of the *Enterococcus*. *Clin Microbiol Rev*, **3**, 46–65.

Stevens DL (1992). Invasive group A streptococcus infections. *Clin Infect Dis*, **14**, 2–13.

Stevens DL (1995). Streptococcal toxic shock syndrome: spectrum of disease, pathogenesis and new concepts of treatment. *Emerg Infect Dis*, **1**, 69–78.

Stevens DL (2004). Streptococcal infections. In: Goldman L, Ausiello D (eds) *Cecil textbook of medicine*, 22nd edition, pp. 1782–7. Saunders, Philadelphia.

Stevens DL, *et al.* (2000). Molecular epidemiology of *nga* and NAD glucohydrolase/ADP-ribosyltransferase activity among *Streptococcus pyogenes* causing streptococcal toxic shock syndrome. *J Infect Dis*, **182**, 1117–28.

Stevens DL, *et al.* (2005). Practice guidelines for the diagnosis and management of skin and soft-tissue infections. *Clin Infect Dis*, **41**, 1373–1406.

Woodford N (1998). Glycopeptide-resistant enterococci: a decade of experience. *J Med Microbiol*, **47**, 849–62.

7.6.3 Pneumococcal infections

Anthony Scott

Essentials

Streptococcus pneumoniae is an encapsulated Gram-positive bacterium that lives almost exclusively in the human nasopharynx. Each pneumococcus expresses one of 91 immunologically distinguishable capsular polysaccharides that are the principal target of systemic human immunity and define its serotype.

Epidemiology

Pneumococci are transmitted through contact with infected nasal secretions or by airborne dissemination, and most preschool children carry them in their nasopharynx. The risk of acquisition is increased by contact with other children, crowded environments, and cold weather. The incidence of pneumococcal disease is highest in young children and elderly people, and also increased in males, certain indigenous populations, smokers, alcoholics, and patients with chronic medical illnesses or immune susceptibility, including HIV infection, sickle cell disease, and splenectomy.

Clinical features

Pneumonia—pneumococci are the commonest cause of severe community-acquired pneumonia at all ages in the developed and developing world. Typical presentation of pneumococcal lobar pneumonia is with abrupt onset of fever, followed by cough, difficulty breathing, pleuritic chest pain, haemoptysis, and purulent sputum. Physical signs include high pyrexia, raised respiratory rate, cyanosis, and chest features of lobar consolidation, namely reduced chest movement, dullness on percussion, fine crepitations, and bronchial breathing over the affected area. The chest radiograph shows a lobar opacity, often with a pleural effusion.

Other diseases—pneumococci cause significant morbidity in adults and children through meningitis and septicaemia, and they can also cause bronchopneumonia and multiple disease syndromes simultaneously (e.g. meningitis and pneumonia). In children, the most common pneumococcal disease is otitis media. Other less common presentations include sinusitis, pleural empyema, pericarditis, endocarditis, septic arthritis, osteomyelitis, peritonitis, and conjunctivitis.

Diagnosis

S. pneumoniae is a fastidious organism that grows successfully on blood agar, producing α-haemolysis. Blood culture is the principal aetiological tool to diagnose pneumococcal pneumonia, but cultures are positive in only 15 to 30% of cases. The capsular serotype is identified by a positive Quellung reaction with specific rabbit antisera. In addition: (1) pneumococci can be observed on microscopy as Gram-positive diplococci in sputum or, in cases of meningitis, in cerebrospinal fluid, and can be cultured from both specimens; (2) a urinary antigen test for the common pneumococcal constituent C-polysaccharide is sensitive and specific for pneumococcal pneumonia in adults, but not in children; (3) PCR is useful in cerebrospinal fluid, especially when the patient is partially treated and cultures are sterile.

Treatment and prognosis

Most pneumococci are sensitive to β-lactam antibiotics, but some are resistant. (1) Pneumonia—when caused by sensitive or intermediately resistant pneumococci, this should be treated with high-dose oral amoxicillin or intravenous cefotaxime, the latter being effective against pneumococci with cephalosporin MICs up to 1 to 2 μg/ml. Macrolides and newer fluoroquinolones may be used to treat infections that are fully resistant to β-lactam antibiotics. (2) Meningitis—when caused by susceptible pneumococci, ceftriaxone is effective; vancomycin should be added as empirical meningitis therapy in areas with resistant pneumococci; dexamethasone is an effective adjunctive treatment for pneumococcal meningitis where HIV prevalence is low.

The case fatality of pneumococcal pneumonia is 5%, but in bacteraemic pneumonia and pneumococcal meningitis it is 30%.

Prevention

A single dose of 23-valent capsular polysaccharide vaccine prevents invasive pneumococcal disease in elderly or high-risk populations. In infants and young children, 7-valent pneumococcal conjugate vaccine is highly effective in preventing invasive pneumococcal disease as well as pneumococcal pneumonia, meningitis and otitis media. It is given routinely as two or three doses in infancy, with a booster dose at 12 to 15 months of age. Immunization of children reduces pneumococcal transmission and prevents pneumococcal disease in older family members.

Introduction

Streptococcus pneumoniae (the pneumococcus) is an ubiquitous yet potentially fatal human pathogen. Its only viable habitat is the human nasopharynx. Throughout the world, most children and a significant minority of adults carry it at any one time. Most people are exposed to the pneumococcus several times a year but only rarely does this result in illness. When it invades it causes a diverse range of disease syndromes of which pneumonia, meningitis, and septicaemia have high case fatalities, and yet its most common disease manifestation, otitis media, is relatively benign. In old age it affects the healthy, but throughout life it is a burden to those with chronic medical illnesses. Pneumococcal disease is common in temperate and tropical climates; however, because the pneumococcus is fastidious in culture, it is rarely observed and the disease burden is frequently underestimated. Its differentiation into 91 serotypes indicates the complexity of its immunological interaction with humans and its need for adaptability in this long-enduring host–pathogen relationship. Microbiologists and physicians have regarded the pneumococcus as a formidable opponent for over 125 years. They have fought it with antibiotics and, more recently, with efficacious vaccines, each of which renders its nasopharyngeal niche a hostile home. Yet, through its capacity to combine DNA from other bacteria into its own chromosome, it has evolved and survived. It has all the fascination of the esoteric yet a busy doctor will not pass a week in practice without seeing a case.

Historical perspective

S. pneumoniae is a Gram-positive bacterium described historically as *Diplococcus pneumoniae* because of its tendency to appear microscopically in pairs. It was first isolated in 1881 by Sternberg in the United States of America and, simultaneously, by Pasteur in France through experiments inoculating the saliva of a patient dying of rabies into rabbits. Serotypes of pneumococcus are defined by the rabbit immune response to its variable capsular polysaccharide. In 1910, Neufeld and Händel described two serotypes; by 2007, 91 serotypes had been defined.

Convalescent sera from surviving pneumonia patients were shown to be protective against pneumococcal disease in rabbit models in 1891. The protective substance was identified as homologous anticapsular antibody and this underpinned the development of serum therapy in the early years of the 20th century. Although successful, serum therapy required knowledge of the serotype of the infecting pneumococcus, usually determined from sputum or lung aspirate cultures, leading to a delay in treatment. With the introduction of sulphonamide antibiotics in 1938, serum therapy was abandoned.

Antibiotic chemotherapy has been the mainstay of management of pneumococcal disease ever since, but the rapid evolution of resistant strains in the 1990s reactivated interest in vaccine development. A polyvalent capsular polysaccharide vaccine had been shown to protect South African miners from putative pneumococcal pneumonia in 1976. It was poorly immunogenic in infants, among whom most episodes of pneumococcal disease occur, but conjugation of the polysaccharide to immunogenic proteins overcame this limitation and a pneumococcal conjugate vaccine (PCV) against seven serotypes was introduced into the childhood immunization programme in the United States of America in 2000.

In 1928, Griffith inoculated rabbits with a suspension of live avirulent unencapsulated pneumococci and heat-killed serotype 3 pneumococci. The rabbits subsequently succumbed to serotype 3 septicaemia. The avirulent isolate was derived from a serotype 2 strain suggesting that it acquired the type 3 capsule, and virulence, from the heat-killed organisms. In 1944, Avery isolated and purified the 'active principle' that brought about this transformation and characterized it chemically as DNA. The sequence of the pneumococcal genome was first described in 2000 and several strains have now been fully annotated. These sequences have been used to identify conserved surface-expressed proteins that may serve as antigens in noncapsular vaccines.

Epidemiology

Incidence

Throughout the world, the risk of pneumococcal disease is highest in infancy and declines throughout the first 5 years of life. The lowest risk is in older children and young adults and from the age of 50 years onwards disease risk rises progressively (Fig. 7.6.3.1).

Among children older than 5 years, the incidence of culture-proven pneumococcal disease (per 100 000 population) was 70 to 100 in the United States of America before vaccine introduction; in Africa it is 110 to 430. In developed countries, the incidence is 15 to 20 among adults of all ages and at least 50 among adults aged 65 or over. There are no measurements from developing countries, although some estimate can be extrapolated from studies of indigenous peoples living in developed countries. Native Australians and Alaskans and White Mountain Apaches have incidence rates (per 100 000 population) of 200 to 1000 among children, 50 to 180 among adults 18 to 59 years old, and 120 to 170 among older adults.

The total burden of pneumococcal disease is frequently underestimated because it is difficult to detect. Studies of 'invasive pneumococcal disease', which rely on cultures of *S. pneumoniae* from specimens of blood, cerebrospinal fluid, and pleural fluid, fail to

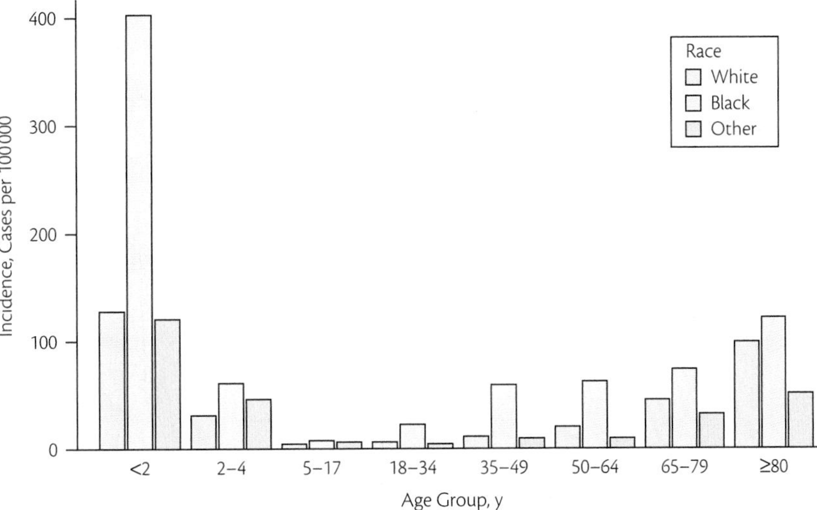

Fig. 7.6.3.1 Incidence of invasive pneumococcal disease in the United States of America between 1995 and 1998 by age and race. The data are taken from the Active Bacterial Core Surveillance of the Centers for Disease Control and Prevention.
(From Robinson KA, *et al.* (2001). Epidemiology of invasive *Streptococcus pneumoniae* infections in the United States, 1995–1998: opportunities for prevention in the conjugate vaccine era. *JAMA*, **285**, 1729–35.)

identify the majority of cases of pneumococcal pneumonia that are not bacteraemic. Lung aspirates obtained by percutaneous fine needle puncture significantly increase the yield of pneumococci from pneumonia cases at all ages but are rarely undertaken. The World Health Organization (WHO) has modelled the incidence of pneumococcal pneumonia, meningitis, and other serious manifestations using global data to derive country-based estimates of disease burden in children aged less than 5 years. In this estimate, there are more than 15 million cases of pneumococcal disease worldwide leading to approximately 800 000 deaths per year. The majority of these deaths take place in Africa and Asia. The global burden of disease in adults is not known.

Carriage, transmission, and serotypes

Viable *S. pneumoniae* have been described in collections of dust and in epizootics of some mammals, but the principal habitat and critical ecological niche of the pneumococcus is the human nasopharynx. Infants can acquire infection within hours of birth and most infants in developing countries become infected in the first 3 months of life. In The Gambia more than 90% of children aged less than 5 years old are colonized by the pneumococcus at any one time. In the United Kingdom, carriage prevalence among children is approximately 50%. Adults also carry *S. pneumoniae* in the nasopharynx but at lower prevalence.

The ratio of the incidence of invasive disease to the incidence of nasopharyngeal acquisition provides an index of the invasiveness of pneumococcal serotypes and can be used to group them. Serotypes 1, 5, 12F, and 46 are found among series of invasive isolates but are rarely isolated in the nasopharynx. These are labelled 'adult' types because they are associated with disease in adults. Other serotypes, including 10A, 11A, 15B, 15C, 16F, and 33F, are found among series of colonizing isolates but are uncommon causes of disease. A third group, which includes serotypes 6A, 6B, 14, 19A, 19F, and 23F, are found very commonly in the nasopharynx but also cause invasive disease. These are labelled 'paediatric' types because they cause the majority of invasive disease episodes among young children.

The duration of carriage can be as short as 3 h or as long as 3 years; in most instances it is between 1 and 6 months. The pneumococcus is transmitted by carriers, particularly preschool children, through direct contact with nasal secretions or by infected fomites. The rapid spread of pneumococcal pneumonia in outbreaks in adults suggests that airborne dissemination, facilitated by cough, is another mechanism of spread.

Risk factors

Risk of pneumococcal disease is a function of exposure to the bacterium, leading to colonization, and of host resistance to invasion. Exposure is increased in crowded environments at home and in institutions (e.g. military barracks, homeless shelters, jails, miners' compounds) and by contact with preschool children. In temperate climates pneumococcal disease follows a consistent seasonal variation with winter peaks and summer troughs. Risk is especially high at New Year when families gather and generations intermingle (Fig. 7.6.3.2).

Throughout life, males have an incidence of pneumococcal disease 1.2 to 1.5 times greater than females. Chronic medical conditions predispose to pneumococcal invasion (see Box 7.6.3.1). Alcoholism is consistently associated with pneumococcal disease and may act directly on macrophage function or, like seizure disorders, by compromising laryngeal defences leading to aspiration. HIV infection increases the risk of invasive pneumococcal disease by approximately 50-fold. Where HIV prevalence is greater than 2%, as in much of Africa, most cases of pneumococcal disease occur among HIV-positive patients. Recurrent pneumococcal disease is especially common in this group.

Antibiotic resistance

Epidemiology

Laboratory isolates of penicillin-resistant pneumococci were first reported in 1967 and by the early 1970s they were being isolated in clinical specimens in Australia and Papua New Guinea. During the 1990s, penicillin resistance spread widely throughout the world reaching a prevalence of 35% in several countries (e.g. France, South Africa, Japan, Hong Kong). Pneumococci are classified as either intermediately resistant (minimum inhibitory concentration (MIC) between 0.12 and 1.0 μg/ml) or fully resistant to penicillin

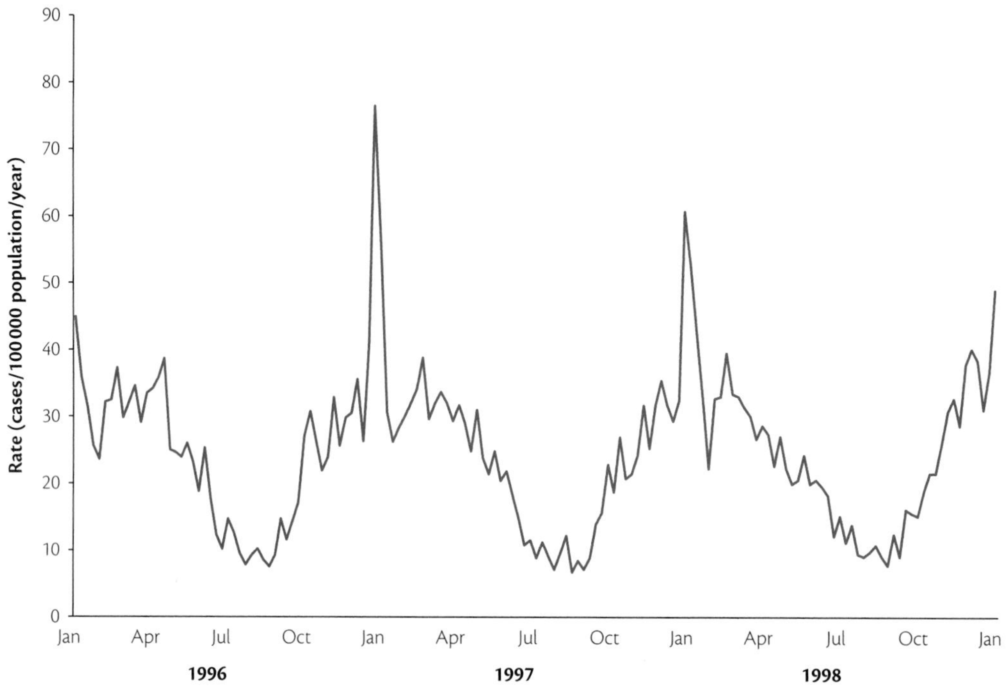

Fig. 7.6.3.2 Annualized weekly incidence of pneumococcal disease among adults in the United States of America between 1996 and 1998 showing a consistent increase in incidence in the winter and a sharp increase in incidence during the Christmas/New Year holiday season. (From Dowell SF, *et al.* (2003). Seasonal patterns of invasive pneumococcal disease. *Emerg Infect Dis*, **9**, 573–9.)

Box 7.6.3.1 Risk factors for pneumococcal disease

Social and demographic
- Older age
- Male sex
- Black race
- Indigenous populations
- Lower level of education
- Unemployment
- Excess alcohol use

Exposure to pneumococci
- Contact with preschool children
- Day care attendance[a]
- Crowding in the home
- Crowded adult environments (homeless shelters, military or occupational barracks)
- Institutionalized care
- Winter season
- Hospital admission

Respiratory tract damage
- Currently smoking
- Passive smoking
- Indoor air pollution
- Chronic obstructive pulmonary disease
- Recent viral respiratory tract infection

Preexisting medical conditions
- Chronic renal failure
- Congestive heart failure
- Cirrhosis
- Cerebrovascular disease
- Dementia
- Seizure disorder
- Asthma
- Diabetes
- Malignancies of the lung

Immune susceptibility
- HIV
- Hypogammaglobulinaemia
- Sickle cell disease
- Asplenia/splenectomy
- Pregnancy
- Not breastfeeding[a]
- Previous pneumococcal disease

[a] These apply only to infants or children.

(MIC 2 μg/ml and above). In developed countries resistance is dominated by fully resistant isolates whereas the reverse is found in developing countries. Resistance to other antibiotic classes, including macrolides, also increased during the 1990s. Use of long-acting macrolides appears to be responsible for increasing resistance to erythromycin.

Multiresistant pneumococci were first observed in South Africa in 1978. Their presence indicates that the use of one antibiotic can select for resistance against another. Penicillin-resistant strains are transmitted more successfully than penicillin-susceptible strains but multiresistant strains spread most successfully within populations. Much of this spread is driven by the expansion of a small number of clones. In the United States of America, 78% of all resistant isolates are represented by just 12 clonal groups.

In the United Kingdom, antimicrobial prescriptions have fallen since 1995 and at the same time there has been a reduction in both penicillin-resistant and macrolide-resistant pneumococci. Use of 7-valent PCV in the United States of America has resulted in a decrease in penicillin-resistant and multiresistant strains, although continued surveillance has revealed disease caused by new strains of pneumococcus some of which are also resistant. Pneumococcal resistance to fluoroquinolones has increased in prevalence but remains less than 5%.

Resistance mechanisms

Pneumococcal resistance to penicillin is entirely due to the accumulation of genetic variations among the six penicillin binding proteins (PBPs) that normally catalyse cross-linkage of the bacterial cell wall. By binding to PBPs, β-lactam antibiotics inhibit cell wall synthesis and promote cell lysis. Resistance to penicillin occurs when a PBP variant arises which has low binding affinity for β-lactams. Sensitive pneumococci have MICs for benzylpenicillin and cefotaxime which are approximately 0.02 μg/ml. Mutations in PBP 2b or 2x genes lead to a 2- to 30-fold increase in MIC. However, isolates that are fully resistant to penicillin usually contain alterations at three PBP genes, 2b, 2x, and 1a. High-level resistance to cefotaxime may be observed with a combination of changes in only two (PBP 2x and 1a).

Resistant strains come about through horizontal transfer and recombination into chromosomal DNA of large sequence blocks of mosaic genes acquired from other streptococci. This transfer may include capsular and resistance genes simultaneously. Pneumococci colonizing the nasopharynx are then exposed to antibiotics, which are commonly prescribed for community-acquired respiratory tract infections, and this selects resistant strains.

Pneumococcal genes *cat*, *erm*(B), and *tet*(M), which confer resistance to chloramphenicol, macrolides, and tetracyclines, respectively, have been found together on DNA elements (conjugative transposons) which spread between pneumococci without involving recombination thus facilitating multidrug resistance. Resistance to fluoroquinolones and trimethoprim/sulfamethoxazole is acquired by point mutations in topoisomerase genes and folate synthesis genes, respectively. Exposure to low levels of antibiotic selects single gene mutants which then acquire higher resistance through additional mutations.

Pathogenesis

Pneumococci exist in two morphologically distinct phenotypes; in the opaque phase they have abundant capsular expression and in the transparent phase they have little. In the nasopharynx, transparent-phase pneumococci predominate as abundant capsule prevents attachment of pneumococcal cell wall structures to epithelial cells. This attachment is mediated by binding of pneumococcal phosphorylcholine and choline binding protein A (CbpA) to human platelet activating factor receptors and polymeric immunoglobulin receptors. Once attached, pneumococci can cause disease by local spread to the middle ear or sinuses, by aerosol inhalation to the lung, or by blood stream invasion to the meninges, joint spaces, or heart valves. Blood stream invasion begins with endocytosis across the mucosal barrier although the components of this pathway are not well understood. In the blood stream pneumococci are found in the opaque phase since capsule is effective in evading opsonophagocytosis.

Pneumococci colonizing the nasopharynx cannot bind to the ciliated epithelium of the bronchi and therefore make their way to the lung in aerosols. However, if the ciliated epithelium is damaged, by antecedent viral infection or by cigarette smoke, it reveals a basement membrane to which pneumococci can adhere easily. Pneumolysin released from pneumococci causes further epithelial damage by direct cytotoxicity and encourages inflammation of the larger bronchioles, which leads to bronchopneumonia.

In the alveoli, pneumococci multiply in serous fluid and spread from one alveolus to another through the pores of Kohn. They adhere to the alveolar type 2 cells, through expression of CbpA, and stimulate production of the inflammatory mediators tumour necrosis factor-α, nitric oxide, and interleukins IL-1, IL-6, and IL-10, which initiates oedema. This creates the first pathological phase of pulmonary consolidation—engorgement.

In the second phase—red hepatization—erythrocytes leak into the alveolar spaces, reducing the compliance of the lung and leading to a liver-like appearance of the gross lung specimen (Fig. 7.6.3.3). Fibrin deposition creates a mesh of erythrocytes, leucocytes, and damaged epithelial cells and the lymphatics become dilated with cells and fibrin. Without ventilation, perfusion declines and the lung becomes maximally consolidated.

CbpA binding stimulates epithelial cells to release chemokines that attract leucocytes to the lung which initiates the third phase of consolidation—grey hepatization. Neutrophils trap pneumococci against the alveolar wall and engulf them by surface phagocytosis. C-reactive protein enhances this process by binding to choline residues on pneumococcal surfaces. The chemokines activate complement that, together with anticapsular antibody, facilitates opsonophagocytosis. Thereafter, lung inflammation begins to decline simultaneously with neutrophil apoptosis, fever declines, and macrophages are recruited to the lung to absorb the debris. Over a period of weeks this leads to complete resolution of the pathology.

Immunity to pneumococcal disease

Historically, the role of anticapsular antibody in recovery from pneumonia and the efficacy of serotype-specific serum therapy suggested that anticapsular IgG was the primary mechanism of immunity to pneumococcal disease. The age groups at highest risk of pneumococcal disease, infants and elderly people, have little anticapsular antibody or have antibody that lacks avidity. The genetic diversity of capsular expression into more than 90 variants suggests the antigen is under considerable immune selection and

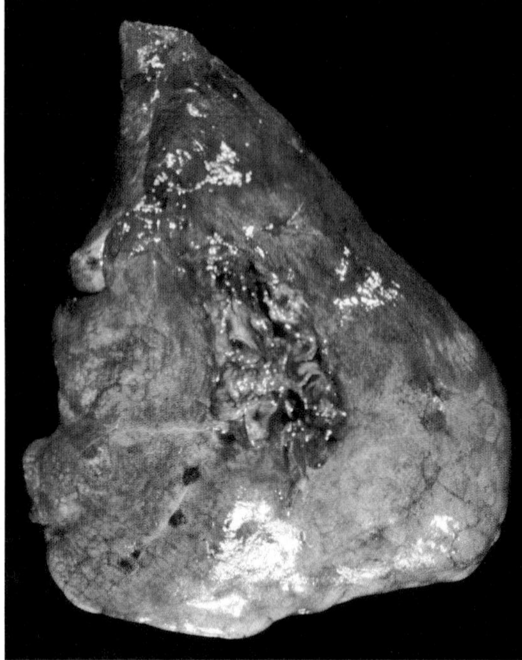
(a)

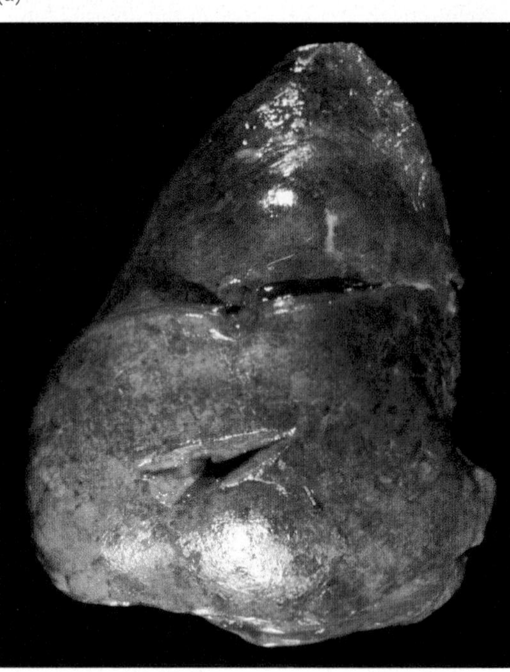
(b)

Fig. 7.6.3.3 Red hepatization in fatal pneumococcal pneumonia. (Copyright D A Warrell.)

the success of polysaccharide antigens as vaccines further reinforces the importance of anticapsular immunity.

Capsular polysaccharides are complex molecules with repeating epitopes that create cross-linkage of antigen receptors on B lymphocytes and which produce antibodies of the IgM and IgG2 isotypes. Antibody production can occur in the absence of T lymphocytes (T-independent) but it does not induce memory responses and can lead to antigen tolerance following repeated stimulation. Pneumococcal capsular and cell wall components both activate the human complement system leading to deposition of C3b and C3d on capsular polysaccharide. In the presence of both anticapsular antibody and complement, encapsulated pneumococci are opsonized and taken up by phagocytes expressing the receptor Fcγ-RIIa (CD32).

In contrast to natural immunity, conjugates of polysaccharides and highly immunogenic proteins (e.g. diphtheria toxoid) induce T-cell-dependent immunity with a predominance of IgG1 antibody and a memory response. These responses are inducible even in very young infants. Anticapsular antibody responses are measured by IgG enzyme-linked immunosorbent assay (ELISA) and a serum concentration of 0.35 μg/ml correlates with vaccine-induced protection in infancy.

In addition to adaptive immunity, innate mechanisms (e.g. lipoteichoic acid stimulation of Toll-like receptor (TLR) 2, or pneumolysin stimulation of TLR4) appear to be important in shaping the inflammatory response to pneumococcal disease and in determining host survival. Furthermore, several lines of evidence suggest that CD4 T cells play an important role in nasopharyngeal immunity that could be exploited by vaccines consisting of pneumococcal proteins or even whole cell killed pneumococci.

Prevention

Pneumococcal polysaccharide vaccine

In 1976, Austrian reported a trial of a 13-valent vaccine among South African gold miners in which the efficacy against putative pneumococcal pneumonia was 78%. This led to the commercialization of a pneumococcal polysaccharide vaccine (PPV), initially with 14 serotypes and later extended to 23 serotypes. Trials of PPV in the older people or in high-risk populations do not provide consistent evidence of protection against pneumococcal pneumonia. Observational studies using case-control designs or the indirect cohort method have more consistently indicated protection against bacteraemic pneumococcal disease. The evidence of effect is greater for older people than for those with chronic disease. On the basis of meta-analyses of the observational studies, PPV is recommended in the United Kingdom for all adults aged 65 years or more and for all persons aged 5 or more years who belong to an at-risk group (e.g. with asplenia, splenectomy, chronic respiratory disease, chronic heart, liver or renal disease, diabetes, or immunosuppression, including HIV infection at all stages). Revaccination of elderly people is recommended at 5-year intervals. Among patients having planned splenectomy, vaccination should take place well before the operation. Although PPV is recommended for United Kingdom patients with HIV this remains controversial. In a study of PPV in HIV-positive individuals from Uganda, the vaccinated group had an elevated risk of pneumonia. PPV is not recommended for HIV-positive populations in the developing world.

Pneumococcal conjugate vaccine

A 7-valent PCV, consisting of separate protein–polysaccharide conjugates for serotypes 4, 6B, 9V, 14, 18C, 19F, and 23F, was licensed in the United States of America in 2000 following successful trials in Californian infants and Native American children. The seven serotypes in the vaccine accounted for 83% of invasive disease in American children less than 2 years old. The efficacy against invasive pneumococcal disease caused by these serotypes was 97% after a four-dose schedule given at 2, 4, 6, and 15 months of age.

The vaccine was also shown to protect against pneumococcal meningitis, bacteraemia, pneumonia, and otitis media.

PCV reduces nasopharyngeal colonization by pneumococci of the serotypes included in the vaccine and increases colonization by other serotypes commensurately. In routine immunization, this has produced two effects. First, the transmission of vaccine-serotype pneumococci has declined providing 'herd protection' for older children and adults whose pneumococcal disease rates have fallen substantially. Second, the incidence of disease caused by serotypes not included in the vaccine has increased slightly. So far this 'serotype replacement disease' has been much smaller in magnitude than the substantial reductions in vaccine-serotype disease. However, to mitigate the effects of serotype replacement disease new vaccines with 10 serotypes (including 1, 5 and 7F) or 13 serotypes (also including 3, 6A and 19A) are being introduced in childhood immunisation programmes.

Vaccine trials in children in South Africa and The Gambia have shown that 9-valent PCV, which includes two additional serotypes (1 and 5), can protect against invasive pneumococcal disease among HIV-infected children and can reduce childhood mortality and admissions to hospital with pneumonia among young children. In 2007, the WHO has recommended introduction of the 7-valent PCV in childhood immunization programmes in developing countries in which the 7 serotypes account for a significant proportion of disease.

In the United Kingdom, the recommended immunization schedule for infants is two doses of PCV given at 2 and 4 months of age followed by a booster dose at 13 months of age. For children 2 to 5 years of age who belong to an at-risk group, the recommendation is for a single dose of PCV followed 2 months later by a single dose of PPV.

Other forms of prevention

For children who are at high risk of invasive pneumococcal disease, including those with sickle cell disease or nephrotic syndrome, or following splenectomy, daily prophylaxis with oral penicillin reduces risk by over 80%. It should be continued until at least 5 years of age.

In developing countries, simple measures such as reducing indoor smoke from cooking stoves and improving nutrition are likely to be effective in prevention. Zinc supplementation can reduce the incidence of pneumonia in children by 40%. In Pakistan, a community intervention to promote hand washing reduced pneumonia incidence in children by one-half.

Diagnosis

Culture of S. *pneumoniae*

Pneumococcal disease is most convincingly diagnosed by culture of *S. pneumoniae* from a normally sterile site in a patient with a compatible illness. Pneumococci are fastidious organisms but they grow readily on 5% blood agar incubated in 5% CO_2. Colonies are small and grey with a draughtsman like central indentation and are surrounded by a greenish zone of α-haemolysis. Species identity is confirmed by sensitivity to optochin (ethylhydroxycupreine), bile solubility, and serotyping. The capsular type of *S. pneumoniae* is differentiated by a change in the refractive index around the cell seen on microscopy in the presence of specific rabbit antisera, the (Neufeld) Quellung reaction (Fig. 7.6.3.4).

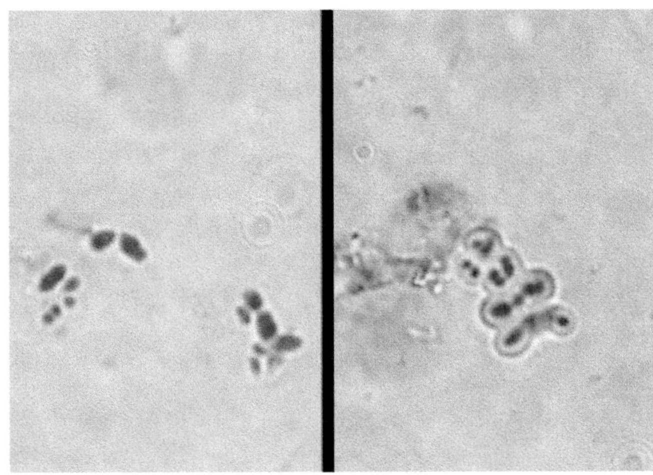

Fig. 7.6.3.4 The (Neufeld) Quellung reaction. Pneumococci show an apparent increase in the thickness of capsule when mixed with homologous anticapsular antibodies. The negative control is shown on the left and the positive reaction on the right.
(From Werno AM, Murdoch DR (2008). Medical microbiology: laboratory diagnosis of invasive pneumococcal disease. *Clin Infect Dis*, **46**, 926–32.)

In pneumococcal meningitis, cerebrospinal fluid frequently yields a positive culture. Pneumococci are also cultured from pleural and joint fluid in thoracic empyema and septic arthritis, respectively. Diagnosis of pneumococcal pneumonia by culture is, however, highly insensitive. Blood culture is a poor diagnostic test for several reasons; infection can be confined to the lungs; episodes of bacteraemia are only intermittent; the density of bacteraemia is too low, especially in children; or the patient can have taken antibiotics that inhibit growth. Sputum culture lacks specificity, since the pharynx is colonized by pneumococci even in healthy individuals, and also has relatively poor sensitivity. Most cases of pneumococcal pneumonia are, therefore, not formally diagnosed. A measure of this insensitivity is obtained from the Gambian trial of PCV where 15 cases of radiographic pneumonia were prevented by vaccination for every two cases of detectable bacteraemic disease prevented.

Antigen detection

Patients with pneumococcal pneumonia excrete pneumococcal breakdown products including C-polysaccharide, a universal component of pneumococcal cell walls, and capsular polysaccharides. Detection of C-polysaccharide in urine has been commercialized in a rapid immunochromatographic test that has a sensitivity of approximately 80% for bacteraemic pneumococcal pneumonia in adults and is highly specific. In children it lacks specificity as positive results may be obtained from healthy individuals who are merely colonized with pneumococci. Antigen detection is a useful adjunct to the testing of cerebrospinal fluid in cases of suspected meningitis.

Polymerase chain reaction

Primers targeting genes encoding the pneumococcal proteins pneumolysin, autolysin, pneumococcal surface adhesin A, and PBPs have been used for polymerase chain reaction (PCR) diagnosis. These assays have the same limitations as culture-based detection. PCR of respiratory specimens does not distinguish colonization from lung infection, and PCR of blood has poor sensitivity for pneumococcal pneumonia. Conversely, PCR of cerebrospinal fluid is sensitive and specific and has proven useful in the investigation of epidemic meningitis.

Clinical features

S. pneumoniae causes pneumonia, meningitis, septicaemia, otitis media, endocarditis, peritonitis, sinusitis, conjunctivitis, and purulent infections of the pleura, joints, and bone. These conditions do not necessarily occur in isolation; pneumococcal meningitis is quite frequently accompanied by pneumonia.

Pneumococcal pneumonia

Symptoms

Typically, the illness starts suddenly although there may be an antecedent upper respiratory tract infection. Fever is usually the first symptom and it is frequently accompanied by rigors. The patient feels weak and anorexic and may have severe headache and myalgia. Cough develops within 24 to 72 h and becomes a prominent symptom. At first the cough is nonproductive but it becomes productive of blood-tinged ('rusty') sputum and later of purulent sputum.

Pleuritic chest pain also develops during the course of the illness. The pain is sharp and stabbing and is aggravated by deep inspiration or coughing. The patient may try to obtain relief by splinting the affected side of the chest or lying on the affected side. Involvement of the diaphragmatic pleura leads to misleading abdominal pain or referred pain in the shoulder.

Among young children, a history of cough and difficulty breathing should raise suspicion of pneumonia. Elderly and immunocompromised patients may present with general malaise and confusion and have few respiratory symptoms and no fever. Prior antibiotic treatment also modifies the classic presentation.

Physical signs

On general examination, adults have tachycardia and pyrexia, with a rectal temperature as high as 40°C. With early presentation the respiratory system may appear normal, but pneumonia patients go on to develop rapid and difficult breathing (of which flaring of the alae nasi is a subtle early sign), cyanosis, and signs of lobar consolidation including reduced chest movement, dullness on percussion, fine crepitations, and, occasionally, bronchial breathing over the affected area. A pleural rub is sometimes audible.

Abdominal distension, upper abdominal tenderness, and guarding suggest involvement of the diaphragmatic pleura. Mild jaundice occurs in a minority. Concomitant herpes labialis ('cold sores') is common. Confusion is a sign of severity and is frequently observed in elderly patients.

In infants, the signs of pneumonia are nonspecific; most will have a raised respiratory rate and nasal flaring but only a minority will have crepitations. In developing countries, most cases of pneumonia are diagnosed and treated by nonmedical health workers. To facilitate diagnosis and promote early treatment, the WHO has designed a simple diagnostic algorithm as part of its Integrated Management of Childhood Illness (IMCI), which defines pneumonia on the respiratory rate (Fig. 7.6.3.5). Severe pneumonia, requiring admission to hospital, is indicated by lower chest wall indrawing; very severe pneumonia, requiring oxygen treatment, is indicated by hypoxia or mental changes (Fig. 7.6.3.6).

Investigations

The pathological process of pneumonia is confirmed by the chest radiograph. This typically shows a homogenous area of opacification confined within the lobar structure (Fig. 7.6.3.7). The lower lobes are affected more frequently than the upper lobes. The area of pathology may be localized to a single lobule or extend over several lobes; early in the presentation there may be no abnormality at all. In children, widespread patchy opacification (bronchopneumonia) is common. Lateral radiographs add to the sensitivity of posteroanterior projections particularly for lower lobe disease hidden beneath the dome of the diaphragm.

In adults, pneumococcal aetiology is defined most sensitively by the C-polysaccharide antigen test in urine. Many patients are severely dehydrated on admission and cannot readily produce a urine specimen. Blood culture is positive for *S. pneumoniae* in about 10 to 30% of adults and about 15% of children. Genuine sputum samples should be differentiated from upper respiratory tract secretions by a high ratio of pus cells to epithelial cells on microscopy. The appearance of large numbers of Gram-positive diplococci on microscopy together with culture of *S. pneumoniae* is diagnostic. However, because prior antibiotic use is common, sputum microscopy is positive in only about one-quarter of patients and sputum culture is positive in only one-half. Young children cannot normally produce a sputum specimen.

Other laboratory investigations determine the prognosis. A Pao_2 less than 8 kPa marks out severe pneumonia but $Paco_2$ is usually unaffected unless terminal ventilatory failure occurs. A plasma urea exceeding 7 mmol/litre is a mark of severity (Fig. 7.6.3.8). The peripheral white blood cell count is elevated in most cases and may be as high as 40×10^9/litre. A low white cell count is a poor prognostic sign.

Differential diagnosis

The abrupt onset of symptoms often leads the patient to seek care before focal signs become established and it is not possible to differentiate pneumonia from other causes of acute febrile illness. In tropical countries, malaria is the main differential at this stage. When localizing symptoms and signs are established, pneumonia must be distinguished from pulmonary infarction. Both conditions lead to chest pain and haemoptysis and are accompanied by tachycardia. Pyrexia and rigors favour a diagnosis of pneumonia, while a very sudden history of chest pain and frank haemoptysis favour pulmonary embolism. Pulmonary oedema (secondary to heart failure), pulmonary atelectasis, pleurisy, lung abscess, tuberculosis, and acute bronchitis should also be considered in the differential diagnosis. Outside the chest, subdiaphragmatic lesions such as cholecystitis, a subphrenic abscess, or an amoebic liver abscess can mimic the clinical picture of lower lobe pneumonia.

Bacterial pneumonia is differentiated from viral or mycoplasma pneumonia by its abrupt onset, severity of symptoms and systemic illness, raised peripheral white blood cell count, and C-reactive protein level exceeding 125 mg/litre in serum. Confusion, signs of multiorgan involvement, lymphopenia, or a low serum sodium should raise the possibility of legionnaires' disease. Tuberculosis occasionally presents with an acute pneumonia in adults. In HIV-infected patients, the differential diagnosis also includes infection by *Pneumocystis jirovecii*, mycobacteria, and cytomegalovirus.

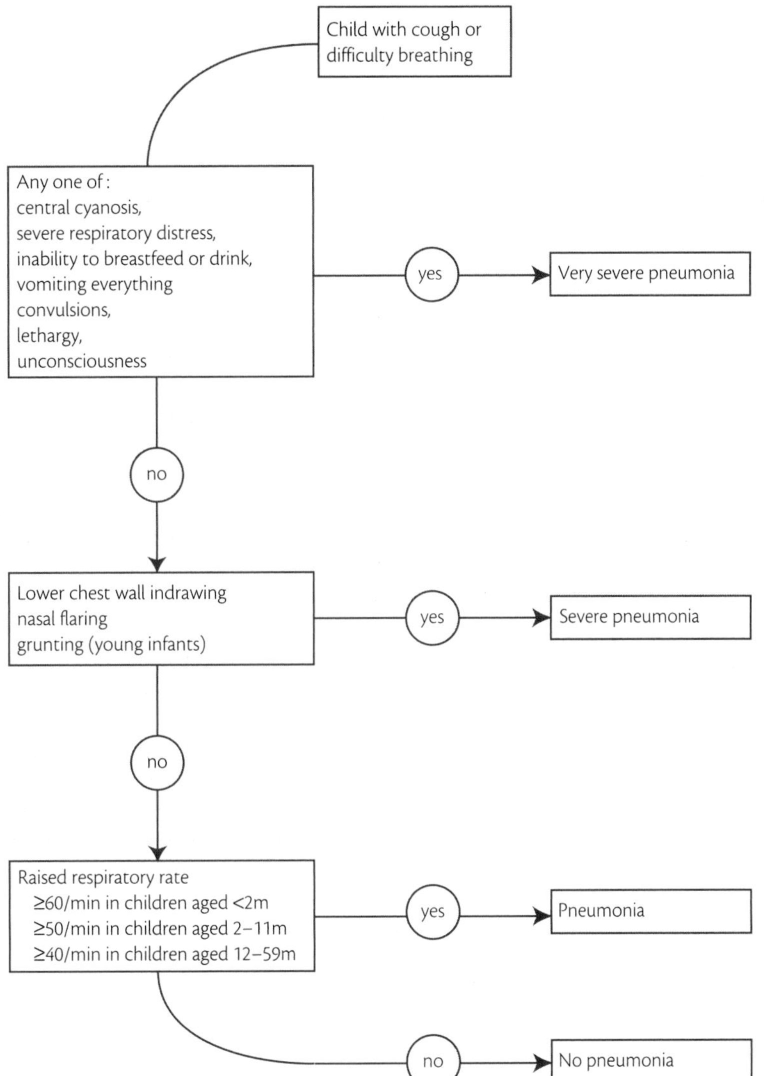

Fig. 7.6.3.5 The WHO classification of pneumonia in developing countries. (Adapted from World Health Organization (2004). *Serious childhood problems in countries with limited resources. Background book on management of the child with a serious infection or severe malnutrition.* World Health Organization, Geneva.)

Treatment

Management of pneumonia first requires an assessment of severity to determine whether the patient should be treated at home, admitted to hospital, or admitted to the intensive care unit. The British Thoracic Society (BTS) recommendations define pneumonia as severe if there are three or more CURB-65 features: **C**onfusion, **U**rea exceeding 7 mmol/litre, **R**espiratory rate equal to or exceeding 30 breaths/min, abnormal **B**lood pressure, either systolic (<90 mmHg) or diastolic (≤60 mmHg) hypotension, and age equal to or exceeding **65** years. Additional features that may influence this assessment include the presence of coexisting disease, hypoxaemia ($Pa\text{O}_2$ less than 8 kPa or $Sa\text{O}_2$ less than 92%), and bilateral or multilobe involvement on the chest radiograph. Bacteraemia is itself an indicator of severity and increased risk of death. Supportive care includes analgesia for chest pain, ample hydration and nutrition, advice to stop smoking, and oxygen for inpatients with hypoxaemia.

Empirical guidelines for pneumonia treatment focus on treatment of pneumococcal pneumonia. High-dose penicillin or amoxicillin therapy will provide serum concentrations sufficiently high to treat pneumonia that is caused by pneumococci with MICs up to 4 µg/ml. Based on efficacy, cost, and acceptability, the optimum antibiotic is amoxicillin. The BTS recommends oral amoxicillin 500 to 1000 mg three times daily for 7 days for nonsevere cases of community-acquired pneumonia treated at home. Erythromycin 500 mg four times daily and clarithromycin 500 mg twice daily are acceptable alternatives. A fluoroquinolone with enhanced pneumococcal activity (e.g. levofloxacin, moxifloxacin) may be considered in outbreaks of resistant pneumococcal disease or in patients unresponsive to first-line antibiotics.

Severe cases of pneumonia requiring admission to hospital should be treated empirically with a broad-spectrum intravenous antibiotic such as co-amoxiclav (1.2 g three times daily), cefuroxime (1.5 g three times daily), cefotaxime (1 g three times daily), or ceftriaxone (2 g once daily) for 10 days. Cefotaxime or ceftriaxone are most active against pneumococci and should be effective against pneumonia caused by pneumococci with high cephalosporin MICs of 1 to 2 µg/ml. Empiric therapy with either erythromycin (500mg four times daily) or clarithromycin (500mg twice daily) should also be given to cover other causes of pneumonia. After 3 days of intravenous antibiotics, clinically stable patients may be safely switched to oral therapy.

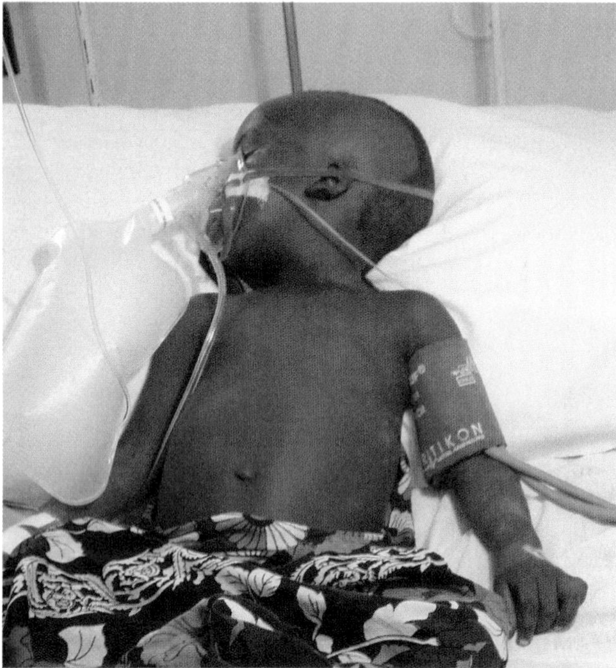

Fig. 7.6.3.6 Kenyan child with very severe pneumonia, as defined by the WHO, receiving high-flow oxygen therapy.
(Taken in the clinical service of Kilifi District Hospital; supplied by Dr Mike English. The patient's parents gave written consent for the taking of this photograph and for its use for educational purposes.)

Course and prognosis

Historically, untreated patients who survived long enough to make specific anticapsular polysaccharide antibody recovered spontaneously by crisis, or by a more gradual lysis, 7 to 10 days after the onset of illness. The significance of the observation, dating from Hippocrates and perpetuated by Osler, that crisis was most likely on uneven days (the 5th and especially the 7th) after the start of fever, remains obscure. However, mortality from pneumococcal pneumonia in the preantibiotic era was 20 to 40%. With antibiotic treatment, mortality is about 5% overall but is 30% among the subset of patients with bacteraemia. Mortality is highest among elderly and very young patients, and among those with an underlying illness such as cirrhosis, alcoholism, or heart disease. Most deaths occur within the first few days of admission to hospital. The causes of death are difficult to establish but include shock, cardiac arrhythmias, and respiratory failure.

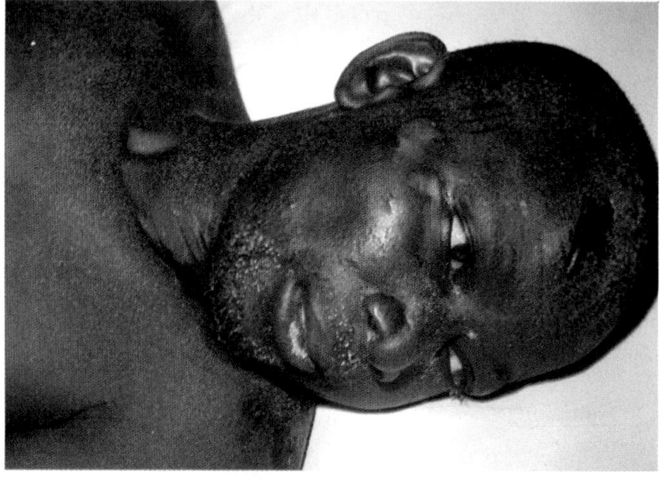
(a)

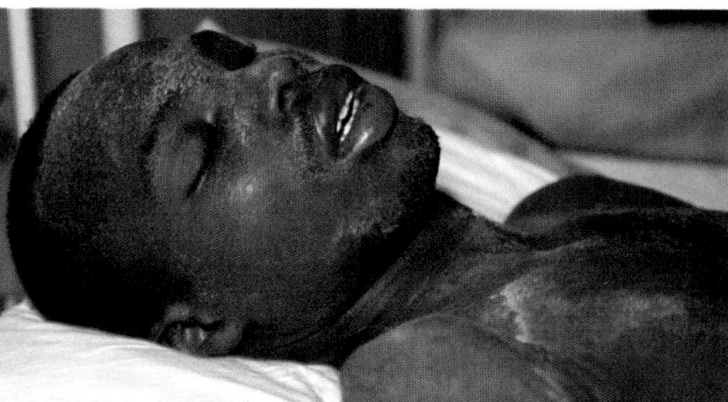
(b)

Fig. 7.6.3.8 Urea frost in two patients with uraemia complicating pneumococcal pneumonia.
(Copyright D A Warrell.)

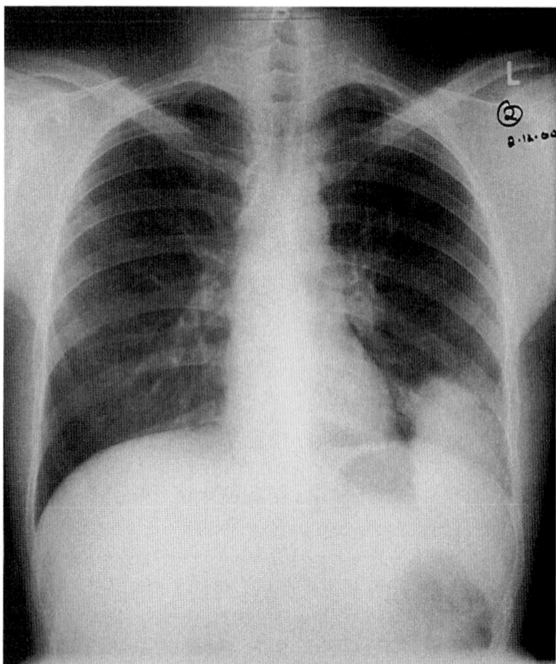

Fig. 7.6.3.7 Chest radiograph of an adult with clinical signs of left lower lobe pneumonia illustrating a well-demarcated area of alveolar consolidation.

Pneumococcal pleural effusion and empyema

A large pleural effusion or an empyema develops during treatment in 2 to 5% of patients with established pneumococcal pneumonia. In children these complications have increased in incidence over recent years and are frequently caused by serotype 1.

Symptoms

Some patients with pneumococcal empyema give a history of recent lung infection but others develop the disease without any previous illness. Hectic fever, rigors, sweats, malaise, anorexia, and marked weight loss are characteristic symptoms, often going back several weeks. Patients with a large pleural collection are breathless and may complain of dull pain on the affected side. A productive cough is unusual unless a bronchopleural fistula has developed.

Physical signs

General examination reveals pyrexia, tachycardia, and evidence of recent weight loss. Examination of the chest usually shows the characteristic signs of a pleural effusion: diminished chest movement, stony dullness on percussion, and diminished breath sounds over the accumulated fluid. The chest wall overlying an empyema may be tender.

Investigations

The effusion will usually be visible on the chest radiograph but loculated effusions may require localization by ultrasonography. On aspiration, turbid fluid or thick pus is obtained which contains pneumococci and degenerate white cells. If antibiotics have been given it may not be possible to culture pneumococci, but the fluid contains detectable pneumococcal antigens. The peripheral white blood cell count is raised predominantly with neutrophils.

Differential diagnosis

The principal differential diagnosis is pulmonary tuberculosis, and pleural biopsy may be required if the pleural fluid is sterile. The absence of copious, purulent sputum differentiates pleural empyema from a lung abscess.

Treatment

Successful treatment requires both intravenous antibiotics and pleural drainage. Appropriate antibiotic treatment for pneumococcal empyema follows the recommendations for pneumococcal pneumonia, with intravenous amoxicillin or a cephalosporin. Because of the frequent coexistence of penicillin-resistant aerobes and anaerobes, a β-lactamase inhibitor or metronidazole should also be given. Antibiotics should be continued for 4 to 6 weeks.

Course and prognosis

If untreated, an empyema may rupture through the chest wall (empyema necessitatis) or into a bronchus causing a bronchopleural fistula. Even when pus is aspirated and healing achieved, subsequent fibrosis and calcification may seriously restrict expansion of the underlying lung.

Pneumococcal meningitis

Pneumococci colonizing the nasopharynx can gain access to the subarachnoid space either by direct spread (from paranasal sinusitis or otitis media), following damage to the base of the skull, or, more commonly, via the bloodstream where they cross the blood–brain barrier at the choroid plexus and cerebral capillaries.

Symptoms

Adults with pneumococcal meningitis usually have fever, headache, neck stiffness, and impaired consciousness. At presentation, one-half of all patients have been ill for less than 24 h. Nausea and photophobia are common and seizures occur before diagnosis in 5 to 10% of patients. Among elderly patients, confusion may be the only symptom. Deterioration in the psychological or neurological state of an elderly patient with community-acquired pneumonia should be investigated with lumbar puncture. The presentation of meningitis in infants may be subtle, beginning with inability to feed and followed by irritability or lethargy.

Physical signs

Patients with pneumococcal meningitis are pyrexial and toxaemic. Classic signs such as nuchal rigidity, Kernig's sign, and Brudzinski's sign are absent in many patients with pyogenic meningitis. Bulging of the anterior fontanelle may be present in infants. Consciousness is often impaired, varying from drowsiness and confusion to deep coma. Raised intracranial pressure due to cerebral oedema or a cerebral abscess may be indicated by bradycardia and hypertension, but papilloedema is rarely seen. A cranial CT or MRI is mandatory before lumbar puncture in the presence of signs of cerebral or cranial nerve damage including a dilated pupil, ocular palsies, hemiparesis, history of focal seizures, decreased or rapidly falling level of consciousness, irregular respiration, tonic seizures, and decerebrate or decorticate posturing.

An associated pneumococcal lesion, such as otitis media or pneumonia, may be detected.

Investigations

Lumbar puncture should be undertaken whenever meningitis is suspected. In pneumococcal meningitis the cerebrospinal fluid is usually turbid and the leucocyte count is equal to or exceeds 1000×10^6/litre. Most of the leucocytes are neutrophils. A few patients have a low leucocyte count ($<100 \times 10^6$/litre) and in patients who present very early the leucocyte count may be normal; a repeat lumbar puncture several hours later will confirm the diagnosis. In pneumococcal meningitis, the concentration of protein in cerebrospinal fluid is increased and the ratio of glucose concentrations in cerebrospinal fluid and plasma is usually less than one-third. In untreated cases, culture of cerebrospinal fluid is usually positive and pneumococci are visible following Gram's staining. In patients who have received less than 48 h of antibiotic therapy the leucocyte count remains high and pneumococcal antigen may be detectable in cerebrospinal fluid. Culture of blood also frequently reveals the pneumococcus. The peripheral white cell count is usually elevated.

Differential diagnosis

Pneumococcal meningitis cannot be differentiated clinically from other forms of meningitis and the aetiology must be defined by investigation of the cerebrospinal fluid. An associated ear infection or pneumonia, or a history of head trauma favours pneumococcal infection. Conversely, rashes are rarely found in pneumococcal meningitis and petechiae or purpura on skin or mucosae strongly suggest meningococcal disease.

Treatment

Standard empirical therapy for meningitis in adults is cefotaxime (300 mg/kg per day divided into three or four doses) or ceftriaxone (100 mg/kg per day divided into two doses) for 10 to 14 days. In parts of the world where strains with intermediate or full resistance to cefotaxime or ceftriaxone have emerged, vancomycin (60 mg/kg per day divided into four doses) should be added to the empiric therapy. Meropenem is a useful alternative to cefotaxime and is active against pneumococci of intermediate but not full cefotaxime resistance. Imipenem increases susceptibility to seizures. Penicillin or ampicillin are effective therapy for culture-proven pneumococcal meningitis caused by penicillin-sensitive strains, but intermediately resistant strains are not adequately treated by these drugs.

In children in developing countries, for several decades the recommended therapy for acute pyogenic meningitis has been chloramphenicol with penicillin. The spread of intermediate penicillin resistance among pneumococci and the expiry of the patent for ceftriaxone have recently led to a change in this policy. In non-epidemic situations, the WHO now recommends treatment with ceftriaxone 100 mg/kg once daily for 5 to 7 days with a maximum daily dose of 2 g.

Treatment with antibiotics should be started as soon as a clinical diagnosis of bacterial meningitis is made. Delay in treatment until after hospitalization is associated with increased mortality. Other supportive therapies include adequate oxygenation, maintenance of normal blood pressure, prevention of hypoglycaemia and hyponatraemia, and control of seizures (which may be covert and unsuspected in an unconscious patient) with anticonvulsants.

The use of dexamethasone in bacterial meningitis in adults has been controversial for many years. In a Cochrane review of five randomized controlled trials, the summary mortality reduction attributable to dexamethasone adjunctive treatment was 43%; the effect was greatest in meningitis caused by *S. pneumoniae*. The summary findings were influenced to a large extent by a single study of European patients. In a more recent study of HIV-infected adults in Africa, among whom case fatality rates were very high, dexamethasone was not beneficial, suggesting that dexamethasone may only be useful in populations with low HIV prevalence who are less sick at presentation. The recommended dose is 10 mg every 6 h for 4 days. Meningeal inflammation facilitates diffusion of vancomycin into the cerebrospinal fluid and the anti-inflammatory action of dexamethasone may lead to suboptimal antibiotic concentrations. Patients on treatment for cephalosporin-resistant pneumococcal meningitis should therefore be monitored both clinically and by repeat lumbar puncture. In children, dexamethasone is highly protective against hearing loss in *H. influenzae* meningitis but also provides some protection in pneumococcal meningitis if given with or before administration of antibiotics. For children in developing countries, however, the evidence suggests there is no benefit to adjunctive dexamethasone.

Course and prognosis

The prognosis of patients with pneumococcal meningitis is poor. Most patients develop complications of which the most important are seizures, brain infarction, brain swelling, hydrocephalus, and cranial nerve palsies. Subdural collections are commonly seen on brain imaging and may require needle puncture to exclude subdural empyema, especially if there is persistence of fever, irritability, neck stiffness, or continued cerebrospinal fluid leucocytosis detected by repeat lumbar puncture.

Over one-third of patients also develop systemic complications such as shock, cardiorespiratory failure, and disseminated intravascular coagulation, and these are frequently the final cause of death among older patients. Among children, supportive therapy to sustain adequate blood pressure is important to maintain cerebral blood flow against the resistance of raised intracranial pressure.

The mortality from pneumococcal meningitis in industrialized countries varies between 10 and 40%, being lower in children than in adults. In developing countries, the mortality range is higher (30–60%). Features on admission that are associated with a poor outcome include advanced age, seizures, cranial nerve palsies, deep coma, low cerebrospinal fluid leucocyte count (below 1000×10^6/litre), low glucose concentration in cerebrospinal fluid, and associated pneumonia. Death is almost inevitable in patients who are in deep coma at the time they are admitted to hospital. Survivors are frequently affected by neurological sequelae: hearing loss occurs in one in five; cerebral damage is common leading to hemiparesis, ataxia, and aphasia; and cranial nerve palsies, particularly of the oculomotor nerve, occur in a small percentage. Among those who appear to make a good recovery from pneumococcal meningitis, one-quarter have residual cognitive slowness.

Otitis media

In young children aged below 2 years, otitis media is one of the commonest reasons for seeking medical advice. The pneumococcus causes a significant fraction of all cases. Following conjugate pneumococcal vaccine introduction in the United States of America, the incidence of all otitis media has fallen by one-fifth. Beyond childhood, otitis media is uncommon.

Symptoms

Acute otitis media starts suddenly, although there may be a history of a recent upper respiratory tract infection. Fever, crying, and extreme irritability are the usual features in young children, in whom febrile convulsions may also occur. Fever and severe pain in the ear are the usual presenting complaints in older children and adults, and patients may also complain of deafness and tinnitus.

Physical signs

On otoscopic examination of the affected ear, the tympanic membrane is red and swollen and lacks the normal light reflection. It may bulge outwards into the external ear and there may be an air–fluid level indicating a middle ear effusion. Pus or blood in the external auditory canal suggests a perforation that is confirmed by observing a ragged hole in the tympanic membrane. The affected ear is usually partially deaf. In children, meningism may be present; if so, meningitis must be excluded by lumbar puncture.

Investigations

Fine needle puncture of the tympanic membrane (tympanocentesis) and aspiration of middle ear fluid is used with variable frequency in different countries but is of most value where antibiotic resistance is prevalent. In complicated cases or in those not responding to initial antibiotics, culture of middle ear fluid may guide therapy. A tympanogram can identify increased middle ear pressure and accumulation of fluid.

Treatment

Most episodes of otitis media are diagnosed clinically without microbiological confirmation. Randomized controlled trials show that otitis media resolves in the majority of otherwise healthy children whether or not they take antibiotics. This evidence underpins a policy of observation without treatment. Immediate antibiotics are indicated in young infants (<6 months) and in older children (>2 years) with a clear bacteriological diagnosis of otitis media or symptoms of severity. The antibiotic of choice for pneumococcal otitis media is oral amoxicillin (90 mg/kg per day) for 5 days. For penicillin-resistant pneumococcal infection the appropriate antibiotic is intravenous ceftriaxone for 3 days.

Course and prognosis

Pneumococcal otitis media normally resolves rapidly and completely. However, rupture of the drum can lead to partial conductive deafness and pneumococcal otitis media can give rise to a chronic discharging ear requiring prolonged or complicated treatment.

The infection can spread to cause acute mastoiditis, meningitis, or a cerebral abscess.

Other clinical syndromes

The pneumococcus is an important cause of bacterial sinusitis resulting from direct spread from the nasopharynx. Sinusitis that does not resolve within 5 to 7 days may require treatment with an antibiotic effective against pneumococcus. A mild form of pneumococcal bacteraemia, variously labelled as 'occult bacteraemia' or 'walk-in bacteraemia', is encountered relatively commonly in children. The child presents with fever or febrile convulsions but without any obvious focus of pneumococcal infection. Although there is a small risk of dissemination to the meninges, the patient is usually successfully treated as an outpatient with oral antibiotics before the culture results are known. Significant bloodstream infection is less common but may lead to septicaemia or purulent localization in meninges, vertebrae, joints, orbits, or testes. Pneumococcal conjunctivitis has been observed in outbreaks among college students and has two unusual features: (1) the causative strain is unencapsulated and (2) the attack rates are high, suggesting little pre-existing immunity.

Septicaemia

Acute septicaemia is a less common form of pneumococcal infection and is encountered most frequently in immunocompromised patients or those without a spleen. Sudden fever, peripheral circulatory collapse, and bleeding (purpura fulminans) are the usual presenting features of this condition, which is indistinguishable from other forms of overwhelming bacterial septicaemia. Leucopenia is usually found. Bleeding is due to disseminated intravascular coagulation. The mortality from septicaemia is very high, even when treatment is started promptly. The pneumococcus has been rarely associated with toxic shock syndrome and with haemolytic uraemic syndrome.

Endocarditis and pericarditis

Cardiac manifestations of pneumococcal infection are well described but where there is good access to antibiotics they are now rare, occurring in less than 1% of all pneumococcal infections. Acute endocarditis may complicate pneumococcal septicaemia to affect healthy heart valves, especially the aortic valve, which may rupture and cause severe aortic incompetence. Emboli derived from cardiac vegetations may reach the brain and other organs. Progressions of the cardiac lesions may be very rapid and the prognosis of this condition is poor. Valve replacement may be necessary for patients who survive the initial episode.

Pneumococci may spread directly from the lower lobes of the lung to produce pericarditis which is clinically silent in some patients or may be manifest only as a transient pericardial rub or an abnormal electrocardiogram. Patients with a pericardial empyema usually complain of dull or pleuritic central chest pain and give a history of persistent fever, malaise, anorexia, and weight loss over several days or weeks. Many patients with a pneumococcal pericardial empyema are critically ill by the time they reach hospital and have pericardial tamponade: a rapid small-volume pulse, pulsus paradoxus, a low blood pressure, elevation of the jugular venous pressure with a further increase during inspiration, peripheral oedema, and ascites. The heart sounds are usually faint and a chest radiograph may show globular enlargement of the heart together with evidence of an associated lung infection. An ultrasonographic examination may help to define the best sites for diagnostic and therapeutic drainage. The electrocardiogram shows low-voltage potentials and ST elevation or depression may be present. Pneumococcal aetiology can be confirmed by culture or antigen detection of drained pus. Mortality is high, and among patients who survive the initial episode constrictive pericarditis may develop within weeks or months of their acute illness.

Peritonitis

Pneumococcal peritonitis is an uncommon condition that is encountered among three risk groups: (1) patients with cirrhosis of the liver or nephrotic syndrome; (2) patients with gastrointestinal disease (e.g. appendicitis), intra-abdominal surgery, or peritoneal dialysis; and (3) otherwise healthy young girls, possibly as a complication of pelvic infection. The condition is characterized by sudden fever and abdominal pain and tenderness. The ascitic fluid is turbid and contains neutrophils and pneumococci. The prognosis of pneumococcal peritonitis is determined principally by the severity of the underlying illness.

Future developments

Of great concern for future treatment of pneumococcal disease is the global spread of multiresistant isolates of *S. pneumoniae.* Resistance to new agents such as fluoroquinolones is established in adult disease and is now reported among paediatric cases in South Africa. Judicious use of antibiotics has curbed the rise in resistance in developed countries but resistant strains still have a competitive advantage in many developing countries where antibiotic use is relatively unregulated. The clinical relevance of *in vitro* resistance to antibiotics, especially intermediate β-lactam resistance in the treatment of pneumonia, remains an area requiring further investigation.

The significance of pneumococcal disease will be shaped to a large extent during the next decade by the global introduction of new vaccines and by the evolutionary response of the pathogen to these interventions. New conjugate vaccines are being introduced that cover 10 and 13 serotypes each. These protect against more cases of pneumococcal disease in developing countries where serotypes 1 and 5, which are not included in the 7-valent PCV, predominate. The potential of PCV to reduce the incidence of childhood pneumonia and reduce childhood deaths is enormous; however, the success of the vaccine will be determined by its population effects, particularly serotype replacement disease. Third-generation vaccines which use surface expressed pneumococcal proteins and virulence factors to stimulate immunity are not restricted to a subset of serotypes and avoid this limitation. These are now beginning to enter clinical trials.

Further reading

Austrian R, Gold J (1964). Pneumococcal bacteremia with especial reference to bacteremic pneumococcal pneumonia. *Ann Intern Med*, **60**, 759–76. [Classic description of the effect of antibiotics on pneumonia mortality.]

Austrian R, *et al.* (1976). Prevention of pneumococcal pneumonia by vaccination. *Trans Assoc Am Physicians*, **89**, 184–94. [Vaccine trial of 13-valent polysaccharide vaccine in South African miners.]

Bentley SD, *et al.* (2006). Genetic analysis of the capsular biosynthetic locus from all 90 pneumococcal serotypes. *PLoS Genet*, **2**, e31, 1–8.

Berkley JA, *et al.* (2005). Bacteremia among children admitted to a rural hospital in Kenya. *N Engl J Med*, **352**, 39–47. [A conservative estimate of invasive pneumococcal disease incidence from Africa.]

Black S, *et al.* (2000). Efficacy, safety and immunogenicity of heptavalent pneumococcal conjugate vaccine in children. Northern California Kaiser Permanente Vaccine Study Center Group. *Pediatr Infect Dis J*, **19**, 187–95.

Briles DE, *et al.* (2000). Immunization of humans with recombinant pneumococcal surface protein A (rPspA) elicits antibodies that passively protect mice from fatal infection with *Streptococcus pneumoniae* bearing heterologous PspA. *J Infect Dis*, **182**, 1694–701. [First study to show human antibodies against pneumococcal proteins are protective.]

British Thoracic Society (2001). BTS guidelines for the management of community acquired pneumonia in adults. *Thorax*, **56** Suppl 4, 1–64. [United Kingdom professional guidelines on management of pneumonia, last updated in 2004 and available at www.brit-thoracic.org.uk/]

Cutts FT, *et al.* (2005). Efficacy of nine-valent pneumococcal conjugate vaccine against pneumonia and invasive pneumococcal disease in The Gambia: randomised, double-blind, placebo-controlled trial. *Lancet*, **365**, 1139–46.

Dowell SF, *et al.* (2003). Seasonal patterns of invasive pneumococcal disease. *Emerg Infect Dis*, **9**, 573–9.

Dowson CG, *et al.* (1989). Horizontal transfer of penicillin-binding protein genes in penicillin-resistant clinical isolates of *Streptococcus pneumoniae. Proc Natl Acad Sci U S A*, **86**, 8842–6. [Early description of the genetic basis of penicillin resistance in pneumococcus.]

Fedson DS, Scott JA (1999). The burden of pneumococcal disease among adults in developed and developing countries: what is and is not known. *Vaccine*, **17** Suppl 1, 11–18.

Giefing C, *et al.* (2008). Discovery of a novel class of highly conserved vaccine antigens using genomic scale antigenic fingerprinting of pneumococcus with human antibodies. *J Exp Med*, **205**, 117–31. [Use of pneumococcal genomics to discover antigenic common pneumococcal proteins.]

Gilks CF, *et al.* (1996). Invasive pneumococcal disease in a cohort of predominantly HIV-1 infected female sex-workers in Nairobi, Kenya. *Lancet*, **347**, 718–23. [Epidemiology and clinical presentation of pneumococcal disease in HIV-positive adults.]

Gordon SB, *et al.* (2000). Bacterial meningitis in Malawian adults: pneumococcal disease is common, severe, and seasonal. *Clin Infect Dis*, **31**, 53–7. [In a setting with high HIV prevalence, pneumococcus caused 18% of bacterial meningitis cases and 32% of bacterial meningitis deaths.]

Greenwood B (1999). The epidemiology of pneumococcal infection in children in the developing world. *Philos Trans R Soc Lond B Biol Sci*, **354**, 777–85.

Heffron R (1939). *Pneumonia with special reference to pneumococcus lobar pneumonia.* The Commonwealth Fund, New York. (Second printing 1979, Harvard University Press, Cambridge, Mass.) [Classic book summarizing the first 60 years of research on pneumococcal pneumonia.]

Hill PC, *et al.* (2006). Nasopharyngeal carriage of *Streptococcus pneumoniae* in Gambian villagers. *Clin Infect Dis*, **43**, 673–9. [Reveals the enormous exposure to pneumococci in a developing world setting.]

Kadioglu A, *et al.* (2008). The role of *Streptococcus pneumoniae* virulence factors in host respiratory colonization and disease. *Nat Rev Microbiol*, **6**, 288–301.

Klugman KP, *et al.* (2003). A trial of a 9-valent pneumococcal conjugate vaccine in children with and those without HIV infection. *N Engl J Med*, **349**, 1341–8.

Malley R, *et al.* (2001). Intranasal immunization with killed unencapsulated whole cells prevents colonization and invasive disease by capsulated pneumococci. *Infect Immun*, **69**, 4870–3.

Mangtani P, Cutts F, Hall AJ (2003). Efficacy of polysaccharide pneumococcal vaccine in adults in more developed countries: the state of the evidence. *Lancet Infect Dis*, **3**, 71–8.

Musher DM (1992). Infections caused by *Streptococcus pneumoniae*: clinical spectrum, pathogenesis, immunity, and treatment. *Clin Infect Dis*, **14**, 801–7.

O'Brien KL, *et al.* (2009). Burden of disease caused by *Streptococcus pneumoniae* in children younger than 5 years: global estimates. *Lancet*, **374**, 893–902.

Ogunniyi AD, *et al.* (2007). Development of a vaccine against invasive pneumococcal disease based on combinations of virulence proteins of *Streptococcus pneumoniae. Infect Immun*, **75**, 350–7. [Illustrates the state of common protein vaccine development and especially the role of vaccines consisting of combinations of different proteins.]

Pallares R, *et al.* (1995). Resistance to penicillin and cephalosporin and mortality from severe pneumococcal pneumonia in Barcelona, Spain. *N Engl J Med*, **333**, 474–80. [Large retrospective study fails to find an increase in mortality from pneumococcal pneumonia caused by penicillin-resistant strains when it was treated with penicillin.]

Prymula R, *et al.* (2006). Pneumococcal capsular polysaccharides conjugated to protein D for prevention of acute otitis media caused by both *Streptococcus pneumoniae* and non-typable *Haemophilus influenzae*: a randomised double-blind efficacy study. *Lancet*, **367**, 740–8.

Reingold A, *et al.* (2005). Direct and indirect effects of routine vaccination of children with 7-valent pneumococcal conjugate vaccine on incidence of invasive pneumococcal disease: United States, 1998–2003. *MMWR Morb Mortal Wkly Rep*, **54**, 893–7. [Illustration of the herd protection provided to older children and adults by pneumococcal conjugate vaccine when children are routinely immunized.]

Scott JA, *et al.* (2000). Aetiology, outcome, and risk factors for mortality among adults with acute pneumonia in Kenya. *Lancet*, **355**, 1225–30.

Siber GR, Klugman, KP, Mäkelä PH (eds) (2008). *Pneumococcal vaccines: the impact of conjugate vaccines.* ASM Press, Washington, DC.

Sleeman KL, *et al.* (2006). Capsular serotype-specific attack rates and duration of carriage of *Streptococcus pneumoniae* in a population of children. *J Infect Dis*, **194**, 682–8. [Provides an estimate of invasiveness of each pneumococcal serotype based on acquisition rates and incidence of invasive disease.]

Tettelin H, *et al.* (2001). Complete genome sequence of a virulent isolate of *Streptococcus pneumoniae. Science*, **293**, 498–506.

Trzcinski K, Thompson CM, Lipsitch M (2004). Single-step capsular transformation and acquisition of penicillin resistance in *Streptococcus pneumoniae. J Bacteriol*, **186**, 3447–52. [Demonstrates in vitro the capacity of pneumococcus to exchange DNA coding for capsular serotype and penicillin resistance in a single genetic step.]

Tuomanen EI, *et al.* (eds) (2004). *The pneumococcus.* ASM Press, Washington, DC. [Modern summaries of research into genomics, pathogenesis, immunity, virulence, colonization, epidemiology, and treatment of invasive pneumococcal disease as well as antibiotic resistance and vaccines.]

van de Beek D, *et al.* (2004). Clinical features and prognostic factors in adults with bacterial meningitis. *N Engl J Med*, **351**, 1849–59.

van der Poll T, Opal SM (2009). Pathogenesis, treatment, and prevention of pneumococcal pneumonia. *Lancet*, **374**, 1543–56.

Watera C, *et al.* (2004). 23-Valent pneumococcal polysaccharide vaccine in HIV-infected Ugandan adults: 6-year follow-up of a clinical trial cohort. *AIDS*, **18**, 1210–3. [In a randomized controlled trial among HIV-infected adults, risk of all causes of pneumonia was, surprisingly, 1.6 times greater in recipients of polysaccharide vaccine.]

Watson DA, *et al.* (1993). A brief history of the pneumococcus in biomedical research: a panoply of scientific discovery. *Clin Infect Dis*, **17**, 913–24.

Weiser JN, *et al.* (1994). Phase variation in pneumococcal opacity: relationship between colonial morphology and nasopharyngeal colonization. *Infect Immun*, **62**, 2582–9.

Weisfelt M, *et al.* (2006). Pneumococcal meningitis in adults: new approaches to management and prevention. *Lancet Neurol*, **5**, 332–42.

Werno AM, Murdoch DR (2008). Laboratory diagnosis of invasive pneumococcal disease. *Clin Inf Dis*, **46**, 926–32. [Up-to-date review of laboratory diagnosis of pneumococcal disease.]

White B (1938). *The biology of pneumococcus.* The Commonwealth Fund, New York. (Second printing 1979, Harvard University Press, Cambridge, Mass.) [Classic book describing the first 70 years of research on the pneumococcus.]

Whitney CG, *et al.* (2003). Decline in invasive pneumococcal disease after the introduction of protein-polysaccharide conjugate vaccine. *N Engl J Med*, **348**, 1737–46. [Surveillance study documenting the large impact of pneumococcal conjugate vaccine on invasive pneumococcal disease among children following routine use in the United States of America.]

World Health Organization (2009) *Integrated management of childhood illness.* http://www.who.int/child_adolescent_health/topics/prevention_care/child/imci/en/index.html

7.6.4 Staphylococci

Bala Hota and Robert A. Weinstein

Essentials

Staphylococci are Gram-positive bacteria that form clusters, but can occur singly, in pairs, chains, or tetrads. They are classically distinguished from other 'Gram-positives' by presence of catalase, an enzyme that degrades hydrogen peroxide (H_2O_2). *S. aureus* is distinguished from other coagulase-negative staphylococci, which are generally less virulent, by the presence of coagulase, an enzyme that coagulates plasma. Many toxins and regulatory elements enhance virulence in staphylococci.

Epidemiology

Colonization—staphylococci are skin commensals. About 20% of adults are persistently colonized by *S. aureus*, 60% are intermittently colonized, and 20% are never colonized. High-risk groups for *S. aureus* colonization include infants, insulin-dependent diabetics, intravenous drug users, HIV-positive patients, and individuals undergoing either haemo- or peritoneal dialysis.

Methicillin-resistant *S. aureus* (MRSA)—risk factors for MRSA colonization and infection among hospitalized patients include antibiotic exposure, surgery, nursing-home residence, or high MRSA 'colonization pressure', i.e. frequent exposure to colonized or infected patients. However, MRSA is no longer only a hospital-related infection, with community-associated MRSA affecting individuals without health care exposures.

Clinical features

S. aureus infection—clinical syndromes can be divided into three groups: (1) Illness due to release of toxins, leading to disease at sites often remote from infection—including (a) staphylococcal scalded skin syndrome—release of epidermolytic toxins leads to bullae and desquamation; (b) food-borne illness due to preformed toxin—a heat-stable superantigen toxin produces sudden vomiting and diarrhoea; (c) toxic shock syndrome—superantigen toxins cause multisystem organ dysfunction; may be menstrual (e.g. tampon-associated) or nonmenstrual. (2) Illness due to local tissue destruction and abscess formation—including (a) impetigo, folliculitis, and cellulitis; (b) furuncles and carbuncles; (c) mastitis; (d) pyomyositis; (e) septic bursitis; (f) septic arthritis; (g) osteomyelitis; (h) epidural abscess; (i) pneumonia; (j) urinary tract infection. (3) Hematogenous infection—including bacteraemia and endocarditis.

Coagulase-negative staphylococci—most infections with these skin commensals are the consequence of medical interventions leading to foreign bodies, e.g. prosthetic joints or heart valves, indwelling intravascular catheters or grafts, or peritoneal catheters. Conditions include endocarditis (5–8% of native valve infections, *c*.40% of prosthetic valve infections), intravascular catheter infections (6–27% of vascular-catheter infections), prosthetic joint infections (up to 38% of arthroplasty infections), peritoneal dialysis, catheter infections, and postoperative ocular infections.

Diagnosis

Diagnosis relies on characteristic clinical and epidemiological features, supported by positive cultures from the relevant clinical site, with identification (when appropriate) of exotoxin-positive strains. Outbreak and epidemiological investigations use molecular fingerprinting techniques to assess relatedness of staphylococci.

Treatment

Aside from supportive care, the mainstays of therapy are (1) prompt drainage of infected foci; and (2) antimicrobials—(a) coagulase-negative staphylococci—vancomycin is the mainstay of therapy because of the high rates of methicillin resistance; (b) *S. aureus*—antimicrobial choice should be based on the local prevalence of MRSA and the clinical severity of illness; a bactericidal agent, preferably a β-lactam, is used whenever possible; oral agents active against MRSA include clindamycin, trimethoprim/sulfamethozaxole, doxycycline, minocycline, linezolid; glycopeptides (i.e. vancomycin or teicoplainin) have been the usual therapy of severe infections due to MRSA, but vancomycin resistance is emerging.

Prevention

Prevention of illness due to *S. aureus*, particularly MRSA, relies on proactive infection control measures, including (1) surveillance for MRSA colonization; (2) imposed grouping (cohorting) of infected and colonized patients; (3) barrier precautions—e.g. gowning and gloving by health care staff; (4) improved hand hygiene; (5) cleaning patients—e.g. with chlorhexidine; (6) improved environmental cleaning; (7) antimicrobial stewardship.

Better strategies for treatment and salvage of infected catheters or methods for treatment of biofilm may improve treatment of coagulase-negative staphylococcal infections. No vaccines are available.

Introduction and historical perspective

Staphylococci are named for their microscopic appearance, the name coming from Greek words meaning 'bunch of grapes' and 'berry'. First described in 1880 by Ogston as an important cause of abscesses in humans, staphylococci are among the most common causes of bacterial colonization and infection in the community and in hospitals.

Staphylococcus aureus, the pre-eminent human staphylococcus, has adapted efficiently to improvements in therapeutics. In the 1940s, shortly after the introduction of penicillin, penicillin-resistant *S. aureus* was noted in the United Kingdom and the United States of America, and by the end of the decade 50% of isolates were resistant. From 1940 to 1960, a particularly invasive clone of penicillin-resistant *S. aureus*, 'phage type 80/81', caused pandemic hospital infections. Following the introduction of methicillin, that strain faded from concern only to be replaced in subsequent decades with endemic health care-associated methicillin-resistant *S. aureus* (MRSA) that frequently was resistant to multiple antimicrobial classes. Most recently, reminiscent of the 1940 to 1960 experience, invasive strains of community-associated MRSA (CA-MRSA) have emerged rapidly in some communities among otherwise healthy individuals. Coagulase-negative staphylococci infections, in contrast, are infecting implanted devices and occurring in association with health care, thereby filling a niche created by medical success.

Microbiology and molecular genetics

Staphylococci stain purple ('positive') with Gram's stain and form grape-like clusters, but can occur singly, in pairs, in chains, or in tetrads. Of 32 staphylococcal species, 16 colonize or infect humans. Classically, staphylococci are distinguished from other 'Gram-positives' by the presence of catalase, an enzyme that degrades H_2O_2. *S. aureus* is distinguished from other staphylococci by the presence of coagulase, an enzyme that coagulates plasma. Most laboratories use latex agglutination tests to detect coagulase; other assays include the tube coagulase and free coagulase tests.

Outbreak and epidemiological investigations use molecular 'fingerprinting' techniques to assess relatedness of staphylococci, i.e. bacteriophage typing, pulsed-field gel electrophoresis (PFGE), multilocus sequence typing (MLST), polymerase chain reaction (PCR), or toxin or 'housekeeping' gene identification.

Pathogenesis

The infectiveness of staphylococci depends in part on bacterial factors that promote growth, colonization, invasiveness (i.e. regulation and virulence determinants), and antibiotic resistance and in part on host susceptibility (e.g. presence of diabetes mellitus).

Regulation and virulence determinants

Regulation determinants 'autoregulate' staphylococci based on environmental conditions or host factors. The major *S. aureus* regulatory gene is the accessory gene regulator (*agr*) that facilitates intercell communication. This and other systems may have roles in tissue destruction (through exoprotein production) and endocarditis (through adhesin regulation).

Virulence determinants, e.g. peptidoglycan, lipoteichoic acids, protein toxins, and biofilm, enhance bacterial pathogenicity but can also activate patient protective mechanisms. Peptidoglycan, an important component of Gram-positive bacterial walls, and lipoteichoic acids, bound to the plasma membrane, are implicated in triggering the inflammatory response in humans that can enhance bacterial killing. Exoproteins and 'superantigens' (i.e. antigens that lead to nonspecific immune activation) can be released by *S. aureus* to cause a severe immune response or disease remote from infection, while local toxins, e.g. Panton–Valentine leucocidin (PVL), may increase bacterial invasiveness. Biofilm, an extracellular complex of polysaccharides, enhances binding to foreign objects (e.g. intravascular catheters) and serves as a bacterial sanctuary from host defences and antimicrobials.

Antimicrobial resistance

S. aureus resistance to β-lactams is mediated by β-lactamases (penicillin resistance) or, more commonly, by altered enzymes responsible for cell wall formation (methicillin resistance). Penicillinases propagate by plasmids or phage transfer; methicillin resistance results from spread of a genomic island of DNA called the staphylococcal chromosomal cassette (SCC). The SCC carries the *mecA* gene (termed SCCmec). The product of *mecA* is penicillin-binding protein 2a (PBP2a), which has low affinity for methicillin and enables cell wall synthesis in spite of active antibiotics. SCCmec type IV primarily is associated with CA-MRSA, while types I, II, and III are associated primarily with hospital strains.

Glycopeptides (i.e. vancomycin or teicoplanin) have been the usual therapy of severe infections due to MRSA. However, vancomycin resistance is emerging among MRSA. Two resistance patterns exist: (1) vancomycin- (or glycopeptide-) intermediate *S. aureus* (VISA or GISA) and (2) vancomycin-resistant *S. aureus* (VRSA). The VISA phenotype has vancomycin minimum inhibitory concentrations (MICs) of 4 to 8 µg/ml, and is thought to arise from thickening of the cell wall, changes in *agr* function, and changes in cell metabolism that arise from subinhibitory exposure to vancomycin. VRSA have higher MICs (≥16 µg/ml) due to a gene (*vanA*) that has been passed from vancomycin-resistant *Enterococcus faecalis* to *S. aureus*. Clinical isolates of VRSA (six so far) have been reported in the United States of America only. Although new agents (linezolid and daptomycin) exist for therapy of MRSA and could be used for VISA/VRSA, fledgling resistance has been reported.

Resistance to antimicrobials in the macrolide–lincosamide–streptogramin (MLS) group is not predictably concordant. Clindamycin resistance can be inducible, producing misleading susceptibility phenotypes in automated testing that are erythromycin resistant and, seemingly but erroneously, clindamycin susceptible, or constitutive (readily detected resistance to erythromycin and clindamycin). The double-disc diffusion test, or D test, will detect inducible clindamycin resistance. Clindamycin therapy is unreliable in organisms with either inducible or constitutive resistance.

Among the coagulase-negative staphylococci, 80% of isolates are resistant to methicillin due to the action of *mecA*. Laboratory testing of coagulase-negative staphylococci is complicated by heterotypic expression of methicillin resistance, which may lead to deceptively low methicillin MICs. PCR testing for *mecA* or slide agglutination testing for PBP2a will reveal resistance; methicillin or oxacillin will not effectively treat such strains.

Epidemiology: *S. aureus*

Colonization

Among staphylococci, as a general rule, colonization precedes infection. *S. aureus* colonizes multiple sites but predominately the anterior nares. Some CA-MRSA may share the ability of coagulase-negative staphylococci to colonize intact skin. Among adults, 20% are persistently colonized by *S. aureus*, 60% are intermittently colonized, and 20% are never colonized. Methicillin-susceptible *S. aureus* (MSSA) colonization prevalence rates are about 30% in the community. High-risk groups for *S. aureus* colonization include infants, insulin-dependent diabetics, intravenous drug users, HIV-positive patients, and patients undergoing either haemodialysis or peritoneal dialysis. Host factors promoting colonization may be antibiotic treatment and polymorphisms in host genes.

Health care-associated MRSA

Health care-associated MRSA infection causes significant morbidity and mortality, and has been associated with 29% longer stays and 36% greater hospital charges for patients with MRSA compared to

MSSA bacteraemia. Among hospitalized patients, risk factors for MRSA colonization and infection include antibiotic exposure, surgery, nursing home residence, or high MRSA 'colonization pressure', i.e. frequent exposure to colonized or infected patients.

There is a large 'resistance iceberg' for MRSA; the ratio of infected-to-colonized patients may reach 1:3, which complicates control measures. Uncleaned hands of health care workers probably represent a major vector for MRSA cross-transmission. Another mechanism of staphylococcal transmission is bacterial shedding from nares of colonized patients or staff, which can be enhanced by rhinitis. Spread via contaminated environmental surfaces may account for an additional 10 to 15% of MRSA transmissions in health care settings.

CA-MRSA

MRSA are no longer exclusively nosocomial pathogens. They have been affecting people without exposure to health care. Although CA-MRSA colonization rates have lagged behind those of MSSA, infection rates for those colonized with CA-MRSA are up to 10 times higher than rates for those colonized with MSSA.

Worldwide, CA-MRSA infections have been mainly due to only a few PFGE types, e.g. USA300 strain. Rates of infection with USA300 CA-MRSA are rising and in some locations have exceeded MSSA infection rates. Risk factors for infection or colonization with CA-MRSA include African American race, HIV infection, drug use, tattooing, and situations and environments associated with increased person-to-person contact such as military service, jails, homosexual contacts, sports activity, and children's day care.

Secular trends and morbidity

Overall trends in hospitalizations for *S. aureus* infections suggest an increasing burden of illness. Trends fostering increases include aging of populations in western societies with increased comorbidities and use of prosthetic devices such as joint replacements; the emergence of CA-MRSA, which is occurring in addition to, not in place of, community-associated MSSA; and use of broad-spectrum antibiotics. In the United States of America, it has been estimated that about 9 of every 1000 hospitalizations may be due to *S. aureus*, and about 43% of *S. aureus* admissions are due to MRSA. Mortality rates among patients infected with *S. aureus* are 15 to 34% in various studies. Clinical factors enhancing the likelihood of death include pneumonia, older age, diabetes, inadequate therapy, and failure to drain infected foci. With spread of CA-MRSA into hospitals, the epidemiology and control of nosocomial MRSA may change.

Prevention: S. *aureus*

General interventions

Prevention of illness due to *S. aureus*, particularly MRSA, relies on proactive infection control measures. These may include surveillance for MRSA colonization to detect the resistance iceberg, barrier precautions (use of gowning and gloving) for care of infected and colonized patients, imposed grouping (cohorting) of infected and colonized patients, isolation wards, improved hand hygiene, antimicrobial stewardship, cleaning patients with chlorhexidine, improved environmental cleaning, and use of intensive care unit 'monitors' to promote adherence to infection control measures.

MRSA

Studies of MRSA control suggest that multiple simultaneous interventions can reduce colonization and infection rates. Highly promoted among packages or bundles of interventions are hospital admission surveillance nasal cultures for MRSA colonization. These are recommended in high-risk units or when other control measures fail to reduce MRSA infection rates. The role of decolonization of patients detected by surveillance is currently controversial. The strongest support for decolonization comes from outbreak investigations, particularly in neonatal units. The risks/benefits of screening and decolonization programmes, and their impact on overall nosocomial infection rates, warrant evaluation.

CA-MRSA

Control of CA-MRSA presents distinct challenges. The feasibility of contact precautions or isolation of infected persons in the community may be limited. Additionally, the role of fomites in transmission of CA-MRSA is unknown, and community environmental decontamination may be difficult. Current guidelines for people with CA-MRSA infections and their community contacts include proper dressings for infected areas, hand hygiene, washing clothes contaminated with infected secretions, and avoiding contact sports while lesions exist. If infection is recurrent or spreading in specific settings, such as families, search for and decolonization of carriers may be useful.

Agents useful for decolonization

Potential agents used for staphylococcal decolonization include topical agents (mupirocin, chlorhexidine, tea tree oil) or short courses of systemic antimicrobials. Mupirocin 2% is effective for decolonization but has not been shown to reduce nosocomial infection rates and is of limited use when mupirocin resistance occurs. Tea tree oil, from the Ti (or Tea) tree (*Melaleuca alternifolia*, Myrtaceae), has been effective for some colonized patients. Chlorhexidine gluconate has potent antibacterial effects for decolonizing skin or as a nasal gel. Assiduous application of approved detergents/disinfectants or bleach can decontaminate the environment.

Clinical features: S. *aureus*

Risk factors for infection

Groups commonly at risk of colonization and infection include AIDS patients, intravenous drug users, and patients with diabetes mellitus. Multiple risk factors for *S. aureus* infection often coexist. For example, haemodialysis and peritoneal dialysis patients are at increased colonization risk and have high-risk foreign bodies. Conditions that predispose specifically to tissue invasion include skin trauma, haematomas, burns, or chronic diseases (e.g. dermatitis or psoriasis); surgical wounds; indwelling vascular catheters; and postviral sequelae such as influenza-related mucosal damage. Rarer conditions associated with increased risks of staphylococcal infection include Chédiak–Higashi syndrome and Job's syndrome (Chapter 5.2).

Clinical syndromes

S. aureus infection syndromes can be divided into three groups: (1) illness due to release of toxins, leading to disease at sites often remote from infection; (2) illness due to local tissue destruction and abscess formation; and (3) haematogenous infection. Therapy for these syndromes is based on the use of active drugs at appropriate dosages with appropriate concern for common side effects and toxicities.

Toxin-related syndromes

Staphylococcal scalded skin syndrome

In 1878, staphylococcal scalded skin syndrome (SSSS), or Ritter's disease, was described in 297 children by the German physician Ritter von Rittershain. After release of epidermolytic toxins by *S. aureus*, patients develop bullae and desquamation. Though clinically impressive (Fig. 7.6.4.1a), this superficial desquamation can be distinguished clinically and histologically from deeper exfoliative illnesses such as toxic epidermal necrolysis (TEN). In SSSS, skin separation occurs within the epidermis, at the stratum granulosum, while in TEN, separation occurs deeper, at the dermal–epidermal junction, leading to more severe skin loss. The absence of mucosal disease in SSSS also distinguishes these syndromes.

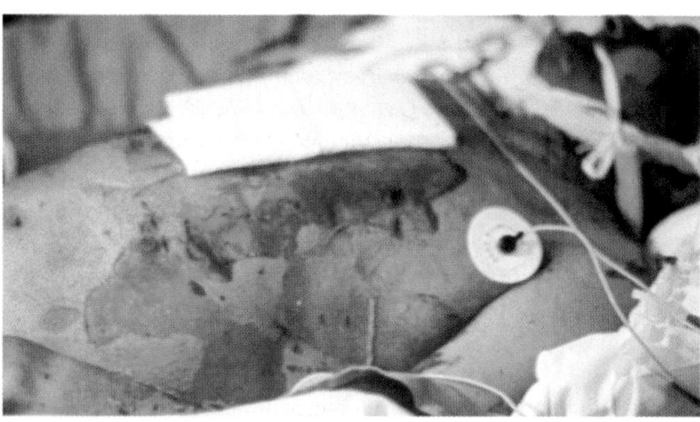

(a)

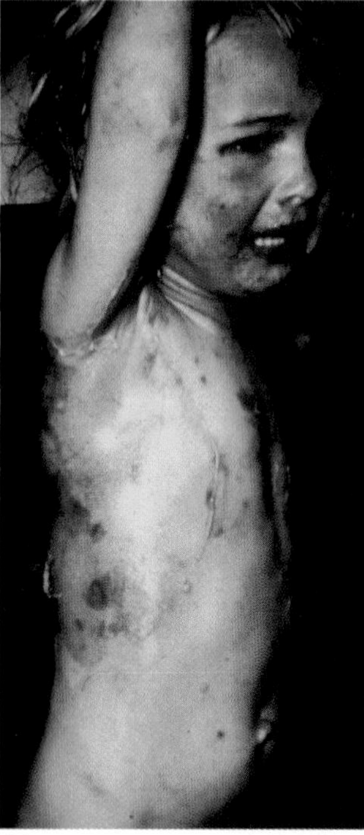

(b)

Fig. 7.6.4.1 Staphylococcal scalded skin syndrome: (a) in an adult; (b) in a child. (a, copyright Professor S J Eykyn; b, copyright Professor W C Noble.)

SSSS occurs more commonly in children (Fig. 7.6.4.1b). Disease may be generalized or localized (i.e. bullous impetigo), and the burden of *S. aureus* may be low. Nasal or mucosal colonization may cause disease. When cases occur in epidemics, such as in neonatal units, patients and health care workers should be screened for carriage. Diagnosis relies on the characteristic clinical and epidemiological features and is supported by identification of exotoxin-positive strains colonizing or infecting clinical sites. Treatment involves topical or systemic antibiotics for infected sites and supportive care for areas of skin/soft tissue destruction.

Food-borne illness due to preformed toxin

S. aureus can produce a heat-stable superantigen toxin that can persist even after cooking has eradicated the organism. Ingestion of toxin in contaminated, often unrefrigerated, food can result in epidemic gastrointestinal disease. There is a short incubation of only 2 to 6 h, followed by sudden vomiting (82%), diarrhoea (68%), and occasionally fever (16%). The differential diagnosis includes other short-incubation toxin-mediated gastrointestinal pathogens such as *Bacillus cereus* and toxins (Chapter 9.2). Treatment involves supportive care, particularly rehydration. The illness is typically self-limited, lasting less than 12 h.

Toxic shock syndrome

Staphylococcal toxic shock syndrome is caused by superantigen toxins released by *S. aureus*, resulting in multisystem organ dysfunction. Staphylococcal toxic shock is clinically similar to streptococcal toxic shock (high fever, mental confusion, erythroderma, diarrhoea, hypotension, and renal failure), but streptococcal toxic shock is typically associated with invasive infection such as necrotizing fasciitis while staphylococcal toxic shock may be precipitated by clinically minor infections that are overshadowed by the systemic effects of the toxin.

Staphylococcal toxic shock occurs in two major forms, menstrual (e.g. tampon-associated) and nonmenstrual. In women with vaginal colonization by *S. aureus*, it is presumably the favourable microenvironment during menses that leads to increased production of toxin (TSST-1).

Management of staphylococcal toxic shock relies on systemic antimicrobial therapy (Table 7.6.4.1), supportive care, and prompt drainage of infected/colonized foci. Common adjunctive therapies such as intravenous immunoglobulin to bind free toxin and antibacterials (especially clindamycin) with activity at the ribosome, which decreases bacterial protein (toxin) synthesis, have a theoretical rationale and some support from animal models; however, clinical data are limited.

Illness due to local tissue invasion/destruction

S. aureus and β-haemolytic streptococci cause approximately 80% of soft tissue infections. *S. aureus* is the aetiological agent of 37 to 65% of native monoarticular joint infections in healthy adults and of 75% of joint infections in rheumatoid arthritis. Osteomyelitis, either of haematogenous or contiguous origin, is caused by *S. aureus* or coagulase-negative staphylococci in more than 50% of cases. Any local infection can lead to secondary bacteraemia and haematogenous seeding of distant sites.

Impetigo, folliculitis, and cellulitis

The most superficial *S. aureus* infections are impetigo, folliculitis, and cellulitis. Impetigo is limited to the epidermis, folliculitis to the hair follicles, and cellulitis to the dermis and/or the subcutaneous fat.

Table 7.6.4.1 Therapy of toxic shock due to *S. aureus*

Drug	Dosage	Duration/comment
For penicillin-susceptible *S. aureus*:		Duration based on focus of infection
Penicillin[a]	2–4 MU IV every 4 h	Adequate drainage is critical
Ampicillin	1–2 g IV every 4–6 h	
Ampicillin + sulbactam	1.5–3 g IV every 6 h	
For methicillin-susceptible *S. aureus*:		Data to support adjunctive use of immunoglobulin and/or clindamycin are needed
Oxacillin/flucloxacillin[a]	1–2 g IV every 4–6 h	
Cefazolin	1–2 g IV every 8 h	
For methicillin-resistant *S. aureus* (or β-lactam allergy):		
Vancomycin[a]	1 g IV every 12 h	
Clindamycin[b]	600 mg IV every 8 h	
Daptomycin	6 mg/kg IV every 24 h	
Teicoplanin	At least 400 mg IV BID	
Linezolid[b]	600 mg IV every 12 h	
Quinupristin/dalfopristin	7.5 mg/kg every 12 h	
Intravenous immunoglobulin	Dosage not standardized	

BID, twice daily; IV, intravenously.
[a] First-line agent.
[b] These agents may be useful for reduction of protein synthesis and toxin production, but require further study.

Impetigo can appear as small round honey-crusted lesions on the skin, primarily on exposed areas (Fig. 7.6.4.2). Impetigo typically is caused by streptococci; in the United Kingdom, *S. aureus* is an infrequent cause. However, bullous impetigo is a clinical variant (caused by *S. aureus* phage type 71), reported in up to 10% of impetigo cases. Initially, the lesions can be vesicles that enlarge into bullae containing clear or yellow fluid.

Cellulitis is typically due to streptococci, but when associated with penetrating trauma, furuncles, or carbuncles *S. aureus* should be considered. Diagnosis depends on the clinical appearance and the presence of purulence that can be cultured. However, aspirates of cellulitic areas are positive in fewer than one-third of cases and bacteraemia is rare.

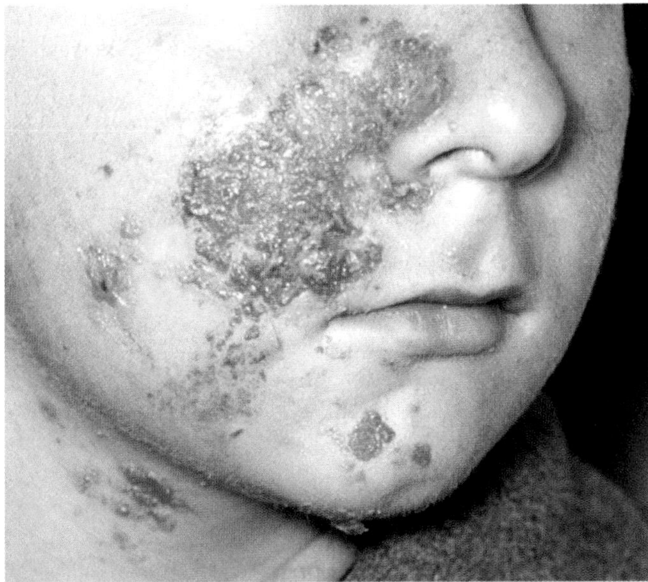

Fig. 7.6.4.2 Staphylococcal impetigo.
(Copyright Dr Renwick Vickers.)

Treatment of impetigo (Table 7.6.4.2) should reflect local antibiotic resistance patterns. Topical therapy may be effective for limited disease, though EMRSA-16, one of two predominant MRSA types in the United Kingdom, often shows high-level mupirocin resistance. Systemic therapy should be used in patients with impetigo who have many lesions or who fail topical therapy. In areas where CA-MRSA prevalence exceeds 10%, initial therapy should be directed by local susceptibility patterns.

Suspicion of more invasive infection, such as necrotizing fasciitis, should be high in cases of soft tissue infections with disproportionate pain, bullae, haemorrhagic or necrotic lesions, cutaneous anaesthesia, rapid progression of lesions, gas in the tissues, presence of risk factors, and when laboratory tests show elevated creatine kinase, acidosis, leucocytosis, or C-reactive protein exceeding 13 mg/litre. Necrotizing infections should prompt inpatient antibiotic therapy assuming MRSA and urgent surgical consultation.

Furuncles and carbuncles

Furuncles and carbuncles are deep suppurative infections that occur in the dermis and originate at hair follicles. Infection can be limited to small lesions that appear as painful nodules, sometimes with necrotic centres (Fig. 7.6.4.3a). Confluence leads to the formation of carbuncles (Fig. 7.6.4.3b). Several members of a family may be affected. Mild lesions cause limited systemic complaints, whereas fever, malaise, or symptoms and signs of sepsis can occur with extensive disease.

Table 7.6.4.2 Therapy of impetigo and mild soft tissue lesions caused by *S. aureus*

Therapy	Drug	Dosage	Duration
Topical	Mupirocin	2% ointment TID	14 days
	Fusidic acid	2% cream TID	
Oral	**For penicillin-susceptible *S. aureus*:**		
	Amoxicillin	250–500 mg PO TID or 875 mg PO BID	5 days
	Amoxicillin + clavulanate	250–500 mg PO TID or 875 mg/125 mg PO BID	
	Penicillin VK[a]	250–500 mg PO QID	
	For methicillin-susceptible *S. aureus*:		
	Dicloxacillin[a]	250 mg PO QID	
	Cefalexin	500 mg PO QID	
	For methicillin-resistant *S. aureus* (or β-lactam allergy):		
	Clindamycin (Ery^S, Clin^S, or D-test negative)	300–450 mg PO QID	
	Trimethoprim/sulfamethoxazole	1–2 double-strength[b] tablets PO BID	
	Doxycycline	100 mg PO BID	
	Minocycline	100 mg PO BID	
	Linezolid	600 mg po BID	

BID, twice daily; Clin^S, clindamycin-sensitive; D, double-disc diffusion; Ery^S, erythromycin-sensitive; PO, by mouth; QID, four times daily; TID, three times daily.
[a] First-line agent.
[b] 160 mg trimethoprim and 800 mg sulfamethoxazole in a double-strength tablet.

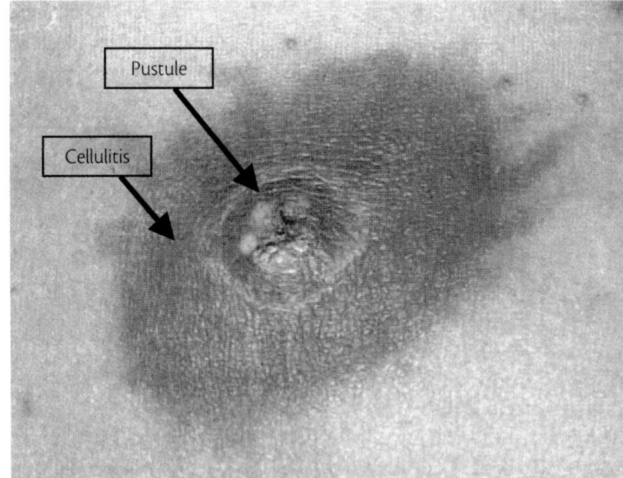

(a)

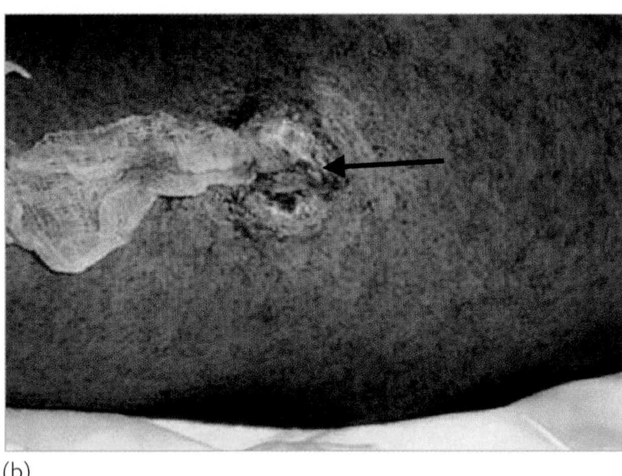

(b)

Fig. 7.6.4.3 (a) Pustule/early furuncle with surrounding cellulitis due to *S. aureus*. (b) Coalescent furuncles, i.e. carbuncle, that required incision and drainage.

Furunculosis is caused increasingly by the emerging pathogen CA-MRSA and has been attributed to the presence of PVL toxin, although the causal role requires validation. Additionally, toxin-containing *S. aureus* has been associated with more fulminant courses in which skin lesions, pneumonia, a sepsis-like picture, or even Waterhouse–Friderichsen syndrome occur. PVL occurs in about 2% of MSSA and most CA-MRSA.

Drainage, spontaneously or surgically, is the mainstay of therapy. Early furuncles may be treated by application of moist heat to stimulate drainage. Lesions on the face, lesions with cellulitis (especially exceeding 5 cm in diameter), or the presence of systemic symptoms and/or signs (fever, chills, or haemodynamic changes) should lead to use of antistaphylococcal antibiotics (Table 7.6.4.3) in addition to drainage. Oral agents are sufficient in most cases, but in severe infections or for bacteraemia parenteral agents should be used.

Mastitis

Mastitis is most commonly caused by *S. aureus*, occurs in 1 to 3% of nursing mothers typically within 3 weeks of birth, and may lead to breast abscesses. Infection can appear as a painful nodule or a draining abscess. Therapy (Table 7.6.4.3) should include topical moist heat, oral antimicrobials with efficacy against *S. aureus* (and MRSA in endemic areas), and abscess incision and drainage.

Pyomyositis

Pyomyositis, or primary bacterial abscess of skeletal muscle, is most common in the tropics where 'tropical pyomyositis' can account for 1 to 4% of hospital admissions (Chapter 24.24.6). In nontropical areas the syndrome is uncommon. *S. aureus* is the cause in about 95% of tropical cases and about 70% of other cases. Associations are with muscle trauma (20–50% of cases), HIV infection, and possibly *Toxocara canis* infection.

Symptoms develop subacutely over 2 to 3 weeks with variable degrees of fever, muscle pain, swelling, and induration. Large lower extremity and trunk muscles are most commonly affected. Regional lymphadenopathy is typically absent. Diagnosis relies on clinical suspicion, helpful radiographic findings (i.e. gas or soft tissue swelling on plain radiographs, abscess or muscle enlargement on ultrasound examination, inflammation, oedema, or focal abscess in muscles on MRI or CT, and the results of aspirating the lesion. Antibacterial therapy for *S. aureus* (Table 7.6.4.3) and open or radiographically assisted percutaneous drainage of abscesses are essential parts of therapy.

Septic bursitis

Infection can occur in any of the approximately 160 bursae found in humans, but septic bursitis usually affects prepatellar or olecranon bursae, usually is a result of trauma. It is due to *S. aureus* in more than 80% of cases but is accompanied by bacteraemia in 8% or less. Diagnosis relies on clinical recognition of the characteristic findings of fever and pain, swelling, redness, and warmth in the area of an affected bursa. Leucocytes and *S. aureus* are found if there is enough bursal fluid to aspirate.

Treatment of septic bursitis includes appropriate antimicrobials (Table 7.6.4.4) and, if possible, drainage. Treatment failures have been described when erythromycin is used as the sole agent. Localized infection with no systemic signs may be treated with oral therapy, since high antimicrobials levels are achieved in bursal fluid. Adequate drainage is important. Patients with systemic signs or symptoms or who are immunocompromised should receive parenteral therapy.

Patients who present within 7 days of developing symptoms may be treated successfully with antibiotics and aspiration every 1 to 3 days. In this situation, bursal fluid may become sterile within 4 days and therapy should be continued for an additional 5 days. Surgical intervention is needed only for patients whose fluid remains infected or cannot be aspirated because the bursa is deep, who have foreign or necrotic material in the bursal space, or who need exploration or removal of the bursa because of recurrences.

Septic arthritis

S. aureus is the most common cause of nonprosthetic monoarticular septic arthritis. The typical pathogenesis is haematogenous seeding, but traumatic direct inoculation can occur. Important differential diagnoses include gonococcal infection in adolescents and adults and urosepsis pathogens and crystal-induced arthropathies in older patients. Because joint destruction is rapid, prompt diagnosis through joint aspiration is essential.

The mainstays of therapy are antimicrobials (Table 7.6.4.4) and prompt joint drainage by serial aspiration; arthroscopy (preferred for knee, shoulder, and ankle) with irrigation, lysis of adhesions, and removal of purulent material; or open drainage (useful for hip or shoulder infections to protect blood supply to femoral or humeral heads, and in instances where repeated aspirates or

Table 7.6.4.3 Therapy of cellulitis, abscess, mastitis, furunculosis, and pyomyositis caused by *S. aureus*

Therapy	Drug	Dosage	Duration/comment
Oral	**For penicillin-susceptible S. *aureus*:**		5 days for cellulitis
	Amoxicillin	250–500 mg PO TID or 875 mg PO BID	For deeper infection duration depends on proper drainage when necessary and clinical response
	Amoxicillin + clavulanate	250–500 mg PO TID or 875 mg/125 mg PO BID	With incision and drainage, lesions with <5 cm of cellulitis in immunocompetent patients may be cured without systemic antibiotics
	Penicillin VK[a]	250–500 mg PO QID	For deeper infection duration depends on proper drainage when necessary and clinical response
	For methicillin-susceptible S. *aureus*:		Early change to oral therapy may be employed in stabilizing, nonbacteraemic patients
	Dicloxacillin[a]	500 mg PO QID	
	Cefalexin	500 mg PO QID	May have a future role
	For methicillin-resistant S. *aureus* (or β-lactam allergy):		
	Clindamycin (Ery[S], Clin[S], or D-test negative)	300–450 mg PO QID	
	Trimethoprim/sulfamethoxazole	1–2 double-strength[b] tablets PO BID	
	Doxycycline	100 mg PO BID	
	Minocycline	100 mg PO BID	
	Linezolid	600 mg PO BID	
	Erythromycin[c]	250 mg PO every 6 h or 500 mg PO every 12 h	
Parenteral	**For penicillin-susceptible S. *aureus*:**		
	Penicillin[a]	2–4 MU IV every 4 h	
	Ampicillin	1–2 g IV every 4–6 h	
	Ampicillin + sulbactam	1.5–3 g IV every 6 h	
	For methicillin-susceptible S. *aureus*:		
	Oxacillin/flucloxacillin[a]	1–2 g IV every 4–6 h	
	Cefazolin	1–2 g IV every 8 h	
	For methicillin-resistant S. *aureus* (or β-lactam allergy):		
	Vancomycin[a]	1 g IV every 12 h	
	Erythromycin[c]	250 mg IV every 6 h or 500 mg IV every 12 h	
	Clindamycin (Ery[S], Clin[S], or D-test negative)	600 mg IV every 8 h	
	Linezolid	600 mg IV every 12 h	
	Daptomycin	4 mg/kg IV every 24 h	
	Quinupristin/dalfopristin	7.5 mg/kg every 12 h	
	Tigecycline	100 mg initially, then 50 mg IV every 12 h	
	Dalbavancin, oritavancin, telavancin		

BID, twice daily; Clin[S], clindamycin-sensitive; D, double-disc diffusion; Ery[S], erythromycin-sensitive; PO, by mouth; QID, four times daily; TID three times daily; IV, intravenously.

[a] First-line agent.

[b] 160 mg trimethoprim and 800 mg sulfamethoxazole in a double-strength tablet.

[c] In many areas high rates of resistance should prevent empiric use of erythromycin.

arthroscopy fail). *S. aureus* can be a cause of infected prosthetic joints, which may have a more indolent atypical presentation.

Osteomyelitis

S. aureus osteomyelitis results from bacteraemia or contiguous spread from a soft tissue focus or chronic ulcer. Risk groups are patients with diabetes mellitus, those with vascular disease or at risk for haematogenous infection (i.e. haemodialysis), children, and elderly people.

Diagnosis usually depends on radiographic studies. Plain radiographs may show evidence of periosteal reaction, and nuclear triple-phase imaging may demonstrate focal persistent uptake in bone. The most sensitive test for osteomyelitis is MRI, which will demonstrate changes within bone and bone marrow. The most specific test is CT, which will reveal the presence of periosteal reaction or other bony changes not evident on plain radiographs. 'Probing to bone' in the case of a chronic ulcer is highly sensitive for a diagnosis of osteomyelitis. The microbiological diagnosis of

Table 7.6.4.4 Therapy of septic bursitis and septic arthritis caused by *S. aureus*

Therapy	Drug	Dosage	Duration/comment
Oral	**For penicillin-susceptible *S. aureus*:**		For septic bursitis, continue therapy for 5 days after aspirates become sterile (with early change to oral therapy in nonbacteraemic patients). For septic arthritis, therapy should be continued for 4 weeks
	Amoxicillin	250–500 mg PO TID or 875 mg PO BID	
	Amoxicillin + clavulanate	250–500 mg PO TID or 875 mg/125 mg PO BID	
	Penicillin VK[a]	250–500 mg PO QID	
	For methicillin-susceptible *S. aureus*:		
	Dicloxacillin[a]	500 mg PO QID	
	Cefalexin	500 mg PO QID	
	For methicillin-resistant *S. aureus* (or β-lactam allergy):		
	Clindamycin (Ery^S, Clin^S, or D-test negative)	300–450 mg PO QID	
	Trimethoprim/sulfamethoxazole	1–2 double-strength[b] tablets PO BID	
	Doxycycline	100 mg PO BID	
	Minocycline	100 mg PO BID	
	Ciprofloxacin or levofloxacin	500 mg PO BID or 500 mg PO once daily	
	With		
	Rifampin	300 mg PO every 12 h	
	Linezolid	600 mg PO BID	
	Erythromycin[c]	250 mg PO every 6 h or 500 mg PO every 12 h	
Parenteral	**For penicillin-susceptible *S. aureus*:**		
	Penicillin[a]	2–4 MU IV every 4 h	
	Ampicillin	1–2 g IV every 4–6 h	
	Ampicillin + sulbactam	1.5–3 g IV every 6 h	
	For methicillin-susceptible *S. aureus*:		
	Oxacillin/flucloxacillin[a]	1–2 g IV every 4–6 h	
	Cefazolin	1–2 g IV every 8 h	
	For methicillin-resistant *S. aureus* (or β-lactam allergy):		
	Vancomycin[a]	1 g IV every 12 h	
	Linezolid	600 mg IV every 12 h	

BID, twice daily; Clin^S, clindamycin-sensitive; D, double-disc diffusion; Ery^S, erythromycin-sensitive; PO, by mouth; QID, four times daily; TID three times daily; IV, intravenously.
[a] First-line agent.
[b] 160 mg trimethoprim and 800 mg sulfamethoxazole in a double-strength tablet.
[c] In many areas high rates of resistance should prevent empiric use of erythromycin.

osteomyelitis relies on positive blood or bone cultures; superficial wound or sinus track culture results are not reliable and may be misleading.

Therapy for osteomyelitis includes drainage of pus (acute osteomyelitis) or debridement of areas of avascular or 'dead' bone (sequestra in chronic osteomyelitis) and antibacterials with activity against the culture-proven pathogen(s). The duration of therapy sufficient to eradicate the organism and prevent relapse is based on common experience and usually is 4 to 6 weeks. Children with acute haematogenous *S. aureus* osteomyelitis may be treated with surgical drainage of purulent collections and short-course intravenous therapy (e.g. 1 week) followed by oral therapy for 4 to 6 weeks as outpatients. Initial choice for therapy is based on the presence of MSSA or MRSA (Table 7.6.4.5); copathogens may require broader therapy. An open-label study showed that for diabetic foot infections, linezolid performed as well as ampicillin–sulbactam for infected ulcers or osteomyelitis.

Epidural abscess

Epidural abscesses occur adjacent to vertebral osteomyelitis and are medical/surgical emergencies (Fig. 7.6.4.4). Enlarging epidural sites can compress the spinal cord or reduce vascular supply through thrombophlebitis. About 50% of cases follow haematogenous spread from known or occult trauma or from parenteral use of illicit drugs, while about 30% result from contiguous spread. *S. aureus* accounts for more than 60% of cases. Risks for MRSA infection include recent health care exposure or rising CA-MRSA rates.

Symptoms and physical findings progress at variable rates, sometimes rapidly, through four stages: (1) back pain at the infected level, (2) pain radiating in the distribution of affected nerve roots, (3) motor weakness (including bladder and bowel dysfunction) and sensory deficit at the appropriate level, and (4) paralysis. The triad of back pain, fever, and neurological findings is highly suggestive of epidural abscess.

MRI or CT scanning is most useful for evaluating epidural abscesses (Fig. 7.6.4.4). For diagnosis and therapy, a space-occupying lesion in the epidural space requires surgical evaluation and emergency laminectomy/decompression or drainage by interventional radiography. Preoperative neurological status predicts outcome. Broad empirical antimicrobial therapy should include coverage for MRSA (Table 7.6.4.6) and Gram-negative bacilli.

Table 7.6.4.5 Therapy of osteomyelitis caused by *S. aureus*

Therapy	Drug	Dosage	Duration
Parenteral	**For penicillin-susceptible *S. aureus*:**		4–6 weeks IV
	Penicillin[a]	2–4 MU IV every 4 h	
	Ampicillin	1–2 g IV every 4–6 h	
	Ampicillin + sulbactam	1.5–3 g IV every 6 h	
	For methicillin-susceptible *S. aureus*:		
	Oxacillin/flucloxacillin[a]	1–2 g IV every 4–6 h	
	Cefazolin	1–2 g IV every 8 h	
	For methicillin-resistant *S. aureus* (or β-lactam allergy):		
	Vancomycin[a]	1 g IV every 12 h	
	Linezolid	600 mg IV every 12 h	

IV, intravenously.
[a] First-line agent.

If MSSA infection is diagnosed, β-lactams are preferred over glycopeptides.

Pneumonia

S. aureus pneumonia can result from haematogenous spread or direct inoculation following mucosal damage. *S. aureus* causes less than 10% of cases of community-acquired pneumonia but causes approximately 20 to 30% of cases of nosocomial pneumonia. Case fatality of *S. aureus* pneumonia ranges from 8% to more than 30%. Risks for a more severe course include MRSA, acute respiratory distress syndrome (ARDS), comorbidities, and renal dysfunction.

S. aureus is a cause of postviral, particularly postinfluenzal, pneumonia. Patients may report a biphasic illness. CA-MRSA may cause a necrotizing pneumonia with more severe course. Additionally, *S. aureus* pneumonia may be associated with complications such as empyema, lung abscesses, and bronchopleural fistulae. Lung abscess must be differentiated radiographically from pneumatocele, a common and relatively benign complication of staphylococcal pneumonia.

Diagnostic studies for patients with pneumonia in the presence of staphylococcal bacteraemia or embolic-appearing lesions on chest imaging (Fig. 7.6.4.5) should seek an intravascular source (e.g. endocarditis or infectious thrombophlebitis). Therapy (Table 7.6.4.7) should include use of an active drug for at least 8 days in less complicated cases or longer if pulmonary involvement is secondary to an intravascular infection, presence of MRSA, or complications such as emboli or empyema. Surgical drainage is indicated for empyema. Daptomycin should be avoided because of its poorer activity in pulmonary infections. Linezolid may emerge as a drug of choice for MRSA pneumonia based on its greater penetration due to smaller molecule size and putative clinical benefit.

Urinary tract infections

S. aureus urinary tract infections (UTIs) result from ascending infection in catheterized patients or haematogenous seeding, which may lead to renal carbuncles (abscesses). Staphylococcal UTIs should prompt consideration of sources of bacteraemia such as endovascular infection. Clinically, patients with renal abscesses have fever and flank pain, but urinary complaints may be absent and urinalyses and urine cultures may be negative. Renal ultrasonography or CT may show a range of findings from 'lobar nephronia' (renal phlegmon) to large multilocular abscesses. Treatment may require percutaneous or open drainage; antimicrobial therapy (Table 7.6.4.8) should reflect results of cultures.

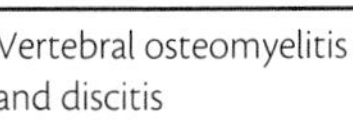

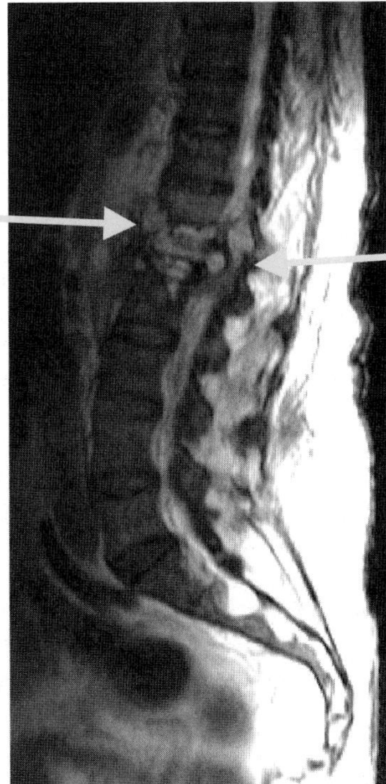

Fig. 7.6.4.4 Epidural abscess and vertebral osteomyelitis due to *S. aureus*.

Table 7.6.4.6 Therapy of epidural abscess caused by *S. aureus*

Therapy	Drug	Dosage	Duration
Parenteral	**For penicillin-susceptible *S. aureus*:**		≥6 weeks IV
	Penicillin[a]	2–4 MU IV every 4 h	
	Ampicillin	1–2 g IV every 4–6 h	
	Ampicillin + sulbactam	1.5–3 g IV every 6 h	
	For methicillin-susceptible *S. aureus*:		
	Oxacillin/flucloxacillin[a]	1–2 g IV every 4–6 h	
	Cefazolin	1–2 g IV every 8 h	
	For methicillin-resistant *S. aureus* (or β-lactam allergy):		
	Vancomycin[a]	1 g IV every 12 h	
	Linezolid	600 mg IV every 12 h	
	Daptomycin	6 mg/kg IV every 24 h	

IV, intravenously.
[a] First-line agent.

Table 7.6.4.7 Therapy of pneumonia due to *S. aureus*

Drug	Dosage	Duration/comment
For penicillin-susceptible *S. aureus*:		8–14 days for uncomplicated infection
Penicillin[a]	2–4 MU IV every 4 h	
Ampicillin	1–2 g IV every 4–6 h	
Ampicillin + sulbactam	1.5–3 g IV every 6 h	
For methicillin-susceptible *S. aureus*:		Requires longer courses if empyema, lung abscess, or bacteraemia present
Oxacillin/flucloxacillin[a]	1–2 g IV every 4 h	
Cefazolin	1–2 g IV every 8 h	
For methicillin-resistant *S. aureus* (or β-lactam allergy):		
Vancomycin[a]	1 g IV every 12 h	
Linezolid	600 mg IV every 12 h	

IV, intravenously.
[a] First-line agent.

Haematogenous infections

Bacteraemia

S. aureus is among the commonest causes of bacteraemia in hospitals and the community. It causes 18 to 27% of endocarditis cases (Fig. 7.6.4.6), is responsible for 13% of nosocomial bloodstream infections, and causes up to 78% of cases of intravascular catheter-related thrombophlebitis. Rates of community-associated *S. aureus* bacteraemia in the United States of America are estimated at 17/100 000 people, similar to rates of invasive *Streptococcus pneumoniae* infection, with mortality of 10 to 20%, depending on underlying illnesses. In Oxfordshire, England, the incidence of nosocomial MRSA bacteraemia increased from 50/100 000 admissions in 1997 to 300/100 000 admissions in 2004, increasing the overall burden of *S. aureus* disease.

S. aureus in blood should always be considered a true pathogen. Bacteraemia has traditionally been categorized as 'health care-associated' (i.e. onset more than 2 days after admission) and 'community-associated' (i.e. onset within 2 days of admission). Complications of bacteraemia include endocarditis (itself a major cause of bacteraemia) and 'metastatic' seeding of distant sites, especially joints, bone, kidney, and skin (Fig. 7.6.4.7). An estimated 13% of nosocomial bacteraemias with *S. aureus* include endocarditis.

The principles of therapy for *S. aureus* bacteraemia include evaluation for endocarditis; use of a parenteral agent; removal of infected foci (i.e. catheters or abscesses); and use of a bactericidal agent, preferably a β-lactam, whenever possible. Occasionally, uncomplicated bacteraemia with drainage of infected foci and no embolic sites may respond to only 14 days of therapy (Table 7.6.4.9); however, more often, prolonged bacteraemia, residual disease, undrained foci of infection, infected clots, or endocarditis all warrant longer therapy (at least 4 weeks).

Endocarditis (Chapter 16.9.2)

Many features of endocarditis are nonspecific (fever, tachycardia, arthralgias and myalgias, wasting, and back pain). Finding a new cardiac (especially diastolic) murmur or septic emboli provides strong supportive evidence. Other suggestive findings include

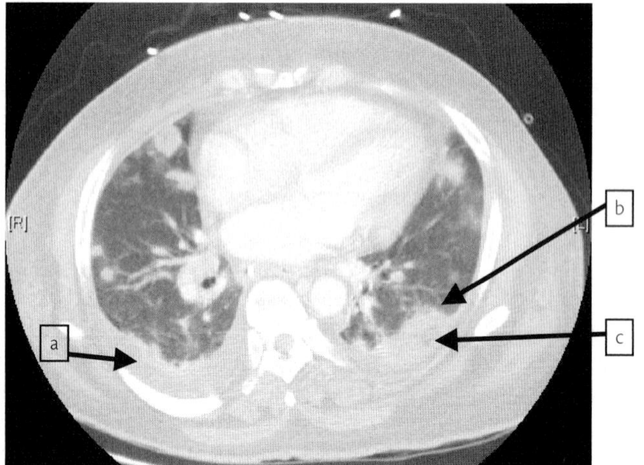

Fig. 7.6.4.5 Pneumonia due to *S. aureus*, from septic pulmonary emboli. Note presence of (a) empyema, (b) nodular (including pleural-based) infiltrate, and (c) early cavitation of abscess.

Table 7.6.4.8 Therapy of urinary tract infection due to *S. aureus*

Drug	Dosage	Duration/comment
For penicillin-susceptible *S. aureus*:		7 days for ascending infection
Penicillin[a]	2–4 MU IV every 4 h	
Ampicillin	1–2 g IV every 4–6 h	≥ 14 days for renal abscess, bacteraemia, or complicated infection (duration is based on resolution of infected foci and/or use of drainage)
Ampicillin + sulbactam	1.5–3 g IV every 6 h	
For methicillin-susceptible *S. aureus*:		
Oxacillin/flucloxacillin[a]	1–2 g IV every 4 h	
Cefazolin	1–2 g IV every 8 h	
For methicillin-resistant *S. aureus* (or β-lactam allergy):		
Vancomycin[a]	1 g IV every 12 h	
Linezolid	600 mg IV every 12 h	

IV, intravenously.
[a] First-line agent.

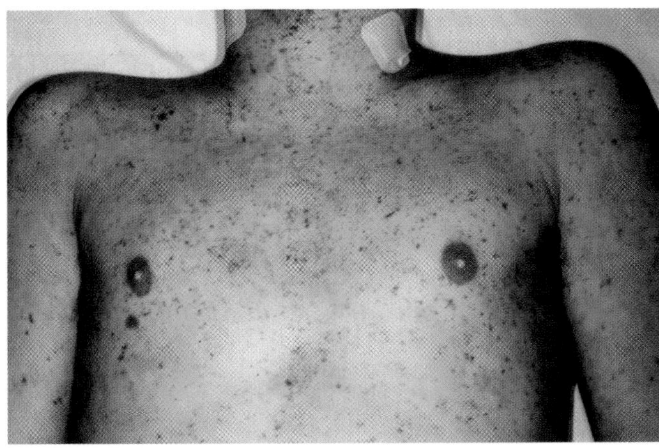

(a)

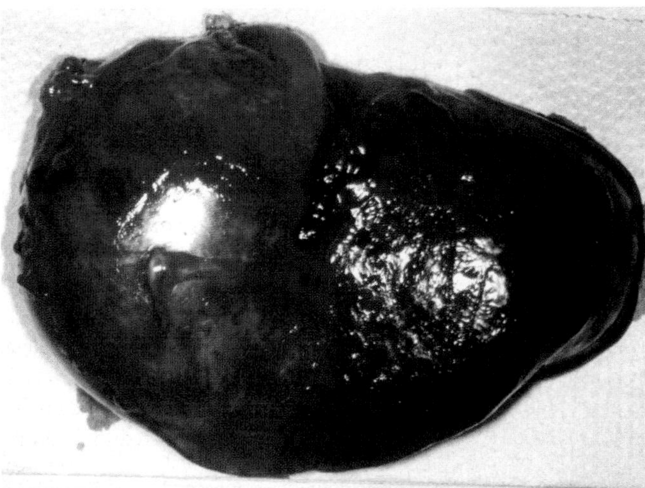

(b)

Fig. 7.6.4.6 *S. aureus* bacteraemia and infective endocarditis. (a) Meningococcal-like rash in a patient with *S. aureus* endocarditis of a bicuspid aortic valve and aortic root abscess. (b) Splenic abscess complicating *S. aureus* endocarditis. (Copyright Professor S J Eykyn.)

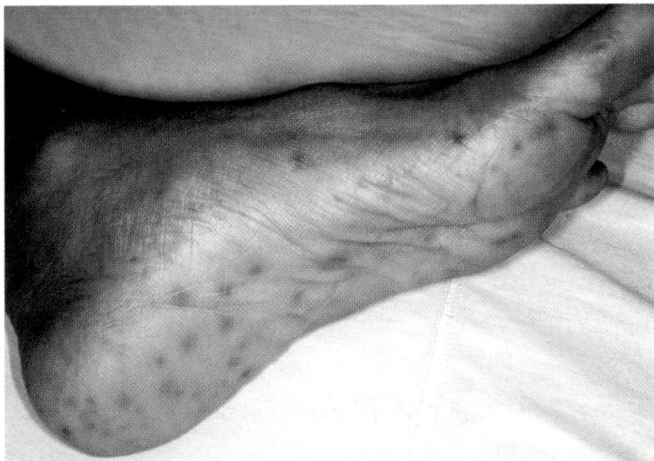

Fig. 7.6.4.7 Seeding of MRSA to the skin in a Vietnamese patient. (Copyright D A Warrell.)

Table 7.6.4.9 Therapy of bacteraemia, without endocarditis, due to *S. aureus*

Drug	Dosage	Duration/comment
For penicillin-susceptible *S. aureus*:		14 days with removable focus of infection Longer course of therapy for complicated infection
Penicillin[a]	2–4 MU IV every 4 h	
Ampicillin	1–2 g IV every 4–6 h	
Ampicillin + sulbactam	1.5–3 g IV every 6 h	
For methicillin-susceptible *S. aureus*:		
Oxacillin/flucloxacillin[a]	1–2 g IV every 4–6 h	
Cefazolin	1–2 g IV every 8 h	
For methicillin-resistant *S. aureus* (or β-lactam allergy):		
Vancomycin[a]	1 g IV every 12 h	
Daptomycin[a]	6 mg/kg IV every 24 h	
Teicoplanin	At least 400 mg IV BID	
Linezolid	600 mg IV every 12 h	
Quinupristin/dalfopristin	7.5 mg/kg every 12 h	
Sodium fusidate	500 mg IV every 8 h	
Dalbavancin, oritavancin, telavancin	May have future role	

BID, twice daily; IV, intravenously.
[a] First-line agent.

petechiae, Janeway's lesions, mycotic aneurysms of arterial vessels (with resultant pain, vascular leak, or adjacent deep venous thrombosis), discitis or osteomyelitis (particularly vertebral disease), and neurological complications such as septic infarcts or mycotic cerebrovascular aneurysms. Conduction abnormalities, e.g. AV delay, may be noted in the presence of myocardial abscess. In the setting of right-sided endocarditis, septic pulmonary emboli are common.

The presence of multiple positive blood cultures is a necessary criterion for diagnosis of endocarditis in the untreated patient. Diagnosis is aided by specific criteria (e.g. modified Duke's criteria). Transthoracic echocardiography is indicated as a noninvasive method to evaluate the presence of cardiac vegetations in those with low pretest probability of disease; individuals with nondiagnostic studies or worsening clinical course should undergo transoesophageal echocardiogram. Patients with high clinical risk, despite nondiagnostic transoesophageal studies, should be restudied after 7 to 10 days.

Therapy for staphylococcal endocarditis requires a bactericidal antibiotic (Tables 7.6.4.10–7.6.4.12). In general, therapy should last for 4 (in uncomplicated disease) to 6 or more (in the setting of metastatic infection, perivalvular abscess, or other complications) weeks. Combination therapies (agents given with either vancomycin or β-lactams) have not been demonstrated to improve outcomes in native valve endocarditis but are commonly used. For example, the addition of gentamicin for 3 to 5 days shortens the duration of bacteraemia by about 1 day but does not influence outcome. Addition of rifampicin for bacteraemic patients with putative failure of therapy (e.g. bacteraemia or fever persisting for more than 4–5 days) is a common strategy. Rifampicin is recommended as part of the standard treatment of prosthetic valve endocarditis.

The average time to clearance of *S. aureus* from the bloodstream is 5 days of β-lactam or 1 week of vancomycin therapy.

Table 7.6.4.10 Therapy of native valve left-sided endocarditis due to *S. aureus*

Drug	Dosage	Duration/comment
For penicillin-susceptible *S. aureus*:		4–6 weeks after negative cultures
Penicillin[a]	2–4 MU IV every 4 h	
Ampicillin	1–2 g IV every 4–6 h	
Ampicillin + sulbactam	1.5–3 g IV every 6 h	
For methicillin-susceptible *S. aureus*:		
Oxacillin/flucloxacillin[a]	2 g IV every 4 h	
Cefazolin	1–2 g IV every 8 h	
For methicillin-resistant *S. aureus* (or β-lactam allergy):		
Vancomycin[a]	1 g IV every 12 h	
Teicoplanin[a]	At least 400 mg IV BID	
Linezolid	600 mg IV every 12 h	
Quinupristin/ dalfopristin	7.5 mg/kg every 12 h	
Daptomycin	6 mg/kg IV every 24 h	
Sodium fusidate	500 mg IV every 8 h	
Trimethoprim/ sulfamethoxazole	320 mg/1600 mg IV every 12 h	
Above therapies can be used with:		
Gentamicin[b] (3–5 days at start of therapy)	1 mg/kg IV every 8 h	

BID, twice daily; IV, intravenously.
[a] First-line agent.
[b] Gentamicin therapy is optional, and has not been demonstrated to change clinical outcomes.

Prolonged bacteraemia should prompt a closer evaluation of antibiotic MICs (especially for vancomycin), a search for sequestered sites of infection or undrained foci, or a myocardial or valvular abscess. Increasing vancomycin dosing has not been demonstrated clearly to improve outcomes, although consensus supports increased trough levels of 15 to 20 mcg/ml (requiring close monitoring of renal function) for strains with upper-end susceptible MICs. Indications for surgical valve replacement include new congestive heart failure (associated with higher mortality), failure to clear the bloodstream, recurrent emboli, and myocardial or valvular abscess.

Table 7.6.4.11 Therapy of native valve right-sided endocarditis due to *S. aureus*

Drug	Dosage	Duration/comment
β-Lactams	As for left-sided disease (Table 7.6.4.10)	4–6 weeks after negative cultures
Vancomycin[a]	As for left-sided disease (Table 7.6.4.10)	
Daptomycin[a]	6 mg/kg IV every 24 h	
Above therapies can be used with:		
Gentamicin[b]	1 mg/kg IV every 8 h	3–5 days at start of therapy, or combined therapy with β-lactam for MSSA infection
Ciprofloxacin/ rifampicin[b]	750 mg/300 mg PO BID	For use in patients with tricuspid valve endocarditis who can not/will not be admitted for intravenous therapy

BID, twice daily; IV, intravenously; PO, by mouth.
[a] First-line agent.
[b] Use is indicated in only limited circumstances. Gentamicin therapy is optional and has not been shown to improve clinical outcomes.

Table 7.6.4.12 Therapy of prosthetic valve endocarditis due to *S. aureus*

Drug	Dosage	Duration/comment
For penicillin-susceptible *S. aureus*:		
Penicillin[a]	2–4 MU IV every 4 h	
Ampicillin	1–2 g IV every 4–6 h	
Ampicillin + sulbactam	1.5–3 g IV every 6 h	
For methicillin-susceptible *S. aureus*:		
Oxacillin/flucloxacillin[a]	2 g IV every 4 h	≥6 weeks
With		
Rifampicin	300 mg PO/IV every 8 h	≥6 weeks
And		
Gentamicin	1 mg/kg IV every 8 h	3–5 days at start of therapy
Cefazolin (second choice for MSSA)	1–2 g IV every 8 h	
For methicillin-resistant *S. aureus* (or β-lactam allergy):		
Vancomycin[a]	1 g IV every 12 h	
With		
Rifampicin	300 mg PO/IV every 8 h	≥6 weeks
And		
Gentamicin	1 mg/kg IV every 8 h	3–5 days at start of therapy

IV, intravenously; PO, by mouth.
[a] First-line agent.

Clinical syndromes: coagulase-negative staphylococci

Coagulase-negative staphylococci are generally less virulent than *S. aureus*. Most infections with these organisms are the consequence of medical progress, related to foreign bodies (e.g. prosthetic joints or heart valves, indwelling intravascular catheters or grafts, or peritoneal catheters), and occur in association with health care. Syndromes caused by coagulase-negative staphylococci include endocarditis (5–8% of native valve infections, *c.*40% of prosthetic valve infections), intravascular catheter infections (6–27% of vascular catheter infections), prosthetic joint infections (up to 38% of arthroplasty infections), peritoneal dialysis catheter infections, and postoperative ocular infections. Production of biofilm by coagulase-negative staphylococci aids infection of both intravascular and peritoneal catheters. Therapy for infections with coagulase-negative staphylococci and side effects and toxicities are outlined in Tables 7.6.4.13 and 7.6.4.14.

Bacteraemia and infected vascular catheters

Clinical features and diagnosis

Coagulase-negative staphylococci are the most commonly reported bacteria in positive blood cultures; however, unlike *S. aureus*,

Table 7.6.4.13 Therapy for coagulase-negative staphylococcal infections

Indication	Drug	Dosage	Duration
Bacteraemia (with prompt catheter removal)	Vancomycin[a]	1 g IV every 12 h	10–14 days
	Oxacillin/flucloxacillin (methicillin-susceptible *S. epidermidis*)	1–2 g IV every 4 h	
Bacteraemia (with attempted catheter salvage)	Vancomycin catheter lock (for catheter salvage)	1–5 mg/ml vancomycin, mixed with 50–100 U heparin or normal saline, to fill catheter lumen (total 2–5 ml of solution) when catheter not in use	14 days
	Vancomycin[a]	1 g IV every 12 h	10–14 days
	Oxacillin/flucloxacillin (methicillin-susceptible *S. epidermidis*)	1–2 g IV every 4 h	
Prosthetic valve endocarditis	Vancomycin[a] with	1 g IV every 12 h	≥6 weeks
	Rifampicin[a] and	300 mg PO/IV every 8 h	
	Gentamicin	1 mg/kg IV every 8 h	
	Oxacillin/flucloxacillin (methicillin-susceptible *S. epidermidis*)	1–2 g IV every 4 h	
Peritoneal dialysis-associated peritonitis	Vancomycin[a]	30–50 mg vancomycin per litre of dialysate given i ntraperitoneally	10–21 days
	Or		
	Vancomycin	1 g IV once, then based on levels (keep trough >10–15 mcg/ml)	10–21 days

IV, intravenously; PO, by mouth.
[a] First-line agent.

coagulase-negative staphylococci are frequently blood culture contaminants. Typical rates of blood culture contamination by skin flora are approximately 2 to 3%; higher rates may be a sign of poor phlebotomy technique.

Infected intravascular catheters are common sources of coagulase-negative staphylococcal bloodstream infections. However, given the association of *S. epidermidis* and contaminated blood cultures, a careful physical examination for signs of catheter infection is critical to determine whether a single positive blood culture represents true infection and/or an infected catheter. Suggestive findings include fever, erythema at or purulence expressible from the site of catheter insertion, or tenderness.

Methods to enhance the identification of true bloodstream infection as opposed to contamination include proper skin preparation and obtaining at least two sets of blood cultures from sites separated by location and time. The use of quantitative catheter tip cultures (more than 15 colonies) or differential time to positivity (more than 2 h) for peripheral compared to catheter-drawn blood cultures helps assess whether a catheter is infected.

Management of bacteraemia and catheter infection

An approach for management of presumed infected catheters is to remove the catheter when the index of suspicion is high and/or the patient is unstable, with insertion of a new catheter at an uninvolved site. When likelihood of infection is unclear and the patient is stable, the catheter can be changed over a guidewire and the tip cultured. Positive tip cultures should prompt removal of the replacement catheter and new catheter insertion at a different site. A negative culture may allow the replacement catheter to remain in place, although its risk of subsequent infection is increased by the exchange process.

Parenteral vancomycin is the mainstay of therapy for vascular catheters infected by methicillin-resistant coagulase-negative staphylococci, and should be continued for 7 to 14 days unless there is metastatic seeding requiring longer treatment. Antibiotic lock therapy (Table 7.6.4.13) may be useful in carefully selected patients for 'line salvage'. The presence of tenderness along the course of a tunnelled catheter is highly predictive of failure of medical management and should lead to catheter removal.

Endocarditis

Multiple positive blood cultures with coagulase-negative staphylococci may indicate the presence of infective endocarditis. More than 80% of patients with prosthetic valve infection have persistent fever, deep valve involvement (e.g. infection of the sewing ring or valve dysfunction, dehiscence, or abscess), and/or cardiac conduction abnormalities. Infections within the first 6 to 12 months following surgery typically reflect acquisition of the organism in the perioperative period and may have a higher likelihood of complicated infection.

Diagnosis of prosthetic valve infection should be sought aggressively when multiple positive cultures with coagulase-negative staphylococci have been obtained in the postcardiac operative period. Physical examination usually shows fever and a new or worsening murmur or valve dysfunction. Evaluation includes serial blood cultures to document degree and persistence of bacteraemia, electrocardiography to search for conduction delay, and

Table 7.6.4.14 Information on indications and toxicity for selected drugs

Drug class	Indications/use	Side effects/toxicities
Semisynthetic penicillins		
Flucloxacillin Oxacillin	Drugs of choice in penicillin-resistant MSSA infection	Interstitial nephritis (which limits methicillin use in adults)
Nafcillin	Not effective in MRSA infection	Neutropenia (nafcillin)
Dicloxacillin	CA-MRSA may equal or exceed 50% prevalence in some areas Range of prevalence of nosocomial MRSA is 2–70% Adequate incision and drainage of infected foci is critical	Elevated transaminases (oxacillin, nafcillin)
First-generation cephalosporins		
Cefazolin Cefalexin	Alternative agents for penicillin-resistant, MSSA infection Not effective in MRSA infection CA-MRSA may equal or exceed 50% prevalence in some areas Range of prevalence of nosocomial MRSA is 2–70% Adequate incision and drainage of infected foci is critical	15% cross-reaction for penicillin-allergic patients Hypersensitivity Eosinophilia
Penicillins and aminopenicillins		
Penicillin Ampicillin Amoxicillin Ampicillin + sulbactam Amoxicillin + clavulanate	Penicillin is the drug of choice in known penicillin-sensitive *S. aureus* infection	Hypersensitivity
	Duration of therapy and indications similar to those of oxacillin	
Glycopeptides		
Vancomycin Teicoplanin Dalbavancin Oritavancin Telavancin	Indicated for MRSA infections or MSSA infections in penicillin-allergic patients	3–11% of patients given vancomycin may develop anaphylactoid reaction (i.e. 'red man' or 'red-neck' syndrome) due to overly rapid infusion
	Indicated for coagulase-negative staphylococcal infections	Nephrotoxicity with vancomycin (0–7% alone, 14–20+% in conjunction with aminoglycoside) and teicoplanin (5%)
	MRSA that are vancomycin susceptible but have increased MIC may require higher doses	Neutropenia with vancomycin (1–2%)
	Vancomycin trough levels should be 10–15 mg/litre and monitored closely in the setting of renal dysfunction; ≥15 if vancomycin MIC >1 mcg/ml Teicoplanin levels should be >10 mg/litre in bacteraemia and >20 mg/litre in endocarditis	Erythematous rash with teicoplanin (7%)
Lincosamide		
Clindamycin	Indicated for nonsevere MRSA infections that are erythromycin and clindamycin susceptible or that are erythromycin resistant and double-disc diffusion (D) test is negative	20% of patients develop diarrhoea
	An option for nonsevere MSSA infections in penicillin-allergic patients	Increased risk of *Clostridium difficile*-associated diarrhoea (10%)
Tetracyclines		
Doxycycline Minocycline Tigecycline	Not recommended in children aged <8 years	Photosensitivity
	Bacteriostatic, not recommended for bacteraemia or severe infections	Eosinophilia
	Recent review in osteomyelitis demonstrated success rate in over 80%; retained foreign body in osteomyelitis may lead to failure	SLE-like reaction with minocycline
	Likely need additional agent for treatment of long duration (i.e. rifampicin or fluoroquinolone) to prevent emergence of resistance	Pseudotumour cerebri or vestibular toxicity
	Potency/activity of drugs: tigecycline > minocycline > doxycycline > tetracycline	Antianabolic

Table 7.6.4.14 (*Cont'd*) Information on indications and toxicity for selected drugs

Drug class	Indications/use	Side effects/toxicities
Dihydrofolate reductase inhibitors		
Trimethoprim/ sulfamethoxazole	Higher failure rate as compared with vancomycin in MSSA endocarditis seen in one study MRSA endocarditis success equivalent to vancomycin TMP/SMX resistance may be common among nosocomial MRSA (up to 50%) but is generally uncommon among CA-MRSA (<10%)	Hypersensitivity, may progress to erythema multiforme and/or Stevens–Johnson syndrome Macrocytic anaemia Photosensitivity Methaemoglobinaemia (rare)
Fluoroquinolones		
Ciprofloxacin Gatifloxacin Gemifloxacin Levofloxacin Lomefloxacin Moxifloxacin Ofloxacin Norfloxacin Pefloxacin Others	Should not be used as monotherapy due to rapid emergence of resistance May possibly be used with other agents (e.g. TMP/SMX, rifampicin) Ciprofloxacin or levofloxacin in combination with rifampicin may be an option for patients with uncomplicated tricuspid valve endocarditis who cannot/will not be admitted; or those with skin/soft tissue infection with CA-MRSA	Neurological (0.9–11% delirium and/or seizures) Arthropathy, tendinitis, tendon rupture Hypoglycaemia
Rifamycins		
Rifampicin	Part of combination treatment of prosthetic valve endocarditis, or in setting of endovascular infection with a foreign body Should be used with another agent given rapid acquisition of resistance	Gastrointestinal complaints Hepatitis Myeloid suppression Acute tubular necrosis or acute interstitial nephritis SLE-like syndrome
Macrolides		
Erythromycin Clarithromycin Azithromycin	May be used in penicillin-allergic patients for skin/soft tissue infections Should be used with caution based on local susceptibility to erythromycin in *S. aureus* and emergence of resistance	Gastrointestinal complaints (prokinetic) QT prolongation in conjunction with other medications
Oxazolidinones		
Linezolid	Comparable indications to vancomycin; of use in therapy for MRSA or VISA/VRSA Data suggest better efficacy than vancomycin for pneumonia and skin/soft tissue infections with MRSA Has been used for bacteraemia in small open label trials Bacteriostatic Limited clinical experience	Myelosuppression Serotonin syndrome Peripheral neuropathy Lactic acidosis (due to mitochondrial toxicity)
Lipopeptides		
Daptomycin	Bactericidal May have use in VISA/VRSA Resistance has been noted to develop on therapy Not indicated for treatment of pneumonia 'Noninferior' to vancomycin for right-sided endocarditis and uncomplicated bacteraemia with *S. aureus* and possibly better for MRSA	Myopathy, especially with higher doses or in the setting of renal insufficiency
Streptogramins		
Quinupristin/dalfopristin	May have use in soft tissue infections, bacteraemia, or osteomyelitis in settings where other agents are not available/ useful May have use in MRSA or VISA/VRSA infections Presence of inducible or constitutive clindamycin resistance (i.e. MLS resistance) may indicate elevated MICs for quinupristin/ dalfopristin	Phlebitis (30%)—limits general usefulness Arthralgias (9.1%) Myalgias (6.6%)

(*Continued*)

Table 7.6.4.14 (*Cont'd*) Information on indications and toxicity for selected drugs

Drug class	Indications/use	Side effects/toxicities
Sodium fusidate	Topical therapy for impetigo	Thrombophlebitis (parenteral use)
	May be used parenterally in therapy of MRSA bacteraemia or endocarditis, depending on susceptibility	Reversible jaundice (parenteral use)
	Should not be used in newborns	Thrombocytopenia (parenteral use)

CA, community-acquired; MIC, minimum inhibitory concentration; MLS, macrolide–lincosamide–streptogramin, MRSA, methicillin-resistant *S. aureus*; MSSA, methicillin-susceptible *S. aureus*; SLE, systemic lupus erythematosus; TMP/SMX, trimethoprim/sulfamethoxazole, VISA/VRSA, vancomycin-intermediate/vancomycin-resistant *S. aureus*.

echocardiography or angiography for documentation of valve function. Therapy for prosthetic valve endocarditis should include parenteral vancomycin (for methicillin-resistant strains), gentamicin, and/or rifampicin (Table 7.6.4.13).

Peritoneal dialysis-associated peritonitis

Peritoneal dialysis catheter infection is characterized by abdominal pain, cloudy exchange fluid, and peritoneal fluid containing predominantly polymorphonuclear leucocytes (more than 100 leucocytes/mm^3). To improve diagnostic yield of peritoneal dialysate fluid cultures, 2 to 3 ml of fluid can be inoculated into thioglycolate broth or blood culture bottles.

Therapy for catheter-associated *S. epidermidis* peritonitis depends on susceptibility results. For susceptible organisms, β-lactams, trimethoprim/sulfamethoxazole, and vancomycin have all been effective, and both parenteral and oral antibiotics have been used. However, if methicillin-resistant *S. epidermidis* is suspected, vancomycin therapy (Table 7.6.4.13) with monitoring of serum levels may be indicated. Therapy can consist of either systemic or intraperitoneal antimicrobial administration. Intraperitoneal therapy is advantageous because it allows continued ambulatory care and therapy directly to the site of infection. Catheter salvage is frequently possible, but relapses may lead to catheter removal.

Other organisms

S. saprophyticus is a common cause of UTIs (20% of UTIs in women 16–35 years old). *S. lugdunensis* has been reported as a cause of endocarditis, including native valves, and bloodstream infection; its true incidence is not clear given the lack of speciation of most coagulase-negative staphylococci in many laboratories. *S. lugdunensis* infections have been characterized by a clinical course more like that of *S. aureus*, with valve destruction a prominent part of the illness.

Likely developments in the near future

Future directions in the management of *S. aureus* infections include vaccine development, new antimicrobials, enhanced understanding of epidemiology and control of nosocomial-associated and CA-MRSA, and evaluation and control of the emergence of VISA/VRSA. A bivalent vaccine containing *S. aureus* polysaccharides 5 and 8 briefly reduced risk of bacteraemia in haemodialysis recipients in a prospective study published in 2002. Further testing of booster doses of the vaccine to demonstrate increased efficacy is in progress. An additional target for vaccine synthesis is the PVL toxin, which may provide protection against CA-MRSA. Another preventive measure may be screening for nasal or skin colonization with MRSA, with subsequent decolonization of colonized persons. However, populations that require screening (i.e. universal or targeted screening), actions to pursue among the colonized, and efficacy and costs of such a programme are all variables that require further clarification. The promise of such a strategy may be control of MRSA and reduction of the costs and morbidity associated with MRSA infection.

New glycopeptides (telavancin, oritavancin, and dalbavancin) and existing agents with evolving indications (daptomycin, linezolid) may improve treatment options for MRSA and VISA/VRSA. Better strategies for treatment and salvage of infected catheters with catheter coating (e.g. with chlorhexidine) or methods for treatment of biofilm may improve treatment of coagulase-negative staphylococci.

Further reading

Baddour LM, *et al.* (2005). Infective endocarditis: diagnosis, antimicrobial therapy, and management of complications: a statement for healthcare professionals from the Committee on Rheumatic Fever, Endocarditis, and Kawasaki Disease, Council on Cardiovascular Disease in the Young, and the Councils on Clinical Cardiology, Stroke, and Cardiovascular Surgery and Anesthesia, American Heart Association: endorsed by the Infectious Diseases Society of America. *Circulation*, **111**, e394–434. [Guidelines in the United States of America for the treatment of infective endocarditis, including staphylococcal endocarditis.]

Darouiche RO (2006). Spinal epidural abscess. *N Engl J Med*, **355**, 2012–20. [Review of clinical features and therapy of epidural abscess.]

Drees M, Boucher H (2006). New agents for *Staphylococcus aureus* endocarditis. *Curr Opin Infect Dis*, **19**, 544–50. [A review of new and soon to arrive therapy for *S. aureus*.]

Elliott TS, *et al.* (2004). Guidelines for the antibiotic treatment of endocarditis in adults: report of the Working Party of the British Society for Antimicrobial Chemotherapy. *J Antimicrob Chemother*, **54**, 971–81. [Guidelines in the United Kingdom for the treatment of infective endocarditis, including staphylococcal endocarditis.]

Fowler VG Jr, *et al.* (2005). *Staphylococcus aureus* endocarditis: a consequence of medical progress. *JAMA*, **293**, 3012–21. [Interesting data regarding the epidemiology of *S. aureus* endocarditis.]

Gemmell CG, *et al.* (2006). Guidelines for the prophylaxis and treatment of methicillin-resistant *Staphylococcus aureus* (MRSA) infections in the UK. *J Antimicrob Chemother*, **57**, 589–608. [United Kingdom review of the evidence for practices in control and treatment of MRSA infection.]

Grundmann H, *et al.* (2006). Emergence and resurgence of meticillin-resistant *Staphylococcus aureus* as a public-health threat. *Lancet*, **368**, 874–85. [A recent review of the emergence of community-associated MRSA infections.]

Heldman AW, *et al.* (1996). Oral antibiotic treatment of right-sided staphylococcal endocarditis in injection drug users: prospective randomized comparison with parenteral therapy. *Am J Med*, **101**, 68–76. [A comparison of oral ciprofloxacin with rifampin vs parenteral agents in the treatment of right-sided endocarditis.]

Huang SS, Datta R, Platt R (2006). Risk of acquiring antibiotic-resistant bacteria from prior room occupants. *Arch Int Med.* **166**, 1945–51. [Evidence to support the risk of nosocomial and environmental spread of MRSA.]

Klevens RM, *et al.* (2006). Changes in the epidemiology of methicillin-resistant *Staphylococcus aureus* in intensive care units in US hospitals, 1992–2003. *Clin Infect Dis*, **42**, 389–91.

Lipsky BA, Itani K, Norden C (2004). Treating foot infections in diabetic patients: a randomized, multicenter, open-label trial of linezolid versus ampicillin-sulbactam/amoxicillin-clavulanate. *Clin Inf Dis*, **38**, 17–24. [A trial examining linezolid in the treatment of diabetic foot infections.]

Markowitz N, Quinn EL, Saravolatz LD (1992). Trimethoprim-sulfamethoxazole compared with vancomycin for the treatment of *Staphylococcus aureus* infection. *Ann Int Med*, **117**, 390–8. [Parenteral trimethoprim/sulfamethoxazole is compared with vancomycin in this double-blind randomized trial.]

Mermel LA, *et al.* (2001). Guidelines for the management of intravascular catheter-related infections. *Clin Inf Dis*, **32**, 1249–72. [Guidelines for the treatment of catheter-related bloodstream infections; includes information about antibiotic lock in coagulase-negative staphylococcal infections.]

Mulligan ME, *et al.* (1993). Methicillin-resistant *Staphylococcus aureus*: a consensus review of the microbiology, pathogenesis, and epidemiology with implications for prevention and management. *Am J Med*, **94**, 313–28. [A review of nosocomial MRSA colonization and infection. Reviews strategies for decolonization of carriers.]

Ruhe JJ, *et al.* (2005). Use of long-acting tetracyclines for methicillin-resistant *Staphylococcus aureus* infections: case series and review of the literature. *Clin Inf Dis*, **40**, 1429–34. [A review of tetracyclines in treatment of MRSA infections.]

Safdar N, Fine JP, Maki DG (2005). Meta-analysis: methods for diagnosing intravascular device-related bloodstream infection. *Ann Int Med*, **142**, 451–66. [Summary of studies and most effective methods for diagnosis of catheter-related bloodstream infections.]

Shorr AF, Kunkel MJ, Kollef M (2005). Linezolid versus vancomycin for *Staphylococcus aureus* bacteraemia: pooled analysis of randomized studies. *J Antimicrob Chemother*, **56**, 923–9. [Pooled data from two randomized trials show efficacy of linezolid.]

Stevens DL, *et al.* (2005). Practice guidelines for the diagnosis and management of skin and soft-tissue infections. *Clin Inf Dis*, **41**, 1373–406. [Guidelines for the treatment of soft tissue infections.]

Wertheim HF, *et al.* (2004). Risk and outcome of nosocomial *Staphylococcus aureus* bacteraemia in nasal carriers versus non-carriers. *Lancet*, **364**, 703–5.

Wertheim HF, *et al.* (2004). Mupirocin prophylaxis against nosocomial *Staphylococcus aureus* infections in nonsurgical patients: a randomized study. *Ann Int Med*, **140**, 419–25. [Two studies that evaluate the impact of nasal colonization, and decolonization, in infection rates of hospitalized patients.]

Wyllie DH, Crook DW, Peto TE (2006). Mortality after *Staphylococcus aureus* bacteraemia in two hospitals in Oxfordshire, 1997–2003: cohort study. *BMJ*, **333**, 281. [Epidemiology of *S. aureus* bacteraemia in the United Kingdom is reviewed in this cohort study.]

Zimmermann B 3rd, Mikolich DJ, Ho G Jr (1995). Septic bursitis. *Semin Arthritis Rheum*, **24**, 391–410. [Review of the treatment of septic bursitis.]

7.6.5 Meningococcal infections

P. Brandtzaeg

Essentials

Neisseria meningitidis is an obligate human Gram-negative diplococcus. It is carried in the nasopharynx by about 10% of people, with most strains being harmless and inducing immunity. Pathogenic strains usually belong to specific clones that are encapsulated, express pili and the major porin, PorA. Serogroups A, B, and C usually account for more than 90% of all invasive isolates.

Epidemiology

Young asymptomatic adults are the main reservoir. Meningococci are transmitted by droplets and susceptible people usually develop the first symptoms within 2 to 4 days. The incidence of disease is highest during the first 4 years of life, with a secondary lower peak in adolescents. Pathogenic strains tend to cause single cases or small clusters in industrialized countries, whereas they cause large outbreaks in developing countries, particularly in the meningitis belt of Africa. Host factors predisposing to invasive disease include (1) lack of protective antibodies, (2) defects in the complement system or mannose-binding lectin, (3) polymorphisms of Fcγ-receptor II (Fcγ-RIIa, CD32) and Fcγ-receptor III (Fcγ-RIIIb, CD16).

Clinical features and prognosis

Initially, *N. meningitidis* induces bacteraemia, with growth velocity in the circulation a major determinant of the clinical presentation and outcome. The two major clinical presentations are meningitis and septic shock.

Meningitis—the commonest presentation; preceded by low grade meningococcaemia ($<10^3$/ml); characterized by fever, subsequently a petechial rash (30–80% of cases) and increasing symptoms of meningitis. If adequately treated with antibiotics, case fatality is <5% in industrialized countries, but higher in developing countries. Brain oedema leading to herniation of the cerebellum is the main cause of death. Neurosensory hearing loss is the major complication.

Septic shock—symptoms develop very rapidly; within 6 to 12 h of initial symptoms the patient may have persistent circulatory failure and severe coagulopathy leading to thrombosis and extensive haemorrhage of the skin, thrombosis and gangrene of the extremities, and impaired renal, adrenal, and pulmonary function. Mortality is high (29–53%).

Mild meningococcaemia—in industrialized countries, 20 to 30% of cases present with fever and petechial or macular rash, but without marked signs of meningitis or shock. Occasional complications include pericarditis, arthritis, ocular infection or chronic meningococcaemia. Prognosis is good (with appropriate antibiotic treatment).

Diagnosis

Intra- and extracellular diplococci can be observed in the cerebrospinal fluid, peripheral blood buffy coat (fulminant septicaemia), and biopsies of haemorrhagic skin lesions using Gram or acridine orange stains. *N. meningitidis* can be grown from blood culture and swabs from the nasopharynx/tonsils. Polymerase chain reaction (PCR) methods are increasingly used to detect and classify *N. meningitidis* in blood, cerebrospinal fluid, and other bodily fluids.

Treatment

Aside from supportive care, appropriate antibiotic treatment should be started immediately in suspected cases of meningococcal infection: this should not be delayed while the patient is transferred to hospital, or for the results of investigations to become available. Benzylpenicillin (intravenously or intramuscularly) remains the drug of choice in most countries; third-generation cefalosporins and chloramphenicol are also effective.

Prevention

Vaccination—conjugate vaccines comprising serogroup A, C, Y, and W135 polysaccharide are effective. A vaccine covering serogroup B strains is still lacking, but the outer membrane vesicle vaccines used during a serogroup B outbreak in Norway and New Zealand, containing the porin A (PorA) of the epidemic strain, induced 57 to 73% protection.

Secondary prophylaxis—health authorities in most countries advise that close contacts of cases of meningococcal disease have eradication treatment, e.g. with a single dose of ciprofloxacin 500 mg or ofloxacin 400 mg.

Introduction

Neisseria meningitidis infection remains a major public health problem worldwide by causing clusters or epidemics of meningitis and acute lethal sepsis. Case fatality has gradually declined from 70 to 90% to approximately 10% but has remained at this level since the introduction of antimicrobial chemotherapy in 1937.

The bacterium

N. meningitidis is an obligate human Gram-negative diplococcus classified as a β-proteobacterium and is a member of the family Neisseriaceae. Meningococci are normally located in the mucous membrane of the nasopharynx and tonsils. Invasive isolates from blood and cerebrospinal fluid or as detected in tissue biopsies are encapsulated and express pili and the major porin PorA. Capsule polysaccharides that inhibit phagocytosis and bacterial adhesion are divided into at least 13 different serogroups (A, B, C, D, E, H, I, K, L, W135, X, Y, and Z). Serogroups A, B, and C usually account for more than 90% of all invasive isolates. Less than 10% of clinical isolates are from serogroups X, Y, and W135.

The cell wall of meningococci consists of an outer lipid bilayer, containing lipopolysaccharides (LPS, endotoxin), lipids, and outer membrane proteins, and an inner thin peptidoglycan layer. LPS is the major inflammatory (toxic) component of *N. meningitidis* (Fig. 7.6.5.1). Lipoproteins and fragments of peptidoglycan are weaker inflammatory molecules. They activate the innate immune system via CD14 and the Toll-like receptors 4 (LPS) and 2 (lipoproteins, peptidoglycan) located on monocytes, macrophages, and to a lesser extent neutrophils (Fig. 7.6.5.2). During growth, meningococci release a large number of outer membrane vesicles containing LPS and other outer membrane molecules that trigger the innate immune system in a dose-dependent manner.

Outer membrane proteins are classified according to electrophoretic mobility into five major classes. PorA (class 1 protein) and PorB (class 2 or 3 proteins) are cation-selective and anion-selective porins, respectively. PorB and PorA define serotype and serosubtype, respectively. Loops 1 and 4 in PorA are surface exposed major epitopes inducing bactericidal and opsonophagocytic antibodies when exposed to the human immune system.

Meningococci are fastidious bacteria that readily autolyse. They grow well on blood agar, supplemented chocolate agar, trypticase soy agar, Mueller–Hinton agar, and selective GC medium. Optimal growth occurs at 35 to 37°C in a humid atmosphere with 5 to 10% carbon dioxide. The convex colonies (diameter 1–4 mm) are transparent, nonpigmented, and nonhaemolytic. They produce cytochrome oxidase and ferment glucose and maltose, but not lactose and sucrose, to acid without gas formation.

Practical handling of clinical specimens

Blood culture (10 ml for adults, 2–4 ml for infants/children) and swabs from the nasopharynx and the tonsils are collected immediately. Media for blood culture and transportation of swabs should be optimal for recovery of meningococci. Cerebrospinal fluid is best cultured by direct plating of 0.1 ml on supplemented chocolate agar or a similar medium. If direct plating is impossible or delayed, the sample should be stored at +4°C to +20°C but preferably at refrigerator temperature. Recovery of live meningococci may increase if some drops of the cerebrospinal fluid are stored on a sterile swab in transport medium or injected into blood culture medium and incubated at 35 to 37°C.

Direct visualization of *N. meningitidis* in clinical specimens

Intracellular and extracellular diplococci can be observed in the cerebrospinal fluid, peripheral blood buffy coat (fulminant septicaemia), and biopsies of haemorrhagic skin lesions using Gram's or acridine orange stains.

Polymerase chain reaction

Polymerase chain reaction (PCR) is increasingly used to detect and classify *N. meningitidis* in blood, cerebrospinal fluid, joint fluid, and pericardial fluid. Real-time PCR has made it possible to quantify the total number of meningococci, i.e. live plus dead bacteria, in plasma and cerebrospinal fluid. In shock plasma, nonviable meningococci outnumber those that can be cultured by a factor 1000:1. The number of *N. meningitidis* DNA copies is closely correlated to the LPS levels, clinical presentation, disease severity, and outcome.

Epidemiology

Industrialized countries

Infection presents as single cases or in small clusters. The incidence is usually 1 to 3 per 100 000 inhabitants per year. Strains belonging to specific clonal complexes may cause a hyperendemic situation characterized by a much higher incidence than usually observed (4 to 30 per 100 000 per year). This epidemiological situation may last for more than a decade in defined geographical areas before slowly declining. Serogroup A has disappeared as a cause of

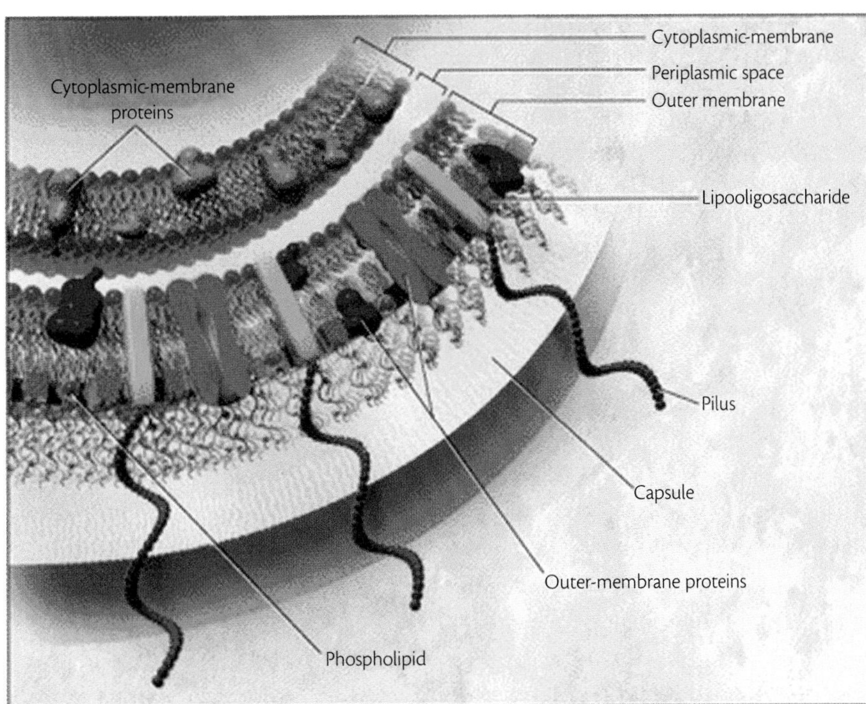

Fig. 7.6.5.1 Cross-sectional view of *N. meningitidis*.
(Reproduced with permission from Rosenstein NE, Bradley BA, Stephens DS, Popovic T, Hughes JM (2001). Meningococcal disease. *N Engl J Med*, **334**, 1378–88.)

significant epidemics. Outbreaks in Finland in the 1970s and in New Zealand in the 1980s were exceptions. In Europe 70% of the cases are presently caused by serogroup B followed by C. In the United States of America serogroups B, C, and Y accounted for approximately one-third of the cases each (Fig. 7.6.5.3).

Developing countries

Large-scale epidemics are confined to developing countries, primarily in sub-Saharan Africa where the incidence approaches 10 to 25 per 100 000 inhabitants per year. During epidemic peaks in Africa, as many as 500 to 1000 per 100 000 inhabitants may contract meningococcal infections. Serogroup A and to lesser extent serogroups W135 and C dominate the isolates of large epidemics (Fig. 7.6.5.3).

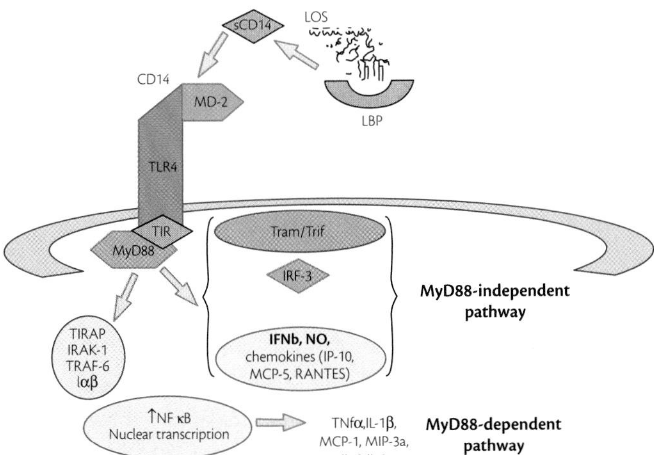

Fig. 7.6.5.2 Activation of Toll-like receptor 4 by endotoxin (lipopolysaccharides or lipooligosaccharides, LOS).
(Reproduced with permission from Stephens DS, Greenwood B, Brandtzaeg P (2007). Epidemic meningitis, meningococcaemia, and Neisseria meningitidis, *Lancet.*, **369**, 2196–210.)

Meningitis belt in sub-Saharan Africa

The area stretches from the Gambia in the west to Ethiopia in the east and includes Senegal, Guinea, Mali, Burkina Faso, Ghana, Togo, Benin, Nigeria, Niger, Chad, Cameroon, The Central African Republic, and Sudan (Fig. 7.6.5.3). Mainly serogroup A strains belonging to a few clonal complexes cause the increased attack rate. In some of these countries large-scale epidemics occur every 8 to 12 years. Recently, serogroup W135 has caused epidemics in West Africa.

Season

In temperate climates most cases occur during the winter and early spring. In the sub-Saharan African meningitis belt the incidence increases from the middle of the dry season and reaches its maximum at the end of that season (harmattan). New cases decline rapidly after the start of the rainy season.

Preceding infections

Influenza A predisposes to invasive meningococcal infections. Mycoplasma infections and rubella have been associated with outbreaks.

Age distribution

Cases are seen in all age groups; however, most occur from 0 to 4 years with a smaller peak from 13 to 20 years. During epidemics the median age appears to increase. Complement-deficient patients may contract the infection at an older age than average.

Genetic diversity

N. meningitidis can exchange and incorporate DNA from other *Neisseria* species or closely related bacteria. Meningococci are genetically more diverse than most other human pathogens. However, strains from certain clonal complexes may persist for many decades

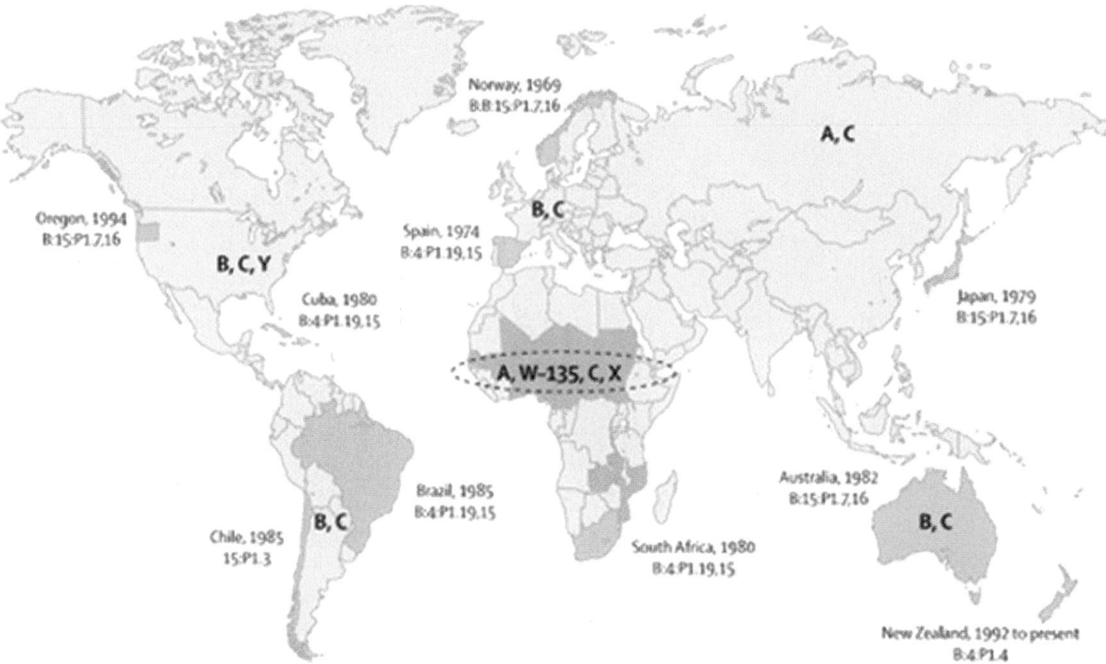

Fig. 7.6.5.3 Outbreaks of different serogroups of *N. meningitidis* since the 1960s. Purple areas indicate countries with serogroup B epidemics.
(Reproduced with permission from Stephens DS, Greenwood B, Brandtzaeg P (2007). Epidemic meningitis, meningococcaemia, and Neisseria meningitidis, *Lancet*, **369**, 2196–210 and Caugant D A (1998). Population genetics and molecular epidemiology of Neisseria meningitides. *APMIS*, **106**, 505–10.)

over wide areas, retaining their pathogenicity. Strains from seven clonal complexes have predominated since the late 1960s.

Nasopharyngeal colonization

Upper respiratory tract mucosa is the natural habitat of *N. meningitidis*. It is spread from person to person by droplets and direct mucosal contact. Most colonizing meningococci are nonpathogenic and are genetically and phenotypically different from virulent invasive strains. Only a minority of those colonized with virulent strains will develop invasive disease. Colonization is asymptomatic; it induces local and systemic immune responses within 1 to 2 weeks.

Carriage

Cross-sectional studies in England and Norway in the 1980s and 1990s indicated that approximately 10% of the population harboured meningococci in the upper respiratory tract. However, only 1% of the healthy normal population carried strains from typical virulent clones prevalent at the time. The acquisition rate leading to carriage appears to be independent of season, whereas invasive meningococcal infections peak in the winter and early spring in temperate countries.

The carriage rate in England is low (2–3%) in the first 4 years of life, rises in children aged 10 to 14 years (9–10%), reaches a maximum among young adults of 15 to 19 years (20–25%), and then gradually declines to less than 15% in persons above 25 years. It increases in closed or semiclosed communities and is particularly high in military camps where strains change frequently. In university communities with bar and catering facilities the carriage rate is high. Smoking increases the carriage rate.

Reservoir of virulent meningococci

Healthy adults carrying virulent strains of *N. meningitidis* are the main reservoir. Household members and kissing contacts of a patient harbour virulent strains more often than the average population. In industrialized countries, infants and children are usually infected by a local adult carrier. Spread from patients to medical staff is very uncommon. In Africa, children may more commonly infect each other with serogroup A strains.

Predisposing factors for invasive disease

These are summarized in Box 7.6.5.1.

Lack of protective antibodies

Antibodies against serogroups A, C, W135, and Y capsule polysaccharides are bactericidal and confer protection at concentrations of 1 to 2 μg/ml of serum. Serogroup B polysaccharide induces a weak transient IgM but no protective IgG response. Bactericidal and opsonophagocytic antibodies recognizing surface-exposed epitopes of the outer membrane protein, in particular PorA, are important for protection. Antilipopolysaccharide antibodies, recognizing commonly shared epitopes among virulent and nonpathogenic neisseria and closely related species, presumably play a role in protection.

Box 7.6.5.1 Factors predisposing for meningococcal infections

- Lack of bactericidal and/or opsonizing antibodies
- Lack of alternative pathway or late complement components, polymorphism of factor H
- Low levels of mannan-binding lectin
- Polymorphism of the Fcγ receptor II (Fcγ-RIIa, CD32) and Fcγ receptor III (Fcγ-RIIIb, CD16)

Defects in the complement system

Reduced function of the complement system caused by defects in the alternative or terminal pathways increases the susceptibility up to 6000 times. Defects in the classic pathway do not predispose to meningococcal infection. Complement defects are rare. They play a minor role in the development of invasive serogroup A, B, and C infections in Europe, but are over-represented in patients with the less common serogroups W135, X, Y, and Z. Polymorphism and high serum levels of factor H appear to increase the risk of invasive meningococcal infections in England.

Defects in the mannose-binding lectin

Mutations in codons 54, 57, and 52 of the mannose-binding lectin gene result in low serum levels and have been associated with one-third of all meningococcal cases in England and Ireland. Low serum levels of mannose-binding lectin combined with properdin defects increase the risk of invasive meningococcal disease.

Polymorphism of Fcγ-receptor II and Fcγ-receptor III

Polymorphisms of Fcγ receptor II (Fcγ-RIIa, CD32) and Fcγ receptor III (Fcγ-RIIIb, CD16) on phagocytic cells are associated with reduced binding of antibodies. They are over-represented in patients with defects in the late complement components (C5–C9) and in children with fulminant meningococcal sepsis. Fcγ-RIIa receptors where arginine has replaced histidine at position 131 are associated with reduced binding of IgG2 subclass (antipolysaccharide) antibodies. The influence of these polymorphisms in adults is uncertain.

Invasive infection

Most patients appear to develop invasive disease 2 to 4 days after acquiring the virulent strain in the upper respiratory tract, but some are carriers for up to 7 weeks before invasive infection develops. *N. meningitidis* adheres to specific molecules on nonciliated epithelial cells in the nasopharynx and on the tonsils (Fig. 7.6.5.4).

During a period of adaptation and proliferation, meningococci presumably alter various surface structures (lipopolysaccharides, pili, outer membrane proteins) by phase variation before starting transepithelial migration. They reach submucosal tissue and, via capillaries, gain access to the circulation (Fig. 7.6.5.5).

The initial bacteraemic phase

Bacteraemia is a prerequisite for systemic meningococcal infection. Meningococci may be eliminated from the blood by lysis induced by bactericidal antibodies and complement and by phagocytosis of opsonized bacteria. Persistent bacteraemia allows meningeal invasion.

Bacterial proliferation and accompanying inflammatory response may occur predominantly in either the subarachnoid space, causing meningitis, or in the circulation, causing meningococcaemia with or without shock.

The rash

Haemorrhagic skin lesions are the hallmark of systemic meningococcal disease, occurring in 70 to 80% of all cases in industrialized countries. They appear as red or bluish petechiae. These lesions are larger and more irregular in size than the petechiae of thrombocytopenic purpura. Each lesion represents a local nidus of meningococci within the endothelial cells, thrombus formation, and extravasation of erythrocytes. The petechial rash indicates meningococcaemia, not necessarily severe sepsis. However, in fulminant meningococcal septicaemia the haemorrhagic lesions are larger (ecchymoses) with a propensity to locate on extremities (Fig. 7.6.5.6). Some patients develop relatively large nonspecific maculopapular lesions, with or without haemorrhagic lesions, at an early stage (Figs. 7.6.5.7, 7.6.5.8). The petechial lesions are difficult to discover on dark skin but may be observed in the conjunctivae (Fig. 7.6.5.9).

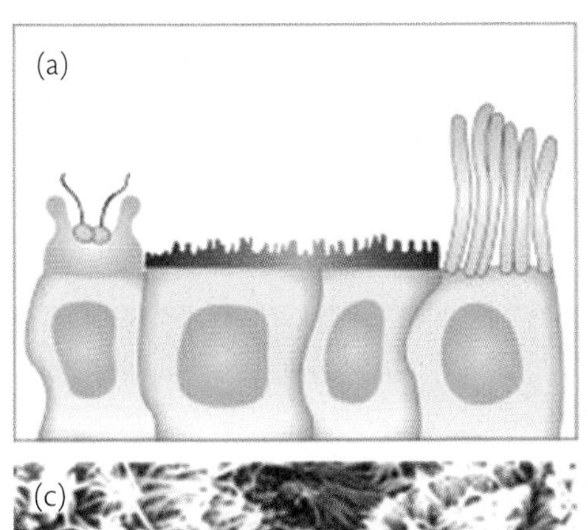

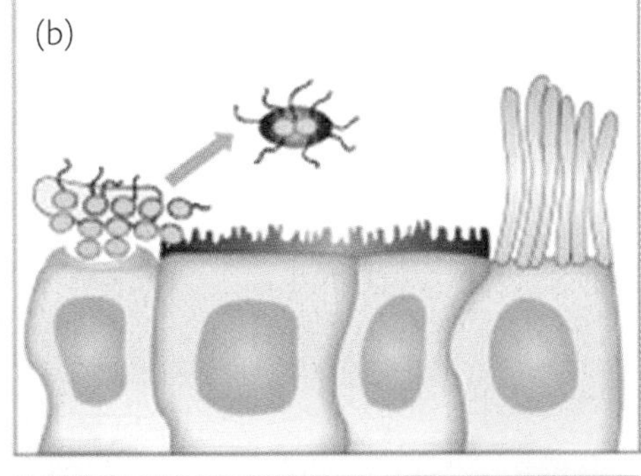

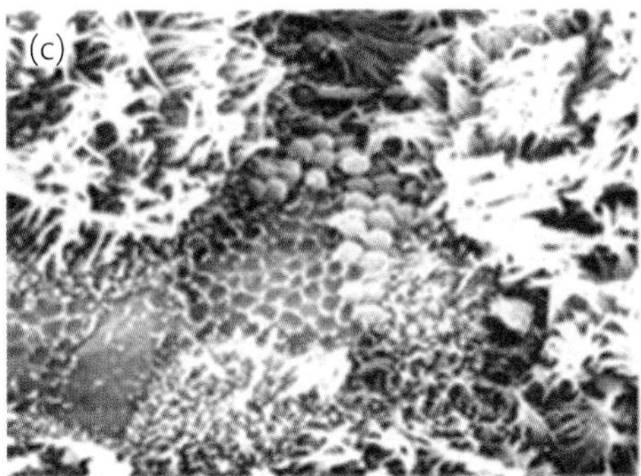

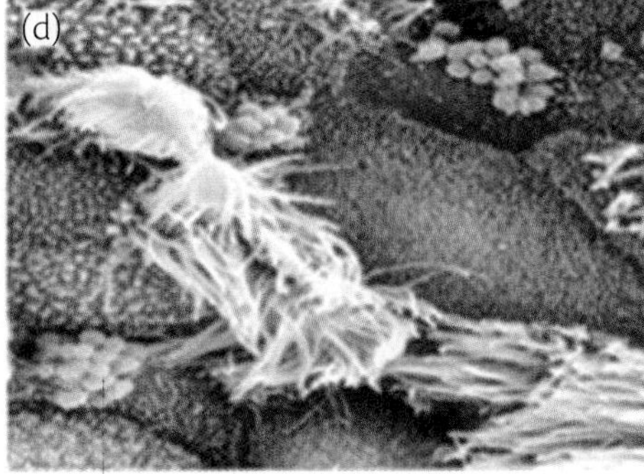

Fig. 7.6.5.4 Attachment to and proliferation of meningococci on nonciliated epithelial cells in nasopharynx.
(Reproduced with permission from Stephens DS, Greenwood B, Brandtzaeg P (2007). Epidemic meningitis, meningococcaemia, and Neisseria meningitidis, *Lancet*, **369**, 2196–210.)

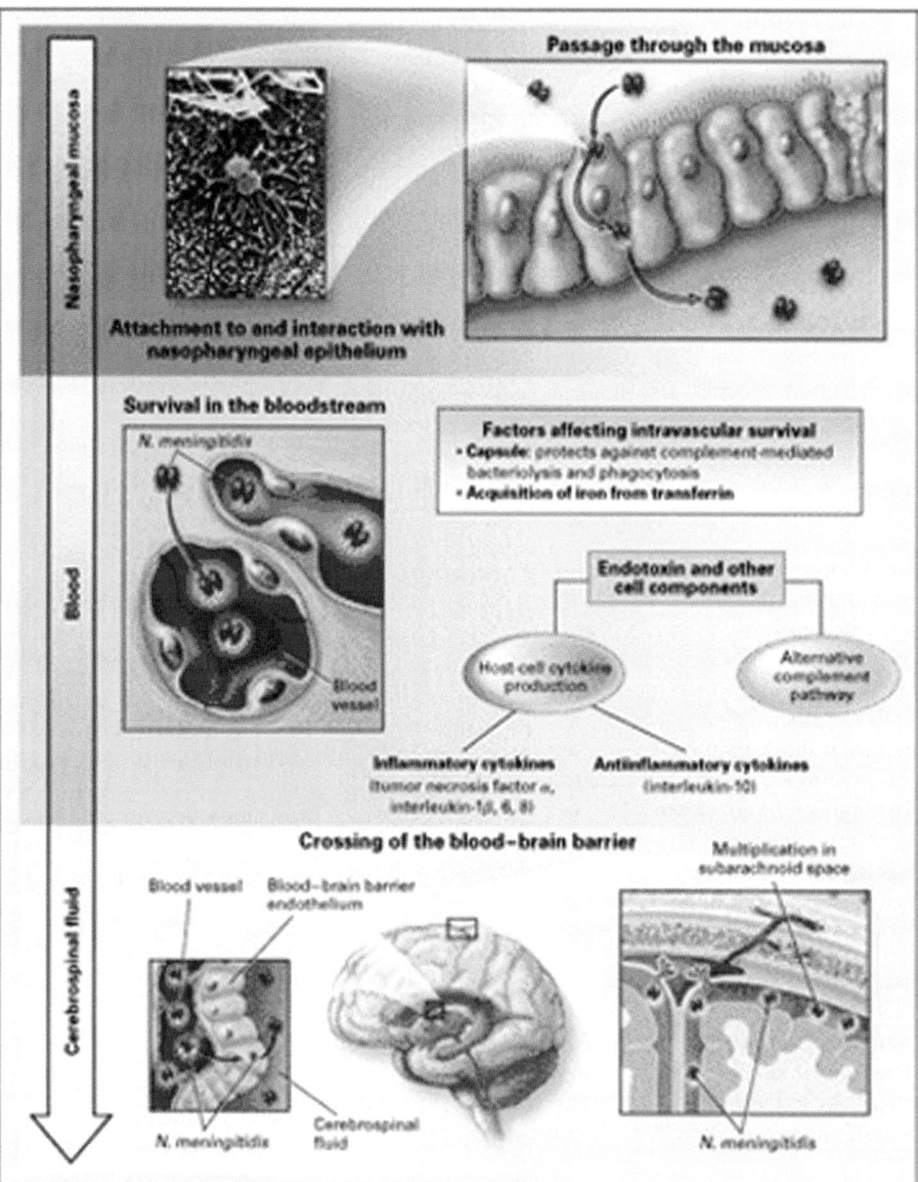

Fig. 7.6.5.5 Events leading to the different clinical presentations of meningococcal infections.
Reproduced with permission from Rosenstein NE, Bradley BA, Stephens DS, Popovic T, Hughes JM (2001). Meningococcal disease. *N Engl J Med*, **334**, 1378–88.

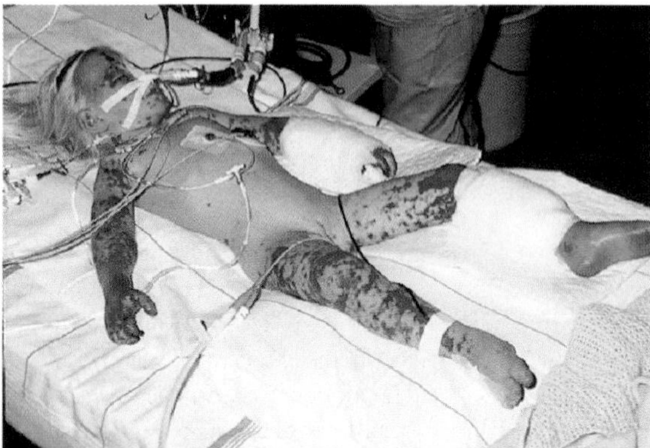

Fig. 7.6.5.6 Massive skin haemorrhage on the extremities of a 4-year-old girl with fulminant meningococcal septicaemia. The infection was caused by *Neisseria meningitidis* group B. The left leg had to be amputated below the knee. She needed extensive skin transplantation and several fingers had to be amputated.

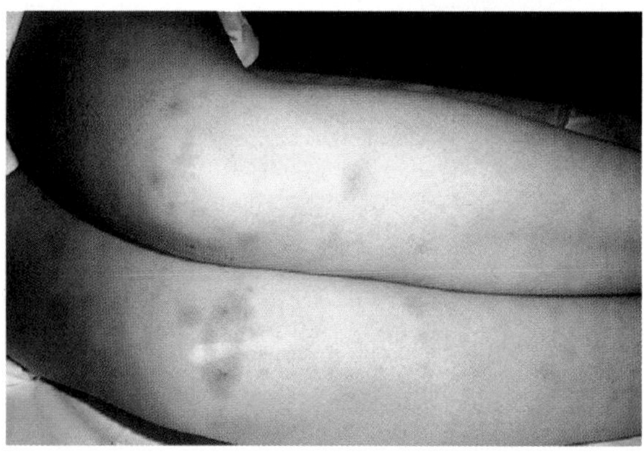

Fig. 7.6.5.7 Macular lesions on the legs, some with a central haemorrhagic spot in a 17-year-old girl with mild meningococcaemia caused by *Neisseria meningitidis* group C. She recovered completely after 5 days treatment with benzylpenicillin.

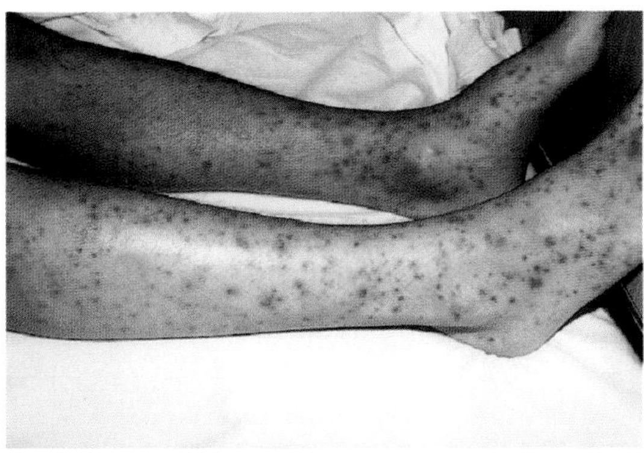

Fig. 7.6.5.8 Macular and haemorrhagic lesions on the legs of a 21-year-old man with mild meningococcaemia caused by *Neisseria meningitidis* group B. He recovered completely after 5 days of penicillin treatment.

Table 7.6.5.1 Levels of *N. meningitidis* DNA, lipopolysaccharides, and inflammatory mediators related to the clinical presentation

	No shock	Shock[a]	Shock	No shock
	Meningitis[b]	No meningitis	Meningitis	No meningitis
Circulation	(+)	++++	++	(+)
Subarachnoid space	+++++	(+)	+++	(+)

[a] Shock denotes persistent hypotension requiring treatment with volume and pressor for 24 h.

[b] Meningitis denotes 100 × 10⁶/litre or more leucocytes in the cerebrospinal fluid or clinically distinct signs of meningism.

Clinical presentations

The initial symptoms of systemic meningococcal infection are attributable to meningococcaemia. This may persist as a low-grade bacteraemia or develop into septic shock in a few hours. Most commonly, the patient develops meningococcaemia without circulatory impairment which gradually evolves to meningitis within 12 to 72 h. Occasionally, patients develop distinct meningitis and persistent shock simultaneously. Based on easily recognizable clinical symptoms, meningococcal infections can be classified as: (1) meningitis without shock, (2) shock without meningitis, (3) meningitis and shock, and (4) meningococcaemia without shock or meningitis. Each clinical presentation is associated with a distinct pathophysiological background and prognosis (Table 7.6.5.1).

Distinct meningitis without persistent shock

Meningism dominates the clinical presentation and the onset is often insidious. The patients, particularly children, may complain of general malaise, nausea, and headache. They vomit and become febrile. The temperature may fluctuate and can be normal at times. Many patients are initially diagnosed as 'gastric flu', gastroenteritis, or upper respiratory tract infection. Gradually, the symptoms of meningitis dominate the clinical picture. The patient complains of headache, vomits, and develops nuchal and back rigidity, photophobia, and in more advanced cases altered consciousness; Kernig's and Brudzinski's signs become positive. Many patients are lethargic and some are agitated. The blood pressure is normal or slightly elevated by stress. Occasionally it is low but can be restored to normal by infusion of a limited volume of fluid. In untreated cases brain oedema develops, the intracranial pressure rises, and the central circulation is increasingly compromised. Finally, herniation of the cerebellum occurs with arrest of the brain circulation. The case fatality rate is usually less than 5% in industrialized countries.

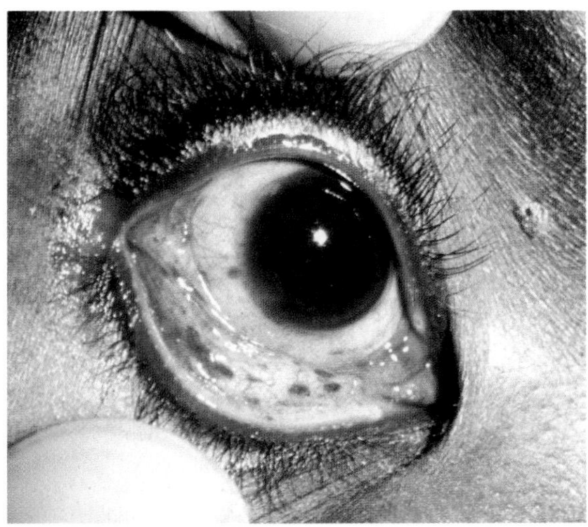

Fig. 7.6.5.9 Conjunctival petechiae in an African child with meningococcal group A meningitis.
(Copyright D A Warrell.)

Meningococcal meningitis without persistent shock accounts for more than 50% of all cases of systemic meningococcal infections in industrialized countries and an even higher proportion of cases reaching hospitals in developing countries. The combination of multiple petechiae and symptoms of meningitis supports a diagnosis of meningococcal meningitis.

Pathophysiological background

N. meningitidis multiply in a compartmentalized manner with the main proliferation occurring in the subarachnoid space. Quantitative PCR indicates that the real number of meningococci is usually less than 10^3/ml in plasma and may increase to 10^9/ml in the cerebrospinal fluid (Fig. 7.6.5.10). This distribution is reflected in the levels of endotoxin and various cytokines which are low in plasma and 100 to 1000 times higher in the cerebrospinal fluid. Meningococci can be cultivated from both compartments in untreated patients. Plasma proteins, mainly albumin, leak into the cerebrospinal fluid, and the influx of mainly neutrophils causes the pleocytosis. The glucose level of the cerebrospinal fluid is reduced mainly as a result of increased central glucose consumption rather than the pleocytosis.

Laboratory findings

The erythrocyte sedimentation rate, C-reactive protein, and leucocyte count in the peripheral blood are markedly elevated with increased numbers of band forms. Sodium, potassium, calcium, and magnesium ions, pH, renal, hepatic, and coagulation parameters are usually within normal range. Cerebrospinal fluid shows a marked pleocytosis (more than 100×10^6 leucocytes/litre), with increased levels of protein and decreased levels of glucose. Intracellular and extracellular Gram-negative diplococci can be detected by direct microscopy.

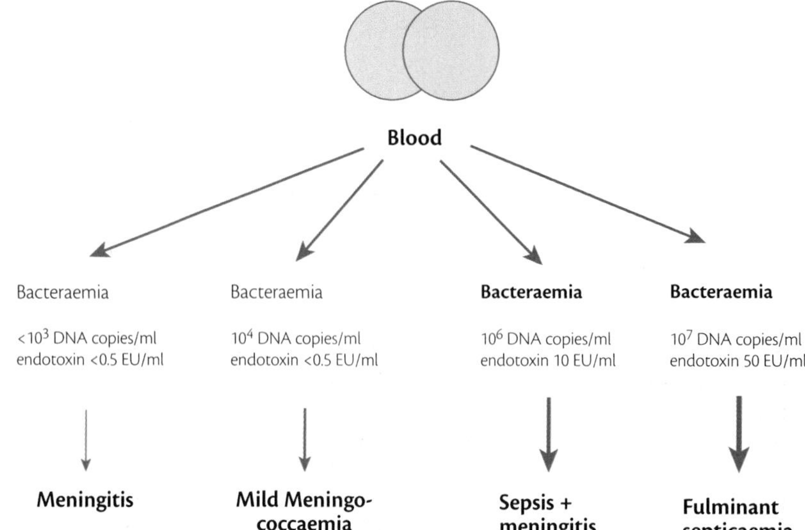

Fig. 7.6.5.10 Median number of *N. meningitidis* (number of DNA copies) as determined by real-time PCR and median level of endotoxin in plasma in the different clinical presentations of systemic meningococcal disease.

Persistent septic shock without distinct meningitis

Fulminant meningococcal septicaemia (Waterhouse–Friderichsen syndrome) is characterized by persistent circulatory failure and severe coagulopathy leading to thrombosis and extensive haemorrhage of the skin, thrombosis and gangrene of the extremities, and impaired renal, adrenal, and pulmonary function.

Symptoms develop very rapidly. Six to 12 h after recognizing their first symptoms the patients are often desperately ill. Initially, they complain of 'flu-like' symptoms such as fever, aching muscle, prostration, abdominal pain, and nausea. The temperature rises rapidly, commonly to between 39.0 and 41.5°C, but occasionally lower. Diarrhoea may occur during the first few hours. The patient appears worryingly sick to relatives. The parents usually recognize cold extremities indicating impaired circulation before the skin haemorrhagic lesions appear but misinterpret the acute symptoms as influenza or acute gastroenteritis.

The haemorrhagic skin lesions are first seen as bluish petechiae, which rapidly increase in size and number. They are distributed all over the body but are often more pronounced and detected earliest on the extremities. Occasionally they are seen on the conjunctivae and other mucous membranes.

The circulation is severely impaired. The extremities are often cold and cyanotic with a capillary refill time of more than 3 s. The blood pressure is low despite tachycardia. The tissue perfusion remains inadequate despite extensive fluid and pressor therapy. Initially, the circulation is hyperdynamic, but gradually becomes hypodynamic from persistent vasodilatation and gradually reduced myocardial performance. The heart becomes dilated with a reduced ejection fraction.

Patients usually lack nuchal and back rigidity, and Kernig's sign is negative. Despite impaired circulation, many patients remain awake and alert on hospital admission, being able to communicate their complaints. They hyperventilate to compensate for the pronounced metabolic acidosis. Urine output gradually dwindles. They may develop acute respiratory distress syndrome (ARDS), i.e. pulmonary oedema after fluid volume repletion of more than 40 ml/kg.

Circulatory collapse dominates the clinical picture during the first 48 to 96 h. Fifty per cent of the nonsurvivors die within 12 h of hospital admission. Few patients die after 48 h. Later, ARDS, renal failure, and the consequences of the diffuse thrombosis of the extremities and the skin dominate the picture. The case fatality rate ranges from 29 to 53%.

Rapidly evolving symptoms with fever, circulatory shock, and extensive skin haemorrhages in a person without a history of splenectomy makes the diagnosis of fulminant meningococcal septicaemia likely. The same clinical picture is, however, observed in cases of overwhelming infections caused by *Streptococcus pneumoniae*, *Haemophilus influenzae*, *Streptococcus pyogenes*, and *Capnocytophaga canimorsus* (after animal bite) and with viral haemorrhagic fevers (Fig. 7.6.5.11).

Pathophysiological background

The pathophysiological changes are explained by the very rapid proliferation of *N. meningitidis* in the circulation. On admission 5×10^5 to 5×10^8 meningococci/ml plasma are detectable by quantitative PCR (Fig. 7.6.5.10). This massive bacterial growth generates very high levels of endotoxin and other bacterial molecules in the blood.

Few meningococci have yet penetrated into the subarachnoid space, which is explained by the short duration of symptoms. The levels

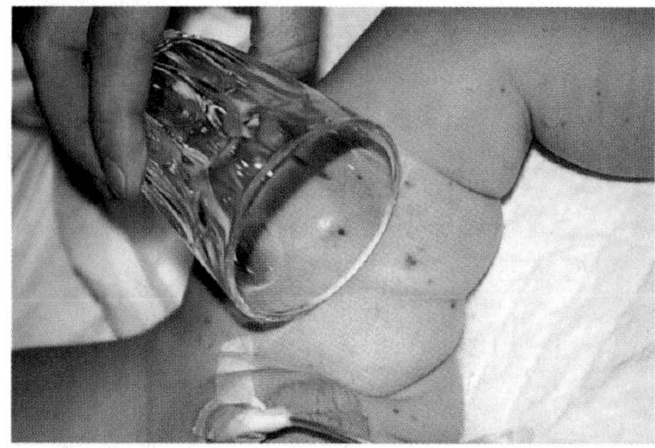

Fig. 7.6.5.11 The 'tumbler test' used to differentiate haemorrhagic skin lesions from viral or drug rash in an infant with meningococcal meningitis caused by *Neisseria meningitidis* group B. There was complete recovery after 5 days treatment with benzylpenicillin.

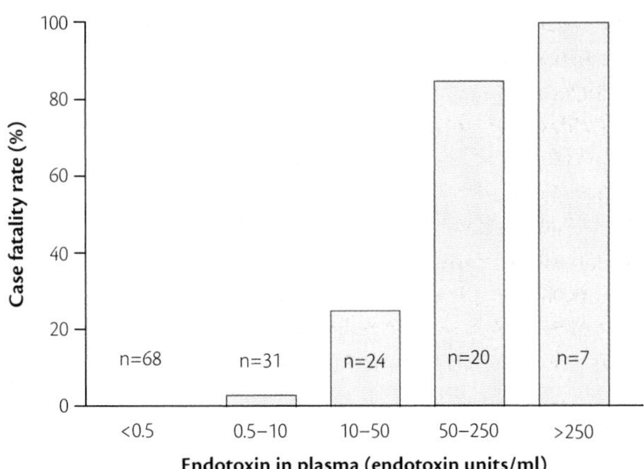

Fig. 7.6.5.12 Relationship between the levels of endotoxin (lipopolysaccharides) in plasma and case fatality rate related to the development of septic shock and multiple organ failure in 150 Norwegian patients with systemic meningococcal disease.

of lipopolysaccharides in the plasma are closely associated with the meningococcal DNA levels and predict the development of persistent septic shock, multiple organ failure, and death. Plasma levels of lipopolysaccharides below 10 endotoxin units/ml were associated with 1% mortality due to circulatory impairment whereas levels above 250 endotoxin units/ml, i.e. 1.4 log higher, were associated with 100% mortality among 150 Norwegian patients (Fig. 7.6.5.12).

Coagulopathy

Coagulation is activated primarily via the extrinsic (tissue factor, FVIIa) pathway. In patients with fulminant meningococcal septicaemia there are increased levels of tissue factor in monocytes and on microparticles released from monocytes. The platelets disappear rapidly and remain at a low level for many days due to extensive consumption at the altered endothelial surface. Thrombopoietin increases in plasma without detectable increase of circulating platelets. The activation of the coagulation system, as measured by formation of fibrin, gradually reduces after antibiotic and fluid therapy is initiated (Table 7.6.5.2).

Inhibited fibrinolysis

Concurrently with activation of coagulation, fibrinolysis is inhibited by high levels of plasminogen activator inhibitor 1 (PAI-1) released from activated endothelial cells and platelets. High levels of PAI-1 are associated with development of persistent septic shock and a fatal outcome. Allelic variations in the promoter region of the PAI-1 gene enhance production and are associated with an increased risk of dying.

Table 7.6.5.2 Factors contributing to the coagulopathy in fulminant meningococcal septicaemia

Procoagulant factor	Tissue factor in monocytes ↑
Anticoagulant factors	Antithrombin ↓
	Protein C ↓↓
	Tissue factor pathway inhibitor ↑
Profibrinolytic factor	Tissue plasminogen activator ↑ ↓
Antifibrinolytic factor	Plasminogen activator inhibitor 1 ↑↑

Thrombus formation

Thrombosis occurs particularly in the vessels of the skin, adrenals, kidneys, muscles, choroid plexus, peripheral extremities, and to some extent in the lungs. The thrombomodulin–thrombin complex on the endothelial cells converting protein C to activated protein C, and the protein C endothelial cell receptor enhancing this activity, are down-regulated. Glycosaminoglycans including heparan sulphate, molecules with an antithrombotic effect, are released from the endothelial surface. Both processes may facilitate formation of thrombi. Concomitantly natural coagulation inhibitors are consumed. Protein C is reduced to 20% and antithrombin to median 50% of normal functional plasma levels. Tissue factor pathway inhibitor increases.

Proinflammatory and anti-inflammatory mediators

A multitude of bioactive proinflammatory and anti-inflammatory mediators are released into the plasma. The complement and the kallikrein–kinin systems generate anaphylatoxins (C3a, C4a, C5a) and bradykinin, which are potent vasodilators. Proinflammatory cytokines, notably tumour necrosis factor-α, interleukin (IL)-1β, IL-6, and various chemokines are massively up-regulated. Concomitantly, high levels of soluble receptors of the same cytokines are released. The anti-inflammatory cytokines IL-10 and IL-1 receptor antagonist are present at high levels and suppress the cell-activating effect of the bacterial lipopolysaccharides and the many proinflammatory cytokines. Nitric oxide production is increased in meningococcal septic shock and is thought to contribute to the vasodilation.

The subarachnoid space

The number of meningococci is very low, if present at all. They can be cultured from cerebrospinal fluid in up to 50% of untreated cases. The inflammatory response is very limited with a leucocyte count usually in the range of 10 to 100 × 10^6/litre and normal contents of protein and glucose.

Laboratory findings

The erythrocyte sedimentation rate and C-reactive protein are only moderately elevated on admission, rising to high levels within 48 h. The leucocyte count is usually low with a marked shift to young band forms of neutrophils. There is evidence of a partly compensated metabolic acidosis with decreased levels of pH and $P\text{CO}_2$. Creatinine and urea are elevated, serum glucose is variable (high, normal, or low), and potassium, calcium, and magnesium are low. Potassium rises with the renal failure. Serum aspartate aminotransferase and alanine aminotransferase are slightly elevated, whereas γ-glutamyl transferase remains normal. Creatine kinase rises within 1 to 3 days, indicating rhabdomyolysis. Prothrombin, activated partial thromboplastin, and thrombin times are prolonged. The levels of platelets, fibrinogen, coagulation factors VII, X, and V, and prothrombin are low. Antithrombin and protein C are low, whereas tissue factor pathway inhibitor is elevated. Fibrin(ogen) degradation products, thrombin–antithrombin complexes, PAI-1, and plasmin-α2-antiplasmin complexes are elevated. Lumbar puncture should be avoided since the procedure may deteriorate the general condition of the patient, particularly the unstable circulation.

Distinct meningitis and persistent shock

There are meningeal and circulatory symptoms. Usually the symptoms from the inflamed meninges dominate the picture. On admission there are classic signs and symptoms of meningitis such as headache and nausea, nuchal and back rigidity, and a positive Kernig's sign. The blood pressure remains low despite fluid volume repletion.

Circulating levels of endotoxin and inflammatory mediators are lower than in patients with fulminant septicaemia, and case fatality is lower (Fig. 7.6.5.12). However, it is higher than in patients with meningitis without compromised circulation.

Meningococcaemia without distinct meningitis and persistent shock

Twenty to 30% of patients with invasive meningococcal disease are hospitalized because of fever and petechial or uncharacteristic rash. They lack distinct signs of meningitis although slight pleocytosis (less than 100×10^6 leucocytes/ml) may be present. The circulation is not severely compromised. They represent a composite group of patients. Many are admitted to hospital early, 12 to 24 h after their first symptoms. Left untreated they might have developed symptoms of meningitis or fulminant shock. The endotoxin level in plasma is less than 7 endotoxin units/ml and the number of *N. meningitidis* DNA copies more than 10^4/ml (Fig. 7.6.5.10). The case fatality rate is close to zero.

Transient benign meningococcaemia

These patients develop fever and often an uncharacteristic rash, but no meningism. They are diagnosed as most likely having a viral infection and receive no antibiotic. When the blood culture results are known, the symptoms have disappeared spontaneously, usually within 1 to 3 days. This syndrome may occur in all age groups.

Subacute meningococcaemia

A few patients develop fever, an uncharacteristic maculopapular rash, general malaise, and arthralgia but no signs of meningitis or shock. They feel uncomfortable but are not severely ill. Meningococci are isolated from blood cultures. Untreated the symptoms may last for days to several weeks but disappear within 1 to 2 days after penicillin therapy is initiated.

Chronic meningococcaemia

The patient develops undulating fever, arthralgia, and maculopapular rash (Fig. 7.6.5.13). The symptoms may last for months, but at times they may disappear completely. Blood cultures are sometimes repeatedly negative. Patients are often treated with corticosteroids because an underlying autoimmune disease is suspected. The fever disappears temporarily before reappearing and at this stage meningococci may well be isolated from blood cultures. Antibiotic treatment clears the symptoms within a few days.

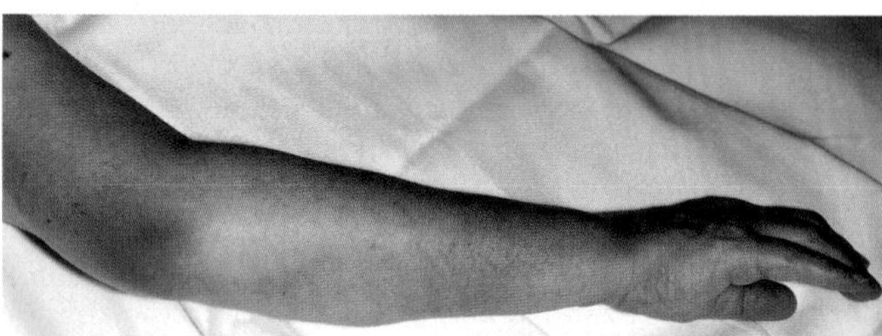

Fig. 7.6.5.13 Maculopapular rash and peri-articular swellings in an adult patient with chronic meningococcaemia.
(Copyright D A Warrell.)

Other organ manifestations

Pericarditis

The pericardium is seeded during a transient meningococcaemia. Subsequent inflammation and exudate may lead to cardiac tamponade if left untreated. The patient is febrile, nauseated, and may complain of epigastric pain. The condition is often misdiagnosed as an acute abdominal condition. Blood cultures may be negative. *N. meningitidis* can be cultured, detected by PCR, and seen in aspirated pus by direct microscopy. Treatment consists of evacuating the pus and administering antibiotics. The condition should be followed daily by ultrasound examination. Serogroup C organisms have been particularly implicated in these cases.

Arthritis

Acute meningococcal arthritis is an uncommon clinical manifestation of a preceding, often low-grade, meningococcaemia. It is usually located to one, or more rarely, several large joints. If the characteristic petechial rash is absent, detection of meningococci in blood or joint fluid is necessary for a correct diagnosis. Arthritis caused by *Neisseria gonorrhoeae* is considerably more common than primary meningococcal arthritis. The symptoms disappear rapidly after penicillin treatment and there are no long-term complications.

Arthritis induced by immune complexes

This is more common than the meningococcal arthritis. One or several large joints become swollen and painful. The symptoms usually develop at the end of the first week of treatment. Blood and joint cultures are negative. The temperature and inflammatory markers may rise after an initial decline. The symptoms disappear gradually after some days of treatment with nonsteroidal anti-inflammatory drugs. Extended antibiotic therapy is not necessary.

Cutaneous vasculitis and episcleritis

This appears simultaneously with the immune complex arthritis and is commonly observed in sub-Saharan Africa (Figs. 7.6.5.14, 7.6.5.15). The vasculitis causes multiple blisters that readily rupture leading to multiple superficial skin ulcers.

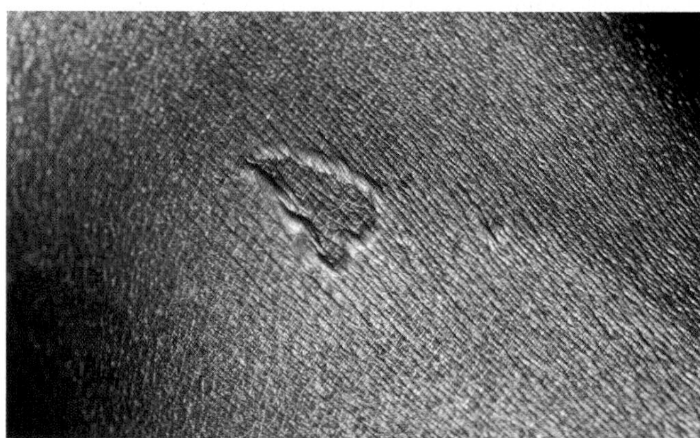

Fig. 7.6.5.14 Vasculitic lesion in an African child with meningococcal group A meningitis.
(Copyright D A Warrell.)

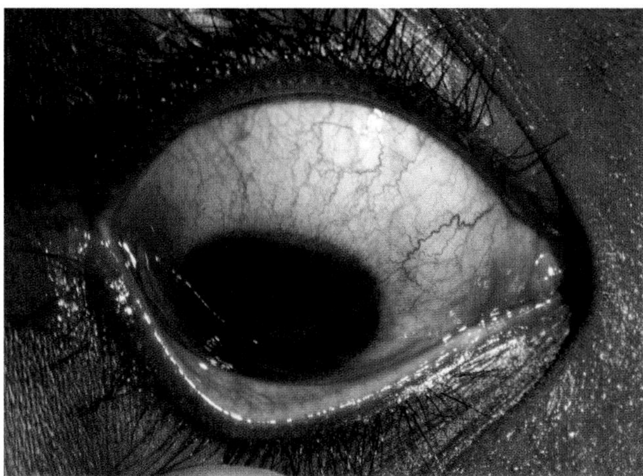

Fig. 7.6.5.15 Episcleritis in an African child with meningococcal group A meningitis.
(Copyright D A Warrell.)

Ocular infections

Conjunctivitis or panophthalmitis may precede other symptoms of invasive meningococcal infection. They are primarily observed in infants and children. The patient develops a red eye which in the case of panophthalmitis becomes painful with impaired vision. Formation of microthrombi and haemorrhage in retina and corpus vitreum, leading to blindness, may complicate the infection.

Pneumonia

Strains belonging to serogroups Y and W135 or more rarely other serogroups may cause pneumonia in adults and children. The diagnosis depends on detecting meningococci in a representative specimen from the low respiratory tract or blood culture. It cannot be differentiated from pneumonia caused by other agents on the clinical symptoms alone.

Treatment

Prehospital antibiotic treatment

Since 10 to 20% of the patients infected with *N. meningitidis* develop fulminant septicaemia characterized by rapidly increasing levels of meningococci and lipopolysaccharides (endotoxin) in the blood, early antibiotic treatment to stop further growth is regarded as vital. Consequently, health authorities in many countries advise general practitioners to start prehospital antibiotic treatment (i.e. benzylpenicillin) in suspected cases of meningococcal infection. The doses in Table 7.6.5.3 rapidly lead to bactericidal concentrations in plasma.

The penicillin is injected intravenously or intramuscularly in one or both thighs. The patients most likely to benefit from this strategy, if applied early enough, are those who are distant from the hospital and have rapidly evolving symptoms leading to a compromised circulation and extensive haemorrhagic skin lesions.

Initial evaluation in hospital

The patients should be regarded as emergency cases. The main clinical presentation and severity should be evaluated immediately. A variety of prognostic scores have been developed. The Glasgow Meningococcal Septicaemia Prognostic Score is the one most commonly used. Scores can be used to select patients for intensive care treatment. They should never be used to justify withholding treatment as they often overestimate case fatality.

Antibiotic treatment

Adequate doses of benzylpenicillin, cefotaxime, ceftriaxone, or chloramphenicol effectively stop further proliferation of *N. meningitidis* in the circulation, cerebrospinal fluid, and other extravascular sites. Induction of an explosive release of bacterial lipopolysaccharides leading to a Jarisch–Herxheimer reaction has never been documented in patients receiving antibiotics for meningococcal infection. Plasma levels of lipopolysaccharides and the levels of important inflammatory mediators decline immediately after treatment with antibiotics is initiated in these patients (Table 7.6.5.4).

Benzylpenicillin, chloramphenicol, cefotaxime, ceftriaxone, and meropenem are bactericidal to *N. meningitidis*. Benzylpenicillin remains the drug of choice in most countries. It is effective, cheap, and nontoxic in high doses as long as renal function is normal. High doses are necessary since it penetrates the cerebrospinal fluid relatively poorly. In patients with fulminant septicaemia and severe renal dysfunction the doses should be reduced after 24 to 48 h.

Strains whose sensitivity to penicillin is reduced because of altered penicillin-binding protein 2 are an increasing problem. In most industrialized countries they account for less than 5% of all meningococcal isolates, but the frequency is higher in Mediterranean countries, particularly Spain. Patients infected with these strains have been adequately treated with benzylpenicillin as long as dosage is adequate. A recent study from the United Kingdom indicated the same outcome among patients infected with fully sensitive strains as compared with strains with reduced sensitivity to penicillin. Penicillinase-producing meningococci remain extremely rare.

Chloramphenicol is a good alternative in patients hypersensitive to β-lactam antibiotics. In developing countries it is the best and cheapest alternative to benzylpenicillin. Meningococcal strains resistant to chloramphenicol occur in certain areas. In many industrialized countries cefotaxime or ceftriaxone is combined with vancomycin as empirical treatment of bacterial meningitis until the aetiological agent has been identified. Cefotaxime and ceftriaxone are highly effective antibiotics that

Table 7.6.5.3 Doses of prehospital antibiotic to be administered in suspected cases of meningococcal infection

Age (years)	Dose
<2	300 mg (0.5 × 10^6 IU) benzylpenicillin intramuscularly
2–7	600 mg (1 × 10^6 IU) benzylpenicillin intramuscularly
>7	1.2 g (2 × 10^6 IU) benzylpenicillin intravenously or intramuscularly

Table 7.6.5.4 Antibiotics in meningococcal meningitis or sepsis

Antibiotic	Dose/24 h		Dose interval (h)
	Adult (g)	Child (mg/kg)	
Benzylpenicillin	14.4 (24 × 10^6 IU)	200 (300 000 IU/kg)	4–6
Cefotaxime	9	200	6–8
Ceftriaxone	4	100	12–24
Chloramphenicol	3	100	6

penetrate the blood–brain barrier better than benzylpenicillin. Nonsusceptible strains have emerged in India. Meropenem is a carbapenem highly active against *N. meningitidis*, *H. influenzae*, and *S. pneumoniae*. It does not induce seizures as observed with the imipenem–cilastatin combination.

In each country the health authorities and microbiological laboratories should recommend the optimal and affordable drug regimen.

Antibiotic treatment should be initiated promptly. Therapy should start immediately after the first clinical evaluation and collection of the necessary samples for microbiological diagnosis. If there are contraindications to lumbar puncture or if it is delayed until after brain imaging, antibiotic treatment should be started immediately. Three to 4 days of treatment is adequate to eradicate sensitive meningococci.

Supportive treatment

Patients with persistent shock should be given extensive volume replacement, whereas patients with meningitis should receive a moderate amount of fluid. All patients should be monitored closely to detect early signs of a deteriorating circulation, renal and pulmonary failure, or increasing intracranial pressure.

Volume treatment

Patients with persistent hypotension and signs of inadequate peripheral circulation require massive fluid volume repletion. The extensive capillary leak syndrome increases the volume required. Children and adults may require an infused volume that is one to several times their circulating blood volume in the first 24 h. NaCl 0.9% is recommended as basic treatment later supplemented with Ringer's solution. In many countries the use of fresh frozen plasma is no longer recommended because of the risk of transmitting pathogens, especially HIV.

Patients presenting with distinct signs of meningitis without shock should receive the basic daily requirement of fluid supplemented with extra volume for dehydration and loss due to vomiting and fever. Excessive hydration should be avoided since it may precipitate irreversible brain oedema and cerebellar herniation. In patients with persistent shock and meningitis, treatment of shock is the priority.

Inotropic support

If initial volume repletion fails to improve the circulation, inotropic support should be added. Dopamine, dobutamine, noradrenaline, and adrenaline are used. Most physicians start with dopamine at 3 to 10 μg/kg per min which at an early stage is combined with noradrenalin at 0.03 to 3.0 μg/kg per min or dobutamine at 1 to 10 μg/kg per min. Ideally, patients should be infused through a central line.

Corticosteroid therapy for shock

In adults with septic shock and reduced adrenal function, low doses of cortisol increased survival in one study but was not confirmed in a larger follow up study. Similar studies do not exist for children. Adrenal haemorrhage is common in patients with fulminant meningococcal septicaemia. Serum cortisol is lower and ACTH higher in nonsurviving than surviving children with meningococcal shock; a relative adrenal insufficiency may therefore exist. Recently many clinicians have treated meningococcal shock with low doses of cortisol.

Corticosteroid therapy for meningitis

The benefit of dexamethasone in meningococcal meningitis is controversial. The studies conducted in industrialized countries have not documented a significant beneficial effect. Dexamethasone did not improve the outcome in any type of bacterial meningitis in a large randomized clinical controlled trial in Malawi. In an open randomized study in Egypt involving 267 patients, dexamethasone injected every 12 h for 3 days did not improve the outcome. Corticosteroid treatment has been associated with relapse of the meningitis in patients who had otherwise been adequately treated. At present, dexamethasone is not recommended for routine use in patients with meningococcal meningitis.

Ventilatory support

Patients receiving volume treatment for profound shock are in danger of developing ARDS. Hyperventilation, increasing oxygen demand, decreased pulmonary compliance, and the appearance of diffuse infiltrates on chest radiograph indicate the development of ARDS. At a partial oxygen pressure in arterial blood ($Pa\text{O}_2$) of less than 8 kPa with the fraction of inspired oxygen ($F\text{IO}_2$) above 0.6 (60% O_2 in the inspiration air), the patient usually requires intubation and artificial ventilation. Infants and children often require mechanical ventilation if the resuscitation fluid volume exceeds 40 ml/kg per 24 h to combat the septic shock, even if the oxygenation is normal.

Renal support

Patients with persistent septic shock and coagulopathy develop renal dysfunction from acute proximal tubular necrosis. Thrombosis in the small peritubular vessels and in glomeruli, and myoglobinaemia may contribute to renal dysfunction. Serum creatinine and urea are elevated on admission and continue to increase for many days without adequate treatment. Hyperkalaemia, which may develop during the first 24 to 48 h, is an immediate threat. Haemodialysis or peritoneal dialysis and continuous haemofiltration are used to treat the renal failure and remove oedema. The renal failure is usually reversible but may last for weeks. Complete kidney failure is uncommon in survivors.

Treatment of disseminated intravascular coagulation

The first priority is to stop further bacterial proliferation with antibiotics. This reduces the thrombin activity by 50% within 2 to 6 h. In the 1970s heparin was extensively used. Two small controlled trials did not document any survival benefit in patients receiving heparin. Infusion of a continuous low-dose unfractionated heparin (10–15 IU/kg per h) has been advocated as supplement to treatment with concentrated protein C. The antithrombin levels should be kept above 35 to 40 IU/ml. Antithrombin does not reduce the fatality rate in other types of severe sepsis.

Infusion of the natural anticoagulant protein C (loading dose 100 IU/kg, followed by 15 IU/kg per h for 4 days to keep the plasma concentration between 0.8 and 1.2 IU/ml) may possibly limit thrombus formation, skin necrosis, and the need for amputation. If used it should be started early. In the few uncontrolled studies that have been published, several patients treated with protein C concentrate still needed amputation. Randomized controlled trials are lacking.

One study with recombinant human activated protein C has shown a reduction in the case fatality rate in adults, but not in children, with severe sepsis and septic shock. It increases the chances of cerebral haemorrhage. Routine transfusion of platelets is controversial. In patients with life-threatening bleeding, massive platelet transfusion can be lifesaving; however, it may also aggravate thrombus formation.

Fibrinolysis

To overcome inhibition by PAI-1, recombinant human tissue plasminogen activator (0.25–0.5 mg/kg in 1.5–4 h) has been infused to enhance fibrinolysis. Retrospective studies suggest that it increases the rate of cerebral haemorrhages. It is not recommended for routine use in severe meningococcaemia.

Plasmapheresis and blood exchange

Plasmapheresis and exchange blood transfusion have been tried to remove pathologically activated plasma and leucocytes; 50 ml plasma/kg body weight has been exchanged with fresh plasma. These techniques do not increase the clearance of bacterial lipopolysaccharide substantially. Results suggest improved survival but adequate control groups are lacking. Even desperately ill patients have tolerated the procedures.

Extracorporeal membrane oxygenation

A limited number of children have been treated with extracorporeal membrane oxygenation in a few centres with apparently good results. However, equally good results have been achieved in another paediatric intensive care unit without using the procedure, suggesting that the experience of the intensive care unit is more important than the procedure *per se*.

Neutralization of bacterial lipopolysaccharides

Three different antiendotoxin principles, the anti-J5 serum, the human monoclonal IgM (HA-1A) antibody, and the recombinant bactericidal/permeability increasing protein (BPI_{21}) have been evaluated in randomized double-blind controlled clinical trials. None increased survival significantly; however, fewer patients treated with BPI_{21} required multiple severe amputations and more patients had a functional outcome similar to that before illness 60 days after treatment. None of the principles are presently commercially available.

Antimediator therapy

Strategies to neutralize tumour necrosis factor-α, IL-1, bradykinin, platelet-activating factor, and prostaglandins in patients with septic shock have not increased the 28-day survival rate. They have not been specifically evaluated in meningococcal septic shock.

Sequelae

Meningitis

Sensorineural hearing loss or impaired vestibular function occurs in 4 to 19% of patients. It develops at an early stage, is usually irreversible, and is more common in adults than children. Epilepsy, hydrocephalus, and diffuse brain damage are at present rare complications in industrialized countries.

Persistent headache, altered sleep pattern, concentration difficulties, irritability, and neurasthenia may persist in 5 to 8% of all patients.

Shock and coagulopathy

Most long-term complications are related to development of gangrene of the extremities requiring amputation and necrotic skin lesions requiring extensive grafting. The renal failure is usually reversible although reduced function may persist. Permanent adrenal insufficiency, i.e. Addison's disease, develops very rarely in survivors. ARDS may lead to permanent pulmonary fibrosis and reduced function.

Prevention

Vaccination

Capsule polysaccharide vaccine (A, C, Y, and W)

The protective effect of these vaccines in infants below 2 years of age is uncertain. When vaccination is required to prevent serogroup A infection, infants of less than 24 months should receive two doses with at least a 1-month interval, whereas those above 2 years should receive one dose. For serogroup C infection, one dose should be given from 18 months. Revaccination with serogroup C polysaccharide may reduce the antibody level. Malaria reduces the immune response. An antibody level of 1 to 2 µg/ml appears to be necessary for protection which lasts for 3 to 5 years.

Conjugate protein capsule polysaccharide vaccines (A, C, Y, and W)

Serogroup C conjugate vaccines are immunogenic from 2 months of age and have been shown to be very effective. Booster doses are required to keep the anticapsule antibodies at a protective level. A combined vaccine containing serogroups A, C, Y, and W135 has been licensed in the United States of America for the age group 11 to 55 years. Serogroup A, combined A–C, and other combinations of conjugate vaccines are under development and will be licensed in the near future for use in infants.

Outer membrane vesicle vaccine (B)

Since the capsule polysaccharide of serogroup B strains induces a short-lived IgM but no lasting IgG response, several groups have developed an outer membrane vesicle vaccine. The protection rate in adolescents after two doses is lower (57–80%) than for the polysaccharide and conjugate vaccines and is relatively strain specific. The immunodominant epitope is the outer membrane protein PorA. Three doses given 6 weeks apart and a fourth dose 8 months later induce a significantly better immune response than two doses. Studies in New Zealand with a strain-specific vaccine has resulted in 73% protection. The duration of the protection is not known.

Indications for vaccination

Routine immunization with the A, C, Y, and W vaccine is advocated for people with documented deficiencies in the alternative pathway and late complement components.

Nonoutbreak situation

Indications for vaccination with A or C vaccine are close contacts of an index case, travellers to high-risk areas, military recruits, persons with asplenia, and alcoholics.

Outbreak situation

Vaccination has been recommended if two or more persons are attacked by the same strain in a school class or day care centre, the attack rate exceeds 10 cases/100 000 population per 3 months, or the attack exceeds 1/1000 with 3 or more cases in a closed group setting.

Epidemic situation

An advocated threshold for mass vaccination is 15 cases/100 000 population per week for 2 consecutive weeks caused by the same strain. A steadily increasing number of cases and an increase in the median age of the patients indicate an epidemic.

Secondary prophylaxis

Antibiotic prophylaxis

Household contacts of an index case have a 100 to 1000 times increased relative risk for developing meningococcal infections. Usually the second case occurs within 2 weeks of the index case if no eradication treatment is given. However, there is doubt about the effectiveness of eradication treatment when the causative strain belongs to serogroup B.

Health authorities in most countries advise that close contacts have eradication treatment. Presently, adults receive 500 mg ciprofloxacin or 400 mg ofloxacin as a single dose. Pregnant women and children of less than 12 years should receive 250 mg and 125 mg ceftriaxone, respectively, as one intramuscular injection. Alternatively children are treated with rifampicin 10 mg/kg, maximum dose 600 mg, every 12 h for 48 h.

Further reading

Brandtzaeg P, van Deuren M (2005). Meningococcal infections at the start of 21st century. *Adv Pediatr*, **52**, 129–62.

Frosch M, Maiden M (eds) (2006). *Handbook of meningococcal disease.* Wiley, Weinheim.

Gardner P (2006). Prevention of meningococcal disease. *N Engl J Med*, **355**, 1466–73.

Rosenstein NE, *et al.* (2001). Meningococcal disease. *N Engl J Med*, **344**, 1378–88.

Snape MD, Pollard AJ (2005). Meningococcal polysaccharide-protein conjugate vaccines. *Lancet Infect Dis*, **5**, 21–30.

Stephens DS, Greenwood B, Brandtzaeg P (2007). Epidemic meningitis, meningococcemia and *Neisseria meningitidis*. *Lancet*, **369**, 2196–3210.

Van Deuren M, Brandtzaeg P, van der Meer JWM (2000). Update on meningococcal disease, with special emphasis on pathogenesis and clinical management. *Clin Microbiol Rev*, **13**, 144–66.

Welch SB, Nadel S (2003). Treatment of meningococcal infection. *Arch Dis Child*, **88**, 608–14.

7.6.6 *Neisseria gonorrhoeae*

D. Barlow, Jackie Sherrard, and C. Ison

Essentials

Neisseria gonorrhoeae is a Gram-negative, intracellular (within the cytoplasm of a leucocyte), diplococcus that primarily colonizes the columnar epithelium of lower genital tract, only occasionally progressing to the upper genital tract or causing systemic disease. It is almost exclusively transmitted by sexual activity.

Clinical features—(1) Oropharyngeal and rectal infections usually produce no symptoms; (2) men—dysuria (50%) and urethral discharge (98%) develop after a median of more than 5 days; complications, e.g. epididymitis, orchitis, are rare; (3) women—there are no specific symptoms in the absent of complications, e.g. salpingitis, bartholinitis; (4) disseminated gonococcal infection—a comparatively benign bacteraemia affecting joints (particularly shoulder and knee) and skin; more common in women than men.

Diagnosis—microscopy of a suitably stained specimen (urethral, cervical, rectal) is the first-line diagnostic technique; culture (48 h) is specific; nucleic acid amplification tests are rapid and sensitive, but plagued by false positives when used in inappropriate (low prevalence) populations.

Treatment—the gonococcus has adapted rapidly to prevalent antimicrobial usage, leading to reduced sensitivity to many antibiotics, notably penicillins, fluoroquinolones, macrolides and tetracyclines. First-line treatment of uncomplicated infection in adults should be a cephalosporin such as ceftriaxone 250 mg intramuscular injection or cefixime 400 mg orally. Spectinomycin 2 g intramuscular injection is suitable for those with penicillin allergy.

Introduction

Gonorrhoea is an ancient disease. Galen coined its name in the 2nd century AD (from Greek works meaning 'semen' and 'flow'), but there are older references including most of Chapter 15 of Leviticus in the Old Testament. The name of the causative bacterium, *Neisseria gonorrhoeae*, credits Albert Neisser with its discovery in 1879 although Hallier had described its characteristic microscopic appearance 7 years earlier.

In the era of HIV/AIDS, this treatable disease plays an important role as an indicator of risky sexual activity.

Epidemiology

In the United Kingdom since the Second World War, the peak incidence in 1946 resulted from a combination of returning infected soldiers and ascertainment bias (Fig. 7.6.6.1). Changing incidence thereafter seemed independent of the availability of effective antibiotics. However, the rising levels since the late 1950s, peaking in 1974, coincided with an increasing availability of different classes of effective antibiotics and was independent of resistance, first to penicillin and then to tetracyclines, macrolides, and quinolones. The rapid fall in incidence in the late 1980s coincided with a self-imposed regime of safer sex in the gay community.

Differences in the incidence of gonorrhoea between ethnic groups is not explained by genetic susceptibility.

Changes in gonococcal infection

Probably as a result of the availability of effective antibiotics, there have been changes in clinical manifestations of gonococcal infection. In men, the incubation period increased during the last century, from 2 to 3 days before the First World War to more than 8 days in recent years. In the 1990s, the median incubation period of 5.5 days lies outside the often quoted '2 to 5 days'. In women, the incubation period cannot be reliably estimated.

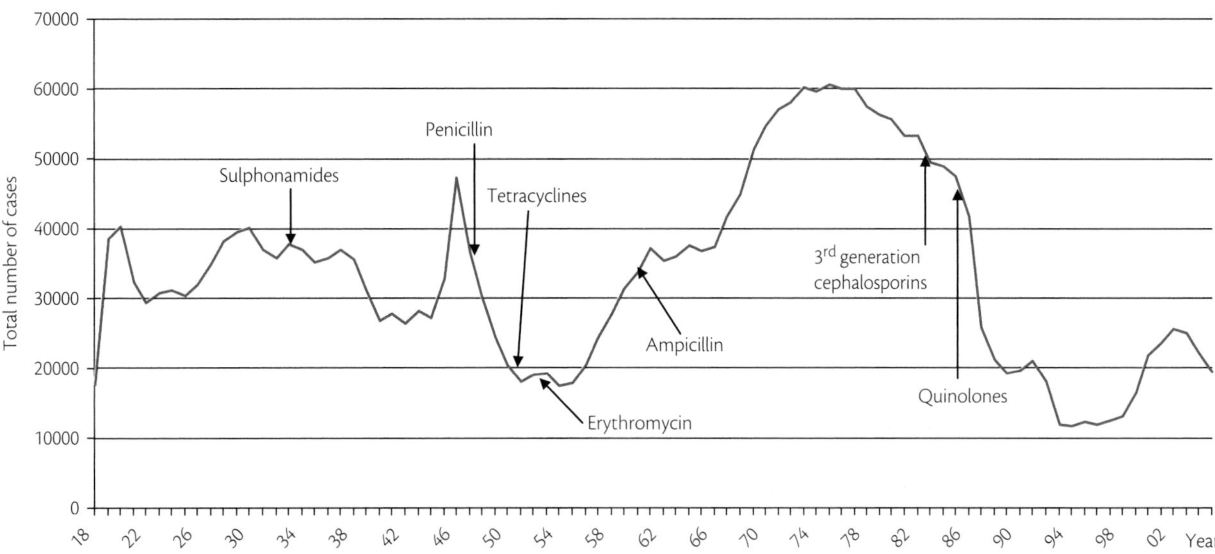

Fig. 7.6.6.1 Reported cases of gonorrhoea in England between 1918 and 2005 (Department of Health).

The time from symptoms to presentation for treatment (the infectious period) increased from under 2 days in 1932 to over 6 days in 1991, possibly because symptoms are less severe. The severe burning dysuria of previous times has been replaced by mild 'stinging' or, in 50% of men with gonococcal urethritis in one large study, no dysuria at all.

The complication rate has declined in parts of the world where management and treatment of sexually transmitted infections (STIs) is readily available. However, antibiotic sensitivity is declining worldwide and there are problems with diagnostic specificity.

Pathogenesis

N. gonorrhoeae has evolved mechanisms of evading host defences and causing repeated infection. Major outer membrane antigens exposed to the immune response are pili, lipo-oligosaccharide (LOS), and three major outer membrane proteins Por, Opa, and Rmp. *N. gonorrhoeae* primarily colonizes the columnar epithelium of the lower genital tract, only occasionally progressing to the upper genital tract or causing systemic disease. To colonize successfully, the organism must attach to and invade the epithelial layer to avoid being swept away by cervical secretions in women or urine in men. Iron is essential to multiplication; *N. gonorrhoeae* expresses transferrin or lactoferrin receptors on its surface. *In vivo*, gonococci resist the bactericidal activity of serum by sialylation of LOS. *In vitro*, most strains become serum sensitive. Pili, Opa, and LOS antigens can alter the part of the molecule exposed to the immune response. This antigenic variation occurs at a frequency higher than the normal mutation rate. On each encounter between the organism and the host, the gonococcus presents a range of immunologically distinct proteins that are not recognized by the host. Host cell receptors are complex carbohydrates, glycosamines, lipoproteins, and glycoproteins.

Gonorrhoea in women

Signs and symptoms

Initially, there are no specific symptoms. Uncomplicated gonorrhoea in women affects the cervix (90%), urethra (75%), rectum (40%), or oropharynx (5–15%). Gonococcal cervicitis results in an increased purulent or mucopurulent exudate from the os, which may present as an increased vaginal discharge (50%). This vaginal discharge has no specific characteristic. Dysuria (12%), without frequency, is not found consistently enough to make it a diagnostically helpful symptom. The occasional urethral discharge is not profuse enough to cause symptoms. Rectal infection may occur without anal intercourse and rarely produces slight dampness or discharge; throat infection is asymptomatic in both sexes. Abdominal pain signifies spread to the pelvic organs.

Complications

Spread to the endometrium, fallopian tubes, and pelvic adnexae is the most common complication (5%). It occurs at or soon after the menstrual period, probably resulting from retrograde flow of menses. Pelvic pain may be unilateral causing confusion with acute appendicitis. Coincidental infection with *Chlamydia trachomatis* is sufficiently common to justify treatment of both organisms. Infection of Bartholin's, Skene's, or periurethral glands is rare in the United Kingdom.

Perihepatitis (Fitz-Hugh–Curtis syndrome) occurs more frequently with *C. trachomatis* than *N. gonorrhoeae*. Right hypochondrial pain, referred to the shoulder, occasionally with pleural effusion and rub, may lead to referral to a surgical or general medical clinician rather than a genitourinary physician.

Disseminated gonococcal infection (DGI) is four or five times more common in women than men, reflecting the lack of genital symptoms in women. It is almost always caused by penicillin-sensitive organisms and is a comparatively benign bacteraemia affecting joints and skin. The shoulder and knee are most commonly affected, followed by wrist, elbow, and small joints of the hands and feet, often with an associated tenosynovitis. The pathognomonic painless usually 4 to 10 skin lesions evolve through vesicular, pustular, and haemorrhagic stages before healing (Figs. 7.6.6.2, 7.6.6.3). Erythema nodosum-like lesions have been described. Systemic symptoms are minimal. White cell count and erythrocyte sedimentation rate are not greatly raised. The response to antibiotic

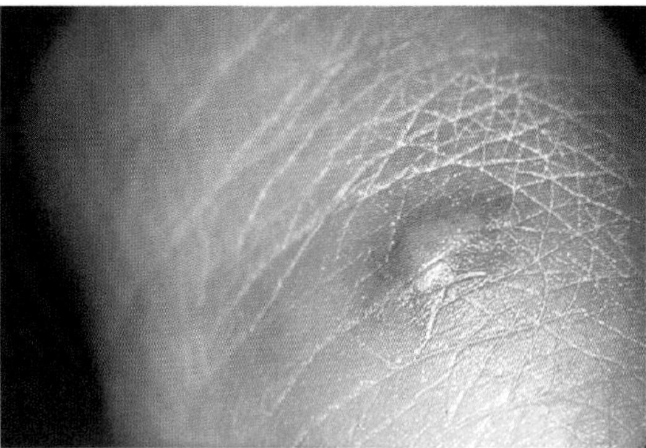

Fig. 7.6.6.2 Disseminated gonococcal infection, haemorrhagic vesiculopustule.

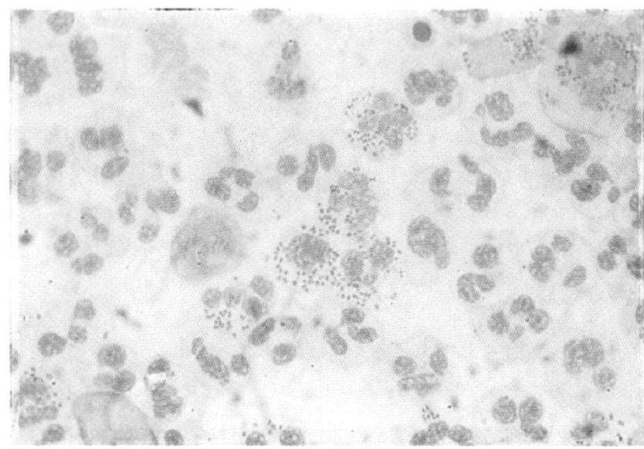

Fig. 7.6.6.4 Gram-stained urethral discharge showing Gram-negative intracellular diplococci.

treatment is rapid, but joints may need to be aspirated. Blood or joint fluid culture may yield gonococci, but the quickest diagnosis comes from anogenital and throat culture.

Gonorrhoea in men

Signs and symptoms

Classically, urethral gonorrhoea causes discharge and dysuria although the severity and frequency of the dysuria has diminished in recent years. The diagnostic thick, profuse, purulent, white or off-white exudate is preceded by a mucopurulent or scanty mucoid discharge. Even if untreated, the discharge may, after some weeks, diminish to a simple clear mucus; therefore, asymptomatic patients (less than 10%) include presymptomatic, postsymptomatic, and unobservant men. Urethral gonorrhoea acquired by fellatio is increasingly seen in gay men practising 'safe' sex. It may be transmitted to a regular partner resulting in rectal gonorrhoea.

Rectal and oropharyngeal infections are asymptomatic in almost all cases. Sore throat after oral sex does not indicate any particular STI.

Complications

Complications are rare in the developed world. Spread to the epididymis and testis is more often due to *C. trachomatis*. Tysonitis, prostatitis, periurethral abscess, or infection of the median raphe are rare in the United Kingdom.

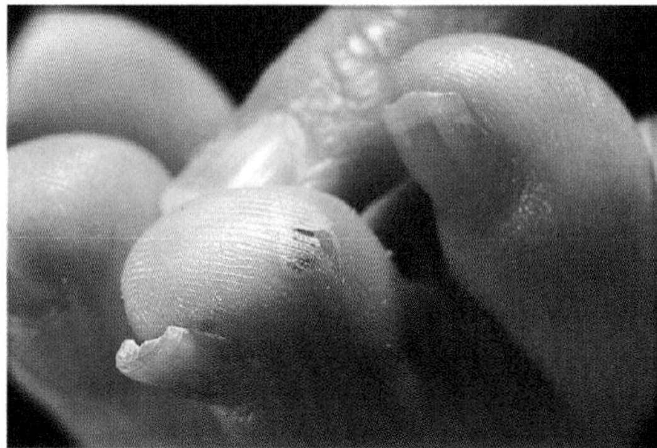

Fig. 7.6.6.3 Disseminated gonococcal infection: healing lesions with desquamation and deposition of haemosiderin.

Diagnosis

Microscopy

Diagnosis is easier in men than in women. Microscopy of a suitably stained specimen is the first line in diagnosis. The organism is a Gram-negative intracellular (within the cytoplasm of a leucocyte) diplococcus (GNID) (Fig. 7.6.6.4). In samples from the male urethra, microscopy is sensitive (identifying 98% of positives in symptomatic men and rather fewer in those without symptoms) and highly specific (<1% will be found on culture to be *Neisseria meningitidis* or other species).

Microscopy of stained samples from the cervix is much less sensitive (55% or less of true positives), but where positive enables immediate treatment. In known contacts of gonorrhoea, microscopy of urethral and rectal samples is indicated. Because of the preponderance of other neisseriae in the oropharynx, microscopy of samples from this site is not helpful.

Laboratory detection of *N. gonorrhoeae*

Isolation of *N. gonorrhoeae* has been the diagnostic gold standard because of its high sensitivity and 100% specificity. However, molecular techniques are now influencing the diagnosis of gonorrhoea. Detection of *C. trachomatis* by nucleic acid amplification tests (NAATs) are more sensitive and specific than previous tests. Since *N. gonorrhoeae* is often concomitant with chlamydial infection, kits which detect both agents are being more widely used.

NAATs for N. gonorrhoeae are now widely used. However, the prevalence of gonorrhoea is variable and in low prevalence populations they may givean unacceptable number of false positives unless the initial test is confirmed using a separate nucleic acid target. In individuals with symptoms consistent with gonorrhoea, or with a positive NAAT test, culture is recommended to obtain a viable organism to allow susceptibility testing.

Isolation and identification of *N. gonorrhoeae*

N. gonorrhoeae requires an enriched medium, such as Thayer–Martin or modified New York City which consist of GC agar base supplemented with a source of iron (lysed horse blood) and essential amino acids and glucose, and incubation in moist conditions with 5 to 7% carbon dioxide at 37°C. Good specimen collection and efficient transport to the laboratory are crucial for successful isolation.

Specimens are taken from appropriate sites using disposable loops or swabs for inoculation in the clinic or transfer to the laboratory in transport medium. Isolation is enhanced by adding antibiotics to the medium to suppress other organisms that colonize the anogenital tract. Vancomycin inhibits Gram-positive organisms, colistin and trimethoprim inhibit other Gram-negative organisms, and amphotericin or nystatin inhibit yeasts.

Gram-negative cocci on primary isolation that are oxidase positive (presence of cytochrome *c* oxidase) are considered to be *Neisseria* spp. In the industrialized world confirmation of identity as *N. gonorrhoeae* is considered normal practice. This is achieved using carbohydrate utilization tests, either alone or in combination with iminopeptidases in commercial kits; *N. gonorrhoeae* differs from other species in that it produces acid from glucose alone. An alternative approach is to use immunological reagents; reagents that are available contain antibodies raised to epitopes on the two types of the major outer membrane protein, Por or PI, and include those linked to fluorescein (GC Microtrak) and to staphylococcal protein A (Phadebact Monoclonal GC OMNI test). These sensitive and specific reagents can identify colonies direct from the primary isolation medium and a result can be obtained on the same day as the organism is isolated. Correct identification of *N. gonorrhoeae* is always desirable but is most important in cases of sexual or child abuse when more than one identification test should be used to confirm an isolate as *N. gonorrhoeae*.

Molecular detection of *N. gonorrhoeae*

NAATS (see above) have not been used as extensively for *N. gonorrhoeae* as for *C. trachomatis*, with which it commonly coexists, because they offer little advantage over Gram staining and culture and they do not provide an organism for susceptibility testing. However, the increasing pressure to screen more patients attending for sexual health care, or asymptomatic individuals in other healthcare settings, has escalated their use recently. The sensitivity and specificity of NAATs is high, they are less affected by suboptimal handling or transport, and can be used with noninvasive specimens as urine or self-taken swabs. No molecular tests are available for determining antibiotic susceptibility and so a representative sample of viable organisms will be required for surveillance purposes to guide antimicrobial therapy.

Typing

This has been used to study reinfection, treatment failure, antimicrobial susceptibility patterns, sexual networks, and for forensic purposes. Molecular typing has largely replaced phenotypic methods (auxotyping, determination of nutritional requirement, serotyping, reactivity with a panel of monoclonal antibodies) because it is more robust and discriminating. However, *N. gonorrhoeae* is nonclonal and highly competent for genetic exchange and therefore exhibits marked genetic diversity. For this reason, genotyping is more appropriate for short-term studies such as analysis of sexual networks, rather than temporal studies or comparisons at different geographical locations. Techniques based on diversity in the *por* gene and sequence-based methods, such as *N. gonorrhoeae* multiantigen sequence typing (NG-MAST) which examines diversity in two genes *por* and *tbp*B1, have proved useful. The combination of a highly discriminatory typing method and detailed epidemiological and behavioural data can provide information on the epidemiology that can be used for public health purposes.

Antimicrobial resistance

N. gonorrhoeae is inherently sensitive to most antimicrobial agents but with increased usage both chromosomally mediated and plasmid-mediated resistance has developed. Resistance is most prevalent in the developing world where the incidence of gonorrhoea is high and appropriate antibiotics are often unavailable or misused. However, in the industrialized world these strains are often imported and then spread by the indigenous population. Penicillin was used as first-line therapy for gonorrhoea for many years, until in 1989 the World Health Organization issued new guidelines for the treatment of gonorrhoea following increasing levels of resistance worldwide. Alternative treatments were recommended: ciprofloxacin (a quinolone), ceftriaxone (a third-generation cephalosporin), or spectinomycin (a macrolide), with penicillin recommended only if the gonococcal population was known to be sensitive. Ciprofloxacin was the treatment of choice in the United Kingdom because it is administered orally and is highly effective and inexpensive, whereas in the United States of America ceftriaxone was more widely used. In 2002 resistance to ciprofloxacin reached levels over 5% in England and Wales resulting in a change in guidelines for first-line therapy to a third-generation cephalosporin, ceftriaxone or cefixime.

Chromosomally mediated resistance

Decreased susceptibility to penicillin was detected as early as 1958 but this could be overcome by increasing the dose of penicillin and by adding probenecid. It was not until the 1970s that strains began to appear with minimum inhibitory concentrations (MIC) to penicillin of more than 1.0 mg/litre and posed a therapeutic problem. Chromosomal resistance to penicillin in *N. gonorrhoeae* (CMRNG) is the result of the additive effects of mutations at multiple loci *penA*, *mtr penB*, *ponA*, and *penC*, the products of which reduce the permeability of the cell wall to penicillin.

Resistance to ciprofloxacin emerged initially in gonococcal strains primarily originating from the Western Pacific with mutations in the DNA gyrase gene *gyrA* and the topoisomerase IV gene *parC*. The level of resistance may be enhanced by additional mutations in the *gyrB* gene or in changes in cell wall permeability possibly due to efflux mechanisms. Ciprofloxacin-resistant gonorrhoea is now endemic in most countries and in many instances is highest among infections in men who have sex with men (MSM).

Therapeutic failure to the oral cephalosporins such as cefixime and ceftibuten is beginning to be reported and is thought to be mediated by apenA mosaic, at least in part. With the increasing use of these highly active agents it is likely that resistance will emerge over time. Spectinomycin may be an alternative choice as resistance, which is high-level and due to a mutation on the chromosome that affects ribosomal binding, has only been reported sporadically. Azithromycin, primarily used for chlamydial infection, is being used for gonorrhoea but resistance has emerged possibly under selective pressure of the lower 1-g dose recommended for chlamydial infection compared to the 2-g dose for gonorrhoea.

Plasmid-mediated resistance

N. gonorrhoeae exhibiting plasmid-mediated resistance to penicillin was first described in 1976. Simultaneous reports appeared of two strains, one from Africa carrying a plasmid of 3.2 MDa and the second from the Far East carrying a plasmid of 4.4 MDa.

Both plasmids encode for the TEM-1 type β-lactamase (penicillinase). The smaller 3.2-MDa plasmid has a deletion from the 4.4-MDa plasmid in a nonfunctional region. Penicillinase-producing *N. gonorrhoeae* (PPNG) carrying the 3.2-MDa and 4.4-MDa plasmids have now disseminated worldwide although their prevalence is greatest in countries of the developing world. PPNG carrying plasmids of differing size (2.9, 3.0, and 4.8 MDa) have been described but have not spread in the same manner.

In 1985, plasmid-mediated resistance to tetracycline was first detected. It is high-level (MIC ≥16 mg/litre) and is due to the acquisition of the *tetM* determinant by the conjugative plasmid of *N. gonorrhoeae* resulting in a plasmid of 25.2 MDa. Strains carrying this plasmid are known as tetracycline-resistant *N. gonorrhoeae* (TRNG). Tetracycline is not the treatment of choice for gonorrhoea but was commonly used, particularly in African countries until the emergence of TRNG, because it was inexpensive and available.

Susceptibility testing

The primary aim of susceptibility testing of *N. gonorrhoeae* is to predict therapeutic failure. However, it is also important to monitor drifts in susceptibility and to detect the emergence of resistant strains to the main first-line therapies. There is much controversy over the correct method for achieving this for gonococci. Determination of zones of inhibition around antibiotic-containing discs has been the method chosen by most clinical laboratories. Gonococci are fastidious organisms that vary in their growth patterns and therefore this method can be difficult to control and interpret. Determination of the full MIC is not necessary for most laboratories and is best performed by reference centres. Etests, which are strips that contain a gradation of concentrations of antibiotics and give a MIC using a similar methodology to disc testing, are very useful for laboratories testing small numbers of strains, albeit still an expensive choice.

Plasmid-mediated resistance to penicillin can be easily detected using the chromogenic cephalosporin (nitrocefin) test. Penicillinase-producing strains change the yellow reagent to a pink/red colour within a few seconds and this can be performed direct from the primary isolation plate. Plasmid-mediated resistance to tetracycline can be detected using either the absence of a zone of inhibition around a 10-μg tetracycline disc or presence of growth on GC agar containing 10 mg/litre tetracycline. Both these screening tests are known to be good predictors of the presence of the 25.2-MDa plasmid and the *tetM* determinant. In a similar manner high-level resistance to ciprofloxacin can be detected by screening for isolates that can grow on agar containing 1 mg/litre ciprofloxacin.

Treatment of gonococcal infection

The choice of treatment will depend on the likely antibiotic sensitivities of the local gonococci. The quinolones recommended in the previous two editions of this book are, like penicillin, no longer first choice unless the organism is known to be sensitive. Because the spectrum of sensitivity/resistance is continuously changing, up-to-date advice may be found at the websites of the Health Protection Agency (HPA) and the British Association of Sexual Health and HIV (BASHH).

First-line treatment of uncomplicated infection in adults should be a cephalosporin such as ceftriaxone 250 mg intramuscularly or cefixime 400 mg orally. Spectinomycin 2 g intramuscularly is an alternative and is suitable for those with penicillin allergy. Ceftriaxone is also suitable for oropharyngeal infection. Ciprofloxacin 500 mg is an alternative if the prevalence of resistant strains is lower than 5% or if the organism is known to be sensitive. It is increasingly common practice to treat any possible chlamydial infection with 1 g azithromycin which has its own antigonococcal effect. This antibiotic should not be used on its own for gonorrhoea because of the presence of high-level resistance (shared with other macrolides). Spectinomycin or ceftriaxone may be used in pregnant or breast-feeding women.

For disseminated gonococcal infection, European guidelines suggest regimens of the above antibiotics: ceftriaxone 1 g intramuscularly or intravenously every 24 h; or cefotaxime 1 g intravenously every 8 h; or spectinomycin 2 g intramuscularly every 12 h continuing for 7 days, which may be switched 24 to 48 h after symptoms improve to an oral regimen such as cefixime 400 mg twice daily or, if quinolone resistance is excluded, ciprofloxacin 500 mg twice daily. Laboratory testing should provide full sensitivities of the causative organism and, unless disseminated gonococcal infection is caused by a resistant strain (an extremely rare occurrence at the time of writing), treatment may be switched to oral amoxicillin 500 mg and probenecid 500 mg, both four times daily.

American and British guidelines suggest that gonococcal pelvic infection or perihepatitis should be treated with parenteral antibiotics, although the evidence for this rather than oral treatment is not strong. Pelvic infection may be due to the gonococcus *C. trachomatis*, mixed anaerobes, or any combination of these, and treatment regimens reflect this. Ceftriaxone (intramuscularly or intravenously) 1 g once daily with doxycycline 100 mg and metronidazole 400 mg, both twice daily intravenously or orally, are recommended.

Infected individuals should be screened for other STIs and their partners identified and, ideally, tested for infection before treatment.

Current national and international guidelines suggest there is no need for a test of cure following treatment. However, several studies from the pre-NAATS era demonstrated a small but significant failure rate in samples from the rectum even when a fully sensitive organism had originally been isolated.

Further reading

Barlow D, Phillips I (1978). Gonorrhoea in women: diagnostic, clinical and laboratory aspects. *Lancet*, **i**, 761–4.

Bignell CJ (2005). *National guideline on the diagnosis and treatment of gonorrhoea in adults 2005.* www.bashh.org/guidelines/ceguidelines.htm

British Association of Sexual Health and HIV (2006). *Sexually transmitted infections: UK National Screening and Testing Guidelines 2006, commissioned by BASHH. Clinical effectiveness.* www.bashh.org/guidelines/2006/sti_screening_guidelines_v14_0806.pdf

Health Protection Agency (2009). GRASP 2008 Report: Trends in Antimicrobial Resistant Gonorrhoea. Health Protection Agency, London. http://www.hpa.org.uk/web/HPAweb&HPAwebStandard/HPAweb_C/1245914959952

Ison CA (1996). Antimicrobial agents and gonorrhoea: therapeutic choice, resistance and susceptibility testing. *Genitourin Med*, **72**, 253–7.

Ison CA (1998). Gonorrhoea. In: Woodford N, Johnson AP (eds) *Methods in molecular medicine*, vol. 15. *Molecular bacteriology: protocols and clinical applications*, pp. 293–308. Humana Press, New Jersey.

Nassif X, *et al.* (1999). Interactions of pathogenic neisseria with host cells. Is it possible to assemble the puzzle? *Mol Biol*, **32**, 1124–32.

Sherrard J, Barlow D (1996). Gonorrhoea in men: clinical and diagnostic aspects. *Genitourin Med*, **72**, 422–6.

Whiley DM, *et al.* (2008). Exploring 'best practice' for nucleic acid detection of *Neisseria gonorrhoeae*. *Sex Health*, **5**, 17–23.

7.6.7 Enterobacteria

Contents

7.6.7.1 Enterobacteria and bacterial food poisoning *727*
Hugh Pennington

7.6.7.2 *Pseudomonas aeruginosa* *735*
G.C.K.W. Koh and S.J. Peacock

7.6.7.1 *Enterobacteria and bacterial food poisoning*

Hugh Pennington

Essentials

The worldwide impact of food poisoning is very great. Such infections kill many children in the developing world, where diarrhoeal diseases stunt their physical and cognitive development. The number of illnesses is also large elsewhere: about 3 to 4% of the population of England and Wales contract food-borne disease every year, with over 20 000 hospitalizations.

The commonest bacterial pathogens are campylobacter and various members of the Enterobacteriaceae, a large family of gram-negative organisms, of which escherichia, shigella, and salmonella are considered in this chapter.

Escherichia coli

Pathogenic *E. coli* include the following:

Enteropathogenic (EPEC)—virulence-positive EPEC are now rare in industrialized countries; food- and water-borne and person-to-person spread occur, resulting in diarrhoeal illness; fewer than 500 cases are recorded annually in the United Kingdom.

Enteroaggregative (EaggEC)—first isolated from malnourished children in Chile suffering from chronic diarrhoea; uncommon in industrialized countries.

Enterotoxigenic (ETEC)—an important cause of mortality in children under 5 in developing countries, and cause travellers' diarrhoea; adhere to the mucosal surface of epithelial cells of the proximal small bowel, a process mediated by at least 12 different kinds of pili encoded by transferable plasmids, and produce enterotoxins.

Enteroinvasive (EIEC)—like shigella, for all practical purposes.

Enterohaemorrhagic (EHEC)—the most important EHEC is *E. coli* O157:H7, which produces a toxin virtually identical to that of *Shigella dysenteriae*. *E. coli* O157 is a normal nonpathogenic inhabitant of the gastrointestinal tract of cattle and sheep; most human infections are contracted either by the consumption of foods contaminated with animal manure or by its direct ingestion, probably from hands that have touched contaminated surfaces. Clinical presentation is with diarrhoea (becoming bloody in 90% of cases) and abdominal pain, with a few cases (15% of children <10) going on to develop haemolytic uraemic syndrome (HUS). Diagnosis is by culture. Management is supportive.

Shigella

Infections are exclusively human, spread by the faecal–oral route from person to person, and with a very low infectious dose. Shigellosis is endemic in developing countries in tropical areas, and it probably kills about 600 000 annually, mostly young children. Presentation is with watery diarrhoea, fever and malaise, with severe infections (most often caused by *S. dysenteriae*) progressing to diarrhoea comprising mucus, blood, and pus, along with severe abdominal cramps and tenesmus. Management of mild cases is supportive; severe cases are given antibiotics (ampicillin, co-trimoxazole, tetracycline, ciprofloxacin, others) as guided by local antimicrobial susceptibility data.

Salmonella

There are over 2000 salmonella serotypes, all belonging to the single species *Salmonella enterica*. Those that cause food poisoning infect both animals and humans, and most infections are food-borne, most often by poultry, with *S. enteritidis* (strictly a serotype rather than a species) the paradigmatic organism. Clinical presentation is typically with headache, vomiting (not usually a prominent feature), diarrhoea, abdominal pain, and fever. Metastatic infection sometimes occurs, particularly osteomyelitis and in atherosclerotic vessels, abnormal heart valves, and joint prostheses. Management of mild cases is supportive; severe cases are given antibiotics, usually ciprofloxacin.

Campylobacter

This is by far the commonest cause of bacterial gastroenteritis in the industrialized world, with an annual incidence of infection perhaps as high as 1 per 100 in the United Kingdom. The organisms are very common in the intestines of wild birds, poultry, cattle, and sheep, but the source of infection in most human cases is unknown. A prodrome of fever and general aching sometimes precedes abdominal pain (sometimes severe) and diarrhoea (frequently bloody). Complications include reactive arthritis (1% of cases) and Guillain–Barré syndrome. Most infections are self-limiting, but aside from supportive care, antibiotics (often erythromycin or ciprofloxacin) are given to severe cases.

Prevention

Prevention of food poisoning depends on Hazard Analysis and Critical Control Points (HACCP), which identifies hazards, identifies the points in a process where they may occur, and decides which points are critical to control to ensure consumer safety, e.g. in milk pasteurization the critical control points are the temperatures reached during heating, its duration, and the measures taken to prevent subsequent contamination.

Introduction

Food poisoning denotes gastrointestinal diseases caused by microbes transmitted in food or by microbial toxins preformed there. Food spoilage by microbes also has important consequences for human health because of its impact on food supply. Each year 10 to 20% of the world's annual cereal crop of approximately 2×10^9 tonnes is lost through spoilage by moulds. Much of this loss occurs in the humid tropics and contributes there to the nutritional deficiencies caused by other factors.

The terms food poisoning and food-borne disease overlap but are not synonymous. Thus variant Creutzfeldt-Jacob disease (vCJD), contracted by eating meat products from cows with bovine spongiform encephalopathy, only fits under the food-borne rubric because of its very long incubation period despite the absence of gastrointestinal symptomatology. It is the same for bovine tuberculosis transmitted by milk.

The worldwide impact of food poisoning is very great, as recognized by the World Health Organization Global Strategy for Food Safety (2002), and is the cause of death of many children in the developing world. Diarrhoeal diseases stunt the growth of children and impair their physical and cognitive development. Mortality rates are much lower in developed countries, but the number of illnesses is still large. Quantitation is difficult because of under-reporting. The largest national study of the number and causes of cases of infectious intestinal disease (IID) was done in England between 1992 and 1996. It found that while 20% of the population had IID in a year, for every 136 cases of IID in the community, 23 presented to a general practitioner, 6.2 had a stool sent routinely for microbiological examination, 1.4 had a positive result, and 1 was reported and appeared in the national statistics. In England and Wales between 1996 to 2000, it has been estimated that each year 1 724 315 people contracted food-borne disease, 21 997 were hospitalized, and there were 687 deaths.

The human intestine is home to 10^{13} to 10^{14} microorganisms. Their collective genome contains at least 100 times as many genes as the human one. They metabolize glycans and amino acids, detoxify xenobiotics, and synthesize isoprenoids and vitamins. A prominent member of the distal gut and faecal flora is the methane synthesizer, *Methanobrevibacter smithii*. However, the taxonomic identity and precise properties of most gut microbes is unknown because they cannot be grown in the laboratory. Cultivable ones that cause disease comprise a small minority, even when those opportunistic pathogens which occur primarily as commensals are included, such as members of the Enterobacteriaceae. This family contains several important causes of disease. *Salmonella typhi* and *S. paratyphi*, the causes of typhoid and paratyphoid fevers, are members of the Enterobacteriaceae. They cause systemic disease and are described in detail in Chapter 7.6.8.

Gastroenteritis caused by non-Enterobacteriaceae, i.e. the Gram-negative organisms *Aeromonas*, *Plesiomonas*, *Vibrio parahaemolyticus* and other noncholera vibrios, and, most important quantitatively by incidence, *Campylobacter*, are included here, together with accounts of food poisoning caused by *Bacillus* spp. For descriptions of diseases caused by *Clostridium botulinum* and *C. perfringens* see Chapter 7.6.24, *C. difficile* see Chapter 7.6.23, and *Staphylococcus aureus* see Chapter 7.6.4. An overview of infections of the intestinal tract is given in Chapter 15.18.

Enterobacteriaceae

The Enterobacteriaceae comprises a large family of Gram-negative bacteria. Many species are free-living, some are associated with plants and can be plant pathogens, and others live in the intestines of animals and humans. The pathogens considered in detail in this chapter belong to the genera *Escherichia*, *Shigella*, and *Salmonella*.

The formal bacteriological definition of the family is that its members are nonsporing Gram-negative rods that are often motile, usually by peritrichous flagella. They are easily cultivable on ordinary laboratory media. They may or may not have capsules. All are aerobes, although many grow anaerobically as well. All ferment glucose with the formation of acid and sometimes gas, and most reduce nitrate to nitrite. They are oxidase negative and, with the exception of one type of *Shigella dysenteriae*, are catalase positive.

For a century, species in the family have been identified by carbohydrate fermentation patterns and by testing the reactivity of the bacteria to antisera prepared against their surface structures.

Salmonella and *Shigella* do not ferment lactose. With the exception of proteus, providencia, and morganella, all other Enterobacteriaceae ferment this sugar freely with acid production. After cultivation on agar medium containing lactose and a pH indicator, nonlactose fermenting colonies stand out because of their colour difference, making the initial detection of salmonella or shigella a fairly straightforward task. A similar approach is used to detect the most frequently occurring enterohaemorrhagic *Escherichia coli* serotype, *E. coli* O157:H7, most isolates of which do not ferment sorbitol. Antigenic epitopes key in identification schemes reside in the thick outer bacterial layer (the O antigens) and in flagella (the H antigens). The outer layer is a complex of lipopolysaccharide (LPS) protein and lipid. The LPS has a hydrophobic lipid A component (responsible for the pathological effects of endotoxin) and a hydrophilic polysaccharide made up of an O-specific polysaccharide and a core oligosaccharide. K-antigen epitopes reside on a capsular polysaccharide which when present covers the O antigens. It can be removed by boiling.

Enterobacteriaceae have a clonal population structure. Each individual pathogen has a common ancestor and the incidence of the disease it causes correlates with the population size of the clone that has grown from it. The task of the diagnostic laboratory is to detect and identify these clones as quickly and as cheaply as possible. In general, the traditional tests described above satisfy these requirements. Enterobacteriaceae clones evolve in real time, however, so markers can often be found to distinguish strains, even those with a recent common clonal origin. Tests that determine the susceptibility of isolates to a range of bacterial viruses, bacteriophage typing, have been widely used for this purpose, particularly in the United Kingdom. Molecular methods that detect DNA sequence differences are widely used internationally and have universal applicability and high discriminatory power.

The Enterobacteriaceae considered here live in the intestines of animals and humans. This environment facilitates gene exchange between individual bacteria. It has been known for many years that plasmids, bacteriophages, and transposons are mobile genetic elements. Studies on *E. coli* virulence factors in the 1990s led to the discovery of pathogenicity islands, large genomic regions that are present in pathogenic strains but not in related nonpathogens. They carry genes associated with virulence, are often associated with tRNA genes, and are frequently flanked by repeat sequences.

Their G+C content is different from the rest of the bacterial chromosome. DNA sequencing studies have shown more recently that similar islands also occur in nonpathogenic strains. The functions they encode contribute to increased adaptability, fitness, and competitiveness. Genomic islands have been acquired from other bacteria, not necessarily closely related ones. With the other mobile genetic elements they form part of a flexible gene pool which confers beneficial traits supplementing the essential functions encoded by the conserved core genome.

Molecular genetics has shown that *Shigella* spp. and *E. coli* are so closely related that formally they belong to a single genus. *Escherichia* has priority; however, *Shigella* is a useful name and is likely to continue in use for the foreseeable future. Likewise, the enthusiasm of those who gave hundreds of specific names to salmonella strains distinguished by serotyping was misplaced. The strains are so closely related they are now referred to as serovars of the single species, *Salmonella enterica*.

Escherichia coli

Theodor Escherich was the first to grow *E. coli* in pure culture. He employed the 'Plattenmethode' described by Robert Koch in 1881 in his investigation in Munich in 1885 of the intestinal bacterial flora of newborns. It was the first detailed study of human commensal bacteria; appropriately so, because an overwhelming majority of the hundred billion billion *E. c*oli bacteria that live in the world at any time are normal inhabitants of the intestines of healthy humans and animals. The perception in the 1940s by molecular biologists of its harmless nature coupled with its nonfastidious cultural requirements and rapid growth (2–3 generations/h in the laboratory) led to its choice as a model organism. The strain most often studied is K12, isolated from the faeces of an American convalescent diphtheria patient in 1922. More Nobel prizes have been won by researchers on *E. coli* than any other species (with the exception of *Homo sapiens*).

The identification of *E. coli* using traditional bacteriological methods is straightforward. It is a nonsporing Gram-negative rod, usually motile with peritrichous flagella, facultatively anaerobic, and a gas producer from fermentable carbohydrates. The methyl red reaction is positive and the Voges–Proskauer reaction negative. Many strains have a polysaccharide capsule or microcapsule and most rapidly ferment lactose. Finding such an organism in a normally sterile site such as cerebrospinal fluid or in larger numbers in urine than can be accounted for by contamination is sufficient to indicate an aetiological role. Different approaches have to be used to detect enterovirulent *E. coli* in stools. Selective indicator media have been developed for *E. coli* O157. Other kinds are not looked for routinely; the best methods for detection use DNA probes or polymerase chain reaction (PCR) amplification procedures that are only available in reference laboratories. Few studies have been done on the carriage of commensal *E. coli* by healthy individuals but it is known that some carry a single clone for long periods, whereas others carry several simultaneously, acquiring and losing different clones rapidly. Some clones have a worldwide distribution; others seem to be only local. The genome sequence of strain K12 was published in 1997 and since then the genomes of representative pathogenic clones have been sequenced. A general principle has emerged that within the species there is an enormous amount of genetic diversity. Comparison of K12, a uropathogenic isolate, and an *E. coli* O157 showed that only 39.2% of the combined set of proteins was common to all. The genomes of the pathogens were as different from each other as each pathogen was from the commensal strain. Another *E. coli* characteristic is that different clones share a common genomic backbone of vertically evolved genes which is punctuated by many islands that have been acquired by different horizontal transfer events in each strain.

All pathogenic *E. coli* are sticky, in that they produce structures on their surfaces that act as organelles of attachment. The proteins that make them sticky are adhesins, which recognize host cell structures—receptors—with stereochemical specificity. This fit is an important determinant of host specificity and tissue tropism. Adhesins are often assembled into hair-like fibres, pili. Some take the form of a fuzzy mass on the bacterial surface, curli. Others form no particular oligomeric structures.

The genomes of uropathogenic strains are also rich in genes coding for autotransporters, phase-switch recombinases, and iron-sequestration systems.

Enteropathogenic *E. coli* (EPEC)

The isolation of antigenically identical *E. coli* strains during the investigation of outbreaks of diarrhoea in young babies in the 1940s in London, Aberdeen, and Liverpool provided the first clear evidence that *E. coli* could be an intestinal pathogen. Subsequent serotyping showed the isolates to be O111 and O55. The disease they caused had a mortality of about 50% and mostly occurred in babies aged 6 months or less. Although volunteer studies in Liverpool showed that isolates from babies caused gastroenteritis in adults, a dose of 2×10^9 organisms only led to a mild short illness.

Typical EPEC cause illness in infants and children under 2 years old; the hospital outbreaks that occurred in the 1940s are no longer seen. Intestinal colonization by typical EPEC involves virulence plasmid-encoded type IV bundle-forming pili which mediate bacterium to bacterium adherence and the formation of compact microcolonies on the surface of host cells, a pattern called localized adherence. EPEC fall into two related groups. Each contains several clones, some of which have been circulating for many years and have been found on several continents. O type does not always correlate with clonal type; thus type O142 marked two clones, one responsible for a high mortality outbreak in a Mexico City hospital in 1965 and the other for much less lethal infections of infants in Indonesia in 1960, hospital outbreaks in England, Scotland, and Ireland from 1969 to 1972, and sporadic cases in Canada in 1972 and Arizona in 1975.

Virulence-positive EPEC are now rare in industrialized countries. Surveys in Brazil showed that they were common there in the 1980s and 1990s. In Europe and North America, EPEC lacking the virulence plasmid are now much more frequent causes of diarrhoea. These atypical EPEC are now becoming proportionally commoner in Brazil as well.

A mechanism central to EPEC pathogenesis is the attaching and effacing (A/E) lesion. At the sites of adhesion in the colon, intestinal cell microvilli disappear. Actin accumulates beneath the bacteria, which become seated on pedestal-like structures. The bacterial genes for the production of attaching and effacing lesions are located on the locus of enterocyte effacement (LEE) pathogenicity island. It codes for intimin, an outer membrane protein responsible for adherence of the bacteria to enterocytes, Esp molecules, which are involved in the machinery that translocates bacterial proteins into enterocytes, and tir, which is translocated and inserts into the enterocyte cell membrane to act as the receptor for intimin.

The incubation period of the diarrhoeal illness caused by EPEC ranges from 12 to 72 h, and the illness can last for several days. Food-borne, water-borne, and person-to-person spread occur. Less than 500 cases are recorded annually in the United Kingdom.

Enteroaggregative *E. coli* (EAggEC)

These adhere to cell cultures in a 'stacked brick' pattern, a property often encoded on a 60-MDa plasmid. EAEC were first isolated from malnourished children in Chile who had chronic diarrhoea and have been found since in Brazil, Mexico, India, and Zaire. They are uncommon in industrialized countries. They have diverse O and H types. Little is known about their virulence factors or their precise pathogenic potential.

Enterotoxigenic *E. coli* (ETEC)

ETEC are an important cause of mortality in children under 5 years old in developing countries, and a significant cause of travellers' diarrhoea; 31 to 75% of Peace Corps volunteers in Africa with diarrhoea have been found to have ETEC in their stools. An incubation period of 12 to 72 h is followed by diarrhoea and vomiting lasting 3 to 5 days. ETEC adhere to the mucosal surface of epithelial cells of the proximal small bowel, a process mediated in different strains by at least 12 different kinds of pili encoded by transferable plasmids. There they produce enterotoxins, either a heat-labile (LT) or a heat-stable (ST) one, or both. LTs resembles cholera toxin in structure, mode of entry into cells, and toxic effects therein (see Chapter 7.6.11). There are different forms but are all made up of one A subunit and five B subunits. There are two kinds of the low molecular weight ST; ST-1 increases intestinal secretion through a route that involves the activation of cyclic guanosine monophosphate. ETEC enterotoxins are often plasmid encoded.

Many *E. coli* O serotypes have ETEC virulence factors; different clones vary in pilus type and in the enterotoxins they express.

Enteroinvasive *E. coli* (EIEC)

For all practical purposes EIEC are like shigella (see below); they have the same virulence factors and cause watery diarrhoea.

Enterohaemorrhagic *E. coli* (EHEC)

The most important EHEC is *E. coli* O157:H7. Because it produces a toxin which is lethal to cultured African green monkey (Vero) cells and is virtually identical to that of *Shigella dysenteriae* serotype 1 it is often called VTEC or STEC.

Epidemiology

E. coli O157 is a new pathogen. It came to notice abruptly and dramatically in the United States of America in 1982 where it infected consumers of beef burgers at a well-known chain of fast food restaurants. The first outbreak in England was in 1983. There is a rough correlation between closeness to the north and south poles and the national incidence of infection, which is higher in Scotland than England, in Canada than the United States of America, and in Argentina than Brazil. Accurate figures on its incidence in tropical countries are not available; it is probably uncommon. *E. coli* O157 is a normal nonpathogenic inhabitant of the gastrointestinal tract of cattle and sheep.

A significant minority of animals, up to 9%, carry it at any one time. The majority of tissue-associated *E. coli* O157 in them adhere to mucosal epithelium in a region extending up to 5 cm proximal to the rectoanal junction characterized by a high density of lymphoid follicles. Transmission of infection in humans is by the faecal–oral route. Person-to-person spread between young children occurs, and most infections are contracted either by the consumption of foods contaminated with animal manure or by its direct ingestion, probably from hands that have touched contaminated surfaces. Prevention of the contamination of carcasses in slaughter houses is difficult, which explains why transmission by meat occurs. Transmission by burgers has been significant in the United States of America because they are often consumed rare; maintaining 60° C for 2 min in their centre makes them safe. Many ready-to-eat foods have been vectors, e.g. lettuce. Poorly pasteurized milk, unpasteurized apple juice, and untreated drinking water have been important vehicles of transmission. Contamination of meats after cooking was important in the big Scottish outbreak in 1996, in which about 500 people were infected and 17 died.

About 80% of infections are sporadic. In North America and Europe they are commoner in people who live in or who have visited rural areas; in a majority of infections a food vehicle cannot be identified and direct transmission probably occurs.

Pathogenesis

E. coli O157 has the locus of enterocyte effacement pathogenicity island and adheres to enterocytes with the production of attaching and effacing lesions. In this respect it resembles EPEC; it may be that the latter was its progenitor. It also produces Shiga toxins (Stx1, Stx2). They are made of a single A subunit and a B pentamer. Stx1 is almost identical to the toxin produced by *Shigella dysenteriae* type 1; there are several allelic variants of Stx2 which are 50% homologous to Stx1 in amino acid sequence. The B subunit binds to the glycosphingolipid globotriaosylceramide on the surface of host cells; the A subunit enters and turns off protein synthesis by disrupting the large ribosomal subunit in a ricin-like fashion. Shiga toxins induce apoptosis in human renal cells as well. Most pathogenic *E. coli* O157 are Stx2 gene positive; about two-thirds are positive for Stx1.

Clinical features

After an incubation period ranging from 2 to 12 days, most commonly 3 days, diarrhoea starts. In up to 90% of cases it becomes bloody after another 1 to 3 days. Asymptomatic infections are not rare. Most symptomatic cases are afebrile; abdominal pain is more severe than in other forms of bacterial gastroenteritis and abdominal tenderness is common. After between 5 and 13 days of diarrhoeal onset, a minority of cases develop haemolytic uraemic syndrome (HUS). The risk is much greater at the extremes of age; about 15% of children under 10 years develop HUS. Other risk factors are antibiotic administration and the use of antimotility agents. Thrombocytopenia is the first abnormality to develop. There is increased activity of plasminogen activator inhibitor 1 and the concentration of fibrin D-dimers and thrombin fragments 1 and 2 becomes high. In full HUS (some cases never progress beyond thrombocytopenia) the kidneys fail. Neurological complications—thrombotic or haemorrhagic strokes, seizures, and coma—occur in 10% of HUS cases and cardiac dysfunctions occur in about the same proportion; they are important determinants of mortality. No treatment has been shown to prevent the development of HUS or specifically affect its course; the vascular damage that causes it is almost certainly well under way when patients present with diarrhoea. There is no bacteraemia and at this time the Shiga toxin has probably already reached its target organs via the blood stream. Management is supportive rather than specific.

Antibiotics, antimotility agents, and nonsteroidal anti-inflammatory drugs should not be given. Fluid balance should be monitored and treated carefully to avoid cardiac overload. Platelet monitoring will indicate whether the HUS risk period has passed. Anaemia sometimes requires transfusion. Renal failure requires specialist management, and renal function returns in a majority. The sequelae of *E. coli* O157 HUS mostly relate to renal function; risk factors for long-term problems are the severity of the HUS itself and the need for dialysis. In most cases of HUS, long-term problems have not been described.

Laboratory diagnosis

The diagnosis of *E. coli* O157 infection is by culture. Growth on selective media containing sorbitol leads to the formation of colourless colonies that are provisionally identified using O157 antiserum. For the detection of small numbers or organisms in, e.g. food suspected to be a vehicle of transmission, enrichment cultures followed by a specific concentration step using magnetic beads covered with O157 antiserum is carried out. Direct tests for Shiga toxin have been developed. Subtyping by phage typing and by pulsed-field gel electrophoresis (for high resolution and in countries where phage typing is not available) is an essential tool in outbreak investigation.

E. coli O157 is the commonest EHEC and cause of HUS. Other serotypes fall into these categories, and O26:H11, O103:H2, O111:H−, and O113:H21 have caused outbreaks in Australia and in continental Europe. Some pathogenic strains of *E. coli* O157 ferment sorbitol. Routinely used selective media detect none of these.

Control

The inability to influence the outcome of EHEC infections once established means that prevention is paramount. The development and implementation of preventive policies has been driven by the impact of big dramatic outbreaks, particularly those associated with burger chains in the United States of America in the 1990s and a butcher's shop in Scotland in 1996. In the United States of America, the Food and Drug Administration classifies *E. coli* O157 as a food adulterant; in consequence its detection has very bad commercial effects. In the United Kingdom and in Europe as a whole, the implementation of Hazard Analysis and Critical Control Points (HACCP)—the evidence-based food safety system—has probably been driven more rapidly than it otherwise would have been. With occasional exceptions these measures have worked well. For example, in Scotland rural/environmental risk factors for infection now far outweigh food ones. Further reductions in the number of cases will be difficult to achieve. No effective measures for reducing *E. coli* O157 in ruminants have been devised, and ruminants shed large numbers into the environment. In north-east Scotland (human population 5×10^5) it has been estimated that cattle and sheep drop about 3×10^{13} live *E. coli* O157 on the ground every day; the infectious dose of *E. coli* O157 for humans is very small, less than 100. Fortunately, the chain of events that leads to transmission from manure to mouth only occurs infrequently. In most years since the mid-1990s the annual incidence of infection in Scotland by *E. coli* O157 has been the highest in the world, but it is usually about 4 per 100 000, so infections are uncommon.

Shigella

Bacteriologists working in Japan, Germany, and the Philippines in the early 20th century demonstrated the bacterial aetiology of many cases of dysentery, and that the causative organisms belonged to a group of related but different nonmotile noncapsulate Gram-negative bacilli closely resembling *E. coli* but differentiated from it by their inability to ferment lactose on overnight incubation. The names of the genus, *Shigella*, and three of the four species, *S. flexneri*, *S. boydii*, and *S. sonnei*, commemorate them. The pioneer was Kiyoshi Shiga, who discovered *S. dysenteriae* in Tokyo in 1898.

Epidemiology

As countries become more affluent there is a fall in the number of shigella types circulating as common causes of disease. There is also a relative shift towards types that cause milder disease. *S. dysenteriae* type 1 causes the most severe disease. In the United Kingdom it had disappeared by the mid-1920s, when several *S. flexneri* types and *S. sonnei* were endemic. In England and Wales after 1950, 95 to 98% of infections were caused by *S. sonnei*, although *S. flexneri* was still commoner in Scotland. In the United States of America *S. flexneri* became less common than *S. sonnei* in 1968; currently in Thailand *S. sonnei* is becoming commoner than *S. flexneri*. However, the propensity of shigella to cause epidemics has meant that the change in incidence of infection has not been one of unremitting reduction. Thus in England and Wales after a postwar peak of 49 000 notifications of *S. sonnei* dysentery in 1956, the incidence declined steadily to an annual average of 3000 notifications between 1970 and 1990. However, they rose sharply in 1991 and again in 1992, peaking at 17 000 cases and then falling again. *S. dysenteriae* type 1 became commoner in Mexico and Central America in 1968, in the Indian subcontinent in 1975, and Central Africa during 1985.

Shigella infections are exclusively human (monkeys are susceptible but very probably catch their infections from humans) and are spread by the faecal–oral route. Volunteer studies and information from outbreaks caused by the faecal contamination of water and food on cruise liners have shown that the infectious dose is very low; dysentery can follow the ingestion of 10 viable organisms. Most spread is person-to-person and infection is greatly facilitated by bringing people close together in institutions and circumstances where unsanitary defaecation and inadequate hand washing is common; well-described examples are prisons in England in the early 19th century, mental hospitals in the United Kingdom, Germany, Denmark, and the United States of America later in the 19th century and in the early 20th century, British soldiers in Greece and Mesopotamia (now Iraq) in the First World War, and children in nursery and primary (elementary) schools in the United Kingdom in the early 1990s. It is considered that those with diarrhoea are by far the most effective transmitters of infection. After recovery many individuals continue to excrete organisms for a few weeks; temporary carriers of this kind are not thought to be important sources of infection, even if they are food handlers. Large and dramatic water-borne outbreaks have occurred occasionally in industrialized countries; milk and ice cream have also been vectors. Vegetables contaminated with human faeces during growth, harvesting, or preparation have also caused outbreaks. Molecular typing has revealed the international nature of some; e.g. more than 100 cases in the United Kingdom, Denmark, Norway, and Sweden in 1994 were shown in this way to be due to lettuce contaminated with an identical strain of *S. sonnei*. Shigellosis is endemic in developing countries in tropical areas; a long-standing estimate is that it kills about 600 000 people—mostly young children—annually.

Pathogenesis

Central to the pathogenesis of shigellosis (including that of enteroinvasive *E. coli*, which can be regarded as a variant of *S. sonnei*) is invasion of the colonic mucosa. Organisms gain access to the basolateral pole of enterocytes through M cells, components of intestinal lymphoid follicles (Peyer's patches). Bacteria infect macrophages in these structures and kill them by apoptosis. Their release allows direct invasion and is associated with a cytokine-induced inflammatory response that facilitates bacterial invasion by disrupting the epithelial architecture. The entry of shigella into intestinal cells is actin-microfilament dependent. Shortly after entry the bacterium lyses its phagocytic vacuole and grows in the cytoplasm at a rate of about 40 min/generation; most of the bacterial proteins responsible are plasmid-encoded. Bacteria then spread from cell to cell. Infected cells die and bacterial spread continues deep into the lamina propria. There is an acute inflammatory response dominated by polymorphonuclear leucocytes. Rectocolitis with epithelial desquamation and purulent necrosis with ulcers leads to the production of bloody mucus. Spread of bacteria from the intestines to other parts of the body is rare.

Shiga toxin is only produced by *S. dysenteriae* type 1 (see above). As with EHEC, infections with *S. dysenteriae* type 1 lead, in a minority of cases, to HUS. The increased severity of *S. dysenteriae* type 1 rectocolitis compared with that caused by other *Shigella* spp. is probably due to the local effects of Shiga toxin on the colonic vasculature.

Clinical features

After an incubation period ranging from 12 h to 7 days, but most commonly 2 to 3 days, symptoms usually start suddenly, often with abdominal colic. Watery diarrhoea follows, usually with fever and malaise. The symptomatology of most *S. sonnei* infections progresses no further and, commonly, the number of watery stools is small. The most severe infections are caused by *S. dysenteriae*. After 1 to 3 days the diarrhoea becomes bloody and very frequent, being composed of mucus, blood, and pus. Abdominal cramps and tenesmus are severe. Serious complications, sometimes lethal, are hyponatraemia, hypoglycaemia, septic shock, and HUS. Recovery in complicated cases is slow. More straightforward but severe illnesses such as those not infrequently caused by *S. flexneri* and *S. boydii* usually last about 4 days but may continue for 10 days or more.

Laboratory diagnosis

Diagnosis is by culture and traditional bacteriological methods work well; faeces are the best samples. Shigella dies rapidly when swabs dry and such samples should be transported to the laboratory quickly. Inoculation of enrichment cultures from broths or direct inoculation onto special media gives colonies recognizable as shigella by morphology. Further identification is by biochemical tests and type-specific antisera. DNA probes for plasmids are available and Shiga toxin can be looked for.

Treatment

S. sonnei infections in healthy individuals other than those at the extremes of age do not benefit from antibiotic treatment. Agents reducing gut motility should be avoided. Antibiotic treatment of severe infections must be guided by antimicrobial susceptibility data; antibiotic-resistant strains are common in areas where these infections have a high incidence. Ampicillin, co-trimoxazole, tetracycline, or ciprofloxacin have worked well; ceftriaxone and pivmecillinam have been successfully used to treat infections in children caused by antibiotic-resistant strains.

Control

The occurrence of urban epidemic shigellosis in countries like the United Kingdom long after the universal provision of treated town water shows that, while the provision of safe water in parts of the world where serious shigella infections are common is a necessary general public health measure, it will not be sufficient. Interrupting faecal–oral spread needs the provision of toilets and wash hand basins in homes—more a concomitant of economic development than of public health programmes.

Salmonella

The number of different salmonella clones is very large, but they all belong to the single species *Salmonella enterica*. Traditional bacteriological methods—serotyping using O and H antigens and simple biochemical tests—have been used to identify different kinds of salmonella since the 1930s and they are good markers of clonal identity. The custom of referring to the entities they define as though they were species, e.g. *Salmonella enteritidis* is taxonomically incorrect (they are serotypes) but operationally useful. A minority of salmonella serotypes has a host range limited to a single species, e.g. for humans *Salmonella typhi* (see Chapter 7.6.8), and these serotypes not considered further here. The serotypes that cause food poisoning infect both animals and humans, and well over 2000 have been described.

Epidemiology

Person-to-person spread is uncommon and the infected/carrier food handler is not an important source; faecal–oral spread after contact with carrier animals such as terrapins and other reptiles occurs from time to time, but most infections are food-borne. In the United Kingdom a big increase in microbiologically confirmed salmonella infection rates and the number of serotypes causing infections occurred in the late 1940s and early 1950s. A common pattern, which continues, is that a serotype appears, persists, and then declines. Their source for humans is food animals. Cattle, sheep, and pigs are far less important than poultry, although S. Typhimurium of bovine origin has remained quite common for many years. However, poultry dominate and the paradigmatic organism is S. Enteritidis. It caused a panzootic in broiler and layer chicken flocks in Europe and the United States of America starting in the 1980s and concomitantly a human pandemic. In England and Wales it peaked in 1993, when 17 257 infections accounted for 56% of all salmonella isolates. In chickens, S. Enteritidis not only grows in the intestines but also invades the reproductive tract leading to egg contamination. Since the early 1990s, control in flocks by slaughter, vaccination, and heightened biosecurity in hen houses has markedly reduced carriage levels in poultry, accounting for the decline in the number of human cases; in England and Wales in 2004 there were 2201 infections. The propensity of certain *Salmonella* serotypes to expand their population size has been enormously facilitated by the scale and nature of the poultry industry. The increase in the number of human infections since the 1940s has followed the expansion of broiler production. In 1950, United States broiler production was 631 million heads and *per capita* consumption was 8.7 pounds ready to cook; in 1990, it was 5864 million and 61.0 pounds, respectively.

Cross-contamination, where organisms from chicken carcasses have been transferred to ready-to-eat foods in the kitchen, has caused large outbreaks. Undercooked egg products are important vectors of *S.* Enteritidis. Many other foods have been vehicles of transmission: unpasteurized milk, dried milk, desiccated coconut, alfalfa sprouts, lettuce, and chocolate. Multicontinental outbreaks occur because of international trade, e.g. 4000 cases of *S.* Agona infection were caused by a contaminated kosher snack in the United Kingdom, Israel, the United States of America, and Canada in 1996.

Pathogenesis

Volunteer studies give an infectious dose ranging from 125 000 to 50 million organisms. For some foods, particularly those with much fat, e.g. cheese, potato chips, peanut butter, and chocolate, it is much less and ranges from fewer than 10 to 100. Organisms attack the distal small intestine and large intestine. At points of contact there is a transient denaturation of brush border microvilli, bacteria are internalized, and they remain in membrane-bound compartments. Replication is necessary for virulence; their presence triggers a transepithelial migration of neutrophils. These processes need the action of many bacterial genes, some of which are in pathogenicity islands.

Clinical features

The incubation period ranges from 4 to 48 h but most commonly it is between 8 and 24 h. Onset is often sudden, with headache, vomiting (not usually a prominent feature), diarrhoea, and abdominal pain; fever is common. The clinical course is usually short, up to 2 to 3 days; in a minority it is severe and prostrating with dehydration. Mortality rates are low but are higher in infants (meningitis sometimes occurs) and elderly people with preexisting pathologies. Some serotypes, e.g. *S.* Dublin are more virulent; bacteraemia with any serotype is usually transient but sometimes leads to metastatic infection, particularly in atherosclerotic vessels, abnormal heart valves, and joint prostheses. Osteomyelitis most frequently occurs in long bones, costochondral junctions, and the spine. Sickle cell anaemia is an important predisposing condition. Arthritis may be septic or reactive; the latter follows more than 1% of infections. It is commonest in those with the HLA-B27 haplotype. Faecal excretion of organisms continues for 4 to 8 weeks and is longer for infants; the number of organisms excreted is usually low. Carriage for longer than 6 months is rare.

Laboratory diagnosis

Diagnosis is by culture. Direct plating of faeces onto selective media and testing of suspicious colonies by slide agglutination for O antigens can give a presumptive diagnosis in 24 h. Enrichment broth cultures increase test sensitivity and are used to search for small numbers of bacteria in faeces or food. Phage typing schemes, available for *S. enteritidis*, *S. typhimurium*, and *S. virchow*, and pulsed-field gel electrophoresis have high resolution and are used to type isolates from patients and other sources in outbreaks.

Treatment

Fluid and electrolyte replacement is the management mainstay. Drugs that reduce gut motility are contraindicated. In uncomplicated cases antibiotics have no place and they may prolong the excretion of organisms. In patients with a high risk of bacteraemia and invasive disease (infants under 3 months, immunosuppressed patients, patients with cancer, and those with haemoglobinopathies) they should be considered. Ciprofloxacin is usually the agent of choice but antibiotic-resistant strains have emerged and therapy must be guided by susceptibility testing. Cefotaxime and ceftriaxone have been of value in treating meningitis in infants.

Prevention

Preventing the infection of food animals is central and it has been successful in poultry in Northern Europe and North America. HACCP has been adopted worldwide; refrigeration and adequate cooking are very important critical control points.

Campylobacter

Campylobacter was discovered as a pathogen of sheep at the beginning of the 20th century, but 70 years elapsed before it was recognized as a common cause of human gastroenteritis. Its high optimum growth temperature (42°C), need for a microaerobic atmosphere, and requirement for help from selective medium to inhibit other competing gut bacteria hindered its detection. *Campylobacter* shares about 50% of its genes with helicobacter; both have a spiral shape and flagella. Most human infections are caused by *Campylobacter jejuni* and some by *C. coli*. Occasional infections are caused by *C. fetus*, an important pathogen of cattle and sheep, and sometimes in patients with immune deficiency.

Epidemiology

Campylobacter is by far the commonest cause of bacterial gastroenteritis in the industrialized world. In England and Wales in 2005 it caused gastroenteritis 4 times more often than salmonella. In the United Kingdom the annual incidence of infection may be as high as 1 in 100.

Campylobacteriosis is a zoonosis. The organisms are very common inhabitants of the intestines of wild birds, poultry, cattle, and sheep. Mechanized processes in chicken abattoirs mean that the majority of carcasses leave with surface contamination. However, the source of infection in most human cases is unknown; outbreaks, an invaluable epidemiological investigative tool, are rare, and the very great genotypic and phenotypic diversity of the *C. jejuni* genome caused by frequent horizontal gene exchange seriously impedes the development of epidemiologically useful typing systems. Multilocus sequence typing allows the identification of genetically related clonal complexes. The commonest, ST-21 has been isolated from human cases and healthy cattle, broiler chickens, wild birds, and sheep.

Unlike *Salmonella*, the organisms do not grow on contaminated food, so outbreaks are uncommon. They have been associated with failures in milk pasteurization and water chlorination. The incidence of sporadic human cases in the United Kingdom rises sharply in weeks 21 to 24 (May and June); the reason for this is unknown.

Pathogenesis

The infectious dose is low, less than 1000 viable organisms. The jejunum and ileum are colonized first, with extension distally, often to the colon and rectum. Infection is invasive; the mesenteric lymph glands enlarge and become inflamed and neutrophil polymorphonuclear leucocytes accumulate in the intestinal mucosa. A cytolethal distending toxin, phospholipase A, and flagellar structural proteins as well as other bacterial proteins with unknown functions are produced by all pathogenic isolates.

Clinical features

The incubation period ranges from 1 to 7 days and averages 3 days. A prodrome of fever and general aching sometimes precedes abdominal pain and diarrhoea; vomiting is not a prominent feature. Abdominal pain may be severe and acute appendicitis is a frequent differential diagnosis. The diarrhoea contains leucocytes, is frequently bloody, and seldom lasts more than 2 to 3 days. Most patients have culture-negative stools after 5 weeks. Ten to 15% of patients have a recurrence of symptoms.

About 1% of patients develop reactive arthritis 1 to 3 weeks after the onset of illness. It is indistinguishable from that which follows *Salmonella* infections. *Campylobacter* gastroenteritis is the commonest event that leads to the development of the Guillain–Barré syndrome (Chapter 24.16); 26 to 41% of cases have a history of its occurring 1 to 3 weeks after the onset of diarrhoea.

Laboratory diagnosis

Laboratory diagnosis is by culture. Stools are plated onto selective media and incubated for 48 h at 42 to 43°C in 5 to 15% oxygen and 1 to 10% CO_2. Infectivity is labile; if delays in transport to the laboratory are expected, faeces should be refrigerated or placed in transport medium. Diagnosis of recent infections is by serology.

Treatment

Most *Campylobacter* infections are self-limiting. Fluid and electrolyte replacement may be needed. Most strains are sensitive to erythromycin; ciprofloxacin and other fluoroquinolones are also effective in more severe infections, but resistant strains are becoming commoner.

Miscellaneous food poisoning bacteria

Listeria monocytogenes

See Chapter 7.10.34.

Vibrio parahaemolyticus

Vibrio parahaemolyticus is the commonest bacterial cause of diarrhoea (usually watery, sometimes explosive) in Japan. Infection follows the consumption of seafoods, particularly those prepared raw in the Japanese style. The incubation period is commonly 10 to 20 h (range 4–9 h) and the illness lasts 1 to 2 days. Pathogenic strains produce a heat-stable toxin and are Kanagawa positive (produce haemolysis on Wagatsuma's agar). Other vibrios that cause seafood-associated gastroenteritis are *V. fluvialis*, *V. hollisae*, *V. mimicus*, and *V. vulnificus*.

Aeromonas hydrophila

This Gram-negative rod is frequently isolated from diarrhoea. Virulence factors remain unidentified.

Exotoxin producers

See Chapters 7.6.23 and 7.6.24 for *Clostridium difficile*, *C. botulinum*, and *C. perfringens*, and Chapter 7.6.4 for *Staphylococcus aureus*.

Bacillus cereus

This Gram-positive saprophyte produces heat-resistant spores. It is common in raw foods, especially rice, and causes two kinds of food poisoning, emetic and diarrhoeic. Vomiting occurs 6 h or less after eating food containing preformed toxin, usually lightly cooked rice that has then been stored at room temperature and reheated, conditions which stimulate the bacterium to produce the low molecular weight heat-, acid-, and protein-resistant peptide toxin. Diarrhoea occurs 8 to 24 h after eating contaminated food. A heat-labile enterotoxin is produced in the intestine. Both kinds of illness are short lived. Other *Bacillus* spp., *B. licheniformis*, *B. pumilis*, and *B. subtilis*, have caused *B. cereus*-like illnesses.

Prevention of food poisoning

The production of safe food rests on evidence-based practical technologies and management systems; HACCP is central to their delivery. The system was developed by the National Aeronautics and Space Administration (NASA) and others in the 1960s to prevent food poisoning in space; the notion of diarrhoea and vomiting in zero gravity was too awful to contemplate. HACCP is now used worldwide and in many countries for some food businesses it is a legal requirement. It identifies hazards, identifies the points in a process where they may occur, and decides which points are critical to control to ensure consumer safety. A good example is milk pasteurization; critical control points are the temperatures reached during heating, its duration, and the measures taken to prevent subsequent contamination.

As a written scheme testable by food law enforcers, HACCP stops at the farm gate and the dwelling door. However, its principles apply on the farm and in the home, and their promulgation there currently exercises all promoters of food safety. Ignorance of them is not restricted to these environments; large food poisoning outbreaks have followed failures of food processors to follow them. Milk pasteurization is again a good example. Political resistance to its implementation in England meant that 65 000 died there from milk-borne bovine tuberculosis between 1912 and 1937. Thirty-nine milk-borne salmonella outbreaks with deaths in Scotland between 1970 and 1981 drove legislation preventing the sale of unpasteurized milk there, and now nearly all United Kingdom milk is pasteurized. However, pasteurization failures or postpasteurization contamination still lead to campylobacter and *E. coli* O157 outbreaks.

Further reading

Advisory Committee on the Microbial Safety of Food (2005). *Second report on campylobacter*. Food Standards Agency, London.

Cheasty T, Smith HR (2005). Escherichia. In: Borriello SP, Murray PR, Funke G (eds) *Topley and Wilson's microbiology and microbial infections (bacteriology)*, pp. 1360–75. Hodder Arnold, London.

Granum PE, Lund T (1997). *Bacillus cereus* and its food poisoning toxins. *FEMS Microbiol Lett*, **157**, 223–82.

Maskell D, Mastroeni P (eds) (2006). *Salmonella infections: clinical, immunological and molecular aspects. (Advances in molecular and cellular microbiology)*. Cambridge University Press, Cambridge, UK.

Nair GB, *et al.* (2007). Global dissemination of *Vibrio parahaemolyticus* serotype 03;K6 and its serovariants. *Clin Microbiol Rev*, **20**, 39–48.

Schroeder GN, Hilbi H (2008). Molecular pathogenesis of shigella species: controlling host cell signaling, invasion and death by type III secretion. *Clin Microbiol Rev*, **21**, 134–56.

Tarr PI, Gordon CA, Chandler WI (2005). Shiga-toxin-producing *Escherichia coli* and haemolytic uraemic syndrome. *Lancet*, **365**, 1073–86.

The Pennington Group (1997). *Report on the circumstances leading to the 1996 outbreak of infection with* E. coli *O157 in Central Scotland, the implications for food safety and the lessons to be learned.* The Stationery Office, Edinburgh.

Threlfall EJ (2005). Salmonella. In: Borriello SP, Murray PR, Funke G (eds) *Topley and Wilson's microbiology and microbial infections (bacteriology)*, pp. 1398–434. Hodder Arnold, London.

Young KT, Davis LM, Dirita VJ (2007). *Campylobacter jejuni*: molecular biology and pathogenesis. *Nat Rev Microbiol*, **5**, 665–79.

7.6.7.2 **Pseudomonas aeruginosa**

G.C.K.W. Koh and S.J. Peacock

Essentials

Pseudomonas aeruginosa is a highly versatile environmental Gram-negative bacterium that can be isolated from a wide range of habitats, including soil, marshes, and the ocean, as well as from plants and animal tissues. It is resistant to many disinfectants and antibiotics, giving it a selective advantage in hospitals, where it rarely causes infection in the healthy host but is a major opportunistic pathogen.

Clinical features—(1) In hospitals—causes a range of infections, including bacteraemia (often in association with neutropenia), ventilator-associated pneumonia, urinary tract infection, skin and soft-tissue infections, and bacteraemia associated with burns. (2) In the community—the largest group of people affected by *P. aeruginosa* are those with cystic fibrosis, who develop long-term colonization of the airways punctuated by episodes of clinical infection.

Diagnosis—this is usually straightforward when samples are available from normally sterile sites, but is often challenging when infection is suspected in sites such as a catheterized urinary tract, burns, or ulcers.

Treatment—*P. aeruginosa* is intrinsically resistant to a broad range of antimicrobial drugs. Appropriate and effective prescribing for high-risk patients requires (1) clinical awareness of risk factors for *P. aeruginosa*, combined with knowledge of the spectrum of diseases caused by this organism; (2) carefully considered empirical regimens based on local antimicrobial susceptibility data—these will typically include an antipseudomonal cephalosporin (e.g. ceftazidime, cefepime), carbapenem (e.g. imipenem, meropenem) or penicillin (e.g. piperacillin, ticarcillin—commonly available in combined preparations with sulbactam or clavulanate); and (3) attention to susceptibility profiles once the causative strain has been isolated and tested.

Genetics and pathogenesis

The *Pseudomonas aeruginosa* genome is composed of a single chromosome of 6.3 Mbp containing around 5700 predicted open reading frames. This is markedly larger that most other sequenced bacterial genomes, and approaches the size of the simple eukaryote *Saccharomyces cerevisiae*, the genome of which encodes around 6200 proteins. The *P. aeruginosa* genome contains a high proportion of regulatory genes and a large number of genes involved in catabolism, transport, and efflux of organic chemicals. The size and complexity of the genome underpins its ability to thrive in diverse environments. Findings from multilocus sequence typing (MLST) of *P. aeruginosa* are indicative of a high rate of genetic recombination, with evidence for clusters of closely related strains or clonal complexes within the population. MLST has also demonstrated distinct phylogenetic clustering of *P. aeruginosa* present in specific environments such as the ocean. *P. aeruginosa* produces a single polar flagellum and numerous fimbriae or pili which allow it to adhere to the respiratory epithelium. More than one-half of all clinical isolates produce pyocyanin (a blue pigment) and pyoverdin (a green pigment), which are responsible for the characteristic blue-green colour of *P. aeruginosa* colonies growing on solid media. Pyocyanin is an exotoxin that has immunomodulatory effects on respiratory epithelial cells, is toxic to neutrophils, and is involved in iron acquisition. Alginate mediates adherence to epithelial surfaces and protects the organism from phagocytosis. The production of alginate exopolysaccharide by mucoid strains of *P. aeruginosa* has been shown to be involved in the colonization of the lungs of patients with cystic fibrosis, and is an adverse prognostic factor.

P. aeruginosa in the environment

P. aeruginosa is ubiquitous in the environment. In homes, it is often found in the aerators and traps of sinks, shower heads, water coolers, contact lens solutions, and cosmetics, as well as in swimming pools, whirlpool baths, and jacuzzis. It may also be cultured from a wide variety of raw fruit and vegetables. It is difficult to eradicate from the hospital environment, where it has been found in soap dishes, dialysis fluid, irrigation fluids, eye drops, disinfectants, ointments, and mechanical ventilators. *P. aeruginosa* is resistant to several commonly used disinfectants. Ammonium acetate-buffered benzalkonium chloride solution will support the growth and division of *P. aeruginosa*, and the organism readily develops resistance to chlorhexidine. *P. aeruginosa* is killed by povidone-iodine, glutaraldehyde, bleach, and alcohol, but may be relatively resistant to these when present in a biofilm or embedded within proteinaceous material.

Human colonization and disease

Colonization

P. aeruginosa is probably consumed regularly and is capable of colonizing the human gastrointestinal tract. It is rarely present on the intact skin or mucous membranes of healthy individuals but often colonizes severely ill patients, particularly those on broad-spectrum antibiotics. *P. aeruginosa* often colonizes areas of chronically broken skin, such as ulcers, and medical devices in contact with the environment, such as long-term urinary catheters.

The organism may cause a broad range of infections, most commonly in patients with one or more risk factors.

Bacteraemia

This occurs primarily in immunocompromised patients, particularly those with haematological malignancies, neutropenia, or severe burns. *P. aeruginosa* accounts for approximately one-quarter of all hospital-acquired bacteraemias, and has a mortality of 18%. In 2007, there were 3823 reported cases of pseudomonas bacteraemia in the United Kingdom (6.9 per 10 000 population), a 20% increase compared to 2003. Clinical features of sepsis associated with *P. aeruginosa* infection do not differ from those associated with other bacterial infections, and empirical antimicrobial prescribing for high-risk patients should include cover for *P. aeruginosa*. A primary source of infection (e.g. a chronic ulcer in a diabetic patient, a urinary catheter, etc.) should be sought and removed wherever possible. In rare cases of *P. aeruginosa* infection, patients may develop a skin lesion called ecthyma gangrenosum (Fig. 7.6.7.2.1) which, although not pathognomonic for *P. aeruginosa*, is rarely a feature of infection by any other organism. This presents as a painful well-circumscribed erythematous lesion anywhere on the body. It progresses to necrosis within hours or days. Ecthyma rarely appears in a non-neutropenic host, and its appearance marks the failure of the host immune response to control the infection. In these patients, *P. aeruginosa* may often be cultured both from blood and from the lesion, but not every patient with ecthyma is detectably bacteraemic.

Pulmonary infection

P. aeruginosa consistently ranks either first or second in frequency as a cause of ventilator-associated pneumonia in United States of America surveys (National Healthcare Safety Network). Diagnosis is complicated by the fact that severely ill patients commonly become colonized by *P. aeruginosa*, and appropriate sampling of patients with suspected ventilator-associated pneumonia requires the use of blind bronchoalveolar lavage or more invasive procedures such as bronchoscopy combined with bronchoalveolar lavage or protective brush sampling of the distal airways. The diagnosis and treatment of ventilator-associated pneumonia is described in Section 18 and Chapter 18.4.3. *P. aeruginosa* commonly colonizes the respiratory tract of people with cystic fibrosis and is the leading cause of respiratory infection in this group. Asymptomatic *P. aeruginosa* colonization is associated with a more rapid decline in lung function and increased mortality from respiratory failure. The distinction between lung colonization and infection is often difficult in cystic fibrosis patients as the organism seldom causes frank pneumonia. Diagnosis is guided by a combination of clinical and laboratory features. Cystic fibrosis is discussed in Chapter 18.10. *P. aeruginosa* may cause a fulminant necrotizing pneumonia in neutropenic patients as part of a syndrome of disseminated infection.

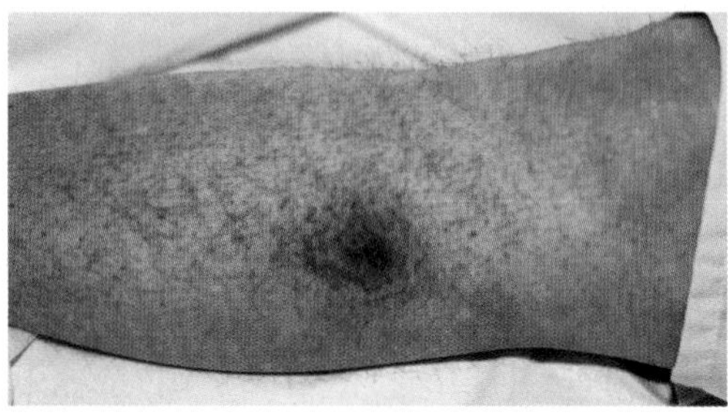

Fig. 7.6.7.2.1 Ecthyma gangrenosum lesion in a patient with Pseudomonas aeruginosa septicaemia.
(Courtesy of the late Dr BE Juel-Jensen).

Skin and soft tissue infection

P. aeruginosa rarely invades healthy skin and a breach of the integument (e.g. skin maceration from chronic immersion in water, a burn, a cut or nick from a razor blade or rose thorn, a surgical wound, or an ulcer) is usually required for infection to become established. 'Hot tub' dermatitis is a self-limiting skin infection in healthy people caused by exposure to water contaminated with *P. aeruginosa* and manifests as folliculitis or vesicular lesions. Outbreaks have been associated with jacuzzis, spas, and swimming pools. *P. aeruginosa* is a cause of surgical wound infections (4.6–11% according to annual National Nosocomial Infections Surveillance System surveys), but is far less common than *Staphylococcus aureus*. *P. aeruginosa* colonization of chronic leg ulcers is common, but it is rarely the only organism found from superficial swabs taken from this type of lesion and is usually a colonizer rather than an invader. Superficial swabs of ulcers are best avoided in the absence of clinical signs of active infection, and, when infection is present (e.g. cellulitis, associated osteomyelitis, bacteraemia), cultures from deep tissue that does not communicate with the ulcer or wound surface should be obtained. Ecthyma gangrenosum is described under the section on bacteraemia (see above). *P. aeruginosa* is an important cause of infection in patients with burns, the other important pathogen being *S. aureus*.

Urinary tract

The initiating event in *P. aeruginosa* urinary tract infection is usually urinary catheterization or instrumentation of the urinary tract, although infection may occasionally occur by haematogenous spread to the kidneys. Patients with long-term indwelling urinary catheters are at particular risk, a combined effect of the presence of prosthetic material that provides a nidus for infection and because frequent antimicrobial therapy for recurrent urinary infection selects for resistant organisms such as *P. aeruginosa*. No specific clinical features distinguish *P. aeruginosa* urinary infections from infection caused by other pathogens. The diagnosis is made on urine culture in the presence of appropriate clinical features, predominant of which is fever. *P. aeruginosa* infection in this patient group is rarely cured without removal/replacement of the urinary catheter on which organisms persist within a biofilm. Catheter change should be performed towards the end of therapy once the burden of planktonic bacteria (bacteria free in urine) is much reduced. Routine urine culture of patients with long-term urinary catheters provides no useful information in the absence of clinical features of active infection. Renal imaging may be useful to exclude renal abscesses or calculi if the reason for the infection is not obvious.

Ear infection

P. aeruginosa is a leading cause of otitis externa, an infection of the external auditory canal that causes inflammation, pain (which is exacerbated by traction on the pinna), and, if severe, a purulent discharge. It is common to find lymphadenopathy just anterior to the tragus. The disease is usually seen in children and the source of infection includes underchlorinated swimming pools or fresh water (lakes or rivers). The diagnosis is based on signs and symptoms, and empiric treatment with eardrops is usually effective. Malignant otitis externa is rare but much more serious. It not a neoplastic process, but is so called because of the risk of localized destructive spread to the central nervous system. It most commonly occurs in elderly patients with diabetes and people with HIV infection, and is essentially an osteomyelitis of the mastoid and petrous temporal bone. Affected patients present with an erythematous oedematous inflamed external auditory canal, and the tympanic membrane is often hidden by oedema. Otoscopy is necessary to make the diagnosis, but is often poorly tolerated because of pain. Lymphadenopathy of the ipsilateral cervical lymph nodes may be present; facial nerve involvement produces an ipsilateral lower motor neuron seventh nerve palsy. Spread to the temporomandibular joint causes pain on mastication, and spread to the apex of the petrous temporal nerve produces Gradenigo's syndrome (trigeminal and trochlear nerve palsies). Features of malignant otitis externa should prompt immediate referral to an ear, nose, and throat surgeon for assessment and debridement of the ear canal and adjacent bone. The diagnosis is made by demonstrating osteomyelitis of the skull base on a technetium-99 bone scintigram or on MRI, along with *P. aeruginosa* cultured from the discharge or from a bone biopsy.

Eye infection

The most common manifestation of *P. aeruginosa* eye infection is keratitis, which occurs following direct inoculation from trauma (e.g. contact sports, industrial accidents) or minor abrasions (e.g. contact lens use). Contact lens keratitis has been associated with contaminated contact lens disinfectant solutions. *P. aeruginosa* keratitis requires prompt ophthalmological referral and treatment since infection may be rapidly progressive and can result in corneal opacification and even perforation within 48 h. Pseudomonal endophthalmitis most commonly occurs as a consequence of penetrating injury or surgery, but there is also a rare syndrome of neonatal endophthalmitis that may be bilateral, the main risk factor for which is prematurity. Clinical features include severe pain, chemosis, loss of the red reflex, hypopyon, and corneal clouding. Neonatal pseudomonal endophthalmitis most commonly arises from haematogenous spread, frequently in association with a syndrome of disseminated disease that includes meningitis and pneumonia, and is commonly fatal. Endophthalmitis is diagnosed on the basis of culture of a sample of vitreous humour.

Bone and joint infection

Patients with diabetes may develop osteomyelitis of the foot following penetrating injury or local extension of an untreated chronic ulcer. Results from superficial swabs are of minimal clinical relevance, and diagnosis should be based on the results of bone biopsy which should be processed for culture and histopathology. Parenteral antimicrobials are not always successful and radical debridement or amputation may be necessary to clear the infection. Intravenous drug users are susceptible to *P. aeruginosa* septic arthritis and osteomyelitis of the axial skeleton.

HIV infection

Patients with HIV infection are more susceptible to *P. aeruginosa* infection, usually when the CD4 count is below 100 cells/μl. The incidence has fallen since the advent of highly active antiretroviral therapy (HAART). The presentation of *P. aeruginosa* infection in HIV patients is more indolent than that in neutropenic patients, but mortality is 22 to 34%. The fever is frequently low grade and ecthyma gangrenosum is rare. It is most commonly intravenous device related. Pneumonia is the most common community-acquired presentation, followed by sinusitis, and infections of the urinary tract, all of which may be associated with bacteraemia.

Antimicrobial therapy

P. aeruginosa elaborates a range of β-lactamases (penicillinases and cephalosporinases) and has a relatively impermeable outer membrane, which makes it intrinsically resistant to a wide variety of antimicrobials, including all first-generation and second-generation cephalosporins, most penicillins, and all macrolides. The antipseudomonal cephalosporins include ceftazidime and cefepime; of the carbapenems, imipenem and meropenem are effective. The antipseudomonal penicillins are piperacillin and ticarcillin (commonly available in combined preparations with sulbactam or clavulanate). The β-lactams are bactericidal and there is good clinical evidence for their efficacy and safety. There is evidence from animal studies that continuous infusions of β-lactam are superior to intermittent dosing. The monobactam aztreonam has not found widespread use because isolates that are resistant to ceftazidime or piperacillin are generally also resistant to aztreonam. However, there are rare metallo-β-lactamase-producing strains of *P. aeruginosa* that may be resistant to carbapenems but sensitive to aztreonam. The aminoglycosides (gentamicin, amikacin, tobramycin, etc.) are effective *in vitro* and may be used in combination with β-lactams in empiric regimens for febrile neutropenic patients and for *P. aeruginosa* ventilator-associated pneumonia. Concern over the efficacy of aminoglycosides in neutropenia has led to the use of other combinations for empirical therapy in the treatment of febrile neutropenia (e.g. β-lactam plus fluoroquinolone). Aminoglycosides remain useful for topical therapy, which may be used for the treatment of otitis externa and superficial eye infections. The fluoroquinolone drug ciprofloxacin is active when administered orally, an attribute that makes it almost unique among the therapeutic options available for *P. aeruginosa* treatment. The newer quinolones (e.g. moxifloxacin and gatifloxacin) are not licensed for the treatment of *P. aeruginosa* infection.

Acquired drug resistance is a problem in patients who are antibiotic experienced (an important example being patients with cystic fibrosis), but resistance to commonly used antibiotics is a problem even outside this patient group. The United Kingdom Health Protection Agency reported that of the *P. aeruginosa* strains isolated from blood during 2007, 12% were resistant to ciprofloxacin, 8% to ceftazidime, 5% to piperacillin/tazobactam, 12% to imipenem, and 9% to meropenem. It is not uncommon for resistance to develop during the course of treatment, an event that is associated with excess mortality. Gentamicin-resistant strains may remain susceptible to kanamycin or neomycin, but cross-resistance to tobramycin is common in strains that colonize patients with cystic fibrosis frequently become multiply resistant and older antimicrobial agents such as colistin and polymyxin B may then be used.

The antimicrobial treatment and management of *P. aeruginosa* infection is complex because the infection types are often system or patient-group specific and so a single guideline is not appropriate. As a general rule, first-line therapy of patients with serious suspected *P. aeruginosa* infection should include a β-lactam (e.g. piperacillin or meropenem) with or without a second agent, and therapy should be altered in the light of culture and susceptibility results. Decisions on empirical antimicrobial therapy should be taken in the light of local information on patterns of resistance. The reader is encouraged to study this section in conjunction with other relevant chapters on the management of conditions including neutropenic sepsis, ventilator-associated pneumonia, cystic fibrosis, and urinary tract, ear, and eye infections.

Prevention

Groups of patients (e.g. neutropenic patients, or patients with severe burns) who are particularly susceptible to invasive pseudomonal infection may be housed in clean units. Such units are equipped with filtered air supplies, and incoming water is chlorinated and continuously heated to 60°C. Attention is paid to the regular maintenance of air conditioning, hydrotherapy units, and water coolers. Visitors and staff are required to wear protective gowns and gloves, and to remove their shoes to avoid contaminating the hospital environment with bacteria brought in from outside the hospital. Fresh flowers and fruit are prohibited for the same reasons, and a rigorous regimen of hand washing is instituted for all visitors and staff. The emergence over the last decade of highly transmissible strains of *P. aeruginosa* in people with cystic fibrosis has necessitated the institution of measures to segregate affected patients. Several vaccine candidates have entered phase I trials, but none are currently licensed for clinical use.

Further reading

Carfrae MJ, Kesser BW (2008). Malignant otitis externa. *Otolaryngol Clin North Am*, **41**, 537–49.

Flume *et al.* (2009). Cystic fibrosis pulmonary guidelines: treatment of pulmonary exacerbations. *Am J Respir Crit Care Med*, **180**, 802–8.

Garau J, Gomez L (2003). *Pseudomonas aeruginosa* pneumonia. *Curr Opin Infect Dis*, **16**, 135–43.

Glasmacher A, *et al.* (2005). An evidence-based evaluation of important aspects of empirical antibiotic therapy in febrile neutropenic patients. *Clin Microbiol Infect*, **11**, 17–23.

Sander R (2001). Otitis externa: a practical guide to treatment and prevention. *Am Fam Physician*, **63**, 927–36.

Shigemura K, *et al.* (2006). Complicated urinary tract infection caused by *Pseudomonas aeruginosa* in a single institution (1999–2003). *Int J Urol*, **13**, 538–42.

Tredget EE, *et al.* (2004). Pseudomonas infections in the thermally injured patient. *Burns*, **30**, 3–26.

7.6.8 Typhoid and paratyphoid fevers

C.M. Parry and Buddha Basnyat

Essentials

Typhoid and paratyphoid fever (the enteric fevers) are caused by specific serovars of the Gram-negative bacillus, *Salmonella enterica*. Sources of typhoid transmission are excreting chronic or convalescent carriers and the acutely infected, with transmission occuring through contamination by carriers of food or water by effluents containing infected urine or faeces. There are an estimated 27 million cases of enteric fever in the world each year, almost all in the developing world, with about 200 000 deaths.

Clinical features—the main symptom is fever (39–40°C); headache and malaise are common; constipation is a frequent early symptom, but most patients will experience diarrhoea; abdominal pain is usually diffuse and poorly localized. Physical examination is often unremarkable, apart from fever, but rose spots and relative bradycardia may be observed. In developing countries, patients may progress in the second to fourth week, with life-threatening manifestations including gastrointestinal bleeding, intestinal perforation, and the syndrome of mental confusion.

Diagnosis—the principal method for confirming the diagnosis is by isolating *S. enterica* ser. *Typhi* or *Paratyphi* from blood or bone marrow. The organisms may also be isolated from stool, urine, and bile aspirates, but such demonstration should be interpreted with caution in areas with many chronic carriers as the acute illness may be due to another cause.

Treatment—aside from supportive care, antibiotic therapy reduces mortality and complications and shortens the illness. Antibiotic resistance is a common and increasing problem, hence the choice of antibiotic should be informed by knowledge of likely local susceptibility. Fluoroquinolones are often given as first-line treatment, although low-level resistance to these agents (marked by nalidixic acid resistance) is widespread in Asia, with extended-spectrum cephalosporins and azithromycin as alternatives.

Prevention—typhoid has been eliminated from industrialized countries by (1) the provision of safe drinking water and safe disposal of sewage; (2) legal enforcement of high standards of food hygiene, and programmes to detect, monitor, and treat chronic carriers; and (3) prompt investigation and intervention when these safeguards are breached. Measures for individual protection are to (1) kill the organism in water by heating to 57°C, iodination, or chlorination; (2) take care with uncooked or reheated food; and (3) immunization—two typhoid vaccines are available and widely used in travellers, but their role as a public health tool in endemic areas is undefined; there is no paratyphoid vaccine.

Acknowledgement: The authors acknowledge the contribution of Dr John Richens to previous editions of this chapter.

Introduction

Typhoid and paratyphoid types A, B, and C are a group of infections in humans collectively known as enteric fever. They commonly present as a prolonged febrile illness with a paucity of physical signs. The spectrum of disease varies from a mild self-limiting febrile illness to severe disease associated with gastrointestinal bleeding, intestinal perforation, or mental confusion with shock. In the 19th century typhoid fever was a leading cause of death in Europe and America. The disease today is predominantly found in developing countries.

Aetiology

The Gram-negative bacilli *Salmonella enterica* subspecies *enterica* serovar Typhi (*S. enterica* ser. Typhi) and *S. enterica* ser. Paratyphi A are the principal causative agents of enteric fever. Three antigens are important for identification: in Typhi the somatic oligosaccharide O antigen (9 and 12), the protein flagellar H-d antigen, and the polysaccharide envelope Vi antigen; in Paratyphi A the relevant O antigens are 1,2,12 and H antigens a:[1,5]. Antibiotic resistance is conferred by R plasmids, usually of the incompatibility group IncH-1 (chloramphenicol, amoxicillin, co-trimoxazole), and by mutations in the chromosomal *gyrA* gene (fluoroquinolones). The sequencing of isolates of *S. enterica* ser. Typhi and Paratyphi A is shedding light on the pathogenicity of these organisms. It is apparent that the genome of *S. enterica* ser. Typhi has a remarkable plasticity compared to other bacteria, with recombination of homologous rRNA operons as well as insertion of nonhomologous DNA.

Transmission

Sources of typhoid transmission are excreting chronic or convalescent carriers and the acutely infected. Transmission occurs through contamination by carriers of food or water by effluents containing infected urine or faeces. 'Typhoid Mary' was a faecal carrier and cook who infected 53 people early last century, while the Aberdeen outbreak in 1964 was traced to a leaking corned beef tin which had been cooled with faecally contaminated river water. Transmission of typhoid has also been attributed to flies, laboratory mishaps, unsterile instruments, and anal intercourse. Hornick demonstrated that 10^7 organisms of Quailes strain of *S. enterica* ser. Typhi given orally infected 50% of experimental subjects. Susceptibility is increased by medicines which decrease the gastric acidic environment or vagotomy. Infection may lead to acute disease, transient symptoms, or a symptomless carrier state.

Multiplication and dissemination

Bacteria are thought to pass from the gut through the cytoplasm of enterocytes and M cells overlying lymphoid tissue (Peyer's patches) of the small intestine to reach the lamina propria from which they are conveyed to the mesenteric nodes before reaching the blood stream via the thoracic duct. During a transient primary bacteraemia the organism is seeded to reticuloendothelial sites where intracellular multiplication occurs during a 7- to 14-day incubation period. A second bacteraemia follows, accompanied by symptoms as the infection spreads throughout liver, gallbladder, spleen, Peyer's patches, and bone marrow. Multiplication occurs mainly in macrophages. Concentrated sites of infection in reticuloendothelial tissues, known as typhoid nodules, are characterized by infiltrates of lymphocytes and macrophages. At postmortem examination, hypertrophy of lymphoid tissue is often visible within liver, spleen, mesenteric nodes, and Peyer's patches. Ulceration of Peyer's patches is seen where the inflammatory process has resulted in ischaemia and necrosis.

Endotoxin plays a central role in stimulating the release of cytokines, such as tumour necrosis factor and interleukin-6, from macrophages and neutrophils by activating the complement cascade and upregulating the adhesive capacity of neutrophils and endothelial cells. Unlike in meningitis and malaria, no clear correlation between levels of tumour necrosis factor and clinical outcome has been demonstrated in typhoid. The capacity of whole blood to produce proinflammatory cytokines following stimulation is reduced in patients with severe typhoid.

Immune response

There is a cell-mediated immune response lasting about 16 weeks, a mucosal immune response lasting for up to 48 weeks, and persistent circulating anti-O and anti-H agglutinins for up to 2 years. The predominance of clinical typhoid among children and young adults in endemic areas suggests a degree of acquired immunity. Only 25% of volunteers given a standard inoculum of *S. enterica* ser. Typhi 20 months after an initial infection developed clinical illness. Prolonged elevation of Vi antibody occurs in typhoid carriers. Immunodeficiency reduces the ability to clear salmonella infections.

Epidemiology

Worldwide, an estimated 27 million cases of enteric fever occur each year with about 200 000 deaths. In affluent countries, enteric fever is seen in returned travellers visiting friends and relatives abroad in areas of endemicity or when food or water safety measures fail. With appropriate antibiotic treatment, death is rare. In the Indian subcontinent, Central and South-East Asia, Indonesia, and sub-Saharan Africa, high rates of transmission are seen and annual incidence rates of 100 to 1600 cases per 100 000 population have been recorded. In these countries, transmission has been exacerbated by antibiotic resistance. Peaks of transmission occur in dry weather or at the onset of rains. Case fatality rates have exceeded 10% in some reports of hospitalized patients in Indonesia and Papua New Guinea.

Prevention

The elimination of typhoid from industrialized countries can be attributed to the provision of safe drinking water, safe disposal of sewage, legal enforcement of high standards of food hygiene, programmes to detect, monitor, and treat chronic carriers, and prompt investigation and intervention when these safeguards are breached. Outbreaks can be investigated using phage typing of isolates, pulsed-field gel electrophoresis and other molecular typing methods, registers of known carriers, and sewer swabs used to trace isolates back to their source.

Measures for individual protection are to kill the organism in water by heating to 57° C, iodination, or chlorination, care with uncooked or reheated food, and immunization. Patients and convalescents with typhoid should be advised to wash their hands after using the toilet and before preparing food and to use separate towels. Western travellers visiting friends and relatives in areas of endemicity are vulnerable to acquiring enteric fever; therefore counselling needs to be targeted on this group. The approach of travel medicine, which has evolved around the tourist industry, will miss this susceptible group.

Clinical features

Typhoid is predominantly an infection of infants, children, and young adults, affecting both sexes equally. The incubation period ranges from 3 to 60 days, but most infections occur 7 to 14 days after exposure. The main focus of typhoid is in the small bowel, but systemic symptoms often overshadow abdominal symptoms. The predominant symptom is the fever which rises gradually to a high plateau of 39 to 40°C, and shows little diurnal variation. Rigors are uncommon, except in late or complicated typhoid or in patients treated with antipyretics. Patients usually complain of headache and malaise, and constipation is a frequent early symptom. Most patients will experience diarrhoea, and typhoid can present as an acute gastroenteritis and occasionally bloody diarrhoea. Severe diarrhoea or colitis has been reported in HIV-infected patients. The abdominal pain is usually diffuse and poorly localized but occasionally sufficiently intense in the right iliac fossa to suggest appendicitis. Nausea and vomiting are infrequent in uncomplicated typhoid but are seen with abdominal distension in severe cases. Other early symptoms include cough, sore throat, and epistaxes. In developing countries, patients with typhoid in its second to fourth week present with accelerating weight loss, weakness, altered mental state, intestinal haemorrhage and perforation, refractory hypotension, pneumonia, nephritis, and acute psychosis. Those infected with multidrug-resistant infections may have more severe disease.

Physical examination is often unremarkable apart from fever. A coated tongue is often observed. Rose spots appear at the end of the first week and form a sparse collection of maculopapular lesions on the abdominal skin, which blanch with pressure and fade after 2 or 3 days (Fig. 7.6.8.1). Osler found them in 90% of white-skinned patients and 20% of patients with black skin. The rash may extend on to the trunk and arms. Melanesian typhoid patients develop purpuric macules that do not blanch (Fig. 7.6.8.2). Petechiae are sometimes visible on the conjunctivae (Fig. 7.6.8.3) Tachycardia is common although temperature–pulse dissociation (relative bradycardia) is considered characteristic. Hypotension has important implications (see below 'Severe typhoid'). Adventitious lung sounds, especially scattered wheezes, are common and may suggest pneumonia. These findings with a normal chest radiograph and high fever should prompt consideration of typhoid. Abdominal examination may reveal the typhoid rash, distension, or a diffuse tenderness, occasionally localized to the area of the terminal ileum. Intra-abdominal inflammation sometimes provokes retention of urine. A moderate soft tender hepatosplenomegaly eventually develops in most patients but it less likely to be found early.

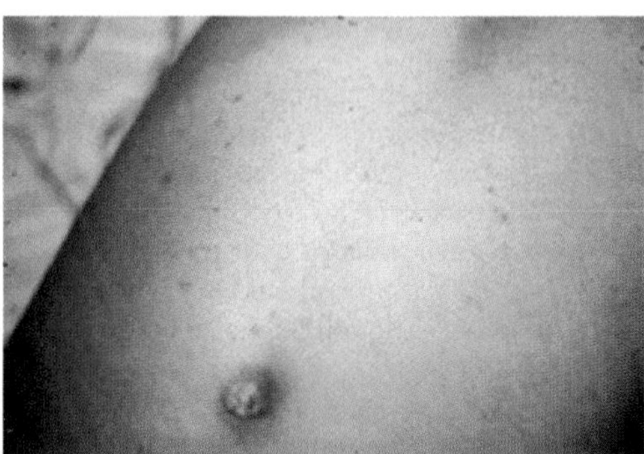

Fig. 7.6.8.1 Rose spots on the abdomen in typhoid fever.

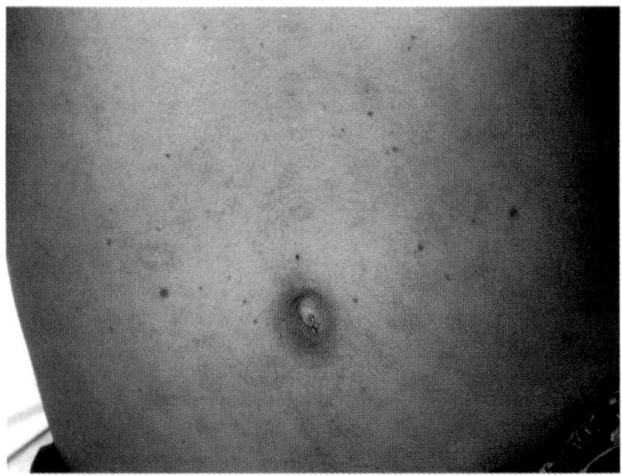

Fig. 7.6.8.2 Typhoid rash in a Melanesian child: sparse purpuric (nonblanching) macules.
(Copyright D A Warrell.)

Patients with advanced illness may display the 'typhoid' facies (Fig. 7.6.8.4), a thin flushed face with a staring apathetic expression. Mental apathy may progress to an agitated delirium, frequently accompanied by tremor of the hands, tremulous speech, and ataxic gait. If the patient's condition deteriorates further the features described in the writings of Louis and Osler make their appearance—muttering delirium, twitchings of the fingers and wrists (subsultus tendinum), agitated plucking at the bedclothes (carphology/carphologia), and a staring unrousable stupor (coma vigil).

Typhoid in children

Community-based studies in highly endemic areas have shown that enteric fever is more common in children less than 5 years old than was once appreciated. The main differences, compared to adults, are a greater frequency of diarrhoea and vomiting, jaundice,

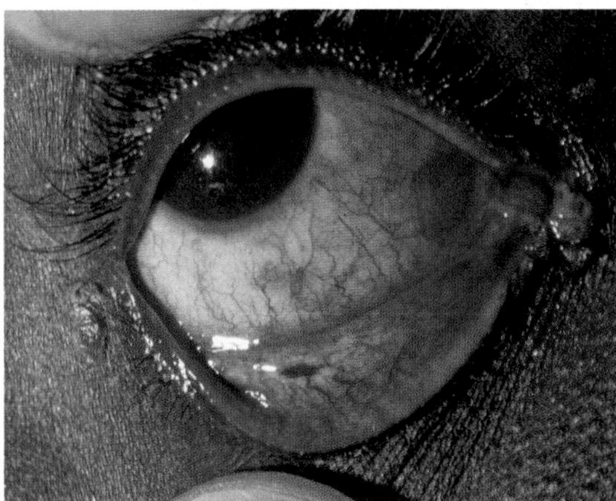

Fig. 7.6.8.3 Conjunctival petechial haemorrhage in an African child with typhoid.
(Copyright D A Warrell.)

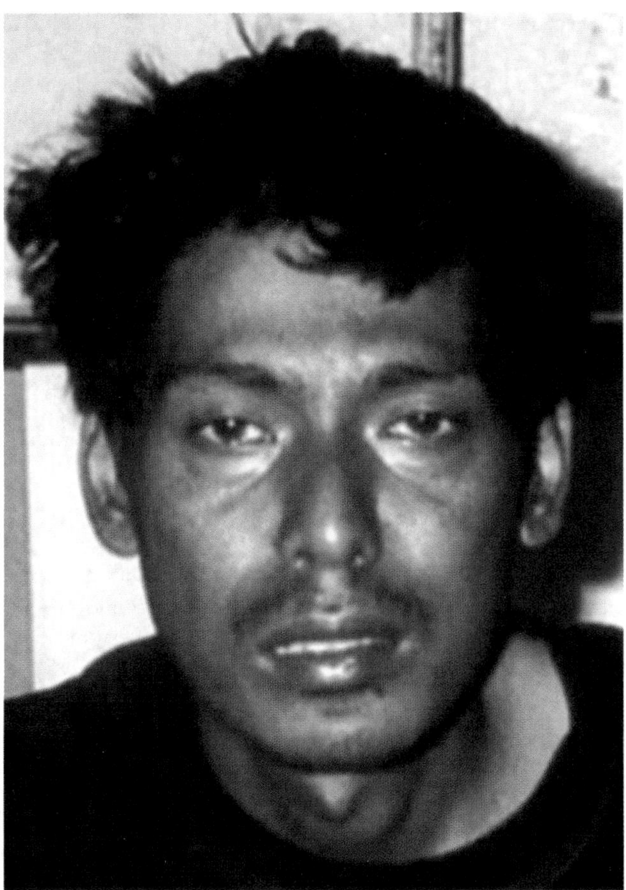

Fig. 7.6.8.4 Typhoid facies: a man with the apathetic expression seen in severe typhoid.

febrile convulsions, nephritis, or typhoid meningitis. Relative bradycardia is of greater diagnostic significance for typhoid in febrile children. In some reports case fatality rates are high in the under-fives. The disease can also take a milder course in very young children, behaving like a mild respiratory illness that is not clinically recognized as enteric fever. Typhoid may also occasionally develop in neonates born to infected mothers.

Differential diagnosis

Many viral, bacterial, and protozoal infections as well as noninfectious conditions characterized by fever, including lymphoproliferative disorders and vasculitides, resemble enteric fever. Typhoid should always be considered when suspected malaria has not been confirmed or has not responded to antimalarial therapy. In areas of endemicity, typhus, leptospirosis, and dengue should be considered in the differential diagnosis.

Diagnosis

Culture

The definitive diagnosis of enteric fever rests on the isolation of *S. enterica* ser. Typhi or Paratyphi from blood, bone marrow, cerebrospinal fluid, and rose spots. In mild typhoid, the number of bacteria in blood may be as low as 1 colony-forming unit/ml. The median number of bacteria in the blood of children is higher than adults and declines with increasing duration of illness. Successful culture from blood can be achieved in up to 80% of patients but depends on taking a generous volume of blood and using the correct volume of blood to broth (1:10). Bone marrow gives the highest yield, including those exposed to antibiotics, but yields only marginally more than blood. Rose spots, when present, can give a positive culture in 70% of patients.

The organisms may also be isolated from stool, urine, and bile aspirates. The number of organisms recoverable from faeces increases through the illness. The results should be interpreted with caution in areas with many carriers, as the acute illness may be due to another cause in chronic carriers. Isolation from urine is more common in areas endemic for schistosomiasis. Culture of bile obtained from an overnight duodenal string capsule gives a similar yield to blood and offers additional means to isolate *S. enterica* ser. Typhi and Paratyphi from children or from carriers.

Serology

The use of a tube or slide agglutination test (the Widal test) to diagnose typhoid is cheaper and simpler than culture but fraught with pitfalls. The demonstration of a fourfold rise in titre of antibodies to *S. enterica* ser. Typhi or Paratyphi antigens suggests enteric fever but is too delayed to help clinical decision-making and is not observed in all patients. Single measurements of antibody titres have been found useful in populations where accurate up-to-date information about the predictive value of the test at specific cut-off points is available. False-positive serological tests are obtained from persons with previous infection, infection with cross-reacting organisms, or following vaccination.

Other tests for typhoid

Many other tests for the detection of antibodies, antigens, and salmonella DNA in body fluids have been described. Few have so far been adopted for routine use. Some new serological tests are now commercially available which, although probably more sensitive the Widal test, are still subject to problems of false-positive and false-negative results.

Other laboratory findings in typhoid

A mild normochromic anaemia, mild thrombocytopenia, and an increased erythrocyte sedimentation rate are common. Most patients have a total white cell count within the normal range. Leucocytosis suggests either perforation or another diagnosis. Laboratory evidence of mild disseminated intravascular coagulation is common but rarely of clinical significance. Common biochemical findings include hyponatraemia, hypokalaemia, and elevation of liver enzymes. The urine often contains some protein and white cells.

Treatment

The aims of management are to eliminate the infection swiftly with antibiotics, to restore fluid and nutritional deficits, and to monitor the patient for dangerous complications. In many parts of the world antibiotic treatment for typhoid fever is started empirically based on the syndrome of fever of 3 or 4 days and constitutional symptoms with no known source of infection and a negative malaria smear. Because there are no reliable clinical predictors, in areas of endemicity concurrent treatment with doxycycline to cover for typhus and leptospirosis may be considered.

Supportive care

Cooling is preferred to antipyretics for relief of fever, and simple analgesics may be used to relieve headache. Most patients can eat and drink normally; special diets do not protect the bowel from perforation. Daily assessment of the patient's mental and circulatory status is required plus examination of the abdomen for signs of impending perforation. Severely ill patients require intensive care with parenteral fluids, intravenous steroids (see below), inotropic support, and sedation.

Antibiotics

Effective antibiotic therapy in typhoid reduces mortality and complications and shortens the illness (see Table 7.6.8.1 for doses). Chloramphenicol was the first antibiotic found to be effective and the standard against which subsequent antibiotics have been measured. Symptom resolution occurs over a period of 4 to 6 days although the antimicrobial should be given for at least 2 weeks to prevent relapse. Ampicillin, amoxicillin, and co-trimoxazole have been shown to have comparable efficacy to chloramphenicol while having less toxicity; they must also be given for at least 2 weeks. In many areas these drugs are no longer used because of the spread of multidrug resistant (MDR) strains of *S. enterica* ser. Typhi and Paratyphi A. Alternative antibiotics active against MDR infections include the fluoroquinolones, although resistance has in turn emerged to these agents, the extended-spectrum cephalosporins (e.g. parenteral ceftriaxone), and azithromycin.

In recent years many physicians have given a fluoroquinolone, ciprofloxacin or ofloxacin, as first-line therapy. Treatment can be completed in a week or less with minimal toxicity. In controlled trials in endemic areas, infections with fully susceptible isolates have resulted in a rapid resolution of symptoms with high cure rates and low relapse and faecal carriage rates. Response rates in endemic areas may be better than those of nonimmune travellers. There have been questions about the safety of fluoroquinolones in children and during pregnancy. Careful follow-up studies of children in Asia following fluoroquinolone therapy have shown no toxicity and there has been a growing consensus that the advantages of therapy outweigh the potential dangers.

Unfortunately strains of *S. enterica* ser. Typhi and Paratyphi A with low-level resistance to the commonly used fluoroquinolones (ciprofloxacin and ofloxacin) have become common in Asia and have sporadically been reported in sub-Saharan Africa. These strains are not detected by current ciprofloxacin disc susceptibility breakpoints but are usually nalidixic acid resistant and this has proved to be a useful, although not a completely sensitive, laboratory marker. Where possible fluoroquinolones should be avoided in patients infected with these strains. They should be treated with extended-spectrum cephalosporins (ceftriaxone) or, in nonsevere cases, with azithromycin. If fluoroquinolones are the only available option they should be used at the maximum dose. Recent data from Vietnam and Nepal suggest that the new fluoroquinolone gatifloxacin is effective in these infections. Cefixime, an oral third-generation cephalosporin, is another alternative although there

Table 7.6.8.1 Guidelines for drug dosages in typhoid

Antibiotic	Daily dose	Route[a]	Doses/day	Duration in nonsevere enteric fever (days)	Duration in severe enteric fever[b]
Acute infection					
Chloramphenicol[c]	50–100 mg/kg	O/IM/IV[d]	4	14	14–21
Co-trimoxazole[e]	Trimethoprim 6.5–10 mg/kg Sulfamethoxazole 40 mg/kg	O/IM/IV	2–3	14	14
Amoxicillin	75–100 mg/kg	O/IM/IV	3	14	14
Ceftriaxone	50–60 mg/kg	IM/IV	2	7–14	14
Cefixime	20 mg/kg	O	2	7–14	
Ciprofloxacin[f]	20–25 mg/kg	O/IV	2	7–14	14
Ofloxacin[f]	15–20 mg/kg	O/IV	2	7–14	
Pefloxacin[f]	800 mg	O/IV	2	7–14	
Fleroxacin[f]	400 mg	O/IV	1	7–14	
Gatifloxacin	10 mg/kg	O	1	7	
Azithromycin	10–20 mg/kg	O	1	7	
Treatment of carriers					
Ampicillin or amoxicillin with probenecid	100 mg/kg 30 mg/kg	O	3–4	90[g]	
Co-trimoxazole	6.5–10 mg trimethoprim	O	2	90	
Ciprofloxacin	1500 mg	O	2	28	

O, oral; IM, intramuscular; IV, intravenous.

[a] Oral therapy is satisfactory for most patients. Parenteral therapy is generally reserved for severely ill patients.

[b] In intestinal perforation, the antibiotic therapy should also cover other aerobic and anaerobic gastrointestinal bacteria contaminating the peritoneum. In severe typhoid (characterized by delirium, obtundation, coma, or shock) dexamethasone is beneficial (see text).

[c] May cause bone marrow suppression.

[d] The oral route is preferred; there are reports of lower blood levels of chloramphenicol in patients given parenteral therapy.

[e] May cause allergic reactions and nephrotoxicity. Not suitable for children younger than 2 years or during pregnancy.

[f] Infection with isolates that have low-level fluoroquinolone resistance (nalidixic acid resistance) may not respond.

[g] The duration of treatment can be shortened if parenteral therapy is given, e.g. 8-hourly intravenous ampicillin for 2 weeks.

have been concerns about its efficacy in some studies. Some areas in the Indian subcontinent now report fully fluoroquinolone-resistant isolates but also an increase in isolates that have regained susceptibility to the old first-line drugs, chloramphenicol, ampicillin, and co-trimoxazole, and in such circumstances these older drugs are appropriate. Some antibiotics such as gentamicin appear sensitive *in vitro* but are ineffective *in vivo* and should not be used in enteric fever.

Ampicillin, amoxicillin, or ceftriaxone are considered safe in pregnancy with enteric fever. There are limited data on the management of immunocompromised patients with enteric fever, but data from patients with nontyphoidal salmonella infections suggest that they may need extended treatment to prevent relapse.

Complications

Box 7.6.8.1 lists the complications of typhoid. Most are rare and only likely to be encountered in patients who present with untreated disease lasting 2 weeks or more. Occasionally, a complication dominates the clinical picture and deflects attention from the underlying diagnosis of typhoid.

Box 7.6.8.1 Complications of typhoid

Abdominal
- Intestinal perforation
- Intestinal haemorrhage
- Hepatitis
- Cholecystitis (usually subclinical)
- Spontaneous splenic rupture
- Rupture and haemorrhage from mesenteric nodes
- Pancreatitis

Genitourinary
- Retention of urine
- Glomerulonephritis
- Pyelonephritis
- Cystitis
- Orchitis

Cardiovascular
- Asymptomatic ECG changes
- Myocarditis
- Pericarditis
- Endocarditis
- Phlebitis and arteritis
- Deep venous thrombosis
- Gangrene
- Shock
- Sudden death

Respiratory
- Bronchitis
- Laryngeal ulceration
- Glottal oedema
- Pneumonia (*S. enterica* ser. Typhi, *Streptococcus pneumoniae*)

Neuropsychiatric
- Delirium
- Psychotic states
- Depression
- Deafness
- Meningitis
- Encephalomyelitis
- Transverse myelitis
- Signs of upper motor neuron lesions
- Signs of extrapyramidal disorder
- Impairment of coordination
- Optic neuritis
- Peripheral and cranial neuropathy
- Guillain–Barré syndrome
- Pseudotumour cerebri

Haematological
- Disseminated intravascular coagulation (usually subclinical)
- Anaemia
- Haemolysis
- Haemolytic uraemic syndrome

Focal infections
- Abscesses of brain, liver, spleen, breast, thyroid, muscles, lymph nodes
- Parotitis
- Pharyngitis
- Osteitis, especially tibia, ribs, spine
- Arthritis

Other
- Myopathy
- Hypercalcaemia
- Decubitus ulceration
- Abortion
- Relapse

Severe typhoid

Studies from Indonesia and Papua New Guinea have revealed an important subgroup of patients with mental confusion or shock (defined as a systolic blood pressure of less than 90 mmHg in adults or less than 80 mmHg in children), with evidence of decreased skin, cerebral, or renal perfusion, who have a 50% fatality rate and account for most typhoid deaths. In one study in Jakarta, high doses of dexamethasone substantially reduced the mortality of such severe cases. The criteria for severe typhoid were marked mental confusion or shock. In adults treated with chloramphenicol, 3 mg/kg dexamethasone infused intravenously over 30 min, followed by eight doses of 1 mg/kg every 6 h, resulted in a 10% case fatality rate compared to 55.6% in controls. It has proved almost impossible to duplicate this study because the number of severe typhoid patients has decreased, probably because of the ready availability of over-the-counter antibiotics.

Intestinal haemorrhage and perforation

Perforation of ileal ulcers occurs in less than 5% of typhoid patients (Fig. 7.6.8.5). The development of acute abdominal signs is often gradual, making diagnosis difficult. Severely ill patients display only restlessness, hypotension, and tachycardia. A chest radiograph may show free gas under the diaphragm. Ultrasonography is useful for demonstrating and aspirating faeculent fluid in the peritoneal cavity. Management includes nasogastric suction, administration of fluids to correct hypotension, and prompt surgery. Simple closure of perforations is adequate but experienced surgeons use procedures to bypass the worst-affected sections of the ileum in order to reduce postoperative morbidity. Closure of perforations should be accompanied by vigorous peritoneal toilet. Metronidazole or clindamycin should be added to the therapy of ceftriaxone or fluoroquinolone-treated patients. Metronidazole and aminoglycosides are recommended for patients receiving chloramphenicol, ampicillin, or co-trimoxazole. The survival of patients undergoing surgery for perforation is generally 70 to 75%, but reaches 97% in the best series. This compares with survival rates of around 30% in conservatively managed patients.

Evidence for silent gastrointestinal bleeding may be sudden collapse of a patient or a steadily falling haematocrit. Most bleeding episodes are self-limiting. Severe bleeding is sometimes seen in advanced typhoid but is rarely fatal. A few require transfusion. In exceptional circumstances surgery or intra-arterial vasopressin have been used to halt haemorrhage.

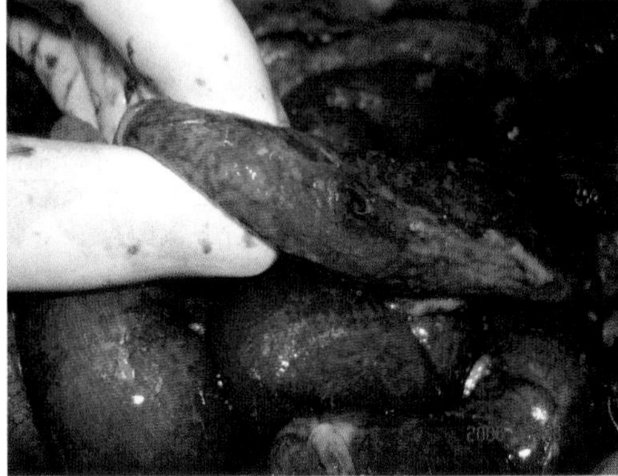

Fig. 7.6.8.5 Typhoid perforation of the distal ileum at operation.

Relapse

Relapse in typhoid is a second episode of fever, usually milder than the first, occurring a week or two after recovery from the first episode. Isolates from relapsing patients usually have identical antibiotic susceptibility to those identified during the first episode. Relapse rates of 10% have been described in untreated typhoid and chloramphenicol-treated patients. Relapse is managed with a similar or abbreviated course of the same therapy used in the initial episode. Reinfection may also occur but can only be distinguished by differences in the sensitivity pattern or molecular typing of isolates.

Carriers

Many patients excrete *S. enterica* ser. Typhi or Paratyphi in their stools or urine for some days after starting antibiotic treatment. Convalescent carriers excrete for periods of up to 3 months. Patients still excreting at 3 months are unlikely to cease and at 1 year meet the formal definition of 'chronic carrier'. Among carriers detected by screening, 25% give no history of acute typhoid. Faecal carriage is more frequent in individuals with gallbladder disease and is most common in women over 40; in the Far East there is an association with opisthorchiasis. Urinary carriage is associated with schistosomiasis and nephrolithiasis. Acute typhoid in carriers has been reported. There is an increased risk of carcinoma of the gallbladder.

Patients discharged after treatment for typhoid with six negative stool and three negative urine specimens and negative Vi serology are considered free of infection. Most patients with positive stools at the completion of treatment excrete temporarily and can be safely followed up. Antibiotic eradication of carriage is advised in those still excreting at 3 months, or earlier in those at particular risk of communicating infection to others. The patient with a persistently elevated or rising Vi antibody titre is likely to be a carrier. Repeated checks of urine and faeces should be made and consideration given to obtaining bile cultures if these are negative.

Eradication of carriage requires prolonged, high-dose antibiotics (Table 7.6.8.1). Ampicillin, amoxicillin, and co-trimoxazole have been used with some success. More recently, good results have been reported with fluoroquinolones. Cholecystectomy and nephrectomy, once used to eliminate carriage (and not without operative mortality), are hard to justify on public health grounds alone, but can be considered if antibiotic methods fail and there are additional indications for operation. The success rates of surgery are increased by giving antibiotics as well.

Vaccines

The greatest need for typhoid vaccination is among infants, children, and young adults in endemic areas, especially where antibiotic resistance is increasing, and among laboratory workers handling the organisms. In practice, vaccines are given mostly to travellers to endemic areas. The most currently available vaccines are the parenteral Vi vaccine, given as a single injection, and the live attenuated Ty21a vaccine, given as three or four oral doses. The Ty21a vaccine should not be given to immunosuppressed persons or those taking mefloquine or antibiotics. Current typhoid vaccines do not protect against paratyphoid infection and the protection afforded by vaccination can be overcome by large inocula of bacteria. Efficacy figures derive largely from trials conducted in partly immune populations and overestimate the benefit in persons without prior exposure.

The risks of typhoid among travellers are low (3 to 30 cases per 100 000) and the precise efficacy of currently recommended doses in previously unexposed adults remains unknown. However, circumstantial evidence indicates typhoid vaccine affords protection to travellers visiting endemic areas. Travellers without the vaccine seem more susceptible to the disease, and this is true for even short-term (less than 1 week) travellers to endemic areas. Several new vaccines are currently being developed or evaluated, notably a Vi conjugate vaccine and single-dose oral vaccines.

Paratyphoid fever

Paratyphoid A occurs chiefly in Asia and Africa, Paratyphoid B worldwide, and paratyphoid C in Asia and the Middle East. Paratyphoid A has recently been increasing in South Asia, including drug-resistant disease. Outbreaks of paratyphoid are more often food-borne than water-borne, probably because larger inocula are needed to establish infection. Paratyphoid has a shorter incubation period (4–5 days). Recent reports suggest that the clinical syndromes caused by Typhi and Paratyphi A are indistinguishable, in particular that Paratyphi A may be as severe as Typhi. The management of paratyphoid is the same as that of typhoid.

Areas of uncertainty and controversy

The recommendation for first-line antibiotic therapy in endemic areas has been debated. Many practitioners have used fluoroquinolones for first-line therapy where multidrug resistance is common. The emergence of low-level resistance to fluoroquinolones has bought that approach into question. The laboratory detection of such isolates has proved problematic. Although nalidixic acid resistance is a useful laboratory marker of low-level resistance, it is not completely reliable and new fluoroquinolone breakpoints are needed. The optimum treatment for such infections is also undefined. The extended-spectrum cephalosporins, such as ceftriaxone, and azithromycin are available options and new fluoroquinolones, such as gatifloxacin, may be effective. In some areas isolates have regained sensitivity to first-line agents and chloramphenicol is being used. Whether isolates with full fluoroquinolone and extended-spectrum cephalosporin resistance become common in the next decade remains to be seen.

A second area of controversy is the use of vaccination as a public health tool in endemic areas. The emergence of multidrug resistance may swing the cost–benefit ratio in favour of vaccination. Several Vi vaccine demonstration trials are in progress to evaluate the cost-effectiveness of vaccination and these projects should provide an evidence base to inform policy. The realization that typhoid is common in children under 5 years has also focused attention on the development of vaccines appropriate for this age group. A Vi conjugate vaccine and single-dose oral vaccine are likely to become available in the near future.

Further reading

Basnyat B, *et al.* (2005). Enteric fever (typhoid) fever in travellers. *Clin Infect Dis*, **41**, 1467–72. [A recent review of issues relating to travellers.]

Bhan MK, Bahl R, Bhatnager S (2005). Typhoid and paratyphoid fever. *Lancet*, **366**, 749–62. [A useful, recent, and general review.]

Butler T, *et al.* (1985). Typhoid fever complicated by intestinal perforation: a persisting fatal disease requiring surgical management. *Rev Infect Dis*, **7**, 244–56.

Christie AB (1987). Typhoid and paratyphoid fevers. In: Christie AB (ed) *Infectious diseases: epidemiology and clinical practice*, 4th edition, vol. 1, pp. 100–64. Churchill Livingstone, Edinburgh. [An outstanding, detailed, and generously referenced monograph on typhoid.]

Forsyth JRL (1998). Typhoid and paratyphoid. In: Smith GR, Easmon CSF (eds) *Topley and Wilson's principles of bacteriology, virology and immunity*, 9th edition, vol. 3, pp. 459–78. Arnold, London. [A useful chapter covering microbiological aspects of typhoid in depth.]

Hoffman SL, *et al.* (1984). Reduction of mortality in chloramphenicol-treated severe typhoid fever by high-dose dexamethasone. *N Engl J Med*, **310**, 82–8.

Sanger Institute. *Bacterial genomes*. www.sanger.uk/Projects/Microbes [Information concerning the S. enterica ser. Typhi genome sequence.]

7.6.9 Intracellular klebsiella infections (donovanosis and rhinoscleroma)

J. Richens

Essentials

There are two rare intracellular species of klebsiella that cause granulomatous disease in humans. *Klebsiella rhinoscleromatis* typically causes bulky growths in the upper respiratory tract of patients with rhinoscleroma. *K. granulomatis* (until recently named *Calymmatobacterium granulomatis*) is associated with the genital ulcers or growths of donovanosis (granuloma inguinale). The histological appearances of both diseases are similar. The observation of vacuoles containing capsulated coccoid bacteria within histiocytes is the key to diagnosis. Both diseases are found in small endemic foci in warm climates and are linked to poverty and poor hygiene. Treatment for donovanosis with azithromycin and for rhinoscleroma with ciprofloxacin is recommended. Both diseases may require surgery for complications.

Donovanosis

Introduction

Donovanosis was first described in Calcutta by Donovan in 1905. It is a sexually transmitted infection best known in Papua New Guinea, India, southern Africa, and Brazil. An important focus among Australian aborigines has recently been eliminated. Donovanosis seems to be retreating, raising hopes of eventual eradication. Dark-skinned people appear to have greater susceptibility. The predilection of lesions for the anogenital region of sexually active adults and the frequent association with other sexually transmitted infections point strongly to sexual transmission. In the past, epidemics of donovanosis in New Guinea were linked to ritual homosexual and heterosexual practices. Perinatal transmission has been observed in a few cases.

Aetiology

An unusual Gram-negative bacillus can be isolated in HEp-2 cells or human peripheral blood mononuclear cells from patients with the characteristic lesions of donovanosis. This organism will not grow on conventional solid media. Previously named *Donovania* and subsequently *Calymmatobacterium* by Aragão and Vianna in 1913, it has now been classed as *Klebsiella granulomatis* on the basis of close DNA homology with other klebsiella species. *K. granulomatis* shows morphological identity with Donovan bodies observed within clinical lesions of donovanosis and patients with characteristic lesions have high levels of antibody that react equally with Donovan bodies and with *K. granulomatis. K. granulomatis* is pathogenic only to humans. Experimental transmission has been reported with lesion material, but to date not with a pure culture of this organism. Donovanosis shows a close macroscopic and microscopic similarity to rhinoscleroma which produces granulomatous lesions of the upper airways. These lesions contain intracellular clusters of the closely related organism *Klebsiella rhinoscleromatis*.

Pathogenesis

The organism has a special tropism for dermal macrophages. The response to infection is characterized by vigorous granulomatous inflammation that damages the skin and subcutaneous tissues. Extension of the infection is a local process of spreading ulceration. The inguinal lesions are probably seeded by lymphatic spread. Haematogenous dissemination and spread to the upper genital tract of women are exceptional. Lesions in women tend to be more extensive and may progress rapidly during pregnancy.

Clinical features

After an incubation period of 3 to 40 days, the disease usually starts with a small genital lesion. A nonspecific papule evolves into a painless ulcer displaying a deep red colour, contact bleeding, and a rolled edge. Hypertrophic lesions that pout outwards from the surrounding skin are frequent. Local lymphoedema is seen commonly in women. Chronic lesions tend to expand gradually along skin folds forming a large continuous area of ulceration with a characteristic serpiginous outline (Fig. 7.6.9.1). Inguinal lesions are common (Fig. 7.6.9.2). They start as a firm, subcutaneous swellings and often ulcerate. The term 'pseudobubo' tends to be applied to any inguinal lesion in donovanosis although it was originally coined to describe a subcutaneous inguinal abscess, which is a rare event. Such lesions have even given rise to suspicion of bubonic plague when Donovan bodies in the aspirate were misinterpreted. Primary lesions of the cervix simulate carcinoma of the cervix. Upper genital tract involvement in women may simulate pelvic inflammatory disease or malignancy and hydronephrosis may ensue. Anal lesions in have been described in homosexual men. Involvement of the rectum seldom occurs.

Oral lesions of donovanosis with extension to cervical nodes have been described. Haematogenous dissemination is associated with pregnancy and causes lesions of bone, liver, and spleen. Lesions in infants tend to involve the ears and nearby lymph nodes.

Complications of donovanosis include extensive scar formation, lymphoedema of the genitalia, penile autoamputation, and the development of squamous carcinoma in active or healed lesions. Secondary infection with fusospirochaetal organisms can cause rapid, extensive, and sometimes fatal tissue destruction.

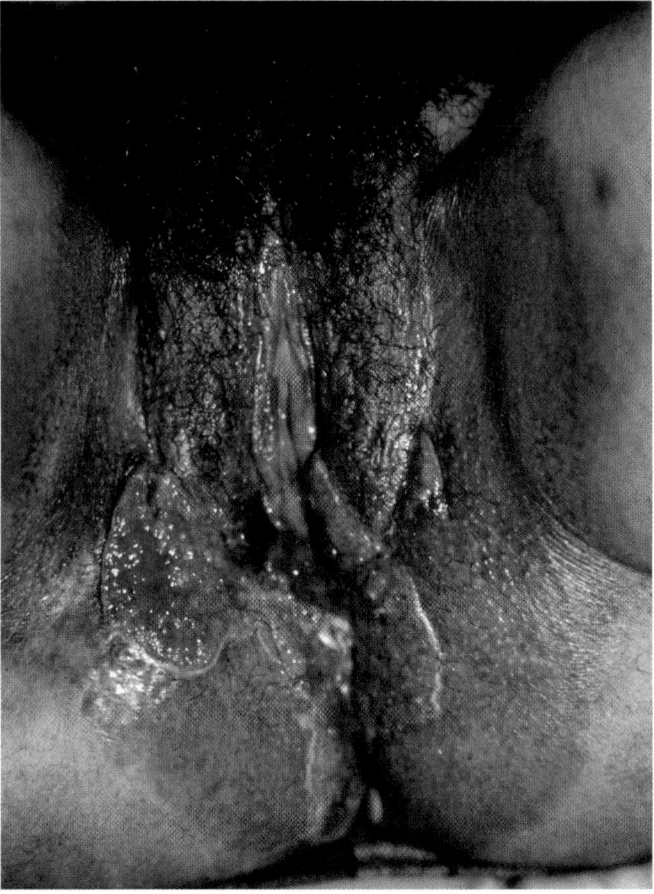

Fig. 7.6.9.1 Characteristic serpiginous ulcer in female patient with long-standing donovanosis.

Diagnosis

Donovanosis is diagnosed by demonstrating Donovan bodies lying within histiocytes in material taken from a typical lesion. Donovan bodies show well with Giemsa's, Leishman's, and Wright's stains but poorly with haematoxylin and eosin. Histology typically shows a heavy plasma cell infiltrate and epithelial hyperplasia in addition to histiocytes containing Donovan bodies (Fig. 7.6.9.3). Common misdiagnoses are squamous carcinoma of cervix, vulva, or penis, secondary syphilis, and conditions that produce genital lymphoedema such as filariasis and lymphogranuloma venereum.

Treatment

In 1913, Aragão and Vianna described the value of trivalent antimony in treating donovanosis (Fig. 7.6.9.2). Current expert opinion suggests that azithromycin gives the best results at a daily dose of 500 mg or weekly doses of 1 g. Erythromycin is safe and gives good results in pregnant women. Women in labour found to have untreated lesions of the cervix should be delivered by caesarean section to reduce known risks of haematogenous dissemination and transmission to the neonate. A week of epidemiological treatment may be offered to healthy contacts to abort incubating infections. Patients with genital deformity may benefit from plastic surgical procedures.

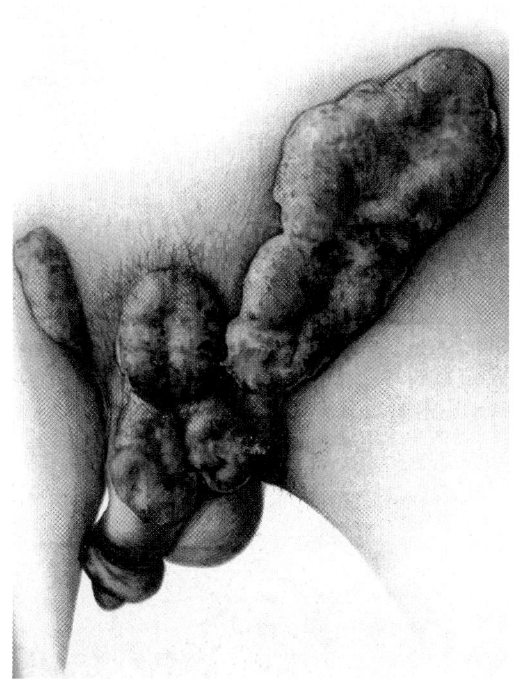

Fig. 7.6.9.2 Inguinal lesion: from Aragão and Vianna's paper on the value of trivalent antimony in treating donovanosis.
(From Aragão H, Vianna G (1913). Resquizas sobre o *Granuloma venereo. Mem Inst Oswaldo Cruz*, **5**, 211–38.)

Rhinoscleroma

Introduction and aetiology

Rhinoscleroma or scleroma is characterized by inflammatory growths of the upper airways. Endemic foci have been described in Africa (especially Egypt and Uganda), Siberia, Turkestan, the Middle East, the Indian subcontinent, China, the Philippines, Indonesia, and Papua New Guinea. There are many foci in South and Central America where it has been identified in terracotta Maya heads of AD 300 to 600. The disease has retreated in Eastern and Central Europe where it was first described by Hebra and Kaposi in 1870.

Klebsiella rhinoscleromatis can be isolated from about 60% of patients.

Pathogenesis

Transmission is believed to occur from person to person in endemic areas. Initially patients infected with this organism may complain of an exudative rhinitis. An atrophic rhinitis may follow. The most characteristic phase of the disease is the nodular stage during which a granulomatous reaction to the organisms within macrophages leads to the development of bulky masses within any part of the respiratory tract from nares to tracheal bifurcation. The process can extend into and destroy neighbouring soft tissues, cartilage, bone, and skin. Fibrosis and strictures are seen in the final stage.

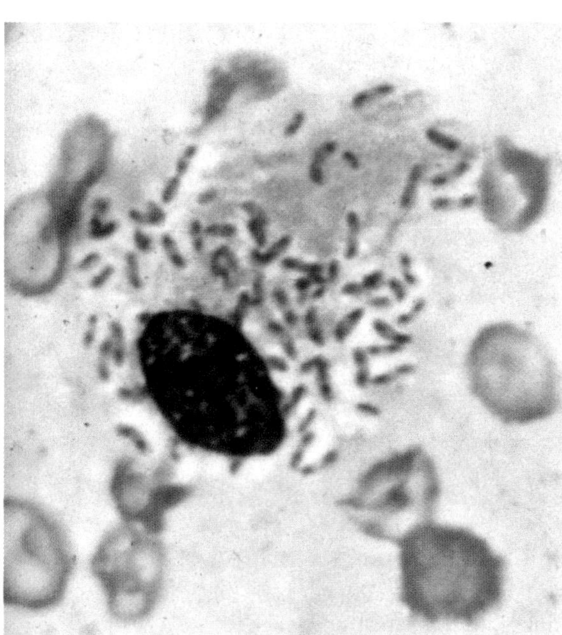

Fig. 7.6.9.3 Donovan bodies: Giemsa-stained smear from donovanosis lesion demonstrating the characteristic 'closed safety pin' appearance of encapsulated organisms within a large histiocyte.

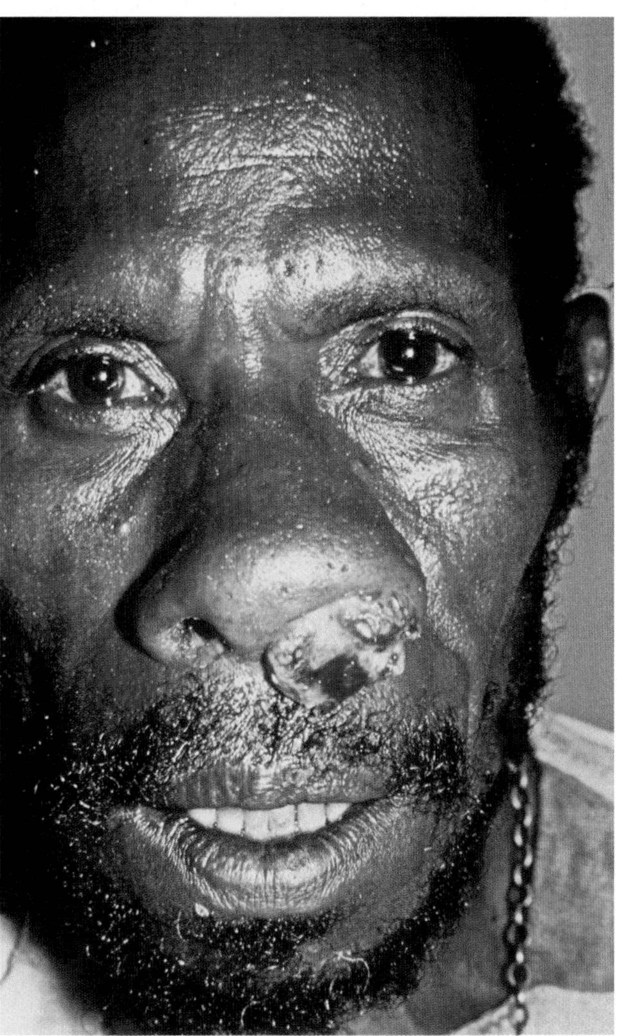

Fig. 7.6.9.4 Rhinoscleroma with characteristic nasal splaying (Hebra nose) and obstruction of the left nostril in a 30-year-old man from Papua New Guinea.
(From Cooke R (1987). *Colour atlas of anatomical pathology*, p. 31. Churchill Livingstone, Edinburgh, with permission.)

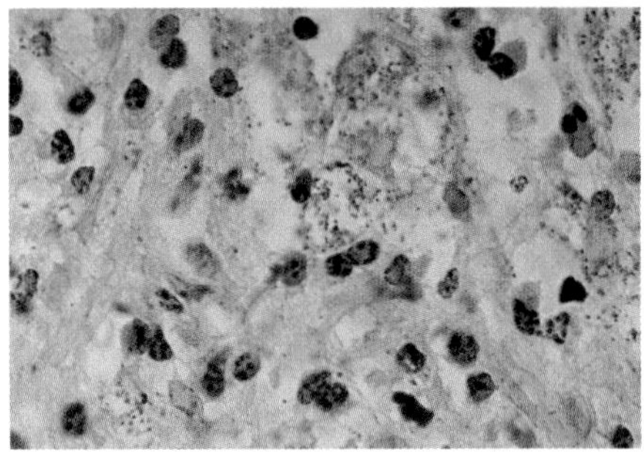

Fig. 7.6.9.5 Rhinoscleroma. Silver-stained preparation showing bacteria. (Copyright J Richens.)

Clinical features

Rhinoscleroma runs a slow fluctuating course over several years, progressing through exudative, atrophic, nodular, and fibrotic stages. Systemic symptoms are not seen. The usual presentations are with nasal obstruction and bleeding and nasal deformity (splaying of the lower nose, often with a visible growth extending down to the upper lip, known as Hebra nose) (Fig. 7.6.9.4). Some patients present with ozaena, which is an atrophic rhinitis accompanied by a foul smell and formation of crusts within the nose. Patients with tracheal involvement may present with stridor. With the help of sinus endoscopy and newer imaging techniques it is not unusual to find evidence of spread into the sinuses, orbits, cranial cavity, middle ear, and regional lymph nodes.

Diagnosis

Histology shows a dense infiltrate of plasma cells among which are seen large foamy histiocytes (Mikulicz cells) containing Gram-negative bacteria and Russell bodies which are thought to be effete plasma cells (Fig. 7.6.9.5). The diagnosis is usually made by demonstrating intracellular organisms in Giemsa-stained or silver-stained sections taken from typical lesions, combined with culture for *K. rhinoscleromatis*. CT scanning and endoscopic techniques provide useful ways to define the extent of the disease.

Treatment

Treatment with ciprofloxacin 250 mg twice daily for 4 weeks appears to be substantially superior to previously used antibiotic regimens (rifampicin, streptomycin, tetracyclines, ampicillin, and co-trimoxazole). Debulking operations may be needed for obstructing nasal and tracheal disease, and tracheostomy may be required as a temporary measure. Reconstructive surgery may be needed to deal with late fibrotic stenosis.

Further reading

Borgstein J, Sada E, Cortes R (1993). Ciprofloxacin for rhinoscleroma and ozena. *Lancet*, **342**, 122.

Bowden FJ, *et al.* (1996). Pilot study of azithromycin in the treatment of genital donovanosis. *Genitourin Med*, **72**, 17–19.

Canalis RF, Zamboni L (2001). An interpretation of the structural changes responsible for the chronicity of rhinoscleroma. *Laryngoscope*, **111**, 1020–6.

Carter JS, *et al.* (1999). Phylogenetic evidence for reclassification of *Calymmatobacterium granulomatis* as *Klebsiella granulomatis* comb. nov. Int J Syst Bacteriol, **49**, 1695–1700.

Richens J (1991). The diagnosis and treatment of donovanosis (granuloma inguinale). *Sex Transm Infect*, **67**, 441–52.

7.6.10 Anaerobic bacteria

Anilrudh A. Venugopal and David W. Hecht

Essentials

Anaerobic bacteria will not grow when incubated with 10% CO_2 in room air, but vary in their tolerance of different levels of oxygen. They are important commensal flora of the skin and oral, intestinal, and pelvic mucosae, and are classified according to their Gram staining characteristics and ability to produce spores: (1) Gram positive—cocci, non-spore-forming bacilli, and spore-forming bacilli (notably clostridium); (2) Gram negative—cocci and bacilli. Many anaerobic bacteria possess virulence factors that facilitate their pathogenicity, e.g. histiolytic enzymes and various toxins.

Clinical features—anaerobes typically cause clinically significant infections when there is tissue compromise, ischaemia or mucosal injury. These infections are often polymicrobial in nature and include (1) bacteraemia; (2) central nervous system infection—intracranial abscesses by contiguous spread, e.g. from chronic otitis media, or haematogenous spread, e.g. from tooth abscess; (3) head and neck infections—periodontal and pharyngeal infections from spread of gingival disease; (4) pleuropulmonary infections—e.g. lung abscess from aspirated oropharyngeal flora; (5) intra-abdominal infections—often caused by mixed colonic flora that have been displaced by bowel injury; (6) gastrointestinal infections—*Clostridium difficile*-associated disease (see Chapter 7.6.23); (7) genitourinary infections; (8) skin and soft-tissue infections—ranging from cellulitis to necrotizing fasciitis; should be considered in cases of infected animal and human bites, and in intravenous drug users; diabetic foot ulcers often have polymicrobial infections that include anaerobes.

Diagnosis—a putrid odour of the affected tissue or discharge is very suggestive of anaerobic infection, as is the presence of gas in tissues. Care must be taken when collecting specimens for anaerobic cultures because many of the organisms are very sensitive to oxygen, and some cannot tolerate more than a few minutes at ambient oxygen levels. However, anaerobic spores are aerotolerant, can survive in harsh oxygen-laden environments, and will germinate under appropriate conditions.

Treatment and prevention—aside from supportive care, treatment requires (1) drainage of abscesses and resection of devitalized tissue; and (2) antibiotics—agents that are active against anaerobes include metronidazole, vancomycin, β-lactam/β-lactamase combinations and carbapenems, but resistance patterns are changing and hence choice of empirical therapy is best guided by knowledge of local susceptibility testing. Prophylaxis against anaerobic bacteria significantly reduces postoperative infection rates following intra-abdominal surgery.

History

In 1690 Antonie van Leeuwenhoek first described anaerobic bacteria as 'animalcules' that could survive in the absence of air. This observation was overlooked until nearly 200 years later. In 1861 Louis Pasteur had observed that the bacteria near the surface of a droplet of water had stopped moving while the organisms at the centre of the droplet continued to move about. He hypothesized that oxygen in the air had caused the death of the surface bacteria. Pasteur's early experiments with bacterial fermentation led to the development of anaerobic bacteriology.

Initially there was uncertainty about the importance of these organisms, but the invention of the anaerobic jar by James McIntosh and Paul Fildes in 1916 allowed the repeated culture and study of anaerobes. This led to the discovery of many anaerobic bacteria responsible for various human diseases.

Definition

Anaerobic bacteria are organisms that cannot grow in the presence of various levels of oxygen. Room air is approximately 20% oxygen and when cultured in this environment, anaerobes will not grow on solid media. Reduced oxygen tensions are required for their growth. Anaerobes are described as strict, moderate, or facultative anaerobes, according to their tolerance of oxygen.

Strict anaerobes may grow only at oxygen levels of less than 0.5%. They are usually catalase negative and lack superoxide dismutase rendering them susceptible to toxic oxygen radicals, although this is not always the case. Moderate anaerobes also grow poorly in air and prefer media that have oxygen levels of 2 to 8%. Facultative anaerobic bacteria are organisms that can grow in various levels of oxygen including normal oxygen tensions.

Taxonomy of important anaerobic organisms

Table 7.6.10.1 lists the species of anaerobes that colonize human mucosal surfaces and skin or produce clinically significant disease. They are classified according to their Gram-staining characteristics and ability to produce spores.

Epidemiology

Limited data about the incidences of anaerobic infections are available. A few well-known anaerobic infections occur frequently enough to deserve mention here.

Clostridium difficile-associated disease (see Chapter 7.6.23) is the single bacterial agent most frequently isolated in diarrhoeal illnesses when a causative agent is established. It is a common cause of hospital-acquired diarrhoea and can present in different ways that are discussed later in this chapter.

Enterotoxigenic *Bacteroides fragilis* (ETBF) is another emerging enteric pathogen causing diarrhoeal illness in humans. It has been known to cause epidemics of diarrhoeal illness in industrialized and developing nations.

Human commensal flora

Commensal bacteria are organisms that live on both mucosal surfaces and skin of humans but under normal circumstances do not cause disease. They play an important role in normal host physiology by colonizing and helping to prevent infections by pathogenic organisms. By producing toxic metabolites, lowering the local pH, and depleting the area of nutrients they make the surrounding area uninhabitable to other pathogenic organisms. Anaerobes make up a large part of this commensal flora in humans, as outlined below.

Skin

The commensal flora of the skin consists predominantly of aerobes, anaerobes, and yeasts. The principal anaerobes present are Gram-positive bacilli of the genus *Propionibacterium*. The three main species are *P. acnes*, *P. granulosum*, and *P. avidum*. They occur mainly in hair follicles and sebaceous glands. *P. acnes* produces free fatty acids from triglycerides, but, while this may control the growth of pathogenic bacteria on the surface of skin, it has also been associated with the development of acne.

Upper respiratory tract and oral cavity

The nasal cavity mucosa tends to be colonized with organisms that are similar to the organisms found on skin surfaces and the sebaceous glands. Oropharyngeal flora typically includes *Peptostreptococci*, *Tannerella forsythensis*, and *Fusobacterium*. In the oral cavity, areas such as the tonsillar crypts, gingival crevices, and the clefts on the tongue have a more favourable atmosphere for anaerobes. Their lower oxygen levels promote colonization with prevotella, *Peptostreptococci*, *Fusobacterium*, and other anaerobic Gram-positive bacilli.

Gastrointestinal tract

The upper gastrointestinal tract from oesophagus to jejunum is relatively free of microorganisms but can become transiently colonized with bacteria following meals or from the swallowed secretions of the upper airway. The terminal ileum tends to have a flora more closely resembling that of the large intestines where anaerobes can outnumber the aerobes 100 to 1000:1. Among a diverse group of

Table 7.6.10.1 Taxonomy of important anaerobic bacteria

Gram-positive anaerobes			Gram-negative anaerobes	
Cocci	Bacilli		Cocci	Bacilli
	Nonspore-forming	Spore-forming		
Peptococcus spp.	*Actinomyces* spp.	*Clostridium* spp.	*Veillonella* spp.	*Bacteroides fragilis* group
Peptostreptococcus spp.	*Bifidobacterium* spp.			Other *Bacteroides* spp.
Streptococcus spp.	*Eubacterium* spp.			*Bilophila wadsworthia*
Finegoldia magna	*Lactobacillus* spp.			*Fusobacterium* spp.
	Mobiluncus spp.			*Porphyromonas* spp.
	Propionibacterium spp.			*Prevotella* spp.

anaerobes, the *Bacteroides fragilis* group predominates. *B. vulgatus* and *B. thetaiotaomicron* are more common than *B. fragilis*. Another group of colonizing anaerobes found in the stool are *Clostridium* spp., including *C. perfringens* and *C. novyi*. Infants have been found to be colonized with *C. difficile* but without symptoms. Infantile intestinal mucosal cells in rabbits lack the receptors to bind the disease-producing *C. difficile* toxin, but they acquire the receptors with increasing age.

Genitourinary tract

The kidneys, ureters, urinary bladder, and proximal part of the urethra are normally free of organisms as they are constantly flushed with urine if the anatomy of the urinary tract is normal. The distal portion of both male and female urethras have a scanty flora including aerobic skin colonizers and some anaerobic organisms including bacteroides, *Fusobacterium*, *Peptostreptococcus*, and clostridium. The vaginal flora can include both aerobes and anaerobes but, by adulthood, anaerobes such as lactobacillus, *Prevotella*, *Fusobacterium*, and *Peptostreptococci* predominate (Fig. 7.6.10.1)

Pathogenesis

Several factors predispose to the pathogenesis of anaerobic infections, including tissue injury and destruction, impaired blood supply, or any breakdown in the integrity of mucosa or skin.

Many anaerobic bacteria possess one or more characteristics that enhance their pathogenic virulence. Histolytic enzymes such as collagenase, fibrinolysin, lipases, and other enzymes are produced by bacteroides and *Prevotella*. These enzymes cause tissue destruction, whereas the α-toxin found in *C. perfringens* can also cause haemolysis. Enterotoxigenic *B. fragilis* is known to produce a metalloproteinase toxin that causes cell proliferation and protein shedding resulting in a diarrhoeal illness. Various organisms including *C. perfringens* and *C. difficile* have also been found to have enterotoxins that alter intestinal cell function and cause cell death leading to diarrhoea. Certain species of clostridium including *C. botulinum* and *C. tetani* produce neurotoxins that block neuromuscular transmissions leading to paralysis or spasms plus rigidity, respectively. Gram-negative anaerobes, like their aerobic counterparts, have a lipopolysaccharide layer in their outer membrane that can act as an endotoxin. Endotoxins can cause macrophage and complement activation leading to fever, hypotension, and oedema from the release of cytokines. However, the endotoxin of the *B. fragilis* group is defective and weak when compared to those of other facultative anaerobic bacteria. *Porphyromonas gingivalis*, *Bacteroides* spp., and *Fusobacterium* produce heparinases that can promote coagulation leading to tissue ischaemia. The capsular polysaccharides associated with the *B. fragilis* group, *Prevotella melaninogenica*, and *Peptostreptococcus*, are associated with impaired phagocytosis by host cells and can lead to abscess formation. *Porphyromonas gingivalis*, *B. fragilis*, and *Fusobacterium*

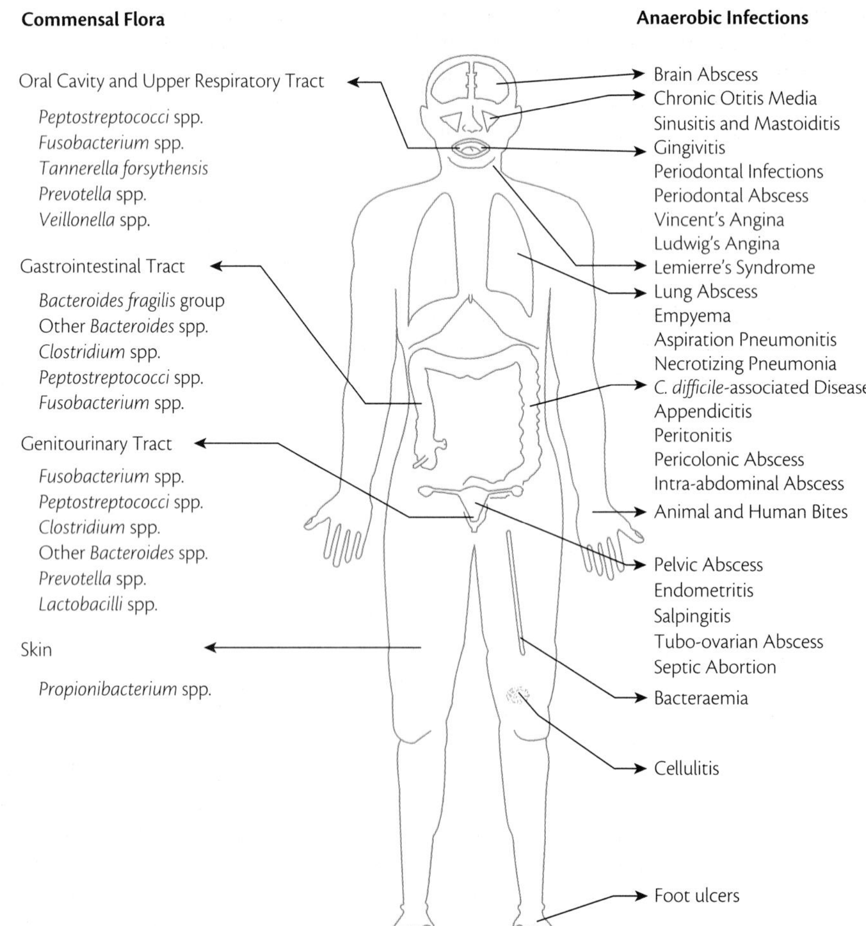

Fig. 7.6.10.1 Human anaerobic commensal flora (left) and clinical spectrum of anaerobic infections (right).

nucleatum produce catalase and superoxide dismutase which is believed to help the organisms tolerate higher levels of oxygen. Spore-producing organisms like the clostridial species can survive in harsh oxygen-laden environments by developing spores that will later germinate when environmental conditions become favourable again. Finally, several organisms produce surface ligands and charges that help to improve mucosal adherence and bacterial aggregation, while others produce metabolites that inhibit the growth of normal flora.

Clinical spectrum

Anaerobic bacteraemia

Anaerobes account for 0.5 to 12% of all positive blood cultures. Underlying risk factors for the development of anaerobic bacteraemia include malignancies, immunosuppression, hepatic failure, and diabetes mellitus. The organism isolated depends on the underlying infectious condition. In cases of gastrointestinal or necrotic skin infections it is usually a member of the *B. fragilis* group. Peptostreptococcus and clostridium are other commonly found blood isolates. The isolation of *Clostridium septicum* or the facultative anaerobe *Streptococcus bovis* in bacteraemic patients should raise the suspicion of underlying cancer, especially of colonic origin.

Central nervous system infections

Intracranial infections with anaerobes can arise by contiguous spread from surrounding structures, e.g. with chronic otitis media, mastoiditis, or sphenoidal sinusitis. This can lead to abscess formation, septic thrombophlebitis, or venous sinus infections. When frontal sinusitis spreads to involve the frontal bone it can lead to osteomyelitis and subperiosteal abscess known as Pott's puffy tumour. Intracranial abscesses may also arise as a result of haematogenous seeding of the brain parenchyma from suppurative distant foci such as dental abscesses and alveolar infections. Abscesses that arise may be single or multiple in number and involve any portion of the brain, although the site involved depends on the mode of infection. Anaerobic organisms commonly associated with infections of the central nervous system include prevotella, *Peptostreptococci*, and *Fusobacterium* spp., although these are often polymicrobial infections involving aerobes.

Head and neck infections

The origin of oral, head, and neck infections is often the anaerobic flora of the oral cavity. Lower oxygen tension in the gingival crevices promotes colonization with anaerobes. When dental hygiene is poor, dental plaque develops leading to gingivitis, periodontal infections, and abscesses. Periodontal infections result from spread of gingival disease to the surrounding tissue. As infection spreads from more superficial gingival disease to deeper infections there is a shift in the pathogenic organisms from Gram-positive cocci and bacilli to Gram-negative bacilli. Anaerobic pharyngeal infections may arise in relation to gingivitis. Complications may arise by contiguous spread of these infections along medial, lateral, or submaxillary spaces. Ludwig's angina is described as a brawny induration of the submaxillary and sublingual spaces with cellulitis usually arising from spread of lower molar dental infections. Severe infections threaten the airway and may extend to the mediastinum. Lemierre's syndrome frequently occurs in young previously healthy patients as the result of spread of an oropharyngeal infection leading to septic thrombophlebitis of the internal jugular vein. Clinical features helpful in diagnosing this condition are recent oropharyngeal infection, clinical evidence of thrombophlebitis including ipsilateral neck tenderness with fevers and chills, as well as isolation of the anaerobic pathogen. Most commonly, the organism isolated is *Fusobacterium necrophorum*, although other organisms have been identified. Early diagnosis is required to reduce morbidity associated with distant septic emboli and mortality. Vincent's angina is an acute necrotizing ulcerative gingivitis manifested by inflamed gingivae, interdental ulcerations, and halitosis. Typically it is not associated with pharyngitis. Otitis media and sinusitis occasionally involve anaerobes, although they are more common in chronic infections of these spaces.

Pleuropulmonary infections

The spectrum of anaerobic lung infections extends to include lung abscesses, empyema, aspiration pneumonitis, and necrotizing pneumonias. The origins of these anaerobes are usually from aspirated oropharyngeal flora. *Peptostreptococcus*, *Fusobacterium*, pigmented *Prevotella*, *Porphyromonas*, and *Bacteroides* spp. are most commonly isolated, often in combination with aerobes and other microaerophilic anaerobes such as *Streptococcus* spp. Patients with an anaerobic lung abscess will often complain of fevers, weight loss, and foul-smelling or foul-tasting sputum. This odour is frequently detectable on entering the patient's room.

Intra-abdominal infections

Intra-abdominal infections are often caused by mixed colonic flora that have been displaced by surgery, penetrating trauma, intestinal malignancy, inflammatory bowel disease, or perforation of colonic diverticula. Intra-abdominal abscesses, pericolonic abscesses, and peritonitis may develop. Isolates are most commonly mixed facultative and strict anaerobes, notably the facultative anaerobe *Escherichia coli* and the anaerobe *B. fragilis* group. Other commonly occurring anaerobes include *Peptostreptococcus* spp., *Fusobacterium* spp., and *Clostridium* spp.

Gastrointestinal infections

C. difficile-associated disease (CDAD) is discussed in Chapter 7.6.23. Risk factors include recent or current antibacterial therapy (especially clindamycin, cephalosporins, and fluoroquinolones), advanced age, recent hospitalization or long-term care residence, and recent gastrointestinal surgery or procedures. Severity of CDAD ranges from diarrhoea to ileus, pseudomembranous colitis, toxic megacolon, and death. Clinical symptoms often include abdominal pain and distension, fevers, and profuse foul-smelling watery diarrhoea. Laboratory findings include leucocytosis (leukaemoid reactions) and hypoalbuminaemia. *C. difficile* produces toxin A, an enterotoxin that causes intestinal fluid secretion and inflammation, and toxin B, a cell cytotoxin that disrupts tight mucosal cell junctions. Diagnosis is achieved by enzyme immunoassay detection of toxins A and B (sensitivity 60–80%), but the most sensitive diagnostic test is the slow and labour-intensive tissue culture assay. Treatment involves first stopping the offending antibiotics and then giving oral metronidazole. Seriously ill patients require oral vancomycin therapy. In the presence of ileus, vancomycin may be given by retention enemas. It is important to perform strict contact isolation measures for patients suspected of *C. difficile* disease to prevent nosocomial transmission.

Genitourinary infections

Like the oral cavity and colon, the female genital tract has an increased colonization ratio of anaerobes to aerobes of nearly 10:1. Disruption of the integrity of the tissues of the female genital tract increases the risk of anaerobic infections such as periurethral and labial pyogenic infections, pelvic abscesses, postpartum endometritis, salpingitis, tubo-ovarian abscess, and septic abortions. *B. fragilis* group, *Prevotella* spp. including *P. bivia*, *P. disiens*, and *P. melaninogenica*, *Peptostreptococci*, and *Clostridium* spp. are commonly isolated. Actinomyces have been associated with intrauterine device-related infections. Bacterial vaginosis (see Chapter 14.15) is an infection characterized by malodorous vaginal discharge caused by a polymicrobial infection often including prevotella, *Peptostreptococci*, *Mobiluncus*, and the facultative anaerobe *Gardnerella vaginalis*. *Clostridium sordellii* is a toxin-producing Gram-positive anaerobe that has been known to cause pelvic infections. This usually presents with vague symptoms causing deep infections following childbirth, medically induced abortions, or trauma. There is rapid clinical deterioration with profound hypotension, an intense leukaemoid reaction, and high mortality rate.

Skin and soft tissue infections

These usually arise after the integrity of the skin has been lost from injury, ischaemia, or surgery and there is contamination by either faecal or oral secretions. These are usually polymicrobial infections with aerobic and anaerobic bacteria. The spectrum of disease ranges from cellulitis to necrotizing fasciitis. Anaerobic skin infections should also be considered in cases of infected animal and human bites, and also with intravenous drug users who clean their needles with saliva and present with cellulitis at previous injection sites. Diabetic foot ulcers often have polymicrobial infections that include anaerobes. Common isolates from soft tissue infections include *B. fragilis* group, *Peptostreptococci*, and *Clostridium* spp.

Bone and joint infections

Osteomyelitis and septic arthritis from anaerobes are rare but can result when infection spreads from surrounding soft tissue, as in the case of diabetic foot ulcers. Diagnosis is made by the careful collection of fluids in anaerobic containers or by bone biopsy cultures. *Fusobacterium* spp. and other *Bacteroides* spp. have been isolated from joint infections on a few occasions.

Diagnosis

Clinical clues

A putrid odour of the affected tissue or discharge is very suggestive of anaerobic infections. Underlying illnesses such as diabetes mellitus, abscess formation, tissue ischaemia, and necrotic tissue are predisposing factors. Another important clue is the location of the infection in relation to mucosal surfaces that are normally colonized by anaerobes such as intra-abdominal and oral infections. Gas in tissues suggests anaerobic infection. It can often be detected on radiographs in cases of skin and soft tissue infections or with CT or MRI in deeper infections. However, gas formation in tissues is not specific to anaerobes and can be found in many aerobic infections as well. Some characteristic anaerobic infections such as actinomycosis may be identified on smears or tissue biopsy by the presence of filamentous Gram-positive bacilli and 'sulphur granules', although these may be easily missed.

Collection of specimens

The greatest barrier to the diagnosis of anaerobic infections (aside from not considering anaerobes) is faulty collection and transport of specimens. Aspirated pus or excised infected tissue should be despatched to the microbiology laboratory under anaerobic conditions as soon as possible. The use of swabs is discouraged because of the low yield of organisms collected with these specimens. Gram's stains and plating of the specimens should be done promptly with minimal exposure to air to minimize the loss of obligate anaerobes during handling. Immediately after inoculation, the media should be kept under anaerobic conditions in either anaerobic jars or chambers at 35 to 37°C. Most microbiology laboratories will not set up anaerobic cultures if the specimens have been collected improperly or were not transported in anaerobic transport media.

Anaerobic blood cultures

The collection of anaerobic blood cultures for the routine surveillance of bacteraemias has been debated for several years. Recent studies have confirmed their importance in detecting both anaerobic and early facultative anaerobic bacteraemias. Paired cultures should be drawn, including both aerobic and anaerobic bottles, and these should be collected from peripheral sources. This is important as positive cultures for anaerobes often occur when not suspected.

Treatment

Susceptibility and resistance

Anaerobic susceptibility patterns have consistently demonstrated resistance by members of the *B. fragilis* group since the late 1970s. Antibiotics vary in their *in vitro* activity against anaerobes. One of the most active agents is metronidazole which is the preferred agent for the treatment of *B. fragilis* and *C. tetani* and demonstrates activity against most species of *Clostridium*. It is effective in the treatment of *C. difficile* infections and is often used as initial therapy in patients with mild to moderate disease. Oral vancomycin must be recognized as the agent of choice for severe cases of *C. difficile* disease. Among 110 isolates of toxigenic *C. difficile*, no resistance to vancomycin and metronidazole was demonstrated.

β-lactam/β-lactamase combinations such as ampicillin/sulbactam, piperacillin/tazobactam, and ticarcillin/clavulanate demonstrate a high degree of *in vitro* activity against anaerobes including members of the *B. fragilis* group. Carbapenems such as imipenem/cilastatin, meropenem, and ertapenem also demonstrate excellent *in vitro* activity against nearly all anaerobes, while chloramphenicol has continued to maintain good *in vitro* activity against most anaerobic isolates due to its limited use.

Moderate antianaerobic *in vitro* activity is seen with cephamycins such as cefoxitin and cefotetan. Among fluoroquinolones, moxifloxacin has demonstrated moderate to good *in vitro* activity against most anaerobes. Over recent years, the *B. fragilis* group has shown the most significant increase in resistance to clindamycin.

Resistance patterns of the *B. fragilis* group members from isolates tested in both the United States of America and Europe are shown in Table 7.6.10.2. Anaerobes from the non-*Bacteroides* group are generally more susceptible to antianaerobic antibiotics. Exceptions to this rule include the resistance of *Prevotella* spp.

Table 7.6.10.2 *In vitro* resistance of six species of the *B. fragilis* group from the United States of America and Europe to selected agents[a] (given in percentages)

Isolate	Cefoxitin		Clindamycin		Imipenem/cilastatin		Piperacillin/tazobactam		Metronidazole		Moxifloxacin	
	USA[b]	Europe[c]	USA	Europe	USA	Europe	USA	Europe	USA	Europe	USA	Europe
B. fragilis	5	3	19	13	0.5	1	0.4	0.7	<0.001	0.5	27	8
B. thetaiotaomicron	17	13	33	15	0.2	0.5	0.4	0.5	0	0	26	8
B. vulgatus	8	9	35	30	0.3	1	0.7	3	0	2	55	19
B. ovatus	17	7	33	25	0.2	0	0.4	2	0	0	38	16
B. distasonis	30	6	30	10	0.4	0	1	0	0	0	29	10
B. uniformis	5	0	29	11	0.5	0	0	0	0	0	39	11

[a] Testing of the isolates was performed using the reference agar dilution method recommended by the Clinical and Laboratory Standards Institute.

[b] Percentage of resistance of six species of the *B. fragilis* group members against six antibiotics, 1997 to 2004, from 10 medical centres in the United States of America.
(Snydman DR, *et al.* (2007). National survey on the susceptibility of *Bacteroides fragilis* group: report and analysis of trends in the United States from 1997 to 2004. *Antimicrob Agents Chemother*, **51**, 1649–55.)

[c] Percentage of resistance of six species of the *B. fragilis* group members against six antibiotics, 1999 to 2001, from 19 European medical centres.
(Hedberg M, Nord CE (2003). Antimicrobial susceptibility of *Bacteroides fragilis* group isolates in Europe. *Clin Microbiol Infect*, **9**, 475–88.)

(clindamycin and moxifloxacin resistance at 38% and 29%, respectively), other *Clostridium* spp. (non-*C. perfringens* show cefoxitin, clindamycin, and moxifloxacin resistance at 30%, 10%, and 20%, respectively), and *P. acnes* (metronidazole resistance 100%). *Peptostreptococcus* spp. demonstrate clindamycin and moxifloxacin resistance of 14% and 17%, respectively, and penicillin resistance in the range of 4 to 8% among tested isolates (personal communication D.W. Hecht, 2007). Antibiotic resistance among anaerobes is less predictable than with aerobic and facultative anaerobes. Institutions should perform susceptibility testing at least annually to establish patterns of resistance to be reported with the hospital's antibiogram. Susceptibility of individual isolates should be performed if they were cultured from otherwise sterile sites and in cases of severe infections or those requiring long-term antibiotics.

Surgery

Often, antimicrobial therapy alone is not sufficient to cure anaerobic infections. Since many infections are associated with abscess formation or occur in areas with tissue ischaemia, surgical intervention frequently becomes imperative with drainage of abscesses and resection of devitalized tissue.

Surgical antimicrobial prophylaxis

In cases where contamination of surgical wounds by the local flora could result in infection, it has become common practice for surgeons to use antimicrobial prophylaxis in the intraoperative and postoperative periods. In intra-abdominal procedures, prophylaxis against anaerobic bacteria significantly reduces postoperative infection rates. The regimens may cover both aerobes and anaerobes. The choice and duration of therapy depends on the nature of the surgery and whether it is an elective or emergency procedure. These decisions are based on timing, type of clinical presentation, and intraoperative findings. The antimicrobials used include cephamycins such as cefoxitin and cefotetan or other more specific antianaerobic agents such as metronidazole. Ertapenem has proved an effective alternative to cefotetan in prophylaxis of infections for elective colorectal surgery.

Further reading

Aldape MJ, Bryant AE, Stevens DL (2006). *Clostridium sordellii* infection: epidemiology, clinical findings and current perspectives on diagnosis and treatment. *Clin Infect Dis*, **43**, 1436–46.

Bartlett JG (2006). Narrative review: the new epidemic of *Clostridium difficile*-associated enteric disease. *Ann Int Med*, **145**, 758–64.

Chow AW (2006). Anaerobic infections. In: Dale DC, *et al.* (eds) *ACP medicine*, pp. 1604–20. Web MD, New York.

Finegold SM, George WL (eds) (1989). *Anaerobic infections in humans.* Academic Press, New York.

Hagelskjaer L, Prag J (2000). Human necrobacillosis, with emphasis on Lemierre's syndrome. *Clin Infect Dis*, **31**, 524–32.

Hecht DW (2004). Prevalence of antibiotic resistance in anaerobic bacteria: worrisome developments. *Clin Infect Dis*, **39**, 92–7.

Hecht DW, Onderdonk A (2007). *Methods for antimicrobial susceptibility testing of anaerobic bacteria*, 7th edition. Clinical and Laboratory Standards Institute, Wayne, PA.

Hecht DW, *et al.* (2007). In vitro activities of 15 antimicrobial agents against 110 toxigenic Clostridium difficile clinical isolates collected from 1983 to 2004. *Antimicrob Agents Chemother*, **51**, 2716–19.

Hedberg M, Nord CE (2003). Antimicrobial susceptibility of *Bacteroides fragilis* group isolates in Europe. *Clin Microbiol Infect*, **9**, 475–88.

Itani KMF, *et al.* (2006). Ertapenem versus cefotetan prophylaxis in elective colorectal surgery. *N Engl J Med*, **355**, 2640–51.

Jenkins SG (2001). Infections due to anaerobic bacteria and the role of antimicrobial susceptibility testing of anaerobes. *Rev Med Microbiol*, **12**, 1–12.

Lassmann B, *et al.* (2007). Reemergence of anaerobic bacteremias. *Clin Infect Dis*, **44**, 895–900.

Snydman DR, *et al.* (2007). National survey on the susceptibility of *Bacteroides fragilis* group: report and analysis of trends in the United States from 1997 to 2004. *Antimicrob Agents Chemother*, **51**, 1649–55.

Solomkin JS, *et al.* (2003). Guidelines for the selection of anti-infective agents for complicated intra-abdominal infections. *Clin Infect Dis*, **37**, 997–1005.

Talan DA, *et al.* (1999). Bacteriologic analysis of infected dog and cat bites. *N Engl J Med*, **340**, 85–92.

Tzianabos AO, Kasper DL (2005). Anaerobic infections: general concepts. In: Mandell GL, Bennett JE, Dolin R (eds) *Principles and practices of infectious diseases*, pp. 2810–16. Elsevier Churchill Livingstone, Philadelphia.

7.6.11 Cholera

Aldo A.M. Lima and Richard L. Guerrant

Essentials

Vibrio cholerae is a Gram-negative organism that can be subdivided into over 200 serogroups based on the somatic O antigen, with only serogroups O1 and O139 causing epidemic and pandemic disease. Historically it has killed millions from dehydrating diarrhoea, encouraged the birth of modern epidemiology, the sanitary revolution, and oral rehydration therapy; it persists today as a glaring reminder of poverty and inadequate water/sanitation. Contaminated food (especially undercooked seafood) is the usual route of transmission in developed countries; contaminated water and street food vendors are more common vehicles in less developed countries.

Clinical features and diagnosis—typical presentation is with sudden onset of voluminous, painless, watery diarrhoea, which can exceed 500 to 1000 ml/h, leading to severe dehydration in a couple hours and risk of death. Definitive diagnosis is by isolating *V. cholerae* from stool or rectal swab samples.

Treatment—oral rehydration therapy with sugar or starch, water, and salts must be provided in the community and at field stations, clinics, and hospitals where most patients present: this reduces the case fatality of untreated severe cholera from about 50% to 1% or less. Antibiotics can shorten the illness and decrease diarrhoeal purging: tetracycline, cotrimoxazole, ciprofloxacin, or azithromycin have been effective, but there is increasing resistance.

Prevention—effective preventive measures include (1) ensuring a safe water supply; (2) improving sanitation; (3) making food safe for consumption by thorough cooking of high-risk foods, especially seafood; and (4) health education through mass media. Two oral cholera vaccines can provide significant (but not complete) protection.

Introduction and historical perspective

Cholera, the dreaded scourge causing death from dehydrating diarrhoea, existed for centuries in South Asia until, in 1817, it broke out along trade routes; since then there have been seven pandemics across all six inhabited continents. Cholera was largely responsible for encouraging the birth of modern epidemiology and for driving the sanitary revolution in Western Europe and North America in the 19th century. In the last one-third of the 20th century, it helped drive scientific discoveries of cell signalling, intestinal ion transport, and oral rehydration therapy (ORT), which have brought global diarrhoea mortality down from over 5 million/year to below 2 million/year. Yet cholera persists today as a disease of poverty, along with other faecally transmitted pathogens, a sign of inadequate water and sanitation among the desperately poor and displaced around the world.

Aetiology, genetics, and pathophysiology

Thirty years before the causative agent *Vibrio cholerae* was discovered during the fifth pandemic in 1884 in Kolkata, India, by Robert Koch, John Snow's classic epidemiological study of cholera in London in 1854 suggested that it was transmitted by contaminated drinking water. Snow even postulated that a toxin might cause the dramatic fluid loss. *V. cholerae* is a halophilic flagellated curved Gram-negative organism classified by biochemical tests and further subdivided into serogroups based on the somatic O antigen. Among over 200 serogroups, only O1 and O139 cause epidemic and pandemic disease. The other strains are classified as non-O1 and non-O139 *V. cholerae*. Serogroup O1 is further subdivided into three serotypes, Inaba, Ogawa, and Hikojima, and into two phenotypically different biogroups, Classical and El Tor (named for the Egyptian village quarantine station where it was first isolated in 1905 from Indonesian pilgrims travelling to Mecca). This strain then became the cause of the seventh pandemic that continues around the world today. The O139 serogroup, first seen in 1992, appears to have emerged from horizontal gene transfer of a fragment of DNA that encodes O-antigen biosynthesis from another serogroup (perhaps O22) into the seventh pandemic *V. cholerae* O1 El Tor strain. O139 and O1 (both Classical and El Tor biotypes) now coexist and continue to cause large outbreaks in India and Bangladesh. *V. cholerae* O1 (biotype El Tor) has two circular chromosomes and the entire genome sequence was recently described. The large chromosome has most of the genes required for growth and pathogenicity and the small chromosome encodes components of several essential metabolic and regulatory pathways. Critical to the pathogenicity of *V. cholerae* (and distinct from environmental isolates) is the acquisition of two distinct phages. The first contains a 'pathogenicity island' (VPI) encoding the 'toxin coregulated pilus' (TCP). Remarkably, TCP serves as both a major intestinal colonization factor and as the receptor for the second phage, CTXφ, that encodes for cholera toxin and accessory proteins (including ACE and Zot) as well as containing genes required for phage replication, integration, and regulation in the RS2 region. Genes encoding colonization factors or toxin are regulated in response to environmental conditions. The 32-kDa transmembrane protein ToxR binds upstream of *ctxAB* to increase transcription and synthesis of cholera toxin. ToxR also regulates the expression of other genes in the ToxR regulon; hence, the expression of ToxR is controlled by environmental factors.

Vibrios are acquired from contaminated water or food and they must pass though the acidic stomach before they are able to colonize the upper small intestine. Colonization occurs with filamentous protein fimbriae, called toxin coregulated pili, which extend from the vibrio wall and attach to receptors on the mucosa. *V. cholerae* adhere to the M cells without causing tissue damage and rapidly multiply to 10^7 to 10^8 cells/g of tissue. Attached vibrios efficiently deliver cholera toxin directly to the epithelial cells (Fig. 7.6.11.1). The A subunit consists of two peptides linked by a disulphide bond. The larger, A1, containing the toxic activity, is endocytosed following toxin binding via its B subunit to GM1 ganglioside. A1 subunit catalyses the covalent bonding of adenosine diphosphoribose from nicotinamide adenosine dinucleotide to the α-subunit of Gs, the heterotrimeric adenylyl cyclase-stimulating G protein, thus activating adenylate cyclase to form cAMP. cAMP then acts to open the cystic fibrosis transmembrane conductance regulator (CFTR) chloride channel causing increased chloride secretion by the intestinal crypt cells and a blockade of neutral sodium and chloride absorption by villous cells. This leads to voluminous fluid efflux into the small intestinal lumen which exceeds the absorptive

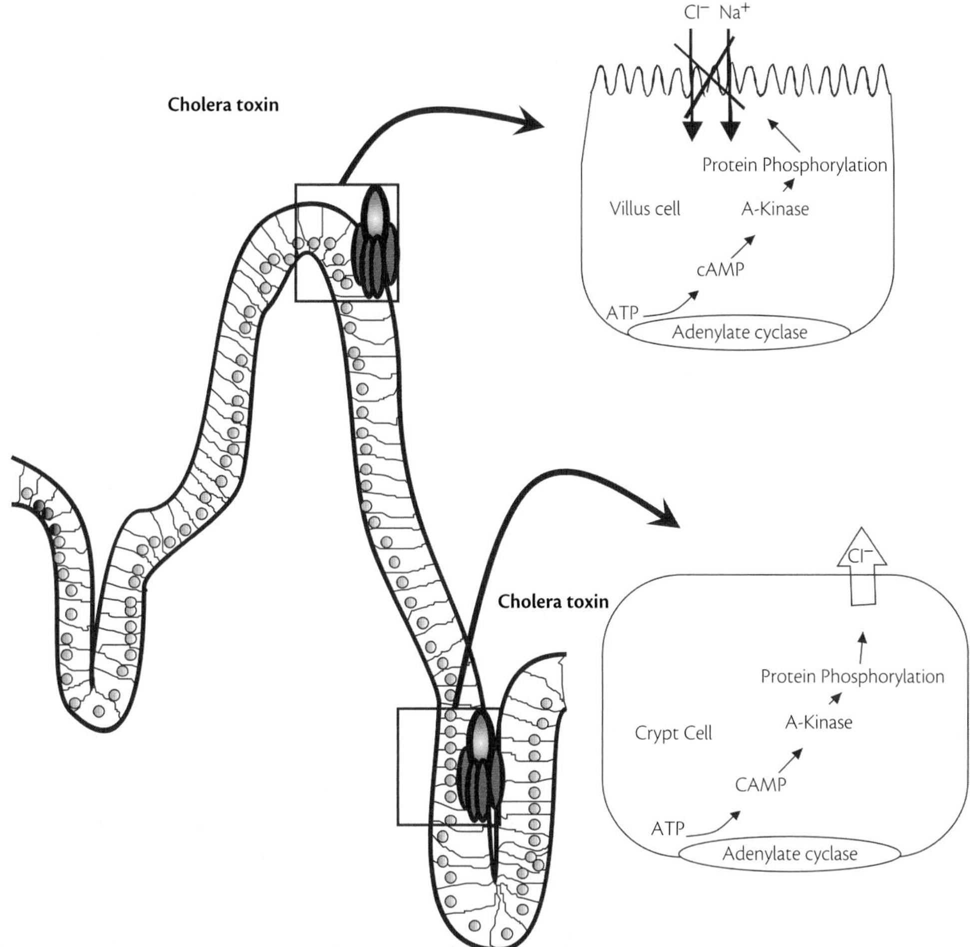

Fig. 7.6.11.1 Pathophysiology of cholera. *V. cholerae* produces a major virulence factor, cholera toxin (CT), an 84-kDa protein consisting of a dimeric A subunit and five identical B subunits. The A subunit consists of two peptides linked by adisulphide bond, the larger, A1, containing the toxic activity. Each of the B subunits binds tightly to the GM1 ganglioside abundant in the intestinal brush border membrane. The toxin's A1 subunit is endocytosed following toxin binding to GM1. A1 subunit covalently modifies the α subunit of Gs, the adenylyl cyclase-stimulating G protein.
Modified from Wachsmuth IK, Blake PA, Olsvik O (eds) (1994) *Vibrio cholerae and cholera: molecular to global perspective*, Figure 3C Mode of action of CT, p. 151 (redrawn), ASM Press.

capacity of the bowel and results in watery diarrhoea. The diarrhoeal fluid contains large amounts of sodium, chloride, bicarbonate, and potassium, but little protein or blood cells. The loss of electrolyte-rich isotonic fluid leads to blood volume depletion with attendant low blood pressure and shock. Loss of bicarbonate and potassium leads to metabolic acidosis and potassium deficiency.

Epidemiology

Ever since Snow's seminal epidemiological treatise, cholera has been described as the classic water-borne disease. However, it is also transmitted by contaminated food, especially undercooked seafood or food mixed with contaminated water. Contaminated food (especially undercooked seafood) is the usual vehicle for transmission in developed countries, and contaminated water and street food vendors are more common vehicles in less developed countries. *V. cholerae* is found in brackish surface water and in shellfish, and survives and multiplies in association with zooplankton and phytoplankton independently of infected human beings. There is no known other animal reservoir for *V. cholerae. V. cholerae* is endemic in the Indian subcontinent and the re-emergence of cholera in other continents is highly dependent on environmental factors. The association of the bacteria with plankton has led to the suggestion that ship ballast is a cause of its global spread. *V. cholerae* has evolved to survive in the aquatic environment and then in the host. In water, *V. cholerae* vibrios are free swimming or attached to plants, green algae, copepods, crustaceans, or insects. In humans, the intestinal milieu fosters the acquisition of genetic elements from the TCP bacteriophage, lacking in most environmental strains. TCP phage encodes type IV fimbria which serves as colonization factor and receptor for the CTX phage that carries genes encoding cholera toxin. Thus both bacteriophages integrate into the bacterial genome and form episomal replication intermediates. The production of cholera toxin and the biogenesis of CTX phage both depend on a type II secretion apparatus, encoded within the bacterial genome. In Bangladesh and Peru, where the disease has been endemic and epidemic, cholera tends to occur in the warm seasons albeit before and after the monsoon rains in Bangladesh.

Most *V. cholerae* infections are asymptomatic (case:infection = 1:3 to 1:100) or associated with mild nonspecific diarrhoea. Since a high inoculum dose is required for infection, person-to-person infection is rare without intervening water or food contamination. Infection and its severity also depend on the gastric acid barrier, local intestinal immunity, and blood group. Those with blood group O are at higher risk of severe El Tor cholera than are those with other blood groups. This susceptibility may explain the lower prevalence of blood group O in the Ganges delta area. In cholera-endemic areas, the highest attack rates are in children aged 2 to 4 years. In newly invaded areas, attack rates are similar for all ages.

First illnesses are often seen in adult men, presumably because of greater exposure to contaminated food and water.

The current seventh pandemic began in 1961, in Sulawesi (Celebes), Indonesia. By 1966 the disease had spread to other countries in eastern Asia including Bangladesh, India, the former Union of Soviet Socialist Republics, Iran, and Iraq. Cholera reached West Africa in 1970, and in 1991 it appeared in Latin America for the first time in more than a century. Until 1992 only serogroup O1 had been implicated in epidemics while other serogroups had caused only sporadic cases of diarrhoea. However, in late 1992 cholera broke out in India and Bangladesh caused by a previously unrecognized serogroup of *V. cholerae*, designated O139. It is unclear whether this new serogroup from Southeast Asia will spread to other regions of the world. It is estimated that 120 000 people die from cholera worldwide each year (Fig. 7.6.11.2).

All cases of suspected cholera should be reported to local and national health authorities, since cholera outbreaks can become massive epidemics. These cases should be confirmed by laboratory investigation. If a patient older than 5 years develops severe dehydration or dies from acute watery diarrhoea, or if there is a sudden increase in the daily number of patients with acute watery diarrhoea, a cholera outbreak should be suspected.

Prevention and vaccines

Since contaminated water and food are the main vehicles of transmission, effective preventive measures include ensuring a safe water supply (especially for municipal water systems), improving sanitation, making food safe for consumption by thorough cooking of high risk foods (especially seafood), and providing health education through mass media (Box 7.6.11.1).

Two safe and well-tolerated oral cholera vaccines that provide significant protection have been licensed for commercial use:

1 Killed whole cell *V. cholerae* plus recombinant B subunit of cholera toxin vaccine given as two doses 1 to 6 weeks apart (rCTB-WC; Dukoral). In Dukoral the A subunit of cholera toxin is deleted.

2 Live attenuated *V. cholerae* O1 strain, CVD 103-HgR vaccine given as a single dose (Orochol; known as Mutachol in Canada). In Orochol, the gene for encoding the A subunit of cholera toxin has been largely deleted.

Neither vaccine is licensed in the United States of America.

Twenty-five trials of oral cholera vaccines were reviewed to assess the effect of cholera vaccines in preventing cases of cholera and preventing deaths. Eighteen efficacy trials of relatively good quality, testing parenteral and oral killed whole cell vaccines and involving over 2.6 million adults, children, and infants were included. Eleven safety trials were conducted using killed whole cell vaccines and involving 9342 people. The efficacy of the killed whole cell vaccines compared to placebo to prevent cholera at 12 months was 49%. Both parenteral and oral administrations were effective, although killed whole cell vaccines had a significant protection extended in older children and adults. Parenteral killed whole cell vaccines were associated with increased systemic and local adverse effects

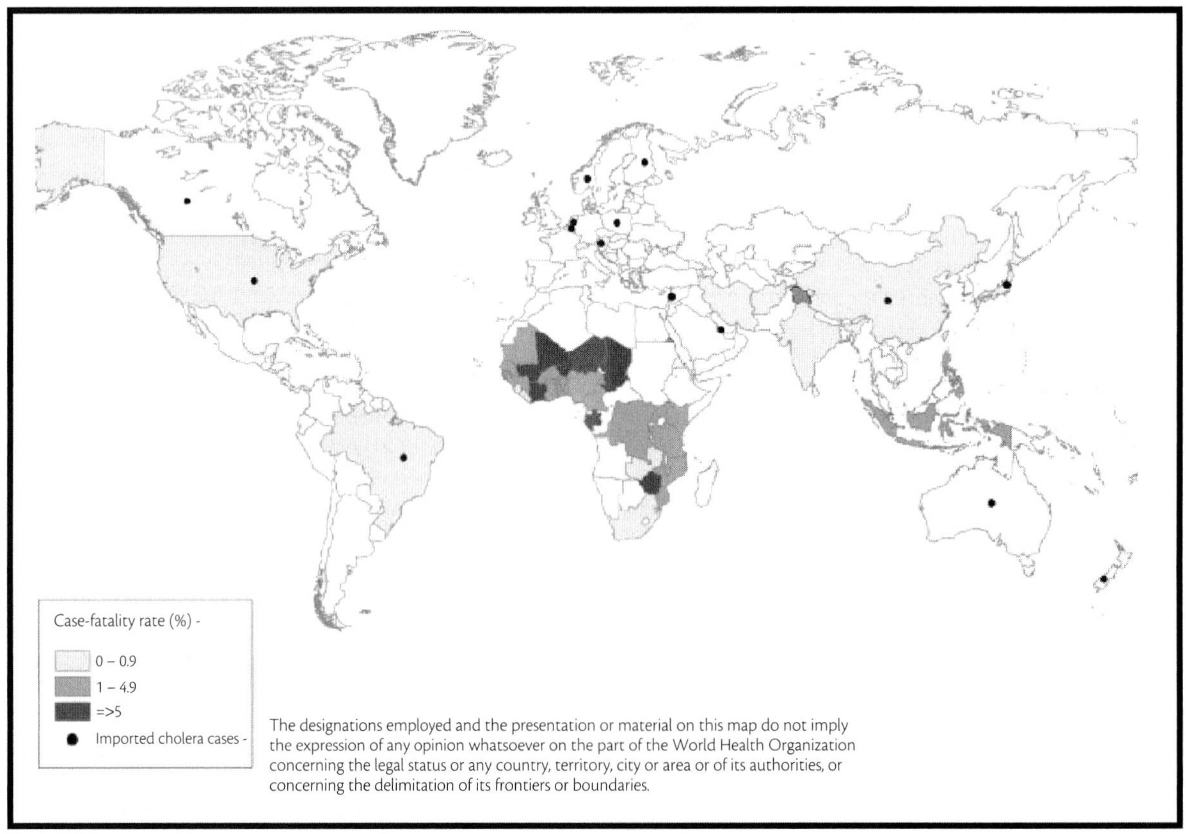
Case-fatality rate (%) -
0 - 0.9
1 - 4.9
=>5
Imported cholera cases -
The designations employed and the presentation or material on this map do not imply the expression of any opinion whatsoever on the part of the World Health Organization concerning the legal status or any country, territory, city or area or of its authorities, or concerning the delimitation of its frontiers or boundaries.

Fig. 7.6.11.2 Countries and areas reporting cholera cases in 2005.
(From Cholera. *Weekly Epidemiological Record* (2006), **81**(31), 297–307.)

Box 7.6.11.1 Prevention of cholera

- Ensure a safe water supply.
- Wash hands after defecation and before food preparation.
- Improve sanitation, making water and food safe for consumption.
- Provide health education through mass media.
- Vaccination and improvements in sanitation work synergistically.

compared to placebo. Oral killed whole cell vaccines were not associated with adverse events compared to placebo. In conclusion, killed whole cell cholera vaccines are relatively effective and safe. Because vaccine efficacy is overcome by larger infectious doses, vaccine should be seen as synergistic with improvements in water and sanitation that reduce the numbers of vibrios ingested.

Recently an oral killed whole cell low cost 2-dose vaccine has been modified to comply with WHO standards, and it was safe and provided 67% protection in 2 years at all ages above 1 year old.

Clinical features

The incubation period of cholera usually ranges from 18 h to 5 days. There is a sudden onset of voluminous watery diarrhoea with occasional vomiting. Diarrhoea is severe in 5 to 10% of those infected. Its most distinctive feature is the painless purging of voluminous stools resembling rice-water with a fishy odour. The vomitus is generally a watery and alkaline fluid. Severe diarrhoea can exceed 500 to 1000 ml/h, leading to severe dehydration in 2 h and risk of death. Dehydration can be classified based on the presence and severity of clinical findings (Table 7.6.11.1). Signs of severe dehydration include absent or low-volume peripheral pulse, undetectable blood pressure, poor skin turgor, sunken eyes, and wrinkled hands and feet. Metabolic acidosis can develop and lead to gasping (Kussmaul) breathing. Urine output is diminished or absent until dehydration is corrected.

Table 7.6.11.1 Assessment of patients with diarrhoea for dehydration

Feature	No dehydration	Some dehydration[a]	Severe dehydration[a, b]
General appearance	Well, alert	Restless, irritable	Lethargy or unconscious; floppy
Eyes	Normal	Sunken*	Very sunken and dry*
Tears	Present	Absent*	Absent*
Mouth and tongue	Moist	Dry*	Very dry*
Thirst	Drinks normally, not thirsty	Thirsty, drinks eagerly	Drinks poorly or not able to drink
Skin pinch[c]	Goes back quickly	Goes back slowly	Goes back very slowly

[a] Two or more of these signs including one indicated by *.

[b] Absence of radial pulse and low blood pressure are also signs of severe dehydration in adults and children older than 5 years.

[c] The skin pinch is less useful in patients with marasmus (severe wasting), kwashiorkor (severe malnutrition with oedema), or in obese patients.

(From Azurin JC, *et al.* (1967). A long-term carrier of cholera: cholera Dolores. *Bull World Health Organ*, **37**, 745–9.)

Complications generally result from inadequate fluid replacement, acute renal failure due to protracted hypotension, hypoglycaemia, hypokalaemia, and cramps due to electrolyte imbalance.

Differential diagnosis

Most cases are indistinguishable from other cases of diarrhoeal diseases, but since the treatment of any dehydrating diarrhoea is the same—fluid replacement—identification of the pathogen is not essential for patient management. However, if an adult patient becomes severely dehydrated and is in the right epidemiological setting or with a history of travelling, the clinician and public health authorities should be alert to the possibility of cholera.

Criteria for diagnosis

Definitive diagnosis is by isolating *V. cholerae* from stool or rectal swab samples on selective media. *V. cholerae* survives in faecal specimens if kept moist. Cary–Blair transport medium should be used for transport to the laboratory for plating onto thiosulphate citrate bile salts sucrose (TCBS) agar that inhibits most other normal faecal flora but supports the growth of the vibrios. Specimens should also be inoculated into alkaline peptone water, an enrichment broth that preferentially supports the growth of vibrios. After 6 to 12 h of incubation, a second TCBS plate is inoculated. These plates are incubated for 18 to 24 h, and *V. cholerae* colonies appear as smooth yellow colonies with slightly raised centres. *V. cholerae* is a Gram-negative polar monotrichous oxidase-positive asporogenous curved rod that ferments glucose, sucrose, and mannitol and is positive in the lysine and ornithine decarboxylase tests. The organism is classified by biochemical tests and is further subdivided into serogroups based on the somatic O antigen. Presumptive identification of *V. cholerae* O1 or O139 can be made on the basis of typical colonies, which are oxidase-positive and agglutinate with O1 or O139 antiserum.

Rapid tests include dark-field microscopy and rapid immunoassays which can be useful for monitoring epidemiological patterns in remote areas where cultures are not readily available. New outbreaks must be confirmed by cultures. Polymerase chain reaction (PCR) and DNA probes are available but are not practicable in many areas where cholera is common.

Treatment

Treatment must be provided at the community and field stations, clinics, and hospitals where most of the patients present. ORT was a major therapeutic breakthrough that has drastically decreased mortality from cholera and other dehydrating diarrhoeal diseases. The case fatality rate of untreated severe cholera approaches 50%, but with ORT it is decreased to 1% or less. The physiological basis for ORT is the Na^+-coupled transport with glucose; transport from the enterocyte to the lateral intercellular space creates a local osmotic gradient that initiates water flow (Fig. 7.6.11.3). The oral rehydration salts (ORS) formulation approved by the World Health Organization (WHO) is based on the electrolyte composition lost in stool in patients with cholera. Table 7.6.11.2 summarizes the electrolyte concentrations from cholera stool and several oral rehydration formulations, including that approved and recommended by the WHO.

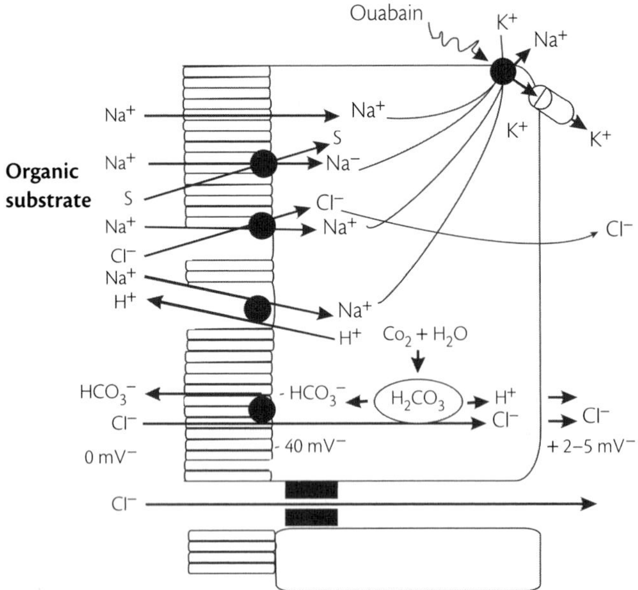

Fig. 7.6.11.3 The pharmacological principle and basis for oral rehydration therapy. Na^+ coupling permits the organic substrate to be transported 'uphill', i.e. from low luminal to higher concentration, a gradient opposite to that for Na^+. The Na^+ gradient is the driving force for sugar and amino acids. As these organic solutes are absorbed, salt is absorbed with them, and water follows osmotically—transport from enterocytes to lateral intercellular space creates a local osmotic gradient that initiates water flow. This coupled transport of Na^+ and organic substrate is the theoretical basis for oral rehydration therapy in cholera and other diarrheal diseases.

Table 7.6.11.1 summarizes the clinical assessment and management of patients with mild, moderate, or severe dehydration. In all cases the key is to rapidly replace fluid deficits, correct metabolic acidosis and potassium losses, and to continue replacing ongoing fluid losses. Because cholera toxin has prolonged effects, it is imperative to continue replacing fluid losses, for which a 'cholera cot' with a central hole, plastic sheet, and bucket to monitor purging can be tremendously helpful to both the patient and medical attendants.

Five to 7.5% of the bodyweight should be given as ORS with additional ORS to compensate for other losses. In patients who are severely dehydrated, having lost at least 10% (5 litres for a 50-kg patient) of their bodyweight, volume replacement must be rapid. Lactated Ringer's solution is an excellent commercially available intravenous fluid. Other polyelectrolyte solutions with added potassium can also be used. Since ORS is the best polyelectrolyte solution to compensate for the acidosis and potassium deficiency, they should be given as soon as possible after initial intravenous fluid resuscitation.

A formulation of ORS that uses rice rather than glucose is better for cholera patients because it reduces the purging rate by providing polymeric glucose with lower osmolarity. ORS have been modified to prevent hypernatraemia (more common with other diarrhoeas) by having a reduced concentration of sodium (75 mmol/litre). This hypo-osmolar solution is also acceptable for cholera. ORS are easily prepared by adding the following simple ingredients to 1 litre water: 2.6 g sodium chloride, 2.9 g trisodium citrate, 1.5 g potassium chloride, and 13.5 g glucose (or 50 g boiled and cooled rice powder).

Adults and children are encouraged to eat, and breastfeeding can continue as there is no scientific basis for resting the gut.

Antibiotics can shorten the illness and decrease diarrhoeal purging. One- to 3-day courses of tetracycline, co-trimoxazole, or ciprofloxacin have been effective but there is increasing resistance. Azithromycin has been used more recently, but growing macrolide resistance may limit its use as well. Antibiotic sensitivity testing is therefore recommended during outbreaks. Antibiotics are not indicated for asymptomatic contacts. Prophylactic use of antibiotics increases the risk of the development of resistance and it is not indicated to prevent cholera.

Prognosis

Case fatality should be 1% or less if adequate ORT is used early in the illness, even at the community level. Adequate fluid and

Table 7.6.11.2 Composition of cholera stools and electrolyte rehydration solutions used to replace stool losses

Fluid	Sodium (mmol/litre)	Chloride (mmol/litre)	Potassium (mmol/litre)	Bicarbonate (mmol/litre)	Carbohydrate (g/litre)	Osmolality (mmol/litre)
Cholera stool						
Adults	130	100	20	44	–	–
Children	100	90	33	30	–	–
Oral rehydration salts						
Glucose	75	65	20	10[a]	13.5[b]	245
Rice	75	65	20	10[a]	30-50[c]	About 180
Intravenous fluids						
Lactated Ringer's	130	109	4	28[d]	–	271
Dhaka solution	133	154	13	48[e]	–	292
Normal saline	154	154	0	0	–	308

[a] Trisodium citrate (10 mmol/litre) is generally used, rather than bicarbonate.
[b] Glucose 13.5 g/litre (75 mmol/litre).
[c] Depending on degree of hydrolysis, 30–50 g rice contains about 30 mmol/litre glucose.
[d] Base is lactate.
[e] Base is acetate.
(From Sack DA, *et al.* (2004). Cholera. *Lancet*, **363**, 223–33.)

electrolyte replacement reverses or prevents complications such as acute renal failure or hypoglycaemia even in moderate or severe cholera. Cholera may well persist in its brackish marine reservoir, but improved water and sanitation and increasingly available vaccines promise to control this dreaded disease.

Other issues (health economics, areas of uncertainty or controversy, and likely developments ahead)

Areas of uncertainty or controversy include the mechanisms and importance of natural reservoirs of cultivable and even noncultivable vibrios and marine organisms from plankton to shellfish in the ecology of cholera. Despite the remarkable advances in understanding the pharmacological mechanisms of cholera toxin action, reliable, effective, and inexpensive means of blocking the effects of the toxin remain elusive.

With molecular genetic understanding of virulence and protective immunity, likely developments in the near future include the promise of new and better vaccines, toxin-blocking or absorption-enhancing drugs, and continued improvements in ORT, perhaps with nutrients, micronutrients, or probiotics that compete with vibrio colonization or deliver proabsorptive drugs or nutrients.

Further reading

Azurin JC, *et al.* (1967). A long-term carrier of cholera: cholera Dolores. *Bull World Health Organ*, **37**, 745–9.

Donnenberg M (2000). Pathogenic strategies of enteric bacteria. *Nature*, **406**, 768–74.

Faruque SM, *et al.* (2003). Reemergence of epidemic *Vibrio cholerae* O139, Bangladesh. *Emerg Infect Dis*, **9**, 1116–22.

Field M (2003). Intestinal ion transport and the pathophysiology of diarrhea. *J Clin Invest*, **111**, 931–43.

Fontaine O, Gore SM, Pierce NF (2000). Rice-based oral rehydration solution for treating diarrhoea. *Cochrane Database Syst Rev*, **2**, CD001264.

Graves P, *et al.* (2000). Vaccines for preventing cholera. *Cochrane Database Syst Rev*, **4**, CD000974.

Guerrant RL (2006). Cholera: still teaching hard lessons. *N Engl J Med*, **354**, 2500–2.

Hill DR, *et al.* (2006). Oral cholera vaccines: use in clinical practice. *Lancet Infect Dis*, **6**, 361–73.

Murphy C, Hahn S, Volmink J (2004). Reduced osmolarity oral rehydration solution for treating cholera. *Cochrane Database Syst Rev*, **4**, CD003754.

Sack DA, *et al.* (2004). Cholera. *Lancet*, **363**, 223–33.

Saha DS, *et al.* (2006). Single-dose azithromycin for the treatment of cholera in adults. *N Engl J Med*, **354**, 2452–62.

Salim A, *et al.* (2005). *Vibrio cholerae* pathogenic clones. *Emerg Infect Dis*, **11**, 1758–60.

Sur D, *et al.* (2009).Efficacy and safety of a modified killed-whole-cell oral cholera vaccine in India: an interim analysis of a cluster-randomized, double-blind, placebo-controlled trial. *Lancet*, **374**, 1694–702.

Trucksis M, *et al.* (1998). The *Vibrio cholerae* genome contains two unique circular chromosomes. *Proc Natl Acad Sci U S A*, **95**, 14464–9.

World Health Organization (1993). *Global Task Force on Cholera Control. Guidelines for cholera control.* World Health Organization, Geneva.

World Health Organization (2006). Cholera 2005. *Weekly Epidemiol Rec*, **81**, 297–308.

7.6.12 *Haemophilus influenzae*

Derrick W. Crook

Essentials

Haemophilus influenzae (Pasteurellaceae) is a Gram-negative bacillus that is an exclusively human pathogen. There are six capsular serotypes (a–f), of which type b (Hib) being a major cause of childhood infectious disease. Transmission occurs by close bodily contact, the main source being other children, and is usually followed by nasopharyngeal carriage, following which susceptible people may develop disease.

Clinical features—in infants Hib causes symptoms ranging from a mild nonspecific febrile illness (occult bacteraemia) to fully blown sepsis with meningitis, epiglottitis, pneumonia, septic arthritis, and cellulitis. Noncapsulate or nonserotypable *H. influenzae* cause otitis media and conjunctivitis in children, and exacerbations of chronic bronchitis, sinusitis, and pneumonia in adults. *H. parainfluenzae*, *H. aphrophilus*, *H. paraphrophilus*, and *H. segnis* are rare causes of infective endocarditis and other sepsis.

Diagnosis and treatment—Gram staining of cerebrospinal, synovial, or pleural fluid is a key investigation, but definitive diagnosis requires culture or detection of specific DNA by polymerase chain reaction (PCR) methods. Aside from supportive care, treatment requires (1) appropriate antibiotics—resistance is an increasing problem: the agent of choice for invasive Hib disease is a third-generation cephalosporin with good cerebrospinal fluid penetration (e.g. ceftriaxone or cefotaxime, but not cefuroxime); chloramphenicol with or without ampicillin remains effective in some developing countries. (2) corticosteroids—except in children in low-income countries, these reduce mortality, severe hearing loss, and neurological sequelae of Hib meningitis. Antibiotic treatment of noncapsulate *H. Influenzae* otitis media, sinusitis, and chronic bronchitis is widely practised but largely uinsupported by evidence.

Prevention—polyribosyl ribitol phosphate (PRP)-conjugate vaccines, often given at 2 to 6 months of age, have virtually eliminated Hib disease from North America, Europe and some other countries.

Introduction

Haemophilus influenzae is a human-adapted pathogen with no other reservoir. Typically, it inhabits the nasopharynx but may also be recovered from other mucosal surfaces including genital and intestinal tracts. Despite being a fastidious organism that is relatively difficult to grow, it was first isolated as early as 1890 by Pfeiffer who mistakenly thought it was the cause of a current influenza pandemic.

Description of the organism

The genus *Haemophilus* (family Pasteurellaceae) includes *H. ducreyi*, which causes chancroid, the sexually transmitted infection (Chapter 7.10.13), and other human-adapted species all of which are commensals: *H. parainfluenzae* (the most abundantly colonizing species), *H. aegyptius*, *H. aphrophilus*, *H. haemolyticus*, *H. paraphrophilus*, and *H. segnis*.

H. influenzae is a small (0.2–0.3 × 0.5–0.8 μm) Gram-negative nonmotile coccobacillus that grows well on rich media under 5% CO_2 and produces 2- to 3-mm-diameter grey translucent colonies after 18 to 25 h incubation. It is fastidious with the following specific growth requirements: it does not grow on nutrient agar, such as Columbia, without growth supplements X factor (haemin) and V factor (NAD). *H. parainfluenzae* requires only V factor. Rich media such as chocolate agar support the growth of *Haemophilus* spp. and is the preferred solid medium for propagation of these organisms. Precise speciation requires sequence analysis, e.g. 16s ribosomal DNA.

H. influenzae are phenotypically and genetically diverse. A minority are capsulate (serotypeable) among the majority of noncapsulate (nonserotypeable) strains. Capsulate strains produce one of six chemically and antigenically distinct polysaccharide capsules a to f. These strains are relatively nondiverse, consisting of few lineages compared to the much more diverse noncapsulate strains. This suggests that genes encoding the capsule were acquired relatively recently. The type b capsule is essential for the pathogenesis of bacteraemia and meningitis, a feature recognized in the early 1930s.

Pathogenicity

H. influenzae expresses several cell surface features essential for colonization of the nasopharynx. These are virulence factors of which the capsule is the most important. Of the six antigenically distinct structures (types a–f), type b accounts for virtually all the invasiveness of *H. influenzae* in children. The serotype b capsule consists of a negatively charged phosphodiester-linked linear polymer of disaccharide units of polyribosylribitol phosphate (PRP) which resists phagocytosis by interfering with binding of serum complement. The capsule also resists desiccation, perhaps promoting host-to-host transmission. Serum antibody directed against serotype b capsular polysaccharide is protective. This simple observation stimulated the development of the highly successful *H. influenzae* type b (Hib) vaccine, now used routinely in national childhood immunization programmes. Modern vaccines contain PRP covalently conjugated to a protein carrier such as tetanus toxoid.

Other cell surface structures involved in pathogenesis, particularly in those strains lacking a capsule (nonserotypeable *H. influenzae*), include lipopolysaccharide, pili, and other adhesion proteins.

Epidemiology

Haemophilus influenzae type b

Hib is a major cause of childhood infectious disease. Acquisition occurs by close bodily contact, the main source being other children, and is usually followed by carriage. The organism dwells harmlessly for months in the nasopharynx. However, in a few susceptible individuals, acquisition immediately precedes invasive disease. Carriage rates increase from birth until 4 years and are higher in developing countries especially where there is crowding, day care attendance, and contact with siblings. Hib immunization virtually eliminates carriage and produces a marked herd effect, protecting against disease. In 2000, it was estimated that as many as 60% of the world's children were unimmunized, but Hib vaccine is now being brought to most parts of the world. However, in some parts of Asia, particularly China, Hib is far less prevalent and so the health benefits of mass vaccination may be insufficient to justify a national vaccination programme.

The main diseases caused by Hib are meningitis, primary bacteraemia, pneumonia, epiglottitis, and arthritis (Table 7.6.12.1); the most important is meningitis. Before the introduction of vaccination, it was the most important cause of childhood meningitis in the United States of America, accounting for 80% of cases (Fig. 7.6.12.1), and in the United Kingdom it accounted for approximately 50% of cases. In contrast, it was a much less prominent cause of meningitis than *Neisseria meningitidis* in the 'meningitis' belt of Africa.

The incidence of Hib infections varies with age. Neonates are protected, after which disease peaks by 9 months of age and declines to very low levels by 4 years. Age-specific disease incidence is inversely related to serum antibodies to Hib. Male gender and ethnicity are risk factors for disease. For example, the incidence among Native Americans less than 4 years old exceeded 150 cases/100 000 per year compared to only 50 cases/100 000 per year in the population as a whole. In western countries, case fatality of Hib meningitis was about 5% and long-term morbidity (deafness and neurological and learning deficits) occurred in at least 10% of cases.

Since the implementation of Hib conjugate vaccination, the disease has virtually disappeared from North America and Europe and there has been a similar dramatic decline in The Gambia and Kenya. A striking but temporary re-emergence of Hib disease in the United Kingdom (Fig. 7.6.12.2) was attributed to the introduction, in 2000, of a combined Hib-acellular pertussis vaccine that induced lower Hib antibody levels.

Noncapsulate or nonserotypeable *H. influenzae*

Noncapsulate *H. influenzae* is acquired soon after birth and is carried by 20 to 80% of the population but it rarely causes bacteraemia and meningitis. However, it does cause otitis media, sinusitis, chronic bronchitis, and pneumonia. In cases of otitis media, one of the commonest childhood diseases, *H. influenzae* was cultured from middle ear fluid of 23%, while 23% and 26% grew *Moraxella catarrhalis* or *Streptococcus pneumoniae*, respectively. Bronchitis and sinusitis are diseases predominantly of adults. Chronic bronchitis and pneumonia associated with *H. influenzae* occur more frequently with advancing age.

Table 7.6.12.1 Clinical manifestations of *H. influenzae* type b disease

Disease	Percentage
Meningitis	52
Pneumonia	12
Epiglottitis	10
Septicaemia	8
Cellulitis	5
Osteoarticular	4
Multifocal	6
Other	3

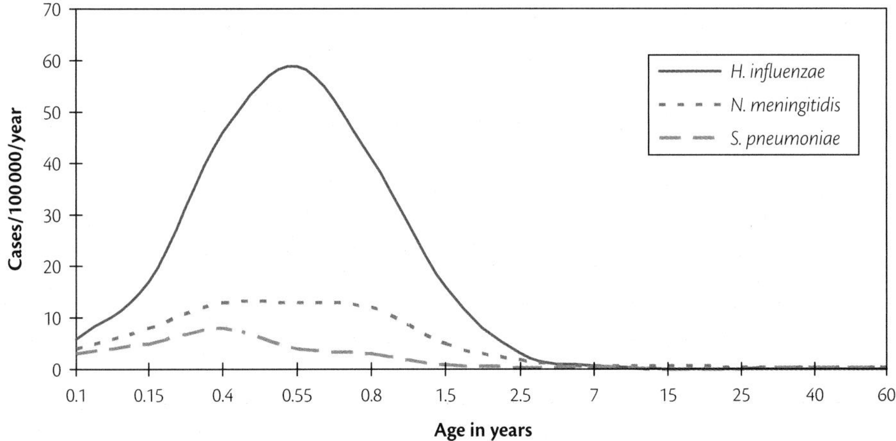

Fig. 7.6.12.1 Incidence of meningitis in the United States of America caused by *H. influenzae*, *N. meningitides*, and *S. pneumoniae* before the implementation of the Hib conjugate vaccine.
(Data derived from various sources.)

Antibiotic resistance

Resistance of *H. influenzae* to antibiotics was first reported in the early 1970s. Since then, the prevalence of ampicillin-resistant β-lactamase-producing strains has risen rapidly in most parts of the world and strains resistant to tetracycline, chloramphenicol, and trimethoprim or multiresistant to these antibiotics have emerged. In recent years, resistance rates have remained reasonably constant in Europe at 10 to 20%.

Clinical features

Hib invasive disease

In infants, clinical features vary from a mild nonspecific febrile illness, reflecting so-called occult bacteraemia, to fully blown sepsis with meningitis. Infants may present with fever and irritability alone but severe cases show typical features of meningitis including altered mental status, stiff neck, and sepsis. In some cases there is disseminated intravascular coagulation with purpuric rash and septicaemic shock, reminiscent of meningococcaemia. Diagnosis is by examination of cerebrospinal fluid and blood culture. In older children, lumbar puncture should not be performed until cerebral oedema can be excluded by CT, but antibiotic treatment must not be delayed.

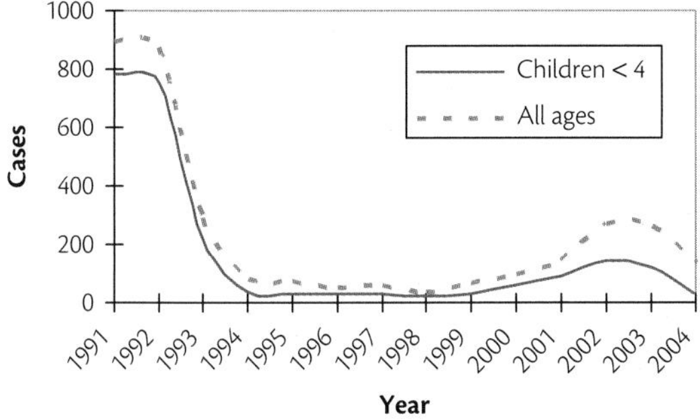

Fig. 7.6.12.2 Number of cases of Hib occurring in the United Kingdom from just before implementation of Hib conjugate vaccine until the end of 2004. The rise in cases between 2000 and 2005 is apparent in children less than 4 years old and all ages.
(Data from the Health Protection Agency available on www.hpa.org.uk/infections/topics_az/Haemophilus_influenzae/data.htm.)

Epiglottitis is an acutely life-threatening medical emergency. Against a background of sepsis (fever, tachycardia, and tachypnoea), pronounced local signs and symptoms evolve rapidly, including sore throat, drooling, dysphagia, hoarseness, barking 'brassy' cough, and stridor. The epiglottis is inflamed and swollen, looking like a red cherry, but attempts to examine the throat may precipitate acute airway obstruction. Pneumonia is an important but relatively unrecognized feature of Hib disease. The main features are fever with signs of respiratory distress including tachypnoea, nasal flaring, and intercostal indrawing. Chest examination and radiography are diagnostic.

The child with septic arthritis shows features of sepsis, is unwilling to use the affected limb, and resists movement of the painful joint. Examination and culture of joint fluid are diagnostic. Cellulitis is rare in children and cellulitis of the neck is unusual in adults. These presentations have been increasingly associated with *H. influenzae* type f infection, especially since the introduction of Hib conjugate vaccine.

Noncapsulate *H. influenzae*

Otitis media is the main clinical presentation. This common childhood illness presents with irritability and, on otoscopy, an inflamed tympanic membrane is visible and may perforate discharging pus. Although not used routinely, tympanocentesis is the most reliable means of aetiological diagnosis. A high proportion of cases of conjunctivitis in children are caused by noncapsulate *H. influenzae*. Historically, *H. aegyptius* has also been associated with conjunctivitis. Culture of conjunctival swabs is the main test for making a diagnosis. Brazilian purpuric fever, a fulminant septicaemic illness with high case fatality, is also caused by *H. aegyptius*.

Noncapsulate *H. influenzae* sinusitis presents with local pain, a sense of pressure in the head, local facial oedema, and visible pus draining from the ostia of the sinuses. Diagnosis is by skull radiography, with special (Towne's and Water's) views, or CT scan, which reveals sinus opacification and a fluid level. Sinus aspiration provides an aetiological diagnosis.

In adults, exacerbations of chronic bronchitis are commonly associated with noncapsulate *H. influenzae*. *H. influenzae* and *S. pneumonia* are cultured from sputum of up to 50% of cases although their precise aetiological role is uncertain.

Noncapsulate *H. influenzae* can cause severe invasive disease such as neonatal sepsis, resembling group B streptococcal neonatal sepsis, and pneumonia in adults, particularly older people. It has also been implicated in meningitis associated with head trauma, particularly skull fracture.

Laboratory diagnosis

Culture or detection of specific DNA is essential for aetiological diagnosis. Direct examination of cerebrospinal, pleural, or synovial fluids by Gram's stain may reveal organisms with the morphological features of *H. influenzae*. This is very helpful in indicating bacterial infection but is nonspecific. Blood culture using most commercial systems yields excellent growth in both anaerobic and aerobic bottles. However, growth on agar and differentiation of *Haemophilus* spp. requires special conditions (see above).

Antibiotic susceptibility testing using antibiotic discs requires supplemented media to support the growth of *Haemophilus* spp. but this may be inaccurate and should be supplemented by measurement of β-lactamase activity. Chloramphenicol disc susceptibility is frequently inaccurate and should be supplemented by an assay for chloramphenicol acetyltransferase activity.

Capsular type b antigen can be rapidly detected in cerebrospinal fluid, sterile site fluid, or urine but is seldom used since the implementation of Hib vaccination. Polymerase chain reaction (PCR) of cerebrospinal fluid has been developed for diagnosing *Haemophilus* spp. meningitis. Capsular typing of *H. influenzae* can be achieved serologically but a PCR-based method has proved more reliable.

Treatment

Antibiotics

A third-generation cephalosporin with good cerebrospinal fluid penetration is the first-line antibiotic treatment for invasive Hib disease. High-dose ceftriaxone or cefotaxime are effective for treating *H. influenzae* meningitis and septicaemia, but cefuroxime must not be used. In developing countries, chloramphenicol alone (depending on the prevalence of chloramphenicol resistance) or in combination with ampicillin is effective therapy.

Antibiotics are commonly prescribed for otitis media, sinusitis, and chronic bronchitis, but large meta-analyses have failed to demonstrate convincing efficacy although some subgroups are benefited. Oral amoxicillin is the first-line drug. Amoxicillin/clavulanate, trimethoprim, tetracycline (adults only), and quinolones (adults only) can also be used.

Corticosteroid treatment

Corticosteroids significantly reduce mortality, severe hearing loss, and neurological sequelae. In adults with community-acquired bacterial meningitis, corticosteroid therapy should be started with the first antibiotic dose. In children, data support the use of adjunctive corticosteroids in children only in high-income countries.

Prevention and control

PRP-conjugate vaccines are the best preventive measure for controlling Hib disease. Highly effective vaccines contain capsular antigen PRP conjugated to tetanus toxoid (PRP-T), outer membrane protein (PRP-OMP), or mutant diphtheria toxoid (PRP-CRM, HbOC). Three doses are given at intervals between the ages of 2 and 6 months. In many countries, a booster dose is given at age 1 to 2 years.

Rifampicin, 20 mg/kg orally once a day for 4 days, eradicates carriage and is believed to prevent secondary cases among close contacts. This is appropriate only where they have not received Hib vaccine.

Other nasopharyngeal *Haemophilus* spp.

H. parainfluenzae

H. parainfluenzae is a well-adapted commensal that colonizes virtually everyone soon after birth but is rarely associated with disease. It has been isolated in cases of infective endocarditis, neurosurgical meningitis, prosthetic device infection, and brain and liver abscesses. It is treated in the same way as *H. influenzae*.

Rare species

H. aphrophilus, *H. paraphrophilus*, and *H. segnis* are implicated in fewer than 2% of all cases of infective endocarditis and in brain or lung abscesses and empyema fluid. Since they are slow growing, they may be missed if blood cultures are not incubated for prolonged periods. Antibiotic treatment is the same as for *H. influenzae*.

Further reading

Adegbola RA, *et al.* (2005). Elimination of *Haemophilus influenzae* type b (Hib) disease from The Gambia after the introduction of routine immunisation with a Hib conjugate vaccine: a prospective study. *Lancet*, **366**, 144–50.

Barbour ML, *et al.* (1995). The impact of conjugate vaccine on carriage of *Haemophilus influenzae* type b. *J Infect Dis*, **171**, 93–8.

Frazer DW (1982). *Haemophilus influenzae* in the community and the home. In: Sell SH, Wright PF (eds) *Haemophilus influenzae*: epidemiology, immunology and prevention of disease. Elsevier Science, New York.

Kim KS (2010). Acute bacterial meningitis in infants and children. *Lancet Infect Dis*, **10**, 32–42.

Morris SK, Moss WJ, Halsey N (2008). *Haemophilus influenzae* type b conjugate vaccine use and effectiveness. *Lancet Infect Dis*, **8**, 435–43.

Murphy TF (2003). Respiratory infections caused by non-typeable *Haemophilus influenzae*. *Curr Opin Infect Dis*, **16**, 129–34.

Peltola H (2000). Worldwide *Haemophilus influenzae* type b disease at the beginning of the 21st century: global analysis of the disease burden 25 years after the use of the polysaccharide vaccine and a decade after the advent of conjugates. *Clin Microbiol Rev*, **13**, 302–17.

Prasad K, Karlupia N, Kumar A (2009). Treatment of bacterial meningitis: an overview of Cochrane systematic reviews. *Respir Med*, **103**, 945–50.

Schaad UB, *et al.* (1990). A comparison of ceftriaxone and cefuroxime for the treatment of bacterial meningitis in children. *N Engl J Med*, **322**, 141–7.

Ulanova M, Tsang RS (2009). Invasive *Haemophilus influenzae* disease: changing epidemiology and host-parasite interactions in the 21st century. *Infect Genet Evol*, **9**, 94–605.

Watt JP, Wolfson LJ, O'Brien KL, *et al.* (2009). Burden of disease caused by *Haemophilus influenzae* type b in children younger than 5 years: global estimates. *Lancet*, **374**, 903–11.

Zwahlen A, *et al.* (1989). The molecular basis of pathogenicity in *Haemophilus influenzae*: comparative virulence of genetically-related capsular transformants and correlation with changes at the capsulation locus cap. *Microb Pathog*, **7**, 225–35.

7.6.13 *Haemophilus ducreyi* and chancroid

Nigel O'Farrell

Essentials

Haemophilus ducreyi, which should on phylogenetic grounds be reclassified as an actinobacillus, is a Gram-negative, facultative anaerobic bacillus that is the cause of chancroid, which is endemic in eastern and southern Africa and the Caribbean, although the overall global incidence of the condition has decreased dramatically since the mid 1990s.

Clinical features—presentation, after an incubation period of 4 to 7 days, is with a tender genital papule that develops into a pustule and then an ulcer with a ragged undermined edge and a yellow base that bleeds readily. The usual sites of infection in men are the prepuce and coronal sulcus, and in women the labia minora and fourchette. Inguinal lymphadenopathy is found in about half the male cases. Chancroid is an important risk factor for the bidirectional transmission of HIV.

Diagnosis and treatment—nucleic acid amplification tests are the optimal method of diagnosing *H. ducreyi*. Treatment is with ciprofloxacin, erythromycin, azithromycin, or ceftriaxone.

Introduction

The causative organism is *Haemophilus ducreyi*, a Gram-negative facultative anaerobic bacillus. Chancroid has also been known as soft sore (*ulcus molle*) and was first differentiated from syphilis by Ricord in 1838 in France. In 1889 in Naples, Ducrey inoculated the forearms of patients with material from their own genital ulcers and maintained serial ulcers through multiple generations. The first successful culture was undertaken by Lenglet in 1898. The Ito-Reenstierna test was developed subsequently using a commercial antigen for intradermal testing and proved positive in 90% of true cases.

Aetiology

Recent phylogenetic studies suggest that the causative organism should be reclassified as an actinobacillus of the Pasteurellaceae. The organism is small, nonmotile, and nonspore-forming, and shows streptobacillary chaining on Gram's stain. Colonies can be seen 48 h after incubation and are greyish in colour. These colonies are cohesive and can be pushed across culture media with a thin wire.

Epidemiology

Chancroid is endemic in eastern and southern Africa and the Caribbean. In Asia, cases in India and Thailand used to be fairly common but have decreased recently and are now only sporadic. Overall, the global incidence of chancroid has decreased dramatically since the mid-1990s when it accounted for 30 to 50% of genital ulcers in southern Africa. This may reflect changes in sexual behaviour, the increased use of and adherence to syndromic management for genital ulcers that included effective antibiotic cover for chancroid, or some other unknown factors.

Sporadic outbreaks have been reported in the West. These have usually been associated with sex work and have been brought under control using intensive partner notification schemes.

The male to female ratio is about 5 to 1. Chancroid is more common in uncircumcised than circumcised men. This may reflect inferior standards of genital hygiene and a tendency for small microabrasions to develop in the subpreputial space that might provide a portal of entry for infection. Asymptomatic carriage has been identified in women but is uncommon.

Pathology and pathogenesis

A human model of experimental infection is available for the study of chancroid pathogenesis. Abrasions are necessary for *H. ducreyi* to penetrate the epidermis and cause infection. Cell-mediated and humoral responses occur. The cutaneous response consists of two components, a polymorphonuclear response and a mononuclear infiltrate component. Virulence factors include a haemolysin and a cytolethal distending toxin. Repeat infections are possible.

Clinical features

The usual incubation period is 4 to 7 days and there are no prodromal symptoms. Lesions start as a tender papule that develops into a pustule and then an ulcer. Classically, ulcers have a ragged undermined edge with a grey or yellow base that bleeds when touched. Lesions may be single or multiple.

The usual sites of infection are the prepuce, coronal sulcus, frenulum, and glans in men, and the labia minora and fourchette in women. Ulcers of the vaginal wall and cervix are uncommon. Extragenital lesions are rare but have been reported on the fingers, breasts, and inner thighs. *H. ducreyi* does not disseminate systemically.

Clinical variants can occur. These include giant phagedenic ulcers, dwarf chancroid similar to herpes, follicular chancroid similar to pyogenic infection, and single painless ulcers not unlike syphilis.

Painful inguinal lymphadenopathy is found in about one-half the male cases but less so in women. These lymph glands may develop into buboes that should be managed by aspiration rather than incision and drainage. Fluctuant buboes may rupture spontaneously causing delayed healing.

The differential diagnosis includes syphilis, genital herpes, lymphogranuloma venereum, and donovanosis. Mixed infections with other causes of genital ulceration should always be considered.

Laboratory diagnosis

Nucleic acid amplification tests (NAATs) are now the optimal method of diagnosing *H. ducreyi* but their availability remains limited in areas where chancroid is found. Primers have been developed to amplify sequences from the *H. ducreyi* 16S ribosomal RNA gene, the rrs (16S) to rrl (23S) ribosomal intergenic spacer region, and the *groEL* gene. Multiplex polymerase chain reaction tests have been developed that can identify infection with *H. ducreyi*, *Treponema pallidum*, and *Herpes simplex* virus types 1 and 2 from genital ulcers.

Antigen detection using fluorescence techniques may be useful but is expensive. Serological tests are unable to differentiate between old and new infections and have limited application.

Culture was the usual method of diagnosis of chancroid until relatively recently but has now been overtaken by NAATs. Culture media must be fresh and may need fine adjustment depending on the characteristics of local strains of *H. ducreyi*. Two culture media are required to achieve a reasonable sensitivity of 50 to 80%. Media used include gonococcal agar base and Mueller–Hinton with various additives and supplements. Vancomycin may be used to inhibit Gram-positive bacteria. Cultures should be incubated at 33°C with 5% carbon dioxide in a humid atmosphere. Thioglycolate haemin-based transport medium may allow storage of viable organisms at 4°C for 24 h or possibly longer. Most strains are β-lactamase producers. *H. ducreyi* reduces nitrate to nitrite and all strains are oxidase positive and catalase negative. Gram-stained smears of material from ulcers may show characteristic Gram-negative coccobacilli in a 'school of fish' or 'railroad track' appearance.

Histology shows superficial necrosis with large numbers of neutrophils, endothelial proliferation, and infiltration with plasma cells, lymphocytes, and fibroblasts.

Treatment

Current treatment of chancroid comprises one of the following regimens: ciprofloxacin (500 mg twice daily for 3 days), erythromycin (500 mg three times daily for 7 days; can be used in pregnant women), azithromycin (a single oral dose of 1 g), or ceftriaxone (a single dose of 250 mg intramuscularly). Trimethoprim/sulphamethoxazole is no longer recommended. Healing of ulcers is usually achieved after 7 to 14 days. Longer courses of treatment are sometimes required in HIV-positive patients who should be followed up until healing is complete. Single-dose treatment should probably not be given to HIV-positive patients.

In the preantibiotic era, circumcision, saline soaks, and improved hygiene were recommended. Initially organisms were sensitive to penicillin but resistance emerged fairly rapidly. Trimethoprim/sulphamethoxazole then became the mainstay of treatment but resistance to this antibiotic emerged in the early 1990s.

Chancroid and HIV

Chancroid has been identified as an important risk factor for the bidirectional transmission of HIV, particularly in eastern and southern Africa. In some high-risk groups it was undoubtedly an important factor in driving the initial spread of HIV. At the biological level, the mechanism for this is likely to be that chancroid ulcers allow a route of entry and exit for HIV and are likely to bleed when subject to trauma. In addition, subpreputial lesions in men that subsequently heal might result in partial phimosis with thinning of the superficial mucosa. This mucosa would then be more susceptible to trauma during sexual intercourse thereby increasing the potential risk of HIV transmission through microulcerations. There are some reports that HIV-positive men have increased numbers of ulcers that heal slowly, although this may be related to low CD4 counts.

Prevention and control

In developed countries intensive partner notification and epidemiological treatment of sexual contacts have formed the basis for managing outbreaks.

The World Health Organization has recently renewed interest in the elimination of chancroid as an additional HIV prevention strategy. In most developing countries genital ulcers have been managed by the syndromic approach. This involves treating for the most likely causes of ulceration that in the past have been syphilis and chancroid. However, the prevalence of chancroid in previously endemic countries has reduced considerably leaving genital herpes as the most frequent cause of genital ulceration. With this emergence of genital herpes, the case for treating empirically for chancroid has weakened and it may be that new epidemics of chancroid will emerge as treatment regimens change.

Further reading

Bong CT, Bauer M, Spinola SM (2002). *Haemophilus ducreyi*: clinical features, epidemiology, and prospects for disease control. *Microbes Infect*, **4**, 1141–8.

Spinola S (2008). Chancroid. In: Holmes KK, *et al.* (eds) *Sexually transmitted diseases*. McGraw-Hill, New York.

Spinola SM, Bauer ME, Munson RS (2002). Immunopathogenesis of *Haemophilus ducreyi* infection (chancroid). *Infect Immun*, **70**, 1667–76.

Trees DL, Morse SA (1995). Chancroid and *Haemophilus ducreyi*: an update. *Clin Microbiol Rev*, **8**, 357–75.

7.6.14 Bordetella infection

Cameron Grant

Essentials

Bordetella are small Gram-negative coccobacilli, of which *Bordetella pertussis* is the most important human pathogen. It is the cause of whooping cough, which is one of the 10 leading causes of childhood death worldwide. Transmission is primarily by aerosolized droplets, and the condition is very infectious.

Clinical features—presentation varies with age, immunization and previous infection: (1) infants—apnoea, cyanosis, and paroxysmal cough; (2) nonimmunized children—cough, increasing in severity with distressing, repeated, forceful expirations followed by a gasping inhalation (the 'whoop'); (3) children immunized in infancy—whooping, vomiting, sputum production; (4) adults—cough, post-tussive vomiting. Complications include pneumonia, pulmonary hypertension, seizures and encephalopathy. Most deaths occur in those less than 2 months old.

Diagnosis and treatment—culture lacks sensitivity; preferred diagnostic methods are polymerase chain reaction (PCR) detection from nasopharyngeal samples and serology (IgG antibodies to pertussis toxin). Aside from supportive care, antibiotics (usually erythromycin) are recommended if started within 4 weeks of illness onset.

Prevention—Pertussis vaccines protect against disease more than infection. Preventing severe disease in young children remains the primary goal, hence schedules consist of a three-dose infant series and subsequent booster doses. Acellular vaccines enable immunization schedules to include adolescents and adults. Antibiotic prophylaxis is given when there is an infant at risk of exposure.

Introduction

Four of nine identified Bordetella species cause human infections. *Bordetella pertussis*, as the principal cause of whooping cough (pertussis), is the most important. Pertussis is one of the 10 leading causes of childhood death.

The epidemiology of *B. pertussis* infection and pertussis disease differ. Immunization has caused a large reduction in pertussis but minimal change in the circulation of *B. pertussis*. Eradication of the disease is not currently possible.

Historical perspective

Before the introduction of immunization, pertussis was a predominant child killer. In the 1930s in the United States of America pertussis caused more infant deaths than measles, diphtheria, poliomyelitis, and scarlet fever combined. Preimmunization, pertussis incidence was not decreasing. With mass immunization, disease incidence decreased dramatically.

Aetiology, genetics, pathogenesis, and pathology

Two of the four *Bordetella* species that infect humans, *B. pertussis* and human-adapted *B. parapertussis*, are strictly human pathogens. In immunocompromised hosts *B. bronchiseptica* causes respiratory illnesses and *B. holmesii* causes respiratory illnesses, bacteraemia, and endocarditis.

B. pertussis is very infectious. Each primary case produces approximately 15 secondary cases. Transmission is primarily by aerosolized droplets. There is an average of 2 weeks between successive cases. In immunized populations the household secondary attack rate remains greater than 80%, although many such infections are asymptomatic.

Pathogenesis is incompletely understood. *Bordetella* spp. have numerous virulence factors including filamentous haemagglutinin, fimbriae, pertactin, pertussis toxin, adenylate cyclase, and lipopolysaccharides. Filamentous haemagglutinin interacts with macrophages, altering cytokine production and inhibiting T-cell proliferation. Pertactin and fimbriae are implicated in attachment to host epithelial cells, and fimbriae interact with monocytes/macrophages. Adenylate cyclase has anti-inflammatory and antiphagocytic functions.

B. pertussis organisms multiply on the ciliated respiratory epithelium. Necrosis occurs within the bronchial epithelium. A necrotizing bronchopneumonia is present in most fatal cases.

Epidemiology

Underestimation and how this varies with age and surveillance intensity is central to understanding pertussis epidemiology. Pertussis affects all ages; however, incidence has always been highest in infants and children. The more recent increase in reported incidence in adults is primarily due to greater awareness and improved laboratory diagnosis.

Mortality

The propensity for pertussis to kill young infants is unique among vaccine preventable diseases, with the exception of tetanus.

Globally the estimated number of pertussis deaths fell from 500 000 in 1990 to 300 000 in 2000. The World Health Organization (WHO) estimated in 2002 that pertussis caused 290 000 of the 1.4 million fatalities from vaccine preventable diseases in children under 5 years old. Estimates are complicated by the relationship between pertussis and malnutrition. Malnutrition contributes to more than one-half of the deaths in this age group. A prolonged period of weight loss frequently complicates pertussis in the developing world.

In the developed world it is estimated that there are 3 times more deaths from pertussis than are reported. Pertussis deaths occur despite intensive care.

Morbidity

Most pertussis incidence estimates are based on passive notification which identifies only 6 to 25% of cases. The proportion of cases notified decreases with increasing age and decreasing severity.

Countries with consistently low pertussis incidence have, in common, high immunization coverage rates sustained over decades. Higher disease rates are due primarily to lower coverage, but also sometimes to lower vaccine efficacy or suboptimal immunization schedules.

Prevention

Neither disease nor immunization confer lifelong immunity. Pertussis vaccines protect against disease more than infection. Schedules consist of a three-dose infant series and subsequent booster doses. Pertussis remains endemic in adolescents and adults. Without boosters it is also endemic in school children.

Whole cell and acellular pertussis vaccines are combined with other antigens. Acellular vaccines contain between one and five *B. pertussis* antigens. The most efficacious whole cell and acellular vaccines induce protection against clinical disease in approximately 85% of recipients.

In order to minimize the pertussis risk to infants the primary series must be completed without delay. However, without booster doses, timely completion of the primary series is insufficient to prevent disease in infants.

Duration of protection following whole cell and acellular vaccines is comparable and somewhat shorter than after natural disease. After the primary infant series the first booster dose is not necessary until approximately 5 years of age. Protection following both disease and immunization is superior to either alone. Hence those who have had pertussis should be immunized.

With the recognition that adolescents and adults spread pertussis to infants, the timing of booster doses has been reconsidered. Randomized trials have confirmed the efficacy and safety of acellular vaccines in adolescents and adults. Several counties have scheduled adolescent booster doses.

Clinical features

Presentation varies with age, immunization, and previous infection. In infants apnoea, cyanosis, and paroxysmal cough are key symptoms. These can occur sufficiently early in the illness that clinical differentiation from other infections is impossible. Thus pertussis must be considered in infants presenting with an acute life-threatening event or apnoea.

Pertussis in the nonimmunized child is a coughing illness increasing in severity over several weeks with distressing repeated forceful expirations followed by a gasping inhalation. Between paroxysms symptoms can be minimal. The contrast between parental descriptions of the previous night's events and the normal appearance the following morning is deceiving. Following pertussis, viral respiratory tract infections can cause the coughing paroxysms to recur.

In school-aged children immunized in infancy, clinical symptoms which distinguish pertussis are whooping, vomiting, sputum production, and the absence of wheezing.

Persistent cough, not infrequently for more than a month, is the cardinal feature in adults. Cough is worse at night and often paroxysmal. Adults describe being woken by a choking sensation. Post-tussive vomiting and whoop are frequent.

Differential diagnosis

Not considering pertussis in someone with prolonged cough is a more important cause of a missed diagnosis than is an atypical presentation. In infants, coinfection with respiratory viruses occurs not infrequently, causing more severe disease and diagnostic confusion.

A careful history of coughing illnesses in other household members is critical. With pertussis, successive household members of varying ages are symptomatic over weeks to months rather than having almost concurrent respiratory illnesses.

Infections with *Mycoplasma pneumoniae*, *Chlamydia pneumoniae*, *C. trachomatis*, adenoviruses, and other respiratory viruses can cause illnesses which overlap clinically with pertussis. Particularly because it is also worse at night, cough from sinusitis can be confused with pertussis.

B. pertussis infection causes approximately 20% of prolonged coughing illnesses in adolescents and adults. Presentation is often delayed until symptoms have persisted for several weeks. Other causes of chronic cough such as asthma, gastro-oesophageal reflux, tuberculosis, and malignancy need to be considered.

Clinical investigation

Laboratory diagnosis of pertussis has improved with the development of polymerase chain reaction (PCR) and serological assays. However, availability remains limited globally.

B. pertussis is a small Gram-negative coccobacillus. It is strictly aerobic and fastidious; special media such as charcoal blood agar are important. Culture lacks sensitivity. Careful collection and rapid transport of the nasopharyngeal sample to the laboratory is required. Immunization and antibiotic treatment both reduce the yield. The organism is most abundant before the onset of paroxysmal cough and is rarely recovered once cough has been present for 3 weeks.

PCR is more sensitive and rapid than culture. Sensitivity decreases with illness duration and less so with antibiotic treatment.

Antibodies to pertussis toxin are specific to *B. pertussis* with measurement of only IgG antibodies recommended. A single antibody titre of 100 U/ml has been shown to be sensitive and specific for recent *B. pertussis* infection.

The preferred laboratory test varies with age and cough duration. PCR is particularly useful in infants. In older children, adolescents, and adults the sensitivity of culture and PCR is lower, and, particularly with later presentation, serology is more useful.

Criteria for diagnosis

The WHO surveillance case definition is a case diagnosed as pertussis by a physician, or a person with cough for 2 weeks with at least one of paroxysms of coughing, inspiratory whoop, or post-tussive vomiting without other apparent cause. During epidemics pertussis should be considered in anyone with paroxysmal cough of any duration, or cough with inspiratory whoop, or cough ending in apnoea, vomiting, or gagging.

Treatment

Antibiotic treatment reduces infectivity. *B. pertussis* cannot be isolated from most patients after 5 days of antibiotics. If started

Table 7.6.14.1 Antibiotics for the treatment or prevention of pertussis

Drug	Dosage	Regimen	Side effects	Contraindications
Erythromycin	Children, 40–50 mg/kg per day Adults, 1–2 g/day	Four divided doses for 14 days[a]	Gastrointestinal irritation, abdominal cramps, nausea, vomiting; hypertrophic pyloric stenosis has been reported in infants	Known sensitivity to any macrolide antibiotic; use with caution in neonates
Azithromycin[b]	10 mg/kg (maximum 500 mg) as a single dose on day 1; 5 mg/kg (maximum 250 mg) thereafter	Lower dose once daily for an additional 4 days	Allergic reactions and hepatic toxicity	Known sensitivity to any macrolide antibiotic
Clarithromycin	20 mg/kg per day (maximum 1 g/day)	Two divided doses daily for 7 days	Allergic reactions and hepatic toxicity	Known sensitivity to any macrolide antibiotic
Trimethoprim/ sulfamethoxazole	Trimethoprim, 8 mg/kg per day (maximum 320 mg/day); sulfamethoxazole, 40 mg/kg per day (maximum 1600 mg/day)	Two divided doses daily for 7 days	Rash, kernicterus in newborns	Known allergy to sulphonamides or trimethoprim; should not be given to pregnant women shortly before delivery, breastfeeding mothers, or infants< 2 months old because of the risk of kernicterus

[a] A 7-day regime of erythromycin estolate has similar efficacy to a 14-day regimen.

[b] Azithromycin is the preferred antibiotic for infants < 1 month old because of risk of idiopathic hypertrophic pyloric stenosis associated with erythromycin.

(From Hewlett EL, Edwards KM (2005). Clinical practice. Pertussis—not just for kids. *N Engl J Med*, **352**, 1215–22.)

within 2 weeks of cough onset, antibiotic treatment may decrease symptom severity.

Antibiotics are always recommended if started within 4 weeks of illness onset. To minimize transmission to young infants, treatment is recommended for 6 to 8 weeks after illness onset for pregnant women in the third trimester and health care workers.

Erythromycin or the newer macrolides are first-line treatment (Table 7.6.14.1). Azithromycin is now the preferred macrolide for infants < 1 month old. Antibiotic resistance is uncommon. A 7-day course of erythromycin estolate has similar efficacy to a 14-day course.

Prophylaxis is most important when there is an infant at risk of exposure. Interruption of household transmission is only possible if treatment is started within 3 weeks of symptom onset in the primary case and before any symptomatic secondary cases.

Prognosis

Pertussis in young infants is unpredictable with the potential for rapid deterioration. Complications include pneumonia, pulmonary hypertension, seizures, and encephalopathy. Most deaths occur in those less than 2 months old.

Pneumonia, seizures, and encephalopathy also complicate pertussis in adults. Complications include cough-induced urinary incontinence and syncope, herniated intervertebral disc, inguinal hernia, hearing loss, angina, carotid artery dissection, and death.

Areas of uncertainty or controversy

Vaccine adverse events

Many adverse events have been attributed to the whole cell pertussis vaccine. Febrile convulsions (risk 1 in 1750 to 1 in 13 400 doses), persistent crying (6 in 100 to 1 in 1000 doses), hypotonic hyporesponsive episodes (1 in 350 to 1 in 28 500 doses), and anaphylaxis (1 in 50 000 doses) are recognized associations. There is no causal relationship between pertussis vaccine and infantile spasms, cot death, brain damage, or death. Although acellular pertussis vaccines are less reactogenic (Table 7.6.14.2), the potential exists for causal relationships to be proposed for temporal associations between vaccine administration and otherwise unrelated events.

Table 7.6.14.2 Frequency of reactions after any doses during immunization with three doses of one of 13 acellular or one whole cell pertussis vaccine

Reaction	Acellular pertussis vaccine (n = 1818) (%)	Lederle whole cell pertussis vaccine (n = 371) (%)
Local reactions		
Redness	35	73
Swelling	24	61
Pain	7	40
Systemic reactions		
Fever≥ 38°C	16	38
Fussiness	17	42
Drowsiness	43	62
Vomiting	13	14
Anorexia	22	35

(From Decker MD, *et al.* (1995). Comparison of 13 acellular pertussis vaccines: adverse reactions. *Pediatrics*, **96**, 557–66.)

Future research

Much remains to be learnt about the pathogenesis. What causes the prolonged cough remains unknown. Vaccines containing antigens with greater efficacy against *B. pertussis* infection would potentially decrease endemic disease. Improved surveillance is required in both developed and developing countries.

Likely developments in the near future

The need to extend the duration of immunization-induced protection will lead to further refinement of immunization schedules.

Further reading

Cherry JD. (2005). The epidemiology of pertussis: a comparison of the epidemiology of the disease pertussis with the epidemiology of *Bordetella pertussis* infection. *Pediatrics*, **115**, 1422–7. [Review of pertussis epidemiology.]

Cherry JD, Heininger U. (2004). Pertussis and other bordetella infections. In: Feigin RD, *et al.* (eds) *Textbook of pediatric infectious diseases*, pp. 1588–608. Saunders, Philadelphia. [Comprehensive review of bordetella infections and of pertussis.]

Crowcroft NS, Pebody RG. (2006). Recent developments in pertussis. *Lancet*, **367**, 1926–36. [Comprehensive review of pertussis.]

Crowcroft NS, *et al.* (2003). How best to estimate the global burden of pertussis? *Lancet Infect Dis*, **3**, 413–18. [This manuscript defines the global pertussis burden.]

Fry NK, *et al.* (2004). Laboratory diagnosis of pertussis infections: the role of PCR and serology. *J Med Microbiol*, **53**, 519–25. [Review of laboratory diagnosis of pertussis.]

Halperin SA, *et al.* (1997). Seven days of erythromycin estolate is as effective as fourteen days for the treatment of *Bordetella pertussis* infections. *Pediatrics*, **100**, 65–71. [Important trial demonstrating that a 7-day course of erythromycin estolate had similar efficacy to a 14-day course.]

Hewlett EL, Edwards KM. (2005). Clinical practice. Pertussis—not just for kids. *N Engl J Med*, **352**, 1215–22. [Comprehensive clinical review of pertussis.]

Langley JM, *et al.* (2004). Azithromycin is as effective as and better tolerated than erythromycin estolate for the treatment of pertussis. *Pediatrics*, **114**, e96–101. [Important trial demonstrating that azithromycin was as effective and better tolerated than erythromycin for the treatment of pertussis.]

Mattoo S, Cherry JD. (2005). Molecular pathogenesis, epidemiology, and clinical manifestations of respiratory infections due to *Bordetella pertussis* and other *Bordetella* subspecies. *Clin Microbiol Rev*, **18**, 326–82. [Comprehensive review of bordetella infections.]

Shepard CW, *et al.* (2004). *Bordetella holmesii* bacteremia: a newly recognized clinical entity among asplenic patients. *Clin Infect Dis*, **38**, 799–804.

Ward JI, *et al.* (2005). Efficacy of an acellular pertussis vaccine among adolescents and adults. *N Engl J Med*, **353**, 1555–63. [Important trial demonstrating efficacy of an acellular pertussis vaccine in adults.]

7.6.15 Melioidosis and glanders

S.J. Peacock

Essentials

Melioidosis is a serious infection caused by the soil-dwelling Gram-negative bacillus *Burkholderia pseudomallei*. It is most commonly reported in north-east Thailand and northern Australia, but is increasingly recognized around the world. Infection is predominantly acquired through bacterial inoculation, often related to occupation, and mostly affects adults between the fourth and sixth decade who have risk factors such as diabetes mellitus and renal impairment.

Clinical features—these are very varied, ranging from a septicaemic illness (the commonest presentation), often associated with concomitant pneumonia (50%) and other features including hepatic and splenic abscesses, to a chronic illness characterized by fever, weight loss, and wasting. Case fatality is 50% in north-east Thailand (35% in children) and 19% in Australia.

Diagnosis and treatment—diagnosis requires culture of *B. pseudomallei* (which is classified as a hazard group 3 biological agent) from any specimen. Serodiagnostic tests should be considered in those with suspected melioidosis who are culture-negative. Aside from supportive care and drainage of collections of pus, prolonged antimicrobial therapy is required, with a parenteral phase of 10 to 14 days (ceftazidime or a carbapenem) followed by oral therapy for 12 to 20 weeks (trimethoprim-sulfamethoxazole with/without doxycycline), but *B. pseudomallei* is difficult to eradicate and recurrence occurs in 6% of cases within the first year.

Glanders—this resembles melioidosis and is caused by *Burkholderia mallei*, which appears to have evolved from a single clone of *B. pseudomallei*.

Genetics and pathogenesis

The *Burkholderia pseudomallei* K96243 genome is composed of two chromosomes of 4.07 Mbp and 3.17 Mbp which show functional partitioning of genes. The large chromosome encodes many of the core functions associated with metabolism and growth, while the smaller chromosome carries more accessory functions associated with adaptation and survival in different environments. At least 6% of the genome is made up of putative genomic islands that have probably been acquired via horizontal gene transfer. Findings from multilocus sequence typing (MLST) of *B. pseudomallei* are indicative of a high rate of genetic recombination, and comparison by MLST of isolates from Thailand and northern Australia has demonstrated intercontinental geographical segregation between the two groups.

Experimental studies indicate a role in virulence for lipopolysaccharide, capsular polysaccharide, flagella, and a type III secretion system (TTSS3) that shares homology with the *inv/spa/prg* TTSS of *Salmonella typhimurium* and the *ipa/mxi/spa* TTSS of *Shigella flexneri*. Other candidate virulence factors include a siderophore for iron acquisition, and secreted proteins such as haemolysin, lipases, and proteases. Data from *in vitro* models and postmortem studies indicate that *B. pseudomallei* is equipped for intracellular survival. The organism survives and replicates within neutrophils and monocytes, and employs multiple mechanisms to escape macrophage killing and evade host immunity.

Epidemiology, aetiology, and prevention

The first reported case of melioidosis occurred in a 40-year-old morphine addict in Rangoon (Yangon), Myanmar in 1911. The incidence of recognized cases is highest in north-east Thailand and northern Australia, but melioidosis also occurs in Sri Lanka, southern India, Mauritius, Myanmar, Cambodia, Laos, Vietnam, China, Hong Kong, the Philippines, Singapore, Indonesia, Malaysia, Central America, Ecuador, and Brazil. The route of infection is most commonly via skin inoculation or bacterial contamination of wounds, but other routes include ingestion, inhalation, and aspiration including near drowning. Factors associated with disease acquisition include adverse weather conditions especially heavy rain, route and size of inoculum, and integrity of the host immune system. Melioidosis incidence peaks between the fourth and sixth decades; children represent one-fifth of infected individuals in north-east Thailand. Diabetes mellitus, excess alcohol consumption, chronic renal failure, and chronic lung disease are independent risk factors. Involvement (either directly or as a bystander) of the 2004 tsunami is a newly described risk factor. One or more risk factors are present in approximately 80% of affected adults but only 30% of children (most commonly penetrating injury). The majority of cases in Thailand occur in rice farmers who work without protective footwear. Avoidance of contact with the environment in which *B. pseudomallei* exists is likely to prove an effective preventive measure, but such strategies are not in place across rural Asia.

Clinical features, differential diagnosis, and criteria for diagnosis

The period between *B. pseudomallei* exposure and onset of clinical manifestations is difficult to define since most patients do not report a specific inoculation event. An incubation period of 1 to 21 days (mean 9 days) was determined for 25% of cases in Australia with a specific inoculation event, but this may not be representative for cases overall. The longest recorded incubation period is 62 years. Time from onset of disease to clinical presentation is also variable; in north-east Thailand, approximately one-third of patients have symptoms for less than 7 days, one-half for 7 to 28 days, and the remainder have symptoms for more than 28 days.

Manifestations range from a fulminant sepsis and rapid death to a chronic illness characterized by fever, weight loss, and wasting. The most frequent clinical picture is a septicaemic illness, often associated with bacterial dissemination to distant sites such that concomitant pneumonia (Fig. 7.6.15.1) and hepatic and splenic abscesses are common. Pneumonia occurs in around 50% of patients. Infection may also occur in bone, joints, skin (superficial pustules and cutaneous abscesses, Fig. 7.6.15.2), soft tissue (pyomyositis), testis, and prostate. A specific syndrome of meningoencephalitis with brain stem involvement and risk of respiratory arrest, flaccid paraparesis, or peripheral motor weakness occurs in 4% of cases in northern Australia. Central nervous system infections occur in around 1.5% of melioidosis patients in Thailand (Fig. 7.6.15.3), although meningoencephalitis

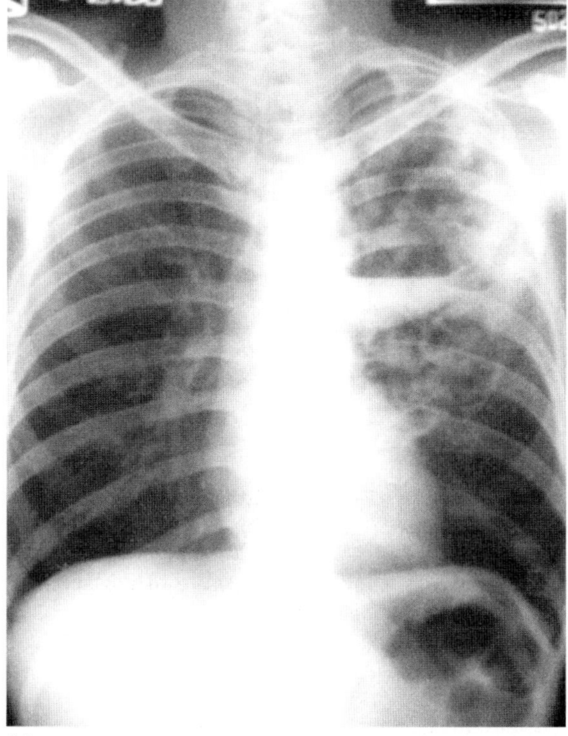

(a)

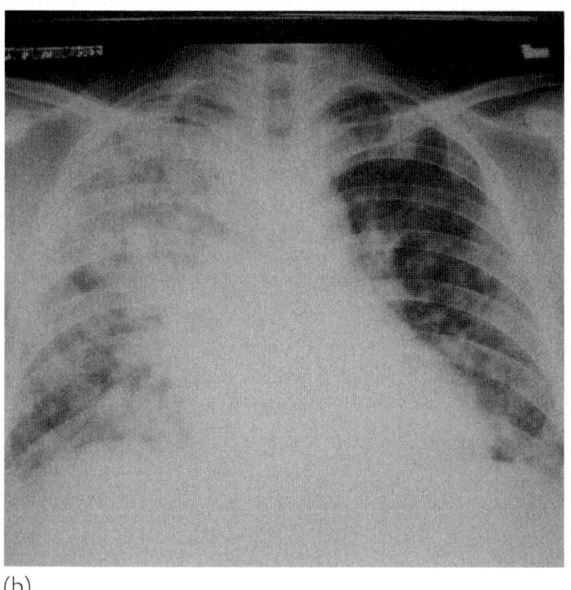

(b)

Fig. 7.6.15.1 Chest radiographs of two patients with melioidosis. (a) Left upper lobe involvement with abscess formation. (b) Diffuse pulmonary involvement with marked radiological changes in the right lung field.

is not recognized in this setting. Involvement of the vascular tree is recognized but unusual. Acute parotitis accounts for one-third of childhood cases in Thailand but is unusual in adulthood. The number of sites involved is variable and possible combinations include positive blood cultures but no other focus, positive blood cultures and one or more distant foci, and negative blood cultures with one or more foci. Classification of patients into different categories based on these observations has been suggested, but it may be more accurate to consider disease as a continuum.

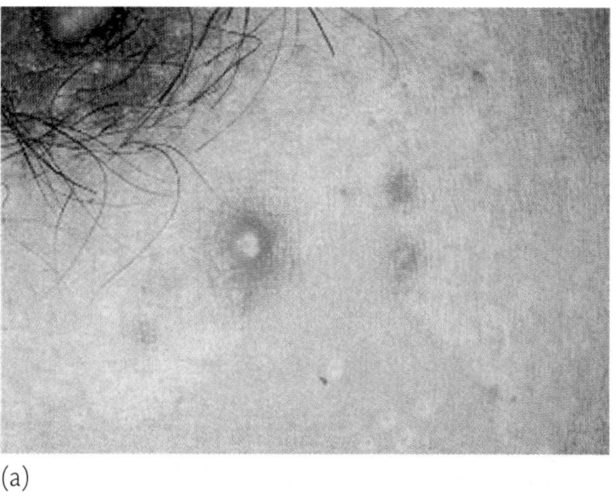

(a)

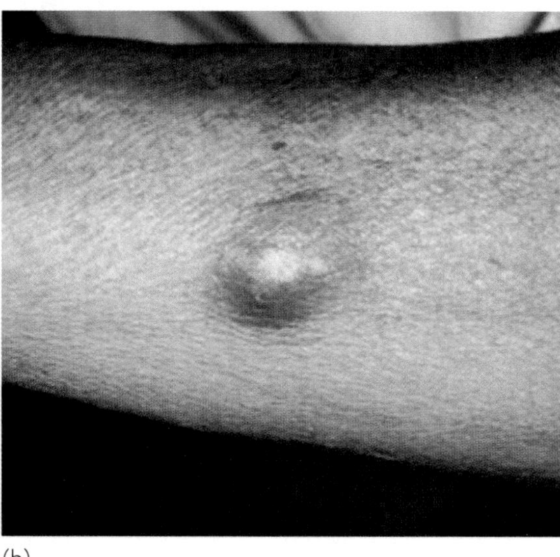

(b)

Fig. 7.6.15.2 Skin and soft tissue involvement in two patients with melioidosis. Skin pustules (a) and subcutaneous abscess (b) occurring as secondary foci of infection associated with disseminated infection.

A high index of suspicion is required in order to diagnose melioidosis in the nonendemic setting. Clinicians should consider the possibility in patients with a fever who have one or more of the following: (1) residency at any time in an endemic region or a relevant travel history; (2) an occupation or other pursuits that may have resulted in contact with soil or water containing *B. pseudomallei* (including military personnel who are on exercise or active service); and (3) the presence of risk factors such as diabetes mellitus or renal disease. The variability in clinical features is such that it is often impossible on clinical grounds to differentiate between melioidosis and other acute and chronic bacterial infections, including tuberculosis. Confirmation of the diagnosis relies on good practices for specimen collection, laboratory culture, and isolation of *B. pseudomallei*.

Clinical investigation and confirmation of diagnosis

Early discussion with the clinical microbiology laboratory is important during investigation of suspected cases. This will raise awareness for the presence of a significant pathogen in a mixed culture.

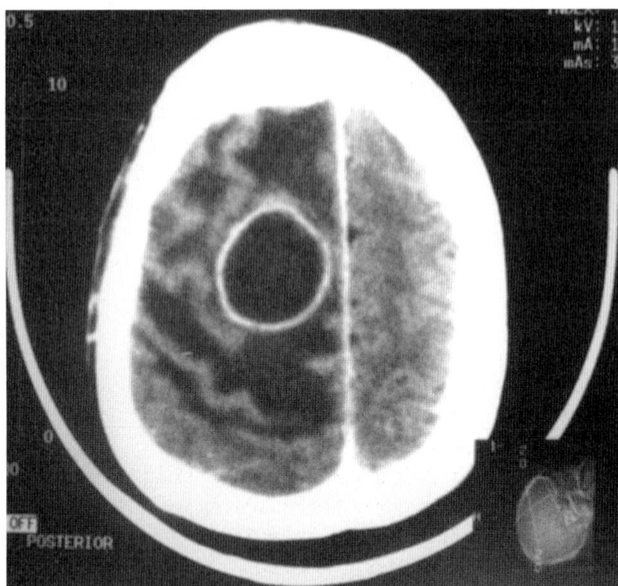

Fig. 7.6.15.3 CT brain scan of a patient presenting with fever, headache, confusion, and hemiparesis. The image shows a ring-enhancing lesion with surrounding oedema in the right frontoparietal lobe, pus from which grew *B. pseudomallei*.

In addition, *B. pseudomallei* is classified as a hazard group 3 biological agent and safe handling requires use of the appropriate containment level. Samples of blood, urine, throat swab, and respiratory secretions should be obtained for culture from all patients, together with pus and wound swabs where relevant. All sample types should be taken where possible since site of culture positivity may not necessarily relate to clinical foci of infection (as an extreme example, it is possible for a throat swab to be positive in a patient with a splenic abscess in the absence of features of respiratory infection). *B. pseudomallei* colonization is extremely rare and isolation of even a single colony from a low quality sample can clinch the diagnosis. Bacterial detection and identification using the polymerase chain reaction is described but is not available in routine microbiology laboratories.

Negative culture does not rule out melioidosis since patients already on effective antimicrobial agents may be culture negative. Serodiagnostic tests should be considered for the investigation of persons with suspected melioidosis who are culture-negative. A rising antibody titre to *B. pseudomallei* in paired serum samples taken 2 or more weeks apart in an individual who does not normally reside in an area where melioidosis is endemic is highly supportive of the diagnosis of melioidosis in the presence of clinical features of disease. This ideal is often difficult to achieve since the potential exposure event may have occurred months or years before presentation and may not be remembered. In this case, a single high antibody titre at presentation is indicative of exposure. A small number of patients with culture-proven melioidosis do not mount a detectable antibody response, and a negative serological result does not rule out exposure or active infection. Serodiagnostic tests in areas where melioidosis is endemic have limited or no value since background seropositivity in the healthy population is high and the detection of antibodies to *B. pseudomallei* has a low diagnostic accuracy for active melioidosis. The most commonly used serodiagnostic method is the indirect haemagglutination assay (IHA). Cut-off points ranging from an IHA titre of 1:10 to 1:40 have been used to indicate exposure.

In patients with melioidosis, laboratory tests should be employed to detect acute renal failure, abnormal liver function tests, and anaemia, all of which are well recognized during severe melioidosis. Arterial blood gases should be taken in patients with lung involvement and/or any evidence of respiratory impairment. Serum C-reactive protein levels do not give an accurate reflection of disease severity. Chest radiographs should be taken in all patients. Features are highly variable and include focal, multifocal, or lobar consolidation, localized patchy alveolar infiltrate, diffuse interstitial shadowing (consistent with blood-borne spread of infection), pleural effusion, and upper lobe involvement which may include cavitation. The radiographic pattern may be indistinguishable from tuberculosis. The development of empyema and/or lung abscess(es) is well recognized, and repeat chest radiographs are indicated for patients with respiratory involvement. Abdominal ultrasound examination or CT scan should be performed to exclude the presence of abscesses in liver and spleen. Clinical evidence of prostatic involvement requires appropriate imaging (transrectal ultrasonography or CT scan). The need for other imaging should be guided by clinical features and organ involvement.

Management, prognosis, and outcome

Appropriate antimicrobial agents should be started immediately on suspicion of the diagnosis of melioidosis. Recommendations are given in Box 7.6.15.1. Treatment is divided into intravenous and oral phases. Initial parenteral therapy is given for 10 to 14 days or until clinical response is seen (which ever is the longer). Ceftazidime or a carbapenem antibiotic is the treatment of choice. Ceftazidime is used as first-line therapy in Thailand, with a switch to a carbapenem antibiotic in the event of treatment failure on ceftazidime. Parenteral treatment at the Royal Darwin Hospital, Australia, consists of ceftazidime or meropenem plus granulocyte colony stimulating factor (G-CSF) if the patient has septic shock. The routine addition of trimethoprim/sulfamethoxazole (TMP-SMX) to ceftazidime or meropenem during the initial intensive therapy phase has recently been discontinued, although this drug is still used in some centres for patients with neurological or prostatic melioidosis in view of its excellent penetration. Intravenous amoxicillin/clavulanate is used to treat children and pregnant women and is second-line empirical treatment for adults. Oral treatment is given for 12 to 20 weeks or longer if clinically indicated, and consists of TMP-SMX alone (Australia) or in combination with doxycycline (adults in Thailand). First-line oral treatment for pregnant women and children is amoxicillin/clavulanate; this is also an alternative for adults who cannot tolerate TMP-SMX.

Collections of pus should be drained wherever feasible. Patients with severe melioidosis associated with septic shock, respiratory failure, acute renal failure, and other manifestations of a severe septic illness require intensive care management, although many cases occur in geographical regions where such resources are scarce. Fever clearance is often slow (median fever clearance time of around 9 days), and without evidence of clinical deterioration is not normally sufficient to indicate a change in therapy. Sputum and draining abscess cultures may remain positive for several weeks in a patient who is otherwise responding to treatment. The benefit of other interventions for critically ill septic patients such

Box 7.6.15.1 Antimicrobial therapy for melioidosis

Initial parenteral therapy

- Ceftazidime 50 mg/kg per dose (up to 2 g) every 6–8 h, or meropenem 25 mg/kg per dose (up to 1 g) every 8 h.
- Intravenous amoxicillin/clavulanate can be used as a second-line agent and is associated with equivalent mortality but a higher rate of treatment failure compared with ceftazidime. Dosage 20/5 mg/kg every 4 h.
- Duration of parenteral therapy: a minimum of 10 days or until clear clinical improvement (which ever is the longer). Extend therapy to 4–8 weeks for deep-seated infection.

Oral eradication therapy

Adults

- Trimethoprim/sulfamethoxazole using a weight-based dosing schedule: 2 × 160/800 mg (960 mg) tablets if more than 60 kg, 3 × 80/400 (480 mg) tablets if 40–60 kg, and 1 × 160/800 mg (960 mg) OR 2 × 80/400 (480 mg) tablets if less than 40 kg
- ± Doxycycline 2.5 mg/kg per dose up to a maximum of 100 mg every 12 h[a]

Children ≤8 years and pregnant women

- Amoxicillin/clavulanate 20/5 mg/kg orally every 8 h.
- For adult patients <60 kg, a dose of 1000/250 mg three times daily is suggested. In regions where amoxicillin/clavulanate is only available in fixed 2:1 combinations, use 500/250 mg three times daily with additional amoxicillin (500 mg three times daily). For patients >60 kg, use a maximum dose of 1500/375 mg three times daily.
- Duration of oral therapy: 12–20 weeks.

[a] Doxycycline is used routinely as a component of oral eradication therapy in Thailand but is not used in Australia. A prospective clinical trial being conducted in Thailand to determine the equivalence of trimethoprim/sulfamethoxazole alone versus trimethoprim/sulfamethoxazole plus doxycycline is to be completed in 2011.

as goal-directed therapy, intensive glycaemic control, and activated protein C has not been evaluated in patients with melioidosis. A randomized placebo-controlled trial of G-CSF for severe melioidosis conducted in Thailand failed to show an outcome benefit.

Several features can be used to predict risk of death. The Acute Physiology and Chronic Health Evaluation II (APACHE II) score is an independent predictor of death from melioidosis. Time to blood culture positivity has prognostic significance, with a mortality rate of 74% for those with a positive culture within 24 h compared with 41% in those with a positive culture after 24 h. In patients who have a positive blood culture, counts of <1 colony-forming unit (CFU)/ml blood have been reported to be associated with a mortality of 42%, compared with a mortality of 96% in those with counts of >100 CFU/ml. *B. pseudomallei* count in urine is also associated with mortality. Patients with melioidosis whose urine culture was negative for *B. pseudomallei* had the lowest death rate (39%). Mortality was 58% in those with positive spun urine pellet only, 61% in those with between 10^3 CFU/ml and 10^5 CFU/ml *B. pseudomallei* in neat urine, and 71% in those with $\geq 10^5$ CFU/ml *B. pseudomallei* in neat urine. Sputum culture positive for *B. pseudomallei* in patients with culture-confirmed melioidosis is associated with a higher mortality (72%) compared with that for melioidosis patients with sputum culture negative for *B. pseudomallei* (42%).

Recurrent melioidosis is not uncommon (6% in the first year and 13% over 10 years). Three-quarters of recurrent cases are due to relapse caused by a strain that has persisted within the host following the primary episode, and the remainder represent reinfection by a different strain. One-quarter of patients with recurrence die as a direct result.

The risk of nosocomial infection between patients or transmission to family or other contacts has not been the subject of specific study. Several case reports have been published. Melioidosis in two infants in northern Australia was related to breast-feeding by mothers with mastitis caused by *B. pseudomallei*, and the wife of a Vietnam veteran with chronic prostatitis caused by *B. pseudomallei* developed an antibody response to the organism in the absence of clinical manifestations of melioidosis. Person-to-person transmission occurred between two siblings with cystic fibrosis and may have occurred between a diabetic brother and sister living in north-east Thailand, and a case of nosocomial infection from a suspected environmental source has been reported from an endemic area.

Likely developments in the near future

The overall incidence of melioidosis is likely to rise among wealthier nations within Asia as the number of susceptible elderly people increases. The number of reported cases worldwide is also likely to increase alongside the dissemination of diagnostic laboratories. Two ongoing therapeutic trials in Thailand will contribute to optimization of treatment regimens; these are a comparison of ceftazidime and meropenem during the initial intravenous phase of therapy, and a comparison of TMP-SMX with or without doxycycline for the oral eradication phase of treatment. Probably the most important strategy required to reduce mortality from melioidosis in rural Asia is early recognition and timely administration of antimicrobial drugs together with adequate fluid resuscitation. Further studies are required to define safe and affordable interventions that improve outcome where intensive care facilities are unavailable, such as protocols to optimize fluid management and glycaemic control in a general ward setting.

Overview of glanders

Burkholderia mallei, the cause of glanders, appears to have evolved through genomic downsizing from a single clone of *B. pseudomallei*. Historically, this pathogen was an important cause of morbidity and mortality in horses worldwide and was occasionally transmitted to humans or other animals. In horses, donkeys, and mules it causes nodules and ulcerations in the upper respiratory tract and lungs. The cutaneous form is known as 'farcy'. The mallein skin test is a sensitive and specific clinical test for equine glanders.

No naturally acquired case has been reported in the United States of America or the United Kingdom since 1938, but it is thought to still occur in the Middle East, Africa, and Asia. An outbreak of equine glanders has recently been documented in the United Arab Emirates. Clinical manifestations of glanders in humans resemble those of melioidosis. The untreated case fatality rate is 95% in

3 weeks. The approach to investigation, diagnosis, and management is as for melioidosis. The organism requires handling in a containment level 3 laboratory; important differentiating bacterial features between *B. mallei* and *B. pseudomallei* are that the former is nonmotile and susceptible to gentamicin. *In vitro* susceptibility is otherwise similar to that for *B. pseudomallei*, and glanders should respond to the regimens used to treat melioidosis.

Further reading

Attree O, Attree I (2001). A second type III secretion system in *Burkholderia pseudomallei*: who is the real culprit? *Microbiology*, **147**, 3197–9.

Chaowagul W, *et al.* (2005). Open-label randomized trial of oral trimethoprim-sulfamethoxazole, doxycycline, and chloramphenicol compared with trimethoprim-sulfamethoxazole and doxycycline for maintenance therapy of melioidosis. *Antimicrob Agents Chemother*, **49**, 4020–5.

Cheng AC, *et al.* (2005). Melioidosis: epidemiology, pathophysiology, and management. *Clin Microbiol Rev*, **18**, 383–416.

Chierakul W, *et al.* (2005). Two randomized controlled trials of ceftazidime alone versus ceftazidime in combination with trimethoprim-sulfamethoxazole for the treatment of severe melioidosis. *Clin Infect Dis*, **41**, 1105–13.

Holden MT, *et al.* (2004). Genomic plasticity of the causative agent of melioidosis, *Burkholderia pseudomallei. Proc Natl Acad Sci U S A*, **101**, 14240–5.

Nierman WC, *et al.* (2004). Structural flexibility in the *Burkholderia mallei* genome. *Proc Natl Acad Sci U S A*, **101**, 14246–51.

Rainbow L, Hart CA, Winstanley C (2002). Distribution of type III secretion gene clusters in *Burkholderia pseudomallei, B. thailandensis* and *B. mallei. J Med Microbiol*, **51**, 374–84.

Stevens MP, *et al.* (2002). An Inv/Mxi-Spa-like type III protein secretion system in *Burkholderia pseudomallei* modulates intracellular behaviour of the pathogen. *Mol Microbiol*, **46**, 649–59.

Wiersinga WJ, *et al.* (2006). Melioidosis: insights into the pathogenicity of *Burkholderia pseudomallei. Nat Rev Microbiol*, **4**, 272–82.

Wuthiekanun V, Peacock SJ (2006). Management of melioidosis. *Expert Rev Anti Infect Ther*, **4**, 445–55.

7.6.16 Plague: *Yersinia pestis*

Michael B. Prentice

Essentials

Bubonic plague is a flea-borne zoonosis caused by the Gram-negative bacterium *Yersinia pestis*, which mainly affects small burrowing mammals including domestic rats. Human disease occurs in endemic countries—currently mainly in Africa (including Madagascar)—following bites from fleas recently hosted by a bacteraemic animal. Historical use of *Y. pestis* as a biological warfare agent has raised fears of its future use in bioterrorism.

Clinical features—the commonest presentation is acute painful lymphadenitis (80–95% of suspected cases), with sudden onset of fever, chills, weakness, headache and development of an intensely painful swollen lymph node (bubo). Spread to the lungs occurs in less than 10% of cases, resulting in pneumonia which can result in onward respiratory transmission by droplet infection. Overall mortality without treatment is 50 to 90%.

Diagnosis and treatment—diagnosis is usually by culture from appropriate specimens (blood culture, bubo aspirate, sputum, cerebrospinal fluid), but rapid confirmation can be provided by detection of *Yersinia pestis* F1 antigen by immunofluorescence in clinical material. Aside from supportive care, early antimicrobial therapy (usually with streptomycin, gentamicin, or doxycycline) greatly improves survival.

Prevention—is by reducing the likelihood of people being bitten by infected fleas, or being exposed to infected droplets from humans or animals with plague pneumonia. Postexposure chemoprophylaxis may be advised for those who have been in unprotected close contact with a person with pneumonic plague. There is no current vaccine.

Introduction and historical perspective

Alexandre Yersin isolated the bacterium now known as *Yersinia pestis* in 1894 from a patient with bubonic plague in Hong Kong, during a plague pandemic when disease spread to ports all over the world from a focus in China. Most mortality in this pandemic was seen in India and China in the late 19th and early 20th century when millions died. Experimental work in India in the early years of the 20th century confirmed the flea–rat cycle of transmission, allowing rational control measures to be developed. This pandemic is called the third plague pandemic because of a retrospective association of bubonic plague with two historical disease pandemics. The second pandemic was the Black Death, which killed one-third of the European population between 1347 and 1352. The first plague pandemic refers to an outbreak which began in the reign of the Roman Emperor Justinian in the 6th century AD.

Aetiology, genetics, pathogenesis, and pathology

Y. pestis strains form a clonal group within *Y. pseudotuberculosis*, an enteric pathogen of mammals spread by the faeco-oral route (this has implications for laboratory identification, see below; see also Chapter 7.6.17). These are Gram-negative bacteria within the family Enterobacteriaceae (Gammaproteobacteria). The change to a two-stage life style alternately parasitizing an arthropod and a mammalian host was very recent in evolutionary terms, and linked to the acquisition of two plasmids, pFra and pPst, with adaptation of preexisting properties of *Y. pseudotuberculosis*.

In the arthropod-parasitizing portion of its life cycle, *Y. pestis* multiplies and forms biofilm-embedded aggregates in the flea midgut after ingestion of a blood meal containing bacteria. Blocked fleas die, but make persistent efforts to feed, regurgitating oesophageal contents and inoculating *Y. pestis* into each bite site. Recent work suggests some fleas may be long-lived successful vectors without blockage. The ability to colonize and multiply in the flea requires a factor encoded by the pFra plasmid. *Y. pestis* dissemination from

Acknowledgement: The author gratefully acknowledges the substantial contribution to this chapter made by Dr Tom Butler based on previous editions.

the fleabite and bubo formation requires plasminogen activator, encoded by the small pPst plasmid.

Y. pestis travels inside macrophages to the regional lymph nodes from the site of inoculation, before switching to extracellular replication in growing necrotic foci which form in infected tissues. Extracellular survival requires expression of a type III secretion system (injectisome) encoded by the yersinia virulence plasmid pCD/pYV to inject virulence effectors (Yop proteins) into mammalian host immune effector cells. This forestalls the usual immune response, preventing phagocytosis. The injectisome component LcrV (V antigen) also has an extracellular anti-inflammatory activity, preventing recruitment of inflammatory cells and granuloma formation which would normally terminate an infection. An antiphagocytic polypeptide capsule (fraction 1 or F1 antigen) is specified by pFra plasmid.

Maintenance of flea transmission requires extreme virulence in the mammalian host. Because of the small volume of blood in a flea meal and a large minimum infectious dose for the flea, a very high level of bacteraemia (10^8/ml) is required in the mammalian host to infect fleas. Few bacteria are transmitted by a flea bite and the organism has a low minimum infectious dose for mammals.

Epidemiology

Between 1987 and 2001, 36 876 cases of plague with 2847 deaths (7.7%) were reported to the World Health Organization, an increase on previous years. The 10 countries reporting most cases over this period (accounting for over 92% of the total) were, in descending order: Madagascar, Tanzania, Democratic Republic of the Congo, Vietnam, Mozambique, Namibia, Peru, Zambia, India (all cases from an outbreak in 1994), and Myanmar. Notably, the very large enzootic focus covering the western United States of America contributed only 125 human cases (12 fatalities) over this period. The plague is seasonal in most endemic countries, with a well-defined geographical distribution correlated with that of the predominant flea vectors and rodent reservoirs and their ecology. Most cases in the United States of America occur from May to October, when people are outdoors in contact with rodents and their fleas. Countries reporting several recent outbreaks include the Democratic Republic of the Congo, Uganda, and China (northern and north western provinces).

Plague is a zoonosis with humans figuring as an incidental host. It is transmitted among animal reservoirs by flea bites and ingestion of animal tissues. The fleas of many major animal reservoirs such as burrowing rodents, including ground squirrels and prairie dogs in the United States of America and tarbagans in Asia, can only contact humans in rural areas. Human infection is more frequent when disease occurs in small mammals in closer contact with humans, particularly urban and domestic rats. The oriental rat flea *Xenopsylla cheopis* is the most efficient vector. Risk factors for acquiring plague include contact with rodents or carnivores in endemic areas and presence of refuges or food sources for wild rodents near homes. Human-to-human transmission of pneumonic plague is limited to rare outbreaks in endemic areas. Although there are no reports of the use of *Y. pestis* as a biological weapon since the Second World War, the possibility of bioterrorism would nowadays be investigated if any cases of plague, particularly pneumonic plague, were diagnosed in a nonendemic area (e.g. Europe, eastern United States of America).

Prevention

Plague prevention measures seek to reduce the likelihood of people being bitten by infected fleas or exposed to infected droplets from humans or animals with plague pneumonia. In plague-endemic areas, monitoring and control of the local plague hosts is important, as well as rat-proofing and insecticide treatment of houses and wearing shoes and garments to cover the legs. Because removing the flea food supply by poisoning their normal hosts can increase human contact with starving fleas, flea control by application of insecticides before vector control in plague outbreak areas is required. Infection control measures for patients with suspected pneumonic plague centre on respiratory isolation with droplet precautions (wearing of disposable masks by medical attendants to reduce the risk from large respiratory droplets) until they have received antibiotic treatment for 48 h. Postexposure chemoprophylaxis is advised for persons who have been in unprotected close contact (defined as coming within 2 m) with a person with pneumonic plague who has not received antibiotic treatment for at least 48 h. Doxycycline, ciprofloxacin, chloramphenicol, or co-trimoxazole can be used as prophylaxis. Standard isolation precautions are recommended for nonpneumonic plague patients. There is no currently available plague vaccine, but a variety of different prospective subunit vaccines are in development and clinical trials, mostly based on combinations of immunogenic plasmid-specified protein antigens LcrV and fraction 1, which in animal models protect against pneumonic challenge.

Clinical features

The most common presentation is acute painful lymphadenitis (80–95% of suspected cases). There is sudden onset of fever, chills, weakness, and headache. At the same time, or shortly afterwards, patients notice the bubo, which is signalled by intense pain in one anatomical region of lymph nodes, usually the groin, axilla, or neck (Fig. 7.6.16.1). The swelling is so tender that patients avoid any motion that might provoke discomfort. If the bubo is in the femoral area, the patient will flex, abduct, and externally rotate the hip to relieve pressure on that area, and will walk with a limp. With an axillary bubo, the patient will abduct the shoulder or hold the arm in a splint. When the bubo is in the neck, patients will tilt their neck to the opposite side.

Buboes are oval swellings varying from 1 to 10 cm in length and elevate the overlying skin, which may appear stretched or erythematous. They may consist of a single smooth uniform mass or an irregular cluster of several nodes with intervening and surrounding oedema. The overlying skin is warm with an underlying tender firm nonfluctuant mass. Patients are typically prostrate and lethargic, but can show restlessness or agitation. Occasionally they are delirious with fever, and seizures are common in children. Fever of 38.5 to 40°C is usual, with a pulse of 110 to 140/min. Blood pressure is characteristically low, 100/60 mmHg, and may be unobtainable if systemic sepsis syndrome occurs as a consequence of the host response to large amounts of circulating bacterial endotoxin. As part of this response, disseminated intravascular coagulopathy (DIC) may occur involving arteriolar thrombosis, skin and serosal haemorrhage, acral cyanosis, and tissue necrosis, as well as multiple organ failure and adult respiratory distress syndrome. A minority of patients (10–20%) develop systemic *Y. pestis* sepsis with no bubo (primary septicaemic plague) and less than 10% develop

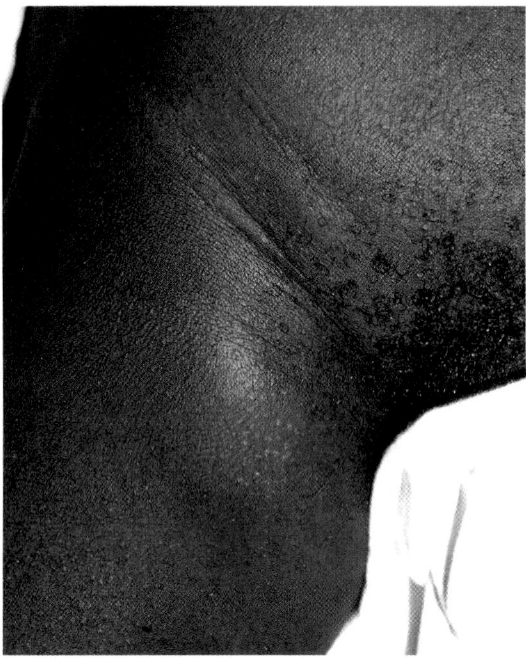

Fig. 7.6.16.1 A right femoral bubo consists of an enlarged tender lymph node with surrounding oedema in a Kenyan patient.
(Copyright D.A. Warrell.)

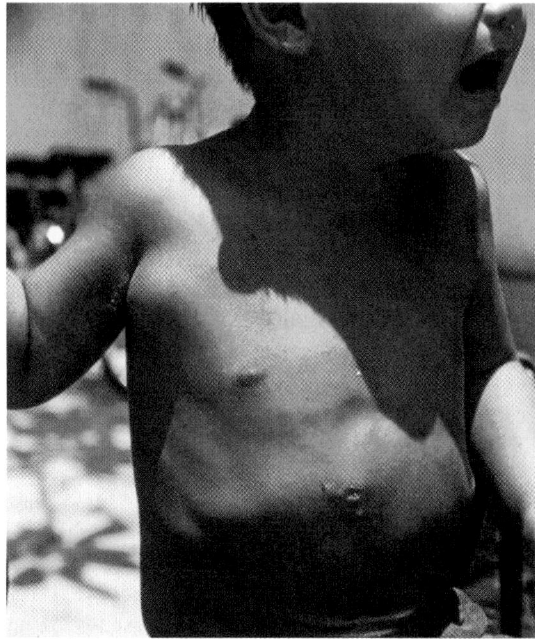

Fig. 7.6.16.2 Right axillary bubo was accompanied by a purulent ulcer on the abdomen, which was the presumed site of the fleabite.
(Copyright Tom Butler.)

secondary pneumonic plague or meningitis as a consequence of bacteraemia.

Differential diagnosis

Other infections producing acute lymphadenitis (streptococcal lymphadenitis, cat-scratch fever, etc.) do not generally share the same suddenness of onset leading to death 2 to 4 days after the onset of symptoms. The plague bubo is also distinctive in the usual absence of a detectable skin lesion or ascending lymphangitis. A minority of patients show various skin lesions (pustules, eschars, or papules) presumably representing the site of flea bite in the skin area draining to the bubo (Fig. 7.6.16.2).

Clinical investigation

The diagnosis should be suspected in febrile patients exposed to rodents or other mammals in endemic areas. *Y. pestis* is on a short list of pathogens to be excluded in any unexplained outbreak of severe respiratory disease which could follow an aerosol release by bioterrorists.

Appropriate diagnostic specimens include blood culture (usually positive in bubonic plague), bubo aspirate, sputum, and cerebrospinal fluid, depending on clinical presentation and, if necessary, taken at postmortem examination. A bubo aspirate is obtained by inserting a 10-ml syringe with a 21-gauge needle containing 1 ml sterile saline through the skin into the bubo. The saline is injected and reaspirated until blood-tinged fluid appears in the syringe. *Y. pestis* grows on standard laboratory media, and standard transport media preserve viability. Cultures should be processed in containment level 3 laboratory conditions.

The organism is characterized as a slow-growing nonlactose-fermenting nonmotile Gram-negative rod, first seen at 24 h on standard laboratory media; it is oxidase negative, catalase positive, urease negative, and indole negative. It may be misidentified as *Y. pseudotuberculosis* or another Enterobacteriaceae species by routine biochemical identification systems and it is important to notify the laboratory if the diagnosis is clinically suspected. In the United States of America *Y. pestis* is a 'select agent' under bioterrorism legislation and diagnostic cultures are strictly notified and controlled.

Gram's stain of smears of sputum, bubo aspirate, or cerebrospinal fluid may show small Gram-negative rods or coccobacilli; bipolar staining may be seen with Wayson's or Giemsa's stains (Figs. 7.6.16.3, 7.6.16.4). Rapid diagnosis is provided by detection of *Y. pestis* F1 antigen by immunofluorescence in clinical material. A dipstick containing F1 antibody has been shown to be a sensitive and specific assay in field conditions in Madagascar on a variety of clinical specimens (sputum, bubo aspirate, cerebrospinal fluid).

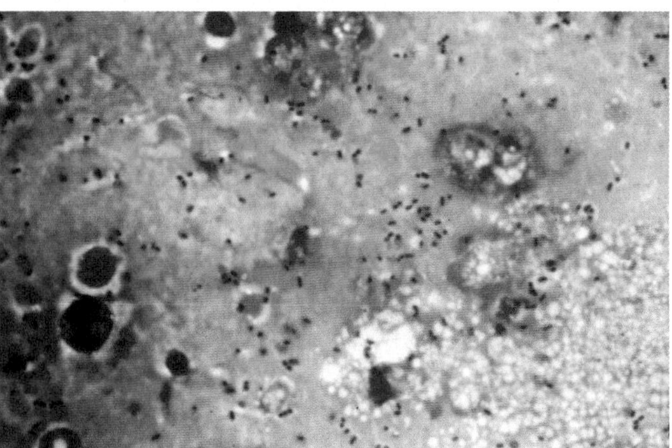

Fig. 7.6.16.3 Bubo aspirate shows bipolar bacilli stained with methylene blue (Wayson's stain).
(Copyright Tom Butler.)

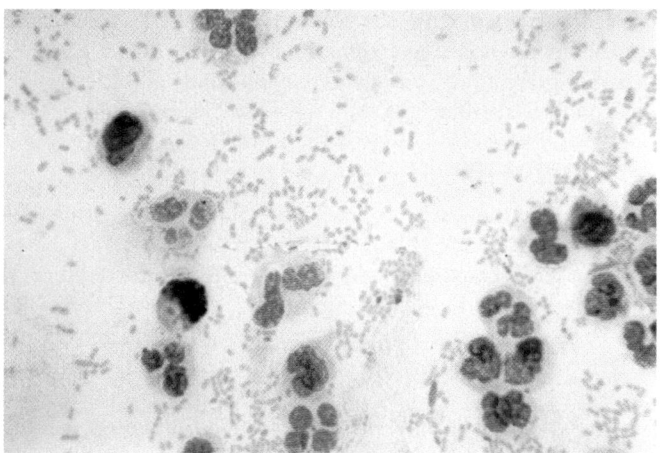

Fig. 7.6.16.4 Gram's stain of cerebrospinal fluid in plague meningitis shows numerous Gram-negative bacilli.
(Copyright Tom Butler.)

Current trials of this dipstick in Africa are ongoing. Polymerase chain reaction (PCR) assays for various targets and an enzyme-linked immunosorbent assay (ELISA) for *Y. pestis* LcrV antigen have also been developed but are not in widespread clinical use, although one real time PCR kit is now licensed by the United States Food and Drug Administration for in vitro diagnosis.

Criteria for diagnosis

Diagnosis is by culture of the organism, F1 antigen detection, or seroconversion (a fourfold or greater titre change) to *Y. pestis* F1 antigen by passive haemagglutination testing of paired serum specimens (PHA test). Specificity of the PHA test requires confirmation with the F1 antigen haemagglutination inhibition test. Seroconversion can occur 5 days after onset of symptoms, but is more usual between 1 and 2 weeks after onset.

Treatment

Streptomycin is traditionally regarded as the most effective treatment for plague at a dose of 1 g IM twice daily (30 mg/kg per day) for 10 days, and was the first antimicrobial shown to be effective against pneumonic plague. The more readily available aminoglycoside gentamicin is as effective as streptomycin in the treatment of human plague when given at standard doses for severe sepsis. Trial data in Africa shows seven-day courses of intramuscular gentamicin 2.5 mg/kg 12 hourly or oral doxycycline therapy 100 mg (adults) and 2.2 mg/kg (children) orally every 12 h are highly effective in adults and children with bubonic, septicaemic, or pneumonic plague (tetracyclines are contraindicated in pregnancy, breastfeeding, and children younger than 7 years because of tooth discoloration). In a mouse septicaemia model, third-generation cephalosporins and quinolones were as effective as streptomycin and tetracycline. In a mouse model of pneumonic plague, β-lactam antibiotics were less effective than aminoglycosides and quinolones. Oral chloramphenicol is recommended for plague meningitis at a loading dose of 25 mg/kg followed by 60 mg/kg per day in four divided doses, reducing to 30 mg/kg per day orally on clinical improvement to complete a total course of 10 days.

General therapeutic measures for systemic bacterial sepsis including intravenous fluids are appropriate, but no available trial data for the use of these in plague are available. A consensus view of treatment for pneumonic plague resulting from biological weapon attack suggests streptomycin, gentamicin, tetracycline, or fluoroquinolones may be effective.

Although still very rare, natural antimicrobial resistance has been detected. A wild-type *Y. pestis* strain resistant to multiple antimicrobials was first reported from Madagascar in 1997, and subsequently a different strain resistant to the first-line antibiotic streptomycin was also identified. Worryingly, both plasmids responsible for these resistance patterns were self-transferrable to other bacteria. Fortunately, no other *Y. pestis* strains with multiple antimicrobial resistance have subsequently been isolated in Madagascar.

Prognosis

Untreated bubonic plague has a mortality of 50 to 90% and untreated meningitis, pneumonia, or septicaemia is fatal in most cases. Diagnosis and appropriate therapy reduce bubonic plague and septicaemia mortality to 5 to 20%, but delay in diagnosis and therapy can be fatal. Primary pneumonic plague mortality approaches 100% untreated and is still over 50% with antimicrobial therapy.

Areas of uncertainty or controversy

There is still controversy whether *Y. pestis* really was the infecting agent in the disease historically described as the Black Death. This is significant in case this fulminant disease re-emerges. Ancient DNA studies looking for *Y. pestis* in the remains of Black Death victims have given variable results.

Likely future developments

Novel subunit vaccines now in clinical trials will come into clinical use. Knowledge of plague evolution and pathogenesis will improve with the completion of numerous genome sequences and intensive genome resequencing of strain collections. Improved ancient DNA technology can be applied to the remains of Black Death victims.

Further reading

Achtman M, *et al.* (1999). *Yersinia pestis*, the cause of plague, is a recently emerged clone of *Yersinia pseudotuberculosis*. *Proc Natl Acad Sci U S A*, **96**, 14043–8.

Dennis DT, *et al.* (1999). Plague manual: epidemiology, distribution, surveillance and control. World Health Organisation, Geneva. www.who.int/csr/resources/publications/plague/WHO_CDS_CSR_EDC_99_2_EN/en/ [Accessed 1/12/09].

Eisen RJ, *et al.* (2006). Early-phase transmission of *Yersinia pestis* by unblocked fleas as a mechanism explaining rapidly spreading plague epizootics. *Proc Natl Acad Sci U S A*, **103**, 15380–5.

Kool JL (2005). Risk of person-to-person transmission of pneumonic plague. *Clin Infect Dis*, **40**, 1166–72.

Mwengee W, *et al.* (2006). Treatment of plague with gentamicin or doxycycline in a randomized clinical trial in Tanzania. *Clin Infect Dis*, **42**, 614–21.

Parkhill J, *et al.* (2001). Genome sequence of *Yersinia pestis*, the causative agent of plague. *Nature*, **413**, 523–7.

Prentice MB, Rahalison L (2007). Plague. *Lancet*, **369**, 1196–207.

Sebbane F, *et al.* (2006). Role of the *Yersinia pestis* plasminogen activator in the incidence of distinct septicemic and bubonic forms of flea-borne plague. *Proc Natl Acad Sci U S A*, **103**, 5526–30.

Sharp S, Shapiro D (2006). Sentinel laboratory guidelines for suspected agents of bioterrorism: Clinical Laboratory Bioterrorism Readiness Plan. American Society for Microbiology, Washington, DC. http://www.asm.org/images/pdf/Ypestis81505.pdf [Accessed 1/12/09].

7.6.17 Other *Yersinia* infections: yersiniosis

Michael B. Prentice

Essentials

Yersiniosis is caused by the enteropathogenic Gram-negative organisms *Yersinia enterocolitica* and *Yersinia pseudotuberculosis*, which are worldwide zoonotic pathogens. Disease is acquired by consumption of contaminated food or water and is commonest in childhood, and in colder climates. Presentation is with diarrhoea, fever and abdominal pain, which may mimic appendicitis. Late complications include reactive arthritis, erythema nodosum, and erythema multiforme. Systemic infection is more likely with *Y. pseudotuberculosis* and a subgroup of *Y. enterocolitica*, and also in patients with diabetes or iron overload. Diagnosis is by culture of the organism or convalescent serology. Most cases of enteritis are self limiting and antimicrobials are not indicated, but septicaemia or focal infection outside the gastrointestinal tract requires antibiotics (usually cefotaxime, ceftriaxone, or ciprofloxacin). Prevention is by standard food hygiene precautions.

Introduction and historical perspective

Yersinia pseudotuberculosis was first identified in 1883 and *Y. enterocolitica* in 1939. Water-borne outbreaks of *Y. pseudotuberculosis* were recognized in Japan and Korea from the 1920s onwards. *Y. enterocolitica* was rarely reported before the 1960s and the first large-scale outbreak of human disease was reported in 1976.

Aetiology, genetics, pathogenesis, and pathology

Enteropathogenic *Yersinia* are Gram-negative organisms of the order Enterobacteriaceae. Ingested enteropathogenic *Yersinia* expressing invasin proteins adhere to and then pass through M cells overlying Peyer's patches. They then multiply in lymphoid tissue, remaining extracellularly located due to the activity of the pYV plasmid-specified injectisome (type III secretion system). This inactivates phagocytic cells by injecting Yop proteins into them. *Y. enterocolitica* classically causes terminal ileitis with or without adjacent mesenteric adenitis (microabscesses inside lymph nodes), while *Y. pseudotuberculosis* causes mesenteric adenitis without terminal ileitis. Some strains of *Y. enterocolitica* (biovar 1B, so-called American strains which are rarely found in Europe) and *Y. pseudotuberculosis* contain a high pathogenicity island (HPI) and produce an additional iron-binding siderophore. These strains are more likely to produce systemic infection and bacteraemia. Correspondingly, patients with iron overload (polytransfused, haemochromatosis) are at risk of serious or fatal consequences if infected by enteropathogenic *Yersinia*, especially when using iron chelators. Recent evidence from mice suggest *Y. enterocolitica* and *Y. pseudotuberculosis* strains penetrating from the gut to the liver and spleen may not be entering via Peyer's patches. Some strains of *Y. pseudotuberculosis* produce a superantigenic toxin, *Y. pseudotuberculosis*-derived mitogen (YPM). *Y. enterocolitica* strains produce a heat-stable enterotoxin. The genome sequence of *Y. enterocolitica* shows the presence of several metabolic operons found in salmonella not present in *Y. pseudotuberculosis*, which may account for epidemiological differences.

Epidemiology

Both enteropathogenic yersiniae are zoonotic pathogens distributed worldwide but commoner in temperate and cold countries. *Y. enterocolitica* commonly colonizes and infects domestic animals, particularly pigs. *Y. pseudotuberculosis* is associated with wild mammals such as rodents, rabbits, and deer, and birds and human infection is more rarely diagnosed. *Y. enterocolitica* infection is commonest in children under the age of 5 years. In Germany 40% of blood donors have anti-*Yersinia* Yop antibodies thought to relate to *Y. enterocolitica* infection, and it is the third commonest cause of bacterial diarrhoea in Scandinavian countries and New Zealand. Seroepidemiology and culture studies suggests human disease is at least 10-fold rarer in the United Kingdom, although United Kingdom animals frequently carry the organism. In the United States of America, high virulence 'American' strains of *Y. enterocolitica* have been displaced by European strains of lower virulence in recent years. Recent outbreaks of yersiniosis involving *Y. enterocolitica* have been mainly pork meat related, for example children in New Zealand consuming cocktail sausages, although large raw and pasteurized milk-related outbreaks have been reported from the USA, Japan and Canada in the past. Recent outbreaks of *Y. pseudotuberculosis* have followed consumption of lettuce and raw carrot (Finland), various raw vegetables (Russia), well water (Korea and Japan) and homogenized milk (Canada).

Prevention

Standard food hygiene precautions are effective including avoiding consumption of undercooked or raw meat (e.g. pork chitterlings), especially by children, and pasteurization of milk. Chlorination of water supplies is important for *Y. pseudotuberculosis* control. *Yersinia* grow (slowly) at refrigerator temperature, and prolonged cold storage of contaminated food or blood products may greatly increase their contamination.

Clinical features

Following an incubation period of 1 to 11 days (usually 4–6 days), enteric *Yersinia* infection usually presents with diarrhoea, fever, and abdominal pain. Abdominal pain in older children and adults is often central or right sided, simulating appendicitis (pseudoappendicitis). Diarrhoea can be minimal or absent. *Y. enterocolitica* diarrhoea contains blood in 25 to 50% of cases. Infection is usually self-limiting, but bacteraemia and systemic spread can occur with subsequent focal infection in various tissues, including mycotic aneurysm. A majority of patients experiencing systemic enteropathogenic *Yersinia* sepsis have diabetes, iron overload, or immunosuppression. Contamination of blood for transfusion with *Y. enterocolitica*, presumably introduced at the time of donation and multiplying on storage, is a rare but usually fatal cause of blood transfusion reactions and systemic sepsis.

Immunological complications of enteric infection are common in northern Europe where HLA-B27 is frequent. Reactive arthritis follows several weeks after diarrhoea with other complications such as erythema nodosum, erythema multiforme, vasculitis and glomerulonephritis. A specific *Yersinia*-associated variant of erythema multiforme has been reported from Germany with localization of eruption to the neck, shoulders and arms, accompanied by erythema nodosum, conjunctivitis and arthralgia.

Y. pseudotuberculosis strains producing superantigenic toxin YPM are associated with Far Eastern scarlet-like fever (FESLF) in eastern Russia, a childhood illness with desquamating rash, arthralgia, and polyarthritis also seen in Japan (Izumi fever) and Korea. There is epidemiological overlap between populations exposed to *Y. pseudotuberculosis* and the incidence of Kawasaki disease, an idiopathic acute systemic vasculitis of childhood.

Differential diagnosis

Differential diagnosis includes appendicitis, other causes of terminal ileitis, mesenteric adenitis (Crohn's disease, tuberculosis), and fever with abdominal pain. Other causes of community-acquired septicaemia should be considered for the rarer systemic infection presentation.

Clinical investigation

Culture of material from normally sterile sites (blood culture, lymph nodes) is carried out on standard media. Selective cefsulodin-irgasan-novobiocin (CIN) agar is used for faeces and other contaminated specimens. Standard biochemical identification to species level is possible in most laboratories, but some *Y. enterocolitica* strains isolated from faeces lack the virulence plasmid and their pathogenicity is uncertain. Reference laboratories separate *Y. enterocolitica* into distinct biotypes and serotypes of more or less established virulence, serotype *Y. pseudotuberculosis*, and provide convalescent serology.

Criteria for diagnosis

Diagnosis is by culture of the organism from a sterile site, biosero-typing of faecal isolates of *Y. enterocolitica* into a pathogenic group, convalescent serology by agglutinating antibodies, enzyme-linked immunosorbent assay (ELISA), or Western blot. *Y. pseudotuberculosis* is rarely isolated from faeces and serology is the usual diagnostic method.

Treatment

Most cases of enteritis are self-limiting and antimicrobials are not indicated. Septicaemia or focal infection or scarlet-like fever (FESLF) outside the gastrointestinal tract require antibiotics. *Y. enterocolitica* strains possess two different β-lactamases and, in the absence of controlled trial data, therapy with cefotaxime, ceftriaxone, or ciprofloxacin are most commonly recommended for acute sepsis. Gentamicin is sometimes given in addition to β-lactams. *Y. pseudotuberculosis* sepsis can be treated by the same agents, although this organism does not produce β-lactamase and is generally ampicillin sensitive.

Prognosis

Acute enteritis is usually self-limiting. Septicaemic illness has a high mortality (up to 50%), probably associated with predisposing illnesses. In northern European countries with high HLA-B27 prevalence, *Yersinia* postinfection complications including reactive arthritis can result in chronic illness which responds poorly to antimicrobials.

Areas of uncertainty or controversy

Virulence plasmid-negative biovar 1A *Y. enterocolitica* strains may have some role in diarrhoea. A Cochrane review is in progress evaluating the evidence of efficacy of antimicrobial treatment of reactive arthritis, including cases caused by *Yersinia*.

Likely future developments

Because chronic oropharyngeal colonization with *Y. enterocolitica* is frequent in apparently healthy domestic animals such as pigs, breaking the transmission chain requires selective breeding of specific pathogen-free herds. This is under way in Norway. Sequencing of more strains of *Y. enterocolitica* (including *Y. enterocolitica* biovar 1A strains) and *Y. pseudotuberculosis* will shed more light on pathogenic mechanisms and organism evolution.

Further reading

Bottone EJ (1997). *Yersinia enterocolitica*: the charisma continues. *Clin Microbiol Rev*, **10**, 257–76.

Carniel E, *et al.* (2006). *Y. enterocolitica* and *Y. pseudotuberculosis*. In: Dworkin M, *et al.* (eds) *The prokaryotes*, vol. 6, *Proteobacteria: Gamma subclass*, pp. 270–398. Springer, New York.

Chain PS, *et al.* (2004). Insights into the evolution of *Yersinia pestis* through whole-genome comparison with *Yersinia pseudotuberculosis*. *Proc Natl Acad Sci U S A*, **101**, 13826–31.

Rimhanen-Finne R, *et al.* (2009). *Yersinia pseudotuberculosis* causing a large outbreak associated with carrots in Finland, 2006. *Epidemiology and Infection*, **137** (Special Issue 03), 342–47.

Sato K, Ouchi K, Taki M (1983). *Yersinia pseudotuberculosis* infection in children, resembling Izumi fever and Kawasaki syndrome. *Pediatr Infect Dis*, **2**, 123–6.

Tennant SM, *et al.* (2005). Homologues of insecticidal toxin complex genes in *Yersinia enterocolitica* biotype 1A and their contribution to virulence. *Infect. Immun.* **73**, 6860–867.

Thomson N, *et al.* (2006). The complete genome sequence and comparative genome analysis of the high pathogenicity *Yersinia enterocolitica* strain 8081. *PLoS Genet*, **2**, 1–13.

Vincent P, *et al.* (2007). Similarities of Kawasaki disease and *Yersinia pseudotuberculosis* infection epidemiology', *Pediatr Infect Dis J*, **26** (7), 629–31.

7.6.18 Pasteurella

Marina S. Morgan

Essentials

Pasteurella multocida is an important human Gram-negative pathogen residing primarily in the oropharynx of mammals and transmitted through bites and scratches. Presentation is typically within 12 h of the injury with rapidly spreading cellulitis or sepsis, leading to serious morbidity and mortality (up to 40%) if untreated. Diagnosis is clinical: fresh bite wound cultures are unhelpful, but the organism may be cultured in cases with established infection. Treatment requires thorough wound debridement, with delayed closure if possible, along with antimicrobials to provide empirical cover against pasteurellae and other expected pathogens, e.g. amoxicillin-clavulanate plus ciprofloxacin, or imipenem plus clindamycin. Prevention is by avoidance of animal bites or scratches and prompt hygienic management of wounds: antibiotic prophylaxis (amoxicillin-clavulanate) should be reserved for high-risk bites (e.g. cat bites) or high-risk wounds that are difficult to debride adequately.

Introduction

Pasteurella multocida (literally 'killer of many species') is a major human pathogen and causes severe morbidity. Pasteurella septicaemia is associated with a mortality of 40% and a propensity for metastatic infection.

Infection usually follows close animal contact or bites. The organism is part of the colonizing oral flora in virtually every species from birds to elephants and water buffalo, but especially in domestic cats.

Historical perspective

The genus *Pasteurella* was named in honour of Pasteur who, in 1880, discovered *P. multocida* to be the cause of fowl cholera. *Pasteurella* spp. cause haemorrhagic septicaemia, 'shipping fever' in cattle, and respiratory infections in goats, sheep, and rabbits.

Aetiology, genetics, pathogenesis, and pathology

Nearly all infected patients have a history of animal exposure. *Pasteurella* spp. such as *P. dagmatis*, *P. pneumotropica*, *P. bettyae*, *P. haemolytica*, and *P. caballi* rarely cause human infection.

Pasteurella spp. are small Gram-negative coccobacilli, often with bipolar staining. Unusually for a Gram-negative rod, *P. multocida* is sensitive to penicillin and fails to grow on MacConkey's agar. An aggressive and opportunistic pathogen, *P. multocida* infection can colonize the oropharynx in those working with animals, and cause invasive infection in those with underlying pathology such as liver cirrhosis or bronchiectasis.

P. multocida is particularly associated with infection following animal bites. Necrotizing soft-tissue infections such as tenosynovitis, septicaemia, and liver and brain abscesses are the commoner manifestations, with very rare reports of epiglottitis, chorioamnionitis, and neonatal sepsis.

Cat-related trauma is particularly likely to result in pasteurella infection, especially septic arthritis and osteomyelitis following hand bites. Small, sharp cat teeth leave a septic focus in deeper tissues, under an apparently innocuous puncture wound.

Inoculation is swiftly followed by a particularly virulent pyogenic inflammatory response. Purulent secretions occur in 40 to 50% of wounds but, paradoxically, regional lymphadenopathy, lymphangitis, or fever occur in less than 20% of patients.

Epidemiology

Infection may be occupationally related, e.g. in veterinary surgeons, farmers, and postmen, but more commonly follows bites from companion animals, accounting for roughly 2% of attendances at Emergency Departments in the United Kingdom. Nearly 60% of cat bites are infected with. *P. multocida*, together with anaerobes.

Prevention

Avoidance of animal bites or scratches and prompt hygienic management of wounds are key to preventing infection.

Antibiotic prophylaxis should be reserved for high-risk bites (e.g. cat bites) or high-risk wounds that are difficult to debride adequately. Oral co-amoxiclav, 625 mg three times daily for 3 to 5 days will cover *Pasteurella* spp. as well as the other 172 other possible oral commensals present.

Patients who have undergone mastectomy and those with diabetes, immunosuppression, cirrhosis, steroid therapy, splenectomy, or prosthetic joints are 'high-risk patients' for whom prophylaxis should be seriously considered. 'High-risk wounds' include puncture wounds, particularly to the hand or wrist, and crush wounds with devitalized tissue.

Erythromycin, clindamycin, and flucloxacillin are ineffective against *Pasteurella* spp. and should not be used for prophylaxis or treatment in the absence of sensitivity information. Numerous reports of breakthrough *P. multocida* septicaemia and meningitis have occurred during erythromycin therapy. Alternative prophylaxis for penicillin-allergic patients includes cefoxitin, tetracycline, or combination therapy (clindamycin and ciprofloxacin or ciprofloxacin and linezolid).

Clinical features of pasteurella infection

Since *Pasteurella* spp. are extremely pyogenic, bite-related or scratch-related infections usually present 8 to 12 h after the incident. Rapidly spreading cellulitis, septic arthritis, and considerable tissue involvement is typical (Fig. 7.6.18.1).

Respiratory tract *Pasteurella* spp. may be commensals or cause infections such as sinusitis, otitis media, conjunctivitis, bronchitis, and pneumonia.

Chorioamnionitis is associated with neonatal sepsis. Pasteurella meningitis occurs at the extremes of age, especially following inappropriate antimicrobial prophylaxis.

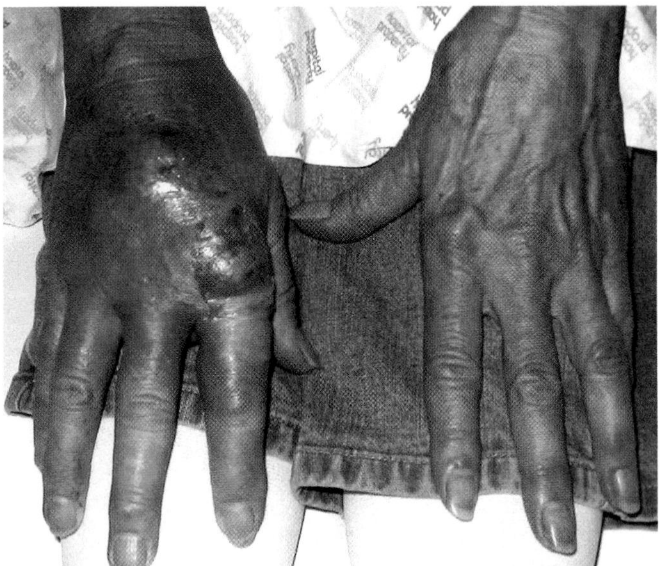

Fig. 7.6.18.1 *Pasteurella multocida* hand infection, preoperative.

Differential diagnosis

Of the hundreds of species contaminating animal bites, other major pathogens to consider include streptococci, staphylococci, and especially anaerobes, the latter more common in deep penetrating wounds.

Clinical investigation

A history of animal bite or scratch preceding any presentation of sepsis should alert the clinician to the possibility of pasteurella infection. Fresh bite wound cultures are unhelpful. Established infections necessitate the taking of blood cultures and culture of any discharge. Prolonged cultures for other fastidious organisms are essential and laboratory staff should be informed of the relevant history.

Treatment

Indications for hospital admission after animal bites include systemic sepsis, involvement of joint or tendon, immunocompromise, bites requiring reconstructive surgery, severe cellulitis, and infection refractory to oral therapy. Hands are especially prone to infection because of the numerous small compartments and lack of soft tissues separating the skin from bone and joint.

Inadequate debridement and incorrect antibiotic prophylaxis are major contributors to the excessive morbidity of *P. multocida* infection. Where adequate debridement of deep wounds, especially cat bites, is not possible, irrigation with 250 ml saline, using a 19- or 20-gauge needle or plastic intravenous catheter on a 30-ml syringe, followed by prophylactic antibiotics may be effective (Fig. 7.6.18.2).

Thorough irrigation and debridement of the wound, and, where possible, delayed closure of limb bites maximizes salvage. Limbs should be elevated and immobilized. Tenosynovitis may be so advanced on presentation that amputation is the only option.

Pus must be drained and affected joints washed out, and the wound left open where possible. Facial bites can be closed primarily since bleeding is profuse and wounds are easily cleaned.

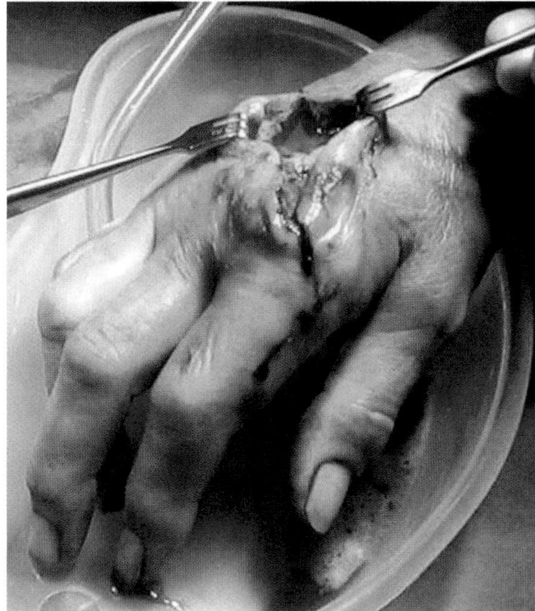

Fig. 7.6.18.2 The same patient: infected area being incised and drained.

Nearly 80% of *P. multocida* are resistant to erythromycin. All are resistant to flucloxacillin and clindamycin.

Treatment of established infections must be aggressive. A combination of intravenous co-amoxiclav 1.2 gm three times daily plus ciprofloxacin, 500 to 750 mg orally twice daily, or intravenous imipenem 500 mg four times daily plus clindamycin 600 to 900 mg four times daily to provide empirical broad cover against *Pasteurella* spp. and other expected pathogens are necessary for rapidly spreading cellulitis, or where involvement of bone or joint is likely. Severely penicillin allergic patients should be given intravenous ciprofloxacin 400 mg twice daily plus clindamycin 900 mg four times daily or ciprofloxacin intravenously plus oral linezolid 600 mg twice daily. Deep-seated infection and tenosynovitis due to *P. multocida* are difficult to treat successfully. Residual damage may be so severe that amputation may be necessary.

For established soft-tissue infection, 10 days therapy is usual, compared with 3 weeks for tenosynovitis, 4 weeks for septic arthritis, and 6 weeks for osteomyelitis. In practice, intravenous therapy until the C-reactive protein (CRP) falls to less than 50 mg/litre is a useful objective guideline for switching to oral therapy.

Prognosis

Established bite-related hand infection often results in permanent impairment of function, justifying aggressive management and thorough documentation. Major factors associated with poor outcome include inadequate initial antimicrobials and inadequate debridement. Pasteurella septicaemia may result from inappropriate therapy with erythromycin or flucloxacillin. *P. multocida* prosthetic joint infection, usually associated with rheumatoid arthritis and female gender, results in loss of the prosthesis in 70% of patients, even with early appropriate antibiotic therapy.

Areas of controversy

The role of antimicrobial prophylaxis following animal bites, in the absence of any other risk factor for infection, is debatable. One meta-analysis of eight randomized trials concluded that the relative risk for infection in patients given antibiotics compared with controls was 0.56 (95% confidence interval, 0.38–0.82), whereas another meta-analysis included trials with few cat bites, resulting in no evidence for the benefit of prophylaxis.

Further reading

Adlam C, Rutter JM (1989). *Pasteurella and pasteurellosis.* Academic Press, London.

Antuna SA, *et al.* (1997). Late infection after total knee arthroplasty caused by *Pasteurella multocida. Acta Orthop Belg*, **63**, 310–12.

Cummings P (1993). Antibiotics to prevent infection in patients with dog-bite wounds: a meta-analysis of randomised trials. *Ann Emerg Med*, **23**, 535–40.

Medeiros I, Saconato H (2001). Antibiotic prophylaxis for mammalian bites. *Cochrane Database Syst Rev*, **2**, CD001738.

Morgan MS (2005). The hospital management of animal bites. *J Infect*, **61**, 1–10.

Talan DA, *et al.* (1999). Bacteriologic analysis of infected dog and cat bites. *N Engl J Med*, **340**, 85–92.

Weber DJ, *et al.* (1984). *Pasteurella multocida* infections: report of 34 cases and review of the literature. *Medicine*, **63**, 133–54.

7.6.19 *Francisella tularensis* infection

Petra C.F. Oyston

Essentials

Fransicella tularensis is a small Gram-negative coccobacillus that circulates in small rodents, rabbits and hares, most frequently in Scandinavia, northern North America, Japan, and Russia. Clinical presentation depends on the route of infection. Most commonly this follows the bite of an infected arthropod vector, resulting in ulceroglandular tularaemia. The most acute and life-threatening disease, respiratory or pneumonic tularaemia, arises following inhalation of infectious aerosols or dusts. The organism is highly fastidious, requiring rich media for isolation and specialized reagents for positive identification; most cases are diagnosed serologically. Treatment is with supportive care and antibiotics (usually ciprofloxacin, doxycycline or gentamicin). There is no vaccine.

Historical perspective

Francisella tularensis was first isolated during an outbreak of a plague-like disease in rodents in California in 1911. Since then it has been recognized as a zoonotic infection of humans capable of causing significant morbidity or death. It is highly infectious by the aerosol route and, as such, has been of concern as a biological threat agent.

Aetiology, genetics, pathogenesis, and pathology

F. tularensis is a small (0.2–0.5 μm × 0.7–1.0 μm) Gram-negative coccobacillus that is nonmotile and an obligate aerobe. For growth it needs an enriched medium such as cysteine glucose blood agar, and it requires 2 to 4 days incubation to produce colonies. The genomes of several strains have been sequenced recently, but there have been very few virulence factors identified.

F. tularensis is able to infect a wide range of hosts including humans to cause tularaemia. An intracellular pathogen, it is one of the most highly infectious bacteria known with an infectious dose in humans as low as 10 bacteria by the inhalational route. It multiplies to high levels within macrophages, and mutants unable to multiply in macrophages are avirulent.

Epidemiology

F. tularensis is mainly isolated in the northern hemisphere, most frequently in Scandinavia, northern America, Japan, and Russia (100–400 cases/year), but has never been isolated in the United Kingdom. It circulates in populations of small rodents, rabbits, and hares, and outbreaks in human populations frequently mirror outbreaks of disease occurring in wild animals. A wide range of arthropod vectors have been implicated in the transmission of the disease within wild animal populations and to humans. Rural populations and especially those individuals who spend periods of time in endemic areas such as farmers, hunters, walkers, and forest workers are most at risk of contracting tularaemia. Outbreaks have also been associated with contaminated water supplies and can involve large numbers of cases. Recent reports of tularaemia have been from Russia (following a sable bite), northern Spain (possibly associated with aerosolized contaminated water), and the United States of America (Utah).

Prevention

No licensed vaccine is available for prevention of tularaemia. Avoidance of contact with infected animals and vectors reduces the risk of infection. Hunters in particular should wear gloves when skinning dead animals, and meat should be thoroughly cooked before eating. Reducing the risk of inhalation of infectious dusts, e.g. during farming activities in endemic areas, by wearing respiratory protection should be considered.

Clinical features

Tularaemia in humans can occur in several forms depending on the route of infection. Although tularaemia can be a severely debilitating and even fatal disease, especially when caused by virulent strains, many cases of disease caused by lower virulence strains go undiagnosed due to the nonspecific nature of the symptoms. The incubation period is normally 3 to 5 days (range 1–21 days), and patients develop flu-like symptoms which may be protracted and relapsing if untreated.

Infection through skin or mucous membranes

Infection through the skin results in ulceroglandular tularaemia (Figs. 7.6.19.1, 7.6.19.2); where no ulcer is reported, this is termed glandular tularaemia. These forms of tularaemia are the most common presentations of the disease and can arise following the bite of an infected vector or through direct contact with the flesh of

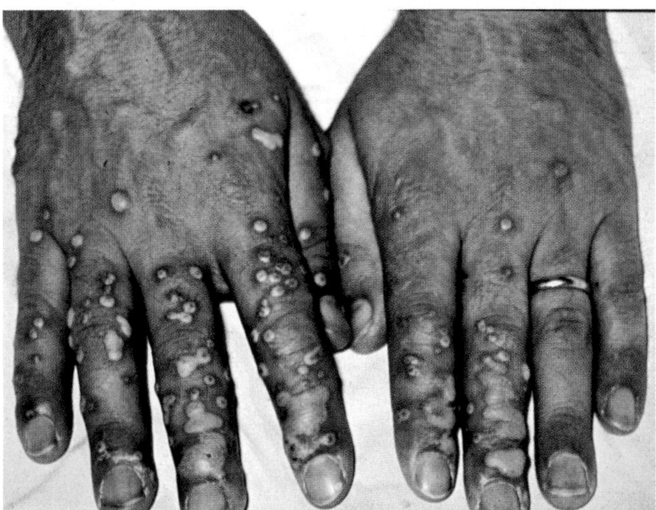

Fig. 7.6.19.1 Hands in a case of ulcero-(cutano-)glandular tularaemia. (Courtesy of A Berglund, Fallund, Sweden.)

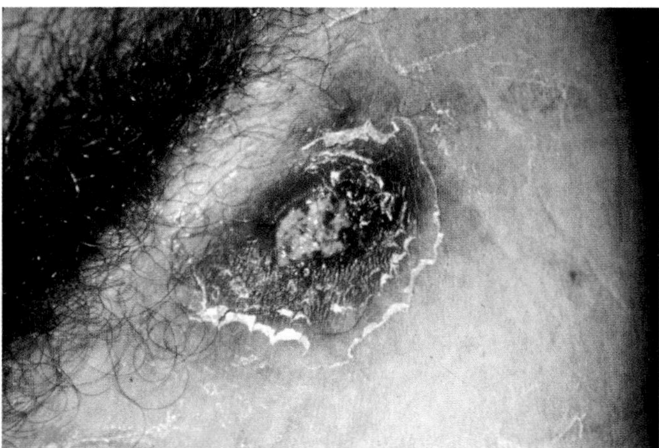

Fig. 7.6.19.2 Inguinal lymphadenopathy in ulceroglandular tularaemia. (Courtesy of A Berglund, Fallund, Sweden.)

infected animal. A lesion develops at the site of infection, often a single papule which develops into an ulcer surrounded by a zone of inflammation. The ulcer is relatively painless and heals within a week. Within 3 to 5 days following infection, the patient develops fever, chills, malaise, headaches, and a sore throat. The local draining lymph nodes become enlarged and painful, like a bubo. Lymphadenopathy can take a significant period to resolve even with treatment, and without treatment suppuration occurs in approximately 30% of patients. Symmetrical rashes have been attributed to hypersensitivity (Fig. 7.6.19.3).

Less commonly, infection can occur through the conjunctiva. This is termed oculoglandular tularaemia and arises following direct contamination of the eye, e.g. through rubbing the eyes after skinning an infected rabbit. The patient develops conjunctivitis in the infected eye, swollen eyelids, and a purulent secretion. Untreated, the infection can spread to the local lymph nodes, in a similar way to ulceroglandular tularaemia.

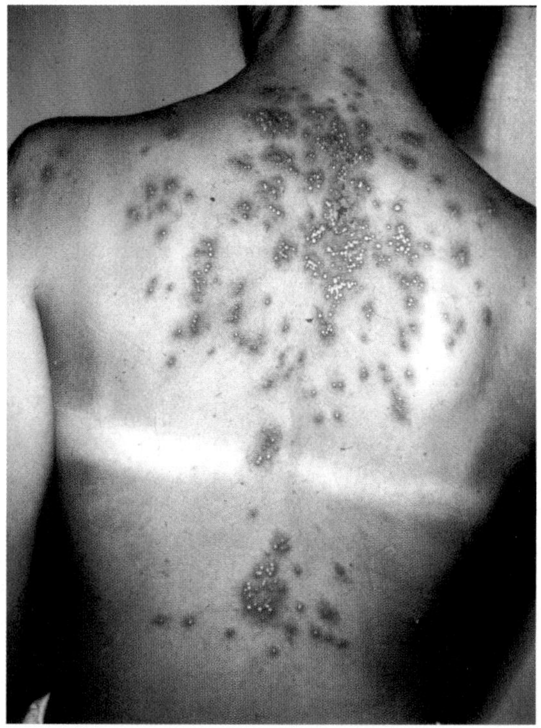

Fig. 7.6.19.3 Hypersensitivity reaction in infection with *Francisella tularensis* (Courtesy of A Berglund, Fallund, Sweden.)

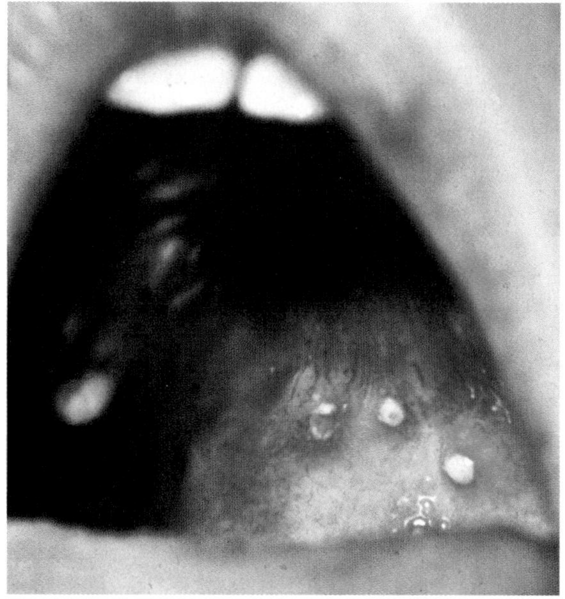

Fig. 7.6.19.4 Oral tularaemia in a case from northern Sweden. (Courtesy of A Berglund, Fallund, Sweden.)

Ingestion of infected meat can result in oropharyngeal (Fig. 7.6.19.4) or gastrointestinal tularaemia. Ulcers, pharyngitis, and swollen cervical lymph nodes develop, and a yellow-white pseudomembrane may be seen in oropharyngeal tularaemia. Gastrointestinal tularaemia can range from a mild but persistent diarrhoea to an acute fatal disease with extensive ulceration of the bowel, depending on the size of the infecting dose.

Any of the above infections may disseminate and progress to systemic disease without the appearance of swollen lymph nodes or ulcers. This is termed typhoidal tularaemia. Severe complications may also occur, such as septic shock.

Infection through inhalation

Inhalation of *F. tularensis* results in respiratory or pneumonic tularaemia. Pneumonia can also arise following haematogenous spread in other forms of tularaemia. Symptoms can be variable and depend on the virulence of the strain involved. Infection with the most highly virulent strains can have a case fatality rate of up to 30% if untreated, but antibiotic therapy reduces this to approximately 2%. Presentation can range from a mild pneumonia to an acute infection with high fever, malaise, chills, cough, delirium, and pulse–temperature dissociation. Radiological examination may reveal parenchymal infiltrates, most commonly in one lobe, and hilar lymphadenopathy may be present.

Differential diagnosis

Diagnosis of tularaemia is difficult due to the nonspecific nature of most of the symptoms, particularly if the ulcer has already healed.

Table 7.6.19.1 Differential diagnosis of tularaemia

Tularaemia	Differential diagnosis
Ulceroglandular	Pyogenic bacterial infection, orf, pasteurella infections, syphilis, chancroid, lymphogranuloma venereum, scrub typhus, streptococcal and staphylococcal cellulitis, mycobacterial infections (including tuberculosis), sporotrichosis, herpes simplex virus, anthrax
Glandular	Pyogenic bacterial infection, cat-scratch disease, toxoplasmosis, mycobacterial infections, sporotrichosis, streptococcal and staphylococcal adenitis, syphilis, plague
Oropharyngeal	Streptococcal pharyngitis, infectious mononucleosis, adenoviral infection, diphtheria
Oculoglandular	Pyogenic bacterial infection, cat-scratch disease, herpes simplex virus, syphilis, adenovirus
Typhoidal	Enteric fever, brucellosis, leptospirosis, malaria, Q fever, rickettsial infection, toxic shock syndrome, endocarditis
Gastrointestinal	Enterohaemorrhagic *E. coli*, GI anthrax, *Clostridium perfringens*, listeriosis
Respiratory	Q fever, other atypical bacterial pneumonias (mycoplasma, *Chlamydia pneumoniae*, Legionnaire's disease, psittacosis), viral pneumonia (influenza, hantavirus, respiratory syncytial virus, cytomegalovirus), tuberculosis, pneumonic plague

A high index of clinical suspicion is therefore required. Other diseases which must be rapidly excluded in patients presenting with acute respiratory distress and fever or influenza-like disease include plague and Q fever (Table 7.6.19.1). Oculoglandular tularaemia may be confused with severe infection caused by a range of viral and bacterial conjunctival pathogens.

Criteria for diagnosis

Most cases of tularaemia are diagnosed on the basis of clinical picture and serology. A range of serological tests for the detection of antibodies against *F. tularensis* are commercially available. The antibody response peaks at 4 to 6 weeks, but can be detected from 2 weeks.

The organism is fastidious but can grow in routine laboratory media, albeit slowly. Due to the infection risk posed to laboratory personnel, the ordering physician should clearly indicate if tularaemia is suspected. In addition, such notification will increase the likelihood of a positive identification as the culture media, incubation conditions, and length of incubation (>48 h) can be tailored to improve recovery of the organism. Polymerase chain reaction (PCR) and enzyme-linked immunosorbent assay (ELISA) can be used to positively identify the bacteria, both following isolation and in specimens. Such direct detection of the pathogen is useful in patients who are serologically negative, e.g. in the early days of infection.

Treatment

Historically, aminoglycosides have been the drugs of choice for the treatment of tularaemia. Although clinically effective streptomycin is rarely used now, and gentamicin is a suitable alternative aminoglycoside, usually given for 7 to 14 days. Due to the requirement for parenteral dosing and monitoring of serum levels, aminoglycosides are now only used for the most serious cases. Doxycycline is effective in treatment of tularaemia and can also be used in children and pregnant women. The tetracyclines have, however, been associated with high relapse rates on withdrawal. Chloramphenicol is usually reserved for treatment of meningitis.

Ciprofloxacin has been shown to be highly effective in oral therapy of tularaemia and can be considered the current drug of choice for uncomplicated tularaemia. It has been shown to be effective in treating tularaemia in children and may be suitable for use in pregnant women.

Supportive care should be provided as appropriate; some patients may require intensive care with respiratory support should sepsis develop. Suppurating nodes should be drained.

Prognosis

Tularaemia responds well to antibiotic therapy, especially if started early in infection. The mortality rate of the more acute forms of the disease is reduced from 30% to 2% if the patient receives suitable antibiotics. Most deaths are associated with pneumonic or typhoidal forms. Relapse may occur when antibiotic therapy is withdrawn (even with aminoglycosides or fluoroquinolones).

Other issues

Patients are not considered an infection risk and do not require isolation. Tularaemia is notifiable in some countries, although not in the United Kingdom.

Autopsies should only be performed by personnel wearing respirators if death from tularaemia is suspected. Bodies should not be embalmed before burial.

Likely future developments

Work is under way to identify a vaccine against tularaemia that will be suitable for licensing. It is highly likely that progress will be made in this area in the next few years, although it can take many years to obtain approval.

Further reading

Centers for Disease Control and Prevention. *Emergency preparedness and response: tularaemia*. www.bt.cdc.gov/agent/tularemia/index.asp

Dennis DT, *et al.* (2001). Tularemia as a biological weapon: medical and public health management. *JAMA*, **285**, 2763–73.

Health Protection Agency (2007) *Tularemia*. www.hpa.org.uk/infections/topics_az/tularemia/menu.htm

Jacobs RF, Condrey YM, Yamauchi T (1985). Tularemia in adults and children: a changing presentation. *Pediatrics*, **75**, 818–22.

7.6.20 Anthrax

Arthur E. Brown and Thira Sirisanthana

Essentials

Anthrax is primarily a disease of herbivorous mammals, caused by the Gram-positive rod *Bacillus anthracis*, which causes human infection when its spores enter the body, most commonly from handling infected animals or animal products. The disease occurs in most countries of the world, but not in those where the condition is controlled in livestock by vaccination programmes. Anthrax is a leading agent of biological warfare.

Pathophysiology—after entry into the body, anthrax spores are phagocytosed by macrophages and carried to regional lymph nodes, where they germinate to produce vegetative bacilli that enter the blood stream. These produce anthrax toxin, which has effects including impairment of cellular water homeostasis and of many intracellular signalling pathways.

Clinical features—anthrax occurs in three clinical forms based on the route of exposure. (1) Cutaneous—lesions are usually found on exposed areas of skin; a small papule develops at the site of infection, enlarges and ulcerates, with the painless ulcer becoming covered with a black leathery eschar surrounded by nonpitting oedema before healing in 2 to 6 weeks; associated systemic symptoms are usually mild. (2) Gastrointestinal—acquired by eating contaminated food and comprising (a) oropharyngeal anthrax, presenting with fever, neck swelling, sore throat, oropharyngeal ulcer, and dysphagia, and (b) terminal ileal/caecal anthrax, presenting with fever, nausea, vomiting, and abdominal pain, followed by rapidly developing ascites and bloody diarrhoea. (3) Inhalation—after a nonspecific viral-type prodrome the disease progresses to a fulminant stage of severe respiratory distress, cyanosis, stridor, and profuse sweating; up to half of patients develop anthrax meningitis; shock and death typically follow in less than 24 h.

Diagnosis—may be very difficult in the absence of a known outbreak, particularly for inhalation anthrax, where a clinical clue is widening of the mediastinum due to lymphadenopathy. Confirmation is by laboratory identification of *B. anthracis*. Serological testing can be used for retrospective diagnosis.

Treatment—this is with supportive care and antibiotics, which are effective against the multiplying (vegetative) form of *B. anthracis*, but not against the spore form. Mild cases of cutaneous anthrax are usually treated with oral penicillin. For gastrointestinal, inhalational and meningeal anthrax, at least two antibiotics should be given intravenously, e.g. ciprofloxacin or doxycycline along with another antimicrobial expected to be effective (e.g. penicillin, ampicillin, rifampin, vancomycin, chloramphenicol, imipenem, clindamycin, and clarithromycin).

Prognosis—the mortality of untreated cutaneous anthrax is 10 to 20%, but fatalities are rare with appropriate antibiotic treatment. Almost all cases of inhalation anthrax and anthrax meningitis are fatal; initiation of treatment after the start of fulminant disease is rarely effective.

Prevention—routine immunization of livestock should be instituted in endemic areas with continuing cases of animal anthrax. Carcasses of animals suspected of dying from anthrax must be disposed of appropriately. Anthrax vaccines should be offered to members of high-risk groups, e.g. those at occupational risk, laboratory workers and some military groups. Postexposure prophylaxis should be given following suspected exposure to aerosolized anthrax spores (e.g. ciprofloxacin for 60 days).

Introduction

Anthrax is a zoonotic disease, primarily of herbivorous mammals, caused by *Bacillus anthracis*. Herbivores are particularly susceptible to anthrax, acquiring the infection via contact with soil-borne spores through oral or gastrointestinal mucosa. The bacteria multiply rapidly to high concentrations and these animals are the common source of exposure to humans. Human infections occur when spores of *B. anthracis* enter the body, most commonly from handling infected animals or animal products. The disease occurs in three clinical forms based on the route of exposure: cutaneous, gastrointestinal, and inhalation. Septicaemia and meningitis may occur from any primary focus. Other names for anthrax include malignant pustule, Siberian ulcer, charbon, malignant oedema, *Milzbrand*, and woolsorters' disease.

Anthrax is present in most countries of the world but has practically disappeared from North America, Western Europe, and Australia since the control of disease in livestock by extensive vaccination programmes. However, it is still prevalent in less developed countries of Asia, Africa, and the Middle East where control programmes are weak or compromised by social disruptions.

Anthrax has gained further importance due to its use as a biological weapon (Chapter 9.5.13). Evidence exists that at least 13 countries have offensive biological weapons programmes and anthrax is one of the most threatening potential agents. Nonstate groups may attempt to use anthrax as a tool of bioterrorism. Recognition of these threats has led to an increase in resources for development of improved methods of diagnosis, therapy, and prevention.

Historical perspective

Anthrax in agricultural settings has been recognized for more than 2400 years. With the industrial revolution, workers processing animal hides and wool became another risk group. Use as a weapon of biowarfare or bioterrorism is now perceived as the major public health threat posed by anthrax. This was made clear by its accidental release from a Soviet military facility in 1979 and its distribution by letter in the United States of America in 2001.

Industrial exposure to anthrax spores carried by animal hides and wool led to cases of cutaneous and inhalation ('woolsorters' disease') anthrax in industrializing countries at the end of the 19th century. In Liverpool, a disinfection station was established where imported wool and other animal fibres were bathed in formaldehyde. This public health measure led to a marked decrease in industrial anthrax in the United Kingdom.

The views expressed in this chapter are those of A E Brown and do not represent the positions of the United States Departments of the Army or Defense.

Anthrax played a central role in the birth of medical microbiology. In the 1870s, Robert Koch and Louis Pasteur carried out complementary studies that proved the causal relation between *B. anthracis* and the disease anthrax. Koch cultured the organism on artificial media, described the vegetative and spore phases of its life cycle, and demonstrated disease causality by fulfilling 'Koch's Postulates'. Pasteur added extensively to the anthrax-based evidence for the germ theory of disease. In the early 1880s, Pasteur in France and Greenfield in England each demonstrated that heat-attenuated strains of *B. anthracis* protected sheep, goats, and cows from anthrax. This disease of livestock had enormous economic importance and by the mid-1890s millions of sheep and cattle had been given this first animal vaccine. In the 1930s, Sterne developed nonencapsulated strains of *B. anthracis* that induce protection within weeks after a single injection. This live attenuated vaccine became the main vaccine in the world for domesticated animals and is still used.

Aetiology, genetics, pathogenesis, and pathology

Anthrax is caused by *B. anthracis*, combining a dormant spore phase in the environment with a rapidly multiplying vegetative phase in animals which resists phagocytosis and produces a lethal toxin-mediated disease. The organism is a large nonmotile Gram-positive rod; in clinical specimens it has a large capsule and occurs singly or in short chains that appear as 'jointed bamboo' rods. Key to the pathogen's life cycle and epidemiology is the property of spore formation outside living animals, related to nutrient depletion in its microenvironment. These spores are resistant to heat, desiccation, ultraviolet light, gamma irradiation, and some disinfectants.

Genetically, *B. anthracis* consists of a 5.2-Mbp chromosome and two plasmids, pXO1 (182 kbp) and pXO2 (96 kbp), which contain hundreds of predicted protein-coding sequences. The nucleotide sequences are highly conserved, with interisolate identity typically greater than 99%. This genetic homogeneity complicates the strain typing needed for molecular epidemiology. Based on the variable copy numbers of tandem repeat markers, six distinct genetic groups have been identified. Since spores long dormant in the environment will cause new disease outbreaks, revision of this initial typing system is expected. Genetic typing of isolates from bioterrorist events has special forensic importance.

Transmission of anthrax to humans is via spores entering the skin or gastrointestinal or respiratory tracts. In the skin, entry is enhanced by abrasion and germination may occur in extracellular tissue fluid. In the respiratory tract, airborne spores reach the alveoli where they are phagocytosed by macrophages and potentially dendritic cells, and are carried to regional lymph nodes. Intracellular spores germinate, producing vegetative bacilli that multiply and activate genes carried on plasmids pXO1 and pXO2 which are the basis of its virulence. pXO1 expresses anthrax toxin, which is made up of three proteins, protective antigen (PA), lethal factor (LF), and oedema factor (EF), expressed from the genes *pag*, *lef*, and *cya*, respectively. pXO2 expresses poly-D-glutamic acid that forms a capsule resistant to phagocytosis. LF and EF impair leucocyte function, and contribute to tissue necrosis, oedema, and relative absence of leucocytes. Multiplying bacteria enter the blood stream, reaching bacteraemias of 10^7 to 10^8 bacilli/ml.

Anthrax toxin causes the massive oedema, organ failure, and immune compromise seen in severe anthrax. Transfer of sterile plasma containing anthrax toxin was shown in the 1950s to be lethal in a guinea pig model. The toxicology of the binding (PA) and active (LF and EF) proteins is complex. PA (83 kDa) binds to cell surface receptors, is cleaved by a furin protease which releases a 20-kDa segment, and oligomerizes into heptamers on cell surface lipid rafts. The final step in forming the toxin–receptor complex is the additional binding of three EF and/or LF proteins. The surface-bound structures are internalized by endocytosis; PA is degraded and EF/LF protected while transported to, and released into, the cytoplasm. EF, a calmodulin-dependent adenylate cyclase, increases intracellular cAMP levels and interferes with water homeostasis. LF, a zinc metalloprotease, cleaves key protein kinases on pathways linking surface receptors to transcription of specific nuclear genes resulting in cellular dysfunction. These toxins also interfere with immune responses, including production of inflammatory cytokines and phagocyte function.

When spores of *B. anthracis* are introduced cutaneously they germinate and multiply, protected by the antiphagocytic capsule. EF and LF impair leucocyte function and contribute to tissue necrosis, oedema, and the paucity of leucocytes in the skin lesion. Spread to draining lymph nodes results in haemorrhagic, oedematous, and necrotic lymphadenitis. Gastrointestinal anthrax follows ingestion of food contaminated with *B. anthracis*. Localization and multiplication of bacilli in the oropharynx and the draining lymph nodes causes oropharyngeal ulcers and neck swelling. Localization and multiplication in the stomach, duodenum, ileum, or caecum cause mucosal inflammation, ulcers, and ascites. Bacteria drain to mesenteric lymph nodes causing haemorrhagic adenitis. Inhalation anthrax follows deposition of spores in alveoli, phagocytosis and transport to tracheobronchial and mediastinal lymph nodes, and intracellular germination. Production of toxins leads to haemorrhagic, oedematous, and necrotic lymphadenitis in the mediastinum.

All primary forms of anthrax can be complicated by septicaemia and, at times, haemorrhagic meningitis. This is especially common with inhalation anthrax; autopsies of untreated cases reveal numerous bacteria in blood vessels, lymph nodes, and multiple organs.

Epidemiology

The natural life cycle of anthrax involves vegetative multiplication in susceptible animals and dormancy of spore forms in soil. Anthrax in animals is usually acquired by exposure of mucous membranes of the mouth and gastrointestinal tract to soil contaminated with spores of *B. anthracis*. Once internalized, the spores germinate to yield vegetative cells which multiply and produce either localized or systemic infection. Animal species vary in susceptibility to infection and disease severity. Herbivores such as horses, sheep, goats, and cattle are most susceptible, dying with overwhelming bacteraemias. They often bleed from the nose, mouth, and bowel, and thereby contaminate soil with vegetative *B. anthracis* which sporulate and can persist for decades. Carcasses of infected animals are additional sources of contamination. *B. anthracis* spores in soil may undergo bursts of vegetative multiplication that increase the local concentration of organisms in the soil of 'hot' zones. The factors controlling this *ex vivo* multiplication of anthrax are poorly understood, but seem associated with major shifts in soil microenvironment after droughts and floods.

Human anthrax may occur in agricultural or industrial settings, or by the intentional use of anthrax spores as biological weapons.

Agricultural cases result from direct contact with infected animals, generally by herders, butchers, and slaughterhouse workers. Industrial cases involve workers in contact (direct or via aerosol) with contaminated animal products such as hides, wool, goat's hair, or bone. No human-to-human transmission of anthrax has been reported. Cutaneous anthrax typically follows skin exposure to infected animals or animal products. Gastrointestinal anthrax follows ingestion of *B. anthracis*-contaminated food, usually meat, and may be more common than appreciated in endemic regions of Asia and Africa. Inhalation anthrax is a result of alveolar deposition of the 1- to 2-μm-diameter spores. Historically, woolsorters and those working with herbivore hides in industrial mills were at risk, but naturally occurring inhalation anthrax is now rare.

The worldwide incidence of human anthrax is not known, but is estimated to be 2000 to 20 000 cases annually, of which some 95% are cutaneous. Based on reporting of anthrax outbreaks in animals, the World Health Organization (WHO) characterizes several countries in Africa, the Middle East, and Asia as hyperendemic/epidemic. Many other countries in these regions, as well as in southern Europe and the Americas, have an endemic level of anthrax, while most remaining countries have at least sporadic cases. The largest reported outbreak of agricultural anthrax occurred in Zimbabwe in the late 1970s during the civil war. Most of the estimated 10 000 human cases were cutaneous and a small number gastrointestinal. Disruption of veterinary health services, especially anthrax vaccination, led to epizootic anthrax in cattle and the associated epidemic in humans.

An outbreak of the oropharyngeal variant of anthrax occurred in Thailand in 1982 when 24 people developed anthrax after eating poorly cooked meat from infected cattle and buffalo. In Switzerland in 1991, 25 workers in one textile factory contracted anthrax, 24 had cutaneous disease and one had inhalation disease. The factory had imported contaminated goat hair from Pakistan. An unnatural outbreak of inhalation anthrax occurred among residents of Sverdlovsk in the former Soviet Union in 1979. Spores accidentally released into the atmosphere from a military laboratory were carried downwind and caused at least 79 cases of inhalation anthrax and 68 deaths. In the United Kingdom and Europe in 2000 and again in 2009, there were infections and deaths among parenteral drug users due to anthrax-contaminated heroin.

State-sponsored biological weapons programmes have often selected anthrax as an ideal organism for tactical use (Chapter 9.5.13). It is easily obtained and cultured, and spores are very stable and small enough to reach alveoli when aerosolized; inhalation infections are usually fatal. In the early 1970s, more than 140 countries signed or ratified the Biological Weapons Convention, agreeing to terminate offensive weapons programmes and destroy existing weapons stockpiles. Monitoring compliance of this convention remains problematic.

Anthrax has also been used by terrorist groups. In the early 1990s, members of the Aum Shinrikyo cult dispersed aerosols of *B. anthracis* (Sterne strain) spores over a Japanese city but caused no disease. In 2001, at least five letters containing anthrax spores (Ames strain) were mailed in the United States of America to several government and news offices, leading to 11 cases of inhalation anthrax with five deaths, and another 11 cases of suspected or confirmed cutaneous anthrax. Thus, in industrialized countries, the threat of human infection due to agricultural and industrial anthrax has lessened while that due to biological warfare has increased.

Prevention

Control of anthrax in animals limits human exposure. Routine immunization of livestock should be instituted in endemic areas with continuing cases of animal anthrax. The most widely used animal vaccine is a live nonencapsulated strain of *B. anthracis* developed in the United States of America by Sterne in the 1930s. Cases of animal and human anthrax should be reported to the appropriate authorities. Carcasses of animals, domestic or wild, suspected of dying from anthrax should be incinerated in a manner that also sterilizes the underlying soil, or buried intact to a depth of six feet and covered with lime to avoid sporulation. Gastrointestinal anthrax can be prevented by public education about proper cooking of meat and avoidance when contamination is suspected. Anthrax vaccines should be offered to members of high-risk groups, such as those at occupational risk, laboratory workers, and some military groups.

Current anthrax vaccines for humans are all produced from attenuated strains of *B. anthracis* that are nonencapsulating. In the United Kingdom and the United States of America vaccines made from cell-free culture supernatants are used to induce antitoxin immunity, PA being the main immunizing antigen. In Russia and China, live spore vaccines have been developed. The licensed vaccine in the United States of America is anthrax vaccine adsorbed (AVA); it is given intramuscularly at 0, 1, 6, 12, and 18 months, with yearly boosters. More than 95% of vaccinees are seropositive after the first three doses. The licensed vaccine in the United Kingdom is anthrax vaccine precipitated (AVP); it is given intramuscularly at 0, 3, 6, and 26 weeks, with yearly boosters. The Russian anthrax vaccine is a suspension of live spores (strain STI-1) in use since 1953; it is given by scarification through a drop of vaccine containing 10^8 spores or subcutaneously at 0 and 3 weeks, with yearly boosters. The Chinese anthrax vaccine is a live spore (strain A16R) product in use since the 1960s; it is given by scarification with a dose of 10^8 colony-forming units and boosted at 6 to 12 months.

Drawbacks of the current cell-free vaccines are the incomplete characterization of the vaccine and the complex immunization regimens. These, along with the increased risk of *B. anthracis* use as a biological weapon, have stimulated renewed efforts to develop improved vaccines. A recombinant PA vaccine is in clinical development. Additional approaches under investigation include antigen and adjuvant modification, live vaccines, and DNA and vectored constructs.

Postexposure prophylaxis is given following suspected exposure to aerosolized anthrax spores. Ciprofloxacin has been approved for this indication in the United States of America (500 mg every 12 h). A 60-day course is recommended because antibiotics are not effective against the spore form that may be dormant in alveoli for many weeks. Antibiotics protect against multiplying organisms, but prevent development of protective immune responses. Therefore, disease may occur if the strain is drug resistant, after cessation of antibiotics, or when compliance is poor. For these reasons, concurrent vaccination may become part of the recommendation.

Clinical features

Cutaneous anthrax

Anthrax acquired its name from the Hippocratic description of the skin lesion's characteristic eschar as being the colour of coal

(Greek *anthrakos* = coal). These cutaneous lesions are usually found on exposed areas of skin, such as the face, neck, arms, or hands, and may be single or multiple depending on the type of exposure. The incubation period ranges from 1 to 12 days, usually 2 to 7 days. Initially a small papule develops at the site of infection, and it then enlarges and ulcerates. The depressed ulcer becomes covered with a black leathery eschar surrounded by nonpitting oedema (Fig. 7.6.20.1) that is occasionally massive ('malignant oedema'). Established lesions are characteristically painless and may be hypaesthetic. Small satellite vesicles, containing many organisms and few white cells, may surround the original lesion; regional lymphadenitis is common. Associated systemic symptoms are usually mild; lesions heal without scarring, although slowly (2–6 weeks), after eschar separation. In 10 to 20% of patients the disease becomes systemic, with bacteraemia and toxaemia. Cutaneous anthrax should be considered in patients with painless ulcers associated with oedema and vesicles, and who have had prior contact with animals or animal products. Differential diagnosis includes staphylococcal or streptococcal skin infections, ulceroglandular tularaemia, bubonic plague, bites of brown recluse spiders, orf, rickettsial pox, and scrub typhus.

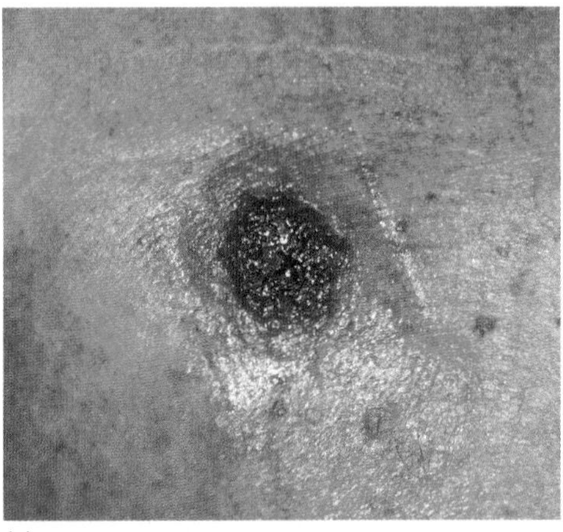

(a)

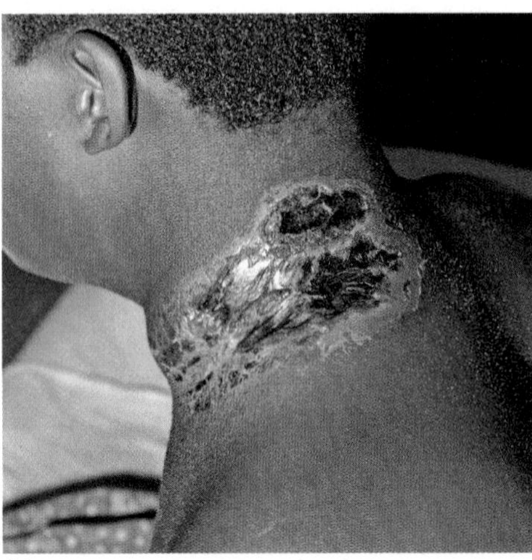

(b)

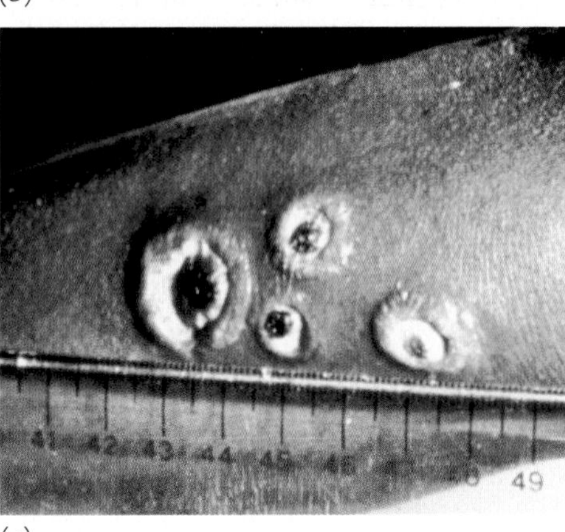

(c)

Fig. 7.6.20.1 Cutaneous anthrax. (a) Early lesion. (b) Large eschar in a Nigerian patient who carried an infected carcass on his shoulder. (c) Ulcer with satellite lesions in a Thai patient.
(a) (Copyright Dr S Eykin.) (b) (Copyright D A Warrell.) (c) (Copyright the late Sornchai Looareesuwan.)

Gastrointestinal anthrax

Gastrointestinal anthrax is acquired by eating contaminated food, and thus may occur in familial clusters. The disease has an incubation period of 2 to 5 days and occurs in two forms. Oropharyngeal anthrax follows deposition of bacteria in the oropharynx. Patients present with fever, neck swelling, sore throat, and dysphagia. The neck swelling is caused by enlargement of the jugular lymph nodes together with subcutaneous oedema as in diphtheria. The lesion in the oral cavity or oropharynx starts as inflamed mucosa, progressing through necrosis and ulceration to formation of a pseudomembrane (no eschar) covering the ulcer (Fig. 7.6.20.2). In severe cases, the subcutaneous oedema extends to the anterior chest wall and axilla, with the overlying skin showing signs of inflammation. Death may result from systemic toxaemia or local airway obstruction. Oropharyngeal anthrax should be considered in patients who present with fever, neck swelling, sore throat, and oropharyngeal ulcer, and who give a history of eating raw or undercooked meat. The differential diagnosis includes diphtheria and peritonsillar abscess.

In the other form of gastrointestinal anthrax, organisms are deposited in the terminal ileum or caecum, and occasionally in

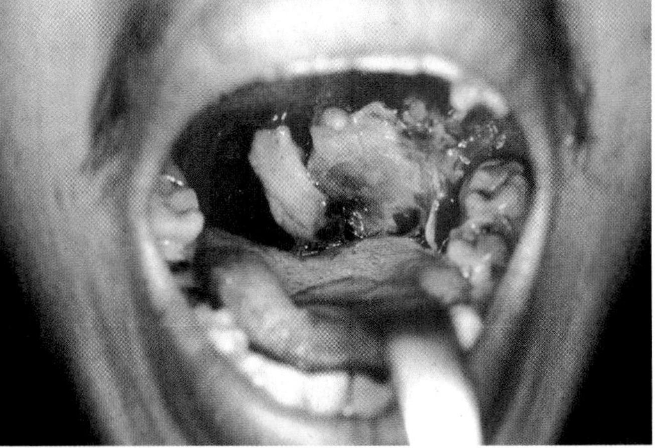

Fig. 7.6.20.2 Oropharyngeal anthrax in a Thai man showing extensive lesion in posterior pharynx.
(From Sirisanthana T, *et al.* (1984). Outbreak of oral-pharyngeal anthrax: an unusual manifestation of human infection with *Bacillus anthracis*. *Am J Trop Med Hyg*, **33**, 144–50.)

more proximal parts of the gastrointestinal tract. Disease onset is nonspecific with fever, nausea, vomiting, and abdominal pain, followed by rapidly developing ascites and bloody diarrhoea. Haematemesis, melaena, haematochezia, and/or profuse watery diarrhoea may occur. In severe cases, toxaemia, shock, and death follow. Early diagnosis is difficult, except in an epidemic setting, and the disease is likely under reported.

Inhalation anthrax

Inhalation anthrax has an incubation period of 1 to 43 days. A prodrome consists of malaise, myalgia, fever, and nonproductive cough, nonspecific symptoms similar to those of viral respiratory diseases. In some patients there is transient improvement after 2 to 4 days. A fulminant stage follows which begins with severe respiratory distress, cyanosis, stridor, and profuse sweating. Subcutaneous oedema of the chest and neck may develop. A characteristic radiographic finding is mediastinal widening with or without pleural effusion. By CT, nearly all patients have mediastinal enlargement secondary to lymphadenopathy, as well as pleural effusions (Fig. 7.6.20.3). Blood cultures collected before the start of antibiotics will grow *B. anthracis*. Up to one-half of patients develop anthrax meningitis. Shock and death typically follow in less than 24 h. During the prodrome, and in the absence of a known outbreak, the disease is very difficult to diagnose. Advanced disease may be suspected in the presence of a characteristically widened mediastinum despite otherwise normal chest radiographic findings. Inhalation anthrax must be distinguished from pneumonic plague.

Meningeal anthrax

Anthrax meningitis, associated with overwhelming *B. anthracis* bacteraemia, may complicate any primary form of anthrax. Rarely, a case of anthrax meningitis has been reported in which the primary site was not identified. Within a few days of the primary lesion the patient suddenly develops confusion, loss of consciousness, and focal neurological signs. The cerebrospinal fluid may be haemorrhagic, but of note is the high concentration of organisms. The disease is almost always fatal.

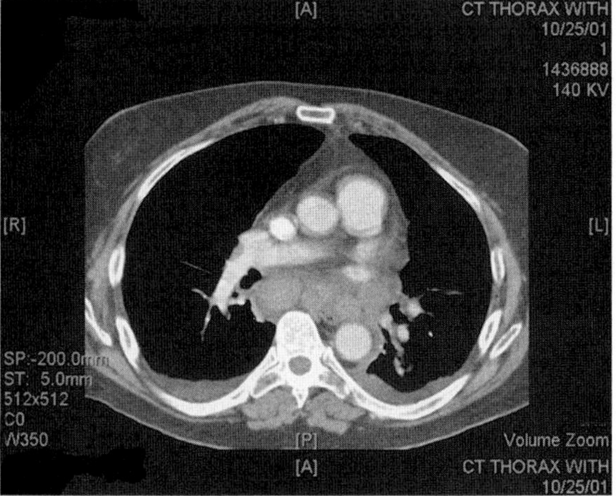

Fig. 7.6.20.3 CT image of an American adult with inhalation anthrax showing mediastinal enlargement secondary to lymphadenopathy. Note small bilateral pleural effusions and nearly clear lung fields.
(From Jernigan JA, *et al.* (2001). Bioterrorism-related inhalational anthrax: the first 10 cases reported in the United States. *Emerg Infect Dis*, **7**, 933–44.)

Criteria for diagnosis

Diagnosis of anthrax may be suspected on clinical and epidemiological grounds, and is confirmed by laboratory identification of *B. anthracis*. Clinical signs and symptoms are discussed above. Clinical specimens containing large Gram-positive rods, singly and in short chains of 2 to 4 cells, should be interpreted as possible *Bacillus* spp. Demonstration of encapsulation of these bacilli by India ink, Giemsa's, or polychrome methylene blue stain leads to a presumptive identification of *B. anthracis*. Culture isolates are identified by classic biochemical and morphological characteristics: Gram-positive broad spore-forming rods, the spores do not swell the vegetative cell and are oval shaped; nonmotile; colonies have a ground-glass appearance and are (nearly always) nonhaemolytic. Standard confirmatory tests include lysis by gamma phage and direct immunofluorescent assays for cell wall or capsular antigens.

Serological testing is not helpful for diagnosis at the onset of symptoms but can be used for retrospective diagnosis. Specific IgG antibodies are detectable by enzyme-linked immunosorbent assay (ELISA), with testing of paired samples preferred. In 2004, the United States Food and Drug Administration approved a rapid blood test for confirmatory diagnosis of anthrax based on antibodies to the anthrax toxin. Delayed-type hypersensitivity is assessed by antigen skin test (Anthraxin) in the former Soviet Union for diagnosis of former infection or response to vaccination. Other technologies include immunohistochemistry, polymerase chain reaction (PCR), and genetic sequencing.

Treatment

Antibiotics are effective against the multiplying (vegetative) form of *B. anthracis*, but not against the spore form. They should be used in combination for all severe anthrax disease. Most strains of *B. anthracis* are susceptible to penicillin, and mild cases of cutaneous anthrax may be treated with oral penicillin at the dosage of 250 mg 6-hourly for 5 to 7 days. For extensive lesions, parenteral penicillin G, 2 million units every 6 h, should be given for a total treatment period of 7 to 10 days. Ciprofloxacin, erythromycin, doxycycline, or chloramphenicol can be used in penicillin-sensitive patients. Antibiotics decrease the likelihood of systemic disease and thus mortality, but the time to resolution of skin lesions is unchanged. The skin lesion should be covered with a sterile dressing and used dressings should be decontaminated.

In gastrointestinal, inhalational, and meningeal anthrax, at least two antibiotics should be given intravenously. If naturally acquired, penicillin G (4 million units every 4 h) has been the drug of choice; ciprofloxacin (400 mg every 12 h) or doxycycline (100 mg every 12 h) are currently recommended in the United States of America. Of note, doxycycline should not be used for meningitis which should be assumed in the management of inhalation anthrax. Many patients will require intensive supportive care.

Anthrax caused by a biological weapon will generally be acquired by inhalation. In this setting, drug resistance due to genetic modification is of concern and drug sensitivity testing is imperative.

Treatment should begin intravenously with ciprofloxacin (400 mg every 12 h) or doxycycline (100 mg every 12 h), along with one or two other antimicrobials expected to be effective (penicillin, ampicillin, rifampicin, vancomycin, chloramphenicol, imipenem, clindamycin, and clarithromycin are candidates). Factors associated with lower mortality are initiation of treatment during the prodrome phase, drainage of pleural fluid, and use of multidrug regimens. Initiation of treatment after the start of fulminant disease is rarely effective.

Prognosis

The mortality of untreated cutaneous anthrax is 10 to 20%. With appropriate antibiotic treatment, fatalities are rare. Almost all cases of inhalation anthrax and anthrax meningitis are fatal. An exception to this is suggested by the recent experience in the United States of America where initiation of multidrug treatment during the prodromal stage, along with drainage of pleural effusions and extensive supportive measures, resulted in a reduction of mortality to about 50%. Mortality of oropharyngeal anthrax is about 15% in treated patients; mortality of the other form of gastrointestinal anthrax is uncertain, but high if disease becomes systemic.

Other issues

The WHO has estimated that 50 kg of *B. anthracis* spores released over a city of 5 million people would infect 250 000 people, killing 40% of them. Numbers would be influenced by the quality of the aerosol, dispersal method, and ambient weather conditions. Cases would be largely inhalation and intensive medical care would be required. Most cities would not have the required medical surge capacity. Antibiotics and vaccine would be needed in great quantities for postexposure prophylaxis. These realities are among the challenges to preparedness planning.

Areas of uncertainty

Specificity of environmental assays will remain challenging, since true-positives will be rare and false-positives disruptive and expensive. The increasing capacity to genetically modify anthrax strains may lead to biological weapons that are resistant to antibiotics or have altered vaccine target sites.

Likely future developments

Methods for detection of spores in the atmosphere will improve. The mechanisms by which anthrax toxins compromise immune responses and cause rapid death will become clear and result in improved therapies. New vaccines with simpler immunizing regimens will become available.

Further reading

Abrami L, Reig N, Gisou van der Goot F (2005). Anthrax toxin: the long and winding road that leads to the kill. *Trends Microbiol*, **13**, 72–8. [Good review of anthrax toxicology.]

Beatty ME, *et al.* (2003). Gastrointestinal anthrax: review of the literature. *Arch Intern Med*, **163**, 2527–31. [Review of gastrointestinal anthrax, clinical, microbiological, and epidemiological aspects.]

Brachman PS, Friedlander AM, Grabenstein JD (2008). Anthrax vaccine. In: Plotkin SL, Orenstein WA, Offit PA (eds) *Vaccines*, pp. 111–126. Saunders, Philadelphia. [Comprehensive and expert review of anthrax vaccines.]

Brachman PS, *et al.* (1962). Field evaluation of a human anthrax vaccine. *Am J Public Health*, **52**, 632–45. [Report of controlled human efficacy study of vaccine against anthrax.]

Brittingham KC, *et al.* (2005). Dendritic cells endocytose *Bacillus anthracis* spores: implications for anthrax pathogenesis. *J Immunol*, **174**, 5545–52. [Evidence for potential role of dendritic cells in pathogenesis.]

Centers for Disease Control and Prevention (2006). Inhalation anthrax associated with dried animal hides: Pennsylvania and New York City, 2006. *MMWR Morb Mortal Wkly Rep*, **55**, 280–2. [Report of first case of naturally acquired inhalation anthrax in the United States of America in 30 years.]

Davies JCA (1982). A major epidemic of anthrax in Zimbabwe, part 1. *Cent Afr J Med*, **28**, 291–8. [First of three articles describing the largest known anthrax outbreak.]

Holty J-EC, *et al.* (2006). Systematic review: a century of inhalational anthrax cases from 1900 to 2005. *Ann Intern Med*, **144**, 270–80. [Retrospective case review of inhalation anthrax showing factors associated with survival.]

Inglesby TV, *et al.* (2002). Anthrax as a biological weapon, 2002: updated recommendations for management. *JAMA*, **287**, 2236–52. [Comprehensive review of bioweapons-related concerns.]

Keim P, *et al.* (2000). Multiple-locus variable-number tandem repeat analysis reveals genetic relationships within *Bacillus anthracis*. *J Bacteriol*, **182**, 2928–36. [Description of genetic groupings of *B. anthracis*.]

Maguina C, *et al.* (2005). Cutaneous anthrax in Lima, Peru: retrospective analysis of 71 cases, including four with a meningoencephalic complication. *Rev Inst Med Trop Sao Paulo*, **47**, 25–30. [Large retrospective review of cutaneous cases.]

Marano N, *et al.* (2008). Effects of reduced dose schedule and intramuscular administration of anthrax vaccine absorbed on immunogenicity and safety at 7 months. *JAMA*, **300**, 1532–43. [Basis for shift to IM administration of vaccine and drop of dose at 2 weeks.]

Meselson M, *et al.* (1994). The Sverdlovsk anthrax outbreak of 1979. *Science*, **266**, 1202–8. [Description of the bioweapons-related outbreak in the former Soviet Union.]

Perl DP, Dooley JR (1976). Anthrax. In: Binford CH, Connor DH (eds) *Pathology of tropical and extraordinary diseases*, vol. 1, pp. 118–23. Armed Forces Institute of Pathology, Washington. [Description and illustrations of gross and microscopic human pathology.]

Plotkin SA, *et al.* (1960). An epidemic of inhalation anthrax, the first in the twentieth century: I. Clinical features. *Am J Med*, **29**, 992–1001. [Landmark description of industrial anthrax.]

Read TD, *et al.* (2002). Comparative genome sequencing for discovery of novel polymorphisms in *Bacillus anthracis*. *Science*, **296**, 2028–33. [Development of genetic typing of isolates, spurred on by the 2001 outbreak in the United States of America.]

Sirisanthana T, *et al.* (1984). Outbreak of oral-pharyngeal anthrax: an unusual manifestation of human infection with *Bacillus anthracis*. *Am J Trop Med Hyg*, **39**, 144–50. [Largest reported outbreak of an unusual variant of gastrointestinal anthrax.]

Vietri NJ, *et al.* (2006). Short-course post-exposure antibiotic prophylaxis combined with vaccination protects against experimental inhalational anthrax. *Proc Natl Acad Sci*, **103**, 7813–6. [Evidence from primates showing benefit of postexposure vaccination with antibiotics.]

7.6.21 Brucellosis

M. Monir Madkour‡

Essentials

There are four species of the Gram-negative, aerobic brucella bacillus, each comprising several biovars: *Brucella melitensis* ('Malta fever', most commonly associated with goats, sheep,and camels), *B. abortus* (cattle), *B. suis* (pigs), and *B. canis* (dogs). The disease that they cause—brucellosis—occurs worldwide, but is especially prevalent in the Mediterranean region, the Indian subcontinent, Mexico, and Central and South America. Transmission is commonly by ingestion of untreated dairy products or other contaminated foods, but can also be by inhalation or inoculation.

Clinical features—symptoms are highly variable, simulating other febrile illnesses, hence travel to endemic areas (with details of drinking and eating behaviour) and occupation are crucial elements in the history. Joint pains, back pain and headache are common (each found in >80% of cases). Signs include spinal tenderness (48%), arthritis (40%), lymphadenopathy (32%), splenomegaly (25%), hepatomegaly (20%), and epididymo-orchitis (21% of men).

Diagnosis and treatment—definite diagnosis requires the isolation of the organism from the blood, body fluids, or tissues. Treatment is with supportive care and antibiotics: regimens containing doxycycline in combination with streptomycin/gentamicin/netilmicin are most effective, incurring fewer therapeutic failures and relapses.

Prevention—human brucellosis can be prevented by eradicating the disease in animals by vaccination. Other preventive measures include avoiding keeping farm animals in close proximity to houses, drinking raw milk and its products, and consumption of raw liver, meat, and bone marrow. There is no effective vaccine for human use.

Aetiological agent

There are four species of *Brucella*, each comprising several biovars: *B. melitensis* ('Malta fever', most commonly associated with goats, sheep, and camels), *B. abortus* (cattle), *B. suis* (pigs), and *B. canis* (dogs). They are small nonencapsulated nonmotile nonsporulating Gram-negative aerobic bacilli. Genomes of *B. abortus*, *B. melitensis*, and *B. suis* have been fully sequenced. They may survive in unpasteurized soft white goat cheese for up to 8 weeks but die within 60 to 90 days in cheese that has undergone lactic acid fermentation. Freezing dairy products or meat does not destroy the organisms but pasteurization or boiling are effective. Organisms shed in animal urine, stool, and products of conception remain viable in soil for 40 days or more.

Epidemiology

The global incidence of human brucellosis is difficult to determine as it is not a notifiable disease in many countries. However, more than 500 000 new cases are reported to the World Health Organization (WHO) each year. In the United States of America, only 4 to 10% of cases are recognized. Illegal importation of unpasteurized dairy products is responsible. Brucellosis is distributed worldwide but is especially prevalent in the Mediterranean region, Indian subcontinent, Mexico, and Central and South America. *B. melitensis* is the commonest cause of brucellosis worldwide. The incidence of human and animal brucellosis is increasing and animal disease has been eradicated in only 17 countries because of the recent expansion of animal industries and lack of scientific and modern methods of animal husbandry. Other factors contribute including traditional eating habits, poor standards of personal and environmental hygiene, methods of processing milk and its products, and the rapid movement of animals both locally and internationally. Control and eradication programmes in animals are expensive and difficult to implement. The ease of modern travel exposes travellers to the disease while visiting endemic countries. In endemic areas, brucellosis affects predominantly young men. Traditionally, farm animals considered as pets are kept in close contact to humans. Childhood disease indicates endemicity in the community. Where animal brucellosis is controlled, human brucellosis is mostly an occupational disease.

Mode of transmission

Ingestion of untreated dairy products, raw meat, liver, or bone marrow are common sources of infection through the gastrointestinal tract. Inhalation is the most frequent occupational hazard in herdsmen, dairy farm workers, meat processers, and laboratory workers. Abattoir workers are commonly infected by pieces of bone penetrating their skin. Veterinary surgeons are vulnerable to accidental autoinoculation or conjunctival contamination by live brucella vaccine while vaccinating animals. Transmission transplacentally or by breast feeding, blood transfusion, marrow or organ transplantation, or sexual intercourse is rare.

Pathogenesis

How brucella survives and replicates inside host macrophages is uncertain. Immunity involves antigen-specific T-cell and humoral responses. Brucella lacks classic virulence factors and typical lipopolysaccharide pathogenicity. However, genes that modify phagocytosis, phagolysosome fusion, cytokine secretion, and apoptosis have been identified. Brucella virulence factor consists of a type IV secretion system responsible for injecting toxins into the cytoplasm of infected cells, resembling the VirB system.

Soon after brucella penetrates the mucosa, there is a polymorphonuclear leucocytosis and migration of activated macrophages to the site of invasion. The initial response is neither antigen nor organism specific (innate immunity), involving γδ T-cell (Vγ9Vδ2), natural killer (NK), and CD4 and CD8 T-cell activation. Lipopolysaccharide on the surface of brucella is recognized by these cells, which activate macrophages and facilitate phagocytosis. Activated γδ T cells may provide the initial γ-interferon (INFγ), tumour necrosis factor-α (TNFα), and other cytokine secretions which become cytotoxic for brucella-infected monocytes and the bacteria, impairing their intracellular survival. Most brucella are rapidly eliminated by phagolysosome fusion. Killing inside macrophages is initiated by cytokines secreted by T-helper cells. Macrophages activate TNFα secretion, initiating a complex cascade of host defence mechanisms, resulting in hydrolytic enzymes and the peroxide–halide system ('oxidative-burst' or 'oxygen-based killing'). Some brucella survive in compartments which are rapidly acidified. Brucella resists being killed by

‡ It is with regret that we report the death of Professor M. Monir Madkour during the preparation of this edition of the textbook.

oxidative-burst using the myeloperoxide–hydrogen peroxide–halide system. Bacteria enter the macrophages through lipid rafts or lipid microdomains. Brucella requires smooth lipopolysaccharide to avoid the bactericidal arsenal of the macrophages.

Impaired Thl immunity, T-cell proliferation, NK-cell cytotoxic activity, and IFNγ production allow invasion. Brucella resists lysosome-mediated killing and phagosome acidification. The mechanism of trafficking of the brucella-containing phagosome within macrophages and the lack of fusion with the lysosome is not understood. Brucella multiplies in the macrophage endoplasmic reticulum without affecting host-cell integrity. The organisms are released by cell lysis and necrosis. Brucella protects infected cells from apoptosis by using IFNγ or TNFα. In the early stage of infection, brucella activates the cAMP/PKA pathway which regulates a variety of mechanisms favouring infection. Brucella later passes through lymphatics to regional lymph nodes, then via the blood stream to all organs of the body particularly those rich in reticuloendothelial tissue. Organ localization is associated with inflammatory cellular infiltrates with or without granuloma formation, caseation, necrosis, or even abscess formation. In the first week of infection, antilipopolysaccharide IgM appears in the serum, followed 1 week later by IgG and IgA which peak during the fourth week. Antilipopolysaccharide antibodies have a limited role in host protection, but are important for diagnosis.

Clinical features

The incubation period ranges from 1 to 3 weeks (maximum several months). Symptoms are highly variable and simulate other febrile illnesses. Travel to endemic areas and occupation are important details in the history. Symptoms may start suddenly (1–2 days) or gradually (1 week or more). Brucellosis is a febrile illness, with or without organ localization. Infection is classified usefully according to whether it is active (i.e. history, clinical features, and significantly raised brucella agglutinins with or without positive blood cultures) and whether it is localized to a particular organ. This determines the treatment regimen and its duration. Classification as acute, subacute, chronic, serological, bacteraemic, or mixed types is not helpful for diagnosis or management. The most frequent symptoms noted in 500 patients with *B. melitensis* who attended the author's clinic are given in Table 7.6.21.1. The fever pattern is neither distinctive nor diagnostic. The patient's temperature is usually normal in the morning and high in the afternoon and evening. Chills or rigors with profuse sweating may simulate malaria. Patients with brucellosis usually look deceptively well. Less frequently, they may look acutely ill. Physical signs may be lacking despite the multiplicity of symptoms. The frequency of physical signs seen in the same group of patients is shown in Table 7.6.21.2.

Table 7.6.21.1 History and symptoms in 500 patients with *B. melitensis* who attended the author's clinic

History/symptoms	Number	Percentage
Animal contact	368	73.6
Raw milk/cheese ingestion	350	70
Raw liver ingestion	147	29.4
Family history	188	37.6
Fever	464	92.8
Chills	410	82.0
Sweating	437	87.4
Body aches	457	91.4
Lack of energy	473	94.6
Joint pain	431	86.2
Back pain	431	86.2
Headaches	403	80.6
Loss of appetite	388	77.6
Weight loss	326	65.2
Constipation	234	46.9
Abdominal pain	225	45.0
Diarrhoea	34	6.8
Cough	122	24.4
Testicular pain (of 290 males)	62	21.3
Rash	72	14.4
Sleep disturbances	185	37.0

Localizations

Septic monoarthritis may result from haematogenous spread to the synovium or via direct extension from neighbouring brucella osteomyelitis (Fig. 7.6.21.1). Knee (Fig. 7.6.21.1), shoulder (Fig. 7.6.21.2a,b), sternoclavicular (Fig. 7.6.21.3), sacroiliac (Fig. 7.6.21.4), and hip (Fig. 7.6.21.5) joints are commonly affected. Joint destruction with loss of function may occur if diagnosis and treatment are delayed. In the spine, infection starts at the superior endplate anteriorly, an area of rich blood supply (Fig. 7.6.21.6). The infection may either regress and heal or progress to involve the entire vertebra, intervertebral disc, and adjacent vertebrae (Fig. 7.6.21.7a,b). Brucella spondylitis may involve single or, less frequently, multiple sites. The lumbar spine, particularly L4, is the most frequent site (Fig. 7.6.21.7a). Extraspinal brucella osteomyelitis is rare but may affect femur, tibia, humerus, or the manubrium sterni (Fig. 7.6.21.8).

Table 7.6.21.2 Signs in 500 patients with *B. melitensis* who attended the author's clinic

Signs	Number	Percentage
Ill looking	127	25.4
Pallor	110	22.0
Lymphadenopathy	160	32.0
Splenomegaly	125	25.0
Hepatomegaly	97	19.4
Arthritis	202	40.4
Spinal tenderness	241	48.0
Epididymo-orchitis (of 290 males)	62	21.3
Skin rash	72	14.4
Jaundice	6	1.2
Central nervous system abnormalities	20	4.0
Cardiac murmur	17	3.4
Pneumonia	7	1.4

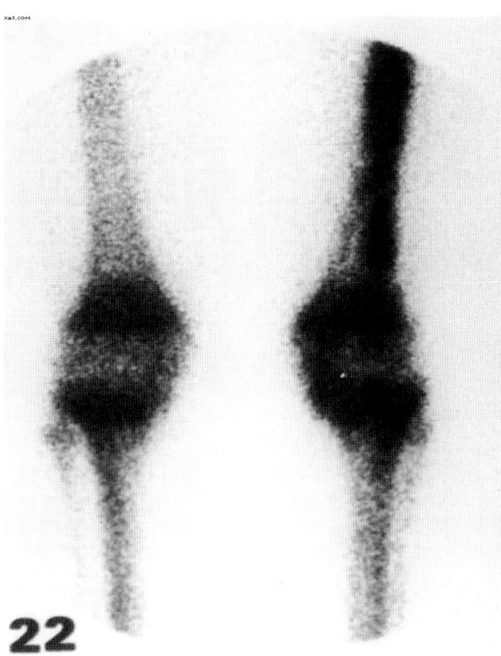

Fig. 7.6.21.1 Brucellar arthritis and osteomyelitis. Scintigram showing increased uptake in the osseous components of the left knee and the distal half of the left femur.

Bursitis, tenosynovitis, and subcutaneous nodules are rare. The peripheral white cell count is normal in brucella septic arthritis and spondylitis. The total white cell count in the synovial fluid ranges from 400 to 40 000/mm^3 with 60% polymorphonuclear cells. Glucose may be reduced and culture is positive in about 50% of cases.

Cardiovascular infections include endocarditis (Fig. 7.6.21.9), myocarditis, pericarditis, aortic root abscess (Fig. 7.6.21.10), mycotic aneurysms, thrombophlebitis, and pulmonary embolism. Patients from endemic areas with 'culture-negative infective endocarditis' should have their blood culture extended for a period of up to 6 weeks. Respiratory symptoms are common but may be missed because they are usually mild. An influenza-like illness with sore throat and mild dry cough is common. Hilar and paratracheal lymphadenopathy, pneumonia (solitary or multiple nodular lung shadows or abscess formation), soft tissue miliary shadowing, pleural effusion, empyema, or mediastinitis are rare.

Gastrointestinal infections are usually mild and are rarely a presenting feature of the disease. They include tonsillitis and hepatitis with mild jaundice (either nonspecific or granulomatous with suppuration and abscess formation); frank cirrhosis is rare. Splenic abscess is rarely reported. Mesenteric lymphadenopathy with abscess formation, cholecystitis, peritonitis, pancreatitis, and ulcerative colitis are described. The liver transaminases, alkaline phosphatase, and serum bilirubin may be mildly raised.

Genitourinary involvement may be the presenting feature of brucellosis: unilateral or bilateral epididymo-orchitis prostatitis or seminal vesiculitis in males; dysmenorrhoea, amenorrhoea, tubo-ovarian abscesses, chronic salpingitis, and cervicitis in female. Acute nephritis or acute pyelonephritis-like features, renal calcifications, and calyceal deformities may occur. Renal granulomatous lesions with abscess formation, caseation, and necrosis may occur, as may cystitis and proximal urethritis.

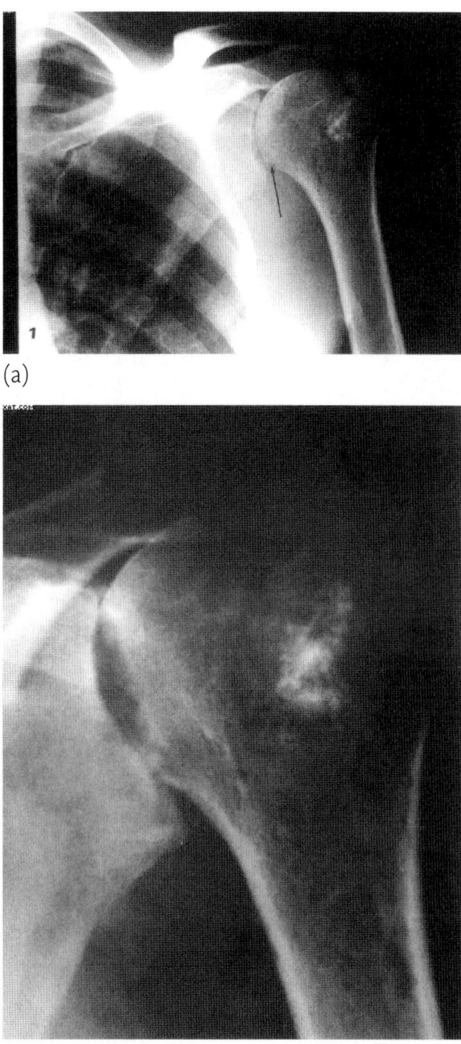

Fig. 7.6.21.2 Destructive brucellar arthritis. (a) Frontal radiograph of the shoulder joint showing diffuse cartilage loss in the glenohumeral joint (arrowed). (b) Radiograph taken 6 months after (a).

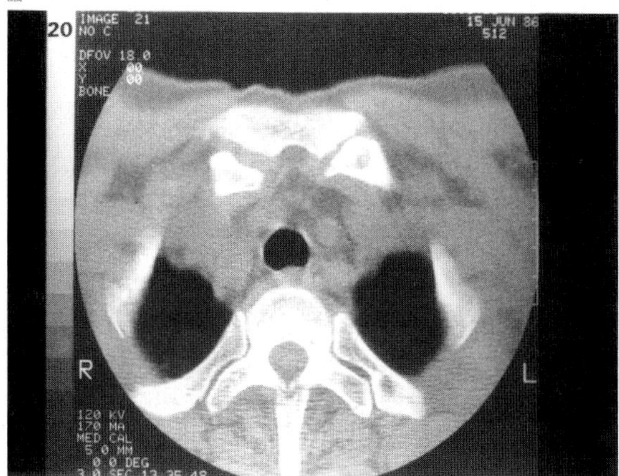

Fig. 7.6.21.3 Destructive brucellar arthritis. High-resolution CT scan showing marked cartilage loss and sternoclavicular erosions in the left sternoclavicular joint.

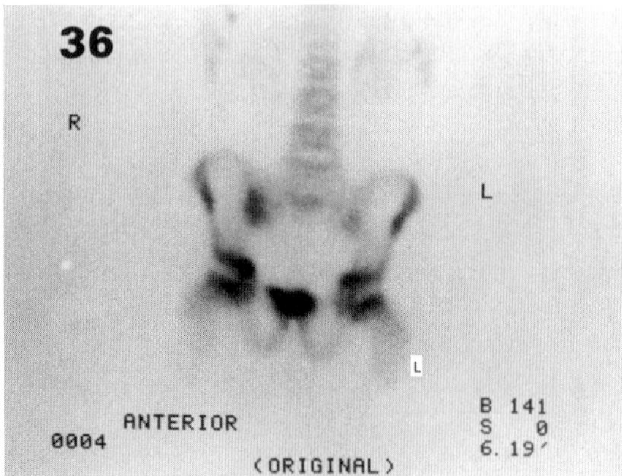

Fig. 7.6.21.4 Brucella sacroiliitis. There is increased uptake in the right sacroiliac joint which can be noted on the anterior view of the scintigram.

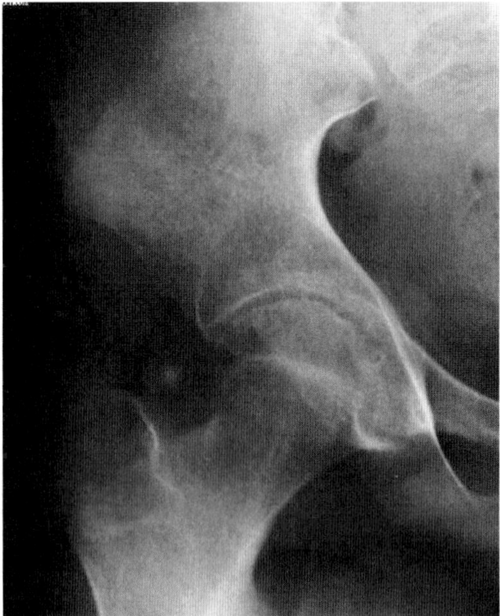

Fig. 7.6.21.5 Destructive brucellar arthritis. Frontal radiograph showing diffuse osteopenia and diffuse cartilage loss in the right hip.

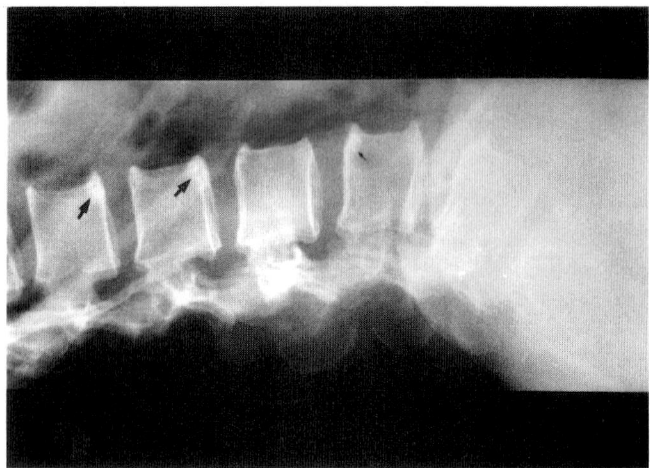

Fig. 7.6.21.6 Early brucellar spondylitis. There is sclerosis at the anterior aspect of the superior endplate of L4 (small arrow). Similar areas are seen in the inferior endplates of L1 and L2 (larger arrows). Note the normal disc spaces.

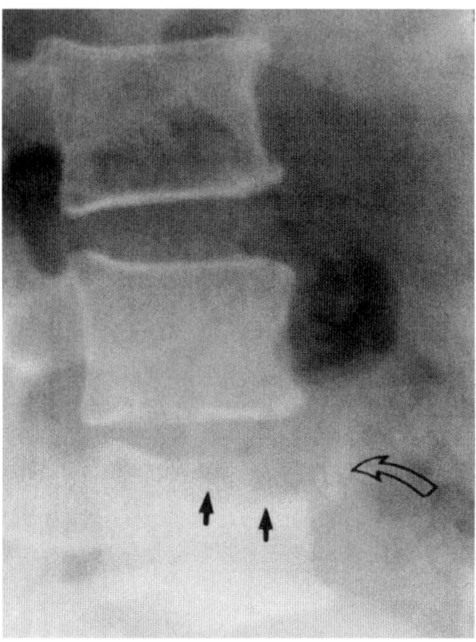

(a)

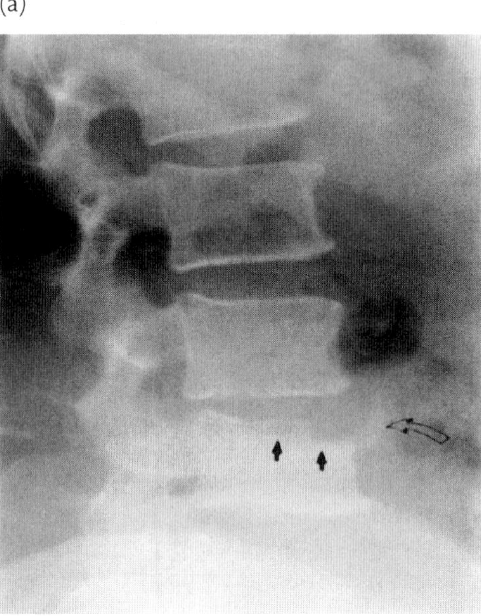

(b)

Fig. 7.6.21.7 (a,b) Progression of brucellar spondylitis to advanced disease. Lateral radiographs show anterior erosions (black arrows), reduction of the L3/L4 disc space and lateral osteophytes (outlined arrow).

Urine culture may be positive in about 50% of patients with brucellosis. Brucella has been isolated from human semen during investigation of possible sexual transmission.

Neurobrucellosis is uncommon but serious and can include meningoencephalitis, multiple cerebral or cerebellar abscesses, ruptured mycotic aneurysm, cranial nerve lesions, transient ischaemic attacks, hemiplegia, myelitis, radiculoneuropathy and neuritis, Guillain–Barré syndrome, a multiple sclerosis-like picture, paraplegia, sciatica, granulomatous myositis, and rhabdomyolysis. Psychiatric features are no more frequent than in other infections. Neurobrucellosis may result from direct blood-borne invasion, pressure from destructive spinal lesions, vasculitis, or an immune-related process.

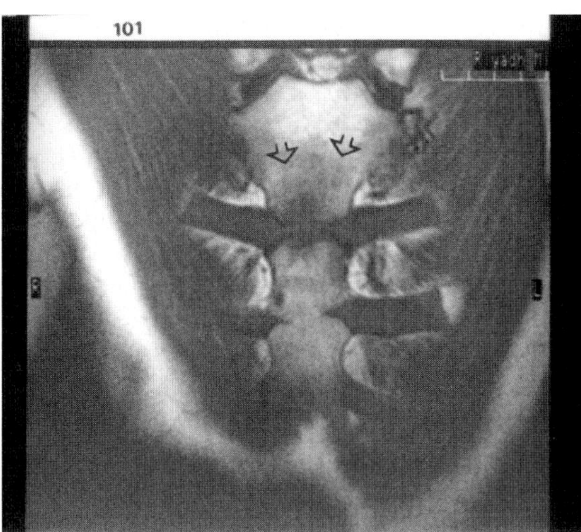

Fig. 7.6.21.8 Brucellar osteomyelitis. MRI of the sternum, coronal cut *T*1-weighted image, showing an area of patchy decreased signal intensity in the lower half of the manubrium (arrows).

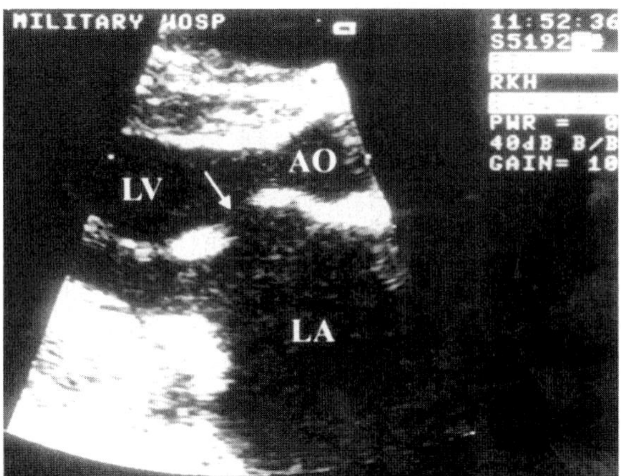

Fig. 7.6.21.9 Brucellar endocarditis. Two-dimensional transthoracic echocardiography showing perforation of the anterior mitral valve leaflet (arrow) due to brucellar endocarditis. AO, aorta; LA, left atrium; LV, left ventricle.

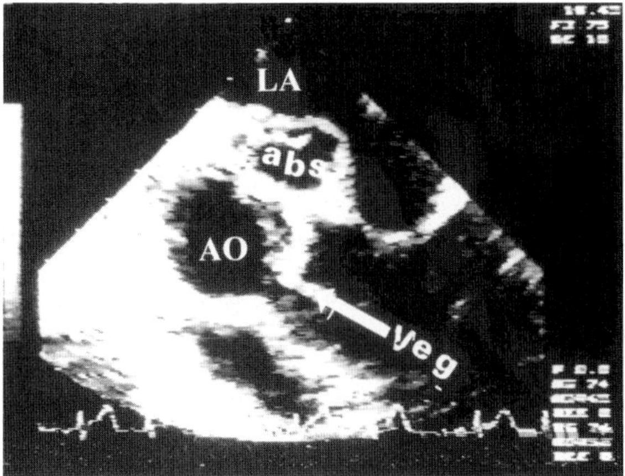

Fig. 7.6.21.10 Horizontal transoesophageal endocardiograph showing brucellar aortic root abscess (abs) and aortic valve vegetation (veg) (arrow). AO, aorta; LA, left atrium.

In meningoencephalitis the cerebrospinal fluid pressure is usually elevated and the fluid may look clear, turbid, or rarely, haemorrhagic. Protein concentration and cells (predominantly lymphocytes) are raised, while glucose may be reduced or normal. Brucella may be cultured from cerebrospinal fluid. Brucella agglutinins in cerebrospinal fluid are usually raised but are sometimes undetectable.

In endemic areas, pregnant women may experience abortion, intrauterine fetal death, premature delivery, and retention of the placenta and other products of conception. They may transmit infection by breast feeding.

The uncommon skin manifestations include maculopapular eruptions, contact dermatitis (particularly among veterinary surgeons and farmers assisting animal parturition), erythema nodosum, purpura, petechiae, chronic ulcerations, multiple cutaneous and subcutaneous abscesses, vasculitis, superficial thrombophlebitis, discharging sinuses, and, rarely, pemphigus.

Splashing live brucella vaccine into the eyes may cause conjunctivitis. Keratitis, corneal ulcers, uveitis, retinopathies, subconjunctival and retinal haemorrhages, retinal detachment, and endogenous endophthalmitis with positive vitreous cultures are well documented.

Diagnosis

Definite diagnosis of brucellosis requires the isolation of the organism from the blood, body fluids, or tissues. Positive blood culture yield ranges between 40 and 70%. Extended culture for up to 6 weeks using biphasic culture media (solid and liquid) or with the Castaneda bottle (incubated at 37°C with and without an atmosphere of carbon dioxide) is commonly used. Automated culture systems are more sensitive and rapid. Bone marrow culture may rarely be required. Brucella species and biotypes are differentiated by their carbon dioxide requirements; ability to use glutamic acid, ornithine, lysine, and ribose; hydrogen sulphide production; growth in the presence of thionine or basic fuchsin dyes; agglutination by antisera directed against certain lipopolysaccharide epitopes; and susceptibility to lysis by bacteriophage. Molecular diagnosis is achieved by polymerase chain reaction (PCR) and 16S rRNA-based fluorescence *in situ* hybridization assay. Many varieties of PCR have been developed, including restriction fragment length polymorphism (PCR-RFLP), nested PCR, real-time PCR, and PCR–enzyme-linked immunosorbent assay (ELISA). They have superior specificity and sensitivity. Identification of specific antibodies against bacterial lipopolysaccharide and other antigens can be detected by the standard agglutination test (SAT), rose Bengal, 2-mercaptoethanol (2-ME), antihuman globulin (Coombs' test), and indirect ELISA. The SAT is the most commonly used serological test in endemic areas. An agglutination titre of 1:160 or higher is considered significant in nonendemic areas and 1:320 or higher in endemic areas.

Since the O-polysaccharide of brucella is similar to that of various other Gram-negative bacteria (e.g. *Francisella tularensis*, *Escherichia coli*, *Salmonella urbana*, *Yersinia enterocolitica*, *Vibrio cholera*, *Xanthomonas maltophilia*), cross-reactions of IgM may occur. The inability to diagnose *B. canis* by SAT due to lack of cross-reaction is another drawback. False-negative SATs may be caused by the presence of blocking antibodies (the prozone phenomenon) in the α_2-globulin (IgA) and in the α-globulin (IgG) fractions. New dipstick assays, based on the binding of brucella IgM antibodies, have proved simple, accurate, and rapid.

ELISAs typically use cytoplasmic proteins as antigens. They detect IgM, IgG, and IgA without some of the shortcomings of the SAT. PCR is fast and specific.

In other laboratory investigations, the peripheral white cell count is normal or occasionally reduced with relative lymphocytosis. Blood biochemistry is commonly normal.

Treatment

Two classic regimens, doxycycline plus streptomycin (DS) or doxycycline plus rifampicin (DR), are recommended by the WHO and have been used all over the world for outpatient management; they have remained effective for many years. Doxycycline (preferred to other tetracyclines) is the most effective agent for the treatment of brucellosis. Its activity is enhanced by the acidic environment of the macrophage phagolysosomes. Regimens containing doxycycline are associated with fewer therapeutic failures and relapses than other regimens. The streptomycin-containing regimen is slightly more efficacious in preventing relapses as rifampicin reduces doxycycline levels in the serum. Doxycycline is given by mouth, 100 mg 12-hourly for 6 weeks; streptomycin is given intramuscularly, 15 mg/kg daily for 2 to 3 weeks; and rifampicin is given by mouth, 600 to 900 mg daily for 6 weeks. Patients with spondylitis, endocarditis, neurobrucellosis, and abscesses may require hospitalization for surgery (urgent valve replacement or drainage of abscesses) and triple antibiotics (doxycycline, aminoglycoside, and rifampicin) for a period of up to 6 months. The overall therapeutic failure rate ranges from 3 to 10%. Parenteral administration of aminoglycoside and the risk of nephrotoxicity and ototoxicity require monitoring. Monotherapy has been abandoned because of unacceptably high rates of therapeutic failure and relapse.

Since 1990, an alternative regimen has been used. Gentamicin or netilmicin are administered intramuscularly or intravenously as a single daily dose of 5 mg/kg for 7 days with doxycycline 100 mg 12-hourly for 45 days. This proved as effective as the DS regimen. In my experience, longer duration of gentamicin plus doxycycline (GD) or netilmicin plus doxycycline (ND) for 14 to 28 days, followed by doxycycline alone for a further 30 to 60 days was associated with no therapeutic failures and only 3% relapse/reinfection rate. Co-trimoxazole by mouth, two tablets (480 mg each) twice daily for 2 months plus doxycycline (CD) or plus rifampicin (CR) have been used; CD proved to be better than CR. In endemic areas, tuberculosis may also be common and the use of rifampicin may be restricted to avoid the emergence of resistance.

Quinolones (ciprofloxacin and ofloxacin) have been used in a limited number of clinical studies in patients without localizations. The activity of quinolones is decreased in the acidic environment of macrophage phagolysosomes but quinolones may have some role in replacing doxycycline or rifampicin when toxicity occurs. Quinolones may be used as second-line regimen in patients who fail to respond or develop relapse after using other regimens. Ofloxacin is given by mouth, 400 mg 12-hourly plus doxycycline or rifampicin combination for 6 weeks. Ciprofloxacin is given by mouth, 500 mg 12-hourly, in combination with doxycycline or rifampicin for 6 weeks. The expense of quinolones is a major draw back. The macrolide azithromycin is rapidly distributed into tissue and cells, particularly phagocytes. However, the acidic macrophage phagolysosomal environment reduces its activity and there were high rates of therapeutic failure and relapses when used against *B. melitensis*.

Children younger than 8 years with brucellosis are treated with the CR regimen. Rifampicin can be given orally or intravenously as a single dose of 10 to 20 mg/kg per day. Co-trimoxazole is given by intravenous infusion, 36 to 54 mg/kg per day in two divided doses. A paediatric suspension is given by mouth, 240 mg/ml 12-hourly.

Oral minocycline 2.5 mg/kg in combination with intravenous rifampicin 10 mg/kg (both given 12-hourly) for 3 weeks proved effective in infants and children in Italy. No dental defects were observed. Pregnant women with brucellosis are treated with the CR regimen. In patients with renal impairment, blood urea, creatinine, and aminoglycoside levels should be carefully monitored or else DR should be used.

Therapeutic response is assessed by improvement of symptoms (within 14 days) and signs (within 2–4 weeks) after starting antibiotics. Lack of clinical improvement 14 days after starting antibiotics until the end of therapy indicates therapeutic failure. Serological tests are not ideal for monitoring response. Titres may not decline and, if the patient develops a Jarisch–Herxheimer reaction with initial worsening of symptoms a few days after starting treatment, the titre may increase. In the first 3 months after completion of treatment, SAT titres decline to less than 1:320 in only 8.3% of patients and in 71.4% after 2 years or more. Of cured patients, 28.6% continue to have a titre of 1:320 or higher, 2 years after completion of clinically successful treatment. Patients receiving doxycycline in the treatment regimen are more likely to achieve serological cure than those who did not. Relapse is indicated by recurrence of clinical features and rise in agglutination titre, with or without positive blood culture, usually in the first 3 to 6 months but may be up to 1 year after completion of treatment. In endemic areas, reinfection may be difficult to differentiate from relapse.

Prevention

Human brucellosis can be prevented by eradicating the disease in animals by vaccination. There are five effective and marketed animal vaccines: *B. abortus* 4-5/20, *B. melitensis* Rev. 1, *B. suis* strain 2, *B. abortus* strain 19, and *B. abortus* RB51. These vaccines offer an animal protection rate of between 65% and 90%. Other preventive measures include changing the habits and traditions of keeping farm animals in close proximity to houses, drinking raw milk and its products, and consuming raw liver, meat, and bone marrow. Currently there is no effective vaccine for human use.

Further reading

Al Dahouk S, *et al.* (2005). Identification of brucella species and biotypes using polymerase chain reaction fragment length polymorphism (PCR-RFLP). *Clin Rev Microbiol*, **31**, 191–6.

Cascio A, *et al.* (2004). No findings of dental defects in children treated with minocycline. *Antimicrob Agents Chemother*, **48**, 2739–41.

Celli J, Gorvel J (2004). Organelle robbery: brucella interactions with the endoplasmic reticulum. *Curr Opin Microbiol*, **7**, 93–7.

Clavijo E, *et al.* (2003). Comparison of a dipstick assay for detection of brucella-specific immunoglobulin M antibodies with other tests for serodiagnosis of human brucellosis. *Clin Diagn Lab Immunol*, **10**, 612–15.

Falagas ME, Bliziotis IA (2006). Quinolones for treatment of human brucellosis: critical review of the evidence from microbiological and clinical studies. *Antimicrob Agents Chemother*, **50**, 22–33.

Ficht TA, *et al.* (2009). Brucellosis: the case for live, attenuated vaccines. *Vaccine*, **27**, Suppl 4, D40–3.

Franco MP, *et al.* (2007). Human brucellosis. *Lancet Infect Dis*, **7**, 775–86.

Ismail TF, *et al.* (2002). Evaluation of dipstick serologic tests for diagnosis of brucellosis and typhoid fever in Egypt. *J Clin Microbiol*, **40**, 3509–11.

Madkour MM (ed) (2001). *Madkour's brucellosis*, 2nd edition. Springer, Berlin.
Mantur BG, Amarnath SK. Brucellosis in India - a review. *J Biosci*, **33**, 539–47.
Maria-Pilar JB, *et al.* (2005). Cellular bioterrorism: how brucella corrupts macrophage physiology to promote invasion and proliferation. *Clin Immunol*, **114**, 227–38.
Morata P, *et al.* (2003). Development and evaluation of a PCR–enzyme-linked immunosorbent assay for diagnosis of human brucellosis. *J Clin Microbiol*, **41**, 144–8.
Oliveira SC, de Oliveira FS, Macedo GC, *et al.* (2008). The role of innate immune receptors in the control of *Brucella abortus* infection: toll-like receptors and beyond. *Microbes Infet*, **10**, 1005–9.
Pappas G, *et al.* (2006). The new global map of human brucellosis. *Lancet Infect Dis*, **6**, 91–9.
Roop RM 2nd, Gaines JM, Anderson ES, *et al.* (2009). Survival of the fittest: how Brucella strains adapt to their intracellular niche in the host. *Med Microbiol Immunol*, **198**, 221–38.
Skalsky K, Yahav D, Bishara J, *et al.* (2008). Treatment of human brucellosis: systematic review and meta-analysis of randomised controlled trials. *BMJ*, **336**, 701–4.
Wellinghausen N, *et al.* (2006). Rapid detection of *Brucellosis* spp. in blood cultures by fluorescence in situ hybridization. *J Clin Microbiol*, **44**, 1828–30.
Whatmore AM (2009). Current understanding of the genetic diversity of Brucella, an expanding genus of zoonotic pathogens. *Infect Genet Evol*, **9**, 1168–84.
Yingst S, Hoover DH (2003). T cell immunity to brucellosis. *Crit Rev Microbiol*, **29**, 313–31.

7.6.22 **Tetanus**

C.L. Thwaites and Lam Minh Yen

Essentials

Clostridium tetani is a Gram-positive, spore-forming anaerobic bacterium that is ubiquitous, being found throughout the world in human and animal faeces, soil, and street dust. In children and adults, superficial skin wounds are the common entry sites, although in 20% no portal of entry can be found.

Pathophysiology—under favourable anaerobic conditions, clostridial spores germinate and bacteria grow and multiply, producing a pathogenic toxin which—either locally or after circulation in the bloodstream—enters motor nerves, with the eventual effect of preventing discharge of γ-aminobutyric acid (GABA) inhibitory interneurons, resulting in unrestricted motor nerve activity, increased muscle tone, and spasms characteristic of tetanus.

Clinical features—after an incubation period of 7 to 14 days the disease presents with symptoms including trismus ('lockjaw', 98%), muscle stiffness (95%), back pain (94%), dysphagia (83%), muscle spasms (46%, with 'risus sardonicus' due to facial muscle spasm), and difficulty breathing (7%). Life-threatening complications include laryngeal muscle spasms and spasm and hypertonus of the respiratory muscles, and in severe cases there are violent autonomic disturbances. Tetanus continues to be a common cause of death in developing countries.

Diagnosis and treatment—tetanus is a clinical diagnosis: the presence of generalized muscle rigidity with trismus being characteristic, and risus sardonicus virtually pathognomonic. Key elements of treatment are (1) wound toilet and antibiotics, usually metronidazole; (2) antitoxin—most commonly human tetanus immune globulin 100 to 300 IU/kg intramuscularly; (3) spasm control—benzodiazepines are the first-line agents, with chlorpromazine, phenbarbitone, and propafol as alternatives; (4) control of any autonomic disturbance. Many patients require intensive care management and nursing.

Prevention—tetanus has largely been eliminated in countries with good immunization programmes and standards of hygiene. The World Health Organization recommendation is for a primary immunization course of three doses in infancy, followed by boosters aged 4 to 7 years and 12 to 15 years, with a further dose given in adult life. All patients with tetanus require a full course of active immunization as the disease itself does not confer long-lasting immunity.

Historical perspective

> Tychon the soldier [was hit by] an arrow in his back ... [He] sounded like someone gnashing his teeth in a fury of rage... He was arched back in opisthotonos, his jaws locked together against his will. A friend forced some wine between his teeth, but Tychon could not swallow, and the liquid was expelled in spurts from his nostrils.
>
> Hippocrates (*c*.425 BC)

Tetanus has been known since ancient times, with the earliest descriptions included in the Edwin Smith papyrus of ancient Egypt (1000 BC). It has been a well-recognized complication of battle injuries (Fig. 7.6.22.1). In 1880, Nicolaier demonstrated that soil contamination of wounds resulted in tetanus and discovered the bacterium responsible when he isolated *Clostridium tetani* bacilli from wounds. Ten years later Faber discovered tetanus toxin, and von Behring and Kitasato produced the first antitoxin. Ramon detoxified tetanus toxin and in 1926 performed the first successful vaccination of humans. Tetanus vaccination was introduced to British armed forces in 1938, and during the 1950s was gradually incorporated into infant immunization programmes throughout the United Kingdom, finally becoming part of the national schedule in 1961.

Aetiology, genetics, pathogenesis, and pathology

Tetanus results from wound inoculation. In neonates the umbilical stump is the usual portal of entry. The bacteria are ubiquitous and have been found throughout the world in human and animal faeces, soil, street dust, and even the air of operating theatres. *C. tetani* is a Gram-positive spore-forming anaerobic bacterium. Under favourable anaerobic conditions the spores will germinate and the bacteria grow and multiply producing the pathogenic toxin. Tetanus toxin (tetanospasmin) is a 150-kDa protein consisting of one heavy and one light chain linked by a disulphide bond. The amino acid sequence is similar to that of the botulinum toxins and the toxins act in similar ways, but as botulinum toxins are not transported into the central nervous system they produce a different clinical picture.

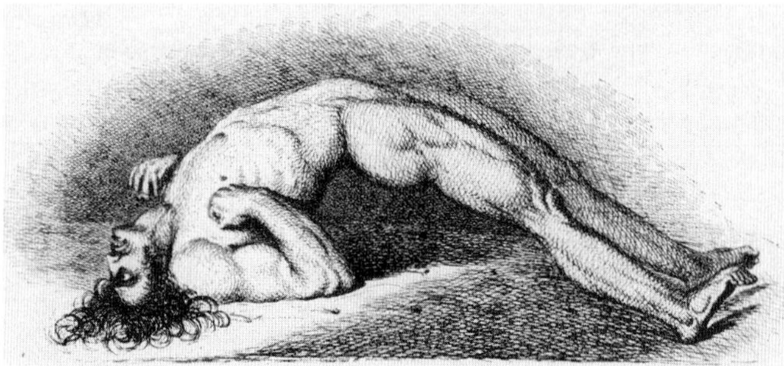

Fig. 7.6.22.1 Opisthotonus in a soldier wounded at the battle of Corunna (1809) and illustrated by Sir Charles Bell in his *The Anatomy and Philosophy of Human Expression* (1832).

The heavy chain of the tetanus toxin mediates toxin entry into the motor nerves, either locally or after circulation in the bloodstream. Its motor specificity is due to binding to specific domains within the motor nerve membrane. The heavy chain is also necessary for the subsequent retrograde axonal transport of the toxin and its passage across the synaptic cleft, where it preferentially enters γ-aminobutyric acid (GABA) inhibitory interneurons. The light chain of the toxin is a zinc-dependent endopeptidase that cleaves vesicle-associated membrane protein II (VAMP II or synaptobrevin) at a single peptide bond. This molecule is essential for synaptic release of neurotransmitters and cleavage disrupts synaptic transmission. By preventing inhibitory discharge, unrestricted motor nerve activity occurs, resulting in the increased muscle tone and spasms characteristic of tetanus. In severe forms of tetanus the autonomic nervous system is also affected giving rise to marked cardiovascular instability.

Epidemiology

In countries with good immunization programmes and standards of hygiene tetanus has largely been eliminated, but in poorer areas tetanus remains a common cause of morbidity and mortality, particularly of neonates but also of children and young adults. In 1988, an estimated 787 000 neonatal deaths occurred, prompting the World Health Assembly to call for the elimination of tetanus by 1995. Slow progress resulted in this goal being postponed until 2000 and then 2005 (when maternal tetanus was added). In 2002, the total number of deaths due to tetanus worldwide was estimated to be 213 000, of which 180 000 were estimated to be neonatal and 15 000 to 30 000 maternal. These numbers are likely to be underestimates as less than 10% of neonatal tetanus cases and deaths are reported and probably similar numbers of tetanus cases in other age groups. Although progress has undoubtedly been achieved, at the end of 2005 there remained 49 countries with incidence rates greater than the target 'elimination' rate (defined as less than one case of neonatal tetanus per 1000 live births in every district).

Neonatal tetanus is usually acquired through contamination of the umbilical stump and is associated with delivery on unclean surfaces or traditional midwifery practices such as cutting the umbilical cord with bamboo or applying soil to the umbilical stump. Mortality rates are high, often greater than 90% in areas with few resources, and even in those with good facilities mortality remains approximately 40 to 50%.

In children and adults, superficial skin wounds are the common entry sites, although in 20% no portal of entry can be found. Mortality is higher with deep entry sites such as postoperative infections, intramuscular injections, or postpartum. Injecting drug users (especially those using the skin 'popping' method of administration) are prone to develop a particularly severe form of tetanus.

Prevention

Tetanus is preventable by immunization and good hygiene. Tetanus vaccines are made from tetanus toxoid adsorbed onto aluminium to increase immunogenicity. They are available as single-dose tetanus toxoid (TT) or combined with diphtheria toxoid. There are two preparations of the latter: (1) DT or high dose for use in children under 7 years and (2) dT or low dose for use in older people. Further combinations of DT or dT are available with whole cell or acellular pertussis (DTwP, DtaP, dTwP, or dTaP). In addition, preparations are now available containing *Haemophilus influenzae* B, hepatitis B, or polio. Tetanus toxoid or standard combinations are safe and effective and adverse events are mild and infrequent. They can be used during pregnancy or in immunodeficient people, including those with HIV, but responses may be diminished. Adequate tetanus vaccination requires a primary course (three doses), boosters (two or three), and further boosters after tetanus-prone wounds.

The World Health Organization (WHO) recommend that five doses of vaccine should be given during childhood: a primary immunization course of three doses in infancy followed by boosters between the ages of 4 and 7 years and 12 and 15 years. They differ from current United Kingdom guidelines by recommending a further booster in adult life, e.g. during a woman's first pregnancy. In the United Kingdom, a total of five doses is recommended. Further doses are deemed necessary only after tetanus-prone wounds (see below).

In nonimmunized adolescents and adults, a three-dose primary course is recommended. The first two doses should be given at least 4 weeks apart and the third at least 6 months after the second. In these people, a total of five doses is expected to confer lifelong protection. This schedule is also recommended for pregnant women with incomplete or unknown vaccination histories who should be given at least two doses (usually dT) at least 4 weeks apart during the pregnancy, a third 6 months later, and two boosters at yearly intervals. If they have had a primary course in infancy, two further doses (at least 4 weeks apart) are recommended. This can be reduced to one dose if they also had a childhood booster. A final (sixth) booster at least 1 year later should confer lifelong immunity.

Booster doses of tetanus toxoid should also be given after certain tetanus-prone wounds (Table 7.6.22.1). In very high-risk situations, additional passive immunization should be given using human or equine tetanus immune globulin.

Clinical features

Symptoms evolve gradually over a period of days and weeks or, in very severe cases, hours, and the time course is divided into specific periods. The incubation period is the period from inoculation to the first symptom (therefore may be unknown if no entry site is found) and is usually around 7 to 14 days. The period of onset is the period from the first symptoms to the first spasm and is usually 2 to 5 days. Both these periods can be shorter in severe disease which tends to progress more rapidly. The initial symptoms complained of on admission by 2422 patients (excluding neonates)

Table 7.6.22.1 Management of tetanus-prone wounds

Wound type		Active immunization	Passive immunization
Clean wound		Only if vaccination history incomplete (i.e. give booster if not up to date or initiate primary course as described in text)	No
Low risk tetanus-prone	**1** Wounds or burns: Requiring surgical intervention or when treatment delayed >6 h With significant degree of devitalized tissue Containing foreign bodies Individuals with systemic sepsis **2** Puncture-type injury, particularly in contact with soil and/or manure **3** Open fractures	Only if vaccination history incomplete (i.e. give booster if not up to date or initiate primary course as described in text)	If vaccination history incomplete, one dose human immune globulin (in different site to vaccination)
High risk tetanus-prone	As above but with heavy contamination with material likely to contain tetanus spores and/or extensive devitalized tissue	Only if vaccination history incomplete (i.e. give booster if not up to date or initiate primary course as described in text)	All one dose human immune globulin (in different site to vaccination, if given)

admitted to the Hospital for Tropical diseases, Ho Chi Minh City, are shown in Table 7.6.22.2.

As tetanus develops, muscle tone gradually increases until spasms occur. In the face trismus ('lockjaw') commonly occurs (Fig. 7.6.22.2) and the characteristic risus sardonicus is seen due to facial muscle spasm. Involvement of the erector spinae group of muscles results in opisthotonus (Fig. 7.6.22.3). Sometimes, tetanus is confined to a local group of muscles producing only local muscle spasm. If this occurs in the head, it is termed 'cephalic tetanus' (Fig. 7.6.22.4). Unlike local tetanus elsewhere, this form is potentially dangerous if laryngeal muscle spasms cause airway obstruction leading to asphyxiation. This occurs commonly in generalized tetanus and is a life-threatening emergency. Respiratory tract secretions are increased in tetanus, due perhaps to a combination of autonomic nervous system stimulation and pharyngeal and laryngeal muscle spasms that prevent swallowing. Spasm and hypertonus of the respiratory muscles is a serious occurrence that, without artificial respiratory support, is a common cause of death in tetanus.

In centres having facilities to control muscle spasm and provide mechanical ventilation, autonomic system effects are responsible for a second group of major complications. The syndrome of autonomic instability usually takes the form of labile hypertension and tachycardia which is difficult to control. However, it may manifest as more sustained hypertension and tachycardia or, less commonly but more seriously, with periods of hypotension and bradyarrhythmias.

Table 7.6.22.2 Presenting clinical features of tetanus

Symptom	Percentage of admissions
Trismus	98
Dysphagia	83
Back pain	94
Muscle stiffness	95
Muscle spasms	46
Difficulty breathing	7
Fever	8

It is associated with acute renal failure (nonoliguric or oliguric) and adult respiratory distress syndrome (ARDS).

The clinical severity of tetanus is commonly described using a modified version of the score described by Ablett (Table 7.6.22.3).

Neonatal tetanus has a similar clinical picture (Fig. 7.6.22.5). Abnormalities of muscle tone usually present as difficulty in feeding and crying and is followed by frank spasms. The WHO define neonatal tetanus as 'an illness occurring in a child who has the normal ability to suck and cry in the first 2 days of life but who loses this ability between days 3 and 28 of life and becomes rigid and has spasms'. Fluctuations in blood pressure and heart rate are common, as are secondary infections and septicaemia.

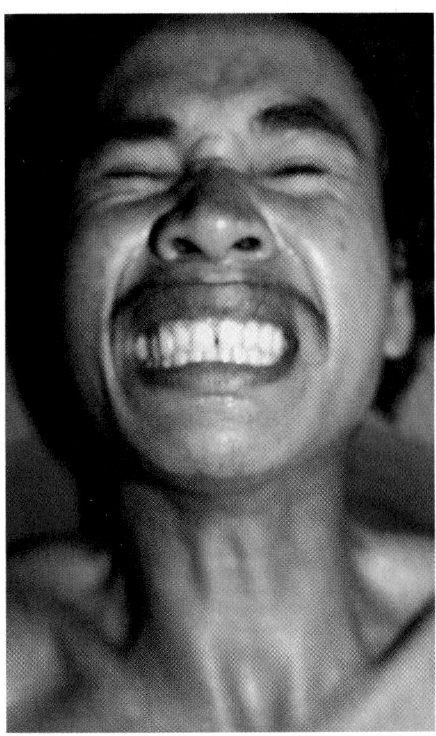

Fig. 7.6.22.2 Risus sardonicus resulting from trismus.
(Courtesy of the late Professor Sornchai Looareesuwan.)

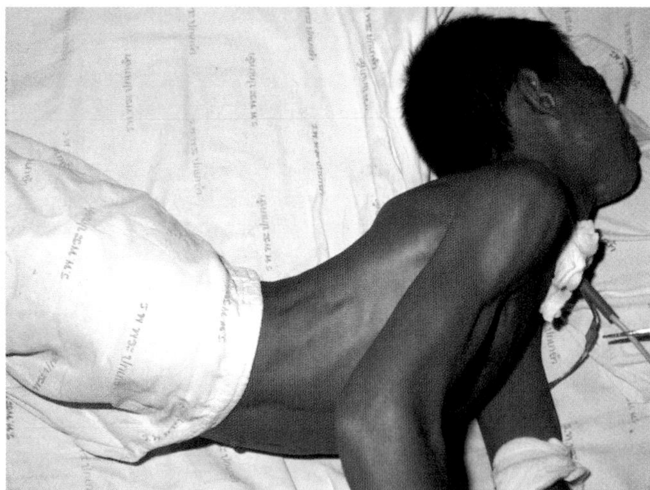

Fig. 7.6.22.3 Opisthotonus.
(Copyright D A Warrell.)

Severity of illness can be predicted on admission from clinical measures. Previously the Dakar (described 1975) and Phillips (described 1967) scores have been used, but the recent tetanus severity score shows superior predictive value. This score (Table 7.6.22.4) is simple to use, is calculated using only baseline observation data and features of the history, and is, therefore, suitable for use in most clinical settings.

Differential diagnosis

Tetanus is a clinical diagnosis. Presence of generalized muscle rigidity with trismus are characteristic, and the risus sardonicus virtually pathognomonic. Wound cultures commonly do not yield *C. tetani*.

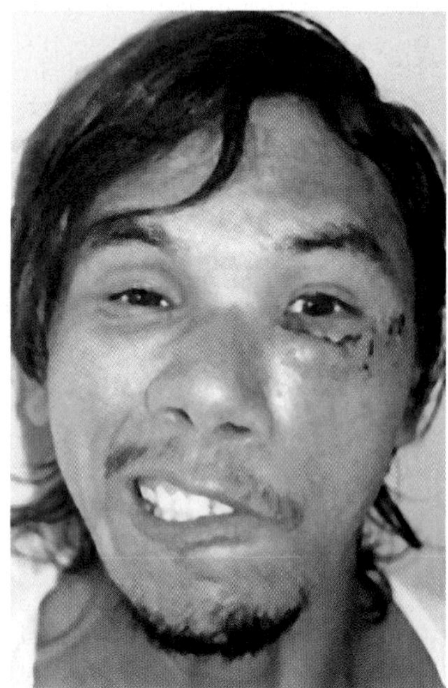

Fig. 7.6.22.4 Brazilian patient with local tetanus confined to muscles innervated by the left VIIth cranial nerve and with trismus, showing the wound causing the infection.
(Courtesy of Dr Pedro Pardal, Belém, Brazil.)

Table 7.6.22.3 Ablett score

Grade	Clinical features
I	Mild to moderate trismus (little or no dysphagia) General spasticity No respiratory embarrassment No spasms
II	Moderate trismus Well-marked rigidity Mild to moderate but short spasms Moderate respiratory embarrassment with an increased respiratory rate greater than 30 breaths/min Mild dysphagia
III	Severe trismus Generalized spasticity Reflex prolonged spasms Increased respiratory rate greater than 40 breaths/min Apnoeic spells Severe dysphagia Tachycardia greater than 120 beats/min
IV	Grade III and violent autonomic disturbances involving the cardiovascular system Severe hypertension and tachycardia alternating with relative hypotension and bradycardia, either of which may be persistent

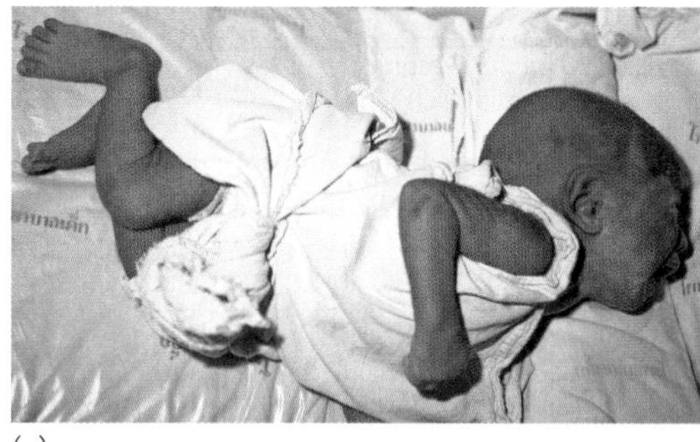

(a)

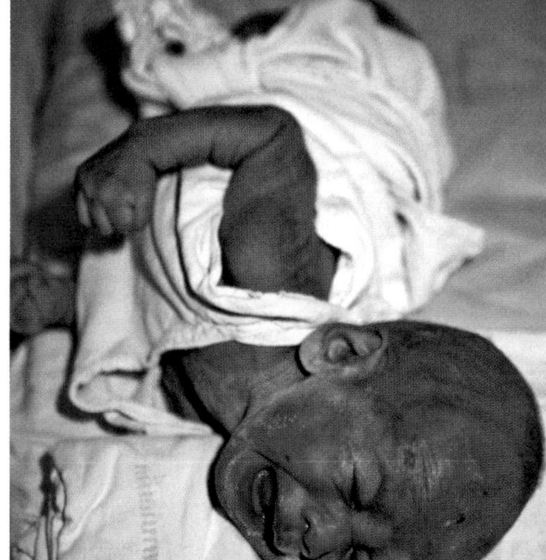

(b)

Fig. 7.6.22.5 (a, b) Neonatal tetanus showing opisthotonus and clenched fist.
(Copyright D A Warrell.)

Table 7.6.22.4 Tetanus severity score (TSS), calculated from the total of individual section scores

		Score
Age (years)	≤70	0
	71–80	5
	>80	10
Time from first symptom to admission (days)	≤2	0
	3–5	−5
	>5	−6
Difficulty breathing on admission	No	0
	Yes	4
Coexisting medical conditions[a]	Fit and well	0
	Minor illness or injury	3
	Moderately severe illness	5
	Severe illness not immediately life-threatening	5
	Immediately life-threatening illness	9
Entry site[b]	Internal or injection	7
	Other (including unknown)	0
Highest systolic blood pressure recorded during first day in hospital (mmHg)	≤130	0
	131–140	2
	>140	4
Highest heart rate recorded during first day in hospital (beats/min)	≤100	0
	101–110	1
	111–120	2
	>120	4
Lowest heart rate recorded during first day in hospital (beats/min)	≤110	0
	>110	−2
Highest temperature recorded during first day in hospital (°C)	≤38.5	0
	38.6–39	4
	39.1–40	6
	>40	8[c]

[a] Defined according to the American Society of Anesthesiologists' physical status scale.
[b] 'Internal' site includes postoperative / postpartum or open fractures; 'injection' includes intramuscular, subcutaneous, or intravenous injections.
[c] Scores ≥ 8 are associated with worse prognosis.

The differential diagnosis includes local causes of trismus and pharyngeal muscle spasm such as oropharyngeal infection or temporomandibular joint pathology.

Rabies, like tetanus, may result from an infected animal bite, but its incubation period is usually much longer (Chapter 7.5.10). Hydrophobic spasms may resemble tetanic spasms, particularly in the case of cephalic tetanus.

Strychnine is a competitive antagonist of the inhibitory neurotransmitter glycine that causes hyperreflexia and severe muscle spasms leading to convulsions. It may be very hard to distinguish this from tetanus. The diagnosis may be suggested by a history of ingestion and confirmed by toxicological tests of urine, serum, or gastric contents. Clinically the continuous muscle rigidity characteristic of tetanus is not present, although this may be difficult to detect with frequent convulsions.

Other causes of muscle tone abnormality are dystonic reactions to antidopaminergic drugs such as metoclopramide or phenothiazines. These may be associated with torticollis or eye and tongue movements which are not features of tetanus. The administration of anticholinergics and withdrawal of the precipitating drug can eliminate these.

In children, hypocalcaemic tetany and meningoencephalitis may present with some of the features of tetanus, but more careful clinical examination and investigation will differentiate these.

Management

The three principal areas of management are wound toilet, spasm control, and control of any autonomic disturbance. Wounds should be cleaned adequately and, if necessary, surgically debrided. Antibiotics are given to prevent further bacterial multiplication, either penicillin or metronidazole. Metronidazole is generally preferred as it does not have penicillin's epileptogenic potential. Patients treated with metronidazole may have fewer spasms than those treated with penicillin.

Antitoxin is given to neutralize any unbound toxin and, if given early enough, may limit the severity of tetanus. Recent debate has centred on whether an intrathecal route would be more effective. An existing meta-analysis failed to show any benefit, but a recent randomized controlled trial showed that patients given intrathecal human tetanus immune globulin (HTIG) had less severe tetanus and a shorter duration of mechanical ventilation and hospital stay. Preparations containing thimerosal must never be given intrathecally. If given by conventional methods, HTIG is given at a dose of 100 to 300 IU/kg intramuscularly. If this is unavailable or too expensive, as is the case in countries where most tetanus occurs, equine antitoxin (500–1000 IU/kg intramuscularly) is an alternative. However, its use is associated with an increased risk of anaphylactic reactions.

Spasms are treated with benzodiazepines as first-line agents. Diazepam is the commonest choice due to its low cost and widespread availability, but other preparations such as midazolam are more suited to long-term administration. High-dose regimes are commonly used, such as diazepam 100 mg/h intravenously. Other agents that may be used include phenobarbitone or chlorpromazine. Chlorpromazine has the potential advantage of α-adrenergic antagonistic activity and has been used alone or as an adjunct. In 1966, Hendrickse reported one of the few randomized trials comparing diazepam, chlorpromazine, and phenobarbitone with chlorpromazine and phenobarbitone alone in 104 neonates and 45 older children. Mortality in the neonates was identical but in the older children the death rate was almost halved in those treated with diazepam, although numbers were too small to reach statistical significance. More modern sedatives such as propofol can also be used, although there are limited data to provide efficacy and safety profiles.

Autonomic disturbance of severe tetanus is difficult to treat. Heavy sedation is used as a means of improving cardiovascular stability. Intravenous morphine is commonly used as it inhibits central sympathetic discharge resulting in peripheral arteriolar vasodilatation. Other authors report the use of calcium antagonists or other vasodilators to reduce blood pressure in hypertension. More recently, several trials have been published using magnesium sulphate to treat tetanus. Initially its use was intended to reduce the autonomic instability of severe tetanus, but it also has muscle relaxant properties that may be beneficial in all patients with tetanus. Results of a randomized controlled trial have shown that intravenous magnesium sulphate (with infusions titrated to produce serum concentrations between 2 and 4 mmol/litre) improves cardiovascular stability and reduces the requirements for sedatives and muscle relaxants. However, those with severe tetanus still required neuromuscular blocking agents and mechanical ventilation. In those with low cardiac output, inotropes such as adrenaline, noradrenaline, or dobutamine may be needed. If bradyarrhythmias occur, cardiac pacing may be necessary.

Patients with severe tetanus are critically ill and require intensive care management and nursing. Fluid balance must be carefully monitored as insensible fluid losses are particularly high in tetanus. Care must be taken to ensure adequate fluid replacement. Patients require regular turning to prevent pressure sores, which can be especially difficult in those with many spasms or high muscle tone. Frequent suctioning is required to maintain airway patency due to the copious secretions, but it provokes spasms. Some authors report high incidence of venous thrombosis in tetanus patients and recommend routine anticoagulant prophylaxis. Almost all units report a high incidence of nosocomial infections, particularly ventilator-associated pneumonia and line-related sepsis. Optimal management of these involves bacterial cultures, appropriate antibiotics, and infection-control procedures and has been associated with improved outcome.

All patients with tetanus require a full course of active immunization as the disease itself does not confer long-lasting immunity.

Further reading

Attygalle D, Rodrigo N (2002). Magnesium as first line therapy in the management of tetanus: a prospective study of 40 patients. *Anaesthesia*, **57**, 811–17.

Attygalle D, Rodrigo N (2004). New trends in the management of tetanus. *Expert Rev Anti Infect Ther*, **2**, 73–84.

Beeching NJ, Crowcroft NS (2005). Tetanus in injecting drug users. *BMJ*, **330**, 208–9.

Blasi J, *et al.* (1993). Botulinum neurotoxin A selectively cleaves the synaptic protein SNAP-25. *Nature*, **365**, 160–3.

Brauner JS, Vieira SR, Bleck TP (2002). Changes in severe accidental tetanus mortality in the ICU during two decades in Brazil. *Intensive Care Med*, **28**, 930–5.

Cook TM, Protheroe RT, Handel JM (2001). Tetanus: a review of the literature. *Br J Anaesth*, **87**, 477–87.

Humeau Y, *et al.* (2000). How botulinum and tetanus neurotoxins block neurotransmitter release. *Biochimie*, **82**, 427–46.

Lipman J, *et al.* (1987). Autonomic dysfunction in severe tetanus: magnesium sulfate as an adjunct to deep sedation. *Crit Care Med*, **15**, 987–8.

Miranda-Filho Dde B, *et al.* (2004). Randomised controlled trial of tetanus treatment with antitetanus immunoglobulin by the intrathecal or intramuscular route. *BMJ*, **328**, 615.

Okoromah CN, Lesi FE (2004). Diazepam for treating tetanus. *Cochrane Database Syst Rev*, **1**, CD003954.

Salisbury DM, Begg NT (2006). Tetanus. In: *Immunisation against infectious diseases (the green book)*. www.doh.gov.uk/greenbook/greenbookpdf-chapter-30-layout.pdf

Thwaites CL, *et al.* (2006). Predicting the clinical outcome of tetanus: the tetanus severity score. *Trop Med Int Health*, **11**, 279–87.

Thwaites CL, *et al.* (2006). Magnesium sulphate for treatment of severe tetanus: a randomized controlled trial. *Lancet*, **368**, 1436–43.

World Health Organization (2006). Tetanus vaccine. *Wkly Epidemiol Rec*, **81**, 198–208.

7.6.23 *Clostridium difficile*

John G. Bartlett

Essentials

Clostridium difficile is a Gram-positive spore-forming anaerobic bacillus found in the environment. Its spores are part of the colonic flora in about 2 to 3% of healthy adults, with colonization rates increasing during hospitalization to 20 to 40%. Disease occurs when the organism shifts to its replicating vegetative form with toxin (A and B) production, this typically happening when there is inhibition of the competing colonic flora by antibiotics. *C. difficile* infection is now recognized as the most important bacterial enteric pathogen in wealthier countries, with a new NAP-1 epidemic strain appearing to produce more toxin than many others.

Clinical features—these range from trivial diarrhoea that subsides rapidly when antibiotics are stopped to fulminant pseudomembranous colitis, which may progress to toxic megacolon; most cases have watery and voluminous diarrhoea, accompanied by evidence of colonic inflammation.

Diagnosis and treatment—the condition should be suspected in any patient who has diarrhoea in association with antibiotic use. Diagnosis is established by demonstrating *C. difficile* toxin in stool by enzyme immunoassay or cytotoxin assay. Treatment is by stopping the implicated antibiotic, supportive care, avoiding antiperistaltic agents, and giving oral metronidazole or vancomycin.

Prevention—the most important issues are avoidance of the major antibiotic causes of *C. difficile*, and infection control in acute and chronic care facilities, including patient isolation and barrier precautions.

Historical perspective

The history of *Clostridium difficile* has three elements: the bacterium, the animal model of the disease, and the clinical features of antibiotic-associated colitis. *C. difficile* was originally described as a component of the normal flora of newborn infants by Hall and O'Toole in 1935. At that time, the organisms was known to produce an exotoxin that was highly lethal when injected intraperitoneally in mice. However, the clinical implications of this were unclear. Review of the relatively rare cases of *C. difficile* infection (CDI) at various anatomical sites showed no unusual clinical features suggesting a histotoxic clostridial syndrome. Work with animal models began during the Second World War, with attempts to determine the efficacy of penicillin for the treatment of gas gangrene in guinea pigs. However, penicillin proved more lethal to rodents than *Clostridium perfringens*. When antibiotics became available in clinical practice, a potentially important complication was staphylococcal enterocolitis, also known as antibiotic-associated colitis. In 1974, a prospective study at Barnes Hospital, St. Louis, by Tedesco *et al.* showed that 10% of patients receiving clindamycin developed pseudomembranous colitis (PMC). In retrospect, this was one of the first outbreaks of *C. difficile* colitis. Unexpectedly, *Staphylococcus aureus* could not be cultivated from the stool despite the ease of recovering this pathogen. This observation stimulated studies to determine the cause of antibiotic-pseudomembranous colitis which had also become known as clindamycin colitis. In 1977–78, *C. difficile* was identified as the agent of antibiotic-associated colitis, presumably involving Hall and O'Toole's *C. difficile* toxin that had been responsible for antibiotic-induced disease in rodents. Retrospectively, stool samples from Tedesco *et al.*'s study of PMC were found to contain *C. difficile* toxin. During the period 1970–80, work from many clinical groups defined the epidemiology, clinical features, methods of diagnosis, and treatment of *C. difficile*. During the 1980s and 1990s, it was recognized as a relatively frequent and important cause of antibiotic-associated diarrhoea. It was readily diagnosed by detecting *C. difficile* toxin in stool and was effectively treated with oral metronidazole or vancomycin. However, occasionally patients had fulminant disease and about 20% relapsed after treatment. Since 2000, the NAP1 strain of *C. difficile* (also known as ribotype 027 or toxinotoxin III), which appears to be a relatively new, has been increasingly recognized in Canada, the United States of America, and much of Europe. NAP1 seems particularly important because it produces large amounts of toxin *in vitro* and, unlike previous strains, is resistant to fluoroquinolones which are now implicated in many cases of antibiotic-associated diarrhoea.

Aetiology, pathogenesis, and pathology

Like all enteric pathogens, *C. difficile* causes a range of clinical and pathological expressions, ranging from asymptomatic carriage that may be accompanied by positive toxin assays to a fulminant and life-threatening PMC. The organism forms part of the colonic flora in about 2 to 3% of healthy adults, but colonization rates increase during hospitalization to 20 to 40%. Under ordinary circumstances, the organism exists as a spore in the colon and presumably shifts to the replicating vegetative form with toxin production when there is inhibition of the competing colonic flora by antibiotics. The organism produces two toxins, designated toxin A and toxin B. Initial studies using intestinal loop assays indicated that toxin A was a cause of a severe inflammatory disease and toxin B was a particularly potent cytopathic toxin, readily detected with tissue culture assays. However, more recent studies with human colonic tissue indicated that both toxin A and toxin B are important causes of colitis in humans. The pathological findings with endoscopy or histopathology show a range of changes from a completely normal colonic mucosa with minimal histological evidence of inflammation to the other end of the spectrum which is PMC. The pseudomembranes are almost always restricted to the colon, and small bowel involvement is rare. This is in contrast to *S. aureus* enterocolitis which generally involves the small bowel as well as the colon.

Epidemiology

Most at risk of *C. difficile* infection (CDI) are older people and those hospitalized in acute or chronic care facilities and exposed to antibiotic treatment. The association with care facilities is presumably due to clustering of large numbers of elderly patients with high rates of antibiotic exposure where there is widespread environmental contamination by spores of *C. difficile*. Almost any drug with antibacterial activity has been implicated, but the most frequently implicated are broad-spectrum β-lactams (third- and fourth-generation cephalosporins, β-lactam–β-lactamase inhibitors, amoxicillin and carbapenems, clindamycin, and fluoroquinolones). Despite these strong associations, some of the more recent studies have defined cases of CDI in substantial numbers of children and adults receiving proton pump inhibitor treatment without any recent history of antibiotic exposure.

Prevention

The most important facets of prevention are avoidance of the major antibiotic causes of CDI and infection control in acute and chronic care facilities. Antibiotic selection is not usually altered by concern for CDI except in institutional epidemics, elderly patients, and patients who have had previous bouts of this complication, especially those who had severe or relapsing disease. Control of implicated antibiotics during institutional epidemics has proven effective. Recommendations for infection control from the Society for Healthcare Epidemiology of America include patient isolation in a single room preferably with a bathroom, barrier precautions, room cleaning with a 1 in 10 solution of bleach, avoidance of rectal thermometers, and the use of soap and water for hand washing.

Clinical features

Clinical symptoms of CDI range from trivial diarrhoea that subsides rapidly when antibiotics are stopped to fulminant PMC, sometimes complicated by toxic megacolon, sepsis syndrome, renal failure, shock, and death. Cardinal features of the disease that apply to most cases are diarrhoea that is frequently watery and voluminous, accompanied by evidence of colonic inflammation, reflected by cramps, fever, leucocytosis, and typical features of colonic inflammation on endoscopy or CT. The small bowel is rarely involved. Three important observations suggest CDI specifically in some cases: hypoalbuminaemia, leukaemoid reactions, and ileus or toxic megacolon, all following recent antibiotic exposure.

Differential diagnosis

The main differential is antibiotic-associated diarrhoea, a common complication of antibiotics that generally resolves with reduction in dose or simply stopping the drug. However, only about 10 to 15% of specimens submitted to laboratories for detection of *C. difficile* toxin are positive. Assuming that most of these are to investigate suspected CDI in patients with diarrhoea following recent antibiotic exposure, the conclusion is that CDI accounts for a relatively small proportion of antibiotic-associated diarrhoea cases. Distinctive features of CDI are evidence of inflammation as summarized above and severity of disease. Diarrhoea is often caused by medications other than antibiotics including many drugs commonly used in hospitals. In patients with inflammatory diarrhoea, other potential causes include enteric pathogens (salmonella, shigella, *Campylobacter jejuni*, etc.), ischaemic colitis, and idiopathic inflammatory bowel disease. Rare cases of antibiotic-associated colitis may be due to *S. aureus*, *Klebsiella oxytoca*, *C. perfringens*, *Salmonella* spp., and *Candida* spp.

Diagnosis

CDI should be suspected in any patient who has diarrhoea that occurs in association with antibiotic use. The probability of this diagnosis increases substantially with clinical evidence of inflammation and exposure to the agents that are most frequently implicated.

The diagnosis is established by demonstrating *in vivo* production of *C. difficile* toxin. This is detected in stool using enzyme immunoassay (EIA) or cytotoxin assay. Advantages of EIA are that it is rapid (results are available in 1–2 h), the reagents are commercially available, it is technically quite easy to perform, and the specificity is good. The disadvantage is lack of sensitivity. The cytotoxin assay is frequently considered the gold standard and has good sensitivity and specificity, but it is technically demanding and gives results only after 24 to 48 h. Perhaps the most sensitive test is the culture–toxin test in which *C. difficile* carriage is demonstrated either by culture or by detection of common antigen. Subsequently, the strain can be tested for toxogenicity either by *in vitro* toxin production or by detecting toxin in stool using the cytotoxin assay. Although detecting *C. difficile* is highly sensitive, the disadvantage is the relatively high carriage rate of this organism without clinical disease in 20 to 40% of hospitalized patients.

Treatment

CDI should be managed by stopping the implicated antibiotic, supportive care, and avoiding antiperistaltic agents such as loperamide and narcotics. Up to one-third of patients will respond to simply stopping the implicated antibiotic. However, in the era of severe disease with hypervirulent NAP1 strain there is often reluctance simply to observe patients without initiating antibiotic treatment that appears effective in the vast majority of patients. However, the drugs for therapy also appear to cause the disease. This may account for one of the major complications of treatment which is relapses. Only two antibiotics have been used frequently, vancomycin and metronidazole. Both are active against virtually all strains of *C. difficile* so that resistance is not an issue. Their pharmacology is very different. Vancomycin given orally is not absorbed but provides levels that are about 100 to 1000 times the minimum inhibitory concentration in the colon where *C. difficile* resides. In contrast, oral metronidazole is almost completely absorbed and so colonic levels are erratic and often undetectable. Comparative trials of metronidazole versus vancomycin have generally shown equivalent responses, but more recently, vancomycin was shown to be superior, especially in patients with severe disease. There is concern about the high cost of oral vancomycin therapy and the fear that its excessive use might lead to vancomycin resistance, not by *C. difficile* but by other organisms such as enterococci. As a result, many authorities now recommend metronidazole (500 mg orally three times a day for 7–10 days) for mild-moderate CDI and oral vancomycin (125 mg orally four times a day for 7–10 days) for those with more serious disease. Patients with fulminant CDI are a special challenge, often because it is so difficult to get antibiotics to the site of infection due to ileus. Recommendations in these cases include oral vancomycin in doses of 500 mg orally or via nasogastric tube four times a day combined with intravenous metronidazole. Many of these patients and especially those with ileus or toxic megacolon may require colostomy.

Another complication of antibiotic treatment of CDI is relapse, which occurs in approximately 20% of patients with their first course of treatment, about 40% treated for a single relapse, and 60% for those treated for two relapses. Several different therapeutic strategies have been recommended for relapses but none is uniformly effective. The most frequently recommended strategy is oral vancomycin in standard dose for 7 to 10 days to control the relapse episode, followed by vancomycin tapered over 2 weeks, followed by a prolonged course of 'pulse vancomycin' (125 mg orally every other day) for a total of 2 to 6 weeks. The presumed mechanism for pulse therapy is to give sufficient vancomycin to maintain the pathogen in spore state, but insufficient to inhibit recolonization by the normal flora which will ultimately control replication and toxin production of *C. difficile*. Other strategies include intravenous immune globulin, probiotics, other antibiotics such as rifamycins, and several experimental agents. Data are inadequate for use of these strategies at present.

Areas of controversy

Diagnostic testing

A range of tests are now used to detect *C. difficile*. Choice is based on speed of results, cost, sensitivity, specificity, and availability of reagents. In the United States of America, 95% of hospital laboratories use EIA as the only diagnostic test. In Europe and Australia, there is much more frequent use of culture–toxin assays based on better sensitivity, but there is an increase in the cost and a delay in receiving results.

Treatment

Most groups have traditionally recommended metronidazole as the drug of choice for CDI, including Centers for Disease Control, Society of Health Care Epidemiology of America, and Infectious Diseases Society of America. However, the use of oral vancomycin is increasingly advocated, especially for patients who are seriously ill, but controversy continues about its cost and the consequences of its excessive use.

Infection control

The recommendation is for a private room and private bathroom to prevent nosocomial spread, but many older hospitals and most chronic care facilities cannot provide these. Another controversy concerns the use of soap and water hand washing, which is favoured because the standard alcohol-based hand cleaning does not eradicate clostridial spores. The problem is lack of easy access to soap and water in many facilities and concern that this is a largely theoretical issue with no demonstrated clinical benefit, while alcohol-based cleaning prevents many other important pathogens.

Antibiotic selection

The most important causative agents have been identified and some workers in the field have felt that their use should be discouraged more aggressively especially during epidemics in which a specific agent has been implicated. Controversy surrounds the definition of an epidemic, clarity in implicating a single agent, and methods of discouraging use while still providing optimal therapy.

Strain identification

The NAP1 strain is implicated as a cause of a particularly severe disease, but most physicians do not know if it is the responsible strain in a particular patient as this would require stool culture with referral to a reference source for *C. difficile* strain typing. This is possibly important in epidemics, but is not important in individual cases since management strategies are based on severity of disease and infection control to prevent spread of the epidemic strain regardless of strain type.

Likely developments in the near future

C. difficile poses many challenges. In recent years there has been progress in diagnosis, treatment, and prevention of CDI. However, recent events have called attention to many deficits in current practice and many now feel that much more attention to diagnosis, treatment, and infection control is needed. For detection, the challenge is to find a test that is fast, cheap, sensitive, and specific. New methods of detecting *C. difficile* or *C. difficile* toxins are unlikely to be developed, with the exception of PCR for detecting strains that produce toxin B. Some current research favours the use of a sensitive method to detect *C. difficile*, such as common antigen detection by EIA or PCR to detect toxigenic strains accompanied by EIA for detection of toxin A and toxin B, with the more sensitive cytotoxin assay to detect those that are *C. difficile* positive and EIA negative for toxin A. For treatment, a drug superior to oral vancomycin for the treatment of acute disease, especially severe acute disease, is unlikely to emerge. The challenge is getting the drug to the site of infection. Future research may define better the role of ancillary methods such as probiotics, indications for colectomy, and the role of intravenous immune globulin. For relapses, the most promising results will be use of nonantibiotic treatment, since the drugs currently in use have the paradox that they cause as well as cure *C. difficile*. Most promising in this category will be antibiotics that selectively inhibit *C. difficile* without altering the colonic flora or the use of nonantibiotics such as anion exchange resins. For infection control, perhaps the biggest challenge is antibiotic stewardship to eliminate abuse of these drugs which is a well-recognized problem, but very difficult to control in terms of physician understanding and patient acceptance.

Further reading

Al-Nassir WN, *et al.* (2008). Comparison of clinical and microbiological response to treatment of *Clostridium difficile*-associated disease with metronidazole and vancomycin. *Clin Infect Dis*, **47**, 56–62.

Aslam S, Hamill RJ, Musher DM (2005). Treatment of *Clostridium difficile*-associated disease: old therapies and new strategies. *Lancet Infect Dis*, **5**, 549–57.

Bartlett JG (2006). Narrative review: the new epidemic of *Clostridium difficile*-associated enteric disease. *Ann Intern Med*, **145**, 758–64.

Blossom DB, McDonald LC (2007). The challenges posed by reemerging *Clostridium difficile* infection. *Clin Infect Dis*, **45**, 222–7.

Dial S, *et al.* (2005). Use of gastric acid-suppressive agents and the risk of community-acquired *Clostridium difficile*-associated disease. *JAMA*, **294**, 2989–95.

Gerding DN, *et al.* (1995). *Clostridium difficile*-associated diarrhea and colitis. *Infect Control Hosp Epidemiol*, **16**, 459–77.

Hall IC, O'Toole E (1935). Intestinal flora in newborn infants with a description of a new pathogenic anaerobe, *Bacillus difficilis*. *Am J Dis Child*, **49**, 390–402.

Hambre LDS, *et al.* (1943). The toxicity of penicillin as prepared for clinical use. *Am J Med Sci*, **206**, 642–52.

Johnson S, *et al.* (1999). Epidemics of diarrhea caused by a clindamycin-resistant strain of *Clostridium difficile* in four hospitals. *N Engl J Med*, **341**, 1645–51.

Lamontagne F, *et al.* (2007). Impact of emergency colectomy on survival of patients with fulminant *Clostridium difficile* colitis during an epidemic caused by a hypervirulent strain. *Ann Surg*, **245**, 267–72.

McFarland LV, *et al.* (1989). Nosocomial acquisition of *Clostridium difficile* infection. *N Engl J Med*, **320**, 204–10.

Monaghan T, Boswell T, Mahida YR (2008). Recent advances in *Clostridium difficile*-associated disease. *Gut*, **57**, 850–60.

Pépin J, *et al.* (2004). *Clostridium difficile*-associated diarrhea in a region of Quebec from 1991 to 2003: a changing pattern of disease severity. *Can Med Assoc J*, **171**, 466–72.

Riegler M, *et al.* (1995). *Clostridium difficile* toxin B is more potent than toxin A in damaging human colonic epithelium in vitro. *J Clin Invest*, **95**, 2004–11.

Tedesco FJ, Barton RW, Alpers DH (1974). Clindamycin-associated colitis. A prospective study. *Ann Intern Med*, **81**, 429–33.

Ticehurst JR, *et al.* (2006). Effective detection of toxigenic *Clostridium difficile* by a two-step algorithm including tests for antigen and cytotoxin. *J Clin Microbiol*, **44**, 1145–9.

Warny M, *et al.* (2005). Toxin production by an emerging strain of *Clostridium difficile* associated with outbreaks of severe disease in North America and Europe. *Lancet*, **366**, 1079–84.

Zar FA, *et al.* (2007). A comparison of vancomycin and metronidazole for the treatment of *Clostridium difficile*-associated diarrhea, stratified by disease severity. *Clin Infect Dis*, **45**, 302–7.

7.6.24 Botulism, gas gangrene, and clostridial gastrointestinal infections

Dennis L. Stevens, Michael J. Aldape, and Amy E. Bryant

Essentials

Botulism

Human botulism is caused by seven serological types of *C. botulinum*, which is ubiquitously distributed in the soil. Poisoning usually results from ingestion of preformed toxin in food, although this is rapidly inactivated at ordinary cooking temperatures, but it can also result from contaminated wounds. *C. botulinum* toxin binds irreversibly to the neuromuscular junction and is the most lethal known microbial toxin.

Clinical features, diagnosis, and treatment—presentation is with symptoms suggesting gastrointestinal tract illness, followed by neurological symptoms including diplopia, blurred vision, dizziness, and difficulty with speech or swallowing, leading on to generalized flaccid paralysis. Diagnosis can be confirmed by testing for botulinum toxin in the patient's serum, urine, or stomach contents, or in the suspect food. Treatment requires (1) supportive care—this, including mechanical ventilation, may be needed for many months until new synapses have developed; (2) antitoxin—this reduces case fatality and shortens the illness.

Acknowledgement: The authors acknowledge inclusion of material from the chapter in the previous edition by Dr H E Larson.

Gas gangrene

Gas gangrene is caused by *C. perfringens* (most commonly), *C. histolyticum*, *C. novyii*, *C. sordellii*, and *C. septicum*, which occur naturally in soil and in the gastrointestinal tracts of humans and animals. Common causes of the condition are severe trauma that interrupts the blood supply to the soft tissues (gunshot wounds, penetrating or crushing injuries) with contamination by dirt, vegetation, or clothing containing vegetative forms of clostridia or spores. Skin popping of black tar heroin is another recently recognized cause. The clostridia responsible elaborate a wide range of toxins with varying effects: the principle toxin of *C. perfringens* is α-toxin, a phospholipase C that cleaves phosphatidylcholine in eukaryotic cell membranes and activates neutrophils, platelets, and endothelial cells, causing obstruction of local blood flow.

Clinical features—severe and sudden pain is the most characteristic symptom. Infection progresses rapidly with local ecchymosis, blistering, massive swelling, and crepitus indicating gas in the tissue as progressive necrotizing soft-tissue infection destroys muscle, fascia, fat, and skin. Without rapid and appropriate treatment, bacteraemia, hypotension, and multiple organ failure ensue.

Diagnosis and treatment—diagnosis must be made on clinical grounds, although Gram stain of the wound discharge or tissue sample may be helpful. Treatment requires (1) early recognition and aggressive surgical debridement of devitalized tissue; (2) antimicrobials—most commonly penicillin and clindamycin (which suppresses α-toxin production); (3) anti-α-toxin serum. The benefit of hyperbaric oxygen (HBO) has not been proven in controlled trials. In an experimental model of gas gangrene, HBO did not improve the efficacy of clindamycin or penicillin.

Prevention—prophylactic antibiotic treatment reduces the risk, but this depends upon factors including the time interval between the injury and surgical debridement.

Particular forms of gas gangrene—(1) *C. septicum* can grow at ambient oxygen tensions, causing 'spontaneous gas gangrene' in normal tissues, most commonly when bacteria spread from a colonic adenocarcinoma to uninjured muscle. (2) *C. sordellii* causes haemoconcentration, leukaemoid reaction without fever, and gradually progressive shock that is fatal in 75 to 80% of patients. Women infected during parturition, after medical abortion, or following gynaecological surgery almost always die.

C. perfringens gastrointestinal infections

Food poisoning—if foods such as meat and heavy gravy infected with type A strains of *C. perfringens* are allowed to sit at room temperature, bacilli can multiply greatly. If the food is then inadequately heated before consumption, preformed heat labile enterotoxin, combined with toxin produced in the gut, causes self-limiting abdominal pain and diarrhoea, usually without fever or vomiting.

Necrotizing enterocolitis—*C. perfringens* type C β-toxin causes fulminating enterocolitis that destroys intestinal mucosa. Epidemic outbreaks occured in postwar Germany (Darmbrand) and New Guinea (enteritis necroticans, 'pig bel') following ingestion of contaminated food, or dramatic change from vegetarian to meat diets. Treatment consists of supportive care and antibiotics (usually benzylpenicillin). Complications, e.g. intestinal perforation, may require surgery, in which case mortality is high. A toxoid vaccine is protective and should be considered in areas of Papua New Guinea where the disease still occurs.

Botulism

Definition

Botulism is an acute symmetrical descending paralysis caused by a neurotoxin produced by *Clostridium botulinum*. Food contaminated by *C. botulinum* spores and elaborated toxin produces illness when ingested. Wound infections with *C. botulinum* or intestinal tract colonization in infants and adults occasionally cause botulism. Although the illness is most commonly described in humans, botulism can occur in wild ducks feeding off the bottoms of alkaline lakes in the western United States of America. The illness is called 'limber neck'.

Occurrence

C. botulinum is ubiquitously distributed in the soil. The surfaces of potatoes, vegetables, and other foods are easily contaminated with spores, which survive brief heating at 100°C. Autoclaving or use of pressure cookers that are appropriately adjusted are very effective at killing spores. In the 1920s in the United States of America, pressure cookers calibrated at sea level which were then used at several thousand feet above sea level in the western states were the cause of outbreaks of botulism among families that home-canned food. The anaerobic conditions characteristic of canning, smoking, or fermentation facilitate clostridial growth and toxin release. Canned food with neutral pH, such as canned corn, is particularly prone to promoting the growth of clostridia. Spores germinate in sausage or cheese kept for extended periods at room temperature. An 18th-century report associated paralytic illness with eating sausages, hence *botulus*, a Latin word for 'sausage'. Cases have been associated with fermented milk in Africa, cheese sauce on baked potatoes in North America, fermented stew in Japan, and imported fish in the United Kingdom.

Although past outbreaks typically involved small groups of people, home-canned peppers served in a restaurant caused two large outbreaks in the United States of America. Outbreaks caused by commercially processed foods are infrequent, but contamination of hazelnut purée added to commercially produced yoghurt caused 27 cases of botulism in Wales and north-west England in 1989, the largest recorded outbreak in the United Kingdom. Most of the contaminated cartons could not be accounted for, suggesting that the attack rate varied or that mild symptoms were not diagnosed as botulism. Commercially prepared chopped garlic in soybean oil caused 36 cases dispersed over 8 provinces and states in North America.

Some outbreaks involved only single contaminated items, such as in the Loch Maree episode in 1922 where eight people died after eating duck paste, the 1978 outbreak in Birmingham involving four people who ate tinned Alaskan salmon, and one case in 1989 following a meal on a commercial airliner. Uneviscerated fresh fish have been associated with botulism, usually where there have been deficiencies in refrigeration.

Purified botulinum toxin has recently come into therapeutic use. Toxin injections produce temporary muscle weakness and are effective in the treatment of strabismus, blepharospasm, and torticollis, and are also used for cosmetic purposes. Treatment doses are considered too small to elicit systemic symptoms. Under experimental conditions, aerosolized botulinum toxin causes illness in monkeys, and the toxin has been utilized as an agent for biological warfare or terrorist activity. For example, botulinum toxin was loaded into

Scud missile warheads by Iraq during the first Gulf War and stockpiled by the Aum Shinrikyo cult in Japan.

The toxin

There are seven serological types of botulinum toxin (A–G). Types A, B, and E account for nearly all human cases. Serotypes implicated in outbreaks of botulism parallel the geographical distribution of soil spores. Type E is nearly always associated with fish, but outbreaks caused by fish products can also involve types A and B.

C. botulinum toxin is heat labile and rapidly inactivated at ordinary cooking temperatures. It is a protein neurotoxin, and a dose as small as 0.1 µg is sufficient to cause death in humans. The 150-kDa molecule is composed of two peptide chains connected by disulphide bonds. One chain binds to and penetrates the neuron, and the other cleaves a protein essential for neurotransmitter release, reducing acetylcholine availability for impulse transmission. Toxin types A, C, and E hydrolyse a protein in the presynaptic membrane while types B, D, F, and G hydrolyse a protein in the synaptic vesicle.

Pathogenesis

Botulinum toxin is absorbed directly across mucous membranes. Locally acting toxin may produce some symptoms but cranial nerve paralysis results from blood stream distribution. Cranial nerves are preferentially affected because botulinum toxin binds more rapidly to sites where the cycles of depolarization and repolarization are frequent. Binding is irreversible and the toxin cannot thereafter be neutralized by antitoxin. Recovery occurs when nerve terminals sprout from the axon to form new motor endplates.

Botulinum toxin blocks impulse transmission mediated by acetylcholine at myoneural junctions, at autonomic ganglia, and at parasympathetic nerve terminals. Nerve stimulus transmission is blocked because the toxin prevents release of acetylcholine from the presynaptic membrane. Impulse conduction within peripheral nerves and muscle contraction are not affected. Synthesis of acetylcholine and impulse transmission within terminal nerve fibrils remain intact. On the other hand, the miniature endplate potentials spontaneously generated by release of acetylcholine in a resting nerve decrease and eventually disappear in the presence of toxin. If a poisoned nerve is stimulated repetitively, temporary summation of acetylcholine release occurs producing an augmented response.

History

The symptoms of botulism vary from mild fatigue to severe weakness and collapse leading to death within a day. Initially, nausea, vomiting, abdominal bloating, and dryness in the mouth and throat may suggest gastrointestinal tract illness. Diplopia, blurred vision, dizziness, unsteadiness on standing, and difficulty with speech or swallowing are common early neurological symptoms. Subsequently, there is progression to weakness or paralysis in the limbs, and generalized weakness and lassitude. The dryness of the mouth and throat may become so severe as to cause pain. Eventually there may be difficulty holding up the head, constipation, urinary hesitancy, and problems in breathing. The incubation period is between 12 and 72 h. Patients with short incubation periods are likely to have ingested large amounts of toxin. However, individuals are known to have ingested large amounts of contaminated food without developing symptoms.

Physical examination

Negative findings in botulism are pertinent. Higher mental functions are preserved, although sometimes patients are drowsy. Sensation is intact. Fever is unusual. The mouth is dry and the tongue is furrowed. Lateral rectus weakness in the eyes produces internal strabismus. Failure of accommodation is common and the pupils may be fixed in mid position or dilated and unresponsive to light. Ptosis, weakness of other extraocular muscles, and inability to protrude the tongue or to raise the shoulders are other early findings. Weakness in the limbs is of the flaccid, lower motor neuron type and deep tendon reflexes are initially preserved. Facial muscles may be spared; gag and corneal reflexes are not lost.

Weakness of the respiratory muscles develops early in relation to other findings and deterioration can be rapid. Paralysis descends symmetrically from cranial nerves to upper extremities to respiratory muscles to the lower extremities in a proximal to distal pattern. Hypotension without compensatory tachycardia, intestinal ileus, and urinary retention are evidence of the widespread autonomic paralysis. Symptoms and signs can be confined to the autonomic nervous system.

Diagnosis

The diagnosis in the first case of an outbreak can be missed because cranial nerve symptoms and signs are ignored in what is apparently a gastrointestinal disturbance. The differential diagnosis usually lies between botulism and the descending form of acute inflammatory polyneuropathy or Guillain–Barré syndrome. There can be similarities in the clinical presentation and progression of symptoms in the two diseases. Patients with botulism have normal cerebrospinal fluid findings and respiratory weakness and failure develop early, before the presence of severe limb weakness. Patients with the Guillain–Barré syndrome have marked limb weakness before the development of respiratory failure. Sensation and mental status are preserved in botulism.

Other diagnoses that may be considered include diphtheria, intoxication with atropine or organophosphorus compounds, myasthenia gravis, cerebrovascular disease involving the brainstem and producing bulbar palsy, paralytic rabies, tick paralysis, and neurotoxic snake bite. Botulism is distinguished from polymyositis and periodic paralysis by its rapid progression and cranial nerve abnormalities. Sometimes patients with other types of poisoning are thought to have botulism, most often with an outbreak of staphylococcal food poisoning. Individuals with carbon monoxide poisoning have been mistakenly been thought to be poisoned by food, but they invariably have headaches and altered consciousness. Poisoning from chemicals or fish produces rapid onset of symptoms. Mushroom poisoning is characterized by severe abdominal pain.

The diagnosis of botulism can be confirmed by testing for botulinum toxin in the patient's serum, urine, stomach contents, or in the suspect food. Mice are inoculated intraperitoneally with 0.5 ml of sample, with and without mixing with polyvalent botulinum antitoxin, and observed for signs of botulism. Electromyography can be helpful in confirming a diagnosis of botulism. Single or low-frequency stimuli evoke muscle action potentials that are reduced in amplitude; tetanic or rapid stimuli produce an enhanced response. Nerve conduction velocities are normal. This result readily differentiates botulism from the Guillain–Barré syndrome. Patients with myasthenia gravis usually have muscle action potentials of normal or minimally decreased amplitude.

Treatment

The priorities in management are assessment of respiratory function followed by administration of antitoxin. Respiration should be monitored closely with a view to elective intubation since deterioration can occur rapidly. Prolonged respiratory support may be required. Profound hypotension can be secondary to hypoxaemia, acidosis, and accumulated fluid deficits or can be a feature of the autonomic paralysis. Treat autonomic paralysis by expanding the intravascular volume using whole blood, protein, and/or saline while monitoring central venous pressure or by infusing a low dose of dopamine.

Trivalent (types A, B, and E) antitoxin reduces case fatality and shortens the course of the illness. To be useful it must be given early, before free circulating toxin has bound to its peripheral targets and before the diagnosis can be confirmed by animal tests. Multivalent equine antitoxin is available from designated regional hospitals in the United Kingdom; one-half of the dose is given intramuscularly and one-half intravenously. An intradermal 0.1-ml test dose is given, but most serum reactions are not predicted by this test. Human botulism immune plasma can be obtained from the Centers for Disease Control, Atlanta, Georgia, United States of America.

Many years ago it was shown that patients dying of botulism carried bacilli in their intestine. The discovery that clinical disease can result from toxin formed within the gastrointestinal tract of infants and adults makes antimicrobial treatment theoretically appealing. Gastric lavage, repeated high enemas, and cathartics have been utilized in an attempt to remove unabsorbed toxin. Drugs capable of reversing neuromuscular blockade have been used to treat patients with botulism, but without any noticeable effect on respiratory muscle weakness or tidal volume.

The mortality from botulism in the early part of the 20th century was 60 to 70%, but this improved to 23% for cases reported between 1960 and 1970 since the use of respiratory support. In a single large outbreak in 1977 there were no deaths among 59 cases. Recovery from botulism depends on the formation of new neuromuscular junctions; clinical improvement thus takes weeks to months. One severe case required respiratory support for 173 days with eventual recovery. Very prolonged fatigue and dyspnoea on exertion can be due to factors other than the neuromuscular blockade.

Wound botulism

Symptoms and signs of botulism can develop in people with injuries. Recognition may be complicated by the presence of fever from wound infection or gas gangrene, or by the absence of gastrointestinal symptoms. The diagnosis is confirmed by electromyography; botulinum toxin is detected in serum in only about one-half of the reported cases. The incubation period averages 7 days with a range of 4 to 17 days. Clinical findings and management are the same as for patients with food-borne botulism. Since 1991, wound botulism has increasingly become a complication of injection drug abuse; small abscesses at injection sites yield *C. botulinum.* An epidemic of wound botulism in the United States of America has been associated with the injection of black tar heroin. *C. botulinum* can be recovered from wounds in the absence of clinical botulism.

Infant botulism

Sporadically, cases of botulism are recognized in infants less than 6 months of age. Previously healthy babies develop constipation, which progresses over 3 to 10 days to poor feeding, irritability, a hoarse cry, and weakness in head control. Examination shows a generally weak, hypotonic, afebrile infant. Abnormalities in eye movements and pupillary reactions are sometimes present and deep tendon reflexes are reduced or absent. There is considerable range in severity; respiratory failure can develop but most recover completely.

The diagnosis can be confirmed by finding *C. botulinum* and toxin in the faeces, and by electromyography. Botulinum toxin is not present in the serum. The disease is thought to follow ingestion of *C. botulinum* spores, which multiply in the infant's gastrointestinal tract and produce toxin. Excretion of *C. botulinum* and toxin may continue for as long as 3 months. Honey has been a source of spores in some cases. Other than supportive measures, no consistent pattern in treatment using antitoxin, antibiotics, cathartics, or enemas has been established.

Gas gangrene

Definition

Gas gangrene is a rapidly developing and spreading infection of muscle caused by toxin-producing clostridial species. Gas gangrene is accompanied by bacteraemia, hypotension, and multiorgan failure and is invariably fatal if untreated.

Aetiology

Clostridia are mainly saprophytes, occurring naturally in soil and in the gastrointestinal tracts of humans and animals. Most cases of gas gangrene are caused by *Clostridium perfringens* type A, but some are due to *C. novyi* and a few to *C. septicum*, *C. histolyticum*, *C. sordellii*, and *C. fallax*; not uncommonly more that one species is isolated. Oxygen inhibits growth of most, although *C. septicum* is quite aerotolerant.

Gas gangrene has been a major cause of wound infection on the battlefield, although recently civilian and iatrogenic traumas have become more common. Disease development requires an anaerobic environment and contamination of the wound with spores or vegetative organisms usually through soil contact. However, proximity to faecal sources of bacteria is also a risk factor for cases occurring after hip surgery, adrenaline injections into the buttock, or amputation of the leg for ischaemic vascular disease. Wound contamination with dirt, shrapnel, or bits of clothing reduces local oxygen concentrations. Traumatic gas gangrene develops in deep wounds involving large muscle masses in the shoulder, hip, thigh, and calf and particularly in those situations where damage to major arteries has occurred. Thus, gunshot wounds, crush injuries, and open fractures account for most of the cases. High-velocity bullets of large calibre are commonly used in contemporary times in civilian and military firearms and these produce extensive tissue damage. Necrotic tissue, foreign bodies, and ischaemia in a wound reduce the locally available oxygen and favour outgrowth of vegetative cells and spores.

The incidence of gas gangrene after trauma reflects the speed at which injured people can be evacuated and receive appropriate treatment. During the Vietnam and Falklands conflicts there were very few cases of gas gangrene among American and British wounded cared for by highly organized surgical teams. This reduction was likely due to more timely cleansing of wounds, maintaining blood flow by vascular surgery, and the use of antibiotics.

In comparison, when a jet airliner crashed in the Florida everglades, eight of the 77 injured survivors developed the disease.

Nontraumatic or 'spontaneous gas gangrene' occurs without a preceding injury. Classically, it presents as a primary infection of the perineum or scrotum or in a limb secondary to seeding from clostridial colonization of a colonic neoplasm. These cases are most commonly caused by the more aerotolerant *C. septicum* where production of superoxide dismutase permits the organisms to survive in the presence of small amounts of oxygen.

Recently, *C. novyi*, *C. sordellii*, and *C. perfringens* have been associated with necrotizing soft tissue infections at injection sites in drug addicts. Outbreaks of these infections were reported in Scotland, Ireland, England, and the United States of America in 2000 and were characterized by extensive soft tissue necrosis, hypotension, severe constitutional toxicity, and a high case fatality rate.

C. sordellii infections have been described in women following natural childbirth or therapeutic abortion, and in men, women, and children following a variety of traumatic and surgical procedures. The infections are perhaps the most aggressive of all clostridial infections, in part because of a unique syndrome of absence of fever, profound hypotension, diffuse capillary leak, haemoconcentration, and leukaemoid reaction resulting in 70% mortality within 2 to 4 days of hospital admission. The toxins responsible for this remarkable infection have not been fully elucidated.

Toxins

The clinical and histological manifestations of gas gangrene are attributable to the production of potent bacterial exotoxins. The clostridia responsible for gas gangrene elaborate a wide range of toxins. More than 12 have been described for *C. septicum*, *C. novyi*, and *C. perfringens*. The principal toxin of *C. perfringens* is α-toxin, a phospholipase C. This toxin cleaves phosphatidylcholine found in cell membrane of eukaryotic cells, releasing diacylglycerol and phosphorylcholine. In small doses, this toxin can hyperactivate a variety of cells including neutrophils, platelets, endothelial cells, and macrophages; in high doses it is cytotoxic. Interestingly, this toxin can cause the rapid and irreversible cessation of blood flow to normal tissue. This perfusion deficit is the consequence of toxin-induced platelet/neutrophil aggregates that irreversibly occlude small to medium-sized vessels. Experimentally, active or passive immunization against α-toxin is protective against active infection. A second toxin, θ-toxin, is a cholesterol-dependent thiol-activated cytolysin that lyses red blood cells and other cells by its ability to form pores in cell membranes. Electron microscopy of θ-toxin-treated cells shows arc and ring structures of 7.5 to 18 nm appearing in the plasma membrane as early as 1 h postexposure. These plasma membrane defects increase with time and can be visualized adjacent to toxin molecules that have been labelled with ferritin. α-Toxin and θ-toxin are not readily detected in the tissues or serum of patients with gas gangrene, possibly because the toxin binds rapidly and irreversibly to lipid moieties in the cytoplasmic membranes.

History

The incubation period of gas gangrene is usually less than 4 days, often less than 24 h, and occasionally as short as 1 to 6 h. Pain is the most characteristic symptom. Patients describe this as severe or excruciating and sudden in onset. Evolution of symptoms and signs can be very rapid. Toxicity may prevent the patient from giving an adequate history.

Physical examination

Early on, it may be difficult to account for the patient's pain by objective physical findings. Swelling, bluish discoloration, or darkening of the skin occurs at the affected site. The traumatic or surgical wounds become oedematous and a thin, serous discharge emerges from the site. Pain steadily increases in severity; the overlying skin becomes stretched and develops a brown or 'bronzed' discoloration. Haemorrhagic vesicles and finally areas of frank necrosis appear. A sweet odour from the wound has been described. Gas is not invariably present early in the course, but radiographs may detect gas earlier than can physical examination. Later, crepitus and exquisite tenderness are present in the wound.

Profound constitutional changes occur. Patients become sweaty and febrile, and though alert and oriented, are very distressed. The pulse is elevated out of proportion to the fever. Death may occur within 48 h. At operation, infected muscle appears dark red with purple discoloration; frank gangrene and liquefaction may be seen. Involved muscle does not bleed when cut or contract when directly stimulated.

Rapidly progressing necrotizing infections of the soft tissue may be monomicrobic, caused by clostridia, *Streptococcus pyogenes*, *Staphylococcus aureus*, *Vibrio vulnificus*, or *Aeromonas hydrophila*. Alternatively, necrotizing infections may be polymicrobic and caused by mixed aerobic and anaerobic microbes. Clostridia and polymicrobial infections are usually associated with gas in the tissue, whereas the others are not. Polymicrobial necrotizing infections occur most commonly following gastrointestinal surgery, penetrating injury to the abdomen, surgical incisions in the vaginal mucosa (episiotomy), or in diabetic patients with peripheral vascular disease. All of these necrotizing infections may destroy fascia, but frequently also destroy muscle, subcutaneous tissue, and skin.

Diagnosis

The diagnosis of gas gangrene must be made on clinical grounds and prompt recognition and treatment improve the prognosis. Sudden deterioration in a postoperative patient or following trauma requires examination of the wound and surrounding tissue. Cases of primary gas gangrene and cases following elective surgery may have a higher fatality because recognition is delayed. Gram's staining of the wound discharge, of an aspirate, or of a needle biopsy may aid diagnosis. In gas gangrene there are many large plump Gram-positive bacilli, usually without spores. Few, if any, polymorphonuclear leucocytes are present in the tissues or exudates, likely due to toxin-induced inhibition of cellular extravasation.

CT scanning can detect gas deep in muscle, but the absence of gas does not exclude the diagnosis. Culture of clostridia does not confirm a diagnosis of gas gangrene as simple colonization without clinical disease occurs in up to 30% of traumatic wounds.

Treatment

Surgical removal of all affected muscle is essential to eliminate the conditions that allow the organism to grow. High-velocity missiles distribute energy radially from their path, producing more extensive tissue damage than missiles at low speeds or with a small mass. Thus, wounds should be excised widely by resection back to healthy, viable muscle and skin. Closure should be delayed for 5 to 6 days until it is certain that the wound is free of infection.

Administration of appropriate antimicrobial agents is also required. Penicillin has been the drug of choice based on *in vitro* susceptibility testing, but experimental evidence has demonstrated that clindamycin or tetracycline is superior to penicillin. This improved efficacy is most likely because these two protein synthesis inhibitors prevent the production of toxins. This has led to the use of penicillin and clindamycin as combination therapy. Ceftriaxone or erythromycin are alternative choices for severely penicillin-allergic patients.

Hyperbaric oxygen therapy (typically 100% oxygen at 303 kPa for 60–120 min, 2–3 times daily) has been used to treat gas gangrene; however, an effect on mortality has never been shown by controlled trials and comparable survival rates have been achieved without using it. Experimental studies have demonstrated that hyperbaric oxygen alone was neither effective in an animal model of *C. perfringens* gas gangrene nor did it improve the efficacy of clindamycin or penicillin.

Therapeutic administration of gas gangrene antitoxin made from horse serum is controversial. Use during the Second World War reduced mortality, but serum sickness and other allergic reactions occurred. It is no longer produced in the United States of America. In recent studies, active immunization of animals with a truncated, nontoxic form (C-domain) of the α-toxin was 100% protective against active muscle infection with *C. perfringens*.

Prevention

Prophylactic antibiotic treatment reduces the risk of gas gangrene but this depends on the time interval between the injury and surgical debridement, the associated vascular deficit, the presence of foreign body, the presence of a compound or open fracture, and the duration of antibiotic administration. Patients have clearly developed gas gangrene after prophylactic administration of β-lactam antibiotics. Gas gangrene can develop from wounds contaminated with either vegetative organisms or spores. Antibiotics may be more effective in the former case since spores, until they germinate, are not affected by antibiotics. Metronidazole or clindamycin may be useful in patients who are hypersensitive to β-lactam antibiotics. Experimentally, active immunization against the α-toxin provides impressive protection against *C. perfringens* gas gangrene, but no active or passive vaccine is currently available.

Clostridial infections of the gastrointestinal tract

Necrotizing enterocolitis

Definition

Necrotizing enterocolitis is a fulminating clinical illness characterized by extensive necrosis of the intestinal mucosa and wall. Terms such as *darmbrand* (Germany), enteritis necroticans, pig bel (Papua New Guinea), or gas gangrene of the bowel describe geographic variants. Cases occur sporadically in adults or as epidemics in all ages. Necrotizing enterocolitis occurs in infants, and some of these cases have demonstrated clostridia in the wall of the intestine.

Aetiology

Gram's staining of the necrotic mucosa and the bowel wall shows many Gram-positive bacilli that are typically identified as *C. perfringens* (*C. welchii*). Sporadic cases usually yield *C. perfringens* type A. However, in the German and especially in the Papua New Guinea outbreaks, there is substantial evidence implicating *C. perfringens* type C. Type C produces large amounts of β-toxin, which has lethal and necrotizing effects. Papua New Guinea highlanders have a high prevalence of antibodies to β-toxin; antibodies are rare in people who live where the disease is uncommon. Patients with pig bel have rising levels of antibodies to β-toxin, and specific passive or active immunization prevents disease. It is not clear whether exogenous human infection with these organisms occurs or whether the lesions are produced by the overgrowth of endogenous clostridia. Sweet potato, a local dietary staple, contains an inhibitor of trypsin. Combined with a low-protein diet this may impair the ability of the intestine to inactivate endogenously produced β-toxin. However, the methods used for roasting the pigs offer many opportunities for clostridial contamination.

History and physical examination

Sporadic cases in patients over 50 years of age or among those recovering from gastric surgery are regularly reported from Scandinavia, Europe, the United States of America, Australia, and the Middle East. Alternatively, epidemic outbreaks as described in post-war Germany and among the highlanders of Papua New Guinea follow ingestion of contaminated food or a dramatic change in eating habits. Severe intermittent abdominal pain is the first symptom and pain rapidly becomes continuous. Bloody diarrhoea and vomiting are common. Patients quickly develop tachycardia, followed by hypotension and evidence of multiorgan failure. On examination there is fever with abdominal distension, localized or diffuse tenderness, and reduced bowel sounds. A tender mass may be palpated. Following resolution of infection, malabsorption and partial small bowel obstruction may develop because of intestinal scarring.

Treatment and prevention

Patients with suspected pig bel should be treated with nasogastric suction and intravenous fluids. Pyrantel is given by mouth and the bowel rested by fasting. Benzylpenicillin, 1 MU, is given intravenously every 4 h and the patient observed for complications requiring surgery. Mild cases recover without surgical intervention, but if surgical indications are present the mortality ranges from 35 to 100%, in part due to perforation of the intestine. As pig bel continues to be a common disease in Papua New Guinea, consideration should be given to the use of a *C. perfringens* type C toxoid vaccine in local areas. Two doses spaced 3 to 4 months apart are preventive.

Clostridium perfringens food poisoning

Occurrence and clinical findings

In the United Kingdom and the United States of America, food poisoning caused by *C. perfringens* is the third most common type of food-borne illness. Meat and poultry are responsible for at least 90% of the outbreaks, which occur where food is prepared in large quantities. Two-thirds of the reported outbreaks are in schools, hospitals, factories, restaurants, or catering establishments, and in a typical outbreak 35 to 40 people are affected. An estimated 12 000 cases were associated with a single outbreak in 1969.

The circumstances surrounding an outbreak repeat themselves with monotonous regularity. A meat dish is prepared by stewing, braising, boiling, or steaming and this is allowed to stand at ambient temperatures for a period of 4 to 24 h. The food is served cold or after rewarming. Six to 12 h after eating the meal, people complain of cramping abdominal pain and then diarrhoea. Vomiting is unusual and fever inconsequential. Twelve to 24 h later the diarrhoea and pain have subsided. Fatal cases occur rarely; at autopsy they show severe enterocolitis.

Undoubtedly many cases of *C. perfringens* food poisoning occur at home but are not reported. Antibodies to the toxin mediating the symptoms are very common and it is likely that nearly everyone has experienced this disease once or more in their lifetime.

Aetiology

C. perfringens is an ubiquitous sporulating anaerobe with an unparalleled virtuosity for production of biologically significant toxins. The clinical effects of infection with any particular strain may depend largely on its toxin-producing capacity. Strains associated with food poisoning have several special characteristics. They are type A, although their production of α-toxin is variable; the organisms are often heat resistant to 100°C. Eighty-six per cent of food-poisoning strains produce a specific heat-labile enterotoxin. Toxin production *in vitro* is closely associated with sporulation rather than with the multiplication of vegetative cells. *In vivo*, toxin probably acts by damaging enterocyte membranes. Free enterotoxin has been detected in diarrhoeal stool after *C. perfringens* food poisoning. Antibody to enterotoxin increases after such episodes, and ingestion of 8 to 12 mg enterotoxin by volunteers produces abdominal pain and diarrhoea.

C. perfringens is a normal human faecal organism, is regularly found in the intestinal tract of domestic animals, often contaminates raw meat, and can be carried by flies. The distribution of enterotoxin-producing strains may be more restricted. However, surface contamination of meat with *C. perfringens* is common and subsequent rolling or grinding distributes these organisms throughout. Spores germinate and multiply to 10^6 to 10^7 cells/g in the anaerobic environment created when meat or meat gravy cools slowly or stands at ambient temperature. Reheating may not kill these cells and, when ingested, they multiply still further, sporulate, and release their toxin.

Enterotoxin-producing strains of *C. perfringens* may sometimes cause diarrhoea by means of overgrowth in the gut. Patients, usually elderly, can experience diarrhoea without known contact with contaminated food. The diarrhoea may be short lived or persist intermittently for several months. Colony counts of 10^8 to 10^{10}/g of faeces are associated with the presence of high titres of free toxin. Previous antimicrobial treatment may encourage the overgrowth and the same strain has been found to cross-infect patients.

Further reading

Botulism

Arnon SS, *et al.* (2006). Human botulism immune globulin for the treatment of infant botulism. *N Engl J Med*, **354**, 462–71.

Cherington M (2004). Botulism: update and review. *Semin Neurol*, **24**, 155–63.

Chertow DS, *et al.* (2006). Botulism in 4 adults following cosmetic injections with an unlicensed, highly concentrated botulinum preparation. *JAMA*, **296**, 2476–79.

Fox CK, Keet CA, Strober JB (2005). Recent advances in infant botulism. *Pediatr Neurol*, **32**, 149–54.

Lalli G, *et al.* (2003). The journey of tetanus and botulinum neurotoxins in neurons. *Trends Microbiol*, **11**, 431–7.

Sobel J (2009). Diagnosis and treatment of botulism: a century later, clinical suspicion remains the cornerstone. *Clin Infect Dis*, **48**, 1674–5.

Gas gangrene

Aldape MJ, Bryant AE, Stevens DL (2006). *Clostridium sordellii* infection: epidemiology, clinical findings and current perspectives on diagnosis and treatment. *Clin Infect Dis*, **43**, 1436–46.

Bryant AE, Stevens DL (1996). Phospholipase C and perfringolysin O from *Clostridium perfringens* upregulate ELAM-1 and ICAM-1 expression, and induce IL-8 synthesis in cultured human umbilical vein endothelial cells. *Infect Immun*, **64**, 358–62.

Bryant AE, *et al.* (1993). *Clostridium perfringens* invasiveness is enhanced by effects of theta toxin upon PMNL structure and function. *FEMS Immunol Med Microbiol*, **7**, 321–36.

Bryant AE, *et al.* (2000). Clostridial gas gangrene I: cellular and molecular mechanisms of microvascular dysfunction. *J Infect Dis*, **182**, 799–807.

Bryant AE, *et al.* (2000). Clostridial gas gangrene II: phospholipase C-induced activation of platelet gpIIbIIIa mediates vascular occlusion and myonecrosis in *C. perfringens* gas gangrene. *J Infect Dis*, **182**, 808–15.

Bryant AE, *et al.* (2006). *Clostridium perfringens* phospholipase C-induced platelet/leukocyte interactions impede neutrophils diapedesis. *J Med Microbiol*, **55**, 495–504.

Centers for Disease Control (2000). Update: *Clostridium novyi* and unexplained illness among injecting-drug users. *MMWR Morb Mortal Wkly Rep*, **49**, 543–5.

Cohen AL, *et al.* (2007). Toxic shock associated with *Clostridium sordellii* and *Clostridium perfringens* after medical and spontaneous abortion. *Obstet. Gynecol*, **110**, 1027–33.

Darke SG, King AM, Slack WK (1977). Gas gangrene and related infection: classification, clinical features and aetiology, management and mortality. A report of 88 cases. *Br J Surg*, **64**, 104–12.

Maclennan JD (1962). The histotoxic clostridial infections of man. *Bacteriol Rev*, **26**, 177–276.

Shouler PJ (1983). The management of missile injuries. *J R Nav Med Serv*, **69**, 80–4.

Stevens DL, Bryant AE (2005). Clostridial gas gangrene: clinical correlations, microbial virulence factors, and molecular mechanisms of pathogenesis. In: Proft T (ed) *Microbial toxins: molecular and cellular biology*, pp. 313–35. Horizon Bioscience, Norfolk, UK.

Stevens DL, *et al.* (1993). Evaluation of therapy with hyperbaric oxygen for experimental infection with *Clostridium perfringens*. *Clin Infect Dis*, **17**, 231–7.

Stevens DL, *et al.* (2004). Immunization with the C-domain of alpha-toxin prevents lethal infection, localizes tissue injury, and promotes host response to challenge with *Clostridium perfringens*. *J Infect Dis*, **190**, 767–73.

Gastrointestinal infections

Abrahao C, *et al.* (2001). Similar frequency of detection of *Clostridium perfringens* enterotoxin and *Clostridium difficile* toxins in patients with antibiotic-associated diarrhea. *Eur J Clin Microbiol Infect Dis*, **20**, 676–7.

Alfa MJ, *et al.* (2002). An outbreak of necrotizing enterocolitis associated with a novel clostridium species in a neonatal intensive care unit. *Clin Infect Dis*, **35**, S101–S105.

Bos J, *et al.* (2005). Fatal necrotizing colitis following a foodborne outbreak of enterotoxigenic *Clostridium perfringens* type A infection. *Clin Infect Dis*, **40**, e78–e83.

Fisher DJ, *et al.* (2005). Association of beta2 toxin production with *Clostridium perfringens* type A human gastrointestinal disease isolates carrying a plasmid enterotoxin gene. *Mol Microbiol*, **56**, 747–62.

Lawrence GW, *et al.* (1990). Impact of active immunisation against enteritis necroticans in Papua New Guinea. *Lancet*, **336**, 1165–7.

Li DY, *et al.* (2004). Enteritis necroticans with recurrent enterocutaneous fistulae caused by *Clostridium perfringens* in a child with cyclic neutropenia. *J Pediatr Gastroenterol Nutr*, **38**, 213–15.

Obladen M (2009). Necrotizing Enterocolitis – 150 Years of Fruitless Search for the Cause. *Neonatology*, **96**, 203–10.

Sobel J, CG Mixter, P Kolhe, A Gupta, J Guarner, S Zaki, NA Hoffman, JG Songer, M Fremont-Smith, M Fischer, G Killgore, PH Britz, and C MacDonald (2005). Necrotizing enterocolitis associated with *Clostridium perfringens* type A in previously healthy north American adults. *J Am Coll Surg*, **201**, 48–56.

7.6.25 Tuberculosis

Richard E. Chaisson and Jean B. Nachega

Essentials

Tuberculosis is caused by organisms of the *Mycobacterium tuberculosis* complex, including *M. tuberculosis* (the most important), *M. bovis*, and *M. africanum*. It has been present since antiquity and is the second leading infectious cause of death after HIV infection. An estimated 2 billion people worldwide carry latent infection, when *M. tuberculosis* persists within cells and granulomas, with the potential to reactivate to cause disease decades later.

Tubercle bacilli are transmitted between people by aerosols generated when an infectious person coughs. Proximity to an infectious person determines the risk of infection. Host immunity and factors affecting it—most importantly HIV infection but also diabetes, cigarette smoking, and alcohol and drug abuse—determine the risk of active disease following infection.

Clinical presentation of active tuberculosis is highly variable, depending on the site and extent of disease and the immune status of the host. Disease is generally classified as pulmonary or extrapulmonary, with considerable clinical heterogeneity within each group.

Clinical features—pulmonary tuberculosis

Following deposition of tubercle bacilli in the alveoli of the lungs, they are ingested by alveolar macrophages, multiply intracellularly and eventually cause cell lysis with release of organisms. Over a period of weeks, infection spreads to regional lymph nodes, elsewhere in the lungs and systemically. Infected people who successfully contain viable bacilli in granulomas retain a latent infection, with lifetime risk of reactivation of about 10%.

Active pulmonary tuberculosis—this is usually a subacute respiratory illness, the most frequent symptoms of which are cough, fever, night sweats and malaise. The cough is initially nonproductive, but often progresses to sputum production and occasionally haemoptysis. Loss of appetite and excessive weight loss are common.

Clinical features—extrapulmonary tuberculosis

This may be generalized or confined to a single organ, and is found in 15 to 20% of all cases of tuberculosis in otherwise immunocompetent adults, more than 25% of cases under 15 years of age, and in more than 50% of HIV-related cases. Children under 2 years of age have high rates of miliary or disseminated tuberculosis and meningeal disease.

Infection spreads from the lungs by lymphatic and haematogenous routes. The tissues and organs most likely to be affected are the pleura, lymph nodes, kidneys and other genitourinary organs, bone, and central nervous system. Tuberculosis bacteraemia is unusual, but seen most often in patients with HIV infection and low CD4 lymphocyte counts.

Pleural tuberculosis—this is usually the result of relatively small numbers of tubercle bacilli invading the pleura from adjacent lung tissue, in which case the duration of symptoms is generally brief, with patients complaining of symptoms including fever, chest pain, and nonproductive cough. Pleural tuberculosis involving larger numbers of bacilli produces frank empyema and is commoner in older patients.

Lymphatic tuberculosis—classic scrofula of the cervical or supraclavicular lymph node chains is the most common presentation, but multiple lymph node groups can be involved in HIV-infected patients.

Genitourinary tuberculosis—the most common manifestation is renal tuberculosis, resulting from haematogenous seeding of the renal cortex during primary infection; this is frequently asymptomatic, but may be evident as sterile pyuria.

Bone and joint tuberculosis—the most common form is vertebral tuberculosis (Pott's disease), resulting from haematogenous seeding of the anterior portion of vertebral bodies during primary infection; presentation is typically with back pain; constitutional symptoms are not prominent in most cases.

Tuberculous meningitis—meningeal and leptomeningeal bacterial replication results in a robust inflammatory reaction that increases cerebrospinal fluid pressure and can cause cranial neuropathies. Common symptoms are headache, stiff neck, meningismus, and an altered mental status, including irritability, clouded thinking and malaise. The condition is not common, but usually fatal if untreated.

Miliary/disseminated tuberculosis—these describe widespread infection with absent or minimal host immune responses, usually arising as a result of primary infection, and seen more frequently in children and immunocompromised adults. Typical presentation is with fever and other constitutional symptoms over a period of several weeks.

Diagnosis

Tuberculin skin testing—intracutaneous injection of purified proteins of *M. tuberculosis* provokes a delayed hypersensitivity reaction which produces a zone of induration in those who are infected, but cannot distinguish disease from latent infection.

Interferon-γ release-based assays—these detect *in vitro* responses to *M. tuberculosis* antigens. These appear to be more specific than tuberculin skin testing because false-positive reactions due to sensitization from BCG vaccination (see below) are less likely to occur. They may also be more sensitive, and are appealing because they do not require patients to return for reading of induration.

Detection of tubercle bacilli—microscopical staining of acid-fast bacilli in sputum or other tissue is the method most widely used to diagnose tuberculosis because it is inexpensive, rapid, and technologically undemanding. However, a relatively large number of bacilli are needed for a positive test, and up to 50% of patients with sputum cultures positive for *M. tuberculosis* have negative acid-fast smears. Culture of *M. tuberculosis* is the gold standard for confirming the diagnosis, but takes 10 to 40 days, depending on the method used. Nucleic acid amplification assays and other rapid diagnostic methods allow faster detection of both the presence of mycobacteria and assessment of drug resistance: these have promise in resource-limited settings, but further validation in endemic countries is needed.

Particular issues—(1) Pulmonary tuberculosis—this can involve any portion of the lungs, hence radiographic findings are usually only suggestive, not diagnostic. (2) Pleural tuberculosis—diagnosis can be inferred from pulmonary findings when pulmonary parenchymal involvement is manifest, otherwise analysis of pleural fluid is essential. (3) Lymphatic tuberculosis—swelling of involved nodes accompanied by a positive tuberculin skin test and typical biopsy findings are strongly suggestive of tuberculosis and warrant presumptive therapy.

(4) Tuberculous meningitis—diagnosis requires a high degree of suspicion; presumptive therapy is frequently necessary.

Treatment

Drug-susceptible tuberculosis—combination therapy with isoniazid and rifampin (and other antituberculosis drugs in the first 8 weeks) is highly effective. Treatment is usually once daily but can be given as infrequently as twice per week, with two major interventions to improve adherence and prevent bad outcomes being directly observed therapy (DOT) and the use of fixed-dose combination tablets. Modern 'short course' combination chemotherapy is curative in 6 months, except for bone and central nervous system tuberculosis, which require 12 months. Second-line agents are reserved for treatment of drug resistant tuberculosis and are generally less potent, more toxic and less readily available.

Drug-resistant tuberculosis—this significant challenge arises both through infection with drug-resistant strains (primary drug resistance) and by selection for drug-resistant strains due to ineffective therapy (secondary drug resistance). Multidrug resistant (MDR) tuberculosis is defined as resistance to at least rifampicin and isoniazid. Extensively drug-resistant (XDR) disease, which has been reported in more than 70 countries, is defined as MDR plus resistance to fluoroquinolones and at least one injectable second-line agent (capreomycin, amikacin, or kanamycin). Patients with drug-resistant tuberculosis should be managed by a physician who is a tuberculosis expert because of the complexity of their regimens and their high risk of failure of death.

Prevention

Strategies to control tuberculosis include: (1) Identification and treatment of infectious tuberculosis cases, which rapidly eliminates infectiousness. (2) Treatment of latent tuberculosis infection—the use of preventive therapy in high-risk individuals known or strongly suspected to be latently infected with *M. tuberculosis* can benefit not only the individual patient who does not fall ill with tuberculosis, but also potential contacts of that patient, who might become secondarily infected were disease to develop. (3) Prevention of exposure to infectious particles in air, especially in hospitals and other institutions—infected patients must be identified and managed in respiratory isolation. (4) Vaccination—the attenuated live vaccine, BCG (bacille Calmette-Guérin), is widely administered throughout the world, but remains controversial. Proponents argue that it provides about 50% protection against active tuberculosis disease and also diminishes haematogenous dissemination of primary tuberculosis infection, thereby reducing the incidence of miliary tuberculosis and tuberculous meningitis in children.

Introduction

Tuberculosis is one of the most important diseases in the history of humanity, and remains an extraordinary burden on human health today. Archaeological evidence demonstrates that tuberculosis was present in antiquity, and large epidemics of the disease emerged in Europe in the Middle Ages. While contemporary physicians consider tuberculosis to be one of the classic infectious diseases, recognition of the clinical manifestations of the disease has evolved over the past two millennia. The Greek term *phthisis* was used by Hippocrates to describe the wasting disease later known as tuberculosis. While the Greeks recognized various clinical manifestations of tuberculosis, understanding of the connection between the forms was limited. In the Middle Ages, the study of anatomy and the correlation of pathological findings with clinical syndromes led to a better understanding of the disease. The term 'tuberculosis' was used first only in the early 19th century, derived from the tubercles characterized in the study of pathological features of the disease.

The impact of tuberculosis on the humans population cannot be overstated, as the disease has killed hundreds of millions of people over the centuries and has had economic and social effects perhaps unparalleled in the history of medicine. Between 1700 and 1950, tuberculosis was a great killer in the developed world, earning the sobriquet "the captain of the men of death" from John Bunyan, and "the White Plague" from René and Jean Dubos. The inspiration that artists have drawn from tuberculosis, portrayed in literature, opera, and art, testifies not only to the importance of the disease within their contemporary societies, but also to the extent to which tuberculosis affected artists themselves. The annals of art are filled with those who succumbed to tuberculosis including Keats, Chopin, the Bronte sisters, Stevenson, Poe, and many, many others.

The conquest of tuberculosis through the development of vaccines, drugs, and diagnostics was a principal goal of biomedical research in the 19th and 20th centuries. The first description of the tubercle bacillus as the cause of tuberculosis by Robert Koch in 1882 was a scientific landmark. The postulates established by Koch for determining the microbial aetiology of disease have continuing influence today, and molecular correlates of those derived by Koch further strengthen the ingenuity of his thesis. Koch also developed the microscopic and culture methods for detecting tubercle bacilli, still widely used today. Calmette and Guérin developed an effective vaccine for tuberculosis in the early 20th century, but use of the vaccine was not broad enough to control the disease and it may no longer be effective (see below). The discovery of streptomycin by Schatz and Waksman in 1943 was a major triumph; both Koch and Waksman received the Nobel Prize for their work. The development of additional antimicrobial agents against tuberculosis in the 1950s, 1960s, and 1970s, and the evaluation of chemotherapy in elegant studies conducted by the British Medical Research Council, the United States Public Health Service, and the United States Veterans Administration led to a marked apathy about tuberculosis in the closing decades of the 20th century.

Despite the availability of curative chemotherapy for more than half a century, however, tuberculosis continues to kill more than 1.5 million people/year, and causes an enormous amount of suffering and disability. In 1994, the World Health Assembly declared that tuberculosis was a global health crisis, and the situation has only grown more serious since then. Epidemics of HIV-related tuberculosis and multidrug-resistant disease have expanded in recent years, and global control of tuberculosis remains a formidable challenge.

The unique biological properties of the causative organism, *Mycobacterium tuberculosis* complex, allow for a long incubation period between the time of infection and the development of symptoms. Latent tuberculosis infection can persist for decades before causing disease, or can persist for the lifetime of an infected person without ever causing clinically evident illness. Because latent infection creates a large reservoir of carriers of the infection, disease elimination is difficult to envisage.

Aetiology

Tuberculosis is a granulomatous disease caused by organisms of the *M. tuberculosis* complex, including *M. tuberculosis*, *M. bovis*, and *M. africanum*, of which *M. tuberculosis* is the most important. *M. tuberculosis* and the other mycobacteria are small rod-shaped or curved bacilli in the order Actinomycetales, family Mycobacteriaceae, with a unique thick cell wall composed of glycolipids and lipids. The lipid-rich coat of the mycobacteria renders these organisms resistant to acid decolorization following carbol-fuchsin staining, hence the term 'acid-fast bacilli'. Classification of the mycobacteria was based for many years on the staining and growth properties described by Runyon, but this unwieldy system has been largely replaced with modern techniques that identify mycobacteria by specific DNA sequences and, to a lesser extent, biochemical assays. Mycobacteria are frequently considered according to the diseases they cause more than their behaviour in the laboratory: *M. tuberculosis* complex causes tuberculosis; *M. leprae* causes leprosy; and the nontuberculous mycobacteria, including rapid growers, are associated with a wide range of manifestations, particularly in immunocompromised hosts.

The organisms of the *M. tuberculosis* complex are remarkably slow growing, with a generation time between 20 and 24 h. The exceedingly slow intrinsic reproductive rate of *M. tuberculosis* contributes both to its behaviour as a pathogen and to difficulties in recovering the organism in cultures. Moreover, *M. tuberculosis* is able to persist in a latent form within cells and granulomas for many years, and can reactivate to cause disease decades after infection is acquired. Tubercle bacilli are not known to form spores, but both typical bacilli and nonstaining forms of the bacteria persist in cells and tissues, as evidenced by detection of DNA, years after infection is acquired, and retain the capacity to replicate and produce clinical illness. These unique biological characteristics make the tubercle bacillus exceedingly difficult to combat and control.

Epidemiology

Global incidence

Despite the widely held belief that tuberculosis was waning during the 1980s, global tuberculosis incidence has been steady or increasing for several decades. In Western Europe and North America, the incidence of tuberculosis peaked in the 1700s and 1800s, and then declined over a period of years before the development of chemotherapy. Improvements in hygiene and nutrition, along with reductions in household crowding, were credited with these trends. Following the introduction of curative treatment for tuberculosis in the era following the Second World War the incidence of disease fell even further, and tuberculosis deaths were greatly decreased. The success in controlling tuberculosis experienced in the western nations was not replicated in developing countries, and increasing epidemics of the disease have been occurring in these areas. In addition, progress in tuberculosis control in the western nations ironically led to neglect of public health programmes that were responsible for reductions in morbidity. As a consequence of inattention to control, the United States of America experienced a resurgence of tuberculosis between 1985 and 1992, with a 21% increase in the annual number of reported cases during that time. In the United Kingdom, tuberculosis incidence has levelled off in recent years, with an annual incidence of 11 cases per 100 000 people since 1991. Worldwide, tuberculosis continues to kill more than 1.5 million people per year, making it the second leading infectious cause of death after HIV infection. In fact, tuberculosis is a leading cause of death in AIDS, and HIV-related tuberculosis deaths are attributed to AIDS not tuberculosis. If these deaths were attributed to tuberculosis, then tuberculosis would remain the leading infectious cause of death worldwide.

The World Health Organization (WHO) estimates that 2 billion people, or one-third of the world's population, are infected with *M. tuberculosis*. From this seedbed of latent infection, 9.3 million new cases of active disease and 1.7 million deaths were attributed to tuberculosis in 2007. The global distribution of tuberculosis case rates is shown in Fig. 7.6.25.1. Disease due to *M. tuberculosis* is most common in developing nations, both in absolute numbers and incidence of new cases. Twenty-two countries account for 80% of all cases of tuberculosis; India and China are responsible for 23% and 17% of cases, respectively. In general, the highest incidence of disease is found in the countries of sub-Saharan Africa where HIV infection has contributed to extraordinary increases in case rates. The greatest number of cases arise in the populous nations of Asia, which have moderately high rates of disease per capita. The global incidence of tuberculosis is increasing slightly, though population growth is resulting in higher numbers of cases each year. Declines in incidence in the developed world have been offset by increasing rates in the HIV-ravaged countries of Africa and by escalating incidence in Eastern Europe in the aftermath of the collapse of communism and its public health infrastructure.

Effect of age

Tuberculosis typically affects young adults, with peak incidence in those aged 25 to 44 years. The dynamics of tuberculosis within a particular country or region, however, reflect both historical trends in tuberculosis transmission and current risk factors and practices of disease control. For example, in Western Europe tuberculosis is seen in two demographic groups: elderly native Europeans who were presumably infected many years ago and who experience reactivation of latent infections as they age or become immunocompromised, and younger immigrants from high-incidence countries in the developing world. In the United States of America tuberculosis is seen in young adults who have immigrated from endemic areas and in those with HIV infection, whereas reactivation tuberculosis in older people is increasingly uncommon. In the developing world, tuberculosis most commonly occurs in young adults, with rapidly escalating rates in those with HIV infection. In all countries where tuberculosis is prevalent, young children who acquire tuberculosis from adults account for a small proportion of all cases. Interestingly, children between the ages of 5 and 15 years have extremely low rates of tuberculosis, even in areas with a high disease burden.

Infection and disease

The epidemiology of tuberculosis can be considered as a function of two distinct but related phenomena: the likelihood of becoming infected with *M. tuberculosis* and the probability of developing disease once infection has occurred. Risk factors for becoming infected relate to exposure to infectious cases. Throughout the world, living with someone who has infectious tuberculosis is the most important risk factor for acquiring infection. The longer the duration of undiagnosed tuberculosis, the greater the severity of disease, and the more intimate the contact, the greater the chance of becoming infected.

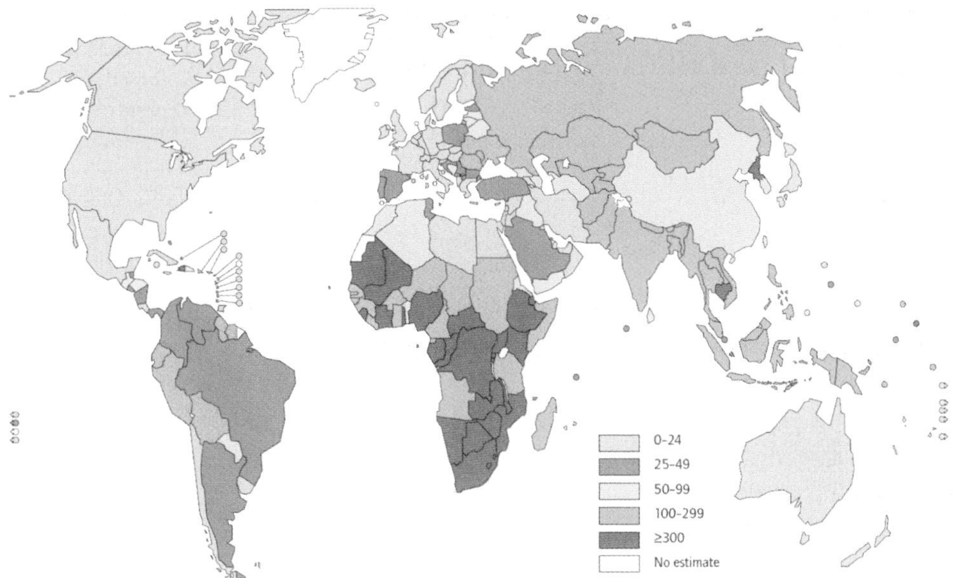

Fig. 7.6.25.1 WHO-estimated global tuberculosis incidence rates in 2005.

Exposure to infectious cases in other environments, including health care facilities, prisons, and the workplace, is another important route of infection. In areas of the world where tuberculosis is relatively widespread, exposure in the community is commonplace and probably unavoidable. In low prevalence countries, community exposure is most likely to occur in distinct pockets of increased incidence, such as poorer areas of large cities or neighbourhoods with high HIV prevalence.

Effect of host immunity

After *M. tuberculosis* infection is acquired, the risk of developing disease is dependent on host immunity. As discussed below, several conditions have been identified that increase the risk of active disease in a person with latent tuberculosis infection, most notably HIV infection. Reactivation from latent tuberculosis infection is an important mechanism for the development of adult tuberculosis. However, studies using DNA fingerprinting techniques show that a significant proportion of tuberculosis cases thought to be due to reactivation are actually recently acquired due to reinfection or new infection, particularly in high HIV prevalence settings.

Effect of *M. tuberculosis* strain

Interestingly, strain differences in *M. tuberculosis* have not been associated with the risk of disease, although inoculum size is associated with probability of becoming ill. For example, household contacts of heavily sputum acid-fast bacilli smear-positive cases of tuberculosis who become infected have a higher incidence of active disease than contacts of acid-fast bacilli smear-negative cases who become infected. On the other hand, while there is some evidence that specific strains of *M. tuberculosis* may more successfully infect contacts than other strains, the risk of disease in those infected with these transmissible strains is not elevated.

Susceptibility

Tuberculosis is a disease traditionally associated with specific population groups, notably the poor, alcohol and drug abusers, and, more recently, those with HIV infection. The increased incidence of tuberculosis in impoverished populations is probably multifactorial, involving increased risk of infection (e.g. due to crowded living conditions and a higher background prevalence of disease in the community) and increased risk of developing disease after infection (e.g. due to malnutrition). Similar reasons may explain the higher rates of tuberculosis seen in cigarette smokers and alcohol and drug abusers, with suppression of host cellular immunity either directly or indirectly caused by substance abuse. The more recent association of tuberculosis and HIV infection is clearly related to development of cellular immunodeficiency in those with HIV, but in many settings those at highest risk for HIV infection are also more likely to be latently infected with *M. tuberculosis* than others.

Effect of the HIV epidemic

The impact of HIV infection on the epidemiology of tuberculosis is striking. As will be discussed below, HIV infection is the most potent known biological risk factor for tuberculosis. The relative risk of tuberculosis in an HIV-infected person is 200 to 1000 times greater than in someone without HIV infection. The risk of tuberculosis increases shortly after HIV seroconversion, doubling within the first year. As a result of the extraordinary risk conferred from HIV infection, the majority of tuberculosis patients in many sub-Saharan countries are HIV seropositive. The incidence of active tuberculosis in HIV-infected patients not receiving antiretroviral therapy in the United States of America, with latent tuberculosis infection defined by a positive tuberculin skin test, is about 10% per year. Of note, an annual incidence rate of about 10% is described in HIV-infected patients in South Africa regardless of tuberculin skin test status. In addition, HIV infection is the unifying theme in many nosocomial outbreaks of tuberculosis, as infection is spread among immunocompromised patients receiving medical care at the same facility. It is increasingly apparent that control of tuberculosis will not be possible globally without control of HIV infection.

Effect of drug resistance

Another very important trend in tuberculosis epidemiology is the growing problem of drug-resistant tuberculosis. Drug-resistant tuberculosis is divided into two categories: primary resistance, which is the presence of drug resistance in someone who has never had treatment for tuberculosis, and secondary resistance, which is the presence of resistance in a patient who has previously been treated for tuberculosis. Primary resistance results from acquiring an infection that is already drug resistant, while secondary resistance is the result of inappropriate therapy that selects for resistant mutants of *M. tuberculosis*. A global survey of resistance performed by the WHO and the International Union Against Tuberculosis and Lung Disease found that the median prevalence of primary drug resistance was 10%, and the median prevalence of acquired resistance was 36%. Moreover, 'hot spots' of drug-resistant tuberculosis were identified on all continents. The most notable of these are in the former Soviet nations where multidrug-resistant (MDR) tuberculosis, defined as resistance to at least rifampicin and isoniazid, is identified in 10 to 20% of all cases. Multidrug-resistant tuberculosis treatment is exceedingly difficult, since the drugs used are less effective, more costly, and poorly tolerated due to drug-related side effects. Furthermore, failure to control the spread of drug-resistant tuberculosis has led to the outbreak of extensively drug-resistant (XDR) tuberculosis, which is defined as multidrug-resistant tuberculosis plus resistance to fluoroquinolones and at least one injectable second-line agent (capreomycin, amikacin, or kanamycin). Extensively drug-resistant tuberculosis been responsible for high rates of mortality in HIV-infected individuals in South Africa and is reported in more than 70 countries globally. Drug-resistant tuberculosis (MDR or XDR) will likely continue without effective implementation of directly observed therapy, short-course (DOTS) and development of more rapid diagnostic tests to detect drug resistance.

Pathogenesis

The development of active tuberculosis, like all infectious diseases, is a function of the quantity and virulence of the invading organism and the relative resistance or susceptibility of the host to the pathogen. Indeed, one lineage of tuberculosis known as the W/Beijing family of strains is predominant in south-east Asia, but widely distributed in India and South Africa. W/Beijing strains of *M. tuberculosis* have been associated with outbreaks of drug-sensitive and drug-resistant tuberculosis and may be more virulent than other strains. Genetic host factors also play a key role in innate nonimmune resistance to *M. tuberculosis*. For example, the human gene *SLC11A1*, which has been mapped to chromosome 2q, may help determine susceptibility to tuberculosis, according to a study in Africa.

Transmission

Tubercle bacilli are transmitted between people by aerosols generated when an infectious person coughs or otherwise expels infectious pulmonary or laryngeal secretions into the air. *M. tuberculosis* bacilli excreted by this action are contained within droplet nuclei, extremely small particles (less than 1 μm) that remain airborne for long periods and are disseminated by diffusion and convection until they are deposited on surfaces, diluted, or inactivated by ultraviolet radiation. Individuals breathing air into which droplet nuclei have been excreted are at risk of acquiring tubercle bacilli by inhaling these nuclei and having them deposited in their alveoli, where a productive infection may occur. Transmission of tuberculous infection by other routes, such as inoculation in laboratories and aerosolization of bacilli from tissues in hospitals, has been documented, but these are an insignificant means of spread. *M. bovis* can be acquired from contaminated milk from tuberculous cows, but modern animal husbandry practices and the pasteurization of milk has virtually eliminated this mode of infection throughout most of the world.

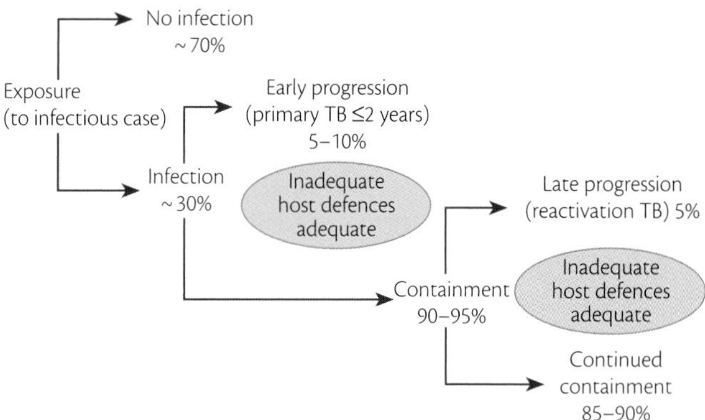

Fig. 7.6.25.2 Natural history of tuberculosis.

Natural history of tuberculosis in humans

People who are in contact with someone with infectious tuberculosis may acquire infection, as described above (see Fig. 7.6.25.2). Factors that affect the likelihood of infection being transmitted include the severity of the disease in the index case (e.g. extent of radiographic abnormalities, cavitation, frequency of cough), the duration and closeness of exposure, and environmental factors such as humidity, ventilation and ambient ultraviolet light. Several studies in diverse locations and circumstances have shown that approximately 20 to 30% of close contacts of an untreated tuberculosis patient become infected with *M. tuberculosis*, as demonstrated by the development of a reactive tuberculin skin test.

Immune response

Deposition of tubercle bacilli in the alveoli results in a series of protective responses by the cellular immune system that forestall the development of disease in the majority of infected people. Alveolar macrophages ingest tubercle bacilli, which then multiply intracellularly and eventually cause cell lysis with release of organisms. Killing of *M. tuberculosis* within macrophages is prevented by inhibition of phagolysosome formation by the tubercle bacilli through a process that is not understood. Additional alveolar macrophages engulf progeny bacilli, resulting in further intracellular growth and cell death. Over a period of weeks as tubercle bacilli proliferate within macrophages and are released, infection spreads to regional lymph nodes, elsewhere in the lungs, and systemically. Foci of tubercle bacilli can be established in multiple organs, including the lymph nodes, brain, kidneys, and bones. In most people, specific immunity is developed after several weeks and consists of activated T lymphocytes mediating a Th1 type response. Macrophages act as antigen-presenting cells, interacting with CD4 lymphocytes primed for *M. tuberculosis* antigens. Activated CD4 lymphocytes produce both IL-2, which promotes activation of additional T lymphocytes, and interferon-γ, which binds with receptors on macrophages and promotes intracellular killing of organisms. Tumour necrosis factor-α production is induced in macrophages, and this too promotes killing of intracellular bacilli. The specific role of CD8 cells in the control of tuberculosis has not been fully elaborated, although there is evidence that cytotoxic T lymphocytes may play a role in containing a tuberculous infection. In addition, CD8 lymphocytes also produce interferon-γ and participate in granuloma formation. Recent evidence also supports a role of innate immunity in combatting tuberculosis infection.

The classic immunological response to infection with tubercle bacilli is the walling off of viable bacilli in granulomas. Granulomas are collections of cells surrounding a focus of *M. tuberculosis*, usually within macrophages but sometimes extracellularly, that serve to contain the infection. Granulomas consist of macrophages, CD4 and CD8 lymphocytes, fibroblasts, giant cells, and epithelioid cells that produce an extracellular matrix of collagenous and fibrotic materials which are continually remodelled and can become calcified. A calcified granuloma at the initial site of infection in the lung is referred to as a Ghon complex, while the combination of a Ghon complex and a calcified regional lymph node is called Ranke's complex.

The development of the cellular immune response to *M. tuberculosis* is accompanied by the development of delayed-type hypersensitivity (DTH) to specific antigens from tubercle bacilli. While DTH is distinct from the cell-mediated immunity that provides protection from disease, this sensitivity to tubercle-derived proteins has proved enormously useful for diagnosing tuberculosis infection. The use of purified protein derivatives (PPD) of tuberculin is the basis for estimating the prevalence of latent tuberculosis infection in populations, is essential in studying the natural history of tuberculosis infection, and is frequently helpful in evaluating patients with suspected tuberculosis disease. The difference between DTH and immunity to tuberculosis is underscored by the observation that 80 to 90% of patients with active disease, and therefore clearly not immune, have positive tuberculin tests.

For the majority of people acquiring a new tuberculous infection, the development of cell-mediated immunity to the organism is protective and holds the bacilli in check, though viability is usually maintained. A small proportion of them will be unable to contain the infection and will progress to active tuberculosis disease, often referred to as primary tuberculosis. Factors associated with early progression of infection to disease include immunosuppression, particularly with HIV infection, a higher inoculum of organisms, malnutrition, and, perhaps, concomitant illness. While rates of active disease in young children who are contacts of cases are no higher than for older contacts, young children with primary tuberculosis do develop more severe forms of tuberculosis than adults, including disseminated disease and tuberculous meningitis.

Reactivation

Those who successfully contain the organism have a latent tuberculosis infection that may reactivate later in life. Based on studies of latent tuberculosis infection acquired in childhood or adolescence, the lifetime risk of reactivation of *M. tuberculosis* is about 10%. Table 7.6.25.1 lists conditions that are associated with an increased risk of reactivating latent tuberculosis infection. The most potent of these is HIV infection, which increases the rate of reactivation by as much as 1000-fold. Immunosuppression from malignancy, cytotoxic therapy, corticosteroids, and other agents that alter cellular immune responses also increase the likelihood that latent tuberculosis infection will reactivate. Other important factors that increase the risk of tuberculosis include diabetes and endstage renal disease, injection drug use (independent of HIV infection), low body weight, gastrointestinal surgery, and silicosis.

Table 7.6.25.1 Incidence of active tuberculosis in people with a positive tuberculin skin test, by selected risk factors

Risk factor	Number of tuberculosis cases/100 person-years
Recent tuberculosis infection:	
Infection <1 year past	2–8
Infection 1–7 years past	0.2
HIV infection	3.5–14
Injection drug use	
HIV seropositive	4–10
HIV seronegative	1
Silicosis	3–7
Radiographic findings consistent with prior tuberculosis	0.2–0.4
Weight deviation from standard:	
Underweight by ≥15%	0.26
Underweight by 10–14%	0.20
Underweight by 5–9%	0.22
Weight within 5% of standard	0.11
Overweight by ≥5%	0.07
Diabetes mellitus	0.3
Renal failure	0.4–0.9
None of the above factors	0.01–0.1

Cigarette smoking is associated with increased tuberculosis incidence, as is alcohol abuse. Recently, the use of inhibitors of tumour necrosis factor-α for the treatment of rheumatoid arthritis or inflammatory bowel disease has been associated with increased risk of tuberculosis. Rates of tuberculosis are usually higher in older people than in younger adults in developed countries, but this may represent a higher prevalence of latent infection in older cohorts, rather than immunological senescence.

Clinical features

Classification of tuberculosis infection and disease

Infection with *M. tuberculosis* can result in clinical manifestations ranging from asymptomatic carriage of latent bacilli to life-threatening pneumonia. Classification of the different stages of *M. tuberculosis* in humans by the American Thoracic Society (ATS) is shown in Table 7.6.25.2. This system is used more for public health purposes

Table 7.6.25.2 American Thoracic Society classification system for tuberculosis

Classification	Description
TB0	No exposure, no infection
TB1	Exposed to tuberculosis, infection status unknown
TB2	Latent infection, no disease (positive PPD tuberculin test)
TB3	Active tuberculosis
TB4	Inactive tuberculosis, healed or adequately treated
TB5	Possible tuberculosis, status unknown ('rule out' tuberculosis)

PPD, purified protein derivative.

than for clinical management, but is useful because it reflects the natural history of *M. tuberculosis* and categorizes patients according to the type of evaluation and treatment they may need.

The ATS category 0 refers to someone without any tuberculosis exposure history and a negative tuberculin skin test (if performed). Category 1 includes those people exposed to an infectious case of tuberculosis but in whom no evidence of infection is found. This is a temporary category used during the evaluation of contacts of tuberculosis cases; repeat tuberculin testing several months after the exposure would result in these individuals being reclassified to another category. Category 2 is defined as latent tuberculosis infection without evidence of disease, and is based on a positive tuberculin skin test without clinical or radiographic signs of illness. Category 3 is confirmed active tuberculosis disease requiring treatment. As discussed below, this category is further divided according to site of disease and laboratory features, including results of acid-fast bacilli smears. Category 4 is defined as inactive tuberculosis. Patients in this category do not have active disease on the basis of clinical and laboratory evaluations, but are known to have previously had tuberculosis. This category includes those who have been treated and cured of active tuberculosis, as well as individuals who have spontaneously recovered from tuberculosis without treatment. Finally, category 5 refers to patients in whom tuberculosis is suspected, but who are still undergoing evaluation. Depending on the degree of suspicion of the diagnosis, such people might be started on presumptive therapy for tuberculosis pending the outcome of cultures and other laboratory assessments. Like category 1, this is a temporary category for patients in the middle of an evaluation, and all patients in this group are reclassified on the basis of diagnostic studies.

Clinical presentation of active tuberculosis

This is highly variable, depending on the site and extent of disease and the immune status of the host. Historically, active tuberculosis has been classified as 'primary' or 'post-primary' on the basis of both the presumed duration of infection and the clinical features of the disease. Recent studies using molecular epidemiological techniques, however, suggest that this classification may be unreliable. For example, the 'classic' presentation of reactivation tuberculosis has been seen in patients whose infection is clearly newly acquired, such as in nosocomial outbreaks where DNA fingerprinting confirms recent transmission. For practical purposes, tuberculosis is generally divided into pulmonary and extrapulmonary forms, with considerable clinical heterogeneity within these categories.

Pulmonary tuberculosis

Pulmonary tuberculosis is usually a subacute respiratory infection with prominent constitutional symptoms. The most frequent symptoms of pulmonary tuberculosis are cough, fever, night sweats, and malaise. Cough in pulmonary tuberculosis is initially nonproductive, but often progresses to sputum production and, in some instances, haemoptysis. The sputum is generally yellow in colour, and is neither malodorous nor thick. Haemoptysis may be seen in patients with untreated tuberculosis, but is also a feature of treated tuberculosis; damage from prior tuberculosis may result in bronchiectasis or residual cavities that can either become superinfected or erode into blood vessels or airways, producing haemoptysis. Extremely advanced tuberculosis may also present with bloody sputum. Rarely, the bleeding is massive leading to shock, asphyxia, and death.

Chest pain is not a prominent symptom in pulmonary tuberculosis, although musculoskeletal pain from coughing may be noted. In patients with tuberculous pleurisy, however, chest pain may be present, particularly on inspiration. Radicular pain across the chest may be associated with spinal tuberculosis. Dyspnoea alone may be a sign of extensive parenchymal destruction, large pleural effusions, endobronchial obstruction, or pneumothorax.

Patients with tuberculosis also experience loss of appetite and weight loss or cachexia, often out of proportion to their diminished intake of food. Elevations in tumour necrosis factor-α are hypothesized to be the cause of cachexia in tuberculosis. Other symptoms with mild severity such as emotional liability, irritability, depression, and headache are frequent.

The duration of symptoms varies greatly, but most patients will report weeks to months of feeling ill before presentation. In surveys of populations with high rates of disease and poor access to medical care, a history of cough for more than 3 weeks was strongly associated with a diagnosis of active tuberculosis. Untreated tuberculosis is associated with high mortality, but many patients may have persistent symptoms for years. A study of untreated pulmonary tuberculosis in the pretherapy era found that after 5 years 50% of patients had died, 25% had spontaneously healed, and 25% were chronically ill with pulmonary disease. A subset of patients has rapidly progressive disease, the so-called 'galloping consumption' of old. Nowadays this is most often seen in patients with HIV infection or other forms of severe immunosuppression. These patients have an escalating course of severe pulmonary symptoms over a period of several weeks, often in the setting of disseminated disease. Failure promptly to diagnose and treat these patients results in death.

Physical findings in pulmonary tuberculosis are limited and not generally helpful in making a diagnosis. Fever is an irregular and unreliable feature, and while most patients complain of fevers before presentation, only one-half to three-quarters of patients with confirmed tuberculosis have a documented fever. Examination of the chest may reveal dullness to percussion and rales, although these findings are highly variable and nonspecific. Signs of consolidation are usually absent. The classic post-tussive rales described in the last century are not often present and are not specific to tuberculosis. Patients with disseminated tuberculosis may have lymphadenopathy, hepatomegaly, or evidence of central nervous system involvement, but these are not generally seen in typical pulmonary tuberculosis. Finger clubbing and cyanosis are findings associated with prolonged and advanced pulmonary disease. Thus, the diagnosis of tuberculosis almost always rests on the patient's history and epidemiological characteristics, in conjunction with laboratory studies described below. The most important step in making a timely diagnosis of tuberculosis is to think of it in the first place.

Radiological evaluations play a critical role in the diagnosis of pulmonary tuberculosis. Disease due to *M. tuberculosis* can involve any portion of the lungs, and radiographic findings are usually only suggestive, not diagnostic, of tuberculosis. The typical radiological manifestations of pulmonary tuberculosis are upper lobe infiltrates that may show cavitation. *M. tuberculosis* exhibits a unique predilection for the upper zones of the lungs for reasons that are not well understood. Latent infection characteristically reactivates in the apical segments of the upper lobes, or the superior segments of the lower lobes. The infiltrates are often fibronodular and irregular, and may be diffuse and associated with volume loss. Cavities, when present, are rarely symmetrical and do not usually have air–fluid levels, such as those seen in pyogenic lung abscesses. Several examples of the radiographic appearance of pulmonary tuberculosis are seen in Fig. 7.6.25.3.

The classic radiographic presentation described above is neither pathognomonic nor highly sensitive for pulmonary tuberculosis. Several other lung infections, notably the pulmonary mycoses, can present with similar findings. More importantly, one-third to one-half of patients with pulmonary tuberculosis lack the classic radiographic findings described. Lower lung zone infiltrates, mid-lung focal infiltrates, pulmonary nodules, and infiltrates with mediastinal or hilar adenopathy are also seen. HIV-infected tuberculosis patients, in particular, most often present with these 'atypical' findings, and up to 5% of them may have a normal chest radiograph in the setting of sputum cultures that yield *M. tuberculosis*. The lack of typical radiographic features should not, therefore, deter the clinician from considering the diagnosis in a patient with a clinical history compatible with and symptoms of tuberculosis.

CT is increasingly used to evaluate pulmonary disorders, including tuberculosis. While the classic findings described above do not usually require confirmation with a more sensitive test, CT scanning is sometimes used to evaluate radiographic findings that are not readily explained after an initial assessment. CT scans of the chest in patients with tuberculosis may reveal a greater extent of involvement than conventional radiographs, including multiple nodules, small cavities, and multilobar infiltrates. However, CT

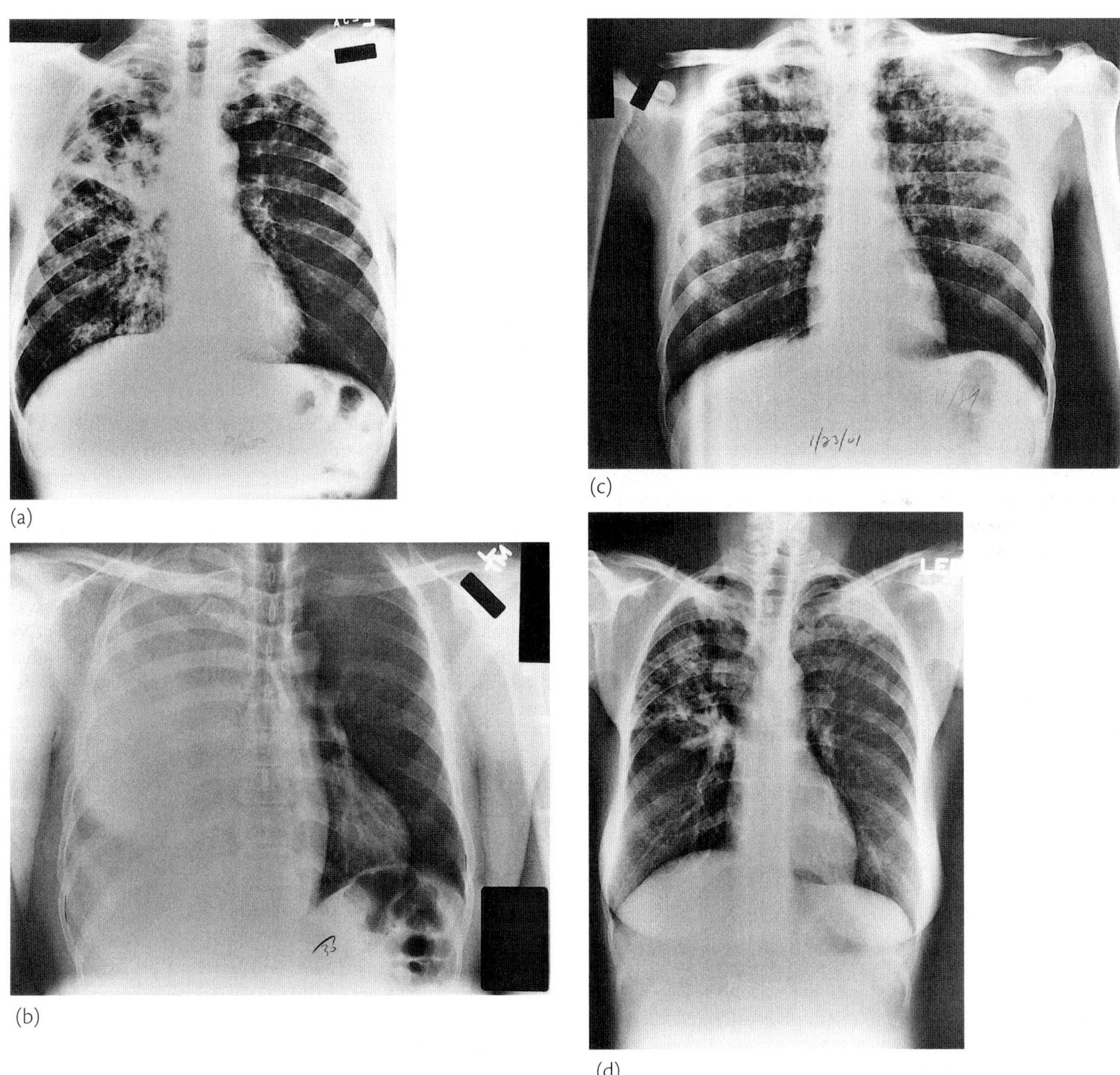

Fig. 7.6.25.3 Radiographic appearance of pulmonary tuberculosis. (a) Extensive tuberculosis with right upper lobe volume loss and multiple small cavities. This patient was the source of at least 14 secondary cases in contacts. (b) A 69-year-old man with right pleural tuberculosis. (c) Diffuse pulmonary nodules in an HIV-infected man with pulmonary tuberculosis. (d) Cavitary upper lobe disease in an HIV-infected woman.

scanning can only suggest the possibility of tuberculosis in a patient with other signs and symptoms consistent with the diagnosis, and further evaluation is still required.

The laboratory diagnosis of pulmonary tuberculosis relies on the microbiological evaluation of sputum or other respiratory tract specimens. A definitive diagnosis requires growth of *M. tuberculosis* from respiratory secretions, while a probable diagnosis can be based on typical clinical and radiographic findings with either acid-fast bacilli-positive sputum or other specimens, or typical histopathological findings on biopsy material. These latter approaches, however, have a variable lack of specificity depending on the prevalence of disease due to nontuberculosis mycobacteria in the population.

Throughout most of the world, sputum acid-fast staining is the sole test used to confirm the diagnosis of pulmonary tuberculosis. In the settings where it is utilized, the positive predictive value of the sputum acid-fast smear is very high, as the likelihood of nontuberculous mycobacterial disease is quite low. In industrialized countries, disease due to the nontuberculous mycobacteria is relatively more common and reliance on smears without cultures is potentially misleading. Despite the best efforts of clinicians, a confirmed diagnosis of tuberculosis cannot be established in some patients who have the disease, and a response to presumptive therapy forms the basis for establishing the diagnosis. Further details on the microbiological approach to diagnosis are provided below.

Extrapulmonary tuberculosis

In the United States of America extrapulmonary tuberculosis is defined as disease outside the lung parenchyma; in the United Kingdom it is defined as disease outside the lungs and pleura. This seemingly subtle distinction has considerable epidemiological impact, however, as pleural tuberculosis is the most common extrapulmonary site of disease in the United States of America.

During the initial seeding of infection with *M. tuberculosis*, described earlier, haematogenous dissemination of bacilli to several organs can occur. These localized infections, as in the lung, can progress into primary tuberculosis or become walled off in small granulomas where bacteria may remain dormant if they are not killed by cell-mediated immune responses. Extrapulmonary tuberculosis, therefore, can either be a presentation of primary or reactivation tuberculosis.

Extrapulmonary tuberculosis may be generalized or confined to a single organ. In otherwise immunocompetent adults, extrapulmonary tuberculosis is found in 15 to 20% of all tuberculosis cases. In young children and immunosuppressed adults, rates of extrapulmonary disease are substantially higher, appearing in more than one-half of HIV-related tuberculosis cases and one-quarter of tuberculosis cases under 15 years of age. Children less than 2 years old have high rates of miliary and meningeal disease.

The organs most frequently involved in extrapulmonary tuberculosis are listed in Table 7.6.25.3. To some extent the frequency with which specific organs are involved reflects the pathophysiology of the disease. Infection spreads from the lungs, the primary site of inoculation, by lymphatic and haematogenous routes. The tissues and organs most likely to be affected are the pleura, lymph nodes, kidneys and other genitourinary organs, bone, and central nervous system. Although infection is transiently spread in the blood, tuberculosis bacteraemia is unusual and is seen most often in patients with HIV infection and low CD4 lymphocyte counts.

Table 7.6.25.3 Common sites of extrapulmonary tuberculosis

Site	Percentage of extrapulmonary cases
Pleura	20–25
Lymphatics	20–40
Genitourinary	5–18
Bone/joint	10
Central nervous system	5–7
Abdominal	4
Disseminated	7–11

The clinical presentation of extrapulmonary tuberculosis depends largely on the organ involved. Both pulmonary and extrapulmonary disease are found in up to 50% of patients with HIV-related tuberculosis, so it is important to consider the possibility of extrapulmonary pathology when pulmonary tuberculosis is diagnosed in an HIV-infected patient (and vice versa). Pulmonary involvement is seen in up to one-quarter of patients with tuberculous meningitis and to lesser degrees with other sites of disease.

Pleural tuberculosis

This is the result of two distinct pathophysiological sequences, which present in strikingly different manners. Most pleural tuberculosis is associated with primary infection and is the result of seeding of the visceral pleura with relatively small numbers of tubercle bacilli via direct extension from adjacent lung tissue. A large proportion of patients with this form of tuberculous pleurisy will have obvious pulmonary disease, although findings may be subtle. The duration of symptoms is generally brief, e.g. several weeks, and patients complain of fever, chest pain, and nonproductive cough. Other constitutional and respiratory symptoms may be present. Unlike pneumococcal pneumonia, which presents abruptly, tuberculous pleurisy starts more insidiously.

The second form of pleural tuberculosis occurs when larger numbers of bacilli invade the pleural space and multiply, producing frank empyema. Tuberculous empyema is seen in older patients, almost all of whom have extensive pulmonary disease. Patients present with prolonged symptoms of cough, chest pain, fever, cachexia, and night sweats. Pneumothorax is a common complication of tuberculous empyema and may be associated with a more rapid disease course.

The radiographic picture in tuberculous pleurisy reflects the underlying pathophysiology of the disease. Patients with the primary type of pleurisy tend to have small unilateral effusions, and up to one-half have visible parenchymal lesions on plain radiographs. In patients with tuberculous empyema, the effusions are larger and more likely to be loculated, and adjacent pulmonary involvement is often evident.

The diagnosis of pleural tuberculosis can be approached along several lines. When pulmonary parenchymal involvement is manifest, sputum smears and cultures have a high yield, and the diagnosis of pleural disease can be inferred from the pulmonary findings. When pulmonary findings are minimal or the initial test results unrevealing, analysis of pleural fluid is essential. Acid-fast stains of pleural fluid are usually negative in patients with primary tuberculous pleurisy as the number of organisms in the pleural space is small.

Repeated sampling will show organisms in less than one-half of cases. Similarly, culture results may be negative. The pleural fluid is usually serous and exudative, with a protein concentration that is more than 50% of the serum level, normal or low glucose, and a slightly acidic pH. The pleural fluid white blood cell count is usually in the range of 1000 to 10 000 per μL with a lymphocytic predominance. Lactate dehydrogenase levels are generally elevated, as are adenosine deaminase levels. All of these tests are nonspecific and cannot reliably distinguish tuberculosis pleurisy from other pleural diseases.

Pleural biopsy is frequently useful in establishing a diagnosis of tuberculous pleurisy. Percutaneous biopsy of the pleura reveals granulomatous inflammation in up to 80% of patients, and cultures obtained at the time of biopsy are positive in over one-half of patients. If a first attempt fails to provide a diagnosis, a second biopsy may be successful. More recently thoracoscopy has been utilized to improve the yield of biopsy by visualizing biopsy targets rather than blindly sampling with a percutaneous pleural needle.

Lymphatic tuberculosis

This can occur in any location, but classic scrofula involving the cervical or supraclavicular chains is the most common presentation. Mediastinal and hilar lymphatic tuberculosis is a feature both of primary and disseminated disease, but discovery of these lesions is usually incidental. The pathophysiology of lymphatic tuberculosis is thought to result from drainage of bacilli in the lungs into supraclavicular and posterior cervical lymph node chains. In contrast, lymphatic disease caused by nontuberculous mycobacteria usually involves anterior cervical, preauricular, or submandibular lymph nodes, suggesting acquisition through the oropharynx. In patients with HIV infection, multiple lymph node groups may be involved including axillary, inguinal, mesenteric, and retroperitoneal.

Symptoms in lymphatic tuberculosis are generally limited, unless the disease is disseminated. Painless swelling of a lymph node is the most common presentation. Constitutional symptoms are not prominent in most cases. Examination of the area may reveal several enlarged lymph nodes, as only about 20% of patients have disease of a solitary node.

The diagnosis of lymphatic tuberculosis usually depends on cultures from affected nodes. Biopsies may show granulomatous changes and acid-fast bacilli. Such findings are nonspecific, however, and cannot distinguish tuberculous from nontuberculosis lymphadenitis. As discussed elsewhere, the presence of a positive tuberculin skin test in the setting of typical biopsy findings is strongly suggestive of tuberculosis; in the setting of suspected lymphatic tuberculosis, these findings warrant presumptive therapy.

Genitourinary tuberculosis

This encompasses a broad array of clinical entities, ranging from disease of the kidneys to endometrial, prostatic, and epididymal disease. The most common of these is renal tuberculosis, which results from haematogenous seeding of the renal cortex during the primary infection. The pathogenesis of other genitourinary sites is either from downstream extension of renal infection over time or from haematogenous seeding at the time of the initial acquisition of *M. tuberculosis*.

Renal tuberculosis is probably underdiagnosed because it is frequently asymptomatic. Many cases of genitourinary tuberculosis are diagnosed as a result of routine urinalyses that detect sterile pyuria. The development of symptoms reflects a more advanced stage of disease, associated with considerable tissue destruction. When genitourinary tuberculosis is symptomatic, the most common symptoms are localized and include urinary symptoms and flank pain. In men, tuberculosis can cause prostatitis and epididymitis, both of which can present with pain resulting from swelling. In women, genital tract tuberculosis may be symptomatic when it involves the ovaries and Fallopian tubes; pelvic pain is also a feature of endometrial tuberculosis. Menstrual abnormalities and infertility may be the only signs of genital disease, however.

The diagnosis of genitourinary tuberculosis depends on the anatomical site of the disease. Renal tuberculosis, as noted, is suggested by sterile pyuria, and the diagnosis rests on isolation of organisms in the urine. Early morning urine samples are more likely to grow *M. tuberculosis* than spot samples obtained at other times. In patients with symptoms of upper urinary tract illness, radiological studies are often helpful. The kidneys may appear calcified on abdominal radiographs. Intravenous pyelography may show distorted or dilated calyces or renal pelvis, papillary necrosis, cavitation or abscesses of the renal parenchyma, or intrarenal or ureteral obstructions. Use of renal ultrasonography or CT scanning may be more sensitive for identifying the abnormalities of renal tuberculosis, but contrast radiography is the technique with which the greatest experience has accrued. When tuberculosis of the bladder is suspected, cystoscopy with biopsy may lead to the identification of granulomas before identification of organisms by culture. Diagnosis of prostatic, testicular, or epididymal tuberculosis is usually accomplished with cultures obtained by fine needle aspiration or transurethral resection of the prostate. Cervical and endometrial tuberculosis can be diagnosed by biopsy with culture.

Tuberculous meningitis (Chapter 24.11.1)

This is the most common central nervous system manifestation of tuberculosis. It is much more likely to occur in children under the age of 15 years and in HIV-infected patients than in immunocompetent adults. Although meningitis accounts for only a small fraction of all cases of tuberculosis, it is a devastating form of the disease that is uniformly fatal if left untreated.

The pathogenesis of meningeal tuberculosis varies with the age and immunological status of the patient. Reactivation of microscopic granulomas in the meninges was found by Rich to cause diffuse meningeal infection. These foci of infection are probably implanted at the time of primary bacillaemia. When these lesions rupture into the subarachnoid space they invoke an inflammatory response leading to tuberculous meningitis. Meningeal disease can also complicate miliary disease, especially in children. Likewise, adults can acquire meningeal disease during bacillaemia of miliary disease, but this is not the usual pathogenesis of meningeal infection. Rarely, invasion into the spinal canal from a paraspinous or vertebral focus can also be the source of central nervous system involvement.

The clinical features of tuberculous meningitis are the consequence of the pathophysiological process underlying the disease. Meningeal and leptomeningeal bacterial replication results in a robust inflammatory reaction, often localized to the base of the brain. The number of bacilli present is usually limited, and the severity of illness is a function of the host response. Meningeal inflammation causes increases in cerebrospinal fluid pressure and can also cause cranial neuropathies. Patients complain of headache, neck stiffness, meningism, and an altered mental status, including irritability, clouded thinking, and malaise; as the disease progresses, symptoms worsen considerably.

The clinical spectrum of tuberculous meningitis has historically been categorized in three stages, defined by the British Medical Research Council in 1948. Stage 1 consists of a prodrome lasting for 1 to 3 months. Nonspecific symptoms such as fever, malaise, and headache predominate. In this stage, patients are conscious and rational, but may have signs of meningism. Focal neurological signs are absent and there are no signs of hydrocephalus. In stage 2 disease, single cranial nerve abnormalities such as ptosis or facial paralysis appear, and paresis and focal seizures may occur. Kernig's and Brudzinski's signs have been noted as well as hyperactive deep tendon reflexes. Prominent signs include alterations in mentation, behavioural change, impaired cognitive ability, and increasing stupor. Headache and fever are also common features of this stage of disease.

In stage 3, patients are comatose (Glasgow coma scale 8 or below) or stuporous and often have multiple cranial nerve palsies and hemiplegia or paraplegia. By this stage, hydrocephalus is common and chronic inflammation in the enclosed space of the skull may result in significant intracranial hypertension. Seizures may be a prominent feature.

Fever, headache, altered level of consciousness, and meningism are present in the majority of patients in most large studies, although no one single sign or symptom has any reliable degree of sensitivity or specificity. Children can be especially difficult to diagnose as symptoms such as fever, vomiting, drowsiness, or irritability are commonly seen in many minor viral illnesses.

Transient tuberculous meningitis that presents as an aseptic meningitis and resolves without treatment has been described. Benign presentations of meningeal tuberculosis are uncommon in clinical practice, and when the diagnosis is made, treatment is mandatory, even in the patient with seemingly trivial symptoms.

The diagnosis of tuberculous meningitis is often difficult and requires a high degree of suspicion. In the setting of disseminated disease, signs of tuberculosis in other organs, particularly the lungs, are often present. Between 25 and 50% of patients with meningitis in most series also have radiographic evidence of pulmonary tuberculosis, either active or healed. The critical features of tuberculous meningitis, however, are found in the cerebrospinal fluid. Patients with tuberculous meningitis usually have elevated cerebrospinal fluid pressure. An exudative fluid with a mononuclear cell pleocytosis is characteristic. Cerebrospinal fluid is usually clear and the protein is generally in the range of 100 to 500 mg/dl. Hypoglycorrhachia is typical, with cerebrospinal fluid glucose less than 50% of the serum value. The white blood cell count rarely exceeds 1000 per μL, and cell counts below 500 are typical. In early meningitis, the cells may be predominantly neutrophils, but mononuclear cells predominate in most instances. Acid-fast stains of concentrated cerebrospinal fluid are only positive in one-third or fewer of patients, and cultures are positive in only one-half, although repeated sampling increases the yield.

The disastrous consequences of failing to diagnose tuberculous meningitis, coupled with the low yield of cerebrospinal fluid acid-fast stains and cultures, has prompted the development of additional tests for establishing a diagnosis. Adenosine deaminase was initially reported to be exceptionally accurate for tuberculous meningitis. Subsequent experience, however, has found it to be insufficiently specific to distinguish tuberculosis from a variety of other acute and chronic meningitides. Several other tests based on identification of mycobacterial antigens or specific antibodies have been evaluated, but none has been found to be reliable. Nucleic acid amplification tests such as polymerase chain reaction (PCR) have great appeal, but the sensitivity and specificity of available assays are only moderately good. Thus, the diagnosis of tuberculous meningitis often rests on the astute judgment of a clinician with a high degree of suspicion based on epidemiological and clinical clues. Presumptive therapy is frequently necessary.

Central nervous system tuberculomas

These are an unusual manifestation and are seen in a small proportion of patients with tuberculous meningitis. Tuberculomas are the result of enlarging tubercles that extend into brain parenchyma rather than into the subarachnoid space. Patients with HIV infection appear to have an increased risk of central nervous system tuberculomas, but the disease is far less common than toxoplasmosis, even in areas where tuberculosis is highly prevalent. Central nervous system tuberculomas may appear with clinical features of meningitis or of intracranial mass lesions. In the absence of meningeal involvement, seizures or headaches may be the only symptoms. The diagnosis is suggested by brain imaging, with MRI scanning being more sensitive than CT scanning. Biopsy of the lesion is required for diagnosis, and material should be submitted for histopathological staining and culture.

Bone and joint tuberculosis

These may affect several areas, but vertebral tuberculosis (Pott's disease) is the most common form, accounting for almost one-half of cases. Haematogenous seeding of the anterior portion of vertebral bone during initial infection sets the stage for later development of Pott's disease. Infection grows initially within the anterior vertebral body, then may spread to the disc space and to paraspinous tissues. Destruction of the vertebral body causes wedging and eventual collapse. Patients usually complain of back pain, with constitutional symptoms less prominent. Neurological impairment is a late complication, but delays in diagnosis are common and many patients experience neurological sequelae. Imaging studies of the spine usually reveal anterior wedging, collapse of vertebrae, and paraspinous abscesses. The diagnosis is established with bone biopsy or curettage, or by culture of the drainage from a paraspinous abscess.

Miliary tuberculosis and disseminated tuberculosis

These are terms used interchangeably to describe widespread infection and the absence of minimal host immune responses. The term 'miliary tuberculosis' is derived from the classic radiographic appearance of haematogenous tuberculosis, in which tiny pulmonary infiltrates with the appearance of millet seeds are distributed throughout the lungs. Miliary tuberculosis is a more common consequence of primary tuberculosis infection than reactivation, and is seen more frequently in children and immunocompromised adults. Primary miliary tuberculosis presents with fever and other constitutional symptoms over a period of several weeks. Clinical evaluation may reveal lymphadenopathy or splenomegaly and choroidal tubercles on retinoscopy. Laboratory tests may show only anaemia. The chest radiograph is initially normal but later develops the typical miliary pattern. Involvement of multiple organ systems is the rule, usually liver, spleen, lymph nodes, central nervous system, and urinary tract. Patients with reactivation of latent infection who present with miliary disease may have a more fulminant course, although progression to severe disease without treatment is the rule in all patients. The diagnosis is made on tissue biopsy and culture, as sputum smears are usually negative, reflecting the small numbers of bacilli typically present in respiratory secretions.

Other forms of extrapulmonary tuberculosis are less common than those listed above, and the diagnosis is based on a combination of clinical suspicion and the results of biopsies and cultures. Abdominal, ocular, adrenal, and cutaneous tuberculosis are all rarely encountered in the modern era, even in immunocompromised patients.

Laboratory diagnosis

Evaluation of patients for *M. tuberculosis* infection or disease relies on both nonspecific and specific tests. Imaging studies, body fluid chemistries and cell counts, and histochemical staining, as described above, are useful and important tests for the diagnosis of tuberculosis. Specific studies for identifying mycobacterial infections include the tuberculin skin test, acid-fast microscopy, and mycobacterial culture.

Tuberculin skin testing

Tuberculin skin testing (TST) involves the intracutaneous injection of purified proteins of *M. tuberculosis* (purified protein derivative, or PPD tuberculin) that provokes a cell-mediated delayed-type hypersensitivity reaction which produces a zone of induration. Tuberculin originated with Robert Koch who prepared a tubercle sensitin that he thought would cure tuberculosis. Administration of Koch's tuberculin, of course, did not cure the disease, and hypersensitivity reactions to the agent were sometimes severe or fatal, bringing Koch great discredit.

Fortunately, it was recognized that because tuberculin induced reactions in people who were infected with tuberculosis the substance might prove a better diagnostic test than treatment. Over a period of years refinements were made in the preparation of tuberculins, and in 1939 Seibert and Glenn produced the reference lot of tuberculin, called PPD-S, which has served as the international standard. Current tuberculin preparations are composed of a variety of small tuberculous proteins derived from culture filtrates and stabilized with a polysorbate detergent to prevent precipitation. The standard dose of tuberculin is 5 tuberculin units (TU) of PPD-S, equivalent to 0.1 mg tuberculin in a volume of 0.1 ml. Commercial and other tuberculin products are standardized against PPD-S to ensure bioequivalence.

Tuberculin testing is used to identify people with *M. tuberculosis* infection, and the test cannot distinguish those who have disease from those with latent infection. Injection of tuberculin into an infected individual invokes a delayed-type hypersensitivity response. Specific T lymphocytes sensitized to tuberculous antigens from prior *M. tuberculosis* infection cause a local reaction at the site of injection. Inflammation, vasodilation, and fibrin deposition at the site result in both erythema and induration of the skin. Induration is the key feature of a tuberculin response, and the result of tuberculin testing is categorized according to the amount of induration measured.

Tuberculin skin testing should be done by the Mantoux method, as this is the only technique that has been standardized and extensively validated. Using a tuberculin syringe and small gauge needle, 0.1 ml of PPD-S is injected intracutaneously in the volar surface of the forearm causing a small wheal. Injection into the subcutaneous space will result in uninterpretable results. Multipuncture devices should not be used. The amount of induration should be measured 2 to 5 days after the injection; measurements performed precisely 48 to 72 h later are not essential. The transverse diameter of induration should be measured in millimetres using a ruler. The edge of the induration can be seen and marked, or the margins can be detected using the ballpoint pen method, in which the pen is rolled over the skin with light pressure and its progress is stopped at the demarcation of the indurated area.

Criteria for the interpretation of tuberculin skin tests vary according to clinical and epidemiological circumstances. Cut-off points for positive tests developed by the ATS and the Centers for Disease Control and Prevention (CDC) are listed in Table 7.6.25.4. A cut-off point of 5 mm induration is used for individuals who are at high risk of tuberculosis infection, or at high risk of disease if infected. Such people include the close contacts of infectious patients and patients with radiographic abnormalities consistent with tuberculosis. The rationale for the 5-mm cut-off in these patients is that the prior probability of infection is high. A 5-mm cut-off is also used for HIV-infected patients and those immunocompromised by corticosteroids or other agents. Failure to diagnose tuberculosis infection in these people could be calamitous, so a lower threshold is used to maximize sensitivity. The use of control antigens such as candida or tetanus toxoid to aid the interpretation of tuberculin tests in HIV-infected patients has been shown to be of no value and is not recommended.

A cut-off point of 10 mm induration is used for people from populations with a high prevalence of tuberculosis or for individuals with conditions that increase the risk of developing active disease if infected. This would include immigrants from endemic areas, residents of some inner cities, and health care workers, as well as patients with diabetes, renal disease, silicosis, and other medical conditions associated with an elevated risk of reactivation of latent tuberculosis. Finally, a cut off of 15 mm is used in people who have no risk factors for tuberculosis infection or disease. In most instances, these patients presumably would not be tested.

Tuberculin testing does have limitations in both sensitivity and specificity. The 5-TU dose of tuberculin used diagnostically is based on studies in the 1940s that showed that 99% of chronic tuberculosis patients responded to this dose, while fewer than 20% of those without disease and no history of tuberculosis exposure had a response. Subsequent research suggested that the lack of specificity of tuberculin testing may be the result of cross-reactions due to exposure to nontuberculous mycobacteria. For example, use of tuberculin derived from *M. avium intracellulare* (PPD-B) induces larger reactions than PPD-S in healthy people from areas where this organism is widespread in the environment. Another important cause of nonspecific reactions to tuberculin is vaccination with bacille Calmette-Guérin (BCG). While the reactogenicity of BCG vaccines differs according to the strain, immunization with BCG can produce falsely positive skin test results. Reactions induced by BCG tend to be smaller than true-positive reactions, and wane over a period of several years. Studies in populations with high rates of BCG coverage indicate that tuberculin testing can still be used to predict those who are most likely to be infected with *M. tuberculosis*, even though precision is reduced because of cross-reactions.

Table 7.6.25.4 Criteria for tuberculin positivity, by risk group

Reaction ≥5 mm induration	Reaction ≥10 mm induration	Reaction ≥15 mm induration
HIV-positive persons	Recent immigrants (i.e. within the last 5 years) from high-prevalence countries or regions	Persons with no risk factors for tuberculosis
Recent contacts of infectious tuberculosis patients	Injection drug users	
Persons with fibrotic changes on chest radiograph consistent with prior tuberculosis	Residents and employees of the following high-risk congregate settings: Prisons and jails Nursing homes and other long-term facilities for older people Hospitals and other health care facilities Residential facilities for patients with AIDS Homeless shelters	
Patients with organ transplants and other immunosuppressed patients (receiving the equivalent of ≥15 mg/day prednisone for 1 month or more)	Persons with the following clinical conditions that place them at high risk: Silicosis Diabetes mellitus Chronic renal failure Some haematological disorders (e.g. leukaemias and lymphomas) Other specific malignancies (e.g. carcinoma of the head or neck and lung) Weight loss of ≥10% of ideal body weight Gastrectomy Jejunoileal bypass	
Others	Mycobacteriology laboratory personnel Children <4 years of age or infants, children, and adolescents exposed to adults at high-risk	

False-negative tuberculin tests result from both errors in applying and interpreting the test and from anergy. Errors in injection of tuberculin are common, and inter-reader variability in measuring results is high. Fortunately, if there is doubt about the interpretation of a skin test, multiple readers can measure the result over a period of days, or the test can be repeated and reinterpreted. Specific anergy to tuberculin is seen in several situations. Approximately 10 to 20% of patients with culture-confirmed pulmonary tuberculosis fail to respond to tuberculin as a result of anergy. These patients often will mount a response after their disease has been treated. HIV-infected patients have a high prevalence of anergy, both to tuberculin and other antigens. Only 10 to 40% of patients with low CD4 counts and confirmed tuberculosis respond to tuberculin. Transient anergy is associated with acute viral infections such as measles, live virus vaccinations, and other acute medical illnesses.

Alternative methods: interferon-γ production by sensitized T cells

Tuberculin skin testing is frustratingly crude and somewhat cumbersome, but despite its limitations has proved superior to numerous more 'modern' assays including antibody tests and other *in vitro* immunodiagnostics. Recently, however, the use of assays to detect interferon-γ production by sensitized T cells in response to challenge with specific antigens from the RD1 region of the *M. tuberculosis* genome has shown promise as an alternative to tuberculin testing. Two commercial assays, one an enzyme-linked immunospot (T-SPOT-TB) and one an enzyme-linked immunosorbent assay (ELISA) (Quantiferon TB Gold-In Tube) are now approved in several countries for *in vitro* diagnosis of tuberculosis infection. These assays are more than 90% sensitive for active tuberculosis and more specific than tuberculin testing in BCG-vaccinated individuals, correlate better than tuberculin skin testing with exposure to a point source of infection, and may not be compromised by immunosuppression related to HIV infection. In some studies, these assays have greater sensitivity than tuberculin skin testing and almost always have better specificity. In evaluating individuals with latent tuberculosis infection, however, the lack of a gold standard of diagnosis makes comparisons difficult. However, emerging evidence suggests that interferon-γ release assays may be more accurate than tuberculin testing in predicting which people are at greatest risk of developing subsequent active tuberculosis disease. Thus, the assays have enormous potential and may contribute to improved detection of both active and latent tuberculosis infections.

Microscopic staining

Microscopic staining of acid-fast bacilli is the method most widely used to diagnose tuberculosis throughout the world. Acid-fast staining is inexpensive, rapid, and technologically undemanding, making it an attractive technique for identifying mycobacterial infections. The waxy glycolipid matrix of the mycobacterial cell wall is resistant to acid–alcohol decolorization after staining with carbol-fuchsin dyes, and red bacilli are visible after counterstaining. Both the Ziehl-Neelsen method (which requires heat fixation) and the Kinyoun method utilize methylene blue or malachite green counterstains, and have similar sensitivities for identifying acid-fast bacilli in clinical specimens.

The major limitation of acid-fast staining is that a relatively large number of bacilli must be present to be seen microscopically. Acid-fast smears are generally negative when there are fewer than

10 000 bacilli/ml of sputum, and many microscope fields need to be examined to identify bacilli even when there are 10 000 to 50 000 bacilli/ml. Thus, up to 50% of patients with sputum cultures positive for *M. tuberculosis* have negative acid-fast smears. In settings where the sputum smear is the only test done to confirm tuberculosis, a large number of smear-negative cases go undetected. This is a serious problem for patients without cavitary tuberculosis, who tend to have fewer bacilli in their sputum, including many HIV-infected tuberculosis patients in developing countries.

Improving the yield of sputum smears

Several techniques can be used to improve the yield of sputum smears. The most important method is enrichment of the specimen through concentration of the sputum. Centrifugation of sputum allows examination of the bacilli-rich pellet, which improves the sensitivity of smears substantially. Treatment of sputum with mucolytic agents is also helpful in identifying organisms by both smear and culture. Use of fluorochrome procedures to identify mycobacteria is more sensitive, but less specific, than acid-fast stains. Auramine O or auramine-rhodamine dyes are used on concentrated smears and examined under a fluorescence microscope. This technique allows much more rapid screening of slides than the traditional methods, but confirmation of positive results with Ziehl-Neelsen or Kinyoun staining is essential, as false-positive fluorochrome results are not uncommon.

The proper collection of specimens is also important for optimizing the results of microscopy and culture. Early morning sputum specimens tend to have a higher yield than specimens collected at other times, and overnight sputum collections have provided even greater sensitivity. Morning gastric aspirates have a moderate yield for acid-fast bacilli in children, who generally have a difficult time producing sputum. Sputum induction with hypertonic saline is useful in evaluating patients with minimal or no sputum production, and the use of fibreoptic bronchoscopy is often advocated for patients with negative sputum smears. In several series, however, the yield of postbronchoscopy spontaneous sputum samples was higher than for the bronchoalveolar lavage fluid. While the goal of sputum collection is to collect a pure lower respiratory tract sample, specimens that appear to consist primarily of upper respiratory tract or oral secretions are often smear or culture positive in patients with pulmonary tuberculosis.

Examination of multiple specimens increases the sensitivity of sputum microscopy for acid-fast bacilli. The first smear identifies 70 to 80% of patients, the second another 10 to 15%, and the third another 5 to 10%. Review of additional specimens has little value.

In addition to the modest sensitivity of acid-fast staining, the specificity of this technique can also present problems. The morphological properties of the mycobacteria are sufficiently similar to make distinguishing *M. tuberculosis* from nontuberculous mycobacteria impossible on the basis of acid-fast smears. This is not a serious problem where tuberculosis is common and nontuberculous mycobacterial infections are unusual. However, in many industrialized countries, disease due to the nontuberculous mycobacteria is relatively common, and distinguishing these types of infections has important therapeutic and public health implications. Thus, while sputum microscopy is useful because of its rapidity and low cost, it should be supplemented with culture or other more sensitive and specific tests whenever feasible.

Culture, nucleic acid amplification, and susceptibility testing

Culture of *M. tuberculosis*

This is the gold standard for confirming the diagnosis of tuberculosis. A variety of media are available that support the growth of mycobacteria, including egg-based and potato-based solid media and several broth-based media. The intrinsic growth rate of *M. tuberculosis* makes the recovery of the organism in culture a slow process. In traditional egg-based media such as Lowenstein–Jensen, growth of colonies of *M. tuberculosis* takes between 3 and 6 weeks, and 7H11 agar requires an average of 3 to 4 weeks to show colonies. Obviously, the slow pace of these traditional culture systems interferes with optimal patient management, and more rapid techniques are required.

Several faster (not rapid) systems for detection of mycobacteria in culture have been commercially developed. The radiometric BACTEC system utilizes ^{14}C palmitate in 7H12 broth to more quickly detect mycobacterial growth. The reliance of this technology on radioisotopes, however, makes it an unattractive approach, and other methods are emerging to take its place.

The Mycobacterial Growth Indicator Tube (MGIT) is a broth-based system that uses fluorescence detection to monitor growth. Both manual and automated systems are available. Once growth is detected, staining to identify acid-fast organisms and species identification need to be performed. The time to detection of mycobacteria using MGIT is considerably faster than conventional solid media, and the yield can be appreciably higher. Contamination of cultures with bacteria and fungi is common, and laboratory cross-contamination remains a concern. Nevertheless, the use of MGIT can increase case detection rates and speed the time to detection of tuberculosis.

Many clinical laboratories use more than one culture system for mycobacteria, both to increase the overall recovery rate and to provide quality control. In addition, if one culture becomes contaminated, alternative cultures can still be utilized.

Preparation of specimens for mycobacterial culture

This follows the same steps as outlined for acid-fast smears. In addition, specimens being submitted for culture also require decontamination to prevent overgrowth by more rapidly multiplying bacteria. Sodium hydroxide (NaOH) and *N*-acetyl-L-cysteine (NALC) are commonly used together for mucolysis and decontamination. By necessity, decontamination also inactivates >50% of mycobacteria in a specimen, thereby reducing the potential yield of the culture. Failure to decontaminate, however, leads to bacterial overgrowth and uninterpretable results. Lack of growth as a result of overdecontamination and bacterial overgrowth resulting from underdecontamination underscore the importance and utility of obtaining multiple specimens for culture, when possible. As with sputum smears, the yield of mycobacterial culture increases with evaluation of additional specimens.

Speciation

After mycobacterial growth has been identified, speciation of the organism is required. Conventional techniques for identification of mycobacterial species involve characterization of colony morphology, pigmentation, rate of growth, and biochemical tests. Niacin reduction, nitrate reduction, and lack of catalase activity at elevated temperatures are all characteristic of *M. tuberculosis*.

Species identification using these methods is time consuming and tedious, and further delays the diagnosis of tuberculosis.

The use of nucleic acid probes has dramatically simplified speciation of mycobacteria in recent years. DNA probes that react with specific mycobacterial rRNA sequences to form DNA–RNA hybrids that can be readily detected by chemoluminescence are commercially available for *M. tuberculosis*, *M. avium* complex, *M. kansasii*, and *M. gordonae*. These probes can be performed within hours of detection of mycobacterial growth, and significantly accelerate the diagnosis of specific pathogens. The sensitivity of these probes is approximately 90 to 95%, depending on the species, with specificities approaching 100%. Cultures that fail to respond to any of the DNA–RNA probes are almost always due to another mycobacterial species, but final identification depends on the laborious biochemical techniques of old.

The difficulties of identifying mycobacteria in patient specimens accentuate the need for rapid and sensitive diagnostic methods for tuberculosis. If any infection seems suited to diagnosis by nucleic acid amplification assays, it would appear to be tuberculosis. Multiple studies of 'in-house' PCR assays for *M. tuberculosis* have shown modest sensitivity and specificity. PCR inhibitors in sputum have been a knotty problem in the molecular diagnosis of pulmonary tuberculosis, although sensitivity has been lower than culture in nonrespiratory specimens as well. Recently, several commercial nucleic acid amplification tests have been introduced or are nearing approval, including assays based on reverse transcription (RT)-PCR, transcription-mediated amplification, ligase chain reaction, and strand displacement amplification. All of these techniques use specific *M. tuberculosis* DNA sequences (most use the *M. tuberculosis* transposon *IS*6110) as targets for nucleic acid amplification. The great advantage of these assays is that they can provide results within 1 day of the collection of specimens. Their disadvantage is that they are uniformly less sensitive than culture, particularly in sputum smear-negative patients. Early studies also suggested that specificity was excellent overall but was reduced in smear-positive samples; further refinements in these assays have resulted in improved sensitivity and specificity, but their diagnostic role in smear-negative sputum or extrapulmonary disease is limited by their moderate sensitivity. Furthermore, the cost of nucleic acid amplification tests may be too high for routine use in resource-limited settings where tuberculosis is endemic.

Evaluations of nucleic acid amplification assays under field conditions have generally shown favourable results. When using these tests, however, clinicians must not forget fundamental clinical and epidemiological principles regarding the diagnosis of tuberculosis: a negative test in a patient suspected of having tuberculosis should not exclude the diagnosis, nor should a positive test confirm it if clinical circumstances do not support the diagnosis. While both the positive and negative predictive values of nucleic acid amplification tests are high (70–90% and >90%, respectively), misclassification of patients does occur, and it is important to use mycobacterial culture to validate the results of these rapid assays.

Drug susceptibility testing

Susceptibility testing of *M. tuberculosis* isolates is essential for both clinical management and public health purposes. Susceptibility tests for the first-line antituberculosis drugs should be performed on at least one culture at the time of diagnosis for all patients. If the initial isolate is susceptible to the first-line agents and treatment proceeds without incident, additional susceptibility tests are not required. Susceptibility testing should be performed for patients who relapse with tuberculosis and for patients who are treatment failures after 3 to 4 months of therapy.

Susceptibility testing for *M. tuberculosis* uses standard concentrations of antituberculosis drugs to measure inhibition of bacterial growth in culture. Drugs tested routinely include isoniazid, rifampicin, pyrazinamide, ethambutol, and streptomycin. Testing of second-line antituberculosis drugs is only done when resistance to the first-line agents is documented or strongly suspected.

Susceptibility testing is generally performed on subcultures of the primary isolate, though direct inoculation of sputum or other specimens can be performed in the case of a strongly positive acid-fast bacilli smear. The standard method for measuring susceptibility to antituberculosis drugs is the proportions method. The organism is grown on agar plates in the presence of known concentrations of specific drugs. Growth on the plates is then compared with growth on control plates. By convention, if the test plate shows a colony count that is >1% of the control value, the isolate is resistant. Laboratories will report the isolate as being susceptible or resistant to the concentration of the drug used in the assay.

Another method for susceptibility testing is to use the MGIT system, in which culture bottles contain antituberculosis drugs. Growth indices are compared to control cultures to determine susceptibility. The MGIT system provides results more quickly than the proportions method, is automated, but is more expensive. Recently, the microscopic examination of growth in wells that are filled with liquid culture medium (MODS) has been reported to enable detection within about 10 days and permit rapid assessment of drug resistance. This technique has some promise in resource-limited settings, but it is labour intensive and needs further validation in endemic countries.

The use of molecular methods to determine drug susceptibility is promising but not currently in routine use. Specific mutations in *M. tuberculosis* have been identified which confer resistance to antituberculosis drugs. For example, mutations in a small region of the *rpo*B gene of *M. tuberculosis* are responsible for more than 90% of all rifampicin resistance. Sequencing of this portion of the genome using a variety of techniques has been shown to be feasible in research laboratories. Rapid identification of rifampicin resistance by molecular methods (line probe assay) would be of enormous clinical benefit, as almost all rifampicin-resistant *M. tuberculosis* isolates are also resistant to isoniazid and are, by definition, multidrug resistant. Thus early detection of resistance mutations would allow early initiation of appropriate treatment and infection control measures. Molecular diagnosis of other types of resistance is more difficult, as the genetic basis of resistance to other drugs is either heterogeneous or not completely understood.

Treatment of active tuberculosis

The treatment of tuberculosis requires the use of a combination of antimycobacterial drugs active against the strain of *M. tuberculosis* causing the patient's disease. The use of multiple agents is necessitated by the emergence of drug resistance when single agents are used. Mutations that confer resistance to antimycobacterial drugs arise spontaneously in wild-type populations of *M. tuberculosis* in frequencies ranging from 1 in 10^5 to 1 in 10^8 bacilli. In the presence of large numbers of organisms, such as are present during active pulmonary disease, a single agent will kill susceptible bacilli, but naturally drug-resistant mutants will survive and eventually emerge to cause drug-resistant disease. Since the mechanisms of resistance are genetically distinct and arise independently, multiple drug resistance within a single organism is exceedingly rare in nature. The use of two or more agents with different mechanisms of action assures that populations of drug-resistant bacilli are not selected for during therapy.

Antituberculosis drugs

These are divided into first-line and second-line agents. The first-line agents are widely available and used routinely in the treatment of tuberculosis, while the second-line agents are generally less potent, more toxic, and less readily available. Exceptions are the newer fluoroquinolones, such as moxifloxacin and gatifloxacin, which appear to have good activity against *M. tuberculosis* in a mouse model. The ability of moxifloxacin to reduce the time to sputum conversion might shorten the duration of tuberculosis treatment, but this remains to be confirmed in ongoing clinical trials. Second-line drugs are reserved for the treatment of drug-resistant tuberculosis. Table 7.6.25.5 lists the first-line antituberculosis drugs, their activity in the treatment of tuberculosis, and common toxicities.

Regimens currently used for the treatment of tuberculosis have been developed on the basis of trials conducted by the British Medical Research Council since the late1970s. By combining drugs that target both rapidly growing bacillary populations and slow-growing or semidormant organisms within cells, modern short-course chemotherapy can successfully cure drug-susceptible pulmonary tuberculosis in 6 months. The regimens recommended for treatment of drug-susceptible tuberculosis are shown in Table 7.6.25.6. Treatment of extrapulmonary tuberculosis is generally for the same duration as for pulmonary disease, with the exceptions of bone and joint and central nervous system tuberculosis, which are treated for 12 months.

The dynamics of mycobacterial growth are such that treatment need be administered only once daily, and can be given as infrequently as twice a week. The long generation time of *M. tuberculosis* and a postantibiotic effect of antituberculosis drugs make more frequent drug dosing unnecessary. The dosages for drugs are listed in Table 7.6.25.7 according to the frequency with which they are administered.

Isoniazid remains a key component of treatment because of its high bactericidal activity. Rifampicin is essential for short-course therapy because it is active against all populations of bacilli, both within and outside of cells. Pyrazinamide is uniquely active during the first 2 months of therapy, but appears to have no activity thereafter. The addition of pyrazinamide to the treatment regimen allows the duration to be reduced from 9 to 6 months, however. Streptomycin has bactericidal activity against *M. tuberculosis*, and ethambutol has bacteriostatic activity at lower doses and bactericidal activity at high doses. These agents primarily are given to prevent the emergence of drug resistance, as they appear to add little activity to combination regimens against drug-susceptible tuberculosis.

Table 7.6.25.5 Drugs for the treatment of tuberculosis

Agent	Activity	Toxicity
Isoniazid	Bactericidal	Liver, peripheral nerve, hypersensitivity
Rifampicin	Bactericidal	Liver, gastrointestinal, discoloration of body fluids, nausea, haematological
Pyrazinamide	Sterilizing	Liver, hyperuricaemia, gout, malaise, gastrointestinal
Ethambutol	Bacteriostatic (dose-dependent)	Liver, optic neuritis, skin
Streptomycin	Bactericidal	Ototoxicity, kidneys

Table 7.6.25.6 Treatment regimens for tuberculosis in children and adults

	Frequency	Drugs
Option 1	Intensive phase, daily	Isoniazid, rifampicin, pyrazinamide, and ethambutol or streptomycin[b] for 8 weeks
	Continuation phase, daily or 2–3 times weekly[a]	Isoniazid and rifampicin for 16 weeks
Option 2	Intensive phase, daily	Isoniazid, rifampicin, pyrazinamide, and ethambutol or streptomycin[b] for 2 weeks
	Intensive phase, twice weekly	Same drugs for 6 weeks[b]
	Continuation phase, twice weekly[a]	Isoniazid and rifampicin for 16 weeks
Option 3	Entire course of therapy, 3 times weekly[a]	Isoniazid, rifampicin, pyrazinamide, and ethambutol or streptomycin for 24 weeks

[a] Intermittent dosing should be directly observed.
[b] In areas where drug resistance is 4%, omit fourth drug.

Drug toxicities

Although antituberculosis therapy is remarkably well tolerated and almost always given on an ambulatory basis, important drug toxicities do exist. The most serious adverse drug reaction during tuberculosis treatment is liver toxicity, which may occur in up to 5 to 10% of treated patients. Isoniazid, rifampicin, and pyrazinamide are all associated with liver toxicity and use of these agents together increases the risk of a reaction. Isoniazid causes more hepatotoxicity than rifampicin or pyrazinamide, however, and is the agent most frequently implicated when reactions occur. Isoniazid can produce an idiosyncratic hepatocellular injury, manifested by elevated liver enzymes and clinical hepatitis. Elevation of transaminases does not always portend the development of hepatitis, but may serve as an important signal to anticipate clinical toxicity. The development of signs and symptoms of hepatitis, such as abdominal pain, nausea, vomiting, or jaundice, requires immediate discontinuation of isoniazid, as continuing treatment may result in death from hepatic failure. Risk factors for developing isoniazid hepatotoxicity include increasing age, chronic liver disease, alcohol abuse, daily dosing of isoniazid, and use of other hepatotoxic drugs, including rifampicin. In addition, individuals with a slow isoniazid acetylation genotype are significantly more likely to develop hepatotoxicity from the drug than intermediate or rapid acetylators. Isoniazid interferes with metabolism of pyridoxine (vitamin B_6) which can result in a sensory neuropathy. Coadministration of pyridoxine with isoniazid abrogates this effect without compromising the antimicrobial activity.

Rifampicin also causes hepatotoxicity, although the characteristic picture of liver disturbances due to rifampicin is cholestasis.

Table 7.6.25.7 Dosage recommendation for the initial treatment of tuberculosis in children and adults

Drugs	Daily dose		Twice-weekly dose		Thrice-weekly dose	
	Children	Adults	Children	Adults	Children	Adults
Isoniazid (mg/kg)	10–20 (max. 300 mg)	5 (max. 300 mg)	20–40 (max. 900 mg)	15 (max. 900 mg)	20–40 (max. 900 mg)	15 (max. 900 mg
Rifampicin (mg/kg)	10–20 (max. 600 mg)	10 (max. 600 mg)	10–20 (max. 600 mg)	10 (max. 600 mg)	10–20 (max. 600 mg)	10 (max. 600 mg)
Pyrazinamide (mg/kg)	15–30 (max. 2 g)	15–30 (max. 2 g)	50–70 (max. 4 g)	50–70 (max. 3.5 g)	50–60 (max. 3.5 g)	50–60 (max. 3.5 g)
Ethambutol (mg/kg)	15–25 (max. 1.5 g)	15–25 (max. 1.5 g)	50 (max. 4 g)	50 (max. 4 g)	25–30	25–30
Streptomycin (mg/kg)	20–40 (max. 1.0 g)	15 (max. 1.0 g)	25–30 (max. 1.5 g)	25–30 (max. 1.5 g)	25–?30 (max. 1.5 g)	25–30 (max. 1.5 g)

However, the incidence of hepatotoxicity when rifampicin is given with isoniazid is substantially greater than when isoniazid is given alone. Rifampicin predictably causes a discoloration of body fluids, resulting in orange-tinted tears, sweat, and urine. Haematological toxicity from rifampicin includes thrombocytopenia and anaemia. Higher doses of rifampicin may produce a hypersensitivity reaction, with fever, rash, and joint swelling. It is for this reason that doses of rifampicin are not escalated during intermittent therapy, whereas the intermittent dosages of the other drugs are increased to deliver weekly doses that are equivalent to daily dosing.

Pyrazinamide is often associated with arthralgias, and may precipitate gout. Pyrazinamide inhibits renal tubular uric acid excretion, resulting in increased serum uric acid levels. Frank gouty arthritis is relatively uncommon with pyrazinamide use, and its frequency is reduced with intermittent dosing. Routine use of allopurinol to prevent gout is not recommended.

The major toxicity of ethambutol is optic neuritis, which is common at doses above 30 mg/kg daily and unusual at doses below 25 mg/kg daily. Patients receiving ethambutol should have baseline tests of visual acuity and colour discrimination, with monthly monitoring while on treatment. Ethambutol use is discouraged in children under 8 years old because of their inability reliably to report visual disturbances. However, the incidence of optic neuritis with the doses of ethambutol typically used is so low that its use in young children is only relatively contraindicated.

Streptomycin was a staple of antituberculosis therapy for many years, but its use has been greatly curbed in recent years. Several studies have demonstrated that regimens containing isoniazid, rifampicin, and pyrazinamide are equally efficacious with or without streptomycin. Streptomycin is given by intramuscular injection, causing discomfort to patients and creating an infection risk for patients and health care workers. In addition, streptomycin can be ototoxic and nephrotoxic. Consequently, ethambutol has replaced streptomycin in many settings around the world.

Monitoring of therapy

Patients receiving therapy for tuberculosis require regular monitoring to assess adherence with therapy, clinical response, and adverse reactions. In the initial phase of therapy, monitoring by a nurse or other trained clinician at least weekly is recommended, and supervision of every dose of medication is suggested by the WHO and other authorities (see below). Patients should be observed for clinical responses, including defervescence, improvement in cough and appetite, and weight gain. Improvement in these symptoms and signs may take several weeks, but usually occurs within 3 weeks after starting treatment. Failure to improve suggests that the patient is not adhering to treatment, has drug-resistant tuberculosis, or has another illness in addition to or instead of tuberculosis.

Treatment response should also be documented with repeated sputum smears and cultures and a follow-up chest radiograph after 2 to 3 months (for pulmonary tuberculosis). All patients should have a repeat sputum smear and culture after 2 months of therapy; those who are smear or culture positive at 2 months should have another at 3 months. Failure to convert sputum smears and cultures to negative with 3 months of therapy is associated with a high risk of treatment failure; patients who are still smear or culture positive at 4 months of treatment are considered treatment failures and should be evaluated for drug-resistant disease. A culture at the end of therapy is recommended to document cure, while an end of therapy radiograph is not necessary.

Monitoring for drug toxicity is also required throughout therapy. At least monthly monitoring for symptoms and signs of liver toxicity is essential, and patients should be advised to stop therapy and seek care if evidence of hepatitis is noted. Routine liver enzyme monitoring is recommended primarily for patients with underlying liver disease or baseline abnormalities in liver enzymes. Patients with symptoms of hepatitis, of course, should have liver studies obtained. As noted above, monthly visual assessment is also recommended when ethambutol is given.

Adherence to therapy and directly observed therapy

Since the 1960s experts in tuberculosis have noted that the success of treatment depends largely on adherence to therapy. Poor adherence to therapy is responsible for treatment failures, early relapses, and the emergence of drug-resistant disease. Two major interventions to improve adherence and prevent poor outcomes are directly observed therapy (DOT) and the use of fixed-dose combination tablets. DOT was first promoted in the 1950s in India, and experience with DOT grew over the ensuing years. Intermittent dosing of tuberculosis therapy, along with the relatively short course of treatment, make supervision of treatment feasible in many settings. Ecological and programmatic studies of DOT programmes have shown that the introduction of DOT improves cure rates for tuberculosis, reduces nonadherence, and reduces the emergence of drug-resistant disease. Two observational studies have shown better survival of HIV-infected tuberculosis patients who receive DOT.

On the other hand, two randomized trials of DOT in developing countries have not found improved treatment completion rates compared with self-administered treatment. These trials have been criticized for demonstrating only that DOT can be done badly, but the lack of randomized studies documenting that DOT *per se* leads to improved outcomes is of some concern. The data from observational studies are compelling, however, and DOT has been shown to be cost-effective in resource-limited settings and, therefore, is strongly encouraged by many experts and professional organizations.

The use of fixed-dose combination tablets is intended to reduce the risk of selecting for drug resistance, as opposed to improving adherence generally. By combining two, three, or four medications in the same tablet, depending on the regimen being used, the opportunity for patients to receive partial treatment that would select for drug resistance is avoided. The bioequivalence of fixed-dose combinations to individual medications has been established for some, but not all, of the combination products on the market.

The catastrophic state of global tuberculosis control led the WHO to develop the directly observed therapy, short-course (DOTS) strategy. This strategy is a series of policies related to national tuberculosis control practices. The five elements of the DOTS strategy are:

1 Governmental commitment to tuberculosis control
2 A reliable supply of tuberculosis drugs
3 Diagnosis of tuberculosis cases microscopically
4 A registration system for tracking the outcomes of treatment
5 Supervision (DOT) of at least the first 8 weeks of treatment

The DOTS strategy has been extremely successful in focusing attention on serious problems in tuberculosis treatment and control, and implementation of the programme in several countries has produced remarkable improvements in clinical outcomes for patients with tuberculosis. There is strong evidence that the use of the DOTS strategy results in lower rates of drug-resistant tuberculosis. Nonetheless, the WHO estimates that in 1999 only 21% of tuberculosis patients in the world were treated within a DOTS programme. Further expansion of the DOTS strategy and improvements in tuberculosis treatment programmes are clearly needed.

Treatment of multidrug-resistant tuberculosis

This is beyond the scope of this chapter. Patients with drug-resistant tuberculosis should be managed by a physician who is a tuberculosis expert. Effective treatment and cure of multidrug-resistant tuberculosis (MDR-TB) requires prolonged use (about 2 years) of a combination of drugs that include second-line drugs which are less effective than first-line agents, have a greater toxicity, or demonstrate both disadvantages. Supervised therapy is considered mandatory for patients with resistant tuberculosis. Physician mistakes remain one of the leading causes of the emergence of multidrug-resistant and extensively drug-resistant tuberculosis (XDR-TB), and the identification of a drug-resistant isolate of *M. tuberculosis* should result in immediate expert consultation. It is also clear that addressing drug-resistant tuberculosis cannot be accomplished without addressing the overall tuberculosis control effort.

Treatment of tuberculosis in HIV-infected people

The United States (ATS/CDC/Infectious Disease Society of America) recommendations for the treatment of tuberculosis in HIV-infected adults are, with a few exceptions, the same as those for HIV-uninfected adults, i.e. standard 6-month rifampicin-based therapy. The continuation phase is extended from 6 to 9 months for any patient with cavitary tuberculosis and positive cultures at 2 months, regardless of the HIV status. The optional continuation phase regimen of isoniazid plus rifapentine once weekly is contraindicated in HIV-infected patients because of an unacceptably high rate of relapse, frequently with organisms that have acquired resistance to rifamycins. The development of acquired rifampicin resistance has also been noted among HIV-infected patients with advanced immune suppression treated with twice weekly rifampicin-based or rifabutin-based regimens. Consequently, patients with CD4 cell counts <100 cells/μl should receive daily or three-times weekly treatment. DOT and other adherence-promoting strategies are especially important for patients with HIV-related tuberculosis. Recent studies show improved survival when antiretroviral therapy is given during tuberculosis treatment rather than afterwards. Timing of combined therapy is challenging, however, due to drug interactions and immune reconstitution inflammatory syndrome (see below).

Drug interactions

There are three possible complications that arise when tuberculosis treatment and antiretroviral drugs are coadministered: shared side effects and toxicity, drug interactions arising from the induction of metabolism (cytochrome P450 enzymes) and efflux pumps by rifampicin, and the immune reconstitution inflammatory syndrome. Rifamycins induce the activity of cytochrome P450 enzymes that are important in drug metabolism. Two key antiretroviral drug classes, protease inhibitors and non-nucleoside reverse transcriptase inhibitors, are substrates of cytochrome P450 enzymes. Protease inhibitors are also substrates of P-glycoprotein, which is also induced by rifamycins. The available rifamycins differ in potency as P450 enzyme inducers, with rifampicin being the most potent and rifabutin the least. Coadministration with rifampicin reduces the concentrations of non-nucleoside reverse transcriptase inhibitors to a moderate extent, but dramatically reduces the concentrations of protease inhibitors. Rifabutin does not significantly affect the concentrations of ritonavir-boosted protease inhibitors and is recommended when protease inhibitors have to be used. However, the use of rifabutin in low resource settings is currently limited due to its very high cost and the widespread use of fixed-dose combination antituberculosis drugs that include rifampicin.

Between 8 and 45% of patients commencing antiretroviral therapy while being treated for tuberculosis develop paradoxical deterioration of tuberculosis, the so-called immune reconstitution inflammatory syndrome (IRIS). Paradoxical deterioration was well known in the pre-HIV era, but occurs much more frequently in HIV-infected patients starting antiretroviral therapy. The pathogenesis of IRIS is not completely understood. The most common manifestations of tuberculosis-related IRIS are focal inflammatory exacerbations of tuberculosis (lymphadenitis, serositis, or abscesses, new infiltrates), 'unmasking' of tuberculosis or other subclinical diseases after antiretroviral therapy initiation, etc. It typically occurs within 2 to 4 weeks after antiretroviral initiation. Risk factors associated with an increased risk of IRIS include shorter intervals between antituberculosis therapy and antiretroviral therapy initiation, low baseline CD4 counts and high baseline viral load, and vigorous CD4/viral load response to antiretroviral therapy. However, new or worsening clinical features should be attributed to IRIS only after a thorough evaluation has excluded other possible causes, notably poor adherence to antituberculosis therapy, multidrug-resistant tuberculosis, new opportunistic diseases, and systemic drug hypersensitivity reactions. The benefit of adjunctive corticosteroids in the management of patients with IRIS is suggested by results of at least one randomized controlled trial.

Duration of therapy

Despite these complications, antiretroviral therapy should not be withheld simply because the patient is being treated for tuberculosis. The optimal timing of initiation of antiretroviral therapy in relation to initiation of antituberculosis treatment is unclear. Treatment for tuberculosis should always be initiated first, and it is prudent to wait at least until it is clear that the patient is improving and tolerating the antituberculosis therapy before beginning antiretroviral therapy. While awaiting the results of ongoing controlled trials, a 2006 WHO expert opinion panel has suggested that the CD4 lymphocyte count should determine the initiation of antiretroviral therapy, unless there is other serious HIV morbidity. These WHO guidelines state that patients with CD4 counts <200 cells/μl should initiate antiretroviral therapy after 2 to 8 weeks of antituberculosis therapy and those with CD4 counts 200 to 350 cells/μl after 8 weeks. Data from recent clinical trials support initiating antiretroviral therapy for all patients with a CD4 count <500 cells/μl within two months of starting tuberculosis therapy, as this reduces mortality by >50%. Until there have been controlled studies evaluating the optimal time for starting antiretroviral therapy in patients with HIV infection and tuberculosis, this decision should be individualized. Possible factors for consideration are a patient's initial response to treatment for tuberculosis, CD4 response to tuberculosis therapy, possible drug interactions, risk of IRIS, adherence, occurrence of side effects, and availability of antiretroviral therapy. For patients who are already receiving an antiretroviral regimen when tuberculosis is detected, antiretroviral treatment should be continued during antituberculosis therapy.

Adjunctive steroid treatment

Corticosteroids are frequently advocated with tuberculosis treatment to reduce inflammation in tuberculosis, but evidence for this practice is often lacking, particularly in HIV infection. Mortality was reduced in a small trial of patients given prednisolone for tuberculous pericarditis. Also, dexamethasone reduced mortality in a large Vietnamese study of adults with tuberculous meningitis. The HIV-infected subgroup of the latter study appeared to gain a similar benefit, but this failed to achieve statistical significance. A Ugandan study of adjunctive prednisolone in HIV-infected patients with pleural tuberculosis found faster resolution with prednisolone, but no mortality benefit. Of great concern, however, was their finding of excess cases of Kaposi's sarcoma in the prednisolone arm. This sobering result is a reminder that the additive immunosuppressant effect of glucocorticoids can have severe consequences in HIV infection. Adjunctive glucocorticoids should only be used in HIV-infected patients when there is likely to be a mortality benefit, which may be the case for tuberculous meningitis and pericarditis, but there is still a need for definitive evidence from larger studies in both conditions.

Treatment of latent tuberculosis infection

Isoniazid chemoprophylaxis

Prevention of tuberculosis with isoniazid therapy was first documented in children in the mid-1950s. Subsequently, several controlled trials of isoniazid chemoprophylaxis were undertaken, and its efficacy firmly established. A meta-analysis of 11 placebo-controlled trials of isoniazid, involving more than 70 000 persons, found that treatment reduced tuberculosis incidence by 63%. Among patients who adhered to >80% of the isoniazid regimen, protection was 81%. These studies also showed that isoniazid chemoprophylaxis reduced tuberculosis deaths by 72%. The efficacy of isoniazid therapy to prevent tuberculosis in high-risk persons is incontrovertible.

Enthusiasm for isoniazid chemoprophylaxis was considerably dampened in the late 1960s and early 1970s when drug-related hepatotoxicity, including deaths, was observed. Several studies based on decision analysis or modelling suggested that the risks of chemoprophylaxis might outweigh the benefits, and use of preventive therapy was curtailed or ignored in many settings. Because the risk of isoniazid-related hepatotoxicity increases with age, use of chemoprophylaxis in people older than 35 years was particularly discouraged.

Preventive therapy in high-risk individuals

The resurgence of tuberculosis in the developed world, particularly HIV-related tuberculosis, and the uncontrolled global epidemic have renewed interest in the use of preventive therapy in high-risk individuals known or strongly suspected to be latently infected with *M. tuberculosis*. The term 'treatment of latent tuberculosis infection' is now preferred, emphasizing that preventive treatment is really targeted at an established infection. The ATS and the CDC published guidelines in 2000 on screening for latent tuberculosis that stress the importance of targeting efforts on populations and patients who would benefit from treatment to prevent active disease. In the past, screening for tuberculosis infection has been unfocused and often directed at patients who, if found to be infected, would have little risk of progressing to active disease. The new guidelines propose that only people with a high risk of disease or high prior probability of latent tuberculosis be tested, and that treatment be offered to infected individuals regardless of age. Individuals who should be targeted for tuberculin testing are those listed in the first two columns of Table 7.6.25.4, i.e. those in whom a positive test is considered equal to or exceeding 5 or equal to or exceeding 10 mm induration. People without risk factors for tuberculosis (those in whom a positive test is equal to or exceeding 15 mm) should not be tested.

Treatment regimens for latent tuberculosis are listed in Table 7.6.25.8, along with the rating given to the regimen by the ATS and CDC. Isoniazid remains a favoured drug for tuberculosis preventive therapy because of its well-documented efficacy, low cost, and relatively low toxicity. The optimal duration of isoniazid therapy for latent tuberculosis has been the subject of extensive debate in

Table 7.6.25.8 Treatment regimens for latent tuberculosis

Drug regimen	Duration (months)	Interval	Rating (HIV−)	Rating (HIV+)
Isoniazid	9	Daily	A II	A II
Isoniazid	9	Twice weekly	B II	B II
Isoniazid	6	Daily	B I	C I
Isoniazid	6	Twice weekly	B II	C II
Rifampicin	4	Daily	B II	B III

A, strongly recommended; B, recommended; C, optional; I, randomized trials; II, data from other scientific studies; III, expert opinion.

recent years. The International Union Against Tuberculosis and Lung Disease conducted a landmark trial in Eastern Europe in the 1970s and 1980s that compared no treatment to 3, 6, or 12 months of isoniazid in adults with fibrotic changes on radiographs. The results showed that, compared to placebo, 12 months of isoniazid reduced the incidence of tuberculosis by 75%, compared to 66% for 6 months and 20% for 3 months. In addition, patients who completed the 12 months of therapy and were judged to be compliant experienced a 92% reduction in tuberculosis risk, compared to a 69% decrease for compliant patients completing a 6-month regimen. A meta-analysis by the Cochrane Collaborative found that 12 months of isoniazid was more effective than 6 months for prevention of tuberculosis. A recent analysis of varying durations of isoniazid therapy in Alaskan natives revealed that the effectiveness of isoniazid therapy was optimal after 9 months, and that further treatment conferred no additional benefit. The new ATS/CDC statement, therefore, recommends 9 months of isoniazid as the preferred regimen, with 6 months considered an alternative, but less effective, course of treatment.

Isoniazid hepatotoxicity

Although isoniazid is a well-tolerated drug, serious hepatotoxicity can occur in a small proportion of patients. Isoniazid may result in asymptomatic elevations in hepatic aminotransferase levels, but this does not always signal impending clinical toxicity. Hepatotoxicity is of concern when symptoms of hepatitis develop, including pain, nausea, vomiting, and jaundice. Continuing isoniazid in the presence of symptoms may lead to death from fulminant hepatic necrosis and liver failure, with a case fatality rate of 10 to 15%. Studies in the 1960s and 1970s found evidence of hepatotoxicity in 1 to 5% of recipients of isoniazid, with higher rates among older patients. More recent experience with isoniazid therapy that is closely monitored shows a risk of hepatotoxicity in the range of 0.1 to 0.3%. Thus, appropriate patient screening and follow-up makes the use of isoniazid for treating latent infection markedly safer.

Alternative regimens

One of the most important new developments in the treatment of latent tuberculosis is the development of alternative regimens that shorten the duration of treatment. A 3-month regimen of rifampicin alone was found to reduce the incidence of tuberculosis by about 65% in men with silicosis, and was more effective than 6 months of isoniazid. The combination of rifampicin and isoniazid given for three to four months is widely used for treatment of latent tuberculosis in children and improves completion rates. This regimen has also been found to be equally effective as isoniazid in studies in adults.

The use of rifampicin does pose the risk of important drug interactions. For example, reduction in methadone concentrations caused by rifampicin can precipitate narcotic withdrawal. Moreover, rifampicin can lower levels of protease inhibitors and non-nucleoside reverse transcriptase inhibitors used to treat HIV infection. Substitution of rifabutin for rifampicin in patients receiving HIV drugs provides equally efficacious treatment of active tuberculosis and less effect on antiretroviral drugs. If multidrug-resistant tuberculosis is suspected, the recommended preventive therapy is pyrazinamide and ethambutol or pyrazinamide and a fluoroquinolone (e.g. moxifloxacin) for 6 to 12 months. Treatment for suspected exposure to multidrug-resistant tuberculosis should be routinely extended to 12 months in HIV-infected individuals.

Candidates for treatment of latent tuberculosis are listed in Table 7.6.25.4. Criteria for treatment include a positive tuberculin test according to the categories in Table 7.6.25.4, elevated risk for developing active tuberculosis if untreated, and exclusion of active tuberculosis by clinical evaluation and chest radiograph. In addition, HIV-infected and other severely immunocompromised persons who are contacts to an infectious tuberculosis patient should be treated for latent tuberculosis regardless of tuberculin skin test results.

Monitoring treatment

Patients receiving treatment for latent tuberculosis should be monitored for drug toxicity, as well as to promote adherence to therapy. As in treatment of active tuberculosis, patients receiving isoniazid should be warned about signs and symptoms of hepatotoxicity and advised to discontinue therapy and seek care if any of these occur. Patients with or at risk of chronic liver disease should have baseline liver enzymes obtained, with monthly monitoring if the results are abnormal. All patients should be clinically evaluated at least monthly to assess. Treatment using other preventive regimens (i.e. isoniazid) and treatment of patients with mild transaminase elevations (3 times upper limits of normal or less) can proceed with regular clinical and laboratory monitoring. Higher elevations of transaminases, or the development of symptoms or signs of hepatitis should be managed with discontinuation of therapy at least temporarily. Patients who complete therapy for latent tuberculosis do not need periodic monitoring for tuberculosis subsequently.

Prevention of tuberculosis

Strategies to control tuberculosis are aimed at the prevention of the spread of *M. tuberculosis* infection and the development of clinical tuberculosis. The principal approaches employed toward this end are:

- identification and treatment of infectious tuberculosis cases
- treatment of latent tuberculosis infection
- prevention of exposure to infectious particles in air, especially in hospitals and other institutions
- vaccination

Identification and treatment of infectious tuberculosis cases

Case identification and treatment reduces transmission by rendering patients with communicable tuberculosis noninfectious. Patients with pulmonary tuberculosis produce infectious aerosols that may transmit tubercle bacilli to contacts breathing the same air. When cases are identified and treated, infectiousness is rapidly eliminated. The duration of treatment required to prevent further transmission of infection is not known precisely, but experimental, clinical, and microbiological data suggest that the level of infectiousness is reduced enormously within several days of beginning effective treatment. The number of secondary infections generated by an infectious tuberculosis patient varies greatly depending on the duration of illness, the extent of pulmonary pathology, the amount of patient coughing, and the environment into which the patient expels infectious aerosols. Early diagnosis and treatment reduces the number of secondary infections, while delays can result in ongoing transmission to large numbers of contacts. Failure to retain patients in treatment until they are cured also contributes to spread of infection.

Treatment of latent tuberculosis infection

This is discussed above. The benefit of treating latent infection is not only to the individual patient who does not fall ill with tuberculosis, but also accrues to the potential contacts of that patient, who might become secondarily infected were disease to develop. Targeting of high-risk groups for screening and treatment of latent tuberculosis thereby reduces tuberculosis incidence within communities. Groups that should be targeted for screening are listed in the first two columns of Table 7.6.25.4.

Prevention of exposure especially in hospitals and other institutions

Control of exposure to infectious aerosols can have a major impact on the spread of tuberculosis. In the late 1980s and early 1990s, transmission of tuberculosis, including multidrug-resistant tuberculosis, was widespread in hospitals, homeless shelters, and correctional facilities in New York City. More recently, the outbreak of extensively drug-resistant tuberculosis in the KwaZulu-Natal province of South Africa is a tragic reminder of the importance of infection control measures in institutions. The congregation of large numbers of highly susceptible people, especially HIV-infected persons, in closed environments with untreated tuberculosis patients has resulted in numerous microepidemics of both drug-susceptible and drug-resistant tuberculosis. Reversal of the resurgence of tuberculosis in New York at that time was attributable in large part to strengthening of infection control practices.

Identification and isolation of infected patients

Tuberculosis infection control involves prompt identification and isolation of patients with suspected tuberculosis. The decision to isolate a patient in a hospital setting is a function of epidemiological and clinical factors. Patients with known tuberculosis risk factors who present with symptoms and signs characteristic of pulmonary tuberculosis should be placed in respiratory isolation. Local epidemiological data should influence isolation practices. In settings where tuberculosis is prevalent, all HIV-infected patients with pneumonia may require isolation, whereas isolation can be more selective and based on individual patient features in low prevalence settings.

Respiratory isolation requires placement of the patient in a room with negative air pressure relative to adjoining areas, ventilation to the room should provide at least six complete air changes per hour, and air should not be recirculated without filtering or irradiation. Patients should be instructed to cover their coughs at all times, and should wear surgical face masks when outside the room to reduce aerosol generation. Anyone entering the patient's room should wear an appropriate face mask or respirator to prevent inhalation of droplet nuclei with tubercle bacilli. A considerable amount of debate has occurred in recent years in the United States of America regarding what constitutes appropriate protection for health care workers exposed to infectious tuberculosis. This debate is influenced as much by philosophy as by science, and will not be detailed here. Use of surgical masks for the protection against tuberculosis is clearly inappropriate, even though these masks are useful when placed on patients to prevent creation of infectious aerosols. Tightly fitting face masks that filter out more than 99.7% of particles less than 0.5 μm in size (high-efficiency particle air (HEPA) filters) are effective. Other devices, including positive air pressure respirators (PAPRs), are also effective.

Box 7.6.25.1 Criteria for discontinuing respiratory isolation for tuberculosis in hospital inpatients

- Alternative diagnosis established
- Infectious tuberculosis ruled out
- Tuberculosis diagnosed and:
  - Treatment given for at least 14 days *and*
  - Clinical response to therapy document, including improvement in fever and cough *and*
  - Acid-fast smears of sputum negative *or*
  - Patient discharged to home

Use of ultraviolet germicidal irradiation can be useful for reducing the number of infectious particles in ambient air in settings where ventilation alone is not sufficient. Ultraviolet light must be concentrated in areas of rooms where exposure to people will not occur, such as upper air zones, in order to prevent skin and ocular toxicity. Areas where ultraviolet lights are often used include bronchoscopy suites, inside air circulation ducts, in emergency rooms, and in homeless shelters.

Criteria for discontinuation of respiratory isolation are listed in Box 7.6.25.1. Guidelines for taking patients out of isolation in the hospital are strict and are intended to protect other vulnerable patients and hospital staff from any exposure to the disease. Respiratory isolation is not usually required or practical in the home setting, and patients with infectious tuberculosis do not need to be hospitalized solely for respiratory isolation. It is assumed that contacts in the home environment will already have had significant exposure to tuberculosis by the time a diagnosis is made, and isolation of the patient affords no measurable benefit. Exceptions to this may include patients living in congregate living facilities or other special situations. The primary protective measures for contacts of cases are a clinical evaluation to identify and evaluate symptoms of tuberculosis and tuberculin skin testing with treatment of latent infection, if present. Instituting infection control measures is likely to be challenging in developing countries where the health care system is already overburdened and where facilities often lack negative pressure isolation rooms and air filtration systems. In such settings, work practice and administrative control measures have been emphasized and are considered to be more effective and less expensive. These measures consist of policies and procedures intended to promptly identify infectious tuberculosis cases so that additional precautions and health care steps can be taken.

BCG vaccination

Vaccination against tuberculosis with the bacille Calmette-Guérin (BCG) vaccine is widely administered throughout the world but is a practice mired in controversy. BCG is an attenuated live bacterial vaccine developed in the early 20th century by Calmette and Guérin at the Institut Pasteur in Paris. After a series of uncontrolled and anecdotal assessments of the vaccine, a series of controlled trials of BCG was begun in the 1930s and continued through to the 1990s.

The efficacy of BCG has varied greatly in these studies, ranging from more than 80% protection to complete lack of protection, with possibly increased risk in vaccine recipients. A meta-analysis of BCG trials performed in the early 1990s found that the weighted protective benefit of BCG was about 50% for both the prevention of active tuberculosis disease and death.

In addition to the protective efficacy observed in trials of BCG, there is evidence that BCG diminishes haematogenous dissemination of primary tuberculosis infection and thereby reduces the incidence of miliary tuberculosis and tuberculous meningitis in children. It is primarily for this reason that BCG is included in the Expanded Programme on Immunization of the WHO.

The current efficacy of BCG for preventing pulmonary tuberculosis is debated on the basis of several recent trials which have failed to show protection. Several hypotheses have been proposed for the variation in efficacy reported in various studies, including differences in susceptibility within populations, environmental exposure to mycobacteria which masks vaccine effect, and attenuation of vaccine immunogenicity. This last explanation is very compelling and fits well with clinical trial data. Unlike most vaccines, BCG is not standardized and there is no seedlot of vaccine from which new batches are derived. BCG is grown in several laboratories around the world and has not been re-passaged in animals since it was derived from cattle a century ago. Multiple commercial and noncommercial BCG products are in use presently, and comparative genomic analysis demonstrates considerable genetic heterogeneity in these strains, with many gene deletions and polymorphisms. One analysis of BCG trials found that protective efficacy was reduced in studies using multiply-passaged vaccine strains. The evidence supports the hypothesis that BCG has become further attenuated over time and no longer promotes immunity to *M. tuberculosis* infection and disease in adults. This position has not been universally accepted, however, and BCG remains one of the most widely administered vaccines in the world, largely for its perceived effects on paediatric tuberculosis.

Areas for further research

Effective global tuberculosis control will require a coordinated set of clinical and public health strategies that are based on a thorough understanding of the epidemiology, pathogenesis, and therapy of infection with *M. tuberculosis*. It appears that the WHO's DOTS strategy, which focuses on finding and effectively treating cases, is not sufficient to control or eliminate tuberculosis, particularly in countries with large HIV epidemics. Improved methods for the diagnosis and treatment of tuberculosis infection and disease, particularly drug-resistant tuberculosis, are urgently needed. Effective regimens for the treatment of multidrug-resistant and extensively drug-resistant tuberculosis, with both existing and new agents, need to be developed. A better understanding of the pathogenesis of and natural immunity to tuberculosis may contribute to the development of a more effective vaccine. The sequencing of the genome of *M. tuberculosis* promises to open the door to a new generation of research on tuberculosis and its control. Scientific progress alone, however, will be insufficient to combat tuberculosis worldwide. The willingness of societies and nations to pay for the deployment of the fruits of biomedical research, both past and future, to combat the disease where it is prevalent will be required for the conquest of tuberculosis.

Further reading

Abdool Karim SS, Naidoo K, Grobler A, *et al.* (2010). Timing of initiation of antiretroviral drugs during tuberculosis therapy. *N Engl J Med*, **362**, 697–706.

American Thoracic Society/Centers for Disease Control and Prevention/ Infectious Disease Society of America. (2003). Treatment of Tuberculosis, 2003 ATS. CDC/IDSA Statement. *Am J Respir Crit Care Med*, **167**, 603–62.

Davies PDO, Barnes P, Gordon SB (eds) (2008). *Clinical Tuberculosis*, 4th ed. Hodder Arnold.

Dooley KE, Chaisson RE (2009). Tuberculosis and diabetes mellitus: convergence of two epidemics. *Lancet Infect Dis*, **9**, 737–46.

Dorman SE, Chaisson RE (2007). From magic bullets back to the Magic Mountain: the rise of extensively drug-resistant tuberculosis. *Nat Med*, 13, 295–8.

Fox W, Ellard GA, Mitchison DA (1999). Studies on the treatment of tuberculosis undertaken by the British Medical Research Council tuberculosis units, 1946–1986, with relevant subsequent publications. *Int J Tuberc Lung Dis*, **3**(10 Suppl 2), S231–79.

Gandhi NR, Moll A, Sturm AW, *et al.* (2006). Extensively drug-resistant tuberculosis as a cause of death in patients co-infected with tuberculosis and HIV in a rural area of South Africa. *Lancet*, **368**, 1575–80.

Hopewell PC, Pai M, Maher D, Uplekar M, Raviglione MC (2006). International standards for tuberculosis care. *Lancet Infect Dis*, **6**, 710–25.

Iseman MD (2000). *A Clinician's Guide to Tuberculosis*. Philadelphia, Lippincott Williams & Wilkins.

Lawn SD, Bekker L-G, Miller RF (2005). Immune reconstitution disease associated with mycobacterial infections in HIV-infected individuals receiving antiretrovirals. *Lancet Infect Dis*, **5**, 361–73.

Maartens G, Wilkinson RJ (2007). Tuberculosis. *Lancet*, **370**, 2030–43.

Pai M, Minion J, Sohn H, Zwerling A, Perkins MD (2009). Novel and improved technologies for tuberculosis diagnosis: progress and challenges. *Clin Chest Med*, **30**, 701–16, viii.

Rangaka M, Wilkinson K, Seldon R, *et al.* (2007). The effect of HIV-1 infection on T cell based and skin test detection of tuberculosis infection. *Am J Respir Crit Care Med*, **175**, 514–20.

Ryan F (1992). The Forgotten Plague: How the Battle Against Tuberculosis Was Won - And Lost. Boston, Little Brown.

World Health Organization (2007). *WHO Report 2007: Global tuberculosis control: surveillance, planning, financing*. Geneva, WHO/HTM/ TB/2007.376

7.6.26 Disease caused by environmental mycobacteria

J.M. Grange and P.D.O. Davies

Essentials

The genus *Mycobacterium* contains over 100 species (in addition to tubercle and leprosy bacilli) that exist naturally as environmental saprophytes, particularly in water, are divisible into slow and rapid growers according to their rate of growth on subculture, and occasionally cause opportunist disease in humans and animals. Infection is acquired from the environment: human-to-human spread is extremely rare. Diagnosis usually requires isolation and identification of the causative organism, but care must be taken to distinguish between primary pathogens, saprophytes and contaminants.

Clinical features—environmental mycobacteria cause four main types of disease. (1) Chronic pulmonary—usually caused by *M. avium* complex or *M. kansasii*, most often in patients with predisposing local lung lesions or generalized autoimmune/immunosuppressive disorders; symptoms resemble those of tuberculosis. (2) Lymphadenitis—principally a disease of young children. (3) Postinoculation—(a) Buruli ulcer—see Chapter 7.6.28; (b) swimming pool (or fish tank) granuloma—*M. marinum* enters cuts and abrasions acquired during aquatic activities and produces warty skin lesions. (4) Disseminated—most commonly seen in the context of HIV disease; usually caused by *M. avium* complex; presents with malaise, fever, night sweats, and weight loss; diagnosis made by culture of blood or of biopsies of liver, lymph nodes, or bone marrow.

Treatment—this depends on the site and severity of the infection, the presence of predisposing conditions, and the species of mycobacterium. Therapy of disease due to slow growers is usually based on regimens containing clarithromycin or azithromycin; that for rapid growers is largely empirical. Antiretroviral therapy is more beneficial than antimycobacterial agents in patients with AIDS-related disease.

Introduction

In addition to the tubercle and leprosy bacilli, the genus *Mycobacterium* contains over 100 described species that exist naturally as environmental saprophytes. Some of these occasionally cause opportunistic disease in humans and animals. The environmental mycobacteria (EM) are divisible into two main groups, the slow growers and the rapid growers, according to their rate of growth on subculture.

Most of the slow growers are able to cause human disease, the commonest being two members of the *M. avium* complex (MAC), i.e. *M. avium avium* and *M. avium intracellulare*. With rare exceptions, the only pathogenic rapid growers are *M. abscessus*, *M. chelonae*, and *M. fortuitum*. The principal pathogenic environmental mycobacteria are listed in Table 7.6.26.1.

Environmental mycobacteria cause two named diseases with characteristic features: swimming pool granuloma caused by *M. marinum* and Buruli ulcer caused by *M. ulcerans*. Disease due to other environmental mycobacteria is much less specific, often resembles tuberculosis, and requires identification of the causative organism for diagnosis.

Ecology and epidemiology

Environmental mycobacteria are particularly associated with water and are found in swamps, ponds, rivers, and piped water supplies. They are thus readily transmissible to humans by drinking water, by inhalation of aerosols, or by traumatic inoculation. Infection of humans by environmental mycobacteria is widespread and common but overt disease is rare. In some regions, subclinical infection may affect immune responses, causing cross-reactions on tuberculin testing and modifying the protective efficacy of subsequent BCG vaccination.

The incidence of overt disease due to environmental mycobacteria is determined by the species and numbers of mycobacteria in the environment, the opportunities for infection, and the susceptibility of the human population. Person-to-person transmission of overt disease very rarely occurs, and the prevalence of such disease is therefore unaffected by tuberculosis control measures designed to break the cycle of person-to-person transmission. In recent years there has been an increase in the incidence of disease due to environmental mycobacteria in many countries because of immunosuppression, notably due to HIV infection.

Table 7.6.26.1 Principal environmental mycobacteria causing opportunistic disease in humans

Species	Principal type of disease
Slow growers	
M. avium avium[a]	Pulmonary disease, lymphadenitis, disseminated disease
M. avium intracellulare[a]	Pulmonary disease, lymphadenitis, disseminated disease
M. scrofulaceum	Lymphadenopathy, pulmonary disease
M. kansasii	Pulmonary disease
M. xenopi	Pulmonary disease
M. malmoense	Pulmonary disease
M. szulgai	Pulmonary disease
M. simiae	Pulmonary disease
M. marinum	Swimming pool granuloma
M. ulcerans	Buruli ulcer
M. haemophilum	Lymphadenopathy, skin granulomas in transplant recipients
M. gordonae	Common in the environment but rare cause of disease
M. terrae	Rare cause of infection of wounds contaminated by soil
Rapid growers	
M. chelonae	Post-traumatic abscesses, pulmonary disease
M. abscessus	Post-traumatic abscesses, pulmonary disease
M. fortuitum	Post-traumatic abscesses, pulmonary disease

[a] These are usually grouped together as the *M. avium* complex (MAC).

Types of environmental mycobacterial disease in humans

Environmental mycobacteria cause four main types of disease: chronic pulmonary, lymphadenitis, postinoculation, and disseminated.

Chronic pulmonary disease

This form of environmental mycobacterial disease usually occurs in patients with predisposing local lung lesions, including industrial dust disease, old tuberculous cavities, chronic obstructive pulmonary disease, cancer, cystic fibrosis, and bronchiectasis, or generalized autoimmune or immunosuppressive disorders. A substantial minority of cases occur, however, in people who otherwise appear healthy. Most patients are middle-aged or elderly and men are much more frequently affected than women. For reasons which are unclear, the infection may be particularly aggressive in younger women with low body mass index. Environmental mycobacterial infection is also commoner in smokers. In some industrially developed regions, the incidence of pulmonary environmental mycobacterial disease in the middle-aged and elderly white population exceeds that of tuberculosis.

The most frequent causes worldwide are MAC and *M. kansasii*. *M. xenopi* is more restricted geographically but frequently occurs in southern England while, for unknown reasons, *M. malmoense* is encountered as a pathogen with increasing frequency in many parts of Europe including northern England. Rarer causes include *M. scrofulaceum*, *M. szulgai*, and *M. chelonae*.

Clinical presentation

Symptoms resemble those of tuberculosis, including cough, malaise, weight loss, and sweats, and develop insidiously over weeks or months.

There are no diagnostically reliable clinical and radiological differences between pulmonary environmental mycobacterial disease and tuberculosis and diagnosis therefore depends on the isolation and identification of the causative organism. In contrast to *M. tuberculosis*, environmental mycobacteria isolated from sputum may not be the primary cause of disease; they may be transitory contaminants of the pharynx or secondary saprophytes of diseased tissue. There are no absolute criteria for distinguishing between these possibilities, but at least two pure cultures from specimens taken at least 1 week apart from patients with compatible symptoms and radiological signs in whom other causes, including tuberculosis, have been rigorously excluded renders the diagnosis very likely. In some cases, a diagnosis is made or confirmed by microbiological examination of washings, brushings, or biopsies obtained by fibreoptic bronchoscopy.

Criteria for diagnosis listed by the American Thoracic Society (ATS) apply to symptomatic patients with infiltrative, nodular, or cavitary disease on plain chest radiograph or multifocal bronchiectasis or multiple small nodules on CT scan. The criteria are:

- Three positive cultures of sputum/bronchial wash samples with negative smear for acid-fast bacilli, or two cultures and one positive smear.
- If only a bronchial wash is available then a 2+ to 4+ smear with positive culture or 2+ to 4+ growth on solid media.
- If sputum/bronchial wash samples are nondiagnostic then either a lung biopsy yielding environmental mycobacteria or a biopsy with consistent histopathological features with one sputum/bronchial washing specimen positive for environmental mycobacteria.

Lymphadenitis

This is principally a disease of young children, occurring most frequently in the second year of life and then declining in frequency up to the fifth year, after which it is seldom encountered. The risk is reduced by neonatal BCG vaccination. The disease usually affects the cervical lymph nodes but other nodes, such as axillary and inguinal, may be involved, especially in older patients. Lymphadenitis is caused by many mycobacterial species, the commonest cause being MAC and *M. scrofulaceum*. Most cases occur in otherwise healthy children with no obvious predisposing cause but some cases, particularly in older age groups, are associated with HIV infection.

In most cases without predisposing causes, a single node is involved and surgical excision, if technically possible, is curative. More limited treatment, such as incision and drainage, may lead to sinus formation and should be avoided. Disseminated disease may develop in a few children, particularly those with some form of congenital immune deficiency, and in HIV-positive people.

Postinoculation mycobacterioses

Buruli ulcer

This is thought to result from inoculation of the causative organism *M. ulcerans* into the skin, principally by spiky vegetation. This disease is described in Chapter 7.6.28.

Swimming pool/fish tank granuloma

The natural habitat of *M. marinum*, the cause of swimming pool granuloma or fish tank granuloma, is water. It enters cuts and abrasions acquired during aquatic activities, such as swimming, or tending to tropical fish tanks. The cutaneous lesions are usually warty, although pustules and ulcers may develop. There may be 'sporotrichoid' spread of lesions along the draining lymphatics (Fig. 7.6.26.1). The lesions usually heal spontaneously after a few months, but chemotherapy (see below) accelerates resolution. There have been occasional reports of tenosynovitis, carpal tunnel syndrome, osteomyelitis, and disseminated disease due to *M. marinum* (Fig. 7.6.26.2).

Other postinoculation environmental mycobacterial diseases

Most other cases of postinoculation disease are caused by the rapid growers *M. abscessus, M. chelonae* and *M. fortuitum*.

Postinjection abscesses

The most common lesions are postinjection abscesses, which may occur sporadically or in miniepidemics due to the use of contaminated multidose vaccines or other injectable materials. Abscesses develop from 1 to 12 months after injection and may enlarge to 7 cm or more in diameter. They tend to be chronic and localized, but multiple abscesses with spreading cellulitis may develop in insulin-dependent diabetics. Localized abscesses usually respond well to excision or curettage but chemotherapy (see below) may be required for multiple or spreading lesions.

Keratitis

Trauma to the cornea predisposes to infection by the rapid growers *M. abscessus*, *M. chelonae*, and *M. fortuitum*. Treatment with topical amikacin and erythromycin may lead to temporary resolution

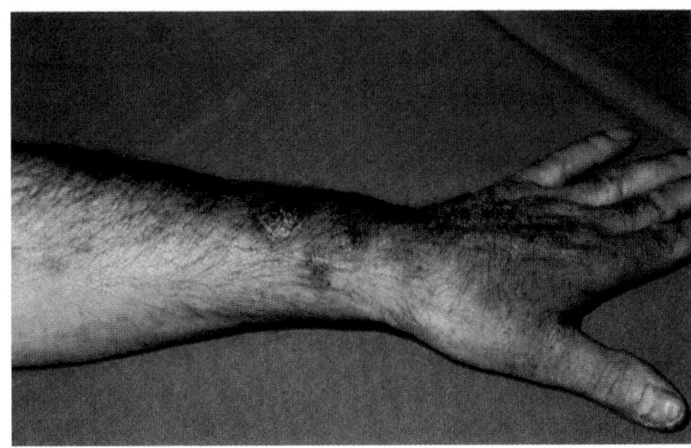

Fig. 7.6.26.1 *M. marinum* infection. A small lesion at the base of the thumb (arrowed) and secondary lesions on the wrist and forearm due to 'sporotrichoid' spread.
(Courtesy of Dr G Haase.)

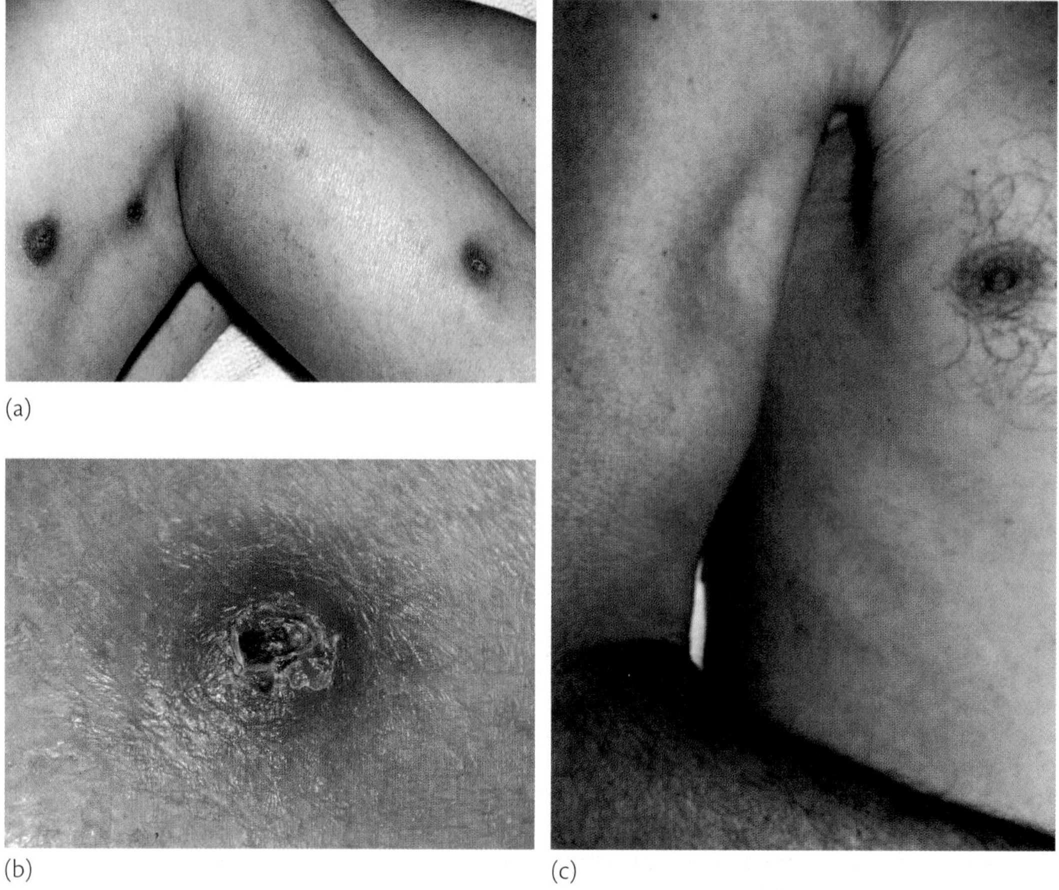

Fig. 7.6.26.2 Disseminated *M. marinum* infection in a patient with a genetic γ-interferon receptor polymorphism who did not respond to conventional chemotherapy. (a) Lesions on leg. (b) Detail of lesion. (c) Ruptured biceps tendon resulting from tenosynovitis.
(Copyright D A Warrell.)

but relapse is common, especially in cases due to *M. abscessus* or *M. chelonae*, and corneal grafting is usually required.

Surgical inoculation

More serious infections have followed accidental inoculation during surgical operations, especially when contaminated materials, including heart valve xenografts, have been inserted. Contamination during cardiac valve surgery has resulted in mycobacterial endocarditis with septicaemia and osteomyelitis of the sternum requiring extensive débridement.

Disseminated disease

Before HIV became widespread, disseminated disease due to environmental mycobacteria was very rare. Some cases, usually due to MAC or rapid growers, occurred in young people with congenital immune deficiencies (Fig. 7.6.26.3) and others, due principally to *M. chelonae*, occurred in renal transplant recipients. *M. haemophilum* was a cause of multiple skin lesions in transplant recipients. As suggested by the name, this mycobacterium requires the addition of blood or other sources of iron in the medium for its *in vitro* cultivation.

However, the situation changed dramatically after the advent of the HIV pandemic and disseminated environmental mycobacterial disease was reported in 30 to 50% of patients with AIDS, particularly in the United States of America. For reasons that are not clear, the great majority of such cases, 90% or more, were caused by

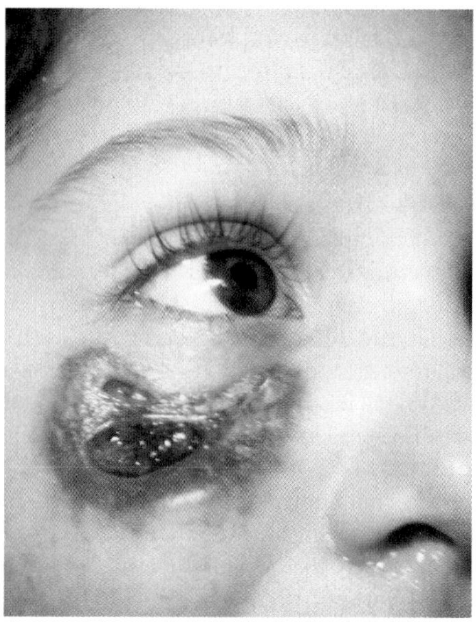

Fig. 7.6.26.3 Ulcer on the face as the initial manifestation of disseminated *M. chelonae* infection in a 4-year-old girl with autosomal IgA deficiency.
(Courtesy of Dr K Schopfer.)

MAC, usually strains identifiable by DNA homology as *M. avium avium* rather than *M. avium intracellulare*. Some cases are due to *M. genavense*, a very slowly growing species which, like *M. avium avium*, has been isolated from diseased birds. The number of cases of disseminated AIDS-related environmental mycobacterial disease has now declined in the wealthier nations following the introduction of antiretroviral therapy. Although HIV infection is common in Africa and MAC is present in the environment, AIDS-related disease due to this species is, for unknown reasons, rare in this continent.

Symptoms include fever, night sweats, weight loss, those of anaemia, and general malaise; they are rather nonspecific and may be caused by other AIDS-related infections. Involvement of the intestine may lead to malabsorption and chronic diarrhoea. The diagnosis of AIDS-related MAC disease is made by culture of blood or of biopsies of liver, lymph nodes, or bone marrow. The bacilli may be isolated from faeces in disseminated disease but they may also be present in the intestinal tract of healthy persons.

Other human disease

Although requiring confirmation, there is some evidence to suggest that *M. avium paratuberculosis*, the causative agent of hypertrophic enteritis or Johne's disease in ruminants, is a cause of Crohn's disease in humans.

Therapy

This depends on the site and severity of the infection, the presence of predisposing conditions such as congenital or acquired immune suppression, and the species of mycobacterium. Too much reliance should not be placed on *in vitro* drug susceptibility tests as these do not always reflect clinical response.

As indicated above, skin lesions may be cured by excision, curettage, or drainage. Surgical excision, when technically possible, is used to treat lymphadenitis and should be considered in cases of localized pulmonary lesions.

Antiretroviral therapy has a greater beneficial impact on MAC disease in AIDS patients than antimycobacterial agents, although the latter improve the quality of the patients' lives. Treatment of disease due to MAC, *M. xenopi* and *M. malmoense* in both HIV-positive and -negative patients is based on rifabutin and ethambutol with the addition of either clarithromycin or ciprofloxacin. The duration of therapy depends on clinical and bacteriological response but is usually 24 months.

Treatment of disease due to *M. kansasii* has been less well evaluated but good responses have been obtained with regimens containing rifampicin, ethambutol and isoniazid. In vitro studies indicate that clarithromycin or azithromycin may be beneficial but this is not yet supported by clinical trials (Box 7.6.26.1).

There have been no comparative trials of drug regimens for disease caused by the rapidly growing species *M. chelonae* and *M. fortuitum*. Therapy is therefore based on anecdotal experience and the results of *in vitro* susceptibility tests. The duration of therapy depends on clinical response. Localized disease often responds to erythromycin with trimethoprim, while spreading or disseminated disease may require the addition of amikacin or a cephalosporin such as ceftriaxone. Limited experience indicates that the fluoroquinolones are effective against *M. fortuitum* and imipenem or meropenem against *M. chelonae*.

Box 7.6.26.1 Recommended regimens for the treatment of pulmonary infections due to the more usually encountered slow-growing environmental mycobacteria

- *M. avium* complex, *M. xenopi*, *M. malmoense* in HIV-positive and -negative patients
  - 24 months' rifampicin and ethambutol plus either clarithromycin or ciprofloxacin. If the patient is not improving at 1 year the drug (clarithromycin or ciprofloxacin) not included in the initial regimen is added.
- *M. kansasii*
  - Rifampicin, ethambutol and isoniazid, continued until sputum has been negative on culture for 12 months.

Skin lesions due to *M. marinum* respond to doxycycline or minocycline, or a combination of rifampicin and ethambutol. In the rare cases of disseminated infection attributable to γ-interferon receptor polymorphisms, adjuvant cytokine therapy with γ-interferon may enhance the response to chemotherapy.

Further reading

Banks J, Campbell IA (2008). Environmental mycobacteria. In: Davies PDO, Barnes PF, Gordon SB (eds). *Clinical Tuberculosis*, 4th edition, pp. 509–18. Hodder Arnold, London.

Corless JA, Stockton PA, Davies PD (2000). Mycobacterial culture results of smear-positive patients with suspected pulmonary tuberculosis in Liverpool. *Eur Respir J*, **16**, 976–9.

Davies PDO, Ormerod LP (1999). Environmental mycobacteria. In: *Case presentations in clinical tuberculosis*, pp. 259–75. Arnold, London.

Evans AK, Cunningham MJ (2005). Atypical mycobacterial cervicofacial lymphadenitis in children: a disease as old as mankind, yet a persistent challenge. *Am J Otolaryngol*, **26**, 337–43.

Greenstein RJ (2003). Is Crohn's disease caused by a mycobacterium? Comparisons with leprosy, tuberculosis, and Johne's disease. *Lancet Infect Dis*, **3**, 507–14.

Griffith DE, Aksamit T, Brown-Elliott BA, *et al.* On behalf of the ATS Mycobacterial Diseases Subcommittee (2007). An Official ATS/IDSA Statement: Diagnosis, treatment, and prevention of nontuberculous mycobacterial diseases. *Am J Respir Crit Care Med*, **175**, 367–416.

Jenkins PA, *et al.* (2008). Clarithromycin vs ciprofloxacin as adjuncts to rifampicin and ethambutol in treating opportunist mycobacterial lung diseases and an assessment of *Mycobacterium vaccae* immunotherapy. *Thorax*, **63**, 627–34.

Karakousis PC, Moore RD, Chaisson RE (2004). *Mycobacterium avium* complex in patients with HIV infection in the era of highly active antiretroviral therapy. *Lancet Infect Dis*, **4**, 557–65.

Marras TK, Daley CL (2002). Epidemiology of human pulmonary infection with nontuberculous mycobacteria. *Clin Chest Med*, **23**, 553–67.

Primm TP, Lucero CA, Falkinham JO (2004). Health impacts of environmental mycobacteria. *Clin Microbiol Rev*, **17**, 98–106.

Zumla A, Grange JM (2002). Infection and disease due to environmental mycobacteria. *Curr Opin Pulm Med*, **8**, 166–72.

7.6.27 Leprosy (Hansen's disease)

Diana N.J. Lockwood

Essentials

Leprosy is a chronic granulomatous disease caused by *Mycobacterium leprae*, an acid-fast intracellular organism not yet cultivated *in vitro*. It is an important public health problem worldwide, with an estimated 4 million people disabled by the disease. Transmission of *M. leprae* is only partially understood, but untreated lepromatous patients discharge abundant organisms from their nasal mucosa into the environment.

Clinical features

These are determined by the degree of cell-mediated immunity towards *M. leprae*, with tuberculoid (paucibacillary) and lepromatous leprosy (multibacillary) being the two poles of a spectrum: (1) tuberculoid—well-expressed cell-mediated immunity effectively controls bacillary multiplication with the formation of organized epithelioid-cell granulomas; (2) lepromatous—there is cellular anergy towards *M. leprae* with abundant bacillary multiplication. Between these two poles is a continuum, varying from the patient with moderate cell-mediated immunity (borderline tuberculoid), through borderline, to the patient with little cellular response, borderline lepromatous.

Presenting symptoms—most commonly (1) anaesthesia—ranging from a small area of numbness on the skin due to involvement of a dermal nerve, to peripheral neuropathy with affected nerves tender and thickened; (2) skin lesions—most commonly macules or plaques; tuberculoid patients have few, hypopigmented lesions that are anaesthetic; lepromatous patients have numerous, sometimes confluent lesions.

Other manifestations—these include (1) type 1 (reversal reactions)—occur in borderline patients; characterized by acute neuritis and/or acutely inflamed skin lesions; often occur in the first 2 months after starting treatment; (2) type 2 (erythema nodosum leprosum reactions)—occur in up to 50% of patients with lepromatous leprosy; (3) neuritis—silent neuropathy is an important form of nerve damage, causing lifelong morbidity; (4) eye disease—blindness occurs in at least 2.5% of patients.

Diagnosis

This is made by recognition of typical skin lesions or thickened peripheral nerves, supported by the finding of acid-fast bacilli on slit skin smears that should be taken from at least four sites (earlobes, and edges of active lesions).

Treatment

There are six main principles of treatment: (1) stop the infection with chemotherapy—first-line antileprosy drugs are rifampicin, clofazimine, and dapsone, given in combination and duration as determined by whether disease is paucibacillary or multibacillary; these are highly effective in killing bacilli but may not halt nerve damage; (2) treat new nerve damage—a 6-month course of steroids should be given to those with nerve damage for less than 6 months; (3) treat reactions—steroids are likely to be required; (4) educate the patient about leprosy; (5) prevent disability; and (6) support the patient socially and psychologically—patients with leprosy the world over are frequently stigmatized; words such as 'leper' should be avoided; the disease can be referred to as 'Hansen's disease'.

Prevention

Vaccination with bacille Calmette–Guérin (BCG) can provide some protection against leprosy (20–80% in different trials).

Aetiology

Leprosy is caused by *Mycobacterium leprae*, an acid-fast intracellular organism not yet cultivated *in vitro*. It was first identified in the nodules of patients with lepromatous leprosy by Hansen in 1873. *M. leprae* preferentially parasitizes skin macrophages and peripheral nerve Schwann cells.

In vivo cultivation of *M. leprae*

M. leprae can be grown in the mouse footpad, but growth is slow, taking over 6 months to produce significant yields. The nine-banded armadillo is susceptible to *M. leprae* infection and develops lepromatous disease. The armadillo and mouse models of *M. leprae* infection have been useful for producing *M. leprae* for biological studies and studying drug sensitivity patterns, respectively.

Biological characteristics

M. leprae is a stable hardy organism that withstands drying for up to 5 months. It has a doubling time of 12 days (compared with 20 min for *Escherichia coli*). The optimum growth temperature is 27 to 30° C, consistent with the clinical observation of maximal *M. leprae* growth at cool superficial sites (skin, nasal mucosa, and peripheral nerves). *M. leprae* isolates from different parts of the world have similar biological characteristics. *M. leprae* possesses a complex cell wall comprising lipids and carbohydrates. It synthesizes a species-specific phenolic glycolipid and lipoarabinomannan. Antibody and T-cell screening have identified numerous protein antigens and peptides that are important immune targets.

M. leprae genome

M. leprae has a 3.27-Mb genome that displays extreme reductive evolution. Less than one-half of the genome contains functional genes and many pseudogenes are present. One hundred and sixty-five genes are unique to *M. leprae* and functions can be attributed to 29 of them. These unique proteins are being identified and analysed to aid in development of new diagnostic tests. Comparison of biosynthetic pathways with *Mycobacterium tuberculosis* is giving new insights into *M. leprae* metabolism. For lipolysis *M. leprae* has only two genes (*M. tuberculosis* has 22); *M. leprae* has also lost many genes for carbon catabolism and many carbon sources (e.g. acetate and galactose) are unavailable to it. This gene loss leaves *M. leprae* unable to respond to different environments and underlies the impossibility of growing the organism *in vitro*. Using comparative genomics and analysis of single nucleotide polymorphisms it has been shown that all extant cases of leprosy can be attributed to a single clone which then disseminated worldwide. Leprosy probably originated in India or eastern Africa and spread with successive human migrations.

Epidemiology

Leprosy continues to be an important public health problem worldwide. In 2004, 407 791 new cases were reported with high rates of childhood cases in the most endemic countries. In 2008, 249 007 new cases were registered. The highest numbers of cases were in India, Brazil, Indonesia, Nigeria and Nepal. India accounts for 64% of the global disease burden. From 1990, the World Health Organization (WHO) led a leprosy elimination campaign but this defined elimination as less than 1 case per 10 000 population. Prevalence figures are highly influenced by operational activities such as reducing the length of treatment. The global focus is now on detecting new cases and providing sustainable care for leprosy patients. An estimated 4 million people are disabled by leprosy. Leprosy has not always been a tropical disease; it was widespread in medieval Europe and was endemic in Norway until the early 20th century. In North America, small foci of infection still exist in Texas and Louisiana. Nearly all new patients now seen in Europe and North America have acquired their infection abroad.

Risk factors

Leprosy is a chronic disease with a long incubation period. An average incubation time of 2 to 5 years has been calculated for tuberculoid cases and 8 to 12 years for lepromatous cases. American servicemen who developed leprosy after serving in the tropics presented up to 20 years after their presumed exposure. Most leprosy patients do not have known contact with a leprosy patient. Age, sex, and household contact are important determinants of leprosy risk; incidence reaches a peak at 10 to 14 years; the excess of male cases is attributed to women's reluctance to present to health workers with skin lesions. Poor nutritional status is cited as predisposing to leprosy but no good evidence substantiates this. Improved socioeconomic conditions, extended schooling, and good housing conditions reduce the risk of leprosy. Subclinical infection with *M. leprae* is probably common but the development of established disease is rare. Little work has been done on the early events in infection with *M. leprae* because there is no simple test that can establish whether an individual has encountered *M. leprae* and mounted a protective immune response.

HIV and leprosy

It was predicted that HIV infection would produce anergic, lepromatous leprosy, However HIV/leprosy coinfected patients have disease types across the leprosy spectrum with typical leprosy skin lesions and nerve involvement. Their skin lesions have typical leprosy histology with granuloma formation even in the presence of low circulating CD4 counts. Patients coinfected with HIV and leprosy appear to be at higher risk of developing leprosy reactions and nerve damage. Leprosy may also present as an immune reconstitution syndrome (IRIS) in patients who have recently started on highly active antiretroviral therapy (HAART) and have rising CD4 counts and a falling viral load. These patients have borderline leprosy which is very immunologically active with inflamed skin lesions and reactions.

Transmission

The transmission of *M. leprae* is only partially understood. Untreated lepromatous patients discharge abundant organisms from their nasal mucosa into the environment. Studies in Indonesia and Ethiopia using polymerase chain reaction (PCR) primers to detect *M. leprae* DNA in nasal swabs have shown that up to 5% of the population in leprosy endemic areas carry *M. leprae* DNA in their noses. The organism is then inhaled, multiplies on the inferior turbinates, and has a brief bacteraemic phase before binding to and entering Schwann cells and macrophages. The combination of an environmentally well-adapted organism, high carriage rates, and a long incubation period means that, even with effective antibiotics, transmission will continue for a long time.

Pathogenesis

Leprosy is a bacterial infection in which the clinical features are determined by the host's immune response (Table 7.6.27.1).

Immune response to *M. leprae* and the leprosy spectrum

The Ridley–Jopling classification (Fig. 7.6.27.1) places patients on a spectrum of disease according to their clinical features, bacterial load, and histological and immunological responses. The two poles of the spectrum are tuberculoid (TT; paucibacillary) and lepromatous leprosy (LL; multibacillary). At the tuberculoid pole, well-expressed cell-mediated immunity effectively controls bacillary multiplication with the formation of organized epithelioid-cell granulomas; at the lepromatous pole there is cellular anergy towards *M. leprae* with abundant bacillary multiplication. Between these two poles is a continuum, varying from the patient with moderate cell-mediated immunity (borderline tuberculoid, BT) through borderline (BB) to the patient with little cellular response, borderline lepromatous (BL). The polar groups (TT, LL) are stable, but within the central groups (BT, BB, BL) the disease tends to downgrade to the lepromatous pole in the absence of treatment, and upgrading towards the tuberculoid pole may occur during or after treatment.

Both T cells and macrophages play important roles in the processing, recognition, and response to *M. leprae* antigens. In tuberculoid leprosy, *in vitro* tests of T-cell function such as lymphocyte transformation tests show a strong response to *M. leprae* protein antigens with the production of Th1-type cytokines such as interferon-γ and interleukin 2 (IL-2). Skin tests with lepromin, a heat-killed *M. leprae* preparation, are strongly positive. Staining of skin biopsies from tuberculoid lesions with T-cell markers shows highly organized granulomas composed predominantly of CD4 cells and macrophages with a peripheral mantle of CD8 cells. This strong cell-mediated immune response clears bacilli but with concomitant local tissue destruction, especially in nerves.

Patients with lepromatous leprosy have no cell-mediated immunity to *M. leprae* with a failure of the T-cell and macrophage response. Tests for lepromin are negative. This anergy is specific for *M. leprae*. Patients with lepromatous disease respond to other mycobacteria such as *M. tuberculosis*, both *in vitro* and in skin tests. Identification of cell types in lepromatous granulomas shows a disorganized mixture of macrophages and T cells, mainly CD8 cells. The T-cell failure may be due to clonal anergy or active suppression. Defects in cytokine production have been demonstrated; intralesional injections of recombinant IL-2 reconstitute the local immune response with elimination of *M. leprae* from macrophages. There is low production of Th2-type cytokines. Macrophage defects described in

Table 7.6.27.1 Major clinical features of the disease spectrum in leprosy

Clinical features	Classification				
	Tuberculoid (TT)	**Borderline tuberculoid (BT)**	**Borderline (BB)**	**Borderline lepromatous (BL)**	**Lepromatous (LL)**
	Paucibacillary			**Multibacillary**	
Skin					
Infiltrated lesions	Defined plaques, healing centres	Irregular plaques with partially raised edges	Polymorphic, 'punched out centres'	Papules, nodules	Diffuse thickening
Macular lesions	Single, small	Several, any size, 'geographical'	Multiple, all sizes, bizarre	Innumerable, small	Innumerable, confluent
Nerve					
Peripheral nerve	Solitary enlarged nerves	Several nerves, asymmetrical	Many nerves, asymmetrical pattern	Late neural thickening, asymmetrical, anaesthesia and paresis	Slow symmetrical loss, glove and stocking anaesthesia
Microbiology					
Bacterial index	0–1	0–2	2–3	1–4	4–6
Histology					
Lymphocytes	+	++	±	++	±
Macrophages	–	–	±	–	–
Epithelioid cells	++	±	–	–	–
Antibody, anti-*M. leprae*	–/+	–/++	+	++	++

+, present, ++, present strongly, –, absent.

lepromatous disease include defective antigen presentation and recognition, defective IL-1 production, a failure of macrophages to kill *M. leprae*, and a macrophage suppression of the T-cell response. Patients with lepromatous leprosy produce a range of autoantibodies that are both organ specific (against thyroid, nerve, testis, and gastric mucosa) and nonspecific, such as rheumatoid factors, anti-DNA, cryoglobulins, and cardiolipin.

Bacterial load

In lepromatous leprosy, bacilli spread haematogenously to cool superficial sites including eyes, upper respiratory mucosa, testes, small muscles, and bones of the hands, feet, and face as well as to peripheral nerves and skin. The heavy bacterial load causes structural damage at all these sites. In tuberculoid leprosy, bacilli are not readily found.

Nerve damage

Neural inflammation is pathognomonic of leprosy. Nerve damage occurs in small nerve fibres, both sensory and autonomic, in the skin and in peripheral nerve trunks. Nerve damage occurs before diagnosis, during treatment, and after treatment. In lepromatous infection, almost all the cutaneous nerves and peripheral nerve trunks are involved. Bacilli are found in Schwann, perineural, and endothelial cells. Extensive demyelination occurs and later wallerian degeneration. Despite large numbers of organisms in the nerve there is only a small inflammatory response, but ultimately the nerve becomes fibrotic and is hyalinized. At the tuberculoid end of the spectrum nerve damage is secondary to a granulomatous response to *M. leprae* antigens. Perineural inflammation and epithelioid granulomas destroy the Schwann cells and axons. In borderline leprosy the combination of *M. leprae* antigens and a cell-mediated immune response results in small granulomas abutting strands of normal-looking but heavily bacillated Schwann cells giving rise to the widespread nerve damage in borderline leprosy. The persistence of *M. leprae* antigens in Schwann cells means that immune-mediated nerve damage can occur after successful antibacterial treatment.

Leprosy reactions

Leprosy reactions are events superimposed on the Ridley–Jopling spectrum. Type 1 (reversal reactions) occur in borderline patients (BT, BB, BL) and are delayed hypersensitivity reactions caused by increased recognition of *M. leprae* antigens in skin and nerve sites. They are characterized by an increase in lymphocytes (CD4 and IL-2-producing cells) within lesions, severe oedema with disruption

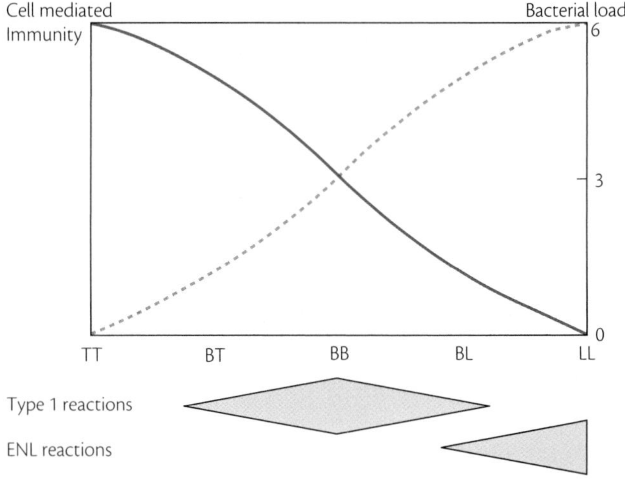

Fig. 7.6.27.1 Ridley–Jopling spectrum of bacterial load, cell-mediated immunity, and reactions.

of the granuloma, and giant cell formation. There is local production of Th1-type cytokines such as interferon-γ and tumour necrosis factor-α.

Type 2 reactions, erythema nodosum leprosum (ENL), are partly due to immune complex deposition and occur in patients with borderline lepromatous and lepromatous leprosy who produce antibodies and have a large antigen load. There is vasculitis with lesional immunoglobulin deposition, complement activation, and polymorphs and circulating immune complexes. There is also enhanced T-cell activity with increased CD8 cells, increased circulating IL-2 receptors, and high levels of circulating tumour necrosis factor-α. After reaction, lepromatous patients revert to a state of immunological unresponsiveness.

Clinical features of leprosy

Patients commonly present with skin lesions, weakness or numbness due to a peripheral nerve lesion, or a burn or ulcer on an anaesthetic hand or foot. Borderline patients may present in reaction with nerve pain, sudden palsy, multiple new skin lesions, pain in the eye, or a systemic febrile illness. The cardinal signs are:

- typical skin lesions, anaesthetic at the tuberculoid end of the spectrum
- thickened peripheral nerves
- acid-fast bacilli on skin smears or biopsy

Early lesions

The commonest early lesion is an area of numbness on the skin or a visible skin lesion. The classic early skin lesion is indeterminate leprosy, which is commonly found on the face, extensor surface of the limbs, buttocks, or trunk. Indeterminate lesions consist of one or more slightly hypopigmented or erythematous macules, a few centimetres in diameter, with poorly defined margins. Hair growth and nerve function are unimpaired. A biopsy may show the perineurovascular infiltrate and only scanty acid-fast bacilli. The indeterminate phase may last for months or years before resolving or developing into one of the determinate types of leprosy.

Skin

The commonest skin lesions are macules or plaques; papules and nodules are more rare. Lesions may be found anywhere although rarely in the axillae, perineum, or hairy scalp. Skin lesions should be assessed for inflammation, colour, and sensation. Tuberculoid patients have few granulomatous hypopigmented lesions while lepromatous patients have numerous, sometimes confluent lesions. The few tuberculoid lesions are usually asymmetrical; more numerous lesions are likely to be distributed symmetrically.

Anaesthesia

Anaesthesia may occur in skin lesions when dermal nerves are involved or in the distribution of a large peripheral nerve. In skin lesions the small dermal sensory and autonomic nerve fibres supplying dermal and subcutaneous structures are damaged causing local sensory loss and loss of sweating within that area.

Peripheral neuropathy

Peripheral nerve trunks are vulnerable at sites where they are superficial or are in fibro-osseous tunnels. At these points a small increase in nerve diameter raises intraneural pressure causing neural compression and ischaemia. Damage to peripheral nerve trunks produces characteristic signs with dermatomal sensory loss and dysfunction of muscles supplied by that peripheral nerve. The predilection sites for peripheral nerve involvement are ulnar nerve (at the elbow) (Fig. 7.6.27.2), median nerve (at the wrist), radial nerve, radial cutaneous nerve (at the wrist), common peroneal nerve (at the knee), posterior tibial and sural nerves at the ankle, facial nerve as it crosses the zygomatic arch, and great auricular nerve in the posterior triangle of the neck (Fig. 7.6.27.3). All these nerves should be examined for enlargement and tenderness. Peripheral nerve function should be assessed by testing the motor function of the small muscles of the hands and feet using the Medical Research Council (MRC) grading scale. Sensory function is best assessed using graded nylon monofilaments (Semmes–Weinstein) as in diabetic screening. Patients should be asked about symptoms of neuropathy.

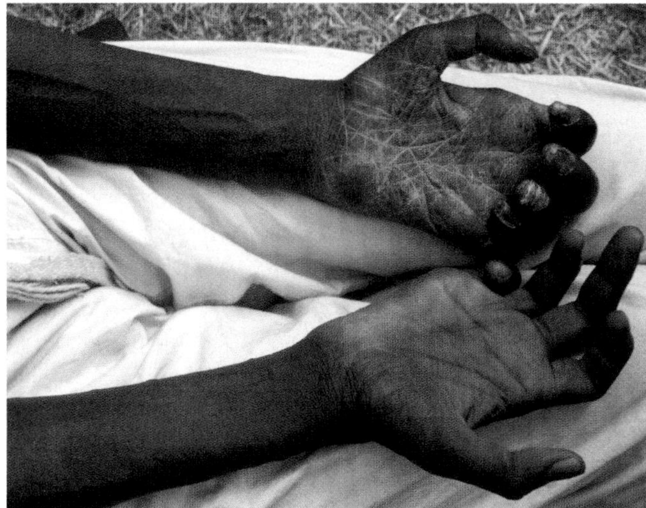

Fig. 7.6.27.2 The effects of ulnar and median nerve paralysis with wasting of the small muscles of the hand and evidence of neuropathic damage.
(Copyright D.A. Warrell).

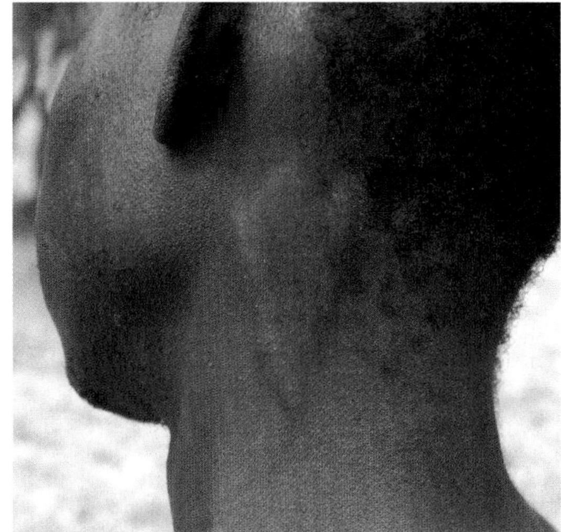

Fig. 7.6.27.3 Thickening of greater auricular nerve.
(Copyright D.A. Warrell.)

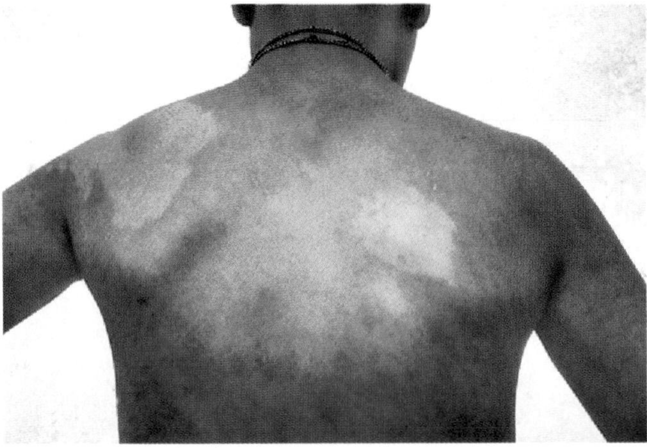

Fig. 7.6.27.4 BT leprosy. This Ethiopian woman was several hypopigmented patches. Testing for anaesthesia will confirm the diagnosis of BT leprosy.

Tuberculoid leprosy (TT)

Infection is localized and asymmetrical. A typical tuberculoid skin lesion is a macule or plaque, single, erythematous, or purple, with raised and clear-cut edges sloping towards a flattened hypopigmented centre. The surface is anaesthetized, dry, and hairless. Sensory impairment may be difficult to demonstrate on the face where there are abundant nerve endings. If peripheral nerve trunk involvement is present, only one nerve trunk is enlarged. No *M. leprae* are found in skin smears. True tuberculoid leprosy has a good prognosis, many infections resolve without treatment, and peripheral nerve trunk damage is limited.

Borderline tuberculoid leprosy (BT)

The skin lesions are similar to tuberculoid leprosy and there may be few or many lesions (Figs. 7.6.27.4, 7.6.27.5). The margins are less well defined and there may be satellite lesions. Damage to peripheral nerves is widespread and severe, usually with several thickened nerve trunks. It is important to recognize borderline tuberculoid leprosy because these patients are at risk of reversal reactions leading to rapid deterioration in nerve function with consequent deformities.

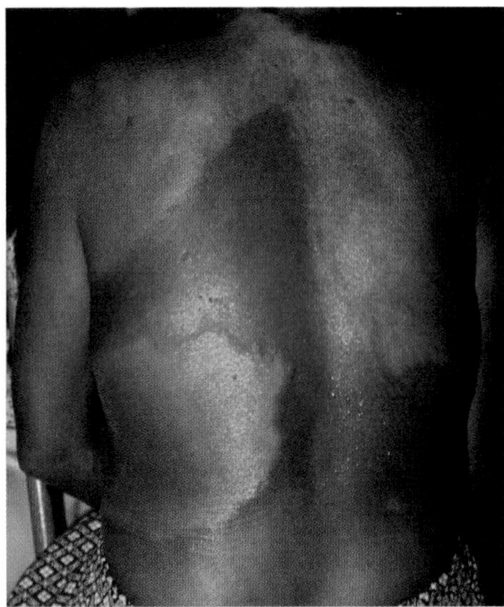

Fig. 7.6.27.5 Active tuberculoid lesions showing the sharp outer edge, thin raised erythematous dry rim, and the broad hypopigmented dry centre. The 'satellite' lesion at the lower outer edge indicates that this is borderline tuberculoid leprosy. Biopsies and smears should be taken from the raised active rim.
(Copyright D.A. Warrell.)

Borderline leprosy (BB)

Borderline disease is the most unstable part of the spectrum and patients usually downgrade towards lepromatous leprosy if they are not treated or upgrade towards tuberculoid leprosy as part of a reversal reaction. There are numerous skin lesions which may be macules, papules, or plaques and they vary in size, shape, and distribution. The edges of the lesions may have streaming, irregular borders. Annular lesions with a broad irregular edge and a sharply defined punched-out centre are characteristic of borderline disease (Fig. 7.6.27.6). Nerve damage is variable.

Borderline lepromatous leprosy (BL)

This is characterized by widespread variable asymmetrical skin lesions. There may be erythematous or hyperpigmented papules, succulent nodules or plaques, and sensation in the lesions may be normal (Fig. 7.6.27.8). Peripheral nerve involvement is widespread. While patients with borderline lepromatous leprosy do not have the extreme consequences of bacillary multiplication that are seen in lepromatous disease, they may experience either or both reversal and ENL reactions.

Lepromatous leprosy (LL)

The patient with untreated polar lepromatous leprosy may be carrying 10^{11} leprosy bacilli. The onset of disease is frequently insidious, the earliest lesions being ill-defined, shiny, hypopigmented, or erythematous macules. Gradually the skin becomes infiltrated and thickened and nodules develop (Fig. 7.6.27.7); facial skin thickening causes the characteristic leonine facies (Fig. 7.6.27.9). Hair is lost, especially the lateral third of the eyebrows (madarosis). Dermal nerves are destroyed leading to a progressive glove and stocking anaesthesia. Position sense is preserved. Sweating is lost, which is uncomfortable

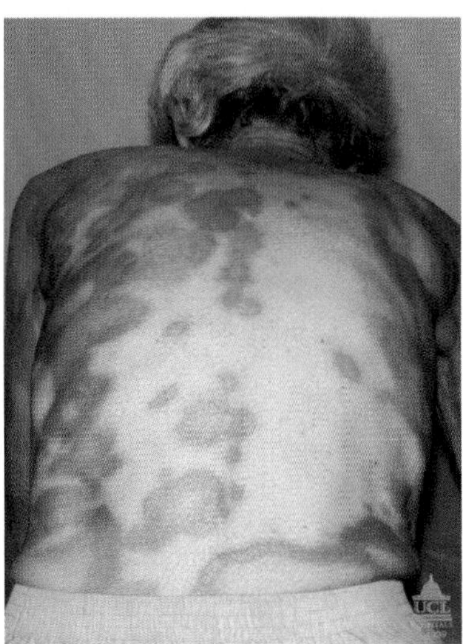

Fig. 7.6.27.6 Multiple, asymmetrical erythematous lesions. Sensation was intact inside the lesions.

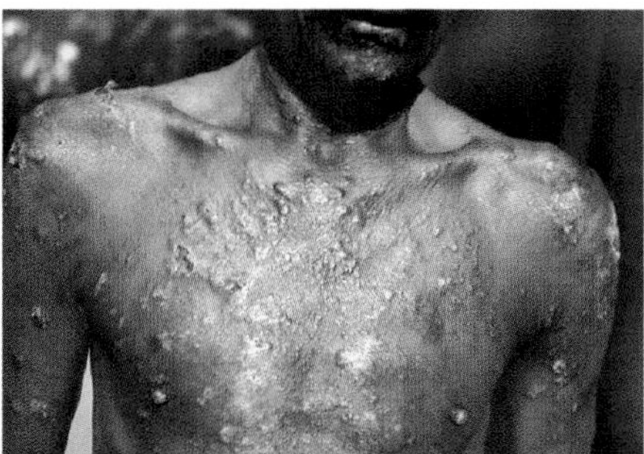

Fig. 7.6.27.7 Advanced nodular lepromatous leprosy. This Indian patient presented with ulcerating nodules all over his body.

in the tropics as compensatory sweating occurs in the remaining intact areas. Damage to peripheral nerves is symmetrical and occurs late in the disease. Infiltration of the corneal nerves causes anaesthesia of the cornea, which predisposes to injury, secondary infection, and blindness (Fig. 7.6.27.10).

Nasal symptoms can often be elicited early in the disease. Septal perforation may occur. There may be papules on the lips and nodules on the palate, uvula, tongue, and gums (Fig. 7.6.27.11). Bone involvement is common, with absorption of the terminal phalanges and pencilling of the heads and shafts of the metatarsals. Testicular atrophy results from diffuse infiltration compounded by acute orchitis that may occur during ENL reactions. The consequent loss of testosterone leads to azoospermia and gynaecomastia (Fig. 7.6.27.12). The extremities become oedematous. The skin of the legs becomes ichthyotic and ulcerates easily.

Other forms of leprosy

There are several variant forms of leprosy. Pure neural leprosy occurs principally in India where it is the presenting form for 10% of patients. There is asymmetrical involvement of peripheral nerve trunks and no visible skin lesions. On nerve biopsy all types of leprosy have been found.

Histoid lesions are distinctive nodules occurring in lepromatous patients who have relapsed due to dapsone resistance or noncompliance with chemotherapy.

Lucio's leprosy is a form of lepromatous leprosy found only in Latin Americans; it is characterized by a uniform diffuse shiny skin infiltration.

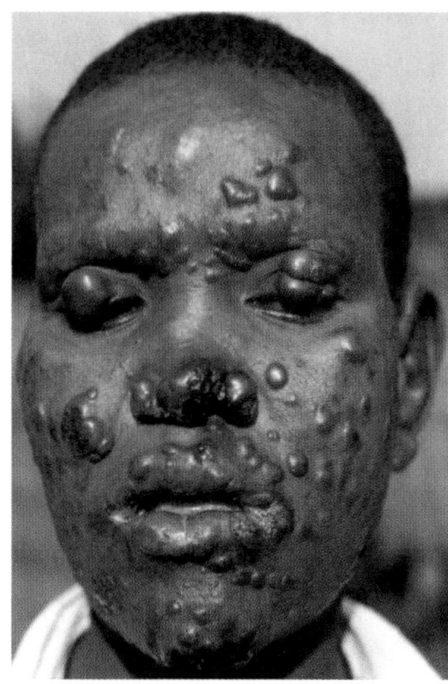

Fig. 7.6.27.9 Lepromatous leprosy.
(Copyright D.A. Warrell.)

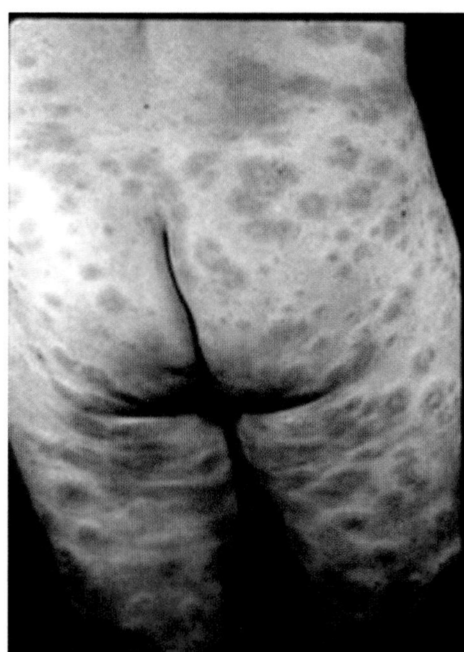

Fig. 7.6.27.8 BL leprosy with multiple erythematous lesions. No anaesthesia was present.

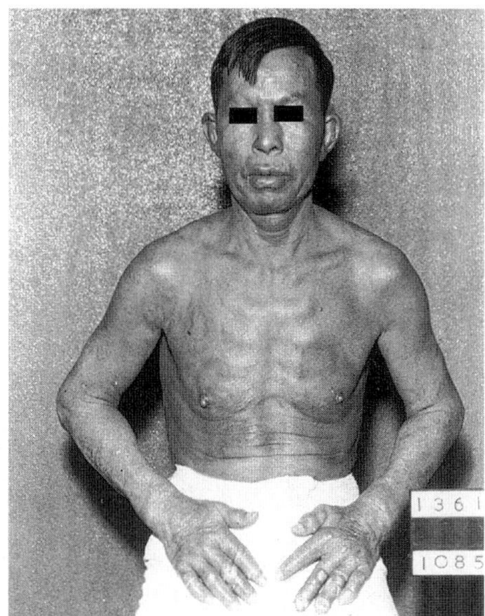

Fig. 7.6.27.10 Active, untreated lepromatous leprosy, showing generalized infiltration of the skin, swelling of fingers and lips, and thinning of eyebrows and eyelashes. The residual annular lesions visible in both pectoral regions indicate that this patient has 'downgraded' from borderline.

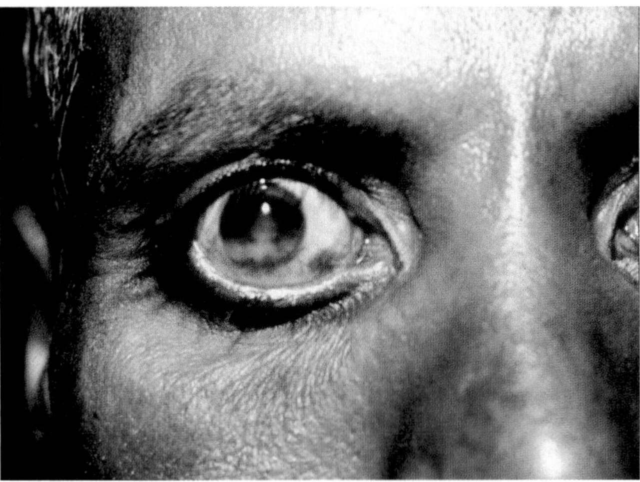

Fig. 7.6.27.11 Corneal damage to eye secondary to lagophthalmos caused by involvement of the zygomatic branch of the facial nerve.

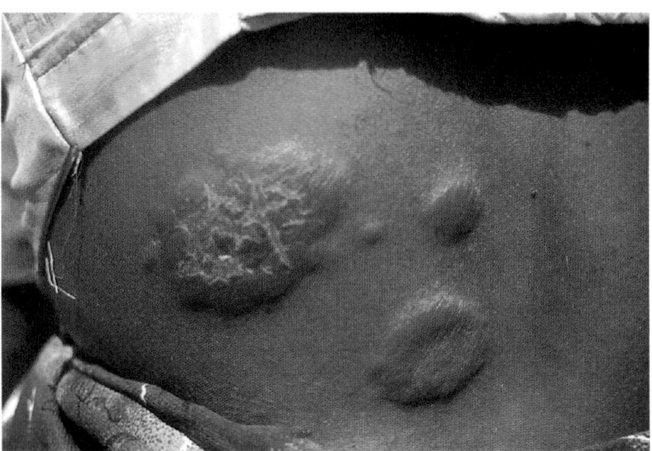

Fig. 7.6.27.13 Severe reversal (Type 1) reaction. This Indian woman has erythematous, oedematous, and desquamating reactional lesions.

Eye disease in leprosy

Blindness due to leprosy, which occurs in at least 2.5% of patients, is a devastating complication for a patient with anaesthesia of the hands and feet. Eye damage results from both nerve damage and bacillary invasion. Lagophthalmos results from paresis of the orbicularis oculi due to involvement of the zygomatic and temporal branches of the facial (VIIth) nerve. These superficial branches are frequently involved in borderline tuberculoid cases, particularly if there are facial skin lesions. In lepromatous disease, lagophthalmos occurs later and is usually bilateral. Damage to the ophthalmic branch of the trigeminal (Vth) nerve causes anaesthesia of the cornea and conjunctiva resulting in drying of the cornea and making the cornea susceptible to trauma and ulceration (Fig. 7.6.27.11). Lepromatous infiltration in corneal nerves produces punctate keratitis and corneal lepromas. Invasion of the iris and ciliary body makes them extremely susceptible to reactions.

Leprosy reactions

Type 1 (reversal reactions)

These are characterized by acute neuritis and/or acutely inflamed skin lesions. Nerves become tender with new loss of sensation or motor weakness. Existing skin lesions become erythematous or oedematous (Figs. 7.6.27.13 and 7.6.27.14); new lesions may appear (Fig. 7.6.27.15). Occasionally oedema of the hands, face, or feet is the presenting symptom, but constitutional symptoms are unusual. Type 1 reactions occur in borderline patients; 35% of borderline lepromatous patients will experience a type 1 reaction. Patients often

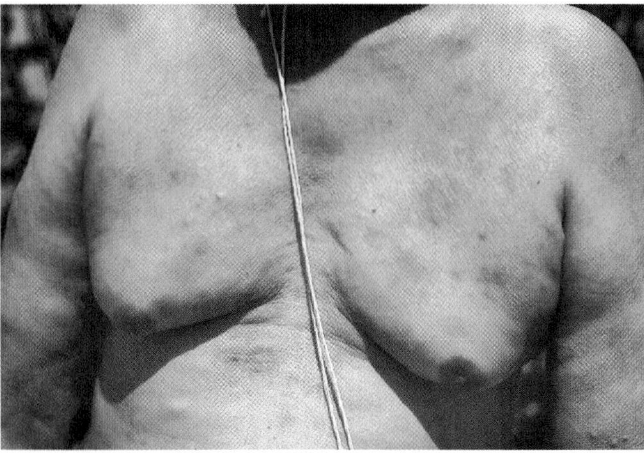

Fig. 7.6.27.12 Complications of lepromatous leprosy. Gynaecomastia is visible in this man, secondary to testicular involvement in lepromatous leprosy. Multiple nodules are present, many dark brown, due to clofazimine pigmentation. He also has new erythematous lesions of ENL.

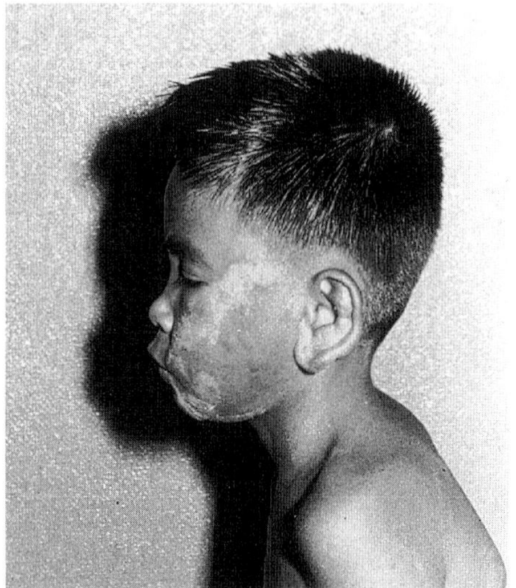

Fig. 7.6.27.14 Reversal-reaction plaque on the left cheek and ear. The edge of this borderline tuberculoid lesion has become very sharply defined, more raised, and erythematous, dry, and scaly. Treatment with corticosteroids is imperative as the patient is at grave risk of rapidly developing lagophthalmos due to associated involvement of branches of the facial nerve.

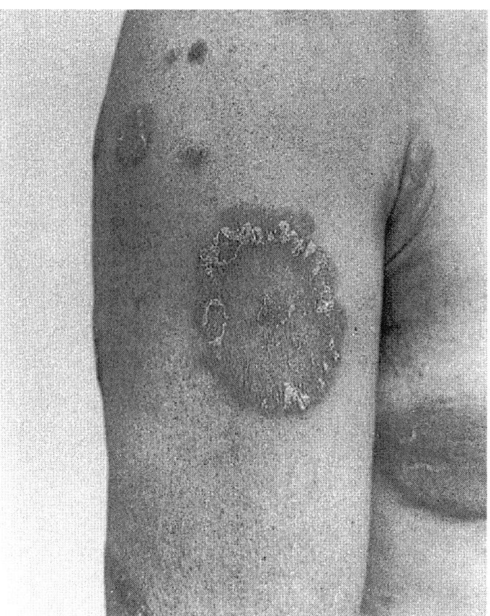

Fig. 7.6.27.15 Type 1 (reversal) reaction: this BL patient developed new, sharp-edged, well-defined, erythematous plaques with desquamating surfaces about 6 months after starting chemotherapy.

present with a skin lesion in reaction since a previously quiescent lesion has become active and visible. The peak time for reactions in the first 2 months after starting treatment and in the puerperium. Late reactions may occur years after finishing multidrug treatment. Some patient experience repeated reactions (Fig. 7.6.27.15).

Type 2 (ENL reactions)

These occur in lepromatous and borderline lepromatous patients. Up to 50% of lepromatous patients will experience ENL reactions and 5 to 10% of borderline lepromatous patients. Attacks are acute and may recur over several years. ENL manifests most commonly as painful red nodules on the face (Fig. 7.6.27.16) and extensor surfaces of limbs (Fig. 7.6.27.17). The lesions may be superficial or deep, with suppuration or brawny induration when chronic. Acute lesions crop and desquamate, fading over several days (Fig. 7.6.27.12). ENL is a systemic disorder producing fever and malaise and may be accompanied by uveitis, dactylitis (Fig. 7.6.27.18), arthritis, neuritis, lymphadenitis, and orchitis. ENL is often not recognized as a complication of leprosy outside endemic areas.

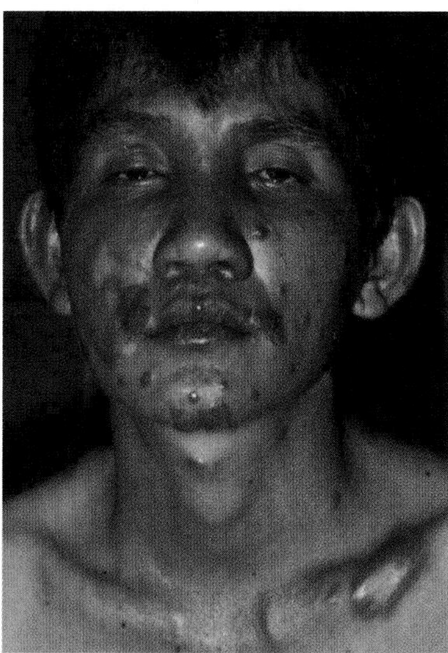

Fig. 7.6.27.16 Erythema nodosum leprosum (ENL) on the forehead of a patient with early lepromatous leprosy. The papules (and nodules) are firm and tender, with rather indefinite edges. In dark-skinned patients the ENL lesions are often easier to feel than to see, especially over the extensor surfaces of the arms and thighs.
(Copyright D.A. Warrell.)

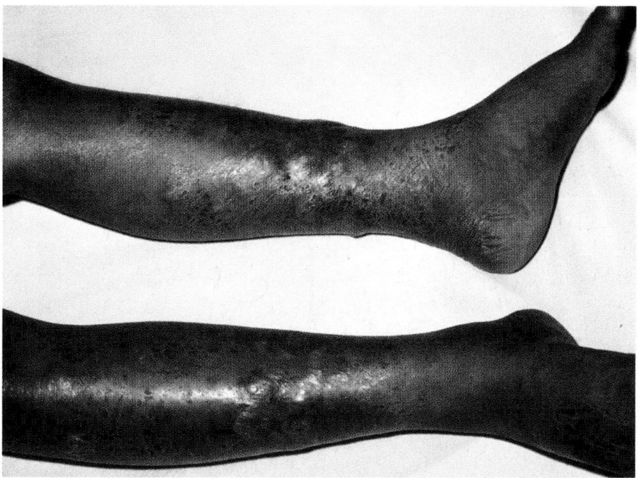

Fig. 7.6.27.17 Erythema nodosum leprosum (ENL) of the shins.
(Copyright D.A. Warrell.)

Neuritis

Silent neuropathy is an important form of nerve damage and presents as a functional neural deficit without a manifest acute or subacute neuritis (Figs. 7.6.27.2, 7.6.27.3, 7.6.27.19, and 7.6.27.20). An Indian study following a cohort of 2608 patients found that 75% of those developing deformity had no history of reactions. In Ethiopian and Bangladeshi cohort studies, silent neuritis accounted for most neuritis. This emphasizes the importance of regular nerve function testing so that new deficits can be detected.

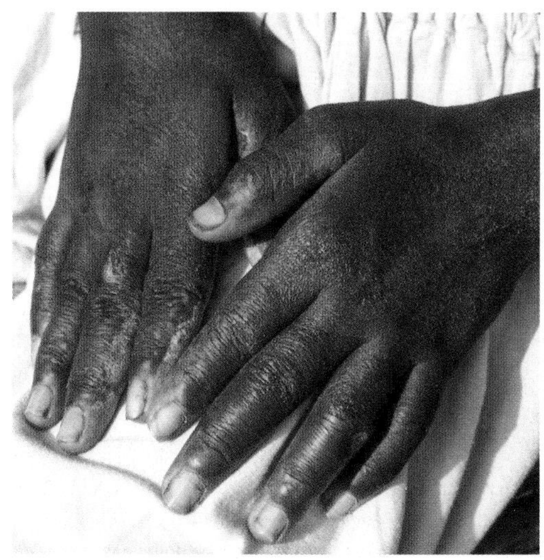

Fig. 7.6.27.18 Dactylitisas part of an ENL reaction.
(Copyright D.A. Warrell.)

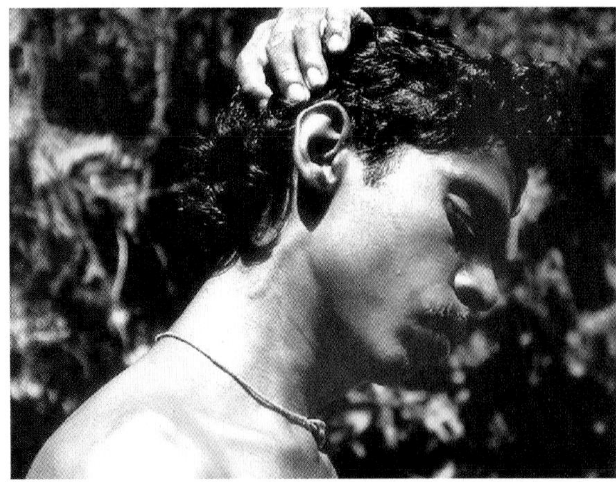

Fig. 7.6.27.19 Peripheral nerve thickening in leprosy. This young man had marked thickening of his great auricular nerve.

Diagnosis

The diagnosis is made on the clinical findings of one or more of the cardinal signs of leprosy and supported by the finding of acid-fast bacilli on slit skin smears. The whole body should be inspected in a good light otherwise lesions may be missed, particularly on the buttocks. Skin lesions should be tested for anaesthesia to light touch, pin prick, and temperature. The peripheral nerves should be palpated systematically examining for thickening and tenderness and peripheral nerve function should be assessed. Histological examination of a biopsy taken from the active edge of a lesion is helpful to support the diagnosis and confirm the classification. The pathologist should be asked to examine for neural inflammation which will differentiate leprosy from other granulomatous conditions. Serology is not usually helpful diagnostically because antibodies to the species-specific glycolipid PGL-1 are present in 90% of untreated lepromatous patients but only 40 to 50% of paucibacillary patients and 5 to 10% of healthy controls. Polymerase chain reaction for detecting *M. leprae* DNA has not proved sensitive or specific enough for routine diagnosis.

Outside leprosy endemic areas, doctors frequently fail to consider the diagnosis of leprosy. Of new patients seen from 1995 to 1999 at The Hospital for Tropical Diseases, London, diagnosis had been delayed in over 80% of cases. Patients had been misdiagnosed by dermatologists, neurologists, orthopaedic surgeons, and rheumatologists. A common problem was failure to consider leprosy as a cause of peripheral neuropathy in patients from leprosy endemic countries. These delays had serious consequences for patients; over one-half of them had nerve damage and disability.

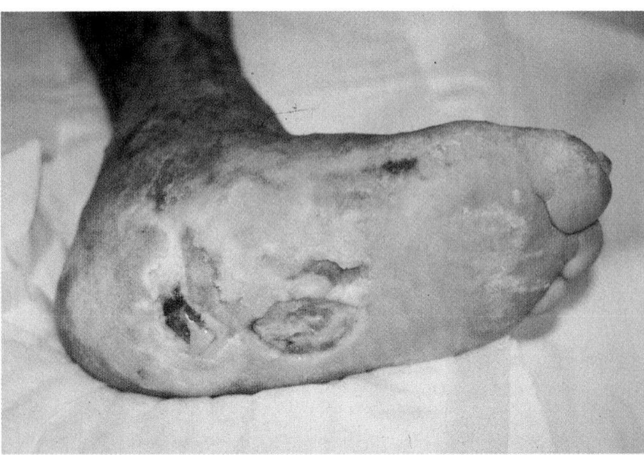

Fig. 7.6.27.20 This foot shows thick, dry cracked skin together with neuropathic damage in an anaesthetic foot. The toes are clawed, the foot arch has collapsed and there is evidence of a Charcot ankle joint.

Slit skin smears

The bacterial load is assessed by making a small incision through the epidermis, scraping dermal material, and smearing evenly onto a glass slide. At least four sites should be sampled (earlobes and edges of active lesions). The smears are then stained and acid-fast bacilli are counted. Scoring is done on a logarithmic scale per high-power field. A score of 1+ indicates 1 to 10 bacilli in 100 fields, 6+ over 1000 per field. Smears are useful for confirming the diagnosis and should be done annually to monitor response to treatment.

Differential diagnosis

Doctors should be aware of the normal range of skin colour and texture in their local population, and also of the common endemic skin diseases, such as onchocerciasis, that may coexist or mimic leprosy.

Skin

The variety of leprosy skin lesions means that a potentially wide range of skin conditions are in the differential diagnosis. At the tuberculoid end of the spectrum, anaesthesia differentiates leprosy from fungal infections, vitiligo, and eczema. At the lepromatous end the presence of acid-fast bacilli in smears differentiates leprosy nodules from onchocerciasis, Kaposi's sarcoma, and post-kala-azar dermal leishmaniasis (Fig. 7.6.27.21).

Nerves

Peripheral nerve thickening is rarely seen except in leprosy. Hereditary sensory motor neuropathy type III is associated with palpable peripheral nerve hypertrophy. Amyloidosis, which can

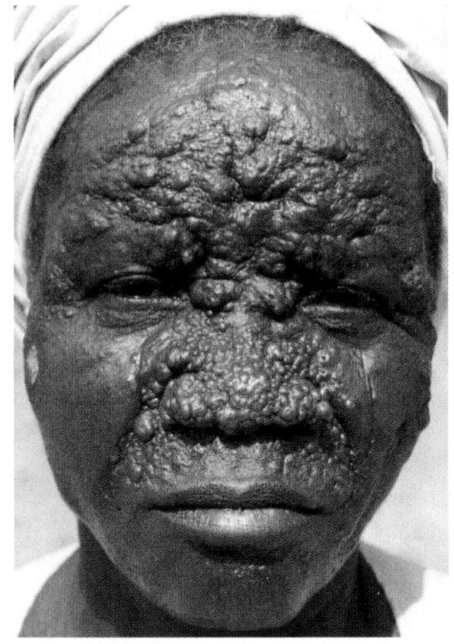

Fig. 7.6.27.21 African woman with facial epidermoid cysts superficially resembling lepromatous leprosy.
(Copyright D.A. Warrell.)

also complicate leprosy, causes thickening of peripheral nerves. Charcot–Marie–Tooth disease is an inherited neuropathy that causes distal atrophy and weakness. The causes of other polyneuropathies such as HIV, diabetes, alcoholism, vasculitides, and heavy metal poisoning should all be considered where appropriate.

Treatment

There are six main principles of treatment:

1 Stop the infection with chemotherapy.

2 Treat new nerve damage.

3 Treat reactions.

4 Educate the patient about leprosy.

5 Prevent disability.

6 Support the patient socially and psychologically.

These objectives need the patient's cooperation and confidence and can be achieved through the leprosy outpatient clinic with appropriate support and patient education. On the first visit there should be a careful assessment of skin and mucosal involvement and accurate evaluation of nerve and eye function. Each patient should be classified using the Ridley–Jopling classification and assessed for evidence of a reaction of new nerve damage.

Chemotherapy

All patients with leprosy should be given an appropriate multidrug combination. The first-line antileprosy drugs are rifampicin, clofazimine, and dapsone. The drug combination and duration are determined by the classification of the patient. The WHO has recommended a simple classification for use in the field determined only by the number of skin lesions. Patients are classified as paucibacillary if they have up to five skin lesions and as multibacillary if they have six or more skin lesions. In the specialist clinic setting, where skin smears and skin biopsies can be combined with clinical data, patients can be classified into paucibacillary (skin smear-negative TT and BT) and multibacillary (skin smear-positive BT, all BB, BL, and LL). Table 7.6.27.2 gives the drug combinations, doses, and duration of treatment. Patients with multibacillary disease and an initial bacterial index greater than 4 will need longer treatment, and the duration should be guided by their clinical status and bacterial index.

Rifampicin is a potent bactericide for *M. leprae*. Four days after a single 600-mg dose, bacilli from a previously untreated patient with multibacillary disease were no longer viable in a mouse footpad test. It acts by inhibiting DNA-dependent RNA polymerase. Because *M. leprae* can develop resistance to rifampicin as a one-step process,

Table 7.6.27.2 WHO recommended multidrug therapy regimens

Type of leprosy[a]	Drug treatment		
	Monthly supervised	Daily self-administered	Duration of treatment
Paucibacillary	Rifampicin 600 mg	Dapsone 100 mg	6 months
Multibacillary	Rifampicin 600 mg	Clofazimine 50 mg	12 months
	Clofazimine 300 mg	Dapsone 100 mg	

[a] WHO classification for field use when slit skin smears are not available: paucibacillary—up to five skin lesions; multibacillary—more than six skin lesions.

this drug should always be given in combination with other antileprotics.

Dapsone (DDS, 4,4-diaminodiphenylsulphone) is weakly bactericidal. Oral absorption is good and it has a long half-life, averaging 28 h. It commonly causes mild haemolysis, but rarely anaemia. Glucose-6-phosphate dehydrogenase deficiency is seldom a problem. The 'DDS syndrome', which is occasionally seen in leprosy, begins 6 weeks after starting dapsone and manifests as exfoliative dermatitis associated with lymphadenopathy, hepatosplenomegaly, fever, and hepatitis.

Clofazimine is a red fat-soluble crystalline dye. The mechanism of its weakly bactericidal action against *M. leprae* remains unknown. The most troublesome side effect is skin discoloration, ranging from red to purple-black, the degree depending on the drug dose and extent of leprous infiltration (Fig. 7.6.27.22(a) and (b)). The pigmentation usually fades within 6 to 12 months of stopping clofazimine, although traces of discoloration may remain for up to 4 years. Urine, sputum, and sweat may become pink. Clofazimine also produces a characteristic ichthyosis on the shins and forearms.

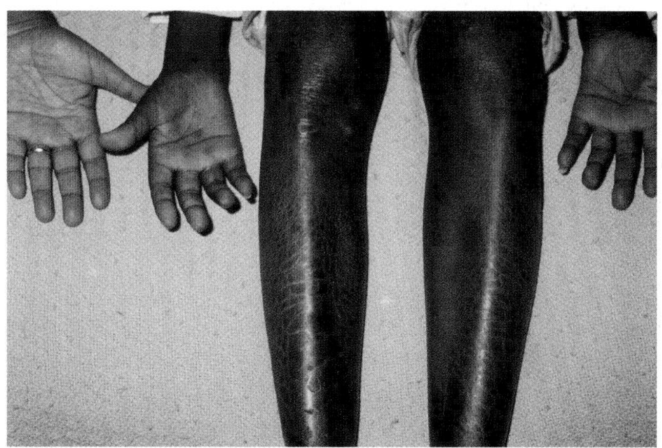

(a)

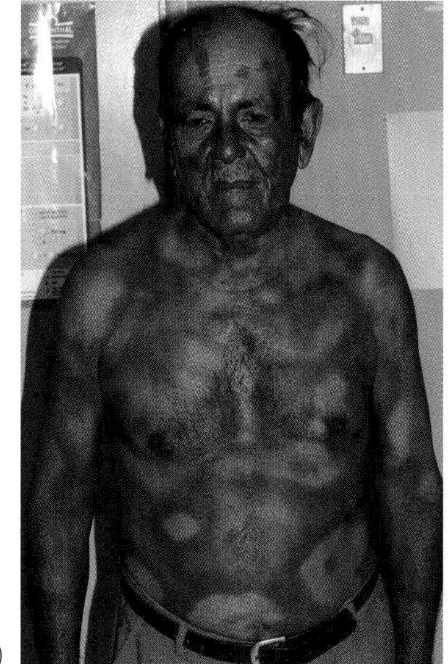

(b)

Fig. 7.6.27.22 Clofazamine pigmentation in Ethiopian (a) and Peruvian (b) patients.
(Copyright D.A. Warrell.)

Other drugs bactericidal for *M. leprae* include the fluoroquinolones pefloxacin and ofloxacin, minocycline, and clarithromycin. These agents are now established second-line drugs. Minocycline causes a black pigmentation of skin lesions and so may not be an appropriate substitute for clofazimine if pigmentation is to be avoided.

A single-dose triple-drug combination (rifampicin, ofloxacin, and minocycline) has been tested in India for patients with single skin lesions and improved 98% of patients. This regimen can also be used in patients who experience adverse effects of dapsone or clofazimine, even in patients with a high BI. Although the study had major flaws and single-dose treatment is less effective than the conventional 6-month treatment for paucibacillary leprosy, it is an operationally attractive field regimen or for use in patients with migrant lifestyles.

The principal outcome of treatment is improvement of skin lesions; nerve damage may also improve but to a lesser extent. At the end of a 6-month treatment of borderline disease there may still be signs of inflammation, which should not be mistaken for active infection. Relapse is uncommon with a cumulative relapse rate of 1.07% for paucibacillary leprosy and 0.77% for multibacillary leprosy at 9 years after completion of multidrug therapy. *M. leprae* is such a slow-growing organism that relapse only occurs after many years. *M. leprae* isolates from relapsed patients who have received multidrug therapy are fully drug sensitive and patients can be retreated with the same regimen. The distinction between relapse and reaction may be difficult.

Since the introduction of multidrug therapy more than 14 million patients have been treated successfully. Clinical improvement has been rapid and toxicity rare. Monthly supervision of the rifampicin component has been crucial to success. Other benefits are reduced deformity rates and increased compliance in control schemes. Reactions may develop months or years after stopping chemotherapy, especially in patients with borderline lepromatous or lepromatous leprosy. It is therefore vital when discharging patients to warn them to return should new symptoms appear, especially in hands, feet, or eyes. Patients with reactions or physical or psychological complications will need long-term care.

Treatment of new nerve damage

Patients with nerve damage present for less than 6 months (assessed by patient history or testing) should receive a 6-month course of steroids starting at a dose of 40 mg prednisolone per day. A randomized controlled trial has shown that nerve damage present for more than 6 months is not improved by steroid treatment.

Management of reactions

Awareness of the early symptoms of reversal reactions by both patient and physician is important because, if left untreated, severe nerve damage may develop. The peak time for reversal reactions is in the first 2 months of treatment. Patients should be warned about reactions because the sudden appearance of reactional lesions after starting treatment is distressing and undermines confidence. The treatment of reactions is aimed at controlling acute inflammation, easing pain, reversing nerve and eye damage, and reassuring the patient. Multidrug therapy should be continued.

Type 1 (reversal) reactions

Simple anti-inflammatory drugs are rarely sufficient to control symptoms. If there is any evidence of neuritis (nerve tenderness, new anaesthesia, and/or motor loss), corticosteroid treatment should be started. Prednisolone should be given, starting at 40 to 60 mg/day, reducing to 40 mg after a few days, and then by 5 mg every 2 to 4 weeks. Patients with borderline tuberculoid leprosy in reaction commonly need 4 months of steroids while borderline lepromatous reactions may need 6 months or more.

Type 2 (ENL) reactions

This is a difficult condition to treat and frequently requires treatment with high-dose steroids (80 mg/day, tapered down rapidly) or thalidomide. Since ENL frequently recurs, steroid dependency can easily develop. Thalidomide (400 mg/day) is superior to steroids in controlling ENL and is the drug of choice for young men with severe ENL (Fig. 7.6.27.16). Women with severe ENL may benefit from thalidomide treatment. This is a difficult decision for the woman and her physician and needs careful discussion of the benefits and risks (phocomelia when thalidomide is taken in the first trimester). Women should use double contraception and report immediately if menstruation is delayed. Unfortunately, the problems with thalidomide mean that it is unavailable in several leprosy endemic countries despite its undoubted value. Clofazimine has a useful anti-inflammatory effect in ENL but takes 6 weeks to become effective and can be used at 300 mg/day for several months. Low-grade chronic erythema nodosum with iritis or neuritis will require long-term suppression, preferably with thalidomide or clofazimine. Acute iridocyclitis is treated with 1% hydrocortisone eye drops given 4 hourly and 1% atropine drops twice daily.

Neuritis

Silent neuritis should be treated similarly to reversal reactions with prednisolone at a dose of 40 mg/day which should be reduced slowly over a period of months.

Education of patients

Stigmatization due to leprosy occurs worldwide. Patients are frightened of social ostracization, physical rejection, and the development of deformities. It is often useful to ask them about their fears so that these can be addressed. They should be reassured that having started treatment they are not infectious to family or friends and can have a sex life. The importance of compliance with antibiotic therapy needs to be emphasized. The patient needs a careful explanation of the diagnosis, aetiology, and prognosis.

Prevention of disability

The morbidity and disability associated with leprosy is secondary to nerve damage. A major goal in prevention of disability is to create patient self-awareness so that damage is minimized. Monitoring sensation and muscle power in patient's hands, feet, and eyes should be part of the routine follow-up so that new nerve damage is detected early. The patient with an anaesthetized hand or foot needs to understand the importance of daily self-care, especially protection when doing potentially dangerous tasks and inspection for trauma. It is helpful to identify for each patient potentially dangerous situations, such as cooking, car repairs, or smoking. Soaking dry hands and feet followed by rubbing with oil keeps the skin moist and supple.

An anaesthetized foot needs the protection of an appropriate shoe. For anaesthesia alone, a well-fitting 'trainer' with firm soles and shock-absorbing inners will provide adequate protection. Once there is deformity, such as clawing, shoes must be made specially to ensure protection of pressure points and even weight distribution.

The patient should be taught to question the cause of an injury so that the risk can be avoided in the future. Plantar ulceration occurs secondary to increased pressure over bony prominences. Ulceration is treated by rest. Unlike ulcers in the feet of patients with diabetes or ischaemia, ulcers in leprosy heal if they are protected from weight-bearing. No weight-bearing is permitted until the ulcer has healed. Appropriate footwear should be provided to prevent recurrence.

Physiotherapy exercises should be taught to maximize function of weak muscles and prevent contracture. Contractures of hands and feet, foot drop, lagophthalmos, entropion, and ectropion are amenable to surgery.

Social, psychological, and economic rehabilitation

The social and cultural background of the patient determine the nature of many of the problems that may be encountered. The patient may have difficulty in coming to terms with leprosy. The community may reject the patient. Education, gainful employment, confidence from family, friends, and doctor, and plastic surgery to correct stigmatizing deformity all have a role to play.

Prognosis

The majority of patients, especially those who have no nerve damage at the time of diagnosis, do well on multidrug treatment with resolution of skin lesions. Left untreated, borderline patients will downgrade towards the lepromatous end of the spectrum and lepromatous patients will have the consequences of bacillary invasion. Borderline patients are at risk of developing type 1 reactions, which may result in devastating nerve damage. Treatment of the neuritis is currently unsatisfactory and patients with neuritis may develop permanent nerve damage despite corticosteroid treatment. It is not possible to predict which patients will develop reactions or nerve damage. Nerve damage and its complications may be severely disabling, especially when all four limbs and both eyes are affected.

Leprosy in women

Women with leprosy are in double jeopardy; not only may they develop postpartum nerve damage but also they are at particular risk of social ostracization with rejection by spouses and family.

Pregnancy and leprosy

There is little good evidence that pregnancy causes new disease or relapse. However, there is a clear temporal association between parturition and the development of type 1 reactions and neuritis when cell-mediated immunity returns to prepregnancy levels. In an Ethiopian study, 42% of pregnancies in borderline lepromatous patients were complicated by a type 1 reaction in the postpartum period. In the same cohort, patients with lepromatous leprosy experienced ENL reactions throughout pregnancy and lactation. ENL in pregnancy is associated with early loss of nerve function compared with nonpregnant individuals. Pregnant and newly delivered women should have regular neurological examination and steroid treatment instituted for neuritis. Rifampicin, dapsone, and clofazimine are safe during pregnancy. Clofazimine crosses the placenta and babies may be born with mild clofazimine pigmentation. Reactions can be managed with the steroid regimens given above but with a more rapid reduction in dose. Women should be warned before becoming pregnant of the risk that their condition may deteriorate after delivery. Ideally pregnancies should be planned when leprosy is well controlled.

Prevention and control

Leprosy control is now becoming more integrated into general services. Different models of providing leprosy control are used depending on the local facilities. In some endemic countries largely vertical programmes are being retained; in others such as Brazil leprosy services are provided within dermatological services. Effective treatment is not merely restricted to chemotherapy but also involves good case management with effective monitoring and supervision and prevention of disabilities. Treating patients with leprosy is a long-term enterprise involving patients, their families, and health workers.

Vaccines against leprosy

The substantial cross-reactivity between bacille Calmette–Guérin (BCG) and *M. leprae* has been exploited in attempts to develop a vaccine against leprosy. Trials of BCG as a vaccine against leprosy in Uganda, New Guinea, Burma, and South India showed it to confer statistically significant but variable protection, ranging from 80% in Uganda to 20% in Burma and this protective effect has been confirmed in a meta-analysis. A case-control study in Venezuela showed BCG vaccination to give 56% protection to the household contacts of patients with leprosy. Combining BCG and killed *M. leprae* has been tried, but in both a large population-based trial in Malawi and an immunoprophylactic trial in Venezuela there was no advantage for BCG plus *M. leprae* over BCG alone.

Areas of uncertainty and controversy

The optimum duration of treatment is a controversial area. The duration of treatment for multibacillary (MB) patients was reduced from 24 months to 12 months without good evidence. However, this occurred after the definition of LL patients was broadened and in India up to 60% of LL patients are smear-negative borderline tuberculoid patients. The concern regards patients with a high initial bacterial load. Data from India show that patients with a high initial bacterial load (bacterial index >4) treated with 2 years of rifampicin, clofazimine, and dapsone had a relapse rate of 8/100 person years, whereas patients treated to smear negativity had a relapse rate of 2/100 person years. The dilemma is that since skin smears are abandoned in many programmes those patients in need of longer treatment courses cannot be identified. A new treatment, uniform multidrug treatment (U-MDT), in which all leprosy patients are given 6-months of rifampicin, dapsone, and clofazimine are taking place. The problem is that this regimen adds in clofazimine for many patients who do not need it and will probably be inadequate for the same number of lepromatous leprosy patients with high bacterial loads who also maintain the infection in the community. These arguments illustrate the difficulty in providing sound evidence for policy decisions when a decade-long wait to establish relapse rates is needed.

Areas where further research is needed

The epidemiology of leprosy still poses unanswered questions. Why are 64% of all patients with leprosy in India? Is this due to living conditions, genetic susceptibility, or particular environmental conditions in India?

Early detection of cases is vital at both an individual and a population level. It is now recognized that substantial nerve damage occurs before diagnosis. A test for early infection might help detect individual cases before nerve damage is established and before the spread of infection. Leprosy-specific peptides for skin tests have been generated and are being evaluated.

The medical management of reactions and nerve damage is currently limited to steroids. These are not effective for about 30% of patients. Trials to determine the effectiveness of established and out-of-patent immunosuppressants such as azathioprine and ciclosporin are taking place.

The WHO started the 1990s with the bold slogan of 'Eliminating leprosy as a public health problem by 2000'. This initiative galvanized leprosy control programmes worldwide, but the unique biology of *M. leprae* and its interaction with the human host rendered this target unattainable. However, there is a strong perception that leprosy has been eliminated and this has hindered research and planning. The WHO policy for 2011–2015 focuses on sustaining leprosy work. Leprosy is a bacterial disease with challenging immunological complications and will be a global and individual problem for many decades. It is unlikely to be eradicated until there is considerable improvement in general health, wealth, living conditions, and education.

Further reading

Britton WJ, Lockwood DN (2004). Leprosy. *Lancet*, **363**, 1209–19.

Fine PE (2007). Leprosy: what is being 'eliminated'? *Bull World Health Organ*, **85**, 2.

International Federation of Anti-Leprosy Associations (ILEP) (n.d.). *Working for a world without leprosy*. www.ilep.org.uk

Monot M, *et al.* (2005). On the origin of leprosy. *Science*, **308**, 1040–2.

Setia MS, *et al.* (2006). The role of BCG in prevention of leprosy: a meta-analysis. *Lancet Infect Dis*, **6**, 162–70.

Ustianowski AP, *et al.* (2006). Interactions between HIV infection and leprosy: a paradox. *Lancet Infect Dis*, **6**, 350–60.

Van Brakel WH, *et al.* (2005). The INFIR Cohort Study: assessment of sensory and motor neuropathy in leprosy at baseline. *Lepr Rev*, **76**, 277–95.

World Health Organisation (2006). *Global strategy for further reducing the leprosy burden and sustaining leprosy control activities 2006–2010*. World Health Organization, Geneva.

7.6.28 Buruli ulcer: *Mycobacterium ulcerans* infection

Wayne M. Meyers and Françoise Portaels

Essentials

Buruli ulcer is caused by *Mycobacterium ulcerans*, which secretes a cytotoxic and immunosuppressive toxin, mycolactone. It is a necrotizing disease of skin, subcutaneous tissue, and bone that is re-emerging as a potentially disabling affliction of inhabitants of tropical wetlands. Major foci are in West and Central Africa, but there are minor endemic foci in Australia, Mexico, South America, and South-East Asia. It is not contagious: environmental sources include water, vegetation, and insects, with humans probably becoming infected by traumatic introduction of the bacillus into the skin from the overlying *M. ulcerans*-contaminated surface in most instances. Clinical presentation may be as a cutaneous nodule, undermined ulcer, plaque or widely disseminated oedematous lesion. Clinical diagnosis is often accurate, but smears for AFB and PCR, culture and histopathology are confirmatory. Treatment is usually by wide surgical excision and skin grafting, but antibiotics (rifampicin with streptomycin) are often effective.

Introduction

Buruli ulcer is an indolent necrotizing infection of the skin, subcutaneous tissue, and bone caused by *Mycobacterium ulcerans*. After tuberculosis and leprosy, Buruli ulcer is the third most common mycobacterial disease and is recognized by the World Health Organization as a re-emerging infection.

In 1962 Clancey and Dodge described many patients from Buruli County, Uganda, with cutaneous ulcers reminiscent of those Cook described in 1897 from the same area, and named the disease Buruli ulcer.

Aetiology

MacCallum and colleagues first isolated the causative agent in 1948 from patients in Australia. *M. ulcerans*, a slow-growing acid-fast bacillus (AFB), grows optimally at 32° C and elaborates mycolactone, a cytotoxic and immunosuppressive polyketide assembled by plasmid-encoded synthases of the aetiological agent. This toxin is the primary virulence factor of *M. ulcerans*. Data from 16S rRNA sequences define four major groups of *M. ulcerans*: African, American, Asian, and Australian strains. Phenolic mycosides of *M. ulcerans* and *Mycobacterium marinum* are identical and the 16S rRNA genes differ only slightly.

Epidemiology and transmission

All endemic foci of Buruli ulcer are near rural freshwater wetlands, especially ponds and swamps. All known foci except those in southern Australia and northern Asia are tropical. Major endemic areas are Benin, Cameroon, Democratic Republic of Congo, Gabon, Ghana,

Ivory Coast, Uganda, and adjacent countries. There are minor foci in South and Central America and south-east and northern Asia.

Documented environmental sources of *M. ulcerans* include irrigation systems and waterbugs dwelling in aquatic plant roots in swamps. In Australia, koalas, possums, and imported alpaca acquire the infection naturally. Cultivation of *M. ulcerans* from the environment was first reported in 2008.

Outbreaks of disease often follow environmental changes that promote flooding or alter water courses, such as deforestation or construction of dams and irrigation systems. Increased farming activities near wetlands and global climatic changes may contribute to the rapid re-emergence of Buruli ulcer. Approximately 75% of new patients are children who often play semi-naked in swamps.

We believe humans become infected by traumatic introduction of the bacillus into the skin from the overlying *M. ulcerans*-contaminated surface. The trauma may be slight (hypodermic injection) or severe (land mine wound or snake bite). Biting insects (e.g. waterbugs) may serve as vectors. Aerosols arising from ponds and swamp surfaces may disseminate *M. ulcerans*. Patient-to-patient transmission is rare.

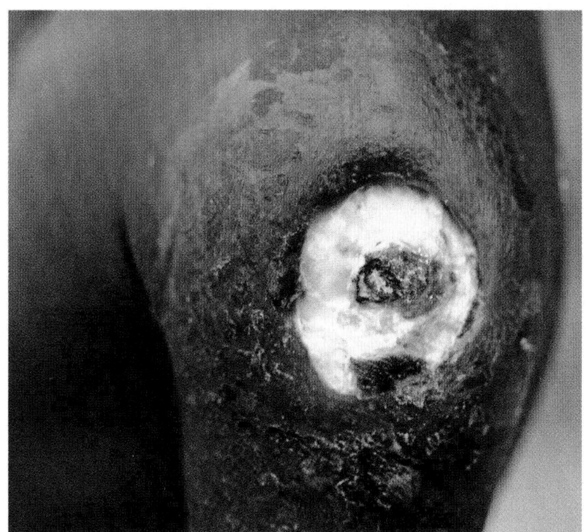

Fig. 7.6.28.1 Buruli ulcer on the left deltoid area in a 12-year-old Congolese boy who had received a hypodermic injection at this site 3 months previously. Note central necrotic slough in the base of the ulcer and undermined edges.

Pathogenesis

Predisposing host factors are poorly understood. Putatively, severity and course of infection are related to pathogen virulence, mode of infection, inoculum size, and immunological response of the host. A Th1 response tends to localize and heal infections while a Th2 type promotes dissemination. Once introduced, the small amount of mycolactone produced by inoculated *M. ulcerans* causes tissue necrosis and apoptosis, and suppresses local immune responses, ensuring survival of the bacillus in niduses of nutrient necrotic tissue. Mycolactone targets subcutaneous fat cells, permitting necrosis to spread just superficial to fascial planes. *M. ulcerans* invades lymphatic and probably blood vessels, causing metastatic spread of the mycobacterium.

Clinical features

Except for those with massive lesions, patients are usually surprisingly well without systemic symptoms or abnormal laboratory findings. Meyers and Portaels published a schema for the natural history and inter-relationships of the forms of Buruli ulcer disease (see Meyers and Portaels 2006). Buruli ulcer may be localized or disseminated.

Localized disease

Typically, the initial cutaneous lesion is a single firm painless non-tender movable subcutaneous nodule up to 3 cm in diameter. Limbs are preferred sites, often around joints. The natural history of the disease is markedly variable, but nodules usually ulcerate within 1 to 3 months of inoculation. A whitish necrotic slough develops in the ulcer base with induration and hyperpigmentation of surrounding skin. Ulcer borders are undermined, sometimes extending widely (major ulcerative disease) (Fig. 7.6.28.1). Some small (1–2 cm in diameter) ulcerated lesions with shallow undermining self-heal (minor ulcerative disease). Without treatment, major ulcerative lesions tend to become inactive, after months or years, and heal by scarring. Scars are depressed and stellate, often causing disfiguring and crippling cicatricial contractures.

Disseminated disease

Disseminated disease may develop from nodules, arise from localized major ulcerative lesions, or disseminate directly and rapidly from site of inoculation, causing indurated plaques covering even an entire limb or vast areas of the trunk. Without treatment, such lesions will eventually slough, leaving a large ulcer with continuing extension of disease at the borders. Eyes, breasts, and genitalia may be damaged or destroyed.

While metastatic spread may arise from localized disease, patients with the highly bacilliferous disseminated disease are most prone to metastatic lesions. Spread may be to distant skin sites or bone, especially bones of the limbs. *M. ulcerans* osteomyelitis develops in approximately 10% of patients and often leads to amputations or other disabilities.

Differential clinical diagnosis

Diagnosis of nodular disease is often perplexing. Differential diagnoses include bacterial, mycotic, and parasitic infections, inflammatory lesions, and tumours. Ulcers resembling Buruli ulcer include tropical phagedenic ulcer (malodorous and not undermined), venous stasis ulcer (not undermined), and venomous snake bite or spider bite (history helpful).

Pathology

Optimal biopsy specimens contain the necrotic base of ulcers and undermined edge of lesions including subcutaneous tissue and fascia. Histopathological sections reveal a contiguous coagulation necrosis (noncaseating) of the deep dermis, panniculus, and fascia. Vasculitis and mineralization are common. Clumps of extracellular acid-fast bacilli are most plentiful in the base of the ulcer; however, intracellular *M. ulcerans* may be seen in inflammatory cells at the edge of necrotic foci. Necrosis extends well beyond the location of bacilli. Local and regional lymph nodes are often invaded and sometimes necrotic. In bone, the marrow is necrotic and contains acid-fast bacilli, and trabeculae are eroded. These features are distinct from those of osteomyelitis of all other known aetiologies.

Development of delayed-type hypersensitivity granulomas heralds healing by fibrosis.

Laboratory diagnosis

Smears stained by the Ziehl-Neelsen method from the ulcer base frequently reveal acid-fast bacilli in clumps. Cultures for *M. ulcerans* are often positive. Polymerase chain reaction provides specific identification of *M. ulcerans*. Histopathological changes are characteristic.

Treatment

The recommended treatment is wide surgical excision followed by skin grafting. Heating the lesion at 40°C is a useful adjunct. Antimycobacterial therapy (rifampicin plus streptomycin) without surgery heals most nodular and minor ulcerative disease, and some advanced lesions; however, controlled trials are needed to establish efficacy. Physiotherapy is essential to prevent contracture deformities.

Prevention and control

Bacille Calmette-Guérin (BCG) vaccination provides short-lived protection. Practical control measures for inhabitants of endemic areas are usually ineffectual; however, use of a protected water supply is important. Tourists can avoid the wetlands in endemic countries.

Socioeconomic impact

Patients are often stigmatized and disabled, and require welfare services for life (services are often locally limited or unavailable). They also require protracted hospital stays, taxing overburdened services.

Further reading

Chauty A, *et al.* (2007). Promising clinical efficacy of streptomycin-rifampicin combination for treatment of Buruli ulcer (*Mycobacterium ulcerans* disease). *Antimicrob Agents Chemother*, **51**, 4029–35. [First extensive trial (224 patients) of antibiotic therapy of Buruli ulcer in West Africa.]

Kiszewski AE, *et al.* (2006). The local immune response in ulcerative lesions of Buruli disease. *Clin Exp Immunol*, **143**, 445–51. [Delineates host response at tissue level.]

Meyers WM (1995). Mycobacterial infections of the skin. In: Doerr W, Seifert G (eds) *Tropical pathology*, pp. 291–377. Springer, Berlin. [Extensive coverage of the clinical and pathological features of Buruli ulcer.]

Meyers WM, Walsh DS (2009). Leprosy and Buruli ulcer: the major cutaneous mycobacterioses. In: Feigin R, Cherry J, Demmler-Harrison G, Kaplan S (eds) *Textbook of Pediatric Infectious Diseases*, 6th edition, vol. 1, pp. 1479–504, Saunders Elsevier, Philadelphia. [Extensive update including classification of Buruli ulcer.]

Portaels F, *et al.* (2008). First cultivation and characterization of *Mycobacterium ulcerans* from the environment. *PLoS Negl Trop Dis*, **2**, e178. [Cultivation and characterization of aetiological agent, in detail.]

Schunk M, *et al.* (2009). Outcome of patients with Buruli ulcer after surgical treatment with or without antimycobacterial treatment in Ghana. *Am J Trop Med Hyg*, **81**, 75–81. [Evaluation of surgical and antibiotic therapy.]

Silva M, *et al.* (2009). Pathogenetic mechanisms of the intracellular parasite Mycobacterium ulcerans leading to Buruli ulcer. *Lancet Infect Dis*, **9**, 699–710. [Comprehensive review of pathogenesis.]

Walsh DS, *et al.* (2009). Buruli ulcer (*Mycobacterium ulcerans* infection): a re-emerging disease. *Clin Microbiol Newsletter*, **31**, 119-28. [Updated comprehensive review.]

7.6.29 Actinomycoses

K.P. Schaal

Essentials

Human actinomycoses are always synergistic polymicrobial infections in which fermentative actinomycetes—predominantly *Actinomyces israelii, A. gerencseriae*, or *Propionibacterium propionicum*—are the principal pathogens, usually needing the assistance of so-called concomitant microbes to produce disease. Nearly all of the members of the mixed actinomycotic microflora belong to the indigenous microbial community of human mucous membranes, hence actinomycoses present as sporadic endogenous infections which are not transmissible.

Clinical features—the initial actinomycotic lesion usually develops in tissue adjacent to a mucous membrane as a subacute to chronic process that is granulomatous as well as suppurative, typically giving rise to multiple abscesses and draining sinus tracts that are preferentially located in the cervicofacial region, thorax or abdomen. These characteristically progress slowly, penetrate tissues without regard to natural organ borders, and spread haematogenously, with symptoms remitting and exacerbating with and without antimicrobial treatment.

Diagnosis—this can be difficult as clinical symptoms, radiographic, or histopathological signs, and the results of serological tests may all be misleading. The finding of so-called sulphur granules is pathognomonic: these are macroscopically visible, yellowish or reddish to brownish particles that exhibit a cauliflower-like appearance under the microscope at low magnifications, and which may be found as free structures in pus or embedded in affected tissue. Reliable diagnosis chiefly rests on bacteriological culture.

Treatment and prognosis—antibacterial drugs used for treatment should be active against both the causative actinomycetes and all concomitant bacteria. For cervicofacial actinomycoses, the rare cutaneous processes, and most thoracic forms of the disease, this requirement is best fulfilled by amoxicillin plus clavulanic acid in medium to high doses: abdominal cases and the presence of unusually resistant concomitant bacteria may require the addition of further antimicrobials (e.g. an aminoglycoside plus either metronidazole or clindamycin). The prognosis of cervicofacial and cutaneous actinomycoses is good provided that treatment is adequate; thoracic and abdominal forms are more serious, with grave prognosis without proper treatment.

Definition

Actinomycoses are sporadically occurring endogenous polymicrobial inflammatory processes in which fermentative (facultatively anaerobic or capnophilic) actinomycetes of the genera *Actinomyces* and *Propionibacterium*, but rarely also *Bifidobacterium*, may act as the principal pathogens. Clinically, the subacute to chronic, granulomatous as well as suppurative disease tends to progress slowly and usually gives rise to multiple abscesses and draining sinus tracts. Because the term 'actinomycosis' denotes a polyaetiological inflammatory syndrome rather than a condition attributable to a single actinomycete species, it should only be used in the plural.

Aetiology of human actinomycoses

Actinomyces israelii and *A. gerencseriae* are by far the most frequent and most characteristic pathogens aetiologically involved in the human form of the disease. *A. gerencseriae* emerged from the former sero- and biovariety 2 of *A. israelii* in 1990. A third species of filamentous fermentative Gram-positive bacteria, *Propionibacterium propionicum* (formerly *Arachnia propionicum*), is a much less common cause of actinomycotic infections (Table 7.6.29.1).

Several other fermentative actinomycetes have occasionally been isolated from actinomycosis-like lesions (Table 7.6.29.1). In a given case, however, it is often difficult to decide whether these organisms are primary pathogens or merely contaminants, especially when the specimen has had contact with mucosal secretions or when two different actinomycete species have been isolated from the same specimen (Table 7.6.29.1). Nevertheless, *A. naeslundii*, *A. odontolyticus*, *A. viscosus*, *A. meyeri*, and *Bifidobacterium dentium* (formerly *Actinomyces eriksonii*) have all been reported to be capable of producing human infections clinically identical to those caused by *A. israelii*, *A. gerencseriae*, or *P. propionicum*, while *A. bovis*, the classic agent of bovine actinomycosis, has never been recovered with certainty from human infective processes (Table 7.6.29.1). Fermentative actinomycetes previously termed *A. naeslundii* and *A. viscosus* underwent considerable taxonomic and nomenclatural changes recently (Henssge *et al.*, 2009). According to these changes, organisms now named *A. viscosus* only occur in animals, particularly in hamsters. Human isolates of the former species *A. naeslundii* and *A. viscosus* have been assigned to *A. naeslundii* sensu stricto and the new species *A. oris* and *A. johnsonii*.

Table 7.6.29.1 Fermentative actinomycetes isolated from human cervicofacial actinomycotic lesions at the Hygiene-Institute of the University of Cologne and the Institute for Medical Microbiology and Immunology of the University of Bonn, Germany, between 1985 and 1999

Species identified	Number	Percentage of cases
One species per specimen:		
A. israelii	421	55.3
A. gerencseriae	111	14.6
A. naeslundii/A. oris/A johnsonii	122	16.0
A. odontolyticus	19	2.5
A. meyeri	5	0.7
A. georgiae	1	0.1
A. neuii subsp. neuii	1	0.1
P. propionicum	7	0.9
Bifidobacterium dentium	3	0.4
Corynebacterium matruchotii	12	1.6
Rothia dentocariosa	5	0.7
Not identified to species level	54	7.1
Two species per specimen:		
A. israelii + A. naeslundii/A. oris/A johnsonii	11	0.8
A. israelii + A. meyeri	2	0.1
A. israelii + A. odontolyticus	1	0.1
A. israelii + P. propionicum	2	0.1
P. propionicum + A. naeslundii/A. oris/A johnsonii	2	0.1
P. propionicum + A. neuii	1	0.1
Total number of isolates	761	100.0

Modified from Pulverer G, Schütt-Gerowitt H, Schaal KP (2003). Human cervicofacial actinomycoses: microbiological data of 1997 cases. *Clin Infect Dis*, **37**, 490–7.

Pathogenesis and pathology

Most of the fermentative actinomycetes pathogenic to humans are found regularly and abundantly in the mouths of healthy adults. However, these microbes occur only sporadically or in low numbers in the digestive, respiratory, and genital tracts, as well as in the mouths of babies before teething and of adults without any natural teeth or tooth implants. Therefore, these actinomycetes may be considered facultatively pathogenic commensals of the human mucous membranes, which, apart from the very rare actinomycotic wound infections following human bite or fist fight traumata, produce disease exclusively as endogenous pathogens.

For active invasion of the tissue, the classic pathogenic fermentative actinomycetes apparently require a negative redox potential, which may result either from insufficient blood supply (caused by circulatory or vascular diseases, crush injuries, or foreign bodies) or from the reducing and necrotizing capacity of other microbes in the lesion. Defective functions of the immune system do not specifically predispose to actinomycotic infections.

Synergistic polymicrobial infection

True actinomycoses are essentially always synergistic mixed infections, in which the actinomycetes act as the specific component, the so-called guiding organisms that decide on the characteristic course and the late symptoms of the disease. The so-called concomitant microbes (Table 7.6.29.2), which may vary considerably in composition (about 100 aerobic and anaerobic species) and number (up to 10 per case) of species from case to case, are often responsible for the clinical picture at the beginning of the infection and for certain complications; they are also part of the resident or transient surface microflora of the mucous membranes of humans.

Particularly pronounced synergistic interactions appear to exist between pathogenic fermentative actinomycetes, especially *Actinomyces israelii* and *A. gerencseriae*, and *Actinobacillus actinomycetemcomitans*, which has recently been reclassified as *Aggregatibacter actinomycetemcomitans*. The latter organism, the species designation of which refers to its characteristic association with actinomycetes (Latin *actinomycetem comitans* = accompanying an actinomycete), may even sustain the inflammatory process under similar clinical symptoms after chemotherapeutic elimination of the causative actinomycete.

Histopathology

Initially an inflammatory granulation tissue develops, which usually breaks down to form either an acute abscess or chronic multiple abscesses with proliferation of connective tissue. The pathognomonic sulphur granules are formed primarily in the infected tissue, but may also appear as free structures in abscess content or sinus discharge. They are then of the highest diagnostic importance.

Sulphur granules, which were originally designated *Drusen* in Harz's first description of *Actinomyces bovis* in 1877, are

Table 7.6.29.2 Concomitant actinomycotic flora isolated from cervicofacial actinomycotic lesions at the Hygiene- Institute of the University of Cologne and the Institute for Medical Microbiology and Immunology of the University of Bonn, Germany, between 1972 and 1999

Species/group identified	Number	Percentage of cases
Aerobically growing organisms		
Coagulase-negative staphylococci	781	39.1
Staphylococcus aureus	99	5.0
α-Haemolytic streptococci	206	10.3
β-Haemolytic streptococci	85	4.3
Other aerobically growing bacteria	104	5.2
Candida spp.	22	1.1
No aerobic growth	943	47.2
Anaerobes and capnophils		
Aggregatibacter (Actinobacillus) actinomycetemcomitans	283	14.2
'Microaerophilic' and anaerobic streptococci	992	49.7
Bacteroides ureolyticus/Campylobacter gracilis/Capnocytophaga spp./*Eikenella corrodens*	370	18.5
Black-pigmented Bacteroidaceae	501	25.1
Other *Bacteroides* spp. and *Prevotella* spp.	419	21.0
Fusobacterium spp.	753	37.7
Leptotrichia buccalis	160	8.0
Propionibacterium spp.[a]	549	27.5
Other anaerobic bacteria	72	3.6
Total number of cases examined	1997	100.0

[a] Other than *P. propionicum*.

Modified from Pulverer G, Schütt-Gerowitt H, Schaal KP (2003). Human cervicofacial actinomycoses: microbiological data of 1997 cases. *Clin Infect Dis*, **37**, 490–7.

macroscopically visible (up to 1 mm in diameter) yellowish or reddish to brownish particles that exhibit a cauliflower-like appearance under the microscope at low magnifications. They consist of a conglomerate of filamentous actinomycete microcolonies formed *in vivo* and surrounded by tissue reaction material, especially polymorphonuclear granulocytes (Fig. 7.6.29.1). At high magnification, a Gram-stained smear of the completely crushed granule reveals the presence of clusters of Gram-positive interwoven branching filaments with radially arranged peripheral hyphae and of a variety of other Gram-positive and Gram-negative rods and cocci, which represent the concomitant flora (Fig. 7.6.29.2). A club-shaped layer of hyaline material may be seen on the tips of peripheral filaments, which can aid in the differentiation of actinomycotic sulphur granules from macroscopically similar particles of various other microbial and nonmicrobial origins.

Clinical manifestations

The primary actinomycotic lesion usually develops in tissue adjacent to a mucous membrane at sites such as the cervicofacial, thoracic, and abdominal areas. The infection tends to progress slowly and to penetrate without regard to natural organ borders, or to spread haematogenously even to distant sites. Remission and exacerbation of symptoms with and without antimicrobial treatment is characteristic. As in other endogenous microbial diseases, the incubation period of actinomycoses is not defined.

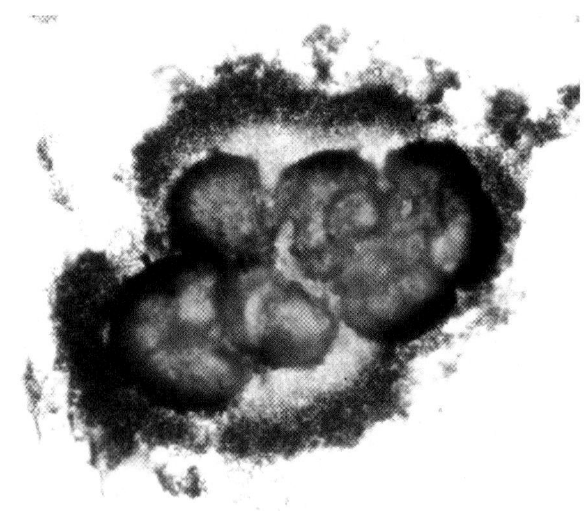

Fig. 7.6.29.1 Actinomycotic sulphur granule. Particle embedded in 1% methylene blue solution, after gently pressing on the coverslip (original diameter 0.8 mm). Note the spherical segment-like structures which represent actinomycete colonies formed *in vivo* and which are coloured brown because the blue dye has been reduced to its leuco base in the anaerobic centre of the particle. The blue-coloured structures surrounding the colonies are polymorphonuclear granulocytes. Magnification × 60.

Cervicofacial actinomycoses

In the vast majority of cases, actinomycotic lesions primarily involve the face or neck. Conditions predisposing to these cervicofacial infections include tooth extractions, fractures of the jaw, periodontal abscesses, foreign bodies penetrating the mucosal barrier (bone splinters, fish bones, awns of cereals), or suppurating tonsillar crypts.

Initially, the cervicofacial actinomycoses present either as an acute, usually odontogenic, abscess or cellulitis of the floor of the mouth, or as a slowly developing chronic hard painless reddish or livid swelling. Small acute actinomycotic abscesses may heal after surgical drainage alone. More often, however, the acute initial stage

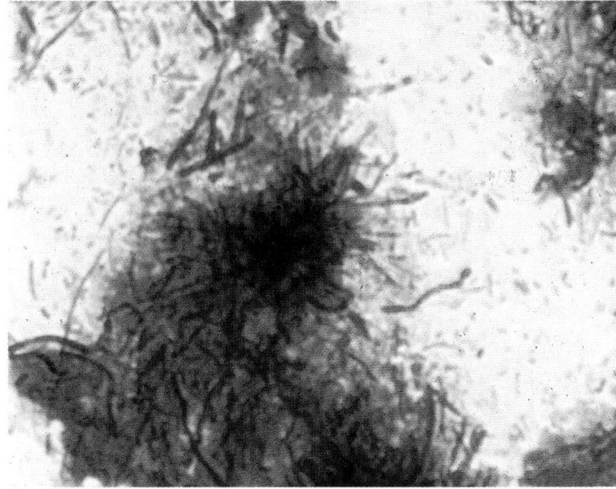

Fig. 7.6.29.2 Gram-stained smear prepared from a crushed sulphur granule. The causative actinomycetes appear as Gram-positive irregularly curved branching filaments which are partially arranged in nest-like structures. In addition, various other bacteria, in particular Gram-negative rods and Gram-positive cocci, can be seen representing the concomitant flora. Magnification ×1200.

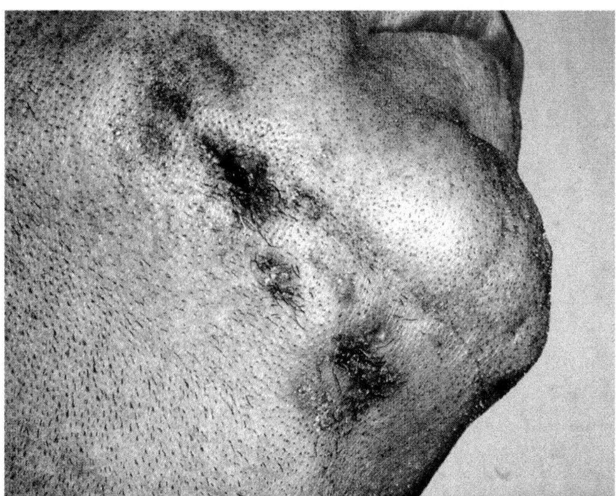

Fig. 7.6.29.3 Primarily chronic cervicofacial actinomycosis with several draining sinus tracts in a 42-year-old man.

is followed by a subacute to chronic course if no specific antimicrobial treatment is given, thereby imitating the primarily chronic form, which is characterized by regression and cicatrization of central suppurative foci while the infection progresses peripherally producing hard painless livid infiltrations. These may lead to multiple new areas of liquefaction, fistulae (Fig. 7.6.29.3), which often discharge pus containing sulphur granules, and multilocular cavities with poor healing and a tendency to recur after temporary regressions of the inflammatory symptoms.

With inappropriate or no treatment, cervicofacial actinomycoses extend slowly, even across organ borders, and may become life-threatening by invasion of the cranial cavity, the mediastinum, or the bloodstream.

Thoracic actinomycoses

Thoracic manifestations, which are much less common than the cervicofacial form (Table 7.6.29.3), usually develop after aspiration or inhalation of material from the mouth (dental plaque or calculus, tonsillar crypt contents) or a foreign body that contains or is contaminated with the causative agents. Occasionally, this form of disease may result from extension of an actinomycotic process of the neck, from an abdominal infection perforating the diaphragm, or from a distant focus by haematogenous spread.

Primary pulmonary actinomycoses present as bronchopneumonic infiltrations that may imitate tuberculosis or bronchial carcinoma radiographically, appearing as single dense or multiple spotted shadows in which cavitations may develop (Fig. 7.6.29.4). If not diagnosed and treated properly, pulmonary infections may extend through to the pleural cavity producing empyema, to the pericardium, or to the chest wall; they may even appear as a paravertebral (psoas) abscess tracking down to the groin. Detailed aetiology, pathogenesis, and clinical relevance of a condition termed 'endobronchial actinomycosis' remain to be definitely clarified.

Table 7.6.29.3 Localization of human actinomycotic infections

Body site involved	Number	Percentage of cases
Cervicofacial area	3197	97.9
Thoracic organs	41	1.3
Abdominal organs including small pelvis	20	0.6
Extremities	4	0.1
Central nervous system	4	0.1
Total number of cases	3266	100.0

Modified from Schaal KP, Pulverer G (1984). Epidemiologic, etiologic, diagnostic, and therapeutic aspects of endogenous actinomycete infections. In: Ortiz-Ortiz L, Bojalil LF, Yakoleff V (eds) *Biological, biochemical, and biomedical aspects of actinomycetes*, pp. 13–32. Academic Press, Orlando.

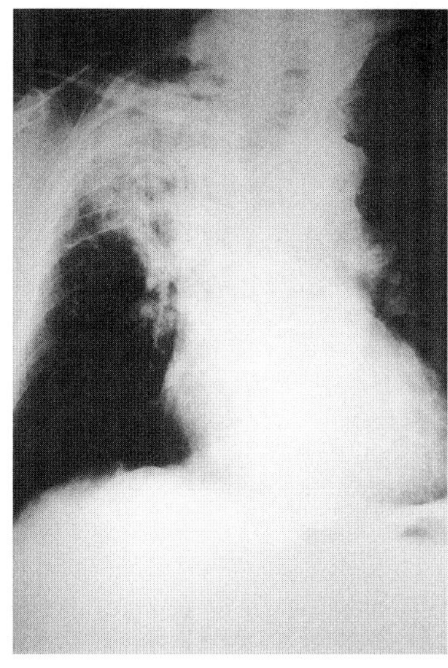

Fig. 7.6.29.4 Chest radiograph of pulmonary actinomycosis of the right upper lobe in a 62-year-old man. Initially, the disease was mistaken for bronchial carcinoma. It was diagnosed only after a huge subcutaneous abscess had developed covering the whole right shoulder blade.

Abdominal actinomycoses

Actinomycoses of the abdomen and pelvis are rare (Table 7.6.29.3). They originate either from acute perforating gastrointestinal diseases (appendicitis, diverticulitis, various ulcerative diseases), from surgical or accidental trauma including injuries caused by ingested bone splinters or fish bones, or from inflammations of the female internal genital organs.

Women who wear intrauterine contraceptive devices (IUCD) or vaginal pessaries for long periods often show a characteristic colonization of the cervical canal and the uterine cavity, but particularly of the thread of the IUCD, by various fermentative actinomycetes and other anaerobes resembling the synergistic actinomycotic flora. However, this colonization only rarely results in an invasive actinomycotic process.

Most abdominal actinomycoses present as slowly growing tumours, which, in the absence of sinus tracts discharging pus with sulphur granules, are difficult to differentiate from malignant neoplasms such as colonic, rectal, ovarian, or cervical carcinomas. By direct extension, any abdominal tissue or organ may be involved including muscle, liver, spleen, kidney, fallopian tubes, ovaries, testes, bladder, or rectum. Haematogenous liver abscesses have been seen, especially associated with genital actinomycoses.

Actinomycotic infections of the central nervous system

Actinomycoses of the brain and the spinal cord are very rare. They may arise from direct extension of cervicofacial infections. Haematogenous spread is also possible, particularly from primary lesions in the lungs or abdomen. The spinal canal may be directly involved from these sites. Brain abscess is much more common than meningitis.

Actinomycoses of the bone

In contrast to bovine actinomycosis which usually affects the skeleton, bone involvement in humans is very rare. It usually develops by direct extension from soft tissue infection resulting in a periostitis with new bone formation visible by radiography. If the bone itself is invaded, localized areas of bone destruction surrounded by increased bone density usually develop. Mandible, ribs, and spine are most frequently involved.

Actinomycotic endocarditis

Endocarditis due to fermentative actinomycetes has occasionally been described. However, detailed bacteriological information on this condition is not yet available so that it remains to be seen whether it may rightly be termed actinomycosis or has merely to be considered an aetiological variant of the common form of endocarditis caused by indigenous oral microbes.

Cutaneous actinomycoses

Actinomycotic lesions of the skin are extremely rare. Usually, they originate from wounds that were contaminated with saliva or dental plaque following human bites or fist fights, but they may also result from haematogenous spread. Symptoms are similar to those of cervicofacial actinomycoses.

Diagnosis

Clinical symptoms are often misleading, especially in the early stages of the disease, histopathological appearances are unreliable, and diagnosis chiefly rests on bacteriological methods.

Radiography

In cervicofacial cases, radiography is useful only for detecting bone involvement. A pulmonary infiltrate associated with a proliferative lesion or destruction of ribs is highly suggestive of either actinomycosis or a tumour. Radiography may also help to locate the abdominal processes and to identify the involvement of organs such as liver, kidney, urinary bladder, or ureter. In general, however, radiographic changes are not diagnostic.

Laboratory diagnosis

Clinical chemistry and haematology

Small localized actinomycotic lesions are not usually associated with abnormalities. In advanced cases, however, especially those in the thoracic or the abdominal area, a raised erythrocyte sedimentation rate and pronounced leucocytosis may be seen. When the central nervous system is involved, a polymorphonuclear or mononuclear pleocytosis is commonly found. The protein content of the cerebrospinal fluid is frequently elevated and the sugar content moderately depressed.

Bacteriology

Pus specimens containing sulphur granules and occasionally looking like semolina should prompt the clinician to ask and the bacteriologist to look specifically for actinomycetes using suitable cultural techniques and other methods.

Pus, sinus discharge, bronchial secretions, granulation tissue, or biopsy materials are suitable specimens. Precautions must be taken to prevent contamination of the specimen by the indigenous mucosal flora. In cases of cervicofacial actinomycoses, pus should therefore be obtained only by transcutaneous puncture of the abscesses or by transcutaneous needle biopsy. When abscesses have already been incised, a sufficient amount of pus should be collected instead of using only a swab. Because sputum always contains oral actinomycetes, bronchial secretions should be obtained by transtracheal aspiration, or material should be collected by transthoracic percutaneous needle biopsy. Percutaneous puncture of suspected abscesses is often the only way of obtaining suitable specimens for diagnosing abdominal actinomycoses.

The transport of specimens to the bacteriological laboratory should be as fast as possible, preferably by messenger. Alternatively, a reducing transport medium such as one of the modifications of Stuart's medium should be used. The specimen should arrive in the laboratory within 24 h, although it has occasionally proved possible to isolate actinomycetes from samples that took 7 days or more to get to the diagnostic laboratory by post.

A quick and comparatively reliable tentative diagnosis is possible microscopically when sulphur granules are present (Fig. 7.6.29.1). The demonstration of concomitant bacteria in Gram-stained smears prepared from crushed granule material (Fig. 7.6.29.2) allows the differentiation of actinomycotic granules from similar particles produced by *Nocardia* spp., *Actinomadura* spp., or *Streptomyces* spp.

Use of transparent culture media and careful microscopic examination of the cultures, preferably on Fortner plates, after at least 2, 7, and 14 days of incubation enables a specialized laboratory to detect possible actinomycete colonies and to subculture them for identification. Isolation and definite identification to the species level may require a further 1 to 2 weeks. Techniques such as the application of gene probes or the polymerase chain reaction for detecting and identifying fermentative actinomycetes are not yet widely used.

Serological diagnosis

None of the routine serological methods has yet provided satisfactory results because sensitivity and specificity have been found to be too low.

Treatment

As the aetiology of human actinomycoses is always polymicrobial, the antibacterial drugs used for treatment should in principle cover both the causative actinomycetes and all of the concomitant bacteria. This usually requires the administration of drug combinations in which aminopenicillins currently represent the therapeutic basis because they are slightly more active against the pathogenic actinomycetes than is penicillin G and because they are able to inhibit *Aggregatibacter (Actinobacillus) actinomycetemcomitans* which is usually resistant to narrow-spectrum penicillins. However, the presence of concomitant β-lactamase producers such as *Bacteroides fragilis*, *B. thetaiotaomicron*, or *Staphylococcus aureus* (β-lactamase producing) may impair the therapeutic efficacy of aminopenicillins and that of many other β-lactams so that the combination with a β-lactamase inhibitor is advisable or even necessary.

For cervicofacial actinomycoses, amoxicillin plus clavulanic acid has proved to be the treatment of choice. Three doses of 2.0 g amoxicillin plus 0.2 g clavulanic acid every day for 1 week and three doses of 1.1 g of the combination for an additional 7 days usually result in complete cure. Thoracic actinomycoses mostly respond to the same regimen. However, it is advisable to maintain doses of 2.2 g 3 times a day for 2 weeks, and to continue treatment for 3 to 4 weeks. Advanced pulmonary cases may require the addition of 2 g ampicillin three times a day in order to increase the tissue concentration of aminopenicillin and, depending on the composition of the concomitant flora, the use of an antimicrobial specifically active against resistant Enterobacteriaceae; the application of drugs such as metronidazole or clindamycin against strict anaerobes is only necessary as an adjunct to the aminopenicillins in chronic cases with reduced blood supply.

Since in abdominal actinomycoses Enterobacteriaceae and β-lactamase producing *Bacteroides* spp. are usually present and the correct diagnosis is mostly established late, suitable antimicrobial combinations for these cases are amoxicillin plus clavulanic acid plus metronidazole plus tobramycin (gentamicin) or ampicillin plus clindamycin plus an aminoglycoside. Imipenem might also be a good choice, but this drug has not yet been widely used for treating actinomycotic infections.

Neither clindamycin nor metronidazole should be used alone. Clindamycin is almost completely ineffective against *Aggregatibacter (Actinobacillus) actinomycetemcomitans* and metronidazole shows no activity at all against pathogenic actinomycetes. The use of further combinations, including additional aminoglycosides, cephalosporins, or β-lactamase-stable penicillins, may be necessary depending on the presence of unusual aerobic organisms. In patients allergic to penicillins, tetracyclines or possibly cephalosporins may be tried instead of aminopenicillins. Incision of abscesses and drainage of pus may still be necessary as an adjunct to the antimicrobial chemotherapy and may help to accelerate recovery and to decrease the risk of relapses.

Prognosis

The prognosis of cervicofacial and cutaneous actinomycotic infections is good provided that the diagnosis is established early and antimicrobial treatment is adequate. However, thoracic, abdominal, and systemic manifestations remain serious conditions that require all possible diagnostic and therapeutic efforts. Without proper treatment, the prognosis is grave.

Epidemiology

Actinomycoses are not transmissible and cannot be brought under control by vaccination or by measures that prevent spread. Sporadically, they occur worldwide. In Germany, the incidence of the disease was estimated to range from 1 in 40 000 (acute and chronic cases together) to 1 in 80 000 (chronic cases alone) per year, but appears to be decreasing in recent years.

Men are affected 2 to 4 times more frequently by cervicofacial actinomycoses than are women. However, the male to female ratio appears to vary with age. Although actinomycoses may be found in patients of any age, men are predominantly affected between their 20th and 50th years and women in the second to fourth decade of their lives. Before puberty and in old age, actinomycoses occur sporadically in patients of both sexes without the pronounced predisposition of men.

Other diseases caused by fermentative actinomycetes

Fermentative actinomycetes play some part in dental caries and periodontal disease, but are clearly not the most important microbes contributing to these important health problems. Lacrimal canaliculitis with and without conjunctivitis is commonly caused by fermentative actinomycetes, in particular *P. propionicum*, but less frequently also by *Actinomyces israelii*, *A. gerencseriae*, *A. naeslundii*, *A. oris*, or *A. odontolyticus*. The concomitant flora, when present, is usually less complex than that of typical actinomycoses. Removal of the lacrimal concretions that are usually present and local application of antimicrobials always result in prompt cure.

Arcanobacterium pyogenes and *A. haemolyticum* (formerly *Corynebacterium (Actinomyces) pyogenes* and *C. haemolyticum*) cause acute pharyngitis, urethritis, or cutaneous or subcutaneous suppurations. The recently described species *Actinomyces neuii* subsp. *neuii* and subsp. *anitratus*, *A. graevenitzii*, *A. europaeus*, *A. radingae*, *A. turicensis*, *A. funkei*, *A. cardiffensis*, *A. hongkongensis*, *A. oricola*, *A. urogenitalis*, and *A. dentalis*, as well as *Arcanobacterium (Actinomyces) bernardiae*, *Actinobaculum schaalii*, and *Varibaculum cambriense* have been isolated from various clinical sources including abscesses and blood cultures, and may also be associated with mixed bacterial flora. *A. turicensis* and possibly *A. urogenitalis* seem to be particularly common in genital infections, while *A. radingae* was found only in patients with skin-related pathologies and *A. nasicola* was isolated from pus from the nasal antrum. *A. europaeus*, *A. turicensis*, and *A. urogenitalis* as well as *Actinobaculum schaalii*, *A. urinale*, and *A. massiliae* were detected in predominantly elderly patients with urinary tract infections, and *A. radicidentis* was isolated from infected root canals of teeth.

Further reading

Henssge U, *et al.* (2009). Emended description of Actinomyces naeslundii and description of Actinomyces oris sp. nov. and Actinomyces johnsonii sp. nov., previously identified as Actinomyces naeslundii genospecies 1, 2 and WVA 963. *Int J Syst Evol Microbiol*, **59**, 509–16.

McNeil MM, Schaal KP (1998). Actinomycoses. In: Yu VL, Merigan TC Jr, Barriere SL (eds) *Antimicrobial therapy and vaccines*, pp. 14–22. Williams and Wilkins, Baltimore.

Pulverer G, Schütt-Gerowitt H, Schaal KP (2003). Human cervicofacial actinomycoses: microbiological data of 1997 cases. *Clin Infect Dis*, **37**, 490–7.

Schaal KP (1986). Genus *Arachnia* Pine and Georg 1969, 269. In: Sneath PHA, *et al.* (eds) *Bergey's manual of systematic bacteriology*, vol. 2, pp. 1332–42. Williams and Wilkins, Baltimore.

Schaal KP (1986). Genus *Actinomyces* Harz 1877, 133. In: Sneath PHA, *et al.* (eds) *Bergey's manual of systematic bacteriology*, vol. 2, pp. 1383–418. Williams and Wilkins, Baltimore.

Schaal KP, Lee HJ (1992). Actinomycete infections in humans: a review. *Gene*, **115**, 201–11.

Schaal KP, Pulverer G (1984). Epidemiologic, etiologic, diagnostic, and therapeutic aspects of endogenous actinomycete infections. In: Ortiz-Ortiz L, Bojalil LF, Yakoleff V (eds) *Biological, biochemical, and biomedical aspects of actinomycetes*, pp. 13–32. Academic Press, Orlando.

Schaal KP, Yassin AF, Stackebrandt E (2006). The family Actinomycetaceae: the genera *Actinomyces*, *Actinobaculum*, *Arcanobacterium*, *Varibaculum*, and *Mobiluncus*. In: Balows A, *et al.* (eds) *The prokaryotes. A handbook on the biology of bacteria: ecophysiology, isolation, identification, applications*, 2nd edition, vol. 1, pp. 850–905. Springer, Berlin.

7.6.30 Nocardiosis

Roderick J. Hay

Essentials

Nocardia species—*Nocardia asteroides*, *N. brasiliensis*, and *N. otidiscaviarum*—are Gram-positive, filamentous, partially acid-fast bacteria. They are occasionally detectable in environmental sources such as soil, but they rarely cause infections in humans, although they can give rise to a variety of different diseases. In generally healthy individuals, most commonly in the tropics, they can present with cutaneous abscesses or subcutaneous infections (actinomycetoma) in which the organisms are present as clusters of filaments or grains. Alternatively, usually in immunocompromised patients following inhalation, they cause a disseminated or localized deep infection, with particular sites affected being the lungs or brain. Diagnosis of nocardial infection depends on culture, although histopathology is very useful in nocardial actinomycetomas. Antibiotic treatment is typically with a sulphonamide (often as co-trimoxazole for lung infections), but combinations of drugs are usually given because the responsiveness of nocardia species is very variable.

Introduction

Nocardiosis (nocardiasis) is the infection caused by *Nocardia* spp., usually *Nocardia asteroides* but, less commonly, *N. brasiliensis*, *N. farcinica*, *N. otitidiscaviarum*, and *N. transvalensis*. The term is most commonly applied to systemic infection due to these organisms but can also be used to describe cutaneous disease that follows the implantation of infection. *Nocardia* spp. are also important causes of actinomycetoma, particularly in Mexico and Central America.

The *Nocardia* spp. are Gram-positive filamentous branching bacteria that ramify in infected tissues. They can also break up into bacillary forms and, in some conditions, aggregate into grains typical of mycetomas. These organisms are aerobic and partially acid fast. They grow readily on ordinary laboratory media.

Pathogenesis

Nocardia spp. are found in soil, particularly where there is decaying vegetation. They can also be isolated from the air and, in most cases, systemic infection is by the airborne route; rarely nocardiosis can be acquired after inoculation into the skin. The characteristic histopathological response to infection is the production of polymorphonuclear leucocyte abscesses without extensive fibrosis. Caseation and palisading granulomas are not generally seen. Dissemination to other organs such as brain and skin can occur. By contrast, in primary cutaneous infections the lesion is usually localized to an abscess containing filaments at the site of inoculation and is accompanied by local lymphadenopathy. Mycetoma grain formation may occur in some of these infections that follow inoculation. It is not known why, in some patients, transcutaneous infection with nocardia results in the development of a mycetoma whereas in others a subcutaneous abscess containing filaments is formed. The formation of mycetomas appears to be more common with *N. brasiliensis* infections.

Epidemiology

Otherwise healthy patients may be infected by nocardia, although the frequency of subclinical exposure and sensitization in normal populations is unknown. However, the majority of patients with systemic nocardiosis are immunocompromised, most commonly with a condition that affects the expression of T-lymphocyte-mediated immune responses. Underlying conditions include:

- malignancies, including cancer and lymphoma
- AIDS and other immunodeficiency states such as chronic granulomatous disease
- solid organ transplantation
- other conditions that require high doses of corticosteroids, such as collagen vascular disease and rheumatoid arthritis
- preexisting pulmonary disease; alveolar proteinosis, in particular, seems to predispose to nocardiosis

The usual site of primary infection is the lung and the disease may remain restricted to this site. It may also be disseminated to other organs, particularly to the brain and skin. Nocardiosis can occur at any age, although it is rare, particularly in childhood.

Clinical features

Primary cutaneous nocardiosis

This is an uncommon infection that appears to follow traumatic inoculation of organisms into a superficial abrasion. The usual primary lesion is a small nodule, ulcer, or abscess at the site of inoculation. There may be a small chain of secondary nodules (as in sporotrichosis, Chapter 7.7.1) along the course of a lymphatic and local lymphadenopathy is common (Fig. 7.6.30.1). Some such cases resolve spontaneously. This form of disease is usually caused by *N. asteroides*.

Nocardia mycetoma

This is discussed in Chapter 7.7.1 *N. brasiliensis* is the usual cause.

Pulmonary nocardiosis

Pulmonary infection is seen in about 75% of cases of systemic nocardiosis, even where there are disseminated lesions elsewhere. Symptoms of pulmonary nocardiosis are variable with cough,

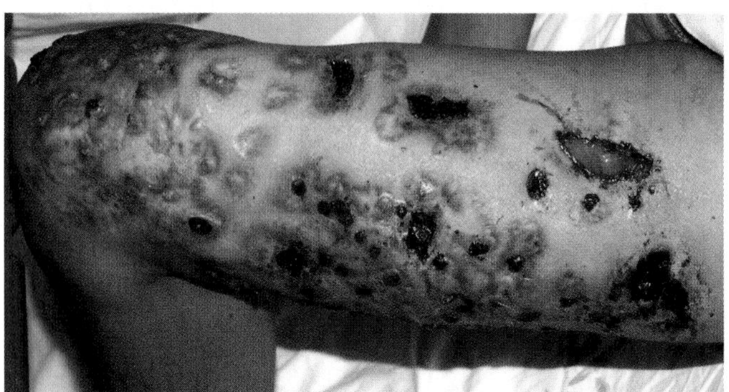

Fig. 7.6.30.1 Extensive chronic nocardiosis at site of injury in a 27-year-old Peruvian man, Instituto de Medicina Tropical 'Alexander von Humboldt', Universidad Peruana Cayetano Heredia, Lima, Peru.

fever, and leucocytosis. In otherwise healthy individuals the changes and signs may be very similar to pulmonary tuberculosis, whereas in the immunocompromised patient the lesions present as rapidly developing, single or multiple lung lesions. In patients with AIDS symptoms are often minimal, even in the presence of extensive disease. These changes are reflected by the course of the disease. In some patients progression is rapid, in others it is chronic.

Chest radiographs may show segmental or lobar infiltrates, cavitation, nodules, or diffuse miliary infiltrates; endobronchial infection has been recorded. Calcification is not common. The infection may spread locally to involve adjacent structures such as the pleural space and diaphragm or may spread to other sites. Very occasionally, *Nocardia* spp. can be isolated from sputum of otherwise healthy patients. Whether this reflects the process of asymptomatic sensitization is not known. Most cases of pulmonary nocardiosis are caused by *N. asteroides*.

Disseminated nocardiosis

Haematogenous spread is common in the immunocompromised patient and may occur without evidence of pulmonary infection. The most common site for dissemination is the brain where it presents with localized abscesses without meningeal involvement. The signs are those due to an intracerebral space-occupying lesion. Spread to other sites is less common, although dissemination to skin, liver, kidneys, and bone may occur.

The acute disseminated forms and those with involvement of the central nervous system have the worst prognosis. Continued therapy with corticosteroids also appears to have bad prognostic significance. Infection in patients with AIDS may not be recognized before death. Rapid diagnosis is therefore a key to successful management. By contrast, pulmonary infection in otherwise healthy patients is usually a chronic process and has to be distinguished from tuberculosis.

Laboratory diagnosis

The infection is often recognized initially by direct microscopy of pus, bronchial washings, or tissue. In Gram's stains the organisms can be shown as fine branching filaments, although distinction from other bacteria may be difficult if short rod-like forms predominate. A modified acid-fast stain using weak acid can be used to demonstrate filaments.

Nocardia spp. grow on ordinary media aerobically. Colonies may take 2 to 3 weeks to appear and cultures need prolonged incubation. Growth is generally more rapid on Lowenstein–Jensen medium.

Histopathological examination is useful in some cases. Filaments stain with modified acid-fast stains using an aqueous solution of a weak acid for decolorization, but can also be highlighted with the methenamine–silver stain (Grocott's modification). The branching nature of the organism is best appreciated in histopathological material. Other pathogens such as *Pneumocystis* spp. may also be present in histopathological material.

Serological tests (usually counterimmunoelectrophoresis or enzyme immunoassay) can be obtained in reference centres and are generally used to monitor the progress of therapy rather than establish the diagnosis.

Therapy

The mainstays of therapy are sulphonamides such as sulfadiazine and sulfafurazole, given in doses of 4 to 6 g daily. Co-trimoxazole is also effective, particularly in pulmonary forms, although the ratio of the trimethoprim to sulphonamide components is not ideal for intracerebral infections. In many cases, drainage of abscesses may hasten recovery. Non-*asteroides* species of nocardia often do not respond as well to sulphonamides. Much of the recommended drug therapy is derived from the personal experiences of a few cases. It is, for instance, the general practice to use two antibiotics.

Other drugs that have been used include amikacin, ampicillin, and minocycline, although testing is necessary before using these. Experience of other drugs is similarly limited. For instance, ciprofloxacin, cefotaxime, and imipenem are all active *in vitro* but clinical experience with them is limited to a few cases.

Clustering of cases may occur occasionally, suggesting exposure to a common source of infection. In two such episodes there had been extensive construction work in the vicinity of the hospital involved. At present, no methods of prevention are known, although the existence of more than two cases in a single or adjacent wards should alert clinicians to the possibility of environmentally acquired infection.

Further reading

Boiron P, *et al.* (1992). Review of nocardial infections in France, 1987–1990. *Eur J Clin Microbiol Infect Dis*, **11**, 709–14.

Brown-Elliott BA, *et al.* (2006). Clinical and laboratory features of the *Nocardia* spp. based on current molecular taxonomy. *Clin Microbiol Rev*, **19**, 259–82.

Filice GA (2005). Nocardiosis in persons with human immunodeficiency virus infection, transplant recipients, and large, geographically defined populations. *J Lab Clin Med*, **145**, 156–62.

Georghiou PR, Blacklock ZM (1992). Infection with *Nocardia* species in Queensland. A review of 102 clinical isolates. *Med J Aust*, **156**, 692–7.

Hay RJ (1983). Nocardial infections of the skin. *J Hyg (Lond)*, **91**, 385–91.

Houang ET, *et al.* (1980). *Nocardia asteroides* infection: a transmissible disease. *J Hosp Infect*, **1**, 31–6.

Kilincer C, *et al.* (2006). Nocardial brain abscess: review of clinical management. *J Clin Neurosci*, **13**, 481–5.

Sakai C, Takagi T, Satoh Y (1999). *Nocardia asteroides* pneumonia, subcutaneous abscess and meningitis in a patient with advanced malignant lymphoma: successful treatment based on *in vitro* antimicrobial susceptibility. *Intern Med*, **38**, 683–6.

7.6.31 Rat-bite fevers

David A. Warrell

Essentials

Rat-bite fever is usually attributable to *Streptobacillus moniliformis* in the Americas, Europe, and Australia; in Asia, *Spirillum minus* is the commoner cause. Bites are increasingly common among child pet owners and pet-shop and laboratory workers. Both bacteria are commensals of rodents and their predators. After an incubation period less than 1 week, *S. moniliformis* causes sudden high fever, rigors, myalgia, petechial rash, and migratory reactive or septic polyarthritis with synovial effusions. Complications include fulminant septicaemia, endocarditis, pneumonia, and metastatic abscesses. *S. minus* infection (sodoku) has a longer incubation period with similarly high fever but concomitant exacerbation of the bite wound, local lymphadenopathy, papular rash, and arthralgia without effusions. In both diseases, fever subsides after a few days but may relapse repeatedly over months. Untreated mortality is about 10% for *S. moniliformis* and 2 to 10% for *S. minus*. *S. moniliformis* can be cultured (with some difficulty) and the diagnosis confirmed by polymerase chain reaction (PCR) methods and serology. *S. minus* cannot be confirmed by culture or serology but can be demonstrated microscopically in the bite wound and other tissues or by isolation in animals. Penicillin is the treatment of choice for both infections. Prevention is by controlling peridomestic rats and avoiding bites by pet or laboratory rodents.

Introduction

Feral rodent populations are increasing worldwide and rat bites occur in impoverished infested rural and urban dwellings. Under these conditions, young children are often bitten while asleep and patients with diabetic or leprous neuropathy are particularly vulnerable. However, increasing numbers of rodents are now kept as pets and as laboratory animals, explaining why bites are becoming more common among pet owners and pet shop and laboratory workers. There are said to be at least 20 000 rat bites in the United States of America each year. Wild rats harbour a variety of other zoonotic pathogens including cryptosporidium, pasteurella, yersinia, listeria, coxiella, salmonella, leptospira, toxoplasma, and hantaviruses.

Streptobacillus moniliformis infection (streptobacillary rat-bite fever and Haverhill fever)

Aetiology

Streptobacillus moniliformis is part of the normal pharyngeal flora of 50 to 100% of wild and 10 to 100% of laboratory rats. It can be recovered from their nasopharynx, middle ear, saliva, and urine. In rodents it can cause septicaemia, pneumonia, conjunctivitis, polyarthritis, and abortion. It has been isolated from rats, mice, guinea pigs, gerbils, squirrels, and animals that feed on rodents such as cats, dogs, pigs, ferrets, and weasels. *S. moniliformis* infection is reported in monkeys, koalas, and turkeys.

S. moniliformis is named after the necklace-like filaments and chains with yeast-like swellings seen in mature cultures on solid media. It is a nonmotile pleomorphic filamentous Gram-negative rod, 1 to 5 μm long. Although it can be grown in ordinary blood culture media, it is ultrafastidious, microaerophilic, and slow-growing making it difficult to isolate. However, it thrives on trypticase soy agar enriched with 20% horse or rabbit blood, serum, or ascitic fluid under 8% carbon dioxide. In liquid media, 'puff ball' colonies appear in 2 to 7 days. In concentrations as low as 0.0125%, sodium polyanethol sulphonate (liquoid), a laboratory anticoagulant added to most commercial aerobic media, inhibits the growth of *S. moniliformis*. On agar, 'fried-egg' colonies appearing after 5 days culture signify L-phase variants that lack a cell wall and are therefore resistant to penicillin.

Epidemiology

S. moniliformis infection occurs worldwide causing rat-bite fever and Haverhill fever.

Streptobacillary rat-bite fever

As a cause of rat-bite fever, *S. moniliformis* is apparently much commoner than *Spirillum minus* in the Americas, Europe, and Australia. Despite its name, there is no history of a bite in 30% of cases. Bites or scratches by rodents or their predators, contact with mucous membranes (e.g. when pet owners kiss or share food with their rodents), or other contact with these mammals whether living or dead may result in infection. In some countries, 10% of those bitten by wild rats are infected. Formerly, most people with rat bites were children of poor families living in urban areas. A bite might not be suspected because it was inflicted while they were asleep. In the United States of America, 55% of those infected are children younger than 12 years old. Increasing numbers of people with rat-bite fever are pet owners and pet shop and laboratory staff. Human-to-human transmission has not been reported.

Haverhill fever

Named after a town in Massachusetts where there was an outbreak involving 86 cases in 1926, Haverhill fever follows ingestion of raw milk, food, or water contaminated by rats. An outbreak in a boarding school in England in 1983 affected 304 people, 43% of the school's population, and was attributed to contamination of the water supply by rats.

Clinical features

Streptobacillary rat-bite fever

If transmission is by bite, the wound usually heals quickly with only trivial local inflammation or pustule formation.

The systemic illness starts suddenly after an incubation period that is usually less than 7 days, is often as short as 1 to 3 days, but is sometimes as long as 7 weeks. There is high fever with rigors, vomiting, severe headache, sore throat, myalgia, and muscle tenderness lasting 3 to 5 days. About 75% of patients develop a rash 1 to 8 days later. Discrete erythematous macules or papules, 1 to 4 mm in diameter, appear symmetrically on the lateral and extensor surfaces and over the joints. They are often most marked on the hands and feet (palms and soles) with associated petechiae, but may also occur on the face. Papules, vesicles, haemorrhagic vesicles, and pustules with scabs may develop. There is desquamation in about 20% of cases. Early in the illness, approximately one-half the patients develop an asymmetrical migratory subacute or chronic polyarthralgia or arthritis which is thought to be reactive (autoimmune). It usually involves the knees, ankles, elbows, shoulders, and hips and is often associated with sterile effusions. Far less commonly, a distinct streptobacillary septic (suppurative) arthritis affects single or multiple distal joints, most often the knee but also the fingers. Severe joint pain and tenderness may be the dominant symptom in patients with rat-bite fever. Diarrhoea and loss of weight are described in young children. Fever and other symptoms subside in a few days in treated cases, but fever may persist for 1 to 2 weeks, relapsing repeatedly over several months, and arthritis may persist for many months in those who are untreated. Severe infections can lead to bronchitis, pneumonia, pleural effusions, metastatic abscess formation (including cerebral abscess), endocarditis, myocarditis, pericarditis with effusion, subacute glomerulonephritis, interstitial nephritis, splenitis or splenic abscess, amnionitis, meningitis, hepatitis, systemic vasculitis, polyarteritis nodosa, and renal and multiorgan failure. Infective endocarditis, usually with underlying rheumatic or other valve disease, has been described.

Haverhill fever

Haverhill fever (erythema arthriticum epidemicum) follows a similar clinical course after the patient has drunk unpasteurized milk or contaminated water. Vomiting, stomatitis, and upper respiratory tract symptoms such as sore throat are said to be more prominent than in rat-bite fever.

Differential diagnosis

Unlike *Spirillum minus* infection (sodoku, see below), the other cause of rat-bite fever, the incubation period is usually short, the bite wound heals permanently with little local lymphadenopathy, the rash is morbilliform or petechial, and arthritis is common. Depending on the geographical area, *S. moniliformis* infection must be distinguished from other acute fevers associated with rodent bites and contact, including lymphocytic choriomeningitis and other arenaviruses, hantaviruses, leptospirosis, melioidosis, tularaemia, plague, murine typhus, trench fever, and *Pasteurella multocida*. The polyarthritis may be confused with acute rheumatic fever, rheumatoid arthritis, systemic lupus erythematosus, or Still's disease. The acute febrile illness and exanthem may suggest other bacterial septicaemias such as meningococcaemia, rickettsial infections, and even secondary syphilis and in children, Kawasaki disease.

Fever after ingestion of raw milk should raise the possibility of brucellosis.

Diagnosis

The diagnosis can be confirmed by culture of bite wounds, blood, synovial and pericardial fluid, skin blister fluid, or pus from abscesses, but the organism is ultrafastidious and slow-growing (see above). In patients with infective endocarditis the differential diagnosis of these slow-growing microaerophilic organism includes *Haemophilus aphrophilus*, *Cardiobacterium hominis*, *Actinomyces actinomycetemcomitans*, and *Eikenella corrodens*. A high or rising titre of agglutinins, complement-fixing or fluorescent antibodies, may be detected between 2 and 3 weeks. Polymerase chain reaction based on 16S rRNA gene sequences, discriminated by BfaI restriction enzyme treatment, is promising. Patients sometimes show a moderate peripheral leucocytosis. The pleomorphic filamentous bacteria may be stained in peripheral blood leucocytes or tissue samples using Gram's, Wright's, or silver stains. In cases of streptobacillary septic arthritis, the synovial fluid contains many leucocytes (neutrophils around 50 000 × 10^9/litre) and bacteria may be visible. False-positive serological tests for syphilis (Venereal Disease Research Laboratory (VDRL) test) are found in 15 to 25% of cases.

Treatment

S. moniliformis is sensitive to penicillin and can be treated with benzyl penicillin 1.2 million units/day for 5 to 7 days followed by oral penicillin or ampicillin 500 mg four times a day for 7 days if there is improvement. Procaine benzylpenicillin (adult dose 600 mg or 600 000 units) by intramuscular injection every 12 h for 7 to 14 days and penicillin V 2 g/day by mouth are also effective. Penicillin-resistant L-variants are susceptible to streptomycin (7.5 mg/kg intramuscularly twice daily), tetracycline (500 mg orally four times a day), and probably erythromycin. For patients hypersensitive to penicillin, erythromycin, chloramphenicol, tetracycline, or cephalosporins can be used. Erythromycin was used successfully in the boarding-school outbreak of Haverhill fever in England in 1983.

Patients with endocarditis should be treated with intravenous benzylpenicillin, 4.8 to 14.4 g (8–24 000 000 units) each day for between 4 and 6 weeks, or 4.8 000 000 units of procaine benzylpenicillin daily by intramuscular injection for 4 weeks if the cultured organism has a sensitivity of 0.1 μg/ml. The addition of streptomycin improves bactericidal activity and eliminates L-forms.

Affected joints may require aspiration or even surgical debridement.

Prognosis

The untreated case fatality was reported to be 10 to 13%. However, the overall mortality in patients with endocarditis, many of whom were untreated or treated late, exceeded 50%. Fulminant and rapidly fatal cases have been reported in immunocompetent children and adults. In survivors, residual arthralgia persisting for as long as 10 years has been described.

Spirillum minus infection (sodoku, sokosha)

Aetiology

The cause of sodoku, *Spirillum minus*, is a relatively thick tightly coiled Gram-negative rod or spirillum (not a spirochaete), between 2.5 and 5.0 μm long, with 2 to 6 (commonly 3) spirals, resembling campylobacters. It darts about under the power of its terminal flagella. Continuous culture on artificial media has not been achieved, but the organism can be demonstrated by inoculating material from the bite wound, regional lymph nodes, or blood intraperitoneally into mice or guinea pigs. Organisms usually appear in the rodent's blood within 5 to 15 days of inoculation. *Spirillum minus* may be found in the blood of up to 25% of apparently healthy rodents and in the eye discharge and mouths of rats with interstitial keratitis and conjunctivitis. In the 1930s, 'sodoku inoculata' (the blood of infected guinea pigs) was used to treat neurosyphilis.

Epidemiology

Sodoku is found worldwide but is particularly common in Japan. In Asia it is commoner than *S. moniliformis* as a cause of rat-bite fever. Infection results from bites, scratches, or mere contact with rodents or their predators including dogs, cats, and pigs.

Clinical features

The initial bite wound usually heals without signs of local inflammation. After an incubation period of 1 to 36 days, but usually 14 to 18 days, there is sudden fever which, in untreated cases, reaches its height in 3 days and resolves by crisis after a further 3 days. At the start of the illness the healed bite wound becomes inflamed, swollen, and indurated; it may break down to become a necrotic or suppurating ulcer. Regional lymph nodes are usually enlarged and tender. Other acute symptoms include rigors, myalgia, and prostration. A rash develops in approximately one-half of patients. It often spreads from the site of the bite and consists of angry purplish or reddish-brown indurated papules, plaques, or macules with urticarial lesions. Arthralgia may be severe but there are no joint effusions. Severe manifestations including meningitis, cerebral abscess, encephalitis, endocarditis, myocarditis, myocardial abscess, pleural effusion, chorioamnionitis, subcutaneous abscesses, and involvement of liver, kidney, and other organs are seen in about 10% of patients. Relapses of fever, rash, and other symptoms lasting 3 to 6 days may occur between remissions of between a week and 2 months and occasionally up to a year in untreated patients.

Differential diagnosis

Sodoku must be distinguishable from streptobacillary rat-bite fever (see above). Its tendency to relapse may suggest relapsing fever (*Borrelia* spp.) or trench fever (*Bartonella quintana*).

Diagnosis

The diagnosis can be confirmed by examining aspirates from the bite wound, lymph nodes, exanthem, or blood (thick and thin films) using dark-field microscopy or Wright's or Giemsa's stains. The organism can be detected in the blood, peritoneal fluid, or heart muscle of inoculated rodents but cannot be cultured on artificial media. No specific serological tests are available. False-positive serological tests for syphilis are found in 50 to 60% of cases, and reactions with Proteus OXK are also common.

Treatment

Penicillin is the drug of choice. For adults, procaine benzylpenicillin 600 mg (600 000 units) should be given every 12 h for 7 to 14 days. Penicillin V, 2 g/day by mouth, is also said to be effective. A Jarisch–Herxheimer reaction may complicate penicillin treatment.

Prognosis

Untreated case fatality is about 2 to 10%.

Prevention of rat-bite fevers

These infections can be prevented by controlling wild peridomestic rodents and by encouraging laboratory and pet shop workers to wear protective gloves and to handle rodents carefully, to avoid hand-to-mouth or hand-to-eye contact, to wash their hands, and to clean all rodent bite wounds. The efficacy of postexposure prophylaxis with antibiotics is unproven. Young children should be supervised when they handle pet rodents to avoid bites, kissing, sharing food, and hand-to-mouth or hand-to-eye contact. An enzyme-linked immunosorbent assay (ELISA) has been developed for surveillance of rodent colonies for *S. moniliformis*. Haverhill fever is prevented by avoiding the consumption of raw milk, by monitoring water supplies (especially those not derived from the mains), and by controlling rat populations.

Further reading

Dendle C, Woolley IJ, Korman TM (2006). Rat-bite fever septic arthritis: illustrative case and literature review. *Eur J Clin Microbiol Infect Dis*, **25**, 791–7.

Elliott SP (2007). Rat bite fever and *Streptobacillus moniliformis*. *Clin Microbiol Rev*, **20**, 13–22.

Gaastra W, Boot R, Ho HT, Lipman LJ (2009). Rat bite fever. *Vet Microbiol*, **133**, 211–28.

Kimura M, Tanikawa T, Suzuki M *et al.* (2008). Detection of Streptobacillus spp. in feral rats by specific polymerase chain reaction. *Microbiol Immunol*, **52**, 9–15.

McEvoy MB, Noah ND, Pilsworth R (1987). Outbreak of fever caused by *Streptobacillus moniliformis*. *Lancet*, **ii**, 1361–3.

Raffin BJ, Freemark M (1979). Streptobacillary rat bite fever: a pediatric problem. *Pediatrics*, **64**, 214–17.

Roughgarden JW (1965). Antimicrobial therapy of rat bite fever. A review. *Arch Intern Med*, **116**, 39–54.

Rupp ME (1992). *Streptobacillus moniliformis* endocarditis: case report and review. *Clin Infect Dis*, **14**, 769–72.

7.6.32 Lyme borreliosis

Gary P. Wormser, John Nowakowski, and Robert B. Nadelman

Essentials

Lyme borreliosis is a zoonotic bacterial infection caused by *Borrelia burgdorferi* sensu lato, a spirochaetal agent transmitted by certain species of *Ixodes* ticks. Small rodents and birds serve as reservoirs. It is the most common vector-borne infection in the United States of America and an important infection in many countries throughout the temperate regions of Europe and northern Asia, where a wider variety of borrelia species account for differences in clinical manifestations in Eurasia compared with the United States.

Clinical features—the commonest and earliest clinical manifestation is erythema migrans, a distinctive cutaneous lesion that occurs at the site of deposition of the spirochaete by the vector tick, beginning 7–14 days later as a red macule or papule, with the rash then expanding over days to weeks, with or without central clearing. This may be associated with 'viral' symptoms, fever and regional lymphadenopathy. Later manifestations include (1) carditis—usually manifested by fluctuating degrees of atrioventricular block; (2) neurological involvement—including cranial neuropathy (typically cranial nerve VII palsy), radiculopathy, and meningitis; (3) arthritis—typically migratory monoarthritis or asymmetric oligoarthritis; (4) acrodermatitis chronica atrophicans—a swollen, bluish-red appearing skin lesion in which the involved skin ultimately atrophies.

Diagnosis—the diagnosis of erythema migrans is purely clinical in geographical areas endemic for Lyme borreliosis: serological testing is not recommended because it is insufficiently sensitive on acute phase serum samples. In patients with suspected later clinical manifestations, serological testing is essential because clinical findings alone lack sufficient specificity. Polymerase chain reaction (PCR) testing of joint fluid and/or cerebrospinal fluid may be helpful in some cases.

Treatment—most people treated for Lyme borreliosis respond well to a 2-week course of antibiotic therapy (preferred oral regimen usually amoxicillin, doxycycline, or cefuroxime). Symptomatic treatment is recommended for patients who have or develop subjective complaints of unclear aetiology despite successful resolution of the objective manifestation of Lyme borreliosis following antibiotic therapy, since randomized double-blind placebo-controlled trials have shown that additional antibiotic treatment is not helpful.

Prevention—measures include avoiding exposure to ticks by limiting outdoor activities in tick-infested locations, using tick repellents, tucking in clothing to decrease exposed skin surfaces, and frequent inspection of the skin for early detection and removal of ticks.

Introduction

Lyme borreliosis (also called Lyme disease) is named after Lyme, Connecticut, United States of America. It is caused by the spirochaete *Borrelia burgdorferi* sensu lato which is transmitted to humans by the usually asymptomatic bite of certain ticks of the genus *Ixodes* (Fig. 7.6.32.1). *Borrelia burgdorferi* sensu stricto (hereafter referred to as *B. burgdorferi*) causes the disease in North America, while in Europe, several species of *Borrelia* in addition to *B. burgdorferi* cause this infection, including *B. garinii* which is probably the most common cause of classic Lyme neuroborreliosis (Bannwarth's syndrome) and *B. afzelii* the most common cause of acrodermatitis chronica atrophicans, a late cutaneous complication. The entire chromosome and associated plasmids of one strain of *B. burgdorferi* have been completely sequenced. Representative strains of other pathogenic species, such as *B. afzelii* and *B. garinii*, have been partially sequenced.

Epidemiology

In North America, more than 20 000 new cases of Lyme borreliosis are reported each year, making it the most common vector-borne disease. It occurs in north-eastern, mid-Atlantic, north-central, and far western regions of the United States of America and in limited foci in Canada (mainly in eastern Ontario). Elsewhere, it occurs in much of the temperate regions of Europe and northern Asia. Ticks acquire this borrelial infection in a complex tick–vertebrate transmission cycle. The white-footed mouse is the most important reservoir for *B. burgdorferi* in North America. White-tailed deer, an important host for adult *Ixodes* ticks, are not a competent reservoir for Lyme borreliae. In Europe a wide variety of small rodents and birds serve as reservoirs. Migrating birds may play a role in the spread of *B. burgdorferi* to new geographical locations.

Lyme borreliosis occurs slightly more frequently in males than in females. There is a bimodal age distribution with the highest rates in children between 5 and 9 years old and in adults 55–59 years old.

Clinical manifestations

The somewhat different manifestations of Lyme borreliosis in Eurasia compared with North America (Table 7.6.32.1) may be explained by the wider variety of species of Lyme borrelia causing infection in Eurasia. Clinical features are similar in adults and children.

Erythema migrans

Erythema migrans (EM) (Figs. 7.6.32.2, 7.6.32.3), the clinical hallmark of Lyme borreliosis, is recognized in approximately 90% of patients with objective clinical manifestations of *B. burgdorferi* infection. Typically, EM begins as a red macule or papule at the site of a tick bite that occurred 7 to 14 days earlier. The rash expands over days to weeks. Central clearing may or may not be present. Secondary cutaneous lesions may develop because of haematogenous spread of spirochaetes to other cutaneous sites. EM must be distinguished from local tick bite reactions, tinea, insect and spider bites, bacterial cellulitis, and plant dermatitis. Lesions eventually resolve spontaneously but may recur if antimicrobial therapy is not given.

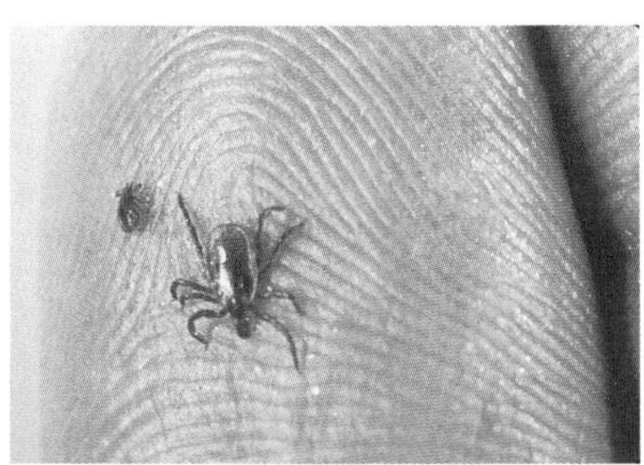

(a)

(b)

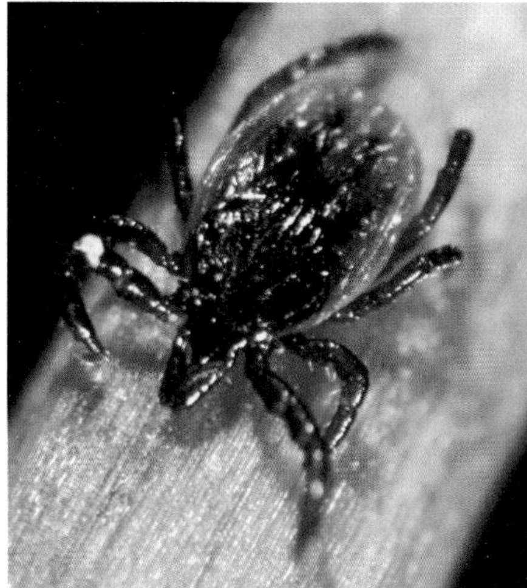

(c)

Fig. 7.6.32.1 (a) Adult female (right) and nymphal (left) *Ixodes scapularis* ticks. (b,c) Nymph of *Ixodes ricinus*, the vector tick in Europe.

Table 7.6.32.1 Lyme borreliosis in North America compared to Eurasia

	North American Lyme borreliosis	Eurasian Lyme borreliosis
Vector	*Ixodes(dammini) scapularis* or *Ixodes pacificus*	*Ixodes ricinus* or *Ixodes persulcatus*
Aetiological agent	*B. burgdorferi* sensu stricto	*B. burgdorferi* sensu stricto, *B. afzelii*, *B. garinii*, *B. spielmanii*
Clinical features	Erythema migrans is the most common manifestation.	Erythema migrans is the most common manifestation
	Systemic symptoms frequently present in patients with erythema migrans (up to 80%) Other skin manifestations such as borrelial lymphocytoma and acrodermatitis chronica atrophicans are much less common than in Europe	Systemic symptoms infrequently present in patients with erythema migrans (<35%) Other skin manifestations such as borrelial lymphocytoma and acrodermatitis chronica atrophicans are much more common than in North America
	Cranial nerve palsy (usually 7th) with or without meningitis is the most common neurological manifestation	Painful meningoradiculoneuritis with or without cranial palsy is the most common neurological manifestation

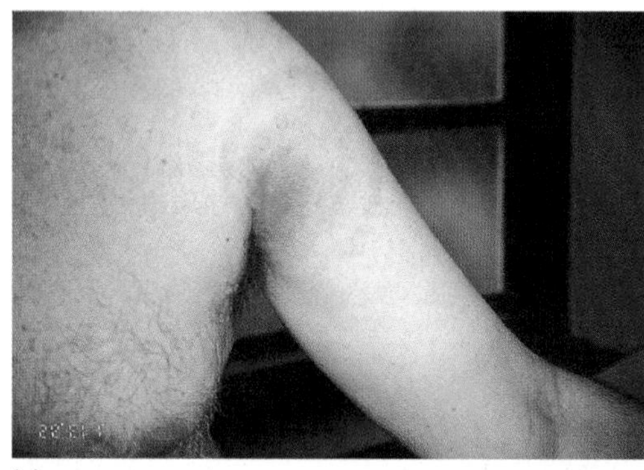

(a)

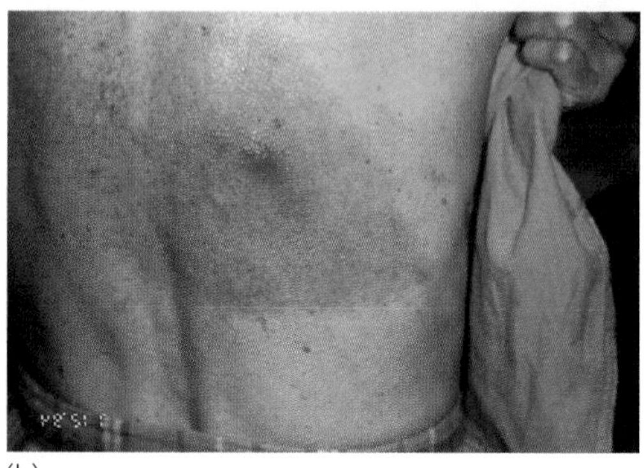

(b)

Fig. 7.6.32.2 (a) Erythema migrans rashes from patients who were culture positive for borrelia: (a) rash with typical central appearance; (b) rash with more homogeneous apparance.

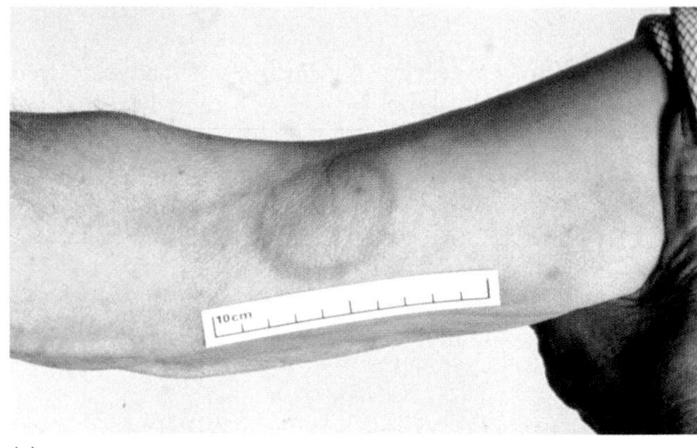

(a)

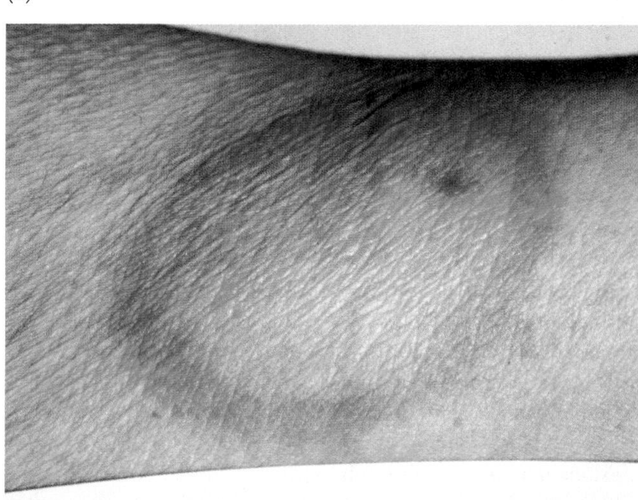

(b)

Fig. 7.6.32.3 English patient with typical erythema migrans. (Copyright D A Warrell.)

Systemic symptoms, such as fatigue, myalgia, arthralgia, headache, fever and/or chills, and stiff neck, are less common in patients with EM caused by *B. afzelii* compared to either *B. burgdorferi* or *B. garinii*. Prominent respiratory and/or gastrointestinal symptoms are so infrequent that their presence should suggest an alternative diagnosis or coinfection with another tick-borne pathogen. Aside from the EM skin lesion itself, the most common objective physical findings are regional lymphadenopathy and fever. Occasional cases of a viral-like illness without EM have been attributed to Lyme borreliosis.

Carditis

Typically, cardiac disease develops within weeks to months after infection, sometimes together with EM. It is usually manifested by fluctuating degrees of atrioventricular block that may cause the patient to complain of dizziness, palpitations, dyspnoea, chest pain, or syncope. Myocarditis may be present but pericarditis with effusion is rarely observed, and endocarditis is absent. The incidence of cardiac manifestations (as measured by ECG confirmed heart block) has been observed to be low in both the United States of America (<1%) and Europe (<4%).

Neurological disease

The incidence of neurological Lyme disease in Europe may be higher than in the United States of America. One explanation may be the greater neurotropism of *B. garinii* (a genospecies which has not been isolated in North America). The principal early neurological manifestations are cranial neuropathy (typically peripheral seventh nerve palsy which can be bilateral), radiculopathy, and meningitis, which may occur alone or together. EM may be present concomitantly. Late neurological manifestations are uncommon and include peripheral neuropathy, encephalopathy, and encephalomyelitis.

Antibiotics appear to hasten the resolution of meningitis but most studies are uncontrolled. The rate of resolution of motor dysfunction, which is fully reversible in the vast majority of cases, is not enhanced by antimicrobial therapy. Symptoms of encephalopathy and peripheral neuropathy improve or do not progress after treatment with antibiotics.

Rheumatological disease

Lyme arthritis occurs in both North America and Europe. In a study of 55 untreated patients with EM diagnosed in the United States of America between 1977 and 1979 and followed for a mean duration of 6 years, objective arthritis developed in more than one-half, occurring within 1 year for 90%. The majority of these patients developed intermittent attacks of migratory monoarthritis or asymmetric oligoarthritis, lasting a mean of 3 months per episode (range 3 days to 11.5 months). The knee was affected at some point in almost all patients, but other large and (less often) small joints could be affected. Temporomandibular joint involvement occurred in 11 (39%) of 28 patients with arthritis in one series. Although large effusions may occur, joint pain and erythema are often minimal. Baker's cysts may develop. Typically, synovial fluid analysis reveals a modestly elevated white cell count (median 24 250 white cells/mm^3 in one study) with a polymorphonuclear predominance and a normal glucose level. Synovitis lasting 1 year or more may ensue for a minority of United States patients, sometimes associated with joint destruction. Although *B. burgdorferi* DNA can be detected by polymerase chain reaction (PCR) in the synovial fluid of up to 85% of untreated patients with Lyme arthritis, *B. burgdorferi* has rarely been successfully cultured from joint fluid.

Acrodermatitis chronica atrophicans (ACA)

This cutaneous manifestation of late Lyme disease develops insidiously on a distal extremity, mainly in elderly women. It is a swollen bluish-red appearing skin lesion in which the involved skin ultimately atrophies. One-third of patients have an associated (usually sensory) polyneuropathy. *B. burgdorferi* has been recovered from a skin biopsy specimen of an ACA lesion of more than 10 years duration. Since the usual causative agent *B. afzelii* does not occur in the United States of America, ACA is essentially a European disease.

Miscellaneous clinical manifestations

Borrelia lymphocytoma, principally caused by *B. afzelii* and *B. garinii*, is a tumour-like nodule which typically appears on the pinna of the earlobe or on the nipple or areola of the breast. Lesions will eventually resolve spontaneously but disappear within a few weeks after antibiotic therapy. This lesion is extremely rare in North America.

Direct involvement of the eye (e.g. uveitis, keratitis, vitritis, optic neuritis) has been attributed to *B. burgdorferi* infection. However, since ophthalmological disorders have almost never been associated with the isolation of *B. burgdorferi* in culture, the actual pathogenesis in these cases is uncertain. Conjunctivitis, originally described in 11% of patients with EM, was rare (<5%) in recent studies of culture-positive patients and may be unrelated to borrelia infection.

Case reports have suggested that adverse outcomes may be associated with pregnancies complicated by maternal Lyme borreliosis. However, prospective and epidemiological studies suggest that the risk of transplacental transmission of *B. burgdorferi* is probably minimal when appropriate antibiotics (Tables 7.6.32.2, 7.6.32.3) are given to pregnant women with Lyme borreliosis. There are no published data to support a congenital Lyme borreliosis syndrome.

Laboratory diagnosis

Where Lyme borreliosis is endemic, the diagnosis of EM is purely clinical. Laboratory testing is neither necessary nor recommended.

In patients with suspected extracutaneous Lyme borreliosis, serological testing is essential to support the diagnosis. Culture of *B. burgdorferi* has been a highly insensitive diagnostic technique for this group of patients, presumably because of inaccessibility of tissues containing the microorganism. PCR testing of joint fluid and sometimes of cerebrospinal fluid may aid in diagnosis, provided appropriate care is taken in performing the assay accurately.

A two-step approach to serological diagnosis is used in both the United States of America and Europe to increase the accuracy of a positive test. A positive or equivocal first-step test (usually an enzyme-linked immunosorbent assay (ELISA) or an indirect immunofluorescence assay (IFA)) is followed on the same serum sample by a second-stage test (immunoblot). Two-step testing, however, is not indicated for those with little or no clinical evidence of Lyme borreliosis because of a low positive predictive value. Since IgM and IgG antibodies to *B. burgdorferi* may persist in serum for years after clinical recovery, serology has no role in measuring response to treatment.

Patients with extracutaneous Lyme borreliosis almost always have diagnostic serum antibodies at time of presentation. In some patients with early neuroborreliosis, however, antibodies to Lyme borrelia may be present in cerebrospinal fluid before they are detected in serum.

Coinfection

Ixodes scapularis ticks (Fig. 7.6.32.1a) are the vectors for several other infections that may be transmitted separately or simultaneously with *B. burgdorferi*, such as *Babesia microti* and the rickettsial agent *Anaplasma phagocytophilum* that causes human granulocytic anaplasmosis (HGA, formerly known as human granulocytic ehrlichiosis (HGE)). In Europe, species of *Babesia* and *Anaplasma* are present in *Ixodes ricinus* ticks (Fig. 7.6.32.1b,c), which are also vectors of the flavivirus causing tick-borne encephalitis. Coinfection may alter the clinical presentation and response to treatment of Lyme borreliosis.

Reinfections

Reinfection with Lyme borrelia can often be recognized clinically by the development of a repeat episode of EM occurring at a different skin site during the months when the vector tick is plentiful in the environment. The clinical manifestations of reinfection in Lyme borreliosis patients who have EM are indistinguishable from initial infection.

Table 7.6.32.2 Recommended antimicrobial regimens for treatment of patients with Lyme borreliosis

Drug	Dosage for adults	Dosage for children
Preferred oral regimens		
Amoxicillin	500 mg three times daily[a]	50 mg/kg per day in three divided doses (maximum 500 mg per dose)[a]
Doxycycline	100 mg twice daily[b]	<8 years: not recommended
		≥8 years: 4 mg/kg per day in two divided doses (maximum 100 mg/dose)
Cefuroxime axetil	500 mg twice daily	30 mg/kg per day in two divided doses (maximum 500 mg per dose)
Alternative oral regimens **The following dosing regimens are specifically for patients with erythema migrans or borrelial lymphocytoma:**		
Selected macrolides[c]	Azithromycin 500 mg orally daily for 7–10 days, clarithromycin 500 mg orally twice daily for 14–21 days (if not pregnant), or erythromycin 500 mg orally four times per day for 14–21 days	Azithromycin 10 mg/kg daily (maximum of 500 mg per day), clarithromycin 7.5 mg/kg twice daily (maximum of 500 mg per dose), or erythromycin 12.5 mg/kg four times daily (maximum of 500 mg per dose)
Preferred parenteral regimen		
Ceftriaxone	2 g intravenously once daily	50–75 mg/kg intravenously once daily (maximum 2 g)
Alternative parenteral regimens		
Cefotaxime	2 g intravenously every 8 h[d]	150–200 mg/kg per day intravenously in 3 or 4 divided doses (maximum 6 g per day)[d]
Penicillin G	3–4 million units intravenously every 4 h[d]	200 000–400 000 units/kg per day divided into six doses given every 4 h[d] (not to exceed 18–24 million units/day)

[a] Although higher dosage given twice daily might be equally as effective, in view of the absence of data on efficacy, twice daily administration is not recommended.
[b] Tetracyclines are relatively contraindicated in pregnant or lactating women and in children less than 8 years of age.
[c] Due to their lower efficacy, macrolides are reserved for patients who are unable to take or who are intolerant of tetracyclines, penicillins, and cephalosporins. Patients treated with macrolides should be closely followed to ensure resolution of the clinical manifestations.
[d] Dosage should be reduced for patients with impaired renal function.
Modified from Wormser GP, *et al.* (2006). The clinical assessment, treatment, and prevention of Lyme disease, human granulocytic anaplasmosis and babesiosis. Clinical practices guidelines by the Infectious Diseases Society of America. *Clin Infect Dis*, **43**, 1089–134.

Treatment

Although most manifestations of Lyme borreliosis resolve spontaneously, antibiotics may speed the resolution of some and will almost certainly prevent the progression of disease. An approach to treatment is summarized in Tables 7.6.32.2 and 7.6.32.3. Presently available fluoroquinolones, sulphonamides, first-generation cephalosporins, rifampicin, and aminoglycosides have no appreciable activity against *B. burgdorferi* and should not be used. There is no evidence to support combination antimicrobial therapy, prolonged (more than 1 month) or repeated courses of antibiotics, and 'pulse' or intermittent antibiotic therapy. Within 24 h after initiation of antibiotics, approximately 15% of patients with EM may develop transient intensification of signs (e.g. rash and fever) and symptoms (e.g. arthralgias) consistent with a Jarisch–Herxheimer reaction. Treatment is symptomatic.

Most people treated for Lyme borreliosis have an excellent prognosis. Although a minority of patients treated for EM in recent series continue to have a variety of mild nonspecific complaints following antibiotic therapy, the development of objective extracutaneous disease after treatment is extremely rare. When such complaints are disabling and last for 6 months or more they have been referred to as post-Lyme disease syndrome (PLDS). Randomized double-blind placebo-controlled antibiotic treatment trials of patients with PLDS have failed to show evidence that the benefit of additional antibiotic therapy outweighs the complications of such treatment. Symptomatic therapy is recommended.

Patients with carditis and neurological disease tend to do well, but may sometimes have residual deficits (e.g. mild seventh nerve palsy) after treatment. In patients with arthritis, clinical recovery occurs typically with oral antibiotic therapy (often in conjunction with a nonsteroidal anti-inflammatory medication (NSAID)). Occasionally patients with Lyme arthritis with subtle signs of neuroborreliosis who are treated with oral antibiotics will develop overt late neuroborreliosis and require parenteral therapy. A small number of American patients with Lyme arthritis continue to have synovial inflammation for months or even several years after the apparent eradication of *B. burgdorferi* from the joint following antibiotic therapy (based on negative PCR testing). Such patients have improved after synovectomy. An immunological mechanism rather than active infection appears to be responsible for the continued inflammatory response in these patients.

In North America predominantly, but also in Europe, several patients with a variety of symptoms of uncertain aetiology, including pain and fatigue syndromes, have been labelled as having 'chronic Lyme disease', irrespective of tick exposure in an endemic area for Lyme borreliosis or credible clinical or laboratory evidence of infection due to Lyme borrelia. There is no scientific evidence that such patients have active infection due to borreliae.

Prevention

Preventive measures include avoiding exposure by limiting outdoor activities in tick-infested locations, using tick repellents, tucking in clothing to decrease exposed skin surfaces, and frequent skin inspections for early detection and removal of ticks. Use of acaricides on property and construction of deer fences have also been proposed.

Table 7.6.32.3 Recommended therapy for patients with Lyme borreliosis[a]

Indication	Treatment	Duration (days)	Range (days)
Tick bite in the USA	Doxycycline 200 mg (4 mg/kg in children ≥8 years of age) *and/or* observation	Single dose[b]	
Erythema migrans	Oral regimen[c,d]	14	10–21[e]
Early neurological disease			
Meningitis or radiculopathy	Parenteral regimen[c,f]	14	10–28
Cranial nerve palsy[g]	Oral regimen[c]	14	14–21
Cardiac disease	Oral regimen[c,h] or	14	14–21
	Parenteral regimen[c,h]	14	14–21
Borrelial lymphocytoma	Oral regimen[c,d]	14	14–21
Late disease			
Arthritis without neurological disease	Oral regimen[c]	28	28
Recurrent arthritis after oral regimen	Oral regimen[c,i]	28	28
	Parenteral regimen[c,i]	14	14–28
Antibiotic-refractory arthritis[j]	Symptomatic therapy[k]		
Central or peripheral nervous system disease	Parenteral regimen[c]	14	14–28
Acrodermatitis chronica atrophicans	Oral regimen[c]	21	14–28
Post-Lyme disease syndrome	Consider and evaluate other potential causes of symptoms, if none found then symptomatic therapy		

[a] Regardless of the clinical manifestation of Lyme disease, complete response to treatment may be delayed beyond the treatment duration. Relapse may occur with any of these regimens; patients with objective signs of relapse may need a second course of treatment.

[b] A single dose of doxycycline may be offered to adult patients and to children ≥8 years of age in the United States of America only when all of the following circumstances exist: (a) the attached tick can be reliably identified as an adult or nymphal *I. scapularis* tick that is estimated to have been attached for ≥36 h based on the degree of engorgement of the tick with blood or on certainty about the time of exposure to the tick; (b) prophylaxis can be started within 72 h of the time that the tick was removed; (c) ecological information indicates that the local rate of infection of these ticks with *B. burgdorferi* is ≥20%; and (d) doxycycline is not contraindicated. For patients who do not fulfil these criteria, observation is recommended.

[c] See Table 7.6.32.2.

[d] For adult patients intolerant of amoxicillin, doxycycline, and cefuroxime axetil, a macrolide may be given (Table 7.6.32.2). Patients treated with macrolides should be closely followed to ensure resolution of the clinical manifestations.

[e] If doxycycline is used, 10 days of therapy is effective; the efficacy of 10-day regimens with the other first-line agents is unknown.

[f] Data from European studies of neuroborreliosis indicate that oral doxycycline and parenteral antibiotic therapy are equally effective in Lyme meningitis. Similar studies have not been conducted in the United States of America. For nonpregnant adult patients intolerant of β-lactam agents, the recommended dosage of doxycycline, 200–400 mg/day orally (or intravenously if unable to take oral medications) in two divided doses, may be adequate. For children ≥8 years of age the recommended dosage of doxycycline for this indication is 4–8 mg/kg per day in two divided doses (maximum daily dosage of 200–400 mg).

[g] Most patients may be treated successfully with an oral regimen. Parenteral antibiotic therapy is recommended for patients with both clinical and laboratory evidence of coexistent meningitis. Systematic studies of oral antibiotic therapy in patients with cranial nerve palsy have only evaluated doxycycline. Other oral agents such as amoxicillin or cefuroxime axetil may be effective in patients who should not receive or cannot tolerate doxycycline, but clinical trials with these antibiotics are lacking. Most of the experience in the use of oral antibiotic therapy is for patients with seventh cranial nerve palsy. Whether oral therapy would be as effective for patients with other cranial neuropathies is unknown. The decision between oral and parenteral antimicrobial therapy for patients with other cranial neuropathies should be individualized.

[h] A parenteral antibiotic regimen is recommended at the start of therapy for patients who have been hospitalized for cardiac monitoring; an oral regimen may be substituted to complete a course of therapy or to treat ambulatory patients. A temporary pacemaker may be required for patients with advanced heart block.

[i] A second course of oral antibiotic therapy is preferred for the patient whose arthritis has substantively improved but has not yet completely resolved. Consideration of retreatment of such patients is often postponed for several months because of the anticipated slow resolution of inflammation after antibiotic treatment. During this interval use of nonsteroidal anti-inflammatory agents (NSAIDs) may be beneficial. Parenteral antibiotic therapy is reserved for those patients whose arthritis failed to improve at all or worsened.

[j] Antibiotic-refractory Lyme arthritis is operationally defined as persistent synovitis for at least 2 months after completion of a course of intravenous ceftriaxone (or after completion of two 4-week courses of an oral antibiotic regimen for patients unable to tolerate cephalosporins); in addition, PCR on synovial fluid (and synovial tissue if available) is negative for *B. burgdorferi* nucleic acids.

[k] Symptomatic therapy might consist of NSAIDs, intra-articular injections of corticosteroids, or other medications. If persistent synovitis is associated with significant pain or if it limits function, arthroscopic synovectomy should be considered.

Modified from Wormser GP, *et al.* (2006). The clinical assessment, treatment, and prevention of Lyme disease, human granulocytic anaplasmosis and babesiosis. Clinical practices guidelines by the Infectious Diseases Society of America. *Clin Infect Dis*, **43**, 1089–134.

Antibiotic prophylaxis with single-dose doxycycline given after recognized *I. scapularis* tick bites has been shown to be 87% effective in reducing further the low (less than 5%) risk of acquiring Lyme borreliosis after tick bites in the United States of America. Vaccination with a single recombinant outer surface protein A (OspA) preparation has been found to be safe and effective for preventing Lyme borreliosis in the United States of America, but this vaccine is no longer available. Canine vaccines for prevention of Lyme borreliosis, however, are widely used in North America.

Further reading

Aguero-Rosenfeld M, *et al.* (2005). Diagnosis of Lyme borreliosis. *Clin Microbiol Rev*, **18**, 484–509.

Feder HM Jr, *et al.* (2007). A critical appraisal of 'chronic Lyme disease'. *N Engl J Med*, **357**, 1422–30.

Günther G, Haglund M (2005). Tick-borne encephalopathies. Epidemiology, diagnosis, treatment and prevention. *CNS Drugs*, **19**, 1009–32.

Halperin JJ, *et al.* (2007). Practice parameter: treatment of nervous system Lyme disease (an evidence-based review). Report of the Quality

Standards Subcommittee of the American Academy of Neurology. *Neurology*, **69**, 91–102.

Kaplan RF, *et al.* (2003). Cognitive function in post-treatment Lyme disease. Do additional antibiotics help? *Neurology*, **60**, 1916–22.

Klempner MS, *et al.* (2001). Two controlled trials of antibiotic treatment in patients with persistent symptoms and a history of Lyme disease. *N Engl J Med*, **345**, 85–92.

Mygland A, *et al.* (2009). EFNS guidelines on the diagnosis and management of European Lyme neuroborreliosis. *Eur J Neurol* (E pub ahead of print).

Nau R, *et al.* (2009). Lyme disease—Current state of knowledge. *Dtsch Arztebl Int*, **106**, 72–82.

Stanek G, *et al.* (1996). European Union concerted action on risk assessment in Lyme borreliosis: clinical case definitions for Lyme borreliosis. *Wien Klin Wochenschr*, **108**, 741–7.

Wormser GP, *et al.* (2006). The clinical assessment, treatment, and prevention of Lyme disease, human granulocytic anaplasmosis, and babesiosis: clinical practice guidelines by the Infectious Diseases Society of America. *Clin Infect Dis*, **43**, 1089–134.

7.6.33 Relapsing fevers

David A. Warrell

Essentials

Louse-borne relapsing fever (LBRF) and tick-borne relapsing fevers (TBRF) are characterized by repeated episodes of high fever separated by afebrile period. They are caused by borrelia spirochaetes distinct from those responsible for Lyme borrelioses. Untreated patients may suffer as many as five (LBRF) or ten (TBRF) febrile relapses of decreasing severity.

Humans are the sole reservoir of epidemic LBRF caused by *Borrelia recurrentis* and transmitted by body lice (*Pediculus humanus corporis*). Endemic TBRFs are caused by at least 15 different borrelia species and have their own particular species of soft *Ornithodoros* tick vectors which also act as reservoirs. Transmission transplacentally, or by needlestick, blood transfusion, or laboratory accident is also possible.

LBRF is a classic historical epidemic disease of war, famine, and refugees, now largely confined to mountainous areas of the Horn of Africa and Peru but still retaining its pandemic potential. TBRF is of increasing endemicity in sub-Sahelian West Africa and is common in Rwanda and Tanzania. It occurs sporadically in parts of North America, Europe, the Middle East, and central Asia.

The most distinctive feature of these infections, the relapse phenomenon, is explained by antigenic variation of borrelial outer-membrane lipoprotein (vmp). Starting 2–18 days after infection, there is acute fever, chills, headache, pain, and prostration. Petechial rash (thrombocytopenia), bleeding, jaundice, hepatosplenomegaly and liver dysfunction are common. In some forms of TBRF, there are neurological manifestations; lymphocytic meningitis, VII and other cranial nerve lesions, myelitis, radiculitis, etc.; and uveitis during relapses.

Dangerous complications are hyperpyrexia, shock, myocarditis causing acute pulmonary oedema, acute respiratory distress syndrome (ARDS), cerebral or massive external bleeding, ruptured spleen, hepatic failure, Jarisch–Herxheimer reactions (JHR), and typhoid or other complicating bacterial infections. Pregnant women are at high risk of aborting and perinatal mortality is high.

Diagnosis by microscopy of blood films is more difficult in TBRF than LBRF. Serology and polymerase chain reaction (PCR) are used increasingly. The most important differential diagnosis in residents and travellers from tropical endemic areas is falciparum malaria.

Untreated mortality, exceeding 40% in some epidemics, can be reduced to less than 5% by treatment with antibiotics such as penicillin, tetracycline, erythromycin, and chloramphenicol, but elimination of spirochaetaemia is often accompanied by a potentially fatal JHR.

Prevention of LBRF is by eliminating lousiness by sterilizing clothing, using insecticides, and improving hygiene. Improved house construction, control of peridomestic rodents, use of residual insecticides, protection of sleepers with impregnated bed nets, and a post-exposure course of doxycyline can reduce the risk of TBRF.

Historical background

A disease characterized by repeated episodes of several days of high fever separated by afebrile periods of about a week was first described by Rutty in Dublin in 1770, but Craigie in Edinburgh coined the name 'relapsing fever' and distinguished it from typhus in 1843. Obermeier discovered the cause, *Borrelia recurrentis* (Fig. 7.6.33.1), in 1867, and transmission by human body lice was proved by Mackie in 1907. The cause of African tick fever was discovered by Ross and Milne in 1904 and, independently, by Dutton and Todd in 1905. Some believe that Dutton died of *B. duttonii* infection (Fig. 7.6.33.2).

Aetiology

The bacteria that cause relapsing fevers are large, loosely coiled, motile spirochaetes (genus *Borrelia*, family Spirochaetaceae), 8 to 20 μm long and 0.2 to 0.6 μm thick, with between 3 and 15 coils and, in some strains, 15 to 30 axial filaments or flagella. They divide by transverse binary fission. Borrelia can be cultured on chick chorioallantoic membrane and maintained in rodents and ticks. *In vitro* culture of borrelia species, including *B. recurrentis*, *B. duttonii*,

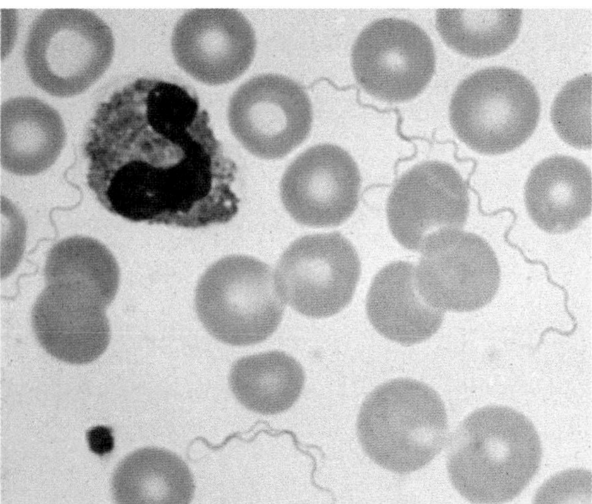

Fig. 7.6.33.1 *Borrelia recurrentis* spirochaetes in a thin blood film. (Copyright D A Warrell.)

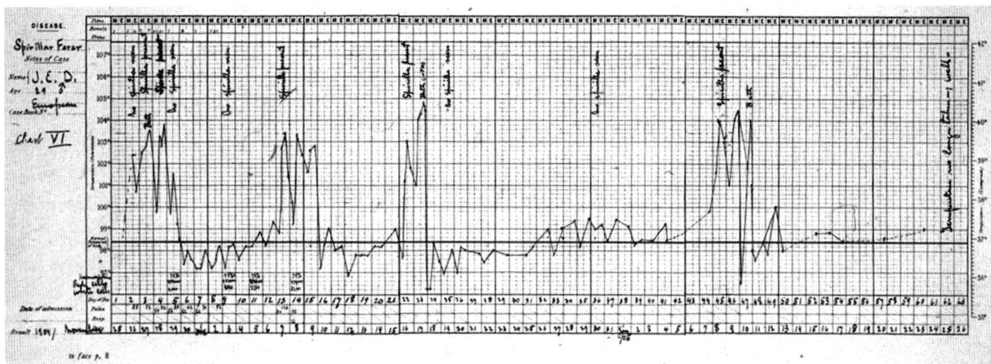

Fig. 7.6.33.2 Temperature chart of J. Everett Dutton who, with J L Todd, discovered the transmission of TBRF in the Congo. Dutton contracted TBRF at the beginning of November 1904. He had relapses of fever and spirochaetaemia on 7 and 16 December 1904 and 8 January 1905. His death on 27 February 1905 has been attributed by some, but not by Todd, to relapsing fever.
(From Dutton JE, Todd JL (1905). The nature of human tick-fever in the eastern part of the Congo Free State with notes on the distribution and bionomics of the tick. *Liverpool School of Tropical Medicine Memoir XVII.*)

and *B. crocidurae*, is now possible using Barbour–Stoenner–Kelly medium. Rapidly increasing amounts of genomic data are available. Sequencing of flagellin and rrs genes suggests that there are three phylogenetic clusters of borrelia: (1) Lyme borreliae (*B. burgdorferi* sensu stricto, *B. garinii*, and *B. afzelii*, Chapter 7.6.32), (2) New World tick-borne relapsing fever borreliae (*B. parkeri*, *B. turicatae*, *B. hermsii*, etc.), and (3) Old World tick-borne relapsing fever and louse-borne relapsing fever borreliae (*B. crocidurae*, *B. duttonii*, *B. hispanica*, *B. recurrentis*, etc.).

Epidemiology

Louse-borne (epidemic) relapsing fever (LBRF)

The vector of *B. recurrentis* is the human body louse *Pediculus humanus corporis* and, to a lesser extent, the head louse *P. humanus capitis*. Body lice, unlike head lice, retreat from the skin after feeding and hide and lay their eggs in clothing seams. More than 20 000 lice have been recovered from the clothes of one person. Lice are obligate blood-sucking human ectoparasites that ingest borreliae while feeding. Under conditions of crowding and poor hygiene they can move from person to person. When the host's body surface temperature deviates far from 37°C as a result of fever, climatic exposure, or death, or when infested clothing is discarded, the louse is forced to find a new host who can then be infected. Transmission of *B. recurrentis* is by scratching, which crushes lice so that their coelomic fluid is inoculated through broken skin or intact mucous membranes such as the conjunctiva, or inoculates infected louse faeces. Transplacental infection explains congenital infection. Blood transfusion, needlestick injuries, and contamination of broken skin by a patient's blood can also result in infection. Unlike ticks, lice cannot infect their progeny and are therefore not reservoirs and, since there is no known animal reservoir, the infection must persist in humans between epidemics in mild or asymptomatic forms.

Wars, famines, and other disasters that generate large numbers of refugees and prisoners favour the spread of lice and epidemic louse-borne infections such as relapsing fever and typhus. The yellow plague in Europe in AD 550, which halved the world's population, and the famine fevers of the 17th and 18th centuries in Ireland and elsewhere were probably LBRF. In the 20th century, a pandemic raged in North Africa, the Middle East, and Africa from 1903 to 1936, causing an estimated 50 million cases with 10% mortality. A second epidemic in 1943–6 created 10 million cases. An endemic focus persists in the Horn of Africa. Poor people with louse-infested clothes crowd together for shelter. In the Ethiopian highlands there are annual epidemics of thousands of cases coinciding with the small (*belg*) and big (*kiremt*) rains, but in the south the disease was perennial before its recent decline. Outbreaks have also occurred in Somalia and southern Sudan. In Ancash in the Peruvian Andes at altitudes above 3800 m, a cluster of 60 clinical cases was reported in 1983; 36 of the patients had *B. recurrentis* in their blood films. Serological evidence of *B. recurrentis* infection has been found in homeless people in Marseille.

Tick-borne (endemic) relapsing fever (TBRF)

In different parts of the world, particular species of borreliae and soft ticks (genus *Ornithodoros*, family Argasidae) are ecologically intimate, forming Borrelia–tick complexes (Table 7.6.33.1). At least 15 borrelia species are known to cause human TBRF. Ornithodoros tick vectors occur in dry savannah areas and scrub, caves, piles of timber and dead trees, or in holes in walls, roof spaces, and beneath the floors of log cabins, anywhere inhabited by small rodents. Unlike LBRF, TBRFs are zoonoses with the possible exception of *B. duttonii* infection that was thought to be transmitted only between humans. However, in central Tanzania, *B. duttonii* may infect domestic chickens and pigs. Vertebrate reservoir species include rodents (rats, mice, gerbils, squirrels, and chipmunks), insectivores, lagomorphs, bats, small carnivores, dogs, and birds. Ticks attack at night, remaining attached for less than 30 min before retreating back to their hiding places. Spirochaetes ingested while the tick sucks blood from an infected animal or human invade the tick's salivary and coxal glands and genital apparatus. Infection is transmitted to a new host either by a bite, introducing infected saliva, or by contaminating mucosal membranes with infected coxal fluid. Borreliae are not excreted in tick faeces. Ticks remain infected for life, even after being starved of blood for as long as 7 years. Spirochaetes can be transmitted venereally from male to female ticks and by females (but perhaps not those of the *O. moubata* complex) transovarially to their progeny. Some borreliae may be transmitted by hard ticks (Ixodidae), such as *B. lonestari* by *Amblyomma americanum* (United States) and *B. miyamotoi* by *Ixodes* spp. (Japan). TBRF, like LBRF, may be transmitted by blood transfusion, needlestick injuries, laboratory accidents, and transplacentally.

Table 7.6.33.1 Borrelia–tick complexes causing TBRFs

Borrelia spp.	*Ornithodoros* spp.	Geographical distribution
New World TBRF borreliae		
B. hermsii	*O. hermsii*	Canada, central and western USA, Mexico
B. turicatae	*O. turicata*	South-western USA, Mexico
B. parkeri	*O. parkeri*	Western USA, Baja California
B. mazzotti	*O. talaje*	Mexico, Central America
B. venezuelensis	*O. (venezuelensis) rudis*	Central America, Colombia, Venezuela, Argentina, Bolivia, Paraguay
Old World TBRF borreliae		
B. duttonii	*O. moubata*	Sub-Saharan Africa, Madagascar
B. crocidurae	*O. (erraticus) sonrai*	North, West, and East Africa, Middle East
B. graingeri	*O. graingeri*	East Africa
B. sp. nov.	*O. porcinus*	East Africa
B. tillae	*O. zumpti*	South Africa
B. persica	*O. tholozani*	Middle East, central Asia from Uzbekistan to western China
B. hispanica	*O. erraticus*	Iberian peninsula, Greece, Cyprus, North Africa
B. sp. nov.	*O. erraticus*	Southern Spain
B. latyschevii	*O. tartakowskyi*	Eastern Europe, Iran, Iraq, Afghanistan, central Asia
B. caucasica	*O. (verrucosus) asperus*	Eastern Europe, Iraq

TBRF is endemic in most temperate and tropical countries except the Arctic, Antarctic, Australasian, and Pacific regions. In Europe, TBRF is caused by *B. hispanica*, especially in Spain, Portugal, and Greece, while *B. crocidurae* and at least three other *Borrelia* spp. are present in Turkey and other adjacent territories. In the West African savannah region, *B. crocidurae* is the most prevalent bacterial infection creating a medical problem second only to malaria. Its prevalence is 1% among children in western Senegal and it is increasing and spreading during the persisting drought (1970–2009). It is a common infection in Rwanda where, in one health centre alone, 1650 proven cases are treated each year (6% of all patients). In parts of East Africa, especially in Tanzania, *B. duttonii* is an important cause of abortion, perinatal mortality, and childhood infection. In Israel, the incidence of *B. persica* infection among military personnel is 6.4/100 000 per year. In North America, isolated sporadic outbreaks of *B. hermsii*, *B. turicatae*, and *B. parkeri* infection occur in mountainous areas of British Columbia, Arizona (especially along the north rim of the Grand Canyon), California (south of Lake Tahoe), Colorado, Montana, New Mexico, and Washington (Browne Mountain). Since the mid-1980s, 280 cases of TBRF have been identified in the United States of America. In Western countries, TBRF is occasionally diagnosed in returned travellers.

Immunopathology and the relapse phenomenon

Symptomatic attacks of relapsing fever are terminated when specific bactericidal IgM antibodies lyse spirochaetes in the blood, independently of complement and T cells. However, some spirochaetes persist between the relapses, extracellularly in various organs including spleen, liver, kidneys, eye, and especially in the brain and cerebrospinal fluid. Relapse of spirochaetaemia and symptoms is explained by antigenic variation, which has been investigated in the greatest detail in *B. hermsii*. Silent gene sequences from an archive stored in extra chromosomal plasmids are transposed to one end of an expression linear plasmid where their recombination leads to synthesis of a new variable major outer membrane lipoprotein (vmp). This new coat allows the borreliae to escape from the host's humoral immune response until antibodies are generated against the new serotypic vmp antigen; this explains the relapse phenomenon and the successive appearance of borreliae expressing different vmps during the course of an untreated infection. Borreliae also possess defences against the host's innate immunity. *B. hermsii* surface protein BhCRASP-1 binds factor H (FH), an inhibitor of the alternative pathway of complement activation, so protecting the pathogen against opsonophagocytosis by inhibiting C3b binding. Plasminogen is also bound and activated to plasmin by BhCRASP-1, stimulating fibrinolysis that frees spirochaetes to spread in the blood stream. Another protective mechanism is rosetting of erythrocytes around spirochaetes. This shields them, by masking or steric hindrance, from host antibody and may cause microcirculatory obstruction that is damaging to the host and reminiscent of cerebral malaria. Antigenic variation may also generate isogenic serotypes with properties that promote the spirochaete's survival in vector and reservoir species, e.g. invasiveness for vertebrates' cerebral vascular endothelium. These same vmps are the principal tumour necrosis factor-α (TNFα)-inducing factors in LBRF.

Pathophysiology

Physiological disturbances during the spontaneous crisis and the Jarisch–Herxheimer reaction (JHR) induced by antimicrobial treatment in LBRF are typical of an endotoxin reaction. Outer membrane vmps of *B. recurrentis* stimulate monocytes to produce TNFα through NF- B. In patients treated with antibiotics, symptoms of the severe JHR are associated with a transient marked elevation in plasma concentrations of TNFα, interleukin (IL)-6, IL-8, and IL-1β (Fig. 7.6.33.3). The stimulus for cytokine release is the phagocytosis of spirochaetes made susceptible by the action of penicillin. Benzylpenicillin attaches to penicillin-binding protein I in *B. hermsii* spirochaetes. Large surface blebs are produced and the damaged spirochaetes are phagocytosed rapidly by neutrophils in the blood and by the spleen. Complement may enhance phagocytosis of spirochaetes, especially in the nonimmune host, but the complement system is not essential for elimination of spirochaetes whether or not specific immunoglobulins are present. *In vitro*, surface contact with spirochaetes induces mononuclear leucocytes to produce inflammatory cytokines and thromboplastin, which could be responsible for the fever and disseminated intravascular coagulation in LBRF. Kinins may be released during the JHR of syphilis and LBRF. The marked peripheral leucopenia that develops during the reaction reflects sequestration, perhaps in the pulmonary blood vessels, rather than leucocyte destruction. Spirochaetes may be found in those organs that bear the brunt of the infection such as liver, spleen (Fig. 7.6.33.4), myocardium (Fig. 7.6.33.5), and brain (Fig. 7.6.33.6), but it is unclear how their

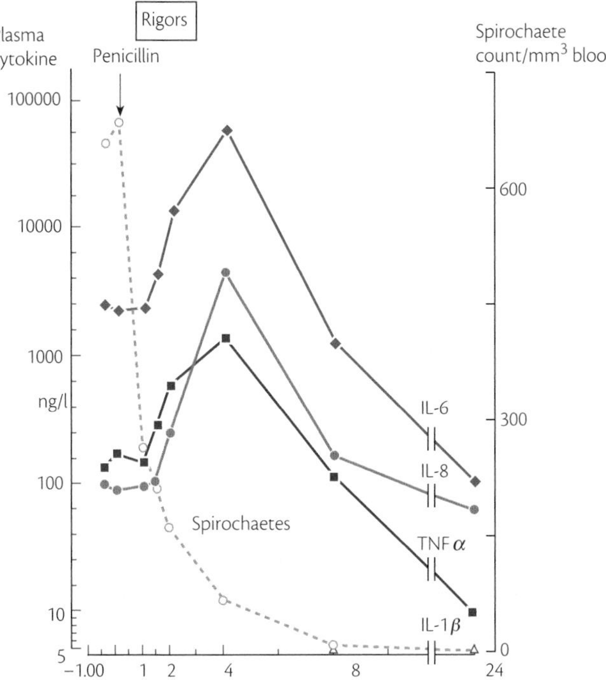

Fig. 7.6.33.3 Typical JRH in a patient with LBRF treated with intravenous penicillin. Following penicillin, the number of spirochaetes (dashed line referring to right hand axis) fell abruptly and circulating levels of TNFα, IL-6, IL-8, and IL-1β started to rise after about 1 h, peaking at 4 h. As cytokine levels were increasing, this patient experienced sustained rigors which subsided before peak levels were achieved.

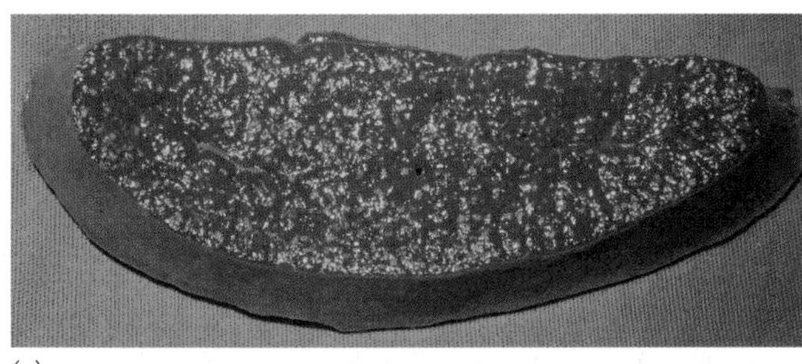

(a)

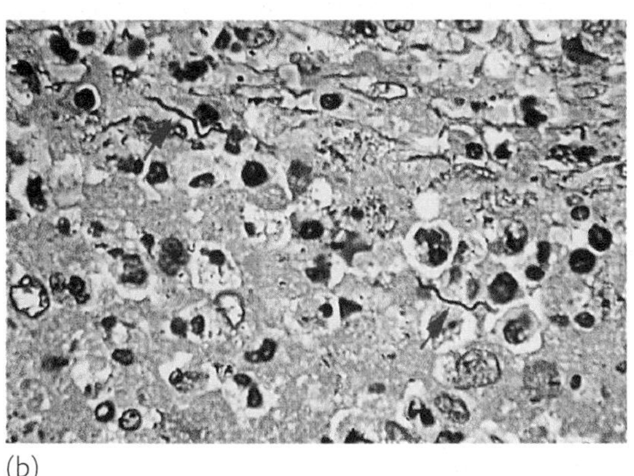

(b)

Fig. 7.6.33.4 Spleen in LBRF: (a) Section of spleen at autopsy; (b) Warthin Starry stain showing *Borrelia recurrentis* (arrows).
(a, copyright D A Warrell; b, courtesy of Dr Ken Fleming.)

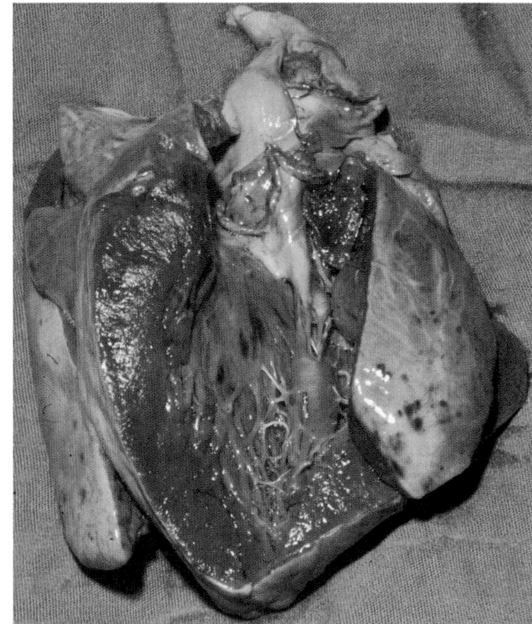

Fig. 7.6.33.5 Epicardial and endocardial haemorrhages.
(Copyright D A Warrell.)

pathological effects are produced. The petechial rash results from thrombocytopenia not vasculitis. The cardiorespiratory and metabolic disturbances in relapsing fever are principally the result of persistent high fever, accentuated by the JHR or spontaneous crisis.

Pathology

The vast majority of spirochaetes are confined to the lumen of blood vessels, but tangled masses are also found in the characteristic splenic miliary abscesses (Fig. 7.6.33.4) and infarcts as well as within the central nervous system adjacent to haemorrhages. Some strains of TBRF borreliae can invade the central nervous system,

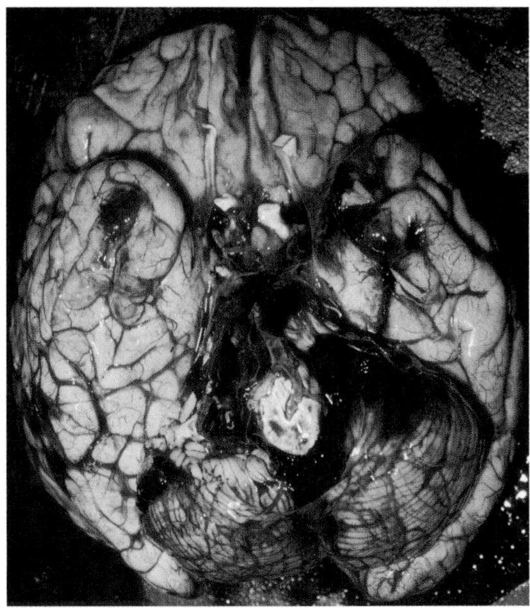

Fig. 7.6.33.6 Cerebral haemorrhage.
(Copyright D A Warrell.)

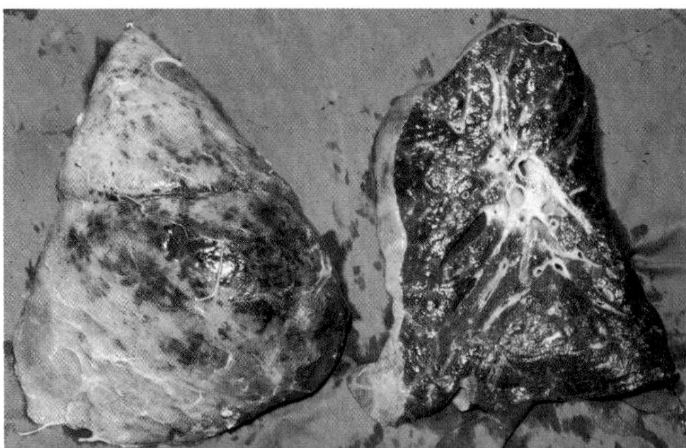

Fig. 7.6.33.7 Pulmonary haemorrhage.
(Copyright D A Warrell.)

aqueous humour, and other tissues. In LBRF, a perivascular histiocytic interstitial myocarditis, found in the majority of cases, may be responsible for conduction defects, arrhythmias, and myocardial failure resulting in sudden death (Fig. 7.6.33.5). Splenic rupture with massive haemorrhage, cerebral haemorrhage (Fig. 7.6.33.6), and hepatic failure are other causes of death. The liver shows hepatitis with patchy midzonal haemorrhages and necrosis. There is meningitis and perisplenitis. Most serosal cavities and surfaces of viscera are studded with petechial haemorrhages (Figs. 7.6.33.5, 7.6.33.6) and there may be massive pulmonary haemorrhage (Fig. 7.6.33.7). Thrombi are occasionally found occluding small vessels, but the peripheral gangrene sometimes found in patients recovering from louse-borne typhus (Chapter 7.6.39, Fig. 7.6.39.7c) is not seen.

Clinical features

Louse-borne relapsing fever

Adults

Prisoners and poor malnourished street-dwellers are most likely to become infected, especially young men. After an incubation period of 4 to 18 (average 7) days, the illness starts suddenly with rigors and a fever that mounts to nearly 40°C in a few days. Early symptoms are headache, dizziness, nightmares, generalized aches and pains (especially affecting the lower back, knees, and elbows), anorexia, nausea, vomiting, and diarrhoea. Later there is upper abdominal pain, cough, and epistaxis. Patients are usually prostrated (Fig. 7.6.33.8) and most are confused. Hepatic tenderness is the commonest sign (about 60%). The liver is palpably enlarged in approximately 50% of patients. Splenic tenderness and enlargement are slightly less common. Jaundice has been reported in 10 to 80% of patients. A petechial or ecchymotic rash is seen in 10 to 60% of patients (Figs. 7.6.33.9, 7.6.33.10); the lesions occur particularly on the trunk. Other sites of spontaneous bleeding include the conjunctivae (Fig. 7.6.33.11), nose in 25% (Fig. 7.6.33.9), and less commonly the lungs (Fig. 7.6.33.7), gastrointestinal tract, and retina. Many patients have tender muscles. Meningism occurs in about 40% of patients; other neurological features include cranial nerve lesions, monoplegias, flaccid paraplegia, and focal convulsions attributable, perhaps, to cerebral haemorrhages. In untreated people, the first attack of fever resolves by crisis in 4 to 10 (average 5) days, followed by an afebrile remission of 5 to 9 days, and then a series of up to five relapses of diminishing severity, occasionally complicated by epistaxis. Petechial rashes are absent during relapses.

Pregnant women are especially susceptible to severe disease and abortions are frequent.

Children

In children older than 5 years, clinical features resemble those in adults but are generally less severe and the case fatality is lower. Fever, chills, headache, abdominal pain and tenderness, vomiting, cough, musculoskeletal pains, tachycardia, and petechial rash are common. In younger children, hepatosplenomegaly, cough, and signs of consolidation may be more common. Reported case fatalities in children range from 1.9 to 5.5%.

Tick-borne relapsing fever

Adults

After an incubation period of 2 to 18 days, the illness starts with sudden fever, chills, headache, muscle and joint pains, extreme

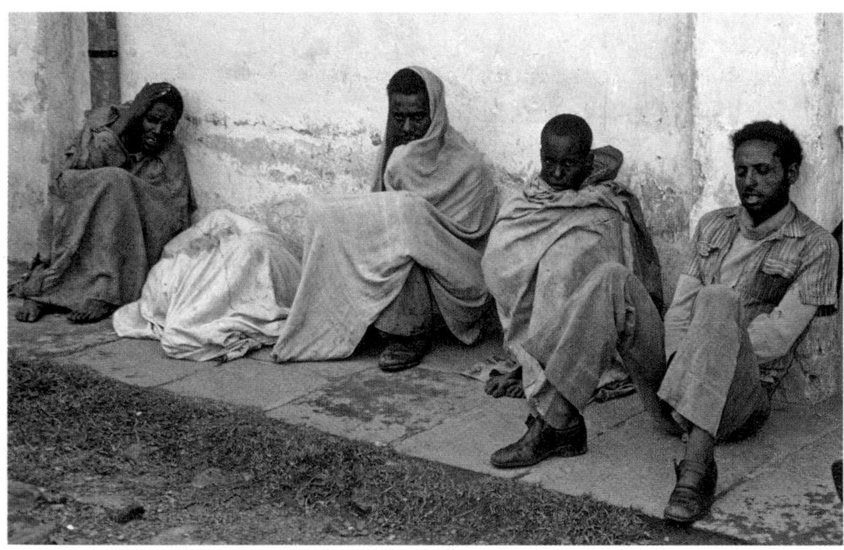

Fig. 7.6.33.8 Patients presenting with relapsing fever at a clinic in Addis Ababa. Most are febrile, confused, and prostrated.
(Copyright D A Warrell.)

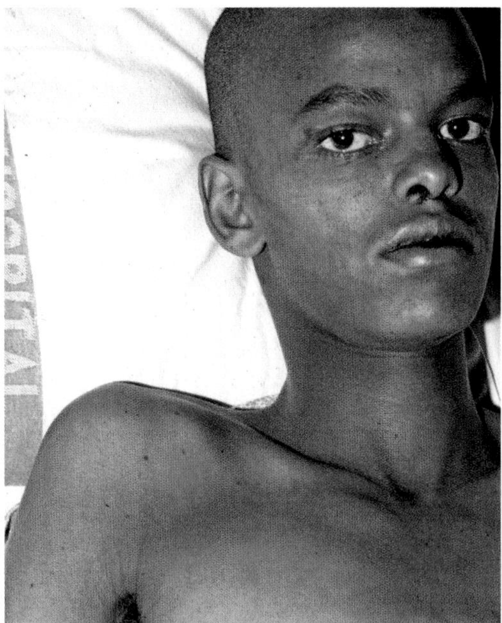

Fig. 7.6.33.9 Ethiopian patient with LBRF showing petechiae on the shoulder and epistaxis.
(Copyright D A Warrell.)

fatigue, prostration, and drenching sweats. These symptoms are similar to those in LBRF but the initial fever usually lasts about 3 days only to recur about 7 to 15 days later. Epistaxis, abdominal pain, diarrhoea, cough, and erythematous or petechial rashes may follow. Jaundice is less common than in LBRF. Several cases of acute respiratory distress syndrome (ARDS) have been described in the United States of America. Neurological disturbances are more common than in LBRF, varying in incidence with the borrelia species involved, from less than 5% in patients with *B. hispanica* and *B. persica* infections to as high as 40% in patients with *B. duttonii*. However, one careful study in northern Tanzania found no focal neurological abnormalities in patients with *B. duttonii* TBRF. The neurological features that have been described are reminiscent of Lyme neuroborreliosis and include paraesthesias, visual symptoms, lymphocytic meningitis, cranial nerve palsies (especially VII),

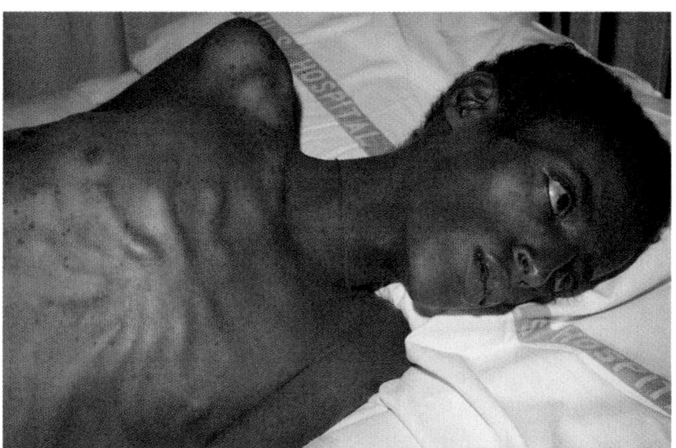

Fig. 7.6.33.10 Ethiopian patient with severe LBRF complicated by typhoid, showing jaundice, petechial haemorrhages, and emaciation.
(Copyright D A Warrell.)

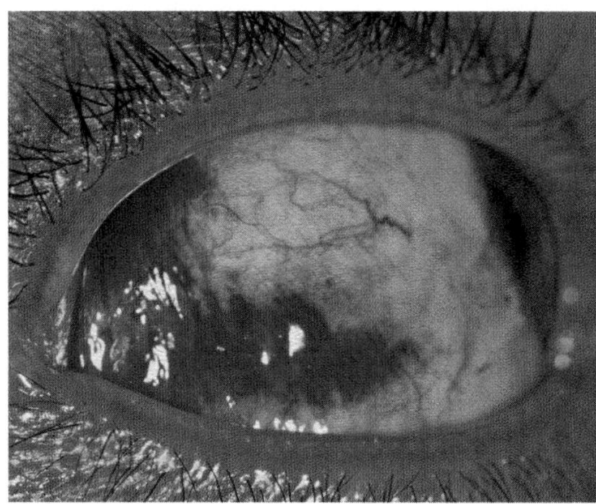

Fig. 7.6.33.11 Subconjunctival haemorrhage in a patient with LBRF.
(Copyright D A Warrell.)

encephalitis, myelitis, sciatica, and radiculitis. Untreated patients may have up to 13 relapses (Fig. 7.6.33.2), becoming sequentially less severe. Ocular complications usually occur during the third and fourth relapses. They include conjunctival injection, eye pain, photophobia, eyelid oedema, keratitis, various degrees of anterior and posterior uveitis, optic neuritis, and blindness.

Spirochaetaemia is higher in pregnant than in nonpregnant women and abortion and perinatal mortality are common. In Tabora, Tanzania, parturition was precipitated in 58% of infected pregnant women. Perinatal mortality was 436/1000 births, its risk related to low birthweight and gestational age, and total fetal wastage was 475/1000.

Children

In endemic areas of *B. duttonii* TBRF in East Africa, most cases are in children, many of them under 5 years old, and pregnant women, implying that older nonpregnant people may acquired some immunity. Fever, splenomegaly, convulsions sometimes recurrent, meningism, petechiae, and jaundice are described. Neonates with congenital infection have fever, inability to suck, jaundice, and features of septicaemia. Reported case fatalities in children less than 1 year old are 2.3 to 73%, compared to 1.6 to 19% in older children.

Severe disease

Severe manifestations include hyperpyrexia, myocarditis with acute pulmonary oedema, ARDS, hepatic failure, ruptured spleen, and haemostatic failure attributable to thrombocytopenia, liver damage, and disseminated intravascular coagulation leading to cerebral, massive gastrointestinal, pulmonary, or peripartum haemorrhage. Dysentery, salmonellosis, typhoid, typhus, tuberculosis, bacterial pneumonia, and malaria are infections that can complicate relapsing fever, increasing the risk of death.

The spontaneous crisis and Jarisch–Herxheimer reaction

Whether or not treatment is given, attacks of relapsing fever usually end dramatically. On about the fifth day of the untreated illness, or about 1 to 2 h after antibiotic treatment, the patient becomes restless and apprehensive and suddenly begins to have distressingly intense rigors that last between 10 and 30 min. The ensuing phenomena have features of a classic endotoxin reaction. During the initial chill phase, temperature, respiratory and pulse rates, and blood pressure rise sharply. Delirium, gastrointestinal symptoms, cough, and limb pains are associated. Some patients die of hyperpyrexia at the peak of fever. The flush phase, which lasts many hours, is characterized by profuse sweating, a fall in blood pressure, and a slow decline in temperature. Deaths during this phase follow intractable hypotension, sudden postural hypotension prompted by the patient's standing up, or the development of acute pulmonary oedema attributable to myocarditis. The incidence of JHRs is highest in adults with LBRF treated with intravenous tetracycline (approaching 100% in some studies). It is lower when low-dose or slow-release penicillin is used and in children. JHR is less commonly observed in TBRF but can be severe and even fatal.

The classic JHR is in secondary syphilis in which the spirochaetes are in the tissues and the reaction is less frequent, more insidious, and much less severe than in relapsing fevers. Milder reactions have been described in Lyme disease and leptospirosis (treated with penicillin), sodoku (treated with arsenicals), *Brucella melitensis* (treated with tetracycline), and even in typhoid and meningococcal infections.

Laboratory findings

Spirochaete densities may exceed 500 000/mm^3 of blood. There is a moderate normochromic anaemia and a neutrophil leucocytosis with marked leucopenia during the spontaneous crisis and JHR. Thrombocytopenia is usual and there is a mild coagulopathy with evidence of increased fibrinolysis. Biochemical evidence of hepatocellular damage (raised levels of aminotransferases, alkaline phosphatase, direct and total bilirubin, low albumin) and mild renal impairment are common. The cerebrospinal fluid shows a lymphocyte or neutrophil pleocytosis without visible spirochaetes.

There is ECG evidence of myocarditis including prolongation of the QTc interval, T-wave abnormalities, and ST-segment depression with transient acute right heart strain after the JHR. Chest radiographs may show pulmonary oedema or pneumonic consolidation.

Diagnosis

Thick and thin blood films should be taken while patients are febrile. Spirochaetes are demonstrated by Giemsa's, Wright's, Field's, or Diff-Quick staining (Fig. 7.6.33.1), dark-field examination, or a quantitative buffy coat technique (acridine orange). The sensitivity of thick films is 20 times greater than thin films. Misidentification of *Plasmodium vivax* microgametes as spirochaetes has led to the diagnosis of 'pseudoborreliosis'. In TBRF, spirochaetes may be difficult or impossible to find even at the height of a relapse and, increasingly, PCR and serology are being used. Lyme disease borreliae may produce cross-reacting antibodies due to expression of conserved antigenic epitopes, but an ELISA using the glycerophosphodiester phosphodiesterase (GlpQ) gene product can distinguish relapsing fevers from Lyme disease. In LBRF, the higher and more persistent spirochaetaemia is more easily detected. Borreliae can be isolated in mice and cultured *in vitro*.

The serum of patients with relapsing fever may give positive reactions with proteus OXK, OX19, and OX2 and false-positive serological responses for syphilis in 5 to 10% of cases.

Differential diagnosis

In a febrile patient with jaundice, petechial rash, bleeding, hepatosplenomegaly, thrombocytopenia, coagulopathy, and elevated serum aminotransferases, the most frequent and urgent differential diagnosis is falciparum malaria. Yellow fever and other viral haemorrhagic fevers such as Rift Valley Fever in the Horn of Africa, viral hepatitis, rickettsial infections (especially louse-borne typhus which shares LBRF's epidemiological predispositions), and leptospirosis may also cause confusion. Trench fever (*Bartonella quintana*) transmitted by lice, and sodoku (*Spirillum minus*) following a rat bite can also cause episodic recurrent fever. Although the diagnosis of relapsing fever can often be confirmed quickly by examining a blood smear, the possibility of complicating bacterial infection, particularly typhoid, or coinfection with malaria should never be forgotten.

Prognosis

During major LBRF epidemics, overall case fatalities of 40% or higher have been reported, but in treated cases they are less than 5%. TBRF is less dangerous and deaths during relapses are most unusual but have been reported. In both LBRF and TBRF, pregnant women and infants are at greatest risk of dying.

Treatment

Antibiotics

LBRF

LBRF is readily cured without relapses by a single oral dose of 500 mg tetracycline or 500 mg erythromycin stearate. However, since few patients with severe LBRF are able to swallow tablets without vomiting them up, a more reliable treatment is a single intravenous dose of 250 mg tetracycline hydrochloride or, for pregnant women and children, a single intravenous dose of 300 mg erythromycin lactobionate (children 10 mg/kg body weight). In mixed epidemics of LBRF and louse-borne typhus, a single oral dose of 100 mg doxycycline proved effective.

Benzylpenicillin (300 000 units), procaine penicillin with benzylpenicillin (600 000 units), and procaine penicillin with aluminium monostearate (600 000 units), all by intramuscular injection, are often effective but may fail to prevent relapses. Long-acting preparations clear spirochaetaemia slowly and the JHR is protracted. Some experienced clinicians prefer to use a low initial dose of penicillin (adult dose, 100 000–400 000 units by intramuscular injection) in severe cases and pregnant women because they believe that the incidence and severity of the JHRs will be less.

Chloramphenicol is effective in a single dose of 500 mg by mouth or intravenous injection in adults.

TBRF

Although TBRF is usually milder than LBRF, it is more difficult to treat because spirochaetes persist in tissues, such as the central nervous system and eye, and produce relapses. Oral tetracycline, 500 mg every 6 h for 10 days is, however, effective. Oral erythromycin can be given to pregnant women (500 mg every 6 h for 10 days) and children (125–250 mg every 6 h for 10 days). In patients unable to swallow tablets, treatment can be initiated with 250 mg intravenous tetracycline hydrochloride or with 300 mg erythromycin lactobionate.

Chloramphenicol is effective in a dose of 500 mg every 6 h for 10 days in adults, and 250 mg every 6 h for 10 days in older children.

JHR

Antimicrobials have reduced the mortality of relapsing fevers from 30 to 70% to less than 5%. However, drugs such as tetracycline, which rapidly eliminate spirochaetes from the blood and prevent relapses, usually induce a severe JHR that may occasionally prove fatal. Clearly, in a disease with such a high natural mortality, treatment cannot be withheld, especially as severe spontaneous crises, which may also prove fatal, occur in a large proportion of LBRF cases after the fifth day of fever. There is no evidence, however, that the shorter and more intense reaction following tetracycline is more dangerous than the more prolonged but apparently milder reaction following slow-release penicillin. Neither hydrocortisone in doses up to 20 mg/kg nor paracetamol prevent the JHR but they reduce peak temperatures, hastens the fall in temperature, and lessens the fall in blood pressure during the flush phase. Pretreatment with oral prednisolone can prevent the JHR of early syphilis, but in LBRF neither an oral dose of 3 mg/kg prednisolone given 18 h beforehand nor an infusion of 3.75 mg/kg betamethasone prevented the reaction to tetracycline treatment. However, meptazinol, an opioid antagonist/agonist, diminishes the reaction when given in a dose of 100 mg by intravenous injection. The discovery of an explosive release of TNFα, IL-6, and IL-8 just before the start of the JHR prompted the testing of a polyclonal ovine Fab anti-TNFα antibody. When infused for 30 min before treatment with intramuscular penicillin, this antibody suppressed the JHR.

Supportive treatment

Patients must be nursed in bed for at least 24 h after treatment to prevent postural hypotensive collapse and the precipitation of fatal cardiac arrhythmias. Hyperpyrexia should be prevented with antipyretics, vigorous fanning, and tepid sponging. Although patients with acute LBRF have an expanded plasma volume, most are dehydrated and relatively hypovolaemic. Adults may need 4 litres or more of isotonic saline intravenously during the first 24 h. Infusion should be controlled by monitoring jugular venous or central venous pressures. Acute myocardial failure may develop, particularly during the flush phase of the JHR or spontaneous crisis. This is signalled by a rise in central venous pressure above 15 cmH_2O; 1 mg digoxin given intravenously over 5 to 10 min has proved effective in this emergency. Because of the intense vasodilatation, diuretics may accentuate the circulatory failure by causing relative hypovolaemia. Oxygen should be given during the reaction, particularly in severe cases. Vitamin K should be given to all patients with prolonged prothrombin times. Heparin is not effective in controlling coagulopathy and should not be used. Complicating infections (typhoid, salmonellosis, bacillary dysentery, tuberculosis, typhus, malaria) must be treated appropriately.

Prevention and control

No vaccines are available.

LBRF: delousing

Infested clothing should be deloused using heat (>60°C), chlorine bleach, or insecticide (10% dichlorodiphenyltrichloroethane (DDT), 1% malathion, 2% temephos, 1% propoxur, or 0.5% permethrin), and patients should be bathed with soap and 1% Lysol (cresol). Lice are abundant in hair, which should be washed or shaved off. Breaking transmission from lice to the susceptible population is essential for the control of an epidemic.

TBRF: tick control

Tick infestation of dwellings can be reduced by improved house construction (e.g. rodent-proofing of cabins on the North Rim of the Grand Canyon), control of peridomestic rodent hosts, and use of residual insecticides (pyrethroids, benzene hexachloride, λ-cyhalothrin, malathion, or DDT). Travellers should avoid sleeping in places where ticks and rodents are abundant, such as poorly maintained log cabins, should apply repellents to their skin (diethyl toluamide (DEET)), and should sleep under insecticide-impregnated bed nets. Postexposure prophylaxis with doxycycline (200mg followed by 100mg on the next 4 days) proved effective against *B.persica* in Israel.

Further reading

Balicer RD *et al.* (2010). Post exposure prophylaxis of tick-borne relapsing fever. *Eur J Clin Microbiol Infect Dis*, [Epub ahead of print] PMID: 20012878.

Barbour AG, Hayes SF (1986). Biology of *Borrelia* species. *Microbiol Rev*, **50**, 381–400.

Brouqui P, Stein A, Dupont HT (2005). Ectoparasitism and vector-borne diseases in 930 homeless people from Marseilles. *Medicine (Baltimore)*, **84**, 61–8.

Bryceson ADM, *et al.* (1970). Louse-borne relapsing fever. A clinical and laboratory study of 62 cases in Ethiopia and a reconsideration of the literature. *QJM*, **39**, 129–70.

Burman N, Shamaei-Tousi A, Bergström S (1998). The spirochete *Borrelia crocidurae* causes erythrocyte rosetting during relapsing fever. *Infect Immun*, **66**, 815–9.

Cadavid D, Barbour AG (1998). Neuroborreliosis during relapsing fever: review of the clinical manifestations, pathology, and treatment of infections in humans and experimental animals. *Clin Infect Dis*, **26**, 151–64.

Fekade D, *et al.* (1996). Prevention of Jarisch-Herxheimer reactions by treatment with antibodies against tumor necrosis factor alpha. *N Engl J Med*, **335**, 311–5.

Felsenfeld O (1971). *Borrelia: strains, vectors, human and animal borreliosis.* Green, St Louis.

Hasin T, *et al.* (2006). Postexposure treatment with doxycycline for the prevention of tick-borne relapsing fever. *N Engl J Med*, **355**, 148–55.

Jongen VH, *et al.* (1997). Tick-borne relapsing fever and pregnancy outcome in rural Tanzania. *Acta Obstet Gynecol Scand*, **76**, 834–8.

LaRocca TJ, Benach JL (2008). The important and diverse roles of antibodies in the host response to borrelia infections. *Curr Top Microbiol Immunol*, **319**, 63–103.

Larsson C, *et al.* (2009). Current issues in relapsing fever. *Curr Opin Infect Dis*, **22**, 443–9.

Mayegga E, *et al.* (2005). Absence of focal neurological involvement in tick-borne relapsing fever in northern Tanzania. *Eur J Neurol*, **12**, 449–52.

McCall PJ, *et al.* (2007). Does tick-borne relapsing fever have an animal reservoir in East Africa? *Vector Borne Zoonotic Dis*, **7**, 659–66.

Negussie Y, *et al.* (1992). Detection of plasma tumor necrosis factor, interleukins 6, and 8 during the Jarisch-Herxheimer Reaction of relapsing fever. *J Exp Med*, **175**, 1207–12.

Parry EH, *et al.* (1970). Some effects of louse-borne relapsing fever on the function of the heart. *Am J Med*, **49**, 472–9.

Perine PL, Teklu B (1983). Antibiotic treatment of louse-borne relapsing fever in Ethiopia: a report of 377 cases. *Am J Trop Med Hyg*, **32**, 1096–100.

Rebaudet S, Parola P (2006). Epidemiology of relapsing fever borreliosis in Europe. *FEMS Immunol Med Microbiol*, **48**, 11–5.

Seboxa T, Rahlenbeck SI (1995). Treatment of louse-borne relapsing fever with low dose penicillin or tetracycline: a clinical trial. *Scand J Infect Dis*, **27**, 29–31.

Vial L, *et al.* (2006). Incidence of tick-borne relapsing fever in West Africa: longitudinal study. *Lancet*, **368**, 37–43.

Vidal V, *et al.* (1998). Variable major lipoprotein is a principal TNF-inducing factor of louse-borne relapsing fever. *Nat Med*, **4**, 1416–20.

Warrell DA, *et al.* (1970). Cardiorespiratory disturbances associated with infective fever in man: studies of Ethiopian louse-borne relapsing fever. *Clin Sci*, **39**, 123–45.

Warrell DA, *et al.* (1971). Physiologic changes during the Jarisch–Herxheimer reaction in early syphilis. A comparison with louse-borne relapsing fever. *Am J Med*, **51**, 176–85.

Warrell DA, *et al.* (1983). Pathophysiology and immunology of the Jarisch–Herxheimer-like reaction in louse-borne relapsing fever: comparison of tetracycline and slow-release penicillin. *J Infect Dis*, **147**, 898–909.

7.6.34 Leptospirosis

George Watt

Essentials

Leptospirosis is a worldwide zoonosis of greatest importance in the tropics that is caused by spirochaetes of the 16 species of the genus *Leptospira*. Rodents are the most important reservoir, with transmission of infection usually occurring through contact with contaminated water or moist soil. Organisms enter the human body through abrasions of the skin or through mucosal surfaces.

Clinical features—subclinical infection is common, but symptomatic disease typically begins with abrupt onset of intense headache, fever, chills, and myalgia. Conjunctival suffusion is a helpful diagnostic clue. Most patients recover within a week, but some then relapse, commonly with meningitis. Less than 10% of symptomatic infections result in severe, icteric illness (Weil's disease) that is characterized by jaundice, renal dysfunction, haemorrhagic manifestations, and high mortality. Leptospirosis-associated severe pulmonary haemorrhage syndrome, which can occur either with or without jaundice and renal failure, has a case fatality rate of about 50%.

Diagnosis—most cases go undiagnosed because serological confirmation is rarely available where most disease transmission occurs. The gold standard microscopic agglutination test is impracticable, and commercially available rapid serodiagnostic kits have unacceptably low sensitivities and lack specificity in regions of high endemic transmission.

Treatment and prognosis—aside from supportive care, antibiotics should be given to all patients with leptospirosis, regardless of age, the stage of their disease, or fear of a possible Jarisch–Herxheimer reaction. High-dose intravenous penicillin is the treatment of choice for adults and children with severe, late disease: doxycycline, ceftriaxone, cefotaxime, and azithromycin are effective in mild disease. Ensuring adequate renal perfusion prevents renal failure in most oliguric patients. Failure to make the diagnosis of leptospirosis is particularly unfortunate: severely ill patients with leptospirosis often recover completely with prompt treatment, but they may die if therapy is delayed or not given.

Introduction

Leptospirosis is a worldwide zoonosis of the greatest public health importance in the tropics. Infection may be asymptomatic, but 5 to 15% of cases are severe or fatal. Most cases go undiagnosed because symptoms and signs are often nonspecific and serological confirmation is rarely available where most disease transmission occurs. Failure to diagnose leptospirosis is particularly unfortunate as severely ill patients often recover completely with prompt treatment, but if therapy is delayed or not given death or renal failure are likely to ensue.

Aetiology

The organism responsible is a tightly coiled spirochaete with an axial filament and hooked ends, 0.1 to 0.2 µm wide, and 5 to 20 µm long. Leptospires are aerobic and travel with a corkscrew-like motion. Unstained organisms can be seen only by dark-field or phase-contrast microscopy. Silver staining is the method of choice for demonstrating leptospires in tissue specimens. Previously, the genus *Leptospira* contained two species, *Leptospira interrogans*, which was pathogenic, and *L. biflexa*, which was saprophytic. Stable antigenic differences allowed subclassification into serotypes, referred to in the literature as serovars (serovarieties). Antigens common to several serovars permitted arrangement into broader serogroups. More than 250 serovars belonging to 24 serogroups were identified for *L. interrogans*. Leptospirosis taxonomy is evolving, however, and the genus *Leptospira* has now been reclassified, based on DNA relatedness, into 16 species including at least 7 pathogenic species: *L. interrogans*, *L. borgpetersenii*, *L. inadai*, *L. noguchii*, *L. santarosai*, *L. weilii*, and *L. kirschneri*. The sequencing of the genome of *L. interrogans* was recently completed, and this advance should facilitate future advances in diagnosis and vaccine development, and provide insights into pathogenesis.

Epidemiology

Measuring incidence by active surveillance confirms that leptospirosis is a surprisingly common disease. Antibody positivity rates of 37% have been recorded in rural Belize and 23% in Vietnam. More than 2527 human cases and 13 deaths were reported for the first 9 months of 1999 by the Ministry of Public Health in Thailand. There was a sustained outbreak between 1998 and 2003. Multilocus sequence typing linked this outbreak to the emergence of a single dominant clone of *L. interrogans* serovar Autumnalis. Bandicoot rats (*Bandicota indica* and *B. savilei*) served as the reservoir. Human leptospirosis is an important disease in China, south-east Asia, India, Africa, and South and Central America. It is also of significance in eastern and southern Europe, Australia, and New Zealand. In the United States of America, the disease is primarily of veterinary importance, with only 50 to 150 human cases reported annually.

Leptospires nest in the renal tubules of mammalian hosts and are shed in the urine. They can survive for several months in the environment under moist conditions, particularly in the presence of warmth (above 22°C) and a neutral pH (pH 6.2 to 8.0). These conditions occur all year round in the tropics but only during the summer and autumn months in temperate climates. Roughly 160 animal species harbour organisms, but rodents are the most important reservoir. Carrier rates of over 50% have been measured in Norway rats, which shed massive numbers of organisms for life without showing clinical illness. Some serovars appear to be preferentially adapted to select mammalian hosts. For example, *L. interrogans* serovar Icterohaemorrhagiae is primarily associated with the Norway rat, *L. interrogans* serovar Canicola with dogs, and *L. interrogans* serovar Pomona with swine and cattle. However, a particular host species may serve as a reservoir for one or more serovars and a particular serovar may be hosted by many different animal species.

The transmission of infection from animals to humans usually occurs through contact with contaminated water or moist soil. Organisms enter humans through abrasions of the skin or through the mucosal surface of the eye, mouth, nasopharynx, or oesophagus. Crowded Asian or Latin American cities that are flood-prone and have large rat populations provide ideal conditions for disease transmission. Escalating migration of the rural poor to urban slums is likely to further exacerbate the risks of leptospirosis transmission. An outbreak in Nicaragua in 1995 and an urban epidemic in Salvador, Brazil in 1999 were associated with particularly heavy rains and flooding. Intense exposure to leptospires has been documented in rice, sugar cane, and rubber plantation workers. Less frequently, leptospirosis is acquired by direct contact with the blood, urine, or tissues of infected animals. Epidemiological patterns in the United States of America and the United Kingdom have changed. Recreational exposure to fresh water (canoeing, sailing, water skiing) and animal contact at home have replaced occupational exposure as the chief source of disease. During the 10-day Eco-Challenge-Sabah 2000 multisport endurance race, 26% of 304 athletes caught leptospirosis.

Pathology and pathogenesis

Leptospires are disseminated by the blood and may be recovered from all organs within 48 h of entering the host. Leptospiraemia lasts from 4 to 7 days and ends when agglutinating antibodies appear. Leptospires can persist for months in the kidneys and ocular tissue. Much of the pathogenesis of leptospirosis remains unexplained. There are only minor histopathological changes in the kidneys and livers of patients with marked functional impairment of these organs. Patients who survive severe leptospirosis have complete recovery of hepatic and renal function, which is consistent with the lack of structural damage to these organs.

Severely ill patients typically have marked leucocytosis but no leucocytic infiltrates in organs, a pattern produced by some toxins. Fatally infected animals and some human patients exhibit changes similar to those produced by the endotoxaemia of Gram-negative bacteraemia. An endotoxin-like substance is present in the cell wall of leptospires but lacks the ketodeoxyoctanoate of a true endotoxin.

Kidney

Renal failure is the most common cause of death in leptospirosis. Leptospires are frequently found in human renal tissue, but their role in mediating kidney damage is unknown. Interstitial nephritis is found primarily in individuals who have survived until inflammation has had an opportunity to develop, but is frequently absent in patients with fulminant disease.

Impaired renal perfusion constitutes the fundamental nephropathic change. Oliguria is rapidly reversed by administration of intravenous fluid in many patients, suggesting that volume depletion is frequent. Hypovolaemia is multifactorial and insensible water loss, diarrhoea, vomiting, reduced fluid intake, and haemorrhage can all contribute. A defect in the kidney's ability to concentrate urine increases fluid loss while renal potassium wasting can lead to hypokalaemia. This unique nonoliguric hypokalaemic renal insufficiency is characterized by impaired proximal sodium reabsorption, increased distal sodium delivery, and potassium wasting. Renal magnesium wasting has been demonstrated more recently but its clinical significance is not known. Widespread endothelial injury causes fluid to move from the intravascular to the extracellular space in some patients. Hypotension of cardiac origin is rare.

Liver

The pathogenesis of jaundice is unexplained; neither haemolytic anaemia nor hepatocellular necrosis are prominent features of leptospirosis. The most severe hepatic pathological changes are seen when organisms are difficult to demonstrate in tissue, suggesting subcellular toxic or metabolic insults.

Striated muscle

Myalgia is typical of early infection, and is presumably due to invasion of skeletal muscle by leptospires. Muscle biopsies in patients with early illness demonstrate vacuolation of the myofibrillar cytoplasm, loss of cellular detail, and fragmentation. Leptospiral antigen can be demonstrated by immunofluorescence within muscle tissue. Muscle pain resolves as antibody appears and organisms are cleared from the blood. Pathological changes are usually absent in muscle tissue from patients who have died, and myalgia is generally waning at the time of death.

Lungs

Localized or confluent haemorrhagic pneumonitis is the usual pulmonary finding, with petechial and ecchymotic haemorrhages noted throughout the lungs, pleura, and tracheobronchial tree. Early life-threatening pulmonary haemorrhage has long been reported from Asia, and is now being increasingly recognized in Latin America. Necropsy findings include massive intra-alveolar haemorrhage with or without diffuse alveolar damage. Leptospires can be demonstrated in lung tissue, but few intact organisms are seen at autopsy suggesting a possible immune-mediated process. Indeed, leptospirosis pulmonary haemmorrhage syndrome was recently shown to be associated with linear deposition of immunoglobulin and complement on the alveolar surface.

Haemorrhage

A progressive severe haemorrhagic diathesis is a prominent feature of experimental leptospirosis. In humans, bleeding is generally restricted to the skin or mucosal surfaces, although occasionally massive gastrointestinal or pulmonary haemorrhage occurs. Coagulopathy and/or thrombocytopenia are common in leptospirosis but do not adequately explain bleeding. By exclusion, capillary damage is the postulated mechanism, and toxins have been suggested as the mediators of endothelial injury.

Meningitis

Organisms easily enter the cerebrospinal fluid during leptospiraemia, and this is thought to explain the high incidence of meningitis. However, signs of meningeal irritation are not due to the invasion of the meninges by leptospires, a process that elicits little reaction. Organisms are frequently isolated from cerebrospinal fluid that is otherwise normal and from individuals without clinically detectable involvement of the nervous system. Symptoms of meningitis coincide with the development of antibody and disappearance of leptospires from the blood and cerebrospinal fluid, suggesting an immunological mechanism. Pathological changes are minimal or absent, and the prognosis is excellent.

Heart

Focal haemorrhagic myocarditis has been reported, but hypovolaemia, electrolyte imbalance, and uraemia are more frequent causes of cardiac dysfunction. Minor electrocardiographic changes such as first-degree heart block are common and reversible, but serious dysrhythmias also occur.

Eye

The aqueous humour provides a protective environment for leptospires, which readily enter the anterior chamber of the eye during the leptospiraemic phase of the disease. There they can remain viable for months, despite the development of serum antibodies. Uveitis is common. Inflammation of the anterior uveal tract begins weeks or even months after the onset of disease and has been attributed to the persistence of organisms in the anterior chamber.

Clinical manifestations

Subclinical infection is common and less than 10% of symptomatic infections result in severe icteric illness. Even relatively virulent serovars such as *L. interrogans* serovar Icterohaemorrhagiae lead more often to anicteric than to icteric disease. Old terms such as pea-picker's disease, swineherd's disease, and canicola fever, which linked specific serotypes with distinct disease manifestations, are misleading and should be abandoned. The median incubation period is 10 days, with a range of 2 to 26 days. The duration of the incubation period has no prognostic significance. Once symptoms develop (see Table 7.6.34.1), they are said to follow a biphasic course. After an initial febrile illness, there is defervescence of fever and symptomatic improvement, followed by a second period of disease. However, a clear demarcation between the first and second stages is atypical of icteric leptospirosis and in mild cases the distinction can be unclear, or the second stage may never occur. The diagnostic usefulness of a history of a biphasic illness has been overemphasized. HIV coinfection does not seem to affect the clinical presentation of leptospirosis in the few coinfected patients described thus far.

Table 7.6.34.1 The most common clinical manifestations of 208 leptospirosis patients in Puerto Rico

Symptoms (% of cases)	Anicteric (106cases)	Icteric (102cases)
Fever	100	99
Myalgia	97	97
Headache	82	95
Chills	84	90
Sore throat	72	87
Nausea	71	81
Vomiting	65	75
Eye pain	54	38
Diarrhoea	23	30
Decreased urine	20	30
Cough	15	32
Haemoptysis	5	14
Signs (% of cases)		
Conjunctival injection	100	98
Muscle tenderness	70	79
Hepatomegaly	60	60
Pulmonary findings	11	36
Lymphadenopathy	35	12
Petechiae and ecchymoses	4	29

(Adapted from Diaz-Rivera RS *et al.* (1963). *Zoonosis Research* **2**, 159.)

Anicteric leptospirosis

Symptoms and signs

Typically, the disease begins with the abrupt onset of intense headache, fever, chills, and myalgia. Fever often exceeds 40°C (103°F) and is preceded by rigors. Muscle pain can be excruciating and occurs most commonly in the thighs, calves, lumbosacral region, and abdomen. Abdominal wall pain accompanied by palpation tenderness can mimic an acute surgical abdomen. Nausea, vomiting, diarrhoea, and sore throat are other frequent symptoms. Cough and chest pain figure prominently in reports of patients from Korea and China.

Conjunctival suffusion is a helpful diagnostic clue which usually appears 2 or 3 days after the onset of fever and involves the bulbar conjunctiva. Pus and serous secretions are absent, and there is no matting of the eyelashes and eyelids. Mild suffusion can easily be overlooked. Less common and less distinctive signs include pharyngeal injection, splenomegaly, hepatomegaly, lymphadenopathy, and skin lesions.

Within a week most patients become asymptomatic. After several days of apparent recovery, the illness resumes in some individuals. Manifestations of the second stage are milder and more variable than those of the initial illness and usually last 2 to 4 days. Leptospires disappear from the blood, cerebrospinal fluid, and tissues but appear in the urine. Serum antibody titres rise, hence the term 'immune' phase. Meningitis is the hallmark of this stage of leptospirosis. Pleocytosis of the cerebrospinal fluid can be demonstrated in 80 to 90% of all patients during the second week of illness, although only about 50% will have clinical signs and symptoms of meningitis. Meningeal signs can last several weeks but usually resolve within a day or two. Uveitis is a late manifestation of leptospirosis, generally seen 4 to 8 months after the illness has begun. The anterior uveal tract is most frequently affected, and pain, photophobia, and blurring of vision are the usual symptoms.

Laboratory findings

The white blood cell count varies but neutrophilia is usually found. Urinalysis may show proteinuria, pyuria, and microscopic haematuria. Enzyme markers of skeletal muscle damage, such as creatinine kinase and aldolase, are elevated in the sera of 50% of patients during the first week of illness. Chest radiographs from patients with pulmonary manifestations show a variety of abnormalities, but none is pathognomonic of leptospirosis. The most common finding is small patchy snowflake-like lesions in the periphery of the lung fields.

Icteric leptospirosis (Weil's disease)

Symptoms and signs

This dramatic and life-threatening illness is characterized by jaundice, renal dysfunction, haemorrhagic manifestations, and a high mortality rate. Although jaundice is the hallmark of severe leptospirosis, fatalities do not occur because of liver failure. The degree of jaundice has no prognostic significance, but its presence or absence does; virtually all leptospirosis renal deaths occur in icteric patients. Icterus first appears between the fifth and ninth days of illness, reaches maximum intensity 4 or 5 days later, and continues for an average of 1 month. Hepatomegaly is found in the majority of patients and hepatic percussion tenderness is a reliable clinical marker of continuing disease activity. There is no residual liver dysfunction in survivors of Weil's disease, consistent with the absence of structural damage seen on pathological examination of this organ.

Bleeding is occasionally seen in anicteric cases but is most prevalent in severe disease. Purpura, petechiae, epistaxis, bleeding of the gums, and minor haemoptysis are the most common haemorrhagic manifestations, but deaths occur from subarachnoid haemorrhage and exsanguination from gastrointestinal bleeding. Conjunctival haemorrhage is an extremely useful diagnostic finding and, when combined with scleral icterus and conjunctival suffusion, produces eye findings strongly suggestive of leptospirosis (Fig. 7.6.34.1). The frequency with which severe pulmonary haemorrhage complicates leptospirosis is variable, but is a cardinal feature of some outbreaks.

Life-threatening renal failure is a complication of icteric disease, although all forms of leptospirosis may be associated with mild kidney dysfunction. Oliguria or anuria usually develop during the second week of illness, but may appear earlier. Complete anuria is a grave prognostic sign, often seen in patients who present late in the course of illness with frank uraemia and irreversible disease. Because renal failure develops very quickly in leptospirosis, symptoms and signs of uraemia are frequently encountered. Anorexia, vomiting, drowsiness, disorientation, and confusion are seen early and progress rapidly to convulsions, stupor, and coma in severe cases. Disturbances of consciousness in a patient with severe leptospirosis are usually due to uraemic encephalopathy, whereas in anicteric patients aseptic encephalitis is the usual cause. Renal function eventually returns to normal in survivors of Weil's disease, although detectable abnormalities may persist for several months.

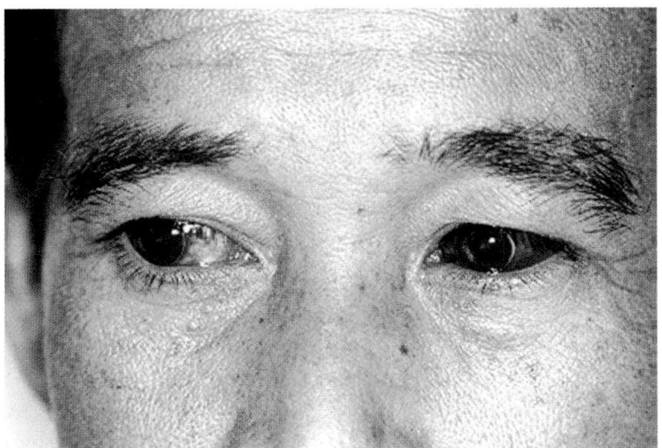

Fig. 7.6.34.1 Jaundice, haemorrhage, and conjunctival suffusion in acute leptospirosis.

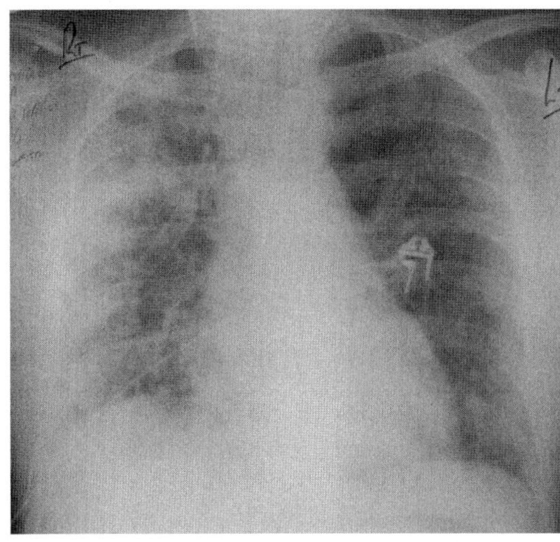

Fig. 7.6.34.2 Chest radiograph of a European traveller with leptospirosis-associated severe pulmonary haemorrhage syndrome acquired in Sabah (Malaysia).
(Copyright D A Warrell.)

Leptospirosis-associated severe pulmonary haemorrhage syndrome (SPHS) is now recognized as a widespread public health problem with a case fatality rate of about 50% (Fig. 7.6.34.2). This lethal complication of leptospirosis can occur either with or without jaundice and renal failure. Haemoptysis is the cardinal sign, but may not be apparent until patients are intubated. Real-time polymerase chain reaction has shown that the apparent critical threshold for severe outcomes such as SPHS and death is a leptospiraemia of 10 000 or more bacteria/ml of blood.

Laboratory findings

Hyperbilirubinaemia results from increases in both conjugated (direct) and unconjugated (indirect) bilirubin, but elevations of the direct fraction predominate. Prolongations of the prothrombin time occur commonly but are easily corrected by the administration of vitamin K; modest elevations of serum alkaline phosphatase are typical. There is mild hepatocellular necrosis; greater than fivefold increases of transaminase (aminotransferase) levels are exceptional.

Jaundiced patients usually have a leucocytosis in the range of 15 to 30×10^9/litre, and neutrophilia is constant. Anaemia is common and multifactorial; blood loss and azotaemia contribute frequently, and intravascular haemolysis less often. Mild thrombocytopenia often occurs, but decreases in platelet count sufficient to be associated with bleeding are exceptional. The specific gravity of the urine is high. Hypokalaemia and hypomagnesaemia due to renal potassium and magnesium wasting can occur.

Diagnosis

Late disease can often be recognized by its typical clinical manifestations, but the presentation of early leptospirosis is usually nonspecific and is therefore difficult to identify clinically. Leptospirosis has long been acknowledged to be a frequent cause of undifferentiated febrile illness in developing countries. Coinfection with diseases such as malaria and scrub typhus have been reported and add to the diagnostic confusion of tropical fevers.

The laboratory diagnosis of leptospirosis remains problematic. The microscopic agglutination test is considered the serodiagnostic method of choice for leptospirosis, but its complexity limits its use to reference laboratories. Dilutions of patient sera are applied to a panel of live pathogenic leptospires. The results are viewed under dark-field microscopy and expressed as the percentage of organisms cleared from the field by agglutination. Inadequate quality controls of the live reference strain panels required can lead to frequent false-negative results. A new generation of commercially available rapid serodiagnostic kits that rely on whole leptospira antigen preparations have been developed. Unfortunately these assays seem to have unacceptably low sensitivities during acute-phase illness and persistent antibody produces low specificity in regions of high endemic transmission. The need for practical and affordable diagnostic kits to be available in areas where leptospirosis is common cannot be overemphasized. Polymerase chain reaction and urine antigen detection are research tools which would be of the greatest potential diagnostic value in patients who present early, before antibodies have reached detectable levels.

Isolation of leptospires from blood or cerebrospinal fluid is possible during the first 10 days of clinical illness, but specialized media are necessary. Serially diluted urine provides the highest yield. Unfortunately, culture results are only known 4 to 6 weeks later, too late to benefit hospitalized severely ill patients.

Treatment

The approach to the patient with possible leptospirosis is summarized in Fig. 7.6.34.3. Placebo-controlled double-blind trials have proved that doxycycline benefits patients with early mild leptospirosis, and that intravenous penicillin helps adults with severe late disease. The outcome of severe paediatric leptospirosis is also improved by penicillin therapy. Antibiotics should therefore be given to all patients with leptospirosis, regardless of age or when in their disease course they are seen. Doxycycline is given at doses of 100 mg orally twice a day for 1 week. Patients who are vomiting or are seriously ill require parenteral therapy. Intravenous penicillin G is administered as 1.5 million units every 6 h for 1 week. Recent trials from Thailand indicate that treatment with ceftriaxone, cefotaxime, and doxycycline had equivalent efficacy to penicillin in patients with mild to moderately severe disease. However, it is not known whether these antibiotics are as effective as high-dose penicillin for treatment of the most severely ill individuals. Doxycycline and azithromycin had comparable efficacy as presumptive treatment of mildly ill patients found later to have leptospirosis, scrub typhus, or duel infections.

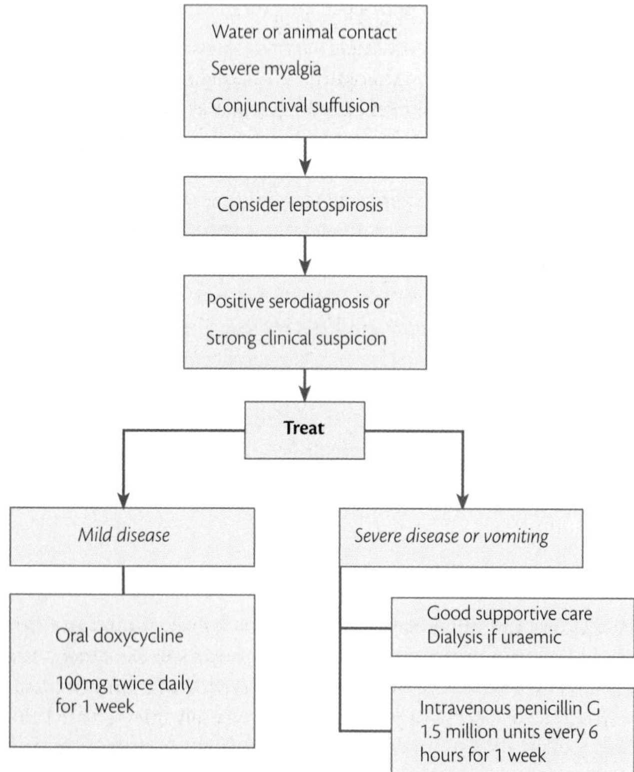

Fig. 7.6.34.3 Management of a febrile patient with possible leptospirosis.

There is controversy regarding the occurrence of a Jarisch–Herxheimer reaction in leptospirosis. If present, it is much less prominent in leptospirosis than in other spirochaetal illnesses. The important practical consideration is that antibiotics should not be withheld because of the fear of a possible Jarisch–Herxheimer reaction.

The management of pulmonary haemorrhage often requires prompt intubation and mechanical ventilation. Patients with SPHS have physiological and pathological evidence of acute respiratory distress syndrome, so ventilation using low tidal volumes and high postexpiratory end-pressures should be provided. Respiratory support to maintain adequate tissue oxygenation is essential because in nonfatal cases complete recovery of pulmonary function can be achieved. Ensuring adequate renal perfusion prevents renal failure in the vast majority of oliguric individuals. Continuous haemofiltration has been shown to be more effective than peritoneal dialysis in treating infection-associated hypercatabolic renal failure. Peritoneal dialysis, however, may be the only option in resource-limited settings. Whichever method of dialysis is chosen, however, it must be started promptly as delays increase mortality.

Prevention

Doxycycline, 200 mg taken once a week, prevents infection by *L. interrogans*. Widespread use of doxycycline prophylaxis is not indicated, but it can benefit those who are at high risk for a short time, such as military personnel and certain agricultural workers.

Infection by leptospires confers only serovar-specific immunity; second attacks due to different serovars can occur. The efficacy and safety of human leptospiral vaccines have yet to be conclusively demonstrated. Prevention of leptospirosis in the tropics is particularly difficult. The large animal reservoir of infection is impossible to eliminate, the occurrence of numerous serovars limits the usefulness of serovar-specific vaccine, and the wearing of protective clothing (e.g. rubber boots in rice fields) is both prohibitively expensive and impractical. Providing proper sanitation in urban slum communities would be the most effective control measure in this setting.

Prognosis

It is imperative to bring affordable tests to areas where leptospirosis is common because treatment (or lack of it) has a substantial impact on outcome. Atypical or mild cases are often confused with other entities such as aseptic meningitis, influenza, appendicitis, and gastroenteritis. Viral hepatitis is a common misdiagnosis in patients with Weil's disease. Leucocytosis, elevated serum bilirubin levels without marked transaminase elevations, and renal dysfunction are typical of leptospirosis but unusual in hepatitis. Malaria, typhoid fever, relapsing fever, scrub typhus, and Hantaan virus infection (haemorrhagic fever with renal syndrome) are important differential diagnoses in the tropics. Leptospirosis with prominent haemorrhagic manifestations is commonly misdiagnosed as dengue fever.

Case fatality rates are over 50% in SPHS and over 10% in Weil's disease. In addition to prompt diagnosis, efficient triage of high-risk patients is critical for the intensive monitoring and therapy required to manage complications. Acute renal failure and especially oliguria is a bad prognostic factor, as are respiratory insufficiency, hypotension, arrhythmias, and altered mental status.

Further reading

Abdulkader RCRM, *et al.* (1996). Peculiar electrolytic and hormonal abnormalities in acute renal failure due to leptospirosis. *Am J Trop Med Hyg*, **54**, 1–6.

Bharti AR, *et al.* (2003). Leptospirosis: a zoonotic disease of global importance. *Lancet Infect Dis*, **3**, 757–71.

Ko AI, *et al.* (1999). Urban epidemic of severe leptospirosis in Brazil. *Lancet*, **354**, 820–5.

McBride AJA, *et al.* (2005). Leptospirosis. *Curr Opin Infect Dis*, **18**, 376–86.

Nicodemo AC, *et al.* (1997). Lung lesions in human leptospirosis: microscopic, immunohistochemical, and ultrastructural features related to thrombocytopenia. *Am J Trop Med Hyg*, **56**, 181–7.

Thaipadungpanit J, *et al.* (2007). A dominant clone of *Leptospira interrogans* associated with an outbreak of human leptospirosis in Thailand. *PLoS Negl Trop Dis*, **1**, 1–6.

Watt G, *et al.* (1988). Placebo controlled trial of intravenous penicillin for severe and late leptospirosis. *Lancet*, **1**, 433–5.

Zaki SR, Shieh WJ, the Epidemic Working Group (1996). Leptospirosis associated with outbreak of acute febrile illness and pulmonary haemorrhage, Nicaragua. *Lancet*, **347**, 535–6.

7.6.35 Nonvenereal endemic treponematoses: yaws, endemic syphilis (bejel), and pinta

David A. Warrell

Essentials

The endemic treponematoses are chronic, granulomatous diseases caused by morphologically and serologically identical spirochaetes of the genus *Treponema*. They are spread by intimate but non-sexual contact and sometimes by fomites, mainly among children. *Treponema pallidum* subsp. *pertenue* causing yaws (framboesia), *T. pallidum* subsp. *endemicum* causing endemic syphilis (bejel) and *T. carateum* causing pinta (carate) are distinguishable from *T. pallidum* subsp. *pallidum*, causing venereal syphilis, by their epidemiology and pathological effects and genomic structure (e.g. the *arp* gene).

Despite the successful WHO/UNICEF mass penicillin treatment campaign (1952–64), there has been a resurgence of yaws, mainly in West Africa. Children living in rural areas in warm, humid climates in tropical countries are most affected by yaws. About 10% of untreated cases develop late, disfiguring, or crippling lesions of skin, bone, and cartilage.

Endemic syphilis occurs in arid areas of the Sahel and Arabian peninsula. It presents with buccal mucocutaneous lesions from contaminated cups. Late systemic effects are much less common than in venereal syphilis. Pinta persists in small foci in southern Mexico and South America, causing hypo- or hyper-pigmented skin lesions. Single-dose benzathine penicillin is effective treatment.

Prevention is by improving hygiene and eliminating the reservoir of infection by mass treatment.

Acknowledgement: The author gratefully acknowledges inclusion of material from previous editions by his late friend and colleague Dr Peter L Perine.

Introduction

Syphilis (Chapter 7.6.36) and the nonvenereal treponematoses are distinguishable by their epidemiological characteristics and the pattern of infection produced in humans and experimentally infected laboratory animals (Table 7.6.35.1). Yaws is caused by *Treponema pallidum* subsp. *pertenue*, a spirochaete that is morphologically identical to *T. pallidum* subsp. *pallidum* (the cause of venereal syphilis), *T. pallidum* subsp. *endemicum* (the cause of nonvenereal syphilis or bejel), and *T. carateum* (the cause of pinta). None is cultivable *in vitro*. They share common antigens so that infection by one species produces varying degrees of cross-immunity to the others. They are serologically indistinguishable. Pathogenic treponemes can be differentiated by polymerase chain reaction using acidic repeat protein (*arp*) gene sequences. The treponemes of yaws, syphilis, and pinta are fragile and readily killed by exposure to atmospheric oxygen, drying, mild detergents, or antiseptics. They cannot penetrate intact skin, but gain entry to the body through small abrasions and lacerations. They prefer cooler temperatures, below 37°C, which may explain their predilection for the skin and bones of the extremities. All cause chronic granulomatous diseases that exhibit primary, secondary, and tertiary (late) stages separated by quiescent or latent periods. Most of their pathological effects are immune-mediated, the peak of the immune response preceding healing. Some spirochaetes survive in tissues and can cause exacerbations as immunity declines.

Yaws

Epidemiology

Yaws is a chronic infection by *T. pallidum* subsp. *pertenue* of skin, bone, and cartilage and periodically the organism spreads systemically. It is nonvenereal and noncongenital and is predominantly a disease of children. Seventy-five per cent of those acutely infected are below the age of 15 years and the peak incidence is between the ages of 6 and 10 years. In endemic areas more than 80% of the population are infected. The organism is transmitted by direct contact of

Table 7.6.35.1 Major features of the treponematoses

Feature	Venereal syphilis	Yaws	Endemic syphilis	Pinta
Organism	*T. pallidum* subsp. *pallidum*	*T. pallidum* subsp. *pertenue*	*T. pallidum* subsp. *endemicum*	*T. carateum*
Age of infection (years)	20–40	5–15	2–10	10–30
Occurrence	Worldwide	Africa, South America, Oceania, Asia	Africa, Middle East	Central and South America
Climate	All	Warm, humid	Dry, arid	Warm, rural
Direct transmission:				
Venereal	Common	No	Rare	No
Nonvenereal	Rare	Common	Rare	Common
Congenital	Yes	No	?	No
Indirect transmission:				
Contaminated utensils	Rare	Rare	Common	No
Insects	No	Rare	No	?
Reservoir of infection	Adults	Infectious and latent cases; ?nonhuman primates	Infectious and latent cases	
Ratio infectious:latent cases	1:3	1:3–5	1:2	?
Late complications:				
Skin	+	+	+	+
Bone, cartilage	+	+	+	No
Neurological	+	No	?	No
Cardiovascular	+	No	?	No

broken skin with an infectious lesion or by fingers or bites contaminated with lesion exudate or rarely indirectly through fomites. Spread is promoted by crowded, unhygienic conditions. In humid, warm environments the early lesion tends to proliferate and teems with spirochaetes, thus increasing the infectious reservoir, whereas in dry, arid climates or seasons the reverse is true. Yaws is rarely fatal but frequently disfiguring and debilitating.

During the 1952–64 World Health Organization UNICEF campaign, an estimated 152 million people were examined and 46.1 million clinical cases, latent infections, and contacts were treated with penicillin in 46 countries, reducing the global prevalence by 95% from 50 to 2.5 million cases and greatly diminishing the yaws reservoir in West and Central Africa, Central and South America, and Oceania. This campaign initiated development of primary health care in many countries. Unfortunately, since the late 1970s there has been a resurgence, initially after control was delegated to national authorities. Seven West African countries started new mass treatment campaigns in the 1980s, but by 1995 the estimated global prevalence of infectious cases was 460 000, with 400 000 of them being in West Africa. Yaws was eliminated in India by 2004, but it persists in rural populations in West Africa (e.g. 26 000 new cases in Ghana in 2005), Ethiopia, South-East Asia (5000 new cases in Indonesia, East Timor), Papua New Guinea (18 000 new cases), Solomon Islands, Vanuatu, and Ecuador. The current worldwide prevalence of infectious cases of yaws may be *c.*500 000. Some African countries such as Nigeria, previously rendered yaws-free by mass treatment campaigns, have experienced a sharp rise in the incidence of venereal syphilis, perhaps reflecting the decline of herd immunity to yaws. Yaws is also prevalent in some gorilla populations.

Pathogenesis

The lesions of yaws and the other treponematoses are due largely to the host's immune response to the treponeme. None of these treponemes carries or produces toxic substances. They have the ability to invade living cells without causing apparent injury. Cell destruction and tissue damage are probably due to the action of immune cells that injure normal tissue in the process of killing treponemes.

Host immunity reaches its highest level after several months of infection, just before disseminated lesions heal and latency begins. Thereafter the host is immune to reinfection and is not contagious, but since not all treponemes are killed, infectious lesions may reappear as immunity wanes over time. Most patients with yaws experience two or three infectious relapses during the first 5 years of infection.

Clinical features

Primary yaws

After an incubation period of 3 to 5 weeks, the initial lesion in yaws usually appears on the extremities. Characteristically, the primary lesion is a single painless papule that appears at the site of infection and enlarges to form a raspberry-like (framboesia) vegetative lesion called a papilloma. This is round to oval, elevated, and not indurated, ranging in size from 1 to 3 cm in diameter (Fig. 7.6.35.1).

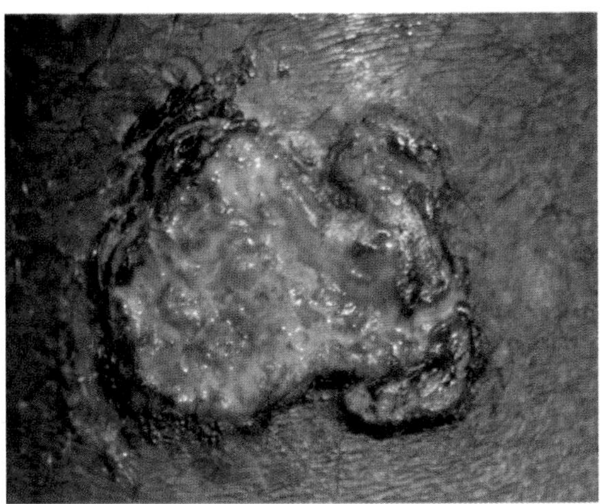

Fig. 7.6.35.1 Primary yaws lesion with ulceration and satellites.
(Courtesy of Dr B Hudson, Sydney, Australia.)

The surface teems with spirochaetes and is often covered by a thin yellow crust that is easily removed. It may ulcerate as it enlarges and becomes secondarily infected with other microorganisms. Lymph nodes draining the initial lesion may enlarge and become tender, but systemic symptoms are rare.

Secondary yaws

Secondary or disseminated ulceropapillomatous or maculopapular lesions appear after 2 to 6 months, often without any intervening latent period, on the skin of moist areas such as the axillae, joint flexures, genitalia, and the gluteal cleft (Fig. 7.6.35.2a,b). They also occur on the soles and palms and, because they are tender, may interfere with gait and use of the hands. Papillomas in different stages of development persist for 6 to 8 months and heal without scars unless they become secondarily infected. Despite the size and number of lesions, children with generalized papillomas experience little discomfort or other constitutional symptoms.

When the climate is arid, yaws lesions are commonly slightly raised scaly pigmented macules measuring between 1 and 4 cm in diameter. They have the same distribution as papillomas and may appear together with lesions of different morphology in the same patient (maculopapular yaws).

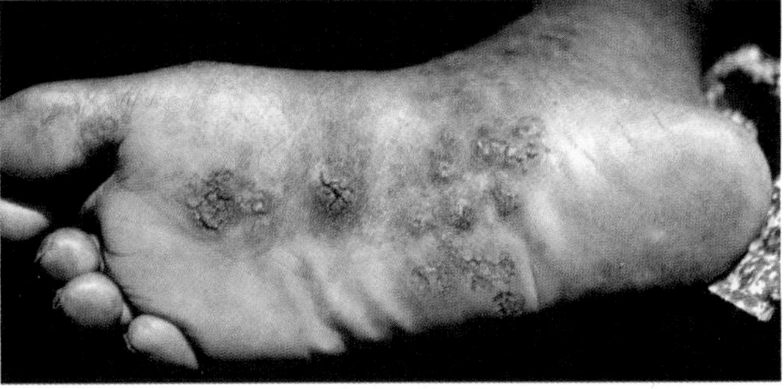

Fig. 7.6.35.3 Plantar papillomas with hyperkeratotic, macular, early plantar yaws ('crab yaws'). These lesions are painful.
(Courtesy of Dr B Hudson, Sydney, Australia.)

The periosteum and bones of the extremities are frequently inflamed during early yaws causing swelling, night pain, and tenderness. There is dactylitis of the proximal phalanges (Fig. 7.6.35.4). Painful osteoperiostitis of the legs, affecting mainly the tibias and fibulas, is especially common (Fig. 7.6.35.5). Hypertrophic osteitis of the maxilla, either side of the bridge of the nose, can cause grotesque swellings ('goundo'). Scaly tender hyperkeratotic lesions of the palms and soles also occur and may be incapacitating. Hyperkeratotic and bone lesions are not contagious, and macular lesions are only minimally so.

One or more relapses of secondary-type lesions usually occur during the first 5 years of infection, each separated by a period of latency. The lesions of late yaws occur thereafter in about 10% of untreated cases.

Late yaws

The lesions are not infectious because they contain few treponemes. Cutaneous plaques produce atrophic scars. Subcutaneous granulomatous nodules erode skin and produce deep ulcers that destroy underlying tissue and cause disfigurement. Hyperkeratotic palmar and plantar yaws (Fig. 7.6.35.3) are incapacitating and often prevent the use of the hands or the ability to walk normally. The weight is placed on the sides of the feet, which produces a gait much like that of a crab ('crab yaws').

The granulomas of late yaws have a histological appearance that is similar to the gummas of syphilis. These proliferative lesions may involve the palate and destroy the soft tissues of the nose, causing a terrible disfiguration called gangosa (Fig. 7.6.35.6a,b). Gummatous

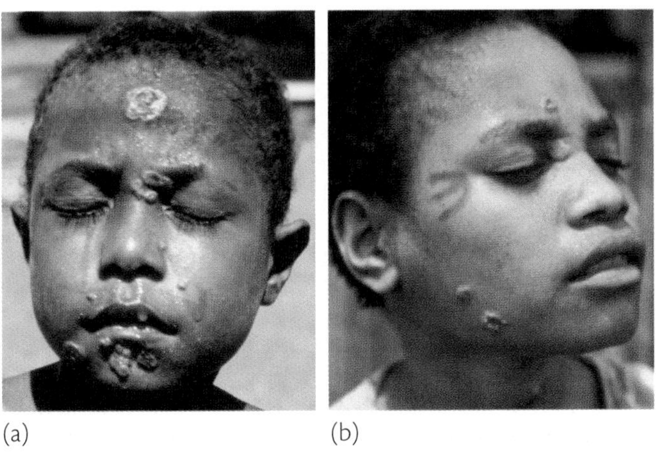

(a) (b)

Fig. 7.6.35.2 (a,b) Early ulceropapillomatous secondary yaws.
(Courtesy of Dr B Hudson, Sydney, Australia.)

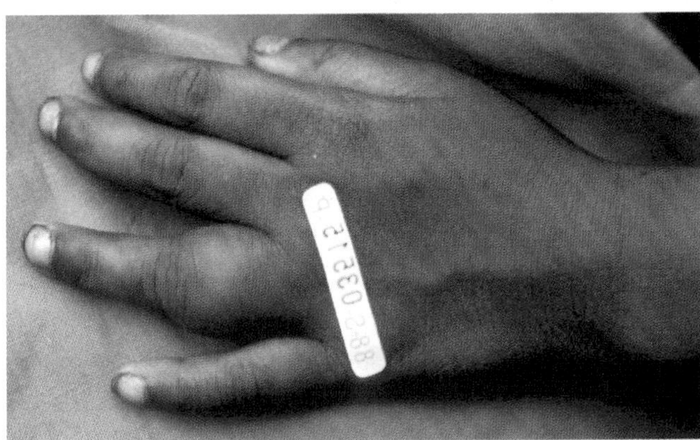

Fig. 7.6.35.4 Dactylitis.
(Courtesy of Dr B Hudson, Sydney, Australia.)

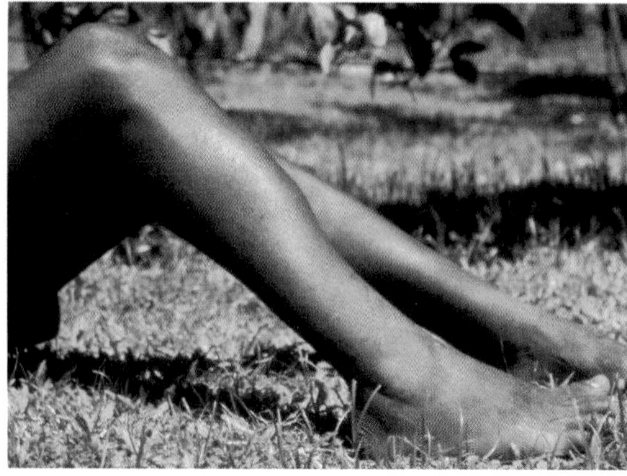

(a)

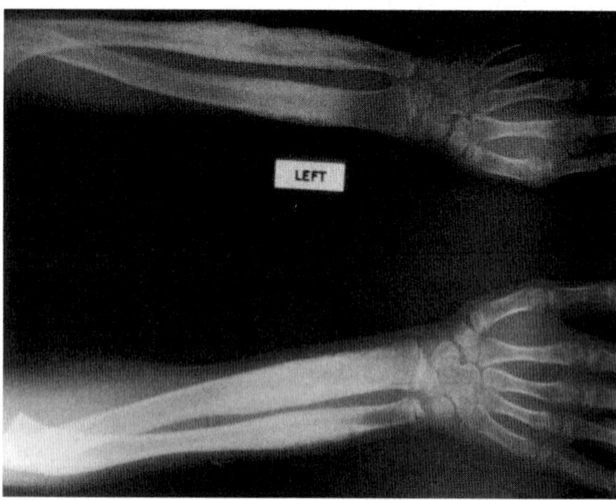

(b)

Fig. 7.6.35.5 (a,b) Osteoperiostitis.
(Courtesy of Dr B Hudson, Sydney, Australia.)

periostitis of the skull, fingers, and long bones is erosive and often retards or stops growth. Active periostitis is occasionally found in young and middle-aged adults who had yaws in childhood. Burnt out osteitis leads to a characteristic deformity 'sabre tibia'.

Endemic syphilis

T. pallidum subsp. *endemicum* is transmitted by nonvenereal contact among children. In contrast to yaws, transmission by contaminated drinking vessels may be more common than by direct contact with infectious lesions. The disease tends to be familial, with spread of infection from children to adults rather than to the community in general. The lesions are virtually indistinguishable from early yaws, and the two diseases may occur at different times in the same population but not in the same person. Venereal syphilis can be acquired by children through social contact with adults who have venereal syphilis, and then be spread by nonvenereal person-to-person contact if levels of sanitation and personal hygiene are low.

Several variants of endemic syphilis are recognized by their geographical distribution: bejel of the eastern Mediterranean, North Africa, and Niger; and njovera or dichuchwa of Africa. Bejel is the only type of endemic syphilis still prevalent. It is found in seminomadic people such as the Tuareg, living in the Sahelian nations of Mauritania, Mali, Niger, Burkina Faso, and Senegal where dramatic increases in the number of cases of endemic syphilis

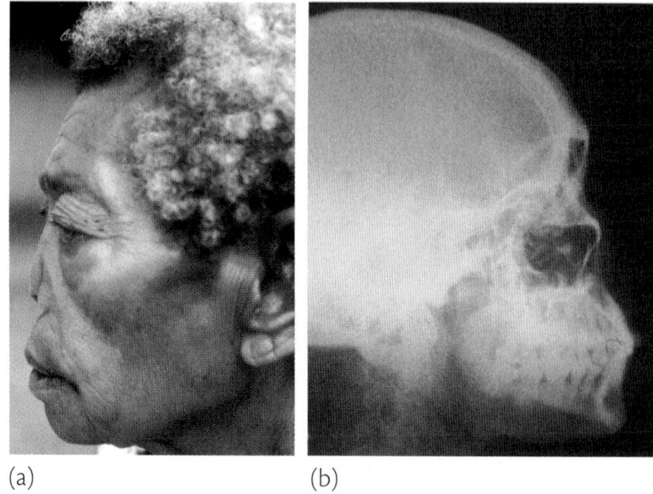

(a) (b)

Fig. 7.6.35.6 (a,b) Gangosa (rhinopharyngitis mutilans) of endemic syphilis and yaws.
(Courtesy of Dr B Hudson, Sydney, Australia.)

have been reported. In Naimey (Niger), seroprevalence was 12% among children under 5 years of age. The disease is also prevalent among the nomadic tribes of the Arabian peninsula, where late complications such as osteoperiostitis predominate.

Clinical features

The initial lesions of endemic syphilis usually appear at the mucocutaneous borders of the mouth or on the oral mucous membranes (mucous patches) as the result of transmission by contaminated drinking vessels. Late ulceronodules and osteoperiostitis are seen in late endemic syphilis, but cardiovascular and neurological complications are extremely rare.

Pinta (carate)

T. carateum resides only in the skin. This peculiar tissue tropism is unexplained. It is probably an inherent property of the treponeme, acting in contact with climatic factors. Pinta is confined to remote parts of Central and South America, principally in the semiarid region of the Tepalcatepec Basin of southern Mexico and focal areas of Colombia, Peru, Ecuador, and Venezuela. Pinta is probably transmitted by direct skin or mucous membrane contact, by insect bites, and perhaps by tribal rituals resulting in skin scratches.

Clinical features

After an incubation period of 15 to 30 days, the primary lesions, single or few in number, are seen on the dorsal surfaces of the limbs, face, chest, or gluteal area, usually of children or young adults (Fig. 7.6.35.7). The lesion is an itchy erythematous papule or depigmented macule that enlarges slowly over a period of several weeks or months to form an erythematous plaque, sometimes with regional lymphadenopathy but without systemic symptoms. Satellite papules form at its edge and undergo a similar type of evolution. The plaques coalesce to form violaceous pigmented plaques that, in several years, slowly depigment from lighter shades of blue to white, leaving symmetrical atrophic depigmented scars.

Rapid dissemination of lesions may occur months or up to about 4 years after the primary lesions, frequently affecting scalp, nails,

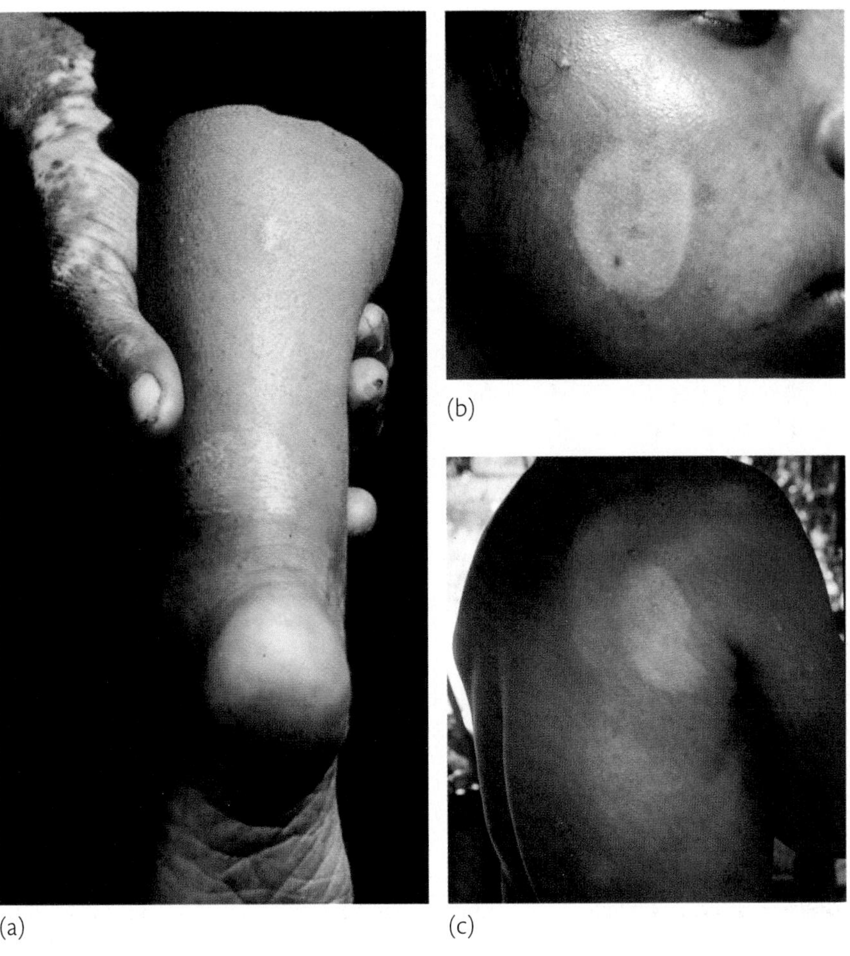

Fig. 7.6.35.7 (a–c) Early lesions of pinta in Yaruro people of northwestern Venezuela.
(Courtesy of Prof. Rolando Hernández Pérez, Hospital Universitario 'Dr. Luis Razetti' Barinas, Universidad de los Andes, Venezuela.)

and mucous membranes (Fig. 7.6.35.8). Depigmented, pigmented, and erythematous-desquamative lesions may occur simultaneously in the same patient. Late lesions are symmetrical, depigmented, atrophic, or hyperkeratotic.

Diagnosis

The diagnosis of yaws and other endemic treponematoses is made by a combination of clinical assessment, of positive dark-ground examination of early lesions and exudates which are usually teeming with treponemes, and of reactive serological tests for syphilis.

Early yaws, endemic syphilis, and pinta are not difficult to diagnose in endemic areas where the disease is familiar. The most difficult diagnostic problem arises when someone who had yaws as a child emigrates to an area of the world where the disease never existed. Such a person usually has reactive serological tests for syphilis and may have a few atrophic scars suggestive of earlier infection. What are the chances that this patient has or has had venereal syphilis? Should they be treated for latent yaws or syphilis? The patient's social and medical history should be carefully reviewed. Clinical findings suggestive of old yaws (scars, inactive tibial periostitis), and the absence of signs of congenital and venereal syphilis support the diagnosis of inactive or treated yaws.

If the patient has a reagin titre (Venereal Disease Research Laboratory (VDRL), rapid plasma reagin (RPR)) of less than 1:8 dilutions, they probably do not have active latent yaws or syphilis. If they received at least one therapeutic dose of long-acting penicillin in their native country during a yaws campaign, they require no further treatment. On the other hand, if the patient is a contact of a case of infectious venereal syphilis, they should be treated as being potentially infected with syphilis because *T. pallidum* subsp. *pallidum* occasionally superinfects people who had yaws as children. If treatment is given, the patient should receive a certificate stating the drug and dosage used and the results of their serological tests to prevent unnecessary future treatment.

Differential diagnosis

Ulceronodular skin lesions of yaws and endemic syphilis resemble tropical ulcers. Yaws lesions are not as painful, necrotic, or deep as tropical ulcers, which are usually singular and restricted to the lower one-third of the leg. Plantar warts are frequently confused with plantar papillomas of yaws, and both conditions may occur in the same patient. Pinta must be differentiated from other hypopigmented and hyperpigmented skin lesions including vitiligo, indeterminate leprosy, pityriasis alba, and psoriasis.

Treatment

Long-acting benzylpenicillin given by intramuscular injection is the recommended treatment for all the endemic treponematoses. The preparation used in previous mass treatment campaigns was penicillin aluminium monostearate (PAM), but benzathine penicillin is currently recommended because it is longer acting and

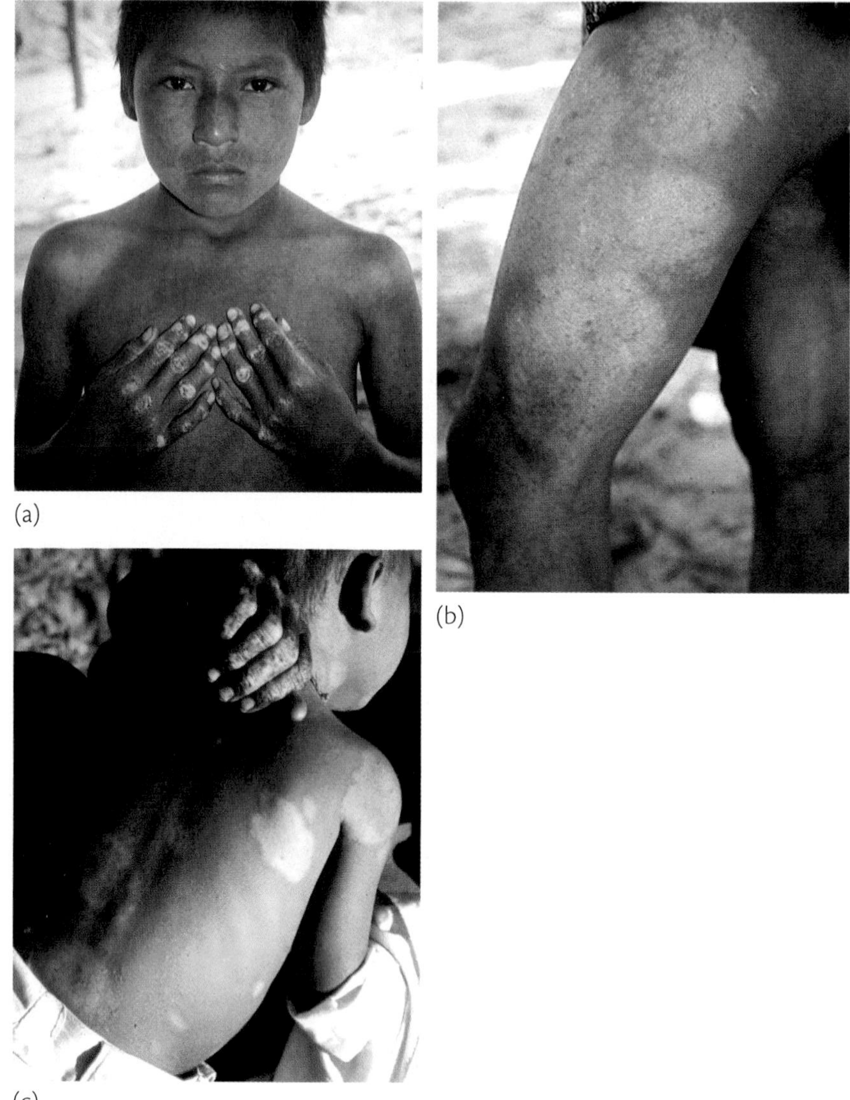

Fig. 7.6.35.8 (a–c) Disseminated lesions of pinta in Yaruro people of north-western Venezuela.
(Courtesy of Prof. Rolando Hernández Pérez, Hospital Universitario 'Dr. Luis Razetti' Barinas, Universidad de los Andes, Venezuela.)

more readily available than is PAM. People who have active infections or who are noninfectious should be given 1.2 mega units in a single intramuscular injection; children under 10 years of age receive 0.6 mega units. Patients allergic to penicillin may be given tetracycline or erythromycin, 500 mg by mouth four times daily for 2 weeks; children under 10 years of age should be given erythromycin in dosages adjusted for their age. Treatment failures have been reported in Papua New Guinea.

Prevention and control

Transmission is reduced as personal hygiene among children improves. Prevention of yaws and other endemic treponematoses in a community requires elimination of the reservoir of infection, often by treating the entire population with penicillin. This has succeeded in some countries, notably recently with yaws in India.

Further reading

Antal GM, Lukehart SA, Meheus AZ (2002). The endemic treponematoses. *Microbes Infect*, **4**, 83–94.

Engelkens HJ, Vuzevski VD, Stolz E (1999). Non-venereal treponematoses in tropical countries. *Clin Dermatol*, **17**, 105–6, 143–52.

Farnsworth N, Rosen T (2006). Endemic treponematosis: review and update. *Clin Dermatol*, **24**, 181–90.

Guthe T (1969). Clinical, serological and epidemiological features of framboesia tropica (yaws) and its control in rural communities. *Acta Derm Venereol*, **49**, 343–68.

Hackett CJ, Loewenthal LJA (1960). *Differential diagnosis of yaws*. World Health Organization, Geneva.

Harper KN, *et al.* (2008). On the origin of the treponematoses: a phylogenetic approach. *PLoS Negl Trop Dis*, **2**, e148.

Harper KN, *et al.* (2008). The sequence of the acidic repeat protein (arp) gene differentiates venereal from nonvenereal *Treponema pallidum* subspecies, and the gene has evolved under strong positive selection in the subspecies that causes syphilis. *FEMS Immunol Med Microbiol*, **53**, 322–32.

Padilha Gonçalves A, Basset A, Maleville J (1992). Tropical treponematoses. In: Canizares O, Harman RRM (eds) *Clinical tropical dermatology*, 2nd edition, pp. 129–50. Blackwell, Boston.

Perine PL, *et al.* (1984). *Handbook of endemic treponematoses: yaws, endemic syphilis and pinta*. World Health Organization, Geneva.

Walker SL, Hay RJ (2000). Yaws: a review of the last 50 years. *Int J Dermatol*, **39**, 258–60.

7.6.36 Syphilis

Basil Donovan and Linda Dayan

Essentials

Syphilis results from infection with the spirochaete *Treponema pallidum* subsp. *pallidum*, for which humans are the only known natural host. In adults it is transmitted primarily by sexual contact. The organism gains entry into the body through small breaks in the skin or the intact mucosal surfaces of the genitals, mouth, or anus, and is able to invade and survive in a wide variety of tissues.

Since the availability of penicillin, syphilis has become primarily (>90%) a disease of less affluent countries or of minority subpopulations in more affluent countries with poor access to health care. It is also a disease of people with rapid rates of partner change, e.g. homosexual men and sex workers.

Clinical features

Syphilis can manifest in three stages: primary within a few weeks to months after infection; secondary after a few months up to a year; and tertiary after years to decades. These stages can overlap, and they are frequently asymptomatic.

Primary syphilis—this appears 9 to 90 days after the organism gains entry via direct inoculation through the thin skin or mucosa of the anogenital tract or mouth during sexual exposure. The resulting lesion is typically a painless ulcer or 'chancre', sometimes indurated, that appears at the site of inoculation and is associated with regional lymphadenopathy, but chancres can be multiple and atypical.

Secondary syphilis—occurs 3 to 6 weeks after the appearance of the chancre, with manifestations including fever, malaise, mucocutaneous lesions (rash, condyloma lata, mucous patches), generalized lymphadenopathy, and (uncommonly) visceral disease. Invasion of the central nervous system is common, but usually asymptomatic.

Latent syphilis—the lesions of both primary and secondary syphilis may wax and wane, but they eventually resolve; there are no signs or symptoms of active syphilis, but serological tests are positive for *T. pallidum*.

Tertiary syphilis—affects around one-third of infected people following a variable period of latent infection, with manifestations including (1) neurosyphilis—can present as (a) aseptic meningitis, with variable features, e.g. focal neurological deficits, cranial nerve palsies, hydrocephalus or psychiatric symptoms; (b) meningovascular disease, with endarteritis leading to cerebral infarction; (c) general paresis, involving changes in the parenchyma of the central nervous system that lead to the gradual onset of cognitive impairment, depression, and personality changes, later progressing to dementia, delirium, seizures, and delusions; (d) tabes dorsalis, with initial symptoms and signs including lightening pains and parasthesias, visceral crises, abnormal deep tendon reflexes, incontinence, ataxia with a wide-based gait, and pupillary abnormalities. (2) Gummatous syphilis—destructive granulomatous lesions most commonly present on skin, mucosal surfaces or in bone. (3) Cardiovascular syphilis—most commonly asymptomatic aortitis, aortic incompetence, aortic aneurysm, and coronary ostial stenosis.

Congenital syphilis—most pregnant women with early syphilis will transmit the condition to the fetus via the placenta, with congenital syphilis often resulting in fetal loss, stillbirth, or neonatal or childhood disease.

Diagnosis and treatment

Diagnosis—the transient nature of the lesions and the spirochetaemia limit the role of direct detection of *T. pallidum*, hence diagnosis usually relies on serology, with tests being (1) nonspecific (or nontreponemal or reagin)—e.g. rapid plasma reagin (RPR) and Venereal Disease Research Laboratory (VDRL) tests; detect phospholipid cardiolipin as an antigen; generally sensitive in early infection but tend to decline over the next several years without treatment; able to quantify disease activity and hence used for follow-up after treatment. (2) specific (or treponemal)—e.g. *T. pallidum* haemagglutination assay (TPHA); use *T. pallidum* as the antigen; may become positive shortly before the nonspecific tests; typically remain reactive for life after successful treatment and therefore have no role in assessing stage of infection, 'cure,' or reinfection.

Treatment—parenteral penicillin G remains the preferred treatment for syphilis, with doxycycline providing an oral alternative. Successful treatment of early disease relies on demonstrating a fourfold decrease in reagin (RPR or VDRL) titres over the next 6 to 12 months. Sexual contacts of early syphilis should be treated presumptively, regardless of their test results, if the contact was within 90 days, usually with a single dose of benzathine penicillin G.

Prevention

The chance of acquiring syphilis following one act of intercourse with an infected person is 1 to 2%, which should be reduced by the use of condoms. Early treatment of disease decreases the duration of infectivity and thereby minimizes transmission to others, hence those at high risk of syphilis should be encouraged to undergo regular syphilis screening (as well as testing for HIV and other sexually transmissible infections).

Prevention of congenital infection and serious outcomes such as stillbirth and neonatal death rely on routine antenatal screening early in the pregnancy, with prompt treatment of infected mothers.

Introduction and historical perspective

In the 1490s, an epidemic of a new and virulent sexually transmitted disease appearance in Europe following the return of Christopher Columbus and his fleet from the Americas. This led many to believe that syphilis originated in the New World. There is now molecular phylogenetic evidence for this 'Columbian hypothesis'. Syphilis spread rapidly through Europe where it was known by a variety of names including *morbus gallicus* (the French disease), *lues venereum* (venereal disease), and the great pox.

The alternative theory proposes that syphilis was simply another variant of a preexisting treponemal infection that had adapted to sexual and congenital transmission and produced greater morbidity (the Unitarian hypothesis). A variety of yaws-like diseases that predominantly affected children were present in Europe and Africa at the time, and a few persisted into the 20th century.

Syphilus (the original spelling) was an afflicted shepherd in a poem by Girolamo Fracastoro published in 1530. The original text described the symptoms of syphilis, hypothesized about its origins, and mentioned the use of early remedies such as guaiacum, a compound derived from a Central American tree, and mercury.

Following an experiment by John Hunter in 1767 it was thought that gonorrhoea and syphilis were different manifestations of the same disease until Philippe Ricord, in 1838, clarified the differences between the two infections. Soon after, the three stages of syphilis were categorized and congenital and neurological syphilis were described.

Because of the toxicity and dubious benefit of the treatments available at the time, a prospective cohort study into the natural history of syphilis was conducted in Oslo between 1890 and 1920. This study followed 1978 initially symptomatic patients and demonstrated that approximately one-third developed late complications. Many of these complications proved fatal.

Rapid advances in knowledge occurred around the beginning of the 20th century. In 1905, Schaudinn and Hoffman demonstrated spirochaetes in secondary syphilitic lesions. One year later, Von Wasserman devised the first serological test for syphilis. In 1910, Paul Erlich announced results for his compound 606 (salvarsan), a form of arsenic that showed activity against syphilis.

The discovery of penicillin by Fleming, its development for therapeutic use by Florey, and the first clinical trial in 1943 by Mahoney revolutionized the treatment of syphilis. During the immediate post-war period the use of penicillin eclipsed other forms of therapy and by the mid-1950s the incidence of syphilis had fallen markedly throughout the industrialized world.

Aetiology, genetics, pathogenesis, and pathology

Treponema pallidum subsp. *pallidum*, a spiral-shaped bacterium, is a member of the order Spirochaetales and the cause of adult acquired and congenital syphilis. Humans are the only known natural host for all *T. pallidum* subspecies, although an unclassified and morphologically indistinguishable simian pathogen, the Fribourg–Blanc treponeme, was isolated from a baboon in Guinea in 1962. The inability to culture *T. pallidum in vitro* has retarded study of its biology.

T. pallidum subsp. *pallidum* is closely related to other pathogenic treponemes that cause nonvenereal disease: *T. pallidum* subsp. *carateum* (pinta), *T. pallidum* subsp. *pertenue* (yaws), and *T. pallidum* subsp. *endemicum* (endemic syphilis or bejel) (see Chapter 7.6.35). Subspecies *pertenue* and *endemicum* and the Fribourg–Blanc treponeme have recently been demonstrated to be genetically distinct from subspecies *pallidum*, consistent with the lack of cross-immunity. The spirochaete is 6 to 20 μm long and only 0.10 to 0.18 μm thick, making it invisible to ordinary light microscopy. Using dark-field microscopy, *T. pallidum* has 6 to 20 characteristic tightly wound spirals and it moves with corkscrew motility or by bending in the middle and popping back into place with a spring. Other nonpathogenic treponemes tend to have fewer coils or a jerkier motion. Commensal species of treponema (*T. denticola* and *T. oralis*) can mimic *T. pallidum*, limiting the usefulness of dark-field microscopy of oral and anal lesions.

The *T. pallidum* DNA genome was first published in 1998. It is small, with a single circular chromosome of 1 138 006 base pairs containing 1041 predicted protein coding sequences, consistent with its limited metabolic capabilities. The organism obtains most of its essential nutrients from the host environment, making it an obligate parasite. *In vivo*, *T. pallidum* has been grown in rabbits and reproduces itself slowly, doubling every 30 to 33 h. *T. pallidum* is able to survive better with low levels of oxygen (3–5%) and is sensitive to heat.

T. pallidum is able rapidly to invade and survive in a wide variety of tissues after gaining entry into the body through small breaks in the skin or the intact mucosal surfaces of the genitals, mouth, or anus. The organism has a reputation as a 'stealth' pathogen because its paucity of surface proteins and lipopolysaccharides helps it to evade the host immune response. *T. pallidum* induces humoral, cell-mediated, and local innate responses that appear to confer immunity to exogenous infection in the chronically infected person (chancre immunity). However, patients treated for early syphilis can become rapidly reinfected.

From the site of inoculation, *T. pallidum* replicates locally and spreads to regional lymph nodes, then into the blood stream from where it can traverse junctions between vascular endothelial cells. Lymphocyte, (CD4+) macrophage, and plasma cell infiltrates accompanied by vasculopathic changes, endarteritis and periarteritis, underlie the histology of syphilitic lesions of all stages. Silver staining of tissues may demonstrate the presence of spirochaetes, usually in the dermal–epidermal junction.

In secondary syphilis, treponemes are found in many sites including visceral organs, the central nervous system, and the skin. *T. pallidum* can remain clinically dormant in the aortic wall, producing an endarteritis in the vasa vasorum and varying degrees of thickening, scarring, and destruction of the arterial wall. This process results in the development of arterial plaques and calcification of the vessels found in cardiovascular syphilis.

In meningitis, perivascular infiltration of lymphocytes and plasma cells causes the meninges to become inflamed. In meningovascular syphilis, thickening of the intima, fibrous changes in the adventitia, and vascular narrowing cause changes in brain blood vessels with resultant infarction and cranial nerve palsies.

The gummas of late syphilis are chronic granulomatous lesions consistent with a hypersensitivity response with few treponemes present. Histologically, central necrosis, peripheral lymphocytosis, perivasculitis, and obliterating endarteritis are seen.

Epidemiology

Since the availability of penicillin, syphilis has become primarily (>90%) a disease of less affluent countries or of minority subpopulations in more affluent countries with poor access to health care. It is also a disease of populations with rapid rates of partner change such as homosexual men and sex workers.

The World Health Organization estimated that in 1999 syphilis continued to infect about 12 million new people a year globally. The greatest number of new infections, 5.8 million, is found in South-East and East Asia. Sub-Saharan Africa accounted for 3.4 million new cases and Latin America and the Caribbean 1.26 million. In Africa, between 4 and 17% of women are seropositive for syphilis in antenatal clinics, and many are coinfected with HIV. About a million pregnancies a year are seriously complicated or aborted by syphilis.

The incidence of syphilis in China has risen following the political and social changes that occurred in the last part of the 20th century. In the former Soviet Union, the incidence of syphilis among the young sexually active population rose rapidly after 1991 with the degradation of the public health system.

Since the beginning of the 21st century, syphilis rates in the United Kingdom, Europe (e.g. in Dublin, Ireland), North America, and other developed countries have risen in homosexual men and especially in those who are HIV positive. Serosorting, the phenomenon of homosexual men of similar HIV status seeking each other for unsafe sex, has been a factor. Oral sex, considered to be relatively safe for HIV infection, readily transmits syphilis.

Prevention

Syphilis in adults is transmitted primarily by sexual contact. The chance of acquiring the infection is estimated to be between 1 and 2% following one act of intercourse with an infected person. Syphilis is found in up to 60% of sexual partners.

As *T. pallidum* is present in mucosal or cutaneous lesions, infected adults are more likely to transmit the disease during primary or secondary stages. The use of condoms to prevent syphilis has not been evaluated in controlled trials. Intuitively, condoms should have some effect in reducing transmission, but they are unlikely to provide 100% protection as they do not cover all areas of anogenital skin during intercourse. Condoms should also be used for oral sex.

Early recognition and treatment of syphilis decreases the duration of infectivity thereby minimizing transmission to others. As symptoms are not always present, those who are at higher risk of syphilis such as homosexual men and sex workers are encouraged to undergo regular syphilis screening, as well as testing for HIV and other sexually transmissible infections. In order to attract those most at risk of syphilis, health services need to be accessible and culturally appropriate, confidential, and provide free or affordable diagnosis and treatment. Presumptive treatment of sexual partners and early recognition and treatment of those who may be core transmitters in a sexual network is essential in any syphilis control programme.

Some authorities now use the Internet to encourage homosexual men to get regular syphilis tests. The Internet can also help these men to inform their sexual partners in a nonthreatening and confidential way.

Syphilis can be transmitted via donated blood or organs, although this is rare. Thus serological screening of donors is routine in most settings.

Mother-to-child transmission of syphilis usually occurs *in utero*. Prevention of congenital infection and serious outcomes such as stillbirth and neonatal death rely on screening and treating for syphilis in the mother early in the pregnancy. In high-incidence populations, rescreening around week 28 to 32 of the pregnancy and again at delivery is also recommended. With timely treatment of the mother, congenital syphilis is almost entirely preventable. Provision of comprehensive antenatal health care with affordable testing for syphilis should form part of a comprehensive syphilis control programme. Community education should encourage women to attend for health care early in pregnancy when treatment can be given with best effect. In high-prevalence areas, if a mother first presents at term, routine treatment of the neonate with a single dose of benzathine penicillin 50 000 units/kg is sometimes recommended if the mother has not been tested or adequate maternal treatment cannot be confirmed.

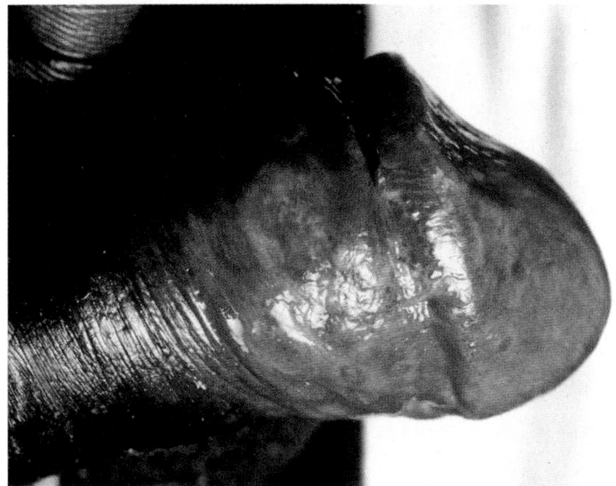

Fig. 7.6.36.1 Multiple painful chronic chancres in a man with HIV infection. (Courtesy of Dr David Bradford.)

Clinical features

Clinical staging of syphilis is important to guide the process of contact tracing or partner notification. Primary, secondary, and early latent syphilis are collectively called 'infectious syphilis'. Late latent and tertiary syphilis are generally regarded as no longer infectious for sexual partners. However, pregnant women may pose an occasional risk to their offspring. Treatment for later stages of syphilis is typically longer than for early syphilis.

Primary syphilis

The chancre, or ulcer of primary syphilis, develops at the site of inoculation within 9 to 90 days (median 3 weeks) of infection, initially as a red macule that soon becomes papular before it ulcerates. The typical ulcer is painless, has fluid or grey slough in its centre, and a well-defined rolled edge. Mature ulcers may have a palpable indurated plaque deep to the lesion. However, chancres can occasionally be painful or multiple, and clinically indistinguishable from other causes of genital ulcers (Fig. 7.6.36.1). Mixed aetiologies are always possible (Fig. 7.6.36.2).

Common sites for chancres in men include the distal penis, while in women the posterior fourchette, labia, and vulva are the

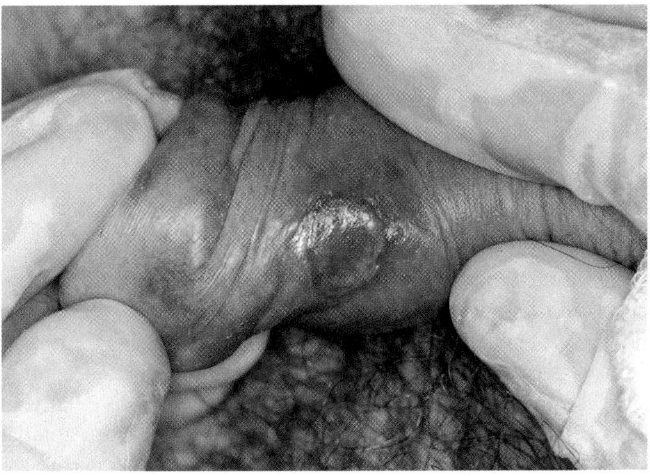

Fig. 7.6.36.2 Chancre against a background of primary genital herpes.

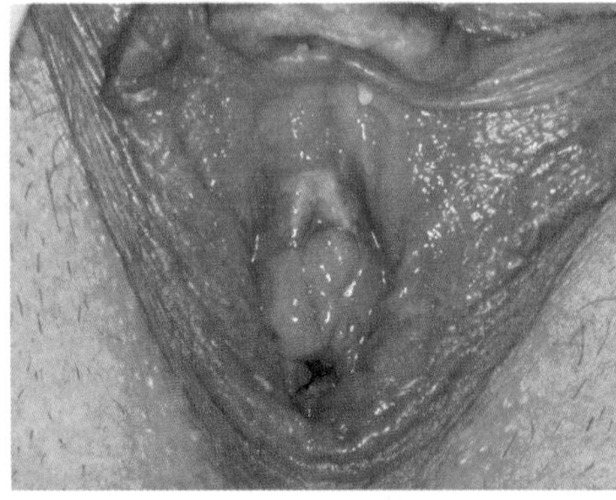

(a)

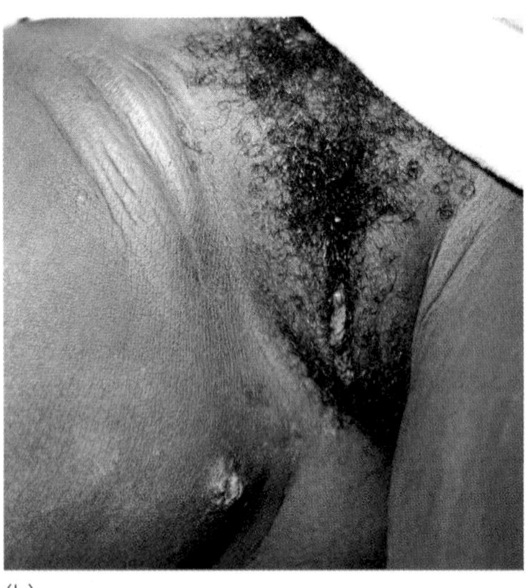

(b)

Fig. 7.6.36.3 (a) A periurethral chancre in a woman who presented with a painless lump. (b) Chancre on thigh and inguinal lymphadenopathy of primary syphilis.
((b) Copyright D A Warrell.)

most commonly diagnosed sites (Fig. 7.6.36.3a). The anal verge, mouth, and lips are all possible sites for chancres, as well as other extragenital sites. If a chancre is small or hidden in the anal canal, vagina, cervix, or mouth, it usually passes unnoticed (Fig. 7.6.36.4). Most patients subsequently diagnosed with secondary syphilis do not recall the lesions of primary syphilis.

Painless and typically rubbery, small lymph nodes are often felt in the affected region within a week of the development of the chancre (Fig. 7.6.36.3b). The chancre usually heals spontaneously in 3 to 6 weeks, but it may occasionally recur ('chancre redux').

Secondary syphilis

This disseminated stage of the infection typically occurs between 3 and 6 weeks following the appearance of the chancre, and the two stages may overlap. However, up to 60% of patients do not recall any signs or symptoms of secondary syphilis at all.

The symptoms and signs of secondary syphilis are often described as protean, as listed in Table 7.6.36.1. Without treatment they resolve spontaneously only to reappear, usually in a milder form, in almost one-quarter (24%) of patients in the following 12 to 24 months (Fig. 7.6.36.5).

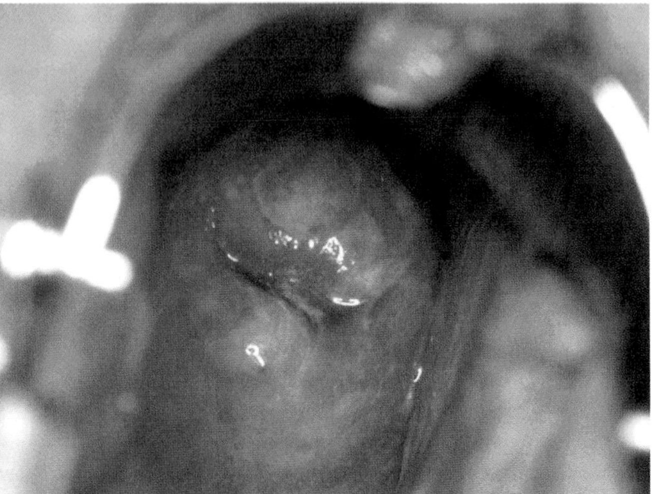

Fig. 7.6.36.4 An asymptomatic chancre on the anterior lip of the cervix in the same woman as Fig. 7.6.36.3a.

Latent syphilis

Latent syphilis is present when there are no signs or symptoms of active syphilis but serological tests are positive for *T. pallidum*. Latent syphilis is arbitrarily divided into early latent syphilis, when the asymptomatic infection has been present for less than 1 or 2 years, and late latent syphilis after this time. In practice, asymptomatic people diagnosed through screening are often deemed to have latent syphilis of unknown duration. As a precaution, such patients are treated with the longer courses of antibiotics that are used for late infections.

Before the antibiotic era, approximately two-thirds of adults remained in the latent phase throughout their lifetime and showed no signs of tertiary syphilis. These days many common antibiotics have some activity against *T. pallidum*, so it is likely that antibiotics used for other conditions are also altering the natural history of, if not accidentally curing, latent syphilis.

Tertiary syphilis

Tertiary syphilis occurred in 15 to 40% of those who remain untreated in the Oslo study, with some modest differences between the sexes (Table 7.6.36.2). In part as a result of the wide availability of antibiotics used for other purposes, gummatous and cardiovascular syphilis are now relatively rare compared to neurosyphilis; most oral antibiotics are unlikely to achieve treponemicidal levels in the central nervous system.

Neurosyphilis

The diagnosis of neurosyphilis frequently raises clinical dilemmas because of the nonspecific nature of its clinical presentations and the absence of definitive tests. Neurosyphilis may manifest as aseptic (basilar pattern) meningitis or meningovascular disease as early as the secondary stage or up to several years after infection. As well as the usual symptoms of meningitis, syphilitic meningitis may also present with focal neurological deficits such as hemiparesis, aphasia, seizures, or psychiatric symptoms. Cranial nerve palsies accompany syphilitic meningitis in about 40% and hydrocephalus in 35% of patients.

Meningovascular syphilis stems from endarteritis leading to infarction, most commonly 5 to 12 years after infection. While any

Table 7.6.36.1 Clinical manifestations of secondary syphilis

	Features	Frequency
Rash	Erythematous or coppery colour Nonpruritic or mildly pruritic Macular or maculopapular (50%) progressing to papular, papulosquamous, psoriasiform, annular (dark-skinned people), pustular, or follicular Usually symmetrical, round to oval lesions, 5 to 20 mm across (Fig. 7.6.36.5a,b) Trunk, palms, soles, and body flexures are most commonly involved Occasionally papules around the forehead hairline ('corona veneris')	Over 70%
Condyloma lata	Pale elevated moist plaques in warmer flexural areas such as perineum, perianal area, groin, axilla, perioral area, and nasolabial folds (Fig. 7.6.36.5c) Appear later than rash	15–50%
Mucous patches	Superficial erosions, papules, or plaques of mucosa of the oropharynx or anogenital area Involvement of the pharynx may result in hoarseness or sore throat	4–17%
Constitutional	Low-grade fever, malaise, headache, myalgias, arthralgias, anorexia, and nausea Occasionally severe	Common, but variable
Lymphadenopathy	Generalized, nontender, and characteristically rubbery and discrete (Fig. 7.6.36.3b)	Over 60%
Hepatitis	Mildly elevated transaminases Usually not clinically important	Up to 10%
Ocular	Iritis or uveitis	Occasional
Alopecia	Follicular disease can lead to patchy 'moth-eaten' alopecia of the scalp or, rarely, loss of the outer part of the eyebrows or beard	Occasional
Central nervous system	Asymptomatic neuroinvasion occurs in up to 25% Symptomatic meningitis or meningovascular disease may be more common in HIV infection Ocular and auditory cranial nerves most commonly involved	Up to 2%
Kidney	Asymptomatic proteinuria Nephritic syndrome Rapidly progressive glomerulonephritis	Rare
Heart	Myocarditis Ventricular arrhythmia	Rare
Parotitis		Rare
Gastritis	Gastritis and stomach ulcers resulting in nausea and abdominal pain	Rare
Periostitis, arthritis, or bursitis	Localized	Rare
Malignant syphilis ('lues maligna')	Rapidly progressive variant with marked constitutional symptoms and disfiguring crusted necrotic ulcers Possibly more common with HIV infection and in alcoholics	Rare

artery may be affected, the middle cerebral is the most frequently involved. Gradual onset and less extensive damage results from smaller arteries being involved than is usual in thrombotic stroke. Psychological changes can mimic the early stages of parenchymal disease (see below).

Confusing the diagnosis, up to 25% of individuals with early syphilis may have *T. pallidum* in the cerebrospinal fluid demonstrated by rabbit inoculation or polymerase chain reaction (PCR). This largely asymptomatic phenomenon is known as neuroinvasion and it is believed that most, but not all, will spontaneously clear *T. pallidum* from the cerebrospinal fluid. Studies in the preantibiotic era demonstrated that the degree of cerebrospinal fluid abnormalities (white cell count, raised protein, and reactive CSF-Venereal Disease Research Laboratory (VDRL) test) in asymptomatic neurosyphilis predicted later progression to symptomatic neurosyphilis.

Rarely, after 20 to 25 years, syphilitic meningitis or meningovascular disease can involve the spinal cord resulting in (often asymmetric) paresis, incontinence, hyper-reflexia, extensor plantar reflexes, and loss of position and vibration sense.

General paresis involves changes in the central nervous system parenchyma, characterized by fibrosis and atrophy, and occurs much later, approximately 15 to 25 years after the initial infection. Parenchymatous central nervous system lesions can present with usually gradual onset cognitive impairment, depression, and personality changes, later progressing to dementia, delirium, seizures, and delusions. Neurological signs can include irregular, often large, pupils that become unresponsive to light and accommodation (Argyll Robertson pupils), dysarthria, facial or hand tremor, loss of facial expression, hypotonia, and hyper-reflexia or loss of reflexes.

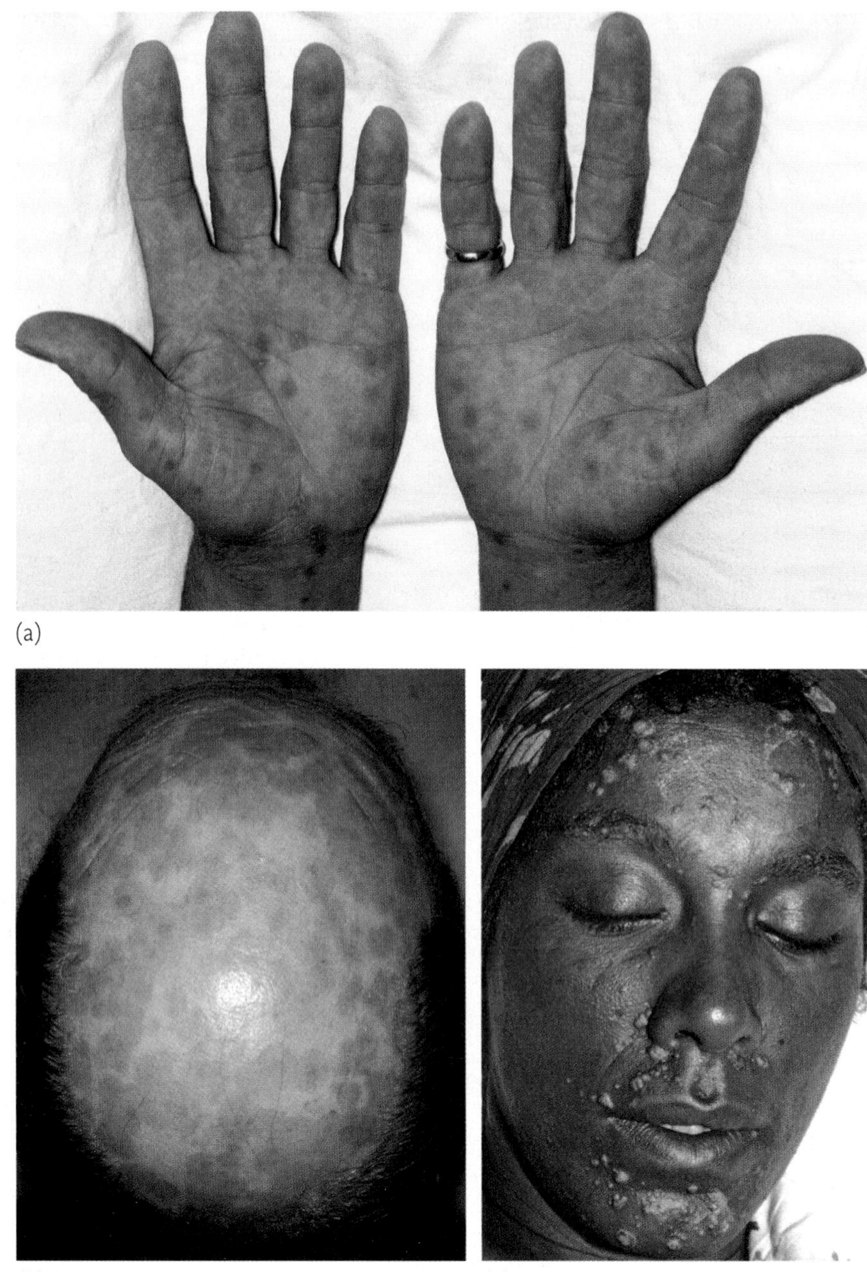

Fig. 7.6.36.5 (a,b) Rash of secondary syphilis on palms and scalp.
(c) Condylomata lata in a woman with secondary syphilis.
(Copyright D A Warrell.)

Tabes dorsalis involves parenchymatous changes in the dorsal root tracts and posterior columns of the spinal cord 15 to 35 years after primary infection. Initial symptoms and signs may include lightening pains and paraesthesias, visceral crises, abnormal deep tendon reflexes, incontinence, ataxia with a wide-based gait, and papillary abnormalities. Rarely, gummas may involve the cerebrum or the spinal cord.

Gummatous (late benign) syphilis

Gummas are destructive granulomatous lesions that most commonly present on skin (70%), on mucosal surfaces (10%), or in bone (10%). They can occur a few years or decades after primary infection. On the skin gummas start as painless nodules that progressively necrose, leaving punched-out ulcers. The face, legs (Fig. 7.6.36.6), buttocks, trunk, and scalp are common sites. Gummatous involvement of the oropharynx can lead to perforations and severe scarring of the palate, pharynx, or nasal septum. Tongue involvement can lead to glossitis, swelling, and leucoplakia. Fractures can occur with gummas of bone.

Table 7.6.36.2 Frequency of late complications of syphilis from the Oslo study in the preantibiotic era

Form of tertiary syphilis	Men (%)	Women (%)
Benign late (gummatous) syphilis	14.4	16.7
Cardiovascular syphilis	13.6	7.6
Neurosyphilis	9.4	5.0

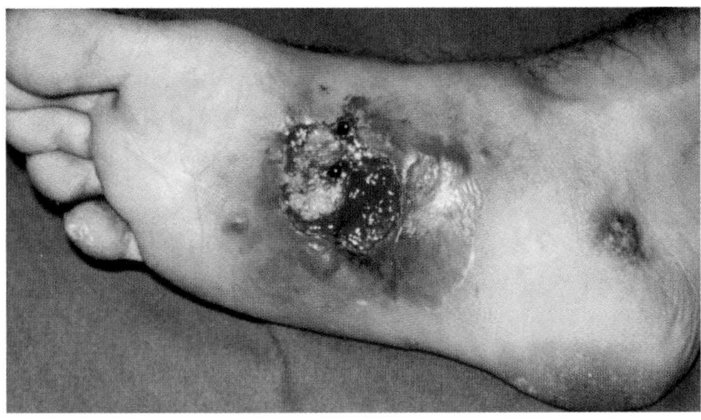

Fig. 7.6.36.6 Ulcerating nodular lesions of gummatous syphilis in a man with HIV infection. Initially thought to be Kaposi's sarcoma, the diagnosis was made by biopsy.
(Courtesy of Professor David Cooper.)

Other organs occasionally affected include the liver, central nervous system, eyes, stomach, lungs, and testes.

Cardiovascular syphilis

Now rare, cardiovascular syphilis develops decades after primary infection. The most common forms are asymptomatic aortitis, aortic incompetence, (usually proximal) aortic aneurysm, and coronary ostial stenosis.

Congenital syphilis

Mother-to-child transmission occurs via the placenta at any stage of gestation. Because the transmission is haematogenous there is no primary lesion (chancre) and it is a disseminated infection from the outset. If the mother has early syphilis, transmission is almost certain; infectivity progressively declines to below 10% in late latent infection.

Fetal wastage from syphilis may manifest as first or second trimester abortion or still birth with a large pale fibrosed placenta or a macerated fetus. Of the infected babies that survive, only 30% have specific symptoms in the neonatal period, though almost all will exhibit symptoms by 3 months. Many of the early (at birth or in the first 2 years) lesions resemble secondary syphilis in the adult (Fig. 7.6.36.7). Failure to thrive in the first few months may be the first sign. Affected infants tend to be small or premature, irritable, snuffly, and cry feebly. The skin is often dry and wrinkled. Generalized rubbery lymphadenopathy is common, often accompanied by hepatosplenomegaly and haematological abnormalities. Early deaths may be due to diffuse pulmonary infiltration.

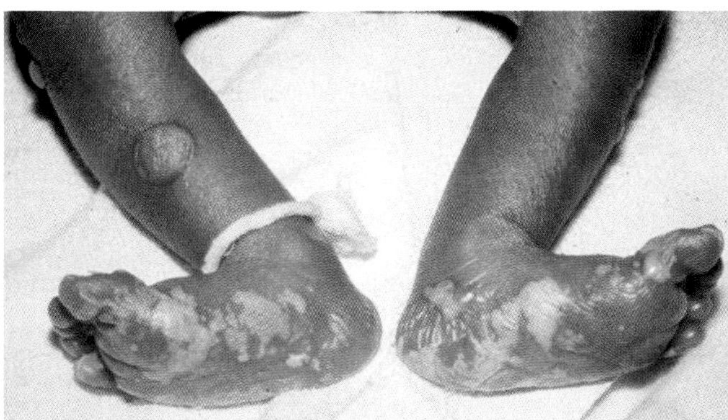

Fig. 7.6.36.7 Bullous syphilis lesions in a neonate.

Painful osteochondritis or epiphysitis of the long bones, and sometimes periostitis, can occur in the first 6 months with characteristic radiological appearances.

Late (after 2 years, but rarely beyond 30 years) congenital syphilis is analogous to tertiary syphilis in adults. However, gummatous disease may be more common while cardiovascular disease is rare compared to adult syphilis. Interstitial keratitis is the most common form of late congenital syphilis. From the fifth year of life onward, the child may develop bilateral eye pain and photophobia, and scleral vascularization. Gumma may lead to perforation of the palate. Periostitis may lead to deformity of the tibia (sabre tibia), the skull (Parrot's nodes), the scaphoid, and the clavicle.

The stigmata of congenital syphilis are permanent deformities or scars left by early or late disease. Sometimes stigmata may help to explain unexpected positive serological tests in adults, as the patient may be unaware of their prior infection. The bony deformities tend to persist, while *T. pallidum* can also invade tooth buds affecting the permanent teeth (Hutchinson's teeth) but not the milk teeth. The molars may be deformed with dwarfed cusps, while the incisors may be small, peg-shaped, and notched at the tip. Previous interstitial keratitis may be demonstrable for life on slit-lamp examination.

Differential diagnosis

Syphilis is often described as the great imitator due to the vast number of illnesses that it mimics. Screening for syphilis was once considered routine for medical and psychiatric hospital admissions. A high index of suspicion is required for the diagnosis.

Primary syphilis

Chancres can resemble anogenital ulcers from any cause, and more than one condition may be present (Fig. 7.6.36.2). Other causes of genital ulcers include herpes simplex virus infections, chancroid, lymphogranuloma venereum, and donovanosis. An anal chancre can be painful and clinical indistinguishable from an ordinary anal fissure. Liberal use of the laboratory to exclude other causes of ulcers is essential. Alternatively, in resource-poor environments that have to rely on syndromic management of genital ulcers, antibiotic combinations need to cover all the common causes of genital ulcers in that region.

Secondary syphilis

The rash of secondary syphilis may resemble a drug eruption, pityriasis rosea, tinea versicolour, seborrhoeic dermatitis, erythema multiforme, scabies, lichen planus, psoriasis, fungal infections, and leprosy. Other infections causing generalized rashes include primary HIV infection, measles, rubella, and meningococcemia. Condyloma lata may be confused with genital warts. Syphilitic alopecia may resemble alopecia areata or fungal scalp infections.

Generalized lymphadenopathy, sore throat, and fever are also seen in infectious mononucleosis, rubella, toxoplasmosis, lymphoma, acute hepatitis, and, most importantly, primary HIV infection. Symptoms of meningitis may also be present in HIV infection, bacterial meningitis, enterovirus infections, and primary herpes simplex virus infection.

Latent syphilis

Childhood treponemal infections such as yaws and pinta, as well as prior congenital syphilis, may be serologically indistinguishable from adult-acquired syphilis and the specific tests are likely to remain positive for life. People from endemic treponemal areas or who may be at risk of congenital infection with positive syphilis serology should be examined for stigmata of these conditions. False-positive nonspecific tests (VDRL and rapid plasma reagin (RPR)) occur in 1 to 2% of the population (see 'Nonspecific serological tests'). Confirmation with a specific treponemal test is essential for asymptomatic people.

Neurosyphilis

Symptoms and signs of meningovascular syphilis are similar to those in other causes of stroke or cerebrovascular accidents due to haemorrhagic or thrombotic mechanisms. Gummas in the brain can be mistaken for tumours and abscesses, particularly in HIV infection. General paresis should be considered in the differential diagnosis of dementia, psychosis, seizures, delirium, and personality changes.

Gummatous syphilis

Other granulomatous diseases such as sarcoidosis, tuberculosis, and neoplastic lesions can be confused with gummatous syphilis.

Cardiovascular syphilis

Signs and symptoms of cardiovascular syphilis are similar to those of atherosclerotic disease and aortic aneurysms are more commonly due to hypertension. Other causes of aortic regurgitation without stenosis include Marfan's syndrome and infective endocarditis.

Clinical investigation

Direct detection of the organism

As with all bacterial infections, ideally *T. pallidum* should be directly detected (Table 7.6.36.3) because a serological response may take days to weeks to evolve. However, the transient nature of the lesions and the spirochaetaemia limit the role of direct detection, leading to reliance on serology or, in resource-poor environments, syndromic management. The role of PCR testing of the CSF has yet to be determined because asymptomatic and transient neuroinvasion by *T. pallidum* correlates poorly with standard criteria for diagnosing neurosyphilis.

Serology

Broadly there are two types of serological tests for syphilis, nonspecific (or nontreponemal or reagin) tests and specific (or treponemal) tests. Although less sensitive for some stages of syphilis as well as being less specific, nonspecific tests require less expertise, are cheaper, and are more indicative of active infection so they are often favoured for screening. Specific tests usually remain positive after treatment, limiting their role in screening in high-prevalence populations (Fig. 7.6.36.8). However, specific tests have an important place in screening in low-prevalence populations and in confirming nonspecific tests.

Nonspecific serological tests

The RPR and VDRL tests are flocculation tests targeting the phospholipid cardiolipin as an antigen. They are relatively sensitive in early infection—77 to 88% for primary syphilis and 100% for secondary syphilis—but tend to decline over the next several years without treatment (Fig. 7.6.36.8). Because they are able to quantify disease activity, nonspecific tests are used for follow-up after treatment. In general, a fourfold change in titre is taken as evidence of cure, relapse, or reinfection. Broadly equivalent, RPR tests can be read macroscopically while VDRL tests require a microscope.

Table 7.6.36.3 Methods of direct detection of *T. pallidum*

Method	Brief description	Role
Animal inoculation	Fresh (or flash-frozen to less than −78°C) lesion material or cerebrospinal fluid is usually inoculated by intratesticular or intradermal means into rabbits. The animals are then monitored for the development of skin lesions, orchitis, or serological response.	The most sensitive test (approaching 100%), but only used as a gold standard to evaluate other tests in the research setting
Dark-field microscopy	Fresh serous fluid with motile organisms is collected by gentle pressure on the lesions and pressed under a coverslip. An on-site microscope with a reflecting dark-field condenser and a skilled microscopist are required. Diagnostic criteria include morphology and motion of the organisms.	Only appropriate for specialist services. Not for oral or anal lesions. Patient must attend service in person. Immediate result
DFA test	Specimen collected as for dark-field microscopy, air dried on a glass slide, and stained with labelled anti-*T. pallidum* globulins immediately before fluorescence microscopy.	Specimen does not need to be fresh, so can be transported to laboratory. High sensitivity (>90%) if the specimen is well collected. Suitable for oral lesions
DFAT test	DFA test adapted to histology specimens, usually transported in 10% buffered formalin.	Skin, brain, placenta, umbilical cord, or gastrointestinal biopsy specimens can be tested
PCR test	Suspected chancres or lightly abraded lesion swabs in PCR transport medium. Possibly cerebrospinal fluid.	Very sensitive for primary and secondary lesions, but only available in referral laboratories

DFA, direct fluorescent antibody; DFAT, direct fluorescent antibody tissue; PCR, polymerase chain reaction.

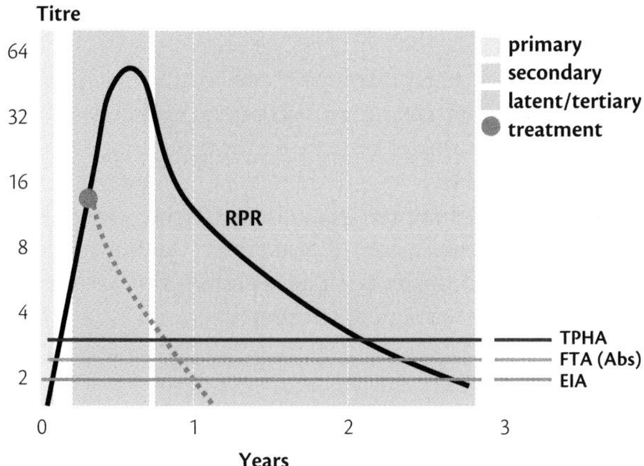

Fig. 7.6.36.8 Serological response to syphilis and its treatment.

The toluidine red unheated serum test (TRUST) is a variant of the RPR test. The VDRL test is the only syphilis test recommended for CSF evaluation.

Such antilipoidal antibodies may be produced by other forms of acute or chronic tissue damage, so confirmation with a specific test is needed if there is no other sign of syphilis. Acute false-positive results are associated with acute infections such as hepatitis, herpes virus infections, measles, and malaria, as well as immunizations and pregnancy. Chronic (exceeding 6 months) false-positive reactions are associated with connective tissue disorders, immunoglobulin abnormalities, drug injecting, ageing, malaria, and malignancy.

Specific serological tests

These tests use *T. pallidum* as the antigen and may become positive shortly before the nonspecific tests. The specific tests typically (more than 85%) remain reactive for life after successful treatment and they do not provide meaningful quantitative results, so they have no role in assessing stage of infection, 'cure', or reinfection. They are technically more difficult and expensive than nonspecific tests, so they may not be available for confirmation in resource-poor environments. Examples of specific tests include the *T. pallidum* haemagglutination assay (TPHA), the *T. pallidum* particle agglutination assay (TPPA), and the microhaemagglutination assay for antibodies to *T. pallidum* (MHA-TP). The fluorescent treponemal antibody absorption (FTA-ABS) test is often used as a confirmatory test and may be the first serological test to become positive in primary syphilis, so it may be added to the nonspecific test to investigate a genital ulcer.

Newer multiantigen enzyme immunoassays (EIAs) for IgG antibodies against *T. pallidum* are becoming increasingly common in high-volume laboratories because they are more objective and can be automated. The EIAs appear to have comparable sensitivity (70–90% for primary and 100% for secondary syphilis) and specificity to the other specific tests. There is considerable overlap in the causes of false-positive specific and nonspecific tests.

As IgM antibodies are large and considered unable to cross the placenta, FTA-ABS and EIA versions of the IgM test have been used on neonates to assess possible congenital infection. The use of IgM tests is not established, and a negative IgM test does not exclude congenital syphilis.

Available only in reference laboratories, western blot can detect IgG or IgM antibodies and appears to be at least as sensitive as other specific tests for syphilis. The IgM western blot looks promising as an aid to diagnosing congenital syphilis with a specificity over 90% and a sensitivity over 83%.

Criteria for diagnosis

Primary syphilis

The direct detection of *T. pallidum* (Table 7.6.36.3) from an ulcer confirms a diagnosis of primary syphilis. Alternatively, a clinically suspicious ulcer and any positive serological test are accepted as a confirmed diagnosis, although more than one serological test is normally ordered if resources permit. If initially seronegative, patients with suspicious ulcers should have repeat serology in 2 to 4 weeks.

Secondary syphilis

Treponemes may be demonstrated in the mucocutaneous lesions of secondary syphilis, although suggestive symptoms or signs (Table 7.6.36.1) plus any positive serological test are sufficient for the diagnosis. The nonspecific tests are normally reactive at high titres.

Latent syphilis

The diagnosis of latent syphilis requires two positive serological tests, at least one of them a specific test. Recent symptoms suggestive of primary or secondary (Table 7.6.36.1) syphilis, or a history of a negative test in the last 1 or 2 years, indicates early latent syphilis. The sexual risk history should be consistent with this clinical staging. Generally, nonspecific reactive test titres are higher in early latent than in late latent infection. In many cases a diagnosis of late latent syphilis or latent syphilis of unknown duration is a diagnosis of last resort after risk and symptom history, clinical examination, and serological picture are judged together. Past childhood treponemal infection can remain a possibility.

Neurosyphilis

Neurosyphilis is defined as a reactive CSF-VDRL or a CSF mononuclear pleocytosis of more than 5 cells/μl, or both. While a reactive CSF-VDRL is very specific it has limited sensitivity (up to 70%) in detecting neurosyphilis. CSF protein concentration may be elevated. Because HIV can cause a CSF pleocytosis anyway, against a background of HIV infection a cut-off of >20 cells/μl has sometimes been used for a neurosyphilis diagnosis. A bloody tap may confound the diagnosis, while symptoms or signs of neurosyphilis add confidence to the diagnosis. CT or MRI of the brain or spinal cord may demonstrate lesions compatible with tertiary syphilis.

Gummatous syphilis

Gumma can be diagnosed clinically (Fig. 7.6.36.6) with reactive serology but, as clinical experience is limited, histological confirmation is usual.

Cardiovascular syphilis

Aortic valve disease or proximal aortic aneurysm with reactive syphilis serology strongly suggest cardiovascular syphilis. However, aneurysm and calcification of the aortic wall are found in other conditions such as hypertension. Coronary angiography demonstrates ostial stenosis.

Congenital syphilis

The diagnosis of congenital syphilis is often problematic, and many neonates are treated before it can be confirmed because of the high risk of serious disease. Direct detection of *T. pallidum* from the placenta or nasal discharge or skin lesions of a newborn infant is definitive but rarely achievable. Usually the diagnosis relies on clinical signs (if present) and serology. Positive serological tests in the neonate may reflect passive antibody transfer from the mother, but a positive nonspecific test is useful if present in higher titres than the mother. An alternative approach to the management of a normal-looking baby of an infected mother is to perform serial quantitative nonspecific serology and treat if the titre rises. More experience is needed with PCR and western blot IgM antibody testing.

As clinically indicated, long-bone and chest radiology, lumbar puncture, cranial ultrasonography, and ophthalmic examination may contribute to the diagnosis where available.

Treatment

Choice of antibiotics

Parenteral penicillin G is the original and remains the preferred treatment for syphilis globally. In most parts of the world this takes the form of long-acting benzathine penicillin G injections, although some prefer daily injections with procaine penicillin, sometimes boosted with probenecid, because treponemicidal CSF levels may be achieved (Table 7.6.36.4). However, daily injections raise adherence and resource issues. No penicillin regime has demonstrated superiority in controlled trials.

Injectable ceftriaxone has been used with short-term success although the exact dose, frequency, and length of course are uncertain. Oral doxycycline provides an alternative for those with an allergy to penicillin, when there is no access to clean needles, or when the patient is averse to injections. Neither of these agents has been well studied.

Macrolides such as erythromycin and azithromycin have also been used. However, treatment failures attributable to a single mutation in the *T. pallidum* genome makes this group of antibiotics a less attractive choice.

Some physicians may use oral corticosteroids to reduce the adverse effects of the Jarisch–Herxheimer reaction (see below) in neurological and cardiovascular syphilis although there is no systematic evidence to support this practice.

Contacts

Sexual contacts of early syphilis should be treated presumptively regardless of their test results if the contact was within 90 days, usually with a single dose of benzathine penicillin G. Contacts beyond 90 days can be treated according to the clinical picture and serology results unless follow-up is uncertain.

Follow up

The goals of treatment are to cure symptoms and signs of infection if present, to render the patient noninfectious, and to prevent late complications occurring or progressing. In primary or secondary syphilis, lesions and constitutional symptoms should be well on the way to resolving within days. However, some symptoms of early neurosyphilis may persist for several months. Antibiotic therapy halts further damage in cardiovascular, neurological, and gummatous syphilis but is usually unable to repair tissue damage that has already occurred.

Follow-up serology can be performed at 3, 6, and 12 months from treatment. Defining successful treatment of early syphilis relies on demonstrating a fourfold decrease in reagin (RPR or VDRL) titres over the next 6 to 12 months. If there is ongoing risk, reinfection

Table 7.6.36.4 Treatment of syphilis

Form of syphilis	US Centers for Disease Control and Prevention (CDC)	Notable variations
Adult, early	Benzathine penicillin G 2.4 million units (equivalent to 1.8 g) intramuscularly in one dose	UK guidelines offer as an alternative: procaine penicillin G 750 mg intramuscularly once a day for 10 days; or if patient averse to injections, amoxicillin 500 mg plus probenecid 500 mg orally four times a day for 14 days; or if allergic to penicillin, doxycycline 100 mg orally twice a day for 14 days
Adult, late; excluding neurosyphilis	Benzathine penicillin G 2.4 million units intramuscularly weekly for three doses	UK alternative: procaine penicillin 750 mg intramuscularly once a day for 17 days; or if patient averse to injections, amoxicillin 2 g plus probenecid 500 mg orally four times a day for 28 days; or if allergic to penicillin, doxycycline 200 mg orally twice a day for 28 days
Neurosyphilis	Aqueous crystalline penicillin G 18–24 million units intravenously per day (as 3–4 million units every 4 h or as a continuous infusion) for 10–14 days	UK alternative: procaine penicillin 2 g intramuscularly once a day plus probenecid 500 mg orally four times a day for 17 days; or if patient averse to injections, amoxicillin 2 g plus probenecid 500 mg orally four times a day for 28 days; or if penicillin allergic, doxycycline 200 mg orally twice a day for 28 days
Syphilis in a pregnant woman	As per stage of adult syphilis	Desensitize if allergic to penicillin (see CDC guidelines); doxycycline is contraindicated in pregnancy
Congenital and childhood syphilis	Aqueous crystalline penicillin G 100 000–150 000 units/kg intravenously in divided doses for 10 days	UK and CDC alternative if active disease: procaine penicillin 50 000 units/kg intramuscularly once a day for 10 days; older children with primary or secondary syphilis, benzathine penicillin G 50 000 units/kg (up to 2.4 million units) in one dose; three doses if late infection or unknown duration of infection; child-protection assessment is essential

CDC, Centers for Disease Control and Prevention (United States of America).

may be impossible to separate from relapse; both are defined as a fourfold rise in reagin titres on at least two occasions. In late infections, where reagin titres are typically low, no drop in titre may be demonstrable. Frequently, a persistently low or nonreactive reagin test, an absence of current symptoms, and a history of adequate treatment have to be accepted as a cure.

Regular reagin testing is recommended for those at ongoing risk of reinfection.

Jarisch–Herxheimer reaction

The Jarisch–Herxheimer reaction may occur in up to 50% of those with primary syphilis and more than 70% of patients with secondary syphilis, but it is uncommon in late syphilis. This transient flu-like reaction occurs between 4 and 24 h (median 8 h) after the first dose of antibiotics and lasts for several hours with malaise, low-grade fever, flushing, and tachycardia. Early and late lesions may transiently flare, secondary rashes may appear for the first time (and be mistaken for penicillin allergy), and cranial nerve and cardiovascular symptoms may worsen. In rare cases, premature labour and fetal distress has been induced. The reaction may result from the release of endotoxin-like substances from killed *T. pallidum*. Patients should be warned in advance and advised to stay home for the first night with paracetamol at hand.

Prognosis

Since the advent of penicillin the late complications of tertiary syphilis are relatively rare and adult mortality is almost never seen. However, in resource-poor environments or where antenatal screening is not routine, fetal wastage and serious congenital disease remain common.

With treatment all mucocutaneous syphilis lesions rapidly resolve, sometimes leaving an atrophic scar. Deformities of bones and teeth generally persist for life. The symptoms of early neurosyphilis usually resolve although this may take several months. The symptoms and signs of late neurosyphilis generally persist but they should not progress. Follow-up CSF examination should document a declining pleocytosis (if present initially) by 6 months, although the CSF-VDRL may take longer to normalize.

Areas of controversy

The role of lumbar puncture

Lumbar puncture is indicated if neurological or ophthalmic symptoms or signs are present. The role of lumbar puncture in the diagnosis, treatment, and follow-up of other patients with syphilis has been debated. Resource and patient consent issues may be difficult. Many experts believe that if using a treatment regimen that is likely to enter the CSF such as daily procaine penicillin, then a lumbar puncture before treatment does not alter management of the case and can be omitted. Lumbar puncture can then be limited to cases where investigation might alter management, such as in cases of differential diagnosis. In the United Kingdom the guidelines recommend lumbar puncture when using a nonpenicillin regimen in HIV coinfection due to the possibly higher rates of neurosyphilis.

HIV infection

HIV and syphilis are both transmitted sexually so it is not surprising that both infections often coexist. Additionally, syphilis lesions can facilitate both the transmission and acquisition of HIV infection. Early syphilis has been reported as leading to a moderate decline in peripheral CD4 cell counts and an elevation of viral load in HIV-infected people; both phenomena seem to resolve with syphilis treatment.

No unique clinical syphilis syndromes have been reported in people with concurrent HIV infection. Limited, largely anecdotal, evidence suggests some more aggressive clinical manifestations of syphilis in HIV infection, but this is the exception rather than the rule. Early neurosyphilis may be more common but the diagnosis is compounded by the HIV infection itself causing neurological symptoms and CSF abnormalities. Higher CSF lymphocyte counts (20 rather than the usual 5 cells/μl) have been used to diagnose neurosyphilis because HIV commonly causes a CSF pleocytosis without syphilis. Higher serum RPR titres (≥1:32) and a lower peripheral CD4 cell count (<350 cells/μl) have been shown to be predictive of neurosyphilis, making these tests relative indications for lumbar puncture particularly if both are present. Some have argued for routine lumbar puncture for HIV-infected people with syphilis, while others, noting that neurosyphilis remains uncommon even in this group, advocate limiting lumbar puncture to people with neurological or ocular symptoms, treatment failure, or late latent syphilis.

Despite some early reports of coinfected patients with negative serological tests in early syphilis, larger studies have failed to show any significant difference and standard syphilis testing procedures are recommended in HIV infection.

In general, authorities such as the United States Centers for Disease Control and Prevention recommend routine treatment with benzathine penicillin G (Table 7.6.36.4) in HIV infection. Some experts advise more aggressive or prolonged penicillin treatment but the value of this strategy is unproven.

A higher rate of serological treatment failure (defined as a fourfold decrease in RPR titre at 6–12 months) has been documented in HIV infection (*c.*20%) compared to HIV-uninfected people (5%). However, the clinical significance of this finding is unknown.

Likely developments in the near future

After further evaluation, nucleic acid amplification tests such as PCR should aid the aetiological diagnosis of genital ulcers if they can be made widely available in multiplex form, i.e. testing for all serious causes of genital ulcers in a single test. PCR testing may also improve the diagnosis of congenital syphilis.

At a more mundane level, improving the availability of low-skill temperature-stable rapid syphilis tests that do not require refrigeration or even electricity could achieve a great deal in resource-poor environments where syphilis is most common. Early experience with immunochromatographic test strips coated with *T. pallidum* antigens that give results in 8 to 20 minutes have been encouraging.

The sequencing of the genome may eventually enable the development of a vaccine, but funding for syphilis research would need to be dramatically increased.

Further reading

British Association for Sexual Health and HIV (2008). *UK national guidelines on the management of syphilis.* www.bashh.org/guidelines

Cates W Jr, Rothenberg RB, Blount JH (1996). Syphilis control: the historical context and epidemiological basis for interrupting sexual transmission of *Treponema pallidum*. *Sex Transm Dis*, **23**, 68–75. [Review of the rationale of syphilis control programmes.]

Centers for Disease Control and Prevention (2006). Sexually transmitted diseases treatment guidelines. *MMWR Recomm Rep*, **55** (RR-11), 1–94.

Centurion-Lara A, *et al.* (2006). Molecular differentiation of *Treponema pallidum* subspecies. *J Clin Microbiol*, **44**, 3377–80. [Evidence of genetic differences between subspecies of T. pallidum.]

Chakraborty R, Luck S (2007). Managing congenital syphilis again? The more things change .... *Curr Opin Infect Dis*, **20**, 247–52. [Up-to-date review of the epidemiology and clinical management.]

Clark EG, Danbolt N (1964). The Oslo study of the natural course of untreated syphilis: an epidemiologic investigation based on a re-study of the Boeck-Bruusgaard material. *Med Clin North Am*, **48**, 613–23. [An analysis of the first natural history study.]

Fraser CM, *et al.* (1998). The genome sequence of *Treponema pallidum*, the syphilis spirochete. *Science*, **281**, 375–88. [First publication of the genome.]

Harper KN, *et al.* (2008). On the origin of the treponematoses: a phylogenetic approach. *PLoS Negl Trop Dis*, **2**, e148.

Hart G (1986). Syphilis tests in diagnostic and therapeutic decision making. *Ann Intern Med*, **104**, 368–76. [Reviews the use and limitations of syphilis tests.]

Holmes KK (2006). Azithromycin versus penicillin for early syphilis. *N Engl J Med*, **354**, 205. [Discusses trial data and implications of macrolide resistance by T. pallidum.]

Hook EW, Marra CM (1992). Acquired syphilis in adults. *N Engl J Med*, **326**, 1060–9.

Larsen SA, Steiner BM, Rudolf AH (1995). Laboratory diagnosis and interpretation of tests for syphilis. *Clin Microbiol Rev*, **8**, 1–21. [Comprehensive review.]

Lin CC, *et al.* (2006). China's syphilis epidemic: a systematic review of seroprevalence studies. *Sex Transm Dis*, **33**, 726–36. [Summarizes 174 studies that track the re-emergence of syphilis in China.]

Lynn WA, Lightmann S (2004). Syphilis and HIV: a dangerous combination. *Lancet Infect Dis*, **4**, 456–66.

Marra CM (2004). Neurosyphilis. *Curr Neurol Neurosci Rep*, **4**, 435–40. [An authoritative review of recent developments in diagnosis and management.]

Morton RS, Rashid S (2001). 'The syphilis enigma': the riddle solved? *Sex Transm Infect*, **77**, 322–4. [Presents the debate on the origins of syphilis.]

Parkes R, *et al.* (2004). Review of current evidence and comparison of guidelines for effective syphilis treatment in Europe. *Int J STD AIDS*, **15**, 73–88.

Peeling RW, Ye H (2004). Diagnostic tools for preventing and managing maternal and congenital syphilis: an overview. *Bull World Health Organ*, **82**, 439–46.

Salazar JC, Hazlett KRO, Radolf JD (2002). The immune response to infection with *Treponema pallidum*, the stealth pathogen. *Microbes Infect*, **4**, 1133–40. [Review of recent developments in the pathophysiology and immunology of syphilis.]

Walker GJA (2001). Antibiotics for syphilis diagnosed during pregnancy. *Cochrane Database Syst Rev*, **3**, CD001143.

Zetola NM, Klausner JD (2007). Syphilis and HIV: an update. *Clin Infect Dis*, **44**, 1222–8.

7.6.37 Listeriosis

H. Hof

Essentials

Listeriosis is caused by the Gram-positive bacillus *Listeria monocytogenes*, whose natural habitat is the soil. Consumption of soft cheeses, other dairy products, meat products, seafood, and vegetables is the principal route of infection. Patients at particular risk include those who are immunocompromised, very young, or very old. Pregnant women are also at risk, although they develop only mild disease, but the bacteria can be transmitted to the child either *in utero* or during birth and cause them serious systemic disease.

Clinical features and diagnosis—the disease varies from a mild, influenza-like illness to fatal septicaemia and meningoencephalitis. Purulent, localized infections of any organ are sometimes seen. Diagnosis is confirmed by culture from blood, cerebrospinal fluid, or organ biopsies using enrichment and selective methods. Immunoassays and nucleic acid amplification techniques are used in specialized laboratories, but serology is nonspecific and not helpful.

Treatment, prognosis, and prevention—aside from supportive care, the usual treatment of choice is high-dose intravenous ampicillin combined with an aminoglycoside, which must be administered for at least 2 weeks. The prognosis is poor, with mortality of up to 30%. Prevention depends upon those that are vulnerable avoiding high-risk foods. There is no vaccine.

Introduction

Exposure of humans to *Listeria monocytogenes* is quite frequent, but infections are rare. Only as small proportion of people are likely to become sick but for them, despite precise diagnosis and adequate therapy, the prognosis remains poor.

Historical perspective

In the 1920s, *L. monocytogenes* was shown to be capable of inducing systemic infections in experimental animals. About 40 years later, it became obvious that epidemics might occur in humans but it took a further 30 years before listeriosis was shown to be a food-borne disease in most instances. Today, listeria is an exciting research tool for studying the biology of intracellular microorganisms that trigger a cell-mediated immune reaction.

Aetiology, genetics, pathogenesis, and pathology

Among the various listeria species, *L. monocytogenes* is the major pathogen for humans (as well as for animals). *L. monocytogenes* has specific requirements for invading and surviving and replicating in host cells. Surface proteins such as internalins are critical for the adhesion to specific receptors on host cells. A pathogenicity island on the chromosome encoding for haemolysin (listeriolysin), phospholipases, and an actin polymerizing protein is crucial for intracellular survival, traffic in the cytoplasm, and cell-to-cell spread. By this means, listeria can cross anatomical barriers such as the intestinal mucosa, the blood–brain barrier, and the placenta. Humoral defence mechanisms are largely ineffective in coping with these bacteria. Rather, a cell-mediated immune response is required to overcome a listeria infection. Eventually, granulomas develop in infected organs, indicating a vigorous immune response. During the acute stage, when a massive multiplication of bacteria takes place intracellularly as well as extracellularly, a purulent inflammatory reaction is seen at the site of infection.

Epidemiology

Listeria species are widespread in nature and their natural habitat is the soil. Various food items of both plant and animal origin, contaminated either during growth or during processing, can give rise to an infection. Consumption of soft cheeses such as Brie, Camembert, and blue-vein types, other dairy products, meat products (e.g. sausages and delicatessen meat), seafood, and vegetables is the principal route of infection. However, tomatoes, apples, and carrots are practically free of listeria. The ability of listeria to multiply at temperatures from 0 to 40° C is of particular concern if infected foods are stored in the refrigerator and consumed without further cooking.

Transmission from infected animals to humans is unusual, but occupational infections in veterinary surgeons or farm workers are reported. Human-to-human transmission occurs only during pregnancy, when the bacteria colonizing the mother infect the fetus *in utero* or the neonate in the birth canal. In most cases disease occurs sporadically, but small epidemics are occasionally observed due to commercially distributed, highly contaminated food items.

Nosocomial infection between neonates has been associated with poor hand hygiene, close contact between infected patients and their mothers, skin care products, and instruments such as rectal thermometers or stethoscopes.

Prevention

A vaccine against *L. monocytogenes* has not yet been developed. Most infections are food-borne; food items are contaminated either intrinsically or during storage in the refrigerator. Foods such as salads should be avoided by people at special risk, and they should also not eat some food items unless they are thoroughly reheated to piping hot temperatures. Food items that commonly carry listeria, such as salads and mushrooms, should be kept separately in the refrigerator from those likely to be free of these bacteria, such as cold meats and other ready-to-eat food, otherwise there will be cross-contamination.

Improvement in the microbiological safety of food production processes and the continued education of the public will further reduce the risk of infection.

Clinical features

Although listeriosis is generally an opportunistic infection of elderly or immunocompromised patients such as those with leukaemia, kidney transplant recipients, patients with severe underlying illness such as liver cirrhosis, severe diabetes mellitus, or iron overload, and pregnant women and newborn babies, some people without these risk factors can be infected. In a few cases, a mild gastroenteritis precedes the systemic infection. The clinical presentation varies from a mild influenza-like illness to fatal septicaemia and meningoencephalitis. Purulent localized infections of any organ occasionally occur.

Recognized syndromes include maternofetal and neonatal listeriosis, septicaemia, meningoencephalitis, cerebritis, gastroenteritis, and localized infections. Outbreaks of gastroenteritis with fever, diarrhoea, nausea, vomiting, and arthromyalgia have been described in immunocompetent adults who have ingested contaminated food. The diagnosis is usually missed because diarrhoeal stools are not cultured selectively for listeria.

Septicaemia occurs mainly in adult patients with malignancies, in transplant recipients, and in immunosuppressed and elderly people. Most present with fever, hypotension, and shock. Many patients also develop meningitis. Meningitis may start abruptly but, in adults, can also develop insidiously, with progressive neurological signs especially meningism. Fever may not be marked, particularly in elderly or immunosuppressed people. A purulent reaction is seen in the cerebrospinal fluid with most of the Gram-positive bacteria lying extracellularly.

Cerebritis in combination with meningitis or separately is increasingly recognized, particularly in immunosuppressed patient. Headache, fever, and varying degrees of paralysis and cerebral disorders such as dizziness or loss of consciousness may be observed. Rhombencephalitis begins with a headache, fever, nausea, and vomiting followed after several days with asymmetrical progressive cranial nerve palsies and decreased consciousness. Infection of the cerebellum may be followed by ataxia and problems of coordination. MRI or CT may show areas of uptake without ring enhancement. Sometimes a brain abscess is diagnosed. In such cases the cerebrospinal fluid may show few, if any, inflammatory cells, and protein and sugar concentrations are normal. Intracerebral foci my be sealed off, so that bacteria or even bacterial DNA are not detected in cerebrospinal fluid or blood, leading to a missed diagnosis.

Localized infections are rare, occurring mainly in immunosuppressed people. They include soft-tissue abscesses, osteomyelitis, septic arthritis, cholecystitis, peritonitis, endocarditis, endophthalmitis, and pneumonia. They usually result from seeding during an initial bacteraemic phase, but focal skin and eye infection can also result from direct occupational exposure.

In maternofetal listeriosis, the mother may develop fever, headache, myalgia, and low back pain due to the bacteraemic phase of the disease. Transplacental infection causes placentitis, amnionitis, and, depending on the time until delivery, spontaneous septic abortion or premature labour with delivery of a severely infected baby.

Neonatal listeriosis of early onset results from intrauterine infection and has a high mortality. The amniotic fluid is greenish and the baby septic and jaundiced, with signs of purulent conjunctivitis, bronchopneumonia, meningitis, and/or encephalitis. Granulomas affect many organs, hence the term 'granulomatosis infantisepticum'. Late-onset disease, developing several days to weeks after birth in a baby who was initially healthy, presents with meningitis. The infection may have been acquired from the mother's genital tract or through cross-infection as a nosocomial infection.

Differential diagnosis

Since various organs may be affected, listeriosis may mimic several quite different local or systemic infectious diseases. The septic manifestations are nonspecific, and particularly in immunocompromised patients and elderly people one should think of listeriosis. Listeria meningitis develops insidiously in most instances, in contrast to other bacterial disorders. In particular, listeria encephalitis is difficult to recognize initially because it can resemble, for instance, a cerebrovascular accident. This infection should be considered in any patient with an acute brain stem or cerebellar disorder associated with fever, particularly if there are no risk factors for cerebrovascular disease.

Bacteraemia as well as meningitis are accompanied by fever and eventually shock. Encephalitis, which may develop slowly, can be confused in elderly people with cerebrovascular disease or even with brain metastases.

Criteria for diagnosis

Listeria are nonsporing, facultatively anaerobic, Gram-positive rods. Enrichment and selective methods are now well established for the isolation of these nonfastidious bacteria from the environment, food, or human specimen. Blood, cerebrospinal fluid, meconium, amniotic fluid, placental tissue, lochia, and swabs from purulent discharge from various organs can yield the pathogens. Gram-positive rods may be seen in a stained smear. Sometimes they are very short and thus can be mistaken for streptococci. A predominance of monocytes among the inflammatory cells, which might lead to early suspicion of listeria, is not regularly seen. Differentiation of the various species is generally possible by means of commercially available biochemical tests. Several typing methods are used to trace food sources, distinguish relapses from reinfections, and investigate outbreaks. Serovars 1/2a, 1/2b, and 4b are the most prominent among human isolates.

L. monocytogenes is the major pathogen, although occasional human infections with *L. ivanovii* and *L. seeligeri* have been reported. *L. welshimeri*, *L. innocua*, and *L. grayi* are not known to cause disease. The crucial difference is that pathogenic isolates display various virulence factors not present in nonpathogenic ones. In various isolates of *L. monocytogenes*, these properties can be differentially expressed, so that the pathogenicity will vary from strain to strain.

Immunoassays and nucleic acid amplification techniques have also been used in specialized laboratories to detect the bacteria. However, serology is nonspecific and does not help diagnosis.

Treatment

Practically all strains of *L. monocytogenes* are susceptible to a large range of common antibiotics including ampicillin, gentamicin (which acts synergistically with ampicillin), co-trimoxazole, erythromycin, tetracycline, chloramphenicol, vancomycin, and rifampicin. On the other hand, *L. monocytogenes* is inherently resistant *in vitro* to the cephalosporins and fosfomycin. It is also resistant to nalidixic acid but susceptible to the newer quinolones such as moxifloxacin. It should be kept in mind, however, that many of the bacteria reside intracellularly where they are protected from some of the active antimicrobial agents.

There are no controlled trials of antibiotic treatment for listeriosis. According to clinical experience, high-dose intravenous ampicillin (i.e. 4×2–3 g/day) in combination with gentamicin (360 mg, or in a dose adjusted with the help of serum concentration measurements, once daily in a 60-min infusion) remains the treatment of choice for adults. This combination should be given for 2 weeks at least. If necessary, ampicillin alone can be continued for another week or even longer, e.g. in case of endocarditis, until clinical resolution. For children, a daily dose of 200 to 300 mg/kg ampicillin, perhaps combined with 3 to 5 mg/kg gentamicin, is recommended. Gentamicin is best avoided in pregnancy, when ampicillin may be used alone, or erythromycin (2 g/day intravenously for 2–3 weeks) if the patient is allergic to penicillin. Intravenous co-trimoxazole (daily dose 20 mg/kg trimethoprim + 100 mg/kg sulfamethoxazole in four divided doses) is the best second-line treatment for meningoencephalitis. This drug can also be considered for oral sequence therapy after an intravenous ampicillin regimen. Since rifampicin is able to attack intracellular bacteria, a combination with this drug (600 mg intravenously daily for 14 days for adults but not for pregnant women) is theoretically helpful for cure.

It is very important to be aware that treatment with cephalosporins is likely to fail. Since acute pyogenic meningitis is usually treated initially with ceftriaxone or cefotaxime until the pathogen is known, ampicillin should also be given with this initial treatment whenever listeriosis is a clinical possibility, unless a Gram-stained cerebrospinal fluid sample shows good evidence of another bacterial cause.

Prognosis

Despite antibiotic therapy, the mortality of systemic listeriosis remains high at up to 30%. Since listeriosis occurs primarily in immunocompromised patients who lack normal defence mechanisms, relapses may occur if the antibiotic regimen is too short, allowing intracellular bacteria to survive. Such endogenous relapses are not attributable to resistant bacteria and so the same regimen can be applied for a second round. Sequelae may be serious.

Food industry

Today, the Hazard Analysis and Critical Control Points (HACCP) management system is now standard in the food industry in Western countries. Once it becomes clear that a working plant is permanently colonized with pathogenic listeria, laborious and expensive intervention and management procedures are necessary. When listeria are detected during screening of food items, the production company must withdraw the affected batches from the market.

Areas of uncertainty or controversy

So far, the infective dose required for induction of overt disease has not been defined. It may depend on cofactors such as concomitant enteric pathogens and in particular on the immune status of the host. Since so many foodstuffs are contaminated, it is practically impossible to guarantee in everyday life that all dishes are free from listeria. Some authorities therefore tolerate certain numbers of bacteria. However, zero tolerance is appropriate for food prepared for babies or sick people. An exact definition of the incubation period is not yet possible. After ingestion of a high inoculum, symptoms appear within a few hours, but it is likely that in some cases days may elapse before invasion occurs.

Likely developments in the near future

At least two different genetic lineages of *L. monocytogenes* isolates have been described in food items or in listeriosis cases. It is a matter of discussion whether this distinction might allow the health risk of contaminated food items to be evaluated.

Although the therapeutic value of moxifloxacin has not yet been assessed in human listeriosis, it can be deduced from cell culture experiments as well as from animal experiments that this quinolone, which is highly active *in vitro*, is able to penetrate into host cells and effectively kill intracellular *L. monocytogenes*, so that rapid cure may be achieved.

Further reading

Gellin BG, Broome CV (1989). Listeriosis. *JAMA*, **261**, 1313–18.
Hamon M, Bierne H, Cossart P (2006). *Listeria monocytogenes*: a multifaceted model. *Nat Rev Microbiol*, **4**, 423–34.
Hof H, Nichterlein T, Kretschmar M (1997). Management of listeriosis. *Clin Microbiol Rev*, **10**, 345–57.
Liu D (2006). Identification, subtyping and virulence determination of *Listeria monocytogenes*, an important foodborne pathogen. *J Med Microbiol*, **55**, 645–59.
Schlech WF (2000). Foodborne listeriosis. *Clin Infect Dis*, **31**, 770–5.

7.6.38 Legionellosis and legionnaires' disease

J.T. Macfarlane and T.C. Boswell

Essentials

Legionellaceae are Gram-negative bacilli, of which *Legionella pneumophila* is the principal cause of human infections. Their natural habitats are freshwater streams, lakes, thermal springs, moist soil and mud, but the principal source for large outbreaks of legionellosis is cooling systems used for air conditioning and other cooling equipment, with infection transmitted by contaminated water aerosols. Middle-aged men, smokers, regular alcohol drinkers, and those with comorbidity are most at risk.

Clinical features and diagnosis—(1) Legionnaires' disease (pneumonia)—typically presents with high fever, shivers, headache, and muscle pains; respiratory symptoms are sometimes minimal; confusion and diarrhoea may dominate the clinical picture. (2) 'Pontiac fever'—an acute nonpneumonic form of legionella infection that presents as a self-limiting, influenza-like illness. Detection of urinary antigen has become the mainstay for diagnosis.

Treatment, prognosis and prevention—aside from supportive care, the first choice antibiotics are macrolides (e.g. erythromycin, clarithromycin) and/or fluoroquinolones (especially levofloxacin). Case fatality is 5 to 15% in previously well adults, but much higher in those who are immunocompromised or develop respiratory failure. Prevention is by the correct design, maintenance, and monitoring of water systems. Notification of a case allows a public health investigation into the likely source and the detection, prompt treatment, and/or prevention of additional cases.

Introduction and historical perspective

In 1976, an outbreak of pneumonia affected 221 and killed 34 members of the American Legion who had attended a convention in a Philadelphia hotel. A newly identified organism, *Legionella pneumophila*, was discovered and named after the outbreak. Since then many different species of the family Legionellaceae have been discovered. Clinical illness is referred to as legionellosis, and there are two principal syndromes: legionnaires' disease (pneumonia) and Pontiac fever (a self-limiting influenza-like illness).

Aetiology and pathology

The organism

The Legionellaceae are aerobic nonsporing Gram-negative bacilli whose cell walls contain distinctive branched-chain fatty acids and lipo-oligosaccharide (LOS). Of the 50 formally recognized legionella species, *L. pneumophila* is the principal cause of human infections. Of the 16 or more serogroups (SG), *L. pneumophila* SG1 is the most pathogenic and responsible for most cases. *L. pneumophila* SG1 can be further subdivided by monoclonal antibody and molecular typing, which is useful for outbreak investigations.

Infections with other serogroups or species (e.g. *L. micdadei* and *L. bozemanii*) can occur in patients who are highly immunocompromised (e.g. transplant recipients). In some parts of Australia, *L. longbeachae* is the commonest species causing legionnaires' disease.

Pathology

Legionellae are intracellular pathogens that are found within protozoa in the environment and in alveolar macrophages in humans. Following inhalation of contaminated aerosol droplets, legionellae reach the alveoli where they are internalized in macrophage endosomes. They block the development of the endosome into a phagolysosome, preventing the normal cellular bacterial killing mechanism through the action of an important virulence factor, the macrophage infectivity potentiator (mip) protein.

The lungs are the principal organ affected and show a severe inflammatory response. The alveoli and terminal bronchioles are distended by fibrin-rich debris, mononuclear inflammatory cells, and neutrophils. Organisms can be demonstrated within alveolar spaces by silver or immunofluorescence stains. In survivors, alveolar and interstitial fibrosis can result.

Epidemiology

The natural worldwide habitats of legionellae are freshwater streams, lakes, thermal springs, moist soil, and mud, where they are found in small numbers. They usually live and multiply within amoebae and other protozoa where they are protected from adverse condition and can survive and disseminate widely.

By contrast, in artificially constructed water systems, legionellae can multiply to extremely high numbers, encouraged by favourable temperatures (20–45°C) and water stagnation. As legionellae are associated with amoebae within the biofilm, complete eradication is difficult once systems are colonized.

The principal source for large outbreaks of legionellosis is wet (or evaporative) cooling systems (cooling towers) used for air conditioning and other cooling equipment. Cooling towers are commonly seen on the outside walls or roofs of buildings such as hotels, office blocks, hospitals, and factories. If poorly maintained, they can become heavily contaminated with legionellae leading to the emission of an infectious aerosol of legionella-containing droplets. Such aerosols can drift 500 m or more, depending on the position of the cooling tower and the climatic conditions.

Within buildings, legionellae commonly multiply in cold-water storage tanks, hot-water calorifiers, and in the hot and cold water distribution pipework, particularly if long and complicated runs of pipework lead to a loss of temperature control, or water stagnation ('dead-legs'). Contaminated aerosols are most commonly disseminated by showers, but other well-recognized sources include:

- whirlpool spas and other warm-water baths
- decorative fountains
- respiratory therapy equipment rinsed or topped up with contaminated tap water
- automatic car washes
- potting compost (for *L. longbeachae* SG1 in Australia).

In temperate countries, legionellosis is seasonal with most cases occurring in the summer and autumn. The same number are related to travel (either within the same country or more commonly abroad) as are acquired locally. A history of recent travel can be an important pointer to legionella infection. Locally acquired legionellosis is increasingly recognized as being domestically acquired.

Hospital-acquired legionellosis is uncommon, but may involve less pathogenic legionella strains affecting a highly susceptible or immunosuppressed patient population in small clusters.

Prevention

Several primary preventive measures can be taken to minimize the risks of acquiring legionellosis from water systems. Cooling towers must be registered with local authorities and regularly maintained, using biocide treatment to inhibit legionella growth; sampling for the presence of legionellae within the recirculating water must be carried out regularly. Hot and cold water systems must be adequately designed and maintained to minimize legionella growth, either through temperature control or use of chemicals, ozonation, or point-of-use filtration. In health care facilities, a balance needs to be struck between adequate water temperature at outlets and risks of scalding. Outlets that are not in regular use should be regularly flushed through to avoid water stagnation.

Although legionellosis is not a formally notifiable disease, even single cases should be reported to public health authorities for investigation of possible environmental sources. Continuing surveillance of legionellosis is important at local, national, and international levels. By collating data, coordinated European surveillance systems have been able to pinpoint outbreaks of legionnaires' disease associated with a particular holiday resort or hotel.

Clinical features

Legionella pneumonia

Legionella infection tends to lead to moderate or severe illness usually requiring hospital admission within 5 to 7 days. It causes 2 to 5% of cases of community-acquired pneumonia admitted to hospital (but with wide geographical and seasonal variation) and is the second commonest community-acquired pneumonia requiring intensive care.

The incubation period is usually 2 to 10 days. Men are 2 to 3 times more frequently affected than women. Infection in children and elderly people is unusual and the highest incidence is in 40- to 70-year-old people, with a mean age of 53 years. People particularly at risk include cigarette smokers, alcoholics, diabetics, and those with chronic illness or who are receiving corticosteroids or immunosuppressive therapy.

Clinical features

Typically, the illness starts fairly abruptly and progresses quickly with high fever, shivers, bad headache, and muscle pains. Respiratory symptoms such as cough and breathlessness can sometimes be minimal, with confusion and diarrhoea dominating the clinical picture, masking the true diagnosis of pneumonia. The patient commonly looks ill, with a high fever over 39°C, signs of pneumonia, and confusion (in one-half of patients).

Differential diagnosis

Table 7.6.38.1 compares features of legionella pneumonia with other types of community-acquired pneumonia. No unique pattern allows the early clinical differentiation of legionella infection from other, more common, causes of pneumonia. Important clues include epidemiological pointers (e.g. recent foreign travel or a local epidemic), high fever, confusion, multisystem involvement, absence of a predominant bacterial pathogen on sputum examination, and lack of response to β-lactam antibiotics.

Clinical investigation

The total white cell count is usually only moderately raised (to 15×10^9/litre), often with a lymphopenia. Hyponatraemia, hypoalbuminaemia, and abnormal liver function tests are detected in more than one-half of the cases (Table 7.6.38.1). Other nonspecific features may include raised blood urea and muscle enzymes, very high C-reactive protein, hypoxaemia, haematuria, and proteinuria. Gram's staining of sputum typically shows few pus cells and no predominant pathogen. Initial blood and sputum cultures are negative.

Radiographic features

Radiographic shadowing is usually homogeneous. Characteristically, radiographic deterioration occurs within the same or opposite lung (Fig. 7.6.38.1). Radiographic improvement is particularly slow. Only two-thirds of radiographs clear within 3 months and some take more than 6 months.

Prognosis and complications

A wide variety of complications have been reported, the most important being acute respiratory failure requiring assisted ventilation which occurs in up to 20% of patients. In addition to confusion, various neurological complications have been reported, leading to the suggestion of a neurotoxin. Acute but usually reversible renal failure may be seen in severe disease. Clinical recovery appears to be very slow in some patients, particularly of symptoms such as tiredness, weakness, breathlessness, memory and concentration impairment, and psychological sequelae. This can have medicolegal implications in those infected through negligent exposure to poorly maintained water systems.

Pontiac fever

This is the acute nonpneumonic form of legionella infection that presents as an influenza-like illness. The attack rate is extremely high, with an incubation period of usually 36 to 48 h. Investigations and chest radiograph are normal, and the illness improves spontaneously, usually within 5 days.

Laboratory diagnosis

A variety of laboratory methods can be used to diagnose legionella infection. In order of usefulness, they are:

1. Antigen detection:
   a. Urinary antigen detection
   b. Direct immunofluorescence
2. Culture
3. Serology
4. Molecular methods (e.g. polymerase chain reaction (PCR))

Table 7.6.38.1 Comparative clinical, laboratory, and radiological features of patients with community-acquired legionella, pneumococcal, staphylococcal, and mycoplasma pneumonia. Values are percentages unless otherwise stated

Feature	**Pathogen**			
	Legionella	Pneumococcal	Staphylococcal	Mycoplasma
Number of patients with data available	79	83	61	62
Patient				
Mean age (years)	53	52	47	34
Men	63	71	57	53
Comorbid disease	35	59	49	19
Symptoms				
Duration of symptoms before hospital referral (days)	7	5	14	13
Urinary tract infection symptoms	14	21	41	40
Productive cough	41	69	86	73
Pleural pain	36	72	56	38
Haemoptysis	14	16	37	3
Headache	27	56	31	26
Confusion	35	17	22	2
Rigors	14	62	7	40
Signs				
Altered mental state	43	25	22	2
Fever >39°C	72	25	43	15
Laboratory				
White cell count >15×10^9/litre	14	60	?	13
Serum sodium <130/dl	55	23	21	5
Blood urea >7 mmol/litre	60	55	52	16
Abnormal liver function tests	59	34	55	16
Radiographic features				
Number of patients with data available	49	91	26	46
Homogeneous consolidation	82	74	60	50
Multilobe involvement	39	39	59	52
Pleural fluid	24	34	32	20
Cavitation	2	4	26	0
Deterioration and spread of shadowing after admission	65	32	64	25

Data adapted from various references including: Macfarlane JT, *et al.* (1984). Comparative radiographic features of community acquired legionnaires' disease, pneumococcal pneumonia, mycoplasma pneumonia, and psittacosis. *Thorax*, **39**, 28–33; Woodhead MA, Macfarlane JT (1987). Comparative clinical and laboratory features of legionella with pneumococcal and mycoplasma pneumonias. *Br J Dis Chest*, **81**, 133–9; Macfarlane JT, Rose D (1996). Radiographic features of staphylococcal pneumonia in adults and children. *Thorax*, **51**, 539–40; Woodhead MA, Macfarlane JT (1987). Adult community acquired staphylococcal pneumonia in the antibiotic era: a review of 61 cases. *QJM*, **245**, 783–90.

Urine is a readily available clinical sample. Diagnosis by urinary antigen detection has now become the mainstay of diagnosis in many centres, usually becoming positive at an early stage of infection and remaining positive for several weeks. Several well-validated commercial enzyme immunoassays and an immunochromatography test are available with excellent specificity and good sensitivity. Immunochromatography can give results in as little as 15 min. It is recommended that legionella urine antigen tests are performed for all patients with severe community-onset pneumonia. Their principal drawback is that only *L. pneumophila* SG1 infection is detected. This is an important limitation, particularly in immunocompromised patients in whom every effort should be made to obtain a positive culture. A negative urine antigen test does not exclude legionella infection and the test should be repeated as clinically indicated.

Direct immunofluorescence with a monoclonal antibody specific for *L. pneumophila* can be used to detect bacteria in suitable respiratory specimens. This technique can provide a diagnosis early in the course of the infection, but is relatively time consuming and relies on the availability of a good respiratory tract sample (e.g. bronchoalveolar lavage (BAL) fluid).

Legionellae can be cultured from suitable respiratory samples (e.g. sputum, endotracheal aspirates, and BAL fluid) using appropriately enriched and permissive agar such as buffered charcoal yeast extract. Culture is diagnostic of infection, as colonization without infection has not been demonstrated, but it is time consuming, expensive, slow

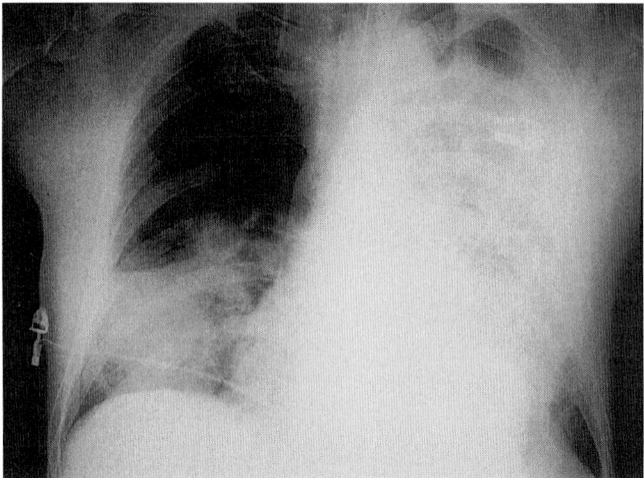

Fig. 7.6.38.1 Chest radiograph of a 58-year-old man who returned from a Mediterranean hotel holiday with legionella pneumonia. There is extensive, bilateral, homogeneous consolidation. He required assisted ventilation for worsening respiratory failure.

(culture can take up to 10 days), and relatively insensitive (especially once legionella active antibiotic therapy has been started). Culture does allow detection of species and serogroups other than *L. pneumophila* SG1, and comparison with isolates from suspected environmental sources. Such speciation and typing, using well-validated methods such as a DNA sequence-based typing scheme, is normally done in reference laboratories.

In the past, serology (i.e. the detection of an antibody response to legionella) was the mainstay of diagnosis, and this is still of value. Properly evaluated serological assays (especially those with sufficient specificity) are based on detecting antibodies to *L. pneumophila* SG1. Antibody responses can be delayed or absent in some patients, but about 40% of patients admitted to hospital will have raised antibodies on admission. A confirmed serological diagnosis involves demonstrating a fourfold or greater rise in antibody titre in suitably timed paired sera. A single high titre suggests infection. False-positive results can occur in some patients with recent campylobacter infection. In these cases, serology should be repeated in the presence of a campylobacter blocking fluid.

The detection of species and subtype-specific legionella DNA in clinical samples by PCR is available in reference laboratories and offers good sensitivity. However, the lack of commercially available assays limits widespread diagnostic value.

Treatment

There are no randomized controlled trials of antibiotic therapy for legionellosis and evaluation of agents has been based on relatively small case studies as well as *in vitro* and animal experiments. Macrolides (erythromycin and more recently clarithromycin) have for many years been regarded as the antibiotics of first choice, mainly based on clinical experience and retrospective analysis of outcome data. One of the key factors is the ability of an antibiotic to reach therapeutic concentrations within alveolar macrophages where the legionella bacteria multiplies. There have been increasing reports of the successful use of fluoroquinolone antibiotics, notably levofloxacin, and even some suggestion that, when combined with early diagnosis using urine antigen detection, they can reduce mortality and morbidity compared to traditional macrolide therapy. Fluoroquinolones demonstrate excellent bioavailability, bactericidal activity against legionellae, and very good intracellular penetration.

For nonsevere community-acquired legionella infection, our practice is to use an oral fluoroquinolone, with a macrolide as an alternative.

For the management of severe or life-threatening legionella pneumonia, we consider the use of a combination of antibiotics including a fluoroquinolone and a macrolide, especially during the crucial first few days, with rifampicin as an alternative if one of these agents cannot be used. Clinicians should be alert to the potential small risk of prolongation of the QT interval on the ECG with the recommended combination, particularly in the presence of other proarrhythmic risk factors. Parenteral rifampicin has a risk of hyperbilirubinaemia, which usually resolves on stopping the drug. There are also reports that the azalide antibiotic azithromycin and tetracyclines (e.g. doxycycline) may be useful.

Prognosis

The patient's previous health and appropriate early therapy are the two most important factors determining outcome. Mortality in previously fit patients is 5 to 15%. It is lower when early diagnosis by urine antigen detection allows prompt treatment. The mortality is approximately 30% in those requiring assisted ventilation, but in immunosuppressed individuals it can approach 75%.

Areas of uncertainty

Three main areas of uncertainty are the pathophysiology of multisystem involvement, (particularly of neuropsychological symptoms), optimal antibiotic management, and the long-term prognosis.

Likely future developments

Advances in bedside urine antigen testing create the possibility of early diagnosis and properly controlled trials of antibiotic therapy, together with controlled follow-up studies to assess long-term sequelae. Near-source rapid testing of water may enhance surveillance of water systems and outbreak investigations, especially if there is progress in detecting species other than *L. pneumophila* SG1.

Further reading

Blazquez Garrido RM, Parra FJE *et al.* (2005). Antimicrobial chemotherapy for legionnaires' disease: Levofloxacin versus Macrolides. *Clinical Infectious Diseases*, **40**, 800–6.

British Thoracic Society (2009). Guidelines for the management of community acquired pneumonia in adults: update 2009. *Thorax*, **64** Suppl III, iii1–55.

Cunha BA (1998). Clinical features of legionnaires' disease. *Semin Respir Infect*, **13**, 116–27.

Den Boer JW, Nijhof J, Friesema I (2006). Risk factors for sporadic community acquired legionnaires' disease. A 3-year national case-controlled study. *Public Health*, **120**, 566–71.

Greenberg D, *et al.* (2006). Problem pathogens: paediatric legionellosis—implications for improved diagnosis. *Lancet Infect Dis*, **6**, 529–35.

Health and Safety Commission (2000). Legionnaires' disease: the control of legionella bacteria in water systems. Approved code of practice and guidance L8. HSE Books, Sudbury, UK.

Lee JV, Joseph C (2002). Guidelines for investigating single cases of legionnaires' disease. *Commun Dis Public Health*, **5**, 157–62.

Lettinga KD, *et al.* (2002). Legionnaires' disease at a Dutch flower show: prognostic factors and impact of therapy. *Emerg Infect Dis*, **8**, 1448–54.
Macfarlane JT, *et al.* (1984). Comparative radiographic features of community acquired legionnaires' disease, pneumococcal pneumonia, mycoplasma pneumonia, and psittacosis. *Thorax*, **39**, 28–33.
Owens RC, Nolin TD (2006). Antimicrobial associated QT interval prolongation: points of interest. *Clin Infect Dis*, **43**, 1603–11.
Pedro-Botet L, Yu VL (2006). Legionella: macrolides or quinolones. *Clin Microbiol Infect*, **12** Suppl 3, 25–30.
Woodhead MA, Macfarlane JT (1985). The protean manifestations of legionnaires' disease. *J R Coll Physicians Lond*, **19**, 224–30.
Woodhead MA, Macfarlane JT (1987). Comparative clinical and laboratory features of legionella with pneumococcal and mycoplasma pneumonias. *Br J Dis Chest*, **81**, 133–9.

7.6.39 Rickettsioses

Philippe Parola and Didier Raoult

Essentials

Rickettsioses are zoonoses caused by obligate Gram-negative intracellular bacteria of the order Rickettsiales, comprising (1) rickettsioses due to bacteria of the genus *Rickettsia*, including spotted fever groups and typhus groups (Rickettsiaceae), (2) ehrlichioses and anaplasmoses due to bacteria of the Anaplasmataceae, and (3) scrub typhus due to *Orientia tsutsugamushi* (see Chapter 7.6.40).

Epidemiology, clinical features, and prognosis of particular rickettsioses

Tick-borne spotted fever group—20 species or subspecies of spotted fever group rickettsiae can infect humans following transmission from their natural vertebrate hosts by ixodid (hard) ticks, with many species having particular geographical restriction. Presentation is typically with fever, headache, muscle pain, rash, local lymphadenopathy, and—for some diseases—a typical inoculation eschar (the 'tache noire') at the tick bite site. These signs vary depending on the rickettsia involved and may allow distinction between different rickettsioses occurring at the same location. Diseases range in severity from mild to severe.

Murine (endemic) typhus—caused by *Rickettsia typhi*, whose natural host is rodents, between whom it is spread by the rat flea. Human infection usually results from contamination of disrupted skin or inhalation of flea faeces containing the organism. Disease is generally mild and self-limiting with non-specific features: less than 15% of cases present with the 'classic' triad of fever, headache, and rash.

Epidemic typhus—caused by *R. prowazekii*, for whom humans are the major (if not only) host, and transmitted by body lice, hence the disease is a particular problem during times of war, conflict, famine, and natural catastrophes. The most recent outbreak, the largest since the Second World War, occurred during the civil war in Burundi in the 1990s. Following a nonspecific prodrome, presentation is with fever, headache, myalgia and a wide range of other symptoms. Most patients develop a macular, maculopapular, or petechial rash. Mortality ranges from 4% (recent series) to 60% (without antibiotics).

Other rickettsioses—include (1) flea-borne spotted fever—cat flea typhus; (2) rickettsialpox—transmitted from mice by house mouse mites.

Diagnosis and treatment of rickettsioses

Diagnosis is by direct evidence of infection by culture or polymerase chain reaction (PCR), or by serological testing. Aside from supportive care, doxycycline remains the drug of choice for immediate empirical treatment of all rickettsioses on clinical suspicion, with many of these infections having high mortality if untreated.

Human ehrlichioses and anaplasmosis

These diseases are tick-borne zoonoses, whose causative agents are maintained through enzootic cycles between ticks and animals. Three species cause human diseases: (1) *Ehrlichia chaffeensis*—causes human monocytic ehrlichiosis; (2) *Anaplasma phagocytophilum*—causes human anaplasmosis; and (3) *E. ewingii*—causes granulocytic ehrlichiosis. These all present as undifferentiated seasonal febrile illnesses, ranging in severity from mild to severe, with multisystem organ failure. Diagnosis is by direct evidence of infection by culture or PCR, or (most commonly) by serological testing. Doxycycline is the antibiotic of choice.

Prevention

Prevention of rickettsioses in general is by (1) avoiding arthropod bites—by applying topical *N,N*-diethyl-*m*-toluamide (DEET) repellent to exposed skin, and treatment of clothing with permethrin; and (2) those staying in infested areas checking their bodies routinely for the presence of arthropods, and promptly removing ticks. In addition, (3) epidemic typhus—louse eradication is the most important preventive measure. No vaccines are available.

Introduction

Rickettsioses are zoonoses caused by obligate intracellular bacteria of the order Rickettsiales. These short Gram-negative rods retain basic fuchsin when stained by Gimenez's method. Their taxonomy has been radically reorganized in recent years. *Coxiella burnetii*, the cause of Q fever (Chapter 7.6.41), has been removed from the Rickettsiales. Currently, three groups of diseases are commonly classified as rickettsioses: (1) rickettsioses due to bacteria of the genus *Rickettsia*, including the spotted fever group (SFG) and the typhus group (Rickettsiaceae), (2) ehrlichioses and anaplasmoses due to bacteria of the Anaplasmataceae, and (3) scrub typhus due to *Orientia tsutsugamushi* (Chapter 7.6.40). Rickettsioses, ehrlichioses, and anaplasmoses are zoonoses associated with arthropods, including ticks, fleas, and mites, which have been implicated as their vectors, reservoirs, or amplifiers.

Rickettsioses (human infections attributable to *Rickettsia* spp.)

Bacteriology

Rickettsiae are 0.3 to 0.5 by 0.8 to 2.0 μm in size. Their cytoplasm contains ribosomes and strands of DNA, limited by a typical Gram-negative trilamellar structure consisting of a bilayer inner membrane, a peptidoglycan layer, and a bilayer outer membrane. Within host cells they are surrounded by an electron-lucent slime layer. The two main groups are the SFG and the typhus group. SFG rickettsiae are mainly associated with ticks, but also with fleas (*Rickettsia felis*) and mites (*R. akari*). Their optimal growth temperature is 32°C, their G+C content is 32 to 33, and they can polymerize actin and thus move into the nuclei of host cells causing spotted fevers in humans. Typhus group rickettsiae are associated with human body lice (*R. prowazekii*) or fleas (*R. typhi*), have an optimal growth temperature of 35°C and a G+C content of 29. They do not enter host cell nuclei but are confined to host cell cytoplasm, causing typhus in humans. Rickettsiae are rapidly inactivated at 56°C. They grow in eukaryotic cells where they live freely and divide by binary fission in the cytoplasm. They must be grown in tissue culture (L929 or Vero cells) or in yolk sacs of developing chicken embryos. Growth in cell monolayers is shown by plaque formation, representing disruption of massively infected cells. SFG rickettsiae form plaques of 2 to 3 mm diameter after 5 to 8 days, whereas typhus group rickettsiae form plaques 1 mm in diameter after 8 to 10 days. The major rickettsial antigens are lipopolysaccharides, lipoproteins, outer membrane proteins of the surface cell antigen (SCA) family, and heat shock proteins. Other antigens include a 17-kDa lipoprotein, and autotransporter family SCA proteins include the 120-kDa S-layer protein (OmpB or Sca5), OmpA (SGF only), and Sca4. Fourteen genes that may encode SCA proteins have been identified in sequenced rickettsial genomes, of which *sca1* is present in all species.

Taxonomy and genomics

Traditional bacteriological identification methods cannot be applied to rickettsiae because they are strictly intracellular. Immunofluorescence serotyping was used but has now been replaced by molecular methods. Genetic guidelines have been proposed for classifying rickettsial isolates at genus, group, and species levels using the sequences of five rickettsial genes, including 16S rRNA (*rrs*), *gltA*, *ompA*, *ompB*. This was validated using 20 uncontested *Rickettsia* spp. identified by serotyping with mouse antisera. Rules have also been proposed for creation of subspecies of rickettsiae that are genetically homogeneous but have distinct genotypic, serotypic, epidemiological, and clinical characteristics. The naming of rickettsiae detected or isolated from patients or arthropods in recent years has also been clarified. Variable intergenic spacers have been identified as the most suitable sequences for genotyping rickettsial strains. In 2001, the first genome of a tick-transmitted rickettsia (*R. conorii* strain Seven) was fully sequenced, revealing several characteristics that are unique among bacterial genomes, including long, irregularly distributed, palindromic repeat fragments. Comparison of their genomes suggests that *R. prowazekii* is a subset of *R. conorii*. The genomes of *R. felis*, *R. typhi*, and *R. bellii* have also been sequenced. These genomic data may provide insights into the mechanism of rickettsial pathogenicity and new tools for diagnostic, phylogenetic, and taxonomic studies.

Pathophysiology

When transmitted to a susceptible human host, pathogenic tick-borne SFG rickettsiae localize and multiply in endothelial cells of small to medium-sized blood vessels, causing a vasculitis which is responsible for the clinical and laboratory abnormalities that occur in tick-borne rickettsioses. Molecular characteristics and expression of particular rickettsial gene products probably contribute to differences in pathogenicity among species of SFG rickettsiae. Expression of OmpA allows adhesion to and entry into host endothelial cells. OmpB and new adhesins also contribute to adherence and invasion. After phagocytosis and internalization, the phagocytic vacuole is rapidly lysed and rickettsiae escape phagocytic digestion to multiply freely in the host's cytoplasm and nucleus (SFG species). Rickettsiae can move between cells by actin mobilization. A gene encoding a phospholipase D may be a key virulence factor. RickA, an *R. conorii* surface protein, activates the Arp2/3 complex *in vitro*, which is essential for actin polymerization.

Tick-borne SFG rickettsioses

Epidemiology

Ixodid (hard) ticks were first implicated as vectors of SFG rickettsioses in 1906, when the Rocky Mountain wood tick (*Dermacentor andersoni*) was shown to transmit *R. rickettsii*, the agent of Rocky Mountain spotted fever in the United States of America. In the 1930s, the role of the brown dog tick (*Rhipicephalus sanguineus*) in transmitting *R. conorii*, the causative agent of Mediterranean spotted fever, was described. However, between 1984 and 2008 at least 13 additional rickettsial species or subspecies causing tick-borne rickettsioses around the world were identified. Nine of these agents were initially isolated from ticks, often years or decades before a definitive association with human disease was established. Keys to the epidemiology of tick-borne diseases are the ecological characteristics of their tick vectors. For example, *Rhipicephalus sanguineus*, which is the vector of *R. conorii*, lives with dogs and has a low affinity for people. However, the human affinity of *Rh. sanguineus* is increased in warmer temperatures. Cases of Mediterranean spotted fever are sporadic and occur mostly in urban endemic areas. In contrast, *Amblyomma hebraeum*, the vector of *R. africae* in southern Africa, actively attack animals and people that enter their biotopes. Numerous ticks can attack several hosts simultaneously, which explains why African tick-bite fever often occurs in groups of people entering the bush together.

However, the life cycles of most tick-borne rickettsiae are poorly understood. In their natural vertebrate hosts, infection may result in a rickettsaemia that allows noninfected ticks to become infected and for the natural cycle to be perpetuated. Ticks may also acquire rickettsiae through transovarial passage. Because ixodid ticks feed only once at each life stage, the rickettsiae acquired can only be transmitted to another host when the tick has moulted to its next developmental stage (trans-stadial passage) and takes its next blood meal. When rickettsiae are efficiently transmitted both trans-stadially and transovarially, the tick serves as a reservoir and the distribution of the rickettsiosis and its tick host will be identical. This has been demonstrated for only for some tick-borne rickettsiae. However, transmission of *R. rickettsii* by *Dermacentor andersoni* diminishes the ticks' survival and reproductive capacity of their filial progenies. *R. rickettsii* has been shown to be lethal for the majority of experimentally and transovarially infected *Dermacentor andersoni*. Similarly deleterious effects have been reported in *Rhipicephalus sanguineus* group ticks experimentally infected by *R. conorii conorii*. This has been suggested as a potential reason to explain a low prevalence of *Rh. sanguineus* infected with R. conorii in nature (usually <1%). However, naturally infected colonies of ticks have been maintained in laboratory conditions over several generations. External factors such as temperature may have an essential role in the survival of *Rh. sanguineus* naturally infected with *R.conorii* compared with uninfected, in liaison with the long-recognized phenomenon known as reactivation – that is, the change in temperature and physiology of the tick host induces the rickettsia to emerge from dormancy and attain infectivity with bad effects on ticks.

Table 7.6.39.1 Characteristics of tick-borne rickettsiae identified in human infections by 2008

Rickettsia sp.	Recognized or potential tick vector(s)	First identification in ticks	Disease (first clinical description)	First microbiological documentation of human cases	Selected clinical and epidemiological characteristics
Confirmed pathogens					
Rickettsia rickettsii	*Dermacentor andersoni* *Dermacentor variabilis* *Rhipicephalus sanguineus* *Amblyomma cajennense* *Amblyomma aureolatum*	1906	Rocky Mountain spotted fever (1899)	1906[a]	Has the reputation of being the most severe tick-borne spotted fever rickettsiosis. However, case fatality has decreased dramatically in recent years in the USA, but fatal cases are still reported in South America. Peak occurrence during spring and summer. Eschars rarely reported. Broadly distributed in the western hemisphere and associated with several species of tick vectors
Rickettsia conorii conorii	*Rhipicephalus sanguineus*	1932	Mediterranean spotted fever (1910)	1932[a]	Disease occurs in urban (66%) and rural (33%) settings. Rash occurs in 97% of cases. Cases generally sporadic. Single eschar. Case fatality ratio approximately 2.5%
Rickettsia conorii israelensis	*Rhipicephalus sanguineus*	1974	Israeli spotted fever (1940)	1971[a]	Compared to Mediterranean spotted fever, eschars are rare (7%). Mild to severe illness
Rickettsia sibirica sibirica	*Dermacentor nuttalli* *Dermacentor marginatus* *Dermacentor silvarum* *Haemaphysalis concinna*	Unknown	Siberian tick typhus (1934)	1946[a]	Disease occurs in predominantly rural settings. Cases occur during spring and summer. Increasing reports of cases. Cases generally associated with rash (100%), eschar (77%), and lymphadenopathy
	Dermacentor sinicus	1974	North Asian tick typhus (1977)	1984[a]	
Rickettsia australis	*Ixodes holocyclus* *Ixodes tasmani*	1974	Queensland tick typhus (1946)	1946[a]	Disease occurs in predominantly rural settings. Cases occur from June to November. Vesicular rash (100%), eschar (65%), and lymphadenopathy (71%). Two fatal cases have been described
Rickettsia japonica	*Ixodes ovatus* *Dermacentor taiwanensis* *Haemaphysalis longicornis* *Haemaphysalis flava*	1996	Oriental or Japanese spotted fever (1984)	1985[a]	Disease occurs in predominantly rural settings. Agricultural activities, bamboo cutting. April to October. Eschar (91%) and rash (100%). May be severe. One fatal case reported
Rickettsia conorii caspia	*Rhipicephalus sanguineus* *Rhipicephalus pumilio*	1992	Astrakhan fever (1970s)	1991[a]	Disease occurs in predominantly rural settings. Associated with eschar (23%), maculopapular rash (94%), and conjunctivitis (34%)
Rickettsia africae	*Amblyomma hebraeum* *Amblyomma variegatum*	1990	African tick-bite fever (1934)	1992[1]	Disease occurs in predominantly rural settings and is associated with international travellers returning from safari, hunting, camping, or adventure races. Outbreaks and clustered cases common (74%). Symptoms include fever (88%), eschars (95%) which are often multiple (54%), maculopapular (49%) or vesicular (50%) rash, and lymphadenopathy (43%). No fatal cases reported
Rickettsia honei	*Aponomma hydrosauri* *Amblyomma cajennense* *Ixodes granulatus*	1993	Flinders island spotted fever (1991)	1992[a]	Disease occurs in predominantly rural settings. Peak in December and January. Symptoms include rash (85%), eschar (25%), and lymphadenopathy (55%)
Rickettsia sibirica mongolitimonae	*Hyalomma asiaticum* *Hyalomma truncatum*	1991	Lymphangitis associated rickettsiosis (1996)	1996[a]	Few cases described in southern France between March and July and in South Africa. Symptoms include eschar (75%), rash (63%), and lymphangitis (25%)
Rickettsia slovaca	*Dermacentor marginatus* *Dermacentor reticulatus*	1968	Tick-borne lymphadenopathy (1997) Dermacentor-borne necrosis and lymphadenopathy (1997)	1997[b] 2003[a]	Fever and rash rare. Typical eschar on the scalp with cervical lymphadenopathy. Illness mild

(Continued)

Table 7.6.39.1 (*Cont'd*) Characteristics of tick-borne rickettsiae identified in human infections by 2008

Rickettsia sp.	Recognized or potential tick vector(s)	First identification in ticks	Disease (first clinical description)	First microbiological documentation of human cases	Selected clinical and epidemiological characteristics
Rickettsia heilongjiangensis	*Dermacentor silvarum*	1982	Far Eastern spotted fever (1992)	1992, 1996[a]	Rash, eschar, and lymphadenopathy. No fatal cases reported
Rickettsia aeschlimannii	*Hyalomma marginatum marginatum* *Hyalomma marginatum rufipes* *Rhipicephalus appendiculatus*	1997	Unnamed (2002)	2002[b,c]	Few cases described in patients from Morocco and South Africa. Symptoms include eschar and maculopapular rash
Rickettsia parkeri	*Amblyomma maculatum* *Amblyomma americanum* *Amblyomma triste*	1939	Unnamed (2004)	2004[a]	One case reported in a patient in the USA. Symptoms include fever, multiple eschars, and rash
Rickettsia massiliae	*Rhipicephalus sanguineus* *Rhipicephalus turanicus* *Rhipicephalus muhsamae* *Rhipicephalus lunulatus* *Rhipicephalus sulcatus*	1992	Unnamed (2005)	2005[a]	The strain was obtained from the blood of a patient from Sicily in 1985, stored, and definitively identified in 2005. A second case has been reported in 2008 in a patient with fever, a chorioretinitis and rash in southern France.
'Candidatus *Rickettsia marmionii*'	*Haemaphysalis novaeguineae* *Ixodes holocyclus*	2003–2005	Australian spotted fever (2005)	2003–2005[a]	Between February and June. Six confirmed cases including one with eschar and two with a maculopapular rash
'Candidatus *Rickettsia kellyi*'	Unknown	Not done	Unnamed (2006)	2006[a,c]	A single case in a 1-year-old boy with fever and maculopapular rash
'Candidatus *Rickettsia raoultii*'	*Dermacentor reticulatus* *Dermacentor silvarum* *Dermacentor marginatus* *Rhipicephalus pumilio*	1999	Unnamed (2006)	2006[b]	Tick-borne lymphadenopathy including eschar on the scalp with cervical lymphadenopathy
'Candidatus *Rickettsia monacensis*'	*Ixodes ricinus*	1998	Unnamed (2006)	2006[a,c]	Two cases in tick-bitten patients from Spain with fever and a maculopapular rash
Rickettsia conorii indica	*Rhipicephalus sanguineus*	1950	Indian tick typhus	2001[b]	Compared to Mediterranean spotted fever, rash usually purpuric. Eschar rarely found. Mild to severe
Potential pathogens					
Rickettsia bellii	Various ixodid and argasid tick species	1966	–	–	None. Suspicions based on its pathogenicity on several animal species
Rickettsia canadensis	*Haemaphysalis leporispalustris*	1967	–	–	Possible Rocky Mountain spotted fever-like disease described in California and Texas. Suspected cause of acute cerebral vasculitis in Ohio
'Candidatus *Rickettsia amblyommii*'	*Amblyomma americanum* *Amblyomma cajennense* *Amblyomma coelebs*	1974	Unnamed (1993)	1993[c]	Possible cause of mild spotted fever rickettsiosis in the USA. Rickettsia also recently identified in Brazilian ticks
'Candiudatus *Rickettsia texiana*'	*Amblyomma americanum*	1943	Bullis fever (1942)	1943[d]	Possible agent of an epidemic which occurred among army personnel at Camp Bullis, Texas during 1942 and 1943. Maybe a strain of 'Candidatus *Rickettsia amblyommii*'
Rickettsia helvetica	*Ixodes ricinus* *Ixodes ovatus* *Ixodes persulcatus* *Ixodes monospinus*	1979	Unnamed (1999)	1999[b]	Although implicated in perimyocarditis and sarcoidosis, the validity of these associations has been debated or not accepted by rickettsiologists. Few cases documented by serology only in France and in Thailand. Rash and eschar seem to occur rarely

[a] Documentation by culture.
[b] Documentation by molecular tools.
[c] Documentation by serology.
[d] Documentation by animal or human inoculation.

Agents and diseases throughout the world

Since 2005, three more SFG rickettsiae, first identified in ticks, have been found to be pathogenic for humans: 'Candidatus *Rickettsia raoultii*', 'Candidatus *Rickettsia kellyi*', and 'Candidatus *Rickettsia monacensis*'. A total of 20 species or subspecies of SFG rickettsiae have now been found to infect humans (Table 7.6.39.1). Geographical distributions are shown in Figs. 7.6.39.1 to 7.6.39.4. There are more rickettsiae 'of unknown pathogenicity' or 'suspected to be pathogens' to be identified as emerging pathogens in the near future.

Clinical features

Symptoms of tick-borne SFG rickettsioses begin 4 to 10 days after the bite and typically include fever, headache, muscle pain, rash, local lymphadenopathy, and, for some diseases, a typical inoculation eschar (the 'tache noire') at the site of the tick bite (Fig. 7.6.39.5). These signs vary depending on the rickettsia involved and may allow distinction between different rickettsioses occurring at the same location (Table 7.6.39.1). For example, there is no eschar in Rocky Mountain spotted fever, whereas they do occur in *R. parkeri* infections which have recently emerged in the United States of America. African tick-bite fever is characterized by the occurrence of multiple inoculation eschars in groups of cases, explained by simultaneous mass attacks by infected amblyomma ticks at a particular geographical location. European Dermacentor ticks that bite humans are most active during early spring, autumn, and occasionally winter and are well known to bite on the scalp. Since *R. slovaca* is transmitted by Dermacentor ticks, the inoculation eschar of *R. slovaca* infection is characteristically located on the scalp during these seasons (Fig. 7.6.39.6).

SFG rickettsioses range in severity from mild to severe and fatal disease. An untreated case fatality exceeding 50% makes Rocky Mountain spotted fever the most dangerous SFG rickettsiosis. The case fatality of Mediterranean spotted fever is usually estimated at around 2.5% in diagnosed cases, but no severe complications or deaths have been reported with African tick-bite fever although the symptoms can be distressing.

Common nonspecific laboratory abnormalities in rickettsioses include mild leucopenia, anaemia, and thrombocytopenia. Hyponatraemia, hypoalbuminaemia, and hepatic and renal abnormalities may also occur. Several specific methods are available to confirm the diagnosis of tick-borne SFG rickettsioses and for other rickettsial diseases. Case definitions and diagnostic scores have been established for African tick-bite fever due to *R. africae* (Box 7.6.39.1) and Mediterranean spotted fever due to *R. conorii* (Table 7.6.39.2).

Flea-borne spotted fever

Flea-borne spotted fever (also called cat flea typhus) is an emerging rickettsiosis due to *R. felis*. It was probably first detected in cat fleas (*Ctenocephalides felis*) in 1918 and rediscovered in 1990. *R. felis* was

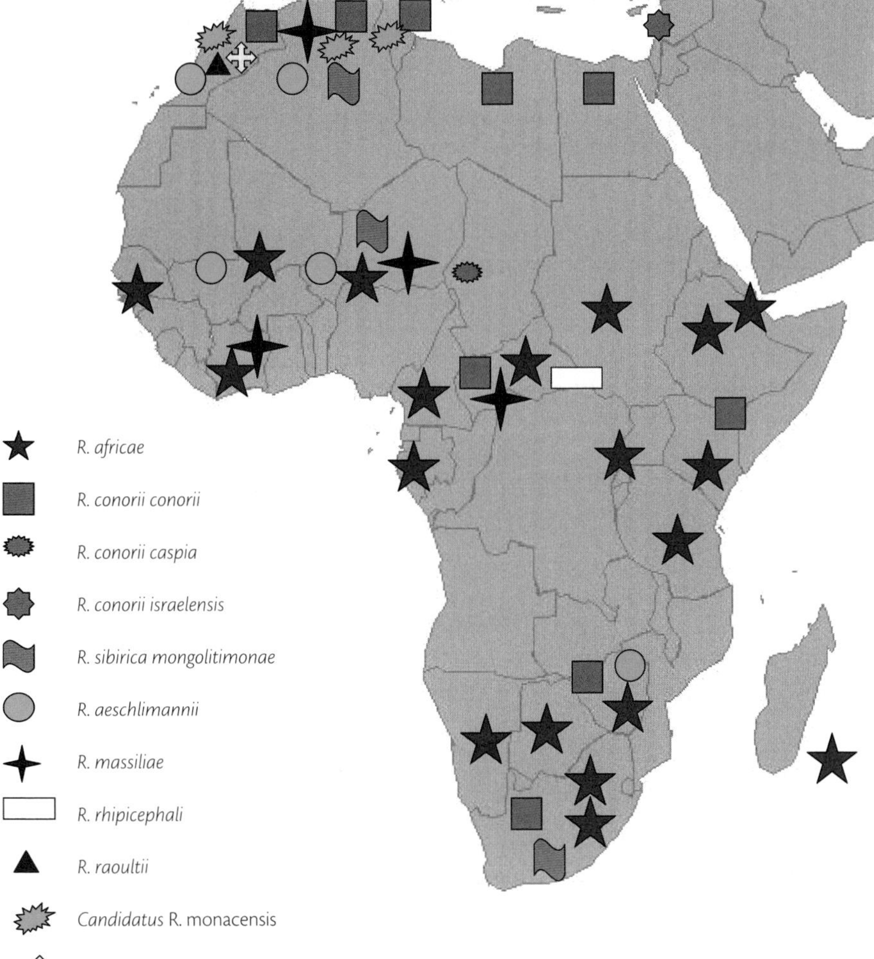

Fig. 7.6.39.1 Tick-borne rickettsiae in Africa. Coloured symbols indicate pathogenic rickettsiae. White symbols indicate rickettsiae of possible pathogenicity and rickettsiae of unknown pathogenicity.

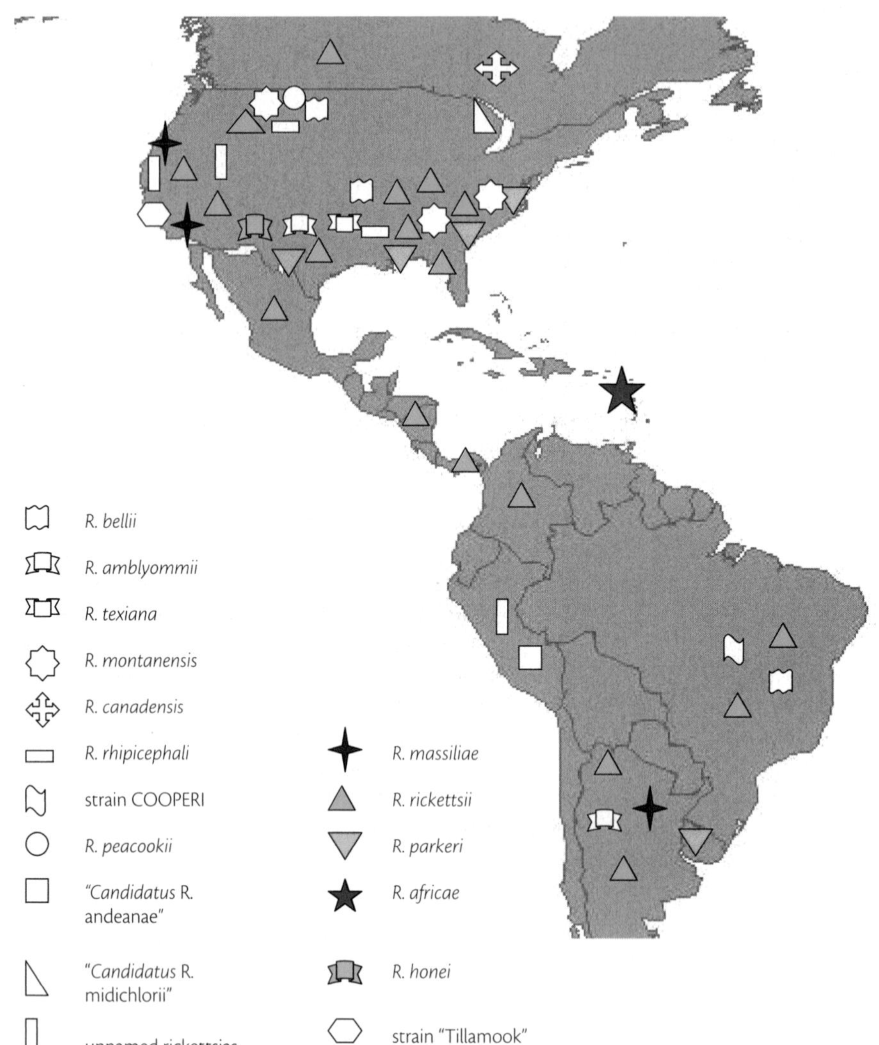

Fig. 7.6.39.2 Tick-borne rickettsiae in the Americas. Coloured symbols indicate pathogenic rickettsiae. White symbols indicate rickettsiae of possible pathogenicity and rickettsiae of unknown pathogenicity.

initially characterized by molecular biology techniques and named the ELB agent for the EL Laboratory (Soquel, California, United States of America). In 1994, ELB agent DNA fragments were detected in blood samples from a Texan patient that had been kept since 1991. In 1994 and 1995, isolation of the ELB agent was reported and the name *R. felis* was proposed, but it was not cultivated definitively at low temperature and fully characterized until 2001 in Marseille, France. More evidence of the pathogenicity of *R. felis* was provided in 2000 in Mexico by three patients whose fever, exanthema, headache, and central nervous system involvement was attributed to *R. felis* infection using specific polymerase chain reaction (PCR) of blood and skin and seroconversion to rickettsial antigens. Two French patients with clinical rickettsial disease and 2 of 16 Brazilian patients with febrile rash showed high antibody titres to ELB agent and specific sequences of ELB agent were identified in the serum of one Brazilian patient. In 2002, two cases of typical spotted fever were reported in a married couple in Germany. Clinical features included fever, marked fatigue, headache, generalized maculopapular rash, and a single black crusted cutaneous lesion surrounded by a livid halo on the thigh and abdomen associated with painful local lymphadenopathy. Serological techniques distinguished *R. felis* infection from several other rickettsiae in one of the patients. *R. felis* infection has been diagnosed serologically in Asia, Tunisia, and the Canary Islands. Rash and/or eschar were reported in most of the documented cases, making it difficult to distinguish from tick-borne spotted fevers.

R. felis is probably cosmopolitan. It has been found in New Mexico, Brazil, Uruguay, Algeria, Ethiopia, Thailand, Indonesia, Europe, New Zealand, and elsewhere in various species of fleas including *C. felis*, *C. canis*, *Pulex irritans*, *Archeopsylla erinacei*, and *Anomiopsyllus nudata*. Transovarial transmission of *R. felis* has been reported, suggesting that fleas could act as reservoirs of the rickettsiae but the role of mammals, including rodents, hedgehogs, cats, and dogs, in its life cycle and circulation remains unclear.

Rickettsialpox

Epidemiology

Rickettsialpox is a cosmopolitan mite-borne spotted fever rickettsiosis caused by *R. akari*. Originally described in New York in 1946, it is still reported mainly in the United States of America. It was studied in the Ukraine in the early 1950s, but few cases have been confirmed in Europe. Serological surveys and occasional case reports identified low *R. akari* antibody titres in a few people in Albania, France, Germany, and Italy, but there have been no confirmed cases. *R. akari* was isolated from the blood of a patient from Zadar, Croatia, in 1991. Recently, rickettsialpox emerged in Turkey. However, the disease is probably ubiquitous but underdiagnosed, particularly in the tropics.

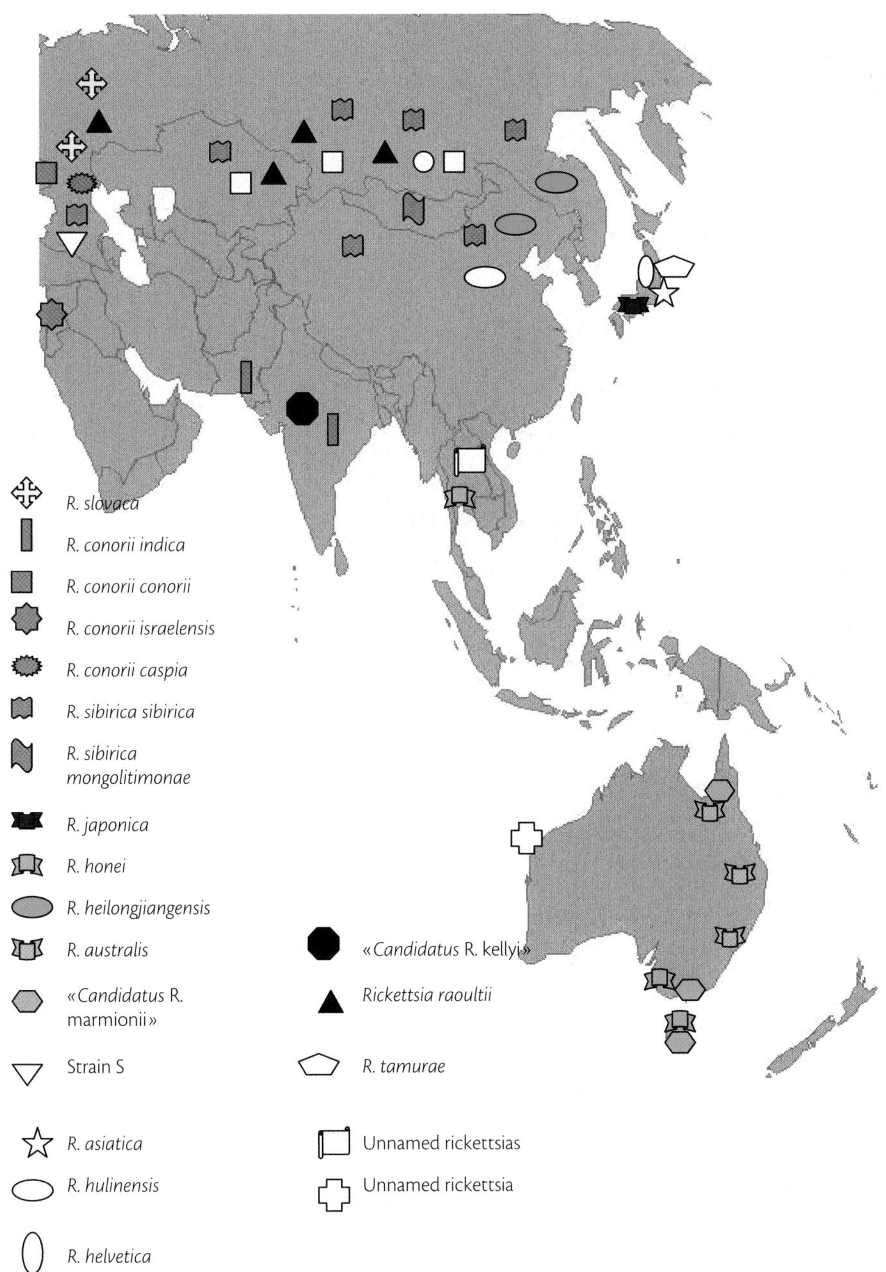

Fig. 7.6.39.3 Tick-borne rickettsiae in Asia and Australia. Coloured symbols indicate pathogenic rickettsiae. White symbols indicate rickettsiae of possible pathogenicity and rickettsiae of unknown pathogenicity.
(From Lepidi H, Fournier PE, Raoult D (2006). Histologic features and immunodetection of African tick-bite fever eschar. *Emerg Infect Dis*, **12**, 1332–7, with permission.)

R. akari is associated with house mouse mites (*Liponyssoides sanguineus*), haematophagous arthropods that maintain *R. akari* in house mice (*Mus musculus*) and may transmit the disease when they bite people exposed by contact with house mice. This mite has been harvested from various other rodents in the United States of America, Eurasia, Africa, and Korea.

Clinical features

The first identified case in New York was an 11-year-old boy who presented with a high fever, a papulovesicular lesion on his back, and axillary lymphadenopathy and, over the next few days, developed a diffuse rash, a temperature of 40.5°C, and remained ill for about 1 week despite penicillin therapy. He made a complete recovery. During the next few months more than 100 more cases were recognized and the causative agent, named *R. akari* from the Greek word for mite, was described.

Rickettsialpox is often described as being like chickenpox because the rash is often vesicular. In 83 to 100% of cases, a primary eschar appears at the site of a mite bite, followed by fever, headache, and development of the papulovesicular rash. The eschar usually starts as a painless vesicle, often described by patients as a pimple, boil, or insect bite. Eventually, the vesicle ruptures and a dark brown or black crust develops over the lesion, forming the characteristic eschar. The exanthem consists of 2- to 10-mm-diameter discrete erythematous maculopapules distributed over the extremities, abdomen, back, chest, and face, but only rarely on palms and soles. After 2 to 3 days some lesions become indurated and develop a small vesicle containing cloudy fluid at their apices, described by the first investigators as 'a window framed in the top of the papule'. Seventeen to 26% of patients have vesicular lesions on their buccal mucous membrane. Two to 7 days after the appearance of the primary lesion there is sudden fever, sweating, lassitude, myalgias, and headache

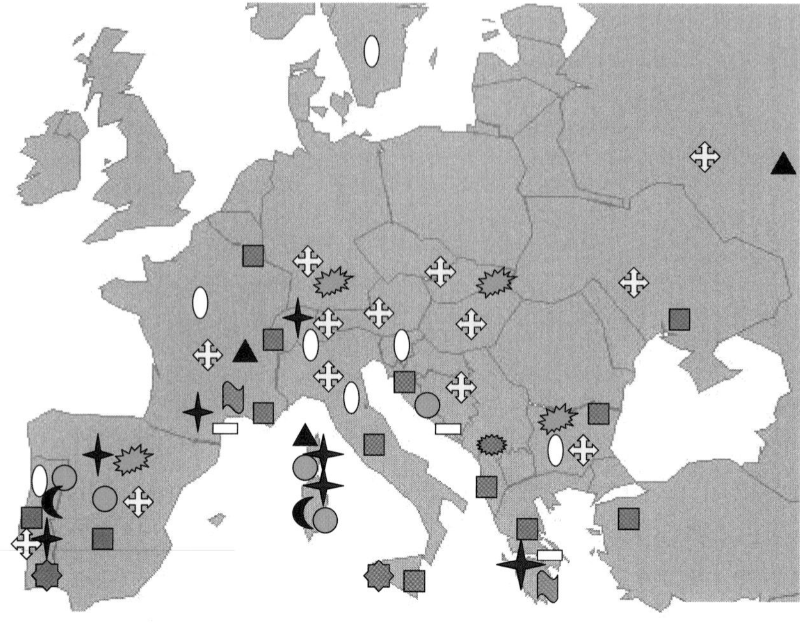

	R. conorii conorii		«*Candidatus* R. barbariae»
	R. conorii israelensis		*R. massiliae*
	R. conorii caspia		«*Candidatus* R. monacencis»
	R. sibirica mongolitimonae		*R. raoultii*
	R. aeschlimannii		*R. rhipicephali*
	R. slovaca		*R. helvetica*

Fig. 7.6.39.4 Tick-borne rickettsiae in Europe. Coloured symbols indicate pathogenic rickettsiae. White symbols indicate rickettsiae of possible pathogenicity and rickettsiae of unknown pathogenicity.

which persist for 7 to 10 days in the absence of antibiotic treatment. Although it is generally described as being relatively benign and self-limiting, neurological symptoms such as photophobia, vertigo, pain on movement of the eyes, and nuchal rigidity may be severe enough to warrant lumbar puncture. *R. akari* has been isolated from eschar biopsy specimens from New York City patients with rickettsialpox.

Murine typhus

Epidemiology

Murine or endemic typhus was probably first reported by Bravo in Mexico in 1570, making it one of the oldest recognized arthropod-borne zoonoses. The first case was described clinically in grain silo workers in Australia and the disease distinguished from epidemic typhus in the 1920s. The causative organism was named *R. mooseri* and thereafter *R. typhi*. Its main vector is the rat flea (*Xenopsylla cheopis*) while rodents, mainly *Rattus norvegicus* and *Rattus rattus*, are its reservoirs. Other fleas or arthropods may also transmit *R. typhi*, including cat fleas (*C. felis*), mouse fleas (*L. segnis*), lice, mites, and ticks, and other rodents and wild and domestic mammals may be hosts. The classic cycle of infection is flea-borne between rats. *R. typhi* is only rarely transmitted transovarially in fleas. Rats are not fatally infected and rickettsaemia persists from day 7 to day 12 after inoculation. Fleas are infected for life, but their lifespan is not shortened. Rickettsiae are excreted in their faeces, where they remain viable for several years. Most people are thought to become infected when flea faeces containing *R. typhi* contaminate disrupted skin or are inhaled into the respiratory tract. Rarely, infections may result from flea bites.

Murine typhus is distributed worldwide but is often unrecognized especially in tropical countries. Cases are regularly documented in the United States of America, Mexico, and Europe, and it recently re-emerged in Japan. Ideas of prevalence are based principally on serosurveys and on cases in travellers from China, Indonesia, India, Morocco, Canary Islands, Africa, Malaysia, Thailand, and Vietnam. Serosurveys suggest that the disease is more prevalent in coastal areas of tropical countries, where rats are particularly common. It has been reported from Tunisia, Brazil (where it may be most prevalent in the south-east), and on the Thailand–Burma border.

Clinical features

Murine typhus is a mild disease with nonspecific features. The incubation period is 7 to 14 days. Fewer than 15% of cases present

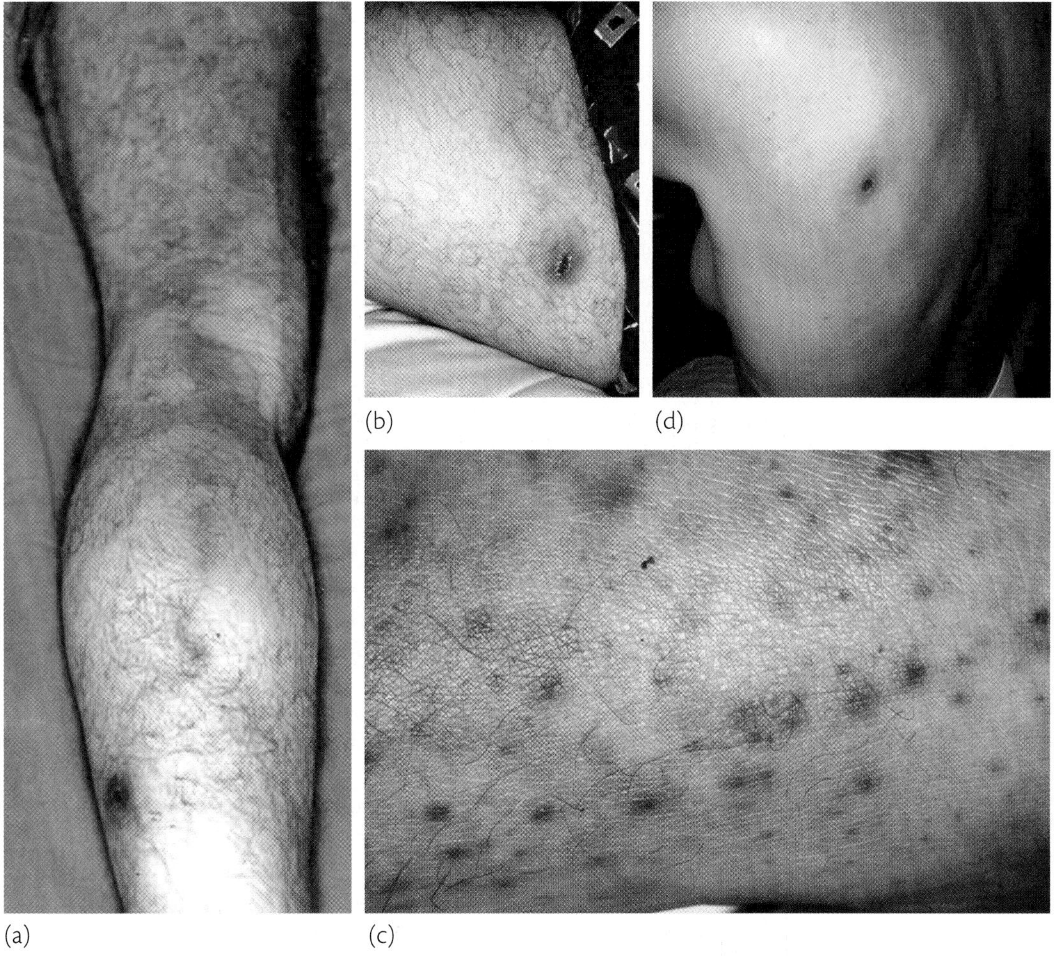

Fig. 7.6.39.5 Inoculation eschar, the hallmark of SFG rickettsiosis which may be absent or uncommon in some specific diseases, such as Rocky Mountain spotted fever, or associated with a lymphangitis, as in the case of *R. sibirica mongolitimonae* (a) and *R. africae* infection (b), or a rash, as in *R. africae* (c) and *R. heilongjiangensis* infection (d).
(a, from Fournier PE, *et al.* (2000). *Rickettsia* mongolotimonae: a rare pathogen in France. *Emerg Infect Dis*, **6**, 290–2, with permission; b, copyright D A Warrell; c, copyright Dr Ed Dunbar, Manchester; d, from Mediannikov O, *et al.* (2004). Acute tick-borne rickettsiosis, caused by *Rickettsia heilongjiangensis* variant in the Russian Far East. *Emerg Infect Dis*, **10**, 810–17, with permission.)

with the 'classic' triad of fever, headache, and rash. Later, fever and headache are more common than the rash, which is present in fewer than 50% of patients and is often transient or difficult to observe. Among 83 patients in Crete, 49 (59%) presented with rash and 17 additional patients (20%) developed rash subsequently. Fever (100%), headache (88%), and chills (87%) were also common. Nausea, abdominal pain, diarrhoea, jaundice, cough, confusion, and seizures have been reported and can lead to misdiagnosis. Fewer than 50% of patients report exposure to fleas or rats. In untreated patients, symptoms last for 7 to 14 days, after which there is usually a rapid return to health.

Epidemic typhus

Epidemiology

Epidemic typhus is caused by *R. prowazekii*, a typhus-group rickettsia. It is suspected to have been responsible for the 'Great Plague' of Athens in the 5th century BC. In 1909, Charles Nicolle

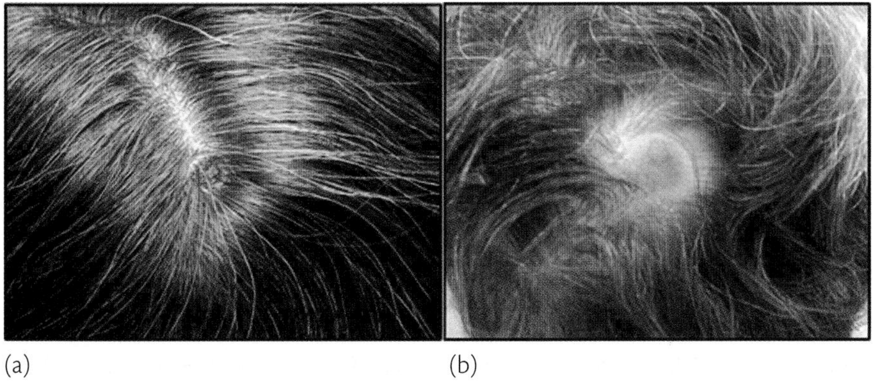

Fig. 7.6.39.6 Patients with *R. slovaca* infection. Inoculation lesion on the scalp (a), residual alopecia (b).
(From Gouriet F, Rolain JM, Raoult D (2006). *Rickettsia slovaca* infection, France. *Emerg Infect Dis*, **12**, 521–3, with permission.)

Box 7.6.39.1 Diagnostic score for African tick-bite fever (ATBF)

A patient is considered as having ATBF when they meet the criteria A, B, or C:

A Direct evidence of *R. africae* infection by culture and/or PCR

Or

B Clinical and epidemiological features highly suggestive of ATBF such as multiple inoculation eschars and/or regional lymphadenitis and/or a vesicular rash and/or similar symptoms among other members of the same group of travellers coming back from an endemic area (sub-Saharan Africa or French West Indies)

and
Positive serology against SFG rickettsiae
Or

C Clinical and epidemiological features consistent with an SFG rickettsiosis such as fever and/or any cutaneous rash and/or a single inoculation eschar after travel to sub-Saharan Africa or French West Indies

and
Serology specific for a recent R. africae infection (seroconversion or presence of IgM >1:32), with antibodies to R. africae greater than those to *R. conorii* by at least two dilutions, and/or a western blot or cross-adsorption showing antibodies specific for *R. africae*.

Table 7.6.39.2 Diagnostic score for Mediterranean spotted fever due to *Rickettsia conorii*

Criteria	Score[a]
Epidemiological criteria	
Stay in endemic area	2
Occurrence in May–October	2
Contact (certain or possible) with dog ticks	2
Clinical criteria	
Fever more than 39°C	5
Eschar	5
Maculopapular or purpuric rash	5
Two of these criteria	3
All three criteria	5
Unspecific laboratory findings	
Platelets less than 150×10^9/litre	1
AST or ALT more than 50 UI/litre	1
Bacteriological criteria	
Blood culture positive for *R. conorii*	25
Detection of *R. conorii* in a skin biopsy	25
Serological criteria	
Single serum and IgG more than 1:128	5
Single serum and IgG more than 1:128 and IgM more than 1: 64	10
Fourfold increase in two sera obtained within a 2-week interval	20

ALT, alanine transferase; AST, aspartate transferase.
[a] The diagnosis is made when the score is 25 or more.

discovered the role of lice in the transmission of typhus and later performed the first successful cultures in animals. He was rewarded with a Nobel Prize.

The vectors of epidemic typhus, body lice (*Pediculus humanus humanus* or *P. humanus corporis*), are a problem particularly during times of war, conflict, famine, and natural catastrophes. They live in clothes and thrive in cold weather when clothes may be washed infrequently and general hygiene declines. After the Second World War, foci persisted in the cooler mountainous countries in Africa but epidemic typhus was considered a disease of the past. However, in recent years, intermittent outbreaks have occurred in Africa (Ethiopia, Nigeria, Burundi), Mexico, Central America, South America, eastern Europe, Afghanistan, northern India, and China. The most recent outbreak, the largest since the Second World War, occurred during the civil war in Burundi in the 1990s.

R. prowazekii is transmitted to people when infected louse feeding sites are contaminate by their faeces, or when the conjunctivae and other mucous membranes are exposed to crushed bodies or faeces of infected lice. Transmission may also result from the inhalation of infected faeces, which is thought to be the main route of infection in health workers attending patients. People who survive epidemic typhus remain infected with *R. prowazekii* for life; when stressed, they may experience a recrudescence (Brill–Zinsser disease), and may be the source of a new epidemic if they become infested with body lice. Humans were long considered the sole reservoir of *R. prowazekii* but its discovery in flying squirrels and their ectoparasites in North America indicates an alternative reservoir. Sylvatic (flying squirrel) typhus has not yet been associated with human fatalities, but North American flying squirrel strains of *R. prowazekii* appear similar to those isolated from patients during louse-borne outbreaks. A non-human typhus reservoir has also been reported in Ethiopia, where 10 isolates of *R. prowazekii* were obtained from hyalomma ticks recovered from livestock. The association of typhus-group rickettsiae with ticks has also been suggested.

Clinical features

After an incubation period of 10 to 14 days, patients develop malaise and vague symptoms before the sudden development of fever (all cases), headache (all cases), and myalgia (70–100%). In Burundi, a crouching attitude was observed, attributable to myalgia. Other common features are nausea or vomiting, coughing, and abnormalities of central nervous system function ranging from confusion to stupor and coma. Diarrhoea, pulmonary involvement, myocarditis, splenomegaly, and conjunctivitis may also occur. Most patients develop a macular, maculopapular, or petechial rash that classically begins on the trunk and spreads to the limbs (Fig. 7.6.39.7a,b). It is difficult to detect in pigmented skins. Gangrene of the distal extremities may occur in severe cases as mentioned in Thucydides' description of the Great Plague of Athens (Fig. 7.6.39.7c).

Case fatality ranges between 4% in the antibiotic era up to 60% before antibiotics were available. Brill–Zinsser disease can appear many years after the acute disease. It is less severe and the rash is less frequent.

Investigation and specific diagnosis

Serology

Serological tests are the most frequently used and widely available methods for diagnosis. The Weil–Felix test, the oldest test, is based

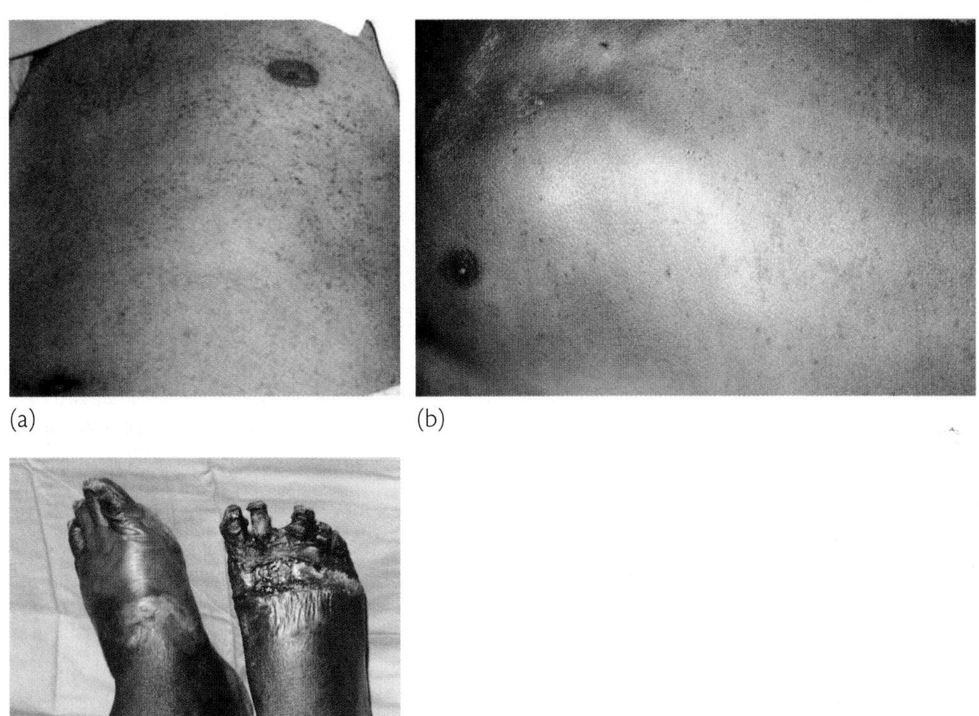

(a) (b) (c)

Fig. 7.6.39.7 (a) Rash in a patient with epidemic typhus due to *R. prowazekii* imported from Algeria to France. (b) Rash of epidemic typhus in an Ethiopian patient. (c) Peripheral gangrene in an Ethiopian patient with epidemic typhus.
(a, from Niang M, Brouqui P, Raoult D (1999). Epidemic typhus imported from Algeria. *Emerg Infect Dis*, **5**, 716–18, with permission; b, courtesy of the late Dr P L Perine; c, copyright D A Warrell.)

on the detection of antibodies to various proteus antigens that cross-react with rickettsiae. Although it lacks specificity and sensitivity, it continues to be used in many developing countries. It has also provided the first diagnostic step towards recognition of emerging pathogens in countries with higher levels of technical development, as in the case of *R. japonica* in Japan. However, immunofluorescence assay (IFA) is currently considered the reference method. Acute-phase and convalescent-phase serum specimens must be collected, several weeks apart. One limitation of serology is cross-reactivity between antigens of pathogens within the same genus, and other genera. Most commercially available IFAs offer a very limited selection of antigens (e.g. *R. rickettsii* in the United States of America and *R. conorii, R. rickettsii*, and *R. typhi* in France). It is important to remind clinicians that IFA may be adequate to diagnose the class of infection (e.g. SFG rickettsiosis), but it is unlikely to provide a specific aetiological agent unless more sophisticated assays are performed. Serology should be considered an initial, but not the sole, method for recognizing and diagnosing 'emerging rickettsioses', particularly if no rickettsiae have been isolated or detected previously in that area. In the Unité des Rickettsies, Marseille, when cross-reactions are noted between several rickettsial antigens, a rickettsia is considered to be causal when titres of IgG or IgM antibody against this antigen are at least two serial dilutions higher than those against other rickettsial antigens. When differences in titres between several antigens are lower than two dilutions, western blot assays and, if necessary, cross-absorption studies are used.

Culture

Rickettsial isolation in culture is the definitive diagnostic method, but can be performed only in P3 facilities that can maintain living host cells or cell cultures. The centrifugation shell-vial technique using HEL fibroblasts has proved effective. Rickettsiae can be isolated from buffy coat preparations of heparinized or ethylenediaminetetraacetic acid (EDTA)-anticoagulated whole blood, skin biopsies, and from arthropods.

Histochemical and immunohistochemical procedures

Rickettsiae can been detected in tissue specimens by various histochemical methods, including Giemsa or Gimenez staining. Immunohistochemical methods are superior for SFG rickettsiae in formalin-fixed paraffin-embedded skin biopsies, particularly eschars (Fig. 7.6.39.8). Most available assays are SFG specific but not species specific.

Molecular tools

PCR and sequencing methods are sensitive and rapid tools for detecting and identifying rickettsiae in blood and skin biopsies. Primers amplifying sequences of several genes have been used. Arthropods are used as epidemiological tools to detect the presence of a pathogen in a specific geographical area. Nested PCR has been reported, but it must be remembered that standard nested PCR assays are highly susceptible to contamination and false-positive results. A PCR assay has been described that has increased sensitivity. This 'suicide PCR' is a nested PCR using single-use primers targeting

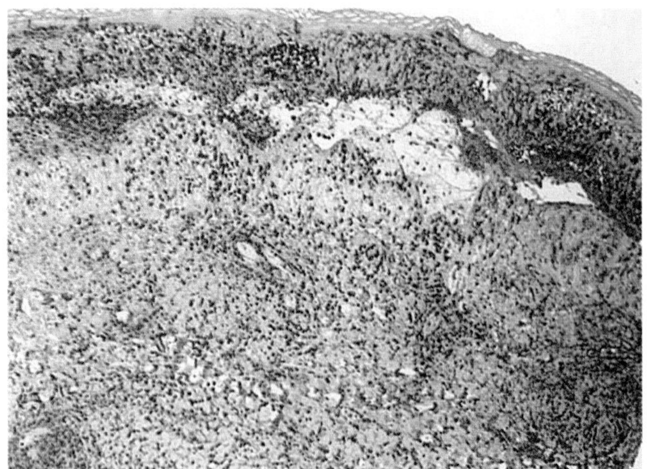

Fig. 7.6.39.8 Inoculation eschar from a patient with African tick-bite fever showing numerous dermal inflammatory infiltrates mainly composed of polymorphonuclear leucocytes. Immunoperoxidase staining with an anti-CD15 antibody; original magnification ×100.
(From Lepidi H, Fournier PE, Raoult D (2006). Histologic features and immunodetection of African tick-bite fever eschar. *Emerg Infect Dis*, **12**, 1332–7, with permission.)

a completely novel gene and so avoiding 'vertical' contamination by amplicons from previous assays, a limitation of the extensive use of PCR. The absence of a positive control does not impair the interpretation of positive results, which are validated by appropriate negative controls. All positive PCR products are sequenced to identify the causative agent. This technique has been successful with EDTA-blood, serum, lymph node specimens, and skin biopsies. Real-time quantitative PCR assays have been developed, as in the case of epidemic typhus. This could aid surveillance in public health programmes, especially for countries where human cases are underdiagnosed.

Treatment and prognosis

Early empirical antibiotic is the rule for any suspected rickettsiosis, before confirmation of the diagnosis.

SFG rickettsioses

Doxycycline (200 mg/day) is the treatment of choice for all SFG rickettsioses, including Rocky Mountain spotted fever in young children. Duration of antibiotic therapy for SFG rickettsioses is governed more by clinical response than a statutory number of days. However, for most of these infections, therapy should continue for at least 3 days after the patient's fever has subsided. A single dose of 200 mg doxycycline has proved adequate for Mediterranean spotted fever, but patients with severe SFG rickettsioses should be given doxycycline intravenously for up to 24 h after they become afebrile. Josamycin has also been used to treat some patients with SFG rickettsioses, including pregnant women with Mediterranean spotted fever. Newer macrolides such as azithromycin and clarithromycin are promising, particularly in children with Mediterranean spotted fever. Chloramphenicol is an alternative, but its use is limited by perceived side effects and it should be considered as empirical treatment of severe cases only if it is the only available drug, as in developing countries. Some fluoroquinolones may be effective against SFG rickettsiae. Many classes of broad-spectrum antibiotics including penicillins, cephalosporins, and aminoglycosides are ineffective against rickettsial diseases.

Murine typhus

Doxycycline is the drug of choice for nonpregnant adults and children. The optimal duration of therapy has not been assessed in clinical studies but 7 to 15 days, or for at least 48 h after the patient has become afebrile, has been recommended. A single dose of 200 mg doxycycline also proved adequate. Response to doxycycline is rapid with defervescence in 2 to 3 days. Chloramphenicol is an alternative, with the reservations discussed above, but relapses have been reported. Fluoroquinolones proved effective *in vitro* against *R. typhi*, but the few clinical studies produced contradictory results. Other antibiotics effective against *R. typhi in vitro*, including rifampicin, thiamphenicol, macrolides, erythromycin, clarithromycin, josamycin, and telithromycin, have no clinical application, and amoxicillin, gentamicin, and trimethoprim/sulphamethoxazole are ineffective.

Epidemic typhus

Tetracycline and chloramphenicol are effective. Chloramphenicol is still widely used as empirical treatment of fever in tropical developing countries since its broad spectrum includes other serious infections such as meningococcaemia and typhoid fevers that can initially mimic epidemic typhus. Most patients improve markedly within 48 h of starting treatment with either of these antibiotics. However, many physicians prefer to use tetracycline for all typhus diseases, as it is cheaper and safer. A single dose of 200 mg doxycycline, the reference treatment, is extremely efficient. Few or no relapses are observed with this treatment, which should be prescribed for any suspected case, including children, as no risk of tooth staining has been demonstrated with this regimen. Ciprofloxacin should be avoided.

Human ehrlichioses and anaplasmosis

These diseases are caused by bacteria of the family Anaplasmataceae, long thought to be of purely veterinary importance. Three species are now implicated in human diseases, *Ehrlichia chaffeensis* causing human monocytic ehrlichiosis, *Anaplasma phagocytophilum* causing human anaplasmosis, and *E. ewingii* causing granulocytic ehrlichiosis. These diseases are tick-borne zoonoses whose causative agents are maintained through enzootic cycles between ticks and animals.

Bacteriology, taxonomy, and genomics

The family Anaplasmataceae consists of intracellular alphaproteobacteria including human and mammal pathogens, whose host cells are of bone marrow or haematopoietic origin including erythrocytes, monocytes or macrophages, neutrophils, and platelets. Members of this family share a high degree of nucleotide sequence similarity in several chromosomal genes, such as *rrs*, *groESL operon*, *gltA*, *RpoB*, and *Ank*. The organisms grow within cytoplasmic vacuoles containing one to many individual organisms which resemble mulberries when observed by light microscopy, and have been called 'morulae' (Fig. 7.6.39.9). *Anaplasma marginale*, a cattle pathogen, was the first discovered, by Theiler in 1910. Since then, others have been described in animals and humans. In 2001, improvements in molecular phylogenetic methods modified the taxonomy of the Anaplasmataceae, based on comparison of sequences obtained from *rrs* (16s rRNA encoding gene) and the *groESL* operon. This contains a spacer region between *groES* and the *groEL* heat shock protein genes and is thought to be more

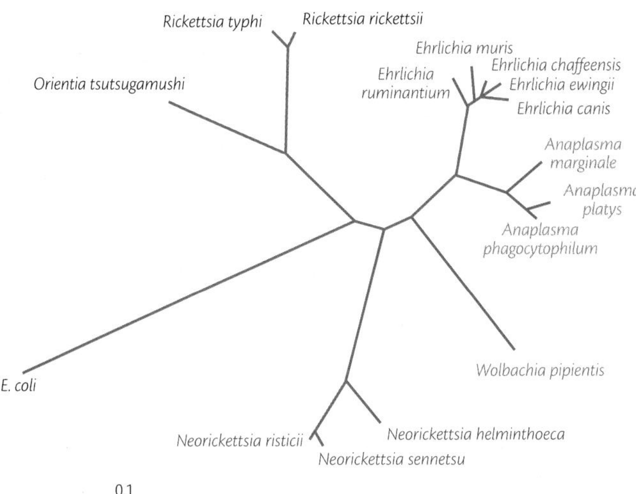

Fig. 7.6.39.9 Current phylogeny and taxonomic classification of genera in the family Anaplasmataceae. The distance bar represents substitutions per 1000 bp. *E. coli*, *Escherichia coli*.

(From Dumler JS, *et al.* (2005). Human granulocytic anaplasmosis and *Anaplasma phagocytophilum*. *Emerg Infect Dis*, **1**, 1828–34, with permission.)

informative phylogenetically than the coding regions. Four clades and four genera have been identified including *Anaplasma*, *Ehrlichia*, *Neorickettsia*, and *Wolbachia*, and some taxa, such as *Cowdria ruminantium* (now called *Ehrlichia ruminantium*) the cause of heart water in cattle, have been reclassified (Fig. 7.6.39.9). Analyses of other gene sequences and the complete genome sequencing of several species of the family (*A. phagocytophilum*, *E. chaffeensis*, *E. ruminantium*, *N. sennetsu*, and *W. pipientis*) have confirmed the new organization of the family Anaplasmataceae. Ehrlichia and anaplasma display a unique large expansion of immunodominant outer membrane proteins, facilitating antigenic variation. Unlike Rickettsiaceae, pathogenic Anaplasmataceae are capable of making all major vitamins, cofactors, and nucleotides, which could be beneficial to the invertebrate vector or the vertebrate host. Ehrlichia and anaplasma lack genes for biosynthesis of the lipopolysaccharide and peptidoglycan activating host leucocytes.

Human monocytic ehrlichiosis

Epidemiology

The first human case of monocytic ehrlichiosis (HME) was identified in 1986, when intracytoplasmic inclusions were seen in monocytes in the peripheral blood smear of a severely ill man bitten by ticks in Arkansas, United States of America. This case was first assumed to be due to *E. canis*, the agent of monocytic canine ehrlichiosis, but *E. chaffeensis* was later isolated.

E. chaffeensis is maintained in nature as a complex zoonosis, involving many vertebrate reservoirs for the bacterium and blood-meal sources for the tick vectors. The Lone Star tick (*Amblyomma americanum*) is its primary vector. All stages of this tick bite people. It is distributed in south, central, south-eastern, and mid-Atlantic areas of the United States of America, in meadows, woodlands, and hardwood forests. Primary hosts include many wild and domestic mammals, although deer are considered to be the definitive host. *E. chaffeensis* has been detected by PCR in other American ticks, but their role as vectors has not been demonstrated. There is no evidence of transovarial transmission, so ticks are not considered to be reservoirs. So far, the white-tailed deer (*Odocoileus virginianus*) is the sole recognized efficient reservoir of *E. chaffeensis* but domestic dogs (with mild to inapparent disease), red foxes, and domestic goats are potential reservoirs.

Between 1986 and 1997, more than 700 presumptive cases were reported to the Centers for Disease Control (CDC), and between 1999 and 2004, more than 1300 cases. Most cases of HME occur in the south, central, and south-eastern regions of the United States of America, where *Amblyomma americanum* reaches its highest prevalence. HME is a seasonal disease whose incidence correlates with the activity of both nymphs and adult ticks. Most cases occur from May to July. Incidence based on active surveillance is 10 times higher than the highest rates reported using passive surveillance. HME seems to be prevalent in Brazil and has been reported from other parts of the world including Latin America, Europe, Africa, and Asia. These diagnoses were based on serological studies, so infection by closely related organism cannot be completely ruled out. Gene fragments closely related to those of *E. chaffeensis* have been detected by PCR in ticks and rodents trapped in continental Asia but, so far, the disease has been clearly identified only in the United States of America.

Clinical diagnosis

Tick bite or tick exposure is reported in 70 to 90% of patients with HME. It is more common in males and can affect individuals of all ages, including children and elderly people. The incubation period is 1 to 2 weeks (median 9 days). It presents as an undifferentiated febrile illness ranging in severity from a mild disease to multisystem organ failure. Apart from immunosuppression due to AIDS or other conditions, the most important risk factor for severe disease is age. The risk of life-threatening complications or death is higher in patients aged 60 years or more, but many severe or fatal cases have been described in apparently healthy children and young adults. More than one-half of patients have to be hospitalized and case fatality is estimated to be 3%.

Clinical features include fever (98%), headache (77%), myalgias (65%), vomiting (36%), rash (35%), cough (25%), and neurological findings with impaired consciousness (20%). The petechial, macular, maculopapular, or diffusely erythematous rash involves trunk, extremities, and, less commonly, the face. Malaise (30–80%), lymphadenopathy, gastrointestinal symptoms, pharyngitis, and, less frequently, conjunctivitis, dysuria, and peripheral oedema may also occur. Leucopenia, thrombocytopenia, and elevated hepatic transaminase levels are the most common laboratory findings. Asymptomatic infection may also occur and, since *Amblyomma americanum* is the vector of other tick-borne agents, coinfection is possible.

E. ewingii granulocytic ehrlichiosis

E. ewingii has been known since 1992 as the agent of canine granulocytic ehrlichiosis, first described in a dog in Arkansas in 1971. The disease was described subsequently in several other states in the south-eastern and south-central United States of America, where the recognized vector is the Lone Star tick, *Amblyomma americanum*. Dogs infected with *E. ewingii* showed fever, lameness, and/or neutrophilic polyarthritis, and/or unexplained ataxia, paresis, or other neurological abnormalities. Laboratory findings include thrombocytopenia, and may include reactive lymphocytes.

White-tailed and South Carolina deer have also been shown to be infected with *E. ewingii*. Human infections with *E. ewingii* were first reported in 1999, when blood samples collected from 413 patients with possible ehrlichiosis in Missouri between 1994 to 1998 were analysed retrospectively. Molecular tools revealed that four tick-exposed patients were shown to be infected with *E. ewingii* and morulae were seen in neutrophils from two others. Clinical signs included fever, headache, and thrombocytopenia, with or without leucopenia. Three of them had underlying diseases and were receiving immunosuppressive therapy. More recently, four male HIV-infected patients from Oklahoma and Tennessee were found to be infected using the same methods. Three were receiving highly active antiretroviral therapy (HAART) and their median CD4+ cell count was 176/μl. Symptoms included fever, malaise and myalgia, headache, and nausea and vomiting. They had leucopenia, thrombocytopenia, anaemia, elevated transaminases, and hyponatraemia. They all survived. It is not clear whether *E. ewingii* can cause disease in immunocompetent people.

Human granulocytic anaplasmosis

Epidemiology

Human granulocytic anaplasmosis was first identified in 1990 in a patient in Wisconsin, United States of America, who died with a severe febrile illness 2 weeks after a tick bite. Clusters of small bacteria, assumed to be phagocytosed Gram-positive cocci, were seen inside neutrophils in the peripheral blood, but a careful review suggested the possibility of human ehrlichiosis. Over the ensuing 2 years, 13 cases with similar intraneutrophilic inclusions were identified in the same region of north-western Wisconsin and eastern Minnesota. In 1994, through application of broad-range molecular amplification and DNA sequencing, the causative agent was recognized as distinct from *E. chaffeensis*. First known as the 'HGE agent', the organism was found to be closely related to *E. equi* and *E. phagocytophila* (pathogens of horses and ruminants, respectively). However, phylogenic studies suggested that they were a single species, *Anaplasma phagocytophilum*. The disease was renamed human granulocytic anaplasmosis (HGA).

HGA is increasingly recognized as an important and frequent cause of fever after tick bite in the upper Midwest, New England, parts of the mid-Atlantic states, and northern California. A total of 2963 cases of HGA have been recorded in the United States of America since 1994, and 700 cases in 2005 alone. Since 1997, the agent and disease have been recognized in Europe, where more than 60 cases have been documented. Seroepidemiological studies confirm that human *A. phagocytophilum* infection is highly prevalent in both the United States of America and in Europe.

Ixodes ticks are the recognized vectors. *A. phagocytophilum* is maintained in a transmission cycle with *Ixodes persulcatus* complex ticks, including *I. scapularis* in the eastern United States of America, *I. pacificus* in the western United States of America, and *I. ricinus* in Europe. A role for *I. persulcatus* in eastern Europe and Asia is also suggested. Tick infection is established after an infectious blood meal. The bacterium is transmitted in ticks trans-stadially but not transovarially, and so ticks are not reservoirs. The major mammalian reservoir for *A. phagocytophilum* in the eastern United States of America is the white-footed mouse *Peromyscus leucopus*, and other small mammals and white-tailed deer *Odocoileus virginianus* can also be infected. Other reservoirs may include ruminants and other mammals. In Europe, horses, cattle, sheep, goats, dog, cats, and small mammals, particularly rodents, may be reservoirs.

Clinical diagnosis

HGA presents most commonly as an undifferentiated febrile illness occurring in spring or summer. Most patients have a moderately severe febrile illness with headache, myalgia, and malaise. A review of clinical date from 10 studies across North America and Europe includes up to 685 patients (Table 7.6.39.3). The most frequent symptoms are malaise (94%), fever (92%), myalgia (77%), and headache (75%). A minority of patients have arthralgia, gastrointestinal symptoms (nausea, vomiting, diarrhoea), respiratory symptoms (cough, pulmonary infiltrates, acute respiratory distress syndrome (ARDS)), and liver or central nervous system disturbances. Rash was observed in 6%, but no specific rash has been described in HGA. A few patients were coinfected with other ixodes-borne agents such as Lyme borreliosis (Chapter 7.6.32) and babesiosis (Chapter 7.8.3) in Europe and the United States of America. Frequent laboratory abnormalities identified in up to 329 patients included thrombocytopenia (71%), leucopenia (49%), anaemia (37%), and elevated hepatic transaminase levels (71%). The case fatality of HGA is estimated as 0.5%.

Diagnosis

Laboratory confirmation of human ehrlichioses and anaplasmosis is based on several tests that are not yet widely available for routine use. Indirect immunofluorescence serology is the most widely available. However, limitations include delay in seroconversion and possible false-positive detection due to cross-reacting bacteria. Laboratory criteria for the diagnosis of both diseases have been defined by the Council of State and Territorial Epidemiologists (www.cste.org). They include a fourfold or greater change in antibody titre to *E. chaffeensis* or *A. phagocytophilum* antigen by IFA in paired serum samples, or a positive PCR assay and confirmation of *E. chaffeensis* or *A. phagocytophilum* DNA, or identification of morulae in leucocytes and a positive IFA titre, or immunostaining *E. chaffeensis* or *A. phagocytophilum* antigen in a biopsy or autopsy sample, or culture of *E. chaffeensis* or *A. phagocytophilum* from a clinical specimen (Fig. 7.6.39.10). Case definitions for HGA have also been proposed by the Study Group for *Coxiella*, *Anaplasma*, *Rickettsia*, and *Bartonella* of the European Society of Clinical Microbiology and Infectious Diseases, whose definition is more restrictive than that of the CDC in requiring sequence determination for confirmation of PCR amplicons (Box 7.6.39.2).

Treatment

Tetracyclines are the reference drugs in treating human ehrlichioses and anaplasmosis but optimal duration of doxycycline treatment has yet to be determined. It is recommended that the treatment be continued for 7 to 10 days, or for at least 3 to 5 days after defervescence. Most patients become afebrile within 1 to 3 days following treatment. *E. chaffeensis* is susceptible *in vitro* to rifampicin (without *in vivo* evidence) but resistant to aminoglycosides, macrolides and ketolides, co-trimoxazole, penicillin, cephalosporin, chloramphenicol, and quinolones. *In vitro* resistance of *E. chaffeensis* to fluoroquinolone was strongly correlated with the presence of a specific amino acid variation in part of the protein sequence of the A subunit of *GyrA*. When antibiotic susceptibilities of eight strains of *A. phagocytophilum* collected in various geographical areas of the United States

Table 7.6.39.3 Meta-analysis of clinical manifestations and laboratory abnormalities in patients with human granulocytic anaplasmosis

Characteristics	All			North America		Europe	
	Median (%)[a]	Mean (%)	Number[b]	Mean (%)	Number	Mean (%)	Number
Symptom or sign							
Fever	100	92	480	92	448	98	66
Myalgia	74	77	514	79	448	65	66
Headache	89	75	378	73	289	89	66
Malaise	93	94	90	96	271	47	15
Nausea	44	38	256	36	207	47	49
Vomiting	20	26	90	34	41	19	49
Diarrhoea	13	16	90	22	41	10	49
Cough	13	19	260	22	207	10	49
Arthralgias	58	46	497	47	448	37	49
Rash	3	6	685	6	289	4	53
Stiff neck	11	18	22	22	18	0	4
Confusion	9	17	211	17	207	0	4
Laboratory abnormality							
Leucopenia	38	49	329	50	282	47	47
Thrombocytopenia	71	71	329	72	282	64	47
Elevated serum AST or ALT	74	71	170	79	123	51	47
Elevated serum creatinine	15	43	72	49	59	0	13

ALT, alanine aminotransferase; AST, aspartate aminotransferase.
[a] Median percentage of patients with feature among all reports.
[b] Number of patients with data available for meta-analysis.
Reprinted from Dumler JS, *et al.* (2005). Human granulocytic anaplasmosis and *Anaplasma phagocytophilum. Emerg Infect Dis*, **1**, 1828–34.

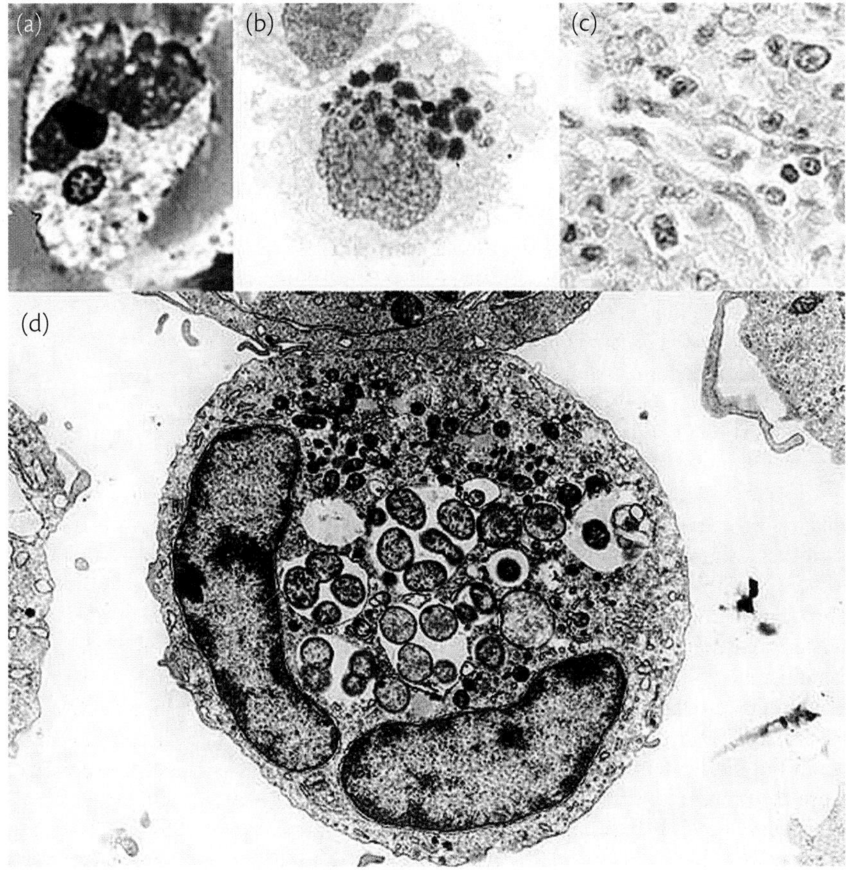

Fig. 7.6.39.10 *Anaplasma phagocytophilum* (a) in human peripheral blood band neutrophil (Wright's stain, original magnification ×1000), (b) in THP-1 myelomonocytic cell culture (LeukoStat stain, original magnification ×400), (c) in neutrophils infiltrating human spleen (immunohistochemistry with haematoxylin counterstain, original magnification ×100), and (d) ultrastructure by transmission electron microscopy in HL-60 cell culture (original magnification ×21 960).
(Courtesy of V Popov. From Dumler JS, *et al.* (2005). Human granulocytic anaplasmosis and *Anaplasma phagocytophilum. Emerg Infect Dis*, **1**, 1828–34, with permission.)

Box 7.6.39.2 Human granulocytic anaplasmosis (HGA) case definitions

Confirmed HGA

- Febrile illness with a history of a tick bite or tick exposure

and

- Demonstration of *A. phagocytophilum* infection by seroconversion or fourfold or more change in antibody titre (IFA)

or

- Positive PCR result (with subsequent sequencing of the amplicons demonstrating anaplasma-specific DNA in blood for European criteria)

or

- Isolation of *A. phagocytophilum* in blood culture

Probable HGA

- Febrile illness with a history of a tick bite or tick exposure

and

- Presence of stable titre of *A. phagocytophilum* antibodies in acute and convalescent sera if titre is more than 4 times above the cut-off value (IFA)

or

- Positive PCR result without sequencing confirmation

or

- Presence of intracytoplasmic morulae in a blood smear

(Bakken JS, Dumler JS (2006). Clinical diagnosis and treatment of human granulocytotropic anaplasmosis. *Ann N Y Acad Sci*, **1078**, 236–47; Brouqui P, *et al.* (2004). Guidelines for the diagnosis of tick-borne bacterial diseases in Europe. *Clin Microbiol Infect*, **10**, 1108–32)

of America were tested *in vitro*, doxycycline and rifampicin proved the most active. Levofloxacin was also active.

Prevention

Currently, no vaccines are available, including the epidemic typhus vaccine developed in the past. Prevention is based first on avoiding arthropod bites. The best method for avoiding tick, flea, and chigger bites is topical *N,N*-diethyl-*m*-toluamide (DEET) repellent applied to exposed skin, and treatment of clothing (including army uniforms) with permethrin, which kills arthropods on contact. Those staying in infested area should routinely check their bodies for the presence of arthropods. Prompt tick removal using blunt rounded forceps is essential for the prevention of tick-borne illnesses. In the case of epidemic typhus, louse eradication (e.g. in refugee camps) is the most important preventive measure and is essential in the control of outbreaks. Since body lice live only in clothing, the simplest method of delousing is to remove and then destroy or wash and boil all clothing. Dusting of all clothing with insecticides kills body lice and reduces the risk of reinfestation. Weekly doxycycline, 200 mg, prevents scrub typhus, but the efficacy against rickettsial infections of doxycycline (100 mg daily), used for malaria chemoprophylaxis, is untested.

Likely future developments

Although they are among the oldest known vector-borne diseases, many new rickettsioses have emerged in recent years. What are the factors influencing their emergence and recognition? The role of the primary physician, including careful history taking and physical and laboratory examinations, has been emphasized, as it was essential for the description of some emerging SFG rickettsioses such as Flinders Island spotted fever, Japanese spotted fever, and Astrakhan fever. Molecular techniques have facilitated epidemiological studies of emerging human rickettsioses all over the world and, with the help of improved culture systems, have incriminated new species as causes of human diseases. People are undertaking more outdoor activities and tourism is developing in rural and remote areas, resulting in increased contact with arthropods and arthropod-borne rickettsial pathogens.

Changes in the host–vector ecology have influenced the emergence of HME, including increasing population densities and geographical distribution of *Amblyomma americanum*, increases in vertebrate host populations (wild turkeys, white-tailed deer) for this tick, the increases in reservoir host population for *E. chaffeensis* (e.g. white-tailed deer), increased human contact with natural foci of infection through recreational and occupational activities, the increased frequency or severity of disease in ageing or immunocompromised people, the increasing proportion of people older than 60 years of age, and immunocompromised people in the population in regions of enzootic infection, as well as available diagnostic procedures and improved surveillance and reporting. HME may occur outside the United States of America and numerous rickettsia, ehrlichia, or anaplasma species have been identified in arthropods, particularly ticks, throughout the world, although their pathogenicity for people has yet to be demonstrated. More studies throughout the world may lead to the description of emerging rickettsioses in the future.

Further reading

Bakken JS, Dumler JS (2006). Clinical diagnosis and treatment of human granulocytotropic anaplasmosis. *Ann N Y Acad Sci*, **1078**, 236–47.

Balraj P, *et al.* (2008). RickA expression is not sufficient to promote actin-based motility of *Rickettsia raoultii*. *PLoS ONE*, **3**, e2582.

Bechah Y, *et al.* (2008). Epidemic typhus. *Lancet Infect Dis*, **8**, 417–26.

Brouqui P, *et al.* (2004). Guidelines for the diagnosis of tick-borne bacterial diseases in Europe. *Clin Microbiol Infect*, **10**, 1108–32.

Chapman AS, *et al.* (2006). Rocky Mountain spotted fever in the United States, 1997–2002. *Vector Borne Zoonotic Dis*, **6**, 170–8.

Civen R, Ngo V (2008). Murine typhus: an unrecognized suburban vector-borne disease. *Clin Infect Dis*, **46**, 913–18.

Dantas-Torres F (2007). Rocky Mountain spotted fever. *Lancet Infect Dis*, **7**, 724–32.

Dumler JS, *et al.* (2005). Human granulocytic anaplasmosis and *Anaplasma phagocytophilum*. *Emerg Infect Dis*, **1**, 1828–34.

Dumler JS, *et al.* (2007). Ehrlichioses in humans: epidemiology, clinical presentation, diagnosis, and treatment. *Clin Infect Dis*, **45** Suppl 1, S45–51.

Dumler JS, *et al.* (2007). Human granulocytic anaplasmosis and macrophage activation. *Clin Infect Dis*, **45**, 199–204.

Fournier PE, Raoult D (2004). Suicide PCR on skin biopsy specimens for diagnosis of rickettsioses. *J Clin Microbiol*, **42**, 3428–34.

La Scola B Raoult D (1997). Laboratory diagnosis of rickettsioses: current approaches to diagnosis of old and new rickettsial diseases. *J Clin Microbiol*, **35**, 2715–27.

Lepidi H, Fournier PE, Raoult D (2006). Histologic features and immunodetection of African tick-bite fever eschar. *Emerg Infect Dis*, **12**, 1332–7.

Mouffok N, Parola P, Lepidi H, Raoult D (2009). Mediterranean spotted fever in Algeria–new trends. *Int J Infect Dis*, **13**, 227–35.

Paddock CD, *et al.* (2004). *Rickettsia parkeri*: a newly recognized cause of spotted fever rickettsiosis in the United States. *Clin Infect Dis*, **38**, 805–11.

Paddock CD, *et al.* (2006). Isolation of *Rickettsia akari* from eschars of patients with rickettsialpox. *Am J Trop Med Hyg*, **75**, 732–8.

Parola P, Raoult D (2001). Ticks and tickborne bacterial diseases in humans: an emerging infectious threat. *Clin Infect Dis*, **32**, 897–928. Erratum: *Clin Inf Dis*, **33**, 749.

Parola P, Paddock C, Raoult D (2005). Tick-borne rickettsioses around the world: emerging diseases challenging old concepts. *Clin Microbiol Rev*, **18**, 719–56.

Parola P, Rovery C, Rolain JM, Brouqui P, Davoust B, Raoult D (2009). *Rickettsia slovaca* and *R. raoultii* in tick-borne rickettsioses. *Emerg Infect Dis*, **15**, 1105–8.

Parola P, Socolovschi C, Jeanjean L, Bitam I, Fournier PE, Sotto A, Labauge P, Raoult D (2008). Warmer weather linked to tick attack and emergence of severe rickettsioses. *PLoS Negl Trop Dis*, **2**, e338.

Parola P, Socolovschi C, Raoult D (2009). Deciphering the relationships between *Rickettsia conorii conorii* and *Rhipicephalus sanguineus* in the ecology and epidemiology of Mediterranean spotted fever. *Ann N Y Acad Sci*, **1166**, 49–54.

Parola P, Labruna MB, Raoult D (2009). Tick-Borne Rickettsioses in America: Unanswered Questions and Emerging Diseases. *Curr Infect Dis Rep*, **11**, 40–50.

Pérez-Osorio CE, *et al.* (2008). *Rickettsia felis* as emergent global threat for humans. *Emerg Infect Dis*, **14**, 1019–23.

Raoult D, Parola P (2007). *Rickettsial diseases*. Informa Healthcare, New York.

Raoult D, Roux V (1999). The body louse as a vector of reemerging human diseases. *Clin Infect Dis*, **29**, 888–911.

Raoult D, Woodward T, Dumler JS (2004). The history of epidemic typhus. *Infect Dis Clin North Am*, **18**, 127–40.

Raoult D, *et al.* (1998). Outbreak of epidemic typhus associated with trench fever in Burundi. *Lancet*, **352**, 353–8.

Rikihisa Y (2006). New findings on members of the family Anaplasmataceae of veterinary importance. *Ann N Y Acad Sci*, **1078**, 438–45.

Roux V, Raoult D (1999). Body lice as tools for diagnosis and surveillance of reemerging diseases. *J Clin Microbiol*, **37**, 596–9.

Silveira I, *et al.* (2007). *Rickettsia parkeri* in Brazil. *Emerg Infect Dis*, **13**, 1111–13.

Vestris G, *et al.* (2003). Seven years' experience of isolation of *Rickettsia* spp. from clinical specimens using the shell-vial cell culture assay. *Ann NY Acad Sci*, **990**, 371–4.

Weissmann G (2005). Rats, lice, and Zinsser. *Emerg Infect Dis*, **11**, 492–6.

7.6.40 Scrub typhus

George Watt

Essentials

Scrub typhus (tsutsugamushi fever) is a zoonosis of rural Asia and the western Pacific islands that is caused by the obligate Gram-negative intracellular bacterium *Orientia* (formerly Rickettsia) *tsutsugamushi*, which is transmitted (typically from rats) to humans by the bite of a larval leptotrombidium mite (chigger). More than a billion people are at risk and more than a million cases are transmitted annually, making it the commonest rickettsial disease.

Clinical features—an eschar and regional lymphadenopathy often develop at the site of the chigger bite, and may by followed by a systemic illness ranging in severity from inapparent to fatal. Many cases go undiagnosed, particularly those in which an eschar cannot be found. Diagnosis may be made serologically, but laboratory confirmation of infection is rarely available in rural areas where the disease is most frequently encountered. Aside from supportive care, treatment is with tetracycline, doxycycline, or chloramphenicol. Before antibiotics, mortality rates up to 35% were reported, but were generally much lower. Chemoprophylaxis with doxycycline can prevent infection. There is no vaccine.

Aetiology and epidemiology

Orientia tsutsugamushi differs in its cell wall structure and genetic makeup from rickettsiae, which it resembles under light microscopy. It is an obligate intracellular Gram-negative bacterium (Fig. 7.6.40.1). Infection with one of the multiple serotypes of *O. tsutsugamushi* confers transient cross-immunity to another. Scrub typhus is a zoonosis. Larval mites (of the *Leptotrombidium deliense* group) usually feed on small rodents, particularly wild rats of the subgenus *Rattus* (Fig. 7.6.40.2). Humans become infected when they accidentally encroach on a zone where there are infected mites (Fig. 7.6.40.3). These zones are often made up of secondary or 'scrub' growth, hence the term 'scrub typhus'. Infected chiggers are generally found in only very circumscribed foci within these zones. Large numbers of cases can occur when humans enter these so-called 'mite islands'. However, mite habitats as diverse as seashores and semideserts have been described. Many scrub typhus patients in south-east Asia are rice farmers. Disease transmission occurs when infected mites burrow into the skin, take a meal of tissue fluid, and inoculate the infectious organisms. Human-to-human transmission of scrub typhus via contaminated blood has never been documented. The endemic area forms a triangle of more than 5 million square miles bounded by northern Japan and

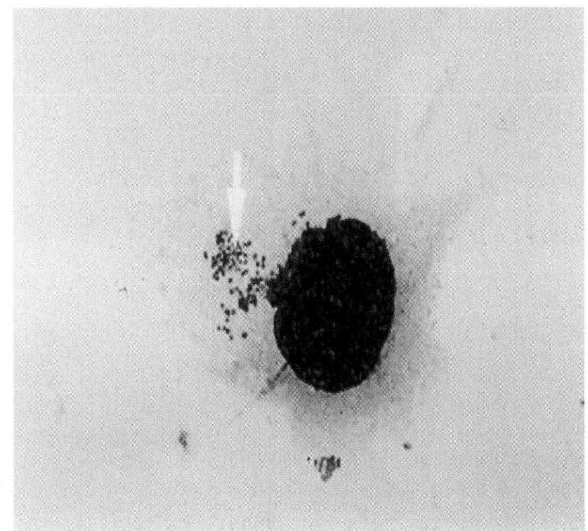

Fig. 7.6.40.1 Perinuclear clusters of Giemsa-stained *O. tsutsugamushi*.
(Courtesy of Dr Kriangrai Lerdthusnee, Department of Entomology, AFRIMS, Bangkok.)

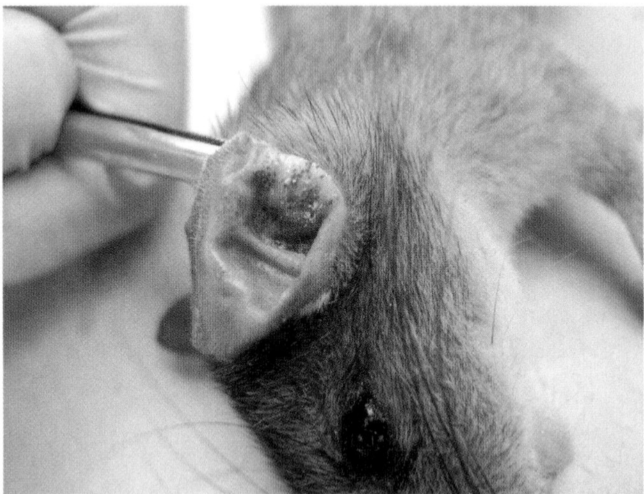

Fig. 7.6.40.2 Numerous reddish coloured chiggers attached to the earlobe of a wild rodent (*Rattus rattus*).
(Courtesy of Dr Kriangrai Lerdthusnee, Department of Entomology, AFRIMS, Bangkok.)

south-eastern Siberia to the north, Queensland, Australia, to the south, and Pakistan to the west (Fig. 7.6.40.4). Disease transmission occurs in rural and suburban areas as well as in villages, but inhabitants of city centres are not at risk.

Pathology and pathogenesis

Much remains unknown about the pathogenesis of scrub typhus, partly because most descriptions of severe cases pre-date advances made in immunohistology since the 1950s. Marked geographical variations in severity of the illness occur but determinants of severity are poorly characterized. Strains which differ in virulence, partial immunity, and regional differences in general health could affect disease presentation, but coinfection with the HIV-1 virus does not. Scrub typhus appears to be a vasculitis, but clinical and pathological findings do not correlate closely. The host cell of *O. tsutsugamushi* in humans has not been defined with certainty. The endothelial cell has been proposed because of findings in experimental animals and by analogy with other rickettsial diseases. However, in human liver infected with scrub typhus examined by electron microscopy, organisms predominate in Kupffer cells and hepatocytes rather than within endothelial cells. *O. tsutsugamushi* is present in peripheral white blood cells of patients with scrub typhus and is found within a variety of cell types. The HIV-1 viral load falls markedly in some AIDS patients who acquire acute *O. tsutsugamushi* infection, and sera from HIV-seronegative patients with scrub typhus inhibit HIV replication *in vitro*.

Clinical features

The painless chigger bite can occur on any part of the body, but is often in difficult to see in locations such as under the axilla or in the genital area. An eschar (Figs. 7.6.40.5, 7.6.40.6) forms at the bite site in about one-half of primary infections, but in a minority of secondary infections. The eschar begins as a small painless papule which develops during the 6- to 18-day (median 10 days) incubation period. It enlarges, undergoes central necrosis, and acquires a blackened scab to form a lesion resembling a cigarette burn. Regional lymph nodes are enlarged and tender. The eschar is usually well developed by the time fever appears and is often healing by the time the patient presents to hospital.

Fever, headache, myalgia, and nonspecific malaise are common symptoms. Hearing loss concurrent with fever is reported by as many as one-third of patients and is a useful diagnostic clue. Conjunctival suffusion (Fig. 7.6.40.7) and generalized lymphadenopathy are common and helpful physical signs. A transient macular rash may appear at the end of the first week of illness but is often difficult to see (Fig. 7.6.40.8). The rash first appears on the trunk and becomes maculopapular as it spreads peripherally. Cough sometimes accompanied by bilateral reticular infiltrates on the chest radiograph is one of the commonest presentations of *O. tsutsugamushi* infection. In severe cases, tachypnoea progresses

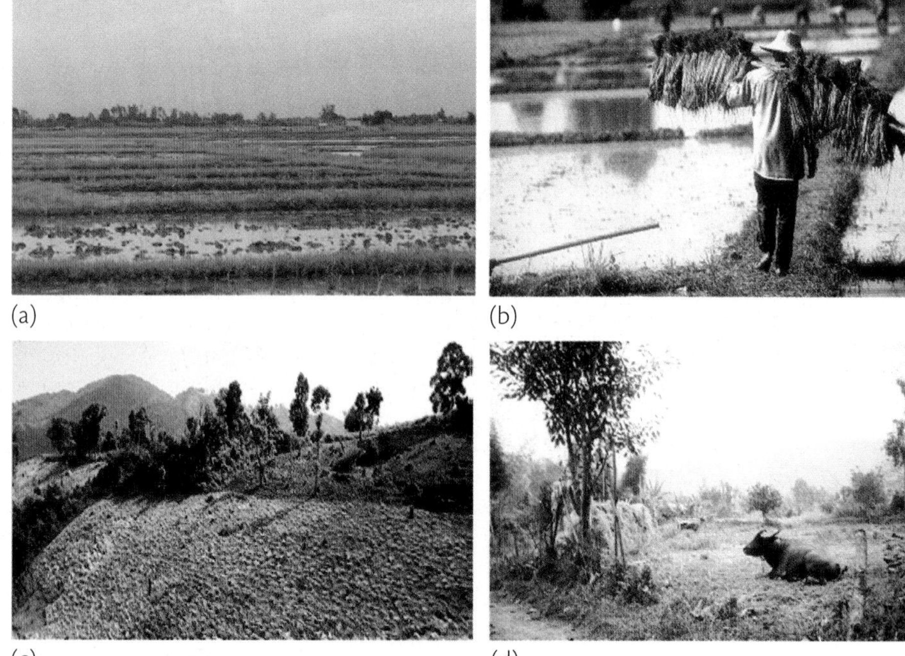

Fig. 7.6.40.3 Scrub typhus habitats. (a) Transmission occurs in active rice fields. (b) Farmers intrude on the chigger–rodent cycle taking place on walkways between flooded fields. (c, d). Typical 'scrub' or secondary vegetation in Thailand.
(a, courtesy of Dr Kriangkrai Lerdthusnee, Department of Entomology, AFRIMS, Bangkok.)

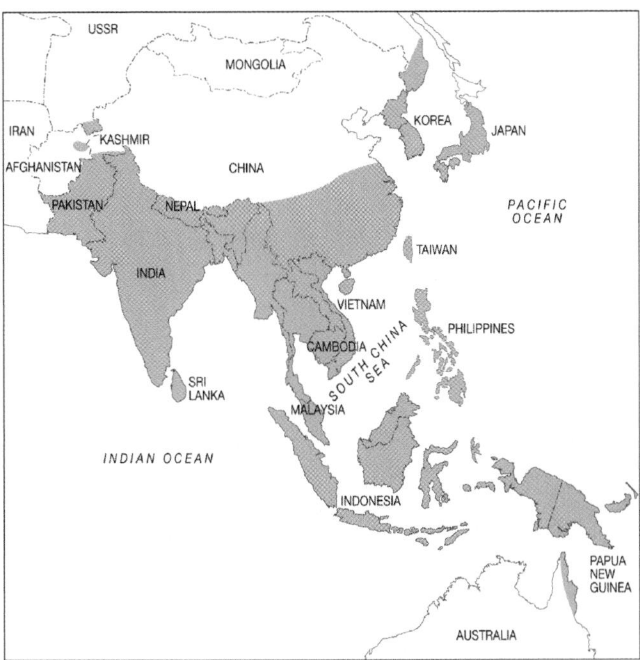

Fig. 7.6.40.4 Geographical distribution of scrub typhus.

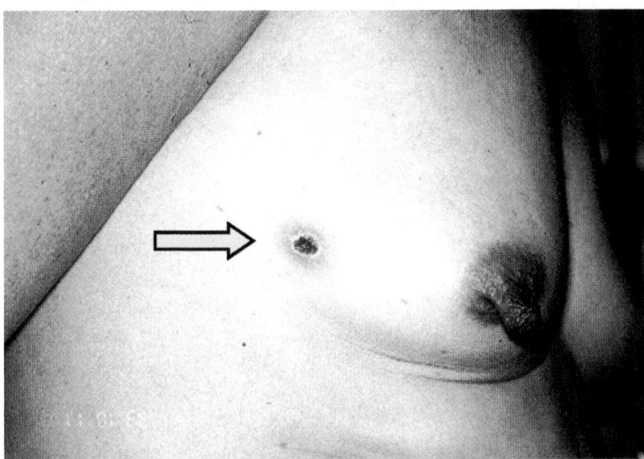

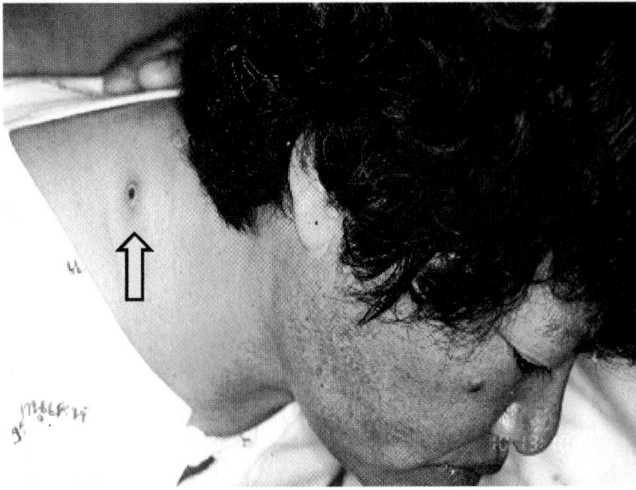

Fig. 7.6.40.5 Two typical eschars (blue arrows).

to dyspnoea, the patient becomes cyanotic, and full-blown acute respiratory distress syndrome (ARDS) may ensue. Apathy, confusion, and personality changes are not uncommon and only rarely progress to stupor, convulsions, and coma. Abnormalities resolve completely in nonfatal cases.

Diagnosis

The eschar is the single most useful diagnostic clue and is pathognomonic when seen by a physician experienced in diagnosis of scrub typhus. Even typical eschars can be overlooked or misdiagnosed, however, and atypical presentations are common. Eschars in the genital area often lose their crust and can be confused with the ulcers of chancroid, syphilis, or lymphogranuloma venereum.

There is no constellation of laboratory test results which strongly suggests *O. tsutsugamushi* infection. Slight increases in the number of circulating white blood cells are common. Atypical lymphocytes and moderately elevated serum transaminase levels are not uncommon. Laboratory findings are chiefly useful to rule out other infections. A low white cell count and thrombocytopenia with a haemorrhagic rash suggest infection with dengue virus rather than *O. tsutsugamushi*. Haemorrhagic manifestations are more common in haemorrhagic fever with renal syndrome (HFRS) than in scrub typhus, and lumbar back pain, flank tenderness, and occult blood in urine suggest HFRS rather than *O. tsutsugamushi* infection. Raised serum creatinine and serum bilirubin levels with marked myalgia suggest leptospirosis rather than scrub typhus. Enteric fever rarely causes generalized lymphadenopathy or conjunctival suffusion.

Some occupations place individuals at increased risk of contracting not only *O. tsutsugamushi* infection but also other infections. For example, in Thailand most cases of scrub typhus and leptospirosis occur in rice farmers. Dual infections with scrub typhus and leptospirosis are not uncommon.

The Weil–Felix test using the proteus OXK antigen is a commercially available serodiagnostic test which has been used for many years, but is insensitive. The indirect immunofluorescent assay and the immunoperoxidase test are the confirmatory tests of choice but their complexity limits their use to a small number of reference centres. An accurate rapid dot blot immunoassay which does not require a microscope has been developed. Such kits would be of enormous benefit if they could be made commercially available and affordable for use in rural tropical Asia where most scrub typhus cases occur. The causative organism can be demonstrated by culture and by PCR, but the sensitivity of currently available techniques is too low for them to be clinically useful.

Treatment

Prompt antibiotic therapy shortens the course of the disease, lowers the risk of ARDS, and reduces mortality. Treatment must often be presumptive, but the benefits of avoiding severe scrub typhus by early antibiotic administration generally far outweigh the risks of a 1-week course of tetracycline, which is the treatment of choice. Either oral tetracycline 500 mg four times daily, or oral doxycycline 100 mg twice daily for 7 days is recommended. Oral chloramphenicol 500 mg four times a day is a cheaper alternative still widely used in endemic areas. Treatment for less than a week is initially curative, but may be followed by relapse. Parenteral doxycycline should be administered to patients who cannot swallow tablets or who are severely ill. Parenteral chloramphenicol (50–75 mg/kg per day) is an alternative if parenteral tetracycline is unavailable.

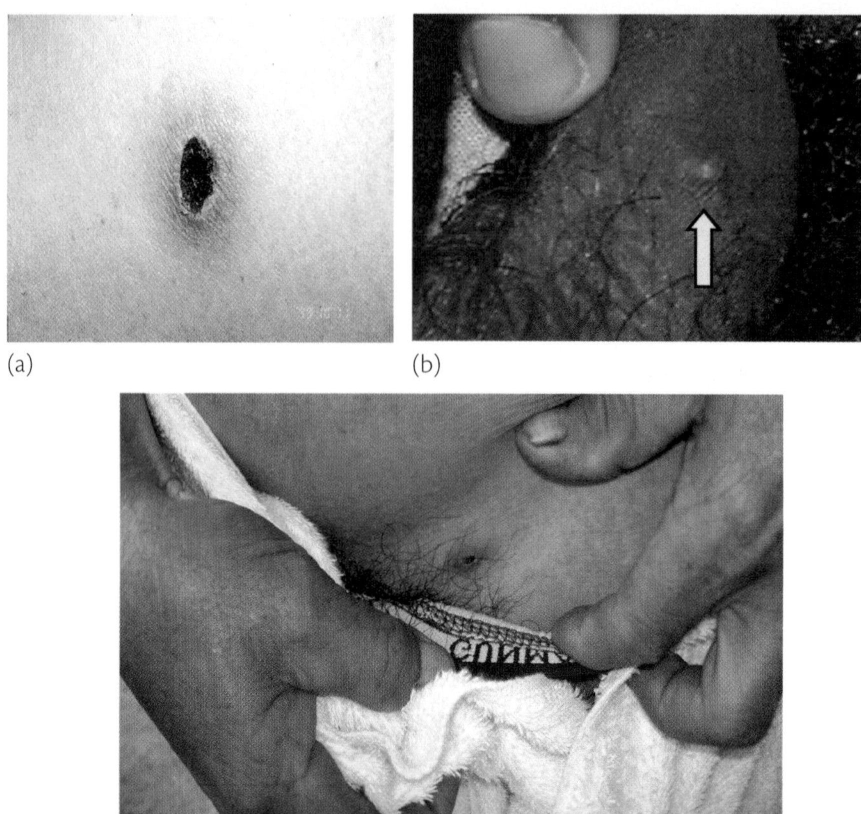

Fig. 7.6.40.6 Typical eschars (a) may be missed because they are located in difficult to examine areas (c). Eschars may be atypical and lose their crust in moist locales such as the scrotum (b). (b,c, courtesy of Dr Kriangkrai Lerdthusnee, Department of Entomology, AFRIMS, Bangkok.)

Scrub typhus cases from northern Thailand which respond poorly to conventional therapy have been described, but neither the mechanism of resistance nor its geographical distribution

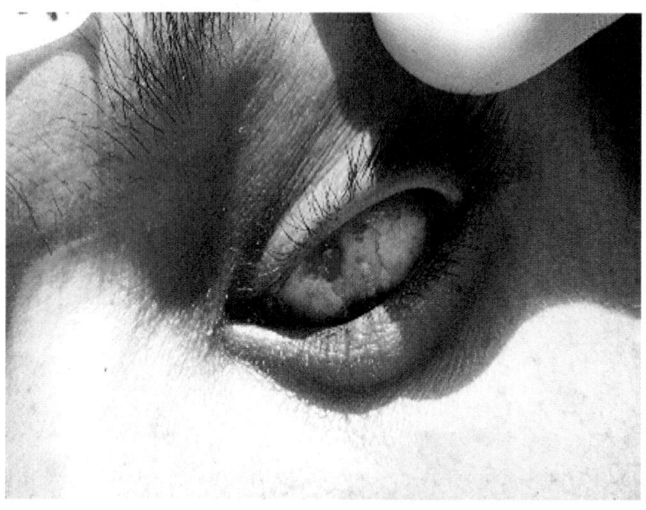

Fig. 7.6.40.7 Conjunctival suffusion in scrub typhus.

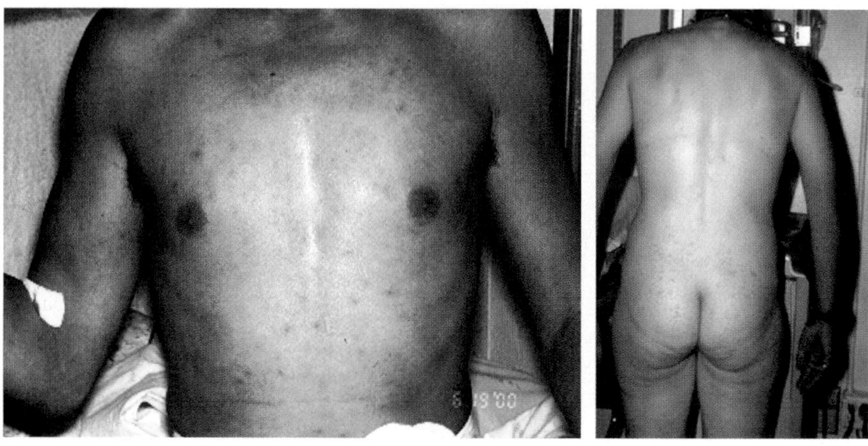

Fig. 7.6.40.8 The subtle rash of scrub typhus predominates on the trunk.

have been defined. Scrub typhus has serious adverse effects on pregnancy but conventional therapy with tetracyclines or chloramphenicol for pregnant women and children poses problems. Both drug-sensitive and drug-resistant scrub typhus cases have been cured by azithromycin and this antibiotic appears to be the treatment of choice during pregnancy and early childhood.

Prevention and control

Weekly doses of 200 mg doxycycline can prevent *O. tsutsugamushi* infection. Chemoprophylaxis should be considered for nonimmune people sent to an enzootic area to perform work that places them at high risk of acquiring scrub typhus. Soldiers and road construction crews are typical examples, but chemoprophylaxis should also be considered in high-risk travellers such as trekkers. Contact with chiggers can be reduced by applying repellent to the tops of boots, socks, and on the lower trousers and by not sitting or lying directly on the ground. There is no vaccine for scrub typhus.

Prognosis

Scrub typhus was a dreaded disease in the preantibiotic era when case fatality rates reached as high as 50%. Prompt antibiotic therapy generally prevents death, but up to 15% of patients still die in northern Thailand. Deaths are attributed to a variety of factors including late presentation, delayed diagnosis, and drug resistance.

Further reading

Kantipong P, *et al.* (1996). HIV infection does not influence the clinical severity of scrub typhus. *Clin Infect Dis*, **23**, 1168.

Olson JG, *et al.* (1980). Prevention of scrub typhus. Prophylactic administration of doxycycline in a randomized double blind trial. *Am J Trop Med Hyg*, **29**, 989.

Watt G, *et al.* (1996). Scrub typhus infections poorly responsive to antibiotics in northern Thailand. *Lancet*, **348**, 86–9.

Watt G, *et al.* (2003). HIV-1 suppression during acute scrub typhus infection. *Lancet*, **356**, 475–9.

7.6.41 *Coxiella burnetii* infections (Q fever)

T.J. Marrie

Essentials

Q fever is a zoonosis caused by *Coxiella burnetii*, an intracellular Gram-negative spore-forming bacterium, the common animal reservoirs of which are cattle, sheep, and goats. It is trophic for the endometrium and mammary glands of female animals, and during pregnancy the organism reaches very high concentrations in the placenta such that at the time of parturition organisms are aerosolized and contamination of the environment occurs. Inhalation of even one microorganism can result in infection.

Clinical features—there are two main forms of the disease: (1) acute—can present as inapparent infection, self-limited febrile illness, pneumonia, and hepatitis, or less commonly with a variety of organ-specific manifestations such as encephalitis, pericarditis, and pancreatitis; Q fever in pregnancy is associated with a high rate of abortion or neonatal death. (2) Chronic—most often 'culture-negative' endocarditis or infection of aortic aneurysms, but occasionally osteomyelitis.

Diagnosis, treatment, and prevention—diagnosis is confirmed by serological testing: in acute disease antibodies to phase II antigen are higher than those to phase I, whereas the reverse is true in chronic disease. Acute Q fever is treated with doxycyline or a quinolone; chronic disease with long-term doxycycline and hydroxychloroquine; and Q fever in pregnancy with co-trimoxazole for the duration of the pregnancy and—for those with a chronic Q fever serological profile—1 year of doxycycline and hydroxyochloroquine after delivery. Vaccination should be offered to those whose occupation places them at high risk for *C. burnetii* infection.

History

In August 1935, Dr Edward Holbrook Derrick, Director of the Laboratory of Microbiology and Pathology of the Queensland Health Department in Brisbane, Australia, was asked to investigate an outbreak of undiagnosed febrile illness among workers at the Cannon Hill abattoir. Derrick realized that he was dealing with a type of fever that had not been previously described—he named it Q (for query) fever. Two years later, Sir Frank Macfarlane Burnet in Australia and Herald Rea Cox in the United States of America isolated the microorganism responsible for Q fever.

Coxiella burnetii

This microorganism, the sole species of its genus, has a Gram-negative cell wall and measures 0.3 × 0.7 µm (Fig. 7.6.41.1). It is an obligate phagolysosomal parasite of eukaryotes that sporulates, stains well with Gimenez's stain, and multiplies by transverse binary fission. *C. burnetii* undergoes phase variation akin to the smooth to rough transition in some enteric Gram-negative bacilli. In nature and laboratory animals it exists in the phase I state. Repeated passage of phase I virulent organisms in embryonated chicken eggs leads to the conversion to phase II avirulent forms. Antibodies to phase I antigens predominate in chronic Q fever, while phase II antibodies are higher than phase I antibodies in acute Q fever. The genome of *C. burnetii* strain Nine Mile Phase I has 1 995 275 base pairs. There are many genes with potential roles in adhesion, invasion, intracellular trafficking, host-cell modulation, and detoxification.

Immune control of *C. burnetii* is T-cell dependent and it does not eliminate *C. burnetii* from infected humans. In 80 to 90% of bone marrow aspirates from those who have recovered from Q fever, polymerase chain reaction (PCR) assays for *C. burnetii* DNA are positive. The use of microarrays allows insight into the complexity of the host microorganism interaction in illnesses such as Q fever. In one such experiment 335 genes in the *C. burnetii*-infected human monocytic leukaemia cell line THP-1 were up- or down-regulated at least twofold.

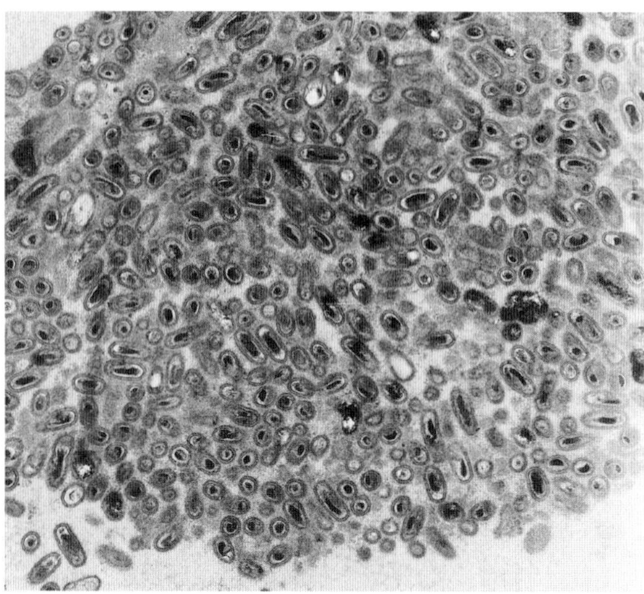

Fig. 7.6.41.1 Transmission electron micrograph showing *C. burnetii* cells within a macrophage in the heart valve of a patient with Q fever endocarditis. The dark material in the centre of each cell is condensed DNA. Magnification ×15 000.

C. burnetii has survived for 586 days in tick faeces at room temperature, 160 days or more in water, 30 to 40 days in dried cheese made from contaminated milk, and up to 150 days in soil.

Epidemiology

Q fever is a zoonosis. There is an extensive wildlife and arthropod (mainly ticks) reservoir of *C. burnetii*. Domestic animals are infected through inhaling contaminated aerosols or by ingesting infected material. These animals rarely become ill, but abortion and stillbirths may occur. *C. burnetii* localizes in the uterus and mammary glands of infected animals. During pregnancy there is reactivation of *C. burnetii* and it multiplies in the placenta, reaching 10^9 infective doses per gram of tissue. The organisms are shed into the environment at the time of parturition. Humans becomes infected after inhaling organisms aerosolized at the time of parturition, or later when organisms in dust are stirred up on a windy day. Infections have occurred up to 18 km downwind from a source. Infected cattle, sheep, goats, and cats are the animals primarily responsible for transmitting *C. burnetii* to humans. There have been several outbreaks of Q fever in hospitals and research institutes due to the transportation of infected sheep to research laboratories. Some studies have suggested that ingestion of contaminated milk is a risk factor for the acquisition of Q fever; volunteers seroconverted but did not become ill after ingesting such milk.

Percutaneous infection, such as when an infected tick is crushed between the fingers, may occur but is rare. Transmission via a contaminated blood transfusion has rarely occurred. Vertical transmission from mother to child has been infrequently reported. A 1988 review documents 23 cases of Q fever in pregnant women. The authors found that Q fever was present in 1 in 540 pregnancies in an area of endemic Q fever in southern France. Person-to-person transmission has been documented on a few occasions. To date, 45 countries on five continents have reported cases of Q fever. Q fever is estimated to cost $A1 million in Australia each year and results in the loss of more than 1700 weeks of work.

There are several studies where young age seems to be protective of infection with *C. burnetii*. In a large outbreak of Q fever in Switzerland, symptomatic infection was 5 times more likely to occur in those over 15 years of age compared with those younger than 15. In many outbreaks of Q fever, men were affected more commonly than women. It had been assumed that this was due to the fact that certain occupations in which men predominate were more likely to be associated with Q fever. However, in France, despite similar exposures, the male to female ratio is 2.45 to 1. The explanation for this gender difference is that female sex hormones are protective against Q fever infection.

Currently Q fever is common in several European countries with ongoing outbreaks in Germany and the Netherlands. There are a considerable number of sporadic cases of Q fever in England, France, and Spain.

Clinical features

Humans are the only species known consistently to develop illness following infection with *C. burnetii*. There is an incubation period of about 2 weeks (range 2–29 days) following inhalation of *C. burnetii*. A dose–response effect has been demonstrated experimentally and clinically. *C. burnetii* is one of the most infectious agents known; a single microorganism is able to initiate infection in humans. The resulting illness can be divided into acute and chronic varieties.

Acute Q fever

Self-limiting febrile illness

The most common manifestation of acute Q fever is a self-limiting febrile illness that is dismissed as a 'cold'. Serosurveys reveal that in most endemic areas 5 to 10% of the population have antibodies to *C. burnetii* but never remember the illness that resulted in seroconversion.

Q fever pneumonia

This is the most commonly recognized manifestation of Q fever. There is often a seasonal distribution, most of the cases occurring between February and May (consistent with the birthing season in the small ruminant reservoirs). The onset is nonspecific with fever, fatigue, and headache. The headache may be very severe, occasionally so severe that it prompts a lumbar puncture. A dry cough of mild to moderate intensity is present in 24 to 90% of patients. About one-third of patients have pleuritic chest pain. Nausea, vomiting, and diarrhoea occur in 10 to 30% of patients. Most cases of *C. burnetii* pneumonia are mild; however, about 10% are severe enough to require admission to hospital and, rarely, assisted ventilation is necessary. Death is rare in Q fever pneumonia and is usually due to comorbid illness. The white blood cell count is usually normal, but is elevated in one-third of patients. Liver enzyme levels may be mildly elevated at 2 to 3 times normal. Alkaline phosphatase is raised in up to 70% of patients and 28% are hyponatraemic. Reactive thrombocytosis is surprisingly common and microscopic haematuria is a common finding.

The chest radiographic manifestations of Q fever pneumonia are usually indistinguishable from those of other bacterial pneumonias (Fig. 7.6.41.2); however, rounded opacities are suggestive of this infection (Fig. 7.6.41.3). Some investigators have reported delayed

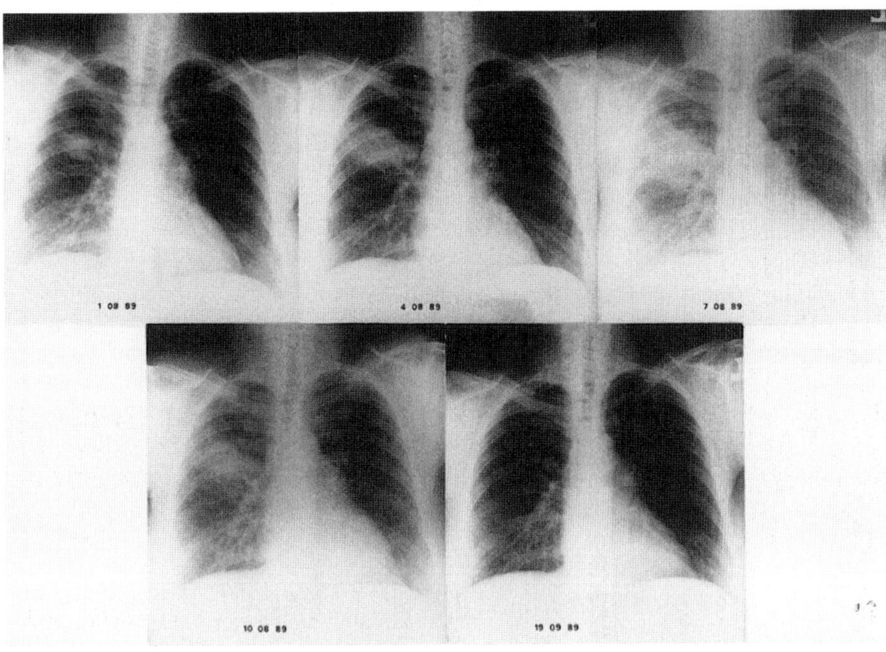

Fig. 7.6.41.2 Serial chest radiographs of a 35-year-old patient with Q fever pneumonia. The first radiograph (1 August 1989) shows a round opacity in the right upper lobe, which increases in size over the next 6 days. The pneumonia has completely cleared by 19 September 1989.

clearing of the pneumonia; however, in our experience resolution is usually complete within 3 weeks.

Hepatitis

The liver is probably involved in all patients with acute Q fever. There are three clinical pictures:

- Pyrexia of unknown origin with mild to moderate elevation of liver function tests.
- A hepatitis-like picture: liver biopsy shows distinctive doughnut granulomas consisting of a granuloma with a central lipid vacuole and fibrin deposits. Prolonged fever unresponsive to antibiotics is common in these patients.
- 'Incidental hepatitis'.

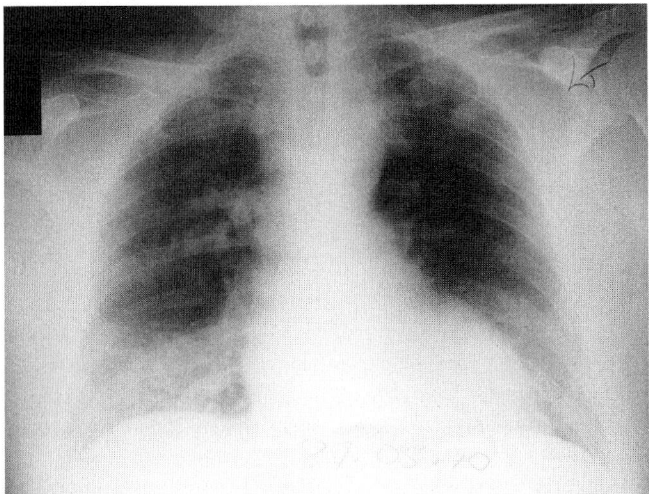

Fig. 7.6.41.3 Portable anteroposterior chest radiograph of a 72-year-old man with Q fever pneumonia. This radiographic picture is indistinguishable from pneumonia due to any other microbial agent.

Q fever in pregnancy

Acute Q fever occasionally complicates pregnancy. In 23 published cases 35% had premature birth, and 43% ended in abortion or neonatal death. In a serosurvey of 4588 pregnant women in Halifax, Nova Scotia, Canada, women seropositive for *C. burnetii* were 3 times more likely to have a current or previous neonatal death.

Neurological manifestations

Encephalitis, encephalomyelitis, toxic confusional states, optic neuritis, and demyelinating polyradiculoneuritis are uncommon manifestations of Q fever.

Rare manifestations

These include myocarditis, pericarditis including constrictive pericarditis, bone marrow necrosis, rhabdomyolysis, glomerulonephritis, lymphadenopathy, pancreatitis, splenic rupture, acalculous cholecystitis, mesenteric panniculitis, erythema nodosum, epididymitis, orchitis, priapism, and erythema annulare centrifugum. Chronic fatigue may be a sequel of Q fever in some patients.

Chronic Q fever

The usual manifestation of chronic Q fever is that of culture-negative endocarditis. Some 70% of these patients have fever and nearly all have abnormal native or prosthetic heart valves. Hepatomegaly and or splenomegaly occur in about one-half of these patients and one-third have marked clubbing of the digits. A purpuric rash due to immune complex-induced leucocytoclastic vasculitis and arterial embolism occurs in about 20% of patients. Hyperglobulinaemia (up to 60 g/litre) is common and is a useful clue to chronic Q fever in a patient with the clinical picture of culture-negative endocarditis.

Other manifestations of chronic Q fever include osteomyelitis, infection of aortic aneurysm, and infection of vascular prosthetic grafts.

The strains of *C. burnetii* that cause chronic Q fever do not differ from those that cause acute Q fever. Peripheral blood lymphocytes from patients with Q fever endocarditis are unresponsive to

C. burnetii antigens *in vitro*, while responding normally to other antigens.

Diagnosis

A strong clinical suspicion based on the epidemiology and clinical features as outlined above is the cornerstone of the diagnosis of Q fever. This suspicion is confirmed by determining a fourfold or greater increase in antibody titre between acute and 2- to 3-week convalescent serum samples. A variety of serological tests are available including complement fixation, microimmunofluorescence, and enzyme immunoassay. The immunofluorescence antibody test is the best test. In acute Q fever the antibody titre to phase II antigen is higher than that to phase I antigen, while the reverse occurs in chronic Q fever. In chronic Q fever, antibody phase I titres are extremely high, in the order of 1:8192 and higher. In acute Q fever, antibody titres to phase I antigen are rarely in excess of 1:512 (usually 1:8 to 1:32), while peak antibody titres to phase II antigen are between 1:1024 and 1:2048. The microorganism can be isolated in embryonated eggs or in tissue culture; however, a biosafety level 3 laboratory is required. The PCR can be used to amplify *C. burnetii* DNA from tissues or other biological specimens.

Treatment

Acute Q fever is treated with a 2-week course of tetracycline or doxycycline. Quinolones can also be used. Any patients who develop acute Q fever and have lesions of their native valves (e.g. congenital bicuspid aortic valve), prosthetic valves, or prosthetic intravascular material should have serological monitoring every 4 months for 2 years, and if the phase I IgG titre exceeds 1:800 further investigation is warranted. Some authorities recommend that patients with valvulopathy who have acute Q fever should receive 12 months of doxycycline and hydroxychloroquine to prevent chronic Q fever.

The duration of treatment for chronic Q fever is determined by monitoring the serum antibody titres to *C. burnetii*, although some authorities recommend lifelong therapy for chronic Q fever. In general, antibiotics can be discontinued when the IgA antibody titre to phase I antigen is less than 1:200. The treatment of choice for chronic Q fever is doxycycline 100 mg twice daily and hydroxychloroquine 200 mg three times daily to maintain a plasma level of between 0.8 and 1.2 μg/ml. This regimen is given for 18 months. Photosensitivity is a potential adverse reaction and patients should be warned to take preventive measures. In addition, an ophthalmologist must examine the optic fundus every 6 months for chloroquine accumulation. We have used rifampicin 300 mg twice a day and ciprofloxacin 750 mg twice a day to treat patients with chronic Q fever. Rifampicin and doxycycline or tetracycline and trimethoprim/sulfamethoxazole have also been used to treat chronic Q fever. Antibody titres should be measured every 6 months for the first 2 years. A progressive decline in antibody titre reflects the successful treatment of chronic fever. Cardiac valve replacement may be necessary as part of the management of chronic Q fever.

Many patients with granulomatous hepatitis due to Q fever have a prolonged febrile illness that does not respond to antibiotics. For these individuals treatment with prednisone 0.5 mg/kg has resulted in defervescence within 2 to 15 days. Once defervescence has occurred the dose of steroids is tapered over the next month.

Q fever occurring during pregnancy should be treated with co-trimoxazole for the duration of the pregnancy. In one retrospective study this approach reduced obstetrical complications from 81 to 44%. There were no intrauterine fetal deaths in the co-trimoxazole-treated group. Those with a chronic Q fever serological profile should be treated with doxycycline and hydroxychloroquine for 1 year following delivery.

Prevention

A formalin-inactivated *C. burnetii* whole-cell vaccine is protective against infection and has a low rate of side effects; 1% of vaccinees developed an abscess at the inoculation site and another 1% had a lump at this site 2 months after vaccination. The vaccine should be offered to those whose occupation places them at high risk for *C. burnetii* infection.

Good animal husbandry practices are important in preventing widespread contamination of the environment by *C. burnetii*. Prevention of zoonotic spread is best accomplished by isolating aborting animals for up to 14 days, raising feeding troughs to prevent contamination of feed by excreta, destroying aborted materials by burning and burying fetal membranes and stillborn animals, and wearing masks and gloves when handling aborted materials.

Only seronegative pregnant animals should be brought into the facilities where research is to be done. In addition only seronegative animals should be used in petting zoos.

Blood donation should be suspended in outbreak areas for up to 4 weeks following cessation of the outbreak.

Further reading

Carcopino X, *et al.* (2007). Managing Q fever during pregnancy: the benefits of long-term cotrimoxazole therapy. *Clin Infect Dis*, **45**, 548–55.

Raoult D, Tissot-Dupont H, Foucault C (2000). Q fever 1985–1998: clinical and epidemiological features of 1,383 infections. *Medicine (Baltimore)*, **79**, 110–23.

Raoult D, *et al.* (1999). Treatment of Q fever endocarditis: comparison of 2 regimens containing doxycycline and ofloxacin or hydroxychloroquine. *Arch Intern Med*, **159**, 167–73.

7.6.42 Bartonellas excluding *B. bacilliformis*

Emmanouil Angelakis, Didier Raoult, and Jean-Marc Rolain

Essentials

Bartonella species are Gram-negative bacilli or coccobacilli belonging to the α2 subgroup of Proteobacteria that are closely related to the genera *Brucella* and *Agrobacterium*. Each persists in particular mammalian hosts, with transmission to humans primarily mediated by haematophagous arthropods. A remarkable feature of the genus *Bartonella* is the ability of a single species to cause either acute or chronic infection with either vascular, proliferative, or suppurative features, the pathological response to infection varying substantially with the host's immunocompetence.

Clinical features

Cat-scratch disease—the most common *Bartonella* zoonosis, caused by *B. henselae*, with transmission usually occurring directly by a cat scratch. Typical presentation is with history of a cat scratch and/or bite and locoregional lymphadenopathy (which may persist for months), sometimes with fever and constitutional symptoms. A few cases present with severe systemic symptoms indicating disseminated infection. Encephalopathy and neuroretinitis are uncommon manifestations.

Trench fever—caused by *B. quintana*; transmitted by the body louse; typically presents as an acute febrile illness often accompanied by severe headache and pain in the long bones of the legs.

Bacillary angiomatosis—caused by *B. henselae* or *B. quintana*, particularly in immunocompromised patients (mainly those with HIV); presents with the gradual appearance of numerous brown to violaceous or colourless vascular tumours of the skin and subcutaneous tissues.

Bacillary peliosis—reported in immunosuppressed patients infected with *B. henselae*; causes vascular proliferation in solid internal organs with reticuloendothelial elements, particularly the liver (peliosis hepatis).

Bacteraemia and endocarditis—'culture-negative' and usually caused by *B. quintana* or *B. henselae*; patients with abnormal heart valves and those with chronic alcohol abuse are at particular risk.

Diagnosis, treatment, and prevention

Diagnosis—this is difficult because of the fastidious nature of bartonella and the nonspecific clinical manifestations; diagnostic techniques include culture from blood and other tissues, detection of organisms in lymph nodes by immunofluorescence, PCR amplification of bartonella genes, and serology.

Treatment—bartonella is susceptible to many antibiotics when grown in the laboratory, but this correlates poorly with *in vivo* efficacy. General recommendations are as follows: (1) cat-scratch disease—symptomatic treatment only, with azithromycin in severe or complicated cases; (2) trench fever—combination of doxycycline with gentamicin; (3) bacillary angiomatosis or peliosis—erythromycin; (4) endocarditis—gentamicin with ceftriaxone with or without doxycycline.

Prevention—*B. quintana* infections can be prevented by delousing, changing, or washing clothes. Immunocompromised patients should avoid contact with cats and cat fleas.

Historical perspective

Until 1990 the genus *Bartonella* contained only two species, *B. bacilliformis*, the cause of Carrión's disease (Chapter 7.6.43), and *B. quintana*, the cause of trench fever. In 1993, following the proposal of Brenner *et al.* based on comparison of 16S rDNA gene sequences, *Rochalimaea* spp. have been reclassified within the family Bartonellaceae and the genus *Bartonella*. In 1995, Birtles and colleagues proposed the unification of the genus *Grahamella* within the genus *Bartonella*. Numerous other bartonella species have been described in humans and several other species. Human infections due to bartonella species include old and newly described human infections. *Bartonella quintana* infection of humans was first described during the First World War as being responsible for trench fever, which caused more than 1 million deaths. Cat-scratch disease (CSD) was initially described in 1931 in France by Debré *et al.* but the aetiological agent (*B. henselae*) was first identified in 1992 and its role in bacillary angiomatosis was demonstrated using molecular methods.

Aetiology, genetics, pathogenesis, and pathology

The bacteria of the genus *Bartonella* are short, pleomorphic, fastidious aerobes that are oxidase and catalase negative. They are closely related phylogenetically to the genera *Brucella*, *Agrobacterium*, and *Rhizobium*. The 1.6-Mb genome of *B. quintana* was found to be a derivate of the 1.9-Mb genome of *B. henselae*. Prophages and horizontally acquired genomic islands have been identified in *B. henselae*, but are absent from *B. quintana*. Because no distinguishing phenotypic characteristics have been described for bartonella species, their identification and phylogenetic classification have been based mainly on genetic studies. Many DNA regions and encoding gene sequences have been used, including the 16S rDNA gene, 16S–23S rRNA intergenic spacer region (ITS), citrate synthase gene (*gltA*), heat shock protein gene (*groEL*), genes encoding the PAP31 and 35-kDa proteins, and cell division protein gene (*ftsZ*). A phylogenetic neighbour-joining tree resulting from comparison of sequences of the concatenated genes of bartonella species is shown in Fig. 7.6.42.1. According to La Scola *et al.*, a new *Bartonella* isolate can be considered a new species if a 327-bp *gltA* fragment shares less than 96% sequence similarity with the existing species and if an 825-bp *rpoB* fragment shares less than 94% sequence similarity with the validated species. Bartonella are considered intracellular bacteria that target endothelial or red blood cells, resulting in a long-lasting intraerythrocytic bacteraemia and angiogenesis. The intraerythrocytic localization of bartonella has been demonstrated in several hosts (Table 7.6.42.1). Although intraerythrocytic infection by bartonella is host-specific,

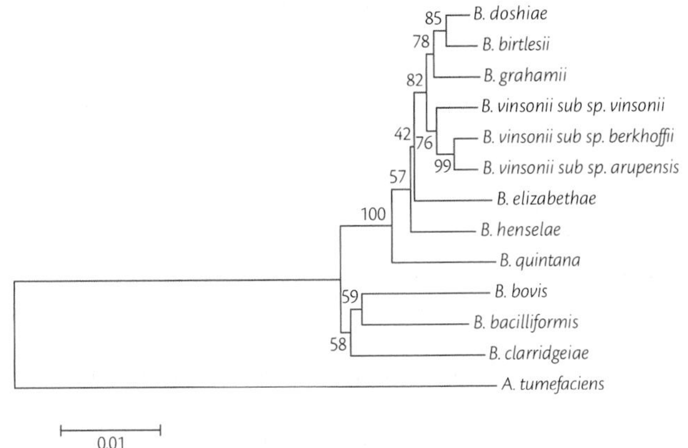

Fig. 7.6.42.1 Neighbour-joining tree based on the combined RNase P RNA, 16S and 23S rRNA sequence alignment.

Table 7.6.42.1 Species of *Bartonella* reported to date: epidemiological and clinical data

Bartonella spp.	Reservoir host	Vector detection in arthropods	Disease in humans	First cultivation	Detection in erythrocytes
B. bacilliformis	Human	Sand fly (*Lutzomyia* spp.)	CSD, END	1919	+
B. talpae	Mole	Unknown	Unknown	1911	
B. peromysci	Unknown	Unknown	Unknown	1942	
B. vinsonii subsp. *vinsonii*	Rodents	Unknown	Unknown	1946	
B. quintana	Human, cats	Human body lice and fleas	TF, BA, BAC, END	1961	+
B. henselae	Cats, rats, dogs	Fleas (*Ctenocephalides felis*)	CSD, BA, BAC, LMF, END, PH, RET	1990	+
B. elizabethae	Rodents, dogs	Fleas	END (1 case)	1993	
B. grahamii	Voles, rodents	Fleas?	RET (1 case)	1995	
B. taylorii	Rats	Fleas?	Unknown	1995	
B. doshiae	Voles	Fleas?	Unknown	1995	
B. clarridgeiae	Cats, dogs	*Ctenocephalides felis*	Unknown	1995	+
B. vinsonii subsp. *berkhoffii*	Dogs, coyotes, grey foxes	Fleas and ticks	END	1995	
B. vinsonii subsp. *arupensis*	Rodents, cattle	Deer ticks	BAC (1 case)	1999	
B. tribocorum	Rats	Unknown	Unknown	1998	
B. koehlerae	Cats	Fleas	END (1 case)	1999	+
B. alsatica	Rabbit	Fleas or ticks	END (1 case)	1999	
B. bovis (weissii)	Cows, cats	Unknown	Unknown	1999	
B. washoensis	Rodents, dogs	Unknown	MYOC (1 case)	2000	
B. birtlesii	Rats	Unknown	Unknown	2000	
B. schoenbuchensis	Wild roe deer	Unknown	Unknown	2001	
B. capreoli	Wild roe deer	Unknown	Unknown	2002	
B. chomelii	Cows	Unknown	Unknown	2004	
B. rattimassiliensis	Rats	Unknown	Unknown	2004	
B. phoceensis	Rats	Unknown	Unknown	2004	

BA, bacillary angiomatosis; BAC, bacteraemia; CSD, cat-scratch disease; END, endocarditis; LMF, lymphadenopathy; MYOC, myocarditis; PH: peliosis hepatis; RET, retinitis; TF, trench fever.

these pathogens can cause localized tissue manifestations in both reservoir and incidentally infected host(s). Bartonella species have the ability to colonize vascular tissues, which is considered to be a crucial step in the establishment of vasoproliferative lesions by *B. henselae* and *B. quintana* (bacillary angiomatosis and bacillary peliosis).

Epidemiology

The most common bartonella zoonosis worldwide is CSD, caused by *B. henselae*. Human cases have been reported from several continents, including North America, Europe, and Australia, and from most countries where investigators looked for that infection. These bacteria are the most common bartonellas detected in cats worldwide and are highly prevalent. Transmission from cat to human mainly occurs directly by a cat scratch and possibly by a cat bite or possibly by cat flea or tick bite. Flea faeces may be the only infected material that can be inoculated by a cat scratch. Other bartonella species have been detected in cat fleas, including *B. clarridgeiae*, *B. koehlerae*, and *B. quintana*.

B. quintana infections are transmitted by the body louse *Pediculus humanus*. Outbreaks of trench fever are linked mainly with poor socioeconomic conditions and wars, which predispose to body louse infestation. *B. quintana* infections decreased after the First World War and re-emerged during the Second World War. There have been sporadic outbreaks in Europe and the United States of America in poor people and alcoholics.

The epidemiology of the other bartonella species is not well understood. They can cause asymptomatic bacteraemia in reservoir hosts: *B. henselae* and *B. clarridgeiae* in cats, *B. bovis* in cattle, *B. alsatica* in rabbits, and *B. tribocorum* in rats (Fig. 7.6.42.2).

Clinical features

A remarkable feature of bartonella is the ability of a single species to cause either acute or chronic infection with either vascular

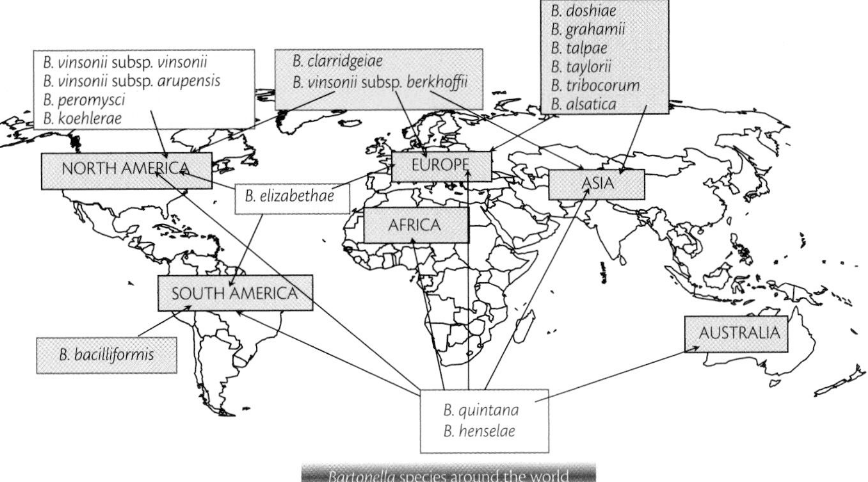

Fig. 7.6.42.2 *Bartonella* species isolated around the world.

proliferative or suppurative features. The pathological response to infection with bartonella varies substantially with the host's immunocompetence. There have been few clinical studies employing a standard case definition, culture confirmation, and rigidly defined disease outcomes in patients with similar immunocompetence. Therapeutic recommendations are often based on a few subjects.

Trench fever

Trench fever is also known as quintan fever, Wolhynia fever (because the disease was first observed by German medical officers on the East German front in Wolhynia), and 5-day fever (because of its tendency to relapse on the fifth day). After the bite of the body louse the incubation period ranges from 15 to 25 days, but in volunteers inoculated with a large volume of crushed infected lice it was less than 9 days. The illness varies from asymptomatic to severe. The classic clinical presentations among troops was an acute febrile illness, often accompanied by severe headache and pain in the long bones of the legs. The interval between attacks of pyrexia ranges from 4 to 8 days, but is usually 5 days. Trench fever often results in prolonged disability, but no fatalities have been recorded. The first 4 to 6 weeks of the illness are the most severe and, in a few cases, chronic fever, anaemia, loss of weight, and neuropsychiatric symptoms develop.

Cat-scratch disease (CSD)

CSD is a common infection. Cats are the main reservoir of *B. henselae*, and the bacterium may be transmitted between cats by the cat flea *Ctenocephalides felis*. Depending on the clinical manifestations, CSD has been characterized in two forms: classic typical clinical CSD with lymphadenopathy and a history of a cat scratch and/or bite, and atypical CSD. Classic CSD usually occurs in children and young adults but may also affect elderly people. Most patients with typical CSD remain afebrile. The main clinical manifestations in an immunocompetent host appear approximately 2 weeks after inoculation, although *B. henselae* DNA can be isolated from the peripheral blood of patients as long as 4 months after infection. One-third of the patients present with a history of fever lasting from 0 to 70 days (mean 14.8 days) with a maximum temperature between 37.9 and 42.0°C. The localization of lymphadenopathy is mainly axillary, cervical, or submaxillary, i.e. the lymph nodes that usually drain the area where the cat scratch occurs (Fig. 7.6.42.3). Lymphadenopathy may sometimes last for months, and in a few cases can be prolonged for as long as 12 to 24 months. Finally, general symptoms including malaise, headache, convulsion, sore throat, otalgia, vomiting, diarrhoea, anorexia, and tiredness can persist for a long time.

Atypical CSD occurs in a minority of cases, most of whom have severe systemic symptoms indicating disseminated infection. Patients with atypical CSD have prolonged fever (>2 weeks), myalgia, arthralgia/arthropathy, malaise, fatigue, weight loss, splenomegaly, and Parinaud's oculoglandular syndrome (POGS). POGS appears to be the most common ocular complication of CSD, affecting approximately 5% of symptomatic patients. Organisms from an infected cat are inoculated indirectly into the eye rather than by direct contact through a scratch.

Encephalopathy and neuroretinitis

These are less common manifestations of CSD. Two-thirds of patients with neuroretinitis have evidence of past infection by *B. henselae*. Other bartonella species causing retinitis include *B. quintana*, *B. grahamii*, *B. clarridgeiae*, and *B. elizabethae*. Retinitis is typically stellar. The onset of neurological complications varies from a few days to 2 months after the onset of lymphadenopathy and tends to occur more often in older school-age children.

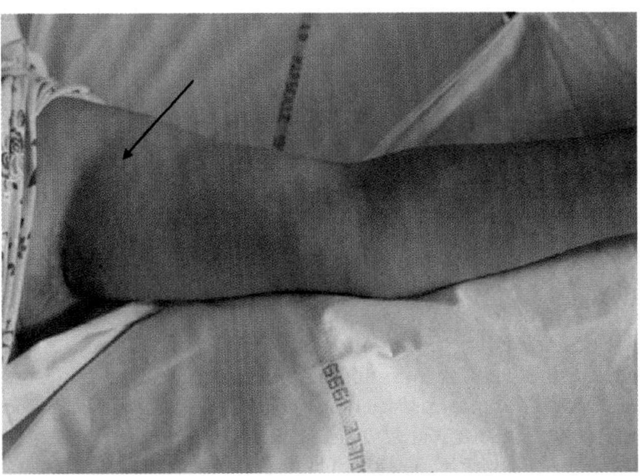

Fig. 7.6.42.3 Axillary lymphadenitis (CSD).

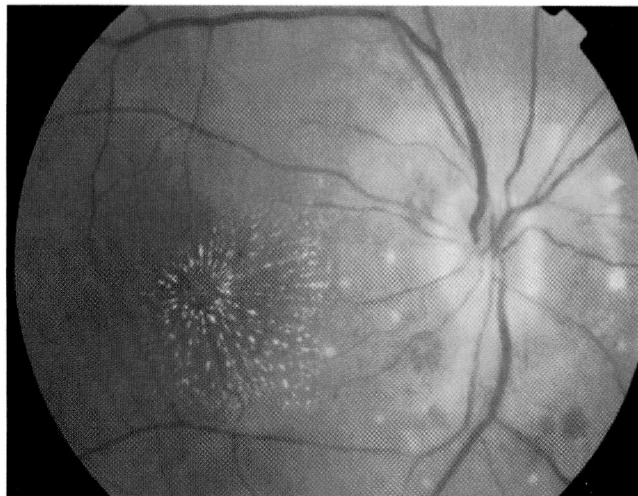

Fig. 7.6.42.4 Stellar retinitis due to *B. henselae*. (Courtesy of Dr M J Dolan.)

Features include headache, malaise, lethargy lasting for one to several weeks, impaired consciousness, acute hemiplegia, optic disc oedema and macular star formation, loss of vision with central scotoma, and glaucoma (Fig. 7.6.42.4).

Bacillary angiomatosis

Bacillary angiomatosis, also called epithelioid angiomatosis, is a vascular proliferative disease most often involving the skin that occurs particularly in immunocompromised patients, mainly those infected with HIV. Without appropriate therapy, infection spreads systemically, can involve virtually any organ, and may be fatal. Rarely, it can also affect immunocompetent patients. Both *B. henselae* and *B. quintana* are considered aetiological agents. In the case of *B. quintana* there are associated subcutaneous and lytic bone lesions, and *B. henselae* is associated with peliosis hepatis. Bacillary angiomatosis is manifested by the gradual appearance of numerous brown to violaceous or colourless vascular tumours of the skin and subcutaneous tissues, numbering a few to several hundred and varying in size from a few millimetres to several centimetres. Three morphologically distinct cutaneous lesions have been described: (1) pyogenic granuloma-like lesions, the most common type; (2) subcutaneous nodules; and (3) hyperpigmented indurated plaques. The clinical differential diagnosis includes pyogenic granuloma, haemangioma, subcutaneous tumours, and Kaposi's sarcoma. The skin lesions are very similar to those reported for verruga peruana, the chronic form of Carrión's disease. Bacillary angiomatosis lesions can also involve the bone marrow, liver, spleen, or lymph nodes.

Bacillary peliosis

Bacillary peliosis is a condition affecting solid internal organs with reticuloendothelial elements, especially the liver in which bacillary peliosis causes vascular proliferation of sinusoidal hepatic capillaries resulting in blood-filled spaces (peliosis hepatis), but also the spleen, abdominal lymph nodes, and bone marrow. The disease was first described in patients with tuberculosis and advanced cancers and was associated with the use of anabolic steroids. It has also been reported in organ transplant recipients and HIV-infected patients with *B. henselae*.

Bacteraemia and endocarditis

Infection due to *B. quintana* should be suspected in indigent, chronic alcoholic patients with culture-negative endocarditis, especially those with a long-standing valve lesion. *B. quintana* bacteraemia has also been reported in other patients with endocarditis. Evidence of bartonella endocarditis was found in 0.5 to 12% of all patients diagnosed with endocarditis tested at reference centres in different countries in the old world, decreasing from north to south. Among cases of bartonella endocarditis in Europe, 75% were associated with *B. quintana* and 25% with *B. henselae*. In North Africa most cases were caused by *B. quintana*, which is also responsible for asymptomatic, prolonged, and intermittent bacteraemia in homeless people in cities both in Europe and in the United States of America.

Endocarditis due to *B. henselae* should be suspected in patients with previous valvulopathy and culture-negative endocarditis, especially those who have contacts with cats.

Endocarditis and/or bacteraemia due to other bartonella species. are unusual but *B. elizabethae*, *B. vinsonii* subsp. *berkhoffii*, *B. vinsonii* subsp. *vinsonii*, *B. koehlerae*, and *B. alsatica* have been isolated from heart valves of patients with culture-negative endocarditis. One case of myocarditis has been attributed to *B. washoensis*.

Prolonged fever

Prolonged fever (>15 days) may occur in patients with atypical CSD.

Diagnosis

Diagnosis is difficult because of the fastidious nature of bartonella and the nonspecific clinical manifestations. Diagnostic techniques for bartonella-related infections include culture and detection of organisms in lymph nodes by immunofluorescence, molecular techniques including polymerase chain reaction (PCR), and serology. Table 7.6.42.2 presents the most common clinical features caused by bartonella and the best techniques for their identification, and Fig. 7.6.42.5 presents the current strategy that could be used for the diagnosis of infections due to bartonella.

Specimen collection

Various specimens, especially serum, blood, biopsy specimens, and arthropods, are useful. They should be sampled as soon as possible after the onset of disease. For serological diagnosis, serum samples should be collected early and during convalescence 1 to 3 weeks later. Serum samples can be stored easily at −20°C or below for long periods without degradation of antibodies. Blood should be sampled before antimicrobial therapy either in citrate-containing vials for culture or in ethylenediaminetetraacetic acid (EDTA) for PCR techniques. EDTA should be avoided for culture since it leads to detachment of cell monolayers. Biopsies of lymph nodes, cardiac valves, vascular aneurysms, or grafts should be taken in two parts, one in absolute alcohol for histopathology and immunodetection and another frozen and stored at −70°C in a sterile vial for culture and PCR analysis. These methods can be also used to detect bartonella in various arthropods including ticks, lice, and fleas (xenodiagnosis). The arthropod should be disinfected with iodinated alcohol and then crushed in medium before being inoculated into a shell vial for culture or processing using molecular methods. Arthropods can be easily stored dry in a box and sent by mail to a reference centre for analysis.

Table 7.6.42.2 Most common clinical manifestations and diagnostic methods for bartonella infections

Disease in humans	Commonly isolated	Rarely isolated	Specimen	Methods
Cat-scratch disease	*B. henselae*	*B. quintana*, *B. clarridgeiae*	Lymph nodes	PCR, serology
Endocarditis	*B. henselae*, *B. quintana*	*B. elizabethae*, *B. koehlerae*, *B. vinsonii* subsp. *berkhoffii*, *B. alsatica*	Blood, serum, valves	PCR, serology
Retinitis	*B. henselae*	*B. grahamii*	Serum, aqueous humour	PCR, serology
Bacillary angiomatosis	*B. henselae*, *B. quintana*		Blood, serum, cutaneous biopsy	PCR
Bacteraemia	*B. quintana*	*B. henselae*, *B. vinsonii* subsp. *arupensis*	Blood, serum	PCR, serology
Peliosis hepatitis	*B. henselae*		Blood, serum, hepatic biopsy	PCR, serology
Osteomyelitis	*B. henselae*		Blood, serum, bone biopsy	PCR, serology
Trench fever	*B. quintana*		Blood, serum	PCR

PCR, polymerase chain reaction.

Direct diagnosis

Culture

The most widely used methods for isolation are direct plating into solid media, blood culture in broth, and cocultivation in cell culture. Bartonella can be grown on blood agar at 37°C in a 5% CO_2 atmosphere, except for *B. bacilliformis* which should be grown at 30°C. Primary isolates are typically obtained after 12 to 14 days, although an incubation period of up to 45 days may be necessary (Fig. 7.6.42.6). Subculture in blood broth in shell vials is the most efficient culture method in patients with endocarditis. Specimens are placed on human embryonic lung cells in shell vials and incubated at 37°C in an atmosphere of 5% CO_2. Culture may be successful using blood samples, skin, lymph nodes, or other organ biopsy samples. Lysis centrifugation and freezing have been shown to enhance the recovery of bartonella from blood. However, despite improved culture methods, the results of blood cultures may be negative if the patient has recently received antibiotics or if the organism is fastidious or requires special culture techniques. A recently described growth medium for the detection and isolation of bartonella, bartonella-Alphaproteobacteria growth medium (BAPGM), may provide an improved or alternative method to isolate these fastidious microorganisms from patient samples.

Immunodetection

Detection of bartonella using specific antibodies has been achieved in various situations. Demonstration of microorganisms in valve tissues by the Warthin–Starry stain (Fig. 7.6.42.7) is a classic criterion for the histological diagnosis of infective endocarditis. Direct immunological detection in lymph nodes has been reported in patients with CSD, for patients with peliosis hepatis, in red blood cells of bacteraemic homeless people, in cardiac valves, and in skin biopsies. Immunohistochemistry is a convenient tool for detecting *B. quintana* in tissues but specific antibodies are often not available.

Molecular biology

PCR is a convenient method for detecting bartonella either in fresh or in formalin-fixed and paraffin-embedded tissues. The current target genes used for the detection and identification of bartonella are the citrate synthase gene (*gltA*), the 16S RNA gene, the 16S–23S rRNA *ITS*, the 60-kDa heat-shock protein (*groEL*), and the *pap31* gene. Although these methods are highly specific, their sensitivity varies according to the type of samples. Thus the current strategy for the diagnosis of bartonella infections is to use two different target genes (e.g. *ITS* gene and *pap31*), and if the results are discordant to use a third gene (*groEL*). Samples should be considered positive only if at least two genes are positive and if sequences obtained give the same identification. Improvement of molecular methods may increase the sensitivity especially the use of real-time PCR with Taqman probes. Recently a new tool has been proposed for the diagnosis of bartonella endocarditis by real-time nested PCR assay performed on a LightCycler apparatus (LCN-PCR) using serum, which could shorten the delay in the diagnosis. For the typing and characterization of *B. henselae* isolates, multilocus sequence typing (MLST) is a relatively new typing method that groups bacteria based on comparison of nucleic acid sequences of

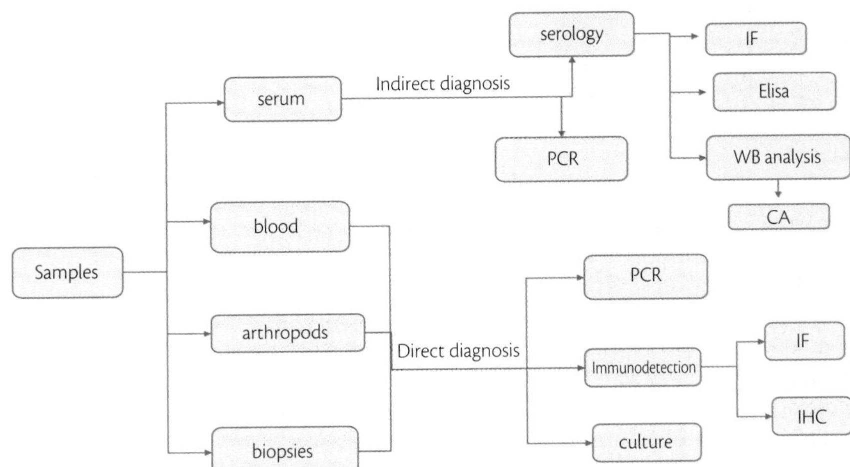

Fig. 7.6.42.5 Strategy for the diagnosis of *Bartonella* spp. infections.

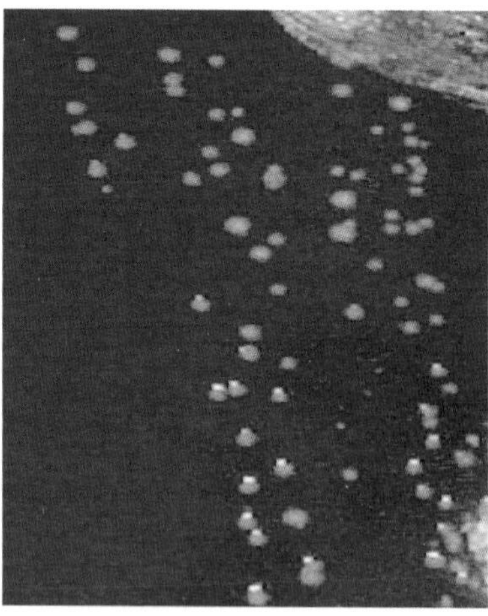

Fig. 7.6.42.6 Colony morphology of *B. henselae* on Columbia 5% sheep blood agar.

450 to 500 bp derived from the internal fragments of a number (typically seven) of housekeeping genes. More recently a molecular typing method based on the sequences of such noncoding zones rather than of housekeeping genes was developed and called multispacer typing (MST).

Indirect diagnosis

Serology is the only useful noninvasive method for the diagnosis of bartonella infections, especially for CSD, bacteraemia, and endocarditis. The sensitivity of serological tests varies between laboratories, from nearly 100% to less than 30% depending on the method used for preparation of antigens. Sources of antigens for serology can be either whole-cell lysates or outer membrane protein preparations and, more recently, recombinant proteins. The most widely used serological test for diagnosis is the indirect fluorescence assay (IFA) to detect antibodies against *B. henselae* whole cells. An IgG anti-*B. henselae* antibody titre of 1:64 or more is considered positive for infection when patients are tested at least 2 to 3 weeks after a suspected infection. Bartonella-associated endocarditis in humans and animals is usually associated with much higher IFA antibody titres (>1:800). False-negative results are due to either antigenic heterogeneity among *B. henselae* species or to other diseases such as mycobacterial infections, lymphoma, or Kaposi's sarcoma. Cross-reactions have been reported either with other bartonella species, or between bartonella species and *Coxiella burnetii* or chlamydia. Lepidi *et al.* have developed autoimmunohistochemistry, which is a peroxidase-based method with the patient's own serum as the source of antibodies directed against the aetiological microorganism, for the diagnosis of infective endocarditis. The rate of detection of bacteria by autoimmunohistochemistry was significantly higher than that by culture but was similar to that by PCR. The most sophisticated serological method, western blot analysis after cross-adsorption, has been shown to be a powerful tool for the identification of bartonella to species level in endocarditis (Fig. 7.6.42.8).

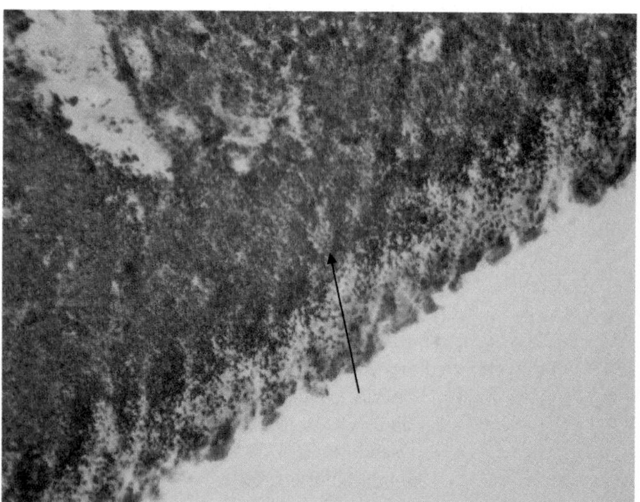

Fig. 7.6.42.7 Warthin–Starry staining of a cardiac valve of a patient with *B. quintana* endocarditis. Arrow shows the clumps of bacilli. Magnification ×400.

Treatment

In vitro susceptibility to antibiotics

This can be performed in either eukaryotic cells or axenic media. Bartonella species are susceptible to many antibiotics when they are grown axenically, including penicillin and cephalosporin compounds, aminoglycosides, chloramphenicol, tetracyclines, macrolide compounds, rifampicin, fluoroquinolones, and co-trimoxazole. However, these results correlate poorly with *in vivo* efficacy because antibiotics are not bactericidal, except for aminoglycosides. This has also been reported in cell-culture models for *B. henselae* in murine macrophage-like cells and for *B. quintana* in red blood cells. Recent *in vivo* data have demonstrated the benefit of a combination of doxycycline with gentamicin in the treatment of bartonella-related infections including endocarditis and bacteraemia in homeless peoples. Mutations in the 23S RNA gene and insertion of nine amino acids in the L4 ribosomal protein for *B. henselae* and *B. quintana*, respectively, can be selected *in vitro* by erythromycin. Mutations such as the A2059G transition have been detected directly in the lymph node of a patient with CSD, suggesting that natural erythromycin-resistant strains may infect humans.

In vivo in human patients

Trench fever

Most cases of trench fever were reported before the antibiotic era. However, successful treatment with tetracycline or chloramphenicol was reported during the Second World War. According to a recent placebo-controlled clinical trial, patients with chronic *B. quintana* bacteraemia should be treated with gentamicin (3 mg/kg intravenously once a day) for 14 days and with doxycycline (200 mg/day orally once a day) for 28 days. Patients with chronic bacteraemia should be carefully evaluated for endocarditis, which requires prolonged therapy under close monitoring. Those with renal insufficiency or obesity need a twice-daily dosing schedule to avoid gentamicin nephrotoxicity.

CSD

CSD typically does not respond to antibiotic therapy. Management consists of analgesics for pain, follow-up, and drainage when necessary. Recent data re-emphasize that patients who do not improve clinically benefit from excision of affected lymph nodes and search for coexistent diseases such as tuberculosis and/or lymphoma. The only double-blind placebo-controlled study for

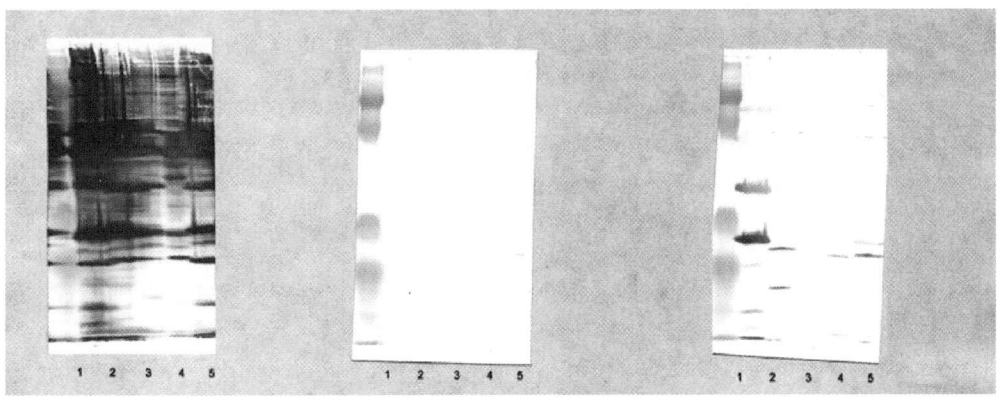

Fig. 7.6.42.8 Western blot of a patient with *B. quintana* endocarditis before (a) and after cross-adsorption with *B. quintana* (b) or *B. henselae* (c). Line 1: *B. quintana*; line 2: *B. henselae*; line 3: *B. elizabethae*; line 4: *B. vinsonii* subsp. *berkhoffii*; line 5: *B. alsatica*.

the treatment of CSD with azithromycin in immunocompetent patients showed only a faster reduction of their lymph node volume as compared to placebo. Thus, the current recommendation for the treatment in mild to moderately ill immunocompetent patients with CSD is no antibiotic treatment. Treatment with azithromycin could help patients with bulky lymphadenopathy or those with complicated CSD with retinitis and central nervous system disease.

Endocarditis

Effective antibiotic therapy for suspected bartonella endocarditis should include an aminoglycoside (gentamicin) for at least 14 days together with ceftriaxone with or without doxycycline for 6 weeks to achieve a bactericidal effect. Valve replacement is necessary in the majority of patients because of extensive damage.

Bacillary angiomatosis and peliosis hepatis

Erythromycin is the first choice for bacillary angiomatosis and peliosis hepatis. Treatment should continue for at least 3 months for bacillary angiomatosis and 4 months for peliosis hepatis. Longer treatment should be given in HIV-infected and immunocompromised patients. An *in vitro* model of *B. quintana* cultured in endothelial cells has shown that erythromycin acts mainly antiangiogenically rather than as an antibiotic, explaining the often dramatic response to this antibiotic in bacillary angiomatosis. Bacillary peliosis hepatis responds more slowly than cutaneous bacillary angiomatosis, but hepatic lesions usually are improved after several months of treatment. Relapses of peliosis hepatis and bacillary angiomatosis lesions in bone and skin have been reported frequently, mostly in severely immunocompromised HIV-infected patients. Finally, patients who have relapses after the recommended treatment should receive secondary prophylactic antibiotic treatment with erythromycin or doxycycline as long as they are immunocompromised.

Prevention

B. quintana infections can be prevented by delousing, changing, or washing clothes. To avoid *B. henselae*, immunocompromised patients should avoid contact with cats and cat fleas. Only seronegative cats should be kept by immunocompromised people, but is better to avoid them altogether or to eradicate cat fleas.

Conclusions

Bacteria of the genus *Bartonella* are responsible for emerging and re-emerging infections worldwide and can present in many different ways, from benign and self-limited infections to severe and life-threatening diseases. Consequently, diagnosis and treatment of these infections should be adapted to each clinical situation, to the species involved, and to whether the disease is an acute or a chronic form.

Further reading

Alsmark CM, *et al.* (2004). The louse-borne human pathogen *Bartonella quintana* is a genomic derivative of the zoonotic agent *Bartonella henselae*. *Proc Natl Acad Sci U S A*, **101**, 9716–21.

Birtles RJ, *et al.* (1995). Proposals to unify the genera *Grahamella* and *Bartonella*, with descriptions of *Bartonella talpae* comb. nov., *Bartonella peromysci* comb. nov., and three new species, *Bartonella grahamii* sp. nov., *Bartonella taylorii* sp. nov., and *Bartonella doshiae* sp. nov. *Int J Syst Bact*, **45**, 1–8.

Biswas S, Raoult D, Rolain JM (2006). Molecular characterization of resistance to macrolides in *Bartonella henselae*. *Antimicrob Agents Chemother*, **50**, 3192–3.

Breitschwerdt B, Kordick D (2000). *Bartonella* infection in animals: carriership, reservoir potential, pathogenicity and zoonotic potential for human infection. *Clin Microbiol Rev*, **13**, 428–38.

Brenner DJ, *et al.* (1993). Proposals to unify the genera *Bartonella* and *Rochalimaea*, with descriptions of *Bartonella quintana* comb. nov., *Bartonella vinsonii* comb. nov., *Bartonella henselae* comb. nov., and *Bartonella elizabethae* comb. nov., and to remove the family *Bartonellaceae* from the order *Rickettsiales*. *Int J Syst Bact*, **43**, 777–86.

Dehio C (2001). *Bartonella* interactions with endothelial cells and erythrocytes. *Trends Microbiol*, **9**, 279–85.

Foucault C, Brouqui P, Raoult D (2006). *Bartonella quintana* characteristics and clinical management. *Emerg Infect Dis*, **12**, 217–23.

Greub G, Raoult D (2002). *Bartonella*: new explanations for old diseases. *J Med Microbiol*, **51**, 915–23.

Houpikian P, Raoult D (2001). 16S/23S rRNA intergenic spacer regions for phylogenetic analysis, identification, and subtyping of *Bartonella* species. *J Clin Microbiol*, **39**, 2768–78.

Houpikian P, Raoult D (2003). Western immunoblotting for *Bartonella* endocarditis. *Clin Diagn Lab Immunol*, **10**, 95–102.

La Scola B, Raoult D (1999). Culture of *Bartonella quintana* and *Bartonella henselae* from human samples: a 5-year experience (1993 to 1998). *J Clin Microbiol*, **37**, 1899–905.

La Scola B, *et al.* (2003). Gene-sequence-based criteria for species definition in bacteriology: the *Bartonella* paradigm. *Trends Microbiol*, **11**, 318–21.

Lepidi H, Fournier PE, Raoult D (2000). Quantitative analysis of valvular lesions during *Bartonella* endocarditis. *Am J Clin Pathol*, **114**, 880–9.

Lepidi H, *et al.* (2006). Autoimmunohistochemistry: a new method for the histologic diagnosis of infective endocarditis. *J Infect Dis*, **193**, 1711–17.

Maurin M, Raoult D (1996). *Bartonella (Rochalimaea) quintana* infections. *Clin Microbiol Rev*, **9**, 273–92.

Maurin M, Rolain JM, Raoult D (2002). Comparison of in-house and commercial slides for detection of immunoglobulins G and M by immunofluorescence against *Bartonella henselae* and *Bartonella quintana*. *Clin Diag Lab Immunol*, **9**, 1004–9.

Meghari S, *et al.* (2006). Anti-angiogenic effect of erythromycin in *Bartonella quintana*: *in vitro* model of infection. *J Infect Dis*, **193**, 380–6.

Musso D, Drancourt M, Raoult D (1995). Lack of bactericidal effect of antibiotics except aminoglycosides on *Bartonella (Rochalimaea) henselae*. *J Antimicrob Chemother*, **36**, 101–8.

Pitulle C, *et al.* (2002). Investigation of the phylogenetic relationships within the genus *Bartonella* based on comparative sequence analysis of the *rnpB* gene, 16S rDNA and 23S rDNA. *Int J Syst Evol Microbiol*, **52**, 2075–80.

Raoult D, *et al.* (2003). Outcome and treatment of *bartonella* endocarditis. *Arch Intern Med*, **163**, 226–30.

Rolain JM, *et al.* (2001). Immunofluorescent detection of intraerythrocytic *Bartonella henselae* in naturally infected cats. *J Clin Microbiol*, **39**, 2978–88.

Rolain JM, *et al.* (2002). *Bartonella quintana* in human erythrocytes. *Lancet*, **360**, 226–8.

Rolain JM, *et al.* (2003). Molecular detection of *Bartonella quintana*, *B. koehlerae*, *B. henselae*, *B. clarridgeiae*, *Rickettsia felis* and *Wolbachia pipientis* in cat fleas, France. *Emerg Infect Dis*, **9**, 338–42.

Rolain JM, *et al.* (2004). Recommendations for treatment of human infections caused by *Bartonella* species. *Antimicrob Agents Chemother*, **48**, 1921–33.

Rolain JM, *et al.* (2006). Lymph node biopsy specimens and diagnosis of cat-scratch disease. *Emerg Infect Dis*, **12**, 1338–44.

Zeaiter Z, *et al.* (2002). Phylogenetic classification of *Bartonella* species by comparing groEL sequences. *Int J Syst Evol Microbiol*, **52**, 165–71.

7.6.43 *Bartonella bacilliformis* infection

A. Llanos-Cuentas and C. Maguiña-Vargas

Essentials

Bartonellosis (Carrión´s disease, verruga Peruana, Oroya fever, Guaitará fever) is caused by the Gram-negative bacillus *Bartonella bacilliformis*. It is endemic in the western Andes and inter-Andean valleys of Peru, and is still occasionally reported in Ecuador, with infection resulting from the bite of various female sandflies.

Clinical features, diagnosis, management, prognosis and prevention—infection of red blood cells manifests with nonspecific 'viral-type' symptoms and haemolytic anaemia in the acute stage of disease. Following an asymptomatic phase, the late 'eruptive' stage is characterized by dermal nodules ('verrugas') that frequently heal spontaneously. Secondary opportunistic infections are common. Diagnosis in areas where the disease occurs is usually by demonstration of bacteria in the blood film. Ciprofloxacin is the treatment of choice in most cases. Mortality is 1.1 to 2.4% in endemic areas and around 9% in patients admitted to hospital. There is no satisfactory prevention for people living in endemic areas; tourists can take the usual precautions against being bitten by insects.

Aetiological agent

Barton, a Peruvian physician, described the causative organism in 1905. *Bartonella bacilliformis* is a small motile aerobic Gram-negative bacillus that stains deep red or purple with Giemsa (Fig. 7.6.43.1). This facultative intracellular haemotropic bacterium varies in morphology and quantity during various stages of the disease. Although it is a pleomorphic organism, two essential types are distinguishable, bacilli or rod-shaped forms and coccoid forms. Rod-shaped forms predominate in the acute stage of the disease and coccoid in the convalescent stage. *B. bacilliformis* may infect red blood cells (Fig. 7.6.43.2), endothelial cells of capillaries, and sinusoidal lining cells. The organism is 2 to 3 μm long and 0.2 to 2.5 μm thick. In cultures, 1 to 10 flagella, 3 to 10 μm long, may originate from one end of the organism. Bartonella can be cultured in Columbia agar supplemented with 5% defibrinated human blood or other supplemented media containing rabbit serum and haemoglobin at 28° C under aerobic conditions for up to 6 weeks.

Epidemiology

Bartonellosis has occurred since pre-Columbian times, as proven by artistic representations in pre-Inca pottery and lesions in an ancient mummy. It is an endemic disease mainly in inter-Andean valleys in west, central, and east Andean areas of Peru (Fig. 7.6.43.3) and increasingly in high jungle areas. This is an emergent disease, extensively distributed in Peru; 142 districts were affected in 2000 and 416 in 2006 (192% increase), and 18 of 24 departments of Peru have been involved (Fig. 7.6.43.4). Some cases have recently been reported in Zumba (Chinchipe), Ecuador. The epidemiological pattern is endemic plus epidemic in the new areas. Transmission is usually in rural towns and around human dwellings. The disease occurs between 500 and 3200 m above sea level. Transmission varies throughout the year, being greatest towards the end of the rainy season (March to May). Interepidemic periods occur every 10 to 15 years. Incidence is greatly influenced by climatic, environmental, and ecological changes such as the El Niño phenomenon.

At present, 11 species and subspecies of the genus *Bartonella* have been associated with human infections but only three have epidemiological importance: *B. bacilliformis*, of which six antigenic

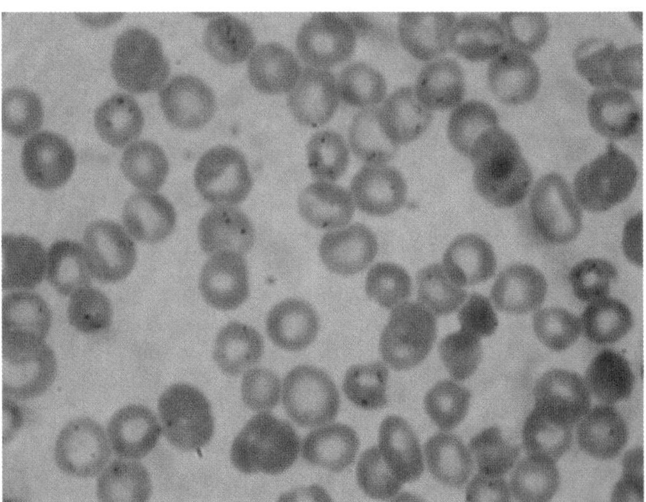

Fig. 7.6.43.1 *B. bacilliformis* in blood smear stained with Giemsa.

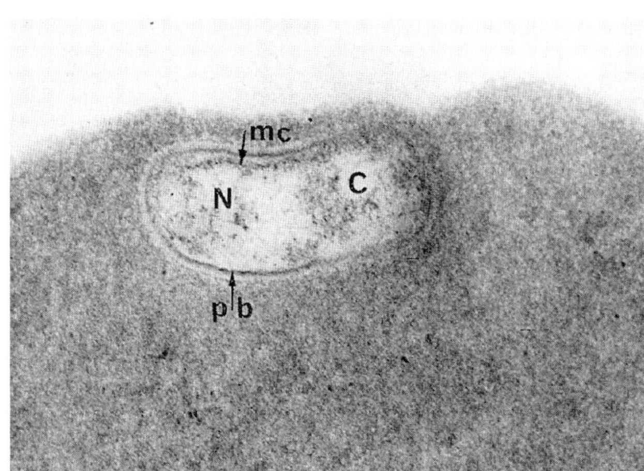

Fig. 7.6.43.2 *B. bacilliformis* in a red blood cell.

variants have been described in Peru; *B. henselae*, the major cause of cat-scratch disease and peliosis (Chapter 7.6.42); and *B. quintana* (formerly *Rochalimaea*), the agent of trench fever (Chapter 7.6.42). Recently, a new bartonella named *B. rochalimae* has been described in tourists infected in Peru. Other bartonellas such as *B. vinsonii* subsp. *berkhoffii*, *B. vinsonii* subsp. *arupensis*, *B. elizabethae*, *B. koehlerae*, *B. alsatica*, *B. grahamii*, and *B. clarridgeiae* occasionally cause disease in humans. In immunocompromised people, especially those with the HIV/AIDS, *B. henselae* and *B. quintana* cause opportunistic infections, frequently manifested as cutaneous bacillary angiomatosis, resembling verruga peruana.

In old endemic areas, the disease appears in childhood and usually produces few symptoms. Outsiders generally develop acute severe forms of the disease (Oroya fever). Large epidemics have occurred when large groups of nonresidents have entered endemic areas. In 1870, an epidemic engulfed workers building the railroad from Lima to Oroya (Fig. 7.6.43.5); the estimated mortality was 7000.

Infection results from the bite of females of several species of sandflies (*Lutzomyia*), especially *Lutzomyia verrucarum*. These vectors frequent human dwellings and, because they are active during twilight hours, humans are infected around sunrise and sunset. Although the reservoir is unknown, humans are regarded as being increasingly important. Asymptomatic *B. bacilliformis* infection has been demonstrated in endemic populations. However, since bartonellosis can be acquired in several Andean areas uninhabited by humans, other reservoirs for the disease may exist. Some domestic animals including horses, donkeys, mules, dogs, and cats are susceptible and develop lesions similar to verrugas. Bartonella-like isolates have been obtained from a mouse (*Phyllotis*, Cricetidae).

Pathogenesis

After inoculation of *B. bacilliformis* by sandfly bite, the bacteria multiply in endothelial cells of small vessels and phagocytic cells near the skin. Systemic invasion and multiplication in endothelial cells and red blood cells follows. In the most serious cases, 95% of red cells are infected with numerous bacteria. The hallmark of the disease is the severe haemolytic anaemia caused by massive infection of red blood cells and subsequent erythrophagocytosis. Several mechanisms contribute to anaemia: increased fragility, form and size alteration, and reduced half-life of infected and noninfected red cells. Some inhibition of haemoglobin synthesis, probably induced by toxic factors, has also been invoked, since red cell production increases dramatically with reduction of bacteraemia. Erythrophagocytosis contributes to lymphadenopathy and hepatosplenomegaly. 'Blockade' of the mononuclear phagocytic system and the presence of the circulating iron leads to superinfection, usually by enterobacteria, during the anaemia stage or early recovery from it. Transient depression of cellular immunity has been reported. During the anaemic phase, mild lymphopenia with a reduction of OKT4, a mild increase of OKT8, and decrease of the polyclonal stimulation of lymphocytes occurs. High levels of interleukin (IL)-10 were found in the acute phase. In Gram-negative sepsis, an uncontrolled production of IL-10 may produce 'immunological paralysis' of antigen-presenting cells.

In endemic areas, 20.5% of those infected with *B. bacilliformis* infection remain asymptomatic, 31.5% will develop the eruptive form (chronic phase) without evidence of an acute illness, 37% develop the eruptive form preceded by some symptoms, but only 11% will develop the classic acute form. The eruptive form appears

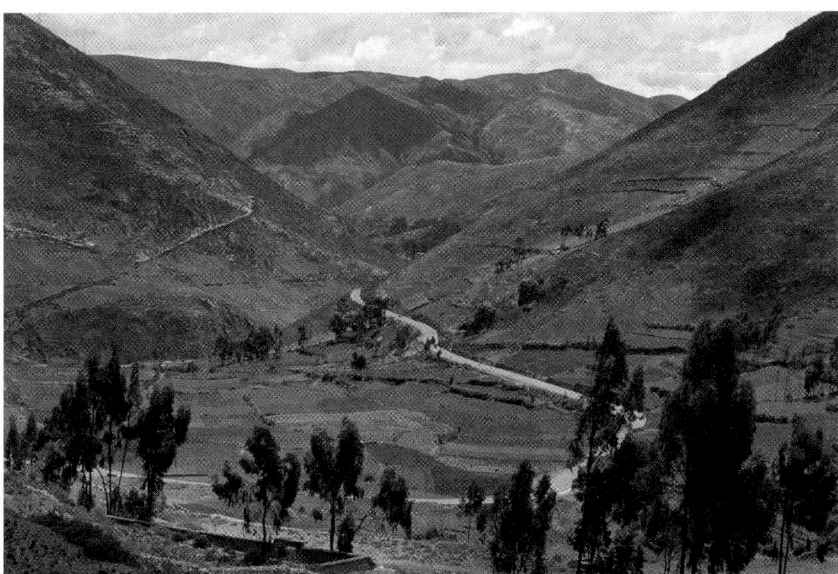

Fig. 7.6.43.3 Endemic area for bartonellosis; near Tarma, Peru. (Copyright D A Warrell.)

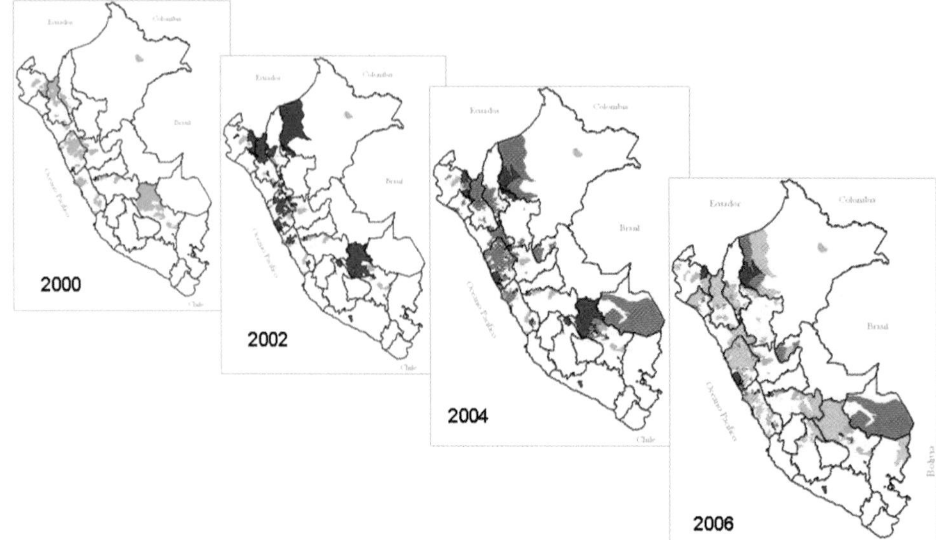

Fig. 7.6.43.4 Extension of the geographical distribution of bartonellosis in Peru between 2000 and 2006.

a few weeks to months after the acute illness has subsided, and in Peru is named 'verruga peruana' (Fig. 7.6.43.6a,b). The vascular skin lesions show endothelial proliferation and histiocytic hyperplasia (the cells contains degenerate organisms; Fig. 7.6.43.7) and later show fibrosis and necrosis. Electron microscopy of verrucous tissue shows *B. bacilliformis* in the interstitial tissues, indicating that the presence of the bacteria is important for this unusual vascular response to occur. Verruga peruana results from persistent infection, an immune response that is probably insufficient, and a peculiar vascular reaction, which could be caused by an angiogenic bacterial factor.

Clinical features

The disease has two stages, anaemic and eruptive, with an asymptomatic intermediate period. After an incubation period of around 60 days (range 10–210 days), nonspecific prodromal symptoms appear. The onset is usually gradual with malaise, mild chills, fever, and headache. Occasionally, high fever may develop rapidly or build up over a few days. It is accompanied by sweating and rigors. Common symptoms include weakness, aching of the head, back, and extremities, prostration, and depression. The clinical picture is dominated by severe (haemolytic) anaemia and the patient rapidly become pale (Fig. 7.6.43.8), dyspnoeic, and jaundiced. There may be hepatosplenomegaly, generalized lymphadenopathy, tachycardia, myocarditis (Fig. 7.6.43.9), purpura, hepatitis, diarrhoea, pericardial effusion, exudates, anasarca, and retinal changes (Fig. 7.6.43.10); sometimes there is generalized oedema, drowsiness, and convulsions, and exceptionally meningoencephalomyelitis. The duration of this state is variable (generally 2–4 weeks). In pregnant women, the disease in this phase may cause abortion, fetal death, and transplacental transmission of the disease; maternal death is common.

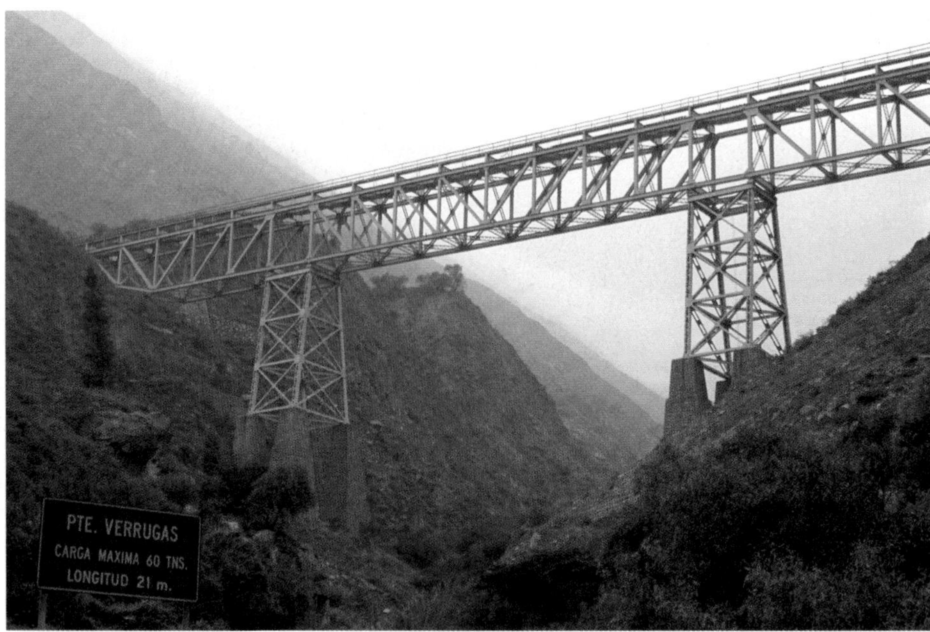

Fig. 7.6.43.5 Endemic area for bartonellosis; Rimac valley, Peru—Puente Verrugas.
(Copyright D.A. Warrell.)

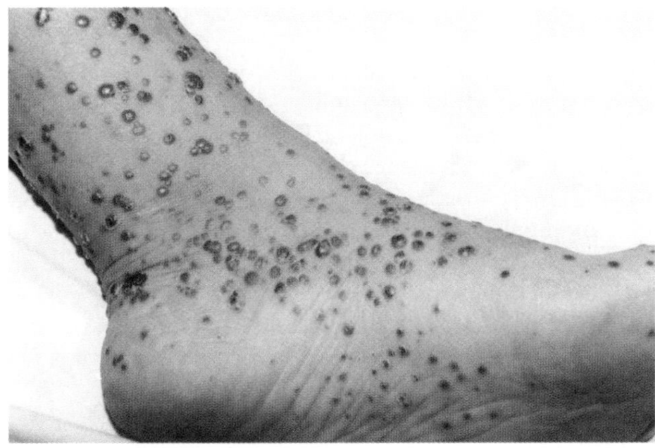

(a)

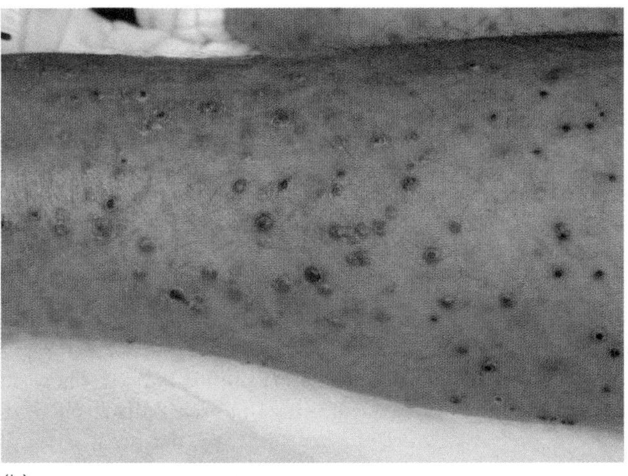

(b)

Fig. 7.6.43.6 Verruga peruana: miliary haemangioma-like lesions.

In the intermediate period, patients are asymptomatic and recover from the anaemia through great bone marrow activity. This pre-eruptive period varies from weeks to months.

In the eruptive stage, many nodular lesions of varying size appear on the face, trunk, and limbs, over a period of a month or more and usually persist for 3 or 4 months. There is accompanying mild arthralgia, myalgia, and sometimes fever. The red or purplish skin lesions are papules a few millimetres across. Most often the eruption is miliary (miliary form) with many haemangioma-like lesions of the dermis (Fig. 7.6.43.6a,b). Nodular lesions (nodular form) are larger but fewer and more prominent on the extensor surfaces of arms and legs (Fig. 7.6.43.11a,b). They are painless and prone to bleeding (Fig. 7.6.43.11c), secondary infection, and ulceration. The appearance may resemble haemangioma, cutaneous bacillary angiomatosis, granuloma pyogenicum, Kaposi's sarcoma, fibrosarcoma, leprosy (histoid form), or yaws. Occasionally one to a few, large, deep-seated ulcerating lesions (mular form) may develop. These tend to appear near joints where they may be painful and limit motion. Apart from skin, the mucous membranes of the mouth, conjunctiva, and nose, serous cavities, and the gastrointestinal and genitourinary tracts may be involved. The eruptive phase frequently tends to heal spontaneously, although the course is often prolonged.

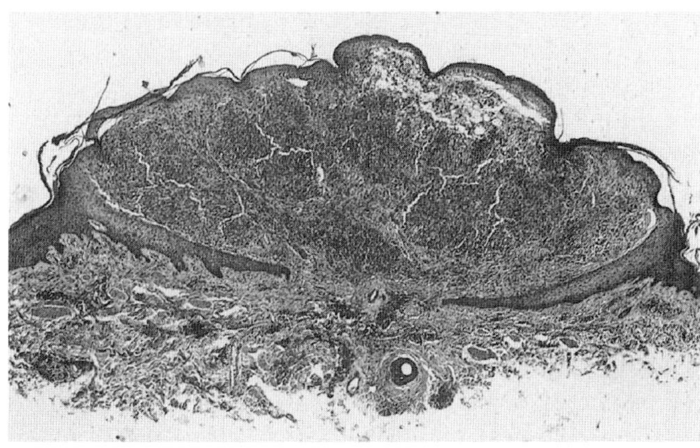

Fig. 7.6.43.7 Verruga peruana: histology.

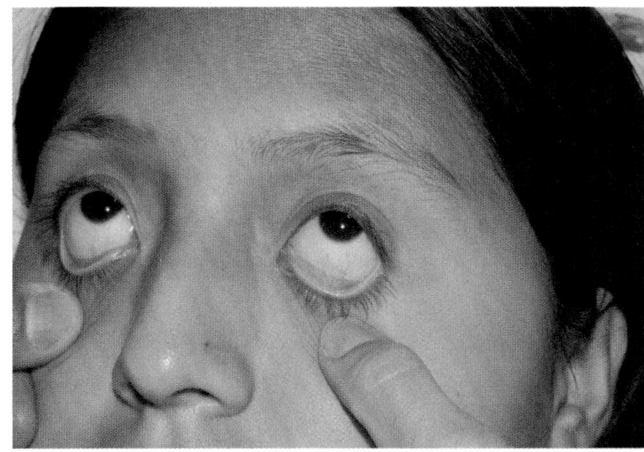

Fig. 7.6.43.8 Severe anaemia (haematocrit 9%) in a patient with acute bartonellosis.
(Copyright D A Warrell.)

The severe acute form can develop infectious and/or noninfectious complications. The principal complication is superinfection leading to septicaemia, which occurs at different stages of the diseases but generally in the later part of the anaemic stage and during the intermediate stage. Formerly, salmonella, *Mycobacterium tuberculosis*,

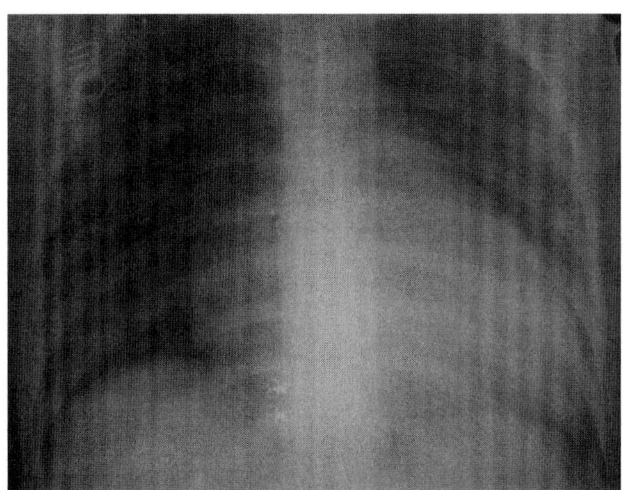

Fig. 7.6.43.9 Cardiomegaly due to myocarditis in a patient with acute bartonellosis.
(Copyright D A Warrell.)

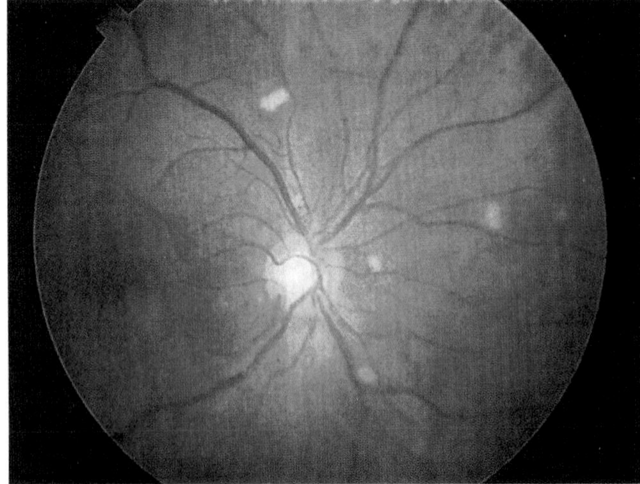

Fig. 7.6.43.10 Retinal changes.

and enterobacter were the most frequent pathogens. Reactivation of toxoplasmosis, histoplasmosis, pneumocystosis, leptospirosis, typhus fever, and staphylococcal infections are some of the other infections that are now frequent. Refractory haemodynamic failure, severe respiratory distress, and renal failure are some of the noninfectious complications.

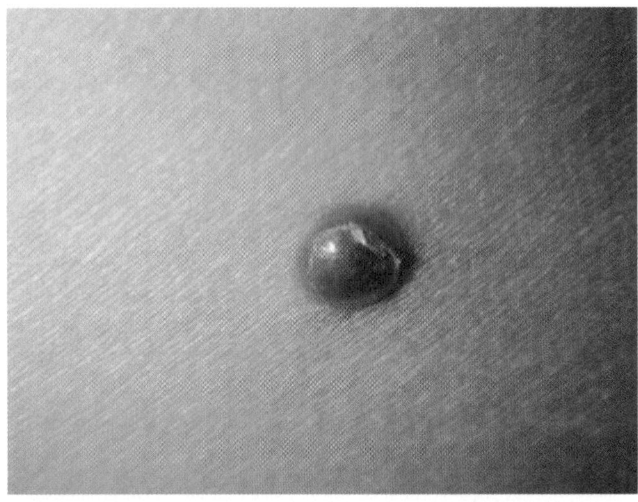

(a)

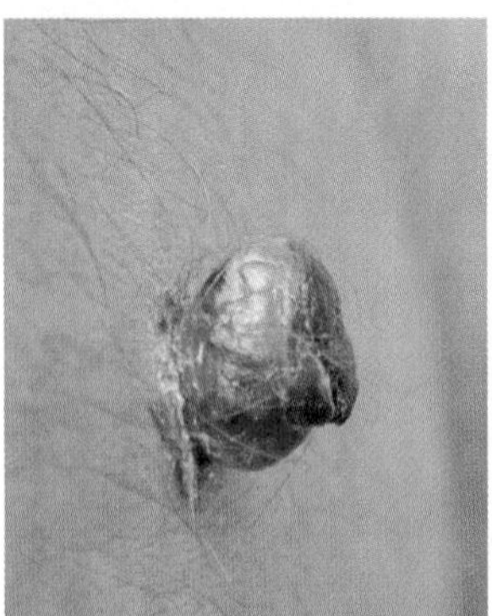

(b)

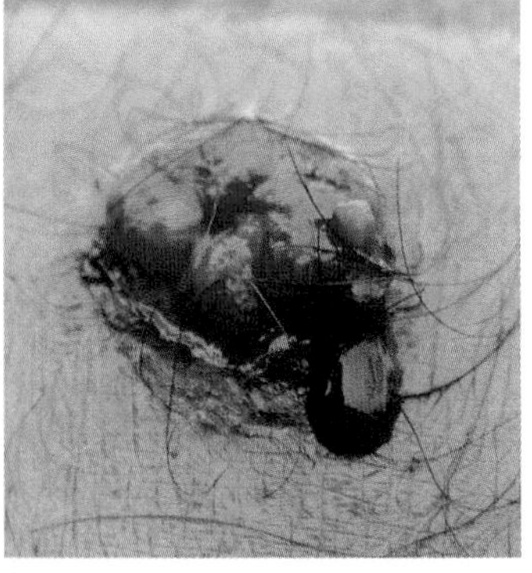

(c)

Fig. 7.6.43.11 Verruga peruana: nodular haemangiomatous lesions.

Diagnosis

Two elements must be considered: (1) travel or residence in an endemic area and (2) a compatible clinical picture with demonstration of the bacteria in the blood film (Fig. 7.6.43.1). Fluorescence antibody test, indirect haemagglutination, immunoblot (94% sensitive to chronic form and 70% sensitive to acute form), enzyme-linked immunosorbent assay (ELISA) and polymerase chain reaction (PCR) are new tests that are not generally available. PCR can detect *B. bacilliformis*-specific DNA from blood samples as well as skin biopsies. Antibodies are nonspecific due a cross-reaction with *B. henselae*, *B. quintana*, *Chlamydia psittaci*, and unknown antigens.

Laboratory features

Bartonella can be isolated from the blood during the anaemic stage and sometimes during the eruptive stage. The enriched media may be positive in 4 to 28 days at 28°C. As fever develops, intraerythrocytic bacteria are visible in thick and thin films stained with Giemsa's, Wright's, or other Romanovsky stains. Organisms can also be seen and cultivated in verrucous skin lesions. The anaemia may be very severe (haematocrit <10%). It is haemolytic but Coombs' test negative. The blood picture is of a macrocytic and hypochromic anaemia with polychromasia, anisocytosis, and poikilocytosis. Reticulocytosis is marked (average 11%). The marrow is hyperactive and megaloblastic with erythrophagocytosis. The white cell count is not markedly elevated unless there is a secondary infection. Thrombocytopenia is quite common. After the crisis, the intracellular organisms become coccoid and later disappear, the white cell count rises, and there is lymphocytosis. Eosinophils, which are usually absent during the acute stage, reappear in the peripheral blood.

Prognosis

Deaths usually occur during the anaemic phase. In the preantibiotic era, case fatality varied between 20 and 95%. At present, it varies between 1.1 and 2.4% in endemic areas and around 9% in patients admitted to hospital. During outbreaks, especially when the disease is not promptly recognized and treated, the case fatality can reach around 88%. Alterations of consciousness (excitement, stupor, and coma) and progressive or focal neurological features, biochemical evidence of hepatic dysfunction (increased transaminases and alkaline phosphatase), pulmonary complications (noncardiogenic pulmonary oedema), severe neurological involvement, anasarca (severe hypoalbuminaemia), pregnancy, and not being indigenous are all associated with a higher mortality.

Treatment

Chloramphenicol, penicillin, erythromycin, co-trimoxazole, and ciprofloxacin are effective, usually eliminating the fever in around 48 h. Because of the common association with salmonellosis, ciprofloxacin is the treatment of choice in a dose of 500 mg orally twice a day for 14 days. The alternative is amoxicillin plus clavulanic acid 1 g orally twice a day for 14 days, which is the treatment of choice in pregnant women and children under 14 years of age. In severe acute disease, the drugs indicated are ceftriaxone 2 g intravenously daily plus ciprofloxacin 400 mg intravenously twice a day for 14 days. Supportive treatment includes transfusion of packed red cells and empirical dexamethasone if there is severe neurological involvement. Azithromycin 500 mg orally once a day for 7 days is the drug of choice for the verrucous form. The dose in children is 10 mg/kg daily orally for 7 days. The alternative is rifampicin (300 mg twice a day in adults or 10 mg/kg daily in children orally for 21–28 days).

Prevention

There is no satisfactory prevention for people who live in endemic areas. Sandflies can be eliminated temporarily by spraying inside and outside with dichlorodiphenyltrichloroethane (DDT) or pyrethroids, and this strategy is recommended during outbreaks. Spraying insecticides inside the house and mass use of long-lasting insecticide-impregnated bed nets are measures that would probably reduce the rate of infection. Tourists can protect themselves with insect repellents, clothes impregnated with pyrethroids, and sleeping with nets impregnated with insecticides, or by avoiding sleeping in highly endemic areas.

Further reading

Birtles RJ, *et al.* (1999). Survey of *Bartonella* species infecting intradomicillary animals in the Huayllacallan valley, Ancash-Perú, a region endemic for human bartonellosis. *Am J Trop Med Hyg*, **60**, 799–805.

Maguiña C (1998). *Bartonellosis o Enfermedad de Carrión*. A.F.A. Editores Importadores S.A. Lima, Peru.

Maguiña C, Gotuzzo E (2000). Bartonellosis new and old. *Infect Dis Clin North Am*, **14**, 1–22.

Ministry of Health of Peru (2006). *Atención de la Bartonelosis o Enfermedad de Carrión en el Perú*. Norma técnica No. 048-MINSA/DGSP-C .01, pp. 10–61.

Walker DH, Maguiña C, Minnick M (2006). Bartonellosis. In: Guerrant RL, Walker DH, Weller PF (eds) *Tropical infectious diseases: principles, pathogens and practice*, pp. 454–62. Elsevier, Churchill Livingstone, Philadelphia.

7.6.44 Chlamydial infections

David Taylor-Robinson and David Mabey

Essentials

Chlamydiae are pathogenic bacteria that probably evolved from host-independent, Gram-negative ancestors and are specialized for an intracellular existence. The chlamydial infectious elementary body binds to and enters the host cell by 'parasite-specified' endocytosis, with a new generation of elementary bodies being released 30 to 48 h later.

There are nine species of genus *Chlamydia* (which some would reclassify based on ribosomal sequence data into two genera, *Chlamydia* and *Chlamydophila*), of which *C. trachomatis* and *C. pneumoniae* are primarily human pathogens, and *C. psittaci*, *C. abortus*, and *C. felis* are species transmitted occasionally from animals.

Trachoma

Caused by *C. trachomatis* serovars A, B, Ba, and C. A disease of poor rural communities, mainly in Africa and Asia, where the reservoir of infection is the eye (and possibly nasopharynx) of children with active disease, with transmission from the eye of one individual to that of another via fingers, fomites, coughing and sneezing, and by eye-seeking flies.

Clinical features and diagnosis—the active (inflammatory) stage is a follicular conjunctivitis with characteristic subconjunctival follicles that are usually seen in children in endemic areas. Repeated infections lead to conjunctival scarring, with turned-in lashes rubbing against the cornea (trichiasis) and eventually causing severe damage (3.6% of global blindness, or 1.3 million cases). In endemic areas diagnosis is made on clinical grounds.

Treatment and prevention—inflammatory trachoma responds to either an appropriate course of 1% topical tetracycline ointment or a single oral dose of azithromycin. Community-based mass treatment is recommended when there is high prevalence of disease in children aged 1 to 9 years. Trichiasis requires surgical correction. A World Health Organization initiative to eliminate blinding trachoma by 2020 is based on the acronym 'SAFE': Surgery for trichiasis; Antibiotics for treatment; Face washing; Environmental improvement to reduce fly populations that transmit the organisms.

Genital tract infections

These are caused by *C. trachomatis* serovars D to K, which exist worldwide. In men they cause up to 50% of symptomatic nongonococcal urethritis and of acute epididymitis. In women they cause up to 50% of (mostly asymptomatic) urethritis and of (often asymptomatic) cervicitis; further spread leads to endometritis, salpingitis and (occasionally) perihepatitis, and infertility follows a single upper genital tract infection in about 10% of women. See Chapter 8.5 for further discussion.

Other diseases caused by *C. trachomatis*

These include: (1) Adult paratrachoma and otitis media. (2) Reactive arthritis—at least one-third of sexually acquired reactive arthritis is initiated by genital *C. trachomatis* infection (see Chapter 19.8). (3) Neonatal infection—babies exposed to serovars D to K at birth often develop conjunctivitis, and some develop pneumonia. (4) Lymphogranuloma venereum—caused by *C. trachomatis* serovars L1, L2 or L3. Endemic in parts of Africa, Asia, South America, and the Caribbean; 2003 saw the start of an outbreak (serovar L2) across western Europe, the United Kingdom, North America, and Australia in homosexual men who were mainly HIV-positive. The clinical course comprises three stages: (a) primary—a small painless papule occurs at the site of inoculation; followed some weeks later by (b) secondary—inguinal and/or femoral lymphadenopathy with systemic features; anorectal involvement is usually seen in homosexual men; sometimes progressing to (c) tertiary—severe fibrosis, which is rarely seen because of earlier broad-spectrum antibiotic therapy. Diagnosis depends on serology or on identification of the organism in appropriate clinical samples. Treatment is usually with doxycycline or erythromycin.

Other chlamydiae

C. pneumoniae—transmitted directly from person to person by droplet spread and causes respiratory disease (pharyngitis, bronchitis, pneumonia), is a possible trigger for reactive arthritis and for some cases of juvenile chronic arthritis, and its DNA has been detected in atheromatous arteries, but without definite evidence that it contributes to heart disease. See Chapter 18.4.2 for further discussion.

C. psittaci—transmitted from psittacine birds and causes psittacosis, which can range from a mild influenza-like illness to a fulminating toxic state with multiorgan involvement.

C. abortus—causes abortion in sheep and may do so in pregnant women exposed to infected animals during the lambing season.

Diagnosis and treatment

Diagnosis—depends on (1) culture—chlamydiae can be grown in cultured cells, but this is slow, labour intensive, and less sensitive than molecular methods; (2) antigen detection—enzyme immunoassays are easy to use, but insensitive; (3) nucleic acid detection—the 'gold standard' for routine diagnosis, screening, and for research into chronic or persistent disease; and—to a much lesser extent—(4) serology.

Treatment—chlamydiae are particularly sensitive to tetracyclines (e.g. doxycycline) and macrolides (e.g. erythromycin, and with azithromycin gaining popularity because it can be effective as a single dose).

Introduction

Trachoma is recognizable in descriptions of blindness in ancient Chinese and Egyptian writings. It was not until 1907 that L. Halberstaedter and S. von Prowazek first described intracytoplasmic inclusions in conjunctival scrapings from patients with trachoma and recognized the involvement of an infectious agent. In 1930, a chlamydial agent (*Chlamydia psittaci*) was first isolated from psittacosis; 27 years later the genomically and biologically different agent associated with trachoma, *C. trachomatis*, was isolated in fertile hens' eggs. The advent of the cell-culture technique paved the way for the isolation of *C. trachomatis* by this means in 1965 and, together with immunological developments, made it possible to explore the nature, range, prevalence, and pathogenesis of clinical conditions associated with chlamydial infection. The complete sequencing of the chlamydial genome in 1998 aided this progress.

Classification

Chlamydiae are ubiquitous pathogens infecting many species of mammals and birds. The family Chlamydiaceae, in the order Chlamydiales, was formerly classified as four species belonging to a single genus, *Chlamydia*. These species comprised *C. trachomatis* causing human ocular and genital infections; *C. pneumoniae* causing mainly human respiratory disease, but with some strains infecting horses and koalas; *C. psittaci* infecting birds and other animals, with occasional transmission to humans; and *C. pecorum*, the cause of pneumonia, polyarthritis, encephalomyelitis, and diarrhoea in cattle and sheep.

In the 21st century, a taxonomic reclassification was based on ribosomal sequence data, and the members of the family Chlamydiaceae were divided between two genera, *Chlamydia* and *Chlamydophila*. However, this official taxonomy has not been fully implemented by researchers who favour a single genus *Chlamydia* now containing nine species: *C. trachomatis*, *C. pneumoniae*, *C. psittaci* (birds), *C. abortus* (sheep), *C. felis* (cats), *C. pecorum* (cattle), *C. suis* (pigs), *C. muridarum* (mice), and *C. caviae* (guinea pigs). The first two are primarily human pathogen; *C. psittaci*, *C. abortus*, and *C. felis* cause zoonotic infections which are transmitted occasionally to humans from infected animals. This classification is used here.

Growth cycle, serovars, and protein profile

Chlamydiae probably evolved from host-independent Gram-negative ancestors with peptidoglycan in their cell walls. They are bacteria specialized to exist intracellularly. The chlamydial envelope possesses bacteria-like inner and outer membranes. The infectious elementary body is electron dense, DNA rich, and approximately 300 nm in diameter. It binds to the host cell and enters by 'parasite-specified' endocytosis. Fusion of the chlamydia-containing endocytic vesicle with lysosomes is inhibited and the elementary body begins its unique developmental cycle within the eukaryotic cell. After about 10 h it differentiates into the larger (800–1000 nm) noninfectious, metabolically active, reticulate body. This divides by binary fission and by 20 h has begun to reorganize into a new generation of elementary bodies (Fig. 7.6.44.1). These reach maturity up to 30 h after entry into the cell and rapidly accumulate within the endocytic vacuole to be released from the cell between 30 and 48 h after the start of the cycle.

All species of *Chlamydia* contain a common heat-stable lipopolysaccharide antigen, which is exposed on the surface of the reticulate body but not on the elementary body. The major outer membrane protein (MOMP) is immunodominant in the elementary body and contains epitopes exhibiting genus, species, and serovar specificity. The serovar-specific epitope is the basis of the microimmunofluorescence (MIF) test by which *C. trachomatis* has been separated into 15 serovars: A, B, Ba, and C are responsible mainly for endemic trachoma; D to K for oculogenital infections; and L1, L2, and L3 for the genital disease lymphogranuloma venereum. Only one

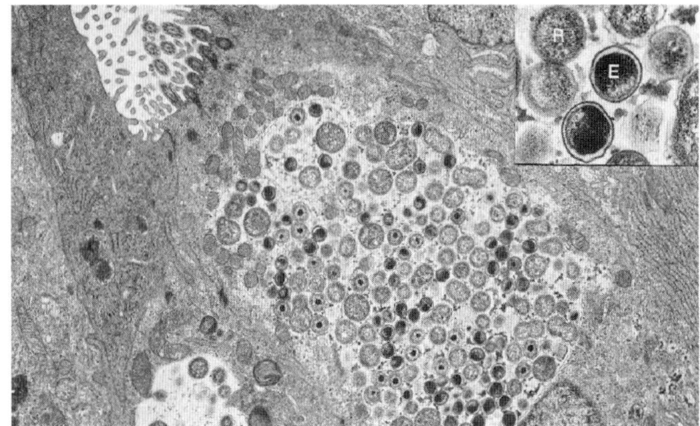

Fig. 7.6.44.1 Elementary bodies (E) and reticulate bodies (R) of *C. trachomatis*, forming an inclusion in an oviduct cell; shown by transmission electron microscopy.

C. pneumoniae serovar has been identified, although minor geographical serovar variations have been described. *C. psittaci* is loosely defined and likely to contain a wide variety of host-related serovars. Amino acid sequences of the MOMPs of all *C. trachomatis* serovars and epitope maps of different antigenic domains have been elucidated. The MOMP genes consist of five highly conserved regions punctuated by four short variable sequences. Serovar-specific epitopes have been demonstrated in variable sequence I and II, while species-specific epitopes have been found in variable sequence IV. It is also probable that these variable sequences influence chlamydial pathogenesis. *C. trachomatis*, *C. psittaci*, and *C. pneumoniae* species have been compared and although there is only 10% DNA homology between each of them, the MOMP genes show up to 65% amino acid homology, indicating a probable common ancestor. A common chlamydial 57-kDa protein has been described; its possible role in disease pathogenesis is considered below.

Trachoma

Trachoma is a chronic keratoconjunctivitis caused by the 'ocular' serovars A, B, Ba, and C of *C. trachomatis*. In the 19th century it was an important and common cause of blindness in Europe and North America, but it disappeared from more affluent parts of the world as living standards improved in the 20th century. In poor communities where hygiene standards are low, there is direct transfer of chlamydial organisms from eye to eye and trachoma is endemic. As standards of hygiene improve, this mode of transmission is no longer possible and trachoma tends to disappear. It is now a disease of poor rural communities, mainly in Africa and Asia, but it remains the leading infectious cause of blindness worldwide. A recent review by the World Health Organization (WHO) estimated that trachoma was responsible for 3.6% of global blindness, or 1.3 million cases.

Clinical features

The active (inflammatory) stage of trachoma is a follicular conjunctivitis, affecting chiefly the subtarsal conjunctiva, but follicles may be elsewhere on the conjunctiva and at the limbus. Such subconjunctival follicles are the characteristic sign of active disease (Fig. 7.6.44.2) and are usually seen in children in endemic areas. Limbal follicles resolve leaving characteristic shallow depressions known as Herbert's pits. New vessels (pannus) may be seen at this stage in the cornea (Fig. 7.6.44.3), usually at the superior margin, and punctate keratitis may also be a feature. Since symptoms are mild or absent, the disease may not be suspected unless the upper

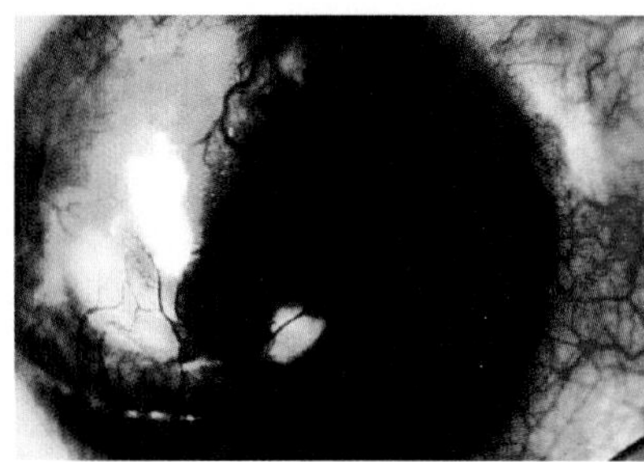

Fig. 7.6.44.3 Extensive neovascularization of the cornea (pannus) due to trachoma.

eyelid is everted. *C. trachomatis* can often be found in active cases, although follicles can persist for some time after infection has been cleared. Intense inflammation is seen in the subtarsal conjunctiva in some cases (Fig. 7.6.44.4) in which the *C. trachomatis* organism loads are higher. The disease may progress over many years and, with repeated infection, result in conjunctival scarring (Fig. 7.6.44.5). As the scars contract, the lid margin turns inwards (entropion), and the lashes rub against the cornea, a condition known as trichiasis (Fig. 7.6.44.6). This damages the cornea, eventually rendering it opaque.

The WHO criteria for the clinical diagnosis of active trachoma, its potentially blinding sequelae, and for grading their severity is as follows:

1. Trachomatous inflammation, follicular (TF)—five or more follicles, each at least 0.5 mm in diameter, in the upper tarsal conjunctiva (Fig. 7.6.44.2)
2. Trachomatous inflammation, intense (TI)—pronounced inflammatory thickening of the tarsal conjunctiva that obscures more than one-half of the normal deep tarsal blood vessels (Fig. 7.6.44.4)
3. Trachomatous conjunctival scarring (TS)—easily visible scarring in the tarsal conjunctiva (Fig. 7.6.44.5)
4. Trachomatous trichiasis (TT)—at least one eyelash rubbing on the eyeball, or evidence of recent removal of inturned eyelashes (Fig. 7.6.44.6)
5. Corneal opacity (CO)—easily visible corneal opacity over the pupil, so dense that at least part of the pupil margin is blurred when viewed through the opacity

Epidemiology

Trachoma is a disease of poverty, which disappears as living standards improve. In the past, it has been endemic in urban communities such as in the East End of London, but it is now a disease of rural

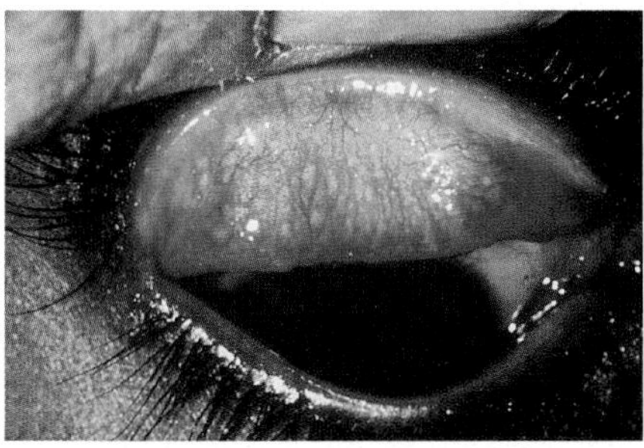

Fig. 7.6.44.2 Everted upper eyelid showing follicular trachoma (TF).

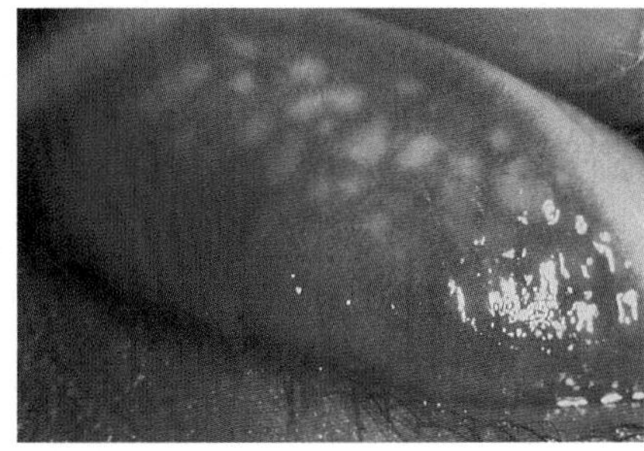

Fig. 7.6.44.4 Everted upper eyelid showing intense inflammatory trachoma (TI).

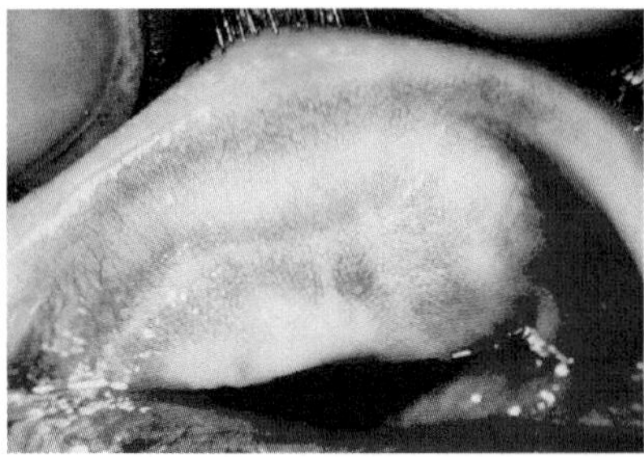

Fig. 7.6.44.5 Everted upper eyelid showing trachomatous scarring (TS).

communities that lack access to water and sanitation, especially affecting marginalized groups. The reservoir of infection in endemic areas is the eye, and possibly the nasopharynx, of children with active disease. *C. trachomatis* may be transferred from the eye of one individual to that of another via fingers, fomites, coughing, and sneezing, and by eye-seeking flies. Active cases tend to cluster in households with prolonged intimate contact within the family. The higher prevalence of active disease and scarring in women than in men is probably due to their closer contact with children. Severe conjunctival scarring is associated with repeated exposure to reinfection.

Diagnosis

In trachoma-endemic areas, the diagnosis is made on clinical grounds, following the simplified WHO grading scheme (Figs. 7.6.44.2, 7.6.44.4–7.6.44.6). Trachomatous follicles (TF) may be confused with the giant papillae of vernal conjunctivitis, in which pannus may also be seen. Several viruses, notably adenoviruses, can cause a short-lived follicular conjunctivitis. Intense cases of trachoma (TI), in which follicles may not be visible, should be distinguished from bacterial conjunctivitis. The diagnosis of trachomatous scarring (TS) is usually obvious, as few other conditions cause conjunctival scarring of the upper lid. Laboratory diagnosis of ocular *C. trachomatis* infection may help to direct treatment to communities with the greatest need, since clinical signs may persist for years after infection has been cleared. *C. trachomatis* may be found in about one-half of the cases of active inflammation (TF or TI), but in only a minority of those with scarring disease (TS). A portable dipstick test for chlamydial antigen detection has given promising results in trachoma endemic regions in Africa. Other diagnostic methods are discussed below.

Treatment

Inflammatory trachoma (TF and TI) responds to antimicrobial treatment (Table 7.6.44.1). The WHO recommends either 1% topical tetracycline ointment, to be applied to both eyes daily for 6 weeks, or a single oral dose of azithromycin (20 mg/kg, to a maximum of 1 g). Community-based mass treatment is recommended when the prevalence of TF exceeds 10% in children aged 1 to 9 years. Reinfection is rapid if individual cases are treated separately. Trichiasis requires surgical correction. Several eyelid operations have been described, but few have been evaluated prospectively. Bilamellar tarsal rotation is probably the operation of choice.

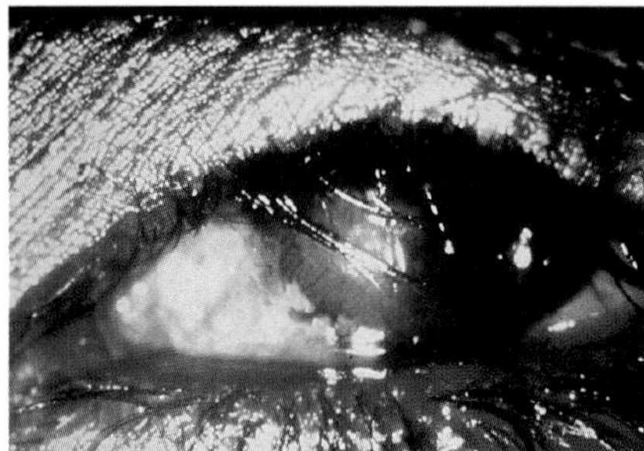

Fig. 7.6.44.6 Trachomatous trichiasis (TT).

Prevention

The WHO has launched a strategy for the global elimination of blinding trachoma by the year 2020, based on the acronym 'SAFE': Surgery for trichiasis, Antibiotics for the treatment of inflammatory disease and the elimination of the reservoir of infection, promotion of Face washing, and Environmental improvement to reduce fly populations. These procedures are likely to reduce the rate of transmission of ocular *C. trachomatis* infection.

Genital tract infections

Genital tract infections due to *C. trachomatis* serovars D to K (Table 7.6.44.2) occur worldwide. The highest prevalence is in women of 15 to 24 years of age and in men of 20 to 24 years of age. In developed countries, they are much more common than gonococcal infections. Their frequency imposes an enormous economic burden on health services. It is estimated that 2.8 million new cases of genital chlamydial infection occurred in the United States of America in the year 2000. In Sweden, widespread and effective diagnostic testing, coupled with aggressive contact tracing and treatment, reduced genital chlamydial infections in the decade from 1984, but subsequently there has been a slow increase. Screening programmes in some other developed countries, including the United Kingdom, have gradually been developed and implemented, but the reported chlamydial incidence has increased in most countries in Western Europe and North America since the mid 1990s. The extent to which this increase is due to more widespread testing using more sensitive assays is not clear.

Nongonococcal urethritis

The incubation period is 7 to 14 days compared to 2 to 5 days for gonococcal disease. *C. trachomatis* is detectable in the urethra of up to 50% of men with symptomatic nongonococcal urethritis and as many as 7% of those who are asymptomatic. It is also likely that chlamydiae are a cause of some cases of chronic (persistent/recurrent) nongonococcal urethritis. Treatment of gonococcal urethritis with an antibiotic ineffective against *C. trachomatis* may result in postgonococcal urethritis, which usually appears about 1 week after the treatment of gonococcal disease. *C. trachomatis* is responsible for 80 to 90% of cases.

In women, chlamydial urethral infection may cause urethritis but, in contrast to men, infection and inflammation are almost always asymptomatic. The 'urethral syndrome' (dysuria and frequency with $<10^5$ organisms/ml urine) is rarely of chlamydial origin.

Prostatitis and epididymitis

There is no evidence that *C. trachomatis* causes acute symptomatic prostatitis. Transperineal biopsies from patients with chronic abacterial prostatitis show chronic inflammation, but chlamydiae have not been detected by culture or direct immunofluorescence

Table 7.6.44.1 Recommended treatment schedules for chlamydial infections and associated diseases

Disease/infection	Antibiotic	Dose schedule[a]	Duration (days)
Trachoma	Topical tetracycline	1% ointment daily	42
	Azithromycin alone	20 mg/kg (up to 1 g)	Single dose
Adult inclusion conjunctivitis	Tetracycline HCl	500 mg 4 times daily	14
	Or doxycycline	100 mg twice daily	14
	Or erythromycin stearate	500 mg 4 times daily	14
	Or azithromycin	1 g	Single dose
NGU	Antibiotics and regimens as for treatment of adult inclusion conjunctivitis		7
Epididymo-orchitis	Ceftriaxone	250 mg	Single dose
	Then antibiotics as for NGU		10
Cervicitis/urethritis	Antibiotics and regimens as for NGU		7
Pelvic inflammatory disease (ambulatory patients)	Ceftriaxone	250 mg intramuscularly	
	Then doxycycline	100 mg twice daily	14
Pelvic inflammatory disease (patients admitted to hospital)	(a) Doxycycline	100 mg twice daily intravenously	≥4
	And cefoxitin	2 g three times daily intravenously	≥4
	Then doxycycline	100 mg twice daily	14
	And metronidazole	400 mg twice daily	14
	Or (b) clindamycin	600 mg 4 times daily intravenously	≥4
	And then Clindamycin	450 mg 4 times daily	10[b]
	And gentamicin	2 mg/kg intravenously	Single dose
	And then gentamicin	1.5 mg/kg 3 times daily	≥4
Neonatal infections	Erythromycin syrup	50 mg/kg daily in 4 divided doses	14
Lymphogranuloma venereum	Antibiotics and regimens as for NGU[c]		21
C. pneumoniae infections	Antibiotics and regimens as for NGU except doxycycline twice daily		7–21[d]
C. psittaci infections	Antibiotics and regimes as for NGU except doxycycline twice daily		≥14

NGU, nongonococcal urethritis
[a] All antibiotics orally unless otherwise indicated.
[b] Total duration of therapy 14 days.
[c] Azithromycin likely to be effective but multiple doses probably required.
[d] Relapse more often with short course.

techniques, although polymerase chain reaction (PCR) tests are positive in about 10%. Such largely negative observations, and the failure to detect chlamydial antibody, suggest that *C. trachomatis* is not often implicated directly in the chronic disease. However, the predominance of CD8 cells in the tissues suggests that some cases of chronic disease might be of chlamydial origin.

C. trachomatis is responsible for up to 50% of cases of acute epididymitis or epididymo-orchitis occurring primarily in young men (≤35 years of age) in developed countries, and has been detected in at least one-third of epididymal aspirates. There is a strong correlation between IgM and IgG chlamydial antibodies, measured by MIF, and chlamydia-positive disease. In developing countries, although chlamydiae are important, *Neisseria gonorrhoeae* is the major cause of acute epididymitis. In patients older than 35 years, epididymitis/epididymo-orchitis tends to be caused by urinary tract pathogens.

There is no good evidence that chlamydial epididymitis or chlamydial urethral infection leads to male infertility.

Bartholinitis, vaginitis, and cervicitis

C. trachomatis has been weakly associated with bartholinitis and should be considered in the absence of other known pathogens. Chlamydiae are often detected more frequently in women with bacterial vaginosis than in those without, but there is no evidence that they contribute to the disease. In prepubertal children, the vaginal epithelium is columnar and susceptible to chlamydial infection. In adults, the squamous epithelium of the vagina is not susceptible and the cervix is the primary target for *C. trachomatis*, where it is an established cause of mucopurulent/follicular cervicitis (Fig. 7.6.44.7) which is often asymptomatic. Women younger than 25 years, unmarried, using oral contraceptives, and who have signs of cervicitis are the most likely to have a chlamydial infection.

Table 7.6.44.2 Assessment of the extent to which *C. trachomatis* is involved in various oculogenital and associated diseases

Disease	Evidence that C. trachomatis is a cause[a]	Proportion of disease due to C. trachomatis
In men		
Acute NGU	++++	Up to 50%
Postgonococcal urethritis	++++	Up to 90%
Persistent and recurrent NGU	++	?
Acute and chronic prostatitis	+	?
Acute epididymo-orchitis	++++	Up to 50%
Infertility	–	
In women		
Urethritis	+++	?
Bartholinitis	+	?
Vaginitis (prepuberty only)	+++	?
Bacterial vaginosis	–	
Cervicitis	++++	About 50%
Cervical dysplasia	+	
Endometritis	+++	?
Salpingitis	++++	? 40–60%
Periappendicitis	++	?
Perihepatitis	+++	?
Infertility	+++	≥10% due to chlamydial salpingitis
Ectopic pregnancy	+++	?
Early miscarriage	+	?
Abortion	–	
In men or women		
Conjunctivitis	++++	?
Otitis media	++	?
Arthritis (Reiter's syndrome)	+++	About 40%
Endocarditis	++	?
Pharyngitis	–	
Proctitis	+++	?
Lymphogranuloma venereum	++++	100% (by definition)
In infants		
Conjunctivitis	++++	Up to 50%
Pneumonia	++++	30%?
Chronic lung disease	++	?
Gastroenteritis	–	

NGU, nongonococcal urethritis.
[a]++++, overwhelming; +++, good; ++, moderate; +, weak; –, none.

(a) 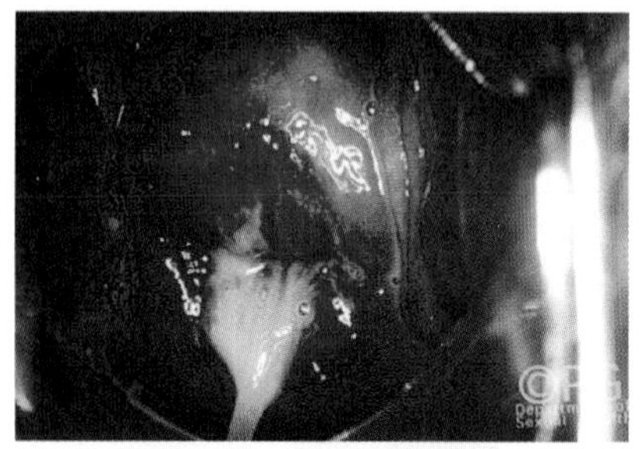

(b) 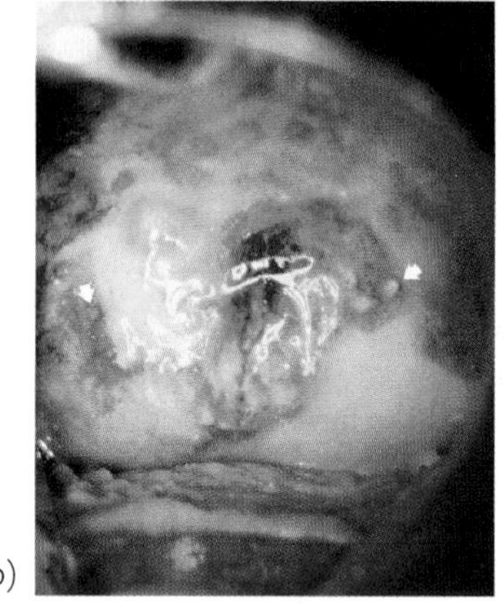

Fig. 7.6.44.7 (a) Mucopurulent cervicitis; (b) follicular cervicitis.

A significant association between cervical chlamydial infection and cervical squamous cell carcinoma, but not adenocarcinoma, has been established and it has been suggested that chlamydial infection may enhance the effect of oncogenic papillomaviruses.

Pelvic inflammatory disease

Canalicular spread of chlamydiae to the upper genital tract leads to endometritis, which is often plasma cell associated and sometimes intensely lymphoid. Further spread causes salpingitis (Fig. 7.6.44.8), seen in about 10% of women with cervical infection. Classic signs often ensue but inflammation may be subclinical. Spread to the peritoneum results in perihepatitis (the Fitz-Hugh–Curtis syndrome) (Fig. 7.6.44.9), sometimes confused with acute cholecystitis in young women, in addition to periappendicitis and other abdominal symptoms. Surgical termination of pregnancy or insertion or removal of an intrauterine contraceptive device may predispose to dissemination of infection.

Chlamydial infection is the major cause of pelvic inflammatory disease in developed countries. Infertility may be the first indication of asymptomatic tubal disease. It occurs in about 10% of

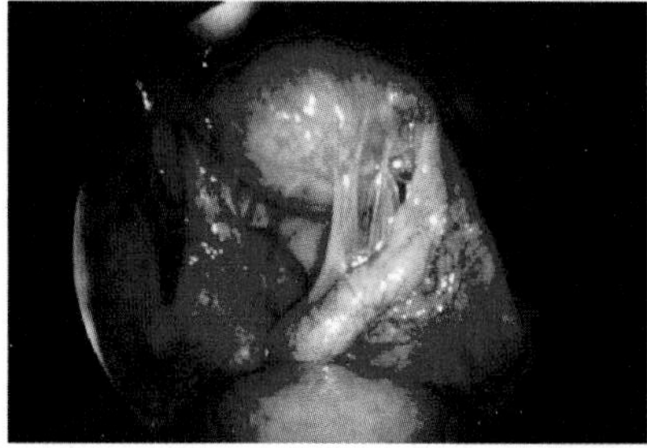

Fig. 7.6.44.8 Laparoscopic view of inflamed fallopian tube due to *C. trachomatis*. (Courtesy of P Greenhouse.)

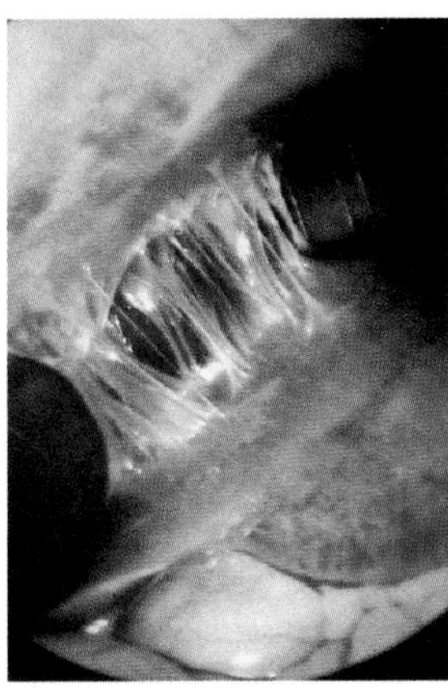

Fig. 7.6.44.9 Adhesions in perihepatitis (Fitz-Hugh–Curtis syndrome). (Courtesy of P Greenhouse.)

women following a single upper genital tract infection and in possibly one-half of those after two or three episodes. Infertility could result possibly from endometritis, and certainly from blocked or damaged tubes, or perhaps abnormalities of ovum transportation. Other consequences of salpingitis are chronic pelvic pain and ectopic pregnancy. Following chlamydial pelvic inflammatory disease, the risk of ectopic pregnancy increases seven- to tenfold.

There is conflicting evidence on the effect of *C. trachomatis* on pregnancy. However, a serological association has been demonstrated between *C. trachomatis* and early miscarriage (before 12 weeks of pregnancy) and recurrent miscarriage, but not late miscarriage (after 12 weeks) or stillbirth (after 24 weeks).

Other diseases associated with *C. trachomatis*

Adult paratrachoma (inclusion conjunctivitis) and otitis media

Adult chlamydial ophthalmia is distinguished from trachoma by its causative *C. trachomatis* serovars D to K. It commonly results from the accidental transfer of infected genital discharge to the eye. In contrast to 'reactive' conjunctivitis seen in Reiter's syndrome (see below), chlamydiae can usually be detected in conjunctival specimens. It usually presents as a unilateral follicular conjunctivitis, acute or subacute in onset, with an incubation period of up to 21 days. The features are swollen lids, mucopurulent discharge, papillary hyperplasia, and, later, follicular hypertrophy and occasionally punctate keratitis. About one-third of patients have otitis media and complain of blocked ears and hearing loss. The disease is generally benign and self-limited. Pannus formation and corneal scarring are rare and not seen if systemic treatment is given. Patients and their sexual contacts should be investigated for genital chlamydial infection and managed appropriately.

Arthritis

Arthritis occurring with or soon after nongonococcal urethritis is termed 'sexually acquired reactive arthritis' (SARA). Conjunctivitis and other features characteristic of Reiter's syndrome are seen in about one-third of patients. Evidence of chlamydial infection, by a specific serological response or by the presence of *C. trachomatis* elementary bodies or DNA and antigen in the joints, is found in at least one-third of patients. *C. trachomatis* has also been associated in the same way with 'seronegative' arthritis in women. Viable chlamydiae have not been detected in the joints of patients with SARA which is probably the result of immunopathology (see below). Despite this, early tetracycline therapy has been advocated by some investigators.

Immunocompromised patients

C. trachomatis has been isolated from the lower respiratory tract of a few immunocompromised adults with pneumonia, some after renal transplantation, but other pathogens are often also present. *C. pneumoniae* is not an especially important respiratory tract pathogen in AIDS patients. Genital *C. trachomatis* infection is likely to increase viral shedding from HIV-positive people, and enhance the susceptibility to HIV in the uninfected. Conversely, HIV infection increases the susceptibility of women to *C. trachomatis* genital infection. In contrast, hypogammaglobulinaemic patients do not appear to be especially prone to infection with any of the chlamydial species.

Neonatal infections

Although intrauterine chlamydial infection can occur, the major risk of infection to the infant is from passing through an infected cervix. The proportion of neonates exposed to infection depends, of course, on the prevalence of maternal cervical infection, which varies widely. Conjunctivitis appears in 20 to 50% of infants exposed to *C. trachomatis* (serovars D–K) infecting the cervix at birth. A mucopurulent discharge (Fig. 7.6.44.10) and occasionally pseudomembrane formation occur 1 to 3 weeks later. It usually resolves without visual impairment. Complications tend to be in untreated infants.

Approximately one-half of the infants who have conjunctivitis also develop pneumonia, although a history of recent conjunctivitis and bulging eardrums are found in only one-half of the infants. Chlamydial pneumonia usually begins between the 4th and 11th week of life, preceded by upper respiratory symptoms. There is tachypnoea, a prominent staccato cough, but no fever, and the illness is protracted. Radiographs show hyperinflation of the lungs with bilateral diffuse symmetrical interstitial infiltration and scattered areas of atelectasis. Finding serum IgM antibody to *C. trachomatis* in infants with pneumonia is pathognomonic. Children infected during infancy are more likely to develop obstructive lung disease and asthma than are those who have had pneumonia of other causes.

The vagina and rectum also may be colonized by *C. trachomatis* at birth, but this has not been associated with clinical disease. Rectal shedding might occur 2 to 3 months after birth, suggesting colonization of the gastrointestinal tract, but there is no evidence of infant chlamydial gastroenteritis.

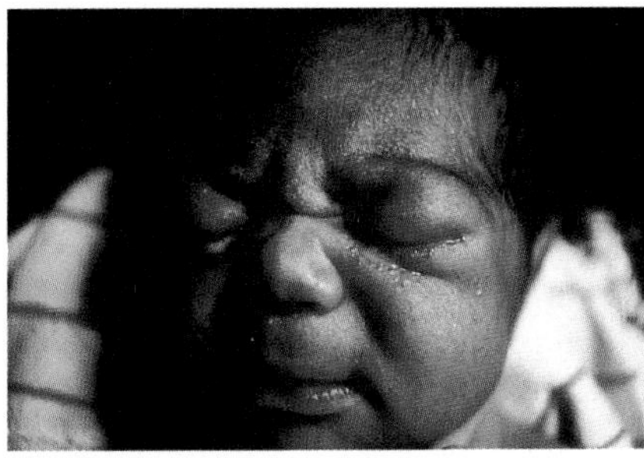

Fig. 7.6.44.10 Mucopurulent neonatal conjunctival discharge due to *C. trachomatis*.

Lymphogranuloma venereum

Lymphogranuloma venereum (LGV) is a systemic, sexually transmitted disease caused by serovars L1, L2, and L3 of *C. trachomatis*. These are more virulent in animal models than serovars A to K, and more invasive in humans. Serovars A to K are largely confined to mucosal columnar epithelial surfaces of the genital tract and eye, but the LGV serovars predominantly infect monocytes and macrophages, which pass through the epithelial surface to regional lymph nodes and may cause disseminated infection.

Clinical features

The clinical course of LGV can be divided into three stages. The primary stage at the site of inoculation, the secondary stage in the regional lymph nodes and/or the anorectum, and the tertiary stage of late sequelae affecting the genitalia and/or rectum.

After an incubation period of 3 to 30 days, the primary stage begins with a small, painless papule which may ulcerate. It occurs at the site of inoculation, usually the prepuce or glans in men; anorectal and rectosigmoid colon sites in homosexual men; or the vulva, vaginal wall, or occasionally the cervix in women. Extragenital primary lesions on fingers or tongue are rare. The primary lesion is self-healing and may pass unnoticed by the patient, especially if it is in the alimentary tract of homosexual men. Among patients with LGV presenting with buboes in Thailand, more than one-half had not been aware of an ulcer.

The secondary stage occurs some weeks after the primary lesion, which has usually healed. Chlamydiae are carried to regional or rectal lymph nodes. The inguinal form is more common in men than women, since the lymphatic drainage of the upper vagina and cervix is to the retroperitoneal rather than the inguinal lymph nodes. LGV proctitis occurs in those who practise receptive anal intercourse, probably due to direct inoculation.

The cardinal feature of the inguinal form of LGV is painful, usually unilateral, inguinal and/or femoral lymphadenopathy (bubo). Adenopathy above and below the inguinal ligament gives rise to the 'groove sign' in 10 to 20% of patients, once believed to be pathognomonic. Enlarged lymph nodes are usually firm and often accompanied by systemic signs of fever, chills, arthralgia, and headache. Biopsy reveals small discrete areas of necrosis surrounded by proliferating epithelioid and endothelial cells. These areas of necrosis may enlarge to form stellate abscesses, which may coalesce and break down to form discharging sinuses, although this phenomenon occurs in less than one-third of patients with inguinal disease. In women, signs include a hypertrophic suppurative cervicitis, backache, and adnexal tenderness. Anorectal involvement is seen predominantly in homosexual men. Clinical features include a purulent anal discharge, anorectal pain and bleeding due to an acute haemorrhagic proctitis or proctocolitis, and there may be pronounced systemic signs of fever, chills, and weight loss. Asymptomatic LGV is rare, according to a large study in the United Kingdom using molecular typing of chlamydial isolates. Early detection of LGV at a 'presymptomatic' stage of disease might be found among people who are regularly screened for rectal *C. trachomatis*. Proctoscopy reveals a granular or ulcerative proctitis from which large numbers of polymorphonuclear leucocytes are seen in rectal smears. CT or MRI scans may show pronounced thickening of the rectal wall, with enlargement of iliac lymph nodes. Enlarged inguinal nodes may also be palpable.

Extragenital infection can cause lymphadenopathy outside the inguinal region. For example, cervical adenopathy due to LGV has been reported after oral sex, and laboratory workers who developed pneumonitis after accidental inhalation of LGV strains of *C. trachomatis* were found to have mediastinal and supraclavicular adenopathy. A follicular conjunctivitis has also been described following direct inoculation of the eye, which may be accompanied by preauricular lymphadenopathy. Other rare manifestations of the secondary stage include acute meningoencephalitis, synovitis, and cardiac involvement.

The tertiary stage appears after a latent period of several years, but all late complications are rare today because of the use of broad-spectrum antibiotics. Chronic untreated LGV leads to fibrosis, which may cause lymphatic obstruction and elephantiasis of the genitalia in either sex, or rectal strictures and fistulae. Rarely, it can give rise to the syndrome of esthiomene (Greek: 'eating away'), with widespread destruction of the external genitalia (Fig. 7.6.44.11).

Epidemiology

LGV is a rare disease in industrialized countries, but is endemic in parts of Africa, Asia, South America, and the Caribbean. The reported sex ratio is greater than 5:1 in favour of men, probably because of the easier recognition of disease. The epidemiology of infection is poorly defined because LGV is often indistinguishable clinically from chancroid and other causes of genital ulceration with bubo formation, and it has been difficult to obtain laboratory confirmation. LGV is an uncommon cause of genital ulceration in Africa. Ten per cent of patients with buboes presenting to a sexually transmitted disease clinic in Bangkok were found to have LGV, and an epidemic of LGV has been found among crack cocaine users in the Bahamas. In 2003, an outbreak of LGV proctitis due to the L2 serovar was reported among homosexual men in the Netherlands, and in the subsequent 3 years over 1000 cases were reported in homosexual men across Western Europe, the United Kingdom, North America, and Australia. The majority of affected men have been HIV positive.

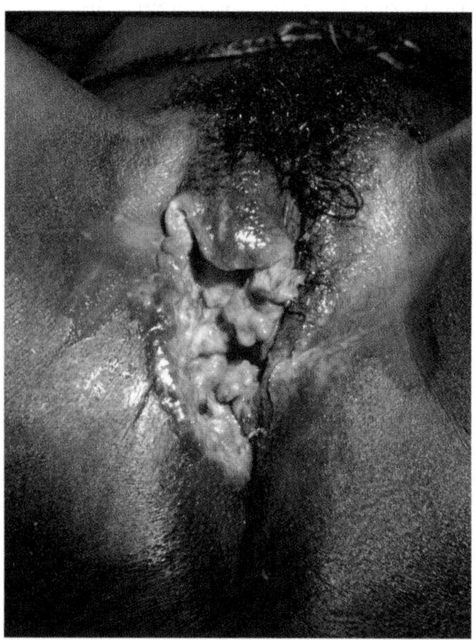

Fig. 7.6.44.11 Esthiomene: destruction of the female genitalia by lymphogranuloma venereum in a Nigerian patient.
(Copyright D A Warrell.)

Diagnosis

LGV may present as a genital ulcer or as inguinal lymphadenopathy (usually painful) without evidence of genital ulceration. The differential diagnosis of sexually acquired genital ulceration also includes chancroid, herpes, syphilis, and donovanosis (granuloma inguinale). Less common causes include trauma, nonvenereal infections such as cutaneous leishmaniasis or amoebiasis, and fixed drug eruption. The differential diagnosis of inguinal adenopathy includes chancroid, herpes, and syphilis, although there is usually a genital ulcer or at least a history of an ulcer in these conditions. Chronic sinus formation in the inguinal region may be due to tuberculosis of the lumbar spine, and bubonic plague should be considered in endemic areas where a patient with inguinal lymphadenopathy is acutely ill. LGV proctitis needs to be distinguished from inflammatory bowel disease due to ulcerative colitis or Crohn's disease, although clinical and histopathological features may be identical.

The laboratory diagnosis of LGV depends on serology or on identification of *C. trachomatis* in appropriate clinical samples. Because it is more invasive, LGV infection induces higher serum antibody titres than do uncomplicated genital infections with *C. trachomatis* serovars D to K. The MIF test can distinguish between infections with different chlamydial species. A MIF titre exceeding 1:128 strongly suggests LGV, particularly in a patient with typical signs and symptoms, although invasive genital infection with *C. trachomatis* serovars D to K, as in pelvic inflammatory disease, can also give rise to high antibody titres.

C. trachomatis can be identified in a smear of bubo material by direct fluorescence microscopy (Table 7.6.44.3) using commercially available conjugated monoclonal antibody, although bacterial contamination impedes detection. *C. trachomatis* can be isolated in cell culture from ulcer material, bubo aspirate, or endourethral or endocervical scrapings, but the success rate is poor. Commercially available nucleic acid amplification methods are much more sensitive and the diagnosis of LGV can be confirmed by amplification and restriction fragment length polymorphism (RFLP) typing or sequencing of the outer membrane protein 1 (*omp1*) gene.

Treatment

There has been no adequately powered study comparing antibiotic regimens for LGV. Recommended treatment for both bubonic and anogenital LGV is doxycycline 100 mg twice daily or erythromycin 500 mg four times daily for 21 days. Azithromycin has been used successfully in some cases, although a 1-g single oral dose is unlikely to be sufficient and the optimal regimen is unknown. Fever and bubo pain subside rapidly after antibiotic treatment is started, but buboes may take several weeks to resolve. Large collections of pus should be aspirated, using a lateral approach through normal skin. Rectovaginal fistulas, rectal strictures, and esthiomene require surgical correction with antibiotic cover.

C. pneumoniae infections

The prototype strains of *C. pneumoniae* were isolated in the 1960s from conjunctival samples collected from a child in Taiwan (strain TW-183) and another in Iran (strain IOL-207). In 1983, a third *C. pneumoniae* strain was isolated, this time from the throat of a patient with acute respiratory (AR) disease, i.e. pharyngitis (strain AR-39). This prompted the name TWAR (TW+AR) being coined for the isolates. The two original isolates (TW-183 and IOL-207) were serologically identical and distinct from *C. trachomatis* and *C. psittaci*. In 1989, *C. pneumoniae* was defined as the third species of the genus *Chlamydia*. Only one serovar of *C. pneumoniae* has been identified, although minor geographical serovar variations are described.

Clinical features

Respiratory tract disease

After an incubation period of approximately 3 weeks, acute disease often begins with pharyngitis. More than 80% of patients with lower respiratory tract disease have a sore throat. A cough may develop later and fever is uncommon. Bronchitis sometimes appears and in young adults about 5% of primary sinusitis is associated with *C. pneumoniae*. Mild respiratory infections are probably frequent but pneumonia is most common. Radiographs usually

Table 7.6.44.3 Advantages and disadvantages of chlamydial detection procedures

Factor considered	Culture	Direct fluorescent antibody	Enzyme immunoassay[a]	Nucleic acid amplification
Speed/temperature for transport of specimen	Rapid or at low temperature	Unimportant if specimen fixed	Unimportant if specimen in buffer	Speed not crucial if at low temperature; may use fixed specimens
Storage requirements	4°C if overnight; liquid nitrogen if long term	4°C if short term; −20°C and fixed if long term	4°C if 3–5 days; freezing if longer	4°C if short term; −70°C if long term
Evaluation of adequacy of specimen	Not practical	Evaluate during test	Not practical	Determine whether DNA present
Special equipment or procedure	Centrifuge	Fluorescence microscope	ELISA reader	Thermocycling machine and electrophoresis equipment
Processing of specimen	Tedious	Simple	Relatively simple	Requires precautions against DNA contamination
Reading of test	Subjective and moderately tedious	Subjective and tedious	Objective and simple	Objective and simple
Duration of test	48–72 h	30 min	3 h	12–24 h
Sensitivity of test	<70%	70–100%	<50–70%	Up to 100%

ELISA, enzyme linked immunosorbent assay.
[a] Now rarely used.

reveal a unilateral pneumonia, but more severe infection causes bilateral signs. This is often difficult to distinguish clinically from *Mycoplasma pneumoniae* and other pneumonias. Up to one-fifth of exacerbations of chronic obstructive pulmonary disease (COPD) are associated with *C. pneumoniae* and it has been implicated in exacerbations of both adult and childhood asthma.

Arthritis

An exaggerated synovial lymphocyte response to *C. pneumoniae* has been found in some adults with reactive arthritis and *C. pneumoniae* DNA and high titres of specific antibody have been detected in synovial fluid from the joints of a few children with juvenile chronic arthritis, suggesting the possibility of a causal role.

Atherosclerosis

Finnish investigators in the 1980s observed an association between chronic coronary heart disease or acute myocardial infarction and antibody to *C. pneumoniae*. The idea of chronic infection was enhanced by the detection of chlamydiae or their DNA in at least 40% of atheromatous plaques in coronaries and other major arteries, but not normal tissue, of people as young as 15 years of age. Specific DNA was also found in peripheral blood mononuclear cells, suggesting that they transmit the organisms from the respiratory tract to the arterial wall. Euphoria about these findings has been dealt a blow by the results of three major antibiotic trials in the United States of America. Subjects who received long courses of azithromycin in two trials and gatifloxacin in the other, subsequently experienced untoward coronary events as often as those given a placebo. This outcome was not completely unexpected in patients with well-established, long-standing disease.

Other diseases

C. pneumoniae has been linked to Alzheimer's disease, stroke, and multiple sclerosis, as well as chronic secretory otitis media, cystic fibrosis, sarcoidosis, and primary biliary cirrhosis, but there is no evidence to suggest a causal association.

Epidemiology

C. pneumoniae genotypes have been detected in horses, koalas, bandicoots, amphibians, and reptiles but there is no evidence of transfer to humans. It is thought that human strains are transmitted directly from person to person. Serological evidence indicates that *C. pneumoniae* is widespread and endemic in many areas, although localized respiratory epidemics have been recorded in both military and civilian groups in Scandinavia, the United States of America, the United Kingdom, and elsewhere. *C. pneumoniae* probably causes many mild respiratory infections that were previously thought to be viral in origin and it is also likely that many infections labelled 'human psittacosis' or 'ornithosis' in the past were due to *C. pneumoniae*.

C. psittaci infections

The *C. psittaci* species forms a diverse group isolated from a variety of mammals, reptiles, and many avian species. There is a relatively low degree of homology between serovars exhibited in DNA–DNA hybridization analyses, with the possibility of further differentiation between organisms assigned to the species. The spectrum of animal diseases caused by *C. psittaci* and other chlamydiae includes conjunctivitis, pneumonia, enteritis, abortion, sterility, arthritis, and encephalitis, all of which result in economic loss. The organisms are occasionally transmitted to humans. Psittacosis is an avian and human infection by *C. psittaci* found in psittacine birds, and ornithosis is infection by strains from other birds. 'Psittacosis' is now often used indiscriminately when referring to infection from psittacine and nonpsittacine birds. It is a potential hazard to those who keep pet birds and those who work in poultry processing plants or in animal husbandry.

Clinical features

After an incubation period of 1 to 2 weeks, the presentation of psittacosis varies from a mild influenza-like illness to a fulminating toxic state with multiple organ involvement. The disease may begin insidiously over a few days, or start abruptly with high fever, rigors, and anorexia. A headache is common, a cough, often dry, occurs in over two-thirds of patients, and arthralgia and myalgia in over one-third of patients. Inspiratory crepitations are more usual than classic signs of consolidation. Chest radiographs show patchy shadowing, often in the lower lobes. Homogeneous lobar shadowing is less frequent, miliary and nodular patterns even less so, and significant pleural effusions are rare. Extrapulmonary complications, mostly rare, include endocarditis, myocarditis, pericarditis, a toxic confusional state, encephalitis, meningitis, tender hepatomegaly, splenomegaly, pancreatitis, haemolysis, and disseminated intravascular coagulation. Improved diagnostic tests should not allow *C. psittaci* infections to be confused with those caused by *C. pneumoniae*.

Other chlamydial infections

C. abortus is endemic among ruminants and colonizes the placenta, causing abortion in sheep and rarely in pregnant women. They are often farmers' wives exposed to sheep with enzootic abortion during the lambing season. *C. felis* is endemic among domestic cats worldwide causing feline keratoconjunctivitis, rhinitis, and pneumonitis, and it can be isolated from the genital tract of female cats. In humans it has caused follicular conjunctivitis similar to that caused by *C. trachomatis* serovars D to K.

Laboratory diagnosis of chlamydial infections

The laboratory identification of chlamydial infection depends on culture, antigen, or nucleic acid detection, and to a much lesser extent on serology. The advantages and disadvantages of the tests are summarized in Table 7.6.44.3. Certain swabs, e.g. those with cotton tips, are superior to others, and swabs provided in commercial enzyme immunoassay kits may be toxic if used for collecting specimens for culture. Examination of two or more consecutive swabs from patients improves the chlamydial detection rate, which may be achieved by pooling cervical and urethral specimens. 'First-catch' urine specimens are unsuitable for chlamydial culture, but the centrifuged deposits are unquestionably valuable samples from both men and women, if tested by molecular methods. This also applies to the use of meatal samples in men and of vulva/vaginal samples.

Culture and staining of chlamydiae

The growth of chlamydiae more than 40 years ago in cultured cells, rather than in embryonated eggs, revolutionized their detection and chlamydial research. *C. pneumoniae* is particularly difficult to isolate, but will grow in selected cell lines including Hep-2. The isolation *C. trachomatis* involves centrifugation of specimens onto cycloheximide-treated McCoy cell monolayers, followed by incubation and then staining with a fluorescent monoclonal antibody or with a vital dye, usually Giemsa's, to detect inclusions. One blind passage may increase sensitivity but cell-culture techniques are slow, labour intensive, and no more than 70% sensitive compared to molecular methods.

Staining of epithelial cells in ocular and genital smears with vital dyes to detect chlamydial inclusions is insensitive and often nonspecific. In contrast, detection of elementary bodies using species-specific fluorescent monoclonal antibodies is rapid, highly sensitive, and specific for *C. trachomatis* oculogenital infections, in the hands of skilled observers. This test is most suitable for dealing with a few specimens and for confirming positive results obtained with other tests.

Enzyme immunoassays and nucleic acid amplification techniques

Enzyme immunoassays that detect chlamydial antigens, usually the group lipopolysaccharide, are easy to use but insensitive. At least 30% of genital swab specimens and a larger proportion of urine samples from women contain less than 10 chlamydial organisms, so many chlamydia-positive patients have remained undiagnosed. Molecular methods have largely replaced these immunoassays.

The enormous amplification of specific nucleic acid sequences with the PCR assay, the strand displacement assay (SDA), and the transcription-mediated amplification (TMA) technique overcomes the lack of specificity and particularly the poor sensitivity of other tests. The first two assays detect the cryptic plasmid, present in multiple copies in each chlamydial elementary body. The TMA reaction is directed against rRNA, also present in multiple copies. These assays have replaced culture as the 'gold standard' and are now important in routine diagnosis, in maintaining effective screening programmes, and for research into chronic or persistent disease. A variant of *C. trachomatis* serovar E that had escaped detection by commonly used nucleic acid amplification systems was found in Sweden in 2006 and subsequently has been found widely throughout the country but scarcely outside. This underlines the importance of taking into account the structure and function of genomes when selecting appropriate target nucleic acid sequences for diagnostic tests.

A sensitive rapid 'point-of-care' dipstick test, mentioned previously in the section on trachoma, is not yet available commercially.

Serological tests

The traditional complement-fixation test (CFT) cannot distinguish between the chlamydial species. Most of the pertinent diagnostic information originates from the MIF test which measures class-specific antibodies (IgM, IgG, IgA, or secretory). A significant increase in IgM and/or IgG titre is so unusual that the test is of little value. The presence of *C. trachomatis* IgG and/or IgA antibody in tears correlates well with isolation from the conjunctiva in endemic trachoma and adult ocular paratrachoma. In genital infections, serum or local IgA-specific antibodies do not necessarily indicate a current cervical chlamydial infection. In pelvic inflammatory disease, especially in the Fitz-Hugh–Curtis syndrome, antibody titres tend to be higher than in uncomplicated cervical infections. A high IgG antibody titre (1:256 or greater), suggests causation in pelvic disease, but high titres do not always correlate with detection of chlamydiae and are associated more with chronic or recurrent disease. Specific *C. trachomatis* IgM antibody in babies with pneumonia is pathognomonic of chlamydia-induced disease.

In primary respiratory infections with *C. pneumoniae*, IgM antibody appears within a few weeks and IgG antibody by 2 months. In repeat infections, IgG but not IgM antibody develops more rapidly and to a greater titre. The interpretation of results on a single serum is confounded by cross-reacting antibodies to the other species. Finding *C. pneumoniae* antibody in a single serum sample is only an assurance of infection in children. It is unwise to use the CFT to diagnose LGV or psittacosis because of its lack of specificity.

Treatment of chlamydial infections: general aspects

Chlamydiae are intracellular and hence insensitive to aminoglycosides and other antibiotics that do not penetrate cells efficiently. They are particularly sensitive to tetracyclines and macrolides, and also to a variety of other drugs. The rifamycins are probably more active than the tetracyclines *in vitro*, but there is evidence of chlamydial resistance to the rifamycins. These have only rarely been used to treat refractory chlamydial infections, and they are reserved for mycobacterial infections. Tetracycline resistance is not widespread enough to cause clinical problems but vigilance is needed to detect resistant strains, which would not be found by the new routine diagnostic procedures.

The macrolide erythromycin is often used particularly to treat chlamydial infections in infants, young children, and in pregnant and lactating women. A single dose of azithromycin is popular because it is effective and enhances compliance. The recent fluoroquinolones are among other active drugs but they are not used regularly.

Table 7.6.44.1 shows details of the doses and duration of antibiotic treatment. Systemic treatment is given as well as, or in preference to, topical treatment to eradicate nasopharyngeal carriage in trachoma and for neonatal chlamydial conjunctivitis, since topical treatment provides no additional benefit. Oral erythromycin should be used to treat conjunctivitis and to prevent the development of pneumonia.

Azithromycin in a single oral dose (20 mg/kg) is as effective as 6 weeks of topical tetracycline for active trachoma and it is the drug of choice. A single 1-g oral dose of azithromycin is recommended for nongonococcal urethritis. Treatment is usually started before a microbiological diagnosis can be established in patients with complicated genital tract infections, including epididymo-orchitis and pelvic inflammatory disease, so additional broad-spectrum antibiotic cover may be needed. Adequate doses of antibiotics, strict compliance, and treatment of patients' partners are all essential to eradicate genital infections.

The treatment of *C. pneumoniae* and *C. psittaci* infections is the same as for *C. trachomatis*.

Immune response and pathogenesis

The immune response to chlamydial infections may be protective or damaging. Active trachoma is uncommon in adults in endemic areas suggesting that protective immunity follows natural infection. Similarly, genital *C. trachomatis* infection is most prevalent in the youngest sexually active age groups, and the chlamydial isolation rate for men with nongonococcal urethritis is lower in those who have had previous episodes. The duration of ocular infection is shorter in adults than in children. Several trachoma vaccine trials in the 1960s used killed whole organism vaccines, which provided some degree of protection. Primate studies suggested that vaccination could provoke more severe disease on subsequent challenge, indicating immunopathological damage by *C. trachomatis*.

The lymphoid follicle is the hallmark of chlamydial infection and follicles contain typical germinal centres, consisting predominantly of B lymphocytes, with T cells, mostly CD8 cells, in the parafollicular region. The inflammatory infiltrate between follicles comprises plasma cells, dendritic cells, macrophages, and polymorphonuclear leucocytes, with T and B lymphocytes. Fibrosis is seen at a late stage, typically in trachoma and pelvic inflammatory disease. T lymphocytes are also present and outnumber B cells and macrophages. Biopsies from patients with cicatricial trachoma and persisting inflammatory changes show a predominance of CD4 cells, but those from patients in whom inflammation has subsided contain mainly CD8 cells.

A chlamydial heat shock protein (hsp 60), homologous with the GroEL protein of *Escherichia coli*, elicits antibody responses which are associated with the damaging sequelae of *C. trachomatis* infections in both the eye and genital tract. *In vitro* studies show that interferon-γ interferes with the chlamydial development cycle, leading to persistent infection with continuing release of hsp 60. It is not known whether the immune response to hsp 60 is itself the cause of immunopathological damage, or merely a marker of more severe or prolonged infection.

Studies in trachoma-endemic communities suggest that T-helper 1 type cell-mediated responses are important in the clearance of ocular *C. trachomatis* infection. Gene expression at the site of infection, the conjunctival epithelium, is used to identify molecular pathways to fibrosis, in which matrix metalloproteinase 9 (MMP 9) appears be important. Case control studies have identified polymorphisms in several immune response genes (encoding tumour necrosis factor-α, interferon-γ, and interleukin-10) associated with the severe scarring of trachoma.

Infectious chlamydial elementary bodies are actively taken up by epithelial cells, and develop inside an intracellular inclusion. Fusion of the chlamydial inclusion with lysosomes is inhibited while the organisms remain viable. Understanding of the pathogenesis of chlamydial infection has been enhanced by sequencing the complete genome of several *C. trachomatis* strains. The serovar D genome contains genes homologous with those coding for virulence factors in other bacteria, including a cytotoxin gene and genes encoding a type III secretion pathway. A conserved chlamydial protease, proteasome-like activity factor (CPAF), is secreted into the host cell cytoplasm where it interferes with the assembly and surface expression of HLA molecules and inhibits apoptosis. The serovar A genome has been found to be 99.6% identical to serovar D. The 'ocular' serovars (A, B, Ba, and C) differ from the 'genital' serovars (D to K) in lacking a functional tryptophan synthase gene, rendering them more sensitive to inhibition by interferon-γ.

Further reading

Bauwens JE, *et al.* (2002). Epidemic lymphogranuloma venereum during epidemics of crack cocaine use and HIV infection in the Bahamas. *Sex Transm Dis*, **29**, 253–9.

Bavoil PM, Wyrick PB (eds) (2006). *Chlamydia: genomics and pathogenesis.* Horizon Bioscience, Norfolk, UK.

Brunham RC, Rey-Ladino J (2005). Immunology of chlamydia infection: implications for a *Chlamydia trachomatis* vaccine. *Nat Rev Immunol*, **5**, 149–61.

Carlson JH, *et al.* (2005). Comparative genomic analysis of *Chlamydia trachomatis* oculotropic and genitotropic strains. *Infect Immun*, **73**, 6407–18.

Chernesky MA (2002). *Chlamydia trachomatis* diagnostics. *Sex Transm Infect*, **78**, 232–4.

Grayston JT, *et al.* (1990). A new respiratory tract pathogen: *Chlamydia pneumoniae* strain TWAR. *J Infect Dis*, **161**, 618–25.

Herrmann B, *et al.* (2008). Emergence and spread of *Chlamydia trachomatis* variant, Sweden. *Emerg Infect Dis*, **14**, 1462–5.

Mabey D, Solomon A, Foster A (2003). Trachoma seminar. *Lancet*, **362**, 223–9.

Michel CEC, *et al.* (2006). A rapid point-of-care assay for targeting antibiotic treatment to eliminate trachoma. *Lancet*, **367**, 1585–90.

Rasmussen SJ (1998). Chlamydial immunology. *Curr Opin Infect Dis*, **11**, 37–41.

Resnikoff S, *et al.* (2004). Global data on visual impairment in the year 2002. *Bull World Health Organ*, **82**, 844–51.

Solomon A, *et al.* (2004). Mass treatment with single-dose azithromycin for trachoma. *N Engl J Med*, **351**, 1962–71.

Stephens RS, *et al.* (1998). Genome sequence of an obligate intracellular pathogen of humans: *Chlamydia trachomatis. Science*, **282**, 754–9.

Taylor-Robinson D (1991). Genital chlamydial infections: clinical aspects, diagnosis, treatment and prevention. In: Harris JRW, Forster SM (eds) *Recent advances in sexually transmitted diseases and AIDS*, pp. 219–62. Churchill Livingstone, Edinburgh.

Taylor-Robinson D, Thomas BJ (1998). *Chlamydia pneumoniae* in arteries: the facts, their interpretation, and future studies. *J Clin Pathol*, **51**, 793–7.

Thylefors B, *et al.* (1987). A simple system for the assessment of trachoma and its complications. *Bull World Health Organ*, **65**, 477–83.

Van der Bij AK, *et al.* (2006). Diagnostic and clinical implications of anorectal lymphogranuloma venereum in men who have sex with men: a retrospective case-control study. *Clin Infect Dis*, **42**, 186–94.

Viravan C, *et al.* (1996). A prospective clinical and bacteriologic study of inguinal buboes in Thai men. *Clin Infect Dis*, **22**, 233–9.

Wang SP, *et al.* (1967). Trachoma vaccine studies in monkeys. *Am J Ophthalmol*, **63**, 1615–20.

7.6.45 Mycoplasmas

David Taylor-Robinson and Jørgen Skov Jensen

Essentials

Mycoplasmas are the smallest self-replicating prokaryotes. They are devoid of cell walls, with the plasticity of their outer membrane favouring pleomorphism, although some have a characteristic bottle-shaped appearance. Mycoplasmas recovered from humans belong to the genera *Mycoplasma* (14 species) and *Ureaplasma* (2 species). They are predominantly found in the respiratory and genital tracts, but sometimes invade the bloodstream and thus gain access to joints and other organs.

Respiratory infection

Clinical features—*Mycoplasma pneumoniae* is the most important mycoplasmal respiratory pathogen, with presentations ranging from inapparent infection and mild, afebrile, upper respiratory-tract disease to severe pneumonia. It is responsible for 15 to 20% of all pneumonias in the United States of America. Extrapulmonary manifestations include Stevens–Johnson syndrome and haemolytic anaemia.

Diagnosis and treatment—diagnosis is made by culture (slow and of limited value in clinical diagnosis), molecular methods (rapid detection by PCR is routine in some settings) and/or serology. Aside from supportive care, treatment is usually with tetracyclines or erythromycin. There is no commercially available effective vaccine.

Genitourinary and related infections

Clinical features—(1) Men—*M. genitalium* causes nongonococcal urethritis (NGU) in men, and ureaplasmas may play a role in some cases. (2) Women—*M. genitalium* causes cervicitis, endometritis, and possibly salpingitis; *M. hominis* and (to a lesser extent) ureaplasmas are associated with bacterial vaginosis; *M. hominis* may contribute to salpingitis. (3) Pregnancy—ureaplasma infection of amniotic fluid is associated with preterm labour; ureaplasmas may be involved in the chronic lung disease of very low birthweight babies.

Diagnosis and treatment—diagnosis of infection by ureaplasmas and *M. hominis* is usually by culture of swabs from the urethra or cervix/vagina; PCR is used to detect *M. genitalium*. Patients with NGU should receive an antibiotic with activity against *C. trachomatis*, ureaplasmas, and *M. genitalium*, e.g azithromycin, with moxifloxacin used if *M. genitalium* becomes resistant and chronic disease develops.

Rheumatological manifestations

(1) Chronic arthritides—*M. fermentans* has been detected in the joints of patients with, e.g. rheumatoid arthritis, but the significance of this is unknown. (2) Reiter's syndrome—sexually acquired reactive arthritis (SARA) is not uncommon after *M. genitalium*-positive NGU, but no causal link has been established. (3) Arthritis in patients with hypogammaglobulinaemia is often caused by mycoplasmas (particularly ureaplasmas).

Introduction

Mycoplasmas, the trivial name for members of the class Mollicutes, are the smallest (0.3 μm diameter) free-living microorganisms. They lack the rigid cell wall of other bacteria, making them resistant to penicillins and related antimicrobials. Instead, they have a pliable trilaminar unit membrane (Fig. 7.6.45.1) enclosing the cytoplasm, DNA, RNA, and other components necessary for propagation in cell-free media. The small size of the mycoplasma genome (as little as 580 kbp) restricts metabolic capabilities, making culture of some mycoplasmas difficult or impossible. Despite their general similarity, mycoplasmas are a heterogeneous group with differing host specificities, nutritional requirements, metabolic reactions, and DNA and antigenic composition. Mycoplasmas are divided into four orders: Mycoplasmatales, Entomoplasmatales comprising those from insects and plants, Acholeplasmatales, and the strictly anaerobic Anaeroplasmatales. The last two do not need sterol for growth. The mycoplasmas isolated commonly from humans belong to the family Mycoplasmataceae within the order Mycoplasmatales. This family includes the genus *Mycoplasma*, the organisms of which metabolize glucose or arginine or both, and the genus *Ureaplasma*, the organisms (ureaplasmas) of which uniquely hydrolyse urea. Ureaplasmas were originally termed T-strains or T-mycoplasmas because of the tiny (T) colonies (15–60 μm diameter) they form on agar medium, in contrast to the larger (≥90 μm diameter) characteristic fried-egg-like colonies produced by most other mycoplasmas (Fig. 7.6.45.2).

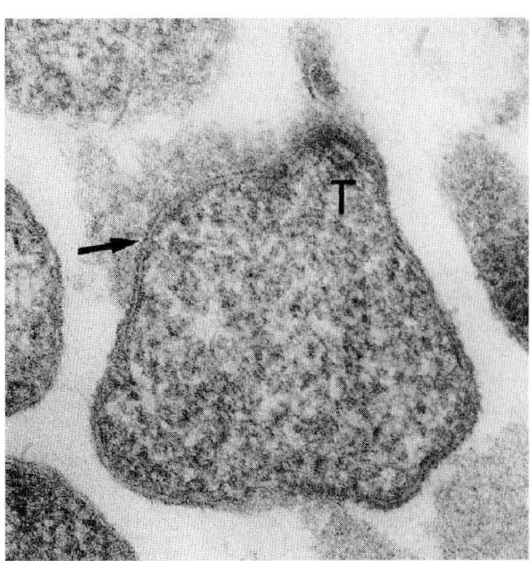

Fig. 7.6.45.1 Electron micrograph of *M. pulmonis* (murine origin), illustrating that the organism does not have a bacterial cell wall but has a trilaminar unit membrane (arrow); also note what appears to be a terminal structure (T). Magnification ×66 000.

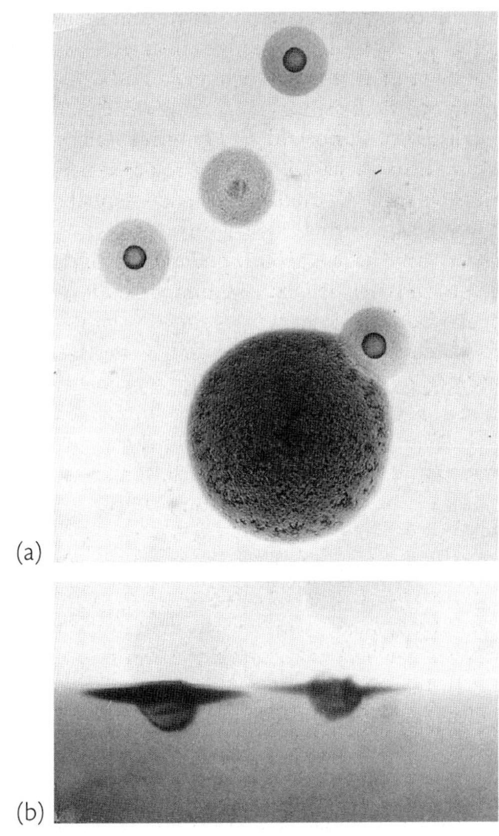

Fig. 7.6.45.2 (a) Fried-egg-like mycoplasma colonies (one ill-formed) and a larger bacterial colony. Transmission light microscopy, magnification ×43. (b) Section through mycoplasma colonies illustrating growth in the depth of the agar. Magnification ×78.

Historical perspective

The first mycoplasma to be recognized, *Mycoplasma mycoides* subsp. *mycoides*, was isolated in 1898 from cattle with pleuropneumonia. As other pathogenic and saprophytic isolates accumulated from veterinary and human sources, they became known as pleuropneumonia-like organisms (PPLO), a term later superseded by mycoplasmas. The first mycoplasma of human origin, *M. hominis*, was recovered from a Bartholin's gland abscess in 1937 and the first of undoubted pathogenicity, *M. pneumoniae*, from the respiratory tract in 1962. Ureaplasmas were first detected in the urethras of men with nongonococcal urethritis (NGU) in 1954 and *M. genitalium* was isolated from this site in 1981. The mycoplasma of human origin recognized most recently is *M. amphoriforme*, isolated in 1995. Over more than a century, numerous other mycoplasmas have been isolated from various animals and have been shown to be of economic importance because of the pneumonia, arthritis, keratoconjunctivitis, and mastitis they cause among livestock and poultry. This is apart from the plant diseases recognized as being due to mycoplasmas in recent years. In humans, as in other animal species, mycoplasmas cause respiratory and genital tract diseases and escape from these sites to cause disease elsewhere, e.g. in joints.

Mycoplasmas are also notorious for contaminating cell cultures, particularly continuous cell lines. Various species of animal or human origin are responsible, e.g. porcine *M. hyorhinis* and human *M. orale* or *M. fermentans*. The contamination may affect almost any property under investigation in a totally unpredictable way and may lead to misinterpretation of any result based on studies in cultured cells.

Occurrence of mycoplasmas in humans

Fourteen species of mycoplasmas and two ureaplasmas have been isolated from humans, and constitute the normal flora or behave as pathogens (Tables 7.6.45.1, 7.6.45.2); in addition, several case reports have described infection with species of animal origin. Most of the human flora is found in the oropharynx. There is little information about the distribution or significance of *M. amphoriforme*, *M. penetrans*, *M. pirum*, and *M. spermatophilum*.

Respiratory infections

Relationship between mycoplasmas and respiratory disease

M. pneumoniae is the most important mycoplasma found in the respiratory tract (see below); most of the others behave as commensals (Table 7.6.45.1). *M. genitalium* was found originally in the male genitourinary tract but was isolated subsequently from a few respiratory specimens, which also contained *M. pneumoniae*. *M. genitalium* is not an important pathogen in the respiratory tract. *M. fermentans* has been detected in the throat more often since the use of polymerase chain reaction (PCR) (see below) and has been recovered from adults with an acute influenza-like illness, which sometimes deteriorates rapidly with development of a rare but

Table 7.6.45.1 Biological features, occurrence, and disease association of mycoplasmas of human origin[a]

Mycoplasma	Metabolism of:	Haemadsorption	Frequency of detection in the:					Cause of disease
			Respiratory tract	Genitourinary tract	Rectum	Eye	Blood	
M. amphoriforme	Glucose	Yes	Rare[b]	–[c]	–[c]	–[c]	–[c]	?Yes
M. buccale	Arginine	No	Rare	–	–	–	–	No
M. faucium	Arginine	Yes[d]	Rare	–	–	–	–	No
M. fermentans	Glucose, arginine	No	Common	Rare	–	–	Rare	?Yes
M. genitalium	Glucose	Yes	Rare	Common	Rare	Rare	?	Yes
M. hominis	Arginine	No	Rare	Common	Common	Rare	Very rare	Yes
M. lipophilum	Arginine	No	Rare	–	–	–	–	No
M. orale	Arginine	Yes[d]	Common	–	–	–	–	No
M. penetrans	Glucose, arginine	Yes	–	Rare	Very rare	–	?	?
M. pirum	Glucose	?	?	–	Rare	?	Very rare	?
M. pneumoniae	Glucose	Yes	Rare[e]	Very rare	–	–	–	Yes
M. primatum	Arginine	No	–	Rare	–	–	–	No
M. salivarium	Arginine	No	Common	Rare	–	–	–	No[f]
M. spermatophilum	Arginine	No	–		?Rare	?	?	?
Ureaplasma parvum[g]	Urea	Serotype 3 only	Rare	Common	Common	Rare	Very rare	Yes
Ureaplasma urealyticum[g]	Urea	No	Rare	Common	Common	Rare	Very rare	Yes

[a] Occasional isolations of mycoplasma species of nonhuman origin not included.
[b] Except in immunocompromised patients.
[c] No reports of detection.
[d] With chick erythrocytes only.
[e] Except in disease outbreaks.
[f] Except in hypogammaglobulinaemia.
[g] Ureaplasmas have been divided into two species formerly described as biovars.

Table 7.6.45.2 Summary of the relationship between mycoplasmas and disease. Evidence for an association (A) between the indicated mycoplasma[a] and disease, and for the causation (C) of disease

	M. pneumoniae		***M. fermentans***		**Ureaplasmas**		***M. hominis***		***M. genitalium***	
	A	**C**	**A**	**C**	**A**	**C**	**A**	**C**	**A**	**C**
Upper respiratory tract disease	+++	+++	–		–		+++	–	–	
Bronchitis	+++	+++	–		–		–		–	
Pneumonia	++++	++++	++	+	–		–		–	
Asthma	++	+	NE		NA		–		–	
Extrapulmonary sequelae of *M. pneumoniae* infection (see text)	+++	+++	NA		NA		NA		NA	
Nongonococcal urethritis	NA		–		+++	+++	–		++++	++++
Chronic prostatitis	NA		NE		++	+	–		+	–
Epididymitis	NA		NE		++	++	–		++	++
Bartholinitis	NA		NE		–		+	–	NE	
Bacterial vaginosis	NA		NE		++	–	++++	+	–	
Cervicitis	NA		–		–		–		+++	+++
Pelvic inflammatory disease	NA		NE		+	–	+++	++	+++	+++
Infertility	NA		NE		++	–	–		++[b]	++
Urinary calculi	NA		–		++	+	–		NE	
Pyelonephritis	NA		NE		+	–	+++	++	NE	
Chorioamnionitis	NA		++	+	++	++	–		NE	
Preterm labour/delivery	NA		NE		+++	++	++	++	+	+
Spontaneous abortion	NA		+	–	+++	+	++	+	+	–
Postabortal fever	NA		NE		++	+	++++	+++	NE	
Postpartum fever	NA		NE		++	+	++++	+++	NE	
Postpartum arthritis	NA		NE		–		+++	+++	NE	
Low birthweight	NA		NE		++	+	–		NE	
Neonatal chronic lung disease	NA		NE		+++	++	++	+	NE	
Rheumatoid arthritis	+	–	+++	–	++	–	–		+	–
Juvenile chronic arthritis	++	+	NE		–		–		NE	
Sexually acquired reactive arthritis/ Reiter's disease	–		–		++	++	–		++	++
Arthritis in hypogammaglobulinaemia	++++	++++	NE		++++	++++	++++	+++	NE	
Wound infections	NA		NE		++	+	+++	+++	NE	
AIDS	–		++	–	–		–		–	

NA, not appropriate to examine; NE, not examined; ++++, strong; +++, good; ++, moderate; +, weak; –, none.
[a] See text for *M. amphoriforme* and other mycoplasmas.
[b] Tubal factor infertility.

often fatal respiratory distress syndrome. *M. hominis* is occasionally recovered from the respiratory tract. However, although it caused a mild pharyngitis in adult male volunteers inoculated orally, it is not known to do this naturally in children or adults. *M. amphoriforme* is a newly described species isolated from patients with chronic bronchitis, primarily those with B-cell deficiencies, and is phylogenetically related to pathogenic species such as *M. pneumoniae* and *M. genitalium*. The clinical importance of *M. amphoriforme* in the general population is unknown.

In the late 1930s, nonbacterial pneumonias or primary atypical pneumonia were distinguished from typical lobar pneumonia. Patients from whom the 'Eaton agent' had been isolated in embryonated eggs often developed cold agglutinins. This agent was presumed to be a virus until it was found to be sensitive to chlortetracycline and gold salts. Its mycoplasmal nature was established by cultivation on a cell-free agar medium. The agent, *M. pneumoniae*, was established as a respiratory pathogen by studies based on isolation, serology, volunteer inoculation, and vaccine protection.

Clinical features of *M. pneumoniae* disease

M. pneumoniae produces a range of effects from inapparent infection and mild afebrile upper respiratory tract disease to severe pneumonia.

The most typical clinical syndrome is tracheobronchitis, often accompanied by upper respiratory tract manifestations such as acute pharyngitis. A clinical diagnosis of *M. pneumoniae* pneumonia is impossible as it shares features of other nonbacterial pneumonias. Malaise and headache often precede chest symptoms by 1 to 5 days, and pneumonia is seen radiographically before physical signs such as rales are detectable. Usually, only one of the lower lobes is involved and the radiograph shows patchy opacities. Pneumonia develops in about one-third of those infected and about 20% of patients have bilateral pneumonia. Pleurisy and pleural effusions are unusual. The course of the disease is variable but often protracted. Symptoms may persist for several weeks and may relapse. The organisms can persist in respiratory secretions despite antibiotic therapy, particularly in patients with hypogammaglobulinaemia where excretion may continue for months or years rather than weeks. Although a few very severe infections have been reported, usually in patients with immunodeficiency or sickle cell anaemia, death is rare. In children, illness may be prolonged with paroxysmal cough followed by vomiting, simulating whooping cough. *M. pneumoniae* has been implicated in bronchial asthma, but this is controversial (see below).

Extrapulmonary manifestations of *M. pneumoniae* infection

Disease caused by *M. pneumoniae* is usually limited to the respiratory tract, but various extrapulmonary conditions may occur during the course of the respiratory illness or subsequently (Table 7.6.45.3). Whether any are due to *M. genitalium* is uncertain. Haemolytic crisis is precipitated by cold agglutinins (anti-I antibodies). Mycoplasmas apparently alter the I antigen on erythrocytes sufficiently to stimulate an autoimmune response. A similar mechanism may be responsible for neurological and other complications. Invasion of the central nervous system cannot be discounted as *M. pneumoniae* has been isolated from cerebrospinal fluid.

Table 7.6.45.3 Extrapulmonary manifestations of *M. pneumoniae* infections

System	Manifestations	Estimated frequency
Cardiovascular	Myocarditis, pericarditis	<5%
Dermatological	Urticaria, erythema multiforme, Stevens–Johnson syndrome, other rashes	Some skin involvement in about 25%
Gastrointestinal	Anorexia, nausea, vomiting, and transient diarrhoea	15–45%
	Hepatitis	?
	Pancreatitis	?
Genitourinary	Acute glomerulonephritis	Insignificant
Haematological	Cold agglutinin production	About 50%
	Haemolytic anaemia	?
	Thrombocytopenia	?
	Intravascular coagulation	>50 reported cases
Musculoskeletal	Myalgia, arthralgia, arthritis	15–45%
Neurological	Meningitis, meningoencephalitis, ascending paralysis, transient myelitis, cranial nerve palsy, poliomyelitis-like illness	<5% in a few studies based on serology

Epidemiology of *M. pneumoniae* infections

Pathology is age dependent. About one-quarter of infections in children aged 5 to 15 years result in pneumonia, whereas only about 7% of infections in young adults do so. Pneumonia is less frequent thereafter, but is more severe the older the patient.

M. pneumoniae causes inapparent or mild upper respiratory tract symptoms more often than severe disease. It is responsible for a minority of all upper tract infections, usually attributable to viruses or streptococci. *M. pneumoniae* causes many lower respiratory tract infections, e.g. about 15 to 20% of all pneumonias in the United States of America. In populations such as military recruits it has been responsible for up to 40% of acute pulmonary illness.

M. pneumoniae infections appear to occur globally. Infection is endemic in most areas and throughout the year, with a predilection for late summer and early autumn. Epidemic peaks have been observed about every 4 to 7 years. The incubation period ranges from 2 to 3 weeks. Spread from person to person occurs slowly, usually where there is continual or repeated close contact, as within a family.

Immunopathological factors in the development of *M. pneumoniae* pneumonia

The crucial step of adherence of *M. pneumoniae* organisms to respiratory mucosal epithelial cells, cytadsorption (Fig. 7.6.45.3), is mediated by P1 and other specialized adhesins on the mycoplasmal surface. In animals, there is peribronchiolar and perivascular pulmonary infiltration mostly by T lymphocytes (Fig. 7.6.45.4). The pneumonia caused by *M. pneumoniae* is largely an immunopathological process since immunosuppression prevents pneumonia or diminishes its severity. A mycoplasmal polysaccharide–protein fraction is involved in the cell-mediated immune response, whereas the main antigenic determinant in complement fixation and other serological reactions is a glycolipid. After the initial lymphocyte response, polymorphonuclear leucocytes and macrophages appear in the bronchiolar exudate. The slow evolution of the primary disease contrasts with an accelerated and often more intense host response to reinfection. Children of 2 to 5 years old show serological evidence of infection at an early age. The pneumonia that occurs in older people is considered to be an immunological over-response to reinfection, with lung infiltration by previously sensitized lymphocytes.

Chronic respiratory disease

Animal mycoplasmas are frequently associated with chronic illnesses, and so the possible role of mycoplasmas has been considered in human chronic respiratory disease. *M. pneumoniae* often persists in the respiratory tract long after clinical recovery and occasionally the disease is protracted but there is no evidence that *M. pneumoniae* is a primary cause of chronic bronchitis, or that it maintains chronic disease other than by possibly causing some acute exacerbations.

M. salivarium, *M. orale*, and perhaps other mycoplasmas present in the oropharynx of healthy people spread to the lower respiratory tract of people with chronic bronchitis. There is no hard evidence that these mycoplasmas cause acute exacerbations, but they may

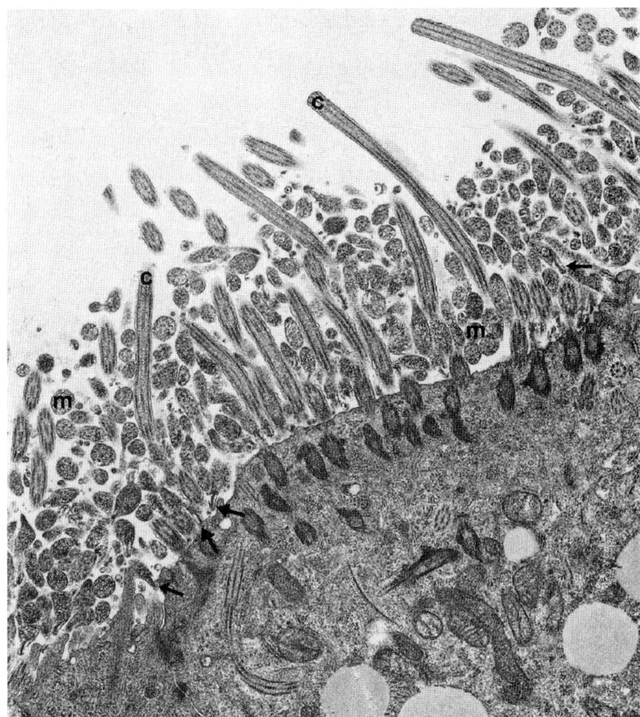

Fig. 7.6.45.3 Electron micrograph of ciliated epithelial cells in the tracheal mucosa of a hamster infected with *M. pneumoniae*. Note cilia (c) and individual organisms (m), some with specialized terminal structure oriented towards the membrane of the host cell (arrows). Magnification ×9880.

perpetuate an episode. Specific antibody responses follow such exacerbations more frequently than at other times, suggesting that mycoplasmas multiply and contribute to the tissue damage that is primarily due to viruses and bacteria.

M. amphoriforme was recovered from the respiratory tract of patients with chronic bronchitis, most of whom were B-cell deficient. Recovery may depend on the eradication of this organism but its role in the general population is unknown.

The role of *M. pneumoniae* in asthma is controversial. Acute *M. pneumoniae* infection is associated with wheezing and the organism has been found, mainly by PCR, more frequently in subjects with asthma than in those without. However, no causal relationship has so far been established.

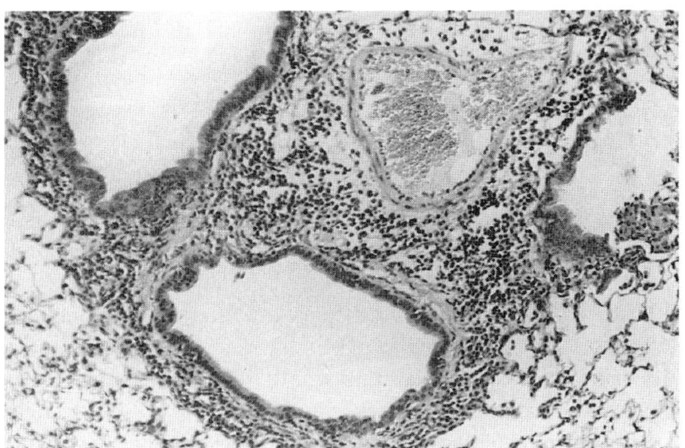

Fig. 7.6.45.4 Pneumonia 2 weeks after intranasal inoculation of a hamster with *M. pneumoniae*. Note peribronchiolar and perivascular infiltration of mononuclear cells, predominantly lymphocytes. Haematoxylin and eosin, magnification ×98.

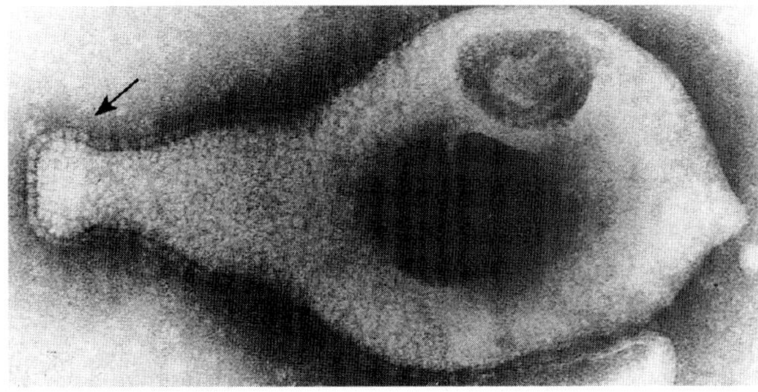

(a)

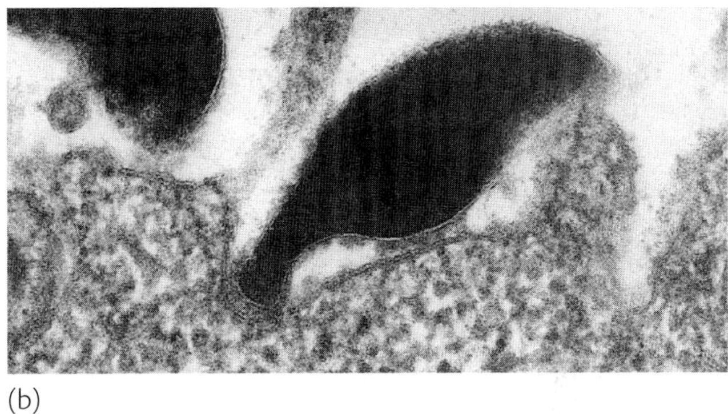

(b)

Fig. 7.6.45.5 (a) Electron micrograph of *M. genitalium*, negatively stained to show flask-shaped appearance and terminal specialized structure (arrow). Magnification ×90 000. (b) Electron micrograph of *M. genitalium* adhering to a Vero cell by the terminal structure. Magnification ×60 000.
(From Tully JG, *et al.* (1983) *Mycoplasma genitalium*, a new species from the human urogenital tract. *Int J Syst Bacteriol*, **33**, 387, with permission.)

Genitourinary and related infections

Nongonococcal urethritis (NGU) and its complications

M. genitalium, a large-colony-forming mycoplasma (Table 7.6.45.1, Fig. 7.6.45.5a), is strongly associated with acute NGU (Table 7.6.45.4). It has been detected almost independently of *Chlamydia trachomatis* by PCR in about 25% of cases compared with significantly fewer (about 6%) healthy controls. It also causes urethritis experimentally in male chimpanzees and adheres to and enters epithelial cells (Fig. 7.6.45.5b). Intracellular *M. genitalium* may be partially protected from antimicrobials, particularly tetracyclines, resulting in persistent or recurrent nongonococcal urethritis.

Although *M. hominis* has been isolated from about 20% of patients with acute NGU, it has not been implicated as a cause.

The role of ureaplasmas in NGU has been contentious for many years. The results of most qualitative studies have failed to demonstrate a significant difference between the prevalence of ureaplasmas in men with or without acute NGU, but there are some quantitative data indicating higher titres of organisms in men with disease. There are two species of human ureaplasmas, *U. urealyticum* and *U. parvum*. PCR assays of clinical specimens tend to show a stronger association between *U. urealyticum* and NGU, but most studies did not consider clinical histories. Intraurethral inoculation of first-passage ureaplasma strains produced a mild

Table 7.6.45.4 Association of *M. genitalium*, *M. hominis*, and ureaplasmas with human genitourinary, reproductive, and perinatal disease

Disease	Evidence suggesting a causal relationship of:			Comments on the relationship
	M. genitalium	*M. hominis*	Ureaplasmas	
Nongonococcal urethritis	Strong	None	Good	The proportion of nongonococcal urethritis caused by ureaplasmas is unknown
Chronic prostatitis	Weak	None	Weak	None of the microorganisms appears to be a cause
Epididymitis	Some (not published)	None	Some	Ureaplasmas involved in one case of acute disease
Urinary calculi	?	None	Weak	Experimentally, ureaplasmas cause bladder calculi in male rats but so far little evidence for a cause of natural human disease
Pyelonephritis	?	Some	None	*M. hominis* possibly causes some cases of acute pyelonephritis and exacerbations
Reiter's disease/sexually acquired reactive arthritis	Some	None	Some	*M. genitalium* detected in joint of one patient; ureaplasmas are related on the basis of lymphocytic response to specific antigen
Bartholinitis	?	Very weak	None	Doubtful whether *M. hominis* is involved
Bacterial vaginosis	None	Weak	None	*M. hominis* and to a lesser extent ureaplasmas are associated with bacterial vaginosis, but a causal relationship is unproved
Cervicitis	Good	None	None	*M. genitalium* is associated with nongonococcal, nonchlamydial cervicitis
Pelvic inflammatory disease	Good	Some	Weak	*M. genitalium* is associated serologically and has been detected in the upper genital tract of patients with endometritis and salpingitis; *M. hominis* probably causes a small proportion of cases, but very doubtful that ureaplasmas do
Postabortal fever	?	Good	Weak	*M. hominis*, and to a much lesser extent ureaplasmas, are responsible for some cases, but the proportion is unknown
Postpartum fever	?	Good	Weak	*M. hominis*, and to a much lesser extent ureaplasmas, are responsible for some cases, but the proportion is unknown
Infertility	Some	None	None	*M. genitalium* is associated serologically to tubal factor infertility; ureaplasmas are associated with reduced sperm motility, but a causal relationship is unproved
Premature labour	Weak	Some	Some/good	*M. genitalium* associated in one study, but not in others. Considerable evidence for the involvement of ureaplasmas, less so for *M. hominis*; both possibly as part of bacterial vaginosis
Spontaneous abortion and stillbirth	?	Weak	Weak	Maternal and fetal infections are associated with spontaneous abortion, but a causal relationship is unproved
Chorioamnionitis	?	None	Some	An association exists with ureaplasmas, but a causal relationship is unproved
Low birth weight	?	None	Weak	An association exists with ureaplasmas in some studies, but a causal relationship is unproved
Neonatal meningitis	?	Some	Some	A rare event
Neonatal lung disease	?	Weak	Some	*M. hominis* has been involved in pneumonia soon after birth; ureaplasmas possibly involved in premature infants weighing less than 1000 g

urethritis and an antibody response in male chimpanzees. The disease responded to tetracycline therapy. Four investigators who inoculated themselves intraurethrally developed urethritis. In one study, two received cloned *U. urealyticum*, serotype 5, isolated from patients with acute NGU in whom no other potentially pathogenic microorganisms could be detected, although *M. genitalium* was not sought at that time. Both developed symptoms and signs of urethritis which responded to treatment with minocycline. Another volunteer experiment suggested that ureaplasmas may cause disease the first few times they gain access to the urethra but later insults result in colonization without disease, accounting perhaps for their frequent occurrence in the urethras of healthy men.

Some patients with hypogammaglobulinaemia develop a prolonged urethrocystitis with persistent ureaplasmal infection. Treatment is often complicated by antimicrobial resistance and a combination of different classes of antibiotics is recommended.

Epididymitis and chronic prostatitis

Ureaplasmas may be a rare cause of epididymitis since they have been recovered from the urethra and epididymal aspirate fluid of a patient with acute nonchlamydial, nongonococcal epididymitis, with a specific antibody response. *M. genitalium* has not been sought in aspirates, but it has been found in the urethra without other known pathogens (Table 7.6.45.4).

Information linking prostatic infection with acute ureaplasmal urethral infection is scanty, although ureaplasmas have been isolated more frequently and in greater numbers from patients with acute urethroprostatitis than from controls. Most of those with more than 10^3 organisms in expressed prostatic fluid responded to tetracycline therapy. In contrast, ureaplasmas have not been found, and *M. genitalium* only rarely, in prostatic biopsy specimens from patients with chronic abacterial prostatitis. *M. hominis* is not associated with prostatitis.

Pelvic inflammatory disease (Chapter 8.5)

Microorganisms in the vagina and lower cervix may ascend to and cause inflammation of the fallopian tubes and adjacent pelvic structures (Table 7.6.45.4). Large-colony-forming mycoplasmas, predominantly *M. hominis*, have been isolated from inflamed fallopian tubes, tubo-ovarian abscesses, and pelvic abscesses or fluid. Laparoscopy samples yielded *M. hominis* from the tubes of about 10% of women with salpingitis but not from those of healthy women. This might occur with bacterial vaginosis since large numbers of the organisms are in the vagina (Chapter 8.4). Hysterosalpingography may also precipitate inflammation of the fallopian tubes in women who carry *M. hominis* in the lower genital tract. *M. hominis* antibody was found in approximately one-half of salpingitis patients, but in only 10% of healthy women. Antibody was found in one-half of the patients who had *M. hominis* present in the lower genital tract.

Although ureaplasmas have been isolated directly from the fallopian tubes of a very small proportion of patients with acute salpingitis, from pelvic fluid, and from a tubo-ovarian abscess, it seems that they are of little importance in acute pelvic inflammatory disease.

PCR testing has established that *M. genitalium* is involved in at least some cases of pelvic inflammatory disease. It is a cause of cervicitis and its presence in the cervix or upper genital tract is associated significantly with histological endometritis. It has rarely been detected in tubes but in one study of women with pelvic inflammatory disease, an antibody response was detected to *M. genitalium* but not to *M. hominis* or *C. trachomatis* in one-third of the patients. Other studies have not shown this association but *M. genitalium* has been related serologically to tubal factor infertility.

Fallopian-tube organ culture, in which the tissues are maintained in a condition similar to that *in vivo*, show that gonococci destroy the epithelium, *M. genitalium* causes some damage, *M. hominis* organisms multiply but only produce swelling of some cilia, and human ureaplasmas cause no damage. This differential effect may be a true reflection of the pathogenic potential of these microorganisms *in vivo* but, as the immune system is not operational, failure to demonstrate damage does not confirm avirulence. Inoculation of *M. hominis* or *M. genitalium* into primates caused a self-limiting acute salpingitis and parametritis with an antibody response, whereas ureaplasmas had no effect.

Effects of mycoplasmas on pregnancy

Preterm labour

The involvement of genital mycoplasmas is debated but ureaplasma infection of the amniotic fluid is associated with preterm labour. *M. hominis* probably plays a part through its involvement with bacterial vaginosis, a known cause of preterm labour. *M. hominis* and ureaplasmas are unlikely to cause low birthweight in otherwise normal full-term infants. *M. genitalium* is probably not pathogenic during pregnancy.

Postabortal and postpartum fever

M. hominis has been isolated from the blood, with an antibody response, in up to 10% of women with fever after abortion but not from those without fever. However, a pure culture of *M. hominis* in blood is needed before it can be accepted as a cause of fever. The role of ureaplasmas is unclear. Patients with postabortal or postpartum fever of mycoplasmal origin usually recover without antibiotic treatment.

Neonatal infections

Whether transmitted *in utero* or during birth, ureaplasmas may be isolated from the throats and tracheal aspirates of some neonates. Ureaplasma-infected infants of very low birthweight (<1000 g) have died or have developed chronic lung disease twice as often as uninfected infants of similar birth weight or those of over 1000 g. However, the pathogenicity of ureaplasmas is uncertain since erythromycin treatment has failed to prevent disease in two trials. *M. hominis* has very rarely been implicated in pneumonia soon after birth but the other bacteria present could be responsible.

Mycoplasmal infection should be considered in cases of neonatal disease of the central nervous system in which the results of bacteriological staining and culture are negative. *M. hominis* or ureaplasmas have been found in the cerebrospinal fluid of neonates with meningitis or brain abscess.

Joint infections

Rheumatoid arthritis

Mycoplasmas cause several animal arthritides, and gold salts (used to treat rheumatoid arthritis) inactivate mycoplasmas. However, the search for mycoplasmal infection of joints was unfruitful until PCR testing showed *M. fermentans* and ureaplasma DNA in more than 20% of patients with rheumatoid arthritis and other chronic inflammatory disorders, in contrast to those with noninflammatory disorders. The significance of these findings is unknown.

M. pneumoniae and other mycoplasmal infections

In mycoplasmal arthritides of animals, organisms isolated from the joints are often found in the respiratory tract. Human *M. pneumoniae* respiratory infection is often accompanied by nonspecific arthralgia or myalgia (Table 7.6.45.3) during the acute phase, and occasionally it leads to migratory polyarthritis affecting middle-sized joints in adults. A fourfold or greater rise in the titre of antibody to *M. pneumoniae* has been seen occasionally in juvenile chronic arthritis, but an aetiological association has not been demonstrated.

M. hominis has been isolated from septic joints, usually hip, that have developed in mothers after childbirth. The arthritis responds to tetracycline therapy and the diagnosis should be considered in a postpartum arthritis which is unaffected by penicillin.

Reiter's disease

Arthritis may occur soon after or concomitant with NGU (sexually acquired reactive arthritis; SARA) or the arthritis may be associated with conjunctivitis and urethritis (Reiter's disease). *M. genitalium* causes uncomplicated NGU and ureaplasmas may do so to a lesser extent, but previous antimicrobial treatment usually prevents adequate investigation of patients with arthritis. *M. genitalium* has been detected in the synovial fluid of a patient with SARA and clinical experience has shown that SARA is not uncommon after *M. genitalium*-positive NGU, but no causal link has been established. The latter is also true in the case of some patients whose synovial lymphocytes have been shown to proliferate *in vitro* in response to ureaplasmal antigens.

Wound infections

M. hominis has rarely been linked to fever in patients with burns, trauma, or wound infections. It is most common in fever after surgery on the urogenital tract; ureaplasmas are also likely to be present, but neither these nor *M. hominis* will be found unless specifically sought. Kidney transplant patients occasionally develop mixed infections with ureaplasmas and *M. hominis*, which in severe cases may create fistulas.

A rare wound infection is 'seal finger' or 'blubber finger' which is well known in Arctic regions where the handling of sea mammals is part of daily living. A few days after a seal bite, oedema of the affected finger develops with swelling of the interphalangeal joint adjacent to the lesion. It is extremely painful, suppuration can occur, extensive surgery may be needed, and residual dysfunction is possible. The infection usually responds rapidly to tetracyclines but macrolides are inefficient. Rapidly growing mycoplasmas, some of which have not been speciated, can be recovered from the lesion.

Mycoplasmas in immunodeficiency states

Arthritis in patients with hypogammaglobulinaemia

Arthritis of mycoplasmal aetiology (Fig. 7.6.45.6a,b) should be considered in patients with hypogammaglobulinaemia who develop an abacterial septic arthritis. *M. pneumoniae*, *M. hominis*, *M. salivarium*, and, in particular, ureaplasmas have been isolated from synovial fluids of at least two-fifths of these patients. Vigilance should be kept for infection by mycoplasmas of nonhuman origin. The arthritis usually responds to tetracyclines or other antimicrobials to which the organisms are sensitive. Intravenous and combination therapy should be considered to avoid antimicrobial resistance developing due to suboptimal drug concentrations at the infection site. Administration of specific antiserum against the mycoplasma in question may be helpful in a few patients when antimicrobial therapy fails.

Mycoplasmas in patients with AIDS

Although *M. fermentans* was distributed widely in tissues taken at autopsy from some patients with AIDS, no association has been found with the stage of the disease, the patients' $CD4^{+}$ count, viral load, or rate of progression of the illness.

M. penetrans, which avidly invades eukaryotic cells, was isolated from urine sediments of a few HIV-1-positive homosexual men.

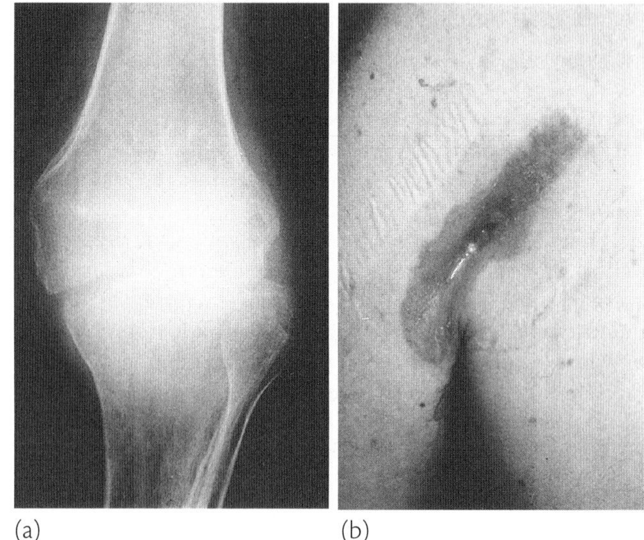

Fig. 7.6.45.6 (a) Damage to the knee joint of a hypogammaglobulinaemic patient caused by *U. urealyticum* infection. (b) Sinus connected with the shoulder joint of a patient with hypogammaglobulinaemia; ureaplasmas were isolated repeatedly from the sinus exudate.
(Courtesy of A D B Webster.)

While it is possible that *M. fermentans*, *M. penetrans*, or other mycoplasmas might proliferate in this immunodeficiency state, there is no convincing evidence that they are important for the development of AIDS.

Conditions of rare or equivocal mycoplasmal aetiology

Bacterial vaginosis (Chapter 8.4)

M. hominis organisms may well have a role in the pathogenesis of bacterial vaginosis in which they occur in very large numbers, but proof is impossible due to the variety of other bacteria present in profusion. Ureaplasmas are less likely to be pathogenic and *M. genitalium* does not seem to be involved at all.

Pyelonephritis

Over 30 years ago *M. hominis* was isolated, sometimes in pure culture, from the upper urinary tract of almost 10% of patients with acute pyelonephritis, occasionally accompanied by an antibody response, but not from patients with noninfectious urinary tract diseases. However, there has never been confirmation that *M. hominis* is responsible for a few cases of acute pyelonephritis or acute exacerbations of chronic pyelonephritis.

Urinary calculi

Animal model and human isolation studies have suggested that ureaplasmas, which have a urease, could be involved in the development of urinary calculi, but proof is lacking.

Other conditions

There is no confirmation that ureaplasmas are associated with male or female infertility. Mycoplasmas are not apparently related to fibromyalgia, chronic fatigue syndrome, or the Gulf War syndrome.

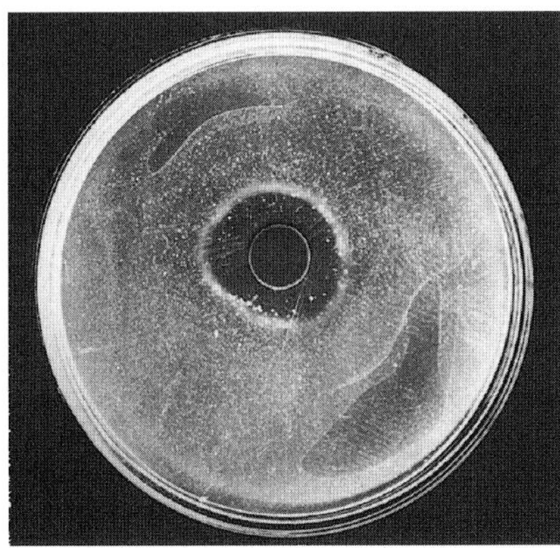

Fig. 7.6.45.7 Mycoplasma identification by agar growth inhibition. Colony development inhibited around a filter-paper disc impregnated with specific antiserum. Note also antibody–antigen precipitation at edge of inhibition zone.

Laboratory diagnosis of mycoplasmal infections

M. pneumoniae infection

The diagnosis is made by culture, molecular methods, and/or serology. The complex culture media for *M. pneumoniae* isolation contain glucose, selective antibiotics, and a pH indicator (phenol red). The fluid medium, inoculated with sputum, throat washing, pharyngeal swab, or other specimen, is incubated at 37°C and a colour change (red to yellow) signals the fermentation of glucose (Table 7.6.45.1) with production of acid, due to multiplication of the organisms. This preliminary identification may be confirmed by subculturing to agar medium and demonstrating inhibition of colony development by specific antiserum (Fig. 7.6.45.7) or by immunofluorescence of colonies with an *M. pneumoniae*-specific antibody.

Culture may take as long as 5 weeks, and consequently it is of limited value in clinical diagnosis. Rapid detection of *M. pneumoniae* by PCR has become routine in some settings. Serological testing by complement fixation is still undertaken in some laboratories. Recent infection is indicated by a fourfold or greater rise in antibody titre with a peak at about 3 to 4 weeks after disease onset, but this occurs in only about 80% of cases. A high titre (1:128 or greater) in a single serum is suggestive but not proof of infection in the previous few weeks or months; a fourfold or greater fall in antibody titre, perhaps over 6 months, may be helpful, but may be difficult to relate to a particular prior illness. The complement-fixation test does not distinguish between *M. pneumoniae* and *M. genitalium*. A more accurate diagnosis is made using a specific IgM microimmunofluorescence test which confirms a current infection or one within the previous few weeks. IgM detection is much less reliable in reinfection, which is most often the case in adults. This also applies to commercially available enzyme immunoassays specific for IgM which are used more routinely. Cold agglutinins, detected by agglutination of O Rh-negative erythrocytes at 4°C, also correlate with specific IgM and are suggestive of a recent *M. pneumoniae* infection, but the test is rarely used as it is not specific.

Genitourinary and other infections

Swabs from the urethra or cervix/vagina provide a slightly more sensitive means of collecting specimens for mycoplasmal isolation than urine specimens. Ureaplasmas and *M. hominis* usually show evidence of growth in culture media within 1 to 5 days. Primary isolation of *M. genitalium* is difficult and may take 50 days or more, so that PCR is used to detect this mycoplasma. A PCR assay also identifies *M. fermentans* and *U. urealyticum*/*U. parvum*.

M. hominis cultured on agar medium produces colonies of ca 200 to 300 µm diameter, whereas ureaplasma colonies are tiny (15–60 µm) (Fig. 7.6.45.8a) but can be seen more easily on medium containing manganous sulphate (Fig. 7.6.45.8b). *M. hominis* may grow on ordinary blood agar where it produces nonhaemolytic pinpoint colonies after extended incubation. Ureaplasma colonies are too small to be detected on blood agar, but occasionally a scrape from the agar surface will yield ureaplasmas when inoculated into ureaplasma medium. In a few research laboratories only, serological tests have been used to detect antibodies to *M. hominis*, *M. genitalium*, and the ureaplasmas.

Treatment

M. pneumoniae infections

M. pneumoniae is sensitive to the bacteriostatic tetracyclines and erythromycin. The newer macrolides, such as clarithromycin and azithromycin, are very active *in vitro*, but their clinical effect is not documented extensively in randomized clinical trials. The newer quinolones, such as moxifloxacin, are also highly active *in vitro*. They should not be used as first-line therapy but, as they are bactericidal, they may have a role in immunosuppressed patients. Recently, a rapid increase in high-level macrolide resistance in *M. pneumoniae* has been reported among infected patients in Asia but there have been only sporadic cases in Europe.

The value of tetracyclines was shown first in a controlled trial in military recruits in the United States of America in whom

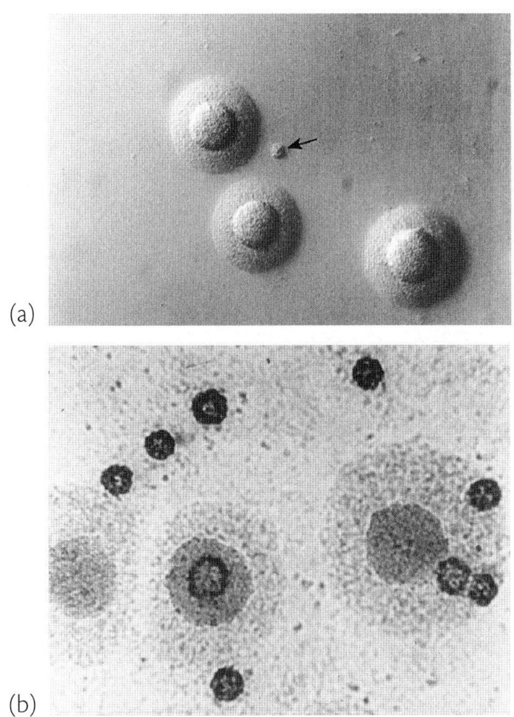

Fig. 7.6.45.8 (a) A ureaplasma colony (15 µm diameter) (arrow) adjacent to colonies of *M. hominis* (90 µm diameter) grown from urethral exudate. Oblique light, magnification ×68. (b) Dark ureaplasma colonies with colonies of *M. hominis* on agar containing manganous sulphate. Magnification ×136.

Table 7.6.45.5 Susceptibility of some genital mycoplasmas to various antibiotics. A combination of *in vitro* susceptibility data and clinical efficacy is given where such experience is available

Antibiotics	*M. hominis*	*M. fermentans*	*U. urealyticum*	*M. genitalium*
Tetracyclines				
Tetracycline	+	+	+	±
Doxycycline	++	++	++	±
Macrolides				
Erythromycin	–	±	+	+
Clarithromycin	–	±	++	++
Azithromycin	–	±	+	+++[a]
Lincosamides				
Clindamycin	+++	++	±	±
Quinolones				
Ciprofloxacin	+	++	+	+
Ofloxacin	+	++	+	+
Moxifloxacin	++	+++	++	+++

+++, extremely sensitive; ++, highly sensitive; +, moderately sensitive; ±, weakly sensitive; –, insensitive; [a], high-level macrolide resistance may be common in settings where azithomycin 1 g single dose is commonly used.

demethylchlortetracycline significantly reduced the duration of fever, pulmonary infiltration, and other signs and symptoms. In civilian practice, antimicrobials may prove less effective, probably because disease is often well established before treatment begins. Nevertheless, treatment with an antimicrobial is worthwhile. Erythromycin rather than a tetracycline is often used for pregnant women and children, although with reluctance by some. The newer antibiotics should not be ignored. Successful treatment of disease with bacteriostatic drugs does not always correlate with eradication of intracellular organisms from the respiratory tract. Relapse may be avoided by giving antibiotics for at least 10 days. It is uncertain whether early treatment prevents complications but it should start as soon as possible, even if there is only clinical evidence and a suggestive single antibody titre.

Corticosteroids in conjunction with antimicrobials appear to have been helpful in patients with severe pneumonia and erythema multiforme.

Genitourinary and other infections

Antimicrobial susceptibility of the mycoplasma species found most commonly in the urogenital tract is presented in Table 7.6.45.5 as a combination of *in vitro* susceptibility data and clinical experience. Treatment must take into account the fact that several different microorganisms may be involved and that a precise microbiological diagnosis is not available. Patients with NGU should receive an antibiotic with activity against *C. trachomatis*, ureaplasmas, and *M. genitalium*. Azithromycin is being used increasingly for chlamydial infections and is also active against a wide range of mycoplasmas, including *M. genitalium* and, to a lesser extent, ureaplasmas. However, in settings where azithomycin 1 g single dose is used as the first-line therapy for NGU and cervicitis, development of high-level macrolide resistance may be common. Such development of resistance is less common where azithromycin is given as 500 mg day 1 followed by 250 mg o.d days 2–5. This is a better option than using one of the tetracyclines since *M. genitalium* is less sensitive to these antibiotics and 10% or more of ureaplasmas are resistant to tetracyclines. If resistance does occur, patients may require a quinolone with a good Gram-positive spectrum, such as moxifloxacin.

A broad-spectrum antibiotic should also be included in the treatment of pelvic inflammatory disease to cover *C. trachomatis*, *M. hominis*, and *M. genitalium*. Since 20% or more of *M. hominis* strains are resistant to tetracyclines, other antibiotics such as clindamycin or fluoroquinolones may be needed.

Prevention of infection

M. pneumoniae infection or disease may occur despite high titres of serum mycoplasmacidal antibody. The correlation between the presence of IgA in respiratory secretions and resistance to *M. pneumoniae* disease endorses the importance of local immune factors in resistance. IgA could prevent attachment of organisms to respiratory epithelial cells. Protective immunity also depends on the severity of infection. Thus, in one study, patients with nonpneumonic illness were susceptible to an epidemic occurring 5 years later, whereas those with *M. pneumoniae* pneumonia were protected until the following epidemic 10 years later.

No efficient antimycoplasma vaccine has been developed for human use. Vaccination against *M. pneumoniae* has been attempted. Formalin-inactivated vaccines prevented mycoplasmal pneumonia in only one- to two-thirds of subjects, perhaps because they failed to stimulate cell-mediated immunity and/or local antibody. Live attenuated vaccines, containing temperature-sensitive mutants of *M. pneumoniae*, have not been considered safe for general human use. Recombinant DNA vaccines involving P1 and other proteins, or a recombinant vaccine developed by cloning part of the *M. pneumoniae P1* gene into an adenovirus vector, may offer greater success in the future.

Further reading

Haggerty CL (2008). Evidence for a role of *Mycoplasma genitalium* in pelvic inflammatory disease. *Curr Opin Infect Dis*, **21**, 65–9.

Herrmann R, Ruppert T (2006). Proteome of *Mycoplasma pneumoniae*. *Methods Biochem Anal*, **49**, 39–56.

Jensen JS (2006). *Mycoplasma genitalium* infections. Diagnosis, clinical aspects, and pathogenesis. *Dan Med Bull*, **53**, 1–27.

Maniloff J (ed) (1992). Mycoplasmas. *Molecular biology and pathogenesis*. American Society for Microbiology, Washington, DC.

McGarrity GJ, Kotani H, Butler GH (1992). Mycoplasmas in tissue culture cells. In: Maniloff J (ed) *Mycoplasmas. Molecular biology and pathogenesis*, pp. 445–54. American Society for Microbiology, Washington, DC

Razin S, Tully JG (ed) (1996). *Molecular and diagnostic procedures in mycoplasmology*, vol. **1**. *Molecular characterization*. Academic Press, London.

Razin S, Yogev D, Naot Y (1998). Molecular biology and pathogenicity of mycoplasmas. *Microbiol Mol Biol Rev*, **62**, 1094–156.

Sutherland ER, Martin RJ (2007). Asthma and atypical bacterial infection. *Chest*, **132**, 1962–6.

Taylor-Robinson D (1996). Infection due to species of *Mycoplasma* and *Ureaplasma*: an update. *Clin Infect Dis*, **23**, 671–84.

Taylor-Robinson D (1996). Mycoplasmas and their role in human respiratory tract disease. In: Myint S, Taylor-Robinson D (eds) *Viral and other infections of the human respiratory tract*, pp. 319–39. Chapman & Hall, London.

Taylor-Robinson D (2007). The role of mycoplasmas in pregnancy outcome. *Best Pract Res Clin Obstet Gynaecol*, **21**, 425–38.

Taylor-Robinson D, Bebear C (1997). Antibiotic susceptibilities of mycoplasmas and treatment of mycoplasmal infections. *J Antimicrob Chemother*, **40**, 622–30.

Taylor-Robinson D, Keat A (2001). How can a causal role for small bacteria in chronic inflammatory arthritis be established or refuted? *Ann Rheum Dis*, **60**, 177–84.

Taylor-Robinson D, Gilroy CB, Jensen JS (2000). The biology of *Mycoplasma genitalium*. *Venereology*, **13**, 119–27.

Tully JG, Razin S (ed) (1996). *Molecular and diagnostic procedures in mycoplasmology*, vol. **2**. *Diagnostic procedures*. Academic Press, London.

7.6.46 A check list of bacteria associated with infection in humans

J. Paul

Essentials

In addition to the relatively small number of well-known pathogenic bacteria that are able to infect otherwise healthy people, e.g. *Staphylococcus aureus*, *Mycobacterium tuberculosis*, and *Streptococcus pyogenes*, there is a steadily growing list of less well known organisms, many of which are able to cause disease only under special circumstances.

All bacteria associated with infections in humans are listed in the table that forms the bulk of this chapter, which has been designed to serve as a single port of call for clinicians who seek concise information on the less well known clinically significant bacteria. Every name in the table has been checked to see that it has 'standing in nomenclature': widely used names that do not have standing in nomenclature (at the time of writing) are included, but written in inverted commas (e.g. *'Spirillum minus'* – one of the causes of rat bite fever). For an up to date check on nomenclature, the reader is referred to http://www.bacterio.cict.fr/. Reported antibiotic susceptibilities and treatments are listed as a rough guide only: for some organisms the only available published information consists of *in vitro* test results for small numbers of strains, or apparent clinical response to therapy for a single case. There is no substitute for the determination of the susceptibilities of organisms as they are cultured on a case by case basis in tandem with the monitoring of therapeutic response.

Geographical restriction and particular exposures—some pathogenic bacteria, e.g. *Burkholderia pseudomallei* (the cause of melioidosis), are associated with special geographical areas; others are associated with particular forms of exposure, e.g. some *Actinobacillus* species with animal bites, and *Rickettsia* species with tick bites.

Bacterial commensals and usually harmless environmental organisms as causes of disease—given the right kind of help, bacteria that live usually as harmless human commensals can cause disease, e.g. skin commensals such as *Staphylococcus epidermidis* can cause line sepsis and infect prosthetic devices; gut commensals such as *Bacteroides* species can grow in abscesses; and oral commensals such as *Streptococcus salivarius* can cause endocarditis. Immunosuppressed patients, ventilated patients, and patients undergoing continuous ambulatory peritoneal dialysis are vulnerable to infection by a wide range of otherwise harmless environmental organisms.

Improved understanding of disease processes and discovery of 'new' pathogens—a refined understanding of, e.g. periodontal disease, has resulted in the characterization of new organisms such as *Pseudoramibacter alactolyticus*, *Johnsonella ignava*, *Centipeda periodontii*, and *Capnocytophaga gingivalis*: some of these have subsequently been identified in systemic infections such as bacteraemia.

Impact of new laboratory techniques—these have revealed the presence of new species and new disease associations, e.g. *Tropheryma whipplei* was associated with Whipple's disease by molecular methods before the organism was cultured; molecular methods have detected oddities like *Bradyrhyzobium elkanii* in aortic aneurysm tissue, although its role as potential pathogen is doubtful.

Changes in nomenclature—amidst the discovery of new bacteria, taxonomic rearrangements and changes in nomenclature pile on additional layers of confusion for the clinician. For example, it has been recognized that organisms formerly known as *Burkholderia cepacia* are actually a complex of several genomospecies, which have been given individual names. It is also confusing when a well-known genus is split to reflect the recognition that its composite species are a number of groups that are only distantly related, e.g. many organisms that were once known as *Bacteroides* species. New organisms will continue to be described and name changes will continue to occur.

For an up-to-date check on nomenclature, the reader is referred to http://www.bacterio.cict.fr/.

Table 7.6.46.1 A check list of bacteria associated with infection in humans

Nomenclature Genus (synonyms, CDC alphanumeric groups)	Species and subspecies	Associated infections	Reported susceptibilities and treatments	Notes
A				
Abiotrophia adiacens—see *Granulicatella adiacens*]				
Abiotrophia	*A. defectiva*	Endophthalmitis, brain abscess, osteomyelitis, peritonitis, endocarditis	Vancomycin, ceftriaxone (plus gentamicin or rifampicin)	Previously known as nutritionally deficient or variant streptococci
[*Abiotrophia elegans*—see *Granulicatella elegans*]				
['*Abiotrophia para-adiacens*'—see *Granulicatella* notes]				
Achromobacter (*Alcaligenes*)	*A. denitrificans* *A. insolitus* *A. piechaudii* *A. ruhlandii* *A. spanius* *A. xylosoxidans*	Septicaemia, CAPD peritonitis, pneumonia, ear infection, pulmonary infection in cystic fibrosis, keratitis, vascular line sepsis	Ureidopenicillins, ceftazidime, carbapenems	
[*Achromobacter* CDC group Vd and *Achromobacter* groups A, C, and D—see *Ochrobactrum*]				
[*Achromobacter* groups B and E—see *Pannonibacter*]				
Acidaminococcus	*A. fermentans*	Abscesses, postsurgical infections	Metronidazole	
Acidovorax (*Pseudomonas*)	*A. avenae* *A. delafieldii* *A. facilis* *A. temperans*	Wound infection, UTI, bacteraemia, meningitis, septic arthritis		
Acinetobacter	*A. baumannii* *A. calcoaceticus* *A. haemolyticus* *A. johnsonii* *A. junii* *A. lwoffi* *A. parvus* *A. radioresistens* *A. schindleri* *A. ursingii*	Septicaemia, UTI, wound infections, abscesses, endocarditis, meningitis, osteomyelitis	Aminoglycosides, ureidopenicillins, ceftazidime, carbapenems, tigecycline	May be multiresistant. Nosocomial outbreaks reported. Infections associated with debilitated patients
Actinobacillus	*A. actinomycetemcomitans* (*Haemophilus actinomycetemcomitans*)	Periodontitis, endocarditis, abscesses, pericarditis, meningitis	Penicillin (plus gentamicin for endocarditis)	Human oral commensal. The genus *Aggregatibacter* has been proposed to accommodate *A. actinomycetemcomitans* and some *Haemophilus* spp.
	A. equuli *A. lignieresii* *A. suis*	Wound infection, abscesses, endocarditis, meningitis	Ampicillin (plus gentamicin for endocarditis)	Associated with animal contact and bites
	A. hominis	Septicaemia, empyema	Amoxicillin–clavulanate	
	A. ureae (*Pasteurella ureae*)	Meningitis, pneumonia, endocarditis, hepatitis, peritonitis	Ampicillin (plus gentamicin for endocarditis), chloramphenicol	Respiratory tract commensal in humans

Actinobaculum	*A. massiliense* *A. schaalii* *A. urinale*	Pyelonephritis, UTI, septicaemia, superficial skin infection	Penicillin, cefuroxime, nitrofurantoin, tetracycline, clindamycin	
Actinomadura	*A. Latina* *A. madurae* *A. pelletieri* *A. vinacea*	Actinomycetoma, Madura foot	Co-trimoxazole, dapsone	
Actinomyces	*A. cardiffensis* *A. dentalis* *A. europaeus* *A. funkei* *A. georgiae* *A. gerencseriae* *A. graevenitzii* *A. hongkongensis* *A. israelii* *A. meyeri* *A. naeslundii* *A. neuii neuii* *A. neuii anitratus* *A. odontolyticus* *A. oricola* *A. radicidentis* *A. radingae* *A. turicensis* *A. urogenitalis* *A. viscosus*	Actinomycosis	β-Lactams	
Advenella	*A. incenata*	Pulmonary infection, bacteraemia		
Aerococcus	*A. sanguinicola* *A. urinae* *A. urinaehominis* *A. viridans*	Endocarditis, UTI, wounds, meningitis, abscesses, CAPD peritonitis, lymphadenitis, spondodactylitis	Penicillin, vancomycin (plus gentamicin for endocarditis)	
Aeromonas	*A. allosaccharophila* *A. bestiarumA. Caviae* *A. enteropelogenes* *A. hydrophila* *A. jandaei* *A. media* *A. salmonicida* *A. schubertii* *A. trota (A. tructi)* *A. veronii*	Wound infection, abscesses, septicaemia, meningitis, leech-bite infection, alligator-bite infection, acute diarrhoea	Aminoglycosides, chloramphenicol, ceftazidime, co-trimoxazole	Infections associated with aquatic exposure. *A. veronii*includes biovars Veronii and Sobria. The taxonomic status of some species is unclear. The status of *A. allosaccharophila* is controversial. *A. trota* may be a synonym of *A. enteropelogenes*

(*Continued*)

Table 7.6.46.1 (*Cont'd*) A check list of bacteria associated with infection in humans

Nomenclature		Associated infections	Reported susceptibilities and treatments	Notes
Genus	Species and subspecies			
(synonyms, CDC alphanumeric groups)				
Afipia	*A. felis*	Cat-scratch disease	Imipenem, aminoglycosides	Cat-scratch disease is associated also with *Bartonella* spp.
	A. broomeae	Bone marrow infection, septic arthritis	Imipenem, aminoglycosides	Role as pathogen uncertain
	A. clevelandensis	Bone infection	Imipenem, aminoglycosides	Role as pathogen uncertain
	A. birgiae *A. massiliensis*	Pneumonia	Imipenem, aminoglycosides	Roles as pathogens uncertain
Agrobacterium	*A. radiobacter* (*A. tumefaciens*)	Endocarditis, CAPD peritonitis, UTI, line sepsis	Co-trimoxazole, gentamicin, amikacin, piperacillin-tazobactam	The nomenclature of this taxon is unsettled. The names *A. tumefaciens* and *A. radiobacter* both have standing in nomenclature. Transfer of *Agrobacterium* to *Rhizobium* has been proposed
[*Alcaligenes denitrificans*—see *Achromobacter denitrificans*]				
Alcaligenes	*A. faecalis* *A. latus*	Pneumonia, otitis, UTI, osteomyelitis, bacteraemia	Amoxicillin–clavulanate, cephalosporins, fluoroquinolones	
[*Alcaligenes xylosoxidans*—see *Achromobacter xylosoxidans xylosoxidans*]				
[*Alcaligenes piechaudii*—see *Achromobacter piechaudii*]				
[*Alcaligenes ruhlandii*—see *Achromobacter ruhlandii*]				
Alishewanella	*A. fetalis*	From fetal necropsy specimen		Clinical significance uncertain
Alistipes	*A. finegoldii* (*Bacteroides finegoldii*) *A. onderdonkii* *A. putredinis* (*Bacteroides putredinis*) *A. shahii*	Appendicitis, peritonitis, abdominal abscess	Metronidazole, ertapenem	β-Lactamase producers. Abdominal infections, found in association with other anaerobes
Alloiococcus	*A. otitis* (Alliococcus otitis)	Otitis media	Vancomycin	
[*Amycolata autotrophica*—see *Pseudonocardia autotrophica*]				
Amycolatopsis	*A. orientalis* (Nocardia orientalis)			Role as pathogen uncertain
	A. palatopharyngis	Palatopharyngeal infection		Clinical significance poorly defined
Anaerobiospirillum	*A. succiniproducens* *A. thomasii*	Diarrhoea, bacteraemia	Cefuroxime, tetracycline, chloramphenicol	Infection may be related to exposure to cat or dog faeces
Anaerococcus (*Peptostreptococcus*)	*A. hydrogenalis* *A. lactolyticus* *A. octavius* *A. prevotii* *A. tetradius* *A. vaginalis*	Mixed anaerobic infections, abscesses	β-Lactams, metronidazole	
Anaeroglobus	*A. geminatus*	From postoperative collection		Role as pathogen uncertain
Anaerorhabdus (*Bacteroides*)	*A. furcosus*	Lung abscess, appendix and abdominal abscesses		

[*'Anguillina coli'*—see *Serpulina pilosicoli*]				
Anaplasma	*A. phagocytophilum*	Anaplasmosis	Doxycycline	Previously known as human granulocytic ehrlichiosis
[*Arachnia propionica*—see *Propionibacterium propionicus*]				
Arcanobacterium	*A. haemolyticum (Corynebacterium haemolyticum)*	Tonsillitis, cellulitis, lymphadenopathy, brain abscess, septicaemia, osteomyelitis	Penicillin, erythromycin	
	A. bernardiae (Actinomyces bernardiae)	UTI, septicaemia, septic arthritis	β-Lactams	Previously known as CDC coryneform group 2
	A. pyogenes (Actinomyces pyogenes)	Septic arthritis	β-Lactams	
Arcobacter (Campylobacter)	*A. butzleri* *A. cryaerophilus*	Abdominal cramps, diarrhoea		Self-limiting
Arthrobacter	*A. albus* *A. creatinolyticus* *A. cumminsii* *A. luteolus* *A. oxydans* *A. scleromae* *A. woluwensis*	UTI, bacteraemia, skin infection	Vancomycin, penicillins	*Arthrobacter* sp. has been implicated in Whipple's syndrome, a disease usually associated with *Tropheryma whipplei*
Atopobium	*A. minutum (Lactobacillus minutus)* *A. parvulum (Streptococcus parvulus)* *A. rimae (Lactobacillus rimae)*	UTI, dental abscesses, pelvic abscesses, wound infection		Isolates from periodontal sites suggest possible role in periodontal disease
	A. vaginae	Bacterial vaginosis		
[*Aureobacterium*—see *Microbacterium*]				
Azospirillum	*A. brasilense (Roseomonas fauriae)*	CAPD peritonitis, line sepsis	Imipenem, aminoglycosides, ceftriaxone, ciprofloxacin	
B				
Bacillus	*B. anthracis*	Anthrax	Penicillin, erythromycin	Ciprofloxacin for postexposure prophylaxis
[*Bacillus brevis*—see *Brevibacillus agri*]				
	B. circulans *B. coagulans* *B. megaterium* *B. mycoides* *B. sphaericus* *B. thuringiensis*	Pneumonia, septicaemia, corneal infections, meningitis, food poisoning, eye infection, lung infection	Vancomycin, clindamycin, aminoglycosides, imipenem, penicillin	Other than the well-known *B. anthracis* and *B. cereus*, *Bacillus* spp. are rare causes of focal and systemic sepsis. Some isolates are resistant to vancomycin. Isolates may represent specimen or laboratory contamination. *B. thuringiensis* is a biological insecticide which has caused corneal infection
	B. cereus *B. licheniformis* *B. pumilus* *B. subtilis*	Food poisoning, wound infection, cutaneous lesions, bacteraemia, endocarditis, eye infection	Clindamycin, vancomycin, gentamicin	Diarrhoea is self-limiting. *B. cereus* is resistant to β-lactams

(*Continued*)

Table 7.6.46.1 (*Cont'd*) A check list of bacteria associated with infection in humans

Nomenclature		**Associated infections**	**Reported susceptibilities and treatments**	**Notes**
Genus	**Species and subspecies**			
(synonyms, CDC alphanumeric groups)				
Bacteroides	*B. caccae* *B. capillosus* *B. coagulans* *B. eggerthii* B. finegoldii *B. fragilis* B. massiliensis B. nordii *B. ovatus* *B. pyogenes* *B. salyersae* *B. splanchinicus* *B. stercoris* *B. tectus* *B. thetaiotaomicron* *B. uniformis* *B. ureolyticus* *B. vulgatus*	Abscesses, bacteraemia, bite infections, wound infections, chronic otitis media, pelvic inflammatory disease, neonatal sepsis	Ureidopenicillins, carbapenems, metronidazole	Resistance to metronidazole and β-lactams has been reported. Many species previously classified as Bacteroides have been transferred to other genera: see *Alistipes*, *Anaerorhabdus*, *Campylobacter*, *Dialister Mitsuokella*, *Parabacteroides*, *Prevotella*, *Porphyromonas*, and *Tannerella*
Balneatrix	*B. alpica*	Pneumonia, bacteraemia, meningitis	Ceftriaxone, ofloxacin, amoxicillin, netilmicin	Infection associated with exposure to hot spring water
Bartonella	*B. bacilliformis*	Oroya fever, verruga peruana	Chloramphenicol, streptomycin	
	B. elizabethae (Rochalimaea elizabethae)	Endocarditis	Gentamicin, imipenem, co-trimoxazole	
	B. clarridgeiae *B. henselae (Rochalimaea henselae)*	Cat-scratch disease, bacillary angiomatosis	Aminoglycosides, doxycycline	Cat-scratch disease is associated also with *Afipia felis*
	B. quintana (*Rochalimaea* quintana)	Trench fever, bacillary angiomatosis	**Aminoglycosides, doxycycline**	
	B. schoenbuchensis	Deer ked dermatitis		Evidence to associate this organism with deer ked dermatitis is circumstantial
	B. vinsonii arupensis	Bacteraemia	Ceftriaxone	Zoonosis from rodents
Bergeyella	*B. zoohelcum (Weeksella zoohelcum)*	Wound infection, septicaemia, meningitis	Cefotaxime, penicillins, ciprofloxacin, tetracycline	Associated with dog and cat bites
Bifidobacterium	*B. adolescentis* *B. angulatum* *B. bifidum* *B. dentium* *B. longum (B. infantis)* *B. pseudocatenulatum*	Bacteraemia, abscesses, peritonitis, otitis, paronychia	Clindamycin, penicillins, cefoxitin	Reported risk factors include surgery, malignancy, steroid therapy, intravenous drug use, and acupuncture. Some strains used as probiotics
[*Bifidobacterium* inopinatum—see *Scardovia inopinata*]				
Bilophila	*B. wadsworthia*	Appendicitis, abscesses, bacteraemia, biliary tract sepsis, mastoiditis	Metronidazole, amoxicillin/clavulanate, ureidopenicillins, cephalosporins	
Bordetella	*B. bronchiseptica*	Respiratory tract infection	Tetracycline, fluoroquinolones	Zoonosis from dogs and other animals
	B. hinzii *B. holmesii* *B. trematum*	Bacteraemia, otitis, wound infection		*B. hinzii* is a pathogen of poultry

	B. parapertussis *B. pertussis*	Whooping cough, respiratory tract infection	Erythromycin	*B. parapertussis* causes less severe disease
Borrelia	*B. afzelii* *B. andersoni* *B. bissettii* *B. burgdorferi* *B. garinii* *B. japonica* *B. lusitaniae* *B. sinica* *B. spielmanii* *B. tanukii* *B. turdi* *B. valaisiana*	Lyme disease	Amoxicillin, doxycycline, ceftriaxone	
	B. caucasica *B. crocidurae* *B. duttonii* *B. graingeri* *B. hermsii* *B. hispanica* *B. latyschewii* *B. mazzottii* *B. parkeri* *B. persica* *B. recurrentis* *B. turicatae* *B. venezuelensis*	Relapsing fever	Tetracycline, erythromycin, chloramphenicol, penicillin	*B. recurrentis* is louse-borne; other agents are tick-borne
Bosea	*B. massiliensis*	Linked with ventilator-associated pneumonia	Doxycycline, telithromycin	Amoeba-resisting bacterium from hospital water supplies
Brachyspira	*B. aalborgi* *B. pilosicoli* (*Serpulina pilosicoli*, '*Anguillina coli*')	Intestinal spirochaetosis		Of uncertain significance
Bradyrhizobium	*B. elkanii*	Detected in tissue from aortic aneurysm		Potential role as pathogen uncertain
[*Branhamella catarrhalis*—see *Moraxella catarrhalis*]				
Brevibacillus	*B. centrosporus*	Bacteraemia	Vancomycin	Previously confused with *B. laterosporus* and reported as such in clinical literature
	B. parabrevis	Bacteraemia, abscess	Vancomycin	
Brevibacterium	*B. casei* *B. epidermidis* *B. luteolum* (*B. lutescens*) *B. mcbrellneri* *B. otitidis* *B. paucivorans*	Bacteraemia, endocarditis, meningitis, chest infection, pericarditis, vascular catheter sepsis	Glycopeptides	

(*Continued*)

Table 7.6.46.1 (*Cont'd*) A check list of bacteria associated with infection in humans

Nomenclature		Associated infections	Reported susceptibilities and treatments	Notes
Genus	**Species and subspecies**			
(synonyms, CDC alphanumeric groups)				
Brevundimonas (*Pseudomonas*)	*B. diminuta* *B. vesicularis*	Septicaemia, endocarditis	Cefazolin, ceftriaxone, piperacillin (plus gentamicin for endocarditis)	
Brucella	*B. abortus* *B. canis* *B. melitensis* *B. suis*	Brucellosis	Doxycycline (plus streptomycin or rifampicin)	The four species names used for clinical purposes represent biovars of a single species, *B. melitensis*
Bulleidia	*B. extructa*	Necrotizing ulcerative periodontitis in HIV patients		
Burkholderia (*Pseudomonas*)	*B. ambifaria* *B. anthina* *B. cenocepacia* *B. cepacia* (*Pseudomonas cepacia*) *B. dolosa* *B. multivorans* *B. pyrrocinia* *B. stabilis* *B. vietnamiensis*	Lung infection in cystic fibrosis, bacteraemia, endocarditis, septic arthritis, UTI	Ureidopenicillins, ceftazidime, aztreonam, carbapenems, fluoroquinolones, co-trimoxazole	*B. cepacia sensu stricto* and other taxa listed are genomospecies of the *B. cepacia* species complex (*B. cepacia sensu lato*). Hard to differentiate by routine methods. Differences in disease progression in cystic fibrosis may relate to different genomospecies
	B. gladioli (*Pseudomonas gladioli*)	Lung infection in cystic fibrosis	Ureidopenicillins, ceftazidime, aztreonam, carbapenems, fluoroquinolones, co-trimoxazole	
	B. fungorum	Septic arthritis, bacteraemia, meningitis	Amoxicillin, cefuroxime, ceftazidime, ciprofloxacin, meropenem, co-trimoxazole	
	B. mallei (*Pseudomonas mallei*)	Glanders	Sulfadiazine, co-amoxiclav, tetracycline, co-trimoxazole	
	B. pseudomallei (*Pseudomonas pseudomallei*)	Melioidosis	Ceftazidime, co-trimoxazole, chloramphenicol, imipenem	
Buttiauxella	*B. agrestis* *B. noackiae*	Appendicitis, wound infection	Aminoglycosides, doxycycline	Cephalosporin resistance reported
Butyrivibrio	*B. fibrisolvens*	Endophthalmitis	Penicillin, chloramphenicol	From rumina of farm animals
C				
[*Calymmatobacterium granulomatis*—see *Klebsiella granulomatis*]				
[*Campylobacter butzleri*—see *Arcobacter butzleri*]				
[*Campylobacter cinaedi*—see *Helicobacter cinaedi*]				
[*Campylobacter fennelliae*—see *Helicobacter fennelliae*]				
[*Campylobacter pyloridis*—see *Helicobacter pylori*]				
Campylobacter	*C. coli* *C. jejuni jejuni* *C. jejuni doylei* *C. mucosalis*	Gastroenteritis, bacteraemia	Erythromycin, fluoroquinolones	Infections are usually self-limiting

	C. concisus *C. curvus* (*Wolinella curva*) *C. gracilis* (*Bacteroides gracilis*) *C. rectus* (*Wolinella recta*) *C. showae* *C. sputorum*	Periodontitis, appendicitis, peritonitis, head and neck infections, abscesses	Ureidopenicillins, amoxicillin/clavulanate, carbapenems, fluoroquinolones, metronidazole	
	C. fetus fetus	Fever, diarrhoea, meningoencephalitis, endocarditis, abscesses	Erythromycin, ampicillin, chloramphenicol, gentamicin	
	C. fetus venerealis	Bacterial vaginosis		Role as human pathogen poorly defined. Reported from faeces of homosexual men
	C. hyointestinalis *C. lari* (*C. laridis*) *C. upsalensis*	Diarrhoea, bacteraemia, abscess	Erythromycin, ampicillin, gentamicin	Zoonoses from mammals and birds
Capnocytophaga	*C. canimorsus* (CDC DF-1) *C. cynodegmi* (CDC DF-2)	Wound infection, septicaemia, abscesses, meningitis, endocarditis	Penicillin	From dog bites
	C. gingivalis *C. granulose* *C. haemolytica* *C. ochracea* *C. sputigena*	Periodontitis, septicaemia	Penicillins, ciprofloxacin, tetracycline, chloramphenicol	From oral flora. Infections associated with malignancy and neutropenia
Cardiobacterium	*C. hominis* *C. valvarum*	Endocarditis, meningitis	Penicillin (plus gentamicin for endocarditis)	
Catonella	*C. morbi*	Periodontitis, endodontic infection		Role as pathogen unclear
CDC EF-4		Bite infections	β-Lactams	
Cedecea	*C. davisae* *C. lapagei* *C. neterii*	Bacteraemia	Chloramphenicol, cefamandole, gentamicin	Two other species (sp. 3 and sp. 5) have been isolated from clinical specimens
Cellulomonas	*C. denverensis* *C. hominis* (CDC coryneform group A-3)	Bacteraemia, meningitis, pilonidal abscess, wound infection, homograft valve infection	Clarithromycin, clindamycin, imipenem, minocycline, rifampicin, vancomycin	
[*Cellulomonas cellulans*—see *Cellulosomicrobium*]				
[*Cellulomonas turbata*—see *Oerskovia turbata*]				
Cellulosimicrobium	*C. cellulans* (*Cellulomonas cellulans*, *Oerskovi xanthineolytica*) *C. funkei*	Meningitis, pyonephrosis, CAPD peritonitis, endophthalmitis	Vancomycin and gentamicin or rifampicin	
Centipeda	*C. periodontii*	Periodontitis		Role as pathogen unclear. Shown to inhibit lymphocytes
Chlamydia	*C. trachomatis*	Trachoma, genital infection, neonatal infection, lymphogranuloma venereum	Erythromycin, tetracycline, azithromycin	Includes 18 serovars clustered into two biovars: trachoma and lymphogranuloma venereum
Chlamydophila	*C. abortus* (*Chlamydia psittaci*)	Abortion		Associated with contact with infected ruminants

(*Continued*)

Table 7.6.46.1 (*Cont'd*) A check list of bacteria associated with infection in humans

Nomenclature Genus (synonyms, CDC alphanumeric groups)	Species and subspecies	Associated infections	Reported susceptibilities and treatments	Notes
	C. pneumoniae (*Chlamydia pneumoniae*)	Chest infection	Tetracycline	Infections in humans associated with biovars TWAR
	C. psittaci (*Chlamydia psittaci*)	Psittacosis	Tetracycline	Zoonosis from birds
Chromobacterium	*C. violaceum*	Septicaemia, osteomyelitis, abscesses, eye infection	Erythromycin, tetracycline, chloramphenicol, gentamicin	Associated with exposure to soil and water
Chryseobacterium (*Flavobacterium*)	*C. gleum* *C. indologenes*	Bacteraemia, abdominal sepsis, vascular catheter sepsis	Piperacillin-tazobactam, minocycline, fluorquinolones, rifampicin	Susceptibilities vary. Often multiresistant
[*Chryseobacterium meningosepticum*—see *Elizabethkingia meningoseptica*]				
[*Chryseomonas luteola*—see *Pseudomonas luteola*]				
Citrobacter	*C. amalonaticus* *C. braakii* *C. diversus* *C. farmeri* *C. freundii* *C. gilenii* *C. koseri* *C. murliniae* *C. rodentium* *C. sedlakii* *C. werkmanii* *C. youngae*	UTI, meningitis, bacteraemia, haemolytic–uraemic syndrome	Aminoglycosides, β-lactams	Variable susceptibility. May be multiresistant. Nosocomial outbreaks of infection reported. *Citrobacter spp. are part of the normal faecal flora*
Clostridium	*C. argentinense* *C. baratii* *C. beijerinckii* *C. bifermentans* C. bolteae *C. butyricum* *C. cadaveris* *C. carnis* *C. celatum* *C. clostridioforme* *C. cochlearium* *C. cocleatum* *C. fallax* *C. ghonii* *C. glycolicum* *C. haemolyticum* *C. histolyticum* *C. indolis* *C. innocuum* *C. irregulare*	Wound infection, bacteraemia, abscesses	Penicillin, clindamycin, metronidazole	Many *Clostridium*spp. have been isolated form clinical specimens. For most, their clinical significance is poorly defined. *C. baratii*and*C. butyricum* are rare causes of botulism. *C. fallax*, *C. histolyticum*, *C. novyi*, *C. septicum*, and *C. sordellii* are gas-gangrene agents. Treatment of gas gangrene includes debridement and penicillin, clindamycin, or metronidazole

	C. leptum *C. limosum* *C. malenominatum* *C. novyi* *C. oroticum* *C. paraputrificum* *C. piliforme* *C. putrefasciens* *C. ramosum* *C. sardiniense* (*C. absonum*) *C. septicum* *C. sordellii* *C. sphenoides* *C. sporogenes* *C. subterminale* *C. symbiosum* *C. tertium*			
	C. botulinum	Botulism		Antitoxin and respiratory support as treatment
	C. difficile	Diarrhoea, pseudomembranous colitis	**Metronidazole, vancomycin**	Infection associated with antibiotic exposure
	C. perfringens	Food poisoning, necrotizing enterocolitis, gas gangrene		Debridement and penicillin, clindamycin, or metronidazole for treatment of gas gangrene
	C. tetani	Tetanus	**Metronidazole, penicillin**	Antitoxin and supportive treatment
Collinsella	*C. aerofaciens*			From faecal flora. Clinical significance is undefined
[*Comamonas acidovorans*—see *Delftia acidovorans*]				
Comamonas (Pseudomonas)	*C. terrigena* *C. testosteroni*	Bacteraemia, UTI, conjunctivitis, endocarditis, wound infection, abdominal abscess, peritonitis, meningitis	Ureidopenicillins, ceftazidime, ciprofloxacin, aminoglycosides, imipenem	Infections in neutropenic patients. Infections associated with animal bite and exposure to tropical fish
Corynebacterium	*C. accolens* *C. afermentans* *C. amycolatum* C. appendicis *C. argentoratense* *C. atypicum* *C. aurimucosum* (*C. nigricans*) *C. auris* *C. bovis* *C. confusum* *C. coyleae* *C. durum* *C. falsenii* C. freneyi	Septicaemia, peritonitis, UTI, eye infection, wound infection, endocarditis, osteomyelitis, septic arthritis, meningitis, abscesses	Glycopeptides, β-lactam, erythromycin, rifampicin	More than 40 *Corynebacterium* spp. have been isolated from clinical specimens. For many of them, clinical significance and empirical therapy are poorly defined. Many isolates are susceptible to β-lactams. Multiresistant, vancomycin-susceptible isolates of CDC coryneform group G-2, *C. jeikeium* and *C. urealyticum*have been reported. Nosocomial outbreaks have been reported. *Corynebacterium*spp. may be specimen or laboratory contaminants. CDC coryneform groups 1, E, F-1, and G-2 await designation of scientific names

(*Continued*)

Table 7.6.46.1 (*Cont'd*) A check list of bacteria associated with infection in humans

Nomenclature: Genus (synonyms, CDC alphanumeric groups)	Species and subspecies	Associated infections	Reported susceptibilities and treatments	Notes
	C. glucuronolyticum *C. imitans* *C. jeikeium* *C. kroppenstedtii* *C. kutscheri* *C. lipophilum* *C. macginleyi* *C. matruchotii* *C. mucifaciens* *C. pilosum* *C. propinquum* *C. renale* C. resistens *C. riegelii* *C. sanguinis* *C. singulare* *C. striatum* *C. sundsvallense* *C. thomssenii* *C. tuberculostearicum* *C. tuscaniense* *C. urealyticum* *C. xerosis*			
	C. diphtheriae	Diphtheria, cutaneous infection	Penicillin, erythromycin	Toxigenic infection requires treatment with antitoxin
	C. minutissimum	Erythrasma, bacteraemia, endocarditis		Role as an agent of erythrasma is poorly defined
	C. mycetoides	Tropical ulcer, septicaemia		
	C. pseudodiphtheriticum	UTI, endocarditis, lymphadenopathy, necrotizing tracheitis	Penicillin	
	C. pseudotuberculosis	Lymphadenitis, pulmonary infection	Penicillin, erythromycin	Associated with sheep contact. May require drainage or excision
	C. ulcerans	Diphtheria-like disease, pharyngitis	Penicillin, erythromycin	Toxigenic infection requires treatment with antitoxin
	C. vitaeruminis	Associated with aortic aneurysm		Role as pathogen uncertain
[*Corynebacterium* group A-3—see *Cellulomonas*]				
[*Corynebacterium* groups A-4 and A-5—see *Microbacterium*]				
[*Corynebacterium* group 2—see *Arcanobacterium bernardiae*]				
Coxiella	*C. burnetii*	Q fever	Tetracycline, ciprofloxacin, co-trimoxazole, rifampicin	
Cryptobacterium	*C. curtum*	Periodontitis		

Cupriavidus (*Ralstonia*) (*Wautersia*)	*C. gilardii* *C. pauculus* *C. respiraculi* *C. taiwanensis*	Meningitis, pulmonary infection in cystic fibrosis, line sepsis	Cephalosporins, imipenem, co-trimoxazole, quinolones, amikacin	
D				
Delftia	*D. acidovorans* (*Comamonas acidovorans*)	Bacteraemia, endocarditis	Ureidopenicillins, fluoroquinolones	
Dermabacter	*D. hominis*	Brain abscess, bacteraemia, wound infection	Cephalosporins, glycopeptides	
Dermacoccus	*D.* sp.	Associated with aortic aneurysm		Role as pathogen uncertain. Found on skin and mucous membranes
Dermatophilus	*D. congolensis*	Cutaneous infection	Penicillin	Zoonosis from cattle, sheep, goats, and horses
Desulfomicrobium	*D. orale*	Periodontitis		
Desulfomonas	*D. piger* (*D. pigra*)	Pilonidal cyst abscess, peritonitis		From faecal flora
Desulfovibrio	*D. desulfuricans* *D. vulgaris*	Bacteraemia, liver abscess	Penicillin, clindamycin	
	'*D. fairfieldensis*'	Cultured from urine of patient with UTI and meningoencephalitis		Proposed name does not have standing in nomenclature
Dialister	*D. invisus* *D. micraerophilus* *D. pneumosintes* *D. propionicifaciens*	Periodontitis, endodontic infection, bacteraemia		
Dichelobacter	*D. nodosus* (*Bacteroides nodosus*)	Pilonidal cyst, rectal fistula, wound infection		Cause of ovine footrot. Isolates reported from humans may not be *D. nodosus*
Dietzia	*D. maris*	Prosthetic hip infection, bacteraemia	Vancomycin, teicoplanin, rifampicin, amoxicillin, gentamicin, clindamycin, co-trimoxazole	Papillomatosis has been associated with '*Dietzia* strain X'
Dolosicoccus	*D. paucivorans*	Bacteraemia	Cephalosporins	
Dolosigranulum	*D. pigrum*	Spinal cord infection, eye infection		Significance as a pathogen poorly defined.
Dysgonomonas	*D. capnocytophagoides* (CDC group DF-3) *D. gadei* *D. mossii*	Diarrhoea, bacteraemia, abscess	Tetracycline, clindamycin, imipenem	
E				
Edwardsiella	*E. hoshinae* *E. ictaluri* *E. tarda*	Wound infection, abscesses, gastroenteritis	β-Lactams, aminoglycosides, fluoroquinolones	Aquatic exposure, penetrating fish injury
Eggerthella	*E. hongkongensis* *E. lenta* (*Eubacterium lentum*) *E. sinensis*	Rectal abscess, bacteraemia	Penicillin, metronidazole	Variable susceptibility to cefotaxime

(Continued)

Table 7.6.46.1 (*Cont'd*) A check list of bacteria associated with infection in humans

Nomenclature Genus (synonyms, CDC alphanumeric groups)	Species and subspecies	Associated infections	Reported susceptibilities and treatments	Notes
Ehrlichia	*E. chaffeensis* *E. ewingii*	Ehrlichiosis	Tetracycline, doxycycline	Antibodies to *E. muris* detected in healthy humans in Japan
[*Ehrlichia sennetsu*—see *Neorickettsia sennetsu*]				
Eikenella	*E. corrodens*	Septicaemia, endocarditis, abscesses, septic arthritis	Penicillin (plus gentamicin for endocarditis)	
Elizabethkingia	*E. meningoseptica* (*Chryseobacterium meningosepticum, Flavobacterium meningosepticum*)	Meningitis, bacteraemia, endocarditis, necrotizing fasciitis, pneumonia	Quinolones, co-trimoxazole, minocycline, rifampicin	Treatment with vancomycin is controversial
Empedobacter	*E. brevis* (*Flavobacterium breve*)	Endophthalmitis, bacteraemia, UTI	Broad-spectrum cephalosporins	Carbapenem-resistant
Enterobacter	*E. aerogenes* *E. amnigenus* *E. asburiae* *E. cancerogenus* *E. cloacae* *E. gergoviae* *E. hormaechei* *E. kobei* *E. ludwigii* *E. sakazakii*	Bacteraemia, respiratory tract infections, UTI	Carbapenems, fluoroquinolones, aminoglycosides, ureidopenicillins	May be multiresistant. Common cause of nosocomial infection
Enterococcus	*E. avium* *E. casseliflavus* (*E. flavescens*) *E. cecorum* *E. dispar* *E. durans* *E. faecalis* *E. faecium* *E. gallinarum* E. gilvus *E. hirae* *E. malodoratus* *E. mundtii* *E. pallens* *E. pseudoavium* *E. raffinosus* *E. solitarius*	Bacteraemia, abscesses, endocarditis, meningitis, UTI, peritonitis, osteomyelitis, wound infection	Penicillins, glycopeptides	May be resistant to penicillins and glycopeptides. Nosocomial outbreaks reported
Erwinia	*E. persicinus*	UTI	Cephalosporins, fluoroquinolones, aminoglycosides	The causative agent of necrosis of bean pods
Erysipelothrix	*E. rhusiopathiae*	Erysipeloid, septicaemia, endocarditis	Penicillin	Animal contact
[*Escherichia adecarboxylata*—see *Leclercia adecarboxylata*]				

Escherichia	*E. albertii*	Diarrhoea		Previously known as *Hafnia alvei*-like strains
	E. coli	UTI, bacteraemia, wound infection, meningitis, enteric infection, haemolytic fluoroquinolones, uraemic syndrome	β-Lactams, aminoglycosides, co-trimoxazole	Susceptibilities variable
	E. fergusonii	Bacteraemia, wounds, UTI	Chloramphenicol, gentamicin	Ampicillin-resistant
	E. hermanii	Wounds	Chloramphenicol, cephalosporins, gentamicin	
	E. vulneris	Wounds	Ampicillin, cephalosporins, gentamicin	
Eubacterium	*E. brachy* *E. combesii* *E. contortum* *E. cylindroids* *E. infirmum* *E. limosum* *E. minutum* *E. moniliforme* E. multiforme *E. nitrogenes* *E. nodatum* *E. plautii* *E. rectale* *E. saburreum* *E. saphenum* *E. sulci* *E. tenue* *E. timidum* *E. tortuosum* *E. ventriosum* *E. yurii yurii* *E. yurii mararetiae* *E. yurii schtitka*	Wounds, abscesses, septicaemia, periodontitis	Penicillins, clindamycin, metronidazole	
Ewingella	*E. americana*	Septicaemia, wounds, UTI	Ureidopenicillins, aminoglycosides	
Exiguobacterium	*E. acetylicum* *E. aurantiacum*	Wound infection, bacteraemia		
F				
Facklamia	*F. hominis* *F. ignava* *F. languida* *F. sourekii*	UTI, bacteraemia, abscess		

(Continued)

Table 7.6.46.1 (*Cont'd*) A check list of bacteria associated with infection in humans

Nomenclature		Associated infections	Reported susceptibilities and treatments	Notes
Genus	**Species and subspecies**			
(synonyms, CDC alphanumeric groups)				
Filifactor	*F. alocis* *F. vilosus*	Gingivitis, periodontitis		
Finegoldia	*F. magna (Peptostreptococcus) magnus*			
[*Flavimonas oryzihabitans*—see *Pseudomonas oryzihabitans*]				
Flavobacterium	*F. mizutaii* (*Sphingobacterium mizutae*)			
[*Flavobacterium gleum*—see *Chryseobacterium gleum*]				
[*Flavobacterium indologenes*—see *Chryseobacterium indologenes*]				
[*Flavobacterium meningosepticum*—see *Elizabethkingia meningoseptica*]				
'*Flexispira*'	'*F. rappini*'	Bacteraemia, diarrhoea		Not in approved lists of bacterial names. There is a growing consensus that 'Flexispira' actually represents several *Helicobacter* spp.
[*Fluoribacter bozemanae*—see *Legionella bozemanae*]				
[*Fluoribacter dumoffii*—see *Legionella dumoffii*]				
[*Fluoribacter gormanii*—see *Legionella gormanii*]				
Francisella	*F. philomiragia* (Yersinia philomiragia)	Septicaemia, invasive systemic infection	Fluoroquinolones, aminoglycosides, chloramphenicol, cefoxitin	
	F. tularensis	Tularaemia	Streptomycin, tetracycline	
Fusobacterium	*F. gonidiaformans* *F. mortiferum* *F. naviforme* *F. necrogenes* *F. necrophorum necrophorum* *F. necrophorum fundiliforme* *F. nucleatum nucleatum* *F. nucleatum fusiforme* *F. nucleatum polymorphum* *F. nucleatum vincentii* *F. periodonticum* *F. russii* *F. ulcerans* *F. varium*	Abscesses, bacteraemia, periodontitis, endocarditis, necrobacillosis	Metronidazole, penicillins, carbapenems, cephalosporins	
G				
Gardnerella	*G. vaginalis*	Intrauterine and neonatal sepsis	β-Lactams, clindamycin	Associated with bacterial vaginosis

Gemella	*G. bergeri* *G. haemolysins* *G. morbillorum* (Streptococcus morbillorum) *G. sanguinis*	Bacteraemia, endocarditis	Penicillin or vancomycin (plus gentamicin for endocarditis)	
Globicatella	*G. sanguinis*	Bacteraemia, UTI, meningitis	Vancomycin	
Gordonia (*Gordona*) (*Rhodococcus*)	*G. aichensis* G. araii *G. bronchialis* G. effuse G. otitidis G. polyisoprenivorans *G. rubropertinctus* *G. sputi* *G. terrae*	Pulmonary infection, cholecystitis, breast abscess, sternal wound sepsis, brain abscess, bacteraemia, otitis	Co-trimoxazole, ceftriaxone, imipenem, fluoroquinolones	
Granulicatella	*G. adiacens* (*Abiotrophia adiacens*) *G. elegans* (*Abiotrophia elegans*)	Endocarditis, septic arthritis, endodontic infection	Penicillin or cefazolin or vancomycin plus gentamicin (plus rifampicin)	Previously known as nutritionally deficient or variant streptococci; the proposed name '*Abiotrophia para-adiacens*' for strains allied to what is now known as *Granulicatella adiacens* does not have standing in nomenclature
Grimontia	*G. hollisae* (*Vibrio hollisae*)	Diarrhoea	β-Lactams, quinolones	Infection associated with ingestion of shellfish
H				
Haemophilus	*H. aegyptius*	Brazilian purpuric fever	Ampicillin, cephalosporins, chloramphenicol	Treated by some authors as a biotype of *H. influenzae*
	H. aphrophilus (*H. paraphrophilus*) *H. parainfluenzae* H. pittmaniae *H. segnis*	Sinusitis, otitis media, pneumonia, abscesses, endocarditis	Cefotaxime, chloramphenicol, ampicillin, aminoglycosides	The genus *Aggregatibacter* has been proposed to accommodate *H. aphrophilus* (including *H. paraphrophilus* as a heterotypic synonym of *H. aphrophilus*), *H. signis*, and *Actinobacillus actinomycetemcomitans*
	H. ducreyi	Chancroid	Macrolides, ceftriaxone, fluoroquinolones	
	H. influenzae	Bacteraemia, meningitis, epiglottitis	Cephalosporins, penicillins, fluoroquinolones	Many strains produce penicillinases
Hafnia	*H. alvei*	Bacteraemia		Doubtful enteropathogen. Susceptibility variable. Includes two genomospecies. '*Hafnia alvei*-like' strains from Bangladesh have been described as *Escherichia albertii*
Helcococcus	*H. kunzii* '*H. pyogenica*' *H. sueciensis*	Sebaceous cyst infection, breast abscess, wound infection	Penicillins, vancomycin	From skin flora. The name *H. pyogenica* does not have standing in nomenclature
Helicobacter	*H. bilis* ('*Flexispira rapinni*' *corrig. taxon 9*)	Cholecystitis, bacteraemia		Zoonosis from rodents
	H. canis	Gastroenteritis		Zoonosis from dogs
	H. cinaedi (*Campylobacter cinaedi*) *H. fennelliae* (*Campylobacter fennelliae*)	Proctitis in homosexual men, septicaemia	Ampicillin, gentamicin	Zoonoses from hamsters

(*Continued*)

Table 7.6.46.1 (*Cont'd*) A check list of bacteria associated with infection in humans

Nomenclature		Associated infections	Reported susceptibilities and treatments	Notes
Genus	**Species and subspecies**			
(synonyms, CDC alphanumeric groups)				
	H. bizzozeronii *H. felis* *H. salomonis* 'Candidatus *H. bovis*' 'Candidatus *H. heilmannii*' ('*Gastrospirillum hominis*') 'Candidatus *H. suis*' ('*H. heilmannii*-like organisms')	Gastritis		Zoonoses from domestic and farm animals. Some organisms known as '*Flexipsira rapini*' may belong to this group of *Helicobacter* spp.
	H. canadensis *H. pullorum*	Gastroenteritis		Zoonoses from birds (or possibly rodents)
	H. pylori (Campylobacter pyloridis)	Gastritis	Omeprazole plus clarithromycin and metronidazole	Numerous similar treatment combinations have been recommended
	'*H. westmeadii*'	Bacteraemia in AIDS		Name does not have standing in nomenclature
	'*H. winghamensis*'	Gastroenteritis		Name does not have standing in nomenclature. Possibly a zoonosis from rodents
Herbaspirillum	*H.* sp.	Associated with aortic aneurism		Detected by 16S gene analysis. Of doubtful clinical significance
Holdemania	*H. filiformis*			From faecal flora. Clinical significance is unclear
I				
Ignavigranum	*I. ruoffiae*	Wound infection, ear abscess		Role as pathogen poorly defined
Inquilinus	*I. limosusI.* sp.	Pulmonary infection in cystic fibrosis, endocarditis	Imipenem, quinolones, gentamicin	
J				
Janibacter	*J. melonis*	Bacteraemia	Vancomycin, β-lactams, fluoroquinolones	An undescribed *Janibacter* sp. was isolated from a leukaemia patient
Johnsonella	*J. ignava*	Periodontitis		
K				
Kerstersia	*K. gyiorum*	Wound infection		
Kingella	*K. denitrificans* *K. kingae* *K. oralis* *K. potus*	Septic arthritis, endocarditis, bite infection	Penicillins (plus gentamicin for endocarditis)	
[*Kingella indologenes*—see *Suttonella indologenes*]				
Klebsiella	*K. granulomatis* (Calymmatobacterium granulomatis)	Donovanosis	Tetracycline, co-trimoxazole	
[*Klebsiella ornitholytica, K. planticola, K. terrigena*—see *Raoultella*]				

	K. oxytoca *K.pneumoniae ssp. pneumoniae* *K. pneumoniae ssp. ozaenae* *K. variicola*	UTI, bacteraemia, wound infection, respiratory tract infection	β-Lactams, aminoglycosides, fluoroquinolones	Susceptibilities vary. Nosocomial outbreaks reported
	K. pneumoniae ssp. rhinoscleromatis	Rhinoscleroma	Ciprofloxacin, rifampicin, co-trimoxazole	
Kluyvera	*K. ascorbate* *K. cryocrescens* *K. georgiana* *K. intermedia (Enterobacter intermedius)*	Bacteraemia, UTI, mediastinitis, line sepsis	Aminoglycosides, ceftazidime, imipenem, ciprofloxacin	
Kocuria (Micrococcus)	*K. kristinae* *K. rosea* *K. varians*	Cholecystitis, line-related sepsis	Penicillin, clindamycin, vancomycin	
[*Koserella trabulsii*—see *Yokenella regensburgei*]				
Kurthia	*'K. bessonii'* *K. gibsonii* *K. zopfii*	Bacteraemia, endocarditis	Penicillin	Not in approved lists of bacterial names Isolated from faeces of patients with diarrhoea
Kytococcus (Micrococcus)	*K schroeteri* *K. sedentarius*	Endocarditis, cerebral cyst infection	Imipenem, vancomycin, rifampicin	
L				
Lactobacillus	*L. acidophilus* *L. brevis* *L. casei* *L. catenaformis* L. coleohominis *L. crispatus* *L. fermentum* *L. gasseri* *L. iners* *L. jensenii* *L. leichmannii* *L. oris* *L. paracasei* *L. paraplantarum* *L. plantarum* *L. rhamnosus* *L. salivarius* *L. vaginalis*	Abscesses, bacteraemia, endometritis, endocarditis, lung infection, UTI	Cephalosporins, vancomycin, penicillins, aminoglycosides, clindamycin	Reported risk factors for infection include surgery, malignancy, diabetes, and immunodeficiency. May be vancomycin-resistant

(Continued)

Table 7.6.46.1 (*Cont'd*) A check list of bacteria associated with infection in humans

Nomenclature		Associated infections	Reported susceptibilities and treatments	Notes
Genus	**Species and subspecies**			
(synonyms, CDC alphanumeric groups)				
Lactococcus (*Streptococcus*)	*L. garviae* *L. lactis*	Bacteraemia, endocarditis, UTI	Penicillin (plus gentamicin for endocarditis)	
Lautropia	*L. mirabilis*			Role as potential pathogen unclear. From oral flora of HIV patients and sputum of cystic fibrosis patient
Leclercia	*L. adecarboxylata* (Escherichia adecarboxylata)	Bacteraemia, wound infection		Variable susceptibility
Legionella	*L. anisa* *L. birminghamensis* *L. bozemanae* (*L. bozemanii*) *L. cincinnatiensis* *L. dumoffii* *L. feeleii* *L. gormanii* *L. hackeliae* *L. israelensis* *L. jordanis* *L. lansingensis* *L. longbeachae* L. lytica *L. maceachernii* *L. micdadei* *L. oakridgemsis* *L. pneumophila* L. quinlivanii L. rubrilucens *L. sainthelensi* *L. tucsonensis* *L. wadsworthia* L. worsleiensis	Legionnaires' disease, Pontiac fever	Macrolides, fluoroquinolones, rifampicin	Infections caused by species other than *L. pneumophila* and *L. micdadei* are seldom reported
Leifsonia	*L. aquatica* *(Corynebacterium aquaticum)*	UTI, endocarditis, meningitis, CAPD peritonitis	Ampicillin, chloramphenicol, gentamicin	Previously confused with *Aureobacterium* (which has been united with *Microbacterium*)
Leminorella	*L. grimontii* *L. richardii*	UTI, bacteraemia, surgical site infection, peritonitis	Imipenem, chloramphenicol, tetracycline, gentamicin	
Leptospira	*L. biflexa* *L. borgpetersenii* *L. broomii* *L. inadai* *L. interrogans* *L. kirschneri* *L. noguchii* *L. santarosai* *L. weilii*	Leptospirosis	Penicillin, tetracycline	*L. interrogans* is composed of severalnamed serogroups, including: australis, bataviae, canicola, copenhageni, cynopteri, hurstbridge, hardjo, grippotyphosa, icterohaemorrhagiae, panama, pomona, pyrogenes, sejroe, tarassovi

Leptotrichia	*L. buccalis* *L. goodfellowii* *L. shahii* *L. trevisanii*	Bacteraemia, endocarditis	β-Lactams, metronidazole	Associated with dental plaque and gingivitis. '*L. amnionii*' from amniotic fluid does not have standing in nomenclature and may belong in the genus Sneathia
Leuconostoc	*L. citreum* *L. lactis* *L. mesenteroides* ssp. *cremoris* *L. mesenteroides* ssp. *dextranicum* *L. mesenteroides* ssp. *mesenteroide* *L. pseudomesenteroides*	Meningitis, bacteraemia, pulmonary infection	Penicillin and gentamicin or clindamycin	Vancomycin-resistant
Listeria	*L. ivanovii* L. grayi *L. monocytogenes* L. seeligeri	Septicaemia, meningitis, intrauterine infection, enteric infection	Ampicillin and gentamicin	
[Listonella damsela—see *Photobacterium damselae]*				
Luteococcus	*L. peritonei* *L. sanguinis*	Peritonitis, bacteraemia		
M				
Massilia	*M. timonae*	Bacteraemia, wound infection		
Megasphaera	*M. elsdenii* *M. micronuciformis*	Endocarditis, abscess	Metronidazole	
Mesorhizobium	*M. amorphae*	Pneumonia		
Methylobacterium	*M. extorquens* *M. mesophilicum* (*Pseudomonas mesophilica*)	Bacteraemia, CAPD peritonitis, UTI, septic arthritis	Ureidopenicillins, imipenem, aminoglycosides, chloramphenicol, fluoroquinolones	Detected in aortic aneurysm
Microbacterium (Aureobacterium)	*M. arborescens* *M. imperiale* (CDC coryneform groups A-4 and A-5) M. liquefaciens (*Aureobacterium liquefaciens*) (*'Corynebacterium aquaticum'*) *M. oxydans* *M. paraoxydans* *M. resistens* *M. trichothecenolyticum*	Endophthalmitis, UTI, endocarditis, soft tissue infection, hypersensitivity pneumonitis, meningitis, CAPD peritonitis, bacteraemia	Glycopeptides, β-lactams, chloramphenicol, gentamicin	*M. resistens* is vancomycin-resistant. *Microbacterium* isolates have been misidentified as *'Corynebacterium aquaticum'* a taxon now known as *Leifsonia aquatica*
Micrococcus	*M. luteus* *M. lytae*	Bacteraemia, endocarditis, septic arthritis	Vancomycin, penicillin, rifampicin	From skin flora. Common specimen contaminants
Mitsuokella	*M. multocida* (*Bacteroides multiacidus*)			Role as human pathogen poorly defined

(*Continued*)

Table 7.6.46.1 (*Cont'd*) A check list of bacteria associated with infection in humans

Nomenclature		Associated infections	Reported susceptibilities and treatments	Notes
Genus	**Species and subspecies**			
(synonyms, CDC alphanumeric groups)				
Mobiluncus	*M. curtisii curtisii* *M. curtisii holmesii* *M. mulieris*	Endometritis, chorioamnionitis	Ampicillin, cephalosporins, clindamycin	Associated with bacterial vaginosis
Moellerella	*M. wisconsensis*	Diarrhoea		Of uncertain significance
Mogibacterium	*M. diversum* *M. neglectum*	Endodontic infection		
Moraxella	*M. atlantae* *M. catarrhalis* (Branhamella catarrhalis) *M. lacunata* *M. nonliquefaciens* *M. osloensis*	Conjunctivitis, wound infection, endocarditis, abscesses, osteomyelitis, respiratory infections, endocarditis, bacteraemia	Penicillin, cefuroxime	Penicillin resistance has been reported. Some authors retain *Branhamella catarrhalis*
[*Moraxella phenylpyruvica*—see *Psychrobacter phenylpyruvicus*]				
[*Moraxella urethralis*—see *Oligella urethralis*]				
Morganella	*M. morganii morganii* *M. morganii sibonii*	Bacteraemia, UTI, wound infection	β-Lactams, aminoglycosides	Susceptibilities vary
Moryella	*M. indoligenes*			
Mycobacterium	*M. abscessus* *M. africanum* *M. alvei* *M. asiaticum* M. arupense M. aubagnense *M. aurum* *M. avium* M. barrassiae M. boenickei *M. bohemicum* *M. bolletii* *M. bovis* *M. branderi* M. brisbanense *M. brumae* M. canariasense *M. celatum* *M. chelonae* M. chimaera *M. chubuense* *M. colombiense* *M. conceptionense* *M. confluentis* *M. conspicuum* *M. cookii* *M. cosmeticum*		Isoniazid, rifampicin, ethambutol, pyrazinamide, streptomycin, azithromycin, clarithromycin, ciprofloxacin, dapsone, clofazimine, imipenem, co-trimoxazole, amikacin	Many *Mycobacterium* spp. have been associated with infection. *M. tuberculosis*, *M. africanum*, and *M. bovis* are the agents of tuberculosis. *M. scrofulaceum* causes cervical adenitis. The agent of Buruli ulcer is *M. ulcerans*. *M. marinum* causes fish-tank granuloma. *M. leprae*causes leprosy. *M. malmoense*, *M. szulgai*, *M. shimoidei*, *M. kansasii*, and *M. xenopi* cause pulmonary infection. *M. intracellulare*and *M. avium* cause systemic infection mainly in immunocompromised patients. The rapid growers, *M. chelonae*,*M. abscessus*, and *M. fortuitum* cause local postinoculation injury and systemic infection

M. doricum
M. elephantis
M. flavescens
M. florentinum
M. fortuitum
M. gadium
M. gastri
M. genavense
M. goodii
M. gordonae
M. haemophilum
M. hassiacum
M. heckeshornense
M. heidelbergense
M. hodleri
M. holsaticum
M. houstonense
M. immunogenum
M. interjectum
M. intracellulare
'M. jacuzzii'
M. kansasii
M. kubicae
M. kumamotonense
M. lacus
M. lentiflavum
M. leprae
M. mageritense
M. malmoense
M. marinum
M. massiliense
M. microgenicum
M. microti
M. monacense
M. mucogenicum
M. neoaurum
M. nebraskense
M. neworleansense
M. nonchromogenicum
M. novocastrense
M. palustre
M. parascrofulaceum
M. parmense
M. peregrinum
M. p hlei
M. phocaicum
M. porcinum

(Continued)

Table 7.6.46.1 (*Cont'd*) A check list of bacteria associated with infection in humans

Nomenclature: Genus (synonyms, CDC alphanumeric groups)	Species and subspecies	Associated infections	Reported susceptibilities and treatments	Notes
	M. saskatchewanense *M. scrofulaceum* *M. seoulense* *M. septicum* *M. shimoidei* *M. simiae* *M. smegmatis* *M. szulgai* *M. terrae* *M. thermoresistibile* *M. triplex* *M. triviale* *M. tuberculosis* *M. tusciae* *M. ulcerans* *M. vaccae* *M. wolinskyi* *M. xenopi*			
Mycoplasma	*M. amphoriforme* *M. buccale* *M. faucium* *M. fermentans* *M. genitalium* *M. hominis* *M. lipophilum* *M. orale* *M. penetrans* *M. pirum* *M. pneumoniae* *M. primatum* *M. salivarium* *M. spermatophilum*	Respiratory infection, postpartum fever, pyelonephritis, pelvic inflammatory disease, myocarditis, pericarditis, meningitis	Tetracycline, macrolides, fluoroquinolones	May be resistant to macrolides. *M. pneumoniae*infection may be complicated by haemolytic anaemia, intravascular coagulation, Stevens–Johnson syndrome, or erythema multiforme
	M. phocicerebrale (*M. phocacerebrale*)	Seal finger	Tetracycline	Other *Mycoplasma* spp. from seals are *M. phocae* and *M. phocirhinis*
Myroides (*Flavobacterium*)	*M. odoratimimus* *M. odoratus*	UTI, wound infection	Minocycline	May be multiresistant
N				
Neisseria	*N. animaloris* (CDC gro up EF-4a) *N. canis* *N. weaveri* (CDC group M-5, 'Neisseria parelongata') *N. zoodegmatis* (CDC group EF-4b)	Wound infections, abscesses, endocarditis, meningitis, bacteraemia	Amoxicillin	Zoonoses from animal bites

	N. bacilliformis *N. cinerea* *N. elongata elongata* *N. elongata glycolytica* *N. elongata nitroreductens* *N. flavescens* *N. lactamica* *N. mucosa* *N. polysaccharea* *N. sicca* *N. subflava*	Meningitis, bacteraemia, endocarditis, osteomyelitis	Penicillin, cephalosporins	Bacteraemia in AIDS reported for several species. Penicillin resistance rarely reported in commensal *Neisseria*spp. N. subflava includes biovars flava, perflava, and subflava
	N. gonorrhoeae	Gonorrhoea, septicaemia, ophthalmia neonatorum	Cephalosporins	Susceptibility varies geographically. The name '*Neisseria gonorrhoeae* ssp. *kochii*' was proposed for isolates from conjunctivitis cases in rural Egypt
	N. meningitidis	Septicaemia, meningitis, conjunctivitis, genital infection, epiglottitis	Penicillin, cefotaxime	Rifampicin, ciprofloxacin, or ceftriaxone to clear carriage
Neorickettsia	*N. sennetsu (Ehalichia sennetsu)*	Sennetsu fever	Doxycycline	Associated with eating raw fish in Asia
Nocardia	*N abscessus* *N. africana* *N. anaemiae* *N. aobensis* *N. araoensis* *N. arthritides* *N. asiatica* *N. asteroides* *N. beijingensis* *N. brasiliensis* *N. brevicatena* *N. carnea* *N. concave* *N. cyriacigeorgica* *N. elegans* *N. exalbida* *N. farcinica* *N. higoensis* *N. inohanensis* *N. kruczakiae* *N. mexicana* *N. niigatensis* *N. ninae* *N. nova* *N. otitidiscaviarum*	Nocardiosis (including bacteraemia, pulmonary and soft tissue infections)	Sulphonamides, co-trimoxazole, amikacin, imipenem	

(Continued)

Table 7.6.46.1 (*Cont'd*) A check list of bacteria associated with infection in humans

Nomenclature		Associated infections	Reported susceptibilities and treatments	Notes
Genus	**Species and subspecies**			
(synonyms, CDC alphanumeric groups)				
	N. paucivorans *N. pneumoniae* *N. pseudobrasiliensis* *N. puris* *N. sienata* *N. takedensis* *N. thailandensis* *N. testaceus* *N. transvalensis* *N. vermiculata* *N. veterana* N. yamanashiensis			
Nocardiopsis	*N. dassonvillei* *N. synnemataformans*	Mycetoma, cutaneous infection, pulmonary infection, conjunctivitis	Fluoroquinolones, piperacillin	
O				
Ochrobactrum (*Achromobacter CDC group Vd; Achromobacter* groups A, C, and D)	*O. anthropi* *O. intermedium*	Bacteraemia, endophthalmitis, liver abscess	Imipenem, fluoroquinolones, aminoglycosides	Nosocomial infections in debilitated patients
Oerskovia	*O. turbata (Cellulomonas turbata)*	Bacteraemia, endocarditis	Amikacin, co-trimoxazole, chloramphenicol	Vancomycin resistance reported
Oligella	*O. ureolytica* (CDC IVe) *O. urethralis (Moraxella urethralis)*	UTI, septicaemia	Aminoglycosides, cephalosporins	Associated with urinary catheters
Olsenella	*O. uli* (*Lactobacillus uli*)			
Orientia	*O. tsutsugamushi (Rickettsia tsutsugamushi)*	Scrub typhus	Tetracycline, chloramphenicol	
P				
Paenibacillus	*P. alvei* *P. macerans* *P. polymyxa* *P. popilliae*	Septicaemia, meningitis, pneumonia	Vancomycin	
Pannonibacter	*P. phragmitetus* (*Achromobacter* groups B and E)			
Pantoea	*P. agglomerans (Enterobacter agglomerans)* *P. ananatis* *P. dispersa*	Bacteraemia, endocarditis, wound infection, cellulitis, alligator-bite infection, endophthalmitis	Carbapenems, fluoroquinolones, ureidopenicillins, aminoglycosides	Susceptibilities vary. May be multiresistant
Parabacteroides	*P. distasonis* *P. goldsteinii (Bacteroides goldsteinii)* *P. merdae*	Abscesses	Metronidazole	

Parachlamydia	*P. acanthamoebae*	Humidifier fever		
Paracoccus	*P. yeei*	Bacteraemia	Ampicillin, cephalosporins, ciprofloxacin	
Parvimonas	*P. micra (Peptostreptococcus micros)*			
Pasteurella	*P. aerogenes* *P. bettyae* *P. canis* *P. dagmatis* *P. gallinarum* *P. haemolytica* *P. multocida multocida* *P. multocida gallicida* *P. multocida septica* *P. pneumotropica* *P. stomatis*	Wound infection, septicaemia, abscesses, pneumonia, endocarditis, meningitis	Penicillin, tetracycline, ciprofloxacin	*Pasteurella* infections in humans relate to species usually associated with animals. There may be no history of an animal bite or contact
[Pasteurella ureae—see *Actinobacillus ureae]*				
Pediococcus	*P. acidilactici* *P. damnosus* *P. dextrinicus* *P. parvulus* *P. pentosaceus*	Bacteraemia, abscesses, pulmonary infection	Imipenem, gentamicin, chloramphenicol	Debilitated hospital patients. Resistant to vancomycin
Peptococcus	*P. niger*	Abdominal sepsis	Penicillin, clindamycin	
Peptoniphilus (Peptostreptococcus)	*P. asaccharolyticus* *P harei* *P. indolyticus* *P. ivorii* *P. lacrimalis*	Mixed anaerobic infections, abscesses	β-Lactams, metronidazole, chloramphenicol	
Peptostreptococcus	*P. anaerobius* P. stomatis *'P. trisimilis'*	Mixed anaerobic infections, abscesses, endocarditis	β-Lactams, metronidazole, chloramphenicol	See also *Peptoniphilus*, *Anaerococcus*, *Finegoldia*
Photobacterium	*P. damselae (Listonella damsela and Vibrio damsela)*	Necrotizing wound infection, bacteraemia	Penicillins, tetracycline, chloramphenicol	Infection associated with penetrating fish injury. May require debridement
Photorhabdus (Xenorhabdus)	*P. luminescens*	Bacteraemia, wound infection	Cefoxitin, oxacillin, gentamicin	
Plesiomonas	*P. shigelloides*	Gastroenteritis, septicaemia, meningitis, endophthalmitis	Ciprofloxacin, trimethoprim, cephalosporins	Infections associated with contaminated food and water
Porphyromonas (Bacteroides)	*P. asaccharolytica* *P. cangingivalis* *P. canoris* *P. cansulci* *P. catoniae* *P. circumdentaria* *P. crevioricanis* *P. endodontalis*	Mixed anaerobic infections at various sites, periodontitis, human and animal bites	Metronidazole, ureidopenicillins, amoxicillin/clavulanate, carbapenems, cephalosporins, chloramphenicol	Members of the oral flora of humans and animals

(Continued)

Table 7.6.46.1 (*Cont'd*) A check list of bacteria associated with infection in humans

Nomenclature: Genus (synonyms, CDC alphanumeric groups)	Species and subspecies	Associated infections	Reported susceptibilities and treatments	Notes
	P. gingivalis *P. gingivicanis* *P. levii* *P. macacae* *P. somerae* *P. uenonis*			
Prevotella (Bacteroides)	*P. bergensis* *P. bivia* *P. buccae* *P. buccalis* *P. corporis* *P. dentalis* *P. denticola* *P. disiens* *P. enoeca* *P. heparinolytica* *P. intermedia* *P. loeschii* *P. melaninogenica* *P. multiformis* *P. multisaccharivorax* *P. nigrescens* *P. oralis* *P. oris* *P. oulorum* *P. tannerae* *P. timonensis* *P. veroralis* *P. zoogleoformans*	Abscesses, bacteraemia, wound infection, bite infections, genital tract infections, periodontitis, endodontic infection	Metronidazole, amoxicillin/clavulanate, ureidopenicillins, carbapenems, cephalosporins, clindamycin, chloramphenicol	A genus that includes the well-known former *Bacteroides melaninogenicus*and allied species of anaerobes
Propionibacterium	*P. acnes* *P. avidum* *P. granulosum* *P. propionicum (Arachnia propionicus)*	Abscesses, endocarditis, bacteraemia, septic arthritis, endophthalmitis	Glycopeptides, penicillin, macrolides	Associated with acne vulgaris
Propionimicrobium	*P. lymphophilum* (*Propionibacterium lymphophilum*)	UTI		Isolated from lymph nodes in Hodgkin's disease
Proteus	*P. mirabilis* *P. penneri* *P. vulgaris*	UTI, bacteraemia, wound infection, abscesses	β-Lactams, aminoglycosides, fluoroquinolones	Susceptibilities vary

Providencia	*P. alcalifaciens* *P. rettgeri* *P. rustigianii* *P. stuartii*	UTI, wound infection, bacteraemia	β-Lactams, aminoglycosides, fluoroquinolones	Susceptibilities vary. *P. alcalifaciens* has been associated with gastroenteritis
[Pseudomonas acidivorans—see *Delftia acidivorans]*				
Pseudomonas	*P. aeruginosa* *P. alcaligenes* *P. chlororaphis* *P. fluorescens* *P. mendocina* *P. monteilii* *P. mosselii* *P. otitidis* *P. pertocinogena* *P. pseudalcaligenes* *P. putida* *P. stutzeri*	Bacteraemia, UTI, wound infection, abscesses, septic arthritis, conjunctivitis, endocarditis, meningitis, otitis	Ureidopenicillins, aminoglycosides, ceftazidime, fluoroquinolones, carbapenems	Nosocomial infections associated with invasive devices in debilitated patients. Nosocomial outbreaks reported. May be multiresistant
[Pseudomonas cepacia—see *Burkholderia cepacia]*				
[Pseudomonas diminuta—see *Brevundimonas diminuta]*				
[Pseudomonas mallei—see *Burkholderia mallei]*				
[Pseudomonas maltophilia—see *Stenotrophomonas maltophilia]*				
[Pseudomonas mesophilica—see *Methylobacterium mesophilicum]*				
	P. luteola (Chryseomonas luteola)	Bacteraemia, endocarditis, CAPD peritonitis	Ureidopenicillins, ceftazidime, ciprofloxacin, aminoglycosides	
	P. oryzihabitans (Flavimonas oryzihabitans)	Septicaemia, eye infection, CAPD peritonitis	Ampicillin, tetracycline, gentamicin, cefotaxime	
[Pseudomonas paucimobilis—see *Sphingomonas paucimobilis]*				
[Pseudomonas pickettii—see *Ralstonia pickettii]*				
[Pseudomonas pseudomallei—see *Burkholderia pseudomallei]*				
[Pseudomonas putrefaciens—see *Shewanella putrefaciens]*				
[Pseudomonas terrigena—see *Comamonas terrigena]*				
[Pseudomonas testosteroni—see *Comamonas testosteroni]*				
[Pseudomonas vesicularis—see *Brevundimonas vesicularis]*				
Pseudonocardia	*P. autotrophica (Amycolata autotrophica)*			Role as pathogen uncertain
Pseudoramibacter	*P. alactolyticus*	Periodontal disease, wound infection, abscesses	Penicillin, clindamycin, chloramphenicol	
Psychrobacter	*P. immobilis* *P. phenylpyruvicus (Moraxella phenylpyruvica)*	Meningitis, bacteraemia, eye infection	Penicillins, aminoglycosides, chloramphenicol	

(Continued)

Table 7.6.46.1 (*Cont'd*) A check list of bacteria associated with infection in humans

Nomenclature		Associated infections	Reported susceptibilities and treatments	Notes
Genus	**Species and subspecies**			
(synonyms, CDC alphanumeric groups)				
R				
Rahnella	*R. aquatilis*	UTI, septicaemia	Ciprofloxacin	Immunocompromised patients
Ralstonia	*R. insidiosa* *R. mannitolilytica* *R. pickettii (Pseudomonas pickettii)* *R. taiwanensis*	Meningitis, peritonitis, bacteraemia, UTI, pulmonary infection	Co-trimoxazole, imipenem, ceftazidime, quinolones	
Raoultella (*Klebsiella*)	*R. ornithinolytica* *R. planticola* *R. terrigena*	Bacteraemia, UTI, surgical sepsis, pancreatitis	Cephalosporins, carbapenems, aztreonam, quinolones, aminoglycosides	β-Lactamase producers. Associated with histamine (scombrotoxin) fish poisoning
'*Rasbo*'	'*R. bacterium*'	Pneumonia, pericarditis		Proposed name does not have standing in nomenclature
Rhodococcus	*R. equi (Corynebacterium equi)*	Bacteraemia, osteomyelitis, lung abscesses	Vancomycin, erythromycin, aminoglycosides	In immunocompromised patients, including AIDS
Rickettsia	*R. africae* *R. akari* *R. australis* *R. conorii* *R. felis* *R. honei* *R. japonica* '*R. mongolotimonae*' *R. prowazekii* *R. rickettsiae* *R. sibirica* *R. slovaca* *R. typhi*	Rickettsial spotted fever, tick typhus, tick-bite fever, rickettsialpox	Tetracycline	Transmitted by arthropods. Agents of Astrakhan fever, Israeli tick typhus, and Thai tick typhus await designation of scientific names. Other *Rickettsia* spp. are of uncertain clinical significance
Roseomonas	*R. cervicalis* *R. gilardii* ssp. *gilardii* *R. gilardi* ssp. *rosea* *R. mucosa*	Bacteraemia, wound infection, peritonitis	Aminoglycosides, imipenem, ciprofloxacin, ticarcillin-clavulanate	
[*Roseomonas fauriae*—see *Azospirillum brasilense*]				
Rothia	*R. dentocariosa*	Endocarditis, abscesses	Penicillin and gentamicin	
	R. mucilaginosa (Micrococcus mucilaginosus) (Stomatococcus mucilaginosus)	Endocarditis, meningitis, neutropenic sepsis, necrotizing fasciitis	Glycopeptides, imipenem, rifampicin, ceftriaxone	

Ruminococcus	*R. flavefaciens* *R. hansenii (Streptococcus hansenii)* *R. luti* *R. productus (Peptostreptococcus productus)*	Abdominal sepsis, abscesses	Penicillins	
S				
Salmonella	*S. bongori* *S. choleraesuis* ssp. *arizonae* *S. choleraesuis* ssp. *choleraesuis* *S. choleraesuis* ssp. *diarizonae* *S. choleraesuis* ssp. *houtenae* *S. choleraesuis* ssp. *indica* *S. choleraesuis* ssp. *salamae* *S. enteritidis* *S. paratyphi* *S. subterranea* *S. typhi* *S. typhimurium* *S. enterica* ssp. *arizonae* *S. enterica* ssp. *diarizonae* *S. enterica* ssp. *enterica* *S. enterica* ssp. *houtenae* *S. enterica* ssp. *indica* *S. enterica* ssp. *salamae* *S. subterranea*	Gastroenteritis, enteric fever, osteomyelitis	β-Lactams, fluoroquinolones, chloramphenicol	Salmonella nomenclature is complicated by the existence of two sets of names, both of which have standing in nomenclature. Both sets of names are listed in the table. The first scheme listed is more helpful for clinicians because it treats the clinically important taxa *S. typhi* (the agent of typhoid fever), *S. paratyphi*, *S. enteritidis*, and *S. typhimurium* as species. As yet, *S. subterranea* has not been associated with infection. It should be noted that bacteriologists widely adhere to the practice of writing serotype names in the form of Linnaean binomials (e.g. '*S. virchow*') and that such names do not have standing in nomenclature
Scardovia	*S. inopinata* (*Bifidobacterium inopinatum*)	Dental caries		
Selenomonas	*S. artemidis* *S. dianae* *S. flueggei* *S. infelix* *S. noxia* *S. sputigena*	Bacteraemia, lung abscess	Clindamycin, chloramphenicol, metronidazole	Malignancy and alcohol abuse reported as risk factors for infection
[Serpulina—*see* Brachyspira]				
Serratia	*S. ficaria* *S. fonticola* *S. grimesii* *S. liquefaciens* *S. marcescens* *S. odorifera* *S. plymuthica* *S. proteamaculans* *S. quinivorans* *S. rubidaea*	Septicaemia, abscesses, burn infections, osteomyelitis	Imipenem, aminoglycosides, fluoroquinolones, ureidopenicillins, ceftazidime	Nosocomial outbreaks reported. May be multiresistant. At time of writing a proposal to use the name *S. rubidae* in place of *S. rubidaea* has not been validly published

(*Continued*)

Table 7.6.46.1 (*Cont'd*) A check list of bacteria associated with infection in humans

Nomenclature		Associated infections	Reported susceptibilities and treatments	Notes
Genus	**Species and subspecies**			
(synonyms, CDC alphanumeric groups)				
Shewanella	*S. algae* *S. putrefaciens (Alteromonas putrefaciens) (Pseudomonas putrefaciens)*	Abdominal sepsis, meningitis, bacteraemia	Ampicillin, cefotaxime, gentamicin, chloramphenicol	Debilitated patients
Shigella	*S. boydii* *S. dysenteriae* *S. flexneri* *S. sonnei*	Enteric infection	Co-trimoxazole, fluoroquinolones	
Simkania	*S. negevensis*	Bronchiolitis, pneumonia		
Slackia	*S. exigua (Eubacterium exiguum)*	Periodontitis		
Sneathia	*S. sanguinegens (Leptotrichia sanguinegens = L. microbii)*			
Sphingobacterium (Flavobacterium)	*S. multivorum* *S. spiritivorum* *S. thalpophilum*	Bacteraemia, pulmonary infection	Co-trimoxazole, chloramphenicol, tetracycline, cephalosporins, quinolones	
[*Sphingobacterium mizutae*—see *Flavobacterium mizutaii*]				
Sphingomonas	*S. parapaucimobilis* *S. paucimobilis (Pseudomonas paucimobilis)* *S. sanguinis (S. sanguis)* *S. yanoikuyae*	Septicaemia, UTI, wound infections, CAPD peritonitis	Ceftazidime, aminoglycosides	Nosocomial infections
Spirillum	*'S. minus'*	Rat-bite fever	Penicillin	*Streptobacillus moniliformis* is also a rat-bite fever agent. The name '*Spirillum minus*' does not have standing in nomenclature
Staphylococcus	*S. aureus* *S. auricularis* *S. capitis capitis* *S. capitis ureolyticus* *S. caprae* *S. cohnii cohnii* *S. cohnii urealyticus* *S. delphini* *S. epidermidis* *S. equorum* *S. gallinarum*	Bacteraemia, wound infection, endocarditis, catheter-related sepsis, UTI, toxic shock syndrome, food poisoning, eye infection, osteomyelitis	Glycopeptides, β-lactams, aminoglycosides, tetracycline, macrolides, rifampicin, fluoroquinolones, daptomycin, linezolid, fusidic acid, mupirocin	Staphylococci are surface commensals of humans and animals. *S. aureus* is also a major pathogen, causing focal and systemic sepsis, toxic shock syndrome, and food poisoning. *S. epidermidis* infection is often associated with foreign bodies (e.g. catheters and implants).*S. saprophyticus* causes UTI. *S. lugdunensis* is a rare cause of endocarditis.*S. intermedius*, *S. hyicus*, and others are from animals. Susceptibilities are variable but glycopeptide resistance is as yet rare

	S. haemolyticus *S. hominis hominis* *S. hominis novobiosepticius* *S. hyicus* *S. intermedius* *S. lugdunensis* *S. pasteuri* *S. saccharolyticus* *S. saprophyticus* *S. schleiferi schleiferi* *S. schleiferi coagulans* *S. sciuri* *S. simulans* *S. vitulinus (S. pulvereri)* *S. warneri* *S. xylosus*			
Stenotrophomonas	*S. maltophilia* *(Pseudomonas maltophila)* *(Xanthomonas maltophila)* *(Stenotrophomonas africana)*	Bacteraemia, meningitis, wound infection, UTI, pneumonia	Fluoroquinolones, chloramphenicol, co-trimoxazole	Resistance to aminoglycosides, penicillins, and carbapenems reported
[Stomatococcus mucilaginosus—see *Rothia mucilaginosa]*				
Streptobacillus	*S. moniliformis*	Rat-bite fever, Haverhill fever	Penicillin, erythromycin	*'Spirillum minus' is also a causative agent of rat-bite fever*
Streptococcus	*S. acidominimus*	Pneumonia, pericarditis, meningitis	β-Lactams	From cattle
	S. agalactiae *S. canis* *S. dysgalactiae dysgalactiae* *S. dysgalactiae equisimilis* *S. equi equi* *S. equi zooepidemicus* *S. iniae (S. shiloi)* *S. porcinus* *S. pseudoporcinus* *S. pyogenes* *S. urinalis*	Pharyngitis, bacteraemia, pyogenic infection, necrotizing infection, septic arthritis, UTI, glomerulonephritis, meningitis	β-Lactams, macrolides	*S. pyogenes* (Lancefield group A), *S. agalactiae* (group B), and *S. dysgalactiae equisimilis* (groups C and G) are commensals and pathogens of humans. *S. iniae* is from fish. Others are from mammals
	S. anginosus *S. constellatus constellatus* *S. constellatus pharyngis* *S. intermedius*	Abscesses, bacteraemia, endocarditis, pharyngitis	β-Lactams, macrolides	Often termed '*S. milleri*' or microaerophilic streptococci. From human oral flora

(*Continued*)

Table 7.6.46.1 (*Cont'd*) A check list of bacteria associated with infection in humans

Nomenclature		Associated infections	Reported susceptibilities and treatments	Notes
Genus	Species and subspecies			
(synonyms, CDC alphanumeric groups)				
	S. equinus (S. bovis) *S. gallolyticus* ssp. *gallolyticus* *S.* gallolyticus ssp. *pateurianus* *S. infantarius* ssp. *coli* *S. infantarius* ssp. *infantarius* *S. lutetiensis* *S. pasteurianus*	Endocarditis, CAPD peritonitis	β-Lactams (plus gentamicin for endocarditis)	Intestinal streptococci from animals and humans. Some taxonomic problems relating to this group (the 'bovis' streptococci) await resolution
	S. criceti *S. mutans* *S. ratti* *S. sobrinus*	Dental caries, endocarditis	β-Lactams	From the tooth-surface flora of humans and mammals
	S. cristatus *S. gordonii* *S. massiliensis* *S. mitis* *S. oralis* *S. parasanguinis* *S. salivarius* *S. sanguinis* *S. sinensis* *S. vestibularis*	Bacteraemia, endocarditis, wound infection	β-Lactams, macrolides	Human oral streptococci including taxa sometimes known as the 'viridans streptococci'
	S. pneumoniae *S. pseudopneumoniae*	Pneumonia, bacteraemia, sinusitis, peritonitis, otitis, conjunctivitis	β-Lactams, macrolides, chloramphenicol	Penicillin resistance locally common
	S. suis	Meningitis	β-Lactams	Associated with pig contact
Streptomyces	*S. albus* *S. anulatus* *'S. paraguayensis'* *S. somaliensis*	Actinomycetoma	Dapsone, co-trimoxazole	
	S. bikiniensis *S. griseus*	Bacteraemia, abscess, pericarditis, endocarditis	Vancomycin, tetracycline, penicillin	Treatment options poorly defined
Succinivibrio	*S. dextrinosolvens*	Bacteraemia, pneumonia	Penicillin	From faecal and gingival flora
Sutterella	*S. wadsworthensis*	Appendicitis, peritonitis, abscesses, osteomyelitis	Amoxicillin/clavulanate, ticarcillin/clavulanate, meropenem, ceftriaxone	One-third of isolates reported to be metronidazole resistant
Suttonella	*S. indologenes (Kingella indologenes)*	Endocarditis, eye infection	Penicillin (plus gentamicin for endocarditis	
T				
Tannerella	*T. forsythensis* *(T. forsythia,* *T. forsythus)*	Endodontic infection		
[*Tatlockia*maceachernii—see *Legionella maceachernii*]				

[*Tatlockia micdadei*—see *Legionella micdadei*]				
Tatumella	*T. ptyseos*	Bacteraemia, UTI	Ampicillin, tetracycline, chloramphenicol, gentamicin	The significance of isolates from sputum is unclear
Tissierella	*T. praeacuta (Bacteroides praeacuta)* *(Clostridium hastiforme)*	Bacteraemia	Metronidazole	
Trabulsiella	*T. guamensis*	Diarrhoea	Co-trimoxazole, gentamicin, chloramphenicol	Role as possible pathogen uncertain
Treponema	*T. amylovorum* *T. denticola* *T. lecithinolyticum* *T. maltophilum* *T. medium* *T. parvum* *T. pectinovorum* *T. putidum* *T. scoliodontum* *T. socranskii* *'T. vincentii'*			Associated with periodontal disease. Role as potential pathogens unclear
	'T. carateum'	Pinta	Penicillin	Name does not have standing in nomenclature
	T. minutum *'T. phagedenis''* *'T. refringens'*			From genital flora. Considered nonpathogenic but have been isolated from genital lesions
	T. pallidum *'T. pallidum endemicum'*	Syphilis	Penicillin	*'T. pallidum endemicum' is the agent of nonvenereal endemic syphilis*
	T. pertenue ('T. pallidum pertenue')	Yaws	Penicillin	
Tropheryma	*T. whipplei (T. whippelii)*	Whipple's disease		Uncultured organism
Tsukamurella	*T. inchonensis* *T. paurometabola* *T. pulmonis* *T. strandjordii (T. strandjordae)* *T. tyrosinosolvens*	Septicaemia, cutaneous infections, lung infections	β-Lactam (plus aminoglycoside)	Line-associated infections in debilitated patients. *T. pulmonis* isolated from the sputum of a tuberculosis patient
Turicella	*T. otitidis*	Otitis, cervical abscess	Glycopeptides, β-lactams	
U				
Ureaplasma	*U. parvum* *U. urealyticum*	Urethritis	Tetracycline, erythromycin	
V				
Vagococcus	*V. fluvialis*		Ampicillin, vancomycin cefotaxime	Possible role as pathogen poorly defined
Varibaculum	*V. cambriensis*	Abscesses		

(Continued)

Table 7.6.46.1 (*Cont'd*) A check list of bacteria associated with infection in humans

Nomenclature		Associated infections	Reported susceptibilities and treatments	Notes
Genus	**Species and subspecies**			
(synonyms, CDC alphanumeric groups)				
Veillonella	*V. atypical* *V. dipsar* *V. montpellierensis* *V. parvula*	Abscesses, bacteraemia	Metronidazole	
Vibrio	*V. alginolyticus*	Wound infection, ear infection	Chloramphenicol, tetracycline	Infection associated with aquatic exposure
	V. cholerae	Cholera	Tetracycline	
	V. cincinnatiensis	Bacteraemia	Moxalactam, chloramphenicol, cephalosporins	Risk factors for infection not defined
[*Vibrio damsela*—see *Photobacterium damselae*]				
	V. fluvialis *V. furnissii* *V. metschnikovii* *V. mimicus* *V. parahaemolyticus*	Diarrhoea, septicaemia	Tetracycline, chloramphenicol	Infection associated with ingestion of contaminated water or shellfish
	V. harveyi (V. carchariae)	Wound infection	Cephalosporins, chloramphenicol, gentamicin	Infection associated with shark bite. May require debridement
[*Vibrio hollisae*—see *Grimontia hollisae*]				
	V. vulnificus	Wound infection, septicaemia, meningitis, endometritis	Tetracycline, penicillins, gentamicin, chloramphenicol	Risk factors include aquatic exposure and penetrating fish injury. May require debridement
W				
Wautersiella	*W. falsenii*	Bacteraemia, wound infection		
Weeksella	*W. virosa*	Peritonitis	Imipenem, ampicillin	From vaginal flora
[*Weeksella zoohelcum*—see *Bergeyella zoohelcum*]				
Weissella	*W. confusa*	Endocarditis		
Williamsia	*W. muralis*	Pulmonary infection		
Wolbachia	*W. sp.*	filariasis	doxycycline	Endosymbiont of filarial nematodes
[*Wolinella curva*—see *Campylobacter curvus*]				
[*Wolinella recta*—see *Campylobacter rectus*]				
X				
Xanthomonas	*X. campestris*	Bacteraemia		
[*Xenorhabdus luminescens*—see *Photorhabdus luminescens*]				

Y				
Yersinia	*Y. aldovae* *Y. bercovieri* *Y. enterocolitica* *Y. frederiksenii* *Y. intermedia* *Y. kristensenii* *Y. mollaretii* *Y. pseudotuberculosis* *Y. rohdei*	Enterocolitis, soft tissue infections, mesenteric lymphadenitis	Tetracycline, chloramphenicol, aminoglycosides, fluoroquinolones, cephalosporins	Medical significance of many *Yersinia* spp. is unclear. Antibiotic treatment is not indicated for uncomplicated enteric infection
	Y. pestis	Plague	Streptomycin, tetracycline	
Yokenella	*Y. regensburgei (Koserella trabulsii)*	Bacteraemia, wound infection	Aminoglycosides, chloramphenicol	

CAPD, continual ambulatory peritoneal dialysis; sp. species; ssp. subspecies; UTI, urinary tract infection.

7.7

Fungi (mycoses)

Contents

7.7.1 Fungal infections *998*
Roderick J. Hay

7.7.2 Cryptococcosis *1018*
William G. Powderly

7.7.3 Coccidioidomycosis *1020*
Gregory M. Anstead and John R. Graybill

7.7.4 Paracoccidioidomycosis *1023*
M.A. Shikanai-Yasuda

7.7.5 *Pneumocystis jirovecii* *1028*
Robert F. Miller and Laurence Huang

7.7.6 *Penicillium marneffei* infection *1032*
Thira Sirisanthana

7.7.1 Fungal infections

Roderick J. Hay

Essentials

The mycoses are disorders caused by fungi, which are saprophytic or parasitic organisms found in every continent and environment. Many are common commensals in nature, but others cause agricultural disease. The mycoses that are human infections include diseases ranging from those that are worldwide and common, such as dermatophytosis and candida infections, to those that are rare and often potentially life threatening, e.g. histoplasmosis. In humans, fungi usually adopt one of two morphologies: (1) the yeast form—where individual cells produce daughter cells by a process of budding and subsequently separate; or (2) the hyphal form—where cells do not separate but multiply to produce chains of cells joined end to end.

Diagnosis

Mycological diagnosis is often complex because many fungi are also commensals or transiently carried in humans, hence it is necessary to show both that the organisms are present and that they are causing disease, which is particularly difficult in the context of opportunistic fungal infection. The main laboratory diagnostic tests involve (1) visualization of fungi in tissue—by direct microscopy or histopathology; (2) culture—often using a glucose peptone agar (Sabouraud's agar); (3) detection of antibody, fungal antigens or DNA fragments—assimilation of genetic tests such as PCR-based methods into routine diagnosis has been slow, and they are offered by few laboratories.

Superficial infections

Superficial fungal infections may reach prevalence rates of 15 to 25% in some communities, with the common infections being dermatophytosis or ringworm, pityriasis versicolor, and superficial candidosis.

Dermatophytoses—otherwise known as tinea infections—commonly affect the feet (tinea pedis), the body (tinea corporis), the scalp (tinea capitis) and the finger and toe nails (onychomycosis). They occur in all climates and usually present in primary care as scaly rashes. Diagnosis is made by direct microscopy of skin scales mounted in potassium hydroxide (20%) to demonstrate hyphae, and by culture.

Pityriasis versicolor—caused by a skin surface commensal, *Malassezia globosa*, and often triggered by sun exposure. Presentation is with hypo- or hyperpigmented scaling on the trunk. Laboratory diagnosis (if required) is by demonstration of the yeasts and hyphae in skin scales removed by scraping.

Superficial candidosis (candidiasis)—these infections affect the mouth, vagina, and body folds, often in the context of some form of predisposition, e.g. recent antibiotic therapy or, in the case or severe oral infection, immunosuppression including that associated with HIV/AIDS. Infections are diagnosed by microscopy and culture, the latter being particularly important where non-*albicans Candida* species may be involved.

Treatment—the main treatments for superficial mycoses are topical agents that include imidazole preparations (e.g. ketoconazole, clotrimazole), but for widespread infections or those involving hair or nails, oral imidazoles (e.g. itraconazole, fluconazole) or the allylamine, terbinafine, are employed.

Subcutaneous mycoses

Subcutaneous fungal infections, e.g. mycetoma (Madura foot), chromoblastomycosis and sporotrichosis, are not common and usually restricted to the tropics and subtropics. They may present in immigrants from tropical areas, sometimes years after the person has left the tropics, and hence cause diagnostic confusion. Diagnosis is by histological examination of affected tissues or culture. Treatment is often difficult, with only partial responses being achieved, but oral imidazole drugs or terbinafine are helpful in some cases.

Systemic mycoses

Systemic mycoses are deep and often disseminated infections that involve many different sites, including the blood and bone marrow. They may be caused by organisms which invade normal hosts (endemic mycoses) and those which only cause disease in compromised patients (opportunistic mycoses).

Endemic mycoses—these include histoplasmosis, coccidioidomycosis (see Chapter 7.7.3) and infections due to *Penicillium marneffei* (see Chapter 7.7.6), all of which may occur in healthy people, although many are also common complications of HIV/AIDS. Initial manifestations are as respiratory infections, but they can spread haematogenously to other sites, e.g. skin, liver, and brain. Diagnosis is made on culture or biopsy of affected areas.

Opportunistic mycoses—these occur in those who are immunocompromised, e.g. patients with neutropenia secondary to cancer. The routes of fungal entry into the body are very variable, e.g. skin, gastrointestinal tract, lung. Infections include systemic candidosis, aspergillosis, and zygomycosis, but in severely compromised patients, e.g. those with profound neutropenia, many organisms not usually associated with human disease can cause invasive infections, e.g. *Fusarium* species. *Cryptococcus neoformans*, a yeast that can invade the lungs, often presents with meningitis or other signs of intracranial infection.

Prognosis and treatment—the endemic mycoses are often fatal if untreated, and even with treatment the mortality of opportunistic fungal infection can be high, e.g. over 40% for the severely neutropenic patient with aspergillosis. Aside from supportive care, oral or parenteral agents such as amphotericin B, fluconazole, itraconazole, voriconazole, posaconazole, and caspofungin are the treatments of choice, but detecting the organisms and successfully treating the infections remains a challenge.

Introduction

Fungi are saprophytic or parasitic organisms that are normally assigned to a distinct kingdom. As eukaryotes, they have the complex subcellular organization and highly organized genetic material seen in both animal and plant cells. The cell wall is a distinctive feature of fungi and has a complex cytoskeleton based on mannan, glucan, or chitin subunits. The arrangement and reproduction of individual cells is also characteristic. Most fungi form new cells terminally, which remain connected to form long, branching filaments or hyphae (the mould fungi). Some reproduce in a similar manner but each new cell separates from the parent by a process of budding (the yeast fungi). It is a feature of certain fungi to be yeast-like during one phase of their life history but hyphal at another, a phenomenon known as dimorphism. In culture, mould fungi usually form a cottony growth on laboratory media while yeasts normally have a smooth, shiny appearance.

Fungi adversely affect humans in a number of ways. They cause disease indirectly by spoilage and destruction of food crops, with subsequent malnutrition and starvation. Many of the common moulds produce and release spores, which may act as airborne allergens to produce asthma or hypersensitivity pneumonitis. Fungi elaborate complex metabolic by-products, some of which are useful to humans, such as the penicillins. However, others are toxic. Disease caused by the ingestion of fungal toxins includes both poisoning by eating certain mushrooms (mycetism) and damage caused by the ingestion of minute quantities of toxin (mycotoxicosis), e.g. in contaminated grain. The contribution of the latter mechanism to human disease remains largely unexplored, as does the question of whether inhalation of toxic fungal spores may cause pathology. Finally, fungi may invade human tissue. Medical mycology is largely concerned with this last group. Invasive fungal diseases are normally divided into three groups: the superficial, subcutaneous, and deep mycoses. In superficial infections, such as ringworm or thrush, fungi are confined to the skin and mucous membranes. Extension deeper than the surface epithelium is rare. Subcutaneous infections are usually tropical: the main site of involvement is within subcutaneous tissue, although secondary invasion of adjacent structures such as bone or skin may occur. In deep or systemic infections, deep organs such as the lung, spleen, or brain are invaded. This classification of mycoses is based on the main 'sphere of involvement' by the causal organisms, but there are exceptions. For instance, brain involvement has been recorded in patients with chromoblastomycosis, which is normally a subcutaneous infection.

The fungi causing systemic mycoses are often classified in two groups: the opportunists and the endemic pathogens. The former cause disease in overtly compromised individuals. These contrast with the true pathogens, which cause infection in all subjects inhaling airborne spores.

Superficial fungal infections

The main superficial mycoses are the dermatophyte infections, superficial candidosis, and tinea versicolor (see Section 23). These are both common and widespread. Rare superficial infections include tinea nigra, and black or white piedra.

Dermatophyte infections (dermatophytoses)

Aetiology

The dermatophyte or ringworm infections are caused by a group of organisms capable of existing in keratinized tissue such as stratum corneum, nail, or hair. The mechanism of invasion is thought to be linked to production of extracellular enzymes; three distinct metalloproteinase genes are found in *Microsporum canis*.

Epidemiology

Some dermatophyte fungi have a worldwide distribution; others are more restricted. The most common and most widely distributed is *Trichophyton rubrum*, which causes different types of infection in different parts of the world. It is commonly associated with athlete's foot (tinea pedis) in temperate areas as well as tinea corporis or tinea cruris in the tropics. This distinction is not based solely on climatic factors, as immigrants from tropical countries, particularly eastern Asia, may still have tinea corporis caused by *T. rubrum* when living in northern Europe. Certain dermatophytes are limited to defined areas. For instance, tinea imbricata caused by *T. concentricum*, is found in hot, humid areas of the eastern Asia, Polynesia, and South America. Scalp ringworm tends to occur in well-defined endemic areas in Africa and elsewhere. In different regions, different species of dermatophytes may predominate. Thus, in North Africa, the most common cause of tinea capitis is *T. violaceum*; in southern parts of the continent, the major agents may be *Microsporum audouinii*, *M. ferrugineum*, and *T. soudanense*. Not all dermatophyte infections are endemic and dominant species may disappear to be replaced by others. *M. audouinii*, once endemic and common in the United Kingdom, is now infrequent but associated with infections in African Caribbean children. By contrast, *T tonsurans* is now established as a major cause of tinea capitis in urban areas in the United Kingdom, parts of Europe, and the United States of America. Dermatophytes may be passed from person to person (anthropophilic infections), from animal to person (zoophilic), or from soil to person (geophilic). Sources of zoophilic organisms in Europe include cats and dogs, cattle, hedgehogs, and small rodents. Rarer sources include horses, monkeys, and chickens. Lesions produced by zoophilic species may be highly inflammatory.

Factors governing the invasion of stratum corneum are largely unknown, but heat, humidity, and occlusion have all been implicated. Susceptibility to certain infection, such as tinea imbricata, may be genetically determined.

Clinical features

The clinical features of dermatophyte infections are best considered in relation to the site involved. Often the term tinea, followed by the Latin name of the appropriate part (such as *corporis*, meaning 'body') is used to describe the clinical site of infection.

Tinea pedis

Scaling or maceration between the toes, particularly in the fourth interspace, is the most common form of dermatophytosis seen in temperate countries. Itching is variable, but may be severe. Sometimes blisters may form both between the toes and on the soles of the feet. The causative organisms are commonly *T. rubrum* and *T. interdigitale*, the latter being responsible for the vesicular forms. Similar appearances can be caused by *Candida albicans* and in the bacterial infection, erythrasma. Gram-negative bacterial infection causes erosive interdigital disease associated with discomfort.

'Dry type' infections of the soles and palms

These are normally caused by *T. rubrum*. Palms (Fig. 7.7.1.1) or soles have a dry, scaly appearance, which in the soles may encroach on to the lateral or dorsal surfaces of the foot. The palmar involvement is often unilateral, an important diagnostic feature. Nail invasion is often seen (see below). Itching is not prominent, and infections are usually chronic.

Tinea cruris

Infections of the groin, most often caused by *T. rubrum* or *Epidermophyton floccosum*, are relatively common. They occur in both tropical and temperate climates, although in the former the infection may spread to involve the whole waist area in both males and females. Tinea cruris in females is uncommon in Europe. An erythematous and scaly rash with a distinct margin extends from the groin to the upper thighs or scrotum. Itching may be severe. Coincident tinea pedis is common, and patients should be examined for this. The rash of crural erythrasma shows uniform scaling without a margin, whereas in candidosis, satellite pustules occur distal to the rim.

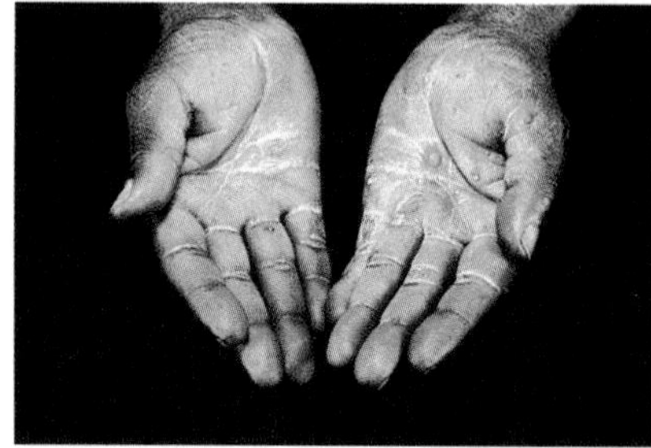

Fig. 7.7.1.1 Palmar scaling due to *Trichophyton rubrum*.

Onychomycosis (caused by dermatophytes)

Invasion of the nail plate is most often seen with *T. rubrum* infections. The plate is invaded distally and becomes thickened and friable with terminal loss of the nail plate. Onycholysis may be seen. More rarely, and most often with *T. interdigitale*, the dorsal surface of the plate is invaded, causing superficial white onychomycosis.

Tinea corporis (body ringworm)

Dermatophyte or ringworm infection on the trunk or limbs may produce the characteristic annular plaque with a raised edge and central clearing (Fig. 7.7.1.2). Scaling and itching is variable. Lesions caused by zoophilic organisms may be highly inflammatory and in certain cases, particularly those caused by *T. verrucosum*, intense itching, oedema, and pustule formation (kerion) may develop. This reaction is seldom secondarily infected by bacteria but is a response to the fungus on hairy skin. Infections of the beard, tinea barbae, are often highly refractory to treatment. Facial dermatophyte infections may mimic a variety of nonfungal skin diseases, including acne, rosacea, and discoid lupus erythematosus. However, the underlying annular configuration can usually be distinguished. The term tinea incognito is used to describe such atypical lesions.

Tinea capitis (scalp ringworm)

In the United Kingdom as in the United States of America, the most common cause of scalp ringworm is *T. tonsurans*, an anthropophilic fungus which mainly occurs in inner cities, particularly in

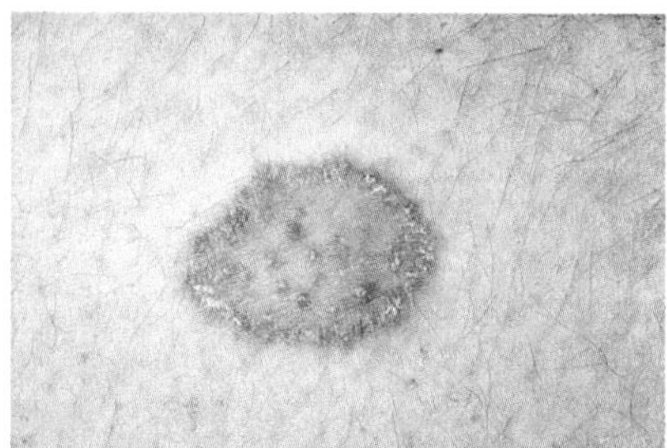

Fig. 7.7.1.2 Tinea corporis due to *Microsporum gypseum*.

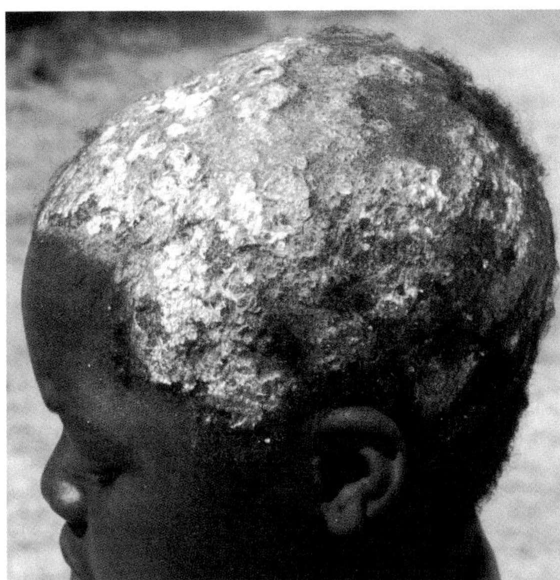

Fig. 7.7.1.3 Advanced favus of scalp in a Nigerian cattle herd caused by *Trichophyton schoenleinii*.
(Copyright D A Warrell.)

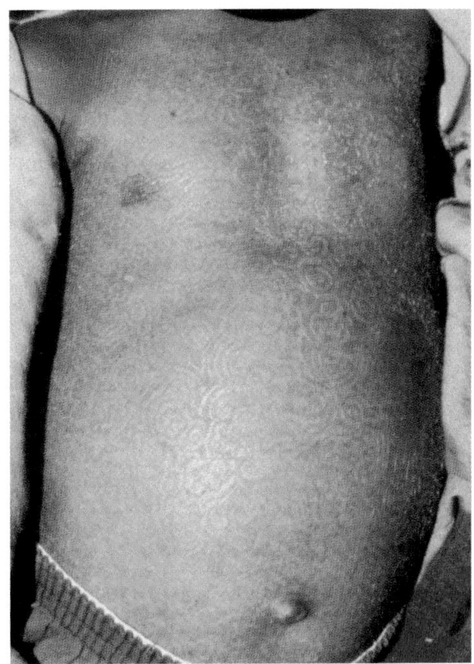

Fig. 7.7.1.4 Tinea imbricata, Papua New Guinea.
(Courtesy of Dr B Hudson, Sydney.)

black Caribbean or African children. This has now replaced *Microsporum canis*, originating from an infected cat or dog, although this dermatophyte is dominant elsewhere in the United Kingdom and Europe. Scalp ringworm is mainly a disease of childhood, but infections may occur in adult women. Spontaneous clearance at puberty is the rule. *M. canis* causes an 'ectothrix' infection where spores form on the outside of the hair shaft and the scalp hair breaks above the skin surface. Scaling, itching, and loss of hair occur. Other causes of ectothrix infection include *M. audouinii*, which is becoming more common in Europe, and is still seen in West Africa. This infection can be spread from child to child and causes serious social handicap. The infection may occur in epidemic form, particularly in schools. By contrast, infections with *M. canis* are acquired from a primary animal source rather than by spread from human lesions. In endothrix infections where sporulation is within the hair shaft, scaling is less pronounced and hairs break at scalp level (black dot ringworm). Examples include *T. tonsurans* and *T. violaceum*, the latter being most prevalent in the Middle East, parts of Africa, and India, although it also is being recognized with increasing frequency in Europe.

Favus, now most often seen in isolated foci in the tropics, is a particularly chronic form of ringworm caused by *T. schoenleinii* or *T. violaceum* where hair shafts become surrounded by a necrotic crust or scutulum (Fig. 7.7.1.3). Individual crusts coalesce to form a pale, unpleasant-smelling mat over parts of the scalp. Such infections may cause extensive and permanent hair loss.

Tinea imbricata (tokelau)

This infection is endemic in parts of eastern Asia, West Pacific, and Central and South America, and is caused by *T. concentricum*. In many cases the trunk is covered with scales laid down in concentric rings producing a ripple effect (Fig. 7.7.1.4). Alternatively, large, loose scales may form (hence the name; *imbricata* is the Latin word for 'tiled'). The infection is often chronic, and may constitute a serious social handicap. There is some evidence that susceptibility of this disease in Papua New Guinea may be inherited as an autosomal recessive trait.

Infection in HIV and immunocompromised patients

While dermatophyte infections are no more common in the immunocompromised patient, they may differ clinically. In patients with HIV infections there may be (1) more tinea facei, (2) more widespread and atypical skin lesions, and (3) a distinct pattern of nail infection characterized by white discoloration spreading rapidly through the nail plate from the proximal nail fold.

Laboratory diagnosis

The mainstays of diagnosis are direct microscopy of skin scales mounted in potassium hydroxide (20%) to demonstrate hyphae, and culture. Scalp hairs may also be examined in a similar way, and the site of arthrospore formation, inside or outside the shaft, determined. Fluorescent whitening agents (Calcofluor) or chlorazol black stain have been used to highlight fungi in scales. Further tests, such as the ability to penetrate hair, may be used to separate similar cultures. Identification of organisms is important, as it will indicate the source of infection in scalp ringworm, for example. When large numbers of children are involved, screening of scalp infections with a filtered ultraviolet lamp (Wood's light) is useful. Certain species, including *M. canis* and *M. audouinii*, cause infected hair to fluoresce with a vivid greenish light. Scalps can also be screened for infection by passing a sterile brush or scalp massager through the hair and plating this directly on to an agar plate.

Treatment

The treatment of dermatophyte infections depends to an extent on the nature and severity of infection. Topical therapy is reserved for circumscribed infections such as athlete's foot and tinea corporis, not involving hair or nail keratin. Scalp and nail infections, severe or widespread ringworm, and failures of topical therapy are usually treated orally with griseofulvin, itraconazole, or terbinafine.

Specific antifungal drugs in topical form are effective and well tolerated. The important compounds in this group are miconazole, clotrimazole, ketoconazole, and econazole, which are imidazole derivatives, undecenoic acid, and tolnaftate and the allylamine, terbinafine. Generally treatment is given for 7 to 30 days. They are all very similar in their clinical efficacy, but topical terbinafine is particularly rapid in foot infection (≤7 days). Adverse reactions are rare.

For oral therapy the main alternatives are terbinafine, itraconazole, or fluconazole. Terbinafine (250 mg/day) is rapidly effective in most forms of dermatophytosis that require oral therapy and also produces rapid responses in toe nail (12 weeks) and sole infections (2 to 4 weeks), without a high rate of relapse. Side effects include headache and nausea, but loss of taste may also occur. Itraconazole is somewhat similar in its profile, but is given intermittently (200 mg twice daily for 7 days). This course is given once for sole infections but repeated three times at monthly intervals for toe nail infections, as pulsed therapy. Side effects include nausea and abdominal discomfort. Fluconazole is also active and is given in a dose of 150 mg weekly; 300 mg may be necessary for toe nail infections. This side effect profile is similar to itraconazole. All three drugs are extremely rare causes of hepatic toxicity. Griseofulvin is still used for tinea capitis in a dose of 10 to 20 mg/kg daily. Treatment should be continued for at least 6 weeks in tinea capitis. Side effects are not common, but include headache, nausea, and urticaria. The drug can also precipitate acute intermittent porphyria and systemic lupus erythematosus in predisposed subjects.

Scytalidium infections

The organisms *Scytalidium dimidiatum* (*Hendersonula toruloidea*) and *S hyalinum*, can cause a superficial scaly condition that resembles the 'dry type' of dermatophyte infection on the palms or soles. Nail plate destruction may also occur, the lateral border of the nail being the initial site of invasion. The disease has been seen in Europe, almost invariably in immigrants from the tropics, particularly the Caribbean, West Africa, India, or Pakistan. Its prevalence in the tropics is unknown, although in some surveys it has been shown to be relatively common. In skin scrapings the tortuous hyphae may resemble those of a dermatophyte, but the organisms do not grow on media containing cycloheximide, which is often incorporated into agar for routine dermatophyte isolation.

Treatment is difficult, but some improvement may follow the use of keratolytic compounds such as salicylic acid. Nail infections do not respond to terbinafine, griseofulvin, or azoles.

Miscellaneous nail infections

Occasionally, fungi other than dermatophytes or *Scytalidium* species are isolated from dystrophic nails. These include *Scopulariopsis brevicaulis*, *Onychocola canadensis*, acremonium, and fusarium species, and certain types of aspergillus. These infections are usually seen in elderly or immunosuppressed individuals. It is often difficult, particularly with aspergillus species, to establish that the organism is playing a pathogenic role.

Pityriasis versicolor (tinea versicolor)

Aetiology

Pityriasis versicolor is a superficial infection caused by *Malassezia* species, usually *M. globosa*. Although most common in tropical countries, it has a worldwide distribution. Dermal penetration does not occur.

There are six species of malassezia that can be found on normal skin, the commonest of which are *M. sympodialis* and *M. globosa*. In pityriasis versicolor there is transformation of yeast cells to produce hyphae. It is likely that the state of host immunity plays some part in pathogenesis and depression; for instance, endogenous or exogenous corticosteroids potentiate the disease in some individuals. However, it is also commonly seen in normal individuals, and climatic factors or sun exposure are believed to trigger the infection in many cases. There is no effective animal model for studies of this disease.

Epidemiology

Pityriasis versicolor is very common in the tropics, where it may be widespread on the body. Its incidence in temperate climates has increased over the last 20 to 30 years. It is not more common in HIV-infected individuals.

Clinical features

The rash of pityriasis versicolor is asymptomatic or mildly pruritic. Its presents with scaling, confluent macules on the trunk, upper arms, or neck. These may be hypopigmented or hyperpigmented. In some people and in the tropics, other areas including face, forearms, and thighs may be involved.

The diagnosis is rarely confused with other complaints, although eczema or ringworm infections are sometimes considered. Patients are often anxious to exclude leprosy, but the two are unlikely to be mistaken. In vitiligo, depigmentation is complete and there is no scaling.

Laboratory diagnosis

The diagnosis is made by demonstration of the yeasts and hyphae of malassezia in skin scales removed by scraping. Culture is difficult and unnecessary.

Treatment

Topical ketoconazole, miconazole, clotrimazole, or econazole is effective. Oral itraconazole may be used in recalcitrant cases. Whatever the treatment, relapse is common.

Other malassezia-associated conditions

Malassezia yeasts have been implicated in the pathogenesis of a number of other skin diseases such as seborrhoeic dermatitis and a form of itchy folliculitis, malassezia folliculitis. The evidence connecting seborrhoeic dermatitis, one of the most common of skin diseases, and malassezia is largely concerned with the response of antifungal drugs and the observation that improvements in the rash mirror disappearance of organisms from the skin. Severity of the skin condition does not appear to reflect the numbers of yeasts on the skin surface.

Superficial candidosis (candidiasis)

Aetiology

Superficial candidosis is a term used to describe a group of infections of skin or mucous membranes caused by species of the genus *Candida*. They range in severity from oral thrush to chronic mucocutaneous candidosis, a chronic infection refractory to conventional antifungal treatment.

Candida albicans is the species most frequently involved. It is a saprophytic yeast often found as a commensal in the mouth

Box 7.7.1.1 Predisposing factors in superficial candidosis

- Local epithelial defects, occlusion, constant immersion in water, e.g. damaged nail folds, beneath dentures
- Defects of immunity (primarily T cell or phagocytosis)
  - Primary immunological disease, e.g. chronic granulomatous disease
  - Immunodefects secondary to intercurrent illness, e.g. leukaemia
  - Immunodefects secondary to therapy, e.g. cytotoxic therapy in organ transplantation
- Drug therapy, e.g. antibiotics
- Carcinoma or leukaemia
- Endocrine disease
  - Diabetes mellitus
  - Hypothyroidism, hypoparathyroidism, hypoadrenalism (all in chronic mucocutaneous candidosis)
- Physiological changes, e.g. infancy, pregnancy, old age
- Miscellaneous disorders, e.g.
  - Iron deficiency
  - Zinc deficiency
  - Malabsorption

and gastrointestinal tract, and is commonly present in the vagina. Several factors may influence the incidence of carriage. For instance, oral colonization is more common in hospital staff than in equivalent nonhospital employees. Vaginal carriage is more common in pregnancy. Other factors (Box 7.7.1.1) are known that predispose to conversion from a commensal to a parasitic role with the causation of disease—candidosis. The list includes factors that influence host immunological response, such as carcinoma, AIDS, or cytotoxic therapy; those that disturb the population of other microorganisms, such as antibiotics; and those that affect the character of the epithelium, such as dentures.

Other species of candida may also cause superficial infections, but are less common. They include *C. glabrata*, *C. dubliniensis*, and *C. parapsilosis*. There is evidence that the first two species are more common in oral infection in patients with HIV and *C. glabrata* in vaginal candidosis.

Epidemiology

Superficial candida infections are seen in all countries.

Clinical features

There are a number of clinically distinct types of superficial infection caused by candida species, as follows.

Oral candidosis (thrush)

Oral infection by candida is fairly common, particularly in infancy and old age, or in association with antibiotic or cytotoxic therapy, or in diseases where the neutrophil or T-lymphocyte responses may be impaired. In older people, the wearing of dentures is a predisposing factor. The lesions present with discomfort both in the mouth and at the corners of the lips. The mouth and buccal mucosa show patchy or confluent, white adherent plaques; less commonly the mucosa and tongue are sore and glazed—erythematous candidosis. Angular cheilitis usually accompanies the oral lesions. In long-standing cases, the plaque may become hypertrophic, with oedema of the mucosal surfaces, or the mucosa may appear glazed and raw.

There is a significant correlation between leucoplakia and oral candidosis, and it has been suggested that the infection may lead to epithelial dysplasia.

The diagnosis is made by the demonstration of yeasts and hyphae of candida in smears, and by culture.

Vaginal candidosis (thrush)

See Chapter 8.4 for further detail.

Paronychia

Infection around the nail fold is seen in people whose occupations involve frequent wetting of the hands (such as cooks) or in those with eczema or psoriasis. The aetiology is complicated and there may be a mixture of bacterial infection and irritant or allergic contact dermatitis as well as candida infection. The condition presents with painful, red swelling of the nail fold. Pus may be discharged. Secondary invasion of the lateral border of the nail plate by candida may occur from this site.

Candida intertrigo

Infection of the moist folds of the skin in the groin or under the breasts causes itching and discomfort. The area becomes macerated and erythematous. Candida may contribute to this condition, but is certainly not the only factor. It may also superinfect the napkin area in infants. The presence of satellite pustules (see above) is a useful indicator of involvement by candida in the disease process.

Direct invasion of toe-web folds by candida closely resembles 'athlete's foot' caused by dermatophytes. A similar erosive infection may occur in the finger webs—interdigital candidosis—and is seen most commonly in the tropics.

Chronic superficial candidosis

Chronic candida infections of the mouth, vagina, and nail present problems in management. Chronic oral candidosis, for instance, is associated with leucoplakia. Predisposing causes should be searched for. The most serious of this group of infections is chronic mucocutaneous candidosis, a rare condition in which chronic skin, nail, and mucosal infection coexist (Fig. 7.7.1.5). A series of underlying genetic, endocrine (hypoparathyroidism, hypoadrenalism, or hypothyroidism), and immunological abnormalities has been found; in some cases it has been associated with mutations in an

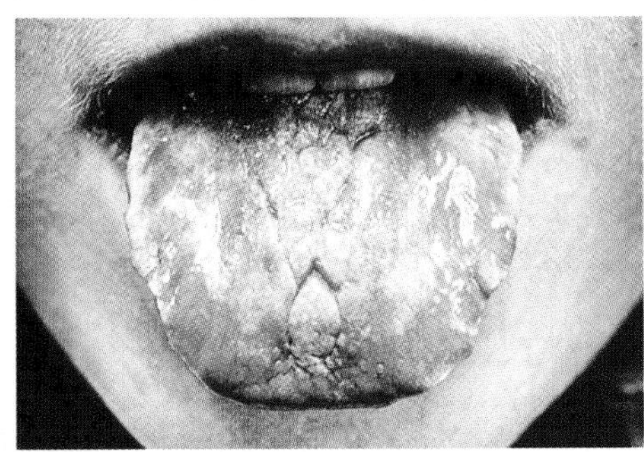

Fig. 7.7.1.5 Oral candidosis in a patient with chronic mucocutaneous candidosis.

autoimmune regulator gene (*AIRE*). Extensive human papillomavirus (wart) or dermatophyte infections may also be present in these patients, whose condition is normally diagnosed in childhood.

Oral candidosis is one of the earliest signs of untreated AIDS, occurring in a high proportion of patients. The appearances are similar to those seen with other groups, although plaque formation may be very extensive. Oesophageal infection is common in this group.

Laboratory diagnosis

All these infections are diagnosed by microscopy and culture. When associated with the condition, candida cells are always evident on microscopy. Culture establishes the specific identity and is important particularly where species other than *Candida albicans* may be involved.

Treatment

Two groups of drugs are effective in superficial candidosis. The polyenes such as nystatin and amphotericin B are topically active in many forms of candidosis. They are often less effective in oral candidosis in immunodeficient patients, including those with AIDS. Likewise, topical azole drugs such as miconazole and clotrimazole are usually effective in superficial candidosis. For unresponsive cases, oral therapy with fluconazole, itraconazole, or ketoconazole may be necessary. Fluconazole resistance can occur and *C. glabrata* is seldom responsive to this drug.

For vaginal infections, topical creams or vaginal preparations should be used—many requiring only a single treatment. Single-dose oral fluconazole is an alternative. In recalcitrant cases it may be necessary to use longer courses of fluconazole or itraconazole.

Miscellaneous superficial mycoses

There are a number of relatively rare, superficial fungal infections such as tinea nigra, and black or white piedra. They never cause invasive disease, and are mainly confined to the tropics.

Tinea nigra

Tinea nigra is a superficial infection confined to the epidermis of the palms or soles, and more rarely elsewhere. The initial lesion is a dark macule without scaling, which resembles a brown stain on the skin and spreads slowly over the palmar or plantar surface. The disease is normally asymptomatic.

On scraping the skin, brown pigmented hyphae can be seen by direct microscopy, and the causative organism, *Phaeoanellomyces werneckii*, isolated.

The lesion responds to Whitfield's ointment.

Black piedra

Black piedra is a disease of the tropics in which small, dark nodules form on hair shafts in the scalp or, less commonly, elsewhere. There are no symptoms. Each nodule consists of a dense mat of hyphae containing the sexual spores (ascospores) of the fungus.

The diagnosis is made by direct microscopy of infected hair, and the isolation of *Piedraia hortae*. Treatment using a 1% azole solution or amphotericin B lotion is usually effective.

White piedra

White piedra occurs in both temperate and tropical climates, and is rare. It produces pale nodules on the hair of the beard, groin, or scalp. The hair shaft may fracture. The nodule consists of hyphae, arthrospores (spores formed by fragmentation of hyphae), and blastospores (budding yeast cells). The organism *Trichosporon* species can be readily cultured. The treatment is similar to that for black piedra.

Subcutaneous mycoses

Subcutaneous infections caused by fungi are rare, and are mainly seen in the tropics. The organisms gain entry via the skin; in mycetoma, organisms may be implanted subcutaneously via a thorn. The majority of the causative organisms in this group of infections can be isolated from vegetation or soil. Involvement of deep viscera is rare. Attempts to establish experimental infections that resemble the human diseases have been largely unsuccessful. A clearer understanding of the pathogenesis therefore awaits such a model system. These infections tend to be chronic, chemotherapy may be lengthy, and in the case of mycetoma, often unsuccessful.

Mycetoma (Madura foot)

Aetiology

Mycetoma is a chronic infection involving subcutaneous tissue, bone, and skin, in which colonies of infecting fungi or actinomycetes (grains) are found within a network of burrowing abscesses and sinuses (Fig. 7.7.1.6).

The more common organisms that cause mycetoma are listed in Box 7.7.1.2. The organisms are divided into two groups, the actinomycetomas and the eumycetomas, caused by actinomycetes and fungi, respectively. The size and colour of the grains (red, pale, or dark) are important clues to their identification. The organisms can be found in the natural environment such as soil, and some have even been identified in association with acacia thorns in an endemic area. The infection is initiated when an infected thorn is implanted in deep tissue. However, many years may elapse before the formation of a clinically apparent mycetoma.

Epidemiology

The disease is seen primarily in the tropics, although rare cases, apart from imported ones, may occur in temperate areas. Countries with the most reported cases include India, Mexico, Senegal, Sudan, and Venezuela. However, the disease is widely distributed in the tropics, particularly in Africa to the south and east of the Sahara Desert.

The pattern of prevalence of infections caused by certain organisms differs strikingly in different parts of the world. For instance, *Streptomyces somaliensis* is most common in the Sudan and Middle East, but *Madurella grisea* is mainly found in the New World. Altogether about 60% of reported infections are caused by

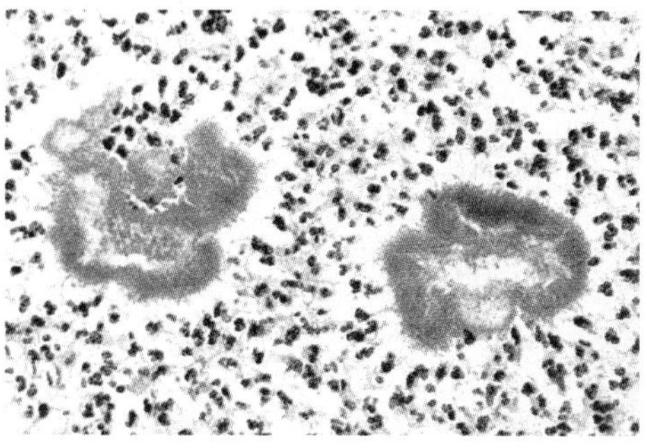

Fig. 7.7.1.6 Grains in abscess in actinomycetoma (*Nocardia brasilensis*) (haematoxylin and eosin stain).

Box 7.7.1.2 Causes of mycetoma

- Fungi, e.g.
  - *Madurella mycetomatis*
  - *Madurella grisea*
  - *Scedosporium apiospermum*
  - *Exophiala jeanselmei*
  - *Leptosphaeria senegalensis*
  - *Species of Acremonium, Aspergillus, Fusarium*
- Actinomycetes, e.g.
  - *Nocardia brasiliensis*
  - *Actinomadura madurae*
  - *Actinomadura pelletieri*
  - *Streptomyces somaliensis*

actinomycetes, of which *Nocardia brasiliensis* is the most common (Chapter 7.6.30).

Clinical features

Early mycetomas may present with a circumscribed area of hard painless subcutaneous swelling (Fig. 7.7.1.7). Later, sinus tracts open on to the skin surface and visible grains may be discharged, along with serosanguinous fluid (Fig. 7.7.1.8). Bone erosion and destruction, leading to deformity, may occur. However, severe pain is rarely a problem. Local lymph node invasion may occur, but more widespread involvement is very rare.

Feet and lower legs are the areas most commonly involved, but the arms, buttocks, chest, and head may all be sites of infection. Mycetoma caused by *N. brasiliensis* may occur in any site, but one favoured area is the chest wall.

The radiological features of mycetoma are cortical erosion, followed by the development of lytic deposits in bone. Periosteal proliferation and destruction, leading to deformity, may follow. MRI provides a clearer picture of bone involvement and may be positive earlier than radiography.

Laboratory diagnosis

The diagnosis is made by the demonstration and identification of grains obtained from the sinus openings by gentle pressure or curettage. If these measures are not successful, tissue should be obtained by deep surgical biopsy. Grains can be mounted in potassium hydroxide and examined microscopically. Those containing filaments 3 to 4 μm or more in diameter are caused by true fungi (eumycetomas), and those with filaments of less than 1 μm by actinomycetes (actinomycetomas). These features can usually be distinguished by direct microscopy.

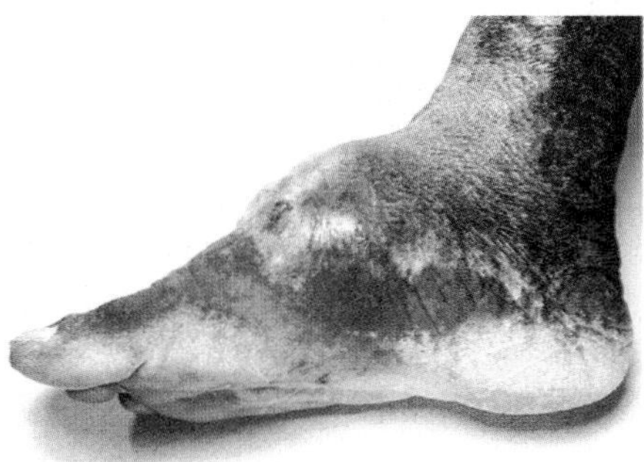

Fig. 7.7.1.7 A mycetoma caused by *Madurella grisea*.

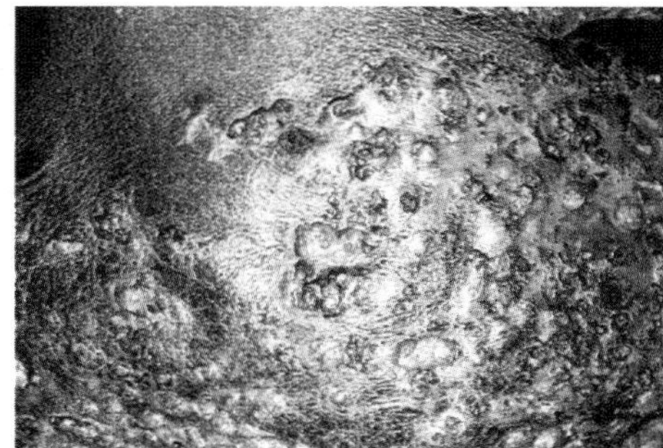

Fig. 7.7.1.8 *Nocardia brasiliensis* actinomycetoma draining sinus.

The morphology of grains fixed, sectioned, and stained with haematoxylin and eosin is typical. Special stains are less helpful. Grains can be used for culture, although several attempts at isolation may have to be made. Serology (such as immunodiffusion) can also be helpful, although the tests are not widely available.

Treatment

Actinomycetomas may respond to sulphones such as dapsone (50-100 mg daily) or sulphonamides such as sulphadiazine. The treatment of choice for many is long-term co-trimoxazole (2-3 tablets twice daily) with an initial 2 to 3 months of streptomycin or rifampicin. Treatment may have to be continued for many months or years. Dapsone is an effective and cheaper alternative to co-trimoxazole. Extensive actinomycetomas may respond poorly and additional treatment with amikacin or fucidin may be necessary. The eumycetomas seldom respond to antifungal therapy. About 20% of *Madurella mycetomatis* infections respond to ketoconazole. In other infections griseofulvin, amphotericin B, voriconazole, ketoconazole, and itraconazole have rarely produced remission or cure. A trial of therapy may be attempted, where the patient can be monitored closely in outpatient departments. Otherwise, radical surgery or amputation is usually necessary. Small, local excisions are rarely successful.

Mycetoma is slowly progressive and increasingly disabling. However, wider dissemination is very rare, and therefore cases are seldom fatal, except where the skull is involved. However, the deformity caused by the disease may be severely disabling.

Chromoblastomycosis (chromomycosis)

Aetiology

Chromoblastomycosis, one of the intermediate subcutaneous mycoses, is a chronic granulomatous fungal infection characterized histologically by the presence of brown, spherical fungal cells known as sclerotic cells or fumagoid bodies. In most cases, the lesions are confined to the skin and subcutaneous tissues. In the past there has been great confusion over nomenclature of the aetiological agents of chromoblastomycosis. At present, five agents assigned to four genera are recognized as causing chromoblastomycosis – most are due to the first two. They are:

- *Fonsecaea pedrosoi*, which occurs in high-rainfall areas and is found worldwide
- *Cladophialophora carrionii*, the sole cause of chromoblastomycosis in arid areas

- *Phialophora verrucosa*, the first agent to be described
- *Fonsecaea compactum*, an uncommon cause and isolated only a few times
- *Rhinocladiella aquaspersa*, a rare cause.

Sporadic cases caused by other dematiaceous fungi such as *Cladosporium trichoides* and *Taeniolella boppii* have been reported from Uganda and Brazil.

Epidemiology

The principal endemic areas for chromoblastomycosis are tropical and subtropical countries including Central and South America, Costa Rica, Africa, Japan, Australia, Madagascar, and Indonesia. Curiously, sporadic cases have been reported from Finland and Russia.

Although soil itself does not seem to be a particularly good substrate, the various agents of chromoblastomycosis occur as saprobic fungi in the environment and have been isolated from soil, decaying vegetation and rotting wood. Strains of *F. pedrosoi* and *P. verrucosa* have been isolated from the atmosphere but proved less virulent than those isolated from human lesions or organic material.

Infection occurs as a result of trauma, however minor, the fungi gaining entrance through a cut, abrasion, or thorn prick. Farmers and labourers in agricultural areas are most likely to be exposed to contaminated material. Although lesions on exposed areas may be accounted for in this way, it was suggested by Wilson in 1958 that lesions on nonexposed areas may result from a previously unrecognized pulmonary focus. Bacquero later demonstrated the presence of *F. pedrosoi* in bronchial washings and subsequently proved their pathogenicity by inoculating those strains into normal skin of human volunteers and recovering the fungus from the ensuing skin lesions. Other methods of transmission have included metal particles from automobiles, and acupuncture. Person-to-person and animal-to-human transmission have not so far been reported. Chromoblastomycosis has rarely been reported in children, and it may be that factors other than trauma and exposure to contaminated material are necessary for its development.

Pathogenesis

Host resistance and virulence of the organism are the two main factors associated with the pathogenesis of this disease. Chromoblastomycosis occurs mainly in healthy individuals. However, it has been found in immunosuppressed patients. Although the mechanism of granuloma formation is not well understood, it appears that lipids extracted from these fungi and cell-wall constituents may be responsible for this reaction.

Clinical features

The initial lesion of chromoblastomycosis is a small papule at the site of trauma, which gradually enlarges (Fig. 7.7.1.9). Nodules and tumours develop, producing a malodorous discharge; eventually, over a period of years, a wide variety of morphological patterns may emerge including dry, hyperkeratotic plaques, verrucose lesions, and large, cauliflower-like masses (Fig. 7.7.1.10). Extensive cicatricial plaques, surrounded by peripherally spreading vegetative lesions, may also be present. Evolution is slow and lesions usually involve the lower limb. However, any part of the body may be involved and the sites may be multiple.

Dissemination occurs by (1) surface spread; (2) the lymphatics, the most common method; (iii) autoinoculation from scratching; and (iv) haematogenously, resulting in subcutaneous lesions at sites distant from the primary. Visceral metastases are known to occur and involvement of the central nervous system, respiratory system, larynx, and vocal chords has been recorded. Therapeutically, therefore, early diagnosis is important.

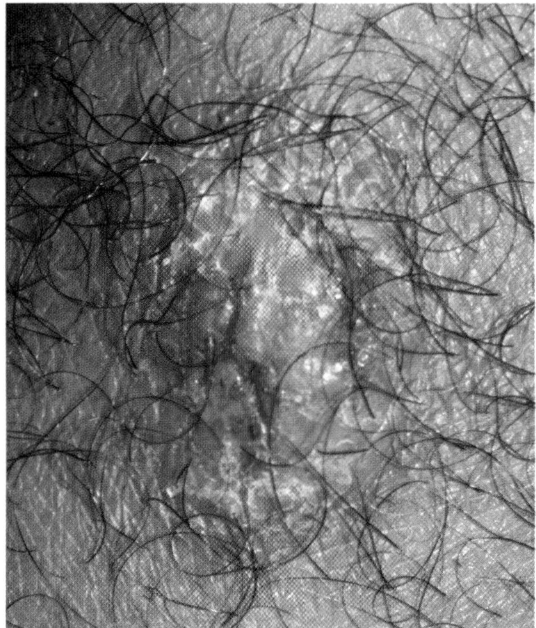

Fig. 7.7.1.9 Chromoblastomycosis. Early lesion in a Brazilian patient. (Copyright D A Warrell.)

Complications of long-standing chromoblastomycosis include lymphoedema, flexion deformity of joints, and development of squamous carcinoma.

Diagnosis

Although the history and clinical presentation may suggest the diagnosis, the varied clinical presentation of chromoblastomycosis necessitates consideration of other granulomatous diseases such as sporotrichosis, cutaneous tuberculosis, Hansen's disease, blastomycosis, candidosis, leishmaniasis, paracoccidioidomycosis,

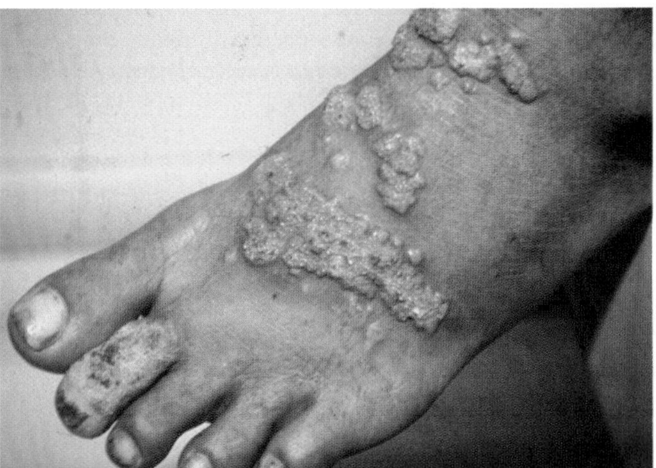

Fig. 7.7.1.10 Chromoblastomycosis: late lesion. (Courtesy of João LC Cardoso, São Paulo, Brazil.)

rhinosporidiosis, tertiary syphilis, squamous carcinoma, and even psoriasis, sarcoidosis, and discoid lupus erythematosus.

Therefore, to establish a definitive diagnosis, histological and mycological investigations are essential. Diagnosis is confirmed by the presence of the characteristic brown, sclerotic bodies in histological sections. From both epidemiological and therapeutic points of view, culture is necessary as *F. pedrosoi* is the most difficult of the causative fungi to eradicate whereas *C. carrionii* responds rapidly to treatment.

Treatment

Small, single, localized lesions are satisfactorily eradicated by cryosurgery, but long-term follow-up is needed to assess accurately the success of this treatment. Thermotherapy has been found effective by some, again principally in the management of small, single lesions, but here the possibility of a burn must be borne in mind. Rapid spread of the disease has been associated with inadequate surgery, curettage, and electrodesiccation.

Oral monotherapy has been unsuccessful in some cases and drug resistance remains a problem. However itraconazole and terbinafine have both been reported as effective agents. A combination of 5-flucytosine with either thiabendazole or itraconazole may also be efficacious, particularly in long-standing disease.

Whatever method of treatment is used, chromomycosis although clinically healed, should be followed-up for at least 2 years before its total eradication can be assumed.

Sporotrichosis

Aetiology

The most common clinical form of sporotrichosis is a subcutaneous infection, which may spread proximally from its initial site in a series of nodules along the course of a lymphatic (Fig. 7.7.1.11a, b). More rarely, systemic involvement is seen, e.g. in the lung (see 'Systemic mycoses', below).

The causative organism *Sporothrix schenckii* can be found in soil, in vegetation, or in association with plants or bark. People who develop the subcutaneous infection may have had contact with material that harbours the organism, such as moss or flowers (e.g. florists). It is assumed that the pathogen gains entry via an abrasion and in some endemic areas there is often a preceding history of a cat scratch or insect bite.

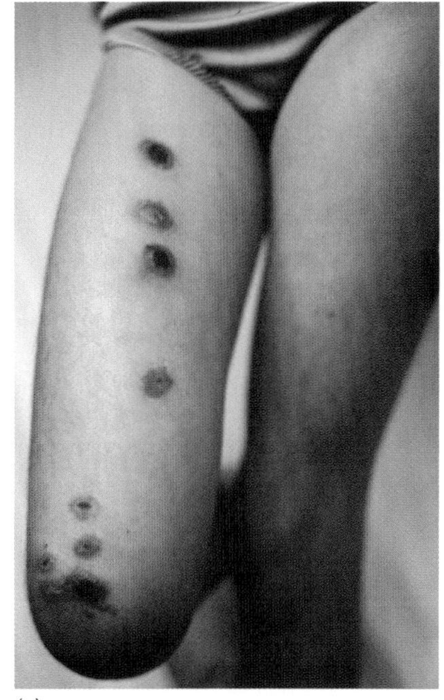

(a)

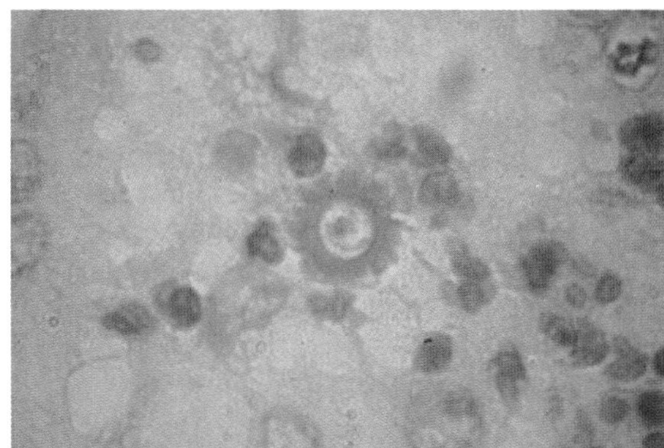

(b)

Fig. 7.7.1.11a (a) Sporotrichosis. (b) Histopathological appearances. (a, courtesy of João LC Cardoso, São Paulo, Brazil; b, copyright Professor R Hay.)

Epidemiology

Although sporotrichosis was once prevalent in Europe, particularly France, nonimported cases are now very rare in this area. However, the disease is seen in the United States of America, Mexico, Central and South America, and Africa. In the late 1930s, there was a remarkable epidemic of sporotrichosis in workers in the Witwatersrand gold mines (South Africa). The source of infection was a large number of wooden pit props contaminated with the organism. Other, smaller 'epidemics' have been described in certain groups, such as Mexican pottery workers packing ceramics in straw. Normally, however, cases are sporadic in incidence. There are also 'hyperendemic' areas where there is an unexpectedly high incidence of this infection.

Systemic sporotrichosis is much rarer, and cases have mainly been described from the United States.

Clinical features

There are two main clinical types of subcutaneous sporotrichosis.

The first, the fixed type, presents with a solitary cutaneous ulcer or nodule. In this form of the disease, infection does not spread along lymphatics. It has been suggested that it is most common in children, and it has been described most frequently in Central and South America.

In the lymphangitic form, an initial nodule forms on a limb or extremity, such as a finger. This may break down and ulcerate. Subsequently, one or more secondary nodules develop along the draining lymphatic channel, which may ulcerate through the skin (Fig. 7.7.1.11a). Other variants include the psoriasiform or verrucous types or a superficial granuloma that resembles lupus vulgaris. These usually represent chronic infection.

Rarer forms include secondary spread via scratching, which may present with multiple widespread ulcers or multiple cutaneous lesions secondary to systemic disease. In HIV-positive individuals, widespread cutaneous lesions may develop.

Fixed-type sporotrichosis may resemble many other forms of cutaneous ulceration. However, in endemic areas a major source of confusion is cutaneous leishmaniasis. The lymphangitic variety may also resemble other infections, notably atypical mycobacterial infections, particularly fish-tank granuloma, or 'sporotrichoid' leishmaniasis.

Treatment

Some cases of sporotrichosis may heal spontaneously. However, treatment is usually advised to prevent scar formation. The cheapest treatment is potassium iodide, which is administered in a saturated aqueous solution. The starting dose is 0.5 to 1 ml, given three times daily, and this is increased drop by drop per dose to 3 to 6 ml, three times daily. The mixture is more palatable if given with milk. Treatment should be given for a month after clinical resolution. However, both itraconazole and terbinafine are also effective; minimal durations of treatment for these agents have not been defined.

Subcutaneous zygomycosis due to basidiobolus

Subcutaneous zygomycosis is an infection primarily seen in children in Africa or eastern Asia (Indonesia). It is characterized by the development of localized woody swellings on the limbs or trunk. The swelling is rarely inflammatory, but has a well-defined leading edge, and is hard. Progression is slow. The causative organism *Basidiobolus haptosporus* can be cultured or demonstrated histologically in biopsy material. Although resolution has been recorded without treatment, therapy is normally given. Potassium iodide solution is the treatment of choice, and is given in as high a dose as possible (see 'Sporotrichosis', above). Itraconazole may also be effective.

Subcutaneous zygomycosis due to conidiobolus (conidiobolomycosis or rhinoentomophthoromycosis)

Conidiobolomycosis is a similar infection confined to subcutaneous tissue and presenting with painless swelling. The infection is mainly seen in West Africa, but a case has been seen in the Caribbean. There are important differences from the subcutaneous zygomycosis caused by basidiobolus. The disease is most common in young adults, and is confined to facial tissues around the nose, the forehead, and the upper lip (Fig. 7.7.1.12). The initial site of infection is in the region of the inferior turbinate in the nose. The diagnosis is established by biopsy or culture. The causative organism is *Conidiobolus coronatus*. Treatment with itraconazole or ketoconazole is effective, but an alternative is high-dose potassium iodide. Relapse after treatment is common, and residual fibrosis may be severely disfiguring.

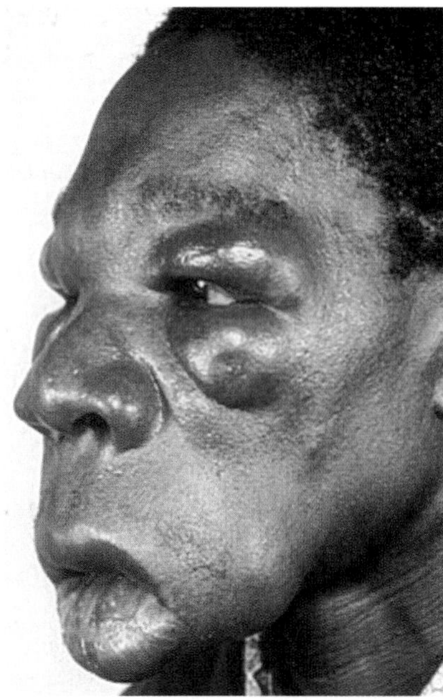

Fig. 7.7.1.12 Subcutaneous zygomycosis (*Conidiobolus coronatus*). (Copyright Professor R Hay.)

Lobo's disease (lobomycosis)

Lobo's disease is a subcutaneous infection. The organism, in tissue, appears to be a yeast. It has a tendency to form chains of four to six yeast cells with prominent nucleoli, joined by a narrow intercellular bridge. However, the organism has never been cultured from human cases and can only be identified by biopsy and histology. The disease is seen in countries of South America around and to the north of the Amazon basin, and cases are also seen in Central America. Apart from humans, the only other species affected are freshwater dolphins. Often, exposed sites (such as earlobes) are invaded and small nodules containing the organisms develop. These may resemble keloids (Fig. 7.7.1.13). More diffuse plaques may also be seen. Deep invasion has not been documented. The treatment is excision, and there is no effective chemotherapy, although there have been recent reports that posaconazole may be effective.

Systemic mycoses

The systemic or deep visceral mycoses include some of the rare and more serious fungal infections. There are two main types of infection in this group: (1) the endemic mycoses, caused by organisms that invade normal hosts, and (2) the opportunistic mycoses, which cause disease only in compromised patients. The fungi associated with these two types of infection differ in their innate levels of pathogenicity, but an element of opportunism, depending on host susceptibility, is usually recognizable in all cases of systemic mycoses.

The endemic pathogens cause infections such as histoplasmosis or coccidioidomycosis. These diseases have well-defined endemic zones and the majority of those exposed remain symptomless but usually develop positive skin tests. However, in certain patients, chronic local or disseminated disease may occur. In the systemic infections caused by opportunistic fungi, there is usually a serious

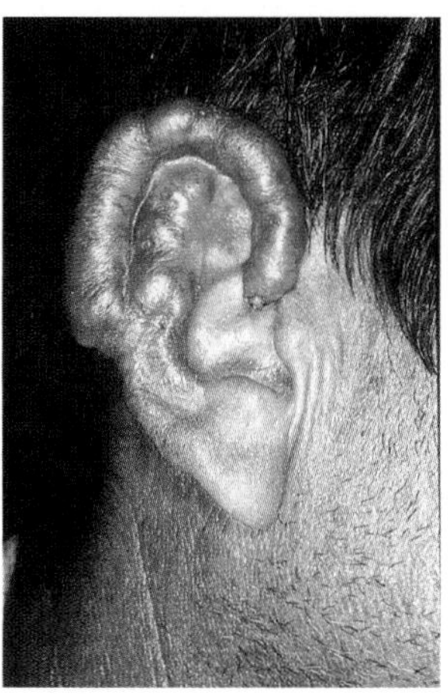

Fig. 7.7.1.13 Lobo's disease in a Brazilian man. (Copyright D A Warrell.)

underlying abnormality in the patient affecting T lymphocytes (such as HIV) or neutrophils (such as cancer chemotherapy). Such infections are worldwide in occurrence: where tissue invasion occurs the mortality is high. Cryptococcosis, a systemic yeast infection, has features of both types of systemic disease and occurs in both normal and immunosuppressed subjects (Chapter 7.7.2).

The systemic endemic infections are histoplasmosis, coccidioidomycosis (Chapter 7.7.3), blastomycosis, paracoccidioidomycosis (Chapter 7.7.4), and infections due to *Penicillium marneffei* (Chapter 7.7.7). The significance of various laboratory tests in these infections is shown in Table 7.7.1.1.

Histoplasmosis (see Chapter 18.4.2)

There are two forms of histoplasmosis. In both types, the organism is present in tissue in its yeast phase. In small-form or classic histoplasmosis, the diameter of the yeast cells is between 3 and 4 μm. Infections are most common in the United States of America, but sporadic cases are reported widely from the New World, Africa, and eastern Asia. By contrast, large-form or African histoplasmosis is most common in Central Africa, south of the Sahara and north of the Zambezi river. Yeast forms in infected tissue are much larger, 10 to 15 μm in diameter. Both infections are clinically distinct (see below), but cultural isolates are indistinguishable.

Histoplasmosis (classic or small-form histoplasmosis)

Aetiology

Histoplasmosis is a systemic infection caused by *Histoplasma capsulatum*. The main route of infection is pulmonary. The majority of those exposed are sensitized without overt signs of infection, but more rarely chronic pulmonary or disseminated forms of the disease are seen.

The organism, *H. capsulatum*, can be found in soil in endemic areas. Its growth is facilitated by the presence of bird excreta, e.g. in old chicken houses, bird roosts, and barns. In tropical and some temperate areas, bat guano plays a similar role. Exposure to a suitable source, such as a cave containing bats, is often recorded in acute epidemic histoplasmosis (see below). It is rarely identified in more slowly evolving cases.

The condition of the host is important in determining the clinical course and manifestations of histoplasmosis. Slowly evolving (chronic), disseminated disease may occur in normal individuals. However, infants, elderly people, or those with untreated AIDS appear to be more likely to develop the more rapidly progressive forms of disseminated infection.

Epidemiology

The major endemic area, as shown by skin testing, is in the central region of the United States around the Ohio and Mississippi valley basins. Prevalence is highest in the states of Tennessee, Kentucky, and Ohio. Up to 95% of those skin-tested in certain parts of these areas have positive delayed reactions to intradermal histoplasmin. Scattered cases of active disease, healed calcified foci in chest radiographs, and foci found at autopsy representing inactive histoplasmosis also provide evidence of spread within this area. However, the disease also occurs in other parts of the United States, Mexico, Central and South America, Africa, eastern Asia, and Australia. Outside the major endemic areas in the United States, human cases are less frequent, and much of the evidence of the endemicity comes from positive skin tests or the presence of the organism in

Table 7.7.1.1 Laboratory tests in systemic mycoses[a]

	Direct microscopy	Significance of positive cultures	Serology	Histopathology
Histoplasmosis				
Classic (small form)	Sometimes positive	Significant	ID, CIE, CFT Urine antigen detection	Yeasts (3–4 μm)
African histoplasmosis	Positive in pus (valuable)	Significant	ID, CFT	Yeasts (10–15 μm)
Coccidioidomycosis	Positive in pus, sputum, etc. (valuable)	Significant NB Handle with caution	ID, CFT, TP, CIE	Spherules(50–150 μm)
Blastomycosis	Positive in pus, sputum, etc. (valuable)	Significant	ID, CFT, CIE (unreliable)	Yeasts (4–10 μm) Broad-based buds
Paracoccidioidomycosis	Positive in pus, sputum etc. (valuable)	Significant	ID, CFT, TP Antigen detection	Yeasts (5–15 μm) Multiple buds
Cryptococcosis	Often positive in CSF (rare in urine, pus) NB Indian ink	Significant	Latex agglutination or ELISA for antigen (ID, CFT, WCA, IF)	Encapsulated yeasts (5–10 μm) Mucicarmine positive
Systemic candidosis	Positive in oral smzears, sputum, etc. (interpret with caution)	Significance depends on site and presence of positive microscopy	ID, CFT, WCA, CIE Antigen detection	Yeasts (5–10 μm) and hyphae
Invasive aspergillosis	Rarely positive, depends on site	Positive sputum cultures not always significant	ID, CIE, rarely positive Antigen detection e.g. Pasteurex	Hyphae—dichotomous branching
Invasive zygomycosis	Rarely positive	Depends on site	Rarely positive	Hyphae—broad and aseptate

CFT, complement fixation test; CIE, counterimmunoelectrophoresis; CSF, cerebrospinal fluid; ID, immunodiffusion; IF, immunofluorescence; RIA, radioimmunoassay; TP, tube precipitation; WCA, whole-cell agglutination.

[a] Molecular diagnostic techniques are increasingly used but are not standardized.

selected sites, such as caves. Although there has been considerable discussion on the nature of soil factors responsible for the growth of *H. capsulatum*, the conditions limiting its occurrence to certain areas are largely unknown.

Clinical features

The clinical forms of histoplasmosis can be placed in several groups:

- asymptomatic
- acute symptomatic pulmonary:
  - acute epidemic
  - acute reinfection
- chronic pulmonary
- disseminated (acute, subacute, and chronic)
- primary cutaneous (by inoculation)

Asymptomatic infection

Over 99% of patients becoming infected in endemic areas record no overt symptoms but develop a positive skin test. The incidence of positive skin tests declines in individuals above the age of 60 years.

Acute (symptomatic) pulmonary histoplasmosis

Acute epidemic histoplasmosis Groups of people exposed to a source of infection, e.g. during cave exploration, or those who may have inhaled a large infecting dose, often develop a symptomatic illness 12 to 21 days after exposure. The main features are pyrexia, cough, chest pain, and malaise. Flitting arthralgia and, less commonly, erythema nodosum or multiforme may occur. The radiological appearances may be much more severe than would be supposed from the symptoms, and enlargement of hilar lymph nodes and diffuse or patchy consolidation suggesting pneumonitis may occur (Fig. 7.7.1.14).

These patients develop precipitating or complement-fixing antibody, but this often follows the peak of illness. About 50% of those with symptoms do not develop positive antibody responses. Likewise, skin-test conversion is often too late to be of diagnostic value, and its use is normally contraindicated, as a single histoplasmin test may cause the development of false-positive serological results. Cultures are often negative. The symptoms and history of exposure to a suitable source, combined with a rising antibody titre, are often the best evidence of infection.

The majority of cases require no specific therapy apart from rest. Those with severe or prolonged symptoms or impaired gas exchange require intravenous amphotericin B or itraconazole. The lung lesions often heal to leave multiple scattered pulmonary calcifications.

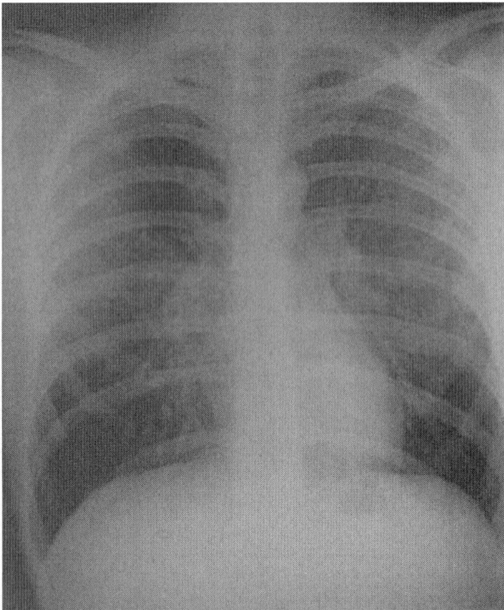

Fig. 7.7.1.14 Acute pulmonary histoplasmosis.
(Copyright Professor R Hay.)

Acute reinfection histoplasmosis Massive acute exposure to *H. capsulatum* in sensitized individuals is believed by some physicians to cause a less severe infection associated with bilateral pulmonary infiltrates. The incubation period is shorter than with acute epidemic histoplasmosis, namely 5 to 10 days.

Chronic pulmonary histoplasmosis

Chronic pulmonary disease caused by *H. capsulatum* is mainly seen in the United States. It is more common in men and smokers, and there is often underlying pulmonary disease such as emphysema. Early cases may present with pyrexia and cough, but malaise and weight loss occur later. Lesions may heal initially, but relapse is common, leading to established consolidation and cavitation. The most common radiological appearance of early lesions is of unilateral, wedge-shaped, segmental shadows in the apical zones. Subsequently, the disease may become bilateral, with fibrosis and cavitation. In some cases, extensive and progressive destruction of lung tissue may occur.

Culture and serology are both helpful methods of diagnosis in this form of histoplasmosis, but repeated attempts may be required before positive results are obtained.

In early cases, resolution may occur on rest alone. However, relapse occurs in at least 25% of cases, and these patients may require amphotericin B therapy or itraconazole. Although chemotherapy may virtually sterilize lesions, fibrosis persists and relapse may occur. Surgical excision or lobectomy is sometimes effective.

Solid lung tumours may persist after the primary infection. These may be single (coin lesions) or multiple, and have to be distinguished from carcinomas. The diagnosis is normally made at surgery, although the presence of calcification may give a clue to the nature of the lesion (histoplasmoma). The organisms can be demonstrated by histopathology, but they are seldom viable.

Disseminated histoplasmosis

There is considerable variation in the rate of progression of histoplasmosis that has spread beyond the initial focus in the lung. In rapid or acutely disseminated cases, widespread infiltration of reticuloendothelial cells of bone marrow, spleen, and liver may occur. Gastrointestinal lesions, endocarditis, and meningitis are less common, and meningitis is more usually associated with a slower course of disseminated disease. Infants, elderly people, or immunosuppressed patients are more susceptible to acute dissemination. The most prominent symptoms are fever and weight loss, with accompanying hepatosplenomegaly. Extensive purpura and bruising secondary to thrombocytopenia may occur. The blood picture may reflect marrow infiltration with organisms, leading to pancytopenia. Disseminated histoplasmosis is also seen in patients with AIDS. The clinical manifestations are not significantly different, although skin papules and ulcers have been reported in many (Fig. 7.7.1.15); isolation of histoplasma from blood has also been reported more frequently in these patients. Cultures, including sputum or bone marrow, should be taken. Serology is often positive, with high titres of complement-fixing antibodies occurring in some patients. However, new antigen detection systems in serum or urine provide a better means of confirming the diagnosis and monitoring treatment.

A much more slowly progressive form of disseminated histoplasmosis may present with fewer localized lesions, such as persistent oral ulcers, chronic laryngitis, or adrenal insufficiency. Granulomas, few of which contain organisms, can be found in the liver in some patients. Such cases may present up to 30 years after the patient has left an endemic area. Outside endemic areas this form is the most widely recognized presentation of histoplasmosis, occurring in Europeans, for instance, who have worked in Africa or eastern Asia.

The diagnosis of disseminated histoplasmosis is made on culture or biopsy of affected areas. Antibodies may only be positive in low titres and in all cases adrenal involvement should be looked for.

Treatment is required in all forms of disseminated histoplasmosis. Itraconazole is preferred by most physicians, although amphotericin B may be necessary in some patients. Posaconazole is an alternative. In patients with AIDS who are acutely ill, the disease is often controlled by a short (2-week) course of amphotericin B and thereafter patients receive continuous itraconazole indefinitely.

Primary cutaneous histoplasmosis

Primary infection sometimes follows accidental inoculation of viable organisms in a laboratory or autopsy room. This type of infection is normally associated with a chancre at the site of inoculation and regional lymphadenopathy. The condition is self-limiting.

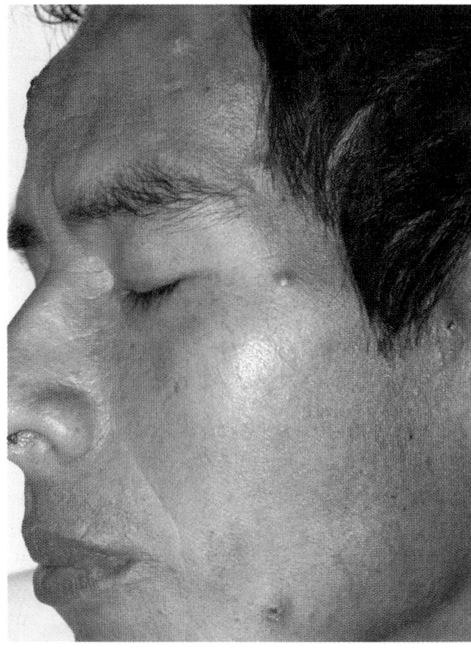

Fig. 7.7.1.15 Histoplasmosis. Molluscum-like skin lesions in an HIV-immunosuppressed Peruvian patient.
(Copyright D A Warrell.)

African histoplasmosis

Overt pulmonary involvement is rare in this form of histoplasmosis, and the normal portal of entry of the pathogen is not known. The most common presenting features are skin lesions (papules, nodules, abscesses, or ulcers) (Fig. 7.7.1.16) or lytic bone deposits. Solitary or multiple foci may be present, and in the latter instances rapid progression and death may occur. In such cases, gastrointestinal and lung lesions may develop.

The diagnosis is normally made by culture, smear, or biopsy. The organism *H. capsulatum* var. *duboisii* is identical to that causing classic histoplasmosis in culture, but in lesions the yeast forms are considerably larger (10–15 μm).

Although local excision of skin nodules has been reported to be curative, treatment with itraconazole, ketoconazole, or amphotericin B is usual. Some patients will respond to co-trimoxazole. A skeletal scan should be made to detect occult foci of infection.

Blastomycosis (see also Section 23)

Blastomycosis (North American blastomycosis) caused by *Blastomyces dermatitidis* is a systemic fungal infection in which skin and lung involvement are common features.

The infective organism, *B. dermatitidis*, has only been isolated from the environment on rare occasions. Positive sites have included soil and rotten timbers. The organism infects humans and domestic animals, particularly dogs.

Epidemiology

Blastomycosis was originally thought to be confined to North America, where it occurs sporadically throughout the south and east-central area, and in areas of central Canada. 'Epidemics' of acute disease are rare, and where these occur a source of infection is rarely demonstrated. There is evidence that sources may include areas exposed to flooding.

More recently, cases have been found in Africa. Again, these are widely scattered from the north coast to the southern parts of the continent, and are rare in all areas. Patients with the disease have also been reported from the Middle East and central Europe.

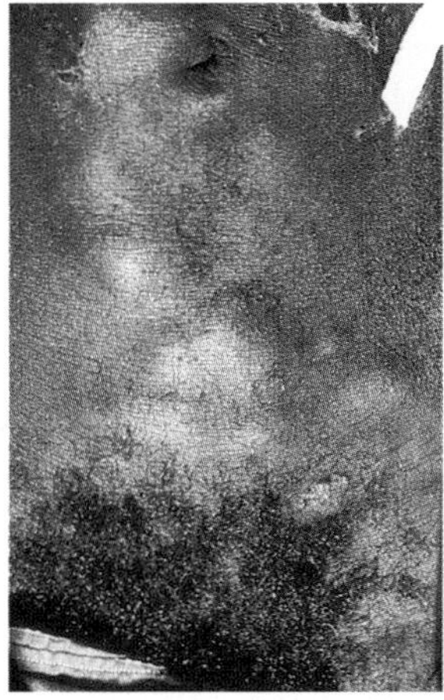

Fig. 7.7.1.16 Nodular subcutaneous lesions of African histoplasmosis in a Nigerian man.
(Copyright D A Warrell.)

Clinical features

The clinical forms of blastomycosis differ from histoplasmosis in a number of important aspects. The existence of an asymptomatic form has not been proved conclusively, because there is no reliable skin test. Acute infections or infections in groups are rare, and the features are often similar to histoplasmosis (acute pulmonary). However, specific serological tests may be negative in 30 to 50% of cases. The demonstration of the organisms in sputum and positive cultures are more reliable diagnostic criteria. Although some cases undoubtedly resolve without sequelae, some physicians advise chemotherapy, with a short course of amphotericin B in acute cases of blastomycosis.

Chronic pulmonary blastomycosis

Chronic consolidation or cavitation of the upper or mid zones occur with chronic pulmonary infections. Fever, malaise, and cough with sputum are seen. Weight loss may be prominent. Culture is again the most reliable method of diagnosis.

The mainstays of treatment are itraconazole or amphotericin B.

Disseminated blastomycosis

Although generalized infiltration in skin, lungs, and liver may occur over a short period, leading to rapid death, signs of chronic extrapulmonary dissemination are more usual.

The skin is an area that is frequently involved (chronic cutaneous blastomycosis). The face or forearms and hands are common sites for skin lesions. These are slow, spreading, verrucose plaques with central scarring. The initial lesion is often a dermal nodule. Many such cases have underlying pulmonary consolidation, or cavities. The diagnosis is established by biopsy and culture. Bone deposits in the form of lytic lesions, and involvement of the genitourinary tract, particularly the epididymis, are also seen in chronic disseminated blastomycosis. Unlike tuberculosis, the kidneys are often spared.

In slowly progressive forms of blastomycosis, itraconazole (200–400 mg daily) has proved to be very effective. Alternatively, amphotericin B can be given intravenously and is indicated where there is rapidly progressive disease.

Coccidioidomycosis

See Chapter 7.7.3.

Paracoccidioidomycosis

See Chapter 7.7.4.

Systemic sporotrichosis

In addition to causing cutaneous disease, *Sporothrix schenckii* may be responsible for a systemic mycosis. The infection is rare and has been mainly reported from the United States of America. Involvement may be confined to a single site such as a lung or a joint, or it may be multifocal. Cavitation in the lung associated with weight loss and pyrexia is probably the most common variety of systemic sporotrichosis. Unlike cutaneous forms of the disease, systemic sporotrichosis responds poorly to potassium iodide, and amphotericin B is the treatment of choice.

Rare systemic infections

These include pulmonary invasion by *Geotrichum candidum* (geotrichosis) and adiaspiromycosis, a respiratory infection caused by *Emmonsia crescens* or *E. parva*. Isolated examples of human disease caused by fungi are consistently reported and almost always occur in the immunosuppressed host. In these patients many fungi that are normally saprophytes in the environment may invade and cause disease.

Systemic mycoses caused by opportunistic fungi

The opportunistic mycoses are a worldwide problem, although fortunately rare in most countries. In recent years they have been recognized more frequently with the increase in transplantations of organs such as heart or bone marrow and in the more effective but immunocompromising regimes of cancer chemotherapy. Opportunistic invasion by organisms such as candida or zygomycetes (mucor, absidia) may also occur in cases of malnutrition. One of the recent trends in the management of the patient with neutropenia has been the emergence of new pathogens such as non-*albicans* species of *Candida* or other organisms such as fusarium, trichosporon, or scedosporium species.

The opportunists present particular problems in diagnosis and management. Because many of the organisms are normally saprophytic, it has to be positively established that they have assumed an invasive role. Mere isolation may not provide sufficient evidence and in some instances low titres of antibody may be present even in normal hosts. The significance of various laboratory tests in these infections is shown in Table 7.7.1.1. Treatment is also difficult and it is important in most cases to attempt to reverse the process that led to the establishment of the infection.

Systemic candidosis

Aetiology

In addition to their role in superficial infections, candida yeasts may also cause invasive systemic disease. The clinical forms described range from bloodstream isolation or candidaemia to disseminated invasive disease, sometimes with involvement of a single organ, site, or body cavity (deep focal candidosis) as may occur in peritonitis or meningitis. Urinary tract infections may also be caused by candida species.

The factors underlying systemic candida infections are shown in Box 7.7.1.3. All these factors are important in disrupting the balance

Box 7.7.1.3 Predisposing factors in deep candida infections

- Local defects, foreign bodies, e.g. prosthetic heart valves, intravenous lines
- Defects of immunity (primarily T cell or phagocytosis), e.g. cytotoxic therapy or systemic lupus erythematosus
- Drug therapy, e.g. antibiotics
- Carcinoma or leukaemia
- Endocrine disease, e.g. diabetes mellitus in urinary tract candidosis
- Physiological changes, e.g. infancy, old age, and pregnancy (urinary tract)
- Miscellaneous disorders, e.g.
    - Malnutrition
    - Surgery such as gastrointestinal resections
    - Drug addiction

by which candida is maintained as a saprophyte. Intravenous or central venous pressure lines may serve as a portal of entry or as a nidus for circulating yeasts in a candidaemia. Antibiotic therapy may upset the balance by inhibiting a potentially competitive bacterial flora.

Candida albicans is the most common species involved but other species may be isolated, particularly in cases of endocarditis, e.g. *C. parapsilosis. C. tropicalis* has been implicated in infections of patients with neutropenia. These non-*albicans Candida* species are now more frequent causes of systemic infection and are important to recognize as their antifungal susceptibility may differ from that of *C. albicans*. Portals of entry include the gastrointestinal tract (common), skin, and urinary tract (rare). However, superficial candidosis or saprophytic colonization of mouth, skin, or airways may also occur in compromised patients and does not necessarily indicate systemic invasion.

Epidemiology

Systemic infections caused by candida species are worldwide in distribution. However, they are particularly associated with a number of predisposing factors such as neutropenia, antibiotic usage, indwelling lines, and abdominal surgery.

Clinical features

Candidaemia

The isolation of candida in blood culture may be linked to any of the factors listed in Box 7.7.1.3. Common predisposing features are the presence of intravenous lines, previous surgery (mainly gastrointestinal), antibiotic therapy, hepatic failure, or neutropenia. Patients develop a swinging fever and feel generally unwell. Clinical shock may occur.

Some such cases resolve following removal of predisposing factors, particularly the intravenous lines. Generally, however, all such patients receive treatment and a careful investigation should be made to identify the presence of established invasive disease. Other sites should be searched for evidence of infection; e.g. urine by culture or the presence of white cells. Signs of muscle invasion (tenderness) or metastatic skin nodules should be excluded (Fig. 7.7.1.17). Other signs of invasion include the development of new cardiac murmurs or of soft, white, retinal plaques caused by candida. Persistently positive blood cultures or serum candida antigen levels or high antibody titres may also indicate possible deep invasion.

Disseminated candidosis

Although multiorgan invasive candidosis may follow candidaemia, at least 50% of disseminated infections develop in patients without initially positive blood cultures. The features of some forms of invasive candidosis are listed above (under candidaemia). Although candida may be isolated from the sputum in these patients, there is rarely objective evidence of lung invasion. Moreover, there is no radiological appearance that is diagnostic of pulmonary candidosis and, indeed, chest radiographs may even appear normal. General localizing signs may be a late feature of disseminated candidosis.

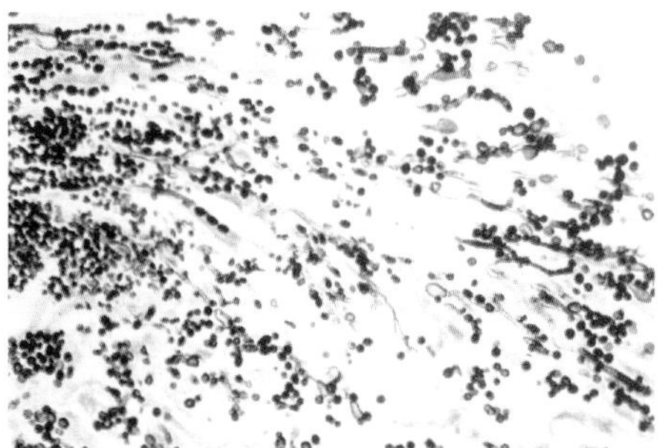

Fig. 7.7.1.17 Candidosis disseminated to skin (methenamine silver, × 516).

Laboratory diagnosis of disseminated candidosis

The diagnosis may be made by culture or PCR, and repeated attempts to isolate should be made where cultures are initially negative. Numerous techniques have been used to detect antibody or antigen in disseminated candidosis. However, in many patients, particularly those with neutropenia, it may not be possible to confirm the diagnosis using laboratory tests and treatment is often initiated on the basis of clinical suspicion (empirical therapy) as the risk of delaying antifungal therapy is great.

By themselves, positive cultures, particularly from sputum, or the presence of antibodies do not necessarily prove the existence of deep-seated candidosis. A positive isolation may simply indicate the presence of colonization and normal individuals may have low titres of antibody to candida. If there is a readily accessible lesion from which to take a biopsy, such as a skin nodule or even a pulmonary infiltrate, this may provide the best evidence of invasion, although such procedures may carry their own risk (Fig. 7.7.1.16).

Treatment of disseminated candidosis

Untreated disseminated candidosis is normally progressive and fatal. The signs must be separated from, for instance, bacterial septicaemia, which may coexist with the candida infection.

The treatment of invasive candidosis is intravenous amphotericin B or caspofungin or intravenous or oral fluconazole given until there is a clinical and mycological response. This may take between 2 and 20 weeks depending on the site of infection and the underlying state of the patient. Fluconazole is usually used in infections where the patient is not neutropenic. Lipid-associated forms of amphotericin B are also useful and carry a lower risk of renal impairment. An alternative approach is to add flucytosine in doses of 150 to 200 mg/kg body weight daily to amphotericin B in serious infections or where cure may be hampered by poor penetration of amphotericin B, such as in the eye. A biologic, Mycograb, which is an antibody against candida heat shock protein 70 has been shown to improve treatment responses in candidaemia when used in combination with amphotericin B.

Deep focal candidosis

Candida infections in the peritoneum or meninges most often follow direct implantation after dialysis or surgery. Alternatively, secondary invasion from the middle ear or a perforated bowel is also possible. The signs and symptoms are similar to bacterial meningitis or peritonitis but candida is isolated. Sometimes these infections clear spontaneously, but normally treatment is instituted with fluconazole, which penetrates areas such as peritoneum, or amphotericin B.

Candida endocarditis

Invasion of heart valves, mainly the mitral or aortic valves, most commonly follows homograft replacement, but it may occur also in patients with neutropenia or drug addicts. The symptoms are similar to bacterial endocarditis. However, candida vegetations may reach considerable size. Embolic phenomena may involve obstruction of large vessels including the femoral artery or large cerebral vessels. The detection of large vegetations using an echocardiography, particularly in cases with negative blood cultures, should raise the possibility of fungal endocarditis. Blood cultures are usually positive at some stage in the illness but repeated sampling may be necessary. High antibody titres are usually seen in such cases and serological tests are therefore of considerable value.

Untreated candida endocarditis is uniformly fatal. There is also a high mortality associated with cases in which early surgical intervention is precipitated by impending heart failure. Normally, treatment consists of amphotericin B given intravenously and, where possible, valve replacement. There is no evidence to suggest that the addition of flucytosine to the regimen increases the effectiveness of treatment. However, the relapse rate is high and combination therapy may therefore be a reasonable approach on theoretical grounds.

Urinary tract candidosis

Candida species may be isolated from the urine, particularly in conditions associated with urinary stasis such as neurogenic bladder or where there is an indwelling catheter. Type 2 diabetes is another predisposing factor. There is no value in using the presence of pyuria or quantitative yeast-colony counts to assess the significance of infection. Treatment is normally given where there are symptoms such as dysuria or frequency or where there is a potential risk of invasion such as in immunosuppressed patients. Fluconazole is very useful in these patients as urinary levels are above inhibitory concentrations.

Aspergillosis (see also Chapter 7.2.4 and Section 18)

Aspergillosis is the name given to diseases associated with species of mould fungi of the genus *Aspergillus*. As such, it comprises a series of clinically distinct infections: aggressive pulmonary infections with angio-invasion and the potential for widespread systemic haematogenous spread (invasive pulmonary aspergillosis); slow but progressive paranasal sinus infection mainly seen in the tropics (paranasal aspergillus granulom); and colonization of a pre-existing space or cavity (aspergilloma) which may give rise to medical problems including severe haemorrhage. They are also associated with both superficial and subcutaneous fungal infections. Aspergillus species cause a number of different allergic disorders including asthma and allergic bronchopulmonary aspergillosis (Chapter 18.14.2). Box 7.7.1.4 indicates the range of diseases associated with aspergillus.

Aspergillus species are ubiquitous and have established themselves in every conceivable terrain and environment. As they propagate through the production of large number of airborne spores, exposure is difficult to avoid. Production of spores is also determined by local and environmental conditions. For example, construction or destruction of buildings and turnover of soil have been associated with focal outbreaks of infection in predisposed and immunosuppressed individuals. Susceptibility to aspergillus infections is dependent, to a large extent, on defective immunity or structural abnormalities, and therefore the major diseases caused by these organisms are usually seen in immunosuppressed individuals, including, in particular, neutropenic patients or people with anatomocal abnormalities such as lung cavities. The incidence of infection can reach high levels in certain populations such as patients following bone marrow transplantation (Chapter 7.2.4).

Aspergillus species can produce a number of potent metabolic byproducts or myxotoxins, such as the aflatoxins produced by *A. flavus* which, if present in contaminated food, can induce liver necrosis.

Box 7.7.1.4 Diseases caused by aspergillus species

Superficial infections

- Onychomycosis
- Otitis externa
- Keratomycosis

Subcutaneous infections

- Mycetoma
- Systemic infections
- Localized invasive aspergillosis:
  - Aspergilloma, chronic aspergillosis of the paranasal sinuses, chromic pulmonary aspergillosis, paranasal aspergillus granuloma
- Invasive aspergillosis with potential for systemic spread:
  - Invasive (pulmonary) aspergillosis (common sites for dissemination are brain, liver, skin)
  - Aspergillus endocarditis

Allergic disease

- Asthma, allergic rhinitis,
- Extrinsic hypersensitivity pneumonitis (*A. clavatus*)
- Allergic bronchopulmonary aspergillosis
- Allergic aspergillus sinusitis

Toxicosis

- Mycotoxin-producing aspergilli, e.g. *A. flavus*—aflatoxins

The commonest human pathogen amongst the aspergillus species is *A. fumigatus*, followed by *A. flavus* which causes infections more commonly in warmer climates. *A. niger* causes aspergilloma rather than invasive disease but *A. nidulans* rarely causes mycetoma. *A. terreus* is sometimes found as a cause of onychomycosis. Hence aspergillus infections may present to a wide range of different specialities and, in the severely immunocompromised patient, dissemination of aspergillus through the blood stream may result in infection of almost any organ.

Cryptococcosis

See Chapter 7.7.2.

Invasive zygomycosis (mucormycosis, phycomycosis)

Aetiology

Invasive disease caused by mucor-like (zygomycete) fungi is rare. In the compromised host it may lead to paranasal destruction, necrotic lung or skin lesions, and disseminated disease.

The causative organisms commonly belong to three genera: *Absidia*, *Rhizopus*, and *Rhizomucor*. More rarely other organisms such as *Cunninghamella* or *Saksenaea* have been implicated. Most of the agents are associated with decaying vegetable matter and are common airborne moulds. The route of infection is highly variable: they may invade via the lungs, paranasal sinuses, gastrointestinal tract, or damaged skin. The predisposing illness may in some way determine the site of clinical invasion. Underlying factors include diabetic ketoacidosis (rhinocerebral involvement), leukaemia and immunosuppressive therapy (lung and disseminated infection), malnutrition (gastrointestinal infection), and burns or wounds (cutaneous invasion). These patterns are not always strictly followed.

Epidemiology

Invasive zygomycosis is rare but has a worldwide distribution. Its invasive nature, particularly the tendency to involve blood vessels and its selection of compromised hosts, distinguishes this form of infection from subcutaneous zygomycosis, which is also caused by zygomycete species.

Clinical features

The most characteristic features of this type of infection are the extensive necrosis and infarction that may follow blood vessel invasion leading to thrombosis. A similar type of invasion may occur with invasive aspergillosis, but is usually less prominent. Invasive zygomycosis follows a number of different patterns.

The infection may initially localize in one of several sites. The most common is in the paranasal sinuses and this is most often seen in diabetic patients with ketoacidosis. The patient presents with fever and unilateral facial pain. Subsequently, there may be facial swelling with nasal obstruction and proptosis. There may be invasion into the orbit leading to blindness, into the brain, and into the palate. Palatal ulceration should be searched for. Widespread dissemination with infarction of major organs or limbs may occur subsequently. A similar pattern of invasion of surgical wounds or burns may occur and has on occasions been associated with contamination of dressing packs. Infections are initially localized causing extensive necrosis around the original wound. Gastrointestinal invasion may be heralded by perforation of viscera, and diarrhoea or haemorrhage.

Alternatively, a patient may present with established pulmonary or widespread dissemination. Such patients are usually leukaemic or are severely immunosuppressed. Neutropenia is often seen.

Once infection has spread beyond the original site, invasive zygomycosis is almost invariably fatal with or without treatment.

Laboratory diagnosis

The diagnosis is suggested by the combination of infection and extensive infarction, particularly if it occurs in any of the sites mentioned. The organisms may be difficult to culture even from biopsy and histology is often the quickest way of establishing the diagnosis. Serology is frequently negative.

Treatment

Treatment should be initiated as soon as possible and extensive surgical debridement combined with intravenous amphotericin B in maximum daily dosage offers the best chance of success. Local instillations of amphotericin B may also be used where appropriate (such as nasal sinuses). Some physicians also recommend anticoagulation with heparin to forestall thrombosis. Despite therapy, the mortality remains high. Liposomal amphotericin B also has been used with some success is cases of mucormycosis.

Rhinosporidiosis

Rhinosporidiosis is an infection found in India, Sri Lanka, parts of East Africa, and South America. It is characterized by polypoid growth from the nose or conjunctiva. The causative organism can be demonstrated in tissue and consists of aggregates of large sporangia containing spores in various phases of development. However, they have never been successfully cultured and they appear to be related genetically most closely to aquatic protista, members of the Mezomycetozoa. The treatment is surgical excision.

Otomycosis and oculomycosis

External otitis is often multifactorial, but in some cases dense fungal colonization can contribute to the picture. In severe cases, the external ear may be plugged by a dense mat of mycelium. Aspergillus species are the most common organisms cultured, particularly *A. niger*, but candida, penicillium, and mucor may all contribute. Intensive ear toilet may eradicate the infection without recourse to antifungal agents.

Infections of the eye, particularly the cornea, caused by fungi (oculomycosis) are rare. They often follow penetrating injuries to the globe or contamination of lacerations. An opacity develops within the cornea with associated pain and chemosis. An exudate is usually present in the aqueous humour. Prompt treatment with intensive topical instillation of drugs containing an antifungal drug such as miconazole or econazole is necessary every 2 to 4 h. Perforation of the eye may occur in advanced cases.

Approaches to management of fungal infections

Antifungal agents can be considered in four main groups: the polyenes, azoles, morpholines, and allylamines, and an assortment of unrelated drugs with specific activity.

Polyenes

The polyene antifungals are macrolide substances derived originally from species of *Streptomyces*. They include amphotericin B, natamycin, and nystatin. More recent additions to this group are partricin and mepartricin. Amphotericin B is the only one widely used as a parenterally administered drug. Nystatin and natamycin are purely topical. Amphotericin B is metabolized in the liver with low penetration of body cavities, cerebrospinal fluid, and urine. The polyenes have broad activity against a wide range of fungi. The mode of action of the polyenes appears to involve inhibition of sterol synthesis in the fungal cell membrane.

The combination of an amphotericin B with a lipid, for instance a liposome, has been proposed as a means of reducing the nephrotoxicity of this drug. Three commercial lipid amphotericins are available: AmBisome (a true liposome), amphotericin B lipid complex—ABLC or Abelcet (a ribbon-like lipid binding amphotericin B), and amphotericin B colloidal dispersion (ABCD) (a dispersion of lipid discs).

Azoles

The imidazoles are synthetic antifungal agents. They include miconazole, clotrimazole, econazole, isoconazole, ketoconazole, tioconazole, and bifonazole. The triazole series contains two potent oral agents, fluconazole and itraconazole. Voriconazole and posaconazole are newer additions Most are used topically except for ketoconazole (oral), itraconazole (oral), voriconazole (oral and intravenous and posaconazole (intravenous). These are metabolized in the liver and, like amphotericin B, affect fungal cell-membrane synthesis and penetrate cerebrospinal fluid and urine in low concentrations. The imidazoles have a broad spectrum of activity against many fungi, particularly those causing superficial infectiond. Fluconazole is less active against moulds and there are instances of both primary (*Candida krusei*, *C. glabrata*) and secondary resistance to this compound. New triazoles, voriconazole and posaconazole, are now available; voriconazole is an effective treatment for invasive aspergillosis. The allylamines such as terbinafine are primarily active against superficial fungi, but *in vitro* appear to have fungicidal activity at low concentrations.

Other antifungals in this category include flucytosine, which is a synthetic pyrimidine analogue. Given either intravenously or orally it is mainly useful for chromomycosis and certain yeast infections. Drug resistance is a major problem with flucytosine, particularly with cryptococcus. The drug shows a number of modes of action including disruption of RNA transcription following uptake by the cell. Caspofungin an echinocandin, is an effective treatment for deep candida, including fluconazole-resistant, infections. Newer echinocandins are anidulafungin and micafungin. Griseofulvin is derived from a species of penicillium. It can be given orally and is only useful against dermatophytes. It is best absorbed when given with a meal and selectively accumulates in stratum corneum in concentrations approximately 10 times greater than serum levels. Griseofulvin acts by inhibiting intracellular microtubule formation.

Management of superficial infections

Specific details of therapy are included under the separate diseases. Benzoic acid compound (Whitfield's ointment), which contains 2% salicylic acid and 2% benzoic acid, acts as a keratolytic agent by causing exfoliation of the superficial layers of the stratum corneum. Other topical agents with only weak antifungal activity include gentian violet (candidosis or dermatophytosis); Castellani's paint, which contains magenta and resorcinol (candidosis or dermatophytosis); and brilliant green (dermatophytosis). Selenium sulphide (2%) remains a highly effective method of treating pityriasis versicolor by application once daily for 2 weeks.

The more specific antifungals such as the polyenes, amphotericin B, nystatin, and natamycin (candidosis) or the imidazoles (candidosis, dermatophytosis, and pityriasis versicolor) are highly effective and probably quicker than the keratolytics or dyes, although more expensive. Local irritancy can be a problem, particularly with Whitfield's ointment, which is usually given as a half-strength preparation. Allergic contact dermatitis is rare but has been recorded from some imidazoles (miconazole, clotrimazole, tioconazole) and tolnaftate. Topical terbinafine is highly active in tinea pedis with cures being effected with less than 1 week of therapy.

Terbinafine or itraconazole is more effective in many forms of dermatophytosis requiring oral therapy than griseofulvin. In onychomycosis they are preferred. Terbinafine has occasional side effects, mainly related to gastrointestinal intolerance, although it may also cause transient loss of taste. It is given in daily doses of 250 mg. Itraconazole is usually given in 'pulses', e.g. 200 mg twice daily for 1 week monthly. Itraconazole likewise can cause gastrointestinal discomfort and nausea. Both drugs rarely cause hepatic injury, with a frequency of less than 1 in 70 000 to 1 in 120 000. This is in contrast with ketoconazole, which also causes hepatitis but in around 1 in 8000 cases. Liver function tests should be monitored if ketoconazole is used extensively over any length of time. In high doses, ketoconazole may block human androgen biosynthesis causing side effects such as gynaecomastia. Fluconazole is also effective in dermatophytosis and is given in weekly doses of 150 to 300 mg. Griseofulvin is still the principal treatment for tinea capitis (10 to 20 mg/kg per day).

In onychomycosis caused by dermatophytes both terbinafine and itraconazole lead to remission of toe-nail infections in only 3 months. Terbinafine is used on a daily basis, whereas itraconazole is given in a pulsed regimen, 200 mg twice daily for 1 week every month for 3 to 4 months. There is one study which shows better responses with terbinafine for toe-nail disease. Amorolfine, a morpholine drug, is used in the topical treatment of nail disease where there is less than complete involvement of the nails. It can be given together with other drugs, such as terbinafine.

Management of deep mycoses

Very few drugs are effective in systemic fungal infections, and those that are used should always be accompanied by supportive measures and, if possible, an attempt to eliminate any predisposing conditions. For instance, if their condition permits, patients who have developed a candidaemia while a central venous line is in place should be managed by removal of the line. However, fluconazole is also usually given as well. In the patient with neutropenia, a positive blood culture would be regarded as evidence of dissemination and antifungal therapy would be required.

Amphotericin B is given intravenously in a 5% dextrose infusion not containing additional drugs, if possible. A test dose of 1 to 5 mg is given over 2 h and this is followed by gradually increasing doses over the next 3 to 9 days to the normal maximum of 0.6 to 1.0 mg/kg body weight daily depending on the infection. In some cases this slow approach may help the patient to tolerate the drug better, or may define the dose at which side effects such as pyrexia start. In severely ill patients, half of the full dose may be given 4 h after a test dose of 5 mg, usually under hydrocortisone cover. The full dose is given 24 h later. Side effects include thrombophlebitis, nausea, hypotension, and pyrexia. Renal clearance may fall in the initial period but this usually returns to normal after a temporary halt in therapy. More permanent renal tubular damage may follow a total dose of 4 g or more. Amphotericin B does not penetrate urine, cerebrospinal fluid, or peritoneal fluid in significant concentrations. Local instillations (such as the peritoneum) can be used, but can be highly irritant. Amphotericin B is normally given until clinical or mycological cure is induced. This is often difficult to judge accurately and in many of the mycoses caused by the systemic pathogens a course of at least 2 g is often used on an empirical basis. In the opportunistic infections, lower total doses are probably effective and the length of treatment should depend on the clinician's judgement.

This approach is not necessary with the lipid-associated amphotericin B formulations, which can be given without the slow build-up. The initial dose is usually 1 mg/kg but standard daily doses of 3 mg/kg are common. Patients are less likely to develop renal impairment although it can occur. There have been a few clinical trials comparing these formulations with amphotericin B and these show equal efficacy with less toxicity; however, these formulations are expensive. The main lipid-associated formulations are given above.

The azole drugs are also used in systemic mycoses. Fluconazole is given in systemic candidosis, urinary tract infections, and as a long-term suppressive, in addition to primary therapy, in cryptococcosis in patients with AIDS. Side effects are uncommon, although it can cause nausea and vomiting. Fluconazole can be given orally or intravenously. It penetrates urine in effective concentrations. Its daily dosage varies from 100 to 200 mg for oropharyngeal infections to 600 to 800 mg for disseminated candidosis. It is highly active in candida infections. It can also be used in some endemic mycoses such as histoplasmosis. Resistance to fluconazole has mainly been recorded with oropharyngeal candidosis, principally in HIV-positive patients, although it can occur with other candida infections; e.g. *C. krusei* and *C. glabrata* are often primarily resistant to this drug.

Itraconazole has been evaluated in a variety of systemic mycoses from aspergillosis to cryptococcosis. Its active range includes histoplasmosis, sporotrichosis, chromoblastomycosis, blastomycosis, coccidioidomycosis, and paracoccidioidomycosis. Itraconazole is used as an oral preparation, but an intravenous formulation is now available. Oral absorption is often defective in individuals with AIDS and patients after bone marrow transplantation and in these groups the mean daily dosage is doubled (200 mg). An itraconazole suspension is also available for treatment of oral infections.

Voriconazole is now the treatment of choice for aspergillosis and for some other systemic mycosis. The indications for posaconazole include fluconazole unresponsive infections but it also appears be effective in some mould infections including some cases of fusarium infection.

Flucytosine (5-fluorocytosine) is an effective oral and intravenous antifungal agent that is primarily active against yeasts such as candida and cryptococcus. It enters urine, cerebrospinal fluid, and peritoneal fluid. Its excretion is reduced in renal failure and the daily dose should be reduced accordingly and blood levels monitored. The main disadvantage of flucytosine is the development of either primary or secondary drug resistance in a significant number of isolates, and when given in toxic doses it may cause bone marrow depression. The serum level should not be allowed to rise above 100 to 120 µg/ml.

Combination amphotericin B and flucytosine therapy may offer an alternative but effective method of treatment. Theoretically, as the drugs synergize, the dose of amphotericin B may be reduced. In cryptococcal meningitis, combination therapy using a dose of 0.3 to 0.6 mg/kg body weight of amphotericin B with the normal dose of flucytosine is more effective at sterilizing the cerebrospinal fluid and preventing relapse. In other forms of systemic infection such as candidosis there is little evidence that it is more effective than amphotericin B alone, although this may be the case. Combinations of other drugs have not been critically evaluated *in vivo*.

Caspofungin is used in fluconazole-resistant deep candidosis.

A new 'biological' antibody therapy (Mycograb) directed against a candida heat shock protein has recently been developed and shows considerable promise as adjunctive therapy for patients with systemic candidosis.

Further reading

General

Dismukes WE, Pappas PG, Sobel J (2006). *Clinical mycology*. Oxford University Press, New York.

Merz W, Hay RJ (eds) (2005). *Mycology. Topley and Wilson's microbiology and microbial infections*, 10th edition, Vol. 4. Arnold, London.

Kibbler CC, MacKenzie DWR, Odds FC (1996). *Principles and practice of clinical mycology*. John Wiley & Sons, Chichester.

Midgley G, Clayton YM, Hay RJ (1997). *Diagnosis in colour. Medical mycology*. Mosby-Wolfe, London.

Dermatophytosis

Aly R (1994). Ecology and epidemiology of dermatophyte infections. *J Am Acad Dermatol*, **31**, S21–25.

Hay RJ (2005). Fungal infections. In: Bos JD (ed.) *Skin immune system (SIS)*, pp. 593–604. CRC Press, Boca Raton, FL.

Hay RJ, *et al.* (1996). Tinea capitis in south-east London—a new pattern of infection with public health implications. *Br J Dermatol*, **135**, 955–8.

Munoz-Perez MA, *et al.*(1998). Dermatological findings correlated with CD4 lymphocyte counts in a prospective 3 year study of 1161 patients with human immunodeficiency virus disease predominantly acquired through intravenous drug abuse. *Br J Dermatol*, **139**, 33–9.

Scytalidium

Hay RJ, Moore MK (1984). Clinical features of superficial fungal infections caused by *Hendersonula toruloidea* and *Scytalidium hyalinum*. *Br J Dermatol*, **110**, 677–83.

Malassezia

Ashbee, H.R (2006). Recent developments in the immunology and biology of *Malassezia* species. *FEMS Immunol Med Microbiol*, **47**, 14–23.

Candidosis

Bodey GP (ed.) (1993). *Candidiasis. Pathogenesis, diagnosis and treatment*. Raven Press, New York.

Greenspan D, *et al.* (2000). Oral mucosal lesions and HIV viral load in the Womens Interagency HIV study (WIHS). *J Acquir Immune Defic Syndr*, **25**, 89–104.

Sobel JD (1992). Pathogenesis and treatment of recurrent vulvovaginal candidiasis. *Clin Infect Dis*, **14**, S148–153.

Mycetoma

Hay RJ (2005). Eumycetomas. In: Merz WG, Hay RJ (eds.) *Mycology. Topley and Wilson's Microbiology and Microbial Infections*, 10th edition, Vol. 5, pp. 385–95. Arnold, London.

Fahal AH (2004). Mycetoma: a thorn in the flesh. *Trans Roy Soc Trop Med Hyg*, **98**, 3–11.

Chromoblastomycosis

Banks IS, *et al.* (1985). Chromomycosis in Zaire. *Int J Dermatol*, **24**, 302–7.

Bayles MAH (1989). Chromomycosis. In: *Tropical fungal infections, Baillière's clinical tropical medicine and communicable diseases*, Vol. 4, pp. 45–70. Baillière Tindall, London.

Esterre P, *et al.* (1997). Natural history of chromo-blastomycosis in Madagascar and the Indian Ocean. *Bull Soc Pathol Exot*, **90**, 312–17.

Minotto R, *et al.* (2001). Chromoblastomycosis: a review of 100 cases in the state of Rio Grande do Sul, Brazil. *J Am Acad Dermatol*, **44**, 585–92.

Silva JP, *et al.* (1999). Chromoblastomycosis: a retrospective study of 325 cases on Amazonic Region (Brazil). *Mycopathologia*, **143**, 171–5.

Sporotrichosis

Carvalho MT, *et al.* (2002). Disseminated cutaneous sporotrichosis in a patient with AIDS: report of a case. *Rev Soc Bras Med Trop*, **35**, 655–9.

Kauffman CA (1999). Sporotrichosis. *Clin Infect Dis*, **29**, 231–236.

Lyon GM. *et al.* (2003). Population-based surveillance and a case-control study of risk factors for endemic lymphocutaneous sporotrichosis in Peru. *Clin Infect Dis*, **36**, 34–9.

Systemic mycoses

de Pauw BE, Meunier F (1999). The challenge of invasive fungal infection. *Chemotherapy*, **45**, Suppl 1, 1–14.

Histoplasmosis

Ashford DA, *et al.* (1999). Outbreak of histoplasmosis among cavers attending the National Speleological Society Annual Convention, Texas, 1994. *Am J Trop Med Hyg*, **60**, 899–903.

Barton EN, *et al.* (1988). Cutaneous histoplasmosis in the acquired immunodeficiency syndrome: a report of three cases from Trinidad. *Trop Geogr Med*, **40**, 153–7.

Khalil MA, Hassan AW, Gugnani HC (1998). African histoplasmosis: report of four cases from north-eastern Nigeria. *Mycoses*, **41**, 293–5.

Wheat LJ, Kaufman CA (2003). Histoplasmosis. *Infect Dis Clin North Am*, **17**, 1–19.

Wheat J, *et al.* (2000). Practice guidelines for the management of patients with histoplasmosis. Infectious Diseases Society of America. *Clin Infect Dis*, **30**, 688–95.

Blastomycosis

Chapman SW, *et al.* (2000). Practice guidelines for the management of patients with blastomycosis. Infectious Diseases Society of America. *Clin Infect Dis*, **30**, 679–83.

Emerson PA, Higgins E, Branfoot A (1984). North American blastomycosis in Africans. *Br J Dis Chest*, **78**, 286–91.

Lemos LB, *et al.* (2000). Blastomycosis: organ involvement and etiologic diagnosis. A review of 123 patients from Mississippi. *Ann Diagn Pathol*, **4**, 391–406.

Opportunistic systemic mycoses

Magill SS, *et al.* (2006). The association between anatomic site of Candida colonization, invasive candidiasis, and mortality in critically ill surgical patients. *Diagn Microbiol Infect Dis*, **55**, 293–301.

De Pauw BE (2006). Increasing fungal infections in the intensive care unit. *Surg Infect*, **7** Suppl 2, S93–6.

Wingard JR (1999). Fungal infections after bone marrow transplant. *Biol Blood Marrow Transplant*, **5**, 55–68.

Aspergillosis

Marr KA (2008). Fungal infections in hematopoietic stem cell transplant recipients. *Med Mycol*, **46**, 293–302.

Pini G, *et al.* (2008). Invasive pulmonary aspergillosis in neutropenic patients and the influence of hospital renovation. *Mycoses*, **51**, 117–22.

Zygomycosis

Nenoff P, *et al.* (1998). Rhinocerebral zygomycosis following bone marrow transplantation in chronic myelogenous leukaemia. Report of a case and review of the literature. *Mycoses*, **41**, 365–72.

Rhinosporidiosis

Fredericks DN, *et al.* (2000). *Rhinosporidium seeberi:* a human pathogen from a novel group of aquatic protistan parasites. *Emerg Infect Dis*, **6**, 272–6.

Therapy

Bassetti M, *et al.* (2006). Candida infections in the intensive care unit: epidemiology, risk factors and therapeutic strategies. *Expert Rev Anti-Infect Ther*, **4**, 875–85.

Bennett JE (2006). Echinocandins for candidemia in adults without neutropenia. *N Engl J Med*, **355**, 1154–9.

Bohme A, Karthaus M, Hoelzer D (1999). Antifungal prophylaxis in neutropenic patients with hematologic malignancies: is there a real benefit? *Chemotherapy*, **45**, 224–32.

Elweski B (ed.) (1996). *Cutaneous fungal infections.* Marcel Dekker, New York.

Gupta AK, *et al.* (2006). Onychomycosis therapies: strategies to improve efficacy. *Dermatol Clin*, **24**, 381–6.

Vanden Bossche H *et al.* (1998). Antifungal drug resistance in pathogenic fungi. *Med Mycol*, **36** Suppl 1, 119–28.

7.7.2 Cryptococcosis

William G. Powderly

Essentials

Cryptococcus neoformans, which is found worldwide as a soil organism and thought to be transmitted by inhalation, most often causes disease in patients with abnormal cell-mediated immunity, notably patients with HIV infection and solid-organ transplant recipients, but the infection also occurs rarely in apparently immunocompetent people in restricted geographical areas, especially involving *C. neoformans* var. *gattii*.

The most common presentation is with subacute meningoencephalitis, but other manifestations, e.g. isolated pulmonary disease, are well described. Diagnosis is by culture or serology. Untreated cryptococcal meningitis is fatal: aside from supportive care (including monitoring for raised intracranial pressure), the therapy of choice is an initial period (at least two weeks) of amphotericin B, followed by at least 3 months of fluconazole. Most immunocompromised patients subsequently require maintenance suppressive therapy, usually with fluconazole.

Aetiology and epidemiology

Infection with the fungus *Cryptococcus neoformans* occurs mainly in patients with impaired cell-mediated immunity. It is the most common systemic fungal infection in patients infected with HIV and is also seen as a complication of solid-organ transplantation, lymphoma, and corticosteroid therapy. *C. neoformans* is found worldwide as a soil organism; it is an encapsulated yeast measuring from 4 to 6 μm with a surrounding polysaccharide capsule ranging in size from 1 to over 30 μm. Two varieties exist, distinguishable by serology: *C. neoformans* var. *neoformans* (serotypes A and D) and *C. neoformans* var. *gattii* (serotypes B and C). Virtually all HIV-associated infection is caused by *C. neoformans* var. *neoformans*. About 5% of HIV-infected patients in the Western world develop disseminated cryptococcosis; the disease is more prevalent in sub-Saharan Africa and South-East Asia. *C. neoformans* var. *gattii* infection is more common in tropical and subtropical areas (Australia, New Guinea, and the Philippines) in apparently immunocompetent people. Recent outbreaks of *C. neoformans* var. *gattii* infection have occurred in the western parts of North America. It has only rarely been reported in HIV-immunosuppressed patients.

The exact mechanism of infection is unknown. It is assumed that transmission occurs via inhalation of the organism leading to colonization of the airways and subsequent respiratory infection. Throughout the world, the excreta of birds such as pigeons are the richest environmental source of *C. neoformans* var. *neoformans*.

The ecological association of *C. neoformans* var. *gattii* is with river red and forest river gum trees (*Eucalyptus camaldulensis* and *E. tereticornis*) and with mammals such as koalas. It has been suggested that infective basidiospores are released at flowering.

In the case of *C. neoformans* var. *neoformans*, the absence of an intact cell-mediated response results in ineffective clearance with subsequent dissemination. The polysaccharide capsule, composed mainly of glucuronoxylomannan, is thought to be its primary virulence factor. It is not clear whether cryptococcal infection in immunocompromised patients represents acute primary infection or reactivation of previously dormant disease.

Clinical features

The most common presentation of cryptococcosis is a subacute meningitis or meningoencephalitis with fever, malaise, headache, and altered behaviour and level of consciousness. Symptoms are usually present for 2 to 4 weeks before diagnosis. Classic meningeal symptoms and signs (such as neck stiffness or photophobia) (Fig. 7.7.2.1) occur in only about a quarter to a third of patients. Papilloedema and cranial nerve palsies (especially VI and VII) are common (Fig. 7.7.2.2). Patients may present with encephalopathic symptoms such as lethargy, altered mentation, personality changes, and memory loss. Analysis of the cerebrospinal fluid usually shows a mildly elevated serum protein, normal or slightly low glucose, and a lymphocytic pleocytosis. India ink staining of the cerebrospinal fluid will usually reveal the yeast. Cryptococcal antigen is almost invariably detectable in the cerebrospinal fluid. The opening pressure in the cerebrospinal fluid is elevated in a majority of patients.

Infection with *C. neoformans* can involve sites other than the meninges. Isolated pulmonary disease has been well described and usually presents as a solitary nodule in the absence of other symptoms. Cryptococcal pneumonia also occurs. In immunocompromised patients, especially those with AIDS, subsequent dissemination is common but presentations such as cough or dyspnoea, and abnormal chest radiographs may be the initial finding. Many patients have positive blood cultures. Skin involvement is common; several types of skin lesion have been described (Fig. 7.7.2.3) but the most common form is that resembling molluscum contagiosum. Osteolytic bone lesions and prostatic involvement have also been described.

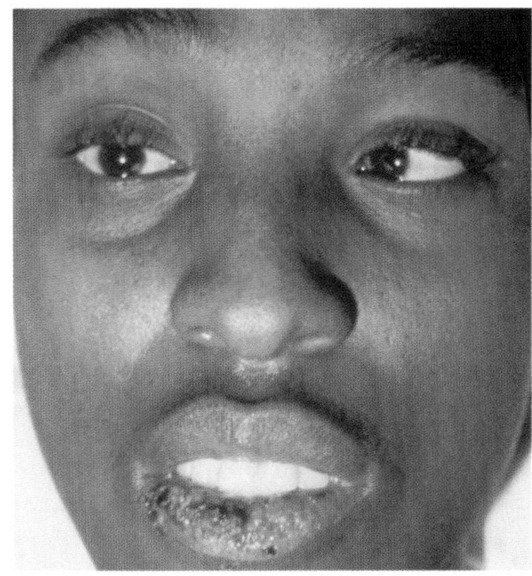

Fig. 7.7.2.2 Right cranial VI (abducens) nerve paralysis in an African HIV-seropositive patient with *Cryptococcus neoformans* var. *neoformans* meningitis. (Copyright D A Warrell.)

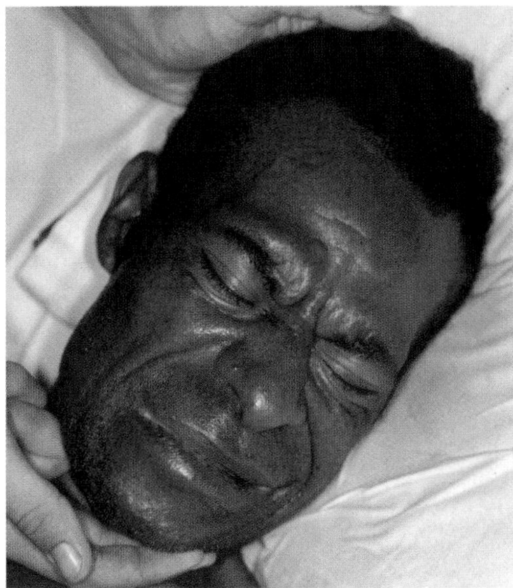

Fig. 7.7.2.1 Neck stiffness in a Papua New Guinean patient with *Cryptococcus neoformans* var. *gattii* meningitis. (Copyright D A Warrell.)

In New Guinea, *C. neoformans* var. *gattii* is the commonest cause of chronic meningitis (Fig. 7.7.2.1). Immunocompetent people are affected. Compared to *C. neoformans* var. *neoformans* meningitis in AIDS patients, patients with *C. neoformans* var. *gattii* have more aggressive retinal involvement with papilloedema and haemorrhagic papillitis in more than a half of patients, leading to blindness in one-third of survivors.

Diagnosis

The latex agglutination test for cryptococcal polysaccharide antigen in the serum is highly sensitive and specific in the diagnosis of infection with *C. neoformans* and a positive serum cryptococcal

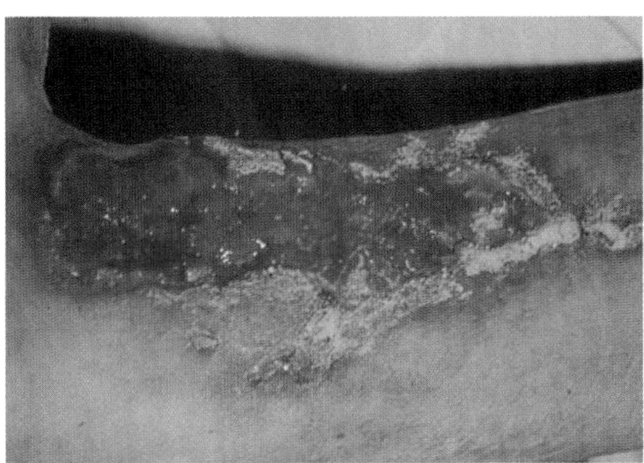

Fig. 7.7.2.3 Cryptococcal cutaneous ulcer. (Courtesy of Professor R Hay.)

antigen titre of greater than 1:8 is presumptive evidence of cryptococcal infection. Such patients should be evaluated for possible meningeal involvement. Culture of *C. neoformans* from any body site should also be regarded as significant and is an indication for further evaluation and initiation of therapy.

Treatment

Management of patients with cryptococcal infection depends on the extent of the disease and the immune status of the patient. The finding of a solitary pulmonary nodule in a normal host may not need treatment, provided patients have careful follow up. Fluconazole (200–400 mg/day) can be given for 3 to 6 months in most patients with localized pulmonary disease. Extrapulmonary disease is generally managed in the same way as meningitis. In patients who are not known to be immunosuppressed, a search for underlying problems should be initiated. An HIV antibody test should be performed, as cryptococcal meningitis may be the initial AIDS-defining event. Additionally, a CD4+ lymphocyte count should be considered, as cryptococcal infection has been described as one of the manifestations of so-called 'isolated CD4 T lymphocytopenia'.

Untreated, cryptococcal meningitis is fatal. In patients with AIDS, amphotericin B (0.7 mg/kg intravenously) given for 2 weeks followed by fluconazole (400 mg orally) for a further 8 weeks is associated with the best outcome to date in prospective trials, with a mortality of less than 10% and a mycological response of approximately 70%. This regimen is also reasonable for treatment of meningitis in other circumstances. Concomitant use of flucytosine (100 mg/kg per day in four divided doses) with amphotericin B may be considered. In patients with AIDS, it does not improve immediate outcome but may decrease the risk of relapse. In other hosts, more prolonged use (4–6 weeks) of amphotericin B and flucytosine may be curative but is also toxic. In this circumstance (e.g. solid-organ transplant patients requiring immunosuppressive therapy), lipid or liposomal formulations of amphotericin B may be less toxic options.

Clinical deterioration in patients with meningitis may be due to cerebral oedema, which may be diagnosed by a raised opening pressure of the cerebrospinal fluid. All patients with cryptococcal meningitis should have the opening pressure measured when a lumbar puncture is performed; if the opening pressure is high (>25 cmH_2O), pressure should be reduced by repeated lumbar punctures, a lumbar drain, or a shunt.

Cryptococcal meningitis in AIDS requires lifelong suppressive therapy unless the immunosuppression is reversed with effective treatment of HIV infection. In that circumstance, treatment can be discontinued if the CD4+ lymphocyte count increases to over 200 cells/mm^3. In other immunocompromised patients, suppressive treatment for 6 to 12 months may be given. Effective antiretroviral therapy may also sufficiently improve the immune system such that there is an immunological response to the fungal infection. This may be associated with clinical deterioration and apparent relapse of symptoms; this immune reconstitution syndrome should not prompt change in antifungal therapy and patients should receive anti-inflammatory therapy, as needed. It has also been described in transplant patients whose immunosuppressive therapy is decreased during management of the cryptococcal infection.

Fluconazole, 200 mg daily, is the suppressive treatment of choice. Fluconazole, in dosages ranging from 400 mg weekly to 200 mg daily, and itraconazole, 100 mg twice daily, are very effective in preventing invasive cryptococcal infections, especially in HIV-positive patients with CD4 counts less than 50 to 100 cells/mm^3. However, because of the relative infrequency of invasive fungal infections, antifungal prophylaxis does not prolong life and is not routinely recommended where antiretroviral therapy is readily available.

Further reading

Bicanic T, Harrison TS (2005). Cryptococcal meningitis. *Br Med Bull*, **72**, 99–118.

Ellis DH, Pfeiffer TJ (1990). Ecology, lifecycle, and infections propagule of *Cryptococcus neoformans*. *Lancet*, **36**, 923–5.

Graybill JR, *et al.* (2000). Diagnosis and management of increased intracranial pressure in patients with AIDS and cryptococcal meningitis. *Clin Infect Dis*, **30**, 47–54.

Perfect JR, *et al.* (2010). Clinical Practice guidelines for the management of cryptococcal disease: 2009 update by the Infectious Diseases Society of America. *Clin Infect Dis*, **50**.

Shelbourne S, *et al.* (2005). The role of immune reconstitution inflammatory syndrome in AIDS-related *Cryptococcus neoformans* disease in the era of highly active antiretroviral therapy. *Clin Infect Dis*, **40**, 1049–52.

Sorrel TC (2001). *Cryptococcus neoformans* variety *gattii*. *Med Mycol*, **39**, 155–68.

Speed B, Dunt D (1995). Clinical and host differences between infection of the two varieties of *Cryptococcus neoformans*. *Clin Infect Dis*, **21**, 28–34.

7.7.3 Coccidioidomycosis

Gregory M. Anstead and John R. Graybill

Essentials

Coccidiodomycosis results from inhalation of arthroconidia of *Coccidioides* spp., which are soil fungi endemic to the south-western United States of America and parts of Latin America. Most infections are asymptomatic, but primary infection may resemble community-acquired pneumonia, sometimes with hypersensitivity manifestations such as erythema nodosum, erythema multiforme, and arthritis. Acute pulmonary infection usually resolves spontaneously, but—especially in immunocompromised patients, African Americans, and Filipinos—it may progress to persistent pulmonary disease or disseminate to skin, soft tissues, osteoarticular tissue, and the central nervous system. Diagnosis is by culture, histopathology or serology. Fluconazole and itraconazole are usually the initial drugs of choice, with amphotericin B reserved for severe pulmonary and disseminated disease, and in pregnancy.

Introduction

Coccidioidomycosis results from inhalation of arthroconidia of dimorphic fungi of the genus *Coccidioides*, of which the two species are *C. immitis* (Californian isolates) and *C. posadasii* (non-Californian isolates). Both species cause similar clinical effects. These soil fungi inhabit semiarid to arid areas in the south-western United States of America and parts of Latin America. Hyperendemic areas include the San Joaquin Valley (California) and Pima, Pinal, and Maricopa counties in Arizona. There are approximately 150 000 infections per year in the United States of America.

Persons at risk

Residence in or travel to endemic areas is the key risk factor for acquiring coccidioidomycosis. At increased risk of more serious disease are people of Filipino or African American descent, those with blood group B, those exposed to soil, and the immunocompromised (organ transplant recipients, patients with AIDS, pregnancy, cancer, and diabetes, and recipients of tumour necrosis factor α antagonists). Outbreaks may follow dust storms, earthquakes, droughts, and activities causing soil disruption, such as archaeological digs.

Pathogenesis

Inhaled coccidioides arthroconidia are ingested by pulmonary macrophages and, over 3 days or more, convert to thick-walled round spherules containing hundreds of endospores. When spherules rupture, the endospores may disseminate to meninges, bones, skin, or other soft tissues. Resolution of coccidioidomycosis depends on intact cell-mediated immunity.

Diagnosis

This is based on clinical findings supported by microbiological, histopathological, and/or serological evidence. Coccidioides mycelia grow readily on many culture media. They are formed by barrel-shaped arthroconidia, with intercalated 'ghost' cells. Histopathological findings may vary, from abscesses with many spherules, large endospores, and neutrophils (in uncontrolled disease) to well-formed granulomas with few organisms (in patients with competent cell-mediated immunity). These findings are readily seen with haematoxylin and eosin staining.

Serological methods are often used to diagnosis of coccidioidomycosis. IgM antibodies detected by the tube precipitin (TP) test or immunodiffusion TP appear within the first few weeks of infection and clear within 1 or 2 months. IgG is detectable by complement fixation (CF) or immunodiffusion CF after several months and persists for years. Serum CF titres of 1:16 or higher suggest deterioration or dissemination. In coccidioidal meningitis, any positive titre confirms the diagnosis; the cerebrospinal fluid IgG titre is positive more than 75% of the time, whereas cerebrospinal fluid cultures are positive in less than 50% of patients.

More recently, enzyme-linked immunosorbent assay (ELISA) has been used for coccidioidal IgG and IgM antibodies. ELISA optical density correlates roughly with immunodiffusion CF titre. ELISA may be falsely negative early in the course of the disease and false positives sometimes occur with histoplasmosis and paracoccidioidomycosis.

Clinical presentation

Primary infection

About 60% of subjects are asymptomatic. Symptomatic primary infection presents from 1 to 3 weeks after exposure, with fever, cough, and pulmonary infiltrates, and may be accompanied by hypersensitivity manifestations, such as erythema nodosum, erythema multiforme, and arthritis. Antifungal therapy is not required. Eosinophilia may occur, or eosinophilic pleocytosis in cases of meningitis. Treatment of primary disease should be undertaken with immunocompromised patients. Recent appreciation that primary coccidioidomycosis makes up a substantial percentage of community acquired pneumonias in Arizona again raises the question whether fluconazole should be used more broadly for primary disease.

In addition to uneventful resolution, there are various outcomes of primary coccidioidomycosis, which include those given below.

Coccidioma formation

Pulmonary infiltrates may contract into an asymptomatic mass (coccidioma), which may persist for years. In an immunocompetent person, antifungal therapy is unnecessary.

Progressive/persistent pneumonia

Heavily exposed immunosuppressed patients may develop acute respiratory failure. Amphotericin B treatment is recommended. Pneumonia persists more than 2 months, with extensive infiltrates and, often, cavitation. Initial treatment is with amphotericin B if the patient is severely ill. IDSA guidelines suggest between 3 and 6 months for the duration of therapy, but we would favour treatment for more than 6 months after resolution of symptoms, and for more than a year with diffuse miliary disease. Conversion to an oral azole is appropriate when the patient is improving.

Chronic pulmonary coccidioidomycosis

This occurs in about 5% of patients with symptomatic primary coccidioidomycosis and may have a fluctuating course over years. Nodular lesions may cavitate, with surrounding infiltrates and fibrosis. Cavitary disease may be asymptomatic or be associated with rupture and pneumothorax, haemorrhage, or secondary infection. Cavities smaller than 2.5 cm in diameter tend to resolve, while cavities larger than 5 cm persist. Cavities may remain stable for years or become infected with *aspergillus*, or fluctuate with intermittent infiltrates and fibrocavitary disease. Chronic pulmonary coccidioidomycosis can progressively destroy the lungs and requires medical therapy with either fluconazole or itraconazole. The appropriate duration of therapy is uncertain. If large asymptomatic cavities persist for several years, resection should be considered.

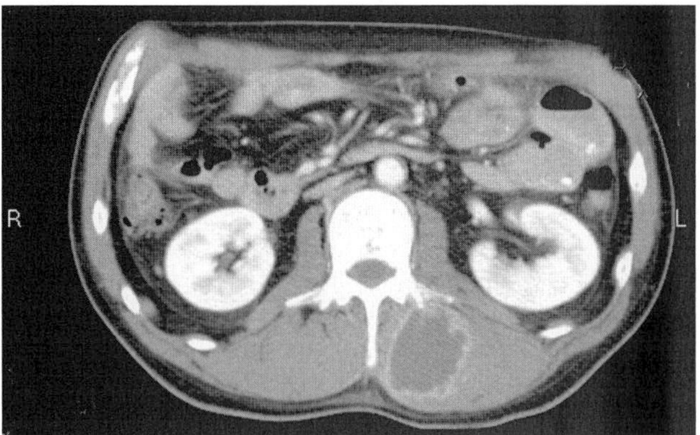

Fig. 7.7.3.1 CT of paraspinous abscess in a patient with coccidioidomycosis.

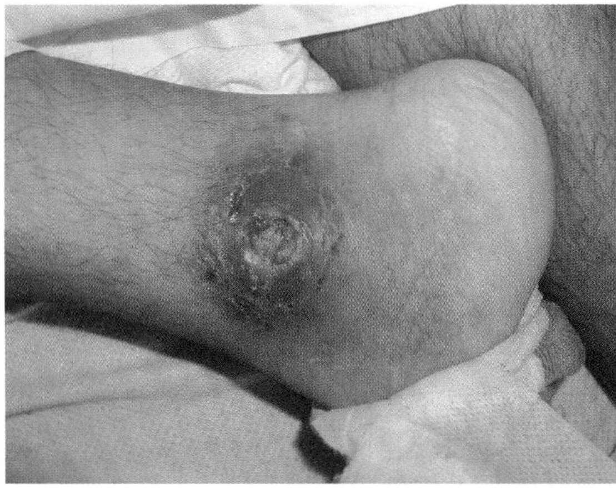

Fig. 7.7.3.2 Ulcerative ankle lesion with underlying osteomyelitis in a patient with coccidioidomycosis.

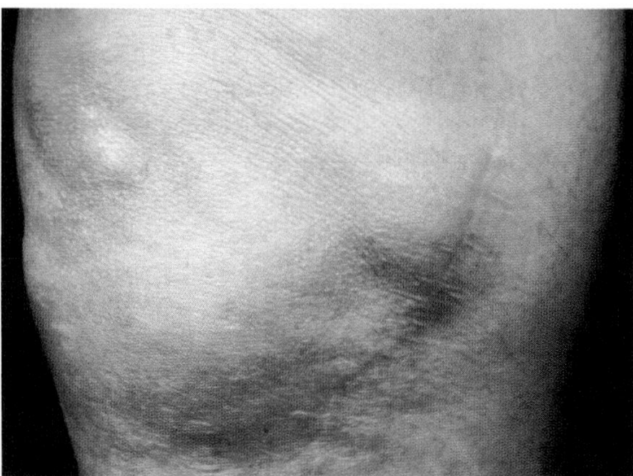

Fig. 7.7.3.4 Coccidioidal arthropathy.
(Copyright R. Hay.)

Coccidioidal mycetoma may occur in pre-existing cavities and is treated by resection.

Disseminated coccidioidomycosis

Pleura and pericardium may be invaded. Haematogenous dissemination occurs within a few months after infection and may involve skin, soft tissue, osteoarticular tissue, and meninges (Figs. 7.7.3.1–7.7.3.3). Papules, nodules, abscesses, verrucous plaques, or ulcers are seen. Medical therapy is often combined with surgical therapy to debulk lesions.

In chronic coccidioidomycosis, fluconazole at 400 or 800 mg/day or itraconazole at 200 mg twice daily are used but death may ensue despite intensive medical and surgical intervention.

Osteoarticular disease

Any bone and joint may be targeted, but those that are weight bearing are more vulnerable (Fig. 7.7.3.4). Infection can destroy the vertebral body, with collapse and joint instability. Paraspinous abscesses should be drained and, if necessary, the joint(s) stabilized.

Central nervous system involvement

Coccidioidal meningitis may be accompanied by coccidioma, vasculitis, infarction, and hydrocephalus. Most clinicians initiate treatment of meningitis with high-dose fluconazole (800–2000 mg/day), which may be reduced as the patient improves. Lifelong treatment is necessary. Obstructive hydrocephalus requires ventriculoperitoneal shunting.

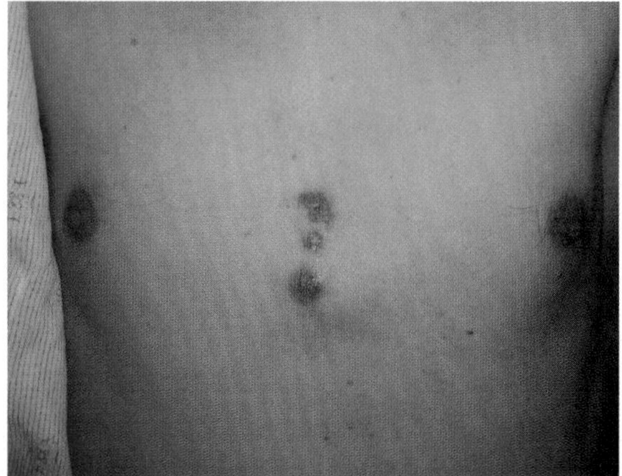

Fig. 7.7.3.3 Abscesses on the chest in a patient with coccidioidomycosis.

Selection of antifungal agents

Azoles are preferred for treating most forms of coccidioidomycosis. In a randomized comparison of fluconazole and itraconazole, between 50 and 60% were cured with both drugs. In small trials, osteoarticular disease responded better on itraconazole than fluconazole. Either drug, 400 mg/day, is usually given for a year or more after clinical cure. In AIDS patients with nonmeningeal disease, antifungal therapy may be stopped if their fungal disease is quiescent and their CD4 count increases above 250 cells/μl by antiretroviral therapy. In meningitis, fluconazole is clearly preferred due to more reliable oral absorption and central nervous system penetration.

Posaconazole is licensed in Europe for salvage therapy of coccidioidomycosis, based on limited clinical experience. Posaconazole may succeed in cases of disseminated nonmeningeal coccidioidomycosis in which other azoles and amphotericin B have failed. The dose is 200 mg 4 times daily, given orally with a lipid containing meal. Voriconazole has been used successfully in a few cases of coccidioidomycosis.

Amphotericin B should be used largely as salvage therapy and in pregnancy, since azoles are teratogenic. After therapy has been stopped, the patient should be observed for years as coccidioidomycosis has an unpleasant propensity to relapse.

Further reading

Anstead GM, Graybill JR (2006). Coccidioidomycosis. *Infect Dis Clin North Am*, **20**, 621–43. [A recent comprehensive review.]

Crum NF, *et al.* (2004). Coccidioidomycosis: a descriptive survey of a reemerging disease. Clinical characteristics and emerging controversies. *Medicine (Baltimore)*, **83**, 149–75. [A recent cohort study of the characteristics of 223 patients with coccidioidomycosis.]

Galgiani JN, *et al.* (2000). Comparisons of oral fluconazole and itraconazole for progressive, nonmeningeal coccidioidomycosis – a randomized, double-blind trial. *Ann Intern Med*, **133**, 676–86. [The only randomized, double-blind trial ever conducted for the treatment of coccidioidomycosis.]

Galgiani JN, *et al.* (2005). Coccidioidomycosis. *Clin Infect Dis*, **41**, 1217–23. [The 2005 guidelines of the Infectious Diseases Society of America for the treatment of coccidioidomycosis.]

Johnson RH, Einstein HE (2006). Coccidioidal meningitis. *Clin Infect Dis*, **42**, 103–6. [A recent review of the clinical characteristics and treatment of the difficult problem of coccidioidal meningitis.]

7.7.4 Paracoccidioidomycosis

M.A. Shikanai-Yasuda

Essentials

Paracoccidioidomycosis is a systemic mycosis caused by the dimorphic fungus *Paracoccidioides brasiliensis*, which is found in soil and in a variety of animals, and transmitted to humans by inhalation. It is restricted geographically to Central and South America, where it is the commonest endemic chronic human mycosis, acquired in rural and periurban areas, equally distributed among prepubescent boys and girls, but more frequent in men than women (10:1).

Clinical features—manifestations range from an asymptomatic course to severe and potentially fatal disseminated disease. (1) Acute form (juvenile type)—1 to 20% of cases; presentation is with progressive lymphadenopathy; fever and weight loss are common; liver and spleen are usually moderately enlarged; other manifestations include mucocutaneous lesions and bone and small bowel involvement. (2) Chronic form—usually occurs in men aged 30 to 50 years who have worked in agricultural areas; frequently involves the lung, skin and mucous membranes (mainly pharynx, larynx, and trachea); may involve lymph nodes and adrenals, also (less frequently) intestine, spleen, bones, central nervous system (brain, cerebellum, meninges) and genitourinary system. Complications include microstomia, laryngeal/tracheal/bronchial stenosis, pulmonary emphysema/fibrosis, respiratory insufficiency and cor pulmonale.

Diagnosis and treatment—diagnosis is by (1) direct microscopy or culture from sputum, pus or other lesions; (2) histopathology—silver or periodic acid–Schiff staining reveals granulomas containing fungal cells with either proliferative and/or exudative reactions; or (3) serological testing. Treatment of mild cases is with sulfamethoxazole–trimethoprim or itraconazole; severe cases of acute or chronic disease require intravenous amphotericin B or other amphotericin formulations, followed by oral drugs. Long courses of treatment (6–36 months) are required until stabilization or disappearance of antibodies detected by immunodifusion or counterimmunoelectrophoresis tests.

Definition

Paracoccidioidomycosis is a systemic granulomatous disease caused by a dimorphic fungus, *Paracoccidioides brasiliensis*, that involves mainly the lungs, phagocytic mononuclear system, mucous membranes, skin, and adrenals.

History

The disease was first described in 1908 by Lutz, a Brazilian scientist. In 1912, Splendore classified the organism as a yeast of the genus *Zymonema* and, in 1928, Almeida and Lacaz suggested the name *Paracoccidioides*. In 1930, Almeida named the fungus *Paracoccidioides brasiliensis*. Formerly, the disease was known as South American blastomycosis or Lutz–Splendore–Almeida disease. In 1977, it was renamed paracoccidioidomycosis.

Epidemiology

Paracoccidioidomycosis is the most common endemic human mycosis in Latin America but is restricted geographically to Central and South America, ranging from Mexico to Argentina. The disease is prevalent in Brazil, Colombia, Venezuela, Argentina, Uruguay, Paraguay, Guatemala, Ecuador, Peru, and Mexico. Imported cases have been recorded in the United States of America, Europe, and Asia. Paracoccidioidomycosis is the eighth most important cause of mortality from chronic infectious diseases in Brazil, the highest among systemic mycoses.

Prevalence, inferred from the result of intradermal paracoccidioidin testing, ranges from 6 to 60.6% among rural and urban populations of endemic and nonendemic areas; lower rates were observed in the same region when a more specific antigen, 43 kDa glycoprotein, was employed in comparison with paracoccidioidin. The disease is equally distributed among prepubescent boys and girls but among adults the sex ratio of clinical cases is 10 or more men to each woman. This may be explained by the ability of oestrogens to inhibit the transformation of mycelium or conidia to yeast. The disease is most common among 20- to 50-year-old agricultural workers or those who have lived in rural endemic areas. Spouses of patients are rarely affected by the disease, which suggests that hormonal and genetic factors play a part in the distribution of this mycosis. Transmission from one person to another has not been shown.

Ecology

The geographical regions where paracoccidioidomycosis is most prevalent are humid with more acidic soils and a temperature range from 15 to 30°C. *P. brasiliensis* has been isolated from soil, animals such as armadillos and bats, dog food, penguin faeces, and the intestinal contents of bats. Efforts to maintain the fungus in bat intestines have been unsuccessful. The saprophytic habitat of *P. brasiliensis* has yet to be discovered.

Aetiology

Phylogenetic studies of eight regions in five nuclear loci of 65 *P. brasiliensis* isolates indicated initially that this fungus consisted of at least three distinct, previously unrecognized species: S1 (species 1 with 38 isolates from Brazil, Argentina, Paraguay, Peru, and Venezuela isolates), PS2 (phylogenetic species 2 with five Brazilian and one Venezuelan isolates), and PS3 (phylogenetic species 3 with 21 Colombian isolates). Additionally, other Brazilian isolate 'Pb01-like' species exhibit great sequence and morphological divergence from the S1/PS2/PS3 species clade and was named as *Paracoccidioides lutzii*.

Mycology

P. brasiliensis is a dimorphic fungus that can be cultivated either as a mould or a yeast. When cultured at 25°C, it appears after 15 to 30 days as white colonies. When Sabouraud's dextrose agar is used, the mycelium shows hyaline septate hyphae with branches.

P. brasiliensis grows as a yeast in human and animal tissues (Fig. 7.7.4.1) and in cultures maintained at 37°C. Colonies can be observed after 7 to 20 days. Under direct microscopy, yeast forms are seen as oval or spherical cells with doubly refractile walls; the cells vary in size from buds of 2 to 10 μm in diameter to mature cells of 20 to 30 μm. Mother cells may produce 10 to 12 uniform or variably sized buds (Fig. 7.7.4.2), forming the characteristic 'pilot wheel' shape observed in biological samples or in infected tissues.

Conidia produced by mycelium represent the infectious form and are inhaled through the respiratory tract.

Analysis of 6022 assembled groups from mycelium and yeast phase expressed sequence tags of about 80% of the estimated genome of *P. brasiliensis*. The transcriptome analysis reported information about sequences related to the cell cycle, stress response, drug resistance, and signal transduction pathways of the pathogen.

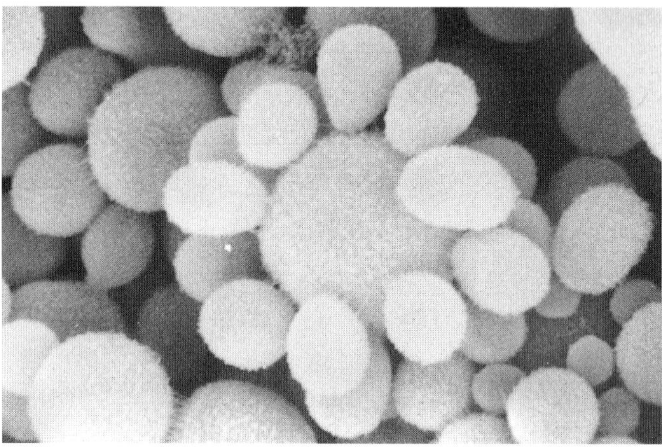

Fig. 7.7.4.2 Scanning electron micrograph of a multiple budding yeast cell of *Paracoccidioides brasiliensis*.
(Courtesy of C S Lacaz.)

Virulence

Virulence, defined as the ability to produce disseminated infection in experimental animals, varies between different fungal isolates but little is understood of the biochemical basis for these differences. The presence of higher levels of α-1,3-glucan in virulent strains of *P. brasiliensis* compared with avirulent strains was initially related to virulence, but no correlation has been shown between glucans and virulence in experimentally induced infections. Binding of laminin to yeast cells (possibly through binding to gp43) enhanced their pathogenicity in the hamster testicle model.

Pathogenesis

Experimental and clinicopathological observations indicate that the respiratory route is the main portal of entry and the lung is the primary site of infection.

The first fungus–host contact occurs through inhalation of airborne conidia. When mice are experimentally infected through the respiratory route, conidia have been observed in the alveoli soon after inoculation. Some 12 to 18 h after the exposure, yeast forms can be observed in the alveoli. There is an initial inflammatory response, which is mediated by polymorphonuclear cells, followed by granuloma formation.

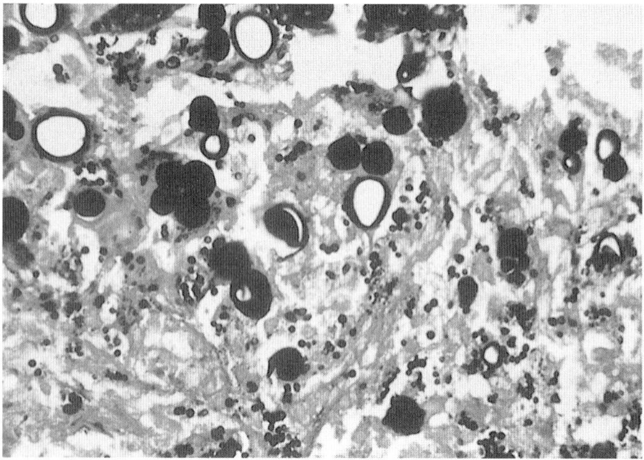

Fig. 7.7.4.1 Small and large yeast forms of *Paracoccidioides brasiliensis* in the lung of a transplant recipient (methenamine silver stain).
(Courtesy of C S Lacaz.)

The primary infective complex develops at the inoculation site and involves the surrounding lymphatic vessels and regional lymph nodes. The fungus spreads to other parts of the lung through peribronchial lymphatic vessels and drains into regional lymph nodes. Haematogenous dissemination to a variety of organs and tissues may occur at this time. The lesions usually undergo involution and the fungi remain dormant if the host's immune response can control their proliferation. A balanced host–fungus relationship is associated with the absence of symptoms, although, in some children or young adults, acute disease may arise, primarily affecting the phagocytic mononuclear system. In adult life, previously quiescent lesions may become reactivated, especially in the lungs, leading to the adult or chronic form of the disease.

Pathology

The characteristic lesion is a granuloma containing *P. brasiliensis* cells. The infected tissue may exhibit a predominantly proliferative, granulomatous inflammatory response and/or an exudative reaction, sometimes resulting in necrosis, with variable numbers of neutrophils and large numbers of extracellular yeast cells, leading to a chronic epithelioid granuloma.

Autopsy studies, mainly of adult patients, indicate that the organs most frequently involved are the lungs (42–96%), adrenals (44–80%), lymph nodes (28–72%), pharynx/larynx (18–60%), and skin/other mucosal surfaces (2.7–64%).

Host–fungus interaction

Nonspecific immune response

The influence of genetic factors on the individual susceptibility to this mycosis is suggested by the observation of higher rates of HLA phenotypes A9, B13, B40, and Cw3 among patients than in controls and higher rates of HLA DRB1*11 in patients with unifocal disease than with other forms of the. In isogenic mice, resistance to *P. brasiliensis* is controlled by a single autosomal gene.

The ability of circulating human neutrophils obtained by bronchoalveolar washing to digest the yeast forms of fungi was impaired in severe cases, while this defect was absent in uninfected family members of patients.

Specific immune response

Host–fungus interaction in infection and disease was analysed through *in vivo* intradermal tests for ubiquitous fungal antigens, *in vitro* lymphoblastic transformation tests, and intra- and extracellular cytokines secretion, chemokines and regulatory T cell activity after stimulation with mitogens or *P. brasiliensis* antigens (PbAg). Infected people (asymptomatic individuals without disease) showed a positive skin test to PbAg, absence of specific antibodies, a vigorous lymphoproliferative response to PbAg, and a typical T-helper (Th) type 1 pattern of cytokines (see Table 7.7.4.1). They had a higher expression of CD80 monocytes and lower expression of CD86 monocytes compared to patients with chronic or acute disease. Patients with acute disease showed impairment of proliferative response to PbAg and Th2 cytokine pattern. This pattern is associated with poor granuloma formation, spreading of the fungus and high levels of antibody production (immunoglobulins IgG 1, IgG 4, and IgE). Patients with chronic disease had intermediate profiles. The specific lymphoproliferative response was lower than in asymptomatic paracoccidioidomycosis-infected patients but higher than in patients with acute disease (see Table 7.7.4.1).

More recent research indicates that regulatory T cells exhibiting suppressive activity in patients' cells seem to play a role in controlling local and systemic immune response. In mice, treatment of dendritic cells with gp43 plus lipopolysaccharide was followed by increase of fungal colony forming units in the lungs in comparison with controls, suggesting that gp43 might reduce effectiveness of the immune response in the primary infection. In pulmonary murine paracoccidioidomycosis, a dual role of interleukin 4 (IL-4, a Th2 cytokine) was observed in IL-4-depleted mice depending on the host genetic pattern: isogenic resistant mice showed better control of the disease. Conversely, susceptible mice showed enhanced pulmonary infection, suggesting a role for IL-4 in the modulation of immune response, not only as Th2 cytokine.

Antibodies may enhance phagocytosis through opsonization of the fungus, but their role in resistance is not established.

Table 7.7.4.1 Host–fungus interaction in paracoccidioidomycosis: cytokine secretion and *P. brasiliensis* antigenaemia/antigenuria in infection and disease

Groups	Cytokine secretion and antigenaemia/antigenuria	Intracellular cytokines
Infection[a]	IFγ, Ab undetectable	IFγ↑, TNFα↑, IL-2↑
Acute disease	IFγ↓, IL-4↑↑, IL-5↑↑, IL-10↑, Ab↑ (IgG 4), antigenaemia/antigenuria↑	IFγ↓, TNFα↓, IL-2↓
Chronic disease	IFγ↓, IL-4↑, IL-5↑, IL-10↑, Ab↑ (IgG 2)	IFγ↓, TNFα↓, IL-2↓
Immunosuppressed patients	? IFγ↓, IL-10↑, ? IL-4, ? IL-5↓, Ab increased or lower levels, antigenaemia/antigenuria ↑	?[b]

Ab, antibodies; IF, interferon; IL, interleukin; TNFα, tumour necrosis factor α; ↓, decrease; ↑, increase.

[a] Asymptomatic individuals sensitized by *P. brasiliensis* antigens without signs and symptoms.

[b] Decrease in lymphoproliferation in response to *P. brasiliensis* antigens: intracellular cytokines unknown.

The importance of late hypersensitivity in protection has been observed recently in patients receiving cytotoxic therapy for associated neoplasms and in those with AIDS presenting severe disease.

Clinical features

The range is from an asymptomatic course to severe and potentially fatal disseminated disease. The incubation period is unknown except in a laboratory worker, who developed a skin lesion some days after an accidental inoculation. The disease has been reported in children 3 years of age or older who had lived for some years in the endemic area.

A proposed classification of clinical forms of paracoccidioidomycosis is shown in Box 7.7.4.1.

Localization in a particular tissue or organ and the degree of severity of the disease according to established criteria make this classification easily and uniformly applicable. General and nutritional debility and organ dysfunction (lung, brain, adrenals, bone marrow) indicate the severity of the disease. In immunosuppressed patients, signs of chronic and acute disease are observed simultaneously, with dissemination of fungi through phagocytic mononuclear cells.

Acute form (juvenile type)

Children, adolescents, and young adults (under 30 years of age) are affected, men and women equally. Only 1 to 20% of patients fall into this group. There is progression for 2 or 3 months or longer, characterized by involvement of the phagocytic mononuclear system. Cervical, axillary, and inguinal nodes are the most commonly enlarged (Fig. 7.7.4.3). Nodes are initially hard but are sometimes fluctuant and drain pus rich in fungi. Less frequently, deep-seated lymph nodes may also be affected. When the hepatic perihilar lymph nodes are enlarged, they may produce symptoms of obstructive jaundice.

The liver and spleen are usually moderately enlarged. Bones (clavicle, scapulae, ribs, skull, long, and flat bones) and, rarely, the bone marrow may be involved. Radiographs show lytic lesions without periosteal reaction. Involvement of the small bowel may be asymptomatic or produce abdominal pain, diarrhoea, constipation, and even intestinal obstruction. Radiological studies of the digestive tract reveal intestinal tract involvement in about 50% of clinical cases. Fever and weight loss are common. Multiple mucocutaneous lesions are more frequent in some geographical areas (Fig. 7.7.4.4). High transient blood eosinophilia (up to 30 000/mm^3) has sometimes been described.

Box 7.7.4.1 Paracoccidioidomycosis: proposed classification of clinical forms

- Paracoccidioidomycosis infection
- Regressive (self-healing) paracoccidioidomycosis
- Paracoccidioidomycosis disease
  - Acute form (juvenile type)—moderate or severe
  - Chronic form (adult type)—mild, moderate, or severe
- Sequelae

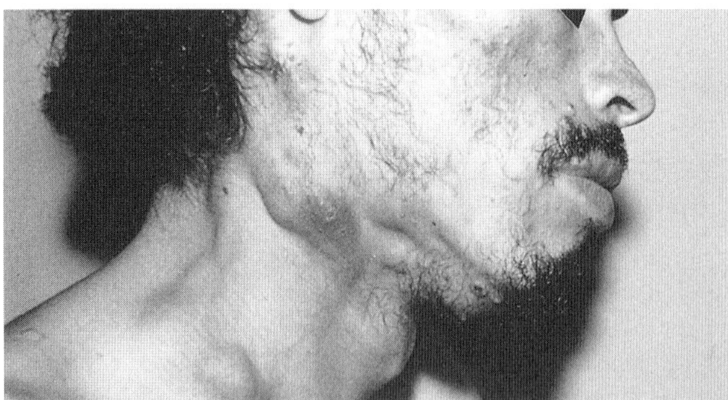

Fig. 7.7.4.3 Lymph node and skin involvement in a patient with the acute form of paracoccidioidomycosis.
(Courtesy of C S Lacaz.)

Clinical lung involvement is rarely described in this form of paracoccidioidomycosis. In some case reports, either bronchopneumonia or primary complex-like disease have been observed.

Chronic form

This form of the disease usually occurs in 30- to 50-year-old men who have worked in agricultural areas. The male:female ratio varies from 10:1 to 25:1. The evolution is insidious and, in many cases, clinically mild.

The organ most frequently involved is the lung, followed by skin and mucous membranes, mainly pharynx, larynx, and trachea. Lymph nodes and adrenals may be compromised. More than one organ or tissue is usually involved. Less frequently, intestine, spleen, bones, central nervous system (brain, cerebellum, meninges), eyes, genitourinary system, myocardium, pericardium, and arteries are involved.

The patients may be asymptomatic or complain of dyspnoea, cough, sometimes purulent sputum, and, rarely, haemoptysis. Fever is unusual. Physical examination is frequently normal or there may be scattered rales. In contrast, chest radiography commonly reveals bilateral, asymmetrical, reticulonodular infiltrates in the middle and lower parts of the lungs (Fig. 7.7.4.5). Apical cavities and pleural effusions are less frequently observed.

Cutaneous lesions include papules, pustules, ulcers, crusted ulcers, vegetations, tuberculoids, verrucoids, or acneiform lesions

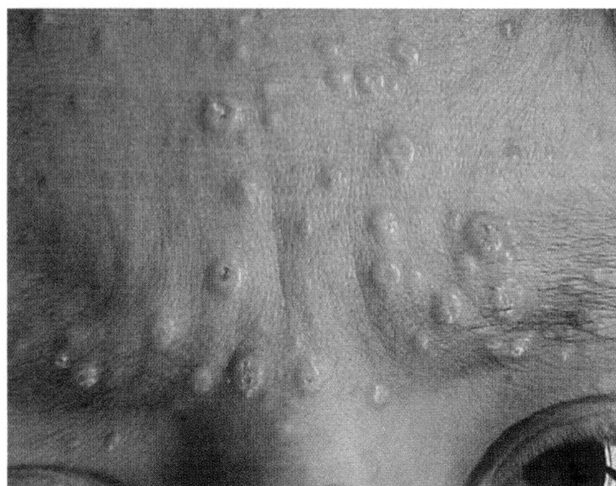

Fig. 7.7.4.4 Multiple molluscum-like lesions in a young Peruvian patient.
(Copyright Francisco Bravo, Lima.)

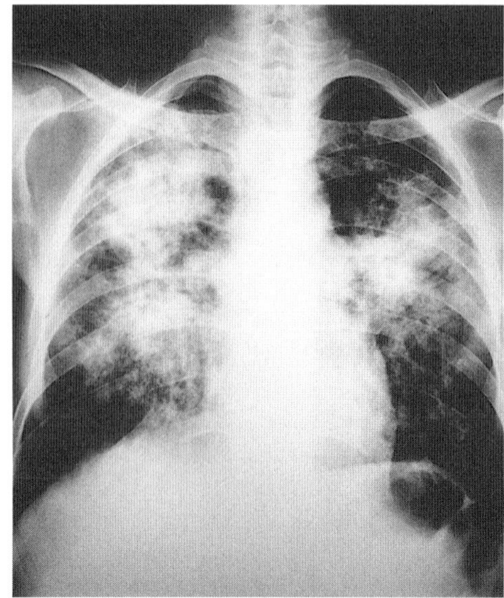

Fig. 7.7.4.5 Alveolar and interstitial infiltrates in both lungs in a patient with chronic paracoccidioidomycosis.
(Department of Infectious and Parasitic Diseases, School of Medicine, University of São Paulo.)

mainly on the face (Fig. 7.7.4.6) or limbs. Multiple, scattered lesions result from haematogenous dissemination (Fig. 7.7.4.7). Subcutaneous cold abscesses, more commonly associated with bone lesions, can occur.

Mucosal lesions are usually in the mouth and/or oropharynx, including the palate (Fig. 7.7.4.8), uvula, and tonsils, or in the respiratory tract, involving mainly the larynx (vocal cords, glottis, and epiglottis) and trachea. Pain is usually intense and may hamper mastication and swallowing. Hoarseness and dysphonia result from laryngeal lesions and may lead to obstruction of the upper respiratory tract. Examination shows ulcerative, verrucous, vegetant, and infiltrative 'moriform' stomatitis, resembling a raspberry, with papules, vesicles, and haemorrhagic spots. The last is characteristic of this mycosis and appears as shallow ulcers, with a granular surface showing multiple, fine, haemorrhagic points.

Few lymph nodes may be involved, in contrast to the acute form of the disease.

Uni- or bilateral lesions in the adrenal glands have been found in about half of patients coming to autopsy. Partial adrenal insufficiency has been documented in about 40% of the cases but only 7.4% were symptomatic.

Concomitant tuberculosis is observed in about 10 to 15% of cases of pulmonary paracoccidioidomycosis and has also been described

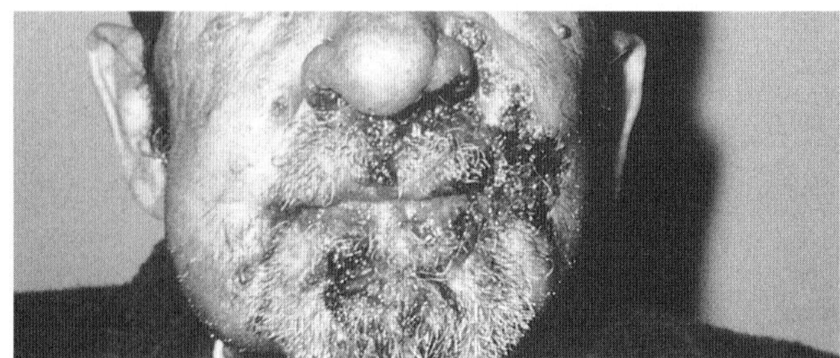

Fig. 7.7.4.6 Mucocutaneous lesions in a patient with chronic paracoccidioidomycosis.
(Courtesy of C S Lacaz.)

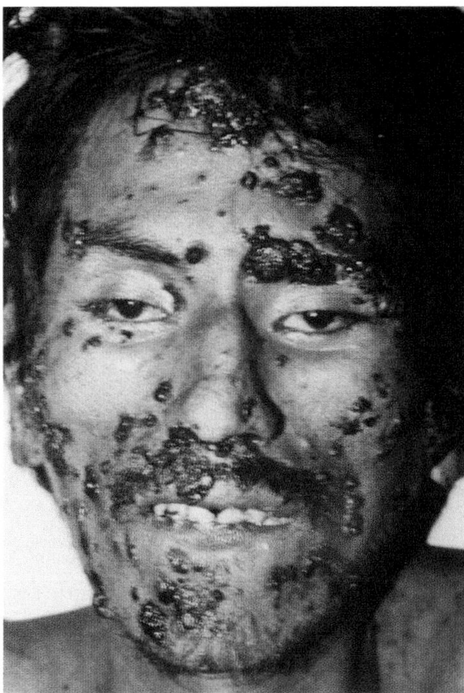

Fig. 7.7.4.7 Disseminated skin lesions.
(Courtesy of Universidad Peruviana Cayetano Heredia.)

in cases of lymph node involvement by *P. brasiliensis*. Carcinomas may arise in pulmonary or mucosal mycotic lesions.

Sequelae

Nowadays, sequelae constitute one of the most important problems in the management of paracoccidioidomycosis. Although fungal multiplication can been controlled by chemotherapy, impairment of vital functions might prove fatal.

Acute form

Lesions in the small intestine and mesenteric lymph nodes may fibrose, causing lymphatic obstruction, intestinal malabsorption, or protein-losing enteropathy. A clinical picture of severe malnutrition and immunodeficiency has been reported (Fig. 7.7.4.9).

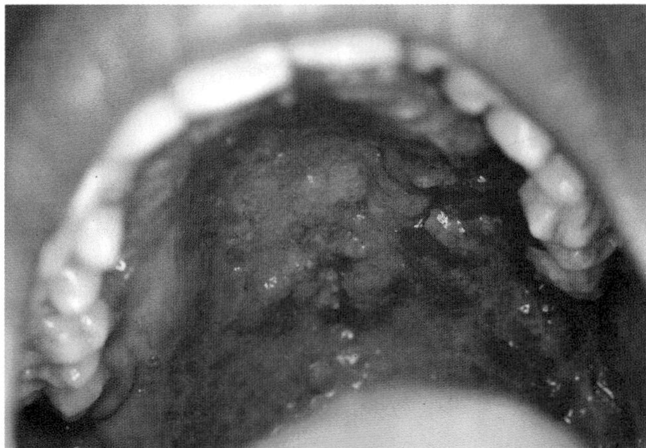

Fig. 7.7.4.8 Palatal lesion.
(Copyright D A Warrell.)

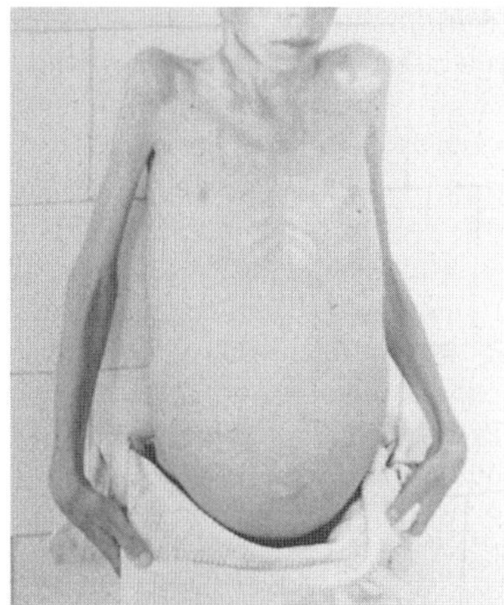

Fig. 7.7.4.9 Ascites, cachexia, and immunodeficiency due to malabsorption and protein-losing enteropathy as sequelae of acute paracoccidioidomycosis.
(Courtesy of M. Shiroma.)

Chronic form

As the lesions usually tend to heal by fibrosis, sequelae such as microstomy and laryngeal, tracheal, or even bronchial stenosis may be observed. Corrective surgery is indicated.

Pulmonary emphysema, fibrosis, respiratory insufficiency, and, finally, cor pulmonale are frequent sequelae. Obstructive and restrictive patterns of ventilatory defect have been found in about 36 and 16% of patients, respectively. As many as 30% of these patients may die as a result of respiratory or cardiorespiratory failure. Adrenal reserve is decreased in 15 to 50% of patients and there is central nervous system dysfunction in about 6 to 25% of patients.

Diagnosis

Microbiological identification

Isolated or budding (single or multiple) mother cells are observed under direct microscopy in sputum, pus from lymph nodes, and material from the skin or mucous membrane lesions.

Specimens are cultured at 37°C on blood, chocolate, or yeast extract agar. The colonies are produced after 7 days, usually in 10 to 20 days. Cultures can be maintained at 25°C on Sabouraud's dextrose agar, where the colonies may be noticed after 15 to 30 days.

Histopathology

Silver or periodic acid–Schiff staining is required to detect the fungus on sputum. Diagnostic features are the variable size (1–30 µm) of the yeast cells, and their multiple budding. Proliferative or exudative reactions, as described in the section on pathology, may be observed.

Immunological tests

Serological reactions

Immunodiffusion (Ouchterlony) and counterimmunoelectrophoresis are the best techniques initially. Sensitivities and specificities are as high as 95%. Cross reactions are mainly with other deep mycoses such as histoplasmosis, aspergillosis, cryptococcosis, and candidiasis.

Complement fixation and indirect immunofluorescence are less reliable tests for diagnosis but they can be employed in patients under treatment.

Recently, enzyme immunoassays employing PbAgs, including a 43 kDa glycoprotein, have shown high sensitivity and specificity. Antibody titres tend to decrease about 3 to 6 months after starting specific therapy and to disappear after 9 months to 5 years or more.

Antigenaemia and antigenuria have been considered useful indications in patients presenting low levels of antibodies in the sera, both for diagnosis and follow-up after treatment, particularly in an immunocompromised host. Circulating gp43 and gp70 antigens were detected in 100% of cerebrospinal fluid and almost all serum samples of patients with neuroparacoccidioidomycosis.

The correlation between immunological and histopathological findings and clinical forms is outlined in Table 7.7.4.1.

Therapy

Clinically active disease is treated for between 6 and 36 months until stabilization or disappearance of antibodies detected by immunodiffusion or counterimmunoelectrophoresis tests. In milder cases, co-trimoxazole (160 mg of trimethoprim and 800 mg of sulphamethoxazole) or imidazoles (itraconazole 100–400 mg/day) have been shown to be effective. In a randomized trial, sulphadiazine (150 mg/kg per day), itraconazole (50–100 mg/day), and ketoconazole (200–400 mg/day) were equally effective in patients with moderately severe disease. Voriconazole has been used in a randomized study in comparison with itraconazole with similar results and, since it achieves high levels in cerebrospinal fluid, it could be useful in neuroparacoccidioidomycosis.

Severe cases of acute or chronic disease should be treated with intravenous infusion of amphotericin B. The daily dose begins at 0.1 to 0.2 mg/kg, increasing up to 1.0 mg/kg. The total dose ranges from 1 to 3 g or more. Toxic reactions to amphotericin B include fever, chills, headache, anaemia, and nephrotoxicity characterized by tubular acidosis and potassium urinary excretion and resultant hypokalaemia and azotaemia. In most cases, these reactions can be controlled until the end of the course of therapy. Liposomal amphotericin has been used in severe cases of paracoccidioidomycosis, but a short period of treatment was followed by relapses.

Prognosis

Even though the disease is easily controlled in the majority of cases, the course of treatment is long and abandonment of treatment is the most important cause of therapeutic failure, e.g. in Brazil. Normalization of cellular specific responses, particularly of the skin test (paracoccidioidin) indicates a good prognosis.

Death may occur in severe acute or chronic cases and severe cases with sequelae.

Further reading

Borges-Walmsley MI, *et al.* (2002). The pathobiology of *Paracoccidioides brasiliensis*. *Trends Microbiol*, **10**, 80–7.

Calich VLG, *et al.* (1985). Susceptibility and resistance of inbred mice to *Paracoccidioides brasiliensis*. *Br J Exp Pathol*, **66**, 585–94.

Felipe MS, *et al.* (2005). Transcriptional profiles of the human pathogenic fungus *Paracoccidioides brasiliensis* in mycelium and yeast cells. *J. Biol Chem*, **280**, 24706–14.

Matute DR, *et al.* (2006). Cryptic speciation and recombination in the fungus *Paracoccidioides brasiliensis* as revealed by gene genealogies. *Mol Biol Evol*, **23**, 65–73.

Oliveira SJ, *et al.* (2002). Cytokines and lymphocyte proliferation in juvenile and adult forms of paracoccidioidomycosis: comparison with infected and non-infected controls. *Microbes Infect*, **4**, 139–44.

Shikanai-Yasuda MA (2005). Pharmacological management of paracoccidioidomycosis. *Expert Opin Pharmacother*, **6**, 385–97. [Critical revision on treatment.]

Teixeira MM, *et al.* (2009). Phylogenetic analysis reveals a high level of speciation in the Paracoccidioides genus. *Mol Phylogenet Evol*, **52**, 273–83.

7.7.5 *Pneumocystis jirovecii*

Robert F. Miller and Laurence Huang

Essentials

The ascomycete fungus *Pneumocystis jirovecii* (previously called *Pneumocystis carinii*) is the cause of pneumocystis pneumonia (PCP) in humans, which occurs largely among people with impaired CD4+ T-lymphocyte function or numbers, e.g those infected with HIV, or organ transplant recipients taking therapeutic immunosuppressive agents. The organism is restricted to humans, and disease is now thought to arise from *de novo* infection by inhalation from an exogenous source.

Clinical features and diagnosis—presentation of PCP is nonspecific, with progressive dyspnoea and nonproductive cough. Examination of the chest is typically normal, but fine bibasal end-inspiratory crackles may be heard. Diagnosis is usually by demonstration of organisms on microscopy (preferably with immunofluorescence staining) of induced sputum or bronchoalveolar lavage fluid.

Treatment and prognosis—aside from supportive care, first-line therapy of PCP is sulphamethoxazole–trimethoprim (co-trimoxazole, which has a high rate of treatment-limiting adverse drug reactions), with adjunctive corticosteroids indicated for those with severe disease. In patients whose disease is failing to respond, or those intolerant of co-trimoxazole, the main alternatives are intravenous pentamidine or clindamycin with primaquine. Among HIV-infected patients, the optimal timing of initiation of antiretroviral therapy after treatment of PCP remains uncertain.

Prevention—primary prophylaxis is recommended for (1) HIV-infected patients—when the CD4 count falls below 200 cells/μl or they have HIV-constitutional features or other AIDS-defining diagnoses; and (2) other at risk groups—e.g. some organ transplant recipients. Secondary prophylaxis is given after an episode of PCP. The first-choice prophylactic agent is co-trimoxazole; alternative options include nebulized pentamidine.

Introduction

What is *Pneumocystis jirovecii*?

Pneumocystis species are ascomycetous fungi which infect a wide variety of mammalian hosts asymptomatically but sometimes cause pneumonia, which is known as pneumocystis pneumonia (PCP). *Pneumocystis jirovecii* (previously called *Pneumocystis carinii*) is the cause of PCP in humans.

Who gets PCP?

Most patients have abnormalities of T-lymphocyte function or numbers but, rarely, PCP develops in patients with isolated B-cell defects and in people without evidence of immunosuppression. In non-HIV-infected people, glucocorticoid administration is an independent risk factor for development of PCP irrespective of the type or intensity of immunosuppression or the nature of the underlying disease process. In HIV-infected people, those at greatest risk of PCP have CD4+ T lymphocyte counts less than 200 cells/μl. In the early years of the AIDS epidemic, PCP was the AIDS-defining diagnosis for almost two-thirds of patients. Since the introduction of highly active antiretroviral therapy (HAART), although there has been a marked decline in incidence of PCP, it remains the most common serious opportunistic infection in HIV-infected people in Europe, the United States of America, and Australasia. Patients living in countries without access to PCP prophylaxis or HAART remain at high risk of PCP.

Aetiology

Pneumocystis cannot be cultured *in vitro*. Pneumocystis organisms from different mammalian host species show antigenic, karyotypic, and genetic heterogeneity. Cross-infection between host species has not been successful, suggesting host specificity and that pneumocystis infection in humans is not a zoonosis. The demonstration of antibodies against pneumocystis in the majority of healthy children and adults has been regarded previously as supportive of the hypothesis that PCP arises in an immunocompromised individual by reactivation of a childhood-acquired latent infection. However, this hypothesis is challenged by the failure to demonstrate pneumocystis in bronchoscopic alveolar lavage (BAL) fluid or necropsy lung tissue of immune competent people and the observation that pneumocystis DNA is detectable only at low levels in less than 25% of HIV-infected people with low CD4+ T-lymphocyte counts presenting with respiratory episodes and with diagnoses other than PCP. Human pneumocystis infection is now thought to arise from *de novo* infection from an exogenous source. Finding different genotypes in each episode in patients with recurrent PCP supports the reinfection model.

Pathogenesis

After inhalation of pneumocystis, the organism reaches the alveoli where the trophic form attaches to type 1 pneumocytes. In an immune competent person, the organism is eliminated; in the immunodeficient, PCP will develop.

The major surface glycoprotein of pneumocystis binds to macrophages and induces T-lymphocyte proliferation and increased secretion of L1 (L1CAM, CD171), L2 and tumour necrosis factor-α. Monocytes respond to major surface glycoproteins by releasing interleukin 8 and tumour necrosis factor α. Pneumocystis induces changes in the quantity and quality of pulmonary surfactant; total cholesterol, glycerol, and phospholipase A2 are increased while phospholipid is reduced.

Clinical presentation

This is nonspecific. Patients typically present with progressive exertional dyspnoea, a nonproductive cough, and fever of several days or weeks duration. They often report an inability to take in a deep breath that is not due to pleural pain. Purulent sputum, haemoptysis, and pleural pain are atypical for PCP and suggest a bacterial or mycobacterial pathogen. In HIV-infected patients, the presentation is usually more indolent than in patients immunosuppressed for other reasons. However, in a small proportion of HIV-infected patients, the disease course of PCP is fulminant with an interval of 7 days or less between onset of symptoms and progression to respiratory failure. Occasionally, PCP may present as pyrexia of undetermined origin.

Examination of the chest is usually normal; occasionally. fine bibasal end-inspiratory crackles are heard. Signs of focal consolidation or pleural effusion suggest an alternative diagnosis.

Pathology

Within the lung, pneumocystis infection is characterized by an eosinophilic, foamy intra-alveolar exudate, associated with a mild plasma-cell interstitial pneumonitis. Morphologically, two forms of pneumocystis may be identified: thick-walled cystic forms (6–7 μm diameter) that lie freely within the alveolar exudate are demonstrated by Grocott's methenamine silver, toluidine blue O, or cresyl violet stains (Fig. 7.7.5.1). The exudate consists largely of thin-walled, irregularly shaped, single-nucleated trophic forms (2–5 μm diameter) that are shown by Giemsa stain but lack distinctive features. Rarely, interstitial fibrosis, diffuse alveolar damage, granulomatous inflammation, nodular and cavitary lesions, and pneumatocele formation may occur. Rarely, pneumocystis infection extends beyond the airspaces; extrapulmonary pneumocystosis involving liver, spleen, gut, or eye may occur and is strongly associated with use of nebulized pentamidine for prophylaxis.

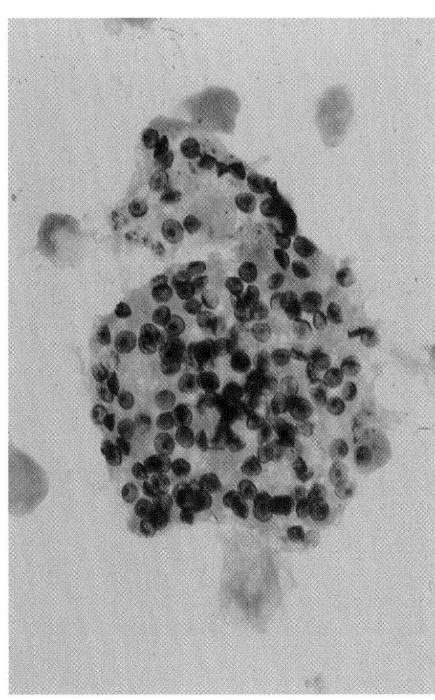

Fig. 7.7.5.1 Cysts of *Pneumocystis jirovecii* in lung tissue. The walls of the cysts are stained black (silver stain).

Investigations

Chest radiograph

The chest radiograph may be normal in early or mild PCP. With more severe disease or later presentation, bilateral perihilar interstitial or reticular infiltrates are seen (Fig. 7.7.5.2). These may progress to diffuse bilateral alveolar (air space) consolidation that mimics pulmonary oedema. In the late stages, the lungs may be massively consolidated and almost airless. Radiographic deterioration from near normal at presentation to being markedly abnormal may occur over 48 h or less. Up to 20% of chest radiographs are atypical, showing intrapulmonary nodules, cavitary lesions, lobar consolidation, pneumatoceles (Fig. 7.7.5.3), or hilar/mediastinal lymphadenopathy. All of these typical and atypical radiographic appearances may also be seen in bacterial, mycobacterial, and fungal infections and in nonspecific pneumonitis and pulmonary Kaposi's sarcoma.

With treatment and clinical recovery, the chest radiograph in some individuals may remain abnormal for many months in the absence of symptoms. In others, postinfectious bronchiectasis or fibrosis occurs.

Arterial blood gases/oximetry

Less than 10% of patients with PCP have a normal $Pa\text{o}_2$ and a normal $P(\text{A–a})\text{o}_2$. These measures are sensitive though not specific for PCP and may also occur in bacterial pneumonia, pulmonary Kaposi's sarcoma, and tuberculosis.

CT

High-resolution CT of the chest may be useful in the symptomatic patient with a normal or equivocal chest radiograph. Areas of 'ground-glass' shadowing indicate active pulmonary disease (Fig. 7.7.5.4). These appearances may be caused by other fungal infection and by cytomegalovirus as well as by PCP.

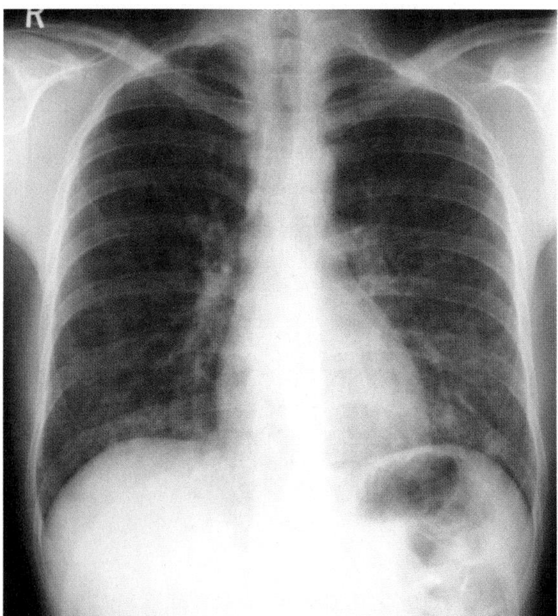

Fig. 7.7.5.2 Chest radiograph showing bilateral interstitial infiltrates typical of pneumocystis pneumonia.

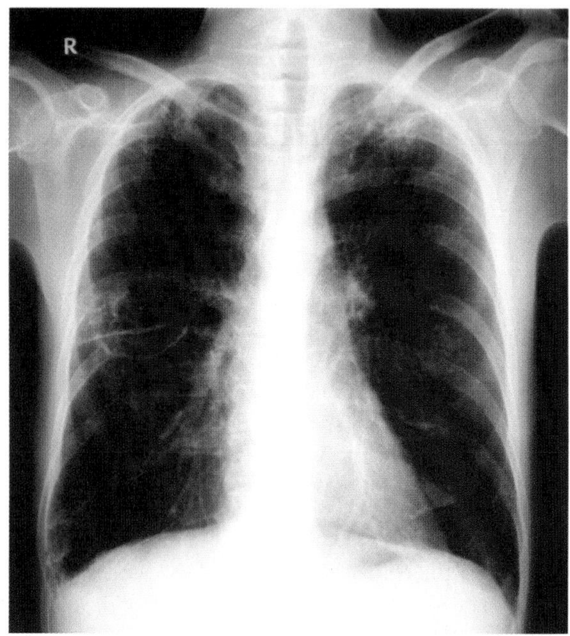

Fig. 7.7.5.3 Chest radiograph showing atypical appearances for pneumocystis pneumonia, including bilateral apical shadowing and a right mid-zone thin-walled pneumatocele.

Induced sputum

Spontaneously expectorated sputum is inadequate for diagnosis of PCP. Sputum induction by inhalation of ultrasonically nebulized hypertonic (2–5 mol/litre) saline may provoke a suitable sample. Pneumocystis is usually found in clear saliva-like samples. Purulent samples suggest an alternative diagnosis. The sensitivity varies between 55 and 90% and a negative result for pneumocystis should prompt further diagnostic tests.

Bronchoscopy

Fibre-optic bronchoscopy with BAL has a sensitivity exceeding 90% for detection of pneumocystis. Immunofluorescence staining

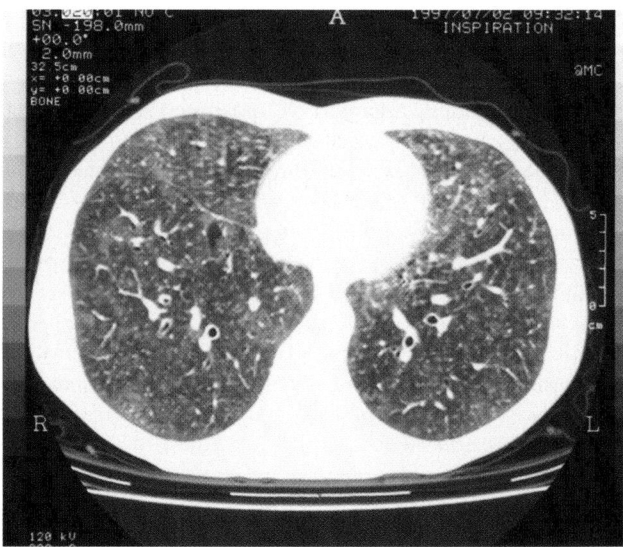

Fig. 7.7.5.4 CT of thorax showing diffuse bilateral 'ground-glass' shadowing typical of pneumocystis pneumonia.

increases the diagnostic yield compared to conventional histochemical staining. Transbronchial biopsies add very little to the diagnostic yield and are associated with a relatively high complication rate (*c.*8%). As pneumocystis persists in the lung for many days (and even weeks) after the start of antimicrobial therapy, bronchoscopy may be performed up to 1 week after commencing antipneumocystis therapy without a reduction in diagnostic yield.

Molecular detection tests

Detection of pneumocystis-specific DNA by the polymerase chain reaction (PCR) on BAL fluid and induced sputum is superior to conventional histochemical methods but specificity is less than 100%. Detection of pneumocystis DNA by PCR may also be achieved on oropharyngeal samples obtained by gargling with 10 ml normal saline. These molecular techniques are not widely available.

Empirical therapy

Many centres in the United Kingdom and North America seek to confirm a diagnosis in every suspected case of PCP. Others treat HIV-infected patients empirically when they present with features typical of PCP: symptoms and signs, chest radiographic abnormalities, and hypoxaemia. Bronchoscopy is reserved for those who fail to respond to empirical therapy by day 5 or who have atypical presentations. Both strategies are equally effective in clinical practice.

Treatment

It is important to stratify PCP as mild (Pao_2 on air >11.0 kPa, Sao_2 >96%), moderate (Pao_2 8.0–11.0 kPa, Sao_2 91–96%), or severe (Pao_2 >8.0 kPa, Sao_2 >91%) as some drugs are unproven or ineffective in severe disease.

First-choice treatment is high-dose co-trimoxazole (sulphamethoxazole 100 mg/kg per day and trimethoprim 20 mg/kg per day, in two to four divided doses orally or intravenously). In HIV-infected patients with PCP, 21 days are recommended; in those with other causes of immunosuppression, from 14 to 21 days are frequently given. In mild disease, oral medication may be given throughout; in moderate or severe disease, intravenous therapy is usually given for the first 7 to 10 days, then orally.

Other treatment in patients with severe disease is clindamycin (450–600 mg three to four times daily orally or intravenously) with primaquine (15–30 mg once daily orally). Despite its toxicity, pentamidine (4 mg/kg per day intravenously) may be used if other treatments have failed. In patients with mild or moderate disease, alternatives to co-trimoxazole include clindamycin with primaquine (doses as above), dapsone (100 mg once daily orally) with trimethoprim (20 mg/kg per day orally), or atovaquone (750 mg twice daily orally). Nebulized pentamidine has no role in treatment of PCP; treatment response is delayed, early relapse is common, and extrapulmonary dissemination of pneumocystosis is not suppressed.

Adjuvant steroids

HIV-infected patients with moderate or severe PCP and Pao_2 less than 9.3 kPa, on air, benefit from adjuvant glucocorticoids, which reduce the need for mechanical ventilation and risk of death. Many non-HIV-infected patients with PCP are already receiving glucocorticoids as part of their regimen of immunosuppression and the benefits of dose increases have not clearly been demonstrated. Adjunctive glucocorticoid regimens include prednisolone (40 mg twice daily orally for 5 days, then 40 mg once daily on days 6 to 10, then 20 mg once daily on days 11 to 21) or methylprednisolone (intravenously at 75% of these doses). An alternative regimen is methylprednisolone (1 g intravenously for 3 days, then 0.5 g intravenously on days 4 and 5) followed by prednisolone (reducing from 80 mg once daily orally to zero over 16 days).

Adverse reactions

Adverse reactions to co-trimoxazole, which usually occur between days 6 and 14 of treatment, are more common in HIV-infected patients than in patients with other causes of immunosuppression. Anaemia and neutropenia (≤40% of patients), rash and fever (≤30% each), and biochemical hepatitis (≤15%) are the most frequent adverse reactions. Coadministration of folic or folinic acid does not attenuate haematological toxicity. Diarrhoea and rash (≤30% each) are the most frequent adverse reactions to clindamycin. Stool should be examined for *Clostridium difficile* in patients developing diarrhoea on clindamycin.

Glucose-6-phosphate dehydrogenase deficiency

Patients with glucose-6-phosphate dehydrogenase deficiency should not receive co-trimoxazole, dapsone, or primaquine.

Prophylaxis

HIV-infected patients are at increased risk of PCP as the CD4+ T lymphocyte count decreases. Primary prophylaxis (to prevent a first episode of pneumocystis pneumonia) is given when the CD4 count falls below 200 cells/µl or the CD4:total lymphocyte ratio is less than 1:5 to patients with HIV-constitutional features (unexplained fever of 3 or more week's duration or oral candida irrespective of CD4 count), and to patients with other AIDS-defining diagnoses, for example Kaposi's sarcoma. Secondary prophylaxis is given after an episode of PCP.

The first-choice agent for primary and secondary prophylaxis is co-trimoxazole (960 mg daily: 800 mg sulphamethoxazole and 160 mg trimethoprim). A lower dose (i.e. 960 mg three times weekly or 480 mg daily) may be equally effective and have fewer side effects. Co-trimoxazole may also protect against bacterial infections and reactivation of cerebral toxoplasmosis. Alternative, less effective options include nebulized pentamidine (300 mg once monthly, or once per fortnight if the CD4 count is 50 µl or less), dapsone (100 mg daily) with pyrimethamine (25 mg once weekly (and folinic acid)), atovaquone (750 mg twice daily), and azithromycin (1.25 g once weekly).

Non-HIV-infected patients with high attack rates of PCP should receive prophylaxis (drug choice and doses as above). At-risk groups include those with acute lymphoblastic leukaemia, severe combined immunodeficiency syndrome, Hodgkin's lymphoma, rhabdomyosarcoma, primary and secondary central nervous system tumours, Wegener's granulomatosis, and organ transplantation including allogenic bone marrow, renal, heart, heart/lung, and liver.

Areas of uncertainty/future research

The mode of transmission of human pneumocystis infection is unclear but recent molecular data suggests that transmission from infected patients to susceptible immunocompromised individuals may occur and that patients with minor immune suppression, including those with moderate to severe chronic obstructive lung disease, and those receiving long-term corticosteroids (prednisolone 20 mg/day or more), irrespective of the cause of underlying immune suppression, may be colonized by pneumocystis, thus acting as a potential infectious reservoir. The drug target for sulphamethoxazole and dapsone is dihydropteroate synthase (DHPS). Mutations in the *DHPS* gene of pneumocystis occur more commonly in individuals who have prior exposure. There is conflicting evidence as to whether *DHPS* mutations are associated with poor outcome (failure to respond to co-trimoxazole or death) from PCP. HIV-infected patients with PCP are recommended to receive HAART but the immune reconstitution inflammatory syndrome (IRIS) has been reported and the optimal timing of instituting this therapy remains unclear.

Further reading

Kaplan JE, *et al.* (2009). Guidelines for prevention and treatment of opportunistic infections in HIV-infected adults and adolescents: recommendations from CDC, the National Institutes of Health, and the HIV Medicine Association of the Infectious Diseases Society of America. *MMWR Recomm Rep*, **58** (RR-4), 1–207. [Evidence-based guidelines for use of prophylaxis against Pneumocystis jirovecii pneumonia.]

Morris A, *et al.* (2004). Current epidemiology of *Pneumocystis* pneumonia. *Emerg Infect Dis*, **10**, 1713–20. [A comprehensive review of the epidemiology of human pneumocystis infection.]

Redhead SA, *et al.* (2006). *Pneumocystis* and *Trypanosoma cruzi*: nomenclature and typifications. *J Eukaryot Microbiol*, **53**, 2–11. [A detailed account of the taxonomy of *Pneumocystis* and the reasons behind the re-naming of infection in humans as *Pneumocystis jirovecii*.]

Thomas CF, Limper AH (2004). *Pneumocystis* pneumonia. *N Engl J Med*, **350**, 2487–98. [A detailed summary of information about human pneumocystis infection.]

Walzer PD, Cushion MT (eds) (2004). *Pneumocystis carinii* pneumonia, 3rd edition. Marcel Dekker, New York. [The definite, fully comprehensive, text on the basic biology, clinical presentation and treatment of pneumocystis infection.]

7.7.6 *Penicillium marneffei* infection

Thira Sirisanthana

Essentials

Penicillium marneffei infection is very rare in the immunocompetent but one of the most common opportunistic infections in HIV-infected people in South-East Asia, north-eastern India, southern China, Hong Kong, and Taiwan. Presentation is usually with fever, chills, lymphadenopathy, hepatomegaly, and splenomegaly, with skin lesions—most commonly papules with central necrotic umbilication—in two-thirds of cases. Diagnosis is made by microscopy of bone marrow aspirate or biopsy specimens. Standard treatment, which is usually effective, is with amphotericin B followed by itraconazole.

Introduction

Penicillium marneffei was first isolated from Chinese bamboo rats *Rhizomys sinensis* in Vietnam in 1956. The fungus is endemic in South-East Asia, north-east India, south China, Hong Kong, and Taiwan. Less than 40 cases of infection with *P. marneffei* were reported before the HIV epidemic. Since then, the incidence of disseminated *P. marneffei* infection has increased markedly. This increase is mainly due to infection in patients immunocompromised by HIV. Most patients have been reported from Thailand, Hong Kong, and Taiwan. Cases have also been reported in HIV-infected individuals from the United States of America, Europe, Japan, and Australia following visits to the endemic region.

Aetiology

P. marneffei is the only dimorphic fungus of the genus *Penicillium*. The fungus grows in a mycelial phase at 25°C on Sabouraud dextrose agar. Mould-to-yeast conversion is achieved by subculturing the fungus on to brain-heart-infusion agar and incubating at 37°C. Microscopic examination of the mycelial form shows typical structures of the genus *Penicillium*; examination of the yeast form reveals unicellular, pleomorphic, ellipsoidal-to-rectangular cells (*c.*2 µm × 6 µm in dimension) that divide by fission and not by budding.

Natural history

Many features of the natural reservoir, mode of transmission, and natural history of *P. marneffei* infection remain unknown. The fungus was isolated from several species of bamboo rats in the endemic area. Since the bamboo rats usually live near the forest and have limited contact with people, it is believed that both humans and bamboo rats are infected with *P. marneffei* from a common source, rather than patients' being infected by rats. By analogy with other endemic systemic mycosis, such as histoplasmosis, it is likely that *P. marneffei* conidia are inhaled from a contaminated reservoir in the environment and subsequently disseminate from the lungs if and when the host becomes immunosuppressed. The disease is significantly more likely to occur in the rainy season, suggesting that there may be an expansion of the environment reservoirs with favourable conditions for growth during these rainy months.

In endemic areas, it is likely that a certain proportion of the population is infected, but remains asymptomatic. Patients have been reported with long periods of asymptomatic infection before presentation with clinical *P. marneffei* infection. In other cases, the clinical manifestation of *P. marneffei* infection occurred within weeks of exposure to the fungus.

Clinical features

The majority of patients with *P. marneffei* infection have already been infected with HIV. Commonly, they present with symptoms and signs of infection of the reticuloendothelial system. These include fever, chills, lymphadenopathy, hepatomegaly, and splenomegaly. Cough, dyspnoea, and lung crepitations may be present. Other manifestations are secondary to dissemination of the fungus via the bloodstream. Cutaneous and subcutaneous lesions are observed in up to two-thirds of the patients. As in other

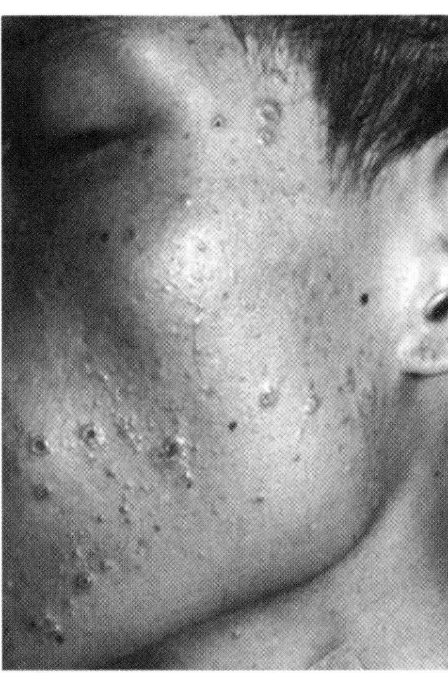

Fig. 7.7.6.1 *P. marneffei* in an HIV-infected Thai patient: typical molluscum-like lesions.
(Copyright G Watt, Bangkok, Thailand.)

systemic mycoses such as histoplasmosis or paracoccidioidomycosis, skin lesions resemble molluscum contagiosum (Fig. 7.7.6.1). They may break down and bleed (Fig. 7.7.6.2) while some larger lesions become indurated and appear infarcted. Mucosal and palatal lesions are also seen (Fig. 7.7.6.3). Arthritis and osteomyelitis are not uncommon. Cases with mesenteric lymphangitis, colitis, genital or oropharyngeal ulcer, retropharyngeal abscess, or pericarditis have been reported.

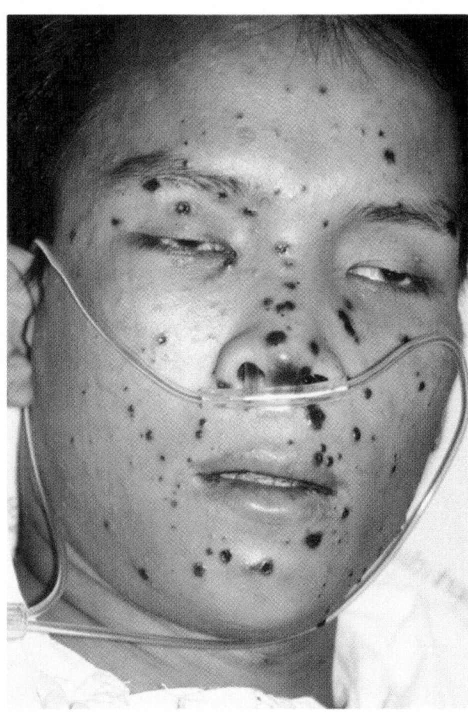

Fig. 7.7.6.2 Bleeding into *P. marneffei* skin lesions.
(Copyright D Walsh.)

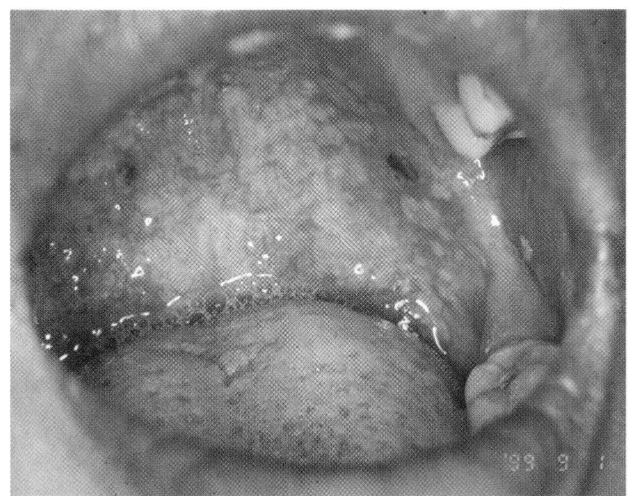

Fig. 7.7.6.3 *P. marneffei* palatal lesions.
(Copyright D Walsh.)

In HIV-infected patients, *P. marneffei* infection occurs late in the course of the disease. The patient's CD4+ cell count at presentation is usually below 50 cells/µl. HIV-infected patients with *P. marneffei* infection have a more acute onset and higher fever. They are more likely to have fungaemia and their skin lesions are more numerous and tend to be papules with central necrotic umbilication. Non-HIV-infected patients are more likely to have one or several subcutaneous nodules, which may develop into abscesses and cause skin ulceration.

Biochemical and haematological laboratory findings are nonspecific and include elevation of liver enzymes, anaemia, and leukocytosis. The chest radiograph may show diffuse interstitial, localized alveolar or diffuse alveolar infiltrates. Cases with chest radiographs showing cavitary lesions or lung masses have been reported (Fig. 7.7.6.4).

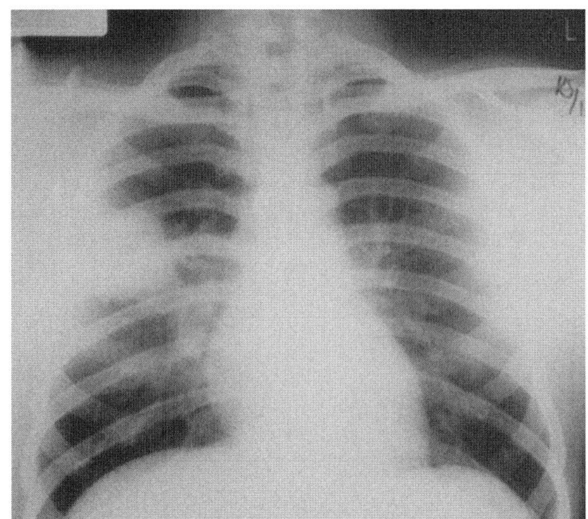

Fig. 7.7.6.4 Pulmonary lesion in an HIV-infected patient from Hong Kong.
(Copyright D A Warrell.)

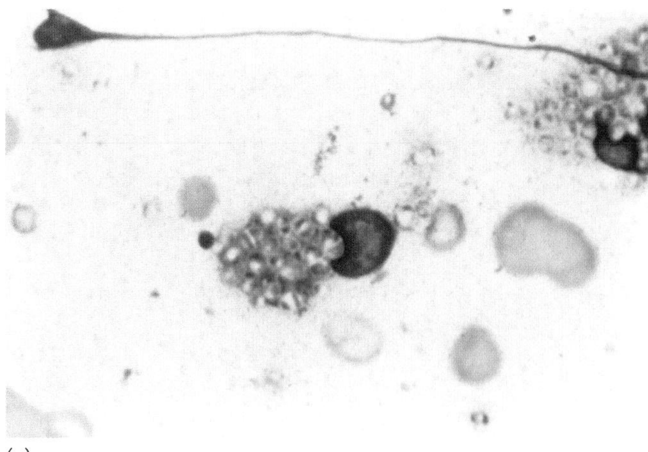

(a)

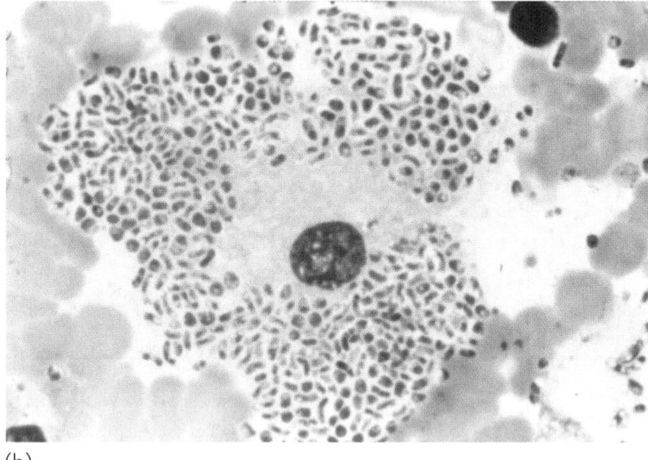

(b)

Fig. 7.7.6.5 Microscopic appearance of *P. marneffei* yeasts in (a) skin biopsy and (b) bone marrow biopsies, showing characteristic septation.
(Copyright Thira Sirisanthana.)

Diagnosis

Diagnosis depends on familiarity with the clinical syndrome and a high index of suspicion. Presumptive diagnosis can be made by microscopic examination of Wright-stained samples of bone-marrow aspirate, touch smears of the skin-biopsy specimen, and/or the lymph-node biopsy specimen. Many intracellular and extracellular basophilic, spherical, oval, and elliptical yeast cells can be seen with this technique, some of which have clear central septation, a characteristic feature of *P. marneffei* (Fig. 7.7.6.5). The diagnosis is confirmed by histopathological sections and/or by culturing the fungus from the blood, skin biopsy specimens, bone marrow, or lymph nodes. Cases of *P. marneffei* infection can clinically resemble tuberculosis, histoplasmosis, and cryptococcosis. Tests to detect the antibody or antigen of *P. marneffei* as well as tests based on the polymerase chain reaction (PCR) have been developed. Clinical trials are needed to show their usefulness in the diagnosis of active *P. marneffei* infection and in predicting relapses. They may also be used to identify HIV-infected individuals, who are infected with *P. marneffei* but are still asymptomatic. These individuals may then benefit from pre-emptive treatment with an antifungal agent.

Treatment

P. marneffei infection is a potentially fatal disease. The mortality rate is high if the diagnosis has not been made promptly. The fungus is sensitive to ketoconazole, fluconazole, itraconazole, and amphotericin B. The recommended treatment is to give amphotericin B intravenously in the dose of 0.6 mg/kg per day for 2 weeks, followed by itraconazole 400 mg/day orally in two divided doses for the next 10 weeks. Patients with less severe symptoms may be treated with itraconazole in the same dosage for 12 weeks without the initial treatment with amphotericin B. The majority of patients respond well, with resolution of fever and other signs of infection within the first 2 weeks. After initial treatment, HIV-infected patients should be given 200 mg/day of itraconazole orally as secondary prophylaxis for life in countries where antiretroviral treatment is not available. In patients who are treated with highly active antiretroviral drugs, secondary prophylaxis with itraconazole can be stopped after their $CD4^+$ cell counts reach 100 cells/μl and remain at or above that level for at least 6 months.

Further reading

Chaiwarith R, *et al.* (2007). Discontinuation of secondary prophylaxis against penicilliosis marneffei in AIDS patients after HAART. *AIDS*, **21**, 365–7. [When can secondary prophylaxis be stopped?]

Deng Z, *et al.* (1988). Infection caused by *Penicillium marneffei* in China and Southeast Asia: review of eighteen published cases and report of four more Chinese cases. *RevInfect Dis*, **10**, 640–52. [A review of *Penicillium marneffei* infection in patients not infected with the human immunodeficiency virus.]

Sirisanthana T, Supparatpinyo K (1998). Epidemiology and management of penicilliosis in human immunodeficiency virus-infected patients. *Int J InfectDis*, **3**, 48–53. [A review of the epidemiology and management of penicilliosis.]

Supparatpinyo K, *et al.* (1994). Disseminated *Penicillium marneffei* infection in Southeast Asia. *Lancet*, **344**, 110–13. [A report of the clinical findings in patients with disseminated *Penicillium marneffei* infection.]

Supparatpinyo K, *et al.* (1998). A controlled trial of itraconazole to prevent relapse of *Penicillium marneffei* infection in patients infected with the human immunodeficiency virus. *N Engl J Med*, **339**, 1739–43. [A report on the means to prevent relapse of *Penicillium marneffei* infection.]

7.8

Protozoa

Contents

7.8.1 Amoebic infections *1035*
Richard Knight

7.8.2 Malaria *1045*
David A. Warrell, Janet Hemingway, Kevin Marsh, Robert E. Sinden, Geoffrey A. Butcher, and Robert W. Snow

7.8.3 Babesiosis *1089*
Philippe Brasseur

7.8.4 Toxoplasmosis *1090*
Oliver Liesenfeld and Eskild Petersen

7.8.5 *Cryptosporidium* and cryptosporidiosis *1098*
S.M. Cacciò

7.8.6 *Cyclospora* and cyclosporiasis *1105*
R. Lainson

7.8.7 Sarcocystosis (sarcosporidiosis) *1109*
John E. Cooper

7.8.8 Giardiasis, balantidiasis, isosporiasis, and microsporidiosis *1111*
Martin F. Heyworth

7.8.9 *Blastocystis hominis* infection *1118*
Richard Knight

7.8.10 Human African trypanosomiasis *1119*
August Stich

7.8.11 Chagas disease *1127*
M.A. Miles

7.8.12 Leishmaniasis *1134*
A.D.M. Bryceson and Diana N.J. Lockwood

7.8.13 Trichomoniasis *1142*
Sharon Hillier

7.8.1 Amoebic infections

Richard Knight

Essentials

Two very different groups of amoebic species infect humans. (1) Obligate anaerobic gut parasites—including the major pathogen *Entamoeba histolytica*, *Dientamoeba fragilis* (which causes relatively mild colonic involvement with diarrhoea), and eight non-pathogenic species including *Entamoeba dispar*. (2) Aerobic free-living, water and soil amoebae—these can become facultative tissue parasites in humans after cysts or trophozoites are inhaled, ingested, or enter damaged skin or mucosae.

Entamoeba histolytica *infection*

The term amoebiasis (when unqualified) generally refers to *E. histolytica* infection, which is common in Mexico, South America, Natal, the west coast of Africa, and South-East Asia; nearly all amoebic disease seen in temperate countries is acquired elsewhere. Transmission is by the faecal–oral route; following ingestion of infective cysts, a population of trophozoites becomes established in the caecum and proximal colon.

Clinical features—clinical features range from minimal changes in bowel habit to severe dysentery. Onset is usually gradual or intermittent, with initially mild constitutional upset, colicky abdominal pain, and foul-smelling stools that always contain visible or occult blood. Less typical presentations of amoebic colitis include (1) fulminant; (2) amoebic colitis without dysentery; (3) amoeboma—presenting as an abdominal mass, most frequently in the right iliac fossa; (4) localized perforation and amoebic appendicitis; (5) rectal bleeding. The most significant complication is hepatic amoebiasis.

Diagnosis, treatment, and prognosis—examination of dysenteric stool, bowel-wall scrapings, liver abscess aspirate, or other samples in temporary wet mounts is critical, with identification of live erythrocytophagous trophozoites confirming the diagnosis of invasive amoebic disease. Other diagnostic methods include (1) demonstration of amoebal DNA in faeces/tissues by PCR; (2) serology—but seropositivity does not distinguish current and past tissue invasion. Aside from supportive care, metronidazole for 5 days is usually the first-choice treatment, with the addition of diloxanide to eliminate infection from the bowel and so prevent recurrence of tissue invasion or transmission to others. Uncomplicated invasive intestinal disease (and uncomplicated hepatic amoebiasis) should have mortality less than 1%, but this may reach 40% for amoebic peritonitis with multiple gut perforation.

Hepatic amoebiasis—less than 50% of patients give any convincing history of dysentery and few have concurrent dysentery. Presentation is typically with fever, sweating, liver or diaphragmatic pain, weight loss, and tender hepatomegaly. Diagnosis is usually achieved by demonstration of a (most often solitary) liver abscess on ultrasonography or CT and positive serological testing, with a therapeutic amoebicide trial generally being preferable to diagnostic needling of the liver.

Prevention—simple hygienic measures and health education provide considerable protection: boiling water for 5 min kills cysts. Travellers to endemic areas may need a medical check on their return; but chemoprophylaxis is not appropriate.

Free-living amoebae

Three genera of free-living amoebae cause human disease: (1) *Naegleria*—causes a primary meningoencephalitis after bathing or diving in fresh water; Amphotericin B an effective drug, but most cases are fatal, partly because of diagnostic delays. (2) *Acanthamoeba*—causes a painful keratitis, mainly in contact lens users, which usually responds to intensive local amoebicides, although corneal grafting may be needed. (3) *Acanthamoeba* and *Balamuthia*—can cause granulomatous encephalitis in both immunocompromised and immunocompetent people; presentation is with headache and meningism or with evidence of a focal brain lesion; survival is rare.

Introduction

The amoebic species infecting humans belong to two very different groups. The obligate anaerobic gut parasites include the major pathogen *Entamoeba histolytica*, which ranks second to malaria as the most dangerous parasite in humans; *Dientamoeba fragilis*, a minor pathogen; and eight nonpathogenic species including the common and important *Entamoeba dispar*. The second group includes certain aerobic free-living, water and soil amoebae which produce cytopathic changes in cultured cell monolayers and cerebral invasion after intranasal inoculation into mice. They can become facultative tissue parasites in humans after or cysts or trophozoites are inhaled, ingested, or enter damaged shin or mucosae.

All motile feeding amoebae are called 'trophozoites'; they move with pseudopodia and divide by binary fission. The hyaline external cytoplasm, the 'ectoplasm', is a contractile gel that surrounds the sol endoplasm containing numerous phagocytic and pinocytic vacuoles. Noninvasive trophozoites feed on bacteria. Most species can form environmentally resistant transmissive cysts by rounding up and secreting a chitinous cyst wall.

The definitive taxonomic separation of *E. dispar* as a nonpathogenic species separate from *E. histolytica* was made in 1993. This was based upon genomic and biochemical differences. This distinction is of fundamental importance because their cysts and noninvasive trophozoites are morphologically indistinguishable, but they are now separated by specific antigen and PCR assays. All strains of *E. histolytica* are now regarded as pathogenic, whereas the commoner *E. dispar* is never pathogenic.

Entamoeba histolytica infection

Biology and pathogenicity

Following ingestion of infective cysts, a population of trophozoites becomes established in the caecum and proximal colon. Some degree of tissue invasion occurs in all subjects with at least low-titre seroconversion. Tissue invasion is frequently mild, self-limiting, and with minimal symptoms, but at the other end of the clinical spectrum it can lead to extensive destruction of the colonic mucosa. Parasite genotype may partly determine clinical outcome. Invasive trophozoites have a characteristic morphology; they may reach 30 to 40 μm in diameter and are very active with apparently purposeful, unidirectional movements during which they become considerably elongated. Their most important diagnostic characteristic is the presence of host erythrocytes within the endoplasm, which otherwise appears clear and contains no bacteria. Trophozoites containing red blood cells are described as erythrocytophagous. Progression through tissues is by active movement, facilitated by secreted collagenase; leucocytes are drawn chemotactically towards the amoebae but most are rapidly destroyed on contact.

The transmissive cystic form of the parasite is derived entirely from a commensal population within the colonic lumen. Live commensal amoebae measure from 10 to 20 μm in diameter, the endoplasm is granular and contains bacteria, and the pseudopodia are blunt and movement is sluggish. Intestinal hurry from any cause, including the use of laxatives, can lead to the appearance of commensal trophozoites in the faeces. Cysts are spherical and measure from 11 to 14 μm in diameter; when mature, they contain four nuclei, several chromatoid bodies that are ribosome aggregates, and a glycogen vacuole.

Host factors may increase susceptibility to overt disease. Steroid therapy given systemically or locally into the rectum carries great risk, as may cytotoxic therapy. Severe amoebic bowel disease is particularly common in late pregnancy and the puerperium. Before puberty, both sexes are equally susceptible to hepatic amoebiasis, but in adults this condition is much more common in males. Local disease can also favour tissue invasion; thus amoebic ulceration may be superimposed upon colonic and rectal cancers, or those of the uterine cervix. Colonic disease is favoured by concurrent *Trichuris* infection or intestinal schistosomiasis. Infection with HIV appears to have little effect on colonic disease but may facilitate liver involvement.

Epidemiology

The incidence of disease is particularly high in Mexico, South America, Natal, the west coast of Africa, and South-East Asia. In most temperate countries, *E. histolytica* is now rare and nearly all amoebic disease seen in such countries will have been acquired elsewhere. Symptomless or convalescent carriers are the main source of infection; patients with dysentery normally pass only trophozoites in their stool and are therefore noninfectious. Cysts remain viable in the environment for up to 2 months. The infection is eventually self-limiting and rarely exceeds 4 years.

Tissue invasion can occur at any time during an infection but is much more common during the first 4 months; the incubation period may be as short as 7 days. *E.histolytica*-associated diarrhoea can retard growth in preschool children.

The incidence of amoebiasis in a population is best estimated from seropositivity surveys. Surveys for cysts are of no value as their differentiation from *E. dispar* is impossible. All modes of faeco-oral transmission occur in amoebiasis. Of special importance are the food handler and contaminated vegetables; transmission by flies and drinking-water is less common. Drinking-water can be contaminated in the home or at surface-water sources. Direct spread can produce outbreaks; it occurs within institutions for children and people with learning difficulties and with contaminated colonic irrigation equipment. Household clustering is common; hand-fed infants are frequently infected from the fingers of their mother. Contamination of piped water supplies can lead to serious disease outbreaks, as happened in the Chicago hotels epidemic in 1933. Interruption of piped water supplies probably caused the recent outbreak in Georgia. *Entamoeba* infections are common among male homosexuals, but most are due to *E. dispar*.

Pathology

The basic lesion is cell lysis and tissue necrosis, which, by creating locally anoxic and acidic conditions, favours further penetration of the parasite; most amoebae are seen at the advancing edge of the lesion with little inflammatory cell response. In tissue sections, amoebae stain indistinctly with haematoxylin and eosin but appear bright red with periodic acid–Schiff stain; iron haematoxylin is necessary to show nuclear detail. Cysts of *E. histolytica* are never seen in tissue.

Amoebic lesions of the gut are most common in the rectosigmoid and caecum but can occur anywhere in the large bowel; involvement may be patchy or continuous. Less commonly, the appendix or terminal ileum are affected. The initial lesions are either small, discrete erosions of the mucosa or minute crypt lesions (Fig. 7.8.1.1). Unrestrained, the lesions extend through the mucosa, across the muscularis mucosa and into the submucosa, where they expand laterally to produce lesions that are typically flask shaped in cross-section (Fig. 7.8.1.2). Further lateral spread of the submucosal lesions leads to their coalescence and, later, to denudation of overlying mucosa. The bowel wall may become appreciably thickened. Blood vessels involved in the disease may thrombose,

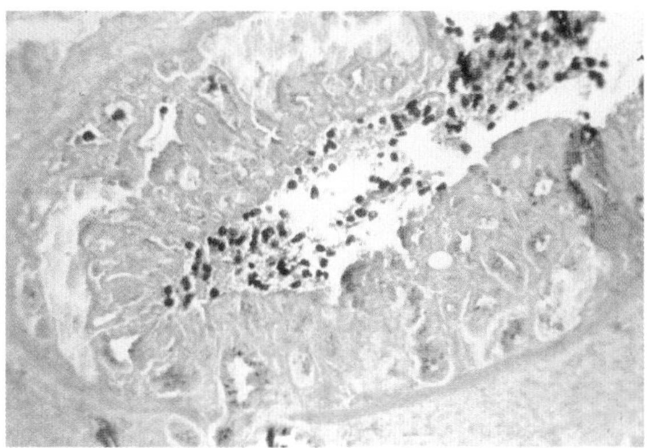

Fig. 7.8.1.1 Amoebic colitis. Crypt abscess. Periodic acid–Schiff stains amoebae red.
(Copyright Viqar Zaman.)

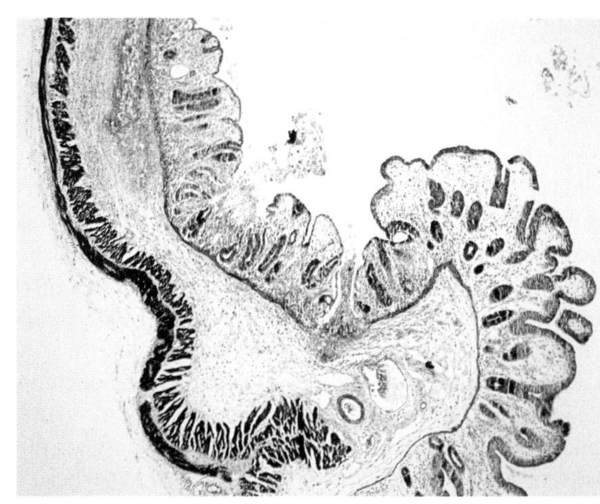

Fig. 7.8.1.2 Amoebic colitis. Superficial ulcer breaching the muscularis mucosae. (Copyright Viqar Zaman.)

bleed into the gut lumen, or, in the case of portal-vein radicles, enable dissemination of amoebae to the liver. In very severe lesions, and usually in association with toxic megacolon, there is an irreversible coagulative necrosis of the bowel wall.

Amoebomas are tumour-like lesions of the colonic wall measuring up to several centimetres in length; they are most common in the caecum and may be multiple. Histologically there is tissue oedema, with a mixed picture of healing and new areas of epithelial loss and tissue destruction; round-cell infiltration is patchy. Lesions may be annular and rarely an amoeboma initiates an intussusception; narrow, stricture-like amoebomas may occur in the anorectal region.

Amoebae reach the liver in the portal vein. Once initiated, the amoebic lesion extends progressively in all directions to produce the liver-cell necrosis and liquefaction that constitute an amoebic liver abscess. The lesions are well demarcated from surrounding liver tissue; untreated nearly all will eventually extend into adjacent structures. Secondary bacterial infection is rare and usually follows rupture or aspiration.

Clinical manifestations

Invasive intestinal amoebiasis

The clinical features show a wide spectrum from minimal changes in bowel habit to severe dysentery. Lesions may be limited to a small part of the large bowel or extend throughout its length. A relapsing course is common.

Amoebic colitis with dysentery

Dysentery, the passage of loose or diarrhoeal stools containing fresh blood, occurs when there is generalized colonic ulceration or when more localized lesions occur in the rectum or rectosigmoid. Onset may be gradual, intermittent, or, much less commonly, acute. Typically, constitutional upset is initially mild and the patient remains ambulant; mild or moderate abdominal pain is common, often colicky and maximal over affected parts of the gut. Tenesmus can occur but is rarely severe. Stools vary in consistency from semiformed to watery. They are foul smelling and always contain visible or occult blood; even when they are watery, faecal matter is nearly always present. Symptoms frequently wax and wane over a period of weeks or even months and such patients can become debilitated and wasted. In a few patients the disease runs a fulminating course. The most frequent physical sign is abdominal tenderness in one or both iliac fossae, but tenderness may be generalized. The affected gut may be palpably thickened. A low fever is common, but dehydration is uncommon. Abdominal distension occurs in the more severely ill patients, who sometimes pass relatively small amounts of stool.

A careful proctoscopy or sigmoidoscopy should be done. The endoscopic appearances may be nonspecific in early, acute, or very severe colitis; the findings are hyperaemia, contact bleeding, or confluent ulceration. In more chronic cases, the presence of normal-looking intervening mucosa is highly suggestive of amoebiasis. Early lesions are often elevated, with a pouting opening only 1 to 2 mm in diameter; later, ulcers may reach 1 cm or more in diameter, with an irregular outline and often a loosely adherent, yellowish or grey exudate. Mucosal scrapings or superficial biopsies taken at endoscopy should be examined immediately by wet-preparation microscopy.

Special forms of amoebic colitis

Fulminant colitis This may arise *de novo*, e.g. in pregnant women or during steroid therapy, or it may evolve during a dysenteric illness. Patients show progressive abdominal distension, vomiting, and watery diarrhoea. Bowel sounds are absent and there may be little or no abdominal tenderness, guarding, or rigidity. Plain radiographs may reveal free peritoneal gas, together with acute gaseous dilatation of the colon; affected segments of bowel may appear relatively narrow and show visible mucosal pathology. Barium enema and full sigmoidoscopy are contraindicated. Stools contain erythrocytophagous trophozoites.

Amoebic colitis without dysentery When ulceration is limited to the caecum or ascending colon, or when early, mild, or localized lesions occur elsewhere in the colon, there may be no dysenteric symptoms. Patients complain of change in bowel habit, blood-staining of the stool, flatulence, and colicky pain. Often the only physical sign is tenderness in the right iliac fossa or elsewhere along the course of the colon. Some patients eventually go into complete remission; others progress to a dysenteric illness.

The most important diagnostic measure is repeated stool examination for erythrocytophagous amoebae; the finding of cysts or commensal trophozoites is of little diagnostic value, especially in endemic areas. Sigmoidoscopy is often normal when the distal bowel is not involved but colonoscopy may reveal typical lesions.

Amoeboma This presents as an abdominal mass, most frequently in the right iliac fossa. The lesion may be painful, tender, and associated with fever. Bowel habit is altered and some patients have intermittent dysentery, especially if lesions are multiple or distal. Evidence of partial or intermittent bowel obstruction may be present, particularly when lesions are distal and annular.

Localized perforation and amoebic appendicitis Sudden perforation with peritonitis can occur from any deep amoebic ulcer; alternatively, leakage may lead to a pericolic abscess or retroperitoneal cellulitis. Amoebic appendicitis is an uncommon but important condition that occurs when amoebic lesions are confined to the appendix and caecum. The clinical presentation can resemble that of simple appendicitis, often with some clinical evidence of dysentery. If it is unrecognized at appendicectomy the outcome can be disastrous, with gut perforation; fresh smears should be made from the resected appendix and examined immediately.

Rectal bleeding Some patients with amoebiasis present with rectal bleeding, with or without tenesmus; this occurs particularly in children. Massive bleeding into the gut lumen can occur in any form of amoebic colitis but is rare.

Differential diagnosis

Amoebic colitis must be differentiated from other causes of infective colitis. High-volume diarrhoea, copious mucus, and severe tenesmus are all uncommon in amoebiasis. In temperate countries, nonspecific ulcerative colitis, *Clostridium difficile* colitis, and colorectal carcinoma create the greatest diagnostic problems. Parasitic conditions to be considered are intestinal schistosomiasis, heavy *Trichuris* infection, and balantidiasis. More chronic amoebic pathology may clinically resemble Crohn's disease, ileocaecal tuberculosis, diverticulitis, or anorectal lymphogranuloma venereum.

Hepatic amoebiasis

Less than half of all patients give any convincing history of dysentery and few have concurrent dysentery. In those with no dysenteric history, the interval between presumed infection and presentation may be as short as 3 weeks or as long as 15 years; for most, it is between 8 weeks and 1 year.

The dominant symptoms are fever and sweating, liver or diaphragmatic pain, and weight loss. Onset of constitutional symptoms is often insidious, but pain may begin abruptly. Most patients seek medical help between 1 and 4 weeks. Fever is typically remittent, with a prominent evening rise, brief rigors, and very profuse sweating. Liver pain may be poorly localized initially and later become pleuritic, referred to the right shoulder tip or localized to the abdominal wall. Within a few weeks, patients lose much weight and often become anaemic; a painful dry cough is common.

The most important clinical finding is liver enlargement (Fig. 7.8.1.3) with localized tenderness, which should be searched for in the right hypochondrium, the epigastrium, and along all the intercostal spaces overlying the liver. Liver pain, on compression or heavy digital percussion, is a less useful sign. Left-lobe lesions can present as an epigastric mass. Hepatomegaly may be difficult to detect by abdominal palpation when enlargement is mainly upwards, but bulging of the right chest wall may be noted, together with a raised upper level of liver dullness on percussion. Reduced breath sounds or crepitations may be heard at the right lung base.

Important radiological findings are a raised or locally upward-bulging right diaphragm (Fig. 7.8.1.4) with immobility on screening, areas of lung collapse or consolidation, and sometimes a pleural effusion. A neutrophil leukocytosis is almost invariable, the ESR is raised, and normochromic normocytic anaemia is common. Liver function tests are frequently completely normal or there may be a raised alkaline phosphatase; less commonly the serum transaminase or bilirubin is elevated. Liver scanning to demonstrate a filling defect is of great value; about 70% of lesions are solitary, but multiple lesions are common in children and those with concurrent dysentery. Ultrasonographic and CT scans are the most useful. Lesions appear round or oval and are usually between 4 and 10 cm in diameter at the time of presentation. On ultrasonography most are hypoechoic with well-defined walls without enhanced echoes. Even when concurrent dysentery is absent, the stools are frequently, but not always, positive for *E. histolytica*. Colonoscopy may reveal unsuspected lesions.

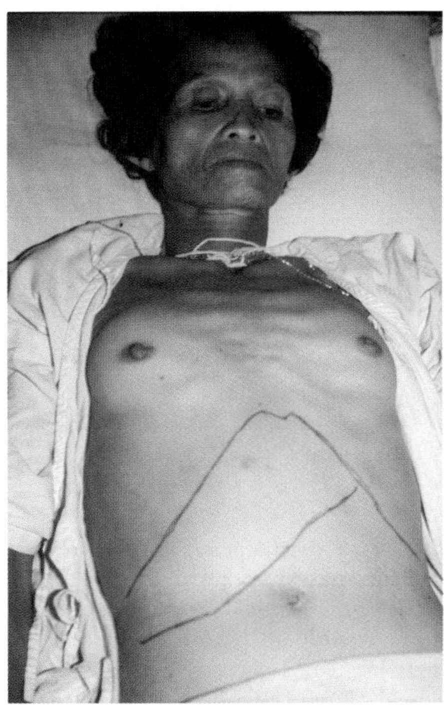

Fig. 7.8.1.3 Amoebic liver abscess. Hepatic enlargement with focal tenderness in a Thai woman.
(Courtesy of the late Professor Sornchai Looareesuwan.)

Complication

Most complications involve extension of hepatic lesions into adjacent structures: usually the right chest, the peritoneum, and the pericardium. Upward extension usually produces adhesions between the liver, the diaphragm, and the lung; in consequence, subphrenic rupture and amoebic empyema are rare, although a right serous pleural effusion is not uncommon. Untreated, the disease process advances upwards through lung tissue leading to hepatobronchial fistula and expectoration of brownish, necrotic liver tissue, the so-called 'anchovy sauce' sputum. Rupture into the peritoneum can occur at any time; it is sometimes the mode of presentation of an amoebic liver abscess, the cause of peritonitis being discovered only at laparotomy. Amoebic pericarditis usually results from upward extension of a left-lobe liver lesion. Initially patients have retrosternal pain and a pericardial friction rub; later rupture or large serous effusion produces cardiac tamponade. The diagnosis is most difficult when an underlying liver abscess was not suspected.

Less commonly the lesion extends through the skin, producing a sinus and cutaneous lesion. The gut, stomach, vena cava, spleen, and kidney are occasionally involved by direct spread. Blood-borne spread to the lung produces a lesion resembling an isolated pyogenic lung abscess. Amoebic brain abscesses due to *E. histolytica* are rare; most are discovered postmortem (Fig. 7.8.1.5). Jaundice occurs when a large lesion compresses the common bile duct or when multiple lesions compress several intrahepatic bile ducts. Rupture into a major bile duct can cause haemobilia. Portal-vein compression occasionally produces portal hypertension and congestive splenomegaly.

Differential diagnosis

Amoebic serology and scanning have now greatly simplified diagnosis. However, a few patients, generally less than 5%, are initially seronegative; scanning patterns may be atypical before lesions have liquefied. Pyogenic abscess, especially when cryptogenic, may be clinically indistinguishable and this condition is quite common in some Asian countries. Other conditions to be distinguished are primary and secondary carcinoma of the liver, lesions of the right lung base and right pleura, subphrenic abscess, cholecystitis, septic cholangitis including that resulting from aberrant *Ascaris* worms, and liver hydatid cysts.

Needle aspiration of the liver (Fig. 7.8.1.6) may be necessary for diagnostic or therapeutic purposes (see below). Suspected pyogenic abscess is the main indication for the former; blood cultures should also be taken. Typically the aspirate in hepatic amoebiasis is pinkish-brown, odourless, and bacteriologically sterile (Fig. 7.8.1.7); a thinner, malodorous, or frothy aspirate suggests bacterial infection. A therapeutic amoebicide trial is generally preferable to diagnostic needling of the liver.

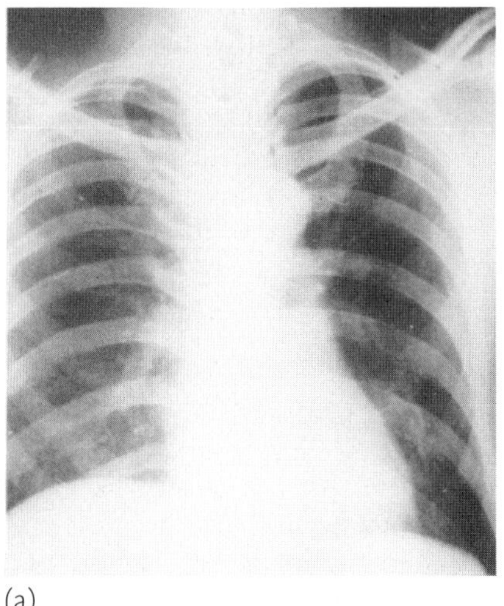

(a)

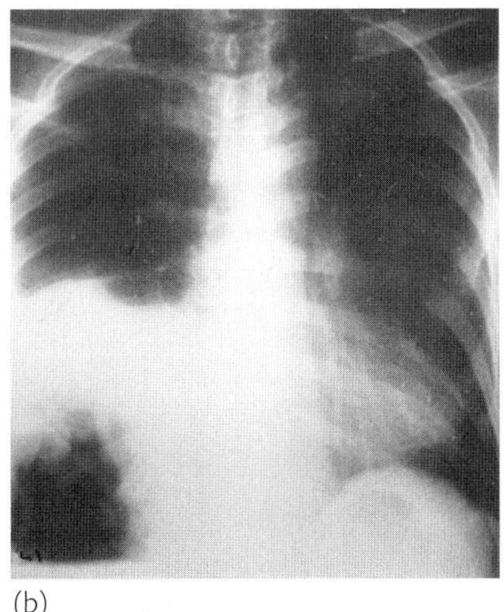

(b)

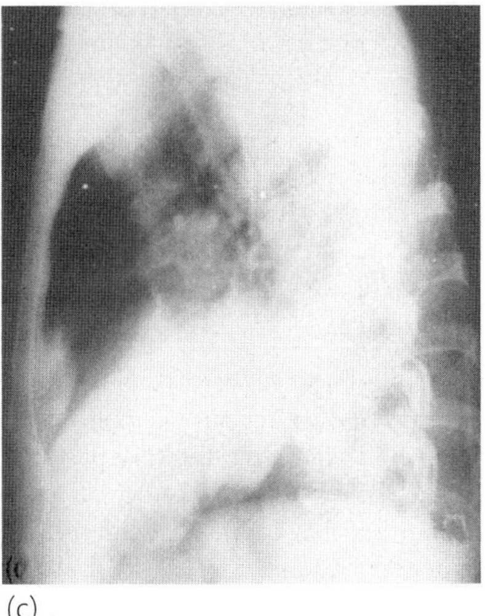

(c)

Fig. 7.8.1.4 Amoebic liver abscess. Radiographic changes showing (a) elevated right diaphragm; (b) enormous abscess in the right lobe of the liver outlined with air (fluid level) and contrast medium introduced during the aspiration of more than 1 litre of pus; and (c) same patient as (b), lateral view.
(Courtesy of the late Professor Sornchai Looareesuwan.)

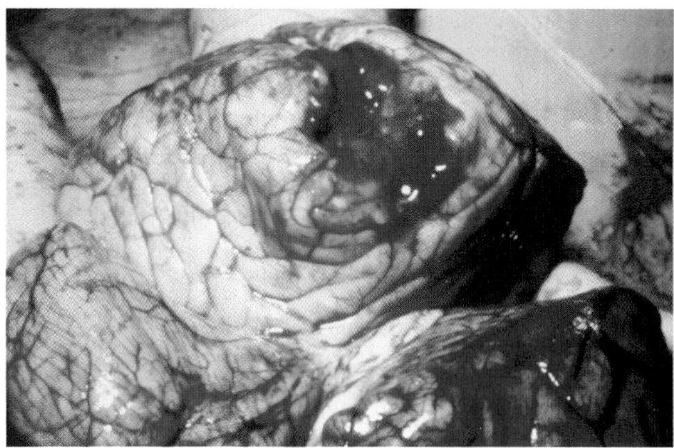

Fig. 7.8.1.5 Metastatic brain abscess in a patient with an amoebic liver abscess. (Courtesy of the late Professor Sornchai Looareesuwan.)

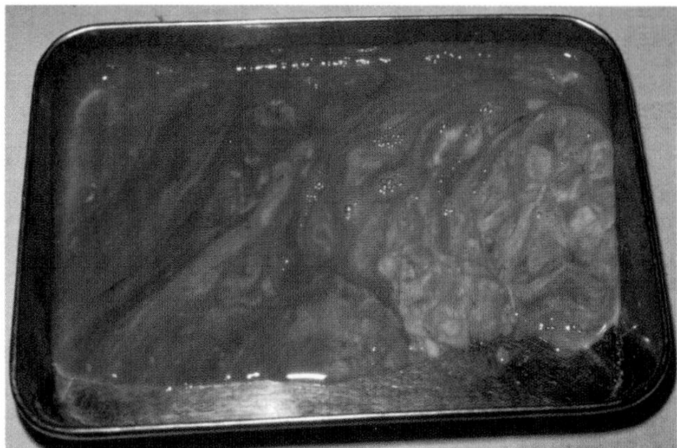

Fig. 7.8.1.7 'Anchovy sauce' pus drained from and amoebic liver abscess. (Copyright Viqar Zaman.)

Cutaneous and genital amoebiasis

Skin ulceration due to *E. histolytica* produces deep, painful, and foul-smelling lesions that spread rapidly. Secondary bacterial infection is common and may mask the amoebic pathology. Lesions are most frequent in the perianal area, but also occur at colostomy stomas, laparotomy scars, and at the site of skin rupture by a hepatic lesion.

Female genital involvement results from faecal contamination, the extension of perianal lesions, or by the formation of internal fistulae from the gut, which can involve the bladder. Lesions of the vulva and uterine cervix may resemble carcinoma. Male genital lesions follow rectal coitus, the lesion beginning as a balanoposthitis and progressing rapidly.

Laboratory diagnosis

Microscopy and culture

The identification of live erythrocytophagous trophozoites in temporary wet mounts is of prime importance because it confirms the diagnosis of invasive amoebic disease. Amoebae should be sought in dysenteric bowel-wall scrapings, the last portion of aspirate from a liver abscess (Fig. 7.8.1.8), sputum, and tissue scrapings from skin lesions. In nondysenteric stools, flecks of pus, blood, or mucus should be looked for and examined. The amoebae remain active for about 30 min at room temperature. Other microscopical features of faeces in amoebic colitis are scanty or absent leucocytes, clumped or degenerating red cells, and, sometimes, Charcot–Leyden crystals. If wet preparations are not made or are negative, a portion of the specimen should be preserved in polyvinyl alcohol or sodium acetate–acetic acid–formalin fixative for later smear preparation; alternatively, drying faecal smears should be fixed in Schaudinn's solution. In either case, fixed smears should be stained with Gomori trichrome or Heidenhain's iron haematoxylin.

Cysts and commensal trophozoites of *E. histolytica* found in wet faecal mounts are indistinguishable from those of *E. dispar*. The cysts of both species are four-nucleated and can be differentiated from the smaller *E. hartmanni* using an eyepiece micrometer. Direct mounts are made by emulsifying a small portion of stool in 1% eosin and in Lugol's iodine; however, the diagnostic sensitivity, per specimen, is only about 30%. Concentration methods for cysts such as formol-ether sedimentation give a 70% sensitivity per specimen. Cultivation of intestinal amoebae from faeces in Robinson's medium is relatively easy. Species identification requires immunofluorescent staining. Amoebae are often difficult to find microscopically in liver aspirates. Positive cultures from extraintestinal sites do confirm invasive *E. histolytica*.

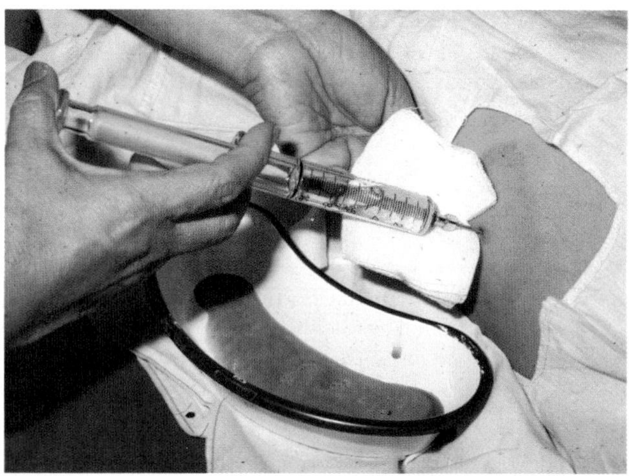

Fig. 7.8.1.6 Diagnostic/therapeutic aspiration of 'anchovy sauce' pus from a patient with amoebic liver abscess. Contrast medium is being injected after aspiration of the abscess.
(Copyright D A Warrell.)

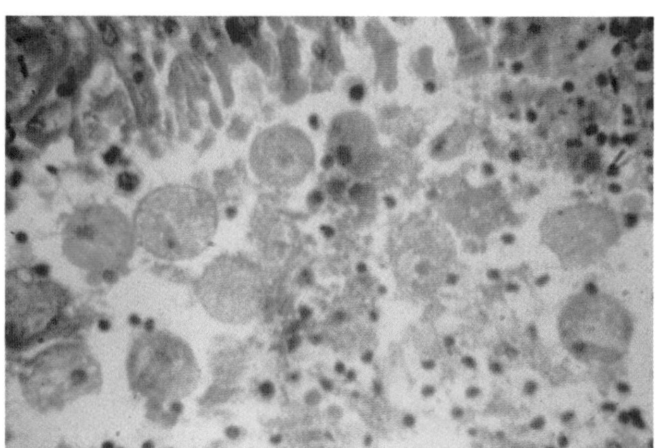

Fig. 7.8.1.8 Aspirate from amoebic liver abscess showing margin of hepatocytes and erythrocytophagous trophozoites of *E. histolytica*.
(Copyright Viqar Zaman.)

DNA and immunological tests

Polymerase chain reaction (PCR) methods can now be used for both *E. histolytica* and *E. dispar* using either faecal or tissue material. *E. histolytica* antigen can be detected in faecal specimens, and assays for antigen in serum have also been used in extraintestinal disease. These new methodologies have excellent sensitivity and specificity. Where they are available, they greatly simplify diagnosis in both amoebic disease and in carriers. They are already revolutionizing our ideas on epidemiology.

Many serodiagnostic methods have been applied to amoebiasis. The most detectable antibody is IgG, with some IgM in active disease. However, seropositivity does not distinguish current and past tissue invasion. The more sensitive methods are indirect haemagglutination, enzyme immunoassay, and indirect immunofluorescence. Latex agglutination and gel-diffusion precipitation are also used, the former being commercially available as a slide test, taking only minutes to perform. Using sensitive tests, over 95% of patients with liver abscess are seropositive, as are about 60% of those with invasive bowel disease; patients with amoeboma are nearly all seropositive. All patients with tissue invasion eventually become seropositive. Titres decline after therapy but may remain positive for 2 years or more with the most sensitive tests.

Patient management

Chemotherapy

Metronidazole for 5 days will be the first choice in most patients. The usual adult dose of metronidazole is 800 mg thrice daily for 5 or 8 days; the paediatric dose is 35 to 50 mg/kg in three divided doses. The alternative is tinidazole, which has the advantage of a single daily dose, 2 g in adults and 50 to 60 mg/kg in children. A 5- or even a 3-day course may be sufficient for tissue amoebae but rates of parasite elimination from the intestine are low. When nitroimidazoles are contraindicated, or not available, erythromycin is useful in nonsevere colitis.

The synthetic derivative dehydroemetine is a potent tissue amoebicide. It has less cumulative cardiotoxicity than the alkaloid emetine and is more rapidly excreted in the urine. Where appropriate nitroimidazoles are unavailable, as continues to be the case in many tropical contexts, this drug will continue to be life saving, especially when a parenteral drug is needed. A daily intramuscular dose of dehydroemetine of 1.25 mg/kg (maximum 90 mg) is given for 5 days.

Cutaneous and genital amoebiasis responds well to metronidazole, partly perhaps because the lesions often contain anaerobic bacteria. Amoebiasis at other sites is nearly always secondary to hepatic lesions and the chemotherapy will be the same. Metronidazole crosses the blood–brain barrier and should be used in the desperate situation of amoebic brain abscess due to *E. histolytica*.

All patients with *E. histolytica* infection treated with a tissue amoebicide should also be given diloxanide to eliminate infection from the bowel and so prevent recurrence of tissue invasion or transmission to others. The dosage of diloxanide for adults is 500 mg thrice daily for 10 days; the daily dose in children is 20 mg/kg daily in three divided doses. Alternatives to diloxanide when it is not available are paromomycin 30 mg/kg daily for 5 to 10 days or iodoquinol 650 mg thrice daily for 20 days, but iodoquinol may cause optic or peripheral neuropathy if the dose is exceeded.

Convalescent carriers, and also infected family contacts, should always be treated. Persons entering temperate countries from the tropics or new residents from such countries should be screened if there is a significant risk of infection; those with *E. histolytica* faecal antigen, or who are seropositive and have four-nucleated *Entamoeba* cysts in their stools, should be treated. In these contexts diloxanide is the drug of choice. Metronidazole is less effective even using an 8-day course and side-effects are troublesome. Unfortunately cure rates with tinidazole are very low when followed up at 1 month.

Supportive and surgical management

Intestinal amoebiasis

Supportive management plays a major role in patients with complicated amoebic colitis, with emphasis on fluid and electrolyte replacement, gastric suction, and blood transfusion as necessary. Gut perforation complicating extensive colitis carries a very poor prognosis; management may have to be medical. Parenteral metronidazole is invaluable in these situations because of its activity against anaerobic bacteria in the peritoneum and blood stream. Gentamicin plus a cephalosporin will normally be given as well.

Amoebomas respond well to metronidazole; a slow response should arouse suspicion that the amoebic lesion is superimposed upon other pathology, particularly a carcinoma. Surgical management is important in several situations. Acute colonic perforation in the absence of diffuse colitis or ruptured amoebic appendicitis may be amenable to local repair. In the case of diffuse colitis, local repair, or end-to-end anastomosis, may not be possible because of the poor condition of the gut wall: temporary exteriorization with an ileostomy may be necessary. In fulminant colitis with multiple perforation the viability of the gut wall is uncertain and the only definitive option is total colectomy.

Hepatic amoebiasis

A favourable response to medical treatment alone can be expected in about 85% of patients. Liver abscesses may rupture before, during, or after oral chemotherapy; this requires parenteral metronidazole or dehydroemetine. Intra-abdominal rupture will always require laparotomy. Extension into the pleural or pericardial cavities necessitates drainage of these structures, together with aspiration of the liver lesion; pericardial drainage is most urgent when tamponade is present. Hepatopulmonary lesions generally require drainage of the liver lesion but medical treatment alone has been successful in some cases. Antibiotics will always be needed when the abscess ruptures into the peritoneum or lung.

The most common management problem is slow response to the amoebicide. Patients whose pain and fever do not subside by 72 h are at significantly greater risk of rupture or therapeutic failure, and aspiration is generally to be recommended. A likely explanation of poor initial response is a tense lesion that restricts drug entry. Regular ultrasonographic monitoring is of great value as it will indicate the risk of rupture and guide the aspiration procedure. No change in lesion size on ultrasound can be expected during the first 2 weeks, although its outline may become clearer. Percutaneous aspiration with a wide-bore needle will be possible in most patients; if unsuccessful or anatomically contraindicated, then surgical help should be sought. Catheter drainage is a possible alternative to repeated needle aspiration with very large abscesses. Resolution times for small or moderate lesions are unaffected by aspiration. All patients with hepatic amoebiasis should be give diloxanide to eliminate bowel infection.

Prognosis

Uncomplicated invasive intestinal disease and uncomplicated hepatic amoebiasis should normally have a mortality rate of less than 1%.

In complicated disease, the mortality is much greater and may reach 40% for amoebic peritonitis with multiple gut perforation. Prognosis is usually better in centres where the disease is common and more likely to be recognized early. Late diagnosis increases the probability of complicated disease and mortality rises accordingly.

Unless parasitological cure is achieved and the gut completely freed of *E. histolytica*, clinical relapse is quite common, although probably limited by immunological responses. There is, so far, no evidence of naturally occurring strains of *E. histolytica* being resistant to normally used drugs. Hepatic scans show that nearly all liver abscesses completely disappear within 2 years; the median resolution time is 8 months. In secondarily infected lesions, bizarre hepatic calcification may be seen years afterwards. Healing of the bowel is remarkably rapid and complete; occasionally fibrous strictures persist after severe dysentery,

Prevention

Chlorination of water supplies does not destroy amoebic cysts, but adequate filtration will remove them. Regular stool screening of food handlers and domestic staff is of no value, but health education is important with encouragement to have a medical check if diarrhoea occurs.

Visitors to the tropics should not attempt chemoprophylaxis; in particular, long-term unsupervised use of hydroxyquinoline drugs must be strongly deprecated. Simple hygienic measures provide considerable protection. Boiling water for 5 min kills cysts. Routine examinations in temperate countries for returning visitors from the tropics or for new residents coming from such countries is of no value unless *E. histolytica* can be differentiated from *E. dispar*. Amoebic serology is particularly useful in those with gut symptoms or a history of dysentery.

Other parasitic gut amoebae including *Dientamoeba fragilis*

The nuclei of *Entamoeba* species have a fine ring of peripheral chromatin and a small central endosome. *E. gingivalis* has no cystic stage and lives in the mouth within gingival pockets and tonsillar crypts. It is spread by kissing or more indirect oral contact. Its possible role in periodontal disease was formerly dismissed but there is now renewed interest following recognition of its high prevalence in individual lesions in people with this condition; it may act as a bacterial vector within the lesions. It has been found on intrauterine devices that have been removed because of symptoms. Both in the uterus and in the mouth, this amoeba occurs in association with the bacterium *Actinomyces israelii*.

Five other *Entamoeba* species are nonpathogenic colonic commensals. *Entamoeba coli* has eight-nucleated cysts and is the commonest species in most surveys. *E. dispar* and *E. hartmanni* both have cysts with four nuclei; the former was previously known as 'nonpathogenic *E. histolytica*' and the latter as 'small race *E. histolytica*'. Size is the only simple diagnostic criterion for *E. hartmanni*; its cysts are less than 10 µm in diameter. The relative prevalence of *E. dispar* and *E. histolytica* varies greatly, but the former is usually much more common, especially where sanitation and water supplies are better. *E. chattoni* is primarily a pig and primate parasite; the cyst has one nucleus and an 'inclusion body'. Human infections are common in highland Papua New Guinea where humans and pigs may share a peridomestic environment; elsewhere it is rare. Lastly there is *E. moshkovskii*, which normally lives in soil and sewage; it infects and can be transmitted between humans. It was previously incorrectly referred to a low-temperature variant of *E. histolytica*.

Endolimax nana and *Iodamoeba bütchlii* both have nuclei with large endosomes and no visible peripheral chromatin. Cysts of the former are oval in shape with four nuclei; those of the latter are somewhat irregular in shape with a single nucleus and a large glycogen vacuole that stains prominently with iodine. Neither species is pathogenic.

Dientamoeba fragilis is overlooked in most parasitological laboratories and most reports are from developed countries. There is good evidence that it can cause colonic inflammation; however, this is not severe and there is no ulceration or systemic spread. It has no cystic stage and, unless this organism is specifically looked for, it will be missed. In fixed stained smears, about 60% of trophozoites have two nuclei; the endosome is large and lobulated and there is no peripheral chromatin. Alternatively it may be identified in faeces or cultures using immunofluorescence with specific antibody or by PCR; some patients are seropositive. Transmission is direct but possibly within eggs of the threadworm *Enterobius*. It causes a relatively mild diarrhoeal illness that may persist for several weeks and sometimes there is a superficial eosinophilic colitis. Irritable bowel syndrome may be suspected. Protein-losing enteropathy is reported and blood eosinophilia is quite common. This infection is frequent in some institutional contexts. It is found within some resected appendices but a causal role is unlikely. Electron micrographs and genetic studies indicate that *D. fragilis* is a trichomonad rather than a true amoeba. The infection responds to metronidazole, but a single dose of ornidazole is also effective.

Free-living amoebae

A shared feature of these species is the very large central nuclear endosome, quite different from that of *E. histolytica*, from which differentiation may be necessary in tissue sections. Under dry conditions, trophozoites form resistant cysts that permit survival and also airborne dispersal; cysts can resist chlorination. Many species are thermophilic and they are one of the causes of 'humidifier fever', a form of extrinsic allergic alveolitis presenting with fever, cough, and dyspnoea. Some bacteria including *Legionella* and *Parachlamydia acanthamoebae* may live symbiotically within these amoebae persisting within the phagosome, being resistant to lysosomal enzymes. Surprisingly, *Legionella* can survive encystment: the amoebae provide a refuge for these bacteria when chlorination or other antibacterial measures are applied. Three genera of free-living amoebae cause human infections:

1 ***Naegleria*** is an amoeboflagellate with two trophozoite forms. The amoeba moves rapidly with a single pseudopodium, it can transform into a nonfeeding flagellate in hypotonic media, and these free-swimming forms facilitate dispersal. Cysts are thin walled and spherical.

2 ***Acanthamoeba*** has no flagellate form. The small pseudopodia are multiple, thin, and spike-like; they are called acanthopodia (Fig. 7.8.1.9). Cysts are thick walled, angulated, and buoyant (Fig. 7.8.1.10); their dispersal may be wind borne. Several species are pathogenic but morphological classification is unsatisfactory; rRNA sequences differentiate 15 genotypes. *Acanthamoeba* is sometimes isolated from throat or nasal swabs or from stool specimens.

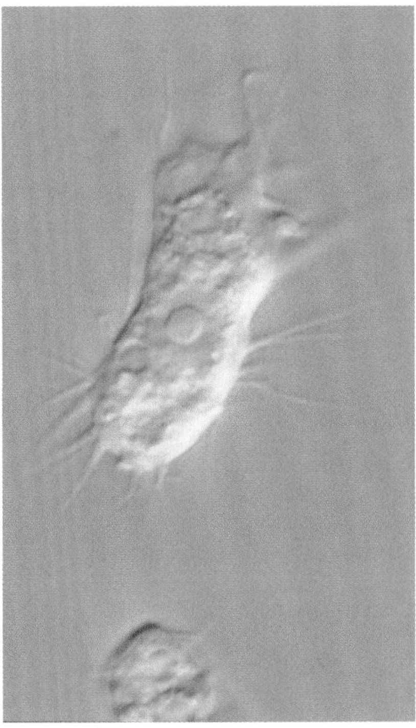

Fig. 7.8.1.9 *Acanthamoeba* trophozoite showing spike-like acanthopodia.
(Courtesy of the late Professor Sornchai Looareesuwan.)

3 ***Balamuthia*** is closely related to *Acanthamoeba* and not a leptomyxid amoeba; it shows little directional movement and has an irregular or branched shape. Cysts are thick walled and spherical. Human infections formerly attributed to *Hartmanella* are now all thought to be due to *Balamuthia mandrillaris*, a species described in 1993 from a mandrill baboon that died of meningoencephalitis in San Diego zoo. *Balamuthia* can only be cultured on tissue culture monolayers. About 100 cases have been reported worldwide, but many are from Latin America.

Primary amoebic meningoencephalitis due to *Naegleria fowleri*

Epidemiology and pathology

Nearly all patients give a history of swimming or diving in warm fresh water or spa water between 2 and 14 days before the illness began. Common-source outbreaks occur during warm summer months in temperate countries. Amoebic trophozoites cross the cribriform plate from the nasal mucosa to the olfactory bulbs and subarachnoid space. At autopsy the brain shows cerebral softening and damage to the olfactory bulbs; cysts are never formed in the tissues. Only about 200 cases have been documented since the first human case was reported in 1965. However, some are missed clinically and are discovered at autopsy or in preserved pathological material. Specific antisera enable amoebae to be recognized by immunofluorescence staining.

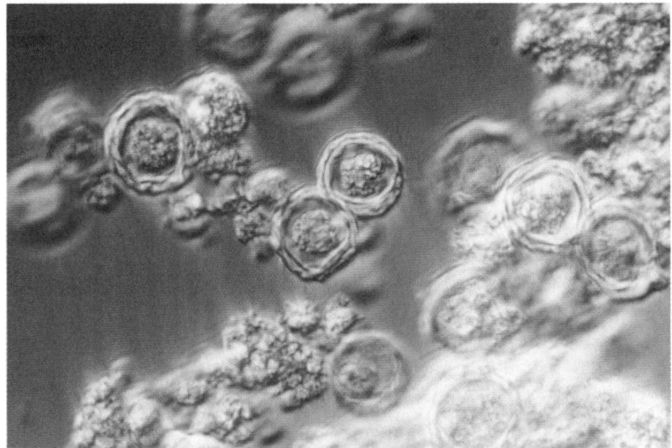

Fig. 7.8.1.10 *Acanthamoeba* cysts.
(Copyright Viqar Zaman.)

Clinical features and diagnosis

Patients are immunocompetant; most are young adults and children. Initial nasal symptoms and headache are soon followed by fever, neck rigidity, coma, and, later, convulsions; most die within a few days. Cerebrospinal fluid is often turbid and bloodstained with high protein, low glucose and neutrophils. Amoebae must be urgently looked for in wet specimens using phase-contrast microscopy. Unless amoebae are seen, bacterial meningitis will be suspected; on Gram staining amoebae appear as indistinct smudges. Fixed preparations stained with iron haematoxylin will show full details of nuclear structure. Confirmation is by culture at 37°C using a bacterial lawn on non-nutrient agar. Amphotericin B is an effective drug, it should be given by daily intravenous infusion, and intrathecally; other additional drugs that have been used are miconazole or fluconazole, and rifampicin; in mouse models, azithromycin is effective. So far, very few patients have survived but this may partly be due to diagnostic delays.

Amoebic keratitis due to *Acanthamoeba*

Most patients, but not all, are contact lens users. Among the latter, annual incidence rates of 1.49 and 0.33 per 10 000 are reported from Scotland and Hong Kong, respectively, but most figures are lower. Risk factors include poor hygiene when handling lenses and their cases, use of chlorine-based disinfectants, swimming or washing eyes while wearing lenses, handling lenses after gardening, and too prolonged use of plastic or unwashed lenses. The most appropriate disinfectants are chlorhexidine and hydrogen peroxide.

Corneal lesions are painful and present as indolent and progressive ulcers leading eventually to perforation. Recognition may be in the context of lesions unresponsive to antibiotics or corticosteroids. Differentiation must be made from commoner causes of microbial keratitis, including *Pseudomonas*, *Staphylococcus*, and herpes simplex. Inflammatory cells are mainly neutrophils. Infection may be by wind-borne cysts upon a damaged epithelium or from contact lenses. Solutions used to store or wash lenses can be contaminated by these amoebae, many of which are resistant to some antiseptics, especially as cysts. Amoebae are found in corneal scrapings or histologically in corneal tissue, but can be missed unless stained with iron haematoxylin or immunofluorescence. PCR methods are now available. Cysts may be seen in tissue. Cultures from fresh material, using a bacterial lawn on non-nutrient agar, should be at 30°C. The majority (90%) of cases are due to genotype T4.

Early aggressive topical treatment using a biguanide together with a diamidine is usually successful, however only the former is cysticidal. Initially, hourly application is needed, and courses may last a month. Additional topical neomycin or chloramphenicol may be necessary. Corneal grafting may be needed.

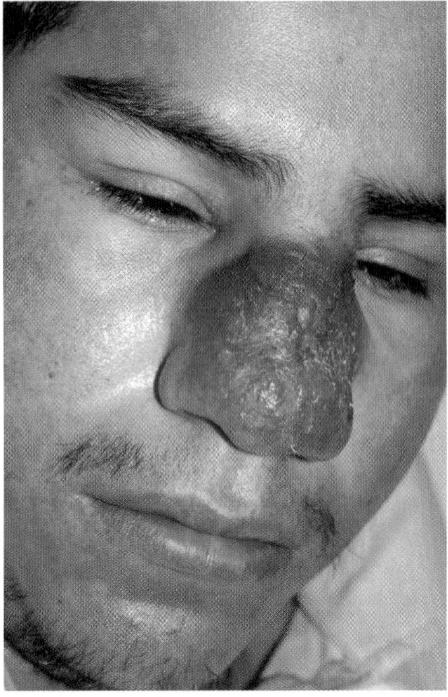

(a)

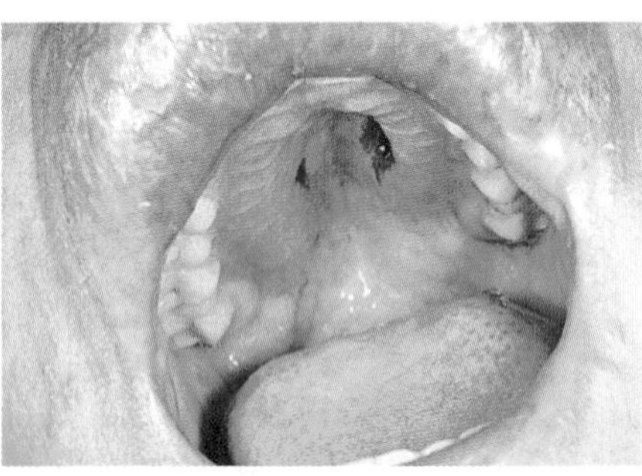

(b)

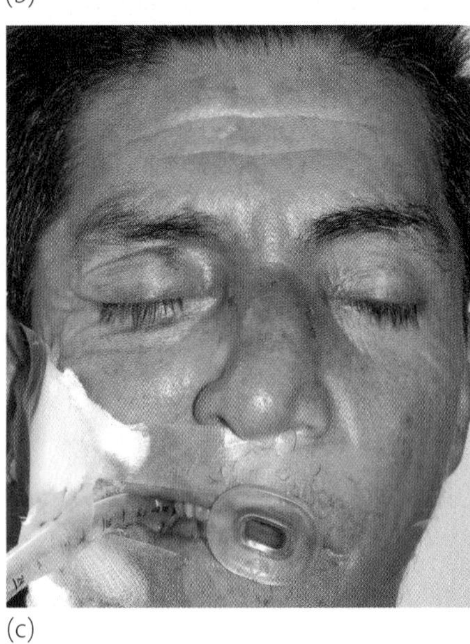

(c)

Fig. 7.8.1.11 *Balamuthia mandrillaris* infection. Cases at Instituto de Medicina Tropical 'Alexander von Humboldt' Universidad Peruana Cayetano Heredia, Lima, Peru: (a) cutaneous lesion in a 26-year-old man from Ica, (b) perforating lesion of palate in 16-year-old boy from Piura, and (c) encephalitis in a 57-year-old man from Piura showing the skin lesion that was the likely portal of entry.
(Copyright D A Warrell.)

Granulomatous amoebic encephalitis due to *Acanthamoeba* and *Balamuthia*

The main route of infection is the lower respiratory tract followed by haematogenous spread to the brain. Other routes of entry are the skin (Fig. 7.8.1.11a), the nasopharynx (Fig. 7.8.1.11b), the lungs and the stomach. Primary lesions have been described at all these sites.

Almost all patients infected by *Acanthamoeba* are immunocompromised, as are about 75% of those with *B.mandrillaris*. Soil contamination of skin and craniofacial wounds is an important risk factor. Causes of immunocompromise include malignancy, collagen disorder, alcoholism, diabetes mellitus, AIDS, and steroid or immunosuppressant therapy. Recently two patients with *B.mandillaris* infection have been described both of whom had received a kidney graft from the same donor. However, in Peru, most of the patients infected with *B. mandrillaris* have no obvious cause for immunosuppression.

Pathologically lesions resemble chronic bacterial brain abscesses or localized subacute haemorrhagic necrosis; involvement of the meninges is common. Some patients present with headache and meningism, others with evidence of a focal brain lesion (Fig. 7.8.1.11c, Fig. 7.8.1.12).

Unless these amoebae are found in wet tissue preparations or cerebrospinal fluid, the diagnosis will be usually based on histology, often at autopsy. Cysts may be seen in tissue but trophozoites may be missed unless stained with iron haematoxylin or immunofluorescence using specific antisera. Cultural diagnosis at 37°C from fresh biopsies or cerebrospinal fluid is sometimes possible. PCR methods are becoming available.

Survival of patients with this condition is still only rarely reported. Total excision of cerebral lesions is occasionally possible. Drug treatment with combinations of fluconazole with pentamidine, 5-fluorocytosine, sulphadiazine, and azithromycin has been successful in a few patients.

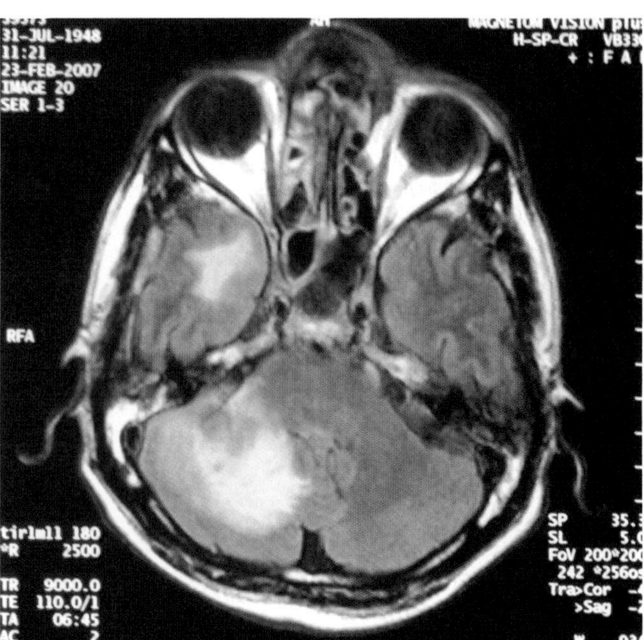

Fig. 7.8.1.12 *Balamuthia mandrillaris* infection. MRI scan in same patient as in Fig. 7.8.1.11c.
(Copyright D A Warrell.)

Further reading

Gut amoebae (*Entamoeba*)

Ali IKM, *et al.* (2007). Evidence for a link between parasite genotype and outcome with *Entamoeba histolytica*. *J Clin Microbiol*, **45**, 285–89.

Barwick RS, *et al.* (2002). Outbreak of amebiasis in Tbilisi, Republic of Georgia, 1998. *Am J Trop Med Hyg*, **67**, 623–31.

Calderaro A, *et al.* (2006). *Entamoeba histolytica* and *Entamoeba dispar*: comparison of two PCR assays for the diagnosis in a non-endemic setting. *Trans R Soc Trop Med Hyg*, **100**, 450–7.

Diamond LS, Clark CG (1993). A redescription of *Entamoeba histolytica* Schaudinn, 1903 (emended Walker 1911) separating it from *Entamoeba dispar* Brumpt, 1925. *J Eukaryot Microbiol*, **40**, 340–4.

Fotedar R, *et al.* (2007). Laboratory techniques for *Entamoeba* species. *Clin Microbiol Rev*, **20**, 511–32.

Mondal D, *et al.* (2006). *Entamoeba histolytica*-associated diarrheal illness is negatively associated with the growth of preschool children: evidence from a prospective study. *Trans R Soc Trop Med Hyg*, **100**, 1032–8.

Pritt BS, Clark CG (2008). Amebiasis. *Mayo Clin Proc*, **83**, 1154–60.

Ravdin JI, ed. (2000). *Amebiasis (tropical medicine: science and practice)*. Imperial College Press, London.

Singh O, *et al.* (2009). Comparative study of catheter drainage and needle aspiration in management of large liver abscess. *Ind J Gastroenterol*, **28**, 88–92.

Stanley SL Jr. (2003). Amoebiasis. *Lancet*, **361**, 1025–34.

Dientamoeba fragilis

Ginginkardesler KO, *et al.* (2008). A comparison of metronidazole and single dose ornidazole for the treatment of dientamoebiasis. *Clin Microbiol Infect*, **14**, 601–4.

Johnson EH, *et al.* (2004). Emerging from obscurity: biological, clinical, and diagnostic aspects of *Dientamoeba fragilis*. *Clin Microbiol Rev*, **17**, 553–70.

Stark D, *et al.* (2005). Detection of *Dientamoeba fragilis* in fresh stool specimens using PCR. *Int J Parasitol*, **35**, 57–62.

Stark D, *et al.* (2006). Dientamoebiasis: clinical importance and recent advances. *Trends Parasitol*, **22**, 92–6.

Windsor JJ, Macfarlane L (2005). Irritable bowel syndrome: the need to exclude *Dientamoeba fragilis*. *Am J Trop Med Hyg*, **72**, 501–2.

Free-living amoebae

Carter R.F. (1972). Primary amoebic meningo-encephalitis. *Trans R Soc Trop Med Hyg*, **66**, 193–208.

Dart JKG, Saw VPJ, Kilvington, S (2009). *Acanthamoeba* keratitis: diagnosis and treatment update 2009. *Am J Ophthalmol*, **148**, 487–99.

Greub GD, Raoult D (2004). Microorganisms resistant to free-living amoebae. *Clin Microbiol Rev*, **17**, 413–33.

Jung SRL, *et al.* (2004). *Balamuthia mandrillaris* meningoencephalitis in an immunocompetent patient: an unusual clinical course and a favorable outcome. *Arch Pathol Lab Med*, **128**, 466–8.

Khan NA. (2008). *Acanthamoeba* and the blood brain-barrier: the breakthrough. *J Med Microbiol*, **57**, 1051–57.

Khan NA, ed. (2009). *Acanthamoeba: biology and pathogenesis*. Caister Academic Press, Norwich, UK.

Matin A, *et al.* (2008). Increasing importance of *Balamuthia mandillaris*. *Clin Microbiol Rev*, **21**, 435–48

Paltiel ME, *et al.* (2004). Disseminated cutaneous acanthamebiasis: a case report and review of the literature. *Cutis*, **73**, 241–8.

Visvesvara GS, Moura H, Schuster FL (2007). Pathogenic and opportunistic free-living amoebae: *Acanthamoeba* spp., *Balamuthia mandrillaris*, *Naegleria fowleri*, and *Sappinia diploidea*. *FEMS Imm Med Microbiol*, **50**, 1–26.

Visvesvara GS, Schuster FL, Martinez AJ. (1993). *Balamuthia mandrillaris*, N.G., N. Sp., *agent of amebic meningoencephalitis in humans and other animals. J Eukaryot Microbiol*, **40**, 504–14.

7.8.2 Malaria

David A. Warrell, Janet Hemingway, Kevin Marsh, Robert E. Sinden, Geoffrey A. Butcher, and Robert W. Snow

Essentials

Malaria has been eliminated from many countries but remains the most important human parasitic disease in sub-Saharan Africa and other tropical and subtropical zones. It causes more than 500 million cases of illness and a million fatalities each year in 100 countries. There is currently a renewed international effort to reduce its impact on populations still at risk.

Human malaria parasites, mosquitoes, and transmission of malaria

Malaria parasites and their impact on the human genome—five species of *Plasmodium* commonly cause malaria in humans: *P. falciparum*, *P. vivax*, *P. ovale*, *P. malariae* and *P. knowlesi*. The genome of *P. falciparum*, the most pathogenic species, has been completely sequenced. This parasite has exercised immense selection pressure on the human genome, as is evident from the global distribution of the many human genes that constrain malarial development, such as a point mutation in position 6 of the β-globin chain (sickle cell haemoglobin), and deletion of α-globin genes (α thalassaemia).

Biology of the parasite and mosquito vector—sporozoites are injected into humans during the female anopheles mosquito's blood meal. They invade hepatocytes. Hepatic schizogony releases merozoites into the blood stream where they invade red blood corpuscles (RBCs) and undergo further asexual multiplications before gametocytes form. If these are ingested by mosquitoes, male and female gametes fuse, resulting in ookinetes that penetrate the mosquito's midgut and develop into oocysts. Daughter sporozoites are released. They invade the mosquito's salivary glands, ready to infect a new human host. Persistent latent forms (hypnozoites) of *P. vivax* and *P. ovale* remain in the liver to give rise to later relapses of parasitaemia and symptoms. All the stages express distinct antigen, repertoires excite different immune responses, and are equipped survive in different microenvironmants.

Mosquito biology—species of the *Anopheles gambiae* complex, the most effective malaria vectors, prefer to feed on humans to whom they are attracted by smell: other species are less particular. They vary in their choice of breeding habitats. MacDonald's equation for vectorial capacity and the related basic reproduction number (R_0) allows prediction of the impact of vector control methods under different conditions. The genome sequence of *An. gambiae* is known. Important mosquito phenotypes that have a genetic basis include blood feeding preference, habitat choice, insecticide susceptibility, and vectorial capacity.

Acknowledgement: The authors and editors acknowledge the inclusion in this chapter of material contributed by Professor D J Bradley to the 4th edition of the *Oxford Textbook of Medicine*.

Other mechanisms of transmission—malaria can be transmitted by transfusion of blood products, marrow transplants, and contaminated needles.

Epidemiology

In 2007, 2.4 billion people were exposed to *P. falciparum* infection across 87 countries, and 3.18 billion people were exposed to *P. vivax* across 63 countries. Intensity of malarial transmission depends on the varying efficiencies of the local anopheline vectors and their frequency of contact with humans.

Malarial endemicity expresses the amount or intensity of transmission in an area or community. Epidemic malaria implies a periodic or sharp increase in the amount of malaria. Stable transmission implies persistently high prevalence, insensitive to aberrations in climate or local habitats as in holoendemic areas of Africa; unstable malaria is characterised by great variability in space and time, as in South-East Asia. Prevalence of infection in children aged 2 to 9 years is described as hypoendemic (<10%), mesoendemic (11–50%), hyperendemic (51–75%), or holoendemic (>75%).

The epidemiological background to clinical malaria—is changing due to population growth, environmental changes (often human-induced, whether local or global), changing resistance of parasites to drugs, the HIV epidemic and the consequences of attempts at malaria control. An estimated 550 million clinical attacks of *P. falciparum* occurred worldwide in 2002: 71% in Africa, 23% in the low-transmission but densely populated countries of South-East Asia, and 3% in the Western Pacific. In Africa in 2005, *P. falciparum* is estimated to have caused 1.1 million deaths directly, 71 000 to 190 000 infant deaths following placental infection *in utero*, and over 3000 newly acquired persistent epilepsies through brain insults among patients surviving an episode of cerebral malaria in childhood.

Innate resistance and immunity

More human genetic polymorphisms have been associated with innate protection from malaria than for any other infectious disease. Duffy blood group negative RBCs are resistant to *P. vivax* infection, explaining the prevalence of the DARC(Fy) −46C/C genotype especially in West Africa, but there may be an associated susceptibility to HIV-1 infection.

In most stably endemic areas, acquisition of immunity, although never complete, ensures that death due to malaria is rare after the age of 5 years and hardly ever occurs in normally immune competent adults. Immunity allows tolerance of levels of parasitisation that would cause illness in a naive individual by neutralizing parasite toxins or down-regulating the cytokine response to challenge. However, a key aspect of immunity to malaria is control of parasite growth by interfering with parasites' replication or accelerating their removal from the circulation. There is progressive acquisition of both 'strain'-specific and cross-protective responses to a range of potential malarial epitopes. Immunity is stage-specific but probably acts predominantly at the blood stages. Antibody-mediated protection against blood-stage parasites is demonstrated by the relative protection of children in endemic areas during their first few months of life by passively transferred maternal antibody and by experimental amelioration of acute malaria by immune gammaglobulin. Malnutrition increases the risk of severe falciparum malaria in children.

HIV–malaria interaction—in pregnant women, HIV and *P. falciparum* infections are mutually synergistic. Consequences of malaria, especially anaemia, are more severe in HIV-positive women. In areas of unstable malarial transmission, HIV-positive nonimmune adults are at increased risk of severe and fatal malaria. In malaria endemic areas, HIV-positive children are at increased risk of severe malaria.

Molecular pathology, organ pathology, and pathophysiology

Molecular pathology—intravascular, asexual forms are responsible for all the pathological effects of malaria in humans. Fever and inflammation are probably initiated by interaction between parasite products and pattern recognition receptors on host cells, leading to cytokine release by macrophages. The relative virulence of *P. falciparum* is attributed to cytoadherence and sequestration of parasitized RBCs to venular endothelium, especially in the lungs, brain, intestines and muscles, resulting in reduced perfusion and tissue damage. Local release of potentially toxic/pharmacologically active compounds such as reactive oxygen species or nitric oxide may also be involved.

Organ pathology—the brain may be oedematous, especially in African children. Small blood are vessels congested with tightly sequestered parasitized RBCs (PRBCs) containing pigmented mature trophozoites and schizonts, making the brain slate-grey in colour. The cerebrovascular endothelium shows pseudopodial projections, closely apposed to electron-dense, knob-like protruberances on the surface of PRBCs. Other changes include petechial haemorrhages in the white matter, ring haemorrhages and Dürck's granulomas. Among other organs and tissues, retina, bone marrow, lung, heart, liver, intestine, spleen, kidney, and placenta show variable evidence of PRBC sequestration and some other distinctive features.

Pathophysiology—anaemia results from destruction/phagocytosis of both normal red cells and PRBCs as well as from dyserythropoiesis; autoimmune haemolysis is rare. Thrombocytopenia is attributable to splenic sequestration, dysthrombopoiesis, and immune-mediated lysis. Cerebral malaria is associated with inappropriately low cerebral blood flow, increased cerebral anaerobic glycolysis and microcirculatory obstruction. In African children, plasma concentrations of TNF-α, IL-1α and other cytokines correlate with disease severity. Cytokines may be involved in hypoglycaemia, coagulopathy, dyserythropoiesis, and leucocytosis in falciparum malaria. Pulmonary oedema may result from fluid overload, but more often there is increased pulmonary capillary permeability associated with neutrophil sequestration in the pulmonary capillaries. In African children, a syndrome of respiratory distress is associated with metabolic acidosis and severe anaemia. Hypoglycaemia is caused by impaired gluconeogenesis, reduced hepatic glycogen or hyperinsulinaemia secondary to quinine/quinidine treatment. In malarial acute renal failure, there is evidence of PRBC sequestration, and pigment (haemoglobin and myoglobin) toxicity may contribute.

Clinical features

Classic periodic febrile paroxysms with afebrile asymptomatic intervals are uncommon unless treatment is delayed.

Severe falciparum malaria—this is defined by (1) clinical features—prostration, impaired consciousness, respiratory distress/acidotic breathing, multiple convulsions, circulatory collapse, pulmonary oedema (radiological), abnormal bleeding, jaundice, and haemoglobinuria; and (2) laboratory tests—severe anaemia, hypoglycaemia, acidosis, renal impairment, and hyperlactataemia, that are of proven prognostic significance.

Cerebral malaria is defined by impaired consciousness in patients with acute *P. falciparum* infection in whom other causes of coma, including hypoglycaemia and transient postictal coma, have been excluded. Convulsions, dysconjugate gaze, retinal changes, symmetrical upper motor neuron signs, and abnormal posturing are common. Neurological manifestations are different in adults and children. African children surviving cerebral malaria may suffer persistent neurological, cognitive, and learning defects.

So-called benign malarias, *P. ovale*, *P. malariae*, and particularly *P. vivax*, can cause even more severe feverish symptoms than falciparum malaria. Splenic rupture is more common with vivax malaria. *P. knowlesi*, one of the monkey malarias, has recently been recognized as an important and potentially fatal zoonosis in humans in several South-East Asian countries.

Malaria in pregnancy—malaria is an important cause of maternal anaemia and death, abortion, stillbirth, premature delivery, low birth weight, and neonatal death. RBCs infected with strains of *P. falciparum* expressing Var2CSA bind to chondroitin sulphate A expressed on the surface of the syncytiotrophoblast. Placental dysfunction, fever, and hypoglycaemia contribute to fetal distress.

Chronic immunological complications of malaria—these include quartan malarial nephrosis, tropical splenomegaly syndrome (hyperreactive malarial splenomegaly) and endemic Burkitt's lymphoma.

Diagnosis

Repeated thick and thin blood smears and rapid antigen detection over a period of 72 h are necessary to confirm or exclude the diagnosis of malaria. Differential diagnoses include other acute febrile illness: falciparum malaria has been misdiagnosed as influenza, viral hepatitis, epilepsy, viral encephalitis, or traveller's diarrhoea, sometimes with fatal consequences.

Laboratory investigation

In falciparum malaria, blood glucose must be checked frequently, especially in children, pregnant women, and severely ill patients, whether or not the patient is receiving quinine/quinidine treatment.

Treatment

The efficacy of antimalarial chemotherapy is threatened by emerging resistance of *P. falciparum* to available drugs. The World Health Organization (WHO) now advocates the combination of two or more different classes of antimalarial drugs with unrelated mechanisms of action to delay emergence of resistance.

P. vivax, *P. ovale*, *P. malariae*, *P. knowlesi* malarias—these are treated with chloroquine. Resistant *P. vivax* (New Guinea, Indonesia) is treated by increasing the dose of oral chloroquine.

Uncomplicated *P. falciparum* malaria in malarious areas—WHO recommends the replacement of monotherapy with the combination of an artemesinin with another drug (artemisinin-based combination therapy, ACT), even in Africa, although this is more expensive and resistance to artemisinins has recently emerged in Cambodia. In South-East Asia, lumefantrine or mefloquine is added to artesunate. In Africa, lumefantrine, amodiaquine, or sulfadoxine–pyrimethamine might be added. For presumed nonimmune travellers returning to nonendemic areas, artemether–lumefantrine, atovaquone–proguanil, or quinine with doxycycline or clindamycin (pregnant women and children) are recommended.

Severe falciparum malaria—urgent appropriate, parenteral chemotherapy is necessary, initiated with a loading dose. Intravenous artesunate is the drug of choice. Intramuscular artemether, or quinine by intermittent or continuous intravenous infusion or intramuscular injection are less effective. Artemisinin by rectal suppository has proved effective. Resistance to artemisinins is emerging in Cambodia, Thailand, and Burma.

Supportive care—patients with severe malaria should be transferred to the highest possible level of care. Convulsions must be controlled; fluid, electrolyte, and acid–base homeostasis restored; and organ/tissue failure treated (e.g. haemofiltration for acute renal failure). Harmful ancillary remedies of unproven value, such as corticosteroids and heparin, have no role in the treatment of cerebral malaria.

Prevention

Modern malaria control and prevention aims to limit human–vector contact by indoor residual spraying (IRS) and insecticide (pyrethroid) treated nets (ITNs). ITNs can reduce all-cause childhood mortality by 17%, averting 5.5 deaths for every 1000 African children protected, preventing over 50% of clinical cases, and reducing prevalence by 13%. Repellents such as diethyltoluamide (DEET) are used for personal protection. Vectors can also be controlled by environmental modification or manipulation, and human contact can be reduced by zooprophylaxis and by modifying human dwellings and behaviour.

Intermittent preventive treatment in pregnant women (IPTp) and infants (IPTi) with sulphadoxine–pyrimethamine—efficacy is likely to decrease because IPTp works less well in HIV-positive women and there is no proven safe alternative to sulphadoxine–pyrimethamine in areas where resistance to this combination is rapidly expanding.

Malarial vaccines—obstacles to developing a malaria vaccine are the multistage complexity of the parasite, polymorphism of potential immune targets, and the parasite's capacity for evolving evasive strategies, such as antigenic variation and diversity. However, candidate pre-erythrocytic, blood-stage, and transmission-blocking vaccines have been developed. A subunit vaccine (RTS,S) comprising a fusion protein combining part of the circumsporozoite protein of *P. falciparum* with HBsAg and a complex adjuvant (AS02) has achieved 53% protective efficacy against malaria disease.

Travellers—prevention of malaria in people from nonmalarious areas who are visiting endemic regions, including those visiting their friends and relatives (VFRs), has become more difficult because of resistance to antimalarial drugs. Travellers are advised to (1) be aware of the risk; (2) prevent exposure to anopheline mosquitoes; (3) take chemoprophylaxis where appropriate—malarone, mefloquine, or doxycycline is appropriate in areas of chloroquine-resistant falciparum malaria; (4) seek immediate medical advice in case of any feverish illness developing while abroad, or within 3 or more months of returning, and to mention malaria as a possibility—regardless of the precautions taken—to any doctor who sees them. Up-to-date advice is important, as the global distribution and intensity of malarial transmission is changing. Pregnant women are best advised to avoid malarious areas.

Introduction

Malaria is the most important human parasitic disease globally and has had large effects on the course of history and settlement in tropical regions. Following the discovery in the 19th century of both the causative protozoan parasite, *Plasmodium*, and its mosquito vector, the disease was brought under control in many countries through the application of antimalarial drugs, insecticides such as dichlorodiphenyltrichloroethane (DDT), and other environmental interventions including urbanization. In the United States of America, Europe, the Mediterranean region, the Middle East, most Caribbean islands, some South American countries, northern Australia, and most of China, elimination or a high degree of control was largely achieved. Even in Sri Lanka in the early 1960s, cases had fallen from 1.1 million annually to just 18, but failure to maintain surveillance and react to outbreaks resulted in a return to previous levels.

In recent years, malaria has been subject to increased control efforts, with varying degrees of success, but the disease was resurgent in the 1980s and 1990s. Malaria remains the dominant tropical vector-borne disease but, after decades of neglect, international interest in its control has recently revived. There is now a global effort to develop new methods to intervene against parasite dissemination, stimulated by the emergence of drug resistant parasites in South-East Asia and Africa, mosquitoes resistant to DDT and other insecticides, and by the recognition that malaria has a considerable economic impact: in Africa, total gross domestic product losses due to malaria amount to US$12 billion per year, and the global cost is US$18 billion. With over 500 million malaria cases annually and more than a million deaths in more than 100 countries, there remains a clear and urgent need for improved control and treatment.

Biology of the malaria parasite

Life cycle and parasite cell strategies

Five of the 147 known species of protozoan parasites genus *Plasmodium* that cause malaria (*mal aria*, Italian, literally 'bad air') commonly infect humans: *P. falciparum*, *P. vivax*, *P. ovale*, *P. malariae*, and *P. knowlesi* (Fig. 7.8.2.1). The biological organization and life cycle of *P. falciparum*, the species most pathogenic to humans, are distinct from that of all but *P. reichenowi*.

Genomic organization of *Plasmodium* and consequences for the human host

Plasmodium is diploid only until the first (meiotic) division of the genome following fusion of the male and female gametes and is haploid for the rest of its life cycle. The 23-Mb genome of *P. falciparum* has been completely sequenced: it contains from 5000 to 6000 genes distributed between 14 chromosomes ranging in size from about 1 Mb to 2.4 Mb. Considering its comparatively small number of genes, it is remarkable that it not only maintains a complex life cycle but survives in the face of the overwhelming number (20 000–30 000) of genes available to its human host. The parasite has exercised immense selection pressure on the human genome as is evident from the global distribution of the many human genes that constrain malarial development (Box 7.8.2.1).

Development in the mosquito

After the blood meal, ingested intraerythrocytic gametocytes (Fig. 7.8.2.2) in the midgut of the female mosquito are triggered to undergo gamete formation (exflagellation) by a drop in temperature of more than 5°C and the presence of raised concentration of mosquito-derived xanthurenic acid. The gametocytes escape out of the red blood cell (RBC) into the lumen of the midgut, where the female gamete can be fertilized within minutes by a microgamete released from microgametocytes (Fig. 7.8.2.2). Major zygote/ookinete surface proteins are detectable on the zygote surface within 1 h of fertilization, particularly P48/45, P230, P25, and P28, which are potential components of a transmission-blocking vaccine.

Within about 8 h of fertilization, the briefly diploid genome has undergone meiosis producing a single nucleus containing four haploid genomes. Over the ensuing 9 to 12 h, the zygote becomes a motile and invasive banana-shaped ookinete (Figs. 7.8.2.2 and 7.8.2.3). The extracellular gametes, zygotes, and ookinetes are exposed to potentially lethal components in the blood meal, such as complement to which the parasite is initially resistant, antibodies, and mosquito proteases. Then, 24 to 36 h after the blood meal was ingested, the ookinete penetrates the chitinous peritrophic membrane, newly secreted by the mosquito to defend itself against parasitic invasion, and the plasma membrane of midgut epithelial cells. Unlike sporozoites and merozoites (Fig. 7.8.2.3), the ookinete lacks rhoptries and consequently does not form a parasitophorous vacuole (PV) when it invades the epithelial cells. On meeting the collagen-containing basal lamina on the outer wall of the midgut, the ookinete transforms into a vegetative replicating form, the oocyst, protected from the mosquito's immune system by a thick proteinaceous wall containing proteins P380 and circumsporozoite protein (CSP). Commonly, fewer than five of the thousands of gametocytes originally present in the blood meal form oocysts (Fig. 7.8.2.4).

Parasite movement

The motile ookinete, merozoite, and sporozoite are impelled by an unconventional actomyosin motor (Fig. 7.8.2.5).

Development of the oocyst into sporozoites

Depending partly on ambient temperature, the oocyst nucleus undergoes from 10 to 13 endomitotic divisions over a period of 10 to 25 days, until finally a single cytokinetic division results in the simultaneous production of between 2000 and 10 000 daughter sporozoites (Fig. 7.8.2.2). Mature sporozoites secrete a protease (ECP-1) to digest the proteinaceous oocyst wall to escape into the mosquito's haemocoelomic fluid. Only those capable of invading the salivary glands survive. They bind to salivary gland receptors via ligands such as CSP, TRAP, and MAEBL (apical membrane antigen/erythrocyte binding-like), penetrate the plasma membrane of the acinar cells, and come to lie in the salivary ducts. *P. falciparum* sporozoites can remain infectious in the glands for up to 55 days, many times longer than the natural lifetime of the infected mosquito, which delivers 10 to 100 sporozoites per bite.

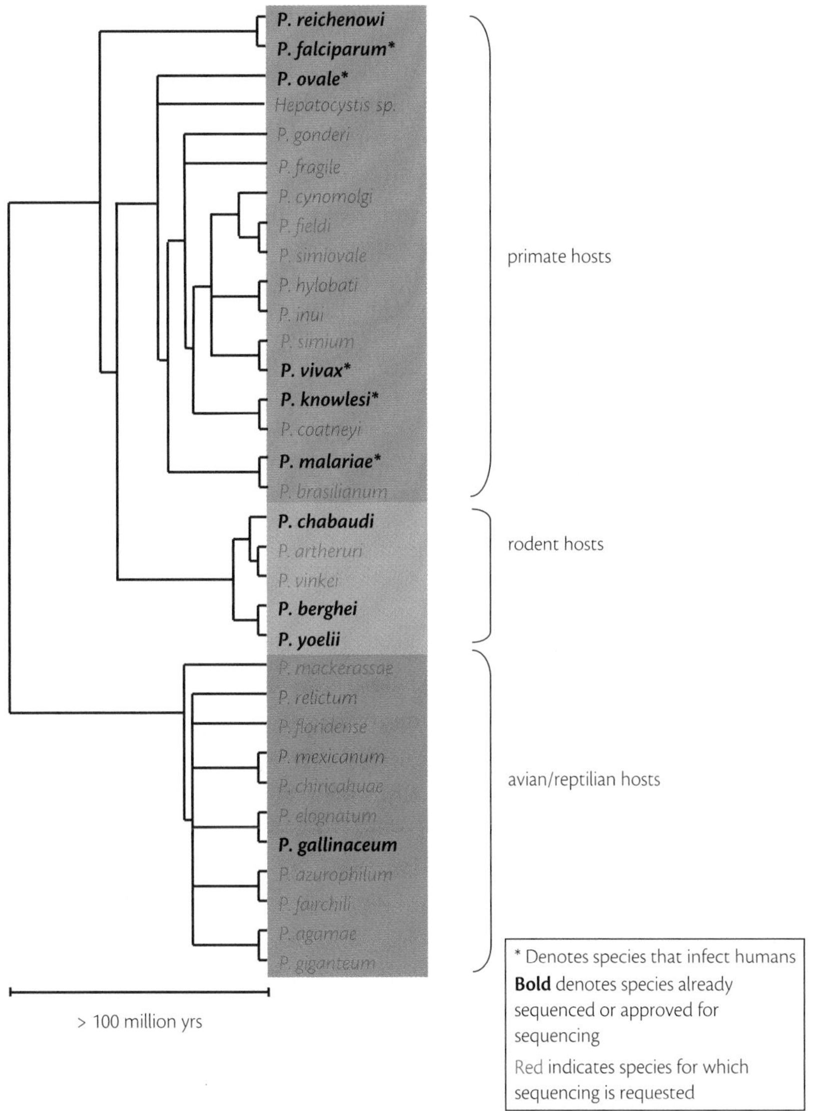

Fig. 7.8.2.1 A cartoon of the evolutionary relationships of malarial parasites derived from analysis of multiple genomes. The branch lengths are not to scale and do not represent the evolutionary distance between species.
(D Neafsey and S Volkman, unpublished data.)

Development of the exo-/pre-erythrocytic (liver) stages

CSP, the dominant surface protein on the sporozoite, is critical to this phase of the life cycle and has been the most popular vaccine candidate. Most of the sporozoites deposited in the dermis by the biting mosquito cross the capillary epithelium and are rapidly transported in the bloodstream to the liver, where they invade phagocytic Kupffer cells. A few sporozoites may enter the lymphatic system, where they may prime antigen-presenting cells in the lymph nodes. Kupffer cells tolerate microbes and their products (portal vein tolerance), but intracellular sporozoites also inhibit phagocytes' oxidative burst. CSP inhibits fusion of lysosomes with the parasite-containing vacuoles (PV). Sporozoites then escape from the Kupffer cells into the space of Disse and invade adjacent hepatocytes. CSP, secreted from the micronemes, binds to heparin sulphate proteoglycans on the hepatocytes and, with TRAP and a perforin-like molecule, enables penetration of the hepatocyte membrane. The parasite may migrate through several hepatocytes, killing them in the process and inducing the production of hepatocyte growth factor that contributes to parasite nutrition. The sporozoites form PVs in hepatocytes where they differentiate into replicating exo-erythrocytic (EE) schizonts.

Parasites inhibit apoptosis, a host cell defence mechanism, so that hepatocyte mitochondria remain available for recruitment by the PV. Down-regulation of hepatocyte proteosomal activity reduces presentation of secreted parasite antigens to major histocompatability complex molecules, compromising recognition of the infected hepatocyte by cytotoxic T cells. However, EE-stage parasites remain a prime target for potential vaccines. Within the infected hepatocyte, sporozoites undergo schizogony, each producing from 10 000 to 30 000 daughter cells (Table 7.8.2.1), or merozoites (Fig. 7.8.2.3). They are released in large cellular masses (merosomes) containing hepatocyte cytoplasm that are attacked by macrophages and neutrophils in the liver. However, individual merozoites escape into the circulation where they invade red blood cells (RBCs). Infection of the liver is without clinical consequences, possibly because only a small number of parasites complete development and little toxic waste is released. The cell cycles of *P. vivax* and *P. ovale* can become arrested with formation of quiescent hypnozoites that can persist in the hepatocyte for long periods, enabling these parasites to survive seasonal absences of mosquitoes. Reactivation of hypnozoites by unknown factors produces 'relapse' infection in the blood. Latencies and frequencies

Box 7.8.2.1 Some human genetic polymorphisms associated with resistance to malaria

- α –Thalassaemia
- β –Thalassaemia
- Haemoglobin S
- Haemoglobin E
- Haemoglobin F
- Haemoglobin C
- South-East Asian ovalocytosis
- Hereditary sphero-, ellipto-, pyropoikilocytoses[a]
- G6PD deficiency
- Pyruvate kinase deficiency
- Duffy blood group
- ABO blood groups
- S-s-U blood group
- Glycophorin B deficiency
- Complement receptor-1
- MHC class I
- MHC class II
- HLA Bw53
- HLA DRB1*1302
- TNF- α promoter
- IFN- γ receptor

G6PD, glucose-6-phosphate deydrogenase; IFN, interferon; MHC, major histocompatibility complex; TNF, tumour necrosis factor (see also http://www.malariagen.net).

[a] *In vitro* evidence only.

of hypnozoite relapses are very variable, suggesting that the strains responsible had their origins in both tropical and temperate zones (Table 7.8.2.1). Hypnozoites do not grow and are therefore susceptible only to 'causal prophylactic' drugs such as primaquine and atovaquone that target mitochondrial enzyme pathways responsible for essential energy metabolism. Relapse must not be confused with a recrudescence, which occurs as a result of the amplification of a chronic subpatent blood-stage infection of *P. falciparum* or *P. malariae*.

Development in the erythrocyte

The underlying mechanism of merozoite invasion of the RBC is highly conserved across *Plasmodium* species, whereas host cell recognition and binding is species limited. Different *Plasmodium* species invade RBCs of different ages. *P. vivax* invades reticulocytes and *P. ovale* also prefers younger RBCs; *P. falciparum* and *P. malariae* invade mature RBCs. Antibodies recognizing the various parasite ligands can inhibit merozoite invasion, thus offering potential targets for prophylactic vaccines. Invasion is a complex active process, taking less than a minute, that involves modification of both the merozoite surface and RBC membrane (Fig. 7.8.2.6). Inside the RBC, a PV is created to contain the merozoite. After successful invasion of the RBC, proteins such as *P. falciparum* reticulocyte-like binding homologue proteins (PfRh) 1 to 4 are released into the PV (Table 7.8.2.2).

Following invasion, phagocytosis of RBC cytoplasm by the growing trophozoite occurs through a cytostome or micropore in the parasite's plasma membrane, forming intracytoplasmic digestive vacuoles into which digestive enzymes such as plasmepsins and dipeptide aminopeptidase are secreted. Digestion of RBC proteins yields toxic haem that is sequestered as haematin crystals in membrane-bound vesicles, to be discarded when schizonts divide into merozoites. The rapid growth of the asexual

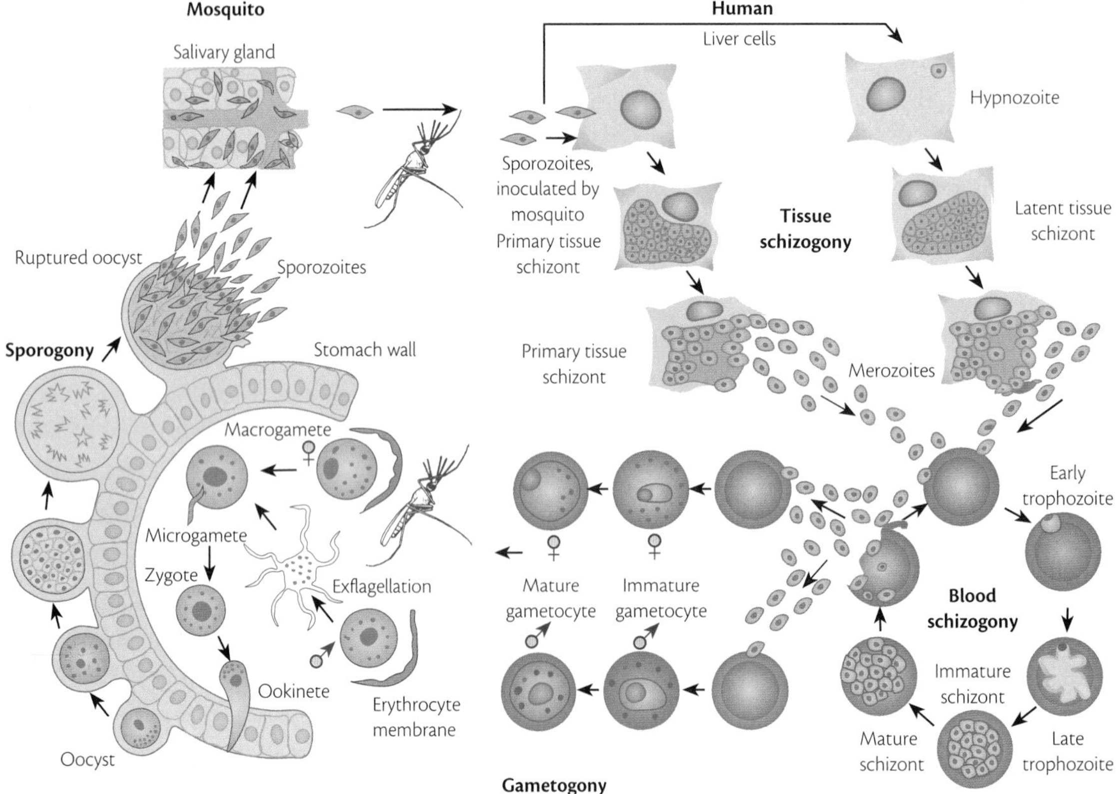

Fig. 7.8.2.2 Developmental cycle of *Plasmodium* species.
(Redrawn by permission of F. Hoffman-la- Roche Ltd, Basel, Switzerland.)

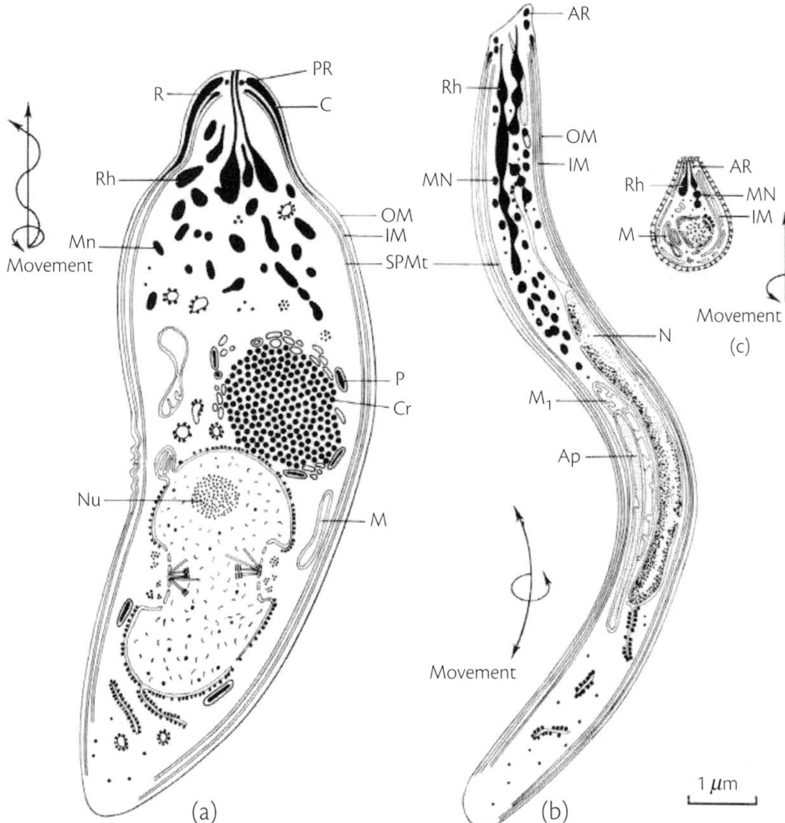

Fig. 7.8.2.3 Diagram of invasive stages, ookinete, sporozoite, and merozoite, illustrating their extensively conserved subcellular architecture.
(From Sinden RE (1978). Cell biology. In: Killick-Kendrick R, Peters W (eds) *Rodent malaria*, pp. 85–168. Academic Press, London.)
Ap, Apicoplast; AR, Apical ring; Co, collar; cr, crystalloid; IM, inner membrane vacuole; M, mitochondrion; MN, micronemes; Nu, nucleus; OM, plasmamembrane; P, pigment; PR, polar ring; R, ring; Rh, rhoptry.

parasite within the RBC demands new permeability pathways in erythrocyte membranes to facilitate entry of essential nutrients and the egress of toxic metabolites, especially lactic acid. *P. falciparum* builds membranous transport structures in the RBC cytoplasm including Maurer's clefts, originally described in 1903, and the recently described tubulovesicular network. Parasite nutrient transporters in the infected RBC (iRBC) membrane are important targets for new antimalarial compounds. *P. falciparum* erythrocyte membrane protein 1 (PfEMP1) is the major parasite protein and is exposed on the RBC membrane as discrete warts (knobs). Energy metabolism of the asexual blood stages is critically dependent upon the mitochondrion. The recently discovered apicoplast is a vestigial chloroplast originating from red algae. It is responsible for pathways in lipid metabolism distinct from those

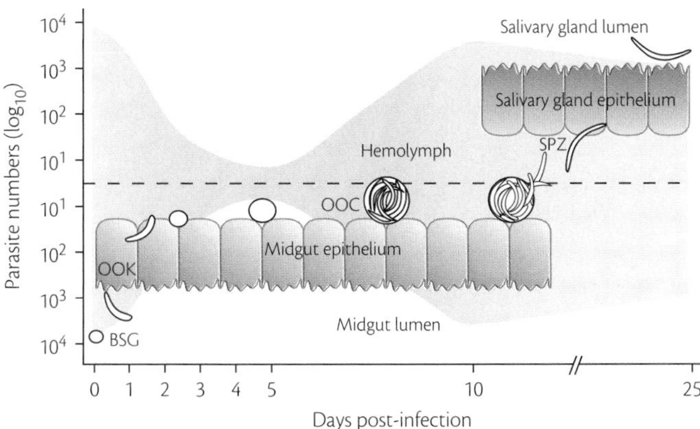

Fig. 7.8.2.4 Diagram illustrating the population bottleneck experienced by *Plasmodium* as it passes from the vertebrate host into the mosquito vector, with the nadir in number being experienced at the oocyst stage.
(Modified from Christophides GK (2005). Transgenic mosquitoes and malaria transmission. *Cell Microbiol*, **7**, 325–33.)

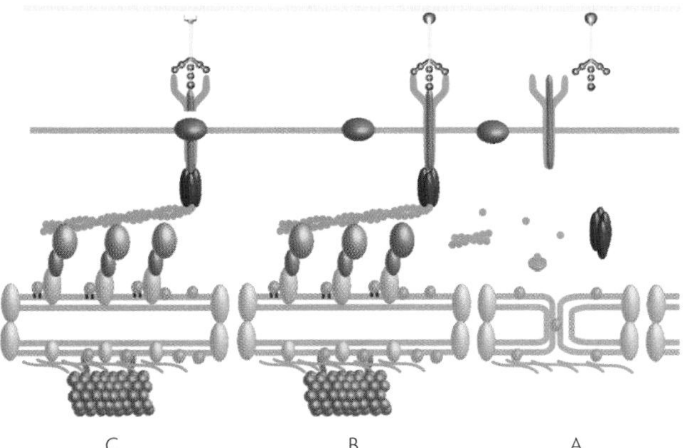

Fig. 7.8.2.5 Mechanism by which the actomyosin motor drives the parasite (ookinete, sporozoite, and merozoite) into host cells and through tissues. (a) On binding the host receptor (yellow), the parasite ligand (green) recruits aldolase (red), which binds to fibrous actin (green spiral). (b) This short actin fibre is moved by myosin A (orange), anchored to the cytoskeleton through myosin A tail domain-interacting protein (purple) and glideosome-associated protein (grey), to the posterior of the cell. (c) At the posterior of the cell, rhomboid protease cleaves the ligand transmembrane domain liberating the parasite from the host cell ligand.

Table 7.8.2.1 Distinguishing characteristics of malaria parasites infecting humans

Parasite	*P. falciparum*	*P. vivax*	*P. ovale*	*P. malariae*	*P. knowlesi*
Development of liver stages (days)	5–7	6–8	9	14–16	5.5
Merozoite number in exo-erythrocytic schizont	<30 000	<10 000	<15 000	<15 000	Unknown
Hypnozoite	No	Yes	Yes	No	No
Maximum period to first relapse	–	<3 yrs	<100 days	–	
Blood parasites detected by microscopy (days)	9–10	11–13	10–14	15–16	9–11[b]
Days/years to first symptoms[a]	12	15/<1[a]	17/<4[a]	28	9–11[b]
RBC Cycle (hours)	48	48	49–50	72	24
Merozoite number in blood schizonts	16	16	8/16[c]	8–12	10
Distinguishing characteristics of species by microscopy[d]	Commonly rings only; Maurer's clefts; crescentic gametocytes,	Schuffner's dots, trophozoites irregular	Large nuclei; Schuffner's dots, trophozoites irregular	Band forms	Light stippling; sometimes band forms; resembles *P. malariae*
Maximum RBC infected (%)	>60	0.01	<0.3	<0.2	12
Oocyst development at 28°C (days)	9–10	8–10	12–14	14–16	8–10
Oocyst size (μm)	55	50	45	40	65

[a] Exceptional cases of *P. vivax* and *P. ovale* took nearly 1 year and 4 years, respectively.

[b] From Chin, *et al.* (1968). Experimental mosquito-transmission of *Plasmodium knowlesi* to man and monkey. *Am J Trop Med Hyg*, **17**, 355–8.

[c] Merozoite numbers in schizonts from relapses of *P. ovale* are increased.

[d] See Garnham PCC (1966). *Malaria parasites and other haemosporidia*. Blackwell, Oxford, and Coatney GR, *et al.* (1971). *The primate malarias*. US Department of Health, Education and Welfare, Bethesda, Maryland, USA.

Data from Garnham PCC (1966). *Malaria parasites and other haemosporidia*. Blackwell, Oxford; Coatney GR, *et al.* (1971). *The primate malarias*. US Department of Health, Education and Welfare, Bethesda, MD; and Bruce-Chwatt LJ (1985). *Essential malariology*, 2nd edition, Heinemann Medical, London.

of either vertebrates or mosquitoes and can, therefore, be targeted by drugs such as fosmidomycin, doxycycline, and clindamycin. These drugs are slow acting, taking two generations of parasite growth (96 h) before inhibition takes effect. Over the next 24 to 72 h, depending on the species, the parasite develops within the PV, eventually forming schizonts containing up to 30 merozoites (Table 7.8.2.1). Just before merozoite release, schizont volume increases and bursts the iRBC explosively. When blood-stage infections are synchronous, iRBC destruction, release of merozoites, and parasite toxic products into the bloodstream result in typical periodic patterns of fever in the human host.

Sexual development (gametocytes)

The asexual parasites themselves are a developmental dead end, but their expansive growth in the blood increases the potential for differentiation into the sexual forms that are responsible for continuing the life cycle by infecting female mosquitoes. Stress on the developing asexual forms, e.g. antimalarial drugs, immune pressure,

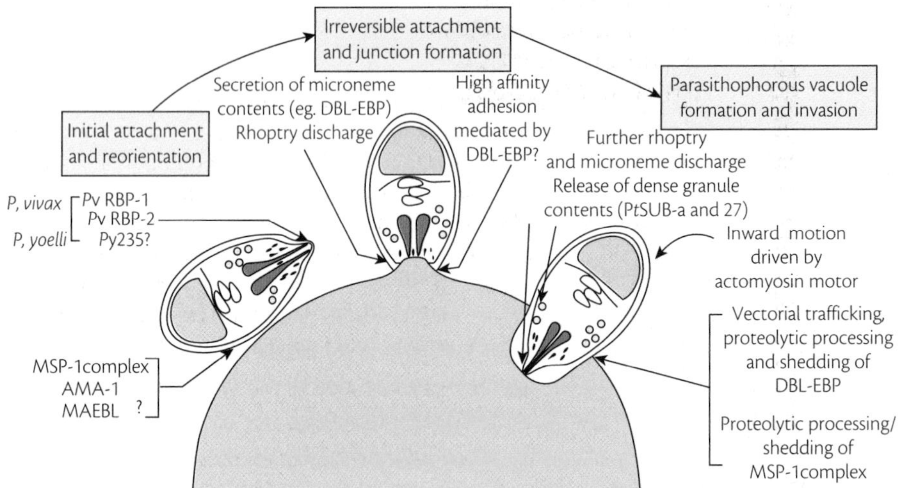

Fig. 7.8.2.6 Merozoite invasion of the red blood cell.
(From Chitnis CE, Blackman MJ. (2000). Host cell invasion by malaria parasites. *Trends Parasitol*, **16**, 411–16.)

Table 7.8.2.2 Some of the major proteins concerned with RBC attachment and merozoite invasion for *P. falciparum* and *P. vivax*

Species	Parasite ligand	Location	Sialic acid	RBC receptor for parasite ligand	RBC receptor sensitivity to trypsin[a]
P. falciparum	PfMSP-1_{42}	MS	Independent	Band 3	–
	PfMSP9	MS	–	Band 3	–
	EBA175	MN	Dependent	Glycophorin A	Sensitive
	EBA140/BAEBL	MN	Dependent	Glycophorin C	Resistant
	EBA181/JESEBL	MN	–	NK	Resistant
	AMA-1	MN/MS	–	–	–
	PfRh1–4	APM/Rhoptries/MN	–	NK	Resistant (1 and 2b)
P. vivax	DBP	–	–	Duffy antigen	–
	PvRBP1	Rhoptries	–	NK	–
	PvRBP2	Rhoptries	–	NK	–
		MS			

AMA-1, apical membrane antigen 1; APM, apical pole of merozoite; DBP, Duffy binding protein; EBA175–181, erythrocyte binding antigen 175, 140, or 181 kDa (BAEBL and JESBEL are alternative names, this group are homologues of *P. vivax* Duffy binding protein); MN, microneme; MS, merozoite surface; NK, not known; PfMSP-1_{42}, *P. falciparum* merozoite surface protein-1 42 kDa fragment; PfMSP-9, *P. falciparum* merozoite surface protein-9; PfRh1–4, *P. falciparum* reticulocyte-like binding homologue proteins 1, 2,2a, 3, and 4; PvRBP1–2, *P. vivax* reticulocyte binding proteins 1 and 2.

This table summarizes: the main parasite ligands thought to be involved in merozoite attachment to, and invasion of, RBC; their location in the merozoite; whether or not they depend on sialic acid residues on the RBC proteins, and the sensitivity of the RBC receptors to trypsin. Other proteins are involved but less is known of their function.

Based on Oh SS, Chishti AH (2005). Host receptors in malaria merozoite invasion. *Curr Top Microbiol Immunol*, **295**, 203–32, and Gaur D, *et al.* (2004). Parasite ligand-host receptor interactions during invasion of erythrocytes by *Plasmodium* merozoites. *Int J Parasitol*, **34**, 1413–29.

and metabolic stress induced by the asexual population itself, stimulates gametocyte production. The progeny of each schizont are all asexual, all male, or all female. Males (microgametocytes) accumulate the proteins required for rapid DNA replication and flagellar motility during gametogenesis and then shut down protein synthesis with the loss of ribosomes and endoplasmic reticulum (ER). In contrast, the mature females (macrogametocytes) retain protein synthetic machinery (ER and Golgi), although shutting down active protein synthesis. Because mature gametocytes of both sexes have ceased protein synthesis, they are less susceptible than asexual parasites to many antimalarial compounds. However, they remain vulnerable to inhibitors of energy metabolism such as primaquine and artemisinin combination therapy. The sexual stages of most malarial parasites mature in the same time as the asexual parasites, but *P. falciparum* is atypical in requiring not 48 h but about 10 days to mature (Table 7.8.2.1). Like the asexual parasites, immature gametocytes of *P. falciparum* express PfEMP1, have knobs, and adhere to receptors. Normally, only mature gametocytes are released into the peripheral bloodstream, where they may persist for 22 days, with a population half-time of 2.2 to 7 days. Most gametocytes are not taken up by mosquitoes but are removed by the spleen, where they stimulate antibody responses to the 'stored' gametocyte proteins, some of which are subsequently expressed on the surface of the gametes (e.g. P230, P48/45) and are now considered possible targets for transmission-blocking vaccines.

Biology of the mosquito vector

The first indication that mosquitoes might be involved in human disease cycles was in 1876, when Patrick Manson found that culex mosquitoes transmitted filarial worms. Ross and Grassi's discoveries of malaria transmission by anopheles mosquitoes followed in the 1890s. The Dipteran order of insects, to which the more than 3500 species and subspecies of mosquitoes belong, has many blood-feeding members and contains the insects of greatest medical and veterinary importance. Mosquitoes have coevolved with their vertebrate hosts, extending their feeding range from reptiles to mammals. The adaptation of malaria parasites to their mosquito hosts probably occurred about 20 000 years ago. From the human perspective, the most devastating link is that between *P. falciparum* and the African mosquito *Anopheles gambiae*, which is estimated to have been in place for as little as 10 000 years.

Blood feeding and host preference

Unlike many haematophagous insects, it is only adult female mosquitoes that have piercing and sucking mouthparts, adapted for taking a blood meal from vertebrate hosts to nourish the development of a single egg batch. Of the three groups of mosquitoes—anophelines, culicines, and aedines—only about 50 anophelines are malaria vectors. Many mosquitoes are part of complexes of sibling species, distinguishable only by modern molecular methods. The *An. gambiae* and *An. funestus* groups contain the most important African malaria vectors. Within the *An. gambiae* complex, *An. gambiae sensu stricto*, the best of the human malaria vectors, prefers to feed on humans, while *An. quadriannulatus*, a nonvector, feeds on cattle and *An. arabiensis*, a secondary vector in many parts of Africa, preferentially feeds on cattle but will take a human blood meal. Olfaction plays a vital role in the host-seeking behaviour of mosquitoes. The segmented antennae and, to a lesser extent, the maxillary palps have numerous sensillae, mostly olfactory, which are responsible for detecting stimuli and eliciting specific behaviour patterns from the mosquito. Feeding selectivity is based on attraction by warmth, moisture, carbon dioxide, and constituents of sweat. Human odour contains 33 chemical signalling compounds, but at least 5 are repellent to mosquitoes.

Preferred habitat for breeding

Mosquitoes have exploited a wide range of aquatic breeding habitats. In Africa, *An. gambiae* breeds extensively in any small, open, clean water body, including standing water in cattle hoofprints, while *An. funestus* breeds in larger, open, clean water bodies such as small ponds. Female mosquitoes lay one to three batches of 30 to 200 eggs during their lifespan, allowing an explosive increase in mosquito numbers from a relatively small number of females once breeding conditions become favourable.

Vectorial capacity and transmissibility

Mosquitoes are most efficient as vectors when the interval between parasite ingestion and its transmission to the next human host (extrinsic incubation period) coincides with the periodicity of female mosquito blood feeds associated with egg production. Vectorial capacity is defined as the average number of potentially infective bites delivered by all the mosquitoes feeding on a single host within 1 day. The numbers of mosquitoes feeding depends on mosquito density in relation to host density and the probability that the mosquito feeds on a host in any 1 day. The feeding frequency on humans is related to the proportion of meals taken on humans compared to other potential hosts. These factors were incorporated into MacDonald's equation for vectorial capacity:

$$V = [ma] \times [p^n] \times [(a/-log_e n(p))]$$

subsequently modified by Garrett-Jones in 1964 and 1974 to

$$V = [ma]^2\ (p^n/-log_e p)$$

where m is relative vector density (i.e. number of mosquitoes per human), a is human-biting frequency (i.e. number of human blood meals per vector per day), ma is the number of bites per person per night, p is the proportion of vectors surviving per day, and n is the latent period (days) of the parasite in the mosquito (extrinsic incubation period).

A measure of the proportion of mosquitoes taking a meal from an infected human that actually become infective is often added to this equation. This is a measure of the genetic and physiological competence of the mosquito. Small changes in the probability that the vector feeds on a host in 1 day (a), the duration of the extrinsic incubation period (n), and the probability that the mosquito will survive 1 day (p) produce large changes in vectorial capacity. This outcome led MacDonald to predict, as early as 1957, that adulticides would be more effective than larvicides in reducing malaria transmission rates, a lesson that has been relearned many times since by successive generations of entomologists. A related measure of the transmissibility or ability of an infectious agent to spread in a population is the basic reproduction number (R_0). R_0 is generally defined as the expected number of hosts who would be infected after one generation of the parasite by a single infectious person who had been introduced into an otherwise naive population. If R_0 is greater than 1, the number of people infected by the parasite increases; and if R_0 is less than 1, the number declines. The value of R_0 and the proportion of the mosquito population that is refractory to infection ultimately explain whether malaria will spread or be eliminated.

To monitor insect infection rates a number of different techniques can be deployed. The gold standard is the dissection and microscopical examination of blood-fed female mosquitoes (Fig. 7.8.2.7), but the polymerase chain reaction (PCR) is used increasingly. The recent discovery of a much higher level of human transmission of *P. knowlesi* in Borneo also shows how reliant techniques such as microscopy are on the ability of microscopists to differentiate between what they believe they should see and what they actually see. New molecular techniques that track specific single nucleotide polymorphism (SNP) patterns now make it practicable to follow the emergence and spread of a disease outbreak and should reduce the level of parasite misclassification in both humans and mosquitoes. However, the specificity and sensitivity of such tests needs careful analysis and is often poorly understood by field practitioners. Sensitivity is the probability that a test will correctly identify an infected host; specificity is the probability that a test will correctly identify organisms. PCR-based tests are available for the four human malaria parasites and *P. knowlesi*. A valid concern with this type of molecular method is that, although they detect the presence of pathogen nucleic acids with great sensitivity, they may not be well correlated with the presence or abundance of viable pathogens. This may be complicated by issues of vector competence, when the mosquito is infected with the parasite but is incapable of transmitting it.

Distribution and density of mosquito populations

Mapping mosquito populations is important for guiding epidemiological activities within a study area. Advances in remote sensing should improve this process. In Kenya, multitemporal meteorological satellites have been used to predict periods when malaria transmission is likely to increase, based on correlations between advanced high-resolution satellite-derived indices of vegetation biomass and mosquito abundance. Use of such remote sensor data will allow studies of large, remote geographical areas to which access is difficult. Logistical growth models have been used to estimate the mosquito population carrying capacity of a given environment. Within this model, the extent to which mosquito births and deaths are conditioned by density is referred to as density dependence. However, the role of density dependence in natural populations is controversial. Other factors, such as predation, interspecies competition, and disease, may intervene to regulate population size long before it reaches its carrying capacity. Density-independent factors that influence population growth include environmental conditions such as food availability, adverse weather, extremes of temperature and relative humidity, and insecticide treatment programmes aimed at changing the age structure/size of mosquito populations. However, some insecticide-based

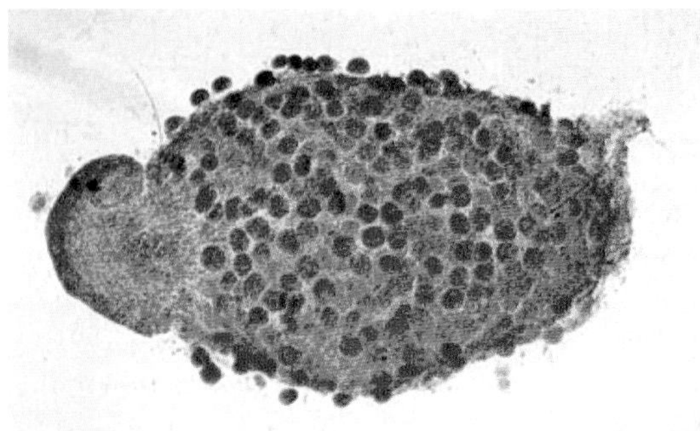

Fig. 7.8.2.7 Dissected *Plasmodium falciparum* oocysts on gut wall of mosquito. (Courtesy of WHO/MAP/TDR.)

interventions act only at a personal level, failing to reduce insect populations sufficiently to produce a herd or population protection effect on humans.

Mosquito genetics and insecticide resistance

The genome sequence of *An. gambiae* was published in 2002. Important mosquito phenotypes that have a genetic basis include blood feeding preference, habitat choice, insecticide susceptibility, and vectorial capacity. Blood feeding involves expression of salivary gland proteins that promote vasodilatation, inhibit platelet aggregation, and prevent blood coagulation in the host. Vector competence is a complex trait involving ingestion, replication, and transmission of plasmodium. The absence of any one of several structural or biochemical properties of the female mosquito could render her incapable of supporting successful completion of the parasite's life cycle. An important advance towards genetic characterization of mosquito refractoriness to parasite invasion in *An. gambiae* was the construction of a microsatellite map for quantitative trait loci. Insecticide resistance is genetically inherited. DNA-based systems are now available for identifying species, determining whether they are infected, identifying the source of their blood meal, and finding the most common insecticide resistance mechanisms. Microarray technology has speeded up the process of identification of metabolic genes that are over- or underexpressed in resistant insects. Different target site resistances can be detected by simple PCR, e.g. a simple SNP-based PCR assay can be deployed to detect the *kdr*-type pyrethroid resistance mechanism, which results from a single nucleotide change in the sodium channel of the insect's nervous system and results in phenotypic resistance to DDT and to all pyrethroids in homozygotes. Heterozygous insects are phenotypically susceptible to all the insecticides. The resistance can be selected by exposure to either DDT or pyrethroids. Retrospective analysis of specimens in laboratory or museum collections demonstrated that the *kdr* mutation was first selected in the 1940s to 1960s by the use of DDT in West and East Africa but remained completely undetected. In West Africa, resistance spread dramatically and was heavily reselected by the introduction of the pyrethroids in the late 1970s. Today, *kdr* in *An. gambiae* in West Africa has been selected almost to completion. It has managed to move between the sibling species of the *An. gambiae* complex and is still spreading. In East Africa, resistance has been confined to small areas of Kenya and has so far shown little evidence of increasing its range. In southern Africa, despite the extensive use of DDT in indoor residual spraying programmes over many years, there is no evidence of *kdr*-type resistance in either *An. gambiae* or *An. funestus*.

There has been spectacular progress in producing transgenic mosquitoes in recent years. At least five mosquito species (*An. gambiae*, *An. stephensi*, *An. albimanus*, *Aedes aegypti*, and *Culex quinquefasciatus*) can be transformed using at least four transposable elements (Fig. 7.8.2.8). Effector genes can abolish the mosquito's vectorial ability. Introduction of such mosquito strains might reduce malaria transmission by replacing wild-type mosquitoes.

Mosquito immunity to malaria

For many years, it was assumed that the insects did not possess an immune system. However, mosquitoes express several elements of vertebrate-specific immune responses. The ookinetes penetrating the mosquito midgut epithelial cells induce some *Anopheles* species to produce nitric oxide synthetase; defensin, a Gram-negative bacterial binding protein; and a thioester-containing protein TEP-1, and to initiate several other enzymatic pathways that may ultimately lead to parasite death. As a result, only a small percentage of mature ookinetes manage to reach the basal lamina to form oocysts, which are themselves vulnerable to melanization and destruction.

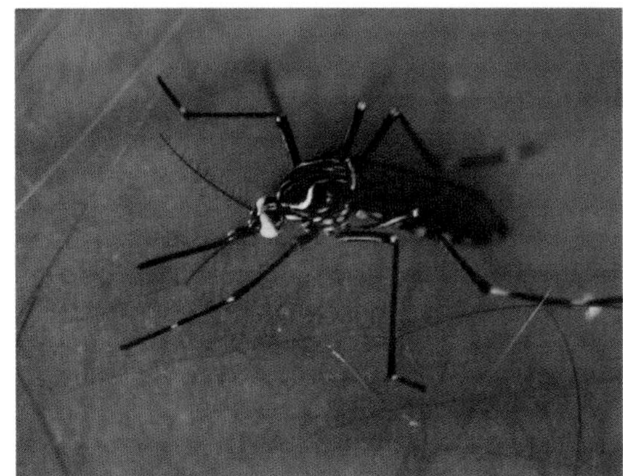

Fig. 7.8.2.8 Transgenic *Aedes aegypti* with green fluorescent protein expressed in the eyes.

Epidemiology

Spatial limits of malaria

The probable maximum preintervention distribution of malaria (*c.*1900) is shown in Fig. 7.8.2.9, reaching latitudinal extremes of 64° north and 32° south. Human efforts to control malaria have restricted its distribution dramatically during the 20th century as shown by the reported limits in 1946, 1965, 1975, 1992, 1994, and 2002. These distribution maps were compiled largely from country reports and expert opinion arising from the network of regional offices of the World Health Organization (WHO). Although they are imperfect representations of the distribution of global malaria infection risk in space and time, they do highlight the progress of malaria control in the 20th century. Between 1900 and 2002, the combined effects of development and control have halved the area of human malaria risk from 53 to 27% of the Earth's land surface. The number of countries and territories with populations of over 100 000 inhabitants exposed to some level of malaria risk fell from 140 to 106 during this time. However, population growth has increased the total number of people exposed to malaria risk from approximately 1 billion in 1900 to approximately 3 billion in 2002.

Renewed interest in global malaria control has been associated with a renaissance in mapping malaria risks. The Malaria Atlas Project has synthesized all available medical intelligence on areas of the world reportedly free from malaria risk and adjusted these limits to other factors that would not support transmission of either *P. falciparum* or *P. vivax*, including human settlement patterns, climate, and altitude. It has been estimated that in 2007 2.4 billion people were exposed to some risk of infection with *P. falciparum* across 87 countries (Fig. 7.8.2.10). The true biological and medical extent of *P. vivax* is harder to map and estimate; adaptations of work published in 2006 suggest that 3.18 billion people may be exposed to *P. vivax* in 2007 across 63 countries. No efforts have yet been made to map the distributions of the other two human malarias, *P. malariae* and *P. ovale*. *P. malariae* is widespread and

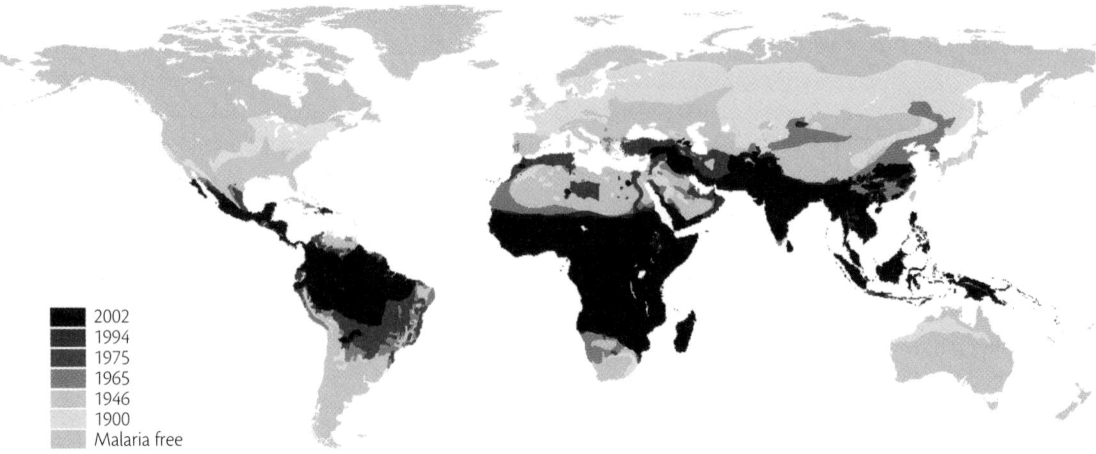

Fig. 7.8.2.9 Global distribution of malaria from pre-intervention to the present (*c.* 1900–2002).
Hay SI, *et al.* (2004). The global distribution and population at risk of malaria: past, present and future. *Lancet Infectious Diseases*, **4**, 327–336.

often overlooked and *P. ovale* largely replaces *P. vivax* in West Africa, where the population is resistant.

The variation in intensity of malaria transmission worldwide

Mosquito-related factors

Only mosquitoes that become infected and then survive for longer than the duration of the extrinsic cycle of the parasite (say 10 days) can pass on the infection. As mosquitoes of a given species have a relatively constant probability of dying during a day, regardless of their age, the longevity may be described by the probability of surviving through 1 day. It varies greatly between mosquito species and environments. Rainfall, temperature, ecology, human settlement patterns, and prevalence of effective control measures largely govern the abundance of malaria mosquito vectors and the development of the parasite in their salivary glands. The behavioural characteristics of mosquitoes make some of them more efficient vectors of malaria than others. The ability of *An. gambiae* to breed opportunistically in small collections of water in rural areas, feed and rest indoors, take frequent blood meals, and live for a relatively long period makes it the world's most efficient malaria vector. However, urban areas provide environments that are less suited to the breeding of *An. gambiae* and so malaria transmission in the rapidly expanding conurbations of Africa is very low. In Africa, *An. arabiensis* is better adapted to semiarid areas but is a less efficient vector than *An. gambiae*, accounting for the lower transmission of *P. falciparum* observed at the fringes of the Sahara, southern Africa, and the Horn of Africa. In South Asia, *An. culicifacies* may feed only every third day. As few as 10% of its meals may be from people, resulting in a human-biting habit that is 15-fold lower than *An. gambiae*. The diversity of vectors is driven by habitat preferences and adapted behaviours ('bionomics'), e.g. *An. sundaicus*, *An. maculatus*, *An. balabacensis*, and *An. subpictus* occupy specific geographical niches in Java (Indonesia). Their varying efficiencies as vectors of malaria account for most of the diversity of malaria in that archipelago.

Transmission and malarial endemicity

Within the geographical ranges of dominant vector species, there are huge variations in the likelihood that a mosquito is infected with malaria and the frequency with which they feed on humans.

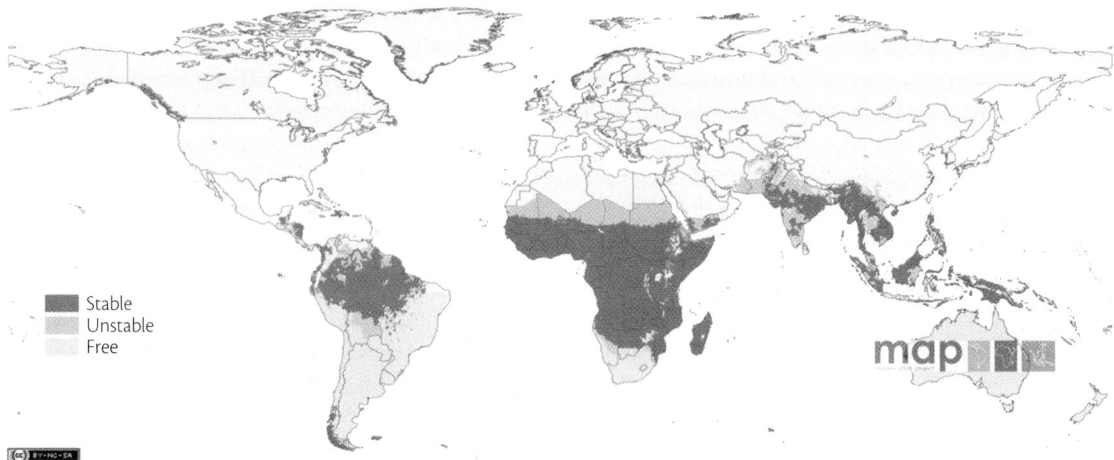

Fig. 7.8.2.10 Spatial limits of *P. falciparum* malaria risk in 2007. Limits are defined by *P. falciparum* annual parasite incidence (*Pf*API) with further medical intelligence, temperature, and aridity masks. Areas were defined as stable (dark red areas, where *Pf*API ≥0.01% per year), unstable (medium grey areas, where *Pf*API <0.01% per year), or no risk (light grey, where *Pf*API = 0).
(From Guerra CA, *et al.* (2008). The limits and intensity of *Plasmodium falciparum* transmission: Implications for malaria control and elimination worldwide. *PLoS Med*, **5**, e38.)

Across the central belt of tropical Africa, individuals may be challenged from less than once to over 1500 times each year. In other parts of the world, where malaria vectors are less efficient than in Africa, an individual might expect to be infected from once a year to every 10 years. Exceptions are found in New Guinea, several states in India, and smaller foci at forest fringes of Thailand, Vietnam, Cambodia, and Burma (Myanmar).

The frequency of contact between humans and malaria-infected vectors is a fundamental epidemiological concept that drives the health impact of malaria and the choice of control strategies. The frequency of malaria parasite encounters experienced by communities (transmission) is expressed using a variety of epidemiological terms and measured using field studies of contact and infection in mosquitoes and humans. The term 'endemicity' is a general expression of the amount or intensity of malaria transmission in an area or community. 'Epidemic malaria' indicates a periodic or sharp increase in the amount of malaria in a given indigenous community. Precise information about the degree of endemicity must be based on quantitative and statistical concepts. Malaria transmission is also classified as stable or unstable. 'Stable' implies equilibrium; the prevalence of infection is persistently high and endemicity is relatively insensitive to aberrations in climate or local habitats. Under stable endemic conditions, variation in transmission is minimal over many years although seasonal fluctuations still do occur and transmission can continue even with very few vectors. Conversely, 'unstable' malaria is characterized by great variability in space and time.

R_0 is often the benchmark epidemiological measure of malaria transmission but it is rarely measured empirically in the field. Two related measures, more commonly used, are derived from sampling mosquitoes or young children. The entomological inoculation rate (EIR) measures the average number of infected bites that an individual might experience from local vectors in a unit of time (often expressed per year) and measured by catching mosquitoes inside and outside people's houses and dissection of mosquito salivary glands to see if they are infected. The parasite rate (PR) represents the proportion of individuals (usually children aged 2–9 years) who have evidence of infection in their peripheral blood when sampled during a cross sectional study in the community. It is not strictly a rate but a proportional ratio of infected persons. The PR has been widely used to classify *P. falciparum* endemicity since the 1950s. Four commonly used terms indicate the prevalence of infection in children aged between 2 and 9 years: hypoendemic (< 10%); mesoendemic (11–50%); hyperendemic (51–75%); and holoendemic (>75%, when measured in infants but routinely measured in children aged 2–9 years). Most measures of malaria transmission are related, often nonlinearly. Classical epidemiological models of malaria transmission, based largely on infection and vectors, are gradually accommodating new concepts related to pathogenesis, virulence, disease outcomes, and heterogeneity of susceptibility and transmission. These new suites of mathematical models should provide a more elaborate framework for understanding the diversity of malaria as a public health problem and how best to tailor control methods to meet specific short and long-term transmission-dependent needs.

The changing epidemiology of malaria

Population growth and environmental change

In most parts of the world, the epidemiological background to clinical malaria is likely to change due to population growth, environmental changes (often the result of human activity, whether local or global), changing resistance of parasites to drugs, and the consequences of attempts at malaria control. Predicting the resources needed to meet international malaria control objectives in the near future must take account of increasing populations at risk of malaria and the changing pattern and intensity of land use. The rate of population growth is significantly higher in urban than rural areas; sometime before 2025, most Africans will live in cities. Urban growth will reduce malaria risk. The pressure on agricultural land as populations grow can lead to deforestation, while increases in irrigation and dams together with poor land management can lead to desertification. In Africa, deforestation rates in the 1990s exceeded those in South America and are projected to increase with the growing capacity of humans to exploit forest habitat. The impact of deforestation on malaria transmission depends on which vector is dominant locally. In Africa, deforestation could create a habitat favouring *An. gambiae*, a more efficient malaria vector than the forest mosquito *An. moucheti*. Deforestation is also benefiting *An. darlingi*, the most efficient malaria vector in the Americas, but in South-East Asia deforestation may reduce malaria transmission by *An. dirus*. In Africa, most of the 525 large and 45 594 small dams have been built since 1950. Their number will increase in the near future and may aggravate malaria transmission, e.g. the restoration of *An. funestus* to the Sahel, after a prolonged period of drought and desertification, has been attributed to irrigation.

Population movements

Human migration has been associated with malaria epidemics when population pressure in hilly areas drives the inhabitants down into malarious regions, when congregation of workers at new sites mixes infected with susceptible people, or when malnourished refugees, with impaired resistance to infection, camp where public health measures have collapsed. Regional conflicts result in large-scale population movements to avoid the ravages of war. During the mid-1990s, the exodus of nonimmune refugees from the nonmalarious highlands of Burundi to endemic areas of Tanzania resulted in an epidemic of severe malaria.

HIV epidemic

In sub-Saharan Africa, an HIV epidemic has been superimposed on an established malaria pandemic. Considering the wide geographical overlap and concurrent high prevalence of both infections, even a modest interaction could have substantial public health implications. HIV-infected adults in malaria-endemic areas and HIV patients of all ages in areas of unstable malaria transmission are at increased risk of malaria infection and death. In endemic areas, the case fatality of malaria is also higher in HIV-infected children. The impact of HIV on malaria depends on the level of malarial endemicity and, hence, the age patterns of clinical malaria and on the geographical distributions of HIV. Populations in southern Africa and urban areas of Africa are most vulnerable to this interaction.

The public health burden of malaria

Direct and indirect consequences of infection

The relationship between *P. falciparum* infection and disease outcome is complex. People born into areas of stable *P. falciparum* transmission frequently have periods when they are being infected with the parasite and periods when they remain uninfected. Most will, at some stage in their lives, develop a clinical response to infection, usually an attack of fever. This may resolve without any medical intervention, progress to severe disease with natural resolution, resolve through medical intervention, or end fatally. In areas where transmission is stable, less than 0.05% of infections prove fatal. This low case fatality is largely a result of combinations of innate genetic protection and acquired clinical immunity. There are, however, indirect consequences of malaria infection that are less effectively controlled by immunity. Chronic subclinical infections, e.g. due to incomplete parasite elimination with failing drugs, may lead to anaemia or other forms of malnutrition that independently increase susceptibility to severe effects of future infections. Subclinical infections may increase the severity of other infectious diseases. Asymptomatic infection of the placenta of a pregnant woman may significantly reduce the weight and hence the chances of survival of her newborn child. Patients who survive severe disease may be left with debilitating sequelae, such as spasticity or epilepsy, or more subtle consequences including behavioural disturbances or cognitive impairment. The combined direct, indirect, and consequential impacts of *P. falciparum* on health are summarized in Fig. 7.8.2.11.

Epidemiological patterns of stable and unstable malaria

The epidemiological features of human malaria differ markedly even between endemic areas. At one extreme, as in holoendemic areas of tropical Africa, everyone is infected shortly after birth, parasitaemia is almost universal throughout childhood, and the brunt of mortality falls in early childhood; epidemics do not occur except at high altitude or during aberrant rainfall in semiarid areas.

Children living in the *An. gambiae* belt of tropical Africa will usually have their first malaria infection during their first 3 months of life when they still have maternal antibodies. The disease is very mild, consisting of just one or two peaks of fever that usually resolve without treatment. When they are between 4 and 6 months old, when maternal antibodies have waned, each new infection leads to more severe febrile illnesses. The repeated infection–fever cycle progressively increases the loss of RBCs to the parasite plus a suppressed ability to replace them. Combined with other severe pathological consequences such as metabolic acidosis and coma, approximately 1% of all children living in these areas will die before their third birthday. The survivors will continue to have frequent attacks of fever until about the onset of puberty. Many will experience between 20 and 50 malaria attacks before reaching their fifth birthday. Thereafter, the frequency of attacks of fever and the intensity parasitaemia slowly wanes until levelling out sometime in early adolescence.

From that point forward, people have an almost constant low parasitaemia despite an almost complete absence of symptoms. In adults, episodes of fever due to malaria occur only once in 2 to 10 years, and last only a few hours even without treatment. The one exception to this rule is malaria in pregnant women, especially those pregnant for the first time.

Malaria in pregnancy

It is estimated that, each year, over 30 million women become pregnant in malarious areas of Africa. In mesoholoendemic areas, pregnant women experience relatively little malaria-specific morbidity but have an increased risk of infection and higher density parasitaemia leading to anaemia and placental sequestration of parasites. Maternal anaemia is an important contributor to maternal mortality and it is estimated that 9% of the excess risk is directly attributed to *P. falciparum* infection. Prematurity and low birth weight (<2500 g) associated with maternal malaria have been

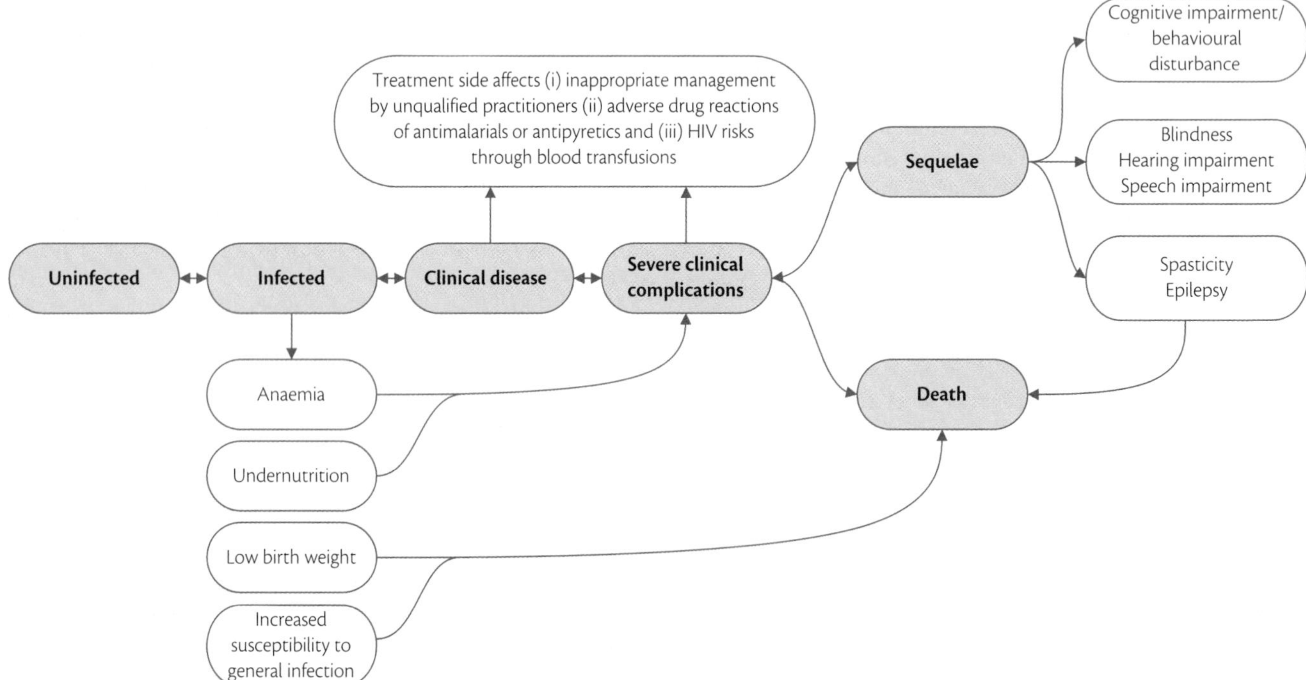

Fig. 7.8.2.11 Direct, indirect, and consequential clinical consequences of *P. falciparum* infection.
(Redrawn from Snow RW, Gilles HM (2002). The epidemiology of malaria. In: Warrell DA, Gilles HM (eds) Bruce-Chwatt's essential malariology, 4th edition, pp. 85–106. Arnold, London.)

reported indirectly to contribute to 3 to 8% of infant mortality. Interactions between malaria and HIV are particularly important among pregnant women who, when coinfected, have an increased risk of clinical attacks of malaria, anaemia and giving birth to a low birth weight baby. It is estimated that 500 000 women will develop clinical malaria in Africa as a result of their HIV infection. It remains uncertain whether malaria during pregnancy increases the vertical transmission of HIV.

Areas of unstable malaria

At the other end of the spectrum, as in parts of South-East Asia, where malaria is unstable or hypoendemic disease affects all ages, the risk of clinical illness is almost directly proportional to the risk of infection, and the risks of acquiring the parasite and developing a clinical event are time and space dependent throughout heterogeneous foci. Despite differences in the age patterns of disease with differing levels of endemicity, there is a much lower overall incidence of clinical disease and death in communities located in areas of low transmission intensity (hypomesoendemic) than in those experiencing moderate-to-high transmission (hyperholoendemic). However, during epidemics, disease burdens in lower transmission areas can be devastating, disrupting livelihoods. Overall, as the annual risk of new infections increases from zero, through to low-to-moderate risks of new infections (say one or two new infections per year), the rates of disease increase proportionately and probably linearly. As transmission intensity increases through hyper- to holoendemic conditions, the relationship between the annual risk of infection and the rates of disease is less clear, probably nonlinear and may reach a plateau after about 10 new infections per year. To understand the clinical spectrum of malaria seen in patients from a given locality, it is essential to understand the local epidemiology.

Global malarial morbidity and mortality

Although it is convenient to classify entire regions of the world by levels of endemicity, the low intensity transmission characteristics of most areas of South-East Asia resemble large swathes of Africa. Similarly, there are areas of South-East Asia that might be regarded as typical of the central *An. gambiae* belt of Africa. Precise estimates of the numbers of clinical cases and deaths due to malaria are notoriously poor in all malaria endemic countries. National data on malarial illness and death are characterized by gaps and inaccuracies due to under-reporting and misdiagnosis. Deaths usually occur outside the formal health sector and many clinical events are self medicated.

Given the weaknesses in international malaria disease reporting, estimations have been made of the public health burden using modified historical and climate-driven maps of malaria transmission, projected population human settlement counts, and endemicity-specific epidemiological survey data of clinical attacks and deaths due to *P. falciparum*. These approaches suggest that there were approximately 550 million clinical attacks of *P. falciparum* worldwide in 2002, distributed by WHO regions as follows: 71% in the Africa region, 23% in the low-transmission but densely populated countries of South-East Asia, 3% in the western Pacific, 0.7% in the Americas; 2.3% in the eastern Mediterranean (including Somalia and Sudan), and 0.1% in the European region. Less is known about global *P. falciparum* mortality and still less about the neglected disease burdens posed by *P. vivax*, despite its wider distribution. In Africa, application of similar epidemiological disease burden models to assess the wider public health consequences of *P. falciparum* (Fig. 7.8.2.11) suggested that in 2005 *P. falciparum* caused 1.1 million deaths directly, between 71 000 and 190 000 infant deaths following placental infection *in utero*, and over 3000 newly acquired persistent epilepsies through brain insults among patients surviving an episode of cerebral malaria in childhood.

Susceptibility to infection and innate resistance

In endemic areas, malaria is thought to account for around one-quarter of all childhood deaths so that this infection has been a major selective force in human evolution. More human genetic polymorphisms have been associated with innate protection from malaria than with any other infectious disease (Table 7.8.2.1). The best known is sickle cell haemoglobin, due to a point mutation in position 6 of the β-globin chain. Here, the mutant-gene frequency is stabilized because the enhanced survival of AS heterozygotes is counterbalanced by the lethal consequences of homozygosity (SS). The protection afforded to AS heterozygotes seems to act predominately on the development of clinical disease. Although infection rates are similar for AA and AS genotypes, the AS genotype is almost completely protected against life-threatening *P. falciparum* malaria. α-Thalassaemia, resulting from deletion of α-globin genes, is less strongly protective against *P. falciparum* malaria but, as most forms are virtually asymptomatic, very high gene frequencies have developed in some parts of the world such as Oceania. However, in Africa, where the selective pressure is greatest, the gene frequency is less (typically *c.*40%). This may be explained by the fact that when sickle cell trait and α-thalassaemia coexist, far from acting synergistically, they cancel out each other's protection, a striking example of negative epistasis.

Many other genetic variants affecting the RBC have been associated with protection from malaria, including other variants of the β-globin gene (HbC and HbE), polymorphisms of the RBC enzymes glucose-6-phosphate dehydrogenase (G6PD) and pyruvate kinase, and variants of structural proteins (erythrocyte band 3), which cause South-East Asian ovalocytosis.

The Duffy (blood group) antigen receptor for chemokines (DARCFy), expressed on the surface of RBCs, is also a receptor for penetration of RBCs by merozoites of *P. vivax*. The extreme rarity of the DARC +46C/C genotype is responsible for the striking resistance to this parasite of people of West African origin. However, these same receptors influence plasma levels of HIV-1 suppressive and proinflammatory chemokines such as CCL5/RANTES and are the site of HIV-1 attachment to RBCs, affecting by HIV adsorption the transinfection of target cells. In African Americans, possession of the prevalent DARC –46C/C genotype was found to be associated with a 40% increase in the risk of acquiring HIV-1. If extrapolated to all Africans, approximately 11% of the HIV-1 burden in Africa may be linked to this genotype.

Many potentially protective polymorphisms affecting other key aspects of malaria–human interaction have now been identified. These include polymorphisms affecting endothelial receptors, cytokines, and other key molecules of the immune system. Any listing of putative protective polymorphisms, such as Table 7.8.2.1, is bound to become quickly out of date. There is now an international coordinated effort to apply whole genome scanning approaches to identify key polymorphisms conferring protection against malaria. Regularly updated information can be found at http://www.malariagen.net.

Acquired resistance

Different aspects of the acquisition of immunity in endemic populations are illustrated in Fig. 7.8.2.12. Such immunity is often described as being slow to acquire and incomplete. From the figure, it can be seen that the prevalence of asymptomatic infection remains high for many years and even in adulthood a substantial proportion of people are infected at a single time point. It is unlikely that anyone ever achieves sterilizing immunity. However, the most important aspects of immunity, the ability to avoid severe disease and death, develop much faster. In most stably endemic areas, death due to malaria is rare after the age of 5 and hardly ever occurs in normally immunocompetent adults.

A characteristic of immunity to malaria is the early acquisition of the ability to tolerate levels of parasitization that would cause illness in a naive individual. This presumably involves either, or both, a immune response to neutralize parasite toxins or a down-regulation of the host's normal cytokine response to challenge. However, it is important to recognize that such 'antitoxic' responses cannot of themselves be the mainstay of protection against serious morbidity, for if the parasite population continued to expand, the host's RBC population would soon be overwhelmed leading to severe anaemia. Thus, even at an early stage, the key aspect of immunity to malaria is an acquired ability to control parasite growth, either by interfering with the replication of parasite or by accelerating the removal from the circulation.

Emphasis is often given to the strain-specific nature of malarial immunity, with the idea that immunity depends on having to acquire a repertoire of responses to different 'strains' of the parasite. However, because the parasite population is constantly outbreeding, it is more accurate to think of polymorphism in key molecular targets of protective immune responses rather than of fixed 'strains'. For some of these polymorphic targets, i.e. parasite-derived molecules expressed on the outside of the infected RBC membrane, children do build up a repertoire of responses. New infections tend to be those that the individual has not yet seen. However, there is also considerable evidence that some protective responses are cross-protective from an early stage. It is likely that the development of immunity involves the progressive acquisition of both strain-specific and cross-protective responses to a range of potential targets.

Potentially, effective immune responses could act at any point in the parasite's life cycle (Fig. 7.8.2.2). Immunity is largely stage specific, i.e. immunity induced by the sporozoite stage that can prevent infection probably has little effect on the blood stages. Similarly the targets and mechanisms responsible for immunity to gametocytes (which prevent transmission) are separate from those responsible for immune response to pre-erythrocytic and erythrocytic stages. Experimental infection of humans and animals with attenuated sporozoites leads under some circumstances to complete immunity to infection (see 'Malarial vaccines', below). However, there is little evidence that such responses play a major role in naturally acquired immunity to malaria and, in fact, adults in endemic areas become infected at similar rates to children (albeit without progressing to clinical illness).

Naturally acquired immunity to malaria probably acts predominantly at the blood stages of the parasite's cycle. Here, the parasite is present briefly as a free merozoite before spending most of its time apparently hidden inside the host RBC. Effective responses are likely to depend either on antibody-mediated mechanisms or on indirect cellular effects involving the release of a range of mediators. The potential importance of antibody mediated responses to blood-stage parasites was demonstrated in classical studies in which gammaglobulin from immune adults was shown to markedly ameliorate attacks of malaria in children. Similarly, the relative protection of children in the first few months of life in endemic area is thought to be due in part to passively transferred maternal antibody. A number of potentially key targets for protective immune responses have been identified. These tend to be either molecules involved in the invasion of RBCs by merozoites or parasite-induced molecules inserted on the surface of the infected RBC during the second half of its blood stage. Most of these antigens show considerable antigenic polymorphism and those growing up in endemic areas develop a wide range of antibodies to many antigenic types. Increasingly it appears that protection from clinical malaria may stem from multiple mechanisms and that the breadth and quality of the immune response to a number of antigens may be more important than responses to any single antigen. Humans also make immune responses to several gametocyte specific antigens. However, although experimental approaches to interrupting transmission in animal models hold promise for transmission blocking vaccines, the evidence that such responses play an important role in nature is controversial.

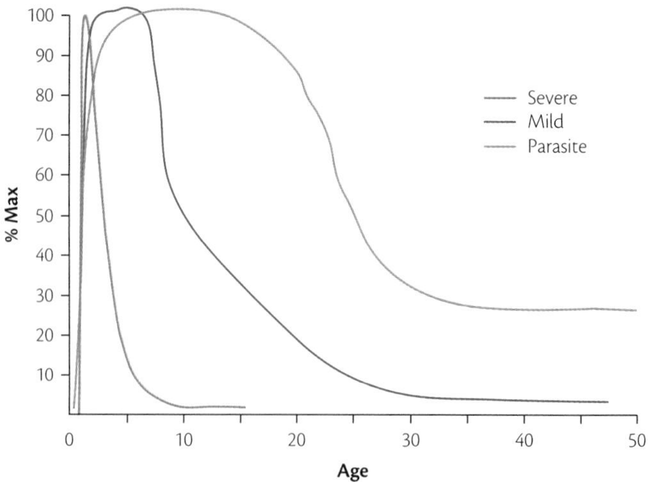

Fig. 7.8.2.12 Acquisition of immunity to malaria with age. The figure shows the period prevalence of three markers of immunity to malaria: the susceptibility to severe (life threatening) malaria, susceptibility to mild febrile episodes due to malaria, and the susceptibility to asymptomatic parasitization. Data are taken from an endemic population in Kilifi District on the coast of Kenya and normalized to a percentage of the maximum achieved in the population.

Immunity is diminished after long periods of absence from endemic areas and in pregnancy. Previously immune pregnant women are at risk of parasitization of the placenta, resulting in spill-over peripheral parasitaemia, increasing anaemia, and impairment of placental function leading to low birth weight babies. This results not from a breakdown in previously established immunity but from the specific appearance of a new site for sequestration of parasites. Parasitized RBCs (PRBCs) recovered from the placenta express a specific subset of PfEMP1 molecules that bind to chondroitin sulphate A (CSA) on the syncytiotrophoblast, leading to the accumulation of sometimes massive numbers of metabolically active parasites. The PfEMP1 molecules responsible for this adhesion are rarely encountered in infections outside pregnancy and so women enter their first pregnancy without specific antibodies. These are acquired during the course of the first and subsequent pregnancies so that effects of placental parasitization and its consequences decrease progressively with ensuing pregnancies.

Malaria and HIV immunosuppression

HIV infection modifies the response to malaria under a number of situations. In pregnant women, the two conditions seem to be mutually synergistic with the prevalence and consequences (particularly anaemia) being more severe in HIV-positive women. In nonimmune adults in areas of unstable transmission, HIV positivity is associated with an increased risk of clinical malaria and with increased risk of death in those who develop it. Recently it has become clear that HIV positivity in children in endemic areas is strongly associated with increased risk of being admitted to hospital with severe malaria.

Malaria and malnutrition

For many years the relationship between malnutrition and malaria was contentious, with claims that it was associated with protection from severe disease. Although there may be situations where very severe nutritional deficiencies may be associated with reduced risk, in general malnutrition is an important risk factor for severe malaria in children in endemic areas.

Molecular pathology

All the pathology associated with malaria infection is attributable to asexual parasite multiplication in the bloodstream. The consequences to the host of the intraerythrocytic multiplication of parasites range from a variety of severe, but not life threatening, symptoms common to all the species that infect humans, to the potentially lethal complications particularly associated with acute *P. falciparum* infection.

The characteristic symptom of malaria is fever and this is probably initiated by a combination of stimuli involving parasite products interacting with pattern recognition receptors, such as Toll-like receptors, and cell surface receptors, such as CD36, on host cells. Parasite products involved include variant parasite molecules expressed on the surface of PRBCs, such as PfEMP1, glycosylphosphatidylinositol anchors which are found on many plasmodium membrane proteins, and haemozoin. These interactions lead to the stimulation of both pro- and anti-inflammatory cytokine cascades, the balance of which may determine the relative outcome in terms of antiparasite effect and host pathology. At one end of the spectrum lies a relatively mild, self-limiting illness; at the other is an attack of severe disease that shares many of the pathological features of sepsis, in which overvigorous or disordered immune responses play a key role. Thus, while tumour necrosis factor (TNF) is protective against the parasite, many studies show an association between severe disease and exaggerated proinflammatory cytokine responses, including TNF, interleukin (IL) IL-1β, IL-6, IL-10, and interferon-γ as well as the macrophage inflammatory protein chemokines MIP1α and MIP1β.

Infection with all species of malaria induces fever, but the acute illness with *P. malariae* or *P. ovale* is relatively self limiting.

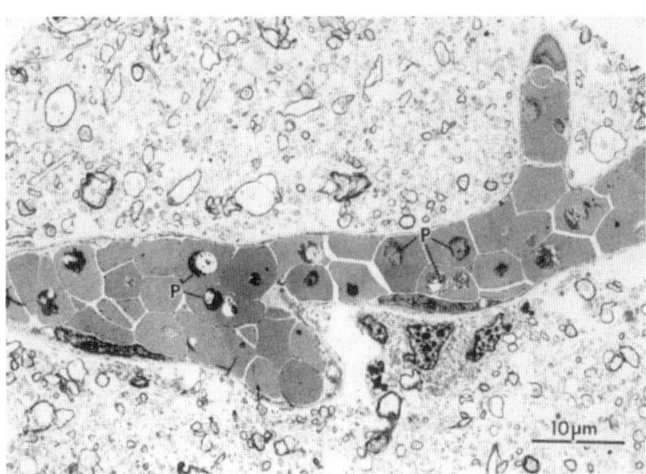

Fig. 7.8.2.13 Brain section of a patient who died of cerebral malaria. The image shows a blood vessel packed with red blood corpuscles, the majority of which were identified as being infected by the presence of parasites (P) or, at a higher magnification, the presence of knobs.
(Courtesy of Professor D Ferguson.)

Although *P. vivax* is traditionally considered a relatively benign parasite, the acute illness can be quite severe and it is increasingly realized that deaths due to *P. vivax* infection do occur. However, it is *P. falciparum* that is responsible for the majority of severe disease and death. The principal life-threatening complications of *P. falciparum* in African children are cerebral malaria and severe anaemia often associated with metabolic acidosis and respiratory distress. The clinical picture in nonimmune adults is more complex and can include single or multiple organ failure. A key difference in the biology of *P. falciparum* believed to play a central role in its enhanced virulence is its propensity to undergo sequestration (Figs. 7.8.2.13–7.8.2.15). Only the younger developmental stages of the parasite circulate, as the more mature forms adhere to specific receptors on venular endothelium. Parasite sequestration occurs in many capillary beds and is often particularly intense in the lungs, brain, intestines, and muscles. The resultant reduction in, or obstruction of,

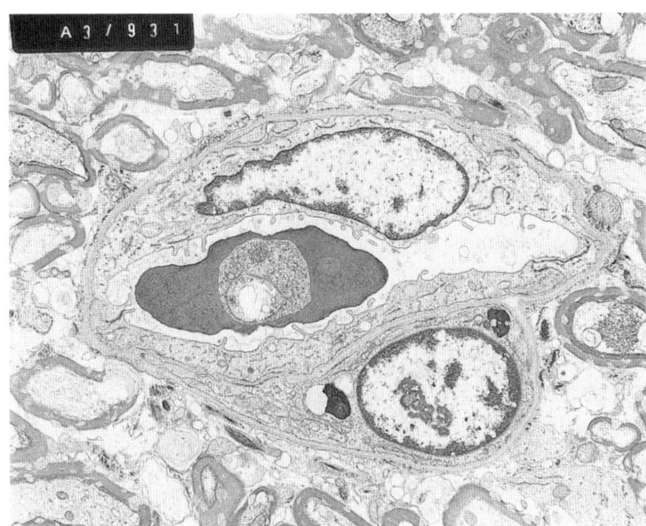

Fig. 7.8.2.14 Human cerebral malaria. Electron micrograph showing endothelial cell microvilli making contact with a parasitized erythrocyte.
(Copyright Dr N Francis.)

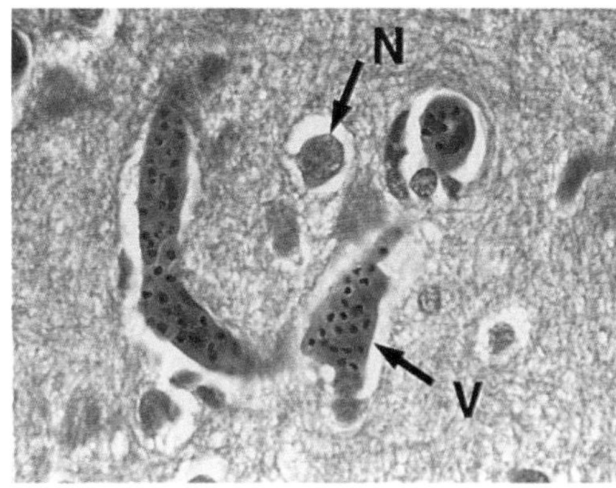

Fig. 7.8.2.15 Section of frontal cortex from a Vietnamese patient who died of cerebral malaria, showing sequestration of parasitized red blood corpuscles in blood vessels. N, neuron; V, vessel.
(Courtesy of Dr Gareth Turner, Oxford.)

local blood flow probably results in reduced perfusion and tissue damage. However it seems likely that this is just one part of a complex set of responses set in train by the interaction of sequestered cells and endothelial cells and the cells of the immune system leading to local release of a number of potentially toxic or pharmacologically active compounds (such as reactive oxygen species or nitric oxide).

Several endothelial receptors for infected RBC cytoadherence have been identified, including CD36 (formerly platelet glycoprotein IV), thrombospondin, ICAM-1, VCAM-1, and E-selectin. No clear correlation has yet emerged between the ability of parasites to bind to individual receptors and disease pattern (other than in the case of pregnancy-associated malaria), though there is suggestive evidence that severe disease in children maybe associated with the ability of parasites to utilize multiple receptors. Some parasite isolates show two other adhesive properties: the rosetting of uninfected erythrocytes around RBCs containing mature developmental forms of the parasite (Fig. 7.8.2.16) and autoagglutination of infected erythrocytes in the absence of immune serum. Both phenomena have been linked to severe malaria and it is presumed that the multicellular aggregates, if they occur *in vivo*, may exacerbate vascular obstruction caused by sequestration.

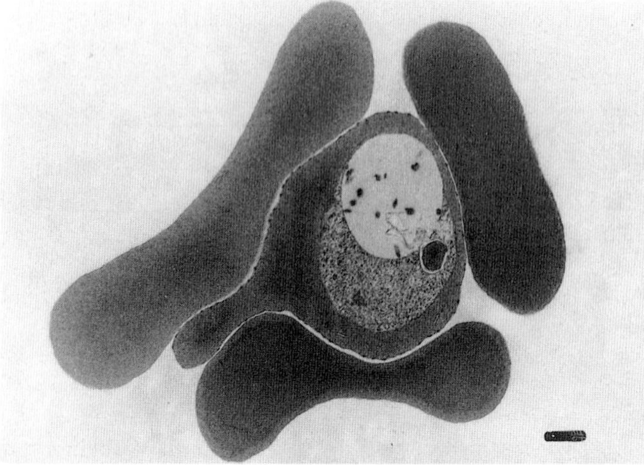

Fig. 7.8.2.16 Rosetting *in vitro*. The central parasitized erythrocyte shows many electron-dense protuberances (knobs) beneath its membrane (bar = 1 μm).
(Copyright Professor D Ferguson.)

On the parasite side of the equation, PfEMP1 plays a key role in cytoadherent interactions, with binding to different receptors localized to different domains of the molecule. The case of pregnancy-associated malaria offers one example where a specific set of PfEMP1 molecules with the ability to bind to a specific receptor (chondroitin sulphate) forms the basis of organ specific biology and pathology. It remains to be seen whether similar subsets of PfEMP1 molecules will be identified associated with other clinical syndromes.

Severe anaemia is a common part of the picture of severe malaria, especially in young children. Although destruction of parasitized RBCs *per se*, especially in a heavy infection, may lead to a significant fall in haemoglobin, it has long been recognized that this cannot account for the often profound degree of anaemia. Two additional processes seem to be important: the sensitization of RBCs with immune complexes and activated components of the complement system leading to immune mediated removal of non-infected cells and a degree of dyserythropoiesis.

Although an episode of *P. falciparum* malaria is potentially life threatening, in endemic areas the large majority of clinical episodes resolve (albeit after an unpleasant illness) without producing severe disease and death. Clearly behavioural factors such as treatment-seeking behaviour are important, but it also seems likely that the wide range of outcomes represent a balance between host and parasite specific factors. In the end, it may be that severe disease represents the unfortunate coincidence of the wrong host with the wrong parasite.

Organ pathology

Brain

Probably only falciparum malaria causes cerebral pathology although *P. vivax*-infected RBCs may also be sequestered. At autopsy, the brain may be oedematous, especially in African children, but there is rarely any evidence of cerebral, cerebellar, or medullary herniation. Small blood vessels, including those of the leptomeninges, are congested with PRBCs. Many of the parasites are schizonts and mature trophozoites containing malaria pigment (Figs. 7.8.2.13 and 7.8.2.14), giving the surface of the brain a characteristic leaden or plum-coloured appearance. Its cut surface is slate grey. In larger vessels, PRBCs form a layer along the endothelium ('margination'). Up to 70% of RBCs in the cerebral vessels are parasitized and are more tightly packed than in other organs. The cerebrovascular endothelium shows pseudopodial projections, closely apposed to electron-dense, knob-like protruberances on the surface of PRBCs (Fig. 7.8.2.14). Numerous petechial haemorrhages are seen in the white matter, the result of bleeding from end arterioles, proximal to occlusive plugs of PRBCs, and fibrin. Ring haemorrhages are centred on small subcortical vessels. They may organize, attracting small collections of microglial cells around an area of demyelination without inflammatory cells (Dürck's granulomas).

Retina

Retinal whitening is associated with swelling of neurons secondary to local hypoxia and haemorrhages are caused by blockage of small retinal vessels with PRBCs and microthrombi.

Bone marrow

In the acute phase of falciparum malaria, there is iron sequestration, erythrophagocytosis, dyserythropoiesis, and cytoadherence with plugging of sinusoids. Maturation defects are present in the marrow for at least 3 weeks after clearance of parasitaemia. Increased numbers of large, abnormal-looking megakaryocytes have been found in the marrow and the circulating platelets may also be enlarged, suggesting dysthrombopoiesis. Malarial pigment and parasites may be found in monocytes and phagocytes in the marrow, even when they are not detectable in peripheral blood.

Liver

The liver is most severely affected in *P. falciparum* malaria. It becomes enlarged and oedematous and is coloured brown, grey, or even black from deposition of malaria pigment. Hepatic sinusoids are dilated, containing hypertrophied Kupffer cells and PRBCs obstructing the circulation. Parasitized and uninfected RBCs are phagocytosed by Kupffer cells, endothelial cells, and sinusoidal macrophages. The small areas of centrilobular necrosis present in severe cases may be attributable to shock or disseminated intravascular coagulation. Hepatocytes appear only mildly abnormal but are depleted of glycogen in some hypoglycaemic patients. Lymphocytic infiltration of portal tracts has been described in some cases of tropical splenomegaly syndrome, a chronic immunological complication of malaria.

Gastrointestinal tract

Cytoadherent, sequestered, PRBCs may be found in the small and large bowel, especially in capillaries of the lamina propria and larger submucosal vessels. The bowel may appear congested, with mucosal ulceration and haemorrhage.

Kidney

Renal failure, with or without 'blackwater fever', is a common and serious complication of severe falciparum malaria in some populations. It is usually associated with acute tubular injury rather than glomerulonephritis. Glomerular lesions consist of mild accumulations of monocytes within glomerular capillaries (acute transient glomerulonephritis) without immune complex deposition. There is PRBC sequestration in glomerular and tubulointerstitial vessels, with fibrin thrombi and pigment-laden macrophages. Tubular pigment casts are prominent in cases of blackwater fever and severe rhabdomyolysis.

Levels of parasite sequestration in the kidney are usually relatively low. They correlates with premortem renal failure, and are significantly higher in malaria-associated renal failure than in fatal cases without renal failure. In quartan malarial nephrosis, a chronic immunological complication of malaria, a distinctive chronic glomerulonephritis develops.

Lung

At autopsy, the lungs are found to be oedematous in almost every case. Pulmonary capillaries and venules are packed with PRBCs and inflammatory cells: neutrophils, plasma cells, and pigment-laden macrophages. The capillary lumen is narrowed by oedema of vascular endothelium and there is interstitial oedema and hyaline-membrane formation. Secondary bronchopneumonia is commonly found.

Spleen

The spleen is enlarged, engorged, and coloured dark red or grayish black. The red and white pulp is congested and hyperplastic, and the splenic cords and sinuses are filled with phagocytic cells containing pigment, PRBCs, and noninfected RBCs. Macrophages may extract the parasites from PRBCs, a process known as 'pitting'. Tropical splenomegaly syndrome is a chronic immunological complication of malaria (see below).

Heart

Myocardial capillaries are congested with pigment-laden macrophages, lymphocytes, plasma cells, and PRBCs but these are not tightly packed or cytoadherent. Subendocardial and epicardial petechial haemorrhages are unusual and there is no myocarditis.

Placenta

Sinusoids are packed with PRBCs and pigment-laden macrophages, giving the placenta a black or slate-grey hue. Necrosis of the syncytiotrophoblast, fibrinoid necrosis, loss of villi, proliferation of cytotrophoblastic cells, and thickening of the trophoblastic membrane may explain impaired fetal nutrition. Although transmission of infection across an intact placenta is considered uncommon, PRBCs are sometimes visible in fetal–placental vessels.

Pathophysiology

Anaemia and thrombocytopenia

Malarial anaemia results from destruction/phagocytosis of PRBCs and dyserythropoiesis. Hyperferritinaemia, an acute-phase reaction, explains the initial iron sequestration and hypoferraemia. Immune-mediated haemolysis occurs in some populations. Erythrocyte survival is reduced even after the disappearance of parasitaemia and there is increased splenic clearance of nonparasitized RBCs and PRBCs. Evidence of Coombs' test-positive haemolysis was found in the Gambia. Intravascular haemolysis occurs in patients whose erythrocytes are congenitally deficient in enzymes such as G6PD in response to oxidant drugs such as primaquine. In classic blackwater fever, G6PD levels are, by definition, normal and the mechanism of haemolysis is unknown. Quinine mediated haemolysis is suspected but has never been satisfactorily demonstrated. Thrombocytopenia is attributable to splenic sequestration, dysthrombopoiesis, and immune-mediated lysis.

Cerebral malaria

In Thai adults with cerebral malaria, global cerebral blood flow was inappropriately low and there was evidence of cerebral anaerobic glycolysis with increased lactate concentrations in the cerebrospinal fluid. Recently, in Bangladeshi patients with severe malaria, orthogonal polarization spectral imaging was used directly to observe the rectal mucosa, as a surrogate for the cerebral microcirculation. Microcirculatory obstruction (proportion of vessels involved and the degree of obstruction) correlated with disease severity and decreased on clinical recovery. Vessels with little or no blood flow were often seen adjacent to vessels with hyperdynamic blood flow.

In African children with cerebral malaria, plasma concentrations of TNFα, IL-1α, and other cytokines correlate closely with disease severity, as judged by parasitaemia, hypoglycaemia, case fatality, and the incidence of neurological sequelae. Cytokines may have other effects on cerebral function, perhaps by releasing nitric oxide, which interferes with neurotransmission, or by leading to the generation of free oxygen radicals. Cytokines may also cause fever, hypoglycaemia, coagulopathy, dyserythropoiesis, and leucocytosis in falciparum malaria.

In South-East Asian adults, the opening pressure of cerebrospinal fluid at lumbar puncture was usually normal. Cerebral oedema was demonstrable by CT during life in only a small minority, usually as an agonal phenomenon. In these patients, there was little evidence of increased blood–cerebrospinal fluid barrier permeability or that brain swelling was responsible for coma. However, in African children with cerebral malaria, intracranial pressure, as reflected by cerebrospinal fluid opening pressure at lumbar puncture, is usually elevated and the majority have swollen brains. In fatal cases, the brain shows evidence of increased vascular permeability. Ischaemic damage, resulting from a critical reduction in cerebral perfusion pressure, hypoglycaemia, and status epilepticus, probably contributes to brain damage in these children.

Pulmonary oedema

This may be provoked by fluid overload, in which case, central venous and pulmonary artery wedge pressures will be elevated. More commonly, the clinical picture is of acute respiratory distress syndrome (ARDS), with normal or low hydrostatic pressures in the pulmonary vascular bed. In these cases, the mechanism is likely to be increased pulmonary capillary permeability resulting from leucocyte products and cytokines, consistent with the histological appearances of neutrophil sequestration in the pulmonary capillaries, increased permeability, and hyaline membrane formation.

Hypoglycaemia and other metabolic disturbances

Cinchona alkaloids (quinine or quinidine) are potent stimulators of insulin secretion by the pancreatic β-cells, causing hyperinsulinaemia. The resulting reduction in hepatic gluconeogenesis and increased peripheral glucose uptake by tissues causes hypoglycaemia. In malaria, glucose consumption is increased by fever, infection, anaerobic glycolysis, and the metabolic demands of the malaria parasites. Glycogen reserves may be depleted, especially in children and pregnant women, as a result of fasting and 'accelerated starvation'. In African children with severe malaria, adult patients with severe disease, and pregnant women, hypoglycaemia develops spontaneously (without treatment with cinchona alkaloids) and is associated with appropriately low plasma insulin concentrations. Plasma lactate and alanine concentrations are elevated and ketone bodies are moderately increased. Counter-regulatory hormone levels are usually very high. The mechanism of hypoglycaemia in these cases may be inhibition of hepatic gluconeogenesis by TNFα and other cytokines. In African children, severe anaemia, tissue hypoxia, hypoperfusion, and increased anaerobic glycolysis by host and parasites contribute to profound metabolic (lactic) acidosis, manifesting clinically as respiratory distress.

Acute renal failure

Oliguria and renal dysfunction reversible by fluid replacement are attributable to hypovolaemia resulting from dehydration. Hyperparasitaemia, jaundice, and haemoglobinuria are risk factors for acute tubular necrosis. Renal cortical perfusion is reduced during the acute stage of the disease but renal cortical necrosis is rare and survivors rarely show evidence of chronic renal impairment. Cytoadherence of PRBCs in the renal microvasculature, deposition of fibrin microthrombi, prolonged hypotension ('algid malaria'), haemoglobinuria in 'blackwater fever' and myoglobinuria may contribute to acute renal failure. Quartan malarial nephrosis is a chronic immunological complication of malaria (see below).

Hyponatraemia

In patients with relatively normal plasma osmolalities, hyponatraemia has been attributed to the inappropriate secretion of ADH triggered by fever or reduced effective plasma volume. However, in Thai patients, ADH levels were appropriate to their gross hypovolaemia. This has been confirmed in Bangladeshi patients. In those who are salt depleted and dehydrated, mild hyponatraemia is often attributable to intravenous therapy with 5% dextrose.

Hypovolaemia and 'shock' ('algid malaria')

Hypotension may be explained by hypovolaemia (dehydration and, rarely, haemorrhagic shock following splenic rupture or gastrointestinal haemorrhage) but is most often associated with a secondary Gram-negative bacteraemia. The source may be an intravenous cannula, urethral catheter, aspiration pneumonia, or invasion of the bloodstream by an enteric pathogen such as salmonella. Transient immunosuppression, impaired macrophage function, or 'blockade' of the reticuloendothelial system may increase the susceptibility of patients to severe secondary bacterial infections.

Clinical features in adults and children

Malaria is typically an acute febrile illness that, if incompletely treated, tends to recrudesce or relapse over periods of months or even years. The classic periodic febrile paroxysms—occurring every 24 h (quotidian), 36 h (subtertian), 48 to 50 h (tertian), or 72 h (quartan) with afebrile asymptomatic intervals—are rarely observed unless treatment is delayed. Severity depends on the species and strain and, hence, on the geographical origin of the infecting parasite, on the age, genetic constitution, state of immunity, general health, and nutritional state of the patients, and on the speed and appropriateness of antimalarial treatment.

Falciparum malaria ('malignant' tertian or subtertian malaria)

The 'prepatent period', the shortest interval between an infecting mosquito bite and detectable parasitaemia, is usually 9 or 10 days but may be as short as 5 days (Table 7.8.2.1). The incubation period, the interval between infection and the first symptom, usually ranges from 7 to 14 days (mean 12 days) but may be prolonged by immunity, chemoprophylaxis, or partial chemotherapy. In Europe and North America, 98% of patients with imported falciparum malaria present within 3 months of arriving back from the malarious area. A few present up to 1 year later, but none after 4 years.

Several days of prodromal symptoms such as malaise, headache, myalgia, anorexia, and mild fever are interrupted by the first paroxysm. Suddenly the patient feels inexplicably cold (in a hot climate) and apprehensive. Mild shivering quickly turns into violent shaking with teeth chattering. There is intense peripheral vasoconstriction and gooseflesh. Some patients vomit. The rapid increase in core temperature may trigger febrile convulsions in young children. The rigor lasts up to 1 h and is followed by a hot flush with throbbing headache, palpitations, tachypnoea, prostration, postural syncope, and further vomiting while the temperature reaches its peak. Finally, a drenching sweat breaks out and the fever defervesces over the next few hours. The exhausted patient sleeps. The whole paroxysm is over in 8 to 12 h, after which the patient may feel remarkably well. These symptoms are typical of a classical 'endotoxin reaction' produced by infection with Gram-negative bacteria or the release of TNFα and other cytokines by other agents. Classic tertian or subtertian periodicity is rarely seen with falciparum malaria. A high irregularly spiking, continuous, or remittent fever or daily (quotidian) paroxysm is more usual. Other common symptoms are headache, backache, myalgias, dizziness, postural hypotension, nausea, dry cough, abdominal discomfort, diarrhoea, and vomiting. Nonimmune patients with falciparum malaria are usually severely unwell. Commonly, there is anaemia and mild jaundice, with moderate tender enlargement of the spleen and liver. Useful negative findings are the lack of lymphadenopathy, rash (apart from herpes simplex 'cold sores'), and focal signs.

Severe falciparum malaria

WHO (2000) has defined severe disease by the clinical and laboratory features shown in Box 7.8.2.2.

Cerebral malaria

The global average case fatality of falciparum malaria is about 1%, or 1 to 3 million deaths per year. Cerebral malaria is an important severe manifestation of *P. falciparum* infection, accounting for a large proportion of adult deaths. Patients who have been feverish and ill for a few days may have a generalized convulsion from which they do not recover consciousness, or their level of consciousness may decline gradually over several hours. High fever alone can impair cerebral function causing drowsiness, delirium, obtundation, confusion, irritability, psychosis, and, in children, febrile convulsions. The term 'cerebral malaria', implying encephalopathy specifically related to *P. falciparum* infection, should be restricted to patients: (1) who are unrousable and comatose, showing no appropriate verbal response and no purposive motor response to noxious stimuli (Glasgow Coma Scale ≤9/14); (2) who have evidence of acute *P. falciparum* infection; and (3) in whom other encephalopathies, including hypoglycaemia and transient postictal coma, have been excluded. Mild meningism may be elicited but neck rigidity and photophobia are rare. Retinal abnormalities (Fig. 7.8.2.17) are best seen with the pupils dilated with 0.5 to 1% tropicamide and 2.5% phenylephrine. Haemorrhages like Roth spots, papilloedema, or exudates are present in about 15% of South-East Asian adults with cerebral malaria. In African children with cerebral malaria, retinal changes include macular and peripheral retinal whitening, vessel changes (orange vessels, tramlining, capillary whitening), retinal haemorrhages, papilloedema, and cotton wool spots. Of these changes, the whitening and vessel changes are specific ('malarial retinopathy') and are associated with a case fatality of about 18%, compared with 44% in children with papilloedema and 7% in those with normal fundi.

In adult patients, pupillary, corneal, oculocephalic, and oculovestibular reflexes are normal. Dysconjugate gaze is common. Muscle tone and tendon reflexes are usually increased and there is ankle clonus. Plantar responses are extensor and abdominal reflexes are absent. In African children, brainstem reflexes may be abnormal and there may be neurological evidence of severe intracranial hypertension with rostrocaudal progression suggesting cerebral, cerebellar, and medullary herniation. Hypotonia is more common than in adults. Patients of all ages may show abnormal flexor or extensor posturing (decerebrate or decorticate rigidity), associated with sustained upward deviation of the eyes, pouting, and grunting respiration (Fig. 7.8.2.18). Hypoglycaemia must be excluded. Most children with cerebral malaria and about half the adult patients experience generalized convulsions. In children, seizures may be covert and difficult to detect. Twitching of the facial muscles or the corner of the mouth, deviation of gaze with nystagmus, irregularities of breathing, and stereotyped posturing of one arm may provide the only clue (Fig. 7.8.2.19). Fewer than 5% of adult survivors have persisting neurological sequelae: these include cranial nerve lesions, extrapyramidal tremor, and transient paranoid psychosis. However, more than 10% of African children who survive an attack of cerebral malaria have sequelae such as hemiplegia, cortical blindness, epilepsy, ataxia, or cognitive and learning disabilities.

Box 7.8.2.2 Features of severe falciparum malaria

Clinical manifestations

- Prostration
- Impaired consciousness
- Respiratory distress (acidotic breathing)
- Multiple convulsions
- Circulatory collapse
- Pulmonary oedema (radiological)
- Abnormal bleeding
- Jaundice
- Haemoglobinuria

Laboratory tests

- Severe anaemia (haemoglobin <5 g/dl or haematocrit <15%)
- Hypoglycaemia (blood glucose <2.2 mmol/litre or 40 mg/dl)
- Acidosis (plasma bicarbonate <15 mmol/litre, or base excess more than −10, or arterial pH <7.35)
- Renal impairment (urine output <12 ml/kg/h, or plasma creatinine above age-related normal range; persisting after rehydration)
- Hyperlactataemia (plasma lactate >5 mmol/litre)

Other severe manifestations and complications

Anaemia (see above) is an inevitable consequence of all but the mildest infections. It is most common and severe in pregnant women, children (Fig. 7.8.2.20), and in patients with high parasitaemia, schizontaemia, secondary bacterial infections, and renal failure. Spontaneous bleeding from the gums (Fig. 7.8.2.21) and gastrointestinal tract is seen in fewer than 5% of adult patients with severe malaria and is rare in children. Jaundice (Fig. 7.8.2.22) is common in adults but rare in children. Biochemical evidence of severe hepatic dysfunction is most unusual and hepatic failure suggests concomitant viral hepatitis or another diagnosis.

Hypoglycaemia is an important complication. Quinine or quinidine treatment can cause hypoglycaemia in pregnant women with

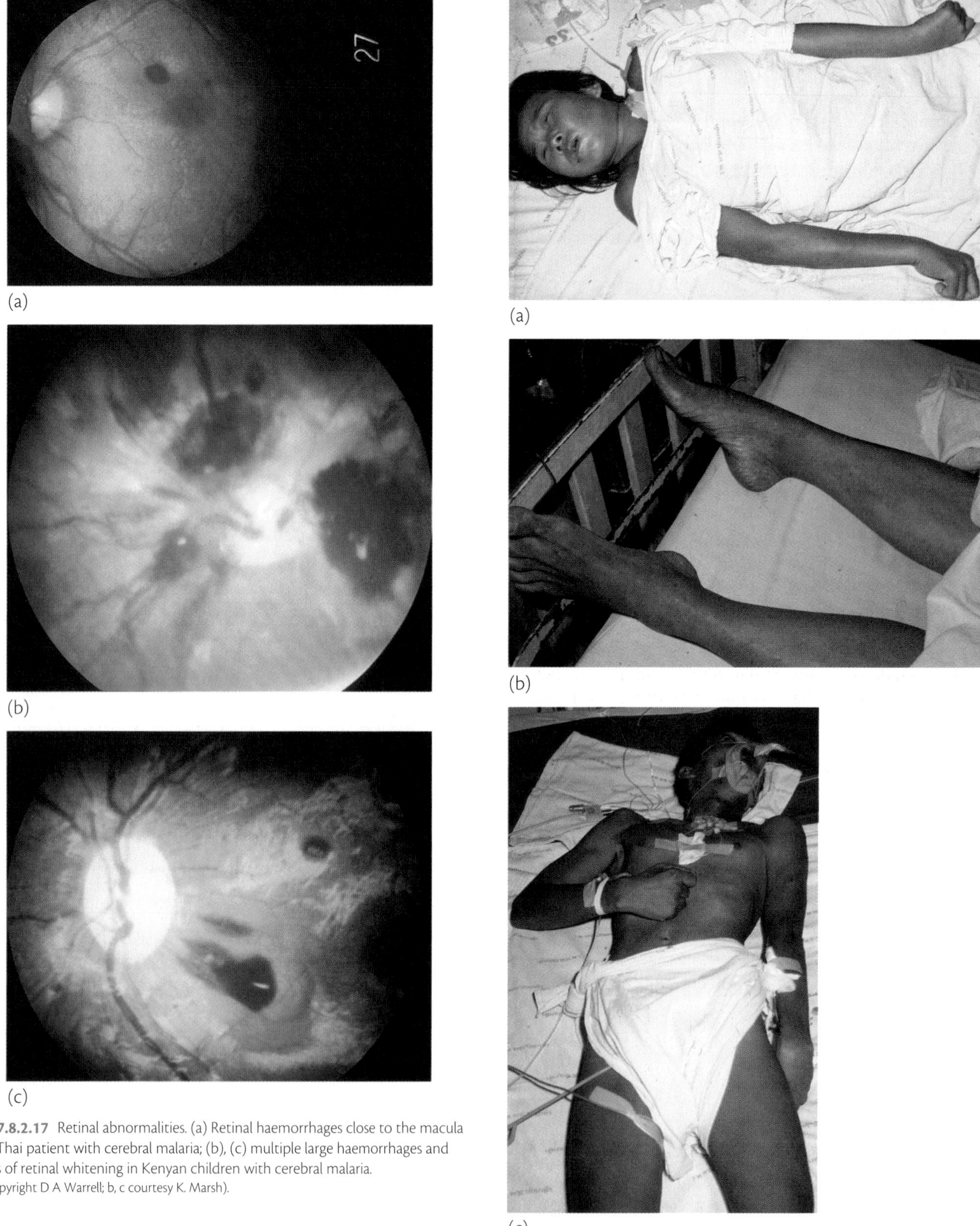

Fig. 7.8.2.17 Retinal abnormalities. (a) Retinal haemorrhages close to the macula in a Thai patient with cerebral malaria; (b), (c) multiple large haemorrhages and areas of retinal whitening in Kenyan children with cerebral malaria. (a, copyright D A Warrell; b, c courtesy K. Marsh).

Fig. 7.8.2.18 (a, b) Extensor posturing (decerebrate rigidity) in a Thai woman with cerebral malaria and profound hypoglycaemia; and (c) extensor posturing (decorticate rigidity) in a Thai man with cerebral malaria. (Copyright D A Warrell.)

severe or uncomplicated falciparum malaria and in any patient with severe disease. This develops a few hours to 6 days after starting this treatment, even after the parasitaemia has cleared. However, even in the absence of quinine or quinidine treatment, pregnant women and children with falciparum malaria and patients with hyperparasitaemia or complicating bacteraemia may become hypoglycaemic

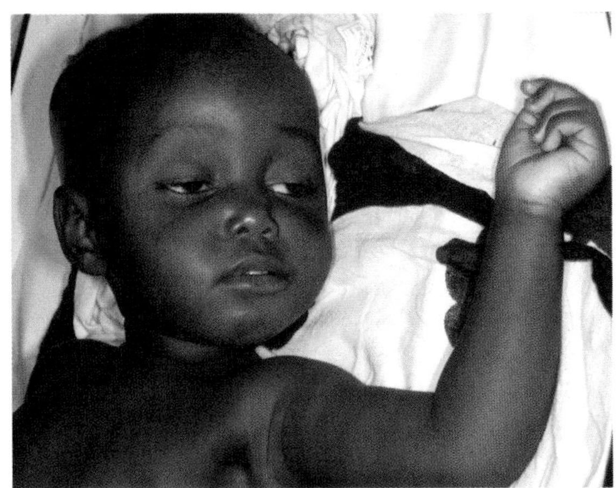

Fig. 7.8.2.19 Covert seizure in a child with cerebral malaria. Note deviation of eyes to the left, retraction of the corner of the mouth, and posturing of the left arm. (Copyright D A Warrell.)

early in their illness. Clinical features of hypoglycaemia include anxiety, tachycardia, breathlessness, feeling cold, confusion, sweating, light-headedness, restlessness, fetal bradycardia or other signs of fetal distress, coma, convulsions, and extensor posturing. All may be misinterpreted as manifestations of malaria *per se*.

Hypotension and shock ('algid malaria') is a consequence of pulmonary oedema, metabolic acidosis, gastrointestinal haemorrhage, and complicating Gram-negative bacteraemias. Mild supine hypotension with postural drop in blood pressure is caused by vasodilatation and relative hypovolaemia. Cardiac arrhythmias are rare but may be precipitated by too rapid intravenous infusion or excessive doses of chloroquine, quinine, or quinidine. Patients with coronary insufficiency may develop angina during febrile crises of malaria.

Renal dysfunction, indicated by oliguria and increased blood urea and serum creatinine concentrations, occurs in about one-third of adults with severe malaria but is uncommon in children. Most patients respond to cautious rehydration, but 10% develop renal failure requiring dialysis.

In patients whose RBCs are congenitally deficient in G6PD or other enzymes, intravascular haemolysis and haemoglobinuria (Fig. 7.8.2.23) may be precipitated by oxidant antimalarial drugs such as primaquine and tafenoquine, whether or not they have malaria. Classic blackwater fever is the association of haemoglobinuria from massive intravascular haemolysis, not explicable by G6PD deficiency, with severe manifestations of falciparum malaria, such as renal failure, hypotension, and coma, in a nonimmune patient.

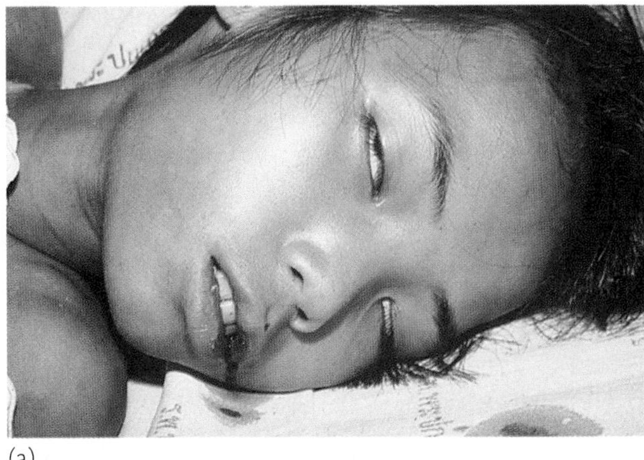

(a)

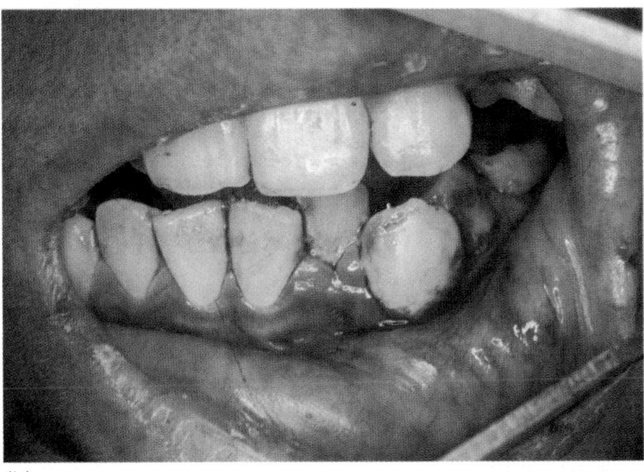

(b)

Fig. 7.8.2.21 Cerebral malaria. (a), (b) Spontaneous systemic bleeding from a gingival sulci in a Thai patient with disseminated intravascular coagulation. (Copyright D A Warrell.)

Metabolic acidosis is seen in association with hyperparasitaemia, hypoglycaemia, and renal failure. It is usually lactic acidosis. In African children, respiratory distress with deep (Kussmaul)

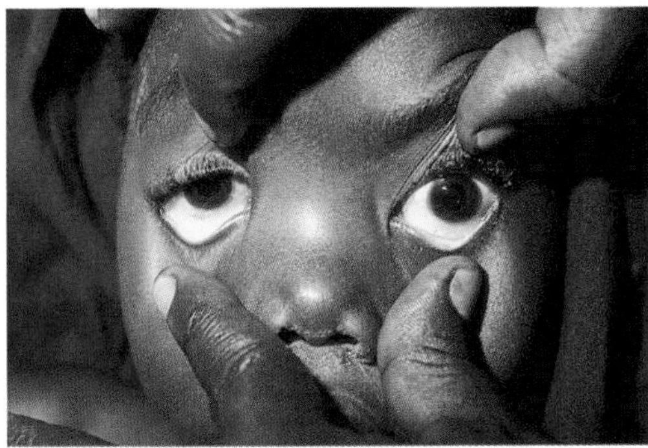

Fig. 7.8.2.20 Profound anaemia (haemoglobin 1.2 g/dl) in a Kenyan child with *P. falciparum* parasitaemia. (Copyright D A Warrell.)

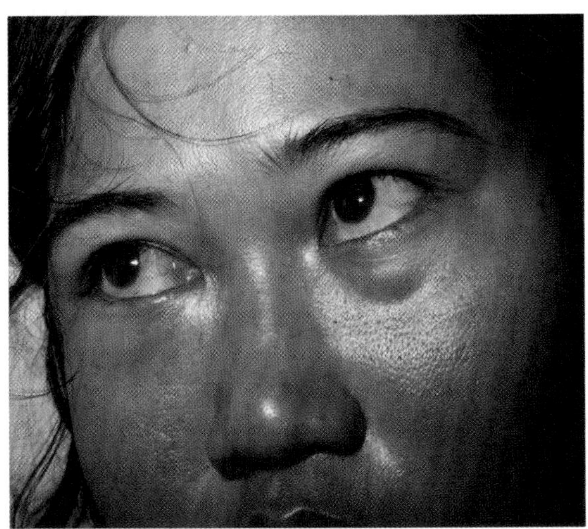

Fig. 7.8.2.22 Jaundice in a Thai woman with severe malaria. (Copyright D A Warrell.)

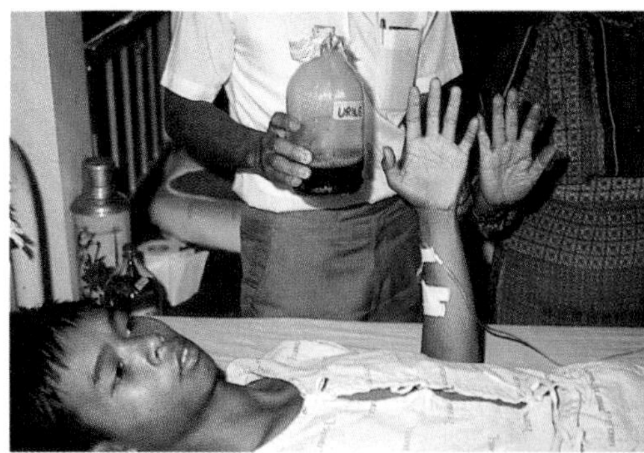

Fig. 7.8.2.23 Intravascular haemolysis in a Karen patient with glucose-6-phosphate dehydrogenase deficiency in whom treatment with an oxidant drug resulted in haemoglobinuria and anaemia (normal hand in comparison).
(Copyright D A Warrell.)

breathing (Fig. 7.8.2.24), associated with severe anaemia and metabolic acidosis, is a syndrome that carries an even higher case fatality than cerebral malaria.

Pulmonary oedema (Fig. 7.8.2.25) is the terminal event in many adults dying of falciparum malaria. It may be precipitated by fluid overload late in the clinical course but pulmonary oedema can also develop in patients with severe disease in normal fluid balance, in which case jugular venous, central venous, or pulmonary artery wedge pressures are normal, as in ARDS. In pregnant women, pulmonary oedema may evolve suddenly after delivery. The earliest sign is an increase in respiratory rate. Without a chest radiograph, pulmonary oedema may be difficult to differentiate from aspiration pneumonia, a common complication in comatose patients, or metabolic acidosis.

Cerebellar dysfunction

A rare presentation of falciparum malaria is cerebellar ataxia with unimpaired consciousness. Similar signs may be seen in patients recovering from cerebral malaria. In Sri Lanka, a syndrome of delayed cerebellar ataxia has been described 3 to 4 weeks after an attack of fever attributed to falciparum malaria. Complete recovery is the rule.

Malarial psychosis

The term 'malarial psychosis' has been uncritically applied, often without proven aetiology. Acute psychiatric symptoms in patients with malaria may be attributable to their drug treatment, including antimalarial drugs such as chloroquine, mefloquine, and the obsolete mepacrine, and to exacerbation of pre-existing functional psychoses. However, in some patients, organic mental disturbances associated with malaria infection have been the presenting feature or, more often, have developed during convalescence after attacks of otherwise uncomplicated malaria or cerebral malaria. Depression, paranoia, delusions, and personality changes associated with malaria are classified as brief reactive psychoses. These symptoms rarely last for more than a few days.

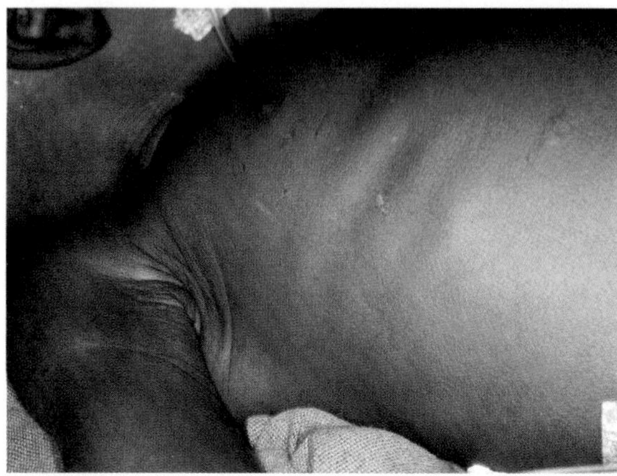

Fig. 7.8.2.24 Respiratory distress with acidotic 'Kussmaul' breathing in a child with severe malaria.
(Copyright D A Warrell.)

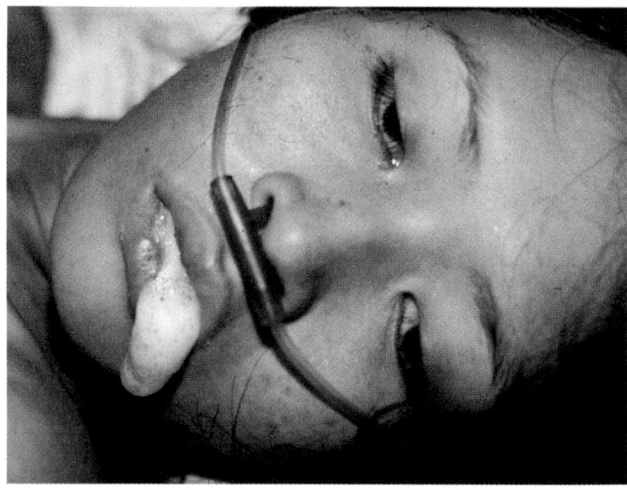

Fig. 7.8.2.25 Pulmonary oedema in a Thai woman developing soon after delivering a stillborn baby.
(Courtesy of the late Professor Sornchai Looareesuwan.)

Vivax, ovale, and malariae malarias

The prepatent and incubation periods are given in Table 7.8.2.1. Some strains of *P. vivax*, especially those from temperate regions (*P. v. hibernans* from Russia, *P. v. multinucleatum* from China) may have very long incubation periods (250–637 days). Only about one-third of imported cases of vivax malaria present within a month of returning from the malarious area; between 5 and 10% will present more than 1 year later.

The inappropriately termed 'benign' malarias cause paroxysmal, feverish symptoms even more hectic and distressing than those of falciparum malaria. Prodromal symptoms may be more severe with *P. malariae* infection. The characteristic tertian interval between fever spikes in *P. vivax* and *P. ovale* infections and the quartan pattern in *P. malariae* infections is established after several days of irregular fever if treatment is delayed. Vivax and ovale malarias have a persistent hepatic cycle, which may give rise to relapses every 2 or 3 months for 5 to 8 years in untreated cases. *P. malariae* does not relapse but a persisting, undetectable parasitaemia may cause recrudescences for more than 50 years.

Vivax malaria

People of West African origin are inherently resistant to *P. vivax* infection. Although symptoms may be severe and temporarily incapacitating, especially in nonimmunes, the acute mortality of vivax malaria is very low. During the 1967–9 Sri Lankan epidemic of predominantly vivax malaria, there were more than 500 000 cases with a case fatality of only 0.1%. Acutely, vivax malaria can cause anaemia, thrombocytopenia, and mild jaundice with tender hepatosplenomegaly. Rarely, the anaemia may be severe enough to be life threatening in debilitated patients and it may contribute to chronic malaise, wasting, malnutrition, and underperformance. Splenic rupture, which carries a mortality of 80%, may be more common with vivax than falciparum malaria. It results from acute, rapid enlargement of the spleen, with or without trauma. Chronically enlarged spleens are less vulnerable. Splenic rupture presents with abdominal pain and guarding, signs of haemorrhagic shock, fever, and a rapidly falling haematocrit. These features may be misattributed to malaria itself. In pregnancy, vivax malaria contributes to maternal anaemia and reduced birth weight. Cerebral vivax malaria has occasionally been reported especially with *P. v. multinucleatum* in China. Mixed *P. falciparum* infection or another encephalopathy must be adequately excluded in such cases. Acute noncardiogenic pulmonary oedema is an increasingly recognized complication of vivax malaria in nonimmune people. Clearly, the pathogenicity and clinical consequences of vivax malaria deserve re-evaluation.

Ovale and malariae malarias

Acute symptoms may be as severe as those of vivax infection, but anaemia is less severe and the risk of splenic rupture is lower although splenomegaly may be particularly gross in areas where *P. malariae* is prevalent. *P. ovale* causes negligible mortality, but *P. malariae* causes chronic morbidity and mortality from nephrotic syndrome and tropical splenomegaly syndrome. The same strictures apply to cerebral *malariae* malaria as to cerebral vivax malaria, especially as *P. malariae* coexists with *P. falciparum* throughout most of its range.

Monkey malarias

Knowlesi malaria

Recently, *P. knowlesi* infection in humans has been recognized as an important zoonosis in several South-East Asian countries. It is probably not new but has been overlooked. It is transmitted among long-tailed macaques *Macaca fascicularis* and related cercopithecine monkeys by jungle mosquitoes of the *An. leucosphyrus* group (notably *An. latens*) and causes fatal malaria in rhesus monkeys *M. mulatta*. *P. knowlesi* was first identified as an important cause of human malaria in Kapit Division, Sarawak (Malaysia), in 2000–2, where 120 (58%) of malaria cases were found to be infected. It had been confused microscopically with *P. malariae* because early trophozoites may appear as band forms, although these are not always seen (Fig. 7.8.2.26). Using *P. knowlesi*-specific PCR primers, about 30% of human cases of malaria in Sarawak, together with cases in Sabah, Palawan (Philippines), Pahang (peninsular Malaysia), Thailand, Burma, and Singapore, have been identified. Increasing human encroachment into the jungle habitat in South-East Asia and possibly an adaptive switch in pathogenicity suggest that *P. knowlesi* infection may become more important. It is currently regarded as a zoonosis because human-to-human transmission has not yet been demonstrated.

Clinical features

There are daily spikes of fever (quotidian periodicity). Four fatal cases in Sarawak had fever and chills, abdominal pain and other gastrointestinal and pulmonary symptoms, jaundice, hypotension,

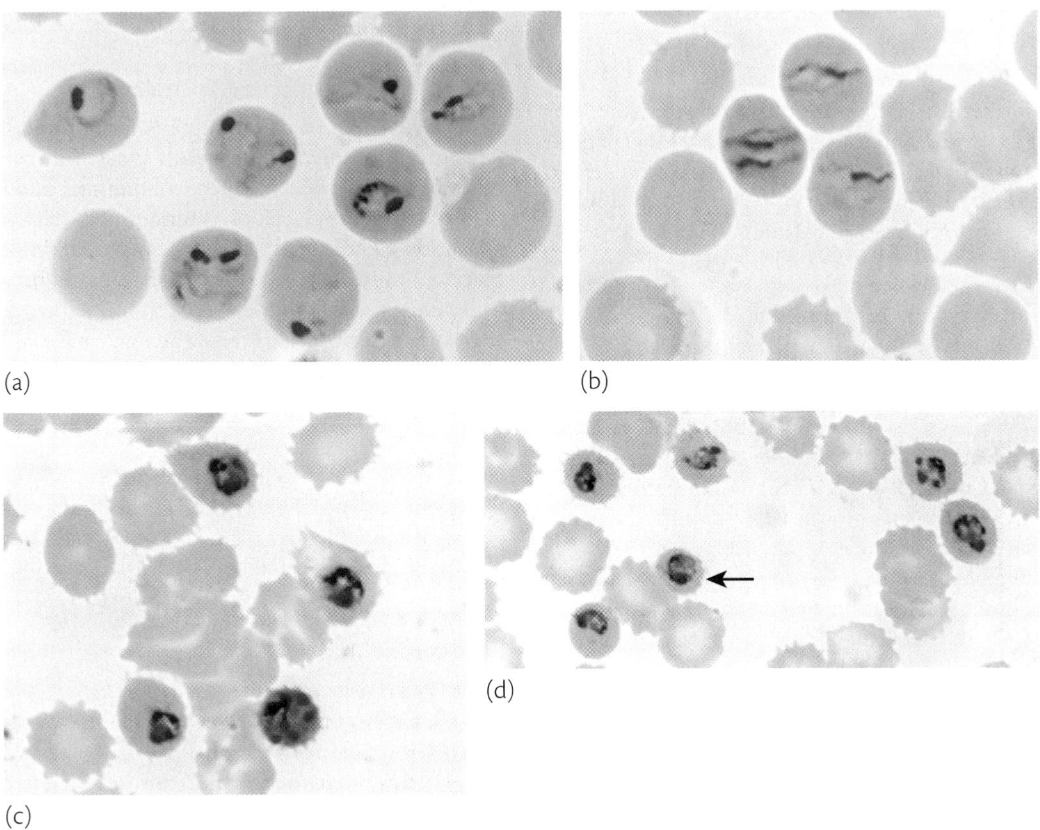

Fig. 7.8.2.26 *P. knowlesi* from human patient on Geimsa-stained blood films. Showing (a) rings and early trophozoites, (b) band forms resembling *P. malariae* (these are not always seen), (c) trophozoites and early schizonts, and (d) trophozoites, early schizonts, and possible gametocyte (arrow).
(Copyright Professor J Cox-Singh.)

acute renal failure, and hyperparasitaemia (764 720 parasites/μl in one case). In Malaysian Borneo, about 10% of patients develop potentially fatal complications and the case fatality is 1.8%.

Other monkey malarias

Human erythrocytes can be infected with at least five other species of simian plasmodia. There have been rare cases of natural infections or accidental laboratory infections by *P. brasilianum*, *P. cynomolgi*, *P. inui*, *P. schwetzi*, and *P. simium*. Severe feverish and systemic symptoms have been described, but no cerebral or other severe complications. No patient has died. Parasitaemia may remain undetectable for 2 to 6 days after the start of symptoms. Periodicity is tertian in *P. simium* and *P. cynomolgi* infections. Infectivity and virulence may be enhanced by repeated passage in humans.

Malaria in pregnancy and the puerperium

Malaria is an important cause of maternal anaemia and death, abortion, stillbirth, premature delivery, low birth weight, neonatal death, and congenital malaria in areas of unstable malaria transmission where women of reproductive age have little acquired immunity. In nonimmune women, hyperpyrexia, hypoglycaemia, anaemia, cerebral malaria, and pulmonary oedema are more common in pregnancy. During the great epidemic of falciparum malaria in Sri Lanka in 1934–5, case fatality among pregnant women was 13%, twice that in nonpregnant women. In Thailand, where malaria was at one time the leading cause of maternal mortality, cerebral malaria in late pregnancy had a case fatality of 50%. In some parts of Africa, one-quarter to one-half of all placentas are parasitized. The incidence is highest in primiparae. Changes in humoral and cell mediated immunity in pregnancy do not explain this vulnerability. It is clear that the placenta is a privileged site for parasite multiplication. RBCs infected with strains (genotypes) of *P. falciparum* expressing Var2CSA, a member of the PfEMP1 family, bind to chondroitin sulphate A, a receptor expressed on the surface of the syncytiotrophoblast. Other host receptors, such as hyaluronic acid and the neonatal Fc receptor, may also support placental binding. This may explain sequestration in the placenta. Placental dysfunction, fever, and hypoglycaemia contribute to fetal distress, which is common when malaria strikes in the last trimester of pregnancy. Painless uterine contractions are often detectable by monitoring. They may subside as the patient is cooled.

Special risks to the mother of malaria during pregnancy

Severe anaemia, exacerbated by malaria, is an important complication of pregnancy in many tropical countries that may persist into the puerperium and beyond. Especially in communities where chronic hookworm anaemia is prevalent, high-output anaemic cardiac failure may develop in late pregnancy.

Asymptomatic hypoglycaemia may occur in pregnant women with malaria, without provocation by cinchona alkaloids, and pregnant women with severe uncomplicated malaria are particularly vulnerable to quinine-induced hypoglycaemia. There is an increased risk of pulmonary oedema, precipitated by fluid overload and the sudden increase in peripheral resistance and autotransfusion of hyperparasitaemic blood from the placenta that occurs just after delivery (Fig. 7.8.2.25).

Interaction between malaria and HIV in pregnancy

In HIV-infected pregnant women, the beneficial effects of parity on severity of malaria are attenuated and peripheral and placental parasitaemia and risk of having an episode of malaria and anaemia during pregnancy are increased. Malaria–HIV coinfection is associated with an increased risk of low birth weight, preterm birth, intrauterine growth retardation, and postnatal infant mortality. Malaria transiently increases peripheral blood and placental HIV viral load but whether this affects the risk of vertical transmission of HIV infection or accelerates HIV disease progression is unknown.

Prevention

Whenever possible, pregnant women should avoid living in and, especially, sleeping in malarious areas. Otherwise, they should sleep under insecticide-treated bed nets, should be monitored for infection in an antenatal clinic and should receive intermittent preventive treatment with sulphadoxine–pyrimethamine or antimalarial prophylaxis extending into the early puerperium.

Congenital and neonatal malaria

Congenital or vertically transmitted malaria is diagnosed by detecting parasitaemia in the neonate within 7 days of birth, or later if there is no possibility of postpartum mosquito-borne infection. Save for a few discordant reports, most evidence from malarious parts of the world indicates that congenital malaria is rarely symptomatic, despite the high prevalence of placental infection. This confirms the adequacy of protection provided by IgG from the immune mother, which crosses the placenta, by active immunization from exposure to soluble malarial antigens *in utero* and by the high proportion of fetal haemoglobin in the neonate, which retards parasite development. Congenital malaria is, however, much more common in infants born to nonimmune mothers. Its incidence increases during malaria epidemics and it can cause stillbirth or perinatal death. All four species can produce congenital infection, but, because of its very long persistence, *P. malariae* causes a disproportionate number of cases in nonendemic countries. Fetal plasma quinine and chloroquine concentrations are about one-third of the simultaneous maternal levels. Thus, antimalarial concentrations adequate to cure the mother may be subtherapeutic in the fetus. Quinine and chloroquine are excreted in breast milk, but the suckling neonate would receive only a few milligrams per day. Maternal hypoglycaemia, a common complication of malaria, or its treatment with quinine may produce marked fetal bradycardia and other signs of fetal distress.

Differential diagnosis

Clinical features of congenital malaria are nonspecific: irritability, feeding problems, hepatosplenomegaly, anaemia, and jaundice. Unless parasites are found in a smear from a heel prick or cord blood, the patient may be misdiagnosed as having rhesus incompatibility or another congenital infection such as cytomegalovirus, herpes simplex, rubella, toxoplasmosis, or syphilis.

Transfusion malaria, 'needlestick', and nosocomial malaria

Malaria can be transmitted in blood from apparently healthy donors. Exceptionally, donors may remain infective for up to 5 years with *P. falciparum* and *P. vivax*, 7 years with *P. ovale*, and 46 years with *P. malariae*. Because the infecting parasites are erythrocytic forms (not sporozoites), no exoerythrocytic (hepatic) cycle will be established and so vivax and ovale malarias will not relapse. Theoretically, parasitaemia might be detectable immediately and, hence, the incubation period should be shorter than with mosquito-transmitted malaria. However, the incubation period tends to be longer because of the time needed to build up parasitaemias sufficient to cause symptoms. Mean incubation periods are 12 days (range 7–29 days) for *P. falciparum*, 12 days (range 8–30 days) for *P. vivax*, and 35 days (range 6–106 days) for *P. malariae*. Whole blood, packed cells (blood products), leucocyte or platelet concentrates, fresh plasma, marrow transplants, and haemodialysis have been responsible for transfusion malaria. As patients requiring transfusion are likely to be debilitated and may be immunosuppressed, and there may be a long delay before making the diagnosis because malaria is not suspected, unusually high parasitaemias may develop with *P. falciparum* and *P. malariae*, but with *P. ovale* and *P. vivax* infections, the parasitaemia is usually limited to 2% because only reticulocytes are invaded. Severe manifestations are common and mortality may be high, e.g. 8 out of 11 infections in a group of heroin addicts and even acute *P. malariae* infections may prove fatal.

Nosocomial malaria has resulted from contamination of saline used for flushing intravenous catheters, contrast medium, and intravenous drugs. Malaria has complicated parenteral drug abuse.

Prevention

Outside the malaria endemic area, donors who have been in the tropics during the previous 5 years should be screened for malarial antibodies (indirect fluorescent antibody). In the endemic area, recipients of blood transfusions can be given antimalarial prophylaxis, or at least they should be watched carefully for evidence of infection. Addition of antimalarial drugs to stored blood is not justified.

Diagnosis

Since malaria can present with a wide range of symptoms and signs, none of them diagnostic, it must be excluded by repeated thick and thin blood smears and rapid antigen detection in any patient with acute fever who has history of possible exposure. Until malaria is confirmed or an alternative diagnosis emerges, at least three smears should be taken over a period of 72 h. However, if the patient has symptoms compatible with severe malaria, a therapeutic trial of antimalarial chemotherapy must not be delayed. Antimalarial drugs may make microscopical diagnosis more difficult and so chemoprophylaxis should be stopped while the patient is under investigation for malaria. A history of travel to malarious areas during the previous year must be obtained. Malaria cannot be excluded just because the patient took prophylactic drugs, for none is completely protective. Short airport stopovers, even on the runway, or working in or living near an international airport may allow exposure to an imported infected mosquito. Small outbreaks of autochthonous malaria (transmission of malaria imported into areas from which malaria has been eliminated but where competent vector mosquitoes exists) have been reported in Europe, North America, and elsewhere. The possibility of transmission by blood transfusion, 'needlestick', or nosocomial infection should be kept in mind. Those who grew up in an endemic area will probably lose their immunity to disease after living for a few years in a temperate zone and they become newly vulnerable on return home to visit friends and relations, especially in rural areas. In malaria endemic regions, a large proportion of the immune population may have asymptomatic parasitaemia and it cannot be assumed that malaria is the cause of a patient's symptoms even if parasitaemia is detected. In malarious countries, the diagnosis of malaria may be missed in the heat of an epidemic of some other infection such as meningitis, pneumonia, or cholera.

Differential diagnosis (Table 7.8.2.3)

Malaria must be included in the differential diagnosis of any acute febrile illness unless it can be excluded by: (1) impossibility of exposure, (2) repeated negative blood smears, and (3) a therapeutic trial of antimalarial chemotherapy. In Europe and North America, imported malaria has been misdiagnosed as influenza, viral hepatitis, viral haemorrhagic fever, epilepsy, viral encephalitis, or travellers' diarrhoea, sometimes with fatal consequences. Cerebral malaria must be distinguished from other infective meningoencephalitides. Examination of the cerebrospinal fluid will identify most of these infective causes (Chapters 24.11.1 and 24.11.2). Abdominal reflexes are absent in cerebral malaria but are brisk in patients with psychotic stupor and hysteria. Overdose of antimalarial drugs (chloroquine and quinine) has been confused

Table 7.8.2.3 Differential diagnosis of malaria

Symptom	Diagnosis
Acute fever	Heat stroke, hyperpyrexia of other causes, other infections, other causes of fever
Fever and impaired consciousness (cerebral malaria)	Viral, bacterial, fungal, protozoal (e.g. African trypanosomiasis, amoebic) or helminthic meningoencephalitis, cerebral abscess. Head injury, cerebrovascular accident, intoxications (e.g. insecticides), poisonings (e.g. antimalarial drugs), metabolic (diabetes, hypoglycaemia, uraemia, hepatic failure, hyponatraemia). Septicaemias, cerebral typhoid
Fever and convulsions	Encephalitides, metabolic encephalopathies, hyperpyrexia, cerebrovascular accidents, epilepsy, drug and alcohol intoxications, poisoning, eclampsia, febrile convulsions, and Reye's syndrome (children)
Fever and haemostatic disturbances	Septicaemias (e.g. meningococcaemia), viral haemorrhagic fever, rickettsial infection, relapsing fevers, leptospirosis
Fever and jaundice	Viral hepatitis, yellow fever, leptospirosis, relapsing fevers, septicaemias, haemolysis, biliary obstruction, hepatic necrosis (drugs, poisons)
Fever with gastrointestinal symptoms	Travellers' diarrhoea, dysentery, enteric fever, other bacterial infections, inflammatory bowel disease
Fever with haemoglobinuria ('blackwater fever')	Drug-induced haemolysis (e.g. oxidant antimalarials in glucose 6-phosphate-dehydrogenase-deficient patient), favism, transfusion reaction, dark urine of other causes (e.g. myoglobinuria, urobilinogen, porphobilinogen)
Fever with acute renal failure	Septicaemias, yellow fever, leptospirosis, drug intoxications, poisonings, prolonged hypotension
Fever with shock ('algid malaria')	Septicaemic shock, haemorrhagic shock (e.g. massive gastrointestinal bleed, ruptured spleen), perforated bowel, dehydration, hypovolaemia, myocarditis

with cerebral malaria. Intravenous drug abusers are at risk from both severe malaria and drug overdose. Alcoholism may be confused with cerebral malaria, whether the patient presents inebriated, with delirium tremens, or with Wernicke–Korsakoff syndrome.

Suspicion of viral haemorrhagic fever may lead to patients with imported fevers being isolated in a high-containment unit where basic investigations, such as examination of a blood smear, may be delayed for fear of infection. Jaundice is a common feature of yellow fever but unusual in other viral haemorrhagic fevers.

Malaria in pregnancy may be confused with viral hepatitis, acute fatty liver with liver failure or eclampsia, and in the puerperium with puerperal sepsis or psychosis.

Laboratory diagnosis

Microscopy

Parasites may be found in blood smears (Fig. 7.8.2.27) taken by venepuncture, finger-pulp or earlobe stabs, and from the umbilical cord and impression smears of the placenta. In fatal cases, cerebral malaria can be confirmed rapidly as the cause of death by making a smear from cerebral grey matter obtained by needle necropsy through the superior orbital fissure, the foramen magnum, the ethmoid sinus via the nose, or a fontanelle in young children. Sometimes no parasites can be found in peripheral blood smears from patients with malaria, even in severe infections. This may be explained by partial antimalarial treatment or by sequestration of parasitized cells in deep vascular beds. In these cases, parasites or malarial pigment may be found in a bone marrow aspirate. Pigment may be seen in circulating neutrophils. A number of Romanowski stains, including Field's, Giemsa, Wright's, and Leishman's, are suitable for malaria diagnosis. The rapid Field's technique, which can yield a result in minutes, and Giemsa are recommended. Smears may be unsatisfactory for any one of a number of reasons: the slides are not clean; stains are unfiltered, old, or infected; the buffer pH is incorrect (it should be pH 7.0–7.4); drying is too slow, especially in a humid climate (producing heavily crenated erythrocytes); or the blood has been stored in anticoagulant causing lysis of parasitized erythrocytes. It is difficult to make a good smear if the patient is very anaemic. Common artefacts resembling malaria parasites are superimposed platelets, particles of stain and other debris, and pits in the slide. Other erythrocyte infections such as bartonellosis and babesiosis may be misdiagnosed as malaria. Parasites should be counted in relation to the total white cell count (on thick films when the parasitaemia is relatively low) or erythrocytes (on thin films). An experienced microscopist can detect as few as 5 parasites/μl (parasites in 0.0001% of circulation RBCs) in a thick film and 200/μl (0.004% parasitaemia) in a thin film.

Fluorescent microscopy

The quantitative buffy coat method involves spinning blood in special capillary tubes in which parasite DNA is stained with acridine orange and a small float presses the PRBCs against the wall of the tube where they can be viewed by ultraviolet microscopy. In expert hands, the sensitivity of this method can be as good as with conventional microscopy of thick blood films but species diagnosis is difficult and the method is much more expensive.

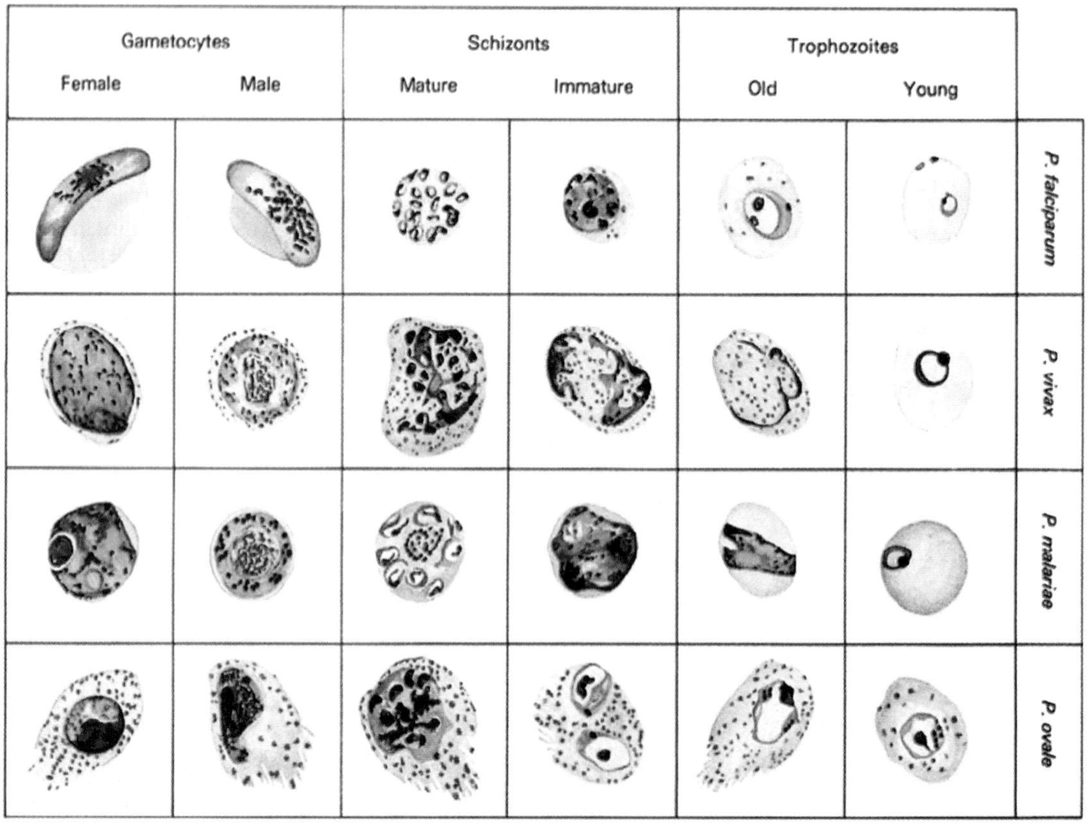

Gametocytes		Schizonts		Trophozoites		
Female	Male	Mature	Immature	Old	Young	
						P. falciparum
						P. vivax
						P. malariae
						P. ovale

Fig. 7.8.2.27 Malaria parasites developing in red blood cells.
(Courtesy of the Wellcome Trust.)

Rapid malarial antigen detection

Malaria dipstick antigen-capture assays employ monoclonal antibodies to detect *P. falciparum* histidine-rich protein 2 (PfHRP-2) or parasite-specific lactate dehydrogenase or aldolase from the glycolytic pathway found in all species. They are a convenient addition or alternative to microscopy as they are quick (taking about 20 min), sensitive (detecting >100 parasites/μl or 0.002% parasitaemia), and species specific. However, false positivity has been a problem and only the parasite-specific lactate dehydrogenase tests detect *P. ovale* and *P. malariae*. The NOW malaria test (Inverness Medical) is available in the United Kingdom. Currently, Paracheck Pf (Orchid Biomedical Systems, Goa, India) and SD Bioline malaria antigen test (Standard Diagnostics, South Korea) are not available in the United Kingdom but are recommended. ParaSight F (Becton-Dickinson), ICT Malaria Pf (ICT Diagnostics), and OptiMAL (Flow Laboratories) are also available.

Other methods

Enzyme- and radioimmunoassays, DNA probes (using chemiluminescence for detection), and PCR now approach the sensitivity of classical microscopy. They take much longer (up to 72 h), are much more expensive, and are unlikely to replace microscopy for routine diagnosis. However, some of these newer methods could be automated for screening blood donors or for use in epidemiological surveys. PCR can distinguish parasite strains.

Serological techniques

Malarial antibodies can be detected by immunofluorescence, enzyme immunoassay, or haemagglutination, for epidemiological surveys, for screening potential blood donors, and occasionally for providing evidence of recent infection in nonimmune individuals. These tests are not useful in making an acute diagnosis of malaria. In future, detection of protective antibodies will be important in assessing the response to malaria vaccines.

Other clinical laboratory investigations

Anaemia is usual, with evidence of haemolysis. Serum haptoglobins may be undetectable. The direct antiglobulin (Coombs') test is usually negative. Neutrophil leucocytosis is common in severe infections whether or not there is a complicating bacterial infection, but the white cell count can also be normal or low. The presence of visible malarial pigment in more than 5% of circulating neutrophils is associated with a bad prognosis. Thrombocytopenia is common in patients with *P. falciparum* and *P. vivax* infections; it does not correlate with severity. Prothrombin and partial thromboplastin times are prolonged in up to one-fifth of patients with cerebral malaria. Concentrations of plasma fibrinogen and other clotting factors are normal or increased, and serum levels of fibrin(ogen) degradation products are normal in most cases. Fewer than 10% of patients with cerebral malaria have evidence of disseminated intravascular coagulation. However, antithrombin III concentrations are often moderately reduced and have prognostic significance. Total and direct (unconjugated) plasma bilirubin concentrations are usually increased, consistent with haemolysis, but in some patients with very high total bilirubin concentrations there is a predominance of conjugated bilirubin, indicating hepatocyte dysfunction. Some patients have cholestasis. Serum albumin concentrations are usually reduced, often grossly. Serum aminotransferases, 5′-nucleotidase, and, especially, lactic dehydrogenase are moderately elevated, but not nearly as much as in viral hepatitis. Hyponatraemia is the most common electrolyte disturbance. There may be mild hypocalcaemia (after correction for hypoalbuminaemia) and hypophosphataemia, especially after patients have been given blood or a glucose infusion. Biochemical evidence of generalized rhabdomyolysis (elevated serum creatine kinase concentration, myoglobinaemia, and myoglobinuria) is sometimes found. In about one-third of patients with cerebral malaria, the blood urea concentration is increased above 80 mg/dl (13 mmol/litre) and serum creatinine above 2 mg/dl (176 μmol/litre). Lactic acidosis is common in severely ill patients, especially those with hypoglycaemia and renal failure. It may be suspected if there is a wide 'anion gap', i.e. $[Na^+] - [Cl^-] + [HCO_3^-]$ is greater than 12 meq/litre.

Blood glucose must be checked frequently, especially in children, pregnant women, and severely ill patients, even if the patient is not receiving quinine treatment and is fully conscious. A bedside dipstick method, with or without photometric quantification, is rapid and convenient. Microscopy and culture of cerebrospinal fluid is important in patients with cerebral malaria to exclude other treatable encephalopathies. In cerebral malaria the cerebrospinal fluid may contain up to 15 lymphocytes/μl and an increased protein concentration. Pleocytosis of up to 80 cells/μl, mainly leucocytes, may be found in patients who have had repeated generalized convulsions. The cerebrospinal fluid glucose level will be low in hypoglycaemic patients and this result may be the first hint of hypoglycaemia. In view of the finding of cerebral compression and high opening pressures in many African children with cerebral malaria, some paediatricians prefer to delay lumbar puncture, while covering the possibility of bacterial meningoencephalitis with empirical antimicrobial treatment. Blood cultures should be performed in patients with a high white cell count, shock, persistent fever, or an obvious focus of secondary bacterial infection. Gram-negative rod bacteria (*Escherichia coli*, *Pseudomonas aeruginosa*, etc.) have been cultured from the blood of adult patients with 'algid' malaria and in African children an association was found between malaria and nontyphoid salmonella septicaemia.

Urine should be examined by microscope and dipsticks. Common abnormalities are proteinuria, microscopic haematuria, haemoglobinuria, and RBC casts. The urine is literally black in patients with severe intravascular haemolysis. Urine specific gravity should be measured: the optical method is most convenient when urine output is small. Monitoring plasma concentrations of antimalarial drugs such as quinine is rarely possible but can be useful.

Treatment

Antimalarial chemotherapy

Classes of drugs that have antimalarial activity are shown in Box 7.8.2.3.

Stage specificity

Among blood schizonticides, artemisinin derivatives can prevent the development of rings or trophozoites, but quinine and mefloquine cannot stop development before the stage of mature trophozoites and pyrimethamine–sulphadoxine combinations do not prevent the development of schizonts.

Box 7.8.2.3 Classes of antimalarial drugs

- Arylaminoalcohols—quinoline methanols (quinine and quinidine extracted from the bark of the cinchona tree), mefloquine, and lumefantrine
- 4-Aminoquinolines—chloroquine and amodiaquine
- Bisquinolines—piperaquine
- Folate-synthesis inhibitors—type 1 antifolate drugs that compete for dihydropteroate synthase (sulphones and sulphonamides); type 2 antifolate drugs that inhibit malarial dihydrofolate reductase (the biguanides proguanil and chlorproguanil and the diaminopyrimidine pyrimethamine)
- 8-Aminoquinolines—primaquine and tafenoquine (Etaquine, WR-238605, or SB-252263)
- Antibiotics—tetracycline, doxycycline, clindamycin, azithromycin, and fluoroquinolones
- Peroxides (sesquiterpene lactones)—artemisinin (*qinghaosu*) derivatives and semisynthetic analogues (artemether, arteether, artesunate, and artelinic acid)
- Naphthoquinones—atovaquone

Antimalarial drugs

Arylaminoalcohols

The antimalarial properties of cinchona alkaloids were discovered in Peru around 1600 but their mode of action remains unknown. Quinine became the first-line treatment of severe falciparum malaria after the emergence of chloroquine resistance but is now being replaced by artemisinin derivatives. Intravenous injection of quinine is dangerous as high plasma concentrations may result during the distribution phase, causing fatal hypotension or arrhythmias. However, quinine can be given safely if it is diluted and infused intravenously over 2 to 4 h, or, if intravenous infusion is not possible and parenteral treatment is needed, it may be given by intramuscular injection divided between the anterolateral parts of both thighs. For intramuscular injection, the stock solution of quinine dihydrochloride (300 mg/ml) should be diluted to 60 mg/ml. It is well absorbed from this site. Historically, intramuscular quinine carried the risk of tetanus but it is safe provided that strict sterile precautions are observed. Because most deaths from severe falciparum malaria occur within the first 96 h of starting treatment, it is important to achieve parasiticidal plasma concentrations of quinine as quickly as possible. This can be accomplished safely with an initial loading dose of twice the maintenance dose (Table 7.8.2.4). The initial dose of quinine should not be reduced in patients who are severely ill with renal or hepatic impairment,

Table 7.8.2.4 Antimalarial chemotherapy in adults or children with uncomplicated malaria who can swallow tablets

Option and age of patient	Chloroquine-resistant *P. falciparum* or where the origin of the infection is unknown	Chloroquine-sensitive *P. falciparum* or *P. vivax*, *P. ovale*, *P. malariae*, or monkey malarias
1	**Artemether with lumefantrine**	**Chloroquine**[a]
Adult	4 tablets (each containing 20 mg artemether and 120 mg lumefantrine)	600 mg base on the 1st and 2nd days; 300 mg on the 3rd day
	Twice daily for 3 days	
Child	<15 kg body weight, 1 tablet	*c.* 10 mg base/kg on the 1st and 2nd days; 5 mg base/kg on the 3rd day
	15<25 kg, 2 tablets	
	25<35 kg, 3 tablets	
	All twice daily for 3 days	
		For radical cure of *P. vivax*/*P. ovale* (except pregnant and lactating women or G6PD-deficient patients), add:
2	**Proguanil with atovaquone**	**Primaquine**
Adult	4 tablets (each containing 100 mg proguanil and 250 mg atovaquone)	15 mg base/day on days 4–17; or 45 mg/week for 8 weeks[b]
	Once daily for 3 days	
Child	11–20 kg, one tablet	0.25 mg/kg per day on days 4–17; or 0.75 mg/kg per week for 8 weeks[b]
	21–30 kg, 2 tablets	
	31–40 kg, 3 tablets	
	All once daily for 3 days	
3	**Quinine**	
Adult	600 mg salt, 3 times daily for 7 days[c]	
Child	Approx. 10 mg salt/kg, 3 times daily for 7 days[c]	

[a] For chloroquine-resistant *P. vivax*, repeat the course.

[b] For Chesson-type strains (South-East Asia, western Pacific), use double the dose or double the duration up to a total dose of 6 mg base/kg in daily doses of 15–22.5 mg for adults.

[c] In areas where 7 days of quinine is not curative (e.g. Thailand), add tetracycline 250 mg four times each day or doxycycline 100 mg daily for 7 days, except for children under 8 years and pregnant women, or add clindamycin 5 mg/kg three times daily for 7 days.

but in these cases the maintenance dose should be reduced to between 3 and 5 mg/kg if parenteral treatment is required for longer than 48 h.

Minimum inhibitory concentrations of quinine for *P. falciparum* in South-East Asia and other areas of the tropics have increased. Longer courses of quinine and combination with pyrimethamine–sulphonamide combinations, tetracycline, or clindamycin have been required for cure. Quinine need not be withheld or stopped in patients who are pregnant. In therapeutic doses, it does not stimulate uterine contraction or cause fetal distress. Hypoglycaemia is the most important complication of quinine treatment. Plasma quinine concentrations above 5 mg/litre cause 'cinchonism': transient high-tone deafness, giddiness, tinnitus, nausea, vomiting, tremors, blurred vision, and malaise. Rarely, quinine may give rise to haemolysis, thrombocytopenia, disseminated intravascular coagulation, hypersensitivity reactions, vasculitis, and granulomatous hepatitis. Self-poisoning with quinine causes blindness, deafness, and central nervous depression. These features are rarely seen in patients being treated for malaria, even though their plasma quinine concentrations may exceed 20 mg/litre. This may be explained by the increased binding of quinine to α_1-acid glycoprotein (orosomucoid) and to other acute-phase reactive serum proteins associated with acute infection.

Quinidine, the dextrorotatory stereoisomer of quinine, is more effective against resistant strains of *P. falciparum* but is more cardiotoxic than quinine. Because it was widely stocked for treating cardiac arrhythmias, quinidine gluconate injection was once more generally available than parenteral quinine. The Centers for Disease Control in the United States of America formerly supplied it for the parenteral treatment of malaria, but it has now been replaced by artesunate.

Mefloquine is a synthetic drug, effective against some *P. falciparum* strains resistant to chloroquine, pyrimethamine–sulphonamide combinations, and quinine. It cannot be given parenterally, but is well absorbed when given by mouth, reaching peak plasma concentrations in 6 to 24 h, with an elimination half-time of 14 to 28 days. The drug can be given as a single dose but, to reduce the risk of vomiting and other gastrointestinal side effects, the dose is best divided into two halves given 6 to 8 h apart. Gastrointestinal symptoms occur in 10 to 15% of patients but are usually mild. Less frequent side effects include nightmares and sleeping disturbances, dizziness, ataxia, sinus bradycardia, sinus arrhythmia, postural hypotension, and an 'acute brain syndrome' consisting of fatigue, asthenia, seizures, and psychosis. These unpleasant symptoms, whose incidence has probably been exaggerated, have made the drug unpopular. Those taking β-blockers or with a past history of epilepsy or psychiatric disease should avoid the drug. Unfortunately, *in vitro* resistance to mefloquine and treatment failures have now been reported in South-East Asia, Africa, and South America. One large observational study in Thailand suggested an increased risk of stillbirth associated with mefloquine but this was not found in Malawi. Mefloquine treatment should be avoided in pregnant women, especially during the first trimester, and pregnancy should be avoided within 3 months of stopping mefloquine.

Lumefantrine (benflumetol) is an arylaminoalcohol that, despite its structural similarity to halofantrine (now withdrawn), is not cardiotoxic. It is combined with artemether as a co-artemether (see below).

4-Aminoquinolines

Chloroquine, a synthetic antimalarial, is concentrated in the parasite's lysosomes where haemoglobin is digested, and may act by inhibiting the haempolymerase that converts toxic haemin into insoluble haemozoin (malarial pigment). Alternatively, the drug may interfere with parasite feeding by disrupting its food vacuole. From the original foci in Thailand and Colombia, chloroquine-resistant *P. falciparum* has spread to most parts of the tropics. The observation that chloroquine resistance could be reversed *in vitro* by high concentrations of calcium channel blockers, which in other situations could reverse the multidrug resistance (mdr) phenotype acquired by tumour cells, focused attention on a malarial homologue of the human *MDR* gene. Genes involved in the development of resistance include *P. falciparum* chloroquine resistance transporter on chromosome 7 and loci on chromosome 5, which harbours the *MDR* gene homologue *PfMDR1*, and chromosome 11. Despite the widespread resistance of *P. falciparum* to this drug and the recent emergence of chloroquine-resistant *P. vivax* in New Guinea and adjacent areas of Indonesia, chloroquine remains the most widely used antimalarial drug worldwide. It is the treatment of choice for *P. vivax*, *P. ovale*, *P. malariae*, and *P. knowlesi* infections and for uncomplicated falciparum malaria acquired in the few areas where the parasite remains sensitive to this drug (Central America northwest of the Panama Canal, Hispaniola (Haiti and the Dominican Republic, and parts of the Middle East). Elsewhere, the emergence of chloroquine resistance has had a devastating effect on malarial morbidity and mortality. In Senegal, mortality from malaria in children under 5 years old increased up to 11-fold between 1984 and 1995. Absorption of chloroquine after intramuscular or subcutaneous injection is very rapid. Unless small doses are given frequently, this can produce dangerously high plasma concentrations, probably accounting for the deaths of some children soon after they had received intramuscular injections of chloroquine. Therapeutic blood concentrations persist for 6 to 10 days after a single dose. Plasma concentrations above about 250 ng/ml cause dizziness, headache, diplopia, disturbed visual accommodation, dysphagia, nausea, and malaise. Chloroquine, even in small doses, may cause pruritus in dark-skinned races. It may exacerbate epilepsy and photosensitive psoriasis. Cumulative, irreversible retinal toxicity from chloroquine has been reported after lifetime prophylactic doses of 50 to 100 g base (i.e. after 3–6 years of taking 300 mg of base per week), although this is most unusual. Chloroquine overdose is described in Chapter 9.1. Chloroquine is safe during pregnancy and lactation.

Amodiaquine, although structurally similar to chloroquine, retains activity against chloroquine-resistant strains of *P. falciparum* in some geographical areas. Unlike chloroquine, it is metabolized to a toxic quinoneimine capable of causing toxic hepatitis and potentially lethal agranulocytosis (which occurred in up to 1 in 2000 people taking amodiaquine prophylactically). Amodiaquine is still used, but, because of its risks and the limited therapeutic advantage over chloroquine, its use for prophylaxis and repeated treatment is now discouraged by WHO.

Bisquinolines

Piperaquine was used extensively as prophylaxis and treatment in China and Indochina from the 1960s until emergence of piperaquine-resistant strains of *P. falciparum* during the 1980s. More recently, it has been combined with artemisinins, as an artemisinin-based combination therapy (ACT) as: dihydroartemisinin (DHA), trimethoprim, piperaquine phosphate, and primaquine phosphate (China-Vietnam (CV), CV4 and CV8); DHA, trimethoprim, and piperaquine phosphate (Artecom), and DHA and piperaquine phosphate only (Artekin, Duo-Cotecxin), which have proved effective and safe in mainland South-East Asia. Piperaquine is highly lipid soluble with a large volume of distribution at steady state/bioavailability, long elimination half-life, and a clearance that is markedly higher in children than in adults. Its tolerability, efficacy, pharmacokinetic profile, and low cost make it suitable as a constituent of ACT.

Folate-synthesis inhibitors

Pyrimethamine–sulphonamide combinations The mode of action of the antifolate drugs is well understood. Pyrimethamine 75 mg and sulphadoxine 1500 mg (Fansidar), once valuable in the treatment of chloroquine-resistant falciparum infections worldwide, is no longer marketed in the United Kingdom, but it and other pyrimethamine combinations such as with dapsone (Maloprim) and with sulphalene (Metakelfin) are still used elsewhere. Unfortunately, resistance to these synergistic combinations has spread to most malarious continents, resulting from mutations at residues 108, 51, 59, 16, and 164 of the parasite's dihydrofolate reductase gene. Pyrimethamine is a folate inhibitor that may cause folic acid deficiency in pregnant women and others unless folinic acid supplements are given. The sulphonamide components of these combinations may cause systemic vasculitis (Stevens–Johnson syndrome), or toxic epidermal necrolysis. Fansidar caused fatal reactions in 1 in 18 000 to 26 000 prophylactic courses. Aplastic anaemia and agranulocytosis can also occur. Both pyrimethamine and sulphonamide cross the placenta and are excreted in milk. In the fetus and neonate, sulphonamides can displace bilirubin from plasma protein-binding sites, thus causing kernicterus. For these reasons, pyrimethamine–sulphonamide combinations are not recommended for treatment during pregnancy or lactation unless no alternative drug is available, and should never be used for prophylaxis.

Chlorproguanil–dapsone This combination was developed as an alternative to pyrimethamine–sulphonamide combinations to replace chloroquine for the treatment of uncomplicated falciparum malaria in Africa. It proved more effective than pyrimethamine–sulphonamide combinations in treating parasites with *DHFR* mutations at bases 108, 51, and 59, but should probably be further combined with an artemisinin to extend its useful therapeutic life.

8-Aminoquinolines

Primaquine is the only readily available drug effective against hepatic hypnozoites of *P. vivax* and *P. ovale*. It is essential for the radical cure of these infections. Primaquine is gametocytocidal for all species of malaria. Mass treatment of patients with *P. falciparum* infection could eliminate the sexual cycle in mosquitoes by sterilizing gametocytes. Its elimination half-time is 7 h. Primaquine causes haemolysis in patients with congenital deficiencies of erythrocyte enzymes, notably G6PD, but severe intravascular haemolysis is unusual except in areas such as the Mediterranean (e.g. Sardinia) and Sri Lanka. Primaquine can cross the placenta and cause severe haemolysis in a G6PD-deficient fetus, most commonly a boy, and is also excreted in breast milk. It should therefore not be used during pregnancy or lactation in areas where G6PD deficiency is prevalent. Like sulphonamides and sulphones (i.e. dapsone), primaquine can produce severe haemolysis and methaemoglobinaemia in patients with congenital deficiency of NADH methaemoglobin reductase. Those affected quickly develop dusky cyanosis, noticed first in the nail beds. In patients with G6PD deficiency, weekly dosage with 45 mg of primaquine is better tolerated than the usual daily dose of 15 mg. In the Solomon Islands, Indonesia, Thailand, and Papua New Guinea, a total dose of 6.0 mg/kg (twice the usual dose) or even more may be needed to eliminate the primaquine-resistant Chesson-type strain of *P. vivax*. This is usually given as 15 mg base/day for 28 days.

Tafenoquine is a newer 8-aminoquinoline; it has a longer half-life (2 weeks) than primaquine and is over 10 times more active as a hypnozoiticide. It is also a potent schizonticide.

Peroxides (sesquiterpene lactones)

Artemisinin Artemisinin or *qinghaosu* (pronounced 'ching-how-soo') from the Chinese medicinal herb *Artemisia annua* (sweet wormwood), family Compositae, has been used to treat fevers in China for more than 1000 years. It is a sesquiterpene lactone, with an endoperoxide (trioxane) active group that was isolated in China in 1971–2. Iron within the parasite probably catalyses the cleavage of the endoperoxide bridge leading to the generation of free radicals, which then form covalent bonds with parasite proteins (alkylation). Artemisinins destroy the blood stages of *P. falciparum* from trophozoite to schizont, including those of multiresistant strains. They clear parasitaemia more rapidly than other antimalarial drug. Resistance is emerging in SE Asia.

Artesunate Dihydroartemisinin (DHA) is the active metabolite, which has a short half-life. In severe falciparum malaria, intravenous artesunate is the treatment of choice but this drug can also be given by intramuscular injection. Multicentre trials enrolling 1461 patients in South-East Asia demonstrated a case fatality of 15% in patients treated with intravenous artemether, compared to 22% in those treated with intravenous quinine, a reduction in mortality of 34.7% in the artesunate-treated group.

Artemether Systematic review of 11 randomized controlled trials comparing intramuscular artemether with parenteral quinine showed lower mortality with artemether, but this was not significant in an analysis of adequately blinded trials. Within these, in an individual patient data analysis of 1919 adults and children, the odds ratio for deaths in artemether recipients was 0.8. In the prospectively defined subgroup analysis of adults with multisystem failure, there was a significant difference in mortality in favour of artemether but intramuscular artemether is erratically absorbed in patients with severe malaria especially those with shock. Artemotil (arteether) is similar to artemether but has been far less used.

Artemisinin suppositories Rectal artesunate proved superior to intravenous/intramuscular quinine in reducing parasite densities 12 and 24 h after administration. Suppository formulations of artemisinin should prove particularly valuable in treating children at peripheral levels of the health service.

Artemether with lumefantrine combination (co-artemether) is effective for the oral treatment of multiresistant falciparum malaria.

The severe neurotoxicity reported in animals given large doses of artemisinins has not been detected in any of the tens of thousands of human patients treated with these compounds. Artemisinins have proved safe in the second and third trimesters of pregnancy but there are insufficient data to support their use in the first trimester.

Hydroxynaphthoquinones

Naphthoquinones, such as atovaquone, act on the electron-transport chain in malarial mitochondria through their structural similarity to coenzyme Q. Atovaquone is marketed in combination with proguanil for the treatment and prevention of multiresistant *P. falciparum*. It inhibits the parasite's mitochondrial respiration by binding to the cytochrome *bc* complex. The drug is poorly and variably absorbed, but bioavailability is greatly enhanced by a fatty meal. Its elimination half-life is between 50 and 70 h.

Antibiotics

All antimalarial antibiotics inhibit ribosomal protein synthesis and probably act on the parasite's mitochondria. Tetracycline, clindamycin, azithromycin, quinolones, and sulphonamides such as co-trimoxazole have some antimalarial activity. They kill parasites too slowly to be used alone but are useful in combination for the treatment of uncomplicated *P. falciparum* malaria.

Treatment of falciparum malaria

Despite discovery of the rapidly effective, easily used, and safe artemisinin derivatives, treatment of falciparum malaria remains challenging in many parts of the world. The use of antimalarial drugs is poorly controlled, there are supply problems resulting from expense, inadequate distribution and erratic and incomplete dosing. Fake antimalarial drugs are penetrating increasingly into the markets in Africa and Asia. A worrying recent development has been the documentation of reduced *in vivo* susceptibility to artemisinins with delayed parasite clearance in Pailin, western Cambodia, and possibly in adjacent countries.

Combination antimalarial treatment

The combination of two or more different classes of antimalarial drugs with unrelated mechanisms of action to delay emergence of resistance was proposed by Wallace Peters in the early 1970s but was not effectively implemented because of the difficulty of identifying drugs that were still active against multidrug resistant *P. falciparum* and whose elimination half-times were similar. To counter the threat of resistance of *P. falciparum* to monotherapies, and to improve treatment outcome, combinations of antimalarials are now recommended by WHO (2006) for the treatment of falciparum malaria.

Artemisinin-based combination therapy (ACT)

The rapid clearance of parasitaemia and resolution of symptoms by artemisinin derivatives provides strong theoretical support for their use in combination with drugs such as mefloquine, amodiaquine, or pyrimethamine–sulphonamide. A meta-analysis of 11 randomized controlled trials confirmed that, in patients with uncomplicated malaria, addition of 3 days of artesunate to these drugs significantly reduced treatment failure, recrudescence, and gametocyte carriage. This lead to WHO's 2006 recommendation to replace monotherapy with ACT. This has proved effective, except in South-east Asia (Cambodia and possibly in Thailand and Burma), where resistance to artemisinins has recently been reported.

Treatment of uncomplicated *P. falciparum* malaria (Table 7.8.2.4)

For treating adults, infants, and children in malarious areas, WHO (2006) recommends ACTs even in Africa, where the deployment of artemisinins cannot yet be justified by published evidence. The drug combined with artesunate depends on the resistance of local strains of *P. falciparum*. In South-East Asia, lumefantrine or mefloquine might be added. In Africa, lumefantrine, amodiaquine, or sulphadoxine–pyrimethamine might be added. For presumed non-immune travellers returning to nonendemic areas, WHO recommends artemether–lumefantrine, atovaquone–proguanil, or quinine + doxycycline or clindamycin. Doxycycline should not be given to pregnant women or children under 8 years old.

Patients with uncomplicated malaria can usually be given antimalarial drugs by mouth. However, feverish patients may vomit the tablets. The risk of vomiting can be reduced if the patient lies down quietly for a while after taking an antipyretic such as paracetamol. Otherwise, the initial dose of antimalarial drug may have to be given by injection or suppository.

Treatment of severe falciparum malaria (Table 7.8.2.5)

Urgent parenteral chemotherapy, initiated with a loading dose, is the priority as there is a highly significant relationship between delay in chemotherapy and mortality. Severely ill or deteriorating patients who have been exposed to malaria should be given a therapeutic trial even if the initial smears are negative. Dosage should be calculated according to the patient's body weight and drugs should be administered parenterally both to patients with severe falciparum malaria and to those who are vomiting and unable to retain swallowed tablets. The treatment of choice is artesunate given by intravenous bolus injection. It can also be given by intramuscular injection. Artemether by intramuscular injection or quinine by intermittent or continuous intravenous infusion or intramuscular injection is less effective. If patients with severe malaria cannot swallow and retain tablets and antimalarial treatment by intramuscular/intravenous injection/infusion is likely to be delayed for several hours, insertion of a single artesunate suppository substantially reduces the risk of death or permanent disability.

Therapeutic response and vital signs must be monitored clinically (temperature, pulse, blood pressure) and by examination of blood films. Patients should be switched to oral treatment as soon as they are able to swallow and retain tablets. They must be watched carefully for signs of drug toxicity. In the case of quinine, the most common adverse effect is hypoglycaemia. Therefore, the blood sugar should be checked frequently.

General management

Patients with severe malaria should be transferred to the highest level of care available, preferably a high dependency area or intensive care unit. They must be nursed in bed because of their postural hypotension and because of the risk of splenic rupture were they to fall. Body temperatures above 38.5°C are associated with febrile convulsions, especially in children, and between 39.5 and 42°C with coma and permanent neurological sequelae. In pregnant women, hyperpyrexia contributes to fetal distress. Therefore, temperature should be controlled by fanning, tepid sponging, a cooling blanket, or antipyretic drugs, such as paracetamol (15 mg/kg in tablets by mouth, or powder washed down a nasogastric tube, or as suppositories) and ibuprofen (tablets or parenteral).

Cerebral malaria

Convulsions, vomiting, and aspiration pneumonia are common, so patients should be nursed in the lateral position with a rigid oral airway or endotracheal tube in place. They should be turned at least once every 2 h to avoid bedsores. Vital signs, Glasgow Coma Score, and convulsions should be recorded. Convulsions can be controlled with diazepam given by slow intravenous injection (adults 10 mg, children 0.15 mg/kg) or intrarectally (0.5–1.0 mg/kg), or with midazolam given initially by intravenous injection of

Table 7.8.2.5 Antimalarial chemotherapy in adults or children with severe malaria who cannot swallow tablets

Chloroquine-resistant P. falciparum or the origin of the infection is unknown	Chloroquine-sensitive P. falciparum or P. vivax, P. ovale, P. malariae, or monkey malarias
1. Artesunate[a]	**1. Chloroquine**[b]
2.4 mg/kg (loading dose) IV on the first day, followed by 1.2 mg/kg daily for a minimum of 3 days until the patient can take oral therapy or another effective antimalarial	25 mg base/kg diluted in isotonic fluid by continuous IV infusion over 30 h (or 5 mg base/kg over 6 h every 6 h)
OR	OR
2. Artemether	**2. Quinine (see left-hand column below)**
3.2 mg/kg (loading dose) IM on the first day, followed by 1.6 mg/kg daily for a minimum of 3 days until the patient can take oral treatment or another effective antimalarial. In children, the use of a 1 ml tuberculin syringe is advisable since the injection volumes will be small	
OR	
3. Quinine	
Adults: 20 mg salt/kg (loading dose)[c] diluted in 10 ml/kg isotonic fluid by IV infusion over 4 h, followed 8 h after the start of the loading dose with 10 mg salt/kg over 4 h, every 8 h until patients can	
Children: 20 mg salt/kg (loading dose)[c] diluted in 10 ml/kg isotonic fluid by IV infusion over 2 h, followed 12 h after the start of the loading dose with 10 mg salt/kg over 2 h, every 12 h until patients can swallow[d]	
The 7-day course should be completed with quinine tablets, approximately 10 mg salt/kg (maximum 600 mg) every 8–12 h[e]	
OR	
4. Quinine (in intensive care unit)	
7 mg salt/kg (loading dose)[c] IV by infusion pump over 30 min, followed immediately with 10 mg salt/kg (maintenance dose) diluted in 10 ml/kg isotonic fluid by IV infusion over 4 h, repeated every 8 h until patient can swallow, etc.[d,e]	
OR	
5. Quinidine (in intensive care unit)	
15 mg base/kg (loading dose)[c] IV by infusion over 4 h, followed 8 h after the start of the loading dose with 7.5 mg base/kg over 4 h every 8 h, until the patient can swallow,[d] then quinine tablets to complete 7 days of treatment[e]	
If it is not possible to give drugs by intravenous infusion	
1 Artesunate	**1. Chloroquine**[b]
Same dosage as for IV above given IM	Total dose 25 mg base/kg given as either:
	IM or SC 2.5 mg base/kg, every 4 h
OR	IM or SC 3.5 mg base/kg, every 6 h
2 Artemether	
As above	
OR	OR
3. Quinine	**2. Quinine**
20 mg salt/kg diluted to 60–100 mg/ml (loading dose)[c] IM into anterolateral thigh (half given into each leg), followed by 10 mg salt/kg, every 8 h until patient can swallow etc.[d,e]	IM (see above left-hand column)
If it is not possible to give drugs by injection (IM/IV) or infusion	
1. Suppositories	**1. Chloroquine**
Artemisinin[f]	
40 mg/kg loading dose as suppositories intrarectally, followed by 20 mg/kg at 4, 24, 48, and 72 h followed by an oral antimalarial drug[g]	10 mg base/kg of body weight as tablets/syrup by mouth or nasogastric tube, then refer the patient to a higher level of healthcare for parenteral treatment
	OR
	Continue 5 mg base/kg 5, 24, and 48 h later[g]

(Continued)

Table 7.8.2.5 *(Cont'd)* Antimalarial chemotherapy in adults or children with severe malaria who cannot swallow tablets

Artesunate[f]	
One 200 mg suppository intrarectally at 0, 4, 8, 12, 24, 36, 48, and 60 h followed by an oral antimalarial drug[h]	
OR	OR
2. Tablets of artemisinin (artesunate, artemether, artemether with lumefantrine), quinine, mefloquine, or other appropriate antimalarials[g] Given by mouth or crushed and given via naso-gastric tube	**2. Suppositories of artemisinin or artesunate, oral quinine, mefloquine, or sulphadoxine/pyrimethamine (see left-hand column)**[g]

IM, intramuscular; IV, intravenous; SC, subcutaneous.

[a] Artesunic acid 60 mg is dissolved in 0.6 ml of 5% sodium bicarbonate diluted to 3–5 ml with 5% (w/v) dextrose and given immediately by intravenous ('push') bolus injection.

[b] Parenteral chloroquine should be used with great caution in young children.

[c] Loading dose must not be used if the patient has received quinine, quinidine, or halofantrine within preceding 24 h.

[d] In patients requiring more than 48 h of parenteral therapy, reduce the dose to 5.7 mg salt/kg every 8 h or 3.75 mg quinidine base/kg every 8 h.

[e] In areas where 7 days of quinine is not curative (e.g. Thailand), add tetracycline 250 mg four times each day or doxycycline 100 mg daily for 7 days except for children under 8 years and pregnant women, or add clindamycin 5 mg/kg three times daily for 7 days.

[f] Artemisinin and artesunate suppositories are registered for use in a few countries. If suppository formulations are not available, tablets of artemisinins should be given orally if possible, or crushed and given by nasogastric tube.

[g] Transfer the patient to hospital as soon as possible after initiating chemotherapy.

[h] In Vietnam, 4 mg/kg of artesunate in suppository form (China) intrarectally as a loading dose, followed by 2 mg/kg at 4, 12, 48, and 72 h followed by an oral antimalarial drug, proved as effective as artemisinin suppositories.

small doses every 2 min and then, when the seizure is controlled, by continuous intravenous infusion diluted in 5% dextrose or normal saline (dosage is adjusted for age and response, in the range of 30 to 300 μg/kg per h). Prophylactic use of phenobarbital was associated with increased case fatality in a placebo-controlled study in African children and is not recommended. Stomach contents should be aspirated through a nasogastric tube to reduce the risk of aspiration pneumonia. Elective endotracheal intubation is indicated if coma deepens and the airway is jeopardized. Deepening coma with signs of cerebral herniation is an indication for CT or MRI, or a trial of treatment to lower intracranial pressure, such as an intravenous infusion of mannitol (1.0–1.5 g/kg of a 10–20% solution over 30 min) or mechanical hyperventilation to reduce the arterial $P\mathrm{co}_2$ to below 4.0 kPa (30 mmHg).

A number of potentially harmful ancillary remedies of unproven value have been recommended for the treatment of cerebral malaria. Two double-blind trials of dexamethasone (2 mg/kg and 11 mg/kg intravenously over 48 h) in adults and children in Thailand and Indonesia showed no reduction in mortality but prolongation of coma and an increased incidence of infection and gastrointestinal bleeding. Low-molecular-weight dextrans, osmotic agents, heparin, adrenaline (epinephrine), ciclosporin A, prostacyclin, pentoxifylline, malarial hyperimmune globulin, anti-TNFα monoclonal antibodies, desferrioxamine, dichloroacetate, and *N*-acetyl cysteine have proved ineffective in the treatment of cerebral and other forms of severe malaria. Some of these interventions were associated with serious side effects. There is some evidence that levamisole inhibits sequestration of PRBCs in patients with falciparum malaria and clinical trials are planned.

Anaemia

Indications for transfusion include a low (<20% or rapidly falling) haematocrit, severe bleeding, or predicted blood loss (e.g. imminent parturition or surgery), hyperparasitaemia, and failure to respond to conservative treatment with oxygen and plasma expanders. When the screening of transfused blood is inadequate and infections such as HIV, HTLV-1, and hepatitis viruses are prevalent in the community, the criteria for blood transfusion must be even more stringent. Exchange transfusion is a safe way of correcting the anaemia without precipitating pulmonary oedema in those who are fluid overloaded or chronically and severely anaemic. The volume of transfused blood must be recorded on the fluid balance chart. Transfusion must be cautious, with frequent observations of the jugular or central venous pressure and auscultation for pulmonary crepitations. Survival of compatible donor RBCs is greatly reduced during the acute and convalescent phases of falciparum malaria.

Disturbances of fluid and electrolyte balance

Fluid and electrolyte requirements must be assessed individually in patients with malaria. Circulatory overload with intravenous fluids or blood transfusion may precipitate fatal pulmonary oedema, but untreated hypovolaemia may lead to fatal shock, lactic acidosis, and renal failure. Hypovolaemia may result from salt and water depletion through fever, diarrhoea, vomiting, insensible losses, and poor intake. The state of hydration is assessed clinically from the skin turgor, peripheral circulation, postural change in blood pressure, peripheral venous filling, and jugular or central venous pressure. The history of recent urine output and measurement of urine volume and specific gravity may be useful. In tropical climates, adult patients with severe falciparum malaria may require 1 to 3 litres of intravenous fluid during the first 24 h of hospital admission. Fluid replacement should be controlled by observations of jugular, central venous, or pulmonary artery wedge pressures. Hyponatraemia (plasma sodium concentration 120–130 mmol/litre) usually requires no treatment, but these patients should be cautiously rehydrated with isotonic saline if they are clinically dehydrated, have low central venous pressures, a high urinary specific gravity, and a low urine sodium concentration (<25 mmol/litre).

Renal failure

Patients with falling urine output and elevated blood urea nitrogen and serum creatinine concentrations can be treated conservatively at first, but established acute renal failure must be treated with haemofiltration or dialysis. Hypovolaemia is corrected by the cautious infusion of isotonic saline until the central venous pressure is in the range +5 to +15 $\mathrm{cmH_2O}$. If urine output remains low after rehydration, increasing doses of slowly infused intravenous furosemide up to a total dose of 1 g and finally an intravenous infusion of dopamine (2.5–5 μg/kg per min) can be tried. If these measures fail to achieve a sustained increase in urine output, strict fluid balance should be enforced with particular emphasis on fluid restriction.

Indications for haemoperfusion/dialysis include a rapid increase in serum creatinine level, hyperkalaemia, fluid overload, metabolic acidosis, and clinical manifestations of uraemia (diarrhoea and vomiting, encephalopathy, gastrointestinal bleeding, and pericarditis). Haemofiltration is the most effective technique in malaria but haemodialysis or peritoneal dialysis is also effective. The initial doses of antimalarial drug should not be reduced in patients with renal failure but, after 48 h of parenteral treatment, the maintenance dose should be reduced by one-third or one-half.

Metabolic acidosis

Lactic acidosis is an important life-threatening complication, especially in anaemic children. It should be treated by improving perfusion and oxygenation by blood transfusion and correcting hypovolaemia, clearing the airway, increasing the inspired oxygen concentration, and by treating septicaemia, a frequently associated complication.

Pulmonary oedema

This must be prevented by propping the patient up at an angle of 45° and controlling fluid intake so that the jugular or central venous pressure is kept below +5 cmH_2O. Those who develop pulmonary oedema should be propped upright and given oxygen to breathe. In a well-equipped intensive care unit, the judicious use of vasodilator drugs can be controlled by monitoring haemodynamic variables, fluid overload can be corrected by haemoperfusion, and oxygenation can be improved by mechanical ventilation with positive end-expiratory pressure.

Hypotension and 'shock' ('algid malaria')

This should be treated as for bacteraemic shock. The circulatory problems should be corrected with blood transfusion (e.g. in anaemic children with respiratory distress and acidosis), plasma expanders, dopamine, and broad-spectrum antimicrobial treatment (such as gentamicin with ceftazidime or cefuroxime plus metronidazole) should be started immediately, bearing in mind that likely routes of infection include the urinary tract, lungs, and the gut. Other causes of shock in patients with malaria include dehydration, blood loss (i.e. following splenic rupture), and pulmonary oedema.

Hypoglycaemia

This may be asymptomatic, especially in pregnancy, and its clinical manifestations may be confused with those of malaria. Blood sugar must be checked every few hours, especially in patients being treated with cinchona alkaloids. Hypoglycaemia may arise despite continuous intravenous infusions of 5 or even 10% dextrose. A therapeutic trial of dextrose (1 ml/kg by intravenous bolus injection) should be given if hypoglycaemia is proved or suspected. This should be followed by a continuous infusion of 10% dextrose. Glucose may be given by nasogastric tube to unconscious patients or by peritoneal dialysis in those undergoing this treatment for renal failure. Among agents that block insulin release, diazoxide was ineffective, but octreotide, a synthetic somatostatin analogue, proved effective in some severe cases of quinine-induced hypoglycaemia.

Hyperparasitaemia and exchange blood transfusion

In nonimmune patients, case fatality exceeds 50% with parasitaemias above 500 000/μl. In Western countries, exchange blood transfusion, haemopheresis (and even plasmapheresis) have been used in presumed nonimmune patients with 'hyperparasitaemia' variously defined as parasitaemias exceeding 5 to 10%. Apart from reducing parasitaemia, these procedures might remove harmful metabolites, toxins, cytokines, and other mediators and restore normal RBC mass, platelets, clotting factors, and albumin. Potential dangers are electrolyte disturbances (e.g. hypocalcaemia), cardiovascular complications including ARDS, and infection from the blood or through infection of intravascular lines. Among more than 100 patients reported, some improved clinically soon after the procedure and most survived. However, there was reporting bias and a meta-analysis discovered no advantage. The efficacy of exchange transfusion is never likely to be put to the test of a randomized controlled trial. Artemisinins clear parasitaemia so rapidly that additional reduction of parasite load by exchange transfusion may not be important.

Splenic rupture

Acute abdominal pain and tenderness with left shoulder-tip pain and haemodynamic deterioration in patients with vivax and falciparum malaria suggests splenic rupture, especially if there is a history of recent abdominal trauma. Free blood in the peritoneal cavity and a torn splenic capsule can be detected by ultrasound or CT examination and confirmed by needle aspiration of the peritoneal cavity, laparoscopy, or laparotomy. Conservative management with blood transfusion and close observation in an intensive care unit is sometimes successful but access to surgical help is essential in case of sudden deterioration.

Disseminated intravascular coagulation

Patients with evidence of a coagulopathy should be given vitamin K (adult dose 10 mg by slow intravenous injection). Prothrombin complex concentrates, cryoprecipitates, platelet transfusions, and fresh-frozen plasma should be considered. Anticoagulants such as heparin and dalteparin are absolutely contraindicated.

Management of pregnant and lactating women with malaria

Chemotherapy

Unjustified fears of abortifacient and fetus-damaging effects of antimalarial drugs have led to the delay or even withdrawal of treatment, but experience since the 19th century has confirmed the safety of quinine in pregnancy. Chloroquine, proguanil, pyrimethamine, and sulphadoxine–pyrimethamine are also considered safe in the first trimester of pregnancy. Inadvertent exposure to other antimalarials in pregnancy is not an indication for termination of the pregnancy. Concerns about mefloquine in pregnancy have not been confirmed but doxycycline and other tetracyclines should be avoided during pregnancy and breastfeeding. Artemisinin derivatives have proved safe in the second and third trimesters of pregnancy, but there are insufficient safety data about their use in the first trimester.

For pregnant women with uncomplicated falciparum malaria, WHO (2006) recommends quinine ± clindamycin in the first trimester and ACTs in the second and third trimesters with artesunate + clindamycin or quinine + clindamycin as alternatives.

For severe falciparum malaria, WHO (2006) recommends artesunate and artemether above quinine in the second and third trimesters of pregnancy because they do not cause recurrent hypoglycaemia. However, blood glucose must be checked at least once a day in pregnant women with malaria, whether or not they are receiving quinine. In the first trimester, the risk of hypoglycaemia associated with quinine is lower, and uncertainties over the safety of the artemisinin derivatives are greater.

In lactating women, only tetracyclines, dapsone-containing antimalarials and possibly primaquine are contraindicated.

Ancillary treatments

Maternal fever should be reduced as soon as possible. Induction of labour, caesarean section, or accelerating the second stage of labour with forceps or vacuum extractor should be considered in patients with severe falciparum malaria. Fluid balance is particularly critical in these patients. If possible, the central venous pressure should be monitored. Exchange transfusion of 1000 to 1500 ml of blood in late pregnancy proved an effective way of managing severe anaemia with high-output cardiac failure in Nigeria. Circulating volume could be reduced and the risk of postpartum pulmonary oedema lessened by replacing exfused blood with a smaller volume of packed cells.

Prevention of malaria during pregnancy

As malaria during pregnancy can result in severe consequences for both the mother and child, therapeutic courses of antimalarials are effective as an intermittent preventive treatment and can be considered (see 'Control and prevention', below).

Treatment of *P. vivax*, *P. ovale*, *P. malariae*, and *P. knowlesi* malarias (Tables 7.8.2.4 and 7.8.2.5)

Chloroquine is the treatment of choice for vivax, ovale, malariae, knowlesi, and uncomplicated falciparum malarias in the few geographical areas where this drug can still achieve a satisfactory clinical response. Severe infections will require parenteral treatment (Table 7.8.2.5). Chloroquine-resistant *P. vivax* (New Guinea, Indonesia) is treated by increasing the dose of oral chloroquine. The usual 3-day course of chloroquine is well tolerated. In patients with vivax or ovale malarias, this should be followed by radical cure with primaquine to destroy hepatic hypnozoites, but caution is needed if there is a risk of a congenital enzyme deficiency (see '8-Aminoquinolines', above), especially in pregnant or lactating women.

Prognosis

Case fatality of acute vivax, ovale, and malariae malarias is negligible except in the circumstances mentioned above. In knowlesi malaria, case fatality appears to be about 2%. Strictly defined cerebral malaria has a mortality of about 10 or 15% when medical facilities are good and may be less than 5% in Western intensive care units. Antecedent factors that predispose to severe falciparum malaria include the lack of acquired immunity or lapsed immunity, splenectomy, pregnancy, and immunosuppression (e.g. HIV infection). There is a strong correlation between the density of parasitaemia and disease severity. Severe falciparum malaria is defined by clinical criteria such as impaired consciousness, renal failure, hypoglycaemia, haemoglobinuria, metabolic acidosis, and pulmonary oedema. The case fatality of pregnant women with cerebral malaria, especially primiparae in the third trimester, is several times greater than in nonpregnant patients. The following laboratory findings carry a poor prognosis: peripheral schizontaemia, malarial pigment in more than 5% of circulating neutrophils, high cerebrospinal fluid lactate or low glucose, low plasma antithrombin III, serum creatinine exceeding 265 μmol/litre or a blood urea nitrogen of more than 21.4 mmol/litre, haematocrit less than 20%, blood glucose less than 2.2 mmol/litre, and elevated serum enzyme concentrations (e.g. aspartate and alanine aminotransferases, lactate dehydrogenase).

Chronic immunological complications of malaria

Quartan malarial nephrosis

In parts of East and West Africa, South America, India, South-East Asia, and Papua New Guinea, epidemiological evidence links *P. malariae* infection to immune-complex glomerulonephritis that leads to nephrotic syndrome. Few of those exposed to repeated *P. malariae* infections develop nephrosis, suggesting that additional factors are involved. Histological changes, which are not entirely specific, are progressive focal and segmental glomerulosclerosis with fibrillary splitting or flaking of the capillary basement membrane, producing characteristic lacunae. Electron microscopy reveals electron-dense deposits beneath the endothelium. Immunofluorescence confirms glomerular deposits of immunoglobulins, C3, and *P. malariae* antigen in about 25% of cases. More than half the patients present by the age of 15 years with typical features of nephrotic syndrome. *P. malariae* is frequently found in blood smears and *P. malariae* antigen in renal biopsies in children but not in adults. The renal lesions may be perpetuated by autoimmune mechanisms. The pattern of immunofluorescent staining has some prognostic significance. Few patients respond to corticosteroids, but some are helped by azathioprine and cyclophosphamide, especially those whose renal biopsies show the coarse or mixed patterns of immunofluorescence. Antimalarial treatment is not effective. This condition could be prevented by antimalarial prophylaxis and has disappeared in countries such as Guyana following malaria eradication.

Tropical splenomegaly syndrome (hyperreactive malarial splenomegaly)

Transient splenomegaly is a feature of acute attacks of malaria in nonimmune or partially immune patients, while progressive splenomegaly is seen in children resident in malarious areas while they acquire immunity. However, a separate entity has been described in Africa (especially Nigeria, Uganda, and Zambia), the Indian subcontinent (Bengal, Sri Lanka), South-East Asia (Vietnam, Thailand, and Indonesia), South America (Amazon region), Papua New Guinea, and the Middle East (Aden). Defining features are: (1) residence in a malarious area, (2) chronic splenomegaly, (3) persistently elevated serum IgM and malarial antibody levels, (4) hepatic sinusoidal lymphocytosis, and (5) a clinical and immunological response to antimalarial prophylaxis. This condition is thought to result from an aberrant immunological response to repeated infection by any of the species of malaria parasite. Though requiring exposure to malaria and responding to antimalarial therapy, there is no association with the actual level of malarial endemicity. However, major differences in incidence in different ethnic groups suggest genetic predisposition.

Immunopathology

The essential feature is the dysregulation of IgM production leading to the formation of macromolecular aggregates of IgM (cryoglobulins), the clearance of which leads to progressive splenomegaly and hepatomegaly. This may stem in part from the production of lymphocytotoxic antibodies specific for suppressor T lymphocytes, which normally control B cell production of IgM. In African patients, there is often an increase in circulating B lymphocytes. Distinction from chronic lymphatic leukaemia may be difficult.

In Ghana, clonal rearrangements of the JH region of the immunoglobulin gene were found in patients with tropical splenomegaly who failed to respond to proguanil chemoprophylaxis, suggesting that the syndrome may evolve into a malignant lymphoproliferative disorder. Some of these patients had features of splenic lymphoma with villous (hairy) lymphocytes.

Clinical features

In malaria endemic areas, patients with tropical splenomegaly syndrome are distinguishable by their progressive splenic enlargement persisting beyond childhood. The spleen may be enormous, filling the left iliac fossa, extending across the midline and anteriorly, and producing a visible mass with an obvious notch. The liver is usually enlarged, especially the left lobe. The massive splenomegaly causes a vague dragging sensation and occasional episodes of severe pain with peritonism, suggesting perisplenitis or infarction. Anaemia may become severe enough to cause the features of high-output cardiac failure. Acute haemolytic episodes are described. These patients are vulnerable to infections, especially of the skin and respiratory system, and most deaths are attributable to overwhelming infection.

Laboratory findings

Severe chronic anaemia is the result of destruction and pooling in the spleen and dilution in an increased plasma volume. Thrombocytopenia may also be caused by splenic sequestration; it rarely causes bleeding. There is neutropenia and, in African patients, peripheral lymphocytosis and lymphocytic infiltration of the bone marrow. Serum IgM is greatly elevated (>2 standard deviations above the population mean, and often very much higher).

The essential histopathological feature is lymphocytosis of the hepatic sinusoids with Kupffer-cell hyperplasia. In some cases, round-cell infiltration of the portal tracts is associated with fibrosis, leading to portal hypertension. In the spleen there is dilatation of the sinusoids, hyperplasia of the phagocytic cells with erythrophagocytosis, and infiltration with lymphocytes and plasma cells. In patients with splenic lymphoma and villous lymphocytes, more than 30% of circulating lymphocytes are villous. These cells can be distinguished from hairy-cell leukaemia by their lack of CD25, CD11c, and tartrate-resistant acid phosphatase markers.

Differential diagnosis

Tropical splenomegaly syndrome must be distinguished from other causes of chronic, painless, massive splenomegaly, including leukaemias, lymphomas, myelofibrosis, thalassaemias, haemoglobinopathies, visceral leishmaniasis (by examination of bone marrow or splenic aspirates), and schistosomiasis (by liver biopsy, rectal snip, and stool examination). Lymphomas (especially chronic lymphatic leukaemia and follicular lymphoma) and even leukaemias may develop in patients with tropical splenomegaly syndrome. Nontropical idiopathic splenomegaly (normal serum IgM) and Felty's syndrome produce a similar histological picture in the liver. Many cases of splenomegaly in the tropics remain undiagnosed.

Treatment

Prolonged antimalarial chemoprophylaxis is the most important element of treatment. The majority of patients improve within 12 months of chemotherapy. The choice of drug will depend on the local sensitivity of whichever species or group of species of malaria parasite are thought to be responsible for this syndrome. The short- and long-term dangers of splenectomy rule out this procedure in the rural tropics. Folic acid may be needed. Diagnosis of patients with splenic lymphoma with villous lymphocytes (Ghana) is important as, in this condition, the risks of splenectomy are outweighed by the benefits.

Endemic Burkitt's lymphoma (Chapter 7.5.3)

Endemic Burkitt's lymphoma, a tumour of the jaw, abdomen, and other areas that spreads to the bone marrow or meninges, is the most common type of childhood malignant disease in many parts of East and West Africa and Papua New Guinea. It has also been reported from Brazil, Malaysia, and the Middle East. Burkitt noticed that its distribution (by altitude, temperature, and rainfall) and even its seasonal incidence followed that of falciparum malaria. Outside malaria endemic areas, Burkitt's lymphoma occurs sporadically. There is a suggestion that the B-cell line in cases in whites comes from lymphoid tissue, whereas in cases in Africans it comes from the bone marrow. Epstein–Barr virus (EBV) produces a lifelong infection of B lymphocytes. Normally this is controlled by specific, HLA-restricted, cytotoxic T cells, which recognize a virus-induced, lymphocyte-detected membrane antigen on B cells. Immunosuppression, as in recipients of renal allografts, allows uncontrolled proliferation of the EBV-infected B-cell line, which may give rise to one of the three chromosomal translocations [t(8;14), t(2;8), t(8;22)] that activate the c-*myc* oncogene on chromosome 8 responsible for malignant transformation. Acute *P. falciparum* infection leads to a reduction in the numbers of suppressor T (CD8) lymphocytes allowing proliferation and increased immunoglobulin secretion by EBV-infected B cells. In highly malaria endemic areas of Kenya, well children aged between 5 and 9 years (the age of maximum incidence of the tumour) have reduced EBV-specific interferon-γ responses. These tumours may grow so rapidly that massive local tissue destruction results in urate nephropathy and acute renal failure. Cyclophosphamide, vincristine, methotrexate, and prednisolone are used in chemotherapy, producing remissions in 80 to 90% of patients and a long-term survival of 20 to 70%. Breakdown of large tumours during the first week of chemotherapy may be so dramatic that the acute tumour lysis syndrome may be precipitated. This consists of metabolic acidosis, hyperuricaemia, hyperphosphaturia, hyperphosphataemia, hyperproteinaemia, and hyperkalaemia, which may result in fatal cardiac arrhythmia and acute uric-acid nephropathy with renal failure.

Control and prevention

General principles of control

The intensity of malaria parasite transmission is spatially heterogeneous. This has important implications for overall risks of disease and the age patterns of disease, disability, and death. Endemicity is a measure of the intensity of malaria transmission in a human population and determines the average age of first exposure, the rate of development of immunity, and, thus, the expected clinical spectrum of disease. It follows that interventions should be tailored to these basic epidemiological foundations, e.g. intermittent preventive treatment in infants (IPTi) is likely to have little impact on the incidence of clinical malaria and anaemia in areas of exceptionally low transmission. Optimizing the introduction of diagnostics to rationalize the use of new, expensive therapies will require better tools to target where this is cost-efficient and where presumptive treatment remains appropriate. Deciding the strategy and optimal mixture of interventions depends on an understanding of the epidemiological patterns in a given area: one size will not fit all.

Across the central belt of sub-Saharan Africa, interventions that minimize loss of life must be directed to young children and their mothers. In addition, careful thought must be given to measures that have a profound impact on the burden of malaria, particularly in the few areas where people might receive one new infection every night and immunity is acquired very early in life. Perhaps reducing human–vector contact might compromise the natural immunity prevalent in the community. In communities infrequently exposed to malaria, a focus on case management alone is a dangerous strategy where the lack of immunity means that each infectious bite carries a far greater risk of severe disease and death compared to many areas of Africa. Preventing the infectious bite carries little risk of compromised immunity and delivers benefit to all in the community.

The cornerstones of contemporary malaria control, case management, indoor residual house spraying (IRS), and insecticide (pyrethroid) treated nets (ITNs) will remain effective only as long as the drugs and pesticides remain effective. Case management is undermined by the evolution of parasite resistance to antimalarial drugs. IRS and ITNs lose their effectiveness as the vectors evolve behavioural or physiological resistance. How we use new chemical agents to minimize resistance is key but there is always a risk that, as resistance develops (or donors lose interest), malaria control will fail and populations that have lost their functional immunity will be more vulnerable to malaria.

Contemporary malaria control has a fundamentally different mission from the Global Malaria Eradication Campaign (1955–69) that was coordinated by WHO. That campaign did not eradicate malaria everywhere, as planned, but did reduce malaria morbidity and mortality and the global extent of the disease. The focus of eradication was on the use of indoor residual spraying with DDT (dichlorodiphenyltrichloroethane) accompanied by effective case detection and management with effective drugs. In some places, malaria remains absent today. In other places, elimination was only a remote possibility because the starting basic reproductive number of infection was so high. After 1974, when resistance began to emerge to widely used insecticides and drugs, the international political and financial commitment to global control waned. In areas where malaria persisted, populations had reduced functional immunity as malaria transmission increased, so malaria morbidity and mortality rebounded. Resistance of *P. falciparum* to most antimalarial drugs had reached epidemic proportions in South-East Asia. In Africa, mortality from malaria in children doubled from the 1980s through to the mid-1990s coincidentally with the rapid expansion of *P. falciparum* resistant to chloroquine and sulphadoxine–pyrimethamine.

Against a rising malaria disease burden, new global programmes such as WHO's Roll Back Malaria (RBM) initiative have emerged and aspire to reduce malaria morbidity and mortality by 75% by 2015. Because of malaria's intrinsic links to development and poverty, malaria also forms part of the United Nations Millennium Development Goal that aims to halt and then reverse the rising incidence of malaria by 2015.

A number of strategies can be combined to reduce the burden of malaria effectively. Most are regarded as cost-effective solutions in resource-poor counties and affordable within the constraints of international financial support. The interventions can be grouped into those that limit human–vector contact (including indoor residual house spraying and insecticide-treated nets), those that aim to reduce vector abundance by targeting breeding sites or adult vector populations and those that target the parasite (including intermittent presumptive treatment and prompt case management).

Limiting human–vector contact

So far, two methods for large-scale operational vector control—indoor residual spraying and long-lasting insecticide-containing nets (LLINs)—have proved capable of reducing malaria transmission. Both are adulticide measures, targeted at reducing the number of adult infective female mosquitoes. Unfortunately, uptake and acceptance of both interventions is poor among local populations in malaria endemic regions, although the situation may be improving. Perversely, coils, aerosols, and insecticide-impregnated mats sold through the private sector have greater acceptance rates, but have little or no demonstrable affect on disease transmission.

Insecticide-treated nets (ITNs)

The use of bed nets impregnated with pyrethroids such as permethrin, cyhalothrin, or deltamethrin gives substantial protection against malaria in endemic areas. In some areas, insecticide-treated door and window curtains are used instead of bed nets. The current combined evidence indicates that ITNs can reduce all-cause childhood mortality by 17%, averting 5.5 deaths for every 1000 African children protected. Over 50% of clinical attacks can be prevented through the wide-scale use of ITNs and infection prevalence can be reduced by 13% in areas of stable endemic transmission. The effect is due to a combination of reduced access of mosquitoes to people because of the net, a repellent and lethal effect of the insecticide on the mosquitoes trying to bite, and, sometimes, an effect on local mosquito densities so that even those outside the nets may get some protection. Thus, health impacts are maximized when large sectors of a community are using ITNs, thereby providing a 'public good' by reducing local transmission. Nets are obviously most effective when mosquito biting is concentrated late at night and indoors.

ITNs appear to be one of the most promising means of control while the development of an operational vaccine is awaited. Although initial coverage in many malaria endemic countries was poor, it has increased in recent years through free distribution linked to mass vaccine campaigns or availability of heavily subsidized nets at clinics. This is crucial for reaching vulnerable and impoverished rural populations. Retreatment of nets has proved difficult to maintain in many parts of Africa. However, the recent launch of two registered brands of permanently treated nets aims to circumvent this problem. LLINs retain 50% of their original anopheline knockdown efficacy after 2 years and cost approximately US$4.80 each in 2005. Currently only one class of insecticides, pyrethroids, are recommended by the WHO Pesticide Evaluation Scheme (WHOPES) for use on nets because of their rapid action, low mammalian toxicity relative to their insect toxicity, and lack of odour. The efficacy of pyrethroids on LLINs is, however, threatened by the rapid increases in pyrethroid resistance among mosquito vectors in many parts of the world. In any insecticide-based vector control activity, insecticide resistance should be monitored at least annually as resistance is dynamic and can evolve rapidly.

Repellents

Repellents are used for personal protection. Compounds such as diethyltoluamide (DEET) applied directly to the skin or to clothes can reduce the amount of mosquito–human biting contact for several hours after they are applied. However, their main use is against day-biting mosquitoes such as *Aedes aegypti* rather than malaria vectors. Some insecticides, such as DDT, have strong repellent properties.

Indoor residual house spraying (IRS)

During the global eradication era, IRS was instrumental in breaking malaria transmission in many parts of the world including Sri Lanka and South America. DDT at 2 g/m^2 will remain toxic to endophilic anophelines for 6 months or more on nonabsorbent wall materials, with cyhalothrin or deltamethrin at a much lower dosage giving up to 4-month protection, while organophosphorus insecticides such as malathion, propoxur, and fenitrothion at the same dosage last about 3 months. This approach relies on killing the mosquito after it has fed and is thus a more community-focused intervention than ITN, requiring coverage of all houses and shelters. It requires a strong national organization to manage the routine spraying of houses and the compliance of householders to allow spray teams access and to remove their possessions from the house before spraying. There are few community-wide randomized controlled trials of IRS across Africa upon which to base an informed choice about the likely benefits of this approach in reducing morbidity and mortality. Most studies have been undertaken in areas of low transmission, with results similar to those with ITN. It is accepted, however, that interruption of transmission is harder to achieve under conditions of intense perennial transmission. In remote rural areas, the logistics of IRS are more difficult, but community cooperation has been achieved and mean parasitaemia was reduced by 80% in one remote area of Mozambique.

Reducing vector abundance

Mosquitoes are highly selective in their choice of larval habitat. The World Health Organization defines environmental management as the implementation of activities related to the modification or manipulation of environmental factors to minimize vector propagation in order to reduce human-vector interaction. Three accepted strategies are as follows:

- Environmental modification—making sites unsuitable for vector breeding by draining, changing the rate of water flow, and adding or removing shade, cutting emergent vegetation, and altering the margins of bodies of water. Near the sea, salinity changes may be relevant. For small reservoirs and irrigation canals, cyclical changes in water level by means of a large siphon may control larvae by alternately stranding and flushing. Intermittent drying out of irrigation channels may also be of value
- Environmental manipulation—filling holes, e.g. with polystyrene beads or soil, or using the Bti toxin derived from the bacteria *Bacillus thuringiensis*
- Reducing human contact—using infective vectors by zooprophylaxis, modifying of human habitations, or purposely changing human behaviour

The basic epidemiology of local mosquito populations must be understood before control programmes are initiated. Mosquitoes cannot be eradicated because of the cost, ecological impact, or logistics and so the target threshold for the vector population is set at or below acceptable levels of potential disease transmission. Where habitats cannot be drained or rendered structurally unsuitable for mosquito breeding, chemical larvicides may be used. Historically, diesel oil, at 40 litre/ha of water surface with or without the addition of insecticides, prevented the larvae breathing when it was applied to the water surface with a spreading agent. Paris Green (1 kg/ha), temephos granules (2–20 kg/ha), or less than one-tenth of the amount of pyriproxyfen are effective and safer.

Intermittent preventive treatment

As an intermittent preventive treatment in pregnancy (IPTp), it was shown during the late 1990s that a therapeutic course of sulphadoxine–pyrimethamine given on two or three occasions during the second and third trimesters of pregnancy was effective in preventing infection of the placenta, reducing the incidence of anaemia in pregnant mothers, and increasing the birth weights of newborn children. This strategy continues to be implemented in many African countries but it is likely to become decreasingly effective because IPTp works less well in HIV-positive women and there is no proven safe alternative to sulphadoxine–pyrimethamine for IPTp in areas where resistance to this combination is rapidly expanding. DHA–mefloquine, DHA–piperaquine, and mefloquine–azithromycin combinations have been proposed as potential replacements subject to successful trials.

The concept of IPT has recently been extended to target infants (IPTi) by providing therapeutic courses of antimalarials at the same time as vaccination. Studies in Africa have shown that sulphadoxine–pyrimethamine or amodiaquine reduces the incidence of malaria and severe anaemia during the first year of life by 50 to 67%. The combined effects of IPTi and ITNs are currently being investigated.

Access to effective medicines

Even though preventive strategies may halve the incidence of clinical malaria, effective and prompt case management remains a fundamental adjunct to control, particularly among African children who experience at least 20 clinical attacks during their first 5 years of life. Cheap drugs such as chloroquine and sulphadoxine–pyrimethamine was the basis of malaria management in Africa and, during the early 1990s, resistance to both drugs increased rapidly and malaria mortality rose to levels similar to those witnessed in the colonial era despite a general decline in childhood deaths not attributable to malaria. Possible replacements for failing drugs are existing drugs combined with artemisinin derivatives. ACTs have the additional public health benefit of reducing transmission, like wide-scale use of ITNs. Introduction of combination mefloquine–artesunate therapy among refugees on the Thai–Burmese border was associated with an 18.5-fold reduction in gametocyte carriage rates, halving frequency of *P. falciparum* transmission in the area.

Control strategies based on case management depend on prompt treatment of appropriate patients with effective medicines. Since clinical criteria for diagnosing malaria have low specificity, parasitological diagnosis remains the gold standard. However, in many remote rural communities diagnostic facilities are inadequate and WHO's Integrated Management of Childhood Illnesses (IMCI) recommends that all children living in malaria endemic areas (where >5% of fevers are due to malaria) should be given presumptive antimalarial treatment if they are febrile. The logic is that misdiagnosis, even in a small proportion of febrile children with malaria, can be serious because of the rapidity of progression to severe disease. Recommendations for older children and adults in malaria endemic areas are more ambiguous, posing a problem at a time when new, more expensive drugs are being deployed and malaria continues to be a diagnosis of convenience or a diagnosis by default, leading to massive overdiagnosis and overtreatment of malaria in these age groups.

Access to medicines remains poor in many malarious countries. In Kenya, less than 5% of children received an antimalarial within 24 h of the onset of symptoms. Increasing accessibility to new ACTs for the most vulnerable groups, largely African children, will require innovative methods of delivery. Operational approaches to improve access to effective medicines include training mothers or community-resource persons to administer medicines in the home, better training of shopkeepers to deliver advice when selling over-the-counter antimalarials, and improving community awareness of the need to get children to clinic early.

The aim of wide-scale use of ACT in Africa by 2015 is confronted by several problems. First, new ACT drugs cost 10 times as much as current failing drugs, putting them beyond the essential drugs budgets of most poor countries. International funding has been assembled through the Global Fund to Fight AIDS, Tuberculosis and Malaria but this will be effective only if there are guarantees of long-term sustainable financing. Secondly, the agricultural sector must produce sufficient *Artemisia annua*, the source of artemisinins. In the longer term, synthetic artemisinin compounds might eventually alleviate the dependence on natural products.

Malarial vaccines

Difficulties facing vaccine development

Vaccines offer one of the most effective public health tools for controlling infectious diseases. The obstacles to developing a malaria vaccine are formidable: the malaria parasite is complex and multistaged, with a large genome (25–30 Mb with 5000–6000 genes). Many of the potential immune targets are polymorphic and the parasite has a large capacity for evolving evasive strategies. Most effort has gone into developing subunit vaccines based usually on single antigens thought to be critical in the parasite's biology. There are now a large number of potential vaccine candidates and one of the barriers to moving from concept to vaccine is the lack of appropriate animal models or *in vitro* correlates of immunity against which to select candidates for field trials. In the case of pre-erythrocytic vaccines, the development of centres for experimental immunization and challenge has offered a way of identifying effective candidates and it is likely that this approach will be extended to blood-stage vaccines.

Pre-erythrocytic vaccines

The aim of a pre-erythrocytic vaccine is either to block the establishment of an infection by preventing sporozoites from invading hepatocytes or to target the intrahepatic parasite to prevent progression to a blood-stage infection. Such infection-blocking immunity can be established in murine and human malaria by the repeated injection of irradiated sporozoites. Although establishing an important proof of principle, the apparent impracticality of using live attenuated sporozoites led to a focus on achieving the same effect using subunit vaccines. This led to the cloning in the 1980s of the first malaria gene, for the circumsporozoite protein, a major component of the coat of the sporozoite. This provided the basis for the development of a subunit vaccine, RTS,S, a fusion protein combining part of the circumsporozoite protein of *P. falciparum* with HBsAg with a complex adjuvant (AS02). RTS,S has consistently provided 30 to 40% protection against sporozoite challenges in nonimmune volunteers. Recent trials in infants and young children in Kenya and Tanzania showed a protective efficacy of 53% against malaria disease and large-scale phase III trials in infants across Africa are underway with results expected by 2011. The demonstration of efficacy (albeit not complete) of a subunit vaccine (RTS, S) based on one part of a single molecule from such a complex parasite has been important in giving confidence to the idea of developing antimalarial vaccines. Many investigators feel that given the complexity of the parasite and the high degree of antigenic polymorphism, the eventual ideal vaccine will involve combinations of antigens, probably from both pre-erythrocytic and erythrocytic stages. An extension of the same idea has recently seen a return of interest in the possibility of whole parasite vaccines. Remarkably, it has been shown that many of the apparent logistic objections to the production of attenuated sporozoite vaccines can in fact be overcome and plans are advanced for first experimental challenges of volunteers.

Blood-stage vaccines

The aims of blood-stage vaccines are to limit parasite replication and prevent clinical disease. A number of candidate vaccines based on key molecules on the merozoite surface or released from the merozoite at the time of RBC invasion (e.g. MSP1, MSP2, MSP3, AMA1) are at various stages of development and several candidate vaccines are in early field trials. Particular problems likely to be faced involve the high degree of antigenic polymorphism shown by most of the candidate vaccine molecules. This has also stood in the way of developing vaccines based on the other obvious target for protective immune responses, the parasite-derived antigens expressed on the infected RBC surface. However, in the particular case of pregnancy related malaria, the RBC expressed parasite molecules are of much more limited diversity and efforts are under way to develop a vaccine based on this subset of PfEMP1 antigens. These efforts have not yet reached the stage of human trials.

Transmission-blocking vaccines (TBVs)

TBVs aim to prevent the transmission of malaria by blocking the parasite's development in the mosquito by inducing antibodies targeting either antigens present on the sexual stages of the parasites or mosquito antigens that are required for the successful development of the parasite in the midgut of its vector. Candidate vaccines have been shown to induce antibodies that completely block transmission of *P. falciparum* and *P. vivax*.

The malaria vaccine field is rapidly changing and updated information on the range of candidate vaccines can be obtained at http://www.malariavaccine.org and http://www.who.int/immunization.

Prevention of malaria in travellers

Advice to travellers

The prevention of malaria in travellers, particularly those usually resident in nonmalarious areas but visiting endemic regions, including those visiting their friends and relatives ('VFR's), has become more difficult because of resistance to antimalarial drugs. As a result, prevention can never be complete. Travellers must be advised to: (1) be aware of the risk; (2) reduce exposure to being bitten by anopheline mosquitoes; (3) take chemoprophylaxis where appropriate; and (4) seek immediate medical advice in the event of any fever or influenza-like illness developing while in the area, or within 3 months or more of leaving it, and to mention malaria as a possibility regardless of the precautions taken.

Preventive advice is subject to uncertainty because unequivocal data on efficacy are often unavailable, published studies are conflicting, the distribution of resistance to many prophylactics is changing and not well mapped, and experts disagree on the balance between the risk of malaria and the risk of side effects. Travellers may obtain conflicting opinions from different sources, jeopardizing their adherence to any one regimen. The WHO list of malarious areas, updated annually, and other publications are inevitably directed towards prophylaxis for areas of greatest transmission. Advice from someone who knows the country and the traveller's itinerary is more specific and therefore more reliable.

No prophylactic regimen will give total protection, but many will reduce substantially the risk of malaria. Strict adherence, even to a suboptimal prophylactic regimen, is more important than vacillation in search of the ideal.

Diagnosis of imported malaria is a medical emergency as, exceptionally, falciparum malaria can be fatal within 24 h of the first symptom and the disease is often misdiagnosed (see Table 7.8.2.3). Several fatal cases are reported in the United Kingdom and the United States of America each year. Expert diagnosis and appropriate drugs may not be readily available. Useful guidelines are published by Centres for Disease Control in the United States of America and the Health Protection Agency and National Travel Health Network and Centre in the United Kingdom.

When falciparum malaria is diagnosed in a traveller, the rest of their tour group should be screened as a matter of urgency, as they can be presumed to have shared the same exposure risk.

Prevention of mosquito bites

Bed nets without tears or other holes through which mosquitoes might enter, impregnated with a pyrethroid insecticide such as permethrin, deltamethrin, or cyhalothrin, should be used and properly tucked in. These also afford protection against other arthropod vectors, ectoparasites and even night-biting kraits (snakes). A well-screened bedroom and other accommodation, combined with use of a knock-down insecticide after the doors have been closed before dusk, gives substantial protection. Clothes (long sleeves and trousers) that deter mosquito bites, repellent sprays and soaps (containing DEET or permethrin), and avoiding exposure to bites in the evenings will also help.

Chemoprophylaxis

Choice and dosage of chemoprophylaxis

Detailed maps of the distribution of malaria in different countries and the recommended chemoprophylaxis for each area are listed in 'Further reading'. Where there is a substantial risk of chloroquine-resistant falciparum malaria, atovaquone–proguanil, mefloquine, or doxycycline are appropriate (Box 7.8.2.4). Of these, mefloquine and atovaquone–proguanil are licensed for children and doxycycline should not be given to children under 8 years old (British National Formulary: 12 years) (Table 7.8.2.6). Pregnant women are best advised to avoid malarious areas. Apart from proguanil–chloroquine, no drug has been proved safe for prophylaxis during pregnancy but, if exposure is unavoidable in a high-risk area, mefloquine is recommended.

Box 7.8.2.4 Recommended malaria prophylaxis (adult dose) in addition to general measures specified in text

- Where chloroquine-resistant *P. falciparum* is absent:
  - Chloroquine 300 mg base weekly (best for short-term visitors)
  - Proguanil 200 mg daily (best for long-term residents)
- Where chloroquine-resistant *P. falciparum* is not widespread and is predominantly of low degree:
  - Chloroquine 300 mg base weekly plus proguanil 200 mg daily
- Where highly chloroquine-resistant *P. falciparum* occurs:[a]

  (1) Atovaquone–proguanil 1 tablet daily

  or

  (2) Mefloquine 250 mg weekly

  or

  (3) Doxycycline 100 mg daily

  or

  (4) [Chloroquine 300 mg base weekly plus proguanil 200 mg daily]

[a]Regimens (1), (2), and (3) are more effective in some areas of South-East Asia, Africa, and South America, but there is a low but significant risk of severe side effects with (2) and (3). Regimen (4) will give only limited protection but is the least likely of the four regimens to cause toxic side effects and is preferred for pregnant women and, at reduced dosage, for young children (Table 7.8.2.6).

Atovaquone–proguanil

This combination has two great advantages: adverse effects are less frequent and less serious than for mefloquine and doxycycline; and it is a causal prophylactic, attacking pre-erythrocytic stages of malarial parasites. Consequently, it need be continued for only 7 days after leaving the malarious area, improving the chance

Table 7.8.2.6 Doses of prophylactic antimalarial drugs for children

Age	Weight (kg)	Drug and tablet size		
		Chloroquine (150 mg) weekly with proguanil (100 mg) daily	Mefloquine 250 mg	Doxycycline 100 mg
Fraction of tablet				
Term to 12 weeks	<6.0	1/4	NR	NR
3–11 months	6.0–9.9	1/2	1/4	NR
1–3 years 11 months	10.0–15.9	3/4	1/4	NR
4–7 years 11 months	16–24.9	1	1/2	NR
8–12 years	25–44.9	1 1/2	3/4	NR
>12 years	>44.9	2	1	1

NR, not recommended.

For children aged under 2 years in areas of chloroquine resistance, the appropriate medication is chloroquine plus proguanil. Chloroquine is available as a syrup but the proguanil has to be powdered on to jam or food. Measures against mosquito bites are specially important.

of adherence. However, resistance is emerging and atovaquone–proguanil is expensive. The cost for short visits is similar to that of mefloquine or doxycycline but the differential cost rises greatly for longer visits.

Mefloquine

Mefloquine has a long half-life and on a weekly dosage schedule the blood level rises to a plateau from about 7 weeks. Most of its side effects, the main problem with its use, are associated with the initial three doses. The drug should therefore be started 2.5 weeks before departure to a malarious area, to allow a switch to an alternative if side effects prove troublesome. It can be used safely for at least 2 or 3 years. The most serious early side effects of mefloquine are neuropsychiatric: anxiety, depression, delusions, fits, and psychotic attacks. Their incidence is disputed. Airline passenger surveys have shown a frequency of 1:10 000, but experienced doctors in the United Kingdom assert a much higher frequency. It is not recommended for those in the first trimester of pregnancy or at risk of pregnancy during the 3 months after the end of chemoprophylaxis. In later pregnancy, the uncertain risk of stillbirth rate must be balanced against the considerable risks of malaria. Mefloquine is contraindicated in people with a history of epilepsy or psychiatric disease. Mefloquine resistance is reported from Africa, South-East Asia, and the Amazon region.

Doxycycline

Doxycycline proved to give good protection against drug-resistant falciparum malaria in trials in Oceania and it is being increasingly used, especially for those who cannot or are unwilling to take mefloquine. It should not be used in children or pregnant women. The main side effects are photosensitization, which occurs in up to 3% of users, a tendency to precipitate vaginal thrush in women (preventable with a one-dose therapy for candidal infections), and the rare risk of *Clostridium difficile* diarrhoea. However, doxycycline may reduce the risk of travellers' diarrhoea. 'Heartburn' and gastrointestinal discomfort from doxycycline itself is not uncommon. The drug is taken daily with food, taking care not to miss any days and avoiding lying down too soon after taking it to avert a real risk of acute pain from ulceration of the lower oesophagus. To get accustomed to taking daily medication, it should be taken a few days before departure.

Chloroquine and/or proguanil

In malarious areas where chloroquine-resistant *P. falciparum* is rare or absent, mainly in western Asia, North Africa, and Central America, chloroquine 300 mg (base), two tablets taken once a week, gives good protection. Since it suppresses only the blood forms, it will not prevent relapses of *P. vivax* or *P. ovale*. Continuous chloroquine prophylaxis is limited to 6 years because of a low risk of irreversible retinopathy. Beyond this, proguanil may be substituted. Proguanil 200 mg daily will act as a true causal prophylactic but is poorly protective against *P. vivax*. The extremely low incidence of adverse effects from proguanil makes it acceptable to long-term residents in endemic areas.

Where the prevalence and degree of chloroquine resistance is low, in parts of India and the rest of South Asia, the combination of chloroquine and proguanil (Table 7.8.2.7) remains effective and has the advantage of low toxicity and safety in pregnant women and in young children. However, it no longer provides adequate protection in sub-Saharan Africa, parts of India, South-East Asia, or the Amazon region.

Continuation after leaving the malarious area

All antimalarial agents except atovaquone–proguanil must be continued for 4 weeks after leaving the malarious area so that merozoites are killed when they emerge late from the liver into the blood stream.

Chemoprophylaxis in people with epilepsy

Proguanil, atovaquone–proguanil, and doxycycline do not increase the risk of fits in people with epilepsy.

Rejected chemoprophylactic drugs

The following drugs are unsuitable for chemoprophylaxis: amodiaquine because of the high risk of agranulocytosis; Fansidar (25 mg pyrimethamine and 100 mg sulphadoxine per tablet) because of the frequency of severe skin reactions; pyrimethamine on its own because it is ineffective in most malarial areas; and halofantrine because of its cardiotoxicity.

Geographical risk of malaria

The risk of malaria is much higher in sub-Saharan Africa than elsewhere. Prophylaxis must be taken except where the altitude is too great for transmission to occur or in the nonendemic southern parts of the continent (Fig. 7.8.2.10). In Asia, the risk is usually much lower. Visitors to the air-conditioned hotels of the larger cities of South-East Asia do not need prophylaxis but elsewhere in Asia there may be urban malaria. Mefloquine does not protect adequately against malaria in South-East Asia; travellers to areas of higher transmission will need regimens (1) or (3) in Box 7.8.2.4. Those living for long periods in such areas may prefer to adopt vigilance and the early treatment of fevers, but awareness of the risk is essential. Freedom from malaria in Asia by travellers does not mean that they will escape infection in Africa!

Travellers in remote areas away from prompt medical assistance should carry a therapeutic dose of atovaquone–proguanil, mefloquine, or lumefantrine-artemether in case they develop an acute fever.

Further reading

General

Russell PF (1955). *Man's mastery of malaria*. Oxford University Press, London.

Warrell DA, Gilles HM (eds) (2002). *Essential malariology*, 4th edition. Arnold, London.

Wernsdorfer WH, McGregor IA (1988). *Malaria. Principles and practice of malariology*. Churchill Livingstone, Edinburgh.

Parasite biology

Coatney GR, *et al.* (1971). *The primate malarias*. US Department of Health, Education and Welfare, Bethesda, MD.

Collins WE, Jeffrey GM (2005). *Plasmodium ovale*: parasite and disease. *Clin Microbiol Rev*, **18**, 570–81.

Collins WE, Jeffrey GM (2007). *Plasmodium malariae*: parasite and disease. *Clin Microbiol Rev*, **20**, 579–92.

Garnham PCC (1966). *Malaria parasites and other haemosporidia*. Blackwell, Oxford.

Gaur D, *et al.* (2004). Parasite ligand-host receptor interactions during invasion of erythrocytes by *Plasmodium* merozoites. *Int J Parasitol*, **34**, 1413–29.

Kats LM, *et al.* (2008). Protein trafficking to apical organelles of malaria parasites—building an invasion machine. *Traffic*, **9**, 176–86.

Kwiatkowski D (2006). Host genetic factors in resistance and susceptibility to malaria. *Parassitologia*, **48**, 450–67.

Loscertales MP, *et al.* (2007). ABO blood group phenotypes and *Plasmodium falciparum* malaria: unlocking a pivotal mechanism. *Adv Parasitol*, **65**, 1–50.

Oh SS, Chishti AH (2005). Host receptors in malaria merozoite invasion. *Curr Top Microbiol Immunol*, **295**, 203–32.

Prugnolle F, Durand P, Neel C, *et al.* (2010). African great apes are natural hosts of multiple related malaria species, including *Plasmodium falciparum*. PNAS published online before print January 19, 2010, doi:10.1073/pnas.0914440107

Sinden RE (1978). Cell biology. In: Killick-Kendrick R, Peters W (eds) *Rodent malaria*, pp. 85–168. Academic Press, London.

Mosquito biology

Fine PEM (1981). Epidemiological principles of vector mediated transmission. In: McKelvey JJ, *et al.* (eds) Vectors of disease agents, pp. 77–91. Praeger Scientific, New York.

Hemingway J, *et al.* (2006). The Innovative Vector Control Consortium: improved control of mosquito borne diseases. *Trends Parasitol*, **22**, 308–12.

James AA, *et al.* (1999). Controlling malaria transmission with genetically engineered *Plasmodium* resistant mosquitoes: Milestones in a model system. *Parassitologia*, **41**, 461–71.

Mongin E, *et al.* (2004). The *Anopheles gambiae* genome: an update. *Trends Parasitol*, **20**, 49–52.

Epidemiology and control

Chandramohan D, Jaffar S, Greenwood BM (2002). Use of clinical algorithms for diagnosing malaria. *Trop Med Int Health*, **7**, 45–52.

Guerra CA, Snow RW, Hay SI (2006). Mapping the global extent of malaria in 2005. *Trends Parasitol*, **22**, 353–8.

Guerra CA, *et al.* (2008). The limits and intensity of *Plasmodium falciparum* transmission: Implications for malaria control and elimination worldwide. *PLoS Med*, **5**, e38.

Guyatt HL, Snow RW (2004). The impact of malaria in pregnancy on low-birth weight in sub-Saharan Africa. *Clin Microbiol Rev*, **17**, 760–9.

Hay SI, *et al.* (2004). The global distribution and population at risk of malaria: past, present and future. *Lancet Infectious Diseases*, **4**, 327–336.

Hay SI, *et al.* (2005). Urbanization, malaria transmission and disease burden in Africa. *Nat Rev Microbiol*, **3**, 81–90.

Hay SI, Snow RW (2006). The Malaria Atlas Project (MAP): developing global maps of malaria risk. *PLoS Med*, **3**, e473.

Hay SI, *et al.* (2009). A world malaria map: Plasmodium falciparum endemicity in 2007. *PLoS Medicine*, **6**, e1000048

Lengeler C (2005). Insecticide treated bednets and curtains for preventing malaria. *Cochrane Database Syst Rev*, CD000363.

MacDonald, G (1957). *The epidemiology and control of malaria*. Oxford University Press, London.

Snow RW, *et al.* (2005). The global distribution of clinical episodes of *Plasmodium* falciparum malaria. *Nature*, **434**, 214–17.

Snow RW, Omumbo JA (2006). Malaria. In: Jamison DT, *et al.* (eds) *Disease and mortality in sub-Saharan Africa*, 2nd edition, pp. 195–214. World Bank, Washington, DC.

Clinical features, immunology, pathology, diagnosis, treatment, and prevention in travellers

Anstey NM, *et al.* (2009). The pathophysiology of vivax malaria. *Trends in Parasitology*, **25**, 20–27.

Artemether-Quinine Meta-analysis Study Group (2001). A meta-analysis using individual patient data of trials comparing artemether with quinine in the treatment of severe falciparum malaria. *Trans R Soc Trop Med Hyg*, **95**, 637–50.

Beare NA, *et al.* (2006). Malarial retinopathy: a newly established diagnostic sign in severe malaria. *Am J Trop Med Hyg*, **75**, 790–7.

Daneshvar C, *et al.* (2009). Clinical and laboratory features of human *Plasmodium knowlesi* infection. *Clin Infect Dis*, **49**, 852–60.

Dondorp A, *et al.* (2005). Artesunate versus quinine for treatment of severe falciparum malaria: a randomised trial. *Lancet*, **366**, 717–25.

Dondorp AM, *et al.* (2008). Direct in vivo assessment of microcirculatory dysfunction in severe falciparum malaria. *J Infect Dis*, **197**, 79–84.

Ekland EH, Fidock DA (2007). Advances in understanding the genetic basis of antimalarial drug resistance. *Curr Opin Microbiol*, **10**, 363–70.

Gomez MF, *et al.* (2009). Pre-referral rectal artesunate to prevent death and disability in sever malaria: a placebo-controlled trial. *Lancet*, **373**, 557–66.

Hanson J, *et al.* (2009). Hyponatremia in severe malaria: evidence for an appropriate anti-diuretic hormone response to hypovolemia. *Am J Trop Med Hyg*, **80**, 141–5.

He W, *et al.* (2008). Duffy antigen receptor for chemokines mediates trans-infection of HIV-1 from red blood cells to target cells and affects HIV-AIDS susceptibility. *Cell Host Microbe*, **17**, 52–62.

Lalloo DG, *et al.* (2007). UK malaria treatment guidelines. *J Infect*, **54**, 111–21.

MacPherson GG, *et al.* (1985). Human cerebral malaria: a quantitative ultrastructural analysis of parasitized erythrocyte sequestration. *Am J Pathol*, **119**, 385–401.

Noedl H, *et al.* (2009). Evidence of artemisinin-resistant malaria in western Cambodia. *N Engl J Med*, **359**, 2619–20.

Marsh K, *et al* (1995). Indicators of life-threatening malaria in African children: clinical spectrum and simplified prognostic criteria. *N Engl J Med*, **332**, 1399–404.

Moody A (2002). Rapid diagnostic tests for malaria parasites. *Clin Microbiol Rev*, **15**, 66–78.

Turner GDH, *et al.* (1994). An immunohistochemical study of the pathology of fatal malaria. *Am J Pathol*, **145**, 1057–69.

Vallely A, *et al.* (2007). Intermittent preventive treatment for malaria in pregnancy in Africa: what's new, what's needed? *Malar J*, **6**, 16.

Warrell DA, *et al* (1982). Dexamethasone proves deleterious in cerebral malaria. A double-blind trial in 100 comatose patients. *N Engl J Med*, **306**, 313–19.

World Health Organization (2000). Severe falciparum malaria. *Trans R Soc Trop Med Hyg*, **94** (Suppl. 1), 51–90.

Internet resources

Centers for Disease Control and Prevention. *Malaria.* http://www.cdc.gov/malaria/index.htm

Chiodini P, *et al.* (2007). *Guidelines for malaria prevention in travellers from the United Kingdom 2007.* Health Protection Agency, London. http://www.hpa.org.uk/webw/HPAweb&HPAwebStandard/HPAweb_C/1203496943315?p=1153846674367

Lalloo DG, *et al.* (2007). UK malaria treatment guidelines. *J Infect*, **54**, 111–21. http://www.hpa.org.uk/web/HPAwebFile/HPAweb_C/1194947343507.

Malaria Atlas Project. http://www.map.ox.ac.uk

Malaria Vaccine Initiative. *Accelerating malaria vaccine development.* http://www.malariavaccine.org

MalariaGen. *Genomic epidemiology network.* http://www.malariagen.net

National Travel Health Network and Centre. *Protecting the health of British travellers.* http://www.nathnac.org/

RDT info. *Commercially available rapid tests for malaria.* http://www.rapid-diagnostics.org/rti-malaria-com.htm

VectorBase. *An NIAID bioinformatics resource center for invertebrate vectors of human pathogens.* http://www.vectorbase.org/index.php

World Health Organization (2006). *Guidelines for the treatment of malaria.* http://www.who.int/malaria/docs/TreatmentGuidelines2006.pdf

World Health Organization (2008). *International travel and health.* http://www.who.int/ith/chapters/en/index.html

World Health Organization. *Immunization, vaccines and biologicals.* Available from: http://www.who.int/immunization

7.8.3 Babesiosis

Philippe Brasseur

Essentials

Babesia are intraerythrocytic, tick-transmitted, protozoan parasites that infect a broad range of wild and domesticated mammals including cattle, horses, dogs, and rodents. Human babesial infection is uncommon, caused by *B. microti* in North America and *B. divergens* in Europe, with most infections occurring in asplenic people. Presentation is typically with nonspecific 'viral-type' symptoms. Haemolytic anaemia is a characteristic feature and can be severe, particularly with *B. divergens*. Diagnosis is by discovering babesia organisms in Giemsa-stained blood smears, or detection of its DNA in blood by PCR. Aside from supportive care, treatment is usually with combinations of clindamycin, quinine, atovaquone and azithromycin. Mortality ranges from 5 to 40%. Prevention is by use of repellents, removing ticks from the skin, and avoidance of exposure for asplenic and immunocompromised individuals: there is no vaccine.

Epidemiology

Although several species of babesia may infect humans, two species, *Babesia microti* and *B. divergens*, are responsible for most cases of human babesiosis. In the United States of America, more than 1000 cases of *B. microti* infections have been reported since 1988, mostly from the north-east coast including Nantucket, Martha's Vineyard, and Block Island. *B. microti* is transmitted by *Ixodes scapularis* (previously *I. dammini*) and its reservoir host is the common white-footed mouse *Peromyscus leucopus*. *B. duncani*, a new species has been identified in 9 patients in United States of America. The zoonotic *Borrelia burgdorferi*, causing Lyme disease, is also transmitted by *I. scapularis* and coinfections are documented. The risk of both babesiosis and Lyme disease is highest in June when nymphal *I. scapularis* are most abundant. More than 20 cases of transfusion-transmitted babesiosis have been reported in the United States of America.

Since the first description of human babesiosis in Europe in 1957, more than 40 cases have been reported. Most of them were due to *B. divergens*, a common cattle pathogen transmitted by *I. ricinus*. France, the United Kingdom, and Ireland account for more than 50% of the cases reported in Europe. Farmers, foresters, campers, and hikers are affected, usually between May and October, the season of activity of *I. ricinus*. Most infections (83%) occur in asplenic people. No transfusion-transmitted case has been reported in Europe, but the risk exists, since *B. divergens* may survive in packed red blood cells for several weeks at 4°C. *B. venatorum*, closely related to but distinct from *B. odocoilei* that infects white-tail deer in United States of America has been isolated in 3 asplenic patients in Italy, Austria and Germany.

Pathogenesis

Ticks infected with babesia inoculate parasites while feeding on a vertebrate. Babesia enter red blood cells directly and multiply by budding to form two or four parasites, rarely more, in 8 to 10 h. They are released and invade other erythrocytes. The spleen plays a major role in resistance to babesial infections, especially in the case of *B. divergens* babesiosis.

Clinical features

B. microti infection

In humans, *B. microti* babesiosis is characterized by gradually developing malaise, anorexia, and fatigue with subsequent development of fever, sweats, and generalized myalgia, starting from 1 to 4 weeks after a tick bite. Headache, shaking chills, nausea, depression, and hyperaesthesia are less frequent. Mild hepatomegaly and splenomegaly may be detected. A mild to severe haemolytic anaemia, thrombocytopenia and normal white blood cell count are generally present. Lactate dehydrogenase, liver enzymes, and unconjugated bilirubin levels may be increased. Parasites are found in peripheral blood of 1 to 20% of patients with intact spleens, but in up to 80% of those who are asplenic. The illness is usually more severe in asplenic and older patients. Complications are more likely in the immunocompromised. Acute illness lasts from 1 to 4 weeks, but weakness and malaise often persist for several months. A low, asymptomatic parasitaemia may persist for several weeks after recovery. Case fatality is about 5%.

B. divergens infection

In Europe, *B. divergens* infections are usually more severe than those caused by *B. microti*, with a case fatality up to 42%. After an incubation period of 1 to 3 weeks, there is sudden severe intravascular haemolysis resulting in haemoglobinuria, severe anaemia, and jaundice, associated with nonperiodic high fever (40–41°C), hypotension, shaking chills, intense sweats, headache, myalgia, lumbar pain, vomiting, and diarrhoea. Peripheral blood *B. divergens* parasitaemia varies from 5 to 80%. Patients rapidly develop renal failure, which may be associated with pulmonary oedema, coma, and death.

Diagnosis

Babesiosis should be suspected in any patient from any area who presents with fever and a history of tick bite. Initially, *Plasmodium falciparum* malaria may be suspected, but lack of recent travel in malaria-endemic areas or recent blood transfusion and lack of a spleen should lead to suspicion of babesiosis. Diagnosis is based on discovering babesia in Giemsa-stained blood smears (Fig. 7.8.3.1). Babesia can be distinguished from plasmodia by the absence of gametocytes and pigment in erythrocytes.

B. microti is characterized by multiple basket-shaped parasites. In some cases, parasitaemia is sparse and detection of antibodies, using an indirect fluorescent antibody assay, may be useful for diagnosis. Antibody titres rise during the first weeks and fall after 5 months, but correlation between antibody titre and severity of the disease is poor.

B. divergens is characterized in Giemsa-stained blood smears by double piriform intraerythrocytic parasites or tetrads, but annular, punctiform, and filamentous forms may also be encountered. Serology cannot be used for a rapid diagnosis of *B. divergens* infection. Amplification of babesial DNA by polymerase chain reaction, using species-specific primers may establish the diagnosis of both *B. microti* and *B. divergens* within 24 h. These assays are more sensitive than, but equally specific as, smear detection. Clearance of DNA seems to be related to disappearance of parasites.

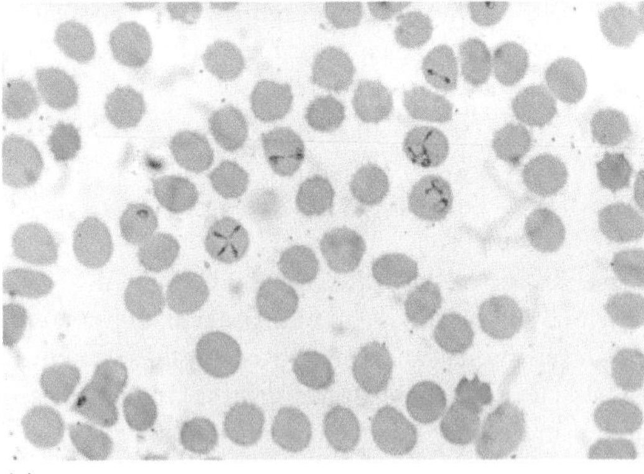

(a)

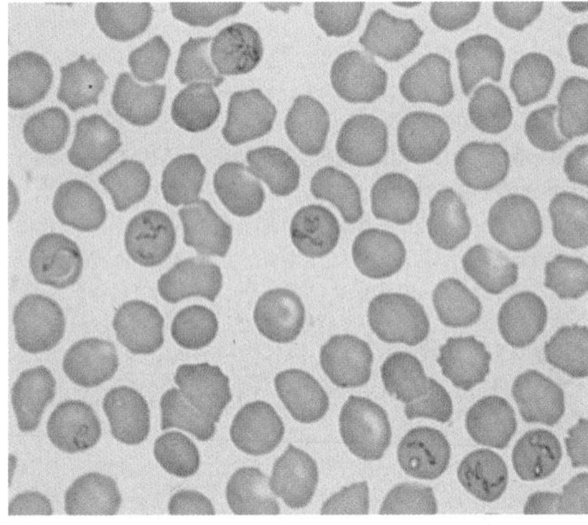

(b)

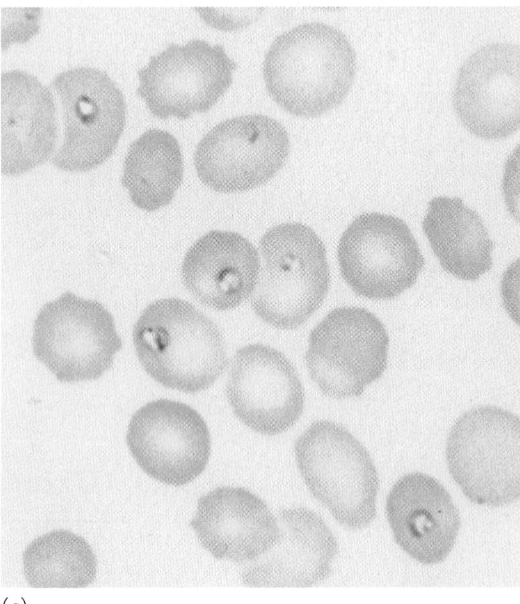

(c)

Fig. 7.8.3.1 (a) *Babesia divergens* infection in a 29-year-old Frenchman infected in Normandy. He had been splenectomized 4 months previously for idiopathic thrombocytopenia . Parasitaemia reached 30%. He was successfully treated with exchange transfusion, clindamycin, and quinine. (b) *Babesia microti* in a male patient, Missouri, United States of America (×100). (c) *Babesia microti* in a 72-year-old female patient, Massachusetts, United States of America (×150). (a, copyright P Brasseur; b, c, courtesy of Centers for Disease Control, Atlanta, GA.)

Treatment and prevention

Chloroquine, sulphadiazine, co-trimoxazole, pentamidine, or diminazene aceturate appear ineffective in completely eliminating babesia parasites. For *B. microti* infection, the standard treatment is a combination of atovaquone (750 mg every 12 h) and azithromycin (500–1000 mg orally on day 1, and 250–1000 mg therafter) for 7 days. Alternatively, a combination of clindamycin (600 mg intravenously or orally) with quinine (650 mg orally) every 6 to 8 h for at least 7 days in adults; treatment for children is atovaquone (20 mg/kg every 12 h, maximum 750 mg/dose) and azithromycin (10 mg/kg per day on day 1 and 5 mg/kg per day thereafter) or alternatively a combination of clindamycin (7–10 mg/kg) and quinine (8 mg/kg) every 6 to 8 h for at least 7 days. For immunocompromised patients, a treatment for 6 weeks and 2 additional weeks after blood parasite clearance is recommended. For patients with high parasitaemias (≥ 10%), haemolysis, or renal failure or those that are immunocompromised, these therapies might not be sufficient and exchange transfusion should be considered.

In Europe, babesiosis should be treated as a medical emergency. Immediate chemotherapy with either a combination of clindamycine and quinine or clindamycin alone reduces parasitaemia and prevents extensive haemolysis and renal failure. Exchange transfusion should be used in fulminating *B. divergens* cases. Imidocarb dipropionate, which has been used for treatment of cattle babesiosis, has been successfully used in two patients in Ireland, although this drug is not approved for human treatment.

Preventive measures consist of use of repellents, removing ticks from the skin, and avoiding exposure for asplenic and immunocompromised individuals. To date, no vaccine against human babesiosis is available.

Further reading

Homer MJ, *et al* (2000). Babesiosis. *Clin Microbiol Rev*, **13**, 451–69.

Vannier E, Krause PJ (2009). Update on babesiosis. *Interdiscip Perspect Infect Dis*; **984568**. Epub 2009 Aug 27.

7.8.4 Toxoplasmosis

Oliver Liesenfeld and Eskild Petersen

Essentials

Toxoplasma gondii is a protozoan parasite with worldwide distribution that infects up to one-third of the world's population. Human infection is acquired through ingestion in water or food of oocysts shed by cats, or by ingestion of bradyzoites released from cysts contained in uncooked or undercooked meat (e.g. sheep, swine, cattle). Following invasion in the intestine, tachyzoites rapidly disseminate throughout the host. Immune mechanisms mediate the formation of cysts, primarily in the brain, eye, and skeletal and heart muscles, where they persist for the life of the host. Presence of infection may be established by direct detection of the parasite in clinical samples (often by polymerase chain reaction, PCR) or by serological techniques.

Clinical features and treatment

Immunocompetent adults and children—primary infection is usually subclinical, but some patients develop cervical lymphadenopathy; specific treatment is not usually required.

Ocular disease—choroidoretinitis; treatment with pyrimethamine and sulphadiazine is usually recommended if there are severe inflammatory responses and/or proximity of retinal lesions to the fovea or optic disk.

Immunocompromised patients—the central nervous system is the most commonly affected site. Reactivation of latent infection can cause life-threatening encephalitis. Empirical anti-*T. gondii* therapy is given to patients with multiple ring-enhancing brain lesions on imaging, positive serology, and advanced immunodeficiency, most commonly with the combination of pyrimethamine/sulphadiazine and folinic acid.

Congenital toxoplasmosis—infection acquired in early pregnancy may cause severe damage to the fetus or intrauterine death; infection in the second and third trimesters goes unnoticed in the newborn in most cases, but signs of disease, e.g. chorioretinitis, may occur later in life. Suspected or established maternal infection acquired during pregnancy must be confirmed by prenatal diagnosis of fetal infection using PCR on amniotic fluid: if this is positive it is highly probable that the fetus is infected and pyrimethamine/sulphadiazine and folinic acid should be given and continued throughout the pregnancy.

Prevention

Prevention of infection by avoiding ingestion is the strategy of choice in seronegative people. Pyrimethamine sulphadiatine can be used for primary and secondary prophylaxis of seropositive immunocompromised patients or seronegative recipients of organ transplants from seropositive donors. Spiramycin can be used for secondary prevention of transmission from the acutely infected mother to her fetus.

Historical perspective

The first human case ascribed to infection with *Toxoplasma gondii* was a child with hydrocephalus reported by Janku in 1923. Sabin reported the first case of encephalitis due to *T. gondii* in 1941. Lymphadenopathy was recognized as a key symptom by Siim and Gard and Magnusson (1951). Encephalitis due to *T. gondii* in immunocompromised patients was first reported from patients with Hodgkin's disease during immunosuppressive treatment in 1967.

Aetiology, genetics, pathogenesis, and pathology

Aetiology

T. gondii is an obligate intracellular protozoan of the phylum Apicomplexa, subclass Coccidiasina. The parasite exists in three basic forms of medical importance: the oocyst ($10 \times 12\,\mu m$ in size), which is the product of the parasite's sexual cycle in the intestine of all members of the cat family; the tachyzoite (2–4 µm wide and 4–8 µm long), which is the asexual invasive form; and the cyst, which contains hundreds or thousands of bradyzoites in tissues (Fig. 7.8.4.1).

Ingestion of *T. gondii* cysts or oocysts (the natural route of infection) results in cyst (or oocyst) rupture and release of bradyzoites (or sporozoites) into the intestinal lumen, followed by rapid entry into intestinal cells and multiplication as tachyzoites. Tachyzoites are spread by disruption of infected cells, invasion of neighbouring cells, and via the bloodstream. In intermediate hosts and extraintestinal tissues of the cat, cysts containing bradyzoites are formed and persist lifelong. Immunodeficiency may result in reactivation of latent infection and severe disease, whereas reinfection does not appear to cause clinically apparent disease.

T. gondii consists of three clonal lineages designated types I, II, III, and archetypes, which differ in virulence and geographical distribution.

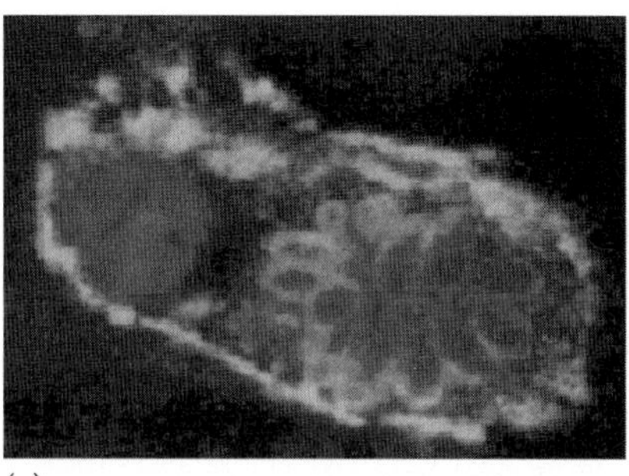

(a)

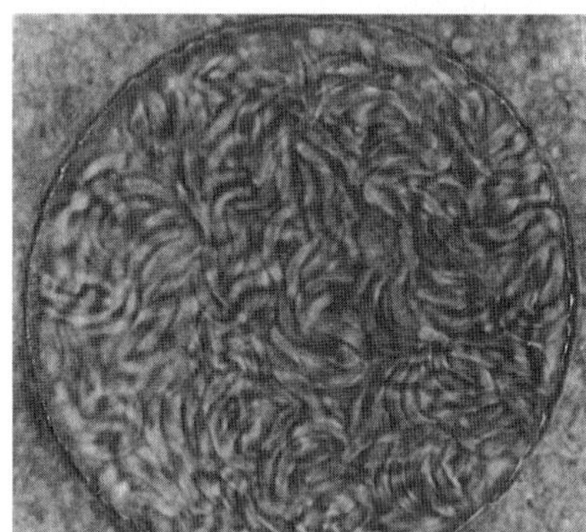

(b)

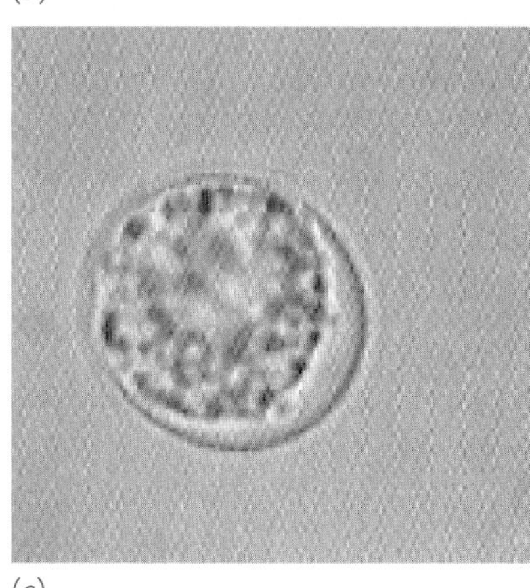

(c)

Fig. 7.8.4.1 *Toxoplasma gondii*: (a) Rosette-forming tachyzoites inside a macrophage, (b) bradyzoites inside a tissue cyst, and (c) oocyst in cat faeces.

Archtypes not belonging to type I, II or III, or more in Brazil compared to Europe and the United States of America, and clinical toxoplasmosis is more severe in Brazil compared to Europe (Gilbert *et al.* 2008). The recent description of strain-specific peptides has allowed typing of strains using serum. The generation of specific gene-deficient strains of *T. gondii* and the sequencing of the *Toxoplasma* genome (http://toxodb.org) will provide further insight into parasite virulence factors and specific host immune responses.

Pathogenesis

The inoculum size and virulence of the organism and the genetic background and immunological status of the individual appear to influence the course of the infection in humans. Following active invasion, *T. gondii* induces the formation of a parasitophorous vacuole containing secreted parasite proteins but excluding host proteins that would normally promote phagosome maturation, thereby preventing lysosome fusion. The molecular characterization and function of a number of proteins from organelles including rhoptries, micronemes, and dense granules have been reported. These molecules and the immunodominant tachyzoite surface antigen SAG1 are among the most promising vaccine candidates. Following intracellular replication and host cell disruption, parasites are disseminated via the blood stream and infect multiple organs including the central nervous system, eye, skeletal and heart muscle, and placenta. The developing immune response causes the formation of cysts in the central nervous system and skeletal muscle during the first week of infection. These persist lifelong. In immunocompromised hosts, cysts may disrupt and cause recrudescence of the infection, which then presents as life-threatening toxoplasmic encephalitis. Infection with *T. gondii* results in a strong and persistent Th1 response characterized by the production of interleukin 12 (IL-12), interferon-γ, and tumour necrosis factor α (TNF-α). Strain-specific differences in the modulation of host-cell transcription are mediated by a protein kinase, ROP16, released from rhoptries and injected into the host, resulting in the activation of signalling pathways and IL-12 production. The combined action of these cytokines and specific antibodies protects the host against rapid replication of tachyzoites and subsequent pathological changes. Dendritic cells and their capacity to produce IL-12 were identified as the main activators of Th1 immune reactions. Granulocytes may also contribute to the early production of IL-12. The activated macrophage inhibits or kills intracellular *T. gondii*, which counteract these actions by down-regulating surface molecules and interfering with apoptosis pathways in antigen-presenting cells, suggesting a role for these cells as 'Trojan horses' in early stages of infection. Sensitized CD4+ and CD8+ T lymphocytes are cytotoxic for *T. gondii*-infected cells. Both proinflammatory (e.g. interferon-γ and TNF-α) and down-regulatory cytokines (e.g. IL-10 and transforming growth factor β) are involved in balancing this response. Within 2 weeks after infection, IgG, IgM, IgA, and IgE antibodies against multiple *T. gondii* proteins can be detected. Reinfection may occur but does not appear to result in disease or in congenital transmission of the parasite. The production of IgA antibodies on mucosal surfaces appears to protect the host against reinfection.

Pathology

Histopathological changes in toxoplasma lymphadenitis in immunocompetent people are frequently distinctive and often diagnostic. They consist of reactive follicular hyperplasia, irregular clusters of epithelioid histiocytes encroaching on and blurring the margins of the germinal centres, and focal distension of sinuses with monocytic cells. Eye infection in immunocompetent patients produces acute choroidoretinitis characterized by severe inflammation and necrosis. The pathogenesis of recurrent choroidoretinitis is controversial. Rupture of cysts may release viable organisms that induce necrosis and inflammation; alternatively, choroidoretinitis may result from a hypersensitivity reaction of unknown cause. Damage to the central nervous system by *T. gondii*, toxoplasmic encephalitis (TE) is characterized by multiple foci of enlarging necrosis and microglia nodules. In infants, periaqueductal and periventricular vasculitis and necrosis are distinctive of congenital toxoplasmosis. The necrotic areas may calcify and lead to radiographic findings suggestive but not pathognomonic of toxoplasmosis. Hydrocephalus may result from obstruction of the aqueduct of Sylvius or foramen of Monro. Tachyzoites and cysts are seen in and adjacent to necrotic foci. The presence of multiple brain abscesses is the most characteristic feature of TE in severely immunodeficient patients and is especially characteristic of AIDS. At autopsy in AIDS patients with TE, there is almost universal involvement of the cerebral hemispheres and a remarkable predilection for the basal ganglia. In cases of congenital toxoplasmosis, necrosis of the brain is most intense in the cortex and basal ganglia.

Epidemiology

Infection with *T. gondii* in humans is naturally acquired through ingestion of cysts or oocysts. Humans can be infected by ingestion of undercooked or raw meat (e.g. sheep, swine, cattle) containing tissue cysts, or of water or food containing oocysts excreted in the faeces of infected cats. The differences in seroprevalence of *T. gondii* depend on eating habits and customs that support the ingestion of cysts as the major source of infection. Epidemics of toxoplasmosis in humans and sheep attributed to exposure to infected cats indicate the importance of oocyst excretion by cats. Several outbreaks of toxoplasmosis through contamination of drinking water by oocysts have been reported. This is a major route of transmission under poor socioeconomic conditions, where untreated surface water is drunk. Transmission of *T. gondii* in organs transplanted from seropositive donors to seronegative recipients remains an important cause of infection in immunocompromised patients. *T. gondii* may also be transmitted by blood or leucocytes from immunocompetent or immunocompromised donors.

In congenital transmission, the parasite gains access to the fetal circulation by infection of the placenta following maternal parasitaemia. The reported birth prevalence of congenital toxoplasmosis ranges from 1 to 10 per 10 000 live births in Europe and North America. The frequency of congenital transmission depends on the time during gestation when the mother acquired her infection (Fig. 7.8.4.2). Maternal infection acquired weeks or a few months before gestation poses little or no risk to the fetus. Infection acquired around the time of conception and within the first 2 weeks of gestation in most cases does not result in transmission, whereas rates of transmission are above 60% in the last trimester. There is an inverse relationship between frequency of transmission and severity of disease. Infection in the first and second trimester, although less frequent than infection in the third trimester, results in severe congenital toxoplasmosis more often (Fig. 7.8.4.3). In contrast, maternal infection during the third trimester, although more frequent

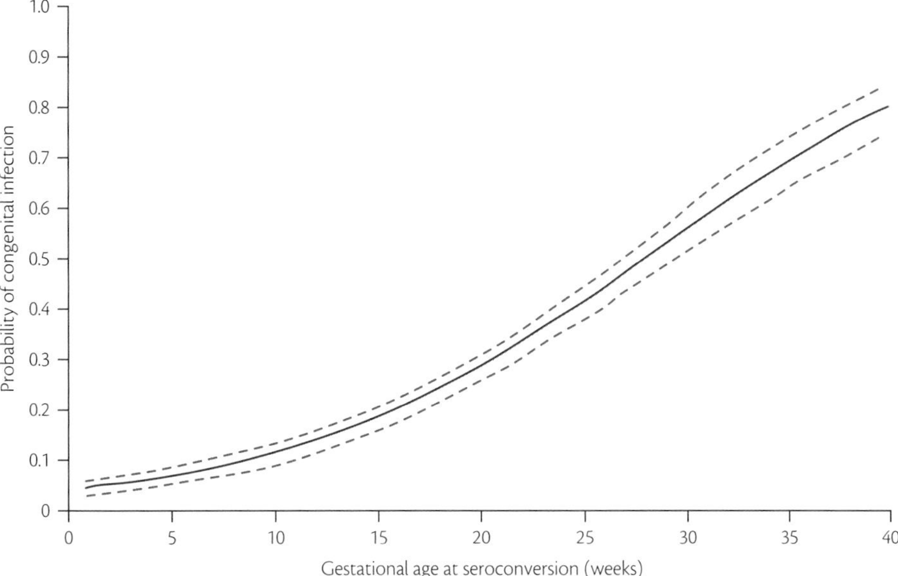

Fig. 7.8.4.2 Risk of mother to child transmission of *T. gondii* by gestational age at maternal seroconversion.
(From Thiebaut R, *et al.* (2007). Effectiveness of prenatal treatment for congenital toxoplasmosis: a meta-analysis of individual patients' data. *Lancet*, **369**, 115–22, with permission).

than infection in the first or second trimester, usually results in subclinical infection of the newborn. It is important to be aware that the overall frequency of subclinical infection in newborns with congenital toxoplasmosis is as high as 85%. The vast majority of these neonatal infections are initially unnoticed, of which a fraction of later develop choroidoretinitis. Treatment of the mother during pregnancy aims to reduce the frequency and severity of fetal infection. However, the efficacy of such treatment is debatable (see below). Treatment aimed at preventing mother-to-child transmission should be given within 3 weeks of infection. In practice, this is very difficult because most infections are asymptomatic.

Seroprevalence increases with age. It does not vary significantly between sexes and tends to be less in cold, hot, and arid areas and at high altitudes. Incidence of infection varies with the population group and geographical location. In El Salvador and France, seropositivity is as high as 40% to 50% by the fourth decade of life, compared with an overall seroprevalence of 15% in the United States of America. In various countries, seroprevalence of *T. gondii* has decreased by approximately one-third over the past decades.

Prevention

Since the infection is naturally acquired through ingestion of undercooked cyst-containing meat or food contaminated with oocysts, infection is preventable in almost all cases. Primary prophylaxis (prevention of infection) by avoiding ingestion is the strategy of choice in seronegative people, whereas in seropositive immunocompromised patients (e.g. people with AIDS) or seronegative recipients of organ transplants (e.g. heart, bone marrow) from seropositive donors, primary prophylaxis using pyrimethamine sulphadiatine has proved effective. Secondary prevention is employed to prevent transmission from the acutely infected mother to her fetus using spiramycin in immunocompromised patients following treatment of reactivated toxoplasmosis (maintenance therapy) using pyrimethamine/sulphadiazine. Systematic serological screening of all pregnant women is performed only in some countries. Uncertainty about the incidence of congenital infection and problems with the sensitivity and specificity of serological tests has hampered attempts to implement screening programmes in several countries. Neonatal screening programmes have allowed the identification of as many as 80% of infected newborns.

Clinical features

Infection with *T. gondii* may go unnoticed (described as '*T. gondii* infection') or it may cause clinical signs and symptoms that vary according to the immune status of the patient and their clinical situation ('toxoplasmosis'). Four clinical situations can be distinguished: the immunocompetent patient, patients with ocular disease, the immunocompromised patient, and the patient with congenital toxoplasmosis.

Immunocompetent adults and children

Primary *T. gondii* infection in children and adults is generally asymptomatic. In approximately 10% of the patients, it causes a self-limited and nonspecific illness that very seldom requires treatment. The most frequently observed clinical manifestation is isolated cervical or occipital lymphadenopathy. Lymph nodes are not tender, do not suppurate, are usually discrete, and stay enlarged for less than 4 to 6 weeks. Very infrequently, chronic lymphadenitis, myocarditis, polymyositis, pneumonitis, hepatitis, or encephalitis can occur in otherwise healthy individuals. Acute toxoplasma infection during pregnancy is asymptomatic in the vast majority of women.

Ocular toxoplasmosis

Toxoplasma choroidoretinitis can be observed in congenital or postnatally acquired disease where it results from acute infection or reactivation. Patients who present with choroidoretinitis as a reactivation of congenital infection are usually in their second and third decades of life. It is uncommon after the age of 40. Bilateral disease, old retinal scars, and involvement of the macula are hallmarks of retinal disease in these cases. In contrast, patients who present with toxoplasma choroidoretinitis in acute toxoplasmosis are more often between the fourth and sixth decade of life. Only one eye is involved, the macula is spared, and there is no old scarring.

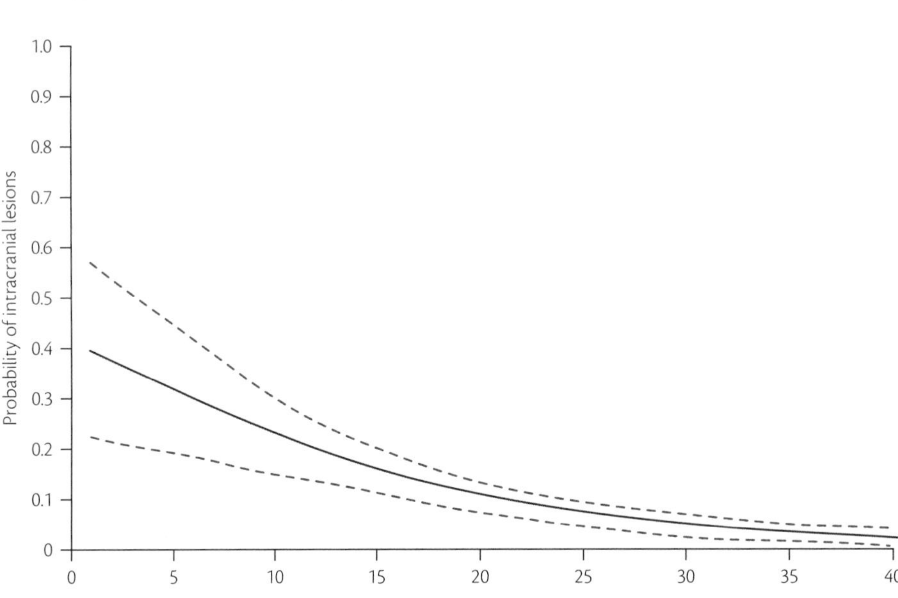

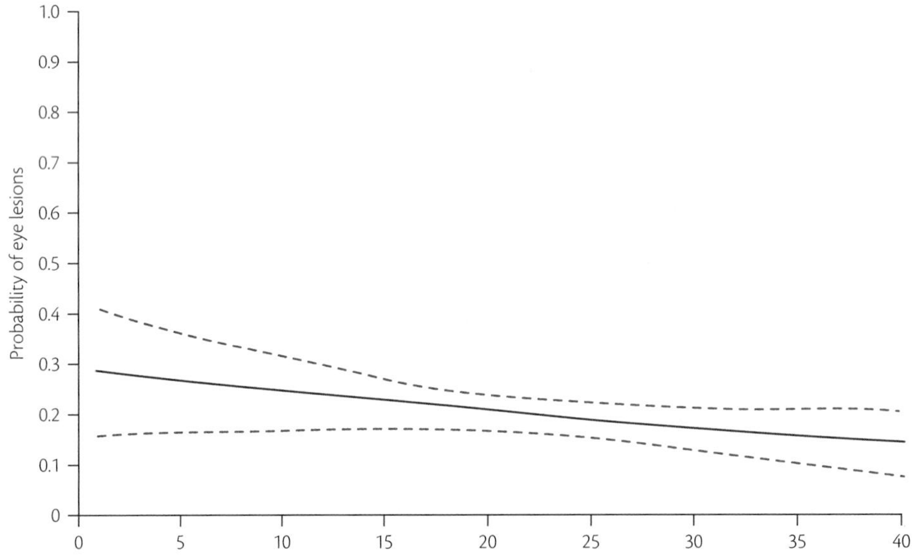

Fig. 7.8.4.3 Risk of intracranial and eye lesions in children infected with *T. gondii* by gestational age at maternal seroconversion.
(From Thiebaut R, *et al.* (2007). Effectiveness of prenatal treatment for congenital toxoplasmosis: a meta-analysis of individual patients' data. *Lancet*, **369**, 115–22, with permission).

AIDS and non-AIDS immunocompromised patients

In contrast to the relatively favourable course of toxoplasmosis in most immunocompetent people, it is life threatening in the immunosuppressed. Toxoplasmosis almost always occurs as a result of reactivation of chronic infection. It occurs when a heart, kidney, or liver from a seropositive donor is transplanted into a seronegative recipient. The central nervous system is the most common affected site. TE may present subacutely, gradually evolving over weeks, or as an acute confusional state with or without focal neurological deficits, evolving over days. Clinical features include changes in level of consciousness, seizures, focal motor deficits, cranial nerve disturbances, sensory abnormalities, cerebellar signs, movement disorders, and neuropsychiatric disturbances. The differential diagnosis of TE lesions includes central nervous system lymphoma, progressive multifocal leukoencephalopathy, and infection with cytomegalovirus, *Cryptococcus neoformans*, aspergillus, and *Mycobacterium tuberculosis*. In immunocompromised patients, toxoplasmosis can also present as choroidoretinitis, pneumonitis, or multiorgan disease, presenting with acute respiratory failure and haemodynamic abnormalities resembling septic shock.

Congenital toxoplasmosis

Prenatal ultrasound examination often fails to detect a fetus with congenital toxoplasmosis. Abnormalities include intracranial calcification, ventricular dilatation, hepatic enlargement, ascites, and increased placental thickness. Approximately 85% of newborns with congenital infection appear normal at birth. Psychomotor retardation and intellectual disability develop only in those children who showed overt features of brain damage at birth. Fetal and neonatal disease is more severe the earlier in gestation the acute infection was acquired. The classic triad of chorioretinitis, hydrocephalus, and cerebral calcification is rather rare. None of the signs described in newborns with congenital disease are pathognomonic for toxoplasmosis and may be mimicked by other congenital infection such as cytomegalovirus, herpes simplex virus, rubella, and syphilis. Early maternal infection may result in death of the fetus *in utero* and spontaneous abortion.

Clinical investigation and criteria for diagnosis

Infection in the immunocompetent host

Immunocompetent adults and children with toxoplasma lymphadenitis are usually not treated unless symptoms are severe or persistent. Characteristic histological criteria and a panel of serological tests (IgG, IgM, IgG avidity) consistent with recently acquired infection establish the diagnosis of toxoplasma lymphadenitis in older children and adults. If required, treatment is usually administered for 2 to 4 weeks, followed by reassessment of the patient's condition. The combination of pyrimethamine, sulphadiazine, and folinic acid for 4 to 6 weeks is the most common drug combination used (Table 7.8.4.1).

Management of maternal and fetal infection

The IgG and IgM antibody status of a pregnant woman should be obtained before or early in pregnancy. The absence of IgG antibodies before or early in pregnancy allows identification of those women at risk of acquiring the infection. The presence of IgG and IgM antibodies indicates recent infection in approximately 40% of patients. The presence of high avidity antibodies essentially rules out an infection acquired in the previous 3 or 4 months, whereas low avidity antibodies can persist for more than 3 months after infection. Detection of IgG and IgM antibodies establishes that the patient has been infected, whereas seronegative women should be provided with necessary information to prevent primary infection (see above). Absence of IgM antibodies during the first two trimesters virtually rules out recently acquired infection unless the sera were obtained too early for the IgM antibody response to be detectable or too late after IgM antibodies had become nondetectable. The definitive diagnosis of acute toxoplasma infection or toxoplasmosis requires demonstration of a rise in titres in serial specimens (either conversion from a negative to a positive titre or a significant rise from a low to a higher titre). Treatment of women with acute acquired infection using spiramycin was thought to reduce the incidence and severity of fetal infection by approximately 60%, but a recent meta-analysis of data from children diagnosed by prenatal screening showed an effect only on intracranial lesions and not on choroidoretinitis at birth. Therapy should be started as soon as possible after diagnosis of recently acquired maternal infection (Table 7.8.4.1). Since maternal infection does not necessarily result in fetal infection, suspected or established maternal infection acquired during pregnancy (based on ultrasonography or serology) must be confirmed by prenatal diagnosis of fetal infection using polymerase chain reaction (PCR) on amniotic fluid. PCR has an overall reported sensitivity of between 64 and 98.8%. When the PCR is positive or it is highly probable that the fetus is infected, pyrimethamine/sulphadiazine is given in combination with folinic acid and continued throughout the pregnancy. If the initial ultrasound reveals no abnormalities, it should be repeated at least monthly until term. Hydrocephalus is an indication for therapeutic abortion. Since fetal infection is undetected in 85% of newborns, serology is commonly performed for neonatal diagnosis. The presence of IgG antibodies in the neonate's serum may reflect maternal and/or its own antibodies. Testing for IgM and IgA antibodies will identify up to 75% of infected newborns. Maternally transferred IgG antibodies usually decline and disappear within 6 to 12 months. Treatment of the fetus is followed by treatment of the symptomatic newborn throughout the first year of life, but the benefit of treating asymptomatic newborns with congenital toxoplasmosis after birth is debatable (Table 7.8.4.1).

Choroidoretinitis

The decision to treat active toxoplasma choroidoretinitis should be based on examination by an experienced ophthalmologist. Low titres of IgG antibody are usual in patients with active choroidoretinitis due to reactivation of congenital *T. gondii* infection. IgM antibodies are usually not detected. Patients with choroidoretinitis due to postnatally acquired disease usually have serological tests results consistent with an infection acquired in the recent past. Most ophthalmologists recommend treatment if there are severe inflammatory responses and/or proximity of retinal lesions to the fovea or optic disk (Table 7.8.4.1). The combination of pyrimethamine and sulphadiazine is the most commonly used regimen. Prednisolone is added if the lesion threatens the macula. The incidence of recurrent toxoplasma choroidoretinitis has been significantly reduced by using long-term intermittent co-trimoxazole.

Infection in the immunocompromised host

In immunocompromised patients with suspected reactivation, PCR rather than serological methods are strongly recommended. Pre-emptive antiparasitic therapy should be considered in all symptomatic seropositive immunosuppressed patients suspected to have toxoplasmosis. If the clinical features suggest central nervous system and/or spinal cord involvement, CT or MRI is mandatory. Empirical anti-*T. gondii* therapy is accepted practice for patients with multiple ring-enhancing brain lesions (usually established by MRI), positive IgG antibody titres against *T. gondii*, and advanced immunodeficiency. Clinical and radiological response to specific anti-*T. gondii* therapy supports the diagnosis of central nervous system toxoplasmosis. The most commonly used and successful regimen continues to be the combination of pyrimethamine/sulphadiazine and folinic acid (Table 7.8.4.1). Clindamycin can be used instead of sulphadiazine in patients intolerant of sulphonamides. Duration of treatment is recommended for 4 to 6 weeks after resolution of all signs and symptoms (often for several months or longer). After treatment of the acute phase (primary or induction treatment) in immunosuppressed patients, maintenance treatment (secondary prophylaxis) should be instituted using the same regimen as for the acute phase but at half the dose. In patients with AIDS, secondary prophylaxis is usually discontinued when the patient's CD4 count has returned to above

Table 7.8.4.1 Suggested regimens for the treatment of infection with *T. gondii*

	Therapy/drug	Dosage	Duration
Acute acquired infection	Symptomatic[a]		
Acute toxoplasmosis in pregnant women[b]	Spiramycin	3 g once a day in three divided doses without food	Until term[c] or until fetal infection is documented
Documented fetal infection (after 12 weeks of gestation)[d]	Pyrimethamine	Loading dose: 100 mg once a day in two divided doses for 2 days, then 50 mg once a day	Until term
	plus		
	Sulphadiazine	Loading dose 75 mg/kg once a day in two divided doses (max. 4 g once a day) for 2 days, then 100 mg/kg once a day in two divided doses (max. 4 g once a day)	Until term
	plus		
	Leucovorin (folinic acid)	5–20 mg once a day	During and for 1 week after pyrimethamine therapy
Congenital Toxoplasma infection in the infant[e]	Pyrimethamine	Loading dose 2 mg/kg once a day for 2 days, then 1 mg/kg once a day for 2–6 months, then this dose every Monday, Wednesday, Friday	1 year
	plus		
	Sulphadiazine	100 mg/kg once a day in two divided doses	1 year
	plus		
	Leucovorin	10 mg three times weekly	During and for 1 week after pyrimethamine therapy
	Corticosteroids (prednisone)[f]	1 mg/kg once a day in two divided doses	Until resolution of signs and symptoms
Choroidoretinitis in adults	Pyrimethamine	Loading dose 200 mg once a day, then 50–75 mg once a day	Usually 1–2 weeks after resolution of symptoms
	plus		
	Sulphadizine	Oral, 1–1.5 g once a day	Usually 1–2 weeks after resolution of symptoms
	plus		
	Leucovorin	5–20 mg three times weekly	During and for 1 week after pyrimethamine therapy
	Corticosteroidsf	1 mg/kg once a day in two divided doses	Until resolution of signs and symptoms
Acute/primary therapy of toxoplasmic encephalitis in AIDS-patients	Standard regimens:		
	Pyrimethamine	Oral, 200 mg loading dose, then 50–75 mg once a day	At least 4–6 weeks after resolution of signs and symptoms
	Leucovorin	Oral, IV, or IM, 10–20 mg once a day (up to 50 mg once a day)	During and for 1 week after pyrimethamine therapy
	plus		
	Sulphadiazine	Oral, 1–1.5 g four times daily	[g]
	or		
	Clindamycin	Oral or IV, 600 mg four times daily (up to IV 1200 mg four times daily)	[g]
	Possible alternative regimens:		
	(1) Co-trimoxazole	Oral or IV, 3–5 mg (trimethoprim component)/kg four times daily	[g]
	(2) Pyrimethamine plus leucovorin	As in standard regimens	[g]
	plus one of the following:		

Table 7.8.4.1 *(Cont'd)* Suggested regimens for the treatment of infection with *T. gondii*

	Therapy/drug	Dosage	Duration
	Atovaquone	Oral, 750 mg four times daily	[g]
	Clarithromycin	Oral, 1 g two times daily	[g]
	Azithromycin	Oral, 1200–1500 mg once a day	[g]
	Dapsone	Oral, 100 mg once a day	[g]

IM, intramuscular; IV, intravenous; q6h, every 6 h; q12h, every 12 h.

[a] Acute acquired infection in immunocompetent patients does not require specific treatment unless there are severe or persistent symptoms or evidence of damage to vital organs. If such signs or symptoms occur, treatment with pyrimethamine/sulphadiazine, and leucovorin should be initiated (for dosages, see 'Toxoplasmic choroidoretinitis in adults').

[b] Practices vary widely between centres.

[c] German and Austrian guidelines recommend to use spiramycin prophylaxis until 17 weeks of pregnancy followed by a 4-week course of pyrimethamine plus sulphadiazine plus leucovorin).

[d] Practices vary widely between centres (pyrimethamine plus sulphadoxine is used in some centres, monthly alternating cycles of pyrimethamine plus sulphadiazine and spiramycin).

[e] Practices vary widely between centres (monthly alternating cycles of pyrimethamine plus sulphadiazine and spiramycin).

[f] When cerebrospinal protein is more than 1 g/dl and when active choroidoretinitis threatens vision.

[g] Duration of treatment as for pyrimethamine in patient with TE.

200 cells/mm^3 and HIV PCR peripheral blood viral load has been reasonably controlled for at least 6 months.

Areas of uncertainty and future developments

- Epidemiology:
  - Sources of infection, relative importance, e.g. water, meat, cats
- Pathogenesis/pathology:
  - Susceptibility of the host to infection, e.g. HLA types
  - Strain differences and clinical presentation
  - Virulence factors
- Diagnosis:
  - Improved avidity testing using recombinant antigens
  - Increased sensitivity of PCR on amniotic fluid
- Treatment/prophylaxis:
  - Clinical treatment trials in different clinical situations, e.g. eye disease and congenital toxoplasmosis using new drugs, e.g. atovaquone
- Prevention strategies/screening:
  - Co-trimoxazole for prevention of multiple episodes of recurrent episodes of chorioretinitis
  - Atovaquone for prophylaxis of toxoplasmic encephalitis
  - Prophylaxis and treatment in bone marrow transplant recipients
  - Effectiveness of prevention strategies in pregnancy
  - Cost-effectiveness of routine screening programmes
  - Vaccination: proteins, DNA, adjuvants, and mucosal strategies

Further reading

Cook AJ, *et al.* (2000). Sources of toxoplasma infection in pregnant women: European multicentre case–control study. European Research Network on Congenital Toxoplasmosis. *BMJ*, **321**, 142–47.

Gilbert RE, *et al.* (2008). The European Multicentre Study on Congenital Toxoplasmosis (EMSCOT). Ocular Sequelae of Congenital Toxoplasmosis in Brazil Compared with Europe. *PLoS Negl Trop Di*, **2**, e277.

Gras L, *et al.* (2005). Association between prenatal treatment and clinical manifestations of congenital toxoplasmosis in infancy: a cohort study in 13 European centres. *Acta Paediatr*, **94**, 1721–31.

Holland GN (2003). Ocular toxoplasmosis: a global reassessment. Part I: epidemiology and course of disease. *Am J Ophthalmol*, **136**, 973–88.

Holland GN (2004). Ocular toxoplasmosis: a global reassessment. Part II: disease manifestations and management. *Am J Ophthalmol*, **137**, 1–17.

Luft BJ, *et al.* (1984). Toxoplasmic encephalitis in patients with acquired immune deficiency syndrome. *JAMA*, **252**, 913–17.

McLeod R, *et al.* (2006). Outcome of treatment for congenital toxoplasmosis, 1981–2004: the National Collaborative Chicago-Based, Congenital Toxoplasmosis Study. *Clin Infect Dis*, **42**, 1383–94.

Montoya JG, Liesenfeld O (2004). Toxoplasmosis. *Lancet*, **363**, 1965–76.

Remington JS, Thulliez P, Montoya JG (2004). Recent developments for diagnosis of toxoplasmosis. *J Clin Microbiol*, **42**, 941–5.

Saeij JP, *et al.* (2006). Polymorphic secreted kinases are key virulence factors in toxoplasmosis. *Science*, **314**, 1780–3.

Schmidt DR, *et al.* (2006). Treatment of infants with congenital toxoplasmosis: tolerability and plasma concentrations of sulfadiazine and pyrimethamine. *Eur J Pediatr*, **165**, 19–25.

Thalib L, *et al.* (2005). Prediction of congenital toxoplasmosis by polymerase chain reaction analysis of amniotic fluid. *BJOG*, **112**, 567–74.

Thiebaut R, *et al.* (2007). Effectiveness of prenatal treatment for congenital toxoplasmosis: a meta-analysis of individual patients' data. *Lancet*, **369**, 115–22.

7.8.5 *Cryptosporidium* and cryptosporidiosis

S.M. Cacciò

Essentials

Cryptosporidia are small coccidian parasites that infect the mucosal epithelia of a variety of vertebrate hosts, including humans, affecting the health, survival, and economic development of millions of people and animals worldwide. Human infection is mainly caused by two species: (1) *Cryptosporidium parvum*—also prevalent in young livestock; can be transmitted from animals to humans (zoonotic transmission, particularly important in children), from person to person ('urban' cycle, due to faecal–oral spread), through contamination of public drinking-water supplies (which can produce massive outbreaks) or food (prepared by a sick food handler), and nosocomially. (2) *C. hominis*—essentially a human parasite; may produce large waterborne outbreaks.

Clinical features—infection involves either children or adults, but is a major cause of diarrhoea in children under 5 years old in both developed and developing countries. Patients may be asymptomatic or experience acute or chronic diarrhoea, depending on their age and immune status: (1) immunocompetent humans—infection usually results in acute self-limiting diarrhoea; (2) patients immunocompromised by drugs or AIDS, and those with concurrent infections such as measles or chickenpox—clinical symptoms are more severe and persistent and may become chronic, leading to electrolyte imbalance, wasting and even death.

Diagnosis and treatment—diagnosis is usually made by detection of oocysts in stool, often by use of direct fluorescent-antibody tests. Detection of soluble *Cryptosporidium* antigens in faecal samples by enzyme-linked immunosorbent assay (ELISA) is useful for the screening of large numbers of specimens. Patients who are immunocompetent are usually managed symptomatically: there is no very effective anticryptosporidial treatment, but those with persistent disease can be given nitazoxanide. Management of patients who are immunocompromised is difficult: aside from supportive care, highly active antiretroviral therapy (HAART) can be effective, both by immune reconstitution (in patients with HIV/AIDS) and by direct inhibition of parasite proteases.

Prevention—primary control is by limiting the opportunity for faecal–oral transmission, both direct and indirect, with maintainence of drinking-water quality and general hygiene (especially in hospitals, wards, etc.) essential for the prevention of the infection. Secondary control, when water supplies are contaminated, can be achieved by boiling water or filtering it (using an appropriate device) before drinking.

Acknowledgement: The author and editors acknowledge the inclusion of material from the chapter by Dr D P Casemore in the 4th edition of this textbook. Plates for this chapter were kindly provided from photographs by A. Curry and D.P. Casemore.

Introduction

The cryptosporidia are obligate intracellular parasites of many vertebrate species. In humans, infection is caused mainly by two species, *Cryptosporidium parvum*, which is also prevalent in young livestock and can be transmitted zoonotically, and *C. hominis*, which is essentially a human parasite. First described in laboratory mice by Tyzzer in 1912, *Cryptosporidium* was recognized as a cause of human infection in 1976. In the 1980s it emerged worldwide as a common cause of severe or life-threatening infection in severely immunocompromised patients, especially those with AIDS, and of acute, self-limiting gastroenteritis in otherwise healthy subjects, especially children.

Biology

Cryptosporidium species have been traditionally considered as members of the coccidia (phylum Apicomplexa), but recent investigations have revealed a closer phylogenetic affinity with the Gregarinae, which are parasites of invertebrates. The oocyst, containing four sporozoites, is an environmentally robust transmissible stage and is fully sporulated and infective upon excretion with the host faeces. Cryptosporidia are monoxenous, i.e. they complete their lifecycle in a single host (Fig. 7.8.5.1). *C. parvum* is not tissue specific but shows a predilection for the lower ileum during the primary stages of infection.

Following ingestion of oocysts, the motile sporozoites are released, through a suture in the oocyst wall, in the lumen of the small bowel. They quickly attach superficially to cells, rounding up to form fixed trophozoites (meronts). The initial site of infection is the brush border of enterocytes in the small bowel, but the parasite is able to infect other epithelial and parenchymal cells. The complex life cycle includes both asexual and sexual stages of replication (Figs. 7.8.5.1 and 7.8.5.2). The endogenous (tissue) stages develop within a parasitophorous vacuole, the outer layer of which is derived from the host cell's outer membranes, in a unique intracellular but extracytoplasmic location.

Molecular biology

The sequences of the genome of both *C. parvum* and *C. hominis* have been described and have revealed many peculiar characteristics. The genomes are very compact, about 10 Mb organized in six chromosomes, and are essentially composed of genes. Unusual biochemical pathways and genes have been described and these may serve as novel targets for drug development.

Protocols based on nucleic acid amplification of specific genes are available to differentiate *Cryptosporidium* species and genotypes in both clinical and environmental samples.

Epidemiology

C. parvum occurs worldwide and is common in humans and in young livestock animals, especially lambs and calves, and has been reported in goats, horses, pigs, and farmed deer as well as in mammalian wildlife. Prevalence in humans varies both geographically and temporally. Because of the diversity of host species that can infect humans, the epidemiology of the infection is complex and involves both direct and indirect routes of transmission from animals to man (zoonotic transmission) and from person to person (urban cycle).

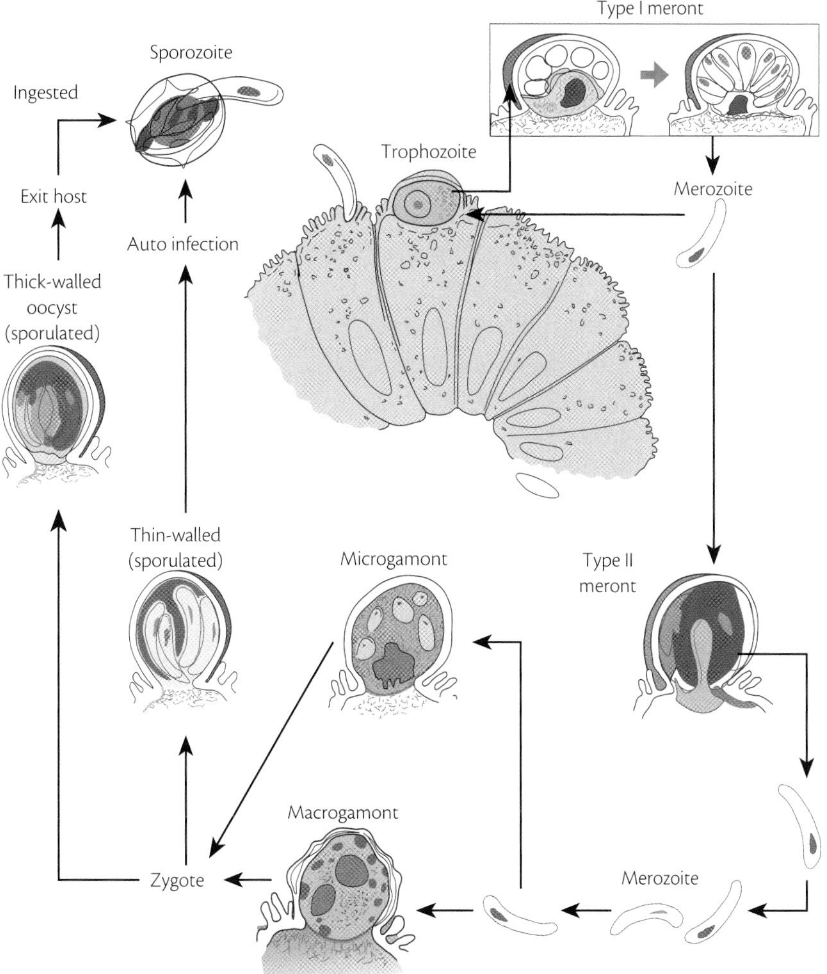

Fig. 7.8.5.1 Diagrammatic representation of the lifecycle of *C. parvum*. Following ingestion of oocysts, the motile sporozoites are released, attach to cells, and develop into fixed trophozoites (uninucleate meronts) in an intracellular but extracytoplasmic location. These undergo schizogony (asexual multiple budding), the first-stage meronts producing 8 merozoites, some of which recycle to form further type I meronts. Type II meronts produce 4 merozoites, which form gamonts (sexual stages) that mature as either macrogametes or as microgamonts containing 16 motile microgametes. Most of the zygotes formed after fertilization develop into thick-walled, environmentally resistant, transmissible oocysts, which then sporulate, usually by the time they are excreted. Some have only a thin unit membrane, which ruptures to release the sporozoites *in situ* to produce an autoinfective cycle.

(Adapted from a drawing by Kip Carter, University of Georgia, and shown by courtesy of W I Current and CRC Press, Inc., Boca Raton, FL.)

Zoonotic transmission

Transmission from livestock is common, particularly in children, including those from urban homes and schools visiting educational farms and rural activity centres. Companion animals have long been considered potential sources for human cryptosporidiosis. However, they appear to be most commonly infected with host-specific nonzoonotic *Cryptosporidium* species; they are therefore not considered important reservoirs of infection. Cryptosporidiosis is rarely seen in adults in rural areas, presumably as a result offrequent exposure and the development of immunity.

Human-to-human transmission

Cases of human-to-human transmission have been reported between family members, sexual partners, children in daycare centres, and hospital patients and staff. Outbreaks in daycare centres have been reported in the United Kingdom and the United States of America, mainly as a result of direct (person-to-person) faecal–oral transmission, although the infection may be introduced in the first instance through zoonotic contact. Affected adults may acquire infection from young children in the home or occupationally. Infection may be transmitted sexually where this involves faecal exposure. *Cryptosporidium* is a cause of traveller's diarrhoea, although apparently not as frequently as *Giardia*.

Waterborne transmission

In the United Kingdom, the United States of America, and elsewhere, there have been numerous well-documented outbreaks resulting from contamination of public drinking-water supplies. Outbreaks, which can be massive, have been associated with *C. hominis*, which indicates contamination of the supply by human sewage, or with *C. parvum*, which suggests an animal source of contamination. Isolates from endemic (sporadic) cases, some of which will be waterborne, fall into both categories. Oocysts have been demonstrated widely in both raw and treated

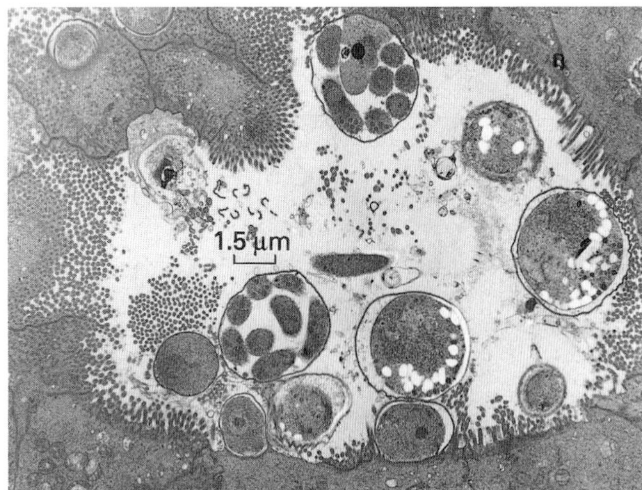

Fig. 7.8.5.2 Electron micrograph of a transverse section of small bowel of a mouse infected with *C. parvum*. The section shows numerous developmental stages: uninucleate meronts (trophozoites); type I meronts (schizonts) containing merozoites in which may be seen the darker granules of the apical complex organelles; the degenerate remains of a schizont and a free-swimming merozoite within the lumen; and macrogamonts showing dark wall-forming granules and electron-lucent amylopectin (polysaccharide) food-storage granules. The parasitophorous vacuole can be clearly seen surrounding the parasite stages. Some of the intracellular stages appear to be free within the lumen because of the plane of sectioning.

water and legislation has been introduced in the United Kingdom and the United States of America in an attempt to limit the latter.

Cryptosporidium is also one of the most commonly recognized causes of recreational waterborne disease. Most outbreaks are the result of faecal accident or cross-connection in swimming pools. Faecal contamination coupled with oocyst resistance to chlorine, low infectious dose, and high bather densities facilitate transmission.

Foodborne transmission

Cryptosporidiosis has been attributed to ingestion of contaminated apple juice, chicken salad, milk, and food prepared by a sick food handler. Food-borne transmission is probably underestimated, because the long incubation period (3–7 days or more) makes the relationship between cryptosporidiosis and a possibly contaminated food item difficult to establish.

Nosocomial transmission

Transmission has been reported between health care staff and patients and between patients, particularly the immunocompromised. Large numbers of oocysts may be present in patients' stools and in vomit; transmission via fomites occurs, although this route is limited by the susceptibility of oocysts to desiccation. Poor handwashing practice has been identified as an important factor. In an outbreak with high mortality in a ward of immunocompromised patients in Denmark, transmission was probably by patients' hands via a ward ice-making machine.

Demography

Age and sex distribution

In the United Kingdom, approximately two-thirds of cryptosporidium-positive samples are from children between 1 and 10 years of age, with a secondary peak in adults under 45 years; the infection is uncommon in infants less than 1 year old and in older people. Distribution appears to be the same in both sexes. A relative increase in adult cases is often seen in waterborne outbreaks. In developing countries, infection is common in infants less than 1 year old and asymptomatic infection is common in older subjects.

Temporal distribution

In the United Kingdom, a marked bimodal seasonal pattern of disease has been described: one peak during spring and the second during late summer/early autumn. The spring peak, which coincides generally with lambing and calving, is almost exclusively due to *C. parvum*, while both *C. parvum* and *C. hominis* occur in the late summer/early autumn peak. In the United States of America, the peak onset of cryptosporidiosis occurs annually from early summer to early autumn and, as it coincides with the summer recreational water season, it might reflect the increased use of communal swimming venues, particularly by susceptible hosts like young children.

Frequency of occurrence

Laboratory rates of detection in immunocompetent subjects average about 2% in developed countries (range <1–5%) and about 8% in developing countries (range 2–30%), and *Cryptosporidium* is about fourth in the list of pathogens detected in stools submitted to the laboratory. In the United Kingdom, from about 5000 to 6000 confirmed cases are reported annually; it is generally somewhat less frequent than giardiasis. Among young children in the United Kingdom, cryptosporidiosis is more common than salmonellosis and detection rates may exceed 20% during peak periods.

Cryptosporidiosis is one of the most common causes of diarrhoea in patients with AIDS and in some studies prevalence has exceeded 50%. The infection rate in patients with AIDS in the United Kingdom has been falling in recent years, which has been attributed to infection control advice and the use of multiple antiretroviral therapy. Infection rates are not generally increased for most other immunocompromised groups.

Clinical aspects

Pathology

Histopathology

There is mucosal involvement of the small bowel, other parts of the gastrointestinal tract, and sometimes beyond. Moderate to severe abnormalities of villous architecture occur, with stunting and fusion of villi and lengthening of crypts. There may be evidence of mild inflammation, with some cellular infiltration into the lamina propria.

The endogenous stages of the parasite in the luminal surface are generally inconspicuous and appear as small (2–8 µm) bodies, apparently superficially attached to the brush border, unevenly distributed over the apical cells, and within the crypts of the villi (Figs. 7.8.5.1 and 7.8.5.2). Peaking and apoptosis of infected cells have been reported. There is usually little intracellular change at the ultrastructural level beyond the attachment zone of the parasite. Rectal biopsy may reveal mild nonspecific proctitis. Extensive and chronic involvement of the bile duct and gallbladder is seen in some patients with AIDS.

Immunological response

The particular immunodeficient conditions in which cryptosporidiosis has been reported to show increased severity or persistence suggest that both humoral and cellular factors have a role in limiting infection. An immune response has been demonstrated in the main immunoglobulin classes, although the initial IgG response may be poor. Serological diagnostic tests are, however, of little clinical value. Seroprevalence studies indicate that the infection is common, even in developed countries, and this may reflect water supply quality or other exposures.

Reports differ on the effect of breastfeeding on incidence in infancy; some studies suggest a protective effect although protection from the environment by breastfeeding may also be important.

Although functioning humoral and cellular immunity seems to be important in limiting or controlling infection, it currently appears that, in animal models, CD4+ and CD8+ T lymphocytes and interferon-γ are especially important in this respect. In humans, CD4 cell counts of fewer than 200 cells/mm^3 probably indicate the need to take special care to avoid exposure to *Cryptosporidium*, and fewer than 100 cells/mm^3 indicates a poor prognosis if infection occurs.

Possible pathogenic mechanisms

The watery diarrhoea is characteristic of noninflammatory infection of the small bowel, especially that associated with toxin-producing organisms and enteric viruses. Several mechanisms have been suggested to explain the symptoms: reduction in absorptive capacity, particularly for water and electrolytes; increase in secretory capacity from crypt hypertrophy; osmotic effects from loss of brush-border enzymes (e.g. disaccharidases) resulting in malabsorption of sugars, increased osmolality of chyme, and subsequent microbial fermentation of sugars in the colon (which may account for the characteristic offensive smell); and toxic activity.

Clinical presentation in otherwise healthy (immunocompetent) people

Cryptosporidiosis in the immunocompetent person is a self-limiting, acute gastroenteritis with a variety of presenting symptoms. In cases where the time of exposure has been known, the incubation period was about 5 to 7 days (range probably 2–14 days; wider limits have been suggested but are unlikely). There may be a prodrome of 1 day to a few days, with malaise, abdominal pain, nausea, and loss of appetite. Gastrointestinal symptoms start suddenly, the stools being described as watery, greenish with mucus in some cases, without blood or pus, and very offensive. Patients may open their bowels more than 20 times a day but more usually 3 to 6 times. Other symptoms include colicky, abdominal pain, especially after meals, anorexia, nausea, and vomiting, abdominal distension, and marked weight loss. Influenza-like systemic effects, including malaise, headache, myalgias, and fever, commonly occur. Gastrointestinal symptoms usually last about 7 to 14 days, but weakness, lethargy, mild abdominal pain, and intermittent loose bowels sometimes persist for up to a further month.

There is no evidence of transplacental transmission but infection during late pregnancy may cause metabolic disturbances in the mother, leading to the infant's failure to thrive. Failure to thrive has also been observed in older infants and children and may be associated with persistent infection and enteropathy, especially in developing countries.

Reported sequelae include pancreatitis (associated with severe abdominal pain), toxic megacolon, and reactive arthritis. In immunocompetent patients, deaths are rarely attributable to cryptosporidiosis.

Recent studied in the United Kingdom have further demonstrated that the impact of cryptosporidiosis on public health extends beyond that of acute diarrhoeal illness. Notably, an increased risk of nonintestinal sequelae (joint pain, eye pains, recurrent headache, and fatigue) is associated with infection with *C. hominis* but not with *C. parvum*.

Clinical presentation in immunocompromised patients

Susceptibility to cryptosporidiosis and the severity of the disease is increased in patients who are immunocompromised as a result of AIDS, hypo- or agammaglobulinaemia, severe combined immunodeficiency, leukaemia, malignant disease, and bullous pemphigoid. Disease susceptibility and severity are also increased during immunosuppressive treatment with cyclophosphamide and corticosteroids, as in patients undergoing bone marrow transplantation, and in children immunosuppressed by measles and chickenpox, especially where there is associated malnutrition. Infection in patients with leukaemia may be unusually severe and has sometimes proved fatal, particularly when associated with aplastic crisis, and may then require modification of chemotherapy to control the infection.

Symptoms of cryptosporidiosis are generally similar to those in immunocompromised patients but often develop insidiously. In those with late-stage AIDS with very low CD4 cell counts or in some other profound deficiency states, diarrhoea may be frequent, profuse, and watery, like cholera. Patients may open their bowels frequently, passing up to 20 litres of infected fluid stool per day; persistent nausea and vomiting is usually associated with severe diarrhoea and suggests a poor prognosis. Associated symptoms include colicky, abdominal pain often associated with meals, severe weight loss, weakness, malaise, anorexia, and low-grade fever. Cryptosporidial infection in immunocompromised patients may involve the pharynx, oesophagus, stomach, duodenum, jejunum, ileum, appendix, colon, rectum, gallbladder, bile duct, pancreatic duct, and the bronchial tree. Cryptosporidial cholecystitis (presenting with severe right upper quadrant abdominal pain), sclerosing cholangitis, pancreatitis, hepatitis, and respiratory-tract symptoms may occur, with or without diarrhoea. The clinical picture may include other features of HIV infection and there is often coinfection with other pathogens such as cytomegalovirus, *Pneumocystis jiroveci*, and *Toxoplasma gondii*.

Patients with less severe impairment of immunity may experience resolution or a more chronic course, with less profuse diarrhoea, sometimes with remission and then recurrence, possibly associated with biliary tract involvement. Except in those patients whose immune suppression can be relieved by stopping immunosuppressant drugs, or, in the case of HIV, intensifying antiretroviral therapy, severe symptoms may persist until the patient dies. This is either as a result of dehydration, acid–base or electrolyte disturbances, and cachexia, from some other opportunistic infection or malignant disease, or a combination of these.

Laboratory investigations

In early acute cases the stools are usually watery, greenish with mucus in some cases, without blood or pus. Peripheral leucocytosis and eosinophilia are found rarely. Serum electrolyte abnormalities will develop in patients who become severely dehydrated. In immunocompromised patients with cryptosporidial cholecystitis, serum alkaline phosphatase and γ-glutamyl transpeptidase levels are raised, while aminotransferase and bilirubin levels may remain normal.

In patients with AIDS, commonly associated infections are with cytomegalovirus and *Isospora belli*. Mixed infection with *Campylobacter*, *Giardia*, and *Cyclospora* species may be found in immunocompetent patients.

In the bowel mucosa, there is histological evidence of enterocyte damage, villous blunting, and inflammatory-cell infiltration of the lamina propria; cell peaking and apoptosis have been reported. Histopathological appearances of the affected biliary tract resembles primary sclerosing cholangitis. Radiographic abnormalities include dilatation of the small bowel, mucosal thickening, prominent mucosal folds, and abnormal motility and, in the biliary system, dilated distal biliary ducts, stenosis with an irregular lumen, and other changes reminiscent of primary sclerosing cholangitis.

Differential diagnosis

The absence of blood, pus, cells, or Charcot–Leyden crystals may distinguish cryptosporidiosis from some acute bacterial diarrhoeas and that associated with amoebiasis and isosporiasis. In immunocompetent patients, the symptoms of cryptosporidiosis resemble those of giardiasis or cyclosporiasis. Intense abdominal pain and cramps are generally more common in cryptosporidiosis, but bloating and weakness less common. In immunocompromised patients, especially in those with AIDS, isosporiasis is clinically indistinguishable, but can be diagnosed by finding the organisms in the stool, where Charcot–Leyden crystals may also be found. This infection responds to treatment with co-trimoxazole, as does cyclosporiasis.

Treatment of cryptosporidiosis

There have been a large number of studies aimed at developing a satisfactory therapy for human cryptosporidiosis, but these investigations have failed to identify a drug of choice. Several groups may

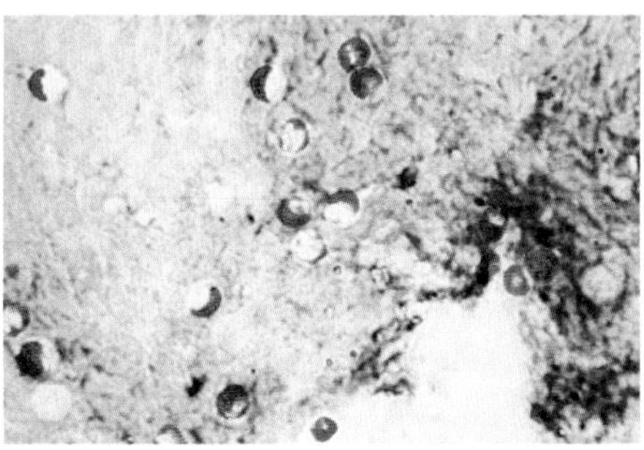

Fig. 7.8.5.4 Modified Ziehl-Neelsenstained faecal smear showing oocysts of *C. parvum* examined with × 100 oil-immersion objective lens. The uniformity of size (4.5-5 μm) but variability of staining of oocysts can be seen.

benefit from an effective therapy, particularly patients with HIV/AIDS, transplant recipients, patients undergoing cancer chemotherapy, and those with severe malnutrition.

Since cryptosporidium infection in the immunocompetent person is a self-limiting disease, a symptomatic antidiarrhoeal treatment is usually sufficient. However, in case of persistent disease, the patients should be given anti-cryptosporidium therapy. Today, the therapy of choice is nitazoxanide (2-acetyloloxy-*N*-(5-nitro-2-thiazolyl) benzamide), a synthetic agent that has a demonstrated activity against a broad range of parasites as well as some bacteria. *In vitro* studies showed inhibition of growth at concentrations of less than 10 μg/ml, and studies in adults have shown that single doses of up to 4 g are well tolerated without important adverse effects.

Immunocompromised patients with persistent severe diarrhoea, malabsorption, and other complications may require prolonged palliative treatment. They should avoid excess milk, as lactose intolerance may develop. Parenteral feeding and fluid, electrolyte, and nutrient replacement may be needed. Antiperistaltic agents such as loperamide, diphenoxylate, or opiates may increase abdominal pain and bloating. Antiemetics may be needed for symptomatic relief. Temporary relief of biliary obstruction has been achieved by endoscopic papillotomy and of cholecystitis by cholecystectomy. Diarrhoea and vomiting may, however, prove intractable.

Highly active antiretroviral therapy (HAART) is the treatment of choice for cryptosporidiosis in immunocompromised patients,

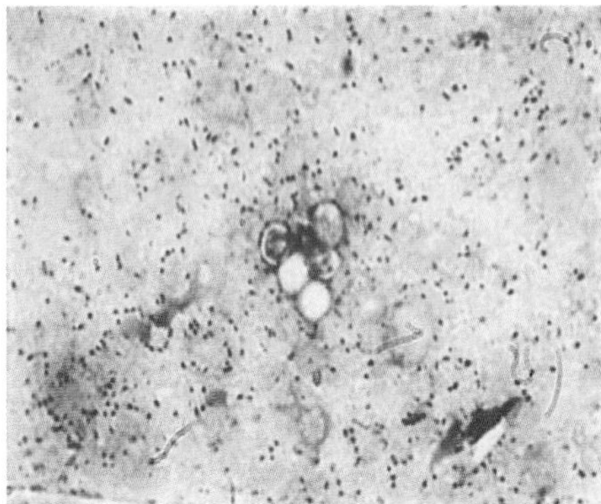

Fig. 7.8.5.3 Modified Giemsa-stained faecal smear showing oocysts of *C. parvum*, examined with × 100 oil-immersion objective lens. The uniformity of size (4.5–5 μm) but variability of staining of oocysts can be seen. The eosinophilic nuclei and basophilic bodies of the sporozoites can be clearly seen within the oocysts that have taken up the stain.

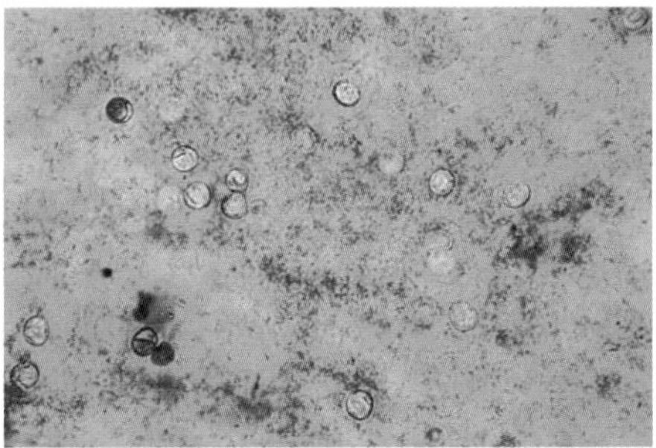

Fig. 7.8.5.5 Modified Ziehl-Neelsen-stained faecal smear showing oocysts of *C. parvum*. The uniformity of size (4.5–5 μm) is apparent but the oocysts in this preparation show a definite increase in refractility and marked failure to take up the stain (identity confirmed by immunofluorescence and electron microscopy).

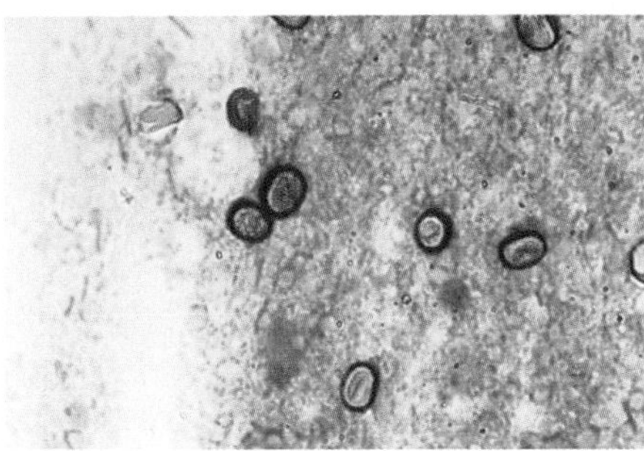

Fig. 7.8.5.6 Modified Ziehl-Neelsen-stained faecal smear showing oocyst-like bodies (mushroom spores) examined with × 100 oilimmersion objective lens (from specimen submitted to Reference Unit for identification).

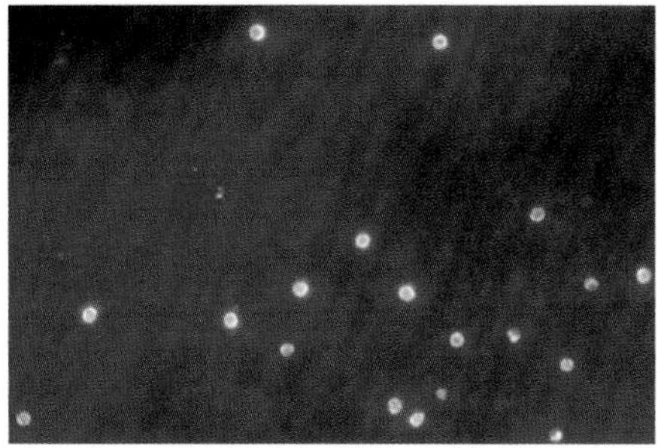

Fig. 7.8.5.8 Phenol-auramine/carbol fuchsin-stained faecal smear showing oocysts of *C. parvum*, examined with × 720 dry objective lens (screening magnification) on a fluorescence microscope.

and can be used not only prophylactically but also as a treatment and secondary prophylaxis for established infections. HAART therapy is effective against cryptosporidiosis and acts both by immune reconstitution and direct inhibition of parasite proteases.

Laboratory detection and diagnosis

The characteristic endogenous stages (Figs. 7.8.5.1 and 7.8.5.2) may be found in histological sections, using light and electron microscopy, but diagnosis is usually by detection of oocysts in stools. Oocysts have also been found in vomit and sputum in some cases, especially those associated with AIDS. The oocysts of *C. parvum* are spherical or slightly ovoid, about 4 to 6 µm, and appear refractile in wet faecal preparations with a highly refractile inner body, the cytoplasmic residuum; the four sporozoites within may be distinguished with difficulty using special optical systems (Figs. 7.8.5.3–12).

Several conventional stains have been adapted for diagnostic purposes, such as the modified Ziehl–Neelsen method and phenol–auramine fluorescent stain.

Direct fluorescent-antibody tests, which detect intact organisms through the use of monoclonal antibodies that label the oocyst wall, are widely used due to their excellent sensitivity and specificity. Detection of *Cryptosporidium* soluble antigens in faecal samples by an enzyme-linked immunosorbent assay (ELISA) is very easy to perform and particularly useful for the screening of large numbers of specimens, albeit its specificity is limited by cross-reactions with other antigens of parasitic and nonparasitic origin that can generate false positives.

Standardization of approach to screening and of reporting is essential for epidemiological purposes. Ideally, all stool samples from cases of diarrhoea should be screened; restriction, where unavoidable, should be based on age group (see demography) and not on factors such as stool consistency. Concentration of stool specimens is not usually required for diagnosis in acute cases.

Fungal spores, yeasts, cysts of *Balantidium*, sporocysts of *Isospora*, and oocysts of *Cyclospora* may readily be mistaken for cryptosporidial oocysts.

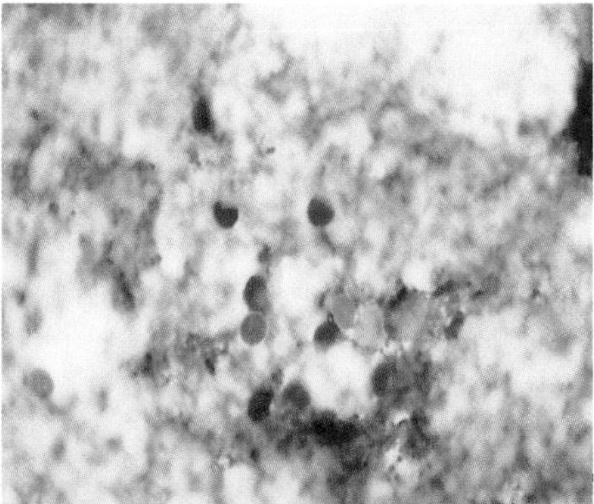

Fig. 7.8.5.7 Modified Ziehl-Neelsen-stained faecal smear showing oocyst-like bodies (mould spores) examined with × 100 oilimmersion objective lens. The spores are uniform in size but a little smaller (4.0 µm) than oocysts of *C. parvum*. They are generally more uniform in their acid-fast staining (identity confirmed by mycological culture and electron microscopy).

Infectivity, resistance, and control

Infectivity

In studies using monkeys and lambs, the infective dose for *C. parvum* was fewer than 10 oocysts. In human volunteer studies in the United States of America, the minimum infective dose for *C. parvum* and *C. hominis* appeared to be similar (ID_{50} was 132 and 83, respectively). In contrast to *C. parvum*, however, *C. hominis* elicted a serum IgG response in most infected persons.

Resistance and disinfection

Oocysts can survive for several months in a cool, moist environment but are highly susceptible to desiccation, prolonged freezing, and moderate heat (pasteurization temperatures). They are remarkably resistant to most disinfectants and antiseptics, including chlorine at concentrations far greater than those used in water

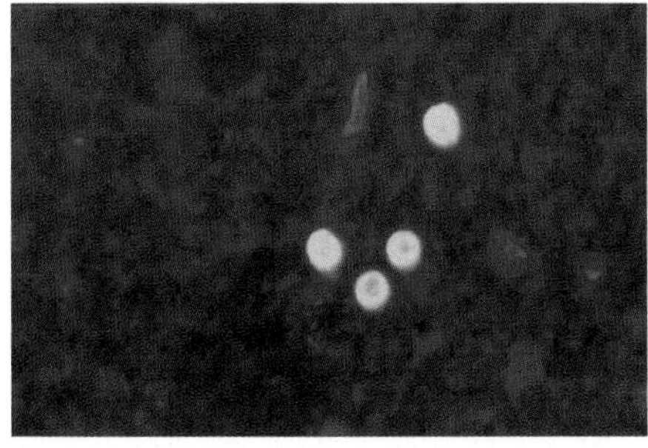

Fig. 7.8.5.9 Phenol-auramine/carbol fuchsin-stained faecal smear showing oocysts of *C. parvum*, examined with × 100 oil-immersion objective lens on a fluorescence microscope.

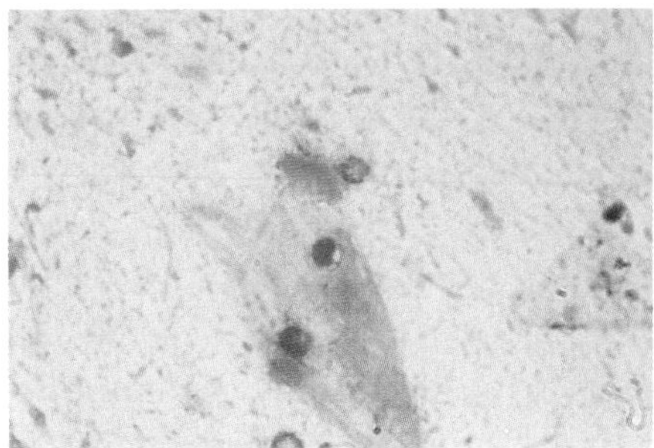

Fig. 7.8.5.10 Fluorescent dye-tagged monoclonal antibody-stained faecal smear showing oocysts of *C. parvum*, examined with × 50 oil-immersion objective lens (screening magnification) on a fluorescence microscope. The suture or associated surface cleft or fold, through which the sporozoites are released, can be seen

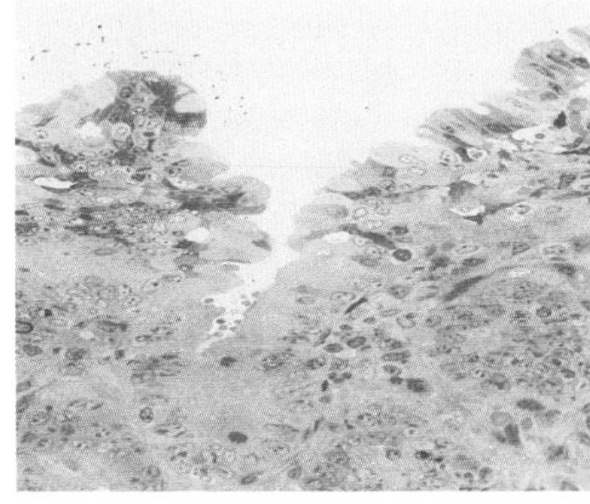

Fig. 7.8.5.12 Toluidine blue-stained semithin section of human rectal biopsy tissue of an AIDS patient with cryptosporidiosis. The apparent pseudo-external location of the parasite can be seen, the true location being intracellular but extracytoplasmic.

treatment and even to glutaraldehyde under normal use conditions. Some disinfectants may be more effective if used at elevated temperature (37°C or higher). Oocysts are sensitive to 10 volume (3%) hydrogen peroxide, to appropriate levels of ozone, and to medium or high-pressure ultraviolet.

In hospitals, adequate disinfection of faecal contamination or of endoscopes is difficult. If such instruments have been used for patients with cryptosporidiosis, prolonged immersion in glutaraldehyde at a temperature higher than 37°C, or in hydrogen peroxide, after careful cleaning, may be required to ensure safety.

Control of transmission

Primary control is by limiting the opportunity for faecal–oral transmission, both direct and indirect. Symptom-free subjects not in contact with immunocompromised patients can normally be permitted to work if their hygiene is scrupulous. Spread via fomites is possible but this route is limited by the susceptibility of oocysts to desiccation. Patients with AIDS are more susceptible to infection with uncommon species or genotypes and advice may be needed to limit exposure.

Contamination of water supplies is inevitable, even in developed countries, and may be the source of some sporadic cases as well as outbreaks. When a public advisory notice is issued to boil water, raising the water just to boiling point is sufficient. In general, bottled water and water from point-of-use filters are unlikely to contain parasites but may carry an increased bacterial load, the health significance of which is uncertain for the immunocompromised. Patients with AIDS and others who are profoundly compromised should be advised never to drink water that has not been boiled or filtered through a suitable device. Users of filters should remember that these devices may concentrate potential pathogens and care is needed in replacing and disposing of filter elements.

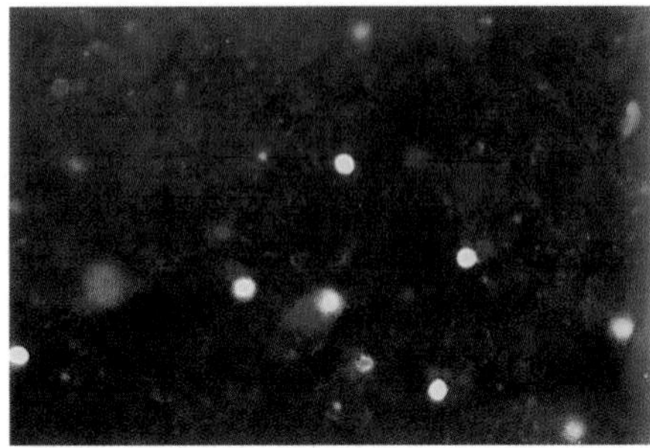

Fig. 7.8.5.11 Modified Ziehl-Neelsen-stained sputum smear from an AIDS patient with respiratory involvement (examined with × 100 oil-immersion objective lens). The *C. parvum* bodies present may include endogenous (tissue) stages attached to exfoliated cells. For this reason, oocyst wall-specific indirect immunofluorescence may show a poor reaction. There may also be less uniformity of size and differences in the staining appearance of the internal structures.

Hospitals involved in the care of profoundly immunocompromised patients should be particularly vigilant in the management of patients with cryptosporidiosis. Long-term arrangements should be made for the provision of safe water for the immunocompromised to avoid difficulties when a notice to boil water is issued.

Further reading

Cacciò SM, Pozio E (2006). Advances in the epidemiology, diagnosis and treatment of cryptosporidiosis. *Expert Rev Anti Infect Ther*, **4**, 429–43.

Casemore DP (1991). ACP Broadsheet 128. Laboratory methods for diagnosing cryptosporidiosis. *J Clin Pathol*, **44**, 445–51.

Coop RL, Wright SE, Casemore DP (1998). Cryptosporidiosis. In: Palmer SR, Soulsby Lord, Simpson DIH (eds) *Zoonoses—biology, clinical practice, and public health control*, pp. 563–78. Oxford University Press, Oxford.

Hunter PR, Nichols G (2002). Epidemiology and clinical features of *Cryptosporidium* infection in immunocompromised patients. *Clin Microbiol Rev*, **15**, 145–54.

Meinhardt PL, Casemore DP, Miller KB (1996). Epidemiologic aspects of human cryptosporidiosis and the role of waterborne transmission. *Epidemiol Rev*, **18**, 118–36.

7.8.6 *Cyclospora* and cyclosporiasis

R. Lainson

Essentials

Most species of *Cyclospora* (Protozoa: Apicomplexa: Eimeriidae) are parasites of various reptiles and mammals. *C. cayetanensis*, which probably infects only humans, is transmitted by way of resistant oocysts voided in the faeces and contaminating food or water. Distribution is worldwide, particularly in regions with a low level of hygiene. Clinical presentation is with explosive outbreaks of acute diarrhoea, with this infection now regarded as an important causative agent of traveller's diarrhoea. Diagnosis is dependent on detection of oocysts in faeces by direct examination or in stained faecal smears. Aside from supportive care, treatment with trimethoprim–sulfamethoxazole has proved effective in eliminating the parasite in immunocompetent patients, but relapses are common in those with AIDS. Prevention is by ensuring good general hygiene, and in areas of high endemicity water should be boiled before drinking or use in preparation of fruits/vegetables that are to be eaten raw.

Introduction

Species of the coccidian genus *Cyclospora* (Protozoa: Apicomplexa: Eimeriidae) have been recorded in invertebrates (millipedes), reptiles (principally snakes), insectivores (moles), rodents, and primates (monkeys and humans).

Endogenous development of most species is within the epithelial cells of the small intestine, culminating in the production of oocysts, which are voided in the faeces and serve as the means of transmission.

Small, bisporocystic coccidial oocysts detected in the faeces of patients with diarrhoea in Papua New Guinea almost certainly represented the first discovery of cyclospora in humans in 1979, but due to difficulties in determining the number of sporozoites in each sporocyst, the parasite was not identified to generic level. What were clearly unsporulated oocysts of the same parasite, seen by other authors in patients with diarrhoea, were for many years referred to as 'cryptosporidium-like oocysts', 'cyanobacterium-like bodies' (bodies resembling blue-green algae), or even 'fungal spores', and it was not until 1992 that the exact nature of the cysts was established and the parasite named as *Cyclospora cayetanensis*.

Life cycle

Cyclospora species have been most extensively studied in nonhuman hosts, in which stages of development are typically intracytoplasmic in the epithelial cells of the small intestine. An exception is *C. talpae* of the mole *Talpa europaea*, which develops within the nucleus of the epithelial cells of the bile ducts and cells of the capillary sinusoids in the liver.

Asexual reproduction (merogony) (Fig. 7.8.6.1a) is followed by the production of female gametocytes (macrogamonts) (Figs. 7.8.6.1b–f) and male gametocytes (microgamonts) that produce a large number of flagellated gametes (Figs. 7.8.6.1g–j). Following fertilization of the female parasites, the zygotes develop a resistant membrane (Fig. 7.8.6.1k). The resulting oocysts are voided, unsporulated, in the host's faeces. The extracellular stages are illustrated in Figs. 7.8.6.2.

During periods varying from a few days to 1 or 2 weeks, depending on the species of *Cyclospora* and the temperature of the contaminated environment, the zygote within the oocyst (Fig. 7.8.6.3a) undergoes division to produce two sporoblasts (Fig. 7.8.6.3b), each of which develops a resistant membrane, the sporocyst (Fig. 7.8.6.3c). Division of each sporoblast then gives rise to two elongate sporozoites, leaving a conspicuous residual body (Figs. 7.8.6.2b and 7.8.6.3c). The sporozoites are the stages that infect further animals of the same species when oocysts are ingested with contaminated food or water.

Epidemiology

Failure to experimentally infect a variety of animals or to detect *C. cayetanensis* in those living in or near houses with human infection has led to the conclusion that humans are the specific host of this coccidian and the sole source of its oocysts.

The parasite is globally distributed, although risk of infection is greatest in developing countries with low standards of hygiene. It is particularly prevalent in Central America and southern Asia. Serious outbreaks of acute diarrhoea have been reported, however, among guests at social events in the United States of America and Canada, with the source of infection traced to imported raspberries from Guatemala. Another outbreak, in Germany, occurred among a group of 34 people who had eaten a salad of imported lettuce spiced with fresh leafy herbs. In other countries, oocysts of *C. cayetanensis* have been detected on green leafy vegetables, in sewage, and even in tap water.

Clinical features

An acute, watery, and nonbloody diarrhoea is variously accompanied by abdominal pain, steatorrhoea, headache, fever, nausea, and general malaise. The diarrhoea may be persistent and last for several weeks. Asymptomatic infections are known to occur, notably in the indigenous population of developing countries.

Diagnosis

Diagnosis is dependent on the demonstration of oocysts of *C. cayetanensis* in the faeces by direct microscopic examination. Flotation methods, using saturated sugar or aqueous zinc sulphate solutions, are useful in concentrating the oocysts, which measure from 8.0 to 10.0 μm in diameter (average 8.6 μm).

The living oocysts are autofluorescent using ultraviolet illumination, which is useful for rapid diagnosis. In addition, most diagnostic laboratories use a variety of staining methods to colour the oocysts in faecal smears fixed in 10% formalin: notably, modified Ziehl–Neelsen acid-fast staining, and safranin stain. These do not reveal details of the oocyst contents (Fig. 7.8.6.4), but their size and

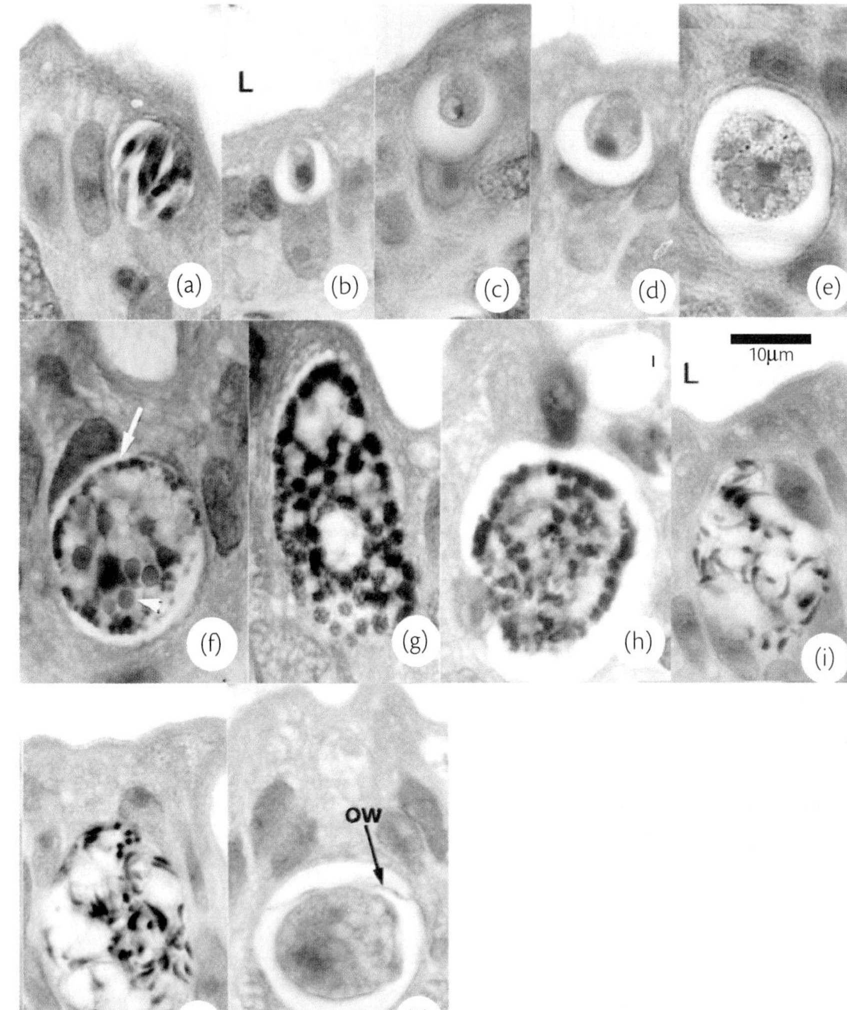

Fig. 7.8.6.1 Intracellular development in epithelial cells of the ileum (haematoxylin and eosin stained sections) in a typical life cycle of a *Cyclospora* species:(a) segmented meronts; (b–e) developing macrogamonts; (f) mature macrogamont with small wall-forming bodies (arrow) and large wall-forming bodies (arrowhead); (g, h) developing microgamonts; (i, j) mature microgamonts shedding microgametes; (k) intracellular zygote, with developing oocyst wall (OW). (From Lainson R (2004). The genus *Cyclospora* (Apicomplexa: Eimeriidae), with a description of *Cyclospora schneideri* n.sp. in the snake *Anilius scytale scytale* (Aniliidae) from Amazonian Brazil—a review. *Mem Inst Oswaldo Cruz*, **100**, 103–110, with permission).

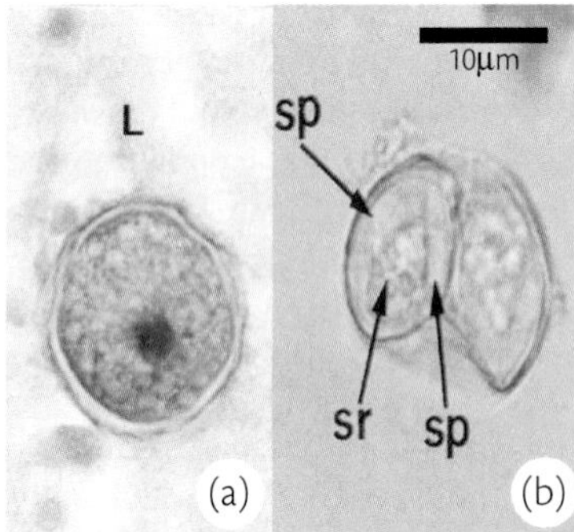

Fig. 7.8.6.2 Extracellular stages in a typical life cycle of a *Cyclospora*: (a) unsporulated oocyst in the intestinal lumen; (b) sporulated and ruptured oocyst in faeces. L, lumen; Sp, sporozoite; Sr, sporocystic residuum. Bar, 10 μm (all figures). (From Lainson R (2004). The genus *Cyclospora* (Apicomplexa: Eimeriidae), with a description of *Cyclospora schneideri* n.sp. in the snake *Anilius scytale scytale* (Aniliidae) from Amazonian Brazil—a review. *Mem Inst Oswaldo Cruz*, **100**, 103–110, with permission).

spherical shape readily distinguishes them from other coccidian oocysts or sporocysts that may be stained by the same methods. The polymerase chain reaction with primers specific for *C. cayetanensis* also affords a highly sensitive, but more costly, diagnostic technique.

There are four other intestinal coccidia that infect humans and may produce similar symptoms, but they are morphologically readily differentiated from *C. cayetanensis* when viewed unstained (Fig. 7.8.6.5). The oocysts of cryptosporidium, also an important cause of acute diarrhoea, are spherical but are only from 4.5 to 5.0 μm in diameter (half the size of *C. cayetanensis* oocysts) and they contain four naked sporozoites. *Isospora belli* oocysts are elongated, measure from 25 to 33 μm in length and from 12 to 16 μm in width, and have two sporocysts, each of which contains four sporozoites. Humans are the definite host of two species of *Sarcocystis*, *S. hominis* and *S. suihominis*: unlike *C. cayetanensis*, their oocysts undergo endogenous sporulation and contain two sporocysts, each containing four sporozoites. The oocysts are very fragile and usually rupture, so that only free sporocysts may be found

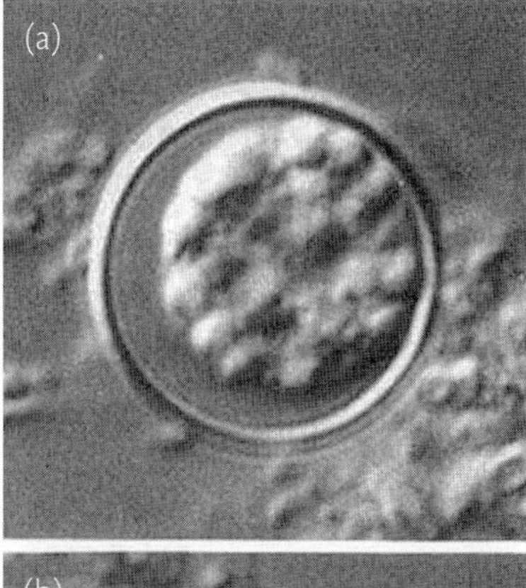

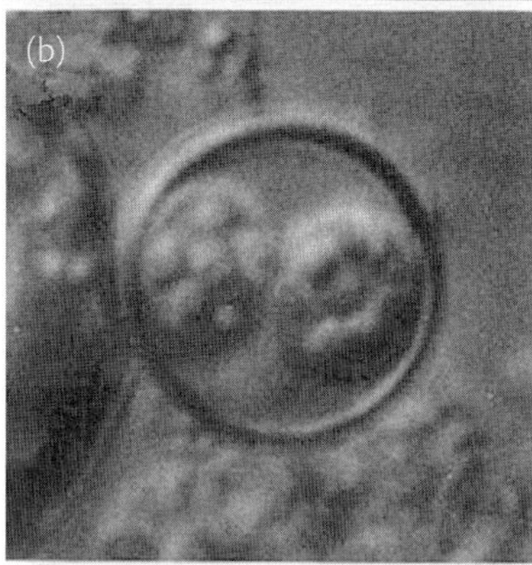

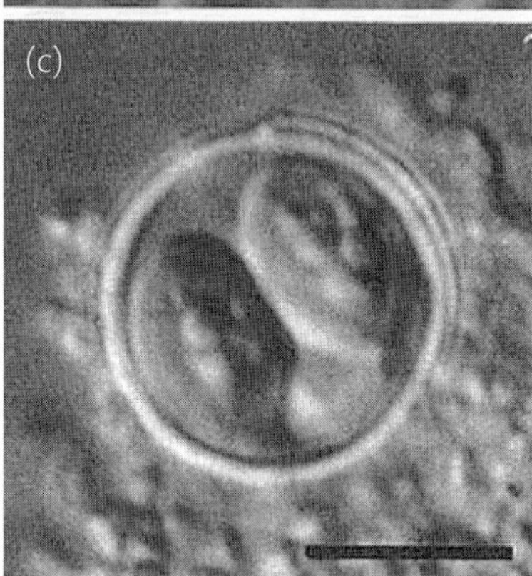

Fig. 7.8.6.3 Developing oocysts of *C. cayetanensis* as seen by Nomarski interference-contrast microscopy: (a) unsporulated oocyst; (b) formation of the two sporoblasts; (c) formation of the two sporocysts. Bar, 5 µm.
(From Ortega YR, Gilman RH, Sterling CR (1994). A new coccidian parasite (Apicomplexa: Eimeriidae) from humans. *J Parasitol*, **80**, 625–9, with permission).

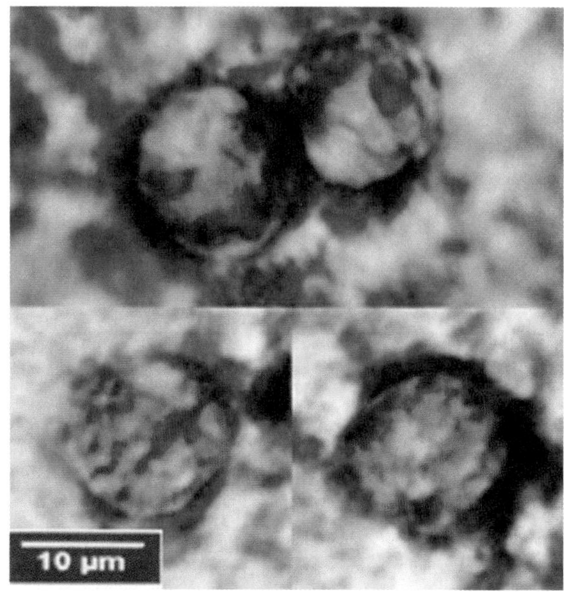

Fig. 7.8.6.4 Safranin-stained oocysts of *C. cayetanensis*. Bar, 10 µm.
(From Eberhard ML, Pieniazak NJ, Arrowood MJ (1997). Laboratory diagnosis of *Cyclospora* infections. *Arch Pathol Lab Med*, **121**, 792–7, with permission.)

in the faeces. These are easily differentiated from *C. cayetanensis* oocysts by their larger size (average 16 µm × 10.5 µm) and ellipsoidal shape.

A well-trained microscopist will have no difficulty in distinguishing other protozoa of the human intestine. Among these are the cystic stages of *Entamoeba histolytica* and *Giardia lamblia* and the non-cystic *Dientamoeba fragilis*, all of which commonly cause abdominal pain and diarrhoea.

Pathology

Histology of jejunal biopsies from patients with cyclosporiasis has shown blunting and widening of infected villi and an intense lymphocytic infiltration in the lamina propria and overlying epithelium (Fig. 7.8.6.6). There is a diffuse oedema, together with reactive hyperaemia and vascular dilation that is accompanied by congestion of the villous capillaries.

Treatment

Co-trimoxazole (960 mg two times daily for 1 week) has proved effective in eliminating the parasite in immunocompetent patients and has been shown successfully to control relapses in those with AIDS by the administration of 960 mg three times a week, indefinitely. Ciprofloxacin (500 mg two times daily for 1 week) is recommended for patients who react badly to sulphonamides.

Prevention

As with all other organisms dependent on faecal–oral transmission, simple precautions will help prevent infection with *C. cayetanensis*. Water should be boiled before drinking or when used to wash fruits (although these are best peeled) or green leafy vegetables that are to be eaten raw. These measures are not only important in the endemic areas of developing countries, but need to be taken when consuming fruit or vegetables that are imported from such regions, as seen with the serious outbreaks of cyclosporiasis in the United States of America due to unwashed raspberries imported from Guatemala.

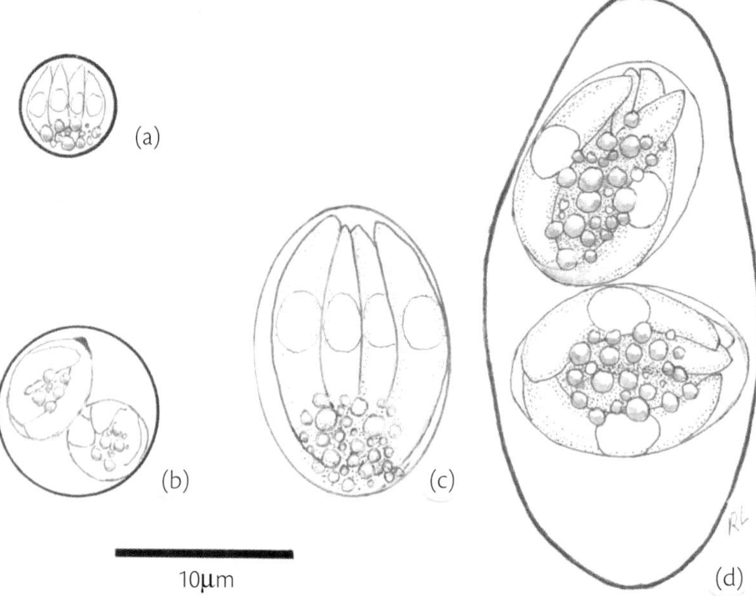

Fig. 7.8.6.5 Faecal stages of the five intestinal coccidia that infect humans: (a) oocyst of *Cryptosporidium parvum*, (b) oocyst of *Cyclospora cayetanensis*, (c) sporocyst of *Sarcocystis hominis* or *S. suihominis* (the two are morphologically indistinguishable), and (d) oocyst of *Isospora belli*. Bar, 10 μm.

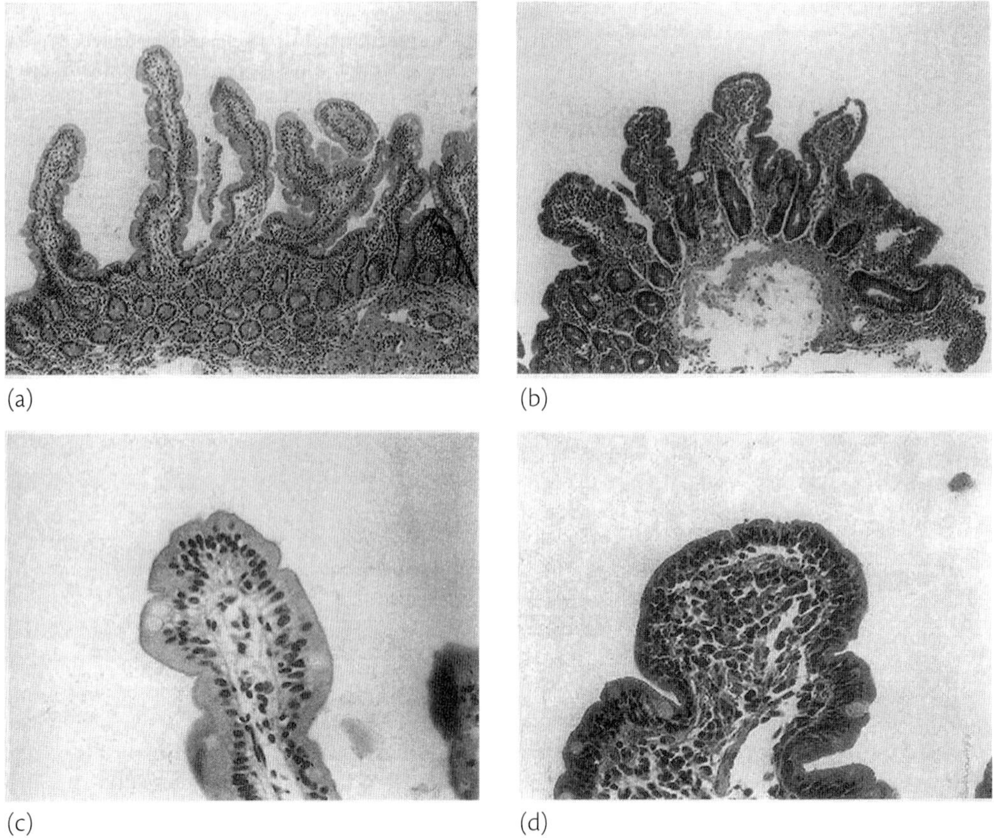

Fig. 7.8.6.6 Comparison of normal human jejunal villi (a,c) and villi infected with *C. cayetanensis* (b,d): low-power appearance (a,b) and high-power appearance (c,d). Note the blunting and widening of the villi, with inflammatory lymphocytic infiltrate in the lamina propria and infiltration of overlying epithelium.
(From Ortega YR, *et al.* (1997). Pathologic and clinical findings in patients with cyclosporiasis and a description of intracellular parasite life-cycle stages. *J Infect Dis*, **176**, 1584–9, with permission.)

Further reading

Ashford RW (1979). Occurrence of an undescribed coccidian in man in Papua New Guinea. *Ann Trop Med Parasitol*, **73**, 497–500.

Eberhard ML, Pieniazak NJ, Arrowood MJ (1997). Laboratory diagnosis of *Cyclospora* infections. *Arch Pathol Lab Med*, **121**, 792–7.

Lainson R (2005). The genus *Cyclospora* (Apicomplexa: Eimeriidae), with a description of *Cyclospora schneideri* n.sp. in the snake *Anilius scytale* scytale (Aniliidae) from Amazonian Brazil—a review. *Mem Inst Oswaldo Cruz*, **100**, 103–110.

McDonald V, Kelly MP (2005). Intestinal coccidia: cryptosporidiosis, isosporiasis, cyclosporiasis. In: Cox FEG, *et al.* (eds) *Topley & Wilson's Microbiology & Microbial Infections: Parasitology*, 10th edition, pp. 399–421. Hodder Arnold ASM Press, London.

Ortega YR, *et al.* (1992). *Cyclospora cayetanensis*: a new protozoan pathogen of humans. Abstract 289 in Proceedings of the 41st Annual Meeting of the American Society of Tropical Medicine and Hygiene. *Am J Trop Med Hyg*, (Suppl), p. 210.

Ortega YR, Gilman RH, Sterling CR (1994). A new coccidian parasite (Apicomplexa: Eimeriidae) from humans. *J Parasitol*, **80**, 625–9.

Ortega YR, *et al.* (1997). Pathologic and clinical findings in patients with cyclosporiasis and a description of intracellular parasite life-cycle stages. *J Infect Dis*, **176**, 1584–9.

7.8.7 Sarcocystosis (sarcosporidiosis)

John E. Cooper

Essentials

Sarcocystosis is characterized by the invasion of muscles and sometimes other tissues by protozoa of the genus *Sarcocystis*, of which *S. hominis* (intermediate host domestic cattle) and *S. suihominis* (domestic pig) are the most significant to humans, to whom they are transmitted by ingestion of uncooked beef or pork. Humans serve as either intermediate or final host: (1) intermediate host—presence of cysts in muscle is usually asymptomatic, but may cause myositis or myopathy; detected on clinical examination or muscle biopsy; (2) final host—may be asymptomatic or cause fever and gastrointestinal upset; oocysts or sporocysts can be detected in faeces. There is no specific treatment. Prevention is by not eating uncooked meat from any animal.

Acknowledgement: I am most grateful to Dr Sarah Cooper for reading and commenting on an early draft of the text.

Introduction

Although often described as uncommon in humans, Sarcocystosis appears to be widespread but undetected. It has been reported from most continents but the exact distribution of the different species remains uncertain, largely on account of the absence of definitive clinical signs in many cases. Over the past decade, veterinary studies, especially serological surveys, have indicated that *Sarcocystis* species are present in a wide range of domesticated and wild mammals and other animals, often at a high prevalence (Fig. 7.8.7.1). Snakes and their rodent prey are definitive and intermediate hosts for many species of *Sarcocystis*; there is evidence of coevolution of the parasites with their vertebrate hosts. Equine protozoal myeloencephalitis, a disease of domestic horses due to *S. neurona*, has prompted a considerable body of research on *Sarcocystis* in recent years because of its great economic importance.

Sarcocystosis presents both actual and perceived public health problems. Some species, such as *S. hominis* and *S. suihominis*, can be transferred from animals to humans but others, while often causing alarm among those who encounter them, do not appear to be transmissible. For example, *S. rileyi*, which commonly affects ducks and geese in North America, presents with readily visible cream-coloured cysts generally running in parallel lines in the

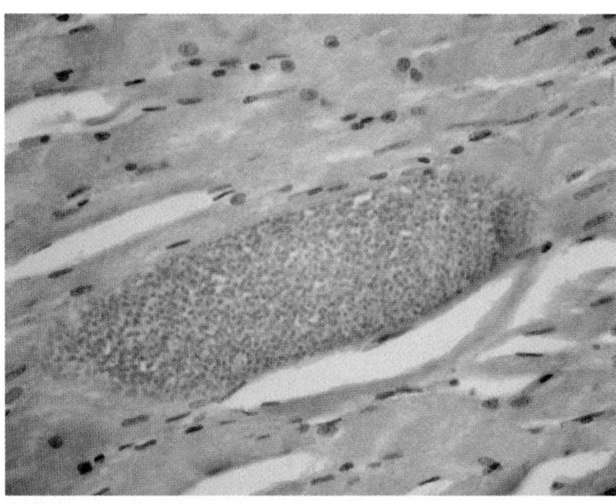

(a)

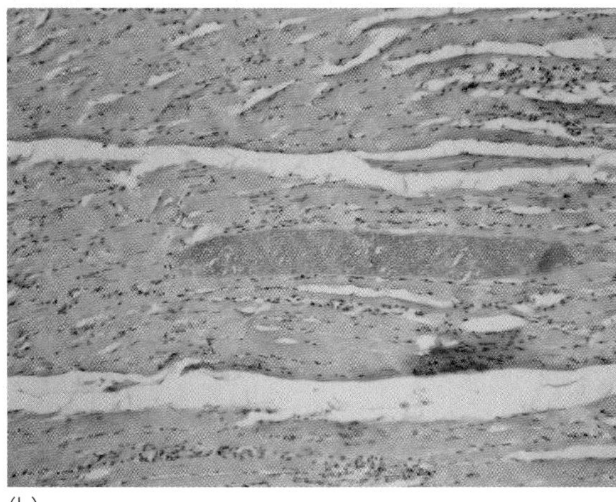

(b)

Fig. 7.8.7.1 *Sarcocystis* in skeletal muscle of a little penguin *Eudyptula minor* (haematoxylin and eosin).
(Courtesy of Dr Richard Norman.)

muscles of affected birds. This condition, often termed 'rice breast disease', is familiar to hunters and to those who skin waterfowl before they are cooked. Many affected carcasses are discarded, but meat containing the cysts presents no known hazard to people who eat it.

However, the role of host resistance in sarcocystosis has not been fully investigated and it is possible that immunosuppression may render humans susceptible to species of *Sarcocystis* that are primarily parasites of wild birds, reptiles, or mammals.

Clinical features

Humans as the final host

Depending on the species of parasite and the previous health of the host, infection in humans who have ingested meat containing cysts of *Sarcocystis* can have effects that range from gastrointestinal disorders and pyrexia to an asymptomatic state.

Humans as the intermediate host

The presence of cysts in human skeletal, visceral, or cardiac muscle is usually not associated with symptoms or clinical signs but it is likely that large numbers may, as in animals, cause myositis or myopathy, especially if calcification occurs, sometimes with vasculitis.

Diagnosis

Humans as the final host

Oocysts or sporocysts can be detected in faeces in smears (especially using Heine's method), in wet saline preparations, or, better, using a sodium chloride or sucrose flotation method (Fig. 7.8.7.2). The oocysts/sporocysts are usually readily recognized by an experienced parasitologist but can easily escape the attention of those who are less familiar with the organism. *Sarcocystis* must be distinguished from other sporozoal organisms that are either being produced in the intestine or are in transit in the lumen following ingestion.

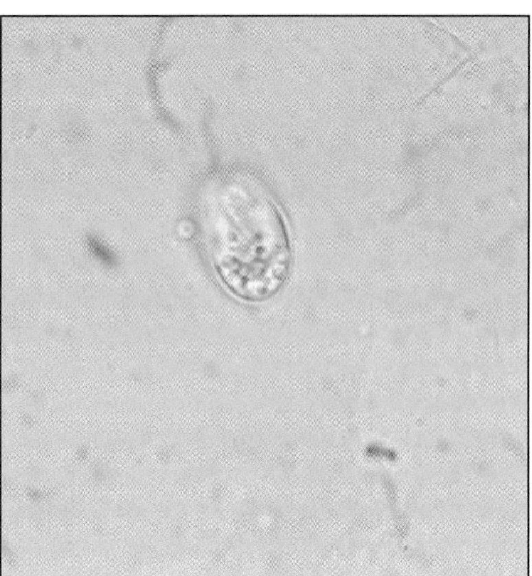

Fig. 7.8.7.2 Sporocyst containing sporozoites in faeces of a fox *Vulpes vulpes*. There are two within the oocyst when freshly passed but single sporocysts are often seen.
(Courtesy of Dr John McGarry.)

Humans as the intermediate host

Occasionally, tissue cysts are detected during routine clinical examination, especially if calcification has occurred. They may also be seen in muscle biopsies, either as an incidental finding or because samples have been taken specifically for diagnostic purposes. Calcified cysts found in biopsies or located at autopsy have a gritty texture when cut.

Sarcocystosis of muscle (Figs. 7.8.7.1 and 7.8.7.3) must be differentiated from toxoplasmosis, in which tissue cysts can also be found. The morphology of the two protozoa differs. In particular, cysts of *Sarcocystis* have a distinct wall, which is thick and striated in some species, and do not stain with periodic acid–Schiff stain, which usually gives *Toxoplasma* cysts a magenta colour.

Treatment

There is no specific therapy for sarcocystosis in humans or animals, although albendazole has been reported to ameleriorate symptoms in a human patient with skeletal cysts and ponazuril has been shown to prevent infection of the central nervous system of mice experimentally given sporocysts of *S. neurona*. When humans are the final host, symptomatic and supportive treatment is indicated.

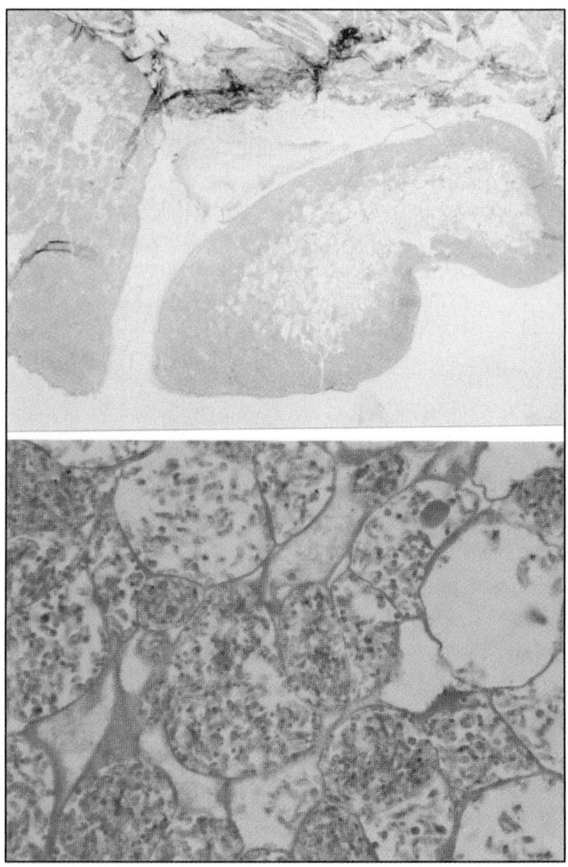

Fig. 7.8.7.3 Cysts of bovine origin, containing crescent-shaped bradyzoites that are infective in the definitive host.
(Courtesy of Dr John McGarry.)

Prevention

Sarcocystosis can be prevented by not eating uncooked meat from any animal. Vaccines, at present experimental, have been shown to produce cellular immunity to certain *Sarcocystis* species in horses.

Further reading

Arness MK, *et al.* (1999). An outbreak of acute eosinophilic myositis attributed to human *Sarcocystis* parasitism. *Am J Trop Med Hyg*, **61**, 548–53.

Bunyaratvej S, Bunyawongwiroj P, Nitiyanant P (1982). Human intestinal sarcosporidiosis: report of six cases. *Am J Trop Med Hyg*, **31**, 36–41.

Fayer R (2004). *Sarcocystis* spp. in human infections. *Clin Microbiol Rev*, **17**, 894–902.

Marsh AE, *et al.* (2004). Evaluation of immune responses in horses immunized using a killed *Sarcocystis neurona* vaccine. *Vet Ther*, **5**, 34–42.

Mehrotra R, *et al.* (1996). Diagnosis of human *Sarcocystis* infection from biopsies of the skeletal muscle. *Pathology*, **28**, 281–2.

Slapeta JR, *et al.* (2003). Evolutionary relationships among cyst-forming coccidia *Sarcocystis* spp. (Alveolata: Apicomplexa: Coccidea) in endemic African tree vipers and perspective for evolution of heteroxenous life cycle. *Mol Phylogenet Evol*, **27**, 464–75.

Velásquez JN, *et al.* (2008). Systemic sarcocystosis in a patient with acquired immune deficiency syndrome. *Hum Pathol*, **39**, 1263–7.

Wong KT, Pathmanathan R (1992). High prevalence of human skeletal muscle sarcocystosis in south-east Asia. *Trans R Soc Trop Med Hyg*, **86**, 631–2.

Zaman V, Colley FC (1975). Light and electron microscopic observations of the life cycle of *Sarcocystis orientalis* sp. n. in the rat (*Rattus norvegicus*) and the Malaysian reticulated python (*Python reticulatus*). *Z Parasitenkd*, **47**, 169–85.

7.8.8 Giardiasis, balantidiasis, isosporiasis, and microsporidiosis

Martin F. Heyworth

Essentials

Giardiasis

Infection with *Giardia intestinalis*, a flagellate protozoan that colonizes the lumen of the small intestine, is acquired by ingesting environmentally resistant cysts of the parasite, typically in water or food. Strains of the parasite that can infect humans are harboured by various mammals, including domestic dogs and cattle.

Clinical features—manifestations include watery diarrhoea, abdominal discomfort and distension, weight loss, and malabsorption, with the infection typically being persistent and severe in individuals with genetic impairment of antibody production.

Diagnosis and treatment—diagnosis is by faecal examination for evidence of *G. intestinalis* infection, including (1) cysts—by microscopy, including immunofluorescence microscopy with fluorescent antibodies; (2) antigen—by enzyme-linked immunoassay; or (3) DNA—by polymerase chain reaction (PCR) amplification. Aside from supportive care, treatment is with metronidazole (although the parasite is becoming increasingly resistant), tinidazole and nitazoxanide.

Prevention—cysts of *G. intestinalis* in water can be killed by boiling or removed by filtration.

Balantidiasis

Balantidium coli is a ciliate protozoan that invades the colonic mucosa. Infection—which may or may not be acquired from pigs or other animals—may be asymptomatic or cause diarrhoea that can be watery or contain blood and mucus. Perforation of the colon can occur, leading to peritonitis, and the parasite can also spread to the liver and lungs. Diagnosis is by recognition of the parasite on microscopic examination of diarrhoeal stools, colonic mucus, or rectal biopsies. Aside from supportive care, treatment with metronidazole or tetracycline has reportedly eradicated infection in some instances. Prevention is by filtration or boiling of drinking water, hand washing before handling food, and careful cleaning and cooking of food.

Isosporiasis

Cystoisospora belli is a coccidian protozoan that colonises epithelial cells of the small intestine. Infection is presumed to be acquired by ingestion of parasite oocysts in water or food, but vehicles for transmission to humans are unknown, although the organism has been found on cockroaches. Clinical features include watery diarrhoea, dehydration, fever, and weight loss, with isosporiasis being an opportunistic infection associated with HIV infection. Diagnosis is by microscopic examination of faecal specimens for oocysts of *C. belli*, which show blue autofluorescence under ultraviolet light. Aside from supportive care, trimethoprim–sulphamethoxazole is partially effective.

Microsporidiosis

Microsporidia are minute intracellular parasites genetically related to fungi, which infect various animals and birds. About a dozen species can cause human infection (some only rarely). In at least some cases this appears to be acquired by ingestion of spores of the causative organism(s) in water.

Clinical features—clinical manifestations are most frequently reported in HIV-infected patients, exemplified by colonisation of the small intestinal mucosa by *Enterocytozoon bieneusi* or *Encephalitozoon intestinalis* leading to watery diarrhoea. Other manifestations of microsporidial infection include acalculous cholecystitis, sinusitis, cough/dyspnoea, urethritis, and keratoconjunctivitis.

Diagnosis, treatment, and prevention—intestinal microsporidiosis is diagnosed by microscopic examination of faecal specimens (after appropriate staining) for microsporidian spores, or by detection of microsporidian DNA in faecal specimens. Aside from supportive care, albendazole is an effective drug for treating encephalitozoon infections, although *Ent. bieneusi* does not respond. In HIV-infected patients, remission of *Ent. bieneusi* infection can be achieved by antiretroviral drug treatment that reduces the HIV load. Prevention can be achieved by killing spores in water by boiling or exposure to ultraviolet light.

Introduction

The organisms that cause the diseases covered in this chapter are not closely related to each other. Of these infections, the first three are caused by protozoa: giardiasis by a flagellate, balantidiasis by a ciliate, and isosporiasis by a coccidian. The term 'microsporidiosis' encompasses a group of infections caused by approximately a dozen species of minute parasites (microsporidia) that are genetically related to fungi and that may have (speculatively) evolved from a fungal ancestor.

Transmission of the organisms covered in this chapter mainly occurs by drinking or eating water or food containing environmentally resistant life-cycle stages of the parasites. Two of the diseases, isosporiasis and, particularly, microsporidiosis, have become much more widely recognized since the start of the HIV/AIDS pandemic in the early 1980s and are included among the opportunistic infections seen in patients with AIDS. The four diseases occur worldwide; although most published reports of balantidiasis and isosporiasis are from tropical countries, these two diseases also occur in nontropical locations.

Historical perspective

Before the 1990s, literature on human giardiasis emphasized a relationship between drinking unfiltered water in wilderness areas and acquiring this infection, as well as occurrence of giardia species in beavers and muskrats (which were presumed to be sources of the human infection). Since then, it has become evident that morphologically indistinguishable giardia organisms colonize a wide variety of mammals, including cattle, horses, and domestic pets (dogs and cats), in addition to human hosts. Genotyping of *Giardia intestinalis* organisms has now enabled morphologically identical parasites to be subclassified into genetic assemblages of particular host preference (in this chapter, the terms 'genetic assemblage' and 'genotype', as applied to *G. intestinalis*, are used interchangeably). This genetic fingerprinting of giardia organisms has helped to clarify the risks of human subjects becoming infected by giardia parasites from particular species of nonhuman host.

Historically, balantidiasis and isosporiasis were recognized sufficiently rarely that they were the subjects of anecdotal case reports. This apparent rarity made it difficult to perform clinical trials to identify drugs useful for treating these diseases. In the 1980s, however, such a trial established the utility of co-trimoxazole in treating isosporiasis.

Before the HIV/AIDS pandemic, most of the literature on microsporidian infections dealt with such infections in nonhuman hosts (e.g. silk moths, honeybees, fish, and rabbits). The burgeoning literature on human microsporidiosis in HIV-infected individuals has been complemented by increased awareness of microsporidia that typically infect immunocompetent people, notably organisms that infect the human corneal stroma.

Because they lack mitochondria and some other features of higher eukaryotic (nucleated) cells, giardia and microsporidia were formerly considered to be extremely primitive. Following the discovery in these organisms of gene sequences homologous with mitochondrial DNA and of organelles (mitosomes) that appear to be derived from mitochondria, the organisms are now regarded as highly specialized rather than primitive. The apparently primitive features are almost certainly adaptations to the parasitic lifestyle, reflecting the colonization of an anaerobic niche (vertebrate intestinal lumen) by giardia species and of host intracellular environments by microsporidia.

Giardiasis

Aetiology, pathogenesis, and pathology

G. intestinalis (synonyms *G. lamblia* and *G. duodenalis*) colonizes the lumen of the small intestine. The parasite's life cycle comprises two stages: motile trophozoites (Fig. 7.8.8.1) and thick-walled ellipsoidal cysts that are excreted in the faeces. *G. intestinalis* trophozoites are dorsoventrally flattened organisms with eight flagella, two nuclei, and a ventral adhesive disc that enables them to become attached to the luminal surface of intestinal epithelial cells. Trophozoites absorb nutrients in the small intestinal lumen and multiply in this environment. New hosts become infected by ingesting *G. intestinalis* cysts; exposure of cysts to gastric acid leads to emergence of trophozoites from the cysts. Trophozoites encyst in the intestinal lumen and the resulting cysts are excreted from the host. The environmentally resistant cyst wall consists of protein and a polymer of *N*-acetylgalactosamine.

The mechanisms responsible for diarrhoea and malabsorption in giardiasis are partially understood. Shortening of microvilli on the luminal surface of intestinal epithelial cells has been observed in small intestinal biopsies from patients with giardiasis. Reduced activity of intestinal disaccharidases has been reported in giardia-infected human subjects and rodents. This functional enzyme deficiency might lead to osmotic diarrhoea (via the presence of undigested disaccharides in the intestinal lumen).

Study of immunity against giardia species has been more feasible in rodents than in human subjects. In mice, clearance of giardia infection appears to be dependent on CD4+ (helper) T lymphocytes and to follow the generation of an intestinal IgA

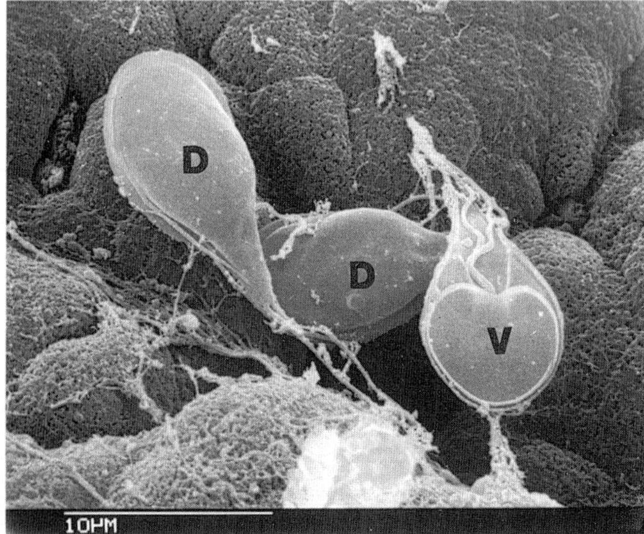

Fig. 7.8.8.1 Scanning electron micrograph of three *Giardia intestinalis* trophozoites on a jejunal biopsy specimen from a patient with giardiasis. The dorsal surfaces of two trophozoites are visible (D), and the ventral adhesive disc of the other trophozoite is shown (V).
(Courtesy of Dr Robert L. Owen; modified from Carlson JR, Heyworth MF, Owen RL (1984). Giardiasis: Immunology, diagnosis and treatment. *Survey of Digestive Diseases*, **2**, 210–23, with permission.)

response against the parasite. Genetically altered knock-out mice that are unable to produce intestinal IgA have an impaired ability to clear giardia infection. In human volunteers who were deliberately infected with *G. intestinalis*, an intestinal IgA response to the parasite occurred. IgA directed against trophozoites binds to these organisms and may, conceivably, inhibit their attachment to the intestinal epithelium, such that they are susceptible to peristaltic expulsion from the host. Giardia infection in mice and in human subjects leads to intestinal hypermotility, which may promote clearance of the parasite.

Epidemiology

G. intestinalis infection is acquired by drinking water that contains cysts. Other modes of spread include faecal–oral transmission of cysts, as in day-care centres for small children, and foodborne transmission of cysts. Waterborne giardiasis occurs as a result of drinking unfiltered, unboiled water from streams and lakes containing *G. intestinalis* cysts. Swimming in (and inadvertently drinking) water in lakes and rivers containing the cysts is also a risk factor for giardiasis. Outbreaks of this infection have resulted from the unintended presence of *G. intestinalis* cysts in public drinking water supplies and in swimming pools. Giardiasis is one of several parasitic and bacterial diseases that are potentially or actually transmitted by eating raw vegetables grown on fields irrigated or contaminated with untreated human sewage or animal manure. Aquatic molluscs, such as mussels grown commercially in estuarine water, concentrate particulate materials (including giardia cysts) from water by filter feeding, thus posing a potential infection hazard to human subjects who eat the molluscs raw.

Genotyping of *G. intestinalis* organisms has revealed genetic similarity between giardia isolates from people and from dogs occupying the same households in India, a finding consistent with transmission of *G. intestinalis* between dogs and people. Approximately 10% of giardia isolates from cattle belong to genotypes that can cause human infection. Flies that feed on garbage and sewage are able to carry giardia cysts on their exoskeletons and in their alimentary tracts and may therefore contaminate human food with viable cysts.

Immunodeficiency predisposes to the occurrence of severe and persistent giardiasis. Human immunodeficiency states that are associated with giardiasis include conditions that impair host antibody responses, notably 'common variable' hypogammaglobulinaemia and X-linked immunoglobulin deficiency. Impairment of intestinal IgA production is a feature of these particular immunodeficiency diseases and may explain how they predispose to chronic giardiasis (via impaired production of antitrophozoite IgA).

Prevention

G. intestinalis cysts can be removed from water by filtration, for example using membrane filters with a pore diameter of less than 5 µm. Cysts in water are killed by boiling. Exposure of water to ultraviolet light can inactivate giardia cysts and other organisms in the water. Water intended for human consumption can be screened for *G. intestinalis* cysts by exposure to magnetic beads coated with an antibody directed against cyst antigens (to capture cysts from suspension) followed by immunofluorescence microscopy using a fluorescent antibody to detect any cysts. Viable and dead cysts retrieved from water can be distinguished by staining with fluorescent dyes that selectively stain living or dead cysts, respectively.

Clinical features

Giardia infection can be asymptomatic (as shown by cyst excretion in the absence of symptoms) and also causes various clinical problems. These include abdominal discomfort, tenderness, and distension, a sensation of fullness, nausea, anorexia, and watery diarrhoea. Other clinical features include heartburn, flatulence, steatorrhoea, and weight loss. In immunologically normal persons, untreated giardiasis typically lasts for several weeks, with symptoms that fluctuate in severity. Clinical sequelae that have occasionally been reported include megaloblastic anaemia resulting from impaired absorption of vitamin B_{12} or folic acid.

Laboratory diagnosis

In a patient suspected of having parasitic infection of the gastrointestinal tract (with one or more species of parasite that might include *G. intestinalis*), faecal light microscopy may be informative. If the patient has giardiasis, *G. intestinalis* cysts may be seen during this examination. Diagnostic sensitivity can be increased by immunofluorescence microscopy of faecal specimens incubated with a fluorescent antibody that binds to *G. intestinalis* cysts. If there is a strong suspicion of infection with *G. intestinalis* (or if the aim is to check the effectiveness of treatment in clearing known giardiasis), immunoassay for *G. intestinalis* antigens is a recommended method. This approach, which involves enzyme-linked immunoassay (ELISA) of faecal specimens with one of several commercially available kits, is more objective and less labour intensive than immunofluorescence microscopy (which detects whole cysts).

Though not widely available in diagnostic laboratories, the ability to detect *G. intestinalis* DNA in faecal specimens by polymerase chain reaction (PCR) is a sensitive and specific method.

Treatment

Table 7.8.8.1 summarizes various drug regimens for treating giardiasis. Metronidazole resistance of *G. intestinalis* is an increasingly recognized problem, which has prompted a continuing search for

Table 7.8.8.1 Various drug regimens for treating giardiasis

Drug	Dose	Treatment duration
Metronidazole	250 mg, three times daily (adult)	5 days
	15 mg/kg body wt per day, in 3 doses (paediatric)	5 days
Albendazole	400 mg daily	5 days
Tinidazole	2 g (adult)	Single dose
	50 mg/kg (paediatric)	Single dose (2 g maximum)
Ornidazole	2 g (adult)	Single dose
Furazolidone	100 mg, four times daily (adult)	7–10 days
	6 mg/kg per day, in 4 doses (paediatric)	7–10 days
Quinacrine	100 mg, three times daily	5 days
Nitazoxanide	500 mg, twice daily (adult)	3 days
	100 mg, twice daily (age 1–3 years)	3 days
	200 mg, twice daily (age 4–11 years)	3 days

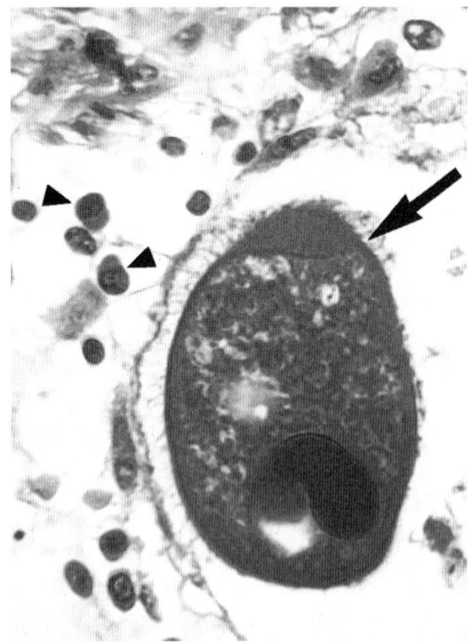

Fig. 7.8.8.2 Light micrograph of *Balantidium coli* trophozoite (arrow) in colonic tissue (×705). Cilia are visible on the surface of the organism. Arrowheads indicate tissue plasma cells.
(Modified from Neafie RC (1976). Balantidiasis. In: Binford CH, Connor DH (eds) *Pathology of tropical and extraordinary diseases*, vol. 1, pp. 325–7. Armed Forces Institute of Pathology, Washington DC, with permission.)

alternative therapeutic agents. In recent years, nitazoxanide has been introduced for treating giardiasis.

Balantidiasis

Aetiology, pathogenesis, and pathology

Balantidium coli, the cause of balantidiasis, is the largest protozoan parasite of man. *B. coli* has a two-stage life cycle comprising motile trophozoites that invade the colonic mucosa (Fig. 7.8.8.2) and nonmotile cysts. Spread of the infection to new hosts occurs by ingestion of the parasite. *B. coli* trophozoites invade and cause ulceration of the colonic mucosa. The mechanisms responsible for tissue invasion by these organisms are not known.

Epidemiology

There is circumstantial evidence that humans can acquire *B. coli* infection from animals. This infection has been described in pigs and in many species of nonhuman primates. A high prevalence of the infection has been seen in human communities that live in close proximity to *B. coli*-infected pigs (e.g. in New Guinea). Consequently, there has been speculation that pigs are a reservoir for spread of *B. coli* to humans. Balantidiasis has also occurred in human subjects who had no known contact with pigs or other animals. Clusters of cases of balantidiasis have been seen in long-stay psychiatric hospitals. In India, *B. coli* cysts have been found in water available for either drinking or use in cooking, and cysts of the organism have been found on cockroaches in Nigeria.

Clinical features

Human subjects with *B. coli* infection can be asymptomatic or can develop diarrhoea with stools that are either watery or that consist of blood and mucus. In severe *B. coli* infection, patients can develop colonic perforation, peritonitis, gangrene of the appendix (resulting from the presence of *B. coli* in the appendiceal wall), and spread of the parasite to the liver or lungs. Balantidiasis is a rare cause of liver abscess. As is evident from the clinical features outlined above, balantidiasis may be clinically indistinguishable from amoebiasis, bacillary dysentery, ulcerative colitis, and Crohn's disease, and can be fatal. *B. coli* infection in the lungs has been described in occasional patients with concurrent malignant disease (including chronic lymphocytic leukaemia).

Laboratory diagnosis

Balantidiasis can be diagnosed by microscopic examination of diarrhoeal stools or colonic mucus obtained at sigmoidoscopy. Examination may show motile trophozoites or, less frequently, cysts of *B. coli*. Histological examination of rectal biopsies may reveal *B. coli* trophozoites. Pulmonary balantidiasis can be diagnosed by bronchoalveolar lavage and finding the parasite in the lavage fluid.

Prevention and treatment

Prevention of balantidiasis involves avoidance of *B. coli* cyst ingestion, via filtration or boiling of drinking water, hand washing before handling food, and careful cleaning and cooking of food.

Patients with balantidiasis have been treated empirically with various antimicrobial drugs. There is, however, little interpretable information about the effectiveness of such treatment, although eradication of *B. coli* has been reported in some individuals treated with metronidazole or tetracycline. Surgical intervention may be necessary in patients with liver abscess or clinical evidence of appendicitis or colonic perforation.

Isosporiasis

Aetiology, pathogenesis, and pathology

The organism that causes isosporiasis was formerly known as *Isospora belli*. Organisms formerly included in the genus *Isospora* that are parasitic to mammals have now been assigned to the genus *Cystoisospora* (the generic name *Isospora* has been retained for avian parasites). *Cystoisospora belli* is a parasite of the human small intestine. There is limited evidence that *C. belli* infects nonhuman hosts: oocysts of *C. belli* have been isolated from dog faeces in India and the parasite has been transmitted experimentally to gibbons.

C. belli oocysts are ellipsoidal structures that are excreted in the faeces of infected individuals (Fig. 7.8.8.3). Studies of cystoisospora species that parasitize nonhuman hosts indicate that infection occurs via ingestion of oocysts and that sporozoites (which emerge from oocysts) penetrate epithelial cells of the small intestine. Subsequent development of cystoisospora species comprises: (1) an asexual pathway, with production of merozoites, which can infect additional epithelial cells; and (2) a sexual pathway, in which fusion of gametes produces oocysts that are excreted from the host.

Mechanisms responsible for the watery diarrhoea that occurs in isosporiasis are unknown. Presumably, the parasitization of epithelial cells in the small intestine contributes to the diarrhoea.

Epidemiology

C. belli infection has been documented in immunosuppressed and, rarely, in immunocompetent individuals. Among 397 HIV-infected

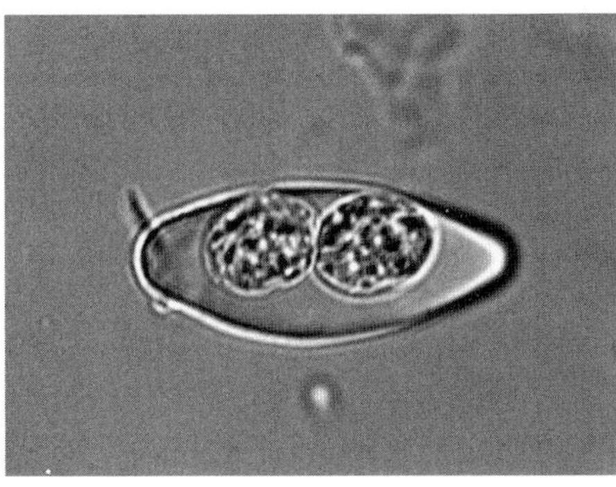

Fig. 7.8.8.3 Light micrograph of a *Cystoisospora belli* oocyst (×2500).
(Courtesy of Dr William L. Current. From Garcia LS (2001). *Diagnostic medical parasitology*, 4th edition. ASM Press, Washington DC, with permission.)

patients in Venezuela, 56 (14%) were found to have *C. belli* infection (as judged by the presence of oocysts in faecal specimens). Of these 56 patients with *C. belli* infection, 98% had diarrhoea. Vehicles for transmission of *C. belli* oocysts to human subjects have not been identified, but presumably include water and food. Oocysts of this parasite are among the human pathogens found on cockroaches in Nigeria.

Clinical features

In patients infected with HIV, *C. belli* infection is associated with chronic watery diarrhoea, abdominal cramps, nausea, fever, and weight loss. Severe dehydration can result from diarrhoea attributable to *C. belli* infection in HIV-infected patients. In immunocompetent individuals, symptoms ascribed to isosporiasis are similar to those that occur in AIDS-associated *C. belli* infection. Isosporiasis has been described in a few patients with haematological malignancy (including Hodgkin's disease, non-Hodgkin's lymphoma, and adult T-cell leukaemia), in whom immunosuppression was presumably a risk factor for *C. belli* infection.

Rarely, extraintestinal *C. belli* infection has been described in patients with AIDS; in the relevant patients, tissues parasitized by *C. belli* have included gallbladder epithelium, liver, spleen, and mesenteric lymph nodes.

Laboratory diagnosis

Isosporiasis can be diagnosed by microscopic examination of faecal specimens for *C. belli* oocysts. Although these structures are relatively large (*c.*20 to 30 µm in length), they are translucent and may be difficult to see in unstained samples. Their visibility is increased by incubation with carbol fuchsin, which stains oocyst internal structures red, or by incubation with lactophenol cotton blue. An alternative approach is to examine faecal smears under ultraviolet light; with this type of illumination, *C. belli* oocysts show blue autofluorescence.

Treatment and prognosis

The efficacy of oral co-trimoxazole in treating *C. belli*-induced diarrhoea was demonstrated in a study of patients with AIDS and isosporiasis in Haiti. Recognition of adverse drug reactions to co-trimoxazole, and less than 100% efficacy of this drug combination in treating isosporiasis, have prompted alternative therapeutic approaches. Diclazuril, albendazole–ornidazole, and pyrimethamine–sulphadiazine are three such alternatives that have shown anecdotal promise in treating isosporiasis associated with HIV infection.

In immunocompetent patients without HIV infection, isosporiasis can persist for weeks or months if untreated. The overall prognosis in patients with isosporiasis and HIV infection is determined by the HIV infection.

Microsporidiosis

Aetiology, genetics, pathogenesis, and pathology

Microsporidia are obligate intracellular parasites, whose lifecycle comprises an extracellular stage (spore) and stages that occur in the cytoplasm of host cells. Spores (Fig. 7.8.8.4) are shed into the environment by infected hosts and infect other members of the host species. The spores induce infection by high velocity extrusion of a hollow tube that penetrates a host cell and forms a channel for delivering sporoplasm (spore contents) into this cell. Replication of the parasite and subsequent production of spores occur in host cells. Some species of microsporidia invade and survive in macrophages and can become anatomically disseminated within the host in these mobile cells. Microsporidia have a small genome (e.g. 2.9×10^6 bp in the case of *Encephalitozoon cuniculi*).

In HIV-infected patients, diarrhoea is the clinical feature that has been most frequently associated with microsporidiosis. In particular, this symptom has been linked to infection with *Enterocytozoon bieneusi* and with *Encephalitozoon intestinalis*. The diarrhoea in these microsporidian infections presumably results from the presence of microsporidia in the small intestinal mucosa. Microsporidian parasitization of the intestinal mucosa can be seen on microscopic examination of biopsy specimens (Fig. 7.8.8.5).

Microsporidia that infect humans are listed in Table 7.8.8.2. Authenticated human infections with microsporidia other than *Ent. bieneusi*, *Enceph.* (*Septata*) *intestinalis*, and *Enceph. hellem*, are rare and some of the microsporidian species have been found in one or two patients only. 'Microsporidium' is a nontaxonomic genus created for microsporidia of unclear identity.

In mice at least, interferon-γ contributes to protective immunity against *Enceph. intestinalis* and *Enceph. cuniculi* infections.

Epidemiology

Most of the documented clinical experience with microsporidiosis has occurred in patients with HIV infection. Among 91 HIV-infected children with diarrhoea in Uganda, 70 were infected with

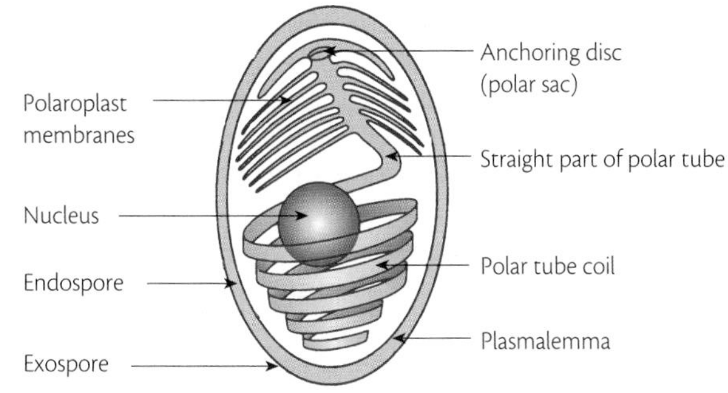

Fig. 7.8.8.4 Diagram of a microsporidian spore, showing internal structure.
(Courtesy of Professor Elizabeth U. Canning. Modified from Canning EU, Hollister WS (1992). Human infections with microsporidia. *Rev Med Microbiol*, **3**, 35–42, with permission.)

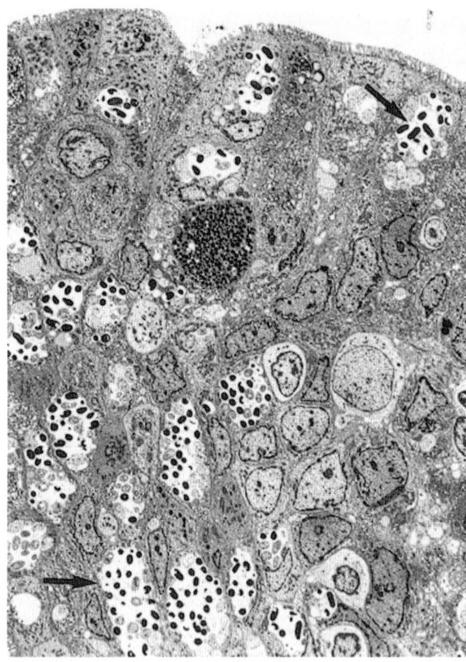

Fig. 7.8.8.5 Transmission electron micrograph of jejunal biopsy from a patient with AIDS and *Encephalitozoon intestinalis* infection. The microvillus border (epithelial surface) is at the top of the photograph. Epithelial cells and lamina propria leukocytes are heavily infected with *Enceph. intestinalis* (arrows). (Courtesy of the Electron Microscopy and Histopathology Unit, London School of Hygiene and Tropical Medicine. From Croft SL, Williams J, McGowan I (1997). Intestinal microsporidiosis. *Sem Gastrointest Dis*, **8**, 45–55, with permission.)

Ent. bieneusi. After its initial description as an intestinal parasite in the HIV-infected population during the 1980s, *Ent. bieneusi* was reported in several HIV-negative, purportedly immunocompetent persons with diarrhoea. Similarly, human encephalitozoon infections have been reported most frequently in HIV-infected patients, but also occur in immunocompetent individuals. Microsporidian infections, sometimes fatal, have been described in immunosuppressed recipients of solid organ or bone marrow transplants.

Experimental work with animals suggests that human infection with some species of microsporidia occurs via ingestion of spores. Environmental sources of microsporidian spores that can infect human subjects include water and, possibly, nonhuman hosts. *Enceph. intestinalis* DNA has been found in drinking water in Guatemala, by PCR amplification. Risk factors for *Ent. bieneusi* infection, in a population of HIV-infected patients surveyed in France, included swimming in a pool in the 12 months before the survey. In rural Mexican households, faecal excretion of *Encephalitozoon* spores was associated with the use of unboiled water for drinking and for preparing food. Heavy parasitization of respiratory tract epithelial cells with *Enceph. hellem*, in at least one HIV-infected patient examined at autopsy, raises the possibility that some microsporidian infections can be acquired by inhaling spores.

Some species of microsporidia listed in Table 7.8.8.2 are known to infect nonhuman hosts: e.g. DNA of three microsporidian species (*Ent. bieneusi*, *Enceph. intestinalis*, and *Enceph. hellem*) has been identified in faecal specimens from urban pigeons in Spain. Spores of *Enceph. intestinalis* have been identified in faecal specimens from nonhuman mammals (dogs, pigs, goats, cows, and donkeys). *Ent. bieneusi* can infect dogs, cats, pigs, goats, and cows.

Table 7.8.8.2 Species of microsporidia that infect humans

Species	Reported sites of infection
Enterocytozoon bieneusi	Small intestinal epithelium, gallbladder epithelium, rarely in respiratory tract and maxillary sinus
Encephalitozoon (formerly *Septata*) *intestinalis*	Intestinal epithelium, gallbladder epithelium, paranasal sinuses, respiratory tract, liver, kidney, pituitary, conjunctiva. Colonizes macrophages
Encephalitozoon hellem	Corneal epithelium, respiratory tract, kidney, paranasal sinuses
Encephalitozoon cuniculi	Kidney, urinary bladder, duodenal mucosa, conjunctiva, respiratory tract, adrenal glands, brain, heart, spleen, lymph nodes, cerebrospinal fluid
Vittaforma corneae (formerly *Nosema corneum*)	Corneal stroma, urinary tract
Trachipleistophora hominis	Skeletal muscle, conjunctiva, corneal stroma, nasopharynx (washings)
Trachipleistophora anthropophthera	Brain, kidney, heart, pancreas, thyroid, parathyroid glands, liver, spleen, lymph nodes, bone marrow, cornea
Pleistophora ronneafiei	Skeletal muscle
Anncaliia algerae[a]	Skeletal muscle, skin, corneal stroma
Anncaliia vesicularum[a]	Skeletal muscle
Anncaliia connori[a]	Generalized
Nosema ocularum	Corneal stroma
'Microsporidium ceylonensis'	Corneal stroma
'Microsporidium africanum'	Corneal stroma

[a] Organisms in the genus *Anncaliia* were formerly designated by the generic names *Brachiola* and *Nosema*.

Prevention

Water can be screened for microsporidian spores by immunocapture of spores on magnetic beads coated with antispore antibody, followed by PCR to detect microsporidian DNA. Microsporidian spores in water can be killed by boiling or by exposure of water to ultraviolet light.

A gene chip method has been developed for detecting and discriminating between DNA of *Ent. bieneusi* and of all three encephalitozoon species simultaneously. This method is potentially applicable to environmental screening of drinking water samples and to diagnostic testing of clinical material, such as human faecal specimens, to look for evidence of microsporidian infection in a patient.

Clinical features

Clinical features of microsporidian infections reflect the anatomical site colonized by the microsporidia (Table 7.8.8.2). Besides watery diarrhoea, weight loss and fat malabsorption have been reported in HIV-infected patients with intestinal microsporidiosis. Microsporidian infection of the gallbladder has been described in occasional HIV-infected patients who had acalculous cholecystitis (characterized by right upper abdominal pain, nausea, and vomiting) and who were treated by cholecystectomy. Symptoms of sinusitis, cough, and dyspnoea have been reported in patients with microsporidian infection of the paranasal sinuses and respiratory tract. Symptomatic urethritis has been ascribed to microsporidian infection in occasional HIV-infected patients. Pulmonary *Ent. bieneusi* infection, though rarely reported, has occurred in patients with HIV infection.

Microsporidian infection of the conjunctiva and corneal epithelium causes symptoms of keratoconjunctivitis (foreign body sensation in the eye, ocular discomfort and redness, photophobia, blurred vision, and sometimes reduced visual acuity). Microsporidian infections of the corneal stroma lead to reduced visual acuity, with or without corneal ulceration. Clinical features in patients with actual or presumed cerebral microsporidiosis have included headache, cognitive impairment, nausea, vomiting, and epileptic seizures. Symptoms of myositis (muscle pain, tenderness, weakness, and wasting) have been described in patients with microsporidian infection of skeletal muscles.

Laboratory diagnosis

Intestinal infection with *Ent. bieneusi* or *Enceph. intestinalis* can be diagnosed by finding microsporidian spores in faecal samples, for example by microscopic examination after exposure to various stains. The spores (which are ovoid) can be detected by microscopy after incubation with crystal violet plus iodine and chromotrope 2R (leading to violet staining of the spores), with optical brighteners such as Uvitex 2B and Calcofluor White M2R (which bind to chitin in the spores, resulting in fluorescence), or with fluorescent antibodies directed against the spores. Spores of *Ent. bieneusi* are smaller (*c.*1.5 µm × 0.9 µm) than those of *Enceph. intestinalis* (*c.*2.5 µm × 1.5 µm). Microsporidian infection of the nasal mucosa and paranasal sinuses can be diagnosed by microscopic examination of nasal secretions for spores after staining. Similarly, microsporidian spores can be found in urine and bile from patients with urinary tract and biliary tract microsporidiosis, respectively.

Detection of microsporidian DNA in clinical specimens (e.g. via the gene chip technique mentioned above) is a more sensitive *ex vivo* method than microscopy for diagnosing microsporidiosis.

Approaches to diagnosis of microsporidian keratoconjunctivitis include examining conjunctival/corneal scrapings or biopsies for spores and (noninvasively) *in vivo* examination of the cornea with a scanning confocal microscope to look for spore-filled epithelial cells.

Treatment and prognosis

Encephalitozoon infections can be treated effectively with albendazole. In a small controlled trial, HIV-infected patients with *Enceph. intestinalis* infection were treated with albendazole (400 mg orally twice daily) or with placebo. Albendazole treatment led to clearance of gastrointestinal *Enceph. intestinalis* infection in this study. Uncontrolled trials and anecdotal case reports describe partial or complete resolution of symptoms (diarrhoea, sinusitis, and keratoconjunctivitis) in patients with *Enceph. intestinalis, Enceph. hellem*, or *Enceph. cuniculi* infection following albendazole treatment. Pregnancy is a contraindication to albendazole treatment.

Albendazole is not an effective treatment for *Ent. bieneusi* infection. In HIV-infected patients with *Ent. bieneusi* infection, remission of this microsporidian infection can be achieved by treatment of the HIV disease with highly active antiretroviral therapy (HAART). This treatment involves simultaneous administration of several drugs directed against HIV, including HIV protease inhibitors. When effective in HIV-positive *Ent. bieneusi*-infected patients, HAART leads to reduction of HIV load, elevation of the circulating CD4+ T-lymphocyte count, clearance of *Ent. bieneusi* infection, and cessation of diarrhoea. Fumagillin is active against *Ent. bieneusi* and *Encephalitozoon* species, although its clinical attractiveness for systemic administration is limited by toxicity to human subjects (manifested by thrombocytopenia and neutropenia).

Microsporidial keratoconjunctivitis has been treated successfully with fumagillin eye drops in HIV-infected patients. HIV-negative patients with microsporidian infection of the corneal stroma have been treated by corneal transplantation, with results that have ranged from failure (opacification of the transplant) to apparent success, as judged by transparency of the graft 6 months after transplantation.

Individual patients infected with *Trachipleistophora hominis* or *Anncaliia vesicularum* reportedly showed some clinical improvement after treatment with albendazole–sulphadiazine–pyrimethamine, or albendazole–itraconazole, respectively.

In HIV-infected patients with microsporidiosis, the overall prognosis is determined by the HIV infection.

Areas of uncertainty or controversy

The importance, if any, of domestic drinking-water supplies in transmitting microsporidian spores is not known. Likewise, it is uncertain whether routine introduction of methods to screen domestic water supplies for microsporidian spores, and to remove/inactivate the spores if present would, be warranted.

Likely future developments

It is likely that the mechanisms by which anti-giardia antibodies protect against *G. intestinalis* infection will be understood during the next 10 years. Such understanding would include the molecular characterization of giardia target antigens that are recognized by protective antibody. Further clarification of the importance of domestic pets and agricultural livestock as sources for human giardiasis and microsporidiosis is likely by genotyping of morphologically identical parasites from human and nonhuman hosts. Selective survival and geographical spread of metronidazole-resistant *G. intestinalis* strains are predictable challenges to the effective treatment of giardiasis.

At least two species of human pathogenic microsporidia, *Anncaliia algerae* and *Trachipleistophora hominis*, can infect mosquitoes and it is not known whether mosquitoes or other insects transmit microsporidia to human subjects. Future work may answer this question.

Further reading

Anonymous (2004). Drugs for parasitic infections. *Med Lett Drugs Ther*, **46**, e1–e12. [Survey of treatment options for parasitic diseases, including the infections discussed in this chapter.]

Didier ES (2005). Microsporidiosis: an emerging and opportunistic infection in humans and animals. *Acta Tropica*, **94**, 61–76. [Review of microsporidian infections, with emphasis on human microsporidiosis.]

Didier ES, *et al.* (2005). Therapeutic strategies for human microsporidia infections. *Expert Rev Anti Infect Ther*, **3**, 419–34. [Review of drug treatment of microsporidiosis.]

Eckmann L (2003). Mucosal defences against *Giardia*. *Parasite Immunol*, **25**, 259–70. [Review of *Giardia* infections, with emphasis on host protective mechanisms against *Giardia* organisms.]

Field AS (2002). Light microscopic and electron microscopic diagnosis of gastrointestinal opportunistic infections in HIV-positive patients. *Pathology*, **34**, 21–35. [Review that includes photomicrographs of *Cystoiospora (Isospora) belli* and of microsporidia in human intestinal mucosa.]

Gajadhar AA, Allen JR (2004). Factors contributing to the public health and economic importance of waterborne zoonotic parasites. *Vet Parasitol*, **126**, 3–14. [Review of waterborne transmission of parasitic diseases.]

Garcia LS (1999). Flagellates and ciliates. *Clin Lab Med*, **19**, 621–38. [Review of human giardiasis and balantidiasis.]

Lindsay DS, Dubey JP, Blagburn BL (1997). Biology of *Isospora* spp. from humans, nonhuman primates, and domestic animals. *Clin Microbial Med*, **10**, 19–34. [Review of *Cystoisospora (Isospora)* species, including the human parasite *Cystoisospora (Isospora) belli*.]

Mathis A, Weber R, Deplazes P (2005). Zoonotic potential of the microsporidia. *Clin Microbial Med*, **18**, 423–45. [Comprehensive review of microsporidian infections in human and nonhuman hosts.]

7.8.9 *Blastocystis hominis* infection

Richard Knight

Essentials

Blastocystis hominis is an anaerobic unicellular colonic parasite of animals and humans. It is transmitted faeco-orally, with human infection associated with travel, institutions, animal handlers and immunodeficiency. Case reports strongly suggest that it causes a self-limited diarrhoeal illness. Diagnosis is by microscopic examination of faecal smears or concentrates. A trial of treatment with metronidazole is justified in patients who are immunocompromised, also when symptoms are prolonged.

Aetiology and biology of the parasite

Molecular and ribosomal RNA studies now indicate that *Blastocystis hominis* is a stramenopile belonging to the kingdom Chromista; other stramenopiles include slime nets, water moulds, and brown algae. The form commonly described in faeces and also in cultures is spherical, from 4 to 15 μm in diameter, with one prominent central vacuole surrounded by peripheral cytoplasm (Fig. 7.8.9.1) that electron microscopy shows to contain a nucleus, a Golgi complex, and mitochondrion-like organelles (Fig. 7.8.9.2). It grows readily in cultures with mixed bacteria but axenic cultures can also be established; division is by binary fission. Transmission is by small, resistant, faecal cysts, from 6 to 8 μm in diameter. The basic life cycle alternates between the univacuolar and cystic stages. However electron microscopy of faeces and cultures may also show multivacuolar, granular, and amoeboid forms of uncertain significance. Bizarre environmentally induced forms with huge vacuoles may develop in cultures (Fig. 7.8.9.3). The common 'univacuolar' form was named *Blastocystis* by Brumpt in 1912 as a yeast, although it was first described by Alexieff in 1911 as a protozoan cyst.

Epidemiology

Prevalence is high in many human populations associated with high faeco–oral transmission. This infection is associated with travel, institutions, animal handlers, and immunodeficiency. *Blastocystis* is genetically diverse and occurs in a wide range of domesticated and wild animals including invertebrates. Currently only one species, *B. hominis*, is recognized. There is now good evidence that this infection can be zoonotic. The resistant cysts can occur in both sewage influents and effluents.

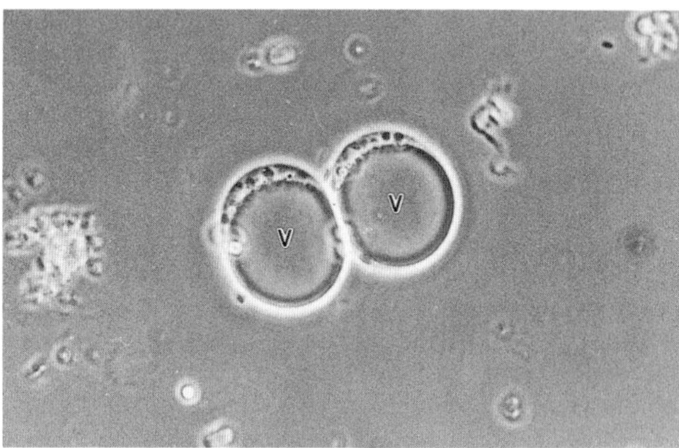

Fig. 7.8.9.1 *B. hominis* from culture showing binary fission; the cytoplasm is at the periphery. v, vacuole. Phase contrast, ×400.

Diagnosis

B. hominis is usually recognized as univacuolar forms in direct wet faecal smears or formol ether concentrates. Wet mounts can be stained with iodine, giving a brownish central body, or with toluidine blue. The organism is often numerous in symptomatic subjects. Permanent mounts stain well with trichrome. *Blastocystis* can resemble amoebic cysts but lack their characteristic nuclei. In fixed smears stained specifically for *Cryptosporidium*, there is no oocyst wall. Special techniques are used to concentrate and identify cysts in environmental samples.

Clinical features and treatment

A diarrhoeal illness lasting from 3 to 10 days is attributed to this organism, sometimes symptoms continue for weeks or months.

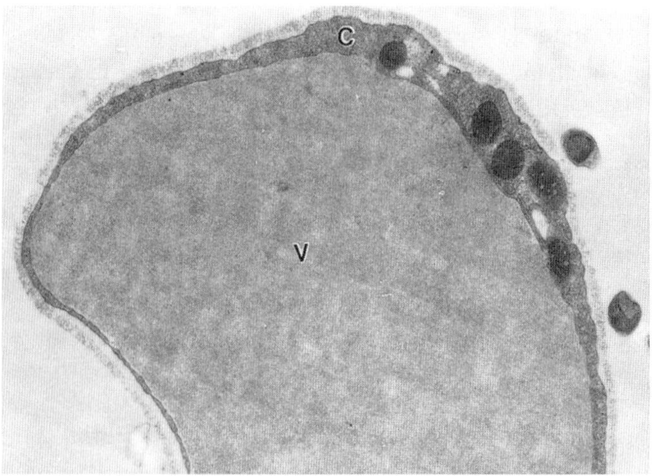

Fig. 7.8.9.2 *B. hominis*. Electron micrograph showing the peripheral cytoplasm (c) and the central vacuole (v); the inclusions in the cytoplasm are mitochondria. ×5000.

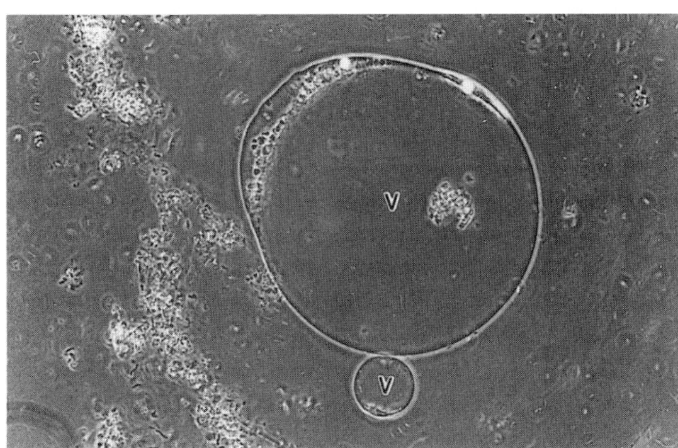

Fig. 7.8.9.3 *B. hominis* from culture showing the great variation in size. v, vacuole. Dark field, ×400.

Associated features are abdominal bloating, flatulence, and anorexia. Symptoms are more prolonged in immunocompromised subjects. There is no definite association with irritable bowel syndrome. Illnesses are self limiting in most persons but infection and symptoms can usually be eliminated with metronidazole or tinidazole; the organism is also sensitive to furazolidine and hydroxyquinoline.

Evidence for pathogenicity

Definite histopathology in humans is still lacking, although serum antibody has been reported in symptomatic subjects. Experimental infections in mice produce mucosal inflammation, but a good laboratory model remains elusive; mice are not normal hosts for this parasite and pathology is not reported in any of its normal hosts. A convincing *in vitro* cytopathic model awaits discovery although cultured colonic epithelial cells release cytokines in the presence of *Blastocystis*.

The genetic heterogeneity between *Blastocystis* isolates correlates weakly with host species. In a recent human study, genotype determined by PCR, correlated with symptoms. Clinical response to metronidazole is hardly compelling evidence for pathogenicity since concurrent infection with other enteropathogens is common and this drug has a wide spectrum of activity including an effect upon small bowel bacterial overgrowth. More well-documented outbreaks and cytopathic evidence are needed.

Further reading

Chen Te-Li, *et al.* (2003). Clinical characteristics and endoscopic findings associated with *Blastocystis hominis* in healthy adults. *Am J Trop Med Hyg*, **69**, 213–16.

Eroglu F, *et al.* (2009). Identification of *Blastocystis hominis* isolates from asymptomatic and symptomatic patients by PCR. *Parasitol Res*, **105**, 1589–92.

Long HY, *et al.* (2006). *Blastocystis hominis* modulates immune responses and cytokine release in colonic epithelial cells. *Parasitol Res*, **87**, 1029–30.

Stensvold CR, *et al.* (2009). Pursuing the clinical significance of *Blastocystis*-diagnostic limitations. *Trends Parasitol*, **25**, 23–9.

Suresh K, Smith HV (2004). Comparison of methods for detecting *Blastocystis hominis*. *Eur J Clin Microbiol Infect Dis*, **23**, 509–11.

Suresh K, Smith HV, Tan TC (2005). Viable *Blastocystis* cysts in Scottish and Malaysian sewage samples. *Appl Environ Microbiol*, **71**, 5619–20.

7.8.10 Human African trypanosomiasis

August Stich

Essentials

Human African trypanosomiasis (HAT, sleeping sickness) is caused by two subspecies of the protozoan parasite *Trypanosoma brucei*: *T. b. rhodesiense* is prevalent in East Africa among many wild and domestic mammals; *T. b. gambiense* causes an anthroponosis in Central and West Africa. The disease is restricted to tropical Africa where it is transmitted by the bite of infected tsetse flies (*Glossina* spp.).

Although well under control in the mid 20th century, HAT has returned to Africa in epidemic proportions since the 1980s, causing a severe public health problem in countries such as the Democratic Republic of Congo, Angola, Sudan, and Uganda. A joint effort by national, international, and nongovernmental organizations, as well as the pharmaceutical industry, is required to reverse this trend.

Clinical features

HAT progresses through distinct clinical stages that invariably lead to death if left untreated. Progress is fast in rhodesiense HAT, often resembling the clinical picture of malaria or septicaemia, and slow—sometimes lasting years—in gambiense HAT.

(1) Trypanosomal chancre—a papule at the site of the bite, surrounded by an intense local erythematous/oedematous reaction and with regional lymphadenopathy, healing without treatment after 2 to 4 weeks.

(2) Haemolymphatic stage (HAT stage 1)—manifests with fever, chills, rigors, headache and joint pains; hepatosplenomegaly and generalized lymphadenopathy are common

(3) Meningoencephalitic stage (HAT stage 2)—insidious onset of headache, sometimes with change in behaviour and personality; convulsions are common; sleep pattern becomes fragmented, eventually leading to somnolence and coma, with inability to drink and eat leading to dehydration and wasting.

Outside Africa, HAT is a rare diagnosis as an imported infection in travellers, but has to be considered in any patient with fever, chronic lymphadenopathy, or neurological changes returning from HAT endemic areas.

Diagnosis, staging, and treatment

Diagnosis—this is established by the detection of trypanosomes (usually by direct microscopy) in chancre aspirate, blood, lymph, or cerebrospinal fluid. Serology is useful for rapid screening under field conditions, but does not necessarily imply overt disease.

Staging—this is crucial for correct management: the cerebrospinal fluid must be examined in every patient found positive for trypanosomes in blood or lymph aspirate.

Treatment—HAT is curable, but many factors make this difficult: the disease is found in remote places, diagnosis is difficult, treatment is costly and complicated, and many drugs are not easily available. Aside from supportive care, specific treatment depends on the trypanosome subspecies and the stage of the disease, including (1) stage 1—pentamidine, and suramin; (2) stage 2—melarsoprol, eflornithine, and nifurtimox. There are no generally accepted recommendations on drug combinations, but—especially in late stages—treatment is difficult and dangerous to the patient; all of the drugs used are toxic and have many side effects, some potentially lethal.

Prevention

Control can be achieved by a combination of mass screening programmes, treatment of patients, and vector control, which together can lead to a complete break of the transmission cycle. There is no vaccine.

Table 7.8.10.1 The principal features of West and East African sleeping sickness

Disease	West African sleeping sickness	East African sleeping sickness
Parasite	*Trypanosoma brucei gambiense*	*Trypanosoma brucei rhodesiense*
Vector	Transmitted by riverine tsetse flies (*Palpalis* group)	Transmitted by savannah tsetse flies (*Morsitans* group)
Clinical course	Insidious onset, slow progression, death in stage II after many months or years	Acute onset, chancre frequent, rapid course, death frequently in stage I (cardiac failure)
Diagnosis	Parasitaemia scanty, Winterbottom's sign, serology	Parasitaemia usually higher and easily detectable, serological tests unreliable
Treatment	See Table 7.8.10.3	
Epidemiology	Tendency for endemicity, humans as main reservoir with evidence for several other mammal species, severe public health problem in many West and Central African countries	Wild (antelopes e.g. bushbuck) and occasionally domestic animals as reservoir and source of case clusters and epidemic outbreaks

Introduction

Sleeping sickness or human African trypanosomiasis (HAT) is caused by subspecies of the protozoan haemoflagellate *Trypanosoma brucei* transmitted to man and animals by tsetse flies (*Glossina* spp.). The distribution of the vector restricts sleeping sickness to the African continent between 14° north and 29° south (Fig. 7.8.10.1). Human disease occurs in two clinically and epidemiologically distinct forms, gambiense or West African and rhodesiense or East African sleeping sickness (Table 7.8.10.1). A third subspecies of the parasite, *T. b. brucei*, causes disease in cattle but is nonpathogenic in humans. In Uganda, the only country where all three forms occur, gambiense and rhodesiense sleeping sickness are currently about to overlap.

The first case reports of the disease go back to the 14th century. In the past, its impact on health in Africa has been enormous. Many areas were long rendered uninhabitable for people and livestock. During the early decades of the 20th century, millions may have died in Central Africa around Lake Victoria and in the Congo basin (Fig. 7.8.10.2). The success of control programmes in the 1960s promised the disappearance of sleeping sickness as a public health problem. However, recent epidemics in the Democratic Republic of Congo, northern Angola, southern Sudan, the Central African Republic, Uganda, and other countries have confirmed a major resurgence of HAT. According to estimates by the World Health Organization (WHO) at the turn of the millennium, the achievements in sleeping sickness control during colonial times had been nearly completely reversed. However, recent successes of control programmes run by national institutions and various non-governmental organizations could again reduce its prevalence and transmission in many accessible areas of central Africa.

Today, about 60 million people in 36 African countries are exposed to the potential risk of HAT. In some 300 currently existing active foci, up to 100 000 people are still believed to be infected, almost all with *T. b. gambiense*. If left untreated, they are doomed. For tourists and expatriates, sleeping sickness has always been a rare disease, although several clusters of cases have been reported

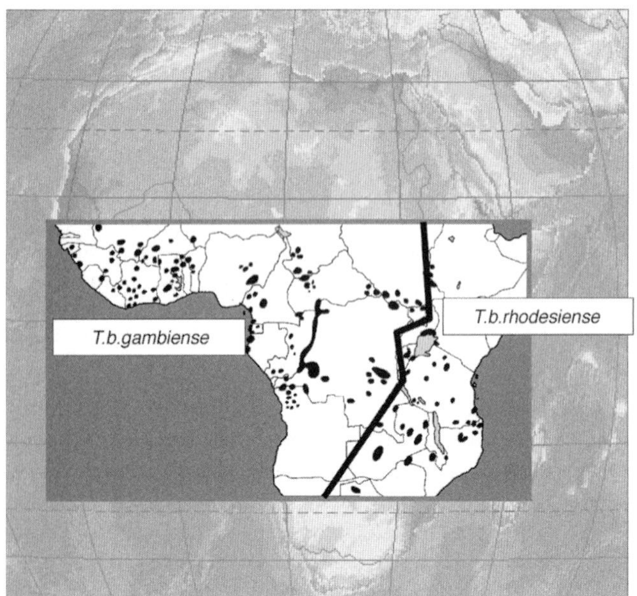

Fig. 7.8.10.1 The geographical distribution of human African trypanosomiasis.

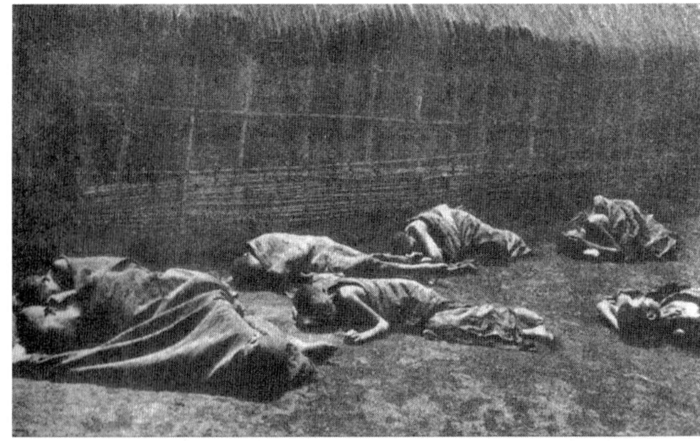

Fig. 7.8.10.2 Sleeping sickness patients on an island in Lake Victoria; historical photograph taken during Robert Koch's research expedition to East Africa.

in tourists to Tanzania, Zambia, and Malawi. The role of trypanosomes recently diagnosed in patients in some areas of the Indian subcontinent caused by *T. evansi* is currently under investigation.

Aetiology

In 1895, Sir David Bruce (1855–1931) suggested an association between trypanosomes and 'cattle fly fever', a major problem for livestock in southern Africa. In 1902, Robert M Forde and Everett Dutton from the Liverpool School of Tropical Medicine identified trypanosomes in the blood of a patient during a research expedition in the Gambia (see Fig. 7.8.10.6b), and in 1903, Aldo Castellani isolated trypanosomes from the cerebrospinal fluid. In the same year, tsetse flies were identified as the vector.

Trypanosoma brucei (phylum Sacromastigophora, order Kinetoplastida) is an extracellular protozoal parasite. Like leishmania, it possesses a centrally placed nucleus and a kinetoplast, a distinct organelle containing extranuclear DNA. The kinetoplast is the insertion site of an undulating membrane, which extends over nearly the whole cell length and ends as a free flagellum.

The three subspecies of *T. brucei* are indistinguishable morphologically. However, they differ considerably in their interaction with their mammalian host and the epidemiological pattern of the diseases they cause. Formerly, *T. b. gambiense* and *T. b. rhodesiense* isolates were characterized either by isoenzyme analysis or by animal inoculation. The advent of molecular techniques created expectations of more reliable tools for their differentiation. However, genomic characterization has revealed several more subdivisions than the three that were expected. Whereas West African isolates proved relatively homogeneous, East African isolates from humans and animals did not simply conform to what is still called *T. b. rhodesiense* and *T. b. brucei* but showed a complex relationship with evidence of sexual genetic exchange in the vector. Further molecular research may lead to a comprehensive phylogenetic tree and a deeper insight into trypanosomal evolution and biology.

Transmission

Although congenital, blood-borne, and mechanical transmission have been reported and may play an occasional role, the main mode of transmission is through the bite of infected tsetse flies (*Glossina* spp., order Diptera; Fig. 7.8.10.3). These are biologically unique insects, which occur only in Africa, with 31 distinct species and subspecies of which less than half are potential vectors of HAT. Their distinctive behaviour, ecology, and chosen habitat explain many epidemiological features of sleeping sickness. Tsetse flies can live for many months in the wild, are viviparous, and give birth to only about eight larvae per lifetime. Both sexes feed on blood.

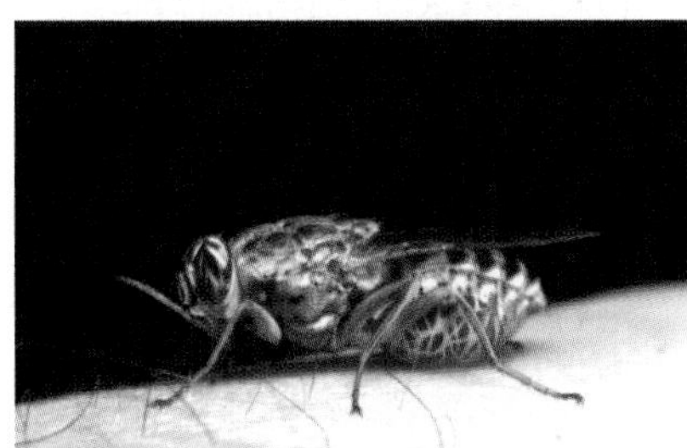

Fig. 7.8.10.3 Adult tsetse fly *Glossina morsitans*.

They are fastidious in requiring warm temperatures, shade, and humidity for resting and larviposition and so their distribution is highly localized. Recently, the mapping and monitoring of possible HAT transmission foci has become possible with the use of satellite imaging techniques.

During the blood meal on an infected mammalian host, the tsetse fly takes up trypanosomes ('short-stumpy form') into its mid-gut, where they develop into procyclic forms and multiply. After about 2 weeks, they migrate to the salivary glands as epimastigotes where they finally develop into infective metacyclic forms. At the next blood meal, they are injected into a new vertebrate host where they appear as 'long-slender' trypomastigotes and multiply by binary fission. In contrast to leishmania and *T. cruzi*, *T. brucei* is an exclusively extracellular parasite.

Molecular and immunological aspects

The cyclic changes of the trypanosome into different developmental stages are accompanied by variations in morphology, metabolism, and antigenicity. Several unique metabolic pathways have been described in trypanosomes, distinct from their host and thus qualifying as potential drug targets.

The bloodstream forms of *T. brucei* are covered with a dense coat of identical glycoproteins with up to about 500 amino acids per molecule. Being highly immunogenic, they stimulate the production of specific antibodies, mainly of the IgM subclass. Once the surface glycoproteins have been recognized by host antibodies, the parasite will be attacked and destroyed through complement activation and cytokine release, giving rise to local and systemic inflammatory reactions.

However, about 2% of *T. brucei* in each new generation change the expression of their specific surface glycoprotein. The 'coat' will then be different in the new clone (thus called variant surface glycoprotein, VSG). This phenotypic switch is done mainly by programmed DNA rearrangements, moving a transcriptionally silent VSG gene into an active, telomerically located expression site. Each *T. brucei* parasite already has the information for hundreds of different VSG genes, and within a whole trypanosome population, the potential repertoire for such different VSG copies seems to be virtually infinite.

Every new VSG copy is antigenically different, thus stimulating the production of a new IgM population. This antigenic variation is the major immune evasion strategy of the parasite, enabling the trypanosome to persist in its vertebrate host. It also reduces parasite load and prolongs the infection. But the inevitable outcome is immune exhaustion of the host (supported by additional immunosuppressive metabolites of the parasites), penetration of trypanosomes into immune-privileged sites such as the central nervous system, and finally death.

Clinical features

Sleeping sickness is a dreadful disease, causing great suffering to patients, their families, and the affected community. The infection often has an insidious onset, but *T. brucei*, whether the East or West African subspecies, will invariably kill unless treated in time. The natural course of HAT can be divided into different and distinct stages. Their recognition and differentiation is important for the clinical management of the patient.

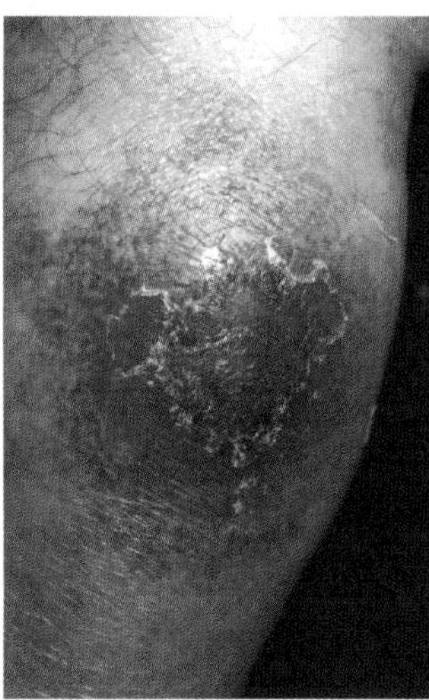

Fig. 7.8.10.4 Trypanosomal chancre on the calf of a missionary returning from the Congo.

Trypanosomal chancre

Tsetse bites can be quite painful, usually leaving a small and self-healing mark. In the case of a trypanosomal infection, the local reaction can be quite pronounced and longer lasting. A small raised papule will develop after about 5 days. It increases rapidly in size, surrounded by an intense erythematous tissue reaction (Fig. 7.8.10.4) with local oedema and regional lymphadenopathy. Although some chancres have a very angry appearance, they are not usually very painful unless they become ulcerated and superinfected. They heal without treatment after 2 to 4 weeks, leaving a permanent, hyperpigmented spot.

Trypanosomal chancres occur in about half the cases of *T. b. rhodesiense*. In *T. b. gambiense*, they are much less common and often go undetected in endemic populations.

Haemolymphatic stage (HAT stage I)

After local multiplication at the site of inoculation, the trypanosomes invade the haemolymphatic system, where they can be detected after 7 to 10 days. There they are exposed to vigorous host defence mechanisms, which they evade by antigenic variation. This continuous battle between antigenic switches and humoral defence results in a fluctuating parasitaemia with parasites frequently becoming undetectable, especially in gambiense HAT. The cyclic release of cytokines during periods of increased cell lysis results in intermittent, nonspecific symptoms: fever, chills, rigors, headache, and joint pains. These can easily be misdiagnosed as malaria, viral infection, typhoid fever, or many other conditions. Hepatosplenomegaly and generalized lymphadenopathy are common, indicating activation and hyperplasia of the reticuloendothelial system.

A reliable sign, particularly in *T. b. gambiense* infection, is the enlargement of lymph nodes in the posterior triangle of the neck (Winterbottom's sign). Other typical signs are a fugitive patchy or circinate rash, a myxoedematous infiltration of connective tissue ('puffy face syndrome'), and an inconspicuous periostitis of the tibia with delayed hyperaesthesia (Kérandel's sign).

In *T. b. rhodesiense* infection, this haemolymphatic stage is very pronounced with severe symptoms, often resembling falciparum malaria or septicaemia. Frequently, patients die within the first weeks after the onset of symptoms, mostly through cardiac involvement (myocarditis). In the early stage of *T. b. gambiense* infection, symptoms are usually infrequent and mild. Febrile episodes become less severe as the disease progresses.

Meningoencephalitic stage (HAT stage II)

Within weeks in *T. b. rhodesiense* and months in *T. b. gambiense* infection, cerebral involvement will invariably follow; trypanosomes cross the blood–brain barrier.

The onset of stage II is insidious. The exact time of central nervous system involvement cannot be determined clinically. Histologically, perivascular infiltration of inflammatory cells ('cuffing') and glial proliferation can be detected, resembling cerebral endarteriitis. As the disease progresses, patients complain of increasing headache, and their families may detect a marked change in behaviour and personality. Neurological symptoms, which follow gradually, can be focal or generalized, depending on the site of cellular damage in the central nervous system. Convulsions are common, usually indicating a poor prognosis. Periods of confusion and agitation slowly evolve towards a stage of distinct perplexity when patients lose interest in their surroundings and their own situation. Inflammatory reactions in the hypothalamic structures lead to a dysfunction in circadian rhythms and sleep regulatory systems. Sleep pattern become fragmented and finally result in a somnolent and comatose state. Progressive wasting and dehydration follows the inability to eat and drink.

In children, HAT progresses even more rapidly towards this meningoencephalitic stage. Parents often notice insomnia and behavioural changes long before the diagnosis is established.

There is no unique clinical sign of late HAT, opening up a wide range of possible neurological and psychiatric differential diagnoses. However, the appearance of the patient with apathy, the typical expressionless face, and swollen lymph nodes at the posterior triangle of the neck, is very suggestive for HAT in endemic areas (Fig. 7.8.10.5).

Diagnosis

HAT can never be diagnosed with certainty purely on clinical grounds alone. Definitive diagnosis requires the detection of the

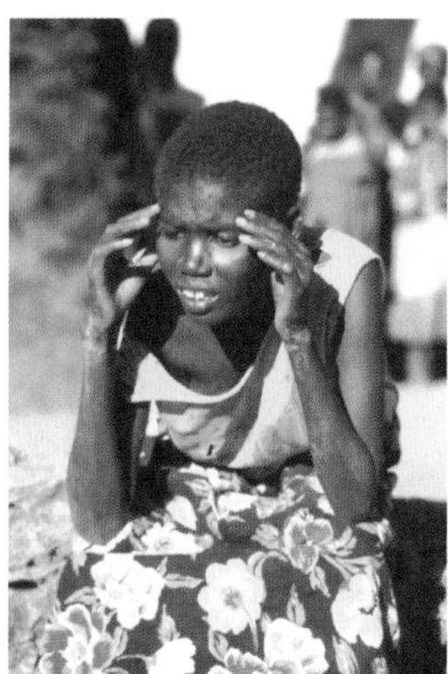

Fig. 7.8.10.5 Patient with late-stage trypanosomiasis.

parasite in chancre aspirate, blood, lymph, or cerebrospinal fluid using various parasitological techniques.

Lymph node aspirate

Lymph node aspiration is widely used, especially for the diagnosis of gambiense HAT. Fluid of enlarged lymph nodes, preferably of the posterior triangle of the neck (Winterbottom's sign), is aspirated and examined immediately at ×400 magnification without additional staining. Mobile trypanosomes can be detected for a few minutes between the numerous lymphocytes.

Wet preparation, thin, and thick blood film

During all stages of the disease, trypanosomes may appear in the blood where they can be detected in unstained wet or in stained preparations. The yield of detection is highest in the thick blood film, a technique widely used for the diagnosis of blood parasites such as plasmodium or microfilaria. Giemsa or Field staining techniques are appropriate (Fig. 7.8.10.6).

Especially in gambiense HAT, parasitaemia is usually low and fluctuating, often even undetectable. Repeated examinations on successive days are sometimes necessary until trypanosomes can be documented.

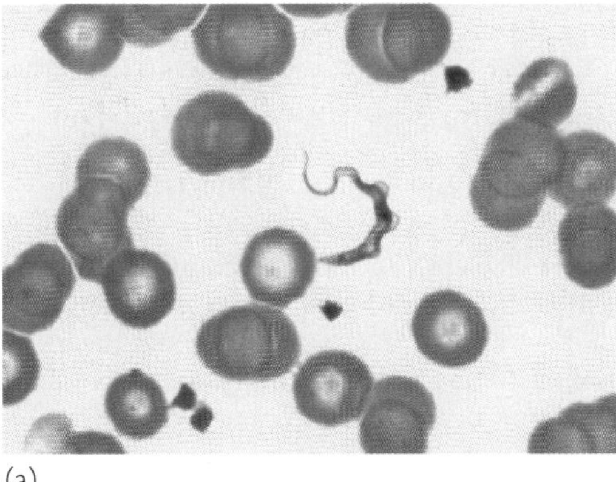

(a)

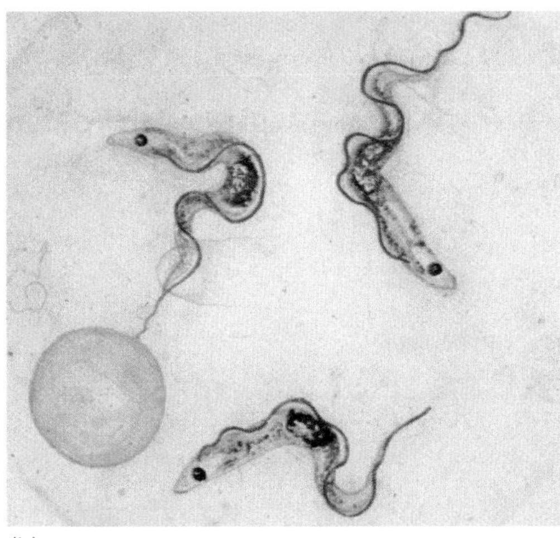

(b)

Fig. 7.8.10.6 (a) Trypanosomes in thin human blood film (Giemsa stain, ×1000). (b) Everett Dutton's painting of trypanosomes.

Concentration methods

To increase the sensitivity of blood examinations, various concentration assays have been developed. Trypanosomes tend to accumulate in the buffy coat layer after centrifugation of a blood sample. The best results have been obtained with the mini anion exchange column technique (mAECT), where trypanosomes are concentrated after passage through a cellulose column, the quantitative buffy coat (QBC) method, which was originally developed for the diagnosis of malaria, or the capillary tube centrifugation (CTC) method, which is widely used in the field.

Nucleic amplification techniques

Several specific primers have been described to detect trypanosomal DNA using the polymerase chain reaction (PCR). They had been successfully applied to samples from blood, lymph, and cerebrospinal fluid, mostly in research laboratory conditions. Although some of these techniques are able to detect fewer than 10 trypanosomes per probe, in the real situation of clinical diagnosis PCR assays are inferior to conventional parasitological techniques.

Serological assays

Serology is a useful tool to detect antibodies against trypanosomiasis. Various test methods have been described, some of them are now commercially available. They are mainly based on the enzyme-linked immunosorbent assay (ELISA) technique or immunofluorescence, but provide reliable results only in gambiense HAT.

For rapid screening under field conditions, the card agglutination test for trypanosomiasis (CATT) is an excellent tool in areas of *T. b. gambiense* infestation. It is easy to perform and delivers results within 5 min. A visible agglutination in the CATT suggests the existence of antibodies, but does not necessarily imply overt disease. Still, any positive serological result requires parasitological confirmation.

Nonspecific laboratory findings

Anaemia and thrombocytopenia are caused by systemic effects of cytokine release, especially of tumour necrosis factor α (TNFα). Hypergammaglobinaemia can reach extreme levels as a result of polyclonal activation of plasma cells. IgM levels detected in HAT are among the highest observed in any infectious disease.

Diagnosis of stage II

Stage determination is crucial for the correct management of a patient. This cannot be done on clinical grounds alone. Cerebrospinal fluid must therefore be examined in every patient found positive for trypanosomes in blood or lymph aspirate. A lumbar puncture should also be performed in all patients in whom HAT is suspected clinically even if peripheral examinations had proved negative. A minimum of 5 ml of cerebrospinal fluid is required to examine for:

- Leucocytes—cerebral involvement in HAT stage II is accompanied by pleocytosis, mostly lymphocytes, in the cerebrospinal fluid. By convention a number of five cells or more per mm^3 cerebrospinal fluid defines central nervous system involvement even if the patient does not (yet) have neurological symptoms. Pathognomonic for HAT is the appearance of activated plasma cells with eosinophilic inclusions in the cerebrospinal fluid, the morular cells of Mott (Fig. 7.8.10.7).

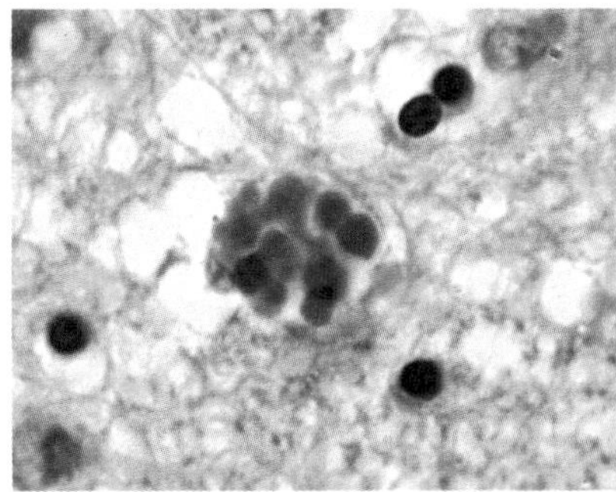

Fig. 7.8.10.7 Morular cell of Mott in a histological brain section of a stage II HAT patient (haematoxylin and eosin stain, ×1000).

- Trypanosomes—the chances of detecting trypanosomes in the cerebrospinal fluid increase with the level of pleocytosis and the technique used. The highest yield is obtained by cerebrospinal fluid double centrifugation and rapid microscopy at the bedside.
- Protein—in patients with HAT, a level of 37 mg of protein per 100 ml cerebrospinal fluid (dye-binding protein assay) or more is highly suggestive of the advanced stage. Stage II HAT is characterized by an autochthonous production of IgM antibodies in the cerebrospinal fluid, which can be selectively detected if suitable laboratory facilities exist (e.g. latex IgM test).

Treatment

General considerations

HAT is curable, especially if the diagnosis is made at an early stage of the disease. In the stark reality of the African situation, however, there are many major obstacles to successful patient management:

- Sleeping sickness is a disease of rural, remote places. The active foci of sleeping sickness are usually in faraway and insecure places, which are difficult to reach. Many treatment centres work under emergency conditions with extremely restricted resources. Numerous affected patients, without proper access to health care, are left unattended.
- The diagnosis is difficult. Initial diagnosis and exact staging of trypanosomiasis requires sophisticated methods that are often dangerous to the patient and justified only in the hands of experienced personnel. Repetitive training programmes, constant supervision, and continuous quality control are necessary but in reality rarely available.
- The treatment of trypanosomiasis is extremely costly, although the drugs themselves are now covered by a donation programme. Invariably, demand exceeds the locally available resources. External funding and sustainable donor commitments for rural Africa are generally decreasing.
- The treatment is complicated. Treatment of HAT is dangerous, prolonged, and usually requires hospitalization. Most patients with late-stage trypanosomiasis are severely ill and malnourished. Adverse drug reactions during treatment are difficult to assess because of concomitant pathologies. Their management requires considerable medical skill and good nursing care. Hospitals in rural Africa are often inadequately equipped and staffed to accomplish good patient care.
- Many drugs are not easily available. Many trypanosomicidal agents are on the verge of disappearance, despite increasing demand. The range of drugs is diminishing, and hardly any new treatments are in sight. This is especially worrying in view of the reported spread of drug resistance.
- HAT treatment is not standardized. Trypanosomiasis treatment regimens vary considerably between countries and treatment centres. Results from different centres are comparable to only a very limited extent. Few properly conducted and sufficiently powered clinical trials are available to evaluate duration, dosage, and possible combinations of drugs. Sufficient infrastructure for carrying out clinical research exists in only a handful of places.

The price for cure of HAT is high: dangerous drugs with limited availability and prolonged treatment schedules administered in many places by poorly trained personnel in rudimentary medical facilities. Little progress has been achieved in the last 30 years.

Stage I drugs

The treatment of HAT depends on the trypanosome subspecies and the stage of the disease (Table 7.8.10.2).

Pentamidine

Since its introduction in 1937, pentamidine has become the drug of choice for gambiense HAT stage I, achieving cure rates as high as 98%. However, there are frequent failures in rhodesiense HAT. Lower rates of cellular pentamidine uptake in *T. b. rhodesiense* may explain these differences. Some cures of stage II infections have also been reported, but cerebrospinal fluid drug levels are usually not sufficiently high to guarantee a reliable trypanosomicidal effect in the central nervous system.

Pentamidine is usually given by deep intramuscular injection, often to outpatients. If hospital care and reasonable monitoring conditions are available, an intravenous infusion, given in normal saline over 2 h, might be used instead. The main advantage of pentamidine over other drugs is the short treatment course and ease of administration. Adverse effects are related to the route of administration or its dose and are usually reversible (Table 7.8.10.3).

Pentamidine is also used as second-line therapy for visceral leishmaniasis and especially in the prophylaxis and treatment of opportunistic *Pneumocystis jiroveci* pneumonia in AIDS. Since the start of the HIV pandemic, the cost of pentamidine has been increased more than tenfold by producers, making it unaffordable by health institutions in low-income countries. After an intervention by

Table 7.8.10.2 The choice of drugs in the treatment of sleeping sickness

	Gambiense sleeping sickness		Rhodesiense sleeping sickness	
HAT	1st line	Pentamidine	1st line	Suramin
Stage I	2nd line	Eflornithine	2nd line	Melarsoprol
HAT	1st line	Eflornithine (+ nifurtimox?)	1st line	Melarsoprol
Stage II	2nd line	Melarsoprol	2nd line	Melarsoprol + nifurtimox

Table 7.8.10.3 Dosage and principal adverse reactions of antitrypanosomal agents

Drug	Dosage regimen	Adverse drug reactions
Pentamidine	4mg/kg body weight intramuscular daily or on alternate days for 7 to 10 injections (3 dose regimen currently under investigation)	Hypotensive reaction with tachycardia, dizziness, even collapse and shock, especially after intravenous administration, close monitoring of pulse rate and blood pressure after injection is mandatory
		Inflammatory reactions at the site of injection (sterile abscesses, necrosis)
		Renal, hepatic, and pancreatic dysfunction
		Neurotoxicity: peripheral polyneuropathy
		Bone marrow depression
Suramin	Day 1: Test dose of 4–5 mg/kg body weight	Pyrexia (very common)
	Day 3, 10, 17, 24, and 31: 20 mg/kg body weight, maximum	Early hypersensitivity reactions such as nausea, circulatory collapse, urticaria
	Dose per injection 1 g	Late hypersensitivity reactions: skin reactions (exfoliative dermatitis), haemolytic anaemia
		Renal impairment: albuminuria, cylinduria, haematuria (high renal tissue concentrations); regular urine checks during treatment are mandatory
		Neurotoxicity: peripheral neuropathy
		Bone marrow toxicity: agranulocytosis, thrombocytopenia
Melarsoprol	New regimen:	Treatment-induced encephalopathy
	Day 1–10: 2.2 mg/kg body weight	Pyrexia
		Neurotoxicity: peripheral motor or sensory polyneuropathy
		Dermatological reactions: pruritus, urticaria, exfoliative dermatitis;
		Cardiotoxicity
		Renal and hepatic dysfunction
Eflornithine	Most commonly used dosage regimen:	Gastrointestinal symptoms such as nausea, vomiting and diarrhoea
	100 mg/kg body weight at 6-hourly intervals for 14 days	Bone marrow toxicity: anaemia, leucopenia, thrombocytopenia
		Alopecia, usually towards the end of the treatment cycle
		Neurological symptoms such as convulsions
Nifurtimox	5mg/kg body weight 3 times daily for 30 days	Abdominal discomfort such as nausea, pains, and vomiting in half of the treated patients, often leading to a disruption of the treatment course
		Neurological complications: convulsions,
		Impairment of cerebellar function, polyneuropathy
		Skin reactions

WHO, a limited amount of pentamidine is now made available for use in HAT as part of a donation programme.

Suramin

In the early 20th century, the development of suramin, resulting from German research on the trypanosomicidal activity of various dyes ('Bayer 205'), was a major breakthrough in the field of tropical medicine. For the first time, African trypanosomiasis, at least in its early stages, became treatable without causing major harm.

Even today, suramin is still used to treat stage I HAT, especially rhodesiense. Like pentamidine, it does not reach therapeutic levels in cerebrospinal fluid. Suramin is injected intravenously after dilution in distilled water.

Adverse effects depend on nutritional status, concomitant illnesses (especially onchocerciasis), and the patient's clinical condition. Although life-threatening reactions have been described, serious adverse effects are rare (Table 7.8.10.3).

Stage II drugs

Melarsoprol

Until the systematic introduction of the arsenical compound melarsoprol in 1949, late stage trypanosomiasis was virtually untreatable. Since then, it has remained the most widely used stage II antitrypanosomal drug both for gambiense and rhodesiense infections. It has saved many lives, but has a high rate of dangerous adverse effects. Increasing frequency of relapses and resistance has been reported in some parts of Congo, Angola, Sudan, and Uganda.

Melarsoprol clears trypanosomes rapidly from the blood, lymph, and cerebrospinal fluid. Its toxicity usually restricts its use to late-stage disease. It is given by slow intravenous injection; extravascular leakage must be avoided.

A new, simpler regimen is based on recently acquired knowledge of the drug's pharmacokinetics (Table 7.8.10.3). The most important adverse effect is an acute encephalopathy, provoked around day 5 to 8 of the treatment course in 5 to 14% of all patients. There are severe headache, convulsions, rapid neurological deterioration, or deepening of coma. Characteristically, the comatose patient's eyes remain open. Most probably, this is an immune-mediated reaction precipitated by release of parasite antigens in the first days of treatment. The overall case fatality under treatment ranges between 2 and 12%, depending on the stage of disease and the quality of medical and nursing care. Simultaneous administration of glucocorticosteroids (prednisolone 1 mg/kg body weight; maximum 40 mg daily) reduces mortality, especially in cases with high cerebrospinal fluid pleocytosis. However, in areas where tuberculosis, amoebiasis, and strongyloidiasis are highly prevalent, corticosteroids have dangers of their own.

Eflornithine (DFMO)

Initially developed as antitumour agent, eflornithine (α-difluoromethylornithine) was introduced in 1980 as an antitrypanosomal drug, in the hope that it might replace melarsoprol for treatment of stage II trypanosomiasis. However, exorbitant costs and limited availability have restricted its use mostly to melarsoprol-refractory cases of gambiense sleeping sickness. *T. b. rhodesiense* is much less sensitive, because of a much higher turnover rate of the target enzyme ornithine decarboxylase, and therefore cannot be treated with eflornithine.

The drug can be taken orally, but intravenous administration is preferred as it achieves a much higher bioavailability and success rate. Eflornithine should be administered slowly over a period of at least 30 min. Continuous 24-h administration is preferable if facilities allow.

The range of adverse reactions to eflornithine is wide, as with other cytotoxic drugs in cancer treatment. Their occurrence and intensity increase with the duration of treatment and the severity of the patient's general condition (Table 7.8.10.3).

In the late 1990s no pharmaceutical company produced eflornithine for use against HAT, despite pressure by WHO. The discovery of its therapeutic effect in cosmetic creams against facial hair helped to restimulate production and thus had a beneficial 'spin-off' effect for HAT. In 2001 agreements were signed between WHO and two major drug companies which led to a 'public–private partnership' (PPP) and helped to assure a sufficient supply of eflornithine and other drugs essential for the treatment of HAT. In 2006, the agreement was prolonged until 2011.

Box 7.8.10.1 Control of human African trypanosomiasis

- Diagnosis and treatment of patients
- Active case finding
- Vector control
- Implementation and continuation of a surveillance system
- Training, health education, and community participation

Nifurtimox

Ten years after its introduction for the treatment of American trypanosomiasis in 1967, nifurtimox was found to be effective in the treatment of gambiense sleeping sickness. It has a place as second-line treatment in melarsoprol-refractory cases or in combination chemotherapies.

Nifurtimox is given orally and generally not well tolerated, but adverse effects are usually not severe. They are dose-related and rapidly reversible after discontinuation of the drug (Table 7.8.10.3).

Combination treatments in HAT

Melarsoprol, eflornithine, and nifurtimox interfere with trypanothione synthesis and activity at different stages. There is also experimental evidence that combinations of suramin and stage II drugs might be beneficial. Therefore, by reducing the overall dosage of each individual component, drug combinations have the

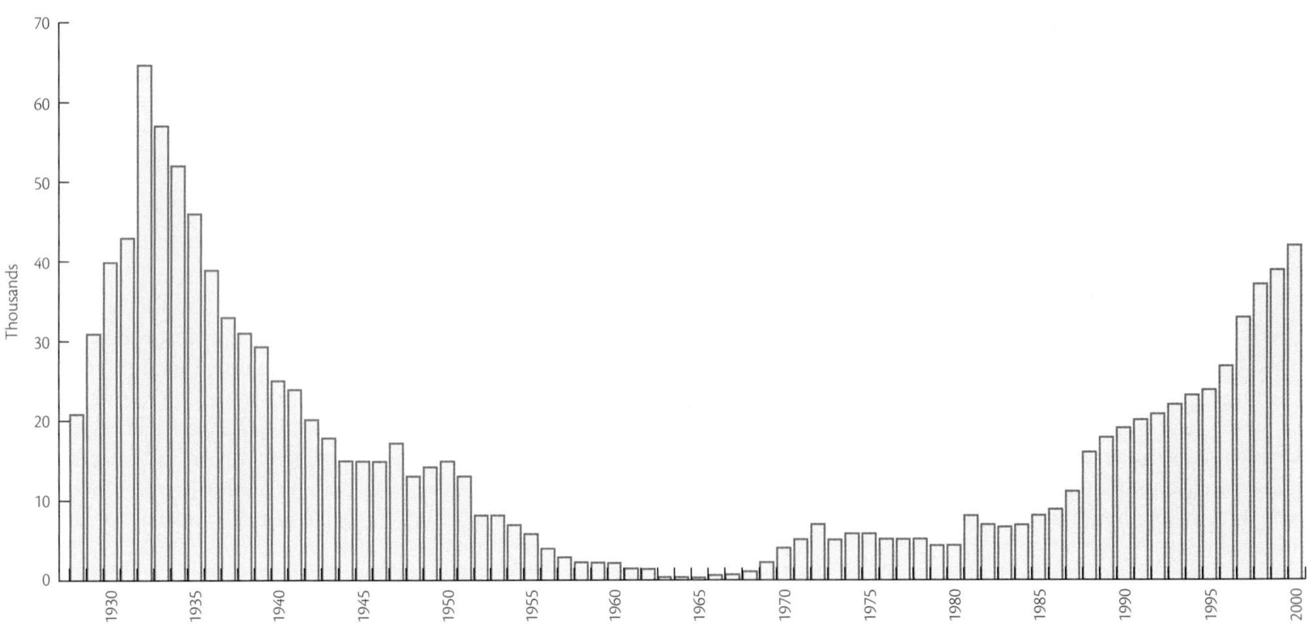

Fig. 7.8.10.8 Number of annually reported cases of human African trypanosomiasis.
(source: WHO Report on Global Surveillance and Epidemic-prone Infectious Diseases); according to WHO, the actual patient numbers are about 10-fold higher.

potential to reduce the frequency of serious side effects and the development of resistance, which are such common problems in the treatment of sleeping sickness.

Recent prospective clinical trials have shown a beneficial effect of nifurtimox eflornithine combination therapy (NECT). This has the potential to develop into the preferred first-line treatment of stage II gambiense HAT in the future.

Individual protection

Tsetse flies have a very patchy distribution. Infested strips of land are often well known to the local population and should be avoided as far as possible. HAT among tourists and occasional visitors to endemic areas is a rare event. Pentamidine or suramin chemoprophylaxis is historical, and can no longer be recommended. Long-sleeved, brightly coloured clothing and insecticide repellents are the best defence against attacking tsetse flies.

Prevention and control

In the past, tremendous efforts were undertaken to control the threat posed by sleeping sickness to human lives and economic development in rural Africa. Control programmes are based on the five complementary pillars given in Box 7.8.10.1.

The most important strategy is active case finding. This requires mobile teams, which regularly visit villages in endemic areas. Mostly based on the results of CATT screening, patients, preferably in the early stage of the disease, are identified and treated. Gradually, the parasite reservoir is depleted. As glossina is a relatively incompetent vector, with infectivity rates usually below 0.1% and susceptible to control measures such as insecticide application, trapping, or even the release of sterile males, the combination of various approaches can lead to a complete break of the transmission cycle. In the past this was achieved in many places. However, the resurgence of sleeping sickness in areas ridden by war and civil unrest during the last decades of the 20th century, in combination with the decreasing availability of drugs on the international market and the general loss of interest in health issues of the developing world, gives rise to the fear that HAT will always be a problem in many rural parts of Africa (Fig. 7.8.10.8).

Trypanosomiasis in the 21st century

There is hardly any other tropical disease that demonstrates more clearly the dichotomy characterizing our modern age. On one side, trypanosomes are kept in culture and studied extensively in numerous research laboratories. Their genome is sequenced, and many molecular, biochemical, and immunological phenomena have been discovered as a result of basic science research.

General interest in this disease is usually restricted only to its research aspects, however. Diagnostic and especially therapeutic tools are increasingly unavailable, because the tens of thousands of infected people in Africa are not commercially viable consumers. The prospects for the fight against trypanosomiasis look grim, although some recent successes have been accomplished usually through the work of committed nongovernmental organizations (e.g. in Sudan and Angola). Global concern about the crisis of human trypanosomiasis in Africa is a question of scientific ethics and international solidarity.

Further reading

Brun R, Balmer O (2006). New developments in human African trypanosomiasis. *Curr Opin Infect Dis*, **19**, 415–20.

Brun R, *et al.* (2009). Human African trypanosomiasis. *Lancet*, doi:10.1016/S0140-6736(08)61345-8.

Burri C, *et al.* (2000). Efficacy of new, concise schedule for melarsoprol in treatment of sleeping sickness caused by *Trypanosoma brucei gambiense*: a randomised trial. *Lancet*, **355**, 1419–25.

Dumas M, Bouteille B, Buguet A (eds) (1999). *Progress in human African trypanosomiasis, sleeping sickness*. Springer-Verlag, Paris.

Jannin J, Cattand P (2004). Treatment and control of human African trypanosomiasis. *Curr Opin Infect Dis*, **17**, 565–70.

Maudlin I (2006). African trypanosomiasis. *Ann Trop Med Parasitol*, **100**, 679–701.

Pepin J, *et al.* (1989). Trial of prednisolone for prevention of melarsoprol-induced encephalopathy in gambiense sleeping sickness. *Lancet*, **i**, 1246–50.

Priotto G, *et al.* (2009). Nifurtimox-eflornithine combination therapy for second-stage African *Trypanosoma brucei gambiense* trypanosomiasis: a multicentre, randomised, phase III, non-inferiority trial. *Lancet*, **374**, 56–64.

Stich A, Barrett MP, Krishna S (2003). Waking up to sleeping sickness. *Trends Parasitol*, **19**, 195–7.

World Health Organization (1998). *Control and surveillance of African trypanosomiasis*. WHO Technical Report Series 881. WHO, Geneva.

7.8.11 Chagas disease

M.A. Miles

A poeira de Curvelo não az mal para ninguém não
Do pulmão lá ninguém morre
O que mata é o coração
The dust of Curvelo does not harm anybody
No one dies there of lung disease
What kills is the heart

(From the poem *O galo cantou na serra* by Luiz Claudio and Guimarães Rosa)

Essentials

Trypanosoma cruzi, the protozoan parasite which causes Chagas disease, is a zoonosis with many mammal host and vector species. It is transmitted to humans by contamination of mucous membranes or abraded skin with infected faeces of bloodsucking triatomine bugs, also by blood transfusion, organ transplantation, transplacentally, and orally by food contaminated with infective forms. It multiplies intracellularly (pseudocysts) as amastigotes in mammalian cells, particularly heart and smooth muscle, from which flagellated trypomastigotes emerge to reinvade cells or circulate in blood. Around 10 million people are infected in Latin America; imported cases and congenital cases may occur elsewhere.

Clinical features

There are classically three phases. (1) Acute—may be asymptomatic, or with manifestations including fever, myalgia, headache, vomiting, diarrhoea, anorexia, facial or generalized oedema, rash, generalized lymphadenopathy, and hepatosplenomegaly; there may be a lesion at the portal of entry; fatal in less than 10%. (2) Meningoencephalitic—rare in adults, excepting those who are immunocompromised (most typically with HIV/AIDS); also seen in congenital cases. (3) Chronic—occurs in up to 30% of those recovering from the acute phase; most often with cardiac involvement (typically cardiomyopathy leading to congestive cardiac failure, with risk of arrhythmia and ECG abnormalities due to focal inflammatory lesions of the conducting system), also megaoesophagus and megacolon. Infection is opportunistic, relapsing in the immunocompromised.

Diagnosis

(1) Acute phase—parasitaemia is scanty, but circulating trypomastigotes may be detectable in the acute phase by microscopy of blood, enhanced by concentration methods. (2) Chronic phase—multiple blood cultures or feeding and subsequent dissection of laboratory-reared triatomines (xenodiagnosis) may reveal infection. (3) Serological testing—can demonstrate evidence of infection, but needs to be standardized with reference sera and by external quality control.

Treatment

(1) Acute phase—proven cases should be treated promptly with nifurtimox or benznidazole, but there is no guarantee that a full course of treatment will eliminate the infection. (2) Chronic phase—the value of drug treatment for adults is still debated; supportive care may include the following (a) for heart disease—conventional drug treatment for cardiac failure and arrhythmias; cardiac pacemaker; (b) for megaoesophagus—dilatation; segmentary removal of stomach muscle; replacement of the distal oesophagus; (c) megacolon—resection and anastomosis with the rectal stump.

Prevention

Proven methods of controlling domestic triatomine bugs include insecticide spraying (with pyrethroids), health education, community support, and house improvement. Serological surveillance of children detects residual endemic foci or congenital transmission and is vital for monitoring the success of control programmes. The Southern Cone programme against *Triatoma infestans* is considered a model for international cooperation in disease control. There is no vaccine.

Introduction and aetiology

In 1907, in the space of a few months, the Brazilian scientist Carlos Chagas discovered the disease that bears his name and described the entire lifecycle of the causative organism. Chagas first found the protozoan agent *Trypanosoma cruzi* in the gut of the large blood-sucking insect vector, the triatomine bug (order Hemiptera, family Reduviidae, subfamily Triatominae) (Fig. 7.8.11.1). Later he returned to bug-infested houses and detected *T. cruzi* in the blood of sick children.

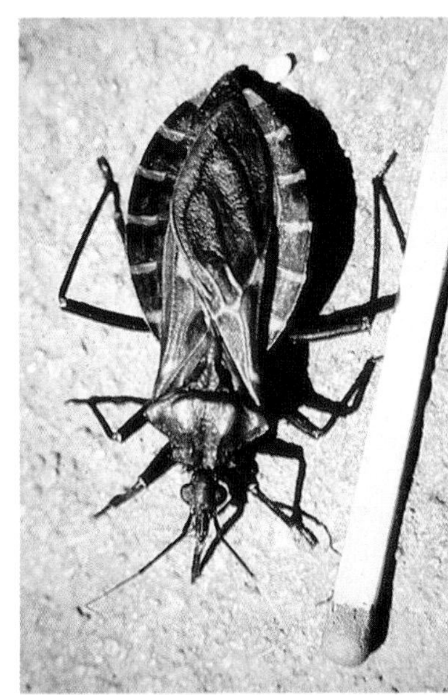

Fig. 7.8.11.1 Adult female triatomine bug (*Panstrongylus megistus*), with a single egg shown adjacent to the tip of the abdomen.
(Courtesy of Dr T V Barrett.)

T. cruzi is a kinetoplastid protozoan. In addition to the nucleus, it has a second, microscopically visible DNA-containing organelle, the kinetoplast. The main lifecycle stages (trypomastigote, amastigote, epimastigote) are distinguished by the position of the kinetoplast relative to the nucleus and by the presence or absence of a free flagellum.

Vector-borne transmission of *T. cruzi* is by contamination of the mammal host with infected faeces of triatomine bugs, not by their bite. During or shortly after feeding, bugs release blackish liquid faeces and urine on to the skin of the host. Infective forms (metacyclic trypomastigotes) penetrate mucous membranes or abraded skin. Inside the mammal, *T. cruzi* is primarily an intracellular parasite. Trypomastigotes enter nonphagocytic or phagocytic cells, in which they transform to ovoid or round aflagellate amastigotes that multiply inside the cell by binary fission to produce a pseudocyst (Fig. 7.8.11.2). After 5 days or more, the pseudocyst ruptures to release numerous new trypomastigotes, which reinvade cells or circulate in the blood. Multiplication may occur at the site of infection, but pseudocysts subsequently predominate in muscle, especially heart and smooth muscle. In the blood, trypomastigotes are small, often C-shaped, with a large terminal kinetoplast (Fig. 7.8.11.3). In fulminating or experimental infections, slender highly motile trypomastigotes may also sometimes be seen. Trypomastigotes do not multiply in the blood. Triatomine bugs become infected by taking a blood meal from an infected mammal; birds and reptiles are not susceptible to infection. Infection in the bug is confined to the alimentary tract, where *T. cruzi* multiplies by binary fission as epimastigotes (kinetoplast adjacent to the nucleus). Metacyclic trypomastigotes are produced in the hindgut and rectum of the bug. All stages of the *T. cruzi* lifecycle can be cultured *in vitro*. *T. cruzi* can also be transmitted by blood transfusion and organ transplantation, across the placenta, via breast milk (rarely), and orally through food contaminated by triatomine faeces and the raw meat of infected mammals. Sexual transmission has not been documented.

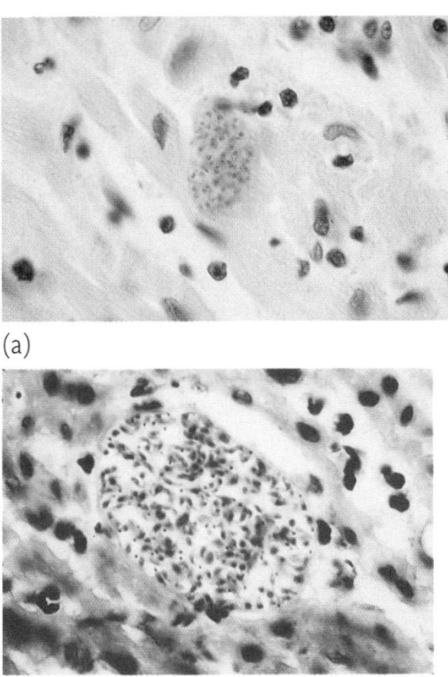

Fig. 7.8.11.2 Pseudocyst of *Trypanosoma cruzi*. Pseudocyst in (a) heart muscle and (b) umbilical cord, from a congenital case of Chagas disease.
(a, courtesy of J E Williams; b, courtesy of Dr Hipolito de Almeida.)

Epidemiology

T. cruzi is confined to the Americas, although closely related organisms of the same subgenus (*Schizotrypanum*) are cosmopolitan in bats. The vast majority of the 140 triatomine bug species are also restricted to the Americas. Their natural habitats are the refuges of mammals, birds, and reptiles, in trees, in burrows, and among rocks. All mammals are thought to be susceptible to *T. cruzi*, which has been reported from at least 150 mammal species. The opossum (*Didelphis* spp.) is the most common sylvatic host. A few triatomine species thrive as domestic colonies. More than 10 000 bugs have been found in a single house. Before the recent Southern Cone initiative to control *Triatoma infestans*, the species was widespread in rural housing of the Southern Cone countries of South America (Argentina, Bolivia, Brazil, Chile, Paraguay, Uruguay, and southern Peru). *Rhodnius prolixus* is the common vector in northern South America and also occurs in Central America, with *Triatoma dimidiata* as secondary vector in the same regions. *Panstrongylus megistus* (Fig. 7.8.11.1) infests central and eastern Brazil, and *Triatoma brasiliensis* north-eastern Brazil. Animals that share human dwellings, such as guinea pigs (cuy), dogs, cats, rats, and mice are domestic reservoirs of *T. cruzi* infection. Chickens, although not susceptible to *T. cruzi*, encourage bug infestation and can sustain large colonies.

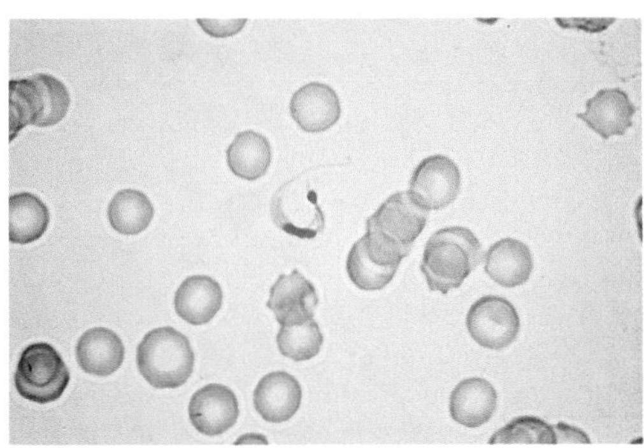

Fig. 7.8.11.3 *Trypanosoma cruzi* C-shaped trypomastigote in blood. Note the large posterior kinetoplast.

Serological surveys suggest that about 10 million people may now be infected with *T. cruzi* in South and Central America, a figure which is reduced from up to 20 million around four decades ago. In some communities, seropositivity rates may still exceed 50%. As expected from the precarious contaminative route of transmission, prevalence rises with age. Based on prevalence, before recent control initiatives, it was estimated that up to 300 000 new infections might occur in Latin America each year; this is now reduced to around 60 000/year. Only approximately 1000 cases are known from the Amazon basin, about half of these due to oral transmission by drinking fruit juices (e.g. from berries of açaí or bacaba palms or cane sugar garapa) in which infected bugs have been accidentally ground up. Oral outbreaks may also occur elsewhere: one among schoolchildren in Caracas, Venezuela, due to guava juice, involved 103 cases. There are relatively few Amazonian cases because the local forest vectors do not colonize houses. For the same reason, autochthonous infection is very rare in the United States of America.

Not surprisingly, sporadic *T. cruzi* infections may be found among migrants from Latin America to the United States of America and elsewhere. This gives rise to occasional cases of transmission by blood or organ donors and to rare congenital cases. Fear of blood transfusion transmission suggests a need to screen some blood donors outside traditional endemic areas. In 2007, the World Health Organization (WHO) launched a 'Global Network for Chagas Elimination' to raise global awareness and coordinate prevention of transmission.

Initial acute infections are frequently asymptomatic or overlooked. It is thought that less than 10% of acute infections in children are fatal. Morbidity due to Chagas disease arises primarily from the chronic infection. Once acquired, infection is usually carried for life. Around 30% of those infected will subsequently display ECG abnormalities and chagasic cardiomyopathy, and a proportion of those have associated megaoesophagus or megacolon.

There are marked regional differences in the epidemiology of Chagas disease. Megasyndromes are common in central and eastern Brazil but seldom described in northern South America and Central America. Research in molecular genetics has shown that *T. cruzi* is not a Single entity, but a species with at least six genetic lineages. Until Recently these were divided into TCI and TCIIa–e, but they have now, more logically, been re-designated as six distinct groups TCI, TCII, TCIII, TCIV, TCV, and TCVI, with differences between ecologies, hosts, vectors, geographical, and disease distributions. The common opossum Didelphis is the most ubiquitous host of TCI, whereas TCIII is associated with the armadillo Dasypus. North of the Amazon the principal agent of Chagas disease is TCI, which causes severe and fatal cardiomyopathy. In contrast, in the Southern Cone countries, where megaoesophagus and megacolon are common, Chagas disease is predominantly caused by TCII, TCV, and TCVI. It has been proved that *T. cruzi* has an extant capacity for genetic exchange, and TCV and TCVI are natural TCII /TCIII hybrids, which are particularly prevalent in humans in Paraguay, Chile, Bolivia, and adjacent regions.

Pathogenesis and pathology

At the portal of entry, local multiplication of *T. cruzi* may lead to unilateral conjunctivitis or to a skin lesion (Fig. 7.8.11.4). Unruptured pseudocysts in muscle apparently generate no inflammatory response. Pseudocyst rupture is followed by infiltration of lymphocytes, monocytes, and/or polymorphonuclear cells. Antigens released from pseudocysts may spread and be adsorbed on to adjacent uninfected cells. Such uninfected cells may be attacked by the immune response of the host and be destroyed. In this way, expanded focal lesions may be produced. Postmortem histology of human hearts and experimental studies in dogs has demonstrated a clear association between ECG abnormalities and focal lesions in the conducting system of the heart. Much damage may occur in the acute phase of infection, particularly if pseudocysts are numerous. Postmortem histology has demonstrated that neuron loss is a feature of chagasic cardiopathy and of megasyndromes that is exacerbated by further disease or age-related loss. Thus, a threshold may be reached, often many years after the acute infection, at which organ function is perturbed. Further ECG abnormalities, aperistalsis, and organ enlargement may ensue. This 'neurogenic' pathogenesis has been linked to sudden death.

It is proposed that pathological exposure of normal host-sequestered antigens, or sharing of antigens between *T. cruzi* and its host, may precipitate autoimmune pathogenesis. Some chronic chagasic cardiomyopathy is said to display a renewed intense inflammatory response and a progressive diffuse myocarditis, and a slow decline in cardiac function.

The contribution of the lifelong infection to the pathogenesis of chronic Chagas disease is somewhat controversial, although published studies suggest that elimination of residual infection may improve long-term prognosis. After the initial acute phase, trypomastigotes are detectable in the blood only by sensitive indirect methods. Similarly, pseudocysts in the tissues are infrequent, but are detectable immunologically and by amplification of *T. cruzi* DNA.

T. cruzi infection is controlled primarily by a cell-mediated immune response, especially the Th1 arm of the immune response.

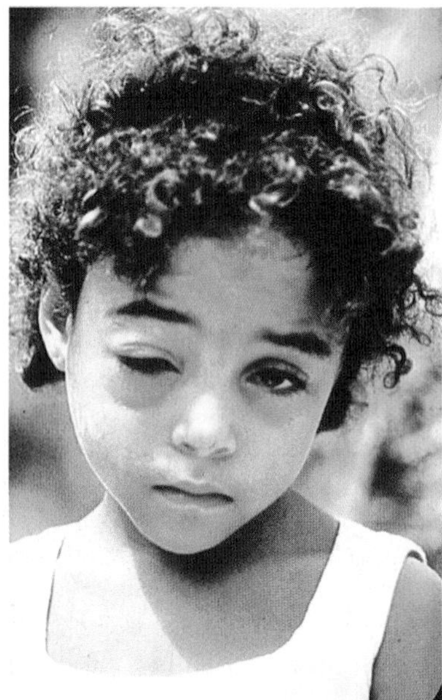

Fig. 7.8.11.4 Romaña's sign in acute Chagas disease.

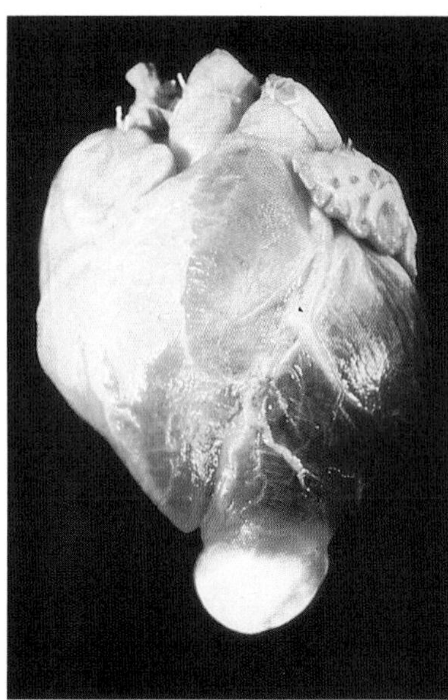

Fig. 7.8.11.5 Apical aneurysm of the left ventricle in chronic Chagas disease. (Courtesy of Dr J S de Oliveira.)

Patients immunocompromised by AIDS have impaired Th1 responses. Thus HIV-positive patients chronically infected with *T. cruzi* may suffer reactivated acute Chagas disease, with microscopically patent parasitaemia and poor prognosis.

At the level of gross pathology, substantial megacardia may be seen. Thinning of the myocardium may be present, with focal aneurysms visible upon transillumination, especially at the apex of the left ventricle (Fig. 7.8.11.5) and thrombus in the right atrial appendage (Fig. 7.8.11.6). Apical aneurysm is considered to be a pathognomonic sign of chronic chagasic cardiomyopathy. Megaoesophagus (Fig. 7.8.11.7) and megacolon (Fig. 7.8.11.8) may show enormous dilatation and thinning of the wall. Chagasic megaoesophagus is more frequent than chagasic megacolon, but both may occur in the same patient and are often accompanied by chagasic heart disease. Chagasic megaoesophagus may be a prelude to carcinoma. Occasionally megasyndromes may arise in infants, following congenital infection.

Clinical features

Classically, there are three clinical phases of Chagas disease. In the acute phase, symptoms include fever, myalgia, headache, hepatosplenomegaly, generalized lymphadenopathy, facial or generalized

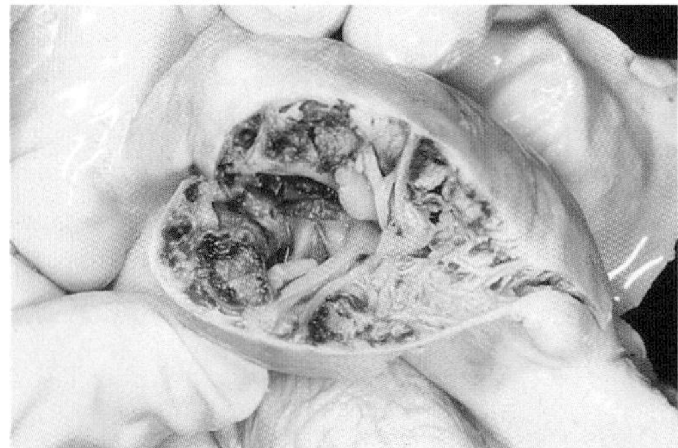

Fig. 7.8.11.6 Mural thrombus filling the right atrial appendage. (Copyright D A Warrell.)

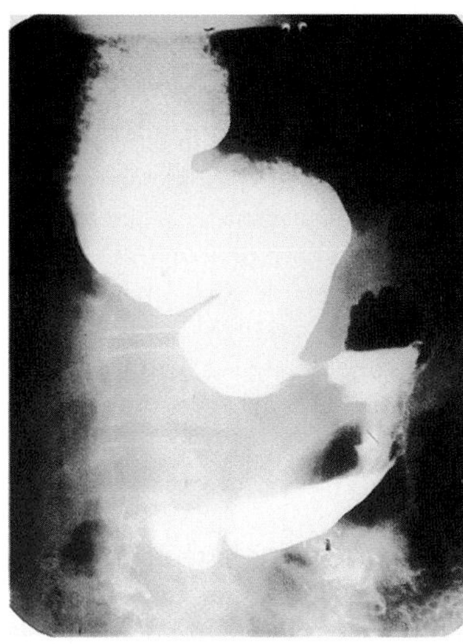

Fig. 7.8.11.7 Megaoesophagus seen by radiography in chronic Chagas disease. (Courtesy of Dr J S de Oliveira.)

oedema, rash, vomiting, diarrhoea, and anorexia. If *T. cruzi* has been inoculated through the conjunctiva, Romaña's sign may be present: unilateral conjunctivitis, chemosis, and periophthalmic oedema (Fig. 7.8.11.4). If the portal of entry is the skin, an indurated oedematous cutaneous lesion (chagoma) may be seen. Regional lymphadenopathy may be present. Multiple chagomas may occasionally occur in acute-phase infections in infants. ECG abnormalities may include sinus tachycardia, increased PR interval, T-wave changes, and low QRS voltage. The incubation period may be as short as 2 weeks or as long as several months if infection is due to transfusion of contaminated blood. General lymphadenopathy and splenomegaly are frequent in blood transfusion-acquired infections.

Congenital acute infection may cause fever, oedema, metastatic chagomas, neurological signs such as convulsions, tremors, and weak reflexes, and apnoea. Hepatosplenomegaly is frequent. The ECG is usually normal but low-voltage complexes, reduced T-wave height, and longer atrioventricular (AV) conduction time may be present.

Meningoencephalitis is rare in adults, more frequent in infants, and common in immunocompromised patients. It carries a poor prognosis.

The clinical picture of AIDS-associated chagasic meningoencephalitis may be similar to toxoplasmosis. Haemorrhagic necrotic encephalitis is described in the nests of trypanosomes in microglia. Congenital infection may resemble toxoplasmosis, cytomegalovirus infection, or syphilis, with an increased likelihood of abortion and premature birth. Congenital infection is well known in Bolivia but less frequently reported from Venezuela and Brazil.

Symptomatic or asymptomatic acute infection may be followed by a symptom-free indeterminate phase of unpredictable length, which may be life long.

Chronic-phase symptoms may emerge in up to 30% of patients recovering from the acute phase. Cardiac symptoms include arrhythmias, palpitations, chest pain, oedema, dizziness, syncope, and dyspnoea. The cardiac enlargement may be massive with chronic congestive cardiac failure, apical aneurysm (Fig. 7.8.11.5), and thrombus in the right atrial appendage (Fig. 7.8.11.6). The cardiac conducting system is involved, especially the sinus node, bundle of His and AV node, in which there is mononuclear and mast-cell infiltration, inflammation, and fibrosis. Characteristic ECG abnormalities are right bundle branch block (RBBB) and left anterior hemiblock (LAH). AV conduction abnormalities, including AV block, may be present. Arrhythmias may include sinus bradycardia, sinoatrial block, ventricular tachycardia, primary T-wave changes, and abnormal Q-waves. The severity of heart disease is graded by the degree of disturbance. Sudden death is attributable, not to ruptured aneurysm, but to arrhythmias often precipitated by exercise (e.g. on the football field). Radiography may reveal megacardia (Fig. 7.8.11.9). Signs of oesophageal involvement include loss of peristalsis, regurgitation, and dysphagia (Fig. 7.8.11.7). Parotid enlargement may be associated.

In megacolon, there may be failure of defaecation, constipation, and faecaloma (Fig. 7.8.11.8). Progressive dilatation of either organ can be graded clinically according to severity and may be detectable by radiography. Megaduodenum and megaureter are also described.

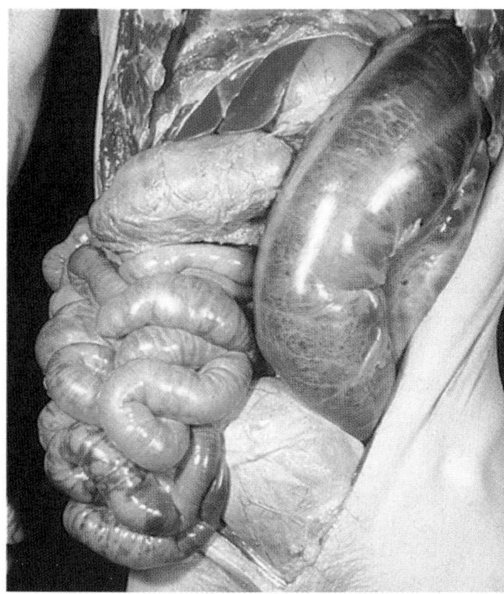

Fig. 7.8.11.8 Megacolon postmortem in chronic Chagas disease. (Courtesy of Dr J. S. de Oliveira.)

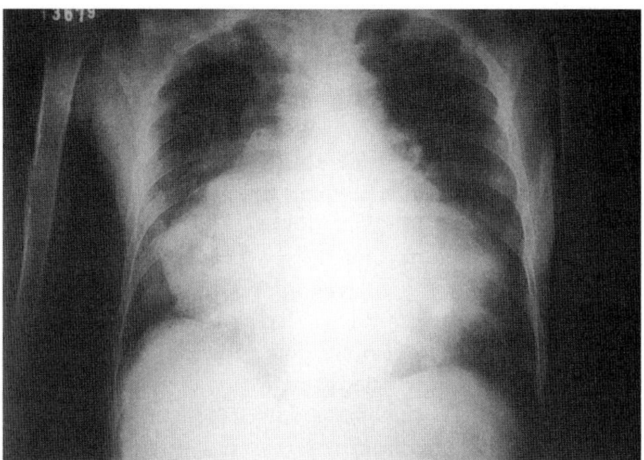

Fig. 7.8.11.9 Chest radiograph showing gross cardiac enlargement in a Brazilian woman with chronic Chagas disease. (Copyright D A Warrell.)

The lymph nodes between the pulmonary trunk and the aorta are frequently enlarged.

The differential diagnosis includes other types of heart disease and causes of ECG abnormalities. RBBB and LAH are indicative, but a history of exposure to *T. cruzi* infection and laboratory diagnostic evidence must be considered (see below).

Laboratory diagnosis

A history of exposure to triatomine bugs, to potentially contaminated transfused blood, or a prolonged stay in endemic regions must be considered.

Motile trypomastigotes might be seen in unstained, wet blood preparations examined by microscopy (Fig. 7.8.11.3). Nevertheless, parasitaemia is often scanty or undetectable by this method. The sensitivity of parasitological diagnosis may be enhanced by microscopy of samples prepared with concentration methods, such as the centrifugation pellet from separated serum (Strout's method), the haematocrit buffy coat layer, Giemsa-stained thick films, or the centrifugation sediment after lysis of red blood cells with 0.87% ammonium chloride. All these tests may be negative if parasitaemia is low. Potentially infected blood must be handled with care, especially during haematocrit centrifugation, as a single trypomastigote can cause infection. Multiple blood cultures may also be performed, with a sensitive blood agar-based medium and physiological saline overlay. Even more sensitive than blood culture is xenodiagnosis, in which hungry fourth or fifth instar bugs from a clean triatomine colony, raised from bug eggs and fed only on birds, are allowed to feed on the patient. Bugs are applied in a plastic pot contained discretely in a black bag, which is tied beneath the patient's forearm. The bugs are dissected 20 to 25 days later. The hindgut and rectum are drawn out into a drop of sterile physiological saline, mixed with a blunt instrument (microspatula), and observed microscopically for motile epimastigotes and trypomastigotes. Dissection should be performed behind a small, Perspex safety screen or in a microbiological safety cabinet. *R. prolixus* is the most avid feeder for xenodiagnosis but may cause delayed hypersensitivity reactions in sensitized patients. Anaphylaxis is rare but two cases are known. The local vector should be used as the susceptibility of triatomine species varies with the strain of *T. cruzi*.

After the acute-phase infection, all the above methods of parasitological diagnosis will fail except xenodiagnosis and, possibly, multiple blood cultures. Up to 50% of patients in chronic phase may yield a positive xenodiagnosis, providing at least 10 triatomine bugs are used. Although polymerase chain reaction amplification of *T. cruzi* DNA is sensitive and specific, it is not yet available as a routine diagnostic test. Serum antibody is produced within a few days of *T. cruzi* infection and persists for life in untreated patients. There is an early IgM response, but it is not sustained at the high levels seen in African trypanosomiasis. Persistent IgG may be detected by the enzyme-linked immunosorbent assay, the indirect fluorescent-antibody test, or the indirect haemagglutination test. Complement fixation, developed in 1913, is effective but now seldom used. Crossreactions may occur with visceral and mucocutaneous leishmaniasis, with treponematoses, and possibly with other hyperimmune responses or autoimmune diseases. Recombinant antigens have been used to improve species specificity and some are commercially available; rapid tests have also been introduced. The majority of diagnostic kits are prepared from *T. cruzi* II preparations but are presumed to be equally applicable to other lineages. Serological assays must be standardized with negative and positive control sera and by reference to experienced external reference centres to check reproducibility. Quality of commercial tests should not be presumed without reference to authoritative comparative studies. Transplacentally acquired IgG may persist for up to 9 months in infants born of seropositive mothers. However, IgM-specific seropositivity in such infants is an indicator of congenital infection. Note that IgM may decline rapidly in filter paper blood spots if they are used as the source of serum. Serology may be performed post mortem using pericardial fluid.

Treatment

Proven acute cases must be treated promptly in an effort to minimize tissue damage and neuron loss. The synthetic oral nitrofuran, nifurtimox was the first successful drug for the treatment of Chagas disease. Bayer has recently safeguarded supply by restarting production in El Salvador. Nifurtimox is given in three divided daily doses at 8 to 10 mg/kg for 90 days, up to double doses for infected children. Adverse effects, which may lead to interruption of treatment, can include anorexia, loss of weight, psychological disturbances, excitability, nausea, and vomiting. Benznidazole is an oral nitroimidazole. The adult dosage is 5 to 7 mg/kg in two divided doses for 60 days; for children, 10 mg/kg also in two divided doses for 60 days. Adverse effects may also demand interruption of treatment. These include rashes, fever, nausea, peripheral polyneuritis, leukopenia, and, rarely, agranulocytosis. Double or even higher doses have been used for immunocompromised patients, especially if meningoencephalitis is present. There is no guarantee that a full course of treatment will eliminate the infection. Although the value of drug treatment for chronic infections is still debated, it is favoured for children under 12 years or by some for those under 15 years, because children tolerate treatment better than adults. Favourable access to these drugs may be obtained via WHO.

Chemotherapy is an important part of supportive treatment. In acute-phase heart failure, sodium intake is restricted and diuretics and digitalis may be indicated. Meningoencephalitis may require anticonvulsants, sedatives, and intravenous mannitol. Heart failure due to Chagas disease may require vasodilatation (angiotensin-converting enzyme inhibitors) and maintenance of normal serum potassium levels; digitalis is a last resort because it may aggravate arrhythmias. A pacemaker may be fitted to improve bradycardia not responding to atropine, or for atrial fibrillation with a slow ventricular response that is not responsive to vagolytic drugs, or for complete AV block. Amiodarone has been suggested as the most useful drug to treat arrhythmias but it may still be aggravating. For ventricular extrasystoles lidocaine, mexiletine, propafenone, flecainide, and β-adrenoreceptor antagonists may be effective. Lidocaine may be used intravenously in emergencies. It is essential to consult detailed WHO expert reports and physicians with substantial experience in the management of chagasic heart disease.

Surgery is a vital part of case management for Chagas disease. Resection of ventricular aneurysms has been suggested. Specialized surgery has been developed in Brazil for the treatment of megaoesophagus and megacolon. Early megaoesophagus may respond to balloon dilatation. The Heller–Vasconcelos operation, in which a portion of muscle at the junction of the oesophagus and stomach is removed, may alleviate megaoesophagus. Severe megaoesophagus requires replacement of the distal oesophagus, e.g. with a portion of jejenum. The modified Duhamel–Haddad operation has been considered the most successful surgery for correction of a megacolon: after resection, the colon is lowered through the retrorectal stump as a perineal colostomy. Subsequent suturing, under peridural anaesthesia, gives a wide junction between the colon and the rectal stump.

Prognosis, even in treated patients who show serological reversion, is unpredictable as the sequelae of damage due to the acute phase of Chagas disease cannot be foreseen.

Prevention and control

There is no vaccine against Chagas disease and no immunotherapy.

Chagas disease flourishes where there is poverty and poor housing conditions. There are proven methods of controlling domestic triatomine bugs. These depend on insecticide spraying, health education, community support, and house improvement. Synthetic pyrethroids are the insecticides of choice and several commercial sources are available. Vector control programmes consist of preparatory, attack, and vigilance phases. In the preparatory phase, the distribution of all dwellings must be mapped, the presence of infested houses assessed, and the attack and vigilance phases costed and planned. The attack phase involves spraying all houses and peridomestic buildings, irrespective of whether bugs have been found. During the vigilance phase, the community plays an essential role in reporting residual bug infestations, which elicit a rapid respraying response for the affected sites. Serology is vital for monitoring the success of control programmes. Children born after control programmes begin should be serologically negative beyond 9 months of age (to exclude transplacental transfer of IgG) except for infrequent cases of congenital transmission.

Blood donors in or from endemic areas should be screened serologically. If conditions demand the use of seropositive blood, it can be decontaminated with crystal violet (250 mg/litre) and storage at 4°C for at least 24 h. Potentially infected organ donors or recipients should be screened serologically. Seropositive immunosuppressed recipients are likely to suffer reactivated acute-phase infection. Prophylactic chemotherapy with benznidazole may be effective.

The Southern Cone programme launched a massive effort to eliminate *T. infestans* from Argentina, Bolivia, Brazil, Chile, Paraguay, Uruguay, and southern Peru. Domestic infestation in Brazil has been reduced by 85%. Uruguay and Chile are essentially free of vector-borne and blood-transfusion transmission. Substantial progress has also been made in the other participating countries. Similar international collaborations have been initiated in Central America and the Andean Pact countries. Reinvasion of sylvatic bugs into domestic habitats may complicate vector control in some regions. One example is *T. brasiliensis* in north-eastern Brazil, which reinvades houses from adjacent rock piles. A second example is *R. prolixus*, which, in some regions of Venezuela and Colombia, has the capacity to reinvade houses from adjacent infested palm trees, as demonstrated by comparative population genetics. A surveillance programme and rapid responses to new domestic triatomine populations has been planned to protect the Amazon against domiciliation of vectors.

Unanswered questions and future research

T. cruzi is of immense research interest. It is not entirely clear how the organism evades the host immune response. Furthermore, the pathogenesis of Chagas disease is not fully understood. Molecular methods have radically changed our understanding of the epidemiology of *T. cruzi* infection. Molecular features unique to trypanosomatids (trypanosomes and leishmanias) make *T. cruzi* an attractive model for molecular biologists. Further research is required to produce a nontoxic, low-cost oral drug, which would eliminate the reservoir of infection in humans, and to clarify further the population genetics and epidemiological significance of diverse strains. The origins and evolution of the organism and its vectors are also of considerable academic interest.

Trypanosoma rangeli

The second human trypanosomiasis in the New World is due to *T. rangeli* infection. *T. rangeli* is also transmitted by triatomine bugs, in particular the genus *Rhodnius*. In *Rhodnius* species, however, *T. rangeli* traverses the wall of the alimentary tract, infects the haemocoel, and reaches the salivary glands, in which the metacyclic infective trypomastigotes are produced. *T. rangeli* is thus transmitted by the bite of the triatomine bug and not by contamination with bug faeces. Although enzootic *T. rangeli* infection is widespread in Latin America, transmission to humans is virtually confined to areas in which *R. prolixus* is the domestic vector of *T. cruzi*. Coinfections of *T. cruzi* and *T. rangeli* may occur. The organism appears to be nonpathogenic in humans. *T. rangeli* can be pathogenic to *Rhodnius* species The importance of *T. rangeli* lies in the fact that it may confuse xenodiagnosis to detect *T. cruzi*. With care and experience, *T. rangeli* can be distinguished from *T. cruzi* either by its long slender epimastigotes (up to 80 μm in length) and its smaller kinetoplast or by its presence in the haemolymph or salivary glands of some xenodiagnosis bugs. The lifecycle in the mammalian host is uncertain, but *T. rangeli* is thought to divide in the peripheral blood. Trypomastigotes are rarely seen in human blood: they are much larger than *T. cruzi*, with a small subterminal kinetoplast (Fig. 7.8.11.10). Antibodies to *T. cruzi* certainly crossreact strongly with *T. rangeli*. Based on experimental work in mice, *T. rangeli* infections are thought to induce very low crossreactive antibody titres to *T. cruzi*. As with *T. cruzi*, there is subspecies genetic heterogeneity, with at least two and up to four distinct *T. rangeli*

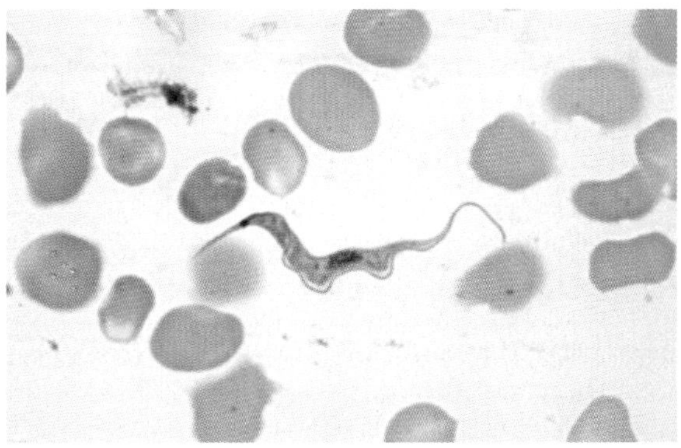

Fig. 7.8.11.10 *Trypanosoma rangeli* in a blood smear from an infected mouse. (Courtesy of J Williams.)

lineages, thought to be linked to two species groups within the triatomine genus *Rhodnius*.

Further reading

Castro JA, de Mecca M M, Bartel LC (2006). Toxic side effects of drugs used to treat Chagas disease (American trypanosomiasis). *Hum Exp Toxicol*, **25**, 471–9. [The potential side effects of treatment.]

Gaunt MW, *et al.* (2003). Mechanism of genetic exchange in American trypanosomes. *Nature*, **421**, 936–39. [The first experimental proof that *T. cruzi* has an extant capacity for genetic exchange.]

Maudlin I, Holmes P, Miles MA (eds) (2004). *The Trypanosomiases*. CABI Publishing, Wallingford, UK. [A detailed review of diverse aspects of both the South American and the African trypanosomiases.]

Miles MA (2004). The discovery of Chagas disease: progress and prejudice. *Infect Dis Clin North Am*, **18**, 247–60. [An account of historical and political aspects of the unusual discovery of Chagas disease.]

Miles MA, Feliciangeli MD, Arias AR (2003). American trypanosomiasis (Chagas disease) and the role of molecular epidemiology in guiding control strategies. *Br Med J*, **326**, 1444–8. [A synthesis of the application of molecular epidemiology to elucidate transmission of *T. cruzi* and guide interventions.]

Raia AA (1983). *Manifestações digestivas da moléstia de Chagas*. Sarvier, São Paulo, Brazil. [For the surgeon, fascinating accounts of the development of lifesaving procedures, especially correction of megaoesophagus and megacolon (in Portuguese).]

Riera C, *et al.* (2006). Congenital transmission of *Trypanosoma cruzi* in Europe (Spain): a case report. *Am J Trop Med Hyg*, **75**, 1078–81. [A case history of congenital transmission in Europe.]

Schmuniz GA (2007). Epidemiology of Chagas disease in non endemic countries: the role of international migration. *Mem Inst Oswaldo Cruz*, **30** (Suppl. 1), 75–85. [Forewarning on the occurrence of Chagas disease outside traditional endemic regions.]

World Health Organization (2002). *Control of Chagas disease*, Technical Report Series 905. WHO, Geneva. [Not strictly on control, but one of the best clinical reviews of Chagas disease in the English language.]

Miles MA, *et al.* (2009). The molecular epidemiology and phylogeography of Trypanosoma cruzi and parallel research on Leishmania: looking back and to the future. *Parasitology*, **136**, 1509–28.

7.8.12 Leishmaniasis

A.D.M. Bryceson and Diana N.J. Lockwood

Essentials

Leishmaniasis is caused by parasites of the genus *Leishmania*, which are transmitted to humans from human or animal reservoirs by the bites of phlebotomine sandflies. In places the disease is common and important, with perhaps 500 000 cases of visceral leishmaniasis and 1.5–2 million cases of cutaneous leishmaniasis worldwide each year. As an imported disease, cutaneous leishmaniasis is common in travellers, military personnel, and immigrants coming from endemic areas, while the diagnosis of the less common visceral leishmaniasis is frequently overlooked.

Cutaneous leishmaniasis

Clinical features—at the site of the infected sandfly bite, an erythematous nodule typically develops into a sore which fails to heal spontaneously in (1) diffuse cutaneous leishmaniasis; (2) leishmaniasis recidivans; and (3) American mucosal leishmaniasis (espundia)—a condition in which mucosal lesions develop in 4 to 40% of patients with untreated cutaneous ulcers due to *L. brasiliensis*; the nose is most commonly involved, and eventually the whole nose and mouth may be destroyed.

Diagnosis and treatment—diagnosis is by demonstration of leishmania organisms in tissue smears or biopsy material by microscopy, culture, or polymerase chain reaction (PCR). Many leishmanial sores can be left to heal naturally, but treatment is indicated for those that are severe, or failing to heal spontaneously, or due to particular species (e.g. *L. brasiliensis*). Treatment may be (1) local—e.g. surgery/curettage; infiltration with a pentavalent antimonial; or (2) systemic—most cutaneous species of leishmania are sensitive to pentavalent antimonials.

Visceral leishmaniasis

Zoonotic disease is common around the Mediterranean littoral, across the Middle East and central Asia, in northern and eastern China, and in South and Central America. Anthroponotic disease causes large outbreaks in North Eastern India and the Sudan.

Clinical features—most infections are subclinical, but clinical presentation is with gradual onset of fever, discomfort from an enlarged spleen, abdominal swelling, weight loss, cough, or diarrhoea. The illness may be associated with HIV infection.

Diagnosis and treatment—diagnosis is by isolation of leishmania from spleen, bone marrow, liver, lymph node, or buffy coat. Serology is useful for diagnosis, and may replace direct demonstration of parasites in remote areas. The best treatment is intravenous liposomal amphotericin B, but (much cheaper) pentavalent antimonials are most often used in countries where visceral leishmaniasis is endemic.

Prevention

Prevention is by controlling reservoir hosts and sandfly vectors, or by avoiding bites by vectors. There is no vaccine.

Introduction

Leishmaniasis is caused by parasites of the genus *Leishmania*, which are transmitted by phlebotomine sandflies. The infection may be anthroponotic or zoonotic, having respectively human or animal reservoirs. In humans, the disease is usually either cutaneous or visceral. The most important variant is mucosal leishmaniasis of South and Central America. In places the disease is common and important, but there are few accurate statistics. The World Health Organization (WHO) estimates 500 000 cases of visceral leishmaniasis and 1.5 to 2 million cases of cutaneous leishmaniasis occur annually, with 200 million people at risk of each disease, but these figures may underestimate the problem. As an imported disease, cutaneous leishmaniasis is common in travellers, military personnel, and immigrants coming from endemic areas, while the diagnosis of the less common visceral leishmaniasis is frequently overlooked.

Aetiological agent and lifecycle

In its vertebrate host, the oval amastigote form of the parasite (2–3 μm in diameter) is found in cells of the reticuloendothelial system (Fig. 7.8.12.1). In the sandfly or in culture medium, it is in the elongated, motile, promastigote form with an anterior flagellum.

The most important species of *Leishmania* that cause disease in humans and their own reservoir hosts are shown in Table 7.8.12.1. Isoenzyme patterns and DNA hybridization are used to distinguish species.

Sandflies require a precise microclimate that is provided in certain places in each endemic focus at particular seasons of the year. Transmission is often seasonal. Amastigotes are ingested from blood or tissues of the mammalian host by the female fly and transform into promastigotes in the gut, rendering the fly infective after about 10 days.

Cutaneous leishmaniasis

Epidemiology

The vectors of *Leishmania major* live in rodent burrows. Visiting hunters, travellers, soldiers, and tourists, and dwellers at oases or in new settlements, are affected. The disease may be sporadic or epidemic, as recently among Afghan refugees in camps in Pakistan. The vectors of *L. tropica* live in crevices in buildings and walls. The disease may be endemic or epidemic. The vector of *L. aethiopica* bites people sleeping in their huts. The disease is endemic and most people are affected by early adulthood. *L. infantum* causes simple, self-healing skin lesions in some parts of southern Europe and North Africa. *L. donovani* causes post-kala-azar dermal leishmaniasis (PKDL) in India.

In the New World, transmission is usually in the forest. *L. brasiliensis*, the major cause of American cutaneous and mucosal leishmaniasis, is the most widely distributed of the New World species. Its vectors are highly anthropophilic and human infection is common. Periurban and urban foci of infection are increasing. Malnutrition is a risk factors for mucosal leishmaniasis. Infection with *L. peruviana* occurs in high Andean valleys, where it may be locally common.

Pathogenesis and pathology

Leishmania, when inoculated by the sandfly, invade and multiply in macrophages in the skin. The parasitized macrophage granuloma is infiltrated by lymphocytes and plasma cells. Piecemeal or focal necrosis destroys parasitized cells. The overlying epidermis shows hyperkeratosis and ulcerates. In chronic lesions, epithelioid cells and Langhans giant cells produce a picture similar to that of noncaseous tuberculosis. Rarely, the cellular immune response is suppressed and histology shows heavily parasitized macrophages with little or no lymphocytic infiltrate, characteristic of diffuse cutaneous leishmaniasis.

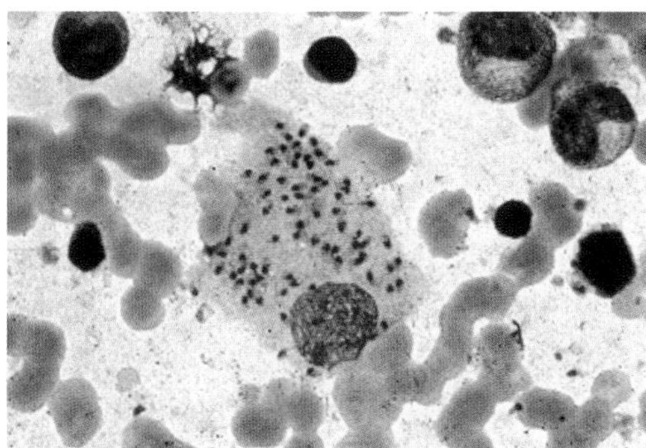

Fig. 7.8.12.1 Amastigotes of *L. donovani* in a reticuloendothelial cell. From the splenic aspirate of a child with visceral leishmaniasis in Kenya. (Copyright A D M Bryceson.)

Table 7.8.12.1 Epidemiology of leishmaniasis

Organism	Geographical location	Reservoir	Vector
Old World			
L. donovani	North-east India, Bangladesh, Nepal	Humans	*Phlebotomus argentipes*
L. infantum	Mediterranean basin, Sudan, Middle East, China, central Asia	Dogs, foxes, jackals	*P. perniciosus, P. major, P. chinensis,* etc.
L. donovani (Africa)	Sudan, Kenya, Horn of Africa, ?Senegal, Gambia	?Rodents in Sudan, ?canines, ?humans	*P. orientalis, P. martini*
L. major	Semideserts in Middle East, north India, Pakistan, North Africa, central Asia	Gerbils (especially *Rhombomys, Meriones*)	*P. papatasi*
L. major	Sub-Saharan savannah, Sudan	Rodents (especially *Arvicanthis, Tatera*)	*P. duboscqi*
L. tropica	Towns in Middle East, Mediterranean basin, central Asia	Humans, ?dogs	*P. sergenti*
L. aethiopica	Highlands of Kenya, Ethiopia	Hyraxes (*Procavia, Heterohyrax*)	*P. longipes, P. pedifer*
New World			
L. chagasi (=*L. infantum*)	Most of Central and South America, especially Brazil	Dogs, foxes opossums (*Didelphis*)	*Lutzomyia longipalpis, Lu. evansi*
L. mexicana	Central and northern South America	Forest rodents (especially *Ototylomys*)	*Lu. olmeca*
L. amazonensis	Tropical forests of South America	Forest rodents (especially *Proechimys, Oryzomys*)	*Lu. flaviscutellata*
L. brasiliensis	Tropical forests and cultivated land throughout South and Central America	?Forest rodents, dogs and equines	*Lu. wellcomei, Lu. whitmani,* etc.
L. guyanensis	Northern South America	Sloths (*Choleopus*), arboreal anteaters (*Tamandua*)	*Lu. umbratilis*
L. panamensis	Central America, Ecuador, Colombia	Sloths (*Choleopus*)	*Lu. trapidoi,* etc.
L. peruviana	West Andes of Peru	Dogs, ?rodents, ?opossums	*Lu. verrucarum, Lu. peruensis*

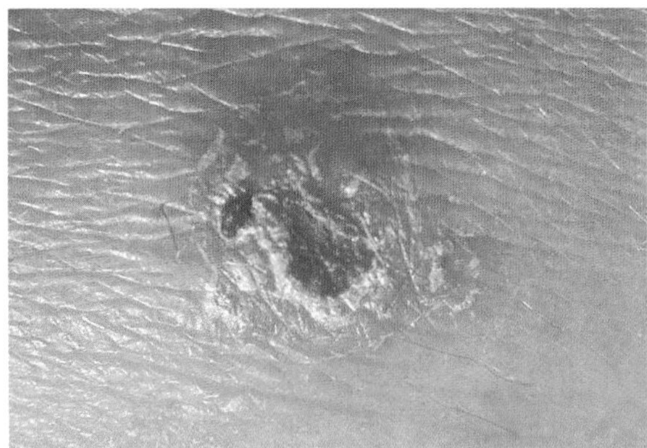

Fig. 7.8.12.2 Nodular lesion of cutaneous leishmaniasis. Showing crusting and small satellite papules, typical of early lesions of all species, in this case *L. brasiliensis*. (Copyright A D M Bryceson.)

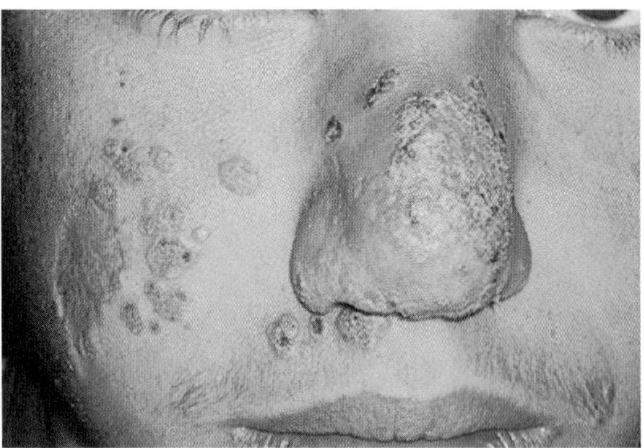

Fig. 7.8.12.4 Cutaneous leishmaniasis due to *L. tropica* in a young man in Kabul. Crusty nodular lesions are spreading on the face. There is a typical depressed scar of a previous lesion on the right cheek.
(Copyright Dr Mark Bailey.)

L. aethiopica, *L. mexicana*, and *L. brasiliensis* may invade cartilage. Cartilaginous lesions are extremely chronic. *L. brasiliensis*, and occasionally *L. panamensis* or *L. guyanensis*, may metastasize through the bloodstream to sites deep in the mucosa of the upper respiratory tract, where they may lie dormant. After months or years a lesion develops, characterized by necrosis, vasculitis, and tissue destruction.

Immunity to a given species of leishmania is usually lifelong. Second infections occur occasionally, especially in older people or immunosuppressed.

Clinical features

After an incubation period of a few days to several months, an erythematous nodule develops at the site of the infected sandfly bite. A golden crust forms (Fig. 7.8.12.2). The sore reaches its final size, usually 1 to 5 cm in diameter, over weeks or months. The crust may fall away, leaving an ulcer with a raised edge (Fig. 7.8.12.3). Satellite papules are common. After months or years, the lesion starts to heal leaving a depressed, mottled scar. Any secondary bacterial infection is superficial and unimportant. The lesion is not normally painful, but may disfigure or disable if scarring is severe or over a joint. Draining lymphatic vessels may be thickened or nodular.

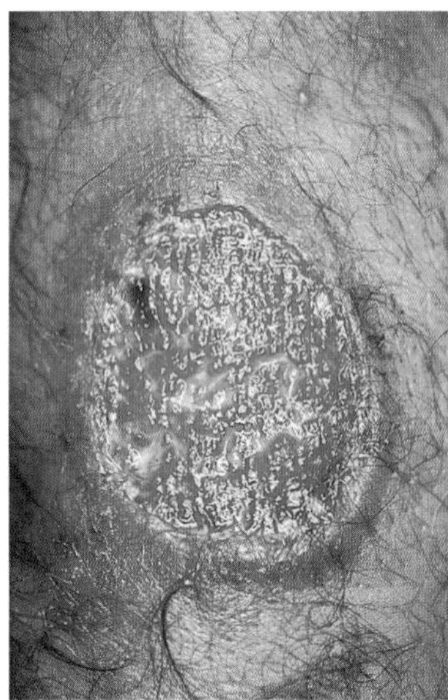

Fig. 7.8.12.3 Cutaneous leishmaniasis due to *L. brasiliensis*. Shallow ulcer with raised edge.
(Copyright A D M Bryceson.)

There are many variations on this classical pattern. Sores due to *L. major* form and heal rapidly (mean 3–5 months) and may be inflamed and exudative: the so-called wet or rural sore. Sores due to *L. tropica* tend to be less inflamed and to heal more slowly (mean 10–14 months): the so-called dry or urban sore (Fig. 7.8.12.4). Lesions due to *L. infantum* have an incubation period of many months and may persist over several years. In *L. aethiopica* infections, lesions are usually central on the face. Satellite papules accumulate to produce a slowly growing, shiny tumour or plaque that may not crust or ulcerate, taking between 2 and 5 years to heal (Fig. 7.8.12.5); mucocutaneous leishmaniasis may develop, producing swelling of the lips and expansion and elongation of the nose. Leishmanial lymphangitis may accompany sores of any species but is commoner in the New World than the Old World (Fig. 7.8.12.6). On occasion, hard thickened lymphatics may accompany an insignificant cutaneous lesion.

L. brasiliensis often causes deep, spreading ulcers, which heal over 6 to 24 months. Up to 15% of patients will relapse after spontaneous or therapeutic cure. *L. mexicana* lesions are commonly on the limbs or side of the face and heal in 6 to 8 months. Sores on the pinna of the ear may invade the cartilage, persist for many years, and destroy the pinna.

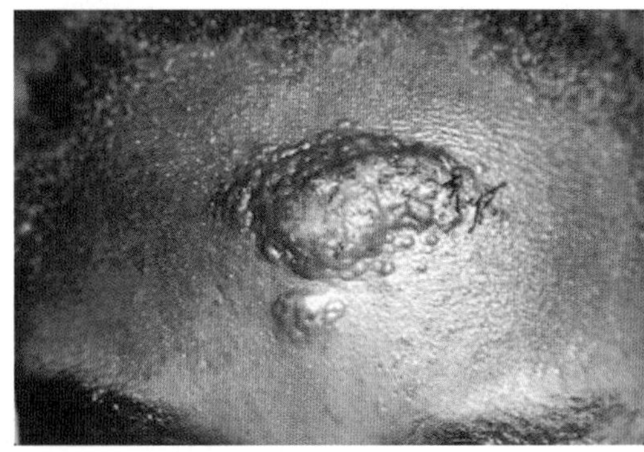

Fig. 7.8.12.5 Spreading nodular lesion typical of *L. aethiopica*, Kenya.

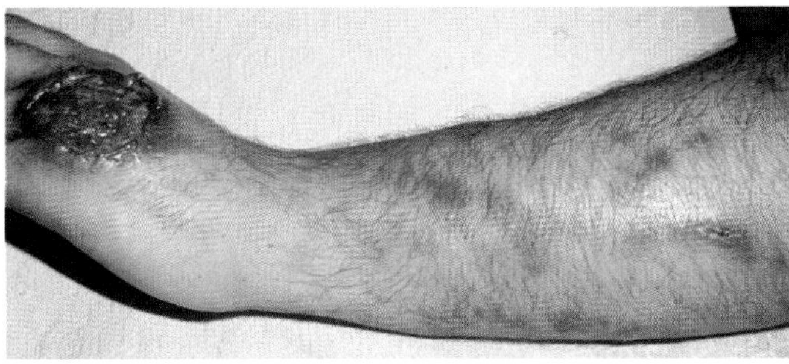

Fig. 7.8.12.6 Leishmanial lymphangitis in a man with cutaneous leishmaniasis from Belize. On occasion, hard thickened lymphatics may accompany an insignificant cutaneous lesion.
(Copyright A D M Bryceson.)

Three forms of cutaneous leishmaniasis do not heal spontaneously: diffuse cutaneous leishmaniasis, leishmaniasis recidivans, and American mucosal leishmaniasis.

Diffuse cutaneous leishmaniasis

This occurs with *L. aethiopica* and *L. amazonensis* infections but is rare. The primary nodule spreads locally without ulceration and secondary blood-borne lesions appear at other sites in the skin, affecting especially the face and the cooler extensor surfaces of the limbs (Fig. 7.8.12.7). The eye, mucosae, viscera, and peripheral nerves are spared, which differentiates it from lepromatous leprosy. The infection proceeds gradually over many years.

Leishmaniasis recidivans (lupoid leishmaniasis)

This is a rare complication of *L. tropica* infection. The initial sore heals, but papules recrudesce in the edge of the scar and the lesion spreads slowly over many years (Fig. 7.8.12.8).

American mucosal leishmaniasis (espundia)

Depending on the geographical location, between 4 and 40% of patients with untreated cutaneous ulcers due to *L. brasiliensis* develop mucosal lesions, half of them within 2 years of the appearance of the original lesion and 90% within 10 years. About one in six patients gives no history of a previous skin lesion. In most cases the nasal mucosa is affected, and in one-third another site is also involved: in order of frequency, the pharynx, palate, larynx, or upper lip. The initial lesion is a nodule and the initial symptom is of nasal obstruction. It commonly presents as protuberant new growth of the nose or lips (Figs. 7.8.12.9 and 7.8.12.10), or cicatrization, which causes an elongated 'tapir' nose. Mucosal leishmaniasis is slowly destructive, the septum perforates, and eventually the whole nose and mouth may be destroyed. Death may result from secondary sepsis, starvation, or laryngeal obstruction.

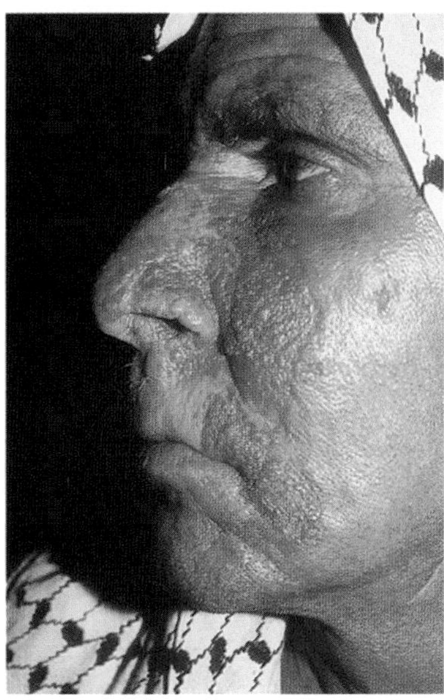

Fig. 7.8.12.8 Lupoid or recidivans leishmaniasis in a citizen of Baghdad.
(Courtesy of Dr Ahmed.)

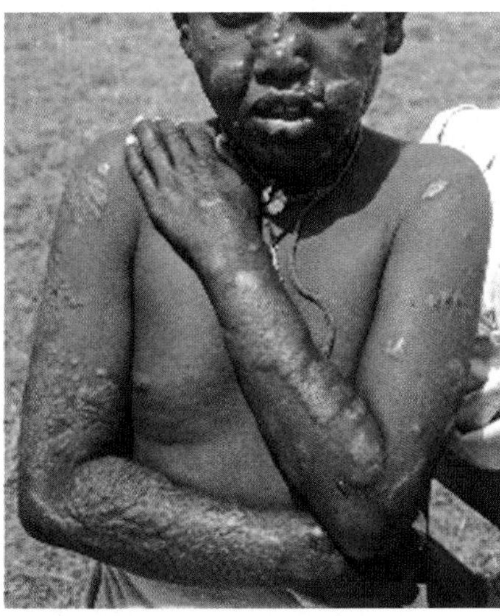

Fig. 7.8.12.7 Diffuse cutaneous leishmaniasis caused by *L. aethiopica*, Ethiopia.

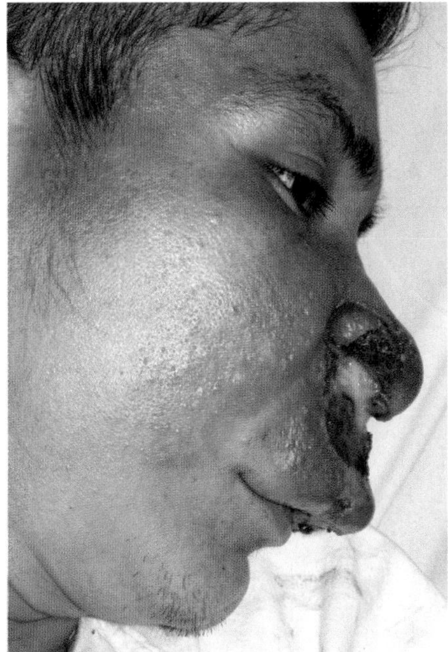

Fig. 7.8.12.9 Espundia. Swollen upper lip and 'tapir' nose due to mucosal leishmaniasis, at Instituto de Medicina Tropical 'Alexander von Humboldt' Universidad Peruana Cayetano Heredia, Lima, Peru.
(Copyright D A Warrell.)

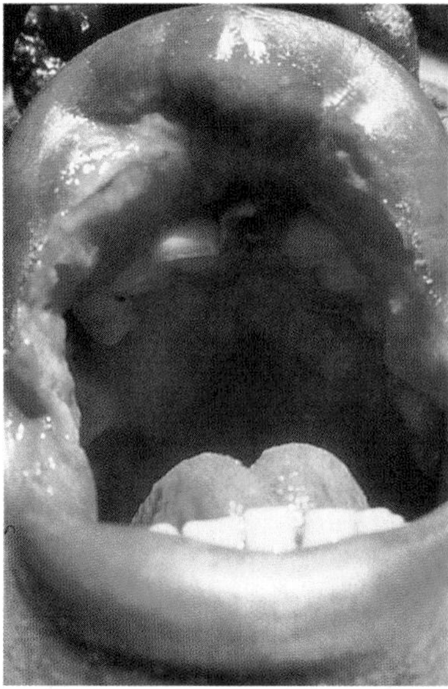

Fig. 7.8.12.10 Infiltration of lip and palate due to mucosal leishmaniasis in Peru.

Mucosal leishmaniasis is occasionally seen in travellers returning from South America.

Mucosal lesions are occasionally seen with Old World species, usually in the mouth or larynx, and tend to be associated with old age, corticosteroid medication, or other forms of mild immunosuppression (Fig. 7.8.12.11).

Laboratory findings

Parasitological diagnosis

Normally, leishmania organisms may be isolated from 80% of sores during the first half of their natural course. The nodular part of the lesion is grasped firmly between the finger and thumb until it blanches. An incision a few millimetres long is made into the dermis with the point of a scalpel, which is used to scrape dermal tissue and juice. Material obtained may be used to inoculate special diphasic culture medium and to prepare smears for staining with Giemsa, Wright's, or Leishman's stains (Fig. 7.8.12.1). Biopsy material may be used to make impression smears, for culture and for histology for differential diagnosis. Polymerase chain reaction (PCR) using kinetoplast DNA primers is nearly 99% sensitive and 93% specific. Diagnosis of mucosal leishmaniasis requires a deep punch biopsy specimen. Species diagnosis by PCR is desirable for American parasites to assess the risk of mucosal leishmaniasis.

Immunological diagnosis

The leishmanin test is occasionally useful in differential diagnosis. It is an intradermal test of delayed hypersensitivity that indicates previous exposure to leishmanial parasites. It becomes positive in over 90% of cases of self-healing forms of cutaneous leishmaniasis and mucosal leishmaniasis. Evaluation of a positive test must take into account naturally acquired positivity in the population at risk. Serology is unhelpful.

Treatment

Old World sores, or those due to *L. mexicana*, *L. amazonensis*, and *L. peruviana* that are not troublesome, may be left to heal naturally. But those that are disfiguring, potentially disabling, inconvenient, or around the ankle where they heal slowly, should be treated either locally or systemically. Systemic treatment is required when there is risk that the sore may be due to *L. brasiliensis*, *L. panamensis*, or *L. guyanensis*, when the sore is too large or badly sited for local treatment, when there is lymphatic spread, and for mucosal leishmaniasis, diffuse cutaneous leishmaniasis, and recidivans leishmaniasis.

Local treatment

Surgery, curettage, CO_2 laser, and cryotherapy are effective methods of removing small sores. Infiltration into the lesion with a pentavalent antimonial, weekly for 2 or 3 weeks or longer, may be successful. The technique needs practice and the infiltration is transiently painful (Fig. 7.8.12.12). An ointment containing 12% paromomycin and 15% methylbenzethonium chloride cures 70% lesions due to *L. major* in 20 days and may be suitable for lesions caused by other species, except *L. brasiliensis*, but is not always well tolerated.

Systemic treatment

All cutaneous species of leishmania are sensitive to pentavalent antimonials in conventional dosage except *L. aethiopica*, where

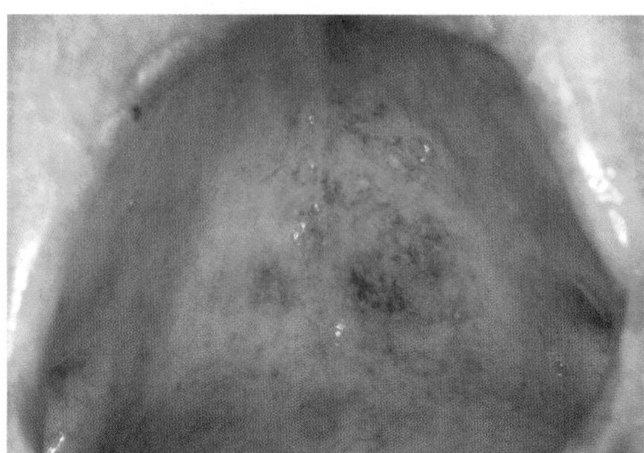

Fig. 7.8.12.11 Mucosal leishmaniasis due to *L. infantum*. Showing erythematous infiltration of the hard palate in an elderly British expatriate living in southern Spain and taking steroids for asthma.
(Copyright A D M Bryceson.)

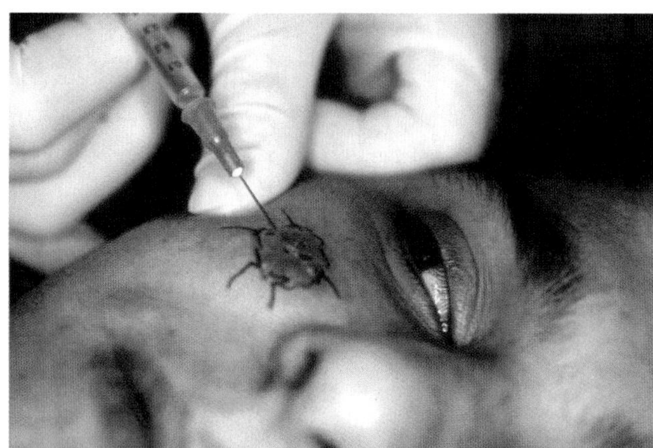

Fig. 7.8.12.12 Infiltrating a lesion of cutaneous leishmaniasis with sodium stibogluconate. The edge of the lesion is demarcated using a ballpoint pen and infiltrated radially from several points on its perimeter using an intradermal syringe and needle.
(Copyright A D M Bryceson.)

Table 7.8.12.2 Dosage regimens for the treatment of leishmaniasis

Drug	Dose
Sodium stibogluconate or meglumine antimoniate	10–20 mg Sb/kg body weight once daily for 21 days (visceral or cutaneous disease) or 28 days (visceral or mucosal disease)—PKDL may need treatment for 2–4 months. See Table 7.8.12.3 for dosage
Amphotericin B desoxycholate	1 mg/kg body weight on alternate days for 2 weeks (visceral disease) or 4–6 weeks (mucosal disease)
Liposomal amphotericin B	Ampoules of 50 mg, 2–3 mg/kg body weight daily for 7–10 doses, using whole ampoules to avoid waste, to total at least 21 mg/kg. In India a total dose of 6–9 mg/kg is sufficient. A 20-day regimen cures PKDL in Sudan
Miltefosine	Adult dose 100–150 mg daily for 28 days; paediatric dose 2.5 mg/kg body weight daily for 28 days
Aminosidine	16 mg/kg body weight daily for 21 days
Pentamidine	4 mg salt/kg body weight once weekly to once monthly
Ketoconazole	60 mg/day (adult) for 4–6 weeks

See text for choice of drug regimen.

pentamidine or paromomycin may be used. Ketoconazole may be useful for *L. major* and *L. mexicana* infections. Miltefosine is effective for *L. major* and *L. panamensis* infections. Patients with diffuse cutaneous leishmaniasis should be treated for at least 2 months, longer than it takes to clear parasites from the skin, and relapses should be treated again promptly. Relapsed cases of mucosal leishmaniasis have usually become unresponsive to antimonials and should be treated with amphotericin B deoxycholate for at least 4 to 6 weeks or liposomal amphotericin B for 3 weeks. See Tables 7.8.12.2 and 7.8.12.3 for dosage regimens. In addition, they may require antibiotics for secondary sepsis, attention to nutrition, and, later, plastic surgery.

Table 7.8.12.3 Simplified dosage regimens for pentavalent antimonials

Nearest weight of patient (kg)	Calculated dose (mg Sb)	Recommended dose (ml (mg Sb))	
		Sodium stibogluconate[a]	Meglumine antimoniate[b]
90	1088	11.0 (1100)	13.0 (1105)
80	1006	10.0 (1000)	12.0 (1220)
70	925	9.5 (950)	11.0 (935)
60	832	8.5 (850)	10.0 (850)
50	737	7.5 (750)	9.0 (765)
40	635	6.5 (650)	7.5 (637)
30	524	5.0 (500)	6.0 (510)
20	400	4.0 (400)	5.0 (425)
10	252	2.5 (250)	3.0 (255)
5	159	2.0 (200)	2.5 (212)

Calculations are based on body surface area according to the formula: body surface area in $m^2 = 0.13/kg^2$, whereby a 20 kg child receives 20 mg Sb/kg at 542 mg Sb/m^2.

[a] Sodium stibogluconate solution containing 100 mg Sb/ml.

[b] Meglumine antimoniate solution containing 85 mg Sb/ml.

(Adapted from Anabwani GM, Bryceson AD (1982). Visceral leishmaniasis in Kenyan children. *Indian Pediatr*, **19**, 819–22.)

Visceral leishmaniasis

Epidemiology

Visceral leishmaniasis is found in four main zoogeographical zones: the Ganges Brahmaputra plains, the Mediterranean basin extending into West and Central Asia, Sudan and East Africa, and Brazil (see Table 7.8.12.1).

Around the Mediterranean littoral, across the Middle East and central Asia, and in northern and eastern China, zoonotic visceral leishmaniasis is endemic in many places, where as many as 50% of domestic and stray dogs may be infected. Children under 5 years of age are especially affected. It is the second most common infectious cause of fever of unknown origin in children in the Balkan countries. HIV infection is a risk factor for adults. In other places, the disease is sporadic. Nonimmune adults such as tourists, hunters, and soldiers are susceptible.

The Ganges and Brahamputra river valleys of India and Bangladesh are the home of epidemic anthroponotic visceral leishmaniasis, or kala-azar, which returns approximately every 15 to 20 years. The majority of cases are in young people under 15 years of age and are found in clusters. The annual incidence is about 250 per 100 000. About 50% of household contacts of cases in Bihar India are seropositive, one in four of whom will develop disease. Malnutrition predisposes to clinical disease. In the interepidemic period, the parasite survives in patients with post-kala-azar dermal leishmaniasis.

Visceral leishmaniasis is endemic in parts of Sudan, where it may be both anthroponotic and zoonotic, and in adjacent parts of Ethiopia and Kenya. Older children and teenagers are most commonly affected. Sporadic cases also occur in nomads and visitors. In Sudan, an epidemic that began in the south in the late 1980s and caused over 100 000 deaths between 1984 and 1994 is still raging. It has been especially severe among refugees from the civil war. In remote areas, half the cases do not reach a medical facility and 90% of deaths go unreported.

In South America, the disease is most common in north-eastern Brazil, where older children are affected. Previously a rural disease, it is becoming increasingly important in towns.

Visceral leishmaniasis may appear unexpectedly in immunosuppressed patients, e.g. after renal transplantation, with haematological malignancies, while receiving immunosuppressive drugs, and in pregnant women. In endemic areas, it is an opportunistic infection in patients with HIV infection.

Visceral leishmaniasis may be transmitted by blood transfusion from subclinical cases; parasites were cultured from 2 to 4% of donor blood samples in endemic areas of France and Spain.

Pathogenesis and pathology

For every case of classical visceral leishmaniasis, there are about 30 subclinical infections that cause leishmanin positivity and lifelong immunity to the infecting species. Established visceral infections are characterized by the failure of specific cell-mediated immunity. The leishmanin test is negative. The parasite multiplies freely in macrophages in the spleen, bone marrow, lymphoid tissues, jejunal submucosa, and Kupffer cells of the liver. Histology shows a variable degree of granuloma formation and interstitial inflammation in the liver that may lead to fibrosis. In the spleen especially, there is massive reticuloendothelial hyperplasia and infiltration with plasma cells. Small splenic infarcts may develop.

Antibodies, polyclonal IgG, and immune complexes circulate at high concentration but rarely cause complications. About half of

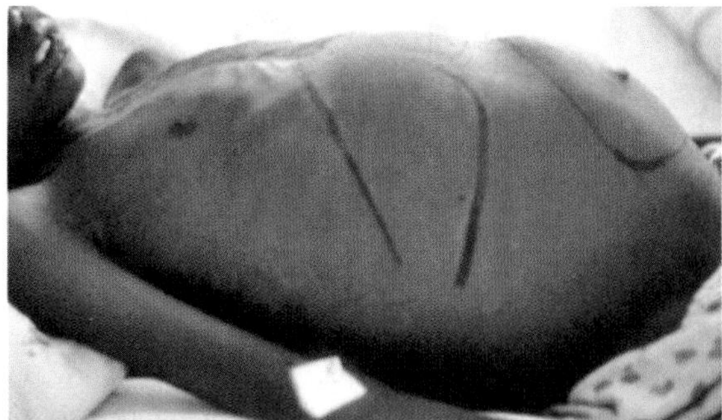

Fig. 7.8.12.13 Visceral leishmaniasis in a Kenyan child. Note the wasting, massive enlargement of liver and spleen, and increased pigmentation.

the patients have mild malabsorption but seldom diarrhoea. When present, jaundice usually has another cause such as viral hepatitis. Spontaneous bleeding is unusual and is associated with hypoprothrombinaemia. Visceral leishmaniasis is characterized by anaemia, leukopenia, thrombocytopenia, and hypoalbuminaemia. The anaemia results mainly from shortened red-cell survival with destruction of cells in the spleen, together with splenic pooling and sequestration (hypersplenism). In young children, profound anaemia may develop rapidly as a result of severe haemolysis. Death is usually due to secondary infection.

Clinical features

The male/female ratio is between 3:1 and 4:1. The incubation period is usually 2 to 8 months. In endemic areas, the onset is usually ill defined. The patient develops fever, discomfort from an enlarged spleen, abdominal swelling, weight loss, cough, or diarrhoea. Classically, the fever spikes twice daily, usually without rigors, but daily, irregular, or undulant fevers are common. During an epidemic or in visitors to an epidemic area, symptoms may start abruptly with high fever and rapid progression of illness with toxaemia, weakness, dyspnoea, and acute anaemia.

Physical examination of early cases may show only symptomless splenomegaly. Patients with advanced disease are wasted, with hair changes and pedal oedema typical of hypoalbuminaemia. Hyperpigmentation is characteristic of visceral leishmaniasis in India (kala-azar means 'black disease'). The spleen is huge, smooth, and nontender unless there has been a recent infarct. The liver is moderately enlarged in one-third of cases. In African patients, a generalized lymphadenopathy is common.

Over months or years the patient becomes emaciated, with a distended abdomen (Fig. 7.8.12.13). Intercurrent infections are common, especially pneumococcal otitis media, pneumonia, septicaemia, tuberculosis, measles, dysentery, other locally important infections, and rarely, cancrum oris. Untreated, between 80 and 90% of patients die.

Post-kala-azar dermal leishmaniasis (PKDL)

About upto 10% of Indian patients and upto 50% of Sudanese patients develop a rash on the face, extensor surfaces of the arms and legs, and trunk after recovery from visceral leishmaniasis. In India, the rash begins after an interval of 1 or 2 years and progresses over many years: pale macules become erythematous plaques, papules, or nodules resembling lepromatous leprosy, and almost the entire body surface may be involved (Fig. 7.8.12.14). In Kenya, the rash usually appears while the patient is still recovering, as discrete nodules, which show a granulomatous histology with

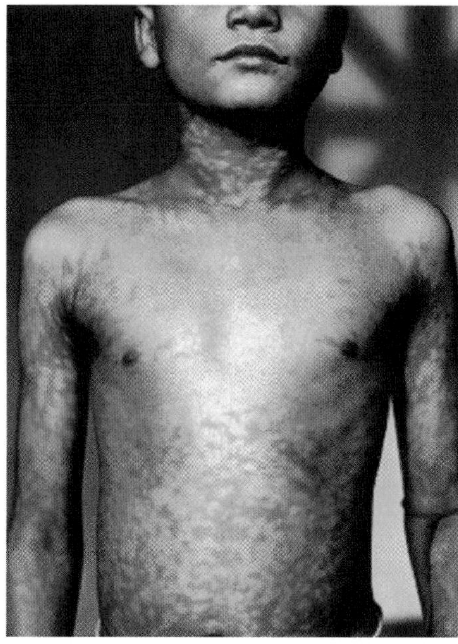

Fig. 7.8.12.14 Post-kala-azar dermal leishmaniasis in an Indian child. Showing the typical hypopigmented macular rash. Note also the nodules on the lower lip.

scanty parasites. It heals spontaneously within 6 months (Fig. 7.8.12.15). Sudanese patients show a mixture of these two forms. PKDL is rarely seen after *L. infantum* infections.

Visceral leishmaniasis and HIV infection

Visceral leishmaniasis may be associated with HIV infection, especially in southern Europe, where it is commonest among intravenous drug users. It may be due to reactivation of latent infection with *Leishmania* or to a recent infection. In Spain, over 50% of adults with visceral leishmaniasis are HIV positive, and it is estimated that 9% of HIV-infected people will acquire visceral leishmaniasis. In northern India, during 2004/05, about 6% of all cases were coinfected with HIV. The presentation may not be typical and there may be unusual skin lesions. Antiretroviral treatment has greatly reduced the clinical impact of coinfection, but in some patients *leishmaniasis* now presents as an immune reconstitution inflammatory syndrome. Often the parasite is found by chance,

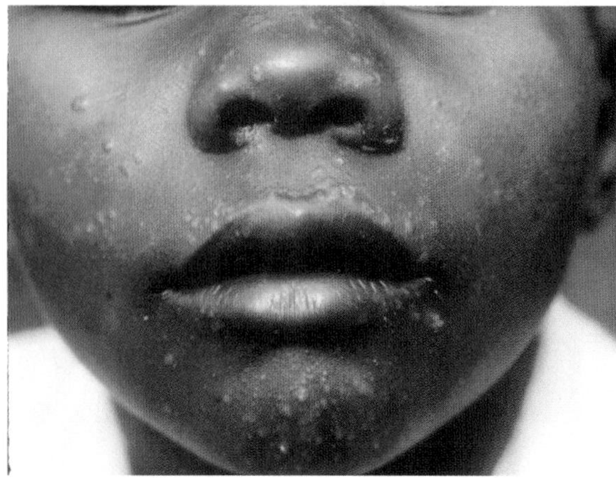

Fig. 7.8.12.15 Post-kala-azar dermal leishmaniasis in a Kenyan child. Showing the typical collection of small discrete nodules on the face.
(Copyright A D M Bryceson.)

e.g. in a rectal or skin biopsy taken for other purposes, or in bronchoscopic lavage. The bone marrow is teeming with parasites but two-thirds of cases have no detectable antileishmanial antibodies. In 90% of cases, the CD4 count is less than 0.2×10^6/litre. Response to treatment is poor and relapse usual (see 'Treatment' below). HIV coinfected people are infective to sandflies and may also transmit parasites by sharing needles.

Laboratory diagnosis

Parasitological diagnosis

Leishmania organisms may be isolated from reticuloendothelial tissue. Yields are of the order of: spleen, over 95% cases; bone marrow or liver, 85%; lymph node in Sudan, 65%; and buffy coat, 70%. Bone marrow aspiration is most commonly used, but splenic aspiration is simple, painless, and safe if the prothrombin time is normal and the platelet count above 40×10^9/litre. Occasionally, the diagnosis is made accidentally on biopsy of bone marrow, liver, lymph node, or bowel mucosa. PCR for leishmanial DNA in bone marrow is even more sensitive. PCR for *leishmanial* DNA in blood is useful for follow up HIV co-infected patients.

Serological diagnosis

Antibodies are present in high titre, useful for diagnosis, and may replace parasite diagnosis in the remote areas. Indirect immunofluorescence is the gold standard but, for fieldwork, it has been replaced by enzyme-linked immunosorbent assay, direct agglutination, and the rK39 antigen dipstick. All give comparable results with sensitivities of about 90% and specificities above 95% (positive predictive value *c.*99% and negative predictive value *c.*70%). The leishmanin skin test is negative.

Other findings

There is normochromic, normocytic anaemia without reticulocytosis, and neutropenia, eosinopenia, and thrombocytopenia. Serum albumin is low (*c.*20 g/litre) and globulin high (*c.*70 g/litre), IgG and IgM being approximately thrice and twice the normal population values. Hepatic enzymes and prothrombin and partial thromboplastin times are usually normal.

Treatment

Chemotherapy

Liposomal amphotericin B by intravenous infusion is the best drug for visceral leishmaniasis in adults and children. It is concentrated and retained in reticuloendothelial cells and is not toxic. Over 99% patients respond promptly, but HIV-coinfected patients relapse. The drug is also effective against PKDL in India and Sudan and it is the drug of choice in pregnancy. At the moment, it is far too costly for most countries where visceral leishmaniasis is endemic, but World Health Organization has recently negotiated a 90% reduction in price. Therefore, a pentavalent antimonial remains the drug of choice in most situations. See Tables 7.8.12.2 and 7.8.12.3 for dosage regimens.

Conventional amphotericin B deoxycholate is cheaper than liposomal amphotericin B and just as effective, though more toxic, and is useful for patients unresponsive to antimonials.

Sodium stibogluconate containing 100 mg Sb/ml and meglumine antimoniate containing 85 mg Sb/ml are of equal efficacy and toxicity. The drug is administered by intramuscular injection, which may be painful, or by intravenous injection through a fine-gauge needle, slowly or by infusion in 50 to 100 ml of 5% dextrose over 20 min to reduce the risk of venous thrombosis. Treatment is given daily for 28 days. Usually the drug is well tolerated but towards the end of treatment there may be malaise, anorexia, nausea, vomiting, and muscle pains. Should toxic effects develop, rest for 1 day and reduce each dose by 2 mg Sb/kg. Hepatic and pancreatic enzyme levels may rise and haemoglobin levels fall, but they return to normal when treatment is stopped. The electrocardiogram develops unimportant T-wave changes. At higher doses, the corrected QT interval may be prolonged, heralding the development of a serious arrhythmia. Cure rates exceed 95% except in Bihar, north of the river Ganges where primary antimony resistance is spreading and up to 60% patients do not respond to antimonials. Secondary resistance develops in patients who relapse.

The aminoglycoside antibiotic paromomycin, or aminosidine, is equally effective and well tolerated, but cure rates vary between countries. It is given by intramuscular injection or intravenous infusion over 90 min. Renal function and hearing should be monitored.

A new oral drug, miltefosine, cures from 90 to 94% of HIV-negative adults and children with visceral leishmaniasis in Sudan and India, even in areas of parasite resistance to antimonials.

Patients who are immunosuppressed as a result of HIV coinfection or immunosuppressive drugs respond slowly, require longer treatment, and are more liable to relapse than immunocompetent patients. Ideally, treatment of such patients should be monitored by splenic aspirate counts of parasites and continued for 2 or 3 weeks beyond parasitological cure. Antimonials cause adverse effects in two-thirds of HIV coinfected patients and may cause pancreatitis. Liposomal amphotericin B and aminosidine are effective and well tolerated. Relapse may be prevented by secondary prophylaxis with pentamidine given every 2 weeks. Highly active retroviral therapy (HAART) reduces the number of relapses and delays their onset.

Supportive treatment

Intercurrent infection must be sought and treated and nutritional deficiencies corrected. Blood transfusion is rarely needed.

Response to treatment

Fever, splenic size, haemoglobin, serum albumin, and body weight are useful monitors of progress. Proof of parasitological cure is not usually necessary. Reassessment at 6 weeks and 6 months will detect over 90% of relapses. Serology is unhelpful in monitoring progress. Relapse rates should be under 4%. Relapsed patients are slower to respond and run a 40% chance of further relapses and of becoming unresponsive to antimony. Primary parasite resistance to antimonials is increasing in India where the next choice lies between miltefosine, aminosidine and amphotericin B deoxycholate. Treatment with two drugs might prevent parasite resistance, and combinations are being tested.

Economic impact

Visceral leishmaniasis is a major economic burden on affected families. The direct costs of an episode of visceral leishmaniasis in rural India or Bangladesh, where the drug is, in principle, provided free, are equivalent to the household's annual income.

Prevention and control of cutaneous and visceral leishmaniasis

Prevention is a matter of controlling reservoir hosts and sandfly vectors or of avoiding bites by vectors. Successful control requires an accurate knowledge of transmission in each ecological focus.

In the Old World, urban cutaneous leishmaniasis is controlled by case-finding and treatment, better housing, and domestic spraying with residual insecticides, while rural leishmaniasis is controlled in the Middle East and North Africa by poisoning or destruction of gerbil colonies. Mediterranean and urban visceral leishmaniasis in South America may be controlled by the destruction or treatment of dogs, but dogs are infectious to flies before they become symptomatic and screening of dogs is problematic. Dog collars impregnated with permethrin reduce the numbers of flies that become infected. In India, mass campaigns to spray houses and cattle sheds are needed. In the interepidemic period, cases of PKDL should be sought and treated. Currently no nation has an effective control programme in place.

In endemic populations, infection may be prevented during the season of transmission by the use of insect repellent creams and fine mesh bed nets, top sheets or chadors (women's outer garments or cloaks) impregnated with permethrin during the hours of biting, usually around dusk and dawn. In endemic foci, a higher level of education in households is associated with lower rates of disease. Vaccines have proved disappointing.

Further reading

Blum J, *et al.* (2004). Treatment of cutaneous leishmaniasis among travellers. *J Antimicrob Chemother*, **53**, 158–66.

Cruz I, *et al.* (2006). *Leishmania*/HIV co-infections in the second decade. *Indian J Med Res*, **123**, 357–88.

den Boer M, Davidson RN (2006). Treatment options for visceral leishmaniasis. *Expert Rev Anti Infect Ther*, **4**, 187–97.

Desjeux P (2001). The increase in risk factors for leishmaniasis worldwide. *Trans R Soc Trop Med Hyg*, **95**, 239–43.

Lockwood DNJ, Sundar S (2006). Serological tests for visceral leishmaniasis. *Br Med J*, **333**, 711–12.

Murray HW, *et al.* (2005). Advances in leishmaniasis. *Lancet*, **366**, 1561–77.

Websites

Centres for Disease Control. http://www.cdc.gov/ncidod/diseases/submenus/sub_leishmania.htm

World Health Organization. *Leishmaniasis.* http://www.who.int/leishmaniasis [Both have good summaries on leishmaniasis and links to new research findings.]

7.8.13 Trichomoniasis

Sharon Hillier

Essentials

Trichomonas vaginalis is a sexually transmitted protozoan pathogen that may cause more than one-half of all curable sexually transmitted genital infections worldwide. Women with trichomoniasis are often asymptomatic, but they may develop vaginal malodour, discharge, erythema, or itching, and their male or female sexual partners may also be infected, although urethritis in men is less likely to cause symptoms. Women with trichomoniasis have an increased risk of HIV acquisition, HIV shedding, pelvic inflammatory disease, and preterm birth. For diagnosis, rapid antigen detection, culture, and polymerase chain reaction (PCR) methods have advantages over conventional microscopy, but are more expensive. Oral metronidazole is usually an effective treatment, with both sexual partners needing to be treated to prevent reinfection.

Acknowledgement: The editors acknowledge the inclusion of material from Dr J P Ackers' chapter in the previous edition of the *Oxford Textbook of Medicine*.

Introduction

Trichomoniasis is an infection of the human urogenital tract caused by the protozoan *Trichomonas vaginalis*. There are about 170 million new cases each year, making it the world's commonest nonviral sexually transmitted infection and, according to the World Health Organization (WHO), it accounts for more than one-half of all curable sexually transmitted infections worldwide. Pregnant women who have trichomoniasis are at increased risk of preterm delivery as well as HIV acquisition and shedding.

Historical perspective

T. vaginalis was first described in 1836. In the preantibiotic era, it was considered a frequent unwanted outcome of sexual activity associated with symptoms but with few adverse health outcomes. With diagnosis and treatment, this infection has become less prevalent in wealthier countries but has remained highly prevalent in the developing world.

Aetiology, genetics, pathogenesis, and pathology

Although there are more than 100 species of this protozoan, only *T. vaginalis* parasitizes the human genital tract. *In vitro*, *T. vaginalis* has a well-defined, contact-mediated, cytotoxic effect, but its relationship to pathogenesis *in vivo* is unknown. It activates complement and attracts neutrophils, which may kill the parasite but, in large numbers, may also contribute to the pathology. The organism produces several proteolytic enzymes which degrade genital tract mucins. In women, *T. vaginalis* may be found in the vagina and the exterior cervix in over 95% of infections, but is recovered from the endocervix in 13%. The urethra and Skene's glands are also commonly infected. In men, the urethra is the most common site of infection but the organism has also been recovered from epididymal aspirates. Dissemination beyond the lower urogenital tract is extremely rare even in severely immunocompromised patients.

Trichomoniasis in women was previously regarded as unpleasant but harmless; however, epidemiological studies have now linked it with a modest increase in the risk of heterosexual HIV transmission, and with complications in pregnancy.

Epidemiology

Understanding the epidemiology of trichomoniasis has been limited by the variability in the sensitivity and accuracy of diagnostic methods used. Although it is often difficult to isolate the organism from male contacts of infected women, epidemiological evidence suggests that *T. vaginalis* is transmitted almost exclusively by sexual intercourse, both during heterosexual intercourse and in sexual activity between female sexual partners. Although the organism can survive for many hours at room temperature if kept damp, there is only limited evidence that this pathogen is transmitted among household members in the absence of sexual exposure. A very small proportion of female babies of infected mothers will become infected during birth, but this infection is transient and trichomoniasis discovered in a child should immediately raise the suspicion of sexual abuse.

Very few studies have been made of genuinely unselected populations; the majority have examined either pregnant women or those attending sexually transmitted disease clinics. Usually cases in women are observed 5 or 10 times more than those in men. *T. vaginalis* has been reported in 18 to 24% of women attending sexual health clinics in the United States of America and in 3 to 34% of women in four African cities. The epidemiology of this pathogen is less well understood among men, but has been reported in 3 to 20% of men attending sexually transmitted disease clinics. Factors associated with trichomoniasis include coinfection with other sexually transmitted pathogens, past infection with *Trichomonas*, being unmarried, having more than one sexual partner, and not using condoms.

In several developed countries, there has been a steady decline in the incidence of trichomoniasis in the past few decades, but this has not occurred in less-developed countries nor in deprived inner-city areas in industrialized nations. Human trichomoniasis is becoming a disease of the underprivileged.

Prevention

Because up to one-half of infected individuals are asymptomatic, the only way to reduce the population prevalence of this pathogen is through screening of individuals and providing treatment to individuals and their sexual partners. Several studies have documented improved cure rates in women whose male partners received treatment. Persons who report use of male or female condoms have a reduced incident of recurrent trichomoniasis. There is no effective vaccine against *T. vaginalis.*

Clinical features

In women, *T. vaginalis* can infect the vagina, urethra, and the Bartholin's and Skene's glands. From 10 to 50% of cases are asymptomatic but acute inflammatory diseases may occur, with copious and malodorous vaginal discharge, vulvovaginal soreness and irritation, dysuria, and dyspareunia. Trichomoniasis is significantly associated with purulent yellow vaginal discharge, vulvar itching, and colpitis macularis (strawberry cervix) detectable by colposcopy, with vulval and vaginal erythema. Vaginal pH is usually elevated and concomitant bacterial vaginosis is common. The discharge fluctuates with time and, if untreated, may disappear spontaneously or persist for months or even years.

Most men with trichomoniasis are asymptomatic, but the parasite is responsible for a small but increasing proportion of cases of nongonococcal urethritis.

Differential diagnosis

In women, vaginal discharge syndromes including bacterial vaginosis, yeast vulvovaginitis, and trichomoniasis should be considered (see Chapter 8.4). Women who present with vaginal discharge, vulvar itching, and/or vaginal malodour may have no infection, or could have any combination of these common vaginal infections. In men, other causes of urethritis should be ruled out.

Criteria for diagnosis

An accurate diagnosis cannot be made based upon signs or symptoms elicited during the clinical evaluation.

Trichomoniasis in women

The most commonly used method for diagnosis is identification of the pathogen in vaginal (not endocervical) secretions examined under the microscope at ×400 magnification. In clinical specimens or culture, *T. vaginalis* is a motile and round or oval flagellate, 10 to 13 μm long and 8 to 10 μm wide. Fixed and stained, it is about 25% smaller (Fig. 7.8.13.1). Diagnostic features include the jerky motility, undulating membrane, and microtubular rod (axostyle), which runs through the body and projects as a thin spine from the posterior end. In contact with vaginal epithelial cells *in vitro*, the organism becomes extremely flattened and adherent. The life cycle is simple; no resistant cysts are formed and there are no intermediate or reservoir hosts. Two other trichomonads, *T. tenax* and *Pentatrichomonas hominis*, are uncommon and probably harmless human parasites of the mouth and large bowel, respectively. All three species are site specific. Urogenital trichomoniasis is not due to contamination from other sites.

Microscopy is inexpensive and can be used as a bedside diagnostic test, allowing immediate treatment of infected people. However, its sensitivity is only 65 to 80% and it requires a microscope. Broth culture methods for detection of *T. vaginalis* have the advantage of greater sensitivity, but require up to 5 days' incubation. Diamond's TYM and the very convenient if rather expensive InPouch system

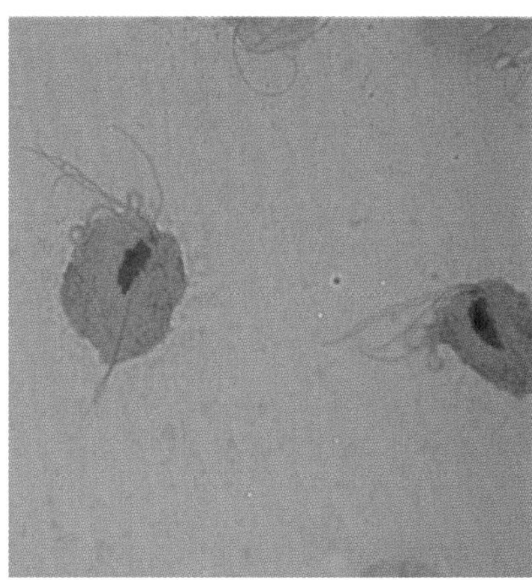

Fig. 7.8.13.1 Trichomonads in vaginal secretions (Giemsa stain). (Copyright J P Ackers.)

are among the best. Rapid antigen tests can be performed within the clinic in a few minutes. Their sensitivity and specificity are equivalent to those of culture, with the advantage of providing results during the clinic visit. The polymerase chain reaction (PCR) has the highest sensitivity and specificity for diagnosis of *T. vaginalis* but is expensive and requires specialized equipment, limiting its implementation. Specimens for PCR can be obtained less invasively with self-administered tampons.

Trichomoniasis in men

For diagnosis of urethritis due to trichomonas in men, culture or PCR is essential as the sensitivity of microscopy with urethral swab or scrapings, centrifuged urine sediment, or prostatic fluid is only 10 to 20%.

Treatment

The first, and the so-far only effective, drugs are 5-nitroimidazoles. A single 2 g dose of oral metronidazole is most widely used. The alternative is 250 mg three times a day for 7 days. Recurrence occurs in 8 to 20% of women in the first month after therapy. About half the occurrences are attributed to reinfection by the same or a new sexual partner. Women who experience treatment failure are more likely to have isolates of *T. vaginalis* that show reduced susceptibility to metronidazole *in vitro*. Single-dose metronidazole may not be adequate to treat these patients. Sexual partners must also be treated. Only the 7-day regimen has been extensively evaluated in men, in whom it appears as effective as in women.

Prognosis

In most women who receive appropriate treatment, symptoms will resolve but they are at increased risk of becoming infected with *Trichomonas* in the future. Men may spontaneously clear their infections, but unless both sexual partners are treated, reinfection is common.

Areas of uncertainty or controversy

Trichomonisis has been linked with preterm birth, pelvic inflammatory disease (Chapter 8.5), and an increased risk of HIV. However, metronidazole treatment has failed to reduce the risk of preterm delivery or acquisition of HIV. No study has yet documented that accurate diagnosis and treatment of trichomoniasis provides a long-term health benefit for men and women.

Likely developments in the near future

Broader implementation of specific and sensitive screening tests and prospective studies of treatment should reveal whether routine screening and treatment of *T. vaginalis* reduces morbidity.

Further reading

Hobbs MM, *et al.* (2008). *Trichomonas vaginalis and trichomoniasis.* In: Holmes KK, *et al.* (eds) *Sexually transmitted diseases*, 6th edition, pp. 773–93. McGraw-Hill, New York.

Honigberg BM (ed) (1989). *Trichomonads parasitic in humans.* Springer-Verlag, New York.

Huppert JS, *et al.* (2007). Rapid antigen testing compares favorably with transcriptase-mediated amplification assay for the detection of *Trichomonas vaginalis* in young women. *Clin Infect Dis*, **45**, 194–8.

Johnston VJ, Mabey DC (2008). Global epidemiology and control of *Trichomonas vaginalis. Curr Opin Infect Dis*, **21**, 56–64.

Kissinger P, *et al.* (2008). Early repeated infections with *Trichomonas vaginalis* among HIV-positive and HIV-negative women. *Clin Infect Dis*, **46**, 994–9.

Petrin D *et al.* (1998). Clinical and microbiological aspects of *Trichomonas vaginalis. Clin Microbiol Rev*, **11**, 300–17.

Krieger JN (1995). Trichomoniasis in men: old issues and new data. *Sex Transm Dis*, **22**, 83–96.

Van der Pol B, *et al.* (2008). *Trichomonas vaginalis* infection and human immunodeficiency virus acquisition in African women. *J Infect Dis*, **197**, 548–54.

7.9

Nematodes (roundworms)

Contents

7.9.1 Cutaneous filariasis *1145*
Gilbert Burnham

7.9.2 Lymphatic filariasis *1153*
Richard Knight and D.H. Molyneux

7.9.3 Guinea worm disease (dracunculiasis) *1160*
Richard Knight

7.9.4 Strongyloidiasis, hookworm, and other gut strongyloid nematodes *1163*
Michael Brown

7.9.5 Gut and tissue nematode infections acquired by ingestion *1168*
David I. Grove

7.9.6 Parastrongyliasis (angiostrongyliasis) *1179*
Richard Knight

7.9.7 Gnathostomiasis *1182*
Valai Bussaratid and Pravan Suntharasamai

7.9.1 Cutaneous filariasis

Gilbert Burnham

Essentials

Filarial infections are transmitted by simulium flies, some of which bite humans almost exclusively, whereas others are to varying degrees zoophilic. They are found worldwide in humans and animals, the filariae which cause cutaneous infections being *Onchocerca volvulus*, *Loa loa*, and the mansonellas.

Onchocerciasis

Onchocerciasis (river blindness), caused by *O. volvulus*, infects perhaps 20 million people, mostly in Africa.

Clinical features—larvae introduced into the body when the vector takes a blood meal develop into male or female adult worms within palpable nodules, commonly located over bony prominences. Other important manifestations are: (1) Eye damage—microfilariae enter the cornea from the skin and conjunctiva; manifestations include sclerosing keratitis, iridocyclitis and (sometimes) choroidoretinal lesions; without treatment permanent visual impairment or blindness are common. (2) Skin disease—ranging from itching with a localized maculopapular rash, to intensely itching with a chronic generalised papular rash or lichenified hyperkeratotic lesions.

Diagnosis, treatment, and prevention—diagnosis is usually made by finding microfilariae in skin snips. Treatment is with ivermectin, often given as a single annual dose, which has dramatically reduced the eye and skin lesions that ravaged many communities in Africa and Latin America. Methods of prevention include adding insecticides to rivers to interrupt simulium breeding and mass distribution of ivermectin.

Loa loa

This filaria, for which humans are the only host, is transmitted by the chrysops fly in West and Central Africa. Clinical manifestations include transient localized inflammatory oedema (Calabar swellings), the appearance of a migrating worm under the skin or (most dramatically) crossing the eye, and (rarely) meningoencephalitis. Diagnosis is based on typical clinical findings, or traditionally by finding microfilariae in a daytime blood sample. Treatment is usually with diethylcarbamazine. The best prevention is avoiding chrysops fly bites.

Mansonellas

This group of filarial infections is transmitted by culicoides midges and is common to many countries, but of negligible clinical importance under most circumstances. Only *Mansonella streptocerca* produces clear-cut manifestations, most typically chronic papular skin lesions. Diagnosis is by finding characteristic microfilariae in the blood or skin. People who are asymptomatic do not require treatment, but *M. streptocerca* responds well to ivermectin.

Onchocerciasis

Onchocerciasis, or river blindness, occurs in 34 countries in Africa, Latin America, and the Arabian Peninsula (Fig. 7.9.1.1). Perhaps 18 million people are infected, the vast majority in Africa. In 1995 it was estimated that infection with *Onchocerca volvulus* had caused blindness in 270 000 people, and left another 500 000 with severe visual impairment. It is likely that mass treatment with ivermectin has now greatly lessened the ocular burden of infection. Besides eye changes, onchocerciasis has chronic systemic effects, causing extensive and disfiguring skin changes, musculoskeletal complaints, weight loss, changes to the immune system, and perhaps also epilepsy and growth arrest. Skin lesions are the most common manifestation of onchocerciasis. Changes include acute and chronic itchy papular disease, and intensely pruritic lichenification. Lesions may be localized or widespread. In the later stages severe degenerative skin disease develops, with a loss of elastic tissue, and extensive pigmentary changes.

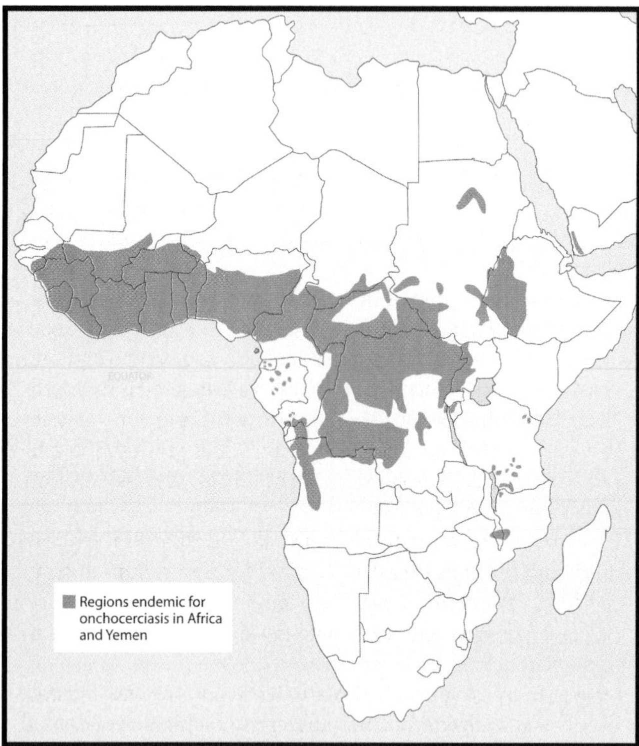

(a)

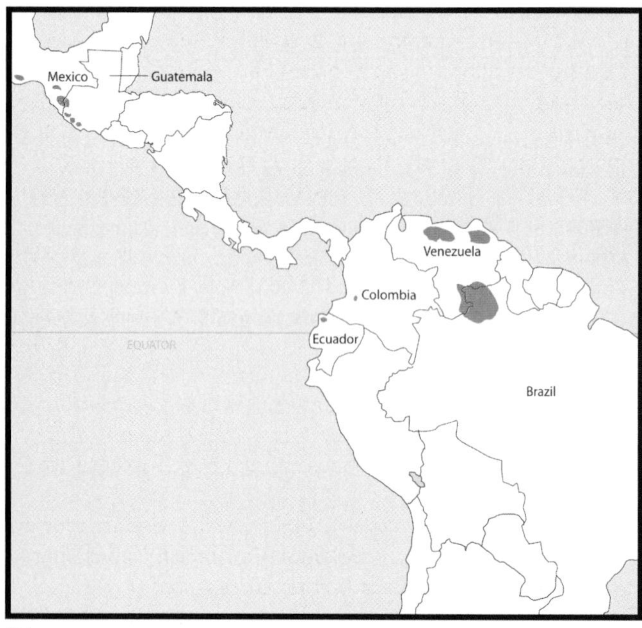

(b)

Fig. 7.9.1.1 Distribution of onchocerciasis in Africa, the Middle East, and Latin America.

The disease, endemic to some of the world's poorest areas, has a great impact on the economic and social fabric of communities. A complex human–parasite tolerance allows people who host millions of parasites to continue daily existence. Mass treatment with ivermectin has blunted the public health consequences of this disease in many heavily infected areas.

Epidemiology

The microfilariae of *O. volvulus* were first observed by O'Neill in Ghana in 1875 in an intensely pruritic chronic skin condition called 'craw-craw'. Leuckart described the adult worm 20 years later, and in 1923 Blacklock in Sierra Leone showed the blackfly *Simulium damnosum* to be the vector. Hissette in the Congo and Robles in Guatemala linked blindness with onchocerciasis. Long before, Ghanaians along the Red Volta river had associated the biting flies with skin lesions and blindness.

The Onchocerciasis Control Programme controlled vector breeding in West Africa's Volta basin between 1974 and 2002, and is thought to have prevented 600 000 cases of blindness. Today, the largest numbers of infected people live in Nigeria, Cameroon, Chad, Ethiopia, Uganda, Angola, and the Democratic Republic of the Congo. In the Americas, onchocerciasis is most common in the highland areas of Guatemala. Other countries with disease foci are Mexico, Venezuela, Colombia, Brazil, Ecuador, and Yemen. Within foci, the disease may be distributed unevenly.

In Africa, blindness was traditionally noted to be more common in savannah and woodland than rainforest areas, but people in forest areas had more depigmented skin disease. Different strains or forms of the parasite were shown to be present in savannah and woodland areas, particularly in West Africa. Environmental changes and migrations have now lessened these distinctions. Onchocercal skin disease reduces marital prospects (and dowry size), disrupts social relationships, and decreases the productivity of agricultural workers.

Parasitology

The larvae of *O. volvulus* enter the human during a blood meal taken by an infected female simulium fly. Within 1 to 3 months, larvae develop into male or female adult worms within palpable nodules commonly located over the bony prominences of the thorax, pelvic girdle, or knees (Fig. 7.9.1.2). Nodules may also be found on the head, particularly among children. These average 3 cm in diameter and are easily palpable, but some are deep, particularly around the pelvis.

A female worm may release 1300 to 1900 microfilariae per day for 9 to 11 years. From the nodules, these microfilariae find their way mainly to the skin and eyes. In the skin they are found predominantly in the subepidermal lymphatics. In the eye, most

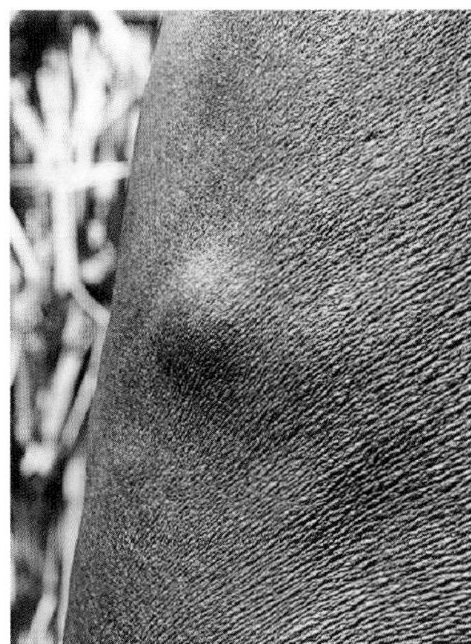

Fig. 7.9.1.2 A 3-cm subcutaneous nodule.

microfilariae are in the anterior chamber, but are also found in the retina and optic nerve. When an infected human is bitten, anticoagulants from the simulium fly create a pool of blood from which blood and microfilariae are ingested. Within the fly, those microfilariae that survive moult twice over the following 6 to 12 days to become infective larvae.

Microfilariae are about 250 to 300 µm in length and may live for up to 2 years. They move easily through the skin and connective tissue, ordinarily remaining within lymphatic vessels and provoking little reaction while alive. They have been seen in blood, urine, cerebrospinal fluid, and internal organs. Millions of microfilariae may be present in a heavily infected person. Although live microfilariae are tolerated by their human hosts, dead and dying microfilariae may evoke intense inflammatory reactions, which are responsible for the eye and skin damage. Tolerance of microfilariae may be regulated by major histocompatibility complex (MHC)-encoded molecules.

Important *Simulium* spp. are complexes made up of sibling species, identifiable through the banding patterns of their larval chromosomes. In Africa, the main vectors are members of the *S. damnosum* complex or *sensu lato* (*s.l.*), which can fly long distances. The vectors in areas of Uganda, Tanzania, Ethiopia, and the Congo are members of the *S. neavei* complex. In the Americas, complexes of *S. ochraceum*, *S. metallicum*, and *S. exiguum* are the principal vectors; these cover shorter distances. Some simulium flies will bite humans almost exclusively, whereas other species are to varying degrees zoophilic.

Simulium develop in water courses varying in size from broad rivers to small streams, depending on the individual sibling species. Rapidly flowing water provides the oxygenation needed for the development of the immature stages. Most larvae and pupae develop on rocks or vegetation just below the water surface, but those of *S. neavei* develop on amphibious *Potamonautes* crabs. During this development period the larvae are susceptible to insecticides. These breeding patterns have made the larviciding of water sources an effective control approach. Unique relationships have developed between the simulium fly and local parasites, so that flies from one geographical area do not efficiently transmit parasites from other areas. Simulium flies of the Americas are in general less efficient at transmission than those of Africa, particularly those in savannah regions.

Clinical features

The manifestations of onchocerciasis are almost entirely caused by localized host inflammatory responses to dead or dying microfilariae. In a heavily infected person, 100 000 or more microfilariae die every day. The predominant immune response in onchocerciasis is antibody mediated, but with an important cellular component. Inflammatory responses may vary considerably between groups of people, depending on the length of exposure to antigens and the down-regulating activities of the host's immune system.

Eosinophils play an important role in the inflammatory response. Cellular proteins derived from eosinophils are deposited in connective tissues throughout the dermis, and bind to elastic fibres causing their destruction and, thereby, skin damage (see 'Skin disease' below).

An important discovery was that filarial parasites host endosymbiotic wolbachia bacteria. The inflammatory response to onchocerciasis seems largely attributable to the wolbachia rather than to the parasite itself. When the parasites were depleted of their wolbachia by doxycycline they did not induce corneal lesions. Further studies showed that inflammatory changes in the cornea in response to wolbachia were dependent on the expression of myeloid differentiation factor 88.

Exposure of the fetus to antigens associated with the parasite *in utero* and through breast milk may induce immune tolerance in residents of endemic areas. This could explain the difference in the disease patterns seen in people from nonendemic areas who become infected.

Among those coinfected with HIV there is a lessened reactivity to *O. volvulus* antigens, but no difference in adverse reactions following ivermectin treatment.

Eye damage

The risk of visual impairment increases as the prevalence and intensity of infection rises in a community. Microfilariae enter the cornea from the skin and conjunctiva. Punctate keratitis develops around dead microfilariae, and clears when inflammation settles. In those exposed to years of heavy infection, sclerosing keratitis and iridocyclitis are likely to develop, causing permanent visual impairment or blindness.

The first sign of sclerosing keratitis (Fig. 7.9.1.3a) is haziness at the medial and lateral margins of the cornea. This is followed by the migration of pigment onto the cornea, accompanied by a progressive ingrowth of vessels. Gradually the cornea becomes opacified. The central and superior areas are the last involved. Although eye lesions can be found wherever onchocerciasis occurs, blindness is most common in the West African savannah. Before control efforts began in Burkina Faso, 46% of men and 35% of women would eventually become blind.

Posterior segment lesions, which can coexist with anterior eye lesions, may be caused by inflammation around microfilariae entering the retina along the posterior ciliary vessels (Fig. 7.9.1.3b). Chorioretinal lesions are commonly seen at the outer side of the macula, or encircling the optic disc. Posterior segment changes are an important cause of loss of vision in Liberia. Optic atrophy has been reported in 1 to 4% of people with onchocerciasis in

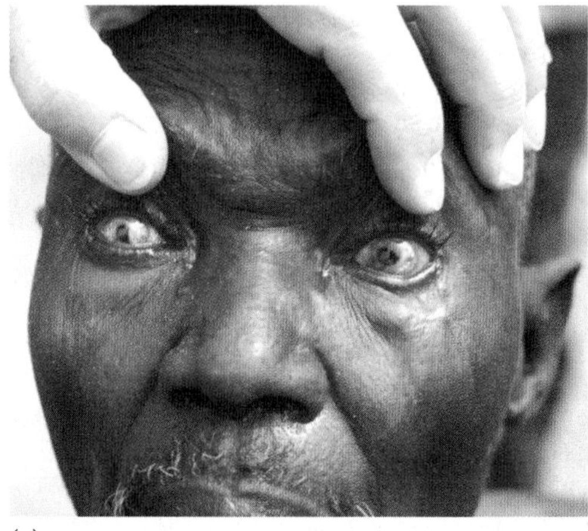

(a)

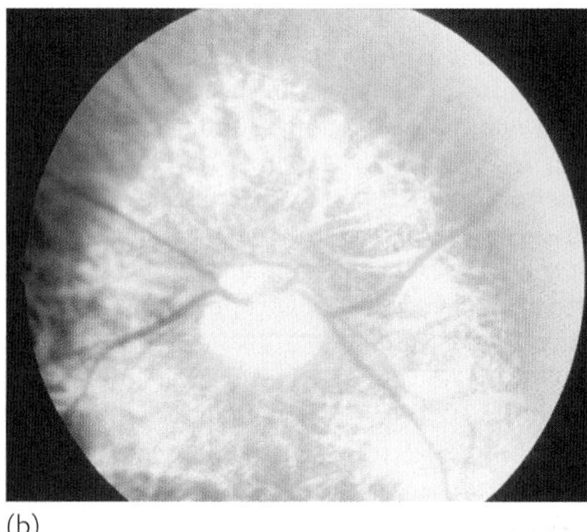

(b)

Fig. 7.9.1.3 (a) Bilateral sclerosing keratitis in a man blinded by onchocerciasis in Nigeria and (b) onchocerciasis producing a Hissette–Ridley fundus and optic atrophy in a person with central keyhole vision remaining.
(a, courtesy of Professor A D M Bryceson; b, courtesy of the Royal Tropical Institute, Amsterdam.)

Cameroon, and 6 to 9% in northern Nigeria. Loss of peripheral vision is well recognized in onchocerciasis.

Skin disease

Of all the consequences of onchocerciasis, skin lesions are the most pervasive. Surveys of seven endemic sites in five African countries found that between 40 and 50% of adults had troublesome itching, which was so intense in some cases that the victims slept on their elbows and knees to minimize the symptom.

In its mildest form, onchocerciasis presents as itching with a localized maculopapular rash (Fig. 7.9.1.4). These reactive lesions and itching may be evanescent, clearing completely without treatment in a few months. In other instances, the papular lesions may become chronic, generalized, and accompanied by severe itching (Fig. 7.9.1.5). Oedema and excoriations can be associated, and lesions may heal with hyperpigmentation. Particularly distressing are lichenified hyperkeratotic lesions, which may be widespread and intensely itchy (Fig. 7.9.1.6). A localized form of chronic papular dermatitis, often confined to one extremity, is known as 'sowda', Arabic for dark. In this condition, first described from Yemen, there is an exceptionally strong IgG antibody response.

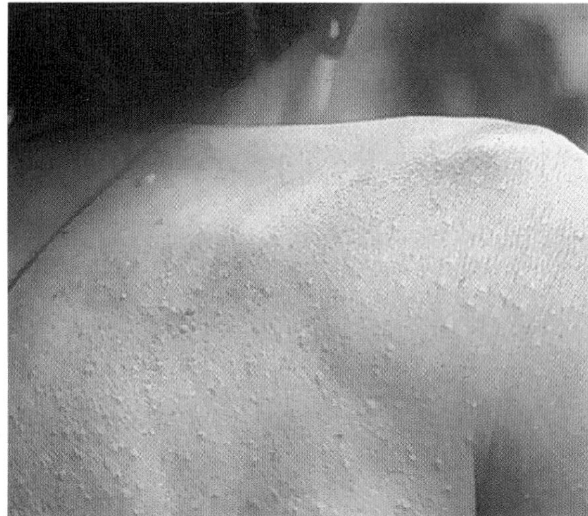

Fig. 7.9.1.4 Maculopapular rash.
Courtesy of Mauricio Sauerbrey.

Light-skinned expatriates infected while visiting an endemic area may present 1 year or more later with intensely itchy and red macular or maculopapular lesions. These may be confined to one area of the body or be more generalized, and may be associated with fever, muscle and joint pain, and sometimes oedema. Rash may sometimes persist for several months following ivermectin treatment.

In endemic areas, degenerative skin changes may develop in some people with long-standing infection. Elastic fibres are destroyed, leaving the skin thinned with a wrinkled cigarette-paper appearance. The atrophied skin begins to sag, the most extreme state being 'hanging groin' with its apron-like skin folds (Fig. 7.9.1.7). Depigmentation of the pretibial areas, or 'leopard skin', is a characteristic finding in older people living in endemic areas (Fig. 7.9.1.8).

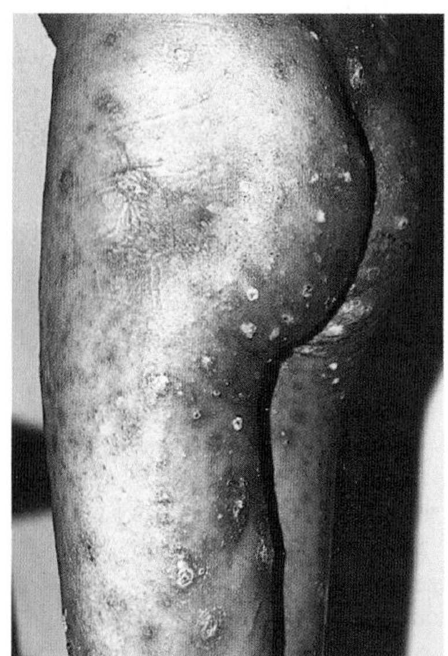

Fig. 7.9.1.5 Excoriated papular lesions of onchocerciasis with hyperpigmentation.

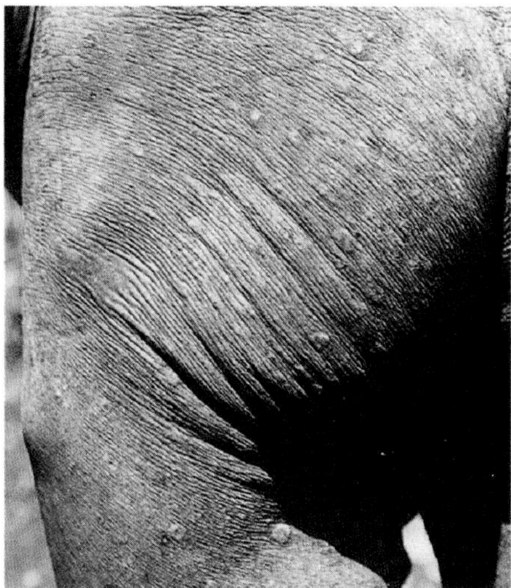

Fig. 7.9.1.6 Lichenified skin lesions with atrophy.

Other conditions associated with onchocerciasis

Both men and women with onchocerciasis weigh less than uninfected people and report more musculoskeletal pains. Evidence, first from Uganda and more recently from other African countries, has suggested a possible association between epilepsy and onchocerciasis. There is also evidence for an association between increasing microfilarial load and excess mortality.

A peculiar pattern of growth arrest beginning around the age of 6 to 10 years was reported from a Ugandan onchocerciasis focus near Jinja in 1951. This Nakalanga syndrome now seems to have disappeared from the area following the elimination of onchocerciasis, but has been noted in western Uganda, and may be present in Burundi.

Diagnosis

Finding microfilariae in skin snips has been the time-honoured method of diagnosis. Microfilariae lie close to the surface, and are most plentiful in the iliac crest area, except in Latin America, where they are more common in the shoulder and scapular areas. Using either a scalpel blade or a sclerocorneal punch, four to six snips (about 5 mg each) are taken under sterile conditions and immersed in normal saline. Microfilariae swimming free of the skin fragments can be counted easily with a dissecting microscope within 24 h. The examination of excised onchocercal nodules shows sections of adult worms. Enzyme immunoassay and polymerase chain reaction (PCR) diagnostic methods have a high degree of sensitivity and specificity. Eosinophilia is common in onchocerciasis.

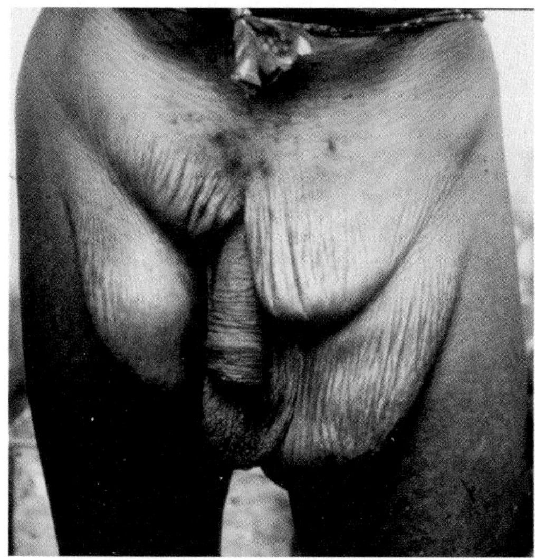

Fig. 7.9.1.7 'Hanging groins'.
(Courtesy of the late Dr B O L Duke.)

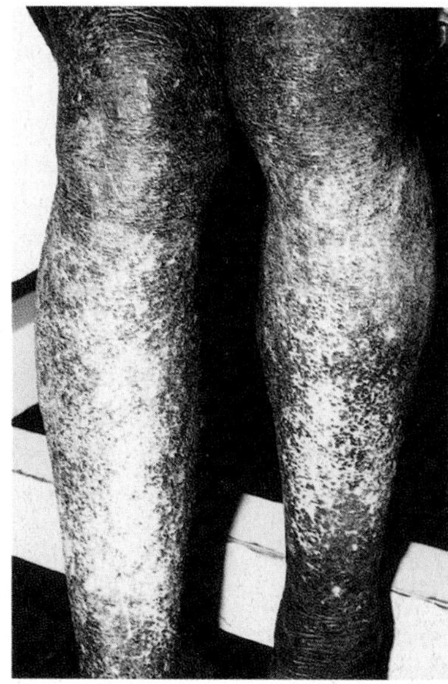

Fig. 7.9.1.8 Depigmented 'leopard skin'.

The Mazzotti test, in which people with onchocerciasis react with itching and a skin rash to 50 mg of oral diethylcarbamazine, is seldom needed for diagnosis, and can be dangerous in heavy infections.

For community assessment, the prevalence of nodules in 30 to 50 men over the age of 20 years, multiplied by 1.5, gives the approximate community prevalence of onchocerciasis. Where the prevalence of nodules is more than 40% the risk of blinding disease is high.

Treatment

The introduction of ivermectin for onchocerciasis in 1987 was one of the milestones of tropical disease treatment. The symptoms of onchocerciasis can be effectively controlled by the treatment of individuals attending clinics, or through the mass treatment of endemic communities.

Ivermectin is derived from *Streptomyces avermitilis*. A single dose of 150–200 μg/kg clears microfilariae from the skin for several months. Annual treatment controls microfilarial counts, and prevents the progression of clinical findings, although in some locations it is given twice yearly, with the intention of interrupting transmission. Treatment can be repeated if itching returns before the next dose is due. In the absence of reinfection, treatment should probably be continued for 10 years or more, or until adult worms stop producing microfilariae. In Nigeria, after 8 years of treatment, gross visual impairment decreased from 16% to 1%, nodule prevalence fell from 59% to 18%, and papular skin dermatitis reduced from 15% to 2%. Treatment in pregnancy and under the age of 5 years is not recommended, although there has been no clear evidence of harm (increased risk of malformations or abortions) where treatment has been given inadvertently.

Limiting the numbers of microfilariae through annual ivermectin treatment improves early and advanced anterior segment eye lesions, halts the development of optic nerve disease, and improves severe onchocercal skin lesions. Adverse reactions to ivermectin commonly consist of increased itching, swelling of the face or extremities, and headache and body pains. Hypotension has been reported rarely after treatment in heavily infected people. Bullae have been seen occasionally. The most pronounced adverse reactions occur after the first ivermectin treatment, decreasing after subsequent treatment cycles. Ivermectin has no adverse effects in uninfected people. Although ivermectin temporarily reduces the release of microfilariae by adult worms, it does not destroy the adults. Those coinfected with *Loa loa*, are at risk of developing potentially fatal central nervous system events after treatment with ivermectin. Although most severe reactions occur with *L. loa* counts more than 30 000 microfilariae/ml, caution should be observed when treating anyone with counts greater than 8000 microfilariae/ml. It has been suggested that treatment with ivermectin in coinfected people be preceded by a 3-week course of albendazole to bring the *L. loa* count to less than 8000 microfilariae/ml.

Ivermectin appears to have three separate actions against the parasite. In microfilariae it acts primarily on parasite neurotransmitters, producing paralysis. This action appears to be mediated by the potentiation or direct opening of glutamate-gated chloride channels. The prolonged disappearance of microfilariae after a single treatment is the result of the drug's effect on embryogenesis in the adult female worm. There is also a slight and poorly understood direct effect on the adult worm.

Resistance to ivermectin has been reported in livestock. In 2007, in an area in Ghana where many treatments had been given, the ivermectin effect of reducing embryogenesis was noted to have lessened, although ivermectin still retained its microfilaricidal effects. This has not been seen elsewhere, and may reflect irregular treatment patterns among some persons in these Ghana foci. As ivermectin is the only agent currently available for the control of onchocerciasis, the development of widespread parasite resistance would be of very serious consequence.

Prevention and control

Methods have included insecticides added to rivers to interrupt simulium breeding, mass distribution of ivermectin, and nodulectomy in an attempt to prevent blindness.

Vector control

Killing simulium larvae by adding the insecticide dichlorodiphenyltrichloroethane (DDT) to rivers eliminated onchocerciasis in Kenya and the Mabari forest of Uganda. In 1974, the Onchocerciasis Control Programme was formed to control simulium by larviciding rivers in the Volta basin of West Africa using ecologically suitable compounds. This highly successful vector control programme, later supplemented with ivermectin distribution, has now permitted tens of millions of people to live free of disease. Mass distribution of ivermectin is now the principal method for onchocerciasis control, although vector control may still be appropriate in a few locations.

Ivermectin mass distribution

After the effectiveness of ivermectin had been shown, its manufacturer Merck & Co. established the Mectizan Donation Program to provide the drug free 'for as long as necessary to as many as necessary'. Between 1988 and 2007, nearly 600 million ivermectin treatments had been administered in endemic countries.

The goal of a control programme may be either complete eradication of the parasite reservoir or elimination of the public health and socioeconomic consequences of continuing infection. In Guatemala, where high population coverage with 6-monthly treatment has reduced parasite transmission by 80 to 100% after 3 years, elimination of infection may ultimately be possible, and this will be true elsewhere in Latin America where sustained treatment is implemented.

The Onchocerciasis Elimination Program in the Americas, and the African Programme for Onchocerciasis Control, are supported by the World Bank and other agencies to eliminate the public health consequences of infection. These programmes focus on regular mass administration of ivermectin through community-based distributors and mobile teams.

Because of the long lifespan of adult worms, ivermectin distribution programmes must be sustained for a period of 15 to 20 years, or perhaps longer. In some places, the duration may be indefinite as a result of the difficulty in achieving good coverage because of continuing insecurity. Taking ivermectin does not prevent new infections.

Nodulectomy

A third form of onchocerciasis control has been the nodulectomy programmes of Mexico and Guatemala. For many years, health workers have moved from village to village removing nodules, especially around the head. The evidence for this preventing blindness is not strong.

Eliminating infections

Although ivermectin brings great relief to the individual, and has a clear impact on the disease in mass distribution programmes, it does not kill adult worms. While symptoms and risks are controlled through annual treatment, the disease itself is not eradicated, and the potential for the development of drug resistance remains. A number of macrofilaricidal drugs capable of eliminating the disease through the killing of adult worms have been tested, but none has so far proved suitable for either individual or mass treatment. It is the availability of a safe, inexpensive macrofilaricidal drug that will make the final elimination of onchocerciasis possible.

Loiasis

Loa loa is a filaria transmitted by *Chrysops* spp. flies in West and Central Africa. The adult worm migrates beneath the skin, and sometimes across the eye, moving at about 1 cm per minute. Periodically, the infection causes sudden but transient localized inflammatory oedema known as Calabar swellings.

Parasitology

The larvae of *L. loa* burrow into human skin during feeding of the chrysops or mangrove fly (*C. silacea* or *C. dimidiata*). In humans, the parasites mature and live in the fascial layers. After 1 year or more, microfilariae are produced. Microfilariae are most heavily present in the blood in the daytime, between 10.00 and 15.00, when the chrysops fly bites. Once taken up by the fly, microfilariae go through developmental stages in the fly's thoracic muscles. After 10 days the fly is able to infect a human, and can do so for another 5 days.

Epidemiology

Infection is most common around the Gulf of Guinea, particularly in Nigeria and Cameroon, but extends through Central Africa into Chad, Sudan, and Uganda, and south to the Congo and Angola (Fig. 7.9.1.9). Humans are the only host, although a similar parasite is found in monkeys in the same areas. The fly lives in the rainforest canopy, and descends to bite humans, attracted perhaps by movement. Transmission may be most intense during the rainy season, when flies are breeding on the muddy banks of forest streams.

Clinical features

The first clinical symptoms of loiasis may appear as soon as 5 months after infection, or as late as 13 years. Calabar swellings appear suddenly, most commonly on the forearms or wrists, and sometimes following heavy exercise or exposure to heat. These oedematous lesions are red and itchy, and may be associated with fever and irritability, but are generally nontender. After several days the affected part returns to normal. However, recurrence is common at irregular intervals. Swellings are not confined to the arms, but may be present in the face, breasts or legs. Calabar swellings are a hypersensitivity reaction to worm antigens, which may be released in the process of migration or perhaps during the maturation of the worm. A high proportion of eosinophils are seen in peripheral blood smears, often exceeding 70%.

A second common feature is the appearance of a migrating worm (Fig. 7.9.1.10). This may be under the skin in any location, but is most dramatic when it crosses the eye ('eye worm'; Fig. 7.9.1.11). Other than local irritation of the conjunctiva while the worm is passing, and the obvious concern of the host, there are no serious consequences. The time of passage may last from 30 min to more than 1 day.

Rare but potentially serious consequences of *L. loa* are meningoencephalitis, renal disease, and endomyocardial fibrosis. Arthralgias have also been noted. The meningoencephalitis may occur spontaneously, although usually after treatment with diethylcarbamazine or ivermectin. Fatalities have been reported following treatment. The renal and endocardial complications of loiasis may have an immune origin.

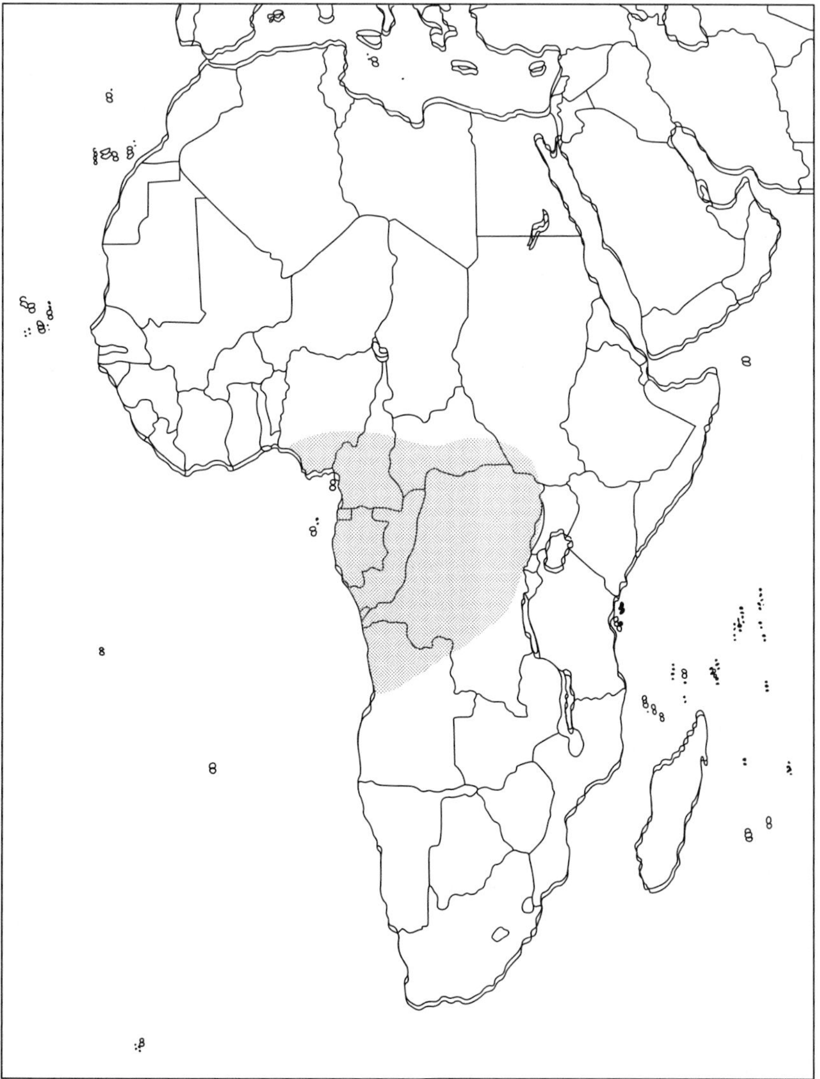

Fig. 7.9.1.9 Map of the approximate distribution of *Loa loa*.

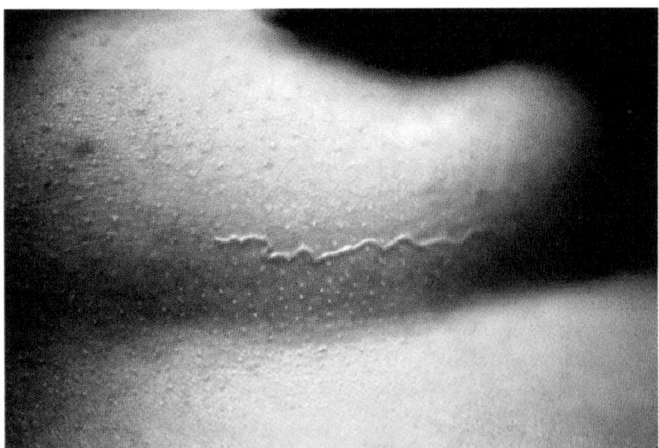

Fig. 7.9.1.10 Migrating *Loa loa*.

Laboratory diagnosis

Diagnosis has traditionally been by the finding of microfilariae in a daytime blood sample, or by a history or typical clinical findings. The use of more sensitive PCR methods has shown that many, even perhaps most, of those infected do not have microfilariae in their peripheral blood.

Treatment

The standard treatment has been diethylcarbamazine, which kills microfilariae and many adult worms. The treatment is commonly given in doses of 5-mg/kg divided into 3 daily doses for 21 days. Fever, arthralgia, and itching can occur during treatment. Ivermectin at 200 µg/kg dramatically decreases the number of microfilariae and some of the loiasis symptoms, but has little macrofilaricidal effect. Two courses of treatment may be required. As with diethylcarbamazine, there is a risk of potentially fatal meningoencephalitis in those with high microfilarial counts. It is prudent not to treat those with concomitant onchocerciasis until *L. loa* counts have been reduced below 8000 microfilariae/ml with albendazole.

Since many people with loiasis also have onchocerciasis, careful monitoring for severe eye and skin inflammation is important when giving diethylcarbamazine. A single treatment is unlikely to eradicate all adult worms, and in endemic areas reinfection is probable. Blood films for microfilariae or PCR tests should be followed to indicate the need for retreatment. Ivermectin is very active against microfilariae, but like diethylcarbamazine, poses the risk of a serious meningoencephalitis. As *L. loa* does not harbour wolbachia, treatment with antibiotics is ineffective.

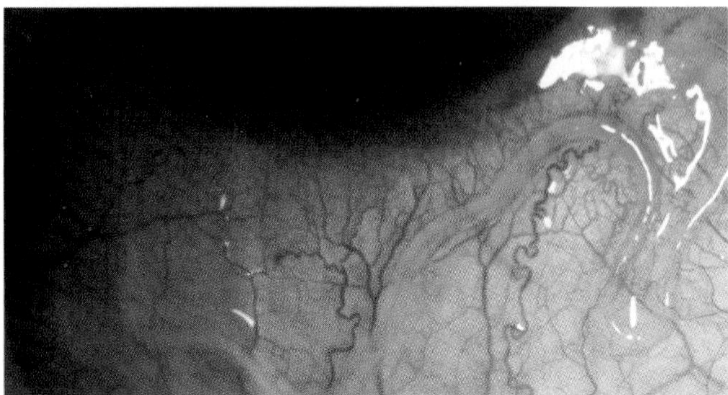

Fig. 7.9.1.11 *Loa loa* crossing the bulbar conjunctiva.

Prevention

The best prevention is avoiding chrysops fly bites. Having window screens on dwellings, wearing clothing to protect the legs and forearms, and avoiding areas where biting is frequent can reduce the risk. Chemoprophylaxis with diethylcarbamazine has been suggested, using either 5 mg/kg on three consecutive days in a month, or a weekly dose of 300 mg while living in an area of transmission.

Mansonellosis

Mansonella spp. are a group of filarial species common to many countries, but are of negligible clinical importance under most circumstances. Infection is transmitted by *Culicoides* spp. midges.

Epidemiology

Mansonella (formerly *Dipetalonema*) *perstans* is found in much of tropical Africa, as well as Trinidad and several parts of South America. The adult worms live free in the abdominal cavity, and microfilariae are found in the blood and skin. *Mansonella ozzardi* is found in the West Indies and Central and South America. In addition to culicoides, simulium flies have been reported to transmit *M. ozzardi* in the Amazon basin. *Mansonella streptocerca* is a common infection in West and Central Africa, extending into western Uganda. Both microfilariae and adult worms are found in the skin, but without the nodules seen in onchocerciasis. Unless *M. streptocerca* microfilariae are differentiated parasitologically from those of *O. volvulus*, inappropriate mass onchocerciasis treatment programmes could be implemented.

Clinical manifestations

Of the mansonellas, only *M. streptocerca* produces clear-cut symptoms, although even these can be confused with those of *O. volvulus*, which may be a coinfection. Chronic papular lesions are commonly present, often associated with postinflammatory hyperpigmentation. Lichenification may occur less commonly. Hypopigmentation has been noted in areas of skin overlying the location of adult worms in the skin. In general, these findings are not easily distinguishable from those of onchocerciasis. Eosinophilia is common.

M. perstans has been reported to produce Calabar-like swellings, pruritus, fever, and headache. *M. ozzardi* infections are generally asymptomatic, although fever, arthralgia, headache, and itching have been associated with infection in the Amazon area.

Diagnosis

Diagnosis is by finding characteristic microfilariae in the blood or skin. The tails of the microfilariae have a distinctive walking-stick shape, and contain four prominent nuclei, distinguishing them from microfilariae of *O. volvulus*. A PCR assay as been described for *M. streptocerca*, and both quantitative buffy coat fluorescent staining and enzyme immunoassay methods for *M. perstans*. Eosinophilia is a characteristic finding.

Treatment

In asymptomatic people no treatment is required. *M. streptocerca* responds well to ivermectin, producing prolonged suppression of circulating microfilariae. Mild reactions similar to those in onchocerciasis may be seen. The treatment of *M. perstans* with diethylcarbamazine reduces microfilarial counts, but repeated treatments have been required to eliminate the infection. Mebendazole 100 mg twice daily for 28 to 45 days appears to be more active than diethylcarbamazine in clearing microfilariae. A combination of both diethylcarbamazine and mebendazole is highly effective against *M. perstans*, while ivermectin has little effect.

Further reading

Boussinesq M (2006). Loiasis. *Ann Trop Med Parasitol*, **100**, 715–31.

Bregani ER, *et al.* (2006). Comparison of different anthelminthic drug regimens against *Mansonella perstans* filariasis. *Trans R Soc Trop Med Hyg*, **100**, 458–63.

Brieger WR, *et al.* (1998). The effects of ivermectin on onchocercal skin disease and severe itching: results of a multicentre trial. *Trop Med Int Health*, **3**, 951–61.

Chan CC, *et al.* (1989). Immunopathology of ocular onchocerciasis. I. Inflammatory cells infiltrating the anterior segment. *Clin Exp Immunol*, **77**, 367–73.

Cooper PJ, *et al.* (1999). Eosinophil sequestration and activation are associated with the onset and severity of systemic adverse reactions following the treatment of onchocerciasis with ivermectin. *J Infect Dis*, **179**, 738–42.

Cupp EW, *et al.* (2004). The effects of long-term community level treatment with ivermectin (Mectizan) on adult *Onchocerca volvulus* in Latin America. *Am J Trop Med Hyg*, **71**, 602–7.

Emukah EC, *et al.* (2004). A longitudinal study of impact of repeated mass ivermectin treatment on clinical manifestations of onchocerciasis in Imo State, Nigeria. *Am J Trop Med Hygiene*, **70**, 556–61.

Fischer P, *et al.* (1997). Occurrence and diagnosis of *Mansonella streptocerca* in Uganda. *Acta Trop*, **63**, 43–55.

Garcia A, *et al.* (1995). Longitudinal survey of *Loa loa* filariasis in southern Cameroon. *Am J Trop Med Hyg*, **52**, 370–5.

Gillette-Ferguson I, *et al.* (2006). *Wolbachia*- and *Onchocerca volvulus*-induced keratitis (river blindness) is dependent on myeloid differentiation factor 88. *Infect Immun*, **74**, 2442–5.

Kaiser C, *et al.* (1996). The prevalence of epilepsy follows the distribution of onchocerciasis in a west Ugandan focus. *Bull World Health Organ*, **74**, 361–7.

Little MP, *et al.* (2004). Association between microfilarial load and excess mortality in onchocerciasis: an epidemiological study. *Lancet*, **363**, 1514–21.

Mectizan and onchocerciasis: a decade of accomplishment (1998). *Ann Trop Med Parasitol*, **92** Suppl 1, S1–174.

Murdoch ME, *et al.* (1997). HKA-DQ alleles associate with cutaneous features of onchocerciasis. The Kaduna-London-Manchester Collaboration for Research on Onchocerciasis. *Hum Immunol*, **55**, 46–52.

Murdoch ME, *et al.* (2002). Onchocerciasis: the clinical and epidemiological burden of skin disease in Africa. *Ann Trop Med Parasitol*, **96**, 283–96.

Osei-Atweneboana MY, *et al.* (2007). Prevalence and intensity of *Onchocerca volvulus* infection and efficacy of ivermectin in endemic communities in Ghana: a two-phase epidemiology study. *Lancet*, **369**, 2021–9.

Ottesen EA (1995). Immune responsiveness and the pathogenesis of human onchocerciasis. *J Infect Dis*, **171**, 659–71.

Thylefors B, Alleman M (2006). Towards the elimination of onchocerciasis. *Ann Trop Med Parasitol*, **100**, 733–46.

World Health Organization (1995). *Onchocerciasis and its control.* Report of a WHO Expert Committee on Onchocerciasis. WHO, Geneva.

Yameogo L, *et al.* (1999). Pool screen polymerase chain reaction for estimating the prevalence of *Onchocerca volvulus* infection in *Simulium damnosum sensu lato*: results of a field trial in an area subject to successful vector control. *Am J Trop Med Hyg*, **60**, 124–8.

7.9.2 Lymphatic filariasis

Richard Knight and D.H. Molyneux

Essentials

Wuchereria bancrofti, Brugia malayi, and *B. timori* are mosquito-borne nematode parasites that are important causes of morbidity, disability, and social stigma in tropical and subtropical countries. Bancroftian filariasis due to *W. bancrofti*, which has no animal reservoir, infects 110 million people; the two *Brugia* species infect about 13 million in South and South-East Asia.

Clinical features

Acute lymphatic filariasis—(1) lymphadenitis and lymphangitis—most common in the inguinal and femoral nodes; (2) acute genital—usually tender fusiform or cylindrical swelling of the spermatic cord; (3) abscess and fever—affected nodes may break down to produce an open ulcer.

Chronic lymphatic filariasis—(1) lymphoedema and elephantiasis—initially transient pitting oedema occurs during acute inflammatory episodes in proximal nodes; eventually brawny, nonpitting oedema becomes permanent; (2) chronic genital—most commonly hydrocele; (3) chronic lymphadenitis and lymphangitis; (4) chyluria and lymphuria; (5) nonlymphatic pathology—including tropical pulmonary eosinophilia, filarial arthritis, and filarial glomerulonephritis.

Diagnosis and treatment

Diagnosis—microfilariae are typically found in Giemsa-stained blood films; the sample best taken at night (22.00–02.00), except in Oceania and parts of Southeast Asia). Microfilariae are also sometimes found in aspirates from lymph varix, hydrocele, lymphocele of the cord, or in urine. A rapid antigen test allows the mapping of prevalence and assessment of the impact of mass drug distribution.

Treatment—diethylcarbamazine, which may provoke both local and systemic reactions, is needed in some situations, including infected visitors, people leaving infected areas, and those with tropical pulmonary eosinophilia or other unusual features where rapid elimination of adult worms is a priority. Concurrent bacterial infection requires prompt treatment with antibiotics, and supportive bandaging can reduce chronic oedema.

Prevention

The Global Programme for the Elimination of Lymphatic Filariasis involves annual rounds of drug administration that interrupt transmission, together with (in appropriate circumstances) vector control.

Introduction

Wuchereria bancrofti, *Brugia malayi*, and *B. timori* are mosquito-borne nematode parasites. They are important causes of morbidity, disability and social stigma in tropical and subtropical countries (Fig. 7.9.2.1). The total population at risk is estimated to be 1.307 billion in some 83 countries where these infections are endemic. Bancroftian filariasis due to *W. bancrofti* infects 110 million people; it was introduced into the Americas from Africa by the Atlantic slave trade. The two *Brugia* species infect about 13 million people in South and South-East Asia. *B. timori* has a localized distribution in Timor Leste and Indonesia.

Aetiology: the biology of the parasite

The adult worms live in the larger lymphatic vessels and lymph nodes. They are smooth, creamy-white, and threadlike; females measure 8 to 10 cm in length and males 4 cm. Their lifespan is estimated to be 4 to 6 years, but may be longer—a critical issue for planning, implementation, and duration of elimination programmes. Mated females produce numerous microfilariae throughout their life; these actively motile embryonic worms are sheathed by the remnants of the egg shell. They are 180 to 290 μm in length and 7 to 10 μm in diameter, with diagnostic species morphologies in stained blood films.

Microfilariae migrate via the lymphatic system to the blood, where they have an estimated lifespan of up to 12 months. Their numbers in the peripheral blood vary during the day and night, a phenomenon known as periodicity, and when not circulating they are sequestered in lung and reticuloendothelial capillaries. Maximum counts in the blood coincide with the biting cycle of the vector. The species and strain of parasite determine the periodicity. Most common is nocturnally periodic, with maximum microfilarial counts between 22.00 and 02.00, and virtual absence during the day. Alternatively, microfilariae may be present throughout the 24-h cycle, with prominent peaks during the day or the night; referred to as diurnal or nocturnal subperiodicity, respectively.

After ingestion by the mosquito, microfilariae penetrate the midgut and migrate to the thoracic muscles, where they mature over 9 to 15 days to infective third-stage larvae. These then migrate to the head of the mosquito and escape through the arthrodial membranes around the proboscis during a blood meal. Larval worms enter the puncture wound made by the vector, enter the peripheral lymphatic system, and most eventually reach the lymph vessels of the proximal limb and male genitalia. Sexual maturity and the appearance of microfilariae in the blood usually take 8 to 18 months, but sometimes only 3 months.

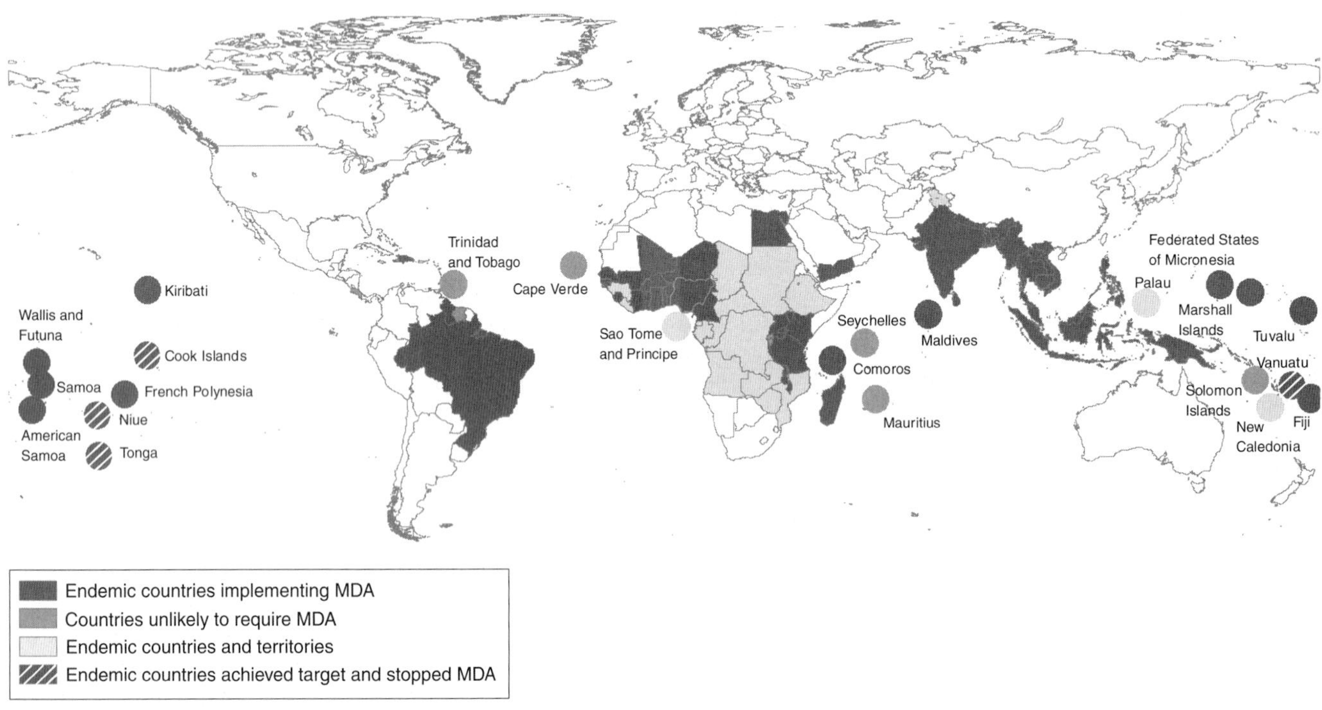

Fig. 7.9.2.1 Lymphatic filariasis endemic countries and territories by mass drug administration (MDA), 2008.
Source: World Health Organization, 2009.

Epidemiology and transmission

In endemic areas microfilaria prevalence rates increase steadily from early childhood to reach a maximum in early adult life, when in highly endemic areas a prevalence of 10 to 30% is not unusual; the prevalence in males is generally higher, perhaps as a result of greater vector exposure. The cord blood of some infants shows microfilariae. Recent studies using an immunochromatographic card test to detect adult worm antigen showed that in a population of Haitian children prevalence reached 25% by the age of 4 years. Using immunochromatographic card test testing as a means of mapping the prevalence of *Wuchereria bancrofti* gives a prevalence double that detected by night blood films. This technique has been used for mapping the prevalence of the disease to assist in defining programme implementation units for the purposes of planning mass drug distribution.

W. bancrofti has no animal reservoir. *Brugia malayi*, however, is a zoonosis in some areas of its distribution (southern Thailand, Malaysia), with a reservoir in cats and leaf monkeys, although their importance in terms of maintaining the cycle in humans is not known; elsewhere it is an anthroponosis with only a human source of infection.

Mosquito vectors and geographical distribution

W. bancrofti infection

Culex spp. transmission

This vector, mainly *C. quinquefasciatus*, breeds mostly in organically polluted water, usually in urban and suburban areas, but also villages where there are suitable latrine and cesspit habitats. *Culex* is the most widely distributed vector and is increasing with urbanization; it occurs in India, Sri Lanka, Central and South America, some Caribbean islands, urban and coastal villages in East Africa and Egypt, and formerly in parts of China, where transmission has been eliminated. *Culex* bites at night; the microfilariae are nocturnally periodic. *Culex* is the most efficient vector and can maintain transmission at low microfilarial densities, making control difficult.

Anopheles spp. transmission

The same *Anopheles* spp. commonly transmit both filariasis and malaria. This occurs in East and West Africa, Papua New Guinea, and Vanuatu. *Anopheles* bites at night, mainly on the legs; microfilariae are nocturnally periodic.

Aedes spp. transmission

This is limited to southern Oceania, especially Fiji, Samoa, Tonga, the Cook Islands, and New Caledonia; but also patchily in Thailand, the Philippines, Vietnam, and the Nicobar Islands. *Aedes* feeds throughout the 24-h cycle, with a daytime biting peak, and bites all over the body; the microfilariae are diurnally subperiodic.

B. malayi infection

Zoonotic *Mansonia* spp. transmission in swamp forests

This occurs in Malaysia, Indonesia, and southern Thailand. *Mansonia* bites mainly by night, but also during the day, usually on the legs below the knee; the microfilariae are nocturnally subperiodic.

Transmission in agricultural areas

In parts of Malaysia, Buru in Indonesia, and southern Thailand a mixed anthroponosis and zoonosis occurs in transitional zones, with monkeys and cats as reservoirs, and both *anopheles* and *mansonia* as vectors. Microfilariae have periodicities intermediate between nocturnally periodic and nocturnally subperiodic.

In India (mainly Kerala), Malaysia, Sulawesi, southern Thailand, and Vietnam infection involves humans only, with *anopheles* as the main vector and *mansonia* as an accessory vector; the microfilariae are nocturnally periodic.

B. timori infection

This is confined to Timor Leste and islands in the Lesser Sundas group in eastern Indonesia. *Anopheles barbirostris* is the vector, and the microfilariae are nocturnally periodic.

Pathogenesis

Local immunological reactions to worm antigens provoke acute and subacute responses, with oedema of lymphatic tissue and infiltration of eosinophils and monocytes. The antigens derive from the moulting fluids of developing worms, excretory products, microfilariae trapped within the lymphatic system, and also dying worms, including those killed by chemotherapy. Dead and disintegrating worms become surrounded by granulation tissue with giant cells and epithelioid cells. Stenosis or blockage of lymph vessels leads to distal dilatation, with varicosities and valve incompetence. Worms also cause local noninflammatory lymph vessel dilatation. Prolonged or recurrent lymph stasis leads to the accumulation of protein-rich interstitial fluid, fibroblast proliferation, dilated dermal lymphatics, and epithelial acanthosis and hyperkeratosis.

Determinants of pathology include the duration of exposure, intensity of transmission, anatomical sites of infective mosquito bites, and species and strain of parasite. Prenatal exposure to filarial antigen is of great importance and induces immunological tolerance. Residents in high-transmission areas often show patent microfilaraemia, but little immunopathology. However, in many adults a later decline in microfilarial prevalence parallels increased host immunological reactivity and pathology. New residents and visitors show marked local reactivity to worms, and often no blood microfilariae; the latter situation was well documented among American troops in the Pacific in the Second World War, and French troops in former Indochina.

Clinical manifestations

Acute lymphatic filariasis

In endemic areas acute episodes are recurrent from the age of 10 years, and most frequent 4 to 8 months after the peak of seasonal transmission. Episodes last several days or weeks; fever and malaise are common, but blood eosinophilia is not marked. Persons leaving endemic areas cease to have acute episodes after 1 year, although they may experience recurrent pain in previously affected tissues, especially after unusual exercise.

Filarial lymphadenitis and lymphangitis

Tender lymphadenopathy is most common in the inguinal and femoral nodes, but axillary and epitrochlear nodes are also affected. Tender retrograde lymphangitis typically spreads peripherally below the node.

Acute genital filariasis

This is uncommon in boys before puberty, but common thereafter. The typical lesion is funiculitis, with a tender fusiform or cylindrical swelling of the spermatic cord; epididymitis and orchitis are less common.

Filarial abscess and filarial fever

Affected nodes in the groin or elsewhere may break down producing an open ulcer that heals slowly leaving characteristic scars. Pelvic and retroperitoneal lymphadenitis can produce a febrile illness that is difficult to diagnose.

Chronic lymphatic filariasis

Lymphoedema and elephantiasis

Initially, transient pitting oedema occurs during acute inflammatory episodes in proximal nodes. Bacterial infection, often caused by *Streptococcus pyogenes*, is common in those with compromised lymphatics, especially when the skin is fissured, breached in an interdigital cleft, or when there is minor injury, an ulcer, or insect bite; this presents as cellulitis and ascending lymphangitis. Later, oedema persists between episodes, becoming distally nonpitting. Eventually, brawny nonpitting oedema becomes permanent (Fig. 7.9.2.2). In patients with leg involvement, epidermal thickening, papillomatosis, and fissuring are common (Fig. 7.9.2.3).

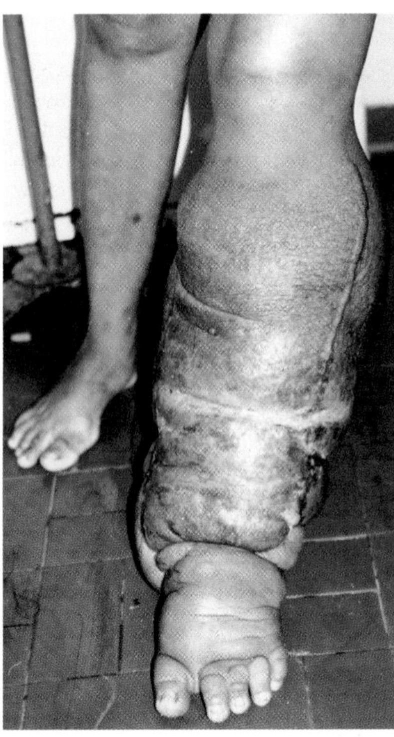

Fig. 7.9.2.2 Chronic elephantiasis in a man in Belém, northern Brazil. Note the scars of unsuccessful surgery.
(Copyright Pedro Pardal.)

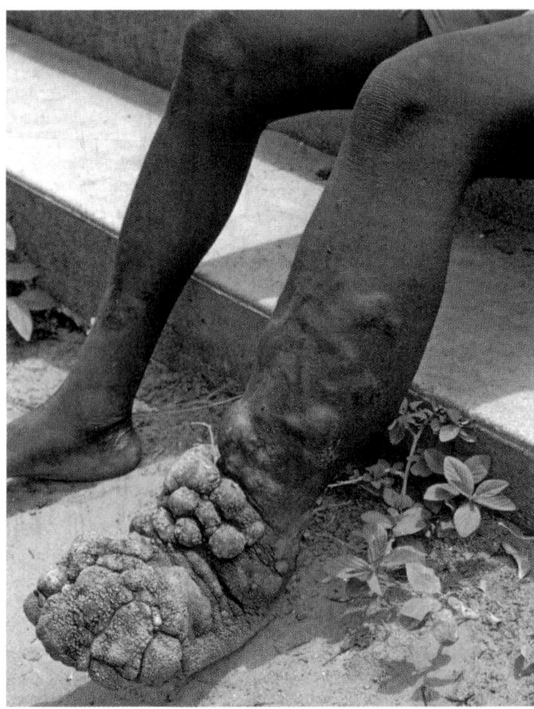

Fig. 7.9.2.3 Chronic elephantiasis with epidermal thickening, fissuring, and papillomatosis in a man in north-east Nigeria.
(Copyright D A Warrell.)

Chronic genital filariasis

Hydrocele (Fig. 7.9.2.4) is the most common lesion, and prevalence rates may reach 30% in men over 35 years in highly endemic areas; many patients give a history of preceding episodes of funiculitis or epididymitis. Hydrocele fluid is usually a transudate, but lymph or blood may be present. The tunica vaginalis is often thickened. Nodular lesions of the spermatic cord and epididymis are common, and the testis itself may become enlarged and indurated. Lymphoceles occur on the cord. Dilated dermal lymphatics in the scrotal wall associated with atrophic epidermis produce lymph scrotum, the skin having a velvety appearance. Rupture of these lymphatics leads to weeping skin lesions and often secondary infection, occasionally complicated by Fournier's gangrene.

Lymphoedema of the scrotum is a late sequel; often the testes are unaffected, and penile lesions are rare. Vulval lymphoedema is underrecognized; it is associated with dilated retroperitoneal lymphatics, and must be distinguished from lymphogranuloma venereum.

Chronic lymphadenitis and lymphangitis

Recurrent episodes of acute inflammation lead to persisting and sometimes massive lymph node enlargement. Thickened lymphatic cords may be palpable connecting the axillary and epitrochlear, or the femoral and popliteal nodes. Varicose lymph vessels may be visible in these areas. Lymph varices are fluctuant sacs of lymphatic tissue derived usually from the capsule of a node, hence the alternative term lymphadenocele. They partially empty when the part is raised, and aspiration reveals lymph or occasionally chyle. They occur in the medial thigh, groin, axilla, and sometimes even the neck.

Chyluria and lymphuria

Dilated pelvic and retroperitoneal lymphatics may rupture into the urinary tract in the renal pelvis, ureter, or bladder. When there is

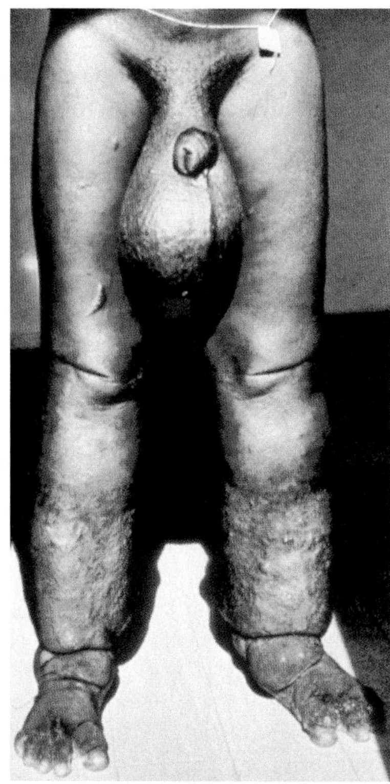

Fig. 7.9.2.4 Cross hydrocele in a patient with chronic filariasis.
(Courtesy of the late P E C Manson-Bahr.)

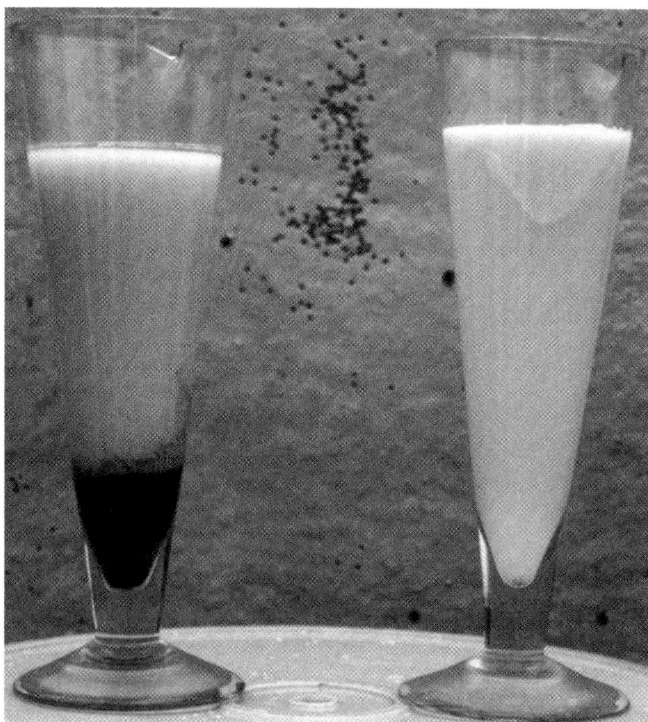

Fig. 7.9.2.5 Chyluria and haematuria in a patient with chronic filariasis.
(Courtesy of the late P E C Manson-Bahr.)

lymph stasis above the cisterna chyli then small-bowel chyle may reflux into the urine postprandially. Chyluria is often intermittent and blood stained (Fig. 7.9.2.5). Continued loss of protein and lipids in the urine may lead to weight loss and cachexia. Chyluria may eventually be self-limiting.

Nonlymphatic pathology

Tropical pulmonary eosinophilia

This presents as a subacute or chronic illness with cough, wheezing, and reticular or miliary pulmonary shadowing. Microfilariae are absent from the blood, but eosinophilia is marked, and titres of filarial antibody are very high. Some patients have features of lymphadenopathic or genital filariasis, but many do not. Loss of lung function is restrictive. The response to antifilarial treatment is good, but untreated the condition can lead to pulmonary fibrosis and pulmonary hypertension. The syndrome is the result of a heightened immunological response to dead microfilariae, which may be found in biopsies of lung and other tissue surrounded by eosinophilic microabscesses. It occurs in most endemic areas, but is rare in Africa. It is more common in men, and rare in children, and many patients are not long-term residents.

Filarial arthritis

Joint involvement is subacute, and often recurrent with effusion; it usually affects the knee.

Filarial glomerulonephritis

This results from filarial and streptococcal immune-complex deposition on the glomerular basement membrane, but there is also tubular damage. Clinical findings include proteinuria and haematuria, which usually respond to chemotherapy. The incidence of clinically significant disease and its prognosis are uncertain.

Diagnosis

Clinical

Many patients will have several clinical features that, together with a history of preceding acute episodes, will be strongly suggestive diagnostically—manifestations such as varicose lymphatics, lymphadenocele, retrograde lymphangitis, and lymph scrotum are highly specific to filariasis. Genital lesions are rare in *Brugia* infections, which usually present with lymphoedema below the knee. In *B. timori* infection lymph node pathology in the legs is often severe, sometimes with skin ulceration. Upper limb and breast lesions are common in diurnally subperiodic *W. bancrofti* infections in the Pacific, but they do occur elsewhere with other strains of this parasite.

Parasitological

Microfilariae (Fig. 7.9.2.6) are typically found in Giemsa-stained blood films, but also in aspirates from a lymph varix, hydrocele, or lymphocele of the cord, or in urine. Blood should be taken to coincide with the expected microfilarial periodicity. For quantitative studies, measured 10- or 20-µl volumes are used to prepare thick blood films. For measuring changes in intensity, larger measured quantities of blood should be used to increase the sensitivity and accuracy of a key parameter. Counting chambers taking 100 µlitres of lysed blood can be used, or larger volumes may be lysed and the spun deposit examined. A sensitive method which allows quantitation of parasite density is filtration of 1–5 ml of heparinised venous blood through a nucleopore filter of pore

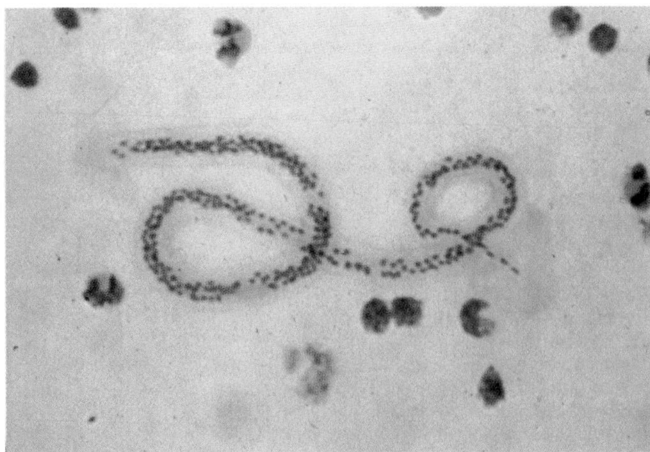

Fig. 7.9.2.6 Microfilaria of *W.bancrofti* on a Giemsa stained blood film showing sheath and row of terminal nuclei (right).

size 5 microns; microfilariae on the filters can then be stained. Nocturnally periodic *W. bancrofti* microfilariae appear transiently in the blood 30 to 60 min after a 100-mg dose of diethylcarbamazine, which forms the basis of the provocation test. Species diagnosis of stained microfilariae is made by their sheath characteristics and the arrangement of caudal nuclei. The microfilariae of *Loa loa*, the tropical eye worm (found only in West and Central Africa) are diurnally periodic and also have a sheath; they must be distinguished from those of lymphatic filariasis.

Immunodiagnosis

Positive filarial antibody and skin tests are common in those exposed to infection, and may be of value in visitors to an endemic area. Several tests are now available for *W. bancrofti* antigen in serum, including a card test for field use. A positive test indicates persisting adult worms; antigen may be present in the absence of microfilaraemia. For *Brugia* infections, techniques for DNA detection by polymerase chain reaction (PCR) are available, and also specific IgG4 antibody tests.

Imaging of lymphatic vessels

Lymphangiography will delineate the anatomical details of abnormal lymphatic tissues, such as lymph varices and lymphatic connections to the urinary tract in chyluria. They are not usually diagnostic for filariasis. Scrotal ultrasonography can show nests of live worms—the 'filarial dance' sign; this can be used to assess chemotherapy.

Lymphoscintigraphy using technetium-labelled dextran or albumin is a less invasive technique for demonstrating lymphatic pathology. Abnormal dermal lymphatics occur in many asymptomatic infected persons in endemic areas.

Filariasis at the community level

The Global Programme to Eliminate Lymphatic Filariasis

A World Health Assembly Resolution in 1997 launched a programme to eliminate lymphatic filariasis as a public health problem by 2020. This resolution was based on new evidence of the impact of two drug combinations on microfilaraemia, and the availability of a rapid antigen test (immunochromatographic card test) that allows mapping of the prevalence of disease and assessment of the impact of mass drug administration (MDA). Clinical studies had demonstrated that the annual distribution of diethylcarbamazine and albendazole, or albendazole and ivermectin, reduced microfilaraemia to levels that would interrupt transmission, provided that treatment with high coverage could be achieved.

The programme was backed by generous commitments by the manufacturers to donate albendazole and ivermectin (for use with albendazole in Africa where diethylcarbamazine cannot be used because of the risks in patients with onchocerciasis and loiasis). A global public–private partnership was formed in 2000, the Global Alliance to Eliminate Lymphatic Filariasis (GAELF). The extensive distribution of lymphatic filariasis required a regional approach to programme management and planning. According to GAELF strategy, countries launched programmes based on World Health Organization (WHO) recommendations on mapping, baseline data collection, and the establishment of evaluation and monitoring based on sentinel-site selection. Training drug distributors; selecting appropriate drug distribution systems; information, education, and communication; social mobilization needs; and reporting systems were recognized as being of great importance.

By the end of 2008, 51 of the 81 lymphatic filariasis-endemic countries had initiated elimination programmes, and were either actively distributing drugs or planning to do so. In 2008, a total of 695 million people were targeted for MDA, of whom 496 million received the recommended WHO two-drug combination of albendazole plus either ivermectin or diethylcarbamazine, or diethylcarbamazine-fortified salt (widely used in China). The rest, mostly in India, received diethylcarbamazine alone. The results of the 8-year MDA programmes are now being published. Apparent success in arresting transmission, based on several measures, is now being reported from Egypt, Togo, Vanuatu, and Zanzibar.

The needs of patients already afflicted with lymphoedema and hydrocele must also be addressed. To this end WHO has issued guidelines for home-based care, whereby lymphoedema patients and their families are taught how to treat lymphatic filariasis -related lymphoedema and prevent acute attacks. WHO also aims to increase access to hydrocele surgery that uses new reconstructive techniques.

Despite resource constraints, particularly in sub-Saharan Africa, there are encouraging signs that the programme is reducing the prevalence of the disease. Egypt is reporting the elimination of transmission in formerly endemic areas of the Nile delta. China claims that earlier campaigns have resulted in the cessation of transmission in a population of some 350 million people. Smaller countries have also demonstrated disease elimination following a range of different interventions. These are Suriname, Costa Rica, Trinidad and Tobago; and also the Solomon Islands, where vector control for malaria, using indoor residual spraying with dichlorodiphenyltrichloroethane (DDT) in the 1970s, appears to have been effective.

Population-based chemotherapy

In the past, different dosage regimens of diethylcarbamazine were used in many endemic areas. Drugs were given annually or 6 monthly, either to the whole population or to those found to be infected; medicated salt being the alternative. The main aim was to eliminate microfilaraemia and hence transmission, but with repeated doses many adult worms are eventually killed.

Ivermectin offers an effective alternative for reducing microfilaraemia, but does not kill adult worms. A single dose of 200 or 400 μg/kg of ivermectin is as effective as a 6 mg/kg dose of diethylcarbamazine. Both will virtually eliminate microfilaraemia for 6 or 12 months, adverse reactions are probably equally common with both drugs. Albendazole is also effective as a microfilaricide, and has some activity against adult worms. A 600 mg dose given annually can replace either diethylcarbamazine or ivermectin in a two-drug annual regimen. Annual dosage with either of these two drug combinations, continued for 4 to 6 years (the lifespan of nearly all adult worms), will interrupt transmission.

It is not recommended that diethylcarbamazine be given in areas where onchocerciasis or loiasis are endemic to avoid dangerous reactions. *Loa*-associated encephalopathy occurs especially in people with *Loa* microfilarial loads of more than 8000/ml of blood. As there are few areas in sub-Saharan Africa where *Loa* and *Onchocerca* do not have potential overlap with *W. bancrofti*, the use of diethylcarbamazine has been discouraged or abandoned there in recent years.

In areas where population-based annual chemotherapy is in progress there is a reduced incidence of worm-related acute manifestations, and often reductions hydrocele size. In addition, there is stabilization or regression in lymphoedema when this is managed by health education, skin hygiene, and antibiotics.

Vector control

The vector control method used depends on the habits of the local vector to be targeted: *Aedes* breeding sites, such discarded tins, tyres, or coconut shells, can be removed; *Culex* numbers can be reduced by improved sanitation, larvicides, and polystyrene beads applied to the water surface of latrines and cesspits. Bed nets and repellents are universally applicable.

However, vector control as part of the GAELF must be planned according to the cost of MDA, the collateral benefits from annual intervention with broad spectrum drugs, and the costs of vector control itself. Thus, vector control targeted specifically at the transmission of lypmhatic filariasis itself is not a major part of the global elimination programme. This is because a lymphatic filariasis specific vector control activity, whilst it may reduce the number of rounds of MDA, is not likely to be a sustainable or cost effective exercise. There is no doubt, however, that where there is vector control in *Anopheles* transmission areas to control malaria (bed nets and indoor residual spraying) there will be an impact on the transmission of *W. bancrofti*. Hence there may be an opportunity to reduce the number of rounds of MDA. There may also be a case for vector control in settings where MDA has not been able to achieve the required reduction in prevalence (<1%) and intensity to reduce transmission below the threshold for parasite elimination.

Management of patients in clinics and hospitals

Chemotherapy

Individual chemotherapy with diethylcarbamazine is still needed in some situations, including infected visitors, people leaving infected areas, and those with tropical pulmonary eosinophilia or other unusual features where rapid elimination of adult worms is a priority. Treatment may provoke both local and systemic reactions, and thus requires care and supervision in the initial stages, especially in *Brugia* infections. Coinfection with *Loa loa* must be treated with great care as both ivermectin and diethylcarbamazine can cause encephalopathy when *Loa* microfilaria counts are high; patients coinfected with *Onchocera volvulus* should not be given diethylcarbamazine (see Chapter 7.9.1).

Diethylcarbamazine treatment should be started at 1 mg/kg on the first day, increasing over 3 days or more to 6 mg/kg daily. In the standard regimen 6 mg/kg is contnued for 12 days; alternatively this dose is given weekly for 12 weeks. These regimens are poorly evidenced based. Ultrasonography reveals the variable killing of adult worms, both within and between individuals, as even a single 600 mg dose will kill most worms in some patients. For tropical pulmonary eosinophilia a full 21 days of treatment is indicated, and may need to be repeated.

Filarial worms harbour *Wolbachia* endosymbionts, which are antibiotic sensitive. In Tanzania an 8-week course of doxycycline 200 mg daily was effective against *Wolbachia bancrofti* adult worms, and reduced morbidity. More recently, in a study in India, a 3 week course produced a significant effect against adult worms and reduced lymphatic dilatation. Doxycycline clearly has therapeutic potential either combined with other filaricides, or alone when the latter are contraindicated; it is also effective against *O. volvulus* which harbour similar *Wolbachia*.

Surgical and supportive management

The acute manifestations of filariasis can mimic strangulated hernia and testicular torsion. The surgical treatment of filarial hydrocele is the same as that for nonfilarial disease. Scrotal lymphoedema can be treated surgically, usually with preservation of the testes. Lymphosaphenous anastomosis is being used for leg elephantiasis; many other procedures have been used in the past, often with disappointing results (Fig. 7.9.2.2).

Bacterial infection is common in those with lymphoedema, especially when skin integrity is breached. Early use of antibiotics, together with resting the affected limb, lessens the risk of increasing lymphoedema; supportive bandaging applied each morning reduces chronic oedema.

Further reading

Beaver PC (1970). Filariasis without microfilaremia. *Am J Trop Med Hyg*, **19**, 181–9.

Bockarie M, Molyneux DH (2009). The end of lymphatic filariasis. *BMJ*, **338**, 1470–72.

Boggild AK, KeystoneJS, Kain KC (2004). Tropical pulmonary eosinophilia. *Clin Infect.Dis*, **39**, 1123–8.

Dreyer G, *et al.* (2006). Efficacy of co-administered diethylcarbamazine and albendazole against adult *Wuchereria bancrofti*. *Trans R Soc Trop Med Hyg*, **100**, 1118–25.

Dreyer G, *et al.* (1999). Acute attacks in the extremities of persons living in an area endemic for bancroftian filariasis: differentiation of two syndromes. *Trans R Soc Trop Med Hyg*, **93**, 413–17.

Dreyer G, *et al.* (2000). Pathogenesis of lymphatic disease in bancroftian filariasis: a clinical perspective. *Parasitol Today*, **16**, 544–8.

Dreyer G, *et al.* (2002). Progression of lymphatic vessel dilatation in the presence of living *Wuchereria bancrofti*. *Trans R Soc Trop Med Hyg*, **96**, 157–61.

Freedman DO, *et al.* (1994). Lymphoscintographic analysis of lymphatic abnormalities in symptomatic and asymptomatic human filariasis. *J Infect Dis*, **170**, 927–33.

Gyapong JO, Chinbuah MA, Gyapong M (2003). Inadvertent exposure of pregnant women to ivermectin and albendazole during mass drug treatment for lymphatic filariasis. *Trop Med Int Health*, **8**, 1093–101.

Helmy H, *et al.* (2006). Bancroftian filariasis: effect of repeated treatment with diethylcarmabazine and albendazole on microfilaraemia, antigenaemaia and antifilarial antbodies. *Trans Roy Soc Trop Med Hyg*, **100**, 656–62.

Jiraamonnimit C, *et al.* (2009). A cohort study of anti-filarial IgG4 and its assessment in good and uncertain MDA-compliant subjects in brugian filariasis endemic areas in southern Thailand. *J Helminthol*, **83**. 351–60.

Kim Y-J, *et al.* (2005). Genetic polymorphisms of eosinophil-derived neurotoxin and eosinophil cationic protein in pulmonary eosinophilia. *Am J Trop Med Hyg*, **73**, 125–30.

Langhammer J, Birk HW, Zahner H (1997). Renal disease in lymphatic filariasis: evidence for tubular and glomerular disorders at various stages of the infection. *Trop Med Int Health*, **2**, 875–84.

Liang JL, *et al.* (2008). Impact of five rounds of mass drug administration with diethylcarbamazine and albendazole on Wuchereria bancrofti (print in italics) in American Samoa. *Am J Trop Med Hyg*, **78**, 924–8.

Mand S, *et al.* (2009) Macrofilaricidal activity and amelioration of lymphatic pathology in bancroftian filariasis after 3 weeks of doxycycline followed by a single dose of diethylcarbamazine. *Am J Trop Med Hyg*, **81**, 702–11.

Molyneux DH (2006). Elimination of transmission of lymphatic filariasis in Egypt. *Lancet*, **367**, 966–8.

Norões J, *et al.* (1996). Occurrence of living adult *Wuchereria bancrofti* in the scrotal area of men with microfilaraemia. *Trans R Soc Trop Med Hyg*, **90**, 55–6.

Nuchprayoon S (2009). DNA-based diagnosis of lymphatic filariasis. *Southeast Asian J Trop Med Health*, **40**, 904–13.

Nutman TB (ed.) (2000). *Lymphatic filariasis*. Imperial College Press, London.

Ong RG, Doyle RL (1998). Tropical pulmonary eosinophilia. *Chest*, **113**, 1673–9.

Ottesen EA (2006). Lymphatic filariasis: treatment, control and elimination. *Adv Parasitol*, **61**, 395–441.

Otteson EA, *et al.* (2008). The global programme to eliminate lymphatic filariasis: health impact after 8 years. *Plos NTD. 2*, **e317**, 1–12.

Supali T, *et al.* (2008) Doxycycline treatment for Brugia (print in italics)-infected persons reduces microfilaraemia and adverse reactions after diethylcarbamazine and albendazole treatment. *Clin Infect Dis*, **46**, 1385–93.

Taylor MG, *et al.* (2005). Macrofilaricidal activity after doxycycline treatment for *Wuchereria bancrofti*: double-blind randomised placebo-controlled trial. *Lancet*, **365**, 2116–21.

Vijayan VK (2007). Tropical pulmonary eosinophilia: pathogenesis, diagnosis and treatment. *Curr Opin Pulm Med*, **13**, 28–33.

Weil GJ, Lammie PJ, Weiss N (1997). The ICT filariasis test: a rapid format antigen test for the diagnosis of bancroftian filariasis. *Parasitol Today*, **13**, 401–4.

Weil GJ, Ramzy RMR (2007). Diagnostic tools for filariasis elimination prgrammes. *Trends Parasitol*, **23**, 78–82.

Wongkamchai S, *et al.* (2006). Diagnostic value of IgG isotype responses against Brugia malayi (print italics) antifilarial antibodies in the clinical spectrum of brugian filariasis. *J Helminthol*, **80**, 363–7.

World Health Organisation (2009). Global programme to eliminate lymphatic filariasis. *Weekly Epidemiological Record*, **84**, 437–44.

7.9.3 Guinea worm disease (dracunculiasis)

Richard Knight

Essentials

Guinea-worm disease (dracunculiasis)—now limited to sub-Saharan Africa—is caused by the nematode *Dracunculus medinensis*, whose life cycle involves water-borne copepod crustaceans and humans, who acquire the infection when they drink water containing infective larvae. Clinical presentation is usually with a skin blister, most often on the leg, sometimes preceded by allergic prodromal symptoms. Bacterial infection is a common complication. Most patients in endemic areas recognize their condition, but irrigation of ulcers can reveal larvae. Treatment is by physical removal of the worm; anthelmintics have no role in management. Provision of safe water for drinking is the key to prevention.

Introduction

The clinical manifestations of Guinea worm and its surgical removal were known in antiquity. Attention was drawn to the seasonal occurrence of painful limb blisters that broke down to reveal a 'worm' in the floor of an ulcer. *Dracunculus medinensis* is the longest nematode infecting humans; in the Bible it is described as the 'fiery serpent'. It was the first human parasite to be shown to have an arthropod intermediate host: in 1870 the Russian naturalist Fedtschenko described the worm's early development *in cyclops*, a 'water flea'. Eradication programmes based on public health measures alone have been very successful. In 1986 3.2 million cases were reported from a total of 20 countries, but by 2008 this had reduced to 6616 in 7 African countries.

Aetiology: the biology of the parasite

The life cycle of the Guinea worm is shown in Fig. 7.9.3.1. Mature female worms, 70 to 120 cm in length, migrate along fascial planes and subcutaneous tissue to reach the skin, usually below the knee. Tissue damage caused by worm products produces a blister that soon ulcerates (Fig. 7.9.3.2). Immersion of the affected part in water causes the worm to contract and expel numerous rhabditiform first-stage larvae from the uterus at the ruptured anterior end of the worm (Fig. 7.9.3.3). The larvae swim vigorously in water for up to 7 days, and some are ingested by predatory copepod crustaceans of the genus *Cyclops*. They penetrate the gut of the intermediate host, and develop with two moults in the haematocele over a period of 14 days to become infective third-stage larvae.

When water containing infected *Cyclops* is swallowed, the released infective larvae burrow though the wall of the duodenum to reach retroperitoneal tissue. After about 60 to 90 days the worms mate, and the females begin their migration towards the limbs; the male worms die and may later calcify. Ten months after infection most female worms, containing fully formed larvae, have reached their destination; within the next month they will rupture through the skin to begin the cycle anew.

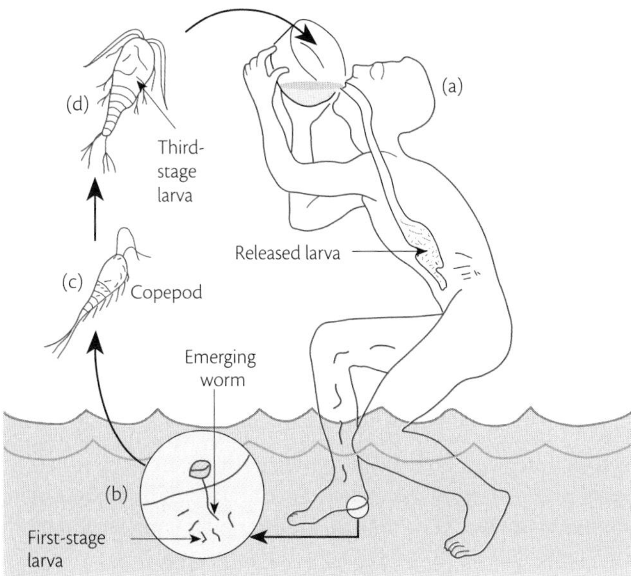

Fig. 7.9.3.1 Life cycle of Guinea worm in humans: (a) copepods infected with third-stage larvae are ingested in drinking water; larvae are released in the intestine, migrate to the body cavity, mature, and mate; (b) gravid female worms migrate to the limbs, cause a blister to form, and release first-stage larvae into water; (c) first-stage larvae are ingested by copepods; and (d) larvae undergo two moults in the copepod and are infective after 2 weeks.

Epidemiology

Guinea worm transmission is predominantly rural, with an annual cycle that often coincides with the planting or harvesting season. Usually, young adults and farmers are most at risk, and there is no immunity. The seasonal morbidity causes great economic hardship. Water sources containing *Cyclops* are easily contaminated by infected persons, including those seeking relief by immersing their painful lesion. In semiarid areas transmission occurs in temporary ponds during the rainy season; in wetter areas flooding and water turbidity limits transmission during the rains, and infection occurs in shallow wells during the dry season. For practical purposes there is no zoonotic reservoir, although infected dogs have been found in endemic areas, and primates can be experimentally infected. Related *Dracunculus* spp. are found in mink, raccoons, and otters in North America.

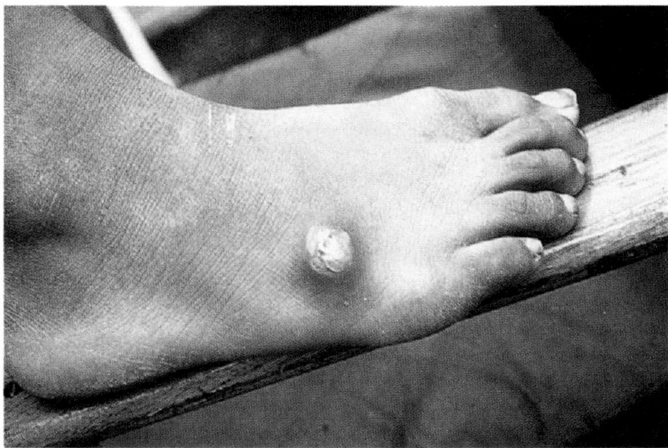

Fig. 7.9.3.2 Blister at site of imminent emergence of the female worm. (Courtesy of the late P E C Manson-Bahr.)

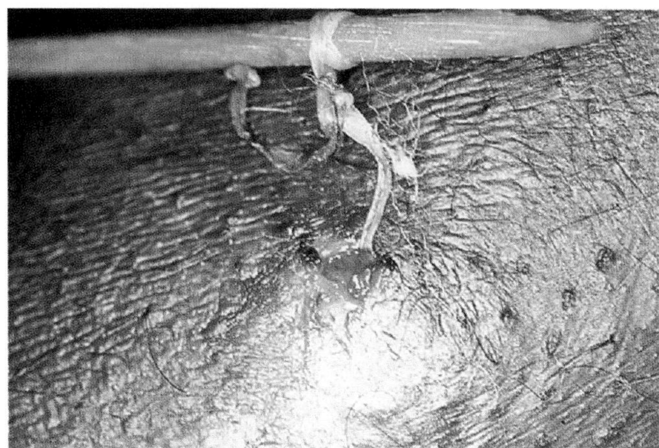

Fig. 7.9.3.3 Emergent female worm being wound out on a stick. (Copyright D A Warrell.)

Geographical distribution

This infection was previously endemic over wide areas of the Middle East and the Indian subcontinent. Largely as a result of improved and protected water sources the infection disappeared from the central Asian republics between 1926 and 1933, from Iran in the 1970s, and from Saudi Arabia in the 1980s. It was eradicated from Pakistan in 1996 and India in 2000. It is now limited to sub-Saharan Africa within the Sahel and Guinea savannah, between latitudes 2° north and 18° north (Fig. 7.9.3.4). It was also present in the Americas, having been introduced with the slave trade, but by the 1880s it had disappeared.

Clinical features

The blister (Fig. 7.9.3.2) is the first sign of infection in most patients. In others, pre-emergent worms may be seen or felt under

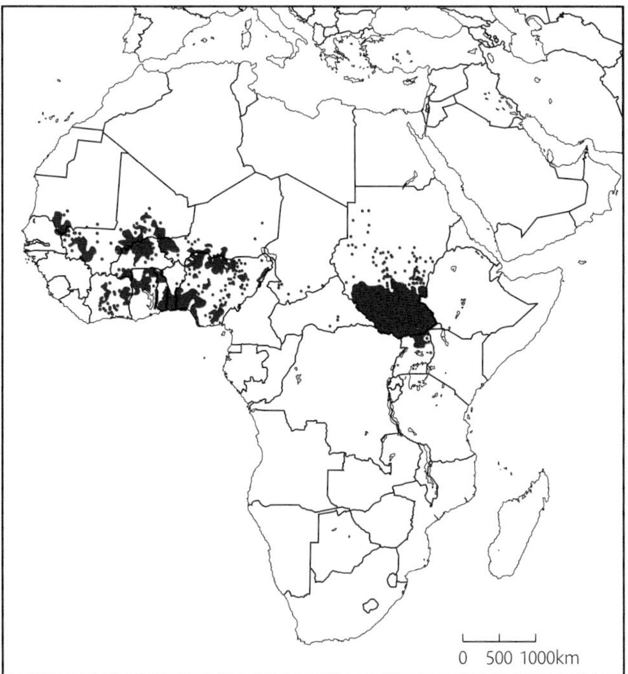

Fig. 7.9.3.4 Distribution of dranunculiasis—endemic villages in Africa.

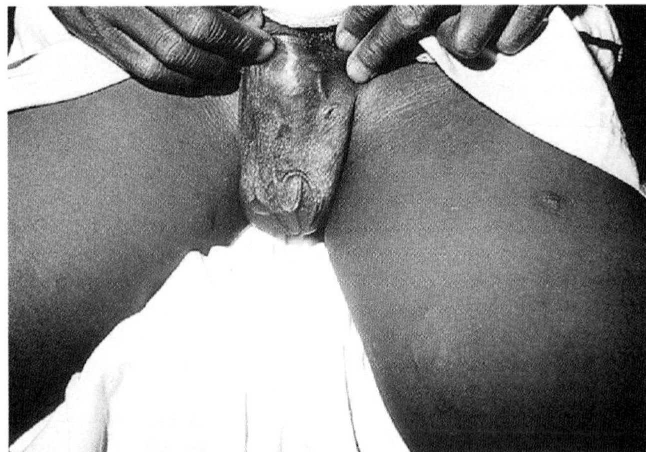

Fig. 7.9.3.5 Guinea worm in the scrotum.
(Copyright D A Warrell.)

the dermis; some are actively motile (Fig. 7.9.3.5). Allergic prodromal symptoms, with urticaria, facial oedema, dyspnoea, and gastrointestinal manifestations, may precede the blister by a few days and disappear when the blister ruptures. Most patients have one or two worms each season, but up to 50 have been recorded. Most gravid worms emerge from the lower limb, but other sites include the buttocks, trunk, arms, scrotum, and vulva.

Uncomplicated cases resolve within 4 weeks. Local complications derive from sensitization to worm products, inappropriate self-treatment, and bacterial infection; these can cause severe pain and prolonged disability. Gravid worms failing to reach the skin release larvae within the host's body, inducing vigorous tissue reactions and abscesses, sometimes presenting as buboes, epididymo-orchitis, or acute arthritis. Joint involvement, often with secondary bacterial infection, is also common near the site of emergence; this leads to ankylosis and tendon contractures, with deformities and permanent disability. Immature female worms may die before reaching the skin and become encapsulated by host tissue; some calcify. They may also enter ectopic sites, including the orbit, pericardium, and central nervous system. Mortality is usually less than 1% and results from systemic or local bacterial infection. Tetanus is a significant risk when spores contaminate open lesions.

Diagnosis

Most patients in endemic areas recognize their condition. Worms release larvae on contact with water, and these can be seen as a milky cloud. When the worm is not visible, ulcers may be irrigated with saline and the centrifuged deposit examined for larvae.

Patient management

Local treatment can be very painful and must often be repeated. Warm moist packs should be applied for several hours, followed by gentle massage along the tract of the worm towards the ulcer. Light traction is then applied to the worm; breakage must be avoided as this greatly aggravates the situation. Analgesics and antibacterial soaks are useful, and oral antibiotics are often necessary. Between local treatments the lesion must be bandaged to reduce the risk of bacterial infection and contamination of water sources.

Pre-emergent worms can be surgically removed, a practice originating in India. A small incision is made adjacent to the worm near its midpoint, and a loop of worm is lifted out with a blunt curved probe. Massage is applied along the length of the worm towards the incision, and by gentle traction the whole worm can usually be removed. In the event of breakage the worm ends should be ligated to minimize contact between host tissue and worm antigens. Deep abscesses require surgical treatment. Anthelmintics have no role in the treatment of Guinea worm.

Control and eradication

Several factors facilitate control: Guinea worm is recognized by local communities as a major health problem, there are no carriers beyond the annual cycle, and there is no animal reservoir. The provision of safe water for drinking is the key to control; it is unrealistic to expect piped water supplies in most endemic areas, but covered tube wells or hand-dug wells provided with parapets are appropriate. Additional measures are filtration of household water with finely woven cloth, and the application of temephos to ponds to kill copepods.

National programmes have played a major role in many endemic areas. Case-detection surveys and health education can be integrated into existing primary health care systems. Unhygienic local treatments such as mud or leaf poultices and crude methods of worm extraction must be discouraged.

Several international health agencies took up the challenge of Guinea worm eradication in the mid 1980s, with an initial target eradication date of 1995. Much has been achieved, but the target was missed. The initial expensive hydrological programmes were later replaced by the training of local cadres who could recruit patients within 24 hours of worm emergence to 'containment centres' for treatment and education to prevent water source contamination. In some areas, private-sector initiatives have been able to gain commercially from the publicity achieved by adopting control in a defined area.

In 2008, 98.6% of the 6616 cases were from southern Sudan, northern Ghana and eastern Mali. Only 4 other countries reported cases: Ethiopia 48, Nigeria 39, Niger 2 and Burkina Faso 1. 70% of the 2008 total were seen in 'containment centres'. The last stages of eradication will be the most difficult, as vertical programmes then become inefficient. Unfortunately, many of the major residual foci are in situations of civil disorder where there are mobile refugees; in others a lack of resources or an absence of democratic institutions may slow progress.

Further reading

Berry M (2007). The tail end of Guinea worm – global eradication without a vaccine. *New Eng J Med*, **356**, 2561–4.

Cairncross S, Muller R, Zagaria N (2002). Dracunculiasis (Guinea worm disease) and the eradication initiative. *Clin Microbiol Rev*, **15**, 223–46.

Glenshaw MT, *et al.* (2009). Guinea worm disease outcomes in Ghana: determinants of broken worms. *Am J Trop Med Hyg*, **81**, 305–12.

Hochberg N, *et al.* (2008). The role of containment centres in the eradication of dracunculiasis in Togo and Ghana. *Am J Trop Med Hyg*, **79**, 722–8.

Muller R (1971). Dracunculus and dracunculiasis. *Adv Parasitol*, **9**, 73–151.

Rhode JE, *et al.* (1993). Surgical extraction of Guinea worm: disability reduction and contribution to disease control. *Am J Trop Med Hyg*, **48**, 71–6.

Ruiz-Tiben E, Hopkins DR (2006). Dracunculiasis (Guinea worm disease) eradication. *Adv Parasitol*, 61, 275–309.

7.9.4 Strongyloidiasis, hookworm, and other gut strongyloid nematodes

Michael Brown

Essentials

Strongyloides stercoralis and hookworms are common soil-transmitted nematodes in tropical and subtropical regions. After the organisms penetrate exposed skin, most infections are asymptomatic, but heavy infections can result in significant morbidity.

Strongyloidiasis

The roundworm *S. stercoralis* infects an estimated 30 million to 100 million people. Clinical manifestations include: (1) skin—often the only clinical manifestation, commonly in the form of larva currens, a serpiginous, pruritic, erythematous eruption at the site of migrating larvae; (2) lungs—cough and tracheal irritation; less commonly wheeze; patchy infiltrates on chest radiography with eosinophilia; (3) intestinal—epigastric pain and diarrhoea; (4) *Strongyloides* hyperinfection—occurs in patients who are immunosuppressed; severe diarrhoea is a common feature; mortality is high. Infection is persistent and may present decades after exposure. Diagnosis is usually by microscopy or culture of stool; serology is useful as a screening test. Treatment is typically with ivermectin or albendazole. Improved sanitation and appropriate footwear may reduce the acquisition of infection.

Hookworms

Hookworm infections, mainly caused by *Ancylostoma duodenale* and *Necator americanus*, affect more than 500 million people, predominantly in sub-Saharan Africa and Asia. Clinical manifestations include: (1) migratory/larval—ground itch (a pruritic, papular, and erythematous rash on the feet or hands); occasionally pneumonitis with eosinophilia; (2) intestinal—occasionally profuse watery diarrhoea, but most people are asymptomatic excepting for iron-deficiency anaemia (sometimes with haemoglobin <2 g/dl) in those with heavy infections, which are a particular problem in infants and pregnant women, in whom it affects pregnancy adversely. Diagnosis of acute infection is clinical and of chronic infection by discovering eggs in the stool by microscopy. A single dose of albendazole will reduce the worm load to levels below those likely to cause disease; complete eradication can be achieved with repeated doses.

Population-based control programmes, using single-dose anti-helmintic therapy, aim to reduce anaemia and improve childhood growth and cognitive development in countries with high prevalence of soil-transmitted helminths. Increasing attention is being paid to the effect of coinfection with hookworm on other diseases such as malaria, tuberculosis, HIV, and asthma.

Nonhuman hookworms

These cannot complete their life cycle in humans but are capable of causing significant morbidity, including: (1) cutaneous larva migrans—usually due to dog hookworms; presents as intensely pruritic lesions on exposed areas of the skin; diagnosis is clinical, although the worm may be visualized in skin biopsies; albendazole is effective; (2) *Ancylostoma caninum*-associated enteritis; (3) oesophagostomiasis; (4) trichostrongyliasis.

Strongyloides stercoralis

Pathogenesis and life cycle

Strongyloides stercoralis is a roundworm that has two alternative life cycles, producing either parasitic or free-living forms. It is one of the few helminths that can complete its life cycle in humans. Filariform larvae in moist soil penetrate exposed skin, and pass via the bloodstream to the lungs and into the alveolar spaces. From there, the larvae ascend the trachea and are swallowed, reaching their final habitat in the crypts of Lieberkühn in the duodenum and upper jejunum, where they mature.

The adult males are rapidly eliminated from the intestine, leaving parthenogenetic adult parasitic females, 2.5 mm in length, attached to the mucosa, where they deposit eggs. One month after infection, the resulting rhabditiform larvae bore through the epithelium into the gut lumen. At this stage, most larvae follow an indirect developmental route—they are excreted in the faeces and develop into free-living adults, which produce eggs from which filariform larvae develop. Some larvae by contrast develop directly via three moults into filariform larvae. These are usually passed in the faeces and can survive in the soil for many weeks. However, some may reinvade the host in the lower gastrointestinal tract or perianal skin before evacuation. It is this process of autoinfection that explains the persistence of chronic *S. stercoralis* infections for decades after exposure, and allows for the multiplication of worms that may lead to the phenomenon of hyperinfection seen in immunosuppressed patients.

Strongyloidiasis, like most helminth infections, is associated with a type 2 immune response, with raised IgE levels and increased circulating eosinophil numbers. In immunosuppressed patients, some elements of this immune response are lacking. The pathogenesis of hyperinfection is not well understood. A possible explanation is that immunosuppression facilitates the direct route of strongyloides development, leading to multiplicative autoinfection, increasing larval intensities, and ultimately, dissemination of larvae beyond the gut mucosa into other organs.

Epidemiology

S. stercoralis infects an estimated 30 to 100 million people, with a distribution throughout tropical and subtropical areas. Prevalence in rural areas of sub-Saharan Africa, South-East Asia, and Central and South America can reach 20%; a lower level of active transmission persists in temperate regions such as southern Europe and the southern United States of America. In highly endemic areas, infection intensities peak in childhood and then plateau or decline. Because of the chronicity of infection, prevalence remains high in immigrants from endemic areas, reaching 30 to 80% in South-East Asian immigrants screened in North America. A prevalence greater than 30% has been observed among former British servicemen who were prisoners of war in the Far East in 1941–5, screened 30 years or more after exposure.

Clinical features

Most infected individuals are asymptomatic. In such patients, diagnosis may only be considered as part of investigation for peripheral eosinophilia.

Cutaneous

Skin symptoms are often the only manifestation of infection, commonly in the form of larva currens, a serpiginous pruritic erythematous eruption on the legs, buttocks, and back, at the site of migrating larvae, that can advance as quickly as 15 cm/h (Fig. 7.9.4.1). The rash is more diffuse and migrates more rapidly than the cutaneous larva migrans associated with hookworm infections. It may occur with the initial infection, but also in people with chronic strongyloidiasis.

Pulmonary

The migratory phase may be associated with cough and tracheal irritation, and less commonly with wheeze, which may be persistent. Patchy infiltrates may be seen on chest radiographs. When larvae become trapped in the lung during migration, eosinophilic pneumonia occasionally occurs. Pulmonary manifestations, including pneumonia, bacterial lung abscesses, and acute respiratory distress syndrome are more prominent in hyperinfected patients (see below).

Intestinal

Intestinal symptoms are generally mild in people with light infection. Epigastric pain mimicking peptic ulcer disease may occur within 3 weeks of infection and persist. Diarrhoea is usually chronic and mild, but may occur early and be associated with bloody stools. In more severe cases, usually associated with hyperinfection, intestinal oedema with malabsorption, mesenteric lymphadenopathy, and ascites may occur. An eosinophilic granulomatous enterocolitis resembling Crohn's disease is well described in older patients on corticosteroids. Subacute intestinal obstruction, biliary stenosis, and necrotizing enteritis are occasionally seen.

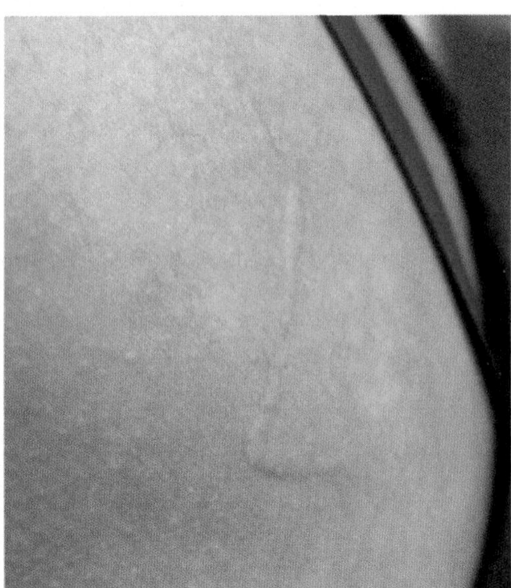

Fig. 7.9.4.1 Characteristic serpiginous rash of larva currens on the shoulder of a traveller with *Strongyloides stercoralis* infection acquired in India. The rash was transient, but recurrent and widespread.
(Courtesy of R H Behrens, Hospital for Tropical Diseases, London.)

Strongyloides hyperinfection

Patients on long-term corticosteroids, and those undergoing chemotherapy or organ transplantation, are at risk from severe manifestations of strongyloidiasis. This also occurs in patients with lymphoma or leukaemia without chemotherapy, most commonly in those with T-cell leukaemia caused by human T-cell leukaemia virus (HTLV)-1 infection. It is also well described in HTLV-1-infected patients without overt malignancy, and less commonly in patients with AIDS. Disseminated disease has a very high mortality rate. Severe diarrhoea is a common feature. Gram-negative pneumonia, bacteraemia, or meningitis caused by enteric pathogens that have breached the mucosal barrier along with the strongyloides larvae are frequent manifestations. Petechial haemorrhages in the skin, especially around the umbilicus, and hepatitis may occur. Peripheral eosinophilia is often absent in disseminated disease.

Diagnosis

Microscopy of stool may reveal rhabditiform larvae, but the sensitivity of direct smears is low. Formol-ether concentration techniques are more useful, but multiple stool samples may be required to detect light infections. Culture techniques have been developed to enhance the diagnostic yield. Agar plate cultures have the highest yield; tracks made by larvae migrating across the plate can be seen. Charcoal culture and filter-paper methods make use of the indirect life cycle: stool is incubated for several days to allow the development of adults and second-generation filariform larvae.

Larvae may also be isolated by duodenal aspiration, or by the string test, although these are of limited sensitivity. In disseminated infection, larvae are found in the sputum and in biopsies from tissues such as the gastrointestinal tract and lung.

Enzyme-linked immunosorbent assays (ELISA) for strongyloides-specific IgG have high sensitivity for strongyloides infection. There is cross-reaction with filarial antibodies, and levels may remain elevated after treatment, so specificity may be limited. It is useful as a screening test, particularly before embarking on immunosuppressive therapy.

Treatment and prevention

Albendazole 400 mg once or twice daily for 3 days is reasonably effective in chronic infections, and is better tolerated than tiabendazole 25 mg/kg twice daily for 3 days. Currently, the treatment of choice is ivermectin 200 μg/kg as a single dose. Prolonged courses of treatment are necessary in patients with severe or disseminated disease. Subcutaneous veterinary preparations have been used when parenteral treatment is required.

Improved sanitation and appropriate footwear may reduce the acquisition of infection. Once established, strongyloides should be eradicated in any patient being considered for immunosuppressive therapy, because of the potentially lethal consequences of hyperinfection.

Strongyloides fuelleborni

Strongyloides fuelleborni fuelleborni is a parasite of primates in tropical Africa and Asia, which can also infect human populations sharing similar habitats. Prevalence rates up to 20% have been reported among forest-dwelling communities. Infections are generally asymptomatic. Unlike *S. stercoralis*, eggs are passed in the stool, and may be confused with hookworm ova. Benzimidazole therapy is effective.

A phylogenetically distinct nematode, *Strongyloides fuelleborni kellyei*, has been found in rural communities in Papua New Guinea. Infection intensities are highest among young children. It is associated with 'swollen belly sickness' in 2-month-old infants, which is characterized by abdominal distension, respiratory distress, generalized oedema, and gastrointestinal disturbance.

Hookworm

Pathogenesis and life cycle

Hookworm infections are principally caused by the two species that can complete their life cycles in humans: *Ancylostoma duodenale* and *Necator americanus*. Their life cycles are similar. Larvae in moist soil penetrate exposed skin, usually on the feet or buttocks. They enter the circulation after 10 days, are carried to the lungs, and cross into the alveolae, from where they are transported to the pharynx and swallowed. The adults, approximately 10 mm in length, attach themselves to the small intestinal mucosa with their buccal cavities, which contain hooked teeth (ancylostoma) or cutting plates (necator). After 3 to 6 weeks the females produce up to 30 000 eggs per day, which are passed in the faeces. The eggs hatch within 48 h, but the larvae can remain viable for up to 6 weeks in appropriate soil conditions. Adult hookworms live for 1 to 9 years. Infection can also be acquired by the ingestion of contaminated soil, and the transmission of infective larvae via breast milk is well recognized.

Infection is associated with tissue and peripheral eosinophilia, and specific IgG and nonspecific IgE responses. Regulatory cytokine responses are probably crucial in limiting immunopathology in established infection. Equally important are a range of worm-derived immunomodulatory molecules that interfere with neutrophil migration and adhesion, inhibit complement, induce T-cell apoptosis, and prevent blood coagulation. Secreted anticoagulants, including serine protease inhibitors of factor Xa, are responsible for anaemia, the main consequence of infection. Radioisotope studies have demonstrated that hookworm infections produce a daily blood loss of up to 0.3 ml per worm per day. This translates into a loss of up to 100 ml per day in heavily infected people. The degree of anaemia is partly a function of worm burden, but also of iron stores. Variations in dietary iron intake, as well as malaria coinfection, account for some of the geographical differences in the incidence of hookworm anaemia.

Epidemiology

Estimates suggest that more than 500 million people are infected with hookworm, predominantly in sub-Saharan Africa and Asia. Although significant overlap occurs, the distribution of *A. duodenale* is more restricted geographically than that of *N. americanus*. Necator is more widespread in sub-Saharan Africa, the Americas, South-East Asia, and India; ancylostoma is also widely distributed in South-East Asia, but is more common in temperate regions, North Africa, and the Middle East. As with other intestinal helminths, most infected people harbour a few adult worms, but a minority are heavily infected. Social, behavioural, and genetic factors determine which individuals within a community are most heavily infected. Unlike most other intestinal helminth infections, the prevalence and intensity of hookworm infection increases with age.

Clinical features

Migratory/larval

Repeated exposure to penetrating hookworm larvae results in ground itch, a pruritic papular erythematous rash on the feet or hands. Larval pulmonary migration is generally asymptomatic, but may result in a pneumonitis characterized by fever, cough, wheeze, haemoptysis, and peripheral eosinophilia. Symptoms may last several weeks, but are rarely severe. Oral ingestion of *A. duodenale* larvae can result in Wakana disease, which presents with nausea, vomiting, cough, pharyngeal irritation, and dyspnoea.

Intestinal

Recently acquired human hookworm infection occasionally causes profuse watery diarrhoea. Most people with established infection are asymptomatic. The major morbidity associated with hookworm infection is iron-deficiency anaemia in those with heavy infections. Haemoglobin concentrations of less than 2 g/dl are not uncommon. Hookworms were first identified in the investigation of anaemic miners in 19th century Europe, notably in Cornish tin mines, where an extreme form of anaemia (chlorosis or 'green disease') was prevalent. Now eradicated in developed countries, hookworm remains a major cause of anaemia in the developing world. It is particularly common among women of reproductive age, and a major contributor towards adverse outcomes in pregnancy, being responsible for 30 to 50% of cases of pregnancy-associated anaemia. Fatigue and listlessness are the principal symptoms, and probably have a significant economic impact in areas of high prevalence. High-output cardiac failure is a major cause of death in patients with severe anaemia. Malabsorption is not a frequent consequence of hookworm infection, but protein loss does occur and may contribute to the oedema seen in severe infections.

Dyspepsia, nausea, and a range of nonspecific symptoms are common in those with heavy worm burdens. Pica, a craving for eating soil, is well described in patients with hookworm anaemia.

Growth and cognitive development

There has been debate about the effect of chronic hookworm infection on growth and cognitive development in childhood. Seminal work in an impoverished community in the southern United States of America in the 1920s demonstrated an inverse association between IQ and hookworm intensity. The results of subsequent studies have been inconclusive. Intervention trials in East Africa have suggested a modest effect of heavy hookworm infection on growth, and the balance of evidence suggests that heavily infected subjects do have impairments of memory and other specific cognitive functions. It is not known to what extent these effects are mediated by or are independent of anaemia. Treatment results in improved cognitive performance and school attendance.

Diagnosis

The diagnosis of acute hookworm infection is clinical. Characteristic symptoms are usually associated with peripheral eosinophilia.

The diagnosis of chronic infection is made by discovering eggs in the stool by microscopy. Symptomatic infection is readily diagnosed by direct microscopy of a single stool sample, as the worm burden is high in these patients. Where diagnosis of lighter infections is required, e.g. in the investigation of eosinophilia, the diagnostic yield is increased by examining multiple stool samples, using concentration methods, or by culture techniques. The latter allow for the development of third-stage larvae, which can be used to identify the infecting hookworm species and differentiate from related nematode species. Semiquantitative techniques, such as the modified Kato smear, can be used to estimate infection intensity. Hookworm eggs degenerate rapidly after excretion, and laboratory processing should be performed as soon as possible.

Treatment, prevention, and control

A single dose of a benzimidazole, such as albendazole 400 mg, will kill more than 80% of adult hookworms and thus reduce the worm load to a level below that likely to cause disease. Complete eradication can be achieved with repeated doses. Treatment is well tolerated, and can safely be given to children and in pregnancy (although not recommended in the first trimester). For patients with anaemia, anthelmintic treatment should be combined with iron replacement. Patients with heart failure or severe anaemia during pregnancy frequently require transfusion of packed red cells.

In developing countries where the prevalence of hookworm and other intestinal helminths is high, the increasing availability of safe, affordable, single-dose anthelmintics makes mass deworming programmes feasible (Fig. 7.9.4.2). The impact of empirical population-based treatment, e.g. in schools, can be sustained in the face of ongoing transmission by repeated treatment at 3- to 12-month intervals. These strategies can be integrated with control programmes for other helminthiases. The World Health Organization has set a target date of 2010 for routine anthelmintic treatment to be provided to 75% of school-age children at risk of infection. A specific impact on hookworm-associated anaemia may not, however, be as great as the effects on other intestinal helminths, because school-based programmes will miss the most vulnerable populations (preschool children and pregnant women).

The age–intensity distribution of hookworm infection is likely to limit any benefit of mass treatment programmes on hookworm transmission. The provision of better footwear and improved sanitation for infected communities probably has only a marginal role, at least in the medium term, in reducing transmission. Vaccines, which are currently undergoing clinical testing, offer potential for better hookworm control.

Consequences of immune modulation by hookworms

Helminth infections have a similar global distribution to other pathogens. Our understanding of the immune response to helminth infection has stimulated interest in the effect of helminths on subjects coinfected with other microorganisms, particularly malaria, tuberculosis, and HIV. Children with heavy hookworm infections mount a reduced febrile response to malaria. There may be effects of hookworm infection on immune responses to mycobacterial antigens, although hookworm does not appear to increase the incidence of tuberculosis or accelerate the progression of HIV infection.

There is evidence that childhood or maternal infection with some helminths, especially hookworm, may protect against the development of atopy. These findings lend support to the 'hygiene hypothesis' that the increasing prevalence of allergy worldwide may partly be a result of reduced exposure to the immunosuppressive effects of helminths, and lead to concerns that mass deworming may have detrimental as well as beneficial effects. A recent trial of experimental hookworm infection as a treatment for asthma did not demonstrate a significant benefit.

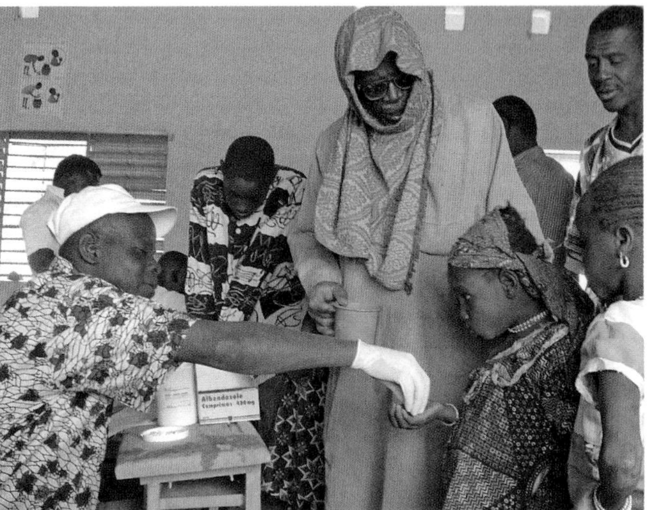

Fig. 7.9.4.2 School-based treatment as part of a mass anthelmintic treatment programme in Burkina Faso.
(Courtesy of A Gabrielli, Schistosomiasis Control Initiative.)

Nonhuman hookworms

Nonhuman hookworms cannot complete their life cycle in the human host, but are capable of causing significant morbidity in the skin and gastrointestinal tract.

Cutaneous larva migrans

Cutaneous larva migrans presents as intensely pruritic lesions on exposed areas of the skin. The rash is commonly seen on the feet or buttocks, but may occur elsewhere (Fig. 7.9.4.3). Dog hookworms such as *Ancylostoma braziliense* are usually implicated. Like human hookworms these species thrive in sandy soil, and frequently infect travellers visiting beaches in the Caribbean, South-East Asia, and Africa. Untreated, the rash can persist for months, with gradual spread through the epidermis leaving serpiginous tracks. Secondary bacterial infection may sometimes occur. Diagnosis is clinical, although the worm may be visualized in biopsies taken from the leading edge of the lesion. Topical albendazole or tiabendazole are usually effective, although short courses of oral albendazole or ivermectin are more effective.

Ancylostoma caninum-associated gastroenteritis

First described in Australia in the 1980s, a distinctive eosinophilic enteritis has been linked to infection with *A. caninum*, a dog hookworm. The global distribution of this disease is unknown. Oral ingestion may be the predominant route of infection. Manifestations range from a limited aphthous ileitis with tissue and peripheral eosinophilia, which may be asymptomatic, to a severe painful eosinophilic gastroenteritis with gut oedema, ascites, and regional lymphadenopathy. Immature hookworm larvae can be identified in the lesions, although the diagnosis may only be made at laparotomy.

(a)

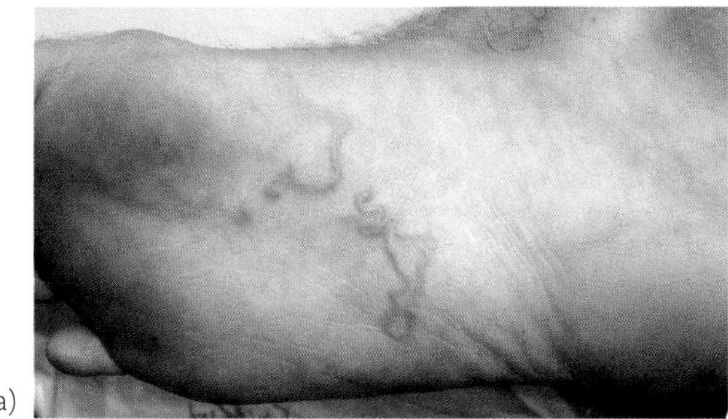

(b)

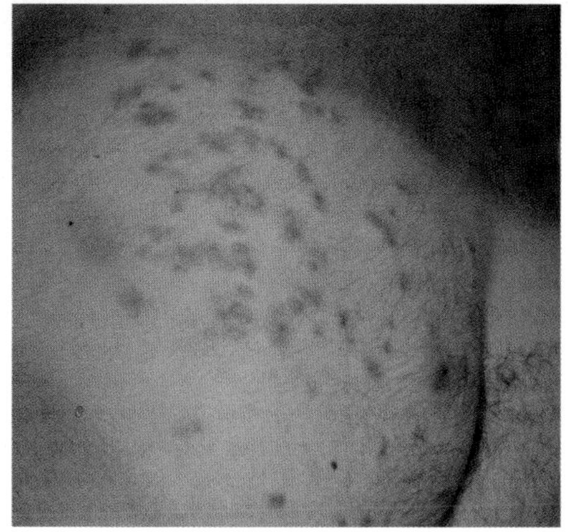

Fig. 7.9.4.3 Cutaneous larva migrans: (a) caused by probable *Ancylostoma braziliense* infection acquired on a beach in the Caribbean, and (b) heavy infection with *Ancylostoma braziliense* acquired in Brazil.
(a, courtesy of D Webster, Oxford Radcliffe Hospitals, United Kingdom; b, copyright D A Warrell.)

Immunodiagnostic tests have been developed, but do not discriminate between human and nonhuman hookworm infections. Mebendazole is effective.

Oesophagostomum spp.

Human oesophagostomiasis, usually caused by *Oesophagostomum bifurcum*, is common in forested areas of West Africa, but rare elsewhere. Prevalence in some areas of Togo and northern Ghana may reach 75%. The nematode can complete its life cycle in humans, and is distinct from related species in primates. Humans probably acquire the disease by ingesting infective third-stage larvae, although a percutaneous route of infection has not been excluded. The larvae migrate to and develop within the colonic wall before returning to the intestinal lumen, where they reach adulthood and excrete eggs.

Intense tissue reactions occur around the larvae, forming nodules along the wall of the (usually ascending) colon. Although these infections are generally asymptomatic, heavy infections may result in the development of multiple pea-sized nodules, with gross mucosal and serosal oedema, and microabscess formation (Fig. 7.9.4.4). Children are most commonly affected, and present with abdominal pain, diarrhoea, and weight loss. Solitary palpable painful inflammatory masses, known as Dapaong tumours, also occur within the bowel wall and in extraintestinal sites such as the mesentery or abdominal wall. Nodules can be detected ultrasonographically. Ova are morphologically indistinguishable from those of hookworm, but can be differentiated by culturing third-stage larvae. Treatment with short courses of albendazole is effective and may obviate the need for surgery.

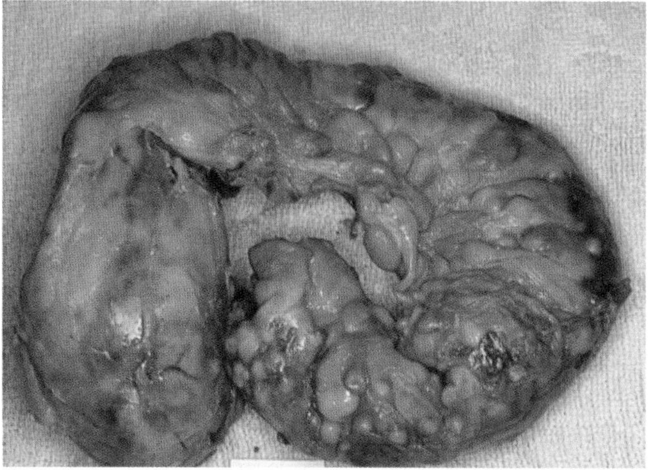

Fig. 7.9.4.4 Excised colon from a young Ghanaian adult with *Oesophagostomum bifurcum*-associated disease. Multiple nodules and serosal oedema are present. The diagnosis was made at laparotomy after the patient presented with abdominal pain and peritonism.
(Courtesy of A M Polderman, Leiden University Medical Center, Netherlands.)

Trichostrongylus spp.

Trichostrongylus spp. are ubiquitous nematode parasites of herbivores, particularly domesticated animals such as sheep, goats, cattle, and donkeys. Human infection occurs most commonly among herders, with a prevalence of more than 80% reported among Iranian nomads. Sporadic human infections occur in urban environments through contact with the faeces of domestic animals. Infective larvae hatch in the soil, and are ingested with contaminated vegetables. There is no migratory phase; the adults develop in the duodenal mucosa, and produce eggs after a long prepatent period. Most infected people are asymptomatic, although eosinophilia is common. Epigastric pain, diarrhoea, and rectal bleeding may occur. Diagnosis is made by finding eggs (which may be mistaken for hookworm ova) by stool microscopy. The adults are occasionally visualized at endoscopy. Benzimidazole anthelmintics may be effective, although resistance is increasing; a single dose of ivermectin 200 µg/kg is usually sufficient.

Further reading

Ashford RW, Barnish G, Viney ME (1992). *Strongyloides fuelleborni kellyi:* infection and disease in Papua New Guinea. *Parasitol Today*, **8**, 314–8.

Croese J, *et al.* (1994). Human enteric infection with canine hookworms. *Ann Intern Med*, **120**, 369–74.

Eziefula AC, Brown M, *et al* . (2008). Intestinal nematodes: disease burden, deworming and the potential importance of co-infection. *Curr Op Infect Dis*, **21**, 516–522.

Gill GV, *et al.* (2004). Chronic *Strongyloides stercoralis* infection in former British Far East prisoners of war. *Q J Med*, **97**, 789–95.

Hotez PJ, *et al.* (2004). Hookworm infection. *N Engl J Med*, **351**, 799–807.

Keiser PB, Nutman TB (2004). *Strongyloides stercoralis* in the immunocompromised population. *Clin Microbiol Rev*, **17**, 208–17.

Leonard-Bee J, Pritchard D, Britton J (2006). Asthma and current intestinal parasite infection: systematic review and meta-analysis. *Am J Respir Crit Care Med*, **174**, 514–23.

Quinnell RJ, Bethony J, Pritchard DI (2004). The immunoepidemiology of human hookworm infection. *Parasite Immunol*, **26**, 443–54.

Siddiqui AA, Berk SL (2001). Diagnosis of *Strongyloides stercoralis* infection. *Clin Infect Dis*, **33**, 1040–7.

Storey PA, *et al.* (2000). Clinical epidemiology and classification of human oesophagostomiasis. *Trans R Soc Trop Med Hyg*, **94**, 177–82.

World Health Organization (2005). *Preventive chemotherapy in human helminthiasis*. WHO, Geneva.

7.9.5 Gut and tissue nematode infections acquired by ingestion

David I. Grove

Ascariasis

Ascaris lumbricoides (the giant roundworm) is widespread in the tropics and subtropics where sanitation is poor and the soil is contaminated with its eggs. Ingested eggs hatch in the small bowel, cycle through the bloodstream and lungs, then return to the small bowel and develop into adult worms 15 to 30 cm long. Most infections are asymptomatic, but there may be pulmonary infiltrates with eosinophilia, abdominal discomfort and—in children with heavy infections—intestinal obstruction. Infection is diagnosed by finding eggs in the faeces. Treatment is with pyrantel, mebedenazole, or albendazole.

Anisakiasis

This is caused by larvae of roundworms in the family *Anisakidae*, which are parasites of marine mammals. After ingestion of larvae in uncooked fish or squid, immature larvae burrow into the gastric or intestinal mucosa and may cause abdominal pain. Diagnosis is usually made at endoscopy, with treatment by endoscopic removal (if possible) of the larvae, although symptoms resolve spontaneously in most cases.

Capillariasis

Intestinal capillariasis—caused by *Paracapillaria philippinensis*, this is acquired by ingestion of undercooked freshwater fish and may cause a severe diarrhoeal disease. Diagnosis is by finding eggs in the stool. Treatment is with mebendazole or albendazole. Prevention is by properly cooking fish.

Hepatic capillariasis—caused by *Capillaria hepatica*, a parasite of rats. Ingested eggs hatch and larvae pass to the liver and cause a syndrome similar to visceral larva migrans (see below). Diagnosis is made by identifying the parasite or eggs in a liver biopsy. Treatment is usually with thiabendazole or albendazole.

Enterobiasis

Enterobius vermicularis (the threadworm) is cosmopolitan. Ingested eggs develop directly into adult worms in the gut; fertilized female worms crawl out of the rectum at night and deposit eggs on the perianal skin. Most infections are asymptomatic, but pruritus ani may be troublesome at night. Diagnosis is made by finding eggs on clear adhesive tape applied to the perianal skin. Pyrantel, mebendazole, and albendazole are effective in combination with sanitary measures.

Toxocariasis

This is due to invasion by larvae of *Toxocara canis* and *T. cati*, acquired by ingestion of eggs from dog and cat stools. It occurs in two clinical forms—visceral and ocular larva migrans.

Visceral larva migrans—usually afflicts children; larvae migrate to the viscera and may be asymptomatic or cause protean manifestations including muscular pain, lassitude, anorexia, cough, urticarial rashes, hepatomegaly, and (occasionally) splenomegaly, lymphadenopathy and skin lesions, and (rarely) central nervous system involvement (convulsions). Eosinophilia is prominent. Definitive diagnosis is by finding larvae on biopsy, usually of the liver; a negative serological test for toxocara antibody rules out the diagnosis. Most patients recover spontaneously; there is no proven therapy.

Ocular larva migrans—more commonly seen in older children and due to granuloma formation around a larva in the retina. Diagnosis depends upon positive serology together with consistent fundoscopic features. There is no proven anthelmintic therapy.

Trichinosis

This is acquired by ingestion of larvae of *Trichinella spiralis* in undercooked meat, usually pork. Adult worms in the small bowel produce larvae which seed the muscles and other tissues, where they develop. Most infections are asymptomatic, but heavy infections typically cause diarrhoea, followed by fever and myositis. Definitive diagnosis depends upon finding larvae in muscle biopsies, although this is usually unnecessary; serological tests become positive several weeks after infection. Treatment is symptomatic. Thorough cooking of pork is the best safeguard against infection.

Trichuriasis

Trichuris trichiura (whipworm) is most prevalent in the tropics and subtropics where sanitation is poor. Ingested eggs hatch in the small bowel and then develop within the gut into adult worms which become embedded in the large bowel mucosa. Very heavy infections may cause dysentery or rectal prolapse. Infection is diagnosed by finding eggs in the faeces. Treatment is with mebedenazole or albendazole.

Ascariasis (giant roundworm infection)

Life cycle

Ascariasis is an infection caused by the giant roundworm, *Ascaris lumbricoides*. Infection is acquired when an egg is ingested (Fig. 7.9.5.1). The infective larva hatches out in the small intestine (Fig. 7.9.5.2) and penetrates the intestinal wall to enter the portal circulation. From here it enters the systemic circulation and reaches the lungs, where it breaks out of the capillaries into the alveoli and undergoes another moult to become a fourth-stage larva. From the

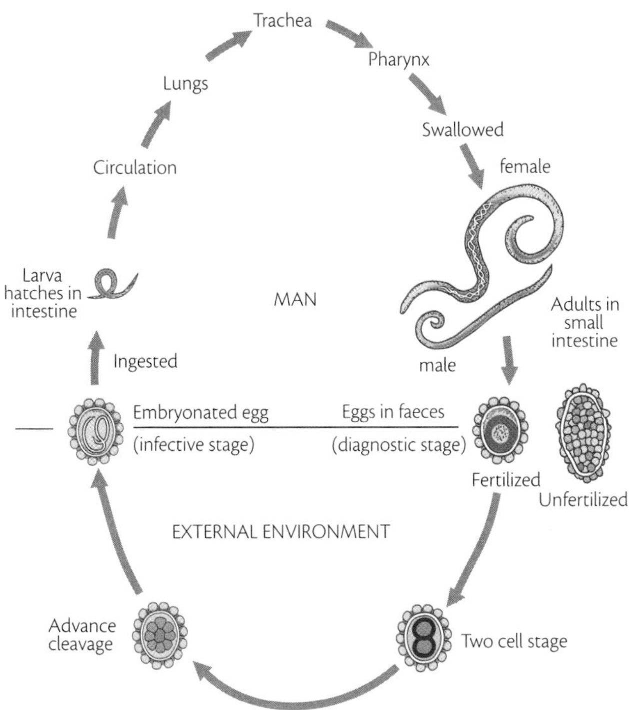

Fig. 7.9.5.1 Life cycle of *Ascaris lumbricoides*.

lungs the larva moves up the bronchial tree to the mouth, and is then swallowed. In the intestine it moults again to become a sexually mature worm about 6 to 8 weeks after ingestion. The mature worm is cylindrical with tapering ends, and creamy white to light-brown in colour (Fig. 7.9.5.3). The female measures 20 to 35 cm in length and 3 to 6 mm in width, whereas the male is 12 to 31 cm long and 2 to 4 mm wide, and has a curved tail.

Normally, the adult worms live in the lumen of the small intestine, primarily the jejunum. The worm is able to maintain its position in the small intestine by the activity of its somatic muscles; if these are paralysed by anthelmintics it is expelled by peristalsis. The lifespan of an adult worm is usually 1 to 2 years, after which it is expelled spontaneously. The worms mate, and eggs are passed in

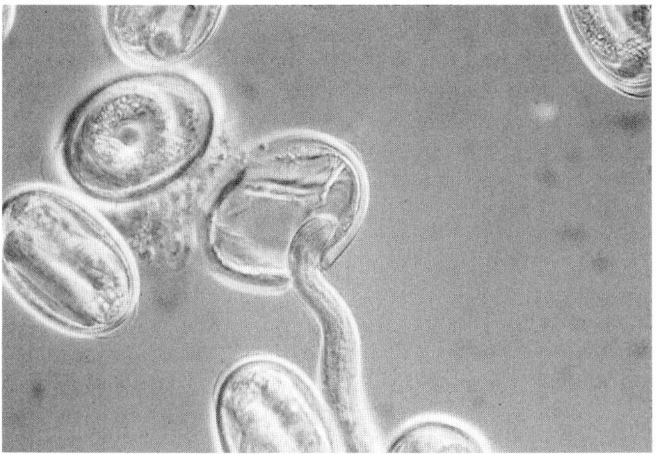

Fig. 7.9.5.2 Decorticated eggs of *Ascaris lumbricoides*, showing emergence of larvae.
(Copyright Viqar Zaman.)

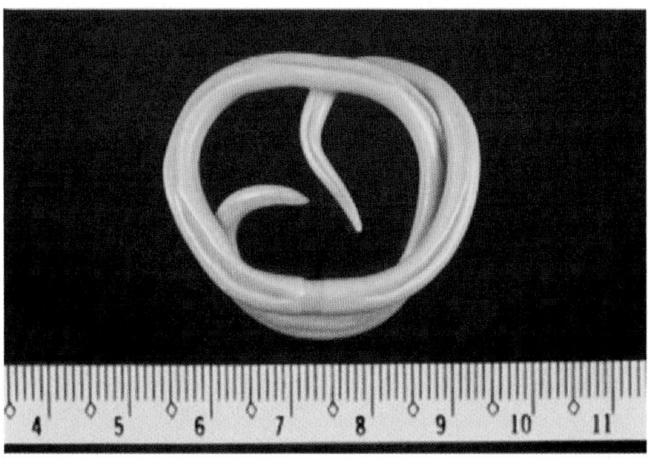

Fig. 7.9.5.3 Adult *Ascaris lumbricoides* (scale in mm).
(Copyright Viqar Zaman)

the faeces, with gravid females producing 200 000 to 250 000 eggs daily. When freshly passed these eggs are not infective, and contain a single cell. This develops in the soil over the next 2 to 6 weeks (faster in warmer temperatures) into an infective larva. The ova are resistant to chemicals and low temperatures, and may remain viable for years in moist soil.

Epidemiology and control

Ascariasis is cosmopolitan, and is probably the most common helminth infection. It is prevalent in areas where there is poor sanitation and contamination of the soil with eggs. Infection is more common in tropical climates, and is particularly prevalent in areas where human faeces are used to fertilize vegetable gardens. Infection is usually acquired by eating contaminated food, or from soil ingested by children when playing, and does not induce resistance to reinfection. It is relatively more common in children, who also carry higher worm loads. In hyperendemic areas with constant warm temperatures and high humidity, children are continuously being infected, so that as some worms are being expelled, others are maturing to take their place. Transmission may only be associated with the rainy season in areas that are generally hot and arid. Environmental sanitation is the best control measure, but when this is not possible mass chemotherapy given at intervals of 6 months reduces the severity and intensity of infection.

Clinical features

The first passage of larvae through the lungs usually causes no symptoms or pathological changes, but subsequent infections may be associated with hypersensitivity reactions, causing ascaris pneumonia (Fig. 7.9.5.4). When this causes fever, cough, dyspnoea, bronchospasm, peripheral eosinophilia, and infiltrates on chest radiograph that are often migratory, this is known as Löffler's syndrome. The condition usually subsides after 7 to 10 days unless reinfection occurs. In areas where pig farming is common, the larvae of *A. suum* may also produce severe pneumonitis and bronchospasm.

Most people with established infection with *A. lumbricoides* are asymptomatic, especially if the worm burden is small. Some may complain of anorexia, nausea, and abdominal discomfort or distension. Heavy infections in children may cause malnutrition, and hinder normal development in terms of both stature and

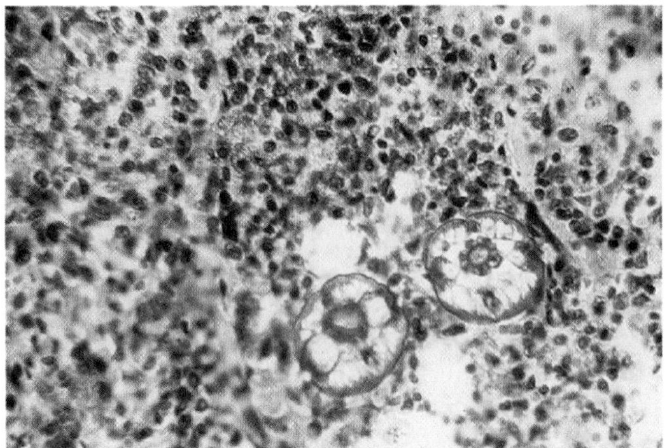

Fig. 7.9.5.4 *Ascaris lumbricoides* in the lungs, surrounded by an inflammatory reaction.
(Copyright Viqar Zaman.)

cognitive performance. Mechanical complications probably occur in less than 1% of infected individuals. Occasionally, usually in children, large numbers of worms may become entangled to form a bolus that blocks the intestinal lumen, usually near the ileocaecal valve, producing signs and symptoms of acute intestinal obstruction. This may be complicated by perforation, intussusception, volvulus, and death. In unusual circumstances, such as fever, irritation caused by drugs, anaesthesia, or bowel manipulation during surgery, the worms may migrate to ectopic sites. Migration into the common bile duct may be complicated with cholangitis and liver abscesses, whereas entry into the pancreatic duct may precipitate acute pancreatitis. Worms may migrate into the appendix, occasionally come out through the mouth and nose, and are rarely found in other ectopic locations.

Diagnosis

Ascariasis is usually diagnosed by finding plentiful numbers of the characteristically oval fertilized eggs measuring 60× 30 to 70× 50 μm in the faeces (Fig. 7.9.5.5). Sometimes the patient brings developing or adult worms that have been passed in the faeces or have emerged from the anus or nose of a sick child. Occasionally, adult worms are outlined in the intestines during barium-meal examination, or are seen at upper gastrointestinal endoscopy.

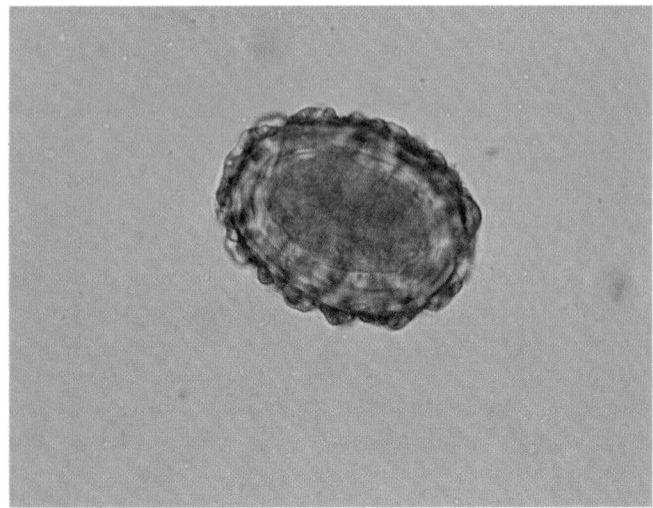

Fig. 7.9.5.5 Egg of *Ascaris lumbricoides*.

Treatment

It is desirable to treat all infected individuals, even when the worm load is small. There are a number of effective drugs (listed below). None of them is recommended by its manufacturer for use in pregnancy, especially in the first trimester, or children under 1 to 2 years of age, although this has been disputed by some authorities.

- Pyrantel embonate (pyrantel pamoate) given in a single dose of 11 mg/kg body weight (maximum 1 g) is effective in curing more than 90% of cases of ascariasis. Side effects are mild, if any, and the drug is well tolerated.
- Mebendazole is given is given as 100 mg twice daily for 3 days in adults and children over 2 years of age. It should not be given to pregnant women.
- Albendazole is given as a single dose of 400 mg in adults and children over 2 years of age. It should not be given to pregnant women.

In cases of intestinal obstruction caused by an ascaris bolus, a piperazine salt given at a dose of 75 mg/kg (maximum 3.5 g) daily for two consecutive days has been recommended as it induces flaccid paralysis of the worms, which may relieve the obstruction. This should be supplemented with decompression of the bowel through an intestinal tube with constant suction, and rehydration and restoration of electrolyte balance with intravenous fluids. In most cases this conservative therapy will relieve the obstruction and the child will rapidly recover. If, however, the signs of obstruction persist and the child's general condition worsens, laparotomy is required. Acute obstructive jaundice or pancreatitis resulting from obstruction of the common bile duct by ascaris also requires urgent surgical intervention.

Anisakiasis

Life cycle

Anisakiasis is an infection caused by the larvae of various species of nematode belonging to the family Anisakidae. Adults live in the lumen of the intestine of marine mammals (cetaceans: whales, dolphins, and porpoises). Eggs are passed in water, and second-stage larvae are ingested by crustaceans, which are then ingested by fish or squid, where they enter the muscles. Cetaceans and humans become infected by eating these saltwater fish or squid.

Epidemiology and control

The adult worms are commonly found in marine mammals in many parts of the world. Humans are infected when they eat raw or improperly cooked fish or squid. The incidence is highest in Japan, countries on the northern European seaboard, and the Pacific coast of the Americas, especially in the South. Infection is prevented by not eating raw, pickled, smoked, or undercooked fish and squid. Larvae are killed by cooking or freezing for 24 h before ingestion.

Clinical features

The larvae do not develop to maturity in humans, but attach themselves to and then burrow into the mucosa of the stomach (especially *Pseudoterranova* species) or small intestine (especially *Anisakis* species), and rarely the large bowel (Fig. 7.9.5.6). Symptoms often develop 4 to 24 h after eating infected fish. Gastric invasion produces severe epigastric pain, nausea, and vomiting, and sometimes haematemesis during the acute stage of the disease. Involvement of the intestine may cause severe lower abdominal pain, which may be misdiagnosed as appendicitis. If symptoms are mild and the patient is left untreated the infection can become chronic, with pseudotumour formation encompassing the parasite. Sometimes infection precipitates an allergic reaction, with urticaria, angio-oedema or anaphylaxis.

Diagnosis

A definitive diagnosis is made by upper gastrointestinal endoscopy, which reveals the lesion and the presence of white or yellow larvae up to 3 cm in size attached to the mucous membrane. Intestinal anisakiasis is more difficult to diagnose, but imaging studies may show thickening of the intestinal wall, and narrowing of the jejunum or ileum.

Treatment

In acute infection, an attempt should be made to remove all the larvae through an endoscope, although in most patients symptoms resolve spontaneously within 2 weeks. In chronic cases, surgical removal of the ulcerated areas or the tumour may be required. No chemotherapy has been proven to be effective, although a trial of albendazole has been suggested.

Capillariasis

There are two forms of capillariasis: intestinal capillariasis caused by *Paracapillaria philippinensis*, and hepatic capillariasis caused by *Capillaria hepatica*.

Intestinal capillariasis

This infection is caused by a worm still generally known as *Capillaria philippinensis* in medical circles, although it has been renamed *Paracapillaria philippinensis*. Fish-eating birds are the definitive reservoir. Adult *C. philippinensis* measure 2.5 to 4.3 mm in length and produce eggs that are deposited in water and ingested by fish, in which they develop into infective larvae. Humans are infected by eating undercooked freshwater or brackish-water fish. In humans, the parasite has the capacity to autoinfect; female worms produce eggs that hatch into larvae that reinvade the intestinal mucosa, resulting in prolonged infection, so that the original source and time of infection may be forgotten. There may be extremely heavy worm loads, especially in immunocompromised patients. The parasite is endemic in parts of South-East Asia, especially the Philippines and Thailand, and has more recently been found in Egypt. Infection is prevented by properly cooking fish.

Intestinal capillariasis may be a severe and even fatal disease. Patients often present with abdominal pain, diarrhoea, and borborygmi. As the worm load increases, diarrhoea becomes more severe, with anorexia, nausea, and vomiting. Prolonged diarrhoea leads to cachexia. There may also be signs of hypotension and cardiac failure. The mortality rate in untreated cases approaches 20%. The diagnosis is made by finding eggs in the faeces, 36 to 45 μm in length by 19 to 21 μm in breadth (Fig. 7.9.5.7), which may superficially resemble those of *Trichuris trichiura*. Larvae or adult worms may also be present, and repeated stool examination may be required in some cases. The parasite may also be found in jejunal aspirate or biopsy. All cases should be treated with either mebendazole or albendazole 200 mg twice daily for 3 weeks. Stools should be re-examined to ensure the eradication of infection; if not, the course of treatment should be repeated. Supportive measures to overcome malnutrition and diarrhoea will be required in severely ill patients.

Hepatic capillariasis

The adults of *C. hepatica* measure 52 to 104 mm in length, and live in the liver of various mammals, especially rats. Eggs are produced that are retained in the liver parenchyma; they measure 28 × 48 to 36 × 66 μm, and have bipolar plugs. The ova eventually reach the soil and embryonate, either by decomposition of a carcass, or when the host is eaten by another animal and the eggs pass through the gut of that animal and are deposited in the faeces. Infective eggs are then ingested by another definitive host, the eggs hatch, and the larvae reach the liver via the portal system. *C. hepatica* is a rare human parasite, and infections occur when eggs in the soil are accidentally swallowed. Clinical features may resemble those of visceral larva migrans, with tender hepatomegaly, fever,

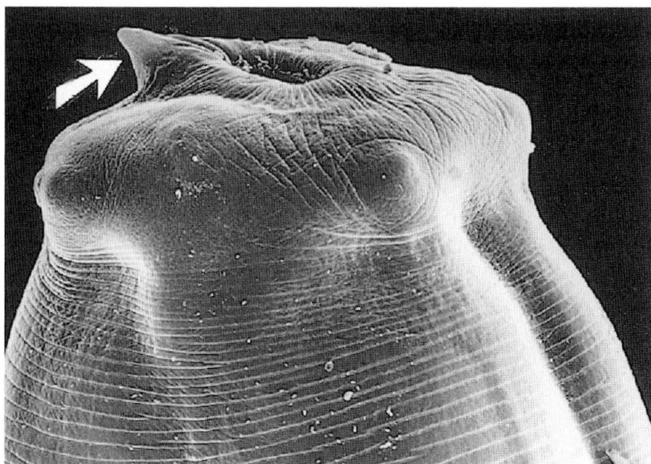

Fig. 7.9.5.6 Third-stage larva of *Anisakis simplex*, showing the tip of the boring tooth (arrow) (×400).

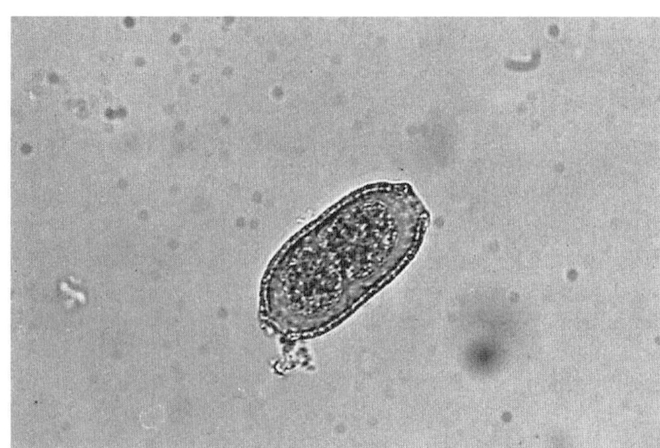

Fig. 7.9.5.7 *Capillaria philippinensis* egg (×1400).

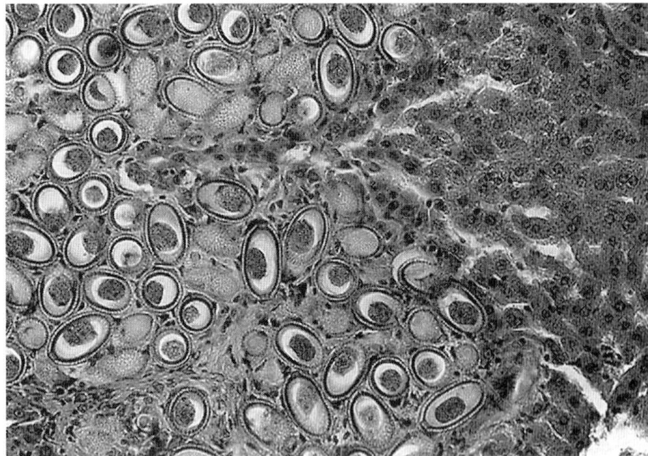

Fig. 7.9.5.8 *Capillaria hepatica* eggs in the liver (×250).

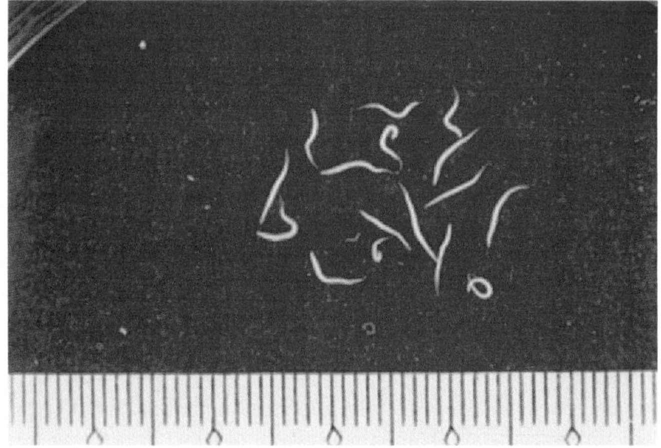

Fig. 7.9.5.10 Adult *Enterobius vermicularis* (scale in mm). (Copyright Viqar Zaman)

and eosinophilia. The diagnosis is made by identifying the parasite or eggs in a liver biopsy (Fig. 7.9.5.8). The most effective treatment is unclear, although cases have been reported to respond to tiabendazole or albendazole; the latter is given as described for intestinal capillariasis.

Enterobiasis (threadworm infection)

Life cycle

Enterobiasis is an infection caused by the threadworm or pinworm, *Enterobius vermicularis.* Infection is acquired by the ingestion of eggs (Fig. 7.9.5.9). Larvae hatch in the upper intestine, and migrate to the region of the caecum, where they mature and copulate. Worms do not invade the tissues. About 1 month after infection, the white thread-like gravid female worms, about 10 to 13 mm long by 0.3 to 0.5 mm in diameter, move down the bowel and pass out of the anus at night (Fig. 7.9.5.10). Each worm each night deposits approximately 10 000 eggs on the perianal skin. The worms then usually die, but sometimes they may re-enter the anus or migrate elsewhere. The eggs are infective within a few hours of deposition.

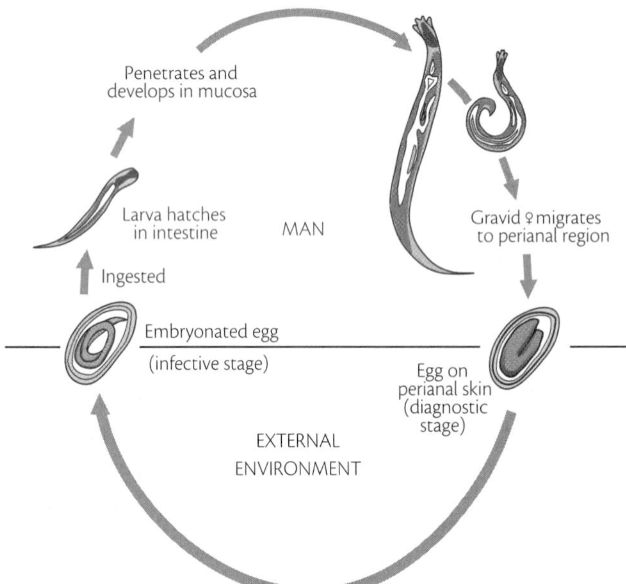

Fig. 7.9.5.9 Life cycle of *Enterobius vermicularis.*

Epidemiology and control

This worm is found worldwide, and is extremely common, being found most frequently in children. Infections are commonly clustered in families and institutions. Humans are the only reservoir of infection. Eggs may remain viable for up to 3 weeks, and can be transmitted via contaminated clothing, bedding, and dust. Resistance to reinfection does not develop, and autoinfection may occur by contamination of the fingers.

Clinical features

Most infected people are asymptomatic. The most common presenting symptom is pruritus ani. This can be very troublesome, and occurs more often during the night, causing restless sleep, especially in children. Persistent itching may lead to inflammation and secondary bacterial infection of the perianal region. Occasionally, adult worms migrate. In females they may enter the female genital tract, causing vulvovaginitis or rarely salpingitis. *E. vermicularis* is sometimes found lodged in the lumen of the appendix (Fig. 7.9.5.11), but whether or not this causes appendicitis is controversial.

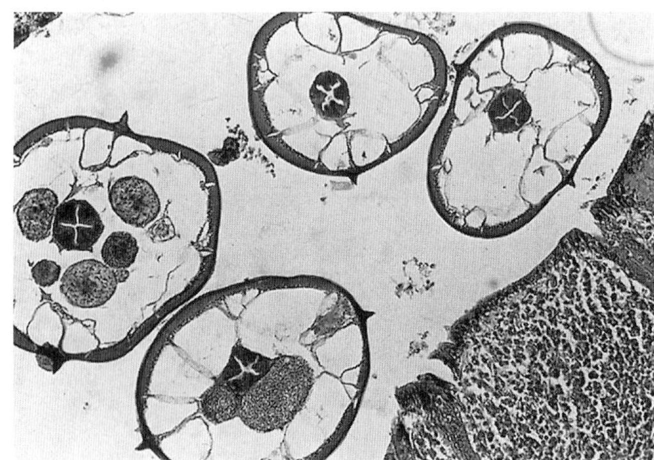

Fig. 7.9.5.11 Histological section of *Enterobius vermicularis* in the lumen of the appendix (×250).

Diagnosis

The eggs are not usually found in the faeces. They are most easily found around the anus first thing in the morning by using cellulose adhesive tape applied with the sticky side against the perianal skin, which is then examined under the microscope; they are 33 × 55 µm in size, and flattened on one side (Fig. 7.9.5.12). Sometimes intact worms are passed in the faeces, and can easily be recognized by their size and shape.

Treatment

All the children and adults in a household should be treated at the same time. Several drugs are available, including mebendazole 100 mg in a single dose, albendazole 400 mg in a single dose, and pyrantel embonate 10 mg/kg in a single dose; pyrantel embonate is recommended for children under 2 years of age and pregnant women. The best results are achieved if the course is repeated after 2 weeks. Attention to personal hygiene is an important part of treatment and prevention. The patient should be instructed to keep fingernails short, and wash hands with soap and water after defaecating. The bed cover and sleeping garments should be washed every day, and the floor in the bedroom kept clean.

Toxocariasis

Toxocariasis in humans occurs in two clinical forms, visceral larva migrans and ocular larva migrans, and is caused mainly by the migrating larvae of *Toxocara canis*, and to a lesser extent *T. cati*, and rarely other nematodes. *T. canis* and *T. cati* are parasites that live in the intestines of dogs and cats, which pass eggs in the faeces. Humans, usually young children, become infected by inadvertently ingesting embryonated eggs in the soil. The larvae hatch in the small intestine, and migrate to various organs of the body, including the liver, lungs, eye, and brain. The larvae, which are about 15 to 20 µm in length, do not mature in humans, but granulomas eventually develop around them (Fig. 7.9.5.13). In a fully formed granuloma the larvae are surrounded by layers of fibrous tissue, and inflammation subsides (Fig. 7.9.5.14). Eggs are never seen in human faeces. Toxocara infection occurs wherever there are large domestic dog and cat populations in close association with humans, and is more common in children. Deworming dogs, and stopping children from eating dirt (pica) when playing in areas frequented by dogs, are important control measures.

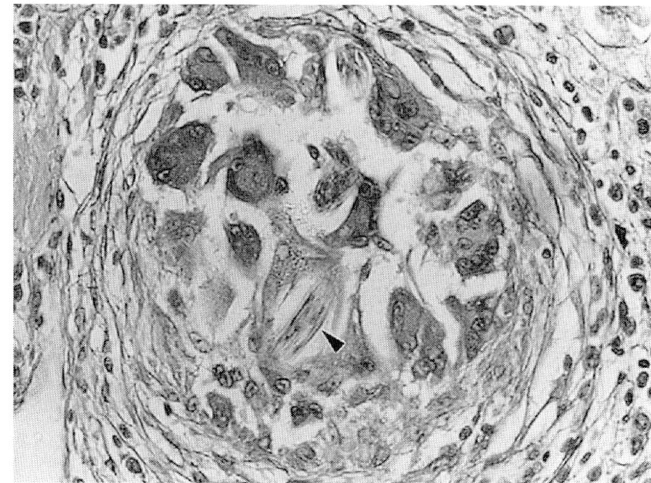

Fig. 7.9.5.13 Histological section. Granuloma formation in a monkey experimentally infected with *Toxocara Canis*, showing a large number of giant cells and some fibroblastic reaction. The arrow marks the larva (×400).

Visceral larva migrans

This disease is most often seen in young children, because of pica. Most people remain asymptomatic. In a minority, symptoms consist of muscular pain, lassitude, anorexia, cough, and urticarial rashes. Physical signs may include wheezing and hepatomegaly. Occasionally there is splenomegaly, lymphadenopathy, and skin lesions. Central nervous system involvement may be manifested by convulsions. The acute phase generally lasts for 2 to 3 weeks, followed by recovery. Sometimes the resolution of all the signs may take up to 18 months. Rarely, the infection may end fatally if a massive dose of parasites has been ingested.

The hallmark of visceral larva migrans is marked eosinophilia, which may reach a level of 75%. Serological tests for toxocara

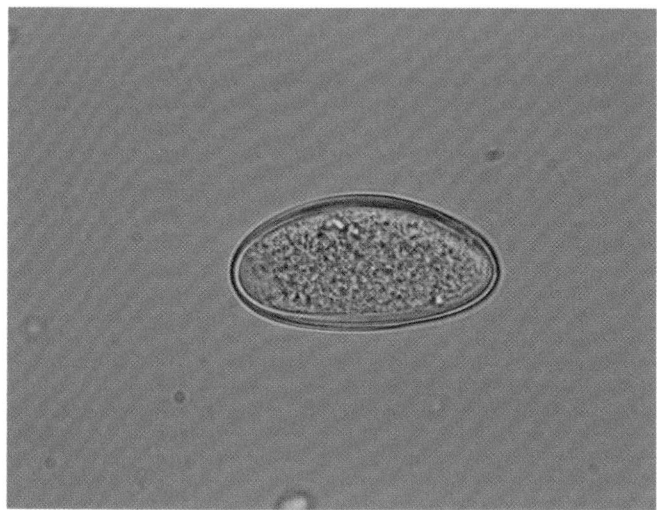

Fig. 7.9.5.12 Enterobius vermicularis egg.

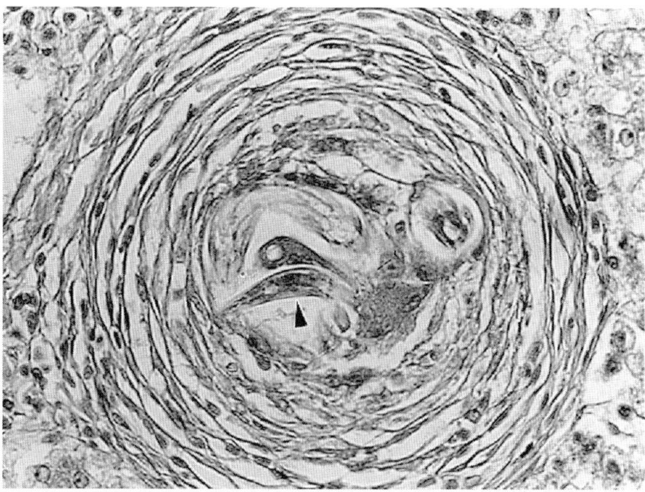

Fig. 7.9.5.14 Histological section. Granuloma formation in the same animal as Fig. 7.9.5.13, at a later stage when the larva is completely surrounded by fibroblasts (×400).

antibody may be helpful; a negative test may rule out the diagnosis, but positive titres are often found in normal individuals. The definitive diagnosis is by finding larvae on biopsy, usually of the liver, but this is not often done because of the large sampling error. Most patients recover spontaneously; the larvae cannot multiply, and they eventually die. There is no proven therapy. Anthelmintics, including mebendazole, albendazole, and diethylcarbamazine, have been tried, but may be ineffective or precipitate an inflammatory reaction. Corticosteroids and nonsteroidal anti-inflammatory agents have been suggested in order to suppress inflammation.

Ocular larva migrans

This condition is caused by granuloma formation around a larva in the eye, and is most commonly seen in older children. If this is near the macula, impairment of vision or even blindness may result. A rounded swelling, often near the optic disc, may be detected on fundoscopy. The features of visceral larva migrans are usually lacking. There is usually no marked peripheral eosinophilia. Diagnosis depends upon positive serology with consistent fundoscopic features; the major differential diagnosis is retinoblastoma. Antibody titres in vitreous or aqueous fluid may be higher than those found in serum. There is no proven anthelmintic therapy, but the agents used in visceral larva migrans may be tried. Visible larvae can be photocoagulated by laser. Vitrectomy has been used in some cases, and local and intraocular steroids also appear to be of some value.

Trichinosis (trichinellosis)

Life cycle

Trichinosis is an infection usually caused by *Trichinella spiralis* and related species. Humans become infected by eating undercooked meat, usually pork or pork products from domestic and wild pigs (boars) (Fig. 7.9.5.15). After ingestion the larvae are liberated in the stomach, then pass into the small bowel, where they invade the columnar epithelium and develop into adult worms living in the cytoplasm of a row of enterocytes. Male trichinellae are about 1.5× 0.05 mm in size, and female worms measure 3.5× 0.06 mm.

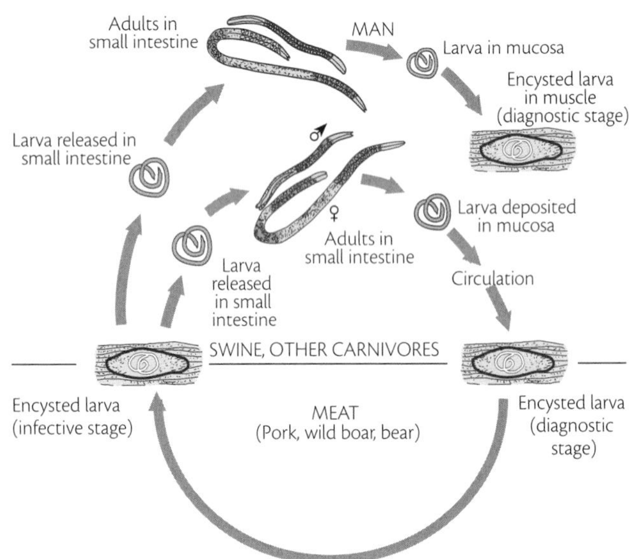

Fig. 7.9.5.15 Life cycle of *Trichinella spiralis*.

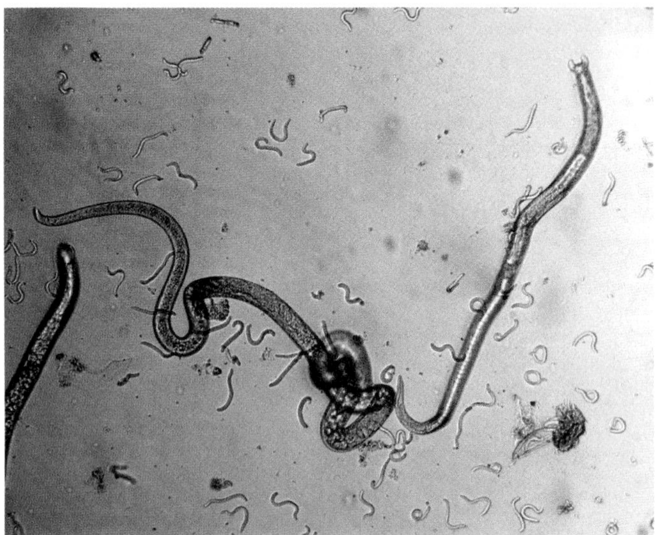

Fig. 7.9.5.16 *In vitro* preparation of infected mouse small bowel, showing adult worms of *Trichinella spiralis* surrounded by newborn larvae.
(Courtesy of D I Grove.)

Over 2 to 3 weeks or so before they are expelled, female worms release about 500 newborn larvae (Fig. 7.9.5.16), which enter the bloodstream and seed the skeletal muscles. Over the next few weeks these larvae in the muscles increase in size, moult, coil, usually develop a cyst wall, and become capable of infecting a new host (Fig. 7.9.5.17); they may remain viable for several years.

Epidemiology and control

Trichinella species are widely distributed in many geographical areas among a large number of carnivorous hosts found in three classes of vertebrate host: mammals, birds, and reptiles (Table 7.9.5.1). Domestic pigs become infected by eating infected scrap from slaughterhouses or farms. Humans are incidental hosts, and are usually infected with *T. spiralis*, but are occasionally infected with other species, depending upon the animal eaten. Infection is best prevented by properly cooking meat.

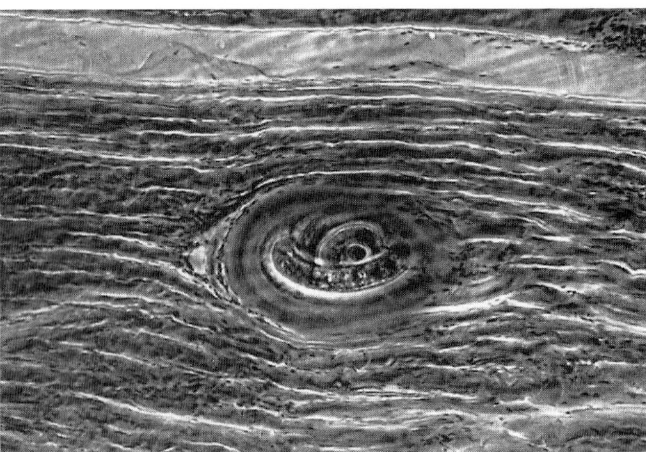

Fig. 7.9.5.17 *Trichinella spiralis* third-stage larvae in human muscle (×100).

Table 7.9.5.1 Major *Trichinella* spp. and their epidemiology

Species	Code	Distribution	Most common hosts	Cyst wall
T. spiralis	T1	Worldwide except Australasia	Pig, horse, bear, rodent, fox	Yes
T. nativa	T2	Arctic, subarctic	Bear, fox, dog	Yes
T. britovi	T3	Temperate, subarctic	Dog, bear, cat, boar	Yes
T. pseudospiralis	T4	Cosmopolitan	Bird	No
T. murrelli	T5	North America	Bear, coyote, dog	Yes
Uncertain	T6	Subarctic	Bear	Yes
T. nelsoni	T7	Sub-Saharan Africa	Hyena, cat	Yes
Uncertain	T8	Southern Africa	Lion, panther	Yes
Uncertain	T9	Japan	Bear	Yes
T. papuae	T10	Papua New Guinea	Pig, crocodile	No
T. zimbabwensis	T11	Central Africa	Crocodile, mammals	No

Clinical features

Most people with light infections are asymptomatic. In heavy infections, diarrhoea develops in the first week and is associated with abdominal discomfort and vomiting. Fulminating enteritis may develop in patients with extremely heavy infections. Symptoms of larval invasion develop during the second week, and include fever, myositis with pain, swelling, and weakness, usually first involving the extraocular muscles, then the masseters, neck muscles, limb flexors, and lumbar muscles. Some patients may develop one or more of cough, dyspnoea, headache, periorbital oedema, subconjunctival haemorrhages, and a petechial rash. These symptoms slowly subside over several weeks, although symptoms persist longer in a minority of patients. In fulminant infections a potentially fatal myocarditis or meningoencephalitis may develop.

Diagnosis

The diagnosis is suggested by a combination of fever, periorbital oedema, myositis, and eosinophilia in a patient who gives a history of eating undercooked meat, often in the context of an outbreak. Elevated creatine kinase and lactate dehydrogenase levels indicate considerable muscle involvement. Serological tests become positive several weeks after infection. A definitive diagnosis depends upon finding larvae in muscle biopsies, although this is usually unnecessary.

Treatment and prevention

Therapy is often unsatisfactory. If the diagnosis is made very early in the illness the administration of mebendazole 5 mg/kg or albendazole 5 mg/kg daily for 1 week may expel adult worms from the gut, and reduce the load of larvae seeding the tissues. In established infections these benzimidazole agents may be tried, but usually have little influence on the course of the disease. In established infections the mainstays of treatment are bed rest and the administration of nonsteroidal anti-inflammatory agents. Corticosteroids may be used in conjunction with anthelmintics in critically ill patients, but evidence of benefit is equivocal. Trichinosis in the pig population can be greatly reduced or eliminated by hygienic rearing methods. Larvae in pork can be killed by freezing at −18 C for 24 h. Thorough cooking of pork is the best safeguard against infection in all endemic areas.

Trichuriasis (whipworm infection)

Life cycle

Trichuriasis is an infection caused by *Trichuris trichiura*. Infection is acquired when an egg is ingested (Fig. 7.9.5.18). The infective larva hatches in the small intestine and enters the mucosal crypts of the caecum, where it moults several times to become an adult worm 30 to 50 mm long. The anterior three-fifths of the worm are thin and elongated, and the posterior two-fifths bulbous and fleshy. The thin end is embedded in a syncytial tunnel in the large-bowel epithelium (Fig. 7.9.5.19). Nearly 3 months after infection the fertilized female worms begin to produce about 10 000 eggs per day. Adult worms live for 1 to 3 years. After passage in the faeces, eggs embryonate in the soil and become infective after several weeks.

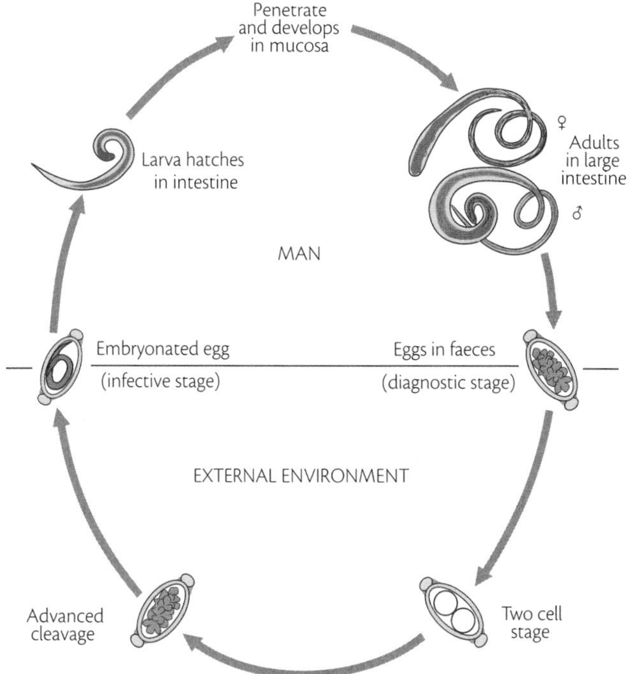

Fig. 7.9.5.18 Life cycle of *Trichuris trichiura*.

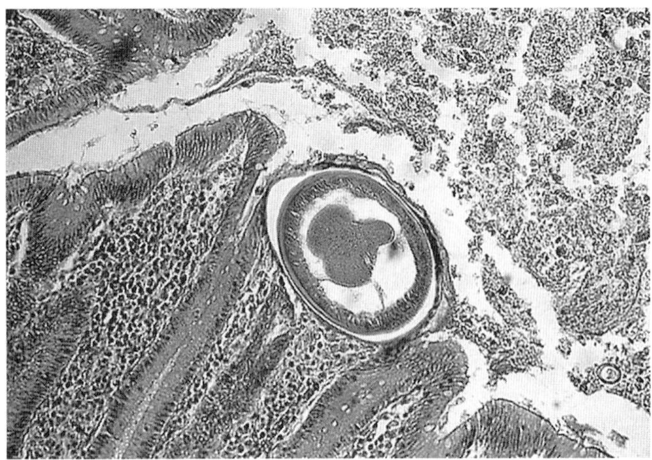

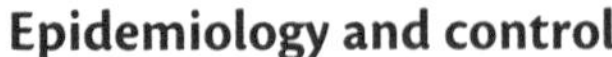

Fig. 7.9.5.19 Histological section. Anterior end of an adult *Trichuris trichiura* embedded superficially in the large bowel mucosa (×250).

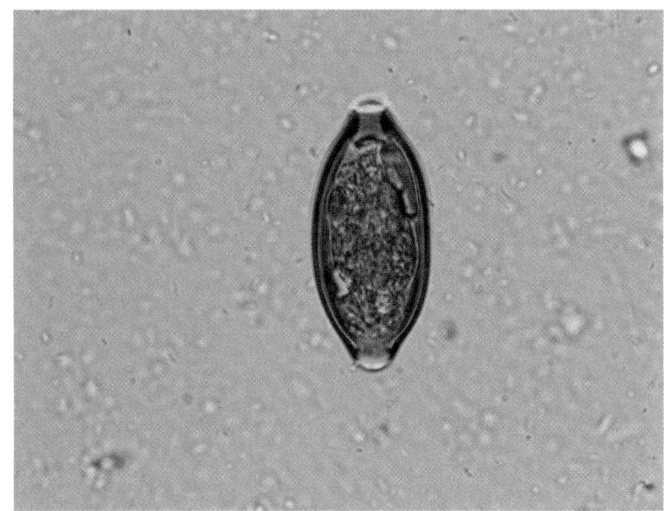

Fig. 7.9.5.20 Egg of *Trichuris trichiura*.
(Courtesy of A R Butcher.)

Epidemiology and control

Trichuriasis has a worldwide distribution, particularly in the warmer parts, and is most common in areas where sanitation is poor, especially where human faeces are used as fertilizer in vegetable gardens. Environmental sanitation is the best control measure. Ground-growing fruits and vegetables should be carefully washed.

Clinical features

Most infections are light and asymptomatic. In heavy infections there is colitis and/or proctitis, with the passage of blood and mucus in the faeces. In some cases prolapse of the oedematous parasitized rectum occurs. Chronic heavy infection may be associated with iron-deficiency anaemia and growth retardation.

Diagnosis

This is based on finding characteristically barrel-shaped eggs 50× 20 mm in size (Fig. 7.9.5.20) in the faeces. Sigmoidoscopy or proctoscopy may show worms attached to the mucous membrane, and sometimes intact worms may be passed in the faeces.

Treatment

Benzimidazole anthelmintics are effective when given for between 1 and 5 days, depending upon the severity of infection. Mebendazole is given is given as 100 mg, and albendazole as 400 mg, to both adults and children. Ivermectin in a dose of 200 μg/kg orally gives similar results.

Uncommon nematode infections acquired by ingestion or other routes

From time to time a patient may be encountered who harbours an unusual nematode. Some of these organisms are free-living parasites, and the patient has a spurious infection, usually as the result of ingesting the worm, or following the *in vitro* contamination of a clinical specimen such as faeces or urine. Other individuals may have true infections, with worms being found in either the gastrointestinal tract or the tissues. Many of these infections are with parasites that are poorly adapted to the human host, and are unable to complete their development in humans. Thus worms in varying stages of development, including larvae, adults, and eggs, may be found in specimens. Some parasites may be recovered from fluids and are viewed intact; if there is uncertainty in identifying the worm help may often be obtained from a veterinary parasitologist, who may be more used to dealing with the species concerned. Sometimes parasites are seen only in histological sections; in these, definitive diagnosis may be very difficult, but the texts by Connor *et al.* and Orihel and Ash may be helpful. A summary of rarely reported nematodes, indicating geographical distribution, usual host, mode of acquisition, stage of development, clinical features, and suggested treatment, is shown in Table 7.9.5.2.

Nematodes found in the gastrointestinal tract may respond to a benzimidazole agent such as mebendazole (100 mg orally twice

Table 7.9.5.2 A summary of rarely reported nematodes found infecting humans, acquired by various routes

Nematode	Geographical distribution	Usual host	Mode of acquisition	Stage of development	Clinical features	Suggested treatment
Agamomermis spp.	?	Free living Grasshoppers	Ingestion?	Larvae, adults	Spurious; worms in mouth, faeces, urethra	Manual removal if necessary
Anatrichosoma spp.	Asia, Africa	Monkeys	?	Larvae	Cutaneous larva migrans	Tiabendazole Albendazole
Ancylostoma caninum	Widespread	Dogs	Cutaneous penetration	Larvae Adults?	Cutaneous larva migrans, myositis, pulmonary infiltrates, eosinophilic enteritis	Mebendazole (enteritis) Tiabendazole (other)

(Continued)

Table 7.9.5.2 *(Cont'd)* A summary of rarely reported nematodes found infecting humans, acquired by various routes

Nematode	Geographical distribution	Usual host	Mode of acquisition	Stage of development	Clinical features	Suggested treatment
Ancylostoma malayanum	Asia	Bear	?	?	?	Mebendazole
Ascaris suum	Widespread	Pigs	Ingestion of eggs	Larvae Adults?	Pneumonitis, abdominal discomfort	Albendazole
Baylisascaris procyonis	North America	Raccoons	Ingestion of eggs in soil	Larvae	Visceral and ocular larva migrans, eosinophilic meningoencephalitis	Albendazole
Bunostomum trigonocephalum	Widespread	Sheep	Cutaneous penetration	Larvae	Cutaneous larva migrans	Albendazole
Brugia spp. (not *malayi, timori*)	Widespread	Monkeys, raccoons, rabbits	Mosquito bite	Larvae, adults	Lymph node swelling	Excision
Cheilospirura spp.	Widespread	Birds	Ingestion of arthropods?	Larvae	Conjunctival nodule	Excision
Contracaecum spp.	Widespread	Fish, birds	Ingestion of undercooked fish	Larvae	See 'Anisakiasis'	See 'Anisakiasis'
Cyclodontostomum purvisi	Asia	Rats	?	Adults	Worms in faeces	Mebendazole
Dioctophyma renale	Widespread	Mammals	Ingestion of aquatic annelids, amphibians, crustaceans, fish	Larvae, adults	Haematuria, retroperitoneal mass, subcutaneous nodule	Excision
Diploscapter coronata	Widespread	Free living	Ingestion with vegetation	Adults	Spurious; worms in stomach contents, urine	Unnecessary
Dirofilaria immitis	Widespread	Dog	Mosquito bite	Larva	Nodule in lung, subcutaneous tissue	Excision
Dirofilaria repens	Europe, Asia	Dog, cat	Mosquito bite	Larva	Nodule in lung, subcutaneous tissue, eye, abdominal cavity	Excision
Dirofilaria tenuis	North America	Raccoon	Mosquito bite	Larva	Nodule in subcutaneous tissue, eye	Excision
Dirofilaria ursi	North America	Bear	Blackfly bite	Larva	Nodule in subcutaneous tissue	Excision
Eustrongylides spp.	Widespread	Fish, birds	Ingestion of undercooked fish	Larvae	Peritonitis	Laparotomy and surgical removal
Gongylonema pulchrum	Worldwide	Ruminants, swine	Ingestion of beetles, cockroaches etc.	Adult	Migrating worm, especially in the oral cavity	Surgical removal
Haemonchus contortus	Widespread	Sheep, cattle	Ingestion of larvae with vegetation?	Adults	?	Mebendazole
Lagochilascaris minor	Central and South America	?	?	Adults, eggs, larvae	Subcutaneous abscess in head and neck, nasopharyngeal or sinus lesions, encephalitis	Surgical removal Levamisole, diethylcarbamazine, tiabendazole
Mammomonogamus (Syngamus) laryngeus	Central and South America	Cattle, felines	?	Adults	Cough, pharyngeal lesion	Endoscopic removal
Meloidogyne (Heterodera) spp.	Widespread	Plant parasite	Ingestion of |vegetation; contamination of faecal specimen	Eggs, larvae	Spurious; eggs and larvae in faeces	Unnecessary
Meningonema peruzzii	Africa	Monkeys	?	Larvae	Meningoencephalitis	Albendazole
Mermis nigrescens	North America	Grasshoppers	Ingestion of adult worm?	Adult	Worm in mouth	Manual removal
Metastrongylus elongatus	Widespread	Pigs	Ingestion of earthworms	Adult	Worm in gut or respiratory tract	Albendazole
Metastrongylid nematode	Italy	?	?	Larvae, adults	Pulmonary arteritis	Anthelmintics?
Micronema deletrix	Widespread	Free living Horses	Trauma or skin lesions	Adults, larvae, eggs	Meningoencephalitis; generalized spread	Albendazole

(Continued)

Table 7.9.5.2 *(Cont'd)* A summary of rarely reported nematodes found infecting humans, acquired by various routes

Nematode	Geographical distribution	Usual host	Mode of acquisition	Stage of development	Clinical features	Suggested treatment
Muspiceoid nematode	Australia	?	?	Larvae, adults	Polymyositis	Albendazole
Necator suillus	Central America	Pigs	Percutaneous	Adults	?	Mebendazole
Onchocerca spp. (not *O. volvulus*)	Widespread	Cattle, horses	Insect borne	Adults	Subcutaneous nodule, eye lesions	Surgical excision
Ostertagia spp.	Widespread	Cattle, sheep	Ingestion of adult worms in undercooked abomasums?	Adults	Spurious? Worms in gut	Mebendazole
Pelodera (*Rhabditis*) *strongyloides*	Widespread	Free living	Cutaneous	Larvae	Papular dermatitis	Albendazole, topical corticosteroid
Philometra spp.	Widespread	Fish	Cutaneous injury	Adults	Worms in laceration	Manual removal
Phocanema spp.	Widespread	Fish	Ingestion of undercooked fish	Larvae	See 'Anisakiasis'	See 'Anisakiasis'
Physaloptera caucasica	Europe, Africa	Primates	Ingestion of beetles, cockroaches?	Adults, eggs	Sometimes spurious; abdominal pain, small bowel gangrene	Mebendazole Surgical removal
Rhabditis spp.	Widespread	Free living	Ingestion	Adults	Spurious; worms in faeces, urine, skin	Unnecessary
Rictularia spp.	Widespread	Mammals, birds	Ingestion?	Adult	Found in an appendix	
Spirocerca lupi	Widespread	Dogs, wolves	Ingestion of beetle?	Adults	Intestinal obstruction and peritonitis in a baby	Surgery
Spiruroid nematode	Japan	Fish, squid	Ingestion of undercooked food	Larvae	Creeping eruption Ileal granuloma	Excision Anthelmintics?
Syphacia spp.	Widespread	Mice	Ingestion	Eggs, adults	Spurious?; worms in faeces	Mebendazole if necessary
Terranova spp.	Widespread	Fish	Ingestion of undercooked fish	Larvae	See 'Anisakiasis'	See 'Anisakiasis'
Tetrameres fissispina	Widespread	Birds	Ingestion of grasshoppers, cockroaches?	Adults	Spurious?; worms in gut	Mebendazole
Thelazia californiensis	North America	Mammals	Deposition on eye by fly	Adults	Conjunctivitis	Manual removal
Thelazia callipaeda	Asia	Dogs, rabbits	Deposition on eye by fly	Adults	Conjunctivitis	Manual removal
Trichuris suis	Widespread	Pigs	Ingestion of eggs	Eggs, larvae, adults	Usually asymptomatic	Mebendazole
Trichuris vulpis	Widespread	Dogs	Ingestion of eggs	Eggs, larvae, adults	Usually asymptomatic	Mebendazole
Turbatrix (*Anguillula*) *aceti*	Widespread	Free living (including vinegar, acetic acid)	Accidental inoculation	Larvae, adults	Spurious; urine, vaginal discharge, blood smears (in stains)	Unnecessary
Uncinaria stenocephala	Widespread	Dogs, cats	Cutaneous penetration	Larvae	Cutaneous larva migrans	Tiabendazole Albendazole

daily for up to 3 days) or albendazole (10 mg/kg orally daily for up to 1 week). Tiabendazole (25 mg/kg twice daily for several days) has been used traditionally for the treatment of systemic larval infections, but its effectiveness is very variable; albendazole may be more active than tiabendazole, and is absorbed better from the gut than mebendazole. If these drugs fail, ivermectin (0.15 mg/kg orally daily for several days) may be tried. Other drugs that have been used in these unusual nematode infections include levamisole and diethylcarbamazine. Unfortunately, some infections are refractory to all to anthelmintics. Nevertheless, these worms generally cannot multiply in humans, and the parasites will die spontaneously after months or years.

Further reading

Bethony J, *et al.* (2006). Soil-transmitted helminth infections: ascariasis, trichuriasis and hookworm. *Lancet*, **367**, 1521–32.

Connor DH, *et al.* (eds) (1997). *Pathology of infectious diseases*, vol 2, pp. 1305–588. Appleton and Lange, Stamford, CT.

Despommier D (2003). Toxocariasis: clinical aspects, epidemiology, medical ecology, and molecular aspects. *Clin Microbiol Rev*, **16**, 265–72.

Nawa Y, Hatz C, Blum J (2005). Sushi delights and parasites: the risk of fishborne and foodborne parasitic zoonoses in Asia. *Clin Infect Dis*, **41**, 1297–303.

Lu LH, *et al.* (2006). Human intestinal capillariasis (*Capillaria philippinensis*) in Taiwan. *Am J Trop Med Hyg*, **74**, 810–13.

Orihel TC, Ash LR (1995). *Parasites in human tissues*. American Society of Clinical Pathologists, Chicago.

Pozio E, Gomex Morales MA, Dupouy-Camet J (2003). Clinical aspects, diagnosis and treatment of trichinellosis. *Expert Rev Anti-infect Ther*, **1**, 471–82.

Websites

Photographs of the various stages of these parasites, and diagrams of their life cycles, may be found at several excellent websites, e.g.:

Centers for Disease Control and Prevention. *Laboratory investigation of parasites of public health concern*. http://www.dpd.cdc.gov/DPDx/

Korean Society for Parasitology. *Web atlas of medical parasitology*. http://www.atlas.or.kr

7.9.6 Parastrongyliasis (angiostrongyliasis)

Richard Knight

Essentials

Parastrongylus cantonensis

The rat lungworm causes eosinophilic meningitis in parts of Oceania and South-East Asia. Human infections follow ingestion of uncooked molluscs, the primary intermediate hosts, or one of several paratenic hosts. Clinical manifestations include headache, meningism, vomiting, cranial nerve lesions, and (less commonly) other neurological features such as seizures. Diagnosis is made by lumbar puncture revealing eosinophilic meningitis, with larval or immature adult worms sometimes seen. Treatment is with albendazole or mebendazole together with prednisolone, or with prednisolone alone. Mortality is 0.5 to 30%. Prevention is by avoidance of raw high-risk dietary items and unwashed salads.

Parastrongylus costaricensis

The cotton rat is the principal reservoir host. Unwitting ingestion of slugs, the intermediate hosts, in salads or fruit leads to human infections, especially in Costa Rica, Nicaragua, Guatemala, and Honduras. The organism causes granulomatous lesions of the right colon: most patients present with right-sided or right iliac fossa pain, with tenderness and sometimes a palpable mass. Diagnosis is usually made histologically on resected material. Surgery may be necessary, but the value of anthelminthics is uncertain. Preventive measures include washing and careful inspection of vegetables, and hand washing before meals by children and those preparing salads.

Introduction

Human disease is caused by two nematode species of the genus *Parastrongylus*. Both parasites normally infect rodents, and molluscs are the primary intermediate hosts. They were previously placed in the genus *Angiostrongylus* but it is now recognized that angiostrongylid worms with rodent hosts belong to the genus *Parastrongylus*. Infection follows accidental or deliberate ingestion of molluscs or paratenic hosts. The epidemiology is complex because of multiple potential routes of transmission.

Parastrongylus cantonensis

This is the rat lungworm. The first known case, reported in 1944, was a 15-year-old Taiwanese boy with meningoencephalitis, in whose cerebrospinal fluid an immature adult worm was found. Detailed clinicopathological studies were made in 1962 during epidemics of eosinophilic meningitis in Tahiti.

Aetiology: the biology of the parasite

Adult worms live in the pulmonary arteries of rats; larvae from hatched eggs ascend the airways, are swallowed, and so reach the faeces. Molluscs ingest these larvae, and after two moults they are infective when eaten by a rodent. In the rat, infective larval worms migrate to the cerebral grey matter, where they start to mature. They then move to the meninges and enter the venous sinuses, thereby reaching the pulmonary arteries, where maturation is completed. Infective larvae from a mollusc can also enter a second or third intermediate host, in which they undergo no further development until they enter a mammalian host. Such supernumerary hosts are termed paratenic hosts, and are important sources of infection in humans.

Development in humans reaches the immature adult stage, measuring 11 to 15 mm in length. Nearly all will die in the superficial cortex, brainstem, and meninges, causing vigorous tissue reactions; very few reach the lungs.

Epidemiology

Human infections occur throughout Oceania, especially Hawaii, Samoa, the Solomon Islands, Papua New Guinea, Indonesia, the Philippines, and northern Australia. In South-East Asia they occur in Thailand, Taiwan, China, south Japan, and rarely India; a few infections are reported from Côte d'Ivoire, Egypt, Madagascar, Cuba, the Caribbean, and South America. All ages can be affected, and outbreaks have occurred after weddings and feasts; infections are often seasonal.

The principal rodent hosts are *Rattus rattus*, *R. norvegicus*, *R. alexandrinus*, and *R. exulans*. The prevalence in rats in endemic areas may be 40% or more. The geographical spread and population increase of these peridomestic rodents has increased the zoonotic reservoir; wildlife is now infected in the southern United States of America. Another factor leading to the increase in human infection has been the dispersal by human agency of the edible giant African snail *Achatina fulica*, from Madagascar in 1800, eastwards across the Indian Ocean and the Pacific, to reach Hawaii in 1936. An edible Brazilian snail, *Ampullaria gigas*, has recently been introduced to Asia, where it has colonized paddy fields and caused disease when served raw in restaurants in China. The popularity of heliculture, the cultivation of exotic snails for food, and keeping them as pets, facilitates the spread of the parasite. Raw snails are eaten as a delicacy and for medicinal purposes; salads may contain small undetected molluscs, their slime trails, or planarians. An outbreak in Taiwan followed the drinking of raw vegetable juice.

Paratenic hosts include freshwater prawns, land and coconut crabs, frogs, and land planarians, which cause infection if eaten raw; drinking-water may contain tiny immature prawns, especially after heavy rains. In Thailand, the yellow tree monitor lizard is an important paratenic host.

The modes of transmission differ geographically, by age and social group, and with time. In Thailand, *Pila* spp. snails are a seasonal delicacy eaten by all the family, but young men take them raw with alcohol; another edible snail, *Ampullaria canaliculatus*, is infected in Taiwan and Japan. In the Ryukyu islands of Japan, patients are usually infected by eating raw snails or toad liver for medicinal purposes.

Pathology

Inflammatory granulomatous lesions, sometimes track-like, occur predominantly in the cortical grey matter and the meninges, but also in the brain stem and cerebellum; nerve roots and the spinal cord may also be affected. Live worms are occasionally found at autopsy, and dead worms are found in many lesions. The number of worms found varies greatly, and may reach several hundred; worm tracks in the tissue and meninges are surrounded by a cuff of eosinophils; Charcot–Leyden crystals derived from eosinophils are numerous. Rarely, adult worms have been found in human lung at autopsy. Ocular infection derives from worms that have migrated across the cribriform plate.

Clinical features

After an incubation period of 2 to 4 weeks the onset is acute, with headache (intermittent at first), together with nausea and vomiting. There is constitutional upset and frequently menigism; fever is unusual. The illness is often self limiting over a period of 4 weeks. Cranial nerve lesions are seen in the optic, abducens, and facial nerves. Less common are seizures, confusion, and radiculopathy (with paraesthesia, root pains, or weakness). Long-tract signs and impaired consciousness are uncommon, except in severe cases, but spinal cord damage can cause sphincter disturbance.

Ocular complications include retinal haemorrhages, and larval worms in the vitreous, anterior chamber, or beneath the conjunctiva (Fig. 7.9.6.1). Rarely, migration to the lungs produces clinical evidence of pneumonitis. Numerous eosinophils occur in the cerebrospinal fluid, and there is blood eosinophilia.

Diagnosis

Lumbar puncture reveals high opening pressure, with a clear or lightly turbid cerebrospinal fluid containing 500 to 2000 cells/mm^3 (of which 10–>90% are eosinophils); protein levels are high, with normal glucose. Detailed examination at low power reveals larval or immature adult worms in up to 25% of cases, measuring 5 to 15 mm in length. Cerebrospinal fluid changes may persist for up to 3 months. CT or MRI may reveal focal cortical abnormalities. Serology using antigens from fourth-stage larvae is useful, but cross-reactions with other nematodes can cause difficulty. Techniques to detect worm antigens in cerebrospinal fluid and serum have also been developed.

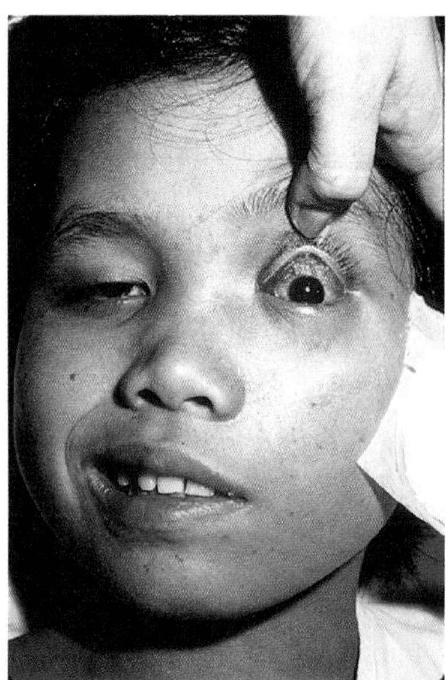

Fig. 7.9.6.1 Parastrongylus under the conjunctiva in a Thai girl with a left facial nerve palsy.
(Copyright D A Warrell.)

Differential diagnosis is from other helminth infections affecting the nervous system, as eosinophils are otherwise rare in cerebrospinal fluid. A detailed geographical and dietary history is essential; conditions to be considered include gnathostomiasis, paragonimiasis, schistosomiasis, and neurocysticercosis. A particular problem in Thailand is confusion with *Gnathostoma spinigerum*, which more commonly causes long-tract signs, bloody or xanthochromic cerebrospinal fluid, neck stiffness, and clouding of consciousness.

Treatment, prognosis, and control

Although worm death might aggravate the clinical condition, clinical studies support the use of the anthelmintics albendazole or mebendazole together with prednisolone. However, in a recent prospective trial prednisolone alone was as effective as prednisolone plus albendazole. Such treatment hastens recovery and relieves headache; it probably improves the prognosis in severe cases. Larvae in the eye chambers should be removed surgically.

Reported mortality rates vary from 0.5 to 30%, and depend mainly on the number of infective larvae ingested; some patients pass into coma after about 2 weeks, and their prognosis is then very poor. Most patients improve in 2 to 4 weeks, but focal neurological deficits can persist for longer; partial relapse after 2 months of illness may represent a reaction to dying worms. Some cases are relatively mild and can be discharged within a few days; during epidemics, mild cases may need only outpatient care.

Control measures include health education to limit the ingestion of raw high-risk dietary items, and unwashed salads. Warnings may be necessary regarding raw molluscs, amphibians, and reptiles used for medicinal purposes. Rodents in vegetable gardens and the peridomestic environment should be controlled.

Parastrongylus costaricensis

This was first recognized in Costa Rica in 1950 in surgical specimens simulating bowel malignancy. The parasite was described from such specimens in 1967, and the complete life cycle in rodents was elucidated during the next 3 years.

Aetiology: the biology of the parasite

In both the rodent and human hosts the worms are located in the ileocaecal mesenteric arteries. The cotton rat *Sigmodon hispidus* is the principal reservoir host, but other species of rodent (including the coatimundi) are also involved, and even dogs and marmosets. In the rodent hosts worm eggs embolize to gut-wall capillaries, and the hatched larvae pass into the gut lumen. Veronicellid slugs, especially *Vaginulus plebeius*, eat rodent faeces containing larvae, and these develop into infective larvae in the fibromuscular tissue of the mollusc after two moults over a period of 18 days. Infective larvae can persist in the slug for several months or be shed in slime trails. The prepatent period in rats eating infected slugs is 24 days.

In human infections the worms reach maturity, but the embryonated eggs do not hatch.

Epidemiology

Infections occur especially in Costa Rica, Nicaragua, Guatemala, and Honduras, but also sporadically elsewhere in the Americas from the United States of America to Argentina, and some Caribbean islands. Recently, infections have been increasingly recognized from southern Brazil. Small veronicellid slugs and their slime trails are the source of infection in man; infection rates in these hosts can reach 85%. Small or chopped slugs may be unnoticed on fallen fruits or in salads; their mucus also contains infective larvae. Many cases are in schoolchildren, but infants and older persons are also affected. Seropositivity in endemic areas suggests that there are unrecognized infections.

Pathology and clinical features

Lesions primarily affect the small arteries, producing subacute or chronic granulomatous inflammatory masses in the wall of the caecum, right colon, and less often the small intestine or elsewhere in the colon. Rarely, the predominant feature is ischaemic infarction. The finding of an adult nematode measuring 18 to 42 mm in length within a gut arterial vessel is diagnostic of infection; eggs may be seen in vessels or in tissue, where they are surrounded by eosinophil granulomas. Lesions also occur in regional abdominal lymph nodes or the omentum. Some larvae enter the hepatic artery and cause granulomatous or necrotic lesions in the liver; others enter testicular arteries causing similar lesions of the testis.

Clinically, most patients present with right-sided or right iliac fossa pain, with tenderness and sometimes a palpable mass in this region. Other features are eosinophilia, fever, diarrhoea, or rectal bleeding. Tender hepatomegaly with high blood eosinophilia occurs in some patients. Serious complications are bowel obstruction and perforation, and rarely testicular infarction.

Diagnosis and treatment

The confirmation of diagnosis is usually made histologically on resected material. The condition can mimic appendicitis, bowel neoplasm, Meckel's diverticulitis, testicular torsion, or other surgical problems. Parasite eggs are not found in faeces, but serology using enzyme immunoassay or latex agglutination is useful. Contrast radiology reveals filling defects and altered motility of the terminal ileum, caecum, or ascending colon. Laparoscopy can reveal the bowel and hepatic lesions; biopsy may be diagnostic.

The value of anthelmintic treatment remains unproven; tiabendazole or high doses of mebendazole have been used. Surgery is often necessary, but can sometimes be deferred in uncomplicated cases when the diagnosis is strongly suspected, as spontaneous remission is common.

Preventive measures include washing and careful inspection of vegetables, and hand washing before meals by children and those preparing salads. Rinsing salads in 1.5% bleach kills larvae.

Further reading

Chotmongkol V, *et al.* (2004). Treatment of eosinophilic meningitis with a combination of albendazole and corticosteroid. *Southeast Asian J Trop Med Public Health*, **35**, 172–4.

Chotmongkol V, *et al.* (2006). Treatment of eosinophilic meningitis with a combination of prednisolone and mebendazole. *Am J Trop Med Hyg*, **74**, 1122–4.

Chotmongkol V, *et al.* (2009). Comparison of prednisolone plus albendazole with prednisolone alone for treatment of patients with eosinophilic meningitis. *Am J Trop Med Hyg*, **81**, 443–5.

Graeff-Teixeira C, *et al.* (1997). Seroepidemiology of abdominal angiostrongyliasis: the standardization of an immunoenzymatic assay and prevalence of antibodies in two localities in southern Brazil. *Trop Med Int Health*, **2**, 254–60.

Kramer MH, *et al.* (1998). First reported outbreak of abdominal angiostrongyliasis. *Clin Infect Dis*, **26**, 365–72.

Lo Re V 3rd, Gluckman SJ (2003). Eosinophilic meningitis. *Am J Med*, **114**, 217–23.

Mackerras MJ, Sandars DF (1995). The life history of the rat lungworm, *Angiostrongylus cantonensis* (Chen). *Aust J Zool*, **3**, 1–25.

Mota EM, Lenzi HL (2005). *Angiostrongylus costaricensis*: complete redescription of the migratory pathways based on experimental *Sigmodon hispidus* infection. *Mem Inst Oswaldo Cruz*, **100**, 407–20.

Pien FD, Pien BC (1999). *Angiostrongylus cantonensis* eosinophilic meningitis. *Int J Infect Dis*, **3**, 161–3.

Punyagupta S, Juttijudata P, Bunnag T (1975). Eosinophilic meningitis in Thailand. Clinical studies of 484 typical cases probably caused by *Angiostrongylus cantonensis*. *Am J Trop Med Hyg*, **24**, 921–31.

Rambo PR, *et al.* (1997). Abdominal angiostrongylosis in southern Brazil—prevalence and parasitic burden in mollusc intermediate hosts from eighteen endemic foci. *Mem Inst Oswaldo Cruz*, **92**, 9–14.

Slom TJ, *et al.* (2002). An outbreak of eosinophilic meningitis caused by *Angiostrongylus cantonensis* in travelers returning from the Caribbean. *N Engl J Med*, **346**, 668–75.

Tsai HC, *et al.* (2003). Eosinophilic meningitis caused by *Angiostrongylus cantonensis* associated with eating raw snails: correlation of brain magnetic resonance imaging scans with clinical findings. *Am J Trop Med Hyg*, **68**, 281–5.

Tsai HC, *et al.* (2004). Outbreak of eosinophilic meningitis associated with drinking raw vegetable juice in southern Taiwan. *Am J Trop Med Hyg*, **71**, 222–6.

Ubelaker JE (1986). Systematics of species referred to the genus *Angiostrongylus*. *J Parasitol*, **72**, 237–44.

Wan KS, Weng WC (2004). Eosinophilic meningitis in a child raising snails as pets. *Acta Tropica*, **90**, 51–3.

7.9.7 Gnathostomiasis

Valai Bussaratid and Pravan Suntharasamai

Essentials

Gnathostomiasis is an extraintestinal infection with larval or immature nematodes of the genus *Gnathostoma* (order Spirurida), the most common mode of human infection being consumption of undercooked freshwater fish. Clinical manifestations include recurrent cutaneous migratory swellings (common), creeping eruption (rare), and neurological deficits (occasional). Definitive diagnosis is by identification of the worm in surgical specimens; serological testing for antibody against gnathostoma antigen can confirm a presumptive diagnosis. Treatment of choice is albendazole or if possible, surgical removal of the worm in accessible areas and when the parasite can be located. Prevention is by avoiding all dishes that contain raw or poorly cooked flesh of animals or fish in or imported from endemic areas.

Aetiology, genetics, pathogenesis, and pathology

Five species of *Gnathostoma* are known to infect humans. Adult parasites live in the upper gastrointestinal tract of the definitive hosts: dogs, cats, and other mammals for *Gnathostoma spinigerum*, the most common infection in Thailand; pigs for *G. hispidum* and *G. doloresi*; weasels for *G. nipponicum*; and canines for *G. binucleatum*. Larvae from ova shed with the host's faeces hatch in water and are ingested by *Cyclops* spp. copepods. These are eaten by freshwater fish, amphibians, reptiles, crustaceans, birds, or mammals; third-stage larvae are found in the walls of the viscera and in the muscles of these second intermediate hosts. Unless the second intermediate hosts are eaten by definitive hosts, the parasites cannot develop into reproductive adults, but they remain infectious to humans and other paratenic hosts.

Consumption of the raw or undercooked flesh of second intermediate and paratenic hosts is the most common mode of transmission. Skin penetration after contact with infected material is less important. Prenatal transmission can occur, as larvae have been recovered in neonates as young as 3 days old.

Genetics

The nucleotide sequence analysis of the gnathostoma genome is incomplete. The 5.8S ribosomal DNAs are almost identical among species, whereas the internal transcribed spacer 2 region is a potential candidate as a genetic marker for the identification of gnathostoma species, because it varies considerably among species. The gene for a 24-kDa diagnostic glycoprotein of *G. spinigerum* has been identified.

Acknowledgement: The authors thank Associate Professor Paron Dekumyoy for the use of unpublished data on serodiagnosis.

Pathogenesis

The ingested larva penetrates the gut wall and migrates to the liver before wandering through almost any tissue except bone. Symptoms and signs vary according to the site and size of the inflammatory or haemorrhagic lesions induced intermittently along the migratory route.

Histopathology

Histopathological findings include mixed eosinophils and other inflammatory cell infiltration, areas of necrosis or haemorrhage, and occasionally parasite tracts. Occasionally, eosinophilic vasculitis or flame figures may be seen in skin biopsy. These findings are not characteristic for gnathostomiasis. The only diagnostic finding is the identification of a parasite. If the biopsy cuts through the bulb or cervical part of the worm, diagnostic features of *G. spinigerum* may be visible: a head bulb bearing eight transverse rows of spines or a cuticle bearing three-toothed spines.

Epidemiology

Isolated *G. spinigerum* infections are reported frequently in Thailand, and sporadically in Japan, China, Bangladesh, India, Sri Lanka, South-East Asia, Cameroon, Zambia, Ecuador, Peru, and Australia. Infections with *G. doloresi*, *G. nipponicum*, and *G. hispidum* have been reported from Japan. In Mexico and Ecuador, *G. binucleatum* is the most common infection.

Gnathostomiasis can present in places far away from these endemic areas as a result of migration of the latently infected human host, or importation of the infective flesh of paratenic hosts. Consumption of a raw fish dish at a party can result in an outbreak.

Prevention

All dishes that contain the raw or poorly cooked flesh of animals in or imported from endemic areas must be avoided. Those who prepare potentially infected flesh should use gloves if prolonged exposure is likely.

Clinical features

Nausea, vomiting, and epigastric pain may develop within 1 or 2 days of consumption of the infective food. Fever, pain in the right upper quadrant of the abdomen, chest pain, dry cough, and hypereosinophilia may develop within 1 to 2 weeks.

The primary invasive illness usually passes unnoticed, and so the incubation period is not known in most cases. General health is scarcely impaired, and fever is uncommon. The illnesses can be categorized according to the affected organs as below.

Cutaneous forms

Gnathostomal creeping eruption

This is rare in *G. spinigerum* infection, but more frequent with the other three species that are prevalent in Japan. The serpiginous track is similar to that caused by dog or cat hookworm larvae, but bigger and more variable in depth. A trail of subcutaneous haemorrhage is sometimes observed.

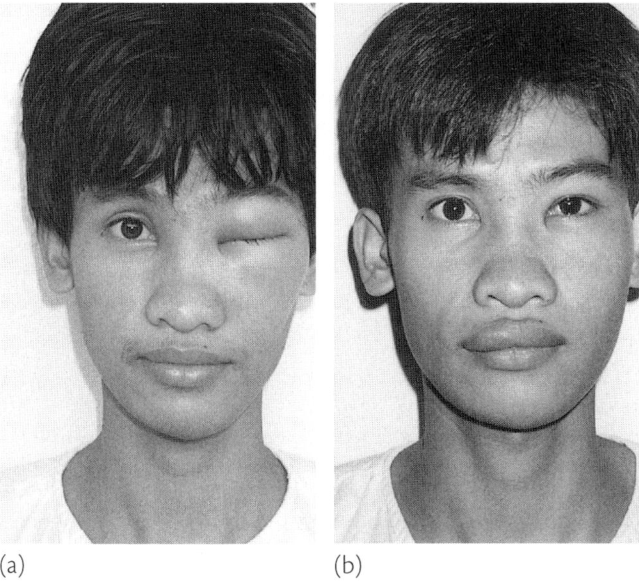

Fig. 7.9.7.1 Migratory swelling in a 23-year-old man. (a) In the left orbital region for 5 days when seen on 5 June 1986. (b) At the right side of the upper lip on 9 June 1986, when the larva was picked out by needle puncture and squeezing.

Cutaneous migratory swelling

The most common manifestation of human gnathostomiasis is intermittent swelling (Fig. 7.9.7.1). The first swelling may develop 3 to 4 weeks after infection, and can occur anywhere; it may recur close to or distant from the original site. The swelling develops rapidly, and usually lasts for about 1 to 2 weeks. Frequently it is extensive, e.g. involving the whole wrist or hand. Swelling of the digits or plantar surfaces can be very painful and incapacitating. Itching is the main associated symptom. Regional lymphadenitis is usually absent. When swelling involves the eyelid, chemosis and conjunctival haemorrhage may be observed.

The worms can escape spontaneously through the skin or the conjunctiva. The interval between episodes of swelling varies from a few days to a few months, and rarely 1 to 2 years. Intermittent cutaneous migratory swelling can persist for more than 5 years.

Visceral forms

Visceral invasion, as described below for *G. spinigerum* infection, has not been reported in infections with other *Gnathostoma* species.

Spinocerebral gnathostomiasis

Involvement of the spinal cord commonly starts with intermittent agonizing shooting pains in a limb or a segment of the trunk, followed by paraplegia with urinary retention, and rarely, quadriplegia. Sensation is correspondingly impaired, and Brown–Séquard syndrome is sometimes seen. A few patients with haematoma and inflammation caused by brain invasion present with severe headache and vomiting, followed very quickly by coma, cranial nerve palsies, and/or hemiplegia. A rapidly advancing or changing pattern of neurological deficits is characteristic. Subarachnoid haemorrhage or eosinophilic meningitis without focal neurological deficit occasionally occurs.

The cerebrospinal fluid can be bloody, xanthochromic, or slightly turbid, with a minor increase in protein content. The proportion of eosinophils is higher than expected from haemorrhage *per se*.

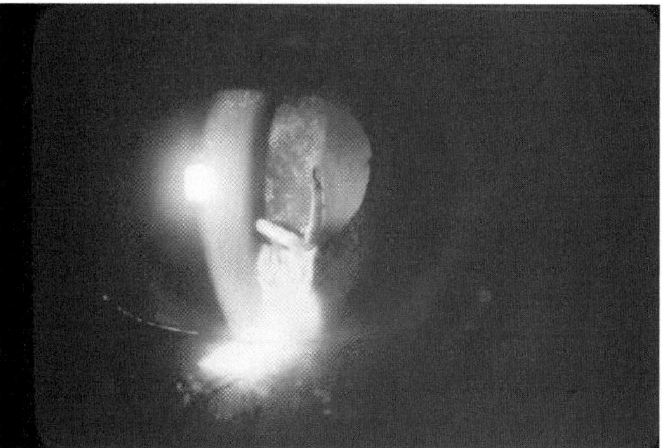

Fig. 7.9.7.2 Gnathostoma larva in the anterior chamber of the eye. (Courtesy of Professor Tiam Lawtiamtong.)

Ocular gnathostomiasis

The parasite can be found in the anterior chamber (Fig. 7.9.7.2) and the vitreous, having migrated through the sclera or the cornea. It can induce uveitis, iritis, intraocular haemorrhage, retinal detachment and scarring, and blindness.

Auditory, pulmonary, intra-abdominal, and genitourinary gnathostomiasis

These uncommon forms can present with hearing loss, productive cough, pleurisy, intestinal obstruction, a painful intra-abdominal mass, and abnormal genital discharge.

Differential diagnosis

The diagnosis of cutaneous forms is based on clinical characteristics, geographical and dietary history, and by excluding other causes. Differential diagnoses include contact dermatitis, angio-oedema and urticaria, Calabar swellings (caused by *Loa loa*), fascioliasis, paragonimiasis, sparganosis, dirofilariasis, and noninfectious causes.

Gnathostoma infection is highly likely if rapidly advancing myelitis follows root pain, or if features of cerebral or subarachnoid haemorrhage occur in a person who is healthy apart from a history of cutaneous migratory swelling. Eosinophil pleocytosis is essential for the diagnosis, as is the exclusion of eosinophilic meningoencephalitis caused by *Angiostrongylus cantonensis*, *Baylisascaris procyonis*, or nonhelminthic encephalomyelitis.

In intraocular infections, the larvae of *A. cantonensis* can be distinguished from Gnathostoma species, as they are thinner, longer, and folding. They usually appear in the eyeball 2 to 3 weeks after the manifestation of eosinophilic meningoencephalitis.

Visceral gnathostomiasis usually depends on identifying the worm in surgical specimens (at autopsy the worms may have migrated away from the site of the main pathological lesion), or in secretions such as sputum, urine, or vaginal discharge.

Clinical investigation

The diagnosis is definitive if the worm can be identified in sections of surgical specimens, as described previously. The whole worm may be available if it emerges through the skin, in excretions and discharges, or from eye operations. Their sizes range from 0.34× 2.2 mm to 1.0× 16.25 mm. Their stage of development does not correlate with the duration of clinical illness. Infections with more than one worm are uncommon.

At present, there is no common serodiagnostic test available for all *Gnathostoma* species. Two serodiagnostic methods are currently used: enzyme immunoassay for *G. binucleatum* infection in Mexico, and immunoblot tests for *G. spinigerum* infection in Thailand. Blood eosinophilia count of (7–76%) occurs irregularly in about 60% of cases, and therefore is not necessary for presumptive diagnosis.

MRI can show tortuous tracks and haemorrhage in cerebral gnathostomiasis.

Criteria for diagnosis

Since the identification of the worm is not always possible, and clinical manifestations overlap with other illnesses, the diagnosis of gnathostomiasis requires the following criteria: (1), clinical presentation described above, and evidence of exposure to gnathostoma larvae, or (2), serological test positive for antibody against gnathostoma antigen, confirming the presumptive diagnosis.

Treatment

Surgical removal is curative, but advisable only in accessible areas such as the eye or skin. Blind exploration of subcutaneous tissues in areas of diffuse swelling is not productive.

Oral therapy with albendazole at an adult dosage of 400 mg twice daily for 2 to 3 weeks induces migration of the parasite to the skin. The worms are frequently recovered between days 2 and 14 of treatment, picked out with a needle, excisional biopsy, or even scratched out by the patient's fingernails. However, the success rate is only 6 to 7%. Recurrence of swelling in patients whose worms do not migrate to the skin is less frequent after albendazole treatment. Aminotransferases should be measured before this treatment, even though hepatotoxicity at this dosage is usually mild and reversible. Oral therapy with a single dose of ivermectin at 200 µg/kg is not superior to placebo or albendazole, but may be considered in patients in whom albendazole treatment fails.

Prognosis

Cerebral gnathostomiasis can be fatal, and blindness is frequent after intraocular infection. Patients can be reassured that central nervous system or intraocular involvement occurs in less than 1% of cases with cutaneous migratory swelling.

Further reading

Bussaratid V, *et al.* (2006). Efficacy of ivermectin treatment of cutaneous gnathostomiasis evaluated by placebo-controlled trial. *Southeast Asian J Trop Med Public Health*, **37**, 433–40.

Bhaibulya M, Charoenlarp P (1983). Creeping eruption caused by *Gnathostoma spinigerum*. *Southeast Asian J Trop Med Public Health*, **14**, 226–8.

Inkatanuvat S, *et al.* (1998). Changes of liver functions after albendazole treatment in human gnathostomiasis. *J Med Assoc Thai*, **81**, 735–40.

Kraivichian K, *et al.* (2004). Treatment of cutaneous gnathostomiasis with ivermectin. *Am J Trop Med Hyg*, **7**, 623–8.

Miyazaki I (1991). *An illustrated book of helminthic zoonoses*, pp. 368–409. International Medical Foundation of Japan, Tokyo.

Nopparatana C, *et al.* (1991). Purification of *Gnathostoma spinigerum* specific antigen and immunodiagnosis of human gnathostomiasis. *Int J Parasitol*, **21**, 677–87.

Rusnak JM, Lucey DR (1993). Clinical gnathostomiasis: case report and review of the English language literature. *Clin Infect Dis*, **16**, 33–50.

Sirikulchayanonta V, Viriyavejakul P (2001). Various morphologic features of *Gnathostoma spinigerum* in histologic sections: Report of 3 cases with reference to topographic study of the reference worm. *Southeast Asian J Trop Med Public Health*, **32**, 302–7.

Suntharasamai P, *et al.* (1992). Albendazole stimulates outward migration of *Gnathostoma spinigerum* to the dermis in man. *Southeast Asian J Trop Med Public Health*, **23**, 716–22.

Swanson VL (1971). Gnathostomiasis. In: Marcial-Rojas RA (ed). *Pathology of protozoal and helminthic diseases with clinical correlation*, pp. 871–9. Williams and Wilkins, Baltimore.

7.10

Cestodes (tapeworms)

Contents

7.10.1 Cystic hydatid disease (*Echinococcus granulosus*) *1185*
Armando E. Gonzalez, Pedro L. Moro, and Hector H. Garcia

7.10.2 Cyclophyllidian gut tapeworms *1188*
Richard Knight

7.10.3 Cysticercosis *1193*
Hector H. Garcia and Robert H. Gilman

7.10.4 Diphyllobothriasis and sparganosis *1199*
David I. Grove

7.10.1 Cystic hydatid disease (*Echinococcus granulosus*)

Armando E. Gonzalez, Pedro L. Moro, and Hector H. Garcia

Essentials

Cystic hydatid disease, caused by *Echinococcus granulosus*, is a zoonotic disease principally transmitted between dogs and domestic livestock, particularly sheep. Humans are infected when they ingest tapeworm eggs, with disease occuring in most parts of the world where sheep are raised and dogs are used to herd livestock.

Clinical features, diagnosis, and treatment—the most common clinical manifestations are cysts in the liver (typically presenting with hepatomegaly) and/or lung (presenting with cough, haemoptysis, and dyspnoea). Diagnosis is usually made on the basis of serological tests in combination with imaging techniques. Treatment options include surgery, chemotherapy with anthelminthic agents, or—for liver cysts—PAIR (puncture–aspiration–injection–reaspiration).

Prevention—echinococcosis is a major public health problem in several countries. Control programmes have been aimed at educating dog owners to prevent their animals from having access to infected offal. Vaccines against sheep hydatidosis and the dog tapeworm stage are promising alternatives.

Introduction

Cystic hydatid disease is a zoonotic disease caused by infection with the larval stage (hydatid cyst) of the tapeworm *Echinococcus granulosus*. Hydatid cysts in liver and lung are frequent causes of human morbidity in endemic zones.

Aetiology

The lifecycle of *E. granulosus* requires two hosts. The adult tapeworm is found in the small intestine of the definitive host, usually dogs or other canids. It consists of only three to five proglottids, and measures between 3 and 7 mm long when fully mature. *E. granulosus* has remarkable biological potential; there may be as many as 40 000 worms in a heavily infected dog, each one of which sheds about 1000 eggs every 2 weeks. Dogs infected with echinococcus tapeworms pass eggs in their faeces that contaminate the soil and vegetation and remain viable for long periods in cold humid places. Intermediate hosts (sheep, cattle, horses, pigs, and other mammals, including humans) acquire hydatid disease by ingesting viable eggs of *E. granulosus*. Eggs hatch in the intestine, freeing oncospheres which penetrate the intestinal mucosa and are transported by the blood and lymphatic systems to the liver, lungs, and other organs, where they develop into cysts.

Molecular studies using mitochondrial DNA sequences have identified 10 distinct genetic types within *E. granulosus*. These include two sheep strains (G1, G2), two bovid strains (G3, G5), a horse strain (G4), the camelid strain (G6), a pig strain (G7) and the cervid strain (G8). A ninth genotype (G9) has been described in swine in Poland, and a tenth genotype (G10) in cervids. The sheep strain (G1) is the most cosmopolitan form that is most commonly associated with human infections. The other strains appear to be genetically distinct. The presence of distinct strains of *E. granulosus* affects clinical aspects and control strategy. The risk of human infection differs as does its localization, clinical expression, and geographical distribution. Shorter maturation time of a given strain in dogs would reduce the duration of infection by the adult intestinal form so that shorter intervals are required between rounds of administration of antiparasite drugs for control.

Epidemiology

Hydatid disease is an important cause of human morbidity, requiring costly surgical treatment. The infection is widely distributed in most parts of the world where sheep are raised and dogs are used to herd livestock. In the Americas, most cases have been reported from Argentina, Chile, Uruguay, Peru, and southern Brazil. Recent studies in Peru have revealed prevalences of hydatid disease ranging from 5.7 to 8.9% in highland villagers, and as high as 32 and 89% in dogs and sheep, respectively. High prevalence of liver hydatid disease, with rates of up to 5.6%, have also been reported in north-western Turkana in Kenya. *Echinococcus* is widespread in the Old World, particularly in Greece, Cyprus, Bulgaria, Lebanon, and Turkey. In the United States of America, most infections are seen in immigrants from endemic countries; however, sporadic autochthonous transmission is currently recognized in Alaska, California, Utah, Arizona, and New Mexico.

Communities at higher risk of infection include those where sheep are raised extensively and where dogs are used to care for large flocks of livestock. Known risk factors for infection include feeding dogs with raw offal and access of dogs to sheep that die in the field (Fig. 7.10.1.1). The risk of infection is also linked to poor hygiene and intimate contact with dogs. In north-western Turkana, dogs are allowed to stay within the house, and are used to clean up women's menses and lick vomit from faces and diarrhoea from the anal regions of their children.

Pathogenesis

The incubation period of human hydatid infections is highly variable and often prolonged for several years. Cysts have been reported to grow continuously. However, recent studies suggest that cyst growth is highly variable. Some cysts grow as much as 1 cm per year while other viable cysts showed no growth during 3 to 12 years of follow-up.

Most human infections remain asymptomatic; hydatid cysts are found incidentally at autopsy much more frequently than the reported local morbidity rates. The locality of the cysts, their size, and their condition determine the particular manifestations.

Clinical features

Hydatid cysts are most frequently seen in the liver (60–70%) followed by the lungs (30–40%). Signs of hepatic hydatid disease include hepatomegaly with or without the presence of a mass in the upper right quadrant. Obstructive jaundice, mild epigastric pain, indigestion, and nausea may occur occasionally. Hydatid cysts may become secondarily infected with bacteria presenting as a hepatic abscess. Features of lung involvement (Fig. 7.10.1.2) are cough, haemoptysis, dyspnoea, and fever. The ratio of liver to lung cysts may vary from one geographical region to another: a liver to lung ratio of 1.4:1 has been observed in Peru, in contrast to the 3:1 to 13:1 ratio reported in Argentina and Uruguay. Differences in echinococcus strains may account for this variation. Brain cysts produce intracranial hypertension and epilepsy. Vertebral cysts compress the spinal cord causing paraplegia; bone cysts produce spontaneous fractures (Figs. 7.10.1.3 and 7.10.1.4) and deformity. Sudden rupture of cysts in the peritoneal cavity may result in peritonitis (Fig. 7.10.1.4), and rupture in the lungs may cause pneumothorax and empyema. Rupture may also cause allergic manifestations such as pruritus, oedema, dyspnoea, anaphylactic shock, and even death.

Diagnosis

Clinical findings such as a space-occupying lesion and residence in an endemic region are suggestive of hydatid disease. Abdominal ultrasonography is an important aid to the diagnosis of abdominal cysts. Portable ultrasonography machines are used with good results in field surveys. Chest radiography is useful for diagnosis of lung cysts. CT scanning is very helpful, especially for diagnosis of nontypical lesions (Fig. 7.10.1.4b).

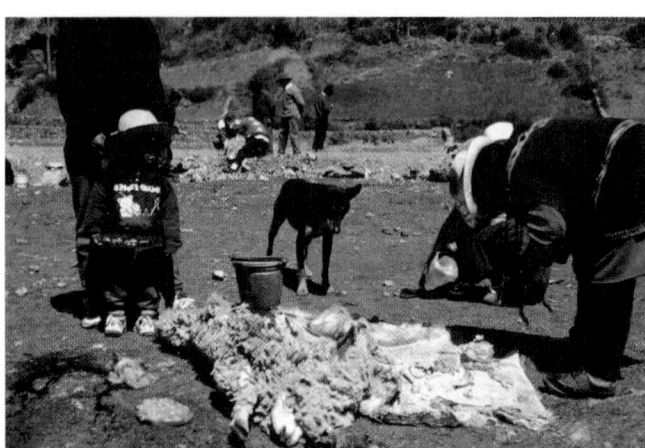

Fig. 7.10.1.1 Epidemiological conditions for completion of the life cycle of echinoccocus: stray dogs waiting for sheep offal outside a slaughterhouse in Peru.

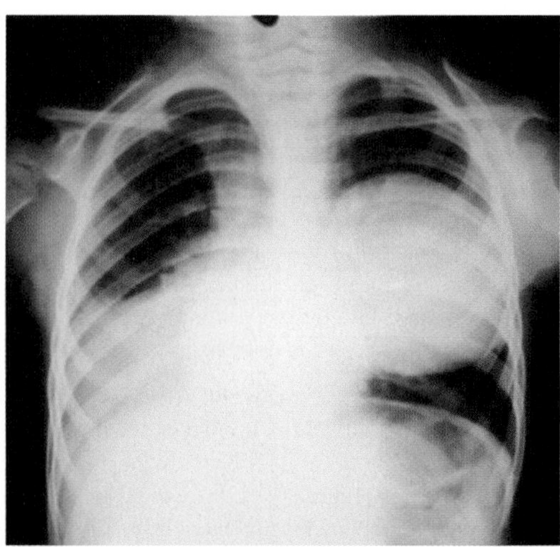

Fig. 7.10.1.2 Plain chest radiograph showing a lung hydatid cyst displacing the heart.

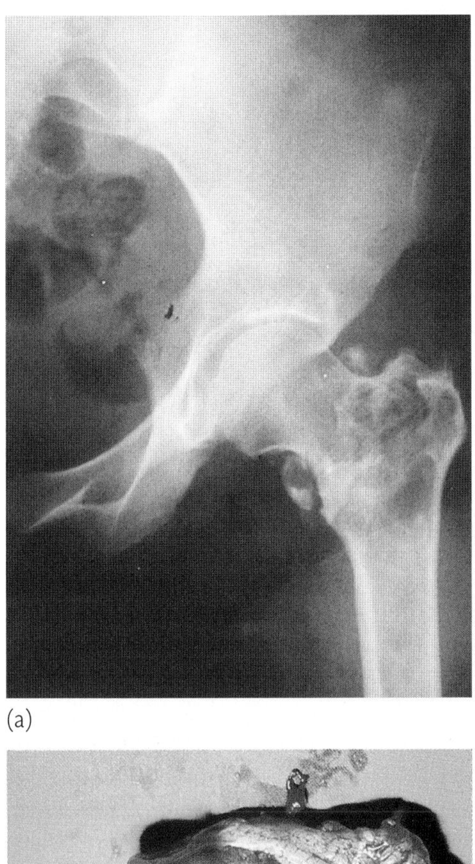

(a)

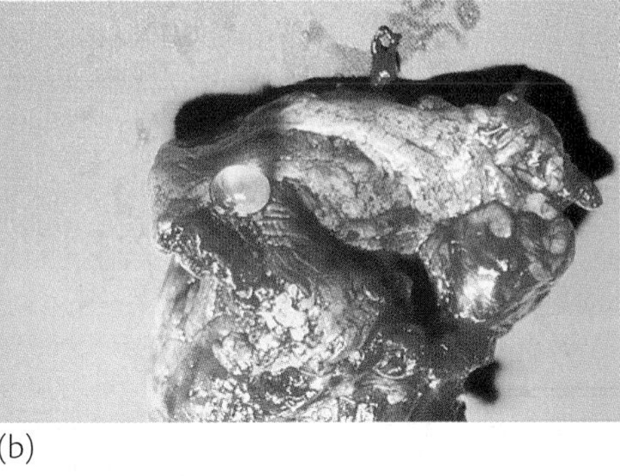

(b)

Fig. 7.10.1.3 (a) Pathological fracture of the femur caused by hydatid infection. (b) Hydatid cyst in muscle excised from around the femoral head (same case as shown in (a)).
(Copyright D A Warrell.)

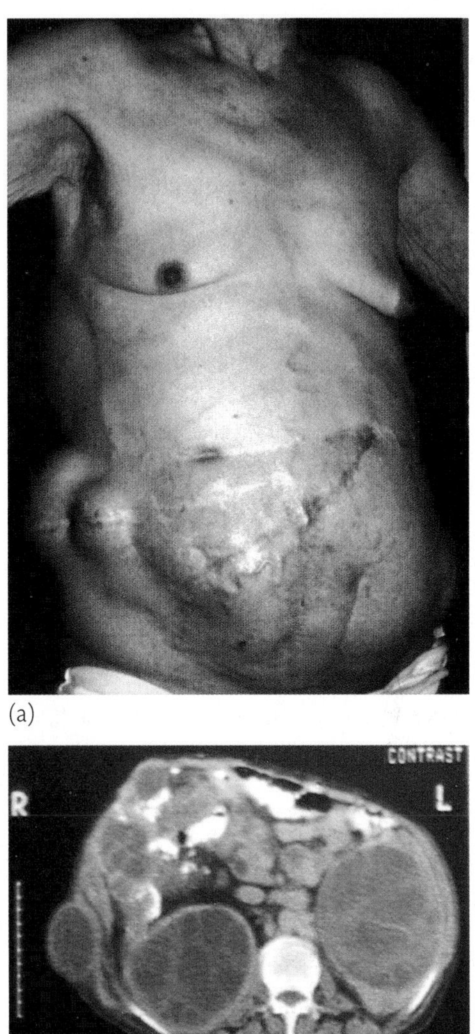

(a)

(b)

Fig. 7.10.1.4 (a) Numerous subcutaneous, peritoneal, and renal hydatid cysts in an Argentine patient. (b) Contrast CT scan of the same patient.(Courtesy of Professor Olindo Adriano Martino, Buenos Aires.)

Serology

A number of serological tests have been developed for diagnosis of hydatid disease, including an enzyme immunoassay, which identifies antibodies against antigen B or components of this antigen. A western blot assay based on the identification of three specific antigens of 8, 16, and 21 kDa is currently used. Major drawbacks in serological diagnosis are low sensitivity for detection of lung hydatid cysts and cross-reactivity with sera of patients with *Taenia solium* infection. Cyst rupture or secondary infection are strongly associated to a positive result in hydatid serology. In field surveys, serological tests should be used in combination with imaging techniques in order to detect most cases of hydatid disease.

Parasitological diagnosis

Although uncommon, this can be done from sputum samples of patients whose lung cysts have recently ruptured. Scolices have four spherical suckers and a rostellum with two rows of hooks.

Treatment

Surgery

Surgical removal of hydatid cysts remains the treatment of choice in many countries. The usual surgical approach involves aspiration of cyst fluid and injection of a protoscolicidal agent into the cyst, usually 20% hypertonic saline solution or 90% alcohol, followed by evacuation of the fluid, prior to surgical excision. Major risks of surgical treatment include accidental spillage of fluid and scolices into the peritoneal cavity, which may lead to anaphylaxis or secondary peritoneal hydatidosis. Recurrence rates following surgery may be as high as 30%. Antihistamines are given as prophylaxis and suction cones have been used to prevent spillage. The efficacy of these methods is uncertain.

Chemotherapy

Benzimidazole compounds have been shown to be effective against hydatid disease. Courses of albendazole in a dose of 10 to 15mg/kg body weight per day for 28 days are interspersed with drug-free periods of 2 weeks. This regime cures approximately one-third of cases of liver hydatid disease and causes partial regression of cysts in another one-third of patients. However, many courses may be needed to achieve complete or partial cyst regression. Small liver or lung hydatid cysts should be treated with albendazole. Because of its high scolicidal activity, albendazole is recommended as a prophylactic agent 1 to 3 months before surgical intervention. Albendazole is indicated when surgery is contraindicated. Mebendazole may also be used, although it is less effective than albendazole. Albendazole, mebendazole, and other benzimidazole compounds should not be used in pregnant women because of their potentially teratogenic effects. The combination of praziquantel and albendazole seems to show a better efficacy than albendazole alone. Since benzimidazoles are potentially hepatotoxic, liver enzymes should be monitored before and during treatment.

Recent experimental studies in animals have shown that another benzimidazole compound, oxfendazole, has strong parasiticidal activity. Intermittent weekly therapy with oxfendazole was effective in sheep hydatid disease, suggesting the possibility that daily therapy as currently used with albendazole may not be needed. Future studies will explore the effect of oxfendazole in the treatment of human hydatid disease.

Percutaneous aspiration, injection, reaspiration (PAIR)

PAIR consists of percutaneous puncture using sonographic guidance, aspiration of substantial amounts of the cyst fluid, and injection of a protoscolicidal agent, usually hypertonic saline for at least 15 min, followed by reaspiration of cyst contents. Albendazole should be administered before PAIR treatment, and antihistamines should be given to reduce the risk of allergic reactions if there is spillage of fluid. Good results have been reported with this procedure with no major complications. A metaanalysis comparing the use of PAIR and surgical treatment for liver hydatid cysts found less complications and a shorter hospital stay in the PAIR-treated group.

Prevention and control

The earliest successful programme against echinococcosis was carried out in Iceland. It was based on a health educational campaign that eradicated the parasite. Control programmes have been aimed at educating dog owners to prevent their animals from having access to infected offal. This approach includes periodic treatment of sheepdogs with praziquantel (every 45 days), reduction in the dog population, close veterinary inspection of slaughterhouse facilities for the presence of dogs, and cremation of infected offal. Control programmes are in force in Argentina, Chile, and Uruguay. Partial success has been achieved. Control programmes in New Zealand and Tasmania have reduced the number of infected animals and the incidence of human infection.

Serological tests such as the western blot for diagnosis of sheep hydatidosis and the coproantigen enzyme-linked immunosorbent assay (ELISA) for canine echinococcosis are potentially useful for measuring the burden of disease and monitoring control programmes in endemic regions. A recent major advance has been the development of a recombinant vaccine (EG95) which seems to confer 96 to 98% protection against challenge infection. Recent trials in Australia and Argentina using this vaccine have reported that 86% of immunized sheep were completely free of viable hydatid cysts when examined 1 year later. The number of viable cysts was reduced by 99.3%. Similarly, a vaccine against the dog tapeworm stage has been developed and conferred 97 to 100% protection against worm growth and egg production in immunized dogs. Although the results of these initial trials seem promising, further research is needed to assess the cost benefit of using these vaccines.

Further reading

Allan JC, *et al.* (1992). Coproantigen detection for immunodiagnosis of echinococcosis and taeniasis in dogs and humans. *Parasitology*, **104**, 347–55.

Craig PS, *et al.* (2007). Prevention and control of cystic echinococcosis. *Lancet Infect Dis*, **7**, 385–94.

Frider B, Larrieu E, Odriozola M (1999). Long-term outcome of asymptomatic liver hydatidosis. *J Hepatol*, **30**, 228–31.

Gavidia CM, *et al.* (2008). Diagnosis of cystic echinococcosis, central Peruvian Highlands. *Emerg Infect Dis*, **14**, 260–6.

Junghanss T, *et al.* (2008). Clinical management of cystic echinococcosis: State of the art, problems, and perspectives. *Am J Trop Med Hyg*, **79**, 301–11.

McManus DP, Thompson RCA (2003). Molecular epidemiology of cystic echinococcosis. *Parasitology*, **127**, S37–51.

Macpherson CNL, *et al.* (1987). Portable ultrasound scanner versus serology in screening for hydatid cysts in a nomadic population. *Lancet*, **ii**, 259–91.

Moro PL, *et al.* (1997). Epidemiology of *Echinococcus granulosus* infection in the Central Andes of Peru. *Bull World Health Org*, **75**, 553–61.

Schantz PM, Williams JF, Posse CR (1973). Epidemiology of hydatid disease in southern Argentina. Comparison of morbidity indices, evaluation of immunodiagnostic tests, and factors affecting transmission in southern Rio Negro Province. *Am J Trop Med Hyg*, **22**, 629–41.

Smego RA, *et al.* (2003). Percutaneous aspiration-injection-reaspiration-drainage plus albendazole or mebendazole for hepatic cystic echinococcosis: a meta-analysis. *Clin Infect Dis*, **27**, 1073–83.

Thompson RCA, McManus DP (2002). Towards a taxonomic revision of the genus *Echinococcus*. *Trends Parasitol*, **18**, 452–7.

Verastegui M *et al.* (1992). Enzyme-linked immunoelectrotransfer blot test for the diagnosis of human hydatid disease. *J Clin Microbiol*, **30**, 1557–61.

Zhang W, *et al.* (2006). Vaccination of dogs against *Echinococcus granulosus*, the cause of cystic hydatid disease in humans. *J Infect Dis*, **194**, 966–74.

7.10.2 Cyclophyllidian gut tapeworms

Richard Knight

Essentials

The cyclophyllidean tapeworms are cestodes that maintain anchorage to the host small-gut mucosa. Humans are an obligatory part of the life cycle in four gut species; in the rest they are an accidental host.

Taenia saginata

The beef tapeworm; prevalent where cattle have access to human faeces and where humans eat undercooked beef. Many people who are infected have no symptoms, except that they experience active exit of single proglottids through the anus. Diagnosis is by finding typical eggs in perianal swabs. Treatment is with niclosamide or praziquantel. Prevention is by health education concerning production and cooking of meat, also by proper sewage treatment and disposal. Mass treatment of selected or whole adult populations is the most effective short-term measure when endemicity is high.

Taenia solium

Adult pork tapeworm infections occur when cysts in undercooked pig meat are eaten. Symptoms, diagnosis and treatment are similar to those of *T.saginata*. The potentially dangerous condition of cysticercosis occurs when eggs from the faeces of persons harbouring adult worms are ingested; this produces cysts in striated muscle, subcutaneous tissue, nervous system and the eye. See Chapter 7.10.3 for further discussion.

Other tapeworms

Hymenolepis nana—the dwarf tapeworm, whose life cycle normally involves only humans. Heavy infection can lead to anorexia, abdominal pain, and malabsorption. Diagnosis is by finding eggs in the faeces. Treatment is with praziquantel or niclosamide.

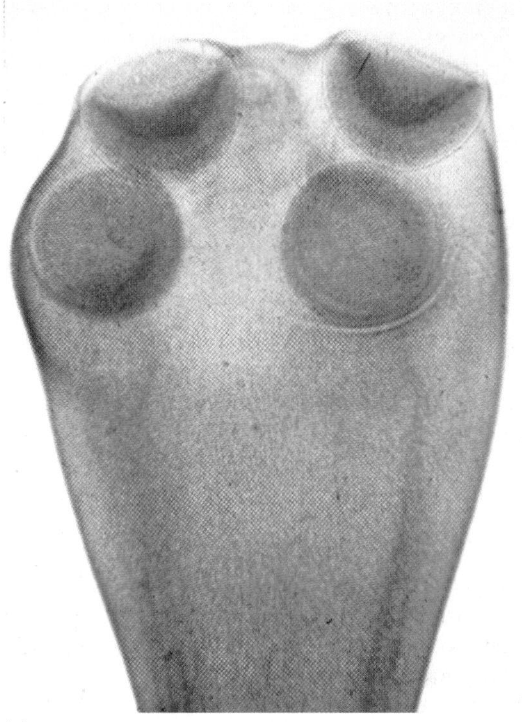

(a)

(b)

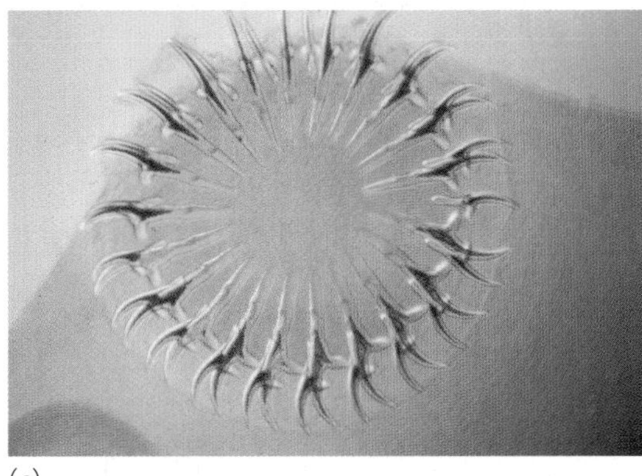

(c)

Fig. 7.10.2.1 (a) *Taenia saginata* showing scolex with four suckers and no hooks. (b *Taenia solium* showing scolex with four suckers and a double row of hooks. (c) *Taenia solium* detail of hooks.
(Courtesy of Professor Viqar Zaman.)

Introduction

The cyclophyllidean tapeworms are cestodes that maintain anchorage to the host small-gut mucosa by means the scolex, a holdfast structure bearing a circlet of four suckers and usually a central evertible rostellum with one or more circlets of minute hooks (Figs. 7.10.2.1a, b, c). The rest of the body forms the strobila and consists of a chain of flattened proglottids, which bud behind the scolex. The worms change their site of attachment regularly, and are surprisingly motile. Gravid proglottids are lost from the end of the worm and are replaced by others that have grown and matured as they pass down the strobila. Each proglottid possesses a complete set of hermaphroditic sex organs and marginal genital openings. Eggs accumulate in the uterus of gravid proglottids and only enter the faecal stream if the proglottids are disrupted. In many species the eggs enter the environment within intact proglottids. In either case the eggs are embryonated and contain a six-hooked hexacanth embryo. The egg shells have two membranes, but in *Taenia* the outer is lost early and the inner forms the thick embryophore.

After ingestion by the intermediate host, eggs hatch and the released hexacanth embryo bores its way into the mucosa. The larval stages of the parasite ('metacestode') are generally cystic with an invaginated embryonic scolex—the protoscolex. The cycle is completed when the larval stage, within the intermediate host or its tissues, is eaten by the definitive host; the protoscolex evaginates and attaches to the gut mucosa.

In four gut species, humans are an obligatory part of the lifecycle (Table 7.10.2.1), in the rest they are an accidental host (Table 7.10.2.2). The three *Taenia* species are anthropozoonoses because the cycle is maintained by an obligatory alternation between human and nonhuman hosts. Patients with *Taenia* infections pass proglottids in their faeces or experience their active migration per anum.

Table 7.10.2.1 Major gut cestodes that infect humans

	Taenia saginata Beef tapeworm	*Taenia asiatica* Asian tapeworm	*Taenia solium* Pork tapeworm	*Hymenolepis nana* Dwarf tapeworm
Larval tapeworm				
Intermediate hosts	Cattle, water buffalo, other bovids, reindeer	Pig, wild boar	Pig, wild boar, humans (cysticercosis)	None but human and murine subspecies perhaps cross-infect
Type and size	Cysticercus 7–10 × 4–6 mm	Cysticercus 2 × 2 mm	Cysticercus 5–8 × 3–6 mm	Minute tailless cysticercoid 50 μm
Location	Muscle, viscera, brain (reindeer only)	Viscera, mainly liver	Muscle, brain, subcutaneous, eye, tongue	Villi of small intestine
Adult tapeworm				
Length	4–12 m	4–12 m	3–5 m	25–40 mm
Number of proglottids	2000 (mean)	2000 (mean)	700–1000	200 (mean)
Gravid proglottid	Longer than wide; 20–30 × 5–7 mm	Longer than wide; 20–30 × 5–7 mm	Longer than wide; 18–25 × 5–7 mm	Wider than long; 0.8 × 0.2 mm
Scolex	No rostellum, no hooks	Rostellum; no hooks	Rostellum with double circlet of hooks	Rostellum with single circlet of minute hooks
Gravid uterus	15–20 lateral branches	15–20 lateral branches	7–12 lateral branches	Bilobed
Egg (contains hexacanth embryo)	Embryophore shell is radially striated and 31–40 μm in diameter	Embryophore shell is radially striated and 31–40 μm in diameter	Embryophore shell is radially striated and 31–40 μm in diameter	Oval, 30–47 μm long; two shell membranes; 4–8 filaments arise from each pole of inner membrane

Table 7.10.2.2 Uncommon gut cestodes that infect humans

Species	Geographic distribution	Definitive hosts	Intermediate hosts	Length and width of tapeworm	Shape of gravid proglottid	Other features
Bertiella mucronata	South America, Cuba	Primates	Oribatid mites	15–45 cm × 5–10 mm	Wider than long	Inner eggshell bears bicornuate knob
B.studeri	South and South-East Asia, Africa, Cuba	Primates	Oribatid mites	27–30 cm × 6–10 mm	Much wider than long	As above
Dipylidium caninum	Worldwide	Dog, cat	Fleas and dog louse	10–70 cm × 2.5–3 mm	Elongate, wider in middle	Double set of sex organs. Egg capsules with 8–15 eggs
Hymenolepis diminuta (rat tapeworm)	Worldwide	Rat	Fleas, beetles, cockroaches	20–60 cm × 3–4 mm	Much wider than long	Egg like *H. nana* but yellow outer membrane and no filaments; 60–85 μm
Inermicapsifer madagascariensis	Madagascar, Africa, Central America, Cuba	Rats	Arthropod	26–42 cm × 2.6 mm	Slightly elongate, white and opaque	Egg capsules with 6–11 eggs
Mathevotaenia symmetrica	Thailand	Rodents	Beetles	13 cm × 1–2 mm	Elongate, wider in middle	Capsule surrounds individual eggs
Mesocestoides lineatus	China, Japan, Korea	Carnivores	Mites (1st host); amphibia, reptiles, birds, rodents (2nd hosts)	40 cm × 1.5–2 mm	Longer than broad	Single medioventral genital opening
Mesocestoides variabilis	Greenland, USA	Carnivores	Mites (1st host); amphibia, reptiles, birds, rodents (2nd hosts)	40 cm × 1.5–2 mm	Longer than broad	Single medioventral genital opening
Raillietina celebensis	East Asia, Polynesia, Australia	Rats	Ant	16–60 cm × 3 mm	As above	Egg capsules with 1–4 eggs
R. demerariensis	Guyana, Cuba, Ecuador	Rats	Cockroach	16- 60 cm × 2–3 mm	As above	Egg capsule with 8–10 eggs

The clinical importance the pork tapeworm relates mainly to cysticercosis, the occurrence of larval forms in human tissue (see Chapter 7.10.3). The dwarf tapeworm *Hymenolepis nana* infects an estimated 9 million people; there is normally no intermediate host.

With any gut cestode, symptoms also result from local hypersensitivity reactions to the worm and its scolex, altered gut motility, and poorly defined systemic symptoms with an immunological basis. A blood eosinophilia up to 10% can occur.

Eggs of the cyclophyllidian tapeworms of the dog and fox can infect humans to produce hydatid and multilocular hydatid disease respectively (see Chapter 7.10.1), here humans are an accidental intermediate host.

Taenia tapeworms

Taenia saginata

Geographical distribution

The beef tapeworm *T. saginata* is prevalent where cattle have access to human faeces and where humans eat undercooked beef. The highest prevalence is in Africa, particularly in eastern and north-eastern parts; it is also common in many countries in the Middle East, South America, and South-East Asia. Prevalence is now very low in the United States of America, Canada, and Australia. It still persists endemically in Europe; but prevalence increases progressively eastwards and into the former Soviet Union.

Epidemiology

Most worms are solitary. Multiple worms are smaller and typically occur in high-transmission areas, probably by simultaneous infection. Viable eggs from human faeces persist on pasture for many months and can survive most forms of sewage treatment. Cattle have access to human faeces on farms, at camp sites and recreation areas, and on railway lines. Infected herdsmen can initiate epizootics. Eggs may be dispersed by flies and dung beetles, and seabirds can ingest proglottids in refuse or estuarine waters and deposit them in their faeces on inland pastures.

In cattle the whitish, ovoid, cysticerci become infective within 12 weeks and remain viable in the living host for 2 years; they are viable in stored, chilled meat for several weeks but are killed at –20°C within 1 week. The prepatent period in man is 3 months and worms may live 30 years. Cattle develop protective immunity to new infection.

Clinical features

The whitish mature proglottids, approximately 2 to 3cm long, are actively motile, elongating and contracting (Fig. 7.10.2.2). Most patients experience active exit of single proglottids through the anus, others pass proglottids at defecation, often in short chains; free eggs also occur in faeces. Many have no other symptoms, but others complain of nausea and upper abdominal pains, often relieved by food. In children, impaired appetite can have nutritional consequences. Some patients have symptoms suggestive of hypoglycaemia, namely dizziness and sweating. Pruritus ani is common. The worm may be visible on small-bowel barium studies.

Proglottids have been found in a variety of surgical specimens, including resected appendices, but a pathogenic role is usually difficult to establish. They occasionally obstruct the small intestine, pancreatic duct, or bile duct. Proglottids are recorded in the gallbladder, and eggs have been found in gallstones.

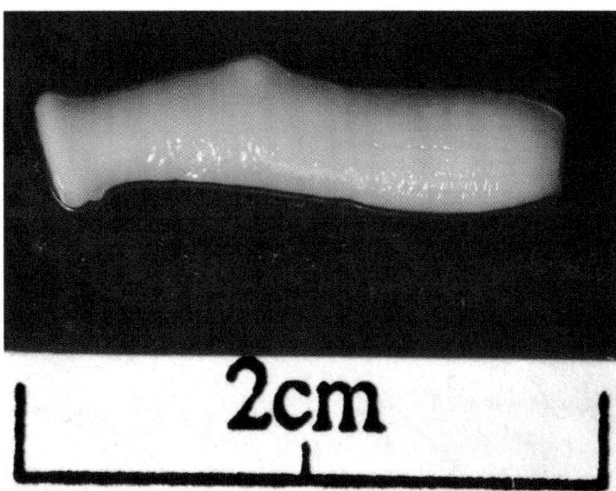

Fig. 7.10.2.2 Actively mobile, contracting proglottid of *Taenia saginata* found by a patient in the stool.
(Copyright D A Warrell.)

Diagnosis

The typical eggs (Fig. 7.10.2.3) may be found in faeces, but this is an insensitive method; perianal swabs are more useful. Eggs are indistinguishable from those of *T. solium* and *T asiatica*; patients should be asked to bring worm specimens. Unless the proglottid is fully gravid the number of uterine branches is an unreliable diagnostic character. A better morphological distinction is the presence of a vaginal sphincter; this is absent in *T. solium*. In human surveys in endemic areas a 24-h faecal collection after an anthelmintic will give the most reliable prevalence.

Treatment

Niclosamide, 2 g, is given to adults and older children as a single morning dose on an empty stomach; the tablets should be chewed. Children aged 2 to 6 years should receive 1 g, and those below 2 years 500 mg. The alternative is praziquantel, 10 to 20 mg/kg as a single dose after a light breakfast. After either drug the proximal part of the worm disintegrates in the gut and the scolex cannot be found. Failure of proglottids to reappear within 3 to 4 months indicates cure.

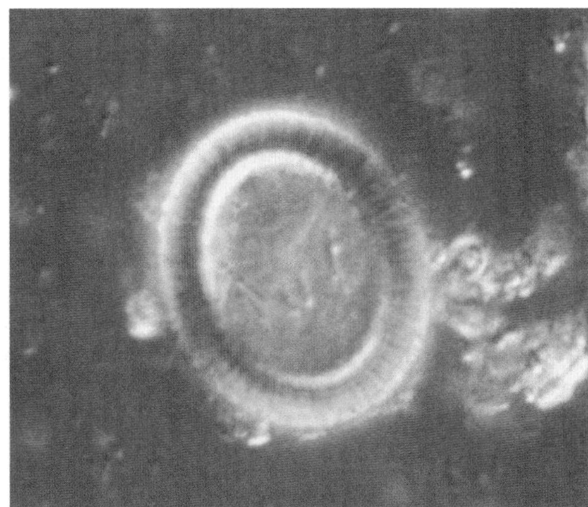

Fig. 7.10.2.3 Egg of *Taenia*.
(Courtesy of Professor Viqar Zaman.)

Control

This includes health education concerning raw beef, meat inspection, sanitation and hygiene on cattle farms, and proper sewage treatment and disposal. Mass treatments of herd contacts, or whole adult populations, are the most effective short-term measures when endemicity is high. *T. saginata* causes great economic loss to the beef industry in some developing countries. Vaccines may soon become available for use in cattle.

Taenia asiatica

This was first described in 1973 as a subspecies *T. saginata* from rural Taiwan, where raw pig or wild boar liver, but no beef, was eaten. It is now recognized as a separate species and known also to occur in Korea, China, northern Sumatra, and Thailand. The cysticerci in pig viscera are very small. In immunodeficient mice *T. asiatica* eggs, but not those of *T. saginata*, produce cysticerci with hooked protoscolices. Eating uncooked pork with viscera from home-killed pigs is a recognized risk factor. Symptoms and treatment are the same as for *T. saginata*.

Taenia solium (see also Chapter 7.10.3)

Generally less common than the beef tapeworm, the pork tapeworm *T. solium* is now very rare in North America and western Europe, but it remains common in much of sub-Saharan Africa, and in China, India, and other parts of Asia. It is highly prevalent in Mexico and other Latin American countries. Two genotypes are now recognized: the European type that has been introduced into the Americas and Africa since the 1500s, and the Asian type. Both types can produce neurocysticercosis, but only the latter causes subcutaneous cysticercosis.

Epidemiology

In pigs, muscle cysticerci produce 'measly pork' (Fig. 7.10.2.4). The cysts are most numerous in the tongue, masseter, heart, and diaphragm, but also occur in the brain. When eaten by humans in undercooked pork, the worms mature in 5 to 12 weeks. The eggs have the same resistant qualities as those of *T. saginata*.

Human cysticercosis arises when eggs from the faeces of people infected with adult worms are ingested and hatch in the upper gut; humans thus become an accidental intermediate host.

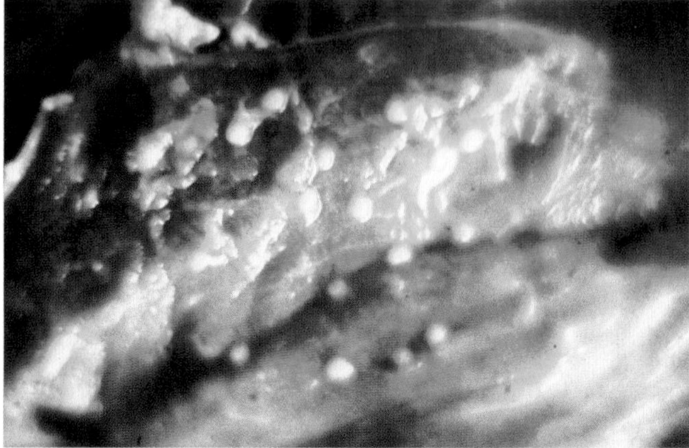

Fig. 7.10.2.4 'Measly pork' showing numerous cysts in the pig's muscle. (Copyright Sornchai Looareesuwan.)

Conditions favouring cysticercosis include poor personal hygiene, which facilitates external autoinfection, and contaminated fingers among food handlers. Faecal pollution of the peridomestic environment, irrigation water, or cultivated vegetables is also important. In parts of Africa, tapeworm proglottids are used in traditional medicine. In the absence of these factors, cases of cysticercosis may be very sporadic even when *T. solium* is common. Cysticercosis is a major health problem in Mexico, some South American countries, and to a lesser extent in Africa and Asia. In 1969, *T. solium* was introduced from Bali into the highlands of Indonesian New Guinea, where the disease is now of great importance.

Pathology of human cysticercosis

Cysts occur especially in striated muscle, subcutaneous tissue (Asian genotype), the nervous system, and the eye. Many remain clinically silent until the parasite dies after 3 to 5 years, when vigorous inflammatory and hypersensitivity reactions can occur; later lesions may calcify. In the brain, particularly in the subarachnoid and the ventricular system, atypical racemose cysts may occur. They appear as irregular or grape-like clusters of cysts that have no protoscolex; they can be mistaken pathologically for nonparasitic cysts.

Clinical features

Symptoms due to the adult worms are similar to those of *T. saginata* but are often milder and not associated with pruritus ani. The proglottids do not migrate actively *per anum*.

Diagnosis

Adult worm infection is detected as for *T. saginata*. Methods for detecting faecal antigen are available and have great potential use in epidemiological studies. Proglottid fragments can be identified using DNA probes.

Treatment and control

Adult worms are treated as for *T. saginata*. Because of the potential risk of internal autoinfection vomiting must be avoided and an antiemetic is often recommended, together with a purgative 2 h after the medication which should be given after a light breakfast. It should be remembered that the faeces will be potentially highly infective for several days, for both the patient and the attendants. Control measures include meat inspection, health education, and population-based chemotherapy. Local risk factors for human cysticercosis must receive special attention. Pigs can be treated with a single dose of oxfendazole and perhaps in the future given recombinant hexacanth vaccines.

Hymenolepis nana

The dwarf tapeworm, sometimes now placed in the genus *Rodentolepis*, is the most common cestode in humans; it is also the smallest. When worm loads are high, it causes more gut pathology than any other species. It is common in most developing and tropical countries. The life cycle normally involves only humans. Fully embryonated infective eggs are passed in the faeces; gravid proglottids normally disintegrate completely in the gut. Infection is commonly direct, but also by the other faeco-oral routes. Eggs hatch in the jejunum and the hexacanth embryo bores into a villus where it transforms into a cysticercoid larva. After 4 to 6 days it re-enters the gut, everts the scolex, and attaches to the mucosa;

eggs appear in the faeces within 12 days. The lifespan is 3 months. The eggs are delicate and survive less than 10 days in the environment. Prevalence is usually much higher in children than adults; outbreaks can occur in families and institutions. External autoinfection is common in high-risk groups and enables high worm loads to build up. In addition, internal autoinfection occurs when there is gut stasis or retroperistalsis. Because of the importance of direct transmission, this infection may be common even in arid environments such as Western Australia.

A similar parasite, recognized as a subspecies *H. nana fraterna*, occurs in the mouse but this has normally has the flour beetle tribolium as intermediate host, although direct mouse-to-mouse transmission can occur. Both human and murine subspecies will infect these beetles. The zoonotic potential of the murine subspecies is uncertain, as at least Australian human strains will not infect mice.

Clinical features

Heavily infected people, especially children, may harbour up to 1000 or more worms. Mucosal damage caused by both larval and adult worms leads to protein loss and sometimes malabsorption. Abdominal pains and anorexia are common.

Immunosuppressant or steroid therapy, particularly in lymphoma patients, can lead to the development of bizarre cystic larval forms in the gut wall, mesenteric nodes, liver, and lungs. A similar condition can be produced in immunosuppressed mice.

Diagnosis and treatment

Eggs can be detected in faeces using concentration methods. Proglottids are rarely found in faeces, except after treatment.

Praziquantel in a single dose of 25 mg/kg is the most effective drug. If niclosamide is used, a 7-day course is needed to ensure that larval stages are killed when they re-enter the gut lumen. The dose on the first day is as for *T. saginata*; on the remaining days one-half of this dose is given. Relapses often result from persistence of eggs in the patient's environment.

Uncommon gut cestodes

Several species have been recorded in humans (Table 7.10.2.2). All have arthropods as intermediate hosts, the larval cysticercoid stage being in the haemocele; the full life cycles of some species are still uncertain. The normal definitive host becomes infected by eating the arthropod, intentionally or accidentally. The means by which humans become infected is sometimes not clear, but fleas, small beetles, and mites are easily overlooked in food. *Dipylidium caninum* infection occurs in children who have groomed their pets. Infections with *Bertiella* are mostly in owners of pet monkeys, but oribatid mites are common in fallen fruit especially mangoes. Children may eat insects deliberately, and this appears to be the mode of infection by *Raillietina* in Bangkok. Beetles are used for medicinal purposes in parts of Thailand and Malaysia, and this is the most likely route by which *Mathevotaenia* is acquired.

In many of these species the eggs are in capsules that are released when the proglottid disintegrates in the gut, or more commonly, in the faecal mass. *Mesocestoides* is unique among these parasites in that two intermediate hosts are required and the genital opening is medioventral. Human *Mesocestoides* infections follow ingestion of raw viscera or blood from game, including birds, or from chickens.

Many patients will present because they have passed proglottids. *D. caninum* actively migrates out of the anus, like *T. saginata*. Faecal examinations of people with abdominal complaints may reveal unusual eggs or egg capsules. Poorly defined systemic and allergic complaints are common. Treatment is as for *T. saginata*.

Recognition of these parasites is of epidemiological interest and may indicate potential transmission of other zoonotic pathogens. It is certain that all these parasites are under-reported. Unusual proglottids or eggs should be preserved in formol saline and sent to a parasitologist.

Further reading

Chitchang S, *et al.* (1985). Relationship between the severity of the symptom and the number of *Hymenolepis nana* after treatment. *J Med Assoc Thailand*, **68**, 424–6.

Fuentes MV, Galan-Puchades MT, Malone JB (2003). Short report: a new case report of human *Mesocestoides* infection in the United States. *Am J Trop Med Hyg*, **68**, 566–7.

Hoberg EP (2006). Phylogeny of *Taenia*: Species definitions and origins of human parasites. *Parasitol Int*, **55** Suppl, 23–30.

Hoberg EP, *et al.* (2001). Out of Africa: origins of the *Taenia* tapeworms in humans. *Proc Roy Soc London B*, **268**, 781–7.

Ito A, Craig PS (2003). Immunodiagnostic and molecular approaches for the detection of taeniid cestode infections. *Trends Parasitol*, **19**, 377–81.

Ito A, Nakao M, Wandra T (2003). Human taeniasis and cysticercosis in Asia. *Lancet*, **362**, 1918–20.

Liu YM, *et al.* (2005). Acute pancreatitis caused by tapeworm in the biliary tract. *Am J Trop Med Hyg*, **73**, 377–80.

Macnish MG, *et al.* (2002). Failure to infect laboratory rodent hosts with human isolates of *Rodentolepis* (= *Hymenolepis*) *nana*. *J Helminthol*, **76**(1), 37–43.

Mason PR, Patterson BA (1994). Epidemiology of *Hymenolepis nana* in primary school children in urban and rural communities in Zimbabwe. *J Parasitol*, **80**, 245–50.

Olson PD, *et al.* (2003). Lethal invasive cestodiasis in immunosuppressed patients. *J Infect Dis*, **187**, 1962–6.

Pawlowski Z, Schultz MG (1972). Taeniasis and cysticercosis (*Taenia saginata*). *Adv Parasitol*, **10**, 269–343.

Subianto DB, Tumada LR, Morgono SS (1978). Burns and epileptic fits associated with cysticercosis in mountain people of Irian Jaya. *Trop Geogr Med*, **30**, 275–8.

7.10.3 Cysticercosis

Hector H. Garcia and Robert H. Gilman

Essentials

Cysticercosis, infection by larvae of the pork tapeworm *Taenia solium* (see Chapter 7.10.2), is the commonest helminthic infection of the human central nervous system. It accounts for up to 30% of all seizures and epilepsy in endemic countries, and travel and immigration now lead to its more frequent presentation in industrialized countries.

Clinical features and diagnosis—manifestations of neurocysticercosis depend on the number, location, size, and stage of the parasite cysts in the brain, as well as on the immunological response of the host. The commonest syndromes are late-onset epilepsy or intracranial hypertension. Diagnosis is based on brain imaging studies (CT or MRI) and supported by highly specific serology.

Treatment and prognosis—treatment is (1) symptomatic—e.g. anticonvulsants; shunts for intracranial hypertension in patients with hydrocephalus; and (2) antiparasitic—albendazole or praziquantel, which are generally given with steroids to control cerebral oedema; but there is no role for these drugs in inactive neurocysticercosis (i.e. calcifications with or without enhancement on CT scan). Prognosis depends mainly on whether the cysts are intraparenchymal (better prognosis) or extraparenchymal (subarachnoid or intraventricular, poorer prognosis).

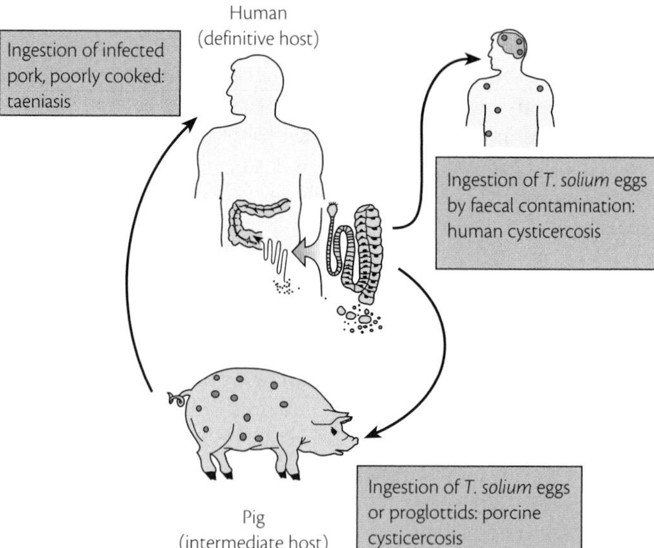

Fig. 7.10.3.1 Life cycle of *T. solium*.

Introduction

Known since the Hippocratic era, cysticercosis is the commonest helminthic infection of the human central nervous system. It is probable that the suspicion of its origins led some religions expressly to forbid the consumption of pork. Socioeconomic improvements eradicated the infection in Europe and North America. However, endemic *Taenia solium* taeniasis/cysticercosis persists in most developing countries, where human cysticercosis is an important cause of epilepsy and other neurological morbidity, and porcine infections cause considerable economic losses to peasant farmers.

Aetiology

Cysticercosis is infection with the larval stage (cysticercus) of *T. solium*, the pork tapeworm (Chapter 7.10.2). In the life cycle of this two-host zoonotic cestode(Fig. 7.10.3.1), humans are the only definitive host and harbour the adult tapeworm, whereas pigs are intermediate hosts. The hermaphroditic adult *T. solium* inhabits the small intestine. Its head or scolex bears four suckers and a double crown of hooks, connected by a narrow neck to a large body (strobila) between 2 and 4 m long, composed of several hundred proglottids (Chapter 7.10.2, Fig. 7.10.3.1b, c). Gravid proglottids, each containing 50 000 to 60 000 fertile eggs, detach from the distal end of the worm and are excreted in the faeces. The cycle is completed when pigs ingest stools contaminated with *T. solium* eggs. Once ingested by the pig, the invasive oncospheres in the eggs are liberated by the action of gastric acid and intestinal fluids and actively penetrate the bowel wall, enter the bloodstream, and are carried to the muscles and other tissues where they develop into larval cysts (Chapter 7.10.2, and see Fig. 7.10.3.4). When humans ingest undercooked pork containing cysticerci, the larva evaginates in the small intestine, its scolex attach to the intestinal mucosa, and it begins forming proglottids. By accidentally ingesting taenia eggs, humans may also act as intermediate hosts for *T. solium* and develop cysticercosis.

Epidemiology

The availability of neuroimaging studies and the subsequent development of specific serodiagnostic tests has resulted in the identification of neurocysticercosis as a frequent neurological disorder in Latin America, Africa, and Asia, where the prevalence of active epilepsy is almost twice that in Western countries. Neurocysticercosis is also an emerging problem in industrialized countries, seen mainly in immigrants from endemic areas, some of whom may spread the infection as tapeworm carriers.

The main sources of human cysticercosis are faecal–oral contamination in those carrying the tapeworm or their contacts and ingestion of food contaminated with *T. solium* eggs. Epidemiological studies suggest that almost every newly diagnosed patient with cysticercosis has been infected by someone in their close environment who is harbouring a *T. solium* and the tendency is to dismiss the role of environment or water in transmission. Airborne transmission of *T. solium* eggs and internal autoinfection by regurgitation of proglottids into the stomach have been suggested but not proved.

Pathogenesis

Any organ may be infected, but parasites survive more frequently in the nervous system, possibly because the immune response there is limited. Signs and symptoms are caused by perilesional inflammation and oedema, mass effect, or obstruction of cerebrospinal fluid circulation. Although complete development of cysts takes 2 to 3 months, symptoms usually develop years after the initial infection. This clinically silent period, and finding inflammation around cysts in symptomatic cases, suggests that in many cases symptoms are due to inflammatory processes associated with the recognition of the parasite by the immune system of the host (presumably progressing towards the death of the parasite) rather than to the presence of the parasite itself.

Subarachnoid cysticerci elicit an intense inflammatory reaction causing thickening of basal leptomeninges. The optic chiasma and other cranial nerves are usually entrapped within this dense exudate, resulting in visual field defects and other cranial nerve dysfunctions. The foramens of Luschka and Magendie may be occluded by the thickened leptomeninges, leading to hydrocephalus. Blood vessels may be affected by the inflammatory reaction. The walls of small penetrating arteries are invaded by inflammatory cells, leading to a proliferative endarteritis with occlusion of the lumen, and which may result in cerebral infarction.

Clinical features

Neurocysticercosis is a pleomorphic disease, whose manifestations vary with the number, size, and topography of the lesions and the intensity of the host's immune response to the parasites. Patients can be classified by the number, stage, and location of the cysticerci, and the presence or absence of associated inflammation or calcifications.

Epilepsy, the most common presentation of neurocysticercosis, is usually the primary or sole manifestation of the disease. Seizures occur in 50 to 80% of patients with parenchymal brain cysts or calcifications but are less common in other forms of the disease. Other focal signs are less frequent and include pyramidal tract signs, sensory deficits, signs of brainstem dysfunction, and involuntary movements. These manifestations usually follow a subacute or chronic course, making neurocysticercosis difficult to differentiate clinically from neoplasms or other infections of the central nervous system. Focal signs may occur abruptly in patients who develop a cerebral infarct as a complication of subarachnoid neurocysticercosis. Subarachnoid cysticerci may reach 10 cm or more in diameter ('giant' cysticercosis, Fig. 7.10.3.2), and exert a mass effect.

Neurocysticercosis may present with increased intracranial pressure, usually from hydrocephalus secondary to basal subarachnoid cysticercosis or intraventricular cysts, cysticercotic arachnoiditis, or granular ependymitis. In these cases, intracranial hypertension develops subacutely and progresses slowly. An encephalitic picture may result from overwhelming inflammation around many parasitic cysts, a syndrome that occurs more frequently in younger people, especially women. In contrast, some patients may tolerate hundreds of intraparenchymal cysticerci with only minor symptoms.

Muscular pseudohypertrophy, a rare presentation, is caused by heavy cysticercal infection of skeletal muscles (Fig. 7.10.3.3) giving a 'Herculean' appearance. The few cases reported are all from India. Other apparent differences in clinical manifestations between Asia and Latin America include a high frequency of subcutaneous cysts and single degenerating brain lesions in Asia.

Pathology

The cysticerci are liquid-filled vesicles consisting of vesicular wall and scolex (Fig. 7.10.3.4). The vesicular wall is composed of an outer or cuticular layer, a middle or cellular layer with pseudoepithelial structure, and an inner or reticular layer. The invaginated scolex has a head or rostellum armed with suckers and hooks, and a rudimentary body or strobila that includes the spiral canal.

The macroscopic appearance of cysticerci varies in different locations within the central nervous system. Cysticerci within the brain parenchyma are usually small and tend to lodge in the cerebral cortex or basal ganglia (Fig. 7.10.3.5). Subarachnoid cysts may be small if located in the depths of cortical sulci, or grow to 5 cm or more in the basal cisterns or sylvian fissures. Ventricular cysticerci are usually single, may or may not have a visible scolex, and may be attached to the choroid plexus or float freely in the ventricle. Spinal cysticerci are usually located in the subarachnoid

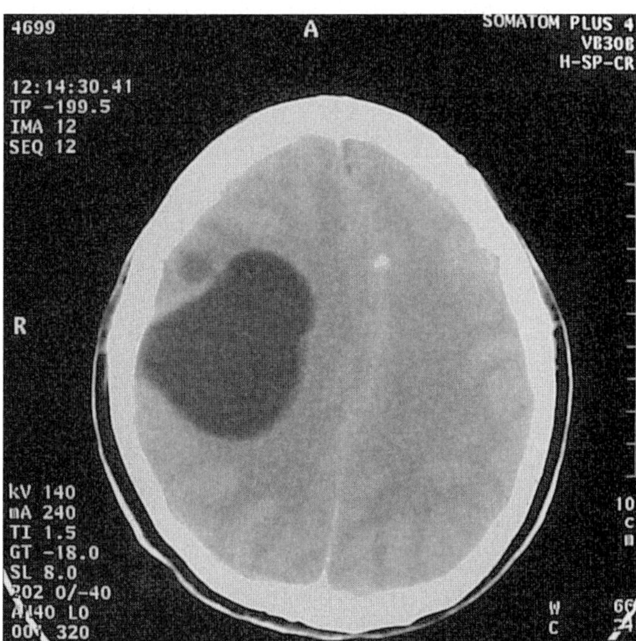

Fig. 7.10.3.2 Giant cysticercotic cyst (brain CT).

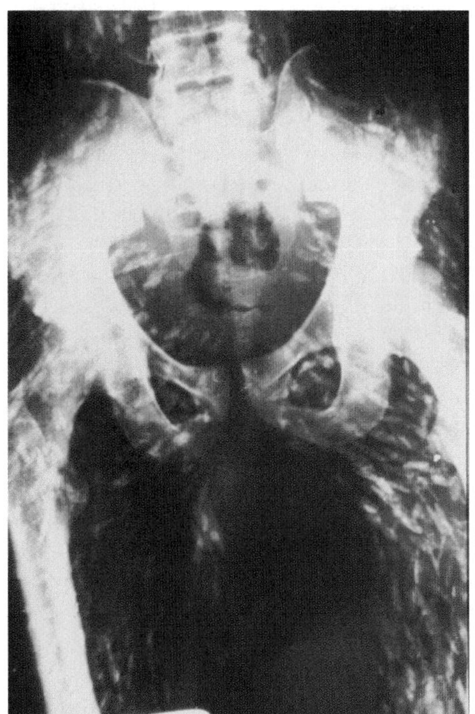

Fig. 7.10.3.3 Heavy cysticercal infection of skeletal muscles.
(Courtesy of the late Professor Sornchai Looareesuwan.)

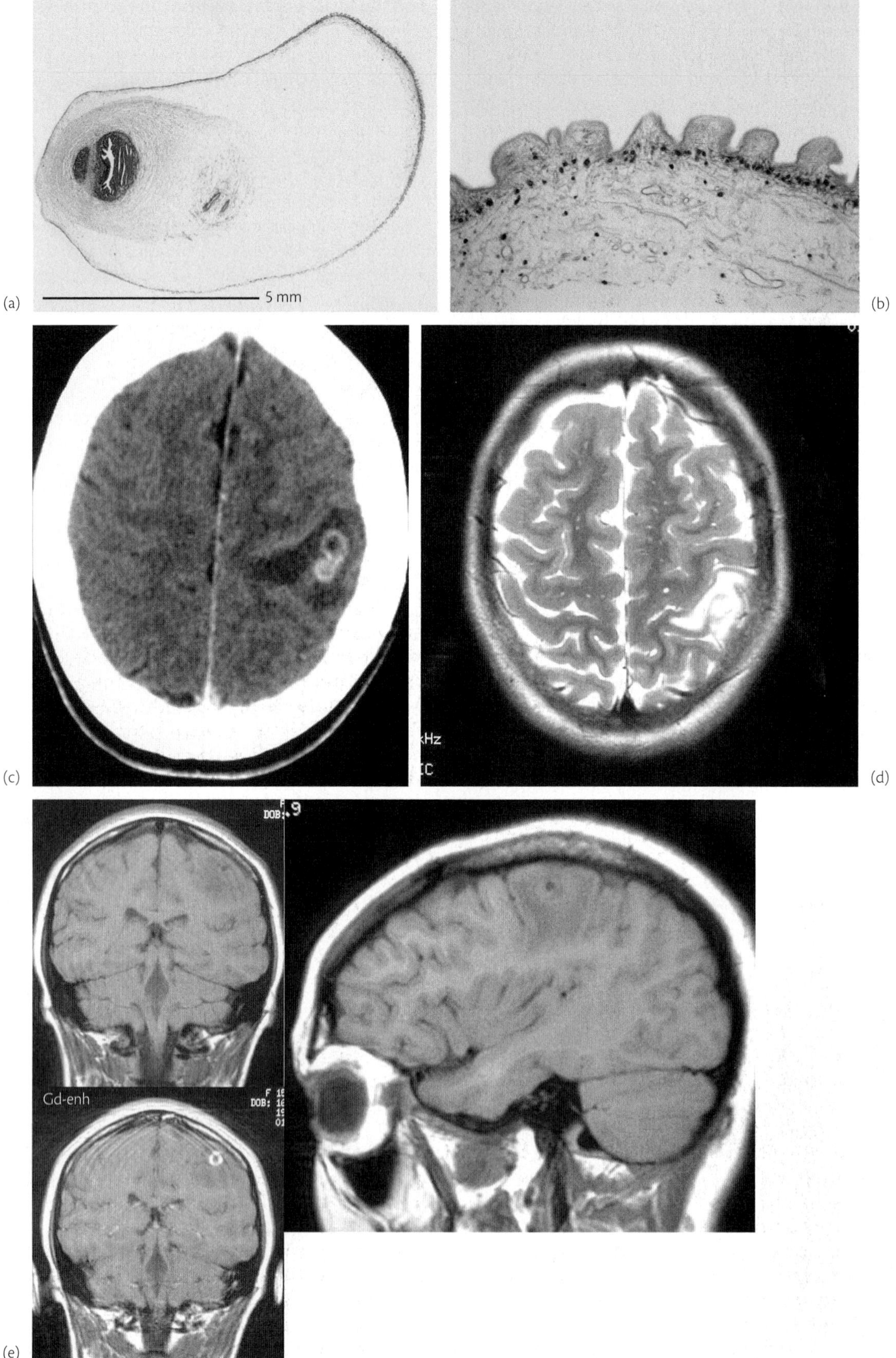

Fig. 7.10.3.4 (a) Histopatholgy of a complete hydatid cyst removed by brain biopsy in a patient with recent onset of focal epilepsy (×4). (b) Structure of the cyst wall (×40). (c) Cerebral imaging CT enhanced. (d) MRI T_2-weighted. (e) MRI T_1-weighted with and without gadolinium enhancement.

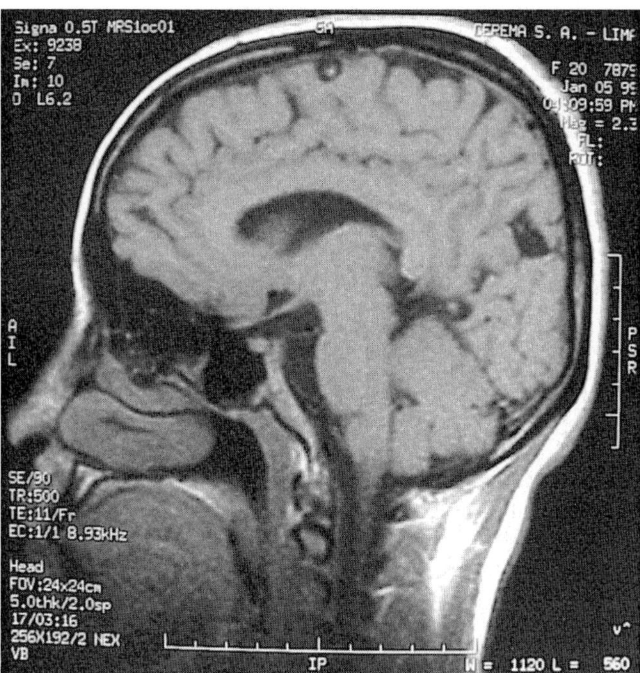

Fig. 7.10.3.5 Uncontrasted T_1 MR image showing two intraparenchymal cysticerci with visible scolices.

space (rarely intramedullary). Their morphology is similar to cysts located within the brain.

Basal cysticerci may undergo a disproportionate growth of their membrane, with extension processes, resembling a brunch of grapes (racemose cysticercosis, Fig. 7.10.3.6). In these cases, the scolex is frequently unidentifiable even by microscopy.

Viable vesicular cysticerci elicit little inflammatory change in surrounding tissues because of active immune evasion mechanisms. The appearance of symptoms is interpreted as the result of immunological attack from the host, in a process of degeneration that ends with the death of the parasite. Inflammatory changes in the parasite membrane and increased density of cyst fluid mark the transition between four defined stages: viable, colloidal, granular nodular, and calcified cyst. Viable cysts may coexist with degenerating cysts or calcifications.

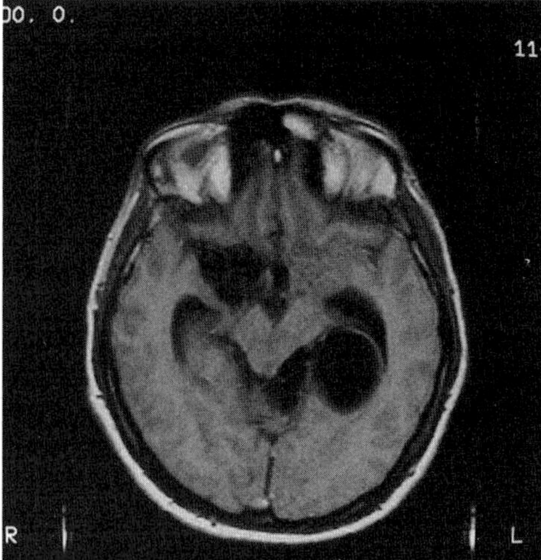

Fig. 7.10.3.6 Basal 'racemose' cysticercosis.

Laboratory/imaging diagnosis

The pleomorphism of neurocysticercosis makes it impossible to diagnose on clinical grounds alone. In endemic regions, late-onset seizures in otherwise healthy individuals are highly suggestive of neurocysticercosis. Most of these patients are normal on neurological examinations. Routine neuroimaging and serological studies are therefore mandatory. Finding cysticerci outside the central nervous system (eye, subcutaneous tissue, muscle) assists the diagnosis of neurocysticercosis. Muscular and subcutaneous cysticerci are far less common in American than in African or Asian patients with neurocysticercosis.

Neuroimaging

CT and MRI have drastically improved diagnostic accuracy by providing objective evidence about the topography of the lesions and the degree of the host inflammatory response to the parasite. Imaging findings in parenchymal neurocysticercosis depend on the stage of involution of cysticerci. Viable cysticerci appear as rounded cystic lesions on CT (Fig. 7.10.3.2), hypointense on T_1 and FLAIR sequences on MRI (Fig. 7.10.3.5), without associated enhancement, whereas degenerating parasites are seen as focal enhancing lesions surrounded by oedema (Fig. 7.10.3.4c–e), and calcifications as hyperdense dots or nodules (Fig. 7.10.3.7). Disappearance of cyst fluid signals the degenerative phase and calcified nodules the residual phase. Single or multiple ring-like or nodular enhancing lesions are non-specific and present a diagnostic challenge. Pyogenic brain abscesses, fungal abscesses, tuberculomas, toxoplasma abscesses, and primary or metastatic brain tumours may produce similar findings on CT or MRI.

CT and MRI findings in subarachnoid neurocysticercosis are less specific. They include hydrocephalus, abnormal

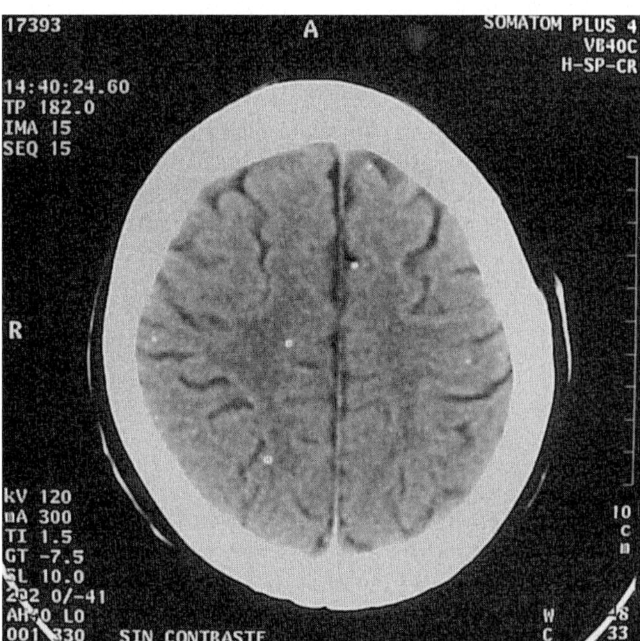

Fig. 7.10.3.7 Calcified neurocysticercosis.

meningeal enhancement, and subarachnoid cysts. Cerebral angiography may show segmental narrowing or occlusion of major intracranial arteries in patients with cerebral infarcts secondary to parasitic vasculitis. In neurocysticercosis there is rarely fever or signs of meningeal irritation; glucose levels in cerebrospinal fluid are usually normal. MRI is generally better than CT for the diagnosis of neurocysticercosis, particularly in patients with basal lesions, brainstem or intraventricular cysts, and spinal lesions. MRI is, however, less sensitive than CT for the detection of calcifications.

Immunological tests

Immunoblot (western blot) using purified antigens is the best available serological test for *T. solium* antibodies. It performs well with serum samples and is 98% sensitive in cases with more than one active lesion, and 100% specific. Its sensitivity may drop in patients with a single cyst. Other assays using unfractionated antigens (e.g. enzyme immunoassay, ELISA) suffer from poor specificity but are more reliable when performed with cerebrospinal fluid than serum. Antigen-detection tests may provide a tool for serological monitoring of antiparasitic therapy. Although results of serology and imaging studies may be similar, they evaluate different aspects of the disease and may be discordant in some patients. Intestinal tapeworm carriers, naturally cured patients, or non-neurological infections may have normal brain images but be positive serologically. Those with only inactive lesions or a single cerebral lesion may be seronegative.

Parasitological diagnosis

A proportion (*c.*10–15%) of patients with neurocysticercosis are tapeworm carriers at the time of diagnosis, and in another 10% or so a carrier can be detected in the household. Parasitological diagnosis is difficult: eggs and proglottids are shed only intermittently in stool and are usually missed by routine stool examination. Stool assays to detect parasite antigens are more sensitive than microscopy, but are not widely available. A recently described serological test for tapeworm carriers may improve detection.

Diagnostic criteria

A set of diagnostic criteria based on neuroimaging studies, serological tests, clinical presentation, and exposure history has been proposed by Del Brutto and colleagues. Besides absolute demonstration of the presence of the parasite, 'major' criteria (including typical findings on neuroimaging, demonstration of specific anticysticercal antibodies, or the presence of typical cigar-shaped calcifications in muscle) are combined with 'minor' criteria and epidemiological data to suggest a probable or possible diagnosis. Application of these criteria should improve the consistency of diagnosis.

Treatment

Because of the clinical and pathological pleomorphism of neurocysticercosis, precise assessment of the viability and size of cysts, the location of parasites, and the severity of the host's immune response is important before planning treatment.

Symptomatic treatment is very important. Seizures secondary to parenchymal neurocysticercosis can usually be controlled with anticonvulsants. However, the optimal duration of anticonvulsant therapy in patients with neurocysticercosis has not been determined, and it is difficult to withdraw this treatment. Prognostic factors associated with recurrence of seizures include the development of parenchymal brain calcifications, and occurrence of recurrent seizures or multiple brain cysts before starting antiparasitic therapy.

Antiparasitic agents destroy viable cysts and are associated with fewer seizures (particularly seizures with generalization) in the long term follow up. Antiparasitic or steroid treatments in patients with a single enhancing lesion seem to independently improve radiological resolution and decrease the chance of seizure relapses, albeit the magnitude of this effect is small. Albendazole is the drug of choice for antiparasitic treatment of cerebral cysticercosis (15 mg/kg per day for 7 days, with steroids), although a recently described single-day praziquantel regimen (75–100 mg/kg, in three doses at 2-h intervals, followed by steroids 6 h later) demonstrated similar cestocidal activity in patients with few cysts. Longer courses may be required in patients with many lesions or subarachnoid cysticercosis. Transient worsening of neurological symptoms can be expected during antiparasitc therapy, secondary to the perilesional inflammatory reaction. There is no role for antiparasitic drugs in inactive neurocysticercosis (i.e. calcifications with or without enhancement on CT scan) since the parasites are dead.

Between the second and fifth day of antiparasitic therapy there is usually an exacerbation of neurological symptoms, attributed to local inflammation caused by the death of the larvae. For this reason, albendazole or praziquantel is generally given simultaneously with steroids in order to control the oedema and intracranial hypertension. Serum levels of praziquantel decrease when steroids are administered simultaneously, an effect that does not occur with albendazole. However, there is no evidence that cysticidal efficacy is decreased. Serum levels of praziquantel or albendazole may be lowered by simultaneous antiepileptic drug (phenytoin or carbamazepine) administration.

Some forms of neurocysticercosis should not be treated with antiparasitic agents. In patients with severe cysticercotic encephalitis, these drugs may result in worsening cerebral oedema and fatal herniation. In this case, the mainstay of therapy is high doses of corticosteroids or mannitol to decrease the inflammatory response. In patients with both hydrocephalus and parenchymal brain cysts, antiparasitic drugs should be started only after placement of a ventricular shunt in case the intracranial pressure increases as a result of drug therapy. Antiparasitic drugs must be used with caution in patients with giant subarachnoid cysticerci. In such patients, concomitant steroid administration is mandatory to avoid cerebral infarction. Albendazole can successfully destroy ventricular cysts, but the surrounding inflammatory reaction may cause acute hydrocephalus if the cysts are located within the fourth ventricle or near the foramens of Monro and Luschka.

Surgery is limited to ventriculoperitoneal shunts to relieve obstructive hydrocephalus, and excision of single cysts (in the fourth ventricle or giant intraparenchymal cysts). However, shunts frequently dysfunction. The protracted course in these patients and their high mortality rates (up to 50% in 2 years) is directly related to the number of surgical interventions required to change the shunts. Recently, neuroventriculoscopy has been employed as a less invasive option for resection of ventricular cysticerci.

Prognosis

Parenchymal cysticercosis has a good prognosis. Appropriately managed, seizures usually subside in time without sequelae. In contrast, extraparenchymal cysticercosis and especially racemose cysticercosis have a poor prognosis, responding poorly to antiparasitic therapy, and leading to progressively deteriorating disease and death. Multiple courses of antiparasitic treatment and careful, prolonged follow-up are crucial in this type of patients.

Prevention and control

Cysticercosis would not exist if pigs had no access to human faeces. However, this approach is hampered in endemic zones by the lack of sanitary facilities and veterinary inspection, and more importantly, because farmers tend to raise pigs under free-range conditions in order to reduce the cost of feeding them. Intervention programmes have concentrated on mass chemotherapy to eliminate human taeniasis, but their results have not been sustained. New tools for control are oxfendazole, an effective and cheap single-dose therapy for porcine cysticercosis, and the candidate porcine vaccines under trial by several groups. TSOL18, an oncosphere-based vaccine developed in Australia, may provide over 99% protection.

Monitoring the effect of an intervention requires suitable indicators. Human seroprevalence does not reflect changes in infection patterns because antibodies persist for years, even after successful treatment. Studies in Peru have shown that serological monitoring of porcine infection is a useful marker for both prevalence and changes in infection intensity over time. Similarly, the rate of infection in uninfected (sentinel) pigs over time can be used to estimate intensity of *T. solium* infection in the community. The prevalences of human and porcine infection are strongly correlated.

Possible future developments

Although most cysts disappear after antiparasitic treatment, the antiparasitic efficacy of currently available regimes is incomplete. Data is missing on whether new drugs, combination therapy, or different schemes of albendazole of praziquantel can improve this efficacy.

Schemes and doses of antiparasitic and steroid therapy need to be assessed in controlled trials targeted to specific types of neurocysticercosis. Some authors suggested an association between brain calcifications secondary to cysticercosis and glial neoplasms. This has not yet been confirmed or rejected. Systematic long-term evaluation is needed to determine whether hydrocephalus is a late complication of anti-parasitic therapy. The efficacy and costs of comprehensive human–porcine eradication programmes must be assessed.

Further reading

Del Brutto OH, *et al.* (2001). Proposed diagnostic criteria for neurocysticercosis. *Neurology*, **57**, 177–83. [A guide to systematic diagnosis.]

Del Brutto OH, *et al.* (2006). Albendazole and praziquantel therapy for neurocysticercosis: a meta-analysis of randomized trials. *Ann Intern Med*, **145**, 43–51.

Evans C, *et al.* (1997). Controversies in the management of cysticercosis. *Emerg Infect Dis*, **3**, 403–5.

Garcia HH, *et al.* (2003). *Taenia solium* cysticercosis. *Lancet*, **362**, 547–56.

Garcia HH, *et al.* (2004). A trial of anti-parasitic treatment to reduce the rate of seizures due to cerebral cysticercosis. *N Engl J Med*, **350**, 249–58.

Garcia HH, *et al.* (2005). Neurocysticercosis: updated concepts about an old disease. *Lancet Neurol*, **4**, 653–61.

Gonzalez AE, *et al.* (1997). Treatment of porcine cysticercosis with oxfendazole: a dose–response trial. *Vet Record*, **141**, 420–2.

Gonzalez AE, *et al.* (2005). Vaccination of pigs to control human neurocysticercosis. *Am J Trop Med Hyg*, **72**, 837–9.

Montano SM, *et al.* (2005). Neurocysticercosis: association between seizures, serology and brain CT in rural Peru. *Neurology*, **65**, 229–33.

Nash TE, *et al.* (2006). Treatment of neurocysticercosis—current status and future research needs. *Neurology*, **67**, 1120–7.

7.10.4 Diphyllobothriasis and sparganosis

David I. Grove

Essentials

Diphyllobothriasis—procercoid larvae of *Diphyllobothrium latum* develop in the gut of people infected by eating undercooked freshwater fish, especially in Scandinavia and Russia (other species cause disease in Japan, Korea, and South America). Adult worms cause mild gastrointestinal symptoms and urticaria, and compete with the host for vitamin B_{12}, leading to pernicious anaemia. Diagnosis is by finding characteristic ova in the stool. Treatment is with niclosamide or praziquantel.

Sparganosis—infection by animal *Spirometra* spp. is by ingestion of water containing infected crustaceans or uncooked meat (frog, snake, poultry, pork). The worm migrates through tissues, often presenting as a lump in subcutaneous tissue or muscle, and more notably in the brain (typically leading to presentation with epilepsy). Diagnosis and treatment is by surgical excision.

Diphyllobothriasis

Life cycle

Diphyllobothriasis is an infection usually caused by adult tapeworms belonging to the genus *Diphyllobothrium*, most commonly the broad fish tapeworm *D. latum* (Table 7.10.4.1). When undercooked freshwater fish are ingested by humans, larvae (known as plerocercoids or spargana) develop in the small intestine into adult worms up to 8 m long and consisting of a string of individual components called proglottids. Eggs begin to be passed in the faeces after about 1 month and large numbers of eggs are excreted each day. If the faeces are deposited in fresh water, the egg embryonates and releases a larva called a coracidium which is ingested by various species of small crustacean copepods in which it further develops into a procercoid larva. When the copepod is ingested by a freshwater fish; the procercoid larvae migrates to the muscles and develops further into a plerocercoid larva up to 2 cm in length.

Table 7.10.4.1 Major species of *Diphyllobothrium* and their epidemiology

Species	Distribution	Usual definitive host
D. latum	Europe, Asia, North and South America	Humans
D. pacificum	Japan, South America	Seals
D. nihonkaiense	Japan	Unknown
D. yonagoense	Japan, Korea	Unknown

Rare human infections have been described with *D.cordatum* (seals, dogs), *D. dalliae, D. dendriticum* (birds), *D. lanceolata, D. ursi* (bears).

Epidemiology and control

Human infections occur where there is a coexistence of infected definitive hosts, susceptible intermediate hosts, deposition of infected faeces in fresh water, and a cultural practice of eating uncooked freshwater fishes such as pike, burbot, perch, salmon, and trout (Table 7.10.4.1). Humans are the usual definitive host for *D. latum*, whereas other fish-eating mammals and birds may be infected with other species that rarely infect humans. Prevention is achieved by freezing fish for 1 day at −18°C or lower.

Clinical features

Infection usually causes no or few symptoms. Abdominal discomfort, fatigue, diarrhoea, and urticaria may be the vague presenting symptoms. Individual proglottids or a strip of gravid segments may pass out through the anus. Pernicious anaemia may be associated with *D. latum* infection because of competition for vitamin B_{12} in the bowel lumen. In these patients, elimination of the tapeworm results in improvement of the anaemia.

Diagnosis

The diagnosis can be confirmed by identifying eggs in the stool by microscopy (Fig. 7.10.4.1) or examination of a discharged proglottid. In endemic areas, all patients with pernicious anaemia should have their stools examined.

Treatment

Niclosamide in a single adult dose of 2 g or praziquantel in a single dose of 10 mg/kg body weight are both very effective drugs for the treatment of infection with all species of *Diphyllobothrium*.

Sparganosis

Sparganosis is an infection usually caused by larval tapeworms belonging to the genus *Spirometra* which are unable to complete their development in humans. *Spirometra* and *Diphyllobothrium* are both classified as pseudophyllidean tapeworms. The usual definitive hosts for *S. mansoni*, *S. mansonoides*, and *S. erinacei* are dogs and cats, with adult worms living in the small bowel and passing eggs. When these are deposited in fresh water, the egg embryonates and releases a larva called a coracidium which is ingested by various species of small crustacean copepods in which it further develops into a procercoid larva. When the copepod is ingested by amphibians (tadpoles and frogs), reptiles (lizards and snakes), birds and some mammals (mice, rats, and humans), it develops further into a white, slender, plerocercoid larva 1 to 30 cm long, otherwise known as a sparganum, in the muscles or connective tissues (Fig. 7.10.4.2). Furthermore, this stage can be transferred from one host to another, e.g. when a snake eats a frog.

Epidemiology and control

Human sparganosis occurs sporadically worldwide. Human infection can be acquired by ingestion of water containing infected crustaceans or infected uncooked frog, snake, poultry, or pork meat where this is a traditional habit. Some people believe that eating raw meat is a tonic or is beneficial for patients with tuberculosis. Rural people in some countries practise applying poultices of infected frog or snake skin to an inflamed eye, in which case a sparganum can directly penetrate the conjunctiva. Infection is prevented by ingesting only treated water or properly cooked meats.

Clinical features

When larvae of *S. mansoni*, *S. mansonoides*, and *S. erinacei* are ingested, they penetrate the intestinal wall and migrate systemically. The worm usually lodges in subcutaneous tissue or muscle of the chest or abdominal walls, breast, limbs, or scrotum. A lump may

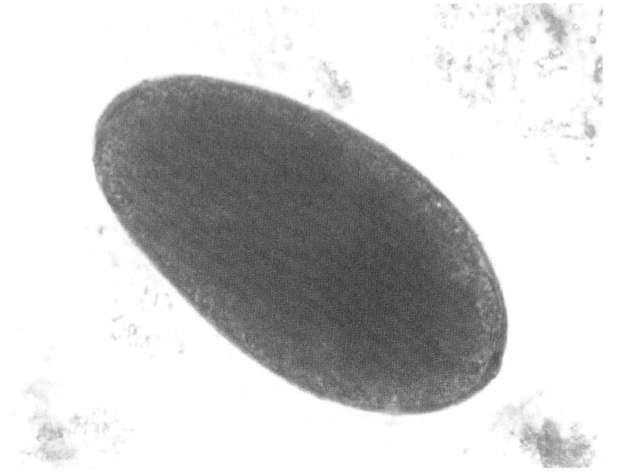

Fig. 7.10.4.1 Egg of *Diphyllobothrium* latum.
(Courtesy of A R Butcher.)

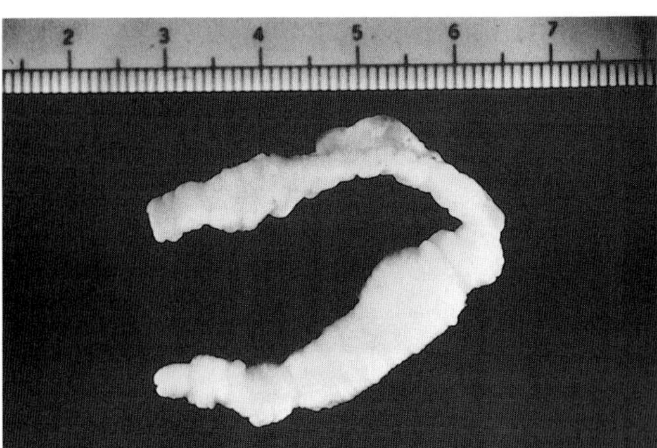

Fig. 7.10.4.2 A sparganum surgically removed from a subcutaneous mass.

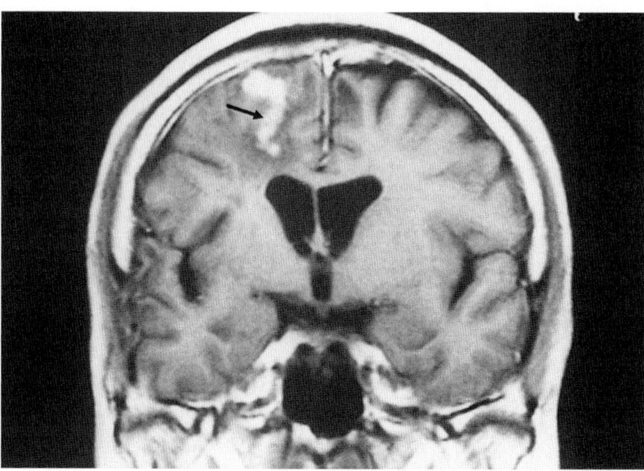

Fig. 7.10.4.3 MRI scan of cerebral sparganosis. Coronal contrast-enhanced T_1-weighted image shows a tortuous curvilinear enhancing lesion (arrows) with surrounding low density of oedema and degeneration in the right frontal lobe.

appear and then spontaneously disappear, only to reappear some weeks or months later at a site remote from the first. Sparganosis of the central nervous system may present with seizures. A granuloma with eosinophilic infiltration is formed along the tortuous migration track (Fig. 7.10.4.3). Suppuration may complicate sparganosis. Ocular infection is the most common presentation of sparganosis in Thailand. Spargana can survive for more than 5 years. In general, one or only a few worms infect each patient.

Sparganum proliferum is a branched, proliferating larva for which the adult worm is unknown. Rare human infections have been described from Japan and the Americas. Thousands of small egg-like larvae may be found in subcutaneous tissues and internal organs.

Diagnosis

The diagnosis of sparganosis is usually made after operative excision. Preoperative diagnosis of cerebral sparganosis is suggested with high confidence when CT or MRI of the brain shows an enhancing nodule with changing shape or position in the sequential images. Serology may be available in some countries.

Treatment

Excision of the mass or removal of the worm from the lesion is curative. Repeated surgery is necessary when the patient has multiple lesions. There are no drugs which are known to be effective against sparganosis. All cases of *S. proliferum* infection have proved fatal.

Further reading

Scholz T, Garcia HH, Kuchta R, Wicht B (2009). Update on the human broad tapeworm (Genus *Diphyllobothrium*), including clinical relevance. *Clin Microbial Rev*, **22**, 146–160.

Dupouy-Camet J, Peduzzi R (2004). Current situation of human diphyllobothriasis in Europe. *Euro Surveillance*, **9**, 31–5.

Wiwanitkit V (2005). A review of human sparganosis in Thailand. *Int J Infect Dis*, **9**, 312–16.

Photographs of various stages of these parasites and diagrams of life cycles may be found at several excellent websites, e.g.: Centers for Disease Control and Prevention. http://www.dpd.cdc.gov/DPDx/HTML/Image_Library.htm

Korean Society for Parasitology. http://www.atlas.or.kr

7.11

Trematodes (flukes)

Contents

7.11.1 Schistosomiasis *1202*
D.W. Dunne and B.J. Vennervald

7.11.2 Liver fluke infections *1212*
David I. Grove

7.11.3 Lung flukes (paragonimiasis) *1216*
Udomsak Silachamroon and Sirivan Vanijanonta

7.11.4 Intestinal trematode infections *1219*
David I. Grove

7.11.1 Schistosomiasis

D.W. Dunne and B.J. Vennervald

Essentials

Schistosomiasis is caused by trematode worms *Schistosoma* spp., whose life cycle requires a definitive vertebrate host and an intermediate freshwater snail host. Transmission to humans occurs through exposure to fresh water containing infectious larvae, which can penetrate intact skin before developing into blood-dwelling adult worms. The disease is patchily distributed in parts of South America, Africa, the Middle East, China, and South East Asia, with about 200 million people infected and 20 million suffering severe consequences of infection.

Clinical features

Most infected people living in endemic areas have few (if any) overt symptoms, but clinical manifestations (when present) depend on the stage of infection.

Stage of invasion—larval invasion causes a transient immediate hypersensitivity reaction with intense itching ('swimmer's itch') and rash (cercarial dermatitis).

Stage of maturation (acute schistosomiasis or Katayama fever)—most marked in primary infections in nonimmune adults; an acute pyrexial illness associated with many non-specific symptoms and signs, and which can (rarely) be fatal. Eosinophilia is almost always present.

Established infection—(1) Urinary schistosomiasis (*Schistosoma haematobium*)—active disease most commonly presents with painless, terminal haematuria; chronic disease is associated with calcification, ulceration, and the development of papillomas in the bladder, and with ureteric fibrosis. (2) Intestinal schistosomiasis (*S. mansoni* and *S. japonicum*)—clinical features are generally encountered in those with high-intensity infections, including diarrhoea, hepatomegaly and splenomegaly; liver disease may progress to presinusoidal periportal fibrosis with portal hypertension. (3) Other manifestations—these include (a) nervous system—myelopathy and radiculopathy; (b) lungs—pulmonary hypertension and/or cor pulmonale; (c) renal—glomerulonephritis.

Diagnosis

A history of exposure to potentially contaminated water in geographically defined areas is important, especially in travellers and immigrants. Definitive diagnosis depends on direct microscopic detection of eggs in urine or stool samples, biopsies or (rarely) secretions such as seminal fluid. Serodiagnosis is not useful within endemic areas, but demonstration of schistosome-specific antibodies is helpful in travellers with a history of exposure and suspected schistosomiasis in whom eggs have not been detected.

Treatment and prognosis

Praziquantel is the drug of choice, with corticosteroids added in cases of Katayama fever to suppress the hypersensitivity reaction. Acute schistosomiasis responds well to early drug therapy, leaving little residual damage: chronic disease responds less well, although some improvement can occur. However, rapid re-exposure and reinfection are common, particularly in young children, unless control measures are implemented at the community level.

Prevention

In areas of high transmission, population-based chemotherapy or treatment of schoolchildren (who have the heaviest worm burdens and contribute most to ongoing transmission) can reduce the prevalence and severity of morbidity. In areas of less intense transmission, treatment can be restricted to diagnosed cases. Health education should be aimed at improving practices of water use and preventing indiscriminate urination and defecation.

Introduction

Schistosomiasis, also known as bilharzia, is caused by infection with parasitic trematode worms (flukes) of the genus *Schistosoma*. Disease is usually associated with chronic infections contracted by exposure to fresh water containing infective cercarial larvae that penetrate intact skin and develop into blood-dwelling worms. Most human infections are caused by one of three species, *S. mansoni*, *S. haematobium*, or *S. japonicum*. Two species, *S. intercalatum* and *S. mekongi*, are less significant. Schistosomiasis is patchily distributed in parts of South America, Africa, the Middle East, China, and South-East Asia (Fig. 7.11.1.1). An estimated 779 million people are at risk of schistosomiasis worldwide, of whom 207 million are infected (Steinmann *et al.*, 2006). Although simple diagnosis and effective drug treatment is available for individual uncomplicated cases, the world disease burden caused by these parasites has increased from an estimated 114 million human infections in 1947. Diagnosis and treatment are often not available to exposed rural populations, and drug-based control programmes are hampered by the continued susceptibility to reinfection of those who have been treated, particularly children. Human schistosomiasis is most often an insidious and chronic disease with a range of pathological manifestations involving the intestine and liver, or the urogenital tract. Mortality estimates are difficult, but 20 000 to 200 000 deaths may be directly associated with schistosomiasis each year.

Parasite life cycle

The schistosome life cycle requires two host species: a definitive vertebrate host, in which adult male and female worms develop and sexual reproduction occurs, and an intermediate freshwater snail host, in which the parasite multiplies asexually. Transmission between these hosts is achieved by two different free-swimming larval stages. For species that infect humans, miracidia hatch from eggs excreted in the faeces or urine of the vertebrate host, and then seek out and infect snails. Cercariae are released from the snail and are able actively to penetrate intact human skin. Different schistosome species have their own, often very restricted, range of snail hosts. Schistosomiasis is thus closely associated with particular freshwater habitats, and its geographical distribution is restricted by the availability of particular snail species. *S. mansoni* and *S. haematobium* are confined to aquatic snails (genera *Biomphalaria* and *Bulinus* respectively) that inhabit ponds, lakes, irrigation canals, slow-flowing streams, and rivers. *S. japonicum* is transmitted by amphibious snails of the genus *Oncomelania* that, in addition to a variety of freshwater habitats, are also present in damp soil and vegetation, such as paddy fields.

Schistosomes that infect humans can also infect other mammals. This is important in the transmission of *S. japonicum*, a zoonotic infection in which cattle, water buffalo, pigs, dogs, and rodents can act as reservoir hosts of the human parasite. *S. mansoni* infects a narrower range of mammals, and only a few rodent species and baboons have any potential to act as occasional reservoirs. In nature *S. haematobium* is essentially specific to humans. The sites of maturation of the adult worms vary between schistosome species, affecting both the transmission of the infection and its clinical sequelae.

Once shed from freshwater snails, cercariae (Fig. 7.11.1.2) live for about 24 h, but their effective period of infectivity is probably shorter under field conditions. Cercarial behaviour and the timing of their release enhance their chance of contacting their vertebrate host of choice. Light and increasing temperature trigger the release of *S. mansoni* and *S. haematobium* cercariae during the day, and they use their tails actively to maintain their position near the water surface. *S. japonicum* cercariae are shed late in the day and are closely associated with the meniscus, perhaps reflecting their wider host range, as species specific for rodents are shed at night. Contact with skin triggers adherence mechanisms, and proteolytic enzymes and muscular movements allow penetration of the skin in minutes. Penetration initiates transformation into a schistosomular larva, with loss of the tail and of the protective outer

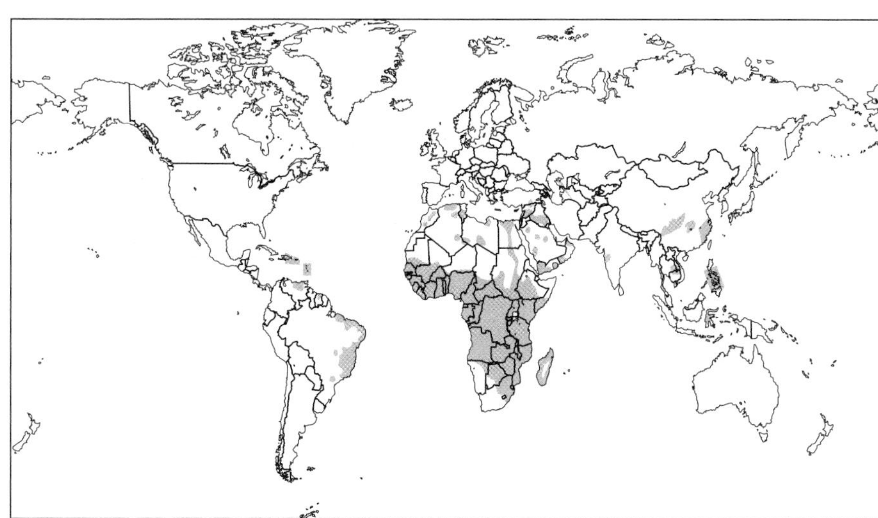

Fig. 7.11.1.1 Global distribution of the schistosomes that affect humans.

glycocalyx layer, and the addition of an extra lipid bilayer to the surface membrane of the parasite's syncytial outer tegument. This tegument now forms the main parasite–host interface and so has physiological and immunological functions vital to long-term survival in the hostile environment of the bloodstream. These include uptake of nutrients, response to injury, and surface adsorption of host antigens to provide an immunological disguise.

Newly transformed schistosomula remain in the epidermis for several days before migrating, via the bloodstream, lungs, and systemic circulation, to the hepatic portal system. Here the schistosomula mature and differentiate into adult worms, pair, and migrate against the portal blood flow to the small venules draining the genitourinary tract (*S. haematobium*) or the large and, to a lesser extent, small intestine (*S. mansoni*, *S. japonicum*, *S. intercalatum*, *S. mekongi*). Male and female worms are 1 to 2 cm long and morphologically distinct. Paired worms remain permanently coupled, with the shorter, flatter, more muscular male gripping the female in its gynaecophoric canal (Fig. 7.11.1.3). Worms ingest blood cells into their blind-ending bifurcated gut, producing a haematin-like pigment that is regurgitated into the blood. Adult worms have average lifespans in humans of 3 years (*S. haematobium*) to 7 years (*S. mansoni*), although active infections are reported in individuals who have left endemic areas more than 20 years previously. Female worms start to produce eggs between 5 and 12 weeks after infection, at rates of 300 (*S. mansoni*) to 3000 (*S. japonicum*) per day. A few days after an egg is laid, a single miracidium develops within the rigid eggshell, the shape and size of which is characteristic for each species. *S. mansoni* (Fig. 7.11.1.4) and *S. haematobium* eggs are ellipsoid, 65 × 150 µm, the former having a lateral spine and the latter a terminal spine. *S. japonicum* eggs are more spherical, 70 × 90 µm, with a small lateral knob that is not always apparent microscopically. Embryonated eggs pass from the venules into the gut or bladder lumen. This is facilitated by host immune responses to secreted egg antigens, as egg excretion is inhibited in immunosuppressed experimental hosts and HIV infected individuals. The passage of the eggs causes tissue damage, as does the granulomatous reactions to eggs that fail to escape from the bloodstream and get swept into the liver by the portal blood flow.

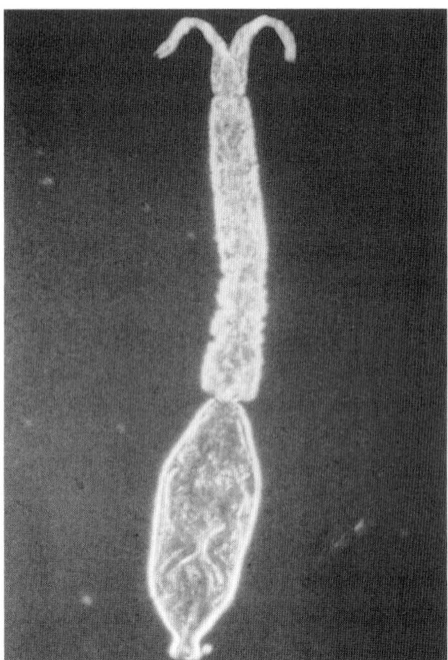

Fig. 7.11.1.2 The infective larva (cerceria) of *Schistosoma mansoni*, length approximately 200 µm. The head region has characteristic suckers; the muscular forked tail propels the free-swimming larva, but is discarded during skin penetration. This larva will develop into an adult worm in a human host.

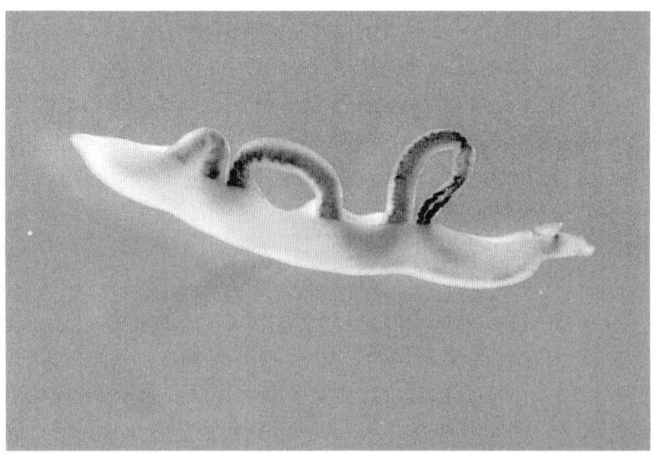

Fig. 7.11.1.3 Adult worms of *S. mansoni*. The shorter male encloses the female in its gynaecophoric canal, the characteristic haematin-like pigment can be seen in the female worm's gut.

Eggs deposited in fresh water rapidly hatch in response to osmotic changes, releasing the miracidium. This ciliated and actively swimming larva lives for about 6 h, and can chemically detect the proximity of snails, modifying its swimming behaviour as it approaches a potential host. The parasite actively penetrates the snail's tissues and transforms into a primary sporocyst. Asexual replication gives rise to daughter sporocysts that migrate to the snail's hepatopancreas where cercariae are asexually generated within each sporocyst. Thus, snails infected with a single miracidium release cercariae that are all of the same sex. Cercariae are first released from snails 3 to 6 weeks after infection, depending on parasite species and ambient temperature. Infected snails can shed hundreds of cercariae daily over several months.

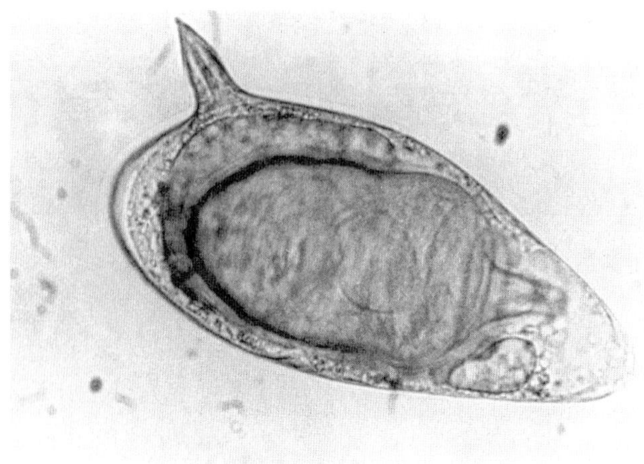

Fig. 7.11.1.4 Egg of *S. mansoni* containing a fully developed miracidium and showing the characteristic lateral spine of this species.

Schistosomiasis is associated with poor living conditions and inadequate sanitation and water supply. Its distribution has changed over the last 50 years. In some areas sustained control strategies have been successful. However, environmental changes, development of water resources, population increases, and migration, have led to its spread into previously nonendemic areas or areas with a low rate of infection. *S. japonicum* and *S. haematobium* have decreased, whereas *S. mansoni* has increased to become the most prevalent and widespread species. *S. japonicum* has been controlled effectively in many areas and is now endemic only in China, where it is much reduced, Indonesia, the Philippines, and Thailand. *S. mekongi* is found in Cambodia and Laos, and *S. intercalatum* is found in 10 countries within the rainforest belt of central Africa. *S. mansoni* is present in most countries of sub-Saharan Africa, and in Madagascar, the Nile delta and valley, as well as Saudi Arabia, Yemen, Oman, Libya, northern and eastern Brazil, Suriname, Venezuela, and some Caribbean islands. *S. haematobium* is widespread in sub-Saharan Africa and Madagascar, and is more prevalent than *S. mansoni* in North Africa and the Middle East.

Clinical features

Stage of invasion: cercarial dermatitis or 'swimmer's itch'

When cercariae penetrate the skin they can cause a skin reaction, called cercarial dermatitis or 'swimmer's itch'. This is frequently seen after exposure to avian schistosomes, and is associated with the death of cercariae in the skin. It is seen both in areas endemic for human schistosomiasis and in non-endemic areas. In people exposed for the first time, the invasion causes a transient immediate hypersensitivity reaction with intense itching. Within 12 to 24 h it is followed by a delayed reaction characterized by a small, red, pruritic, macular rash progressing to papules after 24 h. The rash may persist for up to 15 days and residual pigmentation may persist for months. Following repeated exposure, the signs and symptoms increase dramatically and start earlier. A similar reaction can be seen after re-exposure to human cercariae, predominantly *S. mansoni* and *S. japonicum*. Treatment, if needed, is symptomatic.

Stage of maturation: acute schistosomiasis or Katayama fever

The early stages of a primary infection can be associated with a severe systemic reaction that resembles serum sickness. This acute illness, called acute toxaemic schistosomiasis or Katayama fever, can occur following initial infection with any schistosome infecting humans, although it is more common in *S. japonicum* and *S. mansoni* infections. Acute schistosomiasis is most marked in primary infections in nonimmune adults, but acute *S. japonicum* infection can occur in re-exposed individuals. Symptoms appear 2 to 6 weeks after exposure. The clinical picture resembles an acute pyrexial illness with fever as a prime characteristic. The patient feels ill, and may have rigors, sweating, headache, malaise, muscular aches, profound weakness, weight loss, and a nonproductive irritating cough. Anorexia, nausea, abdominal pain, and diarrhoea can occur. Physical examination may reveal a generalized lymphadenopathy, an enlarged tender liver, and, sometimes, a slightly enlarged spleen and an urticarial rash (Fig. 7.11.1.5). Eosinophilia is almost always present. Patients may become confused or stuporose or present with visual impairment or papilloedema. Severe cerebral or spinal cord manifestations may occur, and this is an indication for urgent investigative measures. Even light infections may cause severe illness and the syndrome can, in rare cases, be fatal.

Differential diagnoses include infections such as typhoid (leucopenia, no eosinophilia), brucellosis, malaria, infectious mononucleosis, miliary tuberculosis, leptospirosis, and other conditions with fever of unknown origin. Fever and eosinophilia occur in trichinosis, tropical eosinophilia, invasive ankylostomiasis, strongyloidiasis, visceral larva migrans, and infections with *Opisthorchis* and *Clonorchis* species.

Established infections

Urinary schistosomiasis (*Schistosoma haematobium*)

The signs and symptoms of *S. haematobium* infection relate to the worms' predilection for the veins of the genitourinary tract, and

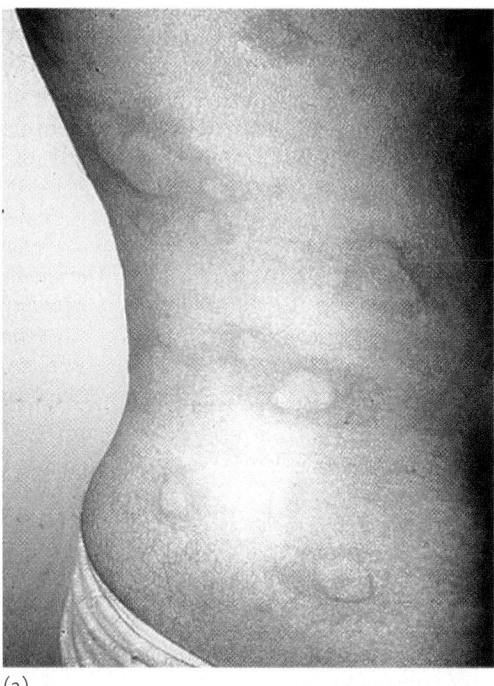

(a)

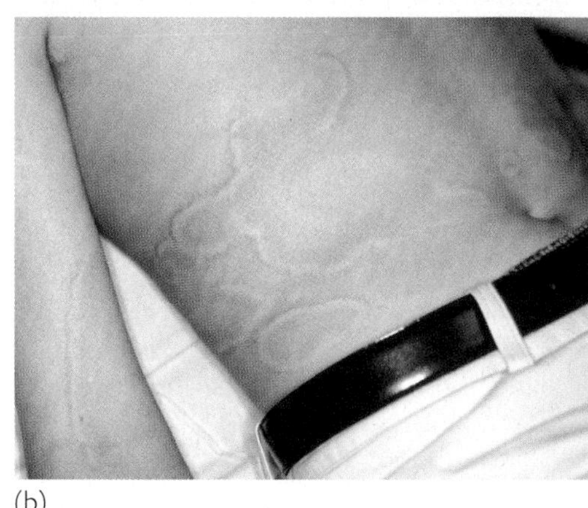

(b)

Fig. 7.11.1.5 Katayama fever (*S. mansoni* infection): (a) giant urticarial rash; (b) rash in a traveller.
(Courtesy of Dr Tom Doherty, London Hospital for Tropical Diseases.)

result from deposition of eggs in the bladder, ureters, and to some extent the genital organs. In the phase of established infection two stages can be recognized:

- an active stage mainly in children, adolescents, and younger adults with egg deposition in the urinary tract, egg excretion in the urine with proteinuria and macroscopic or microscopic haematuria
- a chronic stage in older patients with sparse or absent urinary egg excretion but the presence of urinary tract pathology

In the active stage many patients will have minimal symptoms. The most frequently encountered complaint is a painless, characteristically terminal, haematuria, the prevalence and severity of which is related to the intensity of infection. In communities where *S. haematobium* is highly endemic, macroscopic haematuria among boys is considered a natural sign of puberty. Dysuria, frequency, and suprapubic discomfort or pain is associated with schistosomal cystitis and may continue throughout the course of active infection. Initially the eggs may give rise to an intense inflammatory response in the mucosa. This may cause ureteric obstruction leading to hydroureter and hydronephrosis. Cytoscopy reveals friable masses or polyps extending into the bladder, petechiae, and granulomas. These early inflammatory lesions, including the obstructive uropathy, are usually reversible after treatment with antischistosomal drugs. The bladder lesions and obstructive uropathy can be visualized by ultrasonography (Fig. 7.11.1.6).

As the infection progresses, the inflammatory component decreases, possibly due to modulation by the host immune response, and fibrosis increases. Various changes occur in the bladder, including calcification, ulceration, and the development of papillomas. Cytoscopy reveals 'sandy patches' composed of large numbers of calcified eggs surrounded by fibrous tissue and an atrophic mucosal surface. The bladder lesions may lead to nocturia, precipitancy, retention of urine, dribbling, and incontinence. Calculus formation is common, as is secondary bacterial infection, usually due to *Escherichia coli*, pseudomonas, klebsiella, enterobacter, or salmonella. the ureters are less commonly involved, but ureteric fibrosis can cause irreversible obstructive uropathy which can progress to uraemia. Bilateral ureteric involvement is common, although lesions may predominate on one side. Despite damage to the ureters, symptoms may be absent or minimal.

Egg deposition may also cause granulomas and lesions to develop in the genital organs, most commonly in the cervix and vagina in women and the seminal vessels in men. Dyspareunia, contact bleeding, and lower back pain may result in women, and perineal pain and painful ejaculation in men. Symptoms such as haematospermia and perineal discomfort have been described in travellers returning from Malawi. In some of these patients, eggs have been demonstrated in seminal fluid but not in urine. The impact of genital lesions caused by *S. haematobium* infection on the spread of HIV needs to be elucidated. Although small numbers of *S. haematobium* eggs are frequently detected in faeces and rectal biopsies, intestinal symptoms are uncommon.

In some areas in Africa, an association between *S. haematobium* infection and squamous cell carcinoma of the urinary bladder has been described. The aetiological significance of the parasite in the causation of this cancer is not proven, but is suggested by the finding that the prevalence of carcinoma of the bladder is correlated with intensity of *S. haematobium* infection. In the established stage, *S. haematobium* should be distinguished from renal tuberculosis with haematuria, haemoglobinuria, and cancer of the urogenital tract.

Intestinal schistosomiasis

In most early *S. mansoni* and *S. japonicum* infections, symptoms are mild or absent. Clinical features are generally encountered in those with high-intensity infections. They include diarrhoea, sometimes with blood or mucus in the surface of the stool, abdominal discomfort, and hypogastric pain or colicky cramps. Severe dysentery is rare, but can occur. The liver, especially the left lobe, may be enlarged and tender; the spleen may also be enlarged, but is usually soft. At this stage, the condition is entirely reversible by antischistosomal treatment, but the relative lack of symptoms may cause it to pass unnoticed until irreversible complications set in. Later stages present as intestinal or hepatosplenic disease. Intestinal schistosomiasis is associated with granuloma formation (Fig. 7.11.1.7), inflammation, and fibrosis, primarily in the large intestine. Focal dense deposits of *S. mansoni* or *S. japonicum* eggs in the large intestine can induce the formation of inflammatory polyps. The major clinical manifestation is intermittent diarrhoea with or without passage of blood or mucus, occasionally associated

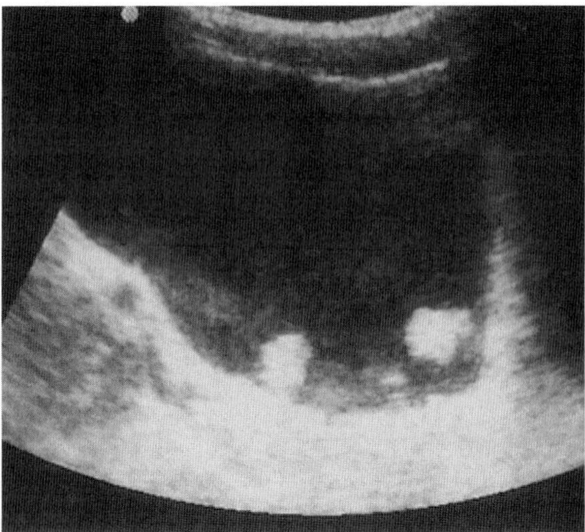

Fig. 7.11.1.6 Bladder pseudopolyps as seen by ultrasound in *S. haematobium* infection.
(Courtesy of Ms Hilda Kadzo, Kenyatta National Hospital, Nairobi, Kenya.)

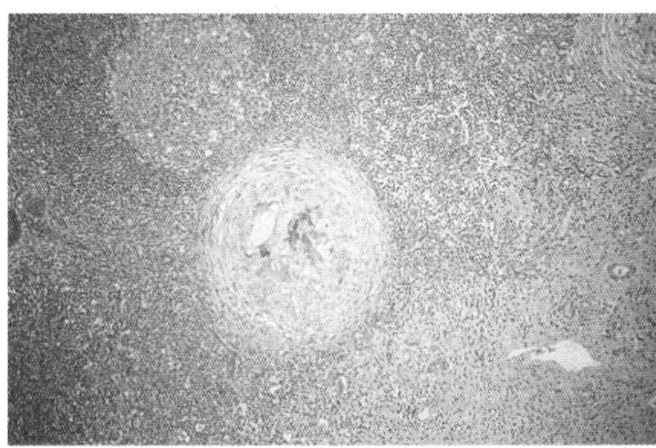

Fig. 7.11.1.7 Schistosomal granuloma in the appendix.

with protein-losing enteropathy and anaemia. Intestinal schistosomiasis in *S. japonicum* infection may also involve the stomach, with gastric bleeding and pyloric obstruction.

Differential diagnosis includes irritable bowel syndrome, amoebiasis, giardiasis, intestinal helminth infection, ulcerative colitis, Crohn's disease, and tuberculosis.

Hepatosplenic schistosomiasis is a chronic manifestation of *S. mansoni* and *S. japonicum* infection. The term covers two distinct clinical entities: early inflammatory and late hepatosplenic disease with periportal fibrosis. Early inflammatory hepatosplenic schistosomiasis is the main cause of hepatosplenic schistosomiasis in children and adolescents. The liver is enlarged, especially the left lobe, and is smooth and firm. The spleen is enlarged, often extending below the umbilicus and firm or hard. Generally no hepatic fibrosis can be demonstrated by ultrasonography. Early inflammatory hepatosplenic schistosomiasis may be found in up to 80% of infected children and the severity is related to intensity of infection (Fig. 7.11.1.8). This type of hepatosplenomegaly may also be associated with concomitant chronic exposure to malaria.

Presinusoidal periportal fibrosis (clay pipe stem or Symmers' fibrosis) (Figs. 7.11.1.9 and 7.11.1.10) develops later in life, generally in young and middle-aged adults with long-standing intense exposure to infection. Patients with periportal fibrosis may excrete very few or no eggs in faeces. During the early stages the liver is enlarged, especially the left lobe; it is smooth, firm, and sometimes tender. Later, in many cases, it becomes small firm and nodular. The spleen is enlarged, often massively, due to passive congestion and reticuloendothelial hyperplasia (Fig. 7.11.1.9). The patient may be asymptomatic or may complain of a left hypochondrial mass with discomfort and anorexia. Anaemia may be present. There may be reduced growth, infantilism, and amenorrhoea, especially in *S. japonicum* infection. Severe hepatosplenic schistosomiasis

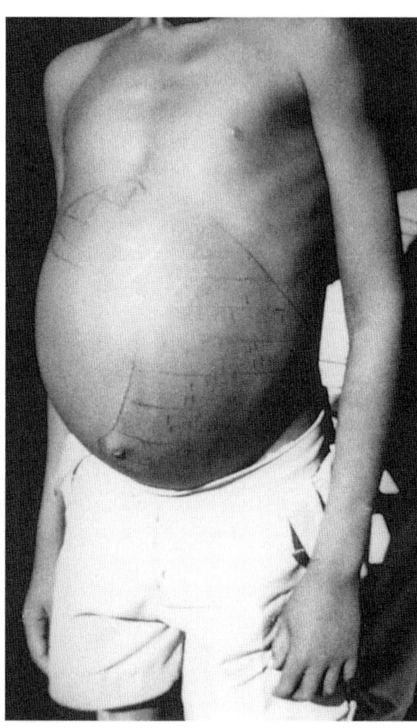

Fig. 7.11.1.8 Kenyan child with severe hepatosplenic schistosomiasis mansoni.

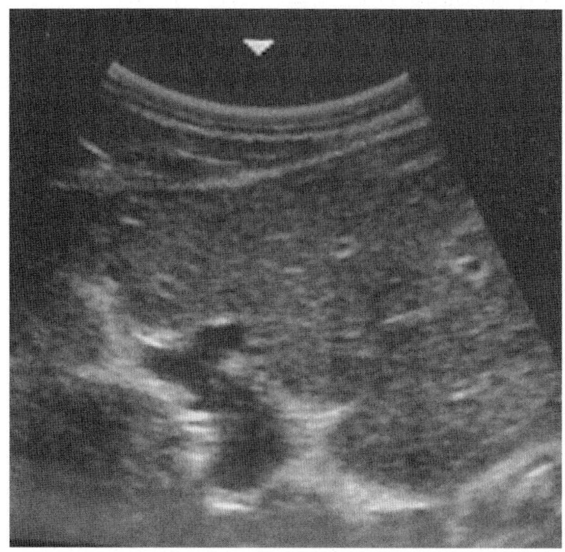

Fig. 7.11.1.9 Hepatic periportal fibrosis as seen by ultrasound in *S. mansoni* infection.

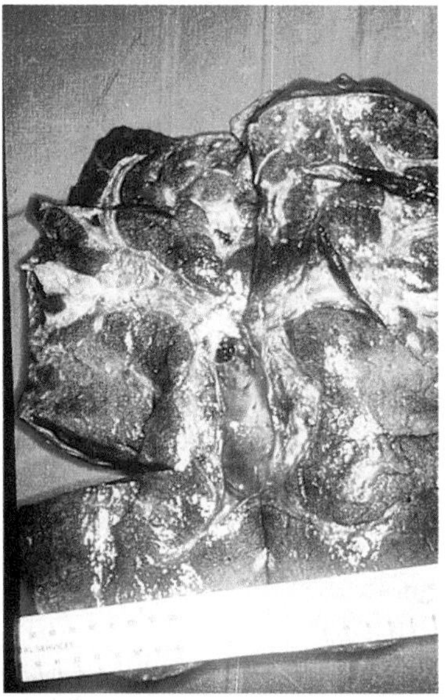

(a)

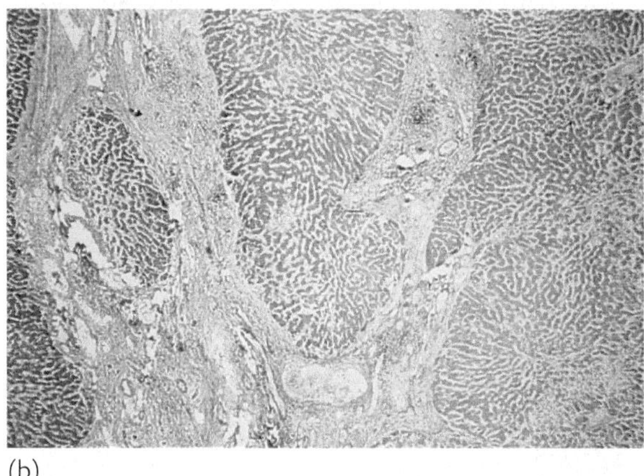

(b)

Fig. 7.11.1.10 The liver in *S. mansoni* infection in South Africa. Clay pipe stem fibrosis: (a) macroscopic views; (b) microscopic view.
(Copyright Gareth Turner.)

may lead to portal hypertension, but hepatic function usually remains normal. Ascites, attributable both to the portal hypertension and to hypoalbuminaemia, may be seen, especially in *S. japonicum* infection. Patients with severe hepatosplenic disease and portal hypertension may develop oesophageal varices detectable by endoscopy or ultrasound (Fig. 7.11.1.11). These patients may experience repeated bouts of haematemesis, melaena, or both. This is the most severe, potentially fatal, complication of hepatosplenic schistosomiasis, and death may result from massive loss of blood.

Differential diagnoses of hepatosplenic schistosomiasis include kala-azar (visceral leishmaniasis), tropical splenomegaly syndrome associated with malaria, leukaemia, lymphoma, alcoholic, or viral cirrhosis, and some of the haemoglobinopathies. Some regression of periportal fibrosis may occur after specific antischistosomal therapy, as judged by ultrasonography examination of the liver, but in most individuals with periportal fibrosis and clinical manifestations of hepatosplenic disease, regression does not occur.

In comparison with *S. japonicum* and *S. mansoni* infections, clinical symptoms of disease in *S. intercalatum* infection are commonly mild or absent, and it is not regarded as a serious public health problem. Active infection is seen in children and adolescents and pathology is detected only in those with egg excretion exceeding 400 eggs/g faeces. The usual clinical presentation is one of diarrhoea, often with blood in the stool and lower abdominal pain or discomfort. *S. mekongi* infections are usually asymptomatic but may produce a clinical picture similar to that of *S. japonicum*, although the infections are usually milder. Hepatosplenomegaly can occur.

Other manifestations

Nervous system manifestations

Nervous system involvement in *S. mansoni* and *S. haematobium* infections most frequently affect the spinal cord following acute infection. This manifestation is not related to the intensity of infection. A myelopathy and radiculopathy results from the inflammatory reaction, caused by the deposition of eggs around the spinal cord, and presents as an ascending flaccid paralysis with sensory level and sphincter involvement. The lesion is usually in the region of the cauda equina. Although paraparesis is seen most commonly during acute schistosomiasis, it may also be a late-stage complication of *S. mansoni* infection in endemic areas with high rates of transmission. Myelography, CT, and MRI are of diagnostic value. In acute cases lesions are seen on MRI scans as a diffuse swelling of the lumbar cord with central softening or cyst formation.

The brain is the major site of central nervous system involvement in *S. japonicum* infections. About 2% of acutely infected patients experience symptoms that mimic acute encephalitis or a focal neurological process. CT shows multiple enhancing lesions. In chronic infections, patients may present with focal brain lesions that can resemble tumours and present as focal epilepsy. These lesions contain masses of eggs and granulomas. Uncontrolled studies suggest that treatment with a combination of antischistosomal drugs and glucocorticoids is effective.

Pulmonary manifestations

Eggs may be deposited in the lungs. Granulomatous reactions and fibrosis develop in the pulmonary vasculature leading to pulmonary hypertension and/or cor pulmonale (Fig. 7.11.1.12). This is normally seen secondary to hepatosplenic schistosomiasis in patients with portal fibrosis and portal hypertension, but pulmonary hypertension may also result from accumulation of *S. haematobium* eggs in the lungs. A syndrome of cough with multiple small radiographic lesions and eosinophilia has been described. Symptoms include fatigue, palpitations, dyspnoea, cough, and sometimes haemoptysis. Patients may progress to decompensation with congestive cardiac failure. In endemic areas schistosomiasis must always be considered as a possible cause of cor pulmonale.

Renal manifestations

Glomerulonephritis is common in chronic *S. mansoni* infection in Brazil, especially in patients with hepatosplenic disease. Immunoglobulins, complement components, and schistosome antigens are deposited in the mesangial area. The condition is manifested clinically as proteinuria and/or nephrotic syndrome, sometimes with hypertension.

Miscellaneous manifestations

Patients infected with any of the three major schistosome species and subsequently infected with salmonella may develop a prolonged intermittent febrile illness. Prolonged excretion of salmonella in the urine and intermittent bacteraemia has been demonstrated in *S. haematobium* infection. Treatment for the

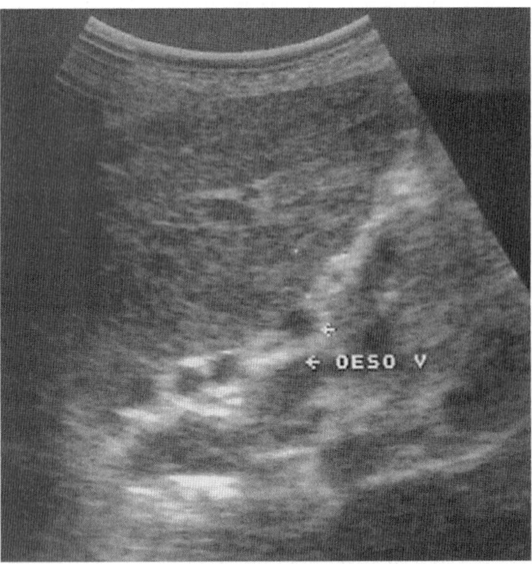

Fig. 7.11.1.11 Oesophageal varices as seen by ultrasound in *S. mansoni* infection.

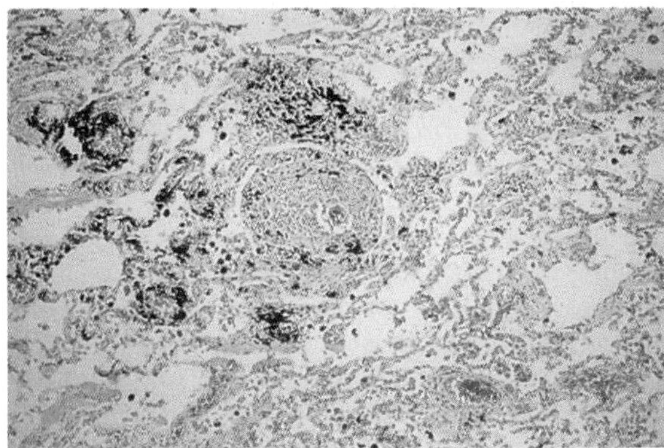

Fig. 7.11.1.12 Schistosomal granuloma in the lung. (Copyright Gareth Turner.)

salmonella infection alone is often not effective without treatment of the underlying schistosome infection.

Diagnosis and investigations

Information about geographical area and history of exposure by wading, bathing, washing, or showering in potentially contaminated fresh water is important for diagnosis of schistosomiasis, especially in travellers and immigrants. This can indicate the likelihood of infection and point to the schistosome species involved. A definitive diagnosis is made by the direct demonstration of schistosome eggs by microscopy of urine or stool samples, biopsies or, on rare occasions, secretions such as seminal fluid. In epidemiological studies it is usually important to obtain quantitative estimates of egg output to provide information about intensity of infection within a population.

Direct parasitological methods

In *S. haematobium* infection, eggs can be detected in urine after filtration, sedimentation, or centrifugation followed by microscopy. Ideally, urine should be passed around midday and the terminal part of the stream examined. The most commonly used method in epidemiological studies in endemic areas is filtration of 10 to 20 ml of urine using a syringe and a polycarbonate (e.g. Nucleopore), polyamide (e.g. Nytrel), or paper filter. Infection intensity is expressed as eggs/10 ml of urine. This may not be sufficiently sensitive for detection of low-intensity infections in travellers. In such cases, diagnosis is often based on filtration of 24-h urine samples.

For *S. mansoni*, *S. japonicum*, *S. mekongi*, and *S. intercalatum* eggs in the faeces, sedimentation of the eggs followed by microscopy is a useful and simple technique. However, the Kato thick smear technique is the most widely used method in epidemiological studies. This is based on microscopic examination of a smear of a small but fixed amount of faecal sample (usually 20–50 mg). Coarse particles and fibrous material are first removed from the sample by passing it through a sieve. A fixed sample volume is obtained by the use of a template. This is placed on a microscope slide and squashed with either a piece of cellophane soaked in glycerol or a glass coverslip. After leaving the slide for 6 to 24 h to allow the preparation to clear, the eggs are counted and the level of infection expressed as eggs/g faeces. Unfortunately, watery or diarrhoeal stools cannot be processed this way, and low-intensity infections may not be detected, since only small faecal samples are examined and eggs may be clumped unevenly in the stool. Increased sensitivity is obtained by increasing the number of samples examined. For diagnosis of light infections in previously unexposed travellers, microscopic examination of a rectal tissue snip crushed between glass slides is often the most sensitive direct diagnostic method. This method can also be used for biopsies. The crushed tissue sample is far better than a sectioned biopsy for the detection and identification of eggs.

Other direct methods

Recently, sensitive enzyme immune assays (ELISA) have been developed to detect circulating schistosome antigens in serum or urine. These antigens, circulating anodic antigen and circulating cathodic antigen, are derived from the gut of the adult schistosomes. The assays have almost 100% specificity and high sensitivity, and are excellent epidemiological tools as they provide a direct estimate of worm burden and can be used to monitor the efficacy of chemotherapy. They are less well suited for diagnosis of light infections in travellers.

Indirect diagnostic techniques

In *S. haematobium* infections, chemical reagent strips for detection of microhaematuria are widely used in endemic areas as a diagnostic measure. The method can be used in areas of both high and low transmission and there is a consistent significant correlation between microhaematuria and intensity of infection. In intestinal schistosomiasis, blood may be found in the stools, but it is not as useful an indicator of infection. In urinary schistosomiasis, eosinophiluria, with high numbers of eosinophil granulocytes in the urine, is a characteristic finding. Recently, detection of the eosinophil granule protein ECP (eosinophil cationic protein) in urine has been used for the qualitative assessment of eosinophil infiltration of the bladder mucosa, and hence local inflammation. Measurement of ECP in urine has proved useful in following post-treatment resolution of urinary tract morbidity in endemic areas. Eosinophilia is often found in acutely infected travellers. In cases where eggs are difficult to find, eosinophilia plus a history of exposure may suggest the need for further examination for schistosomiasis including serodiagnosis.

Immunodiagnosis

In cases of suspected schistosomiasis in which eggs have not been detected, serology can be used to demonstrate specific antibodies. An indirect immunofluorescence test using sections of adult worms for detection of specific immunoglobulins (IgM and IgG) is widely used. For travellers, a positive antibody result combined with a history of exposure should lead to treatment. Serodiagnosis is not useful in endemic areas because of the high levels of specific antibodies found in naturally exposed populations.

Ultrasonography

Ultrasonography is noninvasive, portable, has no biological hazards for the patient, and can be used to either complement or replace many invasive diagnostic techniques. It is the technique of choice for grading schistosomal periportal fibrosis, portal hypertension, hydronephrosis, and urinary bladder lesions. A protocol for standardized investigations and methods of reporting has been produced by the World Health Organization (http://www.who.int/tdr/publications/publications/ultrasound.htm). Ultrasonography is especially useful for monitoring decreases in morbidity after chemotherapy programmes.

Pathophysiology/pathogenesis

Schistosome eggs can be trapped in the tissues, often the walls of the intestines or, depending on species, the urinary bladder or ureters. They may be seen in cone biopsies of the uterine cervix. The eggs of *S. mansoni* and *S. japonicum* are swept into the liver via the portal system, where they embolize into the portal radicles and give rise to vascular and granulomatous changes (Fig. 7.11.1.7). Granulomatous pyelophlebitis and peripyelophlebitis is responsible for development of portal hypertension, while granulomata with subsequent fibrosis may be responsible for the periportal fibrosis. The characteristic lesion in the liver is a presinusoidal periportal fibrosis (Symmers' fibrosis, Fig. 7.11.1.10). There is typically no bridging between the fibrous tracts, no nodule formation, and no hepatic cell damage. Increased portal pressure can result in the development of portosystemic collaterals and eggs may pass directly from the portal vein to the pulmonary circulation (Fig. 7.11.1.12). Here the combination of vascular and granulomatous changes is responsible for pulmonary hypertension.

Treatment

Today the drug of choice is praziquantel, available as 600 mg tablets. It is administered orally, normally in a single dose, 40 mg/kg body weight and is effective against all schistosome species infecting humans. It is also effective for most other trematode infections and against adult cestodes. The drug is safe and well tolerated. After a single dose of 40 mg/kg up to 85% of those treated cease to excrete eggs, and egg counts are reduced by 95% or more in those not cured. In endemic areas, this level of efficacy is generally acceptable since very light residual infections do not lead to severe morbidity. In patients who are not cured by the initial treatment, the same dose can be repeated at weekly intervals for 2 weeks. A repeat dose 6–12 weeks later can be administered to cure prepatent infections, especially if eosinophilia or symptoms persist despite treatment.

Praziquantel has not been shown to be teratogenic in animals and it is now judged to be safe to use for the treatment of pregnant and lactating women and young children. Any side effects are generally mild, resolving spontaneously over a few hours and rarely requiring medication. Gastrointestinal side effects include abdominal pain or discomfort and sometimes vomiting. They occur more frequently in individuals with high infection intensities. Urticarial skin reactions and periorbital oedema may occur in about 2% of treated individuals. General side effects including headache, dizziness, fever, and fatigue can also occur, but less frequently.

As a general principle, all patients with acute schistosomiasis should be treated with praziquantel. Corticosteroids can be added in case of Katayama fever to suppress the hypersensitivity reaction. Since immature schistosomes are not susceptible to praziquantel, treatment should be repeated 4–6 weeks later. Use of praziquantel for cerebral *S. japonicum* infections is effective, resulting in rapid dissipation of cerebral oedema and resolution of cerebral masses. However, corticosteroids and anticonvulsants are sometimes needed in addition to praziquantel in cases with neuroschistosomiasis. Praziquantel should be administered with great caution in the case of concurrent neurocysticercosis. Chemotherapy is only part of the management of schistosomiasis-associated portal hypertension, since the main complications are due to obstructive pathology. Management of portal hypertension and prevention of bleeding from oesophageal varices is beyond the scope of this chapter. Praziquantel has largely replaced other drugs for treatment of schistosomiasis. Oxamniquine (marketed as Mansil in South America) is only effective against *S. mansoni* and is mainly used in Brazil. Artemisinin derivatives are effective against immature stages of *S. mansoni*, *S. japonicum*, and probably also *S. haematobium*. Their use for management of acute schistosomiasis or as prophylaxis is currently under investigation, but they cannot be used in malaria endemic areas due to the risk of inducing artimisinin resistance in malaria parasites.

Prognosis

Most infected people have few, if any, overt symptoms. Acute schistosomiasis can be fatal or can lead to severe residual damage to the nervous system if not treated, but responds well to antischistosomal therapy if started early. Early infections respond extremely well to treatment and the pathological lesions regress leaving little residual damage. However, in endemic areas individuals, particularly young children, are rapidly re-exposed and reinfected unless control measures are taken at the community level. Chronic infections with severe periportal fibrosis respond less well to specific antischistosomal treatment, although some regression of hepatosplenic disease with periportal fibrosis has been seen after treatment. The lifetime prognosis is worst in patients with severe hepatosplenic schistosomiasis and oesophageal varices. Previous episodes of haematemesis indicate a 70%t risk of rebleeding.

Transmission and epidemiology

Each successful cercarial penetration of human skin has the potential to give rise to a single male or female adult worm, but it is probable that many cercariae die naturally in the epidermis. People tend to accumulate worms with continued exposure to infection. However, human populations in endemic areas do not just continue to accumulate worms with age. Intensities of infection increase in children during their younger years (as estimated by numbers of excreted eggs), peaking around the age of 12 years, before falling to lower levels in adulthood (Fig. 7.11.1.13a). This is probably due to the death of older worms, which are not replaced at a similar rate in older people. This age–infection intensity profile is more pronounced if study populations are given chemotherapy to remove existing infections and then monitored for levels of reinfection over several subsequent years. In these circumstances, it is clear that young children are much more susceptible to reinfection than older children or adults, and that a striking change in susceptibility to reinfection occurs after 12 years of age. The slower acquisition of worms in adulthood could be due to reduced exposure to infection or to age-dependent changes in innate resistance or acquired immunity. In many endemic areas children have more contact with water than adults, but careful observation of water-associated behaviour has shown that age profiles of water contact are variable between communities, whereas profiles of reinfection intensities are remarkably consistent (Fig. 7.11.1.13b). This suggests that host-related factors other than exposure influence susceptibility to reinfection. This has been most convincingly shown in fishing communities in areas with high *S. mansoni* transmission on Lake Albert, Uganda. Here occupational water contact results in adults having greater exposure to infection than their children, yet, within 12 months of treatment, it is the children under 12 years of age that suffer much higher reinfection intensities. Current research is focused on assessing the relative roles of innate resistance and acquired immunity in this age-dependent resistance and whether the onset of puberty or the length of time spent living in endemic areas might be important. For example, it is not known if this age-dependent resistance to infection holds true for travellers exposed to infection for the first time. Immune responses to schistosomes also differ between children and adults. Specific IgE and other characteristically Th2-type responses against the parasite are

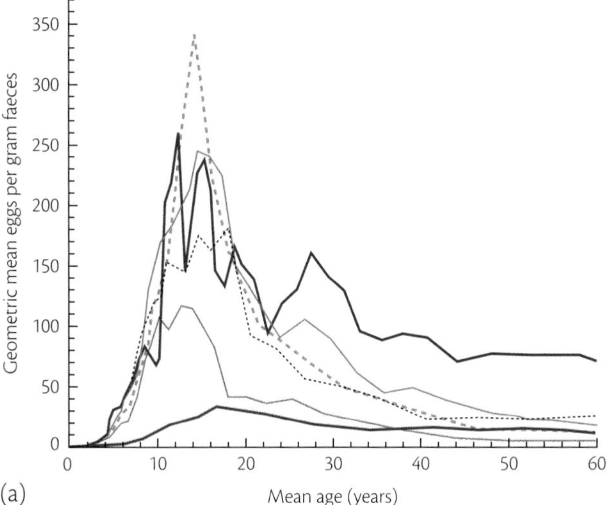

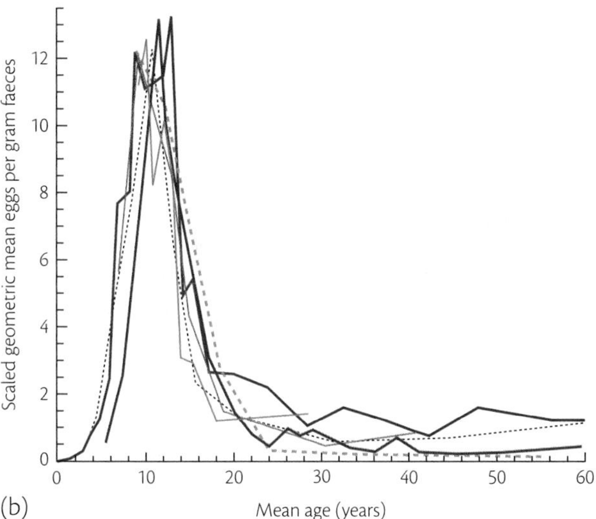

Fig. 7.11.1.13 (a) Age–intensity profiles of *S. mansoni* infection from six communities in Kenya. (b) Age–reinfection intensity profiles of *S. mansoni* after chemotherapy in the same six communities in Kenya, assessed between 12 and 36 months after treatment.

(a, from Fulford, AJ, *et al.* (1992). On the use of age-intensity data to detect immunity to parasitic infections, with special reference to *Schistosoma mansoni* in Kenya. *Parasitology* **105**: 219–227.)

associated with resistance to reinfection. Whatever mechanisms underlie the contrasting susceptibilities of children and adults, continued exposure can be expected to result in reinfection, especially amongst younger children.

Prevention and control

Despite the high risk of reinfection, chemotherapy is usually highly beneficial at both the individual and population levels, as those suffering high intensities of infection are at greatest risk of the more severe forms of schistosomiasis. Furthermore, even low-intensity infections may lead to anaemia and have a negative impact on the well-being of the infected individual. This is specially important among vulnerable groups such as children and pregnant women. Various chemotherapy-based control strategies can be employed depending on intensity of transmission and the available resources. In the Nile delta region of Egypt, injections of tartar emetic were used for mass treatment from the 1960s to the 1980s. Tragically, the needles were not adequately sterilized and, as a result, hepatitis C virus was widely spread in this population to reach its highest recorded prevalence. In areas of high transmission, population-based chemotherapy can avoid the time and expense required for diagnosis and reduce the prevalence and severity of morbidity. Alternatively, schoolchildren can be targeted for treatment, as they invariably have the heaviest worm burdens and contribute most to ongoing transmission. In areas of less intense transmission, treatment can be restricted to diagnosed cases. The provision of safe water supplies and sanitation, where it can be achieved, will make an important additional contribution. Mortality can be prevented and morbidity best controlled by a combination of health education, chemotherapy, provision of safe water supplies and sanitation, and, where appropriate, snail control. Health education should be aimed at improving practices of water use and preventing indiscriminate urination and defecation. The role of molluscicides in control programmes depends on the local epidemiological and ecological circumstances and the resources available. Within the context of a larger concerted intervention, focal mollusciciding of major transmission sites can be useful. Eradication of host snail species is not usually feasible, although modification of the environment to eliminate snails has been successful in parts of China. In general, it has only been through sustained effort with integrated control strategies that disease control has been achieved.

In May 2001 the World Health Assembly passed Resolution 54.19, which called for efforts to reduce morbidity caused by schistosomiasis and soil-transmitted helminths in school-aged children. As a response to this call, the Schistosomiasis Control Initiative (SCI), supported by the Bill and Melinda Gates Foundation, with the objective of encouraging the development of sustainable schistosomiasis control programmes throughout sub-Saharan Africa, was launched in Uganda in March 2003. Five additional countries have now been enrolled: Zambia, Tanzania, Mali, Burkina Faso, and Niger. The goal is to reduce the level of morbidity in schistosomiasis endemic areas throughout sub-Saharan Africa with praziquantel treatment.

Further reading

Danso-Appiah A, Utzinger J, Liu J, Olliaro P. Drugs for treating urinary schistosomiasis. *Cochrane Database Syst Rev*, 2008 Jul 16;(3):CD000053. Review. PubMed PMID: 18646057.

Fairley J (1991). *Bilharzia. A history of imperial tropical medicine.* Cambridge University Press, Cambridge. [A detailed history of schistosomiasis, including developments in research and control up to the 1970s.]

Gryseels B, *et al.* (2006). Human schistosomiasis. *Lancet*, **368**, 1106–18. [Comprehensive review of various aspects of human schistosomiasis.]

Jordan P, Webbe G, Sturrock RF (eds) (1993). *Human schistosomiasis.* CAB International, Wallingford. [The definitive text on human schistosomiasis. Including: A comprehensive review of pathology and clinical aspects of *Schistosoma mansoni* infection by Lambertucci; of *S. haematobium* and *S. intercalatum* by Farid; and of *S. japonicum* and *S. japonicum*-like infections by Gang.]

King CH, Dickman K, Tisch DJ (2005). Reassessment of the cost of chronic helmintic infection: a meta-analysis of disability-related outcomes in endemic schistosomiasis. *Lancet*, **365**, 1561–9. [A systematic review of data on disability-associated outcomes for all forms of schistosomiasis.resulting in an evidenced-based reassessment of schistosomiasis-related disability.]

Mahmoud A (ed.) (2001). *Tropical medicine: science and practice, Vol. 3 Schistosomiasis.* Imperial College Press, London. [Reviews on various aspects of clinical and experimental schistosomiasis.]

Olds GR (2003). Administration of praziquantel to pregnant and lactating women. *Acta Tropica*, **86**, 185–95. [A summary of praziquantel toxicology with data from various studies that suggest that both the pregnant woman and her unborn fetus may suffer consequences from schistosome infection, and the very important conclusion is that pregnant and lactating women should no longer be systematically excluded from praziquantel treatment.]

Richter J (2003). The impact of chemotherapy on morbidity due to schistosomiasis. *Acta Tropica*, **86**, 161–83. [A comprehensive review of the impact of chemotherapy on schistosomiasis morbidity with several tables providing a useful overview of a large number of studies using different treatment regimes and assessment methods.]

Roca C, *et al.* (2002). Comparative, clinico-epidemiologic study of *Schistosoma mansoni* infections in travellers and immigrants in Spain. *Eur J Clin Microbiol Infect Dis*, **21**, 219–23.

Saconato H, Atallah ÁN (2005). Interventions for treating schistosomiasis mansoni. *Cochrane Database Syst Rev*, **3**, CD000528.

Silva LC, *et al.* (2004). Treatment of schistosomal myeloradiculopathy with praziquantel and corticosteroids and evaluation by magnetic resonance imaging: a longitudinal study. *Clin Infect Dis*, **39**, 1618–24.

Steinmann P, Keiser J, Bos R, *et al.* (2006). Schistosomiasis and water resources development: systematic review, meta-analysis, and estimates of people at risk. *Lancet Infectious Diseases*; **6**, 411–425.

Vennervald BJ, Dunne DW (2004). Morbidity in schistosomiasis: an update. *Curr Opin Infect Dis*. **17**, 439–47. [A review of the factors that affect the level of schistosomiasis morbidity in populations living schistosomiasis endemic areas.]

Whitty CJ, *et al.* (2000). Presentation and outcome of 1107 cases of schistosomiasis from Africa diagnosed in a non-endemic country. *Trans R Soc Trop Med Hyg*, **94**, 531–4.

7.11.2 Liver fluke infections

David I. Grove

Essentials

Clonorchiasis and related flukes

Clonorchis (syn. *Opisthorchis*) *sinensis* is a fluke (flatworm) acquired by ingestion of undercooked freshwater fish in eastern Asia. Larvae in the duodenum enter the biliary tree through the sphincter of Oddi and mature. Most patients are asymptomatic, but there may be right upper abdominal discomfort, and infection can be complicated by bacterial cholangitis and perhaps cholangiocarcinoma. Diagnosis is suggested by finding eggs in faeces or in duodenal aspirates, but can only be confirmed by examination of adult flukes. Treatment is with praziquantel.

Opisthorchis viverinni in South-East Asia and *O. felineus* in Eurasia, also acquired from undercooked fish, cause similar infections.

Fascioliasis

Fasciola hepatica and its relative *F. gigantica* are acquired by eating watercress contaminated with cysts. These hatch in the duodenum, from which larvae pass through the peritoneum and track through the liver parenchyma, causing considerable damage before they mature in the bile ducts. This produces a hepatitis-like syndrome followed months or years later by features of biliary obstruction. Diagnosis is made by finding eggs in stool or duodenal fluid. Treatment is difficult, but triclabendazole and nitazoxanide may be effective.

Other liver flukes

Dicrocoelium dendriticum is a rare infection acquired by accidental ingestion of infected ants; *Metorchis conjunctus* infection follows consumption of infected freshwater fish. The clinical features of these infections and diagnostic approaches to them are similar to those of other liver fluke infections. Praziquantel is the treatment of choice.

Introduction

Liver flukes, otherwise known as trematodes, are leaf-like hermaphroditic flatworms. The hepatobiliary system of humans is commonly infected by flukes of the genera *Clonorchis* and *Opisthorchis* and occasionally by other species (Table 7.11.2.1). In addition, *Eurytrema pancreaticum* has been found rarely in the pancreatic duct. These infections are usually diagnosed by finding eggs in the faeces. Unfortunately, eggs of many of these species cannot be differentiated from each other, nor can they be distinguished reliably from the eggs of certain intestinal trematodes. In such cases, definitive diagnosis can only be made if adult worms are recovered from the stools after anthelmintic treatment, at surgery or at autopsy; parasitological texts should be sought for diagnostic details.

Clonorchiasis

Life cycle

Clonorchis (syn. *Opisthorchis*) *sinensis* adult worms, 10 to 25 mm long by 3 to 5 mm wide, are found in the bile ducts or occasionally the gallbladder, attached to the mucosa. They may live for up to 40 years. They produce eggs which are passed in the faeces. The miracidium within the egg hatches after ingestion by a suitable species of aquatic snail; nine species belonging to the families Hydrobidae, Melanidae, Assimineidae, and Thiaridae are known to be susceptible. *Parafossarulus manchouricus* is perhaps the most common. The miracidia develop into sporocysts then in turn become rediae which produce larvae known as cercariae. After 6 to 8 weeks, the cercariae emerge from the snail, swim about in the water until they encounter certain freshwater fishes (>100 species, mostly of the family Cyprinidae, i.e. carp, are susceptible). They attach to the surface of the fish, lose their tails, penetrate under the scales, encyst in the skin or flesh, and develop into infective metacercariae over several weeks. When raw or undercooked infected fish is eaten by humans, the metacercariae excyst in the stomach, enter the common bile duct through the ampulla of Vater and ascend into the biliary passages where they mature in 1 month (Fig. 7.11.2.1).

Epidemiology and control

Fish-eating mammals including humans, dogs, cats, and rats may be infected with *C. sinensis*. Human clonorchiasis is endemic in Japan, Korea, China, and Vietnam where the first and second

Table 7.11.2.1 Liver flukes infecting humans

Species	Geographical distribution	Source of infection	Size of eggs (μm)
Clonorchis sinensis	Eastern Asia	Freshwater fish	28–35 × 12–19[a]
Dicrocoelium dendriticum	Widespread	ants accidentally ingested with food	38–45 × 22–30[b]
Eurytrema pancreaticum	Eastern Asia	Grasshoppers	38–45 × 22–30[b]
Fasciola gigantica	Asia, Africa	Vegetation, e.g. watercress	130–150 × 60–90[c]
Fasciola hepatica	Widespread	Vegetation, e.g. watercress	130–150 × 60–90[c]
Metorchis conjunctus	Canada	Freshwater fish	28–35 × 12–19[a]
Opisthorchis felineus	Europe, Asia	Freshwater fish	28–35 × 12–19[a]
Opisthorchis guayaquilaris	Ecuador	Freshwater fish	28–35 × 12–19[a]
Opisthorchis viverrini	Indochina	Freshwater fish	28–35 × 12–19[a]

[a, b, c] Superscripts indicate that eggs within each group are indistinguishable

intermediate hosts are found and where the population is accustomed to consume raw fish. In endemic areas, fish are kept in ponds and fertilized with human and animal faeces. Over 20 million people are thought to be infected in China. Control programmes include proper waste disposal, measures to control snail numbers, and mass treatment with praziquantel, but the most important is health education to discourage the habit of eating raw or undercooked fish.

Pathology

Pathological changes are related to the intensity and duration of infection. They are produced by mechanical irritation, toxin production, immunological responses, and secondary bacterial infection. Inspection of the cut surface of the liver often reveals dilated, thick-walled bile ducts with adult worms visible within the lumen. Adult flukes may be found in the gallbladder but they are usually killed by bile. Histologically, there is desquamation and hyperplasia of epithelial cells, formation of adenomatous tissue and proliferation of periductal connective tissue, and infiltration with eosinophils and mononuclear cells. This may be complicated by epithelial metaplasia then mucinous cholangiocarcinoma. Recurrent pyogenic cholangitis is a common complication and the worms and eggs act as a nidus for gallstone formation (Fig. 7.11.2.2). Some patients have flukes in the pancreatic duct which may cause pancreatitis.

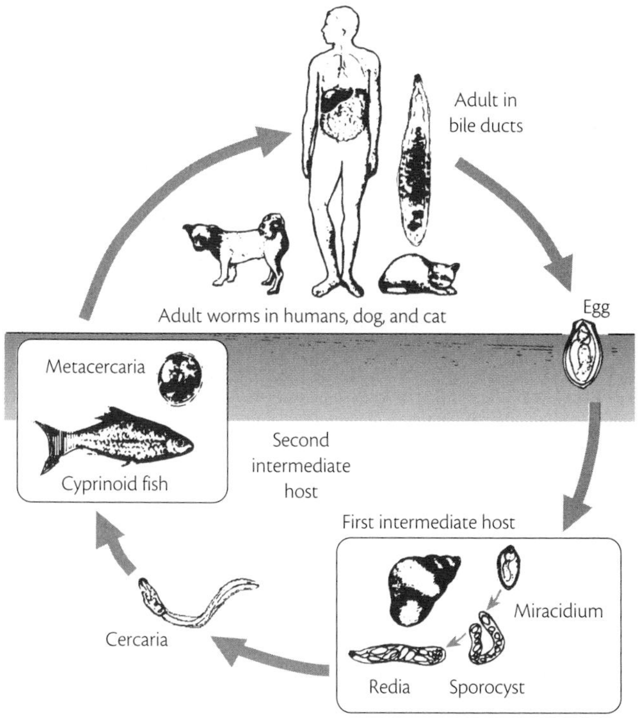

Fig. 7.11.2.1 Life cycle of *Clonorchis* and *Opisthorchis*.

Clinical features

Most patients are asymptomatic and are diagnosed incidentally on stool examination. Symptoms are more common in older patients with heavy worm burdens. It is difficult to differentiate these symptoms from other conditions but they include right hypochondrial or epigastric pain or discomfort, lassitude, anorexia, and flatulence. Some patients complain of a peculiar, hot sensation on the skin of the abdomen or back. Cholangitis causes fever, right upper

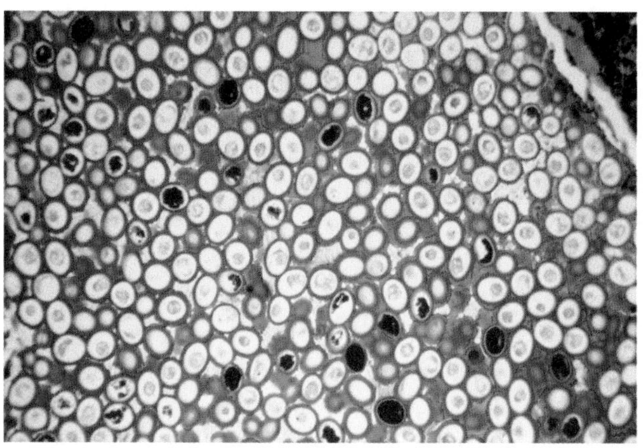

Fig. 7.11.2.2 Histological section of a gallstone showing masses of degenerate *Clonorchis*/*Opisthorchis* eggs.

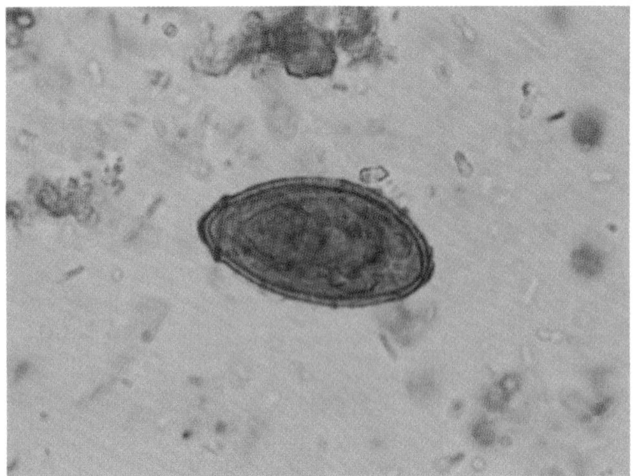

Fig. 7.11.2.3 Egg of *Clonorchis sinensis*: this is identical with that of *Opisthorchis viverrini*.
(Courtesy of A R Butcher.)

quadrant pain, and jaundice. Cholangiocarcinoma is associated with pain, jaundice, and weight loss.

Diagnosis

The diagnosis is suggested by finding eggs in faeces or in duodenal aspirates. They are yellow-brown, 25 to 35 μm long by 12 to 19 μm wide and have a seated operculum with a small knob at the other end (Fig. 7.11.2.3). They cannot be differentiated from ova of *Opisthorchis* species. Furthermore, they are extremely difficult to differentiate from eggs of flukes in the family Heterophyidae (see intestinal trematode infections) although the latter tend to have a smoother egg shell, a less prominent shoulder at the operculum and the knob may be absent. The diagnosis can only be confirmed by examination of adult flukes. Serological tests are not routinely used for diagnosis. Imaging techniques including ultrasonography, CT, and MRI may disclose adult worms or sludge in the gallbladder. The bile ducts are often dilated and contain sludge or calculi and there may be 'too many ducts' on MRI or increased periductal echogenicity on ultrasonography. Liver function tests may be abnormal, often with an obstructive picture.

Treatment

Praziquantel is the treatment of choice and in a dose of 25 mg/kg three times daily after meals for 2 days has a cure rate of close to 100%; eggs should disappear from the stool within 1 week. Biliary tract abnormalities sometimes reverse after treatment. Triclabendazole (see 'Fascioliasis') may prove to be useful, but there is insufficient documentation at present. Bacterial cholangitis is treated with antibiotic therapy such as a combination of amoxicillin, gentamicin, and metronidazole. Surgery may be required in some patients with obstructive jaundice.

Opisthorchiasis viverrini

This infection is very similar to clonorchiasis. The adult *O. viverrini* is smaller than *C. sinensis*, measuring 7 to 12 mm by 1.5 to 3 mm. It may live for over 10 years. The life cycle is similar to that of *Clonorchis*, with various species of snails of the genus *Bithynia* being the first intermediate host. Many species of carp serve as the second intermediate host. Humans, dogs, cats, and other fish-eating mammals are definitive hosts. This parasite is endemic in northern Thailand and adjacent Laos and Cambodia where 10 million people are estimated to be infected because of the popularity of chopped raw cyprinoid fish as a foodstuff.

The pathology and clinical features are similar to those induced by *C. sinensis*. The association with cholangiocarcinoma may be even more striking with this infection. The diagnosis is made as discussed under clonorchiasis. Praziquantel is the drug of choice; 25 mg/kg three times after meals for 1 day gives close to 100% cure rates. Mebendazole (30 mg/kg daily) or albendazole (400 mg twice daily) may be effective if given for several weeks. Triclabendazole may prove to be useful but there is insufficient documentation at present. Control programmes depend heavily on intensive health education.

Opisthorchiasis felineus

This infection is very similar to clonorchiasis. The adult *O. felineus* is morphologically very similar if not identical to *O. viverrini* (the two species have been distinguished by the pattern of flame cells in the cercariae). The life cycle is similar, with *Bithynia leachi* being the only known molluscan intermediate host. Many species of carp serve as the second intermediate host. Humans, dogs, cats, rats, foxes, seals, and other fish-eating mammals are definitive hosts. Infection is acquired by eating raw or undercooked fish; in Siberia, raw, slightly salted and frozen fish is often consumed. This parasite is endemic particularly in Russia and adjacent countries but also in parts of southern Europe and eastern Asia, with several million people probably being infected overall. Eggs are indistinguishable from those of *O. viverrini* and *C. sinensis*. The pathology, clinical features, diagnosis and treatment are similar to *O. viverrini* and *C. sinensis* infections.

Fascioliasis

Life cycle

Fascioliasis is due to infection with the sheep liver fluke *Fasciola hepatica* or with *F. gigantica*. Adult *F. hepatica* flukes 20 to 30 mm by 8 to 13 mm in size live in the large bile ducts and produce eggs which are passed in the stools. The eggs require a period of 9 to 15 days for the miracidia to develop and hatch in water at 22 to 25°C but remain viable for up to 9 months if kept moist and cool. The miracidia penetrate the tissues of various species of amphibious snails of the family Lymnaeidae and develop over the following 4 to 5 weeks through the stages of sporocyst, rediae, daughter rediae, and cercariae. The cercariae emerge from the snails and encyst on various kinds of aquatic vegetation to become metacercariae. A wide range of mammals is susceptible to infection but sheep and cattle are the most important. Human infections are usually acquired by eating watercress or by drinking water contaminated with metacercariae. Metacercariae excyst in the duodenum, penetrate the intestinal wall, and pass into the peritoneal cavity. They then invade the liver capsule and migrate through the hepatic parenchyma to the bile ducts where they mature in about 3 to 4 months. The life span of these flukes is several years.

F. gigantica is large, attaining a size of up to 7.5 cm. The eggs are difficult to distinguish from those of *F. hepatica* and the life cycles of the two parasites are similar.

Epidemiology and control

Because of the wide range of susceptible definitive and intermediate hosts, the infection is geographically widespread. Human infections with *F. hepatica* have been reported from all continents. Fascioliasis gigantica is less frequent and has been seen in Africa and Asia. Infection is prevented by not eating fresh aquatic plants, particularly watercress (*Nasturtium officinale*) and by boiling drinking-water. Veterinary control measures include elimination of the snail intermediate hosts by drainage of pastures and treatment with molluscicides and by eradication of infection from infected herds.

Pathology

In the early stages of infection, larvae migrating through the liver parenchyma may cause considerable destruction with necrosis, abscess formation, and haemorrhage. The number of tunnels lined by ragged walls of necrotic, bleeding and inflamed liver tissue is proportional to the number of worms. In the chronic stages, the walls of the bile ducts become thickened by fibrous tissue and inflammatory infiltration, the epithelium becomes hyperplastic, and the bile ducts dilate. Occasionally the lumina of the bile ducts may become obliterated causing obstructive jaundice. These structural changes predispose to secondary bacterial infection which exacerbates the problem. Sclerosing cholangitis and biliary cirrhosis may follow prolonged heavy infection. There is no apparent association with cholangiocarcinoma.

Clinical features

Human fascioliasis is usually mild and related to the phase of infection. There are three phases.

- Migratory phase—symptoms usually begin about 1 month after infection. Patients may develop abdominal discomfort or pain (especially in the epigastrium and right upper quadrant), anorexia, nausea, vomiting, fever, headache, tender hepatomegaly and urticaria. These initial symptoms may persist for several months.
- Latent phase—this phase is asymptomatic and may last for months to years.
- Obstructive phase—this phase is characterized by the recurrence or appearance for the first time of epigastric and right upper quadrant abdominal pain, biliary colic, anorexia, nausea, vomiting, tender hepatomegaly, fever, and jaundice. These features are frequently due to complicating bacterial cholangitis or cholecystitis and may be associated with bacteraemia.

Flukes occasionally migrate to other sites, especially the anterior abdominal wall. Acute oedematous nasopharyngitis may be an allergic response to larval flukes which attach to the pharyngeal wall after ingestion of infected raw sheep or goat liver (see Chapter 7.13).

Diagnosis

In enzootic areas, early fascioliasis is suspected in patients with fever, tender hepatomegaly, and eosinophilia who give a history of consuming freshwater plants. If available, serological tests may be useful early in the illness before egg production begins. Liver biopsy may be helpful in some cases.

Chronic fascioliasis is diagnosed by finding the characteristic eggs in stools or fluid obtained by duodenal or biliary drainage. The eggs of *F. hepatica* and *F. gigantica* cannot be distinguished reliably from each other or from those of the intestinal fluke, *Fasciolopsis buski*; differentiation of these two infections requires identification of adult flukes. Liver function tests are often abnormal and may show an obstructive picture. Radiolucent shadows of flukes may be seen by cholangiography. Ultrasonography and CT are useful in the demonstration of lesions in the liver and biliary tracts. If the patient has recently consumed infected liver, spurious infection (ingestion of eggs) should be ruled out by placing the patient on a liver-free diet for a few days and repeating the stool examination.

Treatment

Triclabendazole is the drug of choice but its safety in pregnant women has not been proven and resistance has developed in some veterinary populations that may be the source of infection. It is given in a single oral dose of 10 mg/kg although some patients require a second dose after a few weeks. This drug appears to have few side effects. It is available in some countries but not others; further information can be sought from the manufacturer (Novartis, Basle, Switzerland). Flukes are evacuated through the intestinal tract. Nitazoxanide administered in a dose of 100 mg orally twice daily for 7 days cures approximately 50% of patients with fascioliasis; its safety in pregnancy has not yet been established. Praziquantel, which is active against many trematodes, is usually ineffective in fascioliasis but may be tried if other agents are not available.

Dicrocoeliasis

Dicrocoelium dendriticum adult worms measuring 5 to 15 mm by 1.5 to 2.5 mm live in the biliary passages. Eggs passed in the stools are ingested by certain land snails (e.g. species of *Zebrina* and *Helicella*,) in which they develop through two stages of sporocysts with the eventual production of cercariae. The snail leaves slime balls of cercariae on the ground and these are ingested by ants (*Formica* species) in which they develop into metacercariae.

This organism is primarily an infection of sheep, goats, deer, and other herbivores which ingest ants. Humans are rarely infected and are usually accidental. Cases have been reported from Europe, Asia, and Africa. Spurious infections result from the consumption of raw, infected liver. Patients may be asymptomatic but may complain of dyspepsia, flatulence, right upper quadrant pain and diarrhoea. The diagnosis is made by finding the eggs in faeces, bile, or duodenal fluid (Fig. 7.11.2.4); they cannot be differentiated from those of *Eurytrema pancreaticum*. Definitive diagnosis is made by identification of adult worms. Treatment is with praziquantel 25 mg/kg three times after meals for 1 day. Triclabendazole (see 'Fascioliasis') has also been reported to be effective.

Metorchiasis

Many fish-eating mammals of North America serve as definitive hosts for *Metorchis conjunctus*. The aquatic snail *Amnicola limosa* is the first intermediate host; eggs are ingested and hatch miracidia and ultimately release cercariae. Metacercariae develop in the flesh of several species of freshwater fish. Ingested metacercariae hatch in the duodenum and migrate up the biliary tree.

A point source outbreak of this disease has been reported in 19 people who ate raw fish prepared from the white sucker *Catostomus commersoni* caught in a river north of Montreal. The illness was characterized by upper abdominal pain, low-grade fever, eosinophilia, and abnormal liver function tests. Ten days after ingestion of infected

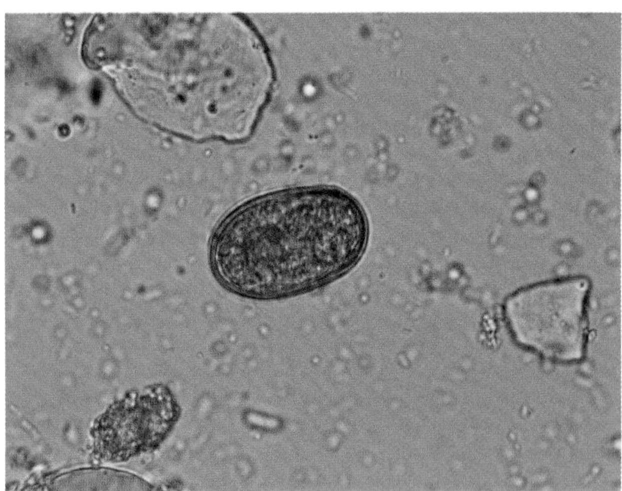

Fig. 7.11.2.4 Eggs of *Dicrocoelium dendriticum*.
(Courtesy of A R Butcher.)

fish, eggs indistinguishable from those of *O. viverrini* were seen in the stools. The patients responded to treatment with praziquantel.

Further reading

Aksoy DY, *et al.* (2005). Infection with *Fasciola hepatica. Clin Microbiol Infect*, **11**, 859–61.

Chai JY, Darwin Murrell K, Lymbery AJ. (2005). Fish-borne parasitic zoonoses: status and issues. *Int J Parasitol*, **35**, 1233–54.

Choi BI, *et al.* (2004). Clonorchiasis and cholangiocarcinoma: etiologic relationship and imaging diagnosis. *Clin Microbiol Rev*, **17**, 540–52.

Keiser J, Utzinger J. (2004). Chemotherapy for major food-borne trematodes: a review. *Expert Opin Pharmacother*, **5**, 1711–26.

Lun ZR, *et al.* (2005). Clonorchiasis: a key foodborne zoonosis in China. *Lancet Infect Dis*, **5**, 31–41.

Rim HJ (2005). Clonorchiasis: an update. *J Helminthol*, **79**, 269–81.

Photographs of various stages of these parasites and diagrams of life cycles may be found at several excellent websites, e.g.: Centers for Disease Control and Prevention. http://www.dpd.cdc.gov/DPDx/HTML/Image_Library.htm

Korean Society for Parasitology. http://www.atlas.or.kr

7.11.3 **Lung flukes (paragonimiasis)**

Udomsak Silachamroon and Sirivan Vanijanonta

Essentials

Paragonimiasis is an infection by flukes of the genus *Paragonimus*, with foci of disease in Asia, Africa, and Central and South America. Humans acquire infection by eating metacercariae in improperly cooked freshwater crabs or crayfish. Acute inflammatory and allergic symptoms are rarely serious and usually resolve spontaneously. Chronic manifestations may be (1) pulmonary—most remarkably with a chronic, productive cough with jam-like, brownish-red sputum; and (2) extrapulmonary—most importantly in the central nervous system, often presenting with seizures. Diagnosis is by demonstrating ova in sputum, stool, or pleural fluid. Serology can be used to support the diagnosis, especially in extrapulmonary paragonimiasis. Treatment with praziquantel is almost always effective. Prevention is by health education and the mass treatment of infected people in an endemic area.

Introduction

Lung fluke infection is caused by *Paragonimus* spp. of which there are more than 40 that cause disease in mammals and about 16 species causing human disease. *Paragonimus westermani* is the most common and widespread. Other species prevalent in some region are *P. heterotremus* in South-East Asia, *P. africanus* and *P. uterobilateralis* in West Africa, *P. skrjabini* in China, and *P. mexicanus* and *P. kellicotti* in Central and South America.

Aetiology and life cycle

Adult flukes are reddish-brown and pea-shaped. They are 0.8 to 1.6 cm in length, 0.4 to 0.8 cm in width, and 0.3 to 0.5 cm thick (Fig. 7.11.3.1). Typically, they are encapsulated in cysts adjacent to the bronchi. Ova (Fig. 7.11.3.2) are expelled through the bronchi and expectorated with sputum or swallowed and passed in the faeces. They hatch in fresh water after a few weeks. The resulting miracidia then infect various species of freshwater snail in which they form sporocysts, rediae, and daughter rediae. Metacercariae develop in susceptible freshwater crabs and crayfish (Fig. 7.11.3.3). Human infection results from ingestion of viable metacercariae in raw or insufficiently cooked crabs and crayfish. Metacercariae excyst in the intestine, then pass through the peritoneal cavity, diaphragm, and pleural cavity, before finally encysting in the lung. Tunnels may be formed during their migration. Encysted flukes mature over a period of 6 to 8 weeks and eggs are produced in 10 to 12 weeks. The circuitous routes of migration allow young flukes to lodge and mature in ectopic locations. The reservoir hosts are wild and domestic mammals. Pigs and wild boars are paratenic hosts in which the flukes remain immature and reside in the muscles. When human consume these meats raw, the young flukes mature into adult worms.

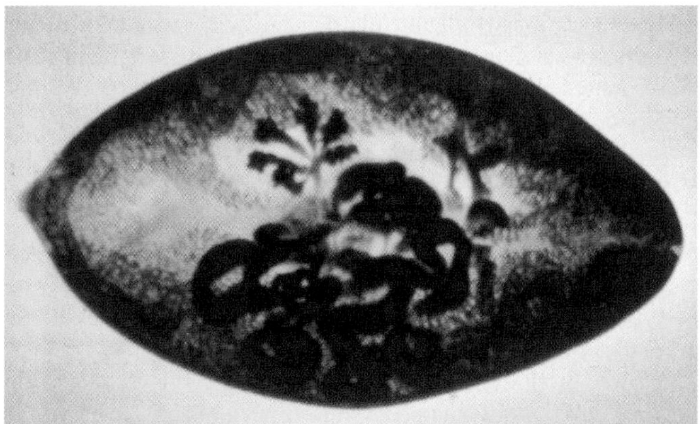

Fig. 7.11.3.1 Adult fluke of *Paragonimus westermani*, approximately 1 cm long.
(Courtesy of Mr Prayong Radamyos, Faculty of Tropical Medicine, Mahidol University, Bangkok.)

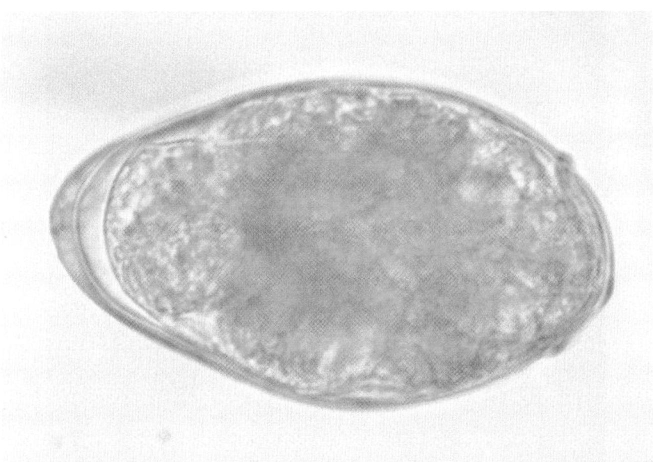

Fig. 7.11.3.2 Ovum of *Paragonimus westermani*, approximately 100 μm long.
(Courtesy of Mr Prayong Radamyos, Faculty of Tropical Medicine, Mahidol University, Bangkok.)

Pathogenesis and pathology

While they migrate, larvae cause irritation, acute inflammatory reactions, traumatic tracts, pressure effects, haemorrhage, and necrosis in affected tissues. Acute, diffuse, fibrinoexudative peritonitis may also occur. Abscess cavities containing young flukes are then formed and become enclosed in a fibrous capsule. Mature cysts adjacent to the bronchi may rupture and their contents then drain into the bronchial system. Single or multiple cysts may occur, usually in the lower lobes of the lungs.

Extrapulmonary pathological changes may be caused by aberrant migratory flukes. Cysts, abscesses, and granulomas may be found in the abdominal viscera, subcutaneous tissue, muscles, genital organs, and brain.

Epidemiology

Paragonimiasis is an important zoonosis. Humans enter the life cycle accidentally. However, in some areas, human paragonimiasis may be common enough for person-to-person transmission. Human infection is limited in its distribution to places where there are contributory factors that facilitate the life cycle: reservoir hosts, suitable environment, intermediate hosts, and permissive dietary habits. The three major foci of this disease are Asia, Africa, and Central and South America.

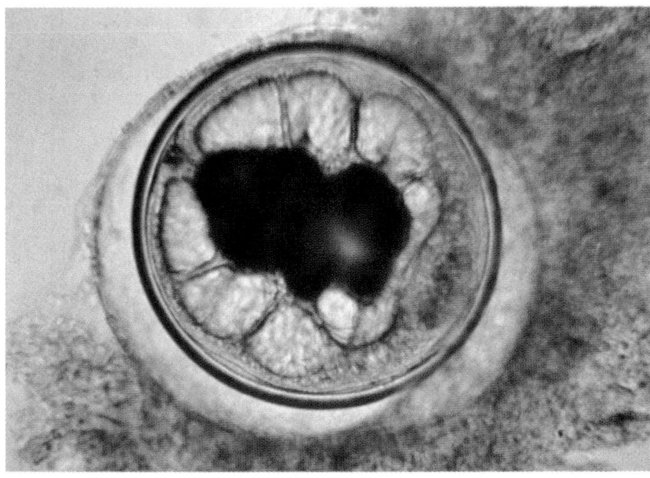

Fig. 7.11.3.3 Metacercaria of *Paragonimus westermani* in a freshwater crab.
(Courtesy of Mr Prayong Radamyos, Faculty of Tropical Medicine, Mahidol University, Bangkok.)

Clinical features

The clinical manifestations are divided into acute and chronic phases. The acute phase occurs after consumption of metacercariae. The incubation period varies from a few days to weeks. The severity of symptoms usually correlates with the worm load. Invasion and migration by young flukes cause inflammatory and allergic responses such as fever, rashes, urticaria, migratory swelling, abdominal pain, cough, and chest pain. Acute symptoms are rarely serious and usually resolve spontaneously.

Chronic manifestations may be pulmonary and extrapulmonary.

Pulmonary paragonimiasis

The most remarkable clinical feature is a chronic, productive cough with jam-like, brownish-red sputum (Fig. 7.11.3.4). Other symptoms include breathlessness and chest pain. Pleural effusion, empyema, or hydropneumothorax may occur. Occasionally, patients may experience haemoptysis following heavy work or exertion. Physical examination usually shows few abnormalities.

Extrapulmonary paragonimiasis

Aberrant migration of young flukes to other organ causes extrapulmonary paragonimiasis. The most common and important site is the central nervous system. Presentation of cerebral paragonimiasis depends on the site of the lesion. Seizures are common. Increased intracranial pressure induces persistent intense headache, nausea, vomiting, papilloedema, diplopia, and loss of visual acuity. Mental disturbances of the schizoid and paranoid type may develop. Involvement of the basal meninges results in increased intracranial pressure, hydrocephalus, arterial thrombosis, and stroke.

Involvement of intrabdominal organs such as spleen, liver, and small and large intestine causes nonspecific symptoms and signs.

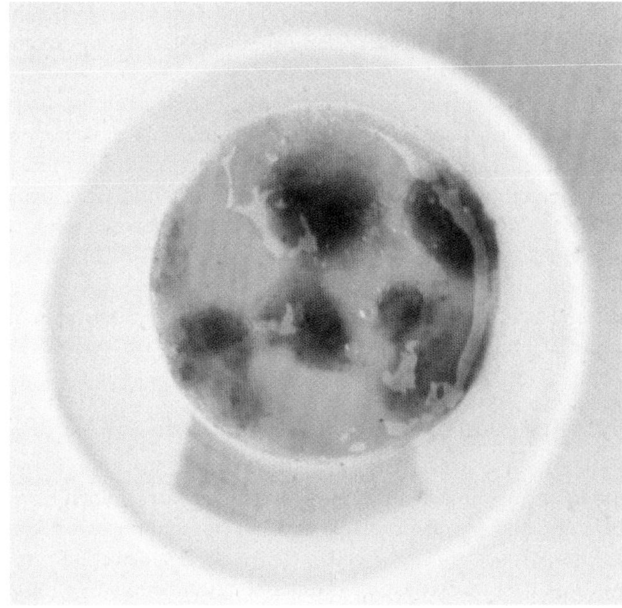

Fig. 7.11.3.4 Typical appearance of sputum coughed up by a patient with pulmonary paragonimiasis.
(Courtesy of the late Professor Sornchai Looareesuwan.)

Migratory subcutaneous nodules may occur. Spinal involvement presents with back pain, paralysis, and sensory impairment of the lower extremities.

Differential diagnosis

Pulmonary paragonimiasis should be differentiated from other conditions presenting with chronic cough productive of bloody or rusty sputum, notably pulmonary tuberculosis, bronchiectasis, lung abscess, and tumour. Paragonimiasis is frequently misdiagnosed as tuberculosis but does not respond to antituberculosis treatment. Patients usually look relatively healthy. A careful history of residence or travel to endemic areas and eating habits aids diagnosis.

Cerebral paragonimiasis should be differentiated from cerebral cysticercosis, hydatidosis, meningoencephalitis, brain abscesses, and tumours. Subcutaneous paragonimiasis may resemble gnathostomiasis, sparganosis, loiasis, or onchocerciasis.

Clinical investigation

Blood counts typically show leucocytosis with eosinophilia. Sputum is thick, gelatinous, rust-coloured or bloody. Microscopic examination shows necrotic tissue, blood, leucocytes, Charcot–Leyden crystals and ova. In pleuropulmonary paragonimiasis, examination of the pleural fluid may be pathognomonic. It is an exudate with eosinophils in variable proportions (12–75%). Typically, it has an elevated protein (6–7 g/dl), low glucose level (<10 mg/dl), low pH (<7.10) and elevated lactic dehyrogenase (>1000 U/litre). Parasite ova may be found in the pleural fluid.

A minority of symptomatic patients have normal chest radiographs. Abnormal findings include linear infiltrations, exudative pneumonia, localized pleural effusion, and nodular or cystic lesions. These lesions are found predominantly in the basilar and peripheral regions of both lower lung fields. Cysts may be single or multiple. The most characteristic radiographic feature is a ring shadow with a crescent-shaped opacity along one side of the heart shadow (Fig. 7.11.3.5). Multiple cysts may aggregate, producing a soap-bubble appearance. Other findings are pleural effusion, pleural thickening, and calcification. Fibroatelectasis resembling tuberculosis may occur.

CT is more sensitive for detecting these abnormalities. Cystic nodules are clearly seen even when they are invisible in plain radiographs (Fig. 7.11.3.6). Focal bronchiectasis is commonly found. Worm migration tracts may be identified. Paragonimiasis is one of the benign lesions that may give an increased uptake in a fluorodeoxyglucose positron emission tomography (FDG-PET) scan and can mimic malignant lung tumour.

Characteristic CT findings in cerebral paragonimiasis are conglomerate, multiple ring-shaped enhancing lesions with surrounding oedema (Fig. 7.11.3.7).

Demonstration of *Paragonimus* infection

Detection of characteristic eggs in sputum, stool, or pleural fluid confirms the diagnosis. *Paragonimus* eggs are golden brown in colour and ovoid in shape with an operculum at one end (size 80–120× 50–60μm) (see Fig. 7.11.3.2). Egg detection rate is low (28–38%) but repeating the examination results in a higher yield. Expectoration of the intact fluke is rare.

Various serological tests have been developed to aid the diagnosis. The complement fixation test is sensitive and can be used for evaluation of treatment response but it is now rarely available. Currently enzyme-linked immunosorbent assay (ELISA) and immunoblot are commonly applied for various kinds of parasitic disease. These tests are highly sensitive (90–100%) and specific (>90%). Species differentiation could be achieved by these tests. They are essential for diagnosis of extrapulmonary paragonimiasis. Positive results persist for some time after successful treatment (4–24 months) so the response to treatment cannot be evaluated.

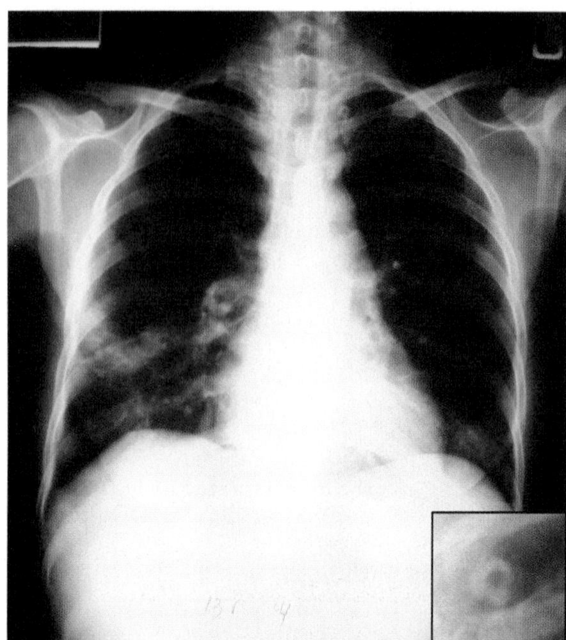

Fig. 7.11.3.5 (a) Posteroanterior radiograph of a patient with pulmonary paragonimiasis showing thick-walled cystic lesions in the right perihilar area and left upper lobe. Patchy infiltration and pleural thickening are also seen in the right lower lobe. (b) Enlargement of the left upper lobe cystic lesion.
(Copyright Dr Udomsak Silachamroon.)

Criteria for diagnosis

Definitive diagnosis can be made by demonstrating ova in sputum, stool, pleural fluid, or tissue biopsy. In cases where eggs are not

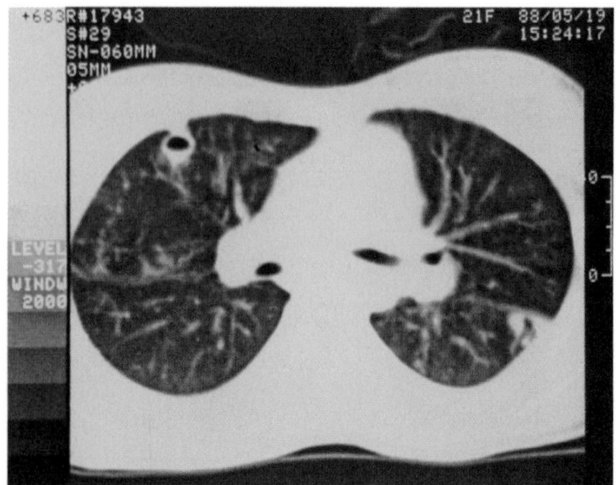

Fig. 7.11.3.6 CT scan of a patient with paragonimiasis,showing multiple cystic lesions in the subpleural region.
(Copyright Professor Sirivan Vanijanonta.)

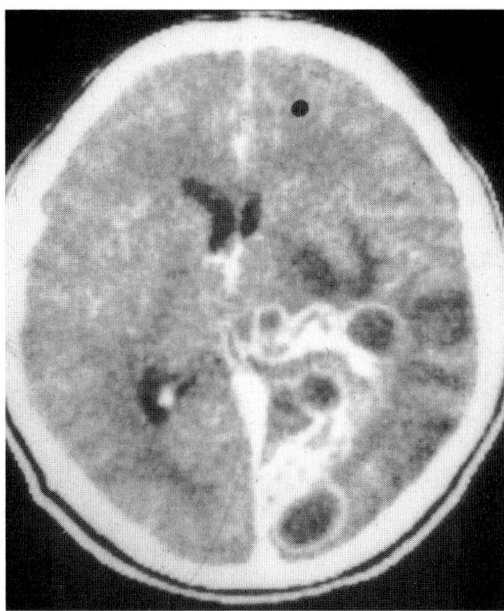

Fig. 7.11.3.7 Cerebral CT scan of a patient with paragonimiasis, showing multiple ring-shaped enhancing lesions with surrounding oedema.
(Courtesy of Professor Seung-Yull Cho, Suwon, Korea.)

detected or paragonimiasis is extrapulmonary, compatible clinical findings with positive serology are accepted as diagnostic.

Treatment

The drug of choice is praziquantel in a dose of 75 mg/kg per day in three divided doses for 2 to 3 days. A cure rate of nearly 100% has been reported in multicentre studies. Symptoms improve within a few days. Eggs disappear from the sputum in a few weeks. Radiological improvement takes months, depending on the extent and chronicity of the disease. Urticaria or transient increase in eosinophilia is occasionally seen, indicating a reaction to dead parasites. Convulsions, coma, and behavioural changes may develop during treatment of cerebral paragonimiasis as a result of brain oedema and increased intracranial pressure. Dexamethasone is suggested for this reaction. Repeated thoracentesis in combination with chemotherapy is required for patients with large pleural effusions. Chronic pleural effusion or empyema may resist chemotherapy because penetration of the drug is limited by pleural thickening. Surgical decortication may be indicated in such cases.

Triclabendazole, a drug for treatment of fascioliasis, was reported to be as effective as praziquantel for pulmonary paragonimiasis and better tolerated by the patients. When available, it may be considered as an alternative to praziquantel. Bithionol and niclofalan are also effective.

Prognosis

Pulmonary paragonimiasis is rarely fatal. The lesions may calcify or resolve completely in a few years. Cerebral paragonimiasis may cause chronic morbidity such as epilepsy, mental changes, and neurological sequelae.

Prevention and control

Effective control measures are directed towards interruption of the life cycle. However, control and eradication of intermediate hosts is impracticable; health education, changes in social and dietary customs, and the mass treatment of infected people in an endemic area are therefore more effective for prevention and control.

Further reading

Dekumyoy P, Waikagul J, Eom KS (1998). Human lung fluke *Paragonimus heterotremus*: differential diagnosis between *Paragonimus heterotremus* and *Paragonimus westermani* infection by EITB. *Trop Med Int Health*, **3**, 52–6. [Development of currently used immunoblot for diagnosis of paragonimiasis.]

Im JG, Chang K, Reeder M (1997). Current diagnostic imaging of pulmonary and cerebral paragonimiasis, with pathological correlation. *Semin Roentgenol*, **32**, 301–24. [A comprehensive review and demonstration of imaging in pulmonary and cerebral paragonimiasis.]

Keiser J, *et al.* (2005). Triclabendazole for the treatment of fascioliasis and paragonimiasis. *Expert Opin Invest Drugs*, **14**, 1513–26. [An overview of triclabendazole including phamacokinetics and phamacodynamics, toxicology and efficacy against the major food-borne trematodes.]

Keiser J, Utzinger J (2009). Food-borne trematodiases. *Clin Microbial Rev*, **22**, 466–483.

Kim TS, *et al.* (2005). Pleuropulmonary paragonimiasis: CT findings in 31 patients. *Am J Roentgenol*, **185**, 616–21. [A recent report of thin section CT scan findings in pleuropulmonary paragonimiasis.]

Kuroki M, *et al.* (2005). High-resolution computed tomography findings of *P. westermani*. *J Thorac Imaging*, **20**, 210–13. [A report of high-resolution CT findings, a useful technique for evaluating lung parenchyma in pulmonary paragonimiasis.]

Nakamura-Uchiyama F, Mukae H, Nawa Y (2002). Paragonimiasis: a Japanese perspective. *Clin Chest Med*, **23**, 409–20. [A comprehensive review of paragonimiasis from the main endemic zone.]

Romeo DP, Pollock JJ (1986). Pulmonary paragonimiasis: diagnostic value of pleural fluid analysis. *South Med J*, **79**, 241–3. [A landmark study of characteristic of pleural fluid profile in pleuropulmonary paragonimiasis.]

Vanijanonta S, Bunnag D, Harinasuta T (1984). *Paragonimus heterotremus* and other *paragonimus* spp. in Thailand: pathogenesis, clinical and treatment. *Drug Res*, **34**, 1186–8. [A review of paragonimiasis caused by *P. heterotremus*, which is prevalent in South-East Asia.]

Velez ID, Ortega JE, Velasquez LE (2002). Paragonimiasis: a view form Columbia. *Clin Chest Med*, **23**, 421–31. [A recent review of paragonimiasis from South America.]

Watanabe S, *et al.* (2003). Pulmonary paragonimiasis mimicking lung cancer on FDG-PET imaging. *Anticancer Res*, **23**, 3437–40. [The first reported case of pulmonary paragonimiasis mimicking lung cancer on FDG-PET imaging.]

7.11.4 Intestinal trematode infections

David I. Grove

Essentials

Intestinal trematode infections are widespread, but most common in Asia as a reflection of cultural culinary factors.

Echinostomiasis and fasciolopsiasis—infection of the intestines with flukes (flatworms) of the family *Echinostomatidae* is acquired by the ingestion of undercooked freshwater fish, molluscs, frogs, or vegetation. Heavy infections with these worms (2–20 mm long) may cause abdominal discomfort and diarrhoea. *Fasciolopsis buski* is a similar fluke (20–70 mm long), acquired by ingestion of contaminated water plants. Diagnosis is by finding eggs in the stool, but ova of these different species are very difficult to differentiate from each other.

Heterophyiasis (including metagonimiasis)—caused by smaller flukes (1–2 mm long), belonging to the family *Heterophyidae*. Infection is acquired by ingestion of undercooked freshwater or coastal fish. Heavy infections may cause abdominal discomfort and diarrhoea. Diagnosis is by finding heterophyid eggs in the stool, but the various species cannot be easily differentiated from each other.

Treatment and prevention—praziquantel is the drug of choice for all of these infections, which can be prevented by thoroughly cooking potentially infected foodstuffs.

Introduction

This chapter is concerned with intestinal trematode infections of humans other than intestinal schistosomiasis. These infections are widespread but are most common in Asia. This is a reflection of cultural factors, particularly the consumption of raw, undercooked, smoked, pickled or dried vectors, most frequently freshwater fish and molluscs but also water plants which contain infective forms of worms called metacercariae that may remain viable for a few days. More than 50 million people are estimated to harbour one or more species of these hermaphroditic flukes. In many instances, the extent of morbidity due to these infections is uncertain.

Diagnosis

The diagnosis of intestinal fluke infections is usually based on recovery of eggs from stools. Unfortunately, ova from species within a given family often look very similar and it may only be possible when using routine laboratory methods to identify an

Table 7.11.4.1 Intestinal trematodes belonging to the family Echinostomatidae that infect humans

Species	Geographical distribution	Definitive hosts other than humans	Source of infection	Size of adults (mm)	Size of eggs (μm)
Acanthoparyphium tyosenense (=kuragamo)	Korea	Birds	Freshwater molluscs	2–4 × 0.5–0.7	84–110 × 60–69
Artyfechinostomum mehrai (=Paryphostomum sufrartyfex)	India	Rats, pigs	Freshwater snails	4.8–8.4 × -	96 × 64
Echinochasmus fujianeusius (= liliputanus)	East Asia	Dogs. cats. foxes, pigs	Water, raw freshwater fish	1.5–2.1 × 0.47–0.56	
Echinochasmus japonicus	East Asia	Cats, dogs, rodents, chickens	Freshwater fish	0.6–0.9 × 0.16–0.18	77–90 × 51–57
Echinochasmus perfoliatus	Asia, Egypt	Cats, dogs, foxes, rats, pigs	Freshwater fish	4.0–5.5 0.85–1.1	99–125 × 58–74
Echinochasmus recurvatum	Egypt, East Asia	Birds, mammals	Amphibians, freshwater molluscs	1.9–7.3 × 0.4–0.9	88–111 × 54–75
Echinostoma cinetorchis	East Asia	Rats	Amphibians, freshwater snails	5.6–21.2 × 1.3–3.7	96–100 × 61–70
Echinostoma hortense	East Asia	Dogs, rats	Freshwater fish, amphibians	8.2–14 × 0.9–1.6	110–126 × 61–70
Echinostoma ilocanum	South-East Asia, China	Dogs, rats, mice	Freshwater snails	4–8 × 0.55–1.0	86–116 × 52–72
Echinostoma melis (= Euparyphium jassyense)	Romania, China		Tadpoles	5.5–7.5 × 1.2	132–154 × 75–85
Echinostoma echinatum (=lindoense)	Indonesia, Brazil	Rats, birds	Freshwater molluscs	13–22 × 2.5–3.0	92–124 × 65–76
Echinostoma macrorchis	Japan	Rats	Freshwater snails	3.3–4.2 × 0.68–0.86	81–89 × 54–58
Echinostoma malayanum	South-East Asia, China	Rats	Freshwater snails, tadpoles, fish	5–10 × 2.5	137 × 75.5
Echinostoma revolutum (=paraulum)	Asia	Ducks, geese, chickens, rats	Amphibians, freshwater molluscs	21–26 × 2.0–3.5	104–112 × 64–72
Episthmium caninum	Thailand	Dogs	Fish	1.0–1.5 × 0.40–0.75	84 × 50–60
Himasthla muehlensi	USA	Birds	Molluscs	11–18 × 0.41-0.67	114–149 × 62–85
Hypoderaeum conoideum	Thailand	Ducks, fowl	Amphibians, freshwater molluscs	6–12 × 1.3–2.0	95–108 × 61–68

Other echinostomes described for which few details are available include *Echinochasmus jiufoensis* and *Echinostoma angustitestis* from China, *Artyfechinostomum malayanum* from Thailand and *A. araoni* from India.

infection to family level such as a heterophyid or echinostomatid egg. Definitive identification relies upon recovery of adult worms after anthelmintic treatment. Identifying characteristics are provided in parasitology texts.

Treatment

Praziquantel has been shown to be effective with a number of these infections and is the drug of first choice. It is given in a dose of 20 mg/kg orally after a meal, perhaps repeated once or twice. Flukes are usually expelled the following day. The role of triclabendazole, perhaps in a dose of 10 mg/kg orally, in the treatment of intestinal trematodiases is not yet clear. Other alternatives which are less likely to be effective include niclosamide 150 mg/kg orally for 1 or 2 days and albendazole 200 mg orally for 2 days.

Prevention

These fluke infections can be prevented by thoroughly cooking potentially infected foodstuffs.

Echinostomiasis

This term may be conveniently used to include all infections with flukes of the family Echinostomatidae. There are more than 30 genera in this family and more than 20 species have been reported to infect humans, although some of these may be synonyms (Table 7.11.4.1). These species vary in size from 1 to 20 mm in length. Echinostomes live in the intestines of various birds and mammals. When eggs are passed in the stools and reach water, the miracidium develops, hatches and enters a snail, the first intermediate host. It then develops through the stages of sporocyst, mother rediae, and daughter rediae to release cercariae. The cercariae in turn infect second intermediate hosts which include various species of gastropod snails, bivalves, tadpoles, frogs, and fish to become encysted metacercariae, or they encyst on vegetation. Humans are infected after ingestion of inadequately cooked food containing these metacercariae.

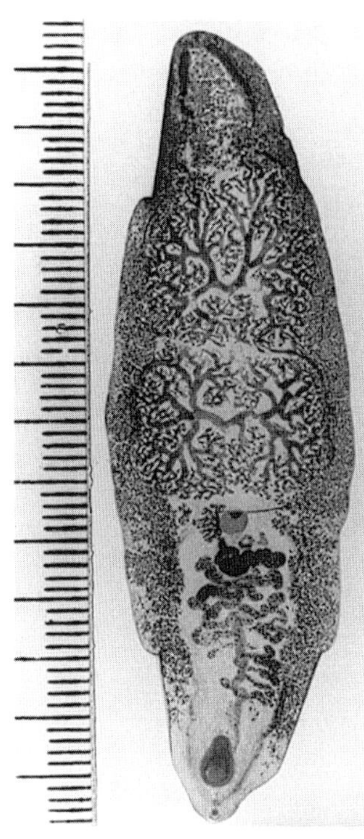

Fig. 7.11.4.2 Adult *Fasciolopsis buski*, 6.5 cm in length.
(Courtesy of P Radomyos.)

In humans, they live in the small bowel, particularly the jejunum, and attach to the mucosa where they may cause a variable amount of damage. Heavy worm loads may cause abdominal discomfort, flatulence and diarrhoea. Eggs (80–150 × 50–75 μm in size) are passed in the stools (Fig. 7.11.4.1). They are yellow-brown, ellipsoidal, thin-shelled and operculate and contain an immature embryo; they cannot be reliably differentiated from each other

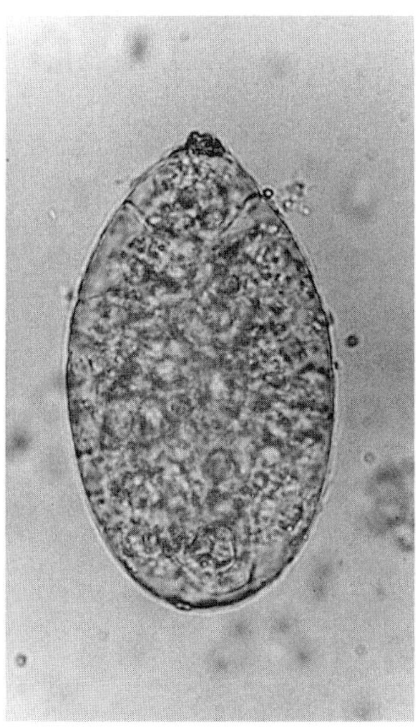

Fig. 7.11.4.1 Egg of *Echinostoma ilocanum*. All echinostome eggs look similar, as do those of *Fasciolopsis* and *Fasciola* species.
(Courtesy of P Radomyos.)

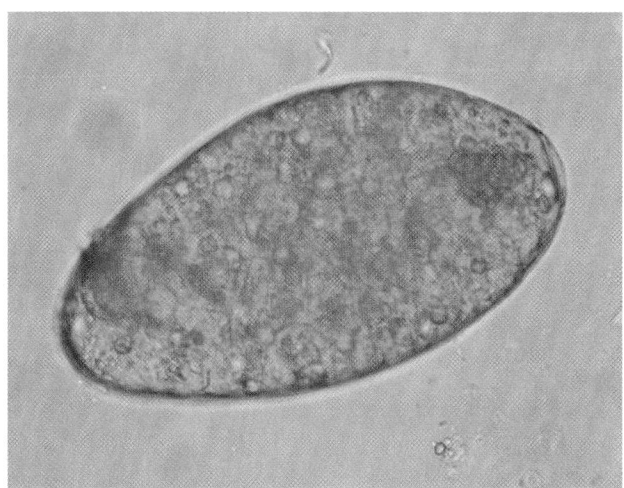

Fig. 7.11.4.3 Egg of *Fasciolopsis buski*. Note its similarity to ova of *Fasciola* species and echinostomes.
(Courtesy of A R Butcher.)

or from those of the intestinal fluke *Fasciolopsis buski* or the liver flukes *Fasciola hepatica* and *F. gigantica*.

Fasciolopsiasis

This infection, caused by *Fasciolopsis buski*, is endemic in Asia. The adult fluke (20–70 × 8–20 mm in size; Fig. 7.11.4.2) is found in the small intestine of humans and pigs. When eggs are passed in the stools and reach water, the miracidium develops, hatches, and enters the first intermediate host which is a freshwater snail, including species of *Segmentina*, *Hippeutis*, and *Gyraulis*. The miracidium then develops through the stages of sporocyst and rediae to release cercariae after 8 weeks or so. The cercariae swim out and encyst on water plants and develop into metacercariae over 4 weeks. Infection is acquired by ingestion of infected uncooked edible plants such as water caltrop (*Trapa* species), water chestnut *Eliocharis tuberosa*, water bamboo *Zizania aquatica*, and watercress *Neptunia oleracea*.

Fifty years ago it was estimated that 10 million people were infected with this parasite. The current prevalence is unknown. Fasciolopsiasis occurs most commonly in areas where people keep pigs and raise and eat freshwater plants.

Table 7.11.4.2 Intestinal trematodes belonging to the family Heterophyidae that infect humans

Species	Geographical distribution	Definitive hosts other than humans	Source of infection	Size of adults (mm)	Size of eggs (μm)
Apophallus donicus	USA	Dogs, cats, rats, foxes, rabbits	Fish	1.1–1.3 × 0.58–0.72	35 × 25
Centrocestus armatus	East Asia	Cats, dogs, rodents, herons	Fish	0.35–0.63 × 0.18–0.29	28–32 × 16–17
Centrocestus caninus	Taiwan	Dogs, cats, rats	Fish	0.4–0.45 × 0.21–0.25	32–35 × 17–20
Centrocestus cuspidatus	Egypt, Taiwan	Chickens, rats	Fish	0.5–0.8 × 0.25–0.35	30–35 × 15–20
Centrocestus formosanus	East Asia	Rats, cats, dogs, chickens, ducks	Fish, frogs	0.42–0.47 × 0.21–0.25	0.24–0.42 × 0.21–0.25
Centrocestus kurokawai	Japan	Dogs, rodents (experimental)	Fish	0.35–0.51 × 0.18–0.23	33–40 × 17–21
Centrocestus longus	Taiwan	Dogs, cats (experimental)	Fish	0.6 × 0.15	41 × 22
Cryptocotyle lingua	Greenland	Cats, dogs, rats	Fish	1.2–2.0 × 0.4–0.9	42–48 × 20–22
Diorchitrema formosanum	Taiwan	Cats, rats	Fish	0.32–0.56 × 0.13–0.21	18–24 × 12–15
Diorchitrema pseudocirratum	Hawaii, Philippines	Dogs, cats	Fish	0.3–0.6 × 0.2–0.3	18–21 × 9–12
Haplorchis microchis	Japan	Dogs, cats,	Fish	0.40–0.76 × 0.17–0.29	27–30 × 14–16
Haplorchis pleurolophocerca	Egypt	Cats	Fish	0.32–0.42 × 0.14–0.17	29–32 × 15–18
Haplorchis pumilio	South-East Asia, Egypt	Dogs, cats, birds	Fish	0.45–0.89 × 0.2–0.4	24–28 × 12–15
Haplorchis taichui	Asia	Dogs, cats	Fish	0.47–0.64 × 0.18–0.22	20–33 × 11–17
Haplorchis vanissimus	Philippines		Fish	0.38–0.51 × 0.25–0.31	25–30 × 18–21
Haplorchis yokogawai	Asia	Dogs, cats	Fish	0.47–0.64 × 0.18–0.22	20–33 × 10–17
Heterophyes heterophyes	Egypt, Asia	Cats, dogs, rats, foxes, weasels, birds	Fish	1.0–1.7 × 0.3–0.4	28–30 × 15–17
Heterophyes katsuradai	Japan	Dogs	Fish	0.61–0.89 × 0.40–0.47	25–26 × 14–15
Heterophyes nocens	East Asia	Dogs, cats, rats	Fish	0.9–1.1 × 0.4–0.5	28 × 15.5
Heterophyopsis continua	East Asia	Dogs	Fish	2.0–2.1 × 0.24–0.28	25–26 × 14–16
Metagonimus minutus	Taiwan	Cats, mice	Fish	0.43–0.50 × 0.25–0.40	21–24 × 12–15
Metagonimus miyatai	Korea		Fish	0.9–1.3 × .04–0.6	28–32 × 16–19
Metagonimus takahashii	Korea	Dogs, cats, rats, birds	Fish	0.84–1.48 × 0.42–0.72	28–34 × 17–21
Metagonimus yokogawai	Asia, Europe	Dogs, cats, pigs, pelicans	Fish	1.0–2.5 × 0.40–0.75	26–28 × 15–17
Phagicola sp.	Brazil	Dogs	Fish		
Procerovum calderoni	Philippines	Cats, dogs	Fish	0.47–0.55 × 0.25–0.26	21–25 × 11–15
Procerovum varium	Japan	Cats, birds	Fish	0.26–0.38 × 0.13–0.16	25–29 × 12–18
Pygidiopsis summa	Korea	Birds, cats, dogs, rats	Fish	0.49–0.76 × 0.25–0.44	21–23 × 11–14
Stellantchasmus (=Diorchitrema) amplicaecus	Taiwan	Dogs, cats, birds	Fish	0.45–0.65 × 0.20–0.34	22–24 × 8–14
Stellantchasmus falcatus	Asia, Hawaii	Dogs, cats	Fish	0.59 × 0.23	21–23 × 12–13
Stictodora fuscata	East Asia	Cats, birds	Fish	0.59 × 0.23	36–38 × 22–23
Stictodora lari	Korea	Seagulls	Fish	0.70–0.86 × 0.27–0.36	28–37 × 17–20

The adult worms attach themselves to the mucosa of the upper small bowel where they may cause inflammation and erosion and provoke a mucous intestinal discharge. Light infections are generally asymptomatic but heavy worm burdens may be associated with anorexia, nausea, abdominal discomfort and diarrhoea, or even intestinal obstruction. Stools may be foul-smelling and contain undigested food. In marked cases, a protein-losing enteropathy is associated with ascites, generalized oedema and prostration.

Eggs (130–140 × 80–85 μm in size) are passed in the stools (Fig. 7.11.4.3). They are yellow-brown, ellipsoid, thin-shelled and operculate and contain an immature embryo; they cannot be reliably differentiated from those of the intestinal echinostomes or of the liver flukes *F. hepatica* and *F. gigantica*.

Heterophyiasis

This term may be conveniently used to include all infections with flukes of the family Heterophyidae, although some infections are more precisely known by the generic name of the infecting organism, e.g. metagonimiasis. These are small flukes, generally less than 1 to 2 mm in length. So far 32 species in this family have been reported to infect humans (Table 7.11.4.2). These infections are found in many places but are most common in Asia and Egypt. *Metagonimus yokogawai* is believed to be the most common heterophyid infection.

Heterophyids live in the intestines of various mammals and birds. When eggs are passed in the stools, they contain a ciliated miracidium which hatches when ingested by a freshwater or brackish-water snail, the first intermediate host. Snails susceptible to *Heterophyes* include *Pirenella conica, Cerithidea cingulata,* and *Tympanotonus micropterus* while *Semisulcospira libertina* and *Thiara granifera* are host to *Metagonimus*. The miracidium then develops through the stages of sporocyst and one or two generations of rediae to release cercariae. The cercariae in turn infect various species of freshwater or coastal salmonoid and cyprinoid fish as the second intermediate hosts. These include mullet (e.g. *Mugil cephalus*) and minnow (*Gambusia* species) for *Heterophyes* species, and carp (e.g. *Carassius carrasius*) and sweet fish *Plecoglossus altivelis* in the case of *Metagonimus* species. Humans are infected after ingestion of inadequately cooked fish containing metacercariae, which mature in the flesh or scales of the fish.

The adult worms attach to or invade the mucosa of the upper small bowel where they may cause granulomatous inflammation and erosion. Light infections are generally asymptomatic but heavy worm burdens may be associated with anorexia, nausea, abdominal discomfort and mucous diarrhoea. Occasionally ova deposited in the bowel wall enter blood vessels and embolize to other tissues. Eggs have been found in the heart and central nervous system and rarely in the blood. In cases of heterophyiasis described in the Philippines, cardiac failure was associated with subepicardial haemorrhages, myocardial damage caused by occlusion of vessels by ova, and eggs stuck to a thickened, calcified mitral valve. Neurological features include focal cerebral disturbances and transverse myelitis.

Eggs (20–40 × 10–20 μm in size) are passed in the stools (Fig. 7.11.4.4). They are yellow-brown, elongated, operculate, and contain a miracidium. Eggs of members of the family Heterophyidae cannot be reliably differentiated from each other. Furthermore, they are extremely difficult to differentiate from eggs of *Clonorchis sinensis* and *Opisthorchis* species although heterophyids tend to have a smoother egg shell and a less prominent shoulder at the operculum, and the abopercular knob may be absent.

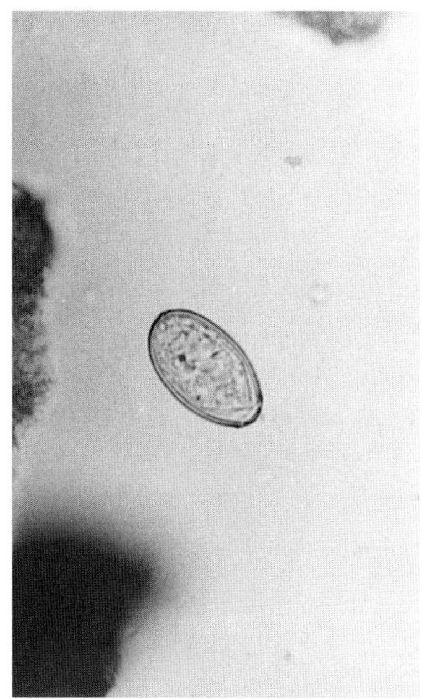

Fig. 7.11.4.4 Egg of *Metagonimus yokogawai*. All heterophyid eggs look similar, as do those of *Clonorchis sinensis* and *Opisthorchis viverrini*.
(Courtesy of P Radomyos.)

Table 7.11.4.3 Families of intestinal trematodes containing species that are uncommon human pathogens

Species	Geographical distribution	Definitive hosts other than humans	Source of infection	Size of adults (mm)	Size of eggs (μm)
Brachylaimidae					
Brachylaima cribbi	South Australia	Mice, birds	Land snails	6–12 × 0.3–0.5	28–30 × 16–17
Gastrodiscidae					
Gastrodiscoides hominis	Asia, Nigeria	Pigs, rats, monkeys, deer	Water plants	4–8 × 3–4	150 × 72
Gastrothylacidae					
Fischoederius elongatus	China	Ruminants	Aquatic plants	9–20 × 3–6	110–140 × 60–80
Gymnophallidae					
Gymnophalloides seoi	Korea	Birds	Oysters	0.4–0.5 × 0.2–0.3	20–25 × 11–15

(Continued)

Table 7.11.4.3 (*Cont'd*) Families of intestinal trematodes containing species that are uncommon human pathogens

Species	Geographical distribution	Definitive hosts other than humans	Source of infection	Size of adults (mm)	Size of eggs (μm)
Lecithodendriidae					
Phaneropsulus bonnei	Thailand, Indonesia	Bats, monkeys	Dragonflies	0.48–0.78 × 0.22–0.35	27–29 × 10–12
Phaneropsulus spinicirrus	Thailand			0.55–0.76 × 0.43–0.63	27–33 × 13–16
Prosthodendrium molenkampi	Thailand, Indonesia	Bats, monkeys, rats	Dragonflies, damselflies		30 × 15
Microphallidae					
Spelotrema (=Carneophallus) brevicaeca	Philippines	Birds	Crabs	0.5–0.7 × 0.3–0.4	15–16 × 9–10
Nanophyetidae (= Troglotrematidae)					
Nanophyetus salmincola (= schickhobalowi)	Russia, North America	Dogs, foxes, birds	Fish	1–2 × 0.3–0.5	80 × 40
Neodiplostomidae					
Neodiplostomum (=Fibricola) seoulensis	Korea	Freshwater snails	Frogs, snakes		
Paramphistomatidae					
Watsonius watsoni	Southern Africa	Monkeys	Water plants?	8–10 × 4–5	120–130 × 75–80
Plagiorchidae					
Plagiorchis harinasutai	Thailand		Insect larvae	1.75–1.87 × 0.60–0.65	32–34 × 16–18
Plagiorchis javensis	Indonesia	Birds, bats	Insect larvae	1.8 × 0.7	36 × 22–24
Plagiorchis muris	Japan	Birds, dogs, rats	Snails, aquatic insects	0.8–2.0 × 0.24–0.84	36 × 21
Plagiorchis philippinensis	Philippines	Birds, rats	Insect larvae	1.5–2.0 × 0.39–0.44	28–30 × 19–21
Strigeidae					
Cotylurus japonicus	China	Birds	Snails		

Other intestinal fluke infections

There are another dozen or so species of intestinal flukes belonging to various families that have been reported to infect humans (Table 7.11.4.3). Diagnosis is suggested by finding eggs in the faeces (e.g. Fig. 7.11.4.5) but as with other fluke infections, definitive diagnosis depends upon recovery of the adult worms; this is most commonly achieved by treatment with praziquantel. *Gastrodiscoides hominis* is unusual in that it attaches to the mucosa of the large bowel.

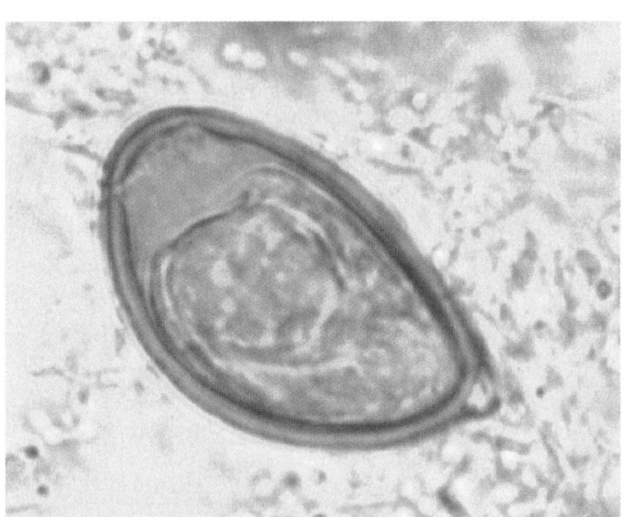

Fig. 7.11.4.5 Egg of *Brachylaima cribbi*.
(Courtesy of A R Butcher)

Further reading

Chai JY, Shin EH, Lee SH, Rim HS (2009). Foodborne intestinal flukes in Southeast Asia. *Korean J Parasitol*, **47**, Suppl S69–S102.

Fried B (2001). Biology of echinostomes except *Echinostoma*. *Adv Parasitol*, **49**, 163–210.

Fried B, Gradczyk TK, Tamang L (2004). Food-borne intestinal trematodiases in humans. *Parasitol Res*, **93**, 159–70.

Keiseer J, Utzinger J (2004). Chemotherapy for major food-borne trematodes: a review. *Expert Opin Pharmacother*, **5**, 1711–26.

Keiseer J, Utzinger J (2009). Food-borne trematodiases. *Clin Microbial Rev*, **22**, 466–483.

Macpherson CN (2005). Human behaviour and the epidemiology of parasitic zoonoses. *Int J Parasitol*, **35**, 1319–31.

Mas-Coma S, Bargues MD, Valero MA. (2005). Fascioliasis and other plant-borne trematode zoonoses. *Int J Parasitol*, **35**, 1255–78.

Muller R (2002). The trematodes. In: *Worms and human disease*, 2nd edition, pp. 3–62. CABI Publishing, Wallingford.

Photographs of various stages of these parasites and diagrams of life cycles may be found at several excellent websites, e.g.: Centers for Disease Control and Prevention. http://www.dpd.cdc.gov/DPDx/HTML/Image_Library.htm

Korean Society for Parasitology. http://www.atlas.or.kr

7.12

Nonvenomous arthropods

J. Paul

Essentials

Most medically important arthropods are insects (including mosquitoes, midges, other flies, bedbugs and other true bugs, lice, fleas, and cockroaches) or arachnids (spiders, ticks, mites, scorpions).

Clinical features

Arthropod-related problems include the following: (1) injuries from direct contact (bites, stings, and other penetrating or crushing injuries from spines, bristles, or pincers) and the consequences of such contact (envenoming, allergic reactions, secondary infection of wounds, and transmission of infectious agents); (2) infestation of the patient's body, skin, hair, clothes, or immediate environment (myiasis, canthariasis, tungosis, pediculosis etc.); (3) inhalant allergy; (4) hygiene and aesthetic issues; and (5) the psychological phenomena of delusion and phobia.

Treatment and prevention—general aspects

Broad principles of management include: (1) Identification of the problem and the kind of arthropod involved. (2) The immediate treatment—if necessary—of allergic reactions or secondary infection. (3) Appreciation of consequences of exposure, such as transmission of infectious agents; many species of dipterans (flies)—including mosquitoes, blackflies, sand flies, tsetse flies, and horse flies—bite humans, and in some regions some of these are important vectors. (4) Use of antimalarials or vaccines and the development of strategies to avoid further contact, including eradication of infestations, changes in behavior, use of repellents and clothing that covers the skin, and bed nets. Travellers and their clinicians should be aware of the risks posed by arthropod-borne infections and ways to prevent them in particular geographical areas.

Particular conditions

True bugs (Hemiptera)—bedbugs infest dwellings and bite at night: patients may complain of mysterious skin lesions and sleeplessness, and a special search may be necessary to find the bugs. In South America, triatomine bugs bite at night and are vectors of trypanosomiasis.

Ticks (Ixodoidea)—these attach themselves while feeding and are noticed by the patient. They are important vectors of many infections, which are often specific to particular genera or species of tick and confined to particular geographical areas. In Europe, tick-related infections include Lyme borreliosis and tick-borne encephalitis.

Infestations—clinically important infestations include the following. (1) Scabies (infestation of the skin by scabies mites) and pediculosis (infestation of the hair or clothing by head or body lice)—these are cosmopolitan in distribution and usually managed by use of topical acaricides or insecticides, although resistance is a growing problem. (2) Fleas—the human flea is now rare in the developed world, but infestation of dwellings with cat fleas is commonly reported. Tungosis is a condition of tropical areas where jigger fleas (not to be confused with similarly named trombiculid mites) burrow into the feet or under the toenails of those who walk about barefoot. (3) Fly and beetle larvae—myiasis, which is the infestation of the body by the larvae (maggots) of dipteran flies, is classified as (a) benign when self-limiting or malign when there is destructive tissue invasion, (b) according to anatomical site (dermal, wound, orbital, ophthalmic, urogenital, intestinal), and (c) according to the species involved. Canthariasis—infestation of the body by beetles or beetle larvae—is clinically similar to myiasis and is rarely reported.

Other aspects—some synanthropic insects, especially certain species of fly, cockroach, and pharaoh's ants, have been implicated in the passive transmission of infections, e.g. shigellosis and hepatitis A. It is generally considered to be in the interests of good hygiene to control these insects in health care settings or where food is prepared.

Introduction

Most arthropods are harmless, but there is a select group of medically significant species. Invertebrates with jointed limbs belong to the phylum Arthropoda. Most of the medically important arthropods are in the classes Insecta (insects) or Arachnida (spiders, ticks, mites, scorpions). Some members of the class Chilopoda (centipedes) may bite humans, and some of the larger members of the Crustacea (crabs, lobsters) may cause injury with pincers or spines. Although they are classified as a separate group, phylum Pentastomida, there is some evidence that the parasitic tongueworms may actually be highly specialized crustaceans (Chapter 7.13). Categories of medical significance include: envenoming by bites or stings (Chapters 5.3 and 9.2); allergic reactions to bites, stings, hairs, or inhaled allergens; transmission of infectious agents; infestation; the pain and trauma from bites or penetrating spines; phobia and delusory parastitosis. Arthropods may cause nuisance by their presence or the noises they may make, or by being perceived as unhygienic. To allow a logical approach to the management of arthropod-related issues it is helpful to identify the species involved, although as this may not always be possible, generic approaches may be developed to the management of problems.

Bites

Arthropod bites are common and often trivial but bites may be important when associated with envenoming (Chapter 9.2), sensitization (leading to pruritus, excoration, and secondary infection), anaphylaxis, or the transmission of infectious agents. Biting insects may simply be a nuisance: e.g. it may be difficult to tolerate swarms of biting flies, making it difficult to work outdoors and dangerous to operate machinery. Immune response varies with age, past exposure, and other factors. Management may be directed towards treatment of the bite, if necessary (topical corticosteroids, systemic antihistamines), considering the risk of transmitted infection and prevention of further bites (eradication of ectoparasites, change in behaviour to avoid exposure, repellents, special clothing, insecticide-impregnated bed nets). It is often possible to associate bites with infesting ectoparasites, such as arthropods which remain attached (ticks) or predatory bloodsuckers that are highly visible (mosquitoes, midges, and blackflies, when swarming) and which cause immediately painful bites (tsetse flies, some mosquitoes, tabanid flies). In is harder to ascribe a cause to bites from arthropods which bite at night or when the patient is asleep (some mosquitoes, sand flies, bedbugs, triatomine bugs) or from arthropods that are inconspicuous and do not cause immediately painful bites (harvest mites, some fleas, some biting flies). Bites of larger arthropods typically have a central punctum and a surrounding area of inflammation and are pruritic. In cases of uncertainty it may be necessary to obtain a dermatological opinion to exclude other diagnoses, including organic disorders, artefact and delusion.

Blood-sucking flies (Diptera)

Many flies are haematophagous (Table 7.12.1). Most blood-sucking flies are in the suborder Nematocera (mosquitoes, sand flies, blackflies, biting midges) and family Tabanidae of the suborder Brachycera (horse flies, deer flies, clegs). The tsetse flies, *Glossina* spp., are in the suborder Cyclorrhapha. Parasitic louse-like flies known as keds, such as the deer ked *Lipoptena cervi*, have been placed in a separate group, Pupipara, although they are considered by many authors to be specialized members of the Cyclorrhapha. All blood-sucking flies are at least a nuisance: the bites are often painful and associated with sensitization. More important, biting flies may transmit infection. Mosquitoes (Culicidae) are vectors of filariasis and numerous viral diseases, including yellow fever and

Table 7.12.1 Blood-sucking flies

Family	Representative genera (and species)	Associated agent or condition
Suborder Nematocera		
Culicidae (mosquitoes)		
Subfamily Anophelinae	*Anopheles*	Malaria, brugian and bancroftian filariasis
Subfamily Culicinae	*Culiseta*	Western equine encephalitis
	Culex	Bancroftian filariasis
	Mansonia	Brugian filariasis
	Aedes	Eastern equine encephalitis, dengue fever, yellow fever, bancroftian filariasis
	Haemagogus	Yellow fever
	Sabethes	Yellow fever
Phlebotomidae (sand flies)	*Phlebotomus*	*Leishmania* spp.
	Lutzomyia	*Leishmania* spp., *Bartonella bacilliformis*
Simuliidae (blackflies)	*Simulium*	*Onchocerca volvulus, Mansonella ozzardi*, haemorrhagic syndrome of Altimira
Ceratopogonidae (biting midges)	*Culicoides*	*Dipetalonema perstans, Mansonella ozzardi*
Suborder Brachycera		
Tabanidae (horse flies, clegs)	*Haematopota*	
	Tabanus	
	Pangonia	
	Chrysops	*Loa loa*
Rhagionidae (snipe flies)	*Symphoromyia*	
	Atherix	
	Spaniopsis	
	Austroleptis	
Suborder Cyclorrhapha		
Glossinidae (tsetse flies)	*Glossina*	African trypanosomiaisis
Calliphoridae (Congo floor maggot)	*Auchmeromyia luteola*	
Muscidae	*Stomoxys calcitrans* (stable fly)	
Hippoboscidae	*Melophagus ovinus* (sheep ked)	
	Lipoptena cervi (deer ked)	

dengue fever. Mosquitoes of the genus *Anopheles* transmit malaria. Depending on species and location, mosquitoes bite at various times of the day. Mosquitoes may be controlled by reducing their access to stagnant water needed for development of their larval stages and by application of insecticides to dwellings. Use of permethrin-impregnated bed nets has been shown to reduce malaria transmission. Sand flies (Phlebotominae) are mainly tropical and subtropical in distribution and transmit leishmaniasis. In South America, sand flies of the genus *Lutzomyia* transmit *Bartonella bacilliformis*. Blackflies (Simuliidae) occur worldwide and are vectors of *Onchocerca volvulus* and *Mansonella ozzardi*. Blackfly larvae require well-oxygenated water. Female blackflies pierce the skin and suck blood from the edge of the puncture. Substances in blackfly saliva inhibit platelet aggregation, impair the final common pathway of the coagulation cascade, and encourage vasodilatation. The bites, oozing blood, have a characteristic appearance and may be associated with severe reaction, sometimes referred to as simuliosis or simuliotoxicosis. Puncture sites often become surrounded by a wide zone of haemorrhagic erythema and oedema. Rarely, haemorrhagic shock may occur. In Brazil, the haemorrhagic syndrome of Altimira has been epidemiologically associated with exposure to blackflies. Blackfly saliva appears to contain immunomodulating substances. In Brazil, the autoimmune condition 'fogo selvagem' (a form of pemphigus foliaceus) occurs in simuliid-infested areas (Fig. 7.12.1a). In Britain, blackflies are rarely troublesome to man except in certain localities. In southern England, the Blandford fly, *Simulium posticatum* occurs on the river Stour, Dorset, on tributaries of the river Thames in Oxfordshire, and on other rivers. In 1993, 16% (22% female, 9% male) of Blandford's inhabitants reported bites. Use of the biological larvicide *Bacillus thuringiensis* as a control measure was associated with a marked drop in the number of people complaining of bites. In Scotland, *S. reptans*, *S. argyreatum*, and other species may bite humans.

Biting midges (Ceratopgonidae) are vectors of the filarial worms *Mansonella (Dipetalonema) perstans* and *M. ozzardi*. In Africa, tabanid flies transmit *Loa loa*. Tsetse flies are vectors of African trypanosomiasis (see Chapter 7.8.10). Deer keds *Lipoptena cervi* are highly evolved louse-like flies with biting mouth parts that feed on deer. Occasionally, deer keds bite people, such as forest workers, hunters, or entomologists (Fig. 7.12.1b). Deer ked dermatitis is a condition where itchy papules exist for weeks to months at the site of bites. Eventually, papules resolve without specific treatment. Recently, it has been suggested that *Bartonella schoenbuchensis* may have a role in the aetiology of the conditions as this agent has been detected in roe deer and in deer keds but not as yet from humans.

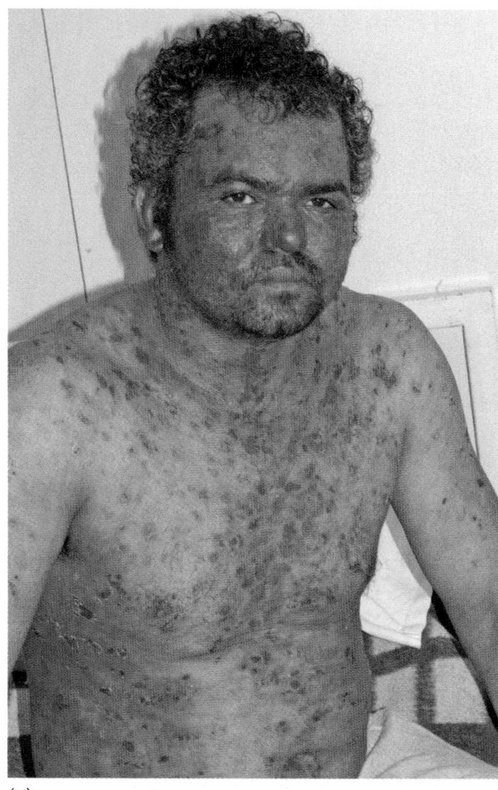

(a)

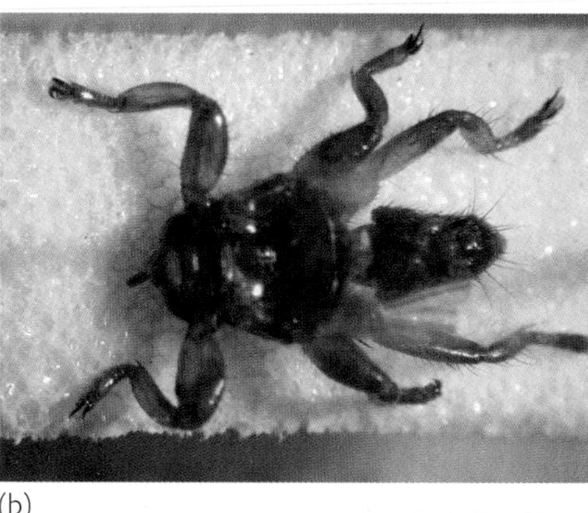

(b)

Fig. 7.12.1 (a) Endemic Pemphigus foliaceus ('fogo selvagem' meaning 'wild fire') in a man from a rural area of São Paulo State, Brazil infested with Simulium flies. (b) Deer ked or deer fly without wings (*Lipoptena cervi* Diptera, Hippoboscidae). (a) (Copyright DA Warrell.) (b) (Copyright J Paul.)

Prevention

When visiting locations where biting flies are troublesome, bites may be avoided to some extent by wearing clothing that covers the skin and by use of repellents.

True bugs (Hemiptera)

Bedbugs

The common bedbug *Cimex lectularius* (Fig. 7.12.2) is cosmopolitan. In recent years, reports of infestations in developed countries such as the United Kingdom have increased. Infestation may be unrelated to lack of general hygiene but associated with translocation of personal effects or furniture. The tropical bedbug *C. hemipterus* occurs in tropical and subtropical countries. Epidemiological studies have failed to produce clear evidence of bedbugs as vectors of infections, such as hepatitis B. They are nocturnal, hiding during the day and feeding at night. Although in some cases bites may go unnoticed and there may be no allergic reaction, bedbugs may cause sleeplessness and the bites may cause pain and swelling and, exceptionally, disseminated bullous eruptions (Fig. 7.12.3). Rooms that are heavily infested may acquire an unpleasant odour. Bugs may be found by making special searches at night or by seeking their hiding places during the day. They resemble lentils superficially, being round and flat. Adults reach a length of about 5 mm. Nymphs pass through five instars to reach adulthood after about 4 months. Bedbugs can live for 6 months without feeding, becoming paper-thin. Related bugs which occasionally bite humans derive

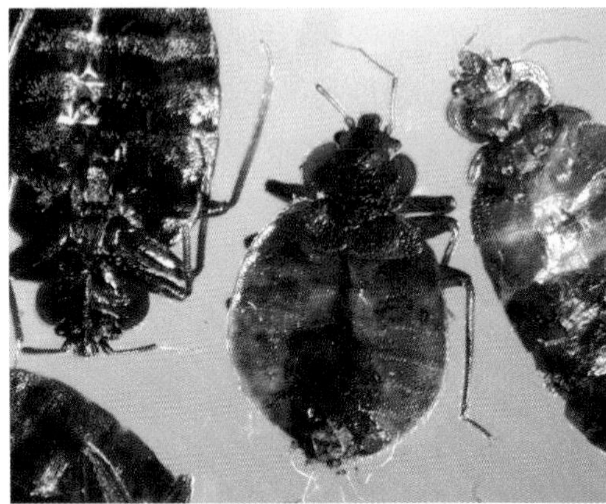

Fig. 7.12.2 Bedbugs *Cimex lectularus*.
(Copyright J Paul.)

from pigeons, bats, and martins (*C. columbarius*, *C. pipistrelli*, and *Oeciacus hirundinis* respectively). Infestation may be managed by restricting access of host species to dwellings, but in the United Kingdom, for example, bats are protected under the Wildlife and Countryside Act.

Prevention Bites are discouraged by keeping the light on all night, sleeping under a permethrin-impregnated mosquito net, and putting newspaper under the undersheet. Eradication is by thorough cleaning of the environment and application of residual insecticides. Sheets should be steam cleaned or exposed to the sun and treated with insecticide. However, insecticide resistance has developed and bedbugs are becoming more abundant.

Cone-nose bugs

Most of the 129 species of cone-nose bugs (family Reduviidae, subfamily Triatominae) occur in the Americas. Seven species occur in Asia and one species, *Triatoma rubrofasciata*, is cosmotropical. Many triatomines are obligate feeders on the blood of vertebrates. Triatomines transmit South American trypanosomiasis. Important vector species are *Rhodnius prolixus*, *T. infestans*, *T. brasiliensis*, *T. dimidiata*, and *Panstrongylus megistus*. The bugs infest dwellings, hiding in crevices during the day and biting at night. Dwellings may be heavily infested: in Columbia, 11 403 specimens of *R. prolixus* were reported from a house occupied by 9 people, all of whom were seropositive for trypanosomiasis. As well as transmitting trypanosomiasis, triatomines may cause significant blood loss to occupants of infested buildings.

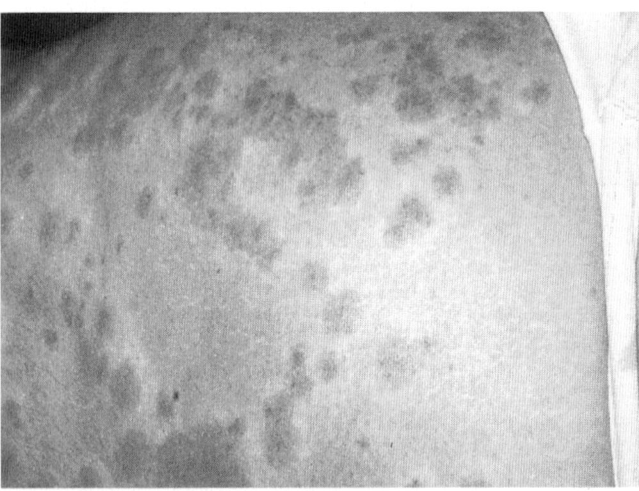

Fig. 7.12.3 Erythematous macules of bedbugs.
(Courtesy of D Hill, Adelaide, South Australia.)

Prevention Dwellings are deinfested with insecticides and constructed to offer few hiding places for the bugs (Chapter 7.8.11).

Ticks (Ixodoidea)

Hard ticks (Ixodidae) and soft ticks (Argasidae) occur worldwide. Stages of the life-cycle are egg, larva (six-legged), and nymph and adult (both eight-legged). Ticks attach and feed with a barbed hypostome and detach when engorged. Smaller stages and ticks in inconspicuous sites, such as the perineum may feed unobserved. Bites are usually painless but may result in local sensitization, secondary infection, and transmission of infectious agents, including numerous viruses, rickettsias, and Lyme disease (Table 7.12.2). Local reaction to bites may be confused with erythema migrans of Lyme disease, (which expands as a ring with a central punctum—see Chapter 7.6.32). Ticks may be removed by gripping with forceps (or, in the field, with finger and thumbnail), between the skin and the tick's head and pulling gently. Special tools for removing ticks have been made widely available by the pet industry and such devices should work just as well with humans. Toothed devices

Table 7.12.2 Ticks and tick-borne diseases

Genus and species	Geographical distribution	Associated infections
Argasidae (soft ticks)		
Ornithodoros spp.	Widely distributed	Endemic relapsing fever
Ixodidae (hard ticks)		
Amblyomma hebraeum	Africa	Tick typhus
Amblyomma cajennense	Americas	Rocky mountain spotted fever
Dermacentor andersoni	North America	Colorado tick fever, Rocky Mountain spotted fever
Dermacentor marginatus	Palaearctic	Tick typhus, Omsk haemorrhagic fever
Dermacentor silvarum	Eastern Palaearctic	Tick typhus, tick-borne encephalitis
Dermacentor variabilis	North America	Rocky Mountain spotted fever
Haemaphysalis concinna	Palaearctic	Tick typhus
Haemaphysalis spinigera	India	Kyasanur Forest disease
Haemaphysalis turturis	India	Kyasanur Forest disease
Hyalomma spp.	Old World	Crimean-Congo haemorrhagic fever
Ixodes scapularis	Eastern North America	Lyme disease
Ixodes pacificus	Western North America	Lyme disease
Ixodes ricinus	Western Palaearctic	Lyme disease, tick-borne encephalitis, louping ill
Ixodes persulcatus	Eastern Palaearctic	Tick-borne encephalitis, Omsk haemorrhagic fever
Rhipicephalus sanguineus	Cosmopolitan	Tick typhus

that work in the manner of combs or forceps that are curved in profile (tick tweezers) have the advantage of allowing removal while avoiding squeezing the tick. Careless removal may detach the head or hypostome, leaving a potential source of inflammation and secondary infection. In the United Kingdom, the ticks most often found on humans are the sheep tick *Ixodes ricinus* (a vector of Lyme disease) and the hedgehog tick *I. hexagonus* (Fig. 7.12.4).

Prevention

When visiting tick-infested places, bites may be avoided by tucking trousers into boots and wearing light-coloured clothing which makes ticks highly visible. After visiting tick-infested habitats, searches of the body allows prompt removal of ticks which reduces the chance of disease transmission.

Harvest mites (Trombiculidae)

In the United Kingdom, larvae of the harvest mite *Neotrombicula autumnalis* are a common cause of bites in late summer, especially in chalk downland. They are tiny and seldom noticed, crawling rapidly on to the body, attaching (often under tight-fitting clothes), injecting proteolytic enzymes, feeding on tissue fluid and then detaching, leaving pruritic, sometimes bullous lesions hours later. For many victims, the cause of irritation remains a mystery. Red bugs or chiggers (confusingly, a term also applied to the flea *Tunga penetrans*) are names given to trombiculids in the Americas. Bites to the penis, associated with swelling and dysuria, have been described in the paediatric literature as 'summer penile syndrome'. In Asia, trombilucids are vectors of scrub typhus.

Prevention

Where trombiculids are troublesome, tucking trousers into boots and applying diethyltoluamide or other repellents may be partially effective. Notorious 'mite islands' densely infested with trombiculids in cleared areas of jungle should be avoided.

Accidental bites

Arthropods which do not normally bite humans but can inflict painful but usually trivial bites when provoked by handling, e.g. by children and entomologists, include predatory true bugs such as the water boatman *Notonecta glauca* and the assassin bug *Reduvius personatus* in the United Kingdom and wheel bugs *Arilus* spp. in the Americas; larger beetles (Coleoptera); dragonflies (Odonata); and bush-crickets (Orthoptera) such as the wartbiter *Decticus verrucivorus*.

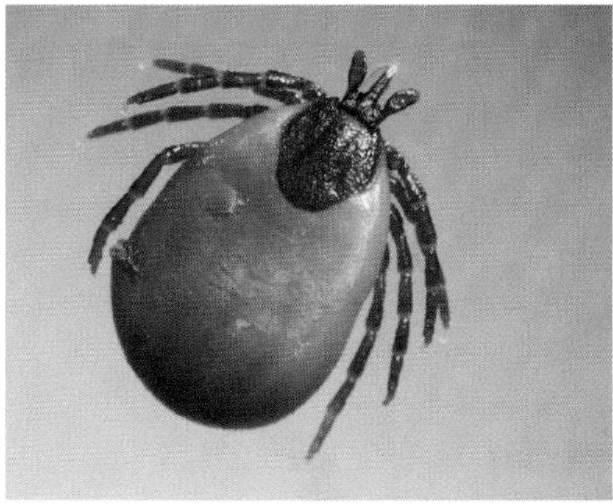

Fig. 7.12.4 Upperside of hedgehog tick *Ixodes hexagonus*, to show sucking mouthparts (hypostome).
(Copyright J Paul.)

Spines used in defence by the great silver diving beetle *Hydrous piceus* and larger tropical grasshoppers of the subfamily Cyrtacanthridinae can cause penetrating injury when handled. Pincers of larger crabs and lobsters (Crustacea) can cause crushing injuries of digits and their spines may cause penetrating injury.

Infestation

Sites of infestation include the hair, body surface, and immediate environment (ectoparasites: lice, fleas); the skin and subdermis (scabies, tungosis, dermal myiasis); wounds, tissues and orifices (myiasis); and the gastrointestinal tract (myiasis, canthariasis). With ectoparasites, the main problems are related to their bites: diagnosis and management may be based on the identification of the ectoparasite.

Delusory parasitosis is a condition in which the patient becomes convinced of infestation by parasites despite reassurance by the doctor and absence of clinical or laboratory evidence.

Scabies

The agent of human scabies, a chronic infestation, is the human scabies mite *Sarcoptes scabiei* var. *hominis*. Scabies mites adapted to other hosts, such as *Sarcoptes scabiei* var. *canis*, cause a self-limiting pruritus in humans. Clinical manifestations of scabies are caused by the adult female mite that burrows through the epidermis. The adult female is oval and about 0.33 mm long (Fig. 7.12.5). The female lives for about 1 month, burrowing and ovipositing daily. The burrow may extend to 1 cm in length. Six-legged larvae hatch after a few days and moult to become eight-legged nymphs and later eight-legged adults. Adult males are smaller than females, do not burrow, and die after mating on the epidermis. Scabies is cosmopolitan in distribution. Prevalence rates vary but may be

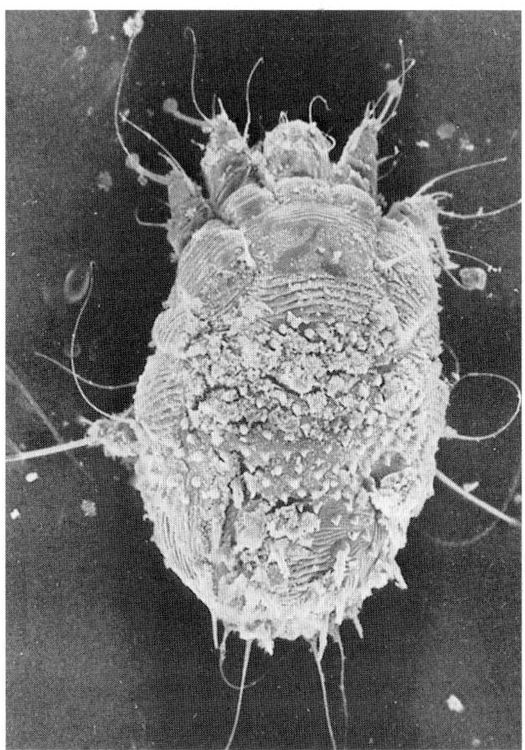

Fig. 7.12.5 Adult specimen of *Sarcoptes scabei*.
(Courtesy of R V Southcott, Adelaide, South Australia.)

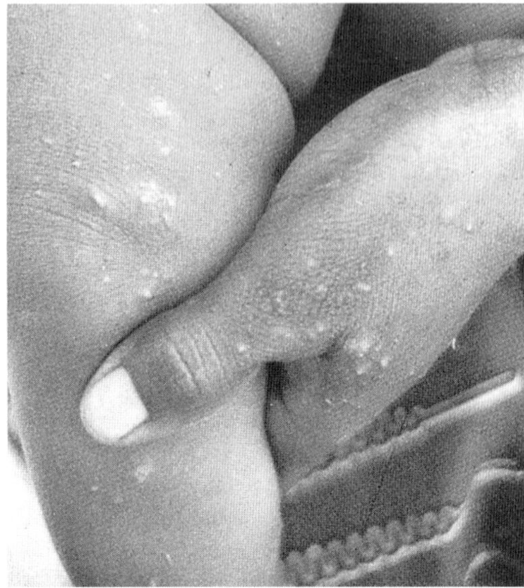

Fig. 7.12.6 Secondarily infected scabies in mother and child.

higher in conditions of overcrowding and following social disruption in wartime. Outbreaks may occur in nursing homes and hospitals. Most cases must be acquired by close contact, as the mites do not survive long away from the body. The main presenting symptom is pruritus which occurs with sensitization about 1 month after the onset of infestation. Symptoms may be worse at night and after a hot bath or shower. Burrows commonly occur in web spaces between the fingers and on the wrists but may be very widespread. There is often evidence of excoriation but the appearance of the skin is variable and may show secondary infection, eczematization, lichenification, and papulovesicles (Figs. 7.12.6 and 7.12.7). Careful examination may reveal burrows and mites. Diagnosis may be confirmed by microscopy of scrapings from affected areas, especially interdigital spaces, but many cases are atypical and a dermatological opinion may be required to exclude other causes. Immunosuppressed patients, including transplant recipients and patients with AIDS, are prone to crusting or so-called Norwegian scabies in which crusting lesions of scales and mites accumulate over the hands, feet, and other sites such as eyebrows, but the patient suffers relatively little discomfort. Such cases, and presumably their fomites, are highly contagious. Occasionally the mites *Dermanyssus gallinae* and *Ornithonyssus* spp., whose normal hosts are birds, bite humans, causing lesions that resemble scabies.

Treatment

Treatment of scabies is by topical application of acaricides. Aqueous lotions of 0.5% malathion or 5% permethrin are currently recommended in the United Kingdom, given as two treatments a week apart. γ-Benzene hexachloride is also effective. The lotion is applied to the whole body surface of all affected people and left on for 24 h before being washing off. Itching may persist for several weeks and requires a topical counter irritant and corticosteroid (e.g. crotamiton and hydrocortisone) and a sedating antihistamine (chlorphenamine at night). Ivermectin (200 µg/kg single dose) is used for Norwegian scabies and in patients whose severe excoriations make topical treatment intolerably irritating and painful. During outbreaks, it may be necessary to treat whole cohorts of patients or health care teams.

Louse infestation

Lice are obligate parasites of animals. They bite using piercing mouthparts to feed on blood or tissue fluids. Three species, of cosmopolitan distribution, are associated with humans: the pubic louse *Pthirus pubis*, the body louse (or clothing louse) *Pediculus humanus* (Fig. 7.12.8), and the head louse *P. capitis*. Body and head lice are morphologically similar and are treated by some authors as subspecies or forms of *P. humanus*. Lice complete their life cycle on their host. Adult females deposit eggs (nits) on hair shafts (pubic and head lice) or on clothing (body louse). Larvae hatch after about 1 week, begin to feed and over the course of about 2 weeks, undergo several moults before reaching adulthood. Adult females live for about 1 month and may lay about 100 eggs. Egg cases remain where attached and may persist after successful treatment of infestation. Most infestations are probably acquired through close contact with an infested case, but some cases may result from contact with clothing, bedclothes, or hairbrushes containing living lice or their eggs, which may be attached to shed hairs. In addition to the aesthetic and social drawbacks of louse infestation, medical problems common to all three taxa relate to sensitization of the host to louse

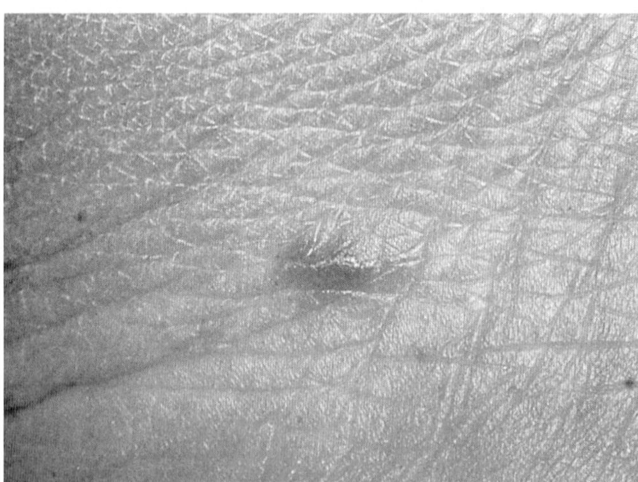

Fig. 7.12.7 Papulovesicular lesions of scabies.

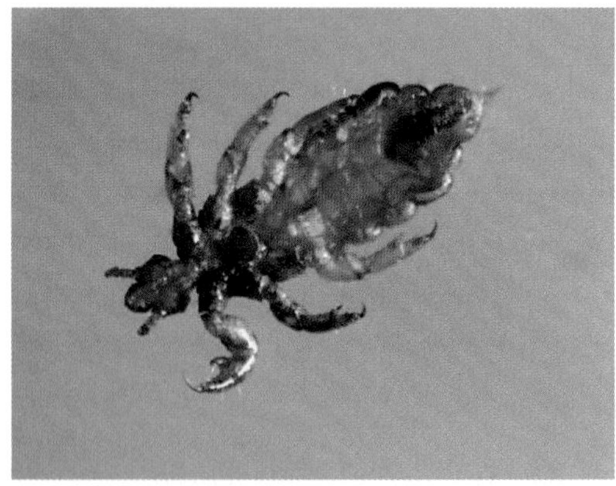

Fig. 7.12.8 Louse *Pediculus humanus*. Head lice and body lice are morphologically similar.
(Copyright J Paul.)

antigens from bites and the resulting pruritus which may lead to excoriation and secondary infection. Louse bites have a central punctum and surrounding small red macule. Body lice may transmit a number of agents, including those of endemic typhus (*Rickettsia prowazekii*), trench fever (*Bartonella quintana*), and relapsing fever (*Borrelia recurrentis*).

Pubic lice (crab lice)

The lice (*Pthirus pubis*) attach themselves to pubic hairs. Rarely, lice may be found on eyebrows, eyelashes (phthirosis palpebrarum), axillary, head, or chest hair. Eggs are deposited on hair shafts. Most infestations are probably acquired through sexual contact with an infested case. Children may acquire phthirosis at atypical sites through close contact with adults. Lice seldom stray from the body. Transmission is possible but unlikely without close contact with an infested case. The main symptom is pruritus, sometimes with excoriation and secondary infection. Grey patches (maculae caeruleae) may occur on the skin. Diagnosis is by observation of the lice, which may be difficult to find, or of eggs or egg cases attached to hair shafts. Adults are 1 to 2 mm long. The anterior legs are smaller than the other two pairs. The body is squat and crablike (body length, excluding head, *c.*1.2 times body width) (Fig. 7.12.9). The original description contained a printing error (pthirus) for phthirus (Greek: louse).

Treatment

Aqueous carbaryl, permethrin, phenothrin, or malathion is applied to the whole body and left on for 1–2 days. This is repeated a week later to kill newly hatched larvae. Sexual contacts must be treated.

Head lice

Head lice infest the scalp and rarely other body sites. They lay their eggs at the base of hair shafts. Infestation is more common in children than in adults and more common in females than in males. Prevalence rates vary but may be very high in certain communities or institutions, such as schools. Prevalence rates may be high despite good standards of hygiene. Most cases probably occur as a result of close contact. The main symptom is pruritus which may be associated with excoriation, secondary infection and lymphadenopathy. Diagnosis is by observation of lice, which generally remain close to the scalp, or of eggs or egg cases, attached to hairs (Fig. 7.9.10). A fine comb (nit comb) may be used to collect material to make the diagnosis. Adults are 3 to 4 mm long.

Treatment

Insecticide lotion (malathion, permethrin, phenothrin, dimeticone, or carbaryl) is applied to the scalp overnight. This is repeated a week later to destroy newly hatched larvae. Permethrin failure has been reported from many parts of the world. Compared with laboratory reference strains, lice collected from infestations failing to respond to permethrin have shown relative resistance to the agent. In Israel, there is evidence that permethrin resistance may be due to monooxygenase plus nerve insensitivity resistance mechanisms. Malathion resistance has been reported and may be due to a malathion-specific esterase. Pediculocides should be used with caution in children and asthmatics. Regular and fastidious use of a nit comb may be used (on its own or in combination with a pediculocide) to treat infestation. There is much anecdotal evidence, that combing can be effective, and it avoids concerns of pediculocide toxicity and resistance, but a study in Wales showed combing to be less effective that chemical treatment. In institutions, coordinated treatment campaigns may be required to prevent reinfestation.

Body lice

Body lice infest clothing and body hair. They lay their eggs on clothing, often along seams. Body lice are morphologically like head lice but slightly larger. Body louse infestation is associated with poor hygiene and social deprivation, as may occur in wartime. Transmission occurs as a result of close contact or through contact with infested clothing. Bites occur on the body, resulting in pruritus which may be associated with excoriation, eczematization, and secondary infection. Diagnosis is confirmed by finding lice, usually on clothing.

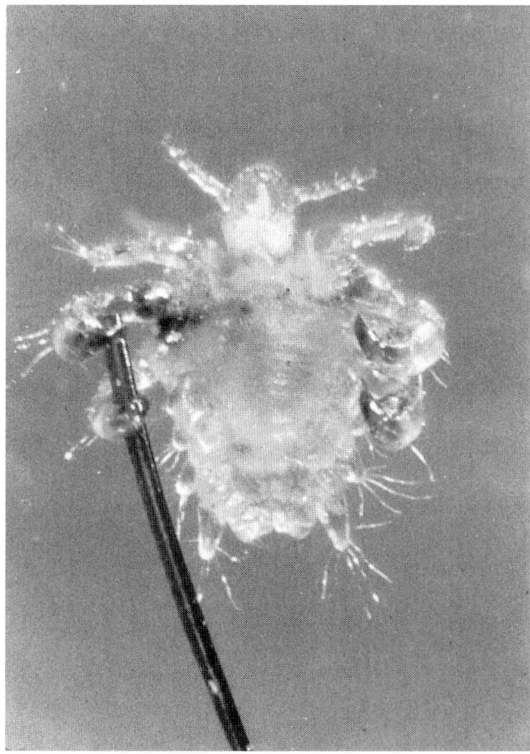

Fig. 7.12.9 Adult specimen of *Pthirus publis*.
(Courtesy of D Hill, Adelaide, South Australia.).

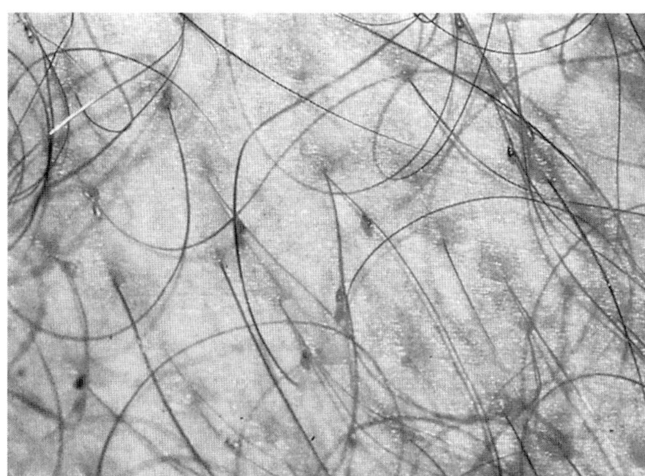

Fig. 7.12.10 Nits attached to hair. Photograph from a patient with pediculosis showing several hair fibres with numerous egg cases attached.
(Courtesy of D Hill, Adelaide, South Australia.)

Treatment

Infestation may be treated by topical application of carbaryl or malathion to the whole body, repeated a week later to kill newly hatched larvae. Hot washing of clothing will destroy adults and early stages.

Fleas (Siphonaptera)

Fleas are bloodsucking ectoparasites. There are thousands of species, adapted to various host animals. Adults are a few millimetres long, brown, laterally compressed and typically very active. Adults move through the fur or under clothing but can survive in the environment for long periods without feeding. Eggs are dropped to the ground, where the larvae develop, feeding on organic matter. The pupa may remain in the environment for long periods before the adult emerges. Increasing standards of hygiene in developed countries have made the human flea *Pulex irritans* a rarity. Most flea bites in Britain are now due to cat and dog fleas, *Ctenocephalides felis* (Fig. 7.12.11) and *C. canis*, either through direct exposure to an infested animal or to an environment exposed to an infested animal, possibly months previously. Flea bites result in intense pruritus at the bite site. There is a central punctum and there may be bulla formation (Fig. 7.12.12). Flea bites often occur in groups.

Although patients may not witness fleas, clues that bites have been caused by fleas include intense pruritus, the appearance of bites in small linear groups, and a history of exposure to a flea-ridden animal or its domain. Troublesome bites may be treated with topical corticosteroids and systemic antihistamines.

Prevention

Good domestic hygiene is important. Infested animals and environments should be treated with insecticides. Certain species of flea are vectors of a number of infectious diseases including plague and murine typhus.

Tungosis

Tungosis is infestation by a flea *Tunga penetrans*, known as the jigger, chigger, or chigoe (but popular names are shared with trombiculid mites). The gravid female, about 1 mm long, burrows into exposed skin (usually the foot), or under a toenail, and swells to about 1 cm in diameter, causing local discomfort. Lesions may be enucleated surgically and the diagnosis confirmed by histology. Local remedies in endemic areas (tropical Africa and the Americas) of shelling out fleas may leave cavities prone to secondary infection and tetanus. The wearing of footwear prevents infestation.

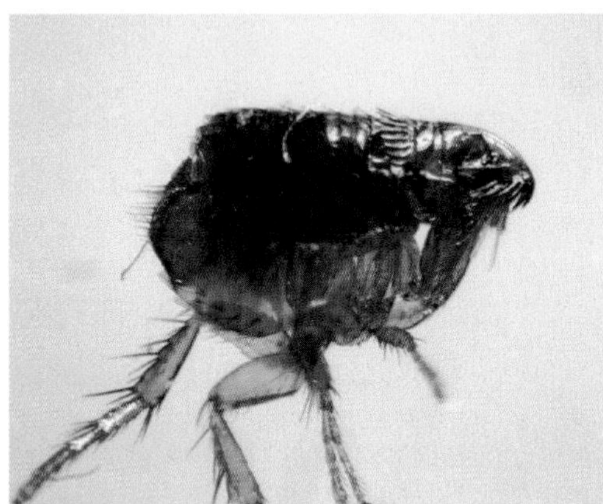

Fig. 7.12.11 Cat flea *Ctenocephalides felis*, a common cause of flea bites in humans. (Copyright J Paul.)

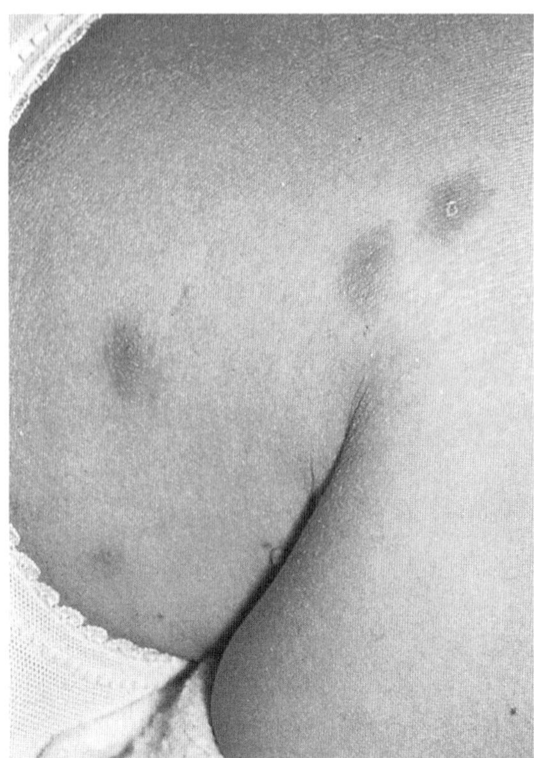

Fig. 7.12.12 Flea bites. Erythematous macropapule with central bite point visible. (Courtesy of D Hill, Adelaide, South Australia.)

Myiasis

Myiasis is the infestation of living animals by the larvae of flies (Diptera). Useful schemes of classification of myiasis include those based on the anatomical site (dermal, subdermal, wound, nasopharyngeal, orbital, ophthalmic, aural, urogenital, pulmonary, intestinal) and on the species of fly involved. Myiasis caused by flies whose larvae are obligate parasites of living tissues may be termed specific or primary myiasis. Myiasis associated with larvae which feed on decaying organic matter may be termed opportunistic or secondary myiasis. Myiasis due to larvae which find there way into the body (especially the gastrointestinal tract) by chance may be called accidental myiasis. Of the many species listed as possible agents (Table 7.12.3), most are opportunists whose saprophagous larvae feed on decaying organic matter, which might include necrotic wound tissue. Opportunists usually confine themselves to dead tissue and may even benefit the healing process. There is no dipterous obligate intestinal parasite of man.

Intestinal myiasis may be caused by coprophagous larvae which invade the rectum or by resilient maggots, such as those of the false stable fly *Muscina stabulans* and the cheese skipper *Piophila casei* which survive when swallowed in food and may cause intestinal disturbance and scarring. Intestinal myiasis may be spurious, following diagnosis based on observation of rapidly hatching larvae on freshly passed faeces. Rat-tailed maggots, larvae of drone flies *Eristalis* spp., are sometimes referred for identification to laboratories and numerous case reports link these maggots to intestinal myiasis. As the maggots naturally live in aqueous

Table 7.12.3 Flies associated with myiasis in humans

Genus and species	Common name	Distribution	Type of myiasis
Psychodidae			
Telmatoscopus albipunctatus	Moth fly	Widely distributed	Intestinal, nasal
Phoridae			
Megasalia	Scuttle flies	Cosmopolitan	Wound, intestinal, urogenital, pulmonary
Syrphidae			
Eristalis tenax	Common drone fly	Widely distributed	Rectal
Piophilidae			
Piophila casei	Cheese skipper	Widely distributed	Intestinal
Muscidae			
Fannia canicularis	Lesser house fly	Cosmopolitan	Urogenital
Musca domestica	House fly	Cosmopolitan	Wound, intestinal
Muscina stabulans	False stable fly	Cosmopolitan	Intestinal
Stomoxys calcitrans	Stable fly	Cosmopolitan	Intestinal
Calliphoridae			
Auchmeromyia luteola	Congo floor maggot	Africa	Sanguinivorous
Calliphora spp.	Bluebottles	Widely distributed	Wound, intestinal
Cochliomyia hominivorax	New World screw worm	Americas	Primary
Cochliomyia macelleria	Secondary screw worm	Americas	Wound
Cordylobia anthropophaga	Tumbu fly	Africa	Subdermal
Cordylobia rodhaini	Lund's fly	Africa	Subdermal
Chrysomya bezziana	Old World screw worm	Africa, Asia	Wound, auricular
Lucilia spp.	Green bottles	Widely distributed	Wound
Sarcophagidae			
Wohlfahrtia magnifica	Wohlfahrt's myiasis fly	Southern Palaearctic	Primary
Wohlfahrtia vigil	Grey flesh fly	North America	Dermal
Wohlfahrtia nuba		Southern Palaearctic	Wound
Sarcophaga spp.	Flesh flies	Widely distributed	Intestinal, wound
Gasterophilidae			
Gasterophilus spp.	Horse bot fly	Widely distributed	Dermal (creeping), tracheopulmonary
Cuterebridae			
Cuterebra spp.	Rabbit bot fly	Americas	Subdermal, nasal, tracheopulmonary
Dermatobia hominis	South American bot fly	Neotropics	Subdermal
Oestridae			
Oestrus ovis	Sheep nasal bot fly	Widely distributed	Ocular myiasis
Hypoderma spp.	Warble flies	Holarctic	Dermal (creeping), ophthalmic, oral

environments that are rich in organic matter, the finding of maggots in latrines may represent spurious association in some cases. Flies from several genera, notably *Fannia*, may cause urogenital myiasis. Scuttle flies (Phoridae) have been reported to cause pulmonary myiasis, possibly following inhalation of the gravid female fly. A small number of flies are obligate parasites of living tissues and a few species are closely associated with, but not specific to, humans. Many cases of myiasis are benign, self-limiting, and relatively harmless, but aural, nasopharyngeal, and malign wound myiasis are potentially lethal entities that may require removal of the larvae and possibly reconstructive surgery. Myiasis is diagnosed by observing dipteran larvae in a lesion. Identification of larvae may require entomological expertise but management of the patient, which depending on the type of lesion, may involve the removal of larvae, surgical exploration, debridement, or treatment of secondary infection, should be based on clinical assessment.

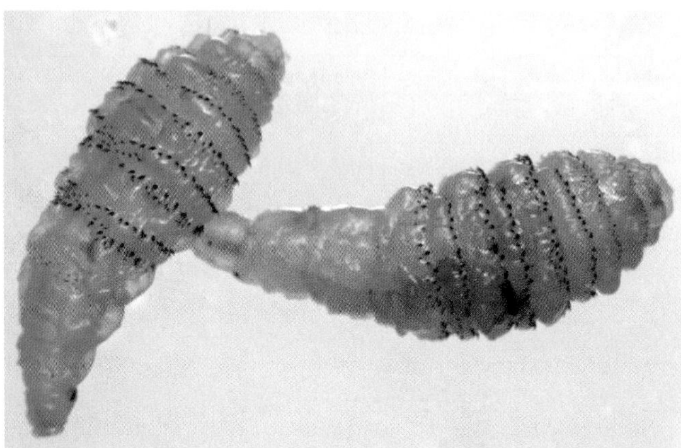

Fig. 7.12.13 Two third larval instars of the human bot fly *Dermatobia hominis* (*c.*13 mm long) extracted form a facial 'boil' in a European who had been visiting Guyana.

Dermal myiasis

The human bot fly *Dermatobia hominis* is a common cause of dermal myiasis in the American tropics. The female fly lays her eggs on biting arthropods, such as mosquitoes. The eggs hatch when in contact with skin into which the larva burrows. The larval stage lasts about 10 weeks, a boil with a small aperture forming as the larva grows. Such boils are not infrequently seen in Europeans returning from the neotropics. The larva may grow to more than 1 cm in length (Fig. 7.12.13). An early symptom is sporadic pain caused by the spiny larva. Unless in an unusual anatomical site, such as close to the eye, infestation is generally harmless. Secondary infection of the wound is the most common complication. Larvae may be removed through a simple incision. Remedies which include application of raw meat or glue to the lesion may not be successful. Squeezing may rupture the larva to evoke a local granulomatous reaction.

The tumbu fly *Cordylobia anthropophaga* is widespread in the Afrotropical region. There have also been rare reports of apparent acquisition in Spain and Portugal. The female oviposits on sand and also on drying clothes. Ironing destroys eggs. Contact with viable ova on clothing leads to infestation. The larvae pierce the skin and grow rapidly. An uncomfortable boil forms which oozes serosanguinous fluid (Fig. 7.12.14). Fever and lymphadenopathy may occur. Larvae reach maturity in about 10 days. Larvae may be removed through a simple incision, but with care it may be possible to express larvae following application of petroleum jelly (Fig. 7.12.15).

The larvae of warble flies *Hypoderma* spp. occasionally cause dermal myiasis in humans. Larvae of horse bot flies *Gasterophilus* spp. cannot complete their life cycle in humans but they can pierce human skin, where they wander for a week or so, causing intense itching (creeping eruption).

Wound myiasis

Many dipterous species are known to cause wound myiasis, but most of them are facultative feeders on necrotic tissue and are rarely destructive to the host although the presence of maggots in a wound may cause distress. Debridement of nectrotic tissue will control such infestation. In contrast, under controlled conditions, clinicians may introduce maggots to promote healing.

Causes of malign myiasis include the New World screw-worm *Cochliomyia hominivorax* in the Americas and the Old World screw-worm, *Chrysomya bezziana* and Wohlfahrt's wound myiasis fly *Wohlfahrtia magnifica* in the Old World. Their larvae are obligate parasites of living tissue. Eggs are laid on wounds, in ears and on mucous membranes. The larvae (Fig. 7.12.16) burrow in groups into healthy tissue, causing widespread destruction which may be mutilating or fatal (Fig. 7.12.17). Secondary bacterial infection or secondary wound myiasis may ensue. All species may cause nasopharyngeal, aural, orbital, genital and malign wound myiasis. Infestation is best avoided by cleaning and dressing wounds as they occur. Treatment involves surgical removal of the larvae, debridement of affected tissue, and treatment of secondary infection. Reconstructive surgery may be required.

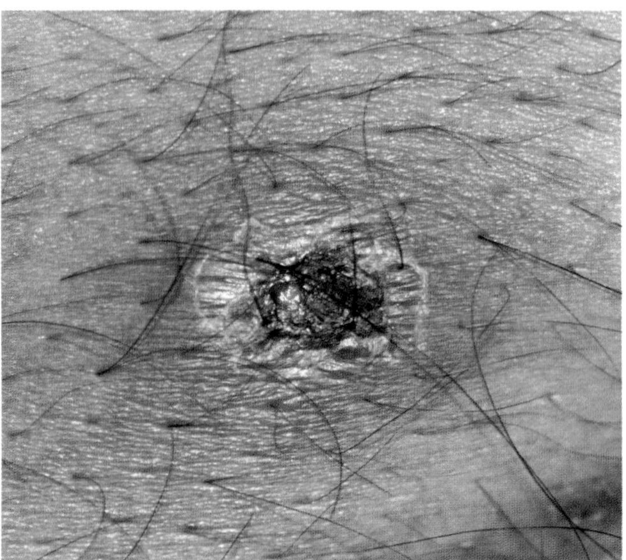

Fig. 7.12.14 Skin lesion caused by larva of the Tumbu fly *Cordylobia anthropophaga* in a Peruvian man who had been working in Zambia. (Copyright DA Warrell.)

Ophthalmic myiasis

The natural hosts of nasal bot flies *Oestrus* spp. are herbivorous mammals. The sheep bot *Oestrus ovis* is common is some sheep-raising areas, although it is now rare in the United Kingdom. Nasal bot flies are larviparous and drop their larvae into the nostrils of the host, where they mature. Occasionally humans act as a temporary

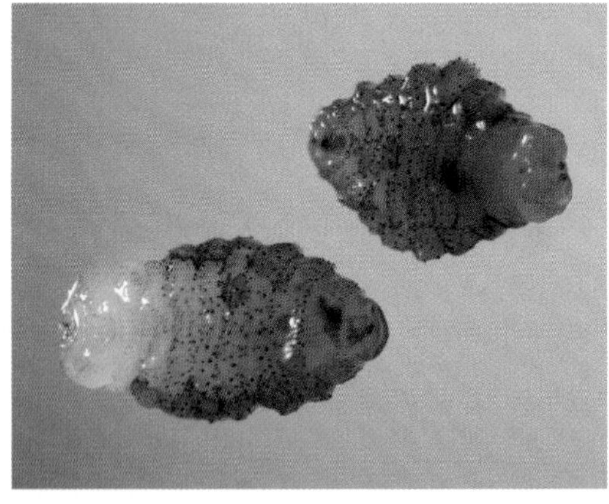

Fig. 7.12.15 Larvae of African tumbu fly *Cordylobia anthropophaga*, a common agent of dermal myosis.

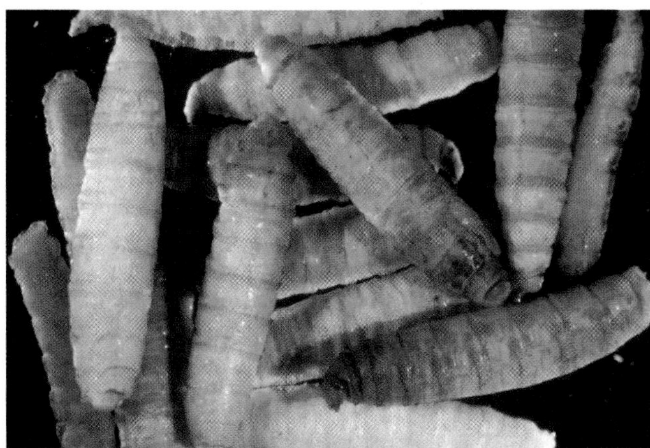

Fig. 7.12.16 Larvae of the New World screw-worm *Cochliomyia hominivorax* (*c.*8 mm long) extracted from the wound illustrated in Fig. 7.12.17. These were sent to the Natural History Museum in London where they were identified. Larvae of the second myiasis species (*C. macellaria*) were also found in the sample and were probably collected from the edges of the wound. (Courtesy of Dr Martin J R Hall, Medical and Veterinary Division, Natural History Museum, London.)

accidental host, when larvae are dropped into the eye. The patient may give a history of having been buzzed in the face by an insect and later of developing symptoms of conjunctivitis. Although the condition is self-limiting, symptoms may be relieved more rapidly by removal of larvae. Patients may be referred to an ophthalmologist. Larvae of warble flies *Hypoderma* spp. are more dangerous: larvae may burrow into the eye, resulting in pain, nausea, and much damage and must be surgically removed.

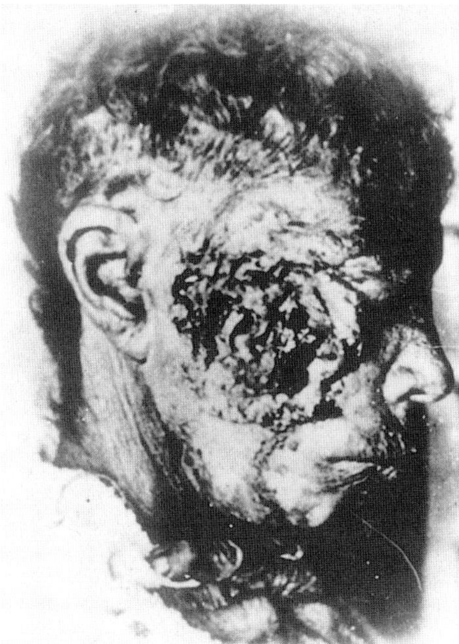

Fig. 7.12.17 Fatal myiasis (New World screw-worm). Historical illustration of a 50-year-old Honduran woman who complained of a small chronic ulcer on the right cheek; on admission to hospital she was found to have a huge ulcer exposing the bones of the face and forehead and he destroying the tissues of the cheek and face, right eye, and orbit. More than 300 larvae were removed (see Fig. 7.12.16). (From Harrison JHH (1908). A case of myiasis. *J Trop Med Hyg*, **XI**, 20.)

Canthariasis

Infestation of the body by beetles (Coleoptera) or their larvae is called canthariasis. Clinically, it may resemble myiasis but is much rarer.

Larvae swallowed with food may dwell temporarilly in the intestines, causing discomfort and may be detected in excreta. Beetles occasionally invade orifices. In Sri Lanka, scarabid dung beetles have been reported to invade the rectum. A specimen of the Asian carabid ground beetle *Scarites sulcatus* was recovered from the vagina of a women complaining of vaginal discharge who had visited Pakistan (Fig. 7.12.18).

In Israel, the dung beetle *Maladera matrida* has been reported to invade the external auditory canal. In Oman, two cases of invasion of the external auditory canal by the ground beetle *Crasydactylus punctatus* were reported. In one case, the beetle reached the middle ear causing sensorineural hearing loss.

(See also venomous coleoptera, Chapter 9.2.)

Allergy

A wide range of immunological responses to arthropod bites has been described, from local pruritus to anaphylaxis. The dead remains, cast skins (exuviae), and faeces of many arthropods include sensitizing agents. They may act as contact or inhalant allergens, following domestic or occupational exposure resulting in dermatitis, conjunctivitis, rhinitis, and asthma. Allergic patients may show specific IgE antibody to a wide range of domestic pests including house flies, clothes moths, cockroaches, carpet beetles *Anthrenus* sp., silverfish *Ctenolepisma longicaudata*, and house dust mites *Dermatophagoides* spp. *Dermatophagoides* spp. are a common cause of allergy in the United Kingdom and exposure to cockroach allergens in household dust has been associated with asthma in the United States of America.

Following mass emergence, nonbiting midges (Chironimidae) and the exuviae of mayflies (Ephemeroptera) and caddis flies (Trichoptera) may act as inhalant allergens. Chironimid midges occur worldwide and are especially troublesome in the Sudan, where *Cladotanytarsus lewisi* (green nimitti midge) breeds in dammed stretches of the Nile, causing seasonal epidemic allergy. Chironimid haemoglobin has been shown to be allergenic. The rearing of chironimid larvae as food for fish has been associated with occupational allergy.

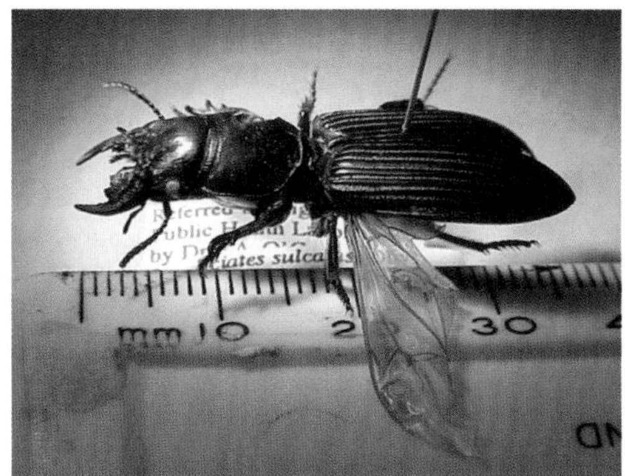

Fig. 7.12.18 An Asian carabid beetle *Scarites sulcatus*, from a patient complaining of vaginal discharge; a rare example of genital canthariasis.

Entomologists who collect insects by sucking them into pooters may develop inhalant allergy to their subject of study. Occupational exposure to deer keds *Lipoptena cervi* has been associated with allergic rhinoconjunctivitis in forest workers in Finland. Larvae of the beetles *Tenebrio molitor* (mealworm) and *Alphitobius diaperinus* (lesser mealworm), which are reared for fish bait and animal food, have been associated with rhinoconjunctivitis, contact urticaria, and asthma. Beetles which infest stored grain, including *Tenebrio molitor*, *Tribolium confusum* (confused flour beetle), *Sitophilus* sp. (grain weevil), and *Alphitobius diaperinus* have been associated with occupational allergy in grain workers or bakers. Allergy has been associated with other beetles, including *Dermestes peruvianus* (hide beetle), *Gibbium psylloides* (mite beetle), and *Harmonia axyridis* (Asian ladybird). Insect allergy can be investigated by skin prick tests, measurement of allergen-specific serum IgE, and monitoring of respiratory function following allergen exposure.

Insects and hygiene

Synanthropic insects which feed or wander over faeces, wounds, and food may serve as passive vectors of bacterial and viral diseases. Such insects include pharaoh's ants *Monomorium pharaonis*, flies, and cockroaches (Dictyoptera). Despite many reports of the isolation of pathogenic bacteria and viruses from these insects, there have been few epidemiological studies to define their importance as passive vectors, although is generally accepted that the presence of these insects in hospitals should be monitored and controlled.

Flies

Many species of fly (especially of the suborder Cyclorrhapha), frequent human and animal food, wounds, eyes, and faeces. Such flies vomit and defecate where they feed. Numerous pathogenic bacteria and viruses have been isolated from flies, suggesting that they may act as passive vectors of bacterial and viral diseases. A controlled study in the Gambia, where fly control was associated with fewer new cases of trachoma, suggested that flies may act as vectors of the trachoma agent *Chlamydia trachomatis*. In the Gambia, *Musca sorbens* is the most common eye-visiting fly. In Pakistan, a controlled study showed fly control to be significantly associated with a reduction in incidence of childhood diarrhoeal illness. In Israel, fly control was associated with a reduction in cases of shigellosis. Flies may be controlled by using insecticides or fly traps in dwellings and latrines.

Ants

Pharaoh's ants *Monomorium pharaonis* L. commonly infest hospitals, where they invade sterile packs and wound dressings. They are potential passive vectors: bacteria including salmonella and staphylococcus have been isolated from these ants, which should therefore be controlled with insecticides. In Iran, ants of the genus *Pheidole* have been associated with sudden localized hair loss from the scalp. Patients in different parts of the country reported awakening to find collections of hair on their pillows and ants on their beds or scalps.

Cockroaches

Cockroaches are omnivorous scavengers. A few of the 3500 described species have become cosmopolitan synanthropes. The main pest species are the common cockroach *Blatta orientalis*, the American cockroach *Periplaneta americana*, the German cockroach *Blattella germanica*, and the banded cockroach *Supella longipalpa*. Other species may be locally important, e.g. *Ectobius lapponicus*, described by Linnaeus as infesting dried fish in Lapland. The common pest species are mostly of tropical origin and require temperatures of 25 to 33°C, but *B. orientalis* will tolerate 20°C. In cooler climates they are restricted to permanently heated areas and can occur in large numbers in hospitals and in sewers. Many pathogenic viruses, including poliomyelitis virus and coxsackie A virus, and bacteria, including *Shigella* spp., have been isolated from cockroaches. There is evidence that cockroaches acted as vectors of hepatitis A during an outbreak in California and of *Salmonella typhimurium* on a paediatric ward in Belgium. Cockroaches are potential allergens, 7.5% of healthy individuals being skin-test positive in one study. Cockroaches wander over sleepers and are attracted to nasal and oral secretions. Herpes blattae is a dermatitis described from Réunion and attributed to cockroach allergy. Cockroaches sometimes wander into ears and nostrils, where they become trapped or reluctant to leave. Lignocaine (lidocaine) spray is reported to hasten the exit of such visitors.

Eye-frequenting moths and beetles

Like the oriental eye fly (*Siphunculina funicola*, Diptera, Chloropidae), some nocturnal moths of the families Pyralidae, Noctuidae, and Geometridae in Africa and South-East Asia habitually feed on the lachrymal secretions of animals. They may visit human eyes, causing a certain amount of discomfort, and may transmit eye infections, including trachoma and viral conjunctivitis. They may also cause mechanical damage to the cornea. The moths stimulate the flow of secretions by vibrating and probing with their probosces. Implicated species include *Lobocraspis griseifulva*, *Arcyophora* spp., and *Filodes fulvidorsalis*. *Calyptra eustrigata* is a skin-piercing, blood-sucking noctuid moth from Malaya. Such Lepidoptera may be avoided by sleeping under a net. In Australia, a beetle, *Orthoperus* sp. has been associated with corneal erosion.

Further reading

Aguilera A, *et al.* (1999). Intestinal myiasis caused by *Eristalis tenax*. *J Clin Microbiol*, **37**, 3082.

Auerbach PS (ed.) (1995). *Wilderness medicine: management of wilderness and environmental emergencies*. Mosby, St. Louis.

Baker AS (1999). *Mites and ticks of domestic animals: an identification guide and information source*. The Stationery Office, London.

Liebold K (2003). Disseminated bullous eruption with systemic reaction caused by *Cimex lectularius*. *J Eur Acad Dermatol Vet*, **17**, 461–3.

Radmanesh M (1999). Alopecia induced by ants. *Trans Roy Soc Trop Med, Hyg*, **93**, 427.

Roberts DT (ed.) (2000). *Lice and scabies: a health professional's guide to epidemiology and treatment*. Public Health Laboratory Service, London.

Rosenstreich DL, *et al.* (1997). The role of cockroach allergy and exposure to cockroach allergen in causing morbidity among inner-city children with asthma. *N Engl J Med*, **336**, 1356–63.

Roth LM, Willis ER (1957). The medical and veterinary importance of cockroaches. *Smithsonian Miscellaneous Collection*, **134**, 1–147.

Smith KGV (ed.) (1973). *Insects and arthropods of medical importance*. British Museum (Natural History), London.

Zumpt, F. (1965). *Myiasis in man and animals in the Old World*. Butterworth, London.

7.13

Pentastomiasis (porocephalosis, linguatulosis/linguatuliasis)

David A. Warrell

Essentials

Pentastomiases or porocephaloses are zoonotic infections caused by maxillopod crustacean parasites (subclass Pentastomida).

Linguatula serrata ('tongueworm')—this is cosmopolitan, infecting upper respiratory tracts of the definitive hosts, canids. Nymphs discharged in nasal secretions are taken up by herbivorous animals, the intermediate hosts, which pass on the infection when they are eaten. Humans may be infected by eating raw liver and other offal of sheep, goats, and other animals, soon after which acute allergic obstructive nasolaryngopharyngitis (halzoun or marrara syndrome) may develop. Larvae can be found in sputum and vomitus.

Armillifer spp.—these are confined to Africa and South-East Asia, where they infect the respiratory tracts of snakes. Humans are infected by drinking snake-polluted water or by eating raw snake, a common practice in some communities. Most infections are asymptomatic, but massive infections may produce symptoms of an acute abdomen and are rarely fatal by causing intestinal obstruction or enterocolitis. Nymphs are detected at laparotomy or autopsy and (calcified) on abdominal radiographs.

Treatment and prevention—aside from standard measures for hypersensitivity phenomena, there is no specific treatment, although mebendazole has been suggested. Prevention is by thoroughly cooking all meat of whatever origin.

Introduction

The Pentastomida are currently regarded as a subclass of maxillopod crustaceans. Common names are 'pentastomes'—because two pairs of hooks above the mouth give the impression of five stomata (Fig. 7.13.1) and 'tongueworms'—because some resemble an animal's tongue. They inhabit the respiratory tracts of vertebrates, feeding on blood and other tissues. There are about 100 living species in the orders Cephalobaenida (e.g. genus *Raillietiella*) and Porocephalida (e.g. genera *Linguatula*, *Armillifer*, *Porocephalus*, *Leiperia*, and *Sebekia*). About 10 species are recognized zoonotic parasites of humans, causing infections termed pentastomiasis, porocephalosis, linguatulosis, or linguatuliasis. In humans, visceral pentastomiasis is most often caused by *Linguatula serrata* or *Armillifer armillatus*. Nasopharyngeal pentastomiasis ('Halzoun' or 'Marrara syndrome') is caused by *L. serrata*.

Aetiology

Linguatula species

Linguatula serrata occurs in Europe, the Middle East, Africa, and North, Central, and South America. The names 'linguatula' and 'tongueworm' describe the numerous annular grooves and flattened shape, particularly of the adult female. Dogs, foxes, and wolves, the definitive hosts, harbour adults and nymphs in their upper respiratory tract and shed them in their nasal secretions, saliva, and faeces. Herbivorous animals ingest the ova, which hatch in the lumen of the gut, releasing larvae that burrow into the tissues and encyst. When these intermediate hosts are eaten by the definitive host, nymphs hatch from the cysts and migrate to the lungs and nasopharynx where they mature.

Clinical features

When humans ingest ova of linguatula, larvae hatch in the gut, burrow through its wall, migrate through the tissues, and encyst especially in the liver. Second- or third-stage larvae cause symptoms only by obstruction or compression, e.g. in biliary, gastrointestinal or respiratory tracts, meninges, or brain. In the anterior chamber of the eye, larvae have caused iritis and secondary glaucoma in the United States of America and elsewhere.

Ingestion of cysts containing third-stage larvae in raw liver or lymph nodes from sheep, goats, cattle, camels, and lagomorphs can cause nasopharyngeal pentostomiasis, known as 'halzoun' in Lebanon and 'marrara syndrome' in the Sudan. This has also been reported from other countries, including Greece, Turkey, North Africa, Egypt, and Jordan. In the human stomach, larvae escape from the cysts and migrate up the oesophagus to the nasopharynx mucosa. Within minutes to a few hours of eating the infected viscera, there is

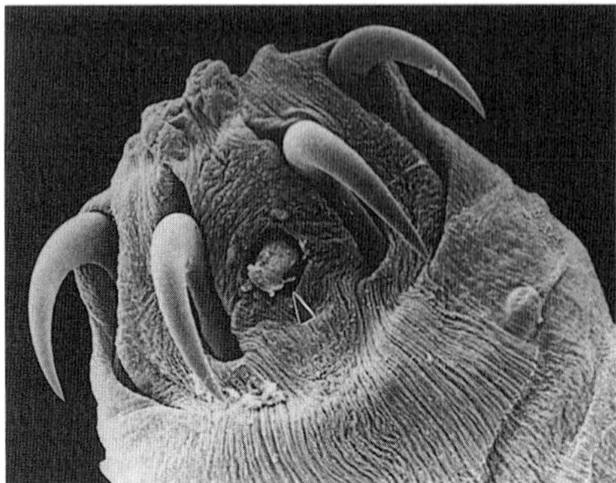

Fig. 7.13.1 Adult pentastomid showing mouth (arrowed) and lateral hooks giving the appearance of five stomata. Scanning electron micrograph, ×400. (Courtesy of Professor Viqar Zaman.)

intense irritation of the upper respiratory and gastrointestinal tracts causing coughing, sneezing, rhinorrhoea, retching, vomiting, lacrimation, haemoptysis, epistaxis, cervical lymphadenopathy, transient deafness, difficulty in speaking, dysphagia, wheezing, dyspnoea, and oedema of the face and oropharynx. The larvae, which are 5 to 10 mm long, can be found in sputum and vomitus. Patients usually recover in 1 or 2 weeks, but fatal acute upper airway obstruction is reported. Clinical features suggest a hypersensitivity reaction. Flukes (*Fasciola hepatica* and *Dicrocoelium dendriticum*) and nematodes (*Mammomonogamus laryngeus*) ingested in raw sheep and goat liver, and aquatic leeches (*Limnatis nilotica* and *Dinobdella ferox*) (see Chapter 9.2) have been implicated in halzoun but cannot explain the classic syndrome. Very rarely, larvae may mature to adulthood in the human nasal cavity, causing bleeding and obstruction.

Armillifer (*Porocephalus*) species

These are also annulated, nonsegmented parasites (Fig. 7.13.2a). Adult males and the much larger females (up to 20 cm long) inhabit the respiratory and digestive tracts of snakes (Fig. 7.13.3), especially those of the genera *Python*, *Lamprophis/Boaedon* (African house snakes), *Naja* (cobras) (Fig. 7.13.4), *Bitis* (African vipers) (Fig. 7.13.2b), *Bothrops* (Latin American lanceheads) (Fig. 7.13.5), and other vertebrates. Ova are shed in the snake's nasal secretions and are picked up by herbivorous mammals. Larvae encyst in the tissues of these intermediate hosts and will develop to the nymph stage if ingested by another animal, but develop to adults only in snakes. Humans may ingest ova by drinking water contaminated by snakes, or they may ingest living encysted larvae in raw or undercooked snake meat. This is eaten habitually or as part of *ju ju* rituals in Africa (Nigeria, Côte d'Ivoire, Benin, Cameroon, and the Democratic Republic of Congo(DRC)) and in South-East Asia, especially by the Temuan tribe of Malaysian aborigines. Ingested eggs hatch in the gut, releasing larvae which burrow into the tissues where they encyst as nymphs. The parasite species are *A. armillatus* and *A. grandis* in Africa and *A. moniliformis* in South-East Asia.

Epidemiology

The prevalence of infection can be judged by discovering calcified nymphs (Fig. 7.13.2) on radiographs of the abdomen and chest (Fig. 7.13.6). These appear as discrete, crescent-shaped, soft tissue calcifications, 4 to 8 mm in size. In West Africa they are seen particularly in the right upper quadrant and are situated beneath the peritoneum covering the liver. In Ibadan, Nigeria, they were seen in 1.4% of randomly selected straight abdominal films (7% in men aged 50–59 years). However, the prevalence of encysted nymphs or larvae at autopsy was 22.5% in DRC, 8% in Cameroon, 5% in West Africa and 45% in Malaysian Orang Asli. Cysts are found most commonly in liver (Fig. 7.13.7), mesentery, gut wall, peritoneum, spleen, kidneys, omentum and lungs. In Ibadan, pentastomiasis was the third most common cause of hepatic cirrhosis.

Human infections with the larvae or nymphs of the following species of *A. Armillifer* have been reported:

- *A. agkistrodontis*—China (in the snake *Deinagkistrodon acutus*)
- *A. armillatus* (18–22 annular rings)—Africa: Egypt, Senegal, the Gambia, Ghana, Benin, Nigeria, Cameroon, DRC, and Zimbabwe

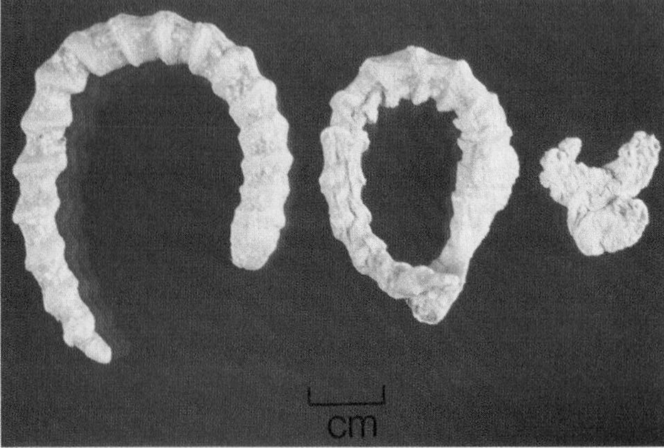

(a)

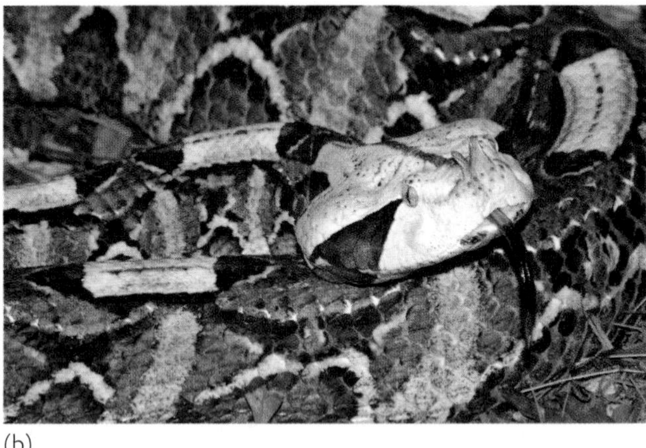

(b)

Fig. 7.13.2 *Armillifer armillatus*. (a) Left: two adults found in the lungs of (b) rhinoceros viper *Bitis rhinoceros*. Right: calcified nymph from the mesentery of a Ghanaian patient.
(Copyright D A Warrell.)

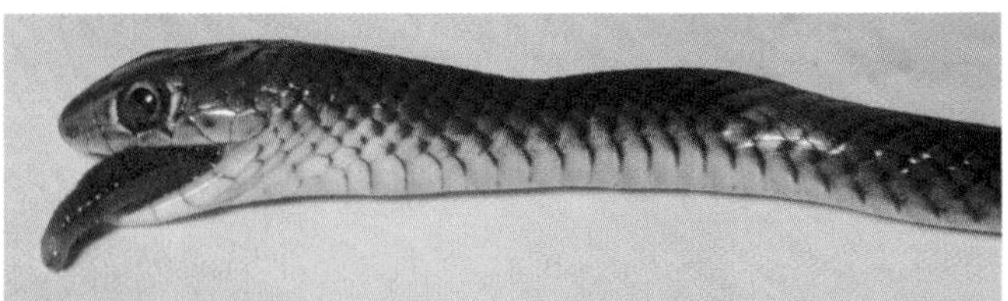

Fig. 7.13.3 Whip snake *Demansia atra* (Papua New Guinea) bringing up a pentastome.
(Copyright Mark O'Shea.)

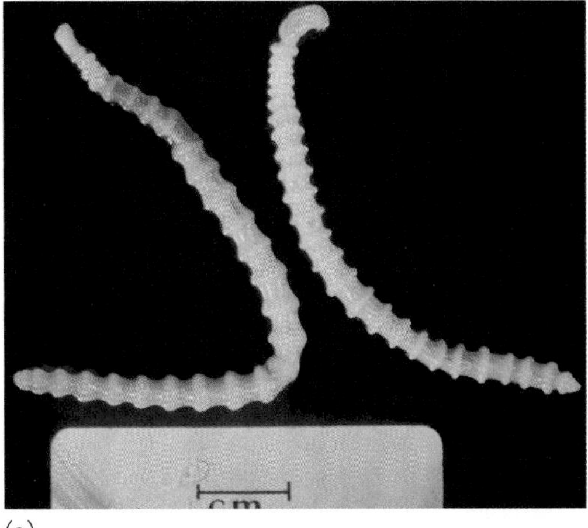

(a)

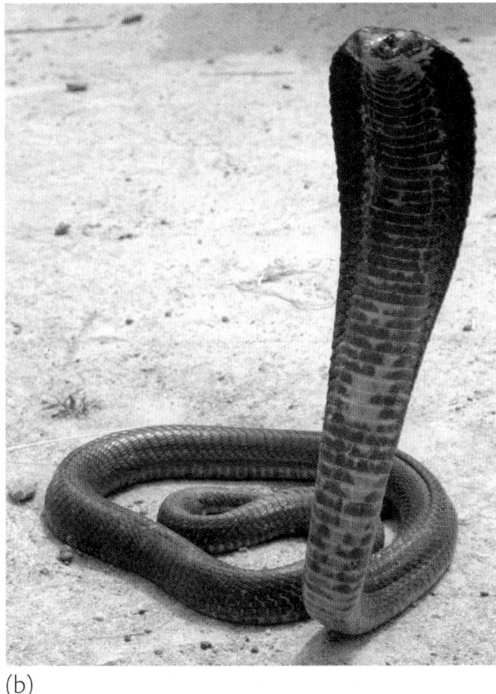

(b)

Fig. 7.13.4 (a) Pentastomes from the lungs of (b) an Egyptian cobra *Naja haje*.

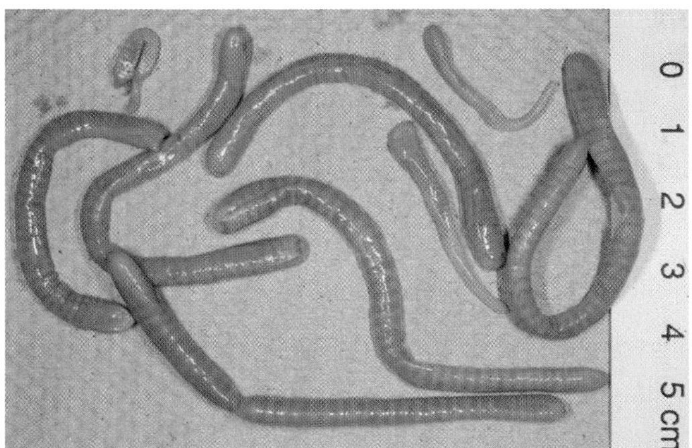

Fig. 7.13.5 Pentastomes found in the respiratory tract of lancehead vipers *Bothrops* spp., Manaus, Brazil.
(Copyright D A Warrell.)

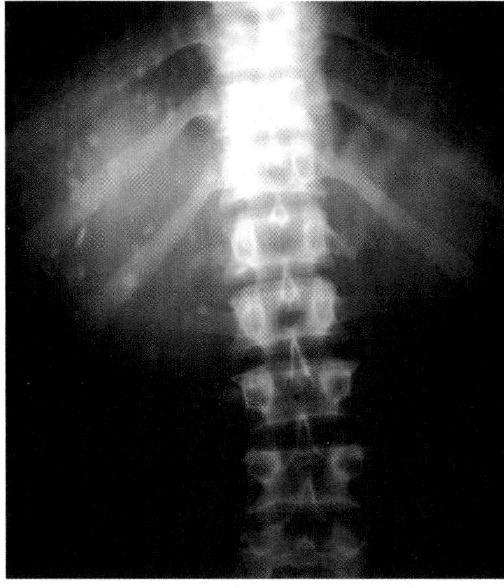

Fig. 7.13.6 Typical radiographic appearance of calcified nymphs of *Armillifer armillatus* in the abdominal cavity of a Ghanaian patient.
(Courtesy of Dr G M Ardran.)

- *A. grandis*—DRC, Côte d'Ivoire
- *A. moniliformis* (30 annular rings)—Malaysia, Philippines, Indonesia, Tibet, and Australia
- *A. najae*—India

Clinical features

Most infections are entirely asymptomatic. Migration of large numbers of larvae from the gut into the tissue may produce

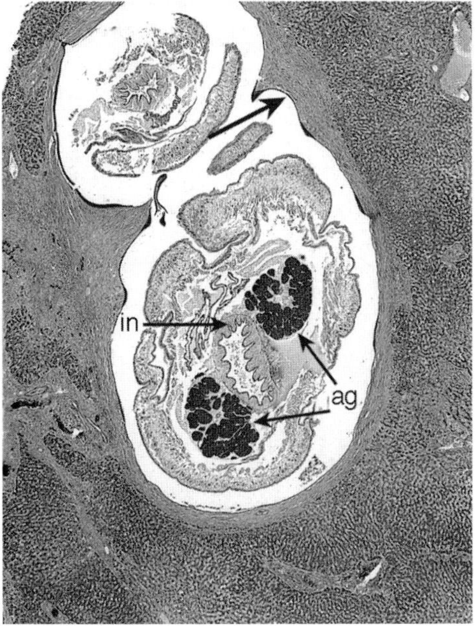

Fig. 7.13.7 Encysted nymph/larva of *Armillifer armillatus* in human liver. The outer layer of the parasite (arrowed) lines the cyst wall. Acidophilic glands (ag), intestine (in), ×21.
(Armed Forces Institute of Pathology photograph, negative number 75–2703.)

abdominal pain and obstructive jaundice. Massive infection, perhaps following ingestion of a gravid female, can cause acute abdominal symptoms prompting laparotomy at which hundreds of wriggling nymphs may be discovered beneath the visceral peritoneum. Serious inflammatory and obstructive effects have been described in the gut, peritoneum, liver and biliary tract, lungs, pleura, pericardium, central nervous system, and anterior chamber of the eye. These may be due partly to hypersensitivity. The few reported fatal cases had intestinal obstruction or haemorrhagic enterocolitis complicated perhaps by secondary Gram-negative septicaemia.

There is no convincing evidence of an association between *Armillifer* infection and colonic or other malignancies.

Other pentastomid infections

Human infections with *Leiperia cincinnalis* have been described in Africa and by *Porocephalus crotali* (from rattlesnakes) in North America. Subcutaneous infections by *Railliettiella gehyrae* and *R. hemidactyli* occur in Vietnam and by *Sebekia* species in Costa Rica. In Vietnam, infection with *Railliettiella* spp. results from swallowing small live lizards for medicinal purposes.

Diagnosis

The radiographical appearances of calcified pentastomid nymphs are distinctive (Fig. 7.13.6). They are not found in muscle, distinguishing pentastomiasis from cysticercosis. Pentastomes may be discovered at surgery or autopsy. In the liver (Fig. 7.13.7), intestinal wall, mesentery, mesenteric lymph nodes, peritoneum, or lung, viable encysted larvae or granulomas containing necrotic pentastomes or their moulted cuticles may be identified. Initially, encysted larvae excite little or no tissue reaction, but the granulomas are surrounded by hyalinized or calcified fibrous tissue. In tissue sections, pentastomes can be distinguished from helminths. Some patients have mild blood eosinophilia. Antibodies to *Armillifer* spp. have been detected by fluorescence in infected patients.

Treatment

There is no specific treatment, although mebendazole has been suggested. Obstruction and compression should be relieved surgically. Hypersensitivity phenomena should be treated with adrenaline (epinephrine), antihistamines, and corticosteroids.

Prevention

Pentostomiasis can be prevented by thoroughly cooking all meat of any origin. Eating sheep's lymph nodes is proscribed by the Shi'ite Muslims of Lebanon.

Other zoonoses transmitted from reptiles to humans

The most important of these is salmonellosis transmitted to humans by the faecal–oral route or by scratches and bites, from chelonians (tortoises, turtles, terrapins) and from snakes and lizards, especially iguanas. In the United Kingdom, 38% of imported tortoises (*Testudo* spp.) contain salmonella. In the United States of America, where 8 million reptiles are kept as pets, contact with reptiles and amphibians accounts for an estimated 74 000 (6%) of the approximately 1.2 million sporadic human salmonella infections that occur there annually. The banning by the United States Food and Drug Administration of commercial distribution of small turtles has prevented an estimated 100 000 cases of salmonellosis among children each year. Although salmonellosis usually causes self-limiting gastroenteritis, septicaemia or meningitis may occur especially in infants and immunocompromised people. Species associated with reptile salmonellosis include *S. enterica* serotype Typhimurium, *S. enterica* serotype Pomona, and *S. enterica* subspecies *diarizonae*.

Other infections transmissible from reptiles to humans include *Arizona hinshawii* (in snake powder, Pulvo de Vibora, made from rattlesnakes), *Plesiomonas shigelloides, Edwardsiella tarda*, leptospirosis, Q fever, sparganosis, capillariasis, strongyloidiasis, mesocestoidiasis, and infestation with the mite *Ophionyssus natricis*. Potential zoonoses include mycobacteria, pseudomonas, other aeromonas species, proteus, and some togaviruses (such as western equine encephalitis in garter snakes in western North America) and herpesviruses.

Further reading

Drabick JJ (1987). Pentastomiasis. *Rev Infect Dis*, **9**, 1087–94.

Haugerud RE (1989). Evolution in the pentastomids. *Parasitol Today*, **5**, 126–32.

Magnino S, Colin P, Dei-Cas E, *et al.* (2009). Biological risks associated with consumption of reptile products. *Int J Food Microbiol*, **134**, 163–75.

Palmer PES, Reeder MM (eds) (2001). Pentastomida. In: *The imaging of tropical diseases with epidemiological, pathological and clinical correlation*, Vol. 2, pp. 389–95. Springer, Berlin.

Riley J (1986). The biology of pentastomids. *Adv Parasitol*, **25**, 45–128.

Schacher JF, Khalil GM, Salman S. (1965). A field study of Halzoun (parasitic pharyngitis) in Lebanon. *J Trop Med Hyg*, **68**, 226–30.

Tappe D, Büttner DW (2009). Diagnosis of human visceral pentastomiasis. *PLoS Negl Trop Dis*, **5**, e320.

Warwick C, *et al.* (2001). Reptile-related salmonellosis. *J Roy Soc Med*, **94**, 124–6.

Yagi H, *et al.* (1996). The Marrara syndrome: a hypersensitivity reaction of the upper respiratory tract and buccopharyngeal mucosa to nymphs of *Linguatula serrata. Acta Trop*, **16**, 127–34.

Yao MH, Wu F, Tang LF (2008). Human pentastomiasis in China: case report and literature review. *J Parasitol*, **94**, 1295–8.

Yapo Ette H, *et al.* (2003). Human pentastomiasis discovered postmortem. *Forensic Sci Int*, **137**, 52–4.

SECTION 8

Sexually transmitted diseases and sexual health

8.1 **Epidemiology of sexually transmitted infections** *1243*
David Mabey

8.2 **Sexual behaviour** *1250*
Anne M. Johnson and Catherine H. Mercer

8.3 **Sexual history and examination** *1253*
Jackie Sherrard and Graz A. Luzzi

8.4 **Vaginal discharge** *1256*
Paul Nyirjesy

8.5 **Pelvic inflammatory disease** *1259*
David Eschenbach

8.6 **Principles of contraception** *1262*
John Guillebaud

8.1

Epidemiology of sexually transmitted infections

David Mabey

Essentials

Although accurate incidence figures are not available in most countries, sexually transmitted infections (STIs) (excluding HIV) are estimated to cause more than 5% of the global burden of disease. The burden falls especially heavily on women and infants, with more than half a million perinatal deaths attributable to syphilis annually. Mobile populations, those with many sexual partners, and those whose partners have many partners are at increased risk, and the prevalence of treatable STIs is many times higher in poor populations, who often lack access to effective treatment. Other STIs, especially those that cause genital ulceration, increase the risk of HIV transmission.

Incidence

In Western countries, the reported incidence of many STIs fell during the 1980s and 1990s, probably as a result of changes in sexual behaviour resulting from the HIV epidemic, but has increased subsequently. The reported incidence of *Chlamydia trachomatis* infection has increased in the general population, especially in teenagers and young adults, and the incidence of syphilis has increased in core groups, including homosexual men.

Strategies to control STIs

These include health education and the promotion of condoms; the provision of accessible, acceptable, and affordable clinical services to provide effective treatment and hence prevent complications and further transmission; and partner notification to reach infected people who may not present to a health facility. Since many STIs are asymptomatic, screening programmes may also play an important role. Screening of pregnant women for syphilis is recommended policy in most countries, and has been shown to be cost-effective even where the prevalence is low. Screening programmes for *C. trachomatis* infection have recently been implemented in some Western countries, but their impact is uncertain.

Introduction

Few countries outside Western Europe and North America have accurate reporting systems for sexually transmitted infections (STIs). As a result, in most of the world's population, the incidence of these infections is unknown. Knowledge of their epidemiology is based on the results of improvised prevalence surveys undertaken in convenient populations (e.g. STI or antenatal clinic attenders), but these are often unrepresentative of the population as a whole.

In an attempt to calculate the worldwide incidence of the curable STIs—syphilis, gonorrhoea, trichomoniasis, and chlamydial infection—the World Health Organization (WHO) estimated the prevalence of each infection by region, on the basis of published surveys, and divided this figure by the estimated duration of the infection. They concluded that, each year, 333 million cases of curable STIs occurred worldwide (Fig. 8.1.1). The most common is trichomoniasis (170 million cases), followed by chlamydial infection (89 million), gonorrhoea (62 million), and syphilis (12 million). In view of the uncertainty surrounding the prevalence estimates, the duration of untreated STIs and the mean duration before effective treatment is received, these figures cannot be considered definitive. In 1993, the World Bank estimated that 5.4% of the worldwide burden of disease resulted from STIs excluding HIV.

Transmission of STIs

The rate at which an STI spreads in a population depends on the average number of new cases of infection generated by an infected individual—the basic reproductive number (R_0). This in turn depends on the mean rate of sexual partner change (c), the average duration of the infection (D), and its infectiousness (i.e. the likelihood of it being transmitted per sexual act, β). This relationship has been described by the simple formula $R_0 = \beta c D$.

When R_0 falls below 1 in a given population, the infection will eventually disappear. However, even when R_0 is less than 1 in the general population, infections may be maintained in core groups

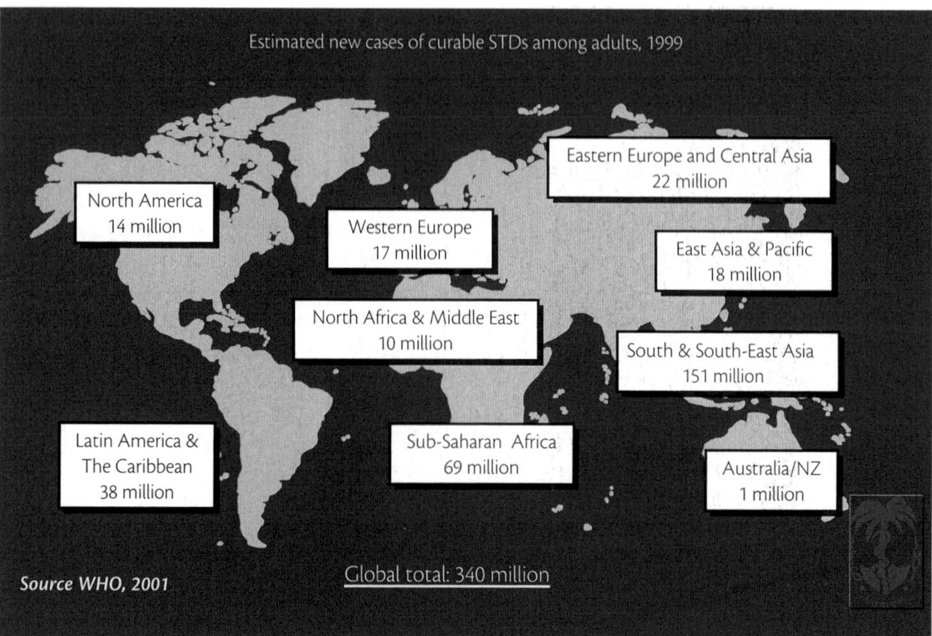

Fig. 8.1.1 The global distribution of five curable STIs (chancroid, syphilis, gonorrhoea, chlamydial infection, and trichomoniasis).

with a high rate of change of sexual partners, and may continue to occur in the general population as a result of sexual contact with members of high-risk groups.

The duration of a curable infection depends on the time that elapses before effective treatment is given. A disease such as chancroid, which almost always causes unpleasant symptoms, is likely to be treated rapidly in populations with access to effective treatment. For this reason, it has almost disappeared in most industrialized countries, but remains endemic in core groups in many developing countries. In contrast, chlamydial infection, which is often asymptomatic in both sexes, is likely to be of longer duration and thus to persist even in affluent populations, unless a comprehensive screening programme is established.

Risk factors for STIs

By definition, STIs are usually transmitted by sexual intercourse, although mother-to-child transmission is also of great public health importance in the case of syphilis and gonorrhoea. Those at highest risk are therefore those with many sexual partners, or those whose partners have many partners—in other words, those who belong to high-risk sexual networks. These include sex workers and their clients, mobile populations such as migrant labourers, truck drivers, fishermen, and soldiers. The youngest sexually active age groups, especially young women, are at particularly high risk.

STIs are more common in poor populations. The incidence of gonorrhoea in inner-city ethnic minorities in the United States of America is at least 30-fold greater than that in middle-class white Americans, and similar to that in many developing countries. Gonorrhoea and syphilis have almost disappeared from affluent countries such as Sweden and Canada, whereas the economic hardship caused by the collapse of the Communist system has led to a dramatic increase in the incidence in reported cases of syphilis in the former Soviet Union.

Poor people are at increased risk of STIs for several reasons. They may have to travel long distances away from their families in search of work. Many poor rural villagers have migrated into cities in developing countries in the last few decades, and many more have been displaced by wars and famines. Poverty and lack of education drive many women into sex work. Health education messages warning of the dangers of HIV/AIDS may be lost on those whose most pressing need is the cost of their next meal. But perhaps most importantly, poor people often lack access to effective treatment for curable STIs.

In China, paradoxically, rapid economic development has coincided with a dramatic increase in the incidence of reported STIs. Syphilis had been virtually eliminated from China in the 1950s, following a massive public health campaign including compulsory screening and treatment for those at risk; but since 1990, its reported incidence has increased more than 20-fold. This reflects the fact that free medical care is no longer available in China, making screening and treatment for syphilis unaffordable for many.

STIs in developed countries

In the United Kingdom, a free and confidential service for people with STIs was established in 1916. Details of patients seen at genitourinary medicine (GUM) clinics are reported to the Health Protection Agency and, since few patients are treated for STIs outside these clinics, the data are believed to be fairly complete and comprehensive. Since the epidemiology of STIs is similar in most countries in Western Europe, the figures for the United Kingdom will be cited as an example (see http://www.hpa.org.uk).

Gonorrhoea

The number of reported cases of both gonorrhoea and syphilis declined steadily from a peak in the early 1980s to the late 1990s, presumably as a result of changes in sexual behaviour following the HIV epidemic (Fig. 8.1.2). The number of cases of gonorrhoea increased in the late 1990s, but has declined in both men and women since 2002 (Fig. 8.1.3). The overall reported incidence in 2005 was 39 per 100 000 total population. The incidence in London was more than twice the national average, and, as in the United

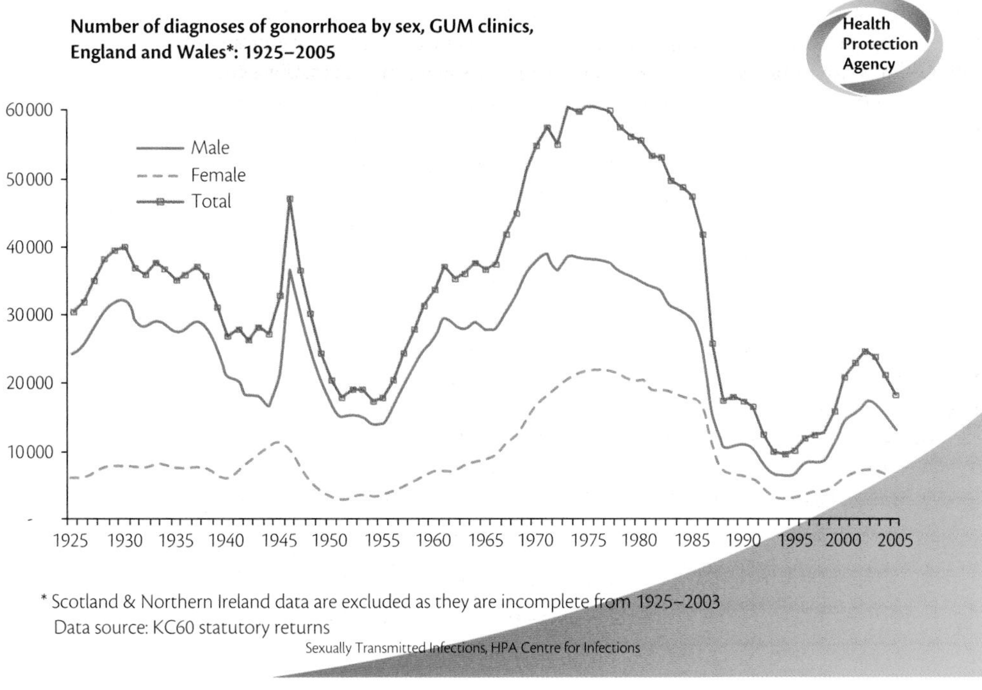

Fig. 8.1.2 The annual incidence of reported gonorrhoea in England and Wales, 1925–2005.
Health Protection Agency
http://www.hpa.org.uk/servlet/Satellite?c=Page&childpagename=HPAweb%2FPage%2FHPAWebAutoListName&cid=1153999752025&p=1153999752025&pagename=HPAwebWrapper&searchmode=simple&searchterm=number+of+diagnoses+of+gonorrhoea+by+sex%2C+GUM+clinics%2C+England+%26+Wales%3A+1925-2005

States of America, was highest in ethnic minorities of African and Caribbean origin.

Syphilis

The number of cases of primary and secondary syphilis increased more than 10-fold in the United Kingdom between 2000 and 2005 (Figs. 8.1.4 and 8.1.5). A high proportion of cases were in homosexual men, in whom HIV was a common coinfection. In 2005, the overall incidence was only 5.7 per 100 000 total population, but it was 19 per 100 000 in men aged 25 to 34 years.

In Eastern Europe, an epidemic of syphilis in the newly independent states of the former Soviet Union was reported in the 1990s. In 1999, the incidence of reported syphilis in these countries ranged from 55 to 180 per 100 000, with increases particularly evident in older adolescents. There was a 20-fold increase in the reported incidence of syphilis in Russia between 1992 and 1996.

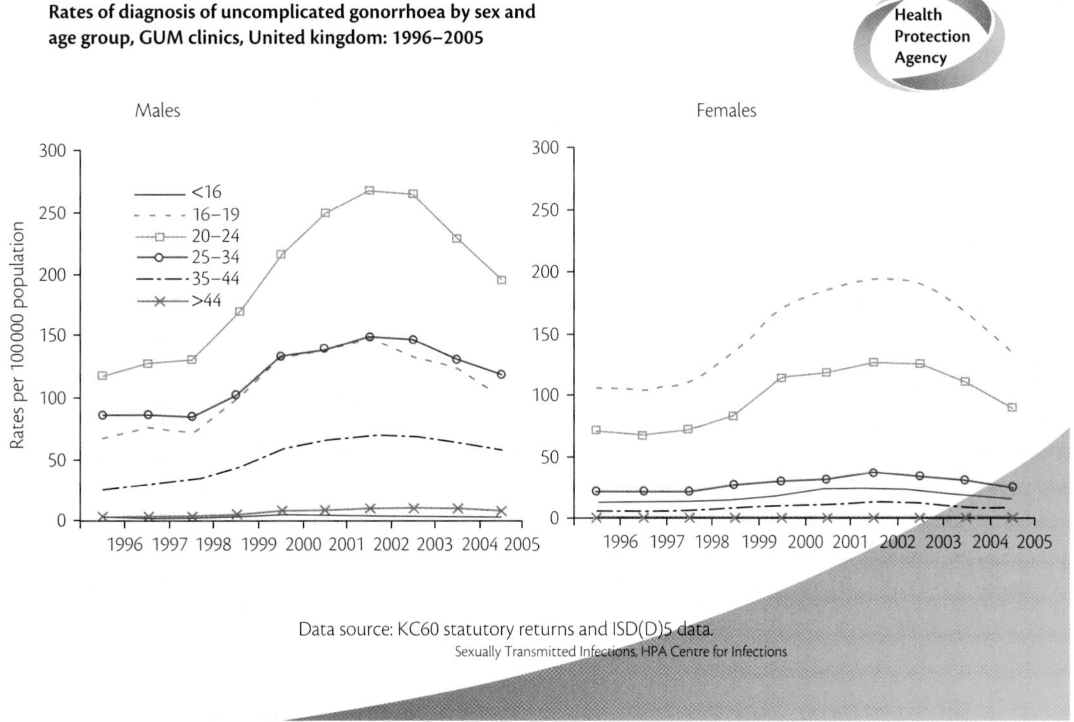

Fig. 8.1.3 The annual incidence of reported gonorrhoea in England and Wales by sex and age group, 1996–2005.
Health Protection Agency

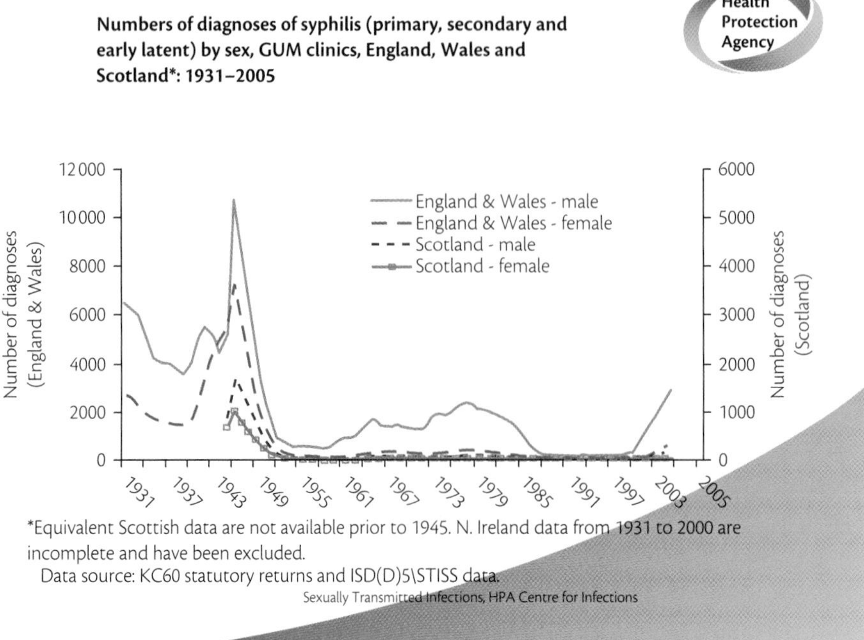

Fig. 8.1.4 The annual incidence of reported early syphilis in England and Wales, 1931–2005.
Health Protection Agency

Chlamydial infection

The number of reported chlamydial infections trebled in the United Kingdom between 1996 and 2005 (Fig. 8.1.6). Similar increases were seen in other Western countries over this period, including Sweden and Canada, despite active screening programmes for chlamydia. It is not clear to what extent this increase is due to an increase in the number of people tested, or to the use of the more sensitive nucleic acid amplification tests, which became widely used in the late 1990s. Paradoxically, the incidence of complications of chlamydial infection, such as pelvic inflammatory disease and ectopic pregnancy, declined in many developed countries over the same period. The overall incidence of reported chlamydial infection in the United Kingdom in 2005 was 223 per 100 000 total population, with the highest rate (1300/100 000) in young women aged 16 to 19 years.

As part of the national survey of sexual attitudes and lifestyles, there was a population-based prevalence survey for *Chlamydia trachomatis* infection in men and women aged 16 to 44 in the

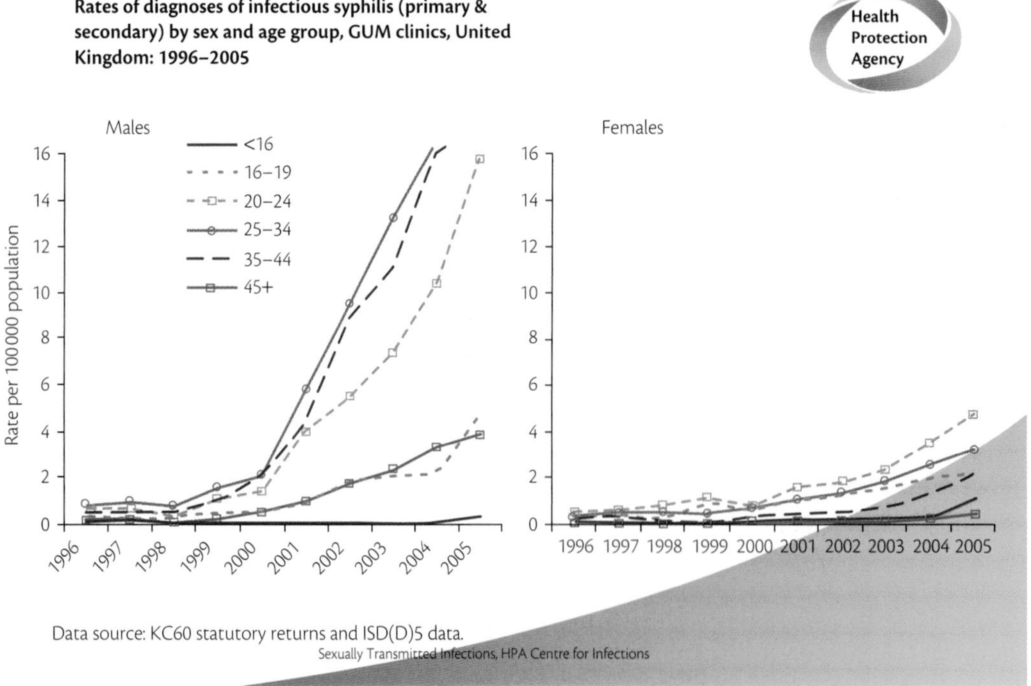

Fig. 8.1.5 The annual incidence of reported syphilis in England and Wales by sex and age group, 1996–2005.
Health Protection Agency

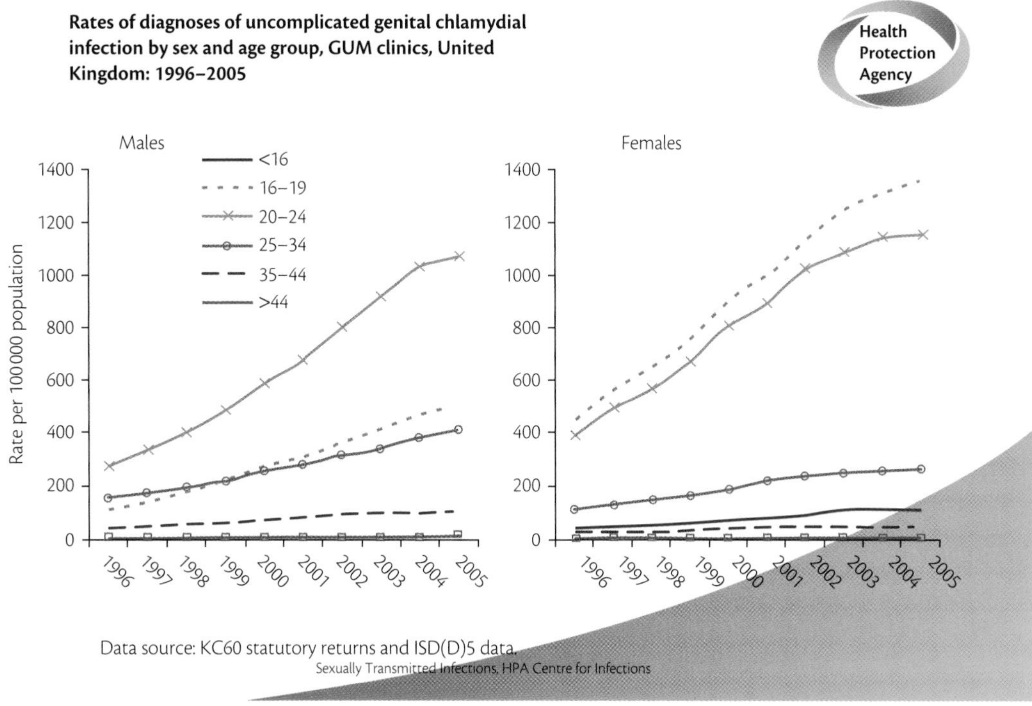

Fig. 8.1.6 The annual incidence of reported chlamydial infection in England and Wales by sex and age group, 1996–2005.
Health Protection Agency

United Kingdom. Infection was found in 2.2% of men, and 1.5% of women, with the highest prevalences in men aged 25 to 34 (3.1%) and women aged 16 to 24 years (3.0%).

Lymphogranuloma venereum (LGV), caused by the more invasive L1, L2, and L3 strains of *C. trachomatis*, is a rare disease in industrialized countries, and is generally considered a 'tropical' STI. In 2003, an outbreak of LGV proctitis due to the L2 serovar was reported among homosexual men in the Netherlands, and in the subsequent 3 years, several hundred cases were reported in homosexual men in Europe and North America, the majority of them HIV positive.

Genital herpes

The incidence of reported genital herpes in women aged 16 to 24 was more than 150 per 100 000 in the United Kingdom in 2005, and in men aged 20 to 24 years it was about half this figure. Classically, genital herpes is due to herpes simplex virus type 2 (HSV2), while herpes simplex type 1 (HSV1) causes oral lesions and is a common childhood infection. Once acquired, these infections persist lifelong, causing recurrent vesicular and ulcerative lesions. In the United Kingdom, the proportion of genital ulcers due to HSV1 is increasing, presumably because of changing sexual practices. More than 50% of episodes in women, and more than 25% in men, are now due to HSV1. The seroprevalence of HSV2 infection is 3% in male blood donors, and 12% in female donors, rising to 16% in pregnant women aged more than 29. In GUM clinic attenders, the seroprevalence exceeds 20% in both sexes.

Human papillomavirus (HPV)

Certain types of HPV (predominantly 6 and 11) cause genital warts, while others (predominantly 16 and 18) cause cervical carcinoma (see Chapter 7.5.19). Genital warts are the most frequently reported viral STI in GUM clinics in the United Kingdom (more than 90 000 cases in 2005), cases increasing by 76% between 1996 and 2005. The incidence in both men and women in the 20- to 24-year-old age group was approximately 700 per 100 000 total population in 2005.

STIs in developing countries

Few reliable data are available on the incidence of STIs in developing countries. Based on numbers of cases seen at health facilities, it is estimated that the incidence of gonorrhoea is at least 50 times higher in sub-Saharan Africa than in the United Kingdom. Several large population-based surveys have confirmed that the prevalence of STIs is high in sub-Saharan Africa, even in rural populations. For example, 5 to 10% of adults were found to be infected with syphilis, 20 to 30% of women, and 10% of men with *Trichomonas vaginalis*, and up to 50% of women were found to have bacterial vaginosis. Syphilis is estimated to cause almost 500 000 stillbirths or neonatal deaths per year in Africa alone.

A population-based study in rural Tanzania found that 50% of women and 25% of men were infected with HSV2 by the age of 20 years. Seropositivity was rare before the age of 16 in both sexes, confirming that HSV2 is mainly transmitted sexually in this population. The proportion of genital ulcers caused by HSV2 has increased in Africa as a result of the HIV epidemic, as recurrences become more frequent and prolonged in the immunocompromised. At the same time, chancroid has apparently become less common in high-risk populations in Africa, perhaps as a result of behavioural change resulting from the HIV epidemic. Cervical carcinoma is the most common malignancy in women in much of the developing world, reflecting the high incidence of sexually transmitted HPV infection.

Interactions between HIV and other STIs

Diseases such as chancroid, syphilis, and herpes, which cause genital ulceration, facilitate sexual transmission of HIV by increasing infectivity and susceptibility. A prospective study of STI clinic attenders in Nairobi, Kenya showed that the likelihood of a man who had acquired a genital ulcer from an HIV-positive sex worker also acquiring HIV was about 1 in 6 after a single sexual exposure. This suggests that the presence of a genital ulcer increases the risk of transmission 50- to 100-fold. STIs such as gonorrhoea that cause genital discharge increase shedding of HIV in both seminal and cervicovaginal secretions.

A community-randomized trial in Mwanza, Tanzania found that improved STI services in rural health centres and dispensaries, using the syndromic approach, reduced the incidence of HIV infection by 40% over a 2-year period. In Uganda, a community-randomized study found that periodic mass treatment for STIs had no impact on the incidence of HIV. In this trial, the HIV epidemic was more advanced, and a high proportion of genital ulcers were caused by HSV2, which was not treated. HIV and HSV2 appear to facilitate transmission of one another, leading to a vicious circle (Fig. 8.1.7). Control of HSV2, perhaps by vaccination, could greatly reduce transmission of HIV in the developing world.

Control of STIs

Strategies for the control of STIs aim to reduce β (transmissibility), c (rate of partner change), or D, the duration of infection.

Primary prevention

Transmissibility can be reduced by the use of condoms. Health promotion and health education aim to encourage the use of condoms, and to persuade people to have fewer sexual partners. This is sometimes referred to as primary prevention, since these measures can prevent people from ever becoming infected. There have been few formal trials of health education in the primary prevention of STIs; but the example of health education in schools suggests that, although education often improves knowledge, it seldom influences behaviour. In Thailand, legislation to close down brothels where condom use was not mandatory, was successful in reducing the incidence and prevalence of HIV infection in the general population.

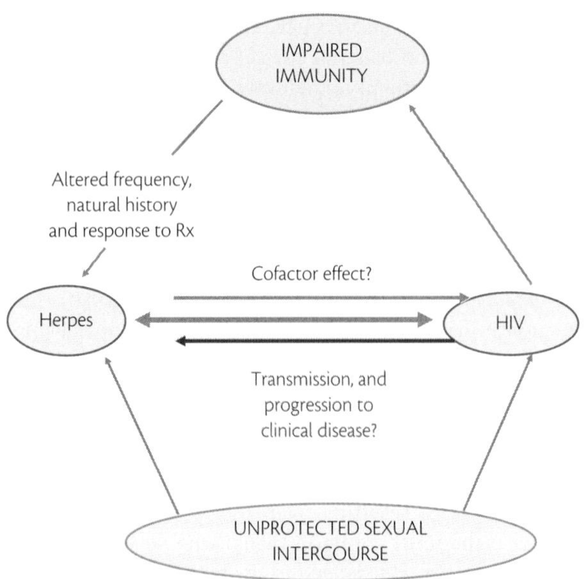

Fig. 8.1.7 Interactions between HIV infections and genital herpes.

Secondary prevention: case management

The duration of treatable STIs can be reduced by the provision of accessible, acceptable, and affordable clinical services, combined with partner notification. Prompt treatment of STIs should be seen as a 'public good', equivalent to the treatment of pulmonary tuberculosis, since it prevents transmission to others, as well as benefiting the person treated.

The aims of patient care are:

- to detect or rule out infection
- to give treatment if necessary
- to educate and counsel on treatment compliance, STD/HIV prevention, and condom use
- to ensure that sexual partner(s) are evaluated and managed (contact tracing)
- to test for other STIs, including HIV

In most developing countries, case management of STIs must be syndromic, because laboratory diagnosis is not available outside a few specialist centres. Syndromic management of genital ulcers and genital discharge in men is straightforward and cost-effective, but syndromic management of vaginal discharge in women is not, because symptoms are poor predictors of the presence of an STI. A cheap, simple, dipstick-type test for gonorrhoea and chlamydial infection in women would be valuable in the control of these infections.

To provide an adequate clinical service, the following components are needed:

- Training should be given to health workers, for instance in the use of flowcharts to simplify the management of STD patients, or to strengthen their health education and counselling skills.
- Laboratory services need to be expanded, depending on the level of health care provided. A reference laboratory should be developed in each country to provide quality control and to support operational research.
- Research should be undertaken to include studies on the aetiology of common syndromes, and assessment of antimicrobial sensitivity.
- Information systems or surveillance are needed to gather epidemiological data, to assess trends, and to provide data for programme planning and monitoring. Various surveillance methods can be used—clinician notification, laboratory notification, sentinel site surveillance (either of syndromes or of aetiological diagnoses), prevalence studies in specific population groups, and aetiological surveys in patients.

Screening programmes

Many people with STIs have no symptoms, and so do not seek medical care. While effective programmes for partner notification may identify some of these, screening programmes have been advocated to identify and treat these people. Because of the severe adverse effects of syphilis on the fetus, screening of pregnant women for syphilis is recommended policy in most countries, and remains a highly cost-effective intervention even when the prevalence of syphilis in pregnant women is less than 0.1%. If universally implemented, it could prevent more than 500 000 perinatal deaths worldwide. The increased resources now available for the prevention of mother-to-child transmission of HIV in many developing countries offer an important opportunity to increase the coverage of antenatal syphilis screening.

Screening of other groups is more controversial. In some countries where sex work is legal or tolerated, screening programmes for sex workers are routinely implemented. A study in the United States of America found that population-based screening for chlamydial infection reduced the incidence of pelvic inflammatory disease. A national screening programme for chlamydial infection in young people seeking health care for any reason has recently been implemented in England, but there is no convincing evidence that such programmes are effective.

Conclusion

A successful STI control programme, by reducing both the incidence and prevalence of STIs, will reduce the morbidity, suffering, and economic cost associated with these diseases. By eliminating STIs as a facilitating factor in HIV transmission, and by contributing to behavioural changes towards safer sex, it will play an important role in the prevention and control of HIV/AIDS. In the longer term, control of STIs will depend on improved living conditions for poor people, particularly women, in both developed and developing worlds.

Further reading

Chen Z-Q, *et al.* (2007). Syphilis in China: results of a national surveillance programme. *Lancet*, **369**, 132–8.

Fenton KA, *et al.* (2001). Sexual behaviour in Britain: reported sexually transmitted infections and prevalent *Chlamydia trachomatis* infection. *Lancet*, **358**, 1851–4.

Fleming DT, Wasserheit JN (1999). From epidemiological synergy to public health policy and practice: the contribution of other sexually transmitted diseases to sexual transmission of HIV infection. *Sex Transm Infect*, **75**, 3–17.

Gerbase AC, Rowley JT, Mertens TE (1998). Global epidemiology of sexually transmitted diseases. *Lancet*, **351** Suppl. III, 2–4.

Grosskurth H, *et al.* (1995). Impact of improved treatment of STD on HIV infection in rural Tanzania: randomised controlled trial. *Lancet*, **346**, 530–6.

Low N (2007). Chlamydia screening programmes: when will we ever learn? *BMJ*, **334**, 725–8.

Obasi A, *et al.* (1999). Antibodies to herpes simplex virus type 2 as a marker of sexual risk behaviour in rural Tanzania. *J Infect Dis*, **179**, 16–24.

Over M, Piot P (1993). HIV infection and sexually transmitted diseases. In: Jamison DT, *et al.* (eds.) *Disease control priorities in developing countries*. Oxford University Press, Oxford.

Schmid G (2004). Economic and programmatic aspects of congenital syphilis prevention. *Bull World Health Organ*, **82**, 402–9.

Peeling RW, *et al.* (2004). Avoiding HIV and dying of syphilis. *Lancet*, **364**, 1561–3.

UK Collaborative Group for HIV and STI Surveillance (2006). *A complex picture: HIV and other sexually transmitted infections in the UK: 2006.* Centre for Infections, Health Protection Agency, London.

Wawer MJ, *et al.* (1999). Control of sexually transmitted diseases for AIDS prevention in Uganda: a randomised community trial. *Lancet*, **353**, 525–35.

8.2

Sexual behaviour

Anne M. Johnson and Catherine H. Mercer

Essentials

Discussion of sexual lifestyle and the ability to take a sexual history are relevant to a wide range of clinical practice. Most of the population is attracted to, and has sex, exclusively with people of the opposite sex. The age at which people first have sex has decreased in recent decades, increasing the time available to accumulate sexual partners and thus be at risk of STIs, including HIV. While many people have few partners, a small proportion of the population has many.

People with many partners are most at risk of STIs, but there are a number of other influences including the gender, age, and ethnicity of their partners and the type of sexual practice. Strategies to reduce the adverse consequences of sexual behaviour (including STIs and unintended pregnancy) tend therefore to encourage reducing partner numbers, using condoms and effective contraception, and engaging in less risky practices.

Sexual function problems are relatively common and need to be considered in a range of clinical consultations.

Introduction

Most men and women are sexually active for a large part of their adult life and sexual fulfilment is important in enhancing the quality of many people's lives. Patterns of sexual behaviour in populations are a key determinant of fertility and transmission of sexually transmitted infections (STIs).

Discussion of sexual lifestyle and ability to take a sexual history are relevant to a wide range of clinical consultations. Common topics include management of genitourinary symptoms, contraceptive advice, sexual dysfunction, and resumption of sexual activity following childbirth, major illnesses, or surgery.

Sexual orientation

Surveys of sexual behaviour in representative population samples show that the majority of men and women are predominantly attracted to, and have experience with, members of the opposite sex throughout their lives. However, sexual orientation is not a simple dichotomy between 'homosexual' and 'heterosexual', but varies from exclusively heterosexual experience through various shades of attraction to and experience with both genders, to exclusively homosexual experience.

In a large British study of adults aged 16 to 44, 6.7% of men and 7.0% of women reported having sexual experience with someone of the same gender at some time. For some, this was a fleeting adolescent experience, followed in many cases by exclusively heterosexual partnerships. A smaller proportion of the British population report homosexual partnerships involving some form of genital contact (5.4% of men and 4.8% of women). Similar findings are reported from France and the United States of America. The majority of those with same-gender partners have had experience of heterosexual intercourse at some time. Exclusively homosexual experience throughout life is thus relatively unusual.

Homosexual experience is more common among men in large metropolitan areas. For example, 8.7% of men sampled in Inner London reported having a homosexual partner in the last 5 years. Capitals and other large cities typically provide a more tolerant atmosphere and better social facilities for those with a homosexual lifestyle. This is reflected in the high proportion of homosexually acquired STIs reported from clinics in London, and the higher rates of homosexually acquired HIV and AIDS reported in many metropolitan areas in Europe and the United States of America.

Age of first heterosexual intercourse

The age of first heterosexual intercourse has been gradually decreasing over recent decades. The proportion of people having sexual intercourse before marriage has rapidly increased, so that sex before marriage has become almost universal in Britain. For men born in the years between 1930 and 1935, the median age of first intercourse was 20 and for women 21. For men and women born between 1975 and 1985, the median age at first intercourse is 16. Similar trends have been observed in other European countries and in the United States of America.

English law gives the age of consent for heterosexual intercourse as 16, and it is illegal for a man to have sex with a woman under 16 in England (and other parts of the United Kingdom). The proportion of men and women in Britain reporting first intercourse before the age of 16 has risen rapidly over recent decades to 29.9% of men and 25.6% of women aged 16 to 19 in 2000. This has important implications for the provision of sex education and the timing of human papilloma virus (HPV) vaccination programmes. Those just embarking on their sexual careers may be most vulnerable to unwanted consequences of unprotected sexual intercourse: STIs and termination of pregnancy are more common in 16- to 24-year-olds than in older men and women.

Heterosexual partners

The number of heterosexual partners is highly variable. While many people have few partners, a small proportion has many. Among men aged 16 to 44 in Britain, 51.6% reported 0 or 1 partners in the last 5 years; 6.4% reported more than 10; and a small proportion reported hundreds or even thousands of partners during their lives.

The risk of acquiring or transmitting an STI increases with the number of sexual partners. For example, in the British survey, 1.2% of men and women with 0 or 1 partners in the 5 years prior to the survey reported STIs, compared to 14.0% of those with at least 10 partners. Those with high numbers of partners may account for a relatively high proportion of STI transmission in a community and for sustaining endemic STI transmission. They are sometimes referred to as a 'core group' for STI transmission. The choice of partner also influences STI transmission in populations. Age, gender, and ethnic mixing are important, as well as the extent to which people choose partners with lifestyles similar to their own (assortative mixing) or different (disassortative mixing), and whether they have serially monogamous or concurrent partnerships.

Commercial sex workers and their clients remain at high risk of HIV and STIs in some parts of the developing world where condom use is infrequent. In some countries, such as Thailand, public health campaigns have succeeded in increasing use of condoms in commercial sex contacts. In many developed countries, although sex workers are at increased risk of STIs, there is evidence that high levels of condom use may protect both them and their clients.

The proportion of men who have commercial sex contacts varies widely between countries. In British survey, 8.9% of men reported paying money for sex at some time, but considerably more frequent exposure is reported in other countries.

Multiple heterosexual partnerships are most common among young people, and among those who are not married or cohabiting. More than 1 in 10 men aged 16 to 24 in Britain reported more than 10 partners during the previous 5 years, even though this group included many individuals who had not yet become sexually active. Age is not the only influence on sexual behaviour. Whatever their age, those who are separated, divorced, or widowed are more likely than married people of similar age to have multiple partners, illustrating the effects of the life course on patterns of partnership. Since the HIV epidemic emerged, public health campaigns have emphasized behaviour change for sexual health promotion. Some evidence suggests that, in the developed world in the late 1980s, there was a reduction in numbers of partners and increased use of condoms resulting in declining rates of STIs. However, since the late 1990s, these trends have been reversed with a return to risky sexual behaviour. In some parts of the developing world, such as Uganda and Thailand, the incidence of HIV has decreased, mainly due to changes in behaviour but also the epidemic stage.

Heterosexual practices

The repertoire and frequency of sexual practices varies between individuals. In heterosexual relationships, vaginal intercourse is the most common practice, but most couples include other practices, particularly mutual masturbation and orogenital contact, in their repertoire.

The frequency of sexual contact varies with age, life stage, and availability of a sexual partner. Among married couples, the median frequency of sexual intercourse is about 4 times per month, but this is highly variable. Frequency declines with age in married and cohabiting couples, depending partly on the duration of the relationship.

Among men and women aged 16 to 44 in Britain, over three-quarters reported orogenital contact during the previous year, both cunnilingus and fellatio. The practices of orogenital stimulation and mutual masturbation have increased in recent decades.

Anal intercourse is a relatively infrequent activity in heterosexual couples. In British survey, 26.0% of men and 24.2% of women had experienced anal intercourse at some time, but only around 11.4% had experienced it in the previous year. Anal intercourse can result in transmission of STIs. Anal intercourse, in addition to vaginal intercourse, may increase the risk of heterosexual transmission of HIV, but since anal intercourse is practised relatively infrequently worldwide, most heterosexual HIV transmission is attributable to vaginal intercourse.

Homosexual behaviour

Male homosexual lifestyles have been more intensively studied than female homosexual lifestyles. Studies of volunteer samples of homosexual men in the United States of America in the 1970s identified a distinctive lifestyle characterized by multiple casual sexual partners, often encountered at gay meeting places such as bars, clubs, and 'bathhouses'. These men were at high risk of STIs and were among the first to suffer high rates of HIV infection. Research in Britain identified a group of homosexual men with similar lifestyles. However, studies of homosexual men recruited from places other than STD clinics and gay meeting places showed smaller numbers of sexual partners, less frequent changes of partner, and lower prevalence of sexually acquired pathogens.

Men who have homosexual partnerships are at increased risk of HIV infection and other STIs, including hepatitis B and syphilis. Female homosexual practices carry a low risk of STI transmission. However, women with homosexual partnerships may be at risk of STIs and HIV as a result of partnerships with men, since a high proportion of these women also have male partners.

Many male–male partnerships are restricted to mutual masturbation or orogenital contact and do not involve penetrative anal intercourse. It is anal intercourse that carries the highest risk of transmission of sexually acquired organisms between homosexual men. Many homosexual men practise both receptive and insertive anal intercourse. Receptive anal intercourse carries the highest risk of HIV transmission. After the HIV epidemic emerged, there was evidence of a reduction in high-risk behaviour among gay men.

Increased use of condoms and reduced partner numbers reduced exposure to unprotected anal intercourse. However, since the late 1990s, risky behaviour has increased and new HIV infections continue to be a significant public-health challenge.

Risk reduction strategies and sexual health

Increasing attention is being paid to promoting sexual health and reducing the adverse consequences of sexual behaviour. Extensive discussion of population strategies is outside the scope of this chapter. However, individuals can reduce their risk of STI and unwanted pregnancy by reducing the numbers of partners with whom they have unprotected intercourse, using condoms, using effective contraception, and enjoying sexual practices with less risk of transmission. Negotiating sexual fulfilment is a more difficult matter, but a greater focus on communication between partners, and on sexual technique, is important.

Problems with sexual function are relatively common. One-third of the men and one-half of the women in the British survey reported some kind of sexual problem for at least 1 month during the previous year. Persistent problems affect approximately 6% of men and 16% of women. The commonest difficulty experienced by both sexes is a lack of interest. Although sexual function problems are common, few people seek help. Most who do consult their general practitioner. Health professionals can help by being capable of taking a tactful sexual history, having the necessary clinical skills, and being informed about sexual health and the need for health promotion.

Further reading

Fenton KA, *et al.* (2001). Sexual behaviour in Britain: reported sexually transmitted infections and prevalent genital *Chlamydia trachomatis* infection. *Lancet*, **358**, 1851–4.

Johnson AM, *et al.* (1992). Sexual behaviour and HIV risk. *Nature*, **360**, 410–12.

Johnson AM, *et al.* (1993). *Sexual attitudes and lifestyles*. Blackwell Scientific, Oxford.

Johnson AM, *et al.* (2001). Sexual behaviour in Britain: partnerships, practices, and HIV risk behaviours. *Lancet*, **358**, 1835–42.

Mercer CH, *et al.* (2003). Sexual function problems and help seeking behaviour in Britain: national probability sample survey. *BMJ*, **327**, 426–7.

Wellings K, *et al.* (2006). Sexual behaviour in context: a global perspective. *Lancet*, **368**, 1706–28.

8.3

Sexual history and examination

Jackie Sherrard and Graz A. Luzzi

Essentials

Sexually transmitted infections (STIs) are common, especially in young people, and it is important that doctors recognize both the need to obtain a sexual history and when to perform genital examination. STIs can present with generalized or extragenital symptoms whose significance may be missed. This chapter gives advice on how to take a sexual history and perform genital examination in both sexes. It also summarizes the common symptoms and syndromes associated with STIs and their causative pathogens, cross-referring to other chapters in the textbook.

Introduction

Sexually transmitted infections (STIs) are a common cause of morbidity, especially in young people. Although many STIs are asymptomatic, important symptoms may be missed because patients are not questioned directly about genital symptoms (Table 8.3.1). If a sexual history is not taken, the risk of an STI may not be appreciated. In general medical practice, it is important that doctors are aware that STIs may present with extragenital symptoms (Table 8.3.2). Examples include secondary syphilis, primary HIV infection, disseminated gonococcal infection, and herpes simplex meningitis. Failure to consider a sexually acquired infection in the differential diagnosis may delay diagnosis and treatment.

Sexual history

A sexual history is essential to establish the patient's risk of an STI, to elicit symptoms that may guide diagnostic tests, and to facilitate treatment of sexual partners who may be at risk (partner notification). If an STI is diagnosed, the discussion is extended to provide relevant information about the condition and to educate on reducing future risk.

The clinician must ask questions that are extremely personal. Initially this can be mutually embarrassing for the doctor and patient. The clinician should endeavour to see the patient alone as they may be reluctant to reveal personal information, especially about previous sexual activity, if their current partner is in the room. It may be difficult for a young person to talk about sexual activity if a parent is present.

Sexual history taking is facilitated by

- being explicit about confidentiality
- asking permission, explaining what to expect and why you are asking the questions
- asking only what is relevant and necessary
- starting with the less intrusive questions, such as symptoms, before asking the ones that are more personal
- using appropriate language and tact
- not making assumptions about sexual orientation or practices

Asking questions

Use open questions such as:

- 'Are you sexually active?'
- 'Are you in a relationship?'
- 'Have you changed partners recently?'
- 'Do you have sex with men, women, or both?'
- 'When was the last time you had any kind of sex?'

The key features of a sexual history are:

- symptoms
- details of sexual partner(s)—gender, timing of last sex, use of condoms or contraception, whether partner is contactable or not, whether partner reported any symptoms
- concurrent illness
- previous STI
- current medication
- in women, assessment of pregnancy risk

However, a number of STIs may present with extragenital symptoms or signs (Table 8.3.2).

Table 8.3.1 Common presentations of STIs

Symptoms	Common causes (see Section 7 and Chapters 8.4 and 8.5)
In women	
Change in vaginal discharge	Candida, TV, BV, less commonly GC, CT
Anogenital sores/ulcers	Herpes simplex, trauma, syphilis
Anogenital lumps	Genital warts, molluscum contagiosum, normal anatomical variants
Pelvic pain/dypareunia and/or irregular menses	Pelvic inflammatory disease: CT, GC
In men	
Urethritis: urethral irritation/ discomfort and/or discharge	Chlamydia, gonorrhoea, nonspecific urethritis
Anogenital sores/ulcers	Herpes simplex, trauma, syphilis
Anogenital lumps	Genital warts, molluscum contagiosum, normal anatomical variants
Scrotal pain/swelling	Chlamydia, gonorrhoea
Additionally in men who have sex with men (MSM)	
Rectal pain/discharge/tenesmus	GC, CT, LGV, HSV

BV, bacterial vaginosis; CT, chlamydia; GC, gonorrhoea; HSV, herpes simplex virus; LGV, lymphogranuloma venereum; TV, *Trichomonas vaginalis*.

Examination

In symptomatic patients, examination is necessary because a visual diagnosis may be possible, examination may suggest the need for further tests, and may also identify complications that need longer or altered treatment regimens (e.g. pelvic examination may suggest pelvic infection requiring a specific treatment regimen). In asymptomatic patients, genital examination is also recommended because patients are often surprisingly unaware of the presence of infection. Although symptoms may be denied, important abnormalities may be found on examination. The increased availability of nucleic acid tests allows noninvasive sampling for many STIs; however, genital examination should always be considered.

Table 8.3.2 Some extragenital symptoms or signs of STIs

System/category	Syndrome/site	Causes (see Sections 7, and 25 and Chapter 19.8)
Eyes	Uveitis, conjunctivitis, optic neuritis, retinitis	Syphilis/HIV/GC/CT/Reiter's syndrome
Joints	Tenosynovitis/septic arthritis especially of small- and medium-sized joints Septic arthritis	Syphilis/GC/Reiter's syndrome (CT associated)/HIV GC
Skin		Reiter's syndrome, GC, HIV, syphilis, scabies, molluscum contagiosum
Cardiac		Syphilis, GC, HIV
Malignancy	Carcinomas: cervix, vulva, penis, anus, lymphoma, Kaposi's sarcoma	HPV, HIV
Gastrointestinal system	Hepatitis, perihepatitis Diarrhoea	Hepatitis B and C, CT HIV, LGV

CT, chlamydia; GC, gonorrhoea; LGV, lymphogranuloma venereum.

Examination involves full inspection of the genitoanal area in both sexes, including palpation of the inguinal nodes and examination of the pubic area. Good lighting is essential.

In patients with syphilis, late HIV disease, Reiter's syndrome, and disseminated gonococcal infection, a full examination is necessary. Some non-STIs may present with genital signs, e.g. lichen sclerosus, lichen planus, psoriasis, eczema, Crohn's disease; in these cases, a full examination may be helpful in making the diagnosis.

In men, examination of the genital area includes palpation of the scrotal contents to detect epididymal or testicular swelling or tenderness. This is best carried out while the patient is standing up. Epididymal cysts are relatively common, especially with increasing age. Acute epididymitis causes tender swelling of the epididymis, usually unilaterally, sometimes with involvement of the testis (epididymoorchitis) causing generalized testicular swelling and hydrocele.

In uncircumcised men, the foreskin should be fully retracted and the subpreputial area inspected for rashes, ulcer, and lumps. The urethral meatus should be everted slightly and inspected for discharge, and lumps such as genital warts. In men who have sex with men (MSM) who report practising anal sex the anal/perianal region should be examined, the rectum inspected by proctoscopy if there are rectal symptoms, and if they report orogenital sex, the oropharyngeal mucosae should be inspected for ulcers and other abnormalities.

In women, examination includes careful inspection of the vulva, which is best performed in the lithotomy position. The vagina and cervix should be inspected by speculum examination and a bimanual examination performed to check for cervical or adnexal tenderness and pelvic masses.

Role of chaperones

In the United Kingdom, the General Medical Council has produced guidance on intimate examinations, which includes:

- the routine offer of a chaperone
- giving the patient privacy to undress and dress
- explaining to the patient why examination is necessary and what it will involve
- obtaining the patient's permission before the examination and discontinuing it if the patient asks you to

Before performing an intimate examination (examination of the genitalia, rectum, or breast), a chaperone should always be offered and the offer recorded in the notes along with a note indicating who the chaperone was. If the offer is declined, this should be recorded, and it may be necessary to reschedule the examination if the doctor does not feel comfortable about proceeding without a chaperone.

During general examination, especially when male doctors examine the heart and lungs of female patients, misunderstandings can arise about perceived inappropriate touching of the breasts. The manner in which the examination is conducted is therefore clearly very important, with appropriate explanation and professionalism.

The general examination is often conducted in the absence of a chaperone, but there are circumstances in which a chaperone should be sought, including when this is requested by the patient, or if the doctor feels that it is appropriate.

A chaperone is present as a safeguard for all parties (patient and practitioner) and is a witness to continuing consent of the procedure. However, a chaperone is not a guarantee of protection for either the patient or the practitioner, and for most patients, explanation, consent, privacy, and a respectful and professional attitude take precedence over the need for a chaperone. When issues arise about individual clinical practice, good record-keeping is very helpful.

8.4

Vaginal discharge

Paul Nyirjesy

Essentials

Vaginal symptoms are a frequent source of discomfort and distress for many women. Bacterial vaginosis, vulvovaginal candidiasis, and trichomoniasis are considered the most common causes in premenopausal women, but atrophic vaginitis and noninfectious disorders seem to occur more often in menopausal women.

Self-diagnosis and syndromic management, although increasingly encouraged in many parts of the world, are fraught with inaccuracy.

A proper diagnosis depends on a thorough history, examination, and readily available tests in the clinic. Ancillary tests to be considered in selective circumstances include cultures for trichomonas or yeast, tests for *Neisseria gonorrheae* or *Chlamydia trachomatis*, and (rarely) Gram stain or maturation index. Once a proper diagnosis is obtained, appropriate treatment can be selected.

Introduction

Vaginal discharge, itching, burning, irritation, and odour are common causes of distress in women, yet they are frequently ignored or trivialized by health care providers. With the availability of over-the-counter antifungals, self-diagnosis and self-treatment of vaginal symptoms have become routine, but questions remain about their accuracy. Appropriate tests in the clinic and laboratory are the only reliable basis for treatment.

The normal vaginal environment

An understanding of the normal vaginal environment is crucial to accurate clinical assessment and interpretation of test results. The normal vaginal environment is controlled by a woman's oestrogen status. By increasing the glycogen content of vaginal epithelial cells, oestrogen fosters the growth of lactobacilli, which in turn seem to inhibit the other growth of other organisms. Thus, a Gram stain of vaginal secretions from a healthy woman in her reproductive years should be dominated by lactobacilli and Gram-positive rods. However, vaginal cultures will yield a broad range of organisms, including skin and faecal flora (e.g. *Staphylococcus epidermidis*, *Staph. aureus*, *Escherichia coli*, anaerobes) and organisms, which in many situations, are considered pathogenic (e.g. *Streptococcus agalactiae* (group B streptococci), *Mycoplasma hominis*, *Ureaplasma urealyticum*, *Gardnerella vaginalis*, and *Candida albicans*). In women who are either prepubertal or postmenopausal, lactobacilli are less numerous, and other bacteria will frequently predominate.

Differential diagnosis and clinical investigation

Most studies suggest that infections such as bacterial vaginosis (30–35% of cases), vulvovaginal candidiasis (20–25%), and trichomoniasis (15–20%) are the most common causes of vaginal symptoms, but many miscellaneous conditions, including atrophic vaginitis, vulvar conditions (e.g. vulvodynia, lichen sclerosus, lichen simplex), or even a physiological discharge can cause symptoms that require assessment. A thorough evaluation will usually allow correct diagnosis.

An accurate diagnosis relies largely on the patient's history. Symptoms are often not limited to discharge alone but frequently include itching, burning, irritation, or malodour. Since patients may be too embarrassed to mention some of these, it is helpful to inquire about each of them in turn. Other pertinent information is about location (vulvar, introital, or vaginal), duration, variation with menstrual cycle, association with sexual activity, and response to previous therapy. A sexual history may identify women at increased risk of a sexually transmitted infection. Pelvic examination should include inspection of the vulva and vestibule; touching the vulva and vestibule with a swab (the 'Q-tip test') may elicit areas of tenderness. Samples should be obtained for further evaluation. Vaginal pH testing, an amine ('whiff') test, and saline and 10% potassium hydroxide microscopy should be practised routinely. If the source of discharge is primarily the cervix, culture or nucleic acid amplification tests for *N. gonorrheae* and *C. trachomatis* should be obtained. Suspected vulvar diseases may require

Table 8.4.1 Testing for vaginal infections

	Vaginal pH	Amine test	Microscopy	Gold standard
Normal	≤4.5	–	Normal	
Bacterial vaginosis	>4.5	+	Clue cells	Gram stain
Trichomoniasis	>4.5	±	Trichomonads	Trichomonas culture
Vulvovaginal candidiasis	≤4.5	–	Pseudohyphae, blastospores	Yeast culture
Atrophy	>4.5	–	Immature epithelial cells	Maturation index

a biopsy for diagnosis. Finally, in situations where the diagnosis is not clear, definitive tests may assist in the diagnosis of bacterial vaginosis, trichomoniasis, and vulvovaginal candidiasis (Table 8.4.1).

Trichomoniasis

Trichomonas vaginalis is a common sexually transmitted protozoan, causing an estimated 180 million infections per year worldwide. Traditionally, it has been considered a minor nuisance, but it is associated statistically with an increased risk of low birth weight or preterm delivery in pregnant women and of HIV transmission in nonpregnant women. Asymptomatic men and women are the primary reservoir for infection. Affected women will complain of an abnormal purulent, frothy or bloody discharge, itching, malodour, dysuria, urinary frequency, dyspareunia, and postcoital bleeding. Examination may reveal, erythema and excoriations of the vulva or vagina, an abnormal discharge, and punctate haemorrhages of the cervix (the 'strawberry cervix'). Saline microscopy may reveal motile trichomonads, but it has limited sensitivity (22–75%). Finding many white blood cells on microscopy, a positive amine test, or an elevated pH may suggest the presence of trichomoniasis but do not prove the diagnosis. The current gold standard is culture. Where available, antigen-based tests at the point of care are much more sensitive than microscopy and provide a more rapid answer than culture.

Treatment is with nitroimidazoles, either metronidazole or tinidazole. A single dose of 2 g of either will cure more than 90% of affected cases. Alternatively, a 7-day course of 500 mg twice daily is recommended. As with other STDs, treatment of the partner is crucial to prevent reinfection. Patients who are allergic to metronidazole should be referred for desensitization and then treated with metronidazole. In cases of treatment failure, patient compliance must first be confirmed and reinfection by her partner excluded. Since tinidazole seems to be more effective than metronidazole, higher doses of tinidazole, such as 2 g daily for 5 days, can be considered. Pregnant women with trichomoniasis should receive metronidazole, as there are no data on tinidazole use in pregnancy.

Bacterial vaginosis

This is considered the most common cause of vaginitis, with a prevalence of 5 to 25%. It represents a polymicrobial infection of the vagina. The vaginal flora is markedly altered. Hydrogen peroxide-producing lactobacilli are absent, and there is an overgrowth of a wide variety of organisms, including *G. vaginalis*, *M. hominis*, *Bacteroides* spp., *Prevotella* spp., *Mobiluncus* spp., and other bacteria that are still being identified. Bacterial vaginosis is associated with a variety of risk factors, including multiple partners, more frequent sexual intercourse, smoking, and douching. Although it may be sexually transmitted in lesbians, treatment of male partners of heterosexual women has failed to reduce recurrence rates and it has been found in sexually inexperienced women. In nonpregnant women, it has been associated with many conditions including pelvic inflammatory disease, infection after abortion or hysterectomy, cervicitis, urinary tract infection, and HIV and herpes simplex virus-2 transmissions. In pregnant women, studies have linked bacterial vaginosis to prematurity, preterm premature rupture of membranes, and postpartum endometritis.

Although up to 50% of women are asymptomatic, affected women will note an abnormal discharge or a fishy odour, which is often worse during menses or after intercourse. Itching and irritation are considered rare. The clinical criteria (Amsel's criteria) which are used to diagnose infection consist of the following:

- a homogeneous grey or white discharge
- a vaginal pH exceeding 4.5
- a positive amine test
- more than 20% clue cells (vaginal epithelial cells stippled with bacteria) on saline microscopy.

Three out of the four criteria are adequate for a diagnosis. Alternatively, a Gram stain (Nugent) score, which evaluates the presence or absence of various bacterial morphotypes, may be used. Because the Nugent score is a permanent record, which can be read by personnel who are blinded to patient information, it is the preferred method of diagnosis in research studies.

Oral or topical treatment seems equally effective.

- Oral regimens, including metronidazole 500 mg twice a day for 7 days, tinidazole 1 g daily for 5 days, or clindamycin 300 mg twice daily for 7 days, tend to be less expensive but may cause gastrointestinal distress; metronidazole and tinidazole are incompatible with drinking alcohol.
- Topical regimens, such as 0.75% metronidazole gel (one 5-g applicator daily for 5 days), 2% clindamycin standard (one 5-g applicator daily for 7 days) or single-dose creams (one 5-g applicator), and 100-mg clindamycin ovules (one ovule nightly, for 3 doses) tend to be more expensive.

In high-risk pregnant women, particularly those with prior preterm birth, as well as nonpregnant women undergoing either hysterectomy or abortion, screening and treating for bacterial vaginosis seems to decrease associated morbidities. To date, low-risk pregnant women do not seem to benefit from screening and treatment for asymptomatic bacterial vaginosis. Apart from tinidazole, pregnant women can be treated with similar bacterial vaginosis regimens as nonpregnant women.

Recurrence after treatment seems to occur commonly, up to 50% within 6 months. For patients with frequent recurrences (3 or more per year), a prolonged 4-month course of suppressive antibiotic therapy, such as metronidazole 0.75% gel, one 5-g applicator twice weekly, was associated with much lower rates of bacterial vaginosis than a placebo group. It is claimed that some commercially available products can repopulate the vagina with lactobacilli, but there are no conclusive data to support their use or efficacy in women with recurrent bacterial vaginosis.

Vulvovaginal candidiasis

About 75% of women will at some time in their lives develop vulvovaginal candidiasis or 'yeast infections'. *C. albicans* causes 90 to 95% of vulvovaginal candidiasis; of the many other species of yeast that are sometimes implicated, *C. glabrata* is thought to be the second most common. Commonly recognized risk factors for candidiasis include the use of oral contraceptives, recent use of broad-spectrum antimicrobials, pregnancy, diabetes mellitus, and immunosuppression. Being sexually active and practising oral receptive sex are associated with vulvovaginal candidiasis, but there are no data to support partner treatment. Patients with vulvovaginal candidiasis complain primarily of vulvar or vaginal pruritus, irritation, burning, dyspareunia, or abnormal discharge. The symptom of discharge is quite unreliable in predicting which women with vaginitis actually have vulvovaginal candidiasis. Examination of affected women may reveal vulvar erythema, oedema, excoriations, or fissures. Vaginal thrush may be present. The vaginal pH is normal. On microscopy, hyphae or blastospores may be seen, but the sensitivity is fairly low (*c*.50%); thus, a simple yeast culture is recommended in women who are symptomatic but with negative microscopy.

For most women with vulvovaginal candidiasis, the infection will be uncomplicated: it is sporadic, associated with relatively mild symptoms, caused by *C. albicans*, and is occurring in an otherwise normal host. Uncomplicated vulvovaginal candidiasis generally responds readily to any available antimycotic treatment. Topical therapies consist primarily of imidazoles, including miconazole, clotrimazole, butoconazole, and terconazole, which are available as creams or suppositories applied for 1 to 7 days. A single150-mg dose of oral fluconazole seems equivalent to topical treatments.

An estimated 5% will suffer complicated vulvovaginal candidiasis, marked by either an underlying medical problem such as diabetes mellitus or HIV infection, severe symptoms, recurrent disease (four or more episodes per year), or an infection caused by a yeast other than *C. albicans*. Most of these women will not have any of the commonly recognized risk factors for infection. Complicated vulvovaginal candidiasis will recur within a month in at least 50% of cases, and is best managed by first obtaining a positive yeast culture to obtain information about the species of the isolate, then by more aggressive therapy and follow-up. In patients with severe vulvovaginal candidiasis, a second dose of fluconazole 3 days after the first, or a second week of topical therapy, improves the chance of complete resolution. Women with recurrent vulvovaginal candidiasis caused by *C. albicans* benefit from prolonged suppressive therapy with weekly oral fluconazole (100–200 mg) after an initial induction phase of 3 doses given 3 days apart. Finally, for *C. glabrata* infections, boric acid capsules (600 mg vaginally), nightly for 14 days, are often curative.

Atrophic vaginitis

Since women are living longer in many countries, larger proportions of their lives are postmenopausal. As a consequence, atrophic vaginitis, which is caused by a lack of oestrogen, is likely to become increasingly common. Women with atrophy may present with a spectrum of complaints, including an abnormal discharge, dryness, itching, and dyspareunia. Signs of labial atrophy, vaginal pallor, or loss of rugal folds may be easily missed. The vaginal pH will usually be elevated above 4.5. On wet mount, immature epithelial cells; either parabasals or intermediate cells, which are rounder, smaller, and have a greater nucleus:cytoplasmic ratio can be seen. Because of its effects on vaginal flora, there may be a decreased normal flora or even a shift to cocci instead of bacilli.

In the absence of contraindications, oestrogen remains the medication of choice. Topical therapy, in the form of cream, tablets, or an oestrogen ring, will give the highest local levels of oestrogen, while minimizing systemic absorption but not eliminating it. Since oestrogen tends to cause slow improvement, patients should be instructed to adhere to treatment for at least 6 weeks before concluding that it will be ineffective.

Conclusions

Vaginitis is a common problem in women of all ages. Effective therapy is available for the many causes of vulvovaginal symptoms, but will depend on an accurate diagnosis.

Further reading

Anderson MR, Klink K, Cohrssen A (2004). Evaluation of vaginal complaints. *JAMA*, **291**, 1368–79.

Centers for Disease Control and Prevention. (2006). Sexually transmitted diseases treatment guidelines 2006. *MMWR*, **55**, 51–8.

8.5

Pelvic inflammatory disease

David Eschenbach

Essentials

Pelvic inflammatory disease (PID) is an infection of the fallopian tubes caused by a wide variety of bacteria, including *Chlamydia trachomatis, Neisseria gonorrhoeae,* and genital tract bacteria, most notably anaerobes.

Manifestations of PID range from mild pelvic pain and tenderness to severe peritonitis. Pelvic abscess formation is a serious infectious complication. However, only about 40% of patients with PID have a fever and even fewer have severe infectious manifestations. Thus, PID is often not diagnosed and it is commonly confused with other pelvic conditions, with a differential diagnosis that most notably includes ectopic pregnancy, appendicitis, and ovarian cyst.

Antibiotic therapy is aimed primarily at *C. trachomatis, N. gonorrhoeae,* and anaerobic bacteria, with prompt identification and treatment of PID recommended in an attempt to reduce the 10% rate of tubal infertility and the 10-fold increased rate of ectopic pregnancy following this infection.

Introduction

Pelvic inflammatory disease (PID) comprises a wide spectrum of female upper genital tract infections, including any combination of endometritis, salpingitis, tuboovarian abscess, and pelvic peritonitis. Salpingitis, or infection of the fallopian tubes, is the most important feature of PID. This is one of the most common and serious infections of the female genital tract because of its long-term effects including infertility, ectopic pregnancy, and chronic pelvic pain.

Aetiology

PID is caused by the canalicular spread of microorganisms along the mucosal surfaces from the cervix, and to a lesser extent from the vagina, into the upper genital tract. Cervical mucus provides a relative barrier to this spread, but virulent microbes can traverse the mucus, which, in any case, is lost during menses. Little is known of local defence mechanisms that might prevent this spread of microorganisms. Certain HLA types appear to be important in chlamydial PID. Factors that appear to influence the ascent of microbes from the cervix into the upper genital tract include surgical procedures such as dilatation and curettage, induced abortion, insertion of an intrauterine device (IUD), and hysterosalpingograms. Vaginal douching with medicated products disrupts the vaginal flora and appears to increase the incidence of PID. Contraceptives can influence the incidence of PID. Barrier contraception reduces the risk of PID by preventing the acquisition of *Neisseria gonorrhoeae* and chlamydia. Oral contraceptives also appear to decrease the incidence of PID, perhaps by reducing the inflammatory response to chlamydial infection. However, bacteria adhere to IUDs, so increasing the risk of PID.

Most initial episodes of PID are attributable to *N. gonorrhoeae* and *Chlamydia trachomatis.* While one or both bacteria can be isolated from the cervix in up to 75% of patients with acute PID, there is a wide variation in the prevalence of these bacteria. In populations where gonorrhoea is highly endemic, there is a 50 to 80% prevalence of *N. gonorrhoeae* in women with PID. A study of 1900 patients with PID, conducted across eight countries, found that the prevalence of *N. gonorrhoeae* varied from 5 to 80%, with a mean of 26%. *C. trachomatis* was isolated from 5 to 50% of these women (mean prevalence of 29%). In Europe, there was a 30 to 50% prevalence of *C. trachomatis* and a 5 to 15% prevalence of *N. gonorrhoeae* in women with PID. Between 10 and 20% of patients with PID harbour both bacteria. However, the use of DNA amplification techniques may reveal even higher numbers of infections with these bacteria.

Mycoplasma hominis and *M. genitalium* cause tubal infection in primates, and *M. genetalium* appears to play a role in human PID. *Ureaplasma urealyticum* has been isolated from the fallopian tubes but appears to play little role in PID.

Facultative and anaerobic bacteria common to the vagina are also isolated from the fallopian tubes of women with PID. In the initial episode of PID, these bacteria appear less frequent than *N. gonorrhoeae* and *C. trachomatis,* but they can become secondary invaders and are important among women with prolonged symptoms. Anaerobic bacteria are virtually always present in pelvic abscesses associated with initial or recurrent episodes of PID. These bacteria are important in recurrent PID, where *N. gonorrhoeae* and *C. trachomatis* are infrequent.

Clinical features

Women with PID have a vast array of clinical symptoms, varying in intensity from negligible to severe. No symptom, clinical sign, or laboratory result is pathognomonic of PID. In women with mild or uncharacteristic manifestations, the diagnosis of PID is usually missed. Perhaps two-thirds of cases of PID go unrecognized, often because the symptoms are mild or suggestive of common, less serious conditions. The diagnostic threshold of PID must be sufficiently low to include women with mild PID, but as the threshold is lowered, diagnostic specificity decreases. However, it is better to overdiagnose than fail to treat mild PID. Most recognized cases of PID present with moderate symptoms and signs such as lower abdominal pain. Symptoms such as abnormal vaginal discharge or bleeding, dysuria, or vomiting do not distinguish women with PID from those whose fallopian tubes are apparently normal at laparoscopy. Among women with PID diagnosed by laparoscopy, only 40% have both a temperature over 38°C and peripheral blood leucocytosis. Women with severe symptoms and signs usually have peritonitis, often from *N. gonorrhoeae* infection, or they have an abscess. Such patients can be very ill. Laparoscopy should be considered both for those with florid peritonitis, to exclude other causes, such as appendicitis and a ruptured abscess, and for those with abscesses greater than 6 cm in diameter, to allow percutaneous drainage.

Perihepatitis (FitzHugh–Curtis syndrome) occurs in about 10% of women with PID. There is often moderate to severe pleuritic pain and tenderness, usually in the right-upper quadrant. These symptoms are often so severe that lower abdominal pain, suggesting PID, may not be noticed. Perihepatitis must therefore be distinguished from other causes of upper quadrant pain and tenderness by careful pelvic examination. Perihepatitis is associated with *N. gonorrhoeae*, *C. trachomatis*, and other aetiologies.

Diagnosis

Cervical samples should be obtained to identify *N. gonorrhoeae* and *C. trachomatis* by culture or DNA technology. Patients with severe manifestations should have peripheral white blood cell counts. Other laboratory tests are usually of little benefit. Ultrasonography is helpful to identify the presence, and particularly the size, of an abscess. Dilated or thickened tubes or fluid within tubes are found in 80 to 90% of women with severe to moderate PID, but in only two-thirds of those with mild PID. Most sonographers have little experience with these findings. Laparoscopy provides an accurate diagnosis and is particularly useful for excluding serious surgical conditions such as ectopic pregnancy, appendicitis, bleeding ruptured ovarian cyst, or a ruptured abscess. Laparoscopy is also useful for difficult cases, such as those unresponsive to antibiotics in which the only objective finding is pelvic tenderness.

Differential diagnosis

Among 814 women who underwent laparoscopy because of a clinical diagnosis of PID, 12% had intraabdominal conditions other than PID: ectopic pregnancy, appendicitis, ruptured ovarian cysts, and endometriosis. In older women, pyelonephritis, gastroenteritis, and diverticulitis can masquerade as PID. A patient with severe clinical signs or peritonitis should be admitted to hospital for ultrasound examination and/or exploratory laparoscopy. A pregnancy

Table 8.5.1 Inpatient and outpatient PID treatment regimens

Inpatient		
Clindamycin 900 mg IV every 8 h	+	Gentamicin loading dose IV, or intramuscular IM (2 mg/kg of body weight) followed by a maintenance dose (1.5 mg/kg) every 8 h. The intravenous IV regimens should be continued for at least 48 h after substantial clinical improvement (but beware of gentamicin toxicity!), then followed by 100 mg doxycycline twice daily or 450 mg clindamycin 4 times daily (both orally) for a total of 14 days of therapy
Outpatient		
Regimen A		
Cefoxitin 2 g intramuscular IM + probenecid, 1 g orally in a single dose concurrently, or ceftriaxone 250 mg intramuscular IM or other parenteral third-generation cephalosporin (e.g. cefotaxime)	±	Doxycycline 100 mg orally 2 times daily for 14 days
Regimen B		
Ofloxacin 400 mg orally 2 times daily or levofloxacin 500 mg orally once daily for 14 days	±	Metronidazole 500 mg orally 2 times daily for 14 days. This regimen should only be used when the risk of gonorrhea is low. (A culture for gonorrhoea is essential because of its resistance to fluroquinolones.)
Other		
Amoxicillin/clavulanic acid with doxycycline, or azithromycin with metronidazole have provided short-term clinical cures		

IM, intramuscular; IV, intravenous.

test is needed. If positive, an ectopic pregnancy or other pregnancy complications must be considered. If the pregnancy test is negative, and a wet mount of vaginal/cervical secretions reveals no neutrophils or bacterial vaginosis, an ultrasound scan is needed to diagnose gynaecological diseases other than PID or a gastrointestinal or urinary disorder. If the wet mount shows more neutrophils than vaginal epithelial cells, PID is probable, but other pelvic conditions are not completely excluded. Ultrasonography or an endometrial biopsy examined for plasma cells is useful to increase the accuracy of diagnosis.

Treatment

Treatment is aimed at eradicating *N. gonorrhoeae* and *C. trachomatis*, and, especially for those with moderate-to-severe disease, anaerobic bacteria (Table 8.5.1). Women with PID who are HIV-seropositive appear less likely to be infected with *N. gonorrhoeae* and *C. trachomatis*, but they are more likely to develop abscesses. These patients respond to treatment as promptly as those who are HIV-seronegative, unless they are severely immunosuppressed.

Complications

Despite prompt treatment, sequelae are common. Tubal infertility is the most common and disturbing complication. About 10% of women develop tubal infertility after a single episode of PID. Tubal infertility is increased by delaying the treatment of abdominal pain by more than 3 days in chlamydial PID, in women aged over 25 years at the time of PID, and particularly by the number of episodes of PID. Tubal infertility occurs in about 20% of women after two episodes and 40% after three episodes of PID. Tubal infertility occurs in about two-thirds of those with a pelvic abscess or severely damaged tubes observed laparoscopically. There is no correlation between clinical manifestations and the degree of tubal damage observed laparoscopically. Thus, women with mild symptoms but severe tubal damage may become infertile from a single episode of PID. About 7 to 10% of women who become pregnant following PID develop an ectopic pregnancy. Chronic pelvic pain of over 6 months' duration occurs in about 15% of patients following PID.

Prevention

Attempts should be made to prevent PID. Ideally *N. gonorrhoeae* and *C. trachomatis* infection should be diagnosed and treated before PID can develop. Reduction of *C. trachomatis* infection has lowered the incidence of PID. This should be the aim of primary care providers, especially since *C. trachomatis* can now be diagnosed more readily using new sensitive DNA detection methods.

Further reading

Centers for Disease Control and Prevention (2006). Sexually transmitted diseases treatment guidelines 2006. *MMWR*, **55**, 51–8.

Cohen CR, *et al.* (1998). Effect of human immunodeficiency virus type 1 infection upon acute salpingitis: a laparoscopic study. *J Infect Dis*, **178**, 1352–8.

Eschenbach DA, *et al.* (1975). Polymicrobial etiology of acute pelvic inflammatory disease. *N Engl J Med*, **293**, 166–71.

Jacobsen L, Westrom L (1969). Objectivized diagnosis of pelvic inflammatory disease. Diagnostic and prognostic value of routine laparoscopy. *Am J Obstet Gynecol*, **105**, 1088–98.

Molander P, *et al.* (2001). Transvaginal power Doppler findings in laparoscopically proven acute pelvic inflammatory disease. *Ultrasound Obstet Gynecol*, **17**, 233–8.

Scholes D, *et al.* (1996). Prevention of pelvic inflammatory disease by screening for cervical chlamydial infection. *N Engl J Med*, **334**, 1362–6.

Westrom L (1980). Incidence, prevalence, and trends of acute pelvic inflammatory disease and its consequences in industrialized countries. *Am J Obstet Gynecol*, **138**, 880–92.

Westrom L, Eschenbach D (1999). Pelvic inflammatory disease. In: Holmes KK, *et al.* (eds.) *Sexually Transmitted Diseases*, pp. 783–809. McGraw-Hill, New York.

8.6

Principles of contraception

John Guillebaud

Essentials

Continued use of any method of contraception is related directly to its acceptability. Advisers should be competent to give information about the efficacy, risks, side effects, advantages, disadvantages, and noncontraceptive benefits of each method.

Ignorance, especially about conditions not yet evaluated by the World Health Organization or the United Kingdom Medical Eligibility Committee, should be admitted during consultations, in which the clinician and the user, or couple, should be on equal terms: a 'consultation between two experts'.

Too often, the combined oral contraceptive ('the Pill') is regarded as being synonymous with contraception. Providers everywhere should promote long-acting reversible contraceptives—injectables, implants and intrauterine methods—which can be forgotten about once administered; an essential attribute of effective continuing contraception.

Introduction

It should be self-evident that:

- Human needs, along with those of all other species sharing the world, will never be met sustainably without stabilizing human numbers: currently increasing, according to the Population Reference Bureau (www.prb.org) by more than 82 million a year and reaching 7000 million in 2011.
- No woman on Earth who wishes to exercise the right to control her own fertility should be denied the means to do so, by her partner or an outside agency, or through lack of correct information or choice of affordable and accessible contraceptives.

To be effective, contraceptives must be used correctly, consistently, and continuously. Continued use of any contraceptive is related directly to its acceptability. Therefore, couples should be given accurate information about all methods that are medically appropriate and helped to choose what is best for them. Health professionals who give advice about contraception should be competent to give information about efficacy, risks, side effects, advantages, disadvantages, and noncontraceptive benefits of each method. Too often, the combined oral contraceptive ('the Pill') is regarded as being synonymous with contraception. Providers too rarely inform women about new, improved, reversible contraceptives, especially the long-acting reversible contraceptives, which are widely misunderstood. Box 8.6.1 presents a 'wish list' for an ideal contraceptive. No available method meets all these criteria, but the levonorgestrel intrauterine system (LNG-IUS) meets more than any other.

Most women who seek contraception are young and healthy. They present fewer problems than over-35s, teenagers, and those with intercurrent diseases or risk factors like high BMI and smoking.

Box 8.6.1 The ideal contraceptive

- 100% effective
- 100% convenient (can be forgotten about once administered, preferably not coitally related)
- 100% safe, free of adverse side effects (neither risk nor nuisance)
- 100% reversible, ideally by the user
- 100% maintenance-free (no potentially uncomfortable intervention by medical personnel required initially, subsequently, or when reversed)
- 100% protective against sexually-transmitted infections (STIs)
- Possesses noncontraceptive benefits, especially against menstrual symptoms
- Cheap, easy to distribute
- Acceptable to every culture, religion, and political view
- Familiar to, or used by woman (ostensibly, women have more to gain than men from its efficacy)

Young people

For young people of both genders, 'sex and relationships education' (SRE) should be promoted rather than 'sex education'. When seeking advice on sex, relationships, contraception, pregnancy, and parenthood, young people are entitled to accessible, confidential, nonjudgemental, and unbiased support and guidance that recognizes the diversity of the traditions of their cultures and faiths. We should listen to their views and respect their opinions and choices. Valid choices include postponing sexual intercourse as well as having safer sex without risk of conception.

However, girls who start having sexual intercourse when they are very young (early coitarche) may escape becoming pregnant for several cycles, partly because a large proportion of early post-pubertal menstrual cycles are infertile. As a result, they often do not seek advice until they have already conceived. Easier access to emergency contraception is an obvious priority. A socially enforced norm must be promoted, as it is in the Netherlands, that relationships may include sex only when contraception is adequate. Wherever mutual monogamy is uncertain, this must include condoms for safer sex. In this age group, long-acting reversible contraceptives should be offered more frequently. Whereas default in using the combined oral contraceptive leads to conception, long-acting reversible contraceptives have the 'default state' of contraception. Intrauterine methods are only relatively contraindicated in this age group, but injectables and implants are usually preferred.

Sexually transmitted infections

Taking a quick and practical sexual history should be part of all contraceptive consultations, not just those involving intrauterine devices or young people.

Ask:

- 'When did you last have sex?' and then immediately
- 'When did you last have sex with anybody different?'

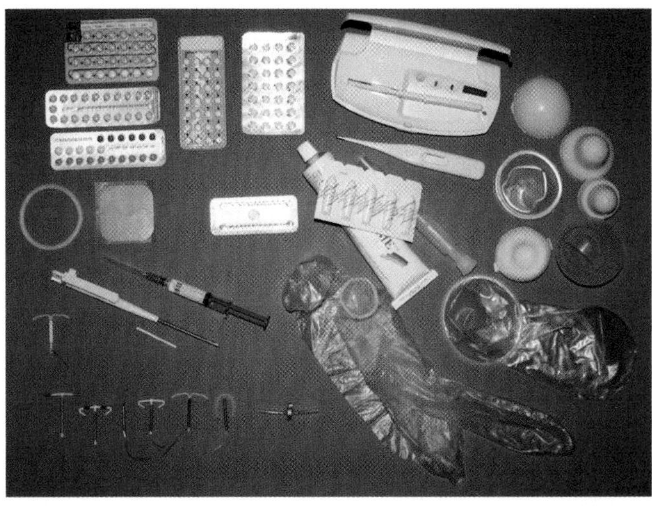

Fig. 8.6.1 The choice of methods available in the UK, 2009. (Reproduced with kind permission of Dr Anne MacGregor.)

Much can be learnt from the second of this pair of open questions, whether the response is 'about 20 years ago …' or '3 months ago' (the latter making it unthreatening to go on and clarify whether this was a change of partner or a one-night stand—and whether there have been others in the past year).

Relative effectiveness of available contraceptive methods (Fig. 8.6.1)

Failure rates are usually expressed as conceptions per 100 woman-years. In Box 8.6.2, 'perfect use' means that the method is used consistently and correctly. 'Typical' use depends on such characteristics as age, social class, acceptability of conception, etc., in the population studied. Note the huge difference in failures between 'perfect' and 'typical' use of the combined pill (0.3 vs 8). The data

Box 8.6.2 Brief overview of contraceptive methods

A. Long-acting and reversible

Contraceptive injection (depot medroxyprogesterone acetate, DMPA)

Failure rates (%)[a]

- Perfect use: 0.3
- Typical use: 3

Mechanism

Two main actions:

- Inhibition of ovulation
- Effect on cervical mucus to prevent sperm penetration

Advantages

- Effective for at least 12 weeks
- Protects against endometrial carcinoma
- Some protection against pelvic inflammatory disease
- Ideal for women on enzyme-inducing drugs who do not need to increase injection frequency
- Good option during lactation

Disadvantages

- The injection cannot be removed, so any side effects may continue for duration of activity (variable)
- Menses may be irregular or prolonged or may cease
- Return of menses and fertility may be long delayed
- Definite risk of weight gain and other progestogenic side effects
- Possible adverse effect on bone density, but also evidence that this reverses on discontinuation of the method
- Committee on Safety of Medicines (UK) recommends consideration of an alternative method every 2 years in all age groups (bone density scanning only where clinically indicated)

(Continued)

Box 8.6.2 (*cont'd*) Brief overview of contraceptive methods

Contraceptive implant (etonogestrel-containing)

Failure rates (%)[b]

- Perfect use: *c.*0.05
- Typical use: *c.*0.05

Mechanism

Single subcutaneous flexible rod releasing etonogestrel; two main actions:

- Inhibition of ovulation
- Effect on cervical mucus to prevent sperm penetration

Advantages

- Phenomenally effective for 3 years but fully reversible at any time by simple removal
- Rapid return of fertility
- No current concerns about bone density

Disadvantages

- Insertion requires local anaesthesia
- Irregular bleeding may be frequent and prolonged; however, at 6 months up to 60% have an acceptable bleeding pattern and 20% have amenorrhoea (a good side effect)
- Not recommended for use with enzyme-inducing drugs

Levonorgestrel intrauterine system (LNG-IUS)

Failure rates (%)

- Perfect use: 0.1
- Typical use: 0.1

Mechanism

Intrauterine release of levonorgestrel (LNG); two main actions:

- Effect on cervical mucus to prevent sperm penetration
- Very high local levonorgestrel levels alter the endometrium to prevent implantation

Advantages

- Effective for 5 years but immediately reversible
- Menses eventually become up to 95% lighter or absent and pain-free, therefore invaluable for women with heavy or painful periods
- Good choice for users of enzyme-inducing drugs

Disadvantages

- Insertion may sometimes be difficult or painful
- Irregular prolonged light bleeding very common for *c.*3 months, sometimes longer; the client should be warned but reassured of good outlook for having very light, painless bleeds or amenorrhoea
- In early weeks there are often temporary hormonal side effects such as headaches, bloatedness, and breast tenderness
- May not be suitable for those at risk of pelvic infection
- Risks include perforation and expulsion
- Not quick-acting enough for use as an emergency contraceptive

Copper intrauterine device (IUD)—the Cu-banded TCu 380A and its variants preferred

Failure rates (%)

- Perfect use: 0.6
- Typical use: 0.8

Mechanism

The copper ion:

- Is lethal to sperm and ova
- Causes changes that prevent implantation

Advantages

- Immediately effective, including postcoitally for emergency contraception up to 5 days after intercourse, or 5 days after calculated day of ovulation (failure rate *c.*0.1% in the cycle of presentation)
- Rapidly reversible on removal
- Usable for 10 years or, if fitted after the age of 40, until 1 year after menopause

Disadvantages

- Insertion may sometimes be difficult or painful
- May not be suitable for those at increased risk of pelvic infection
- Risks include perforation and expulsion
- Menses lengthened by 1 day on average and tend to be *c.*30% heavier. Extra pain with menses in some cases, mainly if small uterus (including nulliparae) or IUD malpositioned

B. Long-acting and permanent

Female and male sterilization

Failure rates (% of procedures, within 10 years)

- Female procedures: 0.5
- Vasectomy, after two azoospermic semen analyses: 0.1 (or 0.05 according to UK data)

Mechanism

The fallopian tubes or the vas deferens are occluded with or without division.

Advantages

- No serious long-term side effects
- Vasectomy is simple and quick under local anaesthesia by the preferred no-scalpel technique

Disadvantages

- Neither method ideal if any doubt about permanence: prospective users must always be informed that some of above reversible alternatives are no less effective
- Pain and some immediate risks, also having to have a surgical procedure

Box 8.6.2 *(cont'd)* Brief overview of contraceptive methods

- Female sterilization has a failure rate 5–10 times higher than vasectomy after azoospermia
- After vasectomy, contraception must be used for 3–4 months before semen testing
- Scrotal pain, usually mild, described by a variable percentage of men after vasectomy
- Small increased risk of ectopic pregnancy if female sterilization fails

C. Oral methods, short-term, not coitally related

Combined pill (also patch and vaginal ring)

Failure rates (%)

- Perfect use: 0.3
- Typical use: 8 (6 for the vaginal ring)

Mechanism

Combination of oestrogen plus progestogen hormones:

- Prevent follicular maturation, the LH surge and ovulation
- Also progestogenic effect on cervical mucus to prevent sperm penetration

Patch

Delivers hormones transdermally, 3 patches for 7 days each, then a 7-day patch-free interval with withdrawal bleeding.

Vaginal ring

Uses transvaginal delivery route, one ring for 21 days, then 7-day ring-free and withdrawal bleed.

Both of these may improve convenience and compliance.

Advantages

- Completely reversible
- Usually reduces heaviness of bleeding, dysmenorrhoea, and other cyclic symptoms
- Protection against ovarian, endometrial, and very probably colorectal carcinoma
- May benefit acne and polycystic ovarian syndrome (some formulations)

Disadvantages

- Low risk of serious side effects including arterial and venous thrombosis
- Not suitable for smokers over 35, women with migraine with aura, and other recognized risk factors
- Possible cofactor in current users in development of breast and cervical cancers
- Enzyme-inducer drugs reduce efficacy

Progestogen-only pill (POP)

Failure rates (%)

- Perfect use: 0.3
- Typical use: 8 (usually lower with desogestrel 75 μg)

Mechanism

- Progestogen hormone alters cervical mucus to prevent sperm penetration
- Also inhibits ovulation: 50% of cycles with old style POPs, but 97% of cycles with desogestrel 75 μg (Cerazette)

Advantages

- Few serious side effects
- Usable when contraindications to oestrogen (WHO 4 or WHO 3)
- Rapid return of fertility
- Ideal in lactation
- Desogestrel is a realistic alternative to combined oral contraceptive in young, highly fertile users

Disadvantages

- Irregular bleeding: but by 6 months, majority have an acceptable bleeding pattern
- Minor hormonal side effects
- Needs to be taken with meticulous regularity: presumed loss of infertility if a tablet is 3 h late (12 h with desogestrel)
- Enzyme-inducer drugs reduce efficacy
- Desogestrel preferred in women weighing over 70 kg

D. Barrier methods, short-term, coitally related

Male condom

Failure rates (%)

- Perfect use: 2
- Typical use: 15

Mechanism

Entrapment of sperm, preventing entry into cervix.

Advantages

- Protection of both partners from sexually transmitted diseases, including HIV
- No major side effects

Disadvantages

- Coitally intrusive, modifies sensations of intercourse
- Must be used meticulously for acceptable efficacy
- May slip off or split
- Oil-based products such as many body lotions may damage the latex (but are usable with polyurethane condoms)
- Latex allergy with cross-reactivity to other allergens (available plastic male or female condoms are alternatives)

(Continued)

Box 8.6.2 *(cont'd)* Brief overview of contraceptive methods

Female condom

Failure rates (%)

- Perfect use: 5
- Typical use: 21

Mechanism

Entrapment of sperm in a lubricated soft polyurethane sac which lines the vagina.

Advantages

- Can be inserted well before intercourse
- Protection of both partners from sexually transmitted infections, including HIV
- Not damaged by oil-based products
- No major side effects

Disadvantages

- Coitally intrusive though can seem less so than male condom
- Essential to ensure the penis enters the condom and not between the vagina and the condom
- 'Perfect' use failure rate found to be surprisingly high

Diaphragm and cervical cap with spermicide, also spermicide-impregnated sponge

Failure rates (%)

- Perfect use: 9 (6 for the diaphragm)
- Typical use: 16

Mechanism

Latex or plastic barrier used with spermicide covering the cervix, but not entrapping sperm.

Advantages

- Not immediately coitally related, can be put in well before intercourse
- May protect against some sexually transmitted infections, but less effective than condoms
- No major side effects

Disadvantages

- Cystitis may occur with diaphragm, lower risk with cervical caps
- 'Perfect' use failure rate unacceptably high for those who must avoid pregnancy

Natural family planning ('sympto-thermal' method)

Failure rates (%)

- Perfect use: 2
- Typical use: High (see 'Disadvantages' below)

Mechanism

Fertile and infertile times of the cycle identified by the well-taught user noting the fertility indicators: changes in cervical mucus supplemented mainly by calendar calculations in the preovulatory and basal body temperature in the postovulatory phases.

Advantages

- No side effects
- Empowering, gives a woman more awareness of her body
- Can also be used to plan a pregnancy

Disadvantages

- Method needs to be learned from a trained teacher (see www.fertilityuk.org)
- Effectiveness depends crucially on compliance with what may seem numerous days of abstinence
- The method is exceptionally unforgiving of imperfect use, except in couples of below-average fertility

Persona is a small handheld computerized monitor with urine test sticks which measures urinary oestrone-3-glucuronide and LH changes. Claimed to have 6% failure rate.

Emergency contraception with levonorgestrel 1500 μg stat postcoitally

Failure rate per 100 women presenting in single cycle (%)

- Use within 24 h: 0.4
- Use within 72 h: c1 (equates to prevention of only *c*.80% of *expected* conceptions, if no treatment were given)

Mechanism

- Inhibition or postponement of ovulation (hence requirement to abstain or use condoms for rest of cycle)
- Effect on cervical and upper genital tract fluid to interfere with sperm transport and fertilization
- Implantation block is weak; stronger with ulipristal acetate (ellaOne 30 mg, new in 2009, licensed for use postcoitally up to 120 hours); strongest with copper IUD

A copper IUD is usable in good faith up to 5 days after estimated earliest ovulation. Failure rate in that cycle: 1–2 in 1000.

[a] Failure rates given here are for 'perfect' users (using the method consistently and correctly) vs typical users. They are expressed as percentages of women unintentionally conceiving within the first year of contraception, except for (1) emergency contraception, where the failure rate is the percentage conceiving in that cycle out of 100 who presented after a single coital exposure, and (2) sterilization, where the failure rate is the percentage experiencing a failure within 10 years after the procedure.

[b] Failures are exceptionally rare and therefore the rate is difficult to estimate (0 failures in the 2500 users prior to marketing).

Table mainly modified from Family Planning Association (2009), with no claims to being fully comprehensive.

Box 8.6.3 WHO classification of contraindications

(A–D is an aide-memoire for the significance of each category)

WHO 1 A is for 'Always usable'

A condition for which there is no restriction for the use of the contraceptive method.
Example: for combined oral contraceptive use, fibroids, or thrush.

WHO 2 B is for 'Broadly usable'

A condition where the advantages of the method generally outweigh the theoretical or proven risks.
Example: nulliparity for IUD use by a monogamous couple.

WHO 3 C is for 'Caution/counselling', if used at all

A condition where the theoretical or proven risks usually outweigh the advantages. Therefore, an alternative method is usually preferred. Yet, respecting the patient/client's autonomy and using expert clinical judgement, if she accepts the risks and rejects or cannot use relevant alternatives, given the risks of pregnancy, the method can be used with caution/sometimes with additional monitoring.
Example: for methods using oestrogen, diabetes mellitus (DM)—but becomes WHO 4 if any known DM tissue damage

WHO 4 'D' is for 'Do not use'

A condition which represents an unacceptable health risk (absolutely contraindicated).
Example: for combined oral contraceptive use, migraine with aura.

come from the United States of America but the 'perfect use' figures can be used anywhere, for comparing methods.

Iatrogenic (doctor-caused) pregnancies frequently result from avoidable errors and omissions by service providers, especially not allowing sufficient discussion time for new users.

Eligibility criteria for contraceptives

In general, contraceptive users are medically fit and can use any available contraceptive method safely. However, certain contraceptives pose health risks for people with medical conditions. Since most trials of new contraceptive methods deliberately exclude subjects with chronic medical conditions, there is little direct evidence on which to base sound prescribing advice.

WHO system for Medical Eligibility Criteria (WHOMEC)

These internationally agreed guidelines, initially devised at a World Health Organization Workshop in Atlanta in 1994, are based on evidence-based systematic reviews and expert opinion. In 2006, the Faculty of Family Planning & Reproductive Health Care (FFPRHC) developed a version of WHOMEC adjusted for British practice (UKMEC), and this is strongly recommended.

The WHO classification is summarized in Box 8.6.3. Clinical judgement is required: (1) In all WHO 3 conditions; or (2) if more than one condition applies. As a working rule, two WHO 2 conditions move the situation to WHO 3; and if any WHO 3 condition applies, the addition of either a WHO 2 or a WHO 3 condition normally means WHO 4, i.e. 'Do not use'.

Prescribers often have to help couples make a decision, despite a frustrating absence of good evidence, or even for conditions not yet evaluated by WHOMEC/UKMEC, a clear statement of expert opinion. Such ignorance should be admitted and strongly underpins the concept that the consultation should always be on equal terms with the user: 'a consultation between two experts'.

Further reading

Campbell M (2006). Consumer behaviour and contraceptive decisions: resolving a decades-long puzzle. *J Fam Plann Reprod Health*, **32**, 241–4.

Guillebaud J (2001). Commentary—Medical-eligibility criteria for contraceptive use. *Lancet*, **357**, 1378–9.

Guillebaud J (2007). *Contraception today*, 6th edition. Informa Healthcare, London.

Guillebaud J (2009). *Contraception—your questions answered*, 5th edition. Churchill Livingstone, Edinburgh.

Family Planning Association (2009). *Your guide to contraception*. Family Planning Association, London.

Websites

Cochrane Collaboration. Cochrane systematic reviews in fertility regulation. www.cochrane.org/reviews/en/topics/64.html

Faculty of Family Planning and Reproductive Health Care (2006). *UK Medical Eligibility Criteria*. http://www.ffprhc.org.uk/admin/uploads/298_UKMEC_200506.pdf [See especially the Summary Table for all Common Reversible Methods 143–8.] Also UK Selected Practice Recommendations www.ffprhc.org.uk/admin/uploads/Final%20UK%20recommendations1.pdf

National Institute for Health and Clinical Excellence (2005). *The effective and appropriate use of long-acting reversible contraception*. www.nice.org.uk/Guidance/CG30.

Royal College of Obstetricians and Gynaecologists (2003). *Male and female sterilization. Evidence-based Guidelines No 4*. http://www.rcog.org.uk

World Health Organization (2004). *WHO Medical Eligibility Criteria (WHOMEC) for contraceptive use*, 3rd edition. http://www.who.int/reproductive-health.

World Health Organization (2005). *WHO Selected Practice Recommendations (WHOSPR) for contraceptive use*, 2nd edition. http://www.who.int/reproductive-health.

SECTION 9

Chemical and physical injuries and environmental factors and disease

9.1 Poisoning by drugs and chemicals *1271*
J.A. Vale, S.M. Bradberry, and D.N. Bateman

9.2 Injuries, envenoming, poisoning, and allergic reactions caused by animals *1324*
David A. Warrell

9.3 Injuries, poisoning, and allergic reactions caused by plants *1361*

9.3.1 Poisonous plants and fungi *1361*
Hans Persson

9.3.2 Common Indian poisonous plants *1371*
V.V. Pillay

9.4 Occupational health and safety *1376*

9.4.1 Occupational and environmental health *1376*
J.M. Harrington and Raymond M. Agius

9.4.2 Occupational safety *1388*
Lawrence Waterman

9.5 Environmental diseases *1393*

9.5.1 Heat *1393*
M.A. Stroud

9.5.2 Cold *1395*
M.A. Stroud

9.5.3 Drowning *1397*
Peter J. Fenner

9.5.4 Diseases of high terrestrial altitudes *1402*
Andrew J. Pollard, Buddha Basnyat, and David R. Murdoch

9.5.5 Aerospace medicine *1408*
D.M. Denison and M. Bagshaw

9.5.6 Diving medicine *1416*
D.M. Denison and M.A. Glover

9.5.7 Lightning and electrical injuries *1422*
Chris Andrews

9.5.8 Podoconiosis (nonfilarial elephantiasis) *1426*
Gail Davey

9.5.9 Radiation *1429*
Jill Meara

9.5.10 Noise *1432*
Syed M. Ahmed and Tar-Ching Aw

9.5.11 Vibration *1434*
Tar-Ching Aw

9.5.12 Disasters: earthquakes, volcanic eruptions, hurricanes, and floods *1436*
Peter J. Baxter

9.5.13 Bioterrorism *1440*
Manfred S. Green

9.1

Poisoning by drugs and chemicals

J.A. Vale, S.M. Bradberry, and D.N. Bateman

Essentials

Poisoning is usually an acute, short-lived event which necessitates immediate care, though complications such as rhabdomyolysis may persist for a few days. Less commonly, symptoms may arise only after prolonged exposure, as occurs with many heavy metals. Rarely, sequelae may not occur until many years after exposure, e.g. with vinyl chloride. It must be stressed that exposure does not necessarily equate with poisoning as uptake of the agent involved is required but, even if this occurs, poisoning does not necessarily result as the amount absorbed may be too small.

Poisoning may be accidental or deliberate; it is usually accidental in small children, but in adults it is almost invariably deliberate. Less commonly, it may be iatrogenic. Occupational poisoning is frequent in developing countries.

Clinical assessment

Assessment of a poisoned patient involves taking an appropriate history and performing a physical examination (including an assessment of the level of consciousness, ventilation, and circulation). Diagnosis is based on the history, circumstantial evidence (if available), the presence of typical features, and, occasionally, on the results of toxicological and other investigations.

Biochemical abnormalities due to disturbed metabolic processes are common in severely poisoned patients. These may be of diagnostic value, but mostly their recognition and treatment are important in management. Acid–base disturbances, particularly respiratory acidosis (due to central nervous system depression or pulmonary toxicity), and metabolic acidosis (due to lactic acidaemia or derangements of intermediary metabolism), are common. Plasma electrolyte abnormalities, particularly hypo- or hyperkalaemia, are observed and are most often due to redistribution of potassium across cell membranes. Hypoglycaemia and, less commonly, hyperglycaemia may also occur.

Management

Initial management involves the treatment of any potentially life-threatening conditions, such as airway compromise, breathing difficulties, haemodynamic instability and clinically significant arrhythmias. Thereafter, convulsions and temperature disturbances should be treated and fluid, acid–base, and electrolyte abnormalities corrected.

There is no evidence that the use of methods to reduce absorption from the gastrointestinal tract—such as activated charcoal, gastric lavage, syrup of ipecacuanha, cathartics, or whole-bowel irrigation—improves the clinical outcome in poisoned patients. However, activated charcoal and gastric lavage may be considered in patients who have ingested life-threatening amounts of a toxic agent up to 1 h previously.

Antidotes exert their beneficial effects by a variety of mechanisms, including forming an inert complex with the poison, accelerating detoxification of the poison, reducing the rate of conversion of the poison to a more toxic compound, competing with the poison for essential receptor sites, blocking essential receptors through which the toxic effects are mediated, and bypassing the effect of the poison. There are, however, only a small number of poisons for which there is a specific antidote, and few antidotes are employed regularly in clinical practice; these include acetylcysteine, naloxone, and flumazenil.

To increase poison elimination, treatment with multiple-dose activated charcoal (in patients who have ingested carbamazepine, dapsone, phenobarbitol, quinine, or theophylline), urine alkalinization (in patients with moderately severe salicylate poisoning) or haemodialysis (which significantly increases the elimination of ethanol, ethylene glycol, isopropanol, lithium, methanol, and salicylate) should be considered, although there is no conclusive evidence that these treatments improve outcome.

Introduction

Poisoning is usually an acute event demanding immediate care and attention, but the consequences of exposure sometimes persist. Distinctive sequelae may not appear until many years have elapsed, e.g. with carcinoma of the oesophagus following ingestion of corrosives or hepatic haemangiosarcoma from vinyl chloride exposure. Symptoms may arise only after prolonged exposure, as with many heavy metals. Exposure by oral, inhalational, dermal, or other routes on their own does not necessarily indicate poisoning. Uptake is required for there to be a toxic effect, but even if this occurs, poisoning does not necessarily result as the amount absorbed may be too small.

If poisoning does occur, the ensuing clinical syndrome may be distinctive: e.g. fixed dilated pupils, exaggerated tendon reflexes, extensor plantar responses, depressed respiration, and cardiac tachyarrhythmias suggest tricyclic antidepressant poisoning; anaemia, constipation, colic, and motor nerve palsies are indicative of lead poisoning. However, with many psychotropic medicines there may only be nonspecific central nervous depression, respiratory impairment, and hypotension.

Poisoning may be accidental or deliberate. It is usually accidental in small children, but in adults it is almost invariably deliberate (deliberate self-harm) or, rarely, it may be with homicidal intent. It may also be iatrogenic in those aged below 6 months, e.g. involving overtreatment with paracetamol. Occupational poisoning is common in developing countries and continues to occur in the developed world. Thus, the medical approach to poisoning should never be confined to the poison and its effects. All the circumstances surrounding the episode must be taken into account, especially in cases where litigation may follow, e.g. in the event of an occupational mishap with a chemical. It is therefore important that the doctor concerned, having instituted any necessary life-saving measures, should take a careful history, retain all pertinent evidence such as a suicide note and biological specimens, make a meticulous record of symptoms, signs, progress and outcome, and remember issues of confidentiality.

Most countries have a poisons information service, which provides advice to medical staff (e.g. in the United Kingdom health care professionals may obtain online advice from www.TOXBASE.org), and in the majority of cases, to the general public as well. Advice should always be sought if unfamiliar poisons are encountered or if there is clinical uncertainty about optimal management.

Epidemiology

Poisoning, either accidental or deliberate, is a common presentation in all countries throughout the world. This phenomenon is, however, a relatively new one. Before the 1950s, hospital admissions from self-harm, now the most frequent cause of poisoning presentation to health care, was extremely rare worldwide. The reasons for this changing pattern of poisoning are poorly understood.

Patients who have suffered toxic exposures present to health care facilities in a variety of ways, including to primary care physicians, hospital emergency departments, and hospital outpatients; rarely, patients are discovered dead. Collecting statistics on poisoning is therefore a complex issue, and there is currently no universally agreed system for documenting and comparing rates of poisoning in different countries. Most statistics refer to hospital admissions (as opposed to hospital presentations in emergency departments) or poisoning-related deaths. Health statistical data from developed countries are usually more sophisticated than those from the developing world, although local surveys suggest that the incidence of self-harm is little different in these different types of society. Poisons information centres also collect information about the types of agent people are exposed to or ingest. Most exposures do not result in clinical ill health, further complicating health statistics.

There are clear age differences in the frequencies and causes of poisoning. In children under the age of 10, accidental poisoning is extremely common, particularly in the very young who are learning to crawl or walk, who tend to place household objects into their mouths. From the age of 10 upwards, self-harm becomes predominant, peaking in the late teens to late twenties and then gradually declining in incidence in higher age groups. The health departments of most developed countries publish data on poisoning mortality on the internet; collection of hospital admission data is less routine and is best represented by countries, such as the United Kingdom, which has centralized health care provision.

Hospital admissions due to poisoning

Poisoning from accidental and deliberate ingestion of drugs or chemicals causes approximately 10% of acute hospital medical presentations in developed countries. The period of most increase was from the mid-1950s to the mid-1970s, and since that time, the numbers have fluctuated slightly year by year. In the United Kingdom there are currently 350 000 to 400 000 per annum. Since deliberate self-harm is a risk factor for further such episodes, approximately 20% of these cases occur in the same patient group.

Self-harm behaviour in women and men is somewhat different. Although hospital admission data suggest that females predominate in all age groups, other than young children, mortality data for out-of-hospital deaths show that young males are more likely to succeed in killing themselves than women. The severity of poisoning depends on the quantities ingested but hospital statistics do not provide adequate data to assess this. Mortality data provide information on the relative toxicity of different compounds if it can be expressed per head of population exposed. This is a technique that is best used for assessing the toxicity of prescription medicines; it is much less easily applied to chemicals and household products when measures of availability are not so readily obtained. Many cases of 'poisoning' in children are more accurately described as 'exposures', since symptomatic poisoning is uncommon in developed countries. The increasing concern is about drug errors causing poisoning; these are extremely difficult data to collect.

Patients who harm themselves often do so because they are acutely stressed. Few of these patients have formal psychiatric diagnoses such as depression or psychosis and few are truly suicidal, since the incident is impulsive rather than planned. Such differences in behaviour affect mortality rates. Mortality is often higher in older age groups where planning of the overdose has been more careful. In addition, older patients often have available prescription medicines, which are more toxic than over-the-counter preparations taken by younger patients. Impulsive behaviour is often associated with ingestion of alcohol, and as many as two-thirds of men and nearly one-half of women may take alcohol in association with an overdose. In many cases of self-harm, more than one drug is included in the cocktail, making clinical management more complex, particularly if two or more agents acting on the same body system are involved. This applies particularly to drugs acting on the brain and cardiovascular system.

The increasing worldwide use of drugs of abuse has also influenced patterns of poisoning. Many cases of poisoning in this population result from variations in quality of supply or experimentation.

Prescription medicines are used in most self-harm episodes in the United Kingdom, and their availability therefore influences the numbers of patients seen. The diagnoses for which the drug is used will also affect how often it is taken as a self-harm agent. Thus, in clinical practice, self-harm with drugs for peptic ulcer disease is very uncommon whereas overdose with antidepressants is much more frequent.

The type of agent taken in overdose is culturally determined. In the United Kingdom, paracetamol contributes approximately one-third of all poisonings seen in hospitals, but although paracetamol is common in North America, the proportion of patients taking this drug is less, as it is in other parts of western Europe. In developing countries such as Sri Lanka and India, drugs are much more expensive and difficult to obtain, and here the agents ingested are either plants, such as yellow oleander, or the widely available pesticides. Agrichemicals cause less than 0.05% of hospital admissions for poisoning in England and Wales whereas in Sri Lanka they are associated with around 70% of all cases of self-harm. Consequently, although the numbers of patients self-harming per head of population are quite similar, the mortality rates in Sri Lanka are orders of magnitude higher than they are in western Europe.

Deaths from poisoning

In developed countries, most deaths from poisoning occur before admission. The quality of hospital care now means than less than 1% of patients presenting to hospital with poisoning are likely to die. The risk of mortality is, however, different with different agents, and the widespread use of drugs of abuse has increased the frequency with which heroin, cocaine, and other high- risk recreational drugs are associated with death. In the United Kingdom, the mortality from drug-related poisoning has been falling; a total of 2967 patients were said to have died in 2000, whereas the figure had fallen to 2598 in 2004. In 2000, 1565 English residents died from drugs of abuse, and in 2004, 1389, the majority in men.

Across the European Union, in young adults aged between 20 and 44 years, external injury and poisoning remain the main causes of death among men, and the second among women. There are marked geographical differences: suicide frequency appears low in the Mediterranean basin (*c.*5/100 000 in Greece, 10 in Italy, 12 in Spain, 13 in Portugal), whereas in Finland (43), Latvia (54), Estonia (55), and Lithuania (90), the rates are much higher. Some of these differences may be determined by the way suicide data are collected.

In previous decades, carbon monoxide (from coal gas) and barbiturates were common causes of death. Substitution of natural gas for coal gas and changes in prescribing patterns have altered the agents most frequently associated with death. Collection of statistics on individual drug-related poisonings is still valuable. For example, the United Kingdom and European Medicines Agencies have enacted legislation on co-proxamol (paracetamol plus dextropropoxyphene) in response to concerns about its toxicity in overdose. Such changes have reduced mortality rates in the United Kingdom.

Childhood poisoning

Accurate data on childhood poisoning are difficult to obtain. Many children with relatively mild features will be managed in emergency departments, where national statistical data are not routinely collected, and so in this population national statistics are unreliable except for agents that cause death. Deaths in children are usually attributable to inappropriate storage of toxic materials, including pharmaceuticals, such as digoxin and quinine; herbicides, such as paraquat; and insecticides, particularly organophosphates. The pattern of poisoning varies in different countries. Herbicide exposures are common in agricultural countries where these materials are stored in the home. In developed countries, exposures often occur when a young child finds a relative's medicines and takes them in an exploratory manner. Child-resistant containers have reduced poisoning rates in children, but tragedies still occur. Increasingly, children are also ingesting drugs of abuse purchased by their parent who then becomes intoxicated leaving material around for the young child to sample.

Diagnosis

Diagnosis of acute poisoning requires that the doctor not only establish that exposure to a poison (whether by ingestion, injection, inhalation, or skin contamination) has occurred, but also its chemical composition and magnitude, so that the features likely to develop can be anticipated and risk assessed. As in any other branch of medicine, diagnosis of acute poisoning is based on the patient's history and on a combination of circumstantial evidence, the findings on physical examination, and appropriate investigations, when a history is not available. However, in acute poisoning, there are many obstacles to establishing the information required. Young children may not be able to give a history; adults are often unreliable; physical signs are rarely diagnostic; circumstantial evidence may be unavailable, tentative, or misleading; and laboratory diagnosis is rarely comprehensive.

History

Since accidental poisoning in childhood is most common between the ages of 9 months and 5 years, an unequivocal history is unlikely to be forthcoming from the victim but may be obtainable from older witnesses. However, statements about quantities must be interpreted cautiously since an accurate assessment of the amounts in original containers is rarely available.

In contrast, since 90% or more of adults presenting with acute poisoning are conscious or drowsy, it should be possible to obtain a history of self-poisoning. A few patients adamantly deny having taken poisons, but most usually admit to it without hesitation, although problems arise in trying to establish precisely the nature and quantity of what has been taken. Comparison of patients' statements with poisons detected by laboratory analysis of blood or urine consistently reveals major differences in about half the cases. Consequently, patients are often thought to be deliberately untruthful. However, self-poisoning is commonly an impulsive act. The patient ingests the contents of the first bottle that comes to hand, often while under the influence of alcohol, and so inaccuracies in the history are not so surprising. Although about 60% of episodes involve drugs prescribed for the victims or their relatives, like many other patients they are often ignorant of the names.

Assessment of the amounts of drugs ingested are even more difficult. Few patients count the number of tablets they consume and neither patient nor doctor can accurately interpret a 'handful', 'bottleful', or similar arbitrary quantity.

Circumstantial evidence

In the diagnosis of acute poisoning, circumstantial evidence becomes important when patients are unable to give a history (as is likely with young children), are confused, or are unconscious, or are unwilling to do so. However, although circumstantial evidence may strongly suggest poisoning, it is seldom incontrovertible. It takes several forms.

Circumstances under which found

In the case of infants, the mother may return to the kitchen or bathroom to find her child with some substance all over their hands, face, and clothing, or surrounded by pills, one of which the child may be eating. The assumption that some has been ingested may not be correct, and the amount swallowed is a matter of speculation.

Self-poisoning is a common cause of coma in previously healthy young adults. Adults may be found unconscious with tablet particles around the mouth or on clothing as the only clue to diagnosis. More often, the presence of empty drug containers with occasional tablets or capsules in close proximity to the patient suggests the diagnosis. Less commonly, they are found unconscious or dead in some remote location. The lack of personal effects to indicate who they are or where they live may suggest a desire not to be identified and should arouse suspicion of poisoning. Protestations by relatives that the patient would never take an overdose are often incorrect and should not prevent full investigation in appropriate circumstances.

Suicide notes

Suicide notes are reliable indicators of poisoning in the absence of physical violence as a cause of coma. The note may specify what has been taken in addition to expressing despair, futility, worthlessness, and remorse.

Features

There are few symptoms or physical signs that cannot be attributed to one poison or another. However, a clinical feature rarely arises in isolation, and clusters of features are of much greater diagnostic value. Those most commonly encountered in present-day practice are given in Table 9.1.1.

Conscious patients with abnormal behaviour, perhaps in combination with auditory and visual hallucinations, may have ingested amphetamines, phencyclidine, lysergic acid diethylamide (LSD), 'magic' (psilocybin-containing) mushrooms (see Chapter 9.3.1), and drugs such as the older antihistamines and tricyclic antidepressants, which have marked anticholinergic actions. Occasionally, a patient with severe salicylate intoxication, who cannot give a history despite being conscious, shows hyperventilation, sweating, flushing, and tachycardia, suggesting a diagnosis that can then be confirmed by the laboratory.

Drowsiness, ataxia, dysarthria, and nystagmus are common after ingestion of benzodiazepines. Coma with hypotonia and hyporeflexia may follow, particularly if alcohol has also been taken. Hypotension, hypothermia, and respiratory depression are rare. In present-day clinical practice, tricyclic antidepressants remain among the most common central nervous system depressants encountered in overdose. They cause hypertonia, hyperreflexia, extensor plantar responses, and dilated pupils. Sinus tachycardia and prolongation of the QRS interval on the electrocardiogram support a diagnosis of intoxication with these drugs; hypotension and hypothermia are uncommon. Tricyclic antidepressants and nonsteroidal anti-inflammatory agents, particularly mefenamic acid, are common causes of seizures. Coma with pinpoint pupils and a reduced respiratory rate is virtually diagnostic of poisoning with opioid analgesics and is an indication for a therapeutic trial of naloxone. Many patients with opioid poisoning will be habitual drug abusers and have venepuncture marks and evidence of venous tracking, particularly in the antecubital fossae. Alcohol may be smelt on the breath as may solvents such as toluene, acetone, or xylene as the result of 'sniffing' glues, cleaning agents, or other preparations. Burns around the lips or in the buccal cavity or pharynx indicate ingestion of corrosives.

Table 9.1.1 Common feature clusters in the poisoned patient

Feature cluster	Likely poisons
Coma, hypertonia, hyperreflexia, extensor plantar responses, myoclonus, strabismus, mydriasis, sinus tachycardia	Tricyclic antidepressants: less commonly antihistamines, orphenadrine, thioridazine
Coma, hypotonia, hyporeflexia, flexor or non-elicitable plantar responses, hypotension	Barbiturates, benzodiazepines and alcohol combinations, severe tricyclic antidepressant poisoning
Coma, miosis, reduced respiratory rate	Opioid analgesics
Nausea, vomiting, tinnitus, deafness, sweating, hyperventilation, vasodilation, tachycardia	Salicylates
Hyperthermia, tachycardia, delirium, agitation, mydriasis	Ecstasy (MDMA) or other amphetamine
Blindness (usually with other features)	Quinine, methanol
Miosis and hypersalivation	Organophosphorus and carbamate insecticides, nerve agents

Skin blisters

Skin blisters may be found after poisoning with a wide variety of drugs including barbiturates, tricyclic antidepressants, benzodiazepines, and nondrug toxins. They often occur over bony prominences that have been subjected to pressure and less frequently at sites where two skin areas have been in contact, e.g. the inner aspects of the knees and are not specific for any poison.

Neurological signs

Lateralizing neurological signs

Since most serious poisonings are associated with impairment of consciousness, neurological signs are particularly important. Lateralizing signs (unless they are attributable to a known neurological disease) virtually exclude a diagnosis of acute poisoning. Such findings have been recorded with barbiturate and phenytoin poisoning, but so rarely that the general rule is not significantly compromised.

Pyramidal tract signs

The usual features of pyramidal tract involvement (hypertonia, hyperreflexia, and extensor plantar responses) are commonly found in tricyclic antidepressant poisoning, and with other drugs with marked anticholinergic actions (e.g. the older antihistamines). However, all of these signs may be abolished in deep coma.

Abnormal movements

Unconscious patients may respond to painful stimuli with flexor and extensor limb movements of the type seen in decorticate and decerebrate states. However, in poisoning, these signs do not indicate irreversible brain damage, and patients showing them can be expected to recover fully; hypoglycaemia must be excluded in these cases. Acute dystonic movements (including acute torticollis, orolingual dyskinesias, and oculogyric crises) are also produced; these are usually caused by metoclopramide, or less commonly by haloperidol, droperidol, prochlorperazine, or trifluoperazine. Choreoathetosis has been reported as a rare presenting feature of poisoning with organophosphorus insecticides.

Pupillary changes in poisoning

Inequality of the pupils is not uncommon in poisoned patients. Widely dilated pupils that react poorly to light may be caused by poisons with anticholinergic actions (e.g. tricyclic antidepressants) or sympathomimetic effects (e.g. amphetamines) or which cause blindness (e.g. quinine, ethanol). Miosis is usually caused by opioid analgesics or poisons with cholinergic or anticholinesterase actions (e.g. organophosphorus insecticides, nerve agents). The degree and speed of reaction of the pupils to light is of no clinical value.

Ocular signs

A variety of ocular signs including strabismus, internuclear ophthalmoplegia, and total external ophthalmoplegia, may be found in acutely poisoned patients.

Strabismus has been described in poisoning with phenytoin, carbamazepine, and tricyclic antidepressants. Usually the optic axes diverge in the horizontal plane, but in some patients there is additional vertical deviation. It is present transiently and only in patients who are unconscious. Dysconjugate, roving eye movements may also be seen if both eyes are observed for a period of time. It is important to know that such abnormalities occur so that they are not misattributed to intracranial vascular lesions or some other pathology requiring surgical intervention.

Dysconjugate eye movements may become apparent only when oculovestibular reflexes are examined by caloric stimuli. Installation of ice-cold water into the external auditory meatus should make both eyes turn to the side irrigated, and failure of one eye to deviate is evidence of internuclear ophthalmoplegia and a lesion of the medial longitudinal fasciculus. This has been reported in poisoning with a variety of drugs including tricyclic antidepressants, phenothiazines, benzodiazepines barbiturates, and ethanol, and can be detected in 10% of cases if caloric tests are carried out. Both sides are usually affected, but internuclear ophthalmoplegia on testing one side only also occurs in acute poisoning.

Loss of oculocephalic and oculovestibular reflexes

It is widely accepted that absence of oculocephalic and oculovestibular responses indicates severe brainstem damage and the likelihood that the patient will not survive. However, this is not the case in acute poisoning where these reflexes may be abolished in patients who subsequently make a full recovery.

Visual impairment

Visual impairment is associated most commonly with quinine and methanol poisoning.

Box 9.1.1 Nontoxicological investigations

- Serum sodium (e.g. hyponatraemia in ecstasy (MDMA) poisoning)
- Serum potassium (e.g. hypokalaemia in theophylline poisoning, hyperkalaemia in digoxin poisoning, rhabdomyolysis, haemolysis)
- Plasma creatinine (e.g. renal failure in ethylene glycol poisoning)
- Blood sugar (e.g. hypoglycaemia in insulin and severe untreated paracetamol poisoning, hypoglycaemia and hyperglycaemia in salicylate poisoning)
- Serum calcium (e.g. hypocalcaemia in ethylene glycol poisoning)
- Serum alanine aminotransferase/aspartate aminotransferase activities (e.g. increased in paracetamol poisoning)
- Serum phosphate (e.g. hypophosphataemia in paracetamol-induced renal tubular damage)
- Acid–base disturbances, including metabolic acidosis
- RBC cholinesterase activity (e.g. organophosphorus insecticide and nerve agent poisoning)

Investigations

Information about the nature of poisons ingested can occasionally be deduced from standard haematological and biochemical investigations, and from arterial blood gas analysis (Box 9.1.1). Emergency measurement of the plasma concentration is essential for the poisons shown in Box 9.1.2; the concentration of these toxins is important to ensure appropriate clinical management. Other agents for which assays should be available on a 24-h basis at specialist laboratories include carbamazepine, digoxin, paraquat, and phenobarbital.

Laboratory screening for poisons in an unconscious patient is often requested when the cause of coma is unknown. Although

Box 9.1.2 Poisons for which emergency measurement of plasma or serum concentration is essential

- Carboxyhaemoglobin
- Digoxin
- Ethanol (when monitoring treatment in ethylene glycol and methanol poisoning)
- Ethylene glycol
- Iron
- Lithium
- Methanol
- Paracetamol
- Salicylate
- Theophylline
- Whole blood methaemoglobin concentration (e.g. in nitrite poisoning)

identification of a toxin may reassure the clinician, this is not a good reason for the request. The clinician should consider how the result of a screen will alter management. The pattern of drugs involved in poisoning in most developed countries is such that specific treatment (e.g. antidotes, techniques to enhance elimination of the poison) is unlikely to be available, and management will therefore be supportive. Screening is labour-intensive, time-consuming, and expensive, and in most cases, cannot be justified on an emergency basis because it will not alter the management of the patient.

A routine ECG is of limited diagnostic value, but is important in patients who are unconscious or thought to have ingested a cardiotoxic drug. Sinus tachycardia with prolongation of the QRS interval in an unconscious patient suggests tricyclic antidepressant poisoning. With increasing cardiotoxicity, it may be impossible to detect P-waves, and the pattern then resembles ventricular tachycardia. Overdose with cardiac glycosides or potassium salts also induces characteristic ECG changes. Q–T interval prolongation is a recognized adverse effect of several drugs in overdose (e.g. quetiapine, terfenadine, and quinine) and predisposes to ventricular arrhythmias, notably torsade de pointes.

Routine radiology is of little diagnostic value. It can be used to confirm ingestion of metallic objects (e.g. coins, button batteries) or injection of globules of metallic mercury. Rarely, hydrocarbon solvents (e.g. carbon tetrachloride) may be seen as a slightly opaque layer floating on the top of the gastric contents with the patient upright, or outlining the small bowel. Ingested packets of illicit substances may be discernible on a plain radiograph, but CT or MRI is more reliable in detecting such objects.

General management

Antidotes and methods to enhance elimination are available for only very small number of poisons, and the management of the great majority of poisoned patients is based on what has been called 'an orderly if unspectacular regimen of supportive therapy'.

Immediate treatment

A small but significant number of poisoned patients arrive at hospital with respiratory obstruction, ventilatory failure, or in cardiorespiratory arrest. In these cases, conventional resuscitation takes precedence over detailed assessment of the patient and attempts to obtain a history. The opioid antagonist naloxone is safe and should be used whenever there is the slightest suspicion that an opioid is involved. Its use intravenously will resurrect a comatose, hypoventilating patient within seconds and, even if it is given inappropriately, it is highly unlikely to have adverse effects.

Unconscious patients need scrupulous attention to respiration, hypotension, hypothermia, and other complications, if they are to survive. Expert nursing is as important as medical measures.

Airway

Establishment and maintenance of an adequate airway is of paramount importance in the management of unconscious poisoned patients. The airway may be obstructed by the tongue falling back, dental plates being dislodged, other foreign bodies, buccal secretions, vomitus, and flexion of the neck. In the first instance, the neck should be extended and the tongue and jaw held forward. Secretions in the oropharynx must be removed, and an oropharyngeal airway should be inserted before turning the patient into a semiprone position. If the cough reflex is absent, an endotracheal tube should be inserted to prevent aspiration into the lungs and allow regular aspiration of bronchial secretions. It is then important to ensure that the inspired air is adequately warmed and humidified.

Ventilation

Once a clear airway has been established, the adequacy of spontaneous ventilation should be assessed. Pulse oximetry can be used to measure oxygen saturation. The displayed reading may be inaccurate when the saturation is below 70%, when peripheral perfusion is poor, and in the presence of carboxyhaemoglobin or methaemoglobin. Only measurement of arterial blood gases, however, indicates the presence both of hypercapnia and hypoxia. The presence of ventilatory insufficiency (as determined by arterial partial pressure of oxygen ≤9 kPa on air and/or arterial partial pressure of CO_2 ≥6 kPa) should lead to consideration of immediate intubation and assisted ventilation, if the central respiratory depression cannot be reversed by administration of a specific antidote such as naloxone.

Unconscious poisoned patients often have a mild, mixed respiratory and metabolic acidosis with CO_2 tensions at the upper limit of normal, and oxygen tensions that fall with increasing depth of coma. Increasing the oxygen contents of the inspired air is often sufficient to correct hypoxia. High inspired oxygen concentrations are imperative in patients with carbon monoxide and cyanide poisoning and in pulmonary oedema resulting from inhalation of irritant gases.

Cardiovascular function

Cardiovascular function should be assessed by measuring pulse, blood pressure, and temperature (core and peripheral). ECG should be monitored in moderately or severely poisoned patients, particularly when a drug with a cardiotoxic action (e.g. a tricyclic antidepressant that produces QRS prolongation) has been ingested.

Hypotension

Although hypotension (systolic blood pressure <80 mmHg) is a recognized feature of acute poisoning, the classical features of shock (tachycardia and pale, cold skin) are seen only rarely because only a minority of patients are severely poisoned.

Hypotension and shock occur in many severely poisoned patients and may be caused by a direct cardiodepressant action of the poison (e.g. β-blockers, calcium channel blockers, tricyclic antidepressants); vasodilatation and venous pooling in the lower limbs (e.g. angiotensin converting enzyme (ACE) inhibitors, phenothiazines); decrease in circulating blood volume because of gastrointestinal losses (e.g. theophylline), increased insensible losses (e.g. salicylates), increased renal losses (e.g. diuretics), and increased capillary permeability. Hypotension may be exacerbated by coexisting hypoxia, acidosis, and dysrhythmias.

Correct management of individual cases depends on accurate identification of the cause. Young patients are generally not at risk of cerebral or renal damage unless the systolic blood pressure falls below 80 mmHg, but in those over the age of 40 years, it is preferable to keep the systolic blood pressure above 90 mmHg.

Hypotension often responds to elevation of the foot of the bed by 15 cm and, if this is unsuccessful, sodium chloride or other plasma expander should be administered. In more severe cases, it is helpful to undertake invasive haemodynamic monitoring to confirm that adequate volume replacement has been administered.

Dobutamine (2.5–10 μg/kg per min) or adrenaline (0.5–2.0 μg/kg per min) is indicated if hypotension is resistant to these measures; dopamine (2–5 μg/kg per min) is an alternative. A vasoconstrictor sympathomimetic drug (e.g. noradrenaline base 6.4–13.3 μg/min) may be necessary in severe cases, but it must be recognized that blood pressure may be raised at the expense of perfusion of vital organs such as the kidneys.

Hypertension

A few drugs when taken in overdose may produce systemic hypertension. If this is mild and associated with agitation, a benzodiazepine alone may suffice. In more severe cases, e.g. those due to a monoamine oxidase inhibitor, there may be a risk of arterial rupture, particularly intracranially. To prevent this, intravenous isosorbide dinitrate 2 to 10 mg/h, up to 20 mg/h if necessary, an α-adrenergic blocking agent (e.g. phentolamine, 5 mg intravenously every 10–15 min) or sodium nitroprusside (0.5–1.5 μg/kg per min by intravenous infusion) should be administered until blood pressure elevation is controlled.

Arrhythmias

Although many poisons are potentially cardiotoxic, the incidence of serious cardiac arrhythmias in acute poisoning is very low. Tricyclic antidepressants, β-adrenoceptor blocking drugs, calcium channel blockers, cardiac glycosides, amphetamines, cocaine, bronchodilators (particularly theophylline and its derivatives), and antimalarial drugs are the most likely causes. Cardiotoxicity usually occurs together with other features of severe poisoning, including metabolic acidosis, hypoxia, convulsions, respiratory depression, and abnormalities of electrolyte balance, which should be corrected before considering the use of antiarrhythmic drugs. The latter have narrow therapeutic ratios and their use may further impair myocardial function.

In general, drug therapy should only be given for persistent, life-threatening arrhythmias associated with peripheral circulatory failure. The drug used must be selected from knowledge of the pharmacology and toxicology of the poison involved and in such a way that it will not further compromise cardiac function. For example, in tricyclic antidepressant poisoning, arrhythmias are due to sodium channel blockade exacerbated by acidosis and are best treated with hypertonic sodium bicarbonate 50 to 100 mmol. Lidocaine (lignocaine) is probably the drug of choice for serious ventricular tachydysrhythmias in poisoning not corrected by reversal of acidosis, particularly where the offending drug is uncertain, since its half-life is short and the dose can be adjusted readily.

Convulsions

Convulsions are potentially life-threatening because they cause hypoxia and metabolic acidosis and may precipitate cardiac arrhythmias and arrest. Short, isolated convulsions do not require treatment but those which are recurrent or protracted should be suppressed with intravenous diazepam 10 to 20 mg in an adult (lorazepam 4 mg is an alternative). This drug is highly effective in adequate doses and alternatives are seldom needed. However, it is important to remember that giving benzodiazepines in this way may potentiate the respiratory depressant effects of other poisons and further complicate management. The combination of convulsions, coma, and vomiting, which may occur with overdosage of theophylline derivatives, is particularly dangerous, and in these circumstances, it may be preferable to paralyse the patient, insert an endotracheal tube, and start assisted ventilation. However, although this ensures control of the airway and oxygenation, thus avoiding the risk of inhalation of gastric contents, it does not suppress seizure activity; cerebral function must therefore be monitored and parenteral anticonvulsants given as required.

Hypothermia

Any poison which depresses the central nervous system may impair temperature regulation and cause hypothermia, especially when discovery of the patient is delayed and environmental temperatures are low. This important complication may be missed unless temperature is recorded rectally using a low-reading thermometer. In severe cases, peripheral and core temperatures should be monitored. Treatment includes nursing the patient in a warm room (27–29 °C) and a heat-conserving 'space blanket'. Cold intravenous fluids should be avoided and bottles for use should be stored in the room or the lines should pass through a heating device.

Hyperthermia

Rarely, body temperature may increase to potentially fatal levels after overdosage with central nervous system stimulants such as cocaine, amphetamines (including ecstasy (MDMA)), monoamine oxidase inhibitors, or theophylline. In such cases, muscle tone is often grossly increased and convulsions and rhabdomyolysis are common. Cooling measures should be instituted, sedation with diazepam should be given and, in severe cases, dantrolene 1 mg/kg body weight should be administered intravenously.

Acid–base disturbances

Acid–base disturbances commonly accompany coma due to drugs. Acute respiratory acidosis is less common than might be expected, but some elevation of arterial CO_2 tensions towards the upper limit of normal is usual. This, in combination with mild hypoxia in the deeper grades of coma, produces overall acidaemia. In general, acidosis should be prevented and managed by ensuring adequate ventilation, oxygenation, and tissue perfusion, and control of convulsions rather than by giving bicarbonate. However, a number of poisons, particularly methanol and ethylene glycol, cause life-threatening metabolic acidosis, which should be corrected by infusion of sodium bicarbonate.

Acute respiratory alkalosis, often in combination with a minor metabolic acidosis, is commonly found in acute salicylate poisoning. The metabolic component may require treatment if it is the dominant feature and is causing overall acidaemia. Respiratory alkalosis should not be treated.

Electrolyte abnormalities

Electrolyte abnormalities may result from acid–base disturbances or the direct effects of poisons. Massive tissue damage, usually rhabdomyolysis, may allow potassium to leak from cells leading to potentially lethal hyperkalaemia. Cardiac glycosides cause hyperkalaemia, secondary to loss from cells due to inhibition of the membrane sodium–potassium pump, while the reverse occurs with sympathomimetic drugs. Oxalic acid and ethylene glycol (which is metabolized to oxalic acid) may cause hypocalcaemia by leading to the formation of insoluble calcium oxalate, which is deposited in tissues. Similarly, ingestion of fluorides is also a possible cause of hypocalcaemia; but the amounts children tend to ingest in the form of tablets to prevent dental caries seldom cause serious problems. Ingestion of potassium salts, even in sustained release formulations, may lead to hyperkalaemia and fatal arrhythmias.

Bladder care

Urinary retention is a common complication of acute poisoning, particularly with tricyclic antidepressants and other drugs, which have marked anticholinergic actions. However, bladder catheterization is all too often an unconsidered measure in unconscious poisoned patients. Coma in inself is not an indication for bladder catheters in poisoned patients, the great majority of whom regain consciousness within 12 h. The bladder can usually be induced to empty reflexively (provided it is not allowed to become grossly over-distended) by applying gentle suprapubic pressure. Catheterization should be reserved for those patients in whom suprapubic pressure is insufficient to empty the bladder, and in those thought to be developing renal failure.

Skin, muscle, and nerve lesions

Bullous lesions should be left intact until they burst, to reduce the risk of infection. De-roofing should be performed when the blister bursts; a nonadhesive dressing is then applied.

Rhabdomyolysis is a further possible result of immobility and may occur in combination with skin lesions or independently. Poisoning is the most common nontraumatic cause of this condition and it may lead to acute renal failure and, rarely, to ischaemic muscle contractures and long-term disability. Urgent orthopaedic referral is indicated if a compartment syndrome is suspected. Peripheral nerves such as the radial, ulnar, and common peroneal may also be damaged by direct pressure while the patient is unconscious.

Unconscious patients should be turned from side to side at least every 2 h.

Antidotes

Antidotes may exert a beneficial effect by:

- forming an inert complex with the poison (e.g. desferrioxamine, D-penicillamine, dicobalt edetate, dimercaprol, digoxin-specific antibody fragments, HI-6, hydroxocobalamin, obidoxime, pralidoxime, protamine, Prussian (Berlin) blue, sodium calcium edetate, succimer (DMSA), unithiol (DMPS))
- accelerating detoxification of the poison (e.g. *N*-acetylcysteine, sodium thiosulphate)
- reducing the rate of conversion of the poison to a more toxic compound (e.g. ethanol, fomepizole)
- competing with the poison for essential receptor sites (e.g. oxygen, naloxone, phytomenadione)
- blocking essential receptors through which the toxic effects are mediated (e.g. atropine)
- bypassing the effect of the poison (e.g. oxygen, glucagon)

The most frequently used antidote in the developed world is *N*-acetylcysteine for paracetamol poisoning. Naloxone for opioid analgesics, oxygen for carbon monoxide, and, possibly, flumazenil for benzodiazepines are the only antidotes commonly needed in the management of unconscious poisoned patients. Other antidotes of proven value are listed in Table 9.1.2. The reader is recommended to read the relevant section in the chapter to obtain further advice. Antivenoms for bites and stings by venomous animals are discussed in Chapter 9.2.

Table 9.1.2 Poisons for which there are specific antidotes

Poison	Antidote
Aluminium	Desferrioxamine (deferoxamine)
Arsenic	Dimercaprol (BAL), succimer (DMSA)
Benzodiazepines	Flumazenil
β-adrenoceptor blocking drugs	Atropine, glucagon
Calcium channel blockers	Atropine
Carbamate insecticides	Atropine
Carbon monoxide	Oxygen
Copper	D-Penicillamine, unthiol (DMPS)
Cyanide	Dicobalt edetate, hydroxocobalamin, oxygen, sodium nitrite, sodium thiosulphate
Diethylene glycol	Fomepizole, ethanol
Digoxin and digitoxin	Digoxin-specific antibody fragments
Ethylene glycol	Fomepizole, ethanol
Hydrogen sulphide	Oxygen
Iron salts	Desferrioxamine (deferoxamine)
Lead (inorganic)	Succimer (DMSA), sodium calcium edetate
Methaemoglobinaemia	Methylthioninium chloride (methylene blue)
Methanol	Ethanol, fomepizole
Mercury (inorganic)	Unithiol (DMPS)
Nerve agents	Atropine, obidoxime, pralidoxime, HI-6
Oleander	Digoxin-specific antibody fragments
Opioids	Naloxone
Organophosphorus insecticides	Atropine, obidoxime, pralidoxime
Paracetamol	Acetylcysteine
Thallium	Prussian (Berlin) blue
Warfarin and other anticoagulants	Phytomenadione (vitamin K_1)

Reduction of poison absorption

Prevention of absorption of volatile poisons through the lungs obviously requires removal from the toxic atmosphere and occasionally removal of soiled clothing as well. The latter is also necessary when absorption is thought to have been percutaneous. In addition, the contaminated skin should be thoroughly washed with soap and water.

Although it appears logical to assume that removal of unabsorbed drug from the gastrointestinal tract ('gut decontamination') will be beneficial, the efficacy of current methods remains unproven, and efforts to remove small amounts of 'safe' drugs are clearly not worthwhile or appropriate.

Activated charcoal

Activated charcoal adsorbs a wide variety of drugs and toxic agents; the exceptions are acids and alkalis, ethanol, ethylene glycol, iron, lithium, and methanol.

In studies in volunteers given 50 g activated charcoal, the mean reduction in absorption was 40%, 16%, and 21% at 60 min, 120 min, and 180 min, respectively, after ingestion. Based on these studies, activated charcoal should be considered in those who have ingested a potentially toxic amount of a poison (known to be adsorbed by charcoal) up to 1 h previously. There are insufficient data to support or exclude its use after 1 h. There is no evidence that administration of activated charcoal improves the clinical outcome.

Gastric aspiration and lavage

Gastric emptying studies in volunteers provide no support for the use of gastric lavage. In the single clinical study in which benefit was claimed for lavage within 1 h of overdose, patients also received activated charcoal. There was also selection bias, and hence conclusions based on these data are limited. Thus, gastric lavage should not be used routinely in the management of poisoned patients as there is no evidence that it improves outcome, and it may cause significant morbidity.

The efficacy with which lavage removes gastric contents decreases with time; therefore, lavage should be considered only in patients who have ingested life-threatening amounts of a toxic agent up to 1 h previously.

Emesis with syrup of ipecacuanha

Syrup of ipecacuanha contains the active alkaloids emetine and cephaeline. Although syrup of ipecacuanha is an effective emetic, there is no evidence that its use prevents significant absorption of toxic material and, moreover, its adverse effects (e.g. persistent vomiting, diarrhoea, lethargy, drowsiness) may complicate diagnosis. It is not recommended.

Whole-bowel irrigation

Theoretically, the more quickly a slowly absorbed poison passes through the gut, the less it is absorbed. The opposite may apply to rapidly absorbed drugs. Whole-bowel irrigation using polyethylene glycol electrolyte solutions does not result in absorption of fluid and electrolytes, even though large volumes are administered rapidly via a nasogastric tube. Some volunteer studies have shown substantial decreases in the bioavailability of ingested drugs, but no controlled clinical trials have been conducted and there is no evidence that whole-bowel irrigation improves outcome. Based on volunteer studies, whole-bowel irrigation may be considered following potentially toxic ingestion of sustained-release or enteric-coated drugs and in body packers.

Cathartics

Cathartics have been used alone and with activated charcoal. Cathartics alone have no role in the management of poisoned patients. Based on available data, routine use of a cathartic with activated charcoal is not endorsed.

Methods to increase poison elimination

Once a poison has been absorbed and providing there is no antidote, it is reasonable to consider the use of treatments that might speed its elimination from the body.

Multiple-dose activated charcoal (MDAC)

Use of MDAC involves repeated administration of oral activated charcoal to increase the elimination of a drug that has already been absorbed into the body. Elimination of drugs with a small volume of distribution (<1 litre/kg), low pK_a (which maximizes transport across membranes), low binding affinity, and prolonged elimination half-life following overdose is particularly likely to be enhanced by MDAC. MDAC also improves total body clearance of the drug when endogenous processes are compromised by liver and/or renal failure.

Activated charcoal adsorbs material in the gut, which may be relevant in cases of poisoning with slow-release drug preparations. It also adsorbs drugs that are secreted in the bile, thereby preventing intestinal reabsorption, and binds any drug that diffuses from the circulation into the gut lumen. After absorption, drugs re-enter the gut by passive diffusion if the concentration in the gut is lower than that in the blood. The rate of passive diffusion depends on the concentration gradient and the intestinal surface area, permeability, and blood flow. Occasionally, drugs such as digoxin may be secreted actively by the intestinal mucosa, though the contribution of active secretion to the effect of MDAC on drug clearance is unlikely to be greater than that of passive diffusion.

Although many studies have demonstrated that MDAC significantly increases drug elimination, it has not been shown to reduce morbidity and mortality in controlled studies in poisoned patients. At present, use of MDAC should be considered only in patients who have ingested a life-threatening amount of carbamazepine, dapsone, phenobarbital, quinine, and theophylline.

Clinical experience in adults suggests that charcoal should be administered in an initial dose of 50 to 100 g and then at a rate of not less than 12.5 g/h, preferably via a nasogastric tube. Smaller initial doses (10–25 g) can be used in children because, generally, smaller overdoses have been ingested and the capacity of the gut lumen is smaller. If the patient has ingested a drug that induces protracted vomiting (e.g. theophylline), intravenous ondansetron is effective as an anti-emetic and thus enables administration of MDAC.

Urine alkalinization

Increasing the urine pH enhances elimination of salicylate, phenobarbital, chlorpropamide, and chlorophenoxy herbicides (e.g. 2,4-dichlorophenoxyacetic acid, mecoprop). However, with the exception of salicylate poisoning, urine alkalinization cannot be recommended as first-line therapy for poisoning with these agents, as MDAC is superior for phenobarbital, and supportive care is invariably adequate for chlorpropamide. A substantial diuresis is required in addition to urine alkalinization to achieve clinically important elimination of chlorophenoxy herbicides.

Urine alkalinization is a metabolically invasive procedure requiring frequent biochemical monitoring and medical and nursing expertise. Before commencing urine alkalinization, it is important to correct plasma volume depletion, electrolytes (administration of sodium bicarbonate exacerbates pre-existing hypokalaemia), and metabolic abnormalities. Sodium bicarbonate is most conveniently administered intravenously as an 8.4% solution (1 mmol bicarbonate/ml). Sufficient bicarbonate is administered (225 mmol was the mean amount required in one study) to ensure that the pH of the urine, which is measured by narrow-range indicator paper or a pH meter, is more than 7.5 and preferably close to 8.5. As the administration of sodium bicarbonate forces potassium into cells, it is important that the patient has a normal serum potassium concentration before sodium bicarbonate is administered. Sodium bicarbonate 8.4% is highly irritant to veins and severe tissue damage can ensue if extravasation occurs. A secure, preferably wide-bore cannula (or control venous line), must therefore be used.

Dialysis, haemodialfiltration, haemofiltration, and haemoperfusion

Haemodialysis significantly increases elimination of ethanol, ethylene glycol, isopropanol, lithium, methanol, and salicylate, and is the treatment of choice in all cases of severe poisoning with these agents. Although haemofiltration and haemodialfiltration are widely available and increase elimination of poisons such as ethylene glycol and methanol, they are much less efficient than haemodialysis, and therefore should not be used unless haemodialysis is unavailable.

Haemodialysis, haemofiltration, and haemoperfusion are of no value in patients poisoned with drugs with large volumes of distribution (e.g. tricyclic antidepressants), because the plasma contains only a small proportion of the total amount of drug in the body. They are indicated in patients with both severe clinical features and high plasma toxin concentrations.

Charcoal haemoperfusion can significantly reduce the body burden of phenobarbital, carbamazepine, and theophylline, but MDAC is as effective and simpler to use.

Drugs (including substances of abuse)

Amfetamines and ecstasy (MDMA)

Amfetamines, particularly metamfetamine ('crystal meth', 'ice') and MDMA, are abused widely. Features of poisoning are related predominantly to stimulation of central and peripheral adrenergic receptors and, in addition, hyperthermia and hyponatraemia (secondary to inappropriate ADH secretion) may develop in severe MDMA toxicity. Poisoning is usually the result of recreational use.

Clinical features

These drugs cause increased alertness and self-confidence, euphoria, extrovert behaviour, increased talkativeness with rapid speech, lack of desire to eat or sleep, tremor, dilated pupils, tachycardia, and hypertension. More severe intoxication is associated with excitability, agitation, paranoid delusions, hallucinations with violent behaviour, hypertonia, and hyperreflexia. Convulsions, rhabdomyolysis, hyperthermia, and cardiac arrhythmias may develop in the most severe cases. Rarely, intracerebral and subarachnoid haemorrhage and acute cardiomyopathy occur and may be fatal.

In the case of MDMA, hyperthermia, disseminated intravascular coagulation, rhabdomyolysis, acute renal failure, and hyponatraemia are observed commonly in severe cases, in addition to those features described earlier. Death occurred in 2 of 17 patients with serum sodium concentrations of 107 to 128 mmol/litre. Their clinical course was remarkably similar; initial vomiting and disturbed behaviour was followed by seizures, drowsiness, a mute state, and disorientation. Severe hepatic damage, including fulminant hepatic failure, has also been reported. The serotonin syndrome has been described.

Management

Intravenous fluids should be given for dehydration. Diazepam 10 to 20 mg intravenously or haloperidol 2.5 to 5.0 mg intramuscularly or intravenously are effective in controlling agitation. The peripheral sympathomimetic actions of amfetamines may be antagonized by β-adrenergic blocking drugs. Although acidification of the urine increases renal elimination of amfetamines, sedation is usually all that is required. Dantrolene 1 mg/kg intravenous should be administered for hyperthermia. In most cases, hyponatraemia responds to fluid restriction alone. Transplantation may be indicated in patients who develop MDMA-induced fulminant hepatic failure.

Angiotensin-converting enzyme (ACE) inhibitors

Clinical features

Overdose commonly causes hypotension and occasional drowsiness. Heart rate is rarely raised above 100 to 120 bpm. Angioedema and metabolic changes, specifically moderate increases in serum potassium, are also seen. The fall in blood pressure is often much greater than from therapeutic doses, and the suggestion that ACE inhibitors have a 'ceiling' effect on blood pressure is clearly incorrect.

ACE inhibitors are likely to bind to activated charcoal, which should be administered in early presentations. The principles of supportive care include volume expansion and subsequent use of inotropes. Since most patients who take this overdose are on treatment for hypertension or heart failure, they may already have impaired myocardial function. Naloxone does not correct hypotension.

Since ACE inhibitors are teratogenic, women exposed in the first trimester of pregnancy need appropriate counselling. They also cause *in utero* growth retardation.

Antibacterial agents

Clinical features and management

Antibiotic overdose is usually asymptomatic and requires no treatment. Transient nausea, vomiting, and diarrhoea may occur, or adverse effects of therapeutic doses may be exaggerated. There have been single case reports of renal failure after overdosage with co-trimoxazole or aminoglycosides, pancreatitis with erythromycin, haemorrhagic cystitis with amoxicillin, and seizures with other β-lactam antibiotics.

Rifampicin

Clinical features

The principal sign of rifampicin poisoning is the colouration of body fluids including sweat and saliva, which become orange-red in colour. These appearances are due to the colouration of the drug and its metabolites, but do not in themselves indicate toxicity. At high concentrations, nausea, vomiting and abdominal pain, and convulsions have been observed. Hepatic induction is seen with rifampicin, and this also results in hepatitis in occasional patients. Changes in liver function tests usually resolve over 72 h.

Management

This is supportive and usually no intervention is necessary.

Anticonvulsants

Carbamazepine

Clinical features

Carbamazepine is structurally related to the tricyclic antidepressants and has similar anticholinergic actions. Overdose causes dry mouth, coma, convulsions, nystagmus, ataxia, and incoordination. The pupils are often dilated, divergent strabismus may be present, and complete external ophthalmoplegia has been reported. Hallucinations may occur, particularly in the recovery phase.

Management

MDAC has been shown to significantly increase elimination of carbamazepine and is as effective as charcoal haemoperfusion. Activated charcoal should therefore be given in severe cases of carbamazepine poisoning in an initial dose of 50 to 100 g for adults, with repeated doses of 12.5 g/h (or the equivalent).

Phenytoin

Clinical features

Acute overdose results in nausea, vomiting, headache, tremor, cerebellar ataxia, nystagmus, and rarely, loss of consciousness.

Management

MDAC may increase elimination though this has not been confirmed.

Sodium valproate

Clinical features

Most frequently there is drowsiness, impairment of consciousness, and respiratory depression. In severe poisoning, myoclonic jerks and seizures may occur and cerebral oedema has been reported. Liver damage and metabolic acidosis, perhaps due to changes in fatty acid metabolism, are very unusual but potential complications.

Management

Treatment is symptomatic and supportive. Haemodialysis is effective in removing sodium valproate and should be employed in severe poisoning, particularly if severe hyperammonaemia and electrolyte and acid–base disturbances are present.

Gabapentin

Clinical features and management

Lethargy, ataxia, slurred speech, and gastrointestinal symptoms may develop. Management is supportive.

Lamotrigine

Clinical features and management

Lethargy, coma, ataxia, nystagmus, seizures, and cardiac conduction abnormalities have been reported. Management is supportive.

Levetiracetam

Clinical features and management

Lethargy, coma, and respiratory depression have been observed. Management is supportive.

Tiagabine

Clinical features and management

Lethargy, facial grimacing, nystagmus, posturing, agitation, coma, hallucinations, and seizures have been reported. Management is supportive.

Topiramate

Clinical features and management

Lethargy, ataxia, nystagmus, myoclonus, coma, seizures, and a normal anion gap metabolic acidosis have been observed; the latter may be due to inhibition of renal cortical carbonic anhydrase. Metabolic acidosis can appear within hours of ingestion and persist for days. Management is supportive.

Antidepressants

These fall into a variety of pharmacological groups but share the common effect of altering central monoamine function. Toxicity is largely affected by other properties of these drugs.

Tricyclic antidepressants

Several different pharmacological actions determine the features of overdose. Reuptake of monoamines (noradrenaline and serotonin) into central and peripheral neurones is blocked. Anticholinergic actions cause reduced gut motility, dry mouth and tachycardia. They are sodium channel blockers with class I antiarrhythmic action prolonging the QRS complex. They are α-adrenergic and histamine antagonists resulting in hypotension and sedation.

Clinical features

Clinical features evolve as the drug is absorbed, usually within 30 to 60 min of ingestion. Patients who remain conscious six hours after ingestion are unlikely to have taken much drug. Early features include drowsiness, sinus tachycardia, dry mouth, and dilated pupils. Urinary retention, increased reflexes, extensor plantar responses, and gaze palsies may then develop. Patients who become unconscious, Glasgow Coma Score (GCS) <8, or are unresponsive to pain, are at increased risk of more serious complications, particularly seizures. Risk of ventricular arrhythmia may be predicted from the length of the QRS complex. Changes in repolarization pattern may also be seen with abnormal T-waves and apparent changes in the ventricular axis. This pattern mimics the Brugada syndrome, the congenital abnormality associated with ventricular fibrillation. Features include ST elevation in leads V1–3, with right bundle block often associated with serious ventricular arrhythmias.

Management

Patients with depressed consciousness and prolonged QRS interval are at risk of fits and arrhythmias. Maintenance of acid–base balance in these patients is crucial. Early and prompt treatment with sodium bicarbonate, even in patients who are not overtly acidotic, ameliorates cardiac effects of tricyclics. Sodium bicarbonate (50 mmol doses, 50 ml of 8.4%) should be administered. If given into a peripheral vein, there is a risk of necrosis if it extravasates. Indications for bicarbonate include QRS duration greater than 120 ms, existing arrhythmias, or hypotension resistant to fluid resuscitation. The aim is to maintain the arterial pH in the range 7.5 to 7.55 without producing greater alkalaemia. Specific antiarrhythmic drugs, such as lidocaine (lignocaine), are also sodium channel blockers, and therefore may worsen arrhythmias. Convulsions should be treated conventionally with diazepam (10–20 mg intravenously, in an adult) or lorazepam (3–4 mg).

The α-adrenoreceptor blocking properties of tricyclics can cause severe hypotension. Noradrenaline is the most appropriate inotrope to use in this situation.

In the past, physostigmine was advocated to counteract the anticholinergic action of tricyclic antidepressants, but most European toxicologists do not recommend this.

During recovery from tricyclic poisoning, there may be a prolonged period of delirium with auditory and visual hallucinations. Sedation with diazepam is appropriate until the patient recovers.

All tricyclic antidepressants may cause these features but dosulepine (dothiepin) is the most toxic in overdose, followed by amitriptyline.

Selective serotonin reuptake inhibitors (SSRIs)

Citalopram, fluoxetine, fluvoxamine, paroxetine, and sertraline, antidepressants that inhibit serotonin reuptake (SSRIs), lack the anticholinergic actions of tricyclic antidepressants.

Clinical features

Clinical features of these agents are principally due to serotonin-like effects, and include nausea and vomiting, agitation, and tachycardia. Convulsions may occur after larger ingestions. Hypertonia and marked clonus are common features of significant poisoning, and increased muscle activity results in rise in serum creatine kinase activity. Citalopram is the most toxic of the group in overdose. All SSRIs cause occasional arrhythmias.

Management

In patients who consume more than one drug affecting serotonin receptors (e.g. tricyclic antidepressants, monoamine oxidase inhibitors, drugs of abuse, including, in particular, ecstasy), the serotonin syndrome may occur. Features include marked agitation and increased muscle activity resulting in hyperpyrexia. About half the patients have central nervous system features including delirium and hallucinations. Other features include autonomic instability with tachycardia and labile blood pressure. Specific serotonin antagonists such as ciproheptadine may be useful. Alternatively, benzodiazepines (e.g. diazepam orally or parenterally) may help reduce agitation.

Venlafaxine

Venlafaxine is a drug that inhibits the reuptake of serotonin and noradrenaline (SNRI). In overdose, it has features of both SSRIs and tricyclic antidepressants but it lacks anticholinergic activity.

Clinical features

Drowsiness and convulsions are the main central nervous system effects. Tachycardia, ventricular arrhythmias, and changes in blood pressure are the main cardiovascular effects.

Management

Management of metabolic acidosis is important to reduce the risk of arrhythmias, which are more common in patients who have had convulsions. Convulsions are managed conventionally with diazepam (10–20 mg intravenously) or lorazepam (3–4 mg intravenously). Activated charcoal should be considered if more than 12.5 mg/kg was ingested within the previous hour. Venlafaxine prolongs the QT interval so that torsades de pointes is a risk that should be treated conventionally by correcting acidosis and with intravenous magnesium.

Monoamine oxidase inhibitors (MAOIs)

These have well-established adverse interactions with foods containing tyramine. The classical MAOIs such as phenelzine, isocarboxacid, and tranylcypramine are now rarely used, and the new more specific inhibitors of MAOI type A (moclobemide) and type B (selegilene) produce less serious adverse effects in overdose.

Classical MAOIs prevent the breakdown of catecholamines within the nerve ending, and result in excess sympathomimetic effects peripherally, and excess adrenergic effects centrally. In patients who are naive to the drugs, onset of inhibition of enzyme takes several hours, and clinical features may not be seen immediately. In patients on chronic therapy, the onset will be more rapid.

Clinical features

Principal effects are central nervous system stimulation with excitement, restlessness, hyperpyrexia, hyperreflexia, convulsions, and coma. These may go on to cause rhabdomyolysis. Cardiovascular effects include tachycardia and changes in blood pressure, depending on whether the effects of adrenaline (vasodilation) or noradrenaline (vasoconstriction) predominate.

Management

Treatment is supportive, with careful monitoring. Patients who develop central excitation should be treated with large doses of diazepam. This will reduce centrally stimulated muscle contraction and hence pyrexia and muscle damage. Cardiovascular monitoring is essential. Changes in blood pressure should be managed where possible with drugs that are not sympathomimetic agonists. Use of β-blockade may result in unopposed α-agonist effect causing large rises in blood pressure. Hypertension is best controlled with an intravenous nitrate such as glyceryl trinitrate.

Antihistamines

First-generation antihistamines include brompheniramine, chlorphenamine, cyclizine, diphenhydramine, promethazine, and trimeprazine. Second-generation drugs include cetirizine, loratidine, fexofenadine, astemizole, and terfenadine.

Clinical features

Older antihistamines have anticholinergic actions but less potent central nervous system toxicity than other anticholinergic drugs. Delirium may be a particular problem in very young children and older people, following a substantial acute overdose. Rhabdomyolysis is a well-recognized complication of severe antihistamine poisoning. The second-generation drugs generally cause less sedation and less psychomotor impairment but some, notably astemizole and terfenadine, have been associated with cardiotoxicity causing QTc interval prolongation and ventricular tachycardia, including torsade de pointes. Astemizole and terfenadine have been withdrawn from use in many countries for this reason.

Management

A 12-lead ECG and cardiac monitoring for at least 12 h is recommended after a substantial overdose. Management should otherwise follow the same principles as for tricyclic antidepressant poisoning (see above).

Antimalarials

Chloroquine

Toxicity can result from doses greater than 1 g (*c.*6 tablets) in adults.

Clinical features

Cardiac arrest is commonly the first clinical manifestation of poisoning, but hypotension usually precedes it and may progress to cardiogenic shock with pulmonary oedema. Electrocardiographic abnormalities, bradyarrhythmias, and tachyarrhythmias are common and are similar to those seen in quinine poisoning. Visual disturbance, agitation, drowsiness, acute psychosis, dystonic reactions, seizures, and coma may ensue. Hypokalaemia is common and is due to potassium channel blockade.

Management

Supportive measures should be employed and hypokalaemia corrected. There is no specific antidote. Sodium bicarbonate 50 to 200 mmol (50–200 ml of 8.4%) is indicated if the ECG shows intraventricular block but will exacerbate hypokalaemia, which should be corrected first. Mechanical ventilation, the administration of epinephrine 1 to 10 µg/kg.min and high-doses of diazepam (1 mg/kg as a loading dose and 0.25–0.4 mg/kg per h maintenance) may reduce the mortality to 10% in severe poisoning. MDAC may enhance chloroquine elimination. Extracorporeal elimination techniques do not have a role. Extracorporeal life support has been utilized successfully in severely poisoned patients unresponsive to conventional measures.

Quinine

Quinine cardiotoxicity is due to sodium channel blockade.

Clinical features

Cinchonism (tinnitus, deafness, vertigo, nausea, headache, and diarrhoea) is common at plasma concentrations greater than 5 mg/litre. In more serious poisoning, collapse with impairment of consciousness (due to ventricular arrhythmias) convulsions, hypotension, pulmonary oedema, and cardiorespiratory arrest may be observed. The latter is often preceded by ECG conduction abnormalities, particularly QT prolongation. Hypoglycaemia, resulting from insulin release, occurs even with therapeutic doses and must be excluded in all cases. About 40% of patients develop ocular features, which may be unilateral, including blindness, contracted visual fields, scotomata, dilated pupils, blurred disc margins, macular oedema, arteriolar spasm, and late optic atrophy. Oculotoxicity is likely when plasma concentrations exceed 10 mg/litre. Visual loss is permanent in about 50% of cases.

Management

MDAC increases quinine clearance. Extracorporeal elimination techniques and stellate ganglion block are of no value. Electrolyte and acid–base disturbances and hypoglycaemia should be corrected. Hypertonic sodium bicarbonate will correct acidosis that persists despite fluid resuscitation and adequate oxygenation and is recommended first-line therapy for conduction abnormalities due to sodium channel blockade, including QRS and QT prolongation. Overdrive pacing may be required if torsade de pointes occurs and does not respond to magnesium sulphate infusion.

Primaquine

Clinical features

The main concern about primaquine is its ability to cause methaemoglobinaemia in overdose. Other adverse effects reported are headache, nausea, abdominal pain, haemolytic anaemia particularly in patients with glucose-6-dehydrogenase deficiency, and leucopenia.

Management

Treatment is supportive. Clinically significant methaemoglobinaemia (generally >30%) is treated conventionally with intravenous methylthioninium chloride (methylene blue) 1 to 2 mg/kg body weight.

Antipsychotics

Antipsychotic drugs are thought to act predominantly by effects on dopamine D_2 receptors. Older antipsychotics were phenothiazines, such as chlorpromazine, and butyrophenones, such as haloperidol. More recent selective antipsychotic drugs were sulpiride and later clozapine, olanzapine, quetiapine, and risperidone (termed 'atypical antipsychotics').

Phenothiazines

These antipsychotics have many actions, including antihistamine and anticholinergic activity. Chlorpromazine blocks α-, β-, and 5HT-receptors *in vitro*. Features such as postural hypotension are likely to be due to the sum of these effects.

Clinical features

In overdose, the predominant clinical features of all of this class of drugs is sedation, loss of consciousness, and hypotension. Respiratory depression may occur in more severe cases. Hypotension and vasodilatation are features of chlorpromazine poisoning. Thioridazine (now withdrawn in many countries) causes prolonged QT syndrome. ECG abnormalities have been seen with some of the newer atypical antipsychotics but they cause less cardiovascular disturbance than the older drugs. Muscle contraction due to central extrapyramidal effects may result in rhabdomyolysis in severe cases. Neuroleptic malignant syndrome, seen during therapeutic use of these compounds, is uncommon in acute poisoning and should be treated conventionally.

Management

Management is supportive. Dystonic reactions may occur, particularly in young adults. These should be treated conventionally with benztropine (1–2 mg intravenously), procyclidine (5–10 mg intravenously), or diazepam (10–20 mg intravenously or oral).

Butyrophenones

Haloperidol is the most widely used of the butyrophenones.

Clinical features

Overdose generally causes drowsiness and hypotension. These drugs are dopamine receptor antagonists and may cause vasodilatation, and there are occasional reports of ECG abnormalities. In young adults, the commonest complication is acute dystonia; parkinsonian effects may be seen in older people. Neuroleptic malignant syndrome is unusual in acute poisoning.

Management

Treatment is supportive, and acute dystonic reactions respond to either anticholinergics such as benztropine (1–2 mg) or procyclidine (5–10 mg) intravenously for an adult, or an intravenous benzodiazepine such as diazepam.

Atypical antipsychotics

These agents cause sedation as their primary effect. Some have caused QT prolongation in overdose. Occasionally fits are reported. Treatment is supportive. A 12-lead ECG should be obtained to check QT duration.

Barbiturates

Except for phenobarbital, barbiturates are now prescribed rarely and therefore overdose with other barbiturates is now rare.

Clinical features

Impairment of consciousness, respiratory depression, hypotension, and hypothermia are typical and potentiated by alcohol. There are no specific neurological signs. Hypotonia and hyporeflexia are the rule and the plantar responses are either flexor or absent. Skin blisters, and rhabdomyolysis may develop. During recovery from coma, with or without hypothermia, it is common to observe a peak of temperature, which cannot be explained by infection. Most deaths result from respiratory complications.

Management

Supportive measures should be used as appropriate. Phenobarbital can be removed efficiently by MDAC; urine alkalinization is less effective.

Benzodiazepines

These are widely used as tranquillizers, hypnotics, and sedatives.

Clinical features

Although many benzodiazepines have active metabolites accounting for their sometimes prolonged sedative effects, all are remarkably safe when taken alone in overdosage. As many as 70 or 80 tablets of any of them is unlikely to produce anything more than mild effects in most adults. However, there is individual variation in response, influenced by habituation and tolerance, which develop during chronic therapy; some otherwise healthy elderly people respond to an overdose with prolonged toxicity. Benzodiazepines potentiate the effects of other central nervous system depressants, particularly alcohol, tricyclic antidepressants, and barbiturates. Dizziness, drowsiness, ataxia, and slurred speech are the usual features; coma, respiratory depression, and hypotension are uncommon and usually mild. Flurazepam is most likely to cause significant central nervous system depression. Amnesia of events during the period of drug effect is also seen.

Management

The use of flumazenil is potentially hazardous in patients who have co-ingested other drugs, particularly tricyclics (risk of fits and lethal arrhythmias), or who are habituated to benzodiazepines from therapeutic use (risk of acute withdrawal and fits). Flumazenil should therefore not be used routinely in benzodiazepine poisoning, nor as a diagnostic test. It should be given to avoid assisted ventilation in a patient who is otherwise going to require intubation, particularly in those with existing chronic airways obstruction. Flumazenil has a relatively short half-life and therefore repeated doses may be required.

β-Adrenoceptor blocking drugs (β-blockers)

β-Adrenoceptor blocking drugs (β-blockers) exert their toxic effects in overdose not only by blocking the β_1- and β_2-adrenoreceptors, but also by virtue of their membrane stabilizing activity, which results in a quinidine-like effect on the action potential as a result of sodium channel blockade; this produces QRS widening, which predisposes to ventricular arrhythmias.

Clinical features

Symptoms usually occur within 6 h of ingestion of non-sustained release preparations. Sinus bradycardia may be the only feature after a small overdose, but if a substantial amount has been ingested, coma, convulsions (particularly with propranolol), profound bradycardia, and hypotension may occur. Other effects include drowsiness, delirium, hallucinations, low-output cardiac failure, and cardiorespiratory arrest (asystole or ventricular fibrillation). Bronchospasm and hypoglycaemia occur rarely.

First-degree heart block, intraventricular conduction defects, right and left bundle branch block, ST segment elevation, ventricular extrasystoles, and disappearance of the P-wave may be noted on the electrocardiogram. Sotalol has been reported to cause QT interval prolongation and ventricular arrhythmias and asystole may follow severe overdose from any β-adrenoceptor blocking drug.

Management

A delay in treatment may be fatal in patients who are severely poisoned. The blood pressure and cardiac rhythm of the patient should be monitored immediately in an intensive care area and supportive measures implemented.

Glucagon is the drug of choice for severe hypotension; it bypasses the blocked β-receptor, thus activating adenyl cyclase and promoting the formation of cAMP (which has a direct β-stimulant effect on the heart) from ATP. It should be given in a bolus dose of 50 to 150 μg/kg (typically 10 mg in an adult) over 1 min, followed by an infusion of 1 to 5 mg/h according to response. Conventional inotropes are less effective than glucagon in severe cases.

If bradycardia is refractory to atropine 0.6 to 1.2 mg intravenously, repeated as necessary, transcutaneous or transvenous pacing should be considered. Sodium bicarbonate may reverse the cardiotoxic effects of β-blockers with membrane stabilizing activity and should be considered for the treatment of ventricular dysrhythmias. Occasionally, diazepam 10 to 20 mg intravenously may be needed for convulsions. If bronchospasm supervenes, salbutamol (albuterol) by nebulizer, should be employed. Hypoglycaemia should be corrected.

β_2-Adrenoceptor agonists

Poisoning with β_2-adrenoceptor stimulants, including fenoterol, pirbuterol, reprobuterol, rimiterol, salbutamol (albuterol), and terbutaline, has followed deliberate and accidental ingestion of these drugs and has also resulted from confusion over the difference between oral and parenteral doses.

Mechanisms of toxicity

β_2-Agonists act on β_2-adrenergic receptors and increase intracellular cAMP. In addition to initiating relaxation of bronchial, vascular, and uterine smooth muscle, β_2-agonists cause glycogenolysis in skeletal muscle and hepatic glycogenolysis and gluconeogenesis. Hypokalaemia is caused by β_2-receptor-mediated activation of Na^+-K^+-ATPase, with extracellular potassium being shifted into the intracellular compartment; hypokalaemia may precipitate supraventricular and ventricular arrhythmias.

Clinical features

Tremor, sinus tachycardia, agitation, convulsions, supraventricular and ventricular arrhythmias, hypokalaemia, hyperglycaemia, and ketoacidosis are the typical features of severe poisoning with β_2-agonists. Psychosis and hallucinations are observed occasionally.

Management

Hypokalaemia should be corrected as soon as possible by the administration of an infusion of potassium at a rate of 40 to 60 mmol/h diluted in 5% dextrose. A non-selective β-blocker, such as propanolol 1 to 5 mg by slow intravenous injection, will also reverse hypokalaemia and sinus tachycardia, but its use may exacerbate pre-existing obstructive airways disease.

Supraventricular tachycardia has been treated successfully with adenosine. If myocardial ischaemia occurs as a result of the tachyarrhythmia, propranolol, 1 to 5 mg intravenously, should be administered. Convulsions are usually single and short-lived but, if necessary, diazepam, 5 to 10 mg intravenously, may be given.

Bismuth chelate (tripotassium dicitratobismuthate)

Although bismuth absorption from bismuth chelate is low after a therapeutic dose, a significant quantity may be absorbed after overdose.

Clinical features

Self-poisoning with large doses of bismuth chelate has caused reversible renal failure 2 and 10 days after overdose and at least one death. During prolonged (and sometimes high-dose) therapy, bismuth-induced encephalopathy has been reported.

Management

Dimercaprol can lower brain bismuth concentrations though there is no evidence that it can prevent nephrotoxicity. DMPS and DMSA are effective oral alternatives.

Calcium channel blockers

Calcium channel blockers act by blocking voltage-gated calcium channels at cardiac conducting and contractile tissue and vascular smooth muscle.

Clinical features

In overdose, calcium channel blockers cause nausea, vomiting, dizziness, slurred speech, confusion, sinus bradycardia and tachycardia, prolonged atrioventricular conduction, atrioventricular dissociation, hypotension, pulmonary oedema, convulsions, coma, hyperglycaemia, and metabolic acidosis. When a sustained release preparation has been ingested, the onset of severe features may be delayed for more than 12 h. Cardiac complications are usually more serious following overdose with verapamil or diltiazem than with the dihydropyridines such as nifedipine and amlodipine. Large overdoses carry a poor prognosis, particularly in patients with ischaemic heart disease and in those taking β-blockers.

Management

Calcium chloride (10%, 5 to 10 ml at 1–2 ml/min) or calcium gluconate (10% solution 10–20 ml intravenously) may reverse prolonged intracardiac conduction times. If significant hypotension persists despite volume replacement, intravenous glucagon 10 mg (150 μg/kg) should be given to an adult and can be followed by an infusion 5 to 10 mg/h depending on response. If hypotension persists, administer a sympathomimetic amine intravenously. Insulin–dextrose euglycaemia has been shown to improve myocardial contractility and systemic perfusion and may be used as an adjuvant to a sympathomimetic amine. There is increasing evidence that intravenous Intralipid is useful in patients who do not respond to other measures. Cardiac pacing may have a role if there is evidence of atrioventricular conduction delay, but there may be failure to capture. Successful use of intra-aortic balloon pumping, cardiac bypass and extracorporeal membrane oxygenation (ECMO) have been reported in extremely severe cases.

Cannabis

Cannabis is obtained from the plant *Cannabis sativa* which contains over 400 compounds including over 60 cannabinoids. The most potent cannabinoid is Δ^9-tetrahydrocannabinol (THC), which is responsible for the psychoactive effects seen with cannabis use; other cannabinoids include Δ^8-tetrahydrocannabinol, cannabinol, and cannabidiol. Smoking is the usual route of use, but cannabis is occasionally ingested as a 'cake', made into a 'tea', or injected intravenously.

Clinical features

Acute use

Features include euphoria, distorted and heightened images, colours and sounds, altered tactile sensations, sinus tachycardia, hypotension, and ataxia. Visual and auditory hallucinations, depersonalization, and acute psychosis are particularly likely to occur after substantial ingestion in naive cannabis users. Cannabis impairs all stages of memory including encoding, consolidation, and retrieval. Memory impairment following acute use may persist for months following abstinence.

Cannabis infusions injected intravenously may cause nausea, vomiting, and chills within minutes; after about 1 h, profuse watery diarrhoea, tachycardia, hypotension, and arthralgia may develop. Marked neutrophil leucocytosis is often present, and hypoglycaemia has been reported occasionally.

Chronic use

Heavy users suffer impairment of memory and attention and poor academic performance. There is an increased risk of anxiety and depression. Regular users are at risk of dependence. Cannabis use results in an overall increase in the relative risk for later schizophrenia and psychotic episodes. Cannabis smoke is probably carcinogenic.

Management

Most acutely intoxicated patients require no more than reassurance and supportive care. Sedation with diazepam, 10 mg intravenously, repeated as necessary, should be administered to patients who are disruptive or distressed. Haloperidol, 2.5 to 5 mg intramuscular repeated as necessary, is occasionally required.

Clomethiazole (chlormethiazole)

Clinical features

In overdose this drug may cause coma, respiratory depression, reduced muscle tone, hypotension, and excessive salivation. The characteristic odour of clomethiazole is often detected on the breath.

Management

Treatment is supportive.

Cocaine

In recent years, there has been a considerable increase in the recreational use of cocaine. It is a powerful local anaesthetic and vasoconstrictor and may be abused by smoking, ingestion, injection, or by 'snorting' it intranasally. Users, body packers, and those who swallow the drug to avoid being found in possession of it ('stuffers'), are at risk of overdose. 'Street' cocaine is cocaine hydrochloride which is water soluble so can be injected or snorted. It may be dissolved in an alkaline solution from which the cocaine is extracted into ether which is then evaporated to leave relatively pure ('freebase') cocaine. 'Crack' (cocaine also without the hydrochloride moiety) is extracted by using baking soda (sodium bicarbonate). Other drugs such as ethanol, cannabis, and conventional hypnotics and sedatives are frequently taken with cocaine to reduce the intensity of its less pleasant effects.

Clinical features

The features of cocaine overdosage are similar to those of amphetamine. In addition to euphoria, it also has sympathomimetic effects including agitation, tachycardia, hypertension, sweating, and hallucinations. Prolonged convulsions with metabolic acidosis, hyperthermia, rhabdomyolysis, ventricular arrhythmias, and cardiorespiratory arrest may follow in the most severe cases. Less common features include dissection of the aorta, myocarditis, myocardial infarction, dilated cardiomyopathy, subarachnoid haemorrhage, cerebral haemorrhage, and cerebral vasculitis.

A number of rare complications of the method of use of cocaine have been reported. These include pulmonary oedema after intravenous injection of freebase cocaine and pneumomediastinum and pneumothorax after sniffing it. In addition, chronic 'snorting' has caused perforation of the nasal septum, rhinorrhoea of cerebrospinal fluid due to thinning of the cribriform plate, and pulmonary granulomata.

Management

Users who are intoxicated may require sedation with diazepam to control agitation or convulsions; very large doses of diazepam may be required. Measures to prevent further absorption are usually irrelevant. Hypertension and severe tachycardia may be controlled with a β-blocker but, in one case at least, the use of propranolol caused paradoxical hypertension. Accelerated idioventricular rhythm should not normally require treatment but ventricular fibrillation and asystole should be managed in the usual way.

Dapsone

Dapsone is predominantly used in the management of leprosy and dermatitis herpetiformis.

Clinical features

Dapsone poisoning is potentially very severe, resulting in methaemoglobinaemia, haemolysis, hepatitis, central effects (including drowsiness, coma, and seizures), and a metabolic acidosis.

Management

Management is supportive. MDAC increases dapsone elimination. Methaemoglobinaemia will reduce the oxygen-carrying capacity of the blood, and at concentrations above 30%, treatment with methylthioninium chloride (methylene blue) 1 to 2 mg/kg intravenously over 5 min should be considered.

Digoxin and digitoxin

Digoxin and digitoxin toxicity occurs in three separate situations:

- in patients on regular therapy who gradually accumulate drug due to excess dosing, or development of incipient renal impairment
- in patients who are receiving digoxin for therapeutic purposes who then take a single, large overdose
- in naive patients who take an overdose of someone else's digoxin

Interpretation of the clinical and biochemical features differs between these situations.

In acute poisoning, the most significant feature normally seen is bradycardia. Since digoxin acts on a Na^+-K^+-ATPase, and subsequent changes in the myocardium develop following this, onset of the effects of digoxin in overdose may take up to 12 h. In very large overdoses, however, severe features may develop sooner than this, although in clinical practice very large overdoses are less common. Because digoxin interferes with Na^+-K^+-ATPase, serum potassium increases, and a very high serum potassium is therefore a useful, rapidly measurable marker for severe digoxin poisoning. Measurement of plasma concentrations of digoxin are also of use. This is particularly the case in patients on chronic therapy who may have less dramatic changes in serum potassium, perhaps because of coexistent diuretic therapy, and where clinical features may be more predominantly tachycardias.

Patients require treatment for cardiovascular compromise, not for blood concentrations. In acute poisoning, blood concentrations may rise to quite high levels (above 5 μg/litre) without necessarily causing particularly severe clinical features. These rises may be transient as the drug redistributes into fatty stores after absorption. In chronic therapy, plasma concentrations give a better indication of the quantities of digoxin present in the body, and in acute overdose in chronically dosed patients, several plasma concentration measurements may need to be taken over a short period to assess the dose absorbed.

Clinical features

Nausea, vomiting, bradycardia, and drowsiness may occur. At high doses, central nervous system features including hallucinations may be present. Sinus bradycardia is the most important and earliest feature in acute poisoning, but in chronic poisoning malignant ventricular arrhythmias are also seen. These will also develop in patients with severe acute poisoning.

Management

In patients who are vomiting, the airway needs to be protected, and consideration should be given to administering charcoal later than 1 h in patients who have ingested significant quantities, as this is such a toxic compound. The temptation to treat moderate hypokalaemia should be resisted as this will interfere with monitoring clinical response. Patients should be treated on the basis of their cardiovascular status, not the plasma concentrations of digoxin alone.

Patients with bradycardia who are symptomatic should receive atropine, and have any acid–base disturbance corrected. In patients with significant bradycardia or malignant ventricular arrhythmias, the most effective therapy is likely to be neutralization of digoxin with digoxin antibody. Doses of antibody recommended by the manufacturers are designed to completely neutralize all digoxin present in the patient. Such an approach is unwarranted, particularly in patients on chronic therapy with digoxin in whom complete reversal of digoxin will unmask the disorder for which they are being treated. It is recommended that half the quantity of the calculated total neutralizing dose be given. Further doses can be given, if necessary. In patients who receive the antibody, clinical improvement will occur rapidly, usually within 20 min. Failure to respond indicates either an incorrect diagnosis or continued absorption of digoxin. Measurement of serum digoxin concentrations is not possible once the digoxin antibody has been administered, since currently available assays measure both bound and free compound. Extracorporeal elimination techniques are ineffective in removing digoxin though MDAC may increase elimination.

Diuretics

Most diuretic overdoses are minor, although inevitably some disturbance of fluid and electrolyte balance will result. When combined diuretic and potassium formulations are ingested, the potassium content is likely to pose the greater risk. More serious consequences are likely if a potassium-sparing diuretic has been ingested.

Clinical features

Symptoms and signs of toxicity include anorexia, nausea, vomiting, diarrhoea, profound diuresis, dehydration, and hypotension. In addition, dizziness, weakness, muscle cramps, tetany, and occasionally, gastrointestinal bleeding may be seen. The electrolyte and metabolic disturbances that may be observed include hyponatraemia, hypoglycaemia or hyperglycaemia, hyperuricaemia, hypokalaemia, and metabolic alkalosis. Hyperkalaemia develops following the ingestion of combined diuretic and potassium preparations and potassium-sparing diuretics, such as amiloride, spironolactone, or triamterene. Small-bowel ulceration and stricture formation has followed poisoning due to diuretics with an enteric-coated core of potassium chloride.

Management

Symptomatic and supportive therapy should be employed with correction of fluid and electrolyte imbalance. Patients with severe hyperkalaemia may need a glucose and insulin infusion followed by oral or rectal administration of an ion-exchange resin.

Ethanol

Ethanol is commonly ingested in beverages before, or concomitantly with, the deliberate ingestion of other substances in overdose. It is also used as a solvent and is found in many cosmetic and antiseptic preparations. It is rapidly absorbed through the gastric and intestinal mucosae. Gastric alcohol dehydrogenase isoenzyme has a role in metabolizing ethanol before absorption, thereby preventing ethanol entering the systemic circulation, particularly following ingestion of moderate amounts of alcohol. Absorbed ethanol is initially and principally converted to acetaldehyde by an NAD-dependent hepatic alcohol dehydrogenase. A small proportion is oxidized by the microsomal ethanol oxidizing system (MEOS) and the catalase pathway. Acetaldehyde is removed by oxidation via the NAD-dependent enzyme aldehyde dehydrogenase, to yield acetate and, subsequently, CO_2 and water. About 95% of ingested ethanol is oxidized to acetaldehyde and acetate; the remainder is excreted unchanged in the urine, and, to a lesser extent, in the breath and through the skin.

Mechanisms of toxicity

Ethanol is a central nervous system depressant that interferes with cortical processes in small doses and may depress medullary function in large doses. The effects of ethanol on the central nervous system are generally proportional to the blood ethanol concentration. Ethanol is also a peripheral vasodilator. In the severely intoxicated, it may cause hypothermia and hypotension. Ethanol metabolism results in accumulation of free NADH, with resulting increase in the NADH:NAD ratio and inhibition of hepatic gluconeogenesis, which may cause hypoglycaemia, particularly in children or when poisoning follows fasting, exercise, or chronic malnutrition. An increase in the lactate:pyruvate ratio may also ensue, with development of hyperlactataemia.

Clinical features

Ethanol is a central nervous depressant that exacerbates the effects of other central nervous system depressants, in particular, hypnotic agents. The fatal dose of ethanol alone is between 300 and 500 ml absolute alcohol, if this is ingested in less than 1 h. The features of ethanol poisoning are summarized in Box 9.1.3.

Severe hypoglycaemia typically occurs within 6 to 36 h of ingestion of a moderate to large amount of alcohol by either a previously malnourished individual or one who has fasted for the previous 24 h; it is common in children 5 years of age or less. The patient is often comatose, hypothermic, and convulsing, with conjugate deviation of the eyes, trismus, and extensor plantar reflexes; the usual features of hypoglycaemia (e.g. flushing, sweating, tachycardia) are often absent. Convulsions are the most common presenting sign in children with hypoglycaemia. Lactic acidosis (usually only mild) is an uncommon but potentially serious complication of acute ethanol intoxication, and occurs particularly in patients with severe liver disease, pancreatitis, or sepsis. Hypovolaemia, which may accompany severe intoxication, predisposes to lactic acidosis.

Box 9.1.3 Clinical features of ethanol poisoning

Mild intoxication (500–1500 mg/litre)

Emotional lability, and slight impairment of visual acuity, muscular coordination, and reaction time

Moderate intoxication (1500–3000 mg/litre)

Visual impairment, sensory loss, muscular incoordination, slowed reaction time, slurred speech

Severe intoxication (3000–5000 mg/litre)

Marked muscular incoordination, blurred or double vision, sometimes stupor and hypothermia, occasionally hypoglycaemia and convulsions

Coma (>5000 mg/litre)

Depressed reflexes, respiratory depression, hypotension, and hypothermia. Death may occur from respiratory or circulatory failure or as the result of aspiration of stomach contents in the absence of a gag reflex

Management

Supportive measures are all that are required for most patients with acute ethanol poisoning, even if the blood ethanol concentration is very high. Particular care should be taken to protect the airway. In more severe cases, acid–base status should be determined. Lactic acidosis requires correction of hypoglycaemia, hypovolaemia, and circulatory insufficiency, if present. An infusion of sodium bicarbonate will be necessary in those patients in whom a lactic acidosis persists.

Blood sugar should be determined hourly in severe cases and the rate of intravenous glucose adjusted accordingly. If blood sugar concentrations decrease despite an infusion of 5 to 10% dextrose, a 50% glucose solution, 50 ml intravenously, should be given because hypoglycaemia is usually unresponsive to glucagon.

Haemodialysis may be considered if the blood ethanol concentration exceeds 7500 mg/litre and if a severe metabolic acidosis is present, which has not been corrected by the measures outlined earlier. Fructose is of negligible clinical benefit in accelerating ethanol oxidation and may cause acidosis; it should not be used.

γ-Hydroxybutyrate

γ-Hydroxybutyric acid (GHB) is a liquid that is abused as a body-building agent (it stimulates growth hormone release) and as an intoxicant in clubs and 'raves'. It is a precursor of γ-aminobutyric acid (GABA) and acts as an agonist at $GABA_B$ receptors as well as at a GHB-specific receptor in the brain.

Clinical features

Low doses cause mild agitation, excitement, nausea, and vomiting with euphoria and hallucinations at higher doses. Coma, bradycardia, and respiratory depression occur in the most severely poisoned. The most unique aspect of GHB poisoning is its very brief duration. Patients may progress from deep coma, requiring intubation, to self-extubation and full alertness over only a few hours.

A GHB withdrawal syndrome can occur in chronic abusers with clinical features occurring within 6 to 12 h of the last dose. Features include insomnia, tremor, and confusion, which may progress to delirium not dissimilar to the alcohol withdrawal syndrome.

Management

There is no role for gastrointestinal decontamination due to the rapid rate of absorption. Supportive measures to maintain adequate ventilation and circulation should be employed, and this is often all that is required. GHB withdrawal should be managed as for acute alcohol withdrawal.

Hypoglycaemic agents

Intentional overdose with insulin and oral hypoglycaemic agents is uncommon. However, deaths from insulin and sulphonylurea poisoning have been reported. Chlorpropamide, because of its long half-life, may induce prolonged hypoglycaemia. In all cases of poisoning with insulin and sulphonylurea, prompt diagnosis and treatment is essential if death or cerebral damage from neuroglycopenia are to be prevented. Metformin rarely causes hypoglycaemia since its mode of action is to increase glucose utilization. Lactic acidosis is a potentially serious complication of metformin overdose.

Clinical features

Features of overdosage include drowsiness, coma, twitching, convulsions, depressed limb reflexes, extensor plantar responses, tachypnoea, pulmonary oedema, tachycardia, and circulatory failure. Hypoglycaemia is to be expected and hypokalaemia, cerebral oedema, and metabolic acidosis might occur. Neurogenic diabetes insipidus and persistent vegetative states are possible long-term complications. Cholestatic jaundice has been described as a late complication of chlorpropamide poisoning.

Management

The blood or plasma glucose concentration should be measured urgently and intravenous glucose given. Glucagon may be ineffective.

Recurring hypoglycaemia is highly likely. A continuous infusion of glucose, together with carbohydrate-rich meals, is required in cases of severe insulin overdosage, though there may be difficulty in maintaining normoglycaemia. In the case of sulphonylurea overdosage, however, further glucose (although its administration may be unavoidable) only serves to increase the already high-circulating insulin concentrations. Diazoxide 1.25 mg/kg body weight intravenously over 1 h, repeated at 6-hourly intervals if necessary, has therefore been recommended since it increases blood glucose concentrations and raises circulating catecholamine concentrations while blocking insulin release.

Iron

Most medicinal preparations of iron are as the ferrous salt. Ferrous iron is oxidized to the ferric state before being absorbed. It is important to differentiate vitamin preparations that contain iron from medicinal preparations, since the former generally do not cause significant clinical problems unless very large amounts are taken. Since iron toxicity is quite closely related to dose per kilogram ingested, serious poisoning is more likely to occur in young children than in adults. The anticipated toxicity of iron is normally estimated by calculating the dose of elemental iron present in the preparation, which varies from salt to salt. Ingestions above 150 mg/kg of elemental iron are generally extremely severe and may be fatal.

Mechanisms of toxicity

Iron salts are both locally corrosive within the gastrointestinal tract and in the cell act as cellular toxins, probably by altering the function of mitochondria. In severe poisoning, patients are unconscious and suffer from circulatory collapse. In this situation hepatic injury is also seen.

Clinical features

Depending on the severity of poisoning features may vary, and in severe cases, features would be expected within the first 6 h and include nausea, vomiting, and abdominal pain. Iron will stain the vomit and diarrhoea and may also cause intestinal ulceration and result in haemorrhage. Large amounts of iron may be visible on a straight abdominal radiograph, but this should not be done routinely to confirm iron ingestion in children. Other reported features include leucocytosis. Following absorption of iron there is often a period of relative calm during which iron is taken into cells before its toxic effects manifest. In severe poisoning, patients may pass into unconsciousness during this phase and develop profound hypotension, metabolic acidosis, and features of hepatic necrosis and renal failure. Such patients require intensive supportive care and mortality rates are high. In patients who recover from significant poisoning, gut strictures following scarring from ulceration may be problematic. The commonest site is around the pylorus, particularly in young children.

Assessment of severity

Although dose is related to toxicity, patients may be sometimes inaccurate in their history, and since vomiting is a frequent early feature it may be difficult to assess exactly how much iron has been absorbed. Plasma concentration measurements on more than one occasion may assist this process. Early, relatively high concentrations (>90 mmol/litre or 5 mg/ml) are more likely to indicate severe poisoning. In this situation, iron will be circulating free in plasma and may result in toxicity.

Management

Iron does not bind to charcoal, and in patients who present early and who have ingested large quantities of iron, consideration should therefore be given to gastric aspiration or lavage. However, in most patients who have ingested such large quantities, vomiting is an early feature, and hence gastric lavage is rarely performed in practice. In the case of ingestion of slow-release preparations of iron, whole-bowel irrigation has been advocated, though data on its efficacy is anecdotal. In patients with significant elevated iron levels and features suggestive of significant poisoning, the specific iron-chelating agent desferrioxamine should be administered. There are few human data to support the usual dose regimen of desferrioxamine (15 mg/kg per hour up to a maximum of 80 mg/kg). It has been shown that giving 15 mg/kg per hour for more than 24 h can lead to pulmonary effects, including ARDS. The toxicity seen from desferrioxamine during its use in the management of chronic disorders, such as haemachromatosis and haemoglobinopathies, is not a normal feature of its use in the management of iron poisoning and should not therefore be used as a guide to limit dosing. Desferrioxamine may cause hypotension as an adverse effect. In addition, there are occasional reports of anaphylactoid reactions. In view of these potential adverse effects, desferrioxamine should not be used unless specifically indicated. Iron desferrioxamine complex colours urine red. Once desferrioxamine has been administered, interpretation of iron concentrations becomes impossible because the iron bound to desferrioxamine is detected in the laboratory assay.

Patients who have not developed features of poisoning within 6 h have probably not ingested very large quantities of iron, unless they have taken a slow release product. The majority of patients merely require treatment for their gastrointestinal disturbance. Since iron preparations are more commonly given to women who are pregnant than other groups of the population, iron overdose may be seen more frequently in pregnant women. There is currently no evidence to suggest these patients should be treated differently because of pregnancy, and desferrioxamine should certainly not be withheld in patients who are deemed to require it.

Isoniazid

Poisoning with isoniazid is potentially very serious, but uncommon.

Mechanisms of toxicity

Isoniazid depresses brain concentrations of γ-aminobutyric acid (GABA), thus leading to seizures.

Clinical features

The ingestion of 80 to 150 mg isoniazid/kg body weight is likely to cause severe poisoning. Nausea, vomiting, slurred speech, dizziness, and visual hallucinations may develop. Stupor, coma, and convulsions follow rapidly and may be associated with hyperthermia, hyperreflexia, extensor plantar responses, and later, rhabdomyolysis. In addition, dilated pupils, sinus tachycardia, and urinary retention may be observed. In severe cases, hypotension, acute renal failure and respiratory failure may ensure. Marked metabolic (lactic) acidosis is common. Less commonly, hyperglycaemia, ketoacidosis, glycosuria, and ketonuria are found.

Management

Supportive measures including the correction of metabolic acidosis should be instituted immediately if the patient is unconscious. Pyridoxine (1 g for 1 g of isoniazid ingested) should be given intravenously to control convulsions. When the ingested dose of isoniazid is unknown, an initial intravenous dose of 5 g pyridoxine should be given. Diazepam alone may be ineffective, but the use of diazepam and pyridoxine is synergistic and both should be used in those with convulsions. Pyridoxine 5 g may be repeated if convulsions persist (in one case, 52 g pyridoxine was given intravenously without ill effects).

Lithium carbonate

Lithium carbonate remains the drug of choice for the treatment of recurrent bipolar illness. It has a low therapeutic index and toxicity is usually the result of therapeutic overdosage (chronic toxicity) rather than deliberate self-poisoning (acute toxicity). Chronic toxicity is usually explained by a reduction in lithium renal clearance without a reduction in dose. However, single large doses are occasionally ingested by individuals on long-term treatment with the drug (acute on therapeutic toxicity).

Clinical features

Features of intoxication include thirst, polyuria, diarrhoea, and vomiting, and, in more serious cases, tremor, impairment of consciousness, hypertonia, and convulsions; irreversible neurological damage may occur. Measurement of the serum lithium concentration confirms the diagnosis. Chronic toxicity is usually associated with concentrations above 1.5 mmol/litre. However, acute massive overdosage may produce much higher concentrations without causing toxic features, at least initially. This is explained by plasma lithium concentrations that are substantially higher than central nervous system lithium concentrations before distribution is complete.

Management

Activated charcoal does not adsorb lithium. Treatment is supportive together with measures to enhance the rate of lithium elimination. Haemodialysis should be considered if neurological features are present, if renal function is impaired, and if chronic toxicity or acute on therapeutic toxicity are the modes of presentation. The efficacy of haemodialysis is limited by the relatively slow movement of lithium ions across cell membranes. It is easy to reduce serum lithium concentrations but they frequently rebound when treatment is stopped and clinical improvement is much slower. Repeated haemodialysis sessions are usually required. Continous haemodiafiltration can be used if conventional haemodialysis is not available, though clearance is less efficient.

Lysergic acid diethylamide (LSD)

Lysergic acid diethylamide acts as an antagonist at peripheral 5-HT receptor subtypes, but as a 5-HT_{2A} receptor agonist in the central nervous system. LSD and MDMA (ecstasy) are sometimes combined ('XL'; 'candyflipping') to increase the response to MDMA.

Clinical features

The ability of LSD to distort reality is well known. Visual hallucinations, distortion of images, agitation, excitement, dilated pupils, tachycardia, hypertension, hyperreflexia, tremor, and hyperthermia are common; auditory hallucinations are rare. Time seems to pass very slowly, and behaviour may become disturbed with paranoid delusions. Panic attacks are relatively common, but frank psychotic episodes (which may result in homicide) are not. The psychoactive effects can last for 48 h.

Episodic visual disturbances ('flashbacks'; hallucinogen persisting perception disorder) occur in which the effects of LSD are re-experienced without further exposure to the drug. The symptoms include false fleeting perceptions in the peripheral fields, flashes of colour, geometric pseudohallucinations, and positive afterimages. These disturbances may persist for several years but are often treatable with benzodiazepines and exacerbated by phenothiazines.

Management

Most patients will require little more than reassurance and sedation. Supportive measures are all that can be offered to those who are seriously ill.

Metoclopramide

Metoclopramide is an antiemetic, which has dopamine receptor antagonist properties, and therefore may cause dystonic reactions at therapeutic doses and after overdose. Such adverse effects are more common in young adults and women.

Management

As the clinical features are normally benign, all that is required is to treat a dystonic reaction with either an anticholinergic (e.g. benztropine 1–2 mg intravenously in an adult) or diazepam (10–20 mg intravenously). Dystonia is extremely distressing for patients and should be treated promptly.

Nitrates

Organic nitrates such as isosorbide mononitrate and isosorbide dinitrate are vasodilators that act by relaxing vascular smooth muscle. These drugs are essentially nitric oxide donors, which increase nitric oxide-induced activation of guanylate cyclase with subsequent elevation of cGMP concentrations. Their effects in overdose are directly related to their therapeutic actions. These drugs undergo extensive first pass metabolism in the liver. Exposure to inorganic nitrates is principally via drinking water.

Clinical features

The symptoms and signs caused by pharmaceutical nitrates in overdose are due primarily to excessive arteriolar and venous dilatation. Headache and vomiting are common, accompanied by flushing of the skin and dizziness. Sinus tachycardia, severe orthostatic hypotension, and syncope may develop. Convulsions and coma may be seen in severely poisoned patients. In contrast to poisoning by inorganic nitrates, methaemoglobinaemia is seen very rarely with organic nitrates. Moreover, methaemoglobinaemia caused by inorganic nitrates is in fact due to conversion of nitrate to nitrite by gastrointestinal bacteria, following ingestion. This is encountered primarily among infants bottle-fed with formula milk that has been made up with water with a high nitrate content.

Nonsteroidal anti-inflammatory drugs

These include a variety of different groups of drugs, all acting by inhibition of cycloxygenase enzymes. The newer, so-called selective, agents are thought to inhibit the inducible form of cycloxygenase more than the other forms of the enzyme. These drugs therefore all tend to inhibit prostaglandin synthesis, and the main toxicity seen in overdose is on the kidney. In very large doses, central nervous system effects may be seen but these are uncommon.

Non-steroidal anti-inflammatory drugs come in different chemical groupings: oxicams (meloxicam, piroxicam, tenoxicam) and phenylpropionic (arylpropionic) acid derivatives (e.g. fenbufen, ibuprofen, naproxen, tiaprofenic acid, mefenamic acid). The COX-2 selective agents are also potentially nephrotoxic in overdose due to inhibition of renal prostaglandin synthesis.

Clinical features

Overdose of mefenamic acid produces nausea, vomiting and, occasionally, bloody diarrhoea. Drowsiness, dizziness, and headaches are common, and hyperreflexia, muscle twitching, convulsions, cardiorespiratory arrest, hypoprothrombinaemia, and acute renal failure have been reported. In a study of 29 cases of mefenamic acid poisoning, convulsions were noted in 38% of patients, although only rarely were they persistent.

Management

Treatment of poisoning with nonsteroidals is generally supportive. It is important to check renal function in patients who have ingested large doses at an interval after ingestion. Changes in serum potassium and elevations in serum creatinine are to be expected in patients ingesting toxic doses. Treatment of renal impairment is conventional. Dialysis may be required in very severe cases. Activated charcoal should only be considered in patients who have ingested very large doses of non-steroidals (generally >20 tablets). Convulsions with mefanamic acid are unlikely to be persistent, but if they are, should be managed by diazepam (10–20 mg intravenously) or lorazepam (3–4 mg intravenously). Other treatments should be symptomatic and supportive.

Opiates and opioids

Opioids are a large group of drugs, which act on opioid receptors and are usually used as analgesics. Widespread abuse of opiates, particularly heroin, causes many patients to present with unintentional overdose, which is normally from intravenous injection (needle marks visible) but may occur from inhalation. Oral ingestion in addicts is less common. Many addicts abuse other drugs in addition to opioids, and the combination of benzodiazepines and opioids are particularly hazardous. Some opioids have other effects not mediated through opioid receptors. Dextropropoxyphene is a sodium channel blocker and causes cardiac arrhythmias; methadone has been shown to inhibit potassium channels at high doses and is also associated with sudden death in susceptible patients due to QT prolongation.

Clinical features

Cardinal signs of opiate overdose are pinpoint pupils, reduced respiratory rate, and coma. Vomiting may also occur, particularly after intravenous injection in naive users, and complicates the clinical pattern due to aspiration pneumonia. Methadone acts slowly (peak effects usually 4–6 h after ingestion) though its onset may be more rapid when given intravenously. Noncardiogenic pulmonary oedema is seen in a proportion of severe opioid overdoses, and is treated by positive pressure ventilation. Hypothermia may occur in patients lying outside. Rhabdomyolysis has also been associated with opioid ingestion.

Buprenorphine, a partial agonist opioid, is now used as an alternative to methadone in replacement programmes. It too is potentially seriously toxic if given intravenously, and in some countries has been combined with naloxone to reduce the acute hazard. Use of dextropropoxyphene has been curtailed in the United Kingdom because of risk of sudden death early after overdose when used in the combination product co-proxamol (paracetamol and dextropropoxyphene). Patients who have ingested dextropropoxyphene should have a 12-lead ECG, particularly if they are unconscious, and any acid–base disturbance corrected to reduce the risk of arrhythmia.

Management

Naloxone is a pure opioid antagonist. It will reverse the effects of all opioids if given in sufficient dose. In the event of veins not being accessible, intramuscular use is an alternative, but the onset will be slower. Use of naloxone by nebulizer has also been used in methadone poisoning. Failure of a suspected opioid poisoning to respond to an adequate dose of naloxone (at least 2.4 mg in an adult) should prompt reassessment of diagnosis. It may indicate co-ingestion of other central nervous system depressants, or ingestion of γ-hydroxybutyrate, which also causes small pupils and loss of consciousness. Naloxone has a half-life of approximately 45 to 90 min so its duration of action is therefore much shorter than that of the opioids being treated. Naloxone may therefore be given by infusion; the normal advised dose is approximately two-thirds of that required to wake a patient, every hour. This dose can be reassessed at regular intervals depending on the expected half-life of the ingested product. Morphine has active metabolites (morphine 6-glucoronide), which may become relevant in large overdoses. This metabolite is renally excreted and more potent than the parent compound, thus poisoning may be prolonged in older people or in patients with renal impairment or renal damage following rhabdomyolysis. Other supportive care should be administered as necessary including respiratory support. Significant hypotension due to pure opioid effects will usually respond to naloxone; patients who are managed just by ventilation may therefore be treated unnecessarily aggressively with fluid replacement. In some patients, high concentrations of opioids, such as codeine, cause histamine release and wealing and itching of the skin. These histamine effects should be treated conventionally with antihistamines.

Paracetamol (acetaminophen)

Mechanisms of toxicity

The toxicity of paracetamol is related to its metabolism (Fig. 9.1.2). In therapeutic doses, 60 to 90% is metabolized by conjugation to form paracetamol glucuronide and sulphate. A much smaller amount (5–10%) is oxidized by mixed function oxidase enzymes to form a highly reactive compound (*N*-acetyl-*p*-benzoquinoneimine, NAPQI), which is then immediately conjugated with glutathione and subsequently excreted as cysteine and mercapturate conjugates. Only 1 to 4% of a therapeutic dose of the drug is excreted unchanged in urine.

In overdose, larger amounts of paracetamol are metabolized by oxidation because of saturation of the sulphate conjugation pathway. As a result, liver glutathione stores become depleted so that the liver is unable to deactivate the toxic metabolite. NAPQI is believed to have two separate but complementary effects. Firstly, it reacts with glutathione, thereby depleting the cell of its normal defence against oxidizing damage. Secondly, it is a potent oxidizing as well as arylating agent; it inactivates key sulphydryl groups in certain enzymes, particularly those controlling calcium homeostasis.

Paracetamol-induced renal damage probably results from a mechanism similar to that which is responsible for hepatotoxicity, i.e. by formation of NAPQI, although in the kidney this is generated by prostaglandin endoperoxide synthetase rather than by cytochrome P450-dependent mixed function oxidases.

Risk factors

As would be expected from the mechanism of toxicity, the severity of paracetamol poisoning is dose-related. An absorbed dose of 15 g (200 mg/kg) or more is potentially serious in most patients. There is, however, some variation in individual susceptibility to paracetamol-induced hepatotoxicity and patients with pre-existing liver disease; those with a high alcohol intake and poor nutrition; those receiving enzyme-inducing drugs; and those suffering from anorexia nervosa or acute starvation should be considered to be at greater risk. Individuals with HIV-related disease also appear to be more susceptible to paracetamol-induced hepatic damage. The mechanisms involved in all these cases have not been elucidated fully, though poor nutrition (and therefore glutathione depletion) plays a major role in some cases.

Clinical features

The features of paracetamol poisoning are summarized in Table 9.1.3. Following the ingestion of an overdose of paracetamol, patients usually remain asymptomatic for the first 24 h, or at most develop anorexia, nausea, and vomiting. Liver damage is not usually detectable by routine liver function tests until at least 18 h after ingestion of the drug, and hepatic tenderness and abdominal pain are seldom exhibited before the second day. Liver damage reaches a peak as assessed by plasma alanine or aspartate aminotransferase (ALT, AST) activity or prothrombin time (international normalized ratio, INR), 72 to 96 h after ingestion. More often there is prolongation of the prothrombin time and a marked rise in aminotransferase activity (activities of several thousand are not uncommon) without the development of fulminant hepatic failure. Renal failure due to acute tubular necrosis develops in about 25% of patients with severe hepatic damage and in a few without evidence of serious disturbance of liver function. Other features, including hypoglycaemia and hyperglycaemia, cardiac arrhythmias, pancreatitis, gastrointestinal haemorrhage, and cerebral oedema may all occur with hepatic failure due to any cause and are not direct consequences of paracetamol toxicity.

Paracetamol can cause metabolic acidosis at two distinct periods after overdosage. Transient hyperlactataemia is frequently found

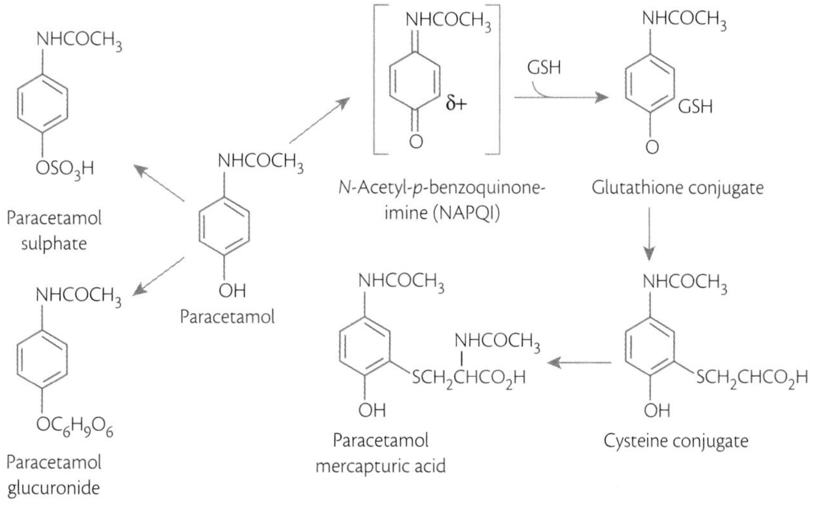

Fig. 9.1.1 Metabolism of paracetamol.

within the first 15 h in all but minor overdoses and appears to be due to inhibition of mitochondrial respiration at the level of ubiquinone and increased lactate production. It is rarely of clinical consequence, although in very severe paracetamol poisoning (plasma paracetamol concentration >500 mg/litre at 4 h after ingestion) the acidosis may be associated with coma. The second phase of hyperlactataemia and acidosis occurs in those patients who present late and go on to develop hepatic damage; in this instance decreased hepatic lactate clearance appears to be the major cause, compounded by poor peripheral perfusion and increased lactate production.

Hypophosphataemia is a recognized complication of acute liver failure, including that due to paracetamol, and may contribute to morbidity and mortality by inducing mental confusion, irritability, coma, and abnormalities of platelet, white cell, and erythrocyte functions. Phosphaturia appears to be the principal cause of hypophosphataemia in paracetamol poisoning; it may occur in the absence of fulminant hepatic failure and indicates paracetamol-induced renal tubular damage; it is a useful prognostic sign.

Prediction of liver damage

In the early stages following ingestion of a paracetamol overdose, most patients have few symptoms and no physical signs. There is thus a need for some form of assessment which estimates the risk of liver damage at a time when the liver function tests are still normal. Details of the dose ingested may be used but, in many cases, the history is unreliable and, even when the dose is known for certain, it does not take account of early vomiting and individual variation in response to the drug. However, a single measurement of the plasma paracetamol concentration is an accurate predictor of liver damage provided that it is taken not earlier than 4 h after ingestion of the overdose. Information gained from several studies has enabled the production of a graph which may be used for prediction of liver damage and which serves as a guide to the need for specific treatment (Fig. 9.1.2). In patients who have taken several overdoses of paracetamol over a short period of time, the plasma paracetamol concentration will be meaningless in relation to the treatment graph. Such patients should be considered at risk and treated. Patients who regularly consume alcohol in excess of currently recommended limits (particularly those who are malnourished); those who regularly take enzyme-inducing drugs (e.g. carbamazepine, phenytoin, phenobarbital, primidone, and rifampicin); and those with conditions causing glutathione depletion (e.g. malnutrition and HIV infection) may be at risk of liver damage from lower plasma paracetamol concentrations than others. The plasma paracetamol concentration for such patients should be considered in relation to the 'high risk' treatment line (Fig. 9.1.2).

Sixty per cent of patients whose plasma paracetamol concentration falls above the line drawn between 200 mg/litre (1.32 mmol/litre) at 4 h and 50 mg/litre (0.33 mmol/litre) at 12 h after the ingestion of the overdose are likely to sustain liver damage (ALT or AST >1000 IU/litre) unless specific protective treatment is given.

Table 9.1.3 Clinical, biochemical, and haematological features of untreated paracetamol poisoning (>200 mg/kg)

Day 1	Day 2	Day 3
Asymptomatic	May become asymptomatic	(in severe untreated poisoning)
Nausea	Vomiting	Jaundice → liver failure → hepatic encephalopathy
Vomiting	Hepatic tenderness ± generalized abdominal tenderness	Back pain + renal angle tenderness → renal failure
Abdominal pain	Occasionally, mild jaundice	Cardiac arrhythmias → cardiac arrest
Anorexia		Disseminated intravascular coagulation
		Pancreatitis

Biochemical abnormalities	Haematological abnormalities
AST/ALT ↑↑	PT ↑
Bilirubin ↑	Platelets ↓
Blood sugar ↓	Clotting factors II ↓ V ↓ VII ↓
Creatinine ↑	
Lactate ↑	
Phosphate ↓	
Amylase ↑	
Potassium ↓	

Prognostic factors

The overall mortality of paracetamol poisoning in untreated patients is only of the order of 5%. The prothrombin time is usually the first liver function test to become abnormal, and for this reason it is of particular value in assessing the prognosis of an individual patient. The more rapid the increase in prothrombin time, the worse the prognosis of the patient. A prothrombin time of more than 20 s at 24 h after ingestion indicates that significant hepatic damage has been sustained, and a peak prothrombin time of more than 180 s is associated with a chance of survival of less than 8%.

Acid–base disturbances are also a good guide to prognosis. Systemic acidosis developing more than 24 h after overdose indicates a poor prognosis; patients with a blood pH below 7.30 at this time have only a 15% chance of survival. In addition, a rise in the serum creatinine concentration is associated with poor survival; patients with a serum creatinine concentration above 300 μmol/litre have only a 23% chance of survival.

A study of prognostic indicators in paracetamol-induced fulminant hepatic failure treated conventionally compared the sensitivity (percentage of patients who died with a positive test), predictive accuracy (percentage of patients whose outcome was predicted accurately), positive predictive value (percentage of patients with a positive test who died), and specificity (percentage of survivors with a negative test) of measurement of factors V and VIII with conventional tests. (factor V is vitamin K-dependent and levels fall in liver failure; levels of factor VIII rise in patients with liver failure.) An admission pH below 7.30 with a serum creatinine concentration above 300 μmol/litre and a prothrombin time above 100 s in patients with grade III–IV encephalopathy has a sensitivity, predictive accuracy, positive prediction value, and specificity of 91, 86, 83, and 91, respectively. However, a factor VIII/V ratio above 30 had comparable values of 91, 95, 100, and 100.

Management

Parenteral fluid replacement should be given for the first 1 or 2 days after overdose if nausea persists or vomiting occurs.

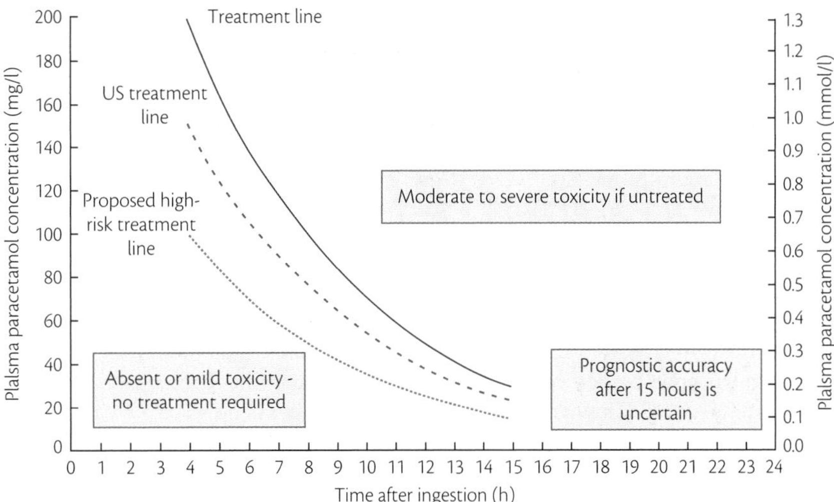

Fig. 9.1.2 Prediction of liver damage after paracetamol overdose.

Patients who have taken staggered overdoses should be treated with an antidote irrespective of the plasma paracetamol concentrations. They can be discharged after antidotal treatment, provided they are asymptomatic and the INR, plasma creatinine concentration, and ALT activity are normal.

Patients who present 15 h or more after ingestion tend to be more severely poisoned and at greater risk of developing serious liver damage and should receive antidotal treatment as the plasma concentration alone may not be an accurate guide of severity, as it may be non-detectable at the time of late presentation. The INR, venous pH, plasma creatinine concentration, and liver function tests are helpful in determining prognosis.

Acetylcysteine

Acetylcysteine acts by replenishing cellular glutathione stores and may also repair oxidation damage caused by NAPQI either directly or, more probably, through the generation of cysteine and/or glutathione. It may also act as a source of sulphate and so 'unsaturate' sulphate conjugation.

The most widely utilized regimen worldwide is a 20.25-h protocol (Box 9.1.4). Provided that acetylcysteine is administered within 8 to 10 h of overdose, the development of hepatic damage is prevented; thereafter, the protective effects decline rapidly. Some 10 to 15% of patients treated with intravenous acetylcysteine (20.25-h regimen) develop rash, angio-oedema, hypotension, and bronchospasm. These reactions, which are due to the initial bolus, are seldom serious and no fatalities have been reported. Antihistamines such as chlorpheniramine or terfenadine may be given if such anaphylactoid reactions do occur, but discontinuing the infusion temporarily is all that is usually required.

Management of severe liver damage

A 10% glucose solution should be administered to prevent the onset of hypoglycaemia. If fulminant hepatic failure supervenes, the use of a continued intravenous *N*-acetylcysteine (the 16-h infusion is continued until recovery or death) will reduce morbidity and mortality. In one prospective study, the survival rate in 25 patients with paracetamol-induced fulminant hepatic failure was 20%, with an incidence of cerebral oedema and of hypotension requiring inotropic support of 68 and 80%, respectively. With *N*-acetylcysteine, the comparable figures in 25 matched patients were 48% (survival rate), 40% (cerebral oedema), and 48% (hypotension).

A proton pump inhibitor will reduce the risk of gastrointestinal bleeding from 'stress' ulceration/erosion. There is no evidence that fresh frozen plasma prevents gastrointestinal haemorrhage in patients with severe coagulation abnormalities (prothrombin time >100 s). If acute renal failure supervenes, then this should be managed conventionally.

Liver transplantation has been performed successfully in patients with paracetamol-induced fulminant hepatic failure.

Salicylates

Despite the introduction of child-resistant packaging, the ingestion of aspirin by children still occurs, iatrogenic overdose is not uncommon, and aspirin remains the drug of choice for many adults who want to poison themselves. Salicylate poisoning may also result from percutaneous absorption of salicylic acid (used in keratolytic agents), and ingestion of methyl salicylate ('oil of wintergreen').

Mechanisms of toxicity

In therapeutic doses, aspirin is absorbed rapidly from the stomach and small intestine, but in overdose, absorption may occur more slowly, and plasma salicylate concentrations may continue to rise for up to 24 h.

The pharmacokinetics of elimination of aspirin are important determinants of salicylate toxicity. Biotransformation to both salicyluric acid and salicylphenolic glucuronide (Fig. 9.1.3) is saturable with the following clinical consequences: (1) the time needed to eliminate a given fraction of a dose increases with increasing dose; (2) the steady state plasma concentration of salicylate, particularly that of the pharmacologically active non-protein-bound fraction,

Box 9.1.4 Dosing regimen for acetylcysteine

Acetylcysteine (intravenous 20.25–21 h regimens)

- 150 mg/kg over 15 min (is sometimes given over 60 min), then 50 mg/kg over the next 4 h and 100 mg/kg over the next 16 h
- Total dose, 300 mg/kg over 20.25 h (or 21 h)

increases more than proportionately with increasing dose; and (3) renal excretion of salicylic acid becomes increasingly important, a pathway, which is extremely sensitive to changes in urinary pH.

When ingested in overdose, salicylates directly stimulate the respiratory centre to produce both increased depth and rate of respiration, thereby causing a respiratory alkalosis (Fig. 9.1.4). At least part of this effect is due to local uncoupling of oxidative phosphorylation within the brainstem. In an attempt to compensate, bicarbonate, accompanied by sodium, potassium, and water, is excreted in the urine resulting in dehydration and hypokalaemia. More importantly, the loss of bicarbonate diminishes the buffering capacity of the body and allows an acidosis to develop more easily. Very high salicylate concentrations in the brain depress the respiratory centre and may further contribute to the development of acidaemia.

Simultaneously, a variable degree of metabolic acidosis develops, not only because of the presence of salicylic acid itself, but also because of interference with carbohydrate, lipid, protein, and amino acid metabolism by salicylate ions (Fig. 9.1.4). Inhibition of citric acid cycle enzymes causes an increase in circulating lactic and pyruvic acids. Salicylates stimulate fat metabolism and cause increased production of the ketone bodies, β-hydroxybutyric acid, acetoacetic acid, and acetone. Dehydration and lack of food intake, because of vomiting, further contribute to the development of ketosis. Protein catabolism is accelerated and synthesis diminished. Aminotransferases (responsible for the interconversion of amino acids) are inhibited. Increased circulating blood concentrations of amino acids result, together with aminoaciduria; inhibition of active tubular reabsorption of amino acids also contributes. Aminoaciduria increases the solute load on the kidneys and, thereby, increases water loss from the body.

A primary toxic effect of salicylates in overdose is uncoupling of oxidative phosphorylation (Fig. 9.1.4). ATP-dependent reactions are inhibited and oxygen utilization and CO_2 production increased. Energy normally used for the conversion of inorganic phosphate to ATP is dissipated as heat. Hyperpyrexia and sweating result, causing further dehydration. Fluid loss is enhanced because salicylates stimulate the chemoreceptor trigger zone and induce nausea and vomiting and, thereby, diminish oral fluid intake. If dehydration is sufficiently marked, low cardiac output and oliguria will aggravate the metabolic acidosis already present which, if severe, can itself diminish cardiac output.

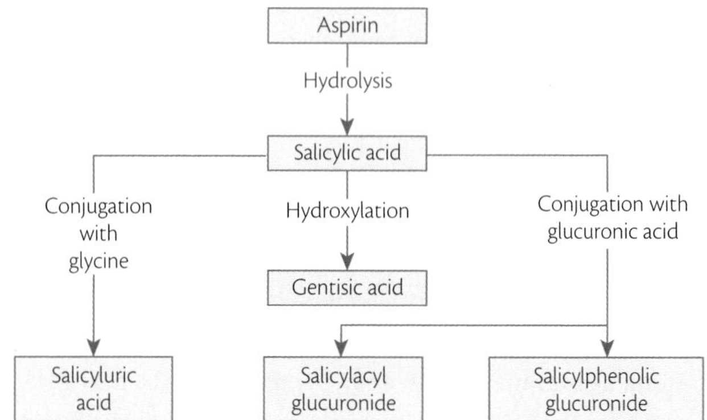

Fig. 9.1.3 Metabolism of aspirin.

Glucose metabolism also suffers as a result of uncoupled oxidative phosphorylation because of increased tissue glycolysis and peripheral demand for glucose (Fig. 9.1.4). This is seen principally in skeletal muscle and may cause hypoglycaemia. The brain appears to be particularly sensitive to this effect and neuroglycopenia can occur in the presence of a normal blood sugar level when the rate of utilization exceeds the rate at which glucose can be supplied from the blood. Increased metabolism and peripheral demand for glucose activates hypothalamic centres resulting in increased adrenocortical stimulation and release of adrenaline. Increased glucose 6-phosphatase activity and hepatic glycogenolysis contribute to the hyperglycaemia, which is sometimes seen following ingestion of large amounts of salicylate. Increased circulating adrenocorticosteroids exacerbates fluid and electrolyte imbalance.

Although this is rarely a practical problem, salicylate intoxication may be accompanied by hypoprothrombinaemia due to a warfarin-like action of salicylates on the physiologically important vitamin K epoxide cycle. Vitamin K is converted to vitamin K 2,3-epoxide and then reconverted to vitamin K by a liver membrane reductase enzyme, which is competitively inhibited by warfarin and salicylates.

Clinical features and assessment of severity of salicylate intoxication

The dose of salicylate ingested and the age of the patient (see below) are the principal determinants of the severity of an overdose. The plasma salicylate concentration should be determined on admission, but it is important to repeat it 2 h later to ensure that the concentration is not rising. If the concentration has risen, the level should be repeated after a further 2 h. Generally speaking, plasma salicylate concentrations that lie between 300–500 mg/litre some 6 h after ingestion of an overdose are associated with only mild toxicity, concentrations between 500 and 700 mg/litre are associated with moderate toxicity, and concentrations in excess of 700 mg/litre confirm severe poisoning.

Salicylate poisoning of any severity is associated with sweating, vomiting, epigastric pain, tinnitus, and deafness (Box 9.1.5).

Young children quickly develop metabolic acidosis following the ingestion of aspirin in overdose, but by the age of 12 years the usual adult picture of a combined dominant respiratory alkalosis and mild metabolic acidosis is seen. To some extent, the presence of an alkalaemia protects against serious salicylate toxicity because salicylate remains ionized and unable to penetrate cell membranes easily. Development of acidaemia allows salicylates to penetrate tissues more readily and leads, in particular, to central nervous system toxicity characterized by excitement, tremor, delirium, convulsions, and stupor and coma. Very high plasma salicylate concentrations cause paralysis of the respiratory centre and cardiovascular collapse due to vasomotor depression.

Pulmonary oedema is seen occasionally in salicylate poisoning, and although this is often due to fluid overload as a result of treatment, it may be noncardiac and occur in the presence of hypovolaemia. In these circumstances, the pulmonary oedema fluid has the same protein and electrolyte composition as plasma, suggesting increased pulmonary vascular permeability.

Although aspirin overdose may be complicated by inhibition of platelet aggregation and hypoprothrombinaemia, gastric erosions and gastrointestinal bleeding are rare following acute salicylate overdose.

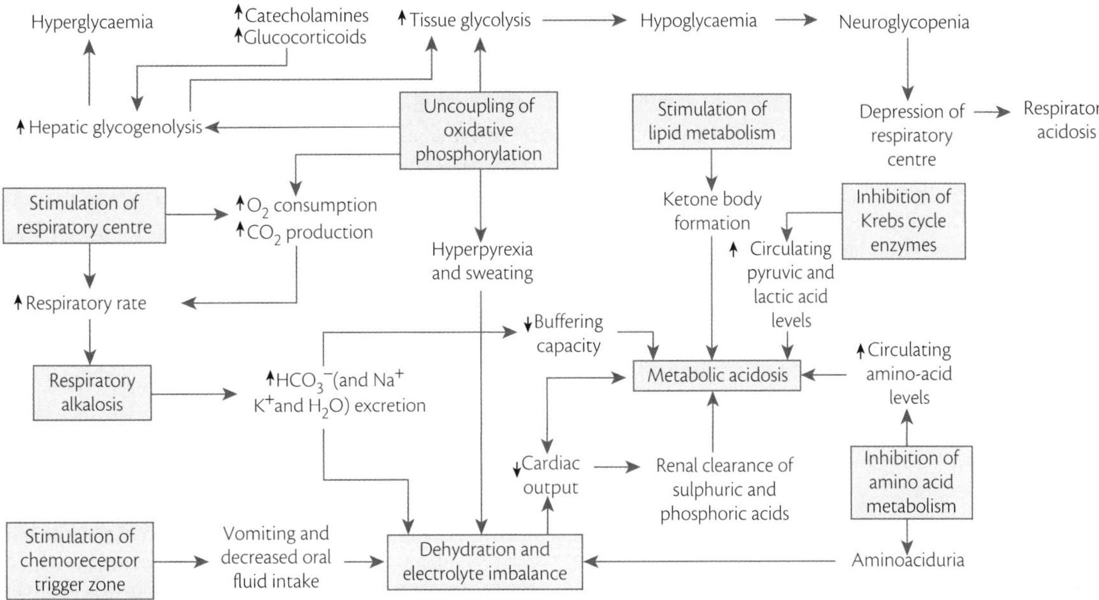

Fig. 9.1.4 Pathophysiology of salicylate poisoning.

Oliguria is sometimes seen in patients following the ingestion of salicylates in overdose. The most common cause is dehydration but, rarely, acute renal failure or inappropriate secretion of antidiuretic hormone may occur.

Although the urinary pH may be alkaline in the early stages of salicylate overdose, it soon becomes acid. Measurement of arterial blood gases, pH, and standard bicarbonate may show a respiratory alkalosis in the early stages of salicylate intoxication accompanied by the development of a metabolic acidosis. The plasma potassium concentration is often low; rarely, the blood sugar may be high.

Management

The plasma salicylate concentration should be re-measured 2 to 3 h after the first measurement. Dehydration, electrolyte imbalance and, most importantly, metabolic acidosis should be corrected.

The role of multiple-dose activated charcoal in increasing salicylate elimination is controversial, and it cannot be recommended on current evidence. As the relationship between renal clearance of salicylates and urine pH is logarithmic, urine alkalinization should be undertaken in patients with a plasma salicylate concentration greater than 500 mg/litre, particularly if an acidosis is present. The therapeutic aim is to make the urine alkaline (ideally, pH 7.5–8.5), and in adults this may be achieved by administration of sodium bicarbonate, 225 mmol (225 ml of 8.4%); further doses of bicarbonate are given as required. Hypokalaemia should be corrected before administration of sodium bicarbonate, because this lowers the serum potassium concentration further. In patients with severe poisoning (plasma salicylate concentration >700 mg/litre or >5.1 mmol/litre), haemodialysis should be considered, particularly when severe acid–base abnormalities are present.

Pulmonary oedema occasionally complicates salicylate toxicity. Fluid overload should be excluded as far as possible but, if increased pulmonary vascular permeability is suspected, measurement of the pulmonary artery wedge pressure may be needed both for confirmation of the diagnosis and to monitor subsequent fluid administration. Positive end expiratory pressure ventilation appears to be beneficial.

Theophylline

Poisoning may complicate therapeutic use as well as being the result of deliberate self-poisoning. If a sustained-released formulation has been ingested, peak plasma concentrations of the drug are frequently not attained until 6 to 12 h after overdose and the onset of toxic features is correspondingly delayed.

Clinical features

Symptoms include nausea, vomiting, and hyperventilation, haematemesis, abdominal pain, diarrhoea, sinus tachycardia, supraventricular and ventricular arrhythmias, hypotension, restlessness, irritability, headache, hyperreflexia, tremors, and convulsions. Hypokalaemia probably results from Na^+-K^+-ATPase activation.

Box 9.1.5 Clinical features of salicylate poisoning

- Nausea, vomiting, and epigastric discomfort
- Irritability, tremor, tinnitus, deafness, blurring of vision
- Hyperpyrexia, sweating, dehydration
- Tachypnoea and hyperpnoea
- Noncardiogenic pulmonary oedema
- Acute renal failure
- Mixed respiratory alkalosis and metabolic acidosis (except in children who usually develop metabolic acidosis alone)
- Hypokalaemia, hypernatraemia, or hyponatraemia
- Hyperglycaemia or hypoglycaemia
- Hypoprothrombinaemia (rare)
- Confusion, delirium, stupor, and coma (in severe cases)

A mixed respiratory alkalosis and metabolic acidosis is common. Most symptomatic patients have plasma theophylline concentrations in excess of 25 mg/litre. Convulsions are seen more commonly when concentrations are greater than 50 mg/litre.

Management

MDAC (e.g. 50 g 4-hourly) enhances the systemic elimination of theophylline. Intractable vomiting may be alleviated by ondansetron, 8 mg intravenously in an adult. Gastrointestinal haemorrhage may require blood transfusion and the administration of a proton pump inhibitor intravenously. Tachyarrhythmias may be induced by the rapid flux of potassium across cell membranes and early correction of hypokalaemia may prevent their development. The plasma potassium concentration should therefore be measured on admission and at hourly intervals thereafter while the patient is symptomatic. Potassium supplements will be needed in almost all cases and doses of up to 60 mmol/h may be required at the outset in severe cases. Non-selective β-adrenoceptor blocking drugs, such as propranolol, may also be useful in the treatment of tachyarrhythmias secondary to hypokalaemia. Convulsions should be treated with diazepam 10 to 20 mg intravenously in an adult.

Thyroxine

Clinical features

Only a small percentage of patients who ingest large amounts of thyroid hormones develop features of toxicity. Symptoms develop within a few hours with tri-iodothyronine (T_3) and after 3 to 6 days with thyroxine (T_4). They tend to resolve in about the same time as they take to develop. Sinus tachycardia, tremor, anxiety, irritability, insomnia, hyperactivity, sweating, diarrhoea and fever, are most common. Atrial fibrillation and convulsions have also been reported. Myocardial necrosis may occur rarely.

Management

Serum T_4 and T_3 concentrations should be measured in blood taken 6 to 12 h after ingestion (this need not be measured as an emergency) since a normal result precludes the possibility of delayed toxicity and allows the patient to be discharged. Those with high T_4 concentrations should be reviewed for evidence of toxicity on the fourth or fifth day after ingestion. Patients who develop toxicity should be given propranolol for 5 days.

Warfarin

Warfarin toxicity is more likely to occur in the setting of therapeutic anticoagulation (as a result of a drug interaction), than as a consequence of acute overdose.

Clinical features

Epistaxis, gingival bleeding, spontaneous bruising, haematomas, haematuria, bilateral flank pain, rectal bleeding, and haemorrhage into any organ. Spontaneous haemoperitoneum has been reported. Severe blood loss may result in hypovolaemic shock, coma, and death.

Management

If major bleeding occurs, give vitamin K_1 10 mg by slow intravenous injection together with prothrombin complex concentrate 50 units/kg or fresh frozen plasma 15 ml/kg.

If the INR is 8.0 or more and there is no active bleeding, and the intention is to continue anticoagulation, discontinue warfarin (restart when the INR $\leq$5.0), give phytomenadione 0.5 mg by slow intravenous injection and repeat the dose if the INR is 8.0 or more 24 h later. If the INR is 6.0 to 8.0, and there is no active bleeding or only minor bleeding, warfarin should be discontinued and restarted when the INR less than or equal to 5.0.

If the INR is 4.0 or less, there is no active bleeding, and continued anticoagulation is unnecessary, treatment with phytomenadione is not required. If the INR is 4.0 or more, phytomenadione 10 mg by slow intravenous injection (100 μg/kg body weight for a child) should be administered.

Metals

Aluminium

Aluminium hydroxide is used as an antacid and as a phosphate binder in the management of chronic renal failure. Aluminium sulphate is employed in water purification and paper manufacture. Aluminium may be absorbed orally and by inhalation. More than 90% of absorbed aluminium is bound to transferrin. Though some accumulates in brain tissue, most body aluminium is stored in bone and the liver. It is excreted mainly via the kidneys so that accumulation may occur in the presence of renal failure.

Clinical features

Acute poisoning

Ingestion of a significant quantity of a soluble aluminium salt such as aluminium sulphate causes burning in the mouth and throat, nausea, vomiting, diarrhoea, abdominal pain, hypotension, seizures, haemolysis, haematuria, and, rarely, hepatorenal failure. Topical aluminium sulphate may be irritant to the skin and eyes. By contrast, insoluble aluminium salts, such as aluminium oxide, do not produce an acute toxic response.

Chronic poisoning

Inhalation of 'stamped aluminium powder' can cause a persistent cough and breathlessness due to lung fibrosis or occupational asthma. Increased death rates from some types of cancer have been observed in aluminium production, but these effects are believed to be the result of exposure to other substances, such as benzopyrene, rather than exposure to aluminium. Aluminium may cause contact allergy.

Aluminium encephalopathy is a potential, though now unusual, complication in patients with chronic renal failure administered aluminium-containing phosphate binders or dialysed using aluminium-contaminated water. The accumulation of aluminium in the brain produces cognitive decline, ataxia, dysarthria, myoclonic jerks, and seizures. A similar clinical picture has been described in patients who intravenously injected oral methadone 'cooked' in an aluminium pot and as a result of reconstructive bone otoneurosurgery using an aluminium-containing cement.

Aluminium intoxication may contribute to renal osteodystrophy and anaemia in patients with chronic renal impairment. Aluminium has also been implicated in Alzheimer's disease with evidence that it plays an active role in the pathogenesis of the neurofibrillary tangles characteristic of this condition.

Management

Desferrioxamine forms a stable complex with aluminium which it mobilizes primarily from bone with subsequent urinary elimination of the chelate. Theoretically 100 mg desferrioxamine can bind

4.1 mg aluminium. Desferrioxamine is absorbed poorly from the gastrointestinal tract and must be administered parenterally.

The desferrioxamine chelate is dialysable and all published clinical studies of aluminium chelation using desferrioxamine have involved patients in renal failure undergoing either dialysis or haemofiltration. As the aluminium–desferrioxamine chelate concentration reaches a maximum between 12 and 24 h after infusion, desferrioxamine should be administered shortly before dialysis for maximum benefit.

There is evidence that desferrioxamine can improve aluminium-induced encephalopathy, bone disease and anaemia in dialysis patients. Desferrioxamine should be prescribed when features of dialysis encephalopathy are present, when there is an increased body aluminium load (serum aluminium concentration >60 µg/litre) and there is clinical evidence of aluminium-related bone disease. In addition, desferrioxamine should be considered in the presence of severe, transfusion-dependant anaemia even in the absence of characteristic clinical or analytical features of aluminium overload. Desferrioxamine is typically administered in a dose of 40 to 80 mg/kg intravenously once a week prior to dialysis. The dose can be reduced to 20 to 60 mg/kg (as indicated by response and adverse effects) if treatment is to be continued for several months.

Arsenic

Arsenic forms both trivalent and pentavalent derivatives. Inorganic arsenical compounds may generate arsine gas (see p. 1307) when in contact with acids, reducing metals, sodium hydroxide, and aluminium. Some 90% of an ingested dose of most inorganic arsenicals is absorbed. The half-life is 1 to 3 days. Excretion is predominantly in the urine. Soluble arsenical compounds can also be absorbed by inhalation but skin absorption is generally poor. In exposed individuals, high concentrations of arsenic are present in bone, hair, and nails.

Clinical features

Acute poisoning

This can follow accidental, suicidal, or deliberate ingestion, the toxicity being largely dependent on the water solubility of the ingested compound. Within 2 h of substantial ingestion of a soluble arsenical compound, severe haemorrhagic gastritis or gastroenteritis may ensue with collapse and death usually within 4 days. A metallic taste, salivation, muscular cramps, facial oedema, difficulty in swallowing, hepatorenal dysfunction, convulsions, and encephalopthy are reported. A peripheral neuropathy (predominantly sensory), bone marrow depression, striate leukonychia (Mee's lines), and hyperkeratotic, hyperpigmented skin lesions are common in those surviving a near-fatal ingestion. In moderate or severe arsenic poisoning, investigations may show anaemia, leucopenia, thrombocytopenia, and disseminated intravascular coagulation. ECG abnormalities have been reported and include QT prolongation and ventricular arrhythmias.

Chronic poisoning

The ingestion of arsenic in contaminated drinking water or 'tonics' has led to progressive weakness, anorexia, nausea, vomiting, stomatitis, colitis, increased salivation, epistaxis, bleeding gums, conjunctivitis, weight loss, and low-grade fever. Characteristically, there is hyperkeratosis of the palms and soles of the feet, 'raindrop' pigmentation of the skin, and Mee's lines on the nails. A symmetrical peripheral neuropathy is typical. Hearing loss, psychological impairment, and EEG changes have been reported. Other chronic effects include disturbances of liver function and ulceration and perforation of the nasal septum. In Taiwan, chronic arsenic exposure has been shown to cause blackfoot disease, a severe form of peripheral vascular disease, which leads to gangrenous changes.

Chronic exposure to arsenic in drinking water has been causally linked to lung, skin, kidney, and bladder cancer, while occupational exposure to arsenic is associated with lung cancer.

Management

Traditionally, dimercaprol (British anti-Lewisite, BAL) has been the recommended chelator. However, DMSA (succimer) may be preferable, if available. DMSA is effective in reducing the arsenic content of tissues and, unlike dimercaprol, does not cause accumulation of arsenic in the brain. DMSA may be given orally in a dose of 30 mg/kg body weight daily, whereas dimercaprol must be given by deep intramuscular injection 2.5 to 5 mg/kg 4-hourly for 2 days, followed by 2.5 mg/kg intramuscularly twice daily for 1 to 2 weeks.

Cadmium

If hygiene is poor, workers can be exposed to cadmium from the smelting and refining of metals, from soldering or welding metal that contains cadmium, or in plants that make cadmium products such as batteries, coatings, or plastics. Itai-itai disease (literally 'ouch-ouch' disease, so named because of the effects of severe pain in the joints), occurred in Toyama Prefecture, Japan in 1950 and was due to mass cadmium poisoning as a result of mining.

Clinical features

Cadmium compounds are poorly absorbed orally but are well absorbed through the lungs. Cadmium is deposited in the liver and kidneys and very slowly excreted in the urine (half-life 10 to 30 years).

Acute poisoning

The ingestion of cadmium salts (>3 mg/kg body weight) may lead to gastrointestinal disturbance which, in severe cases, may progress to circulatory collapse, acute renal failure, pulmonary oedema, and death.

Inhalation of cadmium oxide fumes produced in welding or cutting has led to the development of severe lung damage and death. Often, there are no initial symptoms but after some 4 to 10 h, there is increasing respiratory distress. Dyspnoea, cough, and chest pain are accompanied by chills and tremor. Severe pulmonary oedema may develop, or chemical pneumonitis in less severe cases. Recovery may be complicated by progressive pulmonary fibrosis.

Chronic poisoning

Repeated exposure to cadmium, such as occupationally, leads to renal tubular dysfunction with glycosuria, aminoaciduria, and hypercalciuria, an increased incidence of renal stones and osteomalacia. Less common features include anosmia, anaemia, teeth discoloration and neuropsychological impairment. Later, emphysema may develop. Workers repeatedly exposed to high concentrations of cadmium have developed carcinoma of the prostate or lung.

Management

There is no clinical evidence that a substantial body burden of cadmium may be chelated by any currently available antidote.

Chromium

Naturally occurring chromium exists as chromate ore in which chromium is in the trivalent oxidation state. Industrial applications of chromium use chromium(III) or chromium(VI). Chromium(VI) is the most important toxicologically because it can cross cell membranes readily. In contrast, chromium(III) compounds are confined to the extracellular space. Somewhat paradoxically, the toxicity of chromium(VI) is mediated intracellularly by intermediates formed during the reduction of chromium(VI) to chromium(III), and chromium(III) itself is the final perpetrator of chromium genotoxicity by binding to nuclear DNA. Soluble hexavalent chromium compounds are absorbed mainly by inhalation and, to a lesser extent via the skin or gastrointestinal tract. Chromium is excreted via the kidney.

Clinical features

Acute poisoning

Inhaled soluble chromium(VI) compounds, such as sodium and potassium chromate and dichromate, are highly irritant to mucous membranes and may lead to inflammation of the nasal mucosa. Inhalation of chromium(VI) trioxide (chromic acid) causes cough, headache, chest pain, dyspnoea, and cyanosis.

Ingestion of highly water-soluble chromium(VI) compounds leads within minutes to nausea, vomiting, abdominal pain, diarrhoea, and a burning sensation in the mouth, throat, and stomach; gastrointestinal haemorrhage is a frequent complication. Methaemoglobinaemia, haemolysis, and disseminated intravascular coagulation and renal and hepatic failure have been reported.

Chromic acid splashes produce severe burns. Percutaneous absorption may lead to kidney and liver failure; fatalities have occurred.

Chronic poisoning

'Chrome ulcers' may develop after repeated topical exposure to chromium(VI) compounds. Chromium(VI) compounds are also skin sensitizers and contribute to the development of cement dermatitis and contact dermatitis from paint primer, tanned leather, tattoo pigments, and matches.

Inhalation of chromium(VI) compounds has led to atrophy, ulceration, and perforation of the nasal septum. Pharyngeal and laryngeal ulcers may also occur. Asthma may be precipitated by exposure to fumes. Lung fibrosis, bronchitis, emphysema, and proximal tubular damage result from occupational exposure. Chromium(VI) is carcinogenic in humans.

Management

Ascorbic acid reduces chromium(VI) to the less toxic chromium(III). Topical 10% ascorbic acid, as an ointment or in solution, has improved occupational chromium dermatitis but there is no clinical evidence that the systemic administration of ascorbic acid, or any other reducing agent, lessens morbidity or mortality in severe chromium poisoning. Topical preparations containing sodium calcium edetate may also afford some protection to the skin but there is no evidence that systemic chelation treatment is beneficial in chromium poisoning. Haemodialysis effectively removes chromium from the blood but the high tissue uptake limits the value of this treatment when used alone.

Cobalt

Cobalt is a relatively rare element and usually exists in association with nickel, silver, lead, copper, and iron ores. It is used in steel alloys, in the manufacture of magnets, and in the hard metal industry as a binder for tungsten carbide ('hard metal' is typically 80–95% tungsten carbide and 5–20% cobalt). Cobalt is also an essential dietary trace element available as a component of vitamin B_{12}.

Cobalt can be absorbed orally and by inhalation. Most absorbed cobalt is excreted within days but a small proportion is retained with a biological half-life of approximately 2 years. The normal body burden of cobalt is about 1.1 mg.

Clinical features

Acute poisoning is rare, though ingestion causes gastrointestinal irritation. Occupational exposure to hard metal dust causes 'hard metal pneumoconiosis' with interstitial fibrosis. This usually develops after several years of exposure to high concentrations of dust and may prove fatal. Hard metal lung disease rarely, if ever, occurs following exposure to cobalt alone. In contrast, occupational asthma is recognized among both those working with cobalt alone or in the context of the hard metal industry.

Chronic occupational cobalt exposure also leads to anosmia, auditory nerve damage, visual disturbance, irritability, headache, memory deficit, weakness, peripheral neuropathy, gastrointestinal disturbance, and weight loss. There is no firm evidence that cobalt is carcinogenic, and assessment of its cancer risk is often confounded by a simultaneous exposure to nickel and arsenic.

Chronic ingestion of cobalt has caused polycythaemia, inhibition of tyrosine iodination (and therefore goitre), congestive cardiomyopathy, pericardial effusion and hypertrichosis; most of these effects are reversible if exposure is discontinued.

Simultaneous allergies to nickel and to cobalt are frequent and there is some evidence for mutual enhancing effect of contact sensitization to one metal in the presence of the other. An allergic response to cobalt in surgical prostheses has occasionally been a cause of chronic cobalt poisoning.

Management

In two studies, succimer (DMSA) significantly reduced mortality in mice poisoned with cobalt chloride. No satisfactory human studies have yet been performed.

Copper

Copper is used for pipes and roofing material, in alloys and as a pigment. It is a component of several enzymes, including tyrosinase and cytochrome oxidase, and is essential for the utilization of iron. Copper sulphate is used as a fungicide, an algicide, and in some fertilizers.

Following ingestion, copper transport across the intestinal mucosa is facilitated by cytosolic metallothionein. In blood, copper is initially albumin-bound and transported via the hepatic portal circulation to the liver where it is incorporated into caeruloplasmin. Ninety-eight per cent of copper in the systemic circulation is bound to caeruloplasmin. This renders free copper innocuous, with subsequent excretion via a lysosome-to-bile pathway. This process is essential to normal copper homeostasis and provides a protective mechanism in acute copper poisoning. An impaired or overloaded biliary copper excretion system results in hepatic copper accumulation, as occurs in Wilson's disease (see Chapter 12.7.2) and copper poisoning.

Free reduced Cu(I) can bind to sulfhydryl groups and inactivates enzymes such as glucose-6-phosphate dehydrogenase and glutathione reductase. In addition, copper may interact with oxygen species (e.g. superoxide anions and hydrogen peroxide) and catalyze the production of reactive toxic hydroxyl radicals. Copper(II) ions can oxidize haem iron to form methaemoglobin.

Clinical features

Acute poisoning

Acute copper poisoning usually results from the ingestion of contaminated foods or from accidental or deliberate ingestion of copper salts. Copper salt ingestion causes profuse vomiting with abdominal pain, diarrhoea, headache, dizziness, and a metallic taste. Gastrointestinal haemorrhage, haemolysis, and hepatorenal failure may ensue and fatalities have occurred. Body secretions may have a green or blue discoloration.

Occupational exposure to copper fumes (during refining or welding) or to copper-containing dust causes 'metal-fume fever' with upper respiratory tract symptoms, headache, fever, and myalgia.

Chronic poisoning

Chronic occupational copper poisoning causes general malaise, anorexia, nausea, vomiting, and hepatomegaly. Contact dermatitis, pulmonary granulomata, and pulmonary fibrosis have also been described. There is no convincing evidence that copper is carcinogenic in humans.

Management

Although vomiting occurs invariably following the ingestion of many copper salts, gastric lavage may be of value in reducing copper absorption if presentation is early. Blood copper concentrations correlate well with severity of intoxication following acute ingestion, a value of less than 3 mg/litre indicating mild to moderate poisoning while greater than 8 mg/litre implies severe intoxication. D-Penicillamine 25 mg/kg body weight daily until recovery enhances copper excretion in both acute and chronic poisoning. Chelation with dimercaprol, DMPS, or zinc acetate have also been advocated but there are no controlled data in poisoned patients.

Extracorporeal elimination techniques do not significantly enhance copper elimination.

Lead

Exposure to lead occurs in the reclamation of lead from scrap metal, in the demolition and flame-cutting of structures previously painted with lead paint, and in the manufacture of storage batteries and ceramics. Children with pica who chew on lead-painted railings or toys, or who eat contaminated soil, have developed lead poisoning. Lead poisoning has also been described in individuals who have consumed drinks from lead-glazed mugs. Ingestion of lead-based 'traditional remedies' is an increasingly important cause of lead poisoning, particularly among ethnic minorities. Application of lead-containing cosmetics such as 'surma' to the face in Asian communities has also resulted in lead intoxication. Rarely, lead acetate has been injected intravenously with suicidal intent. Tetraethyl lead, which is used as an antiknock agent in leaded petrol, can be absorbed systemically by inhalation, ingestion, and through the skin. Transplacental transfer of lead results in reduced viability of the fetus, reduced birth weight, and premature birth.

Toxicokinetics

Most (95%) absorbed lead is deposited in the bones and teeth. Of the lead in the blood, 99% is associated with erythrocytes. As the body accumulates lead over many years and releases it into the urine only slowly, even small doses can in time lead to intoxication.

Mechanisms of toxicity

There are two principal mechanisms of lead toxicity. First, lead complexes with important functional chemical groups including –COOH, $-NH_2$, and –SH and so disrupts the function of enzymes and other biologically important molecules. Secondly, lead substitutes for divalent ions, particularly calcium, with the potential for widespread chemical interactions both at cell membranes and within intracellular organelles. The chemical similarity between lead and calcium partly explains why these elements appear to be interchangeable in bone, and why more than 90% of the total body burden of lead is stored in the skeleton.

Lead depresses the enzymes responsible for haem synthesis and shortens erythrocyte lifespan leading to a microcytic or normocytic hypochromic anaemia. For example, lead blocks the conversion of δ-aminolaevulinic acid to porphobilinogen leading to an increase in δ-aminolaevulinic acid in blood and urine. Lead also inhibits ferrochelatase, which results in an elevated free erythrocyte protoporphyrin (FEP) concentration. There is a concomitant increase in urinary coproporphyrins and FEP, commonly assayed as zinc protoporphyrin. Basophilic stippling of erythrocytes is due to nuclear remnants that persist due to inhibition of erythrocyte 5′ nucleotidase by lead.

Clinical features

Mild intoxication may result in no more than lethargy and occasional abdominal discomfort, whereas abdominal pain (which is usually diffuse but may be colicky), vomiting, constipation, and encephalopathy develop in more severe cases. Lead colic was first described by Hippocrates and, on occasions, has been incorrectly managed surgically as a case of an acute abdomen. Encephalopathy (seizures, mania, delirium, coma) is more common in children than in adults. Classically, lead poisoning results in foot drop, attributable to primary motor peripheral neuropathy; wrist drop occurs only as a late sign.

Renal effects include reversible renal tubular dysfunction causing glycosuria, aminoaciduria, and phosphaturia and irreversible interstitial fibrosis with progressive renal insufficiency leading to hypertension. A bluish discoloration of the gum margins due to deposition of lead sulphide is observed occasionally. An elevated zinc protoporphyrin concentration (>350 μg/litre) reaches a steady state in the blood only after the entire population of circulating erythrocytes has turned over (*c.*120 days). Consequently, it lags behind blood lead concentrations and is an indirect measure of long-term lead exposure. Moreover, zinc protoporphyrin is not a good screening test as it is not sensitive at the lower levels of lead poisoning.

Even relatively low blood lead concentrations are of concern in children below the age of 5 years. It has been shown that each increase of 10 µg/dl in lifetime average blood lead concentration is associated with a 4.6-point decrease in IQ. In children whose maximal blood lead concentrations remained less than 10 µg/dl, IQ declined by 7.4 points as lifetime average blood lead concentrations increased from 1 to 10 µg/dl.

Medical surveillance

The current practice in the United Kingdom is to enforce stopping work with lead where a worker's blood lead concentration is shown to be above 60 µg/dl (30 µg/dl for a woman of reproductive capacity and 50 µg/dl for an employee aged <18 years).

Management

Primary prevention aimed at eliminating lead hazards for children and workers must receive due public health attention. As chelation with DMSA did not improve scores on tests of cognition, behaviour, and neuropsychological function in children with blood lead concentrations of 22–45 µg/dl, the importance of primary prevention cannot be overemphasized. The social dimension of the problem must also be recognized: simply giving children chelation therapy and then returning them to a contaminated home environment is of no value. Similarly, if an occupational source of lead exposure is implicated, a thorough evaluation of the workplace, other exposed workers, and the systems for handling lead at work is appropriate.

The decision to use chelation therapy is based on the symptoms present, the blood lead concentration and, if available, an estimate of the total body burden of lead using X-ray fluorescence. Parenteral sodium calcium edetate, 75 mg/kg per day, has been the chelating agent of choice for more than 50 years. However, oral succimer (DMSA) 30 mg/kg per day is also an effective chelator and is considered as an alternative antidote to sodium calcium edetate in patients poisoned with lead, particularly when an oral antidote is preferable.

Mercury

Mercury is the only metal that is liquid at room temperature. It exists in three forms: metallic (Hg^0), mercury(I) (mercurous), and mercury(II) (mercuric). Metallic mercury is very volatile and when spilt has a large surface area so that high atmospheric concentrations may be produced in enclosed spaces, particularly when environmental temperatures are high. In addition to simple salts, such as chloride, nitrate and sulphate, mercury(II) forms organometallic compounds where mercury is covalently bound to carbon, such as methyl-, ethyl-, phenyl-, and methoxyethyl mercury. Nonoccupational mercury exposure occurs principally from dietary intake and, to a minor extent, from dental amalgam. Many foodstuffs contain small amounts of mercury.

Toxicokinetics

The absorption of mercury depends on its chemical form. Inhaled mercury vapour is absorbed rapidly and oxidized to mercury (II) in erythrocytes and other tissues. Prior to oxidation, absorbed mercury vapour can cross the blood–brain barrier, but the divalent ion oxidation product serves to trap mercury in the brain. Mercury vapour is also absorbed via the skin. Less than 1% of an ingested dose of metallic mercury reaches the systemic circulation. Organic mercuric salts are better absorbed following ingestion than are inorganic mercuric salts. Organic mercury compounds cross the blood–brain barrier readily to accumulate in the brain. In contrast, the kidney is the main storage organ for inorganic mercury compounds. *In vivo* mercury is bound to metallothionein, which serves a protective role, since renal damage is caused only by the unbound metal. Mercury is excreted mainly in urine and faeces although a small amount of absorbed inorganic mercury is exhaled as mercury vapour. The half-life of most body mercury is 1 to 2 months but a small fraction has a half-life of several years.

Clinical features

Acute poisoning

Acute mercury vapour inhalation causes headache, nausea, cough, chest pain, bronchitis, and pneumonia. In a few individuals, renal damage from such acute exposure may produce gross proteinuria or nephrotic syndrome. In addition, a fine tremor and neurobehavioural impairment occurs and peripheral nerve involvement has also been observed.

Ingestion of metallic mercury is usually without systemic effects as it is poorly absorbed from the gastrointestinal tract. However, mercuric chloride or other inorganic mercury(II) salts cause an irritant gastroenteritis with corrosive ulceration, bloody diarrhoea, and abdominal cramps and may lead to circulatory collapse and shock. Mercury(I) (mercurous) compounds are less soluble, less corrosive, and less toxic than mercuric salts. Ingestion of mercurous chloride in teething powder has led to 'pink disease' or acrodynia in infants. This is characterized by a desquamating erythematous rash of the extremities, irritability, profuse sweating, tachycardia, and hypertension.

There are reports of deliberate intravenous or subcutaneous metallic mercury injection. Accidental injection also has occurred after injury from broken thermometers. Intravascular mercury may result in pulmonary venous or peripheral arterial embolism. Subcutaneous mercury initiates a soft-tissue inflammatory reaction with granuloma formation. Signs of systemic mercury toxicity are rare following metallic mercury injection.

Chronic poisoning

Chronic poisoning from inorganic mercury compounds or mercury vapour causes anorexia, insomnia, abnormal sweating, headache, lassitude, increased excitability, tremor, gingivitis, hypersalivation, personality changes, and memory or intellectual deterioration. Glomerular and tubular damage may occur and renal tubular acidosis has been described in children.

Exposure to organic mercury compounds usually involves aromatic derivatives such as phenylmercuric acetate and phenylmercuric benzoate, or aliphatic compounds such as methylmercury and ethylmercury chloride. The main features of poisoning are paraesthesiae of the lips, hands, and feet, ataxia, tremor, dysarthria, constriction of visual fields, deafness, and emotional and intellectual changes. There is often a latent period of several weeks between the last exposure and the development of symptoms.

Management

Although there are no controlled clinical data to show that chelation therapy improves outcome in patients with neurological features of mercury poisoning, DMPS 30 mg/kg per day intravenously increases urinary mercury elimination and reduces blood mercury concentrations. Where extracorporeal renal support is required for the management of renal failure, there is some evidence that continuous venous–venous haemofiltration is more effective than haemodialysis at removing DMPS–mercury complexes.

Nickel

Nickel is a ubiquitous trace metal mined in the form of sulphide ore. It is used primarily for producing stainless steel and other alloys. Nickel carbonyl ($Ni(CO)_4$), an intermediate compound in nickel purification, is used as a catalyst in the petroleum, plastic, and rubber industries. Nickel sulphate is used for electroplating and nickel hydroxide is a component of nickel–cadmium batteries.

Nickel can be absorbed both orally and by inhalation and in the blood is transported bound principally to albumin. Nickel is concentrated in the kidneys, liver, and lungs and is excreted primarily in the urine.

Clinical features

Acute poisoning

Nickel carbonyl is a colourless, volatile liquid. Its inhalation leads within a few minutes to dizziness, headache, vertigo, nausea, vomiting, cough, and dyspnoea. In many cases these symptoms disappear and there follows a symptom-free period lasting 12–36 h before the start of tachypnoea, dyspnoea, haemoptysis, cyanosis, chest pain, vomiting, tachycardia, weakness, and muscle fatigue. Paraesthesiae, diarrhoea, abdominal distension, delirium, and convulsions have also been reported. Death may occur 4 to 11 days after exposure from cardiorespiratory failure.

At high concentrations, soluble nickel salts are primary skin, gut, and eye irritants. Workers at an electroplating plant who drank water accidentally contaminated with nickel sulphate experienced nausea, vomiting, diarrhoea, abdominal pain, headache, cough, and breathlessness, which persisted for up to 2 days. A 2-year-old child died 4 h after ingesting 15 g nickel sulphate crystals.

Chronic poisoning

Chronic exposure to aerosols of nickel salts may lead to chronic rhinitis and sinusitis and, in rare cases, anosmia and perforation of the nasal septum. Inhaled nickel can produce a type I hypersensitivity reaction manifest as bronchial asthma with circulating IgE antibodies to nickel. Pulmonary eosinophilia (Loeffler's syndrome) due to a type III hypersensitivity reaction to nickel has also been described.

A significant increase in deaths from non-malignant respiratory disease or pneumoconiosis has also been observed in nickel refinery workers. There is evidence that occupational exposure to nickel may cause cancer of the lung and nasal sinuses.

Metallic nickel and nickel salts cause allergic contact dermatitis in up to 10% of females and 1% of males and is due to a type IV delayed hypersensitivity.

Management

Blood nickel concentrations immediately following exposure to nickel carbonyl provide a guide to severity of exposure and the need for chelation therapy. DMPS (unithiol) enhances the urinary excretion of nickel in nickel-intoxicated animals. Diethyldithiocarbamate and disulfiram (which is metabolized to diethyldithiocarbamate) are effective agents in the treatment of nickel dermatitis, but their role in the treatment of acute severe nickel carbonyl poisoning has not been confirmed in a controlled clinical study.

Zinc

Zinc oxide fumes are emitted in any process involving molten zinc and are the most common cause of metal fume fever. Exposure to zinc chloride occurs in soldering; in the manufacture of dyes, paper, and deodorants; and on military exercises when it is used as a smoke screen. Poisoning has followed the accidental or deliberate ingestion of elemental zinc and zinc chloride and fatal intoxication has followed inadvertent intravenous administration. Inhalation of zinc chloride and oxide may lead to nasopharyngeal and respiratory toxicity. Zinc may be absorbed through broken skin when zinc oxide paste is used to treat wounds and burns.

Clinical features

Acute poisoning

Zinc sulphate ingestion causes gastrointestinal irritation, sometimes in association with headache and dizziness. Zinc chloride is highly corrosive and ingestion has led to erosive pharyngitis, oesophagitis, and haematemesis. Acute renal failure and pancreatitis have also been recorded after ingestion of zinc salts. Topical exposure to zinc chloride causes ulceration and dermatitis of the exposed skin. Zinc chloride is highly irritant to the eye.

Metal fume fever starts up to 24 h after exposure to zinc oxide fumes. It presents as a influenza-like illness with headache, fever, sweating, chest tightness and discomfort, and joint pains. Typically, symptoms appear after a weekend away from work. The illness usually has an excellent prognosis and the symptoms often improve towards the end of the working week as some short-term immunity from further symptoms develops.

In contrast to the relatively mild clinical course after zinc oxide inhalation, exposure to zinc chloride ammunition bombs (hexite) produces a chemical pneumonitis with marked dyspnoea, a productive cough, fever, chest pain, and cyanosis. The adult respiratory distress syndrome may ensue; fatalities have been reported.

Chronic poisoning

Repeated topical exposure to zinc oxide may cause a papular folliculitis. Chronic excessive ingestion of zinc supplements (zinc sulphate) may induce reversible anaemia and leucopenia secondary to a relative copper deficiency.

Management

Management is mainly supportive. Endoscopy should be performed following zinc chloride ingestion to assess the severity of oesophageal or gastric burns. Fluid and electrolyte disturbances should be corrected. There are few data concerning the usefulness of chelation therapy for systemic zinc toxicity. Sodium calcium edetate and dimercaprol increase urine zinc excretion, and some authors have claimed an improvement in neurological status following chelation therapy with these agents, but this remains controversial. The decision to start chelation therapy requires expert advice and should be guided by the severity of the clinical features rather than the plasma zinc concentration.

Pesticides

Aluminium and zinc phosphides

Aluminium and zinc phosphides are highly effective insecticides and rodenticides, which are used to protect grain during transport and storage. The phosphide interacts with moisture in the surrounding air to liberate phosphine, which is the active pesticide. In cases of poisoning by phosphide ingestion, toxic effects are due to phosphine release when the phosphide comes into contact with gut fluids. The gas is absorbed through the alimentary mucosa and widely distributed to tissues. Phosphine toxicity by inhalation may also ensue if phosphides outside the body interact with atmospheric moisture to liberate phosphine. The toxicity of phosphine is discussed on p. 1315.

Clinical features

Ingestion of metal phosphides causes vomiting, epigastric pain, a smell of garlic or onions on the breath, gastric or duodenal erosions causing haematemesis, peripheral circulatory failure (which may be profound), severe metabolic acidosis, and renal failure, in addition to the features induced by inhalation of phosphine. The latter include tachypnoea, dyspnoea, cough, wheeze, pulmonary oedema, and the adult respiratory distress syndrome. Fatalities have occurred.

Management

Treatment is symptomatic and supportive. Gastric lavage should be avoided as it might increase the rate of disintegration of the product ingested and increase toxicity. Activated charcoal is contraindicated as it will not bind metal phosphides.

Anticoagulant rodenticides

Warfarin was widely used as a rodenticide until target species developed resistance to it. The newer anticoagulant rodenticides (sometimes termed 'super warfarins'), such as brodifacoum, bromodialone, chlorophacinone, coumatetralyl, difenacoum, diphacinone and flocoumafen, are more potent and longer-acting antagonists of vitamin K_1 than warfarin. Ingestion of these formulations may result in prolongation of the INR for several weeks or months.

Mechanism of toxicity

These anticoagulants inhibit vitamin K_1-2,3-epoxide reductase and thus the synthesis of vitamin K and subsequently clotting factors II, VII, IX, and X. The greater potency and duration of action of long-acting anticoagulant rodenticides compared to warfarin is attributed to their greater affinity for vitamin K_1-2,3-epoxide reductase, their ability to disrupt the vitamin K_1-epoxide cycle at more than one point, hepatic accumulation, and unusually long biological half-lives due to high lipid solubility and enterohepatic circulation.

Clinical features

Gastrointestinal bleeding, haematuria, and bruising are the commonest features, though the most common site of fatal haemorrhage is intracranial. The onset of bleeding may be delayed for several days.

Management

Routine measurement of the INR is generally not indicated in children as the amounts they ingest are almost invariably small. In all other cases, the INR should be measured on presentation and 36 to 48 h after exposure. If the INR is normal at this time, no further action is required.

If active bleeding occurs, prothrombin complex concentrate (which contains factors II, VII, IX, and X) 50 units/kg, or recombinant activated factor VII 1.2 to 4.8 mg, or fresh frozen plasma 15 ml/kg (if no concentrate is available) and phytomenadione 10 mg intravenously (100 μg/kg body weight for a child) should be given. If active bleeding occurs in a patient who is being prescribed an anticoagulant, warfarin (or other anticoagulant) should be discontinued.

If there is no active bleeding and the INR is less than 4.0, treatment with phytomenadione is not required. If the INR is 4.0 or more, phytomenadione 10 mg by slow intravenous injection (100 μg/kg body weight for a child) should be administered, unless the patient is anticoagulated for therapeutic reasons.

If the patient is prescribed anticoagulants, the INR is 8.0 or more, and there is no active bleeding or only minor bleeding, stop warfarin (restart when the INR ≤5.0), give phytomenadione 0.5 mg by slow intravenous injection and repeat the dose if the INR is 8.0 or more 24 h later. If the INR is between 6.0 and 8.0, and there is no active bleeding or only minor bleeding, warfarin should be discontinued and restarted when the INR is 5.0 or less.

If a patient presents within 1 h of a large ingestion, the administration of activated charcoal (50 g for adults; 10–15 g for children) should be considered as it is known that warfarin is adsorbed to charcoal. In patients with severe poisoning who have ingested a long-acting formulation, oral cholestyramine 4 g three times daily for an adult should be considered in order to shorten the plasma half-life of the rodenticide.

Carbamate insecticides

Carbamate insecticides inhibit acetylcholinesterase, though the duration of this effect is comparatively short-lived as the carbamate–enzyme complex tends to dissociate spontaneously.

Clinical features

Early signs are headache and nausea followed by a sensation of tightness in the chest, coughing, and constriction of the pupils. As poisoning progresses, vomiting, diarrhoea, abdominal pain, blurred vision, muscle fasciculation and weakness, sweating, excessive salivation, and bronchorrhoea develop. Hypotension, sinus tachycardia or bradycardia, and dyspnoea may also be present, while in severe cases, there is muscle twitching, profuse sweating, incontinence, mental confusion, and progressive cardiac and respiratory failure. Carbamates penetrate the blood–brain barrier poorly, and therefore central nervous system effects are usually absent or minimal. Seizures are uncommon, and if they occur, should alert the physician to seek another cause. Symptoms do not usually persist for more than 24 h after exposure.

Management

Symptomatic cases require atropine 0.6 to 2 mg intravenously, repeated as necessary. There is limited experimental evidence to suggest that pralidoxime may increase the toxicity of carbaryl, but insufficient evidence to recommend or prohibit its use in severe poisoning due to other carbamates. Moreover, the use of an oxime is usually unnecessary as rapid recovery within 24 h is the rule.

α-Chloralose

α-Chloralose is marketed for amateur use as cereal or paste baits containing 2 to 4% rodenticide. Technical α-chloralose (*c.*90% pure) is used by professionals against bird pests or rodents. The toxic amount is said to be 1 g for an adult and 20 mg/kg body weight for an infant.

Clinical features

Toxic amounts of α-chloralose cause severe central nervous system excitation with hypersalivation, increased muscle tone, hyperreflexia, opisthotonus, myoclonic jerks, and convulsions. Rhabdomyolysis is a potential complication. Coma, generalized flaccidity, and respiratory depression may follow.

Management

Children who ingest small amounts of baits (amateur formulations) containing α-chloralose are unlikely to develop symptoms. In contrast, patients who have deliberately ingested large amounts of bait or the technical compound are likely to require admission to intensive care for management of convulsions, myoclonus, and coma. Gastric emptying should not be carried out since the procedure may provoke seizures.

Chlorates

Sodium and potassium chlorates are nonselective herbicides. Potassium chlorate is also used in matchstick heads, explosives, and fireworks.

Clinical features

Sodium chlorate and potassium chlorate are powerful oxidizing agents and are highly toxic if ingested. The early features include nausea, vomiting, diarrhoea, abdominal pain, and cyanosis secondary to methaemoglobinaemia. Intravascular haemolysis occurs causing hyperkalaemia, jaundice, and oliguric renal failure.

Management

Methaemoglobinaemia can be corrected by slow intravenous injection of methylthioninium chloride (methylene blue) 2 mg/kg body weight as a 1% solution, although this treatment is less effective in the presence of major intravascular haemolysis. Blood transfusion may be required. Plasma potassium concentrations should be monitored and reduced if necessary. Haemodialysis will remove chlorate and may also be required for the management of renal failure and hyperkalaemia. Plasmapheresis and plasma exchange or exchange transfusion have also been employed to remove chlorate, circulating free haemoglobin, and red cell stroma, and thus help to prevent the development of renal failure.

Chlorophenoxy herbicides

The chlorophenoxy herbicides (Table 9.1.4) include the substances popularly referred to as 'hormone' weedkillers and are used widely in agriculture and by the public. Most instances of serious poisoning have been due to deliberate ingestion, but few cases have been reported. These herbicides exhibit a variety of mechanisms of toxicity including dose-dependent cell membrane damage, uncoupling of oxidative phosphorylation, and disruption of acetylcoenzyme A metabolism.

Clinical features

Ingestion causes burning in the mouth and throat, nausea, vomiting, and abdominal pain. Gastrointestinal haemorrhage may occur. Hypotension, which is common, is due predominantly to intravascular volume loss, although vasodilation and direct myocardial toxicity may also contribute. Coma, hypertonia, hyperreflexia, ataxia, nystagmus, miosis, hallucinations, convulsions, fasciculation, and paralysis may then ensue. Hypoventilation is commonly secondary to central nervous system depression, but respiratory muscle weakness is a factor in the development of respiratory failure in some patients. Myopathic symptoms including limb muscle weakness, loss of tendon reflexes, myotonia and increased creatine kinase activity have been observed. Metabolic acidosis, rhabdomyolysis, renal failure, increased aminotransferase activities, pyrexia, and hyperventilation have been reported.

Management

In addition to supportive care, urine alkalinization with high-flow urine output will enhance herbicide elimination and should be considered in all seriously poisoned patients. Haemodialysis produces similar herbicide clearances to urine alkalinization without the need for urine pH manipulation and the administration of substantial amounts of intravenous fluid in an already compromised patient.

Glyphosate-containing herbicides

Glyphosate-containing herbicides usually contain the isopropylamine salt, together with a surfactant. The latter is often an animal fat derivative (a tallow amine) polyoxyethyleneamine (POEA), which contributes substantially to the toxicity of the formulation. Dilute, ready-to-use glyphosate/POEA preparations are rarely associated with systemic toxicity, which usually requires the deliberate ingestion of a concentrate (typically 41% glyphosate/15% POEA).

Clinical features

Ingestion of more than 85 ml of the concentrated glyphosate/POEA formulation is likely to cause significant toxicity in adults. Fatal ingestions have usually involved more than 200 ml. The most prominent effects are on the alimentary tract with burning in the mouth, throat, nausea, vomiting, dysphagia, and diarrhoea. Upper gastrointestinal haemorrhage is a much less common complication. Renal and hepatic impairment are also frequent and usually reflect reduced organ perfusion. Respiratory distress, impaired consciousness, pulmonary oedema, infiltration on chest radiograph, shock, arrhythmias, renal failure requiring haemodialysis, metabolic acidosis, and hyperkalaemia may supervene in severe cases.

Management

Management is symptomatic and supportive. Intravenous fluids or blood transfusion may be required. Respiratory and renal failure should be managed conventionally.

Table 9.1.4 Chlorophenoxy herbicides

Chemical name	Other names
2,4-Dichlorophenoxy acetic acid	2,4-D
4-(2,4-Dichlorophenoxy) butyric acid	2,4-DB
2-(2,4-Dichlorophenoxy) propionic acid	2,4-DP, dichlorprop
4-Chloro-2-methylphenoxyacetic acid	MCPA
4-(4-Chloro-2-methylphenoxy) butyric acid	MCPB
2-(4-Chloro-2-methylphenoxy) propionic acid	Mecoprop
2-(2, 4-Dichloro-*m*-tolyoxy) propionanilide	Clomeprop

Lindane

Lindane is an organochlorine insecticide containing not less than 99% γ-hexachlorocyclohexane. It was used in agriculture and in topical preparations to treat pediculoses and scabies, though clinical use has now been banned and agricultural use limited in most countries. Lindane is highly lipid-soluble and rapidly absorbed from the skin and gastrointestinal tract. Lindane concentrates in the central nervous system where its effects are predominantly excitatory and related to GABA antagonism. Fatalities have occurred following ingestion or excessive dermal exposure.

Clinical features

The main toxic effects are on the central nervous system with rapid loss of consciousness and the development of myoclonus, hypertonia, hyperreflexia, convulsions, and rhabdomyolysis. Metabolic acidosis, disseminated intravascular coagulation, renal tubular and hepatocellular necrosis, pancreatitis, and proximal myopathy have been reported.

Management

Treatment is symptomatic and supportive. Acid–base abnormalities should be corrected and convulsions controlled.

Metaldehyde

Metaldehyde in the form of pellets is used widely for killing slugs and in some countries as a solid fuel. Exposure usually involves accidental ingestion of a part of a metaldehyde-containing tablet by a child in whom toxicity is unlikely. Cases of deliberate ingestion have also been reported and are the most likely cause of severe metaldehyde poisoning.

Clinical features

Nausea, vomiting, abdominal pain, and diarrhoea often occur 1 to 3 h after ingestion of any amount, while more than 100 mg/kg body weight may cause hypertonia, convulsions, impairment of consciousness, respiratory depression, and metabolic acidosis. Opisthotonos, risus sardonicus, and miosis are recognized. Hepatic and renal tubular necrosis may become apparent after 2 to 3 days. Coma may last several days. Fatalities have occurred.

Management

Treatment is supportive.

Methyl bromide (bromomethane)

Methyl bromide is a colourless, odourless gas at ordinary temperatures and dangerous concentrations may therefore accumulate without warning. Methyl bromide has high penetrating power and is nonflammable. It is used to fumigate soil and a wide range of commodities including grain in warehouses and mills. Its high density causes it to settle at floor level. Poisoning has followed occupational exposures and gas seepage from fumigated structures or stored methyl bromide cannisters adjacent to inhabited areas.

Mechanism of toxicity

Methyl bromide is absorbed readily through the lungs and is excreted largely unchanged by the same route. The remainder is metabolized and inorganic bromide is excreted in the urine. The mechanism of toxicity is uncertain but methyl bromide appears to have an affinity for intracellular proteins, particularly those with sulphydryl groups.

Clinical features

After a latent period of up to 12 h, toxic symptoms occur. Symptoms include dizziness, headache, nausea, vomiting, abdominal pain, malaise, transient blurring of vision, diplopia, and breathlessness. In severe cases, coma, status epilepticus, tremor, myoclonus, ataxia, hyporeflexia, paraesthesiae, hallucinations, acute psychosis, and polyneuropathy may be found. Proteinuria, oliguria (due to renal tubular and cortical necrosis), and jaundice have been described.

Long-term exposure to methyl bromide may lead to a chronic polyneuropathy, pyramidal and cerebellar dysfunction, neuropsychiatric disturbances, and epilepsy.

Management

The casualty should be removed promptly from the contaminated atmosphere and undressed, as methyl bromide can penetrate clothing and rubber gloves. Contaminated skin should be washed with water. Treatment is supportive.

Systemic uptake can be quantified by measuring serum and urine bromide concentrations.

Organophosphorus insecticides

Organophosphorus insecticides are among the most widely used pesticides throughout the world. They vary widely in their toxicity and while some (the phosphates) are directly toxic, others (the phosphorothioates) need biotransformation to become active.

Mechanisms of toxicity

Organophosphorus insecticides inhibit acetylcholinesterase causing accumulation of acetylcholine at central and peripheral cholinergic nerve endings, including neuromuscular junctions.

Clinical features

The features of organophosphorus insecticide poisoning are dose related. Minor exposure may produce subclinical poisoning in which there is reduction of cholinesterase activity but no symptoms or signs. Poisoning is characterized by anxiety, restlessness, insomnia, nightmares, tiredness, dizziness, headache, and muscarinic features such as nausea, vomiting, abdominal colic, diarrhoea, tenesmus, sweating, hypersalivation, and chest tightness. Miosis may be present. Nicotinic effects follow with muscle fasciculation and flaccid paresis of limb muscles, respiratory muscles, and, occasionally, various combinations of extraocular muscles. Respiratory failure ensues and is exacerbated by the development of pulmonary oedema and by the retention in the bronchi of large amounts of respiratory secretions. Consciousness is impaired in severe poisoning and convulsions may occur. Hyperglycaemia and glycosuria have been reported though ketonuria is absent. Though bradycardia would be expected from the mode of action of organophosphates, it is present in only about 20% of cases. Rarely, complete heart block and arrhythmias occur.

Diagnosis

Diagnosis of organophosphorus insecticide poisoning is difficult in the absence of a history of exposure and requires a high index of suspicion. Gastroenteritis is a common erroneous diagnosis and the findings of glycosuria and hyperglycaemia may prompt consideration of diabetes mellitus and its complications. Miosis is an important diagnostic sign but is not invariable. Once raised, the diagnosis can be confirmed by demonstrating reduced plasma, but preferably erythrocyte, cholinesterase activity. Mild, moderate, and severe poisoning are associated with reduction of cholinesterase activity to approximately 20 to 50%, 10 to 20%, and less than 10% of normal, respectively.

Management

Subclinical poisoning does not require treatment other than appropriate measures to prevent further absorption of the poison. The patient should be kept under observation for about 24 h to ensure that delayed toxicity does not develop. The management of symptomatic organophosphorus insecticide poisoning involves supportive measures and judicious administration of antidotes. Soiled clothing should be removed and contaminated skin washed with soap and water to prevent further absorption. Effective removal of respiratory secretions, and correction of hypoxia are essential using endotracheal intubation and assisted ventilation if necessary. The use of diazepam 5 to 10 mg intravenously in an adult may reduce anxiety and restlessness, but larger doses may be required to control convulsions; it may also reduce morbidity and morality.

Atropine 2 to 4 mg intravenously every 5 to 10 min for an adult, depending on the severity of poisoning, should be given to reduce bronchorrhoea and bronchospasm or until signs of atropinization (flushed dry skin, tachycardia, dilated pupils, and dry mouth) develop. In very severe cases, some have advocated doubling the original bolus dose of atropine every 5 min until atropinization has been achieved. As much as 30 mg, and occasionally, much more may be required in the first 24 h. Children should be given 0.02 mg/kg body weight but may require up to 0.05 mg/kg.

Oximes reactivate phosphorylated acetylcholinesterase and should be given together with atropine to every symptomatic patient. For example, pralidoxime mesilate 30 mg/kg body weight (2 g for an adult) should be given by slow intravenous injection; obidoxime 250 mg is an alternative. Preferably, an infusion of pralidoxime 8 to 10 mg/kg body weight per hour (obidoxime 30 mg/h) should be continued; alternatively, further bolus doses of pralidoxime or obidoxime may be given, though this regimen is less effective. Monitoring of erythrocyte (not plasma) cholinesterase activity may be used together with clinical signs to guide the duration of therapy.

Complications

A small number of patients develop what has been called the 'intermediate syndrome', which comprises cranial nerve and brainstem lesions and a proximal neuropathy starting 1 to 4 days after acute intoxication and persisting for 2 to 3 weeks. Respiratory failure secondary to muscle weakness is observed.

The balance of evidence supports the view that neuropsychological abnormalities such as impaired mental agility and attention can occur as a long-term complication of acute organophosphorus insecticide poisoning, if the poisoning is severe. Long-term memory does not appear to be affected. Peripheral neuropathy of a predominantly motor type is a well-recognized complication of poisoning by organophosphorus compounds that inhibit the enzyme lysophospholipase (neuropathy target esterase, NTE). It is possible that peripheral neuropathy can also occur after exposure to organophosphorus insecticides that do not inhibit lysophospholipase.

Paraquat and related herbicides

The bipyridyl herbicides include diquat, morfamquat, and paraquat.

Clinical features

Occupational carelessness in handling paraquat has led to reversible changes in the finger nails and inhalation of spray may cause pain in the throat and epistaxis. Skin splashes that are promptly and thoroughly washed should not cause problems but prolonged dermal exposure may cause burns and, very rarely, may enable enough paraquat to be absorbed to cause serious and fatal systemic poisoning. Splashes in the eye cause blepharospasm, lacrimation, and corneal ulceration.

Potentially lethal poisoning is most common after paraquat ingestion. Probably no more than 5% of the ingested amount is absorbed but absorption is rapid, the volume of distribution is high, and there is energy-dependent accumulation in some organs (particularly the lungs). Elimination is mainly through the kidneys.

The features of toxicity are largely dependent on the amount of paraquat swallowed. Ingestion of 6 g or more of paraquat ion is likely to be fatal within 24 to 48 h while 3 to 6 g is likely to lead to a more protracted, but still fatal, outcome. Nausea, vomiting, abdominal pain, and diarrhoea, rapidly followed by peripheral circulatory failure, metabolic acidosis, impaired consciousness, convulsions, and increasing breathlessness and cyanosis secondary to acute pneumonitis, are the features of ingestion of large amounts of paraquat. With smaller amounts, the cardiovascular and central nervous system complications are not seen, and the course of poisoning is dominated by alimentary features, particularly painful ulceration of the mouth, tongue, and throat, which makes it difficult to swallow, speak, and cough. Perforation of the oesophagus with subsequent mediastinitis has been reported. Mild jaundice may be seen, and renal failure is usually severe. Breathlessness, tachypnoea, widespread crepitations, and central cyanosis may be present by 5 to 7 days after ingestion and progress relentlessly until the patient dies from hypoxia a few days later.

Ingestion of 1.5 to 2.0 g of paraquat causes nausea, vomiting, and diarrhoea, mild renal tubular necrosis, and pain in the throat. Respiratory involvement may not be apparent till 10 to 21 days after ingestion, but may progress till the patient dies of respiratory failure as late as 5 or 6 weeks after taking the paraquat. The features of diquat poisoning are similar. In severe and usually fatal cases, gastrointestinal mucosal ulceration, paralytic ileus, hypovolemic shock, acute renal failure, and coma predominate.

Diagnosis

The diagnosis of paraquat poisoning is usually made on the basis of the history and can be readily confirmed by a simple qualitative test on urine passed within 4 h of ingestion using alkaline sodium dithionite (a blue colour indicates paraquat is present); a negative test indicates that not enough paraquat has been taken to cause problems. The outcome of paraquat poisoning can be predicted with reasonable confidence within a few hours of ingestion by relating the plasma paraquat concentration to the time after ingestion (Table 9.1.5).

In the case of diquat poisoning, the urine goes a green colour in the alkaline sodium dithionite test.

Management

There is no evidence that the outcome of paraquat or diquat poisoning can be altered by any form of intervention. Symptomatic measures including antiemetics, mouth washes, and analgesics are indicated, and intravenous fluids may be necessary to replace gastrointestinal losses.

Pyrethroids

Pyrethroids are used widely as insecticides both in the home and commercially, and in medicine for the topical treatment of scabies and head lice. In tropical countries, mosquito nets are commonly soaked in pyrethroid solutions as part of antimalarial strategies. Despite their extensive worldwide use, severe poisoning with pyrethroids is extremely rare. Pyrethroids modify the gating characteristics of voltage-sensitive sodium channels to delay their closure. A protracted sodium influx ensues, which, if it is sufficiently large and/or long, lowers the action potential threshold and causes repetitive firing which manifests as paraesthesiae.

Clinical features

Pyrethroids are best known for their ability to cause facial paraesthesiae following occupational exposure; these symptoms last only a few hours at most. Coma, convulsions, and pulmonary oedema may occur after substantial ingestion, percutaneous absorption or inhalational exposure.

Management

Symptomatic and supportive measures should be employed and reassurance given that facial paraesthesiae will not be a long-term problem.

Table 9.1.5 Predictive plasma paraquat concentration separating surviving patients and fatalities

Time after ingestion (h)	Plasma paraquat concentration (μg/litre)
4	2000
5	800
6	600
7	480
8	330
10	290
12	230
15	170
20	120
24	100
48	47
72	31

After Proudfoot AT, *et al.* (1979). Paraquat poisoning: significance of plasma-paraquat concentrations. *Lancet*, **1**, 330–1, and Scherrmann JM, *et al.* (1987). Prognostic value of plasma and urine paraquat concentration. *Hum Toxicol*, **6**, 91–3.

Other chemicals

Acetone

Acetone is a clear liquid with a characteristic pungent odour and sweet taste, used widely in industrial and household products.

Clinical features

There is irritation of mucous membranes of eyes, nose, and throat. Acetone can be absorbed through the lungs, gastrointestinal tract, or skin. Following ingestion or inhalation, it can often be smelt on the breath since some is exhaled unchanged. Systemic toxicity causes headache, excitement, restlessness, chest tightness, incoherent speech, nausea and vomiting, and occasionally gastrointestinal bleeding, coma, convulsions, and hyperglycaemia (resulting from the metabolism of acetone via hepatic and extrahepatic gluconeogenic pathways to glucose with subsequent liberation of CO_2).

Management

If toxicity has followed inhalation, remove from exposure, give supportive treatment and correct hyperglycaemia. Gastrointestinal decontamination is not useful after ingestion. Since acetone is a small molecule responsible for toxicity, there may be a role for dialysis in the management of seriously poisoned patients, particularly if plasma acetone concentrations are high.

Acids

Acids commonly involved in cases of poisoning include the inorganic acids hydrochloric, hydrofluoric (see p. 1312), nitric, phosphoric, and sulphuric acids; and organic acids such as acetic, formic, lactic, and trichloroacetic acids. Car battery acid typically contains 28% sulphuric acid. Proprietary cleaning agents and anti-rust compounds often comprise a mixture of hydrochloric and phosphoric acids. Inorganic acids generally are of concentrations more likely to be corrosive at the normally available solution.

Clinical features

On the skin, acids characteristically behave as corrosives leading to erythema, blistering, and features of a burn with ulceration and, in some cases, penetrating necrosis. In the eyes, intense pain and blepharospasm are common, and corneal burns may occur.

When ingested, acids flow rapidly along the lesser curvature of the stomach to the prepyloric region where they pool because of spasm of the pylorus and antrum to cause almost instantaneous coagulative necrosis of one or more layers of the stomach. In some 80% of cases, acids spare the oesophagus because of rapid transit and resistant squamous epithelium. There is immediate pain in the mouth, pharynx and abdomen, intense thirst, vomiting, haematemesis, and diarrhoea. The pain and mucosal oedema cause dysphagia and drooling saliva. Gastric and oesophageal perforation may occur, resulting in chemical peritonitis. Other effects include hoarseness, stridor, and respiratory distress secondary to laryngeal and epiglottic oedema, shock, metabolic acidosis leucocytosis, acute tubular necrosis, renal failure, hypoxaemia, respiratory failure, intravascular coagulation, and haemolysis.

Formic acid ingestion causes systemic acidosis, haematuria, and renal damage.

Management

Acid burns to the skin should be irrigated liberally with water or saline. Dressings are applied as for a thermal burn. Skin grafting may be necessary.

After ocular exposure with acid, the eye should be irrigated preferably with saline for 15 to 30 min. Topical local anaesthetic is usually required to relieve pain and to overcome blepharospasm. Ophthalmic advice should be sought.

After ingestion, a clear airway should be established. Opioids are often necessary for analgesia. Dilution and/or neutralization is contraindicated. Urgent endoscopy is needed. Patients with circumferential ulceration or deep ulcers should be admitted to an intensive care unit. Total parenteral nutrition is often required. Corticosteroids confer no benefit and may mask abdominal signs of perforation; antibiotics should be given for established infection only.

Urgent laparotomy with resection of necrotic tissue and surgical repair should be considered, and may be life saving.

Acid ingestion may result in antral, pyloric, or jejunal strictures, achlorhydria, protein-losing enteropathy, and gastric carcinoma.

Alkalis

Alkali products are commonly found in the home and those commonly encountered in cases of poisoning include sodium hydroxide (drain, lavatory, pipe cleaners), sodium carbonate, sodium silicate, sodium tripolyphosphate (dishwashing detergents), sodium perborate, sodium phosphate, sodium carbonate (denture cleaning tablets), sodium dichloroisocyanurate (water sterilizing tablets), sodium hypochlorite (a bleaching agent), and alkaline batteries.

Clinical features

The features of eye, skin, and laryngeal contamination with alkalis are similar to those produced by acids (discussed earlier). When ingested, alkalis typically damage the oesophagus but usually spare the stomach. There is little immediate oral discomfort, but subsequently, a burning sensation develops in the mouth and pharynx, together with epigastric pain, vomiting, and diarrhoea. Oesophageal ulceration with or without perforation may occur with mediastinitis, pneumonitis, cardiac injury, and aorto-enteric fistula formation as secondary complications of perforation.

Management

The treatment of corrosive injuries caused by alkalis is largely the same as for those produced by acids. High-intensity lavage for eye injuries appears to be effective.

Corticosteroids have been advocated to reduce the incidence of stricture formation and may decrease the need for surgical repair of strictures arising from second- or third-degree burns if they are used in conjunction with either anterograde or retrograde oesophageal dilation. Other authors have questioned the true benefits of this approach and suggested that they may mask symptoms.

Alkali ingestion may result in stricture formation and there is a risk of malignancy. The mean latent period for development of carcinoma of the oesophagus following alkali ingestion is more than 40 years.

Ammonia

Ammonia, a colourless gas with a strong, irritating odour, is used in aqueous solution in industry and in the home. Ammonia is highly soluble in water and causes its toxic and corrosive action as a result of its alkalinity.

Clinical features

Ammonia may be absorbed by inhalation, ingestion, or percutaneously. It irritates the eyes, upper respiratory tract, and pharynx. Exposed surfaces may develop chemical burns, blisters, thrombosis of surface vessels, and severe local oedema, which may lead to respiratory obstruction and death if the larynx and glottis are involved. High inhaled concentrations may cause dyspnoea and pulmonary oedema and persistent lung damage. Ingestion of ammonia water induces caustic lesions in the oropharynx, oesophagus, and stomach. Liquid ammonia is corrosive. Evaporation of liquid ammonia from the eye or skin may cause cold burns.

Management

The casualty should be removed from the contaminated area. The eyes should be irrigated with water or saline 0.9% for 15 to 30 min and an ophthalmic opinion sought as permanent blindness may result. Pulmonary complications should be treated with humidified supplemental oxygen, bronchodilators, and, if necessary, assisted ventilation with positive end-expiratory pressure. Although widely employed, there is no conclusive evidence that diuretics and corticosteroids alter the prognosis. Patients who survive for 24 h are likely to recover fully.

Arsine

Arsine is a colourless, nonirritating gas.

Mechanism of toxicity

Arsine binds with oxidized haemoglobin causing massive intravascular haemolysis. Haemoglobinuria and acute renal tubular necrosis then develop.

Clinical features

There is usually a delay of some 2 to 24 h after exposure before the onset of headache, malaise, weakness, dizziness, breathlessness, migratory abdominal pain, fever, tachycardia, tachypnoea, nausea, and vomiting. A bronze skin colour is noted in some patients, but most have the typical appearance of a jaundiced patient. Acute renal failure is observed by the third day after substantial exposure, and the urine is dark red, then brown, before anuria ensues. Investigations will show leucocytosis, delayed reticulocytosis, elevated plasma haemoglobin, and haemoglobinuria.

Management

If haemolysis is severe, plasmapheresis or exchange transfusion should be undertaken and, if renal failure ensues, haemodialysis/filtration. Patients have survived complete haemolysis (haematocrit 0%). Dimercaprol and DMSA are of no value.

Benzene

Benzene is a colourless, volatile liquid with a pleasant odour. It is an ingredient in many paints and varnish removers and some petrols.

Mechanisms of toxicity

About 10% of inhaled benzene is excreted unchanged in the breath. The remainder is metabolized by mixed function oxidase enzymes predominantly in the liver, but also in the bone marrow, the target organ of benzene toxicity. Benzene is a human carcinogen.

Clinical features

Acute exposure

Following inhalation or ingestion, euphoria, dizziness, weakness, headache, blurred vision, mucous membrane irritation, tremor, ataxia, chest tightness, respiratory depression, cardiac arrhythmias, coma, and convulsions occur. Direct skin contact with liquid benzene may produce marked irritation.

Chronic exposure

The toxic effects of chronic poisoning may not become apparent for months or years after initial contact and may develop after all exposure has ceased.

Anorexia, headache, drowsiness, nervousness, and irritability are well described. Anaemia (including aplastic anaemia), leucopenia, thrombocytopenia, pancytopenia, leukaemia, lymphomas, chromosomal abnormalities, and cerebral atrophy have been reported. There is also an association between occupational benzene exposure and non-Hodgkin's lymphoma. Patients have recovered after as long as a year of almost complete absence of formation of new blood cells. A dry, scaly dermatitis may develop on prolonged or repeated skin exposure to liquid benzene.

Management

Following removal from the contaminated atmosphere, treatment should be directed towards symptomatic and supportive measures. Gastric lavage is hazardous as aspiration is likely to occur.

Benzyl alcohol

Benzyl alcohol has been used as a preservative in intravascular flush solutions and in drug formulations, which has led to severe toxicity in neonates.

Mechanism of toxicity

Benzyl alcohol is metabolized to benzoic acid, which is then conjugated with glycine in the liver and excreted as hippuric acid. The immature liver's capacity to metabolize benzoic acid is limited, and when exceeded, leads to accumulation of this metabolite and metabolic acidosis.

Clinical features

In 1982, a syndrome consisting of metabolic acidosis, convulsions, neurological deterioration (due to intraventricular haemorrhage), gasping respirations, hepatic and renal abnormalities, cardiovascular collapse, and death was described in small premature infants between 2 to 14 days of age. The removal of benzyl alcohol solutions from neonatal units led to a considerable reduction both in morbidity and mortality and in particular there was a reduction in cases of kernicterus and intraventricular haemorrhage. In contrast, healthy adult humans are able to tolerate as much as 30 ml of 0.9% benzyl alcohol by rapid intravenous infusion without signs of toxicity.

Carbon dioxide (CO_2)

CO_2 is a colourless gas that is also available commercially as a solid for refrigeration purposes ('dry ice'). High concentrations may accumulate in wells, silos, manholes, mines and in several volcanic lakes in Africa. In 1986, Lake Nyos in Cameroon emitted a cloud of CO_2 that killed 1700 villagers and 3500 of their livestock.

Clinical features

Dyspnoea, cough, headache, dizziness, sweating, restlessness, paraesthesiae, and sinus tachycardia are features after modest CO_2 exposure. Higher concentrations (>10%) produce psychomotor agitation, myoclonic twitches, eye flickering, coma, and convulsions. Death occurs from acute cardiorespiratory depression, typically at concentrations exceeding 17%.

Skin contact with solid CO_2 (dry ice) may result in frostbite and local blistering.

Management

The casualty should be removed from the contaminated environment and oxygen administered. Thereafter, care is supportive. Dry ice burns are treated similarly to other cryogenic burns, with thawing of the affected tissue and suitable analgesia.

Carbon disulphide

Carbon disulphide is used as a fumigant for grain and as a solvent, particularly in the rayon industry. It is a clear, colourless, volatile liquid with an odour like that of decaying cabbage.

Clinical features

Acute exposure

Acute poisoning is rare. Absorption occurs through the skin as well as by inhalation. Because of its potent defatting activity, carbon disulphide causes reddening, cracking, and peeling of the skin, and a burn may occur if contact continues for several minutes. Splashes in the eye cause immediate and severe irritation. Acute inhalation may result in irritation of the mucous membranes, blurred vision, nausea and vomiting, headache, delirium, hallucinations, coma, tremor, convulsions, and cardiac and respiratory arrest.

Chronic exposure

There is an increased incidence of cardiovascular disease (hypertension, arteriosclerosis, ischaemic heart disease, elevated cholesterol) among workers exposed to carbon disulphide. In addition, sleep disturbances, fatigue, anorexia, and weight loss are common complaints. Intellectual impairment, cerebellar signs, diffuse vascular encephalopathy, parkinsonism, peripheral polyneuropathy, hepatic damage, and permanent impairment of reproductive performance have been described.

Management

Treatment involves removal from exposure, washing contaminated skin, irrigation of the eyes with water, and supportive measures. In the majority of cases, however, preventive measures to keep carbon disulphide concentrations in the workplace as low as possible are more important.

Carbon monoxide

Carbon monoxide is a tasteless, odourless, colourless, nonirritating gas produced by incomplete combustion of organic materials. Normal endogenous carbon monoxide production is sufficient to maintain a resting carboxyhaemoglobin concentration of 1 to 3% in urban nonsmokers and 5 to 6% in smokers.

Common sources of carbon monoxide are car exhaust fumes (in the absence of a catalytic converter), improperly maintained and ventilated heating systems, and smoke from all types of fire. Carbon monoxide derived from domestic heating systems is a major cause of accidental death in the developing world. Inhalation of methylene chloride (from paint strippers) may lead to carbon monoxide poisoning due to breakdown of the parent compound.

Mechanisms of toxicity

Symptoms and signs that follow inhalation of carbon monoxide are the result of tissue hypoxia. The affinity of haemoglobin for carbon monoxide is approximately 240 times greater than that for oxygen. Carbon monoxide combines with haemoglobin to form carboxyhaemoglobin, reducing the total oxygen-carrying capacity of the blood. In addition, the oxygen dissociation curve shifts to the left due to modification of oxygen-binding sites. As a result, the affinity of the remaining haem groups for oxygen is increased, the oxygen dissociation curve is distorted as well as being shifted and the resulting tissue hypoxia is thus far greater than that which would result from simple loss of oxygen-carrying capacity.

Carbon monoxide may also inhibit cellular respiration as a result of reversible binding to cytochrome oxidase a_3. At higher concentrations, carbon monoxide causes brain lipid peroxidation, and it has been suggested this may be relevant to the development of delayed neuropsychiatric sequelae.

Clinical features

The clinical features of carbon monoxide poisoning may be divided into those caused acutely, predominantly due to hypoxia, and those that result from tissue damage by the mechanisms detailed earlier. These later toxicities are therefore related to the initial amounts of carbon monoxide inhaled and length of time before rescue and treatment. In acute poisoning, organs with high oxygen demand are at special risk of damage and this includes, in particular, the heart and brain.

The symptoms of mild to moderate exposure are nonspecific and include headache, nausea, and confusion. These nonspecific symptoms therefore require a high degree of suspicion in patients at potential risk of poisoning with the gas. As concentrations increase, metabolic acidosis ensues from interference with metabolic processes, and central nervous system features progress to cause loss of consciousness with hypertonia and hypereflexia, extensor plantar responses, papilloedema, and convulsions. Cardiovascular changes include arrhythmias, a variety of types, and ischaemic myocardial damage. Other complications tend to be detected later and include persistent neurological damage in any part of the brain, which may result in either paralysis or midbrain damage causing parkinsonism or akinetic mutism, deafness due to central ischaemia of the brain stem nuclei and cochlea, muscle necrosis causing rhabdomyolysis and renal failure, and skin changes (bullae) due to prolonged unconsciousness.

The degree of intoxication is correlated to some extent with carboxyhaemoglobin concentrations, but by the time patients arrive in hospital, they will often have received oxygen in an ambulance, which may lower cabon monoxide concentrations from those present at the scene of the injury. Very severe features are to be expected with carboxyhaemoglobin above 60%, but significant features would not generally be expected at concentrations below 30%.

Neuropsychiatric problems may occur after recovery from carbon monoxide intoxication and are said to develop insidiously over a number of weeks. Defining limits of these changes may be difficult in patients with relatively mild exposure, and ascribing causation is particularly difficult in low-level exposures where formal studies suggest no effect.

Management

Removal from exposure and administration of 100% oxygen using a tightly fitting face mask are essential. If patients are unconscious, endotracheal intubation and mechanical ventilation is required. Prolonged administration of oxygen is necessary to ensure carbon monoxide bound in tissues is released.

Traditionally hyperbaric oxygen has been used in carbon monoxide poisoning, although there remains significant controversy about its efficacy. A trial in the United States of America has shown some suggestion of benefit, but commentators are divided about the relevance of the relatively small changes noted, and the wider application of these results. In part, this is because patients were brought for treatment for quite some distance, and the debate remains as to whether any potential small therapeutic benefit warrants transfer to an expensive treatment facility.

Chlorine

Chlorine is a greenish-yellow gas normally transported as a pressurized liquid. Exposure after spillage may be prolonged because gaseous chlorine is heavier than air, causing it to remain near ground level. Chlorine has a pungent odour that can usually be detected by smell at concentrations of less than 0.5 parts per million.

Mechanisms of toxicity

Molecular chlorine, a strong oxidizing agent, is known to react with many functional groups in cell components. It forms chloramines, oxidizes thiol radicals, reacts with tissue water to form hypochlorite and hydrochloric acid, and may generate oxygen free radicals.

Clinical features

Symptoms begin within minutes and include irritation of the mucous membranes of the eyes, nose, and throat, followed by cough, breathlessness, expectoration of white sputum (which may be bloodstained), chest pain and tightness, abdominal pain, nausea, headache, dizziness, and palpitation due to ventricular ectopic beats. Laryngeal oedema may cause hoarseness of the voice and stridor; cardiac arrest may occur secondary to hypoxia.

Restrictive as well as obstructive ventilatory defects arise in those who have inhaled sublethal amounts. Diffusion is impaired, leading to arterial hypoxaemia. In very severe cases, noncardiogenic pulmonary oedema and respiratory failure may develop. Survival is usually followed by complete resolution of the pulmonary defects. Some workers chronically exposed to the gas become anosmic.

Management

The first priority is to remove the casualty from exposure. Conjunctival skin burns should be treated as for acids (see p. 1306). Patients with respiratory symptoms persisting beyond the period of exposure should be admitted to hospital in case they require bronchodilators and humidified oxygen. Some will require mechanical ventilation, particularly if noncardiogenic pulmonary oedema develops. Corticosteroids and prophylactic antibiotics have not been shown to be of value. Correction of serious metabolic acidosis with intravenous sodium bicarbonate may be necessary, but the use of inhaled sodium bicarbonate to neutralize the hydrogen chloride produced following chlorine exposure remains controversial.

Cyanide

Hydrogen cyanide (HCN) and its derivatives are used widely in industry and are released during the thermal decomposition of polyurethane foams. Cyanide poisoning may also result from the ingestion of the cyanogenic glycoside amygdalin, which is found in the kernels of almonds, apples, apricots, cherries, peaches, plums, and other fruits.

Mechanisms of toxicity

Cyanide reversibly inhibits cellular enzymes which contain ferric iron notably cytochrome oxidase a_3 so that electron transfer is blocked, the tricarboxylic acid cycle is paralysed, and cellular respiration ceases.

Clinical features

Acute poisoning

The ingestion by an adult of 50 ml of (liquid) hydrogen cyanide or 200 to 300 mg of one of its salts is likely to prove fatal. Inhalation of hydrogen cyanide gas may produce symptoms within seconds and death within minutes.

Acute poisoning is characterized by dizziness, headache, palpitation, anxiety, a feeling of constriction in the chest, dyspnoea, pulmonary oedema, confusion, vertigo, ataxia, coma, and paralysis. Cardiovascular collapse, respiratory arrest, convulsions, and metabolic acidosis are seen in severe cases. Cyanosis may occur, and the classical 'brick red' colour of the skin is noted occasionally. There is sometimes an odour of bitter almonds on the breath, but the ability to detect this is genetically determined and some 40% of the population are unable to do so.

Chronic exposure

Chronic exposure results predominantly in neurological damage which can include ataxia, peripheral neuropathies, amblyopia, optic atrophy, and nerve deafness.

Management

The immediate administration of oxygen is of paramount importance, as there is evidence that it prevents inhibition of cytochrome oxidase a_3 and accelerates its reactivation. Treatment thereafter depends on the severity and type of exposure. If HCN has been inhaled and the patient remains conscious 10 min after exposure has ceased, no antidotal treatment is required. In more severe cases an antidote is invariably necessary.

Methaemoglobin binds cyanide, forming cyanmethaemoglobin. Methaemoglobinaemia may be induced efficiently by the administration of intravenous sodium nitrite 300 mg over 3 min. Because the effect of sodium nitrite is relatively rapid and methaemoglobin formation slower, the benefit of sodium nitrite may also be from its vasodilator action and the consequent improved tissue perfusion. Intravenous sodium nitrite is usually given with intravenous sodium thiosulphate; they have been shown to act synergistically in experimental cyanide poisoning by providing sulphane sulphur to enhance endogenous metabolism. Sodium thiosulphate is administered intravenously in a dose of 12.5 g over 10 min.

Dicobalt edetate solutions contain free cobalt, which complexes six times more cyanide than dicobalt edetate. Cobalt is toxic, however, and use of this formulation in the absence of cyanide poisoning may cause cobalt toxicity. Dicobalt edetate should therefore be given only when the diagnosis is certain. Dicobalt edetate is administered intravenously in a dose of 300 mg over 1 min, with a further 300 mg being given if recovery does not occur.

One mole of hydroxocobalamin inactivates one mole of cyanide, but, on a weight-for-weight basis, 50 times more hydroxocobalamin is needed than cyanide because hydroxocobalamin is a far larger molecule. If available, hydroxocobalamin 5 g is given intravenously over 30 min; a second dose (5 g) may be required in severe cases.

Diethylene glycol

Diethylene glycol is used as a coolant, as a building block in organic synthesis, and as a solvent. It can be also found in some hydraulic fluids and brake fluids. Occupational exposure is by the dermal route but the most common route of exposure is ingestion, often unintentionally as a result of contamination of medicines. Diethylene glycol has been responsible for a number of mass poisonings in Australia, Bangladesh, Haiti, India, Nigeria, South Africa, and the United States of America.

Mechanism of toxicity

Diethylene glycol is metabolized in the rat and dog by alcohol dehydrogenase to 2-hydroxyethoxyacetaldehyde and by aldehyde dehydrogenase to 2-hydroxyethoxyacetate (2-HEAA); this is yet to be confirmed in humans. The metabolic acidosis observed in diethylene glycol poisoning is primarily due to 2-hydroxyethoxyacetate, but lactate also plays a part in severe poisoning. The precise aetiology of renal failure has not been elucidated but it is not due to accumulation of oxalate or calcium oxalate crystalluria.

Clinical features

Nausea, vomiting, and abdominal pain occur frequently and are followed by the development of jaundice and hepatomegaly, pulmonary oedema, metabolic acidosis, coma, and renal failure in most cases.

Management

Supportive measures to treat dehydration and to correct metabolic acidosis should be instituted promptly. Management is identical to that for ethylene glycol, with the use of fomepizole or ethanol to prevent metabolism of diethylene glycol and haemodialysis to remove the glycol. It is not known whether 2-hydroxyethoxyacetate is removed by dialysis.

Ethylene glycol (1,2-ethanediol)

Ethylene glycol has a variety of commercial applications and is commonly used as an antifreeze fluid in car radiators. Its sweet taste and ready availability have contributed to its popularity as a suicide agent and as a poor man's substitute for alcohol.

It is thought that the minimum lethal dose of ethylene glycol is about 100 ml for an adult, although recovery after treatment has been reported following the ingestion of up to 1 litre.

Mechanism of toxicity

The toxicity of ethylene glycol depends predominantly on its metabolites though the initial inebriation is due to ethylene glycol itself (Fig. 9.1.5). Central nervous system symptoms coincide with the peak production of glycolaldehyde; aldehydes inhibit many aspects of cellular metabolism. Glycolate is largely responsible for the marked acidosis seen in severe cases; lactate concentrations are generally not very high. Lactate is produced as a result of the large amount of NADH formed by the oxidation of ethylene glycol and by inhibition of the tricarboxylic acid cycle by the condensation products of glyoxylate. There is increasing evidence that calcium oxalate monohydrate crystals are the cause of cerebral oedema and renal failure.

Clinical features

The clinical features of ethylene glycol poisoning may be divided into three stages depending on the time after ingestion (Box 9.1.6). The severity of each stage and the progression from one stage to the next depends on the amount of ethylene glycol ingested. Death may occur during any of the three stages. Typically, hypocalcaemia and severe metabolic acidosis are present, together with calcium

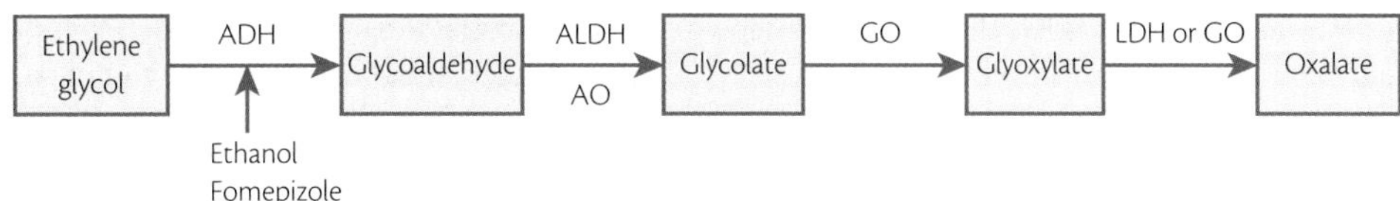

Fig. 9.1.5 Metabolism of ethylene glycol. ADH, alcohol dehydrogenase; ALDH, aldehyde dehydrogenase; AO, aldehyde oxidase; GO, glycolate oxidase; LDH, lactate dehydrogenase.

oxalate crystalluria. A serum ethylene glycol concentration in excess of 500 mg/litre indicates severe poisoning.

Management

Supportive measures to combat cardiorespiratory depression should be employed and metabolic acidosis, hypocalcaemia, and renal failure should be treated conventionally.

If the patient presents early after ingestion, the first priority is to inhibit metabolism using either intravenous ethanol or fomepizole. Fomepizole requires less monitoring, but is substantially more expensive than ethanol.

After a loading dose of fomepizole 15 mg/kg over 30 min, four 12-hourly doses of 10 mg/kg should be given, followed by 15 mg/kg 12-hourly until the glycol concentration is not detectable. If haemodialysis is used, the frequency of dosing should be increased to 4-hourly as fomepizole is dialysable.

Alternatively, a loading dose of intravenous ethanol 50 g for an adult (50 ml of absolute ethanol in 1 litre 5% dextrose, i.e. a 5% ethanol solution) should be given, followed by an intravenous infusion of ethanol, 10 to 12 g/h (most easily given as 1 litre 5% ethanol solution over 4 to 5 h), to achieve a blood ethanol concentration of approximately 1000 mg/litre. Administration of ethanol should be continued until the glycol is undetectable in the blood. If dialysis is used, greater amounts of ethanol (17–22 g/h) must be given, because ethanol is readily dialysable. Ideally, glycol and alcohol concentrations should be measured frequently until recovery.

Haemodialysis removes ethylene glycol, glycolaldehyde, and glycolate, but not oxalate and will also correct acid–base disturbances. Haemodialysis should be employed particularly if presentation is late and marked metabolic acidosis is present. Dialysis should be continued until the glycol and glycolate are no longer detectable in the blood.

Formaldehyde

Formaldehyde is a flammable, colourless gas with a pungent odour. It is most commonly available commercially as a 30 to 50% w/w aqueous solution and is an important raw material in the synthesis of organic compounds such as plastics and resins. It is added to cosmetics and foodstuffs as a preservative and antimicrobial agent and is used in embalming. Formaldehyde also occurs naturally in the environment. It is released during the combustion of organic materials, e.g. in forest fires, wood-burning stoves, and waste incinerators, and is a product of incomplete petrol combustion in internal combustion engines. Absorption may follow ingestion, inhalation, or dermal contact. Once absorbed, formaldehyde is oxidized rapidly to formic acid then converted more slowly to CO_2 and water.

Clinical features

Severe irritation of the mucous membranes of the eyes, nose, and upper airways occurs after minimal exposure to low (<5 ppm) formaldehyde concentrations, which tends to prevent higher exposure in even the most tolerant subjects. Substantial exposure may result in severe bronchospasm, pulmonary oedema, and death. Formaldehyde is a recognized cause of occupational asthma.

Formaldehyde solutions splashed into the eye have caused corneal damage and skin contamination has resulted in dermatitis. Spillage of phenol-formaldehyde resin on to the skin has produced extensive necrotic skin lesions, fever, hypertension, adult respiratory distress syndrome, proteinuria, and renal impairment. Ingestion of formaldehyde solution has resulted in severe corrosive damage to the buccal cavity and tonsils, oesophagus, and stomach with ulceration, necrosis, and subsequent fibrosis and contracture. Shock, metabolic acidosis (due in part to high formate concentrations), respiratory insufficiency, and renal impairment usually ensue. Death may follow ingestion of less than 100 ml in an adult.

Management

Supportive measures, including the correction of acid–base disturbance, should be employed. Haemodialysis is only moderately effective in increasing formate elimination.

n-Hexane

n-Hexane is an extremely volatile liquid that is used as a solvent. It is metabolized oxidatively to a number of compounds, including

Box 9.1.6 Clinical features of ethylene glycol poisoning

Stage 1 (30 min–12 h): gastrointestinal and nervous system involvement

- Apparent intoxication with alcohol (but no ethanol on breath)
- Nausea, vomiting, haematemesis
- Coma and convulsions (often focal)
- Nystagmus, ophthalmoplegias, papilloedema, depressed reflexes, myoclonic jerks
- V, VII, VIII nerve palsies
- Tetanic contractions

Stage 2 (12–24 h): cardiorespiratory involvement

- Tachypnoea, tachycardia
- Mild hypertension
- Pulmonary oedema
- Congestive cardiac failure

Stage 3 (24–72 h): renal involvement

- Flank pain, renal angle tenderness
- Acute tubular necrosis

2,5-hexanedione, which is eliminated through the urine and is implicated in the neurotoxic effect of this solvent.

Clinical features

When ingested *n*-hexane causes nausea, dizziness, central nervous system excitation, and then depression, and presents an acute aspiration hazard. Following inhalation, either inadvertently or deliberately, similar symptoms occur. The development of a progressive sensorimotor neuropathy is the principal hazard of chronic exposure.

Management

Treatment is supportive and symptomatic.

Hydrogen fluoride/hydrofluoric acid

Hydrogen fluoride is a corrosive, fuming, nearly colourless liquid (hydrofluoric acid) at atmospheric pressures and temperatures below 19 °C; above 19 °C it is gaseous. Hydrogen fluoride is very soluble in cold water and for this reason it fumes strongly in moist air. Aqueous solutions dissolve glass.

Mechanisms of toxicity

Hydrogen fluoride is particularly dangerous because of its unique ability among acids to penetrate tissue. The reason for this is the high electronegativity of fluorine, which forms a strong covalent bond with the hydrogen. The result is a weak acid that exists predominantly in the undissociated state. In the undissociated state, hydrogen fluoride is able to penetrate skin and soft tissue by nonionic diffusion. Once in the tissues, hydrogen fluoride dissociates and causes liquefactive necrosis of soft tissue, bony erosion, and extensive electrolyte abnormalities by binding the cations calcium and magnesium.

Clinical features

Hydrogen fluoride can cause severe systemic toxicity from even relatively small dermal exposures. Inhalation or ingestion of hydrogen fluoride causes severe corrosive damage similar to other acids (see p. 1306). Following absorption by whatever route, fluoride chelates calcium and lowers the serum ionized calcium concentration and causes weakness, paraesthesiae, tetany, and convulsions. Hypotension and cardiac arrhythmias, including ventricular fibrillation, may be observed. Central effects of fluoride include confusion, clouding of consciousness, and coma. Hepatic and renal failure may develop.

Skin contact with anhydrous hydrogen fluoride produces liquefactive necrosis and severe burns that are felt immediately. Concentrated aqueous solutions also cause an early sensation of pain but more dilute solutions may give no warning of injury. If the solution is not removed promptly, penetration of the skin by fluoride ion may occur, leading to painful ulcers that heal only slowly.

Management

Following inhalation of hydrogen fluoride, the casualty should be removed immediately from the contaminated atmosphere. Further treatment is symptomatic and supportive. Mechanical ventilation with positive end-expiratory pressure may be needed to treat pulmonary oedema.

If hydrofluoric acid has been ingested, management is as for other acids (see p. 1306). An intravenous injection of 10 ml of 10% calcium gluconate solution should be given.

Skin contact requires thorough washing of the affected area. Contaminated clothing should be removed, with rescuers protecting their hands with suitable gloves. The area should be washed with copious quantities of water for at least 5 to 10 min, even if there is no apparent burn or pain. Skin burns should be coated repeatedly with 2.5% calcium gluconate gel; the gel should be massaged continuously into the skin until at least 15 min after pain is relieved. The area should then be covered with a dressing soaked in the gel and lightly bandaged. If the gel is unavailable, immersion of the skin in iced water until the pain subsides is often helpful. If the pain does not subside, 10% calcium gluconate solution (up to 0.5 ml/cm^2) should be injected under the burn area, though calcium gluconate intraarterially may be more effective.

Hydrogen sulphide

Hydrogen sulphide is a colourless gas that smells of rotten eggs, although high concentrations cause olfactory nerve paralysis. The gas is also found in mines and sewers and is liberated from decomposing fish (a hazard in fishing boats if the hold is filled with 'trash' fish used for making fish meal) and liquid manure systems.

Mechanisms of toxicity

It is now thought that the serious sequelae following exposure to high concentrations of hydrogen sulphide are due principally to inhibition of cytochrome oxidase a_3, in which respect it may be more potent than cyanide.

Clinical features

Exposure to low concentrations leads to blepharospasm, pain, and redness of the eyes, blurred vision, and coloured haloes round lights. Headache, nausea, dizziness, drowsiness, sore throat, and cough may also occur. With exposure to higher concentrations, cyanosis, confusion, pulmonary oedema, coma, and convulsions are common. Death ensues in some 6% of cases.

Management

The casualty should be moved to fresh air from the contaminated atmosphere by a rescuer who has donned breathing apparatus beforehand.

It has been shown in mice that the administration of sodium nitrite is superior to oxygen alone in the treatment of acute hydrogen sulphide poisoning. However, the mechanism of this benefit is disputed and the value of this treatment in humans has not been established.

Isopropanol (isopropyl alcohol; 2-propanol)

Isopropanol is used as a sterilizing agent and as 'rubbing alcohol'. It is also found in aftershave lotions, disinfectants, and window-cleaning solutions. Intoxication can result from both ingestion and skin absorption. The accidental use of an isopropanol-containing enema has resulted in death. Isopropanol is oxidized in the liver to acetone.

Clinical features

Features of toxicity include coma and respiratory depression, the odour of acetone on the breath, gastritis, haematemesis, hypotension, hypothermia, renal tubular necrosis, acute myopathy and haemolytic anaemia; cardiac arrest has occurred.

Management

In addition to supportive measures, haemodialysis should be employed in severely poisoned patients as it removes isopropanol and acetone. No advantage is gained by administering ethanol or fomepizole to block alcohol dehydrogenase, because the toxicity of isopropanol is caused principally by the parent compound and not by acetone. Moreover, such treatment will enhance the toxicity of isopropanol.

Methanol (methyl alcohol)

Methanol is used widely as a solvent. It is also found in antifreeze solutions, paints, duplicating fluids, paint removers and varnishes, and shoe polishes. The ingestion of as little as 10 ml of pure methanol has caused permanent blindness and 30 ml is potentially fatal, although individual susceptibility varies widely. Toxicity may also occur as a result of inhalation or percutaneous absorption.

Mechanisms of toxicity

In humans, methanol is metabolized by alcohol dehydrogenase and catalase enzyme systems to formaldehyde and formic acid (Fig. 9.1.6). The concentration of formate increases greatly and is accompanied by accumulation of hydrogen ions, causing metabolic acidosis.

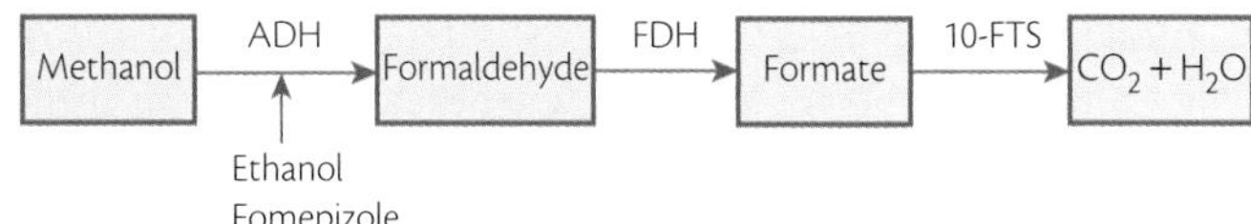

Fig. 9.1.6 Metabolism of methanol. ADH, alcohol dehydrogenase; FDH, formaldehyde dehydrogenase; 10-FTS, 10-formyl tetrahydrofolate synthetase.

Clinical features

Ingested alone, methanol causes mild and transient inebriation and drowsiness. After a latent period of 8 to 36 h, nausea, vomiting, abdominal pain, headaches, dizziness, and coma supervene. Blurred vision and diminished visual acuity may occur and the presence of dilated pupils, unreactive to light, suggests that permanent blindness is likely to ensue. A severe metabolic acidosis may develop and this may be accompanied by hyperglycaemia and raised serum amylase activity. A blood methanol concentration of more than 500 mg/litre confirms serious poisoning. Mortality increases with the severity and duration of the metabolic acidosis. Survivors may show permanent neurological sequelae including blindness, rigidity, hypokinesis, and other parkinsonian-like signs; these features follow the development of optic neuropathy and necrosis of the putamen.

Management

The treatment of methanol poisoning is directed towards (1) the correction of metabolic acidosis; (2) the inhibition of methanol oxidation; and (3) the removal of circulating methanol and its toxic metabolites. Substantial quantities of bicarbonate (often as much as 2 mol) may be required and since this must be accompanied by sodium, hypernatraemia and hypervolaemia may result.

Fomepizole and ethanol inhibit methanol oxidation. These antidotes should be given and monitored as for ethylene glycol. If admission plasma concentrations show that most of the methanol ingested has already been metabolized, ethanol or fomepizole administration will not be of benefit and ethanol might exacerbate the acidosis.

Dialysis is indicated when a patient has ingested more than 30 g of methanol, or develops metabolic acidosis, mental, visual, or fundoscopic abnormalities attributable to methanol, or a blood methanol concentration in excess of 500 mg/litre. Folinic acid 50 mg (1mg/kg in children) intravenously 6-hourly may protect against ocular toxicity by accelerating formate metabolism.

Methylene chloride (dichloromethane)

Methylene chloride is a common ingredient in paint removers and is used as a solvent for plastic films and cements and also as a degreaser and aerosol propellant. Exposures usually follow inhalation, though deliberate ingestion is recognized. Methylene chloride is metabolized to CO_2 and carbon monoxide. Carboxyhaemoglobin concentrations of 3 to 10% (exceptionally 40%) are attained.

Clinical features

Skin contact with liquid methylene chloride can cause a chemical burn. Following inhalation, dizziness, tingling and numbness of the extremities, throbbing headache, nausea, irritability, fatigue, and stupor have been reported. Severe and prolonged exposure may lead to irritant conjunctivitis, lacrimation, and respiratory depression. Hepatorenal dysfunction and pulmonary oedema have also been described. Fatalities have occurred. If high concentrations of carboxyhaemoglobin are present, the features of acute carbon monoxide poisoning may also be present, although these tend to be mild even in the presence of such high concentrations. Methylene chloride ingestion causes corrosive injury to the gastrointestinal tract, agitation, diaphoresis, and drowsiness with rapid progression to coma in severe cases. Consciousness is typically regained after several hours unless hypoxic encephalopathy ensues. Pancreatitis, hepatic dysfunction, and renal and respiratory failure are potential complications. Carboxyhaemoglobin concentrations may remain raised for days.

Management

Prompt removal from exposure prior to death usually results in complete recovery. Thereafter, treatment is supportive and should include the use of supplemental oxygen.

Nitrites

Volatile alkyl nitrites, e.g. amyl and butyl (predominantly isobutyl) nitrite, are popular recreational drugs. They are marketed as aphrodisiacs or 'room odourizers'. These agents are used to improve sexual performance, both enhancing and prolonging orgasm and/or as a smooth muscle relaxant to relax the anal sphincter. They also are claimed to promote a sense of increased well-being with temporary detachment from reality.

The alkyl nitrites cause vasodilatation via nitric oxide mediated vascular smooth muscle relaxation. Vasodilatation accounts for many of the effects observed or described by users following volatile nitrite abuse. However, clinically, the most important mechanism of nitrite toxicity relates to the ability of these agents to cause methaemoglobinaemia via oxidation of haem iron from the ferrous (Fe^{2+}) to the ferric (Fe^{3+}) state.

Clinical features

These reflect the action of nitrites as potent vasodilators with headache, flushing, blurred vision, postural hypotension, and syncope. Vasodilatation is followed by reflex vasoconstriction with sinus tachycardia. With continued exposure, methaemoglobinaemia results. Irritant effects including burning in the nose and eyes; cough and facial dermatitis are recognized; and transient ECG changes (T wave inversion and ST segment depression) have been reported. Methaemoglobin concentrations less than 20% are usually asymptomatic though they cause slate-grey 'cyanosis' due predominantly to the presence of pigmented methaemoglobin. When 20 to 40% total haemoglobin is replaced by methaemoglobin, there may be dizziness and headache, features not dissimilar to those caused by vasodilatation. Higher methaemoglobin concentrations reflect increasing tissue hypoxia and are unusual following volatile nitrite abuse unless inhalation is substantial or ingestion has occurred. However, in these circumstances, life-threatening methaemoglobinaemia may result.

Management

The vasodilatory effects of volatile nitrite abuse are not usually severe and can be managed supportively. In healthy adults, methaemoglobin concentrations less than 30% total haemoglobin are unlikely to warrant specific treatment. At higher methaemoglobin concentrations, or where clinical features suggest tissue hypoxia, antidotal therapy with intravenous methylthioninium chloride (methylene blue) 2 mg/kg body weight as a 1% solution should be given over 5 to 10 min. Treatment is effective within 30 min and a second dose is required rarely.

Nitrogen dioxide

Combustion of fossil fuels yields nitric oxide and nitrogen dioxide (a largely insoluble, brown, mildly irritating gas). Fermentation of silage produces high concentrations of this gas within 2 days of filling the silo. It is also a by-product of many industrial processes.

Clinical features

The clinical features following acute exposure to high concentrations of nitrogen dioxide depend on the concentration and duration of exposure to the gas. Since nitrogen dioxide is only a mild upper respiratory tract irritant, modest acute exposure (<50 ppm) for a short time often produces no immediate symptoms, although throat irritation, cough, transient choking, tightness in the chest, and sweating have been observed. By contrast, exposure to a massive concentration of nitrogen dioxide, such as that found in a silo, can produce severe and immediate hypoxaemia which may be fatal. In less severe cases, the onset of symptoms may be delayed for a few hours (typically 3–36 h) and the patient then develops dyspnoea, chest pain (which may be pleuritic), haemoptysis, tachycardia, headache, conjunctivitis, generalized weakness, and dizziness (which may be due to hypotension). Bronchiolitis obliterans may develop within 2 to 6 weeks.

Management

Bronchodilator and corticosteroid therapy is sufficient in most cases. Pulmonary oedema responds poorly to diuretics; corticosteroids, and mechanical ventilation with positive end-expiratory pressure offer the best hope of reducing the mortality.

Paraffin oil (kerosene)

Paraffin oil has three physical properties accounting for its toxicity. Its low viscosity and surface tension allow it to spread rapidly throughout the lungs when aspirated after ingestion, and its low vapour pressure makes it unlikely to cause poisoning by inhalation.

Clinical features

Repeated local application to the skin results in dryness, dermatitis, and, rarely, epidermal necrolysis. Paraffin ingestion causes a burning sensation in the mouth and throat, vomiting, diarrhoea, and abdominal pain. Pulmonary features may occur within 1 h of ingestion with cough, tachypnoea, tachycardia, basal crackles, and cyanosis. Nonsegmental consolidation or collapse is seen radiologically. Pneumatocoele formation, pneumothorax, pleural effusion, or pulmonary oedema may occur. Other complications include hepatic dysfunction and in severe cases atrial fibrillation and ventricular fibrillation.

Management

Gastric lavage and emesis should be avoided because of the increased risk of chemical pneumonitis. There is no evidence that corticosteroids and antibiotics reduce morbidity or mortality; mechanical ventilation with positive end expiratory pressure may be necessary in severe cases of aspiration.

Petrol (gasoline)

Petrol is a complex mixture of volatile hydrocarbons containing a small proportion of nonhydrocarbon additives.

Clinical features

Following the inhalation of petrol, dizziness and irritation of the eyes, nose, and throat may occur within 5 min followed by euphoria, headache, and blurred vision. If inhalation continues, or if significant quantities of petrol are ingested, then excitement and depression of the nervous system occurs; incoordination, restlessness, excitement, confusion, disorientation, hallucinations, ataxia, nystagmus, tremor, delirium, coma, and convulsions may be seen. Inhalation of high concentrations of petrol may cause immediate death, probably from ventricular fibrillation or respiratory failure. Chemical pneumonitis may occur as in paraffin oil ingestion (see above) and the clinical features and management are then identical. In addition, intravascular haemolysis, hypofibrinogenaemia and cardiorespiratory arrest have been reported, together with (in one patient) epiglottitis so severe that near total airway obstruction resulted.

Management

Following removal from exposure, supportive measures provide the basis of treatment.

Phenol

Phenol ('carbolic acid') is nearly always recognizable by its odour and, distinctively, the pain to which it gives rise is much less than might be expected. This is due to its ability to damage afferent nerve endings.

Clinical features

If phenol is spilt on the skin, pain is followed promptly by numbness. The skin becomes blanched, and a dry opaque eschar forms over the burn. When the eschar sloughs off, a brown stain remains. Phenol penetrates intact skin rapidly and is well absorbed through the lungs. After ingestion, vomiting and abdominal pain occur. Systemic toxicity may follow exposure by any route. Features include coma, loss of vasoconstrictor tone, and hypothermia together with cardiac and respiratory depression. An initial phase of central nervous system stimulation, and rarely convulsions, has sometimes been observed in children. Phenol poisoning is associated with grey or black urine and though this is due in part to metabolites of phenol, Heinz body haemolytic anaemia, as well as methaemoglobinaemia and hyperbilirubinaemia are recognized features. Renal complications are seen frequently.

Management

Skin and eye contamination, renal failure, and methaemoglobinaemia are managed conventionally.

Phosgene

Phosgene is a colourless gas, which is now used in the synthesis of isocyanates, polyurethane and polycarbonate resins, and dyes; it is also produced in fires.

Mechanism of toxicity

Phosgene reacts with glutathione. When glutathione stores become depleted beyond a critical level, covalent binding occurs between phosgene and cell macromolecules with resultant hepatic and renal necrosis.

Clinical features

Exposure to phosgene causes irritation of the eyes, dryness or burning sensation in the throat, cough, chest pain, and nausea and vomiting. There is usually a latent period lasting between 30 min and 24 h (rarely, 72 h) during which the casualty suffers little discomfort and has no abnormal chest signs. Subsequently, pulmonary oedema develops due to increased capillary permeability; circulatory collapse may follow.

Management

Administration of acetylcysteine may confer some protection. Oxygen should be administered. Mechanical ventilation may be life-saving in severe cases.

Phosphine

Phosphine is a colourless gas with a fish-like odour. It is used to treat silicon crystals in the semiconductor industry.

Clinical features

Fatigue, nausea, vomiting, diarrhoea, chest tightness, breathlessness, productive cough, dizziness, and headache are common features of acute phosphine exposure. Acute pulmonary oedema, hypertension, cardiac arrhythmias, and convulsions have been described in severe cases. Ataxia, intention tremor, and diplopia may be found on examination. Focal myocardial infiltration with necrosis, pulmonary oedema, and widespread small-vessel injury were found at autopsy in a child who died.

Management

The casualty should be removed from exposure as soon as possible. Thereafter, treatment is supportive and symptomatic. The value of steroids in preventing pulmonary damage (which may be delayed) has not been established.

Propylene glycol (1,2-propanediol)

Propylene glycol is used widely as a preservative and solvent for oral, intravenous, and topical medications. It is oxidized to lactic acid and pyruvate via hepatic alcohol and aldehyde dehydrogenases in a similar way to the metabolism of other glycols such as ethylene glycol.

Clinical features

The ingestion of substantial quantities of propylene glycol or its administration to neonates, those in renal failure, or in exceptionally large doses (such as patients requiring massive parenteral doses of propylene glycol-containing benzodiazepines in the management of acute alcohol withdrawal) may cause convulsions, coma, cardiac arrhythmias, hepatorenal damage, intravascular haemolysis, metabolic acidosis, and increased serum osmolality.

Management

Metabolic acidosis, renal failure, and respiratory depression should be treated conventionally. Haemodialysis removes propylene glycol efficiently. Ethanol or fomepizole may be used to inhibit propylene glycol metabolism in a similar way to their use in ethylene glycol poisoning, but in practice the diagnosis is often not made until a significant acidosis is present and thus it is too late for antidotal treatment to be useful.

Sulphur dioxide

Sulphur dioxide is a colourless gas, which has a pungent irritating odour. The combustion of fuels for heating and power generation results in environmental pollution from this cause. Sulphur dioxide is also employed in the manufacture of sulphuric acid and is a potential occupational problem in paper mills, steel works, and oil refineries.

Mechanism of toxicity

The irritant effects of sulphur dioxide are thought to be caused by the rapidity with which it forms sulphurous acid on contact with moist membranes.

Clinical features

Following exposure to sulphur dioxide, lacrimation, rhinorrhoea, cough, increased bronchial secretions, bronchoconstriction, and, in severe cases, pulmonary oedema, and respiratory arrest occur. Corneal burns can follow eye exposure and liquefied sulphur dioxide can cause skin burns. Survivors of massive sulphur dioxide exposure have shown a chronic obstructive defect in serial pulmonary studies along with bronchial hyperactivity.

Management

After removal from exposure, admission to hospital for observation is mandatory in severe cases to ensure that delayed pulmonary oedema is treated effectively. Symptomatic and supportive measures should be given and, if necessary, mechanical ventilation with positive end-expiratory pressure should be undertaken if diuretics alone do not control pulmonary oedema; the role of corticosteroids is uncertain. The eyes and skin should be irrigated with water, if exposure has occurred.

Tetrachloroethylene (perchloroethylene)

Tetrachloroethylene is a colourless, nonflammable liquid with a chloroform-like odour. It is used widely as an industrial solvent, particularly for dry-cleaning and degreasing. Poisoning may occur by inhalation or ingestion.

Mechanisms of toxicity

A considerable proportion of an inspired dose is exhaled unchanged, and that retained is excreted only slowly (half-life *c.*144 h) mainly by metabolism to trichloroacetic acid, the major urinary metabolite.

Clinical features

Following inhalation or ingestion, there is depression of the central nervous system; nausea and vomiting may occur and persist for several hours. Irritation of the eyes, nose, and throat may occur. Hepatic and renal dysfunction may also develop and ventricular arrhythmias and noncardiogenic pulmonary oedema have been reported.

Management

After removal from exposure, treatment is supportive and symptomatic.

Toluene

Toluene has much lower volatility and toxicity than benzene. It is used extensively as a solvent in the chemical, rubber, paint, glue, and pharmaceutical industries and as a thinner for inks, perfumes, and dyes.

Metabolism

Following inhalation or ingestion, toluene is oxidized to benzoic acid then to hippuric acid benzoylglucuronates, which are excreted in the urine.

Clinical features

Acute poisoning results in euphoria, excitement, dizziness, confusion, increased lacrimation, headache, nervousness, nausea, tinnitus, ataxia, tremor, and coma.

A review of adults who had abused toluene indicated three major patterns of presentation: (1) muscle weakness, (2) gastrointestinal complaints (abdominal pain, haematemesis), and (3) neuropsychiatric disorders (altered mental status, cerebellar abnormalities, peripheral neuropathy). In addition, hypokalaemia, hypophosphataemia, and hyperchloraemia were common. Rhabdomyolysis occurred in 40% of cases. Distal renal tubular acidosis and urinary calculi were also reported. Cardiac and haematological toxicity due to toluene appears to be uncommon.

Management

If poisoning results from inhalation, whether accidental or intentional, the patient should be removed from the contaminated environment. Thereafter, treatment consists of symptomatic and supportive measures.

1,1,1-Trichloroethane (methyl chloroform)

1,1,1-Trichloroethane is a colourless, nonflammable liquid of high volatility widely used as a solvent in industry, in the office (e.g. typewriter correction fluid), and at home (e.g. aerosol waterproofing products). 1,1,1-Trichloroethane has low systemic toxicity because only small amounts of trichloroacetic acid and trichloroethanol are formed. Most of an inhaled dose is expired unchanged. Concomitant ingestion of ethanol is known to enhance toxicity.

Clinical features

Following inhalation of a sufficiently large dose, central nervous system depression occurs in proportion to the amount inhaled; hepatic and renal dysfunction may also result. Deaths have followed exposure to very high concentrations in unventilated tanks. In such cases, death may either be due to central nervous system depression, culminating in respiratory arrest, or to fatal arrhythmias as a result of myocardial sensitization to circulating catecholamines in the presence of hypoxia. Inhalation of a weatherproofing aerosol containing 96.6% 1,1,1-trichloroethane has been reported to give rise to transient shortness of breath, constricting chest pain, cough, and myalgia.

Management

The casualty should be removed from the contaminated environment. Thereafter treatment is symptomatic and supportive.

Trichloroethylene

Trichloroethylene is a colourless, volatile liquid used widely as an industrial solvent, particularly in metal degreasing and extraction processes. Trichloroethylene is absorbed readily from the gut and through the skin and lungs. Following inhalation, it is excreted unchanged in the breath and metabolized via chloral hydrate to trichloroethanol and trichloroacetic acid, which are excreted in the urine.

Clinical features

Following inhalation, ingestion, or dermal absorption, central nervous system depression occurs with nausea and vomiting, hepatic and renal dysfunction, and death. 'Degreaser's flush' (in which the skin of the face and arms becomes markedly reddened) may occur if ethanol is consumed shortly before or after exposure to trichloroethylene. Cranial nerve damage, cerebellar dysfunction, and convulsions have been described.

Management

Removal from exposure will reduce central nervous system depression, and thereafter, whether trichloroethylene has been inhaled, ingested, or absorbed through the skin, treatment is supportive and symptomatic.

Household products

There is a commonly held belief that household products contain a wide range of highly toxic chemicals, and so the ingestion of these substances by children is a frequent cause for alarm in parents and doctors alike. Even when the toxicity of a household product is high, the risk it poses is usually low, certainly when ingested accidentally. However, adults intent on self-harm may, by deliberately swallowing massive quantities, succeed in killing themselves.

Antiseptics

Antiseptics are chemicals that are applied to living tissue to kill or inhibit microorganisms. The most commonly used are alcohols: ethanol (see p. 1287), isopropanol (see p. 1312), propanol, or mixtures of these alcohols. In addition, chlorhexidine, iodine-containing compounds, and hydrogen peroxide are also employed.

Clinical features

Ingestion of a substantial quantity results in a sensation of burning in the mouth and throat followed by drowsiness, stupor, depression of respiration, and coma.

Management

Management is supportive (see also sections on ethanol, p. 1287 and isopropanol, p. 1312).

Bleaches

Household bleach is normally a 3 to 6% solution of sodium hypochlorite, whereas industrial bleaches contain more than 10%. Some bleaches contain hydrogen peroxide. Household bleach may give rise to toxic gases such as chlorine and chloramine if mixed with other cleaning agents in a lavatory bowl.

Clinical features

Ingestion of hypochlorite may cause a burning sensation in the mouth, throat, and oesophagus, accompanied by a sensation of thirst, vomiting, and abdominal discomfort. Pharyngeal and laryngeal oedema may develop.

Management

Small quantities of household bleach can be managed conservatively with sips of water or milk. In the case of concentrated bleach, endoscopy should be considered. Nasogastric aspiration may be considered providing the airway can be protected. Appropriate management of pain is necessary. Chlorine release in the stomach may also occur and result in toxic injury to the lung.

Dishwashing liquids, fabric conditioners, and household detergents

Most of these products, including carpet shampoo, rinse aid for dishwashing machines, fabric washing powder and flakes, scouring liquids, creams, and powders, contain surfactants that have both hydrophilic and lipophilic groups to allow fat-soluble substances to be dispersed in aqueous media.

There are three types of surfactants of differing toxicity: anionic surfactants, which have a negative electrical charge on the lipophilic groups; cationic surfactants, which have a positive charge; and nonionic surfactants which have no charge.

Dishwasher detergent products are more toxic, particularly for children, as they are alkaline and contain polyphosphates, metasilicate, and sodium hydroxide. Their effects are therefore more akin to that of a moderate alkali (see section on alkalis, p. 1307).

Clinical features

Anionic detergents irritate the skin by removing natural oils and cause redness, soreness, and even a papular dermatitis. Ingestion may cause mild gastrointestinal irritation, nausea, vomiting, and diarrhoea. Nonionic surfactants irritate the skin only slightly and appear to be completely harmless when ingested. Cationic surfactants (e.g. quarternary ammonium compounds) are much more toxic than the others, but are rarely found in household cleaning materials.

Management

After ingestion of products containing either a nonionic or anionic surfactant, liberal amounts of water or milk should be administered.

Disinfectants

These are chemicals that are applied to inanimate objects to kill microorganisms. Once these solutions commonly contained phenol, but this has largely been replaced by either chlorophenol or chloroxylenols (parachlorometaxylenol and dichlorometaxylenol), which, although less toxic than phenol, can still be hazardous if ingested in large quantities. Quarternary ammonium compounds such as benzalkonium chloride, cetyl trimethylammonium bromide, cetylpyridinium chloride, cetylpyridinium chloride, and benzethonium chloride are also used as disinfectants. Sodium hypochlorite (bleach; see above) and formaldehyde are other examples.

Clinical features

Burning in the mouth and throat with nausea and vomiting is typical after ingestion of a phenolic compound. Swelling and superficial ulceration in the mouth and upper alimentary tract develop and the larynx may be involved leading to stridor and breathlessness. Haemorrhagic tracheobronchitis and pulmonary oedema may develop and aspiration has been reported though this may have been due to other ingredients in the formulation. Dermal contact may cause full-thickness burns.

Lavatory cleaners, sanitizers, and deodorants

Solid lavatory sanitizer or deodorant blocks may contain paradichlorobenzene. Ingestion can cause nausea, vomiting, diarrhoea, and abdominal pain. Management is supportive.

Further reading

Epidemiology

Anon (2006). Deaths related to drug poisoning: England and Wales, 2000–2004. *Health Statist*, **29**, 69–76.

Bateman DN, *et al.* (2006). Legislation restricting paracetamol sales and patterns of self-harm and death from paracetamol-containing preparations in Scotland. *Br J Clin Pharmacol*, **62**, 573–81.

Camidge DR, Wood RJ, Bateman DN (2003). The epidemiology of self-poisoning in the UK. *Br J Clin Pharmacol*, **56**, 613–9.

Eddleston M (2000). Patterns and problems of deliberate self poisoning in the developing world. *Q J Med*, **93**, 715–31.

Immediate treatment

Barceloux D, *et al.* (2004). Position paper: cathartics. *Clin Toxicol*, **42**, 243–53.

Chyka PA, *et al.* (2005). Position paper: single-dose activated charcoal. *Clin Toxicol*, **43**, 61–87.

Krenzelok EP, *et al.* (2004). Position paper: ipecac syrup. *Clin Toxicol*, **42**, 133–43.

Kulig K, Vale JA (2004). Position paper: gastric lavage. *Clin Toxicol*, **42**, 933–43.

Tenenbein M (2004). Position paper: whole bowel irrigation. *Clin Toxicol*, **42**, 843–54.

Methods to increase poison elimination

Eddleston M, *et al.* (2008). Multiple-dose activated charcoal in acute self-poisoning: a randomised controlled trial. *Lancet*, **371**, 579–87.

Kay TD, Playford HR, Johnson DW (2003). Hemodialysis versus continuous veno-venous hemodiafiltration in the management of severe valproate overdose. *Clin Nephrol*, **59**, 56–8.

Proudfoot AT, Krenzelok EP, Vale JA (2004). Position paper on urine alkalinization. *Clin Toxicol*, **42**, 1–26.

Proudfoot AT, *et al.* (2003). Does urine alkalinization increase salicylate elimination? If so, why? *Toxicol Rev*, **22**, 129–36.

Vale JA, *et al.* (1999). Position statement and practice guidelines on the use of multi-dose activated charcoal in the treatment of acute poisoning. *Clin Toxicol*, **37**, 731–51.

Drugs (including substances of abuse)

Amphetamines

Barr AM, *et al.* (2006). The need for speed: an update on methamphetamine addiction. *J Psychiatry Neurosci*, **31**, 301–13.

de la Torre R, *et al.* (2004). Human pharmacology of MDMA: pharmacokinetics, metabolism, and disposition. *Ther Drug Monit*, **26**, 137–44.

Derlet RW, *et al.* (1989). Amphetamine toxicity: experience with 127 cases. *J Emerg Med*, **7**, 157–61.

Freedman RR, Johanson CE, Tancer ME (2005). Thermoregulatory effects of 3,4-methylenedioxymethamphetamine (MDMA) in humans. *Psychopharmacology*, **183**, 248–56.

Hall AP, Henry JA (2006). Acute toxic effects of 'Ecstasy' (MDMA) and related compounds: overview of pathophysiology and clinical management. *Br J Anaesth*, **96**, 678–85.

Hartung TK, *et al.* (2002). Hyponatraemic states following 3,4-methylenedioxymethamphetamine (MDMA, 'ecstasy') ingestion. *Q J Med*, **95**, 431–7.

ACE inhibitors

Christie GA, *et al.* (2006). Redefining the ACE-inhibitor dose-response relationship: substantial blood pressure lowering after massive doses. *Eur J Clin Pharmacol*, **62**, 989–93.

Friedman JM (2006). ACE inhibitors and congenital anomalies. *N Engl J Med*, **354**, 2498–500.

Lip GY, Ferner RE (1995). Poisoning and anti-hypertensive drugs; angiotensin converting enzyme inhibitors. *J Hum Hypertens*, **9**, 711–5.

Antibiotics

Holdiness MR (1989). A review of the red man syndrome and rifampicin overdose. *Med Toxicol Adverse Drug Exp*, **4**, 444–51.

Jones DP, *et al.* (1993). Acute renal failure following amoxycillin overdose. *Clin Pediatr*, **32**, 735–9.

Tenenbein MS, Tenenbein M (2005). Acute pancreatitis due to erythromycin overdose. *Pediatr Emerg Care*, **21**, 675–7.

Vannaprasaht S, *et al.* (2006). Ceftazidime overdose-related nonconvulsive status epilepticus after intraperitoneal instillation. *Clin Toxicol*, **44**, 383–6.

Anticonvulsants

Eyer F, *et al.* (2005). Acute valproate poisoning: pharmacokinetics, alteration in fatty acid metabolism, and changes during therapy. *J Clin Psychopharmacol*, **25**, 376–80.

Isbister GK, *et al.* (2003). Valproate overdose: a comparative cohort study of self poisonings. *Br J Clin Pharmacol*, **55**, 398–404.

Thanacoody RHK (2009). Extracorporeal elimination in acute valproic acid poisoning. *Clin Toxicol*, **47**, 609–16.

Antidepressants

Bateman DN (2005). Tricyclic antidepressant poisoning: central nervous system effects and management. *Toxicol Rev*, **24**, 181–6.

Bradberry SM, *et al.* (2005). Management of the cardiovascular complications of tricyclic antidepressant poisoning: role of sodium bicarbonate. *Toxicol Rev*, **24**, 195–204.

Buckley NA, *et al.* (1996). Interrater agreement in the measurement of QRS interval in tricyclic antidepressant overdose: implications for monitoring and research. *Ann Emerg Med*, **28**, 515–9.

Isbister GK, *et al.* (2004). Relative toxicity of selective serotonin reuptake inhibitors (SSRIs) in overdose. *Clin Toxicol*, **42**, 277–85.

Phillips S, *et al.* (1997). Fluoxetine versus tricyclic antidepressants: a prospective multicenter study of antidepressant drug overdoses. *J Emerg Med*, **15**, 439–45.

Thanacoody HK, Thomas SH (2005). Tricyclic antidepressant poisoning: cardiovascular toxicity. *Toxicol Rev*, **24**, 205–14.

Whyte IM, Dawson IM, Buckley NA (2003). Relative toxicity of venlafaxine and selective serotonin reuptake inhibitors in overdose compared to tricyclic antidepressants. *Q J Med*, **96**, 369–74.

Antihistamines

Khosla U, Ruel K, Hunt, DP (2003). Antihistamine-induced rhabdomyolysis. *South Med J*, **96**, 1023–6.

Zareba W, *et al.* (1997). Electrocardiographic findings in patients with diphenhydramine overdose. *AmJ Cardiol*, **80**, 1168–73.

Antimalarials

Clemessy JL, *et al.* (1996). Treatment of acute chloroquine poisoning: a 5-year experience. *Crit Care Med*, **24**, 1189–95.

Jaeger A, *et al.* (1987). Clinical features and management of poisoning due to antimalarial drugs. *Med Toxicol*, **2**, 242–73.

McKenzie AG (1996). Intensive therapy for chloroquine poisoning—a review of 29 cases. *S Afr Med J*, **86**, 597–9.

Antipsychotics

Burns MJ (2001). The pharmacology and toxicology of atypical antipsychotic agents. *Clin Toxicol*, **39**, 1–14.

Hulisz DT, *et al.* (1994). Complete heart block and torsades de pointes associated with thioridazine poisoning. *Pharmacotherapy*, **14**, 239–45.

Isbister GK, Balit CR, Kilham HA (2005). Antipsychotic poisoning in young children. A systematic review. *Drug Saf*, **28**, 1029–44.

James LP, *et al.* (2000). Phenothiazine, butyrophenones, and other psychotropic medication poisoning in children and adolescents. *Clin Toxicol*, **38**, 615–23.

Strachan EM, Kelly CA, Bateman DN (2004). Electrocardiogram and cardiovascular changes in thioridazine and chlorpromazine poisoning. *Eur J Clin Pharmacol*, **60**, 541–5.

Trenton A, Currier G, Zwemer F (2003). Fatalities associated with therapeutic use and overdose of atypical antipsychotics. *CNS Drugs*, **17**, 307–24.

Barbiturates

Vale JA, *et al.* (1999). Position statement and practice guidelines on the use of multi-dose activated charcoal in the treatment of acute poisoning. *Clin Toxicol*, **37**, 731–51.

Benzodiazepines

Hojer J, Baechrendtz S, Gustafsson L (1989). Benzodiazepine poisoning: Experience of 702 admissions to an intensive care unit during a 14-year period. *J Int Med*, **226**, 117–22.

Weinbroum A, *et al.* (1996). Use of flumazenil in the treatment of drug overdose: a double-blind and open clinical study in 110 patients. *Crit Care Med*, **24**, 199–206.

β-Blockers

Bailey B (2003). Glucagon in β-blocker and calcium channel blocker overdoses: a systematic review. *Clin Toxicol*, **41**, 595–602.

DeWitt CR, Waksman JC (2004). Pharmacology, pathophysiology and management of calcium channel blocker and beta-blocker toxicity. *Toxicol Rev*, **23**, 223–38.

Lip GYH, Ferner RE (1995). Poisoning with anti-hypertensive drugs: beta-adrenoreceptor blocker drugs. *J Hum Hypertens*, **9**, 213–21.

β_2-Adrenoceptor agonists

Leikin JB, *et al.* (1994). Hypokalemia after pediatric albuterol overdose: a case series. *Am J Emerg Med*, **12**, 64–6.

Lewis LD, *et al.* (1993). A study of self-poisoning with oral salbutamol—laboratory and clinical features. *Hum Exp Toxicol*, **12**, 397–401.

Minton NA, Baird AR, Henry JA (1989). Modulation of the effects of salbutamol by propranolol and atenolol. *Eur J Clin Pharmacol*, **36**, 449–53.

Bismuth chelate

Akpolat I, *et al.* (1996). Acute renal failure due to overdose of colloidal bismuth. *Nephrol Dial Transplant*, **11**, 1890–1.

Slikkerveer A, *et al.* (1998). Comparison of enhanced elimination of bismuth in humans after treatment with meso-2,3-dimercaptosuccinic acid and D,L-2,3-dimercaptopropane-1-sulfonic acid. *Analyst*, **123**, 91–2.

Stevens PE, *et al.* (1995). Significant elimination of bismuth by haemodialysis with a new heavy-metal chelating agent. *Nephrol Dial Transplant*, **10**, 696–8.

Calcium channel blockers

Holzer M, *et al.* (1999). Successful resuscitation of a verapamil-intoxicated patient with percutaneous cardiopulmonary bypass. *Crit Care Med*, **27**, 2818–23.

Lip GY, Ferner RE (1995). Poisoning with anti-hypertensive drugs: calcium antagonists. *J Hum Hypertens*, **9**, 155–61.

Proano L, Chiang WK, Wang RY (1995). Calcium channel blocker overdose. *Am J Emerg Med*, **13**, 444–50.

Yuan TH, *et al.* (1999). Insulin-glucose as adjunctive therapy for severe calcium channel antagonist poisoning. *Clin Toxicol*, **37**, 463–74.

Cannabis

Ashton CH (2001). Pharmacology and effects of cannabis: a brief review. *Br J Psychiatry*, **178**, 101–6.

Moore THM, *et al.* (2007). Cannabis use and risk of psychotic or affective mental health outcomes: a systematic review. *Lancet*, **370**, 319–28.

Cocaine

Brown E, *et al.* (1992). CNS complications of cocaine abuse: prevalence, pathophysiology, and neuroradiology. *Am J Roentgenol*, **159**, 137–47.

Hollander JE (1996). Cocaine-associated myocardial infarction. *J R Soc Med*, **89**, 443–7.

Kloner RA, *et al.* (1992). The effects of acute and chronic cocaine use on the heart. *Circulation*, **85**, 407–19.

Rubin RB, Neugarten J (1992). Medical complications of cocaine: changes in pattern of use and spectrum of complications. *Clin Toxicol*, **30**, 1–12.

Sporer KA, Firestone J (1997). Clinical course of crack cocaine body stuffers. *Ann Emerg Med*, **29**, 596–601.

Dapsone

Ferguson AJ, Lavery GG (1997). Deliberate self-poisoning with dapsone—a case report and summary of relevant pharmacology and treatment. *Anaesthesia*, **52**, 359–63.

Digoxin and digitoxin

Bateman DN (2004). Digoxin-specific antibody fragments. How much and when?. *Toxicol Rev*, **23**, 135–43.

Kinlay S, Buckley NA (1995). Magnesium sulfate in the treatment of ventricular arrhythmias due to digoxin toxicity. *J Toxicol—Clin Toxicol*, **33**, 55–9.

Williamson KM, *et al.* (1998). Digoxin toxicity: an evaluation in current clinical practice. *Arch Int Med*, **158**, 2444–9.

Diuretics

Lip GY, Ferner RE (1995). Poisoning and anti-hypertensive drugs: diuretics and potassium supplements. *J Hum Hypertens*, **9**, 295–301.

Ethanol

Boba A (1999). Management of acute alcoholic intoxication. *Am J Emerg Med*, **17**, 431.

Ernst AA, *et al.* (1996). Ethanol ingestion and related hypoglycemia in a pediatric and adolescent emergency department population. *Acad Emerg Med*, **3**, 46–9.

Lamminpää A, *et al.* (1993). Alcohol intoxication in hospitalized young teenagers. *Acta Paediatr*, **82**, 783–8.

Zehtabchi S, *et al.* (2005). Does ethanol explain the acidosis commonly seen in ethanol-intoxicated patients?. *Clin Toxicol*, **43**, 161–6.

γ-Hydroxybutyrate

Tarabar AF, Nelson LS (2004). The gamma-hydroxybutyrate withdrawal syndrome. *Toxicol Rev*, **23**, 45–9.

Van Sassenbroeck DK, *et al.* (2007). Abrupt awakening phenomenon associated with gamma-hydroxybutyrate use: a case series. *Clin Toxicol*, **45**, 533–8.

Hypoglycaemic agents

Palatnick W, Meatherall RC, Tenenbein M (1991). Clinical spectrum of sulfonylurea overdose and experience with diazoxide therapy. *Arch Int Med*, **151**, 1859–62.

Quadrani DA, Spiller HA, Widder P (1996). Five year retrospective evaluation of sulfonylurea ingestion in children. *J Toxicol Clin Toxicol*, **34**, 267–70.

Roberge RJ, Martin TG, Delbridge TR (1993). Intentional massive insulin overdose: recognition and management. *Ann of Emerg Med*, **22**, 228–34.

Iron

Anderson BD, *et al.* (2000). Retrospective analysis of ingestions of iron containing products in the United States: are there differences between chewable vitamins and adult preparations?. *J Emerg Med*, **19**, 255–8.

Fine JS (2000). Iron poisoning. *Curr Probl Paediatr Adolescent Health Care*, **30**, 71–90.

Robertson A, Tenenbein M (2005). Hepatotoxicity in acute iron poisoning. *Hum Exp Toxicol*, **24**, 559–62.

Tenenbein M (1996). Benefits of parenteral deferoxamine for acute iron poisoning. *Clin Toxicol*, **34**, 485–9.

Tran T, *et al.* (2000). Intentional iron overdose in pregnancy—management and outcome. *J Emerg Med*, **18**, 225–8.

Isoniazid

Blowey DL, Johnson D, Verjee Z (1995). Isoniazid-associated rhabdomyolysis. *Am J Emerg Med*, **13**, 543–4.

Girnani A, *et al.* (1992). Acute isoniazid poisoning. *Anaesthesia*, **47**, 781–3.

Wilcox WD, Hacker YE, Geller RJ (1996). Acute isoniazid overdose in a compliant adolescent patient. *Clin Pediatr*, **35**, 213–4.

Lithium carbonate

Beckmann U, *et al.* (2001). Efficacy of continuous venovenous hemodialysis in the treatment of severe lithium toxicity. *J Toxicol Clin Toxicol*, **39**, 393–7.

LeBlanc M, *et al.* (1996). Lithium poisoning treated by high performance continuous arteriovenous and venovenous hemodiafiltration. *Am J Kidney Dis*, **27**, 365–72.

Waring WS (2006). Management of lithium toxicity. *Toxicol Rev*, **25**, 221–30.

LSD

Klock JC, Boerner U, Becker CE (1973). Coma, hyperthermia and bleeding associated with massive LSD overdose. A report of eight cases. *West J Med*, **120**, 183–8.

Kulig K (1980). LSD. *Emerg Med Clin North Am*, **8**, 551–8.

Metoclopramide

Bateman DN, *et al.* (1989). Extrapyramidal reactions to metoclopramide and prochlorperazine. *Q J Med*, **71**, 307–11.

Miller LG, Jankovic J (1989). Metoclopramide-induced movement disorders. *Arch Int Med*, **149**, 2486–92.

Nitrates

Bruning-Fann CS, Kaneene JB (1993). The effects of nitrate, nitrite and *N*-nitroso compounds on human health: A review. *Vet Hum Toxicol*, **35**, 521–38.

Sanders P, Faunt J (1997). An unusual cause of cyanosis (isosorbide dinitrate induced methaemoglobinaemia). *Aust N Z J Med*, **27**, 596.

NSAIDs

Turnbull AJ, Campbell P, Hughes JA (1988). Mefenamic acid nephropathy—acute renal failure in overdose. *BMJ*, **296**, 646.

Opioids

Afshari R, *et al.* (2005). Co-proxamol overdose is associated with a 10-fold excess mortality compared with other paracetamol combination analgesics. *Br J Clin Pharmacol*, **60**, 444–7.

Goldfrank L, *et al.* (1986). A dosing nomogram for continuous infusion of intravenous naloxone. *Ann Emerg Med*, **15**, 566–70.

Melandri R, *et al.* (1996). Myocardial damage and rhabdomyolysis associated with prolonged hypoxic coma following opiate overdose. *J Toxicol Clin Toxicol*, **34**, 199–203.

Sachdeva DK, Jolly BT (1997). Tramadol overdose requiring prolonged opioid antagonism. *Am J Emerg Med*, **15**, 217–8.

Paracetamol (acetaminophen)

Keayes P, *et al.* (1991). Intravenous acetylcysteine in paracetamol induced fulminant hepatic failure: A prospective controlled trial. *B M J*, **303**, 1026–9.

Makin AJ, Wendon J, Williams R (1995). A 7-year experience of severe acetaminophen-induced hepatotoxicity (1987–1993). *Gastroenterology*, **109**, 1907–16.

Prescott LF (2000). Paracetamol, alcohol and the liver. *Br J Clin Pharmacol*, **49**, 291–301.

Rivera-Penera T, *et al.* (1997). Outcome of acetaminophen overdose in pediatric patients and factors contributing to hepatotoxicity. *J Pediatr*, **130**, 300–4.

Vale JA, Proudfoot AT (1995). Paracetamol (acetaminophen) poisoning. *Lancet*, **346**, 547–52.

Salicylates

Brubacher JR, Hoffman RS (1996). Salicylism from topical salicylates: review of the literature. *Clin Toxicol*, **34**, 431–6.

Chapman BJ, Proudfoot AT (1989). Adult salicylate poisoning: Deaths and outcome in patients with high plasma salicylate concentrations. *Q J Med*, **72**, 699–707.

Proudfoot AT, *et al.* (2003). Does urine alkalinization increase salicylate elimination? If so, why? *Toxicol Rev*, **22**, 129–36.

Theophylline

Minton NA, Henry JA (1996). Treatment of theophylline overdose. *Am J Emerg Med*, **14**, 606–12.

Shannon M (1999). Life-threatening events after theophylline overdose—a 10-year prospective analysis. *Arch Int Med*, **159**, 989–94.

Thyroxine

Tsutaoka BT, Kim S, Santucci S (2005). Seizure in a child after an acute ingestion of levothyroxine. *Pediatr Emerg Care*, **21**, 857–59.

Warfarin

Yasaka M, *et al.* (2003). Effect of prothrombin complex concentrate on INR and blood coagulation system in emergency patients treated with warfarin overdose. *Ann Hematol*, **82**, 121–3.

Metals

Aluminium

Berend K, van der Voet G, Boer WH (2001). Acute aluminium encephalopathy in a dialysis center caused by a cement mortar water distribution pipe. *Kidney Int*, **59**, 746–53.

Friesen MS, Purssell RA, Gair RD (2006). Aluminium toxicity following IV use of oral methadone solution. *Clin Toxicol*, **44**, 307–14.

McCarthy JT, Milliner DS, Johnson WJ (1990). Clinical experience with desferrioxamine in dialysis patients with aluminium toxicity. *Q J Med*, **74**, 257–76.

Spinelli JJ, *et al.* (2006). Cancer risk in aluminium reduction plant workers (Canada). *Cancer Causes Control*, **17**, 939–48.

Arsenic

Aposhian HV, Aposhian MM (2006). Arsenic Toxicology: Five questions. *Chem Res Toxicol*, **19**, 1–15.

International Agency for Research on Cancer (2004). Arsenic in drinking water. *IARC Monogr Eval Carcinog Risks Hum*, **84**, 41–267.

International Programme on Chemical Safety (2001). *Environmental health criteria 224. Arsenic and arsenic compounds*, 2nd edition. World Health Organization, Geneva.

Cadmium

Greim H, (ed.) (2006). Cadmium and its inorganic compounds. In: *The MAK-collection for occupational health and safety. Part I: MAK value documentations*, pp. 1–41. Wiley-VCH, Weinheim.

Järup L, *et al.* (1998). Health effects of cadmium exposure—a review of the literature and a risk estimate. *Scand J Work Environ Health*, **24**, 1–51.

Chromium

Barceloux DG (1999). Chromium. *J Toxicol Clin Toxicol*, **37**, 173–94.

Bradberry SM, Vale JA (1999). Therapeutic review: is ascorbic acid of value in chromium poisoning and chromium dermatitis. *J Toxicol Clin Toxicol*, **37**, 195–200.

Cobalt

Barceloux DG (1999). Cobalt. *J Toxicol Clin Toxicol*, **37**, 201–16.

Steens W, Von Foerster G, Katzer A (2006). Severe cobalt poisoning with loss of sight after ceramic-metal pairing in a hip—a case report. *Acta Orthop*, **77**, 830–2.

Copper

Barceloux DG (1999). Copper. *J Toxicol Clin Toxicol*, **37**, 217–30.

Takeda T, Yukioka T, Shimazaki S (2000). Cupric sulfate intoxication with rhabdomyolysis, treated with chelating agents and blood purification. *Int Med*, **39**, 253–5.

Lead

Bradberry S, Sheehan T, Vale A (2009). Use of oral dimercaptosuccinic acid (succimer; DMSA) in adult patients with inorganic lead poisoning. *Q J Med*, **102**, 721–32.

Bradberry SM, Vale JA (2009). A comparison of sodium calcium edetate (edetate calcium disodium) and succimer (DMSA) in the treatment of inorganic lead poisoning. *Clin Toxicol*, **47**, 841–58.

Rogan WJ, *et al.* (2001). The effect of chelation therapy with succimer on neuropsychological development in children exposed to lead. *N Engl J Med*, **344**, 1421–6.

Mercury

Bradberry SM *et al.* (2009). DMPS can reverse the features of severe mercury vapor-induced neurological damage. *Clin Toxicol*, **47**, 894–98.

O'Carroll RE, *et al.* (1995). The neuropsychiatric sequelae of mercury poisoning. The Mad Hatter's disease revisited. *Br J Psychiatry*, **167**, 95–8.

Risher JF, *et al.* (1999). Summary report for the expert panel review of the toxicological profile for mercury. *Toxicol Ind Health*, **15**, 483–516.

Nickel

Barceloux DG (1999). Nickel. *Clin Toxicol*, **37**, 239–58.

Bradberry SM, Vale JA (1999). Therapeutic review: do diethyldithiocarbamate and disulfiram have a role in acute nickel carbonyl poisoning. *J Toxicol Clin Toxicol*, **37**, 259–64.

Seet RCS, *et al.* (2005). Inhalational nickel carbonyl poisoning in waste processing workers. *Chest*, **128**, 424–9.

Zinc

Hantson P (2001). Zinc toxicity. *Clin Toxicol*, **39**, 239–40.

Pesticides

Aluminium and zinc phosphide

Gupta S, Ahlawat SK (1995). Aluminium phosphide poisoning: a review. *Clin Toxicol*, **33**, 19–24.

Proudfoot AT (2009). Aluminium and zinc phosphide poisoning. *Clin Toxicol*, **47**, 89–100.

Anticoagulant rodenticides

Watt BE, *et al.* (2005). Anticoagulant rodenticides. *Toxicol Rev*, **24**, 259–69.

Carbamate insecticides

Bradberry SM, Vale JA (2005). Organophosphorus and carbamate insecticides. In: Brent J, *et al.* (eds) *Critical care toxicology: diagnosis and management of the critically poisoned patient*, pp. 937–45. Elsevier Mosby, Philadelphia, PA.

Ecobichon DJ (2001). Carbamate insecticides. In: Krieger RI (ed.) *Handbook of pesticide toxicology. Principles*, Vol 2, 2nd edition, pp.1087–106. Academic Press, San Diego, CA.

Chloralose

Hamouda C, *et al.* (2001). A graded classification of acute chloralose poisoning based on 509 cases. *Presse Med*, **30**, 1055–8.

Chlorates

Helliwell M, Nunn J (1979). Mortality in sodium chlorate poisoning. *Br Med J*, **1**, 1119.

Chlorophenoxy herbicides

Bradberry SM, Proudfoot AT, Vale JA (2004). Poisoning due to chlorophenoxy herbicides. *Toxicol Rev*, **24**, 65–73.

Glyphosate herbicides

Bradberry SM, Proudfoot AT, Vale JA (2004). Glyphosate poisoning. *Toxicol Rev*, **23**, 159–67.

Lindane

Aks SE, *et al.* (1995). Acute accidental lindane ingestion in toddlers. *Ann Emerg Med*, **26**, 647–51.

Davies JE, *et al.* (1983). Lindane poisonings. *Arch Dermatol*, **119**, 142–4.

International Programme on Chemical Safety (1991). *Environmental Health Criteria 124, Lindane.* World Health Organization, Geneva.

Metaldehyde

Shih C-C, *et al.* (2004). Acute metaldehyde poisoning in Taiwan. *Vet Hum Toxicol*, **46**, 140–3.

Methyl bromide

De Haro L, *et al.* (1997). Central and peripheral neurotoxic effects of chronic methyl bromide intoxication. *J Toxicol Clin Toxicol*, **35**, 29–34.

Yamano Y, Nakadate T (2006). Three occupationally exposed cases of severe methyl bromide poisoning: accident caused by a gas leak during the fumigation of a folklore museum. *J Occup Health*, **48**, 129–33.

Zwaveling JH, *et al.* (1987). Exposure of the skin to methyl bromide: A study of six cases occupationally exposed to high concentrations during fumigation. *Hum Toxicol*, **6**, 491–5.

Organophosphorus insecticides

Eddleston M, *et al.* (2005). Differences between organophosphorus insecticides in human self-poisoning: a prospective cohort study. *Lancet*, **366**, 1452–9.

Eddleston M, *et al.* (2008). Management of acute organophosphorus pesticide poisoning. *Lancet*, **371**, 597–607.

Karalliedde L, Baker D, Marrs TC (2006). Organophosphate-induced intermediate syndrome: aetiology and relationships with myopathy. *Toxicol Rev*, **25**, 1–14.

Marrs TC, Vale JA (2006). Management of organophosphorus pesticide poisoning. In: Gupta RC (ed.) *Toxicology of organophosphate and carbamate compounds*, pp. 715–33. Academic Press, Amsterdam.

Pawar KS, *et al.* (2006). Continuous pralidoxime infusion versus repeated bolus injection to treat organophosphorus pesticide poisoning: a randomised controlled trial. *Lancet*, **368**, 2136–41.

Paraquat and related herbicides

Jones GM, Vale JA (2000). Mechanisms of toxicity, clinical features and management of diquat poisoning: A review. *J Toxicol Clin Toxicol*, **38**, 123–8.

Proudfoot AT, *et al.* (1979). Paraquat poisoning: significance of plasma-paraquat concentrations. *Lancet*, **1**, 330–1.

Scherrmann JM, *et al.* (1987). Prognostic value of plasma and urine paraquat concentration. *HumToxicol*, **6**, 91–3.

Vale JA, Meredith TJ, Buckley BM (1987). Paraquat poisoning: clinical features and immediate general management. *Hum Toxicol*, **6**, 41–7.

Pyrethroids

Bradberry SM, *et al.* (2005). Poisoning due to pyrethroids. *Toxicol Rev*, **24**, 93–106.

Other chemicals

Acetone

International Programme on Chemical Safety (1998). *Environmental Health Criteria 207. Acetone.* World Health Organization, Geneva.

Acids

Boyce SH, Simpson KA (1996). Hydrochloric acid inhalation: who needs admission?. *J Accid Emerg Med*, **13**, 422–4.

Cartotto RC, *et al.* (1996). Chemical burns. *Can J Surg*, **39**, 205–11.

Flamminger A, Maibach H (2006). Sulfuric acid burns (corrosion and acute irritation): evidence-based overview of management. *Cutan Ocular Toxicol*, **25**, 55–61.

Singal S, Kar P (2006). Corrosive injuries of esophagus and stomach—issues in management. *Trop Gastroenterol*, **27**, 34–40.

Alkalis

Anderson KD, Rouse TM, Randolph JG (1990). A controlled trial of corticosteroids in children with corrosive injury of the esophagus. *N Engl J Med*, **323**, 637–40.

Brodovsky SC, *et al.* (2000). Management of alkali burns—an 11-year retrospective review. *Opthalmology*, **107**, 1829–35.

Keskin E, *et al.* (1991). The effect of steroid treatment on corrosive oesophageal burns in children. *Eur J Pediatr Surg*, **1**, 335–8.

Winder C (1997). Medical treatment of caustic burns. *Med J Aust*, **167**, 511–2.

Ammonia

De La Hoz RE, Schlueter DP, Rom WN (1996). Chronic lung disease secondary to ammonia inhalation injury. *Am J Ind Med*, **29**, 209–14.

Michaels RA (1999). Emergency planning and the acute toxic potency of inhaled ammonia. *Environ Health Perspect*, **107**, 617–27.

Wibbenmeyer LA, *et al.* (1999). Our chemical burn experience: exposing the dangers of anhydrous ammonia. *J Burn Care Rehabil*, **20**, 226–31.

Arsine

Romeo L, *et al.* (1997). Acute arsine intoxication as a consequence of metal burnishing operations. *Am J Ind Med*, **32**, 211–6.

Wilkinson SP, *et al.* (1975). Arsine toxicity aboard the Asiafreighter. *Br Med J*, **3**, 559–63.

Benzene

Kuang S, Liang W (2005). Clinical analysis of 43 cases of chronic benzene poisoning. *Chem Biol Interact*, **153–4**, 129–35.

Snyder R (2002). Benzene and leukemia. *Crit Rev Toxicol*, **32**, 155–210.

Benzyl alcohol

Gershank J, *et al.* (1982). The gasping syndrome and benzyl alcohol poisoning. *N Engl J Med*, **307**, 1384–8.

López-Herce J, *et al.* (1995). Benzyl alcohol poisoning following diazepam intravenous infusion. *Annf Pharmacother*, **29**, 632.

CO_2

Langford NJ (2005). Carbon dioxide poisoning. *Toxicol Rev*, 24, 229–35.

Carbon disulphide

Greim H (ed.) (2005). Carbon disulfide. In *The MAK-collection for occupational health and safety. Part I: MAK value documentations*, pp. 171–85. Wiley-VCH, Weinheim.

Spyker DA, Gallanosa AG, Suratt PM (1982). Health effects of acute carbon disulfide exposure. *Clin Toxicol*, **19**, 87–93.

Carbon monoxide

Buckley NA, *et al.* (2005). Hyperbaric oxygen for carbon monoxide poisoning: a systematic review and critical analysis of the evidence. *Toxicol Rev*, **24**, 75–92.

International Programme on Chemical Safety (1999). *Environmental Health Criteria 213. Carbon monoxide.* World Health Organization, Geneva.

Thom SR, *et al.* (1995). Delayed neuropsychologic sequelae after carbon monoxide poisoning; prevention by treatment with hyperbaric oxygen. *Ann Emerg Med*, **25**, 474–80.

Varon J, *et al.* (1999). Carbon monoxide poisoning: a review for clinicians. *J Emerg Med*, **17**, 87–93.

Weaver LK, *et al.* (2002). Hyperbaric oxygen for acute carbon monoxide poisoning. *N Engl J Med*, **347**, 1057–67.

Chlorine

Aslan S, *et al.* (2006). The effect of nebulized $NaHCO_3$ treatment on 'RADS' due to chlorine gas inhalation. *Inhalation Toxicol*, **18**, 895–900.

Mvros R, Dean BS, Krenzelok EP (1993). Home exposures to chlorine/chloramine gas: review of 216 cases. *South Med J*, **86**, 654–7.

Schonhofer B, Voshaar T, Kohler D (1996). Long-term sequelae following accidental chlorine gas exposure. *Respiration*, **63**, 155–9.

Sexton JD, Pronchik DJ (1998). Chlorine inhalation: the big picture. *Clin Toxicol*, **36**, 87–93.

Cyanide

Meredith TJ, *et al.* (1993). *IPCS/CEC evaluation of antidotes series. Antidotes for poisoning by cyanide.* Cambridge University Press, Cambridge.

Hall AH, Dart R, Bogdan G (2007). Sodium thiosulfate or hydroxocobalamin for the empiric treatment of cyanide poisoning?. *Ann Emerg Med*, **49**.

Dart RC (2006). Hydroxocobalamin for acute cyanide poisoning: new data from preclinical and clinical studies; new results from the prehospital emergency setting. *Clin Toxicol*, **44**, 1–3.

Borron SW, *et al.* (2007). Prospective study of hydroxocobalamin for acute cyanide poisoning in smoke inhalation. *Ann Emerg Med*,**49**, 794–801.

Diethylene glycol poisoning

O'Brien KL, *et al.* (1998). Epidemic of pediatric deaths from acute renal failure caused by diethylene glycol poisoning. *JAMA*, **279**, 1175–80.

Schep LJ *et al.* (2009). Diethylene glycol poisoning. *Clin Toxicol*, **47**, 525–35.

Woolf AD (1998). The Haitian diethylene glycol poisoning tragedy—A dark wood revisited. *JAMA*, **279**, 1215–6.

Ethylene glycol

Brent J, *et al.* (1999). Fomepizole for the treatment of ethylene glycol poisoning. *N Engl J Med*, **340**, 832–8.

Froberg K, Dorion RP, McMartin KE (2006). The role of calcium oxalate crystal deposition in cerebral vessels during ethylene glycol poisoning. *Clin Toxicol*, **44**, 315–8.

Jacobsen D, McMartin KE (1986). Methanol and ethylene glycol poisonings: mechanism of toxicity, clinical course, diagnosis and treatment. *Med Toxicol*, **1**, 309–44.

Jacobsen D, *et al.* (1988). Ethylene glycol intoxication: evaluation of kinetics and crystalluria. *Am J Med*, **84**, 145–52.

McMartin K (2009). Are calcium oxalate crystals involved in the mechanism of acute renal failure in ethylene glycol poisoning? *Clin Toxicol*, **47**, 859–69.

Formaldehyde

Liteplo RG, *et al.* (eds) (2002). *Concise international chemical assessment document no. 40. Formaldehyde.* Inter-Organization Programme for the Sound Management of Chemicals. World Health Organization, Geneva.

Pandey CK, *et al.* (2000). Toxicity of ingested formalin and its management. *Hum Exp Toxicol*, **19**, 360–6.

n-Hexane

International Programme on Chemical Safety (1991). *Environmental Health Criteria 122. n-Hexane.* World Health Organization, Geneva.

Hydrofluoric acid

Bentur Y, *et al.* (1993). The role of calcium gluconate in the treatment of hydrofluoric acid eye burn. *Ann Emerg Med*, **22**, 1488–90.

Burd A (2004). Hydrofluoric acid revisited. *Burns*, **30**, 720–2.

Dunn BJ, *et al.* (1996). Topical treatments for hydrofluoric acid dermal burns. *J Occu Environ Med*, **38**, 507–14.

Henry JA, Hla KK (1992). Intravenous regional calcium gluconate perfusion for hydrofluoric acid burns. *Clin Toxicol*, **30**, 203–7.

Hydrogen sulphide

Guidotti TL (1996). Hydrogen sulphide. *Occup Med*, **46**, 367–71.

Hall AH, Rumack BH (1997). Hydrogen sulfide poisoning; an antidotal role for sodium nitrite?. *Vet Hum Toxicol*, **39**, 152–4.

Milby TH, Baselt RC (1999). Hydrogen sulfide poisoning: clarification of some controversial issues. *Am J Ind Med*, **35**, 192–5.

Isopropanol

Chan K, Wong ET, Matthews WS (1993). Severe isopropanolemia without acetonemia or clinical manifestations of isopropanol intoxication. *Clin Chemistry*, **39**, 1922–5.

Haviv YS, Safadi R, Osin P (1998). Accidental isopropyl alcohol enema leading to coma and death. *Am J Gastroenterol*, **93**, 850–1.

Pappas AA, *et al.* (1991). Isopropanol ingestion: A report of six episodes with isopropanol and acetone serum concentration time data. *Clin Toxicol*, **29**, 11–21.

Methanol

Barceloux DG, *et al.* (2002). American Academy of Clinical Toxicology practice guidelines on the treatment of methanol poisoning. *Clinl Toxicol*, **40**, 415–46.

Brent J, *et al.* (2001). Fomepizole for the treatment of methanol poisoning. *N Engl J Med*, **344**, 424–9.

Jacobsen D, McMartin KE (1997). Antidotes for methanol and ethylene glycol poisoning. *J Toxicol Clin Toxicol*, **35**, 126–43.

Methylene chloride

Chang Y-L, *et al.* (1999). Diverse manifestations of oral methylene chloride poisoning: report of 6 cases. *Clin Toxicol*, **37**, 497–504.

McDonald W, Olmedo M (1996). Accidental deaths following inhalation of methylene chloride. *Appl Occup Environ Hyg*, **11**, 17–9.

Nitrites

Ringling S, Boo T, Bottei E (2003). Methemoglobinemia from nitrite-contaminated punch. *Clin Toxicol*, **41**, 730–1.

Nitrogen dioxide

Berglund M, *et al.* (1993). Health risk evaluation of nitrogen oxides. *Scand J Work, Environ Health*, **19** Suppl. 2, 1–72.

Karlson-Stiber C, *et al.* (1996). Nitrogen dioxide pneumonitis in ice hockey players. *J Int Med*, **239**, 451–6.

Paraffin (kerosone)

Babar MI, Bhait RA, Cheema ME (2002). Kerosene oil poisoning in children. *J Coll Physicians Surg Pak*, **12**, 472–6.

Tagwireyi D, Ball DE, Nhachi CFB (2006). Toxicoepidemiology in Zimbabwe: admissions resulting from exposure to paraffin (kerosene). *Clin Toxicol*, **44**, 103–7.

Petrol (gasoline)

Cairney S, *et al.* (2002). The neurobehavioural consequences of petrol (gasoline) sniffing. *Neurosci Biobehav Rev*, **26**, 81–9.

Caprino L, Togna GI (1998). Potential health effects of gasoline and its constituents: a review of current literature (1990–1997) on toxicological data. *Environ Health Perspect*, **106**, 115–25.

Phenol

Bentur Y, *et al.* (1998). Prolonged elimination half-life of phenol after dermal exposure. *Clin Toxicol*, **36**, 707–11.

Phosgene

Wyatt JP, Allister CA (1995). Occupational phosgene poisoning: a case report and review. *J Accid Emerg Med*, **12**, 212–3.

Phosphine

Schoonbroodt D, *et al.* (1992). Acute phosphine poisoning? A case report and review. *Acta Clinica Belgica*, **47**, 280–4.

Willers-Russo LJ (1999). Three fatalities involving phosphine gas, produced as a result of methamphetamine manufacturing. *J Forensic Sci*, **44**, 647–52.

Propylene glycol

Bouchard NC, *et al.* (2005). Severe lactic acidemia and systemic toxicity following oral propylene glycol ingestion: a role for fomepizole and hemodialysis. *Clin Toxicol*, **43**, 740.

Peleg O, Bar-Oz B, Arad I (1998). Coma in a premature infant associated with the transdermal absorption of propylene glycol. *Acta Paediatr*, **87**, 1195–6.

Sulphur dioxide

International Program on Chemical Safety (1979). *Environmental Health Criteria 8. Sulfur oxides and suspended particulate matter*. World Health Organization, Geneva.

Tetrachloroethylene (perchloroethylene)

Garnier R, *et al.* (1996). Coin-operated dry cleaning machines may be responsible for acute tetrachloroethylene poisoning: report of 26 cases including one death. *J Toxicol Clin Toxicol*, **34**, 191–7.

Toluene

Bowen SE, Daniel J, Balster RL (1999). Deaths associated with inhalant abuse in Virginia from 1987 to 1996. *Drug Alcohol Depend*, **53**, 239–45.

Deleu D, Hanssens Y (2000). Cerebellar dysfunction in chronic toluene abuse: beneficial response to amantadine hydrochloride. *J Toxicol Clin Toxicol*, **38**, 37–41.

1,1,1-Trichloroethane

House RA, *et al.* (1996). Paresthesias and sensory neuropathy due to 1,1,1-trichloroethane. *J Occup Environ Med*, **38**, 123–4.

Liss GM, House RA (1995). Toxic encephalopathy due to 1,1,1-trichloroethane. *Am J Ind Med*, **27**, 445–6.

Trichloroethylene

Szlatenyi CS, Wang RY (1996). Encephalopathy and cranial nerve palsies caused by intentional trichloroethylene inhalation. *Am J Emerg Med*, **14**, 464–7.

Yoshida M, *et al.* (1996). Concentrations of trichloroethylene and its metabolites in blood and urine after acute poisoning by ingestion. *Hum Exp Toxicol*, **15**, 254–8.

Household products

Arevalo-Silva C, *et al.* (2006). Ingestion of caustic substances: a 15-year experience. *Laryngoscope*, **116**, 1422–6.

Bertinelli A, *et al.* (2006). Serious injuries from dishwasher powder ingestions in small children. *J Paediatr Child Health*, **42**, 129–33.

Chan TYK, Lau MSW, Critchley JAJH (1993). Serious complications associated with Dettol poisoning. *Q J Med*, **86**, 735–8.

Gad-Johannsen H, Mikkelsen JB, Larsen CF (1995). Poisoning with household chemicals in children. *Acta Paediatrica*, **83**, 62–5.

Harley EH, Collins MD (1997). Liquid household bleach ingestion in children: a retrospective review. *Laryngoscope*, **107**, 122–5.

Horgan N, *et al.* (2005). Eye injuries in children: a new household risk. *Lancet*, **366**, 547–8.

Kiristioglu I, *et al.* (1999). Is it necessary to perform an endoscopy after the ingestion of liquid household bleach in children? *Acta Paediatrica*, **88**, 233–4.

Vincent JC, Sheikh A (1998). Phosphate poisoning by ingestion of clothes washing liquid and fabric conditioner. *Anaesthesia*, **53**, 1004–6.

9.2

Injuries, envenoming, poisoning, and allergic reactions caused by animals

David A. Warrell

Essentials

Mechanical injuries

Attacks by wild and domesticated animals are increasing worldwide. They are best prevented by taking local advice. Injuries usually occur in places remote from medical care and may involve extensive trauma, haemorrhagic shock, and a high risk of bacterial contamination. First aid is resuscitation, control of bleeding and perforating injuries, intravenous fluid replacement, and rapid evacuation to hospital for emergency surgery and treatment of infection.

Venomous snakes

Bites by venomous snakes can cause death or permanent disability. This is largely an occupational/environmental hazard of agricultural workers and their children in rural areas of the tropic. Bites are commonly inflicted on the lower limbs and could be prevented by wearing protective footwear, by using lights while walking at night, and by sleeping off the ground or under a mosquito net.

Snake venoms are rich in toxic proteins that cause necrosis, shock, haemostatic disturbances, paralysis, rhabdomyolysis, and acute renal failure. Bites by Elapidae (cobras, kraits, mambas, coral snakes, Australian snakes, and sea snakes) may cause descending flaccid paralysis, starting with ptosis and progressing to respiratory paralysis. Some elapid venoms cause local necrosis, rhabdomyolysis and haemostatic disturbances. Bites by Viperidae (vipers, adders, and pit vipers—rattlesnakes, moccasins, lanceheads) can cause severe local swelling, bruising, blistering, and necrosis together with shock, consumptive coagulopathy, spontaneous systemic bleeding, renal failure, and, with some species, neurotoxicity.

First aid involves reassurance, immobilization of the whole patient, especially the bitten limb, rapid evacuation to the nearest hospital, and avoidance of dangerous traditional methods. When the necessary skills and equipment are available, pressure-immobilization should be applied immediately unless the possibility of a neurotoxic elapid bite can be excluded.

In hospital, specific antivenom (hyperimmune equine or ovine immunoglobulins) is given if there is evidence of systemic or severe local envenoming. Polyspecific antivenoms cover envenoming by medically important snakes in the geographical area for which they are intended. Early anaphylactic or pyrogenic reactions and late serum sickness antivenom reactions are common but not predictable by hypersensitivity tests. After the initial dose, the indication for more antivenom is failure of restoration of blood coagulability after 6 h, or progression of other signs of envenoming. Assisted ventilation, renal dialysis, or cardiovascular support may be required. Necrotic tissue requires surgical debridement. Signs of compartment syndrome may be misleading and fasciotomy is rarely justified.

Venomous arthropods

Many fish of temperate and tropical seas can inflict dangerous stings—stingrays, catfish, weevers, scorpionfish, stonefish, and lionfish. Prevention is by wearing foot protection when wading and avoiding contact with tropical reef fish. Immediate agonizing pain is alleviated by immersing the stung limb in uncomfortably hot but not scalding water (less than 45 °C). Erythematous swelling and necrosis may ensue with the risk of infection by marine bacteria. Stingray spines can cause fatal penetrating injuries. Systemic envenoming is uncommon. Stonefish antivenom is available

Poisonous aquatic animals

Ciguatera poisoning from eating tropical reef fish is prevalent in Pacific and Caribbean regions. Fish acquire polyether toxins from dinoflagellates. Acute gastroenteritis develops 1 to 6 h after ingestion, followed by neurotoxic and cardiovascular disturbances.

Tetrodotoxin poisoning is attributable to the Japanese delicacy 'fugu' (puffer fish). Neurotoxic symptoms caused by this sodium channel blocker develop 10 to 45 min after ingestion. Fatal respiratory paralysis may ensue 2 to 6 h later

Paralytic shellfish poisoning is caused by eating bivalve molluscs contaminated with tetrahydropurine neurotoxins from dinoflagellates. Neurotoxic symptoms appear within 30 min of ingestion, progressing to fatal respiratory paralysis within 12 h

Scrombroid poisoning results when bacterial decomposition of tuna and other dark-fleshed fish generates histamine. Anaphylactic-type symptoms develop within minutes to a few hours after ingestion.

Prevention is by avoiding scaleless (tetrodotoxic) fish, large reef fish (ciguatera-toxic), and shellfish when there is a red tide. Correct processing prevents scrombroid poisoning. Cooking does not destroy any of these toxins.

Venomous marine invertebrates

Cnidarians (jellyfish, stinging corals, sea anemones, etc.) have tentacles studded with stinging nematocysts. Lethal species are Indo-Australian box jellyfish, Irukandji, Portuguese man-o'-war (*Physalia*), and Chinese *Stomolophus nomurai*. Prevention is by observing warning notices on affected beaches, bathing in 'stinger-resistant' enclosures, or wearing protective clothing. Stings produce immediately painful irritant weals. Box jellyfish cause the most severe systemic symptoms: respiratory and cardiac arrest, generalized convulsions, and pulmonary oedema within minutes of the accident. 'Irukandji' syndrome is distinctive: severe persisting musculoskeletal pain, anxiety, trembling, headache, piloerection, sweating, tachycardia, hypertension, and pulmonary oedema starting about 30 min after stings by tiny cubomedusoids. Vinegar inactivates box jellyfish and Irukandji nematocysts. Hot water relieves the pain of *Physalia* stings. Box jellyfish antivenom is available in Australia.

Echinoderm (starfish and sea urchin) spines become embedded in waders' feet, sometimes penetrating bones and joints. Pain is relieved by hot water. Systemic envenoming is rare but there is a risk of marine bacterial infection.

Molluscs—cone shells and small Australasian blue-ringed octopuses can cause fatal envenoming.

Venomous arthropods

Hymenoptera—stings by bees (Apidae); wasps, yellow jackets, and hornet (Vespidae), and ants commonly cause allergic reactions, while rare mass attacks (e.g. by Africanized 'killer' bees) can result in severe envenoming.

People in whom systemic anaphylaxis has been provoked by a hymenopteran sting should always carry—and be competent to use—self-injectable adrenaline (epinephrine). Desensitization with purified venom should be considered if type I hypersensitivity is confirmed by detecting venom-specific IgE. Massive envenoming by Apidae or Vespidae causes histamine toxicity, generalized rhabdomyolysis, intravascular haemolysis, hypertension, pulmonary oedema, myocardial damage, bleeding, hepatic dysfunction, and acute renal failure.

Lepidoptera—stinging hairs of many species of moths and their caterpillars can excite cutaneous irritation and allergy, sometimes causing epidemics. In South America, caterpillars of atlas moths (*Lonomia*) cause many stings. Their venom contains antihaemostatic toxins causing spontaneous bleeding, polyarthralgia, and acute renal failure. An antivenom is available in Brazil.

Coleoptera—contact with 'Spanish fly' and 'Nairobi eye' beetles causes blistering.

Scorpions—stings still cause numerous fatalities in North and South Africa, the Middle East, Mexico, Latin America, and India. Prevention is by excluding scorpions from homes. Severe local pain is the commonest symptom. Systemic symptoms vary according to the species of scorpion involved. 'Autonomic storm' is caused by massive release of acetylcholine and catecholamines by ion channel toxins. Cardiorespiratory effects include hypertension, shock, tachy- and bradyarrhythmias, ECG changes, and pulmonary oedema. Neurotoxic effects include erratic eye movements, fasciculation, and muscle spasms (pseudo-convulsions) causing respiratory distress. Pain is best controlled by local anaesthetic. Antivenom is available in some countries, but pharmacological treatment with prazosin and other vasodilators is preferred elsewhere.

Spiders—bites are common in the Americas, Mediterranean, South Africa, and Australia but there are few fatalities. Only recluse spiders (*Loxosceles*) are reliably associated with necrotic araneism (arachnidism), but many innocent peridomestic species have been vilified. Local pain and swelling develop slowly, followed by the classic 'red-white-and-blue sign' and eventually an eschar, which sloughs leaving a necrotic ulcer. Systemic symptoms, including fever, rash, haemolysis, and renal failure, are unusual. Bites by cosmopolitan black and brown widow spiders, Latin American banana spiders, and Sydney funnel web spiders and their relatives, cause neurotoxic araneism. Immediate pain is followed by sweating with gooseflesh at the site of the bite. Systemic symptoms quickly evolve: headache, nausea, vomiting, profuse generalized sweating, fever, priapism, and painful muscle spasms, tremors, and rigidity that may cause respiratory distress or simulate an acute abdomen. Antivenoms widely used for *Loxosceles* and neurotoxic bites are of uncertain efficacy.

Ticks—mainly in North America and Australia, both ixodid (hard) and argasid (soft) ticks can inject a salivary neurotoxin during their blood meal, causing an ascending flaccid paralysis. The tick must be detached as soon as possible.

Centipedes cause painful stings in tropical countries, while toxic secretions of millipedes may be applied to skin, lips, and eyes by children who are handling or trying to eat them.

Leeches have anticoagulant saliva. Land leeches infest rainforests and can invade clothing while aquatic leeches are swallowed in fresh water or they may penetrate body orifices of swimmers. Prevention is by applying repellents to skin, clothes, and footwear, by boiling or filtering drinking water and by avoiding affected waters. Clinical effects are local pain, itching, blood loss, secondary infection, and phobia. Ingested aquatic leeches may obstruct pharynx, bronchi, or oesophagus. Use of medicinal leeches may be complicated by *Aeromonas hydrophila* infection.

Mechanical injuries caused by animals

Epidemiology

Many species of wild animals have mauled and killed humans. Attacks by wild mammals are increasingly reported. The big cats, wolves, bears, elephants, hippopotamuses, and buffaloes are the most dangerous. Since 2000, about 60 to 80 confirmed unprovoked attacks by sharks with an average of 4.3 fatalities (case fatality *c.*8%) have been reported each year. Other fish, such as barracudas, moray and conger eels, garfish, groupers, stingrays, and piranhas can inflict lethal injuries. Electric 'eels' *Electrophorus electricus* (Gymnotidae) of rivers and coastal waters in Florida and South

American and marine torpedo rays (e.g. *Torpedo* spp., Torpediniformes) can impart fatally stunning electric shocks. Even the 5-cm Amazonian catfish (genus *Vandellia*, Trichomycteridae; Spanish 'canero'; Portuguese 'candirú'), the only vertebrate human ectoparasite, can traumatize humans by burrowing into their urethra, vagina, or anus, causing pain, bleeding, and obstruction. Crocodilians (alligators, caimans, and crocodiles) kill, eat, and scavenge dead humans in Africa, Asia, and Oceania. In the United States of America, especially Florida, alligators *Alligator mississippiensis* are responsible for a few deaths but in Africa, Nile crocodiles *Crocodilus niloticus* kill about 1000 people each year, and in South Asia, northern Australia, and New Guinea the saltwater crocodile *C. porosus* kills hundreds each year. Giant pythons very rarely kill humans in Africa (*Python sebae*), India (*Python molurus*), Indonesia (*Python reticulatus*), Australia (*Morelia amethistina*), and South America (*Eunectes murinus*). To put these nightmares into perspective, in the United States, collisions between vehicles and deer and injuries to horseback riders are much more common than attacks by wild animals.

Bites by domestic dogs are common worldwide. In England and Wales, where the estimated dog population is 6 million, more than 200 000 bite victims attend hospital each year. In the United States, dogs are responsible for 80 to 90% of all animal bites. They bite about 4.7 million people each year (1.8% of the population), 800 000 of whom (0.3% of the population) require medical attention, and 12 are killed. Children are especially vulnerable. Other domestic animals that have caused severe injuries or deaths include camels, cattle, water buffalo, sheep, pigs, cats, and even ferrets.

Prevention

It is essential to obtain local advice about these environmental hazards. Where dangerous wild animals abound, wandering alone and unprotected between dusk and dawn offers the highest risk of attacks. Staying in a vehicle and travelling in groups reduces risk. Pet dogs may attract large predators. In bear country, hikers should travel in groups, making plenty of noise. Bears should never be approached (e.g. for photography), especially if there are cubs. Faced by a charging bear, avoid eye contact and do not attempt to hide, run away, or climb a tree. At a distance of 30 feet (*c.*10 m), a bear may be repelled by discharging a commercial pepper spray (10% capsicum oleoresin) towards its eyes. If attacked by a dog, avoid eye contact, shout, and fight back with sticks and stones. Young children should not be left alone with dogs, even family pets, and notoriously dangerous breeds should be banned. Elephants are dangerous whether wild or tamed. They should be treated with extreme respect or avoided, especially if they are in 'musth'. Swimming or canoeing in hippo-infested waters or blocking their retreat to water is highly dangerous. To prevent crocodilian attacks, keep well away from the water's edge, do not bathe between dusk and dawn, and avoid canoeing in croc-infested waters. If attacked by a crocodilian on land, run; in the water, fight back, hitting the animal on its nose and eyes with any available weapon. To avoid shark attacks, never bathe in shark-infested waters, between sand bars and the deep ocean, where dead fish have been dumped, flocks of sea birds are feeding, or sewage is discharged. If attacked by a shark, fight back, hitting it on the nose and clawing at its eyes and gills. Chemical and electrical-field repellents and chain mail suits have been developed to protect divers.

Clinical features

Teeth, tusks, horns, claws, and spines tear, crush, and puncture soft tissues and break bones. Big cats, bears, pigs, pythons, crocodilians, and sharks will eat their victims. Bovines and elephants trample and kneel on the prostrate body. Body cavities may be punctured, resulting in pneumothorax, haemothorax, herniation and strangulation of bowel, and rupture of liver and spleen. Horse and camel bites and kicks can fracture, dislocate, crush, and concuss. Wild and feral pigs, armed with lethal tusks, can inflict abdominal evisceration, pneumothorax and fractures and lacerations of tendons, arteries, and nerves. Giant pythons asphyxiate by constriction and may swallow the victim. Sharks amputate whole limbs, causing rapidly fatal haemorrhage. Garfish (needle fish) and sting rays can fatally impale. Infection is likely with all these traumas: rabies, tetanus, gas gangrene, cat scratch disease (*Bartonella henselae*), *Pasteurella multocida*, *Capnocytophaga canimorsus*, leptospires, *Spirillum minus*, *Streptobacillus moniliformis*, and aquatic organisms such as *Vibrio vulnificus* and *Aeromonas hydrophila* (see Section 7 Infectious Diseases).

Treatment

Since wild animal attacks are most likely to happen in areas remote from medical care, delayed hospital treatment makes first aid especially crucial for the survival of the victim.

First aid of severe injuries

First, the patient and rescuers must be made safe from further danger and drowning. Bleeding is controlled by local pressure or tourniquets, perforating injuries are closed with pressure dressings, circulating volume repletion is started as soon as possible with intravenous fluids, and the casualty is evacuated promptly to hospital. Some regions have flying doctor services (e.g. AMREF in East Africa). All injuries inflicted by animals must be assumed to be infected by a range of organisms (see earlier paragraphs) and so it may be appropriate to start antibiotic treatment immediately.

Medical treatment in the hospital

Emergency surgery may be required. Blood loss should be replaced and attention given to local mechanical complications such as fractures, tension pneumothorax, damage to large blood vessels, perforation of the bowel, and lacerations of other abdominal viscera. Thorough debridement or amputation of dead tissue may be required with removal of foreign material, teeth, etc., and irrigation and drainage. Except for wounds on the head and neck, which can be sutured immediately, primary suturing should be delayed for 48 to 72 h, after which further debridement, suturing, or covering with split skin grafts should be considered.

Wounds should be thoroughly cleaned with soap and water as soon as possible; suitable antiseptics include iodine and alcohol solutions. Prophylactic antimicrobials such as amoxicillin/clavulanic acid, doxycycline, or erythromycin have proved effective in dog- and cat-bite wounds and are indicated for multiple or severe wounds and bites on the face and hands. For other bites, use penicillin, an aminoglycoside and metronidazole and for marine or aquatic wounds, to cover unusual bacteria such as *Vibrio* and *Aeromonas* spp., doxycycline or co-trimoxazole or, in severe cases, a combination of tetracycline with an aminoglycoside (e.g. gentamicin) and cefotaxime, or tetracycline with aminoglycoside and a fluoroquinolone. Specific infections, such as tetanus, rabies, and herpes simiae virus (from monkey bites) must be considered and treated or prevented appropriately.

Venomous animals

For predation or defence, some animals inject venoms through fangs, chelicerae (venom jaws), stings, spines, hairs, nematocysts, and other specialized venom organs. 'Spitting' snakes, scorpions, and millipedes squirt venom on to absorbent mucous membranes. The flesh or skin of some animals contains poisons acquired through the food chain. Allergic reactions to injected venoms (e.g. of *Hymenoptera* and cnidarians) and ingested poisons (e.g. ciguatera) may cause more frequent and serious medical problems than their direct toxic effects.

Venomous mammals

Male duck-billed platypuses (*Ornithorhynchus anatinus*) have erectile venomous spurs on their hind limbs. These aquatic, egg-laying mammals of eastern Australia sting at least one person each year in Victoria, but only 17 cases have been reported since 1817. There is immediate, agonizing, persistent local pain, as well as prolonged local swelling, chronic pain on movement, hyperaesthesia, wasting, inflammation, and regional lymphadenopathy. These effects are not life-threatening in humans, but dogs have died of envenoming. In the absence of specific treatment, nonsteroidal anti-inflammatory agents (NSAIDs) or corticosteroids have proved effective. The venom contains a C-type natriuretic peptide (which causes mast-cell degranulation), nerve growth factor (NGF), a number of α- and β-defensin-like peptides, enzymes, and other peptides and proteins, including a sildenafil-like phosphodiesterase-5 inhibitor. Male echidnas, the other egg-laying mammal, possess a similar but smaller venom apparatus.

Several species of Insectivora produce venomous saliva conducted into bite wounds by curved and sometimes grooved lower incisors. Venomous species include the Hispaniolan and Cuban solenodons (*Solenodon paradoxus, S. (Apotogale) cubanus*), northern water shrew *Neomys fodiens*, southern water shrew *N. anomalus*, and North American short-tailed shrew *Blarina brevicauda*. Their bites can kill rodents and lagomorphs, but in humans the effect is local pain, swelling, and inflammation.

The saliva of vampire bats (Desmodontinae) contains permeability-increasing factors, a platelet inhibitor, draculin (an inhibitor of activated factors X and IX), and a plasminogen activator which is being developed as a thrombolytic drug.

The slow loris *Nycticebus coucang* (Primates; Lorisidae) possesses brachial glands that secrete a toxin very similar in structure to Fel d 1 cat allergen, which the lorises lick up and can inject when they bite. In humans, slow loris bites may be damaging, infective or toxic, causing pain swelling and even anaphylaxis.

Venomous snakes

Fewer than 200 species of venomous snake (families Colubridae, Atractaspididae, Elapidae, and Viperidae) have been responsible for severely envenoming humans resulting in death or permanent disability. Since it may be difficult to distinguish venomous from nonvenomous species, unnecessary contact with snakes should be avoided, and patients bitten by any species should be assessed carefully.

Distribution

Free from venomous snakes are the Antarctic; most islands of the western Mediterranean, Atlantic, Caribbean, and eastern Pacific (including Hawaii); Chile, Iceland, Ireland, Madagascar, New Caledonia, and New Zealand. Elsewhere, venomous snakes are widely distributed up to altitudes of more than 4000 m in the Himalayas (*Gloydius himalayanus*), within the Arctic Circle (*Vipera berus*), in the Indian and Pacific oceans as far north as Siberia (*Pelamis platurus*), and in some freshwater lakes (*Hydrophis semperi*).

Classification

Medically important species have in their upper jaws one or more pairs of enlarged teeth (fangs) that inject venom into their victims through a groove or closed channel.

Colubridae

The short, immobile fangs are at the back of the maxilla (Fig. 9.2.1). Most of the familiar snakes regarded as nonvenomous, e.g. the British grass snake *Natrix natrix helvetica* and the smooth snake *Coronella austriaca*, belong to this large family. However, many colubrid species have proved capable of causing at least local envenoming and some have caused severe envenoming or death, such as three African species—the boomslang *Dispholidus typus* and the vine, twig, bird, or tree snake or Voëlslang (*Thelotornis kirtlandii* and *T. capensis*); the Japanese yamakagashi *Rhabdophis tigrinus*; the South East Asian red-necked keelback *R. subminiatus;* and possibly the South American green racer *Philodryas olfersii* (Fig. 9.2.1).

Atractaspididae

The African and Middle Eastern burrowing asps, stiletto snakes, or burrowing or mole vipers or adders strike sideways, impaling their victims on a long front fang protruding through the partially closed mouth (Fig. 9.2.2). Three species, *Atractaspis microlepidota,*

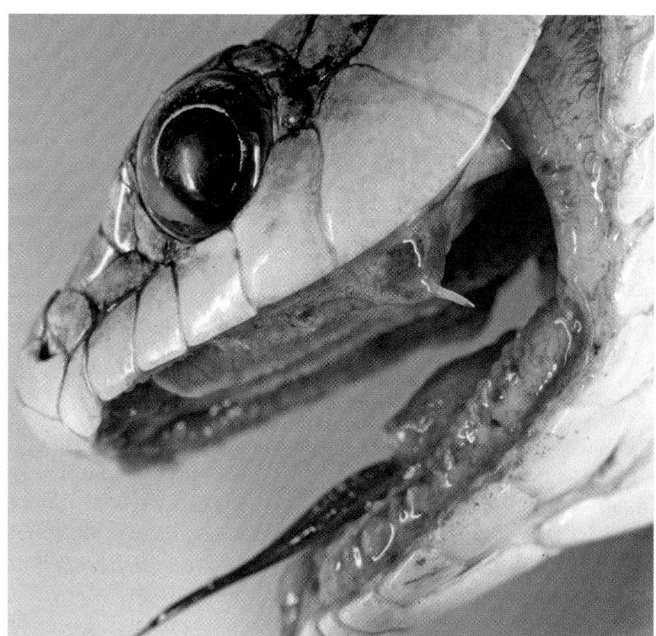

Fig. 9.2.1 Back fangs of the green racer *Philodryas olfersii*, a South American colubrid snake. A possible case of fatal envenoming was reported from Brazil. Copyright D. A. Warrell.

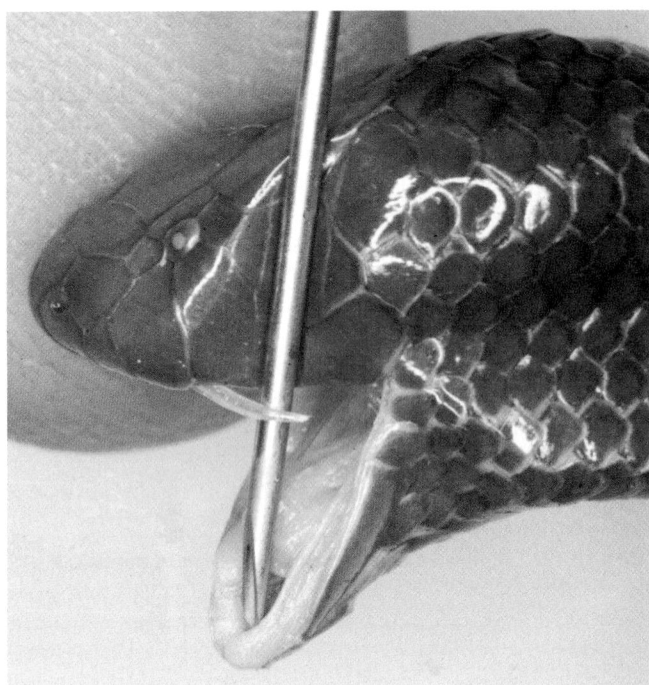

Fig. 9.2.2 Burrowing asp *Atractaspis aterrima*, showing fang.
Copyright D. A. Warrell.

A. engaddensis, and *A. irregularis*, have proved capable of killing humans.

Elapidae

This family includes cobras (Fig. 9.2.3), kraits, mambas, shield-nose snakes, coral snakes (Fig. 9.2.4), garter snakes, all the venomous Australasian snakes (Fig. 9.2.5), and sea snakes (Fig. 9.2.6). The short front fangs are immobile (Fig. 9.2.3a and Fig. 9.2.6). Several African and Asian species (rinkhals and spitting cobras) can eject venom from the tips of their fangs as a fine spray for a distance of a few metres into the eyes of an aggressor.

Viperidae

The front fangs are long, curved, and capable of a wide range of movement (Fig. 9.2.7). The subfamily Crotalinae comprises the American rattlesnakes (Fig. 9.2.8), moccasins, lance-headed vipers, and Asian pit vipers, which possess a heat-sensitive pit organ behind the nostril (Fig. 9.2.9). The Old World vipers and adders (subfamily *Viperinae*) have no pit organ.

Incidence and importance of snake bites

Snake bite is an important medical emergency in some parts of the rural tropics; its incidence is usually underestimated because most victims seek the help of traditional healers rather than practitioners of western-style medicine. In a rural population in Kenya where snake bites cause 6.7 deaths per 100 000 per year (0.7% of all deaths), 68% of bitten people had sought treatment from traditional healers. In Africa, the saw-scaled or carpet viper *Echis* spp., puff adder *Bitis arietans*, and spitting cobras (*Naja nigricollis, N. mossambica*, etc.) are the species of greatest medical importance. In the Benue Valley of north-east Nigeria, *E. ocellatus* (Fig. 9.2.10) causes some 500 bites per 100 000 population per year, with a 12% mortality. Vipers of the genus *Echis*, whose geographical range extends through Africa north of the equator, the Middle East, and eastern Asia to India, are responsible for many bites and deaths. In India, the most important species are cobras *Naja naja, N. oxiana, N. kaouthia* (Fig. 9.2.3), common krait *Bungarus caeruleus*, Russell's viper *Daboia russelii* (Fig. 9.2.7), and *E. carinatus*. An annual snake-bite mortality of 50 000 has been suggested. In Burdwan District, West Bengal, 8000 people are bitten and 800 die each year. In South East Asia, the Malayan pit viper *Calloselasma rhodostoma, D. siamensis*, green pit vipers (e.g. *Cryptelytrops (Trimeresurus) albolabris*), and cobras *N. kaouthia* and *N. siamensis* cause most bites and deaths. In Burma, Russell's viper bite is a common cause of acute renal failure and is responsible for most of the estimated 1000 snake-bite deaths each year. In Central and South America, medically important species include rattlesnakes (e.g. *Crotalus simus, C. durissus*) (Fig. 9.2.8) and the lance-headed vipers *Bothrops atrox* ('barba amarilla' or 'fer de lance'), *B. asper* ('terciopelo'), and *B. jararaca* ('jararaca'). In the United States of America, there are about 45 000 bites and a few deaths each year. Rattlesnakes, especially *Crotalus adamanteus, C. atrox, C. horridus, C.oreganus, C. scutulatus, C. viridis* and *Sistrurus miliaris*, are the most dangerous species. In the Amami and Ryukyu islands of Japan, the habu *Protobothrops flavoviridis* inflicted an average of 610 bites with 5.6 deaths per year during the 1960s. In the United Kingdom, the adder or viper *Vipera berus* is the only venomous species (Fig. 9.2.11). More than 200 people are bitten each year, but only 14 deaths have been reported since 1876, the last in 1975. In Sweden, this species causes between 150 and 200 hospital admissions each year: 44 deaths occurred between 1911 and 1978; and in Finland, 21 deaths in 25 years with an annual incidence of almost 200 bites. *V. aspis* causes most bites in France, and *V. ammodytes* is important in Eastern Europe.

Australia harbours the deadliest snakes in the world, judging by the lethal potency of their venoms. There are about 1000 bites (4.76/100 000 population) and 2 to 5 deaths (0.1–0.2/100 000) per year. Recently, all fatalities have been caused by brown snakes *Pseudonaja* spp. Other important species are tiger snakes (*Notechis scutatus* etc.), taipan *Oxyuranus scutellatus* (Fig. 9.2.5), and death adder *Acanthophis* spp. The highest snake-bite mortalities, up to 24% of all adult deaths, are recorded among hunter–gatherer tribes of Brazil (Kashinawa), Venezuela (Yanomamo), Ecuador (Waorani), Tanzania (Hadza), and Papua New Guinea.

Epidemiology

Most snake bites are inflicted on the lower limbs of farmers, plantation workers, herdsmen, and hunters in rural areas of tropical developing countries. The snake is usually trodden on at night or in undergrowth. Some species such as the Asian kraits *Bungarus* spp. and African spitting cobras *N. nigricollis* enter human dwellings at night and may bite people who roll over on to them while sleeping on the floor. Snakes do not bite without provocation, but may strike if inadvertently trodden upon or touched. In Europe, North America, and Australia, snakes are increasingly popular 'macho' pets: in these countries, bites are inflicted on the hands of men who are picking up their exotic pets. In the United States, 25% of bites result from snakes being attacked or handled. Serious bites by back-fanged (colubrid) snakes usually occur under these circumstances. Seasonal peaks in the incidence of snake bite are associated with agricultural activities, such as ploughing before the annual rains in the West African Sahel and the rice harvest in

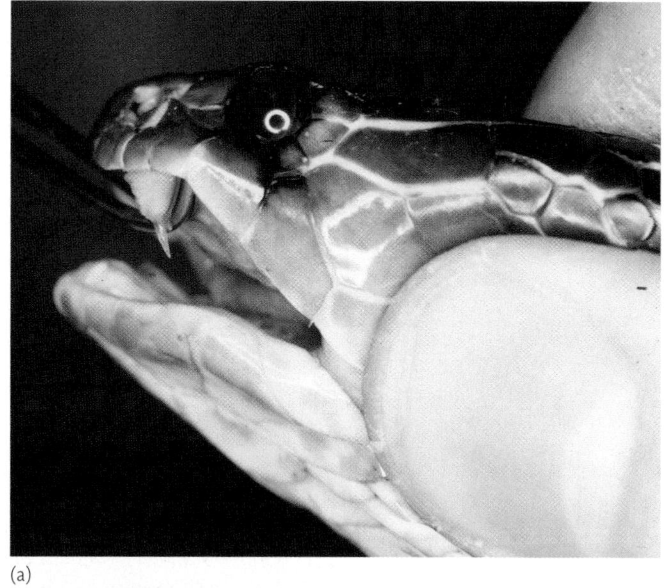
(a)

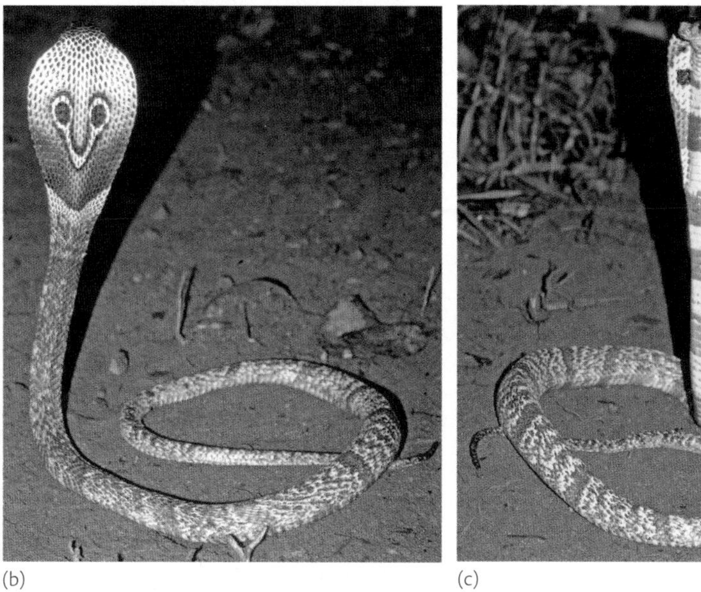
(b) (c)

Fig. 9.2.3 Sri Lankan cobra *Naja naja*: (a) short front fang, (b) and (c) showing defensive posture with open hood with 'spectacle' marking.

South East Asia, or to fluctuations in the activity or population of venomous snakes. Severe flooding, by concentrating the human and snake populations, has given rise to epidemics of snake bite, notably in Colombia, Pakistan, India, Bangladesh, Nepal, Burma, and Vietnam. Invasion of virgin jungle during construction of new highways and irrigation and hydroelectric schemes has led to an increased incidence of snake bite in Brazil and Sri Lanka. Snake bite or injection of snake venom has long been used for murder and suicide.

Venom apparatus

The venom glands of Elapidae and Viperidae are situated behind the eye, surrounded by compressor muscles (Fig. 9.2.7c). A venom duct opens within the sheath at the base of the fang and venom is conducted to its tip through a canal. In Colubridae, venom secreted by Duvernoy's gland tracks down grooves in the anterior surfaces of fangs at the posterior end of the maxilla (Fig. 9.2.1). The average dry weight of venom injected at a strike is approximately 60 mg in *N. naja*, 13 mg in *E. carinatus*, 63 mg in *D. russelii*, and 32 mg in *Daboia palaestinae*. The amount injected when a snake bites a human is very variable. A proportion of bites are 'dry bites', associated with negligible envenoming: more than 50% of those bitten by Malayan pit vipers *C. rhodostoma* or Russell's vipers; less than 10% bitten by *Echis* spp.; but more than 75% bitten by common brown snakes in Australia *Pseudonaja* spp. The Palestine viper *Daboia palaestinae* expends only about one-tenth of the capacity of its venom gland at each consecutive strike, whereas *Daboia siamensis* exhausts more than three-quarters of its reservoir at the first strike. The popular belief that snakes are less dangerous after they have eaten is incorrect.

Prevention of snake bite

To reduce the risk of bites, snakes should never be disturbed, attacked, cornered, or handled, even if they are thought to be a harmless species or appear to be dead. Venomous species should never be kept as pets or as performing animals. In snake-infested areas, boots, socks, and long trousers should be worn for walks in

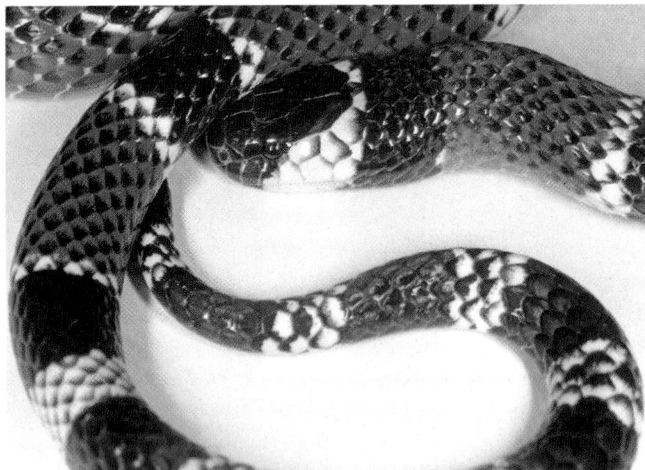

Fig. 9.2.4 Painted coral snake *Micrurus corallinus*, Brazil.
Copyright D. A. Warrell.

undergrowth or deep sand, and a light should always be carried at night. Collecting firewood; dislodging logs and boulders with bare hands; pushing sticks or fingers into burrows, holes, and crevices; climbing rocks and trees covered with dense foliage; and swimming in overgrown lakes and rivers are particularly hazardous activities. Unlit paths and gutters are especially dangerous after heavy rains. Sleeping on the ground carries a risk of nocturnal krait bites in south Asia and of spitting cobra bites in Africa, but mosquito nets are protective. To prevent sea-snake bites, fishermen should not touch these animals when they are caught in nets or on lines. Swimmers and divers should not aggravate them and should avoid wading in the sea, especially in muddy estuaries, in sand, or near coral reefs.

It is futile and ecologically undesirable to attempt to exterminate venomous snakes. Various substances toxic to snakes, such as insecticides and methylbromide, have been used to keep human dwellings free of these animals. However, no effective yet harmless snake repellent has been discovered.

Immunization against envenoming

The idea of inducing protective levels of antibodies against lethal venom components in high-risk populations by pre-exposure immunization has been tried, with inconclusive results, in Japan, against *Protobothrops flavoviridis,* and has been considered in Burma and some other countries. To be effective, high titres of a neutralizing antibody would have to be present at the time of the bite. This has been achieved in animals used for antivenom production but only by frequent immunization, which would not be practicable

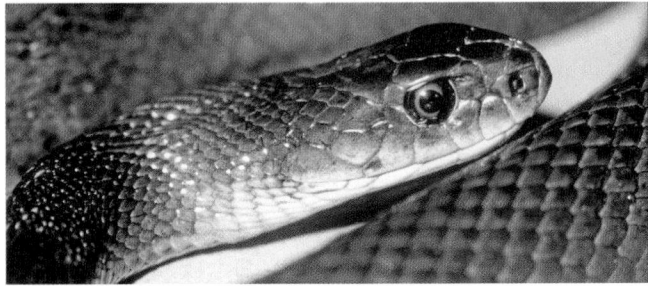

Fig. 9.2.5 Papua New Guinean taipan *Oxyuranus scutellatus canni*, an Australasian elapid snake.
Copyright D. A. Warrell.

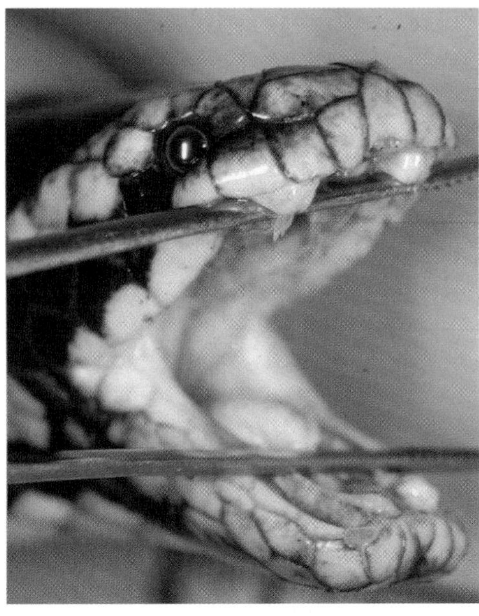

Fig. 9.2.6 Short front fangs of the laticaudine sea snake (sea krait) *Laticauda colubrina*.
Copyright D. A. Warrell.

even in high-risk human populations such as Burmese rice farmers. The accelerated secondary response stimulated by envenoming would be too late to be useful. An anti-rattlesnake vaccine for domestic dogs, of dubious efficacy, is marketed in the United States.

Properties of snake venoms

Snake venoms may contain more than 100 different proteins. More than 90% of the dry weight of venom is protein, in the form of enzymes, nonenzymatic polypeptide toxins, and nontoxic proteins such as nerve growth factor. Enzymes constitute 80 to 90% of viperid and 25 to 70% of elapid venoms. These include digestive hydrolases, hyaluronidase, and activators or inactivators of physiological processes. Most venoms contain L-amino acid oxidase, phosphomono- and diesterases, 5′-nucleotidase, DNAase, NAD-nucleosidase, phospholipase A_2, and peptidases. Elapid venoms also contain acetylcholine esterase, phospholipase B, and glycerophosphatase, while viperid venoms have metalloproteinases, endopeptidase, arginine ester hydrolase, kininogenase, as well as thrombin-like, factor X, and prothrombin-activating enzymes. Phospholipase A_2 (lecithinase) is the most widespread and extensively studied of all venom enzymes. It damages mitochondria, red blood cells, leucocytes, platelets, peripheral nerve endings, skeletal muscle, vascular endothelium, and other membranes, produces presynaptic neurotoxic activity, opiate-like sedative effects, the autopharmacological release of histamine, and may be anticoagulant. The acetylcholinesterase found in most elapid venoms does not contribute to their neurotoxicity. Hyaluronidase promotes the spread of venom through tissues. Proteolytic enzymes (metalloproteinases, endopeptidases, or hydrolases) are responsible for local changes in vascular permeability leading to oedema, blistering, and bruising, and to necrosis. Venom L-amino acid oxidases are homodimeric flavoenzymes that catalyse the oxidative deamination of an L-amino acid substrate to an α-keto acid, ammonia, and hydrogen peroxide. They are widely distributed in venoms of Viperidae and Elapidae. Their reported biological activities include

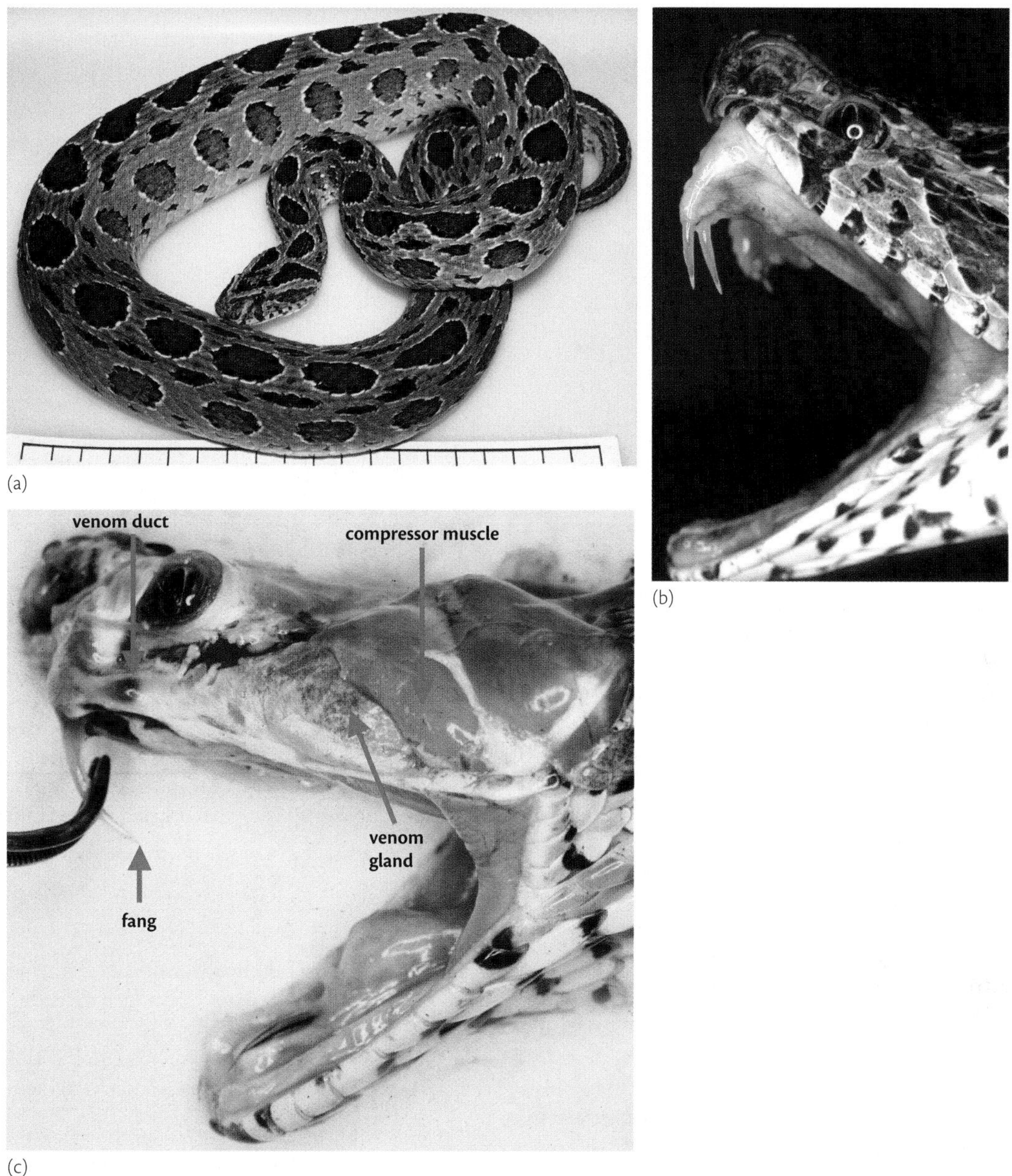

(a) (b) (c)

Fig. 9.2.7 Eastern Russell's viper *Daboia siamensis*, Ban Mi, Thailand: (a) showing 'chain' pattern (scale in cm); (b) showing long, hinged front fangs (reserve fang on the left side) in dental sheath; (c) dissection of venom apparatus.
Copyright D. A. Warrell.

induction of apoptosis, oedema, and haemolysis, antibacterial function, and platelet activation or inhibition.

Polypeptide toxins (neurotoxins)

Postsynaptic (α) neurotoxins such as α-bungarotoxin and cobrotoxin contain about 60 to 62 or 66 to 74 amino acids. They bind to acetylcholine receptors at the motor endplate. Presynaptic (β) neurotoxins, such as β-bungarotoxin, crotoxin, and taipoxin, contain about 120 to 140 amino acids and a phospholipase A subunit. These release acetylcholine at the nerve endings at neuromuscular junctions and then damage the endings, preventing further release of transmitter.

Venom pharmacology

The smaller neurotoxins of the Elapidae are rapidly absorbed into the bloodstream, whereas the larger phospholipase A_2 presynaptic toxins and Viperidae toxins are taken up more slowly through the lymphatics. Venoms of the spitting cobras and rinkhals can be absorbed through the intact cornea, causing systemic envenoming and even death in animals. Envenoming after ingestion of snake venom has not been reported in humans. Most venoms are concentrated and bound in the kidney, and some components are eliminated in the urine. Crotaline venoms are selectively bound in the lungs, concentrated in the liver, and excreted in bile, while polypeptide neurotoxins, such as α-bungarotoxin, are tightly bound at neuromuscular junctions. Most venom components do not cross the intact blood–brain barrier and so central effects of venoms are controversial.

Pathophysiology

Swelling and bruising of the bitten limb result from increased vascular permeability induced by proteases, phospholipases,

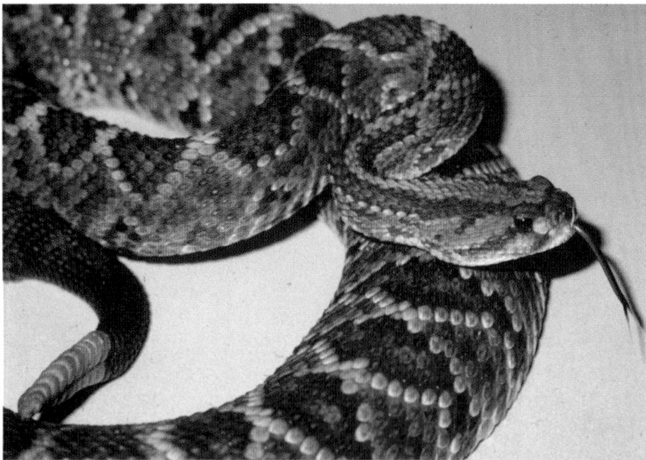

Fig. 9.2.8 South American tropical rattlesnake or cascabel *Crotalus durissus cascavella*.

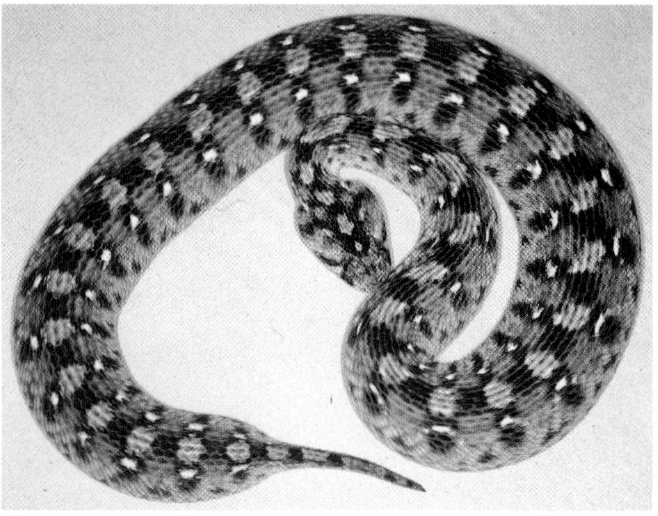

Fig. 9.2.10 Saw-scaled or carpet viper *Echis ocellatus* from West Africa.

membrane-damaging metalloproteinases (haemorrhagins), and endogenous autacoids released by the venom, such as histamine, 5-hydroxytryptamine, and kinins. Venoms of some of the North American rattlesnakes and viperine species cause a generalized increase in vascular permeability resulting in hypovolaemia, haemoconcentration, hypoalbuminaemia, albuminuria, serous effusions, pulmonary oedema, and, in the case of Burmese *D. siamensis*, conjunctival and facial oedema (Fig. 9.2.12). Tissue necrosis near the site of the bite is caused by myotoxic and cytolytic factors: in some cases, ischaemia resulting from thrombosis, intracompartmental syndrome, or a tight tourniquet may contribute. Causes of hypotension and shock include hypovolaemia, vasodilatation, and myocardial dysfunction. Some venoms release vasodilating autacoids such as histamine and kinins. Venom of the Brazilian jararaca *B. jararaca* was found to activate bradykinin and, through a bradykinin-potentiating peptide, to prolong its hypotensive effect by inactivating the peptidyl dipeptidase responsible both for destroying bradykinin and for converting angiotensin I to angiotensin II. This observation led to the synthesis of angiotensin-converting enzyme (ACE) inhibitors. Bradykinin-potentiating and ACE-inhibiting peptides have also been found in a number of other crotaline venoms (genera *Bothrops* and *Agkistrodon*). To date, four sarafotoxins have been isolated from the venom of the Israeli burrowing asp *Atractaspis engaddensis* (Fig. 9.2.2). They show 60% sequence homology with the endothelins, which are also 21-amino acid polypeptides. Sarafotoxins and endothelins are potent vasoconstrictors (including coronary arteries), delay atrioventricular conduction, and are positively inotropic.

Snake venoms can cause haemostatic defects in a number of different ways. Venom procoagulant enzymes, many of them serine proteases, activate the blood clotting cascade at various sites. Some Viperidae venoms contain thrombin-like fibrinogenases, which remove fibrinopeptides from fibrinogen directly. Others activate endogenous plasminogen. Venoms may induce or inhibit platelet aggregation. Spontaneous systemic bleeding is caused by haemorrhagins, metalloendopeptidases, some with disintegrin-like and

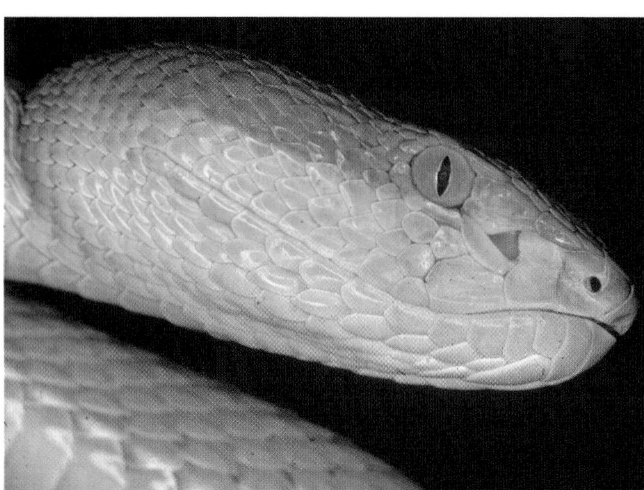

Fig. 9.2.9 Southeast Asian white-lipped green pit viper *Cryptelytrops (Trimeresurus) albolabris* showing heat-sensitive pit organ between eye and nostril.

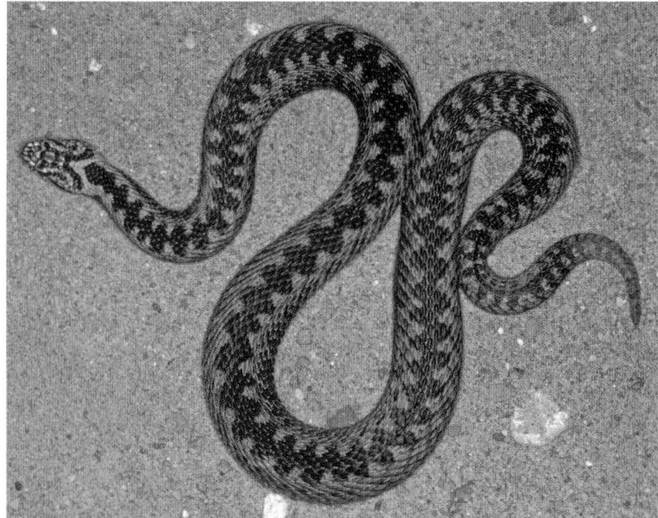

Fig. 9.2.11 European adder or viper *Vipera berus*, the only venomous British snake. This specimen is 50 cm long.

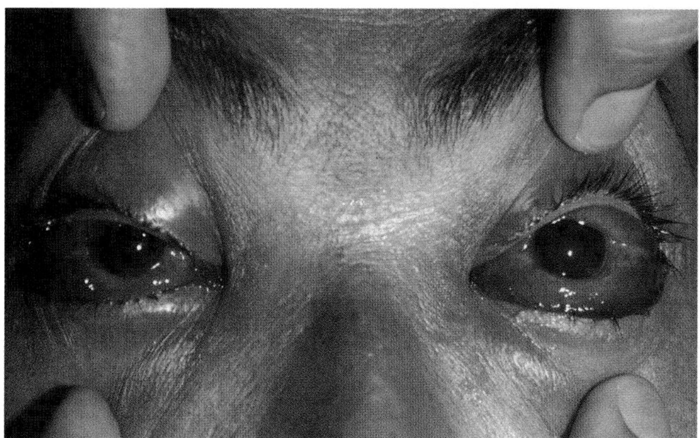

Fig. 9.2.12 Gross bilateral conjunctival oedema (chemosis) in a Burmese rice farmer 48 h after being bitten by a Russell's viper.
Copyright D. A. Warrell.

other domains, which damage vascular endothelium (Fig. 9.2.13). The combination of consumptive coagulopathy, thrombocytopenia, and vessel wall damage can result in massively incontinent bleeding, a common cause of death after bites by Viperidae, Australasian Elapidae, and the few medically important Colubridae. Many venoms are haemolytic *in vitro*, but clinically significant intravascular haemolysis, apart from the microangiopathic haemolysis associated with disseminated intravascular coagulation described in victims of viperine and Australian brown snake *Pseudonaja* bites, is seen only after bites by *D. russelii* (Sri Lanka and India), and some *Bothrops* and colubrid species. Acute renal tubular necrosis may be caused by severe hypotension, disseminated intravascular coagulation (*D. russelii, D. siamensis*), a direct nephrotoxic effect of the venom (*D. siamensis*), and myoglobinuria secondary to generalized rhabdomyolysis (sea snakes, *D. russelii* in Sri Lanka and India, and tropical rattlesnakes). Neurotoxic polypeptides and phospholipases block neuromuscular transmission causing death through bulbar or respiratory paralysis.

Clinical features

Fear, effects of treatment, and the venom contribute to the symptoms and signs of snake bite. Even patients who are not envenomed may feel flushed, dizzy, and breathless and may notice constriction of the chest, palpitations, sweating, and acroparaesthesiae. Tight tourniquets may produce swollen and ischaemic limbs; local incisions at the site of the bite may cause bleeding and sensory loss and herbal medicines often induce vomiting. The earliest symptoms directly attributable to the bite are local pain and bleeding from the fang punctures, followed by pain, tenderness, swelling and bruising extending up the limb, lymphangitis, and tender enlargement of regional lymph nodes. An anaphylaxis-like syndrome of early syncope, vomiting, colic, diarrhoea, angio-oedema, and wheezing may follow bites by European Vipera, Russell's vipers, *Bothrops* spp., Australian elapids, and *Atractaspis engaddensis*. Nausea and vomiting are common early symptom of systemic envenoming.

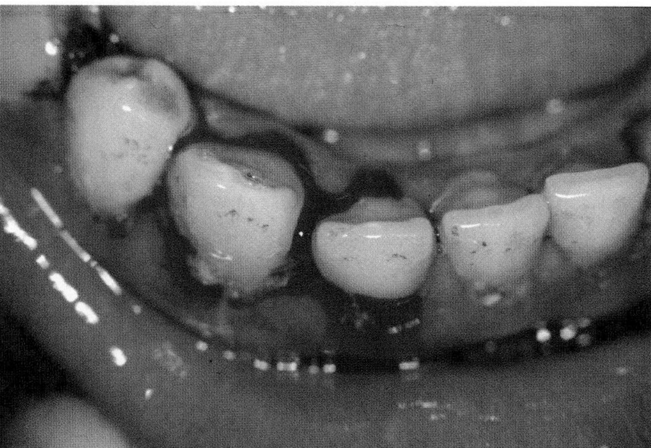

Fig. 9.2.13 Haemorrhagin activity revealed clinically as gingival haemorrhage in a patient bitten by a saw-scaled or carpet viper *Echis ocellatus* in Nigeria.
Copyright D. A. Warrell.

Bites by Colubridae (back-fanged snakes)

Severe envenoming causes repeated vomiting, colicky abdominal pain, headache, widespread systemic bleeding with widespread ecchymoses, incoagulable blood, intravascular haemolysis, and renal failure. Local swelling and bruising may be the only results of envenoming. The first symptoms of envenoming may be delayed for 24 to 72 h after the bite.

Bites by Atractaspididae (burrowing asps or stiletto snakes)

Local effects are pain, swelling, blistering, necrosis, and tender enlargement of local lymph nodes. Violent gastrointestinal symptoms (nausea, vomiting, and diarrhoea), anaphylaxis (dyspnoea, respiratory failure), and ECG changes (atrioventricular block, ST, T-wave changes) have been described in patients envenomed by *A. engaddensis* and *A. microlepidota andersoni*.

Bites by Elapidae (cobras, kraits, mambas, African garter snakes, coral snakes, and Australasian snakes)

Bites by kraits, mambas, coral snakes, and some cobras (e.g. *N. haje, N. nivea* and *N. philippinensis*) produce minimal local effects, but the venoms of African spitting cobras (*N. nigricollis, N. mossambica*, etc.) and Asian cobras (*N. naja, N. kaouthia, N. sumatrana*, etc.) cause tender local swelling, blistering, and superficial necrosis, which may be extensive (Fig. 9.2.14). 'Skip' lesions, separated by apparently normal areas of skin, may occur (Fig. 9.2.15). However, elapid venoms are best known for their neurotoxic effects. Early symptoms, before there are objective neurological signs, include vomiting, 'heaviness' of the eyelids, blurred vision, paraesthesiae around the mouth, hyperacusis, headache, dizziness, vertigo, hypersalivation, congested conjunctivas, and 'gooseflesh'. Paralysis is first detectable as ptosis and external ophthalmoplegia appearing as early as 15 min after the bite, but sometimes it is delayed for 10 h or even more than 24 h. Later the face, palate, jaws, tongue, vocal cords, neck muscles, and muscles of deglutition may become paralysed (Fig. 9.2.16). The pupils are dilated. Respiratory failure may be precipitated by airway obstruction at this stage, or later after paralysis of intercostal muscles and the diaphragm. Neurotoxic effects are completely reversible, either acutely in response to antivenom or anticholinesterases—e.g. following bites by Asian cobras, some Latin American coral snakes *Micrurus* spp., and Australasian death adders *Acanthophis* spp.—or they may wear off spontaneously in 1 to 7 days. Excruciating pain and paraesthesiae radiating up the bitten limb has been described with bites by coral snakes (*Micrurus* spp.) suggesting direct venom action on C (pain) fibres. Severe abdominal pain, perhaps attributable to the smooth muscle stimulating effects of an AVIT toxin, is

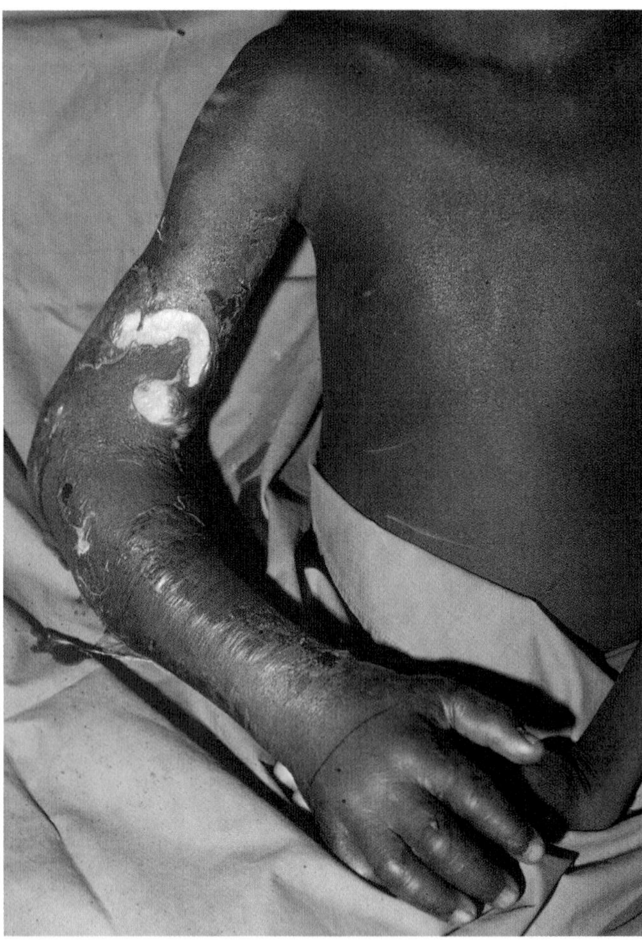

Fig. 9.2.14 Extensive necrosis of skin and subcutaneous tissues in a Nigerian girl bitten 9 days previously on the elbow by a black-necked or spitting cobra *Naja nigricollis*.
Copyright D. A. Warrell.

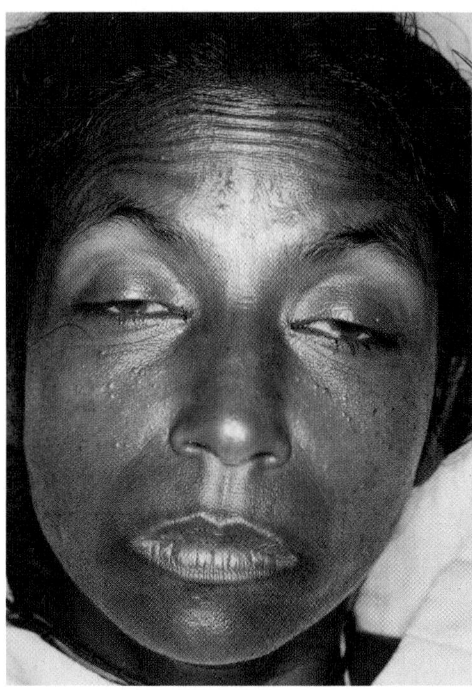

Fig. 9.2.16 Neurotoxic envenoming. Ptosis, external ophthalmoplegia, and facial paralysis in a Sri Lankan patient envenomed by the common krait *Bungarus caeruleus*.
Copyright D A Warrell.

often the most striking initial symptom in victims of krait bites (*Bungarus* spp.).

Envenoming by terrestrial Australasian elapids produces four main groups of symptoms: neurotoxicity (Fig. 9.2.17), haemostatic disturbances and, rarely, generalized rhabdomyolysis, and renal failure. Painful regional lymph nodes are a useful sign of impending systemic envenoming, but local signs are usually mild, except after

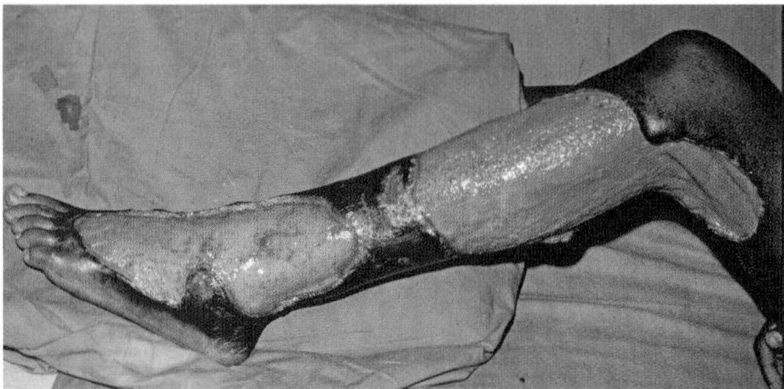

Fig. 9.2.15 Sierra Leonian woman showing 'skip lesion' separated by an area of unaffected skin after envenoming by a black-necked spitting cobra *Naja nigricollis*.
Copyright D. A. Warrell.

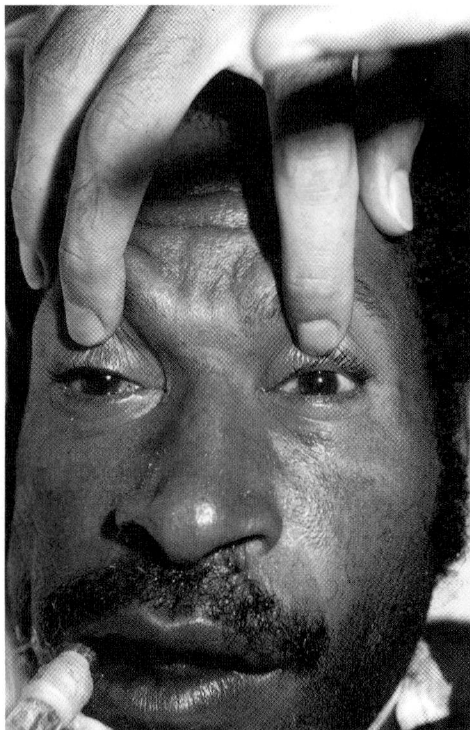

Fig. 9.2.17 Generalized paralysis, including ptosis, external ophthalmoplegia (inability to look upwards), inability to open the mouth, protrude the tongue, swallow or speak, and respiratory paralysis requiring mechanical ventilation in a Papua New Guinean man bitten 24 h previously by a taipan *Oxyuranus scutellatus canni*.
Copyright D. A. Warrell.

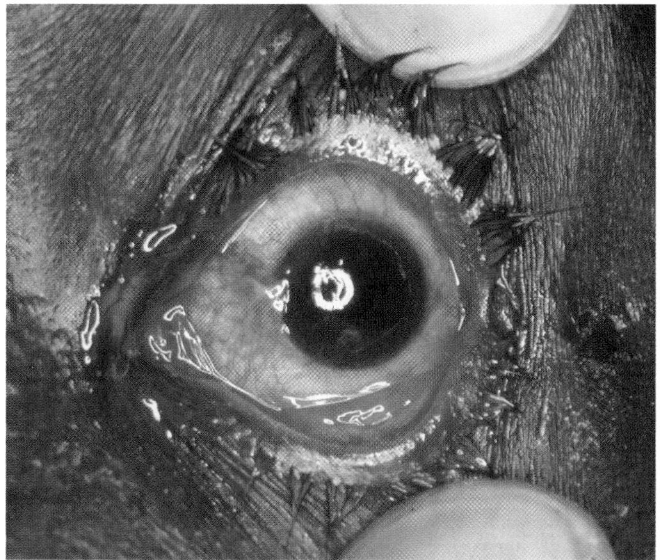

(a)

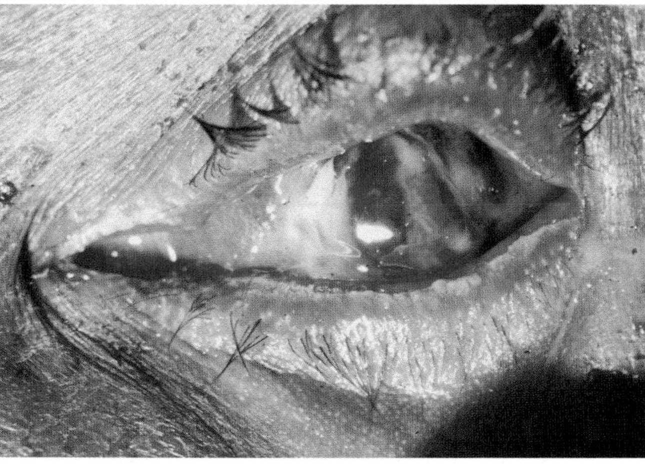

(b)

Fig. 9.2.18 Venom ophthalmia caused by the black-necked spitting cobra *Naja nigricollis*: (a) Acute venom ophthalmia showing intense painful inflammation and discharge. (b) In this case, the corneal injury was neglected and so secondary infection developed, necessitating enucleation of the eye.
Copyright D. A. Warrell.

bites by the king brown or Mulga snake *Pseudechis australis*. Early symptoms include vomiting, headache, and syncopal attacks.

Patients 'spat' at by spitting elapids may develop venom ophthalmia. There is intense pain in the eye, blepharospasm, palpebral oedema, and leucorrhoea (Fig. 9.2.18a). Corneal erosions can be seen by slit-lamp or fluorescein examination in more than half of patients spat at by *N. nigricollis*. Rarely, venom is absorbed into the anterior chamber causing hypopyon and anterior uveitis. Secondary infection of corneal abrasions may lead to permanent blinding opacities or panophthalmitis (Fig. 9.2.18b).

Bites by sea snakes and sea kraits

Patients envenomed by sea snakes notice headache, a thick feeling of the tongue, thirst, sweating, and vomiting. Between 30 min and 3.5 h after the bite, there is generalized aching, stiffness, and tenderness of the muscles. Trismus is common. Later there is generalized flaccid paralysis. Myoglobinuria appears 3 to 8 h after the bite. Myoglobin and potassium released from damaged skeletal muscles can cause renal failure, while hyperkalaemia may precipitate cardiac arrest.

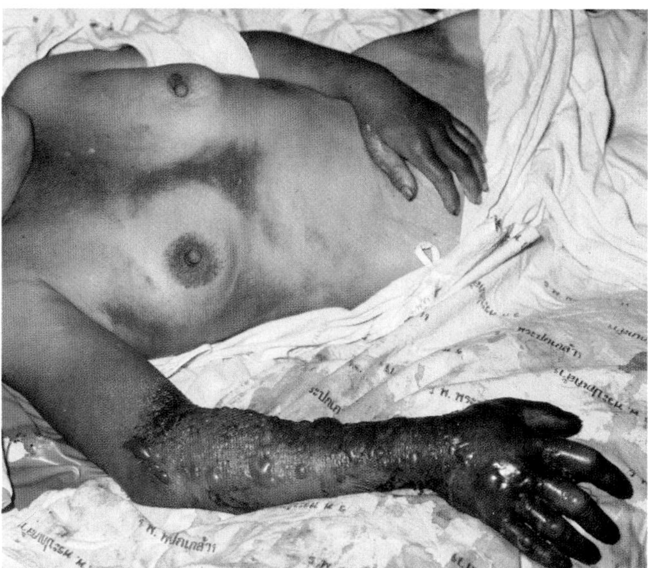

Fig. 9.2.19 Swelling, blistering, and necrosis in a Thai woman bitten on the hand by a Malayan pit viper *Calloselasma rhodostoma*. There is generalized bruising.
Copyright D. A. Warrell.

Bites by Viperidae (vipers, adders, rattlesnakes, lance-headed vipers, moccasins, and pit vipers)

Viper venoms usually produce more severe local effects than do those of other snakes. Swelling may become detectable within 15 min but is sometimes delayed for several hours. It spreads rapidly, sometimes involving the whole limb, adjacent trunk and, in children, the whole body. There is associated pain and tenderness in regional lymph nodes, with bruising of overlying tissues and lymphangitic lines. Bruising, blistering, and necrosis may appear during the next few days (Fig. 9.2.19). Necrosis can be severe following bites by some rattlesnakes, lance-headed vipers *Bothrops* spp., Asian pit vipers, and the large African *Bitis* species. When the envenomed tissue is contained in a tight fascial compartment such as the pulp space of digits or the anterior tibial compartment, ischaemia may result (Fig. 9.2.20). Absence of swelling 2 h after a viper bite suggests that there has been no envenoming. However, fatal envenoming by a few species can occur in the absence of local signs (for example, *C. d. terrificus*, *C. scutulatus*, and Burmese Russell's viper). Haemostatic abnormalities are characteristic of envenoming by Viperidae. Persistent bleeding from fang puncture wounds, venepuncture or injection sites, other new and partially healed

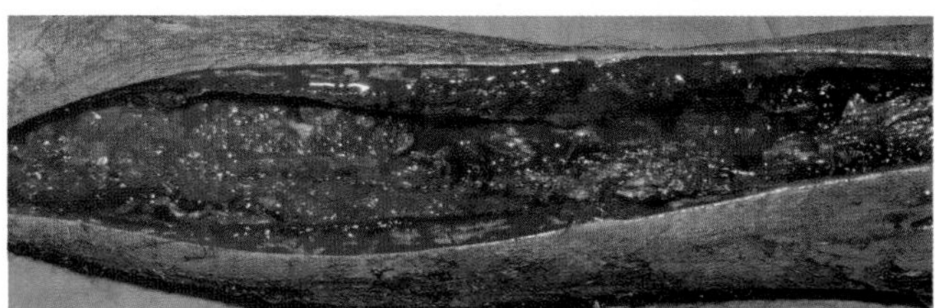

Fig. 9.2.20 Extensive necrosis of skin and muscle including the contents of the anterior tibial compartment in a patient bitten by a lancehead *Bothrops marajoensis* in Brazil 27 days earlier.
Copyright D A Warrell.

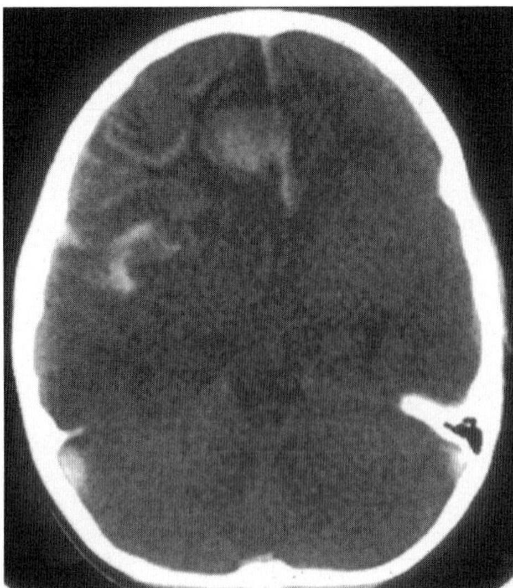

Fig. 9.2.21 CT scan showing intracranial haemorrhage in a child bitten by a common lancehead *Bothrops atrox* in Ecuador. The fluid level in the larger collection of blood indicates that the blood was incoagulable.

wounds, and postpartum, indicates that the blood is incoagulable. Spontaneous systemic haemorrhage is most often detected in the gingival sulci. Epistaxis, haematemesis, cutaneous ecchymoses, haemoptysis, and subconjunctival, retroperitoneal, and intracranial haemorrhages (Fig. 9.2.21) are also seen. Patients envenomed by Burmese Russell's vipers may suffer haemorrhagic infarction of the anterior pituitary (Sheehan's syndrome) (Fig. 9.2.22). Hypotension and shock are common in patients bitten by North American rattlesnakes (e.g. *C. adamanteus, C. atrox*, and *C. scutulatus*), *Bothrops, Daboia*, and *Vipera* species (e.g. *D. palaestinae* and *V. berus*). The central venous pressure is usually low and the pulse

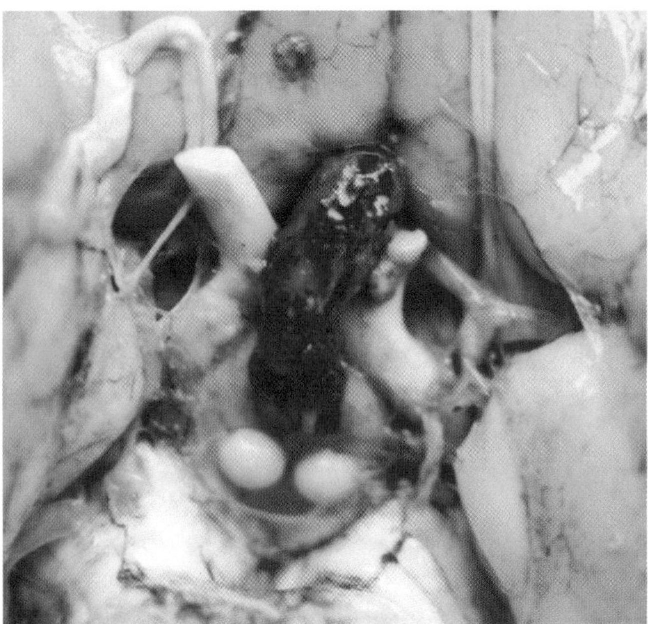

Fig. 9.2.22 Haemorrhagic infarction of the anterior pituitary in a Burmese patient who died after being bitten by a Russell's viper *Daboia russelii siamensis*.
By courtesy of Dr U Hla Mon, Yangon, Myanmar.

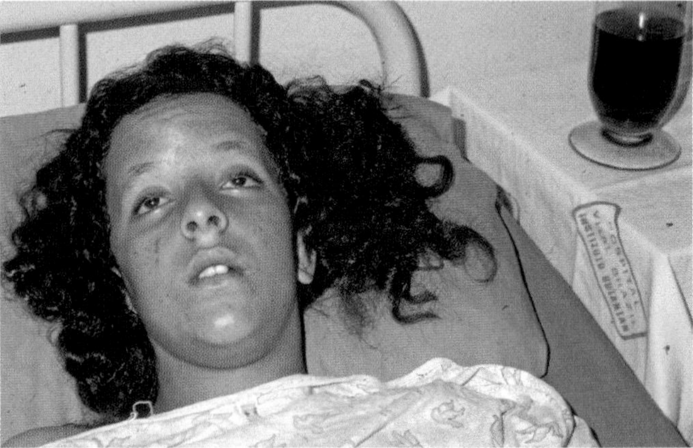

Fig. 9.2.23 Brazilian girl bitten 24 h earlier by a tropical rattlesnake *Crotalus durissus terrificus*. She has bilateral ptosis, paralysis of the facial muscles, and gross myoglobinuria resulting from generalized rhabdomyolysis.

rate rapid, suggesting hypovolaemia resulting from extravasation of fluid into the bitten limb. Patients envenomed by Burmese Russell's vipers and children envenomed by *Vipera berus* show evidence of generally increased vascular permeability. Direct myocardial involvement is suggested by an abnormal ECG or cardiac arrhythmia. Patients envenomed by some species of the genera *Daboia, Vipera, Crotalus*, and *Bothrops* and Australasian elapids may experience early transient and recurrent syncopal attacks, associated with features of an autopharmacological or anaphylactic reaction, such as vomiting, sweating, colic, diarrhoea, shock, and angio-oedema. These symptoms may appear as early as 5 min or as late as many hours after the bite. Early collapse after bites by Australian brown snakes (*Pseudonaja* spp.) and tiger snakes (*Notechis* spp.) has been attributed to coronary and pulmonary thromboembolism but this seems unlikely. Renal failure is a common mode of death in patients envenomed by Viperidae. Victims of Russell's viper may become oliguric within a few hours of the bite and complain of loin pain, suggesting renal ischaemia at a time when their plasma renin activity is high. Neurotoxicity, resembling that seen in patients bitten by Elapidae, is a feature of envenoming by a few species of Viperidae (e.g. *C. d. terrificus, Gloydius* spp., berg adder *Bitis atropos* and other small *Bitis* species, and Sri Lankan *D. russelii*) (Fig. 9.2.23). There is evidence of generalized rhabdomyolysis (Fig. 9.2.23), but progression to respiratory or generalized paralysis is unusual.

Envenoming by European vipers

The common viper or adder *V. berus* (Fig. 9.2.11), the only venomous snake found in the United Kingdom, occurs in England, Wales, Scotland, and northern Europe, extending into the Arctic Circle and through Asia as far east as Sakhalin island and south to northern Korea. There are four other vipers that are widely distributed in mainland Europe: the nose-horned or sand viper *V. ammodytes* in the Balkans, Italy, Austria, and Romania; the asp viper *V. aspis* in France (south of Paris), Spain, Germany, Switzerland, and Italy; Lataste's viper *V. latastei* in Spain and Portugal, and Orsini's viper *V. ursinii* in south-eastern France, central Italy, and eastern Europe. The Montpellier snake *Malpolon monspessulanus* is a large back-fanged colubrid snake whose bite can cause transient mild local symptoms and rarely neurotoxicity.

Clinical features of European viper bite

- Local envenoming: immediate sharp pain is followed by spreading pain, tenderness, and tender enlargement of regional lymph nodes within hours. Reddish lymphangitic lines and bruising appear, and the whole limb may become swollen and bruised within 24 h with involvement of the trunk and, in children, the whole body. Intracompartmental syndromes and necrosis are rare.
- Systemic envenoming: dramatic anaphylactic symptoms may appear between 5 min and many hours after the bite: nausea, retching, vomiting, abdominal colic, diarrhoea, incontinence of urine and faeces, sweating, fever, vasoconstriction, tachycardia, lightheadedness, shock with loss of consciousness, angio-oedema of the face, lips, gums, tongue, throat, and epiglottis, urticaria, and bronchospasm. These symptoms may persist or fluctuate for as long as 48 h in the absence of treatment. Hypotension is a dangerous sign that usually develops within 2 h and may resolve spontaneously, persist, recur, or progress fatally. Clinical features of a bleeding diathesis are unusual, but bleeding from the gums and nose and into the lungs, gastrointestinal and genitourinary tracts, and serosal cavities and retroperitoneally can occur. The risk of bleeding is greatly increased by misguided treatment with heparin. Fatal haemothorax, massive haematemesis and melaena, haematuria, and intrauterine fetal death are rare tragedies. Acute renal failure is not uncommon in children. Increased capillary permeability is reflected by the local and sometimes generalized oedema, as well as the more focal angio-oedema that can lead to fatal occlusion of the upper airway, pulmonary, and cerebral oedema. Coma and seizures are attributable to hypotension, cerebral oedema, hyponatraemia, hypoalbuminaemia, or hypoxaemia secondary to respiratory distress. Cardiac arrest, acute gastric dilatation, paralytic ileus, and acute pancreatitis are other reported complications. Classic mild neurotoxicity (ptosis, external ophthalmoplegia) has been reported after bites by several species of European Vipera, including *V. aspis*, *V. berus*, and *V. ammodytes* in certain geographical areas.
- Laboratory findings: neutrophil leucocytosis is common. Serum creatine kinase, transaminases, urea, and creatinine concentrations may be raised, and bicarbonate may be reduced. Thrombocytopenia and mild coagulopathy; reflected by prolonged prothrombin time, activated partial thromboplastin time, hypofibrinogenaemia, and raised fibrin degradation products or D-dimer; is sometimes detected. Severe coagulopathy is uncommon. Electrocardiographic changes include tachy- and brady- arrhythmias, atrial fibrillation, flattening or inversion of T-waves, ST elevation or depression, second-degree heart block, and frank myocardial infarction.
- Prognosis: most adder bites cause only trivial symptoms, but patients must be assessed individually and deaths have occured between 6 and 60 (average 34) h after the bite. Children may be severely envenomed: in a French series, there were three deaths in a group of seven children aged between 2.5 and 10 years. The dangers of adder bite should not be underestimated. The antivenom treatment of adder bite is discussed in the following paragraphs.

Laboratory investigations

The peripheral neutrophil count may be raised to 20 000 cells/μl or more in severely envenomed patients. The blood film may show evidence of microangiopathic haemolysis. Initial haemoconcentration, resulting from extravasation of plasma (*Crotalus* species and Burmese *D. siamensis*), is followed by anaemia caused by bleeding or, more rarely, haemolysis. Thrombocytopenia is common following bites by pit vipers (e.g. *Calloselasma rhodostoma, Crotalus oreganus helleri*) and some Viperidae (e.g. *Bitis arietans* and Russell's vipers), but is unusual after bites by *Echis* species. A simple bedside test for venom-induced defibrinogenation is the 20-min whole-blood clotting test. A few millilitres of venous blood is placed in a new, clean, dry, glass vessel, left undisturbed for 20 min, and then tipped once to see if it has clotted or not. Incoagulable blood indicates systemic envenoming, either consumptive coagulopathy (plasma fibrinogen concentration below 0.5 g/litre) or effects of an anticogulant toxin (e.g. envenoming by Australian black snake, *Pseudechis* spp.). It may be diagnostic of a particular species (e.g. *Echis* spp. in Africa north of the equator). The only equipment required for the test is a glass tube, but this may be difficult to find in modern hospitals where glass has been replaced by plastics. Glass is essential to contact-activate Hageman factor (factor XII) which initiates the 'intrinsic' coagulation pathway. Laboratory tests of blood coagulation (prothrombin time, activated partial thromboplastin time, fibrinogen concentration) and fibrinolysis (fibrin/fibrinogen degradation products, D-dimer) are useful but take longer. Patients with generalized rhabdomyolysis show a steep rise in serum creatine kinase, myoglobin, and potassium levels. Black or brown urine suggests generalized rhabdomyolysis and/or intravascular haemolysis. Concentrations of serum enzymes, such as creatine kinase and aspartate aminotransferase, are moderately raised in patients with severe local envenoming, due to muscle damage at the site of the bite. High concentrations suggest generalized rhabdomyolysis. Urine should be examined for blood/haemoglobin, myoglobin and protein, and for microscopic haematuria and red cell casts. Electrocardiographic abnormalities such as sinus bradycardia, ST–T changes, various degrees of atrioventricular block, and hyperkalaemic changes may be seen.

Immunodiagnosis

Specific snake venom antigens have been detected in wound swabs, aspirates or biopsies, serum, urine, cerebrospinal fluid, and other body fluids. Enzyme immunoassay (EIA) has been the most widely used. Under ideal conditions, relatively high venom antigen concentrations (wound swabs or aspirates) may be detected quickly enough (15–30 min) to allow the selection of the appropriate monospecific antivenom. A commercial venom detection kit for Australian elapids is produced by the Commonwealth Surum Laboratories (CSL), Melbourne. For retrospective diagnosis, including forensic cases, tissue around the fang punctures, wound and blister aspirate, serum, and urine should be stored for EIA immunodiagnosis.

Management of snake bite

First aid

The patient should be reassured and moved to the nearest hospital or dispensary as quickly, comfortably, and passively as possible. The whole patient should be immobilized and especially the bitten limb, using a splint or sling.

Most traditional first aid methods are potentially harmful and should not be used. Local incisions and suction do not remove venom effectively and may introduce infection, damage tissues, and cause persistent bleeding. Vacuum extractors, potassium permanganate, and ice packs may potentiate local necrosis. Electric shocks are

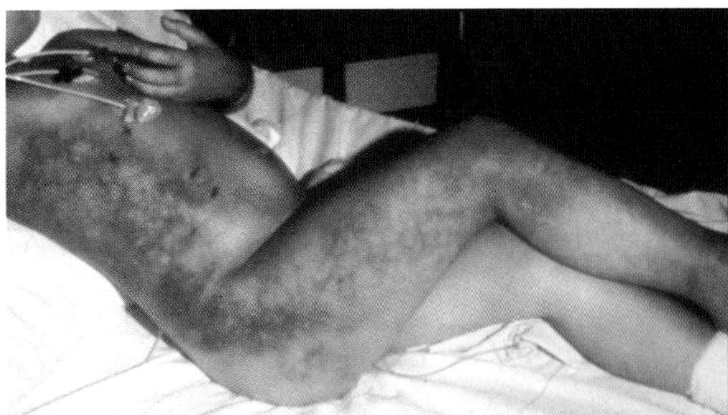

Fig. 9.2.24 Generalized swelling and bruising in a 4-year-old child bitten by a European adder *Vipera berus* in Sweden.
Courtesy of Dr H Persson.

dangerous and have not been proved beneficial. Tourniquets and compression bands are potentially dangerous as they can cause gangrene, increased fibrinolysis, and bleeding in the occluded limb, peripheral nerve palsies, compartmental ischaemia, and intensification of local signs of envenoming.

Pressure-immobilization (P-I)

In animal studies, compressing superficial veins and lymphatics in the bitten limb to a pressure of about 55 mmHg, using a stretchy bandage, reduced the spread of larger molecular weight toxins such as the presynaptic phospholipase A_2 toxins of Australian elapid venoms. In practice, the entire bitten limb is bound firmly, using a long broad elasticated bandage, starting at the toes or fingers and finishing at the groin or axilla. A splint is incorporating to aid immobilization (Fig. 9.2.25).

Anecdotal experience supports the use of the method, but it was not subjected to clinical trial before being recommended by the Australian National Health & Medical Research Council in 1979. The technique has proved difficult to learn and to apply correctly but is recommended for bites by neurotoxic elapids as it is the only available means of delaying the onset of potentially fatal respiratory paralysis until the patient reaches medical care without incurring the unacceptable risks of a tight arterial tourniquet. In cases of bites by snakes whose venoms cause severe local effects, P-I may be harmful by increasing pressure in fascial compartments (risking ischaemic necrosis) and accentuating local necrosis. However, in cases of bites by unknown species, this risk is outweighed by that of early respiratory paralysis. When someone with the necessary skills and equipment is available, P-I should be applied immediately unless a bite by a neurotoxic elapid can, with confidence, be excluded.

Pursuing and killing the snake is not recommended, but if the snake has been killed, it should be taken with the patient to hospital. It must not be handled as even a severed head can inject venom.

Snake bit first aid: pressure-immobilization method

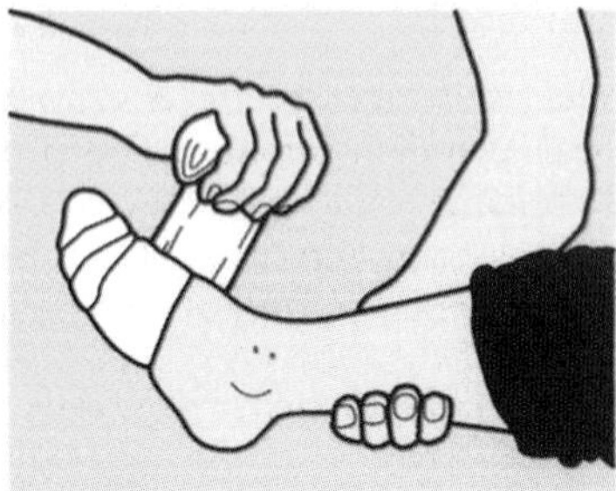

a) Apply a broad pressure bandage from below upwards and over the bite site as soon as possible. Do not remove trousers, as the movement of doing so will assist venom to enter the blood stream. Keep the bitten leg still.

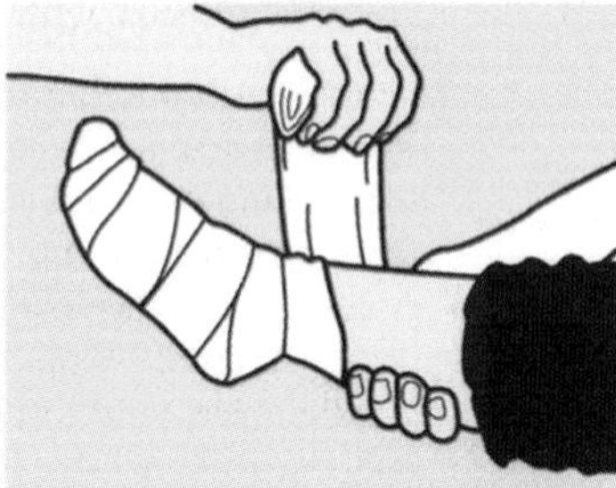

b) The bandage is bound firmly. The patient should avoid any unnecessary movements.

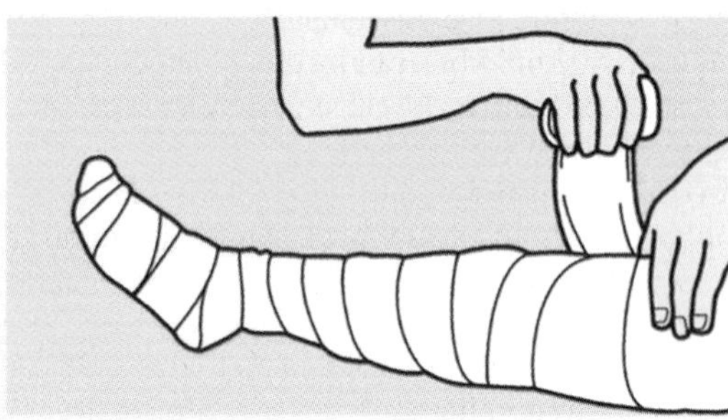

c) Extend the bandages as high as possible (ideally up to the groin).

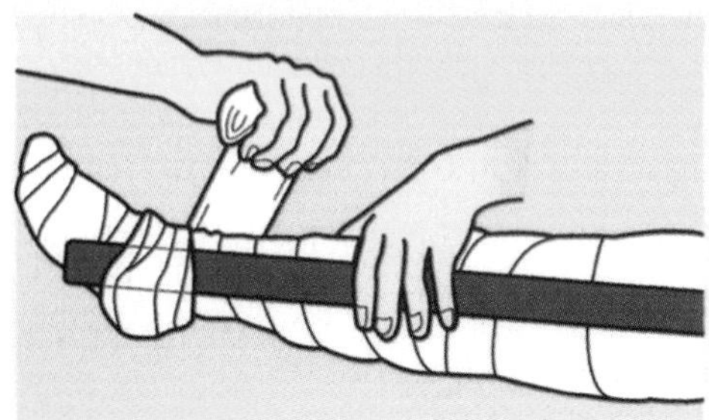

d) Apply a splint to the leg, immobilizing joints either side of the bite.

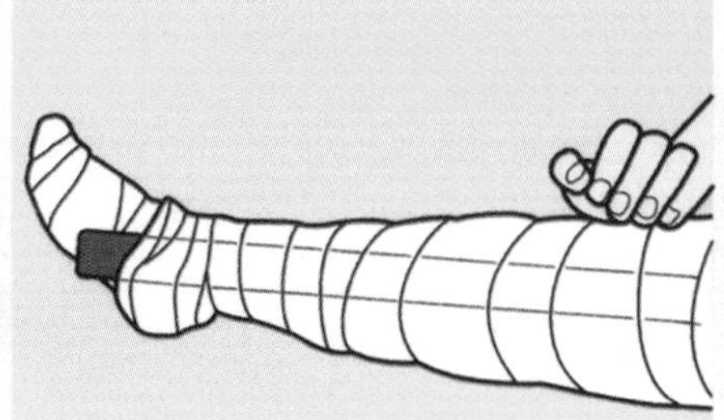

e) Bind it firmly to as much of the leg as possible. Walking should be restricted.

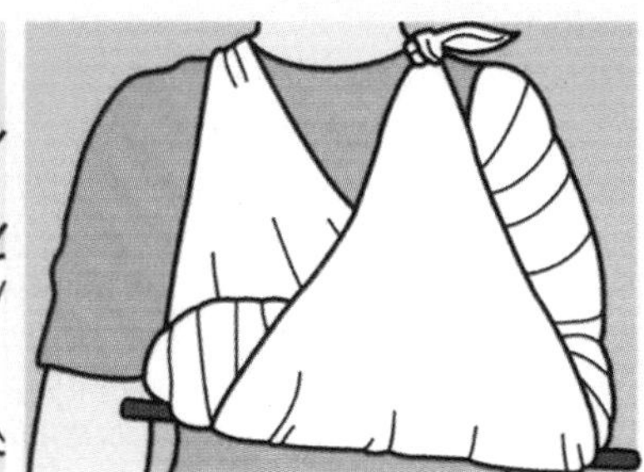

f) Bites on the hand and forearm: bind to the axilla, use a splint to the elbow, and use a sling.

Fig. 9.2.25 Pressure-immobilization method for first aid of patients bitten by neurotoxic elapid snakes.
Copyright DA Warrell.

Patients being transported to hospital should lie on their left side in the recovery position to prevent aspiration of vomit. Persistent vomiting can be treated with chlorpromazine by intramuscular injection (25–50 mg in adults, 1 mg/kg in children; intravenous injection risks hypotension) or chlorpromazine or prochlorperazine by intrarectal suppository. Syncope, shock, angio-oedema, and other autonomic symptoms can be treated with 0.1% adrenaline by intramuscular injection (0.5 ml for adults, 0.01 ml/kg for children) and an antihistamine such as chlorphenamine maleate by intravenous injection (10 mg for adults, 0.2 mg/kg for children). Patients with incoagulable blood will develop haematomas after intramuscular and subcutaneous injections, and so the intravenous route should be used whenever possible except in the case of adrenaline. Respiratory distress and cyanosis should be treated by clearing the airway, giving oxygen, and, if necessary, assisted ventilation. If the patient is unconscious and no femoral or carotid pulses can be detected, cardiopulmonary resuscitation must be started immediately.

Hospital treatment

Clinical assessment

In most cases of snake bite, uncertainties about the species and the quantity and composition of venom injected can be resolved only by admitting the patient to hospital for at least 24 h of observation. Local swelling is usually detectable within 15 min of pit viper envenoming and within 2 h of envenoming by most other vipers, but may not develop in patients bitten by some vipers, colubrids, and elapids such as kraits, coral snakes, and sea snakes. Fang marks are sometimes invisible. Tender enlargement of regional lymph nodes draining the bitten area is an early sign of envenoming by Viperidae and some Elapidae, notably Australasian elapids. All the tooth sockets should be examined meticulously as this is usually the first site of spontaneous bleeding: other common sites are the nose, conjunctiva, skin, and gastrointestinal tract. Persistent bleeding from venepuncture sites and other wounds implies incoagulable blood. Hypotension and shock are important signs of hypovolaemia, vasodilatation, or cardiotoxicity, seen particularly in patients bitten by North American rattlesnakes and some Viperinae (e.g. *V. berus*, Russell's vipers, *D. palaestinae*). Ptosis is the earliest sign of neurotoxic envenoming (Fig. 9.2.16). Respiratory muscle power should be assessed objectively and repeatedly, for example, by measuring vital capacity. Trismus and generalized myalgia with muscle tenderness suggest rhabdomyolysis (sea snakes). If a procoagulant venom is suspected, the coagulability of whole blood should be checked at the bedside using the 20-min whole-blood clotting test.

Antivenom treatment

In managing cases of snake bite, the most important decision is whether or not to give antivenom, the only specific antidote for envenoming. There is abundant evidence that in patients with severe envenoming, the benefits of this treatment outweigh the risks of antivenom reactions (see following paragraphs). Antivenom has reduced the mortality of systemic envenoming by *Echis ocellatus* in Nigeria from 20% to 3% and by *C. d. terrificus* in Brazil from 74% to 12%. Antivenoms are effective in reversing hypotension caused by *V. berus* envenoming and coagulopathies caused by *Bothrops* species, Russell's vipers, *C. rhodostoma*, *Cryptelytrops (Trimeresurus) albolabris*, and *Oxyuranus scutellatus*. Antivenom, also known as antivenin, antivenene, and antisnakebite serum, is the partially purified immunoglobulin (whole IgG, $F(ab')_2$, or Fab fragments) of horses or sheep which have been hyperimmunized with venom. Antivenoms are in short supply in sub-Saharan Africa and New Guinea; elsewhere, they are of variable efficacy and safety and are often used inappropriately.

General indications for antivenom

Antivenom is indicated if there are signs of systemic envenoming such as:

- haemostatic abnormalities: spontaneous systemic bleeding, incoagulable blood, or thrombocytopenia
- neurotoxicity: descending paralysis starting with ptosis and external ophthalmoplegia
- hypotension and shock, abnormal ECG, or other evidence of severe cardiovascular dysfunction
- generalized rhabdomyolysis or massive intravascular haemolysis: black urine

Supporting evidence of severe envenoming is a neutrophil leucocytosis, elevated serum enzymes such as creatine kinase and aminotransferases, haemoconcentration, severe anaemia, myoglobinuria, haemoglobinuria, methaemoglobinuria, hypoxaemia, and acidosis.

In the absence of systemic envenoming, local swelling involving more than half the bitten limb, extensive blistering or bruising, bites on digits, and rapid progression of swelling are indications for antivenom, especially in patients bitten by species whose venoms are known to cause local necrosis (e.g. Viperidae, Asian cobras, and African spitting cobras).

Special indications for antivenom

Some developed countries can afford a wider range of indications.

United States and Canada After bites by the most dangerous rattlesnakes (*C. atrox, C. adamanteus, C. viridis, C. oreganus, C. horridus*, and *C. scutulatus*), antivenom should be given early, even before systemic envenoming has become obvious. Rapid spread of a local swelling is considered an indication for antivenom, as is immediate pain or any other symptom or sign of envenoming after bites by coral snakes (*Micruroides euryxanthus, Micrurus fulvius*, and *M. tener*).

Australia Antivenom should be given to any patient with proved or suspected snake bite if there are tender regional lymph nodes or any other evidence of systemic spread of venom, and in anyone effectively bitten by an identified highly venomous species.

Europe For bites of adder (*V. berus* and other European *Vipera* spp.), Zagreb antivenom, or Protherics ViperaTAb (Table 9.2.1), is indicated to prevent morbidity and reduce the length of convalescence in patients with moderately severe envenoming, as well as to save the lives of severely envenomed patients. Indications are:

1. A fall in blood pressure (systolic to <80 mmHg, or >50 mmHg from the normal or admission value) with or without signs of shock
2. Other signs of systemic envenoming (see earlier paragraphs) including spontaneous bleeding, coagulopathy, pulmonary oedema, or haemorrhage (shown by chest radiograph), ECG abnormalities, and a definite peripheral leucocytosis ($>15\times 10^9$/litre) and elevated serum creatine kinase
3. Extensive local swelling: involving more than half the bitten limb within 48 h of the bite OR rapidly spreading local swelling (beyond the wrist after bites on the hand or beyond the ankle after bites on the foot within about 4 h of the bite).

Table 9.2.1 Guide to initial dosage of some important antivenoms

Species		Manufacturer, antivenom	Initial dose
Latin name	**English name**		**(approximate)**
Acanthophis spp.	Death adder	CSL,[a] monospecific	3000–6000 units
Bitis arietans	Puff adder	Sanofi-Pasteur Fav Afrique and Favi Rept; SAVP;[b] polyspecific	80 ml
Bothrops asper	Terciopelo	Instituto Clodomiro Picado	50–100 ml
Bothrops atrox	Common lancehead	Suero Antiofidico (Instituto Nacional de Higiene y Medicina Tropical 'Leopoldo Izquieta Perez' Guayaquil, Ecuador); Soro Antibotropico (Instituto Butantan, San Paulo, Brazil)	20 ml
Bothrops (Bothriopsis) bilineatus		Same	20 ml
Bothrops jararaca	Jararaca	Instituto Butantan and other Brazilian manufacturers, Bothrops polyspecific	20 ml
Bungarus caeruleus	Common krait	Indian manufacturers,[c] polyspecific	100 ml
Calloselasma (Agkistrodon) rhodostoma	Malayan pit viper	Thai Red Cross, Bangkok, monospecific	100 ml
		Thai Government Pharmaceutical Organization, monospecific	50 ml
Crotalus adamanteus	Eastern diamondback rattlesnakes	Protherics 'CroFab'	7–15 vials
Cryptelytrops (Trimeresurus) albolabris	Green pit viper	Thai Red Cross, monospecific	100 ml
C. atrox	Western diamondback rattlesnakes	Protherics 'CroFab'	7–15 vials
C. oreganus and *C. viridis subspp.*	Western rattlesnakes	Protherics 'CroFab'	7–15 vials
Daboia (Vipera). palaestinae	Palestine viper	Rogoff Medical Research Institute, Tel Aviv, Palestine, viper-monospecific	50–80 ml
Daboia (Vipera) russelii	Western Russell's viper	Indian manufacturers,[3] polyspecific	40 ml
D. siamensis	Eastern Russell's viper	Thai manufacturers, monospecific	100 ml
		Myanmar Pharmaceutical Industry monospecific	50 ml
Echis ocellatus, E. leucogaster, E. pyramidum (Africa)	African saw-scaled or carpet vipers	SAIMR,[b] Echis, monospecific; Aventis-Pasteur 'Fav Afrique'	20 ml
Elapidae (Hydrophiinae)	Sea snakes	CSL,[a] sea snake	1000 units
Naja kaouthia	Monocellate Thai cobra	Thai Red Cross, monospecific	100 ml
N. naja	Indian cobra	Indian manufacturers,[c] polyspecific	100 ml
Notechis scutatus	Tiger snake	CSL,[a] monospecific	3000–6000 units
Pseudechis textilis	Eastern brown snake	CSL,[a] monospecific	3000–6000 units
Oxyuranus scutellatus	Taipan	CSL,[a] monospecific	12 000 units
Vipera berus	European adder	Immunoloski Zavod-Zagreb Vipera, polyspecific	10–20 ml
		Protherics Fab. monospecific'ViperaTAb'	100–200 mg

[a] Commonwealth Serum Laboratories, Australia.
[b] South African Vaccine Producers (formerly SAIMR: South African Institute for Medical Research).
[c] Haffkine, Kasauli, Serum Institute of India, Vins, Bharat, Biological Evans, King Institute, etc.

Patients bitten by European *Vipera* spp. who show any evidence of envenoming should be admitted to hospital for observation for at least 24 h. Antivenom should be given whenever there is evidence of systemic envenoming (see above), even if its appearance is delayed for several days after the bite.

Prediction of antivenom reactions

Skin (intradermal) and conjunctival tests do not predict early (anaphylactic) or late (serum sickness type) antivenom reactions and should not be used.

Contraindications to antivenom

Atopic patients and those who have reacted previously to equine antiserum are at increased risk of developing severe antivenom reactions. In such cases, antivenom should be given only if there is definite systemic envenoming. Reactions may be prevented or ameliorated by pretreatment with subcutaneous adrenaline, antihistamine, and hydrocortisone, or a continuous intravenous infusion of 1:1 000 000 adrenaline while antivenom is being given. However, this prophylaxis is not safe enough to be recommended for routine use. There is no time even for rapid desensitization.

Selection and administration of antivenom

Antivenom should be given only if its stated range of specificity includes the species thought to be responsible for the bite. Whatever the stated expiry date on the ampoule, opaque solutions should be discarded, as precipitation of protein indicates loss of activity and an increased risk of reactions. However, expiry dates quoted on ampoules are often unnecessarily short, for commercial reasons;

provided that the antivenom has been kept refrigerated and the solution is clear, a high proption of its original activity is retained for 5 years or more. Monospecific (monovalent) antivenom is ideal if the biting species is known. Polyspecific (polyvalent) antivenoms are used in many countries because of the difficulty in identifying the species responsible for bites. Polyspecific antivenoms are effective but, depending on their method of preparation, a higher dose may be required. Antivenoms may exhibit a range of paraspecific neutralizing activity. For example, the South African Vaccine Producer's (formerly SAIMR) 'polyvalent antivenom', which is raised against the venoms of 10 species, has paraspecific activity against a further 5 species.

It is almost never too late to give antivenom while signs of systemic envenoming persist, but, ideally, it should be given as soon as it is indicated. Antivenom has proved effective up to 2 days after sea-snake bites and, in patients still defibrinated, weeks after bites by Viperidae. In contrast, local envenoming is probably not reversible unless antivenom is given within a few hours of the bite. The intravenous route is far more effective than intramuscular (Fig. 9.2.26). An infusion of antivenom diluted in approximately 5 ml of isotonic fluid/kg body weight is easier to control than an intravenous 'push' injection of undiluted antivenom given at the rate of about 4 ml/min, but there is no difference in the incidence or severity of antivenom reactions in patients treated by these two methods.

Dose of antivenom

Manufacturers' recommendations are based on mouse protection tests and may be very misleading. Few clinical trials have been performed to establish appropriate starting doses, and in most countries antivenom is used empirically. Many clinical severity grading and scoring systems are in use to guide choice of the initial dose of antivenom but none has been tested for its prognostic significance. The patient's condition may deteriorate suddenly, making these rigid and unproven prescriptions unreliable or even frankly dangerous. Many hospitals in the rural tropics give a standard dose of 1 to 2 ampoules to every patient who claims to have been bitten, irrespective of clinical severity. This practice squanders scarce, expensive antivenom and exposes nonenvenomed patients to the risk of reactions. Some suggested initial doses are given in Table 9.2.1. Children must be given the same dose as adults.

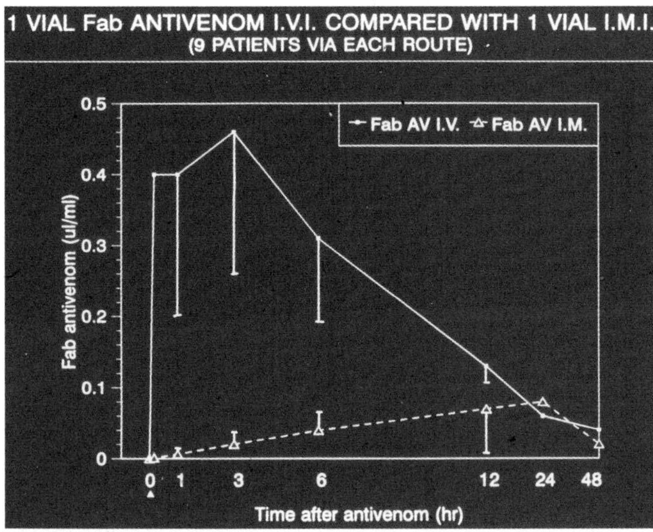

Fig. 9.2.26 Serum therapeutic antivenom concentrations in two groups of patients with mild envenoming given the same dose of a Fab fragment antivenom by intramuscular or slow intravenous injection. Intramuscular administration resulted in delayed peak concentrations (at 24 h) sixfold less than by intravenous injection.
(Theakston RDG, Warrell DA unpublished data)

Response to antivenom

Often, there is marked symptomatic improvement soon after antivenom has been injected. In shocked patients, the blood pressure may rise and consciousness returns (*C. rhodostoma, V. berus, Bitis arietans*). Neurotoxic signs may improve within 30 min (*Acanthophis* spp., *N. kaouthia*), but the response usually take several hours. Spontaneous systemic bleeding usually stops within 15 to 30 min and blood coagulability is restored within a median time of 6 h after antivenom treatment, provided a neutralizing dose has been given. More antivenom should be given if severe signs of envenoming persist after 1 to 2 h, or if blood coagulability is not restored within about 6 h. Systemic envenoming may recur hours or days after an initially good response to antivenom. This is explained by the continuing absorption of venom from the injection site after clearance of antivenom from the bloodstream. The apparent serum half-lives of antivenoms in envenomed patients range from 26 to 95 h. Envenomed patients should therefore be assessed daily for at least 3 or 4 days.

Antivenom reactions

Early (anaphylactic) reactions These develop within 10 to 180 min of starting antivenom in between 3% and 84% of patients, depending on which antivenom is used. The incidence increases with dose and is lowest in antivenoms lacking complement-activating aggregates. Fewer reactions occur when administration is by intramuscular rather than intravenous injection. The symptoms are itching, urticaria, cough, nausea, vomiting, other autonomic manifestations, fever, and tachycardia. Up to 40% of patients with early reactions develop systemic anaphylaxis: hypotension, bronchospasm, and angio-oedema. Deaths are rare, but individual cases, such as the asthmatic boy who died from anaphylactic shock after receiving Pasteur antivenom in England in 1957, have been widely publicized and have led to an unreasonable rejection of antivenom treatment. Early antivenom reactions are unlikely to be type-I, IgE-mediated hypersensitivity reactions to equine serum protein. They result from complement activation by immune complexes or aggregates of IgG.

Pyrogenic reactions Pyrogenic reactions result from contamination of the antivenom with endotoxin-like compounds. Fever, rigors, vasodilatation, and a fall in blood pressure develop 1 to 2 h after treatment. In children, febrile convulsions may be precipitated.

Late reactions Late reactions of serum sickness type may develop between 5 and 24 (mean 7) days after antivenom therapy. The incidence of these reactions and the speed of their development increases with the dose of antivenom. Clinical features include fever, itching, urticaria, arthralgia (sometimes involving the temporomandibular joint), lymphadenopathy, periarticular swellings, mononeuritis multiplex, albuminuria, and rarely, encephalopathy. This is a classic immune complex disease.

Treatment of antivenom reactions

Adrenaline (epinephrine) is the effective treatment for early reactions; 0.5 to 1.0 ml of 0.1% (1 in 1000, 1 mg/ml) is given by intramuscular injection to adults (children 0.01 ml/kg) at the first signs of a reaction. The dose may be repeated if the reaction is not controlled. Patients with profound hypotension, severe bronchospasm, or laryngeal oedema may be given adrenaline by slow intravenous injection (0.5 mg diluted in 20 ml of isotonic saline over 10–15 min). A histamine anti-H_1 blocker, such as chlorphenamine maleate (10 mg for adults; 0.2 mg/kg for children) should be given by intravenous injection to combat the effects of histamine release during the reaction. Pyrogenic reactions are treated by cooling the patient and giving antipyretics. Late reactions respond to an oral antihistamine such as chlorphenamine (2 mg every 6 h for adults; 0.25 mg/kg per day in divided doses for children) or to oral prednisolone (5 mg every 6 h for 5 to 7 days for adults; 0.7 mg/kg per day in divided doses for children).

Supportive treatment

Neurotoxic envenoming

Bulbar and respiratory paralysis may lead to death from aspiration, airway obstruction, or respiratory failure. A clear airway must be maintained and, if bulbar muscle weakness results in pooling of secretions, or respiratory distress develops, a cuffed endotracheal tube or laryngeal mask airway should be inserted or a tracheostomy performed. Provided they are adequately ventilated, patients with neurotoxic envenoming remain fully conscious with intact sensation and can respond to spoken questions by flexing a finger or toe. Lifting their paralysed eyelids so that they can see is very reassuring. Patients have been effectively ventilated manually (by Ambu bag or anaesthetic bag), as in the 1952 poliomyelitis epidemic in Copenhagen, for 30 days and have recovered after 10 weeks of mechanical ventilation. Although artificial ventilation was first suggested for neurotoxic envenoming more than 100 years ago, patients continue to die because they are denied this simple procedure.

Anticholinesterases have a variable but potentially useful effect in patients with neurotoxic envenoming, especially when postsynaptic neurotoxins are involved. The 'Tensilon test' should be performed in all cases of severe neurotoxic envenoming, as with suspected myasthenia gravis. Atropine sulphate (0.6 mg for adults; 50 µg/kg for children) or glycopyrronium is given by intravenous injection followed by edrophonium chloride (Tensilon) by slow intravenous injection in an adult dose of 10 mg, or 0.25 mg/kg for children or neostigmine bromide or methylsulphate (Prostigmin) by intramuscular injection (0.02 mg/kg for adults, 0.04 mg/kg for children). Patients who respond convincingly can be maintained on neostigmine methylsulphate, 0.5 to 2.5 mg every 1 to 3 h up to 10 mg/24 h maximum for adults or 0.01 to 0.04 mg/kg every 2 to 4 h for children by intramuscular, intravenous, or subcutaneous injection.

Hypotension and shock

If the central venous pressure is low or there is other clinical evidence of hypovolaemia, a plasma expander, preferably fresh whole blood or fresh frozen plasma, should be infused. However, the risk of contamination of blood products with various pathogens restricts their use where reliable screening cannot be assured. If there is evidence of increased capillary permeability (e.g. facial and conjunctival oedema, serous effusions, haemoconcentration, hypoalbuminaemia, etc.) it may be safer in the long term to rely on a selective vasoconstrictor such as dopamine (starting dose 2.5–5 µg/kg per min by intravenous infusion). Delayed hypotension developing about 1 week after bites by Burmese *D. siamensis* as a consequence of Sheehan's type syndrome may respond to intravenous hydrocortisone.

Oliguria and renal failure

Urine output, serum creatinine, urea, and electrolytes should be measured each day in patients with severe envenoming, and in those bitten by species known to cause renal failure (e.g. Russell's vipers, *C.d. terrificus, Bothrops* spp., sea snakes). If urine output drops below 400 ml in 24 h, urethral and central venous catheters should be inserted. If urine flow fails to increase after cautious rehydration, diuretics should be tried (e.g. furosemide by slow intravenous injection, 100 mg followed by 200 mg), and then mannitol. Dopamine (2.5 µg/kg per min by intravenous infusion) has proved effective in some patients bitten by Russell's vipers. If these measures are ineffective, the patient should be placed on strict fluid balance. Peritoneal or haemodialysis will usually be required. In Rangoon, Burma, the mortality of established renal failure following *D. siamensis* envenoming has been reduced to less than 30% by using peritoneal dialysis, usually for only 72 h.

Local infection at the site of the bite

After bites by some species (e.g. *Bothrops* spp., *C. rhodostoma*), local infections caused by unusual bacteria derived from the snake's venom or fangs develop in 10% or more cases. A booster dose of tetanus toxoid should be given, but prophylactic antibiotics are not indicated unless the wound has been incised or tampered with in any way. If a local abscess develops, it should be drained and penicillin, chloramphenicol, or erythromycin given. An aminoglycoside such as gentamicin should be given for 48 h if there is evidence of local necrosis.

Management of local envenoming

Bullae are best left intact. The bitten limb should be nursed in the most comfortable position but not elevated excessively as this increases the risk of intracompartmental ischaemia. Once definite signs of necrosis have appeared (blackened anaesthetic area with putrid odour or signs of sloughing), surgical debridement, immediate split-skin grafting, and broad-spectrum antibiotic cover are indicated.

Intracompartmental syndrome and fasciotomy

Increased pressure within tight fascial compartments such as the digital pulp spaces and anterior tibial compartment may cause ischaemia. Necrosis of digits is especially common. This complication is most likely after bites by North American rattlesnakes, *Calloselasma rhodostoma, Protobothrops flavoviridis, Bothrops* spp., and *Bitis arietans.* The signs are excessive pain, weakness and tenderness of the compartmental muscles, and pain when they are passively stretched, hypoaesthesia of skin supplied by nerves running through the compartment, and obvious tenseness of the compartment. Detection of arterial pulses by palpation or Doppler ultrasonograhy does not exclude intracompartmental ischaemia. Intracompartmental pressures exceeding 45 mmHg carry a high risk of ischaemic necrosis. In these circumstances, fasciotomy may be justified, but it did not prove effective in saving envenomed muscle in experimental animals. Fasciotomy is contraindicated until blood coagulability has been restored (by adequate doses of antivenom followed by clotting factors) and must be justified by demonstration that the intracompartmental pressure is consistently raised (to less than 30 mmHg below mean arterial pressure). Early adequate antivenom treatment will prevent the development of intracompartmental syndromes in most cases.

Haemostatic disturbances

Once specific antivenom has been given to neutralize venom procoagulants, restoration of coagulability and platelet function may be accelerated by giving (reliably screened) fresh whole blood, fresh frozen plasma, cryoprecipitates (containing fibrinogen, factor VIII, fibronectin, and some factors V and XIII), or platelet concentrates. Heparin has been used to treat a variety of snake bites, usually with disastrous results. Heparin did not prove beneficial in patients envenomed by *Echis ocellatus*. Recombinant factor VIIa is neither indicated nor necessary.

Other drugs

Corticosteroids, antifibrinolytic agents (aprotinin and ε-aminocaproic acid), antihistamines, trypsin, and a variety of traditional herbal remedies have all been used, but none has proved effective and many are potentially harmful.

Treatment of snake venom ophthalmia

When cobra venom is 'spat' into the eyes, first aid consists of irrigation with generous volumes of water or any other bland liquid such as milk or even urine, which may be available. Unless a corneal abrasion can be excluded by fluorescein staining or slit-lamp examination, treatment should be the same as for any corneal injury: a topical antimicrobial such as tetracycline or chloramphenicol should be applied. Instillation of antivenom is not recommended. A 0.1% adrenaline eyedrop preparation relieves the pain.

Interval between bite and death

Exceptionally, patients may die 'within a few minutes' (reputedly after a bite by the king cobra *Ophiophagus hannah*) or as long as 41 days (*Echis carinatus*) after snake bite. However, most deaths occur about 8 h after cobra bites (*N. naja*), 18 h after krait bites (*Bungarus caeruleus*), 16 h after North American rattlesnake bites (*Crotalus* spp.), 3 days after Russell's viper bites, and 5 days after *Echis* bites.

Venomous lizards

Two species of venomous lizard (genus *Heloderma*) have proved capable of envenoming humans. Venom from glands in the mandible is conducted along grooves in the lower teeth. The Gila monster *H. suspectum* (Fig. 9.2.27), which is striped with a short thick tail and grows to 60 cm in length, occurs in the south-western United States and adjacent areas of Mexico. The Mexican beaded lizard or escorpión *H. horridum*, which is spotted with a relatively long thin tail and reaches 80 cm in length, is found in western Mexico south to Guatemala. *Heloderma* venoms contain lethal glycoprotein toxins, gila and horridum toxins, phospholipase A_2, and 5 bioactive peptides of great interest. Helospectins I and II and helodermin are vasoactive intestinal peptide (VIP) analogues, while exendins -3 and -4 are glucagon-like peptide-1 (GLP-1) analogues that are being developed for the treatment of type 2 diabetes mellitus. Bites are rare. The lizard hangs on with its powerful jaws and is difficulty to disengage but intense heat applied under its chin or instillation of strong alcohol into its mouth may encourage it to release its bulldog-like grip. Radiolucent teeth may be left in the wound. There is immediate severe local pain with tender swelling and regional lymphadenopathy. Symptoms include weakness, dizziness, tachycardia, hypotension, syncope, angio-oedema, sweating, rigors, tinnitus, nausea, and vomiting. Exenatide, a GLP-1 homologue from Gila monster venom used in type 2 diabetes mellitus, can also cause angioedema. There may be leucocytosis, coagulopathy, electrocardiographic changes, myocardial infarction, and acute renal failure. No fatal cases have reliably been reported. Specific antivenom is not generally available. A powerful analgesic may be required. Hypotension should be treated with plasma expanders and perhaps adrenaline or a pressor agent such as dopamine.

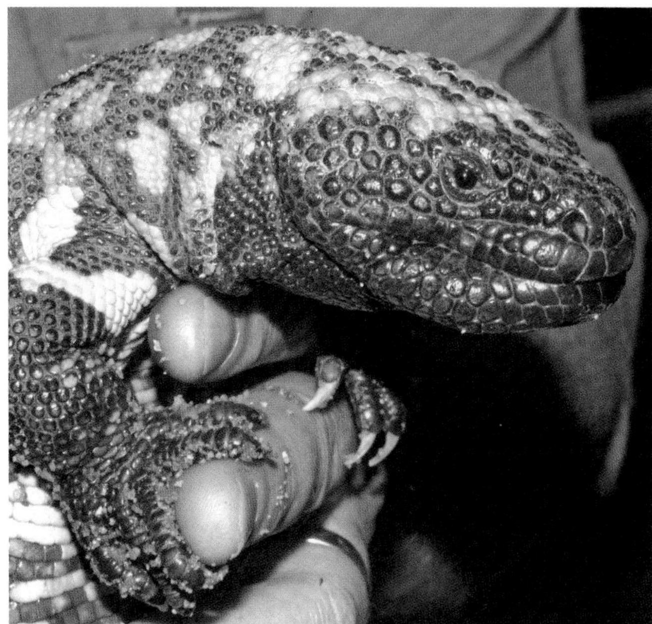

Fig. 9.2.27 Gila monster *Heloderma suspectum*.
Copyright D. A. Warrell.

Recently, venomous salivary secretion have been demonstrated in other groups of lizards such as iguanas (Iguanidae), glass/alligator lizards (Anguidae), and monitors (Varanidae), notably the Komodo dragon *Varanus komodoensis* which has been responsible for human fatalities that were attributed to trauma of infection of the bite wounds.

Poisonous amphibians and birds

Poisonous amphibians

The moist skin of amphibians such as frogs, toads, newts, and salamanders is an accessory respiratory organ, which is protected from microorganisms by highly toxic secretions containing amines, peptides, proteins, steroids, and alkaloids. Some compounds are synthesized *de novo*, while others are sequestered from prey such as ants, beetles, and millipedes. The bitter flavour and lethal effects of these secretions and the vivid warning coloration of many species defend them against predators. The skin of 'poison dart' frogs (Dendrobatidae) of Central and South America secrete lipophilic alkaloids such as batrachotoxins (*Phyllobates* spp.), which activate sodium channels; histrionico toxins (*Dendrobates histrionicus*) (Fig. 9.2.28), which block nicotinic receptors; pumiliotoxins (*D. pumilio*), which affect sodium channels; and epibatidine (*Epipedobates tricolor*), a powerful analgesic and nicotinic receptor agonist. Two Colombian tribes, the Embará and Noanamá Chocó, use the skin poisons of three species of Phyllobates to coat the tips of their blowgun darts. Some toads can squirt from their parotid glands venom containing bufadienolides which affect membrane Na^+, K^+-ATPase. When licked or put in the mouth by dogs or children, or when

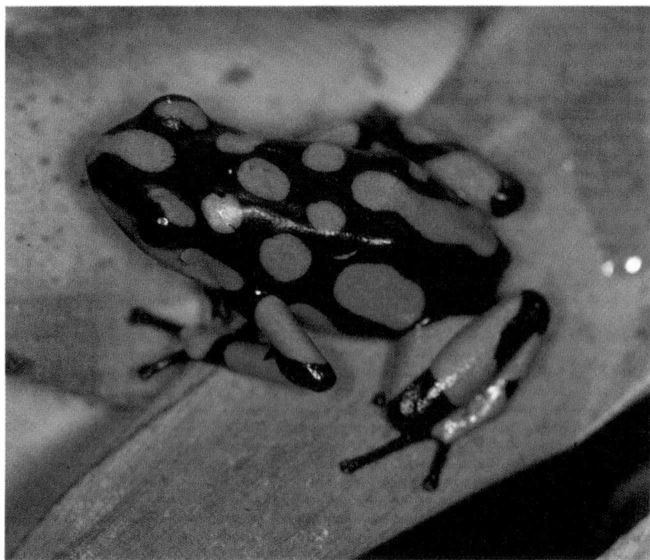

Fig. 9.2.28 Poison frog *Dendrobates histrionicus* (Dendrobatidae) Bahia Solauo, Colombia. Its skin secretion contains potent nicotinic receptor antagonists, histrionicotoxins.
Copyright D. A. Warrell.

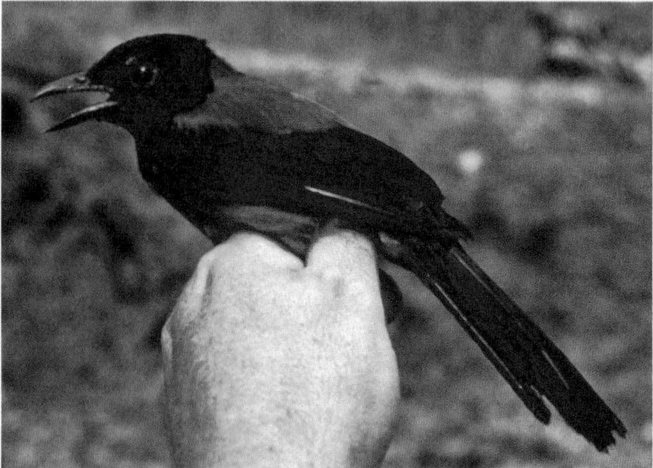

Fig. 9.2.29 Hooded pitohui *Pitohui dichrous*. Varararta National Park near Port Moresby, Papua New Guinea.
By courtesy of Dr Ian Burrows.

ingested as Chinese traditional medicines such as *Kyushin*, *Yixin Wan*, or the topical aphrodisiac *Ch'an-Su*, the poisons can cause fatal digoxin-like poisoning. Symptoms include hypersalivation, cyanosis, cardiac arrhythmias, and generalized convulsions. Antidigoxin antibodies ('Digibind', 'DigiTAb') have some therapeutic effect.

The skin of three species of newts, genus *Taricha*, from the western United States, contains tarichatoxins identical to tetrodotoxin, which also occurs in some toads, frogs, fish, crustaceans, and octopuses (see following paragraphs). Tetrodotoxin can be absorbed through the gastric mucosa, explaining the death of a man who swallowed a 20-cm long Oregon rough-skinned newt *Taricha granulosa*. He developed paraesthesia of the lips, progressing to more generalized numbness and weakness, and had a cardiopulmonary arrest about 2 h after swallowing the newt.

Poisonous birds

The feathers, skin, and breast muscles of five species of pitohui or thickhead, passerine birds from New Guinea (genus *Pitohui;* Pachycephalidae) and the blue-capped ifrita or ifrit (*Ifrita kowaldi;* Cinclosomatidae) contain homobatrachotoxin, a potent steroidal alkaloid that activates sodium channels and was originally isolated from the skin of South American poison-dart frogs (*Phyllobates*—see earlier paragraphs). The birds may acquire the poison by eating melyrid beetles (*Choresine* spp.). Poisonous pitohuis have an unpleasant peppery odour, and their skin has a bitter flavour. Contact with their feathers causes numbness and burning of the tongue, lip or skin wounds, and sneezing. This may be a protective mechanism, and the striking 'warning' coloration of the hooded pitohui (*P. dichrous*) (Fig. 9.2.29) may be the subject of Müllerian mimicry by less poisonous species.

Venomous fish

About 200 species of fish inhabiting temperate and tropical seas possess a defensive venom-injecting apparatus that can inflict dangerous stings, but more than 1200 species are now thought to be venomous. Fatal stings have been reported from cartilagenous fish (class Chondrichthyes), such as sharks and dogfish (order Squaliformes) and stingrays and mantas (order Rajiformes), and from bony fish (superclass Osteichthyes), such as ray-finned fish (class Actinopterygii) of the orders Siluriformes (catfish), Perciformes (families Trachinidae (weever fish), Uranoscopidae (stargazers or stone-lifters), and others) and Scorpaeniformes (scorpion fish, stone-fish, lion fish *Synanceja/Synanceia* spp.) (Fig. 9.2.30). The Indo-Pacific region and other tropical waters have the richest venomous fish fauna, but dangerous species such as sharks, chimaeras, and weevers also occur in temperate northern waters, and a number of large rivers in South American, West Africa, and South East Asia are inhabited by freshwater stingrays *Potamotrygon* spp. (Fig. 9.2.31). Venom glands are embedded in grooves in the spines or, in the case of stingrays, lie beneath a membrane covering the long barbed precaudal spine.

Incidence and epidemiology

Weever fish are common around the coast of the British Isles, especially off Cornwall. Hundreds of stings occur in some years, with a

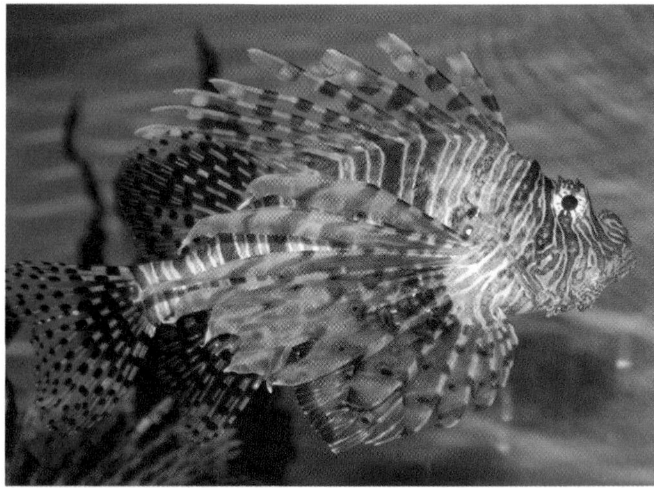

Fig. 9.2.30 Lion fish *Pterois volitans* (Scorpionidae).
Copyright D. A. Warrell.

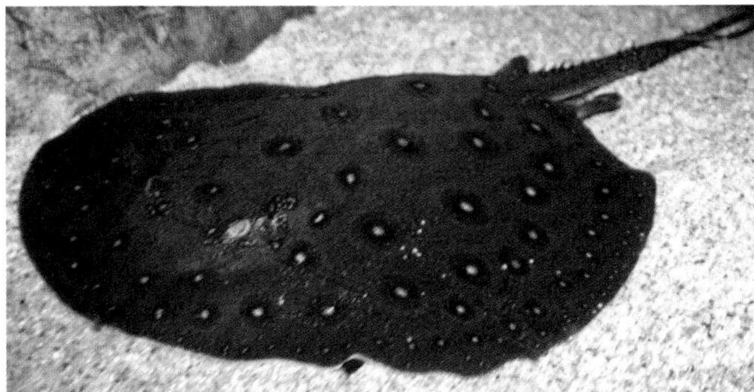

Fig. 9.2.31 Fresh water stingray *Potamotrygon* sp.
Copyright D. A. Warrell.

peak incidence in August and September. A total of 58 cases were seen at one hospital at Pula, Croatia, on the Adriatic coast over a period of 13 years. It has been estimated that there are 1500 stings by rays and 300 stings by scorpion fish in the United States each year. Stings by venomous freshwater rays (*Potamotrygon hystrix, P. motoro*) are common in the Amazon region of Brazil and especially in Acré. In 4 years, 81 cases of stone-fish *Synanceja* spp. sting were seen in Pulau Bukom Hospital near Singapore. Ornate, but aggressive and venomous members of the genera *Pterois* and *Dendrochirus* (lion, zebra, tiger, turkey, or red fire fish) (Fig. 9.2.30), which are popular aquarium pets, often sting their owners on the fingers. Most fish stings are inflicted on the soles of the feet of people wading near the shore or in the vicinity of coral reefs. Venomous fish are effectively camouflaged (*Synanceja* spp.) or lie partly covered by sand. Stingrays lash their tails at the intruding limb and usually impale the ankle (Fig. 9.2.32). Fatal fish stings are very rarely reported.

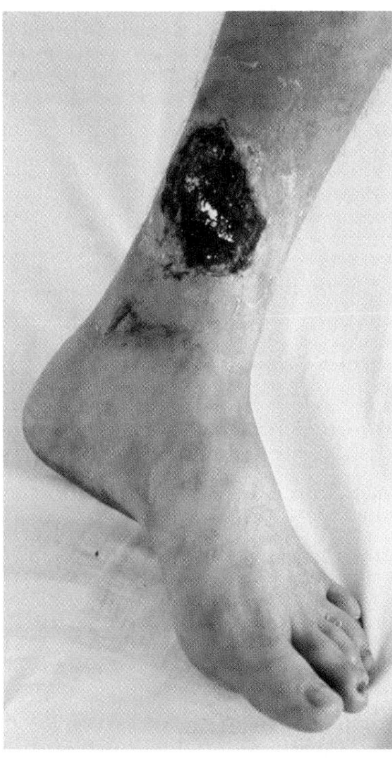

Fig. 9.2.32 Necrotic and secondarily infected wound at the site of a sting by a freshwater ray *Potamotrygon hystrix* in a Brazilian patient.
By courtesy of Dr. João Luiz Costa Cardoso.

Prevention

Fish stings can be prevented by employing a shuffling gait when wading, by avoiding handling living or dead fish, and by keeping clear of fish in the water, especially in the vicinity of tropical reefs. Footwear protects against most species except stingrays.

Venom composition

The instability of most fish venoms at normal ambient temperatures has made them difficult to study. Stingray and weeverfish venoms contain peptides, enzymes, and a variety of vasoactive compounds such as kinins, 5-hydroxytryptamine, histamine, and catecholamines. Pharmacological effects include local necrosis, direct actions on cardiac, skeletal, and smooth muscle, resulting in ECG changes, hypotension, paralysis, and central nervous system depression.

Clinical features

Immediate sharp, agonizing pain is the dominant symptom. Hot, erythematous swelling extends up the stung limb and may persist with pain for several days and be complicated by necrosis (Fig. 9.2.32) and secondary infection by marine *Vibrio* spp. (such as *V. vulnificus*), freshwater species (such as *Aeromonas hydrophila*), and other unusual bacteria, particularly if the spine remains embedded in the wound. Stingray spines, which are up to 30 cm long, can cause severe lacerating injuries, especially to the lower legs, but if the victim inadvertently lies on the ray or falls on to it, the spine may penetrate the thoracic or abdominal cavities with fatal results.

Systemic effects are uncommon after weever stings (Trachinidae), but people stung by rays or Scorpaenidae (scorpion- and stone-fish) may develop nausea, vomiting, signs of autonomic nervous system stimulation; such as diarrhoea, sweating, and hypersalivation; cardiac arrhythmias, hypotension, respiratory distress, neurological signs, and generalized convulsions. Patients have died within 1 h of being stung by *Synanceja verrucosa*.

Treatment

Pain is alleviated by immersing the stung limb in water, which is uncomfortably hot yet not scalding (<45 °C; the 50 °C recommended by some authorities will cause a full thickness scald!). Temperature can be assessed with the unstung limb. Addition of magnesium sulphate is unnecessary. Injection of a local anaesthetic is less effective even when applied as a ring block in the case of stung digits, but a local nerve block with 0.5% of plain bupivacaine does seem to work. The venomous spine (which may be barbed), fragments of membrane, and other foreign material should be removed as soon as possible. Systemic effects must be treated symptomatically. An adequate airway should be established, and cardiopulmonary resuscitation may be needed. Severe hypotension may respond to adrenaline, bradycardia to atropine. CSL in Australia manufacture an antivenom specific for *Synanceja trachynis, S. verrucosa*, and *S. horridus*. This has paraspecific activity against the venoms of the North American scorpion fish (*Scorpaena guttata*) and some other members of the Scorpaenidae. One ampoule (2 ml or 2000 units) is given intravenously for each two puncture marks found at the site of the sting. The dose is increased for patients with severe symptoms. Antibiotic treatment for secondary infections should take into account the range of possible marine pathogens. Doxycycline or co-trimoxazole covers *Vibrio* and *Aeromonas* spp.

Poisoning by ingestion of aquatic animals

Acute gastrointestinal symptoms ('food poisoning') after eating seafood are usually caused by bacterial or viral infections such as *Vibrio parahaemolyticus* (crustaceans, especially shrimps), *V. cholerae* (crabs and molluscs), non-O group 1 *V. cholerae* (oysters), *V. vulnificus* (oysters), *Aeromonas hydrophila* (frozen oysters), *Plesiomonas shigelloides* (oysters, mussels, mackerel, cuttlefish), *Shigella* spp. (molluscs), *Campylobacter jejuni* (clams), *Salmonella typhi* (molluscs), hepatitis A virus (molluscs, especially clams, and oysters), Norwalk virus (clams and oysters), and astro- and caliciviruses (cockles and other molluscs). Botulism has been caused by eating smoked fish and canned salmon; and in Japan and elsewhere, fish and molluscs became contaminated with methyl mercury from industrial waste, causing severe neurological damage and fetal abnormalities ('Minamata disease').

Toxins in seafood may also give rise to gastrointestinal neurotoxic and histamine-like symptoms. Two main syndromes are described.

Prevention of poisoning by ingestion of aquatic animals

Ciguatera toxin, tetrodotoxin, scombrotoxins and some other marine toxins are heat stable, so cooking does not prevent poisoning. Some toxins are fairly water soluble and may be leached out by soaking. Therefore, water in which fish are cooked should not be drunk. In tropical areas, the flesh of fish should be separated as soon as possible from the head, skin, intestines, gonads, and other viscera, which may contain high concentrations of toxin. All scaleless fish should be regarded as potentially tetrodotoxic, and very large fish carry an increased risk of being ciguatera toxic. Moray eels and parrot fish (Scaridae) should never be eaten because of the high risk of unusually rapid and severe ciguatera and scaritoxic fish poisoning. Scrombroid poisoning can be prevented by eating fresh fish or by freezing them as soon as possible after they are caught. Shellfish should not be eaten during the dangerous seasons and when there are red tides.

Gastrointestinal and neurotoxic syndromes

Nausea, vomiting, abdominal colic, tenesmus, and watery diarrhoea may precede neurotoxic symptoms of paraesthesia of the lips, buccal cavity, and extremities, distorted temperature perception (so that cold objects impart a burning sensation like dry ice), myalgia, progressive flaccid paralysis, dizziness, ataxia, cardiovascular disturbances, bradycardia, and rashes. Important causes of this syndrome are:

- Ciguatera fish poisonings: Symptoms develop between 1 and 6 h (extreme range, min to 30 h) after eating fish such as groupers, snappers, parrot fish, mackerel, moray eels, barracudas, and jacks. These are warm-water shore or reef fish. The global incidence is thought to exceed 50 000 cases per year. Up to 1% of the population may be affected each year (e.g. in Kiribati, Tokelau, and Tuvalu in the Pacific region) with a case fatality of 0.1%. The toxins responsible are polyethers such as ciguatoxin (activates Na^+ channels), maitotoxin (activates Ca^{2+} channels), and scaritoxin, ultimately derived along the food chain from benthic dinoflagellates such as *Gambierdiscus toxicus*. They are concentrated in the liver, viscera, and gonads, especially of large carnivorous fish. The increasing market for exotic fish from the Caribbean and elsewhere has led to cases of ciguatera in the United Kingdom. Gastrointestinal symptoms resolve within a few hours, but paraesthesiae and myalgia may persist for a week or even months. Similar symptoms (chelonitoxication) may follow ingestion of marine turtles in the Indo-Pacific area, but the case fatality is much higher.
- Tetrodotoxin poisoning: Scaleless porcupine, sun, puffer, and toad fish (order Tetraodonitiformes) may become highly poisonous at certain seasons, such as May to June, the spawning season in Japan. Tetrodotoxin, an aminoperhydroquinazoline, is one of the most potent nonprotein toxins known. It produces neurotoxic and cardiotoxic effects by blocking voltage-gated sodium ion channels. It is found concentrated in the ovaries, viscera, and skin of tetraodontiform fish; in the skin of newts (genus *Taricha*), frogs, and toads (genera *Colostethus, Atelopus, Bracycephalus*), and salamanders; in the saliva of octopuses; in the digestive glands of several species of gastropod molluscs; in a starfish, flatworm *Planorbis* spp., and nemertine worms in Japan; and is produced by some bacteria *Pseudomonas* spp.

Puffer fish ('fugu') is particularly popular in Japan where, despite stringent regulations, there are still cases of tetrodotoxin poisoning, with about four deaths each year. Neurotoxic symptoms develop within 10 to 45 min, and death from respiratory paralysis usually occurs between 2 and 6 h after eating the fish. There may be no gastrointestinal symptoms. Erythema, petechiae, blistering, and desquamation may appear. Freshwater puffer fish poisoning in northern Thailand has been attributed to saxitoxin.

- Paralytic shellfish poisoning: Bivalve molluscs, such as mussels, clams, oysters, cockles, and scallops (and also xanthid, coconut, and horseshoe crabs) may acquire tetrahydropurine neurotoxins such as saxitoxin from dinoflagellates *Alexandrium* spp. These may be sufficiently abundant between latitudes 30 °N and 30 °S during the warmer months of May to October to produce a 'red tide'. The dangerous season is signalled by the deaths of large numbers of fish and sea birds. Symptoms develop within 30 min of ingestion and may progress to fatal respiratory paralysis within 12 h in 8% of cases. Milder gastrointestinal and neurotoxic symptoms (neurotoxic shellfish poisoning) without paralysis can follow the ingestion of molluscs contaminated by brevitoxins from *Gymnodinium breve*. These microalgae can also cause a 'red tide'. In the United Kingdom, there have been several outbreaks of neurotoxic poisoning by red whelk *Neptunea antiqua* attributable to tetramine.
- Amnesic shellfish poisoning: This develops after ingestion of mussels and other molluscs contaminated with domoic acid from diatoms *Pseudonitzschia* spp. Gastroenteritis starts within 24 h of exposure and, in severe cases, within 48 h there is headache and coma followed by short-term memory loss.

Histamine-like syndrome (scombrotoxic poisoning)

The red flesh of scrombroid fish (tuna, mackerel, bonito, and skipjack) and of canned nonscrombroid fish, such as sardines and pilchards, may be decomposed by the action of bacteria, such as *Proteus morgani* and *Klebsiella pneumoniae*, which decarboxylate muscle histidine into saurine, histamine, cadaverine, and other unidentified toxins: 100 g of spoiled fish may contain almost 1 g of histamine. Histamine absorbed from the gut is normally broken down by *N*-methyl transferase and diamine oxidase (histaminase), but if the histamine concentration is very high, or the patient is taking a diamine oxidase inhibitor such as isoniazid (as antituberculosis chemotherapy), scombrotoxic poisoning may result. Toxic fish may produce a tingling or smarting sensation in the mouth when eaten. Within minutes or up to a few hours after ingestion, flushing, burning, sweating, urticaria, and pruritis may develop with headache, abdominal colic, nausea, vomiting, diarrhoea, bronchial asthma, giddiness, and hypotension.

Diagnosis and treatment

The differential diagnosis includes bacterial and viral food poisoning and allergic reactions.

No specific treatments or antidotes are available, but gastrointestinal contents should be eliminated by emetics and purges if this can be achieved safely and within 1 to 2 h of ingestion. Activated charcoal adsorbs saxitoxin and other shellfish toxins. Atropine is said to improve gastrointestinal symptoms and sinus bradycardia in patients with gastrointestinal and neurotoxic poisoning. Calcium gluconate may relieve mild neuromuscular symptoms. Oximes and anticholinesterases appear ineffective in ciguatera and tetrodotoxin poisoning, respectively. In cases of paralytic poisoning, endotracheal intubation and mechanical ventilation and cardiac resuscitation have proved life saving. In Malaysia, a patient with tetrodotoxin poisoning developed fixed dilated pupils and brain stem areflexia, so appearing brain dead, but made a complete recovery after being mechanically ventilated.

The symptoms of scrombrotoxic poisoning can be alleviated with antihistamines and bronchodilators.

Poisoning by ingesting carp gallbladder

In parts of East Asia, the raw bile and gallbladder of various species of freshwater carp (e.g. the grass carp *Ctenopharyngodon idellus*, 'plaa yeesok' *Probarbus jullienii*) are believed to have medicinal properties. Patients in China, Taiwan, Hong Kong, Japan, Thailand, and elsewhere have developed acute abdominal pain, vomiting, and watery diarrhoea 2 to 18 h after drinking the raw bile or eating the raw gallbladder of these fish. One patient developed flushing and dizziness. Hepatic and renal damage may develop, progressing to oliguric or non-oliguric acute renal failure (acute tubular necrosis). The hepatonephrotoxin has not been identified, but is heat stable and may be derived from the carp's diet.

Venomous marine invertebrates

Cnidarians (Coelenterata)

These include jellyfish, cubomedusoids, sea wasps, Portuguese-men-o'-war or bluebottles, hydroids, stinging corals, sea anemones, etc. Their tentacles are armed with millions of nematocysts (stinging capsules). When triggered by contact or chemicals, stinging hairs are everted at enormous acceleration and force, penetrating the skin as far as the epidermo-dermal junction and producing lines of painful irritant weals. Cnidarian venoms contain peptides and other vasoactive substances such as 5-hydroxyhistamine, histamine, prostaglandins, and kinins, which cause immediate excruciating pain, inflammation, and urticaria.

Epidemiology

The most dangerous species, the box jellyfish, cubomedusoid, sea wasp, or indringa *Chironex fleckeri* of northern Australia, has caused more than 70 deaths since 1883. Most stings occur in December and January. Fatal jellyfish stings in the Indo-Pacific region—from India, north to the Philippines, and east to Bougainville island—are attributable to *Chiropsalmus quadrumanus* and *C. quadrigatus*. Fatal stings have also been inflicted by the Portuguese man-o'-war *Physalia* spp. and the Chinese jellyfish *Stomolophus nomurai*. Many stings in northern Queensland are caused by *Carukia barnesi* and other tiny cubomedusoids (Irukandji stings). Irukandji-like symptoms have been reported from Florida and Guadeloupe in the Caribbean. Hundreds of thousands of swimmers off the northern Adriatic coast were stung by a plague of *Pelagia noctiluca* during the summers of 1977 to 1979. Stings by the sea anemone, *Anemonia sulcata*, are also reported from the coasts of Slovenia and Croatia.

Prevention

Bathers, especially children, should keep out of the sea at times of the year when dangerous cnidarians are prevalent, especially when warning notices are displayed; or they should bathe in 'stinger-resistant' enclosures, although these do not exclude Irukandji. Wetsuits or Lycra garments, nylon stockings, and other clothing will protect against nematocyst stings.

Clinical features

Nematocyst stings may leave a diagnostic pattern on the skin: *C. fleckeri* produces wide, striated brownish-purple weals (Fig. 9.2.33), whereas *Carukia barnesi* causes a transient erythematous macule, and the Portuguese man-o'-war (genus *Physalia*) produces chains of oval weals surrounded by erythema. Immediate severe pain is the commonest symptom. Chirodropids (genera *Chironex* and *Chiropsalmus*) cause the most severe systemic symptoms such as respiratory arrest, generalized convulsions, pulmonary oedema, and cardiac arrest within minutes of the accident. Other systemic effects include cough, nausea, vomiting, abdominal colic, diarrhoea, rigors, severe musculoskeletal pains, and profuse sweating. 'Irukandji syndrome' consists of severe musculoskeletal pain,

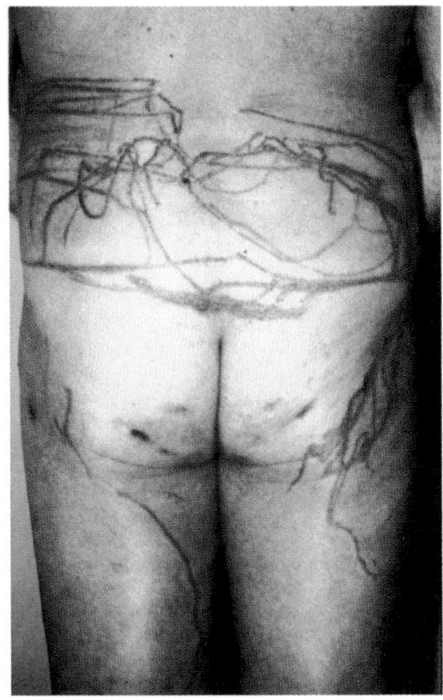

Fig. 9.2.33 Extensive weals from contact with the stinging tentacles of the box jellyfish *Chironex fleckeri* in an Australian stung in Darwin.
By courtesy of Drs B. Currie and P. Nitschke.

anxiety, trembling, headache, piloerection, sweating, tachycardia, hypertension, and pulmonary oedema starting about 30 min after a sting by *C. barnesi* (and at least seven other species of tiny cubomedusoids) and persisting for hours. *Physalia* species can also cause severe systemic envenoming, including intravascular haemolysis, peripheral gangrene, and renal failure.

Treatment

Patients stung by jellyfish must be removed from the water as soon as possible to prevent drowning. The aim is to prevent a further discharge of nematocysts on fragments of tentacles stuck to the skin. The traditional remedy, still recommended by American authorities, is alcoholic solutions such as methylated spirits and suntan lotion. However, these cause massive discharge of nematocysts. Commercial vinegar or 3 to 10% aqueous acetic acid solution inactivates nematocysts of *C. fleckeri* and other cubozoans, including Irukandji, but it is not recommended for stings by *Chrysaora*, *Physalia*, or *Stomalophus* spp. Adherent tentacles should be shaved off the skin using a razor. Hot water treatment (see venomous fish in earlier paragraphs) has proved effective for relieving the pain of stings by *Physalia*. Pressure immobilization is not recommended as it may increase the amount of venom injected. A slurry of baking soda and water (50% weight/volume) is used for stings by the widely distributed Atlantic genus *Chrysaora*. Cardiopulmonary resuscitation has proved life-saving in several Australian patients stung by *C. fleckeri* who became cyanosed, comatose, and pulseless. A specific 'sea wasp' antivenom for *C. fleckeri* is manufactured in Australia but its efficacy is being questioned. Treatment with verapamil is not recommended.

Starfish and sea urchins (Echinodermata)

These animals are protected by hard exoskeletons with numerous long, sharp projecting spines and grapples (globiferous pedicellariae), which can release venom when embedded in the skin (Fig. 9.2.34). Severe pain and local swelling may result, and sometimes systemic effects such as syncope, numbness, generalized paralysis, aphonia, respiratory distress, cardiac arrhythmias, and even death.

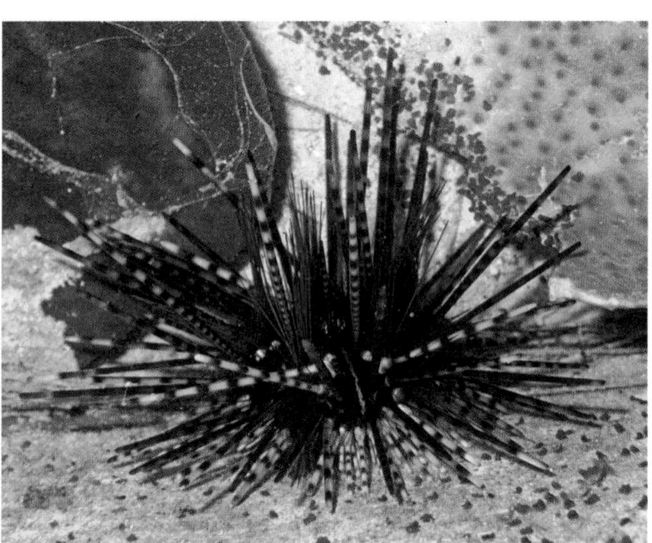

Fig. 9.2.34 Black long-spined sea urchin *Diadema setosum* (Diadematidae) with spines 35 cm long, Madang, Papua New Guinea.
Copyright D. A. Warrell.

Embedded fragments of spines may penetrate bones and joints and lead to secondary infection and chronic granulomas.

Treatment

Hot water (see earlier paragraphs) may relieve the pain. Skin penetrated by the spines, usually the soles of the feet, should be softened with 2% salicylic acid ointment or acetone. An attempt should then be made to squeeze out the spines or removed them surgically but this may prove impossible. No antivenoms are available. There is a risk of marine bacterial infections (see earlier paragraphs).

Cone shells and octopuses (Mollusca)

The 500 species of cone shells (genus *Conus*) are carnivorous marine snails that harpoon their prey (fish, polychaete worms, and other molluscs), implanting a radular tooth charged with venom containing a mixture of small (10–30 amino acid) peptide toxins (Fig. 9.2.35). These include conotoxins, which block acetylcholine receptors and voltage-sensitive calcium and sodium ion channels; conantokins, which are *N*-methyl-D-aspartate receptor antagonists with anticonvulsant activity; and conopressins, which target vasopressin receptors. Cone shells are attractive and valuable collectors' items. People who pick them up may be stung. Symptoms of envenoming are nausea, vomiting, paraesthesia, and numbness of the lips and site of sting, numbness, dizziness, ptosis, diplopia, dysarthria, dyspnoea, and loss of consciousness. In a series of 35 cases mostly stung by *Conus geographus* reported in Japan (1896–1996), 10 died within 2 to 5 h of the sting.

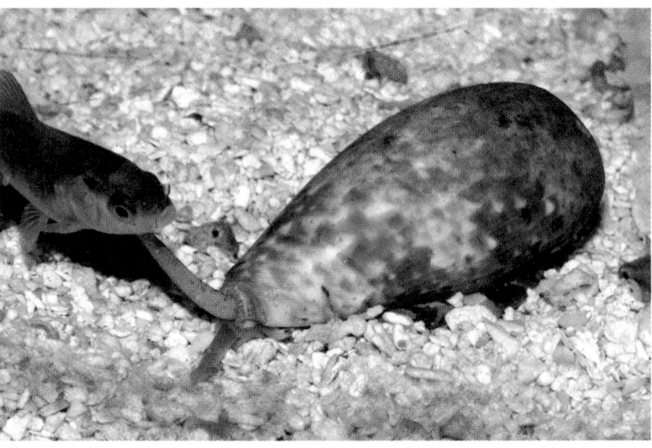

(a)

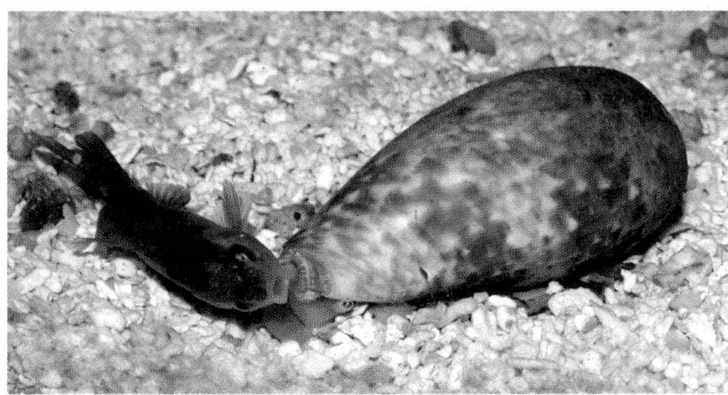

(b)

Fig. 9.2.35 Cone shell *Conus bullatus* harpooning and ingesting a small fish.
Copyright D. A. Warrell.

Several species of small octopus found in the Australian and West Pacific region (blue-ringed octopuses, *Hapalochlaena* spp.) (Fig. 9.2.36) can inject salivary tetrodotoxin when they bite swimmers with their powerful beaks. These bites are painful and cause local bleeding, swelling, and inflammation. Severe neurotoxic symptoms, and even fatal generalized paralysis, may develop within 15 min of the bite.

Treatment

No antivenoms are available. Cardiopulmonary resuscitation and mechanical ventilation may be required.

Venomous arthropods

Bees, wasps, yellowjackets, hornets, and ants (Hymenoptera)

The commonest and most severe stings from hymenoptera are caused by members of the families Apidae (e.g. honey bees *Apis mellifera*, *A. cerania*, *A. dorsata* etc. and bumble bees *Bombus* spp.), Vespidae (e.g. European wasps *Vespula germanica*, *V. vulgaris*; American wasps, yellow-jackets and white-faced 'hornets' *Vespula* and *Dolichovespula* spp. paper wasps *Polistes* spp. and European and Asian true hornets *Vespa* spp.) (Fig. 9.2.37), and Formicidae (e.g. American fire ants *Solenopsis* spp. and Australian bull or bulldog ants *Myrmecia* spp.). Allergic reactions to single stings from hymenoptera are common, whereas envenoming resulting from many stings is rare, except in the Americas. Venom allergens include phospholipases A, hyaluronidase, acid phosphomonoesterases, and polypeptide neurotoxins such as apamin and melittin (*A. mellifera*). Nonallergenic compounds include vasoactive amines, such as histamine, 5-hydroxytryptamine, catecholamines and kinins, cholinesterase (in the venom of *Vespula germanica*), pheromones, 2-methylpiperidine alkaloids (in venoms of fire ants *Solenopsis* spp.), and anti-inflammatory peptides from honey bee venom.

Epidemiology

Fewer than 5 people die from identified hymenopteran sting anaphylaxis in England and Wales each year, 2 to 3 per year in Australia, and between 40 and 50 per year in the United States. The incidence of systemic reactions to stings by hymenoptera has been reported as 0.4 to 0.8% in children. In an adult population in the United States, the prevalence of systemic allergic sting reactions was found to be 4%; 20% of this population showed evidence of venom hypersensitivity (skin tests or radioallergosorbent test, RAST). In the United Kingdom, most patients allergic to bee venom are beekeepers or their relatives. Since the escape of swarms of African honey bees *A. m. scutellata* in Brazil, in 1957, this aggressive strain has spread throughout Latin America and north as far as Las Vegas in the United States. About 30 deaths from mass attacks by these bees have been reported each year. Two species of fire ants, *Solenopsis richteri* and *S. invicta*, were imported into the United States from South America in 1918 and have now spread to 13 southern states where an estimated 2.5 million people are stung each month. The incidence of systemic allergic reactions is about 4 per 100 000 population per year, and there have been fatalities. In Tasmania, and to a lesser extent in southern Australia, the jack jumper ant *Myrmecia pilosula* causes 90% of all ant stings. About 2 to 3% of the population are hypersensitive, and there have been deaths from anaphylaxis in Tasmania.

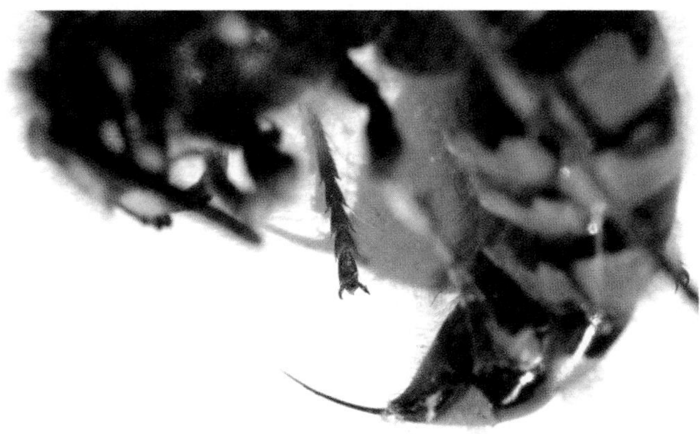

Fig. 9.2.37 Stinger of European wasp *Vespula vulgaris*.
Copyright D. A. Warrell.

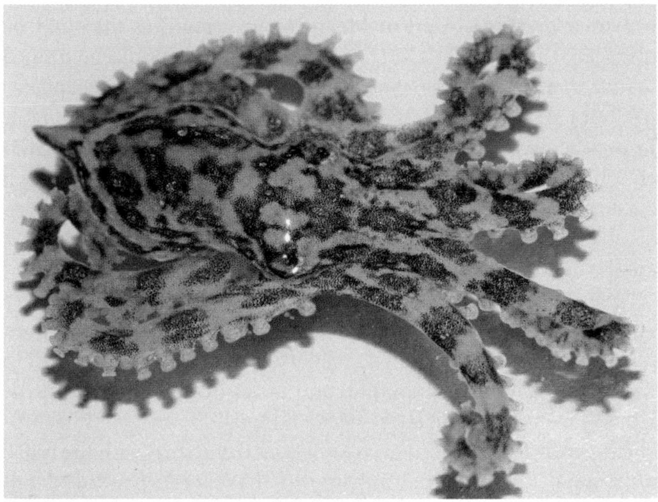

Fig. 9.2.36 Southern/lesser blue-ringed octopus *Hapalochlaena maculosa*, Adelaide, Australia.
Copyright D. A. Warrell.

Prevention

Patients who have a history of systemic anaphylaxis following a sting and who have evidence of hypersensitivity to the venom of the same family of hymenoptera (venom-specific IgE detectable in the serum or a positive skin test) should be considered for desensitization with purified venoms. This treatment proved significantly more effective than placebo or the previously used whole-body extracts of hymenoptera in preventing anaphylactic reactions to sting challenge. Desensitization usually involves weekly visits to hospital for at least 8 weeks for the administration of gradually increasing doses of venom. When protection has been demonstrated by the patient's ability to tolerate 100 μg of venom (equivalent to two stings) they are ready for maintenance therapy, usually 100 μg of venom every 4 to 8 weeks. A period of 2 to 5 years of maintenance desensitization is recommended, after which more than 90% of subjects will remain protected against systemic reactions after stopping treatment. Desensitization is complicated by systemic reactions in 5 to 15% of patients and by local reactions in 50%.

Wasps are attracted by sweet things and meat in kitchens, greengrocers' shops, orchards, vineyards, brightly coloured floral patterns, and perfumes. Hornets are attracted by light. Some hornets (e.g. Asian *Vespa mandarina*) are so aggressive that their nests must be eradicated before the area can be farmed. The risk of mass attacks by apids and vespids can be reduced by vigilance. Observing increasing numbers of vespids can lead to discovery and destruction of their nests. Attacks on farm animals and a tendency for bees to pursue apiarists walking away from the hives are signs of an increasingly aggressive colony, prompting replacement of the queens.

Clinical features

Toxic effects

In nonsensitized individuals, a sting, which, in the case of Vespidae and Apidae, introduces about 50 µg of venom, will rapidly produce a hot, red, painful swelling and weal a few centimetres in diameter, which persists for no more than a few hours. These effects are dangerous only if the airway is obstructed, e.g. following stings on the tongue. As few as 30 stings can cause fatal systemic envenoming in children, but children and adults have survived more than 1000 stings by *A. mellifera*. In some patients, symptoms have suggested histamine toxicity: vasodilatation, hypotension, vomiting, diarrhoea, throbbing headache, coma, and bronchoconstriction. In Latin America, victims of attacks by *A. m. scutellata* have shown evidence of generalized rhabdomyolysis (grossly elevated serum creatine kinase, aminotransferases, and myoglobin), intravascular haemolysis, hypercatecholaminaemia (hypertension, pulmonary oedema, myocardial damage), bleeding, hepatic dysfunction, and acute renal failure. In nonsensitized individuals, stings from *Solenopsis* and *Myrmecia* spp. produce pain, itching, swelling, and erythema around a central weal, which last a few hours, and later vesicles or pustules. In an unsensitized patient, an estimated 10 000 *S. invicta* stings caused no systemic envenoming.

Allergic effects: anaphylaxis

Clinical suspicion of dangerous venom hypersensitivity arises when systemic symptoms follow a sting. Systemic symptoms include tingling scalp; itching, initially of the palms, soles, axillae, and perineum, becoming generalized; flushing; dizziness; syncope; wheezing; abdominal colic (uterine colic in women), violent diarrhoea, incontinence of urine and faeces; tachycardia and visual disturbances; all developing within a few minutes of the sting. Over the next 15 to 20 min, urticaria, angio-oedema of the lips, gums, and tongue, a generalized redness of the skin with swelling, oedema of the glottis, profound hypotension, and coma may develop. The median time to first cardiac arrest is 10 to 20 min after the sting but deaths have occurred after only 2 min. A few patients develop serum sickness a week or more after the sting. Some patients with sting allergy have other evidence of an atopic disposition. Reactions are enhanced by β-blockers.

Diagnosis of anaphylaxis and venom hypersensitivity

Mast-cell tryptase concentrations in serum or plasma peak 0.5 to 1.5 h after the attack but persist for 6 to 8 h. Detection of a raised mast-cell tryptase concentration is useful in confirming the diagnosis of anaphylaxis and excluding panic attacks and other causes of collapse. Type I hypersensitivity is firmed by detecting venom-specific (Vespidae, Apidae, Formicidae) IgE in the serum using RAST or by prick-skin tests. Among hymenoptera venoms, there is strong cross reactivity between bumble bee and honey bee venoms and between wasp, yellow-jacket, and true hornet venoms but not between venoms of Apidae and Vespidae. Patients who have suffered a systemic reaction have a 50 to 60% risk of a reaction to their next sting. Local reactions, even massive ones involving persistent swelling of the whole stung limb, in the absence of systemic symptoms, do not predict a systemic reaction following subsequent stings. Children who have generalized urticaria after a sting have only a 10% chance of a systemic reaction when restung. Hypersensitivity to venom may be lost spontaneously in some children and young adults but this is unpredictable and unreliable. In some countries, live insect sting challenge is used to assess hypersensitivity and response to immunotherapy. The RAST test can be used for a postmortem diagnosis of hymenoptera sting anaphylaxis.

Treatment

The barbed stings of Apidae remain embedded at the site of the sting and continue to inject venom, so they should be removed immediately by any means possible. Vespids can withdraw their stings and sting repeatedly. Wasp stings may become infected because some species feed on rotting meat. Domestic meat tenderizer (papain) diluted roughly 1:5 with tap water is said to produce immediate relief of pain. Ice packs and aspirin are also effective. Systemic but not topical antihistamines can be used for more severe local reactions. Massive local reactions may require aspirin, nonsteroidal anti-inflammatory agents, or even corticosteroids.

Systemic anaphylaxis

First, the patient is laid down and kept flat, ideally in the recovery position. Immediate cardio-pulmonary resuscitation may be needed. Adrenaline should be given as soon as possible: 0.1% (1:1000) (0.5–1 ml for adults; 0.01 mg/kg for children) given by intramuscular injection into the anterolateral thigh, or, if the patient is unconscious or pulseless, diluted 1:100 000, by slow intravenous injection. In rare cases, blood pressure fails to respond to even large doses of adrenaline and plasma expanders. These patients should be given cardiopulmonary resuscitation, selective bronchodilators such as salbutamol, pressor agents such as dopamine, and intravenous histamine H_1 blockers such as chlorphenamine maleate (10 mg for adults; 0.2 mg/kg for children). Corticosteroids probably have no effect in acute anaphylaxis but may prevent relapses a few hours later. Patients who know they are hypersensitive should wear an identifying tag or bracelet (such as provided by Medic-Alert or Medi-Tag in Britain) as they may be discovered unconscious after being stung. They should be trained to give themselves adrenaline using an 'EpiPen' or similar apparatus, but a high proportion of those who carry these kits are unable to use them effectively through lack of training. Adrenaline delivered by a pressurized inhaler ('Medihaler-Epi') or squirted down the endotracheal tube produces transient blood levels insufficient to combat anaphylaxis. Shock and upper- or lower-airway obstruction are the main modes of death following insect-sting anaphylaxis.

Severe envenoming from multiple stings by hymenoptera should be treated with adrenaline, intravenous antihistamines (doses as mentioned earlier), and corticosteroids. Intensive care is essential. Intravenous mannitol and bicarbonate may protect the kidneys from the damaging effects of myoglobinuria and haemoglobinaemia ('pigment nephropathy'), as in patients with the crush syndrome. Experimental antivenoms have been produced but are not yet commercially available. Exchange transfusion or plasmapheresis might be considered to remove venom in severe cases. Renal dialysis is often needed.

Butterflies and moths (Lepidoptera)

The stinging hairs of some species of adult moths can cause contact dermatitis and urticaria ('lepidopterism'), while caterpillars can produce local or even systemic effects ('erucism'). Venomous lepidoptera are found in all parts of the world, but most cases of lepidopterism are reported from Middle and Southern America. Severe cutaneous urticating eruptions can be caused by caterpillars of oak processionary moths *Thaumetopoea processionea* (Thaumetopoeidae) in central/southern Europe and of the genus *Megalopyge* (Megalopygidae—called 'puss caterpillars' in the southern United States) and by adult female moths of the genus *Hylesia* (Saturniidae), which have barbed setae ('flechettes') on their abdomens. Epidemics of stings by these moths have been described, especially from coastal areas of Brazil, Mexico, Peru, and Venezuela. In Brazil, Colombia, Guyane, Paraguay, Peru, and Venezuela, caterpillars of atlas or emperor moths (*Lonomia obliqua, L. achelous*; Saturniidae) cause thousands of stings each year. Venom injected through their bristles contains fibrinolytic (factor XIII activator); anticoagulant; procoagulant (activators of prothrombin, factor X, factor V), kallikrein-like, metalloproteinase, and phospholipase A_2 activities resulting in defibrinogenation and spontaneous bleeding. The case fatality of about 2% is usually attributable to cerebral haemorrhage. Symptoms include local burning, erythema, swelling, inflammation, headache, nausea, vomiting, malaise, bleeding from nose, gums, gut, genitourinary tract, and partly healed scars, polyarthralgia, and acute renal failure. Laboratory findings in envenomed patients are decreased plasma fibrinogen, factor V, factor XIII, and plasminogen concentrations, as well as increased fibrin/fibrinogen degradation products and fibrinolytic activity but a normal platelet count. An effective antivenom ('Soro antilonômico') is produced by Instituto Butantan, São Paulo, Brazil.

In Pará State, Brazil, rubber tappers are frequently in contact with caterpillars (*Premolis semirufa*) whose stinging hairs can cause a disabling arthritis of the hands ('pararama').

Beetles (Coleoptera)

The most notorious vesicating beetle is 'Spanish fly' *Lytta vesicatoria* (Meloidae—blister beetles) (Fig. 9.2.38). Its venom contains cantharidin, which causes blistering 2 to 3 h after application to the skin and priapism (hence its reputation as an aphrodisiac) and renal failure when given systemically or absorbed after eating the legs of frogs which have fed on meloid beetles. Farmed emus are very sensitive to the cantharidin, in blister beetles, which are often found in alfalfa hay on which these birds like to feed.

'Nairobi eye' and similar blistering conditions in Australia and South East Asia are caused by species of the genus *Paederus* (Staphylinidae) 5 to 10 mm in length (Fig. 9.2.39). The typical skin lesions (dermatitis linearis), whose appearance may be delayed 12 to 96 h after contact, consist of erythema, itching, and blistering caused by inadvertently crushing and smearing the beetle. Systemic symptoms such as fever, arthralgia, and vomiting may arise in severe cases. The active principle pederin is the most complex nonproteinaceous insect toxin known. Treatment is palliative. The toxin is easily spread to other sites such as the eye by fingers.

Scorpions (Scorpiones; Buthidae, Hemiscorpiidae)

Species capable of inflicting fatal stings occur in North Africa and the Middle East (*Androctonus*, *Buthus*, *Hemiscorpius* and *Leiurus* spp.) (Fig. 9.2.40); South Africa (*Parabuthus* spp.); India and Nepal (*Mesobuthus tamulus*); North, Central and South America, Trinidad and Tobago (*Centruroides* and *Tityus* spp.) (Figs. 9.2.41 and 9.2.42). Scorpion toxins target sodium, potassium, calcium, and chloride ion channels causing direct effects and the release of neurotransmitters such as acetylcholine and catecholamines.

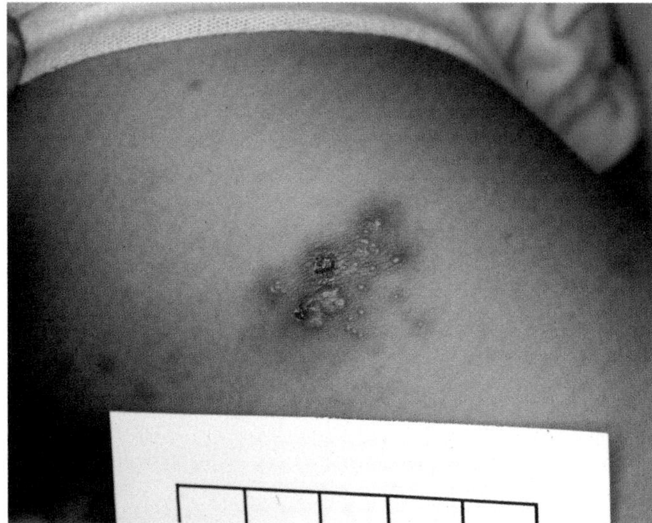

Fig. 9.2.38 Lesions caused by urticating abdominal hairs of female moths *Hylesia* spp. in Brazil.
Copyright D. A. Warrell.

Epidemiology

In Mexico, there were formerly 300 000 stings with 2000 deaths reported each year attributed to *Centruroides limpidus, C. noxius, C. suffusus*, etc., but there are now 250 000 stings with less than 50 deaths/year. In Khuzestan Province, Iran, 25 000 stings (*Hemiscorpius lepturus*, *Androctonus* spp., and *Buthus* spp.) are treated each year and are the fourth major cause of death. In Algeria there were 150 deaths in 1998 and 74 in 2005. In Tunisia, there are about 40 000 stings per year, 1000 hospital admissions and 100 deaths. In the United States 15 000 stings, mainly by *Centruroides exilicauda* (Fig. 9.2.41) are reported inArizona each year but there have been no deaths since 1968. In Trinidad, stings by *Tityus trinitatis* were an occupational hazard of sugar cane and cocoa plantation workers, causing 33 deaths in a group of 698 cases in the 1960s.

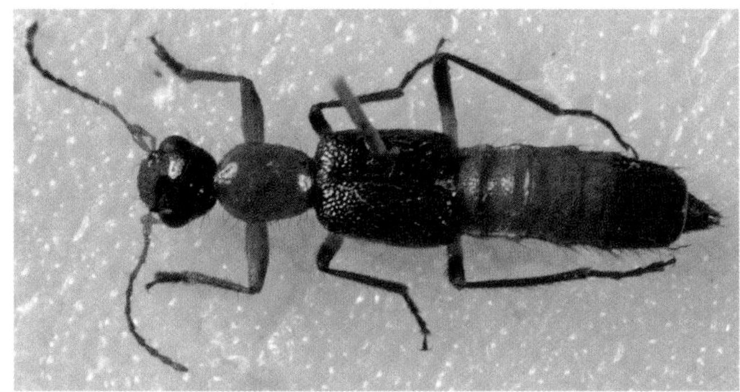

Fig. 9.2.39 Vesicating beetle *Paederus crebripunctatus* (Staphylinidae) responsible for causing 'Nairobi eye'.
Courtesy of Dr John Paul.

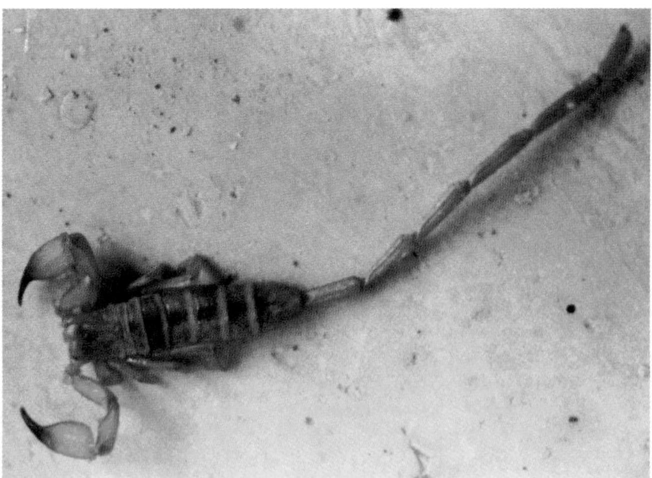

Fig. 9.2.40 *Hemiscorpius lepturus* (Hemiscorpiidae), Iran.
Courtesy of Dr M. Radmanesh.

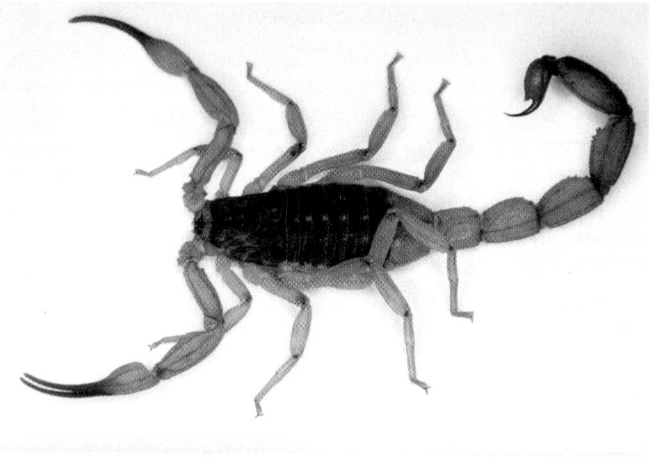

Fig. 9.2.42 South American scorpion *Tityus serrulatus*, São Paulo, Brazil.

Mortality was 25% in children under 5 years compared to 0.25% in adults. In Brazil, where important species are *Tityus serrulatus* (Fig. 9.2.42) and other *Tityus* spp., the case fatality formerly ranged from around 1% in adults to 15 to 25% in children less than 6 years old, but in 2005, among 36 558 reported stings, there were only 50 deaths (case fatality 0.14%). In India, many people are stung by the red scorpion *Mesobuthus tamulus* with fatalities in adults and children.

Prevention

Scorpions can be excluded from houses by incorporating a row of ceramic tiles into the base of the outside wall, making the doorsteps at least 20 cm high, and using residual insecticides, such as carbamate or organophosphate sprays or dusts indoors.

Clinical features

Intense local pain is the commonest symptom. There may be slight local oedema and tender enlargement of regional lymph nodes, but stings by *Hemiscorpius lepturus* (Iran, Iraq, Pakistan, and Yemen) are relatively painless (see next paragraph). Systemic symptoms may develop within minutes or be delayed for as much as 24 h. They vary, according to the species of scorpion involved. Many scorpion venoms stimulate the release of acetylcholine and catecholamines, often resulting in initial cholinergic and later adrenergic symptoms. Early symptoms include vomiting, profuse sweating, piloerection, alternating brady- and tachycardia, abdominal colic, diarrhoea, loss of sphincter control, and priapism. Later, severe life-threatening cardiorespiratory effects may appear: hypertension, shock, tachy- and bradyarrhythmias, ECG changes, and pulmonary oedema with or without evidence of myocardial dysfunction. Severe cardiovascular complications are particularly associated with stings by *Androctonus* spp., *Leiurus quinquestriatus*, *Mesobuthus tamulus*, and *Tityus* spp. (Fig. 9.2.43). Neurotoxic effects such as erratic eye movements, fasciculation and muscle spasms, which can be misinterpreted as tonic-clonic convulsive movements, and respiratory distress are a particular feature of stings by *Centruroides (sculpturatus) exilicauda* in Arizona.

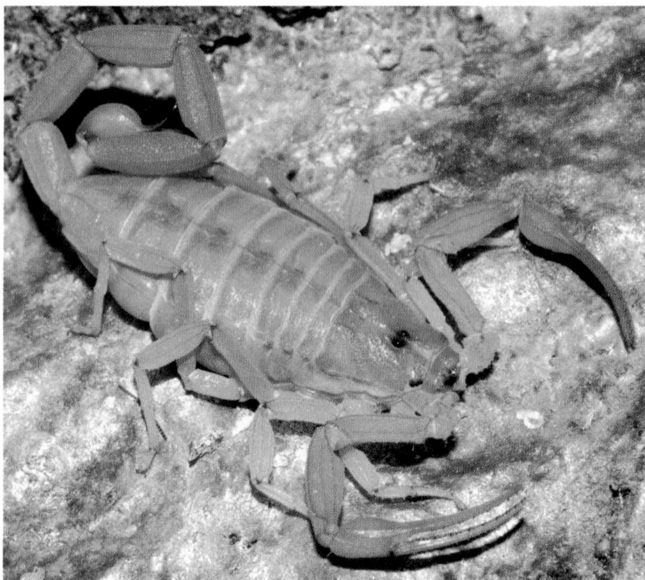

Fig. 9.2.41 Arizona bark scorpion *Centruroides (Sculpturatus) exilicauda*.

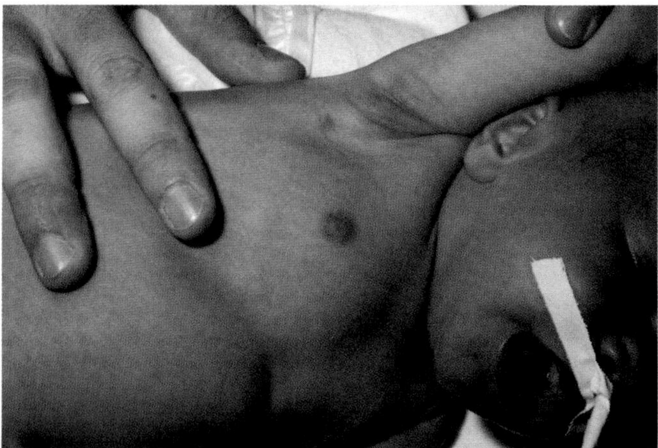

Fig. 9.2.43 Twenty-six-day-old child stung on right axilla in São Paulo, Brazil: showing agitation and pulmonary oedema.

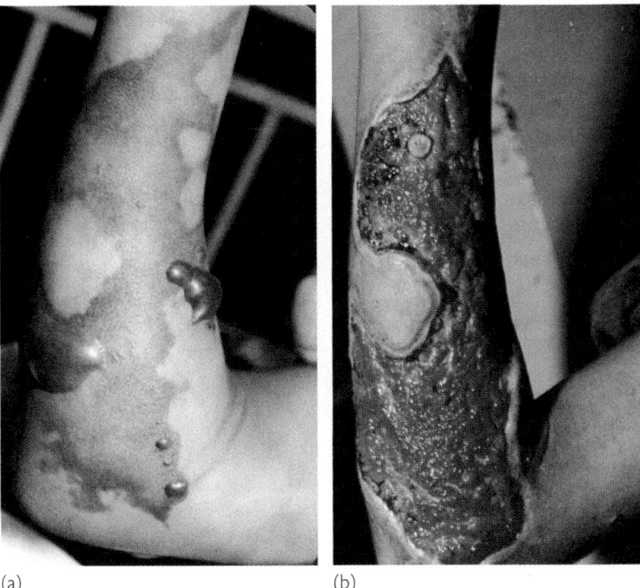

Fig. 9.2.44 (a) Local swelling, blistering, and 'purpuric plaque' caused by the sting of *Hemiscorpius lepturus* in Iran. (b) Progressing to necrosis with granulation tissue. Courtesy of Dr M Radmanesh.

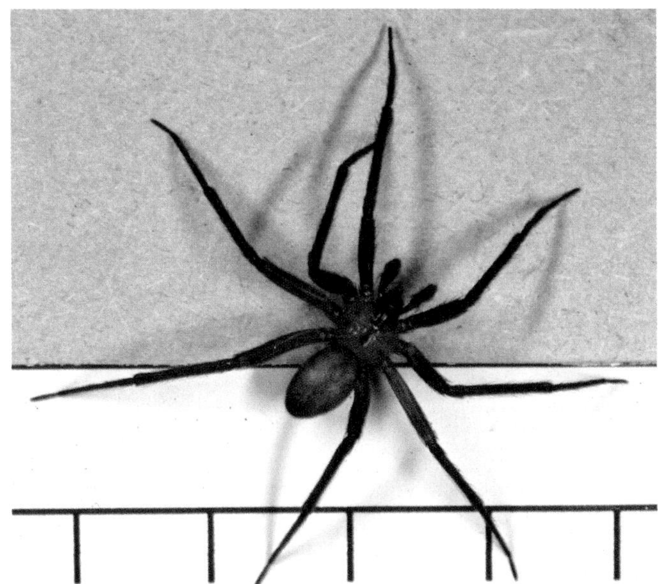

Fig. 9.2.45 South American recluse spider *Loxosceles laeta*, Brazil. Copyright D. A. Warrell.

Parabuthus transvaalicus envenoming in southern Africa is more likely to cause ptosis and dysphagia. Hemiplegia and other neurological lesions have been attributed to fibrin deposition resulting from disseminated intravascular coagulation, for example, after stings by *Nebo hierichonticus* in the Middle East. Hypercatecholaminaemia could explain hyperglycaemia and glycosuria but in the case of stings by the black scorpion of Trinidad (*Tityus trinitatis*) there is severe abdominal pain with nausea, vomiting and haematemesis, hyperglycaemia, and biochemical evidence of acute pancreatitis attributable to simultaneous spasm of the sphincter of Oddi and pancreatic exocrine hypersecretion.

In Iran and Iraq, stings by *Hemiscorpius lepturus* (Hemiscorpiidae) produce a unique clinical syndrome. The sting is painless but macular erythema, pupura, and bullae develop at the site with induration in 39% of cases, swelling and necrosis that requires surgery in 20% of cases (Fig. 9.2.44a, b). Systemic symptoms include dry mouth, thirst, dizziness, nausea, vomiting, fever, cardiac arrhythmias, ST depression on ECG, hypoglycaemia, confusion and convulsions, leucocytosis, thrombocytopenia, coagulopathy, haemolytic anaemia with haemoglobinuria, proteinuria, and renal failure. Twenty per cent of paediatric cases required dialysis. Early treatment with Rhazi Institute antivenom proved effective.

Treatment

Pain responds temporarily to local infiltration or ring block with local anaesthetic. Local injection of emetine or dehydroemetine is said to relieve the pain but may cause necrosis and systemic myotoxic effects. Parenteral opiate analgesics, such as pethidine or morphine, may be required, but are said to be dangerous in victims of *C. exilicauda (sculpturatus)*.

Antivenom is manufactured in a number of countries. Its use is strongly advocated in Africa and the Americas, but ancillary pharmacological treatment is regarded as being much more important in the Middle East and India. However, if specific antivenom is available, it should be administered intravenously as soon as possible in patients with systemic envenoming and in young children stung by dangerous species, even before the development of these symptoms. Patients with cardiovascular symptoms benefit from vasodilator treatment with α-blockers (e.g. prazosin), calcium-channel blockers (e.g. nifedipine), or ACE inhibitors (e.g. captopril). Atropine should not be used except in cases of sinus bradycardia with hypotension. The use of cardiac glycosides and β-blockers is controversial. Bendrodiazepines may be useful in patients with muscle spasms.

Spiders (Araneae)

All but one family of this enormous order are venomous, but few species have proved dangerous to humans. Spiders bite with a pair of small fangs, the chelicerae, to which the venom glands are connected. Medically important genera of venomous spiders include *Loxosceles*, causing necrotic araneism and *Latrodectus, Phoneutria, Atrax, Hadronyche* and *Missulena* spp., causing neurotoxic araneism.

Epidemiology

Spider bites are common in some parts of the world but there are now few fatalities. In Brazil in 2005, 19 634 bites were reported (10/100 000 population) with only 9 deaths (0.05%). In Central and South America, *Loxosceles* spp. such as *L. laeta and L. gaucho* (Fig. 9.2.45) are widely distributed and cause many bites. In Chile, the case fatality of loxoscelism ranges from 1 to 17%. In the southern and south-central United States, the brown recluse spider *L. reclusa* caused at least 200 bites and 6 deaths during the last century. More than 60 cases were reported from Texas between 1959 and 1962. Bites by *L. rufescens* have been reported in the Mediterranean region, North Africa, and Israel. Most bites from *Loxosceles* spp. occur in bedrooms while people are asleep or dressing. In the United States, a number of men were bitten on the genitalia while they sat on outdoor privies in which the spiders had spun their webs.

Black and brown widow spiders are cosmopolitan in distribution. *Latrodectus tredecemguttatus* (sometimes referred to, loosely, as

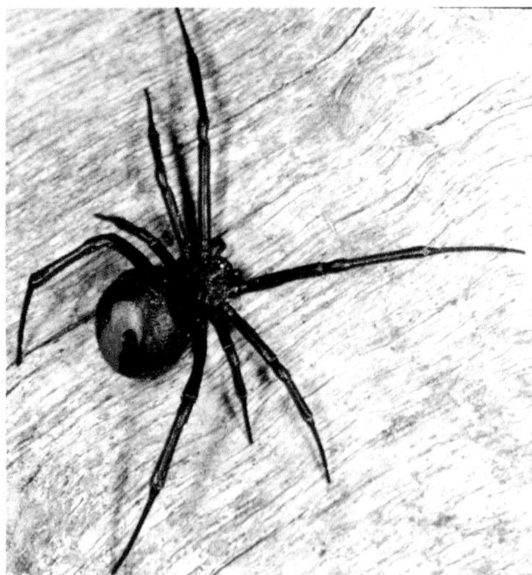

Fig. 9.2.46 Australian redback spider *Latrodectus hasselti*, Adelaide.
Copyright D. A. Warrell.

'tarantula') lives in fields in Mediterranean countries and has been responsible for a series of epidemics of bites. In Italy, 946 cases were reported between 1946 and 1951. the Australian redback spider *L. hasselti* (Fig. 9.2.46) causes up to 340 bites each year in Australia and 20 deaths have been reported. The black widow spider *L. mactans* was responsible for 63 deaths in the United States between 1950 and 1959. Several species of *Latrodectus* occur in Latin America (Fig. 9.2.47).

Wandering, armed, or banana spiders *Phoneutria* spp. (Fig. 9.2.48), cause bites and a few deaths in Latin American countries. They have been imported into temperate countries in bunches of bananas, causing a few bites and deaths.

Highly dangerous funnel web spiders *Atrax* spp. are restricted to south-eastern Australia and Tasmania. The Sydney funnel web spider *A. robustus* is found only within a 160-mile (256-km) radius of Sydney. The aggressive males caused at least 13 deaths between 1927 and 1980. Members of the related genera *Hadronyche* and *Missulena* may be equally dangerous.

In England, mild neurotoxic araneism has been described after bites by *Steatoda nobilis* and *S. grossa* (Theridiidae) and the woodlouse spider *Dysdera crocata*.

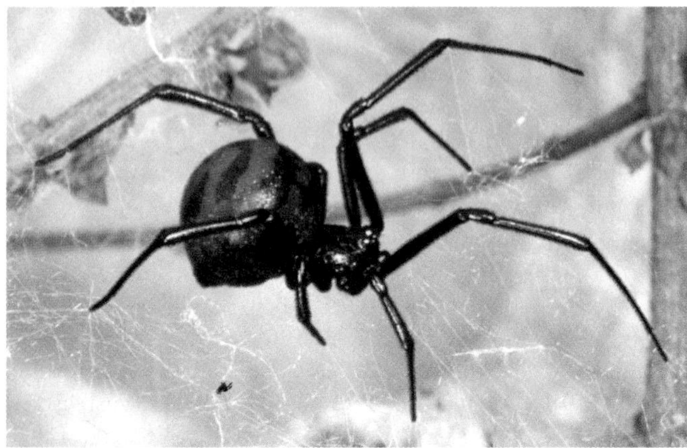

Fig. 9.2.47 South American *Latrodectus curassaviensis*, Brazil.
Copyright D. A. Warrell.

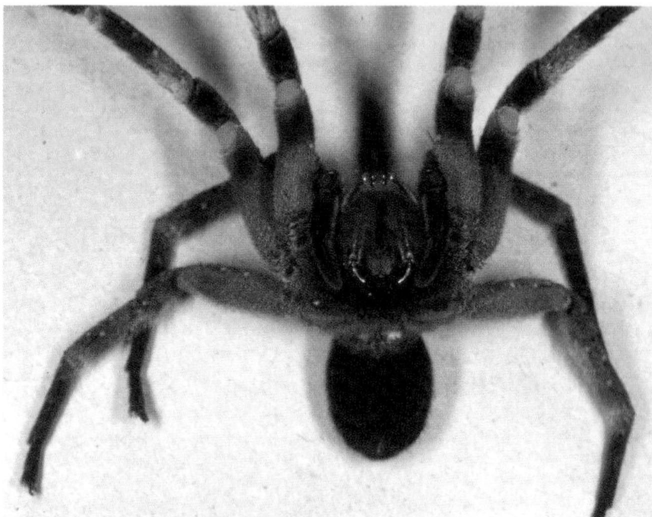

Fig. 9.2.48 Brazilian armed, wandering, or banana spider *Phoneutria nigriventer*.
Copyright D. A. Warrell.

Necrotic araneism

Skin lesions, varying in severity from mild localized erythema and blistering to extensive granulomas and tissue necrosis, have been falsely attributed to a large variety of familiar peridomestic species, such as the Australian white-tailed spider *Lampona cylindrata*, North American hobo spider *Tegenaria agrestis*, European and South American wolf spiders *Lycosa* spp. (including the Italian 'tarantula' *L. terentula*), and cosmopolitan sac spiders *Cheiracanthium* spp. However, only members of the genus *Loxosceles* have proved capable of causing 'necrotic arachnidism/araneism'. Venom sphingomyelinase D is implicated in the pathogenesis of dermonecrosis. Neutrophils adhere to the endothelium of cutaneous capillaries and degranulate. The bite itself is usually painless and unnoticed. Burning develops over several hours at the site of the bite, with swelling and development of a characteristic macular lesion, the red-white-and-blue sign (Fig. 9.2.49) showing

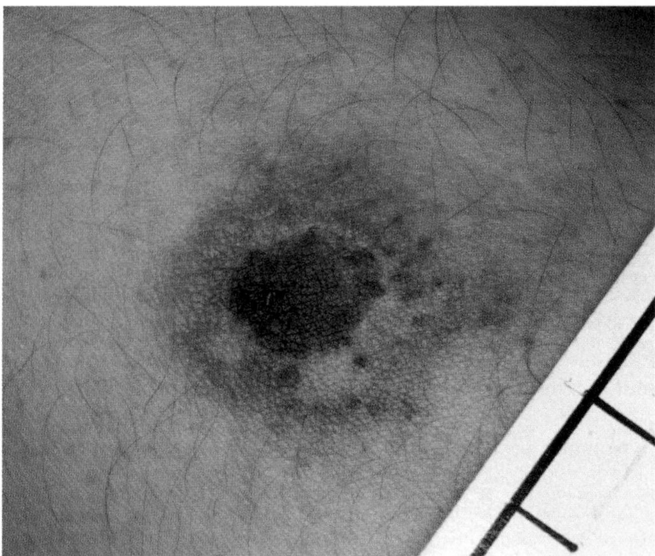

Fig. 9.2.49 'Red-white-and-blue' sign developing 18 h after a bite by the Brazilian recluse spider *Loxosceles gaucho*.
Copyright D. A. Warrell.

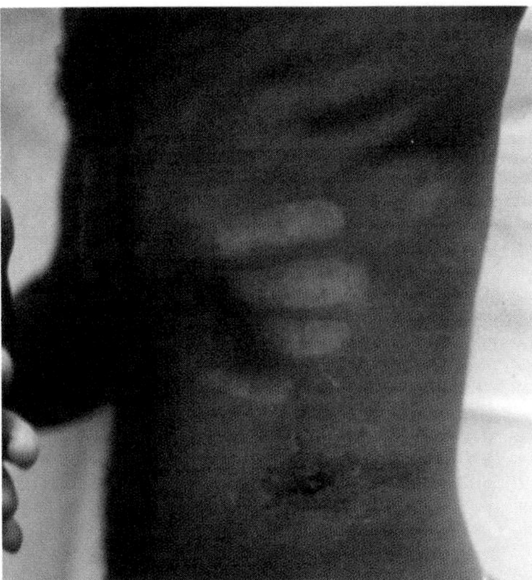

Fig. 9.2.50 Blanching generalised scarlatiniform rash appearing 3 days after a bite above the left hip by a Brazilian recluse spider *Loxosceles gaucho*.
By courtesy of Dr João Luiz Costa Cardoso.

areas of red vasodilatation, white vasoconstriction, and blue prenecrotic cyanosis. A blackened eschar develops, which sloughs in a few weeks, leaving a necrotic ulcer. Sometimes an entire limb or area of the face is involved. Facial bites cause much swelling. Some 13% of cases have systemic symptoms such as fever, headaches, scarlatiniform rash (Fig. 9.2.50), jaundice, methaemoglobinaemia, and haemoglobinuria resulting from intravascular haemolysis. Renal failure may ensue. The average case fatality is about 5%.

Neurotoxic araneism

The bite is very painful immediately but local signs are minimal (*L. mactans*) or moderate (*L. hasselti*). After about 30 min, there is painful regional lymphadenopathy, then headache, nausea, vomiting, and local sweating with piloerection ('gooseflesh'), a sign highly suggestive of neurotoxic araneism (Fig. 9.2.51). In cases of bites by *L. mactans* and *L. tredecemguttatus*, there is profuse generalized sweating and fever with painful muscle spasms, tremors, and rigidity. This may be sufficiently severe to embarrass respiration. The classic 'facies latrodectismica' is an agonized grimace, caused by facial spasm and trismus, associated with swollen eyelids, congested conjunctivae, flushing, and sweating (Fig. 9.2.52). Abdominal rigidity may simulate an acute abdomen and prompt laparotomy. Other features include tachycardia, hypertension, restlessness, irritability, psychosis, priapism, and rhabdomyolysis. A localized or diffuse rash may appear several days later. Envenoming by *Phoneutria* and *Atrax* spp. produces similar features.

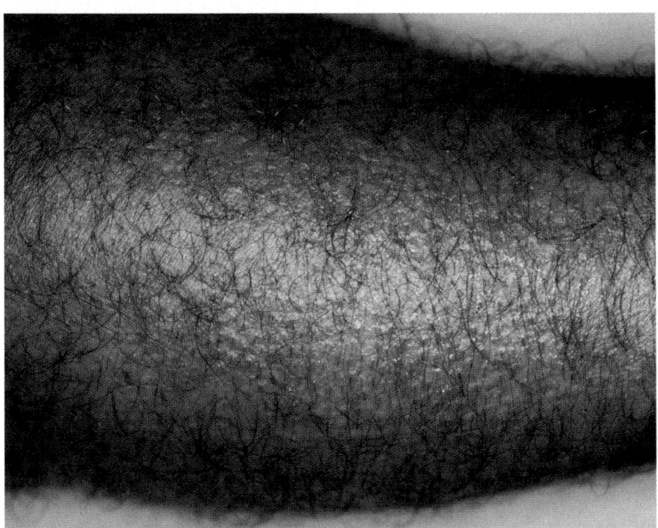

Fig. 9.2.51 Intense local sweating and piloerection at the site of a Brazilian banana spider bite *Phoneutria nigriventer* 30 min earlier.
Copyright D. A. Warrell.

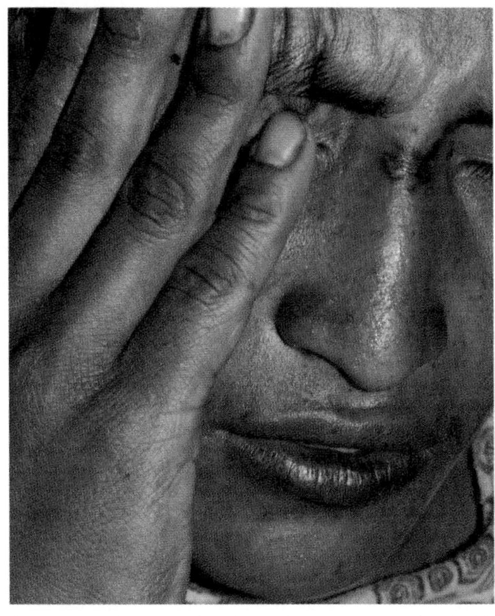

Fig. 9.2.52 'Facies latrodectismica' with profuse sweating and painful muscle spasms, persisting 24 h after a bite by *Latrodectus mactans* ('viuda negra', black widow) near Cusco, Peru.
Copyright D. A. Warrell.

Treatment

First aid

In Australia, pressure-immobilization (see Fig. 9.2.25) is recommended for bites by *A. robustus* and *Hadronyche* species.

Specific treatment

Antivenoms for envenoming by *Latrodectus* spp. are made in Australia, Mexico, South Africa, Brazil, and some other South American countries; for *Atrax* spp. in Australia; for *Loxosceles* spp. in Argentina, Brazil, and Peru; and for *Phoneutria* spp. in Brazil. Despite decades of use, there is no decisive evidenec for the efficacy of *Loxosceles* antivenoms, but neurotoxic araneism is more obviously responsive to antivenom.

Supportive treatment

Oral dapsone (100 mg twice daily) is said to reduce the extent of necrotic lesions by inhibiting neutrophil degranulation and calcium gluconate (10 ml of a 10% solution, given by slow intravenous injection) is said to relieve the pain of muscle spasms caused by the venom of *Latrodectus* spp. rapidly and more effectively than muscle relaxants such as diazepam or methocarbamol. Unfortunately, evidence for efficacy is lacking. Antihistamines, corticosteroids, α-blockers, and atropine have also been advocated. For necrotic araneism cause by *Loxosceles* spp., early surgical debridement, corticosteroids, antihistamines, and hyperbaric oxygen all have their advocates, but there is no basis for recommending their use.

Ticks (Acari)

Taxonomy and epidemiology

Ticks, with mites, form the order Acari of the class *Arachnida*. Adult females of about 34 species of hard tick (family *Ixodidae*) and immature specimens of 9 species of soft ticks (family *Argasidae*) have been implicated in human tick paralysis. The tick's saliva contains a neurotoxin, which causes presynaptic neuromuscular block and decreased nerve-conduction velocity. The tick embeds itself in the skin with its barbed hypostome introducing the salivary toxin while it engorges with blood.

Although tick paralysis has been reported from all continents, most cases occur in western North America (*Dermacentor andersoni*), eastern United States (*D. variabilis*), and eastern Australia from north Queensland to Victoria (*Ixodes holocyclus*) known as the bush-, scrub-, paralysis-, or dog-tick. In British Columbia there were 305 cases with a 10% case fatality between 1900 and 1968. About 120 cases have been reported in the United States, and in New South Wales there were at least 20 deaths between 1900 and 1945.

Clinical features

Ticks are picked up in the countryside or from domestic animals, particularly dogs, in the home. The majority of patients and almost all fatal cases are children. After the tick has been attached for about 5 or 6 days a progressive ascending lower motor neurone paralysis develops with paraesthesiae. Often a child, who may have been irritable for the previous 24 h, falls on getting out of bed first thing in the morning and is found to be weak or ataxic. Paralysis increases over the next few days: death results from bulbar and respiratory paralysis and aspiration of stomach contents. Vomiting is a feature of the more acute course of *Ixodes holocyclus* envenoming.

This clinical picture is often misinterpreted as poliomyelitis. Other neurological conditions, including Guillain–Barré syndrome, paralytic rabies, Eaton–Lambert syndrome, myasthenia gravis, or botulism, may also be suspected. Diagnosis depends on finding the tick, which is likely to be concealed in a crevice, orifice, or hairy area of the body. The scalp is the commonest place. Fatal tick paralysis has been caused by a tick attached to the tympanic membrane.

Treatment

The tick must be discovered and detached without being squeezed. It can be painted with ether, chloroform, paraffin, petrol, or turpentine, or prised out between the partially separated tips of a pair of small, curved forceps. Following removal of the tick there is usually a rapid and complete recovery; but in Australia, patients have died even after the tick had been detached. The antivenoms, raised in dogs and rabbits in Australia, are no longer produced.

Centipedes and millipedes (subphylum Myriapoda)

Centipedes (class Chilopoda)

Epimorph centipedes have 15 to 191 pairs of legs and move rapidly and distractedly. They occur in most parts of the world including the Arctic Circle. The largest, *Scolopendra gigantea* of South America, can grow to more than 30 cm in length. Many species can inflict painful stings through a pair of modified claws (forcipules) on the postcephalic segment (Fig. 9.2.53). More than 3000 stings are reported each year in Brazil. Venoms contain serotonin, histamine, lipids, polysaccharides, proteases, and peptides that are neurotoxic to insects. Stings cause intense radiating pain, swelling, inflammation, erythema, and lymphangitis and sometimes local necrosis. Systemic effects such as vomiting, sweating, headache, cardiac arrhythmias, myocardial ischaemia, rhabdomyolysis, proteinuria, acute renal failure, and convulsions are extremely rare. The risk of mortality was probably greatly exaggerated in the older literature. Hypersensitivity may have played a role in these reactions. Reports of documented fatalities remain elusive but are said to occur on some Indian Ocean islands. The most important genus is *Scolopendra* which is distributed throughout tropical countries. Local treatment is the same as for scorpion stings. No antivenom is available.

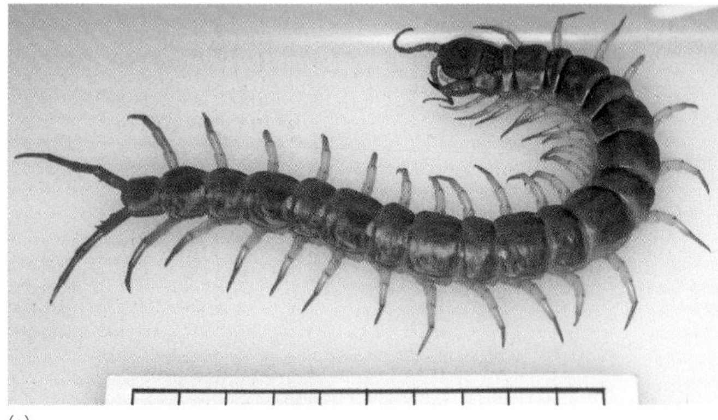

(a)

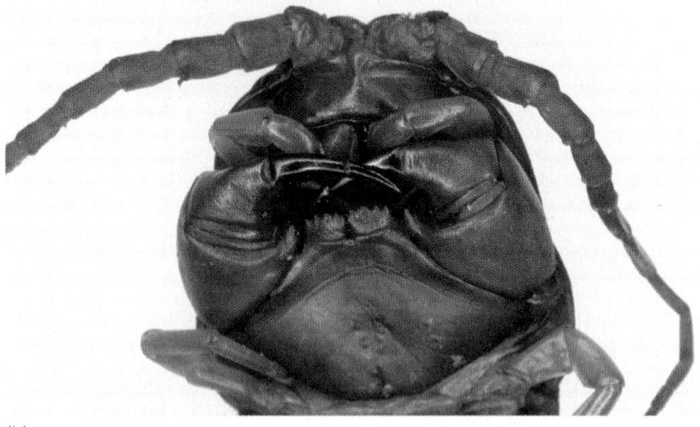

(b)

Fig. 9.2.53 Thai centipede (*Scolopendra* spp.) (a) showing venom 'jaws' (modified limbs) (b).

Millipedes (class Diplopida)

Millipedes are widely distributed. They may exceed 35 cm in length, have hundreds of legs (not a thousand, despite their name), move sluggishly and tend to coil into a ball. Most species possess glands in each of their body segments which secrete, and in some cases squirt out, irritant liquids for defensive purposes. These contain hydrogen cyanide and a variety of aldehydes, esters, phenols, and quinonoids. Members of at least eight genera of millipedes have proved injurious to humans. Important genera are *Rhinocricus* (Caribbean), *Spirobolus* (Tanzania and Papua New Guinea), *Spirostreptus* and *Iulus* (Indonesia), and *Polyceroconas* (*Salpidobolus*) (Papua New Guinea). Children are particularly at risk when they handle or try to eat these large arthropods. When venom is squirted into the eye, intense conjunctivitis results and there may be corneal

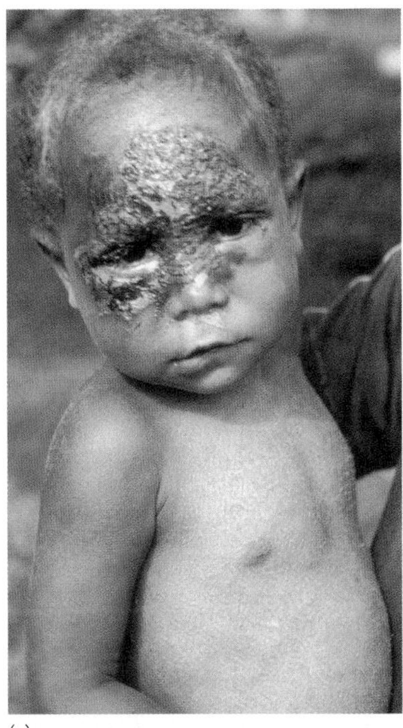
(a)

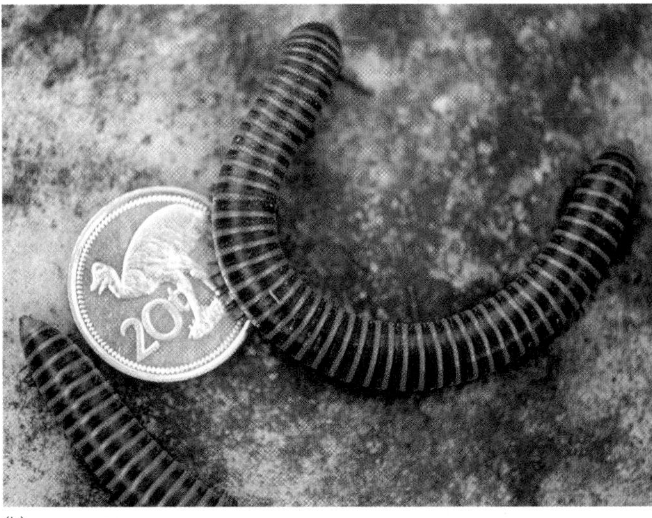
(b)

Fig. 9.2.54 Skin and mucosal lesions (a) caused by application of giant Papua New Guinea millipede (b) (genus *Spirobolus*).

ulceration and, allegedly, blindness. Skin lesions initially stain brown ('mahogany stains') or purple, blister after a few days, and then peel (Fig. 9.2.54). They have been mistaken for signs of child abuse. First aid is generous irrigation with water. Eye injuries should be treated as for snake venom ophthalmia (see p. 1343).

Leeches (phylum Annelida, class Hirudinea)

Leeches are blood-sucking, hermaphroditic, egg-laying annelids, which have elongated annulated bodies. They attach themselves to leaves, rocks, or the host by a posterior sucker. To feed, the leech applies its anterior sucker containing the mouth armed with three radially arranged jaws which make a Y-shaped incision. Blood is sucked out by the action of the muscular pharynx. To prevent blood clotting, the saliva contains a histamine-like vasodilator and anticoagulants, such as: hirudin from the medicinal leech *Hirudo medicinalis*, which inhibits thrombin and factor IXa; hementin from *Haementeria ghilianii*, which is directly fibrinolytic; and hementerin from *H. depressa* (= *H. lutzi*), a plasminogen activator. Other enzymes include esterases, antitrypsin, antiplasmin, and antielastase. Recombinant hirudin is now produced as a therapeutic anticoagulant. The medicinal leech is still used by plastic surgeons to reduce haematomas under skin grafts; the wound may become infected with *Aeromonas hydrophila*, which lives symbiotically in the leech's gut.

Two groups of leeches cause human morbidity and even mortality in tropical countries.

Land leeches

Species of the genera *Haemadipsa* and *Phyrobdella* are 1 to 8 cm long. They infest, often in enormous numbers, the damp, leaf litter and low vegetation of rainforests, choosing game trails and watering places. By standing on the posterior sucker and waving the anterior sucker, they can sense their prey with amazing efficiency. They drop on to the prey or pursue it with a looping or lashing motion. Leeches usually attach themselves to the lower legs or ankles and are adept at penetrating clothing, even long trousers tucked into socks and lace-up boots. The bite is usually painless and infested individuals may not realize what has happened until they hear a squelching sound, notice that their feet are warm and wet, and see blood welling over the tops of their boots. Land leeches ingest about 1 ml of blood in 1 h and then drop off, but the wound continues to bleed for some time and forms a fragile clot.

Aquatic leeches

These species may be swallowed by individuals who drink stagnant water or even mountain stream water, or they may attack bathers, entering the mouth, nostrils, eyes, vulva, vagina, urethra, or anus. *Hirudo medicinalis* can ingest 5 to 15 ml of blood, increasing its initial weight up to 10 times. The enormous brightly coloured buffalo leech *Hirudinaria manillensis* of South East Asia, is up to 16 cm long and can ingest 1 ml of blood in 10 min. *Limnatis nilotica* occurs around the Mediterranean, Middle East, and North Africa. *Myxobdella africana* occurs in East Africa. *Dinobdella ferox* (5 cm long) is found in Asia. Some aquatic leeches are very slow feeders and may remain attached for days or even weeks. *L. nilotica* and *D. ferox* have been implicated in 'halzoun'. However, in Lebanon, leech infestation contracted from spring water ('alack') is distinguished from 'halzoun' following ingestion of raw offal (see Section 7 Infectious Diseases).

Prevention

Leech intrusion can be reduced by impregnating clothing, especially the bottoms of trousers and socks, with repellents such as dibutyl phthalate and diethyl toluamide and applying them to the skin and the inside and outside of footwear. If these compounds are not available, invasion of footwear during jungle walks can be prevented, rather messily, by rolling a rope of tobacco in the tops of the socks and keeping the feet well soaked with water. Women's pantyhose are said to prevent leech attachment but may be damaged by DEET-containing repellents. Children should be discouraged from bathing in leech-infested waters and all drinking water should be boiled or filtered.

Clinical features

The main effect is blood loss, but other symptoms include pain caused by the bite, secondary infection, a residual itching, and phobia. Ingested aquatic leeches usually attach to the pharynx but may penetrate the bronchi or oesophagus. *H. manillensis* entering via the anus can reach the rectosigmoid junction of the bowel causing perforation and peritonitis. Patients with a leech in the pharynx often have a feeling of movement at the back of the throat with cough, hoarseness, stridor, breathlessness, epistaxis, haemoptysis, and haematemesis. Fatal upper-airway obstruction may result. The leech *Limnatis nilotica* is no longer thought to be a cause of 'halzoun' (Lebanon) or 'marrara' (Sudan) (see Chapter 7.13 on pentastomiasis) but aquatic leech infestation could be a differential diagnosis of those dramatic syndromes of pharyngeal obstruction. Bleeding may persist for up to a week after the leech has dropped off. In rural Thailand, vaginal bleeding in girls who have swum in ponds or canals is often attributable to infestation by aquatic leeches. Sexual abuse may be wrongly inferred if this diagnosis is not considered. Transmission of rinderpest and other viruses, leptospirosis, and *Trypanosoma cruzi* has been suggested but not proved. Secondary infection of medicinal leech bites by *Aeromonas hydrophila* has been described.

Treatment

Leeches are best scraped off with a fingernail. Traditional methods such as applying a grain of salt, a lighted match or a cigarette, alcohol, turpentine, or vinegar make the leech regurgitate into the wound, creating a risk of infection. Local bleeding can be stopped by applying a styptic, such as silver nitrate or a firm dressing. Aquatic leeches that have penetrated the respiratory, upper gastrointestinal, genitourinary tracts, or rectum must be removed by endoscope. Spraying with 30% cocaine, 10% tartaric acid, or dilute (1:10 000) adrenaline makes the leech detach from the nasopharynx, larynx, trachea, or oesophagus, while irrigation with a concentrated salt solution may be effective in the genitourinary tract and rectum. Leeches should not be pulled off so roughly that the mouth parts are left in the wound as this will lead to a chronic infection. Antimicrobial treatment of secondary bacterial infections (e.g. of *Aeromonas hydrophila* with cefuroxime or a quinolone) may be required.

Further reading

Mechanical injuries caused by animals

Auerbach PS (ed.) (2007). *Wilderness medicine*, 5th edition, Philadelphia, Mosby Elsevier.

Barss PG (1982). Injuries caused by garfish in Papua New Guinea. *BMJ*, **284**, 77–9.

Barss P, Ennis S (1988). Injuries caused by pigs in Papua New Guinea. *Med J Aust*, **149**, 649–56.

Freer L (2004). North American wild mammalian injuries. *Emerg Med Clin North Am*, **22**, 445–73, ix.

Spotte S (2002). *Candiru. Life and legend of the bloodsucking catfish*. Creative Arts Books Company, Berkely California

Website

Shark attacks: http://www.flmnh.ufl.edu/fish/Sharks/ISAF/ISAF.htm

Venomous mammals

Krane S, *et al.* (2003). 'Venom' of the slow loris: sequence similarity of prosimian skin gland protein and Fel d 1 cat allergen. *Naturwissenschaften*, **90**(2), 60–2.

Whittington CM, *et al.* (2008). Defensins and the convergent evolution of platypus and reptile venom genes. *Genome Res*, **18**, 986–94

Venomous snakes

Gopalakrishnakone P (ed.) (1994). *Sea snake toxinology*, pp. 1–36. Singapore University Press, Singapore.

Meier J, White J (eds.) (1995). *Handbook of clinical toxicology of animal venoms and poisons*. CRC Press, Boca Raton, FL.

Reid HA, *et al.* (1963). Clinical effects of bites by Malayan viper (*Ancistrodon rhodostoma*). *Lancet*, **i**, 617–21.

Sutherland SK, Tibballs J (2001). *Australian animal toxins. The creatures, their toxins and care of the poisoned patient*, 2nd edition. Oxford University Press, Melbourne.

Warrell DA (ed.) (1999). WHO/SEARO Guidelines for the clinical management of snake bites in the South East Asian region. *South East Asian J Trop Med Public Health*, **30** Suppl 1, 1–85.

Warrell DA (2004). Epidemiology, clinical features and management of snakebites in Central and South America. In Campbell J, Lamar WW, Greene H (eds) *Venomous reptiles of the Americas*, 2nd edition, pp. 709–61. Cornell University Press, Ithaca, NY.

Warrell DA (2005). Treatment of bites by adders and exotic venomous snakes. *BMJ*, **331**, 1244–7.

Warrell DA (2010). Seminar snake bite. *Lancet*, **375**, 77–88.

Websites

Antivenoms: general http://www.toxinfo.org/antivenoms/

Envenoming worldwide: http://www.toxinology.com/

Snake bite in South and South East Asia: http://www.searo.who.int/en/Section10/Section17/Section53/Section1024.htm

Venomous snake taxonomy updates: http://sbsweb.bangor.ac.uk/%7Ebss166/update.htm

Venomous lizards

Fry BG, *et al.* (2006). Early evolution of the venom system in lizards and snakes. *Nature*, **439**, 584–8.

Russell FE, Bogert CM (1981). Gila monster, venom and bite—a review. *Toxicon* **19**, 341–59.

Poisonous amphibians

Brubacher JK, *et al.* (1996). Treatment of toad venom poisoning with digoxin-specific Fab fragments. *Chest*, **110**, 1282–8.

Daly JW, Spande TF, Garraffo HM (2005). Alkaloids from amphibian skin: a tabulation of over eight hundred compounds. *J Nat Prod*, **68**, 1556–75.

Myers CW, Daly JW, Malkin B (1978). A dangerously toxic new frog (*Phyllobates*) used by the Emberá Indians of Western Colombia with discussion of blowgun fabrication and dart poisons. *Bull Am Mus Nat History*, **161**(Art 2), 307–66.

Poisonous birds

Dumbacher JP, *et al.* (1992). Homobatracho-toxin in the genus *Pitohui*: chemical defense in birds? *Science*, **258**, 799–800.

Dumbacher JP, *et al.* (2004). Melyrid beetles (*Choresine*): a putative source for the batrachotoxin alkaloids found in poison-dart frogs and toxic passerine birds. *Proc Natl Acad Sci U S A*, **101**, 15857–60.

Venomous fish

Castex MN (1967). Fresh water venomous rays. In: Russell FE, Saunders PR (eds.) *Animal toxins*, pp. 167–76. Pergamon Press, Oxford.

Halstead BW (1988). *Poisonous and venomous marine animals of the world*, 2nd revised edition. Darwin Press, Princeton, NJ.

Smith WL, Wheeler WC (2006). Venom evolution widespread in fishes: a phylogenetic road map for the bioprospecting of piscine venoms. *J Hered*, **97**, 206–17.

Sutherland SK, Tibballs J (2001). *Australian animal toxins. The creatures, their toxins and care of the poisoned patient*, 2nd edition. Oxford University Press, Melbourne.

Williamson JA, *et al.* (eds.) (1996). *Venomous and poisonous marine animals: a medical and biological handbook*. University of New South Wales Press, Sydney.

Poisoning by ingestion of aquatic animals

Bagnis RA, *et al.* (1979). Clinical observations on 3009 cases of Ciguatera (fish poisoning) in the Southern Pacific. *Am J Trop Med Hygiene*, **28**, 1067–73.

Daranas AH, Norte M, Fernández JJ (2001). Toxic marine micro-algae. *Toxicon* **39**, 1101–32.

Halstead BW (1988). *Poisonous and venomous marine animals of the world*, 2nd revised edition. Darwin Press, Princeton, NJ.

International Programme on Chemical Safety (1984). *Aquatic (marine and fresh water) biotoxins. Environmental Health Criteria 37*. World Health Organization, Geneva.

Lin YF, Lin SH (1999). Simultaneous acute renal and hepatic failure after ingesting raw carp gall bladder. *Nephrol Dial Transplant*, **14**, 2011–12.

Williamson JA, *et al.* (eds.) (1996). *Venomous and poisonous marine animals: a medical and biological handbook*. University of New South Wales Press, Sydney.

Venomous marine invertebrates

Halstead BW (1988). *Poisonous and venomous marine animals of the world*, 2nd revised edition. Darwin Press, Princeton, NJ.

Hartwick R, *et al.* (1980). Disarming the box-jellyfish. Nematocyst inhibition in *Chironex fleckeri*. *Med J Aust*, **1**, 15–20.

Olivera BM, Teichert RW (2007). Diversity of the neurotoxic *Conus* peptides: a model for concerted pharmacological discovery. *Mol Interv*, **7**(5), 251–60.

Sutherland SK, Tibballs J (2001). *Australian animal toxins. The creatures, their toxins and care of the poisoned patient*, 2nd edition. Oxford University Press, Melbourne.

Williamson JA, *et al.* (eds.) (1996). *Venomous and poisonous marine animals: a medical and biological handbook*. University of New South Wales Press, Sydney.

Venomous arthropods

Hymenoptera

Brown SG, *et al.* (2003). Ant venom immunotherapy: a double-blind, placebo-controlled, crossover trial. *Lancet*, **361**, 1001–6.

França FOS, *et al.* (1994). Severe and fatal mass attacks by 'killer' bees (Africanised honey bees—*Apis melliferascutellata* in Brazil: clinicopathological studies with measurement of serum venom concentrations. *Q J Med*, **87**, 269–82.

Hunt J Jr., *et al.* (1978). A controlled trial of immunotherapy in insect hypersensitivity. *N Engl J Med*, **2991**, 157–61.

Mueller UR (1990). *Insect sting allergy. Clinical picture, diagnosis and treatment*. Gustav Fischer, Stuttgart.

Piek T (1986). *Venoms of the Hymenoptera. Biochemical, pharmacological and behavioural aspects*. Academic Press, London.

Novartis Foundation (2004). *Anaphylaxis. Novartis Foundation Symposium 257*. Chichester, Wiley.

Soar J, *et al.* (2008). Working Group of the Resuscitation Council (UK) Statement Paper. Emergency treatment of anaphylactic Reactions—guidelines for healthcare providers. *Resuscitation*, **77**, 157–69.

Winston ML (1992). *Killer bees. The Africanized honey bee in the Americas*. Harvard University Press, Cambridge, MA.

Lepidoptera

Da Silva WD, *et al.* (1996). Development of an antivenom against toxins of *Lonomia obliqua* caterpillars. *Toxicon*, **34**, 1045–9.

Kelen EMA, Picarelli ZP, Duarte AC (1995). Hemorrhagic syndrome induced by contact with caterpillars of the genus *Lonomia* (Saturniidae, Hamileucinae). *J Toxicol Toxin Rev*, **14**, 283–308.

Coleoptera

Eisner T, *et al.* (1990). Systemic retention of ingested cantharidin by frogs. *Chemoecol*, **1**, 57–62.

Frank JH, Kanamitsu K (1987). *Paederus sensu lato* (Coleoptera: Staphylinidae): natural history and medical importance. *J Med Entomol*, **24**, 1555–91.

Southcott RV (1989). Injuries from Coleoptera. *Med J Aust*, **151**, 654–9.

Scorpions

Bawaskar HS, Bawaskar PH (1992). Management of the cardiovascular manifestations of poisoning by the Indian red scorpion (*Mesobuthus tamulus*). *Br Heart J*, **68**, 478–80.

Bettini S (ed.) (1978). Athropod venoms. *Handbook of experimental pharmacology*, Vol. **48**, p, 977. Springer-Verlag, Berlin.

Boyer LV, *et al.* (2009). Antivenoms for critically ill children with neurotoxicity from scorpion slings. *N Engl J Med*, **360**, 2090–8.

Brownell P, Polis G (eds) (2001). *Scorpion biology and research*. Oxford University Press, New York.

Fet V, *et al.* (eds.) (2000). *Catalog of the scorpions of the world. (1758–1998)*. New York Entomological Society, New York.

Freire-Maia L, Campos JA, Amaral CFS (1996). Treatment of scorpion envenoming in Brazil. In: Bon C, Goyffon M (eds) *Envenomings and their treatments*, pp. 301–10. Edition Fondation Marcel Mérieux, Lyon.

Ismail M (1995). The scorpion envenoming syndrome. *Toxicon*, **33**, 825–58.

Pipelzadeh MH, *et al.* (2007). An epidemiological and a clinical study on scorpionism by the Iranian scorpion *Hemiscorpius lepturus*. *Toxicon*, **50**, 984–92.

Polis GA (ed.) (1990). *The biology of scorpions*. Stanford University Press, Stanford, CA.

Waterman JA (1938). Some notes on scorpion poisoning in Trinidad. *Trans R Soc Trop Med Hyg*, **31**, 607–24.

Spiders

Clark RF, *et al.* (1992). Clinical presentation and treatment of black widow spider envenomation: a review of 163 cases. *Ann Emerg Med*, **21**, 782–7.

Maretić Z, Lebez D (1979). *Araneism with special reference to Europe*. Novit, Pula-Ljubjan, Yugoslavia.

Southcott RV (1976). Arachnidism and allied syndromes in the Australian region. *Rec Adelaide Child Hosp*, **1**, 97–186.

Sutherland SK, Tibballs J (2001). *Australian animal toxins. The creatures, their toxins and care of the poisoned patient*, 2nd edition. Oxford University Press, Melbourne.

Warrell DA, *et al.* (1991). Neurotoxic envenoming by an immigrant spider (*Steatoda nobilis*) in southern England. *Toxicon*, **29**, 1263–5.

Website

Arachnids: http://www.ufsia.ac.be/Arachnology.

Ticks

Gothe R, Kunze K, Hoogstraal H (1979). The mechanism of pathogenicity in the tick paralyses. *J Med Entomol*, **16**, 357–69.

Murnaghan MF, O'Rourke FJ (1978). Tick paralysis. In: Bettini S (ed.) *Arthropod venoms. Handbook of experimental pharmacology*, Vol. **48**, p. 419. Springer-Verlag, Berlin.

Pearn J (1977). The clinical features of tick bite. *Med J Aust*, **2**, 313.

Stone BF (1987). Toxicoses induced by ticks and reptiles in domestic animals. In Harris JB (ed.) *Natural toxins: animal, plant and microbial*, pp. 56–71. Oxford University Press, Oxford.

Centipedes and millipedes

Bettini S (ed.) (1978). *Arthropod venoms. Handbook of experimental pharmacology*, Vol. **48**, p. 977. Springer-Verlag, Berlin.

Radford AJ (1975). Millipede burns in man. *Trop Geogr Med*, **27**, 279–87.

Radford AJ (1976). Giant millipede burns in Papua New Guinea. *P N G Med J*, **18**, 138–41.

Leeches

Adams SL (1988). The medicinal leech. A page from the Annelids of Internal Medicine. *Ann Int Med*, **109**, 399–405.

Cundall DB (1986). Severe anaemia and death due to the pharyngeal leech *Myxobdella africana*. *Trans R Soc Trop Med Hyg*, **80**, 940–4.

Editorial (1992). Hirudins: return of the leech? *Lancet*, **340**, 579–80.

Keegan HL (1963). Leeches as pests of man in the Pacific region. In: Keegan HL, McFarlane WR (eds.) *Venomous and poisonous animals and noxious plants of the Pacific region*, pp. 99–104. Pergamon Press, Oxford.

Sawyer RT (1986). *Leech biology and behaviour*. Oxford University Press, Oxford.

Snower DP, *et al.* (eds.) (1989). *Aeromonas hydrophila* infection associated with the use of medicinal leeches. *J Clin Microbiol*, **27**, 1421–2.

9.3

Injuries, poisoning, and allergic reactions caused by plants

Contents

9.3.1 Poisonous plants and fungi *1361*
Hans Persson

9.3.2 Common Indian poisonous plants *1371*
V.V. Pillay

9.3.1 Poisonous plants and fungi

Hans Persson

Essentials

Plant poisoning

Many plants contain toxic substances heterogeneous in their chemical composition and diverse in their toxic effects. When classifying plant poisonings, a pragmatic approach is to look at the main clinical effects, but it should be emphasized that few plant toxins produce just one type of symptom, and symptomatology is often multiple, although some features predominate.

Ingestion of, or contact with, poisonous plants is common, but serious plant poisoning is rare worldwide because most plant exposures are accidental: they occur in small children, the ingested dose is usually minimal, and no treatment is required.

Severe plant poisoning is usually the result of intentional exposure. Toxic plants are ingested deliberately as suicidal agents in certain regions, e.g. in Sri Lanka and South India, where cardiac glycosides of yellow oleander *Thevetia peruviana* are responsible for much morbidity and mortality. Other intentional and serious poisonings occur with e.g. *Aconitum* and *Colchicum* spp., and plants with psychotropic and hallucinogenic effects, e.g. *Datura* and *Cannabis* spp., are abused as recreational drugs. Considerable morbidity and mortality results in some regions from the use of herbal medicines or foods containing plant toxins, e.g. aconitine in China and cyanide (cassava) in Africa.

Treatment of severe plant poisoning includes cautious decontamination and symptomatic and supportive care. Specific antidotes are available only for poisoning by plants containing belladonna alkaloids, cardiac glycosides, cyanogenic agents, and colchicine.

Fungal poisoning

Most fungi are nontoxic and most fungal poisonings are not severe. However, in certain regions such as Russia and other Eastern and Central European countries, morbidity and mortality is high. In most places, mushrooms cannot be considered as indispensable for nutrition and so it remains an unacceptable paradox that self-harvested mushrooms, enjoyed as a delicacy, still kill people in the 21st century. Thus, the priority in fungal poisoning is prevention.

Plant poisoning

Aetiology and epidemiology

The most common exposure to toxic plants is semi-accidental in children. Accidental exposures due to senility occur in older people. Herbal medicines containing toxic principles also cause accidental plant poisoning. In teenagers and adults, ingestion may be related to abuse of plants with psychoactive properties. Large amounts, or extractions, of toxic plants are also taken deliberately as suicidal agents. Finally, there is a risk of confusion between toxic and edible plants. Paradoxically, this kind of life-threatening poisoning has mostly affected people on survival courses.

A clinically oriented overview of the main plant toxins is given in Table 9.3.1.1.

Special plant poisonings

Neurotoxic plants

Belladonna alkaloids

Belladonna alkaloids (atropine, hyoscyamine, and scopolamine) occur in deadly nightshade *Atropa belladonna*, henbane *Hyoscyamus niger*, thorn apple/jimson weed *Datura stramonium*, angels' trumpets *Brugmansia suaveolens*, etc. (Fig. 9.3.1.1). They inhibit acetylcholine activity at muscarinic receptors, resulting in central and peripheral anticholinergic effects.

Table 9.3.1.1 Classification of plant toxins

Neurotoxins	Belladonna alkaloids
	Hallucinogenic toxins
	Convulsants
	Agents with nicotine-like effects
Cardiotoxins	Aconitine
	Cardiac glycosides
	Taxin, veratrin, andromedotoxins, phoratoxin
Cytotoxic agents	Colchicine
	Ricin
	Lectins
	Cyanogenic glycosides
Hepatotoxins	Pyrrolizidine alkaloids
Nephrotoxins	Terpenes
	Antraquinone glycosides
Gastrointestinal irritants	Calcium oxalate
	Oxalic acid
	Diterpene esters
	Others
Dermatotoxins	Calcium oxalate
	Oxalic acid
	Phototoxic psoralens

The patient is anxious, excited, warm, flushed (Fig. 9.3.1.2), delirious, and hallucinating. Other symptoms are mydriasis, tachycardia, fever, and urinary retention. The patient may even turn truly psychotic and violent. Rarely, seizures and unconsciousness ensue. Differential diagnoses include poisoning by amphetamines

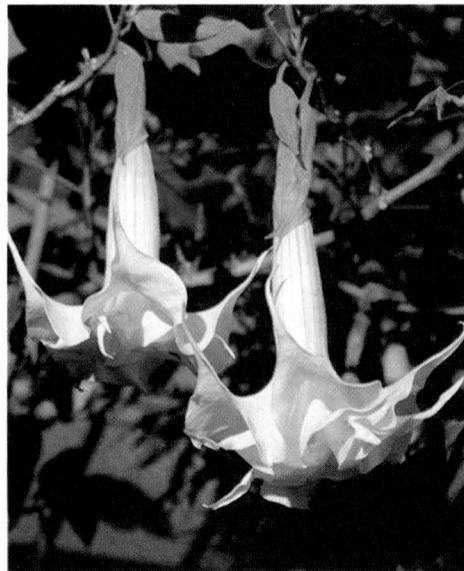

Fig. 9.3.1.1 Angel's trumpet *Brugmansia suaveolens*.
Courtesy of Sven Samelius.

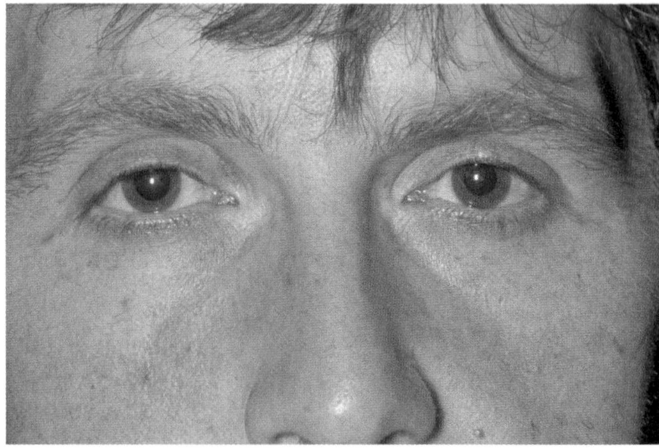

Fig. 9.3.1.2 Accidental deadly nightshade *Atropina belladonna* poisoning showing flushed face and bilateral mydriasis.
Courtesy of D. A. Warrell.

and other central nervous system stimulants, acute organic psychoses, and central nervous system infections.

A quiet environment is beneficial and intravenous diazepam is helpful for sedation. Physostigmine slowly intravenous (adults 1–2 mg, children 0.02–0.04 mg/kg) is the specific antidote, reversing troublesome central anticholinergic symptoms. The dose may be repeated as required. Physostigmine should be withheld if cardiotoxic agents have been coingested, if the patient has a bradycardia, or if there are signs of conduction abnormalities.

Unilateral mydriasis may occur in people (often gardeners, hence 'gardeners' mydriasis') who handle plants of this type and happen to rub their eye. This has more than once caused differential diagnostic problems and unnecessary, expensive investigations. Remember the importance of a proper history!

Hallucinogenic plants

Some plant toxins are particularly popular among abusers because of their hallucinogenic properties. Examples are tetrahydrocannabinols in cannabis *Cannabis sativa*, alkaloids in khat *Catha edulis*, mescaline in peyote *Lophophora williamsii*, and myristicin in nutmeg *Myristica fragrans*. Ingestion of parts of these plants normally results in only mild poisoning. Differential diagnoses include poisoning by other hallucinogenic agents. Treatment is symptomatic.

Plant convulsants

Cicutoxin and oenanthotoxin

Cicutoxin is one of the most potent convulsants known. It occurs in cowbane *Cicuta virosa*, water hemlock *C. maculata*, and western water hemlock *C. douglasii*. Oenanthotoxin in hemlock water dropwort *Oenanthe crocata* has similar effects. Cicutoxin is a potent γ-aminobutyric acid (GABA) antagonist, inducing recurrent seizures, and also causes cholinergic symptoms.

Severe poisoning has occurred in adults mistaking the plants listed above for edible ones. Typical symptoms include gastrointestinal upset, increased salivation, diaphoresis, and violent, recurrent and long-lasting tonic-clonic convulsions. These may result in hypoxia, severe metabolic acidosis, unconsciousness, circulatory instability, rhabdomyolysis, joint dislocations, and even rectal prolapse.

Treatment demands extensive symptomatic and supportive care, with emphasis on combating convulsions (muscle relaxation and

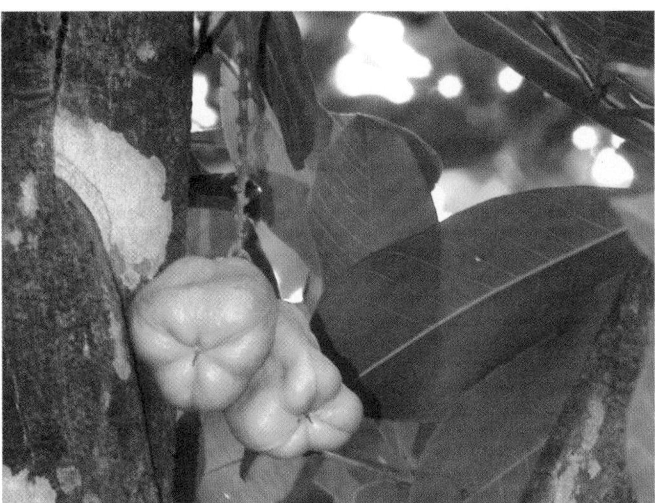

Fig. 9.3.1.3 Ackee fruits *Blighia sapida* (Sapindaceae).
Courtesy of D. A. Warrell.

ventilator support will often be needed), correction of acidosis, and maintenance of urinary output.

Differential diagnoses include other convulsive diseases.

Others

The ackee fruit *Blighia sapida* (Fig. 9.3.1.3) may cause vomiting, hypoglycaemia, and convulsions. Many cases have been reported from Haiti and Jamaica ('Jamaican vomiting disease'). Other convulsants are coriamyrtin in *Coriaria myrtifolia*, terpenes in chinaberry *Melia azedarach*, alkaloids in moonseed *Menispermum canadense*, podophylloresin in may apple *Podophyllum peltatum* (see Chapter 9.3.2), and strychnine in nux vomica *Strychnos nux-vomica*. Treatment is symptomatic and supportive.

Nicotine effects

Apart from the tobacco plant *Nicotiana tabacum*, hemlock *Conium maculatum* (Fig. 9.3.1.4) is the most important plant in this group. Its unpleasant taste should reduce the risk of poisoning by ingestion, but nevertheless it has been confused with parsley. Early symptoms are vertigo, agitation, thirst, tachycardia, hypertension, salivation, diaphoresis, vomiting, diarrhoea, muscle fasciculation, and convulsions. Later on, hypotension, bradyrhythmias, ascending weakness, paralysis, and coma may follow. Symptoms are variable and unpredictable. Extensive symptomatic and supportive care may be required.

Gelsemine in yellow jessamine *Gelsemium sempervirens* exerts nicotine-like effects and has caused fatal poisonings in China. The popular *Laburnum* spp. (e.g. golden chain) contains cytisine, which has mild nicotine-like effects. However, the most common symptoms after ingestion of golden chain are just vomiting and diarrhoea. Childhood exposures are frequent and symptoms mostly mild or moderate. Lobeline in *Lobelia* spp. has similar properties. Treatment is symptomatic.

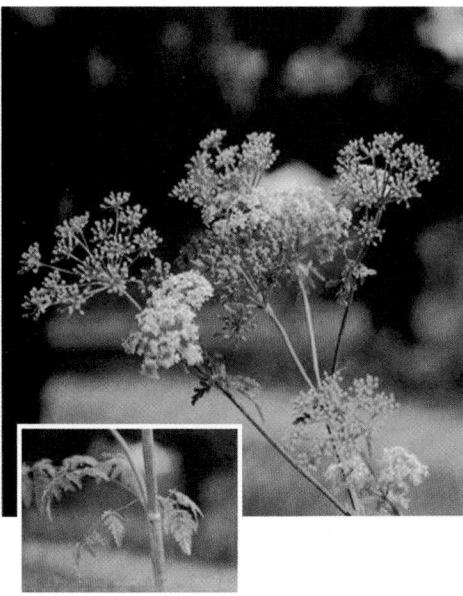

Fig. 9.3.1.4 Hemlock *Conium maculatum*.
Courtesy of Karl Rodhe.

Cardiotoxic plants

Aconitine

Aconitine is one of the most potent plant toxins known. It occurs in *Aconitum* spp., e.g. aconite/monkshood *A. napellus* (Fig. 9.3.1.5). Serious poisoning may result from intentional ingestion of the plant, or it may be accidental through herbal medications.

Ingestion results in rapidly developing burning and tingling sensations of lips, mouth, and pharynx. Numbness and paraesthesia in the extremities, hypersalivation, and gastrointestinal symptoms are also common. Most critical are the cardiac disturbances. Many kinds of arrhythmias occur, but particularly ventricular ectopics (ventricular extrasystole, ventricular tachycardia, and ventricular fibrillation) that may prove refractory to treatment. Myocardial failure and shock often develop. Central nervous system depression, muscular weakness, and seizures may also ensue.

Considering the extreme toxicity of this plant, gastrointestinal decontamination should be rigorous. Treatment includes optimal symptomatic and supportive care, directed at arrhythmias and cardiac failure.

Cardiac glycosides

Cardiac glycosides occur in foxglove *Digitalis purpurea* (Fig. 9.3.1.6), pink/white oleander *Nerium oleander* (Fig. 9.3.1.7), yellow oleander

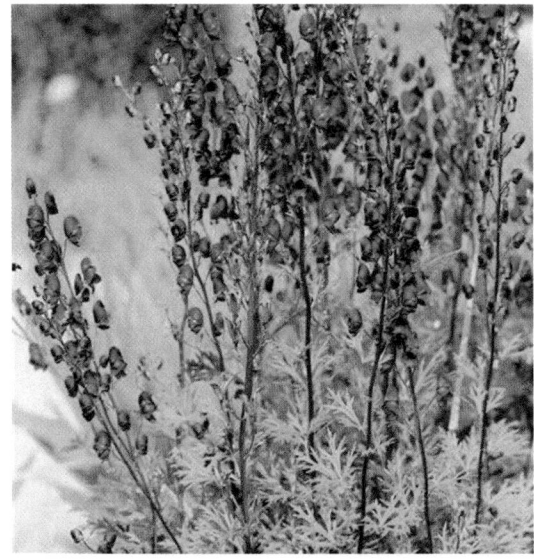

Fig. 9.3.1.5 Monkshood/aconite *Aconitum napellus*.
Courtesy of Karl Rodhe.

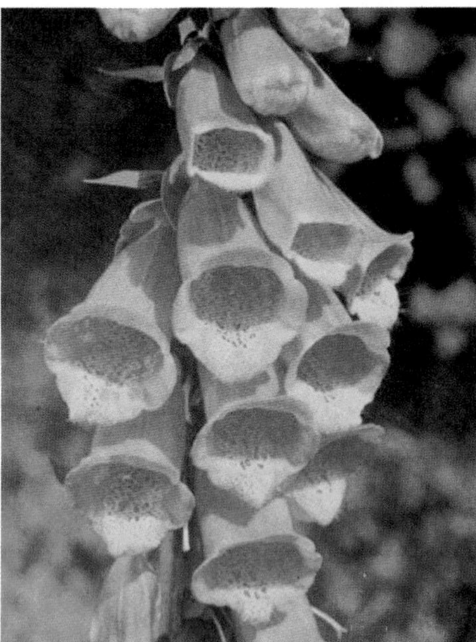

Fig. 9.3.1.6 Foxglove *Digitalis purpurea*.
Courtesy of Karl Rodhe.

Thevetia peruviana (Fig. 9.3.1.8), lily of the valley *Convallaria majalis*, and red squill *Urginea maritima*.

Large ingestions result in symptoms similar to those described for poisoning by digitalis glycosides (Chapter 9.1). Ventricular dysrhythmias are, however, less frequent in oleander poisoning than in digoxin poisoning. Serious poisoning with cardiac glycosides is a life-threatening condition, where the prognosis has improved considerably since the introduction of digitalis-specific antibodies (ovine Fab fragments). Treatment is described in Chapter 9.1.

Others

Taxin alkaloids in yew *Taxus* spp. may induce QRS widening, atrioventricular block, and other arrhythmias. Central nervous system and gastrointestinal symptoms may occur. Veratrine in *Veratrum* and *Zigadenus* spp. may have digitalis-like effects. Other cardiotoxins are andromedotoxins (grayanotoxins) in mountain laurel *Kalmia latifolia*, *Menziesia* spp., *Pieris* spp., and *Rhododendron* spp., and phoratoxin in American mistletoes *Phoradendron* spp.

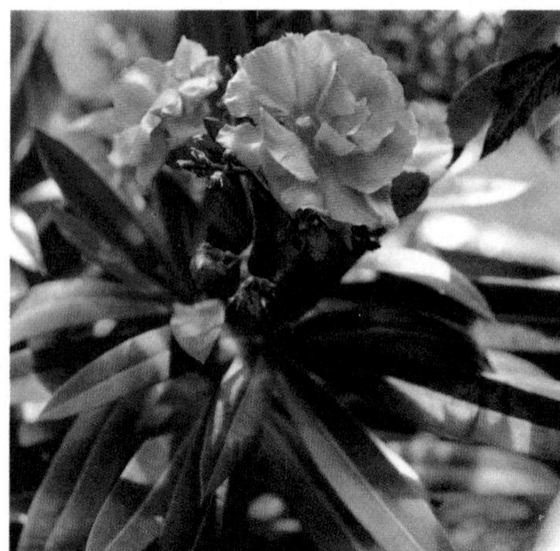

Fig. 9.3.1.7 Oleander *Nerium oleander*.
Courtesy of Bengt Lindåse.

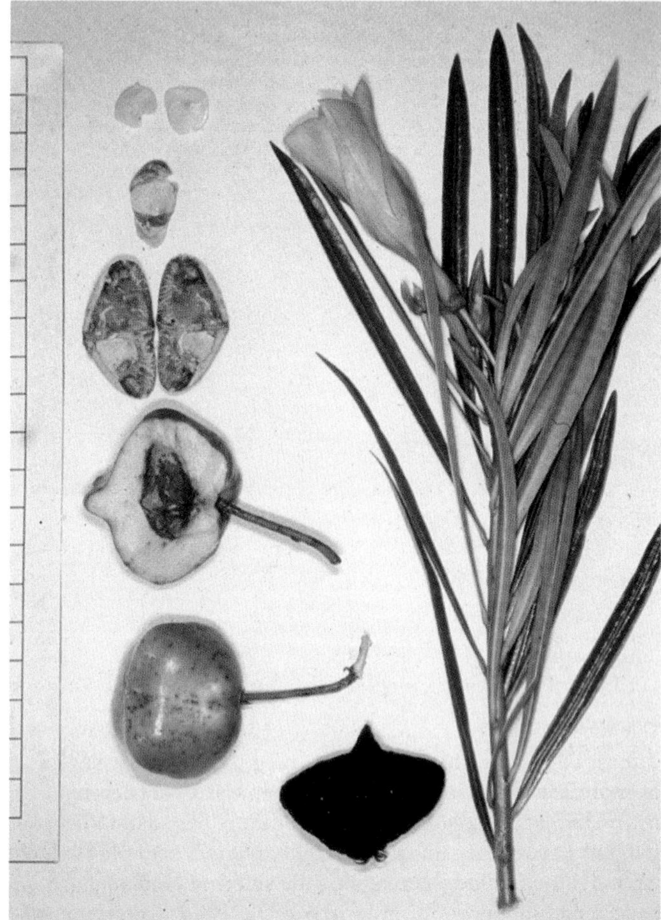

Fig. 9.3.1.8 Yellow oleander *Thevetia peruviana*.
Courtesy of D. A. Warrell.

Cytotoxic plants

Colchicine

Colchicine is the toxin of autumn crocus/meadow saffron *Colchicum autumnale* (Fig. 9.3.1.9) and glory lily *Gloriosa superba*. It has antimitotic effects on cells with high metabolism (e.g. gut and bone marrow), but also exerts direct toxicity on heart, liver, and kidneys. Intentional exposures may result in serious poisoning.

The clinical course has different phases. After an initial delay—sometimes many hours—there is onset of intense and progressive gastrointestinal symptoms, followed by arrhythmias, circulatory failure, seizures, central nervous system depression, and muscular weakness. There may be signs of renal and hepatic damage and, after a few days, bone marrow depression.

Multiple-dose activated charcoal may enhance elimination, but vigorous symptomatic and supportive care is crucial to save the patient. Granulocyte colony-stimulating factor (G-CSF) has been used with promising results in case of severe bone marrow depression. Colchicine-specific antibodies (ovine Fab fragments) will soon become commercially available.

Ricin and lectins

Ricin in castor bean/castor oil plant *Ricinus communis* (see Fig. 9.3.2.1 and Fig. 9.3.2.2 in Chapter 9.3.2) and lectins in jequirity bean/rosary bean/rosary pea *Abrus precatorius* (see Fig. 9.3.2.2) are water-soluble proteins known as toxalbumins. Ricin is on the

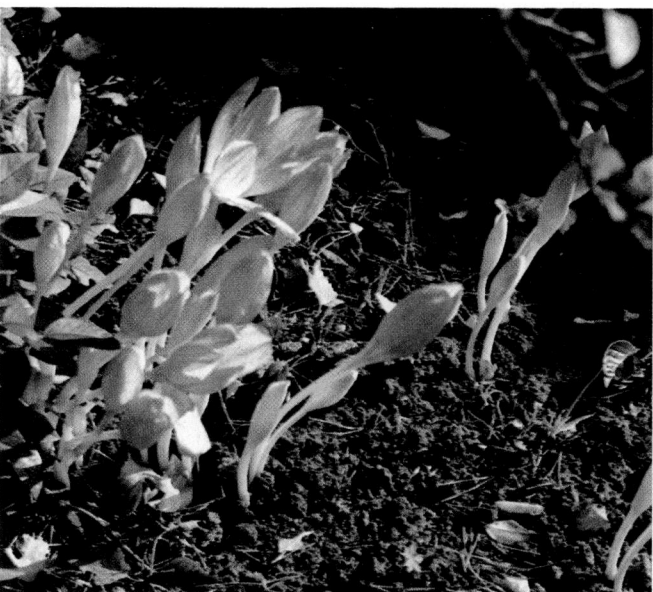

Fig. 9.3.1.9 Autumn crocus/meadow saffron *Colchicum autumnale*.
Courtesy of Ernst Lomenius.

Chemical Weapons Convention List. It blocks protein synthesis, causing cell death. The primary target organ is the gut. A few hours or more after ingestion, a severe gastroenteritis may develop with heavy fluid and electrolyte loss. Renal failure, circulatory instability, and hepatic damage may ensue. Treatment is symptomatic with vigorous fluid replacement, correction of metabolic disturbances, and support of organ dysfunctions.

Cyanogenic glycosides

Cyanogenic glycosides occur in kernels or fruits of *Prunus* spp. such as almonds, apricots, cherries, and peaches. They are also found in loquat *Eriobotrya japonica* and leaves or berries of cherry laurel *Prunus laurocerasus*. Even apple pips *Malus* spp. contain small amounts of cyanogenic glycosides, but large amounts are required to cause poisoning. After the kernels or fruits are chewed and swallowed, cyanide is released in the stomach. This is a slow process, and symptoms of poisoning may be delayed for many hours. Cyanide poisoning from plants is unusual, but should it occur, treatment is as outlined elsewhere for cyanide (see Chapter 9.1).

Inappropriately prepared cassava *Manihot esculenta* represents a special, large-scale problem of chronic cyanide exposure, resulting in neurological disorders such as tropical ataxic neuropathy and konzo. It was observed in Nigeria in the 1930s, and subsequently in other African countries.

Hepatotoxic plants

The liver is not a critical organ in plant poisoning except when plants containing pyrrolizidine alkaloids are involved. They cause veno-occlusive disease and occur in certain *Senecio, Crotalaria, Heliotropium*, and *Symphytum* spp. Cases are reported mainly from Afghanistan, India, and Jamaica. No specific treatment is available. Long-term exposure may induce hepatic cirrhosis. Hepatotoxicity may be caused by cytotoxic plants (see earlier paragraphs) and amatoxin-containing fungi (see following paragraphs).

In recent years, a number of herbal medicines have been reported to be hepatotoxic.

Nephrotoxic plants

Spurge laurel *Daphne laureda*, mezereon *Daphne mezereum*, and savin *Juniperus sabina* contain terpenes that cause intense irritation and blistering in the mouth and gastrointestinal tract, but also renal irritation with haematuria and proteinuria. Anthraquinone glycosides and oxalic acid in rhubarb *Rheum rhabarbarum* cause irritation in the mouth and gastrointestinal tract, and transient renal impairment and moderate metabolic acidosis may follow ingestion of large amounts of raw leaves or stems. *Rumex* spp. (docks and sorrels) also contain oxalates, and food based on these plants may result in similar toxic effects.

Gastrointestinal irritants

Popular plants with sap containing calcium oxalate and oxalic acid are elephant's ear *Philodendron* spp., cuckoo pint *Arum maculatum*, and dumb cane *Dieffenbachia* spp. The needle-shaped calcium oxalate crystals damage mucous membranes mechanically. *Euphorbia* and *Daphne* spp. contain irritating diterpene esters that cause pain, burning sensations in the mouth and pharynx, salivation, reddening, blistering, and possibly nephritis. Dysphagia, vomiting, and diarrhoea may follow. Treatment is rinsing of the mouth and oral fluids for dilution.

Skin damage

Euphorbia and *Dieffenbachia* spp. can damage skin as described earlier for mucous membranes. Hypersensitivity to plant allergens may also cause impressive skin reactions. Examples are poison ivy *Rhus radicans*, western poison oak *Toxicodendron diversilobum*, *Primula obconica*, and citrus plants and fruit (Fig. 9.3.1.10). Treatment is rinsing with water and symptomatic care.

The giant hogweed and other *Heracleum* spp. (Fig. 9.3.1.11), rue *Ruta graveolens*, and the gas plant *Dictamnus albus* contain phototoxic psoralens. Contact with sap and subsequent solar radiation can provoke intense phototoxic reactions with eczematous skin lesions and large, painful bullae (Fig. 9.3.1.12). The best treatment is to rinse the skin directly after exposure and avoid sunlight. When skin damage is already established, treatment is the same as for chemical burns.

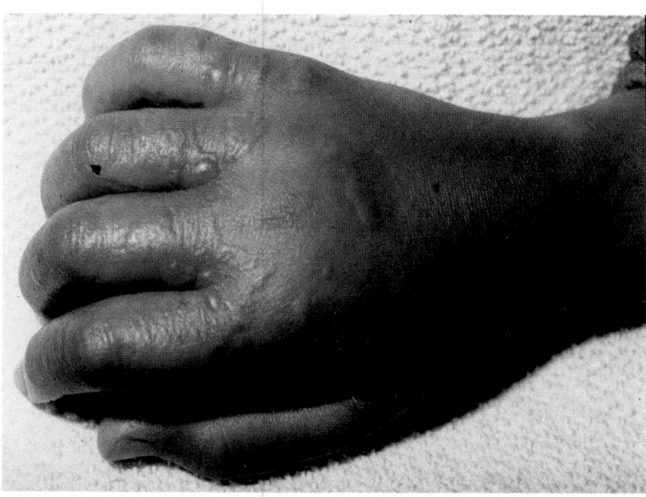

Fig. 9.3.1.10 Phototoxic reaction after immersion in a bowl of soaking citrus fruit.
Courtesy of Sven Samelius.

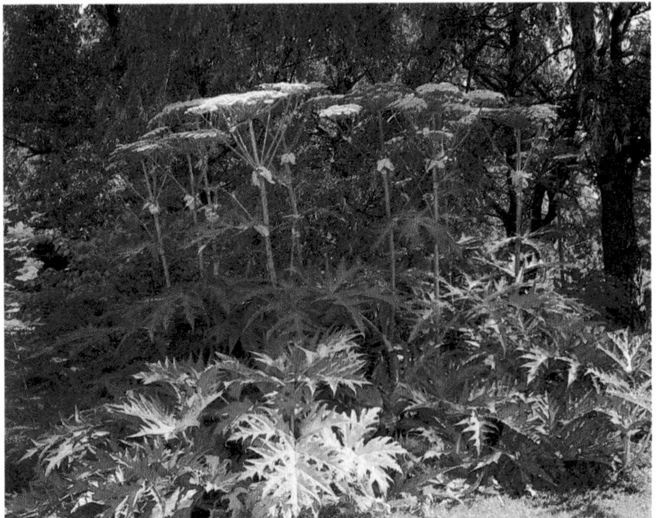

Fig. 9.3.1.11 *Heracleum sibiricum.*
Courtesy of the Department of Dermatology, Karlolinska University Hospital.

Fungal poisoning

Aetiology

The most common cause of fungal poisoning is confusing poisonous mushrooms with edible ones. Safe mushroom hunting requires skill and experience, as there are many possible sources of dangerous confusion. Too many people harvest, cook, and eat mushrooms whose identity is uncertain. Toddlers may accidentally try mushrooms and serious poisoning may occur, but this is fortunately uncommon. Intentional ingestion of toxic fungi is mostly related to abuse of hallucinogenic fungi. Suicidal ingestion is rare.

Illness after eating mushrooms is not necessarily related to poisoning. Large mushroom fragments or raw mushrooms may prove hard to digest, there may be anxiety that toxic mushrooms might have been ingested, and bacterial toxins may be present in mushrooms that have been stored for too long.

There are individual differences in sensibility to some fungal toxins. One example is false morels *Gyromitra* spp. Toxin contents may also vary between mushrooms of the same species.

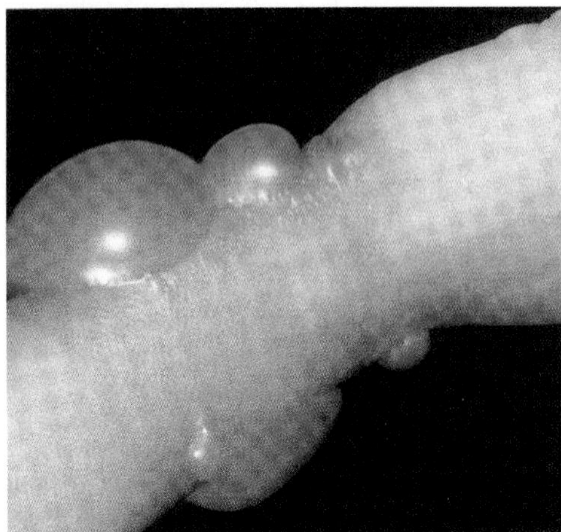

Fig. 9.3.1.12 Phototoxic reaction after contact with *Heracleum* spp.
Courtesy of Ole Högberg.

Epidemiology

The incidence of fungal poisoning varies greatly worldwide. Availability of fungi, depending on climate and geographical conditions, economics, and lifestyle determine different local traditions for harvesting and eating mushrooms. In some parts of the world mushrooms may be a part of the normal diet, but more commonly they are eaten as a delicacy.

Prevention

With a few exceptions, fungal poisoning is accidental. Many people develop severe and life-threatening illness after mushroom meals. Some die; others suffer chronic, irreversible organ damage requiring transplantation.

Since mushrooms are eaten mostly as a delicacy and not as a basic nutritional requirement, it is a paradox that poisoning is so common. The solution is prevention. Information campaigns should be launched to improve knowledge about mushrooms and to raise the awareness of the risks involved in careless harvesting and eating. To many people mushroom hunting is an exciting pleasure, almost a game, but this easy-going attitude must be altered. Because the geographical distribution and appearance of certain fungi are variable, people who are not familiar with the local area tend to be over-represented as victims of fungal poisoning. Educational materials should therefore be multilingual and specifically addressed to immigrants.

Diagnosis

Diagnosis may be difficult, as the circumstances are often confusing. It is important to consider any disease that may mimic fungal poisoning.

The history is crucial. Attention should be paid to the appearance of mushrooms ingested and the habitat where they were harvested. The speed of onset of symptoms and their character, intensity, and duration are often informative.

Some fungal poisonings may present with characteristic symptoms, e.g. those caused by muscarine, psychotropic toxins, and amatoxins (see following paragraphs). Careful observation and evaluation of evolving clinical features may, in combination with the history, allow a diagnosis.

In difficult cases where a dangerous poisoning can not be excluded, macro- and microscopic examination of the fungi, even fragments recovered from vomitus, may prove indispensable. In many countries, poison information centres may assist, either by identifying the mushrooms themselves or by obtaining advice from external experts.

Chemical analysis is available for the identification of amatoxins.

Classification of fungal poisonings

Fungal toxins are a heterogeneous group, chemically and toxinologically. In clinical practice, the most relevant approach is a classification based on toxic effects and related symptoms (see Table 9.3.1.2).

Special fungal poisonings

Gastrointestinal irritants

Fungi solely causing gastroenteritis form the largest subgroup, comprising species from many genera, e.g. *Agaricus, Boletus, Entoloma, Hebeloma, Lactarius, Ramaria, Russula*, and *Tricholoma*. Many of these genera include delicious, popular, and edible mushrooms, increasing the risk of confusion.

Table 9.3.1.2 Overview of fungal toxins, examples of poisonous fungi, and main symptoms

Toxins	Fungi	Symptoms
Gastrointestinal irritants		
Not identified	Certain *Agaricus, Entoloma, Boletus, Hebeloma, Tricholoma, Russula, Lactarius, Ramaria spp.,* etc.	Gastrointestinal symptoms
Neurotoxins		
Muscarine	Certain *Inocybe* and *Clitocybe* spp., etc.	Nausea, diarrhoea, diaphoresis, salivation, miosis, bradycardia, hypotension, lacrimation, chills, tremor, bronchospasm, etc.
Isoxazoles	*Amanita muscaria, A. pantherina, A. regalis, A. strobiliformis*	Inebriation, euphoria, confusion, agitation, anxiety, delusions, hallucinations, violent behaviour, seizures, tachycardia, mydriasis, urinary retention, etc.
Psilocybin	*Psilocybe* and *Panaeolus* spp., etc.	Euphoria, anxiety, agitation, hallucinations, depersonalization, tachycardia, flushing, etc.
Lesional toxins (cytotoxic)		
Amatoxin	*Amanita phalloides, A. virosa, A. verna, Galerina marginata, Lepiota* spp.	Intense gastroenteritis after 8–24 h, liver and kidney damage
Orellanine	*Cortinarius orellanus, C. rubellus (speciosissimus),*	Kidney damage
Gyromitrin	Certain *Gyromitra* spp.	Neurological, gastrointestinal, and hepatic symptoms; haemolysis
Miscellaneous	See text	See text

Few toxins in this group are chemically identified. They cause nonspecific irritation of the gastrointestinal mucosae.

Clinical features

Vomiting and diarrhoea start within a few hours and generally resolve quickly. Intensity and duration may, however, vary. For example, leaden entoloma *Entoloma sinuatum* may cause intense and long-lasting symptoms. Depending on length and duration of symptoms, fluid and electrolyte imbalance may ensue.

Gastrointestinal infection must be considered as a differential diagnosis. Delayed onset of intense symptoms until 8 to 24 h after the mushroom meal suggests potentially dangerous poisoning by amatoxin-containing fungi (see following paragraphs).

Treatment

Admission to hospital is seldom necessary, but if symptoms are more intense fluid and electrolyte replacement may be necessary, especially in children and older people.

Neurotoxic and psychoactive fungi

Muscarine

Toxic amounts of muscarine occur particularly in certain *Inocybe* spp. (e.g. *I. patouillardii)* and *Clitocybe* spp. (e.g. *C. dealbata, C. rivulosa*). Muscarine has also been detected in small, mostly insignificant amounts in other genera. Muscarine stimulates cholinergic receptors in the autonomic nervous system.

Clinical features Symptoms start within 0.5 to 2 h. Nausea, diarrhoea, diaphoresis, hypersalivation, miosis, bradycardia, and hypotension are common and rhinorrhoea, lacrimation, chills, tremor, central nervous system depression, bronchorrhoea, and bronchospasm have been reported. The patient is often pale and feels sick and miserable. The clinical features are fairly diagnostic.

Treatment Intravenous atropine (adults 1–2 mg, children 0.02–0.05 mg/kg) effectively counteracts the cholinergic symptoms. Repeated doses may be required. Symptomatic treatment is given as required.

Isoxazoles

Isoxazoles (ibotenic acid, muscimol, and muscazone) occur in certain *Amanita* species, e.g. fly agaric *A. muscaria* (Figs. 9.3.1.13 and 9.3.1.14), panther cap *A. pantherina* (Fig. 9.3.1.15), *A. strobiliformis*, and *A. regalis*. The toxins act as GABA agonists.

Clinical features Symptoms start within 0.5 to 1.5 h, peak at around 3 h, and vanish gradually over the next 24 h. The symptoms are unpredictable: exhilaration, euphoria, drowsiness, and confusion alternate with anxiety, agitation, delusions, illusions, and hallucinations. Extreme agitation and violent behaviour may ensue. Occasionally myoclonic jerks, muscle fasciculations, and seizures

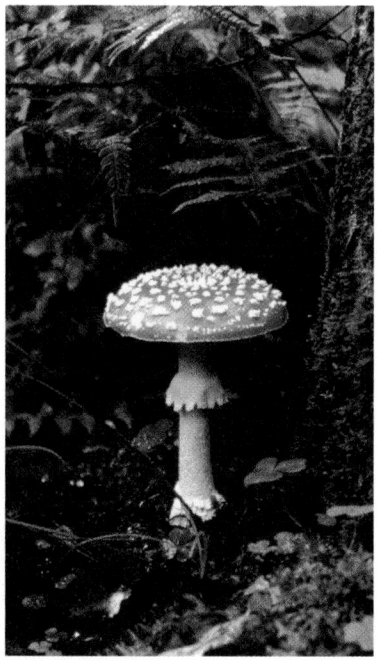

Fig. 9.3.1.13 Fly agaric *Amanita muscaria.*
Courtesy of Ole Högberg.

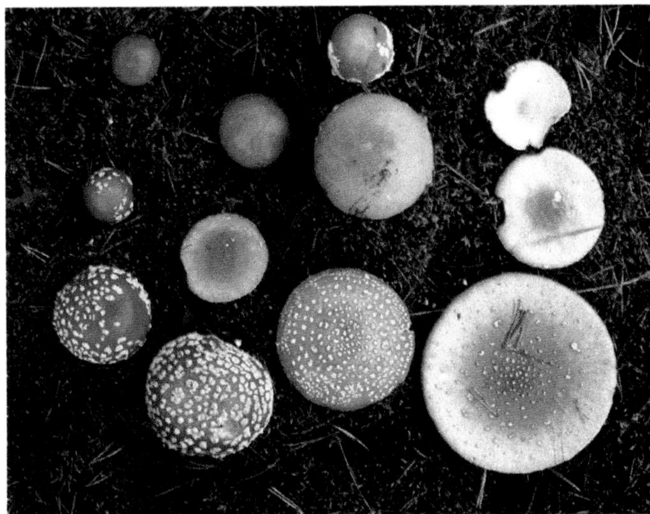

Fig. 9.3.1.14 Possible variations in appearance of fly agaric *Amanita muscaria*—may result in confusion with edible mushrooms.
Courtesy of Hans Marklund.

are observed. Tachycardia, mydriasis, and urinary retention may occur. Cholinergic symptoms are attributable to trace amounts of muscarine in some specimens. Panther cap more often causes central nervous system depression, whereas fly agaric is more likely to trigger excitation and bizarre behaviour.

History and symptoms are often diagnostic. However, the history is often obscure until patients are fit enough to tell their story. Differential diagnoses include organic psychosis and central nervous system infections.

Treatment Treatment is symptomatic and supportive. Intravenous diazepam (adults 5–10 mg, children 0.1–0.2 mg/kg) is given and repeated for sedation. Haloperidol or chlorpromazine may be useful as a complement in delirious and agitated patients.

Hallucinogenic fungi ('magic mushrooms')

Psilocybin and related toxins occur particularly in *Psilocybe* and *Panaeolus* species, e.g. liberty cap *Psilocybe semilanceata* (Fig. 9.3.1.16). The toxins are tryptamine derivatives that increase serotonin levels in the central nervous system and act as potent hallucinogens. The effects mimic those of LSD. Ingestion is almost invariably related to abuse.

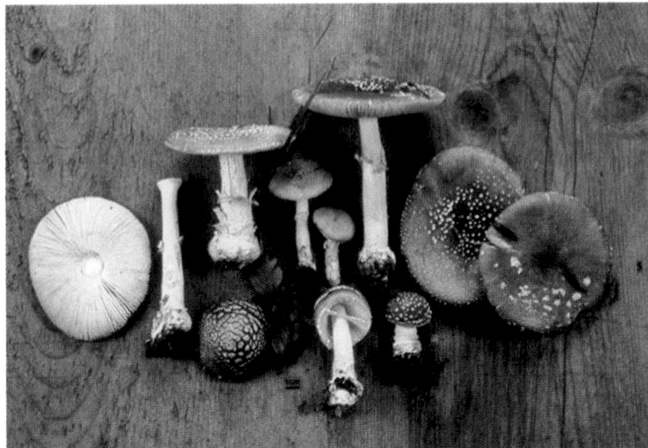

Fig. 9.3.1.15 Panther cap *Amanita pantherina*.
Courtesy of Hans Marklund.

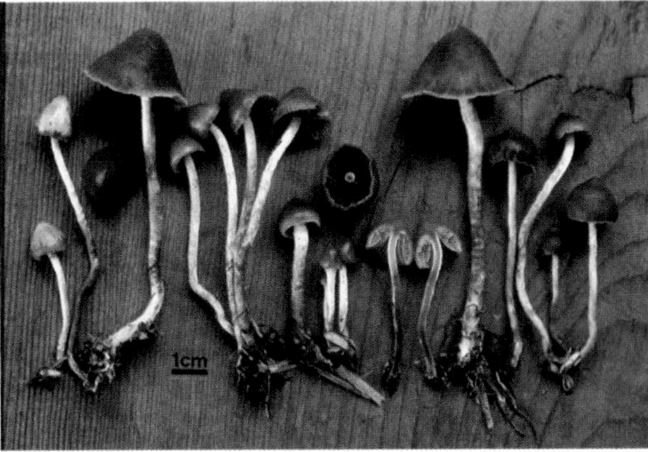

Fig. 9.3.1.16 Liberty cap/'magic mushroom' *Psilocybe semilanceata*.
Courtesy of Hans Marklund.

Clinical features

Within 20 to 60 min, the patient will experience altered sense of time and space, euphoria, hallucinations, and depersonalization. Less pleasurable symptoms are anxiety, agitation, bizarre and terrifying hallucinations, tachycardia, mydriasis, and flushing. Symptoms peak at around 2 h after ingestion and start vanishing after 4 to 6 h. However, symptoms may persist and there may be flashbacks after weeks or months.

Organic psychosis is a differential diagnosis. A reliable history may be available only after recovery.

Treatment

The patient should rest in a quiet environment and be sedated with e.g. diazepam. If this is inadequate, haloperidol or chlorpromazine can be added.

Cytotoxic fungi

Amatoxins

The highly poisonous amatoxins occur in species of the families Amanitaceae (genus *Amanita*), Agaricaceae (genus *Lepiota*), and Cortinariaceae (genus *Galerina*).

The death cap *Amanita phalloides* (Fig. 9.3.1.17), destroying angel *A. virosa* (Fig. 9.3.1.18), fool's mushroom *A. verna*, and *A. bisporigera* are the most commonly involved in human poisoning. Other species such as *Galerina marginata* and certain *Lepiota* spp. may also be implicated.

Epidemiology Amatoxin poisonings are reported from all continents, but are most frequent in Europe, where case fatalities ranged from around 18 to 22% in adults and 33 to 51% in children in the 1970s and 1980s. These figures have improved in Western countries but remain alarmingly high in other parts of the world.

Pathogenesis Amatoxins are cyclic octapeptides that inhibit transcription of DNA to mRNA by blocking nuclear RNA polymerase II activity. This results in defective protein synthesis and cell death. Amatoxins also act with endogenous cytokines to induce apoptosis, and there is glutathione depletion. The main target organs are intestinal mucosa, liver, and kidneys. Hepatotoxicity determines prognosis.

Clinical features After a latent period of 8 to 24 h (mean 12 h) after ingestion, gastrointestinal symptoms start violently with intense,

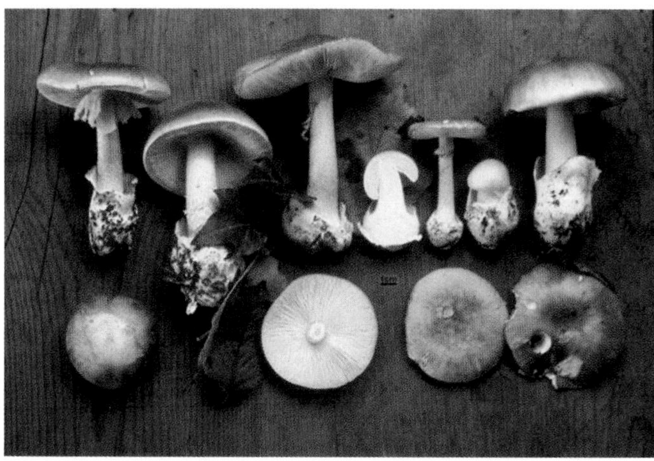

Fig. 9.3.1.17 Death cap *Amanita phalloides*.
Courtesy of Hans Marklund.

watery diarrhoea, and vomiting. This latency has great diagnostic significance. Patients become rapidly dehydrated and develop oliguria, hypoglycaemia, hypokalaemia, and metabolic acidosis. Biochemical signs of liver damage appear after 36 to 48 h and progress over the next few days. Fulminant hepatic failure may develop. Initial disturbances of renal function will resolve after rehydration, but within another 3 to 4 days, renal function may again deteriorate because of toxic kidney damage, a sign of poor prognosis.

Treatment

Decontamination Forced emesis or gastric lavage is performed if the patient is admitted within 4 to 6 h and this can be accomplished safely. Activated charcoal is always given.

Toxin removal

- Multiple-dose activated charcoal is administered for 3 days after ingestion.
- A diuresis of about 200 ml/h (adults) is maintained for the first 24 to 48 h after ingestion.
- Haemoperfusion or haemodialysis is not indicated unless the patient has pre-existing renal disease or is admitted very early and in the asymptomatic period (very rare).

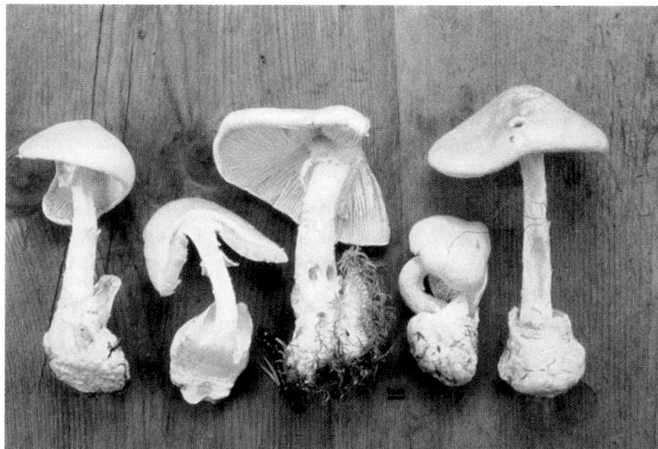

Fig. 9.3.1.18 Destroying angel *Amanita virosa*.
Courtesy of Hans Marklund.

Reduction of hepatic toxin uptake Silibinin in a bolus dose of 5 mg/kg is given as an intravenous infusion over 1 h followed by 20 mg/kg per 24 h as continuous infusion during the 3 days after ingestion. The efficacy of this treatment is not entirely established. Parenteral silibinin is not always available, even in Western countries. High-dose benzyl penicillin is an alternative.

Symptomatic and supportive care

- Symptomatic care is crucial and includes cautious monitoring, fluid replacement, and correction of metabolic disturbances. Hepatic and renal support may be required.
- There is some experimental, theoretical, and clinical support for the use of *N*-acetylcysteine as a liver-protective agent.
- If fulminant hepatic failure is pending, a liver unit should be consulted for advice on treatment and with a view to possible transplantation.

Prognosis and comments The prognosis is related to toxic dose and start of treatment. Case fatality is high after heavy exposure. Vigorous symptomatic and supportive care, maintenance of an adequate diuresis, and multiple-dose activated charcoal are accepted treatments. Silibinin may modify toxicity to some extent through reduction of the hepatic uptake of amatoxin. In some cases, liver transplantation may be the ultimate way of saving the patient.

Orellanine

Orellanine is a potent nephrotoxin present in certain species of the family Cortinariaceae, genus *Cortinarius*. *C. orellanus* and *C. rubellus (speciosissimus)* (Figs. 9.3.1.19 and 9.3.1.20) are responsible for most poisonings. Orellanine is a bipyridine *N*-oxide that may interfere with protein synthesis in the kidneys causing interstitial nephritis, tubular cell damage, basal cell membrane rupture and, eventually, irreversible fibrosis.

Clinical features Orellanine poisoning is the most insidious of all mushroom poisonings. Usually, symptoms do not appear until 2 to 7 (or even 14) days after the mushroom meal, and, by then, reflect established kidney damage. Symptoms evolve insidiously and are difficult for the patient to interpret—headache, fatigue, intense thirst, chills, muscular discomfort, abdominal, lumbar, and flank pain. After a polyuric phase, oliguria and anuria may follow. Laboratory tests on admission reveal elevated serum creatinine and urea, proteinuria, haematuria, and—characteristically—leucocyturia. The acute renal damage may heal or become chronic.

Occasionally, there may be some mild gastrointestinal symptoms within a couple of days after the meal, but as these symptoms are both discrete and inconsistent they are easily overlooked.

Treatment Since patients are normally admitted late, therapeutic interventions can neither prevent nor reduce toxic damage. Renal function is monitored. Therapy is symptomatic with support of renal function and treatment of uraemia, including dialysis while waiting for the kidneys to recover. In case of persistent renal insufficiency, the options are chronic dialysis or transplantation. However, transplantation should not be performed too early, as renal recovery may be considerably delayed.

Very early suspicion of orellanine poisoning should prompt measures to prevent absorption and promote elimination.

Prognosis and comments Endstage renal failure was observed in 11% of Polish, 17% of French, and 40% of Swedish patients. It shall be emphasized that treatment measures discussed above are

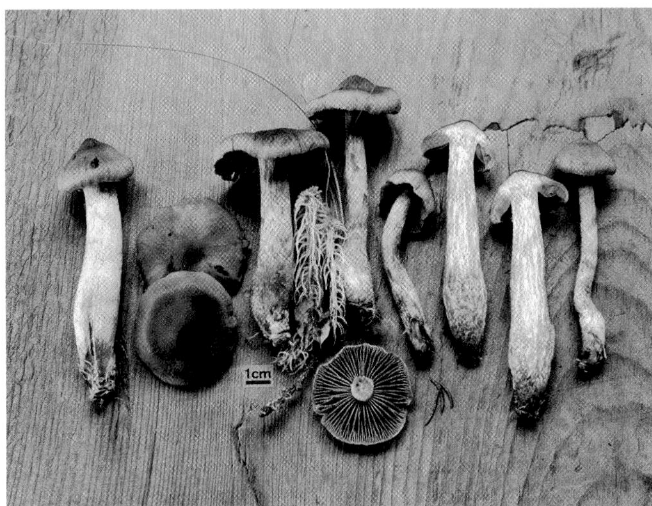

Fig. 9.3.1.19 *Cortinarius rubellus (speciosissimus).*
Courtesy of Astrid Holmgren.

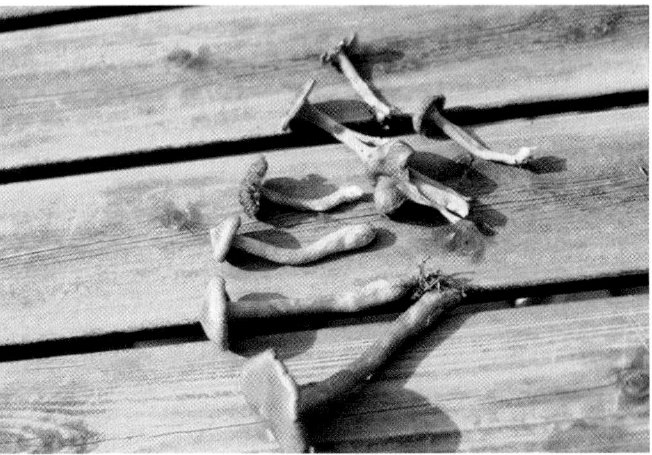

Fig. 9.3.1.20 A common cause of poisoning by nephrotoxic *Cortinarius* spp. is confusion of *Cortinarius rubellus* (the lower three fungi in this picture) and funnel chanterelle *Cantharellus tubaeformis* (above).
(Courtesy of Astrid Holmgren.)

theoretically based and there is so far no clinical support for a rational treatment strategy of this ghostly poisoning, apart from supportive and symptomatic care.

Other possibly nephrotoxic fungi

Renal damage has been reported from North America after ingestion of *Amanita smithiana*, mistaken for *Tricholoma magnivelare*. In a case series from southern France, 53 patients were reported to develop renal dysfunction after eating *Amanita proxima*, mistaken for *A. ovoidea*.

Rhabdomyolysis induced by mushrooms

Over the last few years, rhabdomyolysis has been reported in France and Poland, after ingestion of large or repeated meals of *Tricholoma equestre (flavovirens)*. These puzzling observations, implicating a popular mushroom, have caused considerable attention and concern. The mechanism of possible myotoxicity is under investigation.

Gyromitrin-containing fungi

Gyromitrin occurs in fungi of the family Helvellaceae, genus *Gyromitra*. Most poisonings are caused by the false morel *Gyromitra esculenta*, but the toxin is found also in other *Gyromitra* spp. Gyromitrin decomposes in the stomach to form hydrazines. These are irritating, reduce central nervous system pyridoxine contents, and, hence, GABA synthesis. Glutathione depletion in erythrocytes and damage to hepatic macromolecules has also been postulated. Gyromitrin is water-soluble and volatile, and so can be partly removed from the fungus by drying or boiling.

Clinical features

Systemic symptoms may follow inhalation of vapour, which also irritates eyes and airways. Most common, however, is poisoning by ingestion of false morels that have not been properly prepared. Symptoms are delayed 5 to 8 h. Vomiting and diarrhoea may occur, but more typical features are vertigo, ataxia, nystagmus, diplopia, balance disturbances, diaphoresis, slurred speech, and drowsiness. Rare symptoms are delirium, seizures, and coma. Moderate hepatic damage, haemolysis, and hypoglycaemia have been observed.

Treatment

If neurological symptoms prevail, it is relevant to give pyridoxine at 25 mg/kg as an intravenous bolus infusion over 30 min. Repeated doses may be required. If the patient is convulsing and pyridoxine is not immediately available, diazepam is given initially. It is wise to have a glucose infusion running and maintain an adequate diuresis.

Miscellaneous

Antabuse syndrome

An 'antabuse syndrome' may be induced by *Coprinus atramentarius*, a few other *Coprinus* spp., *Clitocybe clavipes*, and *Boletus luridus*.

The toxin (coprin) acts like disulfiram, blocking acetaldehyde dehydrogenase. Consequently, drinking ethanol after eating these mushrooms will cause an antabuse syndrome—flushing, sweating, nausea, anxiety, tachycardia, hypotension, and dyspnoea. The risk persists for about 1 week after the mushroom ingestion.

If the mistake is discovered early, decontamination and administration of activated charcoal may be useful. Otherwise symptomatic and supportive care is given.

Paxillus syndrome

After repeated ingestion of the roll-rim cap *Paxillus involutus*, its antigens may induce a *Paxillus* syndrome: severe gastroenteritis, haemolysis, and subsequent renal impairment.

Symptomatic and supportive care includes fluid replacement, maintenance of adequate diuresis, and blood transfusions.

Chlorophyllum molybdites

The false parasol or green-spored parasol (*Chlorophyllum molybdites* or *Lepiota molybdites;* also Morgan's mushroom, *Macrolepiota* or *Lepiota morganii*) is the most commonly ingested poisonous mushroom in North America. The toxin is irritant and also exerts α-adrenergic blockade and cholinergic effects.

Within 30 min to 2 (–4) h, intense, watery, and sometimes bloody diarrhoea begins. This may result in dehydration, electrolyte imbalance, shock, and renal impairment. Occasionally miosis, pallor, diaphoresis, and hypotension are observed.

Fluid replacement and other symptomatic and supportive care are given as required. Atropine is given in case of cholinergic symptoms.

Further reading

Bresinsky A, Besl H (1990). *A colour atlas of poisonous fungi. A handbook for pharmacists, doctors, and biologists.* Wolfe Publishing, London.

Cooper MR, Johnson AW (1998). *Poisonous plants and fungi in Britain. Animal and human poisoning*, 2nd edition. The Stationery Office, London.

De Haro L, *et al.* (1999). Syndrome sudorien et muscarinien. Expérience de Centre Antipoisons de Marseille. *Presse Méd*, **28**, 1069–70.

Eddleston M, Warrell DA (1999). Management of acute yellow oleander poisoning. *Q J Med*, **92**, 483–5.

Eddleston M, *et al.* (2000). Anti-digoxin Fab fragments in cardiotoxicity by ingestion of yellow oleander: an randomised controlled trial. *Lancet*, **355**, 967–72.

Enjalbert F, *et al.* (2002). Treatment of amatoxin poisoning: 20-year retrospective analysis. *J Toxicol Clin Toxicol*, **40**, 715–57.

Holmdahl J (2001). Mushroom poisoning: *Cortinarius speciosissimus* nephrotoxicity. Thesis. Institute of Internal Medicine (Department of Nephrology), Göteborg University.

Holmdahl J, Blohmé I (1995). Renal transplantation after *Cortinarius speciosissimus* poisoning. *Nephrol Dial Transplant*, **10**, 1920–2.

Karlson-Stiber C, Persson H (2003). Cytotoxic fungi—an overview. *Toxicon*, **42**, 339–49.

Lin C-C, Chan TYK, Dent J-F (2004). Clinical features and management of herb-induced aconitine poisoning. *Ann Emerg Med*, **43**, 574–9.

9.3.2 Common Indian poisonous plants

V.V. Pillay

Essentials

Common poisonous plants encountered in India include (1) irritant plants, e.g. castor, colocynth, croton, glory lily, marking nut, mayapple, red pepper, rosary pea; (2) cardiotoxic plants, e.g. aconite, autumn crocus, common oleander, yellow oleander, suicide tree; (3) neurotoxic plants, e.g. calotropis, cassava, chickling pea, datura, strychnos; (4) hepatotoxic plants, e.g. neem; and (5) miscellaneous toxic plants and plant products, including arecanut, *Cleistanthus collinus*, and physic nut.

Accidental poisoning with some of these plants or plant products may occur among inhabitants of rural areas, dependent on their farms and gardens for food, due to mistakes in identifying toxic plants, with children being at particular risk. Contamination of foodstuffs and the use of poisonous plants in traditional or folk medicine are other causes of poisoning. Suicide using poisonous plants is fairly common in India, especially in rural areas, most typically with the cardiac glycoside containing fruits of yellow oleander or the suicide tree *Cerbera odollam*, both of which are rarely employed in homicide.

Introduction

India has a rich and varied flora. Inhabitants of rural areas, dependent on their farms and gardens for food, are occasionally poisoned when they fail to identify toxic plants. Contamination of foodstuffs, the use of poisonous plants in herbal remedies, and 'traditional medicines' are other causes of poisoning. Children are especially at risk because they find plants both accessible and attractive.

Box 9.3.2.1 Indian poisonous plants

Irritant plants

Castor, colocynth, croton, glory lily*, marking nut, may apple, red pepper, rosary pea*

Cardiotoxic plants

Aconite*, autumn crocus*, common oleander*, yellow oleander*, suicide tree

Neurotoxic plants

Calotropis, cassava*, chickling pea, *Datura**, *Strychnos**

Hepatotoxic plants

Neem

Miscellaneous toxic plants/plant products

Areca nut, *Cleistanthus collinus*, physic nut

* For accounts of these plants, see Chapter 9.3.1.

Suicide using poisonous plants is fairly common in India, especially in rural areas, but homicide is rare. Since the principles of plant and fungal poisoning are detailed in Chapter 9.3.1, this account is restricted to some aspects of the subject that are of particular importance in India.

Some of the more common poisonous plants encountered in India are listed in Box 9.3.2.1.

Some of the dangerously toxic plants most commonly implicated in poisoning in India are listed in Table 9.3.2.1.

Ricinus communis (castor)

The castor or castor oil plant *Ricinus communis* (Euphorbiaceae: spurges) is also called mole bean, moy bean, or palma christi (Fig. 9.3.2.1). It is an ornamental plant and the oil extracted from its seeds is also used medicinally as a purgative and as a lubricant for engines. In India, castor seed extract is used systemically or

Table 9.3.2.1 Dangerously poisonous Indian plants most often implicated in poisoning

Plant	Main toxic principle	Usual fatal dose
Ricinus communis (castor) (Fig. 9.3.2.1)	Ricin	8–10 seeds
Abrus precatorius (jequirity) (Fig. 9.3.2.2)	Abrin	1–3 seeds
Nerium oleander (common oleander)	Oleandrin	5–15 leaves; 15 g root
Thevetia peruviana (yellow oleander)	Thevetin	8–10 seeds; 15–20 g root
Cerbera odollam (suicide tree) (Fig. 9.3.2.3)	Cerberin	1 kernel
Datura fastuosa (thorn apple)	Atropine, hyoscine	50–100 seeds
Strychnos nux vomica	Strychnine	1–3 g seeds
Cleistanthus collinus (oduvan)	Cleistanthin A and B	A few leaves
Amanita phalloides (death cap mushroom)	Amanitin, phalloidin	1 mushroom

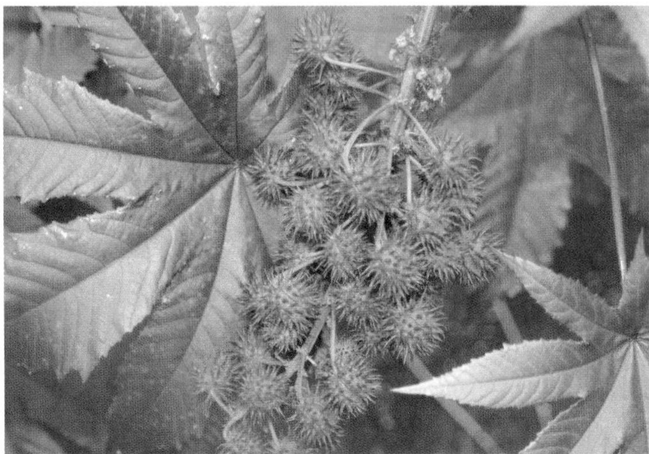

Fig. 9.3.2.1 Castor oil plant *Ricinus communis* (Euphorbiaceae).
(Courtesy of D A Warrell.)

topically as a folk medicine to stimulate breast milk production. Ricin, a toxalbumin, its main active principle, has been used in chemical warfare, as an experimental antitumour and immunosuppressive agent, and to poison moles. Ricin was probably the agent used to assassinate the Bulgarian diplomat Georgi Markov in London in 1978. All parts of the plant are toxic, especially the seeds, but castor oil contains the much milder irritant ricinoleic acid, and not ricin.

Castor seeds (Fig. 9.3.2.2) are harmless when ingested whole, since their outer coating resists digestion, but if the seeds are crushed or chewed before being swallowed, ricin is released. The pulp of the seed contains glycoproteins, which cause allergic dermatitis, rhinitis, and asthma in sensitized individuals.

Clinical features

There is usually a delay of several hours before a burning sensation is felt in the gastrointestinal tract, followed by colicky abdominal pain, vomiting, and diarrhoea. In severe cases, there is haemorrhagic gastritis and dehydration. Delayed central nervous system toxicity may occur, especially involving the cranial nerves. Haematuria and acute renal and hepatic failure may develop. No specific treatment is available. Parenteral injection of ricin can be fatal in doses as low as 1 mg/kg body weight.

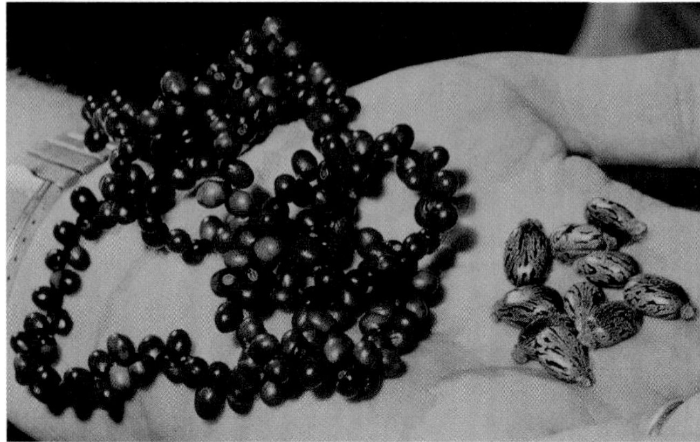

Fig. 9.3.2.2 Castor oil *Ricinus communis* seed (right) and jequirity bean *Abrus precatorius* (left).
(Courtesy of D A Warrell.)

Citrullus colocynthus (colocynth)

The colocynth *Citrullus colocynthus* (Cucurbitaceae: gourds or cucurbits) grows wild all over India. Its dried fruit pulp is used as a purgative by rural people and the root as traditional treatment for jaundice, rheumatism, and constipation. Poisoning causes vomiting, diarrhoea, hypotension, and shock. Treatment is supportive.

Croton tiglium (croton)

Croton tiglium (Euphorbiaceae: spurges) grows well in Assam, Bengal, and the Western Ghats. Its seeds, oil, and root extract are used as a drastic purgative in folk medicine. Plants of this family contain strongly irritant diterpene esters. The stem, leaves, and seeds are most toxic, containing crotin (toxalbumin) and crotonoside (glycoside).

Clinical features

Skin contact with the latex, or chewing the stem causes erythema, swelling, and blistering after 2 to 8 h. Ingestion results in burning pain in the upper gastrointestinal tract, vomiting, tenesmus, watery or blood-stained diarrhoea, hypotension, collapse, coma, and death. Drinking cold milk may alleviate the gastrointestinal irritation. Treatment is otherwise symptomatic.

Semecarpus anacardium (marking nut)

The marking nut tree is a member of the Anacardiaceae, a family that includes cashew, mango, and poison ivy, and grows well in many parts of India. The black, oily juice of the nut is used by dhobis (washermen) in India to mark the laundry after washing.

Extracts of the toxic nut, which contains semecarpol and bhilawanol, are used in folk medicine for various ailments, and the bruised nut is inserted into the vagina as an abortifacient. The fatal dose ranges from 5 to 8 nuts.

Clinical features

Skin contact with the acrid juice results in irritation, inflammation, vesication, and ulceration. Ingestion causes blistering of the mouth and gastrointestinal distress. In severe cases, there is vomiting, abdominal pain, diarrhoea, hypotension, tachycardia, delirium, and coma. Pupils may be dilated. Skin should be decontaminated with soap and water. Milk may ameliorate gastrointestinal symptoms.

Podophyllum spp. (may apple)

Podophyllum spp. (Berberidaceae: barberries), including the may apple or American mandrake (*P. peltatum*) of eastern North America, grow well in the hilly regions of Sikkim, Uttar Pradesh, Punjab, Himachal Pradesh, and Kashmir. Their resins are used as keratolytic agents, as topical treatment of condylomata acuminata (genital warts) and in homoeopathy. The most toxic parts are the leaves and rhizomes which contain at least 50% of podophyllotoxin (lignans and flavonols). Podophyllum and podophyllotoxin have effects similar to colchicines and vinblastine: antimitosis and inhibition of axoplasmic transport protein, RNA and DNA synthesis, and tricarboxylic acid cycle enzymes.

Clinical features

Both ingestion and dermal application can be toxic. About 30 min to several hours after ingestion there is nausea, vomiting, abdomi-

Table 9.3.2.2 Differentiating chilli and datura seeds

Chilli seed	Datura seed
Small	Large
Yellow	Brown
Rounded and smooth	Reniform and pitted
Pungent odour	Odourless
Pungent taste	Bitter taste
On section, the embryo is seen to curve inwards towards the hilum	Embryo curves outwards

nal pain, and diarrhoea, followed by fever, tachypnoea, peripheral neuropathy, tachycardia, hypotension, ataxia, dizziness, lethargy, confusion, and altered sensorium. Seizures may occur. Thrombocytopenia and leucopenia are common. Polyneuropathy generally appears in about a week, and progresses for 2 to 3 months. Consumption of Chinese herbal products containing extracts of podophyllum has caused neuropathies and encephalopathy. Treatment is supportive.

Capsicum spp. (red pepper)

Common Indian species include *Capsicum annuum* and *C. frutescens* (Solanaceae: nightshades). It is also known as chilly, chilli pepper, cayenne pepper, cherry pepper, cluster pepper, Christmas pepper, and cone pepper. Its long tapering fruits, which become red when ripe, contain small, flat yellowish seeds which can be mistaken for datura seeds. Serious poisoning can result from mistaken identity. Table 9.3.2.2 lists salient points of difference.

Capsicum fruit and seeds are very popular in Indian cuisine. In traditional medicine, it is used as an appetite stimulant and carminative. Its main active principle, capsaicin, is used in the treatment of neuralgia and diabetic neuropathy and as a Mace-like repellent to ward off dogs and other dangerous animals. Capsicum vanillyl acids are irritants which deplete nerve terminals of substance P, resulting in local swelling and pain due to dilatation of blood vessels, and intense excitation of sensory nerve endings, followed by relative insensitivity, the basis for the use of capsaicin in analgesic creams. Accidental aspiration of pepper can be fatal. Inhalation has been used as a method of homicide. Forcible introduction of the powder into the anus or vagina has been used by the Indian police during interrogation of suspects, although this has no legal sanction. Cases of child abuse by parents or guardians have also been reported. Robbery, rape, and other crimes may be facilitated by suddenly incapacitating the victim by throwing pepper into their eyes.

Clinical features

Cutaneous exposure causes a burning, stinging, pain and occupational handling of chillies causes 'chilli burns' or 'Hunan hand'. Ocular exposure causes intense pain, lacrimation, conjunctivitis, and blepharospasm, while inhalation or aspiration of chilli powder causes 'chilli workers' cough'. Ingestion results in nausea, vomiting, burning pain, salivation, abdominal cramping, and 'burning' diarrhoea. Topical decontamination is with liberal amounts of water and local and systemic analgesics. Symptoms resulting from ingestion are relieved by sips of cool water or crushed ice.

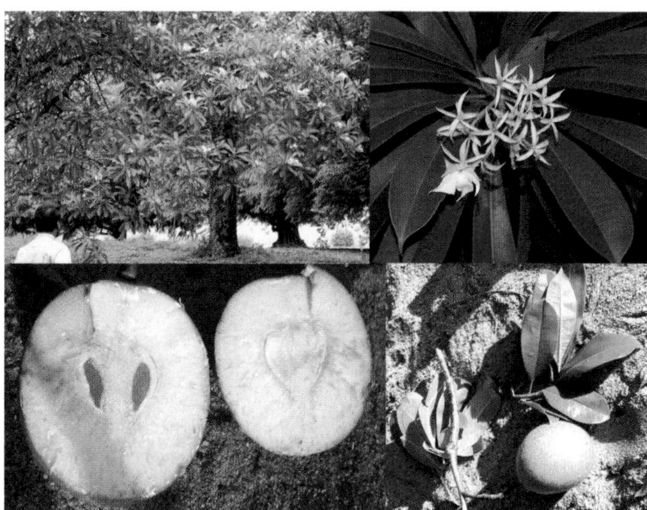

Fig. 9.3.2.3 Suicide tree *Cerbera odollam* (Apocyanaceae) and fruit. (Courtesy of M Eddleston and D A Warrell.)

Cerbera odollam (suicide tree)

The suicide tree *Cerbera odollam* (Apocyanaceae: dogbanes), also known as the Kerala suicide nut, ordeal tree, pong-pong or othalanga (Fig. 9.3.2.3), is endemic to South Asia, growing well in South India, especially in Kerala. Its fruits resemble unripe (green) mangoes. The seeds are used in folk medicine as emeto-cathartics and the kernel of the fruit contains the cardiac glycoside cerberin, which blocks cardiac calcium ion channels.

Clinical features

Manifestations of poisoning and treatment are the same as for oleanders (see Chapter 9.3.1).

Since it is difficult to detect at autopsy, and its flavour can be masked with strong spices, this is a fairly common agent of homicide and suicide in some parts of South India. In Kerala, it is said to be responsible for about 50% of plant poisoning and 10% of all cases of poisoning. Accidental poisoning may result from confusion with unripe mango.

Calotropis spp.

The calotropis, madar, crown flower, giant milkweed, swallow wort, or Sodom apple (*Calotropis procera, C. gigantea*—Apocyanaceae, Asclepiadoideae: milkweeds) grows wild throughout India. It is used by rural practitioners to treat many ailments. The milky juice of the plant was referred to as 'vegetable mercury', as it was said to be effective in the treatment of syphilis. According to Ayurveda, the dried whole plant is a good tonic, expectorant, and anthelmintic. The powdered root is used in asthma, bronchitis, and dyspepsia. The leaves are said to be useful in the treatment of arthralgia, swellings, and intermittent fevers. The flowers are bitter, and are used as a digestive, astringent, and anthelmintic. Calotropis is also used in homoeopathic medicines. All parts of the plant, but especially leaves and juice, contain calotoxin, calotropin, and uscharin.

Clinical features

Contact of the juice with the skin results in intense irritation with redness, swelling, and vesication, and contact with eyes results in severe conjunctivitis. It has been used by malingerers to simulate skin injury or conjunctivitis. Ingestion of leaves or juice causes burning pain and vomiting.

Lathyrus sativus (chickling pea)

The chickling pea, bluesweet pea, grass pea, or Indian pea *Lathyrus sativus* (Fabaceae/Leguminosae: legumes, peas, beans, pulses) grows well in Madhya Pradesh, Bihar, Uttar Pradesh, West Bengal, and the Punjab. The seeds ('kesari dal' in Hindi) are used as a cheap substitute for costlier lentils by the rural people in these states. The toxic principle is β-*N*-oxalyl-l-α,β-diaminopropionic acid (ODAP).

Clinical features

Chronic intake of kesari dal leads to the development of lathyrism, characterized by gradually progressive bilateral spastic paraparesis. Prodromal symptoms include cramps, prickling sensation, and nocturnal calf pain. There are exaggerated tendon reflexes and extensor plantar responses. Complete spastic paraplegia may result eventually. This condition occurs in other parts of the world, notably in the Denbia Depression of Ethiopia.

Azadirachta indica (neem)

The neem or margosa tree *Azadirachta indica* (Meliaceae: mahoganies) grows well in most parts of India and has been introduced into Africa and other tropical countries. It is revered for its medicinal properties. Various parts of the tree as well as the oil have been used in the treatment of a wide variety of ailments. Rural people often clean their teeth by chewing on a twig of this tree. Seed oil (margosa oil) contains aflatoxins and leaves contain stearic, oleic, palmitic, and linoleic acids.

Clinical features

Ingestion of neem leaf extract or an excess of margosa oil results in hepatotoxicity with vomiting, drowsiness, and encephalopathy. Metabolic acidosis is often present. Convulsions, myocarditis (with ventricular fibrillation), and pancreatitis have occurred.

Areca catechu (areca or betel nut)

The areca or betel nut *Areca catechu* (Arecaceae/Palmae: palms) grows well in Kerala, Karnataka, Goa, Assam, and West Bengal. The nuts are chewed for their euphoriant effect by more than 200 million people worldwide. In India it is called 'supari' and is chewed alone or as pan, a mixture of supari, lime, and other ingredients (with or without tobacco) wrapped in betel leaf (*Piper betel*). The Government of India classifies areca nut (supari) as a food item 'injurious to health' because it causes oral squamous cell carcinoma. The leaves and the nut find many therapeutic uses in Ayurvedic medicine. Of the toxic principles in leaf and nut, arecoline is cholinergic and arecaidine is probably carcinogenic. Arecoline is a bronchoconstrictor and can cause exacerbation of bronchospasm in asthmatic patients who chew betel nut. Betel leaf contains a phenolic volatile oil and an alkaloid capable of producing cocaine-like reactions.

Cleistanthus collinus (oduvan)

Cleistanthus collinus (Phyllanthaceae, formerly Euphorbiaceae) grows wild in dry hills of various parts of India from Himachal Pradesh to Bihar and southwards into Peninsular India. It has many names in different Indian languages: oduvanthalai/nillipalai (Tamil Nadu and Puducherry); kadishe (Andhra Pradesh); karlajuri (West Bengal); garari (Hindi-speaking states of India). All parts of the plant contain a multitude of toxic glycosides and arylnaphthalene lignan lactones—cleistanthin A and B, collinusin, and diphyllin ('oduvin').

Clinical features

There is vomiting, epigastric pain, breathlessness, visual disturbances (clouding/blurring/coloured vision), giddiness, drowsiness, fever, tachycardia, hypotension, and/or respiratory arrest. Adult respiratory distress syndrome, distal renal tubular acidosis, and shock secondary to inappropriate vasodilatation may also occur. ECG changes may include QTc prolongation and nonspecific ST-T changes. Rarely, a myasthenic crisis-like syndrome requiring assisted ventilation can occur due to *Cleistanthus collinus* poisoning, which is said to respond to treatment with neostigmine. Cases of suicide accomplished with parts of the *Cleistanthus* plant have been on the increase in several parts of India in recent times, especially in Tamil Nadu and Andhra Pradesh. Accidental poisoning has also been reported.

Jatropha curcas (physic nut)

The black seed of *Jatropha curcas* (Euphorbiaceae: spurges) is known as 'physic nut' or 'purging nut'. It contains curcanoleic acid. Apart from its use as a laxative, the seed oil is applied to painful joints. However, the crude oil when applied externally causes irritation, and when ingested causes severe diarrhoea. The seeds possess the toxalbumin curcin. Ingestion of the seeds results in salivation, sweating, abdominal pain, diarrhoea, weakness, and muscle twitching. Jatropha poisoning is generally not fatal in humans, although it may be so in animals.

Further reading

Ashby J, Styles JA, Boyland E (1979). Betel nuts, arecaidine, and oral cancer. *Lancet*, **i**, 112.

Benjamin SPE, *et al.* (2006). *Cleistanthus collinus* poisoning. *J Assoc Physicians India*, **54**, 742–4.

Dastur JF (1999). *Medicinal plants of India and Pakistan*. DB Taraporewala Sons, Mumbai.

Damodaram P, *et al.* (2009). Myasthenic crisis-like syndrome due to *Cleistanthus collinus* poisoning. *Indian J Med Sci*, **62**, 62–4.

Ellenhorn MJ (1997). Plants, mycotoxins, mushrooms. In *Medical toxicology: diagnosis and treatment of human poisoning*, 2nd edition, pp. 1832–96. Williams & Wilkins, Baltimore, MA.

Eswarappa S, *et al.* (2003). *Cleistanthus collinus* poisoning: case reports and review of the literature. *J Toxicol Clin Toxicol*, **41**, 369–72.

Gaillard Y, Krishnamoorthy A, Bevalot F (2004). *Cerbera odollam*: a 'suicide tree' and cause of death in the state of Kerala, India. *J Ethnopharmacol*, **95**, 123–6.

Ghodkirekar MSG, *et al.* (2005). Mass poisoning with *Jatropha curcas*—a case report. *J Indian Soc Toxicol*, **2**, 44–6.

Jojo VV, Rajesh RR, Pillay VV (2007). Identification of the active principles of *Manihot esculenta* and *Cerbera odollam* by thin layer chromatography: the potential for misinterpretation in forensic cases. *J Indian Soc Toxicol*, **3**, 22–6.

Pinho PMM, Kijjoa A (2007). Chemical constituents of the plants of the genus *Cleistanthus* and their biological activity. *Phytochem Rev*, **6**, 175–82.

Raghunath S, Venkataraghava S, Devadass PK (2009). *Jatropha curcas* poisoning—a case report. *J Indian Soc Toxicol*, **5**, 39–40.

Sivashanmugham R, Bhaskar N, Banumathi N (1984). Ventricular fibrillation and cardiac arrest due to neem leaf poisoning. *J Assoc Physicians India*, **32**, 610–11.

Subrahmanyam BV (2000). *Modi's medical jurisprudence and toxicology*, 22nd edn. Butterworths, India.

Subrahmanyam DKS, *et al.* (2003). A clinical and laboratory profile of *Cleistanthus collinus* poisoning. *J Assoc Physicians India*, **50**, 1052–4.

9.4

Occupational health and safety

Contents

9.4.1 Occupational and environmental health *1376*
J.M. Harrington and Raymond M. Agius

9.4.2 Occupational safety *1388*
Lawrence Waterman

9.4.1 Occupational and environmental health

J.M. Harrington and Raymond M. Agius

Essentials

Occupational health is concerned with managing the health of working people. Occupational health physicians deal with the effects of work on health, and the influence of health on work. Other professional groups, including nurses, hygienists, toxicologists, psychologists, and safety engineers, also have important roles to play in keeping people healthy and at work.

Diseases associated with occupation have been with us since the dawn of history, but it was the vicissitudes of the Industrial Revolution of the 18th and 19th centuries that brought real progress in controlling these diseases through legislation, compensation, and health care.

Occupational health services are not universal, nor are they necessarily comprehensive. National governments in the developed world have approached the question of preventing ill health at work in different ways, with the European Union's directives increasingly dominating the scene in Europe. In general terms prevention involves (1) the recognition of a health problem; (2) an assessment of the workplace risks; and (3) the implementation of control measures in the working environment to eliminate or minimize the risks to human health.

Particular occupational diseases

The most prevalent occupational diseases in developed countries today are musculoskeletal disorders and stress-related conditions, but occupationally related malignancies have the most serious outcomes.

Malignancies—the most significant occupational cancers and relevant exposures are (1) lung—asbestos, ionizing radiation, polynuclear aromatic hydrocarbons, and the compounds of certain metals such as arsenic, chromium, and nickel; (2) bladder—exposure to organic compounds such as aromatic amines; and (3) skin—coal gasification and coke production. Also of note is benzene, widely used in petrochemical industries and the cause of nonlymphocytic leukaemia and aplastic anaemia.

Musculoskeletal disorders caused by the workplace are primarily upper-limb disorders such as tenosynovitis or epicondylitis, mainly due to repetitive movement, bad posture, poorly designed tools, and mechanical stresses in the workplace. Low-back pain and osteoarthritis of the hips and knees are also associated with certain occupations, workplace postures, and weight-bearing activities.

Stress-related conditions—reports of occupational stress have increased dramatically in recent years. Effective management involves both (1) primary prevention, such as ensuring a good match between job demands, job control, and job rewards; and (2) helping those affected to cope with the stresses. Rehabilitation with counselling and behavioural therapies may be required in the last resort.

Skin—most occupational disorders are irritant contact dermatitides, with about one-third due to allergens. Skin care and protection are vitally important components of a preventive health programme to protect workers from the chemicals and dusts to which they may be exposed.

Other systems—the haemopoietic, digestive, nervous, genitourinary, reproductive, and cardiovascular systems can also be damaged by occupational exposures. The effects are extremely variable in type and pathogenesis, ranging from direct toxic damage from heavy metals, such as lead and cadmium, to the bone marrow or kidney, to secondary effects of organic solvents on hepatorenal function. The significant and extensive effects of workplace airborne particulates on the respiratory system are dealt with in Chapter 18.13.

General introduction

Definition and scope

Occupational health is that area of public health concerned with managing the health of working people. This specialty includes physicians; nurses; hygienists who monitor and control exposure to chemical, physical, and biological agents in the workplace; toxicologists, and psychologists able to assess psychosocial aspects of work. Safety engineers are responsible for preventing and investigating accidents at work (Chapter 9.4.2). These specialists will promote occupational health, but for long-term success it is crucial that both managers and the workforce consider it an integral part of their working practices and philosophy.

The medical specialty of 'occupational medicine' deals with effects of work on health, and the influence of health on work, which includes occupational rehabilitation.

History of occupational disease

Stone Age flint knappers were probably exposed to airborne silica (quartz) dust during their work. However, life expectancy then was perhaps shorter than the time course of silicosis. Some industries, such as mining, have always been hazardous. The ancient Egyptians recognized this by restricting such work to slaves and criminals. By the Middle Ages, the plight of the free miner had been recognized by Georgius Agricola (1494–1555) and Paracelsus (1493–1541). Agricola not only described the 'galloping consumption' of Carpathian silver miners but also proposed ways of reducing the dust in mines by improved ventilation.

The first authoritative treatise on occupational disease was written by Ramazzini (1633–1764). His book *De Morbis Artificium* is unsurpassed in its descriptions of many occupational diseases ranging from mercurialism in mirror workers to repetitive strain injury in clerical workers. The Industrial Revolution in the United Kingdom brought occupational diseases to the attention of Parliament, largely through the work of philanthropists like Robert Owen, Robert Peel, and Lord Shaftesbury. Early legislation to control the worst vicissitudes of factory labour was emasculated by Parliament but the process had begun. The First Act of 1802 (which introduced the concept of limiting the hours of work) was followed by others leading to the 1833 Act which saw the start of His/Her Majesty's Factory Inspectorate—the first enforcing authority in this field.

By the early 20th century, the toxic effects of arsenic, mercury, phosphorus, and lead were so common that notification of these diseases became required by law and compensation for ill health was granted. Clearly, working conditions in the Western world have improved greatly since then but working conditions for many in developing countries demonstrate an important tenet of occupational health practice: that is, while occupational disease may be preventable, the continued—often necessary—use of hazardous materials and processes means that many such diseases are not eliminated, only controlled.

Occupational health services

The notion that employers should provide health care for workers is hardly new. During the 14th century, the Pope (not an employer in this connection) decreed that prostitutes should be examined regularly for evidence of sexually transmitted disease. Whether the results were significant epidemiologically is not recorded. The first recognizable occupational health service in England began in the mid 18th century when the London (Quaker) Lead Company recognized the adverse effect of mining on workers and provided health and welfare services in north-west England. Since then, occupational health provision has expanded along different lines in different countries.

The International Labour Organization (Convention 161, 1985) urged members 'to develop progressively occupational health services for all workers. … The provision made should be adequate and appropriate to the specific needs of the undertaking.' Services are not available universally, and interpretation of the requirements varies greatly between countries and employment sectors. Initially, most services arose from a mixture of philanthropy and self-interest; the theory being that the healthy worker was likely to be more productive, a concept that holds sway today. Present-day services range from total health care including primary care and hospital medicine (as in some large multinationals operating in developing countries), to outsourced independent occupational health services. Services in the United States od America and much of Europe may include general health promotion and education, but much inequity in health care exists even between enterprises within the same country.

Recent increase in the provision of occupational health services has followed the enactment of effective health and safety legislation. The Health and Safety at Work etc. Act (1974) in the United Kingdom is an example. Some countries such as the Nordic countries, the Netherlands, and Australia, require the provision of occupational health services by law. Statutory provision of such services in the United Kingdom and the United States is limited to particular industrial sectors and specific occupational exposures such as ionizing radiation, heavy metals, asbestos, and carcinogens. In general, major Health and Safety Acts will 'enable' a variety of government departments to create legislation in the form of 'regulations', requiring action from employers in particular occupational and environmental circumstances.

The European Union (EU), through its directives, increasingly drives the occupational health and safety agenda in member states, requiring them to modify or create legislation in response. The EU philosophy has been to encourage the delivery of occupational health to all by 'competent' persons, although the mode of delivery, even the definition of competent, has been left to member states to interpret. Most important, the level of service provided should be based on a thorough risk assessment of the work processes in that organization and a clear and logical procedure of risk management. To deliver even such a basic service requires multidisciplinary teams including trained physicians, hygienists, and nurses. Few companies have such services and many are too small even to contemplate such provision.

Developments will be tempered primarily by the economic climate, perceptions of what constitutes occupationally mediated disease, and political will. However, an exponential rise in legal action, insurance costs, and compensation will play a significant part in persuading management that competent occupational health services are an absolute requirement of profitable organizations. If this is to encompass small and medium-sized enterprises, provision must come either from larger employers (such as the National Health Service) or from private providers.

Prevention

The prevention of occupational disease depends upon recognition of the condition as occupational, assessment of the level, and duration of 'exposure' and hence its possible effects, control of the problem at source, audit of the risk management procedures, and perhaps health surveillance of those exposed using suitable techniques. These procedures are dealt with in the following paragraphs. Recognition of diseases as occupational may vary from country to country.

Compensation for occupational diseases

In the early years of Western industrialized society, the chances of a worker winning compensation for an occupationally related disease or injury were slim, resting as they did on a successful common law suit for negligence against the employer. Such cases are still notoriously difficult to win. However, by the end of the 19th century, many jurisdictions in Europe and the United States had passed workman's compensation laws of one sort or another. Such schemes were usually restricted to specified diseases or occupations.

The principles underlying such statutory compensation schemes are that they should be 'no fault', that the disease should be, with reasonable certainty, caused by work, and that the benefit claimed should offset job loss, wage-earning deficit, and disability, or provide death benefit to the next of kin. Advice on proposed additions to the list of compensatable diseases is made in the member states by government-appointed advisory groups. In the United Kingdom, this group is the Industrial Injuries Advisory Council, which reports to the Secretary of State for the Department of Work and Pensions.

New EU recommendations propose that national schemes be made uniform. In addition, the EU wishes to see the introduction of a concept to aid those who can prove they have an occupationally related disease which is not on the standard list—the so-called 'individual proof' system. In the United Kingdom such a dual system of specified agents and individual claim opportunities exists only for occupational asthma. No specific agents are listed for dermatitis.

It is important that clinicians are aware of such schemes. If the disease and work exposure seem related, and are scheduled, patients should be advised to claim for compensation. If the disease and/or work exposure are not scheduled, there may still be a case worthy of pursuit under common law.

Assessment of the workforce and their environment

Occupational health comprises recognition, evaluation, and control. Control, including prevention, is paramount; there is no point in knowing what may happen or diagnosing what has happened if no remedial action is taken. For too long, society and industry have relied on occupational physicians to identify failures in control by diagnosing occupational diseases without sufficiently emphasizing the need for control and therefore prevention.

As a result of this realization, current health and safety legislation is driven by risk assessment, i.e. those who generate the risks are responsible for undertaking an assessment, the detail of which must be commensurate with the complexity of the situation and the ultimate risk. It follows from this that the quantified risk must be managed, and hence employers must include risk management in their portfolio of activities.

Before embarking on any evaluation, especially where an occupational cause is suspected, great care must be exercised beforehand to determine what the legislation requires, what the known toxicological/health effects are, previous evidence from similar circumstances/environments, etc. This is the 'recognition' aspect, and highlights the necessity not only to be well informed but also competent to interpret the available information and act appropriately.

Evaluation

To reduce the risk of making wrong decisions and to maximize the usefulness of any information, evaluation of the workforce and workplace must be conducted in a systematic manner. This can be achieved by posing a number of simple questions.

The most fundamental of these questions is why? It is essential that the rationale for evaluating an individual or group is clear and justifiable. However, as occupational health professionals exist to eliminate ill health at work, their priority must always be to eliminate problems in the workplace immediately rather than to delay while quantifying them. The law is prescriptive for only for a limited number of hazards (ionizing radiation, lead, asbestos).

Where large groups are involved, it may be necessary to evaluate a subset—this is the 'who' question. When there is often no other overriding need for selection, such as those working for extended periods (more than 8 h per day), those working at an elevated metabolic/breathing rate, those already unwell, or those likely to undertake unusual or unscheduled tasks (maintenance), individuals should be chosen randomly.

The timing of measurements (i.e. 'when') is often critical. Should health outcome measures be taken before, during, or after the putative exposure, or is there some legislative requirement that dictates the timing? For example, urinary mandelic acid (for styrene exposure) is best collected at the end of a working shift, whereas urinary trichloroacetic acid (for trichloroethylene exposure) is best measured at the end of the working week, this being determined, in part, by the differing half-lives of these compounds.

Often, the issue of 'what' to assess is self-evident, but, as with all other aspects of this systematic approach, answers to the questions are interlinked, certainly with the 'why' question. For example, is biological monitoring or biological-effect monitoring required? The former is the detection of a chemical or its metabolite in a biological sample as a measure of exposure. The latter is measurement of a change in some biochemical or physiological variable to indicate the effect of the contaminant on the body. Sometimes it is not possible to measure uptake or a biological effect short of 'harm', and one can only detect early manifestations of ill health such as asthmatic symptoms from exposure to colophony fume in soldering.

Choice of an appropriate technique for making these measurements should be based, where possible, on indices of sensitivity and specificity, as well as on the economics and acceptability of the technique.

The technique should be both suitable and sufficient for its purpose. For example, in the diagnosis of occupational asthma, suitable techniques include peak-flow meters, simple spirometry (time–volume or flow–volume curves), and whole-body plethysmography, but the simplest of these may be adequate.

Remedial action

The law is clear: the employer must adapt the workplace to be a safe environment for the employees. The employees should not have to adapt themselves to the stresses and strains of their work. Despite this philosophy, it is common for the chain of control to start with ineffective pre-employment medicals whose aim is often only to avoid exposing people to contaminants likely to exacerbate allergies or other diseases, and which may, for example, unscientifically and unethically deny employment to atopic people.

Control is often viewed as a physical alteration of the workplace (engineering) or alteration of the work practice or behaviour of the workforce (administrative). It is preferable for the workplace to be designed appropriately, in the first place. Unfortunately, most control is required remedially, after an unacceptable level of risk has been identified as a result of a formal risk assessment. When exposure to chemical or physical agents is involved, remedial action may involve:

- elimination—removal of the process or agent
- substitution—replacement of the hazardous agent with one carrying a lower risk
- process modification (temperature, agitation, enclosure, etc.)
- substance or agent modification (wavelength, form, size, etc.)
- isolation/segregation (time, distance, shielding)
- local extract ventilation
- minimization of the duration and frequency of exposure
- education and training and the use of personal protective equipment

Occupational cancer (see also Chapter 6.1)

Background

Georgius Agricola's account in 1555 of the illnesses of Carpathian silver miners reveals evidence of a rapidly progressive and fatal lung disorder. The fact that these mines are now known to contain uranium ore suggests that exposure to radon gas may well have been high enough to cause lung cancer in the miners. Nevertheless, it is Percival Pott's description in 1775 of an excess risk of scrotal cancer in postpubertal chimney sweeps that first raised the possibility that chemicals, particularly polynuclear aromatic hydrocarbons (PAH), might cause cancer. Confirmatory evidence from animal experiments did not arrive until 1915, and the first carcinogenic hydrocarbon was identified by Kennaway in 1924 as 1,2,5,6-dibenzanthracene.

While the polynuclear aromatic hydrocarbons were generating interest as skin carcinogens, clinical observations in dyestuff workers were suggesting a link between bladder cancer and certain aromatic amines. In 1895, Rehn described three cases in a group of 45 workers in Germany involved in the preparation of fuchsin. Further reports followed from other countries and the classic studies of Case and his colleagues in the 1950s showed that 2-naphthylamine and benzidine were human carcinogens in manufacturing and user industries. 2-Napthylamine was a contaminant of the antioxidant used in tyre manufacture. Rehn discovered that an organ distant from the point of first contact could bear the main force of the carcinogenic effect if its exposure was most prolonged and intense.

In the same year that Rehn made his discovery, Röntgen discovered X-rays, and 3 years later, the Curies isolated radium. Unfortunately, knowledge of the carcinogenic properties of ionizing radiation came from the skin and bone marrow cancers suffered by these early pioneers. Confirmatory animal data followed soon after. Bone sarcomas were noted in laboratory animals and later, in the 1930s among painters of luminous dials who used radium-235 and mesothorium. The inventor of the luminous paint, Dr von Sochocky, died of aplastic anaemia in 1928. Again in the 1930s, lung cancer, an unusual tumour in those days, was found in 18% of cases of asbestosis. Reports of pleural mesothelioma followed a decade or so later.

Thus, within a century of Rehn's discovery, chemical carcinogenesis had become a well-recognized phenomenon, much of the evidence having come from occupational studies.

Diagnosis

Clinical acumen remains of paramount importance. Clinicians played the major role in discovering new causes of cancer while confirmatory evidence came from epidemiological and laboratory studies.

Such information is collated and interpreted by various national and international agencies. The most reliable source is the extensive monograph series of the International Agency for Research on Cancer (IARC) based in Lyon, France. When a patient is diagnosed as having cancer, it is important that the clinician should review their occupational history and consider an occupational cause. If this seems probable, enquiries should be made to see if state compensation is available for that cancer and that workplace exposure.

Attribution of cancer to occupational causes

The most widely accepted estimates of the proportion of all cancers attributable to occupational exposures is 4%, with a range of 2 to 8% for a developed country like the United States. Occupationally related cancers are almost exclusively concentrated in 20% or so of the population, comprising manual workers aged 20 or over, in mining, agriculture, and industry. In this group, perhaps as many as one lung or bladder cancer in every five may be attributed to workplace exposure.

In addition, it is necessary to consider other exposures which may interact with workplace exposures. These are particularly relevant when considering the relative effectiveness of removing or reducing exposure to one or more jointly acting agents. Few good studies have been completed on interaction, but there is good evidence for the multiplicative effects of cigarette smoking and asbestos exposure in the genesis of lung cancer. Besides asbestos, interactions have been demonstrated to be at least additive for tobacco consumption and exposure to arsenic and nickel compounds as well as ionizing radiation.

Tables 9.4.1.1 and 9.4.1.2 show some important examples of occupational exposures causing cancer.

Polynuclear aromatic hydrocarbons

The PAHs are a large and complex group of compounds mainly generated during the incomplete combustion of carbonaceous products, of which coal and oil result in the most important occupational exposures. Cigarette smoke contains a number of these compounds and so it is often difficult to distinguish lifestyle from

Table 9.4.1.1 Industrial processes causally associated with human cancer. Suspected target organs are in parentheses

Industry	Human target organs
Aluminium production	Lung, bladder (haemopoietic/lymphatic system, oesophagus, stomach)
Auramine manufacture	Bladder
Boot and shoe manufacture and repair	Haemopoietic/lymphatic system, nasal sinus (bladder, digestive tract)
Coal gasification	Skin, lung, bladder
Coke production	Skin, lung, kidney
Furniture and cabinet-making	Nasal sinus
Hairdressers and barbers	Bladder, non-Hodgkins lymphoma, ovary
Haematite mining, underground, with exposure to radon	Lung
Iron and steel founding	Lung (digestive tract, genitourinary tract, haemopoietic/lymphatic system)
Isopropyl alcohol manufacture, strong acid process	Nasal sinus (larynx)
Magenta manufacture	Bladder
Painters (occupational exposure as)	Lung (oesophagus, stomach, bladder)
Petroleum refining	Bladder, non-Hodgkins lymphoma, leukaemia
Rubber industry	Bladder, (haemopoietic/lymphatic system, lung, renal tract, digestive tract, skin, liver, larynx, brain, stomach)
Strong inorganic acid mists containing sulphuric acid	Larynx

Based on IARC Monographs vols. 1–100, 1972–2009.

Table 9.4.1.2 Chemicals and groups of chemicals causally associated with human cancer for which exposure has been mostly occupational. Suspected target organs are in parentheses

Chemical	Human target organ
4-Aminobiphenyl	Bladder
Arsenic and arsenic compounds[a]	Skin, lung (liver, haematopoietic system, gastrointestinal tract, kidney)
Asbestos	Lung, pleura, peritoneum, gastrointestinal tract, larynx
Benzene	Haemopoietic system
Benzidine	Bladder
Beryllium	Lung
Bis (chloromethyl) ether and chloromethyl methyl ether (technical grade)	Lung
Chromium compounds, hexavalent[a]	Lung (gastrointestinal tract)
Coal tars	Skin, lung (bladder)
Coal tar pitches	Skin, lung, bladder (gastrointestinal tract, haemopoietic/lymphatic system)
Cobalt with tungsten carbide	Lung
Erionite	Mesothelioma
Ethylene oxide	Lymphatic and haemopoietic systems
Inorganic acid mists (strong) containing sulphuric acid	Larynx
Ionizing radiation	Haemopoietic/lymphatic system, bone, skin, and other organs depending on exposure and type of radiation
Mineral oils, untreated and mildly treated	Skin (respiratory tract, bladder, gastrointestinal tract)
Mustard gas (sulphur mustard)	Lung, larynx, pharynx
2-Naphthylamine (and other aromatic amines)	Bladder (liver)
Nickel and nickel compounds[a]	Nasal sinus, lung (larynx)
Ortho-toluidine and 4-chloro-*ortho*-toluidine	Bladder
Radon (and its decay products)	Lung
Shale oils	Skin (colon)
Silica (crystalline)	Lung
Soots	Skin, lung
Talc containing asbestiform fibre	Lung (pleura)
2,3,7,8 Tetrachlorodibenzo-para-dioxin (TCDD)	Lung, non-Hodgkins lymphoma, sarcoma
Vinyl chloride	Liver, lung, brain, lymphatic and haematopoietic systems (gastrointestinal tract)

[a] The evaluation of carcinogenicity in humans applies to the group of chemicals as a whole and not necessarily all individual chemicals within the group.

Based on IARC Monographs vols. 1–100, 1972–2009

occupational factors. The site of action of these compounds is mainly the lung, skin, and bladder. The industries most prominently linked to such exposures are coke ovens, gas production, steel industries, aluminium refineries, iron and steel foundries as well as workers exposed to exhaust fumes from soot, pitch, tar, and petroleum products.

Aromatic amines

Aromatic amines are a group of chemically similar compounds which have particular importance as dyestuffs, antioxidants, or intermediates in dye production. Some are known human bladder carcinogens, particularly those in which the amino group is in the *para* position (i.e. on the aromatic ring directly opposite) relative to an aromatic moiety. For a larger number known to be animal carcinogens, human data are limited or lacking. The more potent carcinogens are now banned.

Metals and metalloids

The most important carcinogenic metals are compounds of arsenic, chromium, and nickel. Arsenic and its compounds cause lung and skin cancer, and these risks occur in the extraction of metalliferous ores (which are frequently contaminated by arsenic compounds) and in the now limited use of arsenic in pesticides, wood treatment, and other industrial applications. Hexavalent chromium compounds used in the pigment and plating industries have been shown to cause lung cancer. Lung and nasal cancer are associated with nickel refining, in which the most likely causative agents are sulphidic nickel compounds and possibly oxidic nickel or nickel sulphate. Metallic (elemental) nickel is unlikely to be carcinogenic. Other metals, for which there is evidence of carcinogenicity, at least in some of their compounds, include beryllium and cadmium.

Other organic compounds

Benzene is widely used in industry both as the base compound and as an important building block in the organic chemical industry. It causes nonlymphocytic leukaemia and aplastic anaemia. Vinyl chloride monomer, which is the starting point for synthesis of polyvinyl chloride, causes angiosarcoma of the liver. The most potent lung carcinogens are apparently the chloromethyl ethers, which are used in ion exchange resins. Other suspect organic compounds include acrylonitrile, acrylamide, butadiene, diethyl sulphate, epichlorhydrin, ethylene dibromide, formaldehyde, and styrene oxide. Many of these chemicals or their metabolites are potent electrophiles or alkylating agents and thus can damage DNA.

Industrial processes

Some processes listed in Table 9.4.1.1 are linked to specific exposures, such as PAHs in aluminium production and radon in underground mining. For others, such as boot and shoe manufacture, furniture making, and painting, the specific relevant exposures have not been identified.

Infections

Certain industries, notably health care, are associated with an increased risk of occupational infections. Blood-borne infections such as hepatitis B and HIV pose practical problems for the safety of staff during contact with infected patients, and the safety of patients during contact with infected staff, especially during so-called 'exposure-prone procedures'. Numerous cases of HIV infection have occurred in health care workers following contact with infected blood or body fluids from patients. These have involved needlestick injuries, mainly from contaminated hollow-bore needles, or substantial blood contamination of damaged skin. Cases of HIV transmission from health care workers to patients are also known, but hepatitis B is far more easily transmissible, explaining the higher incidence of outbreaks from doctor to patient and vice versa. Health care staff should be protected from hepatitis B by vaccination but this does not cover other hepatitis viruses. Other occupational infections affecting staff in microbiological laboratories and other health care workers include tuberculosis, salmonellosis, syphilis, and malaria.

Working in tropical environments also exposes workers to the risk of tropical diseases. Occupational and environmental infections involve a range of organisms from viruses, rickettsiae, bacteria, and fungi to larger organisms such as parasites and insects. Occupations involved, together with the diseases involved, are forestry and gamekeeping (Lyme disease), sewage work (leptospirosis—Weil's disease, and some viruses), and farming (brucellosis—of special concern to pregnant workers because of the risk of abortion). Although rare in the United Kingdom, anthrax still occurs and may be responsible for fatalities typically following exposure to infected hides or bones.

Occupation and the skin

Since the skin offers such a large area to physical and chemical exposures in the workplace, it is not surprising that skin damage is a common occupational disease. An occupational dermatosis is a pathological condition of the skin for which occupational exposure can be shown to be a major contributory factor. However, legal definitions vary between countries. The true incidence of occupational skin disease is difficult to ascertain but in the United Kingdom, data from dermatologists' reports suggest an annual incidence of about 1 per 10 000, with approximately sixfold higher incidence rates based on reports from occupational physicians.

Occupational contact dermatitis

Dermatitis, mostly due to irritant contact factors, accounts for 95% of all occupational dermatoses. In the United Kingdom, a million working days a year may be lost from such conditions. In the United Kingdom, the majority are defined by Prescribed Disease D5 as 'non-infective dermatitis of external origin …'. The diagnosis and management is discussed elsewhere (see Chapter 23.6). Some points are worth reiterating. A very detailed chronological occupational and nonoccupational exposure history is essential. About one-third of cases are thought to be allergic in origin. However, in many cases, although it will be easy to decide whether the dermatitis (eczema) is allergic or irritant, this distinction is often difficult to make. Thus a dermatitis that was allergic in origin may be aggravated and sustained by exposure to irritants at work and at home. Atopic subjects are at increased risk of irritant dermatitis.

Employees' and employers' attitudes to dermatitis

Some managers and even some doctors believe that people with dermatitis are out to obtain whatever they can in the way of compensation. However, especially in times of high unemployment, the converse may be true as many people may be reluctant to seek help in case they are labelled as suffering from industrial dermatitis and are then transferred to less skilled work with the loss of bonuses or even their jobs. Once labelled in this way, they are unlikely to find alternative employment.

Many employers believe that dermatitis is not problem in their establishment, but careful inspection of employees' skin shows that the condition may be present in up to one-third of the workforce. Much time is lost because of dermatitis and the burden of suffering, from discomfort to depression and social ostracism, is impossible to quantify.

As with many skin diseases, there are many myths associated with dermatitis. Many people believe that dermatitis is infectious and can be passed on by towels and touching; this results in the social isolation of affected individuals. Dermatitis should not be regarded as contagious, although secondary infections can occasionally arise and need treatment. It can only be acquired by physical or chemical damage to the skin or by the development of an allergy to a substance that has been in contact with the skin. Affected people should not, therefore, have unnecessary restrictions placed on them.

With outbreaks of apparent dermatitis, great care is needed in handling the situation to identify the causes and differentiate those with occupationally related problems from those with other skin diseases.

Causal agents can vary widely. In manufacturing the cause might be an allergen, yet in an office environment rashes could result from low ambient humidity. It may be necessary to ask for the help of a dermatologist with specialist knowledge and to conduct patch tests to identify the cause.

Skin protection

The best form of protection is to control exposure at source by applying the principles described earlier together with a degree of common sense. In industrial situations, the hands and forearms are most at risk. The use of proper gloves (along with gauntlets or arm bands to prevent powders entering under the cuff), coupled with a high standard of hygiene, can minimize contact and provide adequate protection. Where there is moving machinery, wearing gloves may pose a potential danger. Even when gloves are used, they may be taken off for tasks requiring manual dexterity, with the result that contaminated hands are placed back inside the gloves.

Many materials have been used to manufacture gloves, including cotton, leather, nylon, glass fibre, acrylonitrile, rubber, neoprene, butyl rubber, polyurethane, PVC, PVA, and tetrafluoroethylene. These confer specific protection for defined occupational exposures.

No so-called 'barrier cream' actually provides a barrier to penetration of substances into the skin. In fact, in some situations they may actually enhance penetration, and occasionally sensitization may occur to some of the constituents of the cream. The use of a barrier cream may give an employee a false sense of security and lead to increased skin abuse. They may offer some mitigation purely because of their emollient function since they tend to be fatty preparations.

Detergents or solvents will remove fat from the skin, thus damaging its integrity and exposing it to further insults. Frequent handwashing can have the same effect. Emollients containing lanolin may help to improve the hydration and hence suppleness of the skin, with the result that, when cleansers are used, less degreasing of the skin occurs.

There are many 'after-work' creams, essentially moisturizers, which have the benefit of increasing the hydration of the skin following cleaning at the end of the day. They are of particular benefit in occupations where excessive drying of the skin may occur. Their use should be encouraged where hot air dryers are used, as these tend to dry the skin unduly (towels are preferred for hand drying).

When substances remain on the skin after the working day, the risk of irritation or sensitization is increased. The most efficient skin cleaners, however, are often the most irritant of substances due to their solvent or detergent content. If cleaners are too mild for the task, workers will often resort to degreasing agents used in the manufacturing process, e.g. solvents such as paraffins or even turpentine, to obtain adequate cleaning. Although these substances will 'clean', they are potentially very irritating with repeated use. It is often inappropriate to provide one type of product for all jobs. Agents should be chosen that clean adequately in a short period of time without having too strong a degreasing effect.

Nondermatitic occupational dermatoses

These form a minority of occupational dermatoses, but awareness of their existence is important for those involved in managing skin patients. The more important are briefly listed here:

- Psoriasis (see Chapter 23.5) may erupt at sites of injury or as a response to friction in manual workers. When this occurs on the hands, it may be confused with dermatitis although vesicles (blisters) are rarely found in psoriatic skin.
- Urticaria may arise as a consequence of sensitization to agents as disparate as latex or proteins in rat urine. It may be associated with rhinitis, asthma or even anaphylaxis and should therefore be treated with a high index of suspicion. Occupationally induced itching may occur in atopic individuals who exhibit dermographism due to histamine release from mast cells caused by fibres typically around 3 μm in size, which can penetrate the skin. This occurs with exposure to glass fibres, ceramic fibres, and fibreglass.
- Infections include human papilloma virus warts, orf (a poxvirus), and fungal infections such as tinea pedis and cattle ringworm *Trichophyton mentagrophytes*. Chronic paronychia due to candida occurs in those exposed to wet work.
- Acne may be caused by a variety of chemicals including oils, coal tar chlorphenols, and petroleum products. Chloracne is a particularly refractory form of acne caused by halogenated aromatic chemicals, which may also cause systemic toxicity. Mild cases may be difficult to differentiate from conventional acne but multiple comedones (blackheads) are found over the malar regions. Industrial accidents can result in exposure and subsequent symptoms: for example, in 1976, an explosion in a chemical plant near Seveso, Italy resulted in the exposure of the local population to 2,3,7,8-tetrachlorodibenzo-*p*-dioxin which caused severe systemic and cutaneous symptoms.
- Vitiligo may be occupationally acquired. Several substituted phenols including *p*-tertiary-butyl phenol (pTBP) and monobenzyl ether of hydroquinone may cause hypomelanosis indistinguishable from vitiligo. The pTBP molecule is structurally very similar to the essential amino acid tyrosine, which is the staring point for the synthesis of melanin, and it is likely that their competition for the same synthetic enzymes results in chemical vitiligo.
- A scleroderma-like syndrome may be caused by exposure to vinyl chloride (chloroethene), and scleroderma has been reported with exposure to trichloroethylene (trichloroethene) and other organic solvents. Scleroderma-like lesions have also been reported in people exposed to epoxy resin fumes, and silicosis associated with scleroderma has been reported in miners.
- A variety of chemicals may cause alteration of skin pigment, e.g. mercury and silver, which cause argyria. Coal miners may have deposits embedded typically in the skin of their knees or elbows. Usually these are indices of exposure but do not suggest skin 'disease' as such.

Musculoskeletal disorders

In the United Kingdom, musculoskeletal disorders have the highest reported incidence out of the major categories of occupational or work-related ill health, although occupational 'stress' and mental disorders rank a close second. As musculoskeletal disorders are common in the general population, their suspected relationship to specific occupations or activities can often be difficult to confirm and many medically unexplained symptoms may have musculoskeletal manifestations as well as other symptoms such as headache and fatigue. A combination of occupational, psychological, personal, social, and home factors may be involved. The epidemic of so-called 'repetitive strain injury' in Australia during the 1980s highlighted the complex interaction of illness beliefs and behaviour as well as employment in determining the workers' symptomatic complaints.

Work-related upper-limb disorders

A wide range of terms has been coined over time to describe pain and discomfort usually in the wrist and forearm associated with the performance of repeated tasks, mainly at work. These include 'repetitive strain injury', 'cumulative trauma disorder', 'occupational overuse syndrome', and 'work-related upper-limb disorder', some of which restrict the definition to conditions in upper limbs caused by work. Several disorders, such as carpal tunnel syndrome, de Quervain's disease, epicondylitis, and tenosynovitis are often included in the entity, and agreed case definitions have been proposed within the EU. Clusters of cases have been recognized in occupational groups, such as typists, telephonists, computer keyboard operators, musicians, cleaners, hairdressers, butchers, and assembly-line workers. While the wrist and forearm are the anatomical regions most frequently affected, the symptoms are often very diffuse and the shoulder and neck may also be involved. Risk factors common to many cases are:

- constrained postures, sometimes at the extremes of the range of movements, and often against force
- repeated movements at certain joints, often through the full range of movements, for example, flexion and extension at the wrists

Low back pain

This is possibly the commonest musculoskeletal condition experienced by people at work. Poor lifting and manual-handling techniques and sitting for prolonged periods in the course of work activities (e.g. professional drivers) are contributory factors. Nurses, porters, and bricklayers are groups with a high prevalence of low back pain. The total cost of sickness absence, early retirement, and treatment for low back pain in many countries is considerable. Historically this was exacerbated by the belief by patients and their medical attendants that rest was needed for recovery. However, there is now very good evidence that, with the exception of serious spinal diseases and nerve root problems, special investigations are unnecessary and rapid mobilization and return to work should be advocated. Moreover, the rising incidence of back pain reported to be work related, over a period of decades, cannot be adequately explained by physical conditions at work or by work practices. Cultural and psychological factors probably have to be invoked satisfactorily to account for the high frequency of back pain.

Occupations associated with musculoskeletal disorders

Several occupations are associated with a high risk of sustaining an occupationally related musculoskeletal injury. These include fractures and joint damage in construction workers, miners, and deep-sea fishermen; avascular bone necrosis from decompression sickness in tunnellers and divers; acro-osteolysis in workers exposed to vinyl chloride monomer; and septic bone and joint lesions from brucellosis in meat-processing workers. The joints of coalface workers, farmers, and professional dancers are subjected to frequent heavy-impact loading leading to a high incidence of degenerative changes of the hip and knee.

Clinical investigations and management

In all cases, a careful history, including consideration of psychological as well as physical factors, is essential. In a minority of cases, investigations such as measurement of erythrocyte sedimentation rate, acute phase proteins (such as C-reactive protein), and specific serological tests for rheumatoid or related disease, and imaging may help if an underlying medical condition is suspected.

The management of a case of occupational musculoskeletal disorder requires alleviation of symptoms and the consideration of modifications to the system of work or the layout of the workstation. Nonsteroidal anti-inflammatory medication and physiotherapy can reduce pain, discomfort, and limitation of function. Localized areas of inflammation may respond to local injections of corticosteroids. Physical therapy procedures, and rarely surgery, may be considered. There should be an evaluation of ergonomic factors in the design of equipment at the individual's workplace. This requires attention to the adequacy of the workstation, ease of access of the worker to tools, components, and other equipment, and the suitability of the general work environment—its lighting, temperature, humidity, and noise. Training in proper methods of lifting and manual handling is essential.

Musculoskeletal disorders affecting occupation

Patients with known arthritic disease, such as rheumatoid arthritis and systemic lupus erythematosus, need to be assessed for the effect that the condition may have on the performance of their work duties. The fluctuating nature of most forms of chronic arthritis makes precise predictions difficult. Physical disability can improve despite persistence of the disease. This is due both to the beneficial effects of treatment, to the patient's adaptation to the consequences of the disease, and sometimes, to successful rehabilitation at work.

Cardiovascular system

Cardiovascular disease is the major cause of mortality and morbidity in industrialized countries (see Section 16). The association between personal risk factors and cardiovascular disease is well known, but less attention has been paid to occupational and environmental influences.

There is good evidence from the classical studies of bus drivers and conductors that sedentary workers have a higher risk of ischaemic heart disease than those who are more active. There is some evidence linking job stress and heart disease. The Whitehall II studies suggest that control over one's job is an important factor in determining subsequent risk of myocardial infarction.

Since the incidence of cardiovascular disease especially in the developed world is so high, even a small contribution (of the order of say 1%) to adverse outcome as a result of exposure to air pollution could result in a significant health burden and economic cost. Exposure to chemicals may contribute to cardiovascular ill health in a number of ways. Very small particulate pollution (typically with an aerodynamic diameter of substantially less than 1 μm) can cross the alveolocapillary membrane and gain access to the circulation. Through their effects on macrophages and other inflammatory cells they can release cytokines and other mediators, which provoke inflammation, damage to vascular endothelium, and perhaps procoagulant effects. Thus an excess of morbidity and mortality from atheromatous disease has been associated with such exposures. Fine or ultrafine particulate exposure can also affect heart rate and induce dysrhythmias, probably because of effects mediated by the autonomic nervous system. Occupational exposures such as to carbon disulphide, chlorinated organic solvents, nitroglycerine, and vinyl chloride (monomer) may contribute to cardiovascular disease. The cardiovascular effects of exposure to heavy metals are probably largely secondary to their nephrotoxic effects. Toxic industrial gases produce their effect secondary to anoxia. Among physical agents, vibration is known to cause peripheral vascular disease and acute high exposure to noise is known to raise blood pressure. Workers on rotating shifts have an increased risk of ischaemic heart disease.

Genitourinary system

The kidney plays a crucial role in excretion and detoxification. Perhaps the most effective detoxification manoeuvre of the liver is to increase the polarity of the absorbed substance, usually by oxidation to alcohols, aldehydes, or acids, and sometimes followed by conjugation. This, in turn, increases the water solubility of the chemical and hence its renal excretion. The kidney, therefore, bears the brunt of many exposures to toxic chemicals. Some toxic substances reach the kidney unchanged, but most are metabolized to some extent or other. Some, such as cadmium, become sequestered in the renal cortex while others, such as the aromatic amines or their metabolites, can be present in the bladder long enough and at a high enough concentration to induce malignant change in the transitional cell epithelium.

Sudden, severe exposures to some chemicals can cause acute nephropathy. Such compounds may damage the kidney directly due to their intrinsic nephrotoxicity or may induce secondary damage due to prerenal effects, such as the haemolysis following arsine exposure. Hypovolaemic shock can follow acute fluid loss or extreme heat, while post-traumatic renal failure can follow crush injuries or high-voltage electric shock, both of which cause muscle necrosis. Chronic lower-dose exposure leading to nephropathy is more commonly associated with metals or organic solvents.

The metals most commonly implicated in renal disease are mercury, cadmium, lead, and, perhaps, uranium (see Chapter 9.1). Mercury exposure resulting in acute tubular necrosis or the nephrotic syndrome is most unusual these days. Under present-day workplace exposures, the effects of inhaled mercury vapour or absorption of mercury salts are more likely to cause mild proteinuria and limited tubular dysfunction. Biological monitoring of mercury-exposed workers has had to become more sophisticated. Sensitive tests of urinary enzymes, such as *N*-acetyl-β-D-glucosamidase, are necessary to detect those subtle effects. Similarly, modern industrial exposures to cadmium rarely result in the proximal or distal tubular dysfunction or renal cortical damage that was more prevalent in the past. However, cadmium is only slowly leached from the renal cortex and remains a potentially serious long-term cumulative poison. The environmental cadmium contamination which caused widespread tubular dysfunction with hypercalciuria and osteomalacia in multiparous postmenopausal Japanese women (itai-itai disease) has not been described in the West. Lead nephropathy is also a rarity nowadays, but was not uncommon in the early part of this century. Lead is capable of causing damage to all parts of the nephron. More subtle tests of renal enzymes are now needed to assess the effects of lead exposure on the kidney. Soluble uranium compounds such as uranium hexafluoride have been shown to be potent nephrotoxins after acute accidental exposure but this problem is virtually unknown in a well-controlled modern facility.

Chlorinated aliphatic solvents such as carbon tetrachloride and chloroform can cause the hepatorenal syndrome. The renal damage is largely an effect on the proximal tubular epithelium which can lead to tubular necrosis and acute oliguric renal failure. The weight of evidence from case–control studies of workers exposed to solvent suggests an excess risk of chronic proliferative glomerulonephritis. The mechanism is unclear, but the demonstration of antiglomerular basement membrane antibody suggests possible autoimmune damage to the glomerular basement membrane. Parallels may exist between the genesis of scleroderma or similar syndromes, and the renal damage caused by these or similar compounds. They have the propensity to be converted into electrophilic entities or free radicals, which might damage native protein, and thus provoke an autoimmune response.

Although the prostate possesses the curious ability to concentrate (and excrete) heavy metals, little evidence exists of occupationally related prostatic disease. Earlier reports of a link between cadmium exposure and prostatic cancer have not been confirmed. Cancers of the urinary tract associated with occupational exposure to aromatic amines and PAHs were described earlier.

Gastrointestinal tract

The gastrointestinal tract is an uncommon source of occupational exposure, but can be important when skin contamination is transferred to food or cigarettes; it acts as a semipermeable membrane through which ingested pollutants are absorbed. There are defence mechanisms that limit the damage to the gastrointestinal tract from such pollutants, and minimize their absorption. The mucous lining of the gut and diarrhoea and vomiting form part of these defence mechanisms. Hence, systemic absorption via the gastrointestinal tract plays a relatively minor role in causing occupational disease.

Acute gastroenteritis may follow the ingestion of chemicals such as soluble salts of heavy metals.

The liver is frequently at risk from occupational exposures, as it is the target organ for detoxification and metabolism of absorbed compounds. A wide variety of infectious and chemical agents cause different types of hepatocellular injury, which may eventually lead to cirrhosis and liver failure (Table 9.4.1.3), but decline in developed countries, improved working conditions, and perhaps a decline in manufacturing industry has made these manifestations rare.

Haemopoietic system

Damage to cellular precursors in haemopoiesis can result in pancytopenia or anaemia, as well as neoplasia, but these manifestations are rare. Selective damage can result in inhibition of haemoglobin synthesis, typically caused by lead which is probably the commonest occupational disease affecting the blood. Red cell damage resulting in haemolysis is rare.

Lead poisoning is one of the oldest recognized occupational diseases, and is still common especially in the developing world. Exposures are widespread, ranging from nonferrous smelting to burning of old paint. Lead causes anaemia mainly by inhibiting the enzymes involved in haem synthesis, and also by haemolysis. The metal binds to erythrocytes and determination of blood lead levels is used in the monitoring of lead-exposed workers. A diagnosis of lead poisoning is supported by symptoms of malaise, colic, and constipation, signs of anaemia, and peripheral motor neuropathy (rare, usually only in severe cases), and microscopic evidence in the erythrocytes of basophilic stippling (from abnormal

Table 9.4.1.3 Effects of occupationally related hepatotoxins

Effect	Substance	
	Organic	**Inorganic**
Centrilobular necrosis	**Halogenated alkanes/alkenes**	Antimony
	Methyl chloride (chloromethane)	Arsenic
	Carbon tetrachloride (tetrachloromethane)	Boranes
		Phosphorus (yellow)
	1,1,1-Trichloroethane	Selenium
	Vinyl chloride (chloroethene)	Thallium
	Trichloroethylene (trichloroethene)	
	Tetrachloroethylene (tetrachloroethene)	
	Halothane (2-bromo-2-chloro-1, 1, 1-trifluoro-ethane)	
	Halogenated aromatics	
	4,4′-Methylene bis(2-chloraniline)	
	Chlorinated naphthalenes	
	Polychlorinated biphenyls	
	Chlorinated hydrocarbon insecticides	
	Nitrated aromatics	
	Nitrobenzene	
	Dinitrophenol	
	Trinitrotoluene	
Hepatic infections	Viral hepatitis (A,B,C)	
	Leptospirosis	
	Q fever	
	Schistosomiasis	
	Amoebiasis	
Cholestatic cholangiolytic	Methylene dianiline	
	Organic arsenicals	
	Toluene diamine	

Source: Aw TC, Gardner K, Harrington JM (2007). *Occupational health*, 5th edition. Blackwell Scientific, Oxford. With permission.

haemoglobin), elevated blood lead, low haemoglobin, raised free erythrocyte protoporphyrin, and raised urinary δ-aminolaevulinic acid. Indications of excessive lead absorption should lead to removal of the affected worker from further occupational exposure, with full investigation into, and control of, the circumstances of exposure to lead at work.

Massive intravascular haemolysis may be caused by acute exposure to arsine, phosphine, or stibine. These gases are encountered in the smelting and refining of metals, galvanizing processes, and certain soldering procedures. Phosphine also arises when the pesticide fumigants aluminium or magnesium phosphide (usually used for treating grain) are exposed to water. Features of phosphine poisoning include pneumonitis, cardiovascular, and respiratory manifestations. Phosphine, arsine, and stibine are the hydrides of phosphorus, arsenic, and antimony (three elements in group VA of the periodic table), respectively.

Occupational exposure to ionizing radiation can occur following the industrial use of radioactive sources to test the integrity of welds, in the health care industry, and in nuclear power stations (see Chapter 9.5.9).

Benzene is encountered in the petroleum industry, and is used as a starter chemical for the production of other aromatic organic compounds. Its effects on the haemopoietic system include early platelet deficiency, mild haemolysis, and pancytopenia. Major effects are aplastic anaemia and leukaemia.

Methaemoglobinaemia can result from exposure to occupational and environmental agents such as nitrates, and nitro and amino derivatives of aromatic compounds. Specific examples are aniline, aminobenzene, nitrobenzene, and nitrates in drinking water (from soil leachate). Babies are particularly susceptible to this. It is treated by the intravenous administration of methylene blue.

Reproductive system

Occupational and environmental exposures may affect female and male reproductive systems and influence different stages in the outcome of pregnancy. Children can be affected by parental exposure to physical and chemical hazards. There has been much concern that various organic environmental contaminants ranging from pesticides to phthalates and other plasticizers, and compounds with oestrogenic properties might cause reproductive harm to the community. In men it has been postulated that exposure to these 'endocrine disrupters' has resulted in falling sperm counts, and an increased incidence of hypospadias and testicular cancer.

Male reproductive system

Subfertility may result from direct damage to sperm cells or their progenitors or from damage to the supporting (Leydig) cells or other supporting components. Azoospermia and oligospermia have been well documented amongst workers exposed to 1,2-dibromo-3-chloropropane (DBCP) and chlordecone (Kepone). DBCP was used as a nematocide for crops, e.g. in greenhouses. Chlordecone was used as an insecticide. Gynaecomastia has been reported in male workers following prolonged contact with oestrogenic agents such as diethylstilbestrol, and in those involved in the preparation of oral contraceptive products.

Effects on the male reproductive system may also occur following exposure to heat (potentially a problem in workplaces such as foundries), microwave and ionizing radiation, cytotoxic drugs, animal growth promoters, fumigants such as ethylene dibromide, and heavy metals, e.g. lead, manganese, and mercury compounds.

Female reproductive system

Effects on the female reproductive system range from alterations in the menstrual cycle—both the amount of menstrual flow as well as the regularity of cycles—spontaneous abortions, and infertility. Rubella can be a problem for female health care workers and those working in microbiological laboratories, especially if adequate procedures are not in place for occupational health vetting and immunization of this occupational group. Concerns about an increase in spontaneous abortions amongst female anaesthetists exposed to anaesthetic gases were investigated, and reviews of the findings suggest that the evidence was generally weak. Nevertheless, occupational exposure standards have been set in the United Kingdom for limiting workplace exposure to nitrous oxide, halothane, enflurane, and isoflurane. Similar concerns about working with visual display units (such as computer monitors) and spontaneous abortions led to several large-scale epidemiological studies. These studies indicated that the association could well have occurred by chance, given that spontaneous abortions are relatively common events and that there has been a rapid increase in use of visual display units in recent years.

Other occupational and environmental exposures that can affect the female reproductive system are ionizing radiation, cytotoxic drugs, lead, and ethylene oxide.

Neurological disorders

Neurological disorders caused by exposure to chemicals

Central nervous system effects

There is very good evidence that exposure to lead (even if relatively low level by occupational standards), usually through drinking-water but possibly also through inhalation, contributes to cognitive deficiency in children. Exposure to chemicals, primarily encountered by workers in manufacturing, construction, and agricultural jobs, can cause transient and persistent effects on the central nervous system (Table 9.4.1.4). Transient central nervous system dysfunction is most commonly caused by exposure to volatile organic solvents, to organophosphate insecticides, or to carbon monoxide. Many low molecular weight fat-soluble organic solvents, especially if chlorinated, are chemically very similar to the halogen-substituted anaesthetic gases, and it is hardly surprising that they have similar biological effects. In each instance, these substances, acting through different mechanisms, may cause central nervous system dysfunction ranging from acute intoxication manifested by light-headedness and dizziness to loss of consciousness and even death. Persistent central nervous system sequelae may occur following one exposure episode if exposure levels are high and the time of exposure is prolonged.

Persistent central nervous system dysfunction, manifesting as neurobehavioural performance deficits, has been reported, following chronic exposure to moderate concentrations of various agents encountered in the workplace, and occasionally in the environment. This syndrome, chronic toxic encephalopathy, consisting primarily of memory impairment, impaired psychomotor function, and mood disorders, has been seen following chronic exposure to lead, styrene, and certain organic solvents. In more severe cases the deficits persist, but do not progress, following cessation of exposure. If behavioural symptoms are present without evidence of abnormal neurobehavioural test performances (i.e. organic affective syndrome) reversal of these manifestations usually occurs following cessation of exposure. Other rare central nervous system effects include a parkinsonian syndrome which may be a consequence of toxic exposures to manganese.

Table 9.4.1.4 Central nervous system syndromes caused by workplace toxins

Disorders	Manifestations	Causal agent
Acute intoxication	Light-headedness	Carbon monoxide
	Loss of consciousness	Organic solvents
	Death (rare)	Organophosphates
Organic affective syndrome	Fatigue	Organic solvents
	Irritability	Lead
	Depression	Mercury
Chronic toxic encephalopathy	Impaired neurobehavioural function (symptoms as above)	Organic solvents
		Lead (usually organometallic)
Psychosis	Marked emotional instability	Carbon disulphide
		Manganese
		Mercury
		Toluene
Parkinsonian syndrome	Tremor, rigidity, akinesia	Manganese
		Carbon disulphide
		Carbon monoxide
Visual disturbance	Impaired acuity or peripheral field defect	*n*-Hexane
		Methanol
		Organic mercury
	Colour vision loss	Organic solvents
Increased intracranial pressure	Headache	Organotin compounds
Paraplegia	Weakness and spasticity	Organotin compounds
Cerebellar or other damage	Ataxic gait	Acrylamide
		Chlordane
		Chlordecone (Kepone)
		DDT
		Methyl mercury
	Epileptic seizures	Lead (usually organic)
		Organic mercury
		Organochlorine insecticides
		Organotin compounds
	Tremor	Carbon disulphide
		Chlordecone (Kepone)
		DDT
		Mercury

Peripheral nervous system effects

Exposure to certain agents (Table 9.4.1.5) may cause either motor or sensorimotor polyneuropathy. Rarely, exposure to lead at high levels for long periods may cause upper-extremity motor neuropathy, consisting of wrist extension weakness or wrist drop. Certain substances (e.g. acrylamide, hexacarbon aliphatic solvents, and certain organophosphorus compounds) may act as axonal toxins causing a mixed sensorimotor polyneuropathy manifesting assymmetrical, distal sensory loss. The hexacarbon straight-chain solvents are typified by *n*-hexane, which is a good example of how hepatic biotransformation may render a chemical more harmful to

Table 9.4.1.5 Peripheral nervous system syndromes caused by workplace toxins

Disorders	Manifestation	Causal agent
Motor neuropathy	Wrist weakness, foot drop	Lead
Mixed sensorimotor neuropathy	Symmetrical distal sensory loss, mild motor dysfunction	Acrylamide
		Arsenic
		Carbon disulphide
		Carbon monoxide
		DDT
		n-Hexane
		Methyl *n*-butyl ketone
		Mercury
		Organophosphorus compounds (selected agents including triorthocresyl phosphate)
		Thallium
Cranial neuropathy		Carbon disulphide
		Trichlorethylene

the body. Progressive oxidation of *n*-hexane leads to the diketone 2,5;hexanedione, which in turn reacts with the free amino group of the amino acid lysine in the axonal membrane. Upon removal from exposure, the symptoms often, but not invariably, recede over a period of months with modest or no residual damage.

Neurological disorders caused by physical factors

In certain occupations, sustained postures such as working overhead may cause muscular hypertrophy or other changes resulting in entrapment of nerve roots or individual nerves. Such conditions are diagnosed by obtaining a careful work history and are managed by modification of the work environment. The above section on musculoskeletal disorders mentions disorders which may be caused by 'repetitive trauma'—notably median neuropathy in the carpal tunnel. The reader is also referred to Section 19.

Hand–arm vibration syndrome (see also Chapter 9.5.11)

Certain jobs involving the use of vibrating hand tools or pneumatic drills may be responsible for the occurrence of peripheral neuropathy as part of 'hand–arm vibration syndrome'. These disorders may originate from a combination of physical trauma to the nerve itself as well as damage to blood vessels which supply the nerves.

Noise-induced hearing loss is discussed in Chapter 9.5.10.

Respiratory disorders

The respiratory tract is, in many occupations, the most important route of exposure to hazardous substances. In many instances of occupational diseases it is the target organ. These conditions are dealt with in Section 18.

Role of psychology in occupational health

There is growing recognition of the importance of psychological factors in a range of occupational health concerns. The following represents the main areas where psychological factors are now considered to have a significant contributory role.

Occupational stress

The reported incidence of work-related 'stress' and mental disorders in the United Kingdom over recent years has increased dramatically (both in absolute rates as well as in comparison with other work-related ill health). A number of factors in the working environment have been identified as potential psychosocial hazards. These can be categorized as in Table 9.4.1.6. However, the relationship between work and mental well being is a complex one, and it cannot necessarily be assumed that a deterioration in the work environment *per se* is the only explanation for the link between the two.

Prolonged exposure to one or more of these conditions may result in a range of symptoms of psychological distress such as feelings of anxiety, irritability or aggressive behaviour, lack of concentration, lack of confidence and an inability to make decisions, sleep disturbance, and fatigue. There may also be associated physical symptoms such as frequent headaches and nausea. Occupational stress is often identified as a result of the individual's inappropriate (maladaptive) coping strategies such as frequent short-term absences, alcohol and other substance abuse, and poor time-keeping, or by uncharacteristically poor work performance. Effective management of occupational stress usually requires an integrated approach

Table 9.4.1.6 Occupational factors that can act as stressors (psychosocial hazards)

Work overload	Quantitative: too much to do in the given time
	Qualitative: demands beyond the skills or organizational capacity of the worker
Work underload	Quantitative: not enough work to do
	Qualitative: monotonous, boring tasks or below the skills of the worker
Timing and control	Shift work
	Limitations on organizing one's own work
Responsibility	Role ambiguity, conflict
	Unclear responsibility and accountability
Organizational culture, and relationships	Lack of communication, participation
	Bullying and other harassment
Financial and future prospects	Inadequate reward or other recognition of 'worth'
	Job insecurity
	Poor training, personal development, or other prospects for advancement
Hazards and comfort	Physical, chemical, and biological hazards
	Other environmental discomfort or concern at work

which includes attention to both the workplace and the individual and consists of intervention at the three following levels:

- Primary intervention focuses on the identification of particular sources of stress in the working environment and the institution of measures to eliminate or reduce these. These should not be viewed solely as ill health prevention but are generally good management practices.
- Secondary intervention focuses on improving the coping skills of employees by the use of specific forms of stress management training (e.g. relaxation, conflict management, assertiveness, time management) and health promotional activities. These are particularly appropriate where workplace stressors are intrinsic to the particular occupation, and therefore not removable, e.g. the potential for aggressive confrontation with members of the public.
- Tertiary intervention is concerned with rehabilitation of psychologically distressed individuals. When anxiety or depression is manifest, pharmacological intervention and behaviour therapy may be needed. Counselling may help although its evidence base is weak. The source of stress may often be multifactorial, and not therefore solely work-related, but it has an impact upon work performance and may be exacerbated by the demands of work.

Medically unexplained symptoms (see Sections 24 and 26)

The response to hazard exposure

A growing number of occupational health complaints are characterized by a lack of a firm diagnosis or clear occupational causation. These include, in particular, complaints that consist of a range of nonspecific symptoms, typically headache, fatigue, nausea, depressed mood, cognitive confusion, and sometimes eye and nasal irritations. They are reported in diverse situations such as in air-conditioned offices ('sick building syndrome'), proximity to low-frequency electromagnetic fields, and perceived exposure to very low (often undetectable) levels of chemicals. Moreover, the prevalence of musculoskeletal complaints in many workplaces has been shown to be related to the presence of psychosocial hazards. An important element is the structure of health beliefs and attitudes which the individual brings to the situation, as well as the social and cultural environment. These influence their response to real or perceived exposure to hazards by determining their selection of which information to attend to and their subsequent interpretation of that information. Specific examples of syndromes with these features which occur in both an occupational and wider community setting may be 'multiple chemical sensitivity' and 'chronic fatigue syndrome'. Current approaches to effective management of these and other similar conditions favour a 'biopsychosocial' approach, which rejects the artificial distinction between a physically and a psychologically based complaint and treats both physical and psychological symptoms simultaneously.

Conclusion

Clinicians can make important contributions in two ways to 'occupational health' and hence to the health and economic well being of their patients and others. In the first instance they should have a high index of suspicion for occupational (and environmental) causes of disease in their patients. These can manifest to physicians in any specialty. Having reached a clinical diagnosis, especially in the case of work-related ill health, they need to liaise with an occupational physician or other occupational health professional, the relevant enforcing authority, or the employer directly so as to remove their patient from the harmful 'exposure' and to control exposure to prevent similar occurrence in the patient and in other workers. Secondly, whether or not the ill health is work-related, the clinician has an important role in giving advice about return to work and achieving occupational rehabilitation.

Further reading

Adams RM (1999). *Occupational skin disease*, 3rd edition. WB Saunders, Philadelphia, PA.

Agius RM, Seaton A (2005). *Practical occupational medicine*, 2nd edition. Hodder Arnold, London.

Aw TC, *et al.* (2007). *Occupational health*, 5th edition. Blackwell Scientific, Oxford.

Baxter P, *et al.* (eds) (2000). *Hunter's diseases of occupation*, 9th edition. Hodder Arnold, London.

International Labour Office (1998). *Encyclopedia of occupational health and safety*, 4th edition. International Labour Office, Geneva.

Levy BS, *et al.* (2005). *Occupational and Environmental Health*, 5th edition. Lippincott Williams & Wilkins, Philadelphia, PA.

Palmer KT, Cox RAF, Brown I (2007). *Fitness to work; the medical aspects*, 4th edition. Oxford Medical Publications, Oxford.

Parkes WR (ed) (1994). *Occupational lung disorders*, 3rd edition. Butterworth-Heinemann, London.

9.4.2 Occupational safety

Lawrence Waterman

Essentials

Any approach to occupational health must acknowledge that accidents in the workplace result in many injuries. Construction, agriculture, and primary extraction are the main causes of fatalities and serious injuries, but many more minor injuries result from all kinds of work.

Health and safety law has developed with an emphasis on accident prevention that is based on designing and managing the working environment by (1) defining appropriate processes and work practices that are safe; (2) developing and maintaining a health and safety culture; and (3) influencing behaviour so that everyone is focused on the best and safest way to do their work.

Establishing this approach to safety management begins with an organization committing itself to a policy influenced by legal obligations and current good practice, such as the developing standards for corporate governance of risks and public reporting. Management systems based on the formula 'Plan–Do–Check–Act' are central to accident prevention, with detailed decisions driven by risk assessments.

A key ingredient to safety is genuine worker engagement, going beyond the legal obligations for consultation. Organizations can improve their safety culture when they recognize that this is the product of individual and group values, attitudes, competence, and patterns of behaviour that determine the commitment to, and the style and proficiency of, their safety programmes. A positive culture requires appropriate leadership, including genuine commitment of the most senior manager(s) in the organization, and an appropriate emphasis on competence, such that the right people, trained and skilled, are doing the right job in the right way, with their supervisors and managers having ready access to competent health and safety advice when required.

Introduction

Accidents, sometimes fatal, are an important cause of illness at work. In 1995, the World Health Organization estimated that every year, worldwide, there were approximately 120 million accidents leading to 20 000 fatalities. By 2005, the International Labour Organization estimated 270 million accidents each year with 351 500 fatalities. China, whose workforce is expanding quickly through rapid industrialization, has reported a rise in fatal accidents from 73 500 in 1998 to 90 500 in 2001. In industries with a poor safety record, such as mineral extraction and agriculture, the toll of accidental injuries is matched or exceeded by the numbers made ill by exposure to health risks. It is therefore appropriate to give serious consideration to the risks of both accidents and illnesses at work.

Accidents at work occur under varying circumstances. Globally, and in the United Kingdom, the largest group of accidents and fatalities occur in the construction industry. Worldwide, one in six fatal workplace accidents occurs on a construction site. However, in the United Kingdom in 2005/6, 28% of all such fatalities were associated with construction work, the higher proportion reflecting economic development away from traditionally hazardous industries such as heavy engineering and mining. But serious accidents continue to occur: fires and explosions in chemical process plants, transportation disasters, and entanglement in machinery. Most accidents involve everyday events such as slips, trips, and hand-tool injuries that most commonly result in only minor injuries.

Research since the 1950s has demonstrated that in any organization, many minor accidents occur for every serious one. This was developed into a strategy for preventing accidental losses, both financial and human, based on the concept of accident triangles illustrating the relationship between minor events and serious accidents (Fig. 9.4.2.1). Despite the diversity of accidents and their outcomes, their causes and the underlying principles of safety management for their prevention are common to all accidents, and to the control of other health hazards at work. The three elements of safety management are designed to address:

- working environment—encompassing physical arrangements, equipment, materials, and the environment in which they are used
- working processes and practices—the way in which the work is expected to be carried out, often embodied in written standard operating procedures
- culture and behaviour—the human element, that takes the workplace and the procedures and brings them to life, summed up as 'this is the way we do things around here'

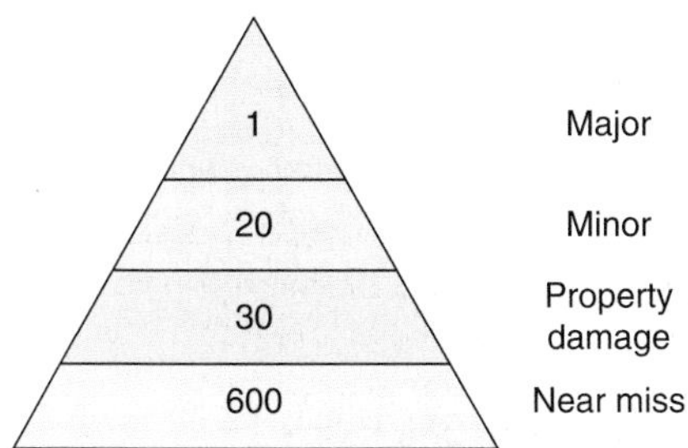

Fig. 9.4.2.1 Accident triangle developed by Frank Bird.

In order to address these elements, employers have increasingly been encouraged to develop formal management systems. The key mechanism adopted for 'encouragement' has been the development of occupational health and safety law. British law from the mid 19th century onwards seemed to reflect Parliament's desire to take action only after a tragedy had happened. As industrial hazards were revealed by research or major accidents, regulators conducted a form of risk assessment and prescribed general control measures. As a result, many different and highly specific sets of regulations ended up on the statute book, with overarching acts, such as the Factories Acts imposing general duties applicable only to defined workplaces, such as factories, workshops, offices, shops, and railway premises. The 1802 Health and Morals of Apprentices Act and subsequent legislation were crucial in driving workplace controls. Many workers were excluded but it was estimated that the 1974 Health and Safety at Work etc. Act brought up to 5 million workers within the ambit of the law.

In the United Kingdom after the First World War, there were developments outside legislation. The Co-operative movement grew into a major developer of social commerce and other organizations, such as the children's organization Woodcraft Folk, were founded on ideas of social improvement. The public began to demand better management of industrial safety, both for moral and economic reasons. The British Industrial Safety First Movement, later the Royal Society for the Prevention of Accidents (RoSPA), promoted accident prevention through committees, workers' participation, the employment of safety officers, joint accident investigations, and the promotion of positive attitudes.

Enlightened industrial management that recognized the cost of accidental losses, legal obligations, and voluntary efforts based on worker engagement and morality was summarized in the 1972 Robens Report, which formed the basis for the Health and Safety at Work etc. Act 1974. Risk assessment, initially implicit, was later made an explicit requirement. Worker engagement, through safety representatives and worker/management committees (at least in the minority of British workplaces with recognized trades unions), was a new element. However, law always seemed to lag behind industrial developments. The 1974 Act established the Health and Safety Commission and the Health and Safety Executive not only to be custodians, developers, and enforcers of the law, but also to be responsible for identifying and disseminating good practice. Although many people accept the need for both enforcement and encouragement in dealing with enlightened and obstinate employers, some call for more prosecutions of companies and individual directors. Employers are no longer expected to adhere slavishly to sets of statutory rules, but to develop their own safety organization and arrangements following good practice. It is now recognized that safety is a key challenge to be addressed by management.

Other events have influenced organizations' approach to risk. Financial scandals (Polly Peck, Mirror Group Newspapers) led to reports from committees chaired by Cadbury (on preventing malpractice), Greenbury (on the role of directors), and Hampel (outlining good governance) that laid the foundations for Turnbull and changes in the rules applying to publicly listed companies in the United Kingdom. Management of risk and safety are essential components of good corporate governance both in the public and voluntary sectors. While these formal risk management requirements were being developed, corporate social responsibility was maturing through the formulation of the Global Reporting Initiative and local ventures such as corporate social responsibility indices, the launch of FTSE4Good, and ethical investment organizations. Their impact should not be underestimated. The history of companies such as Railtrack, where major accidents led to loss of control, should remind directors that they are expected to govern in order to protect the public, the organization, and its shareholders from such disasters.

The size of the problem

During the year 2005/6 212 workers, employees, and self-employed, were killed at work in the United Kingdom. This, the lowest figure on record, reflects both effective accident reduction and a dramatic change in economic activity; there are now many more people working in call centres than in mining. Numbers of nonfatal accidents are less certain, because of under-reporting. Slipping and tripping are responsible for the largest group of major injuries, almost three times the numbers of injuries from moving machinery/objects, from falls, or from direct handling. Of the 2.7 million people on Incapacity Benefit, the largest single group suffer from mental ill health, followed by musculoskeletal disorders. However, an individual's perception of what level of incapacity forces them to be absent from work is clearly influenced by their mental state. The nature of the injuries received and the process of rehabilitation and return to work are clearly important, but the safety practitioner is interested primarily in methods of prevention embodied in safety management systems.

Safety management

Accident prevention requires a safe working environment and safe behaviour, the avoidance of error, by those doing hazardous work. Most practical accident prevention involves physical safeguards or safety rules designed to prevent recurrence of unsafe conditions or acts that have already led to accidents. Similarly, occupational hygienists anticipate, recognize, assess and control hazards to health at work. Accidents usually result from a chain of connected events. Effective safety management addresses the physical conditions and human behaviour that have combined to cause harm. Modern safety management is based on risk assessment and the definition and implementation of methods for preventing harm.

Policy—organizational commitment

Effective health and safety policies set out a clear direction for the organization, indicating what is expected of managers and workers. This may represent no more than a commitment to formal, minimum legal compliance but most bodies express themselves more in the manner of a mission statement. For example, Marks & Spencer is 'committed to ensure the health, safety and well-being of all its employees, customers and others who visit or work on our premises'. The policy is an opportunity clearly to state the responsibilities and arrangements for delivering what is promised.

Planning

The foundation of safety management is planning: to create the right physical conditions and shape the activities undertaken. This includes identifying accident risks inherent in the workplace and the work, assessing their significance and determining suitable precautions. There is a hierarchy of such controls, promulgated across the European Union in the Framework Directive, which targets protection of the whole group of exposed people rather than personal protection:

- Elimination—selection and design of facilities, equipment and processes to prevent exposure to an identified risk. For example, fitting a long-life plastic sign may avoid the need to repaint a high board.
- Minimization—reducing risk. For example, selecting a less-hazardous material, redesigning a tool, or replacing baskets and belts on a conveyor with softer, more resilient materials to reduce noise.
- Personal protection—as a last resort, selecting methods of work and personal protective equipment so that the exposed workers are protected to some extent.

Risk assessment is a critical activity. It requires a degree of knowledge and understanding of the work itself and of the principles of safety management. This means that in practice it is often best conducted by a team made up of workers, managers, and safety practitioners.

Monitoring performance

Residual risks that cannot be wholly eliminated require monitoring. Key performance indicators may be used to explore training courses, supervisory inspections, and accident frequency rates. Accident frequency rates are typically related to workers' hours (i.e. accidents per 100 000 h worked), allowing comparisons between different-sized workplaces and workforces. Active monitoring of key performance indicators is supplemented with reactive monitoring (accident investigations) to determine immediate and underlying causes of failure.

Audit and review

Good organizations learn from their experiences, and apply the lessons. Regular audits check that safety policies are being implemented, that people are discharging their responsibilities, and procedures for safe working are documented and followed. Reviews are more searching and make comparisons with other organizations. They ask the challenging question, 'Are we doing the right or best things?' These processes contribute to an organization's ability to communicate to its stakeholders inside and outside the organization, for example in the annual report. There are three types of corporate report on health and safety:

- minimal reports on injuries and ill health, days lost, comparison with national or sector targets, and information on events such as awards and/or convictions
- comprehensive reports with statistics, trend analysis against performance indicators, director workplace visits, health and safety training days, inspections and audits, emergency drills, etc.
- verified reports, i.e. comprehensive reports that have been reviewed externally

Safety management and safety culture

The effort to create and maintain a physically suitable workplace and equipment, and implement documented safe working practices, will be effective only if it is matched by the engagement of the whole workforce from director to shop floor. A healthy and safe culture is one in which the members of the organization:

- understand and respect the hazards of their operations
- are alert to the many ways in which safe working systems may be breached or bypassed
- are committed to maintaining safe working
- honestly report problems and opportunities for improvement

A key ingredient is real worker engagement, going beyond the legal obligations to consult. Organizations can progress when they recognize that their safety culture is the product of individual and group values, attitudes, competencies, and patterns of behaviour that determine the commitment to, and the style and proficiency of their safety programmes. Those with a positive culture communicate on a basis of mutual trust, share perceptions of the importance of safety, and are confident in the efficacy of preventive measures. This becomes possible only when there is appropriate leadership, including the commitment of the chief executive.

As an example, the strategy adopted by the Olympic Delivery Authority for the planning and construction of venues, test events, and infrastructure for the London 2012 Games, the 2–4–1 approach, has allowed time to establish the right culture. The staff is committed to weaving safe design and construction into all components of London 2012 and its legacy for east London and United Kingdom as a whole. This has been made clear to all the contractors and other suppliers involved in this project.

Competence

Training is an essential part of any company's safety arrangements. How well people have been trained to do what is required, from working safely to conducting risk assessments, is embodied by the term 'competence'. Competence involves having:

- relevant knowledge, skills, and experience
- the ability to apply these appropriately, recognizing the limits of one's competence

Training programmes that include supervision and mentoring, working alongside more skilled people, and attending formal training courses should achieve competence. A personal development plan with skills analysis is required as in the 'Investors in People' standard.

Current issues

Work-related road risk

Work-related road accidents are by far the biggest cause of fatal occupational accidents. Those who drive more than 25 000 miles each year, especially in hazardous industries such as construction or quarrying, have the highest risk of fatal injury. Yet, in most organizations, the prevention of road accidents at work is not treated as part of occupational safety. Employers may increase risk by expecting employees to drive too far; too fast because of time incentives; on routes, under conditions, and in vehicles that are unsafe; when they are tired or untrained to drive an unfamiliar vehicle; when using mobile phones while driving; and in general by encouraging a culture that promotes unsafe driving. Conversely, they can reduce risk levels by avoiding road travel wherever possible, e.g. through videoconferencing; by having clear policies on speed, safe journey planning, vehicle safety, and mobile phone use; by implementing appropriate driver assessment and training; by taking action to combat driver fatigue; and by having clear corporate policies led by the personal example of managers.

What is sensible risk?

Health and safety is under scrutiny. The RSA Risk Commission chaired by Sir Paul Judge is exploring some controversial cases. After a train crash, a major investigation closed railway lines for weeks, diverting traffic onto the roads where many more lives were lost. Health scares over prescription drugs caused thousands of people to stop taking them, leading to far greater damage to health. The press ridiculed the banning of floral hanging baskets and new rules forcing children to wear eye protection while playing conkers. Sensible risk and its management must be defined (see Box 9.4.2.1).

The debate about the extent of legal and other pressures on risk reduction in a complex society is bound to continue.

Box 9.4.2.1 Sensible risk and its management

Sensible risk management should attempt to:

- ensure proper protection of workers and the public
- balance benefits and risks
- enable innovation and learning
- ensure that those who create risks manage them responsibly
- enable individuals to understand that as well as the right to protection, they also have to exercise responsibility

Sensible risk management should not attempt to:

- create a totally risk-free society
- generate excessive bureaucracy and documentation
- scare people by exaggerating or publicizing trivial risks
- stop important recreational and learning activities
- reduce protection of people from risks that cause harm and suffering

The changing world of work

An ageing working population, equality and diversity, and flexible working are some features of the rapidly changing world of work. Over half of the British workforce is now employed in smaller organizations, and over 90% of businesses employ fewer than 10 people. Part-time working has grown, and women now constitute half the workforce. Globalization has intensified competitive pressures, particularly on manufacturers. Public tolerance of accidents is very low and so there is pressure to make further improvements in occupational safety. In the United Kingdom, there will soon be more people over 65 than under 18 and many older people will continue to work past what was regarded as normal retirement age.

Advice and assistance

Those likely to be affected deserve to be properly protected against risks to their health and safety at work. Employers have a duty to protect their employees by sensible risk management. Workers also have a duty to protect their and others' health and safety. Sensible risk management requires effective systems to control those risks that arise frequently and have serious consequences. Balancing benefits and risks often requires expert help. The Management of Health and Safety at Work Regulations require employers to appoint '... one or more competent persons ...' to assist them in meeting their duty of controlling risks. Employers and managers are in the best position to understand the health and safety issues in their business. Coupled with the knowledge of employees, this is often enough to ensure that risks are properly controlled, especially where the hazards are those commonly encountered at work and methods for their control are already established practice. However, if the risks are complex or large numbers of employees are involved, expert help may be needed.

Employers can rely on one or more of their employees to give them competent help, provided the employees have been given enough time, training, and access to information. The employer could:

- train or develop the necessary skills in an existing employee
- recruit someone with the necessary skills
- make use of consultancy support staff

Formally qualified health and safety practitioners can work with a team of risk managers, including occupational-health advisers. In the United Kingdom, the Institution of Occupational Safety and Health sets standards and awards qualifications.

Preventing accidents at work makes an important contribution to the health and well-being of all who may be affected by an enterprise, but achieving this aim requires a systematic approach and leadership.

Further reading

Bird FE, Germain GL (1966). *Damage control (a new horizon in accident prevention and cost improvement)*. American Management Associations, New York.

Eves D, Gummer J (2005). *Questioning performance: the director's essential guide to health, safety and environment*. UK Institution of Occupational Safety and Health (IOSH), Wigston, Leicestershire.

Frick K, *et al.* (eds) (2000). *Systematic occupational health and safety management—perspectives on an international development*. Pergamon, Oxford.

Health and Safety Executive (1997). *Successful health and safety management*, 2nd edition. HSG65. HSE Books, Sudbury.

Reason J (1997). *Managing the risk of organizational accidents*. Ashgate, Aldershot.

Woolf AD (1973). Robens Report—the wrong approach? *Industr Law J*, **2**(1), 88.

9.5

Environmental diseases

Contents

9.5.1 Heat *1393*
M.A. Stroud

9.5.2 Cold *1395*
M.A. Stroud

9.5.3 Drowning *1397*
Peter J. Fenner

9.5.4 Diseases of high terrestrial altitudes *1402*
Andrew J. Pollard, Buddha Basnyat, and David R. Murdoch

9.5.5 Aerospace medicine *1408*
D.M. Denison and M. Bagshaw

9.5.6 Diving medicine *1416*
D.M. Denison and M.A. Glover

9.5.7 Lightning and electrical injuries *1422*
Chris Andrews

9.5.8 Podoconiosis (nonfilarial elephantiasis) *1426*
Gail Davey

9.5.9 Radiation *1429*
Jill Meara

9.5.10 Noise *1432*
Syed M. Ahmed and Tar-Ching Aw

9.5.11 Vibration *1434*
Tar-Ching Aw

9.5.12 Disasters: earthquakes, volcanic eruptions, hurricanes, and floods *1436*
Peter J. Baxter

9.5.13 Bioterrorism *1440*
Manfred S. Green

9.5.1 Heat

M.A. Stroud

Essentials

Rising body temperature triggers behavioural and physiological responses including reduction in physical activity, alterations of clothing, skin vasodilatation, and sweating. Heat-related illness is relatively common, especially with high humidity or prolonged physical activity. Risk can be reduced by acclimatization with repeated heat exposure, but some individuals seem to be particularly susceptible.

Clinical presentations of heat-related illness include (1) 'heat exhaustion'—the commonest manifestation, with symptoms including nausea, weakness, headache, and thirst. Patients appear dehydrated, complain of being hot, and are flushed and sweaty. Treatment requires rest and fluids, given orally or (in severe cases) intravenously. (2) 'heat stroke'—victims often complain of headache, may be drowsy or irritable, and may claim to feel cold. Core temperature is usually 38 to 41 °C, but the patient is shivering with dry, vasoconstricted skin. Treatment requires (a) aggressive rapid cooling—tepid water and fan-assisted evaporation in the first instance, with more invasive measures, e.g. intraperitoneal fluids, if required; (b) close biochemical monitoring; (c) supportive care for organ failure. There is significant mortality.

Thermoregulation in the heat

Most of human evolution took place in Africa and hence all humans are heat tolerant. We try to maintain a near-tropical microclimate against our skin, by using clothing to reduce heat loss to our surroundings. Thermal balance is regulated by the hypothalamus, which integrates information from skin temperature sensors with core temperature data from receptors within walls of large blood vessels and the brain. Rising temperatures trigger both behavioural and physiological responses.

Behavioural changes include reducing physical activity, altering clothing, and seeking shade or cool shelter. Cold drinks are also helpful. Although these responses seem simplistic, decisions may not be straightforward. If physical activity is low and water is in short supply, it is better to increase clothing cover and protect yourself from high radiant heat inputs. If activity must be continued and water is freely available, minimal clothing to permit maximal sweat evaporation is preferable. Immediate physiological responses involve vasodilatation of skin and subcutaneous blood vessels to enhance surface heat loss from radiation, conduction, and convection. The vasodilatation is triggered by a sympathetic cholinergic reflex in response to skin warming, with additional direct effects of heat on arteriolar tone. In a resting person, skin vasodilatation can maintain thermal equilibrium in environmental temperatures up to 32 °C, but with higher temperatures or heat production from activity, core temperatures will rise. This will trigger sweating to promote evaporative cooling.

Heat acclimatization

Repeated heat exposure can increase our capacity to lose heat by about 20-fold. This is partly due to greater skin blood flow from increases in circulating volume and improved vasodilatory responses, but changes in sweating responses are more important. In the nonacclimatized, sweating is triggered by a rise in core temperature of about 1 °C and maximum rates are limited to about 0.5 litre/h. Following acclimatization, a 0.5 °C core rise will trigger the response and sweat rates may exceed 2.0 litres/h. Acclimatization also leads to aldosterone-mediated reductions in sodium loss in both sweat and urine. The acclimatized individual therefore requires no sodium supplementation and giving supplements can delay the acclimatative process. Avoiding them altogether, however, risks salt depletion in nonacclimatized persons during prolonged heat stress. Acclimatization develops swiftly and around 90% of maximum heat tolerance is present after 7 to 10 days on which core temperature has risen by more than 1 °C for more than 1 h. Physical exertion combined with heat makes the changes even more rapid. After returning to cool environments, adaptation is lost in 20 to 40 days.

Susceptibility to heat-related illness

Although we are generally heat tolerant, heat-related illness is relatively common, and a number of factors increase vulnerability. Above an environmental temperature of about 35 °C, we tend to gain heat from our surroundings, and this, along with metabolic heat production, can only be lost via evaporation of sweat. Hot environments with high humidity are therefore the greatest threat. Acclimatization status has a marked influence on heat-related risks, the unacclimatized being prone to hyperthermia and salt depletion, while the fully acclimatized are vulnerable to dehydration from high sweat rates. Dehydration in itself limits sweating capacity and skin blood flow and hence increases risks. It can occur easily since thirst is a poor trigger for adequate drinking. Sweat rates in the acclimatized can also exceed gut capacity for water absorption.

Prolonged physical activity can cause heat illness under quite modest environmental conditions. This is particularly common when individuals are obliged to wear clothing that is insulative or vapour-impermeable. Military heat casualties are sometimes due to these factors, but there have also been fatalities in soldiers who have been susceptible to heat for no obvious cause. Such genetic or constitutional vulnerability should be suspected whenever a heat-related problem occurs following relatively modest heat stress. These people should be strongly advised to avoid similar circumstances in future. Obesity and poor physical fitness are further risk factors in the heat, as is diabetic autonomic dysfunction. Older people are generally heat sensitive and, in addition, are prone to problems from the increased circulatory demands of vasodilatation. Drugs can also induce heat illness (see following paragraphs).

Heat exhaustion

Most casualties in hot environments suffer from heat exhaustion. There is usually a history of prolonged heat stress followed by nausea, weakness, headache, thirst, and sometimes collapse. Patients appear dehydrated with a tachycardia and low blood pressure. If hyperthermic, the casualty should be complaining of feeling hot and should appear flushed and sweaty. The absence of these symptoms and signs, especially with a very high core temperature, suggests heat stroke. Heat exhaustion is ascribable to sodium and/or water depletion, but discriminating between these can be difficult. Sodium depletion tends to be greater if the casualty was poorly acclimatized and hence sweated relatively more sodium than water. Conversely, water depletion is more common in acclimatized individuals. Muscle cramps or whole-body dehydration without marked changes in haematocrit or serum proteins are suggestive of excessive sodium loss, but serum sodium tends to be normal in such cases unless enthusiastic fluid replacement without salt has led to hyponatraemia. This sometimes occurs in runners after completing marathons in hot environments. In predominantly water-depleted heat exhaustion, haematocrit, serum proteins, and serum sodium tend to be high. Renal impairment occurs in either form of heat exhaustion and the treatment of both types often requires 5 to 10 litres of oral or intravenous fluids in the first 24 h. Sodium supplementation is given as appropriate, but if sodium status is uncertain, it is usually safer to provide some than to precipitate acute hyponatraemia.

Heat stroke

Mild heat stroke has occurred when a hot environment or high activity levels have led to pyrexia with cerebral disturbance. Core temperature is usually 38 to 41 °C. The condition frequently follows heat exhaustion but temperature may have risen rapidly allowing no time for salt or water depletion. Sufferers have headaches and may be either drowsy or irritable. They often hyperventilate. The great danger is progression to more severe heat stroke, in which core temperature reaches levels that cause irreversible denaturing of proteins. This usually occurs at above 41.5 °C. Damage is widespread and particularly affects brain, liver, kidney, and muscle. Furthermore, the hypothalamic thermoregulatory centre may fail, switching off vasodilatation and sweating, and switching on cold defences inappropriately. Patients may therefore claim to feel cold and on examination may be shivering with a dry, vasoconstricted skin. A disastrous vicious cycle of increasing temperatures can then ensue.

Treatment for all heat stroke requires early recognition and rapid cooling. Tepid water and fan-assisted evaporation may be more effective than immersion in cold water, which can limit heat loss by stimulating intense peripheral vasoconstriction. Intraperitoneal fluids, paralysis, and ventilation may be needed and, in extreme circiumstances, cooling by cardiac bypass should be considered. Hyperkalaemia, hypocalcaemia, acidosis, rhabdomyolysis, disseminated intravascular coagulation, and hepatic or renal failure are common complications. Ventricular fibrillation is a frequent terminal event. Even if apparently resuscitated and cooled successfully, a 12- to 24-h 'lucid interval' may precede major deterioration. Permanent neurological damage is common.

Drug-induced heat illness

Many drugs can cause mild degrees of pyrexia by inducing local or systemic inflammation or hypersensitivity. Some also increase susceptibility to environmental heat by inhibiting central thermoregulation (e.g. barbiturates and phenothiazines) or reducing sweating capacity (e.g. anticholinergics). Salicylate overdose can generate heat stroke by increasing metabolic heat production while impairing hypothalamic regulation. There are two types of heat-related drug reactions, however, which are particularly dangerous.

Malignant hyperpyrexia

This is usually a dominantly inherited condition, although different gene defects may affect families. Administration of a variety of anaesthetic agents, including halothane and suxamethonium, leads to rapid, massive heat production from generalized increases in skeletal muscle tone. Contraction is triggered at the muscle cell membrane and hence neuromuscular blocking agents are ineffective. Intravenous dantrolene, an inhibitor of muscle calcium flux, is helpful and can be used along with ventilation and cooling/supportive measures. Fatalities are common, and it is therefore important to avoid risks whenever possible. In patients with a relevant personal or family history, in whom an anaesthetic is unavoidable, oral dantrolene should be given prior to the use of low-risk agents.

Neuroleptic malignant syndrome

This condition has similarities to malignant hyperpyrexia but is induced by idiosyncratic reactions to normal doses of antidopaminergic drugs, including phenothiazines and butyrophenones. The onset is less rapid than malignant hyperpyrexia, occurring over a few days. The increased muscle tone is also induced presynaptically and hence neuromuscular blocking agents help. Some recreational drugs, such as ecstasy, may induce this type of response, although most cases of ecstasy-induced hyperthermia are probably cases of heat stroke induced by enthusiastic dancing with limited fluid intake in hot, humid environments.

Further reading

Bouchama A, Knochel JP (2002). Heat stroke. *N Engl J Med*, **346**, 1978–88.

Hodgson P (1991). Malignant hyperthermia and the neuroleptic malignant syndrome. In: Swash M, Oxbury J (eds) *Clinical neurology*, pp. 1344–5. Churchill Livingstone, Edinburgh.

Hubbard RW, Armstrong LE (1988). The heat illnesses: biochemical, ultrastructural, and fluid-electrolyte considerations. In: Pandolf KB, Sawka MN, Gonzalez R (eds) *Human performance physiology and environmental medicine at terrestrial extremes*, pp. 305–59. Benchmark, Indianapolis, IN.

9.5.2 Cold

M.A. Stroud

Essentials

Humans are poorly adapted to cold, which can cause hypothermia, nonfreezing cold injury, and frostbite.

Hypothermia

This occurs especially with wind and wetting, and is seen indoors in older people and those who are thin. At a core temperature of 35 °C, victims complain of cold, act appropriately, shiver, and are peripherally vasoconstricted, but with further cooling they may become confused or drowsy and appropriate physiological responses disappear. Coma occurs at 26 to 32 °C, and death typically at 17 to 26 °C. General investigation and management is as for any comatose patient, but specific issues include (1) accurate measurement of core temperature requires a low-reading rectal thermometer; (2) measurement of serum amylase (risk of pancreatitis) and creatine kinase (risk of rhabdomyolysis); (3) rewarming—if onset of cooling was prolonged, rewarming should generally be slow; (4) diagnosis of death—apparently dead victims should be rewarmed whenever possible before resuscitation is abandoned.

Nonfreezing cold injury

This occurs when skin temperatures below 12 °C are maintained for prolonged periods, particularly in water. This causes paralysis of nerve and muscle, which can be permanent, e.g. trench foot.

Frostbite

Frozen tissues initially appear hard, white, and anaesthetic, but with rewarming become swollen, painful, and blistered. There may be irreversible necrosis, but initial appearances can be misleading and hence early amputation should be avoided. Once thawed, frostbite treatment is similar to that for burns.

Thermoregulation in the cold

It has only been 10 000 to 15 000 years since ancestral humans dwelt exclusively in warm or hot climates. Humans are therefore poorly adapted to cold, and hypothermia occurs quite frequently even in temperate regions. With water immersion it may occur even in the tropics. In truly cold areas, there is also the risk of nonfreezing cold injury and frostbite. Nevertheless, behavioural changes allow us to operate safely even in the coldest environments.

Core temperatures in the cold are usually maintained by adjustments in clothing and physical activity. The latter can increase heat production from a resting 100 W to 1 to 2 kW. This is very effective. Although it takes highly specialized, multilayered clothing to keep warm while inactive in an environment of +5 °C, clothing insulation equivalent to normal office dress (1 clo) will maintain core temperature even in an environmental of −20 °C when working moderately hard.

Our limited physiological cold protection is under hypothalamic control. Falling surface and, to a lesser extent, core temperatures lead to decreased blood flow in the skin due to increased sympathetic adrenergic tone and direct cooling effects of cold on skin arterioles. This minimizes surface heat loss. Unfortunately, vasoconstriction also leads to severe cooling of the hands and feet with problems of temporary skin numbness, muscle weakness, and risks of more permanent peripheral cold injury. It is often this peripheral cooling that limits our capacity to work in the cold.

Falling skin temperatures will also lead to higher resting muscle tone and shivering, especially when declining core temperature releases hypothalamic inhibition of shivering. These mechanisms can only increase resting heat production to around 500 W and, unlike newborn infants and some other mammals, adult humans cannot add significant nonshivering heat production to this figure.

Effects of falling core temperature

Falling core temperature leads to progressive decline in function. At 34 to 36 °C, hypothermic individuals are conscious of feeling cold and try to move around, add clothing, or seek shelter. Simultaneously, physiological defences are activated. With further falls of temperature, mental and physical problems increase. Some people become withdrawn while others exhibit aggression or disinhibition. Once core temperatures reach 33 to 34 °C, victims often stagger and become confused or drowsy. It is also around this point that 'paradoxical undressing' may occur. This phenomenon is well described and appears to be due to hypothalamic dysfunction with alteration of set-point temperature. Victims therefore feel warm or even hot and appropriate behavioural and physiological responses disappear. At core temperatures varying between 26 and 32 °C coma will ensue, and between 17 and 26 °C cardiac output becomes inadequate to sustain life for prolonged periods. The risk of ventricular fibrillation is also high. Nevertheless, successful resuscitations of victims with core temperatures below 15 °C have been reported (see also Chapter 9.5.3).

Causes of hypothermia

A number of factors increase hypothermic risk. Wetting of skin or clothing extracts enormous amounts of heat and reduces insulation of garments. Complete immersion is particularly hazardous and worldwide more than 100 000 people per year die of cold shock or inexorable hypothermia in the water. This far exceeds deaths from drowning without cold. Winds also increase environmental cooling and a still air temperature of +5 °C equates to −50 °C if wind speed is 40 km/h. Coupled with rain, these effects often contribute to hypothermic accidents among hill walkers and mountaineers, although in these cases fatigue may contribute. Prolonged exertion depletes muscle glycogen which reduces heat production capacity from both exercise and shivering. Low blood glucose also impairs hypothalamic temperature control.

Small, thin people cool easily because of their increased surface-to-volume ratios. They also have reduced subcutaneous insulation and low heat-producing mass. A fat person can maintain core temperature at rest, even if mean skin temperature is 12 °C, whereas a thin person struggles to maintain thermal equilibrium with a skin temperature of 25 °C. However, rapid cooling can sometimes have benefits. A small child in cold water may cool so rapidly that vagally triggered bradycardia and lowered brain metabolic demands may permit successful resuscitation after very prolonged immersion.

Older people may also be small and thin and are at risk of so-called 'urban hypothermia'. Poverty, illness, immobility, malnutrition, and a less sensitive regulatory system may contribute but in many cases hypothermia on admission to hospital is secondary to other pathology, e.g. a stroke may have led to prolonged immobility in a cool environment. Drugs that impair consciousness or induce vasodilatation are risk factors, and alcohol is particularly hazardous. Alcoholics with no fixed abode and a tendency to hypoglycaemia are frequent urban cold casualties.

Hypothermic illness

General management of the hypothermic casualty is similar to that for any comatose or semicomatose person. Abnormalities in blood gases, pH, electrolytes, and glucose are common, and pancreatitis or rhabdomyolysis are recognized complications. Accurate measurement of core temperature is surprisingly difficult. Axillary, tympanic, and oral temperatures can all be misleading. A low-reading rectal thermometer is best. Hypothermia has one very specific risk. Pronouncement of death is fraught with difficulty since profound bradycardia, minimal stroke volume, and marked respiratory depression occur. The old adage that you are 'never dead unless warm and dead' must be taken seriously.

A variety of rewarming methods are available. Warm blankets and hot drinks will suffice in many cases but, although they are widely used, metallized 'space blankets' are of no proven benefit. Warmed intravenous fluids are helpful and, in extreme cases, peritoneal warmed fluids or cardiac bypass can be used. Specialized equipment providing heated, humidified air also permits core rewarming. Hot baths are effective but difficult to use safely since a paradoxical fall in core temperature can occur as blood flow is rapidly restored to cold limbs. In general, if cooling was prolonged in onset or duration, rewarming must be undertaken with extreme caution. In critical cases, where rapid rewarming is needed, full resuscitation facilities must be available, although safe defibrillation in the presence of water is impossible.

Careful monitoring during rewarming is vital. Blood volumes are often low due to early cold-induced diuresis, followed by the inability of hypothermic kidneys to retain salt and water. In immersion casualties, hydrostatic effects on the limbs may have promoted additional fluid loss and, if possible, these people must be kept recumbent throughout rescue and rewarming to minimize risks from extreme postural hypotension. Warming cell membranes are extremely unstable, and uncontrollable fluxes in potassium and other electrolytes may occur, although care must be taken in interpreting biochemical results from cold peripheral blood sampling.

Nonfreezing cold injury

Local temperatures of less than 12 °C prevent normal membrane pumping and paralyse nerve and muscle conduction. If such cooling is prolonged, permanent damage may ensue. Immersion in cold water is particularly likely to cause this type of damage and soldiers in military campaigns are frequent victims of 'trench foot'. Long-term damage is likely whenever an anaesthetic, paralysed, cold region becomes hot, red, painful, and swollen after rewarming, although this change may take several days. Degeneration of nerve and muscle can then follow, leading to prolonged anaesthesia, muscle contractures, or inappropriate peripheral vascular control with intolerance to local heat or cold. There may be slow improvement over months or years.

Frostbite

Human tissues freeze at around −2 °C. Ice forms outside cells but the remaining extracellular fluid becomes hyperosmolar and hence severe intracellular dehydration occurs. This denatures proteins. Vascular endothelial cells are particularly vulnerable, and following rewarming, small blood vessels may leak plasma and then become blocked by red cell sludge and clot. Additional ischaemic necrosis is then superimposed on the frost damage.

Frozen tissues appear hard and white and are anaesthetic. Rewarming leads to pain and swelling, often accompanied by blistering. Deep-freezing results in irreversible necrosis but appearances can be misleading, and early amputation of digits should be avoided. If still frozen, rewarming is best achieved rapidly by using immersion in water at 40 to 42 °C, although any thawing should be avoided if refreezing is likely. Once thawed, treatment is similar to that used for burns with prevention of infection paramount. Generous analgesia is required.

Further reading

Dexter WW (1990). Hypothermia. Safe and efficient methods of rewarming the patient. *Postgrad Med*, **88**(8), 55–8, 61–4.

Giesbrecht GG (2000). Cold stress, near drowning and accidental hypothermia: a review. *Aviat Space Environ Med*, **71**, 733–52.

Granberg PO (1997). Cold injury. In: Chant ADB, Barros D'Sa AAB (eds) *Emergency vascular practice*, pp. 119–34. Arnold, London.

Hamlet MP (1988). Human cold injuries. In: Pandolf KB, Sawka MN, Gonzalez R (eds) *Human performance physiology and environmental medicine at terrestrial extremes*, pp. 435–66. Benchmark, Indianapolis, IN.

Stroud MA (1993). Environmental temperature and physiological function. In: Ulijaszek SJ, Strickland SS (eds) *Seasonality and human ecology*, pp. 38–53. Cambridge University Press, Cambridge.

9.5.3 Drowning

Peter J. Fenner

Essentials

Drowning is a major preventable cause of death, most frequently in children and in developing countries. Aspiration (whether of salt or fresh water) is usual in drowning and near-drowning (known as non-fatal, or submersion injury) and leads to cardiac arrest within a few minutes. Death or severe neurological impairment occurs after submersion for more than 5 to 10 min, but much longer durations may be tolerated in hypothermic conditions.

Prevention

Precautions include proper supervision of children in recreation areas such as swimming pools, beaches, and river banks, and of young children and epileptics in baths. Personal flotation devices (life jackets) are the best preventive strategy in boating activities. Prevention and rescue efforts of life-savers are effective in swimming pools and on patrolled beaches.

Clinical features

Prognosis cannot reliably be predicted, but cardiovascular status is a better prognostic indicator than neurological presentation. Patients who are neurologically responsive at the scene of immersion, in sinus rhythm and with reactive pupils, have good outcomes. Those who are asystolic on arrival at hospital and remain comatose for more than 3 h have a poor prognosis unless they are hypothermic. Patients with a normal chest radiograph on admission usually survive.

Management

The factors that influence outcome are (1) immediate management—including rapid rescue; laying the victim on their side for assessment of the airway and breathing to assist drainage of any excess water from the airways and lungs; prompt and effective bystander cardiopulmonary resuscitation, using supplemental oxygen if available, preferably with oxygen of highest concentration possible (e.g. bag–valve–mask) and an oropharyngeal airway, endotracheal tube, or laryngeal mask airway in comatose victims (if suitably skilled personnel are present). (2) Hospital management—important elements are (a) ventilatory support to maintain adequate arterial oxygenation, which may involve the use of extracorporeal membrane oxygenation and/or cardiopulmonary bypass in refractory cases; (b) colloid resuscitation, (c) recognition and treatment of complications, e.g. secondary pneumonia.

Definition

Drowning has most recently been defined as 'the process of experiencing respiratory impairment from submersion/immersion in liquid'. Outcomes of drowning should be classified as death, morbidity, and no morbidity. Recent guidelines suggest that the term 'submersion injury' or non-fatal drowning should replace 'near-drowning', although the latter is still commonly used. The lack of a universally agreed standard definition makes it difficult to evaluate the results of studies of drowning and submersion, particularly as drowning remains difficult to diagnose at autopsy.

Mortality and morbidity

Acute prolonged hypoxia causes haemodynamic effects, cerebral damage, and death. Neurological morbidity in survivors of near-drowning includes difficulties with learning, memory, attention and planning, and cerebral palsy. A large study of childhood immersions has shown that approximately 70% of survivors have no neurological deficit, 30% have some deficit, and 3% will live in a permanent vegetative state.

Epidemiology

The estimated incidence of drowning is 0.5 million per year, making it the fourth most common fatal injury worldwide in the global burden of disease. It is the seventh leading cause of death from unintentional injury in all ages and the second leading cause in children aged 1 to 14 years. Incidences of drowning are highest in children up to 4 years old. In infants and toddlers under 12 months, bathtub and bucket immersions are the highest cause of drowning.

Ten per cent of fatal bucket or tub immersions are attributable to child abuse. Smooth and slippery bathtubs are particularly dangerous and bathtub seats are unsafe, particularly if infants are left unattended. Worldwide, drowning rates in young children, many of whom are unsupervised, have decreased little, despite potentially effective preventive strategies such as fencing of swimming pools, providing education appropriate to the particular circumstances, or increased surveillance. Although there are few such preventive strategies for older children, drowning rates have declined dramatically in the last decade.

Developing countries have the highest rates of drowning. Thirty-eight per cent of the world's drownings occur in the Western Pacific region and Africa, where the drowning mortality rate is 13.1 per 100 000 population per year. Children aged 5 to 14 years suffer the highest mortality rate. Children under the age of 5 years have the highest drowning mortality rate for both sexes. The mothers' age and literacy and family income are identified as risk factors. In Bangladesh, drowning has been shown to be a major cause of childhood mortality: among 1- to 4-year-olds; there are 156 fatal drownings/100 000 population per year. Younger males were at greatest risk of drowning in rural areas, mainly in ditches and ponds. In China, estimated drowning mortality rates for all age groups were 29.8/100 000/year for boys and 29.6 for girls.

In the United States of America in 2000, more than 1400 children younger than 20 years drowned. It is the seventh leading cause of unintentional injury deaths for all ages, the second leading cause of all deaths from injury in children aged 1 to 14 years and the third most common cause of fatality in people under 15 years (after car accidents and asphyxia). Many drownings occur during recreation in swimming pools, spas, hot tubs, lakes, rivers, or oceans. Approximately 53% of victims needed hospitalization or transfer for more specialized care. Drowning rates were highest among children up to 4 years old.

Worldwide, ocean drownings are less common than freshwater drownings, probably because fewer children swim unsupervised in the ocean, and increasing numbers now swim on patrolled beaches in more-developed Countries, where prevention and the rescue efforts of life-saving associations have proved effective. Rate of drowning varies with climate, availability of beaches, lakes, and other natural and artificial water sources, provision of life-saving services, improvements in designs and rules for water craft, and the use of life jackets. Rock fishing carries a high risk of drowning and near-drowning. A genetic basis has been suggested for unexplained drowning or near-drowning.

Ethnicity

White American children aged 1 to 4 years drown twice as often as African-American children of the same age. These accidents usually happen in residential swimming pools. Conversely, in the age group 5 to 19 years, African-Americans drown more often than white Americans. Australian aboriginal children drown more often than nonindigenous children. Worldwide, fatal drowning is generally more prevalent in indigenous races than in others.

Alcohol

Alcohol affects vision, balance, movement, and reasoning and is a major risk factor for drowning in adolescent and adult swimmers, water craft operators, and passengers, who fall overboard while intoxicated. At the time of rescue, resuscitation, or death, 25 to 50% of adult and adolescent victims of drowning had some exposure to alcohol.

Pathophysiology

Aspiration is usual in drowning. Earlier figures had suggested that approximately 10 to 15% of victims of drowning had not aspirated water but recent figures show an incidence of only 2%. In these cases, death may result from laryngeal spasm and asphyxia during submersion. Early animal studies in anaesthetized dogs showed that spontaneous respiratory efforts continued for around 60 s after immersion. Complete cardiac arrest supervenes after 4.5 min (mean 262 s). Recent Chinese bronchoscopic studies in anaesthetized dogs whose lungs were filled with seawater showed that the bronchi fill with bronchoalveolar fluid, causing increasing blood lactate dehydrogenase-L and alkaline phosphatase levels. Electron microscopy shows injuries to type II alveolar epithelial cells, thickened respiratory mucosa, and platelet adherence.

Haemodynamic effects following inspiration of liquid are similar. There is a rapid fall in cardiac output, while pulmonary capillary wedge pressure, central venous pressure, and pulmonary vascular resistance increase. Reduction in the dynamic compliance of the lungs is similar, following inspiration of all types of solutions. However, aspiration of large volumes of hypertonic seawater draws fluid into the lung from the circulation by osmosis, resulting in fluid-filled, nonventilated, but perfused alveoli incapable of normal gas exchange whilst aspiration. However, aspiration of large amounts of hypotonic freshwater may cause sufficient absorption of fluid into the circulation from the alveoli to cause both acute hypervolaemia and haemolysis. Within 1 h, pulmonary oedema develops, resulting in a decrease in circulating blood volume. Early studies suggested that 85% of human drowning victims aspirated 22 ml/kg of water or less, but it has been estimated that about 10% of body weight of water may be absorbed from the lungs during freshwater drowning.

Since the brain has a limited ability to maintain ATP anaerobically when cerebral blood flow is reduced, it suffers irreparable damage within 4 to 6 min. Death or severe neurological impairment occurs after submersion of more than 5 to 10 min. However, in hypothermic conditions, brain activity may be restored after up to 60 min of submersion apnoea. Bystanders' estimates of submersion time are usually inaccurate.

Hypothermia (see Chapter 9.5.2)

A low body temperature generally indicates the severity of the drowning incident. Sudden immersion in ice water causes a reflex cardiorespiratory response, called 'cold shock', causing an initial gasp and hyperventilation despite hypocapnia and also hypertension. Continuous aspiration of cold water results in rapid core cooling, while the circulation is intact. Such victims may survive with little or no neurological deficit after long submersion with extreme hypoxia. After submersion for a maximum of 10 min in water at 16 °C, a good outcome can be predicted in 96.6% of victims. New evidence supports the use of mild hypothermia for periods of 12 to 24 h in comatose drowned victims. A 6-year-old boy, who presented with a rectal temperature of 16.4 °C after a 65-min submersion, survived, apparently neurologically intact when his blood was rewarmed in increments of 3 °C over 96 min. However, later neuropsychological testing revealed cognitive difficulties, especially global memory impairment, despite the fact that MRI and magnetoencephalography were normal. In adults, success is less common. A notable exception was a 31-year-old man with a core temperature of 23 °C who had been asystolic for 80 min but was warmed by cardiopulmonary bypass and recovered.

Despite discouraging data from animal studies, recent reports suggest that in hypothermic submersion-associated cardiac arrest, adrenaline and vasopressin may help to achieve the vasopressor response needed to restore spontaneous circulation prior to rewarming. This treatment could obviate prolonged mechanical cardiopulmonary resuscitation, or the use of extracorporeal circulation. It has proved effective in restoring spontaneous circulation but one patient died of multiorgan failure 15 h later.

In warm-water drowning there appears to be no statistically significant correlation between duration of submersion and survival.

Causes of drowning

Drowning occurs in many different situations: after accidental immersion in people with little or no swimming ability, with head and neck injury, following cardiac and neurological emergencies (including epilepsy), as a result of alcohol and drugs, metabolic disease (including hypoglycaemia), and even child abuse and murder. In countries with long coastlines and many bathing beaches, drowning is common and is often caused by swimmers being caught in 'rip-currents' (also known as 'rips') (large volumes of water returning back out to sea after onshore wave action) (Fig. 9.5.3.1); there is no such entity as the frequently suggested 'undertow'. Swimmers in difficulty may be able to shout for help but, contrary to public opinion, those who are drowning do not. Most drowning victims adopt a characteristic vertical position in the water—legs hanging vertically, head tilted back for quick exhalation and inhalation before bobbing underwater, with no time or sufficient breath to call for help. After only 20 to 60 s, victims may submerge permanently.

Clinical features

Prognostic indicators

None of the recent developments in assessment, treatment, or equipment has improved survival rates among submersion victims. Prevention and rapid rescue remain the most effective means of reducing the toll. The key to a successful outcome and return to productive, full life is early bystander cardiopulmonary resuscitation, early and aggressive advanced life support methods (Fig. 9.5.3.2), induced hypothermia when appropriate, careful rewarming, including extracorporal membrane oxygenation, and extracorporal warming where needed. However, up to 25% of drowning victims presenting to the hospital emergency department will die and a further 6% suffer neurological sequelae. The prognosis cannot be predicted from the initial clinical presentation, laboratory, or electrophysiological examinations, but those with a normal chest radiograph on admission usually survive; Pao_2 may not relate to radiographic appearances. Although the cause and pathophysiological changes of pulmonary insufficiency vary depending on the type and volume of fluid aspirated, serum electrolyte and haemoglobin concentrations (or haematocrit) do not predict survival.

Cardiovascular status

This is a better guide to outcome than neurological status. Mortality is high in victims with circulatory arrest on admission, but those in sinus rhythm with reactive pupils, who are neurologically responsive

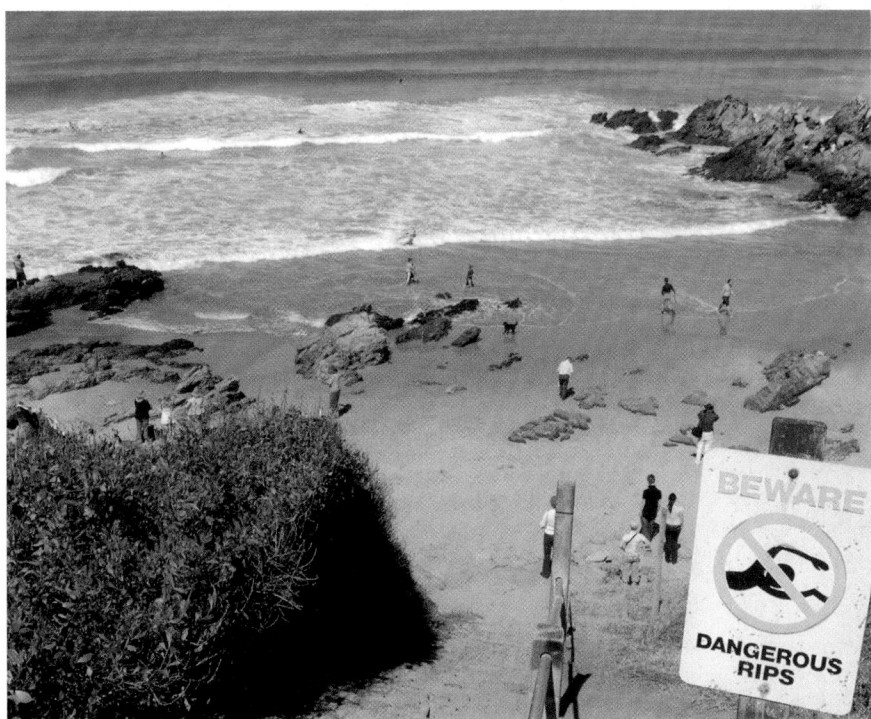

Fig. 9.5.3.1 Australians swimming in the sea at Petrel Cove near Victor Harbour despite notice warning of rip currents.
(Courtesy of D A Warrell.)

at the scene of immersion, have good outcomes. Those who are asystolic on arrival at hospital and remain comatose for more than 3 h have a poor prognosis unless they are hypothermic. Rapid hypothermia from sudden submersion in cold water (see Chapter 9.5.2) carries a relatively good prognosis, compared to insidious hypothermia developed during prolonged submersion that results in cardiac arrest.

Neurological status

Victims who are alert when medical help arrives have a survival rate approaching 100%, whereas the prognosis in those who are comatose with fixed, dilated pupils is poor. Among victims with impaired consciousness, 87% will survive without neurological defects and 2% with minor defects, while 11% will die. Approximately 40 to 50% of victims who are comatose on arrival have incapacitating brain damage. Those with no spontaneous limb movements and abnormal brain stem function 24 h after the accident have a poor neurological outcome.

A modified Glasgow Coma Score is helpful in evaluating neurological injury. A score of 5 or less predicts a mortality risk of over 80%. Pupil reactivity at the time of arrival differentiates survivors from fatalities but could not differentiate between those with minor or incapacitating neurological deficits. Fixed, dilated pupils or total flaccidity are associated with a high mortality. Victims with any motor activity, even posturing or seizures, in the immediate postresuscitation period had a higher incidence of intact survival, but abnormal posturing that persisted or recurred after 12 to 24 h indicated a high probability of severe brain damage.

An abnormal CT scan in the initial 36 h following an immersion incident is associated with a dismal prognosis. MRI with qualitative and quantitative MR spectroscopy data may allow a more accurate prognosis.

The gravity of the early clinical state, the estimated duration of cardiorespiratory arrest, and the severity of the hypothermia, seizures, and paroxysmal EEG activity do not determine the severity of submersion injury encephalopathy. Early EEG patterns with moderate background activity, sleep patterns, response to auditory and painful stimulations, and numerous beta rhythms suggest a good outcome, whereas bad outcomes are suggested by high voltage, rhythmic delta waves; biphasic sharp waves; monotonous EEG, 'burst-suppression' pattern, and absence of beta rhythms. Children who show no spontaneous movements and have abnormal brainstem function 24 h after submersion injury are likely to suffer severe neurological deficits or death.

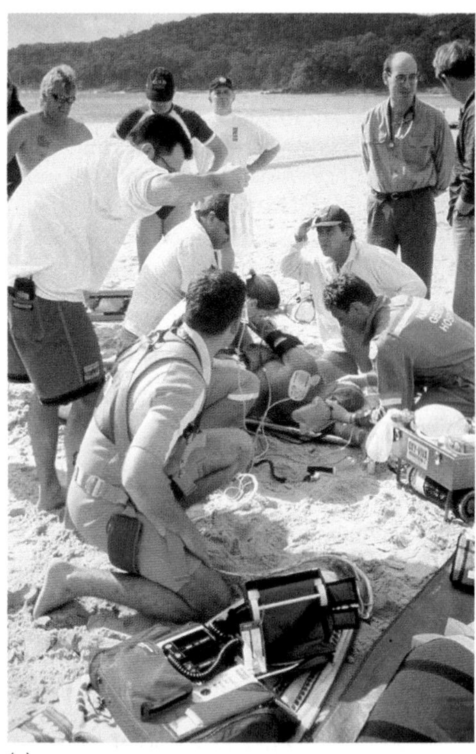

(a)

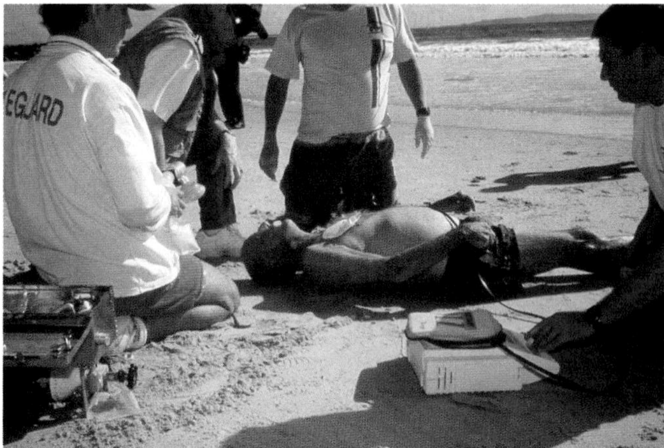

(b)

Fig. 9.5.3.2 Cardiopulmonary resuscitation including defibrillation being carried out on the beach by Australian surf life-savers, in a man who suffered a cardiac arrest while swimming.
(Courtesy of P J Fenner.)

Treatment

Victims of submersion injury must be treated immediately for ventilatory insufficiency, hypoxia, and the resulting acidosis. A successful outcome depends on early effective resuscitation at the scene and on competent intensive life support. In-water resuscitation is effective within 5 mins of the shore, or longer, if the victim shows signs of increased activity after the initial breaths of the shore.

Immediate

Laying victims on their side for assessment of the airway and breathing will assist drainage of any excess water from the airways and lungs (Fig. 9.5.3.2). If necessary, on-site cardiopulmonary resuscitation should be started as soon as possible using supplemental oxygen if available, preferably in the highest concentration (e.g. bag–valve–mask). An oropharyngeal airway, endotracheal tube, or laryngeal mask airway should be inserted in comatose victims, if suitably skilled personnel are present. Pulse oximetry is helpful. Vomiting and regurgitation are significant risks during early resuscitation. Respiratory and cardiopulmonary arrest may occur after an apparently successful rescue, mandating close, uninterrupted monitoring and the early administration of oxygen to all immersion victims.

At the hospital

On arrival at the hospital, after a clear airway and cardio-circulatory support have been established, arterial blood gas tensions and pH should be measured. The pH of the blood will indicate whether there is a residual metabolic acidosis after a substantial period of hypoxia.

Mechanical ventilation may be necessary with positive end-expiratory pressure, or continuous positive airway pressure to maintain arterial oxygen pressure above 10 kPa with an inspired oxygen fraction below 0.6.

After both freshwater and seawater aspiration, large volumes of intravenous colloid are usually needed while circulating blood volume and cardiac output are estimated. Freshwater aspiration is more likely to cause pulmonary oedema. A central venous catheter or pulmonary artery catheter helps to assess the effective circulating blood volume to guide fluid therapy. Failure of response to intravascular replacement with 20 ml/kg of colloid is an indication for starting inotropes. Steroid and prophylactic antibiotic therapy do not appear to increase the chance of survival.

Inpatient treatment

Extracorporeal membrane oxygenation has been proved to be effective after drowning. Patients with severe hypoxaemia may have irreversible cerebral ischaemia. A 3-year-old drowned girl in refractory cardiorespiratory arrest was successfully resuscitated using cardiopulmonary bypass, and then extracorporeal membrane oxygenation for 4 days. Despite a prolonged period in a vegetative state, she later made an almost complete neurological recovery.

If adult respiratory distress syndrome occurs (see Chapter 17.5), it is usually within 6 h of admission. There is evidence that alveolar epithelial barrier function is well preserved even after aspiration of large quantities of hypertonic salt water. Surfactant has been used with some success in refractory respiratory failure in near-drowning but it is expensive.

The risk of secondary pneumonia is high, especially when mechanical ventilation has been used. Although prophylactic antibiotics are not recommended, broad-spectrum antibiotics may be required. Mild reversible renal impairment is rare. Initial serum creatinine, marked metabolic acidosis, abnormal urinalysis, or significant blood lymphocytosis are markers of impending acute renal failure.

Prevention of drowning

Swimming pools and natural bodies of water are the greatest risk to young children. Preventive measures include public media education and campaigns, parental education and supervision, training in cardiopulmonary resuscitation, better safety standards, and safety devices such as the fencing of swimming pools. The number of pool drownings in Brisbane, Australia, decreased after legislation made pool-fencing compulsory. Strategies for the prevention of drowning should also consider hazards in rural areas. Multilingual notices on public beaches are important (Fig. 9.5.3.3) but are often ignored (Fig. 9.5.3.1).

Swimming ability and safety skills of young children may be improved by training. Education of the public is essential. In Australian surf, only 17% of rescues and resuscitations, up to 95% of them successful, occurred within patrolled areas, while 55% (62% of them successfully) occurred outside patrolled areas. Resuscitation success rates fell with increasing distance from patrolled areas. Among nonboating drownings in Australia, 4.7% are among overseas tourists, 89% of whom drown in the ocean.

An adult should supervise all epileptic children and infants aged under 3 while they are in the bath. Currently, up to 89%

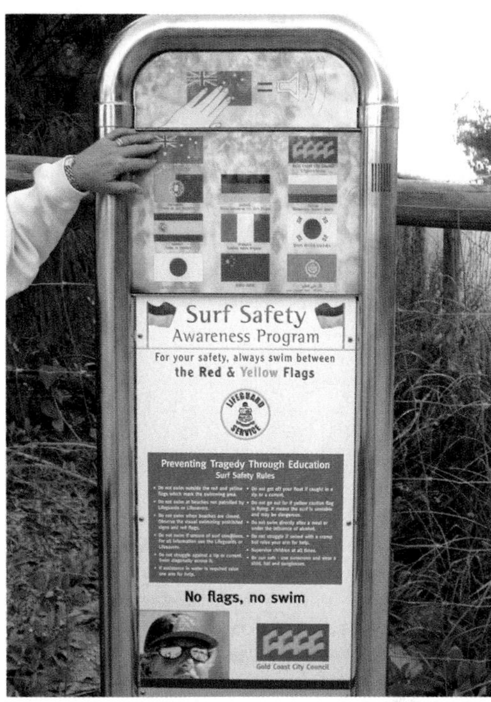
Surf Safety
Awareness Program
For your safety, always swim between
the Red & Yellow Flags
Preventing Tragedy Through Education
Surf Safety Rules
No flags, no swim

Fig. 9.5.3.3 Multilingual talking sign warning of dangers on an Australian beach. (Courtesy of P J Fenner.)

of children aged 35 to 59 months and 6% of those younger than 3 years of age are bathed without adult supervision.

Drownings associated with boating and personalized water craft can be prevented by using life jackets (personal flotation devices), but as many as 50% of boaters do not use them. Efforts to increase their use should target adolescents, adults, and boating enthusiasts, especially those using motor boats. In Alaska's commercial fishing industry, specific measures designed to prevent drowning after vessels have capsized and sunk have proved successful.

In most age groups, more men drown than women. This probably reflects men's overestimation of their abilities, and perhaps greater alcohol consumption. Middle-aged men dominate the group who die of cardiac events (mostly on the surface) (Fig. 9.5.3.2). Fatalities from breath-holding hypoxia during diving tend to occur in young males. Hyperventilation to increase breath-hold time is a dangerous practice that should be discouraged. Drownings are rare at supervised water parks, thanks to the large number of lifeguards on duty.

Further reading

Bierens J, *et al.* (eds.) (2006). *The handbook on drowning*. Springer, Berlin.

Hasibeder WR (2003). Drowning. *Curr Opin Anaesthesiol*, **16**, 139–45.

Idris AH, *et al.* (2003). Recommended guidelines for uniform reporting of data from drowning: the 'Utstein style'. *Resuscitation*, **59**, 45–57.

Papa L, Hoelle R, Idris A (2005). Systematic review of definitions for drowning incidents. *Resuscitation*, **65**, 255–64.

Piette MH, De Letter EA (2006). Drowning: still a difficult autopsy diagnosis. *Forensic Sci Int*, **163**, 1–9.

Salomez F, Vincent JL (2004). Drowning: a review of epidemiology, pathophysiology, treatment and prevention. *Resuscitation*, **63**(3), 261–8.

van Beeck EF, *et al.* (2005). A new definition of drowning: towards documentation and prevention of a global public health problem. *Bull World Health Organ*, **83**, 853–6.

9.5.4 Diseases of high terrestrial altitudes

Andrew J. Pollard, Buddha Basnyat, and David R. Murdoch

Essentials

Ascent to altitudes above 2500 m leads to exposure to hypobaric hypoxia. This affects performance on first arrival at high altitude and disturbs sleep, but physiological changes occur over time to defend arterial and tissue oxygenation and allow the individual to adjust. This process of acclimatization includes (1) an increase in the rate and depth of breathing; and (2) an increase in red cell mass, and in red cell 2,3-diphosphoglycerate. Acclimatization is no longer possible at extreme altitude (>5800 m) and the exposed individual will gradually deteriorate.

Altitude illness results from a failure to adjust to hypobaric hypoxia at altitude. Risk is increased by ascent to higher altitudes, by more rapid gain in altitude, and (in some people) genetic predisposition; the condition may be avoided in most cases by slow, graded ascent. Clinical presentation occurs soon after arriving at a new altitude, most often manifest as one of three conditions:

Acute mountain sickness (AMS)

A common condition that presents with non-specific symptoms, including headache and anorexia. The victim is likely to be apathetic, but clinical examination is generally unremarkable. Mild cases usually resolve with rest and avoidance of further ascent. Those whose symptoms fail to resolve (or worsen) should descend immediately. Treatment with acetazolamide (which can also be used as prophylaxis) or dexamethasone is often given in severe cases.

High-altitude cerebral oedema

An uncommon condition that typically presents with worsening symptoms of AMS and ataxia, with progressive neurological symptoms including behavioural changes, confusion, and impairment of consciousness. Papilloedema and focal neurological signs may be present. Treatment is urgent, with the most important measure being descent. Oxygen or simulated descent using a portable hyperbaric chamber can be helpful. Dexamethasone is widely recommended (and can be used as prophylaxis).

High-altitude pulmonary oedema

A relatively uncommon condition with significant mortality that typically presents with dyspnoea and cough. Signs include low-grade fever, tachycardia, tachypnoea, basal crepitations, and (in late disease) cyanosis. Treatment is urgent, with the most important measure being descent. Oxygen should be given if available. Simulated descent using a portable hyperbaric chamber can be helpful. Nifedipine reduces pulmonary artery pressure, relieves symptoms, and is usually given (and can be used as prophylaxis).

Chronic mountain sickness (Monge's disease) is a disease of adults who reside for prolonged periods at high altitude and develop polycythaemia and eventually cor pulmonale. Symptoms appear to resolve with descent, but treatment with venesection has been attempted in those who remain at altitude. High-altitude pulmonary hypertension has been described in both infants and adults, predominantly native lowlanders who ascend to and reside at high altitude: this also appears to resolve on descent.

Pre-existing medical conditions are mostly little affected by ascent to altitude, but people particularly likely to be affected by hypoxia/altitude include those with (1) coronary ischaemia and a strongly positive exercise treadmill test; (2) sickle cell disease or trait; (3) chronic pulmonary disease, especially pre-existing pulmonary hypertension from any cause.

Introduction

The high-altitude regions of the world are commonly regarded as remote and inaccessible, except to a relatively small number of hardy individuals. However, a surprisingly large number of people live permanently at high altitudes and increasing numbers of low-altitude sojourners visit these regions each year. An estimated 140 million people reside above 2500 m, predominantly in Asia, South America, and North America. In South America, miners and astronomers work at altitudes over 4500 m. Recreational activities, such as trekking, skiing, and pilgrimages, regularly take travellers to altitudes between 3000 m and 5000 m. All these people are susceptible to high-altitude illnesses, which can be fatal.

The high-altitude environment

Although the proportion of oxygen in the air remains constant at 21%, barometric pressure decreases with increasing altitude, and this is accompanied by a corresponding fall in partial pressure of oxygen (Po_2) (Fig. 9.5.4.1). High altitude is a hypoxic environment. At 2500 m, the barometric pressure and inspired Po_2 are about 75% of the sea level values. At 5000 m, which is close to the maximum height for permanent human habitation, Po_2 is about half of the sea-level value. On the summit of Mount Everest (8848 m), Po_2 is about one-third of the sea-level value. In human physiology, the definitions in Box 9.5.4.1 are commonly used

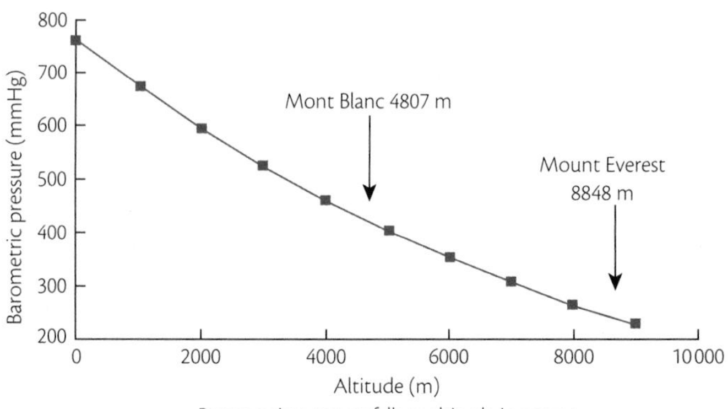

Fig. 9.5.4.1 Change in barometric pressure with altitude.

Box 9.5.4.1 Altitude—definitions

Intermediate altitude (1500–2500 m)

Physiological changes due to hypobaric hypoxia (such as reduced exercise performance and increased ventilation) are detectable, but arterial oxygen saturation remains above 90%. Altitude illness is uncommon, but possible.

High altitude (2500–3500 m)

Altitude illness is common following rapid ascent to this altitude.

Very high altitude (3500–5800 m)

Arterial oxygen saturation falls below 90%. Altitude illness is common and marked hypoxaemia can occur during exercise and sleep.

Extreme altitude (>5800 m)

Further acclimatization cannot be achieved, progressive physiological deterioration occurs, and survival cannot be maintained permanently. Marked hypoxaemia occurs at rest.

In addition to hypoxia, there are several other characteristics of the high-altitude environment. There is a fall in temperature of approximately 1 °C for every 150 m rise in altitude, irrespective of latitude, so that high-altitude areas are considerably colder. Ultraviolet penetration increases by approximately 12% for each 1000-m altitude gain, increasing the risk of sunburn, ultraviolet keratitis, and other sun-related problems. The low humidity contributes greatly to fluid loss and dehydration, as does the increased solar radiation, which may be very much exaggerated by reflection from snow.

Effects of hypobaric hypoxia

Reduction in exercise performance is one of the profound effects of ascent to high altitudes, and is associated with increased fatigue. Maximal oxygen consumption decreases by approximately 10% for each 1000-m gain in altitude above 1500 m, and this does not recover appreciably with acclimatization. This reduced maximal oxygen consumption may be due to a reduction in mitochondrial Po_2, interfering with the function of the electron transport chain, or through central inhibition in the brain. Genetic factors may also be partly responsible for individual variations in exercise performance at high altitudes. For example, mountaineers who perform well at high altitudes tend to have a variant of the angiotensin-converting enzyme gene.

Sleep is also disturbed at high altitude. There is difficulty getting to sleep, frequent arousals, less rapid eye movement (REM) time and decrease in slow-wave sleep. Periodic breathing, characterized by episodes of hyperpnoea followed by apnoea, is relatively common among travellers to altitudes over 2500 m. It is thought to result from instability of the control system through the hypoxic drive or the response to CO_2, and is usually minimized by use of acetazolamide. Hypoxaemia during apnoeic episodes during periodic breathing probably accounts for some of the arousals from sleep that are experienced at high altitude.

Neuropsychological changes at high altitude are often quite subtle, although various changes in mental performance have been documented. At altitudes over 4000 m, there are effects on attention span, short-term memory, arithmetic ability, and decision making.

Acclimatization

Acclimatization is the process by which people gradually adjust to the hypoxia of high altitude. In general, it is a poorly understood physiological process involving a series of adjustments that occur over hours to months. These changes favour increased oxygen delivery to cells and efficiency of oxygen use. In contrast, the term 'altitude adaptation' refers to physiological changes that occur over longer time periods (decades and generations) and confer advantages for life at high altitude. Acclimatization reduces the impact of high-altitude hypoxia, but does not return the body to its sea-level condition.

A few of the principal steps involved in acclimatization to high altitude may be summarized as follows.

Ventilation

Hyperventilation is the most important feature of acclimatization and serves to defend alveolar Po_2. Increases in the rate and depth of breathing occur in response to hypoxic stimulation of the peripheral chemoreceptors, mainly the carotid bodies. Hyperventilation increases alveolar Po_2 in the face of decreased inspired Po_2, and also reduces alveolar Pco_2 leading to a respiratory alkalosis. The alkalosis initially limits increased ventilation, but this is eventually compensated for by a rise in urinary excretion of bicarbonate that returns pH towards normal (but never reaches normal). The degree of hyperventilation in response to high-altitude hypoxia can be profound. Alveolar ventilation increases approximately fivefold on the summit of Mount Everest where inspired Po_2 is less than one-third of its sea-level value.

Blood

Erythropoietin secretion is increased within 2 h of ascent to high altitude, resulting in a relatively slow increase in red cell mass over days to weeks. This, in turn, increases the oxygen-carrying capacity of the blood and permits optimal oxygen transport to tissues. Contrary to popular perceptions, polycythaemia contributes little to initial acclimatization and does not play an important role in acclimatization of people travelling to high altitude for only a week or so. The increase in red cell mass is partly offset by the higher haematocrit, which increases blood viscosity and decreases blood flow. The shift in the oxyhaemoglobin dissociation curve to the right, which occurs on ascent and is due to an increase in red cell 2,3-diphosphoglycerate, favours unloading of oxygen in the tissues, but this particular adjustment is offset by the shift to the left caused by alkalosis.

Circulation

Although there is an abrupt increase in cardiac output on ascent to high altitude, there follows a progressive decrease in stroke volume and maximal cardiac output is reduced at all levels of exercise, including maximal exercise. Although there is no evidence for insufficient myocardial oxygenation, there is disagreement about whether the myocardium is depressed by hypoxia. There is an immediate redistribution of blood flow: coronary and cutaneous flow both fall, cerebral and retinal flow increase, and renal flow decreases initially, and then, with acclimatization, returns to normal.

Fluid balance

Central blood volume increases with ascent to high altitude due to peripheral venous constriction. This, in turn, suppresses antidiuretic hormone and aldosterone and induces a diuresis.

Haemoconcentration and diuresis are normal responses to high-altitude exposure.

Extreme altitudes

Acclimatization in adults seems to be possible up to about 5000 to 5500 m. Above this height, there is a fine balance between adjustment to high altitude and deterioration as a result of chronic hypoxia. The term 'high-altitude deterioration' refers to the general deterioration in physical condition that occurs after lengthy stays at extreme altitudes. Typical features include progressive weight loss, worsening appetite, poor sleep, and increased lethargy.

The most extreme altitudes, such as the summit of Mount Everest, are very close to the limit of human tolerance to hypoxia. Indeed, early estimates indicated that all available oxygen on the summit of Mount Everest would be required for basal oxygen uptake, with none left over for physical exertion. Alveolar gas samples taken near the summit of Everest (8400 m; barometric pressure, 36.3 kPa) show an inspired Po_2=6.27 kPa, and alveolar Po_2=4.00 kPa. Mean arterial gas values at this altitude were: Po_2 3.3 kPa; Pco_2 1.8 kPa; pH 7.5; oxygen saturation 54%. Consequently, it is extraordinary that some humans are able to climb to this height without using supplementary oxygen. A number of reports have suggested mild, possibly permanent, defects in cognition in climbers who have ascended to extreme high altitudes.

Illness due to altitude

Until high-altitude acclimatization has occurred, lack of physiological compensation for hypobaric hypoxia may manifest as altitude illness. Acute mountain sickness (AMS), high-altitude pulmonary oedema (HAPE), and high-altitude cerebral oedema (HACE) are recognized distinct clinical syndromes of altitude illness, although there is substantial overlap between the three syndromes. AMS is the most common.

Development of altitude illness is most likely after a rapid ascent, although there is considerable variation in susceptibility between individuals. Genetic factors are likely to be important in determining susceptibility but a number of other factors are contributory and are discussed in the following paragraphs.

Acute mountain sickness

Incidence rates of AMS vary with the absolute altitude gained and the speed of ascent. Some 30 to 50% of those who ascend to 4500 m on a standard trek in the Himalaya develop AMS. The incidence of AMS is greater at higher altitudes and with greater gains in altitude, and may be precipitated by physical exertion. Some people have a history of recurrent AMS, suggesting individual susceptibility.

Typically, symptoms of AMS begin 6 to 12 h after ascent to altitudes over 2500 m. The familiar features of AMS are non-specific symptoms that are readily confused with many other illnesses and include:

- headache
- nausea
- vomiting
- fatigue
- anorexia
- dizziness
- sleep disturbance

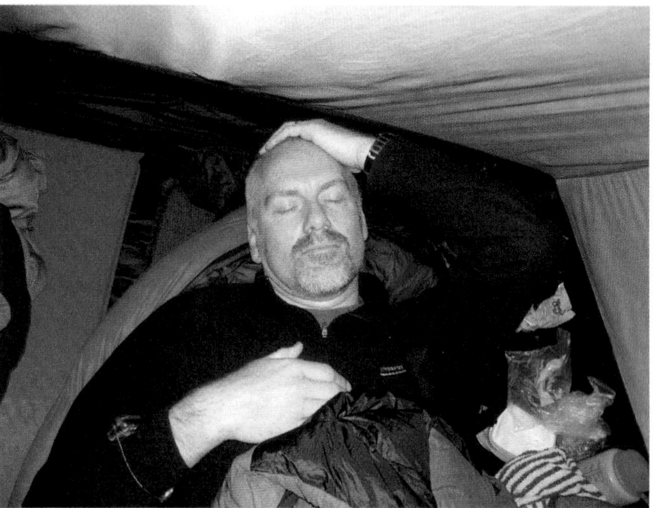

Fig. 9.5.4.2 One of the authors (DM) with symptoms of AMS (headache, anorexia, lethargy, and malaise) on Mount Kilimanjaro in 2006 after rapid ascent to 4100 m.
(Courtesy of J Crump.)

For practical purposes, people ascending to altitude with unexplained symptoms that include the above mentioned should be assumed to have AMS. The headache is typically worse at night, on lying down and with Valsalva's manoeuvre. Anorexia is often pronounced. Clinical examination is typically unremarkable, although it may reveal some peripheral oedema or crepitations on auscultation. There may be tachycardia and elevated core temperature. Typically, the person with AMS is apathetic and withdrawn, seeking solitude in their sleeping bag (see Fig. 9.5.4.2).

The aetiology of AMS is unknown. It has been argued that it is a mild form of cerebral oedema since it often precedes development of HACE, and the symptoms of AMS include symptoms of headache and nausea consistent with a mild increase in intracranial pressure. Brain imaging studies have not found increases in brain volume or oedema in the first 6 to 10 h after exposure to hypoxia despite symptoms of AMS, but it may be that these techniques lack sufficient sensitivity. However, brain volume does increase after longer exposure to hypoxia. Some recent evidence suggests that oxidative stress may be involved in the development of AMS.

Mild AMS usually resolves if the victim avoids further ascent and rests. Paracetamol (acetaminophen) or other analgesics may bring relief from headache. Those, whose symptoms fail to resolve, or worsen, should descend immediately. More severe symptoms of AMS will also resolve with descent but some people will require treatment to facilitate descent. Supplementary oxygen may be beneficial if available. Treatment with acetazolamide (250 mg orally, three times daily), or dexamethasone (4 mg orally, four times daily) can be useful in severe cases. Acetazolamide is a carbonic anhydrase inhibitor, which increases renal excretion of bicarbonate to induce a metabolic acidosis. The hyperventilation induced by the respiratory compensation improves oxygenation to relieve symptoms.

Portable hyperbaric chambers are widely used on trekking routes and can be pressurized to simulate descent and temporarily relieve symptoms, in order to facilitate descent. These chambers are inflated with a hand or foot pump to achieve the barometric pressure of a lower elevation. CO_2 is removed by the airflow generated by the pumping action, and a CO_2 scrubber is included in some models.

AMS can be avoided or prevented in most cases by carefully graded ascent. Above 3000 m, a rate of ascent of 300 to 600 m per day, with a rest day every 1000 m, will avoid symptoms for most people. However, there is considerable individual variation. For some destinations, itineraries are rapid enough to induce symptoms of AMS in a large proportion of travellers. For this reason, prophylaxis with acetazolamide, started on the day before ascent over 3000 m (250 mg twice daily or 500 mg daily of the slow-release preparation) is frequently recommended for prevention and is effective. Since the side effects induced by this drug may be serious (allergic reactions) or intolerable (paresthesiae), test doses should be tried before it is used for prophylaxis during ascent. One meta-analysis suggested that doses of acetazolamide lower than or equal to 750 mg per day were ineffective, but this is not widely accepted by expert interpretation of the available data and total dose of 500 mg per day remains the most widely used. There is evidence that acetazolamide doses of 125 mg twice daily may be effective in some people. Dexamethasone may also be useful for prophylaxis although its mechanism of action is unknown. Ginkgo biloba has been advocated for prevention by some authors, but recent trials do not support its effectiveness. Theophylline reduces periodic breathing during sleep, but not oxygenation and probably has little utility in prophylaxis.

High-altitude cerebral oedema (HACE)

Unlike AMS, which is quite common among travellers to high altitude, HACE and HAPE are relatively uncommon. HACE is more typical after ascent to altitudes over 4000 m, but cases have been described even at the modest elevation of 2100 m. Higher rates are found at the highest altitudes and after more rapid ascent. At 4000 to 5500 m, rates of 1% have been described amongst trekkers. HACE is usually preceded by AMS and frequently associated with HAPE (see following paragraphs). Symptoms of AMS have usually been present for 1 to 2 days before the onset of HACE. Risk factors for the development of HACE are probably similar to those recognized for other forms of altitude illness. HACE may be more common in the presence of intracranial space-occupying lesions such as cysts or tumours.

Worsening symptoms of AMS and ataxia are typical early signs of development of HACE. Behavioural changes (being irrational, withdrawn, or exuberant), confusion, and a change in conscious level leading to coma may ensue. Papilloedema may be present. Both focal neurological signs and cranial nerve lesions may be present. Brain imaging studies show typical signs of cerebral oedema with changes in white matter signal, compression of sulci, and blunting of gyri. Lumbar puncture, if undertaken, reveals raised pressure but is otherwise normal. HACE is indistinguishable clinically from many other causes of compromised cerebral function. There is a very high mortality among those who develop coma.

It is likely that HACE is a vasogenic oedema resulting from injury to the blood–brain barrier, following disturbances in cerebral autoregulation. Cytotoxic oedema from release of mediators in the central nervous system in response to hypoxia may also contribute.

In view of the seriousness of HACE, treatment is urgently required and the most important measure is descent. Oxygen therapy or simulated descent using a portable hyperbaric chamber may improve oxygenation and symptoms and thus facilitate descent. Intravenous dexamethasone (8 mg) followed by 4 mg, orally four times per day may improve symptoms and is widely recommended. HACE tends to recover more slowly than other forms of altitude illness and ataxia is often the last sign to disappear.

HACE is probably prevented by slow, graded ascent (see AMS in earlier paragraph) and prophylaxis with dexamethasone may be beneficial for those with a risk of the condition.

High-altitude pulmonary oedema (HAPE)

HAPE typically occurs within 4 days of ascent to altitudes over 2500 m and may be accompanied by symptoms of AMS or HACE. HAPE presents more frequently with increasing altitude: 1 to 2% of people may be affected at 4500 m, but much higher rates (10%) have been reported after rapid ascent at this altitude. It can also occur in those who have become acclimatized at one altitude and then make a further ascent. HAPE is a serious form of altitude illness and is associated with fatality when not managed urgently and appropriately.

HAPE is more common in men than women. Risk of its developing is increased by cold, rapid ascent, exertion, coexistent viral infection, and possibly by drugs, such as alcohol, that cause respiratory depression. Individual susceptibility is well recognized and those who have previously suffered from HAPE appear to be more susceptible in the future. There are various genetic associations described including pulmonary surfactant protein A, HLA DR6, HLA DQ4, epithelial sodium channel protein, and endothelial nitric oxide synthase genes. People with raised pulmonary blood flow or an exaggerated hypoxic pulmonary vascular response may also be more susceptible (i.e. those with atrial septal defect, absent right pulmonary artery or a chronic respiratory condition). High-altitude dwellers who travel to sea level are at particular risk of re-entry HAPE when they return to high altitude.

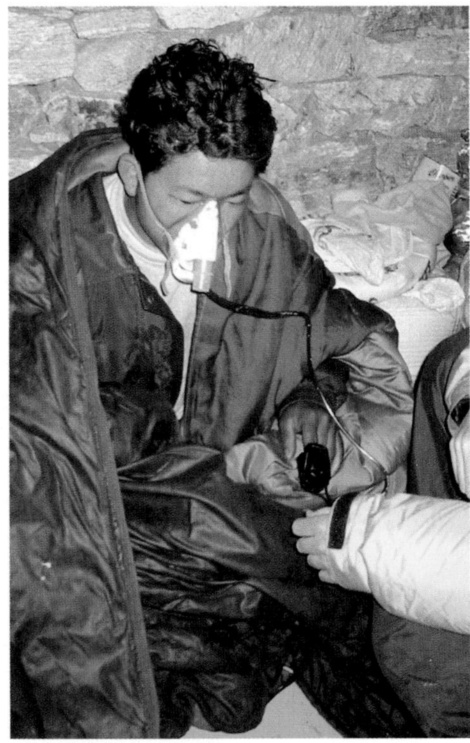

Fig. 9.5.4.3 Hypoxic Nepali porter with HAPE, receiving therapy with supplementary oxygen.
Courtesy of S. Currin and P. Szawarski.

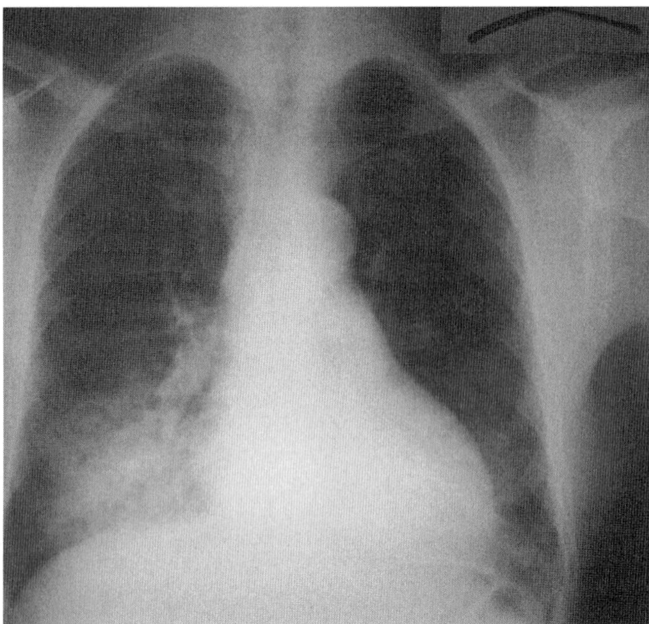

Fig. 9.5.4.4 Chest radiograph showing high-altitude pulmonary oedema with prominent oedema on the right.
Copyright B. Basnyat.

People with HAPE typically present with dyspnoea and cough. The breathlessness is worse on exertion, may be dry or wet, and can present with haemoptysis. Other symptoms include chest pain, orthopnoea, nausea, insomnia, headache, dizziness, and confusion. Low-grade fever is a common finding together with tachycardia, tachypnoea, basal crepitations, and cyanosis in late disease (Fig. 9.5.4.3).

Signs of right ventricular enlargement are present with an accentuated pulmonary second sound and right ventricular heave. Oxygen saturations are decreased, the ECG shows right axis deviation, tachycardia, and peaked P-waves, and the chest radiograph shows oedema, most prominently on the right (see Fig. 9.5.4.4).

In patients who have been studied with cardiac catheterization during HAPE, pulmonary arterial pressure is found to be raised. The majority of people who are susceptible to HAPE show an abnormal rise in their pulmonary arterial pressure at sea level during exposure to hypoxia or on exercise.

The clinical syndrome is not unique, and similar findings occur in other respiratory diseases, including acute bacterial or viral pneumonia. High-altitude cough (see following paragraph) may also cause diagnostic confusion.

As described earlier, HAPE appears to result from an exaggerated hypoxic pulmonary vasoconstrictor response, which leads to capillary leak. The vasoconstriction is heterogeneous, and stress failure of pulmonary capillaries may occur in the overperfused vessels, leading to the patchy oedema.

Once HAPE is recognized, the victim must descend. Even descent of a few hundred metres may be enough to raise the barometric pressure sufficiently to reverse the symptoms. Without appropriate management, HAPE may be fatal, and further ascent should not be undertaken. In a mountain environment, immediate descent may be impossible because of weather, or other circumstances (Fig. 9.5.4.5). The patient may be so breathless that they can not move. Adjunctive therapies may improve symptoms and allow descent. The patient should be encouraged to sit up to prevent orthopnoea. Oxygen should be given if available. Nifedipine (20-mg slow release preparation, four times daily) reduces pulmonary artery pressure and relieves symptoms. Side effects of nifedipine include headache, dizziness, and postural hypotension. Other pulmonary vasodilators such as hydralazine, phentolamine, inhaled nitric oxide, and sildenafil citrate have been used and may be beneficial, but nifedipine is most widely used. Portable hyperbaric chambers are often available on commercial trekking routes. They can simulate descent, improve oxygenation, and relieve symptoms. Devices that help provide positive expiratory airway pressure may also improve oxygenation.

The risk of HAPE is reduced by slow, graded ascent. Above 3000 m, a rate of ascent, of 300 to 600 m per day, with a rest day every 1000 m is recommended. Nifedipine (20-mg slow release preparation, three times daily) and other calcium channel blockers, dexamethasone (8 mg twice daily), inhaled β_2-andrenoceptor agonists, and phosphodiesterase-5 inhibitors are effective for prophylaxis in those known to be susceptible.

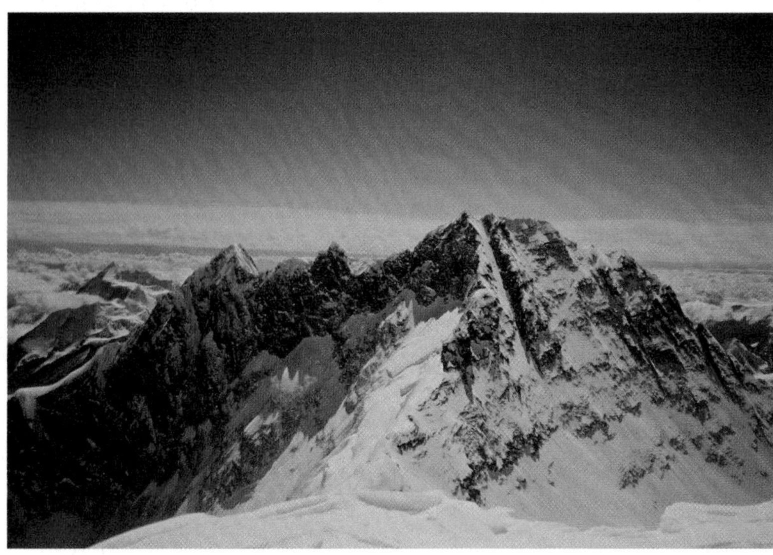

Fig. 9.5.4.5 View of Lhotse (8516 m) from about 8600 m on the South East Ridge of Mount Everest in 1994. Eight climbers died on one day in May 1996, when a storm struck Mount Everest and prevented climbers descending this ridge to the relative safety of Camp IV on the South Col.
Copyright A. Pollard.

High-altitude retinal haemorrhage

Retinal haemorrhages occur frequently at altitudes of 5000 m or higher, even in those without AMS or HACE. Although usually asymptomatic, they can cause visual problems if the macula is involved (Fig. 9.5.4.6). The causes of high-altitude retinal haemorrhage may include increased cerebral blood flow, Valsalva's manoeuvre (during exertion or coughing), polycythaemia, and hypoxia-mediated capillary endothelial permeability. In most instances of high-altitude retinal haemorrhage without altitude illness, descent may not be necessary. The haemorrhages usually resolve within days to weeks. If vision is compromised or there is concomitant altitude illness, descent is mandatory.

Peripheral oedema

Swelling of the hands, face, and ankles commonly occurs at high altitude and may not be related to AMS, HACE, or HAPE. Anasarca is seldom seen. Descent or diuretics will treat the oedema.

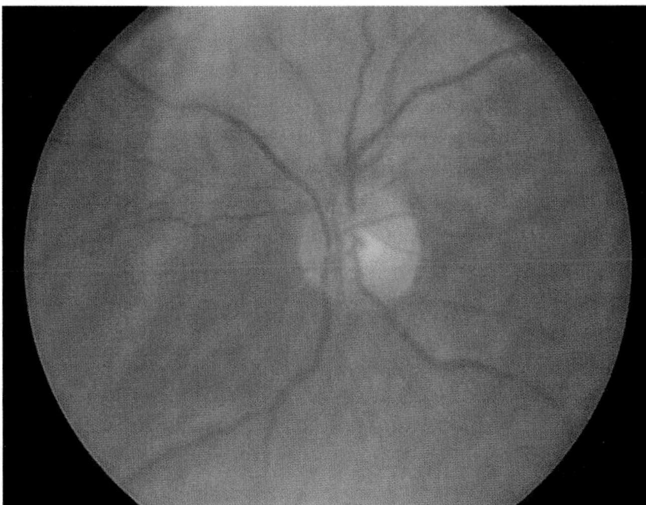

(a)

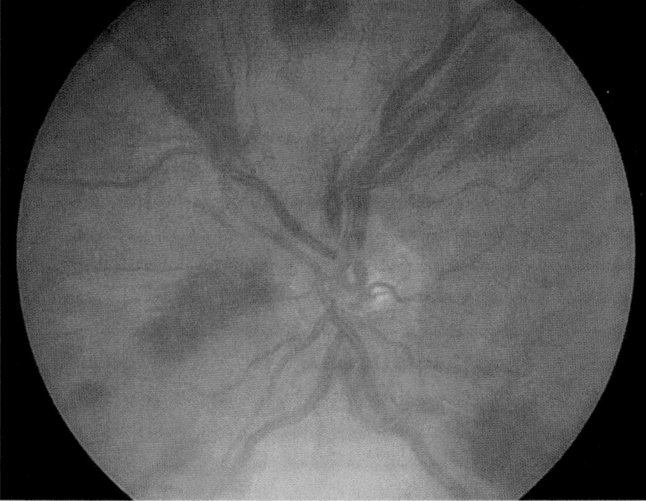

(b)

Fig. 9.5.4.6 Contrasting retinal appearances on Mount Everest. (a) Normal retina of a well-acclimatized and well-oxygenated climber shortly after reaching the summit (8848 m). (b) Retinal haemorrhages in a poorly acclimatized climber at the North Col (7100 m).
Copyright Daniel Morris, Newcastle.

High-altitude cough

Dry hacking cough is a common, bothersome problem at high altitude, and has caused rib fractures in some severe cases. High-altitude cough may be multifactorial in origin: water loss from the airways, post nasal drip, AMS, HAPE, and bronchoconstriction have all been invoked as possible causes of altitude related cough. Breathing through a silk scarf, throat lozenges, and steam inhalation may be helpful. If there is nasal congestion, a decongestant nasal spray is useful.

Effects of high altitude on pre-existing medical conditions

Hypertensive patients should continue their medications at high altitude, and the vast majority of hypertensive skiers and trekkers do very well despite a transient rise in the blood pressure. Some patients with labile hypertension may have a sudden, dangerous rise in their blood pressure at high altitude and, for them, blood pressure monitoring may be necessary. The exaggerated blood pressure response to high altitude is apparently mediated by increased α-adrenergic activity. Hence an α-blocker may be more useful.

People with stable coronary artery disease tolerate intermediate and high altitudes relatively well, even while exercising. This may be partly attributable to the marked reduction in maximal exercise at high altitude, which reduces myocardial oxygen demand and maximal heart rate. Animal experiments at high altitude have also demonstrated down-regulation of the β-receptors of the heart. However, travel to high altitude has precipitated new-onset angina, although it is unclear whether this is related to exertion or to hypobaric hypoxia as such. People with cardiac risk factors or with previous myocardial ischaemia, coronary artery bypass surgery, or angioplasty are considered to be at high risk if they have a strongly positive exercise treadmill test.

Although cold air and exercise are triggers for asthma, many asthmatics remain well at high altitude. This may be due to decreased density of the air, a lack of allergens, or the increase in steroid hormones produced under hypoxic stress. However, it is important for asthmatics going up to high altitude to carry their medicines with them.

Many people with well-controlled epilepsy can venture safely to high altitudes, but there remain some causes for concern. Hyperventilation leading to hypocapnia and hypoxia are themselves triggers for seizure activity.

People with sickle cell disease or trait are at high risk of sickle crises above 2000 m, and should avoid staying at altitude.

Diabetics may find that increased energy expenditure at high altitude alters carbohydrate and insulin requirements. Consequently, rapidly acting insulin, close monitoring, availability of oral and intravenous glucose, and knowledgeable companions are important. Loss of diabetic control due to intercurrent infections, like diarrhoea, is also possible.

Pre-existing pulmonary hypertension from any cause may be a problem at high altitude. Mitral stenosis, kyphoscoliosis, and congenital cardiac defects with pulmonary hypertension may predispose to HAPE and are therefore hazardous at high altitude. Sufferers from chronic obstructive pulmonary disease frequently report increased dyspnoea and reduced exercise tolerance when they ascend to high altitude.

Other illnesses at altitude

Focal neurological problems are occasionally encountered at high altitude. Transient ischaemic attacks and strokes, cerebral venous thrombosis, subarachnoid haemorrhage, high-altitude syncope, delirium, transient global amnesia, cranial nerve palsies, cortical blindness, and amaurosis fugax have all been reported. However, it is unclear whether these deficits are related to hypoxia of high altitude and most need to be distinguished from AMS and HACE.

Venous thrombosis has been reported at high altitude, although its association with high-altitude exposure is uncertain. Cases of cerebral venous thrombosis at high altitude have been reported in previously asymptomatic people with heterozygous protein C and S deficiency and antiphospholipid syndrome. Risk of thrombosis may have been increased by dehydration and polycythaemia. Immobility during inclement weather, coupled with dehydration and polycythaemia, may also predispose to deep vein thrombosis leading to pulmonary embolism. Unanswered questions about the effects of high altitude on blood coagulation include the use of oral contraceptives and whether prophylactic aspirin prevents thrombosis.

Chronic mountain sickness (Monge's disease) and high-altitude pulmonary hypertension (HAPH)

Excessive erythrocytosis, severe hypoxaemia, and, in some cases, moderate to severe pulmonary hypertension leading to cor pulmonale are the features of this disease. Chronic mountain sickness is a disease of long-term residents of altitudes above 2500 m. Besides South America, where this condition was originally described, chronic mountain sickness has also been documented in Colorado and in the Han Chinese population in Tibet. Migration to low altitude cures the problem. Venesection and acetazolamide have been shown to be helpful. It is important to distinguish chronic mountain sickness from chronic obstructive pulmonary disease.

High-altitude pulmonary hypertension (HAPH) is now the accepted term for diseases that include adult subacute mountain sickness and infantile subacute mountain sickness. Unlike chronic mountain sickness, which is characterized by erythrocytosis, the primary feature of this condition is pulmonary hypertension leading to heart failure. The adult form has been described exclusively in Indian soldiers living at extreme altitudes for prolonged periods. The infantile form has been seen mainly in Han Chinese immigrants in Tibet. These conditions bear a striking pathophysiological resemblance to brisket disease in cattle. Descent from high altitude completely cures the problem. HAPH of chronic onset is also well described.

Further reading

Bärtsch P, *et al.* (2004). Acute mountain sickness: controversies and advances. *High Alt Med Biol*, **5**, 110–24.

Bärtsch P, *et al.* (2005). Physiological aspects of high-altitude pulmonary edema. *J Appl Physiol*, **98**, 1101–10.

Basnyat B, Murdoch DR (2003). High-altitude illness. *Lancet*, **361**, 1967–74.

Baumgartner RW, Siegel AM, Hackett PH (2007). Going high with preexisting neurological conditions. *High Alt Med Biol*, **8**, 108–16.

Dehnert C, *et al.* (2005). Identification of individuals susceptible to high-altitude pulmonary oedema at low altitude. *Eur Respir J*, **25**(3), 545–51.

Maggiorini M, *et al.* (2006). Both tadalafil and dexamethasone may reduce the incidence of high-altitude pulmonary edema: a randomized trial. *Ann Intern Med*, **145**, 497–506.

Pollard AJ, Murdoch DR (2003). *The high altitude medicine handbook*, 3rd edition. Radcliffe Medical Press, Oxford.

Roach RC, Hackett PH (2001). Frontiers of hypoxia research: acute mountain sickness. *J Exp Biol*, **204**, 3161–70.

Saxena S, *et al.* (2005). Association of polymorphisms in pulmonary surfactant protein A1 and A2 genes with high-altitude pulmonary edema. *Chest* **128**, 1611–20.

Schoene RB (2004). Unraveling the mechanism of high altitude pulmonary edema. *High Alt Med Biol*, **5**, 125–35.

Schoene RB, Swenson ER, Hultgren H (2001). High-altitude pulmonary edema. In: Horbein TM, Schoene RB (eds.) *High altitude: an exploration of human adaptation*. Marcel Dekker, New York.

West JB (2004). The physiologic basis of high-altitude diseases. *Ann Intern Med*, **141**, 789–800.

9.5.5 Aerospace medicine

D.M. Denison and M. Bagshaw

Essentials

Travel by air is a safe means of transport, but puts people at various physiological risks and is a potential means of spreading infectious disease.

Physiological risks associated with flying include hypoxia—atmospheric pressure falls with altitude. The minimum cabin pressure in commercial passenger aircraft (565 mmHg, 75.1 kPa) brings a healthy individual's arterial Po_2 along the plateau of the oxyhaemoglobin dissociation curve until just at the top of the steep part, but does not cause desaturation. By contrast, people with respiratory disease and a low arterial oxygen pressure may desaturate, which can be overcome by administering 30% oxygen, this being equivalent to breathing air at ground level. Guidance for assessing a passenger's fitness to fly is provided by the websites of the Aerospace Medical Association and the British Thoracic Society. A second physiological risk is increased exposure to cosmic radiation, although there is no evidence that this leads to abnormality or disease.

Other medical problems associated with flying include (1) venous thromboembolism—the relative risk is significant, but the absolute risk is very low. Medical practitioners need to be circumspect in advising preventive measures, taking account of the efficacy and risk profile of any intervention, but compression stockings and/or a single prophylactic dose of low molecular weight heparin may be recommended in high risk cases. (2) Jet lag—there is no simple solution for combating the effects of jet lag: the individual must evolve strategies to suit their particular needs.

Transmission of disease—there is no evidence that the pressurized aircraft cabin itself encourages transmission of disease, and recirculation of cabin air is not a risk factor for contracting symptoms of upper respiratory tract infection. It is important that individuals with a febrile illness should not travel on commercial aircraft. Restricting air travel will not prevent global spread of pandemic influenza, but might delay the spread sufficiently to allow countries time to prepare.

Introduction

Aerospace medicine is a specialized discipline, whose history can be traced back to the descriptions of altered physiology during balloon ascent by Glaisher and Coxwell in 1862. Whereas aviation medicine concerns the welfare of humans flying within the earth's atmosphere, space medicine concerns flight beyond Earth's atmosphere and gravitational pull, involving problems of very prolonged flight times with their associated psychological stresses, life support within a self-contained environment, weightlessness, and exposure to high doses of cosmic radiation. Aviation medicine is relevant to clinicians seeking answers to everyday questions about the effects of flight on the body, but space medicine is of far more limited practical importance. We refer those seeking further information about space medicine to sources such as Clément (2005).

Physics of the flight environment

Earth's atmosphere is an oxygen-rich gas shielding the ground below from solar radiation above. Subjected to gravity, compressed under its own weight, the atmosphere is denser close to the ground than further away. Long waves of infrared light penetrate it easily but heat the ground below. Heated ground reradiates some of this heat at shorter wavelengths, which are absorbed by CO_2 and water vapour, making the air close to the surface much warmer than that higher up. Short waves of ultraviolet sunlight, absorbed by oxygen molecules early in their journey, create a belt of ozone at high altitudes. Some rays intercepted in the same region generate secondary rays that extend lower down, but very few reach the ground. At sea level, the atmosphere exerts a pressure of about 760 mmHg (101 kPa); it is variably moist, has a temperature that ranges from –60 °C to +60 °C, and moves at wind speeds from 0 to 160 km/h. With increasing altitude, the temperature, pressure, and water content of the atmosphere fall, and wind speeds increase (Fig. 9.5.5.1).

Atmospheric pressure

Total gas pressure falls with altitude in a regular manner, halving every 5500 m (18 000 ft) (Fig. 9.5.5.2). The oxygen content of the atmosphere (20.93%) is constant to very high altitudes, so the same curve can be used to obtain the ambient oxygen pressure by rescaling the ordinate (Fig. 9.5.5.2). The oxygen pressure of physiological importance is that which exists in ambient air when it is warmed and wetted on entering the bronchial tree. This raises water vapour pressure to about 47 mmHg, regardless of the total gas pressure outside. The oxygen pressure in moist inspired gas (PiO_2), fully saturated with water vapour at 37 °C, is given by the relationship:

$$PiO_2 = FiO_2\,(P_B - 47)$$

where FiO_2, the fractional concentration of oxygen in the inspirate, is 0.2093 and PB is barometric pressure (mmHg).

Atmospheric temperature

The atmospheric temperature decreases at 1.98 °C/300 m (1000 ft) from the Standard sea level temperature of 15 °C, to the tropopause (12 200 m or 40 000 ft). It remains stable at –56 °C up to about 24 400 m (80 000 ft) and then rises to almost body temperature at about 46 000 m (150 000 ft), but by then air density is so low that its temperature is unimportant.

Atmospheric ozone

Atmospheric ozone is formed by ultraviolet irradiation of diatomic oxygen molecules, which dissociate into atoms. At very high altitudes, all oxygen exists in the monatomic form. Lower down, some of this monatomic oxygen combines with oxygen molecules to form the triatomic gas ozone, with concentrations up to 10 parts per million. The ozonosphere normally exists between 12 200 and 42 700 m (40 000 and 140 000 ft). Below 12 200 m (40 000 ft) the irradiation is normally too weak for significant amounts of ozone

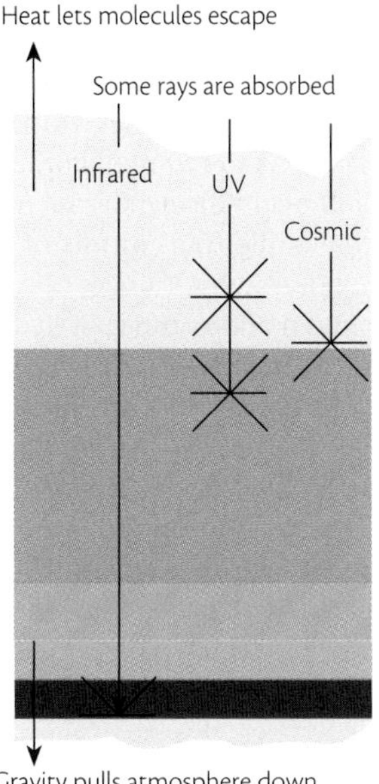

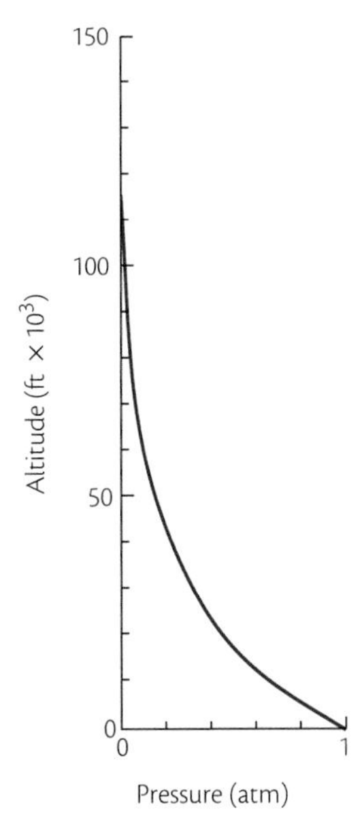

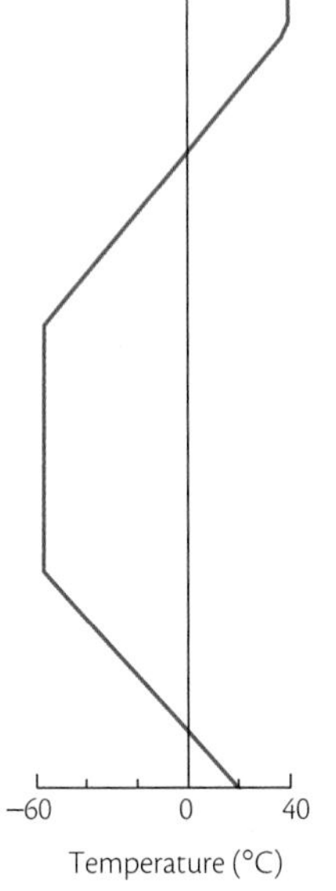

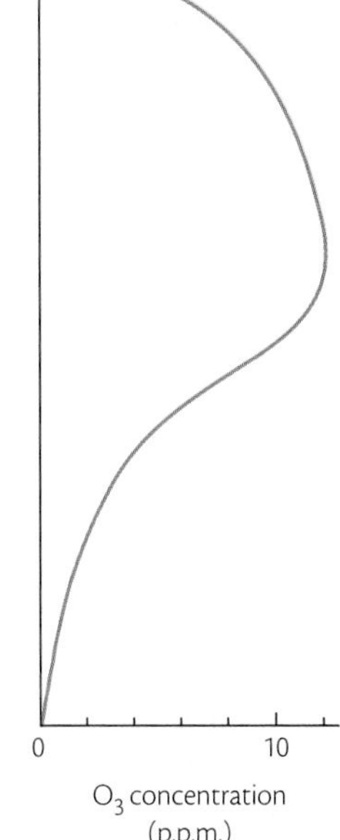

Fig. 9.5.5.1 Some physical features of the Earth's atmosphere, showing the variations in barometric pressure, air temperature, and ozone concentration with altitude. (NB: There is an international aviation safety convention that all altitudes are given in feet.) The shaded diagram on the left illustrates how the Earth's atmosphere is compressed under its own weight. The atmosphere absorbs much solar radiation.

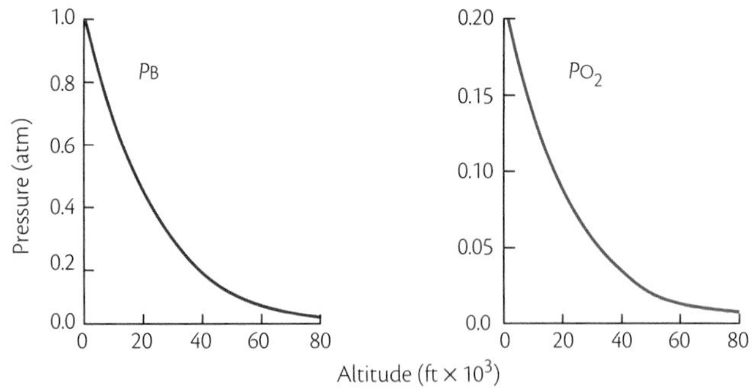

Fig. 9.5.5.2 The variations of barometric pressure (P_B) and ambient oxygen pressure (PO_2) with altitude.

to form. Concentrations of 1 parts per million at sea level can cause lung irritation. However, modern passenger jet aircraft are fitted with catalytic converters in the environmental control system (ECS), which break down the ozone before it enters the pressurized cabin.

Cosmic radiation

Aircraft occupants are exposed to elevated levels of cosmic radiation of galactic and solar origin.

The Sun has a varying magnetic field, which reverses direction approximately every 11 years. Near the reversal, at 'solar minimum', there are few sunspots, and the Sun's magnetic field extending throughout the solar system is relatively weak. At solar maximum, there are many sunspots and other manifestations of magnetic turbulence.

The Earth's magnetic field has a larger effect than the Sun's magnetic field on cosmic radiation approaching the atmosphere. The protective effect is greatest at the equator and least at the magnetic poles. At the altitudes at which jet aircraft operate, galactic cosmic radiation is 2.5 to 5 times more intense in polar regions than near the equator.

The Earth's surface is shielded from cosmic radiation by the atmosphere, the ambient radiation decreasing with altitude by approximately 15% for each increase of around 600 m (2000 ft), dependent on latitude.

Protection against effects of cosmic radiation

The International Commission on Radiological Protection (ICRP) recommended in 1991 that exposure of flight crew members to cosmic radiation in jet aircraft should be considered part of occupational exposure to ionizing radiation.

In May 2000, the Council of the European Union adopted a directive, laying down safety standards for the protection of the health of workers and the general public against the effects of ionizing radiation, incorporating the ICRP recommendations.

The directive applies the ICRP limits for occupational exposure of a 5-year average effective dose of 20 mSv per year, with no more than 50 mSv in a single year. The annual limit for the general public is 1 mSv.

Cosmic radiation doses

The effect of ionizing radiation depends not only on the dose absorbed, but also on the type and energy of the radiation and the tissues involved. These factors are taken into account in arriving at the dose equivalent measured in sieverts (Sv). However, doses of cosmic radiation are so low that figures are usually quoted in millisieverts or microsieverts. Calculated and measured doses are well within the ICRP recommended limits.

Health risks of cosmic radiation

Although it is known that there is no level of ionizing radiation exposure below which effects do not occur, current epidemiological evidence indicates that the probability of airline crew members or passengers suffering any abnormality or disease as a result of exposure to cosmic radiation is very low.

Physiology of flight

The physiological effects of flight are distinguished from those of terrestrial high altitude because exposures are relatively rapid, brief, and not cumulative. Flyers do not adapt to the hypoxic environment, unlike inhabitants of terrestrial high altitudes. However, the aircraft can be a means of transporting an individual to a high-altitude destination.

Hypoxia

Oxygen has a dual role in most animal cells, being simultaneously life-giving and extremely poisonous. In air, or dissolved in simple solution, it is benign and ionized only with difficulty. However, once an electron is successfully attached to an oxygen molecule it becomes a highly corrosive superoxide ion, forming a cascade of other very destructive oxygen radicals. This is an essential feature of oxygen toxicity. Superoxide dismutase and various peroxidases have evolved to protect most cells from the effects of spontaneous formation of oxygen radicals by quenching the ions as rapidly as they appear.

Other enzymes have evolved, which harness this property in a controlled way. There are three types: oxidases, oxygenases, and hydroxylases. Quantitatively, cytochrome a_3 oxidase (EC 1.9.3.1) is the most important because, using oxygen as the ultimate electron sink, it allows many metabolic processes to proceed, at the same time unlocking and trapping most of the energy the body needs (oxidative phosphorylation).

Oxygenases introduce an oxygen molecule into organic molecules, creating new compounds. Although these enzymes consume only a small fraction of the body's total oxygen requirement, they are particularly important for production and dismemberment of many critical compounds, such as the amine transmitters of the brain.

Hydroxylases insert one atom of oxygen and another of hydrogen into organic molecules. They too are responsible for many critical metabolic processes and for the denaturation of many drugs in the liver, kidney, and elsewhere.

These enzymes differ in their affinity for oxygen, described by the Michaelis constant (for oxygen). This constant ($K_m o_2$) is that partial pressure of oxygen which, when all other factors are equal, allows an oxygen-consuming reaction to proceed at half its maximum velocity. The major oxidase (cytochrome a_3), which is the cocatalyst of oxidative phosphorylation, has a very high oxygen affinity, and thus a very low $K_m o_2$ of 1 mmHg or less. Thus, this particular type of oxygen consumption, representing 80 to 90% of the whole, can proceed at high rates down to very low levels of oxygen supply. By contrast (Fig. 9.5.5.3), the other enzymes, which are quantitatively less important but qualitatively critical, have Michaelis constants for oxygen that vary from 5 to 250 mmHg. A fall in oxygen supply

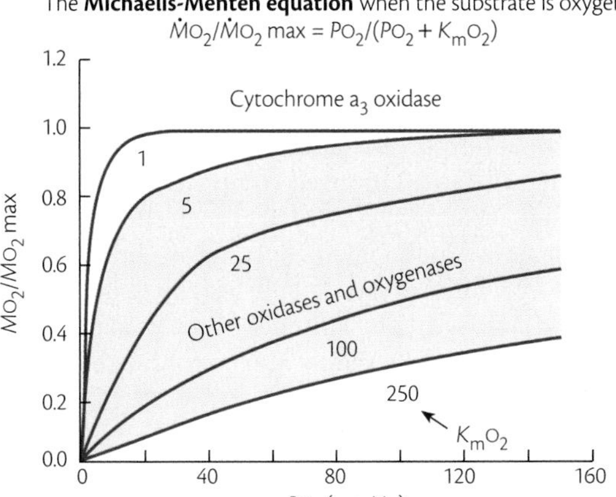

Fig. 9.5.5.3 Curves of oxygen uptake (O_2) as a fraction of the theoretical maximum (O_{2max}) against the partial pressure of oxygen (PO_2) for a family of oxygen-handling enzymes with Michaelis constants for oxygen (K_mO_2) from 1 to 250 mmHg.

will influence these processes long before oxidative phosphorylation is affected, and at times when overall oxygen consumption is diminished little, if at all.

Although Figure 9.5.5.2 describes how ambient oxygen pressure is related to altitude, it does not convey the pressure of oxygen to be found in the lungs. That pressure is determined by two equations (Fig. 9.5.5.4). The alveolar ventilation equation states that alveolar CO_2 pressure ($Paco_2$) depends only on CO_2 excretion and alveolar ventilation (Va), so:

$$Paco_2 = k(CO_2/Va).$$

The alveolar air equation states that since at any one time there is a fixed trading ratio between oxygen uptake and CO_2 excretion ($R = CO_2/O_2$), alveolar oxygen pressure (Pao_2) can be calculated from the moist inspired oxygen pressure ($Pio_2{}^*$) and alveolar Pco_2, so:

$$Pao_2 = Pio_2{}^* - (Paco_2/R).$$

Progressive hypoxia leads to a mild hyperventilation (i.e. a rise in Va and fall in $Paco_2$). Thus, it is possible to plot alveolar oxygen pressure against altitude (Fig. 9.5.5.5a).

The **Alveolar ventilation equation** ignores dead-space, and supposes there is a stream of oxygen-rich CO_2 free gas, V_A and says, for practical purposes:

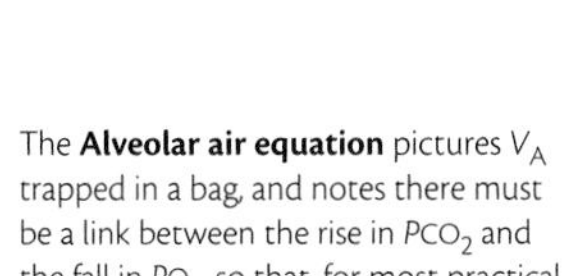

The **Alveolar air equation** pictures V_A trapped in a bag, and notes there must be a link between the rise in PCO_2 and the fall in PO_2, so that, for most practical purposes:

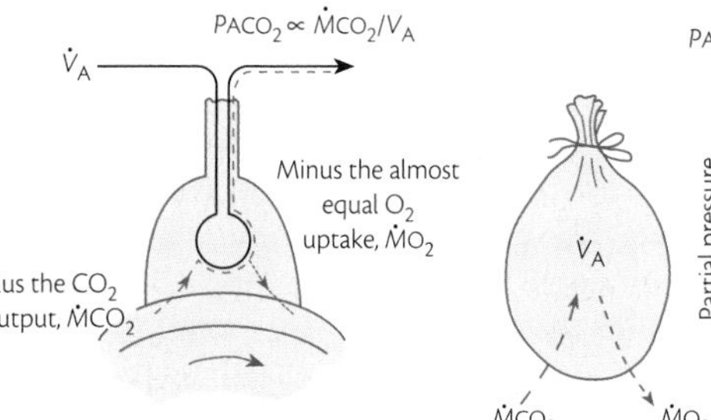

Fig. 9.5.5.4 Graphical representations of the alveolar ventilation and alveolar air equations.

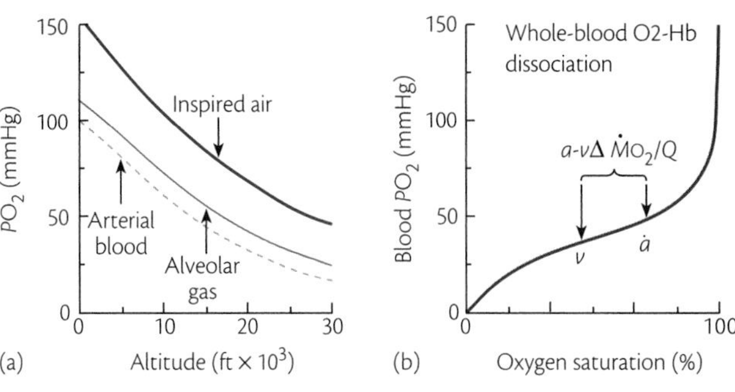

Fig. 9.5.5.5 (a) Variations in moist inspired, alveolar, and arterial oxygen pressure (PO_2) with altitude in normal men. (b) The conventional oxygen–haemoglobin dissociation curve of whole blood plotted to the same pressure scale as the left-hand graph, so that arterial O_2 content can be read directly (at the same horizontal level as the PO_2 curve. It also emphasizes that the arteriovenous oxygen content difference (a − vΔ) is proportional to the ratio of oxygen uptake (MO_2) to local blood flow (Q).

When arterialized blood leaves a healthy lung, the oxygen pressure is about 10 mmHg less than that in the alveoli, due to uneven matching of ventilation to perfusion, some anatomical shunting, and an almost nominal obstacle to diffusion. In resting people, the alveolar–arterial oxygen gradient does not change much with altitude, although the relative importance of the factors contributing to it alter considerably; so subtracting a further 10 to 15 mmHg describes the relation between arterial oxygen pressure and altitude (Fig. 9.5.5.5).

The most important change is the loss of pressure, driving oxygen from the alveoli to blood, as the fall in alveolar Po_2 is much greater than that in mixed venous Po_2 (because of the shape of the oxygen dissociation curve). As a result, the alveolar–venous gradient for oxygen diffusion is smaller and equilibration slower than at ground level.

People ascend to altitude in a matter of minutes, rather than over several days, and adapt to hypoxia by an increase in blood flow and a modest hyperventilation, limiting the effects of hypoxia. The effects are shown in Fig. 9.5.5.6.

Individuals abruptly exposed to altitudes of 3000 m (10 000 ft) and above suffer mental and physical effects, and this is the ceiling over which aviators are provided with oxygen. To allow a margin of safety, the maximum certified cabin altitude in civilian passenger aircraft is 2440 m (8000 ft), at which barometric pressure is 565 mmHg and arterial oxygen pressure is around 55 mmHg (see

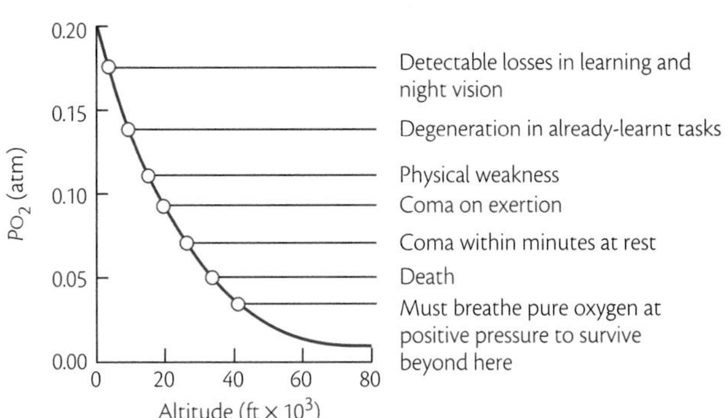

Fig. 9.5.5.6 A summary of the functional consequences of altitude hypoxia.

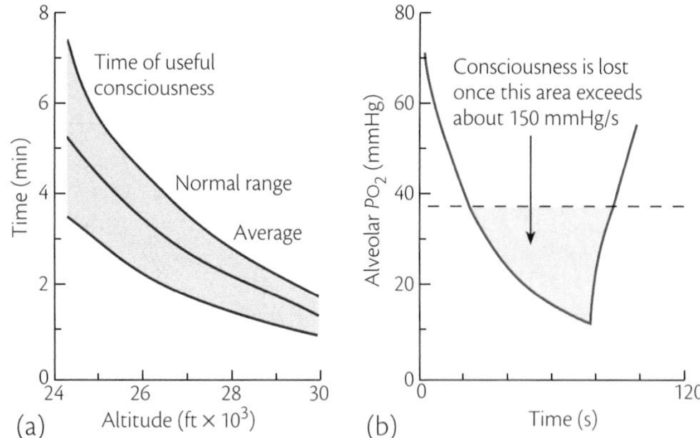

Fig. 9.5.5.7 (a) Variations in the time of useful consciousness with altitude. (b) One way of expressing the dose of hypoxia needed to bring about the loss of consciousness.

Fig. 9.5.5.5b, the oxyhaemoglobin dissociation curve), and venous oxygen pressures have fallen by only 1 to 2 mmHg. Even at this altitude, there is a decrease in performance. The latest generation of passenger aircraft are manufactured from newer materials, which provide greater strength from a given mass, thus allowing a higher differential cabin pressure with a lower cabin altitude.

Two physiological features of altitude hypoxia are important in aviation. The first is the total lack of awareness of cerebral impairment. The second is the time of useful consciousness, describing how rapidly consciousness is lost thus dictating how quickly the condition must be recognized and corrective action taken.

The time of useful consciousness is the interval after the onset of hypoxia during which an individual can carry out some purposeful activity. The general relation between this time interval and the altitude of sudden exposure is shown in Fig. 9.5.5.7a. It diminishes from about 4 min at 7620 m (25 000 ft) to a minimum of roughly 15 s, which is reached at 10 700 to 12 200 m (35 000–40 000 ft). This asymptote represents the sum of the 7 s or so required for blood to travel from the lungs to the brain and the time needed for the brain to utilize the oxygen already dissolved in its substance.

In trained and healthy men breathing normally (i.e. with an alveolar Pco_2 of 35–40 mmHg), the dose of hypoxia acceptable before loss of useful consciousness is equivalent on a curve of alveolar Po_2 against time, to an area of 150 mmHg s, where Po_2 is less than 38 mmHg (Fig. 9.5.5.7b). However, this is sensitive to many other factors, such as the degree of hyperventilation and the acceleration to which the individual is exposed at the time. Hyperventilation causes cerebral vasoconstriction, and positive headwards acceleration ($+G_z$) opposes the upward flow of blood to the brain. Sometimes deterioration in consciousness is quickened by vasovagal syncope, but more often there is tachycardia as consciousness is lost. Exertion also quickens loss of consciousness, because blood transits quickly through the lungs leaving insufficient time for oxygen equilibration.

The minimum cabin pressure of 565 mmHg (75.1 kPa) in commercial passenger aircraft (equivalent to 2440 m or 8000 ft), will bring a healthy individual's arterial Po_2 along the plateau of the oxyhaemoglobin dissociation curve until just at the top of the steep part (Fig. 9.5.5.5), still saturated. At ground level, people with respiratory disease may have arterial oxygen pressures as low as 55 to 60 mmHg. As they ascend to 2440 m (8000 ft), their arterial Po_2 will fall further. If their hypoxaemia at ground level is due to a mismatch of ventilation to perfusion, as is usually the case, the drop in arterial Po_2 will not be as extensive as in healthy people (*c.*40 mmHg), but if it is due to diffusion defect associated with desaturation on exertion, as in some fibrotic conditions, it may be greater. However, in either event, it can be reversed completely by the administration of oxygen, 30% oxygen at 2440 m (8000 ft) being equivalent to breathing air at ground level. Given prior notice, most airlines can provide a personal oxygen supply for any passenger, although there may be a charge. (The altitudes of the patient's destination and transit points en route should also be considered.)

Oxygen equipment and pressure cabins

Aircraft operating below 3000 m (10 000 ft) do not require oxygen equipment. Many sophisticated light aircraft that can cruise above 3000 m do not have pressurized cabins, so oxygen equipment must be provided.

Other aircraft that fly higher usually have reinforced cabins capable of holding a high differential pressure between inside and out. These are the high-differential type, seen in passenger and transport aircraft generally, and the low-differential variety found in military high-performance aircraft. The former, holding a high transmural pressure, maintain cabin pressure above 565 mmHg (the equivalent of 2440 m or 8000 ft). They provide an environment in which the occupants breathe cabin air. However, it is possible for the pressurization system to fail, allowing the cabin pressure to fall to the external ambient value. This can be limited by descent to a lower altitude, but it is not always possible to descend immediately, for reasons of structure or air traffic control. Similarly, it is not always practical to descend below 3000 m (10 000 ft) because, in mid-Atlantic, for example, there may be insufficient fuel for the aircraft to reach the nearest land through the denser air at lower altitudes. Thus, an emergency oxygen supply is available for passengers and crew.

The aircraft environmental control system (ECS) automatically manages the internal cabin environment, providing healthy and comfortable surroundings for all occupants. There are regulatory requirements for minimum cabin air pressure, maximum levels of carbon monoxide, CO_2 and ozone, and minimum ventilation flow rates. The cabin air must also be free from harmful or hazardous concentrations of gases or vapours.

The cabin air supply is bled from the outside air entering the aircraft engine, or may be supplied from the outside air via electrically driven compressors. It is then passed through the air-conditioning packs and mixed with filtered recirculated air before distribution to the cabin. The system provides approximately 566 litres (20 cubic feet) of air per minute per passenger, of which about 50% is recirculated air (compared with up to 80% recirculated in buildings and other forms of public transport), giving a complete cabin air exchange every 2 to 3 min.

These high ventilatory flow rates maintain normal pressurization, as well as temperature control and the removal of odours and CO_2. The high flow rates also ensure that the volume of oxygen far exceeds the requirements of the aircraft occupants (0.34 litres/min at rest and 0.85 litres/min when walking).

The air is distributed to the cabin via overhead ducts and grills running the length of the cabin. The airflow circulates around the cabin rather than along the cabin and is continuously extracted through vents at floor level, as shown in Fig. 9.5.5.8.

Cabin air flow

Fig. 9.5.5.8 Cabin air circulation and distribution.

The recirculated air is passed through high efficiency particulate air (HEPA) filters of the same specification used in hospital operating theatres, giving 99.99% efficiency in the removal of physical contaminants such as microbial particles. Aircraft cabin air has been demonstrated to be bacteriologically cleaner than the air in buildings, trains, or buses.

Although clean, the aircraft cabin air remains dry. During the flight, moisture is derived from the metabolism and activities of the cabin occupants as well as from the galleys and washrooms, giving a maximum relative humidity of the order of 10 to 20%. These levels are associated with surface drying of skin, mucous membranes, and cornea which may cause discomfort. Normal homeostatic mechanisms prevent dehydration and no harm to health has been demonstrated.

A high-differential cabin limits the vehicle's range and manoeuvrability and increases the risk of catastrophic damage if the fuselage is punctured. So, military high-performance aircraft are fitted with low-differential cabins, which prevent cabin pressure falling below 280 mmHg (37.2 kPa) (equivalent to a pressure altitude of 7620 m or 25 000 ft). At this level, decompression illness becomes a potential hazard (see following paragraphs). In such aircraft, oxygen equipment is used routinely.

Mechanical effects of pressure change

In civilian passenger and transport aircraft, the climb to cruise altitude takes about 30 min and involves a maximum decrease of about 200 mmHg (26.6 kPa) in cabin pressure (to the equivalent of 2440 m or 8000 ft). Descent to land takes much the same time. Body fluids and tissues generally are virtually incompressible and do not alter shape to any important extent when such pressure changes are applied. The same is true of cavities such as the lungs, gut, middle ear, and facial sinuses that contain air, provided that they can vent easily. Gas-containing spaces that cannot vent easily behave differently.

The thoracoabdominal wall can develop transmural pressures of +100 mmHg or so briefly, but is normally flaccid and has a transmural pressure of a few millimetres of mercury. Gas within will usually be at a pressure very close to that outside, and must follow Boyle's law. Ascent from ground level (760 mmHg) to 2440 m

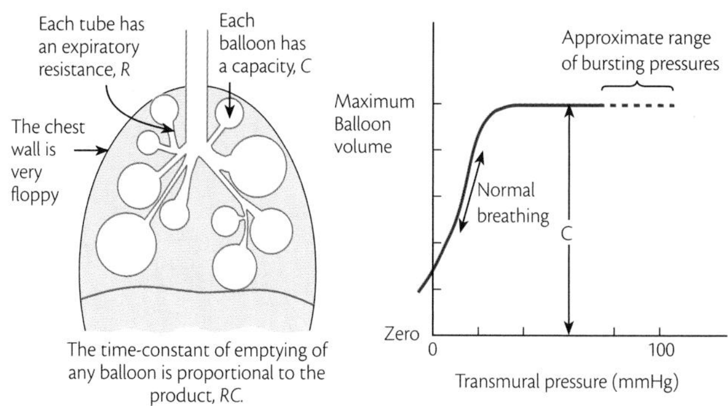

Fig. 9.5.5.9 A graphical summary of the factors determining lung rupture.

(8000 ft) (565 mmHg) will expand a given volume of trapped gas in a completely pliable container by about 35%. This may cause slightly uncomfortable gut distension in healthy people, but it is not an important problem.

Even very diseased lungs can vent themselves over a minute or so. In consequence, the risk of lung rupture in normal flight is extremely rare (Fig. 9.5.5.9).

The cavity of the middle ear vents easily, but sometimes fails to fill because the lower part of the eustachian tube behaves as a non-return valve, especially when it is inflamed. As a result, the cavity equilibrates quite easily on ascent but does not refill on descent, and the eardrum bows inwards, causing pain that can be severe (otic barotrauma).

Altitude-induced decompression illness

If ambient pressure falls quickly to less than half its original value, the gas dissolved in blood and tissue fluids may come out of solution precipitously, forming bubbles and obstructing flow in small blood vessels. The time symptoms take to develop varies widely between individuals and shortens markedly as the altitude of exposure rises. A guide to these times and variability is given in Fig. 9.5.5.10. Symptoms usually resolve quickly after a descent of a few thousand feet and rarely persist after descent to ground level, breathing oxygen. Should they persist, treatment should be along the lines detailed in Chapter 9.5.4.

Atmospheric pressure halves at 5000 m (18 000 ft) and decompression illness occurs rarely, if at all, below this altitude. It is very rare below 7600 m (25 000 ft) and therefore is normally of no concern at normal passenger aircraft cabin altitudes, although the risk

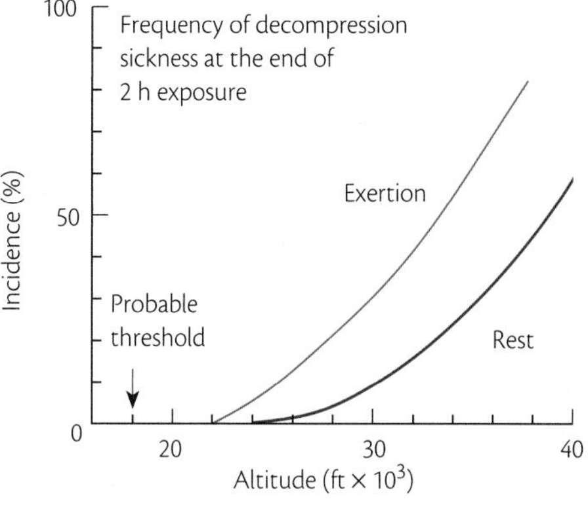

Fig. 9.5.5.10 The incidence of decompression sickness (%) at the end of 2 h of exposure to various altitudes in men at rest, or exerting themselves.

continues to be significant in some military flights. However, it does occasionally occur in those passengers who have been exposed to a hyperbaric environment prior to flight, such as divers and tunnel workers. Subaqua divers (see Chapter 9.5.6) are advised to allow a minimum of 12 h to elapse between diving and flight, or 24 h if the dive required decompression stops.

Clinical aspects of aviation medicine

Travel by air is a safe means of transport. However, from the physiological point of view, flying is a means of putting people at risk, as well as being a potential means of spreading infectious disease. Modern technology, coupled with stringent training requirements for flight crew, minimizes these risks, but clinicians need to be aware of the applications of physics and physiology to the flight environment.

It can be difficult to apply epidemiological principles when considering incidence and outcomes of medical conditions acquired during flight or the spread of infectious disease, because the passengers disperse after the flight before clinical symptoms or signs have become manifest. However, organizations such as the Aerospace Medical Association, the European Civil Aviation Conference, and the World Health Organization have supported or undertaken epidemiological studies to establish the prevalence of conditions such as flight-related deep vein thrombosis (DVT) and venous thromboembolism (VTE), spread of tuberculosis, and spread of newly emerging infectious diseases such as severe acute respiratory syndrome (SARS) and avian flu.

Jet lag

Besides sleep, the major influence on waking performance and alertness is the internal circadian clock. Circadian rhythms fluctuate on a regular cycle which lasts something over 24 h. The circadian rhythms are controlled by the suprachiasmatic nucleus of the hypothalamus. Many body functions have their own circadian rhythm and they are synchronized to a 24-h pattern by 'zeitgebers' (time givers), light being among the most powerful.

Moving to a new light/dark schedule (as in changing time zones) leads to a discrepancy between internal suprachiasmatic nucleus timing and external environmental cues. The internal clock can take days or weeks to readjust, depending on the number of time zones crossed (desynchronosis). Some preventive measures are listed in Box 9.5.5.1.

Box 9.5.5.1 Jet lag: preventive measures

Sleep scheduling

- At home, the best possible sleep should be obtained before a trip.
- On a trip, as much sleep per 24 h should be obtained as would be at home.
- Feelings should be trusted—if the individual feels sleepy and circumstances permit, then they should sleep.

Good sleep habits

- A regular presleep routine should be developed.
- Sleep time should be kept protected.
- The individual should avoid going to bed hungry, but should not eat or drink heavily before going to bed.
- Alcohol or caffeine should be avoided before bedtime.

Fatigue is defined as the likelihood of falling asleep. Therefore, in practical terms, there is little difference between chronic fatigue and acute tiredness. Fatigue can be caused by sleep loss and circadian desynchronosis, but it can also result from low motivation and low levels of external stimulation.

Caffeine consumption may be used to increase alertness. A cup of coffee usually takes about 15 and 30 min to become effective, and the effect lasts for between 3 and 4 h. However, this is less effective for individuals who regularly drink large amounts of caffeine-containing beverages.

Bright light (>2500 lux), used at the appropriate time in the circadian cycle, can help to reset the circadian clock.

After flying east, the traveller should be exposed to evening light, but morning light avoided. Conversely, when travelling west, morning light should be sought and evening light avoided. This makes the best use of the natural zeitgebers in resetting the body clock.

Temazepam is a short-acting benzodiazepine with a short half-life. Many people find this drug helpful in promoting sleep, and if used for two or three days after travel, can assist in resetting the sleep cycle.

Melatonin is secreted by the pineal gland with a rhythm linked to the light/dark cycle through the suprachiasmatic nucleus. It is effective in inducing sleep when taken at the appropriate stage in the circadian cycle. However, if taken at the wrong stage, it can disrupt the sleep/wake cycle and destabilize sleep patterns. This limits its usefulness in treating jet lag.

There is no simple or single solution for combating the effects of jet lag. Individual have to evolve strategies to suit their particular needs.

Traveller's thrombosis (DVT/VTE)

Longhaul travel is associated with prolonged periods of immobility, a recognized risk factor for DVT, first described by Virchow in 1856. However, there have been concerns as to whether there are other factors specific to air travel that further increase the risk.

In the general population, DVT occurs in 1 to 3 per 1000 people per year, of which 20% give rise to pulmonary embolism. Increasing age is known to be a strong risk factor, possibly due to decreased mobility and reduced muscular tone.

The pathogenesis of thrombosis still relies on the basic premise of Virchow, who identified circulatory stasis, hypocoagulability, and endothelial injury as the risk factors.

Several clinical studies have shown an association between air travel and the risk of DVT, with the risk of VTE in travellers increasing with the distance travelled. A recent case–control study showed that all modes of travel increased the risk of venous thrombosis about twofold, with an absolute risk of 1 thrombosis per 6000 journeys.

It has been found that combinations of risk factors synergistically increase the risk of thrombosis. In people with factor V Leiden, the risk of thrombosis after flying was about 14 times increased and in women using oral contraceptives it was around 20-fold increased.

It has also been shown that the risk rises with the number of flights taken in a short time-frame as well as with the duration of the flight. The majority of these clots are asymptomatic and disperse naturally.

Thus, even though the overall risk of venous thrombosis after air travel is only moderately increased, clear subgroups can be identified in whom the risk is higher.

The low humidity of the aircraft cabin does not in itself lead to dehydration. Excessive alcohol consumption may cause dehydration, but there is no evidence that this is a significant risk factor leading to DVT.

Two recent studies of reduced oxygen partial pressure with non-hypoxic control groups found no evidence of coagulation. There is no evidence that hypoxia or the hypobaric environment of an aircraft cabin is a significant risk factor for the development of DVT.

Although there is good evidence for the value of aspirin in preventing arterial thromboembolic disease, its role in the prevention of venous thromboembolic disease is much less clear. The side effect profile is significant.

There is no evidence to support the use of aspirin in preventing the development of DVT during flight.

For those travellers at medium to high risk of DVT, there is evidence that the use of compression stockings appears to substantially lower the risk of asymptomatic DVT, but it remains unclear as to whether this reduction is clinically significant. One study has shown that for 20 to 40% of travellers, the commercially available stockings do not fit adequately. It is essential for stockings to be correctly fitted so as to provide adequate compression to stimulate venous return.

Although the use of low molecular weight heparin for the prevention of DVT in the aviation setting is not supported by direct evidence, in a high-risk traveller consideration may be given to a single prophylactic dose prior to flying.

While the relative risk of developing venous thrombosis when flying is significant, the absolute risk of developing symptomatic DVT is very low. The absolute risk of developing a pulmonary embolus during or after a flight between the United Kingdom and the east coast of the United States of America has been calculated as less than 1 in 10^6.

Medical practitioners need to be circumspect in advising any preventive measures, taking careful account of efficacy and risk profile of the preventive method.

Passenger fitness to fly

Medical clearance is required when:

- Fitness to travel is in doubt as a result of recent illness, hospitalization, injury, surgery, or instability of an acute or chronic medical condition.
- Special services are required (e.g. oxygen, stretcher or authority to carry or use accompanying medical equipment such as a ventilator or a nebulizer).

Medical clearance is not required for carriage of an invalid passenger outside these categories, although special needs (such as a wheelchair) must be reported to the airline at the time of booking.

It is vital that passengers remember to carry with them any essential medication, and not pack it in their checked baggage.

Deterioration on holiday or on a business trip of a previously stable condition, or an accident, can often give rise to the need for medical clearance for the return journey. A stretcher may be required, together with medical support, and this can incur considerable cost. It is important for all travellers to have adequate travel insurance.

Assessment criteria

The passenger's exercise tolerance can provide a useful guide on fitness to fly; if unable to walk a distance greater than about 50 m without developing dyspnoea, there is a risk that the passenger will be unable to tolerate the relative hypoxia of the pressurized cabin.

The websites of the Aerospace Medical Association and the British Thoracic Society provide a good source of guidance.

Spread of infectious disease

There is no evidence that the pressurized cabin itself makes transmission of disease any more likely, and it has been shown that recirculation of cabin air is not a risk factor for contracting symptoms of upper respiratory tract infection. Data suggest that risk of disease transmission to susceptible passengers, by person-to-person droplet spread within the aircraft cabin, is associated with sitting within two rows of a contagious passenger for a flight time of more than 8 h.

Newly emerging infectious disease

SARS is an atypical pneumonia caused by a novel coronavirus, which first appeared in eastern Asia in 2003.

Thousands of flights took place to and from what the World Health Organization defined as 'affected areas' during the outbreak, but transmission occurred only on 5 flights involving 29 secondary cases (24 cases on 1 flight). In addition, a further 40 flights were identified on which one or more probable cases (i.e. symptomatic at the time of travel) travelled but where no secondary cases developed. Thus the risk of transmission on board an aircraft is thought to be low.

Avian influenza ('bird flu') is a highly pathogenic strain A/H5N1 causing an epidemic amongst birds in Asia, Europe, and Africa. Human infection is very rare, but serious when it occurs. During 2006, the World Health Organization reported a total of 109 cases of which 79 died. None of the reported cases occurred within Europe, and air travel is not thought to be a risk factor.

On the other hand, pandemic influenza causes major morbidity and mortality in humans, with serious economic and social consequences. It usually affects a large proportion of the global population due to the absence of immunity, and spreads very rapidly throughout the world. Influenza pandemics occurred in 1918 ('Spanish flu'), 1957 ('Asian flu'), 1968 ('Hong Kong flu') and in 2009 ('Swine flu'), all with high mortality.

The World Health Organization's strategy for rapid containment of an emerging influenza pandemic aims to interrupt disease transmission by isolating and treating infectious individuals, treating and quarantining exposed people, and minimizing the exposure of uninfected persons. Modelling suggests that restricting air travel will not prevent the global spread of pandemic influenza, but might delay the spread sufficiently to allow countries time to prepare. Guidelines can be accessed from http://www.who.int or http://www.cdc.gov.

It is important that individuals should not travel on commercial aircraft with a febrile illness.

Future issues

Aerospace medicine is a subject that is largely understood.

There is concern amongst some flight crew about health effects due to oil pyrolysis products in the cabin air. Evidence is conflicting and research is ongoing.

The major peer-reviewed journal in the field is *Aviation, Space and Environmental Medicine*, published by the Aerospace Medical Association.

Further reading

Campbell RD, Bagshaw M (2002). *Human performance and limitations in aviation*, 3rd ed. Blackwell Science, Oxford.

Clément G (2005). *Fundamentals of Space Medicine (Space Technology Library)*. Springer, Dordrecht.

Coker RK (ed.) (2004). *Managing passengers with respiratory disease planning air travel: British Thoracic Society recommendations*. British Thoracic Society Standards of Care Committee.

Davis JR, *et al.* (eds.) (2008). *Fundamentals of aerospace medicine*, 4th edition. Williams & Wilkins, Philadelphia, PA.

House of Lords Inquiry (2000). *Air travel and health*. The Stationery Office, London.

House of Lords Inquiry (2007). *Air travel and health: an update*. The Stationery Office, London.

Kuipers S, *et al.* (2007). The absolute risk of venous thrombosis after air travel: a cohort study. *PLOS Medicine*, **4**, 1508–14.

Rainford DJ, Gradwell DP (eds.) (2006). *Ernsting's aviation medicine*, 4th edition, Hodder Arnold, London.

Rosenberg CA, Pak F (1997). Emergencies in the air: problems, management and prevention. *J Emerg Med*, **15**, 159–64.

Thibeault C (1997). Special Committee report: cabin air quality. *Aviat Space Environ Med*, **68**, 80–2.

9.5.6 Diving medicine

D.M. Denison and M.A. Glover

Essentials

Diving remains the principal means of exploring and exploiting shallower underwater zones. Immersion and rapid increase in pressure with depth cause most problems unique to diving.

Effects of pressure on gases and ventilation

Gas density, partial pressures, and solubility vary proportionately with ambient pressure. At elevated partial pressure, nitrogen becomes narcotic, as can other inert gases, and contaminants barely detectable at the surface can become toxic as their partial pressures rise with depth. Hyperoxia irritates the lungs and the central nervous system, and sometimes causing generalized seizures. A safe gas mixture at depth can become hypoxic as the partial pressure of oxygen decreases during the return to surface.

Ventilatory effort is impaired at depth and failure of CO_2 elimination increasingly limits activity. Some divers are not distressed by elevated CO_2, but this does not protect them from its toxic effects.

Clinical problems associated with diving and fitness to dive

Immersion hazards include drowning (Chapter 9.5.3), aquatic flora and fauna (Chapters 9.2 and 9.3), water movement, impaired visibility and thermal control (Chapters 9.5.1 and 9.5.2), and enhanced sound and blast propagation. Immersion predisposes susceptible individuals to pulmonary oedema. Aspiration of seawater can cause pulmonary inflammation and systemic manifestations. Water entering the external auditory meati can induce disabling caloric vertigo.

Decompression illness (DCI)—caused during ascent from a dive by bubbles of inert gas, released from tissues or forced intravascularly by pulmonary rupture. Typical symptoms include limb pain and neurological symptoms (often numbness and paraesthesiae, also disturbance of higher cerebral function which can impair the diver's insight). Symptoms develop within a few minutes to 24 h of surfacing in most cases. Management requires exclusion of other diagnoses without delaying first aid treatment of DCI with oxygen (as close to 100% as possible) and rehydration, followed by definitive recompression. Intracardiac right–left shunts, such as patent foramen ovale, predispose to the condition. Extracardiac (pulmonary) shunts can also permit a similar paradoxical embolization of bubbles.

Barotrauma—gas-filled spaces within, or surrounding, the body will be damaged unless they are flexible enough to accommodate pressure-mediated changes in volume, or they are ventilated to prevent distortion. Divers' ears, sinuses, lungs, carious teeth, or their masks and suits are vulnerable.

Long-term consequences of diving—these include aseptic bone infarcts, impaired higher cerebral function, and hearing loss.

Fitness to dive—unrestricted diving demands a high level of physical and medical fitness. Potential disqualifying factors include conditions that might incapacitate, impair, or distract a diver; predispose to DCI or barotraumas; or mimic DCI.

Introduction

Divers are exposed to many hazards while remote from medical care. As a result, diving medicine is largely concerned with prevention. It requires a thorough understanding of the diver's environment and work.

Some dives are conducted in dry pressurized chambers, but most involve immersion in fluids such as seawater. Immersion and rapid change in pressure with depth are responsible for most diving problems. Ambient pressure in seawater rises by 100 kPa for every 10-m descent. Gas densities and partial pressures are proportional to ambient pressure. The amount of a chemically inert gas, such as nitrogen or helium, that can dissolve in the diver's body is proportional to its partial pressure.

A typical shore (Fig. 9.5.6.1) slopes down to between 200 and 300 m at a gradient of about 1 in 50. Diving is largely confined to this continental shelf. Thereafter, the continental slope descends to between 3 and 6 km at a gradient of roughly 1 in 15 to vast flat expanses of soft mud, the abyssal plains, interrupted by occasional mountains and chasms. The deepest point is just over 11 km below the surface.

Currents, arising from differences in water temperature and salinity, course across the abyssal plains and well up the continental slopes as mineral-rich streams supplying plant life in sunlit upper zones. Animals concentrate here to feed on these plants or on each other. Eighty per cent of the ocean biomass lies in the top 200 m, mainly close to the shore. Together, these sites form an area equal to Africa, infinitely more fertile and, as yet, virtually unfarmed.

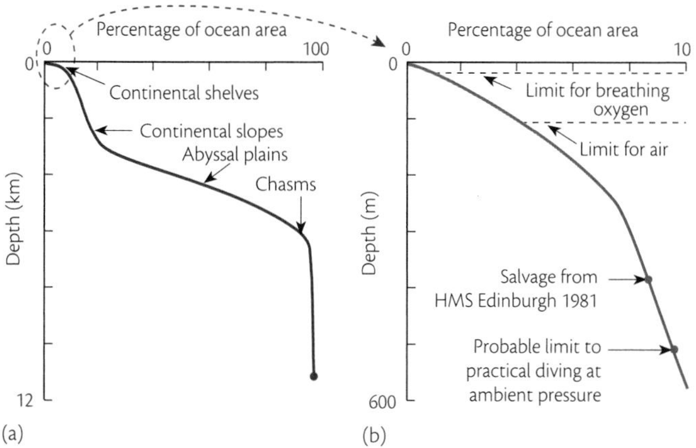

Fig. 9.5.6.1 (a) A cumulative depth versus area plot of the oceans. (b) A similar plot of the top 600 m, including the continental shelves.

Limitations to diving

Currents often exceed swimming speed (Fig. 9.5.6.2a) and may restrict diving to an hour or two each day during slack water. High waves frequently prevent divers from being launched or recovered safely (Fig. 9.5.6.2b). Tidal currents tunnelled along marine canyons, and springs of fresh water or falls of cold ocean water, can carry divers in unexpected directions without them being aware.

Dawn arrives late and dusk comes early to the sea. Light halves in intensity with every 1 or 2 m of descent, and it is effectively 'night' below 80 m. Most recreational diving takes place in clear, shallow, and placid waters. Professional diving occurs throughout the year, alongside or beneath large obstructions, and in turbid waters where finding the task, let alone completing it, may be very demanding. Backscattering often makes artificial illumination ineffective.

Underwater, binaural localization of sound is poor. Sound travels almost five times as fast and many times more efficiently through water than air. This increases susceptibility to blast injury. Loss of air conduction raises auditory thresholds by 30 to 60 dB. Neoprene foam hoods raise thresholds by a further 30 dB or so.

Only the surface waters of tropical seas are warm enough for individuals to remain effective without insulation for any length of time (Fig. 9.5.6.3). Body temperature can be maintained at 37 °C with minimal effort in air at 18 to 24 °C, the zone of thermal neutrality. In water, this zone is high and narrow (35.0 to 35.5 °C). Loss of tactile discrimination and manual dexterity are major problems when working in cold water. Exercise or excessive insulation in warm water rapidly leads to hyperthermia.

Effects of simple immersion

Water resists movement, making most tasks more tiring and less efficient than on land (Fig. 9.5.6.4). A swimmer can sustain about 5 kgf thrust (*c.*50 N), enough for propulsion at 1 to 2 knots (1.85–3.7 km/h). Full inspiration makes an adult swimmer about 2.5 kgf (*c.*25 N) positively buoyant, requiring half of maximum thrust to descend. Breathing out to residual volume results in about 2.5 kgf (25 N) negative buoyancy, requiring half of maximum thrust to ascend. The neutrally buoyant diver can be poised at will but body weight can no longer be used to apply leverage or torque, or to stay in place against a current.

Immersion displaces blood upwards. About 500 ml enters the chest, distending large veins and right atrium. Local stretch receptors interpret this as excess circulating volume and promote diuresis, resulting in hypovolaemia on emersion. The pressure gradient can compromise either inspiratory or expiratory effort, depending on the diver's attitude in the water.

The displaced blood increases cardiac preload. This predisposes susceptible individuals to 'immersion pulmonary oedema' which occurs despite normal cardiac function, and usually after a dive in cold water or involving strenuous exercise. In one study, a history of pulmonary oedema after diving in cold water was associated with elevated peripheral vascular resistance, especially after a cold challenge, and an increased risk of developing hypertension. An acute increase in preload and afterload is presumed to cause the oedema. It typically resolves within hours. Treatment is with oxygen. Diuretics are used in more severe cases.

Aspiration of small amounts of seawater can cause 'saltwater aspiration syndrome', characterized by productive cough, retrosternal discomfort, and haemoptysis during, or within 2 h of, a dive. Fever, aches, malaise, and even impaired consciousness can develop. The casualty is usually normocapnic, often hypoxic and sometimes has a leucocytosis. Treatment is rest and oxygen. Warming often helps extrapulmonary symptoms. Most cases resolve spontaneously within 6 to 24 h.

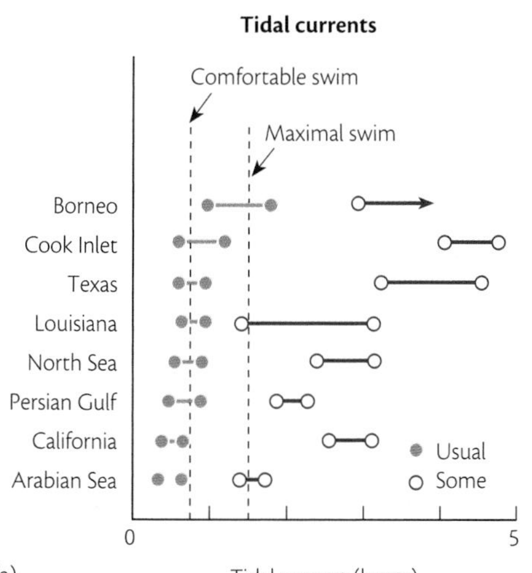

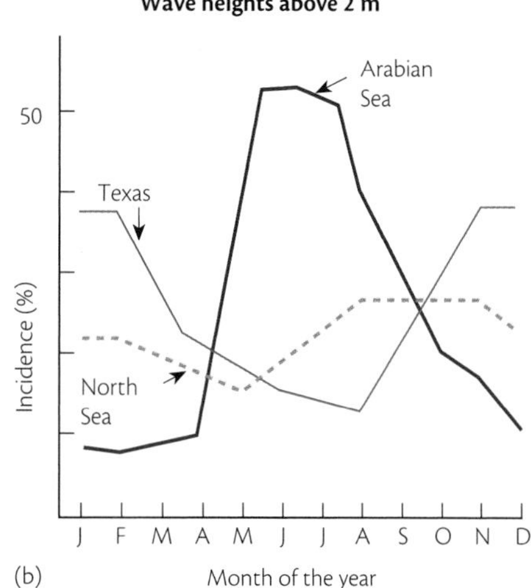

Fig. 9.5.6.2 (a) A plot of the usual and the not uncommonly seen tidal currents in eight diving sites around the world. (b) A plot of the percentage incidence of waves exceeding a height of 2 m at different times of the year in three of the diving sites.

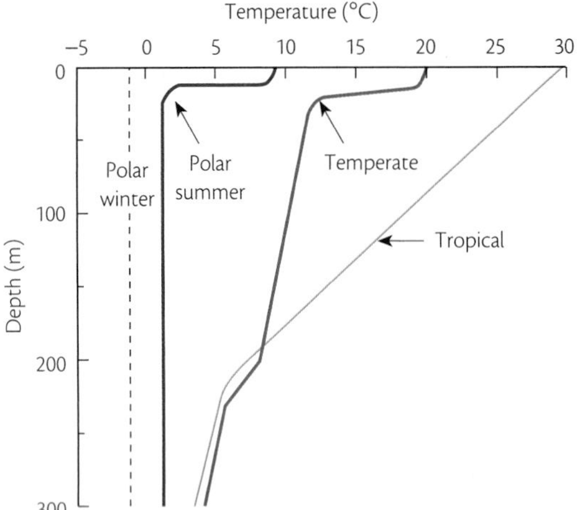

Fig. 9.5.6.3 Variations in sea temperature with site and depth. Note that water temperatures of less than 20 °C are too cold for unclothed individuals to stay in for very long.

If cool water enters one ear canal before the other, then a transient 'caloric vertigo' can result. Recurrent immersion causes problems such as otitis externa and dermatitis.

Problems of descent

The chest wall can maintain a pressure difference equivalent to 1 or 2 m of water, so gas within the body is virtually at the same pressure as the surrounding sea. The lung of a breath-hold diver is compressed from total lung capacity to residual volume at 30 m (400 kPa), so they will need half of their aerobic capacity to ascend. Variation in gas volume in clothing and equipment further complicates buoyancy control.

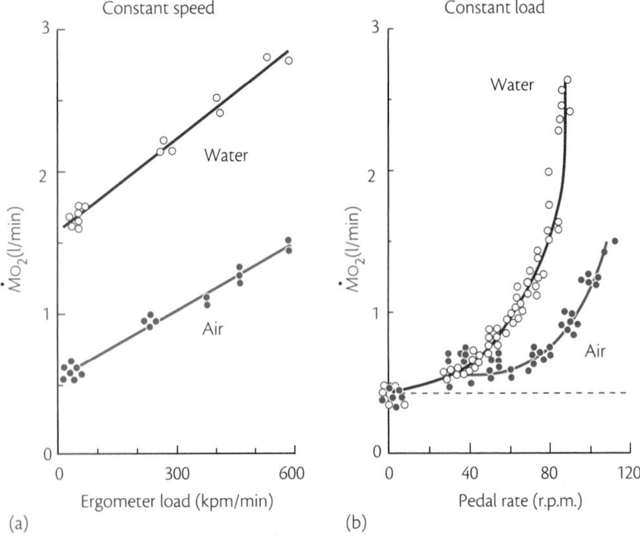

Fig. 9.5.6.4 A comparison of oxygen consumption ($\dot{M}O_2$) when pedalling a cycle ergometer in air and under water, (a) at a constant load (60 rev/min) and (b) at a constant light load. Note the high cost of moving the limbs through water. Most people's aerobic capacity is about 2.5 litres O_2/min.

Barotrauma of descent

Barotrauma is the term used to describe mechanical damage caused by changes in gas volume with pressure.

Compression will force a diver's face into an unvented mask. The resulting facial oedema and subconjunctival haemorrhages usually resolve spontaneously. If gas is not added to a dry suit on descent, particularly if it is poorly tailored, it can pinch the skin resulting in linear wheals, commonly distributed around the neck, axillae, and groins. These require no active intervention but should not be confused with cutaneous signs of decompression illness (DCI). Severe suit squeeze can limit a diver's movements.

Blood is drawn into the chest vessels to compensate for reduced lung volume, so lung injury occurs only at very great depths in breath-hold dives. When gas in obstructed sinuses is compressed, sinus walls become oedematous and may bleed. Epistaxis often occurs on ascent as blood or clot is expelled by re-expanding gas.

Middle-ear barotrauma is the commonest problem in diving. Eustachian tube dysfunction prevents ventilation of the middle ear. Compression of the trapped gas draws the round and oval windows of the inner ear outwards and the eardrum inwards. Eardrum perforations can occur. They normally heal spontaneously but persistent ruptures require surgery. Diving should be avoided until the drums have healed.

Strenuous Valsalva-like efforts to ventilate the middle ear raise thoracic pressure. This transmits to the perilymph and can be sufficient to rupture the oval or, more typically, the round window. This is known as inner-ear barotrauma. Immediate or delayed vertigo, tinnitus, and hearing loss (usually at high frequencies) ensue. Management is bed rest with the head elevated, avoidance of raised intrathoracic pressure, and consultation with an ENT surgeon who might elect to repair the rupture surgically. If the symptoms appear after a dive, they can mimic vestibular DCI. If there is any doubt, a diving medicine specialist should be consulted.

Barotrauma of descent can also affect a blocked external auditory meatus, gas spaces in carious teeth and under fillings or, in the event of loss of breathing gas pressure, the whole body.

Problems at the bottom of a dive

For prolonged dives, compressed gas is delivered to the diver at the same pressure as the surrounding water. This can be via a hose from the surface. A continuous flow through the helmet or face mask is easily engineered but is wasteful of gas. Most divers now use valves that provide gas only on demand. Self-contained underwater breathing apparatus (scuba) allows the diver to carry an on-demand supply of gas independent from the surface. This rarely lasts for more than 1 h. Rebreather equipment achieves greater endurance by replacing oxygen and removing CO_2 from exhaled gas so that it can be recirculated.

Inert gas narcosis

At raised partial pressure, nitrogen and several other inert gases with high solubility in lipids act like anaesthetics. Effects develop within minutes and reverse rapidly because they depend on passive solution. Air is often breathed down to depths of 50 m, although sophisticated tests of cerebral function show impairment starting at 20 m. Below 50 m, effects become more obvious, and divers have been known to offer their mouthpiece to neighbouring fish. Narcosis is completely reversed on ascent. Using a less narcotic gas such as helium allows divers to reach the lowermost parts of the continental shelves without narcosis. Divers can complete routine tasks while narcosed if they have repeatedly rehearsed them at increasing depths. Cognition and problem-solving, however, remain impaired.

Hypercapnia

Work of breathing and physiological dead space increase as gas becomes denser at pressure. Hyperventilation is difficult at depth but can still occur. Breathing air at depths greater than 30 m can cause hypercapnia. Some divers hypoventilate involuntarily and become hypercapnic even in favourable conditions. Although they enjoy good gas economy, hypercapnia increases risk of inert gas narcosis, cerebral oxygen toxicity, and DCI. Use of a less dense mixture, such as oxygen-in-helium, reduces this effect. Hypercapnia can also result from equipment malfunction, contaminated gas, or voluntary hypoventilation.

Oxygen toxicity

Oxygen toxicity is due to complex biochemical interactions and takes time to develop and to reverse. There is a wide range of inter- and intra-individual sensitivity.

Inspired oxygen partial pressures exceeding 50 kPa are toxic to the lungs. Irritation of lung endothelium and epithelium causes a spreading tracheobronchitis and reduction in lung volumes, flows, and gas transfer. Symptoms appear after about 6 h at partial pressures around 79 to 89 kPa and after 3 h at around 200 kPa. Advanced pulmonary changes can be irreversible, but symptoms typically diminish rapidly in 2 to 4 h with complete recovery in 1 to 3 days. Lung function similarly recovers rapidly, although small decrements can persist for more than a week.

Pulmonary damage continues at inspired oxygen partial pressures in excess of 200 kPa, but central nervous system toxicity becomes the primary limit to diving (Fig. 9.5.6.5). Exercise, shivering, hypercapnia, anxiety, immersion, and pyrexia potentiate cerebral oxygen toxicity. As a result, inspired oxygen is usually adjusted between maxima of 130 and 160 kPa when in water, depending on work levels. Manifestations of oxygen toxicity include visual disturbances, tinnitus, irritability, and dizziness. A generalized seizure will usually follow if the oxygen partial pressure is not reduced promptly. Toxicity while immersed can be very dangerous but, in the safety of a hyperbaric chamber, partial pressures up to 300 kPa are used for maximum therapeutic effect.

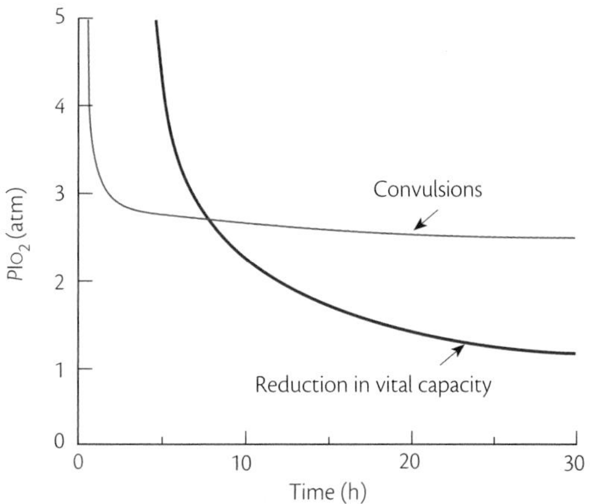

Fig. 9.5.6.5 Commonly observed pulmonary and central nervous O_2 toxicity versus time curves related to inspired PO_2 (PIO_2) (constructed from the data of many workers).

Multiple therapeutic hyperbaric exposures can cause myopic lens changes. They have also been reported in divers breathing oxygen for many hours. Most are reversible within 12 weeks of last exposure.

High-pressure nervous syndrome

Breathing oxygen-in-helium at depths in excess of 100 m causes tremor. Impaired higher function and level of consciousness and, in more severe cases, convulsions, occur at greater depths. The extreme pressures directly compress nerve components and affect their function. Depth and rate of pressurization influence the nature and incidence of symptoms. Slower compressions reduce both incidence and severity. Some habituation occurs during prolonged exposure. Adding a small amount of narcotic gas such as nitrogen to the breathing mixture opposes the compression and reduces some of the manifestations.

Problems of ascent

On ascent, partial pressures of gases fall as they expand, and less gas can remain in solution.

Hypoxia

Hypoxia will occur if breath is held for sufficiently long. Ordinarily, increasing CO_2 stimulates the breath-hold diver to take a breath but predive hyperventilation will delay this, sometimes to a dangerous extent. A frankly hypoxic mixture can be supplied by mistake during a compressed gas dive. In some rebreathers, a hard-working diver can consume oxygen faster than the design delivers it to the mixture (dilution hypoxia). Although the oxygen partial pressure might be sufficient to sustain consciousness at depth in any of these situations, ascent will cause it to fall further.

Barotrauma of ascent

Middle-ear barotrauma can occur on ascent as well as descent. The mechanism of injury is due to expansion of trapped gas. If one ear clears before the other, uneven vestibular stimulation can cause a transient 'alternobaric vertigo'. If gas in sinuses cannot escape, it might eventually burst them. Rupture of the ethmoid sinus is rare but feared because of the risk of cerebral infection. The gut is quite resilient but in some cases, especially on rapid ascent, ruptures have occurred. Dental barotrauma is also reported and rapid ascents can fracture teeth.

In a minority of individuals, the facial nerve or maxillary branch of the trigeminal nerve are exposed to pressure changes in the middle ear and maxillary sinus, respectively. If gas is not vented from the space on ascent, overpressure can impair the nerve's blood flow, and hence cause a cranial nerve deficit a few minutes after ascent. This could be misdiagnosed as DCI. Release of pressure brings about resolution, which is usually within minutes and unlikely to exceed 2 h.

Compressed gas diving allows the diver to fill the lungs at depth and, therefore, to burst them on ascent unless they are adequately vented. About 9.3 kPa overpressure (barely 1 m of seawater) bursts a lung. Ascent at a controlled rate, breathing normally or exhaling, allows the lungs, which have a time constant of emptying close to 0.3 s, to empty and minimizes the risk of rupture.

Ascent at too rapid a rate, or while breath-holding, risks lung rupture. Central tears lead to mediastinal emphysema. Peripheral tears cause pneumothorax. Gas may embolize into the systemic circulation, the most significant targets being central nervous system and myocardium. Escaped gas expands as the ascent continues, making matters worse. The victim may lose consciousness or develop neurological deficit almost immediately. Otherwise dyspnoea, cough, haemoptysis, voice change, or discomfort in the throat or retrosternal region develop a few minutes later. There may be surgical emphysema of the neck and upper chest, increased cardiac dullness or crepitus, and/or evidence of a pneumothorax.

Patients with neurological signs should be recompressed as soon as possible. In the meantime, first aid management is oxygen (as close to 100% as possible) and rehydration. Recompression will also reduce the volume of escaped gas if severe pneumomediastinum or subcutaneous emphysema threatens the airway.

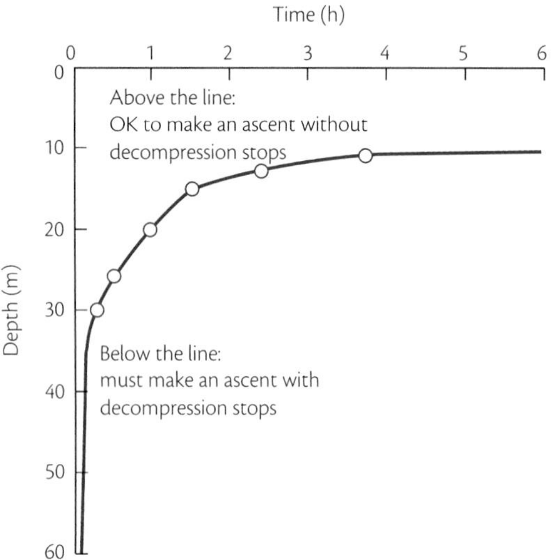

Fig. 9.5.6.6 The 'no-stop' diving curve that determines whether a dive has been shallow and brief enough for the diver to make a free ascent to the surface.

Decompression illness (DCI)

More inert gas dissolves in tissues as dive depth or duration increases. On a safe ascent, this gas comes out of solution, often forming bubbles in the venous circulation, slowly enough for it to diffuse out harmlessly via the lungs. Tissues are said to be 'supersaturated' until all of the excess gas is eliminated. If bubbles are too large or too numerous, they can block blood vessels, damage vascular endothelium, and induce 'foreign body' reactions. More severe decompression can generate extravascular bubbles within solid tissues, causing distortion and even rupturing cells. The term decompression sickness (DCS) describes disease caused by gas coming out of solution. DCI includes both DCS and disease caused by bubbles escaped from a ruptured lung.

The lungs can filter out moderate numbers of venous gas emboli before they reach the systemic circulation. This 'filter' can be circumvented by right–left shunts such as patent foramen ovale (PFO) or pulmonary arteriovenous anastomosis. One in four healthy people has a PFO, but many are only 'probe-patent' with little chance of shunting. Foramina exceeding 10 mm in diameter are found in fewer than 1%. Over half of the victims of neurological DCI have patent foramina, but it is unclear whether that is cause or effect. For instance, a significant pulmonary bubble load could trigger vasoconstriction, raise right heart pressures, and open a previously 'closed' foramen. Increasing intrathoracic pressure by heavy lifting and Valsalva-like manoeuvres to clear ears, could have a similar effect.

It has been estimated that the odds ratio of serious DCS in divers with PFO is around 2.5. Absolute risk of DCS for the whole diving population is low, however, at a little over 2 per 10 000 dives, and primary screening for PFO is not advocated. 'Undeserved' DCI justifies screening with bubble-contrast echocardiography. If a large PFO is found, the usual approach is to advise less provocative diving or percutaneous closure of the defect. Migraine with aura is associated with an increased risk of PFO.

After 24 to 48 h at a constant pressure, no more gas accumulates in tissues. Decompression from this 'saturated' state takes as long as several days but it does not lengthen however much dive duration is extended. This is the basis of saturation diving. A vast amount of experimental work has been done to determine the safe limits to 'no-stop' diving (Fig. 9.5.6.6) and the depth–time profiles that have to be followed on returning to the surface after longer dives.

DCI occurs in about 1% of dives conducted within 'safe' schedules, in some 2 to 3% of dives at the limits of these schedules, and in many badly conducted dives. Signs of arterial gas embolism following pulmonary rupture will usually present within the first 10 min after surfacing; 50% of all DCI cases will develop symptoms within 1 h of surfacing and 90% within 6 h.

The most common presentation in military and commercial diving is limb pain, commonly of the shoulders or elbows in divers and of the knees and hips in tunnel workers. Pain may present a few minutes or as much as 24 h after a dive, often as a dull and poorly localized ache of gradual onset. It is not usually made worse by moving the joint, although weight bearing may make knee pain worse. Signs of inflammation are uncommon. Left untreated, the pain will regress and disappear over 2 or 3 days. Recompression commonly improves the pain quickly.

Although recreational divers also experience limb pain, neurological symptoms are more likely. Sensory disturbance is common, with numbness and paraesthesiae being frequent manifestations. One fulminant form commences with girdle pain followed by loss of sensation and power in the lower limbs. Involvement of the brain is common and may be subtle. This can impair insight and delay a diver's decision to seek assistance. Denial is also a frequent feature. Any of the higher functions can be involved, including loss of short-term memory, altered affect, visual disturbance, and loss of consciousness. Inner-ear DCI can be confused with inner-ear barotrauma. Bubbles do not necessarily respect normal anatomical boundaries, and patchy or multisystem presentations are typical. It is not unusual to exhibit several manifestations, or for them to appear at different times and to evolve in different ways.

Divers developing any manifestation of DCI within 24 h of a dive should be managed as if they have the condition. First aid management is oxygen (as close to 100% as possible) and rehydration. All but trivial cases of DCI should be recompressed as soon as possible. It is an effective treatment. It reduces the size and promotes resorption of existing bubbles before irreversible infarction and oedema occur. It prevents formation of new bubbles. High inspired partial pressures of oxygen facilitate removal of excess inert gas, relieve ischaemia, and reduce oedema, inflammation, and reperfusion injury. The goal is as complete a resolution of symptoms as possible at depth and to avoid recurrence on surfacing. Relapse or residual symptoms require retreatment, so detailed post-recompression examination is necessary. DCI may fail to resolve completely.

Miscellaneous related problems

A diver who ascends more rapidly than the planned decompression schedule has 'omitted decompression'. Risk of DCI is increased. Treatment is oxygen and, in many cases, recompression.

New exposure to an inert gas when saturated with another can increase overall gas burden if there is a mismatch in the rate at which the gases diffuse into and out of a tissue. This can cause a bubble-related disease for which decompression is not the immediate provocation, and is known as 'isobaric counterdiffusion'. The site affected depends on the location of the interface between the two gases. It can cause inner-ear or skin symptoms in saturation divers. Progression can be halted by altering the gas mixture. It can be treated by recompression and prevented by slightly increasing environmental pressure in order to avoid saturation before changing gas mixtures.

Several hours after breathing high fractions of oxygen, a diver can develop an exudate in the middle ear, yet remain able to ventilate the ears. This might be due to consumption of oxygen causing an insidious volume reduction or a direct toxic effect of oxygen upon the middle-ear epithelium. The problem resolves spontaneously within hours. Differential pressure across a restricted aperture can generate large forces with serious, and often fatal, consequences. Examples include the inflow to a culvert or a sudden breach in a pipe containing gas at lower pressure than ambient. Potential mechanisms of injury include entrapment, compromised inspiratory effort, primary trauma, and critical damage to equipment.

Problems after the dive

Autopsies on asymptomatic divers with no history of DCI have revealed that their brains and spinal cords contain considerably more microinfarcts than those of nondiving controls. Although the consequences of such damage are considered slight or subclinical, subjective reports of forgetfulness and poor concentration have been correlated with diving experience. A history of welding increases the probability of a diver reporting these problems. Subjectively forgetful divers, as a group, performed worse than controls in tests of cognitive function, especially memory. They also had structural differences on brain MRI.

Imaging of long bones of divers and caisson workers show aseptic infarcts (dysbaric osteonecrosis) in a sizeable minority (up to 11%). The incidence is higher in those with a history of overt DCI. Lesions can occur after a single decompression, but their incidence rises with age, depth, and diving intensity. Those in the head, neck, or shaft are asymptomatic, but those at juxta-articular surfaces can be disabling. They are more common in caisson workers than divers, but are even seen in professional breath-hold divers, such as the Ama of Japan, in whom the dissolved gas burden must be light. The aetiology is unknown, but gas embolism is the favoured explanation.

Commercial diving, especially saturation diving, enlarges total lung capacity and forced vital capacity (FVC). This is attributed to training effects of prolonged breathing of compressed gases. The FEV_1/FVC ratio falls, due partly to the rise in FVC, but there are also hints of additional small-airway damage. Pulmonary capillary blood volume, as judged by carbon monoxide transfer, also falls. This appears to be due to transient episodes of hyperoxia during saturation-diving procedures, but may also be associated with venous gas emboli on decompression. The effects are slight but definite and may be cumulative. There are no obvious clinical consequences.

Mild high-tone deafness is found in commercial divers and is attributed to the noise of gas flows within their helmets.

Fitness to dive

Fitness assessment balances real and theoretical hazards against employer and physician liability and duty of care, legislation, and the candidate's livelihood or desire to dive. Some organizations adopt didactic standards. Others use guidelines, which leave room for judgement by the physician and, sometimes, for informed risk to be carried by the candidate.

Military and commercial diving is physically demanding and often remote from medical aid. These divers undergo periodic medical examinations. Periodicity and extent of examination depend on local regulations. Many recreational divers simply complete regular health declarations, undergoing examination only if a question is answered 'positively'.

Assessments aim to determine whether candidates:

- are sufficiently physically fit to rescue a fellow diver, to swim in swift currents and rough waters, and to undertake any related nondiving tasks
- are medically fit and have no problems that might incapacitate, impair, distract, predispose to decompression illness or barotrauma, or otherwise make them a liability to themselves or others
- require any restrictions or adjustments

We must avoid understatement of the dangers of diving, especially at its most extreme, but must also assess hazard and risk realistically, enabling imaginative solutions for, and greater acceptability of, disabled divers who can often dive usefully without jeopardizing health or safety of those involved.

An individual who is bodily fit, mentally stable, free of conditions such as epilepsy, obstructive lung disease, ill-controlled diabetes or asthma, alcohol or drug addiction, and has no history of ruptured eardrums or aural surgery is likely to be fit to dive. An acute chest, upper airway, or ear infection would be grounds for temporary unfitness. Diving should be avoided while taking medication that could impair exercise capacity, ability to think clearly, or ability to orientate in space. Medical conditions that can mimic DCI deserve careful assessment. Women are advised not to dive during pregnancy as evidence is suggestive, though not yet conclusive, that the unborn child is at increased risk of developmental defect.

Compromised gas flow or gas exchange could predispose to injury or an inability to cope with the respiratory demands of diving. Risk factors for spontaneous lung rupture such as distortion of lung tissue must be carefully assessed. If a candidate runs several kilometres a day, is a good swimmer, was always good at games at school, and has no history of recent respiratory disease, they are very likely to be fit to dive. FEV_1 multiplied by 35 measures the maximal voluntary ventilation, an indicator of respiratory fitness. FEV_1 should, therefore, be more than 75% predicted. FVC should also be more than 75% predicted because there is good evidence that subjects with a low FVC and, by inference, lungs that are too small for their bodies, are more liable to lung rupture on rapid ascents. The FEV_1/FVC ratio has not been found to be especially helpful. What matters most in diving is the time constant of emptying of the full lungs.

The PEF/FVC ratio is a reasonable measure of this, and PEF should be at least 1.5 times predicted FVC per second.

Past or current asthma used to be an absolute contraindication to diving on theoretical grounds of increased risk of lung rupture on fast ascents. Childhood asthma often disappears, however, and very many people with current mild asthma are known to dive frequently without ill effect. The British Thoracic Society's guidelines permit diving in asymptomatic asthma with normal spirometry, negative exercise test, PEF no more than 10% below best values, and requiring no more than regular inhaled anti-inflammatory agents.

Conclusion

More effective therapies for DCI are sought, either instead of, or to supplement recompression. Surface oxygen is used as a first aid measure but might have a role as a definitive treatment in selected groups. Intravenous perfluorocarbons and lidocaine have both attracted interest but more evidence is required. An intervention as simple as an oral nonsteroidal anti-inflammatory drug showed promise in reducing compression requirements in a recent randomized controlled study. Further meticulous data collection will help to identify subgroups who need minimal or more aggressive treatment from the outset. It will also help to clarify issues of safety of drugs, and of medical conditions, while diving.

Advice on management of diving disorders can be obtained from the British Hyperbaric Association 24-h advice line run by the Institute of Naval Medicine (07831 151523) for England, Wales, and Northern Ireland and by Aberdeen Royal Infirmary (0845 408 6008) for Scotland. There are many helpful organizations around the world. The Divers' Alert Network, for instance, has international coverage, and contact details can be obtained from http://www.diversalertnetwork.org/contact/international.asp

Further reading

Bennett M, Mitchell S, Dominguez A (2003). Adjunctive treatment of decompression illness with a non-steroidal anti-inflammatory drug (tenoxicam) reduces compression requirements. *Undersea Hyperb Med*, **30**, 195–204. [A rare example of a randomized controlled study of a therapeutic aspect of diving medicine.]

Bove AA (2004). *Bove and Davis' diving medicine*, 4th edition. W B Saunders, Philadelphia. [General text with clinical emphasis.]

British Thoracic Society Fitness to Dive Group (2003). British Thoracic Society guidelines on respiratory aspects of fitness for diving. *Thorax*, **58**, 3–13. [A useful summary of the evidence relevant to respiratory fitness to dive and how this has been used to develop fitness standards.]

Brubakk A, Neuman T (eds.) (2003). *Bennett and Elliott's physiology and medicine of diving*, 5th edition. W B Saunders, London. [General text with plentiful details about underpinning investigative work.]

Edmonds C, *et al.* (eds.) (2002). *Diving and subaquatic medicine*, 4th edition. Arnold, London. [General text with practical emphasis.]

Lundgren CEG, Miller JN (eds.) (1999). *The lung at depth*. Dekker, New York. [Detailed chapters on individual interactions between lung and diving environment written by recognized authorities in each area.]

Macdiarmid JI, *et al.* (2004). Co-ordinated investigation into the possible long term health effects of diving at work. In: *Examination of the long term health impact of diving: The ELTHI diving study*. HSE Books, HMSO, Norwich. [A comprehensive and contemporary cross-sectional study on possible long-term effects of diving.]

Slade JB, *et al.* (2001). Pulmonary edema associated with scuba diving. Case reports and review. *Chest*, **120**, 1686–94. [Informative overview of immersion pulmonary oedema.]

UK Health and Safety Executive Research Report RR761—Differential pressure hazards in diving 2009.

Wilmshurst PT, *et al.* (1989). Cold-induced pulmonary oedema in scuba divers and swimmers and subsequent development of hypertension. *Lancet*, **i**, 62–5. [Comprehensive controlled study of cold-induced immersion pulmonary oedema.]

9.5.7 Lightning and electrical injuries

Chris Andrews

Essentials

Lightning

Lightning strikes are rare accidents but carry a 10% case fatality, killing 0.1 to 0.3 per million population each year. During thunderstorms, the risk is increased by sheltering under trees or by being on open water, on tractors, or in open fields or golf courses.

Lightning causes instant asystole. It is suspected clinically if someone is found collapsed in the open with linear or feathered burns, exploded clothing, and ruptured eardrums. Victims are safe to handle, with most victims showing keraunoparalysis (cold, pulseless, mottled extremities). Immediate cardiopulmonary resuscitation (CPR) is mandatory. Survivors may develop complications including pain syndromes and psychological sequelae.

Electrocution

Electrocution is the fifth commonest cause of workplace death, mainly affecting utilities, mining, and construction labourers. Contact with power lines and power tools are the commonest causes, with metal ladders and antennae being particularly dangerous. Prevention is by implementing codes of safe practice.

Victims of electrocution may suffer prolonged attachment to the source of electric current and must be removed or disconnected from the source before resuscitation. Clinical presentations include (1) ventricular fibrillation, sometimes leading to persistent cardiac dysfunction; (2) neurological and muscular manifestations, both early and late, including paraesthesiae, pareses, and generalized convulsions, also tetanic spasm causing respiratory embarrassment and rhabdomyolysis; (3) burns, which may be severe and require expert surgical attention. Electroporation (cell membrane disruption) contributes to cell death; delineation using polaxamers may direct the extent of surgical debridement.

Introduction

Lightning is a powerful force; it provides spectacular displays and has evoked an extensive mythology. The comparatively recent discovery and distribution of electricity have had an equally profound effect, and provide truth to the adage that 'electricity is a good servant and a bad master'.

Epidemiology

Lightning injury

The latest accepted case fatality of lightning shock is around 10% and is around 0.3 per million population in the United States of America each year, but fewer than 0.1 per million in the United Kingdom.

In the early part of the 20th century, most people struck by lightning were outdoor workers (67%) and outdoor recreationalists (28%). Nowadays, the breakdown is 45% and 50%, respectively, explained by changes in social and work habits. Indoor strikes (e.g. by current conducted through communication or power apparatus) continue to account for about 5% of these accidents.

Men are more often injured than women (1.67 males to 0.33 females); the age group most at risk is 20 to 29 years. Risky situations include sheltering under trees, on open water, on tractors, in open fields, and playing golf. Regional differences correlate well with storm activity and population density in that area.

Electrical injury

Electrocution ranks fifth in the causes of workplace death, accounting for the death of 10 000 workers each year in the United States, with a further 10 million being injured. Most of the victims work for utility companies, followed by mining and construction workers. Contact with power lines causes 53% of fatal shocks, and contact with power tools accounts for a further 22%. The most dangerous times of day seem to be between 10.00 a.m. and 3.00 p.m. on Mondays, Tuesdays, and Thursdays. Most of the victims are trade and labouring staff; sales, clerical, and professional categories are at least risk. Metal ladders and antennas are particularly dangerous and can easily be hoisted into overhead power lines. Codes of safe practice are written accordingly.

In domestic situations, contact with overhead lines is again important. Faulty, including amateur, repair of equipment and faulty apparatus, wiring, and especially power and extension cords account for large numbers of deaths and injuries. Children are at particular risk. Death from domestic electric shock has shown a marked decrease with the introduction of residual current devices (RCDs). These sense if current is diverted from the supply main to earth and interrupt it in a matter of milliseconds.

Mechanisms of injury

Lightning injury

Lightning injury may be sustained in five separate ways:

1. A person may be struck directly.
2. A nearby object, such as a tree or a building, may be struck, and someone in direct contact with it may receive a shock.
3. Without direct contact an arc may 'jump' to a nearby person from the struck object, thereby generating a 'side flash'.
4. As current disperses away from the base of a strike to ground, an individual may divert current flowing in the ground to themselves. This is termed 'shock due to increase in earth potential'.
5. A recently documented mechanism is the transient flow of current due to corona and streamer formation.

Both cardiac and respiratory function cease instantaneously under lightning strike, the cardiac arrest being asystolic. Cardiac function restarts under local pacemaker control, but respiratory function does not recommence and secondary hypoxic cardiac arrest supervenes.

The major cranial orifices are portals of entry for lightning current, and from there pathways to the brainstem are short. Respiratory function is thought to be affected there, and thence conduction through the cerebrospinal fluid to neural tissue and bloodstream to the myocardium.

The QT prolongation resulting from lightning injury may predispose to episodic arrythmias. There is no evidence that lightning inhibits body metabolism. Resuscitation is as urgent as with any other injury. There is similarly no evidence that metal on the head, or the presence of a mobile telephone (cellphone), predisposes to being struck.

Electrical injury

With electric shock, it is important to assess the points of entry and exit and the pathway of current through the body. Once the pathway has been determined, a locus for expected injury can be established, and the flow of current can be estimated from the applied voltage divided by the impedance of the proposed pathway. Most impedance is in the skin barriers, and is nonlinear. There is an initial (contact) impedance, which decreases as current flow continues. Impedance also varies with time since application, contact surface area, and frequency.

For currents with a frequency of 15 to 100 Hz, externally applied from hand to hand, or hand to foot, relevant variables are the threshold of perception (0.5 mA) and 'let go' current (10 mA). A 50% chance of fibrillation exists at 2000 mA conducted for 10 ms, or at the other extreme 100 mA conducted for 10 s. Direct internal application of less than 200 μA to the heart muscle may induce fibrillation. Dangerous current levels as well as impedance parameters are documented in standards.

Joule heating may account for tissue damage in the path of the current. It may be calculated from the power dissipation in the tissue—the square of the tissue current (often hard to estimate) times its impedance. The complex phenomenon of electroporation, where cell membranes are breached by the electrical induction of unstable pores in the membrane, may also lead to cell death. The complex nature of internal electric fields leads to internal field damage difficult to quantify and predict.

Presentation of the injured person

Lightning injury

A witnessed strike offers the best chance of resuscitation. The victim is not dangerous to touch, and does not constitute a risk to the rescuer. Immediate cardiopulmonary resuscitation (CPR) is paramount. It has been stated that:

> Any person found with linear burns and clothing exploded off should be treated as the victim of a lightning strike. Feathering burns are pathognomic of lightning injury and occur in no other type of injury. ...Another complex diagnostic of lightning injury includes linear or punctate burns, tympanic membrane rupture, confusion, and outdoor location....
>
> Cooper *et al.* (2000)

In assessing a lightning victim, the following features must be sought.

Cardiovascular and pulmonary consequences

Asystolic arrest is the main cardiac event in lightning injury. ECG signs may take many forms, with ischaemic and infarct forms.

They almost invariably resolve completely over time. Alterations in QT interval and arrythmias of many kinds are seen. ECG changes may not occur until late in the course, and so are poor diagnostic tools. Respiratory arrest is common. A person not suffering cardiopulmonary arrest is highly unlikely to die from lightning strike ($p < 0.0001$).

Neurological consequences

Direct neural injury may occur both centrally and peripherally. All forms of intracranial bleeding have been reported. Direct cerebral damage particularly affects the basal ganglia, cerebellum, and brainstem. Dural tears, scalp haematomata, and fractures are also seen. Seizures occur as a result of anoxia and injury.

Peripheral nerve injury, including autonomic injury, can give prolonged and long-lasting disability, which often develops late. Other late features include spinal cord atrophic paralysis, cerebellar ataxia, incoordination, paraesthesiae, and aphasia. Continuing complex regional pain syndromes may be seen.

Keraunoparalysis and burns

More than 70% of victims demonstrate keraunoparalysis. This is a syndrome of cold, pulseless, mottled, and asensory extremities. The syndrome resembles a compartment syndrome and occurs in the line of passage of the strike current. It resolves spontaneously within 24 h with no sequelae, and requires no surgical intervention.

Burns are of minor consequence in lightning injury, and again require little intervention. Entry and exit burns may be full thickness though small. Arborescent (feathering) burns resemble fern-like patterns on the skin (Fig. 9.5.7.1). Their aetiology is unknown, but they fade within 24 h. Linear burns are due to the passage of hot plasma tongues over the skin. Eschar is simply allowed to separate without further treatment. Flash may be seen, like sunburn or welder's flash, from the profound radiation of the strike. Sheet burns resulting from efflux of hot plasma may be a variant of linear burning, since both seem to follow moisture and sweat lines. There may be contact burns from heated metal such as buckles and coins.

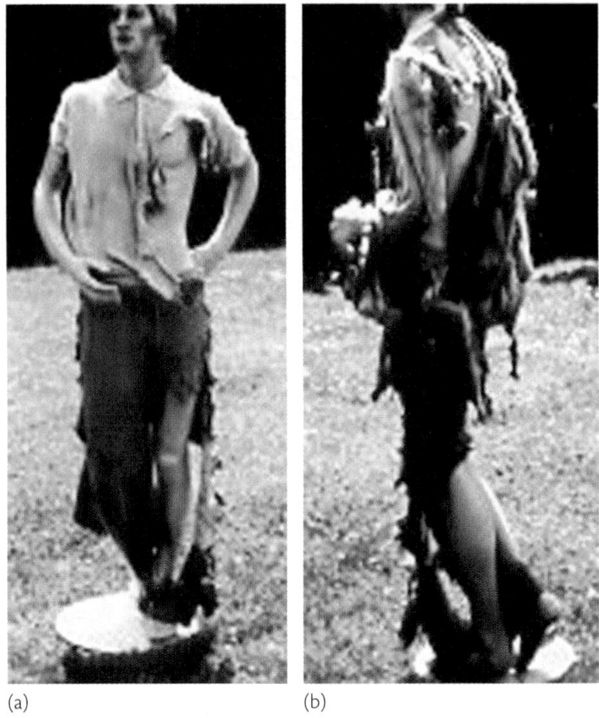

(a) (b)

Fig. 9.5.7.2 Reconstruction of external result of a lightning strike. (Courtesy Professor Mary Ann Cooper, University of Illinois, Chicago.)

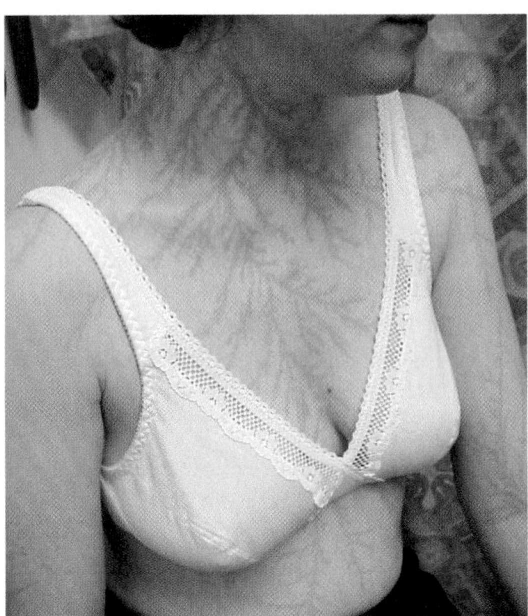

Fig. 9.5.7.1 Example of keraunographic marking. (Courtesy Dr Ajay Mahajan (Mahajan AL, Rajan R, *et al.* (2007). Lichtenberg figures: cutaneous manifestation of phone electrocution from lightning. *J Plast Reconstr Aesthet Surg*, **61**(1), 111–13). Reprinted with permission from Elsevier.)

Eye, ear, and explosive injuries

The explosive force of the lightning insult blasts clothing apart (Fig. 9.5.7.2), and may cause percussive injury to the lungs and abdominal viscera. Tympanic membranes are usually ruptured, perhaps from the explosive force of the strike. Percussive eye injury, particularly retinal, has been reported. Cataracts may develop much later.

Other injuries

Renal and haematological damage have occasionally been reported. In pregnant women, the fetus is unlikely to survive. Menstrual and sexual difficulties have been reported.

Electrical injury

In contrast to lightning injury, victims may suffer prolonged attachment to the source of electrical current, making them dangerous to touch. Before resuscitation, they must be removed from the current source, and this usually means interrupting the current flow at the supply point.

Burns are far more serious, and may merit intense surgical treatment. The likelihood of internal burning (remembering the possibility of electroporation) may require further surgical intervention. Cardiac and respiratory burns may also exist.

Cardiovascular consequences

Fibrillation is the most common cardiac abnormality following electrical injury. Cardiopulmonary resuscitation is urgently required. Electricity suppliers have standard first aid/resuscitation procedures. Cardiac dysfunction may persist for long periods, and ECG signs may not resolve.

Neurological and muscular consequences

Neural injury may be categorized into early and late syndromes, at cerebral, cord, and peripheral levels.

Early tetanic muscular contraction locks the victim on to the electrical conductors. This tetany may compromise respiratory function. Neurological injury may be hard to distinguish from hypoxic and vasospastic injury. Similarly, neural injury is often hard to separate from ischaemic injury due to vessel spasm. Early and late generalized convulsions may occur. Pareses and paraesthesiae may develop, both early and late.

In the long term, complex regional pain syndromes and other chronic pain syndromes must be considered.

Burns

Burns are often severe in electrical injury and merit much treatment effort. Arc and flame burns and contact burns from current entry and exit are seen. For example, tetanic gripping of the electrical conductor causes grasp burns to the hand.

Severe internal thermal or electroporation damage may occur. The management is largely surgical. Joints, ligaments, and tendons may be severely damaged by the heat generated, and osteonecrosis may be seen.

Other aspects

Widespread muscle damage generates myoglobin that must be cleared by the kidney with a severe risk of renal damage. Other metabolic and biochemical disturbances secondary to hypoxia may develop. Massive hyperkalaemia has implications for the use of depolarizing muscle relaxants.

Eye damage includes retinal damage, with punctation and detachment, and thermal damage to other media. During follow-up the possibility of ocular pareses and cataracts must be recognized.

After shock during pregnancy, the prognosis for the fetus is poor. Nonfocal injury is more likely in survivors.

Psychological consequences of electrical and lightning injuries

Although electrical and lightning injuries are fundamentally different in nature and management, their psychological sequelae are similar. Sequelae may be profoundly disabling. They may persist for many years and may never resolve. To a large extent, psychological consequences of persisting pain and dysfunction cannot be separated from organic psychological consequences.

Emotional sequelae include depression, often with organic features. It is hard to separate this from the emotional reaction to injury and continuing disability. Aggression, anxiety, and phobic features are common. Marital disharmony commonly follows social withdrawal, disinterest, and a fatigue state. Loss of interest in sex and in relationships, together with a feeling of fault or guilt, may be associated. Sleep disturbance is common.

There is loss of short-term memory with impaired concentration, higher mental functions, and loss of identity and ability.

Treatment of the injuries

It has been documented that assessment by those unfamiliar with the injury overlooks or wrongly diagnoses over 90% of the resulting syndrome features. First, urgent and life-saving treatment must be administered. Secondly, there must be surveillance for delayed sequelae, and thirdly long-term monitoring for morbidity, including cataract formation and psychological problems.

Lightning injury

First, the casualty is resuscitated and evacuated. Cardiopulmonary resuscitation is continued until medical emergency help is obtained. Ventilation and cardiac support may be required.

ECG monitoring must be used to detect subtle effects like QT prolongation. Associated trauma is treated.

In the long term, patients are observed for development of pain syndromes. Ocular and auditory functions are monitored. Sensitivity to the psychological sequelae is required, and preventive interviewing may be useful.

Carbemazepine, gabapentin, clonazepam, flecainide, and mexilitine are useful to control neurally derived pain and resulting weakness. An antidepressant (see following paragraphs) is a useful adjunct to this.

Electrical injury

Urgent life support is indicated. Ventilatory and inotropic support and correction of arrhythmias may be required.

For burns, progressive debridement and/or amputation may be needed. Renal damage should be prevented.

Associated trauma is treated. Ocular and auditory functions are monitored, and psychological disturbances are reviewed. In the long term, surveillance is similar to lightning injury.

Psychological elements

In all cases, the management of the psychological syndrome is paramount and may be the greatest determinant of long-term functional capability. Awareness of the impact of the injury on employment and relationships and social networks is fundamental. Cognitive and computer aids are being developed.

An antidepressant such as a selective serotonin reuptake inhibitor, possibly citalopram, paroxetine, venlafaxine, or a tricyclic such as clomipramine, may be useful.

Early and continuing neuropsychological assessment is desirable.

Controversy

The place of polaxamers in discovering the extent of electroporation and in delineating debridement levels is of great interest.

The mechanisms of the psychological disability and remote injury remain to be elucidated. Victims are frequently written off as malingering or simply depressed, when a more extensive syndrome exists. Expert evaluation is highly desirable, especially if litigation or compensation is involved. The useful duration of monitoring of otherwise asymptomatic people has not been determined.

Further reading

Andrews CJ (2006). Further documentation of remote effects of electrical injury, with comments on the place of neuropsychological testing and functional scanning. *IEEE Trans Biomed Eng*, **53**, 2102–13.

Andrews CJ, *et al.* (1992). *Lightning injuries: electrical, medical and legal aspects*. CRC Press, Boca Raton, FL.

Cherington M, Cooper MA (eds.) (1995). *Seminars in Neurology* **15** (3, 4). Special issues on lightning and electrical injuries.

Cooper MA (1980). Lightning injuries: prognostic signs for death. *Ann Emerg Med*, **9**, 134.

Cooper MA, Andrews C, Holle R (2005). Lightning injuries. In: Auerbach P (ed.) *Wilderness medicine*, 4th edition, pp. 73–111. Mosby, St Louis, MO.

Cooper MA, Andrews CJ (2005). Disability, not death, is the issue in lightning injury. *Proc Int Conf On Lightn Stat Elec*, Boeing, Seattle, WA.

Hendler N (2005). Overlooked diagnoses in chronic pain: analysis of survivors of electric shock and lightning strike. *J Occup Env Med*, **47**, 796–805.

Lee RC, Capelli-Schellpfeffer M, Kelley K (eds.) (1994). Electrical injury. *Ann N Y Acad Sci*, **720**.

Lee RC, Cravalho EG, Burke JF (1992). *Electric trauma*. Cambridge University Press, Cambridge.

Morse MS, Berg JS, TenWolde RL (2004). Diffuse electrical injury: a study of 89 subjects reporting long-term symptomatology that is remote to the theoretical current Pathway. *IEEE Trans Biomed Eng*, **51**, 1449–59.

9.5.8 Podoconiosis (nonfilarial elephantiasis)

Gail Davey

Essentials

Podoconiosis is an entirely preventable, noncommunicable, geochemical elephantiasis caused by exposure of bare feet to irritant clay soils. It is found across tropical Africa, central America, and north India where such soils coexist with high altitude, high rainfall, and low income. Prodromal symptoms include itching and a burning sensation in the foot; early changes include spreading or 'splaying' of the forefoot, swelling of the sole of the foot, leakage of colourless 'lymph' fluid, and moss-like or velvet-like changes in the skin; in advanced disease there is soft fluid ('water bag') or hard fibrotic ('leathery') swelling. Early stage disease is reversible by good foot hygiene and use of socks and shoes. Late stage disease, which results in considerable economic and social difficulties, is treated with elevation and compression of the leg and (if necessary) debulking surgery. Early stages are reversible given good foot hygiene whereas late stages result in considerable economic and social difficulties and, despite treatment, may never fully resolve.

Historical perspective

The Persian physician Rhazes first distinguished elephantiasis 'of the Greeks' (lepromatous leprosy) from that 'of the Arabs' (most probably nonfilarial elephantiasis) in *c.*905 CE. Towards the end of the 19th century, the discrepancy between the distributions of elephantiasis and filariasis in North Africa, central America, and Europe, prompted investigation by Hirsch and others. In the 1920s, persistently negative tests for filaria led Robles to infer that the elephantiasis he saw in Guatemala was an endemic condition associated with walking barefoot. Ernest Price's extensive work on the ecology and pathogenesis of the condition through the 1970s and 1980s led him to propose the term 'podoconiosis', from the Greek words πoδoσ (foot) and κoνoσ (dust), which has gained widespread acceptance.

Aetiology, genetics, pathogenesis, and pathology

The climatic factors necessary to produce irritant clays include altitudes over 1000 m above sea level, and seasonal rainfall over 1000 mm annually. These conditions contribute to the steady disintegration of lava and the reconstitution of the mineral components into silicate clays with particle size less than 2 μm.

Not everyone exposed to irritant soil develops podoconiosis, but family clustering has long been observed. Recent genetic studies have demonstrated high heritability of the trait and segregation analysis suggests the presence of an autosomal codominant major gene conferring susceptibility to podoconiosis.

Histological examination of the lymph nodes of affected individuals shows a 'starry sky' clustering of small lymphocytes and plasma cells around macrophages in the cortex. Electron microscopy shows that the macrophage phagosomes contain particles of stacked kaolinite ($Al_2Si_2O_5(OH)_4$). The lymph node sinuses are filled with lymphocytes, suggesting that obstruction to lymph flow occurs in the afferent lymphatics rather than the nodes themselves. Light microscopy shows subendothelial oedema and subsequent collagenization of afferent lymphatics reducing and finally obliterating the lumen.

Epidemiology and ecology

Podoconiosis is found in highland areas of tropical Africa, central America, and north-west India. Areas of high prevalence have been identified in Uganda, Tanzania, Kenya, Rwanda, Burundi, Sudan, and Ethiopia, to the east side of Africa, and in Equatorial Guinea, Cameroon, the islands of Bioko, São Tomé and Principe, and Cape Verde to the west (Fig. 9.5.8.1). The condition has been reported in the central American highlands from Mexico, south to Ecuador. Although filarial elephantiasis predominates in India, podoconiosis has been reported from north-west India, Sri Lanka, and Indonesia.

Although studies in Ethiopia suggested gender ratios between 1:1.4 and 1:4.2, the most recent recording was 1:0.98, which was not significantly different from the zonal gender ratio. All major community-based studies have shown onset in the first or second decade and a progressive increase in prevalence up to the sixth decade.

Development of podoconiosis is closely associated with living and working barefoot on irritant soils. Farmers are at high risk, but the risk extends to any occupation with prolonged contact with the soil, and the condition has been noted among gold-mine workers and weavers whose feet operate loom pedals dug into pits in the ground.

Prevention

Evidence suggests that primary prevention should consist of avoiding prolonged contact between the skin and irritant soils through regular use of robust footwear. However, footwear remains an unaffordable luxury for residents of most affected areas. Use of matting on the floors of traditional houses may also diminish risk.

Secondary prevention (prevention of progression of early symptoms and signs to overt elephantiasis) involves training in foot

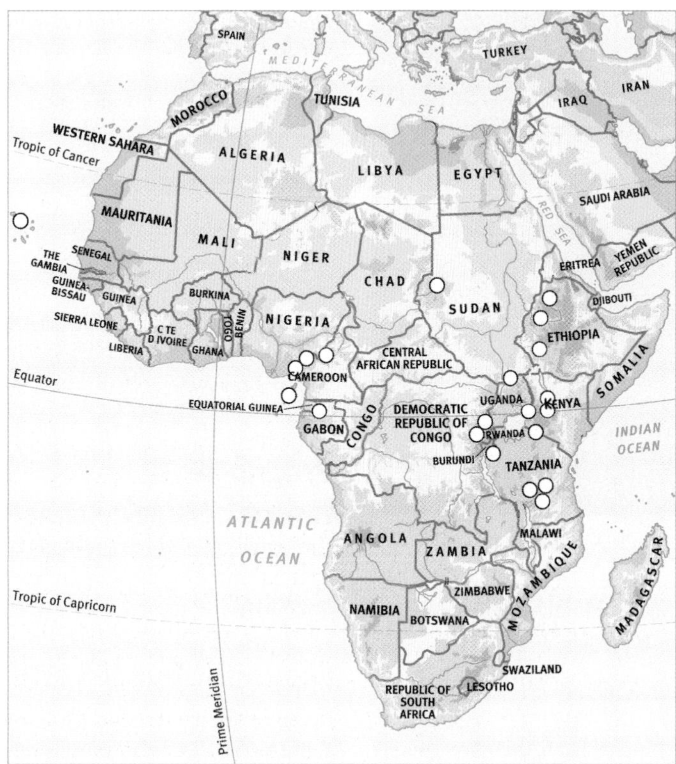

Fig. 9.5.8.1 Distribution of podoconiosis across tropical Africa and islands.

hygiene (washing daily with soap and water), and encouraging the use of socks and shoes. Progression can be completely averted if these measures are strictly adhered to, but compliance must be lifelong. Relocation from an area of irritant soil or adoption of a new occupation are also effective measures, but may not be feasible for the patient.

Clinical features

The disease process is usually described in three phases: prodromal, early, and advanced. Prodromal symptoms include itching of the skin of the forefoot, a burning sensation in the foot and lower leg, 'chills', or generalized joint pains. The affected person may describe exacerbation of symptoms when they try to walk long distances or do hard physical work.

Early changes include spreading or 'splaying' of the forefoot, swelling of the sole of the foot, leakage of colourless 'lymph' fluid from the foot, and changes in the skin so that it looks like moss or velvet (Fig. 9.5.8.2). Sometimes the feet become darker in colour, the toes become less mobile, and lumps with a mossy-looking surface develop on the top of the foot. The affected person may report limb aches, heaviness of the lower leg and foot, and odour from the lymph leak, which may attract flies. Acute episodes (usually asymmetrical and often unrelated to superimposed bacterial or fungal infection), cause fever, rigors, and a rapid increase in pain and swelling of the leg.

As advanced elephantiasis develops, both legs and feet will be affected, though one is usually more severely affected than the other. Even if footwear is available, it is difficult to wear by this stage and may increase discomfort in severely swollen feet. In advanced disease, the swelling persists as one of two types. Soft, fluid swelling is often known as 'water-bag' type, and will typically be linked to lymph fluid leakage (Fig. 9.5.8.3). Hard, fibrotic swelling is termed 'leathery' type, and is often associated with many hard skin nodules (Fig. 9.5.8.4).

Differential diagnosis

Podoconiosis must be distinguished from filarial elephantiasis (see Table 9.5.8.1) and chronic sepsis secondary to plantar ulceration or infected trauma in leprosy.

Clinical investigation

In the community, diagnosis is usually based on the features given in Table 9.5.8.1. However, if surgery is to be considered, filarial

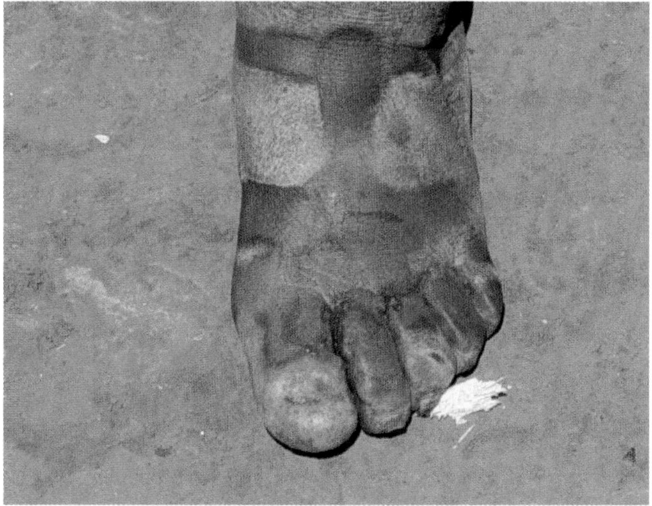

Fig. 9.5.8.2 Early changes—oedema, block toes, changes in skin colour (here related to the pattern of the open sandal worn), lymph ooze, and early mossy changes around interdigital clefts.

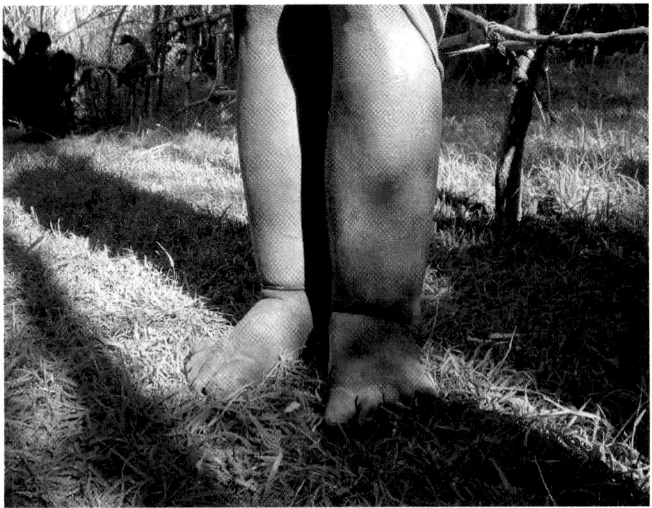

Fig. 9.5.8.3 'Water-bag' type swelling: patient in her early 20s.

disease may be ruled out by examining a midnight blood sample in countries where *Wuchereria bancrofti* is prevalent.

Treatment

Treatment of advanced disease encompasses all the above-mentioned secondary prevention measures, plus elevation and compression of the affected leg, and, if necessary, nodulectomy. To be successful, the legs must be elevated to or above the level of the heart for at least 18 h. Where electricity is available, intermittent compression machines may reduce swelling rapidly, but twice-daily application of elastic bandages is also effective. Charles' operation (removal of skin, subcutaneous tissue, and deep fascia to lay the muscles and tendons bare, followed by grafting of healthy skin), is no longer recommended, as long-term results are disappointing. Nodulectomy may be required if one or two nodules prevent use of footwear. Diathermy has proved particularly useful in treating multiple nodules. Lifelong attention to foot hygiene is mandatory if surgery is performed.

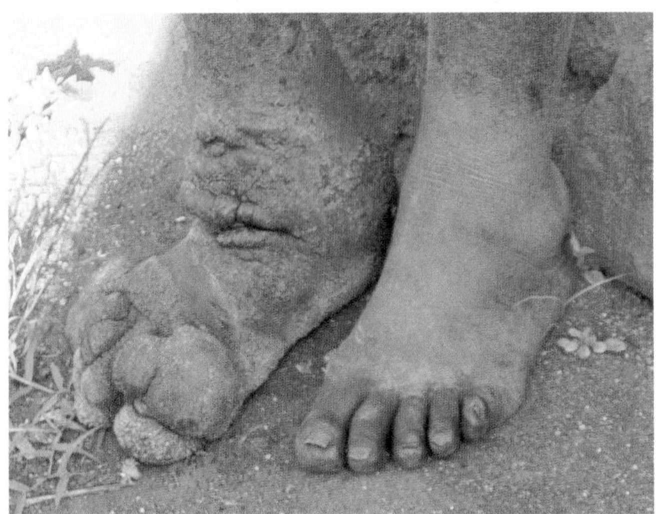

Fig. 9.5.8.4 'Leathery' type advanced podoconiosis in patient aged 14.

Table 9.5.8.1 Criteria for distinguishing of podoconiosis from filarial elephantiasis

Characteristic	Podoconiosis	Filarial disease
Area of residence	>1500 m above sea level	<1000 m above sea level
Mean age of onset	10–20 years	25–30 years
Relation to natural history	Initial symptom	Late complication
Site of first symptom	Toes and foot	Any part of limb except foot
Local lymphadenitis	Follows swelling of limb	Precedes swelling of limb
Typical site of swelling	Distal, below knee	Above and below knee

Prognosis

The excess mortality associated with podoconiosis is unknown. Untreated patients have severely reduced mobility and work capacity by their mid-40s. Episodes of secondary infection cause additional disability.

Economic burden and social stigma

Recent work has detailed the enormous economic burden of podoconiosis on affected communities. In a southern Ethiopian zone of 1.5 million inhabitants, where the prevalence of podoconiosis is known to be 5.4%, the overall cost of podoconiosis was estimated to be in excess of US$16 million per year. In this zone, where the average income is less than US$100 per year, the direct costs to a patient are US$143 per year.

Individuals with podoconiosis are highly stigmatized. They may be excluded from school, rejected by their family, barred from social and religious gatherings, and banned from marriage to any unaffected individual. Siblings of affected individuals are also frequently barred from marriage into unaffected families.

Likely developments

The precise nature of the interaction between host and irritant particles is still unclear. Studies of the genetic basis of podoconiosis continue. Studies examining host immunological and inflammatory responses would be valuable. Adaptation of a clinical scoring system similar to that developed for filarial elephantiasis will permit more accurate staging and assessment of interventions. A pilot study of distribution of footwear to children of affected households is under way.

Further reading

Davey G, Newport M (2007). Podoconiosis: the most neglected tropical disease? *Lancet*, 369, 888–9.

Davey G, *et al.* (2007). Podoconiosis: a tropical model for gene-environment interactions? *Trans R Soc Trop Med Hyg*, **101**(1), 91–6.

Price EW (1990). *Podoconiosis: non-filarial elephantiasis*. Oxford Medical Publications, Oxford.

Tekola F, *et al.* (2006). Economic costs of podoconiosis (endemic non-filarial elephantiasis) in Wolaita Zone, Ethiopia. *Trop Med Int Health*, **11**,1136–44.

Yakob B, *et al.* (2008). High levels of misconceptions and stigma in a community highly endemic for podoconiosis in southern Ethiopia. *Trans R Soc Trop Med Hyg*, **102**(5), 439–44.

9.5.9 Radiation

Jill Meara

Essentials

Ionizing radiation

Ionizing radiation has sufficient energy to break chemical bonds and produce charged ions in living tissue. These changes may cause cell death, but breaks of both strands of a DNA molecule that do not kill a cell may be a precursor of cancer.

Excluding medical exposures, natural radiation accounts for most human exposure, which produces health effects that may be (1) stochastic, where the probability of manifesting the effect depends on the radiation dose, including carcinogenesis and induction of heritable defects; (2) psychological, especially following accidental exposures; and (3) tissue reactions, occurring when sufficient cells are killed after exposure to radiation doses above a certain threshold, including the acute radiation syndrome (radiation sickness) and radiation burns.

Prevention—legislative dose-limits prevent tissue reactions and reduce the risk of stochastic effects, although all doses should be kept as low as reasonably achievable.

Non-ionizing radiation

Ultraviolet radiation affects primarily (1) the skin, causing sunburn in the short term and skin cancer in the long term; and (2) the eye, causing photokeratitis and photoconjunctivitis (arc eye, snow blindness) in the short term, and conjunctival and corneal disorders in the long term, also cataracts.

Information on the health effects of other types of non-ionizing radiation, e.g. radio-frequency microwaves, and power-frequency electric and magnetic fields, is less robust, but controls are recommended to prevent those health effects that are established.

Introduction

The term radiation applies to emissions in the electromagnetic spectrum. Only ionizing radiation is energetic enough to cause ionization of matter. There are natural sources of ionizing radiation, such as radon gas or cosmic rays, and manufactured sources, such as X-rays and radioactive isotopes produced in nuclear reactors. Excluding medical exposures, natural radiation accounts for most human exposure. Some types of nonionizing radiation are also health hazards. These include radiant heat, ultraviolet radiation, radio waves, microwaves, and power-frequency electromagnetic fields.

Historical perspective

The dangers of ionizing radiation became apparent almost as soon as experiments with radioactive materials began. In the early 20th century, radiologists often calibrated their machines by the dose causing erythema on their hands. Many, including Marie Skłodowska-Curie and her daughter Irène Joliot-Curie, died of radiation-induced cancers. Despite universal exposure to natural background radiation, there is a general fear of ionizing radiation, especially that associated with nuclear power and nuclear weapons.

The hazards of certain types of nonionizing radiation such as sunburn and electrical discharge in thunderstorms are well known, but the health of pioneers in nonionizing radiation research was not affected. Recently, the safety of power-frequency and radiofrequency fields—at the levels to which the public are exposed—has been questioned. However, hypotheses about possible long-term health effects, such as induction of cancer, lack biologically plausible mechanisms or confirmation by high-quality epidemiological studies.

Ionizing radiation: mechanism of harm

Atoms, radioactivity, and radiation

Isotopes of some elements are unstable and undergo radioactive decay. The time taken for half of a given quantity to decay is called the half-life, which ranges from fractions of a second to thousands of years, depending on the particular isotope. The unit of radioactivity is the becquerel (Bq). 1 Bq equals 1 atomic disintegration per second. The natural radionuclide potassium-40 (^{40}K), with a half-life of 1.250×10^9 years, makes up 120 parts per million of all potassium on Earth. Since there is about 4000 Bq of ^{40}K in an average person, there are about 14 million radioactive disintegrations per hour from ^{40}K inside the average human body.

Unstable isotopes (radionuclides) decay and release energy as subatomic particles (α- or β-particles) or γ-rays. X-rays are produced by bombarding a metal target with electrons in a vacuum. Neutrons are produced during nuclear fission reactions. These vary in the extent to which they can penetrate the body and can interact with tissues and cells. α-Particles are densely ionizing and are stopped by the dead layer of the skin, but constitute a hazard if taken into the body. β-Particles can penetrate the body to the depth of a few centimetres; X- and γ-rays penetrate the body and, if not absorbed, pass through it. Lead shielding is needed to protect against X-rays and γ-rays. These properties of radiation affect the location and extent of cellular damage following exposure and dictate the protective methods required.

Ionizing radiation has sufficient energy to break chemical bonds and produce charged ions in living tissue. Most of these changes are inconsequential, others may be repaired, but there is a finite probability that damage may cause cell death. Breaks of both strands of a DNA molecule may not kill a cell, but they are known to be a precursor of cancer.

Measuring radiation risk

Acute cell damage depends on the energy imparted by the radiation. The mean energy absorbed per unit mass of tissue (absorbed dose) is measured in gray (Gy). 1 Gy is equal to 1 joule (J) deposited per kilogram of tissue. Radiation and tissue-weighting factors are used to convert the absorbed dose in Gy to an effective dose in sieverts (Sv). This allows external and internal exposures from all types of ionizing radiation to be integrated into one dose, on the basis of equality of stochastic risk. The United Kingdom average annual individual natural background radiation dose is 2.3 mSv. The typical dose from an anteroposterior chest radiograph is 0.02 mSv and that from an abdominal CT scan is 10 mSv.

Health effects of exposure to ionizing radiation

There are three types of health effects associated with exposure to ionizing radiation: stochastic effects, psychological effects, and tissue reactions.

- In stochastic effects, the probability of manifesting the effect depends on the radiation dose and include carcinogenesis and induction of heritable defects. Radiation-induced cancer is clinically and pathologically indistinguishable from idiopathic cases. Risks at low-radiation doses are extrapolated from animal, experimental, and epidemiological studies at higher doses assuming a linear no-threshold model. This implies that there is no 'safe' radiation dose, but very small exposures convey very small risks. The absolute cancer risk per unit of radiation dose (risk coefficient) is estimated to be 5.5%/Sv.
- Psychological effects are found especially following accidental exposures. These are not discussed further in this chapter. Readers are referred to the literature on risk communication.
- Tissue reactions occur after exposure to radiation doses above a certain threshold, when sufficient cells are killed. These include the acute radiation syndrome (radiation sickness) and radiation burns (Fig. 9.5.9.1). Radiation accidents are rare and the initial symptoms of tissue reactions are nonspecific, resembling influenza or food poisoning, so physicians may be involved in diagnosis and treatment before the true cause is appreciated. Patients may present to a range of different medical settings. For example, the theft of a caesium-137 (^{137}Cs) radiotherapy source in Goiânia, Brazil, led to 50 people being overexposed, and resulted in 4 deaths. Many people and large areas of land and property were contaminated before the true cause of the incident was appreciated.

Clinical features of radiation-induced tissue reactions

External exposures, either whole body or partial, do not render patients radioactive and thus pose no radiation risk to medical attendants. If the patient has ingested or inhaled radioactive materials, or has wounds containing them (internal exposure), they and their waste products may pose a persisting radiation or contamination hazard to people working in that environment. Decontamination of radioactive material on skin or clothing is often straightforward, but should not take precedence over life-saving procedures. If contamination is suspected, contact a radiation-protection expert for monitoring and avoid spread of material. Stable iodine can be used to block uptake of radioactive isotopes of iodine. Chelating agents, such as ethylenediamine tetraacetic acid (EDTA), and ion-exchange resins, such as Prussian blue, may be used to enhance excretion of certain internal radionuclides, such as ^{137}Cs and actinides.

Partial-body exposures, especially of the extremities, may not be accompanied by systemic disease if the equivalent whole-body dose does not reach the symptom threshold. Symptoms of radiation burns include erythema, oedema, dry and wet desquamation, blistering, pain, necrosis, and gangrene. There are no pathognomonic features, but margins of ulcers may show epilation. Radiation burns may extend deep into the soft tissue, increasing fluid loss and risk of infection. Skin injuries evolve slowly, usually over weeks to months, may become very painful, and are resistant to treatment. Radiation exposure can be associated with trauma or thermal burns.

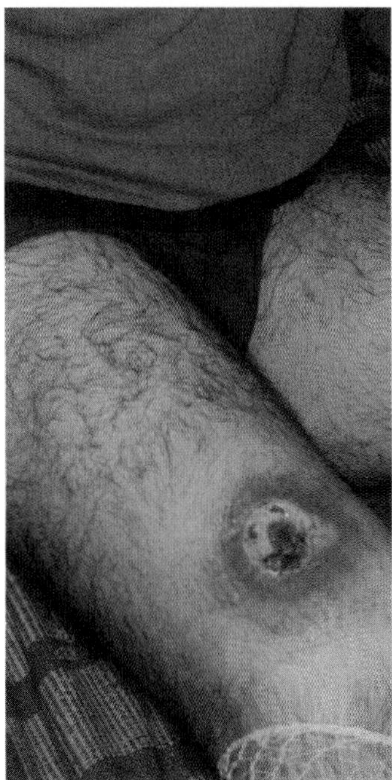

Fig. 9.5.9.1 Mature radiation burn showing central necrosis and annular epilation. Reproduced from *The Radiological Incident in Lilo*, International Atomic Energy Agency, Vienna 2000. ISBN 92 0 101300 0.

Acute radiation syndrome

The acute radiation syndrome is a rare (handfuls of cases per year worldwide), multiphasic illness. The prodrome of high exposure to external ionizing radiation is sudden anorexia, nausea and vomiting, headache, fatigue, fever, and diarrhoea, sometimes with erythema and itching, usually lasting 24 to 48 h. The timing of onset, severity, and duration of prodromal symptoms depend on the radiation dose.

After a latent period of apparent recovery, effects of the killing of cells—especially stem cells—appear. Severity depends on the radiation dose. The main clinical features are:

- haematopoetic syndrome, at whole-body radiation doses exceeding 1 Gy—significant reductions in blood cell counts, infection, haemorrhage, and anaemia
- gastrointestinal syndrome at whole-body radiation doses around 6 Gy—breakdown of the integrity of the gut wall leading to massive fluid and electrolyte loss and ingression of pathogens
- radiation pneumonitis and the cerebrovascular syndrome (at doses exceeding 20 Gy)—respiratory failure, hypotension, and major impairments of cognitive function
- radiation burns if the skin dose exceeds 20 Gy

If the patient survives this phase, recovery is likely. High radiation doses can also lead to permanent sterility.

A number of triage categories have been published, relating the severity and time-course of symptoms and signs to prognosis. Although the threshold radiation dose for symptoms is approximately 1 Gy, lymphocyte dosimetry can detect acute doses down to about 100 mGy. Combined injuries have a worse prognosis. Without medical treatment, an acute dose of approximately 4 Gy is likely to be fatal within 60 days in 50% of those exposed. Doses over 10 Gy are likely to result in earlier death, despite treatment. Similar doses over longer periods (days, weeks, etc.) may cause less severe symptoms as the body has time to repair the damage.

Clinical investigation

This includes full history, examination, cytogenic and regular blood tests. The estimated radiation dose is needed to predict the clinical course of the patient and plan treatment. This dose should be revised as treatment progresses because the heterogeneous nature of accidental exposures makes the scale of radiation damage difficult to estimate.

Vomiting is common about 3 h after acute exposure to doses of about 2 Gy and usually occurs within 2 h of exposure to doses exceeding 4 Gy. However, there is considerable individual variation and vomiting is not invariable even at high doses. Prodromal symptoms last for more than 24 h with doses exceeding 6 Gy. The pattern of fall in blood levels of lymphocytes, granulocytes, platelets, and red cells depends on radiation dose. For pure γ-field exposures, the dose (between 0.1 and 10 Gy), can be estimated by multiplying the lymphocyte depletion rate constant by 8.6.

Chromosome aberration assays, mainly dicentrics (chromosomes with two centromeres) in lymphocytes or other chromosomal abnormalities detected by fluorescence *in situ* hybridization (FISH), can be used to give a more precise estimate of whole-body dose. These assays can be used for several years after exposure.

Treatment of acute radiation syndrome

Good clinical care ensures the best chance of recovery, provided that some stem cells have survived the radiation exposure. Early treatment of associated conventional injuries is important. Routine monitoring should include daily full blood counts, and blood cultures and other infection screens especially in febrile patients.

As a rule of thumb, patients with an estimated dose of 2 Gy or more should be observed in hospital and monitored for onset of acute radiation syndrome, but not all will require intensive treatment. Patients with doses of more than 4 Gy should be presumed to be developing acute radiation syndrome. Early arrangements should be made for specialist treatment.

The mainstays of treatment are:

- symptomatic treatment e.g. antiemetics, analgesics, and fluid replacement
- avoiding infection
- supporting affected organs until surviving stem cells multiply and repopulate the relevant organ/tissue, e.g. antibiotics, blood and platelet transfusions
- stimulating cell repopulation—in recent case studies, cytokines and growth factors have been used early in the progress of the syndrome, but effects on long-term survival are uncertain

Bone marrow transplants have also been used, but have not been proven to be beneficial. Recent reports of stem cell transplants have not yet demonstrated survival benefits.

Haematopoietic syndrome

Reverse barrier nursing and topical treatments to decrease bacterial/fungal colonization should be used. Intravenous lines should be kept to a minimum and sited to decrease infection risk. Febrile neutropenic patients should be given broad-spectrum antimicrobials until they become afebrile. Fungal lung infections can cause late mortality, after all the other effects of radiation have been stabilized. Early use of antifungal agents and γ-globulin for viral infections may be required.

Gastrointestinal syndrome

Use supportive therapy to prevent infection and dehydration. Vomiting should be controlled with antiemetics, such as 5-hydroxytryptamine-3 ($5HT_3$) receptor antagonists. Diarrhoea should be treated with fluids and electrolytes. Food with a low microbial content may minimize infection risk. Elemental diets may help to reduce radiation enteritis, but are unpalatable for oral feeding.

Treatment of radiation burns

Wound contamination is treated by gentle wound toilet and debridement. Wastes arising should be treated as contaminated. Care should be taken not to break intact skin and introduce internal contamination. Systemic corticosteroids may be used in the latent phase to decrease subsequent inflammatory reactions.

Topical treatment includes wet dressings, later alginates and hydrocolloids. Growth factors have been used to foster granulation and epithelialization. In some cases, surgical repair and skin grafting are necessary.

Combined injury

Soft-tissue wounds require biological coverings or skin grafts. Surgical correction of life-threatening and other major injuries should be carried out as soon as possible (within 36–48 h); elective procedures should be postponed until late in the convalescent period (45–60 days), following haematopoietic recovery. Surgical wounds and traumatic lacerations tend to heal more slowly in irradiated tissues.

Health effects of exposures to non-ionizing radiation

Ultraviolet radiation

Ultraviolet radiation primarily affects the skin and the eye. The short-term skin effect is sunburn, with erythema and oedema. In some people, sunburn is followed by increased production of melanin (suntan) but this offers only minimal protection against further exposure. Acute ocular exposure to ultraviolet radiation can lead to photokeratitis and photoconjunctivitis (arc eye, snow blindness, etc.).

The most serious long-term effect of ultraviolet radiation is induction of skin cancer. Nonmelanomatous skin cancers, mainly basal cell carcinomas and squamous cell carcinomas, are common in white populations but are rarely fatal. The overall incidence is difficult to assess because of under-reporting, but is likely to exceed 70 000 cases per year in the United Kingdom. The incidence of malignant melanoma, which is much more likely to be fatal, has increased substantially in white populations for several decades causing about 2000 deaths/year in the United Kingdom. Chronic exposure to solar radiation causes photo-ageing of the skin, characterized by a leathery, wrinkled appearance and loss of elasticity. Suberythemal quantities of ultraviolet radiation are beneficial in stimulating vitamin D synthesis in the skin.

Repeated ocular exposure is a major factor in corneal and conjunctival diseases, such as climatic droplet keratopathy, pterygium, and, probably, pinguecula. Epidemiological data suggest that cumulative exposure to ultraviolet radiation is a major cause of cortical cataracts, but its importance in the general population remains uncertain.

Immune responses

Exposure to ultraviolet radiation can suppress immune responses by complex mechanisms, but the significance for human health and response to vaccinations is uncertain.

Radio-frequency electromagnetic waves

The widespread adoption of radio-frequency microwaves in wireless technology, including mobile phones, has led to concerns about adverse health effects. High exposure to radio frequencies can cause thermal burns. There is no evidence that there is significant risk to the general public from exposure to radio-frequency radiation or from use of micro/radiowave appliances. However, these are new technologies and a cautious approach is appropriate because of the lack of scientific evidence. The Health Protection Agency recommends that children should use mobile telephones (cellphones) only for important calls.

Power-frequency electric and magnetic fields (PFEMFs)

There are concerns that PFEMFs might have adverse effects on health even at levels below those required to interfere with nerves through induced fields and currents. The evidence is controversial. However, epidemiological studies have shown a consistent statistical association—not necessarily indicating causation—between unusually high background magnetic fields in homes and/or residential proximity to power lines and increased risk of childhood leukaemia (possibly 2–5 attributable cases per year in the UK). This prompted the International Agency for Research on Cancer to classify PFEMFs as 'possibly carcinogenic'. In March 2004, the United Kingdom Health Protection Agency recommended that the government should consider precautionary protection from PFEMFs.

Static magnetic fields

Head movements in static magnetic fields stronger than 2 T can cause symptoms such as vertigo, nausea, a metallic taste, and phosphenes (seeing light without light entering the eye). Humans undergoing MRI (magnetic resonance imaging) are exposed to static magnetic fields of this magnitude. There are insufficient data to indicate long-term health effects of exposures to static electric and magnetic fields. In 2008 the HPA advised that individuals being imaged in static magnetic fields in standard operating mode should not be exposed to fields greater than 4 T. Stronger fields can be used in controlled or experimental situations with more rigorous patient monitoring. Limits have also been advised for switched gradient and radiofrequency exposures from MRI.

Further reading

Bennett P, Calman K (eds) (1999). *Risk communication and public health.* Oxford University Press, Oxford.

Berger ME, *et al.* (2006). Medical management of radiation injuries: current approaches. *Occup Med (Lond)*, **56**, 162–72.

Jarrett DG, *et al.* (2007). Medical treatment of radiation injuries—current US status. *Radiat Meas*, **42**, 1063–74.

Levy BS, Sidel VW (eds) (2003). *Terrorism and public health.* Oxford University Press, Oxford.

Mettler F, Upton A (2008). *Medical effects of Ionizing Radiation* (3rd edition) Saunders Elsevier, Philadelphia, PA (2008) (ISBN 978-0-7216-0200-4).

Ricks RC, Berger ME, O'Hara, Jr M (2002) *The medical basis of radiation-accident preparedness, the clinical care of victims.* Parthenon, New York.

Waselenko JK, *et al.* (2004) Medical management of the acute radiation syndrome: recommendations of the Strategic National Stockpile Radiation Working Group. *Ann Int Med*, **140**, 1037–51.

Websites

Advisory Group on Non-Ionising Radiation (2002). *Health effects from ultraviolet radiation.* Documents of the NRPB. Volume 13, No. 1. Advisory Group on Ionizing Radiation (2009). *High Dose Radiation Effects and Tissue Injury.* Documents of the Health Protection Agency RCE-10. http://www.hpa.org.uk/web/HPAwebFile/HPAweb_C/1237362785677 Accessed on 30th Jan 2010. NRPB http://www.hpa.org.uk/web/HPAwebFile/HPAweb_C/1194947340456 Accessed on 30 Jan 2010.

American College of Radiology, Disaster Planning Task Force (2006). *Disaster Preparedness for radiology professionals.* http://www.acr.org/SecondaryMainMenuCategories/ACRStore/FeaturedCategories/QualityandSafety/PracticeManagement/DisasterPreparednessforRadiologyProfessionalsVersion30.aspx Accessed on 30 Jan 2010.

Armed Forces Radiobiology Research Institute (2003). *Medical management of radiological casualties handbook*, 2nd edition. Military Medical Operations, Armed Forces Radiobiology Research Institute, Bethesda, MD. http://www.afrri.usuhs.mil/www/outreach/pdf/2edmmrchandbook.pdf. Accessed on 30 Jan 2010. Health Protection Agency (2008). *Protection of Patients and Volunteers undergoing MRI procedures.* Documents of the Health Protection Agency RCE-7, http://www.hpa.org.uk/web/HPAwebFile/HPAweb_C/1222673275524 Accessed 30 Jan 2010.

International Atomic Energy Agency and World Health Organization (2000). *How to recognize and initially respond to an accidental radiation injury.* http://www-pub.iaea.org/MTCD/publications/PDF/IAEA-WHO-L-Eng.pdf Accessed on 30 Jan 2010.

National Radiological Protection Board (2004). *Advice on limiting exposure to electromagnetic fields (0–300GHz).* Documents of the NRPB, Volume 15, No. 2, http://www.hpa.org.uk/web/HPAwebFile/HPAweb_C/1194947415497 Accessed on 30 Jan 2010.

National Radiological Protection Board (2004). *Review of the scientific evidence for limiting exposure to electromagnetic fields (0–300 GHz).* Documents of the NRPB, Volume 15, No. 3. http://www.hpa.org.uk/webc/HPAwebFile/HPAweb_C/1194947383619 Accessed on 30 Jan 2010.

National Radiological Protection Board (2005). *Mobile phones and health 2004: Report by the Board of NRPB.* Documents of the NRPB, Volume 15, No. 5. http://www.hpa.org.uk/web/HPAwebFile/HPAweb_C/1194947333240 Accessed on 30 Jan 2010.

Radiation Emergency Assistance Center/Training Site, Oak Ridge USA, Publications & Radiation Resources, http://orise.orau.gov/reacts/pubs-resources.htm. Accessed on 30 Jan 2010.

9.5.10 Noise

Syed M. Ahmed and Tar-Ching Aw

Essentials

For clinical purposes, noise is measured in decibels weighted according to the sensitivity of the human ear (dB(A)). Regardless of source, the effects of overexposure to noise are similar. Initially there is a temporary threshold shift, where reversibility of hearing loss is possible with removal away from further noise. Permanent threshold shift occurs following prolonged and/or intense exposure, with poor prospects for improvement of hearing. The classical audiogram for noise-induced hearing loss shows a 4 kHz dip. Prevention is by reducing exposure to noise at source, and in the United Kingdom a limit for exposure has been set at 87 dB(A) averaged over an 8-h day or 140 dB(A) for any instantaneous impulse noise.

Introduction

Noise is any unwanted sound. Excessive noise damages the cochlear outer hair cells, breaking and disrupting the cilia, which act as local electromechanical amplifiers. This can result in physical and psychological harm. In addition to sensorineural noise-induced hearing loss (NIHL), noise contributes to stress and accidents in the workplace.

Exposure

The two important characteristics of sound are its intensity and frequency. The human audible sound intensity range is 0 to 120 decibels. The decibel (dB) scale is logarithmic rather than linear, therefore every increase in sound intensity of 3 dB is equivalent to a doubling of sound intensity. In young adults, the ear sound frequency ranges from 20 Hz to 20 kHz, but its sensitivity is not equal across this range. To mimic the response of the human ear and to allow for the variation in ear sensitivity to different frequencies, noise-meters apply a weighting to the sound intensities, and express the readings as dB(A), i.e. decibels weighted by the A scale (as defined by international standards). Typical sound levels are 65 dB(A) for normal conversation at a distance of 1 m; 140 dB(A) for a jet aircraft taking off 25 m away; and 160 dB(A) for a rivet gun near the ear.

Noisy industries include manufacturing, construction, engineering, printing, motor sports, the military, and entertainment industries. There is a tendency to use more powerful equipment, with increasing potential for generating harmful noise levels. Instantaneous noise levels can be assessed using a noise-meter. For cumulative noise exposure, a personal noise dosimeter provides an 'equivalent noise dose' by averaging the frequencies and intensities over an 8-h shift. In the United Kingdom, the Control of Noise at Work Regulations 2005 stipulate an exposure limit of 87 dB(A) averaged over 8 h/day or 140 dB(A) for any instantaneous impulse noise.

Clinical effects

Exposure to loud noise can cause auditory and nonauditory effects. There is wide variation in individual susceptibility. Massive impulse pressures, e.g. from bomb blasts, can cause perforation of the tympanic membrane. The extent of resulting conductive hearing loss depends on the perforation size. There may be associated otorrhoea or pain. Acute perforations usually heal spontaneously over several weeks unless they are large or complicated by infection. If healing has not occurred by 6 weeks, myringoplasty may be indicated. Attic tympanic membrane perforations need urgent referral to exclude cholesteatoma.

An early response to noise exposure is temporarily increased hearing threshold (temporary threshold shift) often with accompanying tinnitus. This may cause transient dullness of hearing, common in those who work in noisy environments, or those attending loud musical events, and typically lasts up to 24 h after which hearing thresholds return to normal. With continuing exposure, the magnitude of this temporary sensorineural hearing loss and the recovery time increase until, after months or years, there is a permanent shift in threshold accompanied by tinnitus. On audiograms, it is detected as a dip at 4 kHz (Fig. 9.5.10.1). Affected people find it difficult to distinguish between similar sounds, particularly consonants, in the presence of moderate background noise. With severe hearing loss, the listener may experience

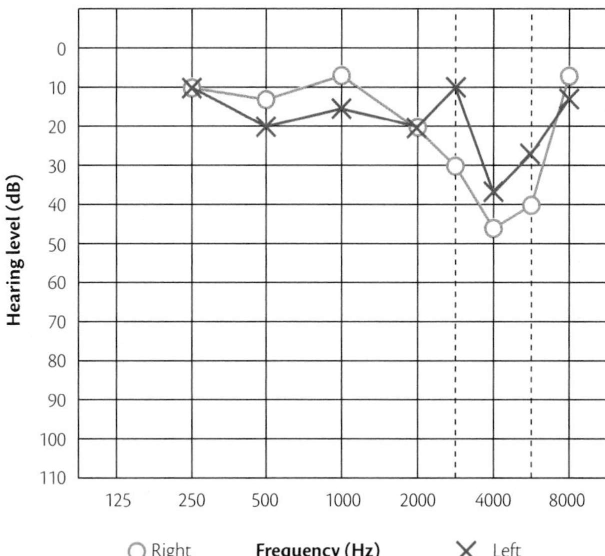

Fig. 9.5.10.1 Audiogram typical of noise-induced hearing loss with a dip at 4 kHz frequency. Red circles, right ear; blue crosses, left ear.

'loudness recruitment', a rapid, uncomfortable increase in sound perceived when intensity increases beyond the already abnormal hearing thresholds. Hearing damage from noise exposure may not be apparent until early middle age. With continued noise exposure, the 4-kHz dip on audiograms extends to lower frequencies and hearing thresholds worsen. This may be combined with presbyacusis (age-related hearing loss) in later years.

The nonauditory effects of noise on health include increased blood pressure, ineffective performance of mental tasks, and symptoms of annoyance, distraction, fatigue, sleep disturbance, and feelings of isolation. These may combine to reduce work output and efficiency. Accidents in noisy workplaces have been attributed partly to inability to hear verbal warnings or instructions clearly.

Diagnosis

A diagnosis of NIHL is from noise exposure assessment, a history of hearing difficulty that may be accompanied by tinnitus, and an audiogram showing the classical 4-kHz dip. Where abnormalities are detected, it is important to establish the history of occupational and leisure noise exposure, exposure to ototoxic drugs and chemicals, previous ear pathology or surgery, other relevant medical history, and the compliance with use of hearing protection. Otoscopic examination, tuning fork tests, and bone-conduction audiometry, should be carried out to exclude conductive hearing loss. Unusual asymmetrical audiograms with vertigo or unilateral tinnitus require otorhinolaryngologist referral to exclude cerebellopontine angle pathology (e.g. acoustic neuroma).

Management, prevention, and surveillance

People with hearing loss and tinnitus may benefit from using hearing aids and a tinnitus masking device.

The emphasis in dealing with noise-induced deafness must be on prevention. Employers whose workplaces are noisy should establish a hearing conservation programme, with commitment to a robust 'noise policy', at the highest level of management. Essential components of such a programme are measures to control noise at source, delineating and controlling access to noisy areas, providing and ensuring use of hearing defenders, and educating and training employees. To control noise at source, less-noisy equipment and engineering controls must be purchased, processes redesigned to reduce noise output. Exposure to noise can be limited by separating its source from the workers using soundproof enclosures or shelters. Hearing protection using ear plugs, ear muffs, or canal caps can reduce noise exposure at the ear by 3 dB(A) to 15 dB(A), but it must be fitted and used correctly to be effective.

The diagnosis of workplace NIHL in a worker should be treated as a sentinel event indicating that other workers were at similar risk and that prompt preventive measures should be implemented. After reduction of noise at source, any residual noise exposure of workers (exceeding 85 dB(A) as defined by the United Kingdom Control of Noise at Work Regulations 2005) warrants health surveillance. This involves symptom review and annual audiometry. In some cases, it may be necessary to consider changing jobs. Clinicians should also advise affected people about benefits available from state compensation schemes.

Further reading

Abbate C, *et al.* (2005). Influence of environmental factors on the evolution of industrial noise-induced hearing loss. *Environ Monit Assess*, **107**, 351–61.

Daniell WE, *et al.* (2006). Noise exposure and hearing loss prevention programmes after 20 years of regulations in the United States. *Occup Environ Med*, **63**, 343–51.

El Dib RP, *et al.* (2006). Interventions to promote the wearing of hearing protection. *Cochrane Database Syst Rev*, **2**, CD005234.

9.5.11 Vibration

Tar-Ching Aw

Essentials

Various occupations can lead to exposure to vibration, which can be transmitted to the whole body or localized to the hands. The main clinical effect of whole body vibration exposure is low back pain. Effects from hand-transmitted vibration can be (1) vascular, with manifestations of secondary Raynaud's phenomenon; (2) neurological, often presenting as paraesthesia and reduced sensory perception; and (3) musculoskeletal, including reduced grip strength and loss of manual dexterity. Management requires exclusion of differential diagnoses, and the identification and reduction of exposure to vibration at source. Diagnosis of an index case should prompt further investigation and (if possible) modification of the workplace to prevent other cases.

Introduction

Vibration is 'the mechanical oscillation of a surface around its reference point'. Workplace exposure to vibration results in local effects, mainly on the hands when the vibration is transmitted to the upper limbs. The clinical syndrome used to be termed 'vibration white finger', highlighting the vascular features, but it is currently referred to as 'hand–arm vibration syndrome', reflecting a combination of vascular, sensorineural, and musculoskeletal components. When vibration is transmitted to the whole body, systemic effects, mainly low back pain, result.

Exposure

Occupational exposure to whole-body vibration occurs in helicopter pilots, and in drivers of heavy vehicles, e.g. tractors, forklift trucks, mobile cranes, and buses. The nature of the surface over which the land vehicles are driven as well as the characteristics of the vehicle cabs contribute to the vibration. Hand–arm vibration exposure occurs in factory workers involved in fettling, chipping, grinding (Fig. 9.5.11.1), riveting, swaging, and using handheld pneumatic hammers, drills, chisels, and rotary tools. Forestry, agricultural, and wood workers using chain saws, miners drilling rock surfaces, and construction and road workers using drills (Fig. 9.5.11.2), and compactors are also at risk. An estimated 3% of the working population of the United Kingdom is occupationally exposed to sources of vibration.

Clinical effects

Whole-body vibration

Exposure to whole-body vibration causes physiological changes to the cardiovascular, respiratory, and musculoskeletal systems. Clinical effects include headache, motion sickness, sleep and visual disturbances, and urinary and abdominal complaints. However, low back pain is the only effect reliably associated with whole-body vibration. In drivers, low back pain may occur as a result of vibration, poor posture within the vehicle cab, and additional tasks such as frequent handling or lifting of heavy loads.

Hand–arm transmitted vibration

This causes secondary Raynaud's phenomenon presenting as prominent episodic digital pallor, usually on exposure to cold or following contact with cold objects (Fig. 9.5.11.3). These symptoms often occur in the morning, or following outdoor activity such as fishing or gardening, especially in cold weather. The vascular changes may be accompanied by neurological and musculoskel-

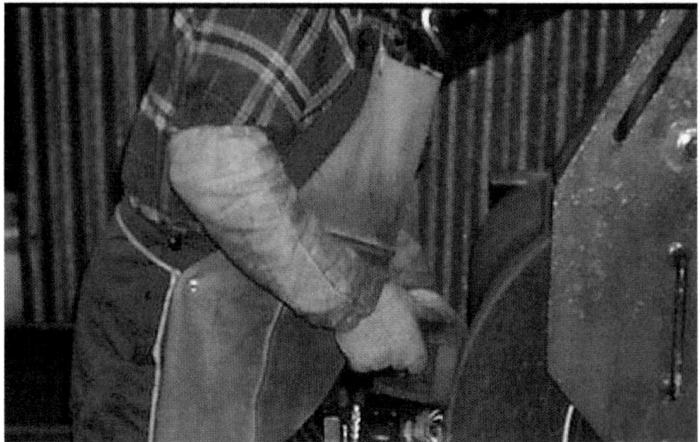

Fig 9.5.11.1 Exposure to vibration from grinding a metal component against a rotating wheel with an abrasive surface.

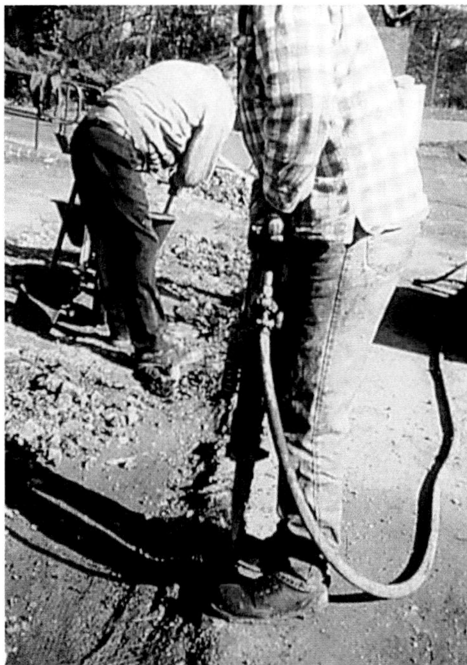

Fig. 9.5.11.2 Exposure to vibration in a road worker from use of a handheld drill.

etal effects that contribute to disability. Vascular and sensorineural effects may appear and progress independently. The latent period between initial exposure and development of symptoms is usually 5 to 10 years, but exceptionally between 6 months and 20 years depending on intensity and duration of exposure. The sequence of colour changes in the affected digits starts with pallor, followed by a bluish hue due to cyanosis, and then redness on spontaneous reversal of the vascular spasm.

Neurological effects include paraesthesia, reduced temperature perception, loss of manual dexterity, and pain. Severe tingling and discomfort often follow rapid warming of the hands. Loss of the ability to distinguish and hold small objects such as coins or to button up clothing causes physical and social disability. Musculoskeletal effects are not as well established, but muscle weakness, bony exostoses, carpal tunnel syndrome, and Dupuytren's contracture have been associated with exposure to vibration.

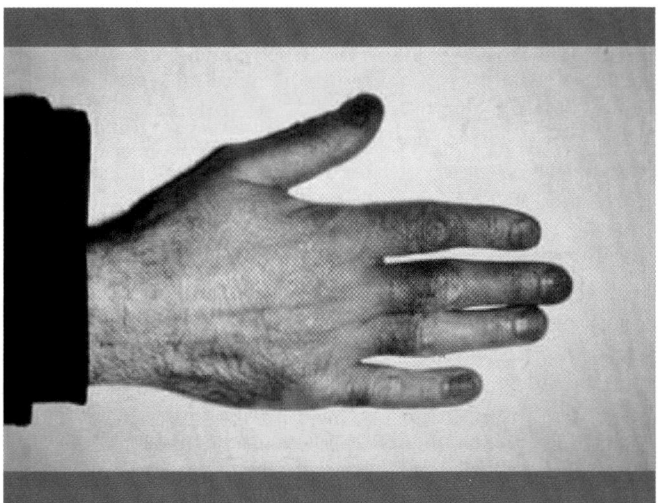

Fig. 9.5.11.3 Patient with hand–arm vibration syndrome showing prominent digital pallor.

Diagnosis

The criteria for a diagnosis of hand–arm vibration syndrome are:

- evidence of sufficient exposure to vibration; guides to the amount of exposure to vibration from various tools are available, e.g. on the National Institute of Working Life website, http://umetech.niwl.se
- confirmed episodic pallor of the digits and/or sensorineural effects
- documented latent period between initial exposure to vibration and onset of symptoms 5 to 10 years
- exclusion of other causes of Raynaud's phenomenon or sensory changes

The presence of associated musculoskeletal features supports the diagnosis. Physical examination may show callosities on the hands, loss of light touch sensation or two-point discrimination in the affected digits, and poor grip strength, although there may be no obvious abnormalities, especially in the early stages of the disease.

Various clinical and special tests have been used in the evaluation of patients with hand–arm vibration syndrome. These include digital blood pressure measurements, vibrotactile thresholds, sensory aesthesiometry, and cold provocation tests. However, the clinical and occupational history is of greater importance than the results of any of these tests in the diagnosis of hand–arm vibration syndrome.

The differential diagnosis should consider other causes of Raynaud's phenomenon. The cause may be constitutional or it may be secondary to rheumatoid arthritis, systemic lupus erythematosus, scleroderma, and other autoimmune disorders, cryoglobulinaemia, frostbite, or thoracic outlet syndrome. Use of ergot, clonidine, and β-blockers, occupational exposure to vinyl chloride monomer, and heavy cigarette smoking may contribute.

Management, treatment, and prevention

The severity of hand–arm vibration syndrome can be staged using the Stockholm Workshop Scale (Table 9.5.11.1). This scale provides separate staging for the vascular and the sensorineural effects. For example, stage '2L(3)/1R(3)' for the vascular component refers to three digits at stage 2 in the left hand; and three digits at stage 1 in the right hand, i.e. stage/hand/number of digits. Further subdivision of stage 2 into early and late effects has recently been proposed.

Engineering controls can minimize the transmission of vibration from machinery to the body or hands. The patient may be able to continue in the same job following such action. Workers with continuing exposure to hand-transmitted vibration should be under regular health surveillance. Where the condition is severe and the source of vibration cannot be eliminated, redeployment should be considered. In early cases, redeployment may arrest or reverse the progression of symptoms. In severe cases, the disease may progress regardless of removal from further exposure to vibration.

Table 9.5.11.1 The Stockholm Workshop scale for hand–arm vibration syndrome

A. Vascular component		
Stage	**Grade**	**Description**
0		No attacks
1	Mild	Occasional attacks affecting only tips of one or more fingers
2	Moderate	Occasional attacks affecting distal and middle (rarely proximal) phalanges of one or more fingers
3	Severe	Frequent attacks affecting all phalanges of most fingers
4	Very severe	As in stage 3, with trophic changes in the fingertips
B. Sensorineural component		
Stage	**Description**	
0_{SN}	Vibration-exposed but no symptoms	
1_{SN}	Intermittent numbness with or without tingling	
2_{SN}	Intermittent or persistent numbness, reduced sensory perception	
3_{SN}	Intermittent or persistent numbness, reduced tactile discrimination and/or manipulative dexterity	

Advice to the patient includes avoidance or reduction of further exposure to vibration, use of appropriate gloves, keeping the body and hands warm especially in cold weather, and cessation of cigarette smoking. Vasodilatory drugs such as tolazoline, inositol, and cyclandelate, and calcium channel antagonists such as verapamil and nifedipine, angiotensin-converting enzyme inhibitors, prostaglandins, and stanazolol have been tried with varying success. The patient should also be advised about entitlement to prescribed diseases benefits, which are awarded according to severity. In the United Kingdom, the scheme is administered by the Department for Work and Pensions through local social security offices.

A diagnosis of Raynaud's phenomenon should always include detailed inquiry into occupational exposure to vibration. Diagnosis of hand–arm vibration syndrome should be viewed as a sentinel event warranting further investigation of the workplace to assess whether improvements in work practices can be implemented to prevent the occurrence of other cases.

Further reading

Department for Work and Pensions (2004). *Hand-arm vibration syndrome. Report by the Industrial Injuries Advisory Council*. The Stationery Office, London.

Health and Safety Executive (2005). *Hand-arm vibration. The Control of Vibration at Work Regulations 2005 & Guidance on Regulation.* HSE Books, Sudbury.

Mason H, Poole K (2004). *Clinical testing and management of individuals exposed to hand-transmitted vibration. An evidence review*. Faculty of Occupational Medicine, London.

9.5.12 Disasters: earthquakes, volcanic eruptions, hurricanes, and floods

Peter J. Baxter

Essentials

Natural disasters (earthquakes, volcanic eruptions, hurricanes, floods) affect the lives of hundreds of millions of people every year, and their impact is increasing year on year because of continuing expansion of human populations into increasingly exposed areas, with environmental degradation making these settlements more vulnerable, especially in heavily urbanized areas. Future climate change may exacerbate matters, with many forecasts predicting an increase in hurricanes, severe wind storms, flooding and droughts.

Disasters are chaotic, but communities can plan and prepare to reduce their impacts. Most deaths in sudden disasters happen before outside aid arrives, hence building local response capacity is crucial. However, international disaster relief can be rapidly and effectively dispatched to needy countries that are politically willing to accept it, and relief teams have an important role in restoring roads and bridges, bringing in potable water, ensuring solid waste management, food protection, vector control, and sanitation. Attendances at medical facilities may return to normal within a few days of a disaster, and restoration of primary care then becomes the priority, rather than emergency treatment.

Introduction

Between 500 and 700 natural catastrophes occur throughout the world each year and the total numbers whose lives are affected is now running into hundreds of millions annually. The numbers of reported natural disasters is increasing almost exponentially (Fig. 9.5.12.1), as are the numbers of people affected globally (Fig. 9.5.12.2). In the past 25 years, floods have killed over 70 000 people and adversely affected more than 300 million throughout the world, while earthquakes, windstorms, volcanic eruptions, and landslides have killed almost 200 000 people and adversely affected more than 60 million. The tsunami that devastated the Indian Ocean region on 26 December 2004 was the greatest recent natural disaster, killing more than 250 000 people and leaving 1.7 million displaced in poor conditions in 10 countries.

Global changes responsible for the worsening impact of disasters include continuing, usually unplanned, expansion of human populations into increasingly exposed areas, and environmental degradation making these settlements more vulnerable, especially in heavily urbanized areas. This reckless development is going on throughout the world, even in areas of well-known risk.

On current trends, climate forecasts of an increase in the world's average temperature of 2 to 3 °C and warming of the oceans could increase the potential for more intense hurricanes over wider areas

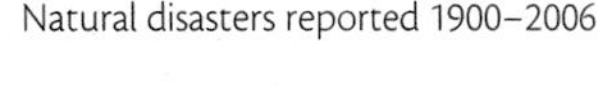

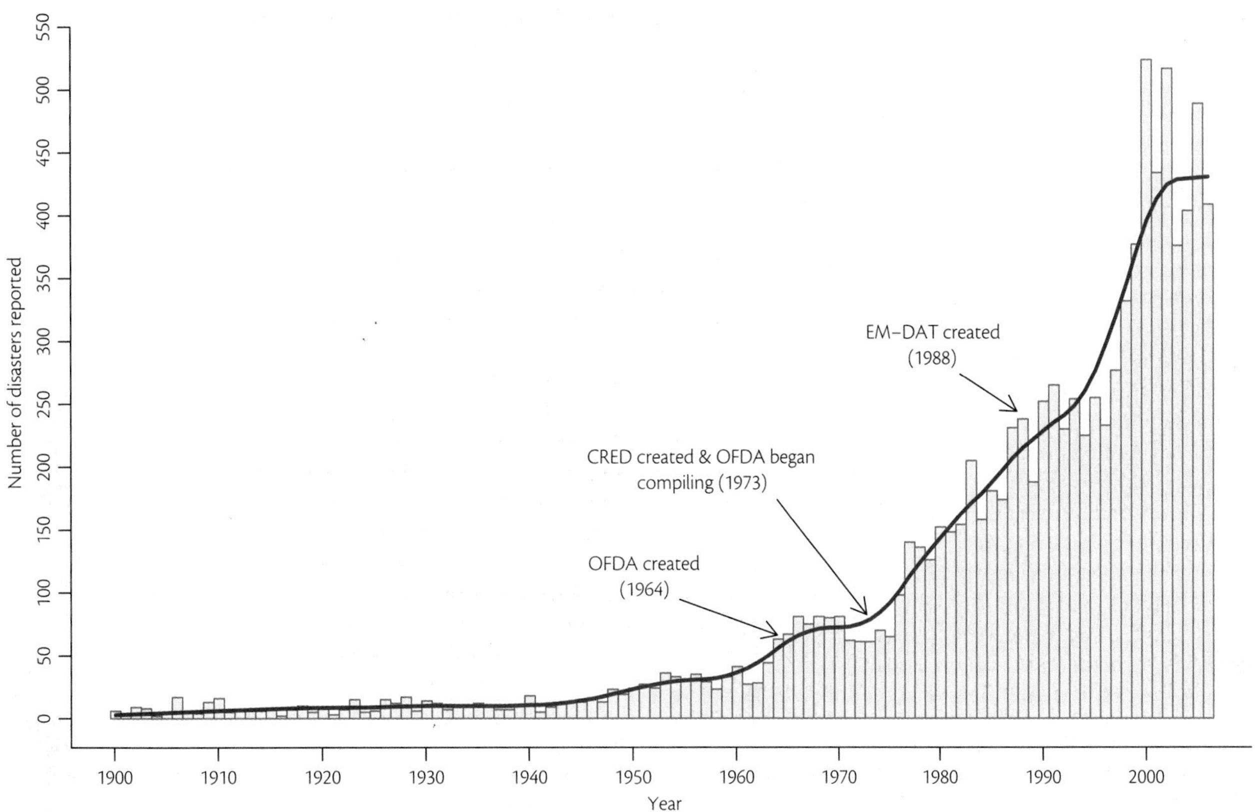

Fig. 9.5.12.1 Reported natural disasters, 1900–2006.
Reproduced from EM-DAT: The OFDA/CRED International Disaster Database – www.emdat.net – Université Catholique de Louvain, Brussels, Belgium.

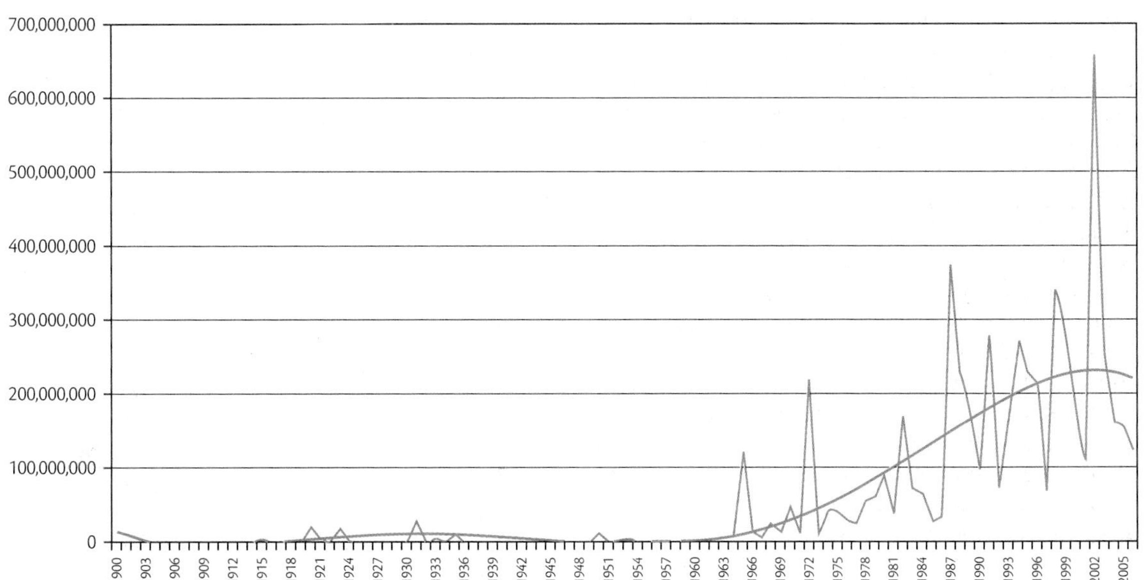

Fig. 9.5.12.2 Total numbers of people affected globally by all types of disasters, 1900–2006.
Reoproduced from EM-DAT: The OFDA/CRED International Disaster Database – www.emdat.net – Université Catholique de Louvain, Brussels, Belgium.

and, in temperate regions, more severe wind storms and fluctuations in rainfall (floods and drought). Rising sea levels will increase the severity and the frequency of coastal floods.

Predisaster measures

Natural disaster results from massive ecological breakdown in the relation between humans and their environment, a serious and sudden (or insidious, as in drought) event on such a scale that the stricken community needs extraordinary efforts to cope with it, often with outside help or international aid. Accurately forecasting the timing and size of natural disasters is rarely possible. This constrains efforts to prevent loss of life by timely evacuation of people from the areas at risk. Disasters are quite different from major incidents in that normal lifelines and infrastructure usually break down. But despite their chaotic elements, disasters are amenable to scientific study and communities can plan and prepare to reduce their impacts. Health workers have a key role in hazard management, risk assessment, predisaster planning, and preparedness, as well as in the emergency response.

Following the agreement leading to the Hyogo Framework of Action 2005–2015, a multihazard, comprehensive approach to disaster risk reduction is slowly becoming accepted and is being enacted in civil protection legislation in many countries. However, poverty and marginalization in developing countries remain potent sources of global vulnerability to natural disasters. Less well publicized are insidious humanitarian crises (complex emergencies) that last for years and can result in the loss of millions of lives, for example, in the eastern Democratic Republic of Congo, Darfur (Sudan), and Eritrea (Ethiopia) They involve conflict and displacement of large populations and are becoming more common, and yet world responses are still poorly prepared for dealing with natural disasters that might occur on top of such pre-existing crises. Thus, in the Asian tsunami, access to some regions of Indonesia and Thailand was prevented by security issues. In 2008, Burmese people living in the Irrawaddy delta had no warning from their government of the approach of cyclone Nargis and hurricane preparedness measures were nonexistent. Over 80 000 people died, most from drowning. The storm of wind, water, and sand was so intense that it blasted away the skin, leaving raw wounds like burns. The disaster was made even worse when, in the immediate aftermath, 1.5 million homeless survivors were left without food, water, or shelter, whilst the Burmese government vacillated for weeks over accepting international aid. In contrast, international disaster relief is nowadays rapidly dispatched to needy countries and is on such a global scale that epidemics and famine are no longer the feared horsemen of the apocalypse they once were.

Earthquakes

Many parts of the world are known to be vulnerable to devastating earthquakes, but it remains impossible to predict where and when a quake will strike. Most deaths and injuries are caused by collapsing buildings and secondary causes such as fires. When timber, masonry, reinforced concrete, and other types of buildings collapse, they inflict injuries in different ways and of different degrees of severity. In masonry buildings, an important cause of death is often suffocation from the weight and dust from the wall or roof material which buries the victims. Falling masonry causes crush injuries to the head and chest, external or internal haemorrhage, and chest compression (traumatic asphyxia). Little is known about the survival times of people trapped in collapsed buildings, but most victims die immediately or within 24 h, depending upon such factors as the severity of aftershocks, fire outbreaks, and rainfall. Rapid extrication of survivors and application of first aid by the uninjured immediately after the event could save up to 25 to 50% of injured victims. The greatest demand for emergency medical services is within the first 24 h and the need for emergency treatment fades after 3 to 5 days. Causes of delayed death include dehydration, hypothermia, crush syndrome, and postoperative sepsis. Most of those requiring medical assistance suffer minor injuries such as lacerations and contusions.

An earthquake of magnitude 9 on the Richer scale off the coast of the island of Sumatra on 26 December 2004 suddenly forced the sea floor upwards by some 10 m, creating a wave that surged through the Indian Ocean. The surface perturbation was initially small but when the water grew shallow, near the coast, the tsunami wave formed. Without warning, the wave hit Indonesia and Thailand within an hour, and then Sri Lanka and India, ultimately reaching as far as East Africa. The province at the north-western end of Sumatra, Aceh, suffered overwhelming devastation. More than 20 000 homes were destroyed, over 100 000 people were killed, and some 700 000 people were displaced. Many victims were health service staff, which hampered the emergency response.

In all countries affected, the main public health infrastructure remained intact as the devastation was limited to coastlines, so the feared epidemics of vector-borne diseases, such as malaria and dengue, as well cholera and dysentery, were able to be prevented. Vast numbers of dead and small numbers of major injuries in survivors are typical of flood disasters, in general, as the severely injured succumb in the water; the injured were mainly treated by local health teams. Many of the patients requiring surgery had infected wounds following contamination by sand and mud. Respiratory tract infections and pneumonias were common among patients who had come close to drowning. Psychosocial needs were identified on a massive scale, but the appropriateness and effectiveness of specific interventions in such disasters remains a controversial area.

An example of the importance of disaster preparedness was the earthquake in Bam, Iran, on 26 December 2003, which resulted in 26 271 deaths and the nearly complete destruction of the city of 80 000 inhabitants. The loss of about one-third of the inhabitants (including 200 out of 500 doctors) was attributable to the weak mud-brick construction. The health infrastructure was destroyed, but within 48 h 11 972 out of 15 000 injured survivors had been air-evacuated by the military to hospitals in the rest of the country and others were transported to facilities by relatives. By the time foreign medical teams arrived, their main task was to provide routine health care to a residual population living in shelters. In contrast, the Pakistan earthquake on 8 October 2005 hit the impoverished mountainous north of the country where access to hundreds of remote villages was hindered by damaged and blocked roads. Over 73 000 people died and 69 400 people had serious injuries; over 3 million people were left homeless. Houses were mostly constructed of weak rubble masonry walls supporting concrete slabs for roofs; the shaking easily razed buildings to the ground or triggered land slides. Roof slabs fell on top of the occupants (Fig. 9.5.12.3) and caused multiple trauma, such as spinal and pelvic fractures. Significant numbers of amputations

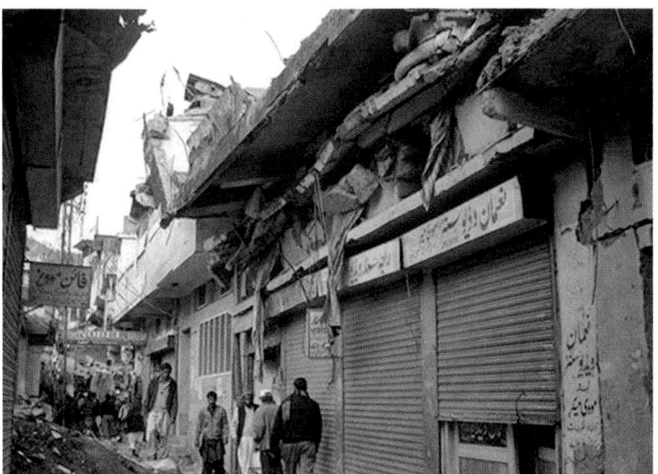

Fig. 9.5.12.3 Pakistan earthquake: collapsed concrete roof slab.
(Source: Emily So)

were performed and postdisaster reconstructive plastic surgery was frequently needed to treat the often severe and localized soft-tissue damage caused by entrapment (Figs. 9.5.12.4). In 2008, the recent rapid economic development and accompanying building boom in China lay behind the destruction by the largest earthquake (7.9 on the Richter scale) to strike the country in recent times, when entire towns collapsed in the mountainous Sichuan province, leaving 80 000 people dead and at least 5 million homeless. Poor building quality has been blamed for the catastrophic failure of homes and schools. Despite the rapid mobilization of thousands of troops to the area, only a few survivors were retrieved from the rubble, sadly emphasizing the country's failure to incorporate seismic resistance in new community developments.

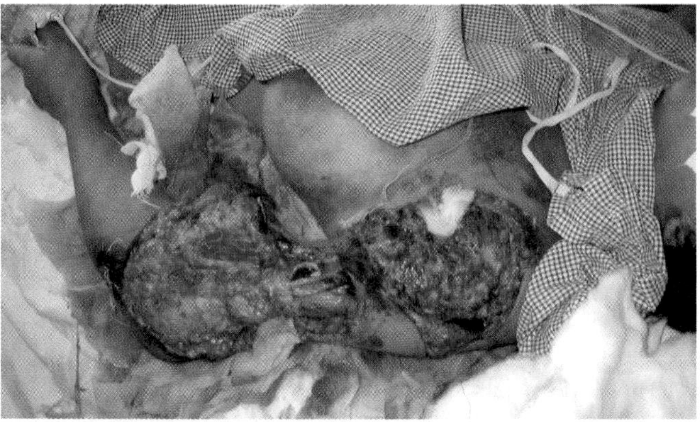

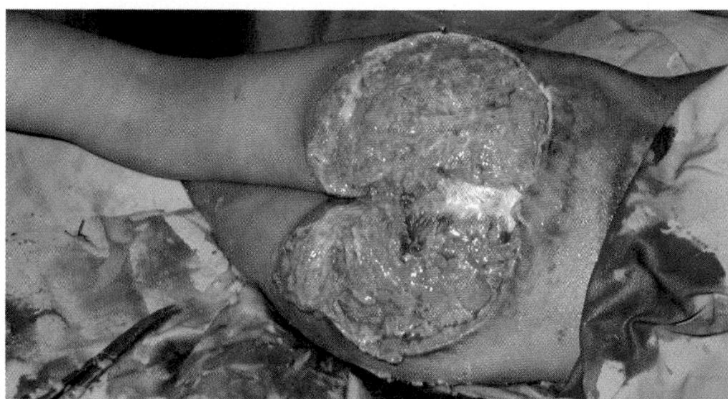

Fig. 9.5.12.4 Pakistan earthquake: severe soft tissue crush injuries.
(Source: Emily So)

Volcanic eruptions

About 500 to 600 quiescent volcanoes around the world are known to be capable of eruptive activity and several major eruptions occur every year. The vast majority of volcanoes are explosive and unpredictable in their behaviour, providing little opportunity for people to escape unless full evacuation measures are taken as soon as premonitory signs develop. In contrast, the less common lava flow eruptions normally allow people to escape by the time the lava heads towards them. Most deaths and injuries in explosive eruptions (such as the one that engulfed ancient Pompeii) are caused by pyroclastic flows and surges, which are clouds of hot ash and gas that can travel at hurricane speeds. Survival is uncommon but victims will have severe, extensive skin burns and inhalation injuries. The worst volcanic disaster in the 20th century was at St Pierre, Martinique, in 1902, when 28 000 people were killed in a laterally directed pyroclastic surge. Mount Vesuvius in Italy remains one of the world's most dangerous volcanoes, but uncontrolled building has resulted in over 1 million people living in an area which could be devastated by pyroclastic flows in a new eruption. Another major cause of death is lahars or wet flows of debris, either ash that has built up on the slopes of the volcano or unstable masses that are mobilized during the eruption, by rain, or rarely by release of water from a crater lake. The eruption of Nevado del Ruiz volcano in Colombia in 1984 triggered a lahar by rapid melting of the glacier at the summit, the melt waters rushing down valleys and mixing with debris as they went. Although adequate warning could have been given to the people below, lack of preparedness meant that the mud flow engulfed towns including Armero, killing around 24 000 people. In one of the largest eruptions of the century, at Mount Pinatubo in the Philippines in 1991, 50 000 people were successfully evacuated from the threat of pyroclastic flows, but over 300 died, from collapse of roofs burdened with accumulated rain and ash, while sheltering in their homes.

The eruption of the Soufrière Hills volcano on the tiny Caribbean island of Montserrat began in July 1995 and gradually escalated, forcing the evacuation of thousands of people from their homes because of the threat of pyroclastic flows. By 1997, these flows had devastated the southern part of the island, evicting three-quarters of the population of 12 000 people. Air pollution from volcanic gases and ash has been a major consideration because of the close proximity of the population to the volcano and the frequent eruption of fine, respirable ash containing hazardous amounts of the crystalline silica mineral cristobalite, which can cause silicosis.

Hurricanes

Hurricanes are one of a broad class of extreme weather phenomena that include winter storms (snow, sleet, freezing rain), thunderstorms (e.g. tornadoes, heavy rains, lightning, wind, and hail), extreme precipitation (e.g. flood and flash floods), and windstorms. Hurricanes (or typhoons as they are called in the western Pacific) are tropical cyclones that form over warm oceans with ocean surface temperatures over 26 °C. Once over land they soon run out of energy and rapidly abate, but can still cause flooding from heavy rain. Very high wind speeds, up to 250 km/h, are restricted to a relatively narrow track, usually no more than 150 km wide, within which localized gusts may even achieve tornado speeds and be extremely destructive. However, most deaths and injuries are not from the effect of wind on people (who normally remain inside for protection) or from building damage (building collapse or being struck by flying debris). Instead, deaths and injuries are commonly the result of flooding from the sea surge as the hurricane strikes land, concurrent heavy rainfall (typically up to 60 cm, over a larger area and extending further inland than wind speed) and resulting landslides. Hurricanes lift the sea, forming a sea surge that typically rises 3 to 4 m above existing tides, and the wind generates waves on top of these. Some storm surges can hit coastal areas well ahead of the landfall of the actual storm and can travel with nearly the same rapidity, and destructiveness, as tsunami waves.

Over 90% of fatalities in hurricanes are drownings associated with storm surges or floods. Other causes of death include burial beneath houses collapsed by wind, penetrating trauma from broken glass or wood, blunt trauma from floating objects or debris, or entrapment in mudslides. The greatest need in the postimpact phase is the provision of adequate shelter, water, food, and clothing, and sanitation. Most victims suffer from lacerations caused by flying glass or other debris, or minor trauma such as closed fractures and puncture wounds.

Katrina was the third most powerful storm ever to make landfall in the United States of America, attaining hurricane category 5 status before it struck the Louisiana coast on the morning of 29 August 2005. It left breaches in the levée system of New Orleans that created catastrophic flooding of an area of more than 400 km^2, submerging half a million homes and trapping tens of thousands of people. Critically, the city's mayor did not issue a mandatory evacuation order until the day before the hurricane hit, which was too late for many, including the poor, who had no means of transport. In Louisana and Mississippi 1700 people died, most by drowning. The emergency response was woeful. Up to 20 000 evacuees were abandoned in the city's Superdome sports stadium for 5 days before being evacuated to other shelters. Two public hospitals were left cut off for days without electrical power, clean water, and medical supplies. The victims were predominantly black and poor. In the aftermath, nearby states were able to absorb several hundred thousand evacuees from the city in a few days. Despite forebodings, epidemics of diarrhoeal diseases, respiratory tract infections and mosquito-borne disease, in particular West Nile virus, did not occur.

Floods

In addition to the major losses of life that can be caused by hurricanes and their associated sea surges, floods mostly result from moderate to large events (rainfall, snow melt, high tides) occurring within the expected range of stream flow or tidal conditions. In the United Kingdom, as in many countries with low-lying coastal land, the hazard of coastal flooding from sea surges and high tides dominates over river flooding, although the latter is more frequent. Flood warning and forecasting, combined with effective land management, community preparedness, and evacuation planning, are as essential as engineered river and coastal defences.

The primary cause of death from floods is drowning, but trauma from impact with floating debris and hypothermia due to cold exposure are also important. The proportion of survivors requiring emergency medical care is small as most injuries are minor, such as lacerations. This absence of victims with severe or multiple trauma is likely to reflect the long delay in reaching survivors, so they die from their injuries or from exposure before search and rescue teams can arrive. Increased morbidity and mortality in survivors who experience flooding was reported in the year after the East Coast Flood in 1953 and a river flood in Bristol in 1968; there was an increase in suicides and mental health problems after the severe flooding caused by heavy rains in central Europe in July 1997.

Postdisaster relief

Myths surrounding postdisaster relief include:

- Any kind of international assistance is needed.
- The affected population is too shocked and helpless to take responsibility for their own survival.
- Natural disasters trigger secondary disasters through outbreaks of communicable diseases.
- Life gets back to normal after a few weeks.

Most deaths in sudden disasters happen before outside aid arrives, and so building local response capacity is most important. However, relief teams have an important role in restoring roads and bridges, bringing in potable water, ensuring solid waste management, food protection, vector control, and sanitation. Attendances at medical facilities may return to normal within a few days of a disaster, and restoration of primary care then becomes the priority rather than emergency treatment. Epidemiology has an important role in postdisaster assessment and health surveillance, particularly when large populations have been relocated, as well as investigating the causes of mortality and morbidity in disasters, including mental ill health and long-term health sequelae.

Further reading

Disasters and humanitarian emergencies. *Epidemiol Rev*, **27**, 2005. [This special issue contains excellent review articles on hurricanes, floods and earthquakes.]

Noji EK (ed.) (1997). *The public health consequences of disasters*. Oxford University Press, New York.

9.5.13 Bioterrorism

Manfred S. Green

Essentials

Bioterrorism is the deliberate use of biological agents to cause illness, death and fear for ideological or personal purposes. Most potential bioterrorism agents occur naturally as known pathogens and are classified as follows: (1) Category A, with greatest risk to the public and national security, comprising (a) infectious and contagious diseases, smallpox, plague, and viral haemorrhagic fevers; (b) infectious but not contagious diseases, anthrax, and tularaemia; and

(c) toxins, botulism; (2) Category B, with intermediate risk—causative agents that are relatively easy to spread and produce diseases with moderately high death rates; (3) Category C—emerging infectious diseases that could be engineered to spread and cause high rates of morbidity and mortality.

Biological agents may be disseminated through aerosolization, food, human carriers, infected insects or water. The incubation periods of potential bioterrorism agents can vary from hours to weeks, with early symptoms mimicking many other disorders. The diagnosis may not be suspected unless cases occur in clusters. Early identification of outbreaks will depend largely on the ability of primary care and emergency room physicians to identify and promptly report cases to the public health authorities. A major concern is that diagnosis of these extremely uncommon diseases may not be considered by physicians who have rarely, if ever, seen such cases. Specific treatment (if available) of affected individuals will depend on the pathogen, but for contagious diseases such as smallpox and plague, isolation of patients and their contacts, barrier nursing, quarantine, and restriction of the movements and social interactions of people are important control measures. Decontamination is relevant mainly for anthrax and smallpox, in the environment of an aerosol attack and at places where patients were treated, .

Public education and effective risk communication are essential in managing a bioterrorism attack: (1) clinicians and public health personnel need access to up-to-date information; (2) the general public requires nontechnical descriptions of the diseases and simple instructions on how to act in an emergency situation. Primary prevention should include addressing the root causes of terrorism, developing comprehensive preparedness programmes and educating health professionals to deal with an outbreak.

Introduction

The potential public health threat posed by bioterrorism could make exceptional demands on clinicians. Rapid diagnosis will have implications far beyond the individual patient. It will initiate a process of preventive actions, which could impact on the lives of hundreds or thousands. Clinicians may have to treat infectious disease casualties en masse under emergency situations, while ensuring the protection of health care workers and other patients. Clinical presentations may be atypical because of the nature of the exposure and the possibility that the organism may have been genetically mutated. Antibiotic resistance and vaccine failure could be encountered and laboratories are likely to be overburdened. Public panic could exacerbate ethical dilemmas in the triage for specialized care in limited facilities.

Historical perspective

The use of biological agents as weapons inspires a special abhorrence and dread. International agreements such as the 'Geneva Protocol' in 1925 and the 'Biological Weapons Convention' in 1972, banned their use and production. However, in the early 1990s, it was revealed that anthrax spores were accidentally released from a military facility in Russia in 1979, causing an outbreak of respiratory anthrax. Evidence emerged that the former Soviet Union had continued a bioweapons programme generating concerns that bioweapon agents and the expertise for their production might reach terrorist groups.

Box 9.5.13.1 Examples of bioterrorism agents by category

Category A

Infectious and contagious diseases

- Smallpox (*Variola major*)
- Plague (*Yersinia pestis*)
- Viral haemorrhagic fevers (filoviruses, e.g. Ebola, Marburg, and arenaviruses, e.g. Lassa, Machupo)

Infectious but not contagious diseases

- Anthrax (*Bacillus anthracis*)
- Tularemia (*Francisella tularensis*)

Toxins

- Botulism (*Clostridium botulinum toxin*)

Category B

- Brucellosis (*Brucella* spp.)
- Epsilon toxin of *Clostridium perfringens*
- Food safety threats (*Salmonella, Escherichia coli* 0157, *Shigella*)
- Glanders (*Burkholderia mallei*)
- Meliodosis (*Burkholderia pseudomallei*)
- Psittacosis (*Chlamidia psittaci*)
- Q fever (*Coxiella burnetii*)
- Ricin from *Ricinus communis* (castor bean)
- Staphylococcal enterotoxin b
- Typhus fever (*Rickettsia prowazekii*)
- Viral encephalitis (alphavirus, e.g. Venezuelan equine encephalitis, eastern equine encephalitis, western equine encephalitis)
- Water-safety threats (e.g. *Vibrio cholerae, Cryptosporidium parvum*)

Category C

- Emerging infectious diseases such as Nipah virus and hantavirus

Source: http://www.bt.cdc.gov/agent/agentlist-category.asp

Biological weapons

Almost all potential bioterrorism agents occur naturally as known pathogens, although many are zoonoses, not normally affecting humans. The United States Centers for Disease Control and Prevention (CDC) classified potential bioterrorism agents into three categories (Box 9.5.13.1). Category A agents have the highest priority since they are considered the greatest risk to the public and national security. These can be subclassified into agents that are infectious and contagious, those that are infectious but not usually contagious, and toxins. Category B includes diseases that are considered an intermediate risk to the public since the causative agents are relatively easy to spread and the diseases result in moderately high death rates. Category C agents include emerging pathogens, which could be engineered to spread and cause high rates of morbidity and mortality.

Since the category A biological agents have been weaponized in past programmes, they are currently of greatest concern. Here they are briefly described but more details about their clinical aspects are provided in Section 7.

Diseases that are both infectious and contagious

Smallpox (Chapter 7.5.4) is the prototype of potential bioterrorism agents that are both infectious and contagious. Although eradicated in 1978, it is believed to have been weaponized by the Soviet Union. Universal vaccination was phased out in the 1970s and since the case-fatality in unvaccinated subjects is around 30%, smallpox is one of the most feared bioterrorism threats. Secondary cases may occur through droplet spread, direct contact with skin lesions or body fluids, and rarely through airborne transmission.

The plague bacillus (*Yersinia pestis*) (Chapter 7.6.16) was included in the bioweapons programmes of both the United States of America and the Soviet Union. Untreated pneumonic plague has a case fatality approaching 100%. The organism can spread from person to person through droplets, causing several generations of the disease.

The viral haemorrhagic fevers caused by the filoviruses (Chapter 7.5.17) and arenaviruses (Chapter 7.5.18) have been weaponized by the former Soviet Union, Russia, and the United States. The Soviet Union is reported to have produced quantities of Marburg, Lassa, Ebola, Junin, and Machupo viruses. Second and later generations of disease can occur through direct contact with body fluids of the patients. Health care workers are at greatest risk.

Infectious but not contagious diseases

Anthrax spores (Chapter 7.6.20) were among the leading agents in biological weapons programmes, since they are highly stable, virulent, resistant to drying, and easily disseminated. Aerosolized spores cause inhalation anthrax, which has an untreated case fatality approaching 100%. The spores can survive in the environment for many years, although once on the ground, they will tend to produce cutaneous anthrax.

The spore-forming coccobacillus *Francisella tularensis* (Chapter 7.6.19), has been weaponized in biowarfare programmes. The untreated case fatality could be 30 to 60%. There is no secondary person-to-person spread.

Toxins

Botulinum toxin, produced by *Clostridium botulinum* (Chapter 7.6.24), is one of the most potent neurotoxins known and has been weaponized. In a bioterrorist incident, it could be disseminated either through food or by aerosol. The untreated case fatality approaches 100%. Ricin (Chapter 8.3.2.2) is a protein cytotoxin produced from the castor bean *Ricinus communis*. There is no antidote. Patients affected by toxins are not contagious at any stage of the disease.

Dissemination of bioweapons

Biological agents may be disseminated through aerosols, food, human carriers, infected insects or water. Aerosolization maximizes the number of people exposed, causing the most damage. Release of contagious agents at different sites could greatly amplify the outbreak. Since most potential agents are not normally aerosol transmitted, the resulting illnesses could occur with shorter incubation periods and atypical clinical manifestations. Clinical effects are likely to depend on the dose.

Epidemiology

Documented contemporary attempts at bioterrorism have employed *Salmonella typhimurium*, botulinum toxin, anthrax spores, Q fever bacteria, Ebola virus and ricin. In 1978, a Bulgarian dissident was assassinated in London by a pellet, probably of ricin, that was inplanted into his leg. In 2001, six envelopes contaminated with powdered anthrax spores were mailed in the United States and infected 22 people. Half suffered from inhalation anthrax and the others from cutaneous anthrax. Thousands of workers received prophylactic therapy, and a large-scale decontamination programme was implemented.

Radiological and chemical terrorism are also potential threats. The only documented incident of radiological terrorism occurred

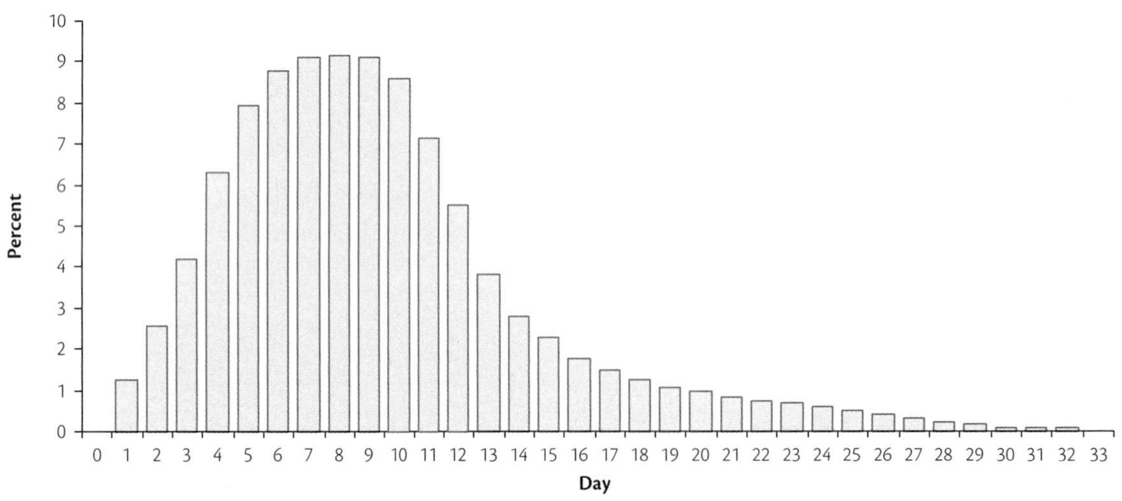

Fig. 9.5.13.1 Simulated epidemic curve for a point-source outbreak of inhalation anthrax without intervention.
Reproduced from Scheulen J, Latimer C, Brown J (2006). Electronic Mass Casualty Assessment and Planning Scenarios (EMCAPS). Johns Hopkins University. Internet http://www.hopkins-cepar.org/EMCAPS/EMCAPS accessed July 14, 2007.

in 2006, when a former officer in the Russian security services was assassinated by exposure to α-emitting polonium-210 ($_{210}Po$), in a public place in London. Although no other cases were detected, others could have been exposed through ingestion of the material from contamination of their hands. The initial symptoms could be confused with an infectious disease.

Prevention

Prevention of bioterrorism includes addressing the causes of terrorism and developing appropriate preparedness strategies. In addition to international condemnation of the development of bioweapons, access to production capabilities must be controlled. Effective preparedness is in itself a deterrent and requires coordination between agencies and specialists from multiple disciplines. Food supplies must be protected from deliberate contamination. Although water is an unlikely vehicle for bioterrorism, drinking-water sources require special security measures.

Preparedness programmes include training and, where indicated, pre-exposure vaccination of 'first responders'. The infrastructure to deal with the impact of different biological agents will require increased clinical surge capacity and patient isolation facilities. Children, pregnant women, and the immunocompromised may have special needs. Dead patients need to be handled using the same barrier precautions as for live patients.

Antivirals and immunoglobulins are currently considered only for treatment and not for prophylaxis. At present, vaccines are relevant only for smallpox and anthrax. In most countries, more than 50% of the population has never been vaccinated against smallpox. Antibody titres have been shown to decline markedly 5 to 10 years following vaccination, although residual immunity may persist for many years. However, previously vaccinated, milder cases in the community could increase the risk of spread.

A number of countries have carried out vaccination programmes against smallpox for military personnel and first responders. Anthrax vaccine is given routinely in some military populations. Some countries have established national stockpiles of pharmaceuticals and vaccines for use in the event of biological or chemical attacks. The global inventory of smallpox vaccine, together with the possibility of diluting vaccine, probably exceeds 3 billion doses.

Secondary prevention depends on comprehensive surveillance and clinical awareness, both for detecting and characterizing the event. This will facilitate prompt implementation of treatment and, where appropriate, postexposure prophylaxis. Rapid implementation of measures such as vaccination, isolation of patients, and quarantine of contacts can ameliorate the spread. Tertiary prevention includes early treatment and rehabilitation of those people who contract the disease and public information campaigns to reduce the long-term psychological impact of the incident.

Clinical features

The incubation periods of potential bioterrorism agents can vary from as little as several hours to weeks. The incubation period for smallpox is between 7 and 14 days, but could be less following exposure to aerosol. Pneumonic plague is likely to develop within 24 h to 2 days after aerosol exposure. Inhalation anthrax has an incubation period of 1 to 6 days, but is probably dose-related and could be as long as 40 days. For inhaled botulinum toxin, the incubation periods is estimated to be between 12 and 80 h and for ricin, perhaps even less.

Diseases such as anthrax, smallpox, and tularemia usually present with influenza-like illnesses, but if exposure is by aerosol, the symptoms may differ from the naturally occurring diseases. Diseases like plague and tularemia may present as pneumonia. Agents such as smallpox will subsequently develop a typical rash. In the later stages, both anthrax and smallpox commonly develop neurological symptoms. The haemorrhagic fevers are characterized initially by high fever and bleeding tendencies. Inhaled botulinum toxin causes acute, afebrile, descending flaccid paralysis starting with ptosis and muscles innervated by cranial nerves. Inhaled ricin causes fever, chest tightness, dyspnoea, nausea, and arthralgia, within 4 to 8 h, followed by acute respiratory distress syndrome and death within 18 to 24 h.

Differential diagnosis

The early symptoms of diseases caused by potential bioterrorism agents can mimic a large spectrum of diseases since influenza-like illness is a common presentation for many. Since diseases such as plague and tularemia may present with pneumonia, cases may not be suspected unless they occur in clusters. Even with the classical sign of widened mediastinum which frequently characterizes inhalation anthrax, it may not be simple to distinguish from other severe pneumonias. Early identification of deliberately caused outbreaks will depend largely on the ability of primary care and emergency room physicians to identify and promptly report cases to the public health authorities. A major concern is that diagnosis of these uncommon diseases may not be considered by physicians who have rarely if ever seen such cases.

Many of the biological agents can be identified by hospital laboratories. However, some may require more specialized laboratories and international collaboration. New techniques, especially those based on the polymerase chain reaction (PCR), are being developed to accelerate specific diagnosis. The safety of laboratory workers must be protected.

Surveillance and early detection

The objectives of surveillance for bioterrorism incidents are twofold. Firstly, early detection of cases can facilitate prompt treatment, identification of the exposure source, rapid introduction of prophylaxis and, where necessary, isolation of cases and imposition of quarantine. Secondly, surveillance systems have a major role in monitoring the progress of an outbreak to support decisions on upgrading and redistributing health services and provide reliable and timely information to the media and the public.

Traditional surveillance, based on routine physicians' reports, could have serious limitations in a bioterrorism incident. Early cases may be missed due to a failure to suspect unusual diseases. Thus there may be considerable delays in alerting public health authorities due to the lag time between the initial symptoms and definitive diagnosis. Furthermore access to timely, processed information during the epidemic may be seriously limited.

Recognizing these limitations, surveillance for symptoms and signs, known as 'syndromic surveillance', has been proposed as a more sensitive method for early detection of an outbreak. Although theoretically appealing, in practice, syndrome surveillance is likely to be most useful to complement early detection and reporting of the index cases by alert physicians. Once an outbreak has been confirmed, syndromic surveillance systems will provide timely data on the location, nature, and evolution of the outbreak.

Sources of data for syndromic surveillance are usually by visits to primary care physicians and emergency rooms and prescription and nonprescription medication. Computer analysis of the data allows temporal and geographical trends to be identified. Clusters in families or in age groups will be useful in locating the exposure source. Surveillance systems must include clear procedures to be followed when a suspected incident is reported. Although syndromic surveillance systems are highly sensitive, they tend to have both low specificity and positive predictive value. Abundant false positive reports could desensitize and paralyse the system. Electronic data systems will, however, be important for confirming and tracking the outbreak, and they can reduce delays in reporting and reliance on reports from individual physicians.

Epidemiological investigation

The main objectives of the investigation are to identify and characterize the outbreak and predict its course. For bioterrorism incidents, the investigators should have specialized knowledge of the possible biological agents and the natural history of the diseases. Close collaboration with the police, public health authorities, and the media is essential. Patient details should include the date and time when symptoms started, signs and symptoms and, when smallpox is suspected, the vaccination history. It is important to establish which public places patients have visited in the incubation period of the suspected agent. Those reported by patients to have similar symptoms and contacts should be interviewed. It is important to document the natural history of the disease for each patient.

Postexposure prophylaxis

Vaccination against smallpox, within 3 to 4 days of exposure, appears to provide protection against clinical disease. However, since the incubation period is usually longer than 4 days, the lag time for recognizing index cases may render postexposure vaccination effective only for contacts of those initially exposed. 'Ring vaccination' involves intensive tracing and vaccination of all primary contacts, followed by vaccination of the secondary contacts as opposed to mass vaccination immediately following diagnosis of the first cases. Ring vaccination accompanied by vaccination in affected regions, followed by countrywide mass vaccination, is likely to be the most effective strategy.

For some agents, postexposure prophylaxis with antimicrobials has a role. Ciprofloxacin, doxycycline, and ampicillin are used for postexposure prophylaxis against anthrax and plague. In the case of anthrax, it can be combined with vaccination. Results of animal studies suggest that postexposure antivirals could be effective in a smallpox outbreak. Ribavirin may have some efficacy in postexposure prophylaxis of RNA viral haemorrhagic fevers such as arenaviruses.

Isolation and quarantine

For contagious diseases such as smallpox and plague, isolation of patients, barrier nursing, quarantine of contacts, and restriction of the movements and social interactions of people are important control measures. Results of modelling studies suggest that closing schools and reducing crowding and the use of public transport would be effective in limiting the spread of diseases. Communicating information about risk is likely to improve compliance.

For contagious diseases, there are specific guidelines for the use of masks by health care personnel and emergency workers. Surgical masks may be adequate for droplet spread whereas N95-type masks would be necessary to protect against aerosols. However, they are more expensive, require special fitting, and cannot be worn for long periods. The efficacy and practicability of the use of masks by the general public are less clear.

Public education and risk communication

The novel and largely unpredictable effects of biological weapons are likely to increase the uncertainty surrounding a bioterrorism incident. Public education and effective risk communication are essential in order to bolster public confidence and improve cooperation with the authorities. Clinicians and public health personnel should have access to up-to-date information. The general public should be provided with nontechnical descriptions of the diseases and simple instructions on how to act in an emergency situation.

Risk communication associated with a bioterrorist event may be divided into five stages: prior to the event, on suspicion of an event, on confirmation of the event, during the event, and following the event. At each stage, the public is likely to ask questions relevant to that stage. Since the authorities may possess very little factual information, the public may suspect that information is being withheld, resulting in hostility. Thus it is important that the public messages be reassuring while sharing uncertainties. Over-reaction or panic should be anticipated. This may be exacerbated by rumours or unsubstantiated statements by professionals or lay people not involved in managing the outbreak.

A variety of problems should be anticipated during an outbreak, including atypical presentations of cases and varying responses to treatment and prophylaxis. Side effects of the medications and vaccines may be reported. Discovery of new exposure foci and reports of disease in apparently unexposed people could cause disquiet and mistrust. There may be inadequate isolation of patients and a breakdown of the implementation of quarantine. Untried, new treatments might be proposed by unauthorized professionals or lay people.

Following a bioterrorist incident, residual public fear and anxiety is likely to persist. Inevitably, there will be questions about the extent to which the authorities were able to control the incident, criticism of actions taken or not taken, and general recriminations. Public messages should be broadcast about the lessons learned from the incident and actions that will be taken to address deficiencies.

Decontamination

Decontamination is relevant, mainly for anthrax and smallpox, in the environment of an aerosol attack and at places where patients were treated. Sodium hypochlorite solution is effective in most settings. Bedding and clothing of patients should be sterilized or disposed of where indicated. Low humidity and temperature prolong survival of the smallpox virus in the environment, and on scab material, it can remain viable for as long as 12 weeks.

Legal and ethical aspects

Bioterrorism preparedness requires the necessary legislation to enable the public health authorities to carry out measures with adequate legal backing. Laws that are of particular importance relate to closing buildings, taking over hospitals, ordering isolation and quarantine, and active surveillance of presumed infected individuals and their contacts. Ethical issues may arise in the triage of patients for admission to overburdened hospital wards and intensive care units.

Areas of uncertainty or controversy

Bioterrorism incidents have so far been very rare, and preparedeness is based on an assumption that the potential risk is both real and severe. There are some concerns that the investment of large resources in bioterrorism preparedness could come at the expense of other essential public health activities. Research should be encouraged to assess the risks, costs, and benefits of the preparedness activities, in order to strike a reasonable balance. New surveillance systems, particular those based on syndromic surveillance, may be insufficiently specific and too much of a burden on the health services to be sustainable for long. Uncertainty remains about the efficacy of vaccines and antimicrobial therapy in the event of an outbreak.

Likely future developments

The threat of bioterrorism is likely to increase, demanding greater resources to deter attacks and improve surveillance, vaccines, and medications.

Conclusions

Bioterrorism is a low-risk but high-impact public health emergency. Deterrence remains the prime goal. Reducing the motivation for terror and banning internationally the use of biological weapons should be promoted at all levels. Sensible preparedness for bioterrorist incidents is a deterrent in itself and ensures that public health systems and society will deal effectively with an incident. Risk communication needs to be strengthened. Such measures will also improve general emergency preparedness and the control of infectious diseases.

Further reading

Arnon SS, *et al.* (2001). Botulism toxin as a biological weapon. Medical and public health management. *JAMA*, **285**, 1059–70.

Barbera J, *et al.* (2001). Large-scale quarantine following biological terrorism in the United States: scientific examination, logistic and legal limits, and possible consequences. *JAMA*, **286**, 2711–18.

Borio L, *et al.* (2002). Hemorrhagic fever viruses as biological weapons. *JAMA*, **287**, 2391–405.

Bozzette SA, *et al.* (2003). A model for a smallpox vaccination policy. *N Engl J Med*, **348**, 416–25.

Centers for Disease Control and Prevention (2006). *Bioterrorism overview. 28 February, 2006.* http://www.bt.cdc.gov/bioterrorism. Accessed 1 July 2007.

Covello VT, *et al.* (2001). Risk communication, the West Nile virus epidemic, and bioterrorism: responding to the communication challenges posed by the intentional or unintentional release of a pathogen in an urban setting. *J Urban Health*, **78**, 382–91.

Dennis DT, *et al.* (2001). Tularemia as a biological weapon. Medical and public health management. *JAMA*, **285**, 2763–73.

Franz DR, *et al.* (1997). Clinical recognition and management of patients exposed to biological warfare agents. *JAMA*, **278**, 399–411.

Henderson DA (1998). Bioterrorism as a public health threat. *Emerg Infect Dis*, **4**, 488–92.

Henderson DA, *et al.* (1999). Smallpox as a biological weapon. Medical and public health management. *JAMA*, **281**, 2127–37.

Ingelsby TV, *et al.* (2002). Anthrax as a biological weapon, 2002. Updated recommendations for management. *JAMA*, **287**, 2236–52.

Kress M (2005). The effect of social mixing controls on the spread of smallpox—a two-level model. *Health Care Manage Sci*, **8**, 277–89.

Leach S (2007). Some public health perspectives on quantitative risk assessments for bioterrorism. In: Green MS *et al.* (eds.) *Risk assessment and risk communication strategies in bioterrorism preparedness.* NATO Security through Science Series A: Chemistry and Biology, Springer, Dordrecht.

Meselson M, *et al.* (1994). The Sverdlovsk anthrax outbreak of 1979. *Science*, **266**, 1202–8.

Mortimer PP (2003). Can post-exposure vaccination against smallpox succeed? *Clin Infect Dis*, **36**, 622–8.

Rotz LD, *et al.* (2002). Public health assessment of potential biological terrorism agents. *Emerg Infect Dis*, **8**, 225–30.

World Health Organization (2004). *Public health response to biological and chemical weapons: WHO guidance.* http://www.who.int/csr/delibepidemics/biochemguide/en/print.html Accessed 1 July 2007.

SECTION 10

Clinical pharmacology

10.1 Principles of clinical pharmacology and drug therapy *1449*
Kevin O'Shaughnessy

10.1

Principles of clinical pharmacology and drug therapy

Kevin O'Shaughnessy

Essentials

The role of clinical pharmacology is to provide the scientific basis for rational prescribing: 'patients may recover in spite of drugs ... or because of them' (Gaddum). This sums up the dilemma facing any doctor who prescribes a drug to a patient: it should certainly be the doctor's explicit intention to do the patient some good, but the drug may actually harm the patient, and on rare occasions it can even kill them.

Principles of clinical pharmacology

Drug therapy can be considered under four headings: (1) pharmaceutical—is the drug getting from the formulation into the patient?; (2) pharmacokinetic—how does the drug dose, formulation, frequency, and route of administration affect the drug concentration in the body, and the way that this concentration changes with time?; (3) pharmacodynamic—how does a drug produce its pharmacological effects?; and (4) therapeutic—is the pharmacological effect being translated into a therapeutic effect?

Adverse drug reactions

Definition and causes—an adverse drug reaction (ADR) can be defined as an unwanted or harmful reaction experienced following administration of a drug, or combination of drugs, under normal conditions of use that is suspected of being related to the drug (or combination). These can be (1) dose related—usually due to an exaggeration of a known pharmacological effect of the drug; or (2) non-dose-related—often caused by immunological or pharmacogenetic mechanisms.

Clinical importance—ADRs are responsible for 1 to 4% of acute hospital admissions, affect 5 to 20% of inpatients at some time during their admission, and are responsible for up to 3% of inpatient deaths. Pharmacovigilance is the subspecialty of clinical pharmacology devoted to the detection and evaluation of ADRs.

Drug interactions

A drug interaction occurs when the effects of one drug are altered by the effects of another drug, usually resulting in an ADR. Drugs likely to precipitate interactions often (1) are highly protein bound, e.g. aspirin and sulphonamides; or (2) induce drug metabolism, e.g. phenytoin, carbamazepine and rifampicin; or (3) inhibit drug metabolism, e.g. cimetidine, metronidazole, and triazole antifungals. The drugs most likely to be affected by drug–drug interactions are those with a steep dose–response curve and a low therapeutic index.

A rational basis for prescribing

This requires that a drug's therapeutic potential is maximized and its side effects minimized. A series of checks and balances for the process of drug prescription is needed. A question checklist that can usefully be applied is as follows: (1) does the patient need a drug at all, that is, do the risks outweigh its benefits? (2) are the benefits of the drug well established, preferably by randomized controlled trials? (3) what drug action is being sought, and what class of drug can best provide it? (4) what is the most appropriate drug in that class, and in what formulation? (5) what is the appropriate dose, and how frequently or in what circumstances should it be taken? (6) for how long should the drug be prescribed?—is it as a single course or for indefinite use? (7) will this drug interact with other drugs the patient is taking? (8) can this drug replace other drugs the patient is taking? (9) what does the patient need to understand about this drug?—and who will communicate this, and how? (10) will it be necessary to review the prescription of this drug?—and if so, when, how, and by whom? (11) does the patient need anything else to derive the most benefit from this drug?

Practical prescribing

Guidelines and formularies—the question checklist above is not completed before every drug is prescribed, many of the questions being addressed by using appropriate therapeutic guidelines and formularies. Guidelines provide prerehearsed decision paths for many of the issues raised in the checklist, whilst formularies specifically tackle the question of which drug to prescribe (from within a therapeutic class).

The patient's drug history—it is essential to obtain a thorough drug history from the patient before prescribing. Key information that should be obtained includes details of: (1) all the medicines currently being prescribed, including their doses; (2) any previous medical treatments; (3) any 'alternative' treatments, e.g. herbal and homeopathic remedies; (4) any self-prescribed medicines; (5) any history of allergy or adverse reactions to drugs.

Prescribing for the particular patient—guidelines, formularies and other prescribing aids are not a substitute for an intelligent clinical approach. The prescriber needs to establish what the patient's experience and expectations of drug therapy are, and the patient needs to know the likely consequences—both good and bad—of taking any drug that is prescribed. This dialogue is important, since it will often decide whether the patient actually takes the drug as prescribed. Patient compliance is a key variable in the prescribing process, and one in which the doctor often has least control.

Balancing a drug's therapeutic benefit with its side effects

The prescriber checklist implies that balancing the expected benefits of a drug against the expected harm is a straightforward process. It is not. By the time a drug reaches the clinic we know a lot about the size of its therapeutic effect, its relation to drug dose, and the proportion of patients likely to show this effect. Measuring harm is a less precise and much slower process. Terms such as 'risk/benefit ratio' are widely used, but can be very misleading. Benefit is often measured in terms of amount and not its probability or frequency. It can also be measured accurately by a single therapeutic endpoint; harm from a drug encompasses a spectrum of side effects that differ in both their frequency and severity.

Some side effects are predictable from the pharmacology of the drug (so-called type A) and are relatively common and dose-dependent. Others are rare and unpredictable (so-called type B or idiosyncratic). Type B side effects are usually more severe with a higher burden of mortality and morbidity and, because of their low frequency, will only come to light after a drug is licensed for clinical use. It is important to remember that only a few thousand patients are exposed to a drug before a license is granted (and for drugs with orphan status, the patient exposure may be very much smaller). The duration of dosing is also inevitably short when the intention is to give the drug to patients indefinitely. Hence, crucial important information about side effects has to be gathered after the drug is licensed, and it may take many millions of patient-years of dosing before some drug side effects emerge.

Perhaps the best way of comparing a drug's benefit with its harm is to define them in terms of the number of patients needed to be treated to observe a certain benefit and cause specific harm. These are referred to as the number needed to treat (NNT) and number needed to harm (NNH), respectively. Take, for example, the drug clopidogrel. It is currently given to patients for 12 months after suffering an acute coronary syndrome (non-ST elevation myocardial infarction, NSTEMI) to prevent myocardial infarction. Because of its antiplatelet action it also causes gastrointestinal bleeding. Used in this way to prevent nonfatal myocardial infarction, the NNT for clopidogrel is about 67 and the NNH to cause a major bleeding episode is 100. So, if 100 patients are treated for 1 year, 1.5 nonfatal myocardial infarctions will be prevented at the expense of causing one major bleeding episode. This is a much more transparent presentation than the relative risk reduction that is often used to highlight drug benefit in clinical trials. These percentage measures inevitably boost the psychological impact of a drug's effect—the NNT for clopidogrel equates to a 22% reduction in the frequency of nonmyocardial infarction!

But even with reliable measures of harm and benefit, how do we decide where the final balance lies? It will depend on other factors such as the severity of the disease and whether there are safer alternative drugs. Hence, if we want to treat a disease with a high fatality rate, using a drug which is highly effective and carries little risk of harm, the balance is clearly in favour of the drug. But if the disease itself carries no mortality or morbidity and we propose using a drug whose effectiveness is low and carries a high risk of harm, the balance is clearly against using the drug. Most clinical decisions to use a drug or not will be in the grey area between these two extremes.

Efficacy, effectiveness, efficiency of drugs

These terms are not synonymous and can be easily confused. Efficacy is a pharmacological term. It refers to the ability of a drug to bring about a certain size of an effect at a given concentration or dose. The effect may not be applicable to clinical practice or is only accurately measured in a clinical trial. Hence the term is best reserved for the performance of a drug in this setting. Effectiveness refers to the performance of a drug in everyday clinical use, and is defined as the likelihood and extent of the therapeutic effect in a given patient. Efficiency weights drug performance against cost: it is the ratio of effectiveness to cost. Clearly, it is more efficient to use the cheaper of two drugs that are equally effective and safe.

The therapeutic index of a drug

The therapeutic index is a term taken from animal pharmacology. It is the dose needed to harm over the dose needed to produce the therapeutic response. However, as harm is measured by a drug's lethality, it is not a useful clinical measure. Instead, the index is employed clinically in a very loose and entirely qualitative way. Drugs that produce side effects at doses well outside the clinical dose range are said to have a high therapeutic index and those where the ranges are much closer or even overlap are said to have a low therapeutic index. Hence penicillins have a high therapeutic index; large doses can be given without the worry of adverse effects unless the patient is allergic to penicillins. In contrast, digoxin has a low therapeutic index; the doses causing toxicity overlap with those producing therapeutic benefit. Drugs with a low therapeutic index include: aminoglycoside antibiotics, anticoagulants, anticonvulsants, antihypertensives, some antiparasitic and antiviral drugs, cardiac glycosides, and cytotoxic and immunosuppressant drugs.

To increase the margin of safety for drugs with a low index, dosing can be guided by measuring drug levels in plasma or serum. Such therapeutic monitoring is mandatory for drugs such as lithium and aminoglycoside antibiotics because of additional pharmacokinetic problems with their use (see pp.1475–1476). Anticoagulants are unusual in being monitored by their effect on clotting rather than as a plasma drug concentration.

Formularies

Formularies are lists of medicines for prescribers and pharmacists, intended to guide the choice and facilitate the dispensing of medicines. Many give details of the formulation and doses of drugs. Each formulary is produced primarily for a particular group, usually the prescribers in one country or region or institution, or even one practice. Most formularies are restrictive, i.e. they make a narrow choice of medicines from all those available. This is typical for the formulary of a hospital, or of a health maintenance organization. A hospital formulary lists only the preparations that are stocked in the hospital pharmacy; a health maintenance organization formulary only those that the organization will pay for. The *British National Formulary* (BNF) is probably the best known and most widely used formulary of all, but is unusual in including all medicines available for prescription in the United Kingdom, whether they are good choices or not. However, every section of the BNF has concise and critical 'notes to facilitate the selection of suitable treatment' that precede the list of available agents. This invaluable resource is revised biannually and available online (http://www.bnf.org).

The WHO 'Model list of essential drugs'

In many developing countries, limited health budgets means that large sections of the population have no access to drugs or health care, and governments cannot afford to provide necessary drugs. To help them to use their limited funds in the best ways, the World Health Organization (WHO) has since 1977 published a regularly updated *Model List of Essential Drugs*. It is currently in its 16th edition (http://www.who.int/medicines/publications/essentialmedicines/en/index.html). Essential drugs on the list are intended to 'provide safe, effective treatment for the majority of communicable and non-communicable diseases'. The WHO list is a 'model' list that can be adapted to meet the needs of the local health economy. Hence, over 150 countries have an essential list based on the WHO model. It is a salient fact that the first WHO list contained 208 drugs and, in the intervening 30 years, it has not doubled in size. There may be some clear lessons here for the drug lists of developed countries.

Medicines management

Because of the rapidly escalating costs of providing drugs within health care systems and the need to maximize drug safety, the concept of medicines management is now widespread. By bringing together clinical, pharmacy, and financial skills, drugs that are considered essential can be prescribed in the most cost-effective and safest way. In the United Kingdom, drugs are assessed at a national level by the National Centre for Health and Clinical Excellence (NICE) before deployment within the National Health Service (NHS). NICE considers in detail the evidence for a drug's alleged benefit and weights this against known side effects and economic modelling of its total cost vs benefit within the NHS.

The principles of clinical pharmacology

Drug therapy can be considered under four headings—pharmaceutical, pharmacokinetic, pharmacodynamic, and therapeutic—each of which addresses a pertinent question about drug therapy (Fig. 10.1.1).

The pharmaceutical process

The pharmaceutical step is concerned with the question, 'Is the drug getting from the formulation into the patient?'

The route of drug administration is usually a more crucial choice than how it is formulated. Nevertheless, formulation can greatly affect the rate and extent of drug absorption. Repackaging short-acting drugs into 'sustained' or 'modified' release formulations to slow release of the drug into the gut allows them to be taken once daily. Morphine, calcium channel blockers (e.g. diltiazem and nifedipine), and L-dopa have been widely reformulated in this way. Other drugs are formulated for specific routes of administration: glyceryl trinitrate is available for sublingual (as a spray and tablets), buccal, and transdermal (as a paste or patch) use. To understand the differences between these various routes, it is necessary to understand the concept of systemic availability.

Systemic availability

Systemic availability, commonly called bioavailability, is the proportion of administered drug that reaches the systemic circulation and is available for distribution to the site of drug action. If a drug is given intravenously, it will enter the systemic circulation directly, i.e. it is said to be 100% bioavailable. The same drug given orally, or by any other route, must be absorbed first (which may be an incomplete process), and possibly metabolized, before entering the systemic circulation.

Metabolism can occur in the gut wall and liver following oral administration, although it can occur at any site of drug administration. Incomplete absorption and this presystemic metabolism ensure that most drugs have a bioavailability of less than 100% when given orally. In some cases, the reduction is so large that a drug has zero bioavailability and is clinically ineffective. Oral insulin or benzypenicillin are good examples of this problem, with their instability in the stomach preventing significant absorption. Complete presystemic metabolism also explains why glyceryl trinitrate and buprenorphine are orally effective only if given sublingually or as a buccal patch. Absorption from the mouth allows the drug to bypass gut wall and liver metabolism.

Special drug formulations

Most drugs are given orally; oral formulations include syrups, ordinary (instant release) tablets, capsules, and modified release formulations. However, drugs can be given by other routes, including sublingually, buccally, rectally, transdermally, by inhalation, and by injection intravenously, subcutaneously, intramuscularly, or locally.

Modified-release formulations

Most conventional instant release tablets are designed to disintegrate in the stomach or proximal small bowel, so that absorption is complete within a few hours on ingestion. Modified or sustained release formulations are oral formulations that allow a drug to be released over long periods (12–24 h typically) relative to the half-life of the drug. The intention of the prolonged and slowed release is to smooth out the concentration profile of the drug in the blood and extend its duration of action. They include formulations of theophylline, nifedipine, diltiazem, morphine, and lithium. Prescriptions of these drugs should specify the exact formulation, as formulations differ in systemic availability and may not be interchangeable.

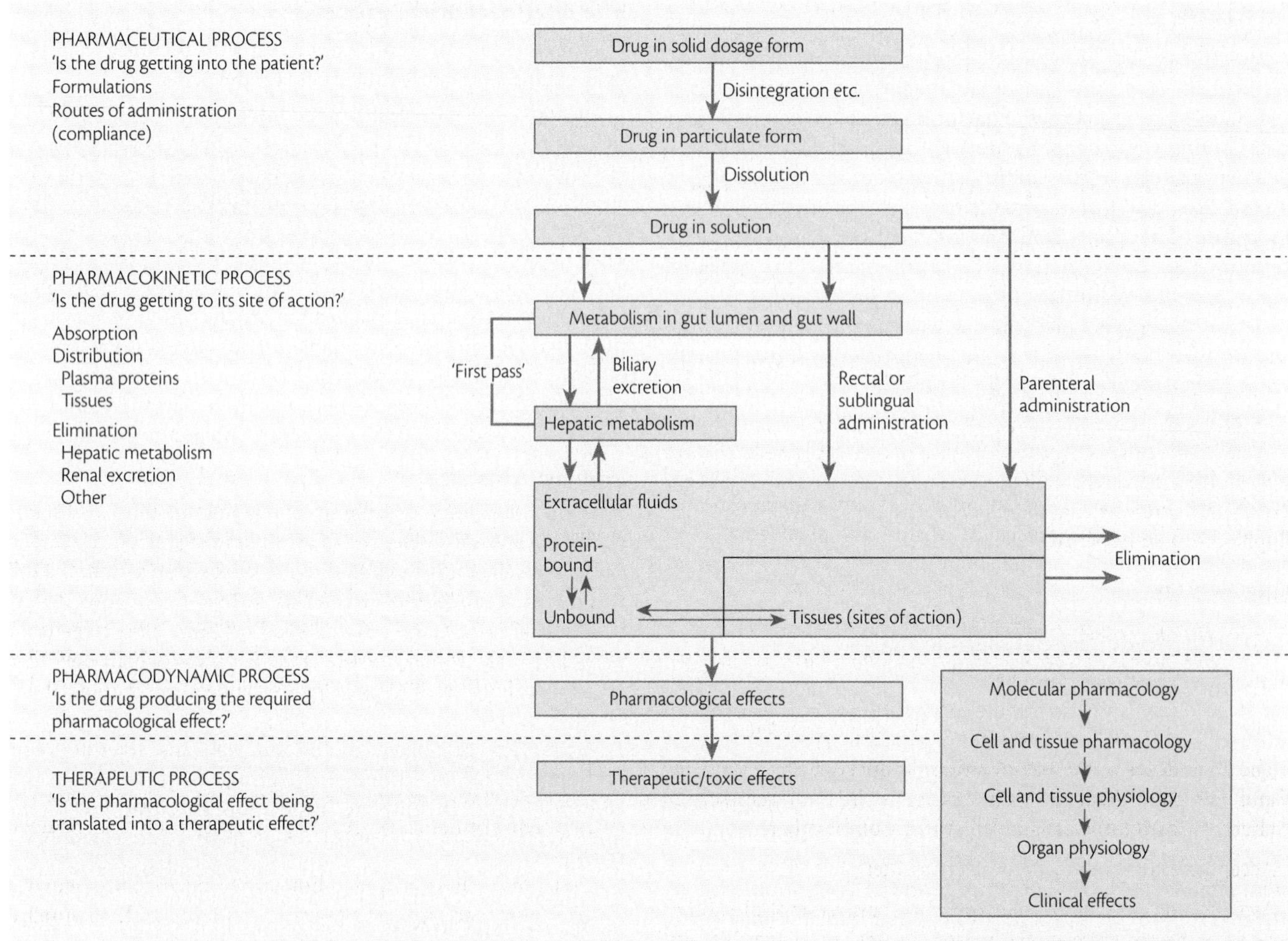

Fig. 10.1.1 The four processes of clinical pharmacology in relation to drug therapy.

Sublingual, buccal, rectal formulations

Drugs that are absorbed through the oral or rectal mucosa avoid first-pass metabolism in the liver by uptake into veins that drain directly into the systemic circulation. For example, sublingual glyceryl trinitrate is rapidly effective as a sublingual tablet, but if the tablet is swallowed, the remainder is not bioavailable because of high presystemic metabolism. Rectal administration achieves a direct effect on the local bowel wall (e.g. corticosteroids in ulcerative colitis), but is also useful for achieving high blood levels rapidly when intravenous access is difficult (e.g. diazepam for seizure control).

Transdermal formulations

Some lipid-soluble drugs are well absorbed through the skin, and their transdermal delivery via 'patches' allows controlled release over many hours or days. Examples are glyceryl trinitrate in the long-term treatment of angina pectoris, transdermal hyoscine for travel sickness, estradiol as hormone replacement therapy, buprenorphine for pain control, and nicotine for smoking cessation.

Inhaled formulations

The lung provides a huge surface area (*c.* 100 m^2) for drug absorption, but to reach the distal airways, a drug for delivery by inhalation must be associated with particles in the 2 to 5 μm range. These can either be solid particles (dry powder devices) or dissolved in small droplets (aerosol devices). For hand-held aerosol inhalers the drug is dissolved in a volatile hydrocarbon, but in nebulizers the drug is in an aqueous solution that is aerosolized by a jet of air or oxygen. Both aerosols and dry powders are widely used to deliver inhaled corticosteroids and bronchodilators used in the management of asthma and chronic obstructive pulmonary disease. Even peptides can be delivered by this route, as demonstrated by the licensing of inhaled insulin. The efficiency of inhalation as a route of administration also explains the 'success' of some drugs of abuse, e.g. nicotine and crack cocaine.

Subcutaneous, intramuscular, and local injections

The rate of absorption of insulin from the site of subcutaneous injection is controlled by its physical state (e.g. monomer, crystalline, or noncrystalline), pH, and the presence of zinc ions or protamine (isophane) in the buffer in which it is suspended. It is also affected by altering the amino acid sequence of insulin; allowing recombinant insulins, which are rapidly (Lispro and Aspart) or slowly released (Glargine or Detemir) after injection. Soluble insulins have a rapid onset (15–30 min) and short duration of action (4–6 h), so they are usually given together with intermediate or long-acting insulin. Long-acting insulins act for more than

24 h and can provide the insulin background as a once daily injection. The isophane insulins have an intermediate duration of action and are usually given twice daily mixed with soluble insulin.

Absorption of a drug after subcutaneous injection is affected by blood flow. Hence, the duration of action of local anaesthetics can be prolonged by vasoconstriction. Adrenaline or felypressin is added to the subcutaneous formulations for this purpose. Smoking also reduces subcutaneous insulin absorption by causing cutaneous vasoconstriction. Reduced absorption also explains why subcutaneous adrenaline is not advised for the treatment of anaphylaxis.

The intramuscular route is a popular parenteral route but can be erratic. Hence, phenytoin and diazepam should not be given by this route for emergency use. Absorption following intramuscular injection may be retarded by esterifying a drug to a large lipid molecule. This gives oily formulations that provide long-lived drug depots in muscle, which are used in the treatment of male hypogonadism (testosterone enantate or undecanoate) and schizophrenia (fluphenazine or flupentixol decanoates).

Combination formulations in oral therapy

Combination products are attractive and may aid compliance (see following paragraphs), but should be used only when at least two criteria are met:

- The frequency of administration of the two drugs is the same.
- The fixed doses in the combination product are therapeutically and optimally effective in most cases, i.e. it is not necessary to alter the dose of one drug independently of the other.

  Acceptable combination products include:

- Aspirin plus codeine (co-codaprin) or paracetamol plus dihydrocodeine (co-dydramol), pairs of drugs that have different analgesic actions (which synergize) and different adverse effects (which do not).
- L-Dopa plus a peripherally-acting dopa decarboxylase inhibitor (benserazide or carbidopa); the peripheral action of the decarboxylase inhibitor blocks peripheral metabolism of L-dopa, which is free to enter the central nervous system, where it is converted to dopamine, producing the therapeutic effect in Parkinson's disease.
- Combined oral contraceptives, which contain an oestrogen and a progestogen.
- Ferrous sulphate plus folic acid, used to prevent anaemia in pregnancy.
- Co-amoxiclav (amoxicillin plus clavulanic acid); the β-lactamase inhibitor, clavulanic acid, prevents the breakdown of amoxicillin by bacterial penicillinase, so broadening its spectrum.

The patient's use of a drug: compliance and concordance

Compliance is the extent to which a patient follows a prescribed drug regimen. Some prefer the term 'concordance', to make it clear that therapeutic decisions are best arrived at jointly between prescriber and patient. Rates of compliance are difficult to measure and can be surprisingly low even in conditions where the drug has a very obvious benefit, such as epilepsy and asthma. Possibly as few as 1 in 6 patients take the drug exactly as prescribed and 1 in 6 take none at all; the remainder take a different dose and/or a different frequency from that prescribed. Poor compliance is still not well recognized by doctors as a cause of therapeutic failure.

The effect of the prescribing regimen

Apart from the financial cost to the patient (which in some countries is substantial), the two factors that determine compliance with drug therapy are the complexity of the regimen and the likelihood of side effects. The complexity of the prescribed regimen reflects frequency of administration and the number of drugs prescribed. Generally speaking, the more frequently a drug is prescribed per day, and the more drugs in total are prescribed, the lower is the rate of compliance. For most chronic diseases, drugs that can be taken once daily are preferred. Obviously, using several drugs (polypharmacy), where one may be adequate, should be avoided wherever possible.

Side effects that a patient attributes to a drug may lead them to stopping the drug completely. It may be necessary then to persuade them to persevere or switch to an alternative drug. However, giving another drug to simply reduce the side effects of the first drug has to be thought through carefully. For example, giving furosemide to a patient who develops ankle oedema on nifedipine, causing in turn gout or hypokalaemia, is nonsensical. But giving omperazole to a rheumatoid patient who develops acid reflux on their nonsteroidal anti-inflammatory (NSAID) is sensible.

The effect of the illness

People with severe mental health problems, e.g. patients with schizophrenia or manic depressive psychosis, often take medicines unreliably.

Physical disability may cause difficulty even in patients who want to take their medicine. For example, patients with rheumatoid arthritis who cannot reach the tablets, or cannot remove the top of a childproof container, cannot take them without help.

Sometimes, a good response to treatment leads patients to stop. For example, patients with tuberculosis need long courses of several drugs to eradicate the infection; once the symptoms have resolved, motivation to continue treatment may decline, risking reactivation and the emergence of resistant tuberculosis.

Some diseases may promote compliance. Patients with insulin-dependent diabetes easily become very ill quite quickly if they forget to take their insulin, and that is likely to make them comply, although they may not use it precisely as advised. Patients in whom a β-blocker or vasodilator has prevented anginal attacks will also be more likely to have good compliance.

The patient's behaviour

People tend to forget to take drugs, or can't be bothered; they may feel no need for treatment (e.g. in asymptomatic hypertension); they may be unclear about the prescribing instructions; they may not want to feel dependent or be thought to be dependent on 'drugs'. There may be social or physical reasons why they cannot reach a pharmacist, financial difficulties, or everyday inconveniences in carrying and taking the medication.

The doctor's behaviour

The enthusiasm and confidence with which a drug is prescribed, and the extent to which these attitudes are transmitted to the patient, may influence not only compliance but also the response to therapy. This is related to the placebo effect of drug taking.

Methods of assessing compliance

It is important to assess compliance both in everyday practice and in clinical trials. The most obvious and usually the easiest approach is to ask the patient whether he or she has been taking the drugs, and whether there have been any problems. If the doctor is nonjudgemental and indicates that difficulties are common, the patient is encouraged to be open.

Less directly, one can ask to see the patient's tablets: this at least confirms that the prescription has been filled. Counting the tablets left in the bottle is a guide to how many have been taken, but some may have been thrown away. Recording devices fitted in the caps of medication containers can record the frequency and exact timing of the opening of the container, and are useful in research.

If a patient is vague or untrustworthy, measurement of the drug level in plasma or urine may give some reassurance of compliance—at least on the day they visit the doctor. The list of drugs for which assays are routinely available is small, but a surrogate marker can be used e.g. the level of thyroid stimulating hormone (TSH) to ensure compliance with thyroxine or the international normalized ratio (INR) for patients on warfarin. Alternatively, a pharmacological effect such as heart rate can be measured directly (to assess β-blocker compliance).

Methods of improving compliance

Compliance can be improved by supervised administration of the drug, by removing barriers to compliance, by simplifying the therapeutic regimen, and by educating the patient on the need to take the medicine, with reinforcement whenever possible.

Supervised administration Administration of a drug by the doctor or nurse ensures compliance. This is possible in hospital or when occasional administration is required (e.g. intramuscular injections of vitamin B_{12}, long-acting intramuscular depot injections of neuroleptics, and supervised twice-weekly antituberculosis therapy). A relative or other carer can give the drug at home and this may be aided by using dosimeter boxes prefilled by a pharmacist.

Removing barriers to compliance Compliance may be encouraged by prescribing pleasant-tasting syrups rather than tablets for children and older people, and by using a drug or formulation that minimizes side effects.

Simplification of the therapeutic regimen The therapeutic regimen can be simplified by reducing both the number of drugs a patient has to take and the frequency of administration. Modified release or combination formulations may be useful here.

Education and reminders Educating the patient about why treatment is necessary (e.g. treating hypertension or diabetes reduces the risk of serious complications) is time-consuming but improves compliance. In the treatment of certain infections (e.g. tuberculosis) and in typhoid carriers, the wider importance to the community should also be explained.

Even in the well-motivated, reminders to take the treatment may improve compliance. Many drugs for long-term use are also now dispensed in a 'calendar pack' to help compliance.

The pharmacokinetic process

Pharmacokinetics concerns the complicated question 'How does the drug dose, formulation, frequency and route of administration affect the drug concentration in the body, and the way that this concentration changes with time?' The answer will depend on the absorption, distribution, metabolism, and excretion of that drug (its ADME). This naturally lends itself to complex mathematical modelling, but the key points can be understood without being overwhelmed by the mathematics.

Basic pharmacokinetic terms and concepts

Before considering the various components of ADME, a few pharmacokinetic terms need to be explained. So, consider a time after administering a drug when its absorption and distribution throughout the various compartments of the body are complete. At this time, there are no concentration gradients across compartments and any further decline in drug concentration reflects drug elimination, that is, excretion and metabolism of the drug. Several parameters characterize this elimination phase of a drug:

Volume of distribution (V_d)

This can be a confusing term, since it is really a mathematical device and not a true physical volume. Hence, it rarely relates to any particular water compartment, e.g. plasma, 3 litres; extracellular water, 16 litres; total body water, 42 litres). It simply allows the amount of drug remaining in the body to be inferred from the drug concentration (concentration = amount/volume). Drugs have a wide range of values for their V_d and sometimes they are much greater than the total water space. This is typical for drugs that bind to tissues or partition into lipid. Amidarone is an extreme example of this behaviour with a V_d of approximately 5000 litres.

Clearance

In the same way that the volume of distribution is a proportionality term, so clearance is used to relate the rate of drug excretion to the concentration of the drug in the body. It is expressed in units of flow (volume per unit time) and is effectively the volume of the V_d cleared of drug per unit time. A drug can be eliminated (or cleared) from the plasma by one or more mechanisms (e.g. through the kidney by filtration and the liver by metabolism). The total clearance of the drug is simply the sum of these different organ-based clearances.

Plasma half-life

During the elimination phase, the drug concentration falls in a predictable way: in a fixed time called the half-life it falls by 50%, and by a further 50% after another half-life and so on. Thus, it takes between four and five half-lives for 95% of the drug to be eliminated (see Fig. 10.1.2). For most drugs the half-life is constant (except if the kinetics becomes nonlinear—see following paragraphs). The half-life is not affected by the starting concentration or amount of the drug, but it is directly affected by the volume of distribution and clearance of a drug (actually proportional to their ratio).

Repeated dosing and the 'plateau principle'

A drug can be given once but it is more common for a drug to be given repeatedly (even indefinitely). After the first dose, the plasma level will rise to its maximum (C_{max}) and fall as shown in Fig. 10.1.2. If the dose is not repeated until all the drug has been eliminated (which means the dose interval must be long, e.g. 10 half-lives), the drug level will oscillate between the C_{max} after a single dose and a trough value of zero. The problem with this regimen is that to give a plasma level that is therapeutic (but not toxic), a large part of the dosing interval is spent with a nontherapeutic drug level. To get around this, the drug is given at smaller doses separated by short

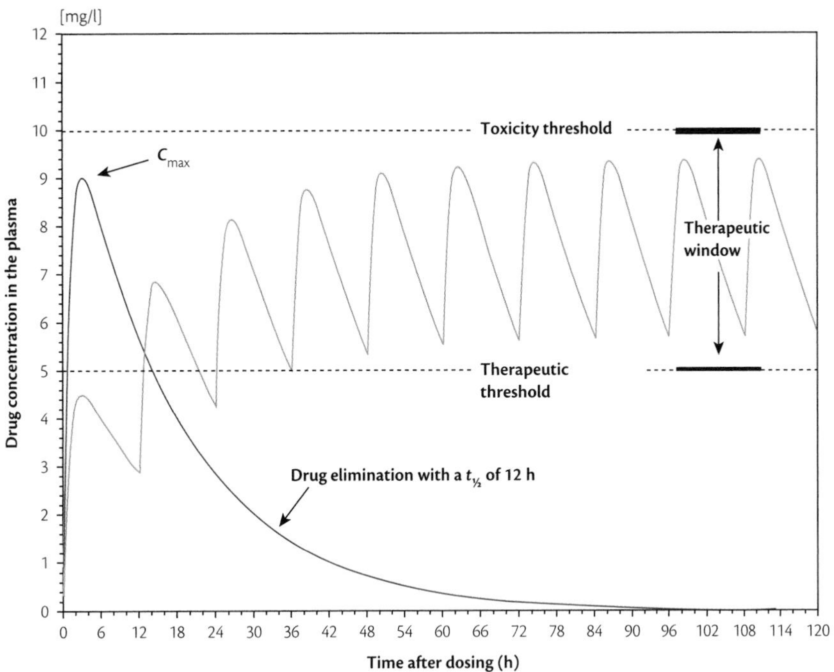

Fig. 10.1.2 Plateau principle. Plasma concentrations of a hypothetical drug after a single oral dose (black line) vs repeated dosing (red line). A smaller dose is used for repeated dosing but the half-life is the same. Both approaches give levels within the 'therapeutic window', but only with repeat dosing are the levels within the window throughout the dose interval.

dose intervals compared to the drug's half-life. Because the dose interval is similar to the drug's half-life, the first dose of drug is not completely eliminated before the second dose is given. The third dose is given before either the second dose, or the remaining fraction of the first dose is eliminated and so on. Hence, the drug plasma level accumulates and eventually it comes to a steady state where it oscillates between a new peak and trough (substantially greater than zero); ideally, the peak is below the toxic threshold and the trough above the therapeutic threshold throughout the dose interval. This is what is known as the plateau principle and the therapeutic and toxic threshold levels for the drug define its 'therapeutic window'.

Loading doses

The half-life also dictates the time it takes for a drug to reach its plateau with repeated dosing. In the same way that it takes almost 5 half-lives to eliminate a drug, it takes almost 5 half-lives to reach plateau. The delay imposed by the drug's half-life in reaching steady state can be unacceptable clinically. Consider, for example, the use of digoxin to treat fast atrial fibrillation. Because of the long half-life of digoxin (40 h), it takes over a week to reach plateau, and over twice this if the patient has renal failure because of the increased half-life. The solution is to give a loading dose of a drug. The loading dose is intended to take the blood concentration rapidly into the therapeutic window. Dosing then resorts to the usual maintenance dose, which is chosen to replace the drug eliminated in each subsequent dose interval.

Absorption and systemic availability

Systemic availability was introduced earlier (see above) and is measured by plotting the blood concentration at various times after dosing. Typical curves are shown in Fig. 10.1.3 for three different formulations (containing the same dose) of a hypothetical drug. The area under each of these curves (abbreviated to AUC) reflects the bioavailability of the formulation and it is actually the same in this simulation. However, it is clear that they produce very different profiles in terms of the maximum concentration (C_{max}) and the time C_{max} occurs after dosing (t_{max}). This reflects the decreasing rate of absorption from left to right for the three formulations, and hence the duration over which absorption occurs. Hence the fastest absorption gives the highest C_{max}, but this would cause transient toxicity as crosses into the toxic range for this drug. The middle curve takes the drug level above the therapeutic threshold for as long as the first curve but remains below the toxicity threshold. The slowest rate of absorption here gives a C_{max} that is too low because the drug concentration is subtherapeutic throughout.

Choosing the optimum concentration profile, and hence the formulation, depends on the therapeutic effect being sought. Hence, a rapid (instant release) formulation of nifedipine would be needed to treat an episode of angina and is typified by the left-hand curve in Fig. 10.1.3. The transient flushing and headache this would cause would be an acceptable side effect. However, when drugs are intended to be given repeatedly, and the therapeutic effect is related to a steady state concentration, the flatter profile of the slowest absorption formulations are preferred (right-hand curve in Fig. 10.1.3). So, for chronic angina prophylaxis, a slow release formulation of nifedipine would be preferred to achieve the smoothest profile of drug level in the blood after dosing.

The rate of absorption

Gastrointestinal motility

Drugs are absorbed mainly in the upper small intestine, so altered gastric emptying can affect absorbance. For example, in migraine, the rate of absorption of analgesics is reduced because of reduced gastric motility, delaying the response to an oral analgesic. In fact, the shift in the drug concentration–time profile is similar to the rightward shift produced by reformulation discussed in Fig. 10.1.3. This delay can be reduced by giving metoclopramide to accelerate gastric emptying. Erythromycin can have a similar effect on gastric emptying. The converse of delayed emptying occurs with antimuscarinics or

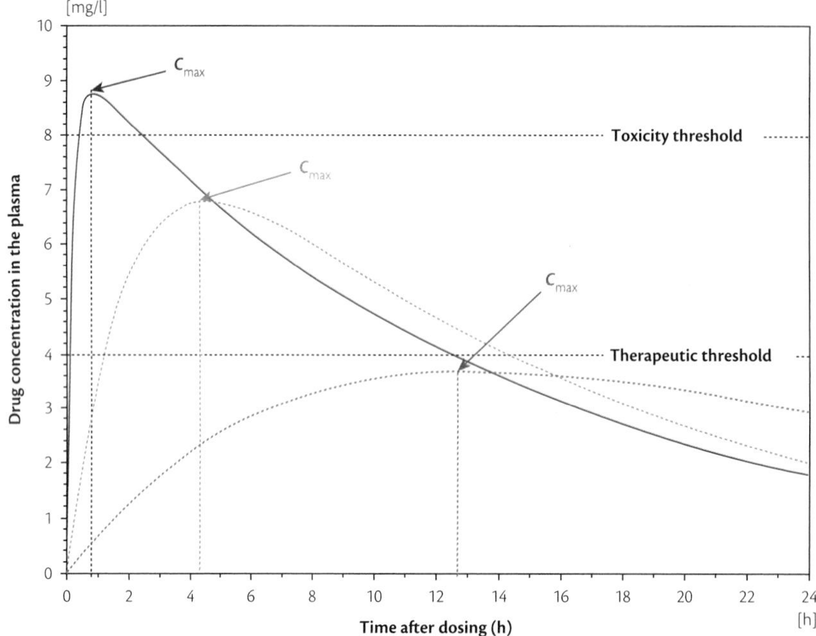

Fig. 10.1.3 Effect of slowed absorption on drug kinetics. Plasma concentration profiles for a hypothetical drug formulated to progressively slow absorption (slows left to right). As the absorption is slowed, the peak concentration (C_{max}) falls and is delayed.

older antihistamines (e.g. promethazine and diphenhydramine) or tricyclic antidepressants (e.g. amitriptyline) that have substantial antimuscarinic actions. This can be particularly important in drug overdoses involving these drugs.

If a drug dissolves more slowly than the stomach empties, increased gastrointestinal motility reduces both the rate and extent of absorption. This effect is exaggerated for sustained release formulations, such that in severe diarrhoea enteric-coated formulations can pass through the gut intact. Proximal ileostomies are also a problem for these formulations.

Malabsorption

Drug absorption is often impaired in patients with malabsorption, but not always. For example, the absorption of propranolol and some antibiotics (co-trimoxazole and cefalexin) is increased in patients with coeliac disease. Digoxin, however, is less well absorbed from tablets in patients with coeliac disease, radiation-induced enteritis, and other gastrointestinal disease, and thyroxine absorption is impaired in coeliac disease.

Food

Food alters the rate and extent of absorption of many drugs. For example, eggs impair iron absorption, and milk (or any calcium, aluminium, magnesium, or ferrous salt) impairs tetracycline absorption by the formation of an insoluble chelate. Such effects are rarely important clinically, unless the drug has a very limited bioavailability, when the effect can be highly significant. Hence, bisphosphonates are only bioavailable in the complete absence of food. Grapefruit juice, but not other citrus juices, can markedly increase the bioavailability of some drugs. These include antihistamines (terfenadine), simvastatin, calcium channel blockers (e.g. nifedipine and verapamil), immunosuppressive drugs (ciclosporin A, sirolimus, and tacrolimus), and PDE5 inhibitors (e.g. sildenafil and vardenafil). Grapefruit juice appears to affect both P450 metabolism (CYP 3A4 principally) and expression of the P-glycoprotein in the gut wall.

Coadministered drugs

Drugs affecting gastric emptying can affect absorption of coadministered drugs as mentioned earlier. Anion exchange resins used for lipid management are avid binders of certain drugs and will reduce the absorption of warfarin, thyroxine, thiazides, and digoxin; so it is usually recommended the resin is taken at least an hour after the drugs. This strategy can of course be put to good effect in drug overdose, where absorption can often be prevented by adsorbing the drug to swallowed activated charcoal (see Chapter 9.1).

First-pass metabolism

First-pass metabolism is metabolism that occurs before the drug enters the systemic circulation. This may happen in the gut lumen itself (e.g. with benzylpenicillin or insulin), the gut wall (tyramine, chlorpromazine), the lungs (various amines and inhaled glucocorticoids), and the liver, which is the most important site.

Many drugs undergo first-pass metabolism in the liver. It is substantial for a number of drugs, including cocaine, desipramine, lignocaine, pethidine, morphine, nicotine, nitroglycerin (and other organic nitrates), propranolol, and verapamil.

When first-pass metabolism results in the formation of compounds with less pharmacological activity than the parent compound, the drug's efficacy is lower after oral than intravenous administration. In some cases, metabolism is so extensive that oral therapy is impossible. However, such a drug given sublingually, rectally, or transdermally, can bypass the liver (see earlier paragraphs).

Distribution

Protein binding

Many drugs are bound to circulating proteins, usually albumin (acidic drugs), but also globulins (hormones), lipoproteins, and α_1-acid glycoprotein (basic drugs). Only free drugs (i.e. not protein bound) can bind to cell surface receptors, cross cell membranes to access intracellular drug targets, or distribute to other tissues where they may be metabolized and excreted (e.g. by the kidney). Thus, changes in protein binding can sometimes cause changes in drug distribution. However, such changes are only important if the drug is extensively bound to plasma proteins (>90%) and not widely distributed to other tissues. Phenytoin and warfarin are the two drugs most frequently affected.

The binding of drugs to albumin may be changed in renal impairment (the explanation for this is unknown), hypoalbuminaemia (drug binding is reduced when the plasma albumin concentration falls below 25 g/litre), the last trimester of pregnancy (during which protein binding is reduced partly because of hypoalbuminaemia), and displacement by other drugs.

Because α_1-acid glycoprotein is an acute-phase protein, its levels are affected by trauma, surgery, inflammatory diseases (e.g. Crohn's disease and rheumatoid arthritis), and infections. Hence, the binding of quinine is increased in malaria.

Tissue distribution

The extent of drug distribution to the tissues of the body varies widely. The drugs with the widest distributions will have the largest volumes of distribution (see earlier paragraphs). Some water-soluble drugs are limited to one or more of the water compartments (vascular and extra- and intracellular), while others are bound extensively in tissues. The distribution of drugs to different tissues is influenced by plasma-protein binding, specific receptor sites in tissues (e.g. the binding of cardiac glycosides to the Na^+,K^+-ATPase in cell membranes throughout the body), regional blood flow (well-perfused organs, such as the heart, kidneys, and liver accumulate drugs more than poorly perfused organs, such as fat and bone), lipid solubility (lipid-soluble drugs enter tissues more readily than charged compounds with poor lipid solubility), and active transport across cell membranes (adrenergic neuron-blocking drugs such as guanethidine accumulate in noradrenergic nerve terminals through the noradrenaline transporter, uptake-1) or active transport across epithelia.

The importance of epithelial transport has been appreciated with the discovery of specific transporters such as P-glycoprotein. This ABC transporter was first identified in tumour cells where it confers multidrug resistance (MDR) by promoting the extrusion of many structurally unrelated anticancer drugs. But P-glycoprotein is widely expressed in normal tissues, typically those involved with excretory function, such as small intestine (brush border membrane of enterocytes), kidney (brush border membrane of proximal tubule cells), liver (canalicular membrane of the hepatocytes), and at the blood–brain barrier (capillary endothelial cells). The latter explains, for example, why drugs such as ivermectin, digoxin, loperamide, and domperidone are rapidly pumped out of the cerebrospinal fluid, so effectively excluding them from the brain.

In some diseases, drug distribution is altered for unknown reasons. In renal failure, for example, the distribution of drugs such as insulin and digoxin is decreased as well as their protein binding. In cardiac failure, the distribution of some antiarrhythmic drugs, such as disopyramide, is also reduced. Obesity and malnutrition influence the distribution of drugs that are highly fat soluble (e.g. inhalational anaesthetics).

Metabolism

Most drugs are metabolized in the liver. Examples of other sites are suxamethonium in the plasma; insulin and vitamin D in the kidneys; and acetylcholine and catecholamines at their corresponding synapses and nerve endings.

Drug metabolism occurs in two phases:

- Phase I metabolism involves chemical alteration of the basic structure of the drug, e.g. by oxidation, reduction, or hydrolysis. This results in free groups such as –OH or $–NH_2$ that are conjugated in phase II. Many phase I reactions are catalysed by enzymes from the P450 family (see following paragraphs). Examples of phase I reactions include the *N*-demethylation of diazepam to desmethyldiazepam, an active metabolite with a long duration of action, and the oxidation of ethanol to acetaldehyde.
- Phase II metabolism involves conjugation, e.g. by sulphation, glucuronidation, methylation, or acetylation. Some drugs are conjugated without prior phase I transformation, while others undergo phase I metabolism before conjugation can occur. The products of conjugation are more water soluble and therefore more easily cleared by the kidney or biliary system. They are usually, although not always, pharmacologically inactive; e.g. morphine-6-glucuronide is an active metabolite of morphine that accumulates in renal failure. Examples of phase II reactions are the glucuronidation of paracetamol and the *N*-acetylation of hydralazine and procainamide. A conjugated product may sometimes be further metabolized. For example, oestrogens are excreted via the bile, deconjugated in the gut by bacteria, and then reabsorbed.

The end result of drug metabolism is inactivation, but during the process, compounds with pharmacological activity are often formed. Alternatively, inactive drugs (prodrugs) may be metabolized to active ones. The antiparkinsonian drug L-dopa, for example, is a typical prodrug. It has no action on dopamine receptors until it enters the central nervous system and is metabolized to dopamine. Other examples include diamorphine and codeine (which are rapidly metabolized to desacetylmorphine and morphine respectively) and many angiotensin-converting enzyme (ACE) inhibitors (e.g. enalapril is converted to its active form enalaprilat).

Some drugs also have toxic metabolites. For example, norpethidine is a metabolite of pethidine that can cause fits, and acrolein is a bladder irritant formed from cyclophosphamide. The normally minor metabolic pathway for paracetamol forming *N*-acetyl-*p*-benzoquinone imine (NABQI) is important in overdose because of the saturation of other detoxification pathways; this metabolite causes the hepatotoxicity that follows paracetamol overdose.

Most of the phase I reactions in the liver are carried out by enzymes of the large cytochrome P450 superfamily of proteins. They are all prefixed by 'CYP' and tens of different isoforms are recognized in the human liver. The commonest is the CYP3A4 isoform through which over 50% of marketed drugs are metabolized. Others such as CYP2D6 have special importance because they are polymorphic, that is, they are encoded by CYP genes that have common variants that affect enzyme activity. The 10 major isoforms and some of the commoner drugs that are substrates for them are shown in Table 10.1.1.

Certain drugs also block CYP isoforms, which reduce the elimination of drugs through these enzymes. Examples of these are cimetidine (1A2), amiodarone (2C9, 2D6, and 3A4), erythromycin (3A4), and ketoconazole (3A4 and 2C19). Conversely, drug elimination through some CYP pathways is enhanced by drugs that act as inducers that increase enzyme activity by directly activating transcription of the corresponding CYP genes. The classical inducers include phenobarbitone (2B6, 3A4), rifampicin (2B6, 2C9, and

Table 10.1.1 The main cytochrome P450 isoforms (in bold) and their common substrate drugs

1A2	**2C9**	**2D6**	**3A4,5,7**
Clozapine	*NSAIDs*	*β-Blockers*	*Macrolide antibiotics*
Imipramine	Diclofenac	Metoprolol	Clarithromycin
Mexilitene	Ibuprofen	Propafenone	Erythromycin
Naproxen	Naproxen	Timolol	NOT azithromycin
Theophylline	Celecoxib	*Antidepressants*	*Antiarrhythmics*
2B6	*Sulphonylureas*	Amitriptyline	Quinidine
Bupropion	Glibenclamide	Clomipramine	*Benzodiazepines*
Cyclophosphamide	Glipizide	Desipramine	Diazepam
Efavirenz	Tolbutamide	Duloxetine	Midazolam
Ifosfamide	*Angiotensin II blockers*	Fluoxetine	Triazolam
Methadone	Irbesartan	Imipramine	*Immune modulators*
2E1	Losartan	Paroxetine	Ciclosporin
Anaesthetics	NOT valsartan	Venlafaxine	Tacrolimus
Enflurane	NOT candesartan	*Antipsychotics*	*HIV protease inhibitors*
Halothane	Phenytoin	Haloperidol	Indinavir
Isoflurane	Sulfamethoxazole	Risperidone	Ritonavir
Methoxyflurane	Tamoxifen	*Opiates*	Saquinavir
Sevoflurane	Warfarin	Codeineoxycodone	*Antihistamines*
	2C19	Tramadol	Astemizole
Paracetamol	*Proton pump inhibitors*		Chlorpheniramine
Ethanol	Omeprazol	Dextromethorphan	*Calcium channel blockers*
2C8	Elansoprazol	Flecainide	Amlodipine
Paclitaxel	Epantoprazole	Mexiletine	Diltiazem
Torsemide	*Antiepileptics*	Ondansetron	Felodipine
Amodiaquine	Diazepam	Tamoxifen	Nifedipine
Repaglinide	Phenytoin		Verapamil
	Phenobarbitone		*Statins*
	Amitriptyline		Atorvastatin
	Clomipramine		Simvastatin
	Cyclophosphamide		NOT pravastatin
	Progesterone		NOT rosuvastatin
			Imatinib
			Methadone
			Pimozide
			Quinine
			Sildenafil

Source: www.medicine.iupui.edu/flockhart/

3A4), and antiepileptics such as phenytoin and carbamazepine (both 3A4). Tobacco and ethanol are also inducers, albeit for minor CYP isoforms (1A2 and 2E1, respectively).

Other factors that affect hepatic drug metabolism are hepatic blood flow (for drugs that are rapidly cleared), liver disease (only important in extensive liver disease or when there is arteriovenous shunting), and age. The metabolism of some drugs is impaired in old people and in babies younger than about 6 months, particularly premature babies. In both cases, this is due to reduced activity of the microsomal enzymes that includes CYP and non-CYP enymes. For example, in neonates uridine diphosphoglucuronyl transferase (EC 2.4.1.7), which conjugates chloramphenicol, is relatively inactive; neonates eliminate chloramphenicol slowly, and may suffer peripheral circulatory collapse (the 'grey syndrome') when given the drug in weight-related doses that do not harm adults.

Excretion

The kidney is a major route of drug excretion. Other, usually minor, routes include the lungs (important for paraldehyde and gaseous anaesthetic gases), breast milk, sweat, tears, and genital secretions (alarming if the orange-red discoloration caused by rifampicin is not mentioned), saliva, and bile. Excretion in bile can be prominent for some drugs and this can lead to the reabsorption of some of the excreted compounds from the gut—a process called enterohepatic recycling. This recycling affects drugs such as oestradiol, rifampicin, and tetracyclines and can substantially prolong their duration in the body. Drugs excreted in bile as water-soluble conjugates (after phase II metabolism—see above) may also be deconjugated by gut bacteria to release parent drug so facilitating enterohepatic recycling (e.g. chloramphenicol, digitoxin, indomethacin, and valproic acid).

Renal excretion of drugs involves three separate processes: glomerular filtration, passive tubular reabsorption, and active tubular secretion. Thus:

Total renal clearance = Clearance by filtration + Clearance by secretion – Retention by reabsorption

If a drug is mainly metabolized to inactive compounds, renal function will have little impact its elimination. However, if the drug itself or an active metabolite is excreted unchanged via the kidneys, changes in renal function will substantially affect its elimination.

Glomerular filtration

All drugs are filtered at the renal glomerulus, although molecules larger than 2 kDa are not freely filtered (e.g. insulin concentration in the ultrafiltrate is 0.89 × plasma) and proteins as large as albumin (69 kDa) are not filtered at all by a normal glomerulus. The extent of filtration is directly proportional to the glomerular filtration rate (GFR = 120 ml/min) and to the fraction of unbound drug in the plasma (f_u), that is, rate of clearance by filtration = $f_u \times$ GFR.

If the total renal clearance of a drug is equal to $f_u \times$ GFR, then it is cleared principally by filtration (it could be affected by the other two mechanisms, secretion and reabsorption, but they would have to cancel each other out). Examples of drugs whose clearance is similar to the GFR (after correction for protein binding) are digoxin, gentamicin, vancomycin, methotrexate, and ethambutol. As creatinine is cleared mainly by filtration, the creatinine clearance is useful in estimating the clearance rates of these drugs; although there is some secretion, which explains its tendency to overestimate GFR.

Passive tubular reabsorption

Drugs are passively reabsorbed by the renal tubules. The elimination of drugs with very low rates of renal clearance (i.e. approaching urine flow rate, or about 1–2 ml/min) will be significantly affected by changes in urine flow rate (because a doubling of flow rate will increase their rate of clearance by 1–2 ml/min, i.e. twofold). However, for weak acids and weak bases that are nonpolar in their unionized form, the main factor affecting passive reabsorption is the pH of the renal tubular fluid (which can vary between 4.5 and 8), because the extent of their ionization (and therefore of their passive reabsorption) depends on the urine pH in relation to the pK_a of the drug. For example, in an alkaline urine, weak acids with a pK_a below 7.5, such as salicylate (pK_a 3), are more highly ionized, and therefore less well reabsorbed. The reverse is true for weak bases with a pK_a greater than 7.5, such as methamphetamine (pK_a 10), whose reabsorption is reduced, and whose clearance is therefore enhanced, by an acid urine. These principles are put to good use in the treatment of overdose (see Section 9). Renal failure alters passive reabsorption indirectly, by changing both urine flow rate and pH.

Active tubular secretion

If the renal clearance of a drug exceeds GFR then there must be active secretion of the drug into the renal tubule. The active transport of organic anions and cations is dependent on specific transporters in the cells lining the proximal tubule. There are broadly two functional groups: organic anion and organic cation transporters. The organic anion transporters are responsible for the secretion of many β-lactam antibiotics, NSAIDs, antivirals, and ACE inihibitors, as well as acidic glutathione and glucuronide-conjugated drug metabolites. Probenecid is a generic inhibitor of anion transport and anionic transport capacity can be measured by *p*-aminohippuric acid (PAH) excretion. Substrates for the organic cation transporters include endogenous cations (e.g. guanidine, choline, *N*-methylnicotinamide, and monoamine neurotransmitters), cationic toxins (e.g. 1-methyl-4-phenylpyridium, MPP^+), and cationic drugs (e.g. cimetidine, procainamide, quinidine, vecuronium, cardiac glycosides). Both cimetidine and trimethoprim can affect cationic transport. Blockade of kidney drug transporters explains a number of drug–drug interactions (see following paragraphs).

Nonlinear kinetics

Most drugs show linear kinetics, i.e. an increase in dose will cause a similar-fold increase in plasma concentration. There are exceptions, however, and when a drug shows nonlinear behaviour (e.g. a 2-fold increase in dose produces a 10-fold increase in plasma level) it implies that some aspect of the drug's elimination pathway has saturated. Some tricylic antidepressants and the selective serotonin re-uptake inhibitor (SSRI) paroxetine show this behaviour. But the best-known example is phenytoin (see Fig. 10.1.4), whose oxidation through CYP 2C19 in the liver is saturated within the therapeutic range. Inspection of the curves in Fig. 10.1.4 shows how small increments in the dose of phenytoin can produce large increments in its plasma level and hence neurotoxicity. In fact, many drugs taken in overdose saturate their elimination pathways, and this is clearly shown by drugs such as ethanol, salicylate, and paracetamol.

The pharmacodynamic process

Pharmacodynamics addresses the question 'How does a drug produce its pharmacological effects?' Of course, this concerns both adverse as well as therapeutic effects.

Drugs have many different mechanisms of action but the overwhelming majority are mediated through receptors, which they either block or activate.

Actions via direct effects on receptors

Receptors are proteins situated either in cell membranes or within the cellular cytoplasm. For each receptor type there is usually an endogenous molecule (or ligand) that binds to the receptor. Drug molecules target the same binding site on the receptor as the

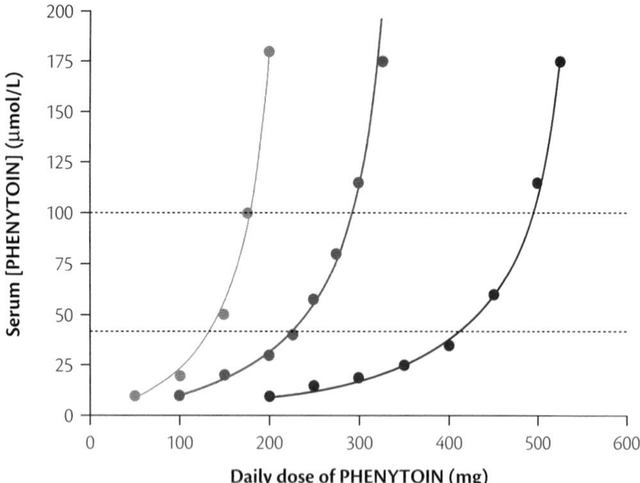

Fig. 10.1.4 Nonlinear kinetics. The plasma level achieved after repeated phenytoin dosing is shown vs the corresponding phenytoin dose for three hypothetical patients. The plots are not straight lines but rise steeply within the therapeutic range (between the dashed lines) as the CYP2C19 metabolic pathway for phenytoin saturates.

endogenous ligand and may activate the receptor, block the binding of the endogenous ligand, or a have mixture of both effects. These actions are referred to as: agonism, antagonism, and partial agonism, respectively.

This terminology is made clearer by considering these actions in terms of the μ opioid receptor. Morphine acts as an agonist at μ opioid receptors to cause analgesia. This μ receptor activation mimics the action of endogenous analgesic peptides such as enkephalin and endorphin. Compare this with naloxone, which behaves as an antagonist at the same receptor and blocks its activation by either morphine or other opiates. Importantly, in the absence of an agonist, a pure antagonist such as naloxone has no pharmacological action through the μ opiate receptor. This contrasts with buprenorphine that behaves as a partial agonist at the μ receptor. Hence, in the absence of an agonist such as morphine, buprenorphine it is able to activate the μ receptor, but it is not able to produce an analgesic effect as large as morphine (this explains the 'ceiling' effect seen clinically). Yet, in the presence of a full agonist such as morphine, buprenorphine can block μ receptor activation (this explains why buprenorphine can trigger opiate withdrawal).

Receptor subtypes

In many cases, a receptor will have subtypes, and drugs may have subtype selectivity. For example, there at least three subtypes of opioid receptors: μ and δ are both involved in analgesia, gastrointestinal motility, and respiratory depression, and κ is involved in analgesia, sedation, and miosis. These receptors are variably distributed in the nervous system. Most opiates act at μ receptors, but none is completely selective and they may act at other subtypes.

Long-term effects of drugs at receptors

During long-term therapy, the effects of a drug may be altered by adaptive responses, usually accompanied by either increases ('up-regulation') or decreases ('down-regulation') in receptor numbers. Such changes may explain both the therapeutic and adverse effects of drugs. Examples include:

- The therapeutic response to antidepressants (e.g. an SSRI) that may involve changes in receptors within the central nervous system secondary to the increased synaptic levels of neurotransmitter caused by these drugs. Also probably explains why the therapeutic response to antidepressants takes a few weeks to emerge.
- The way in which the response to L-dopa in Parkinson's disease changes during long-term administration (e.g. producing the 'on–off' effect).
- Withdrawal syndromes that may occur because long-term changes become unopposed when the drug is withdrawn, e.g. after the long-term use of opiates or benzodiazepines.

Actions via direct effects on second messengers

When an agonist stimulates a membrane-bound receptor, its effect is usually signalled in one of two ways: either through a so-called second messenger (e.g. cAMP, diacylglycerol, or inositol trisphosphate) or by changing the activity of an ion channel linked to the receptor. Some drugs may act by affecting second messengers directly. For example, some drugs block phosphodiesterases that normally metabolize the second messengers cAMP and cGMP. Several types of phosphodiesterases regulate cAMP levels and theophylline and caffeine work by inhibiting them nonspecifically. In contrast, type 5 phosphodiesterase (EC 3.1.4.17) specifically degrades cGMP in smooth muscle and is selectively inhibited by drugs such as sildenafil and vardenafil.

Actions via indirect alterations of the effects of endogenous receptor ligands

Drugs may oppose the physiological effects of the endogenous ligand. For example, glucagon is a physiological antagonist of the actions of insulin; hence its use to treat hypoglycaemia. Other drugs act indirectly on a receptor by altering the levels of the endogenous ligand for that receptor. They can do this in a number of ways:

Increase in endogenous release

Some drugs enhance release of the endogenous ligand. For example, amphetamine and tyramine increase the release of dopamine and noradrenaline, respectively, from nerve terminals.

Prevention of endogenous release or synthesis

The release of many neurotransmitters from nerve terminals is regulated by inhibitory receptors activated by the neurotransmitter itself. Hence, α_2-receptors on noradrenergic nerve terminals reduce noradrenaline release into the synapse. Clonidine and α-methyldopa reduce the release of noradrenaline by activating these receptors (α-methyldopa actually works through its metabolite α-methylnoradrenaline) and is the basis of their antihypertensive action.

Drugs can also reduce the production of the endogenous ligand rather than affect release of a preformed store of the ligand. For example, angiotensin II (which activates the angiotensin II receptor to cause vasoconstriction and aldosterone release) is produced enzymatically from angiotensin I. ACE inhibitors block the converting enzyme and renin inhibitors (e.g. aliskiren) block the enzymatic cleavage of angiotensin I from angiotensinogen.

Inhibition of endogenous reuptake

Many neurotransmitters are pumped back into their corresponding nerve terminals. The transporters that carry out this reuptake are targeted by a number of psychoactive drugs. Many antidepressants, for example, block the reuptake of noradrenaline (such as amitriptyline), or 5-hydroxytryptamine (serotonin, 5HT) (such as fluoxetine), or both (such as venlaflaxine). Reuptake of γ-aminobutyric acid (GABA) is blocked by the anticonvulsant tiagabine.

Inhibition of endogenous metabolism

Drugs can also increase the effect of an endogenous ligand by blocking its metabolism. Examples of these include: cholinesterase inhibitors for acetylcholine (e.g. neostigmine), vigabatrin for GABA, and monoamine oxidase inhibitors (MAO) inhibitors for catecholamines and 5HT (e.g. tranylcypromine).

The MAO inhibitors have some selectivity for the two forms of MAO (types A and B), which explains their use both as antidepressants and antiparkinsonian agents. For example, selegiline selectively inhibits monoamine oxidase type B. This results in blockade of dopamine metabolism in the central nervous system and enhances the action of L-dopa in parkinsonism. However, because MAO in the gut and liver is predominantly type A, selegiline does not produce the 'cheese reaction' (due to tyramine and other amines, see following paragraphs) seen with nonselective MAO inhibitors (e.g. tranylcypromine). In contrast, the antidepressant moclobemide selectively inhibits MAO A. Moclobemide is also unusual in being a reversible inhibitor of MAO. All other MAO inhibitors block MAO irreversibly, so that recovery requires production of new enzyme. This explains the slow offset of their action (7–10 days) and why moclobemide does not produce a 'cheese reaction'.

Actions by inhibiting the movement of ions

Because cations (such as sodium, potassium, and calcium) and anions (such as chloride and iodide) have so many important roles in the maintenance of normal cellular function, inhibition of their transport is an important mechanism of drug action. This movement of cations and anions across membranes can be either through transporters or channels.

Diuretics

Most diuretics reduce sodium reabsorption in the renal tubules by targeting specific transporters or ion channels. Hence, loop diuretics (e.g. furosemide and bumetanide) block the Na–K–Cl transporter in the ascending limb of Henle's loop. Thiazide diuretics inhibit Na–Cl cotransporter (NCCT) in the distal convoluted tubule and potassium-sparing diuretics (amiloride and triamterene) block the epithelial sodium channels in the collecting ducts.

Calcium channel antagonists

The calcium antagonists, such as verapamil, diltiazem, and the dihydropyridines (e.g. nifedipine), inhibit the transport of calcium via voltage-operated calcium channels (of the L-type). They are able to exert different effects in different tissues (e.g. verapamil slows atrioventricular nodal conduction in the heart but nifedipine does not) because of separate binding sites within the L-type calcium channel.

Drugs acting on potassium channels

The potassium permeability of cell membranes affects their membrane potential and is controlled by potassium (K) channels. They are a very large and diverse group of ion channels and drugs may either open or close (or block them).

Drugs that open potassium channels include vascular smooth muscle relaxants, such as minoxidil and nicorandil (targeting K_{ATP} channels). The same K_{ATP} channels are closed by sulphonylureas such as gliclazide. Of the many potassium channels in the heart, the i_{Kr} channel plays a key role as it is involved in repolarization of the myocyte. Blockade of the i_{Kr} channels explains why many drugs cause prolongation of the QT interval and are hence arrythmogenic (e.g. terfendine).

Drugs acting on chloride channels

Intracellular chloride plays a key role in neuronal excitability. Hence, the inhibitory effect of the neurotransmitter GABA on neurons is due to chloride entry into neurons through GABA-activated chloride channels. Progabide behaves as a GABA agonist and GABA-activated chloride currents are increased by benzodiazepines and barbiturates. The antiseizure activity of these drugs is directly attributed the neuronal hyperpolarization that results.

Some anaesthetic agents also probably rely on affects on chloride currents for their general anaesthetic effect. They form a diverse group of agents, such as the halogenated hydrocarbons (halothane, trichloroethylene), and nonhalogenated agents (nitrous oxide, ether, cyclopropane), and were previously thought to influence neuronal excitability by nonspecific effects on the lipid phase of the cell membrane, changing its biophysical properties and hence the kinetics of ion channels. More recent evidence has shown that they specifically affect currents through GABA/glycine-coupled ion channels. Others (such as ketamine) antagonize the excitatory NMDA-coupled ion channel.

Actions via enzyme inhibition

Drugs often act by directly inhibiting enzymes. Inhibitors of cholinesterase and MAO (see earlier paragraphs), for example, have been in therapeutic use for more than half a century.

The metabolism of purines involves the oxidation of xanthine and hypoxanthine to uric acid by xanthine oxidase. Hence, blockade of this enzyme with allopurinol prevents excessive uric acid production during tumour lysis and reduces the frequency of gout.

The cardiac glycosides act by inhibiting the Na/K pump. This changes the distribution of sodium across excitable membranes especially in the heart: and the secondary change in intracellular calcium causes the cells' contractility to increase.

Other drugs that act via enzyme inhibition include warfarin (vitamin K epoxide reductase), aspirin, and other NSAIDs, targeting the cyclo-oxygenase (COX) enzymes involved in prostaglandin synthesis, ACE inhibitors, disulfiram (alcohol dehydrogenase), some anticancer drugs such as cytarabine (DNA polymerase), and imatinib (chronic myelogenous leukaemia-specific tyrosine kinase), and some anti-infective drugs (bacterial or viral enzymes: e.g. trimethoprim inhibits bacterial dihydrofolate reductase, the quinolones inhibit bacterial DNA gyrase, and zidovudine and didanosine inhibit the reverse transcriptase of HIV).

Danazol and stanozolol are examples of drugs that inhibit an enzyme indirectly—they stimulate the production of an inhibitor of C1 esterase and are used to treat hereditary angio-oedema, in which there is reduced plasma activity of the inhibitor.

Actions via enzyme activation or direct enzymatic activity

Some drugs either activate enzymes or are enzymes themselves.

The clotting and fibrinolytic factors are enzymes, and certain drugs that act on clotting and fibrinolysis do so by increasing their activity. Heparin acts by activating antithrombin III. The thrombolytic drugs streptokinase, alteplase, and tenecteplase activate plasminogen.

Deficiencies of clotting factors can be treated by replacing deficient enzymes of the clotting pathway, e.g. factor VIII in patients with haemophilia and fresh frozen plasma in warfarin toxicity. Pancreatic enzymes are used in treating malabsorption in patients with chronic pancreatic insufficiency.

Rasburicase is used to prevent the hyperuricaemia that accompanies the tumour lysis syndrome during the treatment of acute leukaemias and lymphomas. It is recombinant urate acid oxidase that directly catalyses the breakdown of uric acid to the more soluble allantoin.

Actions via other miscellaneous effects

Chelating agents

Drugs that chelate metals can be used to hasten their removal from the body (see Chapter 9.1). Calcium sodium edetate chelates many divalent and trivalent metals and is used to treat poisoning, particularly with lead. Dimercaprol chelates some heavy metals and is used to treat mercury and gold poisoning. Desferrioxamine chelates iron and is used in treating iron poisoning and the iron overload that occurs with repeated blood transfusion (as in thalassaemia). Penicillamine chelates copper and is used in treating hepatolenticular degeneration (Wilson's disease); it is also used to complex cystine and thus prevent renal damage in cystinuria.

Osmotic diuretics

Mannitol is freely filtered at the glomerulus but the renal tubules reabsorb relatively small amounts. It therefore increases the concentration of osmotically active solute in the tubular fluid, the subsequent influx of water massively augments urine flow rates.

Replacement of vitamins and minerals

Some drugs are used simply to replace deficiencies, e.g. ferrous salts in iron deficiency anaemia and hydroxocobalamin (vitamin B_{12}) in vitamin B_{12} deficiency.

Stereoisomerism and drug action

Stereoisomerism (chirality) of organic compounds is due to asymmetry in one or more of their atoms (usually carbon), resulting in two thre-dimensional structures (enantiomers) that cannot be superimposed on each other.

Several different terminologies are used to describe the two chiral partners: *R* and *S* (from the Latin *rectus* = right and *sinister* = left), (+) -*d* and (−)-*l* and D and L (from the Latin *dexter* = right and *laevus* = left). Examples of drug enantiomers are *R*-warfarin and *S*-warfarin, D-glucose (dextrose) and L-glucose (laevulose), and *d*-propranolol and *l*-propranolol.

Of all synthetic drugs used in clinical practice almost 50% are chiral and about 90% of those are marketed in their racemic form (i.e. as an equal mixture of the two enantiomers). Examples include *d,l*-propranolol and *R,S*-warfarin. Naproxen is one of the few examples of a synthetic compound that is marketed as a single enantiomer. In contrast, naturally occurring and semisynthetic compounds are almost all chiral and almost all are marketed as a single isomer. Examples include D-glucose (dextrose) and the naturally occurring amino acids (e.g. L-dopa), *l*-thyroxine, and *l*-noradrenaline.

Enantiomers often have different pharmacological actions. For example, *l*-propranolol is a β-blocker, whereas *d*-propranolol has membrane-stabilizing activity like that of local anaesthetics; *l*-sotalol is a β-blocker, whereas *d*-sotalol has antiarrhythmic effects like those of amiodarone.

Sometimes these differences between the pharmacology of enantiomers can separate the therapeutic and adverse effects of a racemate. For example, *R*-thalidomide is responsible for the sedative effects of *R,S*-thalidomide, while the teratogenic effect resides in the *S* enantiomer. However, this cannot be exploited clinically to limit thalidomide toxicity, because the two enantiomers spontaneously interconvert in the body. This so-called 'chiral inversion' also occurs in some NSAIDs such as ibuprofen.

The interaction of a drug with its target (such as a receptor or enzyme) is often stereo-selective, so enantiomers may show marked differences in potency. For example, *S*-warfarin is some 5 times more potent an anticoagulant than *R*-warfarin, and *S*-citalopram is 30 times more potent as an SSRI than *R*-citalopram. In some cases, one enantiomer is completely inactive therapeutically, e.g. levofloxacin is the active antimicrobial enantiomer in ofloxacin with dextrofloxacin being completely inactive.

Enantiomer may have different pharmacokinetics. For example, the half-lives of *S*-warfarin and *R*-warfarin average around 30 h and 50 h and they are metabolized to 7-hydroxywarfarin and warfarin alcohols, respectively. This is important in some drug interactions with warfarin, because drugs inhibiting warfarin metabolism (such as metronidazole) primarily affect the more potent enantiomer, *S*-warfarin. Omeprazole provides a further example. The single enantiomer of omeprazole, *S*-omeprazole, has almost twice the bioavailability of *R*-omeprazole. Hence, esomeprazole (*S*-omeprazole) gives plasma levels of omeprazole 70 to 90% higher than racemic omeprazole. However, both enantiomers are converted to the same active intermediate and since this lacks a chiral centre the enantiomers are equiactive if they achieve the same plasma level.

Because of these caveats, despite the appeal of prescribing single-drug enantiomers, in most instances, the single enantiomer has failed to show a substantial clinical advantage over the racemate. When comparing racemates to single enantiomers in clinical trials, it is critical they are compared at comparable doses of the active enantiomer.

The therapeutic process

The question associated with the therapeutic process is, 'Is the pharmacological effect being translated into a therapeutic effect?'

Translation of pharmacological effect into therapeutic effect during short-term therapy

The short-term therapeutic and toxic effects of drugs occur as a result of the pharmacological actions discussed earlier. However, the translation of molecular and cellular pharmacological effects into the therapeutic or toxic effect is not a simple process, and involves several translational stages at different pharmacological and physiological levels.

Take, for example, the action of salbutamol, a β_2-adrenoceptor agonist, in the treatment of asthma. Salbutamol stimulates bronchial β_2-adrenoceptors, and so increases the activity of adenylate cyclase; this is its pharmacological effect at the molecular level. The increase in adenylate cyclase activity raises the intracellular concentration of cAMP that leads to relaxation of the bronchial smooth muscle cells; this is the cellular effect. This leads to dilatation of the bronchioles, reduces the resistance to air flow in the bronchial tree, and improves gas exchange; this is the effect on tissue and whole organ function. Finally, the patient feels less breathless and oxygen saturation may improve; this is the desired clinical effect.

This analysis of the short-term effects of a drug teaches us several things about drug action: how drug action may be modified; how therapeutic and adverse effects may be mediated via different pharmacological effects; the relation between the pharmacological effects of a drug and the rate of onset or duration of its therapeutic action; and drug–disease interactions.

How to modify drug action

It is often possible to modify drug action positively or negatively. For example, a methylxanthine derivative, such as theophylline, which blocks cAMP breakdown by its inhibition of phosphodiesterase, should potentiate the action of salbutamol. This turns out to be both a beneficial and an adverse interaction—beneficial because theophylline enhances the therapeutic action of salbutamol, adverse because it enhances the hypokalaemia (by stimulating Na^+/K^+-ATPase) and tachycardia (by activating cardiac β-adrenoceptors) that salbutamol causes.

Different pharmacological actions may mediate therapeutic and adverse or other effects

Some drugs have more than one molecular mechanism of action, and different therapeutic effects of a drug may result from different actions. For example, tetracycline acts against bacteria by interfering with their protein synthesis, but in acne, it helps by interfering with sebum production in sebaceous glands.

Similarly, a therapeutic effect may be brought about by one pharmacological action and an adverse effect by another. For example, the antibacterial action of erythromycin is due to inhibition of bacterial ribosomal function, but its gastrointestinal side effects are due to activation of motilin receptors in the human gut. Other macrolides such as azithromycin are much weaker motilin mimetics and hence produce much less vomiting and diarrhoea.

A drug may also produce therapeutic and adverse effects through the same molecular mechanism but in different tissues. For example, the inhibition of β_2-adrenoceptors within muscle spindles by propranolol reduces benign essential tremor, but blocking the same receptors in the lung causes bronchoconstriction in susceptible individuals and impairs glycogenolysis in the liver (which can delay a diabetic's recovery from hypoglycaemia).

The relation between the pharmacological actions of a drug and the rate of onset and duration of its effects

The rate of onset of a drug's effects depends not only on its pharmacokinetics (i.e. the time it takes for a therapeutic concentration of drug to build up at its site of action), but also on how long it takes for the full pharmacodynamic sequence of events to unroll. In the case of salbutamol, the time between β_2-adrenoceptor stimulation and bronchodilatation is of the order of a few minutes. However, for other drugs, the sequence of events takes much longer. For example, corticosteroids bind to an intracellular receptor protein in the cytoplasm of target cells to form a steroid–receptor complex. This complex translocates to the nucleus, where it binds to regulatory sequences on target genes to effect RNA transcription. The induction of *de novo* protein synthesis by RNA transcription and translation takes several hours, explaining the slow onset of corticosteroid effects.

Similarly, the duration of action of a drug is related not only to the time it takes for the drug to be cleared from the body, but also to the duration of its pharmacological effects. For example, aspirin inhibits COX-1 by acetylating a serine moiety at the active site of the enzyme. As platelets cannot synthesize new protein, the recovery from aspirin requires the appearance of new platelets from the marrow. This process can take 7 to 10 days to restore peripheral platelet function.

Drug–disease interactions

Because of the complex links between the pharmacological effects of a drug and its therapeutic or adverse effects, the pathophysiology of the disease being treated, or of other coincidental diseases, can variously impact the way in which the pharmacological effect is translated into a therapeutic effect.

The use of digoxin in cardiac failure exemplifies this. Digoxin inhibits the activity of the membrane-bound Na^+,K^+-ATPase. Pump inhibition increases the intracellular concentration of sodium, which secondarily raises intracellular calcium to produce a positive inotropic effect. The various steps in this process are affected by drug–disease interactions. Hypokalaemia, for example, is a common side effect of diuretic use to manage fluid overload in heart failure. Low extracellular potassium increases pump block by raising the affinity of digoxin for the sodium pump. This risks calcium overload and hence digoxin toxicity. Coincident diseases also affect digoxin's therapeutic effect. In hyperthyroidism, the nature of the interaction between digoxin and the Na/K pump is altered, resulting in resistance to the inhibitory effects of digoxin. So, increasing the dose may cause digoxin toxicity without ever producing a therapeutic effect. In patients with chronic cor pulmonale, tissue hypoxia digoxin may also lead to Na/K pump inhibition also producing cardiac arrhythmias without increasing myocardial contractility. Digoxin is more likely to produce arrhythmias in myocardium that has failed due to acute myocardial infarction. In patients with hypertrophic obstructive cardiomyopathy, although digoxin increases the rate of myocardial contractility, a rise in cardiac output is prevented because left ventricular outflow remains obstructed.

Thus even when it can be shown that a drug is having its expected action at a particular pharmacological or physiological level, it cannot automatically be assumed that it will have a therapeutic effect.

Interactions with circadian rhythms

Most physiological functions follow a circadian rhythm, so some drug effects are liable to differ at different phases of the rhythm. In some instances, the difference is dramatic. The timing of corticosteroid dosing is a good example. Peak ACTH release from the pituitary occurs at night leading to plasma cortisol peaks at around 08.00 a.m. when ACTH levels are at trough. So, exogenous cortisol in the morning will have no impact on ACTH release. But given in the evening it will completely inhibit night-time ACTH. For this reason, cortisol given once daily in the morning causes much less pituitary inhibition than the same dose given in the evening, or spread throughout the day.

The cholesterol-lowering effect of some statins is also affected by the time of administration because cholesterol synthesis has a circadian rhythm with most synthesis occurring at night. Short-acting statins are hence more effective if given at night (e.g. simvastatin, half-life *c.*3 h). For longer-acting statins there is no discernible difference, as the drug level will still be high enough during the night even with morning dosing (e.g. atorvastatin half-life *c.*20 h with even longer-lived active metabolites).

Translation of pharmacological effect into therapeutic effect: long-term therapy

During prolonged therapy, adaptation may develop to the short-term pharmacological effects of the drug with several consequences.

Therapeutic effects through adaptation

In immunization, by adapting to an initial immunological challenge, the immune system develops the ability to respond to a subsequent similar challenge, e.g. tetanus immunization.

Although tricyclic antidepressants rapidly inhibit reuptake of noradrenaline and 5-HT in the brain, the therapeutic effect of these drugs takes 1 to 2 weeks to become evident. In certain brain regions, there is adaptation to the increased concentrations of neurotransmitters in the synaptic cleft with reduction in numbers of postsynaptic receptors. Part of this adaptive down-regulation probably explains their therapeutic effects.

Tolerance: increasing ineffectiveness of therapy

Tolerance is a state of decreased responsiveness to a drug, resulting from previous exposure, either to the same drug or to one with similar short-term effects.

For example, it can develop to the vasoconstricting effects of ephedrine nose drops, used to treat vasomotor rhinitis: as ephedrine acts by releasing noradrenaline from sympathetic nerve endings, noradrenaline depletion will reduce the effectiveness of ephedrine.

Patients taking long-term glyceryl trinitrate, particularly from transdermal patches, become tolerant to its acute effects. To avoid this, a patch should be applied for no longer than 18 h. This effect probably reflects depletion of tissue sulphydryl groups by oxidation to disulphide groups. Some oral preparations of isosorbide mononitrate are formulated to release their contents over 18 h for the same reason.

Physiological tolerance by homoeostatic mechanisms Secondary hyperaldosteronism is a physiological response to sodium loss produced by loop or thiazide diuretics. The enhanced potassium excretion that it causes may be reduced by using a potassium-sparing diuretic (e.g. amiloride) or the aldosterone antagonist spironolactone.

Another type of physiological tolerance occurs in patients given the carbonic anhydrase inhibitor acetazolamide. This causes both a diuresis and a kaluresis. However, these effects are only sustained for a matter of days, because the large amounts of bicarbonate lost from the kidney causes a metabolic acidosis. Interestingly, topical carbonic anhydrase inhibitors do not show the same tolerance when they are used in chronic glaucoma.

Metabolic tolerance Metabolic tolerance results from faster metabolic clearance of the drug. The commonest cause is induction of hepatic P450 enzymes by drugs such as barbiturates, phenytoin, carbamazepine or rifampicin. Occasionally, drugs may induce their own metabolic clearance—a phenomenon called 'autoinduction', e.g. carbamazepine and artmesinin.

Withdrawal syndromes A common, but not inevitable, outcome of an adaptive response to long-term drug use is a withdrawal response either when the drug is withdrawn or when an antagonist is given.

A withdrawal syndrome occurs in opiate users when the opiate is withdrawn or an antagonist, such as naloxone, is given. The symptoms consist of yawning, rhinorrhoea, and sweating, followed by shivering and goose flesh ('cold turkey'); later, nausea, vomiting, diarrhoea, and hypertension may occur. The acute syndrome subsides within a week, but the anxious and disturbed sleep patterns may last for several weeks or months. This syndrome can be avoided by introducing increasing doses of methadone as the opiate is withdrawn; methadone has a longer half-life than opiates such as heroin and causes much less withdrawal when it is eventually discontinued.

Delirium tremens is a feature of alcohol withdrawal in chronic alcohol abusers. This syndrome consists of disorientation and visual hallucinations. Withdrawal of benzodiazepines after long-term therapy may result in a disturbance of sleep pattern (rebound insomnia associated with abnormal sleep patterns), agitation, restlessness, and occasionally epileptic convulsions.

The risk of angina pectoris, myocardial infarction, and arrhythmias is increased in patients with ischaemic heart disease when β-adrenoceptor antagonists are withdrawn after long-term use. This may be due to up-regulation in the number of cardiac β-adrenoceptors, with increased sensitivity to the β-adrenergic effects of sympathetic stimulation.

Long-term therapy with corticosteroids suppresses pituitary secretion of ACTH, leading to adrenal cortical atrophy. When treatment is suddenly withdrawn, ACTH secretion may take several weeks or months to recover. During this time patients risk an addisonian crisis if stressed, e.g. if they have a myocardial infarction or are operated on.

Adverse effects directly due to adaptation

Patients taking a neuroleptic drug (e.g. fluphenazine or haloperidol) continuously for a period of years commonly develop abnormal movements (known collectively as tardive dyskinesia). The face, mouth, and tongue are often affected, with stereotyped sucking and smacking of the lips, lateral jaw movements, and darting movements of the tongue. Occasionally more widespread dyskinesia may resemble choreoathetosis. The long-term blockade of central dopamine receptors is thought to lead to increased central sensitivity to the effects of dopamine; this partly reflects increases in the number of dopamine receptors. The risk of tardive dyskinesia is much lower in the newer atypical agents such as quetiapine and risperidone; the atypical clozapine has even been suggested to ameliorate established tardive dyskinesia.

Adverse drug reactions

An adverse drug reaction can be defined as 'an unwanted or harmful reaction experienced following administration of a drug, or combination of drugs, under normal conditions of use and is suspected as being related to the drug (or combination)'. Sometimes, the term is broadened to include all adverse reactions whether the drug is dosed appropriately or not. Hence the term 'adverse drug event', which includes drug prescription and dispensing errors and failures of patient compliance, is also used.

Incidence

The scale of the problem is probably still underestimated. Data suggests that:

- 1 to 4% of acute hospital admissions are due to an adverse drug reaction

- 5 to 20% of inpatients suffer an adverse drug reaction at some point in their admission
- up to 3% of deaths in hospital inpatients are due to an adverse drug reaction

In addition to the morbidity and mortality, adverse drug reactions are hugely expensive for health care systems. In the United Kingdom the cost probably amounts to £1 billion annually, and in the United States of America some estimates have exceeded $100 billion annually.

Classification

Dose-related adverse reactions

Dose-related adverse reactions are usually due to an exaggeration of a known pharmacological effect of the drug. The pharmacological effect that produces the adverse reaction may be responsible for the therapeutic effect (e.g. hypoglycaemia following insulin administration), or be a parallel effect (e.g. the anticholinergic action of tricyclic antidepressants, producing a dry mouth or urinary retention).

Dose-related adverse reactions may occur because of variations in the pharmaceutical, pharmacokinetic, or pharmacodynamic properties of a drug, often due to a drug-disease interaction or a pharmacogenetic characteristic of the patient. These mechanisms are illustrated in the following paragraphs.

Pharmaceutical problem

Adverse reactions can be caused by a contaminant, e.g. pyrogens or even bacteria in intravenous formulations. This is obviously a hazard for illicit drugs that are used intravenously: not only are they dissolved under nonsterile conditions, but they may be 'cut' with other drugs, e.g. quinine.

Febrile reactions can occur routinely with some manufactured drugs given intravenously (e.g. amphotericin B and bisphosphonates), but otherwise fever should be treated very suspiciously and the drug and giving set should be sent for microbiological screening.

Out-of-date formulations may sometimes cause adverse reactions because of degradation products. For example, outdated tetracycline may cause Fanconi's syndrome, because it is degraded to anhydrotetracycline and epiandrotetracycline. The omission of the preservative citric acid from tetracycline formulations has reduced the risk of this effect, but has not removed it completely.

Very occasionally a drug has been incorrectly labelled by the manufacturer. Of more concern is the rise of counterfeit medicines. They are thought to account for 15% of drug sales worldwide and in parts of Asia and Africa the figure probably exceeds 50% of sales. Counterfeit agents frequently contain none of the active drug, or subtherapeutic doses, and may also contain additional chemicals or drugs that are harmful. For example, ethylene glycol has been used in the manufacture of fake paracetamol syrups (for its sweetness and viscosity) and caused a number of deaths, especially in children.

Pharmacokinetic variation

There is often enormous variation in rate of drug elimination between individuals. This variation is greatest for drugs cleared by hepatic metabolism and is determined by several factors, which may be genetic, environmental (diet, smoking, alcohol), or hepatic (blood flow and intrinsic drug-metabolizing capacity). On top of this variability, pharmacogenetic or hepatic abnormalities may be associated with specific adverse reactions. In addition, renal and cardiac disease can change drug pharmacokinetics. The impact of pharmacogenetics is discussed in the following paragraphs.

The reserve of the liver parenchyma is large, so adverse reactions due to impaired hepatic metabolism are uncommon. Nevertheless, in patients with severe liver disease caution is needed when a drug has a low therapeutic index or is subject to extensive first-pass metabolism. For example, severely impaired hepatocellular function can reduce the clearance of drugs such as phenytoin, theophylline, and warfarin. The portosystemic shunting seen in advanced cirrhosis can also dramatically increase the bioavailability of drugs normally cleared rapidly by the liver (e.g. morphine and other narcotic analgesics, propranolol, and chlormethiazole). Drugs that the kidneys excrete unchanged, or whose active metabolites are excreted, will accumulate in renal failure. Important examples include digoxin, atenolol, lithium, aminoglycoside antibiotics, and vancomycin.

Pharmacodynamic variation

The variability in pharmacodynamic response to a drug may be compounded by concomitant disease. The patient with cirrhosis is a good example: impaired hepatocellular function can reduce the synthesis of clotting factors; the presence of oesophageal and gastric varices imposes a further risk of upper gastrointestinal bleeding and patients with alcoholic liver disease may have additional thrombocytopenia and impaired platelet function. Judging the response to an anticoagulant, antithrombotic, or antiplatelet drug in this setting is very difficult, and the risk of haemorrhage is high.

A cirrhotic patient is also at risk of exaggerated sedation and encephalopathy from opiates or long-acting benzodiazepines that are cleared by the liver. The hypokalaemic effects of diuretics or amphotericin carry a similar risk. Patients with cirrhosis also have inappropriate salt and water retention that can be worsened by drugs such as NSAIDs, corticosteroids, and carbamazepine.

The pharmacodynamic effects of some drugs may be altered by changes in fluid and electrolyte balance. For example, both hypokalaemia and hypercalcaemia potentiate the toxic effects of digoxin. Hypocalcaemia prolongs the action of muscle relaxants such as tubocurarine. Fluid depletion and hypovolaemia enhances the hypotensive effects of antihypertensive drugs.

Non-dose-related adverse reactions

Non-dose-related adverse drug reactions are caused by immunological and pharmacogenetic mechanisms.

Allergic drug reactions are unrelated to the usual pharmacological effects of the drug, and frequently show a delay between the first exposure to the drug and the subsequent adverse reaction. Very small doses of the drug may elicit the reaction once allergy is established. The reaction disappears on withdrawal; and the illness is often recognizable as a form of immunological reaction, e.g. rash, serum sickness, anaphylaxis, asthma, urticaria, angio-oedema.

Factors associated with an increased risk of allergic drug reactions include a history of allergic disorders (patients with a history of atopic disease and those with hereditary angio-oedema) and HLA status (e.g. the risk of severe skin reactions to carbamazepine and allopurinol is strongly associated with specific alleles of the HLA B locus).

Drug allergy and its manifestations are classifiable according to the classification of hypersensitivity reactions, i.e. into four types, I to IV.

Type I reactions (anaphylaxis; immediate hypersensitivity)

In type I reactions, the drug or metabolite interacts with IgE molecules fixed to cells, particularly tissue mast cells and basophil leucocytes. This triggers a process that leads to the release of pharmacological mediators (a cocktail of histamine, 5-HT, kinins, and arachidonic acid derivatives including leukotrienes), which cause the allergic response.

Clinically, type I reactions manifest as urticaria, rhinitis, bronchial asthma, angio-oedema, and anaphylactic shock. Drugs likely to cause anaphylactic shock include penicillins, local anaesthetics, and iodide-containing radiographic contrast media.

Type II reactions (cytotoxic reactions)

In type II reactions, a circulating antibody of the IgG, IgM, or IgA class interacts with a hapten (drug) combined with a cell membrane constituent (protein), to form a hapten–protein/antigen–antibody complex. Complement is then activated and cell lysis occurs. Most examples are haematological: thrombocytopenia from quinidine or its enantiomer quinine ('gin and tonic purpura'), and occasionally rifampicin; 'immune' neutropenia, which can be difficult to distinguish from neutropenia occurring as a direct toxic effect on the bone marrow—phenylbutazone, carbimazole, tolbutamide, anticonvulsants, chlorpropamide, and metronidazole have all been incriminated; and the haemolytic anaemias that penicillins, cephalosporins, rifampicin, and quinidine can also produce by this mechanism.

Type III reactions (immune-complex reactions)

In type III reactions, antibody (IgG) combines with antigen to form immune complexes that deposit in tissues; complement is then activated, causing capillary endothelial damage. Serum sickness, with fever, arthritis, enlarged lymph nodes, urticaria, and maculopapular rashes, is the typical drug reaction of this type. Penicillins, sulphonamides, and antithyroid drugs may cause it. Another type III reaction is the acute interstitial nephritis caused by penicillins, some NSAIDs, and some diuretics.

Type IV reactions (cell-mediated or delayed hypersensitivity reactions)

In type IV reactions, T lymphocytes are sensitized by a hapten–protein antigenic complex. When the lymphocytes meet the antigen, an inflammatory response ensues. Examples are the contact dermatitis caused by topical local anaesthetics and antihistamines, and topical antibiotics and antifungal drugs. Rashes caused by a type IV mechanism in response to sulphonamides and thiacetazone are more common in people infected with HIV.

Anaphylactoid and pseudoallergic reactions

Anaphylactoid reactions resemble type I allergic reactions clinically, but the mast cell and basophil activation is not IgE-dependent. Instead, the cells are triggered directly, and drugs capable of doing this include: succinylcholine, morphine, *d*-tubocurarine, vancomycin (hence 'red man' syndrome on rapid intravenous administration) and *N*-acetylcysteine. They are generally less severe than allergen-mediated anaphylaxis, and emergency treatment is the same.

Asthma can also trigger an attack of asthma by a nonimmune mechanism. The inhibition of airway COX-1 enzyme by aspirin is thought to remove the inhibitory effect of prostaglandin E_2 and divert arachidonic acid towards production of cysteinyl-leukotriene. This is a very powerful constrictor of airway smooth muscle (*c.*1000-fold the potency of histamine), and this mechanism explains why aspirin-sensitive asthmatics are often sensitive to other NSAIDs (although COX-2 selective drugs may be relatively safe). It does not appear to explain why half of aspirin-sensitive asthmatics are also sensitive to the yellow food dye tartrazine (E102).

In some patients, ampicillin, and its derivative amoxicillin, causes a maculopapular erythematous rash resembling the toxic erythema that can occur in penicillin hypersensitivity. However, this ampicillin rash is not immunological in origin. It can be distinguished from true penicillin hypersensitivity by its later onset after the first dose (typically 10–14 days compared with 7–10 days in penicillin hypersensitivity, though they overlap) and nonrecurrence if re-exposed to ampicillin. Unlike penicillin hypersensitivity, it carries no increased risk of anaphylaxis to penicillin. An ampicillin rash occurs in about 1% of the normal population, but at a much higher frequency in some groups of patients: it occurs almost invariably (and can be a useful diagnostic pointer) in patients with some viral infections (e.g. infectious mononucleosis, cytomegalovirus infection, measles), lymphomas, and leukaemias. The risk is also increased in patients taking allopurinol.

Other manifestations of allergic reactions

Drugs may cause other adverse reactions that do not fit clearly into the earlier hypersensitivity classification, but where there is a strong suspicion of an immune basis.

Drug fever as an isolated phenomenon can occur with antibiotics (penicillins, cephalosporins, isoniazid, sulphonamides, and vancomycin), anticonvulsants (phenytoin and carbamazepine), α-methyldopa, hydralazine, and quinidine. The height or periodicity of the fever is not a useful clue that it is drug-induced, but all drug-induced fevers defervesce rapidly on drug withdrawal (*c.*24–48 h).

Fever is also a manifestation of the neuroleptic malignant syndrome (NMS), a rare and serious idiosyncratic adverse reaction to neuroleptic therapy (either initiation or dose-escalation). In NMS, the fever is accompanied by rigidity, reduced consciousness, and autonomic disturbance. It resembles another rare syndrome, malignant hyperpyrexia, although here the fever and rigidity follows sensitization to volatile halogenated anaesthetic gases (e.g. halothane) or suxamethonium. The aetiology of NMS is still unclear, but patients with malignant hyperthermia have mutations either in the ryanodine receptor or skeletal muscle L-type calcium channel.

A syndrome mimicking systemic lupus erythematosus, often involving joints and skin but generally sparing the kidneys, may follow long-term treatment with hydralazine, procainamide, phenytoin, or ethosuximide. Drug-induced lupus is partly dose-related and, in the case of procainamide and hydralazine, is affected by the acetylator status of the patient. Both drugs are metabolized by *N*-acetylation which is controlled by the polymorphic enzyme NAT2 (see following paragraphs). The two variants cause either slow or fast clearance of the drug and slow acetylators are at increased risk of drug-induced lupus.

Asthma occurring as a pseudoallergic reaction to NSAIDs and tartrazine is noted in the earlier paragraph. Other adverse drug reactions in the lung include pneumonitis associated with drug-induced lupus (see earlier paragraph), pulmonary eosinophilia, and fibrosing alveolitis. The Churg–Strauss syndrome has been associated with the use of cysteinyl-leukotriene receptor antagonists (e.g. montelukast), but it now seems unlikely that the syndrome is actually caused by them. Rather their introduction was frequently accompanied by withdrawal of corticosteroids that probably uncovered a pre-existing disease.

Jaundice may occur as an allergic response to some drugs through either cholestasis (e.g. with phenothiazines, erythromycin, and chlorpropamide) or generalized liver damage (e.g. with halothane, isoniazid, and monoamine oxidase inhibitors).

Long-term effects causing adverse drug reactions

Some adverse effects during long-term therapy are related to both the duration of treatment and the dose.

Adaptive changes

These are the basis of some adverse reactions such as the development of tolerance and physical dependence to opiates, and tardive dyskinesia in patients receiving long-term neuroleptic therapy for schizophrenia.

Rebound phenomena

When adaptive changes occur during long-term therapy, sudden withdrawal of the drug may result in rebound reactions. Examples include the typical syndromes that occur after the sudden withdrawal of opiates or of alcohol (delirium tremens). Sudden withdrawal of barbiturates may result in restlessness, confusion, and convulsions, and a similar syndrome in which anxiety features predominate may occur after the sudden withdrawal of benzodiazepines. Similarly, patients who abruptly stop an SSRI may complain of a constellation of symptoms 3 to 4 days later, which include headache, insomnia, dizziness, paraesthesia, sweating, and flu-like symptoms.

The withdrawal of some antihypertensive drugs may result in rebound hypertension, but is especially common with clonidine. Sudden withdrawal of β-adrenoceptor antagonists may result in rebound tachycardia and arrhythmia, sometimes precipitating myocardial ischaemia.

Acute adrenal insufficiency can occur when corticosteroids are stopped abruptly. The risk depends on the potency and duration of corticosteroids used, but not the route of administration—it has even been reported after stopping high-dose topical or inhaled glucocorticoids.

Reversal of the effects of unfractionated heparin with protamine sulphate may be associated with rebound hypercoagulability and an increased risk of thromboembolism. However, this risk may be justified if heparin overdosage has caused life-threatening haemorrhage. Importantly, protamine sulphate will not reverse the effect of low-molecular-weight heparin and stopping or reversing oral anticoagulants (such as warfarin) does not lead to rebound hypercoagulability.

Other long-term effects

Chloroquine may accumulate in the corneal epithelium (causing a keratopathy) and in the retina (causing a pigmentary retinopathy and blindness). The former occurs in most patients on long-term therapy; the latter is less common but more serious. The risk increases with daily doses of more than 2.5 mg/kg (as the free base) and chloroquine should only be used in inflammatory arthropathies where the safer hydroxychloroquine has failed.

Amiodarone also accumulates extensively in tissues. Almost all patients on long-term amiodarone develop photsensitization from skin deposition. They also develop microdeposits in the cornea, although these are rarely symptomatic. It also accumulates in other tissues but pulmonary alveolitis, neuropathy, and hepatocellular impairment are relatively uncommon.

Delayed effects causing long-term adverse drug reactions

Carcinogenesis

The long-term effects of oestrogen therapy on cancer risk are complex and depend on whether they are administered to pre- or postmenopausal women. Long-term oestrogen exposure through the oral contraceptive pill probably increases the risk of breast cancer but the effect is not consistent across all studies. The administration of hormone replacement therapy (HRT) to postmenopausal woman also increases their risk of breast cancer, although it appears that the breast-cancer risk from combined oestrogen–progesterone HRT is greater than from oestrogen-only HRT (used in women after hysterectomy). The incidence of endometrial carcinoma is also increased in women taking oestrogen HRT for menopausal symptoms. In contrast, the oral contraceptive pill protects against endometrial cancer and the effect persists for many years after taking it. The risk of colon cancer may also be reduced by HRT but not the oral contraceptive pill.

Anabolic steroids carry a risk of both benign and malignant hepatic tumours on long-term administration. The risk is greatest for the 17-alkylated derivatives such as oxymethalone. The later is now largely restricted for palliative use in cachetic states such as HIV wasting syndrome, but is still used illicitly by bodybuilders.

Various anticancer drugs increase the risk of secondary solid tumours and haematological malignancy. For example, cyclophosphamide containing chemotherapy regimens increase the risk of bladder cancer. The risk of secondary acute myeloid leukaemia and myelodysplasic syndromes is substantially increased in patients receiving chemotherapy for Hodgkin's or non-Hodgkin's lymphoma and testicular cancers. Alkylating agents, especially older regimens using the mustard mechlorethamine, carry the highest risk from lymphoma chemotherapy, and etoposide is the greatest risk from testicular cancer chemotherapy.

Immunosuppressive drug regimens are also widely associated with an increased risk of lymphoma and solid tumours in organ transplant recipients. These regimens are typically based on calcineurin inhibitors, such as ciclosporin. Recent data suggests that regimens based on a noncalcineurin inhibitor, sirolimus, may reduce the risk of lymphoma and solid tumours in these patients.

Adverse drug reactions associated with reproduction

Some drugs impair fertility. For example, cytotoxic drugs can cause permanent ovarian failure with amenorrhoea. Sperm production may be reversibly impaired by sulphasalazine (especially in slow metabolizers), gonadotropin hormone antagonists, methotrexate, and androgens. In fact, the reversible azoospermia achieved with depot formulations of testosterone esters and progestogens is being developed for male contraception. Cytotoxic drugs (especially alkylating agents) can reversibly or irreversibly affect sperm production depending on the age of administration (the prepubertal testis is relatively insensitive), the doses used, and duration of exposure.

Teratogenesis

Teratogenesis occurs when a drug taken early in pregnancy causes a developmental abnormality in a fetus. Exposure to a teratogen in the first trimester of pregnancy, and particularly the period of organogenesis (weeks 2–8 of gestation), is most likely to cause structural abnormalities. The central nervous system is vulnerable throughout pregnancy.

For a drug to be teratogenic it must first cross the placenta. As a general rule, the drugs that do this have a low molecular weight, are poorly ionized at physiological pH, and are very lipophilic. Hence, heparin (even low-molecular-weight heparin) is a large, highly charged molecule and *d*-tubocurarine is a small, ionized, and hydrophilic molecule; neither crosses the placenta. The placenta also expresses large numbers of transporter proteins including the ABC efflux pump P-glycoprotein. The efflux pumps are expressed predominantly on the maternal-facing surface of the placental villi and form part of the maternal–fetal barrier. So, whether a drug crosses the placenta depends not just on physiochemical properties, but also its affinity for the efflux pump. The existence of functional polymorphisms in these pumps probably explains the wide variability observed in fetal drug concentrations, incidence of teratogenesis, and drug failure in pregnancies exposed to therapeutic drugs.

Since most drugs that are proven teratogens in animals will not enter human development, it is unclear how well animal teratogenicity testing predicts human teratogenicity. A drug will have been tested for teratogenicity in rodents and one other nonprimate species before it can be registered. However, negative results from animal testing should not reassure anyone that the drug is safe in human pregnancy. Indeed, thalidomide itself is not teratogenic in rodents and the New Zealand rabbit is the only common laboratory mammal that shows similar sensitivity to humans. Women of child-bearing age are excluded from preregistration testing, so the teratogenic risk for humans of a drug at the time its registration is usually unknown. This explains the comments that exist in package inserts and other literature on new drugs, discouraging their use in pregnancy. It also explains why obstetricians often employ drugs that seem to other clinicians to be obsolete. For example, in pregnancy-related hypertension and pre-eclampsia, hydralazine and α-methyldopa are still first-line drugs. In nonpregnant hypertension, they would not even be fourth-line choices. Both drugs have, however, been in obstetric use for over 40 years without associated teratogenicity.

Adverse drug reactions on the fetus during the later stages of pregnancy

Some drugs that are not teratogenic may have adverse effects on the fetus if given later in pregnancy. Table 10.1.2 lists some important drugs that should be avoided or used with care during later pregnancy (some throughout the whole duration of pregnancy).

Given the uncertainty about teratogenic risk, what should be done if a woman of child-bearing potential is given a drug, and then finds out days or weeks later that she is pregnant? First, it is important to identify the drug and the exact time of exposure to it. If it is a known or a likely teratogen, the relation between the time of exposure and the likely time of conception should be determined. Even if the precise date of conception is known, dating the pregnancy by ultrasound is advisable if a suspected teratogen has been taken. If exposure to a known teratogen has occurred during the first 8 weeks of pregnancy, detailed ultrasound examination of the fetus may detect structural abnormalities, and serum and amniotic α-fetoprotein concentrations measured to screen for to neural tube defects. Any advice on termination of a pregnancy should be based on a consideration of the risk of fetal abnormality from both published information and investigation of the individual case.

Table 10.1.2 Drugs with proven or very high teratogenic risk in human pregnancy

ACE inhibitors[a]	Fetal renal toxicity/oligohydraminos
Alcohol	Fetal alcohol syndrome
Carbamazepine	Neural tube defects?/features of hydantoin syndrome
Diethylstilboestrol	Vaginal adenocarcinoma in female offspring
Isoretinoin	Craniofacial and cardiac anomalies
Lithium	Cardiac defects including Ebstein's anomaly
Methotrexate	Fetal aminopterin syndrome
Misoprostil	Moebius syndrome
Phenytoin	Fetal hydantoin syndrome
Tetracyline	Decidual teeth staining
Thalidomide	Phocomelia
Valproic acid	Neural tube defects
Warfarin	Stippled epiphyses/nasal hypoplasia

[a] ATII receptor antagonists carry similar risk.

Adverse reactions to drugs in breast milk

Some drugs cause adverse reactions in babies after ingestion by the mother and excretion in her breast milk. Excretion of drugs into breast milk is important because 90% of women take at least one prescribed drug during the first week after delivery. This may discourage many women from breastfeeding unless they can be reassured that the benefits for the baby of being breastfed far outweigh any risks for the overwhelming majority of drugs (see Table 10.1.3).

The factors affecting drug excretion into breast milk are the same as those that govern drug transfer across the placenta. The only important difference is that breast milk has a lower pH and higher lipid content than plasma. Like the placenta, this passive transfer only explains a fraction of the total transport capacity. Active drug transport also occurs through transporters and efflux pumps expressed in the breast epithelium, which explains why some drugs are present in breast milk at levels higher than expected (e.g. atenolol and benzylpenicillin).

Neonates and young babies may be at risk of adverse drug reactions because clearance pathways for a drug are immature. The GFR is only 25% of the adult value at birth (based on body weight) and only reaches the adult range at 3–6 months. Tubular secretion measured by PAH clearance is also impaired (10% of adult capacity until 6 months), which explains the slow elimination of frusemide in neonates (it is secreted by the PAH transporter). Phase I metabolism through CYP enzymes are isoform dependent: 3A7 is the predominant isoform *in utero*; it is replaced by 3A4 *postpartum*, but it takes more than 1 month to reach adult levels; CYP 1A2 does not appear until 3 months; CYP2D6 and E1 appear after birth but rapidly achieve adult levels within hours of delivery.

Drugs that should be given to breastfeeding mothers with caution are included among the drugs in Table 10.1.3. A more extensive list can be found in the *British National Formulary* and the *Physician's Desk Reference*. If the safety of a drug is in serious doubt and it is not possible to identify an alternative, breastfeeding can be temporarily suspended while the drug is given.

Table 10.1.3 Effects of common maternal drugs on breastfed infants or milk production

Acebutalol/atenolol	Cyanosis, hypotension, bradycardia
Amoxicillin	None
Aspirin	Metabolic acidosis[a]
Bendrofluazide	May reduce milk production
Bromocriptine	Suppresses lactation
Caffeine	Irritability if >2–3 cups of coffee/day
Carbamazepine	None
Carbimazole	Goitre
Ciprofloxacin	None
Digoxin	None
Diltiazem	None
Fluconazole	None
Isoniazid	None
Labetalol	None
Levothyroxine	None
Lithium	Plasma level up to 50% mother
Nalidixic acid/nitrofurantoin	Haemolysis in G6PD deficient infant[a]
Morphine	None
Oestrogen (in oral contraceptive pill)	May reduce milk production
Pethidine	None
Phenobarbitone/primidone	Sedation
Phenytoin	Methaemoglobinaemia[a]
Prednisolone	None
Propylthiouracil	None
Valproic acid	None
Verapamil	None
Warfarin	None

[a] Single case reports.
From American Academy of Pediatrics (2001). *Policy statement.* (http://aappolicy.aappublications.org/cgi/content/full/pediatrics;108/3/776).

Detecting adverse drug reactions: pharmacovigilance

The importance of adverse reactions for drug regulatory bodies and the pharmaceutical industry has led to the evolution of a subspecialty of clinical pharmacology devoted to the detection and evaluation of adverse drug reactions. This specialization is called pharmacovigilance.

Because drugs reach the market based on the experience of dosing just a few thousand patients, capturing as many adverse drug reactions as possible afterwards is of crucial importance. This activity is called postmarketing surveillance, which usually relies on self-reporting by health professionals and in some countries, the general public as well. In the United Kingdom, reporting by health care workers operates through the yellow card scheme run by the Medicines and Healthcare Products Regulatory Agency (MHRA) and the Commission on Human Medicines (CHM). It is a spontaneous reporting scheme in the sense that it is voluntary and relies on the 'yellow card' in the back of every BNF being filled out by the health care worker. The scheme aims to collect (1) serious or fatal adverse drug reactions from all drugs; (2) all adverse drug reactions from newly licensed drugs (designated with a black triangle in the BNF); and (3) all adverse drug reactions in children under 18.

Spontaneous reporting schemes rely on goodwill and are prone to considerable under-reporting. Rare or unusual side effects are easily detected with them (e.g. the withdrawal of cerivastatin because of rhabdomyolysis and pergolide because of valvular heart disease). On the other hand, serious adverse reactions involving effects that occur frequently in the population receiving 3the drug are not so easily detected. The thrombotic risk of COX-2 selective NSAIDs (coxibs), especially rofecoxib(Vioxx), is a timely reminder of this serious flaw in spontaneous reporting schemes. If used over long periods, coxibs cause an excess of stroke and myocardial infarction, but both of these are common events in patients receiving NSAIDs. Most physicians, for example, would not immediately conclude that a 65-year-old patient who died from a stroke or myocardial infarction while on a coxib was the victim of an adverse drug reaction. It is a sobering reminder that rofecoxib was only withdrawn after some 20 million people were exposed to it and many thousand had probably died from taking it.

Despite the limitations of spontaneous reporting, it is a crucial part of the World Health Organization efforts to co-ordinate pharmacovigilance on a global scale as opposed to local efforts such as the yellow card scheme. Their database contained some 4.7 million reports in June 2009, with an annual growth of approximately 400 000, and some 90 countries had signed up to the scheme by January 2009. There is also a Europe-wide (or rather European Union-wide) pharmacovigilance programme run by the European Medicines Agency, called EudraVigilance. The difference in this scheme is that adverse drug reaction notification by the pharmaceutical companies operating within the European Union is not voluntary, by a statutory requirement of their marketing authorization. It is too early to say how the performance of these two systems compares in terms of the early detection of adverse drug reactions.

The probity of the pharmaceutical industry itself has also been seriously questioned recently in the process of alerting the regulatory authorities about suspected adverse drug reactions. Large observational studies commissioned by the pharmaceutical companies to capture adverse reactions have been deliberately hidden (by Bayer in the case of Aprotinin) or methodologically questioned (by Merck in the case of Vioxx) when they confirmed suspected adverse reactions. These and other cases have highlighted the need for regulatory agencies to be able to compel pharmaceutical companies to: (1) carry out the necessary controlled trials to investigate the safety of a new drug and (2) make disclosure of these studies mandatory. Alternatively, health care systems should probably commission the necessary studies. These would certainly be cost-effective considering how much they will have spent e.g. managing the excess of strokes and myocardial infarction that followed the introduction of coxibs.

Prevention of adverse drug reactions: the role of the patient

Most people who take either a prescribed drug or one purchased over the counter do not usually expect unwanted effects from it, although they may have been alerted to potential adverse reactions by the doctor, pharmacist, or packet insert. The information from any of these sources should warn about all potential adverse drug reactions, so that the patient can:

- assess the potential disadvantages of the drug, before deciding to take it
- connect an adverse reaction with the taking of the drug and take appropriate action

However, what is usually lacking is advice about how to minimize or avoid adverse drug reactions. This advice is as relevant for the patient as it is for the prescriber. The prescriber in particular should consider the following:

- First, are there dose-dependent effects? If there are, they can be prevented or minimized by keeping the drug dosage as low as possible. It is always worth considering whether dosing below the pharmaceutical company's recommended range may be appropriate for individual patients. This is especially the case in older people or for non-white ethnic groups (who may metabolize the drug differently) as both are often under-represented in preregistration drug trials. If adverse reactions are more likely with continued use of the drug, then the duration of use should be limited, e.g. with neuroleptic drugs.
- Second, are drug interactions likely? If there are known interactions, they may be prevented by ensuring interacting drugs are avoided. This list should include agents that could be taken by the patient but are not prescribed. For example, it may be necessary to avoid consumption of grapefruit juice or herbal remedies such as St John's wort if the drugs are substrates for CYP 3A4 or P-glycoprotein (and the patient is taking simvastatin bought over the counter).
- Third, there may be serious adverse reactions that are unknown and/or undetected duringpre-registration trials. Drugs that have been prescribed over many years have an established margin of safety and should be used in preference to newer drugs. If there is a compelling reason to use a new drug, the patient should be aware that it is a new drug and there should be closer monitoring for adverse reactions.
- Fourth, adverse reactions are more likely when a prescriber is using a drug they are not familiar with. The prescriber might consider asking for a second opinion about the appropriateness of the drug and problems with its use if they are not sure.
- Fifth, some individuals are predisposed to adverse drug reactions. This is usually a genetic susceptibility. They may, for example, be poor drug metabolizers, porphyriacs, or have G6PD deficiency. If this is known, patients should be aware of drugs they should avoid and they should tell other prescribers of the problem before they take any new drug.

Drug interactions

A drug interaction occurs when the effects of one drug are altered by the effects of another drug. Usually this results in an adverse reaction, but in a few cases, it may actually prove beneficial. Interactions form up to 10% of all adverse drug reactions, but crucially, among patients who die from an adverse drug reaction, about one-third of deaths are due to interactions.

Drugs likely to precipitate interactions often have one or more of the following properties:

- They are highly protein-bound, e.g. aspirin and sulphonamides.
- The induce drug metabolism, e.g. phenytoin, carbamazepine, and rifampicin.
- They inhibit drug metabolism, e.g. cimetidine, metronidazole, and triazole antifungals.

The drugs most likely to be affected by drug–drug interactions are also those with a steep dose–response curve and a low therapeutic index, which includes aminoglycoside antibiotics, warfarin, and other coumarins, anticonvulsants, antihypertensive drugs, cardiac glycosides, cytotoxic and immunosuppressant drugs, oestrogen-containing oral contraceptives, and some centrally acting drugs. The most frequent interactions occur with warfarin and other coumarins.

Drug interactions fall into three basic types (see Table 10.1.4).

Pharmaceutical interactions

These involve physiochemical effects between a drug and the solution it is mixed with or between two drugs when they are mixed together (usually for injection). The interaction results in the drug either precipitating from solution or being inactivated in some other way. There are numerous examples, but some general principles can help to avoid many of them: give intravenous drugs by bolus injection if possible or via an infusion pump; do not add drugs to infusion solutions other than dextrose or saline; only mix drugs in the same infusion solution if they are known to be safe (e.g. potassium chloride with insulin).

Pharmacokinetic interactions

Pharmacokinetic interactions occur when a drug alters the absorption, distribution, or elimination (metabolism or excretion) of another drug.

Absorption interactions

One drug substantially altering the absorption of another is relatively uncommon but there are important examples. Anion exchange resins, for example, bind warfarin, digoxin, and thyroxine very avidly (see earlier paragraphs). Other examples are given in Table 10.1.4.

This type of interaction may occasionally be beneficial. Hence, metoclopramide increases gastric emptying and speeds the absorption of analgesics (such as ibuprofen and paracetamol) used to treat acute migraine. Activated charcoal also binds many drugs in the gut lumen, so preventing their absorption or enteroheptic recycling. This is widely exploited in drug overdoses (see earlier paragraphs and Chapter 9.1). It is also used to accelerate excretion of the antirheumatoid drug leflunomide if it causes a serious adverse reaction because of the extremely long half-life (2 weeks) of its active metabolite.

Protein-binding displacement interactions

Displacement of one drug by another from its binding sites on plasma proteins will cause an increase in the circulating concentration of unbound drug. This is only important if the displaced drug is highly protein bound (>90%) and has a small volume of distribution (that will exaggerate the rise in free drug concentration). The drugs concerned are warfarin, phenytoin, and tolbutamide.

Table 10.1.4 Mechanisms of drug interactions, with important examples

Mechanism		Example	Outcome
Physiochemical		Calcium gluconate plus sodium bicarbonate	Precipitation of calcium carbonate in infusion solution
Pharmacokinetic	Altered absorption	Reabsorption of oestrogens reduced by antibiotics	Contraceptive failure
		Gastric emptying increased by metoclopramide	Increased rate of absorption of simple analgesics
		Fluoroquinolones (e.g. ciprofloxacin) and agents containing divalent/trivalent cations (e.g. antacids or Fe salts) or sulcrafate	Reduced absorption
	Altered protein binding	Displacement of phenytoin by aspirin (not low-dose aspirin)	Phenytoin toxicity (transient)
	Increased metabolism	Oestrogen metabolism increased by carbamazepine, phenytoin, rifampicin	Contraceptive failure
	Reduced metabolism	Warfarin metabolism inhibited by amiodarone, metronidazole, cimetidine	Warfarin toxicity
		Theophylline metabolism inhibited by erythromycin or fluoroquinolones (e.g. ciprofloxacin)	Theophylline toxicity
		Phenytoin /carbamzepine metabolism inhibited by cimetidine, erythromycin, fluconazole, or isoniazid	Phenytoin/carbamazepine toxicity
		Amine metabolism inhibited by monoamine oxidase inhibitors (includes tyramine in foods and phenyl-propanolamine in cold cures)	Acute severe hypertension
	Reduced renal elimination	Penicillin/cephalosporin excretion reduced by probenecid	Prolonged duration of antibiotic action
		Lithium excretion reduced by diuretics or NSAIDs	Lithium toxicity
		Digoxin excretion reduced by amiodarone, quinidine, verapamil	Digoxin toxicity
Pharmacodynamic	Shared mechanisms	Vitamin K competes with warfarin for epoxide reductase	Reversal of the effect of warfarin
		Naloxone displaces opioids from opioid receptors	Reversal of opioid toxicity
		PDE5 inhibitors (e.g. sildenafil) and nitrates	Profound hypotension
		Statin and niacin, fibrates (especially gemfibrozil)	Risk of rhabdomyolysis/renal failure
		SSRIs and tramadol, triptans (e.g. sumatriptan) or monoamine oxidase inhibitors (e.g. selegiline)	Risk of serotonin syndrome
	Parallel mechanisms	Psycoactive drugs and alcohol	Increased sedation
		Cytotoxic drugs acting at different stages of the cell cycle	Therapeutic potentiation in cancer chemotherapy
		Warfarin and antiplatelet drugs (aspirin and other NSAIDs or clopidogrel)	Increased risk of bleeding and impaired haemostasis

The most common precipitant drugs in protein-binding displacement interactions are sulphonamides, salicylates, and chloral hydrate and some of its congeners (because of their metabolite, trichloracetic acid). In addition, valproate specifically displaces phenytoin.

However, displacement interactions are generally relatively unimportant. This is because the rise in free drug concentration increases the drug's clearance, so that the total concentration actually falls if the displacing drug is given chronically. Displacement is only a problem if the initial rise in free drug concentration itself causes toxicity; fortunately, if this is not serious it will be transient.

Interactions through induction of metabolism

Induction of P450 enzymes is a major source of drug interactions. Drugs that induce drug metabolism include barbiturates, carbamazepine, griseofulvin, phenytoin, and rifampicin (see Table 10.1.4). The herbal preparation of St John's Wort also induces P450 isoforms.

Interactions through inhibition of metabolism

Most of the interactions under this heading involve drugs that inhibit specific P450 pathways, for example, through CYP3A4 or 2D6. Some examples are shown in Table 10.1.4.

Metabolism through non-CYP metabolic pathways can also be affected. Hence, the interaction of allopurinol with azathioprine and 6-mercaptopurine results from its inhibition of xanthine oxidase. Both 6-mercaptopurine and azathioprine (which is metabolized to 6-mercaptopurine) are metabolized by xanthine oxidase.

The interaction of MAO inhibitors with dietary tyramine is another example of a non-CYP pathway. Tyramine in the diet usually has very low bioavailability because of degradation by MAO in the gut wall and liver. MAO inhibitors inactivate the enzyme both here and within sympathetic nerve endings, which increase their noradrenaline content. Hence, tyramine ingested after an MAO inhibitor has substantially increased bioavailability, and the resulting plasma levels are sufficient to displace the enhanced noradrenaline stores from sympathetic nerve terminals. The hypertensive crisis this causes is referred to as the 'cheese reaction'.

These interactions may again be sometimes useful. The protease inhibitor ritonavir, for example, is a potent CYP3A4 inhibitor and is added to antiretroviral drug regimens containing other protease inhibitors to specifically inhibit their metabolism and so increase bioavailability (which may otherwise be low). This is referred to as PK-enhanced drug formulation.

Excretion interactions

Most interactions involving drug excretion occur in the kidneys, although secretion into the gut through P-glycoprotein is important for some drugs (e.g. digoxin, cyclosporin). The latter explains drug interactions with substances such as St John's wort and grapefruit juice.

Interactions due to the alteration of active renal drug secretion are shown in Table 10.1.4. Some drugs that are weak acids or bases are passively reabsorbed along the nephron. The extent of reabsorption is pH-dependent and can be exploited following overdose to increase drug elimination in the urine (see earlier paragraphs).

Pharmacodynamic interactions

Pharmacodynamic interactions are very common and occur when one drug alters the effect of another. This can arise because the two drugs act on the same drug target or pathway. Alternatively, the interacting drugs may produce the same effect but by entirely separate mechanisms. Some examples are shown in Table 10.1.4.

Interactions through a shared mechanism

When there is a shared drug target (such as a receptor) the interaction may arise because of antagonism or combined agonism at this site. Many antagonistic interactions are therapeutically beneficial. Examples are the reversal of the effects of benzodiazepines with flumazenil or warfarin with vitamin K. In contrast, synergistic interactions are often adverse. Hence, nitroglycerine and sildenafil are useful drugs to treatment angina and erectile failure, respectively; nitroglycerine being metabolized to nitric oxide (NO) and sildenafil augmenting the effect of endogenous NO. Combining the two, however, causes devastating hypotension.

Interactions through parallel mechanisms

Two drugs may have similar pharmacological or toxic effects but they are achieved through different mechanisms. For example, the bleeding risk of warfarin is increased by drugs that affect platelet function (e.g. NSAIDs, clopidogrel, or glycoprotein IIb/IIIa antagonists), reduce platelet number (drug-induced thrombocytopenia) or cause gastrointestinal ulceration (e.g. NSAIDs).

Exploiting parallel pathways can also be beneficial. Many chemotherapy regimens exploit pharmacodynamic interactions of their component drugs. And combinations of antibiotics are used routinely even when a single organism is being targeted (e.g. penicillin + an aminoglycoside in subacute bacterial endocarditis and multiple-drug regimens for tuberculosis).

Pharmacogenetics and pharmacogenomics

The variability between individuals in terms of both the pharmacokinetics and pharmacodynamics of a drug is partly determined by genetic variation. The variability can occur in a single gene (hence pharmacogenetics) or arise from the interplay of a number of genes (pharmacogenomics).

Pharmacokinetic variability

Several important pathways of drug metabolism can affect drug pharmacokinetics through polymorphic variation in the enzymes involved. These include oxidation, acetylation, *S*-methylation, and suxamethonium hydrolysis (Table 10.1.5).

Oxidation

About 80% of oxidative drug metabolism occurs through the cytochrome P450 or CYP enzyme family of enzymes (see earlier paragraphs). There are some 57 genes in humans encoding these enzymes and they are named with a number and letter for the family and subfamily to which they belong, e.g. *3A4* or *2D6*. Many of these genes are polymorphic, with the common wild-type gene being mutated to produce a change in gene function; usually a reduction. The alleles for these different polymorphisms or gene variants are designated by a number after an asterisk, e.g. *2D6*4* for the commonest variant of *2D6* that reduces enzyme function.

Table 10.1.5 Pharmacogenetic variation affecting drug metabolism

Metabolizer phenotype	Enzyme responsible	Common deficiency gene variant	Frequency in white people	Comments
Suxamethonium apnoea	Butyrylcholinesterase (CHE)	*CHE*70* D>G	1:3000	Many other variants encoding CHE with reduced or no activity
Poor metabolizer	CYP2D6	*2D6*4* (premature stop codon)	5–10%	Commonest allele for PM phenotype
Slow acetylator	*N*-acetyltransferase (NAT2)	NAT2*5B	*c.*40% carry it but compound heterozygotes as likely as **5B* homozygotes	**4* is the fast allele and behaves dominantly
Thiopurine sensitivity	Thiopurine S-methyltransferase (TPMT)	*TPMT*3A* (154A>T, 240T>C)	5% are carriers (homozygous rate *c.*1:250)	20 other variants but 95% of cases due to *2 or *3(A–D)
Irinotican sensitivity	UDP-glucuronyl transferase 1 (UGT1A1)	(TA)7–TATA	*c.*40%	Promoter variant reduces UGT1A1 expression

Drugs that are metabolized through polymorphic CYP enzymes show drug metabolism in the population that has a bimodal (or occasionally trimodal) distribution. An example of this is shown in Fig. 10.1.5, where the metabolic ratios for debrisoquine are shown in the urine of over 1000 patients (debrisoquine is an obsolete antihypertensive but is still used as a 'probe' drug to define metabolic phenotype for CYP enzymes). Most are extensive metabolizers with low-to-intermediate drug:metabolite ratios in their urine, but a significant minority are poor metabolizers with high ratios. In this case, the poor-metabolizer status is due to *2D6* gene variants that reduce 2D6 enzyme activity. Genetically, the defect is very heterogenous with over 70 point mutations, promoter variants, and deletions now recognized (see http://www.imm.ki.se/cypalleles). The frequency of the poor-metabolizer phenotype varies across different ethnic groups: it is around 5 to 10% in northern Europeans but only approximately 1% in the Chinese. Drugs that are commonly metabolized through 2D6 include codeine, dextromethorphan, flecainide, metoprolol, nortriptyline, propafenone, timolol, and tramadol (see Table 10.1.1). The dose-related adverse reactions of these drugs (e.g. central nervous system toxicity with nortriptyline or bradycardia and hypotension with the β-blockers) are more likely in patients with the poor-metabolizer phenotype. Quinidine is an inhibitor of the 2D6 enzyme and is able to convert an extensive to a poor metabolizer.

Some patients even have a super- or ultrametabolizer phenotype. This phenotype occurs through duplication of the *2D6* gene and shortening of the half-life of 2D6-metabolized drugs in these patients is directly related to the degree of duplication (Fig. 10.1.6). They are relatively uncommon compared to the poor-metabolizers (see Fig. 10.1.5), but their status has important clinical consequences. A 2D6 drug will appear to be relatively ineffective in an ultrametabolizer unless very large doses are used, and they may even be suspected of poor compliance. In contrast, if the drug is a prodrug, ultrametabolizers are characteristically very sensitive to its effects. Hence, they may show opiate intoxication from what appear to be low therapeutic doses of codeine because of its rapid and complete metabolism to morphine. Although they are rare in Europe, 30% of East Africans may be ultrametabolizers.

The other CYP enzymes are not as well studied as 2D6, but poor metabolizers have been identified for 2C9 (metabolizing losartan, phenytoin, tolbutamide, and warfarin) and 2C19 (metabolizing omeprazole). There is now a commercial microarray available to genotype individuals for all the known variations in the *2D6* and *2C19* genes (it is called the AmpliChip P450).

Disease associations with polymorphic metabolism

As some diseases may be related to the effects of environmental chemicals that have carcinogenic metabolites, it is of interest that polymorphic acetylation, hydroxylation, and sulphoxidation have other clinical associations. The evidence linking acetylator status with the risk of bladder cancer is probably the best established association; slow acetylators having increased risk. Other weaker associations may exist between debrisoquine metabolizer status (2D6) and risk of parkinsonism in poor debrisoquine hydroxylators, of bronchogenic carcinoma in extensive debrisoquine hydroxylators, and of primary biliary cirrhosis in poor sulphoxidizers.

Acetylation

Some drugs are cleared by acetylation. These include dapsone, hydralazine, isoniazid, procainamide, and some sulphonamides. The enzyme involved is the hepatic enzyme *N*-acetyltransferase (EC 2.3.1.5) and if drug:metabolite ratios for a drug cleared by acetylation are measured, they distribute bimodally in the population. Subjects producing the highest ratios are described as being fast acetylators (cf. extensive metabolizers for the 2D6 pathway). Again the genetic basis for the biochemical phenotype is very heterogenous, and the frequency of fast acetylators varies across different ethnic groups: 40% in northern Europeans, 85% in Japanese, and 5% among the Inuit.

Slow acetylators require lower doses of drugs that are cleared by acetylation than fast acetylators. Slow acetylators are also more likely to develop the lupus erythematosus-like syndrome caused by isoniazid, hydralazine, and procainamide, and the peripheral neuropathy caused by isoniazid (isoniazid actually causes degradation of pyridoxine). The interaction between isoniazid and phenytoin, in which isoniazid inhibits phenytoin metabolism causing phenytoin toxicity, is also more frequent among slow acetylators.

Glucuronidation

The antitumour agent irinotecan is a prodrug. Its active metabolite, SN-38, has about 1000-fold higher activity than irinotecan itself and is inactivated by glucuronidation through UGT1A1. Patients homozygous for a polymorphism in the promoter of UGT1A1 are much more likely to develop severe neutropenia after irinotecan because of defective glucuronidation of SN-38. The same polymorphism is also involved in Gilbert's syndrome.

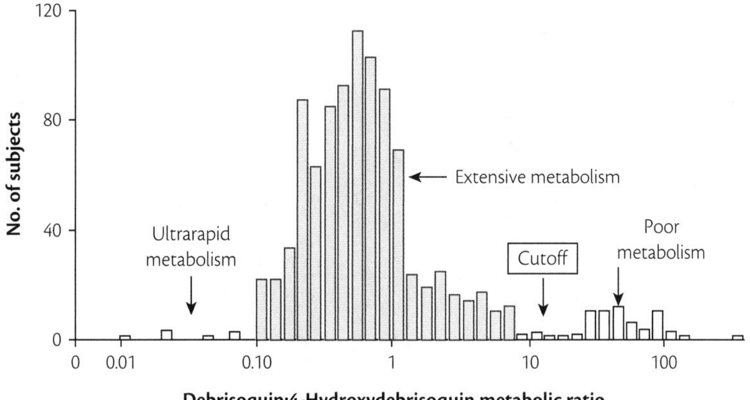

Fig. 10.1.5 Pharmacogenetics of CYP2D6. Urinary metabolic ratios of debrisoquin to its metabolite, 4-hydroxydebrisoquin, for more than 1000 Swedish subjects. Poor metabolizers with no or reduced CYP2D6 activity are separated by the cut-off box from extensive metabolizers.

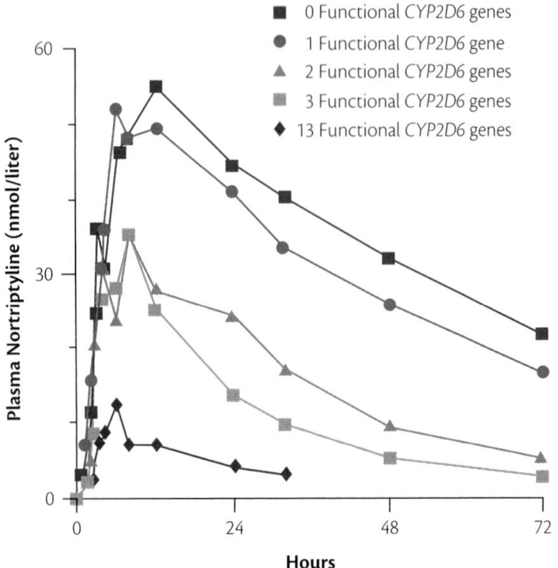

Fig. 10.1.6 Effect of *CYP2D6* gene duplication. Nortripyline is used here as a probe drug. Its clearance is increased (AUC and half-life fall) as the *2D6* copy number increases.

Reprinted by permission from Macmillan Publishers Ltd: Clinical Pharmacology & Therapeutics (1998) 63, 444–452 © 1998.

Methylation

The thiopurines (6-mercaptopurine and 6-thioguanine) are metabolized by *S*-methylation through the enzyme thiopurine *S*-methyltransferase (TPMT, EC 2.1.1.67). The metabolism of azathioprine is also affected by this enzyme as azathioprine is reduced to 6-mercaptopurine after dosing, i.e. it is a prodrug. High levels of TPMT are found in red cells, and the activity is trimodal in the population with high, intermediate, and low levels of TPMT detectable. Because low levels of TPMT (present in *c.*1:300 whites) reduces metabolic clearance of thiopurines, these subjects are exposed to high levels of 6-thioguanine nucleotides. This leads to severe myelosuppression if they are given standard doses of these drugs. Hence, thiopurines can only be used safely in subjects with low TPMT if they are given very low doses.

There are some 20 gene variants that affect the activity of TPMT and carriers for TPMT variants are common—overall frequencies are typically 5 to 10%. The commonest variant (*TPMT**3A*) is actually a double mutant that switches two amino acids and produces an unstable enzyme that explains the low level of TPMT in homozygotes. There is considerable ethnic variation in the frequency of variants, e.g. the **3A* is not seen among the Chinese.

Suxamethonium hydrolysis

Suxamethonium (succinylcholine) is metabolized in the plasma by the nonspecific esterase pseudocholinesterase (EC 3.1.1.8; also called butyrylcholinesterase). Normally this happens quickly, which explains why neuromuscular blockade with this drug lasts only a few minutes. Some patients, however, have very slow clearance of suxamethonium due to low plasma pseudocholinesterase activity. This manifests as prolonged neuromuscular blockade or apnoea after the use of suxamethonium, which can last several hours or longer.

Suxamethonium apnoea is usually very rare, but is common in Inuit (up to 10%). Several different gene defects can cause pseudocholinesterase deficiency: the dibucaine-resistant, fluoride-resistant, and 'silent' gene types. Patients with reduced pseudocholinesterase also show increased sensitivity to the nondepolarizing blocker mivacurium. Interestingly, pseudocholinesterase deficiency does not appear to affect the conversion of the prodrug bambuterol (which is also a substrate for pseudocholinesterase) to its active metabolite terbutaline.

Pharmacodynamic defects

Some biochemical abnormalities make individuals peculiarly sensitive or resistant to the effects of certain drugs. All have a genetic basis.

Red cell enzyme defects (see Section 22)

Adverse drug reactions may affect people whose red cells are deficient in glucose-6-phosphate dehydrogenase (G6PD). If their red cells are exposed to an oxidizing drug, they lose their oxygen-carrying capacity as haemoglobin is oxidized to methaemoglobin and they eventually haemolyse. Drugs commonly implicated are doxorubicin, nalidixic acid, nitrofurantoin, primaquine, and sulphamethoxazole. There is a longer list of drugs that may cause haemolysis in some G6PD-deficient individuals, depending on their genotype. This is because the common African variant gives higher red cell G6PD levels than the Mediterranean form, so mild oxidative stress is better tolerated. This list includes aspirin (low dose is usually safe), chloramphenicol, L-dopa, isoniazid, quinine and related compounds, trimethoprim, and vitamin K.

Porphyria (see Section 11)

The hepatic porphyrias, acute intermittent porphyria and porphyria cutanea tarda, are characterized by abnormalities of haem biosynthesis. Certain drugs may precipitate an attack of porphyria especially cytochrome P450 inducers, e.g. barbiturates, carbamazepine, and rifampicin. The quality of data as to the safety (or not) or other drugs is variable. There is a useful web database that rates drug safety on a five-point scale (http://www.drugs-porphyria.com).

Malignant hyperthermia

This potentially fatal complication of general anaesthesia follows exposure to halogenated anaesthetic gases and suxamethonium (see earlier paragraphs).

Vitamin D-resistant rickets

Three varieties of rickets are resistant to the effects of vitamin D (cholecalciferol): familial hypophosphataemic rickets, vitamin D dependency, and Fanconi's syndrome (see Section 12).

Warfarin sensitivity

Sensitivity to warfarin varies widely in the general population. This has been explained on the basis of common gene variants in its target enzyme vitamin K epoxide reductase (EC 1.1.4.2, encoded by *VKORC1*) and the *CYP2C9* gene responsible for its metabolism.

Pharmacogenomics and the prospect of 'personal prescribing'

The realization that the pharmacokinetics and pharmacodynamics of a drug may be genetically determined has raised the prospect of tailoring the drug to the patient. Predefining the generic variants that a patient has before a drug is given could, in principle, avoid many adverse drug reactions and interactions. The microarray technology to perform the necessary genotyping is now available, and many drug trials now incorporate this technology to identify gene signatures that both affect the therapeutic response to the drugs and predict adverse reactions. However, we are some way off truly 'personalized prescribing'.

Monitoring drug therapy

Monitoring drug therapy usually involves trying to measure the clinical response directly. If this is difficult, or is not related directly in time to a dose of the drug, a surrogate measure of the response may be required. In some cases, it may be necessary to resort to measurement of the plasma concentration of the drug.

Monitoring the therapeutic effects of drugs

Some events can be directly monitored in the individual patient. Examples of therapeutic events that can be monitored in the individual include frequency of seizures during anticonvulsant drug therapy, muscle power during treatment of myasthenia gravis, the frequency of attacks of angina pectoris, and body weight during diuretic therapy.

Preventive measures in medicine often cannot be monitored in the individual patient and their impact has to be predicted from population studies (usually a clinical trial). Examples include the frequency of infections after immunization, the reduction in NSAID-induced peptic ulceration with a proton pump inhibitor, or the prevention of the complications of myocardial infarction by the use of thrombolysis and aspirin.

Monitoring the pharmacodynamic effects of drugs

In some circumstances, the pharmacological effect of a drug can be carefully measured, followed sequentially, and used as a guide to drug therapy even though it may not be correlated precisely with the therapeutic effect. Examples include the effect of insulin on the blood glucose concentration in diabetes mellitus, anticoagulants on the prothrombin time, bronchodilators on FEV_1 and peak flow rate in asthma, and cancer chemotherapy on tumour markers.

Monitoring drug pharmacokinetics (therapeutic drug monitoring)

This is useful for drugs where:

- the clinical evidence of therapeutic or toxic effects is difficult to measure or interpret
- the relation between dose and plasma concentration is unpredictable
- the drug has a low therapeutic index
- the plasma concentration of the drug is a good predictor of response

There are only a handful of drugs that meet these requirements (see Table 10.1.6). For these drugs, monitoring drug levels can be used to individualize therapy (e.g. at the start of drug dosing, when the relation between dose and plasma concentration in the individual is uncertain or rapid changes in renal function alter the relation between dose and plasma concentration), to monitor toxicity and to assess compliance (see page 1454).

Phenytoin

Plasma concentrations of phenytoin in the toxic range are quite well related to its acute neurotoxic effects, but not to its long-term adverse reactions, such as gingival hyperplasia, hirsutism and acne, and folate and vitamin D deficiencies. At low dosages it takes about 2 weeks of maintenance therapy to reach steady state after a change in dose, but because of its nonlinear kinetics (Fig. 10.1.4), the half-life lengthens at higher plasma concentrations; so it can take up to 3 weeks or longer in some patients to reach steady state. For this reason the dosage should not be changed frequently. Provided the sample is not taken too soon after a dose (i.e. within 1 to 2 h), the time of sampling for phenytoin is not critical, as peak–trough fluctuation is small between doses.

Digoxin

Plasma digoxin concentrations correlate well with toxic effects but not with the therapeutic effect within the therapeutic dosage range. The time of blood sampling should be at least 6 h after the last dose. During regular maintenance dosage without a loading dose, steady-state is reached after about 7 days (normal renal function) to more than 14 days (functionally anephric). The pharmacological response to a given plasma level of digoxin is dependent on thyroid function (hyperthyroidism decreases responsiveness and hypothyroidism increases it) and the plasma potassium (hypokalaemia increases responsiveness and hyperkalaemia reduces it). Children younger than 6 months have lower plasma digoxin concentrations at a given dose than older children and adults, and they are also more resistant to the pharmacodynamic actions of digitalis; so plasma digoxin concentrations cannot be clearly interpreted in this age group.

Lithium

The therapeutic range is 0.4 to 1 mmol/litre. In the range of 1 to 1.5 mmol/litre, the incidence of both acute toxicity and long-term adverse effects is increased. Concentrations above 1.5 mmol/litre should be avoided. Blood samples should be taken at least 12 h after the last dose. It takes about 3 days for steady state to be reached during regular maintenance therapy, but patients vary widely. It may take up to a week.

Monitoring the plasma lithium concentration is necessary for several reasons. Lithium is nephrotoxic and excreted by the kidneys, so if toxicity occurs it is self-perpetuating. Systemic availability

Table 10.1.6 Drugs that commonly require therapeutic concentration monitoring and their reference ranges

Drug	Concentration below which a therapeutic effect is unlikely	Concentration above which a toxic effect is more likely
Gentamicin[a]	5 μg/ml (peak)	12 μg/ml (peak), 2 μg/ml (trough)
Digoxin	1.0 nmol/litre	3.8 nmol/litre
Ciclosporin[b]	80–200 nmol/litre	170–300 nmol/litre
Lithium	0.4 mmol/litre	1.0 mmol/litre
Phenytoin	40 μmol/litre	80 μmol/litre
Theophylline	55 μmol/litre	100 μmol/litre

[a] Conventional dosage regimens.
[b] Actual range will vary between laboratories.

varies from person to person and is altered by diarrhoea. It also varies widely between formulations, which cannot be used interchangeably. Sodium balance also affects renal excretion of lithium. For example, diuretic-induced renal sodium loss reduces renal lithium excretion and can precipitate toxicity.

Aminoglycoside antibiotics

Gentamicin is the most widely used aminoglycoside antibiotic, but the principles hold for other aminoglycosides. The relation between the plasma concentration of gentamicin and its therapeutic efficacy is complicated by the fact that different organisms have different sensitivities to the antibiotic. Gentamicin is renally excreted, so in renal impairment it accumulates unless the dose frequency (and eventually the dose itself) is reduced.

The toxic effects of gentamicin on the inner ear and kidneys are related to the 'peak' concentration (usually taken 1 h after an intramuscular injection or the start of an intravenous infusion) and the 'trough' concentration (taken just before the next dose). These should be measured after three or four doses, or sooner if there is renal impairment. A peak plasma concentration of 5 to 9 mg/litre is generally considered necessary, although when gentamicin is used together with benzylpenicillin to treat bacterial endocarditis, lower plasma gentamicin concentrations may be effective. Bacteriological measurement of *in vitro* inhibitory concentrations will help to guide therapy. If there is uncertainty, expert advice on dosing and target plasma concentrations should be sought.

Theophylline

Plasma theophylline concentrations correlate well with therapeutic and toxic effects. Measurement is essential in any patient who has been taking oral theophylline before it is given intravenously. It is also important in smokers who usually have increased theophylline clearance and hence require higher maintenance doses.

Ciclosporin

Ciclosporin is generally measured in whole blood, and the result of the assay may depend on whether the measurement technique is by immunoassay or high-performance liquid chromatography. The time to steady state is about 2 days and samples should be taken at trough (just before the next dose). The whole-blood concentration of ciclosporin can be affected by reduced absorption (due to diarrhoea or reduced bile-salt production) or altered bioavailability (due to liver disease, coadministered drugs such as ketoconazole and rifampicin, grapefruit juice, or St John's wort).

Further reading

Clinical pharmacology

Bennett PN, Brown MJ (2008). *Clinical pharmacology*, 10th edition. Churchill Livingstone, Edinburgh. [Lively and readable, with interesting and stimulating quotations and references. Aimed at clinical medical students and MRCP exam.]

Dollery, CT (1999). *Therapeutic drugs*, 2nd edition. Elsevier, Amsterdam. [A compendium of >800 drug monographs in 2 volumes. Each one details a drug's chemistry, pharmacology, toxicology, clinical pharmacology, pharmacokinetics, metabolism, pharmaceutics, therapeutic use, adverse reactions, high-risk groups, drug interactions, and clinical trials. Although dated, the information on older drugs is invaluable.]

Ritter JM, Lewis LD, Mant TGK (2008). *A textbook of clinical pharmacology*, 5th edition. Arnold, London. [Well organized and illustrated with many clinical case vignettes.]

Pharmacological effects of drugs

Brunton LL, Lazo JS, Parker KL (2006). *Goodman & Gilman's The pharmacological basis of therapeutics*, 11/Eth edition. Mc-Graw Hill, London. [Still the authoritative textbook in the area, now with online access.]

Rang HP, *et al.* (2007). *Rang & Dale's pharmacology*, 6th edition. Elsevier, Amsterdam. [Excellent general introduction aimed at the undergraduate market with online access.]

Pharmacokinetics

Gibaldi M, Perrier D. (1982). *Pharmacokinetics*, 2nd edition. Marcel Dekker, New York. [Very detailed monograph. Examples dated but principles still useful. Not for the mathematically faint-hearted.]

Rowland M, Tozer TN (1995). *Clinical pharmacokinetics. Concepts and applications*, 3rd edition. Lea & Febiger, Philadelphia. [Still the most readable pharmacokinetics textbook. Covers basic concepts, principles of kinetics as applied to drugs, therapeutic regimens, and individualization of therapy. Well illustrated with practical problems.]

Adverse effects of drugs

Aronson JK (ed.) (2006). *Meyler's Side effects of drugs*, 15th edition. Elsevier, Amsterdam. [The definitive encyclopedia of drug side effects. This version is organized into six volumes.]

Websites

UL Cochrane Centre. http://www.cochrane.co.uk/ [Home of the Cochrane database and evidence-based therapeutics.]

Medicines and Healthcare Products Regulatory Agency (MHRA). http://www.mhra.gov.uk/ [Also allows online yellow card reporting.]

World Health Organization (1994). *Guide to good prescribing*. http://whqlibdoc.who.int/hq/1994/WHO_DAP_94.11.pdf

SECTION 11

Nutrition

11.1 Nutrition: macronutrient metabolism *1479*
Keith N. Frayn

11.2 Vitamins and trace elements *1487*
J. Powell-Tuck and M. Eastwood

11.3 Severe malnutrition *1505*
Alan A. Jackson

11.4 Diseases of overnourished societies and the need for dietary change *1515*
J.I. Mann and A.S. Truswell

11.5 Obesity *1527*
I. Sadaf Farooqi

11.6 Artificial nutrition support *1535*
Jeremy Woodward

11.1

Nutrition: macronutrient metabolism

Keith N. Frayn

Essentials

Food intake is sporadic: for most people it occurs in three major boluses each day. Energy expenditure, however, is continuous, with variations during the day that bear no resemblance to the pattern of energy intake, except that over some reasonable period of time (a week or more) the two will, in most people, match almost exactly. Therefore the body has developed complex systems that direct nutrients into storage pools when they are in excess, and that regulate the mobilization of nutrients from these pools as they are needed. The situation is analogous to the fuel tank of a car and the throttle that regulates fuel oxidation, except that in the car there is just one fuel and just one engine: in humans there are three major nutrients and a variety of tissues and organs, each of which may have its own preferences for fuels, that vary with time. Carbohydrate, fat, and protein (made up of amino acids), are the three sources of energy which are variably stored and assimilated from food each day. The fact that we can carry on our daily lives without thinking about whether to store or mobilize fuels, and which to use, attests to the remarkable efficiency of these control systems.

Regulation of macronutrient flux

The principal macronutrient stores are listed in Table 11.1.1 and are related to daily fluxes of energy substrates in the body.

The need for the coordinated control of nutrient storage, mobilization, and flux between tissues and along the many metabolic pathways, is met by a complex series of control mechanisms. These may be viewed on several levels. The simplest involves the effects of substrate concentration, and is dependent upon the kinetic properties of enzymes and transport proteins. Some of these mechanisms are illustrated in Fig. 11.1.1.

The next level involves more specific interaction of nutrients, or pathway intermediates, with enzymes, usually through allosteric effects (binding of the effector alters the conformation of the enzyme and hence its catalytic properties). There are many examples in the metabolism of carbohydrate, fat, and protein. The enzyme 6-phosphofructo-1-kinase (EC 2.7.1.11) in the glycolysis pathway is a good example, subject to allosteric regulation by many compounds that relate to the energy status of the cell. For instance, it is activated by AMP (indicating energy shortage) and inhibited by ATP. Such mechanisms undoubtedly provide important fine tuning of flux along various pathways, entirely in accord with the modern view that control of flux does not reside in certain rate-limiting steps but is distributed among many steps along a pathway. Related to this, the enzyme AMP-activated protein kinase responds to the cellular energy status and regulates a number of metabolic pathways accordingly (see 'Further reading').

These mechanisms operate essentially within tissues. However, the coordination of nutrient metabolism requires considerable interaction between tissues and organs. This coordination is largely brought about by the hormonal and nervous systems. Certain hormones play a particularly important role in regulation of macronutrient flux (Table 11.1.2). The role of the nervous system in metabolic regulation is often difficult to assess. Although the effects of adrenaline are properly regarded as hormonal, liberation of noradrenaline from sympathetic nerve endings in tissues may bring about identical effects and can be difficult to distinguish. The somatic nervous system (motor neurons innervating skeletal muscle) has clear effects, e.g. stimulation of breakdown of muscle glycogen linked to muscle contraction. The autonomic nervous system probably plays multiple roles, but some are indirect, e.g. regulation of blood flow and cardiac output, thus affecting delivery of substrate to tissues, and regulation of the secretion of pancreatic hormones.

The effects of hormones are mediated in many ways, but may be divided into acute effects (usually acting within seconds or minutes), often brought about through reversible phosphorylation of enzymes, and longer-term effects (hours or days), brought about by regulation of gene expression. The former are usually exerted through binding to cell surface receptors linked to a variety of second-messenger systems, the latter through nuclear receptors (e.g. for glucocorticoids and thyroid hormones) (for more details see Chapter 12.1). However, the distinction is not absolute: e.g. insulin brings about both acute and longer-term effects through binding to the same cell surface receptor.

Table 11.1.1 Macronutrient stores in relation to daily intake

Macronutrient	Total amount in body	Energy equivalent (MJ)	Days' supply if the only energy source	Daily intake (g)	Daily intake as percentage of store
Carbohydrate	0.6 kg	8.5	<1	300	60
Free glucose	12 g				
Liver glycogen	100 g				
Muscle glycogen	500 g				
Fat (triacylglycerol)	12–18 kg	550	56	100	0.7
Circulating in plasma	5 g				
Stored in adipocytes	12–18 kg				
Protein and amino acids	12 kg	200	(20)	100	0.8
Free amino acids	100 g				
Protein	12 kg				

Note: These are very much typical rounded figures. Days' supply is the length of time for which this store would last if it were the only fuel for oxidation at an energy expenditure of 10 MJ/day: the figure for protein is given in parentheses since protein does not fulfil the role of an energy store in this way.

A further level of coordination is through the effects of nutrients themselves, or important cellular components such as cholesterol, upon gene expression (summarized in Table 11.1.3). This can be seen as a longer-term mechanism to ensure that metabolism is appropriate to the diet being ingested and the lifestyle followed. A variety of nutrient response elements are known in the promoter regions of genes for enzymes concerned with substrate metabolism. Particular examples are the carbohydrate response element (which up-regulates expression of genes for glucose metabolism such as pyruvate kinase in the glycolysis pathway, and lipogenic genes; see Fig. 11.1.2), the sterol response element (by which insulin activates lipogenic gene expression, as in Fig. 11.1.2, and cellular sterols down-regulate expression of the low density lipoprotein receptor and the enzymes of cholesterol biosynthesis) and response elements for fatty acid derivatives. Fatty acids affect gene expression through a family of transcription factors known as the peroxisome proliferator activated receptors, summarized in Table 11.1.4. The expression of many genes is also regulated by insulin.

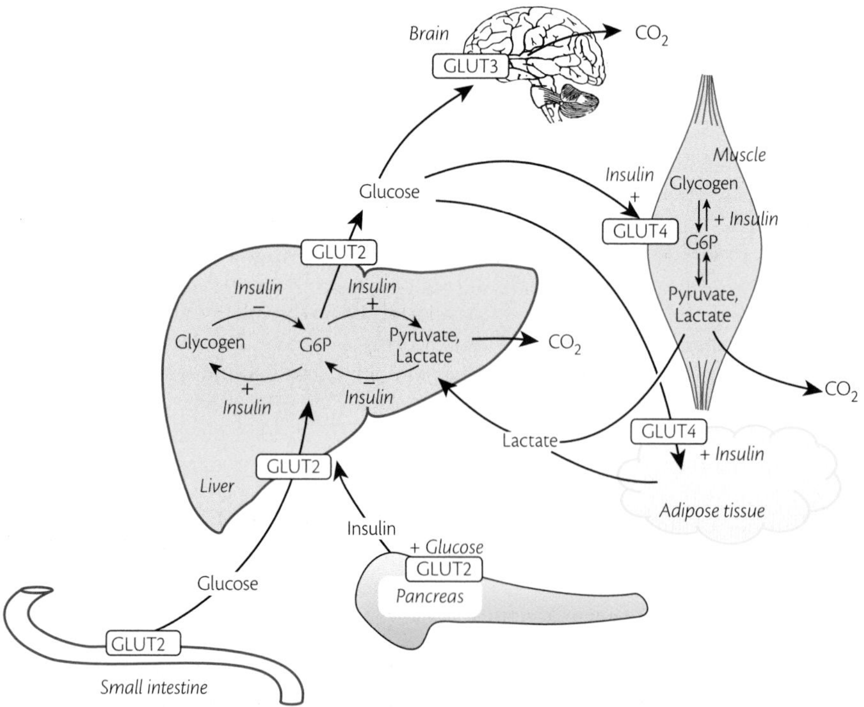

Fig. 11.1.1 Overview of carbohydrate metabolism. Pathways in the liver shown as regulated by insulin are probably controlled by the insulin/glucagon ratio (high in the fed state, low in fasting). In muscle, contraction is an important stimulus for glycogen breakdown and glycolysis. Adrenaline also contributes. Not shown is the significant glucose uptake by red blood cells and other glycolytic tissues, returning lactate to the liver. GLUT2 is the high-K_m noninsulin regulated glucose transporter (i.e. the glucose flux is determined by concentration), GLUT3 is the low-K_m brain glucose transporter (the glucose flux is relatively independent of concentration within the normal range), and GLUT4 the insulin-regulated glucose transporter (insulin brings about movement of GLUT4 to the cell surface from intracellular pools). G6P is glucose 6-phosphate.

Table 11.1.2 Major hormonal effects on intermediary metabolism

Hormone	Origin	Target tissue	Major metabolic effects	Comments
Insulin	Pancreatic islets (β-cells)	Liver	Stimulation of glycogen synthesis/ suppression of glycogen breakdown	Regulates glucose storage in liver
			Stimulation of glycolysis/suppression of gluconeogenesis	Regulates hepatic glucose output
			Suppression of fatty acid oxidation/ ketogenesis	Via malonyl CoA
			Stimulation of triacylglycerol synthesis	
			Stimulation of cholesterol synthesis	
		Skeletal muscle	Stimulation of glucose uptake	Via recruitment of GLUT4 (see Fig. 11.1.1)
			Stimulation of glycogen synthesis	
			Net protein anabolic effect	Suppression of protein breakdown may be more important than stimulation of protein synthesis
		Adipose tissue	Activation of triacylglycerol removal from plasma	Via lipoprotein lipase
			Suppression of fat mobilization	Via hormone-sensitive lipase
Glucagon	Pancreatic islets (α-cells)	Liver	Stimulation of glycogen breakdown/ suppression of glycogen synthesis	In effect the regulation is via the insulin/glucagon ratio
			Stimulation of gluconeogenesis/ suppression of glycolysis	
			Stimulation of fatty acid oxidation/ ketogenesis	
Adrenaline	Adrenal medulla	Adipose tissue	Stimulation of fat mobilization	Via hormone-sensitive lipase
		Skeletal muscle	Stimulation of glycogen breakdown	Acts in concert with muscle contraction
Tri-iodothyronine	Thyroid	All oxidative tissues	Increase in basal metabolism	
Cortisol	Adrenal cortex	Liver	Stimulation of gluconeogenesis	
		Skeletal muscle	Generally catabolic effect on protein	
		Adipose tissue	Promotes site-specific fat deposition (central depots) and fat mobilization (peripheral depots)	
Growth hormone	Anterior pituitary	Liver	Stimulation of gluconeogenesis	Direct effect: other effects are mediated indirectly via insulin-like growth factors
		Adipose tissue	Stimulation of fat mobilization	This is an acute effect: chronically, growth hormone promotes mobilization from central fat depots
Insulin-like growth factors (IGF) I and II	Liver (IGF-I) and other tissues (both)	Several	Generally insulin-like acute effects on metabolism	Physiological role is probably longer-term effects on growth
Leptin	Adipose tissue	Hypothalamus	Suppression of appetite; possibly stimulation of energy expenditure	Latter effect prominent in rodents, may not occur in humans; low leptin levels (signalling starvation) more important than high levels signalling excess
		Reproductive system	Signals sufficient fat stores for reproduction to be possible	As with effects on hypothalamus, low leptin may be a signal of starvation

Carbohydrate metabolism in the postabsorptive and postprandial states

Postabsorptive state

In the overnight-fasted (postabsorptive) state, no glucose enters the plasma from the small intestine. Glucose enters and leaves the plasma at about 2 mg/kg body weight per min (200 g/24 h). About one-half of this will be consumed by the brain. Of the remainder, a considerable proportion will be utilized by blood cells and peripheral tissues by anaerobic glycolysis, thus returning lactate to the liver for reconversion to glucose (Fig. 11.1.1). This is the Cori cycle.

Glucose is produced by hepatocytes from glycogen breakdown and from gluconeogenesis. Net glycogen breakdown is stimulated by the relatively low insulin/glucagon ratio after overnight fasting.

Table 11.1.3 Mechanisms by which nutrients regulate expression of genes involved in macronutrient metabolism

Stimulus	Transcription factor	Examples of proteins whose expression is regulated at the mRNA transcription level	Comments
Glucose	Carbohydrate-response element binding protein	Pyruvate kinase (liver isoform) (+) Acetyl CoA carboxylase 1 (+) Fatty acid synthase (+) SREBP-1c (see below) (+) Insulin (in the pancreatic β-cell) (+)	See Fig. 11.1.2
Insulin	Various, binding to a variety of insulin response elements (see 'Further reading')	GLUT 1, 2, 3, 4 (glucose transporters) (+) Hexokinase, glucokinase (+) Glyceraldehyde-3-phosphate dehydrogenase (+) Glucose-6-phosphatase (−) Acetyl CoA carboxylase 1 (+) Fatty acid synthase (+) SREBP-1c (+)	Glycolysis and lipogenesis are activated, gluconeogenesis suppressed; see 'Further reading' for more information.
Cholesterol (and insulin)	Sterol regulatory element binding proteins (SREBP)	SREBP-1c: Acetyl CoA carboxylase 1 (+) Fatty acid synthase (+) Stearoyl CoA desaturase (+) SREBP2: LDL receptor (+) HMG CoA synthase (+) HMG CoA reductase (+)	The two major isoforms, SREBP-1c and SREBP2, regulate respectively lipogenesis (in response to glucose and insulin) and cellular cholesterol homeostasis (in response to cellular sterol levels; low sterol levels allow mature SREBP2 to migrate to the nucleus)
Fatty acids	Peroxisome proliferator activated receptors (PPARs)	See Table 11.1.4	PPARs act as transcription factors as heterodimers with the retinoid-X receptor; the endogenous ligand is unclear: it might be a fatty acid (weak affinity) or a fatty acid derivate (e.g. a prostaglandin) (higher affinity)
Amino acids	Mammalian target of rapamycin (mTOR); Activating transcription factor 4 (ATF4)	IGFBP-1 (−) Asparagine synthase (−) Amino acid transporters (−) (especially neutral amino acid transport system A; cationic amino acid transporter CAT-1)	Induction of IGFBP-1 (binds IGF-1) when amino acid supply is restricted limits growth; molecular mechanisms are described in 'Further reading'

Note: (+), indicates gene induction; (−), gene suppression.

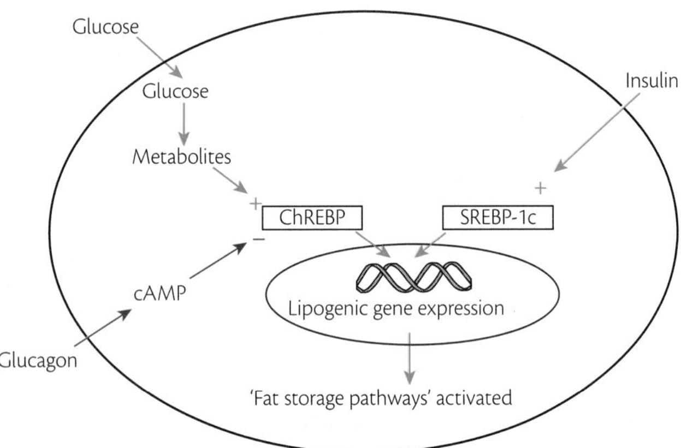

Fig. 11.1.2 Concerted roles of the carbohydrate-response element binding protein (ChREBP) and sterol regulatory element binding protein (SREBP) isoform 1c in activation of expression of lipogenic genes. In addition, ChREBP activates expression of genes of glucose disposal (e.g. glycolysis). The active metabolite from glucose is thought to be xylulose 5-phosphate (produced in the pentose phosphate pathway). This allows movement of ChREBP from cytosol into the nucleus (see 'Further reading').

The major substrates for gluconeogenesis are lactate and pyruvate, released from blood cells and peripheral tissues, together with alanine and glycerol. The pathway of gluconeogenesis predominates over that of glycolysis, again because of the relatively low insulin/glucagon ratio.

Glucose metabolism following a meal

When a meal enters the system, this pattern of metabolism changes rapidly. About 12 g of free glucose are present in the circulation and extravascular space. Typically, a single meal will provide about 100 g of glucose, entering the circulation over perhaps 60 min. In order to minimize variations in plasma glucose concentration, coordinated mechanisms come into play to suppress the production of endogenous glucose and to increase the rate of removal of glucose from the circulation.

Much of the incoming glucose may be taken up by hepatocytes as described earlier, but some enters the systemic circulation and stimulates pancreatic insulin secretion (and somewhat suppresses glucagon secretion). Insulin is liberated into the portal vein. Thus, the liver is exposed to high concentrations of glucose (from the small intestine) and insulin. The net effect is to reverse glycogenolysis, so that glycogen synthesis begins. In addition, gluconeogenesis is suppressed and glycolysis favoured (Fig. 11.1.1). Hepatocyte glucose

Table 11.1.4 Peroxisome proliferator activated receptors (PPARs): tissue distribution and effects of activation

Receptor	Main tissue distribution	Examples of proteins whose expression is regulated at the mRNA transcription level	Comments
PPAR-α	Liver (main site) Kidney, heart, muscle, brown adipose tissue	*Positive:* Apolipoprotein AI Apolipoprotein AII Enzymes of peroxisomal fatty acid oxidation Liver FABP CPT-1 Enzymes of mitochondrial fatty acid oxidation *Negative:* Apolipoprotein CIII	Target for the fibrate lipid-lowering drugs
PPAR-δ[a]	Widespread	*Positive:* Fatty acid transporters (e.g. CD36) Enzymes of mitochondrial fatty acid oxidation Enzymes of mitochondrial oxidation (succinate dehydrogenase, citrate synthase, cytochrome c, cytochrome oxidase) Uncoupling proteins 1, 2, 3	Effects have been documented in adipose tissue, skeletal muscle and heart; agonists are in early clinical trials
PPAR-γ1	Widespread at low levels		
PPAR-γ2	Adipose tissue	*Positive:* Factors involved in adipocyte differentiation Adipose tissue FABP (also known as aP2) Lipoprotein lipase Fatty acid transport protein Acyl CoA synthase GLUT4 Phosphoenolpyruvate carboxykinase *Negative:* Leptin	Target for the thiazolidinedione insulin-sensitizing agents

[a] Also known as PPAR-β, NUC 1, FAAR (fatty-acid activated receptor).
CPT-1, carnitine palmitoyltransferase-1; FABP, fatty acid binding protein; GLUT4, insulin-regulated glucose transporter; HDL, high-density lipoprotein.
Source: Gurr MI, Harwood JL, Frayn KN (2002). *Lipid biochemistry*, 5th edition. Blackwell Scientific, Oxford.

output is therefore rapidly suppressed and converted to an uptake of glucose. At the same time, utilization of glucose by insulin-sensitive peripheral tissues such as skeletal muscle and adipose tissue is increased. The main mechanism of this short-term change is the recruitment of the insulin-regulated glucose transporter GLUT4 to the cell membrane (Fig. 11.1.1). However, the reduction in concentration of plasma nonesterified fatty acids (see following paragraphs) will also remove inhibition of glucose uptake caused by fatty acid oxidation. Within muscle, glycolysis and glycogen synthesis will be stimulated by insulin. In adipose tissue, increased glucose uptake provides glycerol 3-phosphate (formed from glycolysis) for esterification of fatty acids (see following paragraphs). Thus, insulin is the key regulator of the rapid changes that occur in glucose metabolism in the postprandial state: it brings about glucose storage as glycogen, and promotes the utilization of glucose at the expense of fatty acids.

Fat metabolism in the postabsorptive and postprandial states

Forms of fat in the circulation

Fatty acids circulate in various forms: as nonesterified fatty acids, in triacylglycerol (triglyceride), esterified to glycerol in phospholipids, and esterified to cholesterol as cholesteryl esters. The first two are involved in energy metabolism. The main carriers of triacylglycerol in the circulation are the triacylglycerol-rich lipoproteins: chylomicrons secreted from the small intestine and transporting dietary fat, and very low density lipoprotein (VLDL) particles secreted from the liver, transporting endogenous triacylglycerol. In the postabsorptive state, chylomicron triacylglycerol secretion is virtually zero. Secretion of VLDL is a means of exporting fat from the liver to peripheral tissues. In these tissues it is hydrolysed by the enzyme lipoprotein lipase (EC 3.1.1.34) situated in the capillaries of skeletal muscle, adipose tissue, mammary glands, and other tissues that use fatty acids. Lipoprotein lipase acts on the circulating triacylglycerol-rich particles to liberate fatty acids which may diffuse into the parenchymal cells (muscle fibres, adipocytes, etc.). Lipoprotein lipase in skeletal muscle is down-regulated by insulin, whereas that in adipose tissue is up-regulated by insulin. In the postabsorptive state, muscle lipoprotein lipase is likely to predominate as the site of removal of triacylglycerol from the VLDL particles. The fatty acids can then be used as an oxidative fuel by the muscle. In this process, VLDL particles lose their triacylglycerol core and become relatively enriched with cholesterol and phospholipids. After several cycles through such capillary beds, they are reduced to simple particles with a core of cholesteryl ester and an outer phospholipid shell: they become low density lipoprotein (LDL) particles, the main carrier of cholesterol in the circulation.

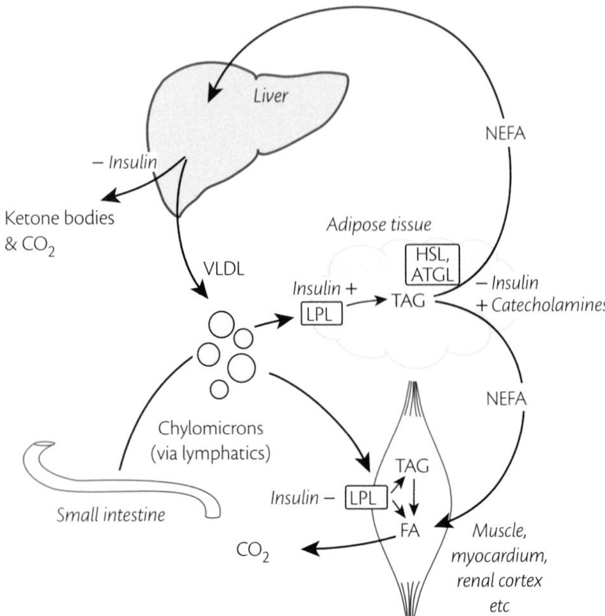

Fig. 11.1.3 Overview of fat metabolism. Dietary triacylglycerol (TAG) enters the circulation in the form of chylomicrons. Fatty acids are taken up by tissues through the action of the enzyme lipoprotein lipase (LPL). Adipose tissue TAG is the major store. It is mobilized in times of energy demand by the enzymes adipose triglyceride lipase (ATGL) and hormone-sensitive lipase (HSL), liberating nonesterified fatty acids (NEFA) into the circulation, from where they may be taken up by a number of tissues and used for synthesis of new TAG and for oxidation. Major points of hormonal regulation are shown (italic).

Nonesterified fatty acids and 'energy transport'

Fat is mobilized from adipose tissue stores in the form of nonesterified fatty acids (Fig. 11.1.3). The adipocyte has a central droplet of triacylglycerol, which is hydrolysed by intracellular enzymes, hormone-sensitive lipase and the newly identified adipose triglyceride lipase (ATGL), releasing glycerol and nonesterified fatty acids. These fatty acids are liberated into the plasma bound to albumin for transport to other tissues, including liver and skeletal muscle. Hormone-sensitive lipase is stimulated by catecholamines but powerfully suppressed by insulin, each exerting control over reversible phosphorylation (see Fig. 11.1.3): insulin leads to dephosphorylation and deactivation. Thus, fat mobilization is active in the postabsorptive state when there is a call upon the body's fat stores. It is also activated during exercise, mainly by catecholamine stimulation. The turnover of nonesterified fatty acids in the plasma is rapid. They are the major oxidative fuel in muscle after overnight fast (glucose supplies only around 5% of the oxidative fuel for resting skeletal muscle in the postabsportive state). In the liver, fatty acids are both a fuel for oxidation and a substrate for synthesis of triacylglycerol that will be exported as VLDL. A typical concentration of nonesterified fatty acids in the plasma after overnight fast is 500 μmol/litre, one-tenth that of glucose, but because of their rapid turnover and their larger molecular mass fatty acids account for about twice the energy turnover of glucose in the circulation.

Disposition of dietary fat

Dietary fat is almost entirely (typically 95% or more) in the form of triacylglycerol. A typical meal might contain 30 to 40 g of fat. The typical plasma triacylglycerol concentration in a healthy subject is 1 mmol/litre, confined to the vascular space; this means that about 3 g of triacylglycerol is present in the circulation. Therefore, as in the case of glucose, the amount in a meal could overwhelm the system unless coordinated mechanisms come into play to ensure its rapid dispersion.

Dietary triacylglycerol is digested in the stomach and small intestine and packaged by the enterocytes of the duodenum and proximal jejunum into chylomicrons, which enter the circulation via the lymphatics (Fig. 11.1.3). Therefore, unlike other nutrients absorbed from the small intestine, they bypass the liver on first passage. The chylomicrons also carry other lipid constituents of food, including cholesterol and fat-soluble vitamins. In the circulation their fate is similar to that of VLDL particles, although the tissue-specific regulation of lipoprotein lipase ensures that adipose tissue (where lipoprotein lipase is up-regulated by insulin) is a major site of clearance of their triacylglycerol. The pathway of triacylglycerol synthesis in adipocytes, as in the liver, is stimulated by insulin. Therefore, there is a short and energy-efficient pathway for storage of dietary fatty acids in adipose tissue (Fig. 11.1.3). The half-life of chylomicron triacylglycerol in the circulation is about 5 min. After hydrolysis of most of the triacylglycerol, the remnant particles are removed by receptors in the liver and other tissues. Thus dietary cholesterol, which remains in the remnant particles along with fat-soluble vitamins, is transported mainly to the liver.

Provided that a meal contains carbohydrate or protein, stimulation of insulin secretion will rapidly suppress the mobilization of adipose tissue fat stores, and concentrations of nonesterified fatty acids in the plasma fall after a meal. Therefore utilization of fatty acids by tissues such as skeletal muscle and liver will be reduced simply by lack of availability. This reduces competition for oxidation in muscle, further increasing glucose utilization. In liver, the lack of nonesterified fatty acids is likely to decrease the secretion of VLDL triacylglycerol. Insulin appears also to suppress VLDL triacylglycerol secretion directly. This is somewhat controversial, and the effects of insulin may be different in the acute, postprandial situation from the situation of prolonged hyperinsulinaemia (as in insulin resistance). Within the liver, insulin powerfully stimulates esterification of fatty acids (for triacylglycerol synthesis) at the expense of oxidation of fatty acids (see following paragraphs), so the suppressive effect of insulin on VLDL triacylglycerol secretion can only be short term. Nevertheless, it seems an exact parallel with the suppression of hepatic glucose output by insulin.

Inter-relationships between carbohydrate and fat metabolism

Links between carbohydrate and fat

In mammals, fat cannot be converted to glucose in a net sense. Glucose can, however, be converted to fat. Acetyl CoA produced by pyruvate dehydrogenase leaves the mitochondrion (it is transported across the mitochondrial membrane as citrate), and is then a substrate for the pathway of *de novo* lipogenesis, which begins with the enzyme acetyl CoA carboxylase (EC 6.4.1.2), forming malonyl CoA. At one time it was believed that *de novo* lipogenesis was a major route for laying down storage fat. Although this may be true in rodents, recent measurements have shown that this pathway makes a quantitatively small contribution to triacylglycerol synthesis in humans. Instead, almost all the triacylglycerol that we deposit in adipose tissue arises from dietary fatty acids, taken up from circulating triacylglycerol-rich lipoproteins by the lipoprotein lipase pathway (Fig. 11.1.3).

The lack of quantitatively significant interconversion of carbohydrate and fat has led to the suggestion that we may view carbohydrate and fat balance as independent. This view is entirely erroneous. Despite the lack of interconversion, carbohydrate balance strongly influences fat balance, and vice versa. These influences occur at a number of levels.

Principal amongst these is carbohydrate-induced insulin secretion. Insulin, as outlined earlier (Fig. 11.1.3), acutely suppresses the release of nonesterified fatty acids from adipose tissue. Therefore, when carbohydrate is readily available, fat stores are conserved. In the longer term, ingestion of a high-carbohydrate diet will induce enzymes of fat synthesis and down-regulate enzymes of fatty acid oxidation, through insulin- and carbohydrate-response elements in the promoter regions of the relevant genes (see Fig. 11.1.2 and Table 11.1.3).

Glucose–fatty acid cycle

Beyond this, there are specific cellular mechanisms that regulate the relative oxidation of carbohydrate and fat. These probably operate in a number of tissues, although they have been most studied in skeletal and heart muscle and in liver. In 1963, Philip Randle and colleagues described the glucose–fatty acid cycle, which encompasses one aspect of this mutual relationship between carbohydrate and fat oxidation. It is summarized in Fig. 11.1.4. The concept was based upon observations that availability of fatty acids reduced the oxidation of glucose in skeletal and cardiac muscle. The precise mechanism has been disputed, but the basic observation has been confirmed many times. The glucose–fatty acid cycle describes both the normal interplay between fat and carbohydrate oxidation, and also pathological situations involving excess availability of fat and insulin resistance (e.g. type 2 diabetes and obesity).

Glucose and the regulation of fatty acid oxidation

An additional mechanism was first described in 1977 by Denis McGarry and Daniel Foster. They were following up a long-standing observation that the generation of ketone bodies by the liver was suppressed by insulin. They showed that malonyl CoA, the first committed intermediate in the pathway of *de novo* lipogenesis (produced by acetyl CoA carboxylase; see above), strongly inhibits fatty acid oxidation. This inhibition is mediated via the enzyme carnitine palmitoyltransferase-1 in the mitochondrial membrane. Carnitine palmitoyltransferase-1 is responsible for the transport of fatty acids from the cytoplasm to the mitochondrion for β-oxidation. Acetyl CoA carboxylase is activated by insulin (both by increased gene transcription and by reversible dephosphorylation). Hence, in a carbohydrate-replete state, malonyl CoA will be formed and fatty acid oxidation inhibited (Fig. 11.1.5).

This is now recognized as a widespread regulatory mechanism. There are two isoforms of acetyl CoA carboxylase. Acetyl CoA carboxylase 1, expressed in lipogenic tissues such as liver and adipose tissue, is involved in *de novo* fatty acid synthesis. Acetyl CoA carboxylase 2 is expressed more in tissues oxidizing fatty acids such as heart and skeletal muscle and is thought to produce malonyl CoA for regulatory, rather than synthetic, purposes. Muscle carnitine palmitoyltransferase-1 is more sensitive to inhibition by malonyl CoA than is the liver enzyme. The ability of glucose to inhibit the oxidation of fatty acids in muscle has been clearly demonstrated *in vivo*, and has been termed the 'reverse glucose–fatty acid cycle'.

Protein and amino acid metabolism and their regulation

Since there are 20 different amino acids incorporated into protein, and a variety of other amino acids that have important biological roles, it is essential here to generalize somewhat about amino acid and protein metabolism.

The body pools of protein and amino acids, and their turnover, are summarized in Fig. 11.1.6. Insulin exerts a net anabolic role on body protein, mainly in skeletal muscle, whereas thyroid hormones and cortisol are generally catabolic. Anabolism is also stimulated

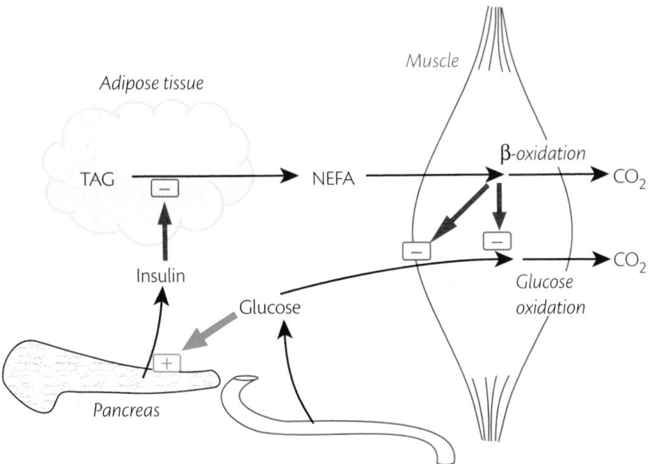

Fig. 11.1.4 The glucose–fatty acid cycle. When glucose and insulin concentrations are high, release of nonesterified fatty acids (NEFA) from adipose tissue is suppressed, and glucose utilization predominates in insulin-sensitive tissues such as skeletal muscle. In the fasting state (glucose and insulin concentrations are low) NEFA utilization predominates, reinforced by inhibitory effects of the products of β-oxidation of fatty acids on glucose uptake and oxidation. This may have pathological significance in that states in which NEFA concentrations tend to be high (e.g. type 2 diabetes) will be associated with resistance of glucose utilization to insulin.

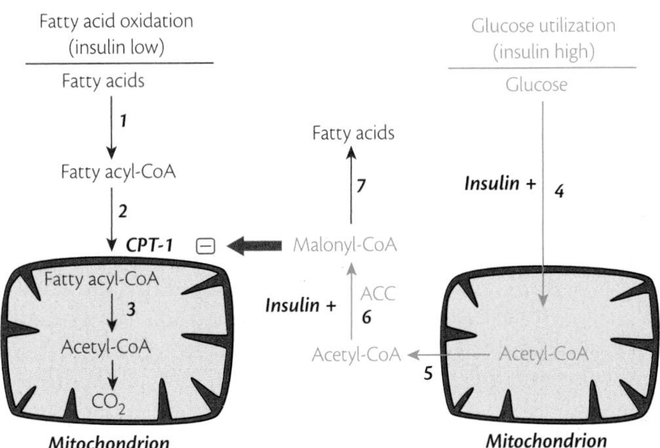

Fig. 11.1.5 The inhibition of fatty acid oxidation when glucose and insulin concentrations are high. Pathways are: (1) fatty acid 'activation' (fatty acyl CoA synthase); (2) transfer of acyl CoA into the mitochondrion via carnitine palmitoyltransferase-1 (CPT-1); (3) β-oxidation; (4) glycolysis (cytosolic) followed by pyruvate dehydrogenase (mitochondrial); (5) transfer of acetyl CoA to the cytosol via citrate (details not shown); (6) acetyl CoA carboxylase (ACC) to form malonyl CoA, which is a powerful inhibitor of CPT-1; (7) fatty acid synthesis (not expressed in all tissues in which this mechanism operates, e.g. skeletal muscle).

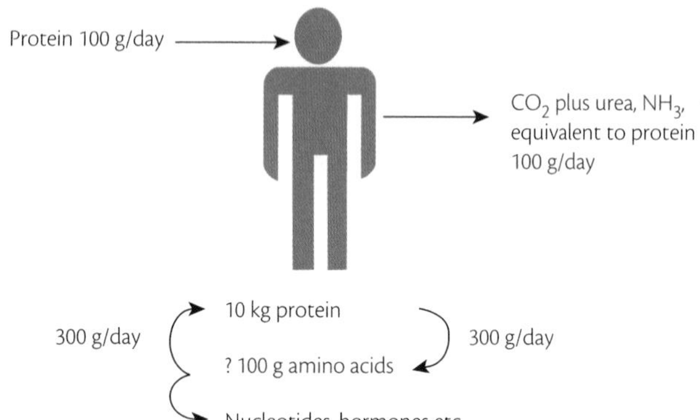

Fig. 11.1.6 The body pools of protein and amino acids, and their turnover. Figures are approximate.

by anabolic steroids, by physical training, and during growth by the insulin-like growth factors.

Dietary protein, digested in the small intestine and absorbed as free amino acids and short peptides, enters the portal vein. In the enterocytes of the small intestine, some amino acids, especially glutamine, are removed for use as an oxidative fuel. The remaining products of digestion next enter the liver, where further preferential extraction takes place. Amino acid oxidation is, under most circumstances, the major oxidative pathway in the liver. About 60% of incoming amino acids may be directed into immediate oxidation. The rate of hepatic protein synthesis is also high, and since much of the protein is secreted (e.g. albumin), this represents a net loss of amino acids from the liver (perhaps a further 20% of the incoming amino acids). The remaining mixture of amino acids, around 20% of those absorbed, enters the systemic circulation. This mixture is enriched in the branched chain amino acids leucine, isoleucine, and valine, which have a special role in muscle.

Urea synthesis takes place only in the liver. (The pathway is present in the brain, but this is not a significant site of blood urea production.) Therefore, amino acids released from proteolysis in peripheral tissues must transfer their amino nitrogen to the liver. This results in considerable interaction between the pathways of amino acid, carbohydrate, and fat metabolism. Measurements of arteriovenous differences across muscle and adipose tissue show that the release of the amino acids alanine and glutamine predominates. Since glutamine carries two nitrogens it is, under most circumstances, the predominant carrier of nitrogen. Arteriovenous difference measurements across the splanchnic bed (by catheterization of the hepatic vein) show an almost identical pattern for uptake: removal of alanine and glutamine far exceeds that of other amino acids. Therefore amino acids in tissues including muscle and adipose tissue must transfer their amino nitrogen to alanine (by transamination with pyruvate) and glutamine (formed from glutamate, itself arising by transamination with 2-oxoglutarate). Aminotransferases (transaminases) bring about this transfer. It is important that the 2-oxoacid acceptors, pyruvate and 2-oxoglutarate, are common metabolic intermediates and thus readily available.

Much of the alanine released from skeletal muscle comes from transamination of pyruvate formed in glycolysis. Within the liver, the amino group can be transferred further, e.g. to oxaloacetate, forming aspartate, which is one of the immediate donors of nitrogen to the urea cycle. The pyruvate thus formed may be a substrate for gluconeogenesis, producing glucose that can be recycled to peripheral tissues. This metabolic cycle has been called the glucose–alanine cycle. It closely parallels the Cori cycle (see Fig. 11.1.1).

The other route of entry of nitrogen into the urea cycle is via ammonia. In peripheral tissues ammonia may be formed by the oxidative deamination of glutamate, catalysed by glutamate dehydrogenase (EC 1.4.1.2). This reaction, in combination with the aminotransferases, can be seen to capture amino nitrogen from a number of amino acids. However, blood ammonia concentrations are very low (it is highly toxic) and instead it seems to be fixed in the amido group of glutamine by the enzyme glutamine synthetase. In the liver, the ammonia required for the urea cycle may be formed from the amido nitrogen of glutamine, removed by the enzyme glutaminase (EC 3.5.1.2), or by the oxidative deamination of glutamate. There is also a supply of ammonia from the small intestine.

An important aspect of the large store of muscle protein is that it represents a potential source of synthesis of new glucose during fasting. In that situation, while the brain continues to require glucose for oxidation, and as glycogen reserves are depleted, new glucose can only be formed from glycerol, released in adipose tissue lipolysis, and from amino acids. The pathways described earlier are for the transfer of nitrogen, but not necessarily of carbon, to the liver. To explain the latter, pathways must exist whereby amino acid carbon can also be exported. Amino acids whose 2-oxoacid can enter the tricarboxylic acid cycle may generate pyruvate (which can also accept amino nitrogen to become alanine). Pairs of amino acids can provide all the carbons necessary for glutamine synthesis.

Further reading

Barish GD, Narkar VA, Evans RM (2006). PPARδ: a dagger in the heart of the metabolic syndrome. *J Clin Invest* **116**, 590–7.

Barthel A, Schmoll D (2003). Novel concepts in insulin regulation of hepatic gluconeogenesis. *Am J Physiol Endocrinol Metab*, **285**, E685–E692.

Feige JN *et al.* (2006). From molecular action to physiological outputs: peroxisome proliferator-activated receptors are nuclear receptors at the crossroads of key cellular functions. *Prog Lipid Res*, **45**, 120–59.

Frayn KN (2010). *Metabolic regulation: a human perspective*, 3rd edition. Wiley/Blackwell, Oxford.

Frayn KN, Arner P, Yki-Järvinen H (2006). Fatty acid metabolism in adipose tissue, muscle and liver in health and disease. *Essays Biochem*, **42**, 89–103.

Jousse C *et al.* (2004). Amino acids as regulators of gene expression: molecular mechanisms. *Biochem Biophys Res Commun*, **313**, 447–52.

Liu Z, Barrett EJ (2002). Human protein metabolism: its measurement and regulation. *Am J Physiol Endocrinol Metab*, **283**, E1105–E1112.

Long YC, Zierath JR (2006). AMP-activated protein kinase signaling in metabolic regulation. *J Clin Invest*, **116**, 1776–83.

McGarry, JD (2002). Banting lecture 2001: dysregulation of fatty acid metabolism in the etiology of type 2 diabetes. *Diabetes*, **51**, 7–18.

Nonogaki K (2000). New insights into sympathetic regulation of glucose and fat metabolism. *Diabetologia*, **43**, 533–49.

O'Brien RM *et al.* (2001). Insulin-regulated gene expression. *Biochem Soc Trans*, **29**, 552–8.

Pégorier JP, Le May C, Girard J (2004). Control of gene expression by fatty acids. *J Nutr*, **134**, 2444S–2449S.

Rosen ED, Spiegelman BM (2006). Adipocytes as regulators of energy balance and glucose homeostasis. *Nature*, **444**, 847–53.

Uyeda K, Repa JJ (2006). Carbohydrate response element binding protein, ChREBP, a transcription factor coupling hepatic glucose utilization and lipid synthesis. *Cell Metab*, **4**, 107–10.

11.2

Vitamins and trace elements

J. Powell-Tuck and M. Eastwood

Essentials

Vitamins

Vitamins are diverse, unrelated organic compounds that some higher animals, humans included, cannot synthesize and which play key roles in metabolism, underpinning the most crucial of biological reactions. They are required in small amounts and have diverse functions, e.g. as:

- activated carriers of biochemical groups—coenzymes (B vitamin derivatives)
- antioxidants (vitamins A, C and E, carotenoids)
- precursors of visual pigments (vitamin A)
- endocrine mediators, especially in calcium and phosphorus metabolism (vitamin D)
- facilitators of blood clotting (vitamin K)

The clinical importance of vitamins lies not only in overt deficiency syndromes, which develop because of persistent inadequate intake or absorption over different periods of time depending upon body storage, but also in the need for optimal intakes to maintain health. This latter role can be difficult to assess for individual nutrients, but is inferred from knowledge of the beneficial and harmful effects of diets containing particular foods.

The traditional classification of vitamins into water and lipid soluble, and by their associated deficiency conditions, becomes less useful as their biochemical roles are better understood. An inadequate dietary vitamin intake will result in specific cellular failure and even death.

Vitamins as biochemical cofactors

Oxygen is the final electron acceptor when food is oxidized, but the transfer from energy substrate to oxygen is not direct; it occurs via intermediaries, important among which are molecules such as nicotinamide adenine dinucleotide (NAD) or flavin adenine dinucleotide (FAD) derived from the B vitamins niacin and riboflavin respectively.

Other metabolically crucial fragments require activated carriage, e.g. thiamine is a carrier for aldehyde groups, folate for one-carbon groups, and coenzyme A (pantothenate) carries two-carbon (acetyl) fragments into the tricarboxylic acid cycle. Thus a small group of molecules derived from the B vitamins is responsible for diverse biochemical interchanges. The stability of these carrier molecules in the absence of catalysts enables enzymes to control the flow of free energy and reducing power.

Vitamins as antioxidants

Although molecular oxygen is an ideal final electron acceptor, 'danger lurks in the reduction of O_2'. Partial reduction, particularly the transfer of single electrons to form superoxide or two electrons to form peroxide, yields potentially damaging products or reactive oxygen species. White cells use this process to kill pathogens, and most cells are protected from it by antioxidants, particularly the enzyme superoxide dismutase—an enzyme that contains manganese in the enzyme's mitochondrial form and copper and zinc in the cytoplasmic forms. The antioxidant vitamins C and E are also important in this process, with fat-soluble vitamin E functioning particularly to protect membranes from lipid peroxidation. NADPH generated by glucose-6-phosphate dehydrogenase maintains levels of reduced glutathione.

Intake of vitamins

There is a dose–response effect of vitamin intake, ranging from the physiological through the pharmacological to the toxic. Recommendations for vitamin intake for different ages, needs, and communities are based on dietary intake, bioavailability, steady-state concentrations in plasma and tissue at defined intakes, urine excretion, adverse effects, biochemical and molecular function, and freedom from deficiency. With increasing intake, either orally or as an infusion, a vitamin is distributed through the body fluids and tissues until the saturation point is exceeded.

Some artificial enteral supplements and feeds and most parenteral feeds are deficient in vitamins unless appropriately supplemented: it is the responsibility of the prescriber to ensure that appropriate vitamin intake is maintained during artificial feeding. The prescription of vitamins parenterally, bypassing the absorptive processes, also has dosage implications.

Trace elements

Trace elements (e.g. magnesium, iron, zinc, copper, manganese, fluoride, selenium, molybdenum, chromium, iodine) are essential nutrients that act as cofactors in enzyme oxidation–reduction reactions. They maintain the specific configuration of proteins, are incorporated into the structure of hormones, and play a structural and catalytic role in gene expression and transcriptional regulation.

Deficiency of trace elements can cause a very wide range of clinical problems, including anaemia from iron deficiency and goitre resulting from iodine deficiency, which is endemic in mountainous areas.

Historical background

Our understanding of the role of vitamins comes from clinical observations, nutritional experiments in animals, and studies using purified preparations of the active principle used to treat deficiency states. Early pioneers differentiated dietary deficiency from infection and other causes of disease. Scurvy was once the scourge of mariners and explorers, but the clinical trials of Lind (1753), confirmed by Captain Cook on his voyages, showed the benefits of citrus fruits. Many years later, Holst and Froelich (1907) produced scurvy in guinea-pigs by dietary deprivation.

Rickets arose in sun-starved urban slums, and Trousseau noted the beneficial effects of cod liver oil (1860). Ejikmann and Grijns fed chickens the same diet as their patients who had beriberi (1897); neuropathy in the chickens resolved when the diet contained whole-grain, rather than polished, rice. In the 1900s, Gowland Hopkins, the discoverer of vitamins, described a fat-soluble, essential growth accessory food factor A in milk. This was differentiated from water-soluble accessory food factor B by McCollum and Davis. Mellanby treated rickets in puppies with a fat-soluble food factor D. In 1931 Lucy Wills described the megaloblastic anaemia of pregnancy, which is now known to be caused by a deficiency of folic acid.

In 1894, Atwater published a table of food composition and dietary standards for the United States of America. The first *USA Recommended Daily Allowances* was published in 1941. Food rationing in the United Kingdom during the Second World War was a triumph for the science of applied nutrition. The natural development of this work was the emergence of recommended daily intakes that recognized the differing requirements of the young and growing, pregnant and lactating, middle-aged and old, and ill; with this, developed the concept of the optimal intake for optimal nutritional status. The isolation and chemical synthesis of the vitamins and their active principles provided formidable challenges to scientists, rewarded by eight Nobel prizes in medicine and physiology and four in chemistry.

The carotenoids illustrate the complexity of vitamins in physiology and pharmacology, and as toxins. Carotenoids are used by archaebacteria to reinforce cell membranes, their long, rigid carbon backbone acting as a rivet across the membrane. The polyene chain of between 9 and 11 double bonds serves to harvest light energy in plants, and, as the pigment retinal, is a visual pigment in animals. The linear system of conjugated C=C bonds make for a high reducing and antioxidant potential. Carotenoids act as the coloration in plants and to protect egg proteins against the enzymatic activity of proteases. Retinoic acid in animals and abscisic acid in plants act as hormones. When retinoids and carotenoids were used in lung cancer chemoprevention trials, the incidence of cancer increased; this was ascribed possibly to the increase in the oxidized products of β-carotene. A mix of vitamins and antioxidants might prevent such oxidation. Such a mix can be found in fruit and vegetables, which emphasizes the benefit of a good diet containing five portions (60 to 150 g) of fruit and vegetables a day.

An inadequate dietary vitamin intake will result in specific cellular failure and even death. There is a dose–response relationship with vitamin intake from the physiological through the pharmacological to the toxic. Recommendations for vitamin intake for different ages, needs, and communities are based on dietary intake, bioavailability, steady-state concentrations in plasma and tissue at defined intakes, urine excretion, adverse effects, biochemical and molecular function, and freedom from deficiency. With increasing intake, either orally or as an infusion, a vitamin is distributed through the body fluids and tissues until the saturation point is exceeded. The prescription of vitamins parenterally, bypassing the absorptive processes, also has dosage implications.

The traditional classification of vitamins into water-soluble and lipid-soluble and by their associated deficiency conditions becomes less useful as their biochemical roles are better understood, but is still widely used and is adopted here for that reason.

Vitamins as biochemical cofactors

Oxygen is the final electron acceptor when food is oxidized, but the transfer of electrons from energy substrate to oxygen is not direct; it occurs via intermediaries, important among which are molecules such as nicotinamide adenine dinucleotide (NAD) or flavin adenine dinucleotide (FAD) derived from the B vitamins niacin and riboflavin respectively. Other metabolically crucial fragments require activated carriage. For example, coenzyme A, derived from pantothenic acid, carries two-carbon (acetyl) fragments into the tricarboxylic acid cycle. Thiamine is a carrier for aldehyde groups, folate for one-carbon groups, and coenzyme A (pantothenate) for acyl groups. Thus, a small group of molecules derived from the B vitamins is responsible for diverse biochemical interchanges. The stability of these carrier molecules in the absence of catalysts enables enzymes to control the flow of free energy and reducing power.

Vitamins as antioxidants

As Stryer and colleagues have noted, although molecular oxygen is an ideal final electron acceptor, 'danger lurks in the reduction of O_2'. Partial reduction, particularly the transfer of single electrons to form superoxide or two electrons to form peroxide, yields potentially damaging products or reactive oxygen species. White cells use this process to kill pathogens. Most cells are protected from this process by antioxidants, particularly the enzyme superoxide dismutase (EC 1.15.1.1)—an enzyme that contains manganese in the mitochondrial form and copper and zinc in the cytoplasmic forms. The antioxidant vitamins, vitamin C and vitamin E, also are important in this process, with fat-soluble vitamin E functioning particularly to protect membranes from lipid peroxidation.

NADPH generated by glucose-6-phosphate dehydrogenase (EC 1.1.1.49) maintains levels of reduced glutathione.

Water-soluble vitamins

Vitamin C (ascorbic acid)

L-Xyloascorbic acid is the naturally occurring form of vitamin C. The active forms are L-ascorbic acid and L-dehydroascorbate to which it is reversibly oxidized. Further oxidation to 2–3 diketo-L-gulonic acid and oxalate is irreversible. Vitamin C is labile; it is oxidized by removal of two electrons, producing the ascorbate free radical and then dehydroascorbate. The fairly unreactive ascorbate free radical acts as a free radical chain terminator. Importantly, it is widely distributed through the body's aqueous fluids. In contact with membranes, it maintains vitamin E, which is fat soluble, in its reduced form. The interaction between ascorbate iron and copper is important. Ascorbic acid is a strong antioxidant and reduces ferric (Fe^{3+}) and cupric (Cu^{2+}) ions to ferrous (Fe^{2+}) and cuprous (Cu^{+}), and reduces oxygen to superoxide (O_2^-) and hydrogen peroxide (H_2O_2). Paradoxically, Fe^{2+} and Cu^{+} act as pro-oxidants by forming OH from superoxide and hydrogen peroxide.

Ascorbic acid:

- is a water-soluble, non-specific radical-trapping antioxidant and reducing agent, which is present in all tissues
- acts synergistically with vitamin E
- is needed to maintain the activity of copper-containing hydroxylase enzymes such as prolyl hydroxylase, an enzyme that requires Fe^{2+} to activate oxygen. (Oxidation of the iron deactivates the enzyme—ascorbate reduces the inactivated enzyme's Fe^{3+}, reactivating it by functioning as an antioxidant. Collagen formed in the absence of ascorbate is less stable than normal collagen, which explains many of the signs of clinical scurvy, e.g. the bleeding gums.)
- is involved in carnitine biosynthesis from lysine, which is necessary for transport of long-chain fatty acids from the cytosol into mitochondria
- is involved in the synthesis of catecholamines
- is involved in the function of cytochrome P450 microsomal enzymes

Dietary sources of ascorbic acid are fresh fruit and fruit juices, especially blackcurrants, guavas, green leafy vegetables, and fresh milk. Ascorbic acid is readily oxidized during cooking—a process accelerated by traces of copper in alkaline solution. Since humans, guinea-pigs, the Indian fruit-eating bat, the red vented bulbul, and some birds are unable to synthesize ascorbic acid, it represents a vitamin in these species.

Ascorbic acid is rapidly absorbed from the small intestine. The plasma concentration (5% as dehydroascorbate) and dietary intake are in a sigmoidal relationship (80 μmol/litre or 100 mg/day) which plateaus at 1000 mg/day intake. The body pool size is 900 mg (5 mmol/litre in the normal adult): approximately 3%, irrespective of pool size, is degraded each day and excreted in the urine as free ascorbic acid, dehydroascorbate, or diketogulonate. High tissue concentrations at birth steadily decline with increasing age.

A shortfall in vitamin C intake without clinical scurvy may be associated with a reduction in the body's water-soluble antioxidant capacity, the consequences of which are still being debated. A large-scale prospective study among a representative sample of people aged 75 to 84 demonstrated blood ascorbate's strong predictive power of mortality over a 4.4 year follow-up. In this British study, 232 of 1175 subjects had plasma ascorbate levels of less than 17 μmol/litre, the lowest quintile. Young people and elderly people are particularly at risk of scurvy, which results from an inadequate intake of ascorbic acid. Clinical scurvy appears after 4 weeks on an ascorbic acid-deficient diet when the body pool is less than 300 mg (1.7 mmol/litre). There is a failure of connective tissue collagen synthesis, and cartilage, bone, and dentine growth are all compromised. Tissues bleed readily, and heal poorly due to defective intracellular linkages between the endothelial cells and capillary basement tissue. Individuals are initially lethargic and irritable. Characteristic livid-coloured, spongy, bleeding gingivitis of the gums develops, and scurvy buds appear in the papillae between the teeth. Large or microscopic haemorrhages occur in the gums, as well as in the eyes (especially bulbar conjunctiva), subcutaneous tissues, synovia of joints, and beneath the periosteum of bones. Perifollicular bleeding occurs in the dependent parts of the body, later becoming more generalized. Fatal haemorrhages may also occur in the brain or heart muscle. Keratin-like material heaps on the surface of hair follicles, through which a deformed corkscrew hair projects. Other signs include dependent oedema, oliguria, depression, megaloblastic or normoblastic anaemia, and superinfection. Infants present with irritability, tender legs, and pseudoparalysis. Scurvy buds, but not gingivitis, occur in edentulous infants. Large subperiosteal haemorrhages develop over the long bones, especially the femur.

Diagnosis requires an awareness of the condition, a careful dietary history, and a clinical examination. The patient can improve on hospital diet alone. Ascorbic acid is measured in plasma or whole blood. While leucocyte or buffy-coat vitamin C concentrations reflect tissue concentrations, this is complicated in disease by different leucocytes types, which vary in number and ascorbic acid content, but a lower limit of 15 μg/10^8 cells is frequently accepted as an indicator of deficiency. Plasma vitamin C is more sensitive to recent change in intake with values less than 11 μmol/litre(0.2 μg/100 ml) indicative of depletion.

Requirements

The optimum dietary intake of ascorbic acid has yet to be defined. The body can be saturated with 1 g/day for 5 days. Recommendations for dietary intake range from 40 to 200 mg per day. An upper limit of intake is recommended at 1 to 2 g/day, based upon body saturation figures rather than toxicity. The dietary reference values for adults of both sexes over the age of 19 are 10 mg/day (lower reference nutrient intake), 25 mg/day (estimated average requirement) and 40 mg/day (reference nutrient intake). During pregnancy and lactation, intake should be increased by 10 mg/day and 30 mg/day, respectively. The ascorbic acid content of breast milk varies between 30 and 80 mg/litre, which provides 25 mg/day; clinical scurvy has not been observed in fully breastfed infants. The pharmacological use of ascorbic acid is extensive and imaginative.

B vitamins

The first two B vitamins to be considered, riboflavin and niacin, function as fundamental electron carriers into and within the mitochondrion. There are four sites of entry of electrons into the electron transport system: one for NADH (complex 1) and three for $FADH_2$ (complex II). Flavoproteins are major components of mitochondrial complexes I and II, which transfer electrons through flavin mononucleotide (FMN) and iron–sulphur complexes to ubiquinone. Ubiquinone transfers electrons to complex III, a cytochrome/iron/sulphur enzyme complex. We shall return to iron later in the chapter. The flow of electrons to oxygen to form water, pumps protons out of the mitochondrion and produces a proton gradient which enables synthesis of ATP.

Storage of B vitamins in the body is poor, with the exception of B_{12}, and deficiencies occur early in the presence of reduced intake. Biochemical, mixed deficiencies of B vitamins are common among patients admitted as an emergency to hospital and also among alcoholics.

Riboflavin (vitamin B_2)

Riboflavin is a substituted alloxazine ring linked to ribotol, an alcohol derived from the pentose sugar ribose. It is light sensitive. Riboflavin links with phosphoric acid as FMN (or riboflavin 5′-phosphate), which, with adenosine monophosphate (AMP), forms flavin adenine dinucleotide (FAD). FMN and FAD are the prosthetic groups of the flavoprotein enzymes. Flavoproteins are involved in redox processes involving the hydrogen transfer chain in the mitochondria and the production of ATP. FAD/FMN acts as a coenzyme in oxidation–reduction reactions, electron transport, oxidative phosphorylation (e.g. succinic dehydrogenases), and β-oxidation of fatty acids.

Dietary sources are liver, milk, cheese, eggs, some green vegetables, and beer. Other sources are yeast extracts (e.g. Marmite) and meat extracts (e.g. Bovril). Riboflavin in the diet exists in either the free form or the phosphorylated coenzyme form. Riboflavin is absorbed from the upper gastrointestinal tract, there is no specific storage tissue, and it is excreted in the urine either free or in small amounts of hydroxylated products. Chronic infection can affect urinary riboflavin excretion. A deficiency of riboflavin causes cheilosis, angular stomatitis, superficial interstitial keratosis of the cornea, and nasolabial seborrhoea. Riboflavin deficiency may impair iron absorption. No toxic effects have been shown for riboflavin.

Riboflavin status can be estimated from the urinary riboflavin:creatinine ratio, which is insensitive at low intakes. The erythrocyte glutathione reductase activation coefficient (EGRAC) is a functional test, which measures tissue saturation.

Requirements

Adults, including elderly people, need between 1 and 1.5 mg of riboflavin per day. The average riboflavin content of breast milk in Britain is approximately 0.3 mg/litre, which is dependent upon maternal intake. Intakes should increase by 0.3 mg/day during pregnancy and 0.5 mg/day during lactation. Recommended intakes for children range from 0.4 mg/day for infants up to 3 months of age and 1.0 mg/day thereafter.

Niacin: nicotinic acid and nicotinamide (vitamin B_3)

The term 'niacin' includes nicotinic acid and niotinamide. It occurs in food as nicotinic acid, as a pyridine nucleotide coenzyme derivative (NAD and NADP), as an amide, nicotinamide (niacinamide), or as a nicotinoyl ester, niacytin, in maize. Nicotinic acid is synthesized from tryptophan, catalysed by kynureninase and kynurenine hydroxylase, which are dependent on vitamin B_6 and riboflavin. A deficiency of either vitamin B_6 or riboflavin may aggravate niacin deficiency. Some 60 mg of dietary tryptophan generates 1 mg of nicotinic acid. The nicotinic acid equivalent is the dietary nicotinic acid content plus 1/60th of the dietary tryptophan. Nicotinamide is a component of the coenzymes nicotinamide adenine dinucleotide (NAD^+) and nicotinamide adenine dinucleotide phosphate ($NADP^+$) NAD coenzymes are biological carriers of reducing equivalents, i.e. electrons, during metabolic oxidation to NADH or NADPH. NAD^+ is a major electron carrier in the oxidation of fuel molecules during which it becomes reduced to NADH. The oxidation of NADH generates ATP. NADPH, the reduced form of $NADP^+$, is the electron donor in most reductive biosyntheses.

Nicotinic acid is found in meat, poultry, fish, wholemeal cereals, pulses, and coffee. The various conjugated forms of niacin are hydrolysed and absorbed in the upper gastrointestinal mucosa as the free acid. Niacytin from maize is neither hydrolysed nor absorbed. In Central America, maize is eaten as tortillas, in which lime water hydrolyses the nicotinoyl ester component. Niacin and tryptophan deficiencies occur in poor populations dependent upon maize for their protein intake. Zein, the principal maize protein, is deficient in tryptophan. Protein energy malnutrition, dietary amino acid imbalances (e.g. an excess leucine intake), anaemia, and other vitamin deficiencies worsen the problem. Dietary fortification with other proteins is necessary.

There is no apparent tissue storage of this vitamin. It is excreted in the urine as nicotinuric acid, nicotinamide-*N*-oxide, and 5′-methylnicotinamide. An inadequate dietary intake of niacin lasting for 1 to 2 months leads to significant tissue depletion and pellagra, which, if untreated, progresses to death. Pellagra is characterized by dermatitis, diarrhoea, and dementia; the disease is chronic, with a seasonal periodicity. Individuals suffer weight and stamina loss, which is worsened by secondary bacterial and parasitic infections. Erythematous dermatitis is symmetrically distributed on skin exposed to sunlight and mechanical irritation. In chronic pellagra, the skin looks sunburnt. In severe cases, gastrointestinal disturbances occur with diarrhoea. There can be glossitis, angular stomatitis, cheilosis, an inflamed tongue, and secondary infection of the mouth. Mild mental changes include anxiety and irritability progressing to manic depressive illness. There may be paraesthesia in the lower limbs, with loss of vibration sense and proprioception leading to ataxia and spasticity.

Pellagra can occur in alcoholism, malabsorption syndromes, and Hartnup disease. Mild cases rapidly improve on treatment with niacin or a suitable dietary protein supplementation. Oral nicotinamide (100 mg every 4 h) results in symptom resolution within 24 h, although mental symptoms, especially dementia, may be unresponsive to treatment. Nicotinic acid may cause unpleasant flushing and burning sensations. A supplementary diet containing good-quality protein and all of the vitamins is important. Nicotinic acid, but not nicotinamide, is used therapeutically for hyperlipidaemias at a dose of 2 to 6 g/day, but it can be hepatotoxic.

Microbiological methods provide the most sensitive means of measuring niacin and nicotinamide in serum, urine, and food. Alternatively, urinary nicotinamide, *n*-methyl nicotinamide (NMN), is measured over a defined time or as a ratio of creatine in urine. Urinary *N*-methyl-2-piridone-5-carboxamide (2-pyridone) excretion is a more sensitive measurement in borderline cases of nicotinamide deficiency, and is expressed in relation to urinary creatinine excretion.

Requirements

These are related to dietary tryptophan intake. A protein intake of between 60 and 85 g/day contains approximately 13 mg tryptophan/g, equivalent to between 13 and 18 mg/day of niacin. The recommended intake as niacin equivalents is 6.6 mg (54 µmol/litre)/4185 J (4.185 J = 1 kcal). Hormonal changes during pregnancy affect tryptophan metabolism, so that 30 mg of tryptophan is equivalent to 1 mg of dietary niacin. Breast milk should provide not less than 3.5 mg preformed niacin/4185 J. Mature human milk provides preformed niacin (2.7 mg/litre), therefore an increment of 2 mg/day niacin for the nursing mother is suggested.

Clinical use

Nicotinic acid is used pharmacologically in doses of 1.5 to 3.0 g/day as an adjunct to statins in dyslipidaemias. It lowers both cholesterol and triglyceride plasma concentrations by inhibiting synthesis and increases high density lipoprotein (HDL) concentrations. Caution is required in the clinical circumstances of unstable angina, acute myocardial infarction, diabetes mellitus, gout, history of peptic ulceration, hepatic impairment, renal impairment; and pregnancy. The dominant side effect is cutaneous flushing, with variable severity among patients; in addition, infrequent hepatic toxicity, hyperglycemia, gout, and rare retinal macular oedema have been reported Side effects can include diarrhoea, nausea, vomiting, abdominal pain, dyspepsia; flushing; pruritus, rash; less commonly tachycardia, palpitation, shortness of breath, peripheral oedema, headache, dizziness, increase in uric acid, hypophosphataemia, prolonged prothrombin time, and reduced platelet count; rarely hypotension, syncope, rhinitis, insomnia, reduced glucose tolerance, myalgia, myopathy, and myasthenia; very rarely anorexia, rhabdomyolysis. Niacin is experiencing renewed interest because it is the most effective currently available agent for raising HDL cholesterol and increasing lipoprotein particle size, it is the only lipid drug that lowers lipoprotein(a), and it is comparable with fibrates in achieving striking reductions in triglyceride levels.

The β-oxidation of fatty acids depends upon initial linkage to coenzyme A to form an acyl-CoA before being degraded to acetyl-CoA. Coenzyme A and carnitine shuttle acyl groups into the mitochondrion where acyl-CoA is degraded by a recurring sequence of reactions: oxidation by FAD, hydration, oxidation by NAD^+, and thiolysis by coenzyme A. In this way, the fatty acid chain length is shortened by two carbons and $FADH_2$, NADH, and acetyl-CoA are formed—an interplay of B vitamin functions. Niacin and riboflavin have already been discussed. A major component of coenzyme A is phosphopantetheine, a direct derivative of pantothenic acid.

Pantothenic acid (vitamin B_5)

Pantothenic acid functions as a crucial acyl (including acetyl) group carrier. Pantothenic acid is the dimethyl derivative of butyric acid joined by a peptide linkage to α-alanine. The active form, 4′-phosphopantetheine, is present in all tissues. 4′-Phosphopantetheine is a constituent of both coenzyme A and acyl carrier protein. As a major constituent of coenzyme A and acyl carrier protein. Pantothenic acid derivatives play a central role in metabolism. As acetyl Co A, it carries two carbon groups into the carboxyxlic acid cycle, thereby forming the final common pathway of the metabolism of fats, sugars, and most amino acids, As part of both coenzyme A and acyl carrier protein, it is also intimately linked with fatty acid synthesis.

It is widely available in foods of animal origin, especially liver, although cereals and legumes are also sources. Pantothenic acid is found in food as the coenzyme CoA or acyl carrier protein form and is hydrolysed by a pancreatic enzyme before absorption. It is not stored in the body. Urinary excretion is in the free acid form. Experimental pantothenic acid deficiency in humans results, within a few weeks, in symptoms including personality changes, fatigue, malaise, sleep disturbances, numbness, paraesthesiae, and muscle cramps. There is impaired motor coordination with an abnormal gait. Gastrointestinal complaints include nausea, abdominal cramp, occasional vomiting, and increased passage of flatus. Pantothenic acid deficiency may occur as part of the overall problem in people who are severely malnourished. No toxic intakes have been recorded. There is no biochemical method for measuring pantothenic acid status in humans.

Requirements

British diets provide a median intake of 6.1 mg/day (adult men) and 4.4 mg/day (adult women). A safe and adequate intake is between 3 and 7 mg per day, including during pregnancy and lactation. Infants require 1.7 mg/day; human milk provides 2.6 mg/day. Infant formula milk should contain at least 2 mg/litre.

Thiamine (vitamin B_1)

Thiamine functions principally (in the form of thiamine diphosphate), as a carrier of aldehyde groups. Its major importance is in carbohydrate metabolism, most notably in the pyruvate dehydrogenase system that generates acetyl-CoA from pyruvate. It is needed also as a cofactor in the oxidative phosphorylation of α-ketoglutarate, the common portal of entry into the tricarboxylic acid cycle of many amino acids. It is needed for the carboxylation of the ketoacids of the branched chain amino acids, so that it is important in the metabolism of nearly all amino acids as well as carbohydrates/sugars. Its involvement in the pentose phosphate pathway (hexose monophosphate shunt), at the transketolase stage, links it closely to the supply of NADPH and the synthesis of ribose 5-phosphate; this pentose and its derivatives are components of RNA and DNA, as well as ATP, NADH, FAD, and coenzyme A.

Thiamine hydrochloride consists of a substituted pyrimidine ring linked by a methylene group to a sulphur-containing thiazole ring. Thiamine may also play a role in neural excitation mechanisms.

All animal and plant tissues contain thiamine, usually in the phosphorylated form. The important sources are plant seeds and cereal germ, nuts, peas, beans, pulses, and yeast. Losses occur with cooking and alkaline pH. Absorption is from the upper gastrointestinal tract, followed by phosphorylation to the active diphosphate form. There is no body store and the only reserve is the vitamin functionally bound to enzymes. Multiple end products are excreted in the urine. Beriberi is caused by dietary thiamine deficiency, a disease that was endemic in east Asia as a result of the ingestion of polished rice which is deficient in the vitamin. Carbohydrate metabolism is impaired by a deficiency of thiamine pyrophosphate, a coenzyme necessary for the decarboxylation of pyruvate to acetyl-CoA. Pyruvic and lactic acid accumulate in the body.

Clinical aspects

The clinical presentations of thiamine deficiency are:

- wet beriberi (high-output cardiac failure)
- dry beriberi (polyneuropathy)

- infantile beriberi
- neuropathy and cardiomyopathy in chronic alcoholism
- Wernicke–Korsakoff syndrome
- lactic acidosis associated with artificial feeding

Initially, the symptoms are of nonspecific malaise and evidence of early cardiac failure and neuropathy. Wet beriberi is characterized by left- and right-sided high-output cardiac failure, cardiomegaly, hypotension, rapid deterioration, and death. Dry beriberi is a polyneuropathy affecting motor and sensory nerves. Initially, there is paraesthesia progressing to painful muscle wasting and polyneuritis. Total sensory loss occurs and patients become immobile and emaciated; they are at a high risk for the development of Wernicke–Korsakoff encephalopathy. Infantile beriberi occurs in breastfed infants of thiamine-deficient mothers, usually when they are between 2 and 5 months old. In the acute form, the child is restless and distressed with evidence of high-output cardiac failure; convulsions may develop, and the child becomes comatose. In the chronic form, the child is fretful, sleeps poorly, and the muscles may be flaccid. Cardiac failure, gastrointestinal symptoms, and sudden death are common. Alcoholic neuropathy presents with a sensory and motor neuropathy sometimes complicated by cardiomyopathy. Sensory nerve dysfunction includes paraesthesia and severe nerve pain ('causalgia'). Motor nerve lesions are of both upper and lower motor neuron type. A patient with Wernicke–Korsakoff syndrome is disorientated and apathetic. Nystagmus, ataxia, and confabulation are not infrequent consequences of lesions in the brainstem, diencephalon, and cerebellum.

Treatment is with intramuscular thiamine 25 mg twice daily for 3 days, and thereafter 10 mg two or three times daily. The reversal of the wet type of beriberi is rapid. Improvement is slow for dry beriberi, especially for the neurological abnormalities. In infantile beriberi, both mother (10 mg thiamine twice daily) and the infant (thiamine intramuscularly 10 to 20 mg/day for 3 days, and thereafter 5 to 10 mg twice daily) are treated. Beriberi can be prevented by eating thiamine-containing foods, unmilled or thiamine-fortified rice, or thiamine supplements.

Long-term intakes in excess of 50 mg/kg body weight per day are toxic, leading to headaches, irritability, insomnia, rapid pulse, weakness, contact dermatitis, pruritus, and even death. Thiamine status can be measured by urinary thiamine and the thiamine:creatinine ratio with or without a loading dose, or by the reactivation of the cofactor-depleted red-cell enzyme transketolase *in vitro*.

Requirements

Thiamine requirements are related to energy and carbohydrate metabolism. The average requirement for adults, normal pregnancy or lactation, and children is 0.4 mg/4185 J and not less than 0.8 mg/day for adults with a supplement of 0.6 mg/4185 J during pregnancy and lactation. Human breast milk contains the equivalent of 0.3 mg/4185 J. Older people may require 1 mg/day.

Pyridoxine (vitamin B_6)

Pyridoxine is to be found in several forms: pyridoxal, pyridoxamine, and pyridoxine. Pyridoxal phosphate enzymes are involved in a wide range of amino acid transformations—transamination, decarboxylations, deaminations, racemizations, and aldol cleavages—so pyridoxal 5′-phosphate is a coenzyme that plays a major role in the intermediary metabolism of amino acids. Pyridoxal 5′-phosphate acts as a coenzyme with glycogen phosphorylase in muscle, and has a role in the actions on hormones which modulate gene expression.

This family of vitamin B_6 compounds is found in many foods: cereals, meat (particularly liver), fruits, and leafy and other vegetables. The free form is common in plants, the phosphorylated form, pyridoxamine phosphate, in animal tissues. Vitamin B_6 is absorbed in the free form and phosphorylated for use in enzymes. There is no specific storage in tissues and it is excreted in urine largely as 4-pyridoxic acid.

Clinical aspects

Primary dietary deficiency has not been reported in adults, largely because of the wide availability of the vitamin, but deficiency has been seen in infants exposed to formula milk with antivitamin properties. These infants suffered seizures that responded to pyridoxine replacement. Experimental restriction of pyridoxine intake causes fatigue and headaches as early symptoms. A biochemical deficiency occurs commonly in alcoholics and in patients admitted to hospital as an emergency. Plasma concentrations tend to decrease with age. Patients taking isoniazid may develop a pyridoxine deficiency and neuropathy.

Clinical signs of deficiency include glossitis, stomatitis, peripheral neuropathy, microcytic hypochromic (sideroblastic) anaemia, It can be difficult to know how specific these signs are or whether they relate to combined deficiencies of other B vitamins.

Hyperhomocystinaemia is a result of reduced pyridoxine intake.

Evidence that vitamin B_6 supplementation can improve premenstrual symptoms and premenstrual depression exists but is limited by the quality of the trials performed.

High-dose (gram) intakes of pyridoxine have been reported to produce ataxia and glove–stocking sensory neuropathy, largely reversible on withdrawal of supplementation.

There is no single marker that is sensitive at all levels of dietary intake. Biochemical markers include plasma pyridoxal phosphate concentrations, red-cell aspartate aminotransferase activation, and the urinary excretion of vitamin B_6 degradation products. Metabolic loading tests also measure vitamin B_6 status, including the tryptophan- and methionine-load tests.

Requirements

The total body pool of vitamin B_6 is 15 μmole (4 mg)/kg, 80% of which is in muscle, with a half-life of 33 days. Adults, pregnant and lactating women, and older people require a daily intake of 13 μg/g of protein (*c.*4 mg/day). The vitamin B_6 content of human breast milk is low at between 40 and 100 μg/l (or 3–8 μg vitamin B_6/g protein). Infants under 3 months of age require 6 μg/g protein, increasing to up to 13 μg/g protein at 7 to 10 years.

Folate (folic acid, folacin; vitamin B_9)

Folates are derivatives of folic acid (pteroylglutamic acid) including the folylpolyglutamate found in foods. Folic acid is a pterin ring (2-amino, 4-hydroxypteridine) attached to *p*-aminobenzoic acid conjugated to L-glutamic acid (PteGlu). Variants include:

- di-(7,8-tetrahydrofolic acid) (DHF) and tetra-(5,6,7,8-tetrahydrofolic acid) (THF) reduced forms of the pteridine ring
- one-carbon substitution (methyl, formyl, methenyl, methylene, or formimino) at positions N5 or 10: 5-formyl-THF, 10-formyl-THF, 5-formimino-THF, 5,10-methenyl-THF, 5,10-methylene-THF, and 5-methyl-THF
- a chain of 4 to 6 glutamates attached to the l-glutamate

Folic acid gives and receives one-carbon groups on the N5 or N10 position in nucleic acid and amino acid biosynthetic reactions.

Sources of folate include liver, yeast extract, and green leafy vegetables. Most dietary folate is in the polyglutamyl form, which is hydrolysed to monoglutamate before being absorbed from the duodenum. A brush-border glutamyl carboxypeptidase is inhibited by alcohol, which is of relevance in alcoholic folic deficiencies. Folate bound to a milk protein is absorbed from the ileum. Folic acid is stored in the liver. Plasma folates are mainly 5-methyl-THF monoglutamate. Within cells, 5-methyl-THF is converted to THF polyglutamates, the main cellular forms of folic acid.

Folate polyglutamates do not readily cross cell membranes. The polyglutamate form has two functions: storage; and as a coenzyme for normal one-carbon metabolism (for which it is the most efficient coenzyme). The 5-methyl group is transferred to homocysteine (creating methionine and THF); the enzyme is the vitamin B_{12}-dependent methionine synthase, wherein methionine, folic acid, and vitamin B_{12} interlink.

Reactions in which folate is involved include:

- methylation of amino acids
- serine reversibly interconverting with glycine
- methionine interconverting with homocysteine (Methionine is the precursor of *S*-adenosyl-l-methionine (SAM), a methyl donor in the methylation of lipids, hormones, DNA, cell division, and proteins.)
- thymidine and purine synthesis

Folic acid deficiency may arise:

- as a dietary deficiency
- in malabsorption syndromes
- where there are excessive demands, as with increased cell proliferation (e.g. in leukaemias and haemolytic anaemias)
- where drugs interfere with folic acid metabolism
- in the rare inborn errors of folic metabolism

Folic acid deficiency is an important cause of megaloblastic anaemia, never to be confused with vitamin B_{12} deficiency. This anaemia was first described in poor Indian textile workers during pregnancy by Lucy Wills and reflected the increased demands for folate during pregnancy.

Neural tube defects are congenital deformities of the spinal cord and brain: spina bifida, anencephaly, encephalocele, and iniencephaly. Folic acid is involved in the aetiology of these defects. The precise mechanism is unclear, but there may be an underlying genetic predisposition involving a variant of 5,10-methyl-THF reductase (EC 1.5.1.20). Closure of the neural tube occurs early in pregnancy, thereby making aetiological studies difficult. It is clear from a major randomized controlled trial that folate replacement in pregnancy reduces the incidence of neural tube defects by about 72%. Food fortification with folate has been in place in the United States of America since 1998 and has now been recommended in the United Kingdom, though concerns have been expressed that it might have an adverse effect in older people in whom there is a high prevalence of subclinical vitamin B_{12} deficiency. Concern has also been expressed over the links of folic acid with bowel cancer.

Folic acid supplementation for 3 years in 50- to70-year-old members of the general population may improve domains of cognitive function that tend to decline with age, but the evidence does not yet provide adequate evidence of an effect of vitamin B_6 or vitamin B_{12} or folic acid supplementation, alone or in combination, on cognitive function testing in people with either normal or impaired cognitive function.

Epidemiological studies suggest an increased risk of vascular disease associated with hyperhomocysteinaemia. Homocysteine is reversibly methylated to methionine, a step which involves folate, vitamin B_{12}, and vitamin B_6. Supplementation of these vitamins has been proposed to reduce the putative dangers of hyperhomocysteinaemia. Folic acid supplementation is beneficial in primary prevention of stroke and is associated with reduction in plasma homocysteine concentrations, but has not yet been confirmed as effective in preventing cardiovascular diseases.

Folic acid supplementation does not reduce the risk of colonic adenoma formation, and may increase it.

Folate status is measured by the folate concentration in serum and red cells. Red-cell folate levels reflect body stores. A coincidental measurement of serum vitamin B_{12} is important.

Requirements

Children and adults, including elderly people, need a folate intake of 200 µg/day. Women planning a pregnancy should increase their intake of folic acid to 0.4 mg/day by capsule supplement. If a previous pregnancy has been affected by a neural tube defect, then 5 mg of folic acid/day before conception is suggested. A problem is that some pregnancies are unplanned. Dietary supplementation is impractical. Total folic acid excretion in breast milk averages 40 µg/day, and an additional maternal intake of 60 µg per day is required.

Cobalamin (vitamin B_{12})

Vitamin B_{12} is a cobalt-containing corrinoid—four linked pyrrole rings (corrin) coordinating with a central cobalt atom. The cobinamides necessary for human well-being are methylcobalamin, adenosylcobalamin, hydroxycobalamin, and cyanocobalamin. Microorganisms, including colonic flora, synthesize cobalamin. Yeast is a source of cobalamin, primarily as adenosyl- and hydroxocobalamin. Methyl cobalamin is found in egg yolk, cheese, and cow's milk. A vegan diet carries a risk of vitamin B_{12} deficiency.

The reactions requiring vitamin B_{12} include:

- isomerization of methylmalonyl-CoA to succinyl-CoA (methyl malonic acid concentrations increase in cases of vitamin B_{12} deficiency
- methyltransferase reactions, e.g. homocysteine to methionine, i.e. the transfer of a methyl group from 5-methyl-TFH to homocysteine, which converts homocysteine to methionine

Vitamin B_{12} has an important role in the maintenance of myelin. Deoxyadenosyl B_{12} is essential for propionyl-CoA reactions by transmutation of methylmalonyl-CoA to succinyl-CoA.

Vitamin B_{12} binds to food proteins and is released by saliva, acid pH, and pepsin, depending upon the mode of cooking and type of food protein. Vitamin B_{12} at stomach pH forms complexes with glycoproteins, transcobalamin, haptocorrin, and intrinsic factor. In the duodenum, cobalamin is released by pancreatic enzymes and alkaline pH and binds solely to intrinsic factor. The vitamin B_{12}–intrinsic factor complex is absorbed from the ileum through a specific receptor. Cobalamin is released from intrinsic factor, converted (80% to methyl and also adenosyl and hydroxy forms) and carried in the blood by transcobalamins I, II, and III. Of these, transcobalamin II releases vitamin B_{12} to the tissues to be stored in the adenosyl form. The total body cobalamin content in adults is between 2 and 5 mg, most of which is stored in the liver. Turnover is 0.1% of the body pool each day. There is efficient conservation by the kidneys and the enterohepatic circulation. Most vitamin B_{12} is excreted in urine and small amounts in faeces, including unabsorbed bacterially synthesized vitamin B_{12}. The relationship between dietary intake and serum concentrations is not linear because the body stores of vitamin B_{12} are largely in the liver.

Vitamin B_{12} deficiency is common in older people and results in megaloblastic anaemia and neurological disorders, especially in the posterolateral columns of the spinal cord. Causes of deficiency are dietary (vegans), lack of intrinsic factor (Addison's pernicious anaemia, gastric resection), intestinal colonization by bacteria and parasites (e.g. tapeworms), and ileal resection. The megaloblastic anaemia is due to a lack of vitamin B_{12} for methionine synthase, insufficient methionine regeneration, and 5,10-methylene-THF and deficient thymidylate synthesis. In vitamin B_{12} deficiency, odd number (15- and 17-carbon) fatty acids and branched chain fatty acids are synthesized and incorporated into an unstable myelin nerve sheath. An inability to regenerate methionine from homocysteine, for the *S*-adenosylmethionine generation necessary for myelin proteins, leads to demyelination.

The efficiency of vitamin B_{12} absorption is measured by the Schilling test or by a whole-body scanner.

Requirements

A dietary intake of between 1 and 2 μg/day for adults of all ages is protective. In pregnancy there is a compensatory increased absorption so that 1.5 μg/day is sufficient. During lactation, an increment of 0.5 μg/day should ensure an adequate supply in breast milk (0.2–1.0 μg/litre). The requirement for infants is of the order of 0.1 μg/day and for children aged 3 to 10 years, 0.5 to 1.0 μg/day. Vitamin B_{12} has extremely low toxicity and as much as 3 mg/day may be taken.

Biotin (vitamin B_7)

Biotin contains a ureido group in a five-membered ring fused with a tetrahydrothiophene ring with a five-carbon side chain terminating in a carboxyl group. Dietary biotin is found in yeast, bacteria, liver, kidney, egg yolks, cooked cereals, pulses, nuts, chocolates, and some vegetables, and biotin is synthesized by intestinal flora. Biotin is a carrier for activated CO_2 and a cofactor for the acetyl-CoA, propionyl-CoA, and pyruvate carboxylase systems involved in the incorporation of bicarbonate as a carboxyl group (activated CO_2/carboxyphosphate) into substrates in fatty acid synthesis and gluconeogenesis. Biotin is absorbed from the upper gastrointestinal tract. Raw egg white contains the glycoprotein avidin (molecular weight 68 000 kDa), which binds biotin with a high affinity and, in large amounts, prevents biotin absorption. Biotin is transported in plasma to the liver for storage. It is metabolized before excretion in the urine as biotin, bisnorbiotin, and biotin sulphoxide.

Biotin deficiency results in fatigue, depression, sleepiness, nausea, loss of appetite, muscle pain, hyperaesthesia and paraesthesia, hallucinations, alopecia, dermatitis, conjunctivitis, smooth tongue, and dry skin. It has been described in the joint contexts of (deficient) parenteral nutrition and short bowel and occurs rarely in individuals unable to absorb the vitamin due to a genetic deficiency of biotinidase. Individuals receiving treatment for epilepsy are at risk of biotin deficiency. There are no indications that excess biotin is toxic. Body stores are measured by plasma biotin concentrations, and lymphocyte propionyl-CoA carboxylase (PCC) and its activation index (ratio of enzyme activity incubated with and without biotin) or urinary 3-hydroxyisovalerate. Egg white feeding results in lower than normal biotin status as judged by PCC within 14 days and activation coefficient is increased by 28 days.

Requirements

The dietary requirement of biotin is not known with certainty. The average intake of a British man is 39 μg/day, ranging from 15 to 70 μg/day, and for women it averages 26 μg/day, ranging between 10 and 58 μg/day. This prevents deficiency. In infants, preterm to 5 years, an intake between 5 and 25 μg/day is suggested.

Vitamins and coronary heart disease

Homocysteine metabolism by vitamin B_6, vitamin B_{12}, and folate

Elevated levels of homocysteine are associated with increased prevalence of coronary heart disease. Dietary supplementation with folic acid and vitamin B_{12} reduces plasma homocysteine levels. Homocysteine is derived from methionine. Conversely, in remethylation it accepts a methyl group from methyl tetrahydrofolate to form methionine. In trans-sulphuration, homocysteine combines with serine to form cystathionine catalysed by a vitamin B_6-dependent enzyme, cystathionine synthase. After adjustment for known risk factors for coronary heart disease, reduction in blood homocysteine by 25% resulted in a decrease of 11% in coronary heart disease and of 19% in stroke.

Interest has focused on coronary heart disease, stoke, depression, cognitive function, and depression. Randomized controlled trials are currently being assessed together to increase their power; however, to date, no evidence for reduction in coronary heart disease or stroke has emerged, though reductions of 10% for myocardial infarction and 20% for stroke cannot be excluded.

Large trials have established either no or an adverse effect on coronary heart disease in patients given these vitamins as supplements, despite effective lowering of plasma homocysteine concentrations. Meta-analysis has demonstrated reductions in stroke with folic acid supplementation. No effect on cognitive function has yet emerged in meta-analysis of the vitamins used singly or in combination.

Fat-soluble vitamins

Vitamin A

The vitamin A family (retinoids) are related to the plant pigment carotene. Dietary vitamin A comes in two forms: preformed vitamin A fatty acid esters from animal sources, or provitamin A carotenoids from plant sources. β-Carotene, a provitamin A carotenoid, consists of two retinol molecules. Retinol is vitamin A alcohol, a hydrocarbon chain with a β-ionone ring at one end and an alcohol group at the other, usually esterified with a fatty acid (retinyl esters) as the *all-trans* stereoisomer. The *cis* configuration isomer (11 or 13 position) is less potent. Retinol can be oxidized to an aldehyde (retinal) or acid (retinoic acid). Retinol and carotene are readily oxidized and are protected by vitamin E.

Retinol is present in dairy products, liver, and fatty fish liver oils. Carotenes are found predominantly in green vegetables as well as in yellow and red fruits and vegetables. Vitamin A is essential for the maintenance of epithelial tissue, visual function, and the immune system. Most actions of vitamin A in development, differentiation, and metabolism are mediated through retinoid receptors of the nuclear steroid receptor family of proteins that bind retinoic acid and regulate gene expression.

The photopigment rhodopsin is formed by the protein opsin and 11-*cis* retinal. A photon of light converts the *cis* retinal to the *trans* form, which reversibly dissociates from the opsin and is seen as light. Retinyl esters are hydrolysed by pancreatic hydrolases and the enteric mucosa. β-Carotene is cleaved to two retinols by β-carotene 15,15′-deoxygenase, and carotenoids oxidatively cleave to retinal and apocarotenoids. Retinal is reduced to retinol, esterified with long-chain fatty acids, and transported to the liver as retinyl long-chain fatty esters in chylomicrons through the lymph. Retinol is a major liver storage form and circulates to tissues, bound to retinol-binding protein. There is an enterohepatic circulation of retinoids.

Vitamin A deficiency is a major worldwide cause of blindness, due to a poor dietary intake of green vegetables, fruit, and dairy produce. Malabsorption is a less common cause. Vitamin A deficiency results in reduced rhodopsin in the retinal rods resulting in loss of vision. Xerophthalmia causes blindness in 500 000 young children each year, especially amongst bottlefed infants and breast-fed infants with vitamin A-deficient mothers. Protein calorie malnutrition compounds the problem during weaning. Vitamin A deficiency aggravates damage from other causes of keratoconjunctivitis, e.g. measles. Epithelial surfaces undergo squamous metaplasia, followed by corneal ulceration and irreversible visual damage. Clinical forms are:

- conjunctival xerosis (Bitots's spots are white plaques of thickened conjunctival epithelium indicative of vitamin deficiency in the young)
- corneal xerosis
- keratomalacia, leading to blindness
- night blindness, an early symptom with or without xerophthalmia
- xerophthalmia fundi
- corneal scars

Vitamin A is important in epithelial metabolism. Deficiency leads to epithelial metaplasia and inappropriately keratinized epithelium in the mucous membranes of the respiratory, gastrointestinal, and genitourinary tract. Sebaceous glands become blocked, thereby causing follicular keratosis.

Prophylaxis demands education in the eating of dark green vegetables. Where xerophthalmia is endemic, vitamin A is given prophylactically in capsule form or by food fortification. Frank deficiency is treated by high-potency Vitamin A: 200 000 IU for 2 days, and a third dosage at least 2 weeks later. Thereafter, improved diet and supplementation are obligatory. Corneal ulceration is treated by antibiotics, and the response is rapid. Vitamin A deficiency is a putative risk factor for childhood morbidity and death, especially for the underweight and premature infant.

β-Carotene is not toxic, but high intakes lead to a yellow appearance sparing the eyes (hypercarotenaemia). Polar bear liver, rich in retinol, is toxic; ingestion can cause drowsiness, headache, vomiting, and excess peeling of the skin. Large intakes of retinol are teratogenic. Pregnant women should be careful not to exceed the recommended intake of vitamin A in the first trimester.

Plasma retinol is an insensitive indicator of vitamin A status. The relative dose–response (RDR test), which measures retinol transport by the retinol-binding protein, is used as a functional test for calculating retinol stores. The concentration of plasma carotenoids reflects short- to medium-term intakes. The following are equipotent to 1 μg of *all-trans*-retinol equivalents/day: 3.33 IU vitamin A, 3.5 nmol retinol or retinyl ester, or 6 μg *all-trans*-β-carotene.

Requirements

Adults require 500 μg retinol equivalents/day; infants, 250 to 350 μg retinol equivalents/day; children, 350 μg retinol equivalents/day; pregnancy, an increment of 100 μg retinol equivalents/day, particularly during the third trimester. Lactation requires an increment of 300 μg retinol equivalents/day. Breast milk vitamin A concentration should exceed 1.5 mmol/litre.

Vitamin D

Insertion the term 'vitamin D' as a keyword into Medline retrieves in excess of 30 000 references. The vitamin D family of sterols includes vitamin D_3 (cholecalciferol) and vitamin D_2 (ergocalciferol). Cholecalciferol is to be regarded as a hormone rather than a vitamin, and is produced by the ultraviolet irradiation of dietary 7-dehydrocholesterol (provitamin D_3) in the skin. The extent of exposure to sunlight determines production. Cholecalciferol is also available in fatty fish (e.g. cod), eggs, and chicken liver. Ergocalciferol is also the result of the exposure of ergosterol (provitamin D_2) to ultraviolet light. Ergocalciferol differs from cholecalciferol in having an extra methyl group at C-24 and a double bond at C-22,23. Although not a steroid, vitamin D acts similarly in that it binds to steroid-like receptor and forms a complex which, as a transcription factor, regulates gene expression through 'zinc fingers'. 1,25-dihydroxycholecalciferol vitamin D (1,25$(OH)_2$D, calcitriol) regulates calcium and phosphate absorption, metabolism, and export into the bloodstream. Such regulation is through steroid:thyroid hormone nuclear receptors. Calcitriol is also a developmental hormone inhibiting proliferation and promoting differentiated function in cells.

Though hitherto vitamin D has been regarded principally in the context of bone metabolism its broader roles are emerging. Vitamin D supplementation is demonstrated in meta-analysis to reduce overall mortality rates. Brain, prostate, breast, colon, and immune cells have a vitamin D receptor and respond to calcitriol. Calcitriol controls more than 200 genes, including genes responsible for regulation of cell proliferation, differentiation, apoptosis, and angiogenesis. 25-Hydroxyvitamin D (calcidiol) reduces cell proliferation of normal cells and cancer cells and favours terminal differentiation. Vitamin D deficiency inhibits innate immunity (monocytes and macrophages). Calcitriol increases insulin production, inhibits renin synthesis, and enhances myocardial function. Vitamin D deficiency has been associated with increased risks of Hodgkin's lymphoma, colon, prostate, and breast cancer. Vitamin D deficiency is associated with insulin resistance and with diabetes mellitus. As with the epidemiology of these cancers, living at high latitude is associated with an increased risk of diabetes, multiple sclerosis, and Crohn's disease. Vitamin D supplementation has been reported to reduce risks of multiple sclerosis, rheumatoid arthritis, osteoarthritis, and type 1 diabetes. Supplemental vitamin D in a dose of 700-1000 IU a day reduces the risk of falling among older individuals. The latter seems to be related to the ability of vitamin D to reduce islet cell antibody production.

Dietary vitamin D is absorbed in the small intestine, as a lipid, transported to the liver bound to α-globulin (*trans*-calciferol) in chylomicrons. Both vitamin D_2 and vitamin D_3 are inactive. They are converted in the liver by a P450 inducible microsomal enzyme into 25-hydroxyvitamin D (calcidiol), which has modest biological activity, before plasma transport on a specific globulin. The active form of vitamin D is calcitriol, formed in the kidney by a mitochondrial D-1-αhydroxylase acting on calcidiol. Production of calcitriol is tightly regulated by plasma parathormone, calcium, and phosphorus concentrations. The half-life of calcidiol is less than 24 h. All forms of vitamin D are stored in fat. Vitamin D is 24-hydroxylated and inactive calcitroic acid formed and excreted.

The standard measure of vitamin D status is the plasma calcidiol concentration, and deficiency is defined by plasma levels of less than 20 ng/ml (50 nmol/litre). Levels of calcidiol are inversely related to parathormone levels until the parathormone level reaches a minimum at calcidiol levels of 75 to 100 nmol/litre (30–40 ng/ml). Hypomagnesaemia results in a blunting of the response of parathormone to vitamin D and calcium deficiency. 30 ng/ml (75 nmol/litre) is regarded as evidence of vitamin D sufficiency when optimal absorption of calcium transport is achieved.

The prime consequence of vitamin D deficiency is rickets, caused by a failure to mineralize the bony skeleton. The epiphyseal cartilage replacement is defective, leading to an overgrowth of subperiosteal osteoid tissue and poor mineralization of the bone matrix, resulting in soft bones. The type of bony abnormalities depends on the age of onset and the weight-bearing bones involved. The appearance of the rachitic child is deceptive; the child may appear quite well or be restless with hypotonic muscles and twisted limb postures. The abdomen is swollen and the child suffers from diarrhoea, respiratory infection, and delayed tooth development. In the infant, the commonest abnormality is enlargement of the end of the radius and the costochondrial junction, termed the 'ricketic rosary'. Later there is bossing of the frontal and parietal bones and delayed closure of the anterior fontanelle. So-called 'pigeon chest' can occur, which is an undue prominence of the sternum and a transverse depression from the costal margins towards the axillae. All are due to pressure on the soft bones when the child is supine. In the walking child, the weight-bearing bones bend, and kyphosis of the spine and bowing of the lower ends of the femur, tibia, and fibula result. Pelvic deformity can make delivery difficult in subsequent pregnancies. Tetanic spasm can occur, whereby spasm of the hands, feet, and vocal chord result in high-pitched cries and breathing problems.

Diagnosis is based on the clinical appearance and measurements of plasma alkaline phosphatase (although interpretation of the results is difficult in the growing child) and plasma calcidiol levels. There are several risk factors:

- inadequate exposure to sunlight (dependent on latitude; in the United Kingdom 30- to 90-min exposure of the face and legs per day will restore calcidiol concentrations)
- strict vegetarianism
- a vitamin D-deficient mother breastfeeding her baby
- high melanin content in the skin, which screens the metabolically active skin sites
- malabsorption

Prevention of vitamin D deficiency requires a supplement of 10 μg of vitamin D daily or regular exposure to sunlight in well-nourished individuals.

Osteomalacia may present with muscular weakness and a waddling gait. Bone pain, tetany, and spontaneous fractures may develop. Radiographic features include bone rarification, pseudofractures, and Looser's zones at points of compression stress. Renal disease, from many causes, may be associated with impaired renal synthesis of calcitriol. A failure of 25-hydroxylation of vitamin D can occur in hepatic disease. Dietary vitamin D intake may be important in immunity to tuberculosis, and calcidiol deficiency may contribute to the occurrence of tuberculosis. Hypervitaminosis occurs during infant supplementation and replacement therapy. Plasma calcium concentrations increase with tetany, ECG changes with resultant convulsions, and occasionally death. Vitamin D in milligram amounts is poisonous, and is used as a rodenticide.

The best measure of the vitamin status in humans is the plasma calcidiol concentration.

Requirements

No minimum dietary intake has been identified for adults exposed to ample sunlight. However, 10 μg/day vitamin D is recommended for those with poor sun exposure. Vitamin D concentrations in breast milk are low (0.25–1.25 μg/litre) and are reduced in the winter. Vitamin D intakes are a problem for the 6- to 12-month-old baby dependent upon modestly fortified weaning foods. The diet thereafter expands, and the plasma calcidiol concentrations are usually satisfactory. Pregnant and lactating women should receive supplementary vitamin D at 10 μg/day. Where older people are insufficiently exposed to the summer sun, their stores may be reduced and a supplement of 10 μg/day vitamin D is recommended.

Clinical use

Supplementation of people over the age of 50 with calcium and vitamin D increases bone mineral content and reduces fracture risk.

Vitamin K

Vitamin K, a naphthoquinone, occurs in two forms in human nutrition: vitamin K_1 and vitamin K_2. Vitamin K_1 of plant origin is a phytylmenaquinone (also known as phylloquinone or phytylmenadione) and consists of 2-methyl-1,4-naphthoquinone (menadione or menaquinone) attached to a 20-carbon phytyl side chain. Vitamin K_2 is one of several homologues produced by bacteria with 4 to 13 isoprenyl units in the side chain (menaquinone-4 to -13). Vitamin K_1 is present in fresh green vegetables (e.g. broccoli, lettuce, cabbage, and spinach) and beef. Vitamin K is involved in the synthesis of proteins central to blood coagulation, namely prothrombin and factors VII, IX, and X. Vitamin K is necessary for the post-translational carboxylation of glutamic acid in the coagulation proteins. γ-Carboxyglutamate allows the binding of calcium and phospholipids in the formation of thrombin.

Vitamin K is absorbed as a lipid, and is transported from the intestine in the blood in chylomicrons as β-lipoproteins. Vitamin K_2 of bacterial origin is absorbed from the colon. When there is vitamin K deficiency, the blood clotting time is prolonged and factor VII, IX, and X activities are reduced. Deficiency is uncommon in adults. However, in infants, deficiency results from a sterile intestinal tract and the inadequate vitamin K content of human and cow's milk. The problem is compounded by the immature liver of the infant being slow to synthesize prothrombin. Acquired deficiencies occur as a result of any cause of lipid malabsorption and after bowel sterilization with broad-spectrum antimicrobial agents. Vitamin K deficiency may also result from the regular ingestion of liquid paraffin, since the vitamin partitions preferentially into this nonabsorbed, nonpolar hydrocarbon oil and is excreted rather than absorbed. Liquid paraffin is still used in many parts of the world as a regular aperient, principally by older people.

Natural vitamin K preparations are free from toxic effects. There are naturally occurring vitamin K antagonists—e.g. spoilt sweet clover produces a dicoumarol that prolongs the prothrombin time of the cow, thereby causing a bleeding condition. Drugs designed to prolong prothrombin time were developed as a result of this observation. Vitamin K deficiency can be detected by the prothrombin time test, which measures prolongation of clotting time.

Requirements

The children and adult dietary requirements of phylloquinone are between 0.5 and 1.0 μg/kg body weight per day. Vitamin K in human breast milk is as the phylloquinone and the concentration varies between 1 and 10 μg/litre. An adequate intake for breastfed infants is 8.5 μg phylloquinone/day. Vitamin K is given as supplements in malabsorption syndromes and prophylactically for haemorrhagic disease of the newborn.

Vitamin E

The vitamin E family consists of fat-soluble biologically active tocopherols and tocotrienols. The tocopherols are the most potent, their activity depending upon the position and number of methyl substitutions. α-Tocopherol, is the most potent; γ-tocopherol and γ-tocotrienol have activity of 48% and 20%, respectively, when compared to α-tocopherol.

The free-radical scavenging properties of vitamin E are a function of the fused chroman ring system; the phytyl side chain facilitates entry into the hydrophobic environment of the membrane. Ascorbic acid may reduce tocopheroxyl radicals formed by the scavenging of free radicals during metabolism. This enables a molecule of tocopherol to scavenge many radicals.

Vegetable oils—wheat germ, sunflower seed, cottonseed, safflower, palm, rape seed, and other oils—are abundant sources of vitamin E. The absorption of the vitamin is incomplete and varies between 20% and 80%. Vitamin E enters the systemic circulation in chylomicrons and very low-density lipoproteins (VLDL) and coincidentally protect the polyunsaturated fatty acids (PUFA), which are also transported. Lipoprotein lipase controls uptake by the liver or transfer to other lipoproteins. The normal lipoprotein concentrations of vitamin E as α-tocopherol range from 11 to 37 μmol/litre. α-Tocopherol forms 90% of the vitamin E found in tissues, including all cell membranes where it inhibits the nonenzymatic oxidation of PUFA by molecular oxygen.

Clinical aspects

Biochemical deficiency may occur as a result of gastrointestinal malabsorption and in premature infants. Vitamin E deficiency has been implicated in peripheral neuropathy associated with malabsorption syndromes and often accounts for the acanthocytosis, retinitis pigmentosa, and neurological features in Bassen–Kornzweig disease (abetalipoproteinaemia). Patients with fat malabsorption due to cystic fibrosis, coeliac disease, prolonged cholestasis, and after massive small intestinal resections are particularly at risk from vitamin E deficiency. Supplements prevent and may slowly ameliorate the neurological deficit. Homozygosity for inactivating mutations in the α-tocopherol transfer protein is a cause of isolated vitamin E deficiency and ataxia, which closely resembles the spinocerebellar ataxia of Friedreich's disease. Patients with Friedreich's ataxia in the absence of frataxin mutations should be investigated for vitamin E deficiency and defects in the tocopherol transfer protein; vitamin E supplements may slowly improve this condition. Longstanding profound deficiency of vitamin E is associated with progressive spinocerebellar ataxia, visual loss due to retinitis pigmentosa, haemolysis (with red cell acanthocytosis), upward visual gaze palsies, dementia, and muscle weakness. If detected, vigorous long-term vitamin E supplementation is indicated as well as attention to the primary cause of the deficiency. There appears to be no adverse effects from large doses of vitamin E up to 3200 mg/day.

Vitamin E status can be measured from the plasma tocopherol concentration, or expressed as a ratio of total blood lipids or vitamin E:cholesterol. A functional test of vitamin E status is the hydrogen peroxide haemolysis test (erythrocyte stress test).

Requirements

The average intake in Britain is 6 mg/day, most of which is derived from fats, oils, and cereals. The dietary requirement is determined by the PUFA content of membranes and tissues and the PUFA content of the diet. The relationship between PUFA intake and vitamin E requirements is not a simple linear relationship. Intakes of 4 mg and 3 mg of α-tocopherol equivalents per day, respectively, for men and women have been regarded as adequate, but may be too low. Alternatively, and better, would be 0.4 mg α-tocopherol equivalents per gram of dietary PUFA/day, thereby increasing the recommendation to 7 mg. This formula might also be used for infants. Human breast milk contains 10 mg of α-tocopherol equivalents/litre in colostrum, reducing to 3.2 mg/litre at 12 days and thereafter.

Trace elements

Trace elements are required in small amounts ranging between milligram amounts (magnesium, iron, zinc, copper, manganese, fluoride) and microgram amounts (selenium, molybdenum, chromium, iodine). They are essential nutrients and, as with vitamins, artificial feeding must contain sufficient amounts of them. They act as cofactors in enzyme oxidation–reduction reactions. Trace elements maintain the specific configuration of proteins; are incorporated into the structure of hormones; and play a structural and catalytic role in gene expression and transcriptional regulation of genes.

The trace elements contained in soil and drinking water vary from area to area, which determines the variation in intake seen in different communities. The amount and chemistry of dietary constituents eaten with the trace elements affects the absorption efficiency of the essential elements. The absorption of calcium and trace metals (e.g. zinc) can be inhibited by dietary phytate. Copper absorption is reduced by competitive interactions affecting its solubility. A mild degree of iron depletion increases not only iron absorption but also that of lead, zinc, cadmium, cobalt, and manganese.

Some properties of trace elements are listed in Table 11.2.1.

Table 11.2.1 Properties of trace elements

Element	Atomic weight[a]	Valency	Natural isotopes[b]	Abundance (%)[c]
Cobalt	59	2, 3	59	0.0018
Chromium	52	2, 3	50, 52, 53, 54	0.033
Copper	64	1, 2	63, 65	0.010
Iodine	127	1	127	6×10^{-6}
Magnesium	24	2	24, 25, 26	1.94
Manganese	55	2, 4	55	0.085
Molybdenum	96	2, 3, 4	92, 94, 95, 96, 97, 98, 100	7×10^{-4}
Nickel	59	2, 3	58, 60, 61, 62, 64	0.018
Phosphorus	31	3, 5	31	0.12
Selenium	79	2, 4	74, 76, 77, 78, 80, 82	8×10^{-5}
Silicon	28	4	28, 29, 30	25.8
Sulphur	32	2, 4	32, 33, 34, 36	0.048
Zinc	65	2	64, 66, 67, 68, 70	0.02

[a] Rounded to the nearest integer.
[b] Atomic numbers of natural isotopes.
[c] Natural abundance in Earth's crust as a percentage of the total.

Cobalt

Sources are wholemeal flour and seafoods. Cobalt's role is as a component of vitamin B_{12}. Uncomplexed cobalt can be absorbed and subsequently excreted in urine. Intakes of cobalt are approximately 0.3 mg or 5 μmol/day and the total body content is 1.5 mg (7.5 μmol). In Quebec, a cobalt-containing beer improver (15 μmol of cobalt/litre) proved to be toxic; its best customers developed severe cardiomyopathy.

Chromium

Chromium potentiates the action of insulin and may participate in lipoprotein metabolism, in maintaining the structure of nucleic acids, and in gene expression. The cationic trivalent form is biochemically active. Chromium is present in most foods especially meat, brewer's yeast, wheat germ and whole grains, legumes, and nuts. Dietary intake in adults vary between 13 and 49 μg/day, more in older people, but absorption is meagre at 1%. Requirements are calculated to be about 23 μg (0.38 μmol/day) and a safe intake of above 25 μg/day has been given for adults. The plasma concentration of chromium is 0.3 μg/ml bound to transferrin, and it is excreted in urine. Deficiency increases the risk of type 2 diabetes and cardiovascular disease. The recommended adult intake is 0.5 μmol/day and between 2 and 19 nmol/kg per day for children and adolescents. The adult body contains 100 to 200 μmol. The chromium content of human milk is 0.06 to 1.56 ng/ml. Chromium in high dosage is well tolerated. Chromium deficiency has been reported in patients on long-term unsupplemented parenteral nutrition in whom glucose intolerance developed.

Copper

Copper is a component of mitochondrial complex IV, cytochrome *c* oxidase and other oxidase enzymes, and cuproenzymes involved in the synthesis of haem. It is also a component of many other enzymes, including superoxide dismutase. Cuproenzymes are involved in the synthesis of a range of neuroactive amines. Copper is required by the immune, nervous, and cardiovascular systems for skeletal development, iron metabolism, and red-cell formation.

Good sources of copper include green vegetables, fish, oysters, and liver. Between 35% and 70% of ingested copper is actively absorbed, but this is affected by age and the chemistry of accompanying food. Copper is concentrated in the liver, excreted in bile, and lost in faeces. In plasma, copper is bound to caeruloplasmin and albumin. The total amount of copper in an adult is approximately 2 mmol (50–120 mg). Copper accumulates in the fetal liver for early extrauterine life; premature birth results in depleted copper stores. Copper deficiency in adults results in anaemia and neutropenia, and a myelopathy presenting with a spastic gait and sensory ataxia, which is similar to the subacute combined degeneration of B_{12} deficiency. There may be hyperzincaemia even in the absence of excess zinc intake. Patients taking large doses of zinc, or the chelator penicillamine for cystinuria and as a second-line agent in rheumatoid arthritis, are at risk from copper deficiency, as are patients post-gastrectomy or with malabsorption. Copper has been implicated as related to the development of Alzheimer's disease. Poisoning with copper presents with haemolysis and brain and hepatocellular damage. The requirement for adults (including during pregnancy) is 1.5 to 3 mg/day, with a proposed reference nutrient intake (RNI) of 1.2 mg (19 μmol)/day. Children range 0.6 to 1.5 mg/day with RNI of 36 μg (0.6 μmol)/kg per day at 9 months to 17 μg (0.3 μmol)/kg per day at age 15 years.

Iodine

Iodine is present in modest amounts in most food and drinking water. Seafood, milk, and meat are good sources. Iodine is required for thyroxine 3,5,3′,5′-tetraiodothyronine (T_4) and 3,5,3′-tri-iodothyronine (T_3). Selenium and zinc are important in the conversion of T_4 to the active T_3, catalysed by selenium-dependent iodothyronine deiodinase. Dietary iodine from food and water is absorbed as inorganic iodide and transported to the thyroid gland. The body content of iodine is between 20 and 50 mg (160–400 μmol).

Goitre results from iodine deficiency and is endemic in mountainous areas. Some 800 million people are at risk of iodine deficiency, of whom 190 million may develop goitres and more than 3 million are cretinous. These populations have an iodine intake less than 25 μg/day—the required intake being 80 to 150 μg/day. Iodine replacement is essential for these populations and may be added to food, salt, or water or by the direct administration of iodine. Goitre may also arise through eating plants containing goitrogens (e.g. thiocyanate in cassava, maize, bamboo shoots, etc.) Maternal iodine deficiency is associated with perinatal death, stillbirths, spontaneous abortions, endemic cretinism, and congenital abnormalities. Thyroxine is essential for brain development during the first 2 years of life. A modest increase in the incidence of hyperthyroidism occurs following the ingestion of iodized salt preparations in individuals over 40 years of age.

Thyroid hormone and urinary iodine measurements reflect iodine status. Adults require 140 μg/day, babies 40 μg/day, infants 50 μg/day, and children 50 to 140 μg/day. Intake should increase to 175 μg/day during pregnancy and 200 μg/day with lactation. Breast milk contains 44 to 93 μg/litre, an adequate iodine intake.

Magnesium

Magnesium is present in most foods, particularly chlorophyll-containing vegetables (it is necessary for photosynthesis). Magnesium is said to be absorbed by a saturable transport system and passive diffusion, but recent studies have shown no change in magnesium fractional intestinal absorption over the typical range of dietary magnesium intakes. Excretion through the kidneys is the primary mechanism for magnesium regulation. This regulation occurs in response to plasma magnesium concentrations in the distal tubule and the ascending loop of Henle. Magnesium reabsorption is also governed by potassium depletion, the rate of salt and water excretion, parathyroid hormone, calcitonin, glucagon, vasopressin, and acid–base changes. Magnesium homeostasis includes reabsorption of endogenous magnesium from enteric secretions. The plasma concentration varies between 0.6 and 1.0 mmol/litre, and adult whole-body magnesium is 1 mol or 25 g—two-thirds in bone with phosphate and calcium, the remainder being complexed with ATP. Magnesium is the second most prevalent intracellular cation (after potassium).

Magnesium is a cofactor for cocarboxylase and is involved in the replication and transcription of DNA and translation of RNA. Restriction enzymes require magnesium for catalytic activity, and it is essential to the function of restriction endonucleases.

Magnesium is also important in energy metabolism. Nucleoside monophosphate kinases catalyse the transfer of a phosphoryl group from a nucleoside triphosphate such as ATP to the phosphoryl group on a nucleosyl monophosphate, e.g. AMP. These enzymes require divalent metal ions such as magnesium or manganese for activity, which bind to the nucleotide (e.g. ATP). Essentially, all nucleoside triphosphates are present as magnesium complexes. Magnesium assists in catalysis by 'induced fit' in which induced structural changes bring two substrates (e.g. AMP and ATP) in close apposition. Hexokinase, which catalyses the transfer of phosphoryl from ATP to six-carbon hexoses, is another important example of a magnesium- (or manganese-) dependent enzyme. Deficiency in dietary magnesium may predispose to type 2 diabetes.

Magnesium has an important role in skeletal development and the maintenance of electrical potential in nerve and muscle membranes.

Magnesium deficiency is manifested by progressive muscle weakness, failure to thrive, neuromuscular dysfunction, arrhythmias, hallucinations, positive Chvosteck's and Trousseau's signs, coma, and death. It results in glucose intolerance and hyperinsulinaemia. Cardiovascular abnormalities associated with hypomagnesaemia include widening of the QRS complex, prolongation of the P–R interval, inversion of the T wave, ventricular arrythmias, and increased sensitivity to cardiac glycosides. Hypomagnesaemia is commonly associated with hypocalcaemia and hypokalaemia, and correction of the magnesium depletion may be necessary to restore plasma levels of the other two ions. Magnesium supplementation leads to a rise in parathormone level under these circumstances.

Hypomagnesaemia results most commonly from gastrointestinal losses in diarrhoeal states, malabsorption, and primary intestinal hypomagnesaemia, and renal losses in volume overexpansion, hypercalcaemia, and osmotic diuresis. It may result from drugs such as diuretics, alcohol, aminoglycosides, cisplatin, amphotericin, ciclosporin, foscarnet, and pentamidine. Primary renal tubular magnesium wasting occurs in two conditions: one is characterized by hypercalciuria, nephrocalcinosis, and a tubular acidification defect; the other, Gitelman's syndrome, is associated with hypocalciuria and a defect in the gene encoding for the thiazide-sensitive sodium–chloride cotransporter. A low plasma magnesium concentration results in a state of functional hypoparathyroidism with parathormone resistance. Hypomagnesaemia can occur after parathyroidectomy, phosphate depletion, correction of chronic acidosis, obstructive nephropathy, and the diuretic phase of acute tubular necrosis. It may also occur during the refeeding of the malnourished patient as part of the refeeding syndrome.

Intravenous infusion of magnesium is beneficial in atrial fibrillation, and in the management of drug-induced ventricular tachycardia/fibrillation—torsade de pointes. Intravenous and nebulized magnesium salts are beneficial in asthma. Intravenous magnesium has been used in pre-eclampsia.

Urinary magnesium is an approximate measure of dietary intake. Typically, a diet in the United Kingdom contains between 8 and 17 mmol of magnesium/day (200–400 mg). Reference nutrient intakes for adult men and women are 12.3 mmol (300 mg) and 10.9 (270 mg) per day, with an increment during lactation of 50 mg (2.1 mmol). Human breast milk contains 0.12 mmol (2.8 mg)/litre. The lactating mother should increase her magnesium intake by 2.0 mmol/day (50 mg). Babies require 30 mg/day, infants 75 mg/day, and children 80 to 200 mg/day.

Therapeutically, magnesium can be administered intravenously in the acute management of tetany or cardiac arrythmias or orally in more chronic deficiency. Oral preparations can cause diarrhoea and the preparations most commonly used are either magnesium glycerophosphate or magnesium oxide tablets, providing 4 mmol per tablet. Doses of 24 mmol/day or more may be needed. Intravenous magnesium is given as magnesium sulphate, 4 to 8 mmol given over 15 to 60 min, depending on the situation.

Manganese

Tea, cereals, legumes, and leafy vegetables are good sources of manganese. Manganese absorption is only 3 to 4% efficient. Calcium, phosphorus, fibre, and phytate interact with and reduce manganese absorption. Manganese is a cofactor and enzyme activator. In animals, manganese is present in enzymes, such as hexokinase, mitochondrial superoxide dismutase, and xanthine oxidase. The plasma concentration is between 1 and 2 µg/g bound to transferrin, the body pool contains 0.3 mmol, and excretion is in bile. In children receiving parenteral nutrition, manganese toxicity has been associated with chronic liver disease and cholestasis. Manganese deficiency has not been reported in humans. The average intake in the United Kingdom is 2 to 5 mg/day, half from tea. Safe intakes for adults are more than 1.5 mg (25 µmol)/day and for children and infants more than 16 µg (0.3 µmol)/kg per day. Breast milk contains 15 µg/litre. A syndrome similar to Parkinson's disease is associated with manganese toxicity and 'manganese madness' was the term used to describe the psychiatric syndrome of manganese toxicity (compulsive behaviour, emotional lability, hallucinations).

Molybdenum

Important dietary sources are wheat flour and its germ, legumes, and meat. Molybdenum is a cofactor for oxidases important in the metabolism of DNA and sulphites, such as xanthine oxidase, xanthine dehydrogenase, aldehyde oxidase, and sulphite oxidase.

Intestinal absorption efficiency is high, at 40 to 100%. Plasma concentration is 1 μg/100 ml, and molybdenum is bound to protein. Storage is in the liver and excretion in urine. There are no clinical reports of molybdenum deficiency in humans, but functional defects responsive to molybdenum occur in adults taking 25 μg/day. Gout has been attributed to high molybdenum intakes of 10 to 15 mg/day. Safe intakes for adults lie between 50 and 400 μg/day (0.5 to 4 μmol/day). Breastfed infants require 0.5 to 1.5 μg/kg per day.

Nickel

It has not been established whether nickel is essential in humans. Absorption is 3 to 6% of the dietary intake. Plasma concentrations are between 2 and 4 μg/100 ml, some of which is bound to albumin. Nickel is excreted in urine. Nickel deficiency might result in depressed growth and haemopoesis. Requirements are unknown, but intakes in the United Kingdom are about 140 μg/day (2.4 μmol/day).

Phosphorus

Phosphorus is present in all natural foods, the usual diet in the United Kingdom providing 1.5 g of phosphorus daily. Phosphorus is an important physiological component: with calcium, of the bony skeleton; of ATP in oxidative phosphorylation; in nucleic acids through phosphorylation of nucleotides; and in enzyme control through phosphorylation by protein kinases. Phosphorus is absorbed as free inorganic phosphorus from the diet (controlled by calcitriol) at both the brush-border and basolateral membranes. The plasma concentration of phosphorus is between 0.8 and 1.4 mmol/litre and it is excreted in both urine and faeces. The bony skeleton contains 80% of the body content of phosphorus as the calcium salt, 19 to 29 mmol (600–900 g). Recommended phosphorus requirements are equimolar to calcium.

Selenium

Selenium is said be 'the only trace element to be specified in the genetic code'. Selenocysteine, which has been dubbed 'the 21st genetically coded amino acid', is a vital component of 35 or more selenoproteins, some of which are important enzymes. Selenium functions as a redox centre, an example of which is the reduction of hydrogen peroxide and lipid and phospholipid hydroperoxides to nondamaging water and alcohols by the glutathione peroxidases. Functions of this kind help maintain membrane integrity, and protect prostacyclin production. Prevention of the oxidative chain reactions in this way prevents further damage to lipids, lipoproteins, and DNA; hence its antioxidant function helps prevent atheroma and cancer, among other things. Selenium is also a cofactor of certain enzymes (e.g. iodothyronine deiodinase and glutathione peroxidases).

Selenium is found in food as selenoamino acids or selenoproteins, and as selenide, selenite, or selenate. Brazil nuts are a rich source, but the main sources of selenium are cereals, meat, and fish. The selenium content of food depends upon soil content and varies regionally and nationally, with soil levels relatively high in Canada, Venezuela, the United States of America, and Japan, and low in most European countries including the United Kingdom. Soil conditions have been associated with clinical selenium toxicity in animals (selenosis) in some areas with very high selenium content, and with selenium deficiency syndromes in animals and humans in areas of low soil selenium. Soil levels in China vary notoriously, with some being exceptionally high, but low level areas associated with the endemic cardiomyopathy, Keshan disease.

Absorption is efficient at 35 to 85%. Population minimum mean intakes likely to meet basal requirements and prevent overt deficiency disease for adult males and females are estimated to be 21 and 16 μg/day, respectively. The RNI for adult men is 75 μg/day (0.9 μmol/day) and for women 60 μg/day (0.8 μmol/day). This intake optimizes the activity of glutathione in plasma and this optimization occurs at plasma levels of 95 μg/litre (range 89–114 μg/litre). However, current intakes in the United Kingdom are about half the RNI. The plasma concentration of selenium is between 7 and 30 μg/100 ml protein bound. Excretion is in urine and possibly bile. Urinary selenium output, red-cell selenium levels, or glutathione peroxidase activity are markers of recent and medium-term dietary intake. Fertility requires an adequate selenium intake, but pregnant women have no additional dietary selenium requirements. Lactation requires an increase in dietary intake of 15 μg/day (0.2 μmol/day). Breast-fed infants should receive approximately 10 μg/day (0.1 μmol/day) and children 15 to 30 μg/day (0.2–0.4 μmol/day). Breast milk contains 20 to 60 μg/litre of selenium.

Clinical applications

Selenium deficiency results in impaired immunity, and supplementation is immune stimulant. Selenium deficiency increases the virulence of some viruses (see Keshan disease in the following paragraphs) by altering their genome to a more virulent one. In veterinary practice, selenium deficiency is well known to result in fetal loss in pregnancy and this may be true in humans too. Selenium is important for male fertility through testosterone synthesis and spermatozoa function. Deficiency may be associated with low mood, increased cognitive decline in older people, and susceptibility to epilepsy. Selenium deficiency exacerbates hypothyroidism in iodine deficiency and may be protective against cardiovascular disease and cancer. It may also be beneficial in a variety of inflammatory conditions by reducing oxidative stress.

Clinical interest in selenium lies in four main areas:

- overt deficiency syndromes
- clinical toxicity
- optimal intakes for health
- use in critical care as an antioxidant

Deficiency syndromes

Keshan disease is a cardiomyopathy associated with enlarged and swollen mitochondria in cardiac muscle. It occurs in selenium-deficient areas of China, and selenium supplementation is beneficial and preventive. It may be the result of an interaction between selenium deficiency and some other factor, perhaps viral (coxsackievirus).

Kashin–Beck disease, first described in 1849, is estimated to affect more than 3 million people worldwide. It is a disabling osteoarticular disease of the epiphyseal growth plate and articular cartilage, which presents at about the age of 5 and involves increasing numbers of joints up the age of 25, following which osteoarthritic degeneration of the affected joints occurs. There is enlargement of the metaphyseal area and shortening of the diaphysis giving rise to arthropathy and growth retardation. Radiologically, the disease affects distal aspects of the limb, especially the lower limb, most with the foot and ankle involved very commonly. The disease is usually bilateral.

Its aetiology is probably multifactorial: factors include selenium and iodine deficiency, fungal contamination of grain, and water contamination with organic material. Kashin–Beck disease is endemic in parts of south-eastern Siberia, Tibet, and China.

Toxicity

The acute ingestion of selenious acid is almost invariably fatal, preceded by stupor, hypotension, and respiratory depression. Prolonged (months, years) intakes of selenium of more than 1000 μg/day are potentially toxic and can result in hair and nail brittleness and loss. The breath smells of garlic as a result of the expiration of dimethyl selenide and there may be a rash, nausea and vomiting, irritability, and fatigue.

Optimal intakes for health

If the intake of selenium in many countries in the world, including the United Kingdom and Europe, are naturally depleted such that they do not achieve optimal plateau levels of glutathione peroxidase or selenoprotein P, what intakes should we aim at in order to optimize health? There is growing evidence that selenium supplementation in such populations may reduce risks of cancer, particularly prostate and gastrointestinal cancer, and cardiovascular disease. Putative anticancer mechanisms include the induction of apoptosis, blocking of cell cycle progression, and inhibition of angiogenesis, reduction in DNA damage, and reduction in oxidative stress, particularly in the context of concomitant low intake of vitamin E. Optimal glutathione peroxidase levels can be achieved an oral intakes close to 100 μg/day but to achieve maximal selenoprotein P concentrations may require larger intakes, which are as yet not fully known. Optimization requirements in individuals may depend upon selenoprotein gene polymorphisms.

Sepsis and critical care

Enzymes such as superoxide dismutase, catalase, and gluthathione peroxidase protect against reactive oxygen species. Selenium is a critical cofactor in the activity of gluthathione peroxidase and is also important in the management of peroxynitrite.

The acute-phase response can reduce circulating levels of selenium, via redistribution out of the blood stream. Studies of patients with burns or systemic immune response syndrome (SIRS) have shown that without supplementation selenium levels can be depleted for a period of 10 to 14 days.

Various doses of selenium have been prescribed in clinical trials to see if this can reduce oxidant stress and mortality in critical illness. The 500-μg dose has been shown to significantly reduce the need for haemodialysis in patients with SIRS and reduce pulmonary infections in patients with burns. Meta-analyses of selenium supplementation trials in critical illness have demonstrated reduction in mortality and that studies using higher than the median dose of selenium(500–1000 μg/day) were associated with a trend toward reduced mortality, whereas studies using a dose less than the median(<500 μg/day) were found to have no effect on mortality. However, a Cochrane meta-analysis in 2005 concluded that there was insufficient evidence to recommend the supplementation of critically ill patients with selenium, except in the setting of randomized clinical trials.

Silicon

Cereal grains and other sources of dietary fibre are important sources of silicon. The role of silicon in human nutrition may be important in cartilage and connective tissue as the human aorta, trachea, lungs, and tendons are rich in silicon. Silicic acid is readily absorbed. The body storage pool is approximately 3 g (1 mol) in a 60-kg man; the plasma monosilicic acid concentration is 500 μg/100 ml. The dietary requirements for silicon are unknown.

Sulphur

Sulphur occurs in proteoglycans; dermatan, chondroitin, and keratin sulphate; glutathione; and coenzymes including coenzyme A. Cysteine, methionine, and disulphide crosslinkage are important in proteins, and sulphate is involved in detoxification processes. Sulphur is absorbed as amino acids, which are subsequently desulphated, and excreted in urine as sulphates. Dietary intake is of the order of 0.7 mg (22 μmol)/day. The dietary requirements for sulphur are unknown.

Zinc

Zinc is an essential nutrient, whose biological functions include cellular integrity and function, growth, immunity, antiapoptotic effects, antioxidant effects through metallothionein induction, and protection against vitamin E depletion. Zinc is an important component of many metalloenzymes, of which carbonic anhydrase was the first to be described; included are over 200 enzymes such as alcohol dehydrogenase, superoxide dismutase, DNA polymerase, RNA polymerase, and alkaline phosphatase. Zinc is therefore required in many processes including nucleic acid synthesis, cell division, protein synthesis and digestion, carbohydrate metabolism, oxygen transport, protection from free radical damage, dark adaptation. It is essential in immune defence: leucocyte-mediated, antibody-mediated, cell-mediated and delayed immune responses. Zinc finger proteins are important as gene transcriptional regulators. It has long been believed that zinc is important for wound healing.

Dietary sources are meats, cheese, whole grains and, to a lesser extent, unrefined cereals, legumes and shellfish. Approximately 20% of dietary zinc is absorbed complexed with amino acids, phosphates, and organic acids. The daily intake of zinc in developed countries is around 9 to 12 mg per day and the RNI for men and women respectively is 9.5 mg and 7.0 mg/day. Deficiency is predicted on long-term intakes below the lower reference nutrient intake (LRNI) of 5.5 and 4.0 mg/day in adult men and women respectively. Phytates and oxalates form insoluble complexes, which inhibit absorption. The normal plasma concentration of zinc is between 80 and 110 μg/100 ml, complexed with albumin. The adult body content of zinc is over 2 g (30 mmol). Bone, the prostate, semen, and the choroid of the eye all contain high concentrations of zinc. Loss of zinc from the body is in faeces.

Deficiency of zinc has been recognized for over 30 years as an important component in growth failure and delayed maturation in populations whose diet is marginal. Zinc replacement can enhance growth and immune competence and reduce infant morbidity, e.g. by reducing acute and chronic diarrhoea and respiratory illness. In hospital practice, deficiency is seen in diarrhoeal states, particularly in the context of short bowel when the duodenal secretions of zinc are insufficiently reabsorbed. Zinc deficiency has been reported as a feature in a number of diseases, including the florid deficiency state and skin condition acrodermatitis enteropathica, an autosomal recessive trait leading to selective impairment of zinc uptake by the upper small-intestinal mucosa. It is also reported in incomplete parenteral nutrition and in patients with severe malabsorption due to Crohn's disease and other intestinal disorders, especially those associated with a loss of inflammatory cells in the gut lumen.

Table 11.2.2 Dietary reference values: RNI (United Kingdom) and USDA goals (United States)

Nutrient	Age/gender	LRNI units	EAR (UK)	RNI[a]	Age/gender	USDA RDA
Thiamin	M 11–50+	0.23 mg/1000 kcal	0.3	0.4	M 14–70+	1.2 mg/day
	F 11–50+	0.23 mg/1000 kcal	0.3	0.4	F 19–70+	1.1 mg/day
Riboflavin	M 11–50+	0.8 mg/day	1.0	1.3	M14–70+	1.3 mg/day
	F 11–50+	0.8 mg/day	0.9	1.1	F 19–70+	1.1 mg/day
Niacin	M11–50+	4.4 mg niacin equiv per 1000 kcal	5.5	6.6	M 14–70+	16 mg/day
	F11–50+	4.4 mg niacin equiv per 1000 kcal	5.5	6.6	F 14–70+	14 mg/day
Vitamin B_6	M11–50+	11 µg per g protein	13	15	M 50+	1.7 mg/day
	F11–50+	11 µg per g protein	13	15	M/F 19–50	1.3 mg/day
Vitamin B_{12}	M 15–50+	1.0 µg/day	1.25	1.5	M/F 14–70+	2.4 µg/day
	F 15–50+	1.0 µg/day	1.25	1.5		
Folate	M 11–50+	100 µg/day	150	200	M/F 14–70+	400 µg/day
	F11–50+	100 µg/day	150	200		
Vitamin C	M 15–50+	10 mg/day	25	40	M 19–70+	90 mg/day
	F 15–50+	10 mg/day	25	40	F19–70+	75 mg/day
Vitamin A	M 15–50+	300µg retinol equivalent/day	500	700	M 11+	1000 µg retinol equivalents
	F 11–50+	250µg retinol equivalent/day	400	600	F 11+	800 µg retinol equivalents
Vitamin D	M/F 11–50	0	0	0		
	M/F 50+	-µg/day	–	10		
Vitamin E	M	- mg/day			M/F 14–70+	15 mg/day
	F					
Vitamin K	M/F	-µg/kg per day				
Calcium	M/F 19–50+	400 (10) mg/day (mmol/day)	525 (13.1)	700 (17.5)	M/F14–70+	1000–1300 mg/day
Magnesium	M 15–50+	190 (7.8) mg/day (mmol/day)	250 (10.3)	300 (12.3)	M 14–70+	400–420 mg/day
	F 19–50+	150 (6.2) mg/day (-mmol/day)	200 (8.2)	270 (10.9)	F 14–70+	310–360 mg/day
Phosphorus		Equal to calcium in mmol				
Sodium	M/F 15–50+	575 mg/day(25 mmol/day)	–	1600 (70)	M/F 14–70+	<2300 mg/day(<101 mmol)
Potassium	M/F 15–50+	2000 mg/day (50 mmol/day)	–	3500 (90)	M/F 14–70+	4700 mg/day (121 mmol)
Chloride	M/F	Equal to sodium in mmol				
Iron	M 19–50	4.7 mg/day (80 µmol/day)	6.7 (120)	8.7 (160)	M 14–70+; F 51–70+	8–11 mg/day
	F 19–50	8.0 mg/day (140 µmol/day)	11.4 (200)	14.8 (260)	F 14–50	15–18 mg
	M/F 50+	4.7 mg/day (80 µmol/day)	6.7 (120)	8.7 (160)		
Zinc	M 15–50+	5.3 mg/day (80 µmol/day)	7.3 (110)	9.5 (145)	M14–70+	11 mg
	F 15–50+	4.0 mg/day (60 µmol/day)	5.5 (85)	7.0 (110)	F 14–70+	8–9 mg
Copper	M/F 18–50+	-mg/d (µmol/day)	–	1.2 (19)	M/F 14–70+	890–900 µg/day
Selenium	M 15–50+	40 µg/d (0.5 µmol/day)	–	70 (0.9)		
	F 15–50+	40 µg/d (0.5 µmol/day)	–	60 (0.8)		
Iodine	M/F 15–50+	70 µg/d (0.6 µmol/day)		140 (1.1)		

[a] UK RNI (units as per LRNI).

The clinical signs are growth retardation, hypogonadism, bullous-pustular dermatitis, paronychia, lethargy, hepatosplenomegaly, and iron-deficiency anaemia, which responds to zinc supplements (15 mg three times daily). Excessive zinc can lead to nausea, vomiting, and fever.

The plasma concentration of unhaemolysed zinc is a measure of a person's current zinc status. Zinc in the red blood cells and hair gives a long-term assessment of zinc status. Adults of all ages (and during pregnancy and lactation) require between 12 and 15 mg of zinc (110–145 µmol)/day. Infants need between 4 and 5 mg/day; however, human milk is not a rich source of zinc (2–3 mg/litre) and the infant depends very much on the stores obtained during its last 3 months of interuterine life. Children require 10 to 15 mg/day.

Clinical applications of micronutrient mixtures

Immunonutrition and micronutrient supplementation in critical illness and surgery

Clinical controlled trials have used 'immune enhancing' enteral feeds, which combine arginine with other 'nutriceuticals' such as antioxidants, glutamine, anti-inflammatory fatty acids, and nucleotides. Most of the clinical trials have employed mixtures of these nutrients in enteral feeds. Since these mixtures vary, results can be difficult to analyse. Meta-analyses have been performed, but provide different interpretations dependent upon which trials are included and which trials are taken together. 'Immunonutrition' feeds tend to be associated with a lower number of infectious complications in critically ill patients and a significantly shorter length of hospital stay, most notably in interventions using a high content of arginine. However, the same meta-analysis drew attention to the significantly higher mortality associated with immunonutrition in trials with high (good) methodological scores. At present, routine use cannot be recommended in critical care, but there may be a place for limited use in the context of complicated surgery.

Oxidant stress can be viewed as pivotal to a gradual amplification of the generalized immune response, to the point where it becomes harmful and progresses to multiple organ failure. The use of large doses of antioxidants might prevent this. In critically ill surgical patients a combination of α-tocopherol and ascorbic acid reduced the risk of developing multiple organ failure. Other antioxidants which have been employed include *N*-acetyl cysteine, vitamin A, and selenium. A meta-analysis showed that aggregation of 11 randomized clinical trials demonstrated reduction in mortality but not infectious complications when antioxidants were tested in critical illness. High-dose parenteral selenium appeared to emerge as the most effective. It is of interest to note that selenium could, through glutathione peroxidase activation, enhance the clinical effect of glutamine.

Preventive antioxidant preparations

Should diet be routinely supplemented? A systematic review of the published literature examined the efficacy of multivitamin and mineral preparations in the primary prevention of chronic disease, specifically cancer, cardiovascular disease, hypertension, cataracts, or age-related macular degeneration. Data for other chronic diseases were lacking. Evidence suggested potential benefit in the primary prevention of cancer in persons with poor nutritional status or suboptimal antioxidant intake. Multivitamin and mineral supplementation had no significant effect on the primary prevention of hypertension, cardiovascular disease, and cataracts, but may slow progression of age-related macular degeneration among persons at high risk for advanced stages of the disease.

Dietary reference values

The dietary recommendations in this chapter are derived from the United Kingdom Department of Health Report on Health and Social Subjects No 41, *Dietary Reference Values for Food and Energy and Nutrients for the United Kingdom*. The estimated average requirement (EAR) is the mean intake which satisfies the needs for an individual nutrient in a normal population of individuals. The requirements are regarded as being normally distributed and the interindividual variability can be expressed as standard deviations of this mean. The reference nutrient intake (RNI) is set two standard deviations above the EAR and represents a level of intake that is very likely to be adequate for this nutrient. The lower reference nutrient intake (LRNI) is set two standard deviations below the EAR and represents a level below which intake of the nutrient is very likely to be inadequate. These can be compared with the United States Institute of Medicine recommendations, the dietary reference intakes (DRIs), which include estimated average requirements (EARs), recommended daily allowances (RDAs), adequate intakes (AI), and tolerable upper intake levels (ULs). The EAR is the average daily nutrient intake level estimated to meet the requirement of half the healthy individuals in a particular life stage and gender group; the RDA is the dietary intake level that is sufficient to meet the nutrient requirement of nearly all (97–98%) healthy individuals in a particular life stage and gender group; the AI is a recommended average daily intake level based on observed or experimentally determined approximations or estimates of mean nutrient intake by groups of apparently healthy people, which is used when the RDA cannot be determined. The UL is the highest average daily nutrient intake likely to pose no risk of adverse health effects for nearly all individuals in a particular life stage or gender group. As intake increases above the UL, the potential risk of adverse effects increases. Table 11.2.2 shows EARs and RNIs for the United Kingdom and compares them with the American RDA.

Further reading

General

Cox DN *et al.* (1998). Take five, a nutrition education intervention to increase fruit and vegetable intakes. *Br J Nutr*, **80**, 123–31.

Eastwood M (1997). *Principles of human nutrition*. Aspen, Gaithersburg, MD.

Panel on Dietary Reference Values of the Committee on Medical Aspects of Food Policy (1991). *Report on Health and Social Subjects 41. Dietary reference values for food energy and nutrients for the United Kingdom*. HMSO, London.

Powers HJ (1997). Vitamin requirements for term infants: considerations for infant formulae. *Nutr Res Rev*, **10**, 1–33.

Sadler MJ, Strain JJ, Caballero B, (eds) (1999). *Encylopedia of human nutrition*. Academic Press, San Diego, CA.

Ziegler EE, Filer LJ Jr (eds.) (1996). *Present knowledge in nutrition*, 7th edition. ILSI Press, Washington DC.

Vitamin C

Benzie IFF (1999). Vitamin C: prospective functional markers for defining optimal nutritional status. *Proc Nutr Soc*, **58**, 469–76.

Sauberlich HE (1994). Pharmacology of vitamin C. *Annu Rev Nutr*, **14**, 371–91.

Thiamin, biotin, and pantothenic acid

Bender DA (1999). Optimum nutrition: thiamin, biotin and pantothenate. *Proc Nutr Soc*, **58**, 427–33.

Folate

Butterworth CE Jr, Bendich A (1996). Folic acid and the prevention of birth defects. *Annu Rev Nutr*, **16**, 73–97.

McNulty H (1997). Folate requirements for women. *Proc Nutr Soc*, **56**, 291–303.

Scott JM (1999). Folate and vitamin B12. *Proc Nutr Soc*, **58**, 441–8.

Selhub J (1999). Homocysteine metabolism. *Annu Rev Nutr*, **19**, 217–46.

Vitamin B_{12}

Scott JM (1999). Folate and vitamin B_{12}. *Proc Nutr Soc*, **58**, 441–8.

Vitamin A/carotenoids

McClaren DS (1980). *Nutritional ophthalmology*. Academic Press, London.

Semba RD (1997). Vitamin A and human immunodeficiency virus disease. *Proc Nutr Soc*, **56**, 459–69.

Thurnham DI, Northrop-Clewes CA (1999). Optimal nutrition: vitamins and the carotenoids. *Proc Nutr Soc*, **58**, 449–57.

Vershinin A (1999). Biological functions of carotenoids—diversity and evolution. *Biofactors*, **10**, 99–104.

Wang XD, Russell RM (1999). Procarcinogenic and anticarcinogenic effect of β-carotene. *Nutr Rev*, **57**, 263–72.

Vitamin D

Bischoff-Ferrari HA *et al.* (2009). Fall prevention with supplemental and active forms of vitamin D: a meta—analysis of randomised controlled trials. *BMJ*, **339**, b3692.

Nutritional aspects of bone; a symposium (1997). *Proc Nutr Soc*, **56**, 903–87.

Wilkinson RJ *et al.* (2000). Influence of vitamin D deficiency and vitamin D receptor polymorphisms on tuberculosis among Gujarati Asians in west London: a case control study. *Lancet*, **355**, 618–21.

Vitamin E

Gabsi S *et al.* (2001). Effect of vitamin E supplementation in patients with ataxia with vitamin E deficiency. *Eur J Neurol*, **8**, 477–81.

Halliwell B (1996). Antioxidants in human health and disease. *Annu Rev Nutr*, **16**, 33–50.

Moreno-Reyes R *et al.* (1998). Kashin–Beck osteoarthropathy in rural Tibet in relation to selenium status. *N Engl J Med*, **339**, 1112–20.

Morrisey PA, Sheehy PJA (1999). Optimal nutrition: vitamin E. *Proc Nutr Soc*, **58**, 459–68.

Stevenson VL, Hardie RJ (2001). Acanthocytosis and neurological disorders. *J Neurol*, **248**, 87–94.

Traber MG, Sies H (1996). Vitamin E in humans: demand and delivery. *Annu Rev Nutr*, **16**, 321–47.

Trace elements

Arthur JR, Beckett GJ, Mitchell JH (1999). The interactions between selenium and iodine deficiencies in man and animals. *Nutr Res Rev*, **12**, 55–73.

Cousins RJ (1994). Metal elements and gene expression. *Annu Rev Nutr*, **14**, 449–69.

Failla ML (1999). Considerations for determining 'optimal nutrition' for copper, zinc, manganese and molybdenum. *Proc Nutr Soc*, **58**, 497–505.

Goyer RA (1997). Toxic and essential metal interactions. *Annu Rev Nutr*, **17**, 37–50.

Lukaski HC (1999). Chromium as a supplement. *Annu Rev Nutr*, **19**, 279–302.

11.3

Severe malnutrition

Alan A. Jackson

Essentials

Severe malnutrition is the consequence of systemic deficiency of energy and nutrients over a prolonged period: in children development is stunted and the individual is at risk of fatal (often clinically 'silent') infection and other illnesses. It is a medical and societal emergency: mortality is high, despite attempts to provide appropriate care.

When severe malnutrition affects several individuals in a society, it reflects a state in which basic needs and justice are not met. Severe malnutrition may also result from clinical disorders affecting a single person with gastrointestinal disease, poor appetite or reduced food intake for other reasons.

Classification

The World Health Organization has produced guidelines for facility-based care of patients suffering severe malnutrition. Prompt classification into groups of differential risk assists in the identification of those requiring the most immediate clinical care (severe acute malnutrition, defined as weight for height more than 3 standard deviations below the reference mean, or the presence of oedema of both feet) and in monitoring the outcomes of intervention. Low height for age indicates long-term malnutrition or poor health (stunting); low weight for height indicates recent or continuing severe weight loss (wasting); low weight for age implies stunting and/or wasting.

Prevention

Malnutrition is a preventable condition and the early identification of those at risk (e.g. by regular weighing) and the implementation of interventions (e.g. advice and demonstration of best practice in child care and feeding) which correct underlying problems and prevent further deterioration is central to strategies for effective care.

Childhood malnutrition is a clinical problem for the individual, but also a symptom of ineffective public health policy. Aside from feeding, important aspects are to recognize and treat infection, immunize against infection, enhance the child-rearing skills of the parents, and strengthen general hygienic practices.

Severe acute malnutrition

Severe malnutrition results from the interaction of three distinct but related processes: (1) reductive adaptation, which is a general response to preserve essential function that takes place when the demands of the body for energy and nutrients are not adequately met; (2) inflammatory/immune responses and healing, which are impaired as a result of reductive adaptations; (3) specific nutrient deficiencies, when failure because of marginal diet to correct excessive losses of nutrients (e.g. through diarrhoea and vomiting) leads to major imbalances. These combine to put the child at risk of the deadly triad of infection, hypothermia, and hypoglycaemia, often compounded by marked fluid and electrolyte disturbances.

Sick malnourished individuals have no appetite for food, with loss of appetite being an important protective mechanism against consuming food which is likely to stress the systems of the body. Attempts (well meaning) to force feed are dangerous: the potentially fatal 'recovery syndrome' (manifest as heart failure, progressing to circulatory collapse, often with severe secretory diarrhoea) must be avoided. Aside from the provision of a sympathetic and quiet environment during treatment, key aspects of management include: (1) resuscitation—management of infection, fluid and electrolyte imbalances, and shock, also treatment of vitamin A deficiency; (2) stabilization—give small frequent meals (every 3–4 h throughout 24 h; 100 kcal/kg per day; 1–1.5 g protein/kg per day), add specific nutrients to food to correct deficiency (potassium, magnesium, folic acid, zinc, copper, multivitamin), treat infections, transfuse for severe anaemia, treat skin lesions, exclude tuberculosis; (3) weight gain (rapid catch up growth)—*ad libitum* intake, continue with micronutrient supplements, add supplemental iron.

Introduction

Severe malnutrition occurs in societies that are not able to meet basic needs for health care and survival. It is characterized by underdevelopment, poverty and deprivation, an insanitary environment, frequent infections, and food that is poor in quality or limited in availability. A series of vicious cycles operate within individuals and across generations, limiting the ability of vulnerable groups, families, and individuals to cope with the harsh realities of a hostile environment, either through the exigencies of nature or a human unwillingness to share the available resources with greater equity. Across the globe, severe malnutrition is a common condition during childhood. It is most prevalent amongst the poorest in developing countries, but it is also found with uncomfortable frequency amongst the most deprived of every society, including those in Europe and North America. It is a frequent aspect of clinical medicine in patients who, for any reason, have a loss of appetite or a reduction in food intake. The same principles of management and care apply wherever the problem is found.

Malnutrition at any age impairs the ability to perform and function. Children with severe malnutrition are at risk of life-threatening diseases, which require urgent attention. More insidiously, malnutrition during childhood stunts development and leaves a scar that remains for the rest of that person's life. This lost potential can express itself as an increased risk of ill health, as impaired intellectual development leading to poor school performance, or in limited physical development leading to poorer work performance. Once part of an individual's potential for development has been lost, the clinical and social implications tend to be cumulative. On a global scale, the sum total of the loss of individual capability represents a fundamental brake on aspirations for social and economic development. Most recent estimates indicate that globally, 35% of the disease burden for children under 5 years of age can be attributed directly or indirectly to malnutrition, at least 3.5 million deaths and 11% of total global disability-adjusted life years (DALYs) This burden is not spread evenly between different parts of the world. For the worst-affected countries, as many as 50% of children under 5 have malnutrition, which is severe enough to threaten life, with the highest prevalence in sub-Saharan Africa and the greatest numbers in South-East Asia. This is representative of the day-to-day situation, and is not a peculiarity of special emergencies. There are at least 200 million children in the world for whom severe deprivation, indexed as stunting or survival on less than $1/day, has limited their potential for normal physical and neurocognitive development.

Notwithstanding the large number of children with severe malnutrition, over the past 20 years there has been a shift to the right of the curve for the distribution of the height and weight of children, indicating a general success for specific interventions. Thus, change is possible, and when suitable measures are put in place sustained improvement can be achieved. However, there is absolutely no basis for complacency, as recent figures suggest a slowing down, or even a reversal, of this improvement. This may relate to an inability to control infections effectively, with tuberculosis, malaria, and diarrhoea continuing to play a major role and the HIV epidemic making a significant contribution. The world's population continues to increase, so an improvement in percentage terms does not necessarily mean a decrease in the absolute numbers of malnourished people across the globe.

Table 11.3.1 The case mortality for complicated severe malnutrition has failed to improve because of four major errors of management (from Scholfield C and Ashworth A (1996). Why have mortality rates for severe malnutrition remained so high? *Bulletin of the World Health Organization* **74**, 223–9)

1.	The assumption that a low plasma albumin concentration is the basis of oedema and can be effectively treated with a high-protein diet
2.	Uncomplicated cases can be treated effectively in the community, but those with complications, indexed by poor appetite and oedema, require care in a facility
3.	The use of diuretics for the treatment of oedema
4.	Early use of iron supplements to treat anaemia
5.	Failing to differentiate that the acute illness should be managed before any attempts to correct weight loss

Severe malnutrition is a late stage in a process where an individual has had inadequate access to sufficient energy and nutrients for a period of time. During this time, the function of the body changes until a point is reached where severely malnourished children are significantly different from normal children in their response to medical treatment. This stage differentiates those who might be readily treated in a community setting from those who require more skilled care in a facility. If this group is treated in the same way as normal children, they will very likely die. Based upon best practice, mortality would be expected to be around 5 to 10%, but in many centres, case mortality has remained unchanged for 50 years, around 40 to 50%. Sometimes, this can be attributed to poor case management, with four major errors in care occurring in about 80% of centres (Table 11.3.1). However, frequently, the organization of systems of care is poor or the availability of simple, basic resources are limited or insecure.

The World Health Organization (WHO) has produced guidelines for community and facility-based care with effective facility-based treatment using a 10-step approach (Fig. 11.3.1). During the early period of care, the order in which different aspects of treatment

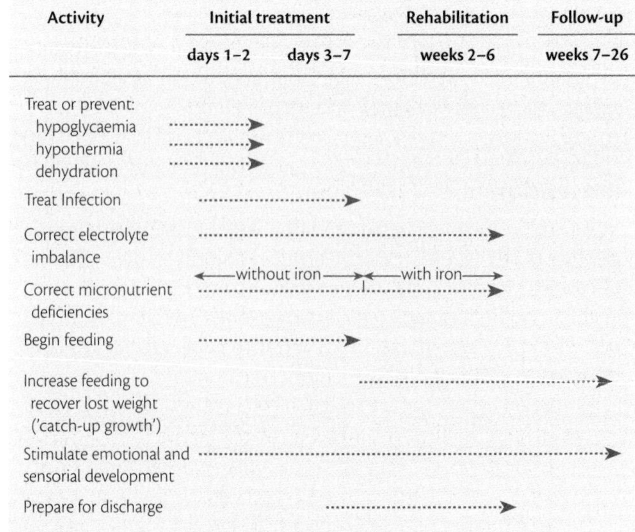

Fig. 11.3.1 WHO recommendations for the 10-step approach to the management of severe malnutrition.

Table 11.3.2 Important clinical features to enable immediate clinical decisions for emergency management of severe malnutrition

Feature	Details/relevance
Anthropometry	Stunting, wasting, presence of pitting oedema
Gastrointestinal	History of anorexia, poor appetite, vomiting, diarrhoea. Appearance of mouth. Distended or scaphoid abdomen, with succussion splash
Liver	Degree of enlargement, jaundice, petechiae
Cardiovascular	Circulatory collapse, anaemia, shock (depleted intravascular volume, cold hands and feet, weak radial pulse, diminished consciousness) ± signs of 'dehydration' (sunken eyes, sunken fontanelle, decreased skin turgor)
Infection	Hypothermia, fever, localizing signs (respiratory distress, broken skin, mouth, ears)
Specific deficiencies	Eye signs of xerophthalmia, vitamin A

are carried out is critical for a successful outcome. A central feature is that, as a first step, the body's cellular machinery has to be repaired if function is to be restored. Silent infections are common. There have been unusual losses of nutrients from the body, which cannot be corrected adequately on a standard diet. The damaged systems of the body are not able to cope with excess energy or further stress. Effective treatment requires the ordered correction of the underlying problems before any attempts are made to correct the tissue deficits.

Clinical syndromes

Severe malnutrition can present with an array of clinical symptoms and signs, which depend upon the duration of the illness, the extent of coinfection, the particular pattern of nutrient deficiencies and metabolic disturbances, and other associated complications such as diarrhoea and vomiting with attendant disturbances in fluid and electrolytes (Table 11.3.2). All descriptions of the condition emphasize one or other feature of the presentation. The archetypal descriptive terms for childhood malnutrition—kwashiorkor, marasmus, or marasmic kwashiorkor—were originally used to characterize clinical syndromes.

The first description of the kwashiorkor syndrome emphasized the development, location, and timing of the skin lesion, with progression from friable hyperpigmented skin, which stripped to reveal hypopigmented skin, which ulcerated easily to provide a ready portal for infection—lesions distinct from pellagra. Other features such as abnormal affect and hepatomegaly were noted, but were less remarkable. Placing emphasis upon variability in clinical presentation has made comparison difficult and encouraged the idea that the underlying pathophysiology, and hence its treatment, differs in important ways between locations. This has diverted attention from similarities in the fundamental changes that take place across the range of clinical presentations.

The function of the body is controlled through the integration of many systems. A fault in any one has implications for the function of all the others. Thus, there is the need for adequate amounts of energy, energy-generating nutrients (carbohydrate, lipid, and protein), minerals, and a range of micronutrients for the body to function effectively in a harmonized way. Lack of any one component, or an imbalance, leads to deranged handling of other components. By adopting an agreed classification, relevant comparisons have been drawn, and it is clear that the range of clinical features represent varying manifestations of a clinical disorder with the interaction of qualitative and quantitative factors. The quantitative change results from an inadequate intake of food and leads to a wasting syndrome, classically marasmus, with the progressive loss of tissue, especially marked for subcutaneous fat and muscle. The result is a thin appearance, with pinched features, thin arms and legs, and a scaphoid abdomen. Qualitative changes are usually associated with unusual losses of nutrients from the body, for example through diarrhoea or infection, reordered metabolism to deal with metabolic stress, or the toxic effects of a range of noxious exposures. The end result of this process is likely to be the loss of cellular integrity and control, leading to oedema.

Classification

An effective classification differentiates those at greatest risk, guides suitable interventions, and helps determine the extent to which interventions have successfully corrected the problem. The more severely malnourished an individual, the greater the risk of complications, and the risk of an adverse outcome is related to the severity of the weight deficit or the extent to which normal function is deranged. The term 'severe acute malnutrition' (SAM) has been introduced to differentiate those who are in need of immediate clinical care associated with wasting, from the more chronic problems associated with stunting. These changes can all be marked either quantitatively or qualitatively. SAM is defined as severe wasting (a score of less than -3 standard deviations weight for height, or on screening a mid-upper arm circumference of less than 110 mm), or the presence of oedema of both feet, or clinical signs of severe malnutrition (Table 11.3.3). Recently, WHO have introduced new growth standards for infants and children up to 5 years of age and their use in practice will have to be compared with the current reference.

Table 11.3.3 Classification of malnutrition. The diagnoses are not mutually exclusive

Moderate malnutrition	Severe malnutrition
Symmetrical oedema	
No	Yes (oedematous malnutrition)*
Weight for height	
SD score between −3 and −2† (70 to 79%)‡	SD score below −3 (< 70%) (severe wasting)§
Height for age	
SD score between −3 and −2 (85 to 89%)	SD score below −3 (< 85%) (severe stunting)

*This includes kwashiorkor and marasmic kwashiorkor in older classifications. To avoid confusion with the clinical syndrome of kwashiorkor, which includes other features, the term 'oedematous malnutrition' is preferred.

†Below the WHO growth standard; the SD score is defined as the deviation of the value for the individual from the median value for the reference population, divided by the standard deviation of the reference population.

‡Percentage of the median WHO growth standard.

§This corresponds to marasmus (without oedema) in the Wellcome clinical classification, and to grade III malnutrition in the Gomez system. To avoid confusion the term severe wasting is preferred.

Quantitative measures indicate the extent to which the expected pattern of growth in height and weight has not been achieved: low height for age, low weight for height, and low weight for age. Low height for age (shortness or stunting) is indicative of longer-term malnutrition or poor health. Low weight for height (thinness or wasting) implies recent or continuing current severe weight loss. Low weight for age (insufficient weight relative to age) implies stunting and/or wasting. Weight is more easily measured than height, and assessing weight for age is the simplest way of excluding severe malnutrition in the absence of oedema. Weight for age is influenced by both height for age and weight for height. Where deprivation is common, there is a high prevalence of low height for age. Weight for age is more strongly influenced by stunting than by wasting, and requires broader public health approaches for its alleviation, being unlikely to respond in the short term to aggressive clinical intervention. The prevalence of stunting starts to increase at around 3 months of age, and the process of stunting slows down at around 3 years of age, after which mean heights run parallel to the reference. Weight for height has the advantage that it can be used when age is not known reliably and suggests recent severe weight loss, indicating those children who are most likely to benefit from immediate aggressive nutritional intervention and support. The rate at which weight improves is used to assess progress during recovery, and success of care is indicated by the achievement of a weight that is appropriate for the individual's height. The measurement of mid-upper arm circumference provides simple, robust indication of the degree of wasting in this age group and is recommended in screening for SAM.

In places where SAM is common there is the need to differentiate those who can be effectively and reliably managed by supervised care in the community, and those who require the level of care that can only be provided in a facility. This differentiation is made using qualitative criteria on the basis of appetite, the presence of oedema, or other identifiable serious comorbidity. Qualitative criteria are more difficult, because of their variability and uncertainty about whether they mark any particular pathophysiological process. It has been agreed that the presence of pitting oedema is the archetype of qualitative change, identified as kwashiorkor in the Wellcome classification and now called oedematous malnutrition. In milder forms, oedema might be restricted to the limbs, but in more severe forms it embraces the entire body. Obtaining a reliable measure of body weight is difficult in the presence of oedema, because of the uncertain contribution of oedematous fluid. The overall appearance might be of a child who superficially appears full, but has evident wasting below the oedema when examined carefully with the clothes removed. The extent of poor appetite or anorexia may be elicited by history, although in some situations, a formal trial of feeding has been used.

Multiple infection is common and often silent, so that specific sites of infection may be difficult to identify or localize. A high index of suspicion is required for the presence of silent infections, which should be presumed to be present. Infection is not part of the diagnostic criteria.

Natural history and clinical presentation

Inadequate nutrition slows the pace of growth and development and the greater the severity of the limitation or insult, or the longer its duration, the greater the difference between the achieved development and that expected. The stress of an insult of greater severity evokes a metabolic response that is associated with a loss of body weight and a reordering of function, so that resources and effort devoted to growth and development are diverted to maintain the integrity of the individual. The nutritional health of the infant is critically determined by how well prepared the mother was to carry the pregnancy, and the effectiveness with which breastfeeding is established and maintained. During pregnancy and for the first months of life, the infant is totally dependent upon the mother for its nutrient supply. During early pregnancy, there is the elaboration and maturation of function in the fetus. The last trimester is of critical importance as it is when the fetus accumulates effective reserves of nutrients, helping survival and facilitating development during the first year of life. The fetus accumulates reserves of energy, as subcutaneous lipid, and of minerals and vitamins, such as iron, zinc, copper, vitamin A, riboflavin, and pyridoxine, in liver and muscle. At birth, the relative protection of the intrauterine environment is replaced by the many hazards of the external world. Gastrointestinal and respiratory infections are amongst the serious dangers to survival, and breastfeeding provides effective protection from both. Even in affluent societies, breastfeeding provides the infant with a level of protection against ill health that identifies effective breastfeeding as a singularly important feature in any rational policy in public health nutrition. There is a massive increase in the risk of ill health for infants who are not breastfed during the early months of life. This risk is magnified enormously for infants exposed to unsanitary environments with limited access to health care. Anything that limits the growth of the fetus, impairs its development, or causes it to be delivered early will limit its ability to cope with extrauterine life, and increase the risk of problems, infections, and malnutrition. There is enhanced mother–infant bonding and emotional development with breastfeeding, and other special benefits include the remarkable bioavailability of energy and nutrients, the presence of non-nutritional factors, protective factors, and growth factors.

Screening: identification and prevention

Malnutrition is a preventable condition, and the early identification of those at risk and the implementation of interventions that correct underlying problems and prevent further deterioration are central to strategies for effective care. Early growth failure can be detected by regular weighing, as an integral part of immunization and other health programmes. A series of plotted weights is most valuable, and intervention is required for those whose weight crosses two growth centiles on successive measurements. If measurements are only available for a single time point, then height for age, weight for height, or mid upper-arm circumference provides an indication of any past or ongoing growth failure. Advice and demonstration of best practice in child care and feeding may be sufficient to correct a mild degree of growth failure, but persistent or more severe growth failure requires closer investigation to exclude underlying problems. Poor anthropometry, with a history of poor appetite and weight loss, should always be taken very seriously and pursued until a cause has been identified and corrected. Severe malnutrition is a medical emergency.

Childhood malnutrition is a clinical problem for the individual, but is also a symptom of ineffective public health policy. Targeted interventions should address the immediate needs of the child, but should also embrace broader considerations. For the child, there is the need to effectively immunize against infection, recognize and treat infection in a timely way, and ensure an effective period of nutritional support following infection. For the family, there is the need to enhance the child-rearing skills of the parents, create a stimulating environment, acquire and practice simple skills in hygiene and food preparation, and strengthen family dynamics and coping strategies. For the community, there is the need to improve the economic base of households, increase food purchasing power, increase food security or household food availability, and treat specific nutrient deficiencies. Sound hygienic practices have to be strengthened at the group or household level, and where necessary, the amount and quality of water and the safe and effective removal of solid waste improved. Each activity can exert a beneficial effect on growth and development. Any one might be relatively easy to introduce, but the real difficulty is to ensure that all are sustained. The need is for a fundamental change in the health culture and the creation of a framework of behaviour in which development activities become rooted and take place as a matter of course. A failure to establish and maintain an effective system of health care leads to a progressive deterioration in the clinical state of the most vulnerable infants, leading eventually to severe malnutrition. The World Bank has identified the severe limitation this places on national development, and the need to have effective interventions before 2 years of age if this critical potential is not to be lost.

Aetiology and pathophysiology

Children may become malnourished simply because there is not enough food available. Community-based interventions place emphasis on providing adequate amounts of food of high nutritional value, if necessary as ready-to-use therapeutic-foods (RUTF), but sick malnourished individuals have no appetite for food. It seems paradoxical that a child who has obviously lost weight and needs to eat may refuse food even when it is readily available. If food is forced, there is the possibility that the child will become worse, or even die. In managing severe malnutrition, appetite is one of the most important symptoms. A loss of appetite is an important protective mechanism against consuming food, which is likely to stress the systems of the body. In experimental studies, there are two major biological reasons why appetite is lost: a deficiency of a specific nutrient and infection. Severe malnutrition is a disorder that results from the interaction of three distinct but related processes, each of which appears to be related directly to the food consumed, but none of which can be easily understood simply by a consideration of food:

- reductive adaptation
- inflammatory and immune responses
- specific nutrient deficiencies

Food helps meet the many needs for normal function, growth, and development in childhood, but also the ability to cope with environmental challenge. A diet that is adequate, but marginal under normal circumstances, is inadequate for the increased demands during recovery from frequent intercurrent illness with the double burden of the need to catch up growth and to make good the unusual losses of nutrients during the infective episode itself. The time available for successful convalescence before the next bout of infection is too short to adequately make up the deficit.

Reductive adaptation: failure to meet the body's usual demands for macronutrients

Reductive adaptation takes place when the demands of the body for energy and nutrients are not adequately met by the dietary intake. The general features are similar, regardless of the basis for the inadequate intake. It is a general response to preserve essential function, but carries a cost. Normal metabolism takes place within a highly regulated environment, through the control and integration of exchange and turnover amongst cells and tissues. For the cellular machinery of the body to remain functionally intact and operationally effective, it requires a constant supply of energy and other nutrients. An estimated one-third of resting energy expenditure may be consumed through the synthesis and degradation of macromolecules such as protein, and a further one-third is associated with the movement of material across membranes, e.g. through the pumping activity of the sodium/potassium pump, Na^+,K^+-ATPase. These processes represent the internal work of the body at cellular level and underlie the functioning of all the organs and tissues. They take place continuously, and the total activity can be measured as energy expenditure. As food consumption is intermittent, the processes are independent of the immediate food intake. However, a sustained lack of food leads to progressive impairment of the cellular machinery as damage due to the wear and tear of normal use can no longer be replaced effectively.

Structure

When food consumption is significantly reduced, metabolic processes continue to enable the body to function, and the energy to support these processes is derived from reserves within the body. The body is in negative energy balance, and tissue mass cannot be maintained, leading to loss in weight. The losses are uneven between tissues, with major losses in subcutaneous fat and muscle, and relative preservation of the metabolically more active visceral tissues. One important consequence is that heat generated by muscle is reduced, and at the same time, insulation in the skin is impaired leading to greater heat loss. The altered body composition underlies all anthropometric methods that are used to assess nutritional status. In addition to the changes in mass, efficiencies in the utilization of energy have to be found.

Function

Efficiencies are achieved by reducing the amount of work carried out by the body. External work is reduced by decreasing physical activity. Internal work is reduced by decreasing cellular metabolic activity, with subsequent effects upon tissue function. Significant efficiencies might be achieved for the major energy-consuming processes such as membrane pumping, protein turnover, and cellular replication. The relative distribution of potassium in the intracellular space and sodium in the extracellular space is fundamental to maintaining the chemical environment of cells. As potassium tends to leak out of the cell and sodium tends to leak into the cell, for the cell membrane to maintain the effective partitioning of electrolytes requires that sodium is pumped out of the cell in exchange for potassium, consuming ATP. The cell membrane tends to become more 'leaky' in malnutrition as its lipid composition changes, and the Na^+,K^+-ATPase is down-regulated as one way in which to reduce energy expenditure. Therefore, compared with normal, all people with malnutrition have reduced intracellular potassium and increased intracellular sodium, hence decreased total body potassium and increased total body sodium, which is not necessarily identified on standard biochemical tests. The ability to maintain protein synthesis is fundamental but energetically expensive; energetic efficiency requires a reduction in protein synthesis, which is not divided equally among tissues. Liver normally accounts for about 25% of protein synthesis, with the synthesis of nutrient transport proteins playing a critical role in the delivery of lipid, minerals, and vitamins to the other tissues. Reduced synthesis of nutrient transport proteins may save energy, but at the cost of reduced delivery to peripheral tissues; e.g. limited synthesis of apolipoproteins limits the delivery of lipid to peripheral tissues and enhances the accumulation of lipid in liver. Cellular replication is energetically demanding, requiring the ready availability of all nutrients. A reduction in cellular replication provides efficiencies in energy and nutrient use but impairs the function of systems critically dependent upon cellular replication: the skin, gastrointestinal tract, respiratory tract, and immune system.

Functional and metabolic cost of reductive adaptation

The function of the cells in all tissues is affected by reductive adaptation. With relative protection of more vital functions, the cost is a reduction in those functions that are not immediately vital, but which provide the functional reserve capability that enables the metabolic flexibility to respond to a changed internal environment or a challenge from the external environment. As a consequence, changes that would be readily managed in the normal state present a metabolic stress in the reductively adapted state. What would normally be a modest challenge can induce a major metabolic perturbation. Reductive adaptation represents the loss of reserve capacity, which leads to increased metabolic brittleness and vulnerability. The cellular machinery is no longer capable of responding effectively to the usual challenges. There is a change in the function of all systems.

Gastrointestinal tract

There is loss of mucosa and submucosal tissues, loss of gastric acidity, and a reduced capacity for digestion and absorption. This leads to impaired bioavailability of nutrients from food, decreased transit time, and predisposition to small bowel bacterial overgrowth. An impaired ability to repair and maintain the integrity of the endothelium predisposes to bacterial translocation and overexposure to endotoxins.

Skin

The skin wastes, loses its ability to retain heat, and readily becomes breached and infected.

Immune system

There is increased exposure to pathogens and a decreased capacity to respond (inflammation and immune response—see following paragraphs).

Liver

There is down-regulation of synthetic and excretory processes. The reduced functional reserve makes it more difficult to maintain glucose homeostasis in the face of increased bacterial exposure. Intermediary metabolism is impaired, and transport proteins for the delivery of lipid, vitamins, and minerals to other parts of the body are reduced. The formation of clotting factors is impaired. Reduced bile and bile salt formation affect digestion. Metabolism and clearance of drugs, toxins, and xenobiotics is also reduced.

Cardiovascular system

A reduction in the functional reserve of the heart, slower pulse, and increased circulation time make heart failure more likely if excess fluid is given intravenously. There is poor circulatory control, with a tendency to reduced intravascular volume with an expanded interstitial fluid space.

Iron is an integral part of haemoglobin in red blood cells, involved in the transport of oxygen from the lungs to the tissues. The mass of red cells is related to the amount of oxygen that has to be transported, which, in turn, relates to the mass of active lean tissue. As part of reductive adaptation, there is a decrease in the lean tissue of the body with an associated decrease in the red cell mass. The iron that is released from haemoglobin is not required immediately for the formation of more red cells. The level of iron in the body is controlled by the rate at which it is absorbed from the gastrointestinal tract, as, once in the body, there are no recognized mechanisms through which iron can be lost. The iron released from red cells therefore cannot be excreted and is placed into storage. Free iron is highly reactive and acts as a focus for uncontrolled excess generation of free radicals, thereby damaging other cellular components. Excess iron is stored in the liver, bound to ferritin. A demand for ferritin synthesis is energetically expensive and diverts amino acids from the formation of other proteins. As part of reductive adaptation, the ability to effectively sequester iron in a chemically quiescent state is impaired.

Renal

There is decreased functional capacity of the kidney, with an impaired ability to concentrate, dilute, or acidify urine.

Muscle

Muscle mass is reduced, and muscle function impaired by reduced potassium, which together lead to reduced generation of heat.

Brain

Brain function is relatively well preserved. Nevertheless, there is blunting of higher functions with decreased mentation, apathy, and depression, and impaired control of hormonal and integrative responses. There is a decrease in activity, poor work performance, and a decrease in discretionary activities, which together contribute to a slowing of learning.

Infection: the inflammatory and immune responses

Survival in a potentially hostile world requires effective nonspecific and specific defence mechanisms. Nonspecific physical barriers (skin and mucous membranes) and chemical protection (gastric acidity, secretions such as tears and mucins) depend upon cellular replication, which is less well maintained during reductive adaptation, and even minor damage leads to a breach that is not repaired. Local damage with bacterial invasion usually elicits local inflammation, a systemic or acute phase response, and a specific immune response. The mounting, coordination, and regulation of an effective response require energy, increased cellular replication, and protein synthesis. The changes in hormones and cytokines associated with reductive adaptation impair the establishment and control of normal inflammatory and immune responses. The localized signs of tissue damage or infection—enlarged lymph nodes, enlargement of the spleen or liver, and the normal features of the acute-phase response (fever, rapid pulse, and respiration)—are blunted or lost in malnutrition, making diagnosis more difficult.

Loss of appetite is a central feature of a more severe acute-phase response, as the body raids its own tissues for the nutrients it requires to satisfy this unusual demand. There is a shift from the usual pattern of protein synthesis, with less emphasis on growth. As muscle wastes, the amino acids are made available for the synthesis of proteins for the immune system, and the liver shifts from synthesizing large amounts of nutrient transport proteins to the formation of acute-phase response proteins, which limit cell damage and help repair. Intravascular albumin is redistributed to the third space, leading to a reduced plasma albumin concentration. A low plasma albumin is frequently seen in malnourished people and is indicative of ongoing infection rather a dietary deficiency of protein. Correcting the problem requires that the underlying infection be effectively treated, not that dietary protein be increased. The cells of the inflammatory and immune systems increase their utilization of glucose, with increased gluconeogenesis from amino acids. A feature of the acute phase response is a profound change in the handling of micronutrients. There is a block in the absorption of iron. Net tissue breakdown releases components for which there is no immediate use. The circulating concentrations may be reduced (iron and zinc, which are sequestered in the liver), or increased (copper), and there may be increased losses from the body in urine or stools (zinc and vitamin A). In childhood, diarrhoea is a frequent accompaniment of infection, which adds an excessive loss of nutrients from the body, especially potassium, magnesium, zinc, and vitamin A.

Specific nutrient deficiencies

Deficiency of specific nutrients is the most difficult aspect of severe malnutrition to manage effectively. Whereas in classical deficiency states, inadequate dietary intake is usually the major underlying cause, in severe malnutrition, it is the failure to correct excessive losses of nutrients, which leads to major imbalances. Major losses of intracellular nutrients can be difficult to identify reliably, for three reasons:

- Losses of intracellular content may not be readily identified using standard biochemical tests on blood (e.g. potassium).
- Bone acts as a very effective buffer for many nutrients and therefore severe total body depletion can develop without obvious biochemical change or loss of function (e.g. magnesium).
- During an inflammatory response, redistribution of nutrients within the body makes standard tests for nutrient deficiency very difficult to interpret (e.g. vitamin A, zinc, or iron).

Infection causes an unbalanced loss of nutrients, which may be obvious in association with diarrhoea and vomiting, or may be more subtle as in the increased urinary losses of vitamin A and zinc which are an integral feature of the acute-phase response. For an individual consuming a diet that is marginal in one or other nutrient, increased losses may make the critical difference to achieving balance, which cannot be restored unless additional nutrients are provided during the convalescent period. All cellular functions are likely to be affected to a greater or lesser degree by specific deficiencies, but one process that is of special importance is the ability to cope with free radicals or oxidation-induced cell damage.

Antioxidant protection

In severe malnutrition, there is a major imbalance between the potential for damage induced by free radicals and protective antioxidant systems. Infection, oxidative burst, and free iron all contribute to an increased potential for damage. Mortality is greatest in those with an obvious impairment of the antioxidant defences. Children with oedematous malnutrition have severely reduced concentrations of glutathione in blood, and mortality is highest in those with impaired activity of glutathione peroxidase. Although the pattern varies with location, deficiencies of micronutrients are common and result in impaired cell function and membrane damage. The many layers of antioxidant protection, which are specific for each compartment of the cell, provide a measure of safety. However, the system is potentially vulnerable to deficiencies or limitations in multiple micronutrients, e.g. niacin, folate, thiamine, riboflavin, cobalamin, ascorbic acid, carotenoids, tocopherol, selenium, zinc, copper, magnesium. A deficiency might not be readily identifiable, either clinically or biochemically, and a high index of suspicion is required.

Oedema

Oedema reflects an inability to maintain the correct distribution of fluid in the intracellular space, the vascular space, and the interstitial space, and is a final common pathway representing a loss of metabolic control. Incorrect approaches to the management of oedema—the use of diuretics or of high-protein diets—are among the commonest reasons for increased mortality. The rationale behind the incorrect approach to management presumes that oedema is simply the consequence of hypoalbuminaemia, itself the result of inadequate dietary protein. There are profound perturbations of protein metabolism in kwashiorkor, but these are due to concurrent infection, loss of appetite, and increased losses of nitrogen in stools rather than a diet deficient in protein. A low plasma albumin usually indicates an acute-phase response to an unrecognized infection. Treatment with a high-protein diet or infusions of albumin does not correct the oedema, but does increase mortality. A low plasma concentration of albumin might contribute to formation of oedema, but is seldom the sole or primary cause. Although diuretics exert a direct effect on cell membranes, giving a diuretic is less likely to be effective if the intravascular space is reduced. Diuretics that lead to increased urinary losses of potassium make the underlying problem of a deficiency of body potassium even worse.

The normal distribution of water between the different body compartments is tightly controlled through a number of interlinked factors. Disruption of one or more of these factors may lead to the development of oedema, and will need to be corrected for the oedema to be effectively cleared (Table 11.3.4).

Potassium deficiency leads to retention of sodium. Altered membrane structure and reduced activity of Na^+,/K^+-ATPase allows intracellular potassium to fall and intracellular sodium to rise. All malnourished individuals should be presumed to be deficient in potassium and to have excess intracellular sodium, regardless of the composition of the plasma measured on routine biochemistry. Indeed, plasma sodium concentrations might be low and it is tempting to give extra sodium, which is absolutely the wrong thing to do. There is more than enough sodium in the body, but it is in the wrong place. A direct approach that seeks to correct the disordered

Table 11.3.4 Major factors which contribute to the development of pitting oedema in severe malnutrition

Hypoalbuminaemia	Associated with impaired protein metabolism, infection or stress, impaired hepatic function, toxic damage
Salt and water retention	Potassium deficiency, phosphate deficiency, acid–base imbalance, impaired renal function
Impaired membrane function	Altered composition (phospholipid composition and fatty acid profile). Impaired or downregulation of $Na^{+}K^{+}$- ATPase. Free radical induced damage

biochemistry is less likely to succeed than an approach which recognizes that the fundamental problem is disordered cellular function. Similar factors lead to cellular damage in any severely undernourished person, and by treating the malnutrition and repairing the metabolic machinery of the cells of the body, oedema will be effectively treated. What is required are generous supplements of potassium and correction of the underlying membrane dysfunction, which enables fluid and electrolyte balance to be restored. There is a close metabolic interdependence of potassium and magnesium, both of which are readily lost from the body in diarrhoea. It is extremely difficult to correct potassium deficiency in the presence of an associated magnesium deficiency, or to correct a magnesium deficiency in the face of a potassium deficiency. They have to be corrected together.

Table 11.3.5 Outline clinical management of severe malnutrition.

1. Resuscitate
Manage infection, fluid and electrolyte imbalance and shock: oxygen, glucose, reduce heat loss, give antibiotics, maintain circulation, treat vitamin A deficiency
2. Stabilize
Control energy and protein intake at maintenance: 400 kJ/kg/day (100 kcal/ kg/day), 1 to 1.5 g protein/kg/day
Small frequent meals: eight meals every 3 h, or six meals every 4 h, throughout 24 h
Correct deficiencies of specific nutrients by addition to food: potassium (4 mmol/kg/day), magnesium (0.4 mmol/kg/day), folic acid (1 mg/day), zinc (2 mg/kg/day), copper (0.3 mg/kg/day), multivitamin supplement
Treat bacterial infection: broad spectrum antibiotics, cotrimoxazole or ampicillin with gentamycin
Treat small bowel overgrowth with metronidazole
Treat helminth infections with mebendazole
Transfuse for severe anaemia
Topical treatment and care for skin lesions
Exclude tuberculosis
Give sensory stimulation and emotional support
3. Weight gain (rapid catch-up growth)
Ad libitum intake to achieve at least 600 kJ/kg/day (150 kcal/kg/day), 4 g protein/kg/day
Continue with micronutrient supplements
Add supplemental iron
Give sensory stimulation and emotional support

Principles of facility-based care

Phases of treatment: the 10 steps (Fig. 11.3.1, Table 11.3.5)

One of the important reasons why mortality from malnutrition has not been reduced in many centres is because the primary objective of treatment has been to try to correct the obvious weight deficit. In attempting to replace the lost tissue as soon as possible, generous intakes of food have been provided, encouraged, and even forced. If appetite is poor, or anorexia is a feature, then generous force-feeding by nasogastric tube has been used. This can be very dangerous. The 10-step approach to treating malnutrition clearly identifies that treatment must be divided into different phases: the cellular machinery has to be repaired before it can be used to enable tissue growth.

Two clinical features that are directly related to specific nutrient deficiencies and are particularly difficult to manage are oedema and persistent diarrhoea. Any specific nutrient deficiency impairs cellular function and increases the risk of infection. Infection increases nutrient losses through tissue wasting as an intrinsic feature of the acute-phase reaction and as vomitus or diarrhoea. Increased generation of free radicals is part of the body's attempts to deal with infecting organisms, and deficiencies of specific micronutrients directly impair the ability to cope with free-radical generation. Even if an individual recovers from an infection, nutrients which have been depleted from the body are not easily replaced. This has two important effects. First, the individual is deficient in a specific nutrient and carries the specific and general features of the deficiency, importantly loss of appetite. Secondly, if the deficiency is severe it may be very difficult for it to be corrected by consuming a normal diet without the addition of specific nutrient supplements. Under this circumstance, poor appetite, persistent reductive adaptation, and continued risk of further infection are maintained.

If energy is provided in excess of the requirements for maintenance, there are few ways in which it can be excreted or handled metabolically. Any significant excess is deposited as new tissue, either as cells or as cells filled with fat. There is a considerable underlying drive to form new cells, but in addition to energy this requires the availability of all the nutrients contained within the cell structure. When specific deficiencies have not been corrected individual nutrients are limiting for cell formation and it is not possible to handle the excess energy through the formation of new tissue. The excess energy creates a very serious metabolic upset (see 'Recovery syndrome' below). Therefore, during the period when nutrient deficiencies are being corrected and infections treated, it is important to give sufficient energy to cover the needs of the body, but not so much that the body is forced to make new tissue. This is the basis for identifying the different phases of treatment: first to repair the machinery and gain control of metabolism by providing only enough energy to satisfy the needs for maintenance, but not enough to drive growth. Managing reductive adaptation, specific nutrient deficiencies, infection, and free radical-induced membrane and cellular damage lie at the heart of the problems associated with immediate care during the resuscitation period.

A loss of appetite is an important protective mechanism limiting food consumption, which is likely to stress the systems of the body. Hence the loss of appetite is a cardinal sign of an underlying metabolic problem that is ongoing. If the problem is identified and corrected, then appetite is restored very quickly. Severely malnourished children may have a profound loss of appetite due to a combination of infection and deficiencies of specific nutrients, which interact to make the problem worse. Correcting the loss of appetite is central to effective care. The restoration of appetite marks the restoration of metabolic control and is a key component of therapy and a marker of progress. Once the emergency treatment required to resuscitate the child has been completed, the emphasis of care is to treat the underlying problems that are associated with a loss of appetite.

Resuscitation

Severely malnourished children present a medical emergency because of two sets of problems: the deadly triad of infection, hypothermia, and hypoglycaemia, and marked fluid and electrolyte disturbances (Table 11.3.5).

The deadly triad: hypoglycaemia, hypothermia, and infection

Brain cells are absolutely dependent upon a regular supply of glucose and oxygen to maintain the availability of ATP. Death occurs within 5 min if the supply of either is impaired, through poor circulation, reduced respiration, or low blood glucose. The glucose required is either made in the liver or taken in the diet. Reductive adaptation limits the capacity for glucose formation and delivery, and a regular dietary supply is required if blood concentrations are to be maintained. The availability of glucose for the brain can be impaired if there is competition from other tissues or functions, e.g. in order to maintain body temperature or to deal with infection. Malnourished individuals generate less heat and have reduced thermal insulation and therefore cool rapidly when exposed. Any attempt to generate more heat consumes glucose and other energy-providing fuels. A normal effective response to infection is a burst of activity in white blood cells, which places heavy demands on available glucose, competing with the brain and leading to hypoglycaemia, and increasing the rate of heat loss leading to hypothermia. Therefore, the triad of hypoglycaemia, hypothermia, and infection indicates a very serious situation in which the body is no longer able to adequately maintain the supply of glucose to support essential functions. The treatment is to increase the supply by giving oral or intravenous glucose, reducing competing demands through decreasing the amount of heat lost, and by effectively treating infections. To deliver glucose and oxygen to the brain effectively requires an adequate circulation, which is compromised by intravascular dehydration. The correction of dehydration is closely associated with the correction of electrolyte imbalances, with energy homeostasis, and with normal cellular function. Care has to be taken to ensure that each is corrected in concert with the other to ensure that imbalances do not arise. All malnourished individuals are deficient in potassium and carry excess sodium.

Specific micronutrients: vitamin A, zinc, and iron

Iron is highly reactive chemically, and fulfils many important functions related to the generation of energy for normal cellular function. High reactivity, if not adequately controlled, carries the potential for cell damage. Red cell mass reduces in malnutrition as the lean body mass decreases. The iron is not used for further haemoglobin formation and cannot be excreted, so has to be stored innocuously, as any unbound iron is liable to increase oxidative cell damage. In severe malnutrition, there is increased stored iron and free iron. The available iron is not used for haemoglobin formation, and giving iron supplements to treat anaemia simply adds to the load, stresses the system further, and increases mortality, especially in the presence of infection such as malaria. Initially, it is more important to repair and restore the capacity to cope with free radicals by improving vitamin and trace element status. Later, when the acute problems have been resolved, the iron will be removed from storage and used to form new tissue. As stored iron is used up, supplemental iron will have to be provided to keep pace with the rate of tissue demand.

Blindness and other eye signs of overt vitamin A deficiency are common in many parts of the world. Less obvious changes lead to impaired integrity of mucosal surfaces in the gastrointestinal and respiratory tracts, lowering resistance to gastroenteritis and respiratory infections. During infection, vitamin A is lost from the body, severe deficiency may develop rapidly, and the eye signs often deteriorate during early treatment. In areas where vitamin A deficiency is common, a large dose of vitamin A given very early in the treatment is an urgent necessity.

Zinc is required for the function of a wide range of enzymes, and a deficiency has widespread effects. A shortage of zinc impairs the replication of cells such as the gut mucosa, leading to further mucosal damage and increased diarrhoea. Zinc deficiency leads to diarrhoea, and diarrhoea leads to zinc deficiency. Similar changes take place in damaged skin leading to ulcerated skin which is readily damaged with mild trauma.

Persistent diarrhoea

Many malnourished children have diarrhoea, which can take time to settle. The diarrhoea may be infective in origin or have an infective component, due to viruses, bacteria, fungi, or helminths. However, diarrhoea that has persisted for any time will also have an element due to specific nutrient deficiencies (zinc and vitamin A) or chemical injury (bile salt deconjugation). With continued diarrhoea, there are ongoing losses of nutrients. Few bacteria exist in the healthy small intestine, but small-bowel overgrowth develops readily in malnutrition, due to a combination of gastric achlorhydria, reduced motility (potassium and magnesium deficiency), leading to bile salt deconjugation, damaged mucosa, and bacterial translocation. For the bowel to repair and re-establish its resistance requires adequate nutrients, especially zinc, vitamin A, and folates. Thus, the effective treatment of chronic diarrhoea requires a three-pronged approach: correction of potassium deficiency, treatment of bacterial overgrowth (with metronidazole), and effective repletion of specific nutrient deficiencies (such as zinc, vitamin A, and folate).

Management

The objectives of the resuscitation phase are to stabilize vital functions, by giving oxygen, supporting respiratory and cardiac functions, and correcting fluid imbalance, to ensure that adequate amounts of glucose are delivered to the brain. Body temperature must be maintained by maintaining glucose supply to the system, limiting heat loss through the skin, and starting to control infection. As the capacity for the body to carry out metabolic functions is impaired, external support has to be supplied regularly on a 24-h cycle. The regular intake of small amounts over 24 h (especially at night) is a very effective way of achieving this (Table 11.3.5). All infections must be treated. Specific nutrient deficiencies must be corrected, but no iron or extra sodium should be provided. The metabolic state must be controlled by limiting the intake of energy and protein to that required to maintain body weight, and ensuring that there is no excess (see following paragraphs). These steps will enable the repair of the metabolic machinery and allow cellular function to move towards normal. The response to a successful intervention will be a return of appetite; the patient will feel better, and smile.

Recovery syndrome

Limited availability of one or more nutrients leads to competition between all cells for the little available. Some nutrients become relatively more deficient, upsetting the balanced function between tissues, and the clinical signs of a deficiency become more obvious. There is a similar explanation for why the clinical signs of a deficiency are not always apparent, even though the body might be particularly deficient. During reductive adaptation, the demand for nutrients is decreased, and the signs of a deficiency are masked. Signs of deficiency become exposed in rapidly dividing tissues, when the demand for nutrients is greatest. Vitamin A and zinc are examples, but the same principles apply to many other nutrients, especially the B vitamins. The recovery or refeeding syndrome develops when individuals who have undergone reductive adaptation are suddenly provided with a relative excess of food. Excess energy drives metabolism while specific nutrient deficiencies are inadequately corrected, and the metabolic machinery is still compromised. The syndrome may vary in its details, but consists of left- and right-sided heart failure associated with an overloaded circulation. This may progress to vascular collapse with abdominal distension as the circulating vascular volume is poured into the bowel as profound secretory diarrhoea. The first sign of the onset of the recovery syndrome is an increase in pulse and respiratory rate. If food continues to be consumed at the same rate, the load on the heart will progress to heart failure. This is a medical emergency, and it is vitally important that the food intake is reduced or stopped. If the changes are identified early and are relatively mild, then food intake should be reduced. If the condition has advanced and is severe, then it may be necessary to stop all food for 12 to 24 h. The problem will then resolve.

Replacing lost weight

The ultimate objective of treatment is to replace the lost tissue. Cellular hypertrophy and hyperplasia are critically dependent upon and limited by the available energy and nutrients. For tissue of average composition, the formation of 1 g tissue requires 20 kJ of energy. A normal 1-year-old infant gains 1 g/kg body weight per day, but for catch-up weight gain during recovery from malnutrition weight, it is possible to form tissue at up to 20 g/kg per day, by consuming an additional 400 kJ/kg per day. Achieving this requires an energy-dense diet, which is consumed throughout the 24 h of the day. Energy is necessary but not sufficient for new tissue formation. The nutrients needed for the formation of cell membranes and protoplasm are required in adequate amounts and suitable proportions. As the lean body mass grows it has an increased need for oxygen, and the red blood cell mass increases. Iron is taken out of storage to form new red cells, and eventually these stores are depleted with the need to add supplemental iron to the diet. There is an increased demand for amino acids to meet the needs of new tissue formation. It is safe to allow quite large intakes of protein. As the amino acids are deposited in tissue and do not accumulate in the free form, there is no risk of toxicity. However, meeting the pattern of amino acids required by the body will require the endogenous biosynthesis of relatively large amounts of the 'nonessential' amino acids in the body, which in itself will require the generous availability of minerals and vitamins.

Important general aspects of care

The physical care that is provided to correct the biochemical, metabolic, and infective problems is critical for success. However, there is also a need to address the broader needs of the child for healthy development. In part, this is provided by creating a warm, caring environment; in part, by suitably structured activities that provide an appropriate level of stimulation to encourage brain function to recover and develop.

All aspects of care need skill and sympathy. The severely malnourished child is desperately sick and must be nursed as a critically ill child with minimum physical disturbance. With correct treatment, progress can be very rapid, and it is desirable to involve the parents and siblings, to encourage and demonstrate preferred childcare practices. This will facilitate the transfer between hospital and home, and make it more likely that the practices become embedded. Less seriously ill children can be effectively managed as outpatients, using the same principles and approach to the management decisions.

Further reading

Black RE *et al.* (2008). Maternal and child undernutrition study group. Maternal and child undernutrition: global and regional exposures and health consequences. *Lancet*, **371**, 243–60.

de Onis M *et al.* (2007). Comparison of the WHO child growth standards and the CDC 2000 growth charts. *J Nutr*, **137**, 144–8.

Grantham-McGregor S *et al.* (2007). Developmental potential in the first 5 years for children in developing countries. *Lancet*, **369**, 60–70.

Valid International (2006). *Community-based Therapeutic Care: A Field Manual.* http://www.validinternational.org/docs/CTC%20Field%20Manual%20First%20Edition,%2020065.pdf

Waterlow JC (2006). *Protein-energy malnutrition.* Smith-Gordon, London.

WHO (1995). *Physical status: the use and interpretation of anthropometry. Report of a WHO Expert Committee*, WHO Technical Report Series 854. World Health Organization, Geneva.

WHO (1999). *Management of severe malnutrition: a manual for physicians and senior health workers.* World Health Organization, Geneva.

WHO/UNICEF (2000). *Management of the child with a serious infection or severe malnutrition: guidelines for care at the first-referral level in developing countries.* World Health Organization, Geneva.

World Bank (2006). *Repositioning nutrition as central to development: a strategy for large scale action. Directions in Development.* World Bank, Washington, DC.

www.intf.org

11.4

Diseases of overnourished societies and the need for dietary change

J.I. Mann and A.S. Truswell

Essentials

The nutritional problems of a country depend more upon the stage of technical and economic development than geographical location. People in affluent societies do not have to worry about the problems of getting food and keeping it uninfected. Food is cheap for them, and they can eat their favourite foods all year round: the diet is energy-dense, high in fat and often also in sugar. There are multiple sources of nutritional advice and concerns, with breakthroughs and scares, science and pseudoscience, about all food. Nutrition related disorders are the principal causes of death and serious morbidity and reliable advice regarding nutrition is an important component of the care of individuals and public health.

Obesity (see Chapter 11.5) is the most obvious and important nutritional disease in affluent societies, with comorbidities including type 2 diabetes, coronary heart disease, hypertension, some cancers, gallstones, osteoarthritis, and obstructive sleep apnoea. Obese people may also be disadvantaged by social, economic, and psychological effects. Particular dietary constituents promote or protect against coronary heart disease by their effect on cardiovascular risk factors, and some promote or protect against various cancers.

While those at the highest personal risk are likely to show the greatest individual benefit from dietary and lifestyle changes, rates of many chronic disease will best be reduced if changes are made by the population at large. The main purpose of such recommendations is to reduce the risk of morbidity and mortality from these disease in those who are in the prime of life. Even greater reduction in morbidity and mortality and an improvement in life expectancy may occur in succeeding generations if they have reduced lifetime exposure to risk factors related to lifestyle.

Dietary guidelines for which there is almost complete agreement are:

- Eat a nutritionally adequate diet composed of a variety of foods.
- Ensure a low intake of saturated (less than 10% total energy) and trans unsaturated (less than 1% total energy) fats. Goals for total fat intake vary from 15 to 35 % total energy.
- Adjust energy balance for body weight control—if necessary fewer energy dense foods which are generally high in fats and or sugar and smaller serving sizes, more exercise.
- Eat plenty of wholegrain cereals, vegetables and fruits.
- Intake of salt and foods rich in salt should be restricted to a maximum of 100mmol/l day (6gNaCl).
- Drink alcohol in moderation (1 to 2 drinks/day), if you do drink.

Introduction

Nutrition issues at different stages of technical and economic development

The nutritional problems of a country depend more upon the stage of technical and economic development than geographical location (Table 11.4.1). Until about 10 000 years ago, our ancestors were hunter-gatherers. There are few contemporary hunter-gatherers left, but some of these have been studied, e.g. Kung bushmen. Hunter-gatherers collected a wide range of plant foods, but also ate meat and fish. They ate little or no salt, alcohol, or milk (other than breast milk as infants), little cereal, and no refined sugar apart from honey. Studies of contemporary hunter-gatherers indicate that they do not become obese but may experience seasonal hunger. We infer also that malnutrition was uncommon unless illness or injury supervened. High blood pressure or coronary heart disease would have been rare and plasma cholesterol was low. Teeth were worn down by hard food and caries was rare. With prolonged lactation, births were spaced fairly widely. The weaning period of childhood was precarious but general nutritional health was good. *Homo sapiens* evolved as hunter-gatherers and it is unlikely there has been sufficient time to adapt genetically to many modern foods.

Many contemporary people in developing countries are peasant agriculturists living a way of life similar to that of the rural population of western Europe and North America before the Industrial Revolution. They tend to rely on the one crop with the best yield and are vulnerable to crop diseases or crop toxins and droughts. Milling and refining cereals increases the risk of malnutrition. Though some foods are stored, diet is seasonal. Malnutrition can

Table 11.4.1 Nutrition issues at different stages of technical and economic development

Hunter-gatherers	Occasional seasonal hunger
	Malnutrition uncommon
	General nutritional health good
	No obesity
	No hypertension
	Low serum cholesterol
Peasant agriculturists	Single crop staple
	Clinical disorders may result from single or multiple nutrient deficiencies
	Hypertension may occur
	Obesity rare
Urban slum and periurban shanty town dwellers	Inadequate breastfeeding
	Inadequate food security
	Diarrhoea and other infective disorders, especially in young children
	Marasmus
	Obesity and alcoholism may occur
Affluent societies	High-fat, energy-dense diets
	Physical inactivity
	Obesity, coronary heart disease, and hypertension common
	Malnutrition may occur in frail elderly and sick people

occur from lack of essential nutrients in the staple food, e.g. vitamin A deficiency, pellagra, kwashiorkor, and iodine deficiency disorders. Hypertension occurs (salt is available), but coronary heart disease is rare. A small number of people at a similar stage of technical development are nomadic pastoralists, e.g. Lapps, Tibetans, Mongolians, Taureg, Fulani, Masai. They follow their grazing animals as suitable pasture changes with the seasons. They rely heavily on animal food, especially milk products.

Urban slums and periurban shanties are homes for an increasing proportion of the growing populations of developing countries who are pouring into overcrowded, insanitary accommodation in vast, polluted cities. Conditions are reminiscent of the slums of London, Manchester, and New York in the 19th century. These people have lost their contact with the land and food traditions and, for them, food is expensive. Mothers of young children have to go out to work. Breastfeeding is almost impossible and it is very difficult to keep bottle feeds hygienic. Young children are most susceptible to diarrhoeal and other infectious diseases; these, with the mothers' absence and inadequate food, can lead to marasmus. Among adults, increasing numbers are becoming obese; others may be alcoholics or dependent on psychotropic drugs.

In affluent societies, the prosperous people of developed countries do not have to worry about the problems of getting food and keeping it uninfected. Food is cheap for them, and they can eat their favourite foods all year round. There is a multiplicity of nutrition advice and concerns with breakthroughs and scares, science, and pseudo-science about all food. The diet is high in fat and, often, also in sugar and dense in energy. Obesity and its related disorders, coronary heart disease, and hypertension (with its complications), are the principal causes of death. While sports are watched on television by millions, many ordinary citizens do not undertake any physical activity that promotes health. Obesity is unfashionable but difficult to avoid and increasing. Malnutrition occurs in frail elderly people and the sick, but this malnutrition is usually subclinical and identified mainly by biochemical tests.

As mortality due to infectious disease is reduced by antibiotics and immunization in most developing countries, and as their people are living longer and increasingly adopting Western foods and labour-saving techniques, noncommunicable diseases are becoming major causes of death. These noncommunicable diseases formerly affected only the ruling and merchant elite of developing countries but there are now epidemic of obesity, diabetes, hypertension, and heart disease. Health authorities in all but the least developed countries have the formidable task of coping with a dual burden of disease, providing education and food policies to prevent malnutrition and at the same time to prevent overnutrition.

Epidemiological methods used to study nutrition-related diseases

The nutritional component of noncommunicable diseases is more difficult to study than classical nutrition deficiency diseases, because noncommunicable diseases develop slowly and are multifactorial. The dietary factor may be a 'risk factor' rather than a direct cause. However, there is now convincing evidence that dietary change can appreciably reduce the risk of some important noncommunicable diseases. Although studies aimed at describing pathology and mechanisms have contributed much to our understanding of these diseases, the epidemiological approach has been pivotal in establishing the extent of the disease burden and the potential for risk reduction. Often, the first clue to the association between a food, or nutrient, and a disease comes from observing striking differences in disease incidence between countries (or groups within a country) that correlate with differences in nutritional intake. Sometimes, dietary changes over time in a single country have been found to coincide with changes in disease rates. Such observations give rise to hypotheses about possible diet–disease links, rather than proof of causation, because many potential causative factors may be confounded by parallel dietary changes.

Case–control studies have sometimes been used as a rapid and inexpensive way of testing hypotheses. A series of people who have been diagnosed e.g. with cancer of the large bowel are asked what they usually eat, or what they ate before they became ill. These 'cases' are compared with at least an equal number of 'controls'—people without bowel cancer, matched for age, gender, and, if possible, social condition. Weaknesses of the method include the possibility that the disease may affect food habits, the fact that cases cannot recall their diet accurately before the cancer was diagnosed, that controls may have some condition that affects dietary habits, or that food intakes are recorded from cases and controls in a different way. Furthermore, it is conceivable (and for coronary heart disease and cancer, likely) that dietary factors may operate many years before the condition comes to light.

Prospective or cohort studies avoid the biases involved in asking people to recall past eating habits. Information about food intake and other characteristics are collected well before onset of the disease. Large numbers of people must therefore be interviewed and examined; they must be of an age at which bowel cancer (say) starts to be fairly common (i.e. middle aged) and in a population that has a fairly high rate of this disease. The healthy cohort thus examined and recorded is then followed up for five or more years. Eventually, a proportion will be diagnosed with bowel cancer and the original dietary details of those who develop cancer can be compared with the diets of the majority who have not developed the disease. Usually, a number of dietary and other environmental factors are found to be more, or less, frequent in those who develop the disease. These, then, are apparent risk factors, or protective factors. However, they are not necessarily the operative factor. Fruit consumption may appear to be protective but perhaps, in this cohort, smokers eat less fruit and smoking may be more directly related. This confounding has to be quantified by analysing the data to see the relationship of fruit to the disease at different levels of smoking.

Definitive proof of a causal association as well as evidence for the benefit of intervention typically comes from one or more randomized controlled trials. Trials involving nutritional interventions and clinical endpoints such as cancer and coronary heart disease are much more difficult to undertake than those involving drugs. Although it is possible to study the effects of a food component given like a pharmaceutical (e.g. antioxidant nutrients), and some trials have been undertaken to study the effects of dietary manipulations on relatively common nutrition related diseases (e.g. diabetes, hypertension), a clinical trial to demonstrate that a particular dietary manipulation will reduce the risk of cancer may be impractical. The magnitude and duration imply huge cost, and long-term compliance with dietary interventions would be very difficult to achieve.

Much research involving the role of diet in chronic degenerative disease has centred around the effects of diet on modifying risk factors rather than the disease itself. For many chronic diseases there are biochemical or clinical markers of risk. High plasma cholesterol is an important risk factor for coronary heart disease, for example, and high blood pressure is a major risk factor for strokes. Innumerable studies have examined the role of different nutrients and foods on plasma cholesterol, blood pressure, or other risk factors. Such studies are easier to undertake and cheaper than population-based studies because far fewer people are studied over a relatively short period of time. They have helped to find which foods lower cholesterol and so should help protect against coronary heart disease. Thus, a decision as to whether or not to recommend dietary change will need to be based on a portfolio of evidence. Such evidence might include consistent and strong associations in longitudinal studies, biological plausibility, and corroborative experimental evidence in animals and humans.

In case–control and cohort studies dietary intake of individuals is assessed by means of food-frequency questionnaires, diet records, or recalls— all of which have different strengths and weaknesses. A weakness of most methods of assessing dietary intake is that some people, especially those who are overweight or obese, tend to underestimate their intake. Food composition tables or nutrient databases are required to convert information gathered regarding food intake to consumption of energy and nutrients. Sometimes, it is more reliable to assess the intake of a nutrient by measuring biomarkers. Thus, level of the nutrient in blood or urine or activity in the body is preferable to attempting to calculate intake from a diet record or food-frequency questionnaire. Intakes of iodine and sodium are assessed by measuring amounts in 24-h urine collections. Measurement of folate concentration in the serum or red blood cells provide a good estimate of intake, since the amounts in fruit and vegetables vary enormously and are also dependent upon shelf-life and method of preparation. Fatty acid composition of serum or red cell membrane provides an indication of the nature of dietary fat intake. For some nutrients that are not always readily bioavailable, adequacy of intake must be assessed by alternative means. In the case of iron, measurement of ferritin in the blood (indicating iron stores) is a more useful indicator of iron status than dietary intake (see also Chapter 22.4.4). Glutathione peroxidase activity provides a measure of assessing selenium status in those with a relatively low intake.

Obesity (see also Chapter 11.5)

Obesity is the most obvious and important nutritional disease in affluent societies, its comorbidities including type 2 diabetes and the many consequences of insulin resistance, coronary heart disease, hypertension, some cancers, gallstones, osteoarthritis, and obstructive sleep apnoea. Obese people may also be disadvantaged by social, economic, and psychological effects. The psychological well-being of children may be particularly affected, and childhood obesity has recently been recognized as a risk factor for fractures in children. Most of the adverse consequences of obesity are appreciably reduced by weight loss, though gallstone formation may not be reduced. Although the genetic component of obesity is acknowledged, its dramatic increase in virtually all westernized countries and many developing countries in recent years provides ample evidence of overwhelming environmental factors. Physical inactivity is unquestionably an important cause but frequent consumption of large portions of readily available energy-dense foods (high in fats and/or sugars) also often contributes to an energy intake in excess of expenditure. Frequent consumption of sugar-sweetened soft drinks and fruit juices appears to enhance excessive weight gain, especially among children. Whole-grain cereals and cereal products, nonstarchy vegetables, and dietary fibre help to reduce the energy density of the diet, promote satiety, and thus reduce the risk of inappropriate weight gain. It seems unlikely that the epidemic of obesity will be reversed unless the environment in which we live is altered by creating more opportunities for physical activity, improving availability of appropriate food choices, and providing supportive health education. Nevertheless, there is some cause for optimism in that obesity rates are relatively low among those of a higher socioeconomic status who are more likely than those of lower socioeconomic status to make healthy food choices and exercise regularly.

Coronary heart disease

Experimental, epidemiological, and clinical trial data provide strong evidence for the role of nutritional factors in the aetiology of coronary heart disease and the potential for dietary modification to reduce cardiovascular morbidity and mortality in the population as a whole, in individuals at high risk, and in those who have already experienced a cardiovascular event. Prospective and experimental studies suggest a wide range of foods and nutrients that may be involved (Table 11.4.2). Foods that increase the risk of coronary heart disease when consumed in large amounts probably

Table 11.4.2 Foods and nutrients which may promote or protect against coronary heart disease

Promoting		Protective	
Foods	**Nutrients**	**Foods**	**Nutrients**
High-fat dairy products Fatty meats	Saturated fatty acids (especially myristic and palmitic acids)	Fruits Vegetables	Antioxidant nutrients[b], folate[b] Dietary fibre (nonstarch polysaccharide)
Eggs	Dietary cholesterol	Whole-grain cereals	Dietary fibre (non-starch polysaccharides) Unsaturated fatty acids
Some margarines[a],cooking oils, confectionery, and manufactured foods	Trans-unsaturated fatty acids Saturated fatty acids	Vegetable oils (e.g. sunflower, safflower, olive, and canola)	Unsaturated fatty acids (linoleic, oleic, linolenic)
		Oily fish	Eicosapentaenoic and and docosahexaenoic acids
		Nuts	Unsaturated fatty acids (oleic, linoleic), vitamin E[b]
		Alcohol (moderate amounts only)	

[a] When containing appreciable quantities of *trans*-unsaturated fatty acids.
[b] When present in foods, not supplements.

do so because they are rich in saturated or *trans*-unsaturated fatty acids, and dietary cholesterol. 'Protective' foods contain several different nutrients that may reduce cardiovascular risk. Oily fish is rich in very long-chain polyunsaturated fatty acids (eicosapentaenoic and docosahexaenoic acids). Fruit and vegetables are good sources of antioxidant nutrients, folate, and other biologically active substances. Nuts contain several potentially 'protective' fatty acids (oleic and linoleic acids) as well as vitamin E. Whole-grain cereals are good sources of dietary fibre as well as of some unsaturated oils. Data presented in Table 11.4.3, derived from two of the best-known prospective studies of cardiovascular disease provide an indication of the extent of the potential cardioprotection afforded by some foods and nutrients. Each of the nutrients mentioned has an appropriately favourable or adverse effect on one or more of the cardiovascular risk factors (Table 11.4.4). As the global prevalence of obesity increases, risk factors associated with excess adiposity (notably dyslipidaemia and insulin resistance) contribute increasingly as 'causes' of coronary heart disease. Thus, it may be appropriate to also consider nutrition-related causes of obesity as causes of coronary heart disease.

Clinical trials have shown that when diet is modified to facilitate appropriate changes in the nutrients mentioned earlier, levels of risk factors are altered in a favourable direction and cardiovascular events are reduced, even when the intervention is started in middle age with cardiovascular disease already present. The various

Table 11.4.3 Age-adjusted relative risk of coronary heart disease according to quintile of intake of certain foods or nutrients

Study population	Relative risk according to quintile of intake					*p* for trend
	1	2	3	4	5	
43 757 male health professionals (40–75 years) (Rimm *et al.* 1996)	Total dietary fibre 1.00	0.97	0.91	0.87	0.59	<0.001
75 521 female nurses (38–63 years) (Liu *et al.* 2000)	Whole- grain consumption 1.00	0.87	0.82	0.72	0.67	<0.001
87 245 female nurses (34–59 years) (Stampfer and Rimm 1995)	Total vitamin E intake[a] 1.00	0.90	1.00	0.68	0.59	<0.001
39 910 male health professionals (40–75 years) (Rimm *et al.* 1996)>	Carotene intake[a] 1.00	0.93	0.93	0.86	0.71	0.02

[a] These nutrients may be a marker for the foods in which they are found, for other components in the foods, or may only confer protection when eaten together with other nutrients which occur in foods, since no evidence of benefit has emerged from randomized controlled trials in which they have been administered in pharmacological doses.

Table 11.4.4 Some effects of nutrients which promote or protect against coronary heart disease on cardiovascular risk factors

Nutrient	Effect
Promoting	
Saturated fatty acids	↑ total and LDL cholesterol
	↑ thrombogenesis
	↓ insulin sensitivity
Trans unsaturated fatty acids	↑LDL cholesterol and Lp(a)
	↓HDL cholesterol
Dietary cholesterol (when taken in large amounts)	↑ total and LDL cholesterol
Protective	
Dietary fibre	↓ total and LDL cholesterol
	↑ insulin sensitivity
Folic acid	↓ homocysteine
Antioxidant nutrients	↓ oxidation of LDL
Unsaturated fatty acids[a]	↓ total and LDL cholesterol
	↓ arrythmias, thrombogenesis

↑ increase; ↓ decrease.
[a] C18:1, $n-9$, oleic acid; C18:2, $n-6$, linoleic acid; C18:3, $n-3$, linolenic acid; C20:5, $n-3$, eicosapentaenoic acid; C22:6, $n-3$, docosahexaenoic acid.

trials have involved different dietary interventions so that formal meta-analysis is inappropriate; nevertheless, it is possible to draw certain general conclusions regarding likely benefit from various dietary changes. Most aimed for a reduction in plasma cholesterol by manipulation of fat intake. For every 1% reduction in plasma cholesterol a 2 to 3% reduction in cardiovascular events occurs. Thus an 8 to 10% reduction in cholesterol, which can be achieved by modifying the types of dietary fat (replacing foods rich in saturated and *trans*-unsaturated fatty acids with those containing mono- and *cis*-polyunsaturated fatty acids and cereals, vegetables, and fruit) will result in appreciable benefit. Trials that have examined potential benefits of dietary manipulations other than those designed to lower plasma cholesterol suggest that further clinical benefit might accrue from favourable changes in other risk factors. Consumption of oily fish two or more times per week, or a small amount of fish oil taken as a supplement, has been shown to reduce cardiovascular death in those with pre-existing coronary artery disease. Although increased intakes of vegetables and fruit may confer a cardioprotective effect, there is, at present, no convincing evidence from clinical trials of benefit associated with the use of folic acid and antioxidant nutrient supplements. The role of margarines rich in plant sterols and stanols, which may further lower dietary cholesterol by preventing absorption and reabsorption of dietary cholesterol, is yet to be established with certainty.

Community programmes aiming to change diet along the lines indicated here have been shown to reduce cardiovascular risk factors and one—the North Karelia Project in Finland—has shown that cardiovascular disease mortality in the intervention county decreased to a greater extent than might have been expected on the basis of experience in other Finnish counties. The availability of appropriate food choices at reasonable cost is an essential component of any programme aimed at reducing cardiovascular risk, since rates are highest in people of the lowest socioeconomic status. While those at the highest personal risk are likely to show the greatest individual benefit from dietary and lifestyle changes, national coronary heart disease rates will best be reduced if changes are made by the population at large. The main purpose of such recommendations is to reduce the risk of morbidity and mortality from coronary heart disease in those who are in the prime of life. Even greater reduction in morbidity and mortality and an improvement in life expectancy may occur in succeeding generations who will have reduced lifetime exposure to risk factors related to lifestyle.

Hypertension and stroke

Three dietary factors are well established as raising blood pressure. The longest known is salt, sodium chloride. In a few isolated communities salt was not available until recently, and there high blood pressures were rare or absent. Usual sodium intakes of around 150 mmol/litre or more per day are about six times more than the physiological requirement (human milk contains only 7 mmol sodium/litre). Salt used to be important for preserving food before canning, refrigeration, and rapid transport and people are now habituated to its flavour in foods like bread. There are technical problems with research examining the relationship between sodium intake and blood pressure. Most of the salt consumed (*c.*85%) is added at the time of manufacture, rather than during food preparation or at the table; thus, 24-h urinary sodium excretion rather than dietary intake measurements are needed to assess salt intake. Sodium excretion (reflecting intakes) and blood pressures fluctuate markedly and some individuals are more salt-sensitive than others. Nevertheless, surveys within one country (e.g. the 1986–1987 British National Dietary and Nutrition Survey) and internationally (the Intersalt Study involving 10 000 people in 32 countries) have shown a clear relationship between urinary sodium and blood pressure, and a Finnish cohort study found an increased risk of cardiovascular disease in those who had high 24-h urinary sodium. There is strong confirmation from carefully controlled primate research that salt is causally related to essential hypertension. Blood pressure rose significantly over an 18-month period when salt was added to the diet of chimpanzees that normally eat a vegetarian and fruit diet, and fell again when the salt was stopped. Several controlled clinical trials in humans have shown that when salt intakes are reduced to around 70 mmol/litre, blood pressure falls—more in people with mild to moderate hypertension. Salt restriction can be used to treat hypertension, but because so much is derived from manufactured food, a major dietary change is needed, emphasizing unprocessed foods and low-salt bread (ordinary bread contains over 100 times more salt than wheat flour).

Overweight and obese people have higher blood pressures than those who are lean and, if they lose weight, blood pressure falls even if the usual salt intake is maintained. An Australian trial showed, in a clinical trial setting, that weight reduction (maximum loss 7.4 kg) compared favourably with metoprolol in the treatment of mild hypertension, and diet was associated with an improved plasma lipid profile not seen on the drug.

Alcohol intake is emerging as the third of the important environmental factors associated with raised blood pressure. In epidemiological studies, blood pressure, especially systolic, increases progressively when reported alcohol intake increases above three drinks per day. Several intervention studies have shown that reduction of alcohol intake can produce an appreciable reduction in blood pressure among hypertensive heavy drinkers. For example, one study showed that replacing standard beer (5% alcohol) with a reduced-alcohol beer (0.9% alcohol) produced a reduction in alcohol intake from 450 to 64 ml/week and a significant fall in blood pressure. It is noteworthy that while small regular alcohol intakes (1–2 drinks/day) appear protective against coronary heart disease, an adverse effect on blood pressure starts above this level.

Other components that may lower blood pressure are not as clearly established. Potassium, probably acting as an antagonist to sodium, has been shown in repeated controlled trials to lower blood pressure modestly, but this was given in pharmacological doses. Potassium may have been one of the operative factors in the few dietary trials that have shown a hypotensive effect. Substantial quantities of fruits and vegetables were found to be effective in lowering blood pressure in the large American DASH trials. In these trials, the addition of low-fat dairy foods produced additional blood pressure lowering, but the effects of calcium have been less effective in controlled trials.

Blood pressure is an important determinant of ischaemic stroke and cerebral haemorrhage, so that all the nutritional determinants of hypertension may be regarded as relevant. In addition, prospective studies have consistently demonstrated that fruit and vegetables protect against ischaemic stroke. Although it appears that most categories of fruit and vegetables are protective, the effect is particularly striking for cruciferous vegetables, green leafy vegetables, and citrus fruits.

Diabetes mellitus and the metabolic syndrome

Rates of type 2 diabetes have escalated in most affluent societies to the extent that the condition is considered to have reached epidemic proportions in many countries. The constellation of abnormalities (including central obesity, raised blood pressure, dyslipidaemia, increased insulin levels, and hyperglycaemia), which constitutes the metabolic syndrome identifies people likely to develop type 2 diabetes and who are at appreciably increased risk of cardiovascular disease. Where information is available, it appears that the frequency of the 'syndrome' has also increased and that risk factors are the same as for type 2 diabetes.

Epidemiological evidence suggests that type 2 diabetes is uncommon in people eating a range of 'traditional diets' high in fresh fruit, vegetables, and cereals, and relatively low in fat. Diabetes prevalence seems to increase rapidly when traditional lifestyles are exchanged for the Western way of life, particularly when such transitions occur over a short time span. Such changes have occurred in China and India, the world's most populous countries, where type 2 diabetes has already created an enormous public health problem. Similar findings had been noted earlier in Micronesians, Polynesians, American Indians, and Aboriginal Australians, as well as in Asian Indian immigrants to Fiji, South Africa, and the United Kingdom, and Mauritius and among Chinese in Singapore, Taiwan, Hong Kong, and Mauritius.

The change from traditional to a Western way of life is generally associated with a reduction in physical activity and an increase in the energy density of the diet, resulting from increased intakes of fats and sugars, with the resultant energy imbalance leading to increasing rates of overweight and obesity. Lack of physical activity and increasing degrees of obesity (especially central adiposity) have consistently been shown in longitudinal studies to be associated with the risk of developing type 2 diabetes. Globally and nationally, rates of type 2 diabetes have increased in parallel with increasing rates of obesity. Genetic determinants of diabetes should not be underestimated, but they clearly cannot explain the exponential increase in so many countries.

While any cause of energy imbalance leading to excessive weight gain will increase the risk of type 2 diabetes, there is less certainty regarding the role of individual macronutrients in the aetiology. Excess sucrose has been largely exonerated as an important dietary factor in the aetiology of type 2 diabetes, except when high intakes contribute to an increase in energy density and excessive energy intakes. A high intake of saturated fatty acids undoubtedly decreases insulin sensitivity, an underlying abnormality in type 2 diabetes and the metabolic syndrome, independently of an effect of excess adiposity. Thus, saturated fats are regarded as a probable cause of the conditions. One large prospective study of health professionals in the United States of America has found that a high intake of low glycaemic index foods (i.e. predominantly carbohydrate-containing foods producing a relatively low glycaemic excursion after ingestion when compared with a comparable amount of glucose) tends to protect against type 2 diabetes and that the effect is independent of other individual dietary attributes. A high intake of dietary fibre has been shown to enhance insulin sensitivity in insulin-resistant individuals, so that foods rich in dietary fibre and with a low glycaemic index are probably protective. Thus, it seems most likely that a combination of factors is responsible. Although we do not fully understand the complex mechanisms by which genes and environment interact to result in type 2 diabetes, randomized controlled trials among individuals with impaired glucose tolerance carried out in Finland, the United States, China and India provide strong support for the suggestion that lifestyle modification can help to prevent or at least appreciably delay the onset of type 2 diabetes. Interventions in the Finnish Diabetes Prevention Study (Box 11.4.1) resulted in an approximately 60% reduction in rates of progression from impaired glucose tolerance to type 2 diabetes, a benefit which has persisted for at least 8 years. Of particular interest is the fact that remarkably few of those individuals who complied with at least four of the five target interventions progressed from impaired glucose tolerance to type 2 diabetes. The benefits appear to accrue principally from reduction in excess body fat, but reduction in saturated fat intake and increase in dietary fibre also account for the risk reduction. The United States, Chinese and Indian studies have reported comparable results. Similar lifestyle interventions have been shown to increase insulin sensitivity in insulin-resistant individuals prior to the development of impaired glucose tolerance or diabetes.

Box 11.4.1 Lifestyle modification targets for the intervention group in the Finnish Diabetes Prevention Study

- Weight loss of 5 to 7% initial body weight (5 to 10 kg depending upon degree of obesity)
- Reduce total and saturated fat by encouraging low-fat dairy and meat products
- Prefer unsaturated soft margarines and vegetable oils rich in monounsaturated fatty acids
- Increase whole grains, vegetables, and fruit
- Physical activity, at least moderate intensity for a minimum of 30 min daily

Many studies in affluent societies have shown that weight reduction in overweight people with type 2 diabetes can often result in normal, or near normal, blood glucose levels without the need for oral hypoglycaemic therapy. Furthermore, diets high in soluble forms of dietary fibre, and in which low glycaemic index carbohydrate-containing foods predominate, can improve glycaemic control in those with diagnosed diabetes, independent of an effect on body mass. However, in people who are not overweight, sufficient improvement to reduce the need for drug therapy and achieve even near-normal blood glucose concentrations is seen only with extreme dietary change (i.e. diets consisting largely of raw and unprocessed foods and exceptionally low in fat).

Although diet is important in the management of type 1 diabetes, nutritional factors do not appear to have contributed to the aetiology of the disease to the same extent as for type 2 diabetes. Genetic and other environmental factors are believed to be more important. Some studies have suggested, however, that infants who have been breastfed may have a reduced risk of type 1 diabetes in later life and this observation could be linked with immune mechanisms known to be associated with this condition.

Cancers

The development of cancer involves several stages and occurs over a long period of time. Nutritional factors may operate at one or more of these stages. During the first stage of initiation, the DNA of the healthy cell is damaged by chance mutation or a carcinogen. During the promotion (second) stage, the 'initiated' cells may be exposed to promoters, environmental factors, which create conditions that favour their growth over that of normal cells. This phase tends to be prolonged and may be delayed or accelerated by environmental factors. Genetic factors also operate. Ultimately, preneoplastic cells are formed, which differ in appearance and function from normal cells. During the final stage of progression, additional mutations tend to occur leading to the transformation of preneoplastic to neoplastic cells. Nutritional factors may act as carcinogens or promoters. Given this long natural history of the disease process, it is hardly surprising that few data from intervention trials are available, and data relating dietary factors to various cancers are derived from epidemiological associations and animal experiments. Despite the difficulty in assessing dietary intake over the prolonged period during which cancer develops, Doll and Peto have estimated that about one-third of all cancers in Western countries may be attributed to diet. The dietary and nutritional factors that may play a role in human cancer are listed in Table 11.4.5. Restriction of total energy intake, provided that nutrient requirements are met, has been clearly shown to reduce the risk of cancer in experimental animals, and obesity in humans is one of the most powerful and consistent epidemiological associations with cancers. Obesity is associated with insulin resistance and increased levels of inflammatory markers and insulin-like growth factors, which may increase cancer risk. These effects are reversed by weight loss.

Table 11.4.5 Nutritional determinants of various cancers

Factor	Causal (↑) Protective (↓)	Cancers
Obesity	↑	Postmenopausal breast, colorectum, endometrium, gallbladder, kidney, oesophagus, pancreas
Processed and red meat	↑	Colorectum
Alcohol	↑	Liver, breast, mouth, larynx, pharynx
Salt	↑	Stomach
Salted fish (Cantonese style)	↑	Nasopharynx
Hot drinks (maté)	↑	Oesophagus
Vegetables	↓	Colorectum, lung, stomach
Fruits	↓	Lung, stomach
Nonstarch polysaccharide/ dietary fibre	↓	Colorectum
Selenium	↓	Prostate
Fish and poultry	↓	Colorectum

Note: In addition to the well-documented causal or protective nutrition-related factors presented in the tables, there are many other possible associations under investigation. In particular, tomatoes, probably because of their lycopene content, and vitamin E, may reduce the risk of prostate cancer and animal products may increase the risk. Folate and calcium are possible protective factors against cancer of the cervix and colorectal cancer, respectively.

High intakes of red meat have been associated with an increased risk of colon cancer. Haem rather than iron *per se* is one possible explanation since it is susceptible to endogenous nitrosation by bacterial flora in the colon. Nitroso compounds can increase the likelihood of neoplastic change. Such effects are not seen with fish or poultry, which appear to be protective against colorectal cancer. Processed meats have also been linked with colorectal cancer, and the relative risk appears to be higher. The definition of 'processed meat' differs in different countries. High intakes of total fat are strongly correlated with colorectal, breast, prostatic, and pancreatic cancer in ecological (between countries) studies. In animal models, high intakes of n – 6 fatty acids (especially linoleic acid) promote tumour progression, an effect reduced by increasing intakes of n – 3 fatty acids. However, these findings are not substantiated in large prospective cohort studies so that definitive conclusions regarding fat intake are not possible at present. The effects of alcohol as a risk factor for breast cancer as well as cancer of the mouth, larynx, and pharynx are consistent and strong. Alcohol probably increases the risk of liver cancer because large intakes lead to cirrhosis of the liver, which is associated with liver cancer, regardless of cause. Other clearly established nutrition-related promoters of cancers tend to operate regionally: salt and salted fish increase the risk of stomach and nasopharyngeal cancer in Japan and China, and maté, consumed at high temperatures in Brazil, is an important cause of oesophageal cancer.

Vegetables and fruit are generally accepted as important protective factors, particularly against lung, stomach, and colorectal cancers. Antioxidants (especially vitamin C, vitamin E, carotenoids, and flavonoids), glucosinolates (found in brassica vegetables), sulphur components (in *Allium* species—onions and garlic) and folates have all been shown to have anticancer properties, which may explain the protective effects that have been demonstrated mainly in case–control studies. Possibly of even greater importance is the protection (particularly against colorectal cancer) conferred by dietary fibre (nonstarch polysaccharide) present in many minimally processed cereal foods, as well as fruits and vegetables. Dietary fibre and resistant starches escape digestion in the small intestine and are fermented in the large bowel by the colonic microbial flora. Short-chain fatty acids are produced, one of which, butyrate, is an antiproliferative agent. Dietary fibre may further reduce the risk of large-bowel cancer by increasing stool bulk and decreasing transit time, which in turn reduces the opportunity for colonocytes to be in contact with carcinogens.

While there is renewed interest in the potential protective effects of selenium, tomatoes, and lycopene against prostate cancer and possible protection of folate and calcium against cervical and colorectal cancers, respectively, it seems likely that reducing rates of obesity may have a more marked effect on reducing nutrition-related cancers than modifying intakes of individual nutrients or foods.

Diverticular disease of the colon

The first suggestion that deficiency of dietary fibre in the diet may be implicated in the aetiology of diverticular disease of the colon came from striking geographical variations in its prevalence and the documented increase in disease rates in several European countries since the 1920s. These variations and trends in rates are certainly compatible with a causative link with low-fibre diets but could also be explained by several alternative dietary and other environmental influences. The best-documented evidence comes from comparisons of asymptomatic groups of vegetarians and meat eaters who volunteered to have a barium meal. Radiological diverticular disease was found more frequently among nonvegetarians than vegetarians, who had appreciably higher intakes of dietary fibre. Furthermore, when comparing individuals with and without diverticular disease, in both the vegetarian and nonvegetarian groups those with diverticular disease had appreciably lower intakes of dietary fibre than those with no evidence of diverticulae following barium meals. Animal experiments provide support (e.g. rats given a low-fibre diet have been shown to develop diverticulae, as do rabbits fed with white bread, sugar, and vitamins, and given prostigmine). An increase in dietary fibre intake is widely recommended to patients with symptomatic diverticular disease, a treatment justified by the findings of some (but not all) controlled clinical trials.

Plausible theories concerning pathogenesis have been suggested; small, hard faeces, undoubtedly seen with a fibre-deficient diet, are associated with narrowing of the colon and the formation of closed segments in which pressure increases. Additional work is needed by colonic muscles to provide the pressure to move the more solid faeces, producing muscular hypertrophy in addition to the diverticula at sites of weakness, where blood vessels penetrate the muscular coat.

Dental caries

Archaeological evidence shows that in ancient times dental caries was exceptionally rare in young people. In contrast, surveys over the past 15 years have suggested that as many as 80% of 5-year-olds in the United Kingdom today require treatment for dental caries and about 10% of all children enter school with more than half their teeth seriously decayed. Some 5% of the adult population in England and Wales and 15% of that in Scotland are edentulous by the age of 30 years. Several strands of evidence suggest a nutritional cause. Among the indigenous population of many countries, where unrefined foods form the bulk of the diet (e.g. China, Uganda), dental caries once had a very low prevalence. Within a few years of the addition of sugar and other refined foods, the frequency showed a rapid increase. A similar change has been shown experimentally in monkeys. In a classical experiment carried out in a Swedish mental hospital, volunteers given toffee apples, chocolate, and caramel in addition to their controlled diet had a 13-fold greater number of tooth surfaces becoming carious each year, compared with those eating the controlled diet alone. While frequency, timing, and amount of free sugars may be important in the aetiology, fluoride in the water at 1 part per million or in toothpaste can profoundly reduce the risk of dental caries.

Constipation and the irritable bowel syndrome

Ninety-nine per cent of a large population sample studied in the United Kingdom reported that they defecated at least three times per week but perceived constipation as a frequent complaint. Approximately 3% of all prescriptions written in the National Health Survey (also in the United Kingdom) were for purgatives and laxatives, at a cost of around £4 000 000, and many times this amount must have been spent in buying these preparations over the counter. In another survey, 6% of people aged between 18 and 80 years described straining when passing stools. On the other hand, constipation is uncommon in populations with a high intake of dietary fibre. In Britain, stool weights in nonvegetarians are usually around 100 g (with a very wide range), whereas in vegetarians with a high fibre intake, the average stool weight is over 200 g. Furthermore, vegetarians and nonvegetarians with high average daily fibre intakes have transit times of less than 75 h and rarely report constipation, whereas those with lower fibre intakes have transit times ranging from 20 to 124 h and frequently complain of constipation. Controlled clinical trials confirm that increasing dietary fibre (especially that derived from cereals) relieves the symptoms of constipation. Diets rich in dietary fibre are widely recommended in the treatment of irritable bowel syndrome, despite the absence of formal clinical trials.

Osteoporosis

Osteoporosis is an important cause of morbidity among elderly people, especially women, and the incidence of osteoporotic fractures is increasing steadily as people are living longer. By the year 2025, it is projected that there will be 1.16 million hip fractures in men and 2.78 million in women due to osteoporosis. The aetiology of osteoporosis is complex; women have a lower peak bone mass in their twenties than men and then lose bone rapidly after the menopause in association with a decline in oestrogens. Women lose approximately one-half their trabecular bone and one-third of their cortical bone, while men lose one-third of their trabecular bone and one-fifth of their cortical bone. Genetic factors influence peak bone mass and bone loss and these may operate by some of the well-known risk factors: strong family history of osteoporosis, short stature, early menopause, and white or Asian race. However, there are also clearly established environmental factors, including leanness, cigarette smoking, excessive salt and alcohol intakes, and lack of vitamin D, especially in elderly housebound people with little exposure to the sun. The role of dietary calcium has been uncertain but there is now convincing evidence that the best way of avoiding osteoporotic fractures in later life is to achieve optimal skeletal mass for one's genetic potential and to retain this as long as possible. The best means of doing so is by ensuring lifelong adequate consumption and maximum absorption and retention of calcium. The need for substantial amounts of dietary calcium, taken in conjunction with physiological amounts of vitamin D, is particularly important during the periods of growth, pregnancy, lactation, and in the postmenopausal years. Fruit and vegetables and adequate levels of physical activity have also been identified as protective factors.

Other diseases

Gallstones, appendicitis, haemorrhoids, varicose veins, and hiatus hernia all occur frequently in developed countries and rarely in developing countries but the evidence linking these diseases to a nutritional cause is tenuous. Gallstones are undoubtedly associated with obesity. Both gallstones and appendicitis are more common in nonvegetarians than vegetarians, and there are some rather indirect data suggesting an association with diets high in sugars and deficient in dietary fibre. The addition of bran to the diet can make bile less saturated, and experimentally induced gallstones in animals tend to be reduced if fibre-rich foods rich are given. Data from the United Kingdom and South Africa taken together provide interesting information concerning appendicitis; appendicitis rates were compared in two matched groups of South African whites, the privileged group living in university halls of residence and the other living in establishments for the indigent, where the diets contained more fibre. Annual rates were 7.8/1000 and 1.8/1000, respectively. Of course, factors other than diets might explain this, but the rates were similar to those found in an almost identical study in Bristol (7.6/1000 in a fee-paying boarding school and 0.8/1000 in an orphanage).

The case for dietary change

Nutrition research often generates results that may be translated by researchers, self-styled 'experts', or the media into potentially confusing and conflicting messages. It is therefore critically important for governments who develop food and nutrition policies, for doctors and others involved in health and nutrition education, and for consumers to have authoritative recommendations that represent consensus opinions of nutrition scientists. Terminology regarding such recommendations has been confusing, but a British government publication in 1991 suggested that the term 'dietary reference values' should be used to describe nutrition recommendations intended for policy makers and health professionals who recommend diets for individuals. Dietary reference values will be largely meaningless to the population at large. For the general public, dietary guidelines have been developed to translate dietary reference values into practical advice.

The British dietary reference values for macronutrients were based to a considerable extent on the evidence-based data, which suggest that alteration of dietary fat intake from that typical of most Western countries is likely to reduce population and individual risk of coronary heart disease. The 1991 recommendations were slightly modified and extended in a 1994 publication relating specifically to coronary heart disease. Table 11.4.6 compares the United Kingdom recommendations for population nutrient intakes with those more recently recommended (2003) by a World Health Organization/Food and Agriculture Organization Expert Consultation on Diet, Nutrition, and the Prevention of Chronic Diseases. There is emphasis on substantial reduction from present levels of intake of saturated and *trans*-unsaturated fatty acids. Assuming that alternative vegetable fat sources replace at least some of the saturated fatty acids, mono- and polyunsaturated fatty acids will increase with potential benefits accruing from some increase in both n – 3 (derived from plant or fish sources) and n – 6 (principally linoleic acid from vegetable oils). The apparent discrepancy between the two sets of recommendations regarding total fat reflects different local and international requirements and the observation that a relatively wide range of total fat intakes appears to be compatible with a low risk of most chronic diseases. The World Health Organization recommended range acknowledges that on the one hand, many countries have a low total fat intake and there is no justification for an increase. On the other hand, for countries with a high fat consumption at present, reduction to an intake of 30% may be a target achievable in the long term. In the United Kingdom, the figure given is considered to be

Table 11.4.6 Ranges of population nutrient intake goals as recommended by WHO/FAO and in the United Kingdom (unless otherwise stated, the goals are expressed as percentage total energy)

	WHO/FAO[a]	UK[b]
Total fat	15–30%	35%
Saturated fatty acids (SFA)	<10%	<10%
Cis-polyunsaturated fatty acids	6–10%	[c]
n – 6 PUFA	5–8%	< 10%
n – 3 PUFA	1–2%	1.5 g/week[d]
Cis-monounsaturated fatty acids	By difference[e]	[c]
Trans fatty acids	<1%	<2%
Dietary cholesterol (mg/day)	<300 mg/day	*c.*245 mg/day
Total carbohydrate	55–75%	50%
Free sugars[f]	<10%	Fruits and vegetables encouraged
Dietary fibre (NSP)	From foods	Complex carbohydrates encouraged
Protein	10–15%	[c]
Sodium chloride	<5 g/day	6 g/day (100 mmol/day)
Potassium		3.5 g/day
Fruit and vegetables	>400 g/day	Encouraged

[a] *Source:* WHO (2003). *Diet, Nutrition and the Prevention of Chronic Diseases.* Report of a Joint WHO/FAO Expert Consultation. Technical Report Series 916, World Health Organization, Geneva.

[b] *Source:* Department of Health (1994). *Report on health and social subjects: 46. Nutritional aspects of cardiovascular disease.* Report of the Cardiovascular Review Group Committee on Medical Aspects of Food Policy. HMSO, London.

[c] No specific recommendation.

[d] Mainly from oily fish.

[e] Total fat – (SFA + PFA + TFA).

[f] All monosaccharides and disaccharides added to foods by manufacturer, cooked, or consumed, plus sugars naturally present in honey, syrups, and fruit juice.

a reasonable short-term goal. A substantial reduction in total fat may facilitate a reduced intake of energy-dense foods and reduced risk of obesity, as well as more directly reducing coronary heart disease by reducing saturated and *trans*-unsaturated fatty acids.

About 50 g of carbohydrate daily is required to avoid ketosis, but many populations maintain an adequate nutritional status when carbohydrate provides up to 80% total energy. A relatively high intake of carbohydrate facilitates a reduction in total and saturated fat and potentially promotes the consumption of vegetables, fruit and wholegrain cereals. Most Western societies are unaccustomed to a high carbohydrate intake and are reluctant to accept substantial increases. A modest increase in total carbohydrate has therefore been recommended in the United Kingdom with a much wider range for international use. A recent FAO/WHO Scientific Update on Carbohydrates suggested that a modestly lower intake of carbohydrate (50% total energy) is acceptable so it seems likely that WHO recommendations will be altered to endorse a wider range (50 and 75% total energy). A high intake of free sugars (principally sucrose and, in the United States, high-fructose corn syrup) increases the risk of obesity by increasing the energy density of the diet, or simply by increasing total energy intake (and energy imbalance) when sugary drinks are consumed in excess. Sugars are also associated with dental caries and in large amounts may enhance the metabolic derangements in people with insulin resistance. Foods with a high intake of free sugars are frequently nutrient poor (i.e. contain relatively few essential nutrients), so limiting such foods has no adverse nutritional consequences. On the other hand, intrinsic sugars (i.e. those incorporated into the cellular structure of foods), milk sugars, and starches are not restricted and generally provide the balance of dietary energy not provided by protein, fat, and free sugars.

There has been much discussion regarding the most appropriate carbohydrate-containing foods. Intact fruit and vegetables and minimally processed cereals tend to be rich sources of dietary fibre, essential micronutrients, and some essential fatty acids. Some of these foods (e.g. some varieties of fruit or hot cooked potato) are largely digested in the small intestine and provide an immediate or fairly rapid source of energy, depending upon the speed of digestion. Others that are high in dietary fibre or starch, which is resistant to digestion in the small intestine (e.g. cooked dried beans, chickpeas, some whole-grain products) enter the colon in a largely undigested state. Resistant starch, oligosaccharides, and some components of dietary fibre (e.g. gum, pectins, mucilages) undergo fermentation that leads to the production of fatty acids, which provide a fuel source (via conversion to glucose in the liver), and may also reduce the risk of colon cancer because of their antiproliferative effects. Other components of dietary fibre remain largely intact and act as stool-bulkers (e.g. cellulose and hemicellulose). Thus a wide variety of fruits and vegetables, whole grains, and minimally processed cereals are particularly appropriate sources of carbohydrate. Free or added sugars in jams and manufactured foods (e.g. confectionery products) or added by the consumer to food and beverages are also rapid sources of energy, but increase energy density and promote obesity, so that foods rich in them should be restricted by most people. The benefits of synthetic forms of dietary fibre or fibre extracted from plant material have not yet been established.

While appropriate distribution of macronutrients and good food choices might be expected to reduce cardiovascular risk, improve bowel function, and probably also reduce the risk of certain cancers and other diseases of the large bowel, the importance of ensuring energy balance cannot be overstated. Obesity and its comorbidities, especially type 2 diabetes, account for a public health problem of enormous magnitude throughout the world. Increasing carbohydrate-containing bulking foods rich in dietary fibre, at the expense of saturated fat, is likely to enhance satiety. Such positive advice, along with the recommendations to reduce frequent consumption of large portions of all energy-dense foods and sugary drinks, is likely to help reduce excessive energy intake.

Table 11.4.7 Reference nutrient intakes for selected major vitamins and minerals

Age	Vitamin B_{12} μg/day	Folate μg/day	Vitamin A μg/day	Vitamin D μg/day	Calcium mmol/day	Sodium[a] mmol/day	Iron μmol/day	Zinc μmol/day	Iodine μmol/day
0–3 months	0.3	50	350	8.5	13.1	9	30	60	0.4
4–6 months	0.3	50	350	8.5	13.1	12	80	60	0.5
7–9 months	0.4	50	350	7	13.1	14	140	75	0.5
10–12 months	0.4	50	350	7	13.1	15	140	75	0.5
1–3 years	0.5	70	400	7	8.8	22	120	75	0.6
4–6 years	0.8	100	500	–	11.3	30	110	100	0.8
7–10 years	1.0	150	500	–	13.8	50	160	110	0.9
Males									
11–14 years	1.2	200	600	–	25.0	70	200	140	1.0
15–18 years	1.5	200	700	–	25.0	70	200	145	1.0
19–50 years	1.5	200	700	–	17.5	70	160	145	1.0
50+ years	1.5	200	700	d	17.5	70	160	145	1.0
Females									
11–14 years	1.2	200	600	–	20.0	70	260[b]	140	1.0
15–18 years	1.5	200	600	–	20.0	70	260[b]	110	1.1
19–50 years	1.5	200	600	–	17.5	70	260[b]	110	1.1
50+ years	1.5	200	600	d	17.5	70	160	110	1.1
Pregnancy	c	+100	+100	10	c	c	c	c	c
Lactation									
0–4 months	+0.5	+60	+350	10	+14.3	c	c	+90	c
4+ months	+0.5	+60	+350	10	+14.3	c	c	+40	c

[a] 1 mmol sodium = 23 mg, 1mmol calcium = 40mg, 1 umol iron = 56ug, 1umol zinc =65ug, 1umol iodine = 127ug.

[b] Insufficient for women with high menstrual losses where the most practical way of meeting iron requirements is to take iron supplements.

[c] No increment.

[d] After 65 years of age the reference nutrient intake is 10 μg/day for men and women.

However, increasing energy output by increasing physical activity is an equally essential component of energy balance and public health measures designed to stem the tide of the global obesity epidemic.

Reference nutrient intakes (adequate for most individuals) are provided for vitamins and minerals (Table 11.4.7). They are set at a level of two standard deviations above the average of all individual requirements, so that requirements for the vast majority in the population are assured. Clinical vitamin deficiencies, discussed in detail in Chapter 11.2, are uncommon in affluent societies except in at-risk subgroups within populations. For example, immigrants who have migrated from sunny tropical regions to cloudy high-latitude countries may be at risk of vitamin D deficiency; strict vegetarians (who consume no animal or dairy products) may become deficient in vitamin B_{12}, and disadvantaged groups (especially the very young, pregnant and lactating women, and older people) may have generally inadequate intakes.

On the other hand, inappropriate intakes of certain minerals are fairly common. Many groups are particularly vulnerable to iron deficiency, due to high physiological requirements (infants and toddlers, adolescents, pregnant women), high losses (menstruating women), or poor absorption (older people and those consuming foods high in inhibitors of absorption, such as fibre and tannin in tea). Vegetarians are also at increased risk of iron deficiency even when total intake of iron appears to be adequate, since nonhaem iron from plant foods is less bioavailable than haem iron from animal sources. Bioavailability is enhanced by the consumption, at the same time, of foods rich in vitamin C. Iodine and selenium are deficient in soils in various parts of the world. Clinical selenium deficiency has only been reported from China, though the consequences of lesser degrees of selenium deficiency have yet to be established with certainty, especially in regions where soils are known to be deficient. Endemic iodine deficiency is widespread, especially in the Himalayas and the Andes, and clinical deficiency states are largely avoided by the use of iodized salt and sanitizers containing iodine used by the dairy industry. In New Zealand, where goitre due to iodine deficiency had virtually been eliminated, mild iodine deficiency appears to be re-occurring possibly as a result of reduced use of iodized salt and the introduction by the dairy industry of alternative sanitizers. Young women often have insufficient calcium to help achieve peak bone mass, and older women may have an inadequate intake to help reduce an age-related bone loss.

Excessive intakes of sodium, to such an extent that it probably contributes to hypertension and its consequences, are common throughout the world. Targets for reduction may be more important than reference nutrient intakes for sodium. An intake of 100 mmol/day (2.3 g sodium/day, roughly equal to 6 g NaCl), a level currently exceeded in most countries, might be an appropriate maximum.

Reference nutrient intakes need to be reviewed regularly. In the 1990s, a value of 200 µg/day for folate was widely recommended. It is now acknowledged that intakes of 400 µg/day can appreciably reduce the risk of neural tube defects. Most countries, though not yet the United Kingdom, have altered their recommended intake to 400 µg/day. Recent evidence from large randomized controlled trials has not confirmed the suggestion from observational studies and experiments suggesting that high intakes of folic acid or antioxidant nutrients, taken as supplements, may be cardioprotective. It is conceivable that these micronutrients are protective against coronary heart disease only when consumed as food constituents rather than as individual supplements.

Box 11.4.2 Dietary guidelines for which there is almost complete agreement

- Eat a nutritionally adequate diet composed of a variety of foods
- Eat less fat, particularly saturated fat
- Adjust energy balance for body weight control—less energy intake, more exercise
- Eat more whole-grain cereals, vegetables, and fruits
- Reduce intake of salt and foods rich in salt
- Drink alcohol in moderation, if you do drink

Substantial changes in what have become traditional eating habits of many affluent societies are required in order to achieve the advised changes in distribution of macronutrients and recommended intake of all essential micronutrients. A multifocal approach is necessary if there is to be a real chance of achieving dietary change. At the policy-making and government level, there needs to be a serious commitment to enabling the population as a whole to make appropriate food choices. Fatty cuts of meat, high-fat products (e.g. meat pies), and convenience foods (e.g. fish and chips, burgers) are relatively inexpensive and therefore frequently eaten by those of lower socioeconomic status who have the highest rates of coronary heart disease. Policies are required which ensure that more appropriate food choices are available at reasonable cost. This is not easy to achieve in many Western countries, where farmers may have considerable political influence, and subsidies may be available for some high-fat dairy products such as butter and cheese. Governments and intergovernmental agencies also have the responsibility for ensuring that food labels and health claims are accurate, interpretable, and likely to facilitate health-promoting food choices, a particularly important issue given the increased consumption of packaged food.

Dietary guidelines are necessary to provide clear directions to individuals and families who wish to aim for a healthy diet pattern. These guidelines vary slightly from country to country though some are almost universal (see Box 11.4.2). Others are less consistent (see Box 11.4.3). The public also need education regarding food groups and the nutrients they contain, the interpretation of food labels, the meaning of health claims, and the methods of

Box 11.4.3 Additional dietary guidelines in some countries

- Recommendation regarding sugar and sugary foods may vary from 'no increase' to 'decrease'
- Drink plenty of fluids each day
- Make sure you get enough calcium or milk
- Eat foods containing iron
- Drink fluoridated water
- Preserve the nutritive value of food (by good food preparation)
- Eat three good meals a day

food preparation. The increased use of convenience and packaged food has meant that many people no longer possess basic cooking skills. They also need (and usually want) to know the merits and demerits of obtaining certain essential micronutrients by taking supplements or fortified food products rather than conventional foods.

Doctors are frequently asked to give nutritional advice but may lack the necessary expertise. Dietitians, nutritionists, and appropriately trained practice nurses play an invaluable role in providing the public with practical advice to facilitate changes from the typical Western diet as well as providing instruction regarding therapeutic diets for those with diseases requiring specific diet therapy. The enormous potential for dietary change to reduce the effects of a wide range of diseases should encourage physicians to approach the nutritional management of their patients with enthusiasm.

Further reading

COMA–CHD Panel on Dietary Reference Values of the Committee on Medical Aspects of Food Policy (1991). *Report on health and social subjects: 41. dietary reference values for food energy and nutrients for the United Kingdom.* HMSO, London.

de Deckere EAM *et al.* (1998). Health aspects of fish and n – 3 polyunsaturated fatty acids from plant and marine origin. *Eur J Clin Nutr*, **52**, 749–53.

Department of Health (1994). *Report on health and social subjects: 46. Nutritional aspects of cardiovascular disease.* Report of the Cardiovascular Review Group Committee on Medical Aspects of Food Policy. HMSO, London.

FAO/WHO (2007). Scientific Update on Carbohydrates, *European Journal of Clinical Nutrition*, **61** supplement: S1–S138.

Food, Nutrition, Physical Activity and the Prevention of Cancer (2007): *A global perspective.* World Cancer Research Fund Second Report.

Liu *et al.* (2000). *J Am Med Assoc*, **284** ,1534–40.

Mann J, Truswell AS (eds) (2007). *Essentials of human nutrition*, 3rd edition. Oxford University Press, Oxford.

Rimm *et al.* (1996). *J Am Med Assoc.* **275**, 447–51.

Stampfer and Rimm (1995). *Am J Clin Nutr*, **62**, 1355–1395.

Truswell AS (2003). *ABC of nutrition*, 4th edition. BMJ Books, London.

WHO (2003). *Diet, Nutrition and the Prevention of Chronic Diseases.* Report of a Joint WHO/FAO Expert Consultation. Technical Report Series 916, World Health Organization, Geneva.

WHO/FAO (1998). *Carbohydrates in human nutrition.* FAO Food and Nutrition Paper 66. Report of a Joint FAO/WHO Expert Consultation. Food and Agriculture Organization, Rome.

11.5

Obesity

I. Sadaf Farooqi

Essentials

Obesity is defined as an excess of body fat that is sufficient to affect health adversely. It is associated with an increased risk of type 2 diabetes, cardiovascular disease, and some forms of cancer and is a serious medical disorder. In routine practice, body mass index (BMI) is most often used to define obesity in population studies and in the clinic: overweight, BMI 25 to 29.9 kg/m^2; obese, BMI 30.0 to 39.9 kg/m^2; morbid obesity, BMI >40 kg/m^2. By this definition about 20% of men and 25% of women in the United States of America and Europe are obese.

Causes of obesity

The rising global prevalence of obesity is driven by environmental factors including the increased availability of palatable energy-dense foods and the reduced requirement for physical exertion during working and domestic life.

The heritability of body weight and fat mass is very high and genetic variation determines the inter-individual differences in susceptibility or resistance to the 'obesogenic' dietary environment. Studies of genetic obesity syndromes have revealed mutations that all arise in molecules involved in the leptin–melanocortin pathway, which plays a key role in the regulation of body weight. Genome wide association studies, which have proved to be an extremely valuable tool for unravelling the aetiology of complex diseases, have shown that variants in the *FTO* gene are strongly associated with increased BMI.

Management of obesity

Management of patients with severe obesity is a challenge, but success is enhanced by a sympathetic approach from the physician, with realistic weight loss goals and monitoring of the effects of treatment. Interventions include (1) low-calorie diets, energy-deficit diets and diets that are low in fat, which should initially provide a 600 kcal/day (2.5 MJ/day) energy deficit, based on estimated energy requirements; (2) behavioural approaches to help subjects to implement and sustain changes to their eating and activity behaviour; (3) drug treatment—which should always be regarded as a therapeutic trial and stopped if weight loss is not apparent after one to two months—with agents used including pancreatic lipase inhibitors (orlistat); (4) surgery—an option for carefully selected patients with morbid obesity, with procedures including laparoscopic gastric banding, gastric bypass, and duodenal switch.

Introduction

Obesity is frequently considered to be a 'modern' disease—a reflection of the excesses of urbanized society. However, artefacts dating from the Palaeolithic age clearly represent subjects with an excess of body fat, and descriptions of obese individuals in medical texts from many of the ancient civilizations, suggest that, throughout history, certain individuals have harboured the tendency to store excess energy as fat. Hippocrates recognized that obesity posed a threat to health when he wrote that, 'sudden death is more common in those who are naturally fat than in the lean'. Galen elaborated upon earlier descriptions of the obese state, distinguishing between different degrees of obesity, 'moderate' or common obesity and 'immoderate' or morbid obesity. Many Greek and Roman physicians documented some of the clinical complications associated with obesity, including reduced frequency of menses and infertility. The first known description of obesity and sleep apnoea dates from Roman times; Dionysius, the tyrant of Heracleia of Pontius who reigned from about 360 BC, was described as 'an enormously fat man who frequently fell asleep'. The obesity-related changes in respiratory function, which are most prominent during sleep, are now recognized as the obesity–hypoventilation or Pickwickian syndrome.

Definition of obesity as a medical disorder

The recognition that obesity represents a serious medical disorder at a population level came with pooled life insurance data from the United States of America, showing that increasing degrees of overweight and obesity were important predictors of decreased longevity, much of which was attributed to cardiovascular disease. Subsequently, a number of epidemiological studies, including the Framingham Study and the Build and Blood Pressure Study have shown that the adverse effects of excess weight tend to be delayed, sometimes for 10 years or longer. These observations led to the recognition that obesity should be defined as a disorder in which excess body fat has accumulated such that health may be adversely affected. We now recognize that obesity is associated with substantially increased mortality from cardiovascular and cerebrovascular disease, type 2 diabetes, and certain cancers. Obesity is also associated with increased morbidity from musculoskeletal, gastrointestinal, psychiatric, and reproductive diseases (Table 11.5.1) and is associated with lowered quality of life, self-esteem, and socioeconomic performance.

The precise measurement of body fat is quite challenging, and accurate methods are not applicable to large populations; therefore, surrogate markers such as the body mass index (BMI—weight in kilograms divided by the square of the height in metres) are most often used to define obesity in population studies and in the clinic. The underlying assumption is that most variation in weight for persons of the same height is due to fat mass and there is a close correlation between BMI and the incidence of type 2 diabetes, hypertension, and coronary heart disease. A World Health Organization Expert Committee has proposed a classification of overweight and obesity (Table 11.5.2) using BMI.

Worldwide prevalence of obesity

Obesity, defined as a BMI of more than 30 kg/m^2, is a common condition in Europe and the United States of America. The most comprehensive information in Europe comes from the data collected between 1983 and 1986 for the MONICA study. On average, 15% of men and 22% of women were found to be obese and more than 50% of the adult population in Europe were either overweight or obese. The striking increase in prevalence between 1980 and 1994 confirms that population-wide increases in overweight and obesity have taken place over a short time interval. The most recent data from the United States of America shows about 20% of American men and about 25% of American women to be obese. In South-East Asia and the Middle East, a dramatic rise is being seen in all populations.

Table 11.5.1 Medical complications associated with obesity

Type 2 diabetes	90% of type 2 diabetics have a BMI of >23 kg/m^2
Hypertension	60–80% of hypertension is linked to excess weight
Coronary artery disease (CAD) and stroke	3.6-fold risk of CAD for each unit change in BMI
Respiratory effects	Neck circumference of >43 cm in men and >40.5 cm in women is associated with obstructive sleep apnoea, daytime somnolence, and development of pulmonary hypertension
Cancers	10% of all cancer deaths among nonsmokers are related to obesity (30% of endometrial cancers)
Reproductive function	6% of primary infertility in women is attributable to obesity
	Impotency and infertility are frequently associated with obesity in men
Osteoarthritis (OA)	Frequent association in older people with increasing body weight
Liver disease	Nonalcoholic fatty liver disease and nonalcoholic steatohepatitis (NASH); 40% of NASH patients are obese
Gallbladder disease	Threefold risk of gallbladder disease in women

Table 11.5.2 Cut-off points proposed by a World Health Organization Expert Committee for the classification of overweight and obesity

BMI	WHO classification
<18.5	Underweight
18.5–24.9	Normal weight
25–29.9	Overweight
30.0–39.9	Obesity
40.0 or greater	Morbid obesity

In children the relationship between BMI and body fat varies markedly with age and with pubertal maturation; however, when adjusted for age and gender, BMI is a reasonable proxy for fat mass. BMI percentile charts using national BMI reference data have now been published in several countries and facilitate the graphical plotting of serial BMI measurements in individual patients. The International Obesity Task Force (IOTF) has recommended the use of BMI data derived from six countries, which extrapolate risk from the adult experience to children. These age- and gender-specific BMI cut-offs (overweight as approximately 91st percentile or greater and obesity as approximately 99th percentile or greater) allow the comparison of obesity prevalence in different populations. Using these criteria, it is clear that the prevalence of overweight and obesity in childhood is a global concern (Table 11.5.3). Although there is no accepted definition for severe or morbid obesity in childhood, a BMI of more than 2.5 standard deviations from the mean (weight off the chart) is often used in specialist centres, and the crossing of major weight percentile lines upwards is an early indication of risk of severe obesity.

Aetiology of obesity

Body weight is determined by an interaction between genetic, environmental, and psychosocial factors acting through the physiological mediators of energy intake and expenditure. By definition, obesity results from an imbalance between energy intake and energy expenditure and, in any individual, excessive caloric intake or low energy expenditure, or both, may explain the development of obesity. A third factor, nutrient partitioning, a term reflecting the propensity to store excess energy as fat rather than lean tissue, may contribute.

A physiological system for the homeostatic regulation of body weight was first proposed by Kennedy, who envisaged a mechanism that monitored changes in energy stores and initiated compensatory changes in food intake and energy expenditure to maintain fat mass at a physiological set point. This adipostatic model of body weight regulation is consistent with the observation that adipose tissue mass remains relatively stable over long periods of time and a decrease in adiposity from fasting causes hyperphagia and

Table 11.5.3 Childhood prevalence (% of population) of overweight (including obesity) in selected countries, by WHO region using IOTF definitions

WHO Region	Year of survey	Age (years)	Boys	Girls
Africa				
Algeria	2003	7–17	6.0	5.6
Mali	1993	5–17	0.2	0.5
South Africa	2001–2004	6–13	14	17.9
Americas				
Brazil	2002	7–10	23.0	21.1
Chile	2000	6	26.0	27.1
USA	2003/2004	6–11	31.7	37.5
Eastern Mediterranean				
Bahrain	2000	12–17	29.9	42.4
Iran	1995	6	24.7	26.8
Saudi Arabia	2002	5–17	16.7	19.4
Europe				
Czech Republic	2001	5–17	14.7	13.4
Portugal	2002/3	7–9	29.5	34.3
Spain	1998–2000	5–16	31.0	19.5
England	2001	5–17	21.8	27.1
South-East Asia				
India	2002	5–17	12.9	8.2
Sri Lanka	2002	10–15	1.7	2.7
Thailand	1997	5–15	21.1	12.6
Western Pacific				
Australia	1995	7–17	21.1	21.3
China	1999–2000	11, 15	14.9	8.0
Japan	1996–2000	6–14	16.2	14.3
New Zealand	2000	11, 12	30.0	30.0

a decrease in energy expenditure, thereby restoring body weight. Thus, marked increases in the prevalence of human obesity over a 10-year period may be the consequence of relatively minor changes in food intake and physical activity and current trends could readily be explained by an increase in the mean weight of an individual of 10 kg over 30 years.

Environmental factors

There are some obvious candidates for increase in obesity prevalence, including the increased availability of palatable energy-dense foods and the reduced requirement for physical exertion during working and domestic life. Globally, as the proportion of a population with a low BMI decreases, there is an almost reciprocal increase in the proportion of the population who are overweight or obese. Further evidence for the critical role of environmental factors in the development of obesity comes from migrant studies, where a marked change in BMI is frequently witnessed where populations with a common genetic heritage live under new and different environmental circumstances. Pima Indians living in the United States are on average 25 kg heavier than Pima Indians living in Mexico. The two priority areas for public health strategies aimed at preventing obesity are increasing physical activity and improving the quality of the available diet within a community. However, such strategies must address the need to improve the population's understanding of the nature of obesity and its management and reduce exposure to an environment that promotes obesity. Achievement of these aims requires the involvement of individuals, their families, health professionals, health services, and a commitment from all sectors of the community.

Genetic factors

Obesity represents a heterogeneous group of conditions with multiple causes. Twin studies, adoption studies, and studies of familial aggregation confirm a major contribution of genes to the development of obesity. Indeed, the heritability of fat mass and of body weight is equivalent to that of height and exceeds that of many disorders for which a genetic basis is generally accepted. As with other common, complex traits, the genetic determinants of interindividual variation in body fat mass are likely to be multiple and interacting, with each single variant producing only a moderate effect. Recently, genome-wide association studies have proved to be an extremely valuable tool for unravelling the aetiology of complex diseases. Variants in the *FTO* gene are strongly associated with increased BMI, a finding that has been replicated in multiple studies. It is likely that genome-wide approaches in larger cohorts and/or those with early-onset disease will result in the identification of other common variants that contribute to obesity risk in populations. To date, the common variants that have been identified explain less than 5% of the heritability of increased BMI. It is likely that rare variants that are more highly penetrant will explain more of the missing heritability of obesity.

Genetic obesity syndromes

Classically, patients affected by genetic obesity syndromes have been identified as a result of their association with developmental delay, dysmorphic features, or other developmental abnormalities. More recently, several single gene disorders resulting from disruption of the hypothalamic leptin–melanocortin signalling pathway have been identified. In these disorders, obesity itself is the predominant presenting feature, although frequently accompanied by characteristic patterns of neuroendocrine dysfunction that will only become apparent on investigation. For the purposes of clinical assessment, it remains useful to categorize the genetic obesity syndromes as those with dysmorphism and/or developmental delay, and those without these features. There are about 30 Mendelian disorders with obesity as a clinical feature but often associated with mental retardation, dysmorphic features, and organ-specific developmental abnormalities (Table 11.5.4).

Several genetic disorders result in severe obesity commencing in childhood without developmental delay (Table 11.5.5). These mutations all arise in molecules involved in the leptin–melanocortin pathway, which plays a key role in the regulation of body weight. Energy homeostasis is tightly regulated, with the hypothalamus playing a pivotal role in integrating signals from adipose tissue stores, such as leptin and short-term meal-related signals from the gut (peptide-YY, glucagon like peptide-1 (GLP-1), cholecystokinin, and ghrelin) (Fig. 11.5.1). Leptin stimulates the expression of

Table 11.5.4 Obesity syndromes with developmental delay

Name of syndrome	Gene/genetic region involved	Clinical characteristics
Prader–Willi	Deletion or uniparental maternal disomy of chromosome 15q11.2–-q12	Hypotonia, short stature, hypogonadotropic hypogonadism, feeding difficulties <2 years of age, then hyperphagia with pica behaviour
Bardet–Biedl	Mutations in multiple genes affect the function of cilia	Polydactyly, retinitis pigmentosa, and hypogonadism are consistent features
Fragile X	Unstable expansion of trinucleotide repeats in the *FMR1* gene	Moderate to severe developmental delay, macro-orchidism, prominent jaw, and high-pitched jocular speech
Cohen	*COH1* mutations	Microcephaly, characteristic facial features, progressive retinochoroidal dystrophy, myopia, and a cheerful disposition
Albright hereditary osteodystrophy	*GNAS1* mutations	Short stature, round facies, brachydactyly, and ectopic soft tissue ossification (osteoma cutis), variable hormone (TSH, PTH) resistance, short fourth metacarpal
BDNF/TrkB deficiency	Mutations/deletions in BDNF or its receptor TrKB	Delayed speech and language development, impaired short term memory and loss of nociception

BDNF, brain-derived neurotrophic factor; PTH, parathyroid hormone; TrkB, neurotrophic tyrosine kinase, receptor, type 2; TSH, thyroid-stimulating hormone.

pro-opiomelanocortin (POMC), which is cleaved by prohormone convertases to yield the melanocortin peptides, which act as suppressors of feeding through the melanocortin 4 receptor (MC4R) (Fig. 11.5.2). Mutations in several of these molecules cause severe obesity associated with specific neuroendocrine abnormalities (Table 11.5.5). One rare genetic disorder, leptin deficiency, is entirely treatable with daily subcutaneous injections of recombinant human leptin, and another, MC4R deficiency, is relatively common, with a population prevalence of 1 in 1000 unselected individuals and 1 in 100 obese people.

Programming and epigenetics

Recent evidence suggests that undernutrition of the fetus during intrauterine development can influence the later onset of obesity, hypertension, and type 2 diabetes, independent of genetic factors. Such a phenomenon suggests the possibility of long-term programming of genetic expression as a consequence of altered intrauterine growth. The influence of maternal diet and other factors on the regulation of genes in their offspring, referred to as epigenetics, is the focus of much current research.

Table 11.5.5 Obesity syndromes in the absence of developmental delay

Name of syndrome	Clinical characteristics
Alstrom	Progressive nephropathy, photophobia, retinitis pigmentosa, deafness, diabetes mellitus due to marked insulin resistance
Leptin	Severe hyperphagia, frequent infections, hypogonadism
Prohormone convertase 1	Neonatal diarrhoea, postprandial hypoglycaemia, multiple endocrine abnormalities
Leptin receptor	Severe hyperphagia, frequent infections, hypogonadism
POMC	Isolated ACTH deficiency, hypopigmentation
MC4R	Increased linear growth, severe hyperinsulinaemia, 'big-boned' appearance

ACTH, adrencorticotrophic hormone; MC4R, melanocortin 4 receptor; POMC, pro-opiomelanocortin

Clinical history, examination, and investigation

For the assessment of severely obese patients, the consultation room should be properly equipped with larger than average chairs, access for wheelchairs for patients with mobility problems, and medical equipment of appropriate size (examination couch, blood pressure cuff, weighing scales, stadiometer, and tape measure). In addition to a general medical history, a specific weight history should be taken carefully establishing the age of onset (clinical photographs are helpful here), as it is useful to distinguish obesity that began in childhood (stronger genetic component) from that occurring later in life either in relation to specific physiological 'critical periods' such as pregnancy, illness, or concomitant medications. A history of previous treatment for obesity, diet, and levels of physical activity should be noted. The assessment of severely obese children and adults should include screening for potentially treatable endocrine and neurological conditions and identifying genetic conditions so that appropriate genetic counselling and, in some cases, treatment can be instituted. In most patients, these specific causes can be excluded by a careful clinical history (Box 11.5.1), examination, and investigations (Table 11.5.6), which should also address the potential hidden complications of severe obesity such as sleep apnoea, coronary heart disease, type 2 diabetes, gynaecological abnormalities, osteoarthritis, gallstones, and stress incontinence. Height should be measured accurately using a stadiometer and weight measured by accurate scales calibrated against known weights. Fat distribution is assessed by measurement of the waist circumference and is used to refine an assessment of risk for patients with a BMI of 25 to 34.9. Waist circumference is taken as the mid point between the lower rib margin and the iliac crest. An examination of the skin is important: thin, atrophic skin is a feature of excess corticosteroids; acanthosis nigricans (pigmented 'velvety' skin creases, especially in the axillae) suggests insulin resistance; severe hirsutism in women may indicate polycystic ovary syndrome. A neck circumference of more than 43 cm indicates a likelihood of obstructive sleep apnoea.

Clinicians should use laboratory testing to evaluate overweight and obese patients who may be at high risk for cardiovascular disease, diabetes, and thyroid disease. Some useful tests to consider are fasting plasma glucose or 2-h postprandial glucose levels and serum lipid levels. Thyroid-stimulating hormone (TSH) may be helpful

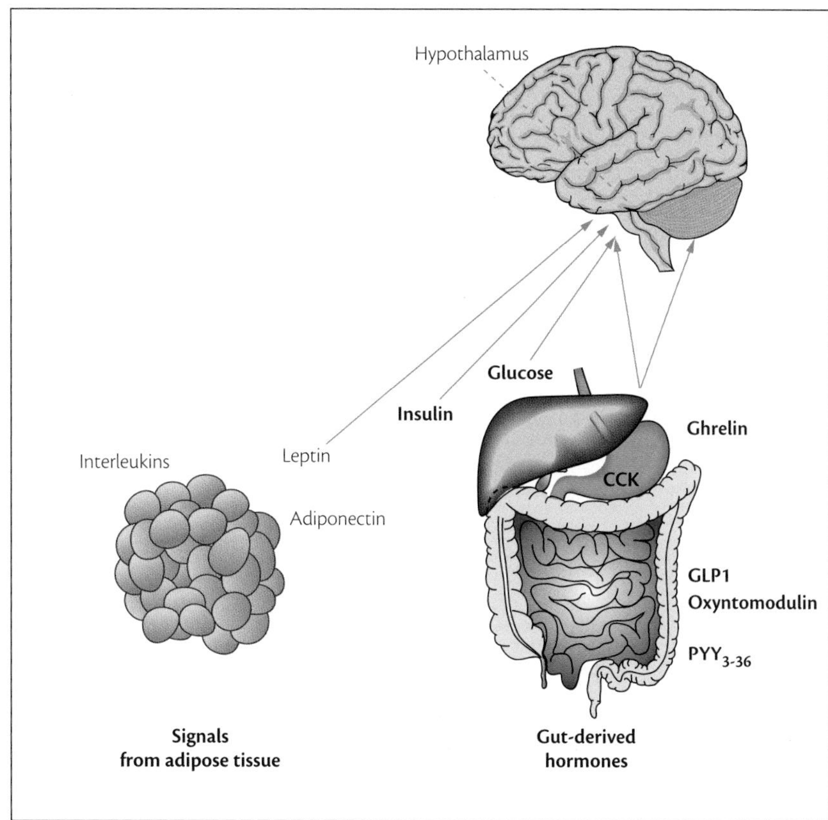

Fig. 11.5.1 Peripheral homeostatic regulators of energy balance include adipocyte-derived hormones, particularly leptin, which is responsible for signalling long-term energy stores; and gut-derived hormones, which are concerned with short-term control of food intake. These peripheral signals are sensed by the brain, particularly the hypothalamus, and to a lesser extent the brainstem, where the long- and short-term nutritional signals are integrated resulting in the regulation of food intake and energy expenditure.

in excluding hypothyroidism. Urinary free cortisol can be obtained if hypercortisolism is suspected. Other tests to consider depend on clinical assessment and include ultrasonography for hepatic steatosis, gallstones, and the polycystic ovary syndrome; electrocardiography in patients at high risk for cardiovascular disease; polysomnography for patients with possible sleep apnoea; and head CT or MRI when pituitary or hypothalamic disorders are suspected. Genetic testing is needed to confirm the diagnosis in patients with rare genetic disorders. The measurement of serum leptin is not recommended as a routine examination, but should be undertaken in cases of severe early onset obesity, since, although it is rare, congenital leptin deficiency is a potentially treatable disorder.

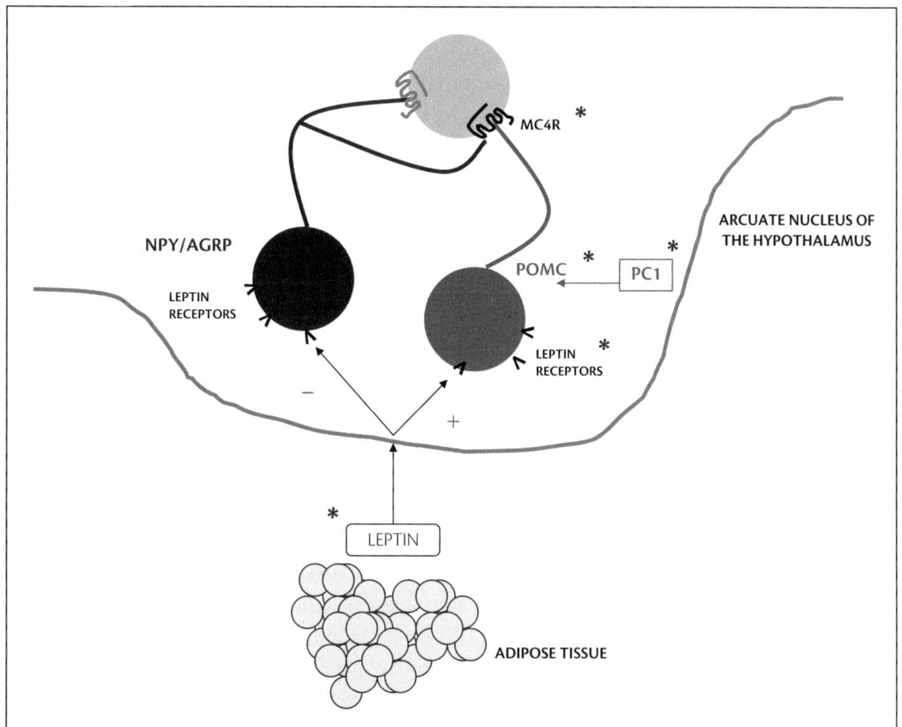

Fig. 11.5.2 Several single-gene defects that disrupt the molecules in the leptin–melanocortin pathway cause severe obesity (indicated by *). Leptin is released from adipose tissue to act on receptors expressed on the surface of distinct populations of neurones in the arcuate nucleus of the hypothalamus. Leptin stimulates a neuropeptide called pro-opiomelanocortin (POMC), which is then cleaved by the enzyme prohormone convertase 1 (PC1) to yield the melanocortin peptides. Leptin inhibits the expression of neuropeptide Y (NPY) and agouti-related peptide (AgRP). Both sets of neurons project to synapse, with second-order neurons expressing the melanocortin 4 receptor (MC4R), ultimately leading to an inhibition of food intake.

Box 11.5.1 History

- Age of onset—use of growth charts and family photographs. Early onset (<5 years of age) suggests a genetic cause.
- Duration of obesity—short history suggests endocrine or central cause.
- A history of damage to the CNS (e.g. infection, trauma, haemorrhage, radiation therapy, seizures) suggests hypothalamic obesity with or without pituitary growth hormone deficiency or pituitary hypothyroidism. A history of morning headaches, vomiting, visual disturbances, and excessive urination or drinking also suggests that the obesity may be caused by a tumour or mass in the hypothalamus.
- A history of dry skin, constipation, intolerance to cold, or fatigue suggests hypothyroidism. Mood disturbance and central obesity suggests Cushing's syndrome. Frequent infections and fatigue may suggest ACTH deficiency due to POMC mutations.
- Hyperphagia—often denied, but sympathetic approach needed and specific questions, such as waking at night to eat, demanding food very soon after a meal suggest hyperphagia. If severe, especially in children, suggests a genetic cause for obesity.
- Developmental delay—milestones, educational history, behavioural disorders. Consider craniopharyngeoma or structural causes (often relatively short history) and genetic causes.
- Visual impairment and deafness can suggest genetic causes.
- Onset and tempo of pubertal development—onset can be early or delayed in children and adolescents. Primary hypogonadotropic hypogonadism or hypogenitalism associated with some genetic disorders.
- Family history—consanguineous relationships, other children affected, family photographs useful. Severity may differ due to environmental effects.
- Treatment with certain drugs or medications. Glucocorticoids, sulphonylureas, oral contraceptives, antidepressants, and antipsychotics.

Approach to the treatment of obesity

The recommendation to treat obesity is based on evidence that relates obesity to increased mortality and the results from randomized controlled trials, which demonstrate that weight loss reduces the risk of disease. Professional, governmental, and other bodies have drawn up guidelines for obesity management and its advisable to seek out the latest national and international guidelines as newer evidence is incorporated. These strategies provide useful evidence-based guidance for clinical management, but it is important to remember that an individually tailored approach is often required and that any treatment programme for obese patients should address weight reduction and the maintenance of the lowered weight and take account of individual circumstances.

Table 11.5.6 Key points in the examination and investigation of an obese patient

Examination	Height, weight—calculate BMI
	Blood pressure
	Waist circumference
	Neck circumference
	Acanthosis nigricans
	Body fat distribution
	Secondary sexual characteristics
	Any evidence of cardiac disease
	Signs of hyperlipidaemia
	Signs of thyroid disease
	Ophthalmic evidence of diabetes or sustained hypertension
Investigations	Fasting and postprandial blood glucose
	Fasting lipid profile
	Strip test for urine glucose and protein
	Free thyroxine and thyroid-stimulating hormone

Goals of weight loss

Achievement of normal or ideal body weight is not a necessary goal in the management of obesity, and is rarely reached in practice. There is evidence from epidemiological studies of intentional weight loss that modest weight loss, of the order of 5 to 10% from presentation weight, is associated with clinically worthwhile reductions in comorbidities, such as hypertension, dyslipidaemia, and diabetes risk (Table 11.5.7). In some patients, particularly in those with severe comorbidity, prevention of weight gain may be a reasonable aim of treatment. Weight loss should be approached incrementally, with new goals for weight loss negotiated with the patient once the original target has been achieved.

Dietary treatment of obesity

A number of dietary approaches have been advocated for the treatment of obesity. Recent evidence-based reviews support the use of low-calorie diets, energy-deficit diets, and diets that are low in fat as being most likely to be effective for modest weight loss. A review of 48 randomized control trials shows that an average weight loss of 8% of the initial body weight can be obtained over 3 to 12 months with a low-calorie diet, and that this weight loss can lead to a decrease in abdominal fat. Such a treatment may require a period of supervision for at least 6 months. The weight-reducing dietary regimen tailored to an individual's need should initially provide a 600 kcal/day (2.5 MJ/day) energy deficit, based on estimated energy requirements. After 6 months, the rate of weight loss usually declines and a further adjustment of calorie intake may be indicated at this stage. The use of very low-calorie diets can be considered, but their use should follow all of the recommendations from the Committee on Medical Aspects of Food Policy, in particular

Table 11.5.7 Potential health benefits that may accrue from the loss of 10 kg from the initial body weight

Mortality	20–25% fall in total mortality
	30–40% fall in diabetes-related deaths
	40–50% fall in obesity-related cancer deaths
Blood pressure	*c.*10 mmHg fall in both systolic and diastolic values
Diabetes	>50% reducution in risk of developing diabetes
	30–50% fall in fasting glucose
	15% fall in haemoglobin A1c
Lipids	10% fall in total cholesterol
	15% fall in LDL cholesterol
	30% fall in triglycerides
	8% increase in HDL cholesterol

HDL, high-density lipoprotein; LDL, low-density lipoprotein.

that such preparations must provide a minimum of 400 kcal (1.7 MJ) per day for women and 50 kcal (2.1 MJ) per day for men. Evidence from randomized trials confirms that over the longer term (more than a year), weight loss following very low-calorie diets is no different from that obtained with low-calorie diets.

Behavioural therapy and exercise

Behavioural approaches aim to help subjects to implement and sustain changes to their eating and activity behaviour and require trained health professionals with good interpersonal skills to use the approach appropriately and in a supportive manner. There is evidence that combining a behavioural approach with more traditional dietary and activity advice leads to improved short-term weight loss. However, these studies are of relatively short duration, so the evidence base is limited to 1 year at present. In general, weight loss with these approaches is modest (about 4 kg or 4% of body weight on average).

Although modest physical activity has undoubted health benefits and can contribute to weight loss, it is not usually advocated as a sole treatment option. Many studies, however, do suggest that it can be helpful to improve weight loss maintenance, although activity levels equivalent to 45 to 60 min of brisk walking each day may be needed to achieve this. The results from randomized controlled trials suggest that a combination of diet and exercise generally produces more weight loss than diet alone.

Principles of drug therapy

Despite the availability of evaluated and approved obesity drugs, doctors have been reluctant to prescribe drugs. The reasons for this may include memories of the adverse events with amphetamine and amphetamine-like drugs and the serious complications from combining phentermine and fenfluramine. The use of obesity drugs should follow the same principles as for any condition and be prescribed after assessment of the potential benefits and risks with appropriately informed patients, and with medical monitoring of the results of treatment. Many people, including doctors, still believe that a short course of drug treatment might 'cure' obesity or that efficacy is measured only by ever-continuing weight loss. These ideas are inconsistent with the known biology, as people who become obese have a lifelong tendency both to defend their excess weight and to continue to gain extra body fat. Effective management must be lifelong and focused on weight loss maintenance in a similar fashion to the effective treatment for hypertension or diabetes. Starting drug treatment should always be regarded as a therapeutic trial and stopped if weight loss is not apparent after 1 or 2 months.

The initiation of drug treatment will depend on the physician's judgement about the risks to an individual from continuing obesity. A drug should not be considered ineffective because weight loss has stopped, provided that the lowered weight is maintained. However, continuation of the drug should depend on the balance between the health benefits of maintained weight and the potential adverse effects of the drug.

Types of drug treatment for obesity

Drugs acting on the gastrointestinal system (pancreatic lipase inhibitors)

Orlistat inhibits pancreatic and gastric lipases decreasing the hydrolysis of ingested triglycerides. It produces a dose-dependent reduction in absorption of dietary fat that is near maximum at a dose of 120 mg, three times daily. It leads to 5 to 10% weight loss in 50 to 60% of patients, and in clinical trials, the loss (and related clinical benefit) is largely maintained up to at least 4 years. Adverse effects of orlistat are predominantly related to malabsorption of fat. These include loose or liquid stools, faecal urgency, and oily discharge; they can be associated with malabsorption of fat-soluble vitamins. As the consumption of a high-fat meal will inevitably lead to severe gastrointestinal symptoms, it is possible that some of the weight loss with orlistat treatment results from an 'antabuse effect', leading to behavioural change.

Centrally acting antiobesity drugs

Sibutramine Sibutramine inhibits the reuptake of noradrenaline and serotonin, promoting and prolonging satiety. It may also have an enhancing effect on thermogenesis through the stimulation of peripheral noradrenergic receptors. Sibutramine is well absorbed following oral ingestion and undergoes first-pass metabolism in the liver to produce two active metabolites that have long elimination half-lives. This enables sibutramine to be given on a single daily basis at a starting dose of 10 mg. Adverse effects include nausea, dry mouth, rhinitis, and constipation. It produces 5 to 10% weight loss in 60 to 70% of patients, and in clinical trials, it is well maintained for at least 2 years. If weight loss is less than 2 kg at 4 weeks, the dose can be increased from 10 mg to 15 mg. The noradrenergic action increases heart rate by 1 to 2 beats/min and attenuates the fall in blood pressure expected with weight loss. Some patients, especially if they fail to lose weight, may record a rise in their blood pressure; it is therefore essential to monitor blood pressure during the first 12 weeks of treatment. Controlled hypertension is not a contraindication for prescribing sibutramine. Recent concerns about increased cardiovascular morbidity associated with Sibutramine have led to prescribing restrictions, particularly relevant to those patients with established cardiovascular disease. Current guidelines in Europe and the USA vary and physicians should consult local guidelines where available.

Rimonabant Rimonabant is the first cannabinoid-1 receptor antagonist to be licensed for obesity treatment. Blockade of cannabinoid-1 receptors in the brain produces weight loss, which is maintained for up to 2 years in clinical trials. However, adverse effects on mood and an increased risk of depression and suicide risk have recently led to this drug being withdrawn in many countries.

New drugs in development

Clinical trials are now well advanced for several drugs with different modes of action. Many of the hormones and hormone receptors that contribute to regulation of appetite or satiety are targets for drug treatment and under active development in preclinical and early clinical trials. Newer agents primarily designed to treat diabetes, such as the synthetic amylin pramlintide and GLP-1 analogue exenatide, are licensed in some countries and lead to clinically important weight loss. There is also interest in gut-derived peptides such as oxyntomodulin to improve satiety.

Most obese people have high concentrations of leptin, and early trials of leptin supplementation in common obesity were disappointing. However, leptin may prove to be useful in combination with other drugs and as an adjunct to weight maintenance strategies.

Surgical treatment of obesity

Randomized controlled trials confirm that surgery for obesity is an option for carefully selected patients with severe obesity 0(BMI >40 kg/m^2 or BMI >35 kg/m^2 with comorbid conditions). The nature of the surgical procedures necessitates long-term hospital follow-up for such patients. The initial findings from the Swedish Obese Subjects study of severely obese subjects (those with a BMI >40) indicate that weight loss of approximately 30 kg over 2 years is associated with a 60% reduction in plasma insulin, a 25% decrease in plasma glucose and triglycerides, and a 10% reduction in blood pressure with associated effects on the risk of cardiovascular disease. Poor health-related quality of life was dramatically improved after gastric restriction surgery, while only minor fluctuations in health-related quality of life were observed in subjects treated by conventional dietary methods. Most surgical treatment is now carried out laparoscopically. Three approaches are widely used.

Laparoscopic gastric banding

This operation involves gastric restriction with the creation of a small compartment (<20 ml) by either a combination of vertical stapling and a constrictive band opening or a gastric band pinching off a small proximal pouch. A modification of the latter procedure is an inflatable gastric band attached to a subcutaneous reservoir which allows access by a hypodermic syringe to inject or withdraw fluid thereby tightening or enlarging the band width. This method mainly works by restricting how much food patients can eat. The average weight loss is around 15 to 20% of body weight, although some weight regain occurs over time. Morbidity and mortality are relatively low (mortality <0.2%), but patients do need to return for band adjustments.

Gastric bypass

This involves creating a small-volume gastric pouch and producing a Roux-en-Y diversion so that food bypasses the duodenum and upper jejunum. This works by both restricting food intake and causing a modest degree of malabsorption. Weight loss is generally greater than with the band. Operative mortality is less than 0.2% for laparoscopic procedures and 0.5% for open procedures.

Duodenal switch

A variant of the older biliopancreatic diversion, this involves a partial (sleeve gastrectomy) and bypass of a long loop of jejunum. Weight loss is greatest with this procedure, but malabsorption is more likely and patients need careful follow-up and attention to their diet, vitamin, and mineral supplementation.

Concluding remarks

As the prevalence of obesity is rising, we are seeing a greater proportion of patients with severe obesity. It is important to have a practical approach to the investigation and management of these vulnerable patients who have considerably increased morbidity and mortality. The clinical evaluation of severely obese patients will become increasingly sophisticated, and novel biochemical and molecular genetic diagnostics will need to be combined with the more traditional nutritional and behavioural approaches to optimize treatment for individual patients.

Further reading

Barsh GS, Farooqi IS, O'Rahilly S (2000). Genetics of body weight regulation: applications and opportunities. *Nature*, **404**, 644–51.

Goldstone, AP (2004). Prader-Willi syndrome: advances in genetics, pathophysiology and treatment. *Trends Endocrinol Metab*, **15**, 12–20.

Kopelman PG (2000). Obesity as a medical problem. *Nature*, **404**, 635–43.

Padwal RS, Majumdar SR (2007). Drug treatments for obesity: orlistat, sibutramine and rimonabant. *Lancet*, **369**, 71–7.

Schwartz MW *et al.* (2000). Central nervous system control of food intake. *Nature*, **404**, 661–71.

Wilding J (2007). Treatment strategies for obesity. *Obes Rev*, **8** Suppl 1, 137–44.

11.6

Artificial nutrition support

Jeremy Woodward

Essentials

The prevalence and importance of malnutrition in affluent societies is under-recognized, and nutritional status is a major predictor of outcome for most diseases.

Nutrition screening identifies patients at risk of malnutrition and should be performed in all clinical areas: this requires evaluation of events in the past (recent weight loss); present (current body mass index (BMI) and clinical signs of malnutrition); and future (current nutrient intake and foreseeable likely causes of reduced intake). A BMI of less than 18.5 kg/m^2, or weight loss of more than 10% over 3 to 6 months, or BMI of less than 20 kg/m^2 with weight loss of more than 5% over 3 to 6 months, is indicative of malnutrition.

Nutrition support is indicated for malnourished patients or those at risk of malnutrition in view of inadequate oral intake or malabsorption. Timing of intervention depends on the pre-existing nutritional status and the likelihood of restoring adequate intake. Nutrient requirements are calculated using weight-based formulae for basal energy and protein requirements, with additional factors for physical activity, severity of illness, or desired weight gain. Increased requirements due to disease are often counterbalanced by reduced activity.

Proper provision of appetizing food of appropriate quantity, texture, temperature, and variety in a conducive environment, with facilities for assistance and encouragement, can obviate the need for artificial nutrition support. Artificial nutrition support can be provided by oral (supplements), enteral, or parenteral routes, but enteral is preferable to parenteral feeding when possible—it maintains gut integrity, appropriately stimulates hormonal regulation of metabolism and gastrointestinal functions, and delivers nutrients to the liver via the portal circulation. Enteral feeding is also cheaper and safer than intravenous nutrition.

Both enteral and parenteral nutrition can be associated with significant complications relating to the means of access or the delivery of nutrients. Catabolic patients are unable to utilize excess protein or energy, and overfeeding results in an increased rate of complications. Oral nutrition support is associated with improved outcomes and significant reductions in mortality in selected patient groups. A multiprofessional team is essential to coordinate and monitor artificial nutrition in the hospital environment, and to provide support for patients fed long-term in the community, most of whom now die from their underlying disease, rather than complications of nutrition support.

Introduction

Undernutrition in societies where food is plentiful is predominantly disease-related and the extent of the problem is underestimated. More than 10% of adults over the age of 65 years in the community are affected, and this figure rises to around 40% of all hospital inpatients and elderly care-home residents. Surveys suggest little change to these proportions over the last 25 years in the United Kingdom. Malnutrition profoundly affects the outcome of all disease states and their treatment, by altering physiological responses and effects on immunity and healing as well as psychology and motivation. Although nutritional requirements are undoubtedly increased by chronic illness, associated anorexia or inability to feed orally contributes more significantly to the malnutrition and is directly amenable to intervention by nutrition support.

Nutritional screening and assessment of nutritional status

Weight loss is easier to prevent than to reverse, and early weight gain after illness or starvation comprises significant components of fluid and fat rather than muscle mass. Therefore, although assessment of a patient's immediate nutritional status is important, it is also crucial to determine the nutrition trajectory—the rate of weight loss and the likelihood of future weight loss due to increased requirements or inadequate intakes—in order to determine a nutrition 'risk score'. Such scores are routinely used to screen for malnutrition in all clinical settings and provide a valuable tool for the prioritization of intervention, for prevention as well as treatment (Fig. 11.6.1).

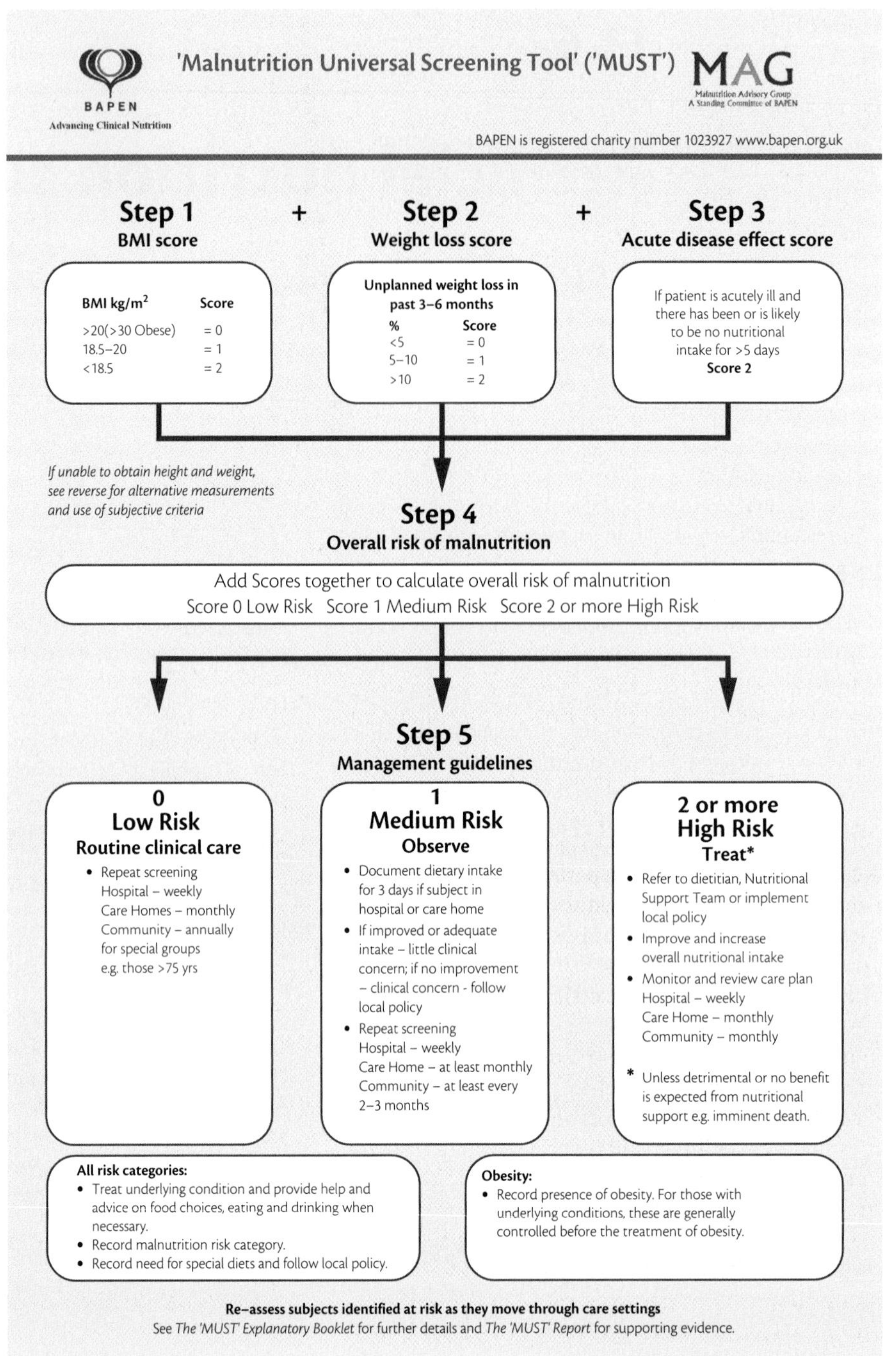

Fig. 11.6.1 The 'Malnutrition Universal Screening Tool' (MUST)—an example of an algorithm for the screening and identification of malnutrition and the appropriate actions to be taken based on risk score. (This tool is reproduced with the kind permission of BAPEN (British Association for Parenteral and Enteral Nutrition). http://www.bapen.org.uk/pdfs/must/must_full.pdf

A good nutrition history will include the nature of the baseline diet—not only for vegans or vegetarians (low in vitamin B_{12} and haem iron), but also for poor fresh fruit and vegetable intake (vitamin C, folic acid), and dairy avoidance (calcium) or other dietary restrictions due to intolerances or dislikes. Excessive alcohol intake can result in thiamine and folic acid deficiency. Oral conditions may make ingestion painful, and abdominal symptoms such as nausea, bloating, or pain can affect dietary intake, but changes in appetite might not be volunteered. Medications can affect nutrition by reducing appetite or inducing nausea. Intake can be significantly affected by psychosocial circumstances such as depression, bereavement, social isolation, impaired mobility, or poverty.

Patients may not be able to quantify weight loss, but this is often clear on clinical examination—e.g. prominent cheekbones, muscle wasting, redundant skin folds, and a concave abdomen. Ill-fitting clothing, belt notches, and loose finger rings provide clues in the clinic. Certain of these signs can be present with recent weight loss even in patients who remain obese. Signs suggestive of specific nutritional deficiencies can be apparent on examination (see Chapter 11.2), particularly of the hair, eyes, skin, nails, teeth, and tongue.

The ratio of weight (in kg) to the square of the height (in m^2) is known as the body mass index (BMI). This provides a useful indication of nutritional status, but is difficult to apply in some cases such as young adults with cerebral palsy or elderly patients with osteoporosis. A BMI of less than 18.5 kg/m^2 is considered indicative of malnutrition, as is weight loss of more than 10% in the preceding 3 to 6 months, or a BMI of less than 20 kg/m^2 in the setting of recent or ongoing weight loss (>5%). The use of centile charts in children is valuable, as sustained undernutrition results in reduced height velocity and failure to meet expected height. Weight-for-age charts will reflect the current nutritional status more accurately. Clinically important changes in lean body mass can be masked by shifts in fluid distribution and adipose tissue, reducing the value of weight measurements in assessing and monitoring nutritional status. Modern bio-impedance scales provide measurements of extracellular water and estimates of fat-free mass from which lean body mass can be calculated, but validation in disease settings is still required. A reasonable estimate of changes in lean mass can be derived from sequential measurements of the mid upper-arm circumference and the triceps skinfold thickness using a tape measure and calipers, respectively. Simple hand-grip dynamometry can similarly provide an objective sequential indication of functional muscle mass. However, wide reference ranges make single measurements of these anthropometric parameters unreliable for nutritional assessment.

Indications for artificial nutrition support

Malnutrition can often be prevented in patients at risk by simple measures to optimize appetite and reduce symptoms such as pain and nausea that can lead to anorexia. In institutions such as hospitals, the range of menus and the presentation and temperature of meals clearly affect the amount consumed. 'Nil by mouth' orders for investigations or procedures, or mealtimes disturbed by interventions, also reduce food intake. Hospital catering needs to accommodate the requirements of patients with altered feeding patterns—e.g. after upper gastrointestinal surgery or with gastrointestinal dysmotility—and older people often prefer to snack rather than take large meals. Patients with disabilities frequently require assistance with feeding, and sufficient staff and time dedicated to helping such patients can maintain nutrition. Altering the food texture may be required in some conditions—puréed or liquid diets benefit patients with oesophageal strictures or gastroparesis, whereas thickening fluids with starch reduces the risk of pulmonary aspiration in neurological causes of dysphagia.

If despite such measures, patients are unable to take sufficient oral food to meet requirements, then artificial nutrition support is required. If swallowing remains intact and palatability is acceptable, this can be in the form of liquid oral nutrition supplements. Unconscious patients, and those unable to swallow or with upper gastrointestinal obstruction, can receive enteral nutrition support if intestinal function is preserved. Access can be achieved by pernasal or transabdominal feeding tube to the stomach or intestine. Patients without adequate intestinal function require total or partial parenteral nutrition support via an intravenous catheter. Common indications for enteral and parenteral artificial nutrition support are given in Table 11.6.1.

The timing of nutrition support intervention depends on the pre-existing nutritional status of the patient. A young well-nourished patient undergoing gastrointestinal surgery may tolerate starvation for up to a week, but a malnourished patient will require nutrition support from the onset of being 'nil by mouth'.

Table 11.6.1 Common indications for enteral and parenteral artificial nutrition support

Enteral	Parenteral
Coma	Intestinal failure: inability of the gastrointestinal tract to absorb sufficient fluid and/or nutrients to maintain life
Ventilated, sedated patients in critical care setting	Anatomical short gut secondary to:
Neurological dysphagia	Trauma
Cerebrovascular disease	Infarction (superior mesenteric artery or vein thrombosis)
Motor neuron disease	Volvulus
Multiple sclerosis	Desmoid tumour
Bulbar palsy	Surgical resections for:
Cerebral palsy	Crohn's disease
Head and neck cancer	Vasculitis
Mucositis due to chemo/radiotherapy	Radiation enteritis
Obstructive lesions	Gastrochisis
Oesophagogastric malignancy	Necrotizing enterocolitis
Acute pancreatitis	Long segment Hirschprung's disease (children)
Dysmotility	Congenital malabsorption
Oesophageal dysmotility	Microvillous inclusion body disease
Gastroparesis	Protracted diarrhoea of infancy
Postsurgical	Autoimmune enteropathy
Oesophagectomy	Intestinal dysmotitily
Gastrectomy	Visceral neuropathy
Liver transplantation	Visceral myopathy
Pancreatectomy	Systemic sclerosis
Inability to meet requirements due to malabsorption, increased requirements or anorexia secondary to chronic illness: overnight feeding to maximize gastrointestinal tract use	Peritoneal disease
Cystic fibrosis	Sclerosing peritonitis due to peritoneal dialysis
Severe pulmonary or cardiac disease (particularly children)	Ovarian or metastatic lobular breast cancer undergoing chemotherapy
Borderline short gut	Postoperative/critical illness
	Prolonged ileus
	High-output enterocutaneous fistula
	Pancreatic fistula
	Chyle leak

Estimating nutrition requirements

Energy

Energy expenditure under basal conditions reflects physiological cellular metabolic functions and hence correlates with body mass. Derivative equations based on weight alone provide estimates of energy consumption that adequately match measurements based on oxygen uptake and CO_2 production (indirect calorimetry) for most clinical purposes. To this basal rate, additions are required for activity and the thermal effect of food. Energy expenditure is increased by disease states such as burns, sepsis, or trauma—however, it is easy to overestimate such contributions, which are often negated by reduced physical activity in illness and may amount to only 10 to 20% of resting energy expenditure. Difficulties arise in estimating the requirements for patients with oedema or obesity based on weight alone, and adjustments based on ideal body weight or a proportion of current weight can be used. Most hospital patients' requirements lie within the range of 25 to 40 kcal/kg per day (105–168 kJ/kg per day).

Fluid

Fluid balance must be factored into estimating nutrition requirements. Most hospitalized adults require 30 to 35 ml/kg per day with additions for replacement. Losses can be high from the kidneys due to diabetes insipidus or recovering from acute tubular necrosis, and can exceed 8 litres a day from the gastrointestinal tract via a proximal jejunostomy or enterocutaneous fistula (Table 11.6.2). Fluid restriction is indicated in overloaded states or in renal or cardiac failure, and diluents for intravenous drugs and line flushes can reduce the fluid allowance available for the feed in ill patients. Most enteral feeds provide 1 kcal/ml but specialized feeds with up to 2 kcal/ml are available for such circumstances.

Electrolytes

Average requirements for sodium and potassium are of the order of 1 mmol/kg per day for most adults. However, significant sodium losses can occur through the gastrointestinal tract and require replacement. Potassium deficits may be large in patients receiving thiazide diuretics, with secretory diarrhoea, during recovery of metabolic acidosis, and during refeeding of malnourished patients. Similarly, phosphate requirements increase greatly during refeeding from a baseline of approximately 0.3 mmol/kg per day. Feeds with minimal electrolyte content are required in renal impairment where solute clearance is reduced. However, the commonest cause of excessive electrolyte administration in hospitals is the use of normal saline and salt-rich colloid solutions for maintenance fluid requirements.

Table 11.6.2 Electrolyte composition of gastrointestinal fluids (in order to calculate replacement of losses)

Fluid	Na^+ (mmol/litre)	K^+ (mmol/litre)	HCO_3^- (mmol/litre)	Cl^- (mmol/litre)	Approximate volume secreted in 24 h (ml)
Gastric juice	60	15	–	90	2500
Pancreatic juice	140	5	90	75	1500
Bile	140	5	35	100	500
Small intestinal contents	100	10	25	100	1000 (succus entericus)
Diarrhoea	60	30	45	45	

Macronutrients

Protein

Protein is required to meet obligatory catabolic losses (minimal requirement) and to stimulate protein synthesis (optimal requirement). The World Health Organization (WHO) recommendation of minimal requirement is 0.75 g protein/kg per day (0.12 g N/kg per day) based on nitrogen balance studies on a protein-free diet (see Fig. 11.6.2). Increasing the dietary protein intake will increase protein synthesis in depleted patients as long as sufficient calories are taken, and the optimal calorie:nitrogen ratio may vary on the disease state. Although net protein synthesis can be achieved by increasing dietary protein in malnourished patients, the same is not true in the catabolic state induced by sepsis, burns, or trauma where excess amino acids can exert detrimental effects. Intakes of above 1.5 g protein/kg per day (>0.24 g N/kg per day) are not generally recommended. Amino acids have physiological roles beyond protein synthesis, and individual amino acid levels vary significantly between different disease states. Most artificial feeds provide standard amino acid solutions that do not cater for such differences and may result in relative imbalances of amino acids that could compromise nitrogen utilization. Histidine levels are low in renal impairment, and branched chain amino acids (valine, leucine, isoleucine) are reduced in chronic liver disease. Glutamine is

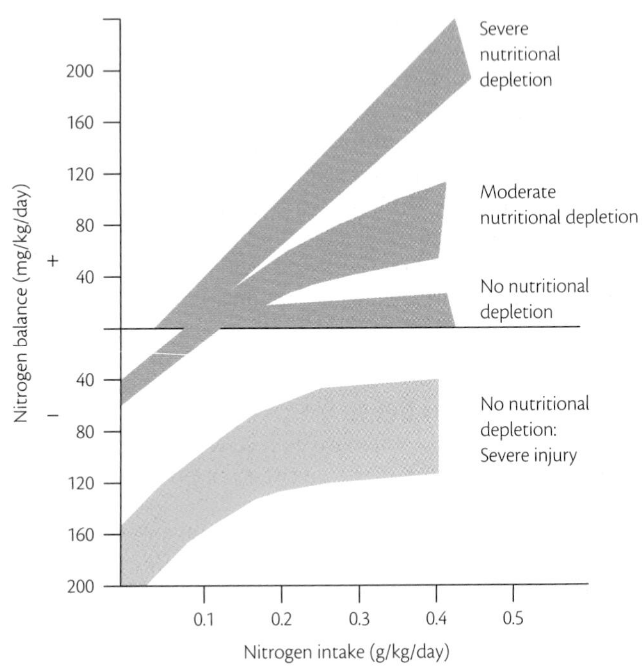

Fig. 11.6.2 Relationship of nitrogen intake and nitrogen balance in patients receiving sufficient energy. Normal subjects reach nitrogen balance at approximately 0.1 g/kg per day nitrogen intake; positive nitrogen balance can be achieved in malnourished patients. Severe illness (trauma, sepsis, burns) results in net catabolism. Patients with a combination of depletion and severe illness react in an intermediate fashion.

(Reprinted from Clinical Nutrition, Vol 1, Elia M, 'The effects of nitrogen and energy intake on the metabolism of normal, depleted and injured man. Considerations for practical nutrition support', pp. 173–192, 1982, with permission from Elsevier.)

significantly depleted in critical illness, and improvement in nitrogen balance has been demonstrated with supplementation.

Carbohydrate

Carbohydrates should make up 50 to 65% of calories in a healthy diet. In excess of 5 g/kg per day, glucose is stored as glycogen up to a maximum storage capacity of about 15 g/kg. Continued administration of glucose results in lipid synthesis. In disease states, however, maximal glucose oxidation rates are frequently lower due to insulin resistance, and excessive glucose administration results in hyperglycaemia.

Lipid

The lower limit constraint on lipid provision is the need for essential fatty acids (linoleic and α-linoleic acids), which can be provided in 3 to 4.5% of the total energy requirements as fat. Lipid is used in artificial nutrition to provide the energy that cannot be supplied as carbohydrate due to the limit of glucose oxidation. The amount of CO_2 produced by oxidation of lipid is 30% less than that of glucose, and could theoretically help patients with respiratory failure or weaning from a ventilator; however, clinical benefits are small in practice.

Micronutrients

Vitamins

Vitamin requirements differ between health and disease, and patients may have pre-existing deficiencies, particularly of the water-soluble vitamins for which there are no body stores. As deficiencies can have profound effects on cellular metabolism and few vitamins are toxic in excess, levels of vitamins in commercial feed preparations are often above estimated requirements. This also helps to compensate for the degradation that occurs in solution—vitamin A and riboflavin are photosensitive (hence parenteral nutrition at the bedside is light-protected), thiamine reacts with preservatives required to maintain shelf life, and vitamin C and vitamin E are ineffective when oxidized. The latter is used in parenteral nutrition solutions in excess to prevent lipid peroxidation. Vitamin K is normally not required in artificial nutrition, due to enteric bacterial synthesis, and its addition could affect therapeutic anticoagulation. Other fat-soluble vitamins—vitamin A, vitamin D, and vitamin E—can be provided in a water-miscible solution in parenteral nutrition.

Minerals and trace elements

In contrast to vitamins, toxicity is associated with excessive delivery of some trace elements. The enterocyte regulates iron uptake, and relatively small amounts of trace elements are absorbed from the intestine. Overadministration is therefore easier in parenteral than enteral nutrition delivery. Manganese and copper undergo biliary excretion, and accumulation can occur in parenterally fed patients with cholestasis—basal ganglia deposition can be detected on brain MRI scanning, but neurological effects are rarely reported. Chromium is excreted in the urine and can accumulate in renal failure. Zinc is lost through the intestine in high output states and in wound exudates; additional replacement may be required. Selenium as a cofactor in glutathione peroxidase plays a key role in cellular redox maintenance, and some authorities recommend supplementation in critical illness. Unfortunately, trace elements are difficult to measure accurately, levels are affected by acute-phase response, and serum albumin concentration and interpretation of low levels is complicated by the possibility that it reflects a physiological response to acute illness, as in the case of iron sequestration.

Complications of artificial nutrition support

The ease with which full nutritional requirements can be delivered by artificial means results in a risk of 'refeeding syndrome' on initiating feeding in chronically malnourished patients. Features include electrolyte imbalance (hypokalaemia, hypophosphataemia, hypomagnesaemia) and an associated risk of cardiac arrhythmia and sudden death, hyperglycaemia, and fluid shifts that can precipitate heart failure. Rapid depletion of available thiamine, an essential cofactor of pyruvate decarboxylase, results in inhibition of glycolysis on refeeding and damage to glucose dependent cells such as neurons—the clinical presentation of Wernicke–Korsakoff syndrome. This is preventable by the administration of high-dose intravenous thiamine prior to refeeding (or glucose administration) in patients considered at risk. Other complications of artificial nutrition support are specific to the route of delivery. Access devices in common use, with their advantages and disadvantages, are listed in Table 11.6.3.

Enteral

Complications of access

Nasogastric tubes

Incorrectly placed nasogastric tubes can result in fatality. Inadvertent pulmonary placement is the most common, but insertion into cranial, pleural, and peritoneal cavities has occurred. Feeding should only be initiated after confirmation of gastric placement by pH measurement of aspirated stomach contents, or radiography. Interruptions due to frequent tube displacement cause a significant reduction in feed delivery—as little as 55% of prescribed feed in one study. This can be prevented by the use of a loop of tape that can be safely and simply passed around the nasal septum to secure the tube. Modern tube materials do not cause significant erosion or irritation of the face, nares, or mucosal surfaces, even with long-term use. However, the difficulty of managing these tubes in the community makes them undesirable for long-term use.

Gastrostomy tubes are used for the majority of enterally fed patients in the community. Percutaneous endoscopically guided gastrostomy (PEG) and radiologically inserted gastrostomy (RIG) are now the commonest techniques used for placement (Fig. 11.6.3). A high fatality rate early after PEG insertion may be due to cardiorespiratory complications in patients sedated for endoscopy who are already at risk of pulmonary aspiration. Asymptomatic pneumoperitoneum is common after PEG insertion, but feed leakage into the peritoneal cavity can result in a chemical peritonitis. Superficial infections at the PEG site are commonly due to methicillin-resistant *Staphylococcus aureus* (MRSA) and are usually easily treated. Growth of gastric mucosa over the internal bolster of the device (the 'buried bumper') can result in blockage, external feed leakage, and infection, but may only be detected at the time of attempted PEG removal.

Complications of feeding

The role of the intestine in regulating nutrient uptake is demonstrated by the reduced metabolic complications of enteral compared to parenteral feeding, and nutritional deficiencies in patients fed appropriately with commercial preparations are highly unusual.

Patients who require enteral feeding often have impaired conscious level or swallowing and are therefore at risk of pulmonary aspiration.

Table 11.6.3 Types of enteral and parenteral access devices in common use

Type of tube	Description	Use	Advantages	Disadvantages
Enteral (EN)				
Nasogastric	Fine bore (6–8F) polyurethane tube; can be secured with a 'nasal bridle' (loop of tape around the nasal septum)	Short- to medium-term intragastric feeding due to inability to swallow; nutritional supplementation: bolus or drip feed	Bedside placement without sedation; well tolerated	Risk of malposition; easily displaced; difficult to manage in community
Nasojejunal	Fine-bore polyurethane tube with tip passed into distal duodenum/proximal jejunum	Inability to swallow complicated by gastro-oesophageal reflux or gastroparesis; gastric outlet obstruction; acute severe pancreatitis	Can be placed noninvasively at bedside; accurate delivery into proximal intestine; drip feed only.	May require endoscopic or fluoroscopic placement; easily displaced;
PEG (percutaneous endoscopically placed gastrostomy)	Tube passed into stomach through abdominal wall using endoscopic technique, retained by internal bumper or balloon; available in lumen sizes up to 24F	Long term intragastric feeding; mucositis due to head and neck cancer therapy; palliative venting use in terminal intestinal obstruction	Difficult to displace; reliable in long term use; can be exchanged for skin-level ('button') device, ideal for younger or ambulant patients	Requires endoscopy for placement; local complications (infection/leakage/granulation tissue) balloon - retained tubes require regular replacement (3–6 monthly); endoscopy is required to change bumper retained PEGs: every 2–3 years
RIG (radiologically placed gastrostomy)	Radiologically placed trans-abdominal gastrostomy tube	Intragastric feeding where endoscopic placement is not possible due to risks of endoscopy or anatomical considerations	Safer than PEG in high-risk patients	Require gastric insufflation via nasogastric tube; some centres report higher rates of local complications than with PEG
PEG-J (PEG with jejunal extension)	Transgastric tube positioned with tip in distal duodenum/proximal jejunum through existing gastostomy	Long-term intestinal feeding where gastric feeding is not available due to gastric dysfunction or outlet obstruction	Minimally invasive route for long-term postpyloric feeding	Jejunal tube can be easily refluxed back into stomach; inner jejunal tube can be displaced from PEG tube
DPEJ (direct percutaneous enteroscopic jejunostomy tube)	PEG tube placed directly into the proximal small intestine rather than stomach	Long-term intestinal feeding	Reliable intrajejunal feeding	May require prolonged endoscopic procedure under deep sedation or general anaesthetic High risk of complications including intestinal volvulus and intractable pain
Surgical jejunostomy	Feeding tube placed surgically into the jejunum and retained by external sutures	Postoperative feeding in upper gastrointestinal surgery and liver transplantation	Permits early enteral feeding in postoperative setting	Not designed for long term use; can be displaced; can result in adhesional intestinal obstruction
Parenteral (PN)				
Midline catheter	Short peripheral (22G) cannula placed into antecubital vein	Short-term parenteral nutrition support	May allow effective parenteral nutrition support or supplementation without risks and delays of central venous access	Limited range of available feeds due to osmolality and pH considerations; thrombosis or thrombophlebitis usually limits use to 7–14 days
PICC (peripherally inserted central venous catheter)	'Long-line': tube placed via the cephalic vein into large central veins	Short- to medium-term parenteral nutrition support (suitable for majority of inpatient PN episodes)	Reduced risk of infection;preserves central venous access points	Thrombophlebitis and thrombosis (avoided with low-dose anticoagulation); not practical for long-term use in ambulant patients or for patients to manage at home
Triple lumen venous catheter	Multilumen direct-puncture central venous access tube	Fluid and drug delivery; central venous pressure monitoring (severely ill patients)	Ease of access in critically ill patients with pre-existing central access	High risk of infection and local complications; In view of this, usage for PN should be discouraged except via a dedicated lumen for limited periods of time
Tunnelled Hickman catheter	Single or double lumen line tunnelled subcutaneously to the skin surface with a Dacron cuff for retention	Medium–long-term parenteral nutrition support	Low risk of infection if properly maintained; low risk of displacement once cuff is 'enmeshed'	Care needs to be taken with the external tube to prevent damage and maintain asepsis, and with the exit site to prevent infection
Implantable subcutaneous port device	Line accessed via a hub placed in a subcutaneous pocket	Long-term parenteral nutrition	Invisible from exterior with no external parts: ideal for active patients requiring long-term parenteral access	Skin puncture required for access: not ideal for frequent/daily use; more difficult than a tunnelled line to reposition; risk of blockage with lipid-containing feeds

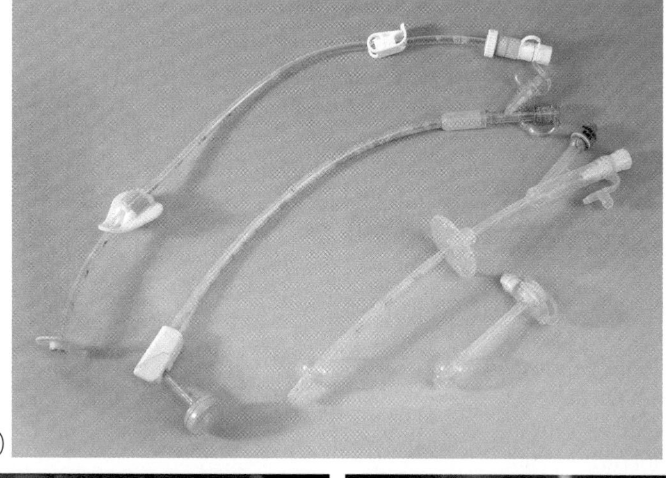

(a)

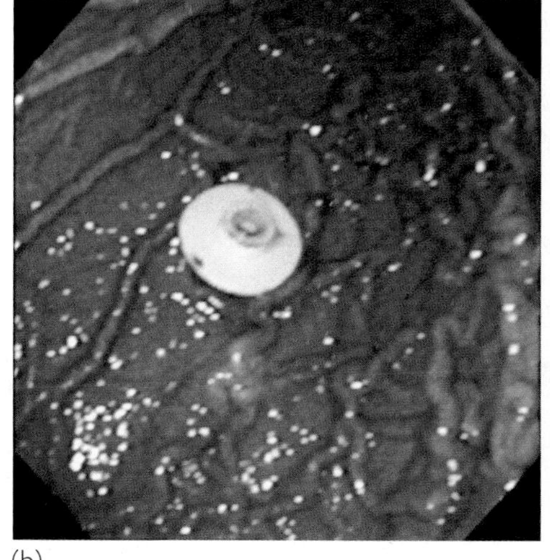

(b)

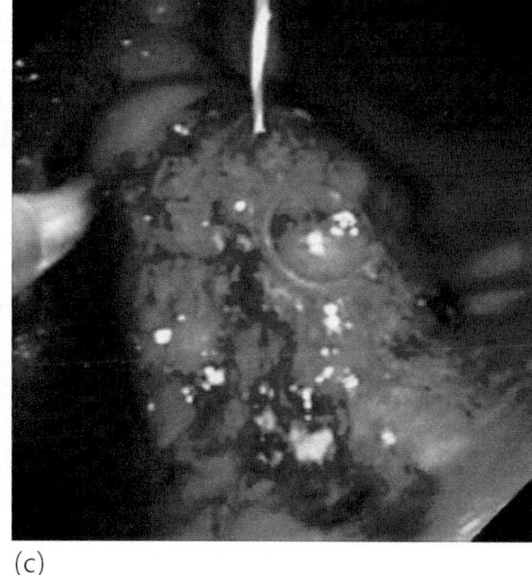

(c)

Fig. 11.6.3 (a) A range of endoscopically placed gastrostomy tubes—from left to right—bumper-retained gastrostomy; traction-removable bumper-retained gastrostomy; balloon-retained gastrostomy; and skin-level 'PEG-button' device (balloon retained). (b) Endoscopic photograph of PEG tube with bumper in place in the stomach. (c) 'Buried bumper'—the bumper of the gastrostomy has eroded into the gastric mucosa as a result of pressure necrosis and the mucosa has overgrown the bumper. A wire has been passed through the lumen of the tube.

Delayed gastric emptying—as frequently occurs in the critically ill—increases the likelihood of aspiration of stomach contents and pneumonia, but this can occur due to gastro-oesophageal reflux even with normal gastric emptying. Reflux may be exacerbated, rather than reduced, by PEG feeding compared to nasogastric delivery. Patients should be fed continuously by infusion pump rather than feed bolus and at a 30° tilt to reduce this risk. Those with high gastric aspirate volumes and no evidence of intestinal ileus or obstruction should be fed by a tube passed beyond the pylorus.

Diarrhoea is common in enterally fed hospital patients, and is often due to the concomitant use of antibiotics. Liquid feed empties rapidly from the stomach compared to solids and can result in an osmolar load that precipitates fluid influx and intestinal hurry, and neuroendocrine mechanisms have been described that result in right colonic fluid secretion with intragastric feeding.

Constipation is a more frequent accompaniment of enteral feeding in the community and is helped by the use of fibre-containing feeds, but may require osmotic laxatives.

Parenteral

Complications of access

Intravenous delivery via peripheral cannulae is limited by the propensity for thrombosis and thrombophlebitis and available preparations are constrained by pH and osmolality requirements. Central venous access is required for longer-term parenteral nutrition with attendant risks of pneumothorax and haemothorax that can be reduced but not eliminated by insertion under ultrasound guidance. Peripherally inserted central lines are convenient for parenteral nutrition in hospital. Infection is the major hazard of intravenous feeding catheters in hospital patients and is reduced by strict asepsis and using a single dedicated line or lumen for feed. Patients predicted to require more than a few days of intravenous feeding should have a peripherally inserted central line or a subcutaneous tunnelled line placed. Staphylococci (coagulase negative and positive strains), Gram-negative bacilli, and candida are common infecting organisms. Infection can present insidiously with low-grade fever, and be complicated by dissemination resulting in bacterial endocarditis, discitis, osteomyelitis, or fungal endophthalmitis.

With longer-term parenteral feeding in the community, catheter-related infections average one every 2 years. Venous thrombosis can occur despite anticoagulation and may limit available venous access for feeding. Creative solutions such as transhepatic caval cannulae or intracardiac lines may be required.

Complications of feeding

Metabolic complications are more likely to occur with parenteral than enteral feeding for a number of reasons:

- Parenteral feeding bypasses the enterocyte, which actively regulates uptake, metabolizes nutrients, and re-exports them via the portal circulation to the liver.

- Insulin and glucagon secretion and other enteroendocrine hormones are controlled by the presence or absence of nutrients in the gut.
- Parenteral feeds cannot replicate the complexity of circulating nutrient molecules, being constrained by requirements of chemical stability.

The metabolic risks of parenteral nutrition have previously been overestimated as a result of 'hyperalimentation', reflecting the ease of nutrient delivery by this route. Hyperglycaemia is especially common, due to insulin resistance associated with critical illness, and results in increased risk of infection and adverse outcomes if not treated with exogenous insulin. Imbalances of other nutrients may occur as a result of variable losses associated with the underlying condition and require regular monitoring and replacement.

The gut derives a proportion of its nutrient requirements from the lumen rather than the bloodstream, therefore parenteral nutrition may result in intestinal mucosal atrophy and impaired barrier function. Physiological and anatomical changes have been described, but sepsis due to bacterial translocation appears to be rare from this cause in humans.

Intestinal failure-associated liver disease (IFALD)

Patients requiring parenteral nutrition are at risk of liver complications. Asymptomatic elevation of liver enzymes is common, but can progress rapidly to cholestasis and cirrhosis in children. Cholestasis also occurs in adults but liver disease normally progresses more insidiously through steatohepatitis to cirrhosis. The underlying disease is responsible for reduced portal inflow in patients with short bowel, and lack of enteral stimulation of cholecystokinin production results in impaired choleresis, gallbladder stasis, and calculi formation. A number of factors associated with the feed—in both excess and deficiency—have been implicated in the aetiology of IFALD (Table 11.6.4). Maintaining oral intake, cyclical rather than continuous feeding, and keeping average exogenous lipid delivery under 1 g/kg per day appears to reduce the risk of advanced liver disease in adults during long-term feeding.

Intestinal failure-associated bone disease

Metabolic osteopenia is common in intestinal failure requiring long-term parenteral nutrition. Prolonged bed rest and immobilization, and vitamin D malabsorption and intestinal loss contribute prior to initiation of parenteral nutrition; however, a low bone turnover state is reported, resembling osteoporosis. Maintenance treatment with intravenous bisphosphonates and in the most severe cases, teriparatide is indicated.

Table 11.6.4 Aetiological factors implicated in intestinal failure-associated liver disease (IFALD)

Cholestasis	Steatosis
Reduced enteral stimulation	Excess provision of calories as carbohydrate or lipid
Phytosterols present in soy-based formulae	Choline deficiency
Infection	Carnitine deficiency
Bacterial translocation	Reduced VLDL synthesis
Taurine deficiency	Inadequate glucagon secretion
Methionine toxicity	

Long-term artificial nutrition support

Patients can receive oral, enteral, or parenteral nutrition support in the community. In the United Kingdom, the British Artificial Nutrition Survey (BANS) carries out an annual survey of the number of tube-fed patients. Approximately 25 000 British adults receive enteral feeding in the community, but only about 600 are fed parenterally (2005 data). Quality of life is often significantly impaired by the underlying disease rather than the nature of the maintenance therapy, and infusing feed overnight helps to minimize disruption to lifestyle. Life expectancy is similarly dictated by the underlying disease with few deaths being attributable to complications of feeding. Recent surveys suggest 10-year survival rates on parenteral feed of 71% in adults, 81% in children. Patients receiving enteral feed at home are generally older and more infirm than parenterally fed patients, with a 5-year survival rate as low as 25%.

Intestinal transplantation

Patients with irreversible intestinal failure who experience life-threatening complications of parenteral nutrition—recurrent catheter-associated infections, IFALD, or loss of venous access through thrombosis—can be considered for intestinal transplantation, which can include other organs such as liver, stomach, pancreas, and kidney ('multivisceral' transplantation). Recent advances in immunosuppression using anti-CD25 or antilymphocyte induction therapy followed by tacrolimus-based protocols have resulted in 5-year survival rates of over 50% and independence from parenteral nutrition in the majority of successful cases (Fig. 11.6.4).

Ethics of artificial nutrition support

Nutrition and starvation are understandably emotive topics. Although it is a basic human right not to be deprived of food and fluid, the same is not true of artificial nutrition support, which involves the invasive placement of tubes for feeding that are associated with risk of morbidity and mortality in their own right. Ethically and legally, withdrawing and withholding nutrition are considered equivalent in view of the ultimate outcome. However, in practice, cessation of feeding through an established feeding tube is rarely practicable, and the natural history of a condition can be significantly altered by nutrition support. This may prolong the process of dying or maintain an intolerable quality of life. The placement of tubes such as PEGs to facilitate nutrition support must be carefully considered in all cases, preferably by a multidisciplinary approach involving clinicians, nutrition nurse specialists, dietitians, speech and language specialists, and carers and relatives or appointed surrogate, taking into the account the patient's wishes or advance directives when stated. The United Kingdom General Medical Council's advice for clinicians on withholding or withdrawing nutrition support has been tested in court.

Special situations in nutrition support

Critical illness—burns, trauma, and sepsis

The metabolic response to stress is characterized by hypermetabolism and rapid tissue catabolism with resulting insulin resistance and hyperglycaemia. Direct effects of inflammatory mediators and cytokines such as tumour necrosis factor α(TNFα) and interleukins IL-1 and IL-6 are responsible. Protein loss can be rapid, particularly in the case of burns, where exudates add to catabolic loss.

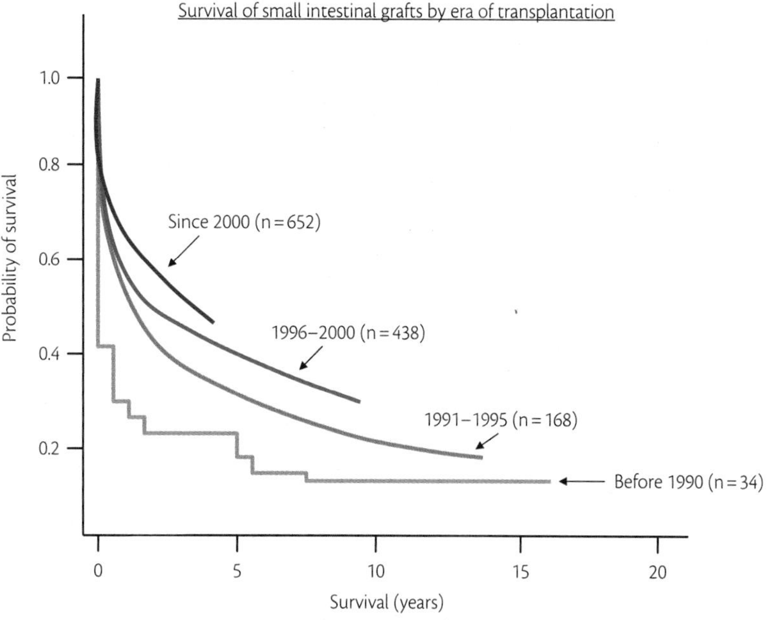

Fig. 11.6.4 Graft survival following intestinal transplantation, showing improvements in outcomes with successive advances in technique. (Data supplied by the International Intestinal Transplant Registry, 2005, with kind permission of Dr David Grant.)

Feeding during acute metabolic decompensation can be detrimental and should be withheld for 24 h; otherwise, early initiation of feeding is likely to be beneficial in the majority of settings. Gastric stasis occurs for 2 to 4 days in severe burns, but longer with head injury, and intestinal ileus is also common in circulatory failure requiring inotropic support. The use of prokinetics such as metoclopramide may maintain gastric emptying in mild cases, but where gastric aspirate volumes remain high or increase during intragastric feeding, postpyloric or parenteral feeding avoids the risks of pulmonary aspiration and ensures nutrient delivery. Adverse outcomes are associated with overfeeding in the acute stages, despite control of hyperglycaemia with insulin infusion, but requirements can be increased for weight gain during recovery—appropriate recognition of the transition from catabolic to anabolic phases remains a challenge. Unfortunately, attempts at reversing catabolism by the use of inflammatory cytokine inhibitors, or anabolic agents such as growth hormone have been unsuccessful. However, nutrients themselves can modulate inflammatory and immune functions. For instance, the use of feeds enriched with n − 3 fatty acids can reduce the production of pro-inflammatory eicosanoids by competing with arachidonic acid, and early studies have demonstrated encouraging benefits in septic and surgical patients.

Renal disease

Renal failure results in wasting, electrolyte and fluid imbalances, and anorexia with resultant malnutrition. Patients undergoing dialysis lose protein into the dialysate—up to 10 g/day on haemodialysis and up to 15 g/day on peritoneal dialysis. Water-soluble vitamins—folic acid, pyridoxine, and vitamin C—are lost in dialysis and require supplementary replacement. Adequate energy intake is essential to minimize catabolism of endogenous protein, and appropriate protein sources are required to replace losses. Specialized artificial feeds are available to meet these requirements with minimal electrolytes and in reduced fluid volumes for renal patients. Parenteral nutrients are often given at the time of dialysis to replenish some of the losses. The use of a reduced (but high-quality) protein diet in predialysis chronic renal failure may delay the requirement for dialysis but this should not be at the cost of inadequate nutrition.

Liver disease

Malnutrition is common in patients with established liver disease due to reduced appetite, altered carbohydrate and lipid metabolism, and in severe cases, impaired urea synthesis from ammonia leading to increased muscle catabolism. In addition, cholestasis results in fat malabsorption. Glucose intolerance may limit glucose intake, and complex polysaccharides may provide the regular supply of glucose required as a result of diminished glycogen stores. Both oral and enteral nutrition support have been shown to improve outcomes in cirrhosis and in alcoholic hepatitis. High-protein feeds may precipitate encephalopathy in cirrhotic patients, but restricting protein is nutritionally undesirable, and an intake of 1.2 to 1.5 g protein/kg per day is recommended. An alternative to restricting protein intake is to optimize the amino acid composition of the feed, as patients with severe cirrhosis have a relative deficiency of branched chain amino acids. Specially enriched formulae exist and are indicated for patients developing encephalopathy while receiving enteral nutrition.

Gastrointestinal disease

Nutrition support is required in a variety of gastrointestinal conditions where access to the gut is impaired as a result of proximal gastrointestinal obstruction or dysmotility, or intestinal failure due to short-bowel syndrome or malabsorption (see Chapter 15.10). Liquid, oral, or enteral feeds can be used to induce remission in active Crohn's disease with a slightly lower efficacy than oral steroids—the mechanism of action may relate to altered bacterial flora rather than improvement of nutritional status.

Patients with enterocutaneous fistulae are often malnourished due to sepsis and increased losses (see Table 11.6.2). A high fistula output in the absence of distal obstruction usually indicates a proximal fistula, and parenteral nutrition may be required to provide sufficient nutritional intake and reduce effluent that may compromise wound healing or complicate stoma management.

Table 11.6.5 Examples of disease-specific and therapeutic feeds designed to have disease-modifying activity ('nutraceuticals')

Feed composition	Intended use	Rationale
Low protein, high in essential amino acids and histidine, low electrolytes, high calorie density (2 kcal/ml)	Renal impairment	Appropriate matching of amino acid composition to requirements may improve protein metabolism; low protein reduces urea synthesis; high calorie density allows lower volumes
Low protein, reduced aromatic and increased branched chain amino acids, low sodium	Hepatic impairment	Reduced risk of encephalopathy with low protein: appropriate amino acid mix to allow optimal protein metabolism
High lipid, low carbohydrate	Pulmonary disease, weaning from artificial ventilation	Reduced CO_2 production
High lipid (especially monounsaturated fatty acids), low carbohydrate, high fructose	Diabetes	Reduced glycaemia, improved diabetic control
Oligopeptides, medium chain triglycerides	Severe pancreatic exocrine deficiency	Reduced dependence on luminal digestion for absorption
Arginine, n−3 fatty acids, nucleotides	'Immune enhancing': critical illness/ perioperative nutrition	Substrates for rapidly dividing cells such as lymphocytes and competitive inhibition of pro-inflammatory eicosanoid production may enhance immune response and reduce inflammatory response
Glutamine	Critical illness	Glutamine levels severely depleted in critical illness: supplementation may improve nitrogen balance, and act as a fuel to rapidly dividing cells such as lymphocytes and enterocytes: maintaining immune responses and gut mucosal integrity

However, in patients who are able to maintain their requirements through enteral intake with a manageable fistula output, there is no evidence that parenteral nutrition and 'bowel rest' results in higher fistula closure rates.

In severe acute pancreatitis, nutrition requirements are increased by the systemic inflammatory response, and there are theoretical concerns of stimulation of pancreatic secretion by enteral feeding. In practice, enteral feed tolerance is limited by gastric stasis that occurs in severe cases, and intrajejunal enteral feeding is often required and preferred to parenteral feeding, which is associated with higher complication rates.

Perioperative nutrition

Malnourished patients undergoing surgery experience up to three times as many complications and a fourfold increase in mortality rate compared to well-nourished individuals. Patients may be at risk of malnutrition as a result of prolonged starvation due to obstruction or postoperative ileus. Surgery should be delayed where feasible in severely malnourished patients, in order to provide a minimum of 10 to 14 days of adequate preoperative nutrition. Recent findings have challenged traditional surgical dogma with regard to perioperative nutrition. Starvation immediately before surgery results in increased insulin resistance and increased complications postoperatively. The simple expedient of providing a 50 g oral carbohydrate load 2 h before surgery can speed postoperative recovery. Similarly, early reintroduction of feeding after routine abdominal surgery is feasible and results in more rapid rehabilitation than waiting for (unreliable) clinical signs of gastrointestinal function.

The hospital nutrition support team

A multiprofessional team comprising clinician, specialist nurse, dietitian, and pharmacist as its core members is required to provide the full range of nutrition support services. By appropriate use of nutrition support, reducing catheter-related complications, and monitoring patients receiving parenteral nutrition, such teams have also been shown to provide significant cost savings.

Cost-effectiveness of nutrition support

The estimated additional annual cost of treating patients with moderate and high risk of malnutrition compared to those with low risk is approximately £5 billion in the United Kingdom (2005 figures)—around 6% of the entire health care budget. Oral nutrition support has been shown to reduce mortality by upto 24% compared to unsupplemented patients in certain hospital and community settings. In addition, the reduced complications (odds ratio 0.29—confidence intervals 0.18–0.47) and lengths of hospital inpatient stay result in significant cost savings with oral nutrition support. Perhaps unsurprisingly (given that comparator groups are likely to be significantly undernourished), studies have demonstrated even greater outcome benefits with the use of enteral nutrition support where indicated.

Future developments

Most importantly, an increased awareness of the critical importance of nutrition in clinical care is likely to improve the recognition of malnutrition and lead to the institution of appropriate preventive measures—with significant benefits in all areas of clinical medicine.

Few innovative nutritional interventions (including novel nutrient substrates that modulate disease processes and disease-specific feeds—Table 11.6.5) are yet in routine clinical use despite considerable theoretical promise, due to the lack of adequately powered trials. Much potential still remains to be unlocked in the field of therapeutic nutrition.

Further reading

Beath SV, Woodward JM (2007). Intestinal failure associated liver disease. In Langnas A (ed.) *Intestinal failure, diagnosis, management and transplantation*. Blackwell, Oxford.

Bozzetti F *et al.* (2002). Central venous catheter complications in 447 patients on home parenteral nutrition: an analysis of over 100,000 catheter days. *Clin Nutr*, **21**, 475–85.

Campbell SE, Avenell A, Walker AE (2002). Assessment of nutritional status in hospital in-patients. *Q J Med*, **95**, 83–7.

Elia M (1982). The effects of nitrogen and energy intake on the metabolism of normal, depleted and injured man. Considerations for practical nutrition support. *Clin Nutr*, **1**, 173–92.

Elia M (2003). *The 'MUST' report: nutritional screening of adults: a multidisciplinary responsibility. Development and use of the Malnutrition Universal Screening Tool (MUST) for adults.* A report by the Malnutrition Advisory Group of the British Association for Parenteral and Enteral Nutrition. BAPEN, Redditch.

Elia M *et al.* (2005). *The cost of disease*-related *malnutrition in the UK and economic considerations for the use of oral nutritional supplements (ONS) in adults.* BAPEN, Redditch.

ESPEN (2006). Guidelines on adult enteral nutrition. *Clin Nutr*, **25**, 177–360.

Frankenfield D, Roth-Yousey L, Compher C (2005). Comparison of predictive equations for resting metabolic rate in healthy nonobese and obese adults: a systematic review. *J Am Diet Assoc*, **105**, 775–89.

General Medical Council. (2002). *Withholding and withdrawing life-prolonging treatments: good practice in decision-making.* General Medical Council, London.

Heyland DK (2000). Parenteral nutrition in the critically ill patient: more harm than good? *Proc Nutr Soc*, **59**, 457–66.

Intestinal Transplant Registry. http://www.intestinaltransplant.org

Jones B *et al.* (2006). *Artificial nutrition support in the UK 2005. A report by the British Artificial Nutrition Survey (BANS).* http://www.bapen.org.uk/res_bans_arch.html

Lewis SJ *et al.* (2001). Early enteral feeding versus 'nil by mouth' after gastrointestinal surgery: systematic review and meta-analysis of controlled trials. *BMJ*, **323**, 773–6.

Ljungqvist O, Nygren J, Thorell A (2002). Modulation of post-operative insulin resistance by pre-operative carbohydrate loading. *Proc Nutr Soc*, **61**, 329–36.

Lloyd DA *et al.* (2006). Survival and dependence on home parenteral nutrition: experience over a 25-year period in a UK referral centre. *Aliment Pharmacol Ther*, **24**, 1231–40.

Malnutrition Advisory Group (2000). *MAG guidelines for detection and management of malnutrition.* British Association for Parenteral and Enteral Nutrition (BAPEN), Maidenhead.

McClave SA *et al.* (2006). Nutrition support in acute pancreatitis: a systematic review of the literature. *J Parenter Enteral Nutr*, **30**, 143–56.

McWhirter JP, Pennington CR (1994). Incidence and recognition of malnutrition in hospital. *BMJ*, **308**, 945–8.

Middleton SJ, Jamieson NV (2005). The current status of small bowel transplantation in the UK and internationally. *Gut*, **54**, 1650–7.

NCCAC (2006). *Nutrition support in adults. Oral nutrition support, enteral tube feeding and parenteral nutrition.* National Collaborating Centre for Acute Care, London.

NCEPOD (2004). *Scoping our practice. The 2004 report of the National Confidential Enquiry into Patient outcome and Death.* http://www.ncepod.org.uk/2004report/index.htm

Parenteral and Enteral Nutrition Group of the British Dietetic Association (PEN Group) (2004). *A pocket guide to clinical nutrition.* PEN Group Publications, London.

Payne-Jones, Grimble GJ, Silk D (eds) (2001). *Artificial nutrition in clinical practice.* Greenwich Medical Media, London.

Royal College of Physicians (2002). *Nutrition and patients: a doctor's responsibility.* Royal College of Physicians, London.

Stratton RJ, Green CJ, Elia M (2003). *Disease*-related *malnutrition—an evidence based approach to treatment.* CAB International, Wallingford.

Veteran Affairs Total Parenteral Nutrition Co-operative Study Group (1991). Peri-operative total parenteral nutrition in surgical patients. *N Engl J Med*, **325**, 525–32.

SECTION 12

Metabolic disorders

12.1 The inborn errors of metabolism: general aspects *1549*
Richard W.E. Watts and Timothy M. Cox

12.2 Protein-dependent inborn errors of metabolism *1559*
Georg F. Hoffmann and Stefan Kölker

12.3 Disorders of carbohydrate metabolism *1596*

12.3.1 Glycogen storage diseases *1596*
Philip Lee and Kaustuv Bhattacharya

12.3.2 Inborn errors of fructose metabolism *1604*
Timothy M. Cox

12.3.3 Disorders of galactose, pentose, and pyruvate metabolism *1610*
Timothy M. Cox

12.4 Disorders of purine and pyrimidine metabolism *1619*
Richard W.E. Watts

12.5 The porphyrias *1636*
Timothy M. Cox

12.6 Lipid and lipoprotein disorders *1652*
P.N. Durrington

12.7 Trace metal disorders *1673*

12.7.1 Hereditary haemochromatosis *1673*
William J.H. Griffiths and Timothy M. Cox

12.7.2 Inherited diseases of copper metabolism: Wilson's disease and Menkes' disease *1688*
Michael L. Schilsky and Pramod K. Mistry

12.8 Lysosomal disease *1694*
P.B. Deegan and Timothy M. Cox

12.9 Disorders of peroxisomal metabolism in adults *1719*
Anthony S. Wierzbicki

12.10 Hereditary disorders of oxalate metabolism—the primary hyperoxalurias *1730*
Christopher J. Danpure and Dawn S. Milliner

12.11 Disturbances of acid–base homeostasis *1738*
R.D. Cohen and H.F. Woods

12.12 The acute phase response, amyloidoses and familial Mediterranean fever *1752*

12.12.1 The acute phase response and C-reactive protein *1752*
M.B. Pepys

12.12.2 Hereditary periodic fever syndromes *1760*
Helen J. Lachmann and Philip N. Hawkins

12.12.3 Amyloidosis *1766*
M.B. Pepys and Philip N. Hawkins

12.13 α_1-Antitrypsin deficiency and the serpinopathies *1780*
David A. Lomas

12.1

The inborn errors of metabolism: general aspects

Richard W.E. Watts and Timothy M. Cox

Essentials

Historical perspective—inborn errors of metabolism were first recognized by Archibald Garrod, whose studies illustrated the dynamic aspects of human biochemistry and how unitary hereditary factors caused variation in the turnover of physiological metabolites derived from dietary components. He proposed that the activity of enzymes involved in human metabolism (e.g. of tyrosine degradation) were subject to control by specific genes, and several of the disorders studied by him were subsequently shown to be the result of block at some point in normal metabolism. He also noted the importance of consanguinity in the clinical expression of rare genetic variants which behave as recessive human disease traits.

Definition—the inborn errors of metabolism are those inherited diseases in which the phenotype includes a characteristic constellation of chemical abnormalities related to an alteration in the catalytic activity of a single specific enzyme, activator or transport protein. About 1500 such disorders have been characterized, and these are now recognized in an evolutionary context as paradigmatic examples of the interplay between the constitutional and environmental aspects of disease.

Genetic basis and pathogenesis

Site of mutations—almost all the inborn errors of metabolism arise from mutations in the nuclear genome and have Mendelian patterns of inheritance, but 13 genes are encoded by the mitochondrial genome, and when these are mutated the cognate diseases are thus maternally transmitted.

Mechanism of diseases—mutations in the proteins giving rise to the inborn errors of metabolism affect primary, secondary, tertiary or quaternary structure. This can lead to an enormous variety of consequences, including (1) abolishing, decreasing, or (occasionally) increasing protein activity; (2) affecting activator proteins, or binding of hormones and other ligands to cell surfaces or other structures; (3) impeding intracellular trafficking of proteins; (4) affecting the transport of metabolites across cellular membranes.

Clinical features and future prospects

Clinical presentation—the symptoms of metabolic disease are protean and may appear vague, hence a high index of suspicion may be required to make a correct diagnosis. In an appropriate clinical context—e.g. unexplained acute neonatal illness and/or failure to thrive in early infancy, developmental slowing and arrest followed by retrogression, unusual physiognomy—the critical clue often comes from taking an appropriate family history, with specific inquiries about affected siblings, possible parental consanguinity, paternity, miscarriages, perinatal deaths, abortions, about the sexes of possibly affected relatives and their placement on the maternal or paternal side of the family, the ages at death of relatives, as well as the ethnic and geographical origins of the parents. Impaired function of proteins that are localized to the mitochondria, lysosomes, and peroxisomes are associated with particular clinical and biochemical characteristics that reflect the compartmentalized functions of these organelles.

Prevention and screening—there is a strong case for mass population screening for some inborn errors of metabolism at the presymptomatic stage to allow early detection and introduction of treatment before irreversible damage occurs. Specific methods, including mass spectroscopy and molecular analysis of genomic DNA, are increasingly used identify those at risk.

Treatment—cure of the underlying abnormality is reserved for a few spectacular disorders, but precise characterization of the biochemical disturbance often permits a rational treatment to be developed. General approaches include (1) restriction of a dietary substrate that cannot be metabolized; (2) replacement of a missing metabolic product; (3) removal of toxic metabolites; (4) administering pharmacological doses of a cofactor; (5) replacement of a missing gene product, usually by enzyme replacement therapy; (6) transplantation of cells (e.g. bone marrow) or organs (e.g. liver) as a 'gene replacement therapy'.

Future prospects—the developments of treatments for inborn errors of metabolism will continue to be assisted by the recent capacity to develop credible models of specific disorders in genetically modified animals. The concept of pharmacological chaperones—based on the ability of small molecules to bind to mutant proteins to prevent their inactivation by abnormal folding, intracellular aggregation and mistargeting—is receiving much attention, but has yet to produce treatments of clinical utility. Numerous trials of gene therapy are planned and after many vicissitudes there are signs of success in patients suffering from several inborn errors of metabolism: it is likely that this strategy will enjoy wider clinical application over the next decade.

Introduction

Inborn errors of metabolism were the brainchild of the physician Archibald Garrod in the early 20th century. In the century since their discovery, this brilliant concept has proved to have far-reaching implications in biochemistry, genetics, evolutionary biology, and medical practice. William Bateson, a biologist and early champion of Mendel, showed Garrod that central to his idea of the 'inborn' was the concept of the gene. Garrod proposed that genetic determinants specify the activity of enzymes which catalyse particular metabolic reactions. Thus Garrod was the first biochemist who, with Bateson, applied mendelian genetics to humans: he recognized the segregation of recessive traits in pedigrees affected by hereditary metabolic diseases and the role of consanguinity in rare inherited disorders. Since Garrod's original description, the term 'inborn error' has broadened to include mutations affecting the function of other proteins, such as the structural proteins fibrillin and collagen, in which mutations are also implicated in disease.

Garrod considered that some 'simple' biochemical traits inherited as Mendelian recessive characters, such as alkaptonuria, appeared to have little, if any, apparent effect on health (in fact, in this emblematic disorder, the focus of much of his early experimentation, the great man was mistaken: alkaptonuric subjects develop severe arthritis and die prematurely from the consequences of cardiovascular disease (see Chapter 12.2)). In other conditions, such as albinism or porphyria, environmental factors (e.g. sunlight, barbiturates) cooperate with host determinants in the development of clinical manifestations. Thus Garrod promulgated the notion of 'chemical individuality' and genetic predisposition to disease; in so doing, he adduced a strong theoretical underpinning to the concept of 'diathesis'—a hitherto pervasive term of the 19th century, largely concealing prejudice and ignorance but persistent in clinical thinking long afterwards. Indeed, years after the publication of Garrod's work, the great American geneticist Thomas Hunt Morgan stated in his Nobel lecture of 1934:

> I am aware, of course, of the ancient attempts to identify certain gross physical human types—the bilious, the lymphatic, the nervous, and the sanguine dispositions, and of more modern attempts to classify human beings into the cerebral, respiratory, digestive and muscular, or, more briefly into asthenics and pycnics. Some of these are proposed to be more susceptible to certain ailments or diseases than are other types, which in turn have their own constitutional characteristics. These well-intended efforts are, however, so far in advance of our genetic information that the geneticist may be excused if he refuses to discuss them seriously.

In fact, by 1931 Garrod had developed his ideas in a prescient essay, *Inborn Factors in Disease*, which has prodigious implications for a modern synthesis of the concept of disease; he had advanced his logic from the inborn error to chemical individuality—a universal quality of the whole species, as opposed to the single individual. It is clear that Garrod had in mind the operation of Darwinian principles: in the example of infectious disease, he refers to the individuality of the human individual and the microbe:

> In our fight against infective diseases we are not confronted with blind forces, acting at random, but with the disciplined offensive of highly trained foes. Whilst on the one hand the weapons of attack have been improved by evolution, there has been a corresponding evolution of protective mechanisms of great ingenuity, and of no small efficiency, for the defence of the individual attacked.

To understand the diverse manifestations of disease, including those clearly due to infectious agents such as *Mycobacterium tuberculosis*, and variable responses to drugs (many of which were metabolized by enzymes in the liver), Garrod further considered the idea of individual uniqueness and interactions with the environment: he realized that an infinite multitude of responses to environmental factors was determined by constitutional (genetic) variation in the individual and, in effect, that the operation of selection in human evolution is also played out within the microcosm of disease. While it has been pointed out that while Garrod did not employ the terms 'multifactorial' or 'susceptibility' and had an incomplete appreciation of contemporary genetics, his ideas foresaw how we might understand 'complex' diseases with their dynamic gene–environment interactions, as well as the so-called monogenic disorders, through the immense technological power available for molecular analysis of the human genome. It now seems that the discovery, characterization, and quantification of environmental factors and their interactions with human genetic variants is a major challenge for the mechanistic understanding of pathology.

To summarize: through the study of rare human phenotypes, and like many others before and after him, Archibald Garrod was able to make observations of astonishing relevance to the large field of medicine. Perhaps the greatest, most penetrating—and lasting—insight to emerge from the concept of the 'inborn' has been the realization that disease can no longer be viewed solely in the context of the 'broken machine' metaphor, but rather, the consequence of interactions between individual uniqueness and an environment for which that individual is, at a given time, maladapted—or 'unfit'. Although the constraint of space prevents full consideration of this theme here, the Darwinian perspective clearly has far-reaching consequences for the teaching and practice of medicine; from it the new field of evolutionary medicine emerges directly (see Chapter 2.1.2).

Inherited diseases of metabolism

There are nearly 12 700 known human gene sequences and estimated to be more than 19 000 potential human phenotypes, the inheritance of which can be described as being autosomal recessive, autosomal dominant, sex-linked, or transmitted maternally through the mitochondrial genome (as noted in the comprehensive Online Mendelian Inheritance in Man, http://www.ncbi.nlm.nih.gov/Omim/). The inborn errors of metabolism are those inherited diseases in which the phenotype includes a characteristic constellation of chemical abnormalities related to an alteration in the catalytic activity of a single specific enzyme, activator, or transport protein: about 1500 of these disorders have been characterized. There are unifactorially inherited diseases in which the current techniques are too insensitive for a chemical abnormality to be identified, so that the syndrome has to be defined in clinical, gross structural, and/or pathological terms; further study is likely to demonstrate that many of these fall into the category of inborn errors of metabolism.

Almost all the unifactorially inherited diseases arise from mutations in the nuclear genome which spans about 3 billion base pairs of DNA. A few mitochondrial proteins have their structures encoded in the mitochondrial DNA (mtDNA). This genetic information is transmitted only through the female line and the category of inborn errors of metabolism includes this group. The nuclear and the maternally inherited diseases stem from mutations of DNA which directs the synthesis of a single specific polypeptide chain. The molecular changes in the enzyme protein may affect the primary, secondary, tertiary, or quaternary structure, decreasing, increasing, or abolishing its catalytic activity. Some mutations affect the function of an activator protein, others reduce the binding of hormones and paracrine factors to cell surfaces and/or subcellular structures, and some derange the migration of proteins within cells; another group impairs the transport of metabolites across cellular and subcellular membranes (Table 12.1.1). Most intracellular enzymes are located in the cytosol where they are correctly orientated in relation to one another, sometimes as macromolecular complexes, and to their substrates. Some are linked to cellular membranes and several are located in anatomically defined subcellular structures or organelles: the mitochondria, lysosomes, and peroxisomes.

Mitochondrial diseases

The mitochondrial genome is a circular double strand containing 16.5 kb of DNA. It encodes 13 of the respiratory chain enzymes, the remainder of which (*c.*60) are encoded in the nuclear DNA. Hitherto, mutations in 26 genes in the mitochondrial genome are associated with defined human phenotypes (see Chapter 24.24.5). Abnormal mitochondrial function impairs the supply of energy for biochemical work in all tissues and therefore has wide-ranging effects. Each mitochondrion also contains 24 RNA genes that participate in intramitochondrial protein synthesis. Transcription and translation of mtDNA are regulated by the nucleus through the noncoding D-loop region of the mitochondrial genome. Human cells contain about 1000 copies of mtDNA, but the individual mitochondria in a cell may not all carry a given specific mutation and different cells carry different proportions of mutated mitochondria (heteroplasmy). The proportion of mutant mtDNA must exceed a critical level before the mitochondrial respiratory chain disease declares itself. This variability, as well as tissue-specific differences in dependence on oxidative metabolism, explains, at least partially, why some tissues are preferentially affected in patients with mtDNA diseases. Postmitotic tissues (e.g. neurons, muscle, endocrine tissues) have high levels of mutated mtDNA and are often clinically affected, whereas rapidly dividing tissues (e.g. bone marrow) are less often clinically affected. Differences in the proportions of mutated and nonmutated mtDNA between and within family members also contribute to the wide phenotypic range encountered in the mitochondrial diseases. The spermatozoal cytoplasm, including its mitochondria, is entirely lost at fertilization and for this reason mitochondrial diseases are only transmitted through the female line. Clinically affected women rarely transmit a mtDNA deletion to their children. However, a woman with a heteroplasmic mtDNA point mutation or duplication may transmit a variable amount of mutated mtDNA to her progeny. The number of mtDNA molecules in each oocyte is reduced and then amplified to a total of about 105 during early development of the oocyte; this presumably random process contributes to the different amounts of mutated mtDNA in different children in the same family. Women whose gametes contain high concentrations of mtDNA are more likely to have clinically affected children than mothers with lower concentrations of mtDNA. The general clinical manifestations of the mitochondrial diseases are shown in Table 12.1.2 and specific examples of mitochondrial diseases are given in Table 12.1.3.

Table 12.1.1 Examples of diseases in which there is defective transport of an enzyme or metabolite within cells or across cell membranes

Disease	Metabolic abnormality
Cystinuria	Failure to transport cystine, lysine, ornithine, arginine, and homoarginine across the plasma membrane of the proximal renal tubular epithelium and the small intestinal mucosa
Cystinosis (cystine storage disease, Lignac's disease)	Failure to transport cystine produced by intralysosomal proteolysis across the lysosomal membrane and into the cytosol
Salla disease	Failure to transport *N*-acetylneuraminic acid (sialic acid) across the lysosomal membrane and into the cytosol
The mucopolysacchridoses	Failure to degrade glycosaminolycans (mucopolysaccharides), the undegraded mucopolysaccharides being neither transportable across lysosomal membranes nor capable of being removed from the lysosomes by exocytosis
Tay–Sachs disease	Defective post-translational processing of the alpha chain of β-*N*-acetylhexosaminidase (hexosaminidase A). This prevents the enzyme from migrating from the endoplasmic reticulum, where it is glycosylated, to the Golgi apparatus for phosphorylation of its mannosyl residues and hence to lysosomes and the exterior of the cell
Primary hyperoxaluria type 1 (some cases)	Mislocation of alanine: glyoxylate aminotransferase in mitochondria as opposed to its normal location in peroxisomes. This arises because a rare mutation (Gly 170 → Arg) is present simultaneously with the common polymorphism (Pro 11 → Leu). The mutation (Gly 170 → Arg) prevents dimerization of the molecule which, in turn, allows the weak mitochondrial targeting sequence generated by the polymorphism (Pro 11 → Leu) to direct the molecule to mitochondria instead of peroxisomes

Table 12.1.2 The main clinical manifestations of diseases due to mitochondrial dysfunction

Disease group	Clinical manifestations
Defects of fatty acid oxidation	Hypoglycaemia
	Hepatic dysfunction
	Cardiac failure
	Myopathy
	Sudden infant death
Respiratory chain disorders	Lactic acidosis
	Encephalopathy
	Hypotonia
	Poor feeding
	Failure to thrive
	Convulsions

Table 12.1.3 Some mitochondrial diseases. (Data from Chinnery PF and Turnbull DM (1999) *The Lancet* **354** (supplement 1), S17–S21)

Mitochondrial DNA defects
Rearrangements (deletions and duplications)
◆ Chronic progressive external ophthalmoplegia
◆ Kearns Sayre syndrome (hypoparathyroidism with deafness)
◆ Diabetes and deafness
Point mutations in protein encoding genes
◆ Leber's hereditary optic neuropathy
◆ Leber's hereditary optic neuropathy/dystonia
◆ Neurogenic weakness, ataxia, and retinitis pigmentosa
◆ Leigh's syndrome*
Point mutations in tRNA genes
◆ Mitochondrial encephalopathy with lactic acidosis and stroke-like episodes
◆ Myoclonic epilepsy with ragged-red fibres
◆ Myopathy
◆ Cardiomyopathy
◆ Diabetes and deafness
◆ Encephalomyopathy
◆ Leigh's syndrome*
Point mutations in rRNA genes
◆ Non-syndromic sensorineural deafness
◆ Aminoglycoside-induced non-syndromic deafness
Nuclear DNA defects
Nuclear genetic disorders with a mitochondrial basis
◆ Friedreich's ataxia (frataxin)
◆ Autosomal recessive hereditary spastic paraplegia
Nuclear genetic disorders of the mitochondrial respiratory chain
◆ Leigh's syndrome (complex I deficiency)*
◆ Optic atrophy and ataxia
◆ Leigh's syndrome (complex IV deficiency)*
Nuclear genetic disorders associated with multiple mtDNA deletions
◆ Autosomal dominant external ophthalmoplegia
◆ Mitochondrial neurogastrointestinal encephalomyopathy (thymidine phosphorylase deficiency)

* An example of different mutations providing the same clinical syndrome (phenocopies). Abbreviations: tRNA = transfer RNA; rRNA = ribosomal RNA; mtDNA = mitochondrial DNA.

Peroxisomal diseases

Some enzymes that are encoded in the nuclear DNA are specifically expressed in peroxisomes, to which they are imported soon after translation. Mutations in these genes result in the peroxisomal diseases listed in Table 12.1.4. Diseases due to defects in peroxisomal proteins are discussed in Chapters 12.9 and 12.10.

Table 12.1.4 Peroxisomal diseases

Zellweger syndrome (absent peroxisomal membranes)
Pseudo-Zellweger syndrome
Adrenoleucodystrophy
Pseudo-neonatal adrenoleucodystrophy
Acatalasia
Infantile Refsum's disease
Refsum's disease (classical form)
Hyperpipecolic acidaemia
X-linked adrenoleucodystrophy
Chondrodysplasia punctatum rhizomelia
Primary hyperoxaluria type 1

Lysosomal storage diseases

Lysosomes are subcellular organelles containing hydrolases with low optimum pH values ('acid hydrolases') which catalyse the degradation of cellular macromolecules. The macromolecules are either derived from the metabolic turnover of structural cellular components or have entered the cell by endocytosis. The products of this macromolecular degradation process leave the lysosomes by specific efflux processes.

In most of the lysosomal storage diseases an inborn error of metabolism affects a specific lysosomal enzyme so that either undegraded or partially degraded macromolecules accumulate in the lysosomes (see Chapter 12.8). The engorged lysosomes distort the internal architecture of the cell, disturb its function, and inhibit the activities of other lysosomal enzymes so that macromolecules other than those related to the primary enzyme deficiency also accumulate.

Cystinosis (cystine storage disease) and Salla disease (*N*-acetylneuraminic (sialic) acid storage disease) are due to metabolic lesions involving the specific efflux processes by which these small molecules generated by the intralysosomal hydrolysis of macromolecule (cystine and sialic acid respectively) leave the lysosome (see Table 12.1.1).

Lysosomal enzymes are glycoproteins which are subject to exocytosis and reuptake by endocytosis. Their protein moieties are synthesized on the rough endoplasmic reticulum and the oligosaccharide side chains are added in the Golgi apparatus. The addition of a terminal mannose 6-phosphate residue recognition marker is necessary if the enzyme molecule is to be correctly routed into the lysosomes, and if it is to be available for receptor mediated reuptake from the interstitial fluids. The types of lysosomal storage diseases and the nature of their metabolic defects together with examples of each group are presented in Table 12.1.5.

Heterogeneity in the inborn errors of metabolism

The individual inborn errors of metabolism are defined on the basis of the phenotype, including the specific enzyme lesion, and by their pattern of inheritance. Close study of any particular inborn error of metabolism reveals unexpected heterogeneity and we are increasingly recognizing diverse patterns of inheritance due to a variety of mechanisms, including somatic mosaicism, dominant

Table 12.1.5 Lysosomal storage diseases other than cystinosis and Salla disease (a complete listing of these diseases and their biochemistry is given in Watts and Gibbs (1986))

Name	Defect	Example
Sphingolipidoses	Failure to degrade compounds containing a sphingoid [sphinoglipids, ceramides, sphingomyelins and glycosphingolipids including the gangliosides (sialoglycosphingolipids)]	Tay-Sachs disease (GM2-gangliosidosis) Gaucher disease (glucocerebrosidosis)
Mucopolysaccharidoses	Failure to degrade the glycosaminoglycans: dermatan, heparan, and keratan sulphates. Incompletely degraded glycosaminoglycan fragments accumulate in the lysosomes as well as extracellularly. This causes secondary deficiencies of other lysosomal enzymes and other undegraded macromolecules, particularly sphingolipids, accumulate	Hurler disease Hunter disease Morquio disease
Glycoproteinoses	A group of enzyme defects in the catabolism of glycoproteins in which characteristic abnormal macromolecules accumulate	Fucisidosis Mannosidosis
Acid lipase deficiency	Two clinically distinct variants. Cholesteryl esters and triglycerides accumulate in most tissues due to deficiency of lysosomal acid lipase	Wohlman's disease Cholesteryl ester storage disease
Glycogenosis II	Lack of intralysosomal hydrolysis of glycogen	Glycogenosis type II (only member of this group)
Mucolipidoses	Originally defined as being clinically intermediate between the sphingolipidoses and mucopolysaccharidoses but without mucopolysacchariduria (abnormal glycosaminoglycan excretion). Subsequently shown to include patients with (i) deficient neuraminidase activities with respect to either glycoprotein substrates (mucolipidosis I, also classified as a glycoproteinosis and termed sialidosis) or ganglioside substrates (mucolipidosis IV); (ii) clinically mild and severe variants of uridine-diphosphate-*N*-acetylglucosamine: lysosomal enzyme precursor *N*-acetylglucosamine phosphate transferase (mucolipidoses II (I-cell disease) and III (pseudo-Hurler polydystrophy) respectively)	See opposite

negative effects in complex multimeric pathways as well as transcriptional silencing of imprinted genes. This may be due to:

- multiple allelism
- mutations at different gene loci affecting the structure of different polypeptide chains in a single enzyme protein
- mutations at different gene loci affecting different proteins with similar catalytic functions
- differences in the overall genetic background against which the single mutation acts
- environmental factors

Clinical pointers towards a diagnosis of an inborn error of metabolism

Although the symptoms of metabolic disease may appear vague and protean, and an inherited disease cannot be diagnosed in the absence of an appropriate family history, some clinical settings suggest the presence of an inborn error of metabolism (Table 12.1.6). In taking the family history special inquiries should be made about affected siblings, possible parental consanguinity, paternity, miscarriages, perinatal deaths, abortions, the sexes of possibly affected relatives and their placement on the maternal or paternal side of the family, and the ages at death of relatives, as well as the ethnic and geographical origins of the parents.

General approaches to the treatment of inborn errors of metabolism

The treatments available for the individual inborn errors of metabolism cover a wide range and may need to be specially developed for individual patients. However, the principles involved can be broadly classified as in Table 12.1.7. Palliative surgical and other measures may be needed to deal with specific complications (e.g. corneal grafting to restore vision in patients with corneal clouding due to one of the mucopolysaccharidoses). Consideration should also be given to meeting the educational and social needs of these patients as well as to optimizing their overall clinical state and correcting the biochemical parameters. The successful management of patients with inborn errors of metabolism requires a multidisciplinary approach which utilizes the special skills of dietitians, social workers, educationalists, and occupational therapists as well as those of physicians, surgeons, biochemists, and geneticists. It is particularly important to plan for the handover of specialist care from the paediatrician to the most appropriate adult physician when follow-up in a paediatric department becomes inappropriate. The perfect outcome is to achieve a physically and mentally healthy adult who is capable of begetting healthy children. Unfortunately the nature of many of the inborn errors of metabolism militates against this ideal so that treatment has to aim at optimizing the child's potential in all its physical, mental, and social aspects. Treatment and support also have to be extended to the parents and siblings who, if not overtly affected themselves, may be carriers of the abnormal gene concerned and require appropriate advice about the transmission of the disease to other offspring and other aspects of the condition.

In many instances inborn errors lead to enzymatic or functional deficiency of a metabolic pathway with either (1) accumulation of toxic intermediates and by-products due to abnormal biochemical fluxes through the pathway, such in the acute porphyrias or the lysosomal storage disorders; the by-products may have secondary inhibitory effects on other biochemical reactions due to their effects on key metabolic enzymes or the operation of negative

Table 12.1.6 Clinical presentation which, in the absence of acquired or other congenital causes, suggest an inborn error or metabolism

- Unexplained acute neonatal illness and/or failure to thrive in early infancy. (Marked muscle hypotonia, recurrent fits, comas, acidosis, and vomiting, especially if withholding milk feeds causes temporary improvement, are especially suggestive)
- Developmental slowing and arrest followed by retrogression
- Developmental slowing and arrest leading to unexplained mental handicap
- Unusual physiognomy, multiple skeletal deformities with developmental delay and retrogression
- Multiple skeletal deformities alone (dysostosis multiplex especially suggests a lysosomal storage disease)
- Gross visceromegaly
- Specific dietary intolerances
- Haemolytic anaemia
- Unusual body odour*
- Urolithiasis
- Cataracts in early life†
- Dislocation of the optic lens‡
- Persistent jaundice and hepatic cirrhosis in infancy.
- Abnormal cutaneous photosensitivity
- Hypopigmentation
- Abnormal drug sensitivity
- A history of recurrent perinatal deaths and/or stillbirths
- Hydrops fetalis in the absence of blood group incompatibility between mother and fetus (red cell enzyme defects)

* Examples are: phenylketonuria (mousy, musty) branched chain ketoacidosis (maple syrup), methionine malabsorption (oast house, dry celery), isovaleric acidaemia (sweaty feet), methylaminuria (stale fish), multiple carboxylase deficiency (tom cat's urine), Hawkinsinuria (swimming pool).

† Examples are: Fabry's disease, galactosaemia, galactokinase deficiency, Lowe's syndrome, mannosidosis, osteogenesis imperfecta, Refsum's disease, Wilson's disease.

‡ Examples are: Ehlers–Danlos syndrome, homocystinuria, hyperlysinuria, Marfan's syndrome, sulphite oxidase deficiency.

Table 12.1.7 General approaches to the treatment of inborn errors of metabolism

Method	Examples
Restriction of a dietary substrate which cannot be metabolized	Phenylalanine restriction in phenylketonuria
	Protein restriction in the hyperamonaemias
	Elimination of galactose in galactosaemia
	Ultraviolet radiation (congenital erythropoietic and variegate porphyrias, and in albinism)
	Ionizing radiation in the DNA repair enzyme defects (xeroderma pigmentosum, ataxia telangiectasia)
	Infections (agammaglobinaemia).
	Medications (oestrogens, barbiturates etc. in acute intermittent porphyria)
Replacement of a missing metabolic product	Orotic aciduria: treatment by uridine which is metabolized to uridylic acid
	Hartnup disease: nicotinic acid to control skin manifestations
Removal of toxic metabolite	Haemodialysis and peritoneal dialysis as temporary treatment of an acute metabolic crisis due to a diffusible toxic metabolite, and to correct certain secondary biochemical abnormalities quickly
	Either specific chemical detoxication (e.g. penicillamine in Wilson's disease) or solubilization (e.g. penicillamine in cystinuria)
Pharmacological doses of a cofactor (only some cases of each disease respond)	Propionic acidaemia: biotin Ubidecarenone (respiratory chain disorders due to coenzyme Q10 deficiency Homocystinuria: pyridoxine Primary hyperoxaluria (type I): pyridoxine Methylmalonic acidaemia: vitamin B12
Replacement of a missing gene product	Adenosine deaminase deficiency Gaucher disease: β-glucocerebosidase Haemophilia: clotting factor VIII
Bone marrow transplantation	Adenosine deaminase deficiency
Haematopoeitic stem cell transplantation	Adenosine deaminase deficiency
Liver transplantation	Hereditary tyrosinaemia (type I) Antitrypsin deficiency Primary hyperoxaluria (type I) Urea cycle disorders Criglar Najjar syndrome (type I)
Gene replacement	Adrenoleukodystrophy Adenosine deaminase deficiency

The examples chosen are situations in which either the proposed treatment is established or in which it can be recommended as elective therapy even though the results of prolonged evaluation are still awaited.

feedback regulation or (2) absence or reduced availability of an essential precursor, e.g. in hormone synthesis; (3) defective active transport of metabolites across cell membranes. Given these basic but by no means universal mechanisms, functional complementation (enzyme replacement or provision of enhancing vitamin cofactors as with pyridoxine in homcystinuria); reduction of the accumulating substrate (as in dietary treatment of phenylketonuria or substrate reduction of cholesterol biosynthesis in low-density lipoprotein (LDL) receptor defects by inhibiting the formation of the first committed precursor, mevalonate, with statin drugs); supplying the missing product (uridine in orotic aciduria or arginine in urea cycle defects). Removal of sundry toxic molecules is also effective in many disorders: e.g. as cystine in the urine and intracellular cystine with thiol agents such as penicillamine and cysteamine; metal chelation with desferrioxamine for iron in haemochromatosis and trientine for copper in Wilson's disease.

The ability to clone human genes into bacteria and eukaryotic cells for ectopic expression which can then produce large amounts of the human gene product is opening the horizons for treatment by protein replacement. The development of macrophage-targeted β-glucocerebosidase enzyme replacement therapy for Gaucher's disease (glucosylceramidase deficiency) type I is a notable recent development in this field and is now regarded as the definitive treatment. Attempts to utilize transplanted fibroblasts and amniotic cells as a source for enzyme replacement therapy have not been successful. Bone marrow transplantation has been used for the treatment of two groups of inherited metabolic disorders: those in which it is desired to replace a particular type of nonfunctioning bone marrow cell by its normally functioning counterpart and those in which an attempt has been made to utilize the fact that the bone marrow produces 50 to 100 g of polymorphonuclear leucocytes per day and that these cells exocytose (release) their lysosomal enzymes for endocytic uptake by enzyme-deficient cells in the body tissues generally. This strategy has been more successful with the first group of diseases, which includes disorders of neutrophil function (e.g. cyclic neutropenia), functional abnormalities of lymphocytes, and osteopetrosis. The beneficial effect on the last disease is due to the introduction of normal osteoclast precursors. The results in the second group of diseases, namely those in which the white cell lineage derived from the transplanted bone marrow is used to supply normal enzyme to enzyme-deficient tissues, e.g. Hurler's disease (mucopolysaccharidosis 1) and Krabbe's disease. In the latter case, recent courageous studies have shown that transplantation of HLA-matched umbilical cord blood in the first 10 days of life has been moderately successful in promoting neurological development in infants born to couples with previously affected offspring and detected by screening early for this otherwise rapidly progressive neurodegenerative disorder. Haematopoietic stem cells have been implanted into the fetus *in utero* to correct severe congenital immunodeficiency but this has not, so far, been applied to diseases without immunodeficiency. This procedure takes advantage of the immunological tolerance of the fetus. The possibility of using liposomes and resealed erythrocyte envelopes as carriers of therapeutic enzymes is also being explored; linking purified or recombinant therapeutic enzymes, such as adenosine deaminase to polymers such a polyethylene glycol, many usefully prolong their survival in circulating plasma.

Definitive enzymatic augmentation with receptor-targeted therapies has attracted much attention: in Gaucher's disease this strategy has proved to be very effective and commercially successful—global sales of the mannose-terminated glucocerebrosidase for about 5000 patients worldwide has enabled the Genzyme corporation to rise to a leading position in the biotechnology industry (see Chapters 2.4.4 and 12.8). Substrate-reduction therapy with the use of specific inhibitors to regulate the flux of key degradative pathways by partial blockade of the rate-limiting step is useful in LDL receptor deficiency (heterozygous familial hypercholesterolaemia as well as the very rare homozygous variant) and thus was born the pharmaceutical star of the statin drugs, which are in wide general use; this approach is at a late experimental phase in the glycosphingolipid diseases. In alkaptonuria, a disease in which Garrod maintained a lifelong interest, the use of substrate-reduction therapy is also far advanced. Nitisinone, a triketone inhibitor of the precursor to homogentisic acid at the level of hydroxyphenylpyruvate dioxygenase in the tyrosine degradation pathway, is a licensed agent for tyrosinaemia type 1. In very small doses, this agent has a striking effect on the formation of toxic oxidative metabolites of homogentisic acid which lead to the life-shortening manifestations of alkaptonuria and it appears likely that at last a well-tolerated and definitive treatment for this landmark disorder is within sight. Gene therapy, and organ and cell-based therapies including liver and bone marrow transplantation, are at various stages of clinical evaluation and development—assisted by the recent capacity to develop credible models of specific disorders in genetically modified animals. The concept of pharmacological chaperones, based on the ability of small molecules to bind to mutant proteins to prevent their inactivation by abnormal folding, intracellular aggregation and mistargeting, is receiving much attention in but has yet to be validated in practice. The chaperone approach is in late-phase clinical development in Fabry's disease and Gaucher's disease; despite much promise, its application to another misfolding disorder, α_1-antitrypsin deficiency (Chapter 12.13), has yet to be proven.

Liver transplantation is used as a form of enzymatic complementation in some inborn errors of metabolism where this organ is the specific site of the metabolic lesion. Liver transplantation has the advantage that the enzyme is introduced in the correct organ, in the correct cell with its correct subcellular location, and correctly orientated with respect to its substrate and other enzymes with which it must act in concert. Liver transplantation can also be regarded as a form of gene replacement therapy in that the donor liver contains the normal gene which will direct the synthesis of a normal enzyme protein. Prenatal transplantation of fetal liver stem cells has potential in the treatment of some inborn errors of metabolism. Successful engraftment at the 12th to 24th week after fertilization with partial correction of the metabolic defect has been demonstrated in β-thalassaemia.

Treatment by gene replacement, using retroviral vectors and gene constructs to introduce the desired DNA sequence into the patient's explanted haematopoietic stem cell genome, these genetically corrected cells being cultured and then returned to the patient's circulation, may have some potential in diseases where expression of the metabolic lesion in the haematopoietic system determines the phenotype, or in those situations where genetically corrected migratory cells of haematopoietic origin can deliver normal enzyme to the enzyme-deficient tissues. Although somatic cell gene therapy using viral vectors and/or gene constructs to introduce the desired DNA sequences into other cell types is currently being investigated extensively in *in vitro* model systems and in animal models of some human inborn errors of metabolism, e.g. using hepatocytes, few of these have reached application in clinical practice. However this approach, using lentiviral vectors which have the advantage that they can be used to transduce by nuclear integration of viral sequences in mitotic cells, has had qualified therapeutic success in trials in children with combined immunodeficiency: unfortunately several patients in this Anglo-French trial developed a late-onset T-cell lymphocytosis leading to leukaemia, later shown to be related to the integration of vector sequences at a genomic 'hot spot' leading to activation of a vicinal endogenous proto-oncogene. At the time of writing these patients are all alive with satisfactory control of the complication—and their disabling immunodeficiency disease—but safety considerations have retarded clinical development until improved vector systems can be utilized. Promising results of a gene therapy trial using a lentiviral vector to correct the enzymatic abnormality in leucocytes derived from haematopoietic precursors in a very rare immunodeficiency disease, adenosine deaminase deficiency, have also been recently been reported—so far with no mutagenic effects. Eight years after the procedure, eight of ten patients with severe combined immunodeficiency no longer require enzyme-replacement therapy and live normally. After two years of using a third-generation lentiviral vector to insert the corrective gene (ABC1) into autologous haematopoietic stem-cell precursors, progression of adrenoleukodystrophy in the brains of two seven-year-old boys has been largely arrested and there have been no signs of neoplastic change or of preferential integration of vector at specific sites in the host genome.

The possibility of using adeno-associated viral vectors as a means of introducing corrected genes for into nonmitotic cells of the nervous system is being explored in human patients; these vectors are maintained as episomal elements which do not integrate readily into the host genome (with the attendant risk of mutagenesis) but persistently express the corrective protein. Adeno-associated vectors have been successfully used in early gene therapy trials of the retinal disease, Leber's congenital amaurosis, with direct intraorbital gene delivery; recent administration of gene therapy by direct injection of vector into striatal tissue in patients with Parkinson's disease was shown to have therapeutic efficacy over a 1-year period without unwanted effects, and opens up the field for further exploration of gene therapy in the human brain. The unique capacity for complementation of soluble lysosomal proteins to be secreted by cells and taken up at a distance by others ('secretion–recapture') renders those lysosomal diseases in which neurological manifestations are excellent targets for clinical exploration of gene therapy (see Chapter 12.8). Here, the principle of allowing a proportion of neural cells to be stably transduced by vector, thus to serve as a source of a given corrective protein that can be taken up into the lysosomes that lack the enzyme in nearby neurons, is an attractive strategy for therapeutic exploration.

Although there are some prospects of correcting some enzyme defects in the somatic cell genome, the correction of defects in the germ line seems remote although the development of advanced *in vitro* fertilization techniques, preimplantation DNA analysis, gene transfer, insertion or conversion, and embryo implantation procedures may render this judgement premature. Ethical objections to human germ-line modifications are also being raised, and could lead to this research being discontinued.

Screening for inborn errors of metabolism

The realization that very early diagnosis is essential in order to achieve good results in the treatment of many inborn errors of metabolism, such as phenylketonuria and galactosaemia, has stimulated interest in the possibility of examining either whole populations or selected groups of predisposed individuals for the biochemical differences which characterize particular inherited metabolic diseases. Diagnosis is needed at a stage which is not only presymptomatic but which precedes the onset of self-perpetuating secondary pathological changes.

Screening for inborn errors of metabolism may be either nonselective (whole population) or selective. The latter, which includes carrier detection studies, aims to cover a part of the population. This may be defined on clinical, genetic, ethnic, or geographical grounds. Phenylketonuria and congenital hypothyroidism are the only members of this group of disorders for which neonatal whole-population screening is generally practised, although the inclusion of galactosaemia, cystic fibrosis, and congenital adrenal hyperplasia (21-hydroxylase deficiency) has been proposed. Whole-population screening should only be established for treatable or preventable diseases, and the consistency of the association of the proposed biochemical or other marker and the serious clinical phenotype must have been proved beyond any doubt. There must be a reliable and robust analytical method suitable for use with a sample of blood or urine which can be obtained without distressing either the parents or the baby. The possibility that metabolic screening will bring to light previously unrecognized variants, which are either mild and do not require treatment, or which by virtue of a fundamentally different biochemical lesion will resist the currently established therapies, has to be borne in mind. Phenylketonuria illustrates these problems. Here, beside classical phenylketonuria, whole-population screening has identified both the clinically unimportant essential (mild) hyperphenylalaninaemia, and the devastatingly serious, but treatable, inborn errors of tetrahydrobiopterin synthesis which produce the 'malignant' hyperphenylalaninaemia syndrome. It is also possible that in some cases immediate postnatal screening and treatment may be too late to prevent minor manifestations of the disease (e.g. in congenital hypothyroidism).

The incidence of disease which merits whole-population screening should be at least similar to that of phenylketonuria in white Europeans (between 1 in 6000 and 1 in 12 000). Cystic fibrosis has an incidence of 1 in 2500 (gene frequency l in 25) in white persons of European ancestry and would merit neonatal whole-population screening on this basis. Molecular genetic approaches are potentially useful. If the disease is not too genetically heterogeneous and when the full range of possible causative mutations is known the specific mutation could be sought directly. Otherwise, after DNA amplification the mutational change in the DNA structure could be detected either by the presence of a restriction endonuclease site or by probing with another primer that hybridizes with only one of the alleles. An appreciable proportion of individuals classified as being homozygotes on the basis of classical genetic analysis prove to be double heterozygotes, that is they carry two different mutations in the same gene. The number of inborn metabolic errors in which the affected individuals and the heterozygous carriers can be identified by molecular genetic analysis is increasing rapidly. It includes such numerically important diseases as sickle cell anaemia, β-thalassaemia, haemophilia, Duchenne muscular dystrophy, cystic fibrosis, and phenylketonuria, as well as rarer but devastating conditions such as the Lesch–Nyhan syndrome.

Prenatal diagnosis

The procedures used in prenatal diagnosis are:

- direct examination of the fetus by ultrasonography and fetoscopy
- chemical analysis of amniotic fluid
- biochemical and cytological analysis of cultured amniotic cells (amniocytes) obtained by amniocentesis at weeks 15 to 16 of pregnancy
- DNA analysis on uncultured amniocytes
- karyotypic enzymological and DNA analysis of chorionic villi obtained by biopsy at weeks 8 to 10 of pregnancy
- similar studies conducted with fetal DNA recovered from the maternal circulation
- biochemical studies on tissue obtained by fetal biopsy *in utero*.

Carrier state diagnosis

Carriers are either individuals carrying the gene for a recessive disorder, which does not express itself in the heterozygous state (e.g. phenylketonuria), or those who carry the gene for a dominant disorder, that is one which does express itself in the heterozygous state, but in which symptoms occur in later life (e.g. Huntington's disease).

The general approaches to carrier state diagnosis are:

- detection of minor clinical, radiological, and clinicopathological abnormalities

- demonstration of levels of enzyme activity in tissue (e.g. leucocytes or cultured fibroblasts) which are intermediate between those observed in individuals homozygous for the abnormal and the normal forms of the enzyme respectively (the observed level of activity may not be exactly 50% of the normal value)
- demonstration of intermediate levels of a characteristic metabolite in an accessible body fluid
- demonstration of mosaicism with respect to the product of the mutant gene on the X chromosome in the case of sex-linked recessive disorders
- direct gene analysis using either a specific gene probe or a linked restriction fragment length polymorphism (RFLP)

The ability to recognize asymptomatic carriers of serious recessive diseases and presymptomatic individuals in the case of dominant disorders raises major ethical and social issues with respect to the psychological impact that this information will have on the affected individuals and their families. This is especially so with the clinically normal carriers of a crippling, lethal, and untreatable disease such as Huntington's disease.

In vitro fertilization and the inborn errors of metabolism

The human embryo produced by *in vitro* fertilization can be biopsied at a very early stage of development (i.e. at the eight-cell stage). A single cell is removed and examined for the DNA mutation responsible for the disease which the parents are known to be carrying. This enables only fertilized ova which do not carry the mutant gene to be implanted.

Animal genetic models of inborn errors of metabolism in humans

Animal models of the inborn errors of metabolism occur spontaneously and have been used in therapeutic research for many years; but the capacity to generate models of genetic disease by transgenic techniques has advanced this avenue of exploration. Not only do such models offer the hope of shedding important light on the mechanisms of disease, they have much to offer in the development of innovative treatments before attempting to transfer these to patients—now referred to as translational medical research. The discovery of embryonic stem cells in the mouse (see Chapter 4.7) and the ability to manipulate the mammalian genome by targeted homologous recombination has been instrumental in generating 'knock-out' models of human genetic diseases. Once the cognate nuclear gene of the mouse has been disrupted in embryonic stem cells, these cells are injected into the inner cell mass of individual host blastocysts. In a proportion of the resultant chimeric embryos, the embryonic stem cells harbouring the mutant locus contribute to the development of the gonads in the adult progeny; ultimately, when this is the case, offspring can be bred to homozygosity for the disrupted locus and studied. Refinements of this technology based on the use of regulatory sequences and tissue-specific promoter elements permit the target locus to be manipulated at will in the whole animal at a predefined stage of development by the administration of small molecules that bind to control elements (inducible knock-out model) or allow the genetic locus of interest to be deleted in particular tissues (conditional knock-out model). Murine and other living experimental models of human diseases are valuable in medicinal research but limitations to the methodology remain when cognitive and behavioural abnormalities are critical features of the clinical phenotype in patients; even with the constraints of recruitment in individually rare diseases, the experimental system by which innovative treatments are best tested for use in human patients, is the clinical trial.

Further reading

Alison MR, Islam S, Lim SM (2009). Cell therapy for liver disease. *Current Opinion in Molecular Therapy*, **11**, 364–74.

Altshuler D, Daly MJ, Lander ES (2008). Genetic mapping in human disease. *Science*, **322**, 881–8. [A powerful, comprehensive and up-to-date discussion of the foundations of disease mapping of mendelian and other traits.]

Bainbridge JWB, *et al.* (2008). Effect of gene therapy on visual function in Leber's congenital amaurosis. *N Eng J Med*, **358**, 2231–9. [Encouraging and well-studied gene therapy trial using rAAV vectors in a rare disease causing blindness—one of two back-to-back reports, this from the Institute of Ophthalmology in the United Kingdom (see Macguire below).]

Bearn, AG (1993). *Archibald Garrod and the individuality of man*. Oxford University Press, Oxford. [The definitive biography of Garrod—full of fascinating insights.]

Billings PR, Hubbard R, Newman SA (1999). Human germ line modification: a dissent. *Lancet*, **353**, 1873–5. [A critical review.]

Buckley B (2008). Clinical trials of orphan medicines. *Lancet*, **371**, 2051–5. [Survey of issues surrounding the development, testing and delivery of orphan drugs in Europe.]

Cartier N, Aubourg P, (2008). Haemopoietic stem cell therapy in Hurler's syndrome, globoid cell leukodystrophy, metachromatic leukodystrophy and X-adrenoleukodystrophy. *Current Opinion in Molecular Therapy*, **10**, 471–8. [Good evaluation of the pitfalls of a much-used transplantation strategy and its therapeutic position in lysosomal diseases with severe neurodegenerative features.]

Cartier N, *et al.* (2009). Haemopoietic stem cell therapy with a lentiviral vector in X-linked leukodystrophy. *Science*, **326**, 818–23. [Sentinel publication and study for a particular application of lentiviral vectors which have been modified to minimize the risk of transformation.]

Childs B (2004). A logic of disease. In Scriver CR *et al.* (eds) *Metabolic and molecular bases of inherited disease*, 8th edition. http://www.ommbid.com. McGraw-Hill, New York. [A brilliant analysis of Garrod's contribution and its implications for understanding human biology and medicine in evolutionary terms.]

D'Costa J, Mansfield SG, Humeau LM (2009). Lentiviral vectors in clinical trials: current status. *Current Opinion in Molecular Therapy*, **11**, 554–64. [Contemporary review of current use of these important vectors after long development.]

Endo A (2008). A gift from nature: the birth of the statins. *Nat Med*, **14**, 1050–2. [A modest but compelling account of this Lasker award-winning discovery and development of a major class of drugs, now used throughout the world but originally developed and tested in a patient with the extremely rare inborn error of metabolism—homozygous familial hypercholesterolaemia. A vindication of substrate reduction therapy and of the information obtained from the study of rare disorders.]

Enquist IB, *et al.* (2006). Effective cell and gene therapy in a murine model of Gaucher disease. *Proc Nat Acad Sci U S A*, **103**, 112–9. [A splendid example of an ingenious inducible and conditional murine model of Gaucher's disease—and its successful cure by gene therapy.]

Fan JQ (2003). A contradictory treatment for lysosomal storage disorders: inhibitors enhance mutant enzyme activity. *Trends Pharmacol Sci*, **24**, 355–60. [Development of the pharmacological chaperone concept.]

Fischer A, Cavazzano-Calvo M (2008). Gene therapy of inherited diseases. *Lancet*, **371**, 2044–7. [Contemporary appraisal supportive of recent developments in this tantalizing field ripe for clinical application.]

Gahl WA, Balog JZ, Kleta R (2007). Nephropathic cystinosis in adults: natural history and effects of oral cysteamine therapy. *Ann Intern Med*, **147**, 242–50. [Important account of an innovative and successful treatment that improves outcome and life quality in this challenging lysosomal transport defect.]

Garrod AE (1909). *Inborn errors of metabolism*. Oxford University Press, Oxford. [Essential source material.]

Garrod AE (1931). *The inborn factors in disease: an essay*. Clarendon Press, Oxford. [Deep insights from Garrod's many years of reflection on the problem of diathesis—'liability' to disease.]

Gooptu B, Lomas DA (2009). Conformational pathology of the serpins: themes, variations, and therapeutic strategies. *Annual Reviews in Biochemistry* **78**, 147–76. [Review of a particular class of protein aggregation disease and the challenges for treatment.]

Grabowski GA (2008). Phenotype, diagnosis, and treatment of Gaucher's disease. *Lancet*, **372**, 1263–71. [A moderately balanced account of developments in this rare disease in which a successful ultra-orphan treatment has been profitable, thus providing enhanced incentives for commercial therapeutic exploration.]

Grieger JC, Samulski RJ (2005). Adeno-associated virus as a gene therapy vector: vector development, production and clinical applications. *Advances in Biochemical Engineering and Biotechnology* **99**, 119–45. [Comprehensive review: the senior author was instrumental in developing these most promising non-pathogenic viruses as episomal vectors with distinct cellular tropisms for long-term transduction of non-mitotic cells and 'designer' applications.]

Haffner ME (2006). Adopting orphan drugs—two dozen years of treating rare diseases. *N Engl J Med*, **354**, 445–447. [The long journey to pharmaceutical exploration and development of treatments for rare diseases—of which, conventionally, inborn errors are a major component.]

Khanna A, *et al.* (1999). Liver transplantation for metabolic liver disease. *Surg Clin North Am*, **79**, 153–62. [Review concentrating on general principles as exemplified by hereditary haemochromatosis and Wilson's disease.]

Leonard JV, Schapira AHV (2000). Mitochondrial respiratory chain disorders. *Lancet*, **355**, 299–304; 389–94.

MacFarland R, Turnbull DM (2009). Batteries not included: diagnosis and management of mitochondrial disease. *Journal of Internal Medicine* **265**, 210–28. [Practical guidance for clinicians faced with these complex diseases.]

Maguire AM, *et al.* (2008). Safety and efficacy of gene transfer in Leber's congenital amaurosis. *N Engl J Med*, **358**, 2240–8. [Encouraging gene therapy trial using rAAV vectors in a rare disease causing blindness—one of two back-to-back reports, this one from the United States of America and Italy (see Bainbridge *et al.*, above).]

Phornphutkul C, *et al.* (2002). Natural history of alkaptonuria. *N Engl J Med*, **347**, 2111–2121.[The burden of alkaptonuria and early studies into its specific treatment.]

Reeve AK, Krishnan KJ, Turnbull DM (2008). Mitochondrial DNA mutations in disease, aging and neurodegeneration. *Annals of New York Academy of Sciences*, **1147**, 21–9.

Suwannarat P, *et al.* (2005). Use of nitisinone in patients with alkaptonuria. *Metabolism*, **54**, 719–728. [Substrate inhibition for the first reported inborn error of metabolism.]

Thomas CE, Erhardt A, Kay MA (2003). Progress and problems with the use of viral vectors for gene therapy. *Nat Rev Genet*, **4**, 346–58. [An excellent and detailed review.]

Vogler C, *et al.* (1998). Murine mucopolysaccharidosis VII: the impact of therapies on the clinical course and pathology in a murine model of lysosomal disease. *J Inherit Metab Dis*, **21**, 575–86.

Worgall S, *et al.* (2008). Treatment of late infantile neuronal ceroid lipofuscinosis by CNS administration of a serotype 2 adeno-associated virus expressing CLN2 cDNA. *Hum Gene Ther*, **19**, 463–74. [Recent trial of gene therapy in infants and children with a severe neurodegenerative disease.]

Zhang KY, Tung BY, Kowdley KV (2007). Liver transplantation for metabolic liver diseases. *Clinics in Liver Disease*, **11**, 265–81.

Zschocke J (2008). Dominant versus recessive: molecular mechanisms in metabolic disease. *J Inher Metab Dis*, **31**, 599–618. [Diverse mechanisms of inheritance associated with the clinical expression of inborn metabolic disorders.]

12.2

Protein-dependent inborn errors of metabolism

Georg F. Hoffmann and Stefan Kölker

Essentials

Protein-dependent inborn errors of metabolism are caused by inherited enzyme defects of catabolic pathways or intracellular transport of amino acids. Most result in an accumulation of metabolites upstream of the defective enzyme (amino acids and/or ammonia), causing intoxication.

Protein-dependent metabolic diseases usually have a low prevalence except for some high-risk communities with high consanguinity rates. However, the cumulative prevalence of these disorders is considerable (i.e. at least >1:2000 newborns) and represents an important challenge for all public health systems.

Types of protein-dependent inborn errors of metabolism

Amino acid disorders—enzyme deficiencies in the proximal part of amino acid catabolism result in accumulation of precursor amino acids which are detectable by ninhydrin (a chemical used to detect ammonia or primary and secondary amines) and thus are called amino acid disorders. Phenylketonuria (PKU) is the most frequent such condition in white people.

Organic acid disorders—distal enzyme defects of amino acid degradation result in pathological accumulation of organic acids but not the precursor amino acid. These disorders became detectable after the introduction of gas chromatography–mass spectrometry (GC/MS) and are called organic acid disorders.

Urea cycle defects—breakdown of amino acids results in the release of ammonia that is detoxified by the urea cycle, which is composed of five catalytic enzymes, a cofactor producer, and at least two transport proteins. The biochemical hallmark of urea cycle defects is hyperammonaemia.

Understanding of the protein-dependent inborn errors is based on the observation that some pathological metabolites impair key intracellular functions, such as energy metabolism, and thus when elevated may become toxic. These metabolites are excreted by urine or following conjugation to L-carnitine or L-glycine. However, in some diseases, such as disorders of tetrahydrobiopterin (BH_4) metabolism, clinical symptoms result from inadequate production of essential metabolites, such as the monoaminergic neurotransmitters.

Clinical presentation

Children with inherited disorders of amino acid, organic acid, or the urea cycle are usually born at term after an uneventful pregnancy and are initially asymptomatic. The onset of the first symptoms is varied, ranging from neonatal metabolic decompensation to onset of symptoms during adulthood. Irreversible organ damage and/or early death often follow if the diagnosis is delayed or missed. Metabolic decompensations in childhood are triggered by excess intake of protein and—most importantly—secondary to breakdown of body protein during episodes that induce catabolism.

Family history—if carefully taken, this may reveal important clues to the diagnosis of protein-dependent inborn metabolic errors. Most disorders are inherited as autosomal recessive traits, which may be suspected if the parents are consanguineous or the family has a confined ethnic or geographic background. Carriers for particular disorders and affected children may be more frequent in certain communities (e.g. Amish), ethnic groups (e.g. Ashkenazi Jews, Arabic tribes), or countries that have seen little immigration over many centuries (e.g. Finland). Specialist investigations are often started only after a second affected child is born into a family: older siblings may be found to suffer from a similar disorder as the index patient or have died from an acute unexplained disease.

Disease spectrum—this is broad, but follows a distinct pattern in specific disorders, for instance: (1) Untreated patients with classical PKU and cerebral organic acid disorders characteristically present with neurological symptoms. (2) Acute life-threatening decompensation is common in classical organic acid and urea cycle defects and maple syrup urine disorder; the young infant vomits or refuses to feed and then deteriorates rapidly. (3) Asymptomatic protein-dependent inborn metabolic errors are rare, but there are a few known enzyme defects, such as histidinaemia, which do not produce disease.

Investigation and management

Every infant presenting with symptoms of unexplained metabolic crisis, intoxication, or encephalopathy requires urgent evaluation of metabolic parameters, including analyses of arterial blood gases, serum glucose and lactate, plasma ammonia and amino acids, acylcarnitine profiling in dried blood spots, and organic acid analysis in urine.

Acute emergency therapy—basic principles are to (1) suppress muscle and liver protein catabolism and ensure a glucose supply above the basal metabolic demand; (2) treat the precipitating illness; (3) reduce increased production of toxic metabolites by reduction or omission of natural protein; (4) enhance detoxifying mechanisms and urinary excretion of pathological metabolites; (5) aggressively treat dehydration and acidosis; (6) prevent secondary carnitine depletion; (7) provide alternative routes of ammonia disposal in hyperammonaemia.

Long-term treatment—this aims principally to mitigate the metabolic consequences of enzyme deficiencies by compensating for them, including: (1) reduction of toxic metabolites by dietary restriction of precursor amino acids, prevention of catabolism, stimulation of residual enzyme activity and detoxification strategies; and (2) substitution with depleted substrates, such as biotin, cobalamin, or L-dopa. However, efficacy is often low in patients in whom diagnosis is made after the onset of symptoms, hence newborn screening programmes have been introduced in many countries, the criteria for implementation of which include: (1) reliable presymptomatic disease detection, (2) treatability of the disease, and (3) starting of treatment in presymptomatic children.

Successful treatment of affected individuals is often difficult to achieve. Careful supervision in metabolic centres involving an experienced multidisciplinary team is invaluable for the best outcome. Treatment is time- and cost-intensive, often lifelong, and mostly performed at home, hence regular training and support of patients and their families is essential to prevent irreversible complications. All patients should carry an emergency card that gives details of their condition and relevant contact numbers. Parent and patient organizations can offer useful support.

Detailed description of individual disorders is to be found in the text of this chapter, and further information on diagnosis, genetic testing, treatment and follow-up is available from several online databases (see 'Further reading').

Introduction

Humans depend on dietary protein as a source of amino acids; they are the metabolic basis of all functional and structural proteins in the body. Some amino acids—termed essential—cannot be synthesized by the human body, such L-isoleucine and L-phenylalanine. Renal conservation of amino acids is extremely effective, with clearance values mostly less than 1%. Stool nitrogen losses are about 1 g/day and are mostly of bacterial origin.

In contrast to glucose and fatty acids, amino acids taken in excess of requirement cannot be stored but are used for energy. The initial step of degradation is the removal of the amino group. Ammonia enters the urea cycle for conversion to urea. The remaining carbon skeletons are degraded via multistep individual pathways to central metabolic intermediates such as acetyl coenzyme A (CoA) or tricarboxylic acid cycle intermediates. Some enzymes require coenzymes, and inherited disease may be due to defects of the apoenzymes or their vitamin coenzymes, e.g. biotin, pyridoxine (vitamin B_6), or cobalamin (vitamin B_{12}).

Amino acids can be specifically detected by the ninhydrin reaction, which became available in the late 1940s, resulting in the identification of disorders such as phenylketonuria (PKU) or maple sugar urine disease. Breakdown of many amino acids occurs mostly intramitochondrially through degradation of CoA-activated carbonic acids, the so-called acyl-CoA compounds. These nonamino organic acids are not detectable by amino acid analysis. Since defects of the latter phases of amino acid degradation induce accumulation of organic acids but not amino acid precursors, these disorders became detectable after the introduction of gas chromatography, especially gas chromatography–mass spectrometry (GC/MS) in the 1960s and have been termed organic acid disorders. Thus the terminology amino acid and organic acid disorders is not based on pathophysiological differences but simply on the different analytical approaches.

Here amino acid disorders, urea cycle defects, and organic acid disorders are described; defects in mitochondrial metabolism and amino acid transport in the kidney tubule and small intestine are not considered.

Historical perspective

In 1902, Archibald Garrod introduced the term 'inborn errors of metabolism'. An extraordinary scientist and paediatrician, he used consanguinity and distribution of cases in families to introduce the hypothesis that autosomal recessive inheritance according to Mendel's rediscovered laws would explain the occurrence of the alkaptonuria phenotype, a defect in tyrosine degradation. Soon afterwards he also recognized albinism, cystinuria, and pentosuria as inborn errors.

Metabolic medicine is closely linked with advances in laboratory techniques. The use of paper chromatography by Bickel and Dent and of automated column chromatography by Moore and Stein opened the field of amino acid disorders. In the late 1960s, Tanaka discovered isovaleric aciduria by GC/MS, and this was followed by the identification of numerous organic acid defects. More recently the rise of molecular biology has revolutionized the field, and now tandem mass spectroscopy is proving a powerful tool in screening and diagnosis. Monogenic defects have been identified for almost every known enzymatic step of protein metabolism. Often it was the discovery of patients with enzyme defects which unravelled individual steps in human metabolism.

Until the early 1950s no treatment of any genetic disorder existed; destiny would take its course, and genetic counselling about recurrence risks was all that could be offered. That changed when, in 1953, Bickel showed that PKU is treatable and that early diagnosis and dietary treatment change the outcome from severe learning difficulties to normal psychosocial development. Subsequently, many other metabolic diseases became manageable in a similar way using the substrate deprivation strategy. Pharmacological doses of vitamins proved useful in defects of cobalamin and biotin metabolism, homocystinuria, and others. Simultaneously with the perception that identification of children before the onset of clinical symptoms was indispensable to improve the outcome, reliable and cheap screening methods have been developed. In the United States of America, Guthrie set the cornerstone for newborn screening by developing a bacterial inhibition assay to detect PKU. Despite early disagreement and resistance by the medical profession, newborn screening has proven its worth over the years and the test is still called the 'Guthrie test' worldwide.

In 1999, the World Health Organization announced orphan diseases as a major future health challenge. Among these diseases, disorders of amino acid and organic acid metabolism are especially important because of their cumulative prevalence (>1 in 2000 newborns) and because successful therapy is available. Inborn metabolic diseases have become a significant challenge for health care systems, particularly in countries where infectious diseases and other perinatal problems are receding in importance.

Aetiology, genetics, pathogenesis, and pathology

The clinical manifestations of most protein-dependent inborn errors is thought to result from toxicity of the accumulating key metabolites to specific organs inducing selective or multiple organ failure. This 'toxic metabolite hypothesis' has influenced research and allowed the development of effective treatment.

Despite increasing knowledge of pathophysiology the most relevant concepts are derived from clinical research. For example, defects of all six enzymes in the degradation pathway of phenylalanine and tyrosine are known (see also 'Defects of phenylalanine and tyrosine metabolism'). Defects in the first enzyme, phenylalanine hydroxylase, cause PKU (learning difficulties, seizures, ataxia, paresis, behavioural problems) and deficiency of tyrosine aminotransferase, the next enzyme, induces tyrosinaemia type 2 (corneal erosions, painful hyperkeratotic lesions, behavioural problems). A defect of 4-hydroxyphenylpyruvate dioxygenase is the cause of tyrosinaemia type 3 which is apparently a nondisease although a few patients develop neurological manifestations. A block in the next step of the pathway, 4-hydroxyphenylpyruvate dioxygenase, results in alkaptonuria (ochronosis, arthritis, heart disease), whereas deficiency of the last enzyme, fumarylacetoacetase, produces a disease deadly in early childhood, tyrosinaemia type 1, presenting with failure to thrive, liver failure, hepatosplenomegaly, hepatocarcinoma, and porphyria-like crises. The distinct syndromes resulting from defective breakdown of aromatic amino acids could never have been inferred simply by biochemical exploration of the metabolic pathway.

Epidemiology

As a group, protein-dependent disorders are by far the most common, acutely life-threatening inborn errors of metabolism (estimated prevalence >1 in 2000 newborns). However, reliable epidemiological data are scarce as all reports suggest a significant portion of patients who evade diagnosis and are considered to have neonatal sepsis or sudden infant death syndrome. All disorders can not be reliably ascertained clinically, and until recently population neonatal screening has only been implemented for PKU. Most epidemiological data are available from European countries, Japan, and the United States of America highlighting variations based on ethnic background, migrations, and/or genetic isolation. In a few communities, the prevalence of individual disorders may increase up to five times the cumulative prevalence of amino acid and organic acid disorders in European countries, Japan, and the United States of America. For example, glutaric aciduria type I is found in up to 1 in 300 newborns in the Amish Community (United States of America) and the Oji-Cree Indians (Canada), and in Qatar the prevalence of classic homocystinuria is 1 in 600 newborns.

Prevention

With the first successful treatment of a young girl with PKU the need for timely diagnosis and implementation of treatment became imperative. In most inborn errors affected neonates are completely asymptomatic, and onset of irreversible symptoms during infancy and childhood can often be prevented if treatment is started while the child is asymptomatic. Since inborn errors of metabolism are rare, only neonatal mass screening can guarantee timely detection. However, which diseases are the most appropriate for screening remains debatable. The criteria of Wilson and Jungner (1968) for an implementation to newborn screening include: (1) reliable disease detection in a presymptomatic state of the disease, (2) treatability of the disease, and (3) the start of treatment in the presymptomatic children. In the 1960s these criteria were achieved for PKU screening, which developed into one of the most important programmes of preventive medicine. Additional inborn errors such as maple syrup urine disease, galactosaemia, congenital hypothyroidism, and biotinidase deficiency were incorporated into the neonatal screening programme of some countries.

In the 1990s a revolutionary technology, tandem mass spectroscopy (MS/MS), was adopted for newborn screening. The possibilities of multianalyte detection by MS/MS led to a change in the screening paradigm, i.e. one test for many diseases (instead of one test for one disease). MS/MS improved screening for diseases from the conventional screening panels and opened the chance for inclusion of many other inborn errors of metabolism. However, each novel candidate disease has to be evaluated with respect to whether this disease fulfils the criteria for a disease to be screened (see Chapter 3.3.2), taking into consideration differences in national health care systems. As a consequence, the number of screened inborn errors of metabolism varies considerably ranging from 2 disorders (United Kingdom, Switzerland) up to more than 50 disorders (some parts of the United States). Notably, the United States screening panel also includes conditions that can be regarded as nondiseases or have at least a doubtful pathological meaning, such as the 3-methylcrotonyl CoA carboxylase deficiency. It should be appreciated that a liberal expansion of the screening panel burdens the health care system, the affected individuals, and the increasing number of false-positive individuals and their families. Given these difficulties, it is to be hoped that screening politics will become harmonized in a joint international effort.

Clinical considerations and diagnostic work-up

Family history

A careful family history may reveal important clues to the diagnosis of protein-dependent inborn metabolic errors. Most disorders are inherited as autosomal recessive traits which may be suspected if the parents are consanguineous or the family has a confined ethnic or geographic background. Carriers for particular disorders and affected children may be more frequent in certain communities (e.g. Amish), ethnic groups (e.g. Ashkenazi Jews, Arabic tribes), or countries that have seen little immigration over many centuries (e.g. Finland). Often specialist investigations are started only after a second affected child is born into a family. Older siblings may be found to have a similar disorder to the index patient, or to have died from an acute unexplained disease classified as 'sepsis with unidentified pathogen', 'encephalopathy', or 'sudden infant death syndrome'. Notably, the disease course of the same disorder may vary considerably even within families depending on genotype–phenotype correlation (if any), varying X-inactivation in female carriers (e.g. ornithine transcarbamylase deficiency), and dominant disorders with variable penetration (e.g. Segawa's disease).

As a result of the successful treatment of inborn errors of metabolism, an increasing number of affected women are reaching reproductive age. If they become pregnant, there may be a risk for their fetuses to be harmed by toxic metabolites from the mother. Especially important is maternal PKU, which is likely to become a major health problem. Other maternal conditions may cause 'metabolic' disease in the neonate or infant postnatally, e.g. methylmalonic aciduria and hyperhomocystinaemia, in fully breastfed children of mothers who have pernicious anaemia or who are on a vegan diet, which causes nutritional vitamin B_{12} deficiency.

Clinical spectrum

The range of clinical and biochemical manifestations of the protein-dependent metabolic errors is wide. Here we focus on the clinical manifestation and differential diagnosis of disorders presenting with acute metabolic decompensations (Boxes 12.2.1 and 12.2.2). There is only a limited repertoire of pathophysiological sequences in the response to metabolic intoxication and, consequently, a limited number of therapeutic measures. Timely and correct intervention during the initial episode is an important prognostic factor.

Many protein-dependent metabolic errors already manifest in the first days of life with progressive irritability or drowsiness. Most typically, a young infant may vomit or refuse to feed and then rapidly deteriorates. The initial erroneous diagnoses are usually neonatal sepsis or intracranial haemorrhage: a presumptive diagnosis of a protein-dependent inborn error should be considered with equal priority. Children with milder forms may be repeatedly admitted, e.g. with unusual metabolic acidosis, hypoglycaemia, or neutropenia in the course of common infections especially gastroenteritis, before an inborn disorder of metabolism is considered, and routine clinical chemistry may be normal in between crises.

A substantial number of patients with protein-dependent inborn errors of metabolism may present differently with acute encephalopathy or chronic and fluctuating progressive neurological disease. The so-called cerebral organic acidaemias (e.g. glutaric aciduria type I) characteristically present with (progressive) neurological symptoms such as ataxia, myoclonus, extrapyramidal symptoms, and metabolic stroke. Routine clinical chemistry is often unrevealing. Important diagnostic clues such as progressive disturbances of myelination, cerebellar atrophy, frontotemporal atrophy, hypodensities, and/or infarcts of the basal ganglia can be derived from MRI of the brain. Chronic subdural effusions, haematomas, and retinal haemorrhages in infants and toddlers are characteristic findings in glutaric aciduria type I, although they are more commonly due to child abuse.

Box 12.2.1 Presentation of organic acidurias

Intoxication

- Kussmaul tachypnea/ acidotic breathing
- Peculiar smell
- Refusal of/ adverse reaction to feeding
- Protracted episodic vomiting
- Erroneous diagnosis of pyloric stenosis (with acidosis)
- Reye's syndrome presentation
- Hepatomegaly/ liver failure
- Rhabdomyolysis
- Sudden infant death syndrome (SIDS) or 'near miss' SIDS

Acute encephalopathy

- Coma
- Seizures (myoclonic, intractable)
- Acute profound dyskinesia
- Pseudotumor cerebri
- Cerebral/intraventricular haemorrhage in full-term babies
- Stroke-like episodes

Chronic encephalo(myelo)pathy

- Progressive psychomotor deterioration
- Macrocephaly
- Ataxia (progressive)
- Hypotonia
- Dystonia, athetosis
- Myoclonus
- Seizures (myoclonic, intractable)
- Peripheral neuropathy
- Pyramidal signs—'cerebral palsy'
- Pronounced deficiency of speech
- Congenital cerebral malformations

Laboratory investigations

The early consideration of metabolic diseases is of the utmost importance. Basic evaluation of metabolic parameters including analyses of blood gases, serum glucose and lactate, plasma ammonia and amino acids, acylcarnitine profiling in dried blood spots (MS/MS), and organic acid analysis in urine (GC/MS) should be performed on an emergency basis in every patient presenting with symptoms of unexplained metabolic crisis, intoxication, or encephalopathy.

Routine laboratory parameters

Diagnostic clues can be obtained from routine laboratory investigations such as electrolytes (also required for the calculation of the anion gap), urinary ketones, serum transaminases, and creatine kinase.

Box 12.2.2 Clinical chemical indices of organic acidurias

- Metabolic acidosis
- Increased anion gap
- Hyperglycaemia
- Ketosis and ketonuria (especially suggestive in newborns)
- Lactic acidosis
- Hyperammonaemia
- Hyperuricaemia
- Hypertriglyceridaemia
- Increase of transaminases
- Granulocytopenia, thrombocytopenia, anaemia
- Hypoketotic hypoglycaemia (fatty acid oxidation defects)
- Increased creatine kinase (fatty acid oxidation defects)
- Myoglobinuria (fatty acid oxidation defects)

Any child admitted to an intensive care unit with life-threatening nonsurgical illness should be tested for these parameters.

Amino acid analysis

Many metabolic parameters show considerable diurnal fluctuations. For example, plasma amino acid concentrations are highly dependent on the metabolic status, and standard samples should be obtained at least 4 h postprandially. Many amino acids can be reliably quantified in dried blood spots by MS/MS, e.g. for PKU and maple sugar urine disease. Homocysteine and tryptophan require specific methods (usually high-performance liquid chromatography, HPLC) for exact quantification. Regular amino acid analyses are required in patients on specific dietary treatments to adjust intake of amino acids and to recognize a deficiency of essential amino acids and micronutrients. For optimal results it is important to separate plasma as soon as possible and to ship samples frozen on dry ice. Haemolysis or shipment of whole blood results in useless values for some amino acids. Some potential problems are summarized in Box 12.2.3.

Quantitative urinary amino acid analysis is indicated only if a renal tubular reabsorption defect such as cystinuria is suspected, and (in addition to plasma analysis) in hyperammonaemia when increased urinary excretion of specific metabolites (e.g. argininosuccinate) may be diagnostic.

Organic acid analysis

Organic acid analysis is best performed on early morning urine specimens. Complete information of the clinical status and recent management of the patient is indispensable for correct interpretation, which is based on key diagnostic metabolites or characteristic biochemical patterns. Repeated analyses may be necessary, preferably during exacerbation of metabolic decompensation, since analyses may be intermittently normal. Characteristic metabolites may, however, also become masked in severe metabolic decompensation and ketosis. Some patients with organic acid disorders may exhibit only slight elevations of diagnostic metabolites that may be underestimated by conventional analysis, such as in 4-hydroxybutyric aciduria, glutaric aciduria type I, and *N*-acetylaspartic aciduria. In these disorders, quantification by stable isotope dilution assays is preferred. This is also the method of choice for biochemical prenatal diagnosis of organic acid disorders in amniotic fluid, providing more rapid diagnosis than enzyme analysis of cultured amniocytes.

Box 12.2.3 Some pitfalls of amino acid analysis

- Shipping/storage without adequate cooling: ↓ glutamine, asparagine, cysteine, homocysteine; ↑ glutamate, aspartate
- Haemolysis: ↓ arginine, glutamine; ↑ aspartate, glutamate, glycine, ornithine
- Postprandial changes: all amino acids

Acylcarnitine analysis

A complementary and rapid diagnostic technique for some organic acid disorders is the analysis of acylcarnitine by MS/MS—by analogy to newborn mass screening—since accumulating acyl-CoA esters are in equilibrium with corresponding acylcarnitines.

Principles of treatment

General aspects

Protein-dependent metabolic disorders are chronic conditions that involve various organ systems and thus require a multidisciplinary approach to care and treatment. Patients with genetic diseases that are prone to acute decompensations should carry an emergency card. Vaccinations should be carried out as recommended and should also include vaccinations against varicella, hepatitis A, pneumococcus, and influenza. Special precautions must be taken before, during, and after surgery/anaesthesia.

Dietary treatment

In many protein-dependent errors of metabolism therapy is based on reduced intake of precursors in deficient pathways, prevention of catabolism, and an intensification of therapy during intercurrent illnesses. This aims to diminish the supply of toxic metabolites and restore energy supply. Dietary treatment must meet the general, age-dependent, and individual requirements for energy and essential nutrients to ensure normal growth and development (Table 12.2.1). Protein deficiency induces catabolism, failure to thrive, and growth retardation, and secondary depletion of essential amino acids and micronutrients may induce life-threatening complications such as lactic acidosis (thiamine or biotin depletion) or pellagra (niacin depletion). Supplementation of precursor-free mixtures of amino acids and semisynthetic supplements of minerals and trace elements minimizes the risk for malnutrition.

Pharmacotherapy

Carnitine at daily doses of 50–200 mg/kg body weight is essential for the elimination of accumulating toxic acyl-CoA compounds and for the restoration of intramitochondrial free CoA-SH in organic acid disorders. In cofactor-responsive disorders, enzyme activity may be restored by specific vitamins, e.g. in biotinidase deficiency, cobalamin-responsive methylmalonic acidurias, and riboflavin-responsive multiple acyl-CoA dehydrogenase deficiency. The accumulation of toxic metabolites derived from gut bacteria,

Table 12.2.1 Protein requirements

Age	Revised safe values (g/kg per day)
0–1 months	2.69
1–2 months	2.04
2–3 months	1.53
3–4 months	1.37
4–5 months	1.25
5–6 months	1.19
6–9 months	1.09
9–12 months	1.02
1–3 years	1.0–0.92
4–10 years	0.88–0.86
11–18 years	0.86–0.77

Data from Dewey KG, *et al.* (1996). Protein requirements of infants and children. *Eur J Clin Nutr*, **50** Suppl 1, S119–47.

such as propionic acid, can be reduced by intestinal antibiotics (e.g. metronidazole).

Emergency treatment

Treatment of intercurrent illness at home

Protein-dependent inborn errors of metabolism often present with acute life-threatening decompensation requiring prompt decisions and measures. A limited number of therapeutic measures have to be taken immediately (Box 12.2.4, Table 12.2.2).

It is imperative to decrease catabolism at an early stage of decompensation. As this usually happens at home, it is essential to educate the family adequately. Home treatment should include adequate control of fever and vomiting, moderate protein restriction, and ample calories, glucose, and fluid (Table 12.2.4). Intake of natural protein can be completely eliminated for the first 24 h of illness, especially if the patient receives precursor-free supplements of amino acids. After 24 h, stepwise reintroduction of natural protein is necessary to prevent protein catabolism. Immediate hospital admission and intravenous treatment is indicated when vomiting persists, fluid and dextrose intake remain poor, the clinical condition deteriorates, or the disease course is prolonged. On admission to hospital, these patients must be assessed and treated without delay. If emergency management is carried out in peripheral hospitals, this should ideally be supervised in consultation with a knowledgeable and experienced physician or paediatrician.

Box 12.2.4 Basic principles for acute emergency therapy

1. Suppress muscle and liver protein catabolism and ensure a glucose supply above the basal metabolic demand
2. Treat the precipitating illness
3. Reduce increased production of toxic metabolites by reduction or omission of natural protein
4. Enhance detoxifying mechanisms and urinary excretion of pathological metabolites
5. Aggressively treat dehydration and acidosis
6. Prevent secondary carnitine depletion
7. Provide alternative routes of ammonia disposal in hyperammonaemia

Table 12.2.2 Home and outpatient emergency treatment

A. Glucose polymer/maltodextrin solution[a]			
Age (years)	**%**	**kcal/100 ml**	**Daily amount**
0–1	10	40	150–200 ml/kg
1–2	15	60	95 ml/kg
2–10	20	80	1200–2000 ml/day
>10	25	100	2000 ml/day
B. Protein intake			
Natural protein	Stop (if amino acid supplements are administered) or reduce to 50% of maintenance therapy (if no amino acid supplements are administered). Reintroduce and increase within 1–2 days		
Amino acid mixtures	If tolerated, amino acid supplements should be administered according to maintenance therapy, e.g. 0.8–1.0 g/kg body weight/day[c]		
C. Pharmacotherapy			
L-Carnitine	Double carnitine intake: 200 mg/kg body weight/day orally (if tolerated)		
Antipyretics[b]	If temperature > 38.5°C, e.g. ibuprofen (10–15 mg/kg body weight per dose, 3–4 doses daily)		

[a] Maltodextran/dextrose solutions should be administered every 2 h day and night. If neonates and infants already receive a specific dietary treatment, protein-free food can be continued but should be fortified by maltodextran. Patients should be re-assessed every 2 h.

[b] Paracetamol administration may be dangerous in acute metabolic decompensation (risk for glutathione depletion).

[c] All calculations should be based on the expected weight, not the actual weight.

Emergency treatment in hospital

Provision of ample quantities and control of fluid and electrolytes is indispensable and must be continued before any laboratory results are available. Glucose infusions must be adapted to age to provide adequate energy supply. For example, in neonates glucose infusion is usually started at 10 mg/kg per min (i.e. 14.4 g glucose/kg body weight per day). Insulin drip may be necessary to prevent hyperglycaemia and to induce an anabolic state. Overhydration is rarely a problem in metabolic crises as they are mostly accompanied by dehydration. Electrolytes, glucose, lactate, and acid–base balance should be checked at least every 6 h and serum sodium should be maintained at no less than 138 mmol/litre. If lactate is constantly increasing while glucose supply is increasing, one should consider a primary defect or secondary inhibition or energy metabolism, such as in classic organic acid disorders. Antibiotics should be started if there is evidence for an infectious cause. Antipyretics should be administered liberally since they help to reduce the additional bioenergetic costs of fever.

Carnitine is essential for the elimination of toxic acyl-CoA esters in organic acidaemias, to prevent secondary carnitine depletion, and to replenish the intracellular CoA pool. Carnitine should be administered intravenously at 100 to 200 mg/kg per day. In hyperammonaemia, nitrogen-disposing drugs are used:

- Sodium benzoate, 250 mg/kg as bolus initially over 1 to 2 h, then 250 (to 500) mg/kg per 24 h.
- Sodium phenylacetate, 250 mg/kg as bolus initially over 1 to 2 h, then 250 (to 600) mg/kg per 24 h; alternatively, sodium phenylbutyrate at the same concentration is administered orally.
- Arginine hydrochloride, 420 mg/kg (i.e. 2 mmol/kg) as bolus initially over 1 to 2 h, then 420 mg/kg per 24 h.

If the response to emergency treatment is poor, the patient deteriorates, or the ammonia concentration exceeds 400 μmol/litre (neonate, infant) or 200 μmol/litre (child, adult), haemofiltration or haemodialysis should be urgently considered. If persisting lactic acidosis is present, thiamine (100–500 mg/day) and biotin (10–20 mg) should be given empirically.

Monitoring of treatment

Dietary treatment without adequate monitoring is dangerous since disease-specific complications, therapy-specific side effects (e.g. malnutrition), and developmental delay might be overlooked.

Anthropometric parameters such as weight, height, and head circumference should be recorded at each visit. Psychomotor development must be regularly assessed with appropriate tests. Weight loss or insufficient weight gain in affected children is often caused by inadequate dietary treatment and may herald impending metabolic decompensation.

The major aim of biochemical monitoring is to ensure that nutrition is not compromised. Biochemical evaluation includes blood count, serum electrolytes, calcium, phosphate, magnesium, ferritin level, liver and kidney function tests, alkaline phosphatase, total protein, albumin, prealbumin, transferrin, cholesterol, triglycerides, zinc, copper, retinol (plasma), carnitine, ammonia, lactate, and plasma amino acids. Although analyses of specific metabolic parameters are required to confirm the diagnosis of an inborn error of metabolism, these parameters are often not informative for biochemical follow-up monitoring since the relationship between the metabolic parameters and outcome is unclear for most disorders. However, regular monitoring of some metabolic parameters is necessary since they are directly related to the outcome. For example, plasma phenylalanine is monitored in PKU, plasma leucine in maple sugar urine disease, plasma glutamine and arginine in urea cycle defects, and plasma homocysteine in trans-sulphuration and remethylation defects.

Likely future developments

The scientific and technological advances described above have offered much benefit to patients with inborn errors of metabolism. To implement and utilize them properly, much remains to be done. Initially, metabolic physicians and scientists need to combine their efforts and concentrate on well-conducted international studies and development of evidence-based guidelines. Significant differences still exist in the diagnostic procedures, treatment, and monitoring of many diseases, resulting in a wide variation in outcome. Even for PKU, the disease with the greatest and longest experience in successful therapy, current international guidelines recommend different cut-offs for the indication of treatment ranging from 400 μmol/litre in the United Kingdom to 360 to 600 μmol/litre in the United States of America and 600 μmol/litre in France and Germany. The knowledge of the academic community must be combined and structured, transferred to the physicians and other medical staff, and implemented in health care systems. Nowadays, this process has become much easier by means of numerous recommendations, information, and even projects available on the internet, permanent professional e-mail round tables, internet editions of book and journals, and open-access databases. In the necessary implementation process, regional differences such as availability of funds, local pathology, and religious and geographic factors must be taken into account. Accordingly, specialized national metabolic centres and appropriate metabolic networks should be established and properly maintained. Unfortunately, novel diagnostic and therapeutic possibilities (Box 12.2.5), such as extended newborn screening or enzyme replacement therapy, are relatively expensive and are still unrealistic for many countries where there are no screening programmes and perhaps no well-organized health care system.

Individual disorders

A summary of protein-dependent inborn errors of metabolism including the enzyme defect, incidence, gene locus, EC number, and OMIM number is given in Table 12.2.3.

Urea cycle defects

Aetiology/pathophysiology

The major source of ammonia is catabolism of protein, which is detoxified to urea in the liver (Fig. 12.2.1). The efficiency of hepatic ammonia detoxification is enhanced through the action of glutamine synthase. Hyperammonaemia (plasma ammonia >80 μmol/litre in newborns; >50 μmol/litre after the newborn period) is caused by increased production (e.g. by intestinal urease-producing bacteria) or decreased detoxification of ammonia. Decreased detoxification results from inherited or acquired deficiency of key enzymes and transporters of the urea cycle, or bypassing of the liver (e.g. open hepatic duct). Secondary impairment of ammonia detoxification results from conditions where glutamate or acetyl-CoA are decreased, such as in organic acid defects, β-oxidation defects, carnitine depletion, or valproate therapy, or where toxic acyl-CoAs are increased, such as propionyl-CoA in

Box 12.2.5 New treatment strategies in inborn errors of metabolism

- Supplementation with end products
- Anaplerotic therapy
- Enzyme replacement
- Chemical chaperones
- Specific blockade of biosynthetic pathways
- Specific blockade of degradation pathways
- Specific blockade of pathophysiological signalling
- (Stem) cell therapy
- Gene therapy

Table 12.2.3 Summary of protein-dependent inborn errors of metabolism

Disease	Enzyme defect	Incidence*	Gene locus	EC number	OMIM
Defects of the urea cycle					
Argininaemia	Arginase I	1/100 000	6q23	3.5.3.1	207800
Argininosuccinic aciduria	Argininosuccinate lyase	1/50 000	7cen-q11.2	4.3.2.1	207900
Citrullinaemia	Argininosuccinate synthetase	1/50 000	9q34	6.3.4.5	215700
Deficiency of	Citrin	< 1/200 000	7q21.3		603471
Deficiency of	N-Acetylglutamate synthetase	< 1/200 000	17q21.3	2.3.1.1	237310
Deficiency of	Carbamoylphosphate synthetase I	1/50 000	2q35	6.3.4.16	237300
Deficiency of	Ornithine carbamoyltransferase	1/30 000	Xp21.1	2.1.3.3	311250
Dibasic amino aciduria II, lysinuric protein intolerance		< 1/200 000	14q11.2	SLC7A7 gene	222700
HHH syndrome	Ornithine transporter	< 1/200 000	13q14	SLC25A15	238970
Defects of branched chain amino acid metabolism					
Isovaleric aciduria	Isovaleryl-CoA dehydrogenase	1:80 000	15q14-q15	1.3.99.10	243500
Maple syrup urine	Branched chain keto acid dehydrogenase (lipoamide)	1:215 000			
	type Ia E1 component α-chain		19q13.1-q13.2	1.2.4.4 ODBA	248600
	type Ib component β-chain		6p21–22	1.2.4.4 ODBB	248611
	type II dihydrolipoamide branched chain transacylase (E2 component)		1p31	2.3.1.– ODB2	248610
3-Methylcrotonylglycinuria	3-Methylcrotonyl-CoA carboxylase	1:60 000		6.4.1.4	210200
	α-subunit		3q25-q27		
	β-subunit		5q12-q13		
3-Methylcrotonyl aciduria type I	3-Methylglutaconyl-CoA hydratase	< 1:200 000	9q22.31	4.2.1.18	250950
3-Methylglutaconic aciduria type II (Barth syndrome)	Tafazzin	< 1:200 000	Xq28	TAZ	302060 300069 300183
3-Methylglutaconic aciduria type III (Costeff optic atrophy)		< 1:200 000	19q13.2-q13.3	OPA3	258501
3-Methylglutaconic aciduria type IV		< 1:200 000			250951
2-Methyl-3-hydroxybutyryl-CoA deficiency	2-Methyl-3-hydroxybutyryl-CoA dehydrogenase	< 1:200 000	Xp11.2	1.1.1.178	300438
Methylmalonic aciduria(Mut^0/Mut$^-$ defects)	Methylmalonyl-CoA mutase	1:100 000	6p12.3	5.4.99.2	251000
Propionic aciduria	Propionyl-CoA carboxylase	1:200 000			
	α-chain		13q32	6.4.1.3	232000
	β-chain		3q21–q22	6.4.1.3	232050
Defects of lysine, hydroxylysine, and tryptophan metabolism					
2-Aminoadipic aciduria					204750
2-Oxoadipic aciduria					245130
Glutaric aciduria type I	Glutaryl-CoA dehydrogenase	1:100 000	19p13.2	1.3.99.7	231670
Gyrate atrophy of choroid and retina	Ornithine-oxoacid/ ornithine aminotransferase	< 1:200 000	10q26	2.6.1.13	258870
Hyperlysinaemia,	Saccharopine dehydrogenase/lysine:α-ketoglutarate reductase	< 1:200 000		1.5.1.7	238700
saccharopinuria,					247900
lysine intolerance					268700
Multiple carboxylase deficiency					
Biotinidase deficiency	Biotinidase	1:80 000	3p25	3.5.1.12	253260

(Continued)

Table 12.2.3 *(Cont'd)* Summary of protein-dependent inborn errors of metabolism

Disease	Enzyme defect	Incidence*	Gene locus	EC number	OMIM
Holocarboxylase synthetase deficiency	Holocarboxylase synthetase	<1:200 000	21q22.1	6.3.4.10	253270
Other organic acidurias					
N-Acetylaspartic aciduria (Canavan's disease)	Aspartoacylase; aminoacylaseII	<1:200 000	17pter-p13	3.5.1.15	271900
Ethylmalonic encephalopathy	Mitochondrial matrix protein	<1:200 000	19q13.2	ETHE1	602473
D-2-Hydroxyglutaric aciduria	D-2-hydroxyglutaric acid dehydrogenase	<1:200 000	2p25.3	D2HGD	600721
L-2-Hydroxyglutaric aciduria	FAD-dependent L-2-hydroxyglutarate dehydrogenase	<1:200 000	14q22.1	L2HGD	236792
Defects of phenylalanine and tyrosine metabolism					
Alkaptonuria	Homogentisate 1,2-dioxygenase	<1:200 000	3q21-q23	1.13.11.5	203500
BH$_4$ deficiency, dopa-responsive dystonia (dominant)	Guanosine-5-triphosphate cyclohydrolase	1:100 000	14q22.1-q22.2	3.5.4.16	128230
BH$_4$ deficiency					
Deficiency of	Dihydropteridinreduktase	<1:200 000	4p15.31	1.6.99.7	261630
Deficiency of	Guanosine-5-triphosphate cyclohydrolase	<1:200 000	14q22.1-q22.2	3.5.4.16	233910
Deficiency of	6-Pyruvoyltetrahydropterin synthase	<1:200 000	11q22.3-q23.3	4.6.1.10	261640
Deficiency of	Sepiapterin reductase	<1:200 000	2p14-p12	1.1.1.153	182125
PKU	Phenylalanine hydroxylase	1:10 000	12q24.1	1.14.16.1	261600
Type I	(Classical PKU = Phe > 1200 μmol/litre) ~ 50%				
Type II	(Mild PKU = 360–600 ≤μmol/litre ≤ Phe ≤ 1200 μmol/litre) *c.*30%				
Type III	(Non-PKU HPA/ MHP = Phe < 360–600 μmol/ litre) *c.*20%				
Types II+III	(BH$_4$-PAH = Phe < 1200 μmol/litre + BH$_4$-responsive) *c.*35%				
Primapterinuria dehydratase	Pterin-4α-carbinolamine	<1:200 000	10q22	4.2.1.96	264070
Tyrosinaemia type I	Fumarylacetoacetase	1:100 000	15q23-q25	3.7.1.2	276700
Tyrosinaemia type II	Tyrosine aminotransferase	<1:200 000	16q22.1-q22.3	2.6.1.5	276600
Tyrosinaemia type III	4-Hydroxyphenylpyruvate dioxygenase	<1:200 000	12q24-qter	1.13.11.27	276710
Neurotransmitter diseases and related disorders					
Deficiency of	Aromatic L-amino acid decarboxylase	< 1:200 000	7p11	4.1.1.28	608643
Deficiency of	Dopamine β-hydroxylase	< 1:200 000	9q34.3	1.14.17.1	223360
Deficiency of	GABA transaminase	< 1:200 000	16p13.3	2.6.1.19	137150
Deficiency of	3-Phosphoglycerate dehydrogenase	< 1:200 000		1.1.1.95	601815
Deficiency of	Tyrosine hydroxylase	< 1:200 000	11p15.5	1.14.16.2	191290
Folinic acid responsive seizures	Unknown	< 1:200 000			
4-Hydroxybutyric aciduria		< 1:200 000	6p22	1.2.1.16	271980
Hyperprolinemia type II	L-Δ^1-pyrroline-5-carboxylate dehydrogenase	< 1:200 000	1p.36		239510
Nonketotic hyperglycinaemia		1:60 000			
	H-protein deficiency		16q24	GCSH	238330
	P-protein deficiency		9p22	1.4.4.2	238300
	T-protein deficiency		3p21.2–21.1	2.1.2.10	238310
	Other				605899
	Transient				605899
Pyridoxal-phosphate- dependent epilepsy	Pyridox(am)ine 5′-phosphate oxidase	< 1:200 000	17q21.32		610090
Pyridoxine-dependent epilepsy	Piperideine-6-carboxylate dehydrogenase	< 1:200 000	5q31.2–3	ALDH7A1 gene	266100

(Continued)

Table 12.2.3 *(Cont'd)* Summary of protein-dependent inborn errors of metabolism

Disease	Enzyme defect	Incidence*	Gene locus	EC number	OMIM
Defects of trans-sulfuration and remethylation					
Deficiency of	Adenosyl-homocysteinase/S-adenosyl-homocysteine hydrolase	< 1:200000	20cen-q13.1	3.3.1.1	180960
Deficiency of	γ-Cystathionase	< 1:70000	16		219500
Deficiency of	Glycine *N*-methyltransferase	< 1:200000	6p12		606664
Deficiency of	Methionine adenosyltransferase I	< 1:200000	10q22	2.5.1.6	250850
Deficiency of	Methionine synthase reductase (cobalamin E)	< 1:200000	5p15.3-p15.2		236270
Deficiency of	Methionine synthase (cobalamin G)	< 1:200000	1q43	2.1.1.13	250940
Deficiency of	5,10-Methylene-tetrahydrofolatreductase	< 1:200000	1p36.3	1.5.1.20	236250
Homocystinuria	Cystathionine-β-synthase	1:100000	21q22.3	4.2.1.22	236200

*Incidences as estimated in the white population; they vary between populations of different ethnic background. < 1:200000 indicates incidence very low but uncertain because not specifically determined. Of some disorders only two or three families are as yet known worldwide.

BH_4-PAH, BH_4-responsive phenylalanine hydroxylase deficiency; Phe = phenylalanine; PKU, phenylketonuria.

propionic and methylmalonic aciduria or isovaleryl-CoA in isovaleric aciduria.

Hyperammonaemia is neurotoxic resulting in brain oedema, convulsions, and coma. Neuropathological evaluation reveals an alteration of astrocyte morphology including cell swelling (acute hyperammonaemia) and Alzheimer type II astrocytosis (chronic hyperammonaemia). Brain relies on energy-dependent glutamine synthesis by astrocytic glutamine synthase for the removal of excess ammonia. As a consequence, increased brain ammonia is considered to amplify glutamatergic signalling, redistribution of cerebral blood flow and metabolism, impairment of brain energy metabolism affecting the glutamate/glutamine cycle, and increased serotonin secretion. Hyperammonaemia exerts reversible (mostly serotoninergic) and irreversible effects. Blood ammonia concentrations exceeding 180 μmol/litre or a coma lasting more than 2 to 3 days appear to be associated with irreversible defects which worsen with the duration of the coma. All inherited urea cycle defects follow an autosomal recessive trait except for ornithine carbamylase deficiency which is X-linked.

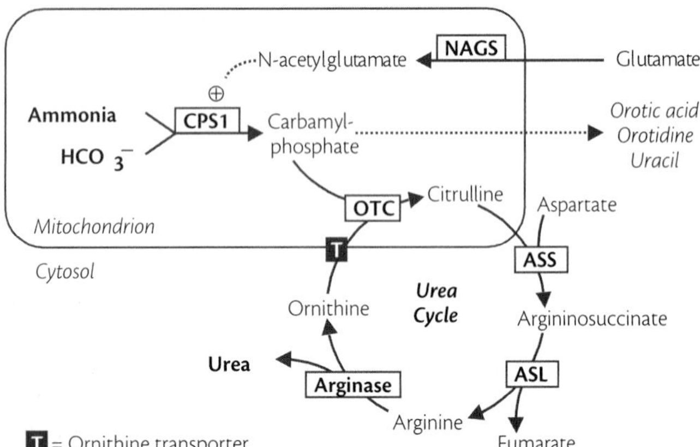

Fig. 12.2.1 The Urea Cycle. Abbreviations: CPS1, carbamylphosphate synthase; NAGS, N-acetylglutamate synthase; OTC, ornithine transcarbamylase; ASS, argininosuccinate synthase; ASL, argininosuccinate lyase; T, ornithine transporter. Adapted with permission from Zschocke and Hoffmann 2004.

Clinical presentation

Urea cycle defects are among the most common inborn errors of metabolism (cumulative incidence is approximately 1 in 30 000 newborns). Six inherited urea cycle defects are well described, i.e. deficiencies of *N*-acetylglutamate synthetase, carbamoyl-phosphate synthase, ornithine transcarbamylase, argininosuccinate synthetase and lyase, and arginase (Fig. 12.2.1). Deficiency of glutamine synthetase has also been identified but is not described here. Five urea cycle defects share a common but variable clinical presentation due to hyperammonaemia. Arginase deficiency and defects of cellular transport including transporter proteins for the dibasic amino acids ornithine (hyperornithinaemia–hyperammonaemia–homocitrullinuria (HHH) syndrome) and aspartate (citrullinaemia II) result in a more subtle disease with predominantly neurological symptoms.

Onset of symptoms may occur at any age; however, it is particularly frequent during the neonatal period, late infancy, and puberty, and is precipitated by excess protein or episodes that induce catabolism such as infectious diseases, trauma, or cortisone therapy. In general, symptoms are less severe with increasing age at onset. Neonatal presentation starts after a short asymptomatic interval with poor feeding, vomiting, lethargy, tachypnoea, and/or irritability which cannot be distinguished clinically from neonatal sepsis. Untreated, acute encephalopathy rapidly progresses to death. In infancy, the symptoms are less acute and more variable than in the neonatal period including anorexia, vomiting, developmental delay, and behavioural problems. In X-linked ornithine transcarbamylase deficiency, female carriers may also be affected due to variable inactivation of the X chromosome (the Lyon hypothesis). Clinical presentation ranges from acute hepatic failure, cognitive deficits, and behavioural problems to psychiatric disease. In arginase deficiency, patients usually present with progressive spasticity which is often mistaken for cerebral palsy, seizures, and learning difficulties. Dystonia and ataxia may develop. Acute decompensation occurs rarely.

Diagnosis

The emergency analysis of ammonia must be part of the basic investigations in all patients at all ages with unclear encephalopathy or acute hepatic failure.

Among the inherited hyperammonaemias, two-thirds are due to urea cycle defects and one-third to organic acid and other inborn errors. Blood gas analyses and anion gap determinations may show alkalosis and normal anion gap in urea cycle defects and acidosis and increased anion gap in organic acid disorders. Characteristic biochemical changes (glutamine, alanine, citrulline, ornithine, arginine, argininosuccinic acid, orotic acid, uracil) can be identified by plasma amino acid analysis, GC/MS analysis of urinary organic acids, or HPLC analysis of orotic acids and orotidine. The diagnosis can be confirmed by enzyme analysis in liver tissue (all urea cycle defects except for *N*-acetylglutamate synthetase deficiency), fibroblasts (argininosuccinate synthase and lyase), or molecular genetic studies. Prenatal diagnosis is possible. Autosomal recessive inherited urea cycle disorders can be identified by molecular genetic studies on chorionic villus biopsy. Enzyme analysis can be performed for deficiencies of argininosuccinate lyase and synthase. Arginase deficiency can also be diagnosed biochemically by fetal blood analysis.

Therapy and outcome

The aim of treatment is to correct the biochemical disorder (glutamine in plasma <800–1000 µmol/litre, ammonia <80 µmol/litre, arginine 80–150 µmol/litre) and to ensure the patient grows normally and thrives. The major metabolic strategies are: (1) reduction of natural protein to decrease ammonia production, (2) supplementation with essential amino acids to prevent malnutrition and to reutilize nitrogen for the synthesis of nonessential amino acids, (3) replacement of arginine or citrulline which become essential amino acids in all urea cycle disorders except for arginase deficiency, and (4) utilization of alternative pathways for nitrogen excretion. This last includes application of sodium benzoate (250–500 mg/kg per day) and sodium phenylbutyrate or phenylacetate (250–600 mg/kg per day) to conjugate glycine or glutamine, resulting in urinary excretion of waste nitrogen in alternative compounds (hippurate, phenylacetylglutamine). In *N*-acetylglutamate synthetase deficiency, *N*-carbamylglutamate can be used as an alternative allosteric activator of carbamoyl-phosphate synthase.

All patients with urea cycle defects are at risk of acute metabolic decompensation precipitated by metabolic stress such as protein load, infection, anaesthesia, or surgery. To prevent or reverse metabolic crises, a stepwise implementation of an intensified emergency treatment is required (see also 'Emergency treatment'). If diet and pharmacotherapy is insufficient to improve hyperammonaemia significantly and rapidly, haemofiltration or haemodialysis should be considered.

The main factors that determine outcome are not fully clear but duration and severity of hyperammonaemia are considered as most important. Thus a beneficial outcome critically relies on rapid diagnosis and immediate start of treatment after the onset of first symptoms. Furthermore, the prognosis is negatively correlated to the time of onset of first symptoms.

Defects of branched chain amino acid metabolism

Maple syrup urine disease

Maple syrup urine disease was first reported in 1954 by Menkes, Hurst, and Craig, who noticed an unusual odour reminiscent of maple syrup in the urine of four infants who died from a rapidly progressive neurological disease. In neonatal screening programmes a prevalence of approximately 1 in 200 000 newborns is encountered but in the Mennonites in Pennsylvania the prevalence is as high as 1 in 200. Maple syrup urine disease is frequent in other ethnic groups and isolates such as persons of French Canadian origin.

In maple syrup urine disease, the branched chain amino acids leucine, isoleucine, and valine, their corresponding α-keto acids and hydroxy acid derivatives as well as L-alloisoleucine are increased in physiological fluids. These amino acids and their metabolites accumulate due to inherited deficiency of the thiamine-dependent branched chain α-keto acid dehydrogenase complex, consisting of subunits $E_{1\alpha,\beta}$, E_2, and E_3 (Fig. 12.2.2). L-Alloisoleucine results from racemization of the 3-carbon of L-isoleucine during transamination. Its elevation is pathognomonic for maple syrup urine disease.

Presentation

Several clinical presentations have been delineated but there is considerable overlap in many patients, particularly if they survive. Most frequently the condition comes to light in the first few days of life with lethargy, irritability, poor feeding, and neurological deterioration. Later-onset forms of maple syrup urine disease are slower with failure to thrive, developmental delay, and sometimes seizures; episodic ataxia and stupor sometimes progressing to coma may be precipitated by high protein intake or intercurrent illness. In patients showing a response to thiamine, the condition tends to resemble later-onset maple syrup urine disease. A rare type of maple syrup urine disease due to deficiency of lipoamide dehydrogenase presents after the neonatal period with lactic acidosis, hypotonia, developmental delay, and abnormal movement with progressive neurological deterioration.

Most patients with maple syrup urine disease have the classic form. If untreated, these neonates quickly deteriorate, developing lethargy, hypotonia alternating with muscular rigidity, opisthotonic posturing, and seizures (Fig. 12.2.3). Despite giving its name to the disease, the characteristic odour may be absent. Neuroimaging shows localized or diffuse generalized cerebral oedema. Convulsions appear regularly and electroencephalography reveals abnormalities with comb-like rhythms (5–9 Hz) of spindle-like sharp waves over the central regions and multiple shifting spikes and sharp waves with suppression bursts. Untreated patients succumb within a few days. Prominent neuropathological signs of untreated maple syrup urine disease are cerebral atrophy, including neuron loss in pontine nuclei and the thalamus and myelin deficiency; spongy degeneration and astrocytic hyperplasia occur. Hypodensities may be present in globus pallidus and thalamus. In a few patients, mostly with intermittent or intermediate variants, the metabolic defect can be corrected by thiamine ('thiamine-responsive' variant). Effective doses vary from 10 mg up to 300 mg per day.

Diagnosis

Maple syrup urine disease is strongly suggested when an odour of maple syrup is present (most noticeably in the ear). Immediate confirmation by positive 2,4-dinitrophenylhydrazine testing is sufficient justification to initiate treatment in families at high risk. Diagnosis is confirmed by detection of increased plasma concentrations of leucine, isoleucine, and valine and/or by increased urinary excretion of α-keto and hydroxy acids. The detection of L-alloisoleucine is pathognomonic. Reduced enzyme activity of the branched chain α-keto acid dehydrogenase complex in leucocytes, lymphoblasts, cultured fibroblasts, or amniocytes confirms the diagnosis. Except for the common Mennonite mutation, the molecular genetics of maple syrup urine disease are too complex

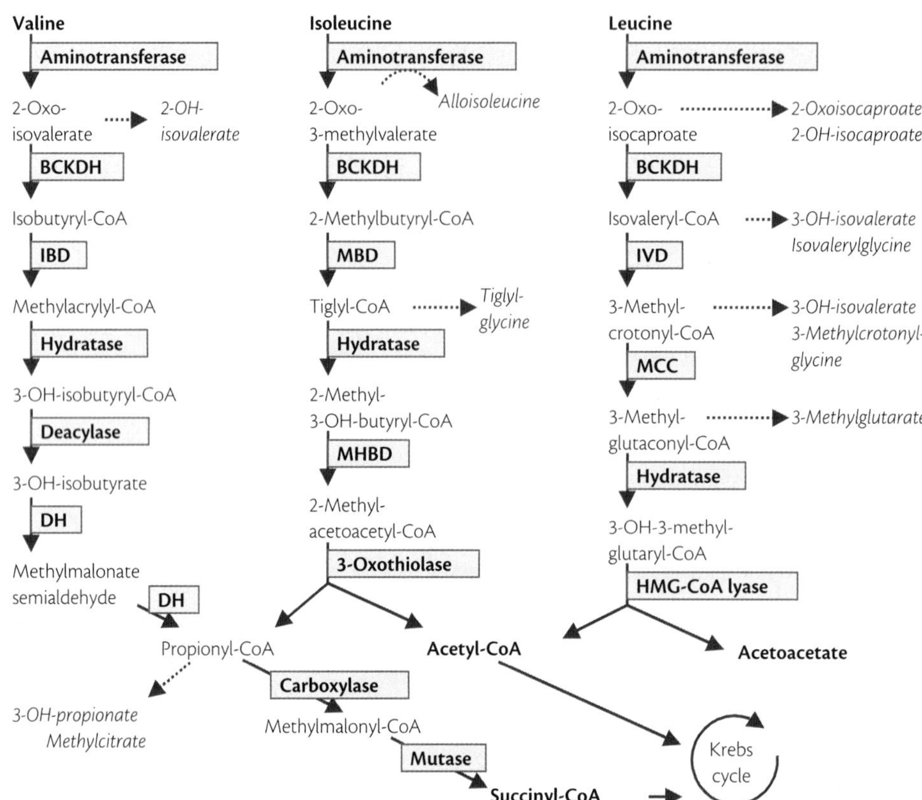

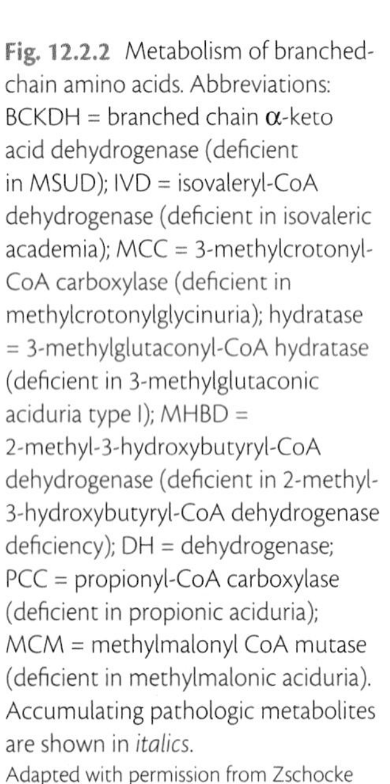
Fig. 12.2.2 Metabolism of branched-chain amino acids. Abbreviations: BCKDH = branched chain α-keto acid dehydrogenase (deficient in MSUD); IVD = isovaleryl-CoA dehydrogenase (deficient in isovaleric academia); MCC = 3-methylcrotonyl-CoA carboxylase (deficient in methylcrotonylglycinuria); hydratase = 3-methylglutaconyl-CoA hydratase (deficient in 3-methylglutaconic aciduria type I); MHBD = 2-methyl-3-hydroxybutyryl-CoA dehydrogenase (deficient in 2-methyl-3-hydroxybutyryl-CoA dehydrogenase deficiency); DH = dehydrogenase; PCC = propionyl-CoA carboxylase (deficient in propionic aciduria); MCM = methylmalonyl CoA mutase (deficient in methylmalonic aciduria). Accumulating pathologic metabolites are shown in *italics*.

Adapted with permission from Zschocke and Hoffmann 2004.

for diagnostic use. Prenatal testing is available by enzymatic analysis of amniotic cells.

Treatment and outcome

Emergency treatment aims to reduce branched chain amino acids, particularly leucine. To induce anabolism, high calorie intake is required. Most importantly, glucose stimulates endogenous insulin secretion activating protein synthesis. If required, insulin should be started early. In parallel, supplements free of branched chain amino acids should be administered by nasogastric drip feeding. Since low plasma concentrations of isoleucine and valine limit protein synthesis, cautious supplementation to decrease leucine concentrations may be required.

Extracorporeal detoxification (haemodialysis, haemofiltration) may be required if leucine exceeds 20 mg/dl (1500 μmol/litre). Liver transplantation may be considered a reasonable treatment option for patients with classic maple syrup urine disease. The decision of medical treatment vs transplantation, however, is very complex and must be reached for each patient individually.

Long-term treatment of maple syrup urine disease is based on dietary restriction of branched chain amino acids and supplementation of thiamine, if proven beneficial. Management requires close and lifelong regulation of diet.

Children with the classic form of maple syrup urine disease have a satisfactory prognosis only if they are diagnosed and treated before symptom onset; for this reason MS/MS-based newborn screening has been introduced in some countries.

Isovaleric aciduria

Aetiology/pathophysiology

Isovaleric aciduria was described by Tanaka in 1966. It is caused by deficiency of isovaleryl-CoA dehydrogenase, an enzyme located proximally in the catabolic pathway of the essential branched chain amino acid leucine (Fig. 12.2.2). The encoding *IVD* gene is localized on 15q14–q15. Due to the metabolic block, isovaleryl-CoA accumulates, and the pathognomonic metabolite isovalerylglycine is formed by conjugation of isovaleryl-CoA to the amino group of glycine through the activity of the mitochondrial enzyme glycine-*N*-acylase. It is suggested that accumulating acyl-CoA esters sequester CoA, thereby disturbing energy metabolism. Specifically, isovaleryl-CoA inhibits pyruvate dehydrogenase and *N*-acetylglutamate synthetase causing lactic acidosis and hyperammonaemia. Furthermore, isovaleric acid inhibits granulopoiesis and occurs during metabolic decompensations.

Clinical presentation

Half of the patients with isovaleric aciduria present in the neonatal period with severe metabolic crises that may lead to coma and

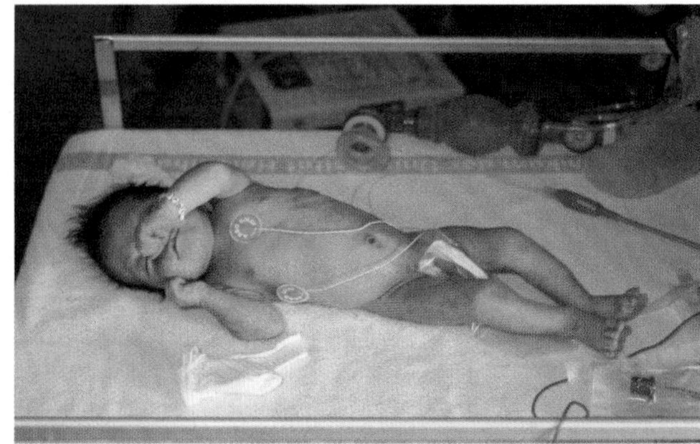
Fig. 12.2.3 Opisthotonic hypertonic comatose infant with MSUD.

death, whereas the remainder experience chronic intermittent disease with episodes of metabolic acidosis and psychomotor retardation. Both phenotypes can occur within the same family suggesting a modifying role of environmental and epigenetic factors. A mild, potentially asymptomatic phenotype exists due to a common mutation (932C-T; A282V). This mutation was detected in one-half of mutant alleles in patients identified by newborn screening and also in older, healthy siblings.

During metabolic crisis patients present with the typical features of classic organic acid disorders, i.e. acidosis, ketosis, vomiting, progressive alteration of consciousness, and, finally, overwhelming illness, deep coma, and death if not given appropriate therapy. Clinical abnormalities often develop within the first days of life. A pathognomonic foul odour reminiscent of sweaty feet, caused by isovaleric acid, occurs. Abnormalities of the haematopoietic system such as thrombocytopenia, neutropenia, or pancytopenia develop; hyperammonaemia is usually mild.

In the chronic intermittent form, children slide into recurrent metabolic crises because of high intake of protein or minor infections inducing a catabolic state. Cytopenias develop as described above, and hyperglycaemia may develop, most likely due to stress-induced counter-regulatory hormonal effects. Pancreatitis may be a complication of isovaleric aciduria. Older patients may have normal psychomotor development or mild to severe learning difficulties, depending on the frequency of decompensation and the age of diagnosis and institution of treatment.

Diagnosis

The clinical symptoms of isovaleric aciduria resemble other organic acidaemias; even the suggestive odour may be shared by similar disorders (see Boxes 12.2.1 and 12.2.2). The combination of ketoacidosis, dehydration, and hyperglycaemia has led to erroneous diagnosis of diabetic ketoacidosis, and persistent vomiting in infancy to the wrong suggestion of hypertrophic pyloric stenosis and unnecessary surgery. A reliable way to accomplish the diagnosis is quantitative analysis of urinary organic acids and acylglycines by GC/MS or the analysis of acylcarnitine profiles by MS/MS.

During metabolic decompensation, the urinary organic acid profile reveals high excretion of isovalerylglycine which remains elevated. 3-Hydroxyisovaleric acid only increases during metabolic decompensation. Isovalerylcarnitine is the characteristic acylcarnitine of this disease and its urinary excretion increases following supplementation with L-carnitine. The diagnosis of isovaleric aciduria can be confirmed by enzyme analysis in fibroblasts or mutation analysis in specialized laboratories. Several methods have been successfully used for prenatal diagnosis including stable isotope dilution analysis of isovalerylglycine, MS/MS detection of isovalerylcarnitine in amniotic fluid, or macromolecular labelling from (1–^{14}C)-isovaleric acid in cultured amniocytes. Molecular diagnosis is only available in a research setting.

Treatment and outcome

Total natural protein intake is restricted according to the patient's leucine tolerance and is adjusted to age-specific requirements. To provide a complementary source of the other amino acids, a leucine-free formula is available. Beyond childhood, a protein-restricted diet allowing a moderate restriction of leucine intake is usually sufficient. In addition, urinary excretion of isovaleryl-CoA as nontoxic glycine and carnitine conjugates is activated by supplementation with carnitine (50–100 mg/kg per day) and glycine (150 mg/kg per day). The glycine dosage can be augmented up to 600 mg/kg per day during metabolic crisis.

During acute decompensation, isovaleric aciduria is treated following the general principles for other organic acid disorders (see 'Emergency treatment', above).

Aspirin is contraindicated in patients with isovaleric aciduria because salicylic acid is a competing substrate for glycine-*N*-acylase, interfering with isovalerylglycine synthesis.

Most children will survive the first life-threatening episode if correct treatment is set in place early. If efficient treatment can be installed before any severe metabolic decompensation, it will significantly improve outcome. Therefore, in some countries isovaleric aciduria is screened for in newborns using MS/MS.

3-Methylcrotonylglycinuria

3-Methylcrotonylglycinuria is an inborn error of leucine catabolism due to deficiency of 3-α-methylcrotonyl-CoA carboxylase (Fig. 12.2.2). It appears to be the most frequent inborn organic acid disorder, with a frequency of 1 in 50 000 newborns. The 3-methylcrotonylglycinuria enzyme requires biotin as a cofactor, and the isolated enzymatic defect must be differentiated from primary deficiencies in the biotin pathway (see 'Biotinidase deficiency' and 'Holocarboxylase synthetase deficiency'). As a consequence of 3-methylcrotonylglycinuria deficiency, 3-hydroxyisovaleric acid, 3-hydroxyisovalerylcarnitine, 3-methylcrotonylcarnitine, and 3-methylcrotonylglycine accumulate.

Clinical presentation

From the follow-up of individuals identified by newborn screening it has become evident that deficiency of 3-methylcrotonylglycinuria is a genetic condition with low clinical expressivity and penetrance, representing largely (*c.*90%) a nondisease. Less than 10% of affected individuals may develop mostly mild neurological symptoms which are often not clearly attributed to 3-methylcrotonylglycinuria deficiency. However, a few patients may develop acute metabolic decompensation (ketoacidosis, hypoglycaemia, hyperammonaemia, Reye-like syndrome) precipitated by febrile illness during infancy; this may be fatal if untreated.

Diagnosis

The diagnosis is confirmed biochemically by identification of 3-hydroxyisovaleric acid and 3-methylcrotonylglycine in urine (GC/MS) or 3-hydroxyisovalerylcarnitine in dried blood spots or plasma (MS/MS). Notably, elevations of 3-hydroxybutyric acid can also be seen in ketotic patients or secondary to valproate treatment, whereas in patients with additionally increased 3-hydroxypropionic, methylcitric, or lactic acids multiple carboxylase deficiency or biotinidase deficiency should be considered. In particular, 3-hydroxyisovalerylcarnitine concentrations which spontaneously decrease to normal values in follow-up investigations of any neonate should prompt the investigation of 3-methylcrotonylglycinuria deficiency in the mother.

Significantly reduced enzyme activity in fibroblasts or leucocytes confirms the diagnosis. It is important to exclude multiple carboxylase deficiency by demonstrating normal enzyme activities of propionyl-CoA carboxylase, pyruvate carboxylase, as well as biotinidase. Prenatal diagnosis is possible by stable isotope dilution analysis of amniotic fluid or by enzymatic and molecular analyses in cultivated amniocytes or chorionic villi.

Treatment and outcome

Most affected individuals do not require specific treatment, with the exception of carnitine supplementation if secondary carnitine depletion is found. However, moderate protein restriction and administration of leucine-free amino acid supplements has been tried. 3-Methylcrotonylglycinuria is usually unresponsive to biotin whereas, in those with the R385S mutation, biotin responsiveness has been reported. If acute metabolic decompensation occurs, affected patients are treated as with other organic acid disorders (see 'Emergency treatment' above). Most affected individuals remain asymptomatic without specific treatment and thus the benefit of newborn screening remains to be elucidated.

3-Methylglutaconic acidurias

Increased urinary excretion of 3-methylglutaconic acid is the biochemical hallmark of a heterogeneous group of inborn errors termed 3-methylglutaconic acidurias types I to IV. Increased urinary concentrations of 3-methylglutaconic acid are also found in patients with primary mitochondrial disorders, e.g. Pearson's syndrome and ATP synthase deficiency, and in plasma of patients with Smith–Lemli–Opitz syndrome.

3-Methylglutaconic aciduria type I

Aetiology/pathophysiology 3-Methylglutaconic aciduria type I is caused by deficiency of 3-methylglutaconyl-CoA hydratase (Fig. 12.2.2) required for the conversion of 3-methylglutaconyl-CoA to 3-hydroxy-3-methylglutaryl-CoA in leucine catabolism. The hydratase is identical to an RNA-binding protein (designated AUH) possessing enoyl-CoA hydratase activity. The defect leads to an accumulation of 3-methylglutaconic, 3-methylglutaric, and 3-hydroxyisovaleric acids.

Clinical presentation The clinical phenotype of affected individuals is variable and also includes asymptomatic disease course. Patients present with neurological symptoms including delayed speech and motor development. Metabolic decompensation with hypoglycaemia and metabolic acidosis is rare but can occur following catabolic state.

Diagnosis Urinary excretion of large amounts of 3-methylglutaconic, 3-methylglutaric, and 3-hydroxyisovaleric acids but normal excretion of 3-hydroxy-3-methylglutaric acid points to hydratase deficiency. Increased 3-hydroxyisovalerylcarnitine is a hint for either type of 3-methylglutaconic aciduria. The definitive diagnosis is made by enzyme analysis in fibroblasts or by mutation analysis.

Treatment and outcome The need for treatment has not been established, especially for dietary treatment. The outcome appears favourable as a significant number of untreated patients have never developed symptoms.

3-Methylglutaconic aciduria type II: Barth's syndrome

Aetiology/pathophysiology The molecular basis of Barth's syndrome is deficiency of tafazzin which is localized in the inner mitochondrial membrane affecting phospholipid metabolism, in particular cardiolipin. The origin of elevated levels of 3-methylglutaconic and 3-methylglutaric acids in Barth's syndrome is unknown.

The identification of the causative gene allowed the retrospective classification of different families labelled in the past as X-linked endocardial fibrosis, severe X-linked cardiomyopathy, or Barth's syndrome. All these entities have been shown to share the same molecular pathology.

Clinical presentation In 1983, Barth and colleagues described an X-linked neuromuscular disease characterized by dilated cardiomyopathy, skeletal myopathy, retarded growth, and neutropenia. Patients may present at birth or during the first weeks of life, usually with congestive cardiac failure. With long-standing cardiac disease endocardial fibroelastosis may develop. Delayed gross motor milestones, myopathic facies, a waddling gait, and a positive Gower's sign are common. Occasionally patients may show moderate lactic acidosis. Postnatal growth retardation may be severe, and beyond 2 years of age patients are usually very stunted but with normal head circumferences.

Diagnosis Barth's syndrome should be considered in any male presenting with dilated cardiomyopathy. If neutropenia, idiopathic myopathy, and growth retardation are also present, the diagnosis of Barth's syndrome is almost certain. Biochemically, increased 3-methylglutaconic acid is usually found in urine but is not a constant feature. 2-Ethylhydracrylic acid may be also elevated. Muscle disease and lactic acidaemia may initiate a work-up for mitochondrial disorders. Muscle biopsy may reveal involvement of deficient respiratory chain complex I and IV. The diagnosis is confirmed by cardiolipin analysis in thrombocytes or mutation analysis. Mutation analysis makes prenatal diagnosis now available.

Treatment and outcome Children affected by Barth's syndrome need to be carefully managed mainly by expert cardiologists; immunologists and neurologists should also be involved. Cardiac arrhythmias carry a poor prognosis and may require implantation of an internal cardiac defibrillator. Successful heart transplantation has been carried out. Due to increased susceptibility to severe bacterial infections, infectious diseases need to be treated promptly and aggressively. Protein restriction and carnitine supplementation has been employed with unclear benefit. About 25% of patients with Barth's syndrome succumb during infancy and early childhood due to cardiac complications or overwhelming bacterial infections.

3-Methylglutaconic aciduria type III: Costeff's syndrome

Aetiology/pathophysiology Costeff's syndrome is caused by mutations in the *OPA3* gene resulting in a defect of a putative mitochondrial protein with yet unknown function. The origin of elevated levels of 3-methylglutaconic and 3-methylglutaric acids is also unknown. So far the disorder has only been reported in Iraqi Jews.

Clinical presentation The determining clinical presentation is early onset optic atrophy, which may be accompanied by nystagmus. In later childhood or adolescence, patients may develop extrapyramidal signs and moderate cognitive impairment. In about one-half of the patients spasticity develops and progresses over years.

Diagnosis Costeff's syndrome should be suspected in patients presenting with early onset optic atrophy if additional neurological symptoms develop. 3-Methylglutaconic aciduria is a biochemical indicator of Costeff's syndrome, which may now be proven by molecular analysis.

Treatment and outcome Effective treatment has not been reported. Treatment is symptomatic and focuses on the prevention of disabilities due to progressive spasticity. The disease appears stationary but the long-term outcome is unknown.

3-Methylglutaconic aciduria type IV: unclassified

Aetiology/pathophysiology 3-Methylglutaconic aciduria type IV is undoubtedly heterogeneous. As unexplained 3-methylglutaconic aciduria, i.e. type IV, was also found incidentally in asymptomatic adults, it appears doubtful that this biochemical feature by itself is of pathophysiological relevance.

Diagnosis Patients are identified by elevated urinary concentrations of 3-methylglutaconic and 3-methylglutaric acids. Classification of type IV methylglutaconic aciduria is made by exclusion of known causes of 3-methylglutaconic aciduria (see above), primary mitochondrial disorders (e.g. Pearson's syndrome), and Smith–Lemli–Opitz syndrome.

Treatment and outcome No effective treatment has been reported. Treatment is symptomatic and focuses on the prevention of neurological deterioration. The identification of type IV 3-methylglutaconic aciduria is not yet of prognostic relevance.

2-Methyl-3-hydroxybutyryl-CoA dehydrogenase deficiency

Aetiology/pathophysiology

2-Methyl-3-hydroxybutyryl-CoA dehydrogenase deficiency is a rare cerebral organic acid disorder. This mitochondrial enzyme is involved in the catabolism of isoleucine and branched chain fatty acids (Fig. 12.2.2). Retrospectively, patients were misdiagnosed as having 3-oxothiolase deficiency until Zschocke and colleagues (2000) recognized the separate distinct clinical and biochemical presentation. Inheritance is X-chromosomal semidominant (females may be symptomatic). Disease-causing mutations were identified in the *HSD17B10* gene. The pathophysiology of this disease is unknown. The enzyme is identical to an amyloid β-peptide-binding protein which is implicated in Alzheimer's disease.

Clinical presentation

2-Methyl-3-hydroxybutyryl-CoA dehydrogenase deficiency mostly results in a progressive neurodegenerative disease. Regression usually becomes obvious in late infancy or early childhood but is variable. Affected boys usually develop truncal hypotonia with spasticity of the limbs, dyskinesia and athetosis, a horizontal nystagmus, and retinal blindness. Motor and mental skills are completely lost, as are sensory modalities. Epilepsy is frequently found and is usually difficult to treat. When hypertrophic cardiomyopathy was diagnosed, deterioration was rapid with death due to progressive heart failure. Neuroimaging documents progressive generalized atrophy, basal ganglia injury, periventricular white matter abnormalities, and occipital infarctions in individual cases. Heterozygous female patients may be asymptomatic or may have variable stationary psychomotor retardation with impaired hearing.

Diagnosis

The disease should be considered in children presenting with early-onset progressive encephalopathy, especially if X-linked inheritance is suggested. The biochemical hallmark of this disease is increased urinary excretion of 2-methyl-3-hydroxybutyric acid and tiglylglycine. Elevations of 2-ethylhydracrylic acid and 3-hydroxyisobutyric acid in urine may also be found. These abnormalities may be subtle.

Treatment and outcome

No effective rationale treatment is known. Care of patients with this disease should repeatedly entail: (1) assessment of muscle and cardiac function, (2) neurological examination including EEG and MRI, and (3) assessment of visual and hearing system. The prognosis is mostly poor, with death in early childhood.

Propionic aciduria

Aetiology/pathophysiology

In 1961, Childs and co-workers described the index patient with propionic aciduria. Since ketosis and hyperglycinaemia were the biochemical hallmarks recognized, the disorder was lumped together with methylmalonic acidurias as 'ketotic hyperglycinaemia' to distinguish it from nonketotic hyperglycinaemia. Implementation of GC/MS analysis to metabolic diagnostic work-up allowed the differentiation of these disorders in the 1970s. Propionic aciduria is caused by an autosomal recessive inherited deficiency of biotin-dependent duodecameric propionyl-CoA carboxylase, the first step in propionate metabolism, in which propionyl-CoA is converted to methylmalonyl-CoA (Fig. 12.2.2). Over 100 disease-causing mutations have been identified in the *PCCA* gene (13q32) and the *PCCB* gene (3q21–22).

Propionyl-CoA is formed from the catabolism of isoleucine, threonine, methionine, valine, odd-numbered fatty acids, and the side chain of cholesterol, and from gut bacteria. Deficiency of propionyl-CoA carboxylase gives rise to accumulation of propionyl-CoA and metabolites of alternative propionate oxidation such as 2-methylcitric acid, 3-hydroxypropionic acid, tiglic acid, propionylcarnitine, and propionylglycine. All of these can be detected and quantified by GC/MS (urine, plasma) or MS/MS (dried blood spots, plasma).

Elevated propionyl-CoA and its pathological derivatives interfere with a variety of metabolic pathways including inhibition of: (1) the glycine cleavage enzyme resulting in hyperglycinaemia, (2) *N*-acetylglutamate synthase resulting in hyperammonaemia, and (3) pyruvate dehydrogenase complex as well as several enzymes of the tricarboxylic acid cycle resulting in lactic acidaemia and hyperketosis, and severe impairment of energy metabolism.

Clinical presentation

Propionic aciduria usually presents with severe neonatal metabolic decompensation characterized clinically by multiorgan failure and biochemically by hyperammonaemia, metabolic acidosis, hyperketosis, lactic acidaemia, hyperglycinaemia, and hyperalaninaemia. Propionic aciduria may be misinterpreted as sepsis or ventricular haemorrhage. Acute metabolic decompensation and long-term complications usually involve organs with a high energy demand, including the brain, heart and skeletal muscle, liver, and bone marrow. Frequent signs and symptoms are failure to thrive, microcephaly, mild to severe motor disabilities and learning difficulties, truncal hypotonia, extrapyramidal symptoms (dystonia, chorea), seizures, cardiomyopathy, myopathy, hepatomegaly, acute or chronic pancreatitis, leucopenia, thrombocytopenia, anaemia, or pancytopenia, whereas renal complications are uncommon. Metabolic decompensations in infancy or childhood are similar to those in the neonatal period. The first symptom is often vomiting; this has led to erroneous diagnosis of pyloric stenosis or duodenal obstruction, resulting in a number of pyloromyotomies or other explorations. Basal ganglia injury, mostly affecting the putamen, occurs (Fig. 12.2.4); generalized cerebral atrophy and white matter disease is common.

A small subgroup of patients exhibit almost exclusively encephalopathy and progressive neurological disease, resembling a lysosomal storage disorder. A milder form of propionic aciduria

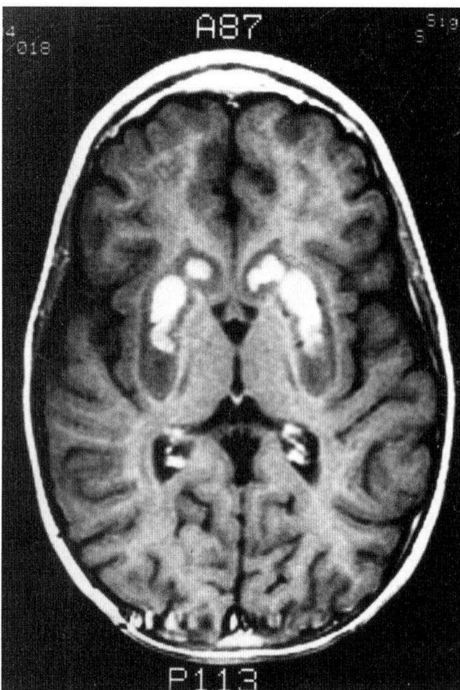

Fig. 12.2.4 Transveral NMR image of a 7-year-old girl, who had been diagnosed with propionic aciduria in infancy and had been successfully treated since then. While in good metabolic control, she suddenly became comatose. Massive infarction of the basal ganglia had occurred, and the child died a few days later. Spin echo technique.
Courtesy of Drs. R. Haas and W.L. Nyhan, Department of Pediatrics, University of California, San Diego, USA.

reported in Japan manifests from childhood with mild learning difficulties or extrapyramidal symptoms, and only occasionally with metabolic acidosis. Finally, some individuals remain asymptomatic until teenage years and are identified during family studies.

Diagnosis

The method of diagnosis is GC/MS analysis of organic acids (urine) or MS/MS analysis of acylcarnitines (dried blood spots, plasma, urine). Characteristic metabolites are 2-methylcitric acid, 3-hydroxypropionic acid, tiglic acid, propionylglycine, and propionylcarnitine. The absence of methylmalonic acid excludes methylmalonic acidurias, and the absence of β-hydroxyisovaleric acid and β-methylcrotonylglycine rules out multiple carboxylase deficiency. In plasma and urine, increased concentrations of glycine and ketone bodies may be present. Confirmation of diagnosis is made by enzyme analysis in leucocytes or fibroblasts, or by mutation analysis. Prenatal diagnosis can be made by mutation analysis, enzyme analysis, or quantitative GC/MS analysis of 2-methylcitric acid.

Treatment and outcome

Prevention of metabolic decompensation is the most important determinant of outcome. During acute decompensation, propionic aciduria is treated like other organic acid disorders (see 'Emergency treatment' above). Long-term treatment is based on lifelong dietary restriction of the precursors isoleucine, valine, methionine, and threonine, as well as by supplementation with L-carnitine. As significant propionate production occurs in the gut, intermittent decontamination (10–14 days/month) with metronidazole or colistin as well as measures preventing constipation are often used. Some patients exhibit recurrent or almost chronic hyperammonaemia, especially during infancy. This may necessitate additional supplementation with arginine or citrulline and/or administration of sodium benzoate or phenylbutyrate. However, benzoate treatment may aggravate the depletion of free carnitine and CoA. Biotin responsiveness in propionic aciduria is very rare, if present at all. Close to 20 children with propionic aciduria have undergone orthotopic liver transplantation, but the outcome has been disappointing. Auxiliary as well as living-related liver transplantations have been successfully performed, but liver transplantation in propionic aciduria seems to be much more complicated than in patients with urea cycle defects.

Patients with neonatal onset of symptoms still have a poor outcome. Patients with late onset of symptoms reach adulthood but often have physical and mental disabilities; nonetheless some patients can survive to adulthood with normal intellects.

Methylmalonic aciduria

Aetiology/pathophysiology

Methylmalonic aciduria is the biochemical hallmark of a heterogeneous group of inborn metabolic errors with a cumulative prevalence of at least 1 in 100 000 newborns in Europe. Index patients were first described in 1967 by Oberholzer and Stokke. This chapter focuses on isolated methylmalonic aciduria caused by mutations in the *MUT* gene localized on 6p21 encoding the apoenzyme methylmalonyl-CoA mutase. Methylmalonyl-CoA mutase can alternatively be impaired by defects in the biosynthesis of 5′-deoxyadenosylcobalamin, deficient cobalamin transport, or by acquired cobalamin deficiency as in pernicious anaemia.

In infancy, severe progressive disease may develop in breastfed infants of mothers who have (undiagnosed) pernicious anaemia or adhere to a strict vegan diet. Methylmalonic acid is a more reliable index of body stores of cobalamin than cobalamin levels in blood.

D-Methylmalonyl-CoA is formed in propionate metabolism by carboxylation of propionyl-CoA. L-Methylmalonyl-CoA is formed from D-methylmalonyl-CoA by D-methylmalonyl-CoA racemase and, subsequently, is converted to succinyl-CoA by the dimeric 5′-deoxyadenosylcobalamin-dependent mitochondrial enzyme methylmalonyl-CoA mutase (Fig. 12.2.2).

As with propionic aciduria (see above), impairment of energy metabolism by propionyl-CoA and 2-methylcitric acid plays a key role in the pathophysiology of methylmalonic acidurias, resulting in multiorgan failure. In addition, methylmalonic acid may exert additional toxic effects.

Clinical presentation

Patients with severe methylmalonyl-CoA mutase deficiency (mut^0) usually present with neonatal metabolic crises which are clinically and biochemically (except for methylmalonic acid) indistinguishable from those of patients with propionic aciduria. In patients with residual methylmalonyl-CoA mutase activity (mut^-), the onset of symptoms is more variable. Neonatal onset of symptoms is found as is a chronic intermittent form, i.e. precipitation of recurrent metabolic crises in infancy and children following high intake of protein or catabolic state. Long-term complications are frequent, in particular in mut^0 patients. These include failure to thrive, chronic neurological symptoms such as extrapyramidal movement disorder, motor disabilities, learning difficulties, and epilepsy, cardiomyopathy, myopathy, and pancreatitis. Neuroradiological studies demonstrate lesions of globus pallidus, generalized cerebral atrophy, and white matter disease. The development of chronic renal failure in a large proportion of patients is unique.

Diagnosis

The best way to make the diagnosis is GC/MS analysis of urinary organic acids or MS/MS analysis of acylcarnitines showing elevated concentrations of methylmalonic acid as well as of metabolites of alternative propionate oxidation (e.g. propionylglycine, 3-hydroxypropionic acid, 2-methylcitric acid, propionylglycine, and propionylcarnitine; as in propionic aciduria). These biochemical abnormalities have a considerable interday and intraday variation and are influenced by responsiveness to cobalamin and metabolic state. Differential diagnosis of methylmalonic aciduria is acquired cobalamin depletion or inherited cobalamin deficiencies, transient mild methylmalonic acidurias of unknown origin in infants, and methylmalonic encephalopathy due to deficiency of succinyl-CoA synthase. Concomitant megaloblastic anaemia and an increase of plasma homocysteine indicates disturbed cobalamin metabolism as the cause of methylmalonic aciduria.

Standardized criteria to define responsiveness to hydroxocobalamin are not established. The determination of methylmalonyl-CoA mutase activity in fibroblast extracts, mutation analysis or the investigation of labelled propionate incorporation following transfection by a vector containing cloned mutase cDNA in intact patients' fibroblasts may be required to differentiate primary defects of methylmalonyl-CoA mutase (mut^0, mut$^-$) from primary defects of 5′-deoxyadenosylcobalamin (cblA and cblB defects). Prenatal diagnosis is available by enzyme or mutation analyses as well as by quantitative stable isotope dilution assay of 2-methylcitric acid.

Treatment and outcome

Metabolic maintenance and emergency treatment follows the treatment principles for organic acid disorders in general and propionic aciduria in particular (see above). In addition, substitution with cobalamin may be beneficial, since partial or complete response to cobalamin has been demonstrated (except for mut^0 patients). In neonates and infants, intramuscular hydroxocobalamin is required; children and adults may be treated with oral cyanocobalamin. Chronic renal failure may progress, necessitating haemodialysis or peritoneal dialysis. Kidney transplantation has only rarely been performed in these patients. Liver transplantation could provide enzyme activity to ameliorate the metabolic defect and the idea of combined liver–kidney or isolated liver transplantation has emerged. The benefit remains doubtful, however, as mortality is high; also liver transplantation does not reliably protect against severe neurological and renal complications.

Defects of lysine, hydroxylysine, and tryptophan metabolism

The common catabolic pathway of lysine, hydroxylysine, and tryptophan is summarized in Fig. 12.2.5.

Hyperlysinaemia I/hyperlysinaemia II or saccharopinuria

Hyperlysinaemia/saccharopinuria is caused by a recessive deficiency of the bifunctional protein 2-aminoadipic semialdehyde synthase. As hyperlysinaemia/saccharopinuria is considered a non-disease, affected individuals do not require specific treatment.

Glutaric aciduria type I

Aetiology/pathophysiology

Glutaric aciduria type I was described in 1975. It occurs with an estimated frequency of 1 in 100 000 newborns, but considerably higher (up to 1 in 300) in genetically consanguineous communities,

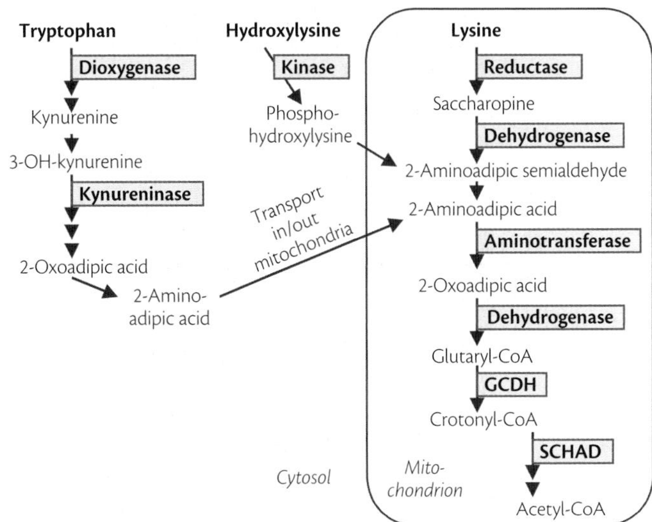

Fig. 12.2.5 Catabolic pathway of lysine, tryptophan and hydroxylysine. 2-Aminoadipic semialdehyde synthase (deficient in hyperlysinaemia/saccharopinuria); 2-aminoadipate aminotransferase/2-oxoadipate dehydrogenase (deficient in in 2-amino-/2-oxoadipic aciduria); glutaryl-CoA dehydrogenase (GCDH; deficient in glutaric aciduria type I).
Adapted with permission from Zschocke and Hoffmann 2004.

e.g. the Amish in Pennsylvania and the Oji-Cree Indians in Canada. Glutaric aciduria type I is caused by deficiency of flavin adenine dinucleotide-dependent glutaryl-CoA dehydrogenase, a mitochondrial enzyme in the catabolic pathway common to tryptophan, lysine, and hydroxylysine (Fig. 12.2.5). Glutaryl-CoA dehydrogenase is encoded by the *GCDH* gene localized on 19p13.2. More than 150 disease-causing mutations have been described. There is no genotype–phenotype correlation. As a consequence of glutaryl-CoA dehydrogenase deficiency, glutaric, 3-hydroxyglutaric, and (inconsistently) glutaconic acids as well as glutarylcarnitine accumulate. The limited permeability of the blood–brain barrier to dicarboxylic acids (such as glutaric acid) leads to their accumulation in the brain (trapping hypothesis). Some of these metabolites are neurotoxins. Candidate mechanisms are stimulation of excitotoxic cell damage via activation of *N*-methyl-D-aspartate receptors, and inhibition of 2-oxoglutarate dehydrogenase and the dicarboxylate shuttle between astrocytes and neurons.

Clinical presentation

Newborns are often asymptomatic but may present with transient and subtle neurological symptoms such as truncal hypotonia or asymmetric posturing. (Progressive) macrocephaly occurs in 75% of patients. Neuroimaging in infancy often reveals hypoplasia of the temporal pole, subependymal pseudocysts, and delayed myelination; subdural fluid collections may be found which may be mistaken as nonaccidental trauma.

The prognostically relevant event of glutaric aciduria type I is the onset of an acute encephalopathic crisis which is usually precipitated by a catabolic state (e.g. febrile illness) during infancy and early childhood. Encephalopathic crises characteristically result in acute striatal injury and, subsequently, dystonia. Approximately 15% of patients with glutaric aciduria type I follow a chronic disease course and develop the same neurological symptoms as the acutely injured children over the first 2 years of life without overt crisis (insidious-onset variant) or during adolescence/adulthood

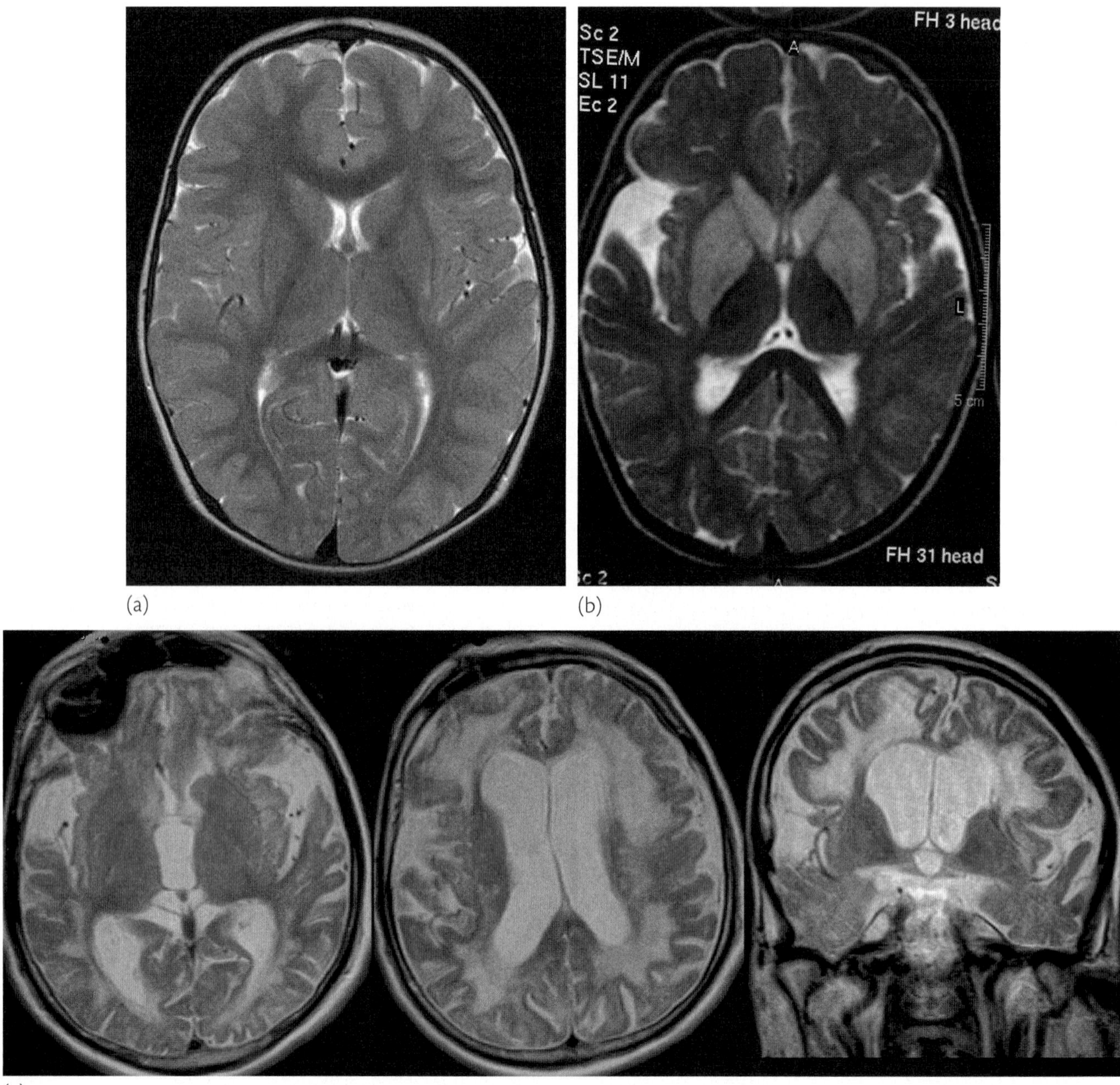

(a) (b) (c)

Fig. 12.2.6 (a) Axial T2-weighted NMR spin echo image of a 2½-year-old boy with glutaryl-CoA dehydrogenase deficiency. He was diagnosed neonatally, never suffered an encephalopathic crisis and developed no major neurological deficit. Extension of Sylvian fissures which was mild during early infancy had slowly regressed. He did not develop characteristic frontotemporal atrophy and showed a normal myelination. (b) Axial T2-weighted spin echo image of a 15-month-old boy with glutaryl-CoA dehydrogenase deficiency two weeks after acute encephalopathic crisis. In addition to extension of sylvian fissures, hyperintensity of putamen, caudate and pallidum are obvious. (c) T2-weighted axial and coronal MR images of a 66-year-old man with glutaryl-CoA dehydrogenase deficiency demonstrating confluent white matter changes, wide temporo-polar and insular CSF spaces, and cortical atrophy, but normal signal of basal ganglia. The previously healthy man presented from the age of 50 with slowly progressive neurologic disease, including seizures, dementia and speech problems. Aggressive behaviour as well as acoustic and visual hallucinations led to the suggestion of psychiatric disease.
(Reproduced with permission from Külkens et al. 2005).

presenting with leukoencephalopathy (late-onset variant). Asymptomatic individuals occur occasionally. Neuroradiological abnormalities are frequently found, including widening of the sylvian fissure due to reduced opercularization (Fig. 12.2.6a), ventriculomegaly and striatal lesions which develop after the encephalopathic crisis (Fig. 12.2.6b), and leukoencephalopathy which is mostly periventricular but may also affect subcortical U fibres (Fig. 12.2.6c).

Diagnosis

Glutaric aciduria type I should be suspected in patients with macrocephaly and an extrapyramidal movement disorder starting in infancy or childhood. The diagnostic process can be guided by further clinical features. Diagnosis is ascertained by the GC/MS detection of glutaric and 3-hydroxyglutaric acids in organic acid analysis (urine, plasma, or cerebrospinal fluid) or by the MS/MS detection of elevated glutarylcarnitine (dried blood spots, plasma, urine). Confirmation by enzymatic analysis in leucocytes or fibroblasts or demonstration of two pathogenic mutations is advisable. A subgroup of patients presents with a mild biochemical phenotype (low excretors) and thus may be missed if diagnostic work-up does not include quantitative methods (e.g. stable isotope dilution assay). Examination of the carnitine status usually reveals low total and free carnitine.

Prenatal diagnosis is possible by determining glutaric acid with stable isotope dilution techniques and by enzymatic and/or molecular testing.

Treatment and outcome

The principal aim of treatment is the prevention of encephalopathic crises and neurological deterioration. Strict adherence to the emergency protocol is especially important (see 'Emergency treatment' above). During the vulnerable period (i.e. until age 6 years), lysine-restricted dietary treatment (including lysine-free amino acid supplements) and carnitine supplementation is recommended. Riboflavin is widely used but is of doubtful benefit. Treatment efficacy of movement disorders is still poor. Baclofen, benzodiazepines, and trihexyphenidyl are widely used to treat dystonia. Botulinum toxin and intrathecal baclofen are valid additions. If diagnosed presymptomatically, treatment prevents brain degeneration in 65% (Amish community) to about 90% (Germany) of patients. In contrast, more than 90% of affected individuals will develop neurological disabilities. Life expectancy is markedly reduced following encephalopathic crises.

Hyperornithinaemia (ornithine-5-aminotransferase): gyrate atrophy

Autosomal recessive hyperornithinaemia associated with gyrate atrophy of the choroid and retina is caused by deficiency of ornithine-5-aminotransferase.

Clinical presentation

Progressive myopia is the first clinical symptom, followed by progressive chorioretinal degeneration with night blindness starting late in the first decade. Loss of peripheral vision proceeds to tunnel vision and eventually blindness by the third or fourth decade. The principal abnormality is an atrophy of choroid and retina. Cataracts also develop but optic discs, cornea, and iris remain normal. A few patients develop mild proximal muscle weakness.

Diagnosis

Severe isolated hyperornithinaemia is usually discovered by amino acid analysis with plasma ornithine concentrations ranging from 400 to 1400 μmol/litre (normal <200 μmol/litre). The disease can be confirmed enzymatically by decreased activity of ornithine-5-aminotransferase in fibroblasts as well as by identification of disease-causing mutations in the *OAT* gene, but the diagnosis is usually evident.

Treatment and prognosis

Permanent reduction of plasma ornithine into the normal range (<200 μmol/litre) is required to stop or at least slow chorioretinal degeneration. Only a small proportion of patients responds to pharmacological doses of the ornithine-5-aminotransferase cofactor pyridoxine. Additional therapeutic approaches to reduce ornithine are the augmentation of renal losses by administration of pharmacological doses of L-lysine or α-aminoisobutyric acid (which is not metabolized), or substrate deprivation by dietary arginine restriction.

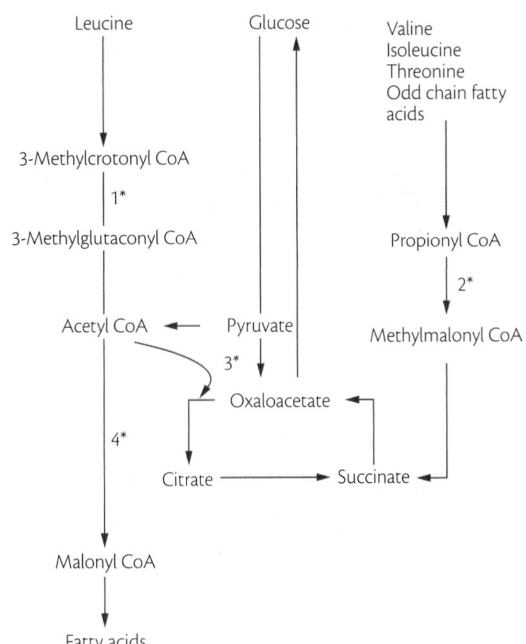

Fig. 12.2.7 Important carboxylases in amino acid metabolism. Asterisked enzymes are: 1, 3-methylcrotonyl coenzyme A carboxylase; 2, propionyl coenzyme A carboxylase; 3, pyruvate carboxylase; and 4, acetyl coenzyme A carboxylase.

Combined treatment appears to be necessary since no single therapy is unequivocally effective.

Multiple carboxylase deficiency

The water-soluble vitamin biotin is a cofactor of four important carboxylases that take part in gluconeogenesis, fatty-acid synthesis, and the catabolism of several amino acids and odd-chain fatty acids (Fig. 12.2.7). The covalent binding of biotin with apocarboxylases forming the active holocarboxylases is catalysed by biotin holocarboxylase synthetase. In the biotin cycle, biotin is recycled after proteolytic degradation of holocarboxylases (Fig. 12.2.8). Biotin in small amounts is widely present in natural foods. Within the body, biotin bound to holocarboxylases represents the major source. In dietary and in endogenous sources, biotin is protein-bound as biocytin or short biotinyl peptides. Liberation of biotin from its protein conjugates is catalysed by biotinidase.

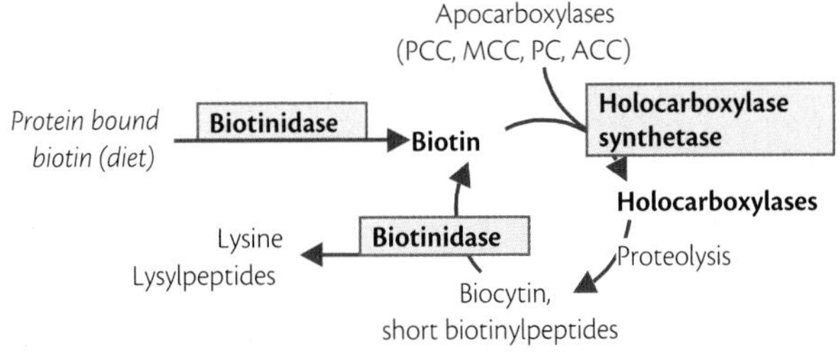

Fig. 12.2.8 The Biotin Cycle. Biotin is cleaved from biocytin (biotinyl-lysine) or small peptides by biotinidase. Activation of the apoenzymes resulting in functioning carboxylases (3-methylcrotonyl-CoA, propionyl-CoA, acetyl-CoA and pyruvate carboxylases) is carried out by holocarboxylase synthetase. Abbreviations: ACC = acetyl-CoA carboxylase; MCC = 3-methylcrotonyl-CoA carboxylase; PC = pyruvate carboxylase; PCC = propionyl-CoA carboxylase. Adapted with permission from Zschocke and Hoffmann 2004.

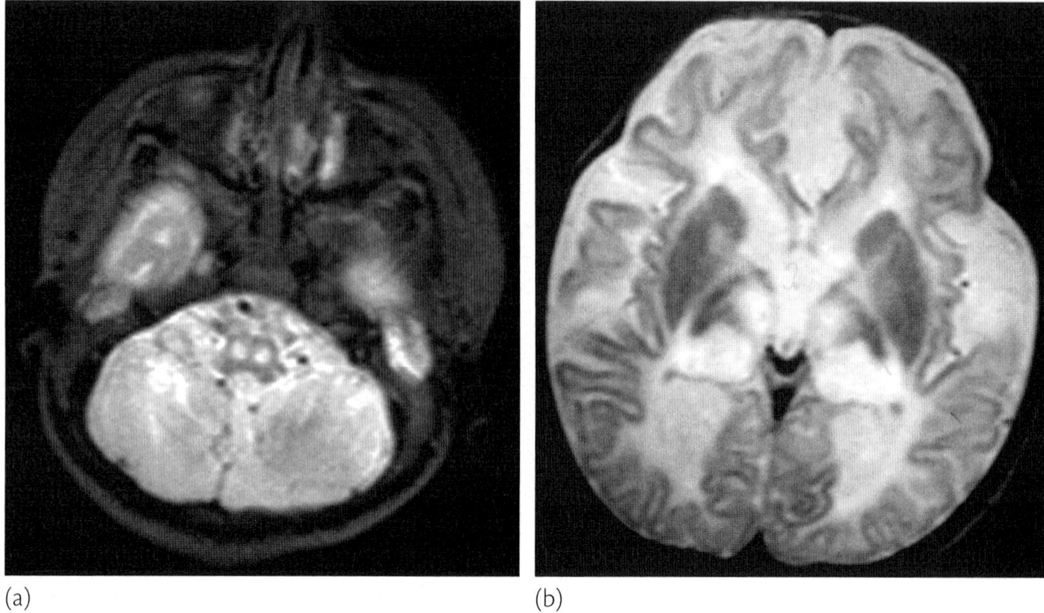

Fig. 12.2.9 Two T2-weighted images of a 7-month-old boy with biotinidase deficiency. The image on the right shows absence of normal myelin signal, cerebral atrophy and symmetrical hyperintense lesions of both thalami. The image on the left displays absence of normal myelin signal in the cerebellum as well as hyperintense signal in both pyramidal tracts.
Courtesy of Dr. T. Bast, Department of Pediatric Neurology, University of Heidelberg, Heidelberg, Germany.

Biotinidase deficiency

Aetiology/pathophysiology

Biotinidase regenerates biotin from endogenous sources and liberates protein-bound biotin, which derives from natural foodstuffs and the holocarboxylases. Free biotin is recycled and used for the re-formation of holocarboxylases by the action of holocarboxylase synthetase through the biotin cycle (Fig. 12.2.8). The primary biochemical defect in most patients with late-onset multiple carboxylase deficiency was shown in 1983 to be a profound deficiency of serum biotinidase encoded by the *BTD* gene (3p25). The metabolic abnormalities caused by deficiency of the respective biotin-dependent carboxylases are as follows: lactic acidosis due to pyruvate carboxylase deficiency; hyperammonaemia and accumulation of metabolites of alternative propionate metabolism (see also 'Propionic aciduria') due to propionyl-CoA carboxylase deficiency; and elevation of 3-hydroxyisovaleric acid, 3-methylcrotonylglycine, and 3-hydroxyisovalerylcarnitine (see also '3-Methylcrotonylglycinuria') due to methylcrotonyl-CoA carboxylase deficiency.

Clinical presentation

Onset of first symptoms is variable, ranging from 1 week to 10 years of age. The mean age of presentation is between 3 and 6 months. Provision of biotin by the mother *in utero* delays symptoms and biochemical abnormalities in newborns with biotinidase deficiency. The most frequent symptoms are lethargy, hypotonia, seizures, and ataxia often in combination with stridor, episodes of hyperventilation, and apnoea. If undiagnosed and untreated, progression of the disease can be potentially fatal (Fig. 12.2.9). In older children progressive neurological disease is often the leading presentation, including ataxia, (myoclonic) epileptic encephalopathy, and developmental delay. Neurosensory hearing loss and ophthalmic disorders, such as optic atrophy, develop in most untreated patients. Skin rash and/or alopecia are hallmarks of the disease.

Diagnosis

Urinary organic acid analysis is useful for differentiating isolated carboxylase deficiencies from the multiple carboxylase deficiencies that occur in biotinidase deficiency and holocarboxylase synthase deficiency. However, metabolic abnormalities are highly variable and are absent at birth when the patient is not biotin-depleted. Whereas accumulation of abnormal organic acid metabolites may show characteristic metabolites of propionic aciduria (see also 'Propionic aciduria'), pyruvate carboxylase deficiency, and 3-methylcrotonylglycinuria (see also '3-Methylcrotonylglycinuria') (Fig. 12.2.2), only 3-hydroxyisovaleric acid may be found elevated, especially in the early stages of the disease. Notably, 3-hydroxyisovaleric acid is also the most commonly elevated urinary metabolite in holocarboxylase synthetase deficiency, 3-methylcrotonyl-CoA carboxylase deficiency, and acquired biotin deficiency. Biotin is decreased in plasma and urine and biocytin is increased in urine.

Diagnosis is made by analysis of serum biotinidase activity. Enzymatic activity less than 10% is classified as profound biotinidase deficiency and activity between 10 and 30% as partial biotinidase deficiency. Furthermore, few patients with decreased affinity of biotinidase for biocytin (K_m variants) exist. They may show erroneously high residual activity on *in vitro* testing. Prenatal diagnosis is feasible by measurement of biotinidase activity but may not be necessary because of effective treatment and favourable clinical outcome. Newborn screening for biotinidase deficiency is now established in many countries.

Treatment and outcome

Biotinidase deficiency is effectively treated by daily oral administration of pharmacological doses of biotin. Restriction of protein is not necessary. Administration of 5 to 10 mg oral biotin per day promptly reverses or prevents all clinical and biochemical abnormalities. Biotin treatment has to be maintained lifelong and has no side effects. Most patients with biotinidase deficiency known today were detected by newborn screening. Patients with K_m variants have an increased risk of becoming biotin deficient and thus must also be treated with biotin. After early detection and consequent treatment, the outcome of biotinidase deficiency is excellent.

Holocarboxylase synthetase deficiency

Aetiology/pathophysiology

Holocarboxylase synthetase deficiency is a rare autosomal recessive disease. Several disease-causing mutations have been identified at the *HLCS* gene (21q22.1). Only about 40 patients have been reported. Residual activity has been observed in all affected individuals suggesting that complete enzyme deficiency may be lethal *in utero*. The coenzyme biotin is attached to the various apocarboxylases by the enzyme holocarboxylase synthetase. The carboxyl group of biotin is linked by an amide bond to an ε-amino group of a specific lysine residue of the apoenzymes. Deficiency of holocarboxylase synthetase leads to failure of synthesis of all carboxylases, causing biochemical and clinical abnormalities attributable to the dysfunction of each respective carboxylase.

Clinical presentation

Although holocarboxylase synthetase deficiency was initially termed early-onset multiple carboxylase deficiency, the age of onset of symptoms varies widely, from a few hours after birth to 6 years of age. Nevertheless, about one-half of patients present acutely in the first days of life with severe metabolic decompensation, lethargy, hypotonia, vomiting, seizures, and hypothermia. Patients with early-onset presentation exhibit severe metabolic acidosis with lactic acidaemia, ketosis, and hyperammonaemia in analogy to biotinidase deficiency (see also 'Biotinidase deficiency'). The metabolic derangement may quickly progress from lethargy to coma and early death. Skin rashes, feeding difficulties, vomiting, muscular hypotonia and hypertonia, seizures, and the odour of male cat urine are other symptoms. Ataxia, tremor, hyporeflexia, or hyperreflexia are neurological manifestations of the disease.

Diagnosis

Biochemical abnormalities of holocarboxylase synthetase deficiency are analogous to those described for patients with biotinidase deficiency (see also 'Biotinidase deficiency'). Importantly, plasma biotin is normal in holocarboxylase synthetase deficiency as is serum biotinidase activity. Holocarboxylase synthetase is characterized by deficient activities of carboxylases in peripheral blood leucocytes prior to biotin administration; the activities of these enzymes increase to near-normal or normal values after biotin treatment. Indirect confirmation of holocarboxylase synthetase deficiency and differentiation from biotinidase deficiency is feasible by measurement of activities of the mitochondrial carboxylases in skin fibroblasts showing residual activity of 0 to 30% when incubated in low-biotin (10^{-10} mol/litre) medium and an increase, sometimes to normal values in biotin-supplemented medium (10^{-6} to 10^{-5} mol/litre). In biotinidase deficiency, the activity of mitochondrial carboxylases in fibroblasts is normalized even under low-biotin conditions. Definite diagnosis of holocarboxylase synthetase deficiency is not routinely available. Prenatal diagnosis is feasible either by demonstrating decreased carboxylase activities in cultured amniocytes or by demonstration of elevated 3-hydroxyisovaleric acid and/or methylcitrate in amniotic fluid. Prenatal molecular diagnosis can be offered in families with previously known disease-causing mutations in the *HLCS* gene.

Treatment and outcome

Holocarboxylase synthetase deficiency can be treated effectively with pharmacological doses of biotin. The required dose of biotin is dependent on the severity of the enzyme defect and has to be assessed individually. In most patients 10 to 20 mg biotin per day is sufficient, but some need higher doses, i.e. 40 to 100 mg/day. In spite of apparently complete recovery, biochemical and clinical abnormalities persist in some patients owing to the high K_m for biotin in the defective holocarboxylase synthetase. In case of acute decompensation, treatment according to the emergency protocol in organic acidurias (see 'Emergency treatment' above) has to start without delay. It is unclear whether prenatal treatment with biotin is beneficial. The prognosis is good if treatment is initiated immediately, except for affected individuals with K_m variants.

Other organic acidurias

D-2-Hydroxyglutaric aciduria

Aetiology/pathophysiology

D-2-Hydroxyglutaric aciduria is a rare autosomal recessively inherited cerebral organic acid disorder first described by Chalmers and colleagues in 1980. The molecular basis of this disease has been unravelled only recently, and found to be deficiency of D-2-hydroxyglutarate dehydrogenase, a mitochondrial enzyme converting D-2-hydroxyglutarate to 2-oxoglutarate. Pathogenic mutations have been identified in the *D2HGD* gene on 2p25.3. Neurodegeneration in D-2-hydroxyglutaric aciduria is explained by activation of *N*-methyl-D-aspartate receptors and inhibition of respiratory chain complexes (cytochrome *c* oxidase, ATP synthase) by D-2-hydroxyglutaric acid.

Clinical presentation

Patients with D-2-hydroxyglutaric aciduria exhibit variable phenotypes. They have been divided into two subgroups based on clinical and neuroradiological findings. One group includes severely affected children who present with encephalopathy of early infantile onset demonstrating a combination of catastrophic epilepsy, hypotonia, cerebral visual failure, and severe psychomotor retardation. Facial dysmorphism, macrocephaly, and cardiomyopathy may also be present. Moderately affected children follow a much milder clinical course with variable symptoms including learning difficulties, hypotonia, and macrocephaly. Rarely individuals remain almost asymptomatic, i.e. presenting only with well-treatable oligoepilepsy or even with no neurological symptoms.

Neuroimaging findings in the severely affected patient group show ventriculomegaly, enlarged subarachnoid spaces, subdural effusions, subependymal cysts, and delayed cerebral maturation (Fig. 12.2.10). Recently, agenesis of the corpus callosum, bilateral involvement of the striatum, and cerebral artery infarctions were added to the spectrum.

Diagnosis

The biochemical hallmark of this disease is the accumulation of D-2-hydroxyglutaric acid in all body fluids. Demonstration of elevated levels of 2-hydroxyglutaric acid must be followed up by differential quantitation of the two isomers L- and D-2-hydroxyglutaric acid. 2-Oxoglutaric acid and other tricarboxylic acid cycle intermediates are usually also elevated in urine. γ-Aminobutyric acid and total protein concentrations may be elevated in cerebrospinal fluid. D-2-Hydroxyglutaric acid can also be elevated in multiple acyl-CoA dehydrogenase deficiency, succinic semialdehyde

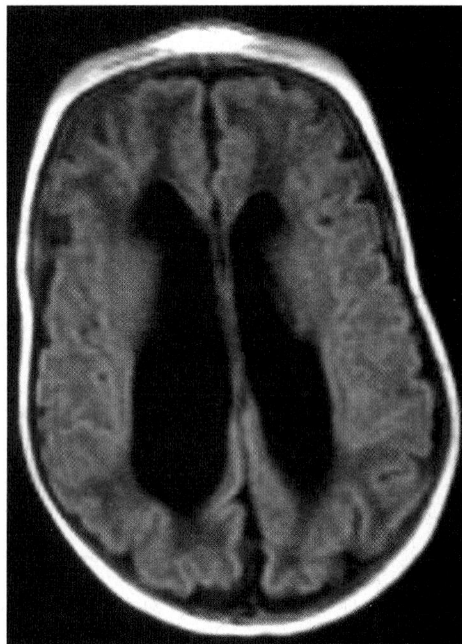

Fig. 12.2.10 Axial T1-weighted spin echo image of a 2-month-old girl with D-2-hydroxyglutaric aciduria. The lateral ventricles are highly dilated, occipital more than frontal, the cerebral maturation is delayed.
(Reproduced with permission from Kölker *et al.* 2002).

dehydrogenase deficiency, and following bacterial overgrowth of the urine specimen. However, due to characteristic additional parameters these differential diagnoses are usually easy to exclude. Prenatal diagnosis can be performed either through genetic testing or by metabolite determination in amniotic fluid by stable isotope dilution GC/MS assay.

Treatment and outcome

No specific therapy exists to date. Long-term care of patients should entail regular evaluation of cardiomyopathy and the progression of neurological disease. The prognosis of D-2-hydroxyglutaric aciduria is extremely variable. Severely affected children may die in infancy, while moderately affected patients have a better prognosis up to an unimpaired life.

L-2-Hydroxyglutaric aciduria

Aetiology/pathophysiology

L-2-Hydroxyglutaric aciduria is a rare autosomal recessively inherited cerebral disorder. The metabolic base of this disease has recently been described. The disease is caused by deficiency of the flavin adenine dinucleotide-dependent mitochondrial enzyme L-2-hydroxyglutarate dehydrogenase converting L-2-hydroxyglutarate to 2-oxoglutarate. This enzyme is encoded by the *L2HGDH* gene on 14q22.1. The pathophysiology of this disease is unknown.

Clinical presentation

L-2-Hydroxyglutaric aciduria was first described by Duran and coworkers in 1980. It is characterized by progressive loss of myelinated arcuate fibres and a spongiform encephalopathy. In the first 2 years of life, mental and psychomotor development may be normal or slightly delayed. Febrile seizures, nonspecific developmental delay, and muscular hypotonia are the presenting symptoms. Progressive ataxia, variable extrapyramidal and pyramidal signs, epilepsy, and progressive learning difficulties eventually develop. By adolescence, patients are usually bedridden and severely mentally disabled (IQ 40–50). Two patients have developed cerebral tumours.

Two patients presented at birth with depressed vital signs, severe epileptic encephalopathy, and an abnormal CT scan showing cerebellar involvement; however, the disease course is usually slowly progressive without metabolic decompensation.

The neuroimaging findings in L-2-hydroxyglutaric aciduria are unique and mostly uniform comprising a progressive loss of arcuate fibres combined with progressive cerebellar atrophy and signal changes in globus pallidus and the dentate nuclei (Fig. 12.2.11a,b).

Diagnosis

L-2-hydroxyglutaric aciduria results in a rather homogenous clinical picture and characteristic abnormalities on neuroimaging. Clinical or neuroradiological suspicion should prompt GC/MS analysis of urinary organic acids and differentiation of L-2- and D-2-stereoisomers. Lysine is often increased both in plasma and cerebrospinal fluid. Prenatal diagnosis is based on the analysis of L-2-hydroxyglutaric acid in amniotic fluid samples or molecular analysis.

Treatment and outcome

No specific therapy exists to date. Epilepsy can generally be controlled by antiepileptic medications. Patients with L-2-hydroxyglutaric aciduria can be expected to reach adult life. The oldest known patients are close to 40 years of age, bedridden, and severely disabled.

N-Acetylaspartic aciduria (Canavan's disease)

Aetiology/pathophysiology

N-Acetylaspartic aciduria is a devastating infantile neurodegenerative disorder. In 1931, a child with spongy matter degeneration was described by Canavan. In 1986, it was recognized that *N*-acetylaspartic aciduria was caused by deficient aspartoacylase in a child with a similar clinical presentation. In 1988, aspartoacylase deficiency was definitely linked to Canavan's disease.

Canavan's disease is found in all ethnic populations but reveals a much higher frequency in Ashkenazi Jews (1 in 5000 to 1 in 14 000 newborns). The frequent missense mutation E285A in the aspartoacylase gene, localized on 17p13-pter, accounts for more than 80% of alleles in Ashkenazi Jews and for 60% of alleles in patients of non-Jewish origin. In healthy individuals high concentrations of *N*-acetylaspartic acid (8 mmol/g tissue) are exclusively found in brain tissue.

Aspartoacylase is localized in oligodendrocytes catalysing the deacetylation of *N*-acetylaspartic acid to produce acetate, a substrate for the synthesis of myelin lipids including cholesterol. It has been proposed that *N*-acetyl-L-aspartate may function as a molecular water pump in myelinated neurons, transporting water against its gradient from neurons to oligodendrocytes. Thus aspartoacylase deficiency may cause both accumulation of metabolic water causing spongiform white matter changes, and deficiency of acetyl groups needed for cholesterol biosynthesis, causing demyelination; both are characteristic of Canavan's disease.

Clinical presentation

Canavan's disease mostly manifests at age 2 to 4 months with delayed development. Hypotonia with prominent head lag, epilepsy, loss of previously acquired skills, as well as progressive megalencephaly are regularly found. Seizures and optic nerve atrophy develop during

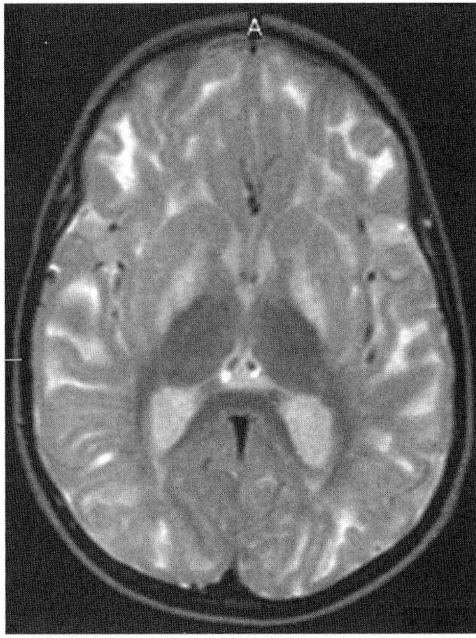

(a)

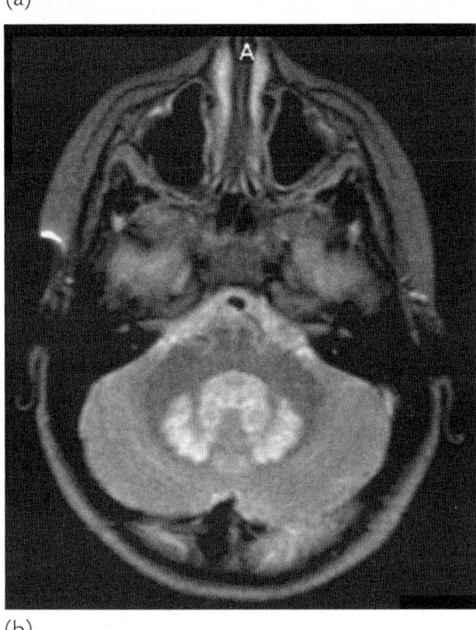

(b)

Fig. 12.2.11 (a) Axial T2-weighted spin echo image of an 8½-year-old boy with L-2-hydroxyglutaric aciduria. Subcortical white matter is severely deficient with much less involvement of the internal capsule and the periventricular white matter. Please note signal changes in the putamen.
(Reproduced with permission from Kölker *et al.* 2002).
(b) Axial T2-weighted spin echo image of an 8½-year-old boy with L-2-hydroxyglutaric aciduria. Please note hyperintense lesions in both dentate nuclei.

the second year of life. As the disease progresses, affected children develop pyramidal signs, and finally decerebration.

Neuroimaging reveals characteristic symmetrical leukodystrophic changes with loss of arcuate fibres; histology demonstrates spongiform degeneration, in particular of the cortex and subcortical white matter (Fig. 12.2.12) with less involvement in the cerebellum and brain stem. In infancy, changes may be subtle and misinterpreted as delayed myelination or periventricular leukomalacia.

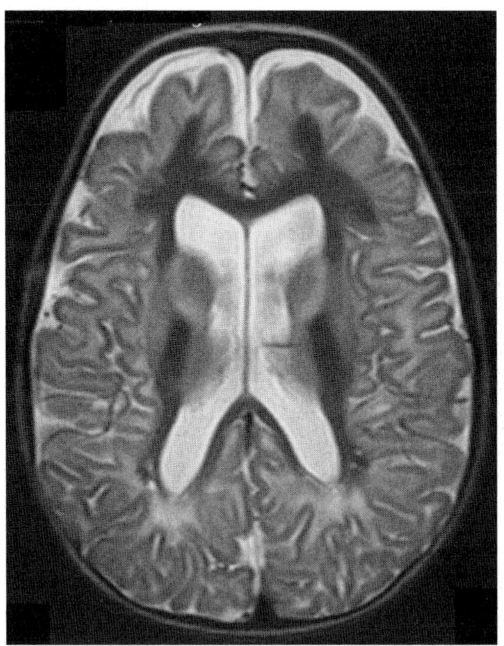

Fig. 12.2.12 Axial fast spin echo image of an 6½-year-old girl suffering from aspartoacylase deficiency. Note the marked discrepancy between the severely affected subcortical white matter and the relatively spared central white matter, at least frontally.
(Reproduced with permission from Kölker *et al.* 2002).

Variant Canavan's disease has been described and partially been proven to be caused by the same metabolic defect.

Diagnosis

Muscular hypotonia, head lag, and progressive megalencephaly in infancy is the classic clinical triad of Canavan's disease.

The identification of the accumulating *N*-acetylaspartic acid by GC/MS analysis and confirmation of the suspected diagnosis by enzyme analysis (skin fibroblasts) or mutation analysis has obviated the need for brain biopsy for the diagnosis of Canavan's disease.

Prenatal diagnosis is possible by quantitative GC/MS analysis of *N*-acetylaspartic acid in amniotic fluid or by mutation analysis. In contrast, enzyme activity is unsuitable for reliable prenatal diagnosis.

Treatment and outcome

Management is symptomatic (antiepileptics) and palliative. Special care is needed to prevent recurrent aspirations. Many patients need tube or gastrostomy feeding. Dietary therapies have not been shown to be beneficial and are potentially harmful. A promising protocol for gene therapy was published in 2002 involving the transfer of human aspartoacylase cDNA intraventricularly; however, the clinical changes were not pronounced and were relatively transient. The prognosis of infantile Canavan's disease is rapidly fatal, whereas milder disease has been described with survival beyond the teenage years.

Ethylmalonic encephalopathy

Aetiology/pathophysiology

Ethylmalonic encephalopathy is a devastating infantile autosomal recessive neurometabolic disorder affecting the brain, gastrointestinal tract, and peripheral veins. The underlying metabolic defect was identified in a beta-lactamase-like, iron-coordinating metalloprotein of the mitochondrial matrix encoded by the *ETHE1* gene. Only recently, it was elucidated using Ethe1-deficient mice that the deficient protein is a mitochondrial sulfur dioxygenase which is involved in the catabolism of sulfide in ethylmalonic encephalopathy. As a consequence, toxic levels of sulfide and thiosulfide are found causing powerful inhibition of cytochrome c oxidase, short-chain fatty acid oxidation, and exerting vasoactive and vasotoxic effects. This explains deficient mitochondrial energy metabolism, the abnormal accumulation short-chain organic acids, acylglycines and acylcarnitines, as well as microangiopathy.

Clinical presentation

Ethylmalonic encephalopathy is characterized biochemically by ethylmalonic aciduria and methylsuccinic aciduria, lactic acidaemia, and clinically by severe psychomotor retardation, acrocyanosis, petechiae, and chronic diarrhoea.

Newborns present with muscular hypotonia followed by progressive neurological deterioration, especially pyramidal dysfunction, learning difficulties, orthostatic acrocyanosis with distal swelling, chronic diarrhoea, and recurrent petechiae (Fig. 12.2.13). Haematuria is often present. MRI scans show signal changes in cerebellar white matter and lesions in the basal ganglia, the latter appearing suddenly.

Diagnosis

The biochemical hallmark is increased urinary excretion of ethylmalonic and methylsuccinic acids associated with abnormal excretion of C4- and C5- (*n*-butyryl-, isobutyryl-, isovaleryl-, and 2-methylbutyryl-) acylglycines and acylcarnitines as well as intermittent lactic acidosis. Since primary mitochondrial disorders are an important differential diagnosis, enzymatic analyses of respiratory chain enzymes in muscle biopsy specimen have been performed in some patients revealing secondary cytochrome c oxidase deficiency. Mutation analysis of the *ETHE1* gene provides the definitive diagnosis including prenatal diagnosis. Increased ethylmalonate in urine is also found in multiple and short-chain acyl-CoA dehydrogenase deficiencies, primary respiratory chain deficiencies, and Jamaican vomiting sickness.

Treatment and outcome

No effective treatment is known. The prognosis is poor and ethylmalonic encephalopathy is usually lethal in early childhood.

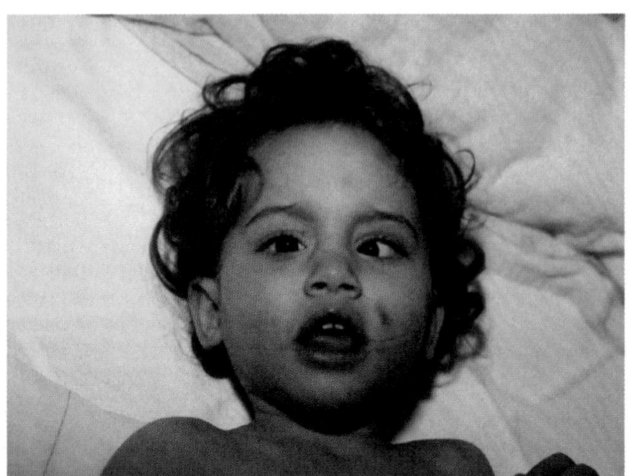

Fig. 12.2.13 Patient with ethylmalonic encephalopathy.

Defects of phenylalanine and tyrosine metabolism

Phenylketonuria (PKU)

The hyperphenylalaninaemias are a group of disorders characterized by defective hydroxylation of phenylalanine to tyrosine resulting in plasma phenylalanine values above the normal fasting range of 40 to 80 µmol/litre. PKU was first identified by the Norwegian Asbjorn Folling in 1934 in several severely disabled individuals. Folling determined the urinary excretion of phenylpyruvic acid which led to the previously used term 'phenylpyruvic oligophrenia'. In 1947, Jervis localized the metabolic error as an inability to oxidize phenylalanine to tyrosine. In 1953, Bickel and colleagues demonstrated that a phenylalanine-restricted diet was beneficial, and was thus the first successful treatment of an inborn error of metabolism and one which led the way to early diagnosis by newborn screening and treatment. The worldwide overall incidence of PKU is approximately 1 in 10 000, with a large national and ethnic variability.

Aetiology/pathophysiology

PKU is an autosomal recessive disorder caused by a severe defect of phenylalanine hydroxylase which converts phenylalanine into tyrosine (Fig. 12.2.14). Tetrahydrobiopterin is required as a cofactor and thus hyperphenylalaninaemia may also be caused by inappropriate generation of tetrahydrobiopterin. Through mechanisms still not completely understood, the excess phenylalanine is toxic to the central nervous system. Phenylalanine competes with the transport of large neutral amino acids through the blood–brain barrier using the sodium-independent system L and induces cerebral depletion of these amino acids and, subsequently, reduced

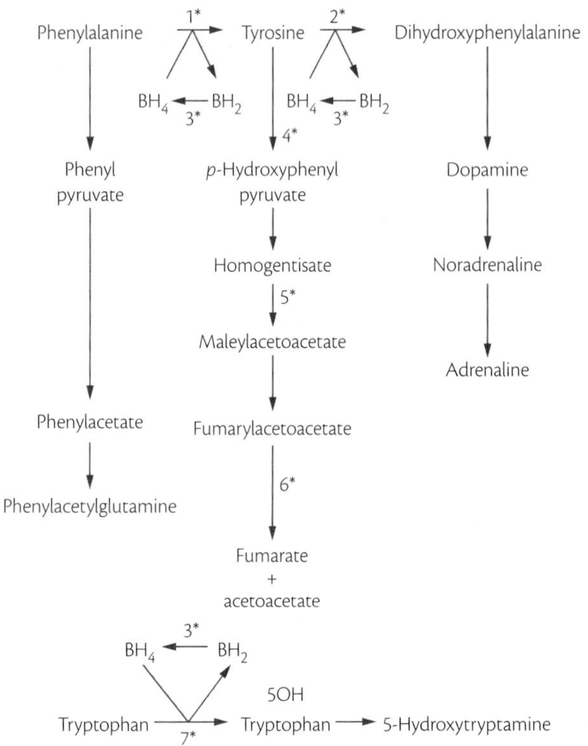

Fig. 12.2.14 The metabolism of phenylalanine and tyrosine and the role of tetrahydrobiopterin. The asterisked enzymes are: 1, phenylalanine hydroxylase; 2, tyrosine hydroxylase; 3, dihydrobiopterin reductase; 4, tyrosine aminotransferase; 5, homogentisic acid oxidase; 6, fumaryl acetoacetate hydrolyase; and 7, tryptophan hydroxylase.

synthesis of proteins and neurotransmitters (large neutral amino acid hypothesis of PKU). In addition, phenylalanine competes with glycine and glutamate at their binding sites in *N*-methyl-D-aspartate and α-amino-3-hydroxy-5-methyl-4-isoxazolepropionic acid receptors, thus impairing glutamate signalling and, subsequently, synapse formation and cognitive function. Furthermore, phenylalanine inhibits the rate-limiting enzyme of cholesterol biosynthesis, 3-hydroxy-3-methylglutaryl-CoA reductase, and switches forebrain oligodendrocytes to a nonmyelinating state.

Clinical presentation

Untreated, PKU almost invariably causes severe learning difficulties. Newborns with PKU are asymptomatic since fetal phenylalanine is metabolized by the mother's liver. On regular intake of natural protein, phenylalanine levels quickly rise. Constitutional abnormalities (80–100% of patients) such as hypopigmentation of the skin and hair (fair) and iris (blue) develop rapidly because synthesis of melanin from tyrosine is impaired. Elevated phenylacetate excretion gives the urine an odour reminiscent of mice and can cause an eczematous skin eruption.

Delayed psychomotor development may become evident from the third month of life. It has been estimated that one IQ point is lost for each week of delay in diagnosis and treatment. Cognitive function is severely compromised in untreated children (IQ <40). Microcephaly and movement disorders are frequent, as are hyperexcitability as well as hypoexcitability and seizures; some patients develop autistic behaviour or aggressiveness. Most patients with untreated PKU cannot be managed by their families and require institutional care.

Diagnosis

Neonatal screening In many countries, newborns are screened for increased phenylalanine levels in dried blood spots during the first days of life (newborn screening). Originally, neonatal screening of phenylalanine was performed by a bacterial inhibition assay (Guthrie test). The implementation of MS/MS techniques has, however, significantly improved the early identification of affected individuals by newborn screening. Confirmation of a positive screening result is performed by quantitative amino acid analysis and mutation analysis. Liver biopsy and subsequent determination of the hepatic activity of phenylalanine hydroxylase is not indicated.

Defects in the metabolism of tetrahydrobiopterin (BH_4), the cofactor of phenylalanine hydroxylase, have to be differentiated from classic PKU by urinary pterin analysis and enzyme analysis of dihydropteridine reductase in dried blood spots. In many centres, an oral dose of 20 mg/kg BH_4 is administered. To perform this test accurately, the initial plasma phenylalanine concentration should be more than 400 μmol/litre (6.7 mg/dl). Following BH_4 administration plasma samples are collected for phenylalanine and tyrosine analysis at defined time points as well as urine samples for pterin analysis. Notably, BH_4 normalizes phenylalanine concentrations in patients with a primary disorder of BH_4 (see below). This test has the advantage that it may also identify BH_4-responsive individuals with PKU.

Treatment and outcome

The most important therapeutic intervention in PKU is phenylalanine-restricted dietary treatment. Regular phenylalanine determinations are used for monitoring. Unfortunately, recommendations for PKU treatment differ considerably with regard to cut-off levels to begin dietary treatment, age-dependent recommendations for phenylalanine concentrations, frequency of clinical examinations, and phenylalanine monitoring (Table 12.2.4). There is no rational explanation for this.

The concept of dietary treatment has four components: (1) complete avoidance of food containing abundant phenylalanine (e.g. meat, fish, milk, etc.); (2) calculated intake of natural food with low phenylalanine/protein ratio (e.g. vegetables and fruit) and low-protein products; (3) adequate intake of energy substrates; and (4) calculated intake of phenylalanine-free amino acid supplements, vitamins, minerals, and trace elements. During catabolic states phenylalanine concentrations may increase, which is counteracted by dietary reduction of phenylalanine intake. In contrast, during growth spurts in childhood and adolescence the requirement for phenylalanine may transiently increase.

When a very strict diet is begun early and is well maintained, affected children can expect normal development and lifespan. Regression of IQ when diets were stopped in later childhood has led to continuation of dietary treatment into the teenage years and adulthood. Patients generally have not suffered when the diet was stopped at or after 15 or 16 years of age. However, there is no follow-up with respect to IQ change of a substantial number who have been off diet for 20 years or more. Most recommendations and centres have adopted a philosophy of 'diet for life'. However, the urgent need for more detailed information remains.

Maternal PKU

In 1980, Lenke and Levy reported the severe effects of maternal hyperphenylalaninaemia in the fetus (Table 12.2.5). The clinical features are similar to the fetal alcohol syndrome, and severity of the manifestations depends on the maternal phenylalanine level. In addition to learning difficulties and behavioural disorders, the adverse effects include malformations such as cardiac defects (usually conotruncal), microcephaly, dysmorphic features, intrauterine growth retardation, neuronal migration disorders, and agenesis of the corpus callosum.

Treatment and outcome

Because of active placental transport, the ratio of fetal to maternal phenylalanine plasma levels is 1.5 to 1.7. Maternal phenylalanine values should be between 120 and 360 μmol/litre, which requires a strict diet and very careful monitoring twice weekly. Microcephaly and congenital heart disease in the offspring of mothers returning to diet at the seventh or eighth week emphasizes the need for preconception diet and training. Lowering maternal plasma phenylalanine concentrations during pregnancy to a level between 120 and 360 μmol/litre results in a favourable outcome in virtually all cases.

Defects of biopterin metabolism

In the hydroxylation of phenylalanine the cofactor BH_4 is consumed and must be regenerated. BH_4 is formed in a three-step pathway from guanosine triphosphate. The first and rate-limiting reaction is catalysed by guanosine triphosphate cyclohydrolase and leads to the production of dihydroneopterin triphosphate. A deficiency of BH_4 does not only impair phenylalanine hydroxylase in the liver, resulting in hyperphenylalaninaemia, but also tyrosine hydroxylase, tryptophan hydroxylase, as well as nitric oxide synthases (Fig. 12.2.15). Tyrosine hydroxylation is needed for the synthesis of noradrenaline and dopamine, and tryptophan hydroxylation for the production of serotonin. BH_4 is therefore crucial to the production of neurotransmitters. The supply of this

Table 12.2.4 Guidelines for treatment and monitoring of PKU: international comparison

	Germany 1999	UK 1993	USA 2000
Indication for dietary treatment	>600 µmol/litre	>400 µmol/litre	>360–600 µmol/litre
Start of dietary treatment	As soon as possible	≤ day 20 of life	≤ day 7 of life

Recommendations for phenylalanine levels and frequency of phenylalanine monitoring

Germany 1999	UK 1993	USA 2000	Age	Germany 1999	UK 1993	USA 2000
40–240 µmol/litre (0.7–4 mg/dl)	120–360 µmol/litre (2–6 mg/dl)	120–360 µmol/litre (2–6 mg/dl)	0	2–4×/month	4×/month	4×/month
			1	1–2×/month		2×/month
			2			
			3			
			4			
			5		2×/month	
	School age:		6			
	120–480 µmol/litre (2–8 mg/dl)		7			
			8			
			9			
40–900 µmol/litre (0.7–15mg/dl)			10	1×/month	1×/month	
			11			
	Adolescence and adulthood		12			
		120–600 µmol/litre (2–10 mg/dl)	13			1×/month
	120–700 µmol/litre (2–11.7 mg/dl)		14			
			15			
40–1200 µmol/litre (0.7–20 mg/dl)			16	4–6 ×/year		
			17			
		120–900 µmol/litre (2–15 mg/dl)	18			
			18+			

Recommendations for clinical monitoring

Germany 1999	Germany 2004	UK 1993	USA 2000
Dietary training	Amino acid profile	Nutrition	No details
Anthropometric data	Blood count	Growth	
Health status	Minerals, trace elements	General health status	
Neurological status	Calcium and phosphorus metabolism		
Psychological development	Enzymes: AP, GOT, GPT		
	Vitamins and serum lipid status		

coenzyme is impaired in five recessively inherited enzyme defects. Most produce hyperphenylalaninaemia, which may not be marked. All but pterin carbinolamine dehydratase deficiency cause progressive neurological disease. In about 1% to 2% of newborns a raised phenylalanine value detected by newborn screening is due to a defect of biopterin metabolism.

The enzyme defects lead to reduced levels of BH_4 within the central nervous system without significantly affecting phenylalanine metabolism in the liver (normal plasma phenylalanine). However, turnover of serotonin and the catecholamines in the brain can still become severely compromised. Fasting plasma phenylalanine levels are always normal in the dominantly inherited guanosine triphosphate cyclohydrolase deficiency (Segawa's disease) and the autosomal recessive sepiapterin reductase deficiency.

Clinical presentation

Except for pterin carbinolamine dehydratase deficiency, which is mostly benign, autosomal recessive defects of biopterin metabolism

Table 12.2.5 Incidences (%) of abnormalities in the offspring of mothers affected with classical PKU

Congenital abnormalities	Maternal PKU	Unaffected mothers
Mental disability	92	5
Microcephaly	73	4.8
Intrauterine retardation	40	9.6
Congenital heart defects	12	0.8

Adapted from Lenke R, Levy HL (1980). Maternal PKU and hyperphenylalaninemia: an international study of treated and untreated pregnancies. *N Engl J Med*, **303**, 1202–8.

result in severe encephalopathies. Common but variable symptoms are progressive learning difficulties, dystonia, chorea, oculogyric crises, convulsions, tremor, spasticity, microcephaly, growth retardation, swallowing difficulties, and depressive and aggressive behaviour. Diurnal variation is often present. Onset of symptoms is in the first months of life with hypotonia; sometimes affected newborns have difficulties in postnatal adaptation. Signs of autonomic dysfunction include hypersalivation, temperature instability, lethargy, hypersomnolence, and episodes of sweating and pallor. Less frequently reported are 'bulbar' signs (drooling, dysarthria, abnormal tongue movements), 'ataxia', probably not cerebellar ataxia or sensory ataxia but dystonic gait, and Gower's sign.

In later infancy and childhood, defects in the metabolism of the biogenic monoamines may be suspected in patients with (fluctuating) extrapyramidal disorders, in particular parkinsonism dystonia or more general 'athetoid cerebral palsy', and vegetative disturbances. A severe epileptic encephalopathy and progressive learning difficulties may be present.

Diagnosis

Every infant with hyperphenylalaninaemia detected in a population newborn screening programme or in the course of other diagnostics later in life must be carefully investigated for possible defects of biopterin metabolism (see also 'Phenylketonuria'). Differential diagnosis requires the analysis of urinary pterins as well as the determination of enzyme activity of dihydropteridine

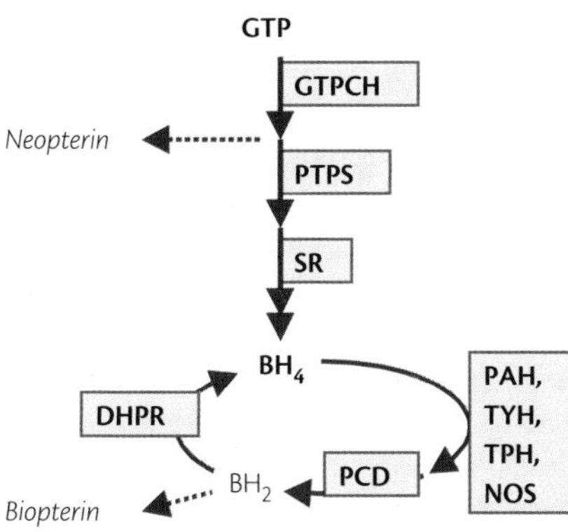

Fig. 12.2.15 Biopterin Metabolism. BH_4 is synthesised and regenerated by five enzymes. BH_4 is consumed as a cofactor in the hydroxylation of tyrosine and tryptophan as well as phenylalanine (see also PKU) and nitric oxide synthase (NOS). BH_2 = dihydrobiopterin. Relevant enzyme defects: GTPCH = GTP cyclohydrolase; PTPS = 6-Pyruvoyl-tetrahydropterin synthase; SR = Sepiapterin reductase; DHPR = Dihydropteridine reductase; PCD = Pterin carbinolamine dehydratase. Adapted with permission from Zschocke and Hoffmann 2004.

reductase in dried blood spots. If the initial plasma phenylalanine concentration is above 400 μmol/litre (6.7 mg/dl), oral loading with BH_4 (20 mg/kg) will result in normalization of phenylalanine values within 4 to 8 h. Urinary biopterin and neopterin values are low in the guanosine triphosphate cyclohydrolase deficiency, whereas 6-pyruvoyltetrahydrobiopterin synthase deficiency has high neopterin values and low biopterin values. In patients with dihydropteridine reductase deficiency, neopterin is normal or slightly elevated and biopterin very high. After the biochemical diagnosis all defects should be ascertained enzymatically and, if available, by mutation analysis. Following a diagnosis of a defect of biopterin metabolism a lumbar puncture becomes necessary for analysis of the neurotransmitter metabolites 5-hydroxyindoleacetic acid and homovanillic acid as well as neopterin, biopterin, and 5-methyltetrahydrofolic acid. This allows differentiation between severe and mild forms of BH_4 deficiencies and sets the indication for treatment with the neurotransmitter precursors L-dopa and 5-hydroxytryptophan. In patients with suggestive encephalopathies and normal phenylalanine values, analysis of neurotransmitters in cerebrospinal fluid is the only way of diagnosis.

Treatment and outcome

Blood phenylalanine concentrations should be more rigidly controlled than in classic PKU patients. In patients with guanosine triphosphate cyclohydrolase deficiency and 6-pyruvoyltetrahydrobiopterin deficiency, administration of BH_4 appears to be the most efficient therapy in controlling blood phenylalanine levels. Patients with dihydropteridine reductase deficiency need a low-phenylalanine diet as in PKU.

Deficiency of neurotransmitters requires treatment with the neurotransmitter precursors L-dopa (3–15 mg/kg per day) and 5-hydroxytryptophan (2–9 mg/kg per day) in combination with carbidopa (10% or 25% of L-dopa). Lumbar punctures must be repeated regularly to adjust doses. In patients revealing L-dopa-induced peak-dose dyskinesia slow-release forms of drugs can be used, and reaching the upper therapeutic limits of L-dopa may be an indication for the use of monoamine oxidase and/or catechol-*O*-methyltransferase inhibitors. Patients with dihydropteridine reductase deficiency, in addition, need administration of folinic acid to restore normal cerebrospinal fluid folate concentrations.

Normal long-term psychomotor development can be achieved but outcome strongly depends on the age when the diagnosis is made and how rigidly therapy is followed, especially in early life.

Dominantly inherited guanosine triphosphate cyclohydrolase deficiency

Clinical presentation

Dominantly inherited guanosine triphosphate cyclohydrolase deficiency, often called Segawa's disease, is an eminently treatable condition. Early recognition is therefore of crucial importance. Presentation in children usually occurs within the first decade of life with a mean age of onset of symptoms being about 7 years (range 16 months to 13 years). The first symptom is usually postural dystonia of one leg with progression to all limbs followed by action dystonia and hand tremor within the next 10 to 15 years, during which time cognition remains intact. Occasionally, in older children, the first signs may start in the arms with torticollis or writer's cramp (focal dystonia). The dystonia is frequently asymmetrical and accompanied by reduced facial expression or slowing of fine finger movements. Diurnal fluctuation is normally present, with symptoms improving after night-time sleep or bed rest. The variation in presenting symptoms is large. Penetrance is reduced and many carriers of a mutant gene are asymptomatic.

Diagnosis

In classic cases with prominent dystonia of the lower limbs, marked diurnal variation, as well as worsening of the symptoms after exercise, the clinical diagnosis of the deficiency is easily made, in particular in the presence of dramatic and sustained response to L-dopa. However, the diagnosis can be a real challenge in atypical cases, in which it can be ascertained by determining BH_4, and decreased levels of neopterin and homovanillic acid in cerebrospinal fluid. Confirmation of the diagnosis can be achieved by enzyme analysis in cultured skin fibroblasts or by mutation analysis.

Treatment and outcome

Treatment relies on L-dopa in combination with 10% to 25% carbidopa. Amounts administered have varied between 3 and 10 mg/kg per day divided into one to four doses with the effectiveness of treatment being monitored by the clinical outcome. The long-term prognosis is usually excellent.

Tyrosinaemias

The steps in tyrosine metabolism starting with the rate-limiting step—the conversion to *p*-hydroxyphenylpyruvic acid by tyrosine aminotransferase—are outlined in Fig. 12.2.14. Intermediates of this tyrosine metabolism are used for production of catecholamines, dopamine, and the principal pigment of hair and skin, melanin.

Tyrosinaemia type 1 (fumarylacetoacetase deficiency)

Clinical presentation Tyrosinaemia type 1 is also known as hepatorenal tyrosinosis. About one-third of patients present acutely in the early weeks of life with failure to thrive, vomiting, hepatomegaly, fever, oedema, and epistaxis; by the end of the first year of life 90% have developed symptoms. The disease can progress rapidly and death from hepatic failure often occurs in infancy.

A milder more chronic presentation is compatible with survival for several years with chronic liver disease, a renal tubular Fanconi syndrome with hypophosphataemic rickets, and episodic abdominal pain and neuropathy suggestive of acute porphyria. The most serious complication is hepatocellular carcinoma which develops in early childhood in one-third of untreated patients.

Diagnosis Raised plasma tyrosine (often together with methionine), succinylacetone, and 5-aminolaevulinic acid excretion as well as a renal Fanconi syndrome are the biochemical markers of tyrosinaemia type 1 caused by a deficiency of fumarylacetoacetate hydrolyase, the last enzyme in the pathway of tyrosine degradation (Fig. 12.2.14). Serum α-fetoprotein is usually strikingly elevated. Succinylacetone, formed from fumarylacetoacetate, is the most specific diagnostic metabolite. Plasma tyrosine values may be normal, resulting in insufficient specificity of this parameter for newborn screening.

Fumarylacetoacetate hydrolyase can be assayed in lymphocytes or fibroblasts. It is nonspecifically depressed in the liver in a variety of liver diseases. The measurement of succinylacetone in amniotic fluid and activity of fumarylacetoacetate hydrolyase in cultured amniocytes or chorionic villus samples forms the basis of prenatal diagnosis, if informative mutations are not available.

Treatment and outcome Restricted intake of tyrosine and phenylalanine may reduce the excretion of succinylacetone and produce regression of the Fanconi tubular defects, but does not cure the liver disease. The risk of hepatocellular carcinoma remains and early liver transplantation was the treatment of choice until nitisinone (2-(2-nitro-4-trifluoromethylbenzoyl)1–3-cyclohexanedione) was introduced by Lindstedt and colleagues in 1991. Nitisinone almost completely blocks 4-hydroxyphenylpyruvate dioxygenase thus turning tyrosinaemia type 1 into tyrosinaemia type 3 and reducing the production of toxic metabolites. Treatment with nitisinone should start as soon as the diagnosis is made with a dose of 1 mg/kg per day. In most patients there is a rapid improvement in liver and renal function; succinylacetone should disappear from the urine within 1 week of treatment. Patients need to be treated with a diet low in phenylalanine and tyrosine at the same time as introducing nitisinone. Plasma levels of tyrosine should be kept between 250 and 500 µmol/litre.

The long-term results of nitisinone treatment are encouraging with greatly reduced incidence of liver damage and hepatic carcinoma. Liver transplantation remains the treatment of choice for a few patients who do not respond to nitisinone and if there is any suggestion of malignant change.

Tyrosinaemia type 2 (tyrosine aminotransferase deficiency)

Clinical presentation Corneal erosions and dendritic ulcers may form within a few months of birth with later scarring, nystagmus, and glaucoma. Skin lesions may begin after the eye lesions with blistering, painful palms and soles, and hyperkeratosis. Tongue changes have been described. Learning difficulties are an inconstant feature in about 50% of patients, but language defects may be more common with possible impaired coordination and self-mutilation.

Diagnosis Tyrosine aminotransferase, which is deficient, catalyses the formation of *p*-hydroxyphenylpyruvic acid (see Fig. 12.2.14). Plasma tyrosine values reach 20 times normal (normal 40–100 µmol/litre) in younger patients and 10 times normal in others. There is increased excretion of tyrosine, *N*-acetyltyrosine, tyramine, and of phenolic acids; there is no Fanconi syndrome and no increase in succinylacetone.

The clinical features and amino acid analyses are usually sufficient for diagnosis, which may be confirmed either by measuring the enzyme activity in liver or by molecular genetic studies.

Treatment and outcome A low-tyrosine, low-phenylalanine diet has been used to produce rapid improvement of skin and eye manifestations. Corneal transplants can be valuable. The neurological symptoms appear to improve less. The degree of dietary control needed to sustain clinical improvement is uncertain. Plasma tyrosine concentrations less than 500 µmol/litre are considered desirable.

Tyrosinaemia type 3 (4-hydroxyphenylpyruvate dioxygenase deficiency)

4-Hydroxyphenylpyruvate dioxygenase deficiency (see Fig. 12.2.14) appears to be very rare and possibly without clinical pathology, i.e. a nondisease. It may be associated with learning difficulties and possibly other neurological complications. The biochemical findings are similar to those in tyrosinaemia type 2, but the plasma values of tyrosine are usually less than 1200 µmol/litre. Enzyme and molecular genetic studies can prove the diagnosis. Most patients are treated with a low-tyrosine, low-phenylalanine diet.

Alkaptonuria

Clinical presentation

In 1902, alkaptonuria was the first disorder to be recognized as an inborn error of metabolism by Garrod. It is caused by a deficiency of homogentisate dioxygenase resulting in the accumulation of homogentisic acid and its oxidized derivative benzoquinone acetic acid. The latter can then be polymerized to form a dark pigment which is deposited in connective tissue. The disorder is extremely rare in most populations but occurs with greatly increased frequency in the Dominican Republic and in Slovakia. Presentation in infancy occurs only if discoloration of the urine is noticed. It is usually normal when passed but darkens on standing (more rapidly at alkaline pH) to deep brown or almost black. Back pain begins in the second and third decade with increasing stiffness due to intervertebral disc degeneration. Involvement of the hips, knees, and shoulders follows. Greyish discoloration of cartilage is seen in the pinna, and pigment is deposited in the sclera. Abnormal pigmentation is seen in the heart valves and joint cartilages, and pigmented stones are common in the prostate. Valvular calcification is prominent, especially in the coronary arteries. Recent studies of the natural course of alkaptonuria indicate that it is associated with premature heart disease and premature death with long-standing impairment of quality of life. Pigment deposition with involvement of the fibrolipid components of atherosclerotic plaques cause calcific stenosis of the aortic valve. In 58 patients studied by Phornphutkul and colleagues, life-table analysis showed that joint replacement occurred at a mean age of 55 years, renal stones at 64 years, and cardiac valve involvement at 54 years; coronary calcification occurred at a mean age of 59 years.

Diagnosis

Homogentisic acid can be demonstrated by urinary organic acid analysis. Enzymatic as well as molecular confirmation is possible. Plasma tyrosine concentrations are normal.

Treatment and outcome

So far no treatment has been shown to prevent the long-term complications. The prognosis for the joints is poor. By the fifth decade the lumbar spine is likely to be rigid and other joints will be seriously affected. Patients often require large amounts of analgesic and risk the complications of long-term consumption of nonsteroidal anti-inflammatory agents, which may exacerbate incipient coronary heart disease.

Homogentisic acid can be decreased by a low-protein diet. It is very probable that specifically designed low-phenylalanine and low-tyrosine diets would lower the production still further. Nitisinone, the triketone inhibitor of 4-hydroxyphenylpyruvate dioxygenase introduced by Lindstedt in 1991, greatly reduces overproduction of homogentisic acid in alkaptonuria. Early studies from Gahl's group at the National Institutes of Health showed that in adults of both sexes with alkaptonuria an oral dose of 1.05 mg twice daily reduced urinary homogentisic acid excretion from a mean of 4 g to 0.2 g per day. More than 220 patients with hereditary tyrosinaemia type 1 have received the drug at daily doses of 0.5 to 2.0 mg/kg body weight and even at these doses it is generally well tolerated, apart from mild blood cytopenias. In alkaptonuria nitisinone, as predicted, may elevate the plasma tyrosine concentrations (in the early trial from *c.*70 to 760 μmol/litre) and there is thus a theoretical risk of lens opacities, which can be avoided by careful slit-lamp monitoring, plasma amino acid measurement, and dietary adjustment. In alkaptonuria the outcome of nitisinone treatment will take many years to evaluate fully, but comprehensive therapeutic study is justified by the clear relationship between overproduction of a single metabolite and life-shortening tissue manifestations with disabling joint disease.

Neurotransmitter diseases and related disorders

Monogenic defects of neurotransmission have become recognized as a cause of early-onset, severe, progressive, and often treatable encephalopathies. The diagnosis is based on the quantitative determination of the neurotransmitters or their metabolites in cerebrospinal fluid, i.e. glycine and γ-aminobutyric acid, the acidic metabolites of the biogenic monoamines, and individual pterin species (Box 12.2.6). Determinations of metabolites in blood or urine are neither sensitive nor specific. In contrast to inborn errors in catabolic pathways, neurotransmitter defects are determined by the interplay of biosynthesis, degradation, and receptor status. Even borderline abnormalities can be diagnostic and their recognition requires a strictly standardized sampling protocol and adequate age-related reference values.

Disorders of monoamine metabolism

Defects in the metabolism of the biogenic monoamines affect serotonin and/or catecholamine (dopamine and norepinephrine) metabolism (Fig. 12.2.16). They present from infancy or childhood with (fluctuating) extrapyramidal disorders, in particular parkinsonian dystonia or more general 'athetoid cerebral palsy', and vegetative disturbances. A severe epileptic encephalopathy and progressive learning difficulties may be present. A folinic acid-responsive seizure disorder is considered in the context of other monoamine disorders as a marker for the disease appears in the analytical system used to measure monoamine metabolites. The underlying aetiology in this disorder remains to be elucidated.

Tyrosine hydroxylase deficiency

Tyrosine hydroxylase catalyses the hydroxylation of L-tyrosine to L-dopa, the rate-limiting step in the biosynthesis of the catecholamines dopamine, norepinephrine, and epinephrine (Fig. 12.2.16). The iron-containing mixed function oxidase requires molecular oxygen and the cofactor BH_4. Tyrosine hydroxylase is expressed only in catecholaminergic neurons and the adrenal medulla.

Tyrosine hydroxylase deficiency has become incorporated into concepts and classifications of dystonias as the cause of recessive L-dopa-responsive dystonia, but can also present as L-dopa-nonresponsive dystonia or progressive early-onset encephalopathy.

Clinical presentation Clinical symptoms often develop between 3 and 7 months of age. Most patients show a substantial clinical improvement on low doses of L-dopa together with the decarboxylase inhibitor carbidopa, although in contrast to L-dopa-responsive dystonia due to haploinsufficiency of guanosine triphosphate

Box 12.2.6 Cerebrospinal fluid: investigation for neurotransmitter disorders

- Cells, protein, immunoglobulin classes and glucose (plus plasma glucose and evaluation of blood–brain barrier)
- Lactate, pyruvate
- Amino acids (plus plasma obtained simultaneously)
- Biogenic monoamine metabolites
- Individual pterin species
- 5-Methyltetrahydrofolate

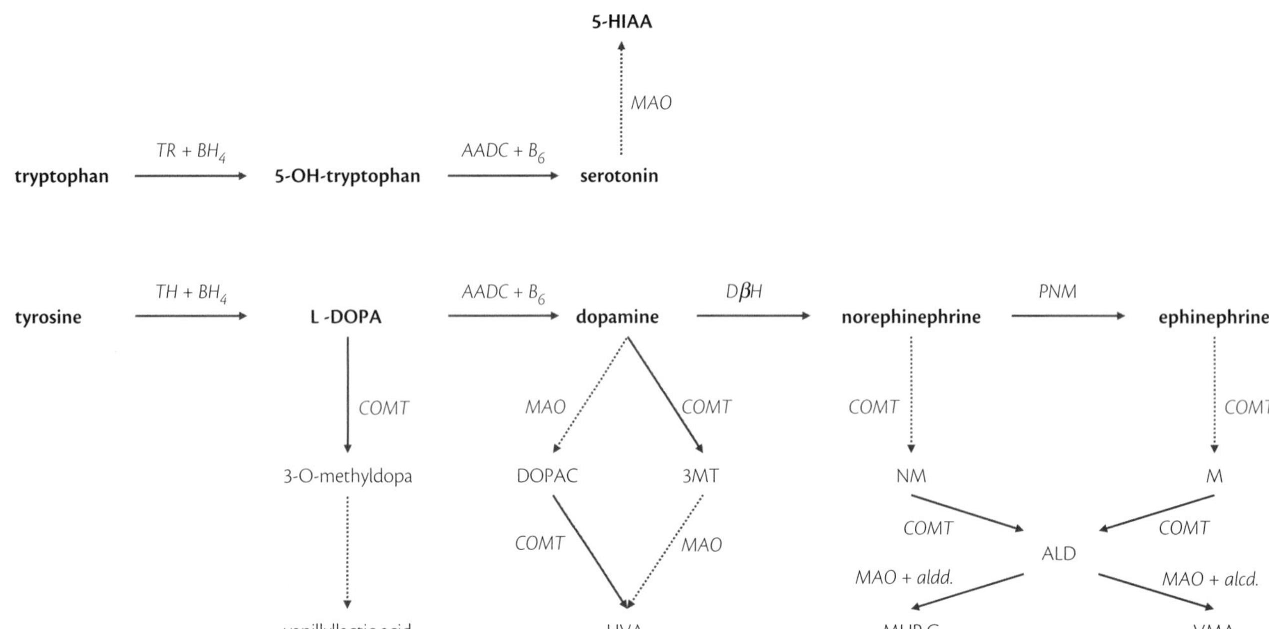

Fig. 12.2.16 Metabolism of Biogenic Monoamines. Abbreviations (in alphabetical order): AADC = aromatic L-aminoacid decarboxylase, alcd. = alcohol dehydrogenase, ALD = intermediate aldehyde (3-methoxy-4-hydroxyphenyl- hydroxyacetaldehyde), aldd. = aldehyde dehydrogenase, BH_4 = tetrahydrobiopterin, COMT = catechol-ortho-methyltransferase, DOPAC = 3,4-dihydroxyphenylacetic acid, DβH = dopamine-β-hydroxylase, 5- HIAA = 5-hydroxyindolacetic acid, HVA = homovanillic acid, M = metanephrine, MAO = monoaminooxidase, MHPG = 3-methoxy-4-hydroxy-phenylglycol, MT = 3-methoxytyramine, NM = normetanephrine, PNM = phenylethanolamine-N-methyltransferase, TH = tyrosin hydroxylase, TR = tryptophan hydroxylase, VMA = vanillylmandelic acid, . . . = several steps involved.

cyclohydrolase I often neither the neurological status nor the catecholamine levels in cerebrospinal fluid can be completely normalized.

At the severe end of the spectrum virtually no movements are observed, not even dystonic movements. Some patients are more severely affected and present with a progressive neurometabolic disorder from early infancy with a progressive infantile encephalopathy characterized by abnormal extrapyramidal movements and affecting several cerebral and possibly cerebellar systems. It is important to stress that such patients also show symptoms of significant catecholamine deficiency, such as hypoglycaemia and inadequate stress responses. There is an obvious tendency to preterm birth with troublesome cardiorespiratory perinatal adaptation.

Most infants with tyrosine hydroxylase deficiency develop surprisingly normally until an arrest of motor development with a characteristic combination of neurological symptoms around 1 year of age. Hypokinesia, marked truncal hypotonia, a mask face, oculogyric crises, myoclonic jerks, and an extrapyramidal tremor can progressively develop. The last three symptoms can be mistaken as epileptic phenomena. Oculogyric crises are present but, as with the miosis, may go undiagnosed because of prominent ptosis. Contractures, failure to thrive, and immobilization may develop. It appears likely that life expectancy is significantly reduced; (dystonic) cerebral palsy is a likely descriptive (mis-)diagnosis. Some patients did not develop extrapyramidal symptoms in the first year of life, were able to walk independently, and followed a clinical course best summarized as spastic paraplegia. Their symptoms fully resolved following L-dopa supplementation, and they are now healthy adults living independently.

Diagnosis The diagnosis of tyrosine hydroxylase deficiency can only be made via cerebrospinal fluid analysis following a standardized lumbar puncture protocol. A characteristic metabolite constellation is found: low concentrations of metabolites of dopaminergic neurotransmission homovanillic acid and 3-methoxy-4-hydroxyphenylethyleneglycol in the presence of normal concentrations of metabolites belonging to the serotonin neurotransmission system such as 5-hydroxyindoleacetic acid (Fig. 12.2.16). Urinary determinations of catecholamines and homovanillic acid turned out to be inconclusive in several affected individuals.

Enzyme analysis is not possible in tyrosine hydroxylase deficiency because tissues expressing enzyme activity—brain and adrenal medulla—are difficult to obtain. Thus mutation analysis is the only way to confirm the diagnosis.

Treatment and outcome Therapeutic interventions with L-dopa together with the decarboxylase inhibitor carbidopa and selegiline were able to improve and or even normalize the clinical picture in most patients but not all. Despite all therapeutic interventions, the disease course can be lethal.

Treatment with L-dopa has to be started slowly and carefully, with doses as low as 0.5 mg/kg per day in two to six divided doses to avoid dyskinesias due to hypersensitivity and up-regulation of dopamine receptors in dopamine-deficient patients. In such patients L-dopa can only be increased very slowly, sometimes over several years. Slow-release preparations may be useful to ensure constant L-dopa levels. In general, incremental steps of L-dopa/carbidopa should not be more than 1 mg/kg per day.

Aromatic L-amino acid decarboxylase deficiency

Aromatic L-amino acid decarboxylase deficiency is caused by autosomal recessively inherited mutations in the *DDC* gene. The enzyme is required for the synthesis of both serotonin and the catecholamines.

Clinical presentation Clinical symptoms are indistinguishable from those of patients with tyrosine hydroxylase deficiency. The severity seems to fall into two groups. About half of the patients present with feeding difficulties, autonomic dysfunction, and hypotonia in the neonatal period. In the first few months of life dystonia or intermittent limb spasticity, axial and truncal hypotonia, extreme irritability, oculogyric crises, and psychomotor retardation become obvious. More mildly affected patients may initially develop unremarkably or only slightly delayed and present with motor retardation, hypokinesia, rigidity, and truncal hypotonia from early childhood.

Diagnosis The enzyme deficiency leads to accumulation of 3-*O*-methyldopa, 5-hydroxytryptophan, and L-dopa (Fig. 12.2.16). 3-*O*-Methyldopa is formed by methylation of L-dopa. Confirmation of the diagnosis is by enzyme assay in plasma and finally by mutation analysis.

Treatment and outcome Different approaches using dopamine agonists (pergolide, pramipexole, bromocriptine, and ropinirole) and/or nonselective monoamine oxidase inhibitors (tranylcypromine, phenelzine) have been attempted. Response to treatment is variable but outcome appears to be better in more mildly affected and later-presenting patients. The overall prognosis is guarded. About half of the patients improve on individual treatment regimens and acquire different degrees of motor and psychosocial skills. Others do not show any improvements.

Dopamine β-hydroxylase deficiency

Clinical presentation Recessively inherited mutations in the dopamine β-hydroxylase gene lead to lowered levels of norepinephrine within central and autonomic noradrenergic neurons (Fig. 12.2.16). The disorder is characterized by sympathetic noradrenergic denervation and adrenomedullary failure. The central consequences appear minimal. Syndromes become obvious in adolescence with noradrenergic failure, severe orthostatic hypotension, and ptosis of the eyelids. During childhood fatigue, episodes of fainting, syncopes, and exercise intolerance are generally present. Physical and cognitive function is normal. In males autonomic neuropathy leads to retrograde ejaculation.

Diagnosis Dopamine β-hydroxylase deficiency is classified as a primary autonomic neuropathy. Conditions that lead to chronic failure of the autonomic nervous system are, therefore, the primary differential diagnosis. Biochemically, dopamine β-hydroxylase deficiency is different from other conditions with orthostatic hypotension or autonomic dysfunction. Failure to produce norepinephrine and the consequent lack of end-product inhibition of tyrosine hydroxylase leads to a norepinephrine/dopamine ratio of less than 0.1, and such a finding is pathognomonic for the disease. An increase in blood pressure and correction of the orthostatic hypotension in response to dihydroxyphenylserine is also diagnostic. Some 3 to 4% of the normal adult population have near zero levels of the enzyme in plasma, therefore plasma enzyme determination alone cannot be used to make a positive diagnosis, it requires mutation analysis.

Treatment and outcome Dopamine β-hydroxylase deficiency is treated with dihydroxyphenylserine. This compound is decarboxylated by L-amino acid decarboxylase to form norepinephrine. Administration of 250 to 500 mg twice daily results in an increase in blood pressure and sustained relief of the orthostatic symptoms. Without appropriate treatment postural hypotension can lead to significant injuries or even death.

Disorders of pyridoxine metabolism

In 1954 Hunt and colleagues described a patient with a seizure disorder that was successfully treated solely by administration of pyridoxine (vitamin B_6) and coined the term 'pyridoxine dependency'. It became good clinical practice to test for pyridoxine responsiveness in every child with 'difficult-to-treat' seizures starting before 2 years of age. Recently the enzymatic defect has been pinpointed to a piperideine-6-carboxylate dehydrogenase located in the lysine degradation pathway in the brain, which results in the accumulation of an intermediate scavenging pyridoxal phosphate. A similar pathogenic mechanism again resulting in intractable seizures is responsible for pyridoxal deficiency in hyperprolinaemia type II and during treatment with the tuberculostatic drug isoniazid.

Another monogenic defect in humans is directly located within the synthesis of pyridoxal 5′-phosphate: pyridox(am)ine 5′-phosphate oxidase deficiency resulting in pyridoxal phosphate-responsive seizures (Fig. 12.2.17).

Each newborn with severe neonatal/infantile epileptic encephalopathy should have a lumbar puncture and then immediately receive consecutive therapeutic trials with vitamin B6, pyridoxal 5′-phosphate, and folinic acid.

Pyridoxine-dependent epilepsy and folinic acid-responsive seizures: alpha-aminoadipic semialdehyde dehydrogenase deficiency

Aetiology/pathophysiology Pyridoxine-dependent epilepsy and folinic acid-responsive seizures are two treatable causes of neonatal epileptic encephalopathy. The genetic base of the former is autosomal recessive inheritance of pathogenic mutations in the *ALDH7A1* (antiquitin)gene causing deficiency of the enzyme alpha-aminoadipic semialdehyde dehydrogenase (Δ^1-piperideine-6-carboxylate dehydrogenase) located in the pipecolic acid pathway, the major route of cerebral lysine oxidation. As a consequence of accumulating alpha-aminoadipic semialdehyde and the cyclic compound Δ^1-piperideine 6-carboxylate, which spontaneously forms an adduct with pyridoxal phosphate via a Knoevenagel reaction, pyridoxal phosphate is inactivated resulting in cerebral

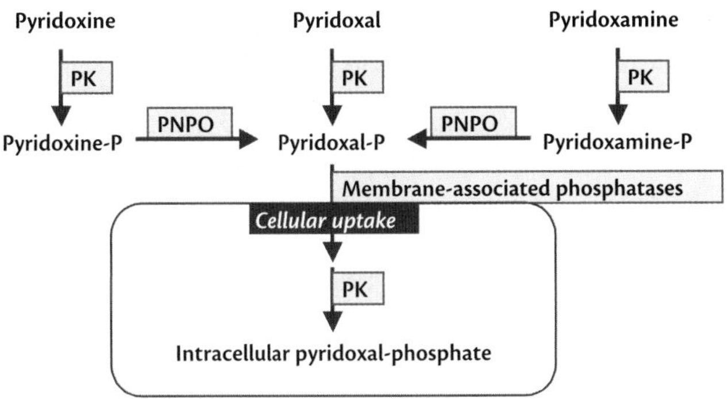

Fig. 12.2.17 Pyridoxine metabolism. Pyridoxal phosphate (PALP; vitamin B_6) is cofactor of transamination and decarboxylation reactions in various pathways including serotonin and dopamine biosynthesis. It is synthesised from dietary pyridoxal, pyridoxamine and pyridoxine; enzymes involved include pyridoxal kinase (PK) and pyridox(am)ine 5-phosphate oxidase (PNPO).
Adapted with permission from Zschocke and Hoffmann 2004.

depletion of pyridoxal phosphate. Pyridoxal phosphate-dependent enzymes such as glutamate dehydrogenase, gamma-aminobutyric acid (GABA) transaminase and aromatic L-amino acid dehydrogenase (AADC) are inactivated by pyridoxal phosphate depletion causing significant disturbance in the metabolism of the neurotransmitters dopamine, serotonine, glutamate and GABA and thus a severe epileptic encephalopathy. The conversion of pyridoxine, pyridoxal and pyridoxamine to pyridoxal phosphate however remains unaffected. Recently, it has been elucidated that folinic acid-responsive seizures which was considered a separate disease entity is genetically and biochemically identical to the major form of pyridoxine-dependent epilepsy.

Clinical presentation Pyridoxine-dependent epilepsy can be heterogeneous in its presentation, and sometimes idiopathic epilepsies respond to treatment with pyridoxine. Classical patients with pyridoxine-dependent epilepsy present with an intractable seizure disorder within the first 2 days of life, and at the latest within 28 days. In some patients intrauterine convulsions are reported. There is no consistent electrographic pattern. Continuous and discontinuous backgrounds, suppression burst-like patterns, and hypsarrhythmia have all been observed. There are additional atypical presentations: 1) late onset, i.e. later than 28 days; 2) neonatal onset but with an initial response to conventional anticonvulsant therapy; 3) neonatal onset with initially negative, but a later sustained positive response to pyridoxine.

Folinic acid-sensitive seizures have been an enigmatic clinical and biochemical entity until it has been elucidated recently that they are alleic to pyridoxine-dependent epilepsy. Patients present with myoclonic or clonic seizures, apnea, and irritability within 5 days after birth. The electroencephalogram shows a discontinuous background pattern with multifocal spikes and sharp waves. Without specific treatment seizures will only be partially controlled. Psychomotor development will become severely impaired. It is therefore recommended that all patients with 'difficult-to-treat' seizures starting before 2 years should have a trial of pyridoxine and folinic acid (usually given orally in this circumstance).

Diagnosis The diagnosis of pyridoxine-dependent epilepsy and folinic acid-responsive seizures should be suspected clinically in patients with neonatal epileptic encephalopathy or "difficult-to-treat" seizures starting before 2 years of age who respond to pyridoxine and/or folinic acid. Because it is a treatable condition a high index of suspicion is warranted. Both pyridoxine and pyridoxal phosphate may cause apnoea and prolonged cerebral depression after the initial dose, and resuscitation equipment and intensive care facilities should be available.

The suspected diagnosis can be confirmed by measurement of alpha-aminoadipic semialdehyde in body fluids. Elevated CSF and plasma pipecolic acid is also used as a biomarker. Furthermore, CSF analysis may reveal a monoamine pattern similar to AADC deficiency, elevated glutamate and decreased GABA concentrations. Enzyme assay and mutation analysis of the *ALDH7A1* gene is the most definitive prove of diagnosis.

Treatment and outcome Treatment requires 5 to 30 mg/kg body weight per day of pyridoxine in one dose. Successful treatment with folinic acid can be achieved with 3 to 5 mg/kg body weight per day of folinic acid given in three doses. Doses need to be increased and adjusted to body weight during growth. Breakthrough seizures are an obvious criterion for increasing the dose. There is evidence that lower doses of pyridoxine and folinic acid, while controlling seizures, may still not prevent the development of cognitive impairment. High doses of pyridoxine carry the risk of developing skin photosensitivity as well of a peripheral sensory neuropathy. Doses up to 1 g/day can be regarded as safe in older children. Serial cognitive assessment is therefore recommended. If there is a positive family history of pyridoxine-dependent seizures, maternal treatment in utero is indicated.

Since pyridoxine-dependent epilepsy and folinic acid-sensitive seizures appear to be genetically and biochemically identical, this new understanding requires a reevaluation of optimal strategies such as combined use of pyridoxine and folinic acid as well as of low lysine diet aiming to reduce the accumulation of alpha-aminoadipic semialdehyde and Δ^1-piperideine 6-carboxylate.

Hyperprolinaemia type II: L-Δ^1-pyrroline-5-carboxylate dehydrogenase deficiency

Clinical presentation For a long time hyperprolinaemia type I, which has no clinically relevant phenotype, was not separated from hyperprolinaemia type II. Also, as individuals with hyperprolinaemia type II often have no clinical manifestations, hyperprolinaemia was considered a nondisease. However, on investigation of larger cohorts of affected individuals it became obvious that hyperprolinaemia type II can lead to epilepsy in more than 50% of patients. The epilepsy usually disappears in adulthood.

Diagnosis Plasma concentrations of proline are highly elevated, exceeding 1500 µmol/litre. Whereas proline is the only amino acid elevated in plasma and cerebrospinal fluid, glycine and hydroxyproline are also found elevated in urine as these three amino acids share a common renal tubular transport system. Hyperprolinaemia type II must be distinguished from hyperprolinaemia type I by demonstration of elevated levels of L-Δ^1-pyrroline-5-carboxylate and/or by enzyme assay or molecular analysis.

Treatment and outcome Unless a seizure disorder is present no specific treatment is required. In a child with a seizure disorder, treatment with 5 to 30 mg/kg body weight per day of pyridoxine in one dose should be started. There are usually no adverse sequelae.

Pyridoxal phosphate-responsive seizures: pyridox(am)ine 5′-phosphate oxidase deficiency

Clinical presentation Pyridoxal phosphate responsive seizures due to pyridox(am)ine 5′-phosphate oxidase deficiency (Fig. 12.2.17) results in a most severe early neonatal encephalopathy with convulsions, myoclonus, rotatory eye movements, sudden clonic contractions, hypoglycaemia, and (lactic) acidosis. Seizures are resistant to conventional anticonvulsant therapy. Many patients are born prematurely, and fetal distress is common, including 'signs of asphyxia' and low Apgar scores. Early (lactic) acidosis and hypoglycaemia may be observed. Thus pyridoxal phosphate-responsive seizures must enter the differential diagnosis of hypoxic–ischaemic encephalopathy in prematurely born infants.

Diagnosis The deficiency of pyridox(am)ine 5′-phosphate oxidase results in combined deficiencies of L-amino acid decarboxylase, threonine dehydratase, ornithine δ-aminotransferase, and the glycine cleavage enzyme with the concomitant biochemical findings. In addition, some patients display variable lactic acidaemia as well as a tendency to hypoglycaemia. However, no biochemical abnormality is 100% specific or sensitive, and a positive response to the drug remains the most reliable indication of pyridoxal phosphate-responsive seizures. The diagnosis is confirmed by mutation analysis.

Treatment and outcome Pyridoxal 5′-phosphate given by nasogastric tube is dramatically effective in stopping seizures and improving the appearances of the electroencephalogram. Long-term treatment requires 30 to 60 mg/kg body weight per day of pyridoxal 5′-phosphate in four doses. Doses need to be increased and adjusted to body weight during growth. Patients probably require lifelong supplementation. Breakthrough seizures are an obvious criterion for increasing the dose. So far many questions remain open with regards to prognosis. Serial cognitive assessment is recommended.

Defects of glycine and serine metabolism

Nonketotic hyperglycinaemia

Nonketotic hyperglycinaemia is the second most common disorder of amino acid metabolism, second to PKU, with an overall worldwide frequency estimated at 1 in 60 000 births. It is caused by deficient activity of the glycine cleavage system which represents the main catabolic route of glycine (Fig. 12.2.18) and is present at high levels in liver, brain, and placenta. In brain, it keeps glycine levels very low, resulting in a typically low cerebrospinal fluid to plasma glycine ratio.

Glycine is connected to multiple biochemical pathways. Most important is the generation of methylenetetrahydrofolate. The glycine cleavage system is made up of four mitochondrial proteins, P, H, T, and L. The P protein is a decarboxylase requiring pyridoxal phosphate. The heat-resistant H protein contains lipoic acid and carries the aminomethyl moiety. Both proteins are needed to generate CO_2 from the carbon-1 of glycine. The T protein requires tetrahydrofolate and produces methylenetetrahydrofolate from carbon-2 of glycine. The fourth protein (L protein) is needed to transfer hydrogen from the lipoic acid moiety of the H protein to nicotinamide adenine diphosphate.

Clinical presentation Symptoms of nonketotic hyperglycinaemia are exclusively neurological. Pregnancy and delivery are generally uneventful. Hiccupping *in utero* maybe recognized retrospectively. Lethargy, convulsions, anorexia, poor feeding, and vomiting progress to coma and unresponsiveness 24 to 48 h after birth. Patients are severely hypotonic. Seizures with hiccupping and myoclonic spasms are prominent, and there is a burst suppression pattern on electroencephalography. Apnoea worsens during the third day of life, mostly requiring ventilation. The mortality rate at this stage is high, especially, if the children are not ventilated. After 2 to 3 weeks the patients improve slightly and no longer require intensive care. However, intellectual development does not occur in survivors, seizures persist, and tendon reflexes are increased. Microcephaly, poor head control, profound retardation, and a picture of spastic cerebral palsy develop.

Up to 15% of patients with neonatal presentation have a better recovery after the neonatal period. They have a milder seizure disorder, usually controlled by benzoate therapy or by a single anticonvulsant. Most of these patients make some developmental progress, but they are still mentally disabled with developmental quotients varying between 10 and 60.

Variant forms of nonketotic hyperglycinaemia present in later infancy or childhood with severe seizures, spastic paraparesis, clonus, and extensor plantar responses with modestly raised plasma and cerebrospinal fluid glycine values. Optic atrophy with cerebellar signs has also been described. The outcome is similar to that of patients with the severe form of neonatal nonketotic hyperglycinaemia.

Diagnosis Confirmation of diagnosis by enzyme assay and/or molecular analysis is highly advisable and should be pursued to facilitate future prenatal diagnosis.

Biochemically, nonketotic hyperglycinaemia is characterized by elevated glycine in plasma and in cerebrospinal fluid, with the glycine being more elevated in cerebrospinal fluid than in plasma. Plasma glycine is elevated to values of 600 to 1200 μmol/litre but may vary throughout the day, and can be normal at times. Normal values for cerebrospinal fluid levels of glycine are around 4 to 5 μmol/litre, the normal cerebrospinal fluid to plasma ratio being less than 0.04. In nonketotic hyperglycinaemia patients, the cerebrospinal fluid to plasma glycine ratio is between 0.07 and 0.30.

Great care must be taken to obtain simultaneous plasma and cerebrospinal fluid samples. Diagnostic pitfalls can arise due to postprandial blood sampling, blood contamination of the cerebrospinal fluid, profound liver dysfunction, and treatment with valproate. Urine organic acids must be determined to exclude propionic aciduria and methylmalonic aciduria, as well as glyceric aciduria. Activity of the glycine cleavage system can only be reliably measured on liver biopsies and in direct uncultured chorionic villi for prenatal diagnosis.

So far the molecular structures of the P protein, the T protein, and the H protein have been elucidated, allowing molecular diagnosis of defects of these three proteins. Molecular studies have demonstrated a defect of the P protein in about 50 to 60% of patients and in the T protein in about 30% of patients; a few patients were found to have mutations in the *GLDC* gene leaving approximately 15% of patients with no mutations found after all three genes had been analysed.

Treatment and outcome Therapeutic interventions are unsatisfactory. Some damage to the central nervous system may be prenatal. Withdrawal of artificial ventilation and intensive care support should be discussed with the parents of neonates in the apnoeic phase. Once breathing resumes, most patients survive for many years.

Plasma glycine can be lowered by exchange transfusion or peritoneal dialysis but without clinical improvement. Low-protein

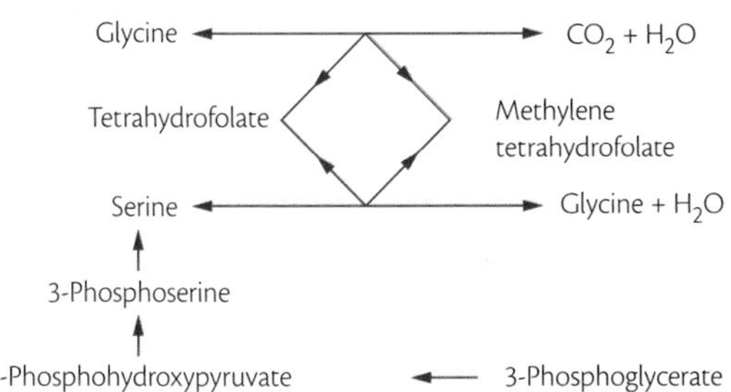

Fig. 12.2.18 Reversible glycine cleavage to carbon dioxide and water is illustrated together with reversible interconversion of serine and glycine. These reactions also serve to generate 1-carbon units. 3-phosphoglycerate (glycolysis) is the ultimate source.

diets have only a limited effect on decreasing plasma glycine concentrations. Supplying one-carbon units in the form of methionine or *N*-formyltetrahydrofolate has not helped. The combination of sodium benzoate to increase glycine excretion and diazepines, which compete for inhibitory glycine receptors in the central nervous system, has lowered plasma and cerebrospinal fluid levels of glycine and reduced seizures. Doses up to 600 to 750 mg/kg per day may be required to lower glycine sufficiently to values between 120 and 280 μmol/litre. At such high doses monitoring of benzoate levels is advised, nevertheless gastric irritation is very frequent and gastric protection with H_2-antihistamine or proton pump inhibitors is preventively recommended.

Most patients need gastric tube feeding or gastrostomy. Gastro-oesophageal reflux develops frequently, and many patients benefit from a Nissen fundoplication. Recurrent bronchitis is a major problem and bronchopneumonia is frequently the cause of death. For patients with mild nonketotic hyperglycinaemia, management of the hyperactivity can be a major challenge.

3-Phosphoglycerate dehydrogenase deficiency

Serine is synthesized from the glycolytic intermediate 3-phosphoglycerate by 3-phosphoglycerate dehydrogenase yielding 3-phosphohydroxypyruvate (Fig. 12.2.18). Deficiency of this enzyme leads to serine deficiency.

Clinical presentation Patients with serine deficiency due to 3-phosphoglycerate dehydrogenase deficiency have congenital microcephaly. They develop severe psychomotor retardation with spastic tetraparesis and severe microcephaly. Seizures usually start in infancy as West's syndrome with hypsarrhythmia. The MRI scan is characterized by striking delayed or absent myelination, with subsequent cortical and subcortical atrophy. Variable symptoms include cataract, hypogonadism, megaloblastic anaemia, and nystagmus.

Diagnosis Serine deficiency in 3-phosphoglycerate dehydrogenase deficiency is most reliably diagnosed in cerebrospinal fluid with values less than 14 μmol/litre (normal cerebrospinal fluid serine 42–86 μmol/litre in infancy). Serine values in fasting plasma are also reduced (28–64 μmol/litre, controls 70–187 μmol/litre). However, nonfasting plasma levels can be normal.

Treatment and outcome L-Serine should be administered orally until normalized (300–500 mg/kg per day). If seizures persist glycine should be added up to 300 mg/kg per day. A very satisfactory outcome was achieved by antenatal treatment in one patient.

Defects of γ-aminobutyric acid metabolism

γ-Aminobutyric acid is formed from glutamate in the brain by the cytosolic enzyme glutamate decarboxylase, which requires pyridoxal phosphate (Fig. 12.2.19). Glutamate can be regenerated from γ-aminobutyric acid by transamination with ketoglutarate (γ-aminobutyric acid transaminase), which is also pyridoxal phosphate dependent. The other product is succinic semialdehyde, which is dehydrogenated to succinate and enters the citric acid cycle. Deficiency of succinic semialdehyde dehydrogenase leads to formation and excretion of 4-hydroxybutyric acid.

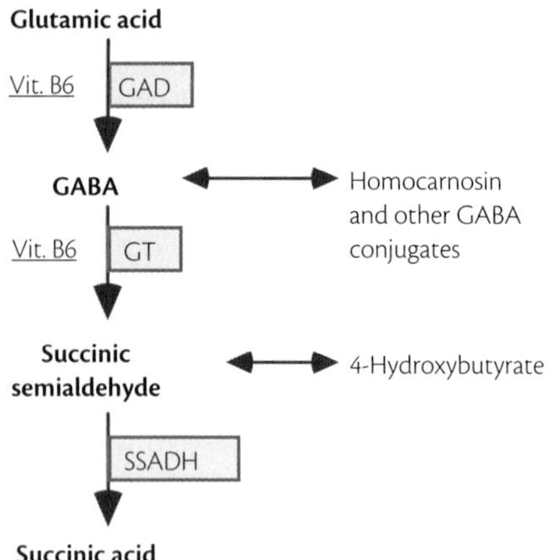

Fig. 12.2.19 Synthesis and catabolism of 4-aminobutyric acid (GABA). The enzymes recognized for known monogenic disorders in humans are shown in boxes: GAD = glutamic acid decarboxylase deficiency, GT = GABA transaminase deficiency, SSADH = succinic semialdehyde dehydrogenase deficiency. The cofactor vit. B6 = vitamine B6 is underlined.
Adapted with permission from Zschocke and Hoffmann 2004.

γ-Aminobutyric acid transaminase deficiency

The few patients described with γ-aminobutyric acid transaminase deficiency presented with a fatal neonatal encephalopathy, characterized by seizures, hypotonia, hyperreflexia, a high-pitched cry (cat cry), and accelerated growth. The diagnosis can be suspected from significantly elevated levels of γ-aminobutyric acid (both free and total), as well as β-alanine and homocarnosine in cerebrospinal fluid. Plasma levels of these amino acids are also increased, but not as significantly. The diagnosis must be confirmed by enzyme assay and possibly mutation analysis, both of which can also be used for prenatal diagnosis. Unfortunately, there is no rational treatment available.

Succinic semialdehyde dehydrogenase deficiency (4-hydroxybutyric aciduria)

Clinical presentation The clinical presentation of succinic semialdehyde dehydrogenase deficiency is highly heterogeneous, even within sibships. The cardinal manifestations are complex and rather nonspecific: hypotonia, delay of motor, mental, and fine motor skills and language. Ataxia and/or seizures occur in about half of the patients. Hyperkinesis and aggressive and autistic behaviour are additional features. MRI studies show bilateral globus pallidus abnormalities but again not constantly.

Diagnosis Diagnosis is usually suspected by demonstrating increased levels of γ-hydroxybutyrate by organic acid analysis. It is confirmed by enzyme assay and preferentially additional mutation analysis.

Treatment and outcome A common treatment for succinic semialdehyde dehydrogenase deficiency is the antiepileptic drug vigabatrin. The results have been encouraging in some patients, but of little value or even detrimental in others. Seizures respond to conventional anticonvulsants. A ketogenic diet shows promise. Succinic semialdehyde dehydrogenase deficiency is a slowly progressive encephalopathy in childhood; it eventually stabilizes in most patients.

Defects of trans-sulphuration and remethylation

The trans-sulphuration pathway transfers the sulphur of methionine to serine, thus generating cysteine (Fig. 12.2.20). Methionine adenosyltransferase, with widely distributed isoenzyme forms, produces *S*-adenosylmethionine, the donor in a variety of methylation reactions. *S*-Adenosylhomocysteine is cleaved to homocysteine,

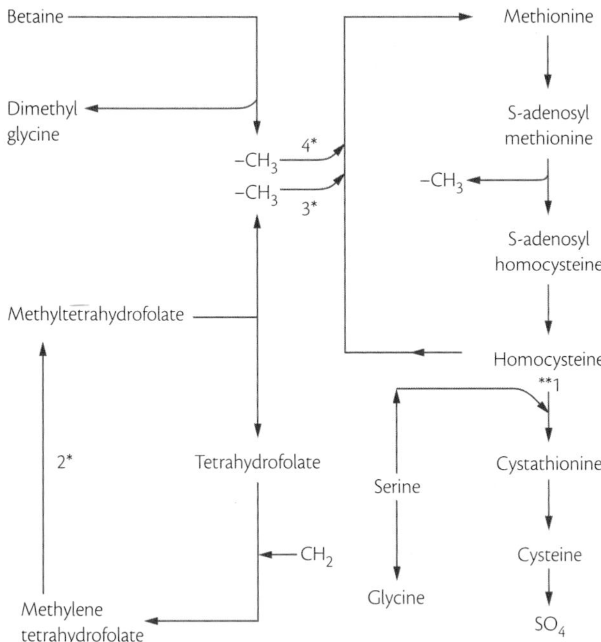

Fig. 12.2.20 The trans-sulphuration pathway from methionine to cysteine is shown on the right and the remethylation of homocysteine on the left. Asterisked enzymes are: 1, cystathionine synthase; 2, methylene tetrahydrofolate reductase, 3, methionine synthase; and 4, betaine methyltransferase.

the sulphydryl compound that exists in reversible equilibrium with its disulphide homocystine. Half of the homocysteine formed goes through the trans-sulphuration pathway and the other half takes a methyl group from betaine (betaine methyltransferase) or 5-methyltetrahydrofolic acid (methionine synthase). The latter is a cobalamin-dependent enzyme which is functionally impaired in defects of vitamin B_{12} metabolism. In addition, methionine synthase reductase is necessary to keep the methionine synthase-bound cobalamin in a functional state. The remethylation of homocysteine is also impaired if the activity of the reductase that generates 5-methyltetrahydrofolate is inadequate. When accumulation of homocystine results from defects of homocysteine remethylation, plasma methionine concentrations are low. They are high when homocystine accumulates from impaired activity of cystathionine β-synthase.

Classic homocystinuria: cystathionine β-synthase deficiency

Clinical presentation

Untreated classic homocystinuria is a slowly progressive devastating multiorgan disorder. First symptoms in childhood are a rapidly progressive myopia and lens dislocation. Lens dislocation usually occurs in preschool years, but later dislocation is well recognized in pyridoxine-responsive patients, and a few have not developed it even in adult life. Monocular and binocular blindness has been relatively frequent due to secondary glaucoma, staphyloma formation, buphthalmos, and retinal detachment.

In the older child skeletal abnormalities and learning difficulties become obvious. Genu valgum and pes cavus are usually the first signs of skeletal changes, which include osteoporosis and spontaneous crush vertebral fractures. The common abnormalities seen in Marfan's syndrome—high arched palate, pectus excavatum or carinatum, genu valgum, pes cavus or planus, scoliosis—are all well recognized in homocystinuria. Arachnodactyly is less common and the fingers not infrequently (and elbows occasionally) show mild flexion contractures. Skeletal disproportion with a crown–pubis length less than the pubis–heel length is usual (Fig. 12.2.21). Learning difficulties affect two-thirds of patients. Patients responsive to pyridoxine (vitamin B6) (see below) have generally higher IQ values than nonresponsive patients. Seizures affect about one-fifth of patients and a few show extrapyramidal features, sometimes with severe involuntary movements. Psychiatric disturbances have also been described.

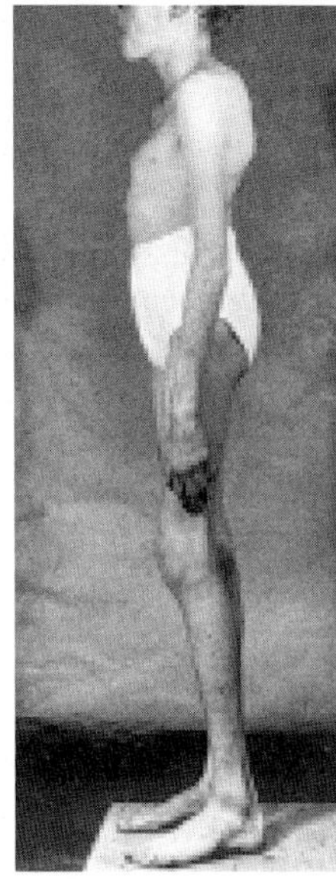

Fig. 12.2.21 Child with cystathionine synthase deficiency. Note the kyphosis and disproportionate short trunk.

Thromboembolism is a major cause of morbidity and the main cause of high premature mortality. Thromboses have been described in a wide variety of arteries and veins: cerebral, coronary, mesenteric, renal, and peripheral.

Diagnosis

Elevated plasma methionine values between 100 and 500 µmol/litre (sometimes higher) are seen with plasma homocystine values of 50 to 200 µmol/litre. A mixed disulphide (half homocysteine, half cysteine) is always present at concentrations somewhat below those of homocystine. Diagnosis requires the determination of fasting quantitative plasma amino acids, as well as plasma total homocysteine. Total homocysteine measured by HPLC includes both homocysteine moieties of homocystine, the homocysteine moiety of the mixed disulphide, and the homocysteine bound to plasma proteins. The urine gives a positive nitroprusside test (it is also positive in cystinuria). However, this test can be falsely negative. Unfortunately, methionine elevation is unreliable in the early days of life, hampering the possibility of neonatal screening. It detects exclusively the more severely pyridoxine nonresponsive patients, and only one-half of them. Confirmation of the diagnosis can be performed by enzyme assay using cultured skin fibroblasts and/or mutation analysis, which allows prenatal diagnosis.

Treatment and outcome

Optimal outcome of treatment depends on its earliest possible introduction. Treatment is focused on correcting homocysteine levels; lifelong monitoring is essential. In about one-half of the patients oral pyridoxine rapidly reduces methionine and homocystine to near normal values. The first treatment should be to try using doses from as low as 50 mg in infants to 1000 mg/day in older children or adults and reducing the dose if a response is achieved; 5 to 10 mg/day of folic acid should also be given. Very large sustained doses (1000 mg/day or more) in adults can cause peripheral neuropathy.

Those responding only partially or not at all to pyridoxine require a very low-protein diet supplemented with a methionine-free amino acid supplement, minerals, and vitamins. Biochemical control may only be achieved in older children and adults on natural protein intakes of 5 to 10 g/day. Plasma cystine should be maintained in the normal range and supplementation should be considered. Both folic acid (5–10 mg/day) and betaine (up to 12 g/day) can further reduce plasma homocystine levels but may produce large elevations of plasma methionine. Low red-cell folate values occur and even megaloblastic anaemia. Low serum vitamin B12 values also occur and should be corrected. Treatment started early can prevent or reduce the clinical sequels and lower the incidence of vascular events throughout life; many patients have a normal life expectancy.

Methylene tetrahydrofolate reductase deficiency

Clinical presentation

Neurological features predominate with psychomotor retardation, seizures, abnormalities of gait, and psychiatric disturbance. The age of symptom development varies widely from infancy with a progressive encephalopathy with apnoea, seizures, and microcephaly to adulthood with ataxia, motor abnormalities, psychiatric symptoms, subacute degeneration of spinal cord, and cerebrovascular events. Demyelination occurs and the changes may resemble the classic findings of subacute combined degeneration seen in vitamin B12 deficiency. The risk of vascular disease is high.

Diagnosis

Plasma methionine concentrations are below normal and plasma homocystine concentrations are in the range 20 to 200 μmol/litre with an elevated excretion of 15 to 600 μmol/day. As homocystine is easily missed on amino acid analysis, quantitative determination of total homocysteine by HPLC is the most important clue to diagnosis. There is no megaloblastic anaemia. The enzyme can be assayed in liver, leucocytes, lymphocytes, or fibroblasts also allowing prenatal diagnosis.

Treatment and outcome

Betaine in large doses (20–150 mg/kg per day) effectively lowers plasma homocystine and raises plasma methionine. Other treatments tried alone or in combination include folinic acid, vitamin B12, pyridoxine, and methionine. Some have suggested a cocktail of all these treatments. It is difficult to be sure of clinical success.

Deficiencies of methionine synthase reductase (cobalamin E defect) and methionine synthase (cobalamin G defect)

Clinical and biochemical findings of methionine synthase reductase (cobalamin E defect) and methionine synthase (cobalamin G defect) deficiencies are virtually identical. Characteristic findings are developmental delay and megaloblastic anaemia, but the onset may be in later in childhood with dementia and spasticity. Retinal degeneration, cardiac defects, and haemolysis have been described.

Megaloblastic anaemia occurs in almost all patients. Biochemical findings include low plasma methionine and raised homocysteine as well as homocystine in plasma and urine. Methylmalonic acid should be measured in urine to exclude other cobalamin defects (see 'Methylmalonic aciduria'). Methionine synthase can be assayed in liver or fibroblasts and antenatal diagnosis has been carried out on cultured amniocytes. Cells with the cobalamin E defect require specific reducing conditions to demonstrate the deficient enzyme activity. Molecular diagnosis is possible for both conditions. Treatment involves large doses of hydroxocobalamin with betaine and possibly folinic acid. Success of therapy and outcome is variable and often unfavourable.

Other defects of sulphur amino acid metabolism

Among several additional defects known, cystathioninuria due to cystathionase deficiency is probably clinically harmless. Cystathionine in excess of 1 g/day may be excreted at clearance values close to the glomerular filtration rate.

Methionine adenosyltransferase deficiency causes raised plasma methionine levels (up to 1200 μmol/litre; normal 15–30 μmol/litre) and appears to be harmless in most patients. The enzyme defect is partial. Severe deficiency of methionine adenosyltransferase I/III may be associated with demyelination and neurological features. In such patients treatment with *S*-adenosylmethionine (400 mg of the toluene sulphonate, twice daily) is an option.

Glycine *N*-methyltransferase deficiency is very rare and was demonstrated in children with mild liver disease. Biochemical findings included elevated plasma methionine and *S*-adenosylmethionine levels.

Similarly rare appear to be patients affected with *S*-adenosylhomocysteine hydrolase. Pathology and clinical findings are significant in liver, muscle, and the nervous system. Biochemical findings are complex, with elevated plasma methionine, *S*-adenosylhomocysteine, and *S*-adenosylmethionine levels. Total homocysteine and cystathionine may also be slightly elevated.

Further reading

Ando T, *et al.* (1971). Propionic acidemia in patients with ketotic hyperglycinemia. *J Pediatr*, **78**, 827–32.

Bickel H, Gerrard J, Hickmans E (1953). Influence of phenylalanine on PKU. *Lancet*, **2**, 812–13.

Blau N, *et al.* (eds) (2003). *Physician's guide to the laboratory diagnosis of inherited metabolic disease*, 2nd edition. Springer, Heidelberg.

Canavan MM (1931). Schilder's encephalitis perioxalis diffusa. *Arch Neurol Psychiatry*, **25**, 299.

Dewey KG, *et al.* (1996). Protein requirements of infants and children. *Eur J Clin Nutr*, **50** Suppl 1, S119–47.

Dixon MA, Leonard JV (1992). Intercurrent illness in inborn errors of intermediary metabolism. *Arch Dis Child*, **67**, 1387–91.

Ensenauer R, *et al.* (2004). A common mutation is associated with a mild, potentially asymptomatic phenotype in patients with isovaleric acidemia diagnosed by newborn screening. *Am J Hum Genet*, **75**, 1136–42.

Fernandes J, *et al.* (eds) (2006). *Inborn metabolic diseases*, 4th edition. Springer, Heidelberg.

Garrod AE (1902). The incidence of alkaptonuria. A study in chemical individuality. *Lancet*, **2**, 1616–20.

Garrod AE (1909). *Inborn errors of metabolism*. Oxford University Press.

Goodman SI, *et al.* (1975). Glutaric aciduria: a 'new' disorder of amino acid metabolism. *Biochem Med*, **12**, 12–21.

Guthrie R, Susi A (1963). A simple phenylalanine method for detecting PKU in large populations of newborn infants. *Pediatrics*, **32**, 338–43.

Hoffmann B, *et al.* (2006). Impact of longitudinal plasma leucine levels on the intellectual outcome in patients with classic MSUD. *Pediatr Res*, **59**, 17–20.

Hoffmann GF (1994). Selective screening for inborn errors of metabolism—past, present and future. *Eur J Pediatr*, **153** Suppl 1, S2–8.

Hoffmann GF, *et al.* (1994). Neurological manifestations of organic acid disorders. *Eur J Pediatr*, **153** Suppl 1, S94–100.

Hoffmann GF, Surtees RA, Wevers RA (1998). Cerebrospinal fluid investigations for neurometabolic disorders. *Neuropediatrics*, **29**, 59–71.

Hoffmann GF, *et al.* (eds) (2002). *Core handbook in pediatrics: inherited metabolic diseases*. Lippincott Williams & Wilkins, Philadelphia.

Hörster F, *et al.* (2007). Long-term outcome in methylmalonic acidurias is influenced by the underlying defect (mut0, mut–, cblA, cblB). *Pediatr Res*, **62**, 225–30.

Hunt AD Jr, *et al.* (1954). Pyridoxine dependency: report of a case of intractable convulsions in an infant controlled by pyridoxine. *Pediatrics*, **13**, 140–5.

Jakobs C, ten Brink H, Stellaard F (1990). Prenatal diagnosis of inherited metabolic disorders by quantitation of characteristic metabolites in amniotic fluid: facts and future. *Prenat Diagn*, **10**, 265–71.

Koch R, *et al.* (2003). The maternal PKU international study: 1984–2002. *Pediatrics*, **112**, 1523–9.

Kölker S, *et al.* (2006). Natural history, outcome, and treatment efficacy in children and adults with glutaryl-CoA dehydrogenase deficiency. *Pediatr Res*, **59**, 840–7.

Lenke R, Levy HL (1980). Maternal PKU and hyperphenylalaninemia: an international study of treated and untreated pregnancies. *N Engl J Med*, **303**, 1202–8.

Ly TB, *et al.* (2003). Mutations in the AUH gene cause 3-methylglutaconic aciduria type I. *Hum Mutat*, **21**, 410–17.

Menkes JH, Hurst PL, Craig JM (1954). New syndrome: progressive familial infantile cerebral dysfunction associated with an unusual urinary substance. *Pediatrics*, **14**, 462–7.

Millington DS, *et al.* (1990). Tandem mass spectrometry: a new method for acylcarnitine profiling with potential for neonatal screening for inborn errors of metabolism. *J Inherit Metab Dis*, **13**, 321–4.

Nyhan WL, Barshop BA, Ozand PA (2005). *Atlas of metabolic diseases*. Hodder Headline, London.

Oberholzer VG, *et al.* (1967). Methylmalonic aciduria: an inborn error of metabolism leading to chronic metabolic acidosis. *Arch Dis Child*, **42**, 492–504.

Phornphutkul C, *et al.* (2002). Natural history of alkaptonuria. *N Engl J Med*, **347**, 2111–21.

Prietsch V, *et al.* (2002). Emergency management of inherited metabolic disease. *J Inherit Metab Dis*, **25**, 531–46.

Schaefer F, *et al.* (1999). Dialysis in neonates with inborn errors of metabolism. *Nephrol Dial Transplant*, **14**, 910–18.

Schulze A, *et al.* (2003). Expanded newborn screening for inborn errors of metabolism by electrospray ionization-tandem mass spectrometry: results, outcome, and implications. *Pediatrics*, **111**, 1399–1406.

Scriver CR, *et al.* (eds) (2001). *The metabolic and molecular bases of inherited disease*, 8th edition. McGraw-Hill, New York.

Strauss KA, *et al.* (2006). Elective liver transplantation for the treatment of classical maple syrup urine disease. *Am J Transplant*, **6**, 557–64.

Surtees RA, Matthews EE, Leonard JV (1992). Neurologic outcome of propionic acidemia. *Pediatr Neurol*, **8**, 333–7.

Suwannarat P, *et al.* (2005). Use of nitisinone in patients with alkaptonuria. *Metabolism*, **54**, 719–28.

Tanaka K, *et al.* (1966). Isovaleric acidemia: a new genetic defect of leucine metabolism. *Proc Natl Acad Sci*, **56**, 236–42.

Wilson JMG, Jungner G (1968). *Principles and practice of screening for disease*. Public Health Papers No. 34, World Health Organization, Geneva.

Wolf B, *et al.* (1983). Biotinidase deficiency: the enzymatic defect in late-onset multiple carboxylase deficiency. *Clin Chim Acta*, **13**, 273–81.

Wolf B, *et al.* (1983). Deficient biotinidase activity in late-onset multiple carboxylase deficiency. *N Engl J Med*, **308**, 161.

Zschocke J, Hoffmann GF (2004). *Vademecum metabolicum. Manual of metabolic paediatrics*, 2nd edition. Schattauer, Stuttgart.

Zschocke J, *et al.* (2000). Progressive infantile neurodegeneration caused by 2-methyl-3-hydroxybutyryl-CoA dehydrogenase deficiency: a novel inborn error of branched chain fatty acid and isoleucine metabolism. *Pediatr Res*, **48**, 852–5.

12.3

Disorders of carbohydrate metabolism

Contents

12.3.1 Glycogen storage diseases *1596*
Philip Lee and Kaustuv Bhattacharya

12.3.2 Inborn errors of fructose metabolism *1604*
Timothy M. Cox

12.3.3 Disorders of galactose, pentose, and pyruvate metabolism *1610*
Timothy M. Cox

12.3.1 Glycogen storage diseases

Philip Lee and Kaustuv Bhattacharya

Essentials

Glycogen metabolism is regulated by a number of different enzymes, defects in any of which result in several types of glycogen storage disease.

Types I, III, VI, and IX have predominantly hepatic manifestations: they typically present in infancy with failure to thrive and hepatomegaly, and they are associated with fasting hypoglycaemia. Diagnosis can be made in many cases by detection of gene mutation or functional tests of red blood cells or white blood cells. Most patients require an intensive dietary regimen providing a constant source of exogenous glucose, particularly in childhood. In illness, glucose requirements increase and it is necessary to continue to provide glucose either enterally or intravenously to prevent hypoglycaemia and secondary metabolic disturbances.

Skeletal muscle is affected predominantly in type II, IIIa, V, VII, and (muscular) IX. Patients generally present in childhood or as young adults with muscle cramps and sometimes myoglobinuria after exercise. Definitive diagnosis is made by assay of the enzyme from muscle or by identifying mutations in the relevant gene. Myopathy in several of these diseases is progressive, with no evidence of long-term benefit from any therapy.

Introduction

Most mammalian cells require glucose as a fundamental energy source. Glycogen, which comprises up to 60 000 glucose molecules, enables organs to temporarily store glucose in an insoluble form that contributes little to cytosolic osmolarity. Defects preventing the normal flux of glucose molecules in the synthesis and degradation of glycogen have widespread consequences affecting many organs. The glycogen storage diseases are a heterogeneous group of disorders caused by enzymatic deficiencies of glycogen metabolism. Qualitative and quantitative deficiencies of each of the enzymes within a given organ, determine the individual phenotype.

The process of synthesis and degradation of glycogen is indicated in Fig. 12.3.1.1. Pathogenesis of disease is determined by either the failure to produce sufficient glucose and/or the abnormal storage of glycogen. There are several classifications of the diseases: a numerical chronological order of identification, eponymous, by enzyme deficiency, or by gene affected (Table 12.3.1.1).

Historical perspective

Identification of the causes of glycogen storage diseases has been intertwined with the unravelling of essential biochemical processes of glucose metabolism and intracellular structure. In 1929, von Gierke initially described the pathological findings of glycogen storage within the liver and kidney as 'hepatonephromegalia glykogenica'. Two decades later, CF and GT Cori showed that the activity of glucose-6-phosphatase was deficient in this disease but only recently have all the genes encoding the catalytic subunits and transport components of this enzyme complex been identified. Soon after the enzymatic defect was described, it was noted that some patients followed a similar course but did not have deficiency of glucose-6-phosphatase. This led to the identification of the glucose 6-phosphate transporter defect in 1968. Over this period it was also noted that other diseases resulted in storage of abnormal forms of glycogen within different intracellular compartments

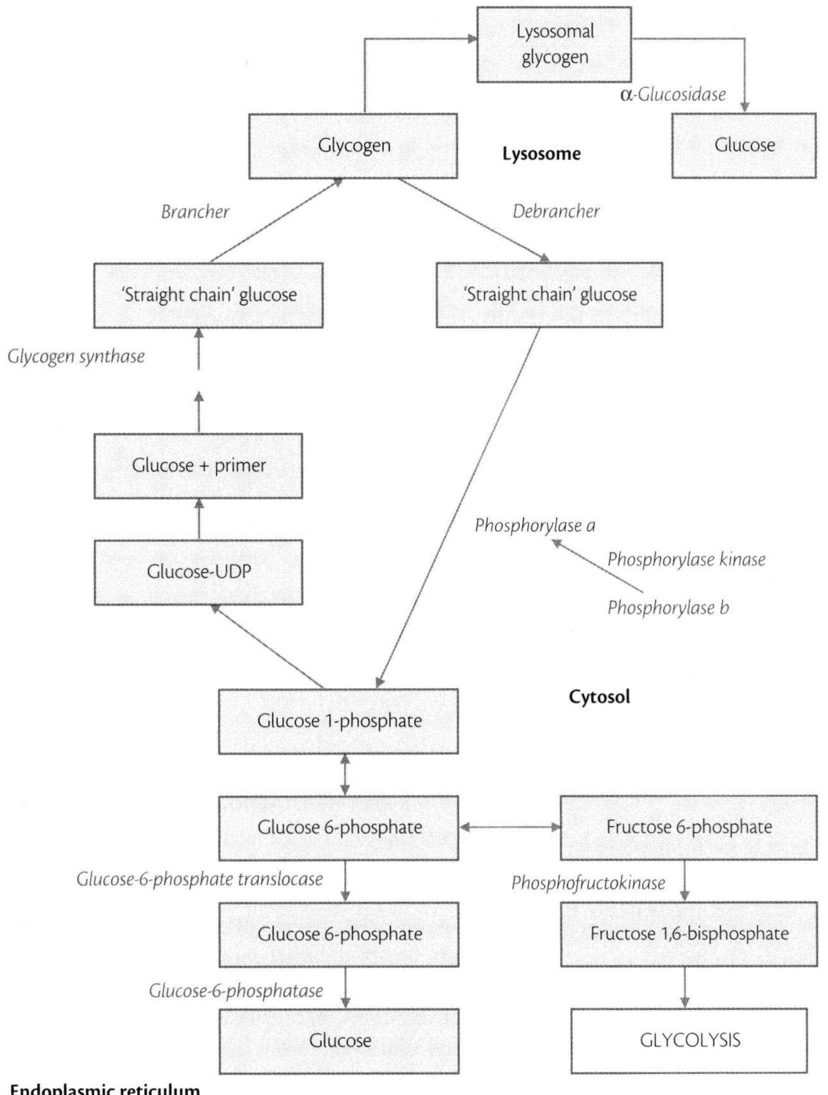

Fig. 12.3.1.1 Enzymatic causes of glycogen storage disease.

(leading to the identification of the first of many lysosomal storage diseases) and within organs such as skeletal muscle where glucose-6-phosphatase is not expressed. Consequently, a quite disparate group of diseases was recognized. This chapter will describe the aetiology and features of the individual diseases grouped into predominantly hepatic presentation or predominantly skeletal presentation, with a guide to diagnosis and treatment after each section.

Incidence

The incidence of all forms of glycogen storage disease (GSD) has been widely cited as 1 in 20 000 with the commonest GSD IX, followed by GSD I, II, and III. The recognition of new phenotypes and improvements in diagnostic methodology mean that this is likely to be an underestimate.

Hepatic glycogen storage diseases

GSD I, III, VI, and IX are associated with predominant hepatic expression leading to hepatomegaly and hypoglycaemia in early childhood. GSD IV is discussed later.

Glycogen storage disease type I

Aetiology

Glucose-6-phosphatase is an endoplasmic reticular enzyme complex that enables production of glucose from glucose 6-phosphate and is deficient in GSD Ia. In the liver it facilitates export of glucose, which is controlled by counter-regulatory hormones such as adrenaline or glucagon (Fig. 12.3.1.2). The endoplasmic reticular transmembrane protein glucose-6-phosphate translocase is deficient in GSD Ib. Glycogenolytic and gluconeogenic processes create ionic glucose 6-phosphate, but this cannot be exported in the form of glucose. Consequently the blood glucose cannot be raised and there is increased flux of glucose 6-phosphate through other pathways (Fig. 12.3.1.3). Many of the short-term problems of GSD I are related to hypoglycaemia, while the long-term problems are a consequence of the products of glucose 6-phosphate metabolism.

Clinical presentation

Patients typically present in the first year of life with failure to thrive, symptoms of hypoglycaemia, and hepatomegaly. Before the use of dietary treatments, patients were susceptible to frequent

Table 12.3.1.1 The glycogen storage diseases

Type	Eponym	Enzyme deficiency	Gene	Gene locus	Affected tissue
Ia	von Gierke	Glucose-6-phosphatase	*G6PC*	17q21	Liver, bowel, kidney
Ib		Glucose 6-phosphate transporter 1	*G6PT1*	11q23	Liver, bowel, kidney, marrow
II	Pompe	α-1,4-Glucosidase (acid maltase)	*GAA*	17q25.2–25.3	Heart, muscle (generalized)
III	Cori/Forbe	Debrancher (amylo-1,6-glucosidase)	*AGL*	1p21	Liver (muscle, heart)
IV	Andersen	Glycogen branching enzyme	*GBE1*	3p12	Liver (generalized)
V	McArdle	Muscle phosphorylase	*PYGM*	11q13	Muscle
VI	Hers	Hepatic phosphorylase	*PYGL*	14q21–q22	Liver
VII	Tarui	Muscle phosphofructokinase	*PFKM*	12q13.3	Muscle
IX		Phosphorylase kinase	*PHKA1*	Xq13.1–q21	Muscle
			PHKA2	Xp22.2–p22	Liver
			PHKB	16q12–q13	Generalized
			PHKG1	7p12–q21	Muscle
			PHKG2	16p12.1–p11.2	Liver and testis
			PHKD	Various	Generalized
XI	Fanconi–Bickel	Glucose transporter 2	*SLC2A2*	3q26.1–q26.3	Liver, kidney
0		Hepatic glycogen synthase	*GYS2*	12p12.2	Liver

episodes of hypoglycaemia which resulted in permanent neurodisability, seizures, or death. Patients also have impaired growth, muscle weakness, and increased subcutaneous fat deposition leading to a 'doll's face' appearance. Meticulous dietary management has altered the course of the disease, such that many of the immediate life-threatening complications are avoided. As survival has improved, multisystem complications have become more apparent (Fig. 12.3.1.4). Biochemical hallmarks include hypoglycaemia and hyperlactataemia after relatively short fasts (2–4 h) and elevations in plasma urate, triglyceride, and cholesterol.

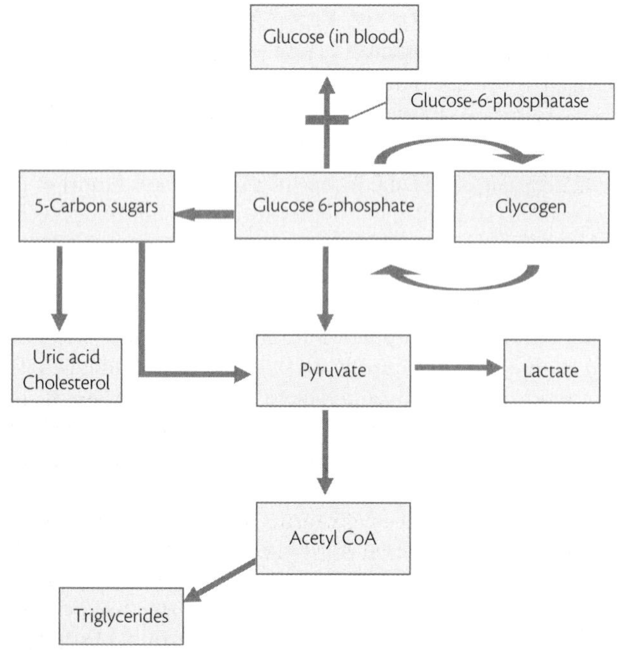

Fig. 12.3.1.2 Regulation of glycogen phosphorylase.

Glycogen storage disease type III

Aetiology

The *AGL* gene coding for the glycogen debrancher enzyme is large, containing 35 exons and spanning 85 kb of DNA, and translates to a monomeric protein product of 1532 amino acids. This enzyme complex is unusual in having two distinct catalytic sites that perform different functions on the same glycogen polymer. Phosphorylase breaks down glycogen to a structure with four glucosyl units remaining before each α-1- 6 branch point : the 1,4-α- D-glucan, 4- α-D-glucosyltransferase activity of debranching enzyme transfers three glucose residues from the shortened branch to the end of another branch so that then the remaining glucose at the α-1,6 branch point can be hydrolyzed by the debranching (amylo-1,6-glucosidase) activity. Deficiency of this enzyme consequently results in accumulation of a short-chain form of glycogen, limit dextrin. Glycogen debrancher deficiency differs from GSD I in that some glucose can be synthesized by gluconeogenesis. The infantile presentation is very similar to GSD I and it is sometimes difficult to discriminate the two clinically (Table 12.3.1.2). Ketosis is present in GSD III but absent in GSD I. Glycogen debrancher deficiency limited to the liver is known as GSD IIIb, while the majority (85%) that have deficiency in liver, skeletal, and cardiac muscle are labelled as GSD IIIa.

Clinical features

Presentation is similar to GSD I. Reduced bone density is seen in patients with both GSD IIIa and b. Motor developmental delay is not uncommon. Typically, by adult life the hypoglycaemic tendency diminishes, but may become more apparent at times of stress such as pregnancy or perioperatively. The myopathy of GSD IIIa is distal and slowly progressive and some patients also develop hypertrophic cardiomyopathy. There are a few reports of cirrhosis occurring in adult patients, mostly in the French and Japanese literature.

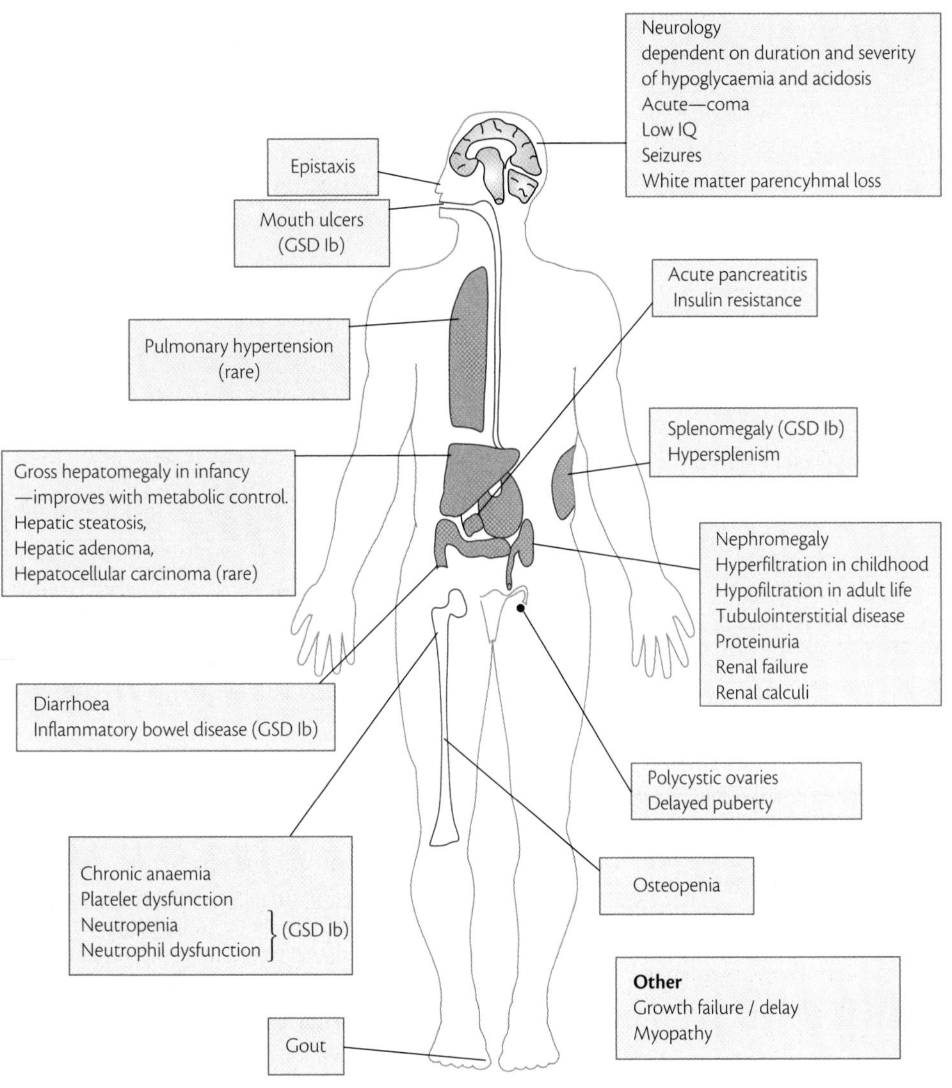

Fig. 12.3.1.3 Intrahepatic utilization of glucose 6-phosphate in GSD I.

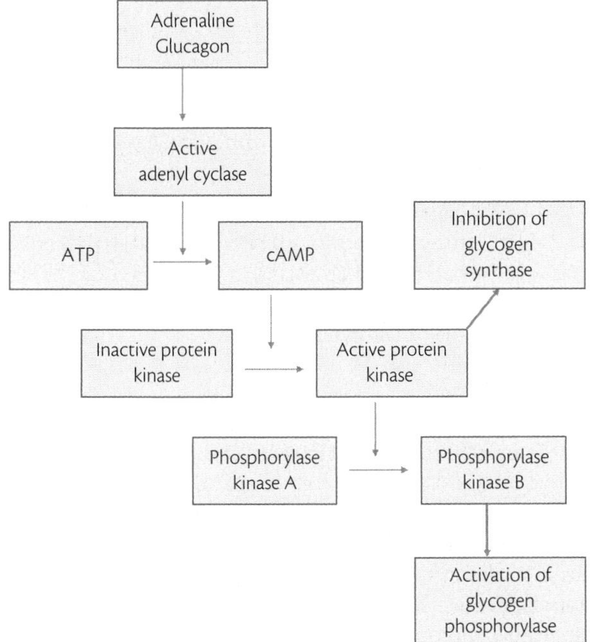

Fig. 12.3.1.4 Complications of GSD I.

Glycogen storage disease type VI

Hepatomegaly, hypoglycaemia, and growth delay are features of this disease. Typically patients present after the first year of life and hypoglycaemia is less pronounced than either GSD I or III and resolves by adult life. There may be mild hyperlipidaemia and ketosis during hypoglycaemic episodes. Hypoglycaemia can be prevented with uncooked cornstarch, which can also stimulate catch-up growth.

Glycogen storage disease type IX (including types VIII and VIa)

Defects of the phosphorylase system have been subject to some confusion in nomenclature. With improved understanding, it is now possible to describe its genetic and enzymatic basis and hence clarify the numerical classification. In the past, some patients were thought to have deficiency of hepatic phosphorylase with involvement of the brain, skeletal muscle, or heart. Many, in fact, had defects of the phosphorylase kinase system, currently classified as GSD IX. The sex-linked variant had alternatively been classified as GSD VIII by some, while others classified the neurological form as GSD VIII.

Table 12.3.1.2 Differential diagnosis of hepatic glycogenoses presenting with hepatomegaly, failure to thrive, and hypoglycaemia

	GSD Ia	GSD Ib	GSD III	GSD VI	GSD IX	GSD XI
Fasting hypoglycaemia	+++	+++	++	+	+ (+)	++
Fasting hyperlactataemia	+++	++	–	–	–	–
Elevated plasma uric acid	+++	++	–	–	–	++
Elevated plasma triglyceride	+++	++	++	+	++	++
Elevated plasma cholesterol	++	+	+	+	+	+
Fasting ketosis	–	–	+++	+	+	+
Glucagon response:						
Glucose	↓	↓	↑	↑	↑	↑
Lactate	↑	↑	–	–	–	–
Elevated creatine kinase	–	–	+++ (IIIa)	–	Variable	–
Nephromegaly	+	+	–	–	–	–
Renal tubular dysfunction	++	+	–	–	–	+++
Neutropenia	–	+ (?cyclical)	–	–	–	–
Definitive diagnosis	*G6PC* gene mutation	*G6PT* gene mutation	Abnormal glygogen and debrancher activity in liver, muscle – enzyme assay in fibroblasts, lymphocytes or red cells; mutation analysis of cognate gene.	Red cell assay: phosphorylase	Red cell phosphorylase kinase assay: mutation of gene indicated from pedigree and phenotype	Mutation of *GLUT2* gene

GSD, glycogen storage disease.

Aetiology

Phosphorylase kinase is the final important step of the regulatory cascade controlling glycogen metabolism (Fig. 12.3.1.2). The active enzyme is a complex tetramer comprising four different monomers: α, β, γ, and δ. The α-subunit is encoded by two different genes which confer expression in a particular organ: *PHKA1* in muscle and *PHKA2* in liver. Similarly the γ-subunit is encoded by *PHKG1* for expression in muscle and *PHKG2* for liver and testis. The β- and δ-subunits are coded for by single genes. The α- and β-subunits are large, enabling regulation of the enzyme. The γ-subunit contains the active site and the δ-subunit is part of the calmodulin group of proteins that bind and respond to calcium. Phenotypic variability is not surprising with deficiencies of this enzyme as corresponding mutations could be in any of these genes; it is also dependent on the tissue expression of the enzyme. GSD IX is the most common glycogen storage disease, but it is probably still underdiagnosed.

Clinical presentation

X-linked hepatic glycogen storage disease type IX

Patients present in infancy or early childhood with similar clinical manifestations to GSD Ia, but there are some differences in biochemistry (Table 12.3.1.2). Symptoms generally resolve by adult life. Most affected individuals are boys, but there are also reports of girls with mild symptoms. Diagnosis can usually be made by enzyme assay in erythrocytes. A few patients have normal or elevated enzyme activity. The former X-linked glycogenosis type I is distinguished from the latter X-linked glycogenosis type II. Both have mutations in the *PHKA1* gene.

X-linked muscular glycogen storage disease type IX

This is a very rare cause of exercise intolerance, myoglobinuria, and myopathy. The course of the disease in those described is similar to GSD V (see below).

Glycogen storage disease type IX due to defect in β-subunit

While the expression of the β-subunit is ubiquitous, the cases reported have a hepatic phenotype with a few having a combined liver and muscle involvement.

Glycogen storage disease type IX due to defect in hepatic γ-subunit

This very rare autosomal recessive form of hepatic glycogenosis has a more severe phenotype than the other forms of GSD IX. Several patients originated from consanguineous families and three had evidence of cirrhosis in childhood.

Diagnosis

Diagnosis has traditionally relied on assay of the appropriate enzyme from affected tissue. However, it is now possible to make a definitive diagnosis for many glycogen storage diseases without invasive procedures. Table 12.3.1.2 indicates features that may be elicited in young children that present with hypoglycaemia, failure to thrive, and hepatomegaly. With appropriate dietary treatment, typical biochemical features can improve. Some patients may need a preprandial and postprandial glucose and lactate profile to assist with diagnosis. Even then it may still be difficult to discriminate the type of glycogen storage disease and biopsy may be necessary. It is prudent to liaise with the laboratory performing the assay prior to biopsy as erroneous handling of samples can lead to false results.

Treatment

Dietetic treatment of hypoglycaemia in glycogen storage disease types I, III, VI, and IX

Historically, these diseases were associated with a very poor outcome until the implementation of intensive but relatively simple dietary measures in the 1970s and 1980s. The principle of such treatment was to maintain a constant exogenous supply of glucose to meet basal requirements. The use of continuous nocturnal nasogastric glucose pump feeds combined with frequent daytime meals clearly improved clinical and biochemical parameters. Subsequently, regular use of uncooked cornstarch enabled longer fasting intervals in the day and allowed some to discontinue overnight feeds. In GSD I, there are some data to indicate that monosaccharides such as fructose (in most fruits) and galactose (in milk) promote hyperlactataemia, in the short term. Consequently some centres restrict these in the diet, but the long-term impact of either an inclusive or a restricted diet is not known. The maintenance of constant blood glucose from exogenous sources requires a diet with about 65% of dietary energy as carbohydrate. Regular dietetic review is important to minimize excessive weight gain, insulin resistance, and ensure the diet is nutritionally complete.

Patients with GSD III, VI, and IX do not often require cornstarch or overnight pump feeds after childhood, except at times of metabolic stress such as pregnancy.

Medical treatment

Glycogen storage disease type I

Intercurrent illness can rapidly provoke hypoglycaemia. It is essential that oral or intravenous glucose is provided (0.2 g/kg per h in adults) and maintained until recovery is complete. Intramuscular glucagon is ineffective in GSD I. Long-term complications need to be managed expectantly. Investigations should be performed on a regular basis so that intervention is timely. We regularly monitor plasma urate, lipid profile, and urine protein excretion. These may require a specific treatment such as allopurinol or an angiotensin-converting enzyme inhibitor. 'Statins' such as atorvastatin are not required to treat atherosclerosis risk but rather to reduce risk of pancreatitis associated with hypertriglyceridaemia. Low-dose human granulocyte colony-stimulating factor is often required in patients with GSD Ib to control recurrent infections and inflammatory bowel disease due to neutropenia. Long-term use of granulocyte colony-stimulating factor is associated with splenomegaly and hypersplenism and there are reports of bone marrow-related malignancies. Ultrasound surveillance of hepatic adenomas is necessary to assess their size and number, but prediction of the rare cases of malignant transformation is difficult. Dual-energy X-ray absorptiometry (DEXA) is used to assess bone density as osteopenia is common. Treatment with calcium and vitamin D may be necessary. Hypertension, renal impairment, and renal calculi are features of adults with GSD I and should be identified and treated appropriately.

Due to a tendency to bleed in GSD I and neutrophil dysfunction associated with poor wound healing in GSD Ib, surgery should be avoided if possible. If performed, preoperative and postoperative fasts need to be managed with intravenous glucose.

Liver transplantation may be required if there is failure of medical treatment in GSD I, such as growth failure, persistent severe hyperlactataemia, multiple growing hepatic adenomas, as well as severe and recurrent infections (GSD Ib). Hepatocyte transfer has been attempted in a single case but this patient went on to require orthotopic liver transplantation. Combined liver and renal transplantations have also been performed in selected cases.

Glycogen storage disease types III and IX

Surveillance of these forms of glycogen storage disease are also necessary. Lipids, liver function tests, and creatine kinase should be monitored. Osteopenia is recognized and so regular DEXA scans and treatment with calcium and vitamin D may be required. In both GSD III and IX, patients may occasionally develop cirrhosis and so biochemical and ultrasound surveillance is indicated. Similarly some patients with GSD IIIa and IX may develop cardiomyopathy and this should be monitored accordingly. In rare cases, liver or heart transplantation has been performed for end-stage disease.

Glycogen storage diseases affecting skeletal muscle

Glycogen storage disease type II

GSD II due to lysosomal acid α-1,4-glucosidase deficiency is discussed in Chapter 12.8. Danon described a similar syndrome with normal acid α-1,4-glucosidase. Deficiency of a lysosome-associated membrane protein (LAMP2) has subsequently been shown to cause this disease.

Glycogen storage disease type V

Aetiology

In 1951, McArdle described a 30-year-old patient with myalgia after exercise. He found that plasma lactate decreased with exercise as opposed to increasing, suggesting dysfunctional glycogenolysis. He also demonstrated a normal increase in both glucose and lactate after infusion of epinephrine, postulating that this was a specific muscle glycogenolytic defect.

Clinical features

Patients generally present as young adults with muscle cramps and sometimes myoglobinuria after exercise. Many describe a 'second wind', whereby exercise becomes less tiring and painful after about 10 min. Rarely myoglobinuria can cause renal impairment. There are a few case reports of a rapidly progressive neonatal variant myopathy with mutations in the *PYGM* gene, as well as a slowly progressive limb girdle dystrophy phenotype in adulthood.

Glycogen storage disease type VII

Aetiology

In 1965, Tarui described three Japanese siblings in their twenties who had exercise intolerance, similar to patients with GSD V. Muscle phosphorylase activity was found to be normal. Elevations in glucose 6-phosphate and fructose-6-phosphate led to identification of complete deficiency of muscle phosphofructokinase and partial deficiency in erythrocytes. Mammalian phosphofructokinase is a tetramer made from three different subunits: muscle (PFK(M)), liver (PFK(L)), and platelet (PKL(P)), encoded by separate genes. The muscle isoform is a homotetramer of M_4, the liver isoform a homotetramer of L_4, while erythrocytes contain a random combination of M and L subunits. Because GSD VII is caused by mutations in the *PFKM* gene, symptoms relate both to skeletal muscle and haemolytic anaemia.

Clinical features

Patients tend to develop muscle cramps, myopathy, and rhabdomyolysis in childhood. There may be mild hyperuricaemia, as well as hyperbilirubinaemia and reticulocytosis, in keeping with haemolysis.

Diagnosis

GSD V, VII, and muscle variants of IX result in impaired glycolysis within skeletal muscle. The ischaemic forearm test identifies an increase in ammonia but not lactate in GSD V, VII, and IX. However, this test can provoke rhabdomyolysis and should be avoided. An exercise tolerance test could be used as an alternative. Definitive diagnosis is made by assay of the enzyme from the muscle or by identifying mutations in the relevant gene.

Treatment of skeletal muscle variants: glycogen storage disease types V and VII (IIIa and IX)

Generic treatments of myopathic diseases apply to these forms of glycogenoses. Low-impact exercises maintain use of affected muscles and care is needed if more strenuous activities are performed. For GSD V, Haller and Vissing have shown short-term improvement in symptoms and energy expenditure by giving glucose intravenously or the disaccharide sucrose orally. Conversely, for GSD VII there are some data indicating symptoms are worse after a glucose load. Furthermore, some suggest a ketogenic diet for these patients. Others address the myopathic problems of these glycogen storage diseases by administering gluconeogenic precursors or high-protein diets. The effects of these dietary regimens have not been evaluated systematically and there is no evidence of long-term benefit from any therapy.

Other forms of glycogen storage disease

Glycogen storage disease type IV

GSD IV is caused by glycogen branching enzyme deficiency. The enzyme is widely expressed with different isoforms in liver, heart, skeletal muscle, brain, leucocytes, and fibroblasts. A very broad range of clinical presentations has subsequently been identified, but there is no clear correlation between phenotype, genotype, and enzyme activity. The storage of a poorly soluble polysaccharide with few branches (similar to amylopectin) in the liver causes a chronic inflammatory response, interstitial fibrosis, and then cirrhosis. This disease is not typically associated with hypoglycaemia. Diagnosis is generally made histopathologically, demonstrating findings of amylopectinosis or polyglucosan bodies. Subsequent enzyme assay or genotype confirms the diagnosis.

Clinical presentation

Classic childhood progressive liver disease

This form was originally described by Andersen in 1956. Patients present in the first 18 months of life with hepatomegaly. Liver biopsy demonstrates typical histopathological findings. It progresses through the development of portal hypertension, splenomegaly, and varices to end-stage liver failure by 5 years. Some patients develop nonprogressive liver disease.

Perinatal neuromuscular form

This pattern of disease is characterized by the fetal akinesia deformation sequence including arthrogryposis multiplex congenita and hydrops fetalis. Some of these cases have had fetal onset as early as 12 weeks gestation and perished *in utero*. The congenital form presents at birth with profound hypotonia and muscle wasting with some having cardiomyopathy and death in infancy.

Juvenile myopathy or cardiomyopathy

The juvenile form presents with either progressive myopathy and/or cardiomyopathy. There is great phenotypic variability in the course with some rapidly progressing to death and others taking a more gradual course.

Adult polyglucosan body disease

This disease is confined to the peripheral and central nervous system and presents with peripheral neuropathy, extrapyramidal symptoms, pyramidal tetraparesis, cognitive impairment, or seizures. Progression of the disease is over many years.

Fanconi–Bickel syndrome

Aetiology

This rare disease is not a glycogenolytic disorder, as originally postulated, and current consensus is not to label this condition as GSD XI. It is caused by deficiency of glucose transporter 2, which is a transmembrane protein facilitating glucose transport across the cell membrane. It is expressed in hepatocytes, pancreatic β cells, basolateral cells of the intestine, and renal tubular cells. Impaired export of intracellular glucose leads to glycogen synthesis and storage within liver and kidney. There is a generalized tubulopathy with exaggerated glycosuria as well as dietary intolerance of glucose and galactose. Both postprandial hyperglycaemia and fasting hypoglycaemia occur due to impaired uptake and release of glucose and impaired pancreatic islet function.

Clinical features

Patients usually present in infancy with failure to thrive, vomiting, and rickets. Profound growth impairment is typical and hepatomegaly is acquired in early childhood. Therapy is support of plasma glucose with slow-release glucose polymers and renal tubular replacement therapy.

Glycogen synthase deficiency

Glycogen synthase deficiency (GSD 0) is a very rare cause of ketotic hypoglycaemia. In contrast to other glycogenoses there are reduced levels of liver glycogen due to impairment of hepatic glycogen synthesis. Fasting ketotic hypoglycaemia, postprandial hyperglycaemia and hyperlactataemia, failure to thrive, osteopenia, and hyperlipidaemia are typical features. A diet rich in complex carbohydrates ameliorates fasting and postprandial secondary metabolic disturbance. Diagnosis can be made by mutational analysis of the *GYS2* gene.

Future developments

Glycogen storage diseases are individually rare and present to a wide range of physicians. This had led to discrepancies in management between centres, with few data demonstrating the best therapeutic strategies. International disease registries will assist in identifying beneficial treatments in the future. For many of these disorders, manipulation of the metabolic milieu by diet can have quite dramatic effects. Starches that are more efficacious than cornstarch for glycogen storage diseases associated with hypoglycaemia have been developed.

The phenotypes of these diseases are broad and there is ongoing work looking at the pathogenesis of disease, including studies looking at the aetiology of hepatic tumours in GSD I as well as cardiomyopathy and cirrhosis in GSD III. Recognition of predictive factors could guide therapy. Patients that have defective or deficient enzymes may be amenable to treatment with 'chaperone' molecules. These can protect and help sustain activity of such enzymes but are ineffective if null mutations mean that no enzyme is produced.

For some diseases, such as GSD Ia, there are animal models of disease. These have facilitated better understanding of the pathophysiology and are being used to evaluate gene therapy. As with many other diseases, this strategy has yet to demonstrate sustained enzyme activity in recipients without complications. However, as techniques improve this may become a therapeutic option in the future.

Further reading

Bhattacharya K, *et al.* (2007). A novel starch for the treatment of glycogen storage diseases. *J Inherit Metab Dis*, **30**, 350–7. [Discussion of new starch for hepatic glycogenosis.]

Bruno C, *et al.* (2004). Clinical and genetic heterogeneity of branching enzyme deficiency (glycogenosis type IV). *Neurology*, **63**, 1053–8. [Review of different forms of GSD IV with novel mutations presented.]

Burwinkel B, *et al.* (2003). Muscle glycogenosis with low phosphorylase kinase activity: mutations in PHKA1, PHKG1 or six other candidate genes explain only a minority of cases. *Eur J Hum Genet*, **11**, 516–26. [Description of the molecular genetic complexity of GSD IX.]

Chen YT (1993). Type I glycogen storage disease: nine years of management with cornstarch. *Eur J Pediatr*, **152** Suppl 1, S56–9. [Discussion of long-term management with cornstarch.]

Chen YT (2001). Glycogen storage diseases. In: Scriver CR, *et al.* (eds) *The metabolic and molecular bases of inherited diseases*, pp. 1521–51. McGraw-Hill, New York. [Detailed description of all forms of glycogen storage disease and molecular basis of disease.]

Correia CE, *et al.* (2008). Use of modified cornstarch therapy to extend fasting in glycogen storage disease types 1a and 1b. *Am J Clin Nutr*, *88*, 1272–6. [A small randomized double-blinded crossover trial, the results of which favourably compared a novel uncooked but modified cornstarch preparation with uncooked raw cornstarch - which is commonly used (see Bhattacharya *et al.*, 2007). The experimental preparation was superior in its capacity to sustain blood glucose; it induced lower peak glucose concentrations with a less rapid decline when administered to patients after fasting. The treatment holds promise for improved metabolic control of patients with glycogen storage disease, but large trials are needed.]

Davis MK, Weinstein DA (2008). Liver transplantation in children with glycogen storage disease: controversies and evaluation of the risk/benefit of this procedure. *Pediatr Transplant*, **12**, 137–45.

Dixon M (2007). Disorders of carbohydrate metabolism. In: Shaw V, Lawson M (eds) *Clinical paediatric dietetics*. 3rd edition, pp. 390–99. Blackwell Publishing, Oxford. [Practical guide to dietetic management of glycogen storage disease.]

Fernandes J (1974). The effect of disaccharides on the hyperlactic acidemia of glucose-6-phosphatase deficient children. *Acta Paediatr Scand*, **63**, 695. [Biochemical study of sucrose and lactose loads in patients with glycogen storage disease.]

Hendrickx J, *et al.* (1999). Complete genomic structure and mutational spectrum of PHKA2 in patients with X-linked liver glycogenosis type I and II. *Am J Hum Genet*, **64**, 1541–9. [Comprehensive discussion of GSD IX with particular emphasis on X-linked mutations.]

Hogrel JY, *et al.* (2001). A non-ischemic forearm exercise test for the screening of patients with exercise intolerance. *Neurology*, **56**, 1733–8. [Discussion of diagnostic testing of muscular glycogenosis.]

Kishnani PS, Koeberl D, Chen Y-T (2007). Glycogen storage diseases. In: C Scriver, *et al.* (eds) *Metabolic and Molecular Bases of Inherited Disease*, 8th ed. OMMBID. www.ommbid.com, New York, McGraw-Hill, Chap. 71. [This is the most complete and authoritative review of the subject – a comprehensive textbook now available in this online version and continually subject to updating].

Koeberl DD, Kishnani PS, Chen YT (2007). Glycogen storage disease types I and II: treatment updates. *J Inherit Metab Dis*, **30**, 159–64. [Review of recent developments in GSD I and II.]

Lee PJ, Leonard JV (1995). The hepatic glycogen storage diseases: problems beyond childhood. *J Inherit Metab Dis*, **18**, 462–72. [Review of complications of GSD I, III, VI, and IX.]

Lee PJ, Dixon MA, Leonard JV (1996). Uncooked cornstarch: efficacy in type I glycogenosis. *Arch Dis Child*, **74**, 546–7. [Discussion of problems with cornstarch therapy.]

Lucchiari S, *et al.* (2002). Clinical and genetic variability of glycogen storage disease type IIIa: seven novel AGL gene mutations in the Mediterranean area. *Am J Med Genet*, **109**, 183–90. [Discussion of genotype and phenotype of GSD III.]

Martens DH, *et al.* (2009). Renal function in glycogen storage disease type 1, natural course, and renopreservative effects of ACE inhibition. *Clin J Am Soc Nephrol*, **4**, 1741–6. [Important information of relevance to the long-term treatment of the renal disorder complicating glycogen storage disease].

Melis D, *et al.* (2005). Efficacy of ACE-inhibitor therapy on renal disease in glycogen storage disease type 1: a multicentre retrospective study. *Clin Endocrinol*, **63**, 19–25.

Rake JP, *et al.* (2002). Glycogen storage disease type I: diagnosis, management, clinical course and outcome. Results of the European Study on Glycogen Storage Disease Type I (ESGSD I). *Eur J Pediatr*, **161** Suppl 1, S20–34. [Comprehensive discussion of European Registry outcome data for GSD I.]

Rake JP, *et al.* (2002). Guidelines for management of glycogen storage disease type I: European Study on Glycogen Storage Disease Type I (ESGSD I). *Eur J Pediatr*, **161** Suppl 1, 112–9. [Consensus guidelines for management of GSD I.]

Reddy SK, *et al.* (2009). Liver transplantation for Glycogen storage disease type 1a. *J Hepatol*, **51**, June 17. Epub ahead of print. [A useful review of the radical management of glycogen storage disease by transplantation].

Santer R, *et al.* (1998). Fanconi-Bickel syndrome: the original patient and his natural history, historical steps leading to the primary defect, and a review of the literature. *Eur J Pediatr*, **157**, 783–97. [Comprehensive review of genotype and phenotypes of Fanconi–Bickel syndrome with follow-up of original patient.]

Spiegel R, *et al.* (2007). The variable clinical phenotype of glycogen synthase deficiency. *J Pediatr Endocrinol Metab*, **20**, 1339–42.

Visser G, *et al.* (2000). Neutropenia, neutrophil dysfunction, and inflammatory bowel disease in glycogen storage disease type Ib: results of the European Study on Glycogen Storage Disease Type I. *J Pediatr*, **137**, 187–91. [Description of outcomes and features of patients with GSD Ib.]

Vissing J, Haller RG (2003). The effect of oral sucrose on exercise tolerance in patients with McArdle's disease. *N Engl J Med*, **349**, 2503–9. [Primary study of simple intervention in GSD V with sucrose. Detailed discussion comparing GSD V and VII.]

Weinstein DA, *et al.* (2006). Hepatic glycogen synthase deficiency: an infrequently recognized cause of ketotic hypoglycaemia. *Mol Genet Metab*, **87**, 284–8. [Review of glycogen synthase deficiency.]

Weinstein DA, *et al.* (2010). AAV-mediated correction of a canine model of glycogen storage disease type 1A. *Hum Gene Ther*, Feb 17. Epub ahead of Print. [A hint of powerful developments current in the field of gene therapy for this group of disorders].

12.3.2 Inborn errors of fructose metabolism

Timothy M. Cox

Essentials

Most people in developed countries ingest 50 to 150 g fructose equivalents daily in their diet. These are absorbed rapidly by a carrier mechanism that facilitates transport across the intestinal epithelium, metabolized (mainly in the liver) by the enzymes ketohexokinase (fructokinase), aldolase B, and triokinase, and eventually converted into glucose or glycogen. Dietary sugar has particular effects on those whose capacity to metabolise fructose is limited. Fructose occurs either as a free monosaccharide, as a component of sucrose, a disaccharide from which it is released by digestion; fructose may also be derived from the metabolism of the sugar alcohol, sorbitol.

'Fructose malabsorption'—describes incomplete absorption of fructose that is associated with abdominal symptoms and diarrhoea reminiscent of intestinal disaccharidase deficiency after ingestion of fructose- or sorbitol-rich foods and drinks such as apple juice, but this condition does not have a defined genetic cause. Symptoms improve when these sugars are excluded from the diet.

Three inborn errors of fructose metabolism are recognized: (1) essential or benign fructosuria due to fructokinase deficiency—a very rare disorder with no ill effects; (2) hereditary fructose intolerance (fructosaemia) caused by deficiency of aldolase B; and (3) fructose-1,6-diphosphatase deficiency.

Hereditary fructose intolerance—an autosomal recessive disease; typically presents at weaning but may come to light at any age with postprandial abdominal pain and vomiting, symptomatic hypoglycaemia (which may induce seizures), hypophosphataemia, acidosis and other metabolic disturbances after consumption of offending foods and drinks. Unrecognized disease causes failure to thrive/growth retardation, a Fanconi-like renal syndrome with nephrocalcinosis, and jaundice with lethal liver injury. Parenteral infusion of fructose or its congeners can be fatal. Diagnosis depends upon demonstration of deficient aldolase B isozyme activity in biopsy material from liver, small intestine, or kidney, or molecular analysis of the aldolase B gene. Treatment requires institution of a strict sugar-exclusion diet supplemented by water-soluble vitamins. Early diagnosis and dietary modification are critical for well-being and normal development.

Fructose-1,6-diphosphatase deficiency—a very rare disease of infancy and childhood associated with failure of hepatic gluconeogenesis causing bouts of severe hypoglycaemia, ketosis, and lactic acidosis that are provoked by infection and starvation, and aggravated by dietary fructose, related sugars and ketogenic fat. Diagnosis depends on identification of a gluconeogenic defect and enzymatic assay of fructose-1,6-diphosphatase in fresh liver biopsy samples. Treatment requires prompt control of intercurrent illnesses and scrupulous attention to nutrition, with a fructose-exclusion diet containing abundant carbohydrate energy, restricted fat and protein. Acute episodes of acidosis or hypoglycaemia are controlled by intravenous infusion of glucose, with bicarbonate if required.

Metabolism of fructose

Fructose is an important component of the modern diet; it occurs as a free monosaccharide in fruit, nuts, honey, and some vegetables. Free fructose is released from the disaccharide sucrose in the gut lumen by the sucrase–isomaltase complex at the brush-border membrane of the mucosal epithelium. Finally, the sugar alcohol sorbitol (a constituent of medicines and tablets, as well as some foods for diabetics) is converted quantitatively to fructose in the liver and intestine. Most people in developed countries ingest 50 to 150 g fructose equivalents daily in the diet. Global production of sugar (sucrose from cane and beet) is rising, but over the last three decades manufacture of fructose as a high-fructose syrup, enzymatically derived from starch in maize (corn), has also burgeoned. This intensely sweet sugar is now used extensively as a sweetener in drinks and processed foods.

The pathways of fructose metabolism are summarized in Fig. 12.3.2.1. Phosphorylated forms of fructose are critical intermediates in the glycolytic and gluconeogenic metabolic pathways in all cells. Fructose is absorbed rapidly by a carrier mechanism that facilitates transport across the intestinal epithelium; this process is mediated by the glucose transporter isoforms GLUT5 and GLUT2, the latter probably contributing to efflux across the basolateral membrane of the enterocyte.

Fructose is then conveyed via the portal bloodstream to the liver, where it is assimilated. The jejunal mucosa and proximal tubule of the kidney are subsidiary sites of fructose metabolism. Assimilation of fructose depends on the concerted activities of the enzymes ketohexokinase (fructokinase), aldolase B, and triokinase, which are expressed specifically in these tissues. Uptake of fructose occurs independently of insulin and its incorporation into intermediary metabolism bypasses the regulation of glycolysis at the level of phosphofructokinase-1. For these reasons, solutions of fructose or sorbitol were advocated and, in the past, extensively used for parenteral nutrition. However, the occurrence of lactic acidosis, hyperuricaemia, and other serious consequences has led to their withdrawal from hyperalimentation regimens in most, if not all, countries.

Fructokinase rapidly phosphorylates fructose at the 1-carbon position. This enzyme has a high affinity for its substrates and the intestinal mucosa and liver rapidly convert fructose to fructose

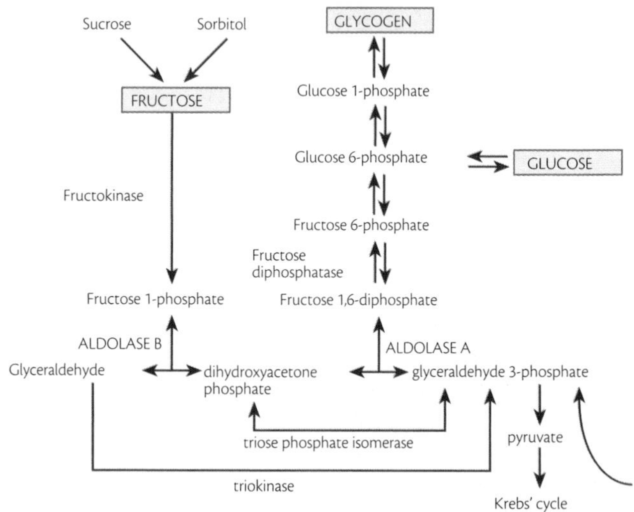

Fig. 12.3.2.1 Fructose metabolism.

1-phosphate; in other tissues, the capacity of hexokinase to phosphorylate fructose at the 6-carbon position is limited. Similarly, the fate of fructose 1-phosphate in the fructose-metabolizing tissues is dependent on a specific isozyme of aldolase, aldolase B. This has greater activity towards fructose 1-phosphate than does its ubiquitous counterpart aldolase A, the natural substrate of which is fructose 1,6-diphosphate. Cleavage of fructose 1-phosphate generates glyceraldehyde and dihydroxyacetone phosphate. These trioses enter the intermediary pools of carbohydrate metabolism, and, as a result of triokinase activity, glyceraldehyde is phosphorylated so that the two triose phosphates may be condensed by aldolase A to form the glycolytic and gluconeogenic intermediate fructose 1,6-diphosphate.

Gluconeogenesis from triose phosphates, lactate, glycerol, amino acids, and Krebs' cycle intermediates such as oxaloacetate, requires reversal of the committed reactions of glycolysis. It is the enzyme fructose-1,6-diphosphatase that releases the glucose precursor fructose 6-phosphate from fructose 1,6-diphosphate. Thus, when the remaining reactions of glycolysis are reversed, exogenous fructose provides a source of glucose or glycogen. Fructose-1,6-diphosphatase is active in the liver, kidney, and intestine, and it is a key enzyme of gluconeogenesis.

Fructose malabsorption

The occurrence of abdominal symptoms and diarrhoea, reminiscent of intestinal disaccharidase deficiency, in response to ingested fructose is well recognized by gastroenterologists and often attributed to incomplete absorption of fructose: it is therefore called 'fructose malabsorption'. The symptoms occur in adults and children after ingestion of fructose-rich or sorbitol-rich foods and drinks such as apple juice, and usually recede when the sugars are excluded from the diet. Many such individuals, as well as a high proportion of healthy control subjects, have findings suggestive of fructose malabsorption based on hydrogen breath tests, but definitive evidence of true malabsorption is usually lacking. Unfortunately, the molecular basis of this syndrome and of the wide variation of tolerance to dietary fructose and its congeners is not known. Moreover, in several patients complaining of fructose-related intestinal symptoms, molecular analysis of the human *GLUT5* gene, which encodes a major intestinal fructose transporter, has so far failed to identify causal mutations. Other studies have suggested that the distal small intestine and colon of patients who experience abdominal flatulence and diarrhoea after ingesting fructose-containing foods contain a bacterial population with enhanced uptake and anaerobic metabolism of fructose. No conclusive evidence has yet been provided to support these observations and more investigative studies are needed in those patients who experience symptoms attributed to malabsorption of this sugar, including measurement of intestinal fructose absorption, metabolism, and transport.

Essential (benign) fructosuria (OMIM 229800)

This is a rare disorder (estimated frequency 1 in 130 000) of little clinical consequence. The abnormality is transmitted as an autosomal recessive condition and is demonstrated by the presence of a reducing sugar in the blood and urine, especially after meals rich in fructose. The abnormality is caused by the deficiency of fructokinase activity in the liver and intestine, significantly reducing the capacity to assimilate this sugar. Mutations in the human ketohexokinase gene on chromosome 2p23.3–p23.2 have been identified in patients with essential fructosuria, thus confirming the suspected molecular defect in this condition. Fructose metabolism occurs slowly in essential fructosuria as a result of conversion to fructose 6-phosphate by hexokinase in adipose tissue and muscle, but, while plasma concentrations remain high postprandially, large amounts of fructose appear in the urine. Essential fructosuria may be confused with diabetes mellitus if the nature of the mellituria is not defined; with the use of glucose oxidase strips in preference to the older chemical methods for urinalysis, such confusion is now unlikely. No treatment beyond recognition and explanation appears to be necessary.

Hereditary fructose intolerance (fructosaemia) (OMIM 229600)

This disorder, first recognized in 1956, is the most common inherited defect of fructose metabolism with an estimated frequency of about 1 in 20 000 births in the United Kingdom and several populations of European origin. The disease has been reported in several diverse populations, including China and Israel. Hereditary fructose intolerance is transmitted as an autosomal recessive trait and, although it manifests itself first in early infancy, the effects of clinical disease may not be recognized until late childhood or adult life. Provided the diagnosis is made before visceral damage occurs, hereditary fructose intolerance responds completely to an exclusion diet and patients can survive to old age.

The cardinal features of the illness are vomiting, diarrhoea, abdominal pain, and hypoglycaemia, and are induced by the consumption of foods, drinks, or medicines that contain fructose, or the related sugars, sucrose or sorbitol. There is a generalized metabolic disturbance with lactic acidosis, hyperuricaemia, and hypophosphataemia. Hypoglycaemia causes trembling, irritability, and cognitive impairment. Attacks are associated with pallor, sweating, and, when severe, loss of consciousness sometimes accompanied by generalized seizures. These episodes usually occur within 30 min of meals that contain large quantities of fructose or sucrose. Continued ingestion of noxious sugars is associated with renal tubular disease, liver damage with jaundice, and defective blood coagulation. There is failure to thrive and growth retardation. Persistent exposure to fructose and the related noxious sugars in infants leads to structural liver injury with cirrhosis, aminoaciduria, coagulopathy, and coma leading to death. The infant is first exposed to the offending sugars at weaning or on transfer from breast milk to artificial feeds. Survival is dependent on recognition of the effects of fruit and sugar by the mother or, especially in older infants, by vomiting or forcible rejection of food.

Infants who survive the stormy period of weaning, develop a strong aversion to sweet-tasting foods, vegetables, and fruits. This usually affords protection against the worst effects of fructose and sucrose, but abdominal symptoms with bouts of tremulousness, irritability, and altered consciousness due to hypoglycaemia usually continue. It has become clear that many cases escape diagnosis in infancy and childhood, but the risk of illness, related to dietary indiscretion, remains throughout life. Characteristically, children and adults with hereditary fructose intolerance show a striking reduction in, or absence of, dental caries.

Recently, a syndrome of chronic sugar intoxication has been recognized in older children and adolescents with hereditary fructose intolerance. General lack of vigour and developmental retardation are prominent features. Hypoglycaemia, though obvious after heavy fructose loading, may be insignificant after chronic low-level exposure in older children. Similarly, tests of hepatic and renal function may be only mildly abnormal. Persistent ingestion of fructose and sucrose is toxic to the kidney and liver, so that renal tubular acidosis (occasionally with calculi) as well as hepatosplenomegaly occur in younger patients. Severe growth retardation may be accompanied by rachitic bone disease that complicates the Fanconi-like syndrome of proximal renal tubular disturbance with bicarbonate wasting. Growth retardation responds to dietary treatment and is usually accompanied by regression of the other disease manifestations.

Provided that organ failure and serious tissue injury do not supervene, patients with hereditary fructose intolerance recover rapidly when the toxic sugars are withdrawn. Children who survive by acquiring the protective pattern of eating behaviour avoid foods which provoke abdominal symptoms. The aversion extends to most sweet-tasting items of food and drink as well as fruits and vegetables; it remains lifelong and consumption of fructose (and sucrose) is usually reduced to less than 5 g daily. It has been shown that normal growth and development can be assured in growing children and adolescents if less than 40 mg/kg fructose equivalents are ingested daily.

Metabolic defect

Hereditary fructose intolerance is caused by a deficiency of aldolase B in the liver, small intestine, and proximal renal tubule. These tissues experience injury as a result of persistent exposure to fructose in patients affected by the disorder. In the absence of the fructose 1-phosphate-splitting activity of aldolase B, the intracellular pool of inorganic phosphate is depleted. Studies *in vivo* by ^{31}P magnetic resonance spectroscopy show that 80% of hepatic free phosphate is sequestrated as sugar phosphates after the infusion of small quantities of fructose (250 mg/kg body weight). The secondary metabolic disturbances are initiated by the accumulation of fructose 1-phosphate in a milieu where free inorganic phosphate is reduced: there is competitive inhibition of aldolase A and inhibition of phosphorylase activity so that glycogenolysis and gluconeogenesis are impaired. Thus, challenge with fructose leads to hypophosphataemia and hypoglycaemia that is refractory to glucagon or the infusion of gluconeogenic metabolites such as glycerol or dihydroxyacetone. During challenge with fructose, high concentrations of fructose 1-phosphate cause feedback inhibition of fructokinase, thereby limiting the incorporation of fructose in the liver. As a result, fructosaemia occurs and, when the blood concentration exceeds about 2 mmol/litre, fructosuria is apparent. Although the assimilation of fructose by the specialized pathway is blocked, only a small fraction of the fructose load is recovered in the urine. Studies show that 80% to 90% of the fructose is taken up under these circumstances by adipose tissue and muscle, where it can serve as an alternative substrate for hexokinase with conversion to fructose 6-phosphate.

Electrolytic disturbances occur during challenge with fructose. Hypokalaemia results from acute renal impairment with defective urinary acidification. There is a defect of proximal tubule function with bicarbonate wasting and acidosis. Occasionally, acute flaccid weakness due to hypokalaemia accompanies the other effects of fructose exposure. In patients with hereditary fructose intolerance, the administration of fructose reproducibly increases serum magnesium concentrations. This is probably explained by the breakdown of magnesium–ATP complexes, releasing intracellular magnesium ions as a result of nucleotide degradation by adenosine deaminase. Significant ingestion of fructose is thus also accompanied by marked hyperuricaemia in patients with hereditary fructose intolerance.

In the absence of acute exposure to fructose, only minor abnormalities of blood analytes are detectable and the blood glucose concentration is normal, even after prolonged fasting. Often trivial elevation of serum transaminase activities occur; red-cell folate and white-cell ascorbate concentrations may be reduced as a result of restrictive dietary habits.

Pathology and molecular genetics

Persistant ingestion of fructose and related sugars in hereditary fructose intolerance causes hepatic injury; there is diffuse fatty change and increased glycogen deposition. Hepatocyte necrosis with intralobular and periportal fibrosis occurs and fully developed cirrhosis results from continued exposure to fructose. After acute experimental challenge, electron microscopy has shown irregular electron-dense material surrounded by membranous structures, suggesting a florid lysosomal reaction to intracellular deposits of fructose 1-phosphate. Parenteral administration of fructose or sorbitol may induce the abrupt onset of hepatorenal failure associated with bleeding. Histological examination shows hepatic necrosis in these cases (Fig. 12.3.2.2). Loss of cellular functions, e.g. in the proximal renal tubule, is probably caused by depletion of ATP resulting from the arrested metabolism of fructose by the specialized pathway. The source of the severe abdominal pain that follows ingestion of fructose is unknown, but stimulation of visceral afferent nerves by the local release of purine nucleotides or lactate may be responsible.

The genetic basis of aldolase B deficiency has been studied intensively and numerous mutations responsible for hereditary fructose intolerance have been identified. The human aldolase B gene maps to chromosome 9q22.3. Several point mutations affecting the function of the enzyme are sufficiently widespread in patients of European origin to merit focused diagnostic investigation. One particular mutation, $Ala^{149}\rightarrow Pro$, which disrupts residues in a substrate-binding domain of aldolase B, is prevalent in populations of European descent. This mutation accounts for most alleles responsible for fructose intolerance, but others, including $Ala^{174}\rightarrow Asp$, $Asn^{334}\rightarrow Lys$, and a four-base deletion in exon 4, are sufficiently frequent and widespread to merit initial examination in a specialized molecular diagnostic laboratory (see below). The intragenic deletion

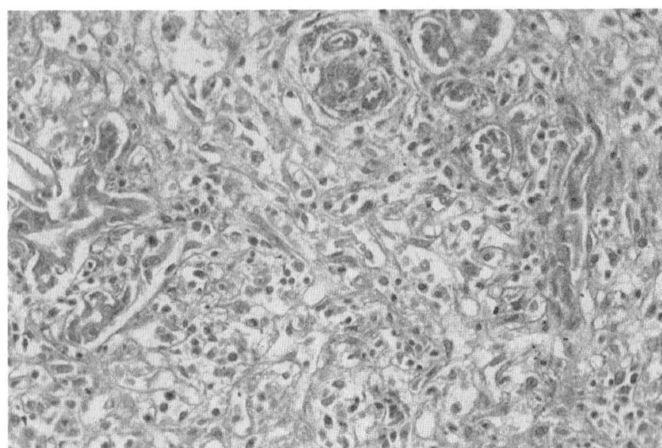

Fig. 12.3.2.2 Effects of fatal perioperative infusions of fructose and sorbitol in a 16-year-old Italian girl.

has also been reported from China. Biochemical and structural studies of the expressed mutant enzymes reveal two main classes of aldolase B in hereditary fructose intolerance, active tetrameric variants which are unstable and readily lose their quaternary structure and mutant aldolases that retain their normal tetrameric structure but are catalytically impaired.

Diagnosis

In infancy and childhood, hereditary fructose intolerance most characteristically causes persistent vomiting, with failure to thrive, acidosis, hypoglycaemia, and jaundice. The symptoms occur rapidly after ingestion of inappropriate foods and drinks. Clearly in very young infants there is a wide differential diagnosis, including Reye's syndrome, but fructose intolerance may be indicated by the nutritional history and feeding difficulties. The differential diagnosis includes pyloric stenosis, galactosaemia, Reye's syndrome, hepatitis, renal tubular disease, Wilson's disease, and tyrosinosis.

A carbohydrate-deficient glycoprotein syndrome may be suspected on the basis of biochemical screening tests carried out in paediatric investigations, since untreated patients with hereditary fructose intolerance almost invariably show a type I pattern of carbohydrate-deficient serum transferrin on isoelectric focusing; this is corrected within a few weeks of fructose exclusion and is due to transient inhibition of phosphomannose isomerase implicated in glycoprotein processing and biosynthesis.

The presence of reducing sugar in the urine may indicate that fructosuria and amino acids may also be present. Older children and adults report food aversion and may show a striking absence of dental caries. If fructose intolerance is considered, then sucrose, sorbitol, and fructose should be excluded completely before definitive tests can be carried out. Striking improvement, suggestive of hereditary fructose intolerance, may be seen within a few days.

Since the prompt institution of strict dietary treatment has beneficial and, in infants and children, life-saving effects in those with fructose intolerance, every reasonable effort should be undertaken to make a definitive diagnosis. This will have important consequences for relatives of the propositus and will provide information critical for the introduction of a rigorous and life-long exclusion diet. Rigorous diagnosis of fructose intolerance requires the demonstration of fructose 1-phosphate aldolase deficiency in visceral tissue or the presence of two causal mutant alleles of the human aldolase B gene.

The intravenous fructose tolerance test was formerly useful for diagnosis, particularly in adults; however, preparations of fructose suitable for intravenous use are now difficult to obtain and direct diagnosis by molecular analysis of the aldolase B gene is preferred. In any event, failure to obtain fructose solutions suitable for parenteral use should *not* encourage the administration of fructose or sucrose orally, since administration by this route may induce catastrophic effects with severe pain, acidosis, and even shock.

If no other method for investigating the patient is available, then the intravenous tolerance test should be carried out under controlled conditions with medical personnel at hand. It requires the infusion of 0.25 g/kg (0.2 g/kg in infants) of D(+)-fructose as a 20% solution over a few minutes; blood samples for potassium ions, magnesium ions, phosphate ions, and glucose are taken before the administration and at regular intervals over a 2-h period. In fructose intolerance, epigastric and loin pain usually accompany the infusion, and hypoglycaemic coma may occur; hypophosphataemia is characteristic. The hypoglycaemia does not respond to glucagon, therefore glucose for parenteral injection must be available. Responses differ between individuals, and hypoglycaemia is usually milder in adults; typical responses in hereditary fructose intolerance and a control subject are shown in Fig. 12.3.2.3. The tolerance test should not be carried out in patients with overt signs of liver disease where it may occasionally yield misleading results, particularly in infants and children.

Aldolase B deficiency may be demonstrated definitively by enzymatic analysis of biopsy samples obtained from the liver or small intestinal mucosa. Biochemical assay of fructaldolases characteristically demonstrates markedly reduced or absent fructose 1-phosphate cleavage activity with a partial deficiency of fructose 1,6-diphosphate aldolase. Since fructaldolase deficiency may accompany other parenchymal disease of the liver, and because liver biopsy for biochemical analysis is invasive, these assays are of limited value in the acutely ill or jaundiced patient.

Tests for fructose intolerance based on the analysis of DNA are increasingly used for diagnosis so that invasive or hazardous investigations using tissue biopsy procedures or parenteral challenge with sugar solutions can be avoided. Direct genetic diagnosis of hereditary fructose intolerance is now possible and is the preferred method, particularly for patients of European ancestry. Molecular analysis of aldolase B genes for the presence of common mutations responsible for the disease can be carried out by specialized laboratories equipped for genetic testing; useful practical protocols for hierarchical mutation screening have been reported. Failure to identify two of the more frequent mutant alleles in patients with

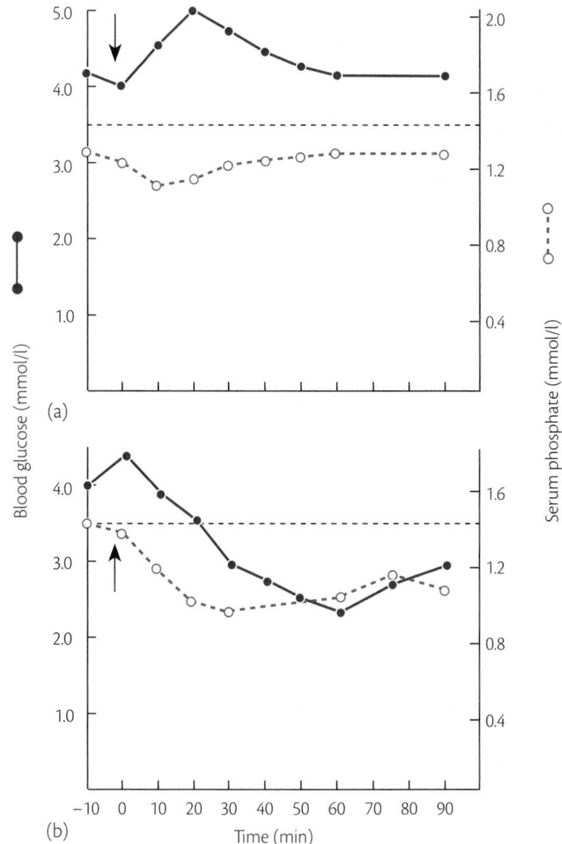

Fig. 12.3.2.3 (a) Intravenous fructose tolerance tests in a 39-year-old woman with hereditary fructose intolerance proved by fructaldolase assay and DNA analysis. (b) An age-matched and sex-matched control subject with alcohol-related episodic hypoglycaemia.

suspected hereditary fructose intolerance should encourage a systematic approach to molecular diagnosis, if necessary to include definitive sequencing of the aldolase B gene.

The ability to identify disease alleles by analysing genomic DNA obtained from very small samples of blood or tissue may not only be beneficial for the investigation of infants with this disorder but also for neonatal testing before dietary exposure occurs. There is a strong case for trials in which the utility of mass population screening for fructose intolerance, a preventable nutritional disease, is investigated.

Treatment

Dietary treatment of fructose intolerance mitigates the disorder but requires the almost complete exclusion of sucrose, fructose, and sorbitol. The daily consumption of sugar should be reduced to less than 40 mg fructose equivalents per kilogram body weight (i.e. 2–3 g for an adult) in order to reverse the disease manifestations and establish normal development in affected infants and children. The ubiquity of fructose and its congeners in the western diet presents serious difficulties. Adult patients have usually restricted their consumption of fructose to less than 20 g daily and the source of the residual sugar may be difficult to establish. For this reason, the advice of an experienced dietitian should be sought (Box 12.3.2.1). Particular care needs to be taken with sugar-coated pills and especially with liquid medications for paediatric use, as large amounts of fructose, sucrose, and sorbitol are frequently present. Children and adults with hereditary fructose intolerance may tolerate the taste of confectionery that contains large quantities of noxious sugars but in which the sweetness is masked by other flavours, such as peppermint, which they enjoy. This behaviour may lead to unexplained hypoglycaemic symptoms and other signs of sugar toxicity. Occasionally, patients are unable to tolerate certain foods that are permitted on their diet sheets; in doubtful cases it is advisable to avoid the offending item or to have it analysed.

Box 12.3.2.1 Food items not allowed for patients with hereditary fructose intolerance and fructose diphosphatase deficiency[a]

- Table sugar
- Fruit sugar, all fruit and fruit products, including tomatoes
- Sorbitol
- Honey, syrup, treacle, molasses
- Diabetic foods
- Chocolate, sherbet
- Preserves, jams, and marmalade
- Frankfurters, honey-roast, and sweet-cured ham
- Processed cheese spreads
- Cream and cottage cheese with chives, pineapple, etc.
- Flavoured milks and yoghurts
- Wheatgerm, brown rice, bran
- Breakfast cereals
- Coffee essence, powdered milk
- Carbonated sweet drinks
- Allspice, nuts, coconut, carob, peanut butter
- Mayonnaise, pickles, salad dressings, sauces
- Some potatoes (especially stored, new potatoes)
- Most legumes

[a] Further information is provided in the Further reading list.

Patients with hereditary fructose intolerance may lack folic acid and vitamin C. Supplements of these vitamins in particular are recommended, especially during pregnancy, but, as with other medicines, care has to be taken to avoid harmful sugars contained in the preparation. Although the use of fructose-containing or sorbitol-containing preparations for intravenous nutritional supplementation has now been stopped, some medicines that are given parenterally are reconstituted in solutions containing harmful quantities of sorbitol or fructose. Hepatorenal failure has recently been reported after the administration of amiodarone in a polysorbate solution to a patient with hereditary fructose intolerance, with dire consequences.

Prognosis

Untreated hereditary fructose intolerance is a potentially fatal disease in infants and young children in whom it generally causes irreversible liver disease and episodic, life-threatening hypoglycaemia. Occasionally, adolescents and adult patients may succumb to the inadvertent use of parenteral fructose or sorbitol, but this practice, which until recently was popular in German-speaking countries, is now obsolete. With the introduction of a strict exclusion diet, the disorder is compatible with a normal quality and duration of life.

Fructose diphosphatase deficiency (OMIM 229700)

Description

This very rare, recessively inherited disorder presents with hypoglycaemia, ketosis, and lactic acidosis in early infancy. Fewer than 100 cases have been reported since its original description in 1970. Severe, sometimes fatal, acidosis is associated with infection and starvation, and most cases present within the first few days of life or in the neonatal period. Onset during the first year of life is the rule.

In newborn infants, the severe metabolic disturbance shows itself by acidotic hyperventilation, which may be accompanied by irritability, disturbed consciousness, seizures, or coma. The unusual combination of ketonaemia, lacticacidaemia, and hypoglycaemia is induced by fasting, the administration of fructose, sorbitol, and glycerol, and by ingestion of a diet rich in fat. Episodes in the neonatal period respond well to infusions of glucose and bicarbonate but, after an interval, further attacks occur, often provoked by intercurrent infection. Lethargy accompanied by hyperventilation is followed abruptly by prostration, coma, and seizures. Investigations reveal hypoglycaemia, ketosis, and profound lactic acidosis; there is also hyperuricaemia, aminoaciduria, and ketonuria. If the infant survives, hepatomegaly due to fatty infiltration may be detected but overt clinical disturbances of hepatic or renal tubular function are not seen. The untreated disease is associated with growth retardation.

The first infant to be affected by fructose diphosphatase deficiency in a given family may succumb before the diagnosis is established and in any case fares worse than siblings for whom the appropriate diet and prompt control of the condition are instituted. The response to treatment is favourable, however, and fructose diphosphatase deficiency is ultimately compatible with a benign course and with normal growth and development.

Metabolic defect

Deficiency of fructose-1,6-diphosphatase causes failure of gluconeogenesis in the liver, although the abnormality may be detected in intestinal mucosa, kidney, and in cultured mononuclear cells from peripheral blood. The muscle isozyme of fructose-1,6-diphosphatase is not affected.

Between meals, blood glucose is maintained by glycogenolysis and hence the onset of disturbed metabolism in fructose diphosphatase deficiency depends on the availability of hepatic glycogen. Since febrile illnesses accelerate the consumption of liver glycogen, the accompanying anorexia with or without vomiting may deplete glycogen stores critically. Acidosis results from the accumulation of gluconeogenic precursors including lactate, pyruvate, and alanine as well as ketone bodies, which cannot be utilized. Hypoglycaemia that is unresponsive to glucagon and associated with exhaustion of glycogen stores occurs; it does not respond to normal gluconeogenic substrates (e.g. glycerol, amino acid solutions, dihydroxyacetone, sorbitol, or fructose); indeed administration of these aggravates the metabolic disturbance.

The pathogenesis of hypoglycaemia and accompanying disturbances in fructose diphosphatase deficiency is complex and not completely explained by exhaustion of hepatic glycogen stores. Well-fed patients have a normal response to glucagon but are intolerant of high-fat diets, as well as fructose, sorbitol, alanine, glycerol, and dihydroxyacetone administration. Challenge with these nutrients induces hypoglycaemia, hyperuricaemia, and hypophosphataemia, accompanied by an exaggerated rise in blood lactate levels. The hypoglycaemia is then unresponsive to glucagon, indicating a secondary inhibition of phosphorylase activity in the liver, which results from the build-up of phosphorylated sugar intermediates that cannot be further metabolized in the context of reduced intracellular free inorganic phosphate. Adenosine deaminase is activated primarily because of reduced phosphate concentrations, so that purine nucleotides are broken down to uric acid. Failure to utilize glucogenic amino acids and metabolites such as dihydroxyacetone and glycerol appears to stimulate triglyceride formation in the liver, which induces steatosis. Unlike hereditary fructose intolerance (see above), high concentrations of hepatic fructose 1-phosphate do not occur, and profound disturbances of blood coagulation or hepatic or renal tubule function with progressive structural damage are absent in fructose diphosphatase deficiency. Similarly, aversion to foods that aggravate the disorder does not develop in affected infants and children; this may be explained by the absence of pain and abdominal symptoms in the condition.

Diagnosis

The importance of establishing the diagnosis of fructose diphosphatase deficiency cannot be overemphasized. Proper dietary control and protocols for the institution of appropriate therapy depend on recognizing the complex disturbance that underlies this disease.

Fructose diphosphatase deficiency should be considered in otherwise normal infants who develop unexplained severe acidosis or hypoglycaemia associated with episodes of infection. The combination of ketosis and lactic acidosis with hypoglycaemia is highly suggestive of a disorder affecting the gluconeogenic pathway, including deficiency of glucose 6-phosphatase, pyruvate carboxylase, pyruvate dehydrogenase, and phosphoenolpyruvate carboxykinase. The absence of abdominal distress, haemolysis, jaundice, coagulopathy, and disturbances of the proximal renal tubule differentiates the condition from hereditary fructose intolerance, tyrosinosis, and Wilson's disease. Confusion may arise with disorders associated with secondary defects in gluconeogenesis, especially the Reye's-like syndrome caused by deficiencies of long-chain, medium-chain, and short-chain acyl coenzyme A dehydrogenase activities, as well as defects of carnitine metabolism. Organic acidaemias are also readily distinguished by biochemical screening methods.

Provocative tests using food deprivation and the administration of infusions of fructose, sorbitol, or glycerol should be avoided in the acutely ill infant or child with suspected deficiency of fructose-1,6-diphosphatase (or fructose intolerance). The definitive diagnosis depends on the demonstration of selectively decreased fructose diphosphatase activity in tissue samples. Most frequently, the enzymatic defect will be identified by biochemical assay of a freshly obtained liver biopsy specimen, which allows other metabolic disorders and gluconeogenic defects to be confidently excluded. The defect may also be demonstrated in biopsy samples of jejunal mucosa and in cultured monocyte-derived macrophages obtained from peripheral blood. However, the presence of fructose-1, 6-diphosphatase in these tissues is metabolically inconsequential and, although useful for confirmation of the diagnosis where it is strongly suspected, in practice decisive identification of this disorder normally depends on a systematic biochemical analysis of liver tissue in an experienced laboratory. The human fructose-1, 6-diphosphatase (*FBP1*) gene maps to chromosome 9q22.2–q22.3, and inactivating mutations have been identified in the disease. Unlike fructose intolerance, however, these mutations tend to be private and thus individually of less diagnostic significance for routine laboratory use in this disorder since mutational heterogeneity appears to be the rule. However, a minor exception to this occurs in the Japanese population, where one mutation (960–961 ins G) appears to account for almost one-half of mutant *FBPI* alleles.

Treatment

Dietary control and avoidance of starvation with rapid relief of febrile illnesses are the mainstays of management. Minor infections and injuries require prompt attention, and intravenous glucose therapy should be instituted early in acute episodes to avoid hypoglycaemia and acidosis. Fasting should be avoided as far as possible, while night-time feeding may be needed in infants during recovery from injuries or infections, and after strenuous exercise in older children. The habit of taking meals at regular 4-h intervals is best inculcated when the patient is young. The diet should exclude excess fat; sorbitol, sucrose, and fructose must be strictly avoided. Breast milk is rich in lactose, which is readily assimilated, but difficulties arise on transfer to artificial feeds during weaning. In addition, medications and syrups containing fructose, sucrose, or sorbitol present a special danger to patients with fructose diphosphatase deficiency. A diet excluding these sugars but containing 56% calories as carbohydrate, with 32% calories as fat and 12% as protein, has produced normal growth and development. Acute episodes of acidosis or hypoglycaemia are controlled rapidly by intravenous administration of glucose with or without bicarbonate as required.

Further reading

Ali M, Cox TM (1995). Diverse mutations in the aldolase B gene that underlie the prevalence of hereditary fructose intolerance. Independent segregation of four mutant alleles in ten affected members of a large kindred. *Am J Hum Genet*, **56**, 1002–5.

Ali M, Rellos P, Cox TM (1998). Hereditary fructose intolerance. *J Med Genet*, **35**, 353–65.

Baerlocher K, *et al.* (1978). Hereditary fructose intolerance in early childhood: a major diagnostic challenge. Survey of 20 symptomatic cases. *Helv Paediatr Acta*, **132**, 605–8.

Baker L, Wingrad AI (1970). Fasting hypoglycaemia and metabolic acidosis associated with deficiency of fructose-1,6-diphosphatase deficiency. *Lancet*, **ii**, 13–16.

Bell L, Sherwood WG (1987). Current practices and improved recommendations for treating hereditary fructose intolerance. *J Am Diet Assoc*, **87**, 721–8.

Boesinger P, *et al.* (1994). Changes of liver metabolite concentrations in adults with disorders of fructose metabolism after intravenous fructose by ^{31}P magnetic resonance spectroscopy. *Pediatr Res*, **36**, 436–40.

Chambers RA, Pratt RTC (1956). Idiosyncrasy to fructose. *Lancet*, **ii**, 340.

Cox TM (1993). Iatrogenic deaths in hereditary fructose intolerance. *Arch Dis Child*, **69**, 413–15.

Cox TM (1994). Aldolase B and fructose intolerance. *FASEB J*, **8**, 62–71.

Cox TM (2002). The genetic consequences of our sweet tooth. *Nat Rev Genet*, **3**, 481–7.

Cox TM (2009). Hereditary fructose intolerance (fructosaemia). In: Lifton R, *et al.* (eds) *Genetic diseases of the kidney*, pp. 619–43. Elsevier, New York.

Curran BJ, Havill JH (2002). Hepatic and renal failure associated with amiodarone infusion in a patient with hereditary fructose intolerance. *Crit Care Resusc*, **4**, 112–15.

Gibson PR, *et al.* (2007). Review article: fructose malabsorption and the bigger picture. *Aliment Pharmacol Ther*, **25**, 349–63.

Greenwood J (1989). Sugar content of liquid prescription medicines. *Pharm J*, **243**, 553–7.

James CJ, *et al.* (1996). Neonatal screening for hereditary fructose intolerance: frequency of the most common mutant aldolase B allele (A149P) in the British population. *J Med Genet*, **33**, 837–41.

Kikawa Y, *et al.* (2002). Diagnosis of fructose 1,6-bisphosphatase deficiency using cultured lymphocyte fraction: a secure and noninvasive alternative to liver biopsy. *J Inherit Metab Dis*, **25**, 41–6.

Krishnamurthy V, *et al.* (2007). Three successful pregnancies through dietary management of fructose-1,6-bisphosphatase deficiency. *J Inherit Metab Dis*, **30**, 819.

Mock DM, *et al.* (1983). Chronic fructose intoxication after infancy in children with hereditary fructose intolerance: a cause of growth retardation. *N Engl J Med*, **309**, 764–70.

Odièvre M, *et al.* (1978). Hereditary fructose intolerance in childhood. Diagnosis, management and course in 55 patients. *Am J Dis Child*, **132**, 605–8.

Pagliara AS, *et al.* (1972). Hepatic fructose-1,6-diphosphatase deficiency. A cause of lactic acidosis and hypoglycaemia in infancy. *J Clin Invest*, **51**, 2115–23.

Pronicka E, *et al.* (2007). Elevated carbohydrate-deficient transferrin (CDT) and its normalization on dietary treatment as a useful biochemical test for hereditary fructose intolerance and galactosemia. *Pediatr Res*, **62**, 101–5.

Reimers A, Spigset O (2003). Declaration of fructose and fructose-related adverse effects in commercial drug preparations in European countries. *Drug Saf*, **26**, 1057–9.

Sachs B, Sternfeld L, Kraus G (1942). Essential fructosuria: its pathophysiology. *Am J Dis Child*, **63**, 252.

Santer R, *et al.* (2005). The spectrum of aldolase B (ALDOB) mutations and the prevalence of hereditary fructose intolerance in Central Europe. *Hum Mutat*, **25**, 594.

Steinmann B, Gitzelmann R, Van den Berghe G (2001). Disorders of fructose metabolism. In: Scriver CR, *et al.* (eds) *The metabolic and molecular bases of inherited disease*, 8th edition, vol. II, pp. 1489–520. McGraw-Hill, New York, www.ommbid.com [updated January 2008].

Thabet F, *et al.* (2002). Severe Reye syndrome: report of 14 cases managed in a pediatric intensive care unit over 11 years. *Arch Pediatr*, **9**, 581–6.

Wasserman D, *et al.* (1996). Molecular analysis of the fructose transporter gene (GLUT5) in isolated fructose malabsorption. *J Clin Invest*, **98**, 2398–402.

12.3.3 Disorders of galactose, pentose, and pyruvate metabolism

Timothy M. Cox

Essentials

Inborn errors of galactose metabolism

Galactose is principally found as free lactose in dairy products; the sugar moiety also occurs as a dietary component in glycoproteins and complex lipids. Three inborn errors of galactose metabolism are recognized:

Galactokinase deficiency ('galactose diabetes')—a very rare condition which impairs the assimilation of dietary galactose that is normally initiated by phosphorylation, principally in the liver; the free sugar and its metabolites, galactonic acid and galactitol, appear in plasma and the urine. Conversion of galactose to osmotically active galactitol in tissues causes premature bilateral cataracts and occasionally pseudotumor cerebri in infants. The abnormalities may be ameliorated by early institution of a galactose- and lactose-free diet.

Galactose 1-phosphate uridylyltransferase deficiency (classical galactosaemia)—the most important disorder, with an overall estimated frequency of 1 in 47 000 births. High concentrations of galactose in the plasma and tissues lead to aberrant glycosylation of glycoproteins and other glycoconjugates, including lipids. The clinical features are diverse and the pathogenesis remains ill understood. The principal manifestations are a bacteriocidal defect associated with neonatal *E. coli* sepsis. There is failure to thrive and—in older patients—growth retardation, mental retardation, and hepatomegaly, which without dietary treatment may cause cirrhosis. Disease of the proximal kidney tubule causes the renal Fanconi syndrome and osteomalacia. The diagnosis is made by plasma galactose, galactose 1-phosphate, and red-cell transferase determinations in blood spots obtained after birth. Visceral disease and stunting are mitigated by institution of a lactose- and galactose-free diet, but ovarian failure leading to premature menopause and osteoporosis is common in young girls and women and occurs irrespective of dietary exclusion therapy. Prompt institution of an appropriate diet allows survival into late adult life, but disabling neurological manifestations persist.

Uridine diphosphate-4-epimerase deficiency—a rare but largely harmless disorder, usually discovered at neonatal screening for galactosaemia.

Pentosuria

Essential pentosuria is an asymptomatic autosomal recessive disorder of glucuronate metabolism (principally affecting Ashkenazi Jews) caused by deficiency of hepatic xylitol dehydrogenase which causes the daily appearance of several grams of L-xylulose in the urine.

Disorders of pyruvate metabolism

Deficiency of the pyruvate dehydrogenase complex is the most common inherited disorder which causes lacticacidaemia. Hereditary defects affect the five principal components of this macromolecular complex, most often producing deficiency of the E1α subunit, which is inherited as an X-linked character. Presentation is with overwhelming neonatal acidosis; moderate lactic acidosis with progressive neurological features; or—in male children and young adults—an indolent neurological course without overt acidosis but with episodes of cerebellar ataxia induced by carbohydrate administration.

Pyruvate carboxylase is a biotin-dependent gluconeogenic enzyme deficiency that mainly causes lactate/pyruvate acidosis with a necrotizing encephalopathy resembling Wernicke's encephalopathy. Hypoglycaemia may complicate intercurrent infections and starvation.

Galactose metabolism

Galactose is derived from the disaccharide lactose (present in milk and dairy products in the diet) by the action of mucosal lactase in the small intestine. The concentration of lactose in human breast milk is approximately 200 mmol/litre. Newborn infants normally receive about one-fifth of their dietary energy supply in the form of galactose, which is derived from the breakdown of this lactose to galactose and glucose in equimolar amounts. Galactose is also complexed with other molecules present in food; it is a component of membrane glycoproteins and glycolipids, and galactosylated sphingolipids are abundant in nervous tissue.

The interconversion of galactose and glucose involves reactions (known as the Leloir pathway) requiring nucleoside (uridine) diphosphate sugar intermediates that lead to the formation of galactose 1-phosphate, which directly enters the main pathways of carbohydrate metabolism (Fig. 12.3.3.1). These intermediates, especially uridine diphosphoglucose, uridine diphosphogalactose, and their aminated derivatives such as uridine diphosphogalactosamine, are critical substrates for the biosynthesis of glycoproteins and glycolipids, including glycosphingolipids; intracellular concentrations of these activated metabolites are influenced by the activity of the enzymes of the Leloir pathway.

Galactose obtained from lactose and other glycoconjugates is present as the β-D-galactose isomer and before it can be further metabolized it must be converted to α-D-galactose in a reaction catalysed by the bidirectional enzyme mutarotase, the crystal structure of which has recently been reported.

The first step in the Leloir pathway involves phosphorylation to form galactose 1-phosphate, which is converted to glucose 1-phosphate and uridine diphosphate-galactose after reaction with the nucleoside diphosphate sugar, uridine diphosphoglucose. Uridine diphosphoglucose is regenerated by the action of uridine diphosphate-galactose-4-epimerase. The presence of this epimerase enables galactose to be produced from glucose for the synthesis of complex glycoconjugates and renders the individual potentially independent of exogenous galactose. Enzymatic defects in the interconversion of these metabolites increase blood and tissue concentrations of galactose, especially after meals containing milk or dairy products.

While the Leloir pathway is clearly the predominant route for galactose metabolism in humans, minor pathways that do not utilize the transferase, epimerase, or galactokinase enzyme system are known to operate: reduction of galactose to galactitol and oxidation to galactonic acid can occur independently, thereby potentially bypassing the metabolic block at the level of the transferase that is responsible for classic galactosaemia. When high concentrations are present, galactose serves as a substrate for enzymes of the polyol pathway catalysed by aldose reductase or L-hexonate dehydrogenase, the former enzyme being responsible for the direct reduction of galactose to galactitol, which is not metabolized any further in the polyol pathway and thus may accumulate in tissues. Raised concentrations of galactitol in blood and urine occur in classic galactosaemia, galactokinase deficiency, and epimerase deficiency. If the transferase is absent, reduction of galactose to galactitol cannot dispose of galactose; rather, it appears likely that formation of galactitol contributes significantly to the pathological effects of galactosaemia. Galactose that accumulates in patients with galactosaemia is in part oxidized to galactonic acid, which may be further degraded to carbon dioxide by the pentose phosphate shunt. A final minor route for galactose breakdown is the pyrophosphorylase pathway, which may dispose of the sugar at about 1% of the rate of the Leloir pathway.

Although they may account for the less severe manifestations of disease in adults who survive with classic galactosaemia, the metabolic capacity of these default pathways is insufficient to mitigate the clinical disease and at the time of writing no effective means to circumvent the defect by this means has been identified.

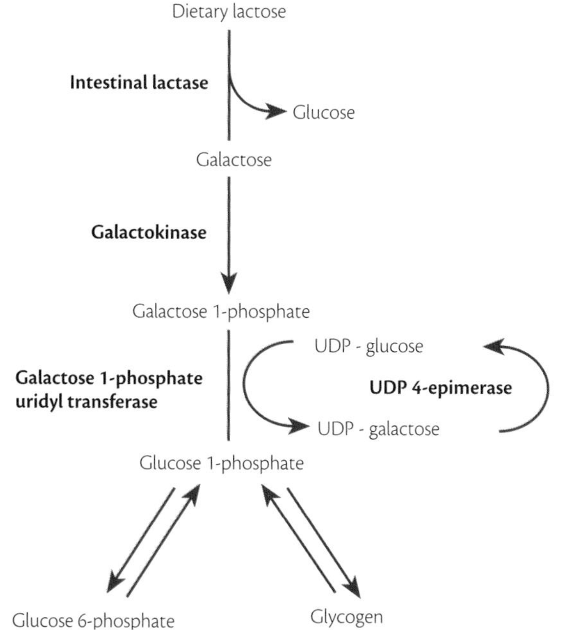

Fig. 12.3.3.1 Galactose metabolism.

Galactokinase deficiency: 'galactose diabetes'

Failure to phosphorylate galactose in the liver and other tissues impairs its clearance from the blood so that the free sugar, as well as its metabolites galactonic acid and galactitol, appear in the urine. Homozygous deficiency of galactokinase occurs with an approximate frequency of 1 in 1 000 000 live births, but it is more frequent in some groups, such as the European Roma gypsy population, in which a single mutant allele of the human galactokinase gene, a (P28T) mutation in *GALK1*, is prevalent.

Clinical features

Precocious formation of bilateral cataracts in infants and children is characteristic, with some heterozygotes developing cataracts before the age of 40 years. When blood concentrations are high, galactose is taken up by the lens and converted to the end-product galactitol by the action of aldose reductase: subsequent toxic or osmotic effects lead to swelling and irreversible damage to lens fibres. Several infants have presented with benign intracranial hypertension (pseudotumour cerebri), possibly as a result of comparable osmotic effects of galactitol in the brain. Patients with galactokinase deficiency persistently excrete reducing sugar in their urine, but, apart from possible confusion with diabetes mellitus, this has no apparent significance.

Diagnosis and treatment

Galactokinase deficiency should be suspected in infants or children with cataracts, and reducing sugar should be sought in the urine. This sugar will not react with glucose oxidase test strips. Definitive diagnosis by enzymatic assay of galactokinase in erythrocytes or cultured fibroblasts differentiates the disorder from classic galactosaemia and hypergalactosaemia due to vascular disease in the liver. In populations with newborn surveillance for high blood galactose concentration, the deficiency may be detected as a result of finding an abnormal blood galactose concentration with normal transferase and epimerase activities. Definitive enzymatic measurements can be conducted on amniocytes and on cultured skin fibroblasts. Neonatal screening that depends on tests for galactose in the blood will not detect galactokinase deficiency. The human gene for galactokinase maps to chromosome 17q24, with a putative second locus on chromosome 15. Numerous mutations responsible for galactokinase deficiency have been identified in the *GALK1* gene at its chromosome 17 locus. Many of these are private, but the so-called Osaka variant, a missense mutation (A198V), was first identified through mass neonatal screening and has a prevalence of 4.1% in Japanese individuals and 2.8% in Koreans; it is uncommon among individuals of Taiwanese and Chinese ancestry. The Osaka *GALK1* variant has been reported to occur in 7.8% of Japanese adults with bilateral cataracts, in whom it may represent a true population risk factor.

Lifelong treatment with a lactose-exclusion and galactose-exclusion diet prevents cataract formation, and early cataract formation in infants may be reversed; otherwise surgical removal may be required. Urinary galactitol concentrations, which have been reported to exceed 2500 mmol/mol creatinine, fall to within the reference range for healthy subjects (<3 mmol/mol creatinine) after some weeks of dietary treatment. Although there are numerous reports of bilateral cataracts in heterozygotes for galactokinase deficiency, it remains unclear whether any propensity to cataract formation in later life is prevented by dietary restriction; some authors have suggested that cataracts are more frequent in otherwise healthy individuals who consume abundant dairy products, but have no galactokinase deficiency. In the face of this controversy, it appears to be most prudent to recommend modest restriction of lactose intake in heterozygotes for galactokinase deficiency.

Galactose 1-phosphate uridylyltransferase deficiency: galactosaemia

Unlike individuals in whom galactokinase is deficient, when those who lack uridylyltransferase activity ingest lactose, there is a significant rise in intracellular galactose 1-phosphate as well as blood galactose concentrations. The severe consequences of classic galactosaemia result from the toxic effects of galactose 1-phosphate principally in cells of the liver, proximal renal tubule, and brain. Although the exact mechanism of toxicity is unknown, as in hereditary fructose intolerance, the accumulation of galactose 1-phosphate in a milieu with depleted inorganic phosphate probably inhibits other enzymatic reactions involving phosphorylated intermediates and may lead to purine nucleotide depletion.

Recognition of galactosaemia in early infancy is of paramount importance since the acute effects of galactose poisoning may be reversed by the institution of a lactose-exclusion diet; the birth frequency is about 1 in 50 000 live births but varies greatly according to the population examined. It is notable that the ability of dietary therapy to promote a completely healthy long-term outcome has now been questioned by follow-up studies in large cohorts of patients with classic galactosaemia, and more research is needed to improve our understanding of the pathogenesis of tissue injury in this nutritional disease with neurodevelopmental manifestations.

Clinical and pathological features

Affected infants appear normal at birth, but vomiting or diarrhoea, jaundice, and hepatomegaly usually occur in the first few weeks. There is failure to gain weight, spontaneous bruising, and progressive enlargement of the liver. Cataracts may be apparent at 1 month of age, by which time abdominal distension with ascites has developed. Learning difficulties do not become apparent until later in the first year of life and vary greatly in severity. Many patients with galactosaemia develop severe infections with *Escherichia coli* during the neonatal period: gram-negative bacterial sepsis may be the first indication of this disorder in young infants. A bactericidal defect in circulating leucocytes has been postulated. In adult patients after reversal of the acute galactose toxicity syndrome, the most obvious sequelae are growth failure, neurological deficit, and, in women, primary ovarian failure with infertility.

A few patients with galactosaemia remain asymptomatic while ingesting milk, but eventually fail to gain weight. Such patients may come to light during childhood or even adult life with varying degrees of learning difficulties and cataracts. Hepatomegaly and intermittent galactosuria are usually present, and often there is a history of feeding difficulties on institution of modified formula feeds during the neonatal period.

The neurological manifestations of classic galactosaemia are highly variable but, despite prompt institution of dietary therapy, a degree of intellectual disability is common in affected children and adults. Characteristic learning difficulties in mathematics and spatial relationships with behavioural deficits have been observed. Children with galactosaemia have a particularly high risk for language impairment. Early dietary lactose may increase the risk for cognitive and language impairments; however, the lack of significant associations of language impairment with days of milk consumption, and other familial and educational risk factors, is consistent with prenatal causation. It appears that the galactose-free diet fails to confer benefit on mental development when instituted beyond the age of 2 years. In follow-up studies of galactosaemic children and adults, a range of neurological deficits, including seizures, apraxia, extrapyramidal disorders, and cerebellar signs, have been documented despite strict dietary measures. In adult galactosaemic patients, recent studies of brain metabolism using positron emission tomography with [^{18}F]-fluorodeoxyglucose revealed extensive regions in which cerebral and cerebellar glucose metabolism was decreased when compared with controls.

Serum tests of liver function are nonspecifically deranged: histological examination shows lobular fibrosis, fatty change, bile ductular proliferation, and progression to frank cirrhosis. A haemorrhagic tendency is an early feature of galactosaemia and the diagnosis should be considered in jaundiced infants with signs of a bleeding diathesis. In the untreated state, biochemical screening tests may suggest a diagnosis of carbohydrate-deficient syndrome since hypoglycosylation and other qualitative abnormalities of serum transferrin *N*-glycans occur; these abnormalities are largely corrected on transfer to a lactose-exclusion diet.

Involvement of the proximal renal tubule is shown by generalized aminoaciduria and occasionally a full-blown Fanconi syndrome with vacuolation of tubular epithelial cells. Histological examination of the brain shows nonspecific signs of injury with gliosis and Purkinje cell loss in the cerebellum; it appears plausible that the deficiency of uridine diphosphate-galactose will affect the biosynthesis of key galactosphingolipids by uridine diphosphate-galactosylceramide transferase in neural cells. Follow-up studies of female patients with galactosaemia have shown a high incidence of gonadal failure with ovarian atrophy; although this complication appears to be more common in patients in whom dietary therapy was delayed, no clear cause-and-effect relationship has been established. A toxic effect on the fetal ovary due to maternal hypergalactosaemia has been postulated to account for the hypergonadotropic hypogonadism in affected women and girls, but abnormal glycosylation of follicle-stimulating hormone has also been postulated. Pregnancies have occurred in a significant minority of women with classic galactosaemia and they have usually resulted in the birth of healthy infants. No evidence of gonadal failure has been found in male patients.

Genetic studies

Galactosaemia is transmitted as an autosomal recessive trait with an overall estimated frequency of 1 in 47 000 in liveborn infants. Classic galactosaemia is rare in Japan but frequent in some isolated groups, most notably in the modern Traveller population of Ireland. In this group, screening methods indicate a birth frequency of 1 in 480 compared with 1 in 30 000 in the non-Traveller Irish population. In African American patients from the United States of America a relatively mild disorder has been reported that is probably due to an unstable enzyme variant; uridylyltransferase activity is absent from the red cells of these patients but amounts to some 10% of normal in samples of liver and small intestinal tissue. Patients with the so-called Duarte variant possess about one-half of the normal enzyme activity in erythrocytes but remain asymptomatic.

The human galactosyl-1-phosphate uridylyltransferase gene maps to human chromosome 9p13 and encodes a protein of molecular weight 43 kDa, which exists as a functional homodimer. Molecular analysis of the transferase gene indicates that most patients with classic galactosaemia harbour missense-type mutations and are compound heterozygotes. Numerous variant transferase enzymes are known and, by early 2008, more than 200 disease-associated mutations were reported. Molecular analysis of the transferase gene has identified several widespread mutations; for example one mutant allele (Q188R) is in linkage disequilibrium with a restriction fragment-length polymorphism flanking exon 6 of the gene sequence in multiple populations worldwide, including those of European descent and Irish Travellers. A less frequent mutation of diagnostic significance in white populations is designated R333W; the Duarte transferase mutation has been identified as N314D. Molecular analysis of the transferase gene now renders prenatal diagnosis of at-risk pregnancies possible.

Diagnosis

Galactosaemia may be suspected in an infant with growth failure, cataracts, liver disease, aminoaciduria, learning difficulties, and especially where reducing sugar is present in the urine. The occurrence of unexplained bacterial sepsis, especially if due to *Escherichia coli* infection in a newborn infant, may indicate galactosaemia. Cataracts may be detected by slit-lamp examination in the first few days of life.

Since the clinical manifestations of galactosaemia are not specific, it is necessary to consider the diagnosis, especially in countries where neonatal screening for galactosaemia is not routinely carried out. The finding of hypergalactosaemia is not specific for those hereditary galactosaemias due to inherited deficiencies of galactose-metabolizing enzymes. Recent studies in infants show that persistent hypergalactosaemia may commonly be due to portosystemic venous shunts that are often associated with patent ductus venosus or other congenital vascular abnormalities in the liver. Doppler ultrasonography is a convenient noninvasive investigation to search for such shunts in infants.

Definitive diagnosis of hereditary galactosaemia is mandatory, and relies on the determination of galactose 1-phosphate uridylyltransferase activity and other galactose-metabolizing enzymes in red cells, skin fibroblasts, or leucocytes by means of a specific enzymatic assay. This procedure is required to confirm the results of initial screening tests conducted on dried blood spots (Beutler assay); transferase activity in patients with classic galactosaemia is generally less than 1% of the normal reference range. Reliable enzymatic or genetic testing for heterozygotes can be conducted in the parents of a child who died before the diagnosis was confirmed. In particular populations, neonatal screening for elevated blood galactose and galactose 1-phosphate concentrations is carried out routinely. Molecular analysis of the gene encoding galactose 1-phosphate uridylyltransferase in at-risk pregnancies has been requested by some affected families. Neonatal screening for galactosaemia is available in the United States of America and in Europe, but only a small percentage of newborns in the United Kingdom are tested. At the time of writing, no prospective studies have demonstrated whether newborn screening programmes lead to an earlier diagnosis and reduce early morbidity and mortality from galactosaemia, and it seems unlikely that screening will prevent or reduce the late complications in adults. However, several retrospective studies indicate that neonatal screening prevents early deaths in this disease; in one survey 80% of patients who underwent newborn screening were diagnosed by 14 days of age, compared with only 35% of patients who were not tested but who had manifest disease.

Treatment

Without strict dietary treatment, most patients with galactosaemia die in early infancy, although some may survive with liver disease and learning difficulties beyond childhood. The course of galactosaemia is strikingly altered on withdrawal of lactose (and galactose), although the outcome of neurological disease is often disappointing.

Lactose is present in many nondairy foods, and advice from an experienced dietician, as well as meticulous attention to detail, is required to eliminate it completely. In infants, soybean milks or commercial casein hydrolysates are used as milk substitutes, and therapy is monitored by periodic assay of red-cell galactose 1-phosphate concentrations. Soya milk contains galactose equivalents complexed to other molecules (about 15 mg/litre) and there is a trend to adopt a completely galactose-free artificial formula in the treatment of affected infants; however, proof that this biochemically successful strategy induces better long-term outcomes in classic galactosaemia is not available. Despite reports that galactose may be reintroduced as the patient develops, lifelong strict adherence to the exclusion diet should be strongly advocated. In the untreated state, the concentration of red-cell galactose 1-phosphate is above 5 mmol/litre but with close adherence to the diet it falls within a few months to less that 0.25 mmol/litre. Although biochemical monitoring has not been shown closely to predict outcomes, as a rule expert centres recommend that the desired long-term target for blood galactose 1-phosphate concentrations should be about 0.15 mmol/litre of erythrocytes and monitoring 2 to 3 times per year in the first decade is usually practised.

In subsequent pregnancies of heterozygous mothers who have had affected children, there is evidence that premature cataracts can be avoided in the fetus if the maternal intake of lactose is restricted. In late pregnancy, lactosaemia and lactosuria are common findings and result from the physiological induction of lactose biosynthesis in mammary tissue. In rare cases (see below) there is a risk of self-intoxication when women with homozygous deficiency of the transferase become pregnant and breastfeed, so that additional dietary precautions are needed to maintain metabolic control during lactation.

Maintaining appropriate lifelong care for patients with galactosaemia in specialist clinics shows benefits in the provision of dietary management with expert advice as well as developmental monitoring and assessment of cognitive function that can be matched to educational needs. Regular review in paediatric, transitional, and then adult metabolic specialist centres is critical for many patients who have overt or hidden difficulties with speech or cognition. Review allows for regular metabolic monitoring and serial evaluation of bone mineralization density and vitamin D status, with opportunities to intervene where appropriate to avoid the risk of fragility fractures. Women with galactosaemia will also benefit from the ability to discuss matters related to reproductive health and fertility and obtain the necessary referrals for gynaecological and endocrinological treatment.

Prognosis

The acute manifestations of galactosaemia and growth failure respond quickly to dietary therapy and cataract formation is prevented. Unfortunately, a proportion of patients have significant neurological deficits despite prompt and conscientious treatment. An international survey of the long-term outcome in 350 patients receiving dietary therapy has been published by Waggoner and colleagues. The presence of ovarian failure and elevated galactose 1-phosphate concentrations in patients apparently ingesting no lactose or galactose raises the possibility that an endogenous pathway of galactose 1-phosphate formation from the pyrophosphorylysis of uridine diphosphate-galactose may occur. This may also explain the late emergence of neurological disease in treated patients. Long-term follow-up and periodic neuropsychiatric as well as physical monitoring is recommended. Recently, several pregnancies have been reported in women who have classic galactosaemia, including subjects homozygous for the Q188R mutation. In such pregnancies, high concentrations of galactitol are found in amniotic fluid but cord blood values have been determined to be within the range found in galactosaemic patients receiving strict dietary therapy. Thus, although maternal galactitol traverses the placenta, it probably does not harm the heterozygous fetus.

Uridine diphosphate-4-epimerase deficiency

Epimerase deficiency is very rare but may be identified during screening for classic galactosaemia. In most cases no symptoms attributable to galactosaemia are apparent and follow-up studies have confirmed the usually benign nature of this anomaly. However, a few cases of marked deficiency of uridine diphosphate-4-epimerase have been discovered in patients otherwise manifesting the classic features of galactosaemia. In the absence of epimerase activity, the individual is dependent on exogenous sources of galactose, since this cannot be derived from glucose. The autosomal recessive nature of this inherited disorder has been confirmed by demonstrating a partial epimerase deficiency in the healthy parents of an affected infant. As a complete deficiency of the epimerase would lead to an absolute lack of uridine diphosphate-galactose for galactosphingolipid synthesis, the ingestion of very small quantities of galactose has been recommended in this unusual disorder so that brain development and biosynthesis of essential galactosides can proceed. Because of the dual activity of the epimerase towards uridine diphosphate-acetyl glucosamine as well as uridine diphosphate-glucose, it has been suggested that small supplements of the aminoacetyl galactosamine should also be provided in the diets of patients with uridine diphosphate-galactose-4-epimerase deficiency. This condition may be contrasted with the transferase deficiency that allows the formation of small amounts of endogenous galactose in the presence of an intact epimerase. The gene for human uridine diphosphate-galactose-4-epimerase has been mapped to chromosome 1p36–p35, and numerous mutant alleles have been identified.

Pentosuria

Pentosuria is caused by the excessive renal excretion of L-xylulose. This has no clinical significance except that it may lead to the incorrect diagnosis of diabetes mellitus should tests for reducing sugar be carried out on the urine. Xylulose does not react with urinary test strips based on the glucose oxidase method.

The disorder has historical significance as one of the original inborn errors of metabolism cited by Garrod in his classic study. Although pentosuria is a rare autosomal recessive trait, its frequency in Ashkenazi Jews may be as high as 0.05%. It is caused by deficiency of L-xylulose reductase, a nicotinamide adenine dinucleotide phosphate-dependent enzyme in the oxidative pathway of glucuronate metabolism, which results in 1 to 4 g xylulose and L-arabitol continuously appearing in the urine; output is greatly enhanced by the ingestion of glucuronic acid or drugs that are excreted as glucuronides. The enzyme is present in many cells including red cells and hepatocytes. Several reactions remove the carboxyl carbon atom of D-glucuronic acid to generate the pentose L-xylulose, which is converted to its stereoisomer, D-xylulose.

D-Xylulose is phosphorylated to D-xylulose 5-phosphate, which can be converted to hexose phosphates in the reactions of the pentose phosphate shunt. The diagnosis is made definitively in specialized laboratories by confirming the enzymatic defect in erythrocytes, but pentosuria is most readily confirmed by paper chromatographic analysis of urine using *n*-butanol, ethanol, and water (50:10:40) as the partitioning solvent and orcinol-trichloroacetic acid as a detection agent; the sugar has a high mobility (R_F 0.26) and is identified by its red colour on development. Long-term monitoring of 40 individuals with pentosuria over more than 16 years showed no decrease in life expectancy.

Inborn errors of pyruvate metabolism

The organic acids, pyruvate and lactate, are key interconvertible intermediates in energy metabolism. Breakdown of pyruvate proceeds by oxidation, first by pyruvate dehydrogenase, then the Krebs cycle, and finally the respiratory chain; anabolic assimilation of pyruvate is mediated by pyruvate carboxylase. Lactate is the product of anaerobic glycolysis and is generated entirely from reduction of pyruvate by lactate dehydrogenase; lactate is disposed of by the reversal of this reaction. Defective metabolism of pyruvate readily leads to the accumulation of lactate and the development of lacticacidaemia.

Pyruvate dehydrogenase deficiency

Deficiency of pyruvate dehydrogenase is the most common cause of lactic acidosis in newborn infants and children, but it is also associated with neurodegenerative syndromes in later life. Pyruvate dehydrogenase exists as a multienzyme complex representing the products of 10 distinct genes. However, defects in one subunit of pyruvate dehydrogenase itself (E1α) account for most patients so far investigated; other defects in dihydrolipoyl transacetylase (E2), dihydrolipoyl dehydrogenase (E3), X-lipoate, or the pyruvate dehydrogenase phosphatase component of the complex have also been reported.

Biochemical defect

The pyruvate dehydrogenase complex catalyses the conversion of pyruvate to acetyl CoA within mitochondria and is rate-limiting for aerobic metabolism of glucose in the brain; in the adult brain, daily glucose consumption is 125 g. Thus the pyruvate dehydrogenase complex is critical for brain metabolism since this is normally entirely dependent on the oxidative breakdown of glucose. Where the activity of the complex is impaired, accumulated pyruvate may either be reduced to lactate or transaminated to alanine, so that hyperalaninaemia and varying degrees of lacticacidaemia occur. Very rare defects in dihydrolipoyl dehydrogenase are associated with deficiency of branched-chain keto acid dehydrogenase. Failure to carry out oxidative reactions in regions of the cortex and midbrain causes neuronal death; deficiency of four-carbon intermediates may critically impair synthesis of neurotransmitter molecules.

There are three main activities associated in the complex: (1) pyruvate dehydrogenase, a thiamine pyrophosphate-dependent complex (E1); (2) dihydrolipoyl transacetylase (E2); and (3) dihydrolipoyl dehydrogenase (E3). Also associated are a pyruvate dehydrogenase-specific kinase and phosphatase (both involved in overall metabolic regulation of the complex) as well as an essential lipoate-containing protein other than dihydrolipoamide transacetylase in the pyruvate dehydrogenase complex (X-lipoate), which possesses an acyl transfer function.

The combined molecular mass is about 8.5 million and the complex comprises 30 units of E1, 60 units of E2, and 6 units each of E3 and X. The E1 unit is an $\alpha_2\beta_2$ tetramer with subunits of 41 and 36 kDa.

Clinical features and prognosis

The extent of clinical expression of the enzymatic defect is highly variable. There may be fulminant lactic acidosis in the newborn infant; intrauterine development is impaired, marked acidosis (blood lactate >10 mmol/litre) is present at birth, and this disorder is rapidly fatal. In others, lacticacidaemia may not be apparent and the disease comes to light because of intrauterine growth failure, neonatal hypotonia asphyxia, and feeding difficulty; the principal abnormality is progressive psychomotor retardation often accompanied by brainstem injury and disease of the basal ganglia. There is dysgenesis with structural abnormalities of the olivopontocerebellar tract and periventricular grey matter. Cortical atrophy and agenesis of the corpus callosum have also been reported in association with spastic quadriplegia, especially in patients presenting with neonatal acidosis. Blood lactate concentrations do not exceed 10 mmol/litre. Without intensive treatment, death usually occurs in infancy; however, should feeding by gavage be instituted, there is a protracted course with failure of neurological development, microcephaly, quadriplegia, seizures, and blindness. Intermittent cerebellar ataxia or torsion dystonia have been recorded and choreoathetoid movements occur. Involuntary eye movements in children are associated with a progressively deteriorating course.

A milder form of the disorder occurs in defects of the X-linked E1α gene (*PDHA1*) but because pyruvate dehydrogenase deficiency is of key importance in brain metabolism, expression of disease is observed in females and affected males; this form of pyruvate dehydrogenase complex deficiency is an X-linked dominant disorder. In boys, however, episodic cerebellar ataxia may be induced by feeding carbohydrate-rich foods or medicinal glucose; the disorder responds to introduction of a ketogenic diet. In these patients, some of whom are otherwise unimpaired and have normal intelligence, blood lactate concentrations may only be trivially elevated. In contrast, in other patients a progressive brainstem disorder occurs, characteristic of Leigh's disease, with haemorrhagic necrosis and symmetrical spongiform appearances in the periventricular grey matter, thalami, midbrain, pons, medulla, and spinal cord; the mammillary bodies are spared.

There are fascinating similarities between pyruvate dehydrogenase complex deficiency and diseases related to thiamine deficiency with or without induction by exposure to alcohol (ethanol). About one-third of patients with pyruvate dehydrogenase complex deficiency have facial appearances reminiscent of the fetal syndrome due to maternal consumption of excess alcohol; this dysmorphism is characterized by a narrow head, retroussé nose, flared nostrils, and an elongated philtrum; there is frontal bossing of the skull and a broad nasal bridge. In the acquired syndrome, acetaldehyde from the maternal circulation is believed to inhibit pyruvate dehydrogenase in the fetus, and Robinson and colleagues have suggested that low endogenous activity of the pyruvate dehydrogenase complex due to genetic deficiency in the fetus is responsible for the developmental abnormalities. A striking connection between agenesis of the corpus callosum, usually in patients with neonatal pyruvate dehydrogenase deficiency, has been made with the Marchiafava–Bignami syndrome, a condition characterized by degeneration of the corpus callosum and associated with longstanding abuse of alcohol. Finally, in Wernicke's encephalopathy, the effects of thiamine deficiency and deficiency of the pyruvate dehydrogenase complex on the brain occur principally in the regions of the greatest metabolic activity, especially in the brainstem and basal ganglia. Diminished activity of the pyruvate dehydrogenase complex caused thiamine pyrophosphate deficiency, possibly combined with inhibition by the ethanol metabolite, acetaldehyde, as a plausible common factor in neuropathogenesis.

Recently, mild forms of pyruvate dehydrogenase deficiency due to defects in lipoamide dehydrogenase (E3 component) have been observed. Hereditary spinocerebellar degeneration appearing in early adult life has been attributed to the deficiency of pyruvate dehydrogenase but there is no direct relationship to Friedreich's ataxia. In patients who present with severe acidosis at birth, subacute necrotizing encephalomyelopathy of the Leigh type has been confirmed at necropsy with cystic appearances principally in the cerebral cortex, basal ganglia, and brainstem.

Genetics

The most common cause of pyruvate dehydrogenase deficiency is due to a defect in the E1α subunit, a protein encoded on the X chromosome. Although the disease is characteristically more severe in males, manifestations in the heterozygous female are unusually frequent for an X-linked disease and probably reflect the low functional reserve of the enzyme complex in the brain. Neonatal lactic acidosis is more frequent in males. An auxiliary gene for the E1α subunit is localized as a result of retroposition from the X chromosome to the long arm of chromosome 4, but is expressed only during spermatogenesis; its presence, however, indicates the critical need for activity of the complex in nearly all tissues. Causal mutations in the *PDHA1* gene on the X chromosome have been described; most appear to be short deletions or duplications and, at present, are not generally applicable for diagnosis. However, analysis of X-chromosome inactivation patterns, by determination of methylation status, has proved useful for the evaluation of enzymatic assays of fibroblasts obtained from obligate carriers or female patients in whom the diagnosis is suspected.

Diagnosis and treatment

The diagnosis is suspected from the presence of severe acidosis at birth. It may also emerge during the investigation of neurological deficits, especially where they are associated with intrauterine growth failure. Routine screening of urine samples for organic acids may identify excessive pyruvate and lactate; hyperammonaemia with citrullinaemia, hyperlysinaemia, and hyperalaninaemia may be found on blood analysis. In patients without clinically evident acidosis, cerebral disease is accompanied by striking elevations of lactate and pyruvate in the cerebrospinal fluid. Mutation analysis of the X-linked *PDHA1* gene and determination of the abundance of immunoreactive pyruvate dehydrogenase protein now permits decisive diagnosis of this disease.

The diagnosis of lacticacidaemia may be very challenging, especially when an inborn error of metabolism is responsible. Lactic acid is the product of the anaerobic metabolism of glucose, principally in circulating erythrocytes, skin, kidney medulla, and white skeletal muscle. Excess production of lactic acid is a consequence of numerous disorders that do not have an overt hereditary basis. These include drug overdose (e.g. biguanide antidiabetic agents); hypoxia, ischaemia, and hypotensive shock; overwhelming sepsis; bacterial overgrowth colonization of the small intestine; and liver disease.

Determination of lactate and pyruvate concentrations in cerebrospinal fluid are of critical value and require special conditions for collection, transport, and storage before assay; measurement of glucose, lactate, pyruvate, 3-hydroxybutyrate, and acetoacetate in whole blood, as well as plasma amino acid concentrations should be carried out. Urine organic acid analysis requires the assistance of a specialized laboratory equipped for gas chromatography; increasingly, mass spectrometry is used in major centres. Muscle biopsy for mitochondrial studies and determination of the redox state in cultured skin fibroblasts using the lactate:pyruvate ratio may also be valuable, but further specialized studies will require advice from a biochemical and genetics service with experience in the diagnosis of inborn errors of metabolism. The value of referral to an appropriate clinical specialist cannot be overemphasized.

Neuroradiological procedures, including cerebral ultrasonography and CT, reveal ventricular dilatation and cerebral atrophy. In several infant girls with pyruvate dehydrogenase deficiency, MRI showed hypoplasia of the corpus callosum as well as loss of normal white matter signal intensity. Proton magnetic resonance spectroscopy revealed high-abundance signals for brain lactate with decreased intensity of *N*-acetylaspartate, while phosphorus magnetic resonance spectroscopy of skeletal muscle showed abnormally low muscle phosphorylation potentials, in keeping with the predicted biochemical disturbance. Pathological examination of previously affected siblings shows shrinkage of gyri, with involvement of the medulla shown by loss or hypoplasia of the pyramids. The pathological features of Wernicke's encephalopathy may be present. The corpus callosum may be absent. Definitive diagnosis, however, depends on genetic and enzymatic studies in skin fibroblasts or blood leucocyte samples.

Institution of a high-fat, low-carbohydrate, ketogenic diet may ameliorate the biochemical abnormalities, but, given the degree of neurological impairment that is normally present at diagnosis, modest clinical improvement can be expected. Therapeutic responses to the administration of high-dose thiamine have been reported in patients with partial enzymatic deficiency, notably where ataxia and abnormal eye movements reminiscent of Wernicke's encephalopathy or features indicative of Leigh's disease were conspicuous. Dichloroacetate, an analogue of pyruvate, has been proposed for the treatment of primary lacticacidaemia, particularly in patients with pyruvate dehydrogenase deficiency. Clinical trials indicate that correction of the biochemical abnormality depends on the molecular defect, and heterogeneity in patient selection may explain the equivocal clinical responses observed in long-term studies. Nonetheless, dichloroacetate appears to be quite well tolerated and deserves consideration in patients who fail to respond to other measures, including the recommended ketogenic diets with high-dose thiamine supplementation.

In patients with the rare autosomally recessive condition due to dihydrolipoyl dehydrogenase deficiency, oral administration of lipoic acid has been reported to correct the organic acidaemia with clinical improvement.

Pyruvate carboxylase deficiency

Inborn defects in pyruvate carboxylase, a key gluconeogenic enzyme, cause hypoglycaemia or profound metabolic acidosis with neurodegenerative features. Neuronal loss is prominent, although the enzyme is principally expressed in astrocytes and other non-neuronal cells; this suggests that a defect impairs the supply of nutrients that are essential for neuronal survival but which are derived from metabolic activity in astroglia. The manifestations closely resemble those caused by deficiencies of pyruvate dehydrogenase activity and appear to be determined by the degree of residual pyruvate carboxylase activity. A severe form associated with hyperammonaemia, hyperlysinaemia, and citrullinaemia is also recognized, particularly in patients of French descent; survival beyond a few months of age in this variant is rare.

Metabolic defect

Pyruvate decarboxylase is a biotin-dependent enzyme which catalyses the first step in the formation of oxaloacetate from pyruvate and is activated allosterically by acetyl CoA. Thus, hypoglycaemia would be expected only after glycogen stores had been depleted. Krebs cycle intermediates may become depleted so that synthesis of neurotransmitters is impaired. There may also be a reduced supply of aspartate for the arginosuccinate synthase reaction of the urea cycle, and hence the association with hyperammonaemia.

Clinical features

Patients with severe deficiency of pyruvate carboxylase may present with Leigh's syndrome (necrotizing encephalomyopathy with lactate/pyruvate acidosis) or hypotonia and neurological retardation. The presence of ataxia and abnormal ocular movements in life suggest the occurrence of midbrain disease resembling Wernicke's encephalopathy. Hypoglycaemia frequently occurs during intercurrent infection or during starvation and acidosis, requiring bicarbonate therapy. The most severe form, originally reported from France, progresses rapidly with evidence of liver damage, hyperammonaemia, hyperlysinaemia, and citrullinaemia.

Genetics

This disorder is transmitted as an autosomal recessive trait. In severely affected patients with hyperammonaemia, pyruvate carboxylase protein and its mRNA are absent in the liver. A partially inactive variant enzyme is detectable in other patients.

Diagnosis and treatment

The condition is suspected when acidosis and neurological disease occur in infants, especially in the presence of hypoglycaemia. As discussed above in relation to lactic acidosis, specific diagnosis requires enzymatic assay in fibroblasts, which can also be used for carrier detection. Disorders of pyruvate metabolism may be mimicked biochemically by mitochondrial diseases and acquired deficiencies of thiamine or biotin. Although biotin therapy has been disappointing in pyruvate carboxylase deficiency, occasional responses to high-dose lipoic acid and thiamine treatment, which may stimulate pyruvate metabolism by the dehydrogenase complex, have been recorded.

Therapy

Episodes of acidosis are treated with intravenous sodium bicarbonate, and glucose may be required for hypoglycaemia. There is evidence that ketogenic diets containing 50% fat and 20% carbohydrate ameliorate the biochemical disturbance and delay the onset of neurological disease. The administration of glutamate and aspartate, which may act as a source of oxaloacetate, appear to have been beneficial in some patients.

Further reading

Inborn errors of galactose metabolism

Bosch A (2006). Classical galactosaemia revisited. *J Inherit Metab Dis*, **29**, 516–25.

Coman DJ *et al.* (2009). Galactosemia, a single gene disorder with epigenetic consequences. *Pediatr Res*, **67**, 286–92.

Cornblath M, Schwartz R (1991). Disorders of galactose: metabolism. In: Cornblath M, Schwartz R (eds) *Disorders of carbohydrate metabolism in infancy*, 3rd edition, pp. 295–324. Blackwell Scientific, Boston.

Dubroff JG, *et al.* (2008). FDG-PET findings in patients with galactosaemia. *J Inherit Metab Dis*, **31**, 533–9.

Elsas LJ, Lai K (1998). The molecular biology of galactosemia. *Genet Med*, **1**, 40–8.

Fridovich-Keil JH, Walter JH (2001). Galactosemia. In: Scriver CR, *et al.* (eds) *Metabolic and molecular bases of inherited disease*, 8th edition. McGraw-Hill, New York. www.ommbid.com [updated January 2008].

Gitzelmann R (1967). Hereditary galactokinase deficiency; a newly-recognized cause of juvenile cataracts. *Pediatr Res*, **1**, 14–23.

Gubbels CS, Land JA, Rubio-Gozalbo ME (2008). Fertility and impact of pregnancies on the mother and child in classic galactosemia. *Obstet Gynecol Surv*, **63**, 334–43.

Holton JB, *et al.* (1981). Galactosaemia. A new severe variant due to uridine diphosphate galactose-4-epimerase deficiency. *Arch Dis Child*, **56**, 885–7.

Kaufman FR, *et al.* (1986). Gonadal function in patients with galactosaemia. *J Inherit Metab Dis*, **9**, 140–6.

Murphy M, *et al.* (1999). Genetic basis of transferase-deficient galactosaemia in Ireland and the population history of Irish Travellers. *Eur J Hum Genet*, **7**, 549–54.

Potter NL, *et al.* (2008). Correlates of language impairment in children with galactosaemia. *J Inherit Metab Dis*, **31**, 524–32.

Ridel KR, Leslie ND, Gilbert DL (2005). An updated review of the long-term neurological effects of galactosemia. *Pediatr Neurol*, **33**, 153–61.

Robinson BH *et al.* (1996). Disorders of pyruvate carboxylase and pyruvate dehydrogenase complex. *J Inherit Metab Dis*, **19**, 452–62.

Robinson BH (2001). Lactic acidemia: disorders of pyruvate carboxylase and pyruvate dehydrogenase. In: Scriver CR, *et al.* (eds) *Metabolic and molecular bases of inherited disease*, 8th edition. McGraw-Hill, New York. www.ommbid.com, [updated January 2008].

Rubio-Gozalbo ME, *et al.* (2006). The endocrine system in treated patients with classical galactosemia. *Mol Genet Metab*, **89**, 316–22.

Schweitzer S, *et al.* (1993). Long-term outcome in 134 patients with galactosaemia. *Eur J Paediatr*, **152**, 36–43.

Tyfield L, *et al.* (1999). Classical galactosemia and mutations at the galactose-1-phosphate uridyl transferase (GALT) gene. *Hum Mutat*, **13**, 417–30.

Tyfield L (2000). Galactosaemia and allelic variation at the galactose-1-phosphate uridyltransferase gene. A complex relationship between genotype and phenotype. *Eur J Pediatr*, **159**, S204–7.

Waggoner DD, Buist NRM, Donnell GN (1990). Long-term prognosis in galactosaemia: results of a survey of 350 cases. *J Inherit Metab Dis*, **13**, 802–18.

Pentosuria

Hiatt HH (2001). Pentosuria. In: Scriver CR, *et al.* (eds) *Metabolic and molecular bases of inherited disease*, 8th edition, vol 1, pp. 1590–9. McGraw-Hill, New York. www.ommbid.com [updated January 2008].

Inborn errors of pyruvate metabolism

Brown GK, *et al.* (1994). Pyruvate dehydrogenase deficiency. *J Med Genet*, **31**, 875–9.

Dahl H-M, *et al.* (1992). X-linked pyruvate dehydrogenase E1-alpha subunit deficiency in heterozygous females: variable manifestation of the same. *J Inherit Metab Dis*, **15**, 835–47.

Hinman LM, *et al.* (1989). Deficiency of pyruvate dehydrogenase complex in Leigh's disease fibroblasts: an abnormality in lipoamide dehydrogenase affecting PDHC activation. *Neurology*, **39**, 70–5.

Liu YM, *et al.* (2003). A prospective study of growth and nutritional status in children treated with the ketogenic diet. *J Am Diet Assoc*, **103**, 707–12.

Lissens W, *et al.* (2000). Mutations in the X-linked pyruvate dehydrogenase (E1) alpha subunit gene (PDHA1) in patients with a pyruvate dehydrogenase complex deficiency. *Hum Mutat*, **15**, 209–19.

Mellick G, Price L, Boyle R (2004). Late-onset presentation of pyruvate dehydrogenase deficiency. *Mov Disord*, **19**, 727–9.

Naito E, *et al.* (2002). Diagnosis and molecular analysis of three male patients with thiamine-responsive pyruvate dehydrogenase complex deficiency. *J Neurol Sci*, **201**, 33–7.

Robinson BH (2006). Lactic acidemia and mitochondrial disease. *Mol Genet Metab*, **89**, 3–13.

Shevell MI, *et al.* (1994). Cerebral dysgenesis and lactic acidemia: an MRI/MRS phenotype associated with pyruvate dehydrogenase deficiency. *Pediatr Neurol*, **11**, 224–9.

Stacpoole PW, *et al.* (2008). Evaluation of long-term treatment of children with congenital lactic acidosis with dichloroacetate. *Pediatrics*, **121**, e1223–8.

Wexler ID, *et al.* (1997). Outcome of pyruvate dehydrogenase deficiency treated with ketogenic diets. Studies in patients with identical mutations. *Neurology*, **49**, 1655–61.

12.4

Disorders of purine and pyrimidine metabolism

Richard W.E. Watts

Essentials

These disorders are due to abnormalities in the biosynthesis, interconversion and degradation of the purines—adenine and guanine—and of the pyrimidines—cytosine, thymine and uracil. All are heterocyclic bases which exist in tri-, di-, and mono-phosphorylated forms, and as either deoxyribosylated or ribosylated derivatives (deoxyribose and ribose are pentose carbohydrates). The phosphorylated deoxyribosylated and ribosylated derivatives are termed 'nucleotides', and the purely ribosylated derivatives, which lack the phosphate group, are 'nucleosides'.

The purine nucleotides, their cyclic derivatives (cAMP and cGMP), and their more highly phosphorylated derivatives have functions in many aspects of intermediary metabolism. Purine compounds also function as signal transducers, neurotransmitters, vasodilators and mediators of platelet aggregation.

The polynucleotide deoxyribonucleic acid (DNA) contains equimolar amounts of adenylic acid (adenosine monophosphate, AMP), guanylic acid (guanosine monophosphate, GMP), thymidylic acid (thymidine monophosphate, TMP) and cytidylic acid (cytidine monophosphate, CMP). Uridylic acid (uridine monophosphate, UMP) replaces TMP in the polynucleotide ribonucleic acid (RNA).

Disorders of purine metabolism

Most human disease connected with disorders of purine metabolism is due to uric acid and sodium urate monohydrate, crystallization of which *in vivo* from supersaturated body fluids causes gout (see Chapter 19.10). This results from either overproduction or underexcretion of urate, or from a combination of these defects:

Decreased net tubular urate secretion—the commonest cause of primary ('idiopathic') gout and for gout secondary to a wide variety of renal disorders, ranging from simple reduction in glomerular filtration rate (chronic kidney disease) to specific defects, e.g. familial juvenile hyperuricaemic nephropathy caused by mutations in the gene for uromodulin (Tamm–Horsfall protein).

Identifiable enzymatic defects that accelerate *de novo* urate synthesis, e.g. (1) X-linked hypoxanthine-guanine phosphoribosyl transferase (HPRT) deficiency—which produces a clinical spectrum extending from hyperuricaemia alone to hyperuricaemia with profound neurological and behavioural dysfunction (Lesch–Nyhan syndrome); (2) X-linked recessive hyperuricaemia and phosphoribosyl pyrophosphate (PRPPS) synthetase superactivity—both of which present with uric acid lithiasis or gouty arthritis in childhood or early adult life. Treatment with newly emerging and established urate-lowering agents as well as anti-inflammatory drugs, is constantly improving;management of these conditions is reviewed here with respect to acute and chronic syndromes of hyperuricaemia and gout.

Hypouricaemia—this may be caused by inherited disorders of uric acid and pyrimidine biosynthesis, e.g. xanthine oxidase deficiency, or to inherited or acquired renal tubule transport defects.

Other diseases of purine metabolism—these cause diverse abnormalities and are generally the result of single gene defects, e.g. adenosine deaminase (ADA) and purine nucleoside phosphorylase (PNP) catalyse sequential steps in the metabolism of purine ribonucleosides and deoxyribonucleosides and are highly expressed in lymphoid cells; their deficiency causes lymphotoxic substrates to accumulate and leads to lymphopenia and immunodeficiency.

Disorders of pyrimidine metabolism

The *de novo* synthesis of pyrimidine nucleotides involves a series of six reactions beginning with the formation of carbamyl phosphate and concluding with orotidylic acid, which then undergoes a series of interconversion and salvage reactions. The inherited disorders of pyrimidine metabolism (e.g. orotic aciduria) are much less common, or possibly much less easily recognized, than disorders of purine metabolism.

Purine biosynthesis, interconversion, degradation, and salvage

The purine nucleotides are built up in a stepwise manner (*de novo* synthesis) and undergo a series of interconversion and salvage reactions and a final degradative process to yield uric acid, as shown in Fig. 12.4.1. Most human conditions connected with diseases of purine metabolism are due to sodium urate monohydrate and to uric acid, although the role of uric acid in relation to oxidative stress is currently a field of active research. The dietary intake of nucleoproteins is also an important factor in diseases due to sodium urate and uric acid. Ingested adenine and guanine nucleotides are

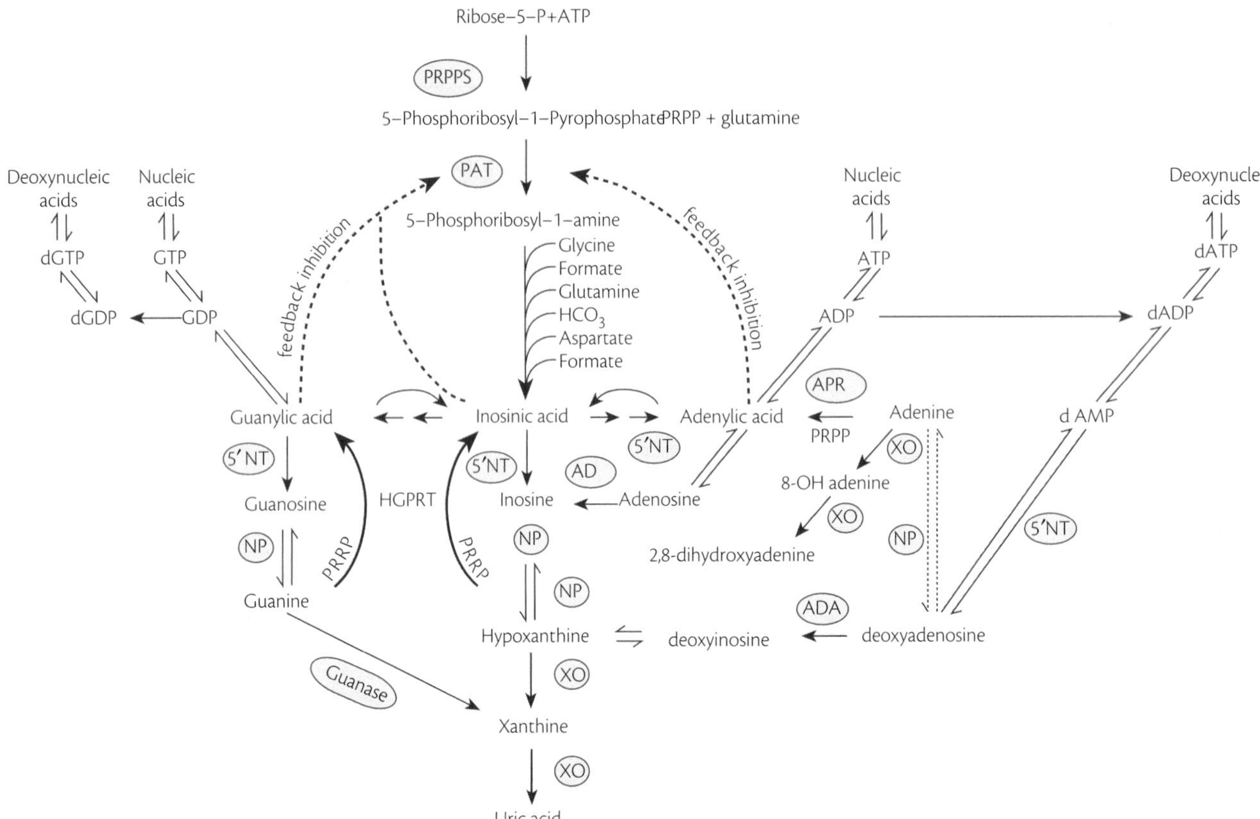

Fig. 12.4.1 Pathways of purine metabolism in humans. ADA, adenosine deaminase; APRT adenine phosphoribosyltransferase; HPRT, hypoxanthine-guanine phosphoribosyltransferase; 5-NP, nucleoside phosphorylase; 5′-NP, 5′-nucleotidase; PAT, PRPP amidotransferase; PRPP, phosphoribosylpyrophosphate; PRPPS, PRPP synthetase; XO, xanthine oxidase.

degraded to free purine bases and, hence, to uric acid by enzymes in the intestinal fluids and in the mucosa of the small intestine, so that the products of their metabolism do not mix with the corresponding endogenous metabolic pools except at the final uric acid stage.

De novo synthesis contributes about 300 to 600 mg (1.8–3.6 mmol/day) and dietary purines about 600 to 700 mg (3.6–4.2 mmol/day) to the dynamic urate metabolic pool of about 1200 mg (7.2 mmol) expressed as uric acid. Each day about two-thirds of the uric acid is excreted in the urine and about one-third is destroyed, mainly by bacterial uricolysis in the gut.

Renal handling of urate

The urate anion is freely filterable at the renal glomerulus, only 5 to 10% being very loosely bound to the plasma proteins (α_{1-2}-globulin fraction). The physiologically important pK_a value of uric acid is 5.75, so that it exists mainly as the monovalent urate anion in plasma (pH 7.4) and assumes more of the free acid form when it passes into regions of the renal tubule, the contents of which are at lower pH values.

The kidney handles urate by:

- glomerular filtration of virtually 100% of the filtered load
- proximal tubular reabsorption by a urate/chloride exchanger in the endothelial brush border (99% of the filtered load)
- tubular secretion (equivalent to about 50% of the filtered load)
- postsecretory reabsorption (equivalent to about 40% of the filtered load)

Thus, the net renal clearance of uric acid is approximately 10% of the filtered load and is in the range of 6 to 11 ml/min per $1.73m^2$ ($1.73\ m^2$ = average body surface area of an adult). The exact location of the reabsorptive, secretory, and postsecretory reabsorptive processes within the distal nephron is unclear.

Some advances have been made in the understanding of this complex process at the molecular level. A urate-anion transporter, URAT1, has been identified. It is encoded by a gene *SLC22A12* on chromosome 11q13. URAT1 belongs to a family of organic anion transporters encoded by a 1659-base pair cDNA; the predicted secondary structure of the protein harbours 12 transmembrane domains with six intracellular loops and one large extracellular loop between the C- and N-termini. A renal-specific urate transporter has been identified in the mouse; it has 74% identity with URAT1 and its study has been valuable. URAT1 is involved in urate reabsorption along the whole proximal tubule and is expressed apically in the brush border epithelium. It is a sodium ion independent anion exchanger stimulated by an outwardly directed chloride gradient. It is inhibited by organic anions, e.g. lactate, and by drugs known to increase urate excretion, e.g. benzbromarone and probenecid.

The *UMOD* gene which encodes uromodulin, as discussed elsewhere, also encodes for a urate channel for urate excretion and mutations lead to familial hyperuricaemic nephropathy. Uromodulin could interfere with postsecretory reabsorption in more distal parts of the nephron.

The urate anion transporter gene (1546 base pairs of cDNA) encodes for a 322-amino acid protein designated galectin 9, which in addition to being a specific urate transporter also has eosinophil–chemotactic cell, apoptosis, and thymocyte–epithelial interactions. It is suggested that the functions of this urate anion transporter, which is expressed in multiple tissues, is to transport urate formed intracellularly by purine catabolism and so maintain intracellular urate concentrations below the solubility limit and prevent intracellular crystallization. The urate anion transporter also acts as a urate transporter channel in polarized epithelial cells where it is expressed in both apical and basolateral membranes promoting urate excretion in both kidney and intestine. Thus it could be responsible for tubular secretion or for the postsecretory phases in the renal tubular handling of urate.

Plasma urate concentrations

The currently quoted overall reference range for plasma urate (expressed as uric acid) in adults is 3.5 to 8.1 mg/dl (210–480 µmol/litre) for men and 2.5 to 6.5 mg/dl (150–390 µmol/litre) for women. The corresponding value for children is 1.0 to 4.0 mg/dl (60–240 µmol/litre) with the lowest values in infancy. It rises to adult values at puberty with values being lower in women than in men until the menopause, after which they gradually rise to the male value. Extrinsic factors, particularly diet, plumbism, the prevalence of a high ethanol intake in the community, and the prevalence of diseases such as malaria and thalassaemia, which lead indirectly to either increased purine biosynthesis or decreased excretion (Box 12.4.1), affect the plasma urate distribution in different populations.

The plasma urate concentration decreases during pregnancy, the reference range being 1.7 to 4.5 mg/dl (100–270 µmol/litre). Hyperuricaemia is a characteristic and often an early feature of pre-eclampsia, preceding the proteinuria and hypertension, and it is a diagnostically valuable parameter. It results from a reduced renal urate clearance and tends to be associated with hypocalciuria.

Epidemiological studies show significant variations in plasma urate concentrations between different ethnic groups, e.g. Maoris and Polynesians have higher values than Western Europeans and Americans. This illustrates the genetic, presumably polygenic, aspects in the control of serum uric acid. Other epidemiological studies emphasize the importance of the environmental factors of purine, protein, and alcohol intake. For example, Gresser and Zöllner showed that the cumulative frequency of plasma urate, expressed as uric acid, rose from approximately 6.2 mg/dl (370 µmol/litre) to about 9.0 mg/dl (536 µmol/litre) between 1962 and 1971 in association with the improved nutritional state of the Bavarian population from the near starvation conditions following the Second World War (Fig. 12.4.2). This effect was not apparent in the female population. Similarly, the plasma urate levels of immigrant communities with low values in their homelands rise towards the values prevailing in the host country as they adopt the lifestyle and dietary habits of that country, e.g. Filipinos migrating to the United States of America. Migrants with genetically determined high urate levels become even more hyperuricaemic.

The frequency distribution of plasma urate values based on asymptomatic populations is only approximately Gaussian, with an excess of higher values due to the inclusion of some asymptomatic hyperuricaemic subjects. Although plasma is saturated with monosodium urate at a concentration of 7.0 mg/dl (420 µmol/litre), higher concentrations of urate can remain in a stable

Box 12.4.1 Causes of hyperuricaemia and gout

Reduced renal excretion of uric acid

If there is an inherited genetic defect in renal tubule excretion which underlies the causes of hyperuricaemia and gout, previously referred to as 'idiopathic' or 'primary', the effect of this genetic lesion may be aggravated by environmental factors. It is the sole determinant in familial autosomal dominant gout or familial juvenile hyperuricaemia with reduced excretion of uromodulin and the medullary cystic kidney disease (the MCKD/FJHN syndrome)

- Renal glomerular disease
- Renal tubule dysfunction
  - Tubulointerstitial nephritis
  - Competition for tubule excretory mechanisms (e.g. hyperlactic acidosis and ketoacidosis from any cause)
  - Drug administration (e.g. diuretics, pyrazinamide, ethambutol, cyclosporin)
- Other conditions in which renal tubule dysfunction has been proposed
  - Hypertension
  - Sickle cell anaemia (there will also be increased metabolic turnover of purines)
  - Myxoedema
  - Bartter's syndrome
  - Down's syndrome
  - Lead nephropathy
  - Sarcoidosis

Increased uric acid production

- Dietary sources
- HGPRT deficiency
- PRPP-synthetase superactivity
- Ribose 5-phosphate overproduction
- AMP deaminase deficiency
- Glycogen storage disease type I
- Glycogen storage diseases types III, V, and VII
- Hereditary fructose intolerance
- Myeloproliferative diseases (NB polycythaemia rubra vera)
- Secondary polycythaemia
- Lymphoproliferative diseases
- Waldenström's macroglobulinaemia
- Chronic haemolytic anaemia of any cause
- Carcinomatosis
- Extensive psoriasis
- Gaucher's disease

HPRT, hypoxanthine phosphoribosyltransferase (hypoxanthine-guanine phosphoribosyltransferase); PRPP, phosphoribosylpyrophosphate; AMP, adenosine monophosphate (adenylic acid).

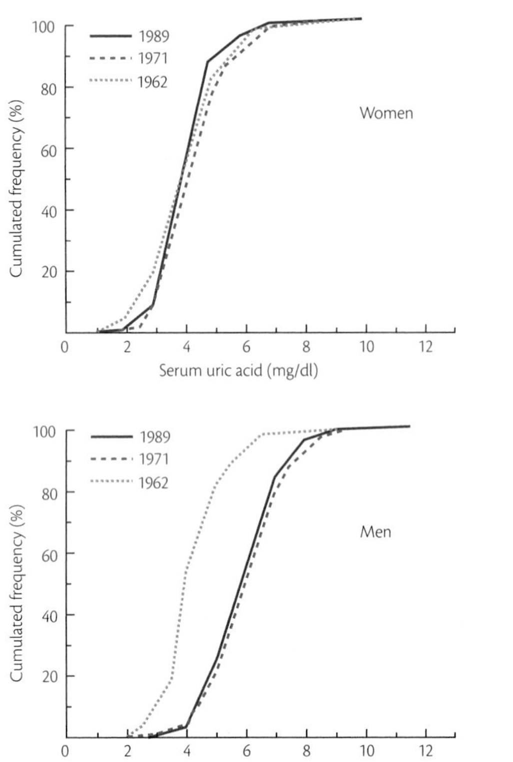

Fig. 12.4.2 Differences in the cumulative frequencies in urate levels in female and male blood donors in Bavaria between 1962 and 1989.
From Gresser U, Zöllner N (1991). *Urate deposition in man and its clinical consequences.* With kind permission of Springer Science + Business Media.

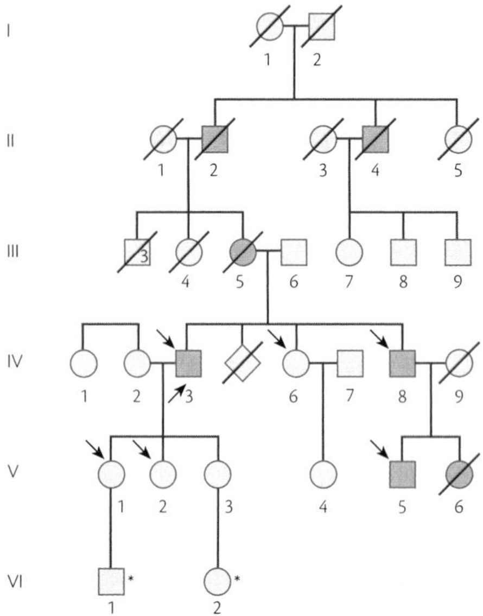

Fig. 12.4.3 Pedigree chart of a family showing autosomal dominant inheritance of gout complicated in some cases by renal failure (hyperuricaemia nephropathy). ■, ●, male and female subjects, respectively, with hyperuricaemia and renal failure; □, ○, male and female subjects not known to be affected; ⊠, ∅, deceased male and female subjects; ↗, propositus; ↘, subjects whose rates of mononuclear cell *de novo* purine synthesis were measured and shown to be normal; *, babies who were examined clinically but not further investigated.
Reproduced with permission from McDermott, *et al.* (1984). *Clin Sci*, **67**, 249–58. ©Biochemical Society and Medical Research Society (http://www.clinsci.org).

supersaturated solution in plasma without producing any symptoms. Ignoring the slight asymmetry of the frequency distribution and defining normality as the mean value ±2 standard deviations about the mean, normal values of 7.0 mg/dl (420 μmol/litre) for men and 6.0 mg/dl (360 μmol/litre) for women have been widely adopted and this has led to considerable overtreatment of patients with quite innocuous plasma urate concentrations. This conclusion may have to be reconsidered when the possible role of urate in relation to oxidative stress and cardiovascular disease is established (see 'Uric acid, oxidative stress, and cardiovascular disease').

Gout and hyperuricaemia

The incidence of gout has been estimated at about 0.2 to 0.35 per 1000. The incidence increases with age and is higher in men than in women, although the incidence in women rises with age after the menopause. In men the first attack has usually occurred by 50 years of age and in women by 70 years of age.

Gout is a classic example of a multifactorial disease in which there is an interplay of genetic and environmental factors. The overall effects of this interplay are wide, extending from cases where there is a clear-cut family history with autosomal dominant inheritance (Fig. 12.4.3) to those where environmental factors may be major determinants, although often against a genetic background that may be either unifactorial or multifactorial. Gout *per se* does not shorten life, although some of its complications may do so in the absence of treatment.

Gout is defined as the syndrome brought about by the crystallization of monosodium urate monohydrate *in vivo* from body fluids supersaturated with this salt. This results from either overproduction or underexcretion of urate, or from a combination of these defects. The underlying causes of hyperuricaemia and gout are:

- Decreased net tubular urate secretion: This occurs in those cases of gout previously described as being idiopathic (or primary), and the hereditary predisposition is often compounded by environmental factors (e.g. high dietary purine intake and alcoholism).
- Identifiable enzymatic defects that accelerate *de novo* urate synthesis: X-linked hypoxanthine-guanine phosphoribosyltransferase deficiency, if complete or virtually complete, causes the Lesch–Nyhan syndrome (see 'The Lesch–Nyhan syndrome and its variants'). Lesser degrees of deficiency cause X-linked recessive hyperuricaemia, gout, and uric acid stones with minor neurological abnormalities in some cases.
- Phosphoribosylpyrophosphate (PRPP) synthetase superactivity: This also presents as X-linked recessive hyperuricaemia, gout, and uric acid stones and, in some cases, neurological manifestations (e.g. deafness and autism).

Secondary causes of hyperuricaemia and gout are shown in Box 12.4.1.

The following abnormalities (features of the 'metabolic syndrome') are commonly associated with, but not causally related to hyperuricaemia and gout:

- obesity
- dyslipidaemia (usually type 4) with raised very low density lipoproteins and normal cholesterol levels, and sometimes hypercholesterolaemia with elevated low-density lipoprotein–cholesterol and low high-density lipoprotein–cholesterol
- hypertension

- insulin resistance with hyperinsulinaemia and impaired glucose tolerance
- ischaemic heart disease

Thus, these patients may display the features of the 'metabolic syndrome X'.

There is no evidence that uric acid is directly toxic to the myocardium. Hyperuricaemia may be a marker of coincident cardiac disease. The elevated plasma uric acid concentrations observed in patients with ischaemic heart disease could arise from up-regulated vascular adenosine synthesis associated with ischaemia and subsequent degradation of adenosine to uric acid. However, the relationship of urate to endothelial function is complex (see 'Uric acid, oxidative stress, and cardiovascular disease'). Plasma uric acid accounts for 60% of the free-radical scavenging activity in human plasma, e.g. it interacts with peroxynitrile to form a stable nitric oxide donor, so promoting vasodilatation and reducing the potential for peroxynitrile-induced oxidative damage. Conversely, it could have an adverse effect on endothelial function by promoting leucocyte adhesion to the endothelium.

The fractional excretion of urate is the ratio of urate clearance to the glomerular filtration rate. In the presence of normal overall renal function, this can be measured on a random urine sample with a simultaneous plasma sample. The equation simplifies to

$$\text{fractional clearance of urate} = U_{\text{urate}} \times P_{\text{creatinine}} / P_{\text{urate}} \times U_{\text{creatinine}}$$

where U and P represent urate and plasma concentrations. The fractional clearance can be used to assess the role of renal tubular dysfunction in the production of hyperuricaemia provided that the overall renal function is normal.

Acute gouty arthritis

Acute gout is a sodium urate monohydrate-induced crystal inflammation of joints, bursae, and tendon sheaths. Clinically the affected structures—classically the first metatarsophalangeal joint is the first joint affected—become acutely inflamed, exquisitely tender, warm to the touch, and the overlying skin becomes red, shiny, and itchy and may desquamate as the inflammation subsides spontaneously over the course of 5 to 15 days in the absence of treatment. Inflammation is usually maximal within 24 h of onset and is accompanied by pyrexia and malaise.

The American College of Rheumatology criteria for the clinical diagnosis of acute gout are shown in Box 12.4.2. The presence of 6 of the 11 criteria has a 95% specificity in differentiating gout from pseudogout (calcium pyrophosphate gout) and an overall sensitivity of 85%. The final confirmation is the demonstration of negatively birefringent sodium urate monohydrate crystals, as opposed to the positively birefringent crystals of calcium pyrophosphate.

Although acute gouty arthritis is typically a monoarthritis, some patients have short, recurrent, mild attacks of discomfort and swelling of other affected joints. Some 10% of attacks affect more than one joint, and typical attacks may provoke migratory attacks in other joints. Multiple, simultaneous attacks are rare. Some attacks are triggered by trauma, intercurrent illness, surgery, alcohol, dietary excess, diuretics, and other medications (see Box 12.4.1). An acute septic arthritis is the most important differential diagnosis of acute gouty arthritis. The joint fluid contains negatively birefringent sodium urate monohydrate as opposed to the positively birefringent crystals of calcium pyrophosphate in pseudogout. Attacks of acute gouty arthritis usually occur when the plasma urate is rising or falling. The cells in the joint fluid are a mixture of monocytes, macrophages, and polymorphonuclear leucocytes.

Box 12.4.2 American College of Rheumatology criteria for the diagnosis of acute gouty arthritis

- More than one attack of acute arthritis
- Maximum inflammation developing within 1 day
- Monoarthritis
- Redness over the affected joint
- The first metatarsophalangeal joint painful and swollen
- Unilateral first metatarsophalangeal joint involved
- Unilateral tarsal joint attack
- Tophus (proven or suspected)
- Hyperuricaemia
- Asymmetrical swelling of a joint on radiography
- Subcortical cysts with an erosion on radiography
- Joint fluid culture negative for microorganisms during an attack

The patient must have at least six of the above criteria or have either proven sodium urate monohydrate crystals in the joint fluid or a proven tophus.

Reproduced with permission from Hochberg MC (2001). Gout. In: Silman AJ, Hochberg MC (eds) *Epidemiology of the rheumatic diseases*, 2nd edition, pp. 230–42. Oxford University Press.

The spontaneous resolution of an attack of acute gouty arthritis depends on the differentiation of monocytes to macrophages that efficiently phagocytose crystals. This conclusion is based on studies of the changing pattern of proinflammatory cytokines tumour necrosis factor (TNF), interleukin-1 (IL-1), and interleukin-6 (IL-6) secreted by monocyte/macrophage cells at different degrees of differentiation and their ability to phagocytose monosodium urate crystals *in vitro*. The crystals are removed by mature phagocytes. It is proposed that this mechanism prevents the development of acute gouty arthritis in stable asymptomatic hyperuricaemic patients. TNFα, IL-1β, and IL-6 secretion promote E-selectin expression and secondary neutrophil capture. Differentiation over 3 to 5 days leads to development of a noninflammatory phenotype with lack of proinflammatory cytokine secretion, lack of endothelial cell activation, and lack of secondary neutrophil recruitment. Acquisition of the noninflammatory phenotype correlates with expression of macrophage antigens but not with dendritic cell marker or activation marker.

Monocytes and macrophages are similarly phagocytic and control particle, zymosan-elicited secretion of all the cytokines in both cell types. Coincubation with monosodium urate suppressed zymosan-induced TNFα secretion from macrophages but not monocytes. In summary, differentiated macrophages provide the mechanism for removal of sodium monohydrate crystals.

Chronic tophaceous gout

Large deposits (tophi) containing monosodium urate monohydrate crystals produce firm nodules over affected joints on the extensor surfaces of the fingers, hands, olecranon bursas (commonly bilateral), extensor surfaces of the forearm, Achilles tendon, the helix of the ear, and in the renal parenchyma. Tophi may discharge white chalky material, containing sodium urate monohydrate.

They cause the bone erosions and joint destruction with secondary degenerative arthritis that is seen on radiographs. Tophus formation can be regarded as an attempted, but disordered, healing process in response to the presence of sodium urate monohydrate crystals in tissues.

Treatment of gout

Acute attack

Full doses of any of the nonsteroidal anti-inflammatory drugs (NSAIDs) are effective in terminating attacks of acute gout. Indomethacin is particularly favoured by some clinicians. Colchicine remains a very effective remedy; an initial dose of 1.0 mg is followed by 0.5 mg every 6 h until either the attack subsides, a total dose of 6.0 mg has been achieved, or symptoms of toxicity (nausea, vomiting, and diarrhoea) occur. More frequent doses of colchicine, 0.5 mg every 2 to 3 h, deliberately inducing symptoms of toxicity, were previously recommended. This is unnecessary now that the NSAIDs are available. Intense regimens of colchicines therapy are not now favored and consensus guidelines issued by European experts recommend a maximum of three 0.5 mg doses in a 24 hour period – a view strongly supported by the results of a large, randomized multicentre trial. Lower total doses (1.5-1.8 mg) have comparable efficacy to higher doses in acute gout but appear to be without the unwanted gastrointestinal toxicity. Heavy dosage with colchicine can cause gastrointestinal haemorrhage and favour the development of other severe side effects, including profuse diarrhoea, rashes, renal hepatic damage, and, more rarely, peripheral neuropathy, myopathy, and alopecia in the long term. Intravenous colchicine is no longer recommended.

An attack of acute gout can be effectively terminated by the adrenocorticotropin analogue, tetracosactrin, or by a single intravenous dose of hydrocortisone. Rebound attacks of acute gout tend to occur unless the situation is covered by either colchicine or an NSAID.

Pharmacological doses of colchicine disrupts the microtubular function in inflammatory cells. This mode of action gives it the potential to do more widespread damage. Short intensive courses of colchicine should not be repeated at less than 3-day intervals, although lower doses (0.5–2 mg/day) can be used for longer periods, as in the treatment of familial Mediterranean fever.

Rasburicase (dosage 200 mcg/kg per day) is a recombinant uricase derived from a modified *Saccharomyces cerevisiae*. It catalyses the oxidation of urate to allantoin which is 5 times more soluble than uric acid at urinary pH values and is the purine metabolite excreted by nonmammalian species. Acute hypersensitivity reactions have been reported in 5% of patients who do not have a history of allergy. It should not be used in pregnancy or in glucose-6-phosphate dehydrogenase deficiency. It can be used to terminate an attack of acute gouty arthritis, but this seems unnecessary with the availability of well-established methods. However, it may have a place in the treatment of acute uric acid nephropathy in the tumour lysis syndrome and in patients who are allergic to allopurinol and the other drugs used to treat hyperuricaemia and gout.

The cytokine inhibitors of TNFα, such as infliximab, will also cut short an attack of acute gouty arthritis but it is unlikely that they will find general application in this context.

Interval treatment

Asymptomatic hyperuricaemia should not be treated with urate-lowering drugs unless the patient experiences more than one acute attack of gout per year (Box 12.4.3). This restriction may have to be relaxed if further work confirms recent studies suggesting that reducing serum urate concentrations by allopurinol has a protective effect in situations involving oxidative stress. Allopurinol, a xanthine oxidase inhibitor, is effective in preventing acute gout by reducing the serum urate concentration to a value below the solubility of sodium urate monohydrate in plasma so that tophaceous deposits are mobilized and healing occurs. This applies to the tophi in bones as well as elsewhere. The drug should be introduced at a low level (e.g. 100–200 mg daily) and increased under cover of either colchicine or an NSAID, which should be continued until the serum urate concentration has stabilized at a normal level. Allopurinol is then continued indefinitely.

Box 12.4.3 Hyperuricaemia detected on routine biochemical screening

- Search for an identifiable cause (e.g. dietary factors, myeloproliferative disease, medications)
- Check renal function
- Imaging to detect the presence of uric acid urinary calculi
- Measure uric acid excretion after eliminating dietary and medication factors
- Treat if:

  More than one attack of acute gouty arthritis per year

  Chronic joint damage attributed to gout

  Tophi

  Hyperuricaemic nephropathy

  Uric acid urolithiasis

  Serum urate concentration:[a] >800 μmol/litre (13 mg/dl in men), >600 μmol/litre (10 mg/dl in women)

[a] This criterion is not universally accepted and may have to be modified if the current work on oxidative stress and uric acid is substantiated.

Initiating allopurinol without cover may cause attacks of acute gout as the serum urate concentration falls. Moderately severe gout may require as much as 300 to 600 mg allopurinol daily and occasionally as much as 700 to 900 mg/day given in divided doses. Between 10 and 20 mg/kg body weight per day is an appropriate dosage for children.

The incidence of adverse reactions to allopurinol is low but they can be severe and occasionally fatal. Reactions include erythema multiforme progressing to the Stevens–Johnson syndrome and toxic epidermal necrolysis, exfoliative dermatitis, vasculitis, interstitial nephritis, eosinophilia, hepatocellular damage, polyneuropathy, bone marrow depression, disturbances of vision and taste, as well as gastroenteropathy. Allopurinol potentiates the effect of coumarin anticoagulants (e.g. warfarin), azathioprine, and 6-mercaptopurine, and predisposes to an ampicillin or amoxicillin rash. At high dosage and in the presence of greatly increased purine synthesis it may cause radiotranslucent xanthine and oxypurinol urinary stones. There is also increased risk of toxicity with captopril (especially in the presence of renal failure) and with cyclosporine.

Much of the overall toxicity of allopurinol is due to the metabolite oxypurinol, which has a much longer half-life *in vivo* than the parent compound. Special care is necessary in the presence of renal failure and a dose of 100 to 150 mg is usually sufficient in this circumstance. Patients with hyperuricaemia due to renal failure rarely develop gout, possibly due to their immunoparesis.

Patients in whom allopurinol produces adverse reactions

Patients for whom the treatment of hyperuricaemia and gout is essential and who have developed severe adverse reactions to allopurinol present a special problem, especially if they have impaired overall renal function. The uricosuric drugs sulphinpyrazone, probenecid, and benzbromarone, together with a sufficiently high fluid intake to provide a measured urine output of at least 3 litres/24 h and alkalization of the urine with sodium or potassium bicarbonate or sodium or potassium citrate, represent an approach to this problem, but may be inappropriate in the overall clinical context, e.g. in patients with cardiac or renal failure. Only sulphinpyrazone is readily available in the United Kingdom. Uricosuric drugs may be inefficient in the presence of renal failure and are contraindicated in the presence of uric acid urinary stones.

The uricosuric agent benzbromarone is sometimes effective in patients with renal failure when other uricosuric agents have lost their efficacy. The use of oxypurinol (at low dosage) has also been proposed. Protocols are also available for the desensitization of patients who have experienced adverse reactions to allopurinol and in whom the risk of uric acid stone formation, with the potential for further reduction of renal function, presents a problem. A new non-purine xanthine oxidase inhibitor, febuxostat, has been recently approved by the European Commission and by the United States Food and Drug Administration for the treatment of chronic gout in which it rapidly decreases serum urate concentrations. Febuxostat is appropriate for patients hypersensitive to, or intolerant of allopurinol; in those in whom this agent has failed to control symptomatic hyperuricaemia – and in patients with chronic kidney disease where uricosuric therapy is contraindicated. As with allopurinol, suitable prophylaxis against exacerbation of acute gout is indicated (eg with colchicine) for six months when treatment with febuxostat is started.

The drug is approved in European countries at 80 and 120 mg daily; in the United States, the label is for a daily dose of 40 mg increasing to 80 mg after at least two weeks if the serum urate concentration remains elevated. Since it is an inhibitor of xanthine oxidase, febuxostat, like allopurinol, has the potential for highly toxic drug interactions with azathioprine, 6-mercaptopurine and theophylline and its derivatives.

Recent phase 3 clinical trials have recently been undertaken in severe chronic gout with a parenteral preparation of recombinant uricase from porcine-baboon, which is combined with polyethylene glycol (PEG) to yield a PEGylated from of the enzyme with prolonged plasma half-life and with less potential for the development of antibodies. The agent appears to has powerful hypouricaemic effects with debulking of tophi in severely affected patients resistant to other therapies; unfortunately infusion reactions are frequent, although frank anaphylaxis appears to be uncommon. Rapid breakdown of plasma urate by uricase has been associated with a high frequency of acute exacerbations of gout in the early weeks after its introduction. Moreover, since all putative treatments of hyperuricaemia based on the action of uricases have the potential to generate abundant hydrogen peroxide and other oxidants, their introduction for long-term use carries with it an appreciable risk of tissue injury (see contraindication for use of rasburicase, below). Although PEGylated and other preparations of uricases from various sources demonstrate clear efficacy *in vivo* and remain attractive for therapeutic research, at the time of writing, this approach does not yet have an established place for the treatment of severe chronic gout.

Asymptomatic hyperuricaemia

Routine biochemical screening frequently identifies patients with hyperuricaemia. Guidance on their management is given in Box 12.4.3.

Acute uric acid nephropathy

This complicates the treatment of widespread malignant disease, particularly chemotherapy and/or radiotherapy of leukaemias and lymphomas. The nephropathy is of multifactorial origin and may form part of the acute tumour lysis syndrome with accompanying tubular necrosis. These patients are usually underhydrated, acidotic, and have high rates of uric acid production from nucleoprotein degradation in the apoptotic tumours. Acute uric acid nephropathy has occasionally been reported after extremely severe muscular exercise, after severe epileptic seizures, and in patients with gout and grossly increased rates of *de novo* purine synthesis.

The renal lesion is the intratubular precipitation of uric acid crystals. In addition, the renal pelvis and ureters may also be blocked by crystal aggregates and/or uric acid stones. Acute uric acid nephropathy can be avoided by giving allopurinol for several days before starting the chemotherapy or radiotherapy. The condition presents as acute oliguric renal failure. Imaging techniques should be used to exclude the presence of bilateral ureteric obstruction by radiotranslucent uric acid stones. Treatment is by:

- induction of an alkaline diuresis
- haemodialysis, peritoneal dialysis, or haemofiltration
- percutaneous nephrostomy and/or ureteric catheterization may be needed if there is an element of postrenal obstruction due to impacted aggregates of sodium urate crystals or uric acid stones
- disruption or removal of impacted stones

After many years of experimentation with the use of heterologous uricases, one preparation of the recombinant fungal enzyme, rasburicase (from *Aspergillus niger*) has been licensed for use as a single-course therapy for hyperuricaemia in the acute paediatric tumour lysis syndrome. The enzyme has a plasma half-life of 18-24 hours and is markedly antigenic; it thus has little application as an off-label agent in severe tophaceous gout and certainly cannot be sustained for more than a few months. On account of its capacity to induce oxidant injury and thus haemolysis in susceptible individuals, rasburicase is contraindicated in patients with glucose 6-phosphate dehydrogenase deficiency.

Chronic sodium urate nephropathy

Between 20% and 30% of patients with untreated chronic tophaceous gout die from renal failure. Clinically these patients form an identifiable subgroup of the gouty population and an autosomal dominant inheritance is sometimes clearly apparent (Fig. 12.4.3). The term 'familial juvenile gouty nephropathy' is sometimes used for patients presenting in early life. Environmental factors exacerbate this hereditary predisposition. Clinically there is another group of gout patients (20–30%) with mild intermittent proteinuria and a good prognosis. Significant renal disease due to sodium urate deposition is very rare in asymptomatic hyperuricaemia. Patients with chronic sodium urate nephropathy have shrunken kidneys containing interstitial monosodium urate microtophi and show segmental destruction of the renal parenchyma due to tubular blockage by aggregates of uric acid crystals (microcalculi). These areas of segmental destruction have been referred to, inappropriately, as 'uric acid infarcts'.

Familial juvenile hyperuricaemic nephropathy and uromodulin

Although genetic factors with an autosomal dominant pattern of inheritance are generally recognized as contributing to hyperuricaemia and gout, and Fig. 12.4.3 shows an extreme example of such a pedigree where a single mutant gene is having a large effect. Different mutations in the same gene but with a relatively small effect could be a contributory factor to gout in other individuals in whom an inherited trait is less apparent. Occasional cases of familial gout presenting in early adulthood, or before, have been identified for a long time. It is now known that familial hyperuricaemic nephropathy is associated with medullary cystic renal disease and a specific syndrome 'medullary cystic kidney disease: familial juvenile hyperuricaemic nephropathy' (MCKD/FJHN) is now recognized. These patients show impaired urine concentrating ability, hyperuricaemia and hypouricosuria due to a reduced net tubular excretion of uric acid, cysts, specifically at the corticomedullary junction, interstitial fibrosis, and ultimately renal failure. These cases are associated with mutations in the gene directing the synthesis of the glycoprotein uromodulin, also known as Tamm–Horsfall protein, which occurs in the cells of the thick, ascending segment of Henle's loop and in renal collecting tubule cells. Uromodulin excretion is diminished. The *MCKD/FJHN* gene is located in the overlapping region of chromosome 16p11–13 and extends over a 22-centimorgan interval flanked centromerically by D316S40 and telomerically by D16S3069. Five heterozygous missense gene mutations (Cys77Tyr, Cys126Arg, Asn128Ser, Cys252Tyr, and Cys300Gly) that alter evolutionary conserved residues in the gene encoding uromodulin have been demonstrated, and it is proposed that these produce changes in the tertiary structure with conformational changes in the protein due to reduction in the intramolecular disulphide bonding, which alters the folding pattern of the protein. Uromodulin is an 85-kDa glycoprotein which also has a role in preventing renal stone formation, the modulation of immune responses, and urothelial cytoprotection. Mutations in the *UMOD* gene can be found in patients presenting with glomerular cystic kidney disease where there is also hyperuricaemia, decreased urine osmolality, and ultimately renal failure.

It is possible that familial diseases such as the example shown in Fig. 12.4.3 are principally due to *UMOD* gene mutations of large effect and that other mutations in this gene with only a small expressivity are at least partially responsible for the genetic component in the common hyperuricaemic and gout patients.

Polycystic renal disease

It can be expected that the progressive destruction of renal tubule function in classic autosomal dominant polycystic renal disease would be associated with disordered renal tubule handling of urate. Hyperuricaemia before the onset of renal failure occurs in autosomal dominant polycystic renal disease, but coincidence between mutations in the *APDKD* gene and in the gene causing decreased net tubular reabsorption in classic hyperuricaemia/gout patients cannot be excluded and, indeed, the two abnormalities might summate to produce early onset hyperuricaemia/gout. There have been reports of a 57% incidence of uric acid urinary stones and a 12% incidence of hyperuricosuria in the uric acid stone-formers.

Similar transport disorders may operate in medullary sponge kidney disease.

Ethanol and hyperuricaemia

Ethanol is oxidized to acetaldehyde by the liver. This raises the ratio of reduced nicotinamide adenine dinucleotide to nicotinamide adenine dinucleotide, which in turn promotes the reduction of pyruvate to lactate in the hepatocytes. Lactate competes with urate in the renal tubular excretory mechanisms and thereby promotes urate retention. There is often an element of starvation ketoacidosis in chronic alcoholics, with acetoacetate and β-hydroxybutyrate also competing for the renal tubular excretory mechanisms which subserve urate tubular secretion. In addition, there is increased urate production associated with ethanol intake, first due to the high purine content of some alcoholic beverages (e.g. beer) and second because the metabolism of alcohol involves increased dephosphorylation and degradation of adenine nucleotides in the liver. The free adenine produced is further metabolized to urate.

Uric acid urolithiasis

Pure uric acid stones account for 5% of all urinary stones in patients in the United Kingdom. There is a much higher incidence elsewhere, e.g. in the Middle East. Uric acid urolithiasis occurs in 10% of patients with gout. In Israel, about 40% of urinary calculi are composed of uric acid and 75% of patients with primary gout develop renal calculus disease. Uric acid stones are more common in secondary than in primary gout and are sometimes associated with an impaired ability to alkalinize the urine. Ileostomy predisposes to uric acid urolithiasis because of: (1) chronic bicarbonate loss, which leads to a persistent acidification of the urine, and (2) a concentrated urine due to excessive water loss. Urinary uric acid concentrations close to or more than those at which spontaneous crystallization begins are frequent in these circumstances. The genetic causes of uric acid urolithiasis are rare: (1) hypoxanthine-guanine phosphoribosyltransferase deficiency, (2) phosphoribosylpyrophosphate (PRPP) superactivity, and (3) congenital renal hyperuricaemia (congenital failure of the renal tubular reabsorption of urate). Renal hypouricaemia may be due to renal tubular damage by other genetic diseases or by toxic damage (Box 12.4.4), and this may be associated with other features of the Fanconi syndrome.

The urinary uric acid concentration is the main determinant of uric acid stone formation. The concentration depends on the state of hydration, the rate of *de novo* purine synthesis, the rate of metabolic turnover of purine compounds, the dietary intake of purines and alcohol, and the action of uricosuric drugs (e.g. sulphinpyrazone). Calcium oxalate stone formation is increased 30-fold in patients with gout, and hyperuricosuria is common in nongouty stone-formers. Uric acid microcrystals may act as epitaxial nucleation sites

Box 12.4.4 Causes of hypouricaemia

Inherited disorders of uric acid and pyrimidine biosynthesis

- Genetic defects in the molybdoflavoprotein enzymes:

  Xanthinuria type I (xanthine oxidase deficiency only)

  Xanthinuria type II (combined xanthine oxidase and aldehyde oxidase deficiencies)

  Sulphite oxidase deficiency (xanthine oxidase, aldehyde oxidase, and sulphite oxidase deficiency)

- Purine nucleoside phosphorylase deficiency
- PRPP synthetase deficiency

Secondary reduction in uric acid biosynthesis

- Allopurinol and oxypurinol medication
- Hepatic failure
- Acute intermittent porphyria

Inherited renal hypouricaemia (isolated renal tubule reabsorption defect)

Inherited causes of the Fanconi syndrome and its variants (the syndrome of multiple renal tubule reabsorption defects)

- Cystinosis (accumulation of intralysosomal cystine)
- Galactosaemia (galactose 1-phosphate toxicity)
- Hereditary fructose intolerance (fructose 1-phosphate toxicity)
- Glycogen storage disease type I (glucose 1-phosphate toxicity; hypoglycaemia may prevent the glycosuria which is part of the syndrome)
- Wilson's disease (copper toxicity)
- Cytochrome *c* deficiency

Acquired causes of the Fanconi syndrome and its variants

- Metal poisoning (Cd, Zn, Cu, Pb, Hg, Ur)
- Multiple myelomatosis
- Nephrotic syndrome
- Malignant disease (paraneoplastic syndrome)
- Autoimmune disease (i.e. Sjögren's syndrome)
- Thermal burns
- Primary hyperparathyroidism
- Acute renal tubular necrosis
- Renal transplant rejection

Drugs

- Drugs used either as uricosuric agents or to block other aspects of renal tubule excretion (sulphinpyrazone, probenecid, benzbromarone)
- NSAIDs with uricosuric properties
- Phenylbutazone
- Azapropazone
- Aspirin dosage >4 g/day
- Coumarin anticoagulants (e.g. warfarin)
- Outdated tetracycline (5α-6-anhydro-4-epitetracycline)

Nutritional deficiencies

- Vitamins B_{12}, C, D
- Kwashiorkor

for calcium oxalate crystallization. It is also possible that colloidal uric acid adsorbs urinary glycosaminoglycan inhibitors of crystallization and crystal growth.

Uric acid stone disease is treated by hydration to maintain a urine volume of at least 3 litres/24 h, alkalization of the urine, and allopurinol if there is hyperuricosuria. The use of sodium and potassium salts for alkalization has to be carefully reviewed in the light of concurrent diseases, particularly impaired renal and cardiac function. The standard imaging techniques (particularly ultrasonography) are required for the diagnosis of these radiotranslucent stones. They can be fragmented or removed by standard procedures.

Congenital renal hypouricaemia and uric acid stones

Reduced net tubular reabsorption of urate occurs as an isolated renal tubular reabsorption defect due to mutations in the gene directing the synthesis of the urate carrier URAT1. Changes in URAT1 affect either the presecretory or the postsecretory phases of the urate handling by the renal tubule. The presecretory type appears to be the commoner, and multiple different mutations have been identified. Reduced tubular urate reabsorption can occur in other inherited or acquired renal tubule transport defects (Box 12.4.4). Congenital renal hypouricaemia is inherited in an autosomal recessive manner. The hyperuricosuria may amount to 1000 mg (5.9 mmol) per 24 h in the homozygote. Lesser degrees of hyperuricosuria occur in heterozygotes. About 30% of the homozygotes have an associated hypercalciuria. Uric acid urolithiasis occurs in about 25% of the homozygotes, most commonly in patients with combined hyperuricosuria and hypercalciuria. The causes of hypouricaemia are summarized in Box 12.4.4.

The Lesch–Nyhan syndrome and its variants

The Lesch–Nyhan syndrome results from mutations in the gene that directs the synthesis of hypoxanthine-guanine phosphoribosyltransferase, an enzyme which normally catalyses the salvage of hypoxanthine and guanine to inosinic and guanylic acids—inosine monophosphate and guanosine monophosphate (GMP), respectively, as shown in Fig. 12.4.1. The clinical spectrum extends from hyperuricaemia alone to hyperuricaemia with profound neurological and behavioural dysfunction. The biochemistry and molecular genetics of this disorder have been studied extensively. Hypoxanthine-guanine phosphoribosyltransferase assay on cultured fibroblasts rather than erythrocyte lysates gives better correlation between the degree of residual enzyme activity and clinical phenotypes. Mutation analysis does not provide precise information for predicting disease severity, but it is a valuable tool

Box 12.4.5 Clinical manifestations of the Lesch–Nyhan syndrome (complete or virtually complete absence of hypoxanthine phosphoribosyltransferase (HPRT) deficiency)

- Sex-linked recessive inheritance
- Failure of overall growth
- Muscle hypotonia
- Delayed motor development
- Torsion dystonia
- Aggressive behaviour
- Dysarthria
- Variable degree of intellectual deterioration in later childhood
- Megaloblastic anaemia (in some cases only)
- Hyperuricaemia and hyperuricaciduria with gout and tophus development after puberty and urolithiasis occasionally during the first decade of life
- Failure of pubertal development and testicular atrophy at the age when puberty would be expected to occur

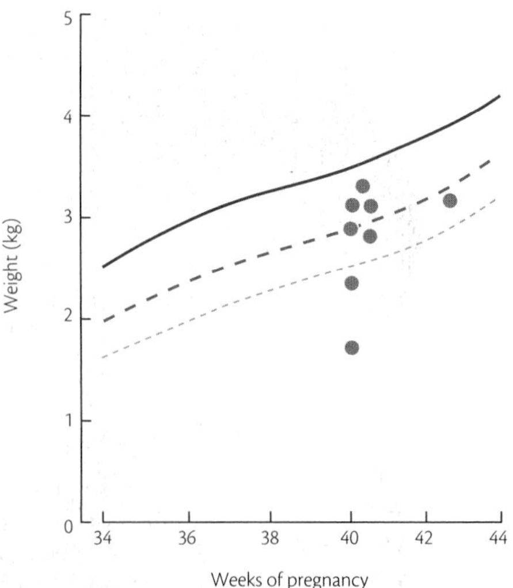

Fig. 12.4.4 Birth weight in eight boys who later developed the Lesch–Nyhan syndrome: the 50th (bold line), 10th, and 3rd (interrupted lines) centiles are shown.
From Watts RWE, *et al.* (1987). Lesch-Nyhan syndrome; growth delay, testicular atrophy and a partial failure of 11β-hydroxylation of steroids. *J Inherit Metab Dis*, **10**, 210–23, with kind permission from Kluwer Academic Publishers.

for genetic counselling in terms of confirming the diagnosis, the identification of carriers, and prenatal diagnosis.

The clinical features of the most severely affected patients who are correctly referred to as having the classic Lesch–Nyhan syndrome or as having 'complete or virtually complete hypoxanthine-guanine phosphoribosyltransferase deficiency' in the fibroblast assay are summarized in Box 12.4.5. In some cases the enzyme has altered kinetics or is unstable but has 1 to 5% residual activity. Patients with partial enzyme defects of 0 to 5% hypoxanthine-guanine phosphoribosyltransferase activity in red cell lysates but more than 8% activity in the fibroblast assays have gout and renal complications but no neurological manifestations. The disease frequency is about 1 in 380 000 births.

Infants affected by HRPT deficiency have a lower than average birth weight, indicating some degree of intrauterine growth retardation (Fig. 12.4.4). The first clinical sign may be the presence of red grit (uric acid crystals with absorbed urinary pigments) on the nappy. Affected infants are hypotonic from birth, although this is frequently not remarked on before poor head control becomes apparent at the age of about 3 months.

Postnatal growth, which becomes more marked after the second year of life, is also subnormal (Fig. 12.4.5) as indicated by sequential measurement of body weight, accurate assessment of body length being impossible due to the dystonic posturing. The overall pattern of weight growth follows centile lines for the first 2 years of life and thereafter slows to about 1 kg/year, or about half normal; a pubertal growth spurt is not observed. Head growth and bone development are less affected than weight. The poor weight gain cannot be attributed to either renal failure or malnutrition.

Torsion dystonia, with its two components of abnormal posturing and episodic rigidity, is superimposed on the basic hypotonia that is present between the dystonic episodes. Severe dysarthria is associated with dyskinesia of the face, mouth, pharynx, and the larynx, which greatly limits communication and even the ability to point accurately, leading to great frustration. The self-injurious behaviour and dyskinesia are eliminated or much reduced when the child is concentrating on a self-selected activity, such as watching an interesting television programme. Self-injury and dyskinesia are exacerbated by excitement, such as the arrival of a visitor, fear, frustration, and unsuccessful attempts at volitional motor activity. The children also appear to be aware of the value of this behaviour as an attention-seeking manoeuvre, and sometimes appear to use it in a manipulative manner. This mixture of involuntary and volitional abnormal motor activity with an apparent interplay of unconscious and consciously meditated behaviour patterns should be common ground for behavioural scientists, neurochemists, and neuropharmacologists.

Although learning difficulties have been stressed as a feature of the Lesch–Nyhan syndrome, they are of inconstant severity and are neither marked nor specific. The apparent degree of intellectual

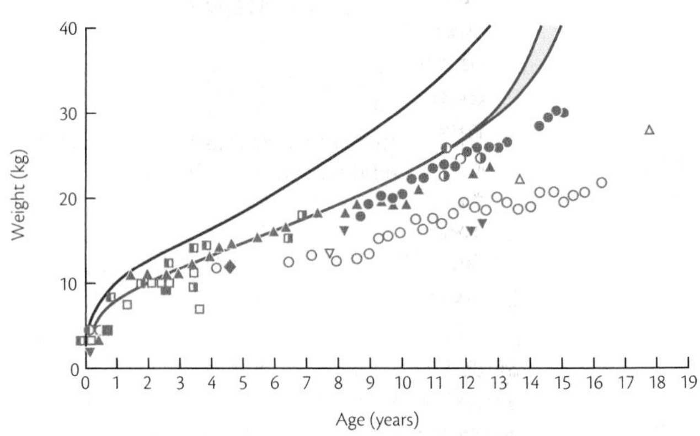

Fig. 12.4.5 Patterns of growth in the weight of 13 boys with the Lesch–Nyhan syndrome: each patient is shown by a different symbol. The 50th and 3rd centiles are shown.
With kind permission from Springer Science+Business Media: *J Inherit Metab Dis*, Lesch-Nyhan syndrome: Growth delay, testicular atrophy and a partial failure of the 11β-hydroxylation of steroids, 10, 3, 1987, 210–223, R. W. E. Watts.

disability may be affected by the extensive disorder of expressive motor functions that exceeds the comprehension defect, by the lack of basic social and educational opportunities, and by the lack of intelligence tests for older children who have lacked these opportunities. However, for whatever combination of reasons, there does appear to be a decline of intellect from the age of 8 to 10 years.

Self-injurious behaviour usually begins at about 2 years of age. Its severity and the ingenuity with which the patients exploit new ways of self-injury exceed that encountered in any other clinical situation. It is not a constant feature and some patients never show it; in the majority its severity waxes and wanes. Self-injury can produce very severe damage, such as complete destruction of the lower lip or traumatic amputation of a fingertip. The patients feel pain normally and are aware of their compulsion; they are afraid of it but are unable to control it. Nyhan and his colleagues consider it to be the clinical hallmark of complete hypoxanthine-guanine phosphoribosyltransferase deficiency, as opposed to those patients with some residual enzyme activity (which may or may not be measurable in erythrocyte lysates).

The severe dystonic spasms with violent extension of the neck can produce damage to the cervical spinal cord and produce motor pyramidal tract signs in the legs. The phenotypes associated with appreciable residual hypoxanthine-guanine phosphoribosyltransferase activity vary from the neurological deficit described for the complete Lesch–Nyhan syndrome but without self-mutilation, to patients with only X-linked gout and/or urolithiasis and only very subtle, if any, neurological features.

There are no structural or ultrastructural changes in the brain as judged by light and electron microscopy or on electroencephalography. Reduction in the size of the caudate nucleus, the putamen, and total cerebral volume have now been demonstrated by refined MRI. Dopamine transporter reduction and hence dopamine deficiency has been demonstrated by positron emission tomography.

Both the *de novo* purine synthesis and the hypoxanthine-guanine phosphoribosyltransferase-catalysed purine salvage pathways are present in all parts of the normal brain. Hypoxanthine-guanine phosphoribosyltransferase activity is absent or defective but the *de novo* synthesis pathway remains active in patients with the Lesch–Nyhan syndrome.

The most recent imaging studies support the concept that hypoxanthine-guanine phosphoribosyltransferase deficiency constrains brain development with particular emphasis on the basal ganglia, and defective function of dopaminergic neurons is specifically involved. The possibility that a postulated postsynaptic transmitter function for cGMP, or a related compound has not been substantiated. The possibility that GTP deficiency might constrain tetrahydrobiopterin synthesis, and hence dopamine synthesis, has not been substantiated.

Evidence has been advanced for some aspects of the Lesch–Nyhan phenotype being related to dysfunction of the small central, but widely projecting, aminergic pathways involved in learning. Thus it has been suggested that the self-injurious behaviour in the Lesch–Nyhan syndrome is due to an imbalance between the activities of catecholaminergic neurons and 5-hydroxytryptaminergic neurons. The catecholaminergic neurons are largely concerned with learning by reward and the 5-hydroxytryptaminergic pathways with learning by punishment. Patients with the Lesch–Nyhan syndrome are insensitive to punishing stimuli and do not learn when such stimuli are used to reinforce the desired behaviour, which in this case is to refrain from self-injury. The ability to learn from rewarding stimuli is impaired. Psychotherapeutic techniques that are effective in eliminating self-injurious behaviour in other situations fail in patients with the Lesch–Nyhan syndrome. They could be modified by a programme of positive reinforcement of abstaining from self-injury and 'time out', but this has proved difficult to achieve in the long term. The reinforcement strategy was found to be unsuitable for use at home because it involved apparently ignoring the self-injury and only paying attention to the child in the absence of self-injurious behaviour. This was misinterpreted by friends and relations as unkindness or indifference.

The present view is that the neurological manifestations are brought about by a neurotransmitter imbalance (probably mainly in the basal ganglia). This imbalance is possibly due to a deficient supply of metabolic energy resulting from the nonsalvage of hypoxanthine and guanine causing a deficiency of adenine nucleotides that provide energy for short bursts of neurotransmitter synthesis. However, the positron emission tomography evidence of dopamine receptor deficiency is the main concrete evidence for a neurotransmitter defect either directly or indirectly because of guanosine triphosphate deficiency underlying the Lesch–Nyhan syndrome. There is increased excretion of the serotonin metabolite 5-hydroxyindoleacetic acid and decreased cerebrospinal fluid homovanillic acid, a major metabolite of dopamine in the cerebrospinal fluid. Deficiency of basal ganglia dopamine systems emerging during the first 2 months of life has been demonstrated in a mouse model of Lesch–Nyhan disease.

Failure of pubertal development and testicular atrophy in hypoxanthine-guanine phosphoribosyltransferase deficiency are attributed to an inadequate supply of purine nucleotides to meet the increased metabolic energy requirement in the testis at this time. A similar inability to meet energy requirements may underlie the neurological manifestations. A partial defect in adrenocortical 11β-hydroxylation of steroids is demonstrable in patients with the Lesch–Nyhan syndrome after ACTH stimulation and is thought to be linked with a failure to modulate mitochondrial function for this hydroxylation due to a deficiency of purine nucleotides.

Patients with Lesch–Nyhan syndrome whose hyperuricaemia has been controlled and who have not had renal damage, die in their teenage years, often with postmortem evidence of gastric aspiration during sleep.

Treatment

Sufficient allopurinol should be administered to reduce the plasma urate and urine uric acid concentrations to normal in order to prevent gouty arthritis, urate nephropathy, and renal calculi. Relatively large doses of allopurinol are needed and the patient should be kept well hydrated to minimize the risk of xanthine and/or oxypurinol (the metabolic oxidation product of allopurinol) stones formation. Both types of stone are, like uric acid stones, radiotranslucent. Allopurinol treatment from birth does not prevent the behavioural phenotype. All therapeutic attempts at neuropharmacological manipulation have been unsuccessful.

Dental extraction, physical restraints with splints and bandages, and strapping the patient into a specially designed padded wheelchair fitted with a firm padded head support to prevent cervical spine injury during violent opisthotonic spasms, are usually needed to limit the effects of compulsive self-mutilation.

Children whose restraints have been temporarily released ask or indicate their wish for the bandages, straps, etc. to be replaced so that they are less able to damage themselves. Every effort should be made to exploit the intellect of these patients and to keep them in a stimulating environment.

Clinical genetic aspects

The Lesch–Nyhan syndrome and its variants are inherited in a sex-linked recessive manner with no clinical manifestations in the female carriers. However, subtle alterations in purine metabolism, with small increases in the rates of *de novo* purine synthesis and increased uric acid excretion and occasionally mild asymptomatic hyperuricaemia, have been reported in females. There are extremely rare reports of female Lesch–Nyhan cases. These have been attributed to either nonrandom inactivation of the X chromosome or to a mutation in the maternally derived X chromosome. In affected male hemizygotes the lack of hypoxanthine-guanine phosphoribosyltransferase is accompanied by an elevated level of PRPP. Genomic analysis is also possible. Carrier females are identified by the demonstration of mosaicism with respect to $HPRT^+$ and $HPRT^-$ hair roots due to random inactivation of the X chromosome, the hair roots being clonal in origin. Autoradiographic techniques can be used to demonstrate two cell populations ($HPRT^+$ and $HPRT^-$) in fibroblast cultures.

Early prenatal diagnosis is possible using chorionic villus samples obtained during the ninth week of pregnancy; this permits elective abortion of an affected fetus before the end of the first trimester of pregnancy. *In vitro* fertilization with enzymatic assay on a cell removed at the four-cell stage to ensure that only unaffected embryos are implanted is possible.

PRPP synthetase superactivity

This enzyme catalyses the production of PRPP, which is required for the first specific and rate-limiting reaction on the *de novo* pathway of purine synthesis. It is subject to feedback inhibition by purine nucleotides. The known mutations in the gene regulating the synthesis of PRPP synthetase diminish its sensitivity to this feedback inhibition, thereby leading to hyperuricaemia, hyperuricosuria, and gout. The condition is inherited in an X-linked recessive fashion.

Affected males develop uric acid lithiasis or gouty arthritis in childhood or early adult life. Hyperuricaemia is often severe and in the range 0.5 to 1 mmol/litre, with uric acid excretion of 5 to 15 mmol/24 h. Heterozygotes remain asymptomatic, although some degree of increased purine synthesis *de novo* has been demonstrated.

In some families, the disorder presents in childhood with associated neurological features such as motor retardation and learning difficulties, ataxia, deafness, hypotonia, disturbed speech, and the development of polyneuropathy, intracerebral calcifications, and dysmorphic facial features. The constellation of associated disorders varies in different families.

Heterozygotes can be identified by studies in cultured skin fibroblasts. Amniocentesis, prenatal diagnosis, and preventive termination of pregnancy are not justified in this condition unless one of the unusually severe phenotypes is known to be segregating in the family. The hyperuricaemia, primary purine overproduction, and uricosuria can be well controlled with allopurinol.

2,8-Dihydroxyadeninuria

These patients lack adenine phosphoribosyltransferase activity; adenine accumulates behind the metabolic block and is oxidized under the catalytic influence of xanthine oxidase to the very insoluble compound, 2,8-dihydroxyadenine. This compound is excreted in the urine along with adenine itself, where it forms radiotranslucent stones that are white or pale fawn in colour. These rough and friable calculi have, in the past, been widely misdiagnosed as uric acid stones because 2,8-dihydroxyadenine reacts as if it were uric acid in colorimetric assays. The use of enzymatic uric acid assays has obviated this confusion. The three-dimensional structure of the enzyme has been establish and several mutations have been identified.

Adenine phosphoribosyltransferase deficiency has an autosomal recessive pattern of inheritance and is clinically silent in heterozygotes. There are two subtypes (I and II). Type I patients have no detectable enzyme activity, being homozygotes or compound heterozygotes for null alleles. Type II patients have between 5 and 25% residual enzyme activity. Whereas type I patients are encountered in many racial groups, the type II subtype has so far only been identified in the Japanese population. Heterozygotes for type I and type II can only be distinguished from one another by enzyme assays on extracts from cultured peripheral blood lymphocytes; both types show no activity in the red cell lysates that are generally used diagnostically.

This condition often presents in early life because of the extremely low solubility of 2,8-dihydroxyadenine in renal tubule fluid and urine. Severe obstructive uropathy and renal failure may occur in infancy.

Treatment is by hydration and xanthine oxidase inhibition with allopurinol, and with standard measures to disrupt or remove the stones and to manage urinary infections and renal failure.

Type I glycogenosis

Type I glycogenosis (hereditary glucose 6-phosphatase deficiency) is associated with hyperuricaemia. This is due to chronic hyperlacticacidaemia which leads to urate retention, and to increased urate production due to the reduced serum phosphate concentrations. The phosphate ion inhibits adenosine monophosphate deaminase, the enzyme which catalyses the rate-limiting step in the metabolic pathway for the conversion of adenine nucleotides to uric acid. Thus, hypophosphataemia increases adenine nucleotide degradation to uric acid and adds to the accumulating urate burden; gouty arthritis may develop in childhood.

Treatment is by maintaining the blood glucose concentration in the normal range with frequent small meals and intragastric glucose infusion at night. Gout is treated in the standard manner with colchicine and/or NSAIDs for the acute attacks, and with long-term allopurinol.

Xanthinuria

Xanthine stones occur in patients with xanthinuria (congenital xanthine oxidase/reductase deficiency) and occasionally in those who are being treated with the xanthine oxidase inhibitor, allopurinol. The latter is particularly likely in patients with accelerated *de novo* purine synthesis, as in patients with the Lesch–Nyhan syndrome. Xanthinuria is inherited in an autosomal recessive manner, and hypoxanthine and xanthine accumulate behind the metabolic block. The plasma urate concentration and urine uric acid excretion are less than about 0.06 mmol/litre (1.0 mg/dl) and 0.30 mmol/24 h (50 mg/24 h), respectively, when the patient is taking an unrestricted diet. It is a very rare condition. The plasma and urine oxypurine (hypoxanthine plus xanthine) concentrations are characteristically elevated. Normal subjects have plasma levels between 0.00 and 0.15 mmol/litre (0.00–0.25 mg/dl) and urine levels of 0.07 to 0.13 mmol/24 h (11–22 mg/24 h); patients with xanthinuria typically have plasma levels between 0.03 and 0.05 mmol/litre (0.00–0.90 mg/dl) and urine levels of 0.60 and 3.5 mmol/24 h (100–600 mg/24 h). Xanthine accounts for 60 to 90% of the total xanthine plus hypoxanthine excreted, presumably reflecting the more active metabolic turnover of hypoxanthine and its efficient salvage by hypoxanthine phosphoribosyltransferase. Hypoxanthine and xanthine are mainly derived from adenine and guanine nucleotides, respectively (see Fig. 12.4.1). Hypoxanthine has a relatively high solubility and causes no problems. Xanthine oxidase functions mainly as a dehydrogenase under physiological conditions but it can convert to an oxidase using molecular oxygen as its cosubstrate producing free radical species which lead to oxygen stress and the subsequent complications.

At any age, about one-third of cases present with radiotranslucent xanthine stones. These stones are usually smooth, soft, and yellow-brown. Xanthinuric myopathy is a rare complication.

Xanthine stones also occur when there is a combined deficiency of the three molybdoflavoprotein enzymes, xanthine oxidase, sulphite oxidase, and aldehyde oxidase, because of defective molybdopterin cofactor synthesis. The clinical picture in these patients is overshadowed by the sulphite oxidase deficiency that produces severe brain damage and dislocation of the ocular lenses. Another subgroup of patients with xanthinuria only lack xanthine oxidase and aldehyde oxidase activity. These patients present with xanthine stones and are detected by their inability to convert allopurinol to oxypurinol, a reaction normally catalysed by aldehyde oxidase.

Adenylosuccinase deficiency

Adenylosuccinase (adenylate succinate lyase) catalyses the eighth step on the 10-step *de novo* purine synthesis pathway and the second step in one of the purine nucleotide interconversion pathways, the formation of ATP from inosine monophosphate.

The patients present in infancy with severe psychomotor disabilities, autism, and axial hypotonia with normal tendon reflexes. Self-mutilation has been recorded in some cases and cerebellar hypoplasia is present on CT scans.

The presence of aspartic acid and glycine in body fluids suggests the diagnosis, and this is confirmed by finding succinyl adenosine and succinyl aminoimidazole carboxamide riboside in plasma, cerebrospinal fluid, and urine. There is gross purine overproduction with high levels of nucleosides in the urine. Urine and plasma uric acid levels are normal. Partial enzyme deficiencies have been demonstrated in liver, kidney, muscle, lymphocytes, and fibroblasts. Mutation analysis has shown a homozygous mutation in one family.

Adenylosuccinase deficiency is inherited as an autosomal recessive. The growth retardation has been improved by adenine (10 mg/day) and allopurinol. The latter promotes purine conservation by blocking hypoxanthine oxidation to xanthine and uric acid, and prevents the oxidation of administered adenine to 2,8-dihydroxyadenine.

Myoadenylate deaminase deficiency

Myoadenylate deaminase is the muscle-specific isoenzyme of adenylate deaminase which catalyses the deamination of adenylic acid to inosinic acid during muscle contraction. This reaction is necessary for normal muscle function. Myoadenylate deaminase deficiency may be congenital, due to a mutation in the gene directing the synthesis of the protein, or associated with a wide range of muscle diseases including the muscular dystrophies, polymyositis, and dermatomyositis.

Patients with congenital myoadenylate deaminase deficiency present at any age including early childhood with a syndrome of muscle weakness and muscle cramps during and after exertion. There is some decrease in muscle mass, some hypotonia, and a little muscle weakness. There may be a modest rise in plasma creatine phosphokinase levels and nonspecific electromyographic changes. The lack of ammonia and inosine monophosphate acid occurs normally in the venous outflow from the affected muscles during exercise, and the enzyme deficiency can be demonstrated histochemically. The pattern of inheritance is autosomal recessive, not all of the homozygotes have clinical symptoms, and the heterozygous carriers are clinically silent. A single mutant allele contains a nonsense mutation that leads to the production of a severely truncated enzyme. The acquired disorder may be due to the coincidental disease arising in a patient whose inherited myoadenylate deaminase deficiency would otherwise be silent. Genetic testing for the mutant allele can be utilized to determine whether congenital myoadenylate deaminase could be contributing to the patient's clinical presentation.

Oral ribose (2–60 g/day, or taking a dose before vigorous exercise, e.g. skiing) has been reported to produce symptomatic improvement. The risk of rhabdomyolysis has led some authors to recommend the avoidance of vigorous exercise, myoglobinuria following strenuous exercise having been reported in a few cases. Such advice is only appropriate if exertion-related myoglobinuria has occurred or been suspected.

Inborn errors of purine metabolism and immunodeficiency

Adenosine deaminase and purine nucleoside phosphorylase catalyse sequential steps in the metabolism of purine ribonucleosides and deoxyribonucleosides. These enzymes are highly expressed in the lymphoid cells and their deficiency, which causes the lymphotoxic substrates 2′-deoxyadenosine and 2′-deoxyguanosine to accumulate, leads to lymphopenia and immunodeficiency.

Most patients with adenosine deaminase deficiency lack both cell-mediated (T cell) and humoral-mediated (B cell) immunity resulting in severe combined immunodeficiency disease. Although purine nucleoside phosphorylase deficiency causes defective T-cell-mediated immunity, these patients may posses either normal, hyperactive, or reduced humoral immunity. Most patients with these enzyme deficiencies present in infancy or early childhood, with severe infections caused by pathogens or opportunistic organisms. About 50% of patients with severe combined immunodeficiency disease have X-linked agammaglobulinaemia (Bruton's disease), a disease that is unrelated to adenosine deaminase and purine nucleoside phosphorylase deficiencies and which displays an autosomal recessive pattern of inheritance.

Adenosine deaminase deficiency

About 85% of patients with adenosine deaminase deficiency are infants with severe combined immunodeficiency disease. Among all severe combined immunodeficiency disease patients, adenosine deaminase deficiency accounts for a minority, possibly about 15% of all severe combined immunodeficiency disease patients and about 50% of all autosomal recessive severe combined immunodeficiency disease patients. Although adenosine deaminase deficiency classically presents in infancy, a minority of patients have a clinically less severe variant and are diagnosed later. The prevalence of adenosine deaminase deficiency has been estimated at between less than 1 in 10^6 and 1 in 2×10^5 live births.

Adenosine deaminase deficiency is inherited in an autosomal recessive fashion, the gene having been mapped to 20q13.11. The diagnosis is made by measuring adenosine deaminase activity in erythrocytes. Heterozygote detection and prenatal diagnosis are best done by using molecular probes for the *ADA* gene; more than 67 mutations have been described and these are mainly missense mutations.

In addition to immunoparesis, about one-third of patients have multiple skeletal abnormalities including fraying of the long bones, abnormally thick growth arrest lines, and chondro-osseous dysphasia at the costochondral junctions. Other occasionally reported comorbidities are renal tubular acidosis, choreoathetosis, spasticity, and fine sparse hair.

The prognosis in untreated adenosine deaminase-deficient severe combined immunodeficiency disease is very poor with death due to multiple recurrent infections during the first year of life.

Adenosine and 2′-deoxyadenosine, derived from the breakdown of DNA due to cell death, accumulate proximal to the metabolic block; 2′-deoxyadenosine is the primary lymphotoxic precursor in adenosine deaminase deficiency and elevated levels are present in plasma and urine. Erythrocytes contain markedly raised levels of deoxyadenosine triphosphate and reduced activity of *S*-adenosylhomocysteine hydrolase due to inactivation by 2′-deoxyadenosine; erythrocyte ATP is reduced. The level of deoxyadenosine triphosphate in erythrocytes correlates with clinical expression and with the level of adenosine deaminase activity expressed in *Escherichia coli* by mutant adenosine deaminase alleles.

There are several mechanisms by which adenosine deaminase deficiency can impair immune function. Accumulation of deoxyadenosine triphosphate can induce apoptosis in lymphoid cells. This may be related to deoxyadenosine triphosphate-induced inhibition of ribonucleotide reductase blocking DNA replication in dividing cells and to deoxyadenosine triphosphate-induced DNA strand breaks in nondividing lymphocytes. Deoxyadenosine triphosphate also activates the protease (caspase 9) involved in apoptosis. *S*-adenosylhomocysteine hydrolase blocks *S*-adenosylmethionine-mediated transmethylation reactions. The formation of deoxyadenosine triphosphate from 2′-deoxyadenosine activates inosine monophosphate dephosphorylation thereby leading to depletion of cellular ATP. It has also been suggested that lymphocyte function may be impaired by aberrant signal transduction mediated by deoxyadenosine acting through G-protein-associated receptors or from an altered costimulatory function of T-cell-associated adenosine deaminase complexing protein CD26/dipeptidyl peptidase IV.

Treatment

This is by bone marrow transplantation from a histocompatible donor. Repeated blood transfusions can provide temporary benefit although repeated transfusion leads to iron overload. More sustained clinical improvement follows the weekly or twice weekly administration of polyethylene glycol-modified bovine adenosine deaminase.

Transplantation of T-cell-depleted marrow from an HLA-haploidentical donor has been tried but is associated with greater morbidity and is less effective than bone marrow transplantation in restoring immune function.

The *ex vivo* retrovirus-mediated transfer of adenosine deaminase cDNA is the first attempt at somatic cell gene therapy in humans. The efficacy of transducing stem cells has been low, but persistence of the vector myeloid cells and T lymphocytes has been demonstrated. The long-term evaluation of this approach is still awaited. Self-inactivating lentivirus vectors for gene transfer correct the immunological and metabolic phenotypes in adenosine deaminase-deficient severe combined immunodeficiency disease mice and may be tried in humans.

Purine nucleoside phosphorylase deficiency

Purine nucleoside phosphorylase deficiency occurs less frequently than adenosine deaminase deficiency. In addition to the clinical results of immunoparesis, more than 50% of these patients have neurological abnormalities including disorders of muscle tone, delayed motor and intellectual development, ataxias, tremors, spastic tetraparesis, and behavioural difficulties. Autoimmune haemolytic anaemia and megaloblastic bone marrow have been occasional associations.

There appears to be a particular susceptibility to virus infection such as varicella, vaccinia, and cytomegalovirus. The tonsils and the thymus are small or absent and the lymph nodes are deficient in the thymus-dependent areas. Circulating lymphocyte counts are usually very low with a low percentage of T lymphocytes and depressed or absent responsiveness to mitogen-induced transformation. Serum immunoglobulin levels and antibody responses to pneumococcal polysaccharide and keyhole limpet haemocyanin are typically increased in these children with purine nucleoside phosphorylase deficiency, and the occasional finding of monoclonal IgG paraprotein strongly suggests that the changes in antibody production are secondary to T-cell defects.

Purine nucleoside phosphorylase deficiency is associated with the accumulation and excretion of 2′-deoxyguanosine and deoxyinosine as well as guanosine and inosine. Paradoxically there is massive purine overproduction and excretion although all patients are severely hypouricaemic.

Erythrocyte concentrations of deoxyguanosine triphosphate are markedly raised in purine nucleoside phosphorylase-deficient cells. T cells but not B cells appear to be particularly susceptible to 2′-deoxyguanosine toxicity, probably as a result of accumulation of deoxyguanosine triphosphate, inhibition of ribonucleotide reductase, impairment of DNA synthesis, and eventually cell death. Analysis of the gene encoding purine nucleoside phosphorylase shows several recurring mutations.

The prognosis in children with purine nucleoside phosphorylase deficiency is often much better than that in adenosine deaminase deficiency. Since some children have remained healthy and free from viral infection until the age of 6 years, high-risk procedures such as bone marrow transplantation are currently not thought to be justified in all cases. Conservative treatment with γ-globulin replacement and attempts at enzyme replacement with red cell transfusions in children with recurrent infections are the current approaches to management, although the use of umbilical cord blood has been reported to correct the immunodeficiency.

Purine 5′-nucleotidase deficiency

Deficiency of the ectoenzyme 5′-nucleotidase is found in some patients with X-linked and 'acquired' adult onset hypogammaglobulinaemia. There is no evidence that the enzyme deficiency causes the immunodeficiency in either case. It is currently thought much more likely simply to reflect an arrested stage of lymphocyte development in these patients.

Other disorders of purine metabolism

There are two unrelated conditions: (1) a regulatory mutation in liver adenylic deaminase as a case of uric acid overproduction and gout in a single patient; and (2) erythrocyte adenylic acid deaminase deficiency in Japanese and Chinese individuals, which has no clinical phenotype.

Uric acid, oxidative stress, and cardiovascular disease

Oxidative stress is a situation in which the rate of production of reactive oxygen species (superoxide anions, nitric oxide, hydrogen peroxide, hydroxyl radicals, and peroxynitrite) exceeds the rate at which they are destroyed. Xanthine oxidase uses molecular oxygen as its electron acceptor and generates reactive oxygen species and, therefore, oxygen stress. Uric acid is reported to be a scavenger for reactive oxygen species. Oxygen stress and hyperuricaemia may thus be related. Epidemiological studies suggests that hyperuricaemia is a risk factor for cardiovascular disease where oxidative stress is an important pathophysiological factor. Reducing serum urate levels by xanthine oxidase inhibition with allopurinol has been reported to have a protective effect in situations associated with oxidative stress, such as ischaemic reperfusion injury and cardiovascular disease. The current position with respect to the effect of hyperuricaemia, on oxidative stress remains unresolved.

The application of advanced statistical techniques to epidemiological data in relation to small elevations of the serum uric acid concentration in patients with cardiovascular disease has led to the detection of myocardial and endothelial cell dysfunction by the production of reactive oxygen species where there is no or minimal, clinical evidence of cardiovascular disease. Thus, there are reports of mild hyperuricaemia being linked to microalbuminuria which is itself predictive of cardiovascular disease. It is also said to be predictive of hypertension with or without other features of the metabolic syndrome and in nonmetabolic syndrome patients with increased coronary artery disease, demonstrated by electron beam tomography. A rising uric acid level has been reported as a bad prognostic sign in terminally ill cancer patients. The use of allopurinol to inhibit xanthine oxidase has been advocated in all of these circumstances and to reduce oxidative stress particularly in relation to cardiovascular disease.

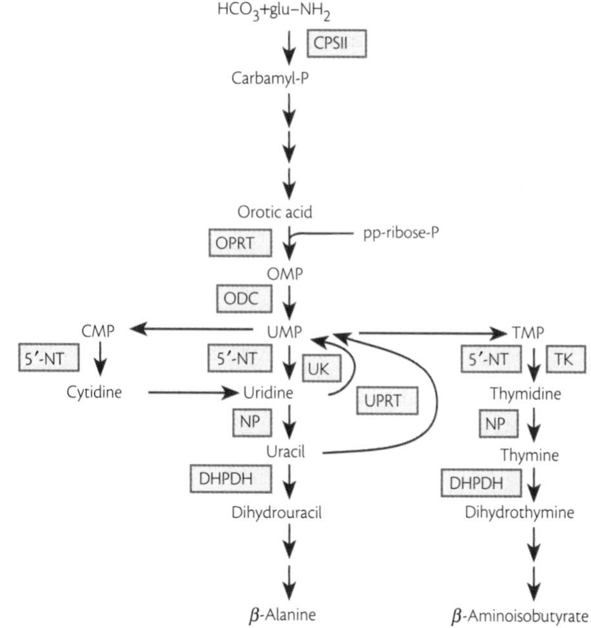

Fig. 12.4.6 Pathways of pyrimidine metabolism in humans. CPSH, carbamyl phosphate synthetase II; OPRT, orotate phosphoribosyltransferase; ODC, orotidine decarboxylase (OPRT + ODC form uridine monophosphate synthase); 5′-NT, pyrimidine 5′-nucleotidase; NP, pyrimidine nucleoside phosphorylase; DHPD, dihydropyrimidine dehydrogenase; UK, uridine kinase; UPRT, uracil phosphoribosyltransferase; TK, thymidine kinase.

Disorders of pyrimidine metabolism

The pathways of pyrimidine biosynthesis interconversion and degradation are shown in Fig. 12.4.6. The *de novo* synthesis of pyrimidine nucleotides involves a series of six reactions beginning with the formation of carbamyl phosphate and concluding with orotidylic acid, which then undergoes a series of interconversion and salvage reactions, as summarized in Fig. 12.4.6. The first three steps on the *de novo* synthesis pathway are encoded in a gene directing the synthesis of the multifunctional protein that encompasses carbamyl phosphate synthetase, aspartate transaminase, and dihydro-orotase. The fourth step is catalysed by dihydro-orotate dehydrogenase which is encoded in a single gene. The fifth and sixth steps are catalysed by the gene directing the synthesis of the bifunctional protein encoding orotate phosphoribosyltransferase and orotidine 5′-monophosphate decarboxylase which reside in separate regions of the protein. The pyrimidines are degraded to β-alanine and β-aminobutyrate (Fig. 12.4.6).

The inherited disorders of pyrimidine metabolism are much less common, or possibly much less easily recognized, than disorders of purine metabolism.

Orotic aciduria

Orotic aciduria is due to point mutations in the gene on chromosome 3q13 directing the synthesis of the bifunctional protein that catalyses the last two steps on the pyrimidine biosynthetic pathway. There is massive overproduction of orotic acid due to loss of feedback inhibition of carbamyl phosphate synthase, which is the first and rate-limiting step on the metabolic pathway.

Orotic aciduria presents during infancy with severe megaloblastic hypochromatic anaemia, orotic acid crystalluria, and occasionally, radiotranslucent orotic acid urinary stones. Cardiac malformations, mild intellectual impairment, and strabismus have been reported. Orotic aciduria is inherited as an autosomal recessive gene.

Enzyme assays on erythrocyte lysates show either low levels of orotate phosphoribosyltransferase and orotidine 5′-monophosphate decarboxylase (type 1 orotic aciduria) or a deficiency of orotidine 5′-monophosphate decarboxylase only (type 2 orotic aciduria). Administration of uridine (100–150 mg/kg per day), which is converted to uridine monophosphate (Fig. 12.4.6), produces a prompt haematological response. Treatment needs to be started as soon as the diagnosis is made during infancy in order to minimize the possibility of persistent neurological deficits.

Some degree of orotic aciduria has been found in urea cycle defect, lysinuric protein intolerance, purine nucleoside phosphorylase deficiency, normal pregnancy, and during allopurinol administration.

Pyrimidine 5′-nucleotidase deficiency

This autosomal recessive disorder leads to nonspherocytic haemolytic anaemia. Uridine triphosphate and cytidine triphosphate accumulate in the red cells which show basophilic stippling and reticulocytosis. There is hepatosplenomegaly. The enzyme is assayed in erythrocytes and activities between 0 and 30% of normal have been reported. The human gene has been cloned and 15 different mutations identified. A wide range of neurological features has been reported for which there is no effective treatment. Lead poisoning can also be associated with acquired erythrocyte pyrimidine 5′-nucleotidase deficiency and it has been reported in myeloproliferative disorders.

Pyrimidine 5′-nucleotidase superactivity

Pyrimidine 5′-nucleotidase superactivity has been reported in four unrelated families with developmental delay and neurological abnormalities. Treatment with uridine is said to have been beneficial.

Deficiency of dihydropyrimidine dehydrogenase

This autosomal recessive disorder presents with variable degrees of microcephaly, hypertonia, epilepsy, learning difficulties, and autism. Some cases have only presented during adult life when they have developed severe adverse side effects following cancer chemotherapy with 5-fluorouracil. Uracil and thymine are elevated in the body fluids, including urine. Absent enzyme activities have been demonstrated in blood, cerebrospinal fluid, leucocytes, liver, and fibroblasts. There is no effective treatment for this condition and the prognosis for life is very variable; very few cases have been reported.

N-Carbamyl-β-aminoaciduria

To date, just one patient has been detected with ureidopropionase deficiency causing *N*-carbamyl-β-aminoaciduria. This patient presented with choreoathetosis, hypotonia, and microcephaly.

Further reading

Anuti A (2004). Gene therapy for adenosine-deaminose-deficient severe combined immunodeficiency. *Best Prac Res Clin Haematol*, **17**, 505–16.

Breese GR, *et al.* (1990). Evidence that lack of brain dopamine during development can increase the susceptibility for aggression and self-injurious behaviour by influencing D1-dopamine receptor function. *Prog Neuropsychopharmacol Biol Psychiatry*, **14** Suppl, S65–80.

Bruce SP (2006). Fibuxostat a selective xanthine oxidase inhibitor for the treatment of hyperuricaemia and gout. *Ann Pharmacother*, **40**, 2187–94.

Cameron JS, Simmonds HA (2005). Hereditary hyperuricaemia and renal disease. *Semin Nephrol*, **25**, 9–18.

Chiarelli LR, *et al.* (2006). Hereditary erythrocyte, pyrimidine 5′-neuclotidase deficiency: a biochemical genetic and clinical overview. *Haematology*, **11**, 67–72.

Cingolani HE, *et al.* (2006). The effect of xanthine oxidase inhibition upon ejection fraction in heart failure patients, La Plata Study. *J Card Fail*, **12**, 491–508.

Corry DB, Tuck ML (2006). Uric acid and the vasculature. *Curr Hypertens Rep*, **8**, 116–19.

de Bont JM, Pieters R (2004). Management of hyperuricaemia with rasburicase review. *Nucleosides Nucleotides Nucleic Acids*, **23**, 1431–40.

de Ruiter CJ, *et al.* (2002). Muscle function during repetitive moderate-intensity muscle contractions in myoadenylate deaminase-deficient Dutch subjects. *Clin Sci*, **102**, 531–9.

Desaulniers P, *et al.* (2001). Crystal induced neutrophil activation. VII: Involvement of Syk in the responses to monosodium urate crystals. *J Leukoc Biol*, **70**, 659–68.

Fam AG (2001). Difficult gout and new approaches for control of hyperuricaemia in the allopurinol-allergic patient. *Curr Rheumatol Rep*, **3**, 29–35.

Glantzounis GK, *et al.* (2005). Uric acid and oxidative stress. *Curr Pharm Des*, **11**, 4145–51.

Goldstein M, *et al.* (1985). Self mutilation in the Lesch-Nyhan disease is caused by dopaminergic denervation. *Lancet*, **1824**, 338–9.

Gresser U, Zöllner N (1991). *Urate deposition in man and its clinical consequences*. Springer, Berlin.

Harkness, *et al.* (1988). Lesch-Nyhan syndrome and its pathogenesis: purine concentrations in plasma and urine with metabolite profiles in CSF. *J Inherit Metab Dis*, **11**, 239–52.

Harris JC, *et al.* (1998). Craniocerebral magnetic resonance imaging measurement and findings in Lesch-Nyhan syndrome. *Arch Neurol*, **55**, 547–53.

Hart TC, *et al.* (2002). Mutations of the UMOD gene are responsible for medullary cystic kidney disease 2 and familial juvenile hyperuricaemic nephropathy. *J Med Genet*, **39**, 882–92.

Hochberg MC (2001). Gout. In: Silman AJ, Hochberg MC (eds) *Epidemiology of the rheumatic diseases*, 2nd edition, pp. 230–42. Oxford University Press.

Hochberg J, Cairo MS (2008). Rasburicase: future directions in tumor lysis management. *Expert Opin Biol Ther*, **8**, 1595–604.

Hosoya T, *et al.* (1993). A study of uric acid metabolism and gouty arthritis in patients with polycystic kidney. *Nippon Jinzo Gakkai Shi*, **35**, 43–8.

Hyland K, *et al.* (2004). Tetrahydrobiopterin deficiency and dopamine loss in a genetic mouse model of Lesch-Nyhan disease. *J Inherit Metab Dis*, **27**, 165–78.

Jinnah HA (1994). Dopamine deficiency in a genetic model of Lesch-Nyhan disease. *J Neurosci*, **14**, 1164–75.

Kang DH, Nakagawa T (2005). Uric acid and chronic renal disease: possible implication of hyperuricaemia on progression of renal disease. *Semin Nephrol*, **25**, 43–9.

Keenan RT, Pillinger MH (2009). Febuxostat: a new agent for lowering serum urate. *Drugs Today (Barc)*, **45**, 247–60.

Kojima S, *et al.* (2005). Prognostic usefulness of serum uric acid after acute myocardial infarction (the Japanese Acute Coronary Syndrome Study). *Am J Cardiol*, **96**, 489–95.

Landis RC, Haskard DO (2001). Pathogenesis of crystal-induced inflammation. *Curr Rheumatol Rep*, **3**, 36–41.

Landis RC, *et al.* (2002). Safe disposal of inflammatory monosodium urate monohydrate crystals by differentiated macrophages. *Arthritis Rheum*, **46**, 3026–33.

Lin SD (2006). Association between serum uric acid level and components of the metabolic syndrome. *J Chin Med Assoc*, **69**, 512–16.

Lipkowitz MS, *et al.* (2001). Functional reconstitution, membrane targeting, genomic structure and chromosomal localisation of a human urate transporter. *J Clin Invest*, **107**, 1103–15.

Liu R, *et al.* (2000). Extracellular signal-regulated kinase 1/extracellular signal regulated kinase 2 mitogen-activated protein kinase signalling and activation of activator protein 1 and nuclear factor kappa β; transcription factors play central roles in interleukin-8 expression stimulated by monosodium urate monohydrate and calcium pyrophosphate crystals in monocytic cells. *Arthritis Rheum*, **43**, 1145–55.

Liu R, *et al.* (2001). Src family protein tyrosine kinase signalling mediates monosodium urate crystal-induced 1L-8 expression by monocyte THP-1 cells. *J Leukoc* Biol, **70**, 961–8.

Madsen TE, *et al.* (2005). Serum uric acid independently predicts mortality in patients with significant angiographically defined coronary disease. *Am J Nephrol*, **25**, 45–9. Epub 21 Feb 2005.

Morel A, *et al.* (2006). Clinical relevance of different dihydropyrimidine dehydrogenase gene single nucleotide polymorphisms on 5-fluorouracil tolerance. *Med Cancer Ther*, **5**, 2895–904.

Mortellaro A, *et al.* (2006). *Ex vivo* gene therapy with lentiviral vectors rescues adenosine deaminase (ADA) deficient mice and corrects their immune and metabolic defects. *Blood*, **108**, 2979–88.

Mount DB, *et al.* (2006). Renal urate transport. *Rheum Dis Clin North Am*, **32**, 313–31.

Myers LA (2004). Purine nucleoside phosphorylase deficiency (PNP-def) presenting with lymphopenia and development delay: successful correction with umbilical cord blood transplantation. *J Pediatr*, **145**, 710–12.

Nyhan WL (2000). Dopamine function in Lesch-Nyhan disease. *Environ Health Perspect*, **108** Suppl 3, 409–11.

Ozdemir O (2006). Severe combined immune deficiency in an adenosine deaminase-deficient patient. *Allergy Asthma Proc*, **27**, 172–4.

Rampoldi L, *et al.* (2003). Allelism of MCKD, FJHN, and GCKD caused by impairment of uromodulin export dynamics. *Hum Mol Genet*, **12**, 3369–84.

Roneo C, Rodeghiero E (2005) *Hyperuricaemic syndromes: pathophysiology and therapy*. Karger, Basel.

Santos RD, *et al.* (2007). Relation of uric acid levels to presence of coronary artery calcium detected by electron beam tomography in men free of symptomatic myocardial ischaemia with versus without the metabolic syndrome. *Am J Cardiol*, **99**, 42–5.

Scriver CA, *et al.* (eds) (2001). *The metabolic and molecular basis of inherited disease*. McGraw–Hill, New York.

Shi Y, *et al.* (2003). Molecular identification of a danger signal that alerts the immune system to dying cells. *Nature*, **125**, 516–21.

Shin HS, *et al.* (2006). Uric acid as a prognostic factor for survival time: a prospective cohort study of terminally ill cancer patients. *J Pain Symptom Manage*, **31**, 493–501.

Silva M, *et al.* (2004). Three-dimensional structure of human adenine phosphoribosyltransferase and its relation to DHA-urolithiasis. *Biochemistry*, **43**, 7663–71.

Sood AR, Burry LD, Cheng DK (2007). Clarifying the role of rasburicase in tumor lysis syndrome. *Pharmacotherapy*, **27**, 111–21.

Speigel EK, Colman RF, Patterson D (2006). Adenylosuccinate lyase deficiency. *Mol Genet Metab*, **89**, 19–31.

Sperling O (2006). Hereditary renal hypouricaemia. *Mol Genet Metab*, **89**, 14–18.

Terkeltaub R (2009). Gout. Novel therapies for treatment of gout and hyperuricaemia. *Arthritis Research and Therapy*, **11**, 236–57.

Terkeltaub RA, *et al.* (2010). High-vs low-dosing of oral colchicine for early acute gout flare: Twenty-four hour outcome results of the first randomized, placebo-controlled, dose comparison colchicine trial. *Arthritis and Rheumatism*, Jan 21 (Epub ahead of print).

Turner JJ, *et al.* (2003). Uromodulin mutations cause familial juvenile hyperuricaemic nephropathy. *J Clin Endocrinol Metab*, **88**, 1398–1401.

Van Kullenburg AB, *et al.* (2004). Beta-ureidopropionase deficiency: an inborn error of pyrimidine degradation associated with neurological abnormalities. *Hum Mol Genet*, **13**, 2793–801.

Waring WS, Webb DJ, Maxwell SRJ (2000). Uric acid as a risk factor for cardiovascular disease. *QJM*, **93**, 707–13.

Watts RWE, *et al.* (1987). Lesch-Nyhan syndrome; growth delay, testicular atrophy and a partial failure of 11β-hydroxylation of steroids. *J Inherit Metab Dis*, **10**, 210–23.

Wong DF (1996). Dopamine transporters are markedly reduced in Lesch-Nyhan disease *in vivo*. *Proc Natl Acad Sci U S A*, **93**, 5539–43.

Yagnik DR, *et al.* (2000). Non-inflammatory phagocytosis of monosodium urate monohydrate crystals by mouse macrophages. Implications for the control of joint inflammation in gout. *Arthritis Rheum*, **43**, 1779–89.

Yagnik DR, *et al.* (2004). Macrophage release of transforming growth factor β1 during resolution of monosodium urate monohydrate crystal-induced inflammation. *Arthritis Rheum*, **50**, 2273–80.

Yamada, *et al.* (1994). Molecular mechanisms of a second female Lesch-Nyhan patient. *Adv Exp Med Biol*, **370**, 337–40.

Yukawa T, *et al.* (1992). A female patient with Lesch-Nyhan syndrome. *Dev Med Child Neurol*, **34**, 534–46.

Zanella A, *et al.* (2006). Hereditary pyrimidine 5′-nucleotidase deficiency from genetics to clinical manifestations. *Br J Haematol*, **133**, 113–23.

Zhang W, *et al.* (2006). EULAR evidence based recommendations for gout. Part II: Management Report of a task force of the EULAR Standing Committee for International Clinical Studies Including Therapeutics (ESCISIT). *Ann Rheum Dis*, **65**, 1312–24.

12.5

The porphyrias

Timothy M. Cox

Essentials

The porphyrias are metabolic disorders characterized by overproduction of haem precursors, principally in the liver and bone marrow. Most porphyrias are inborn errors that affect enzymatic steps in a tightly regulated biosynthetic pathway for haem; nonacute acquired forms also occur.

Hepatic synthesis of haem undergoes rapid and wide oscillations, but haem formation for erythropoiesis is generally constant; it may increase as the erythron expands to meet the demands of blood loss or destruction, or as a consequence of ineffective erythropoiesis.

Acute porphyrias

Clinical presentation—life-threatening neurovisceral attacks occur in four of the porphyrias: acute intermittent porphyria, variegate porphyria, hereditary coproporphyria and Doss porphyria (5-aminolaevulinate dehydratase deficiency). These present with abdominal pain, psychiatric symptoms, signs of sympathetic and hypothalamic autonomic overactivity, sometimes accompanied by convulsions and motor and sensory deficits. They typically develop on exposure to environmental or endogenous factors that place a demand for hepatic haem biosynthesis, the most frequent being changes in reproductive steroid hormones either due to natural hormone cycles or the administration of exogenous gonadal steroids, starvation, intercurrent infection, alcohol and drugs. Acute porphyrias may also be associated with overproduction of photoactive metabolites and thus long-term photosensitivity, which is aggravated during acute attacks.

Diagnosis—this is key to survival of an acute attack of porphyria, which can be suspected on the basis of the past history, in particular of photosensitivity or the intermittent discoloration of urine, and family history, and is confirmed by finding excess water-soluble haem precursors in urine. Enzymatic studies can later be used to verify the exact type of suspected porphyria, with molecular analysis of genes encoding relevant haem synthetic enzymes used to identify at-risk individuals in affected pedigrees.

Management—treatment of an acute porphyric attack mandates immediate withdrawal of inappropriate drugs and other precipitating factors; infusions of haem arginate or other licensed preparations of haem shorten life-threatening episodes and may be effective prophylaxis for recurrent porphyria in women with periodic attacks.

Nonacute porphyrias

The nonacute porphyrias are photosensitivity syndromes caused by excess photoactive macrocyclic porphyrins. The classic manifestations are of severe blistering lesions on sun-exposed skin, particularly of the hands and face, with the formation of vesicles and bullae that may become infected. Healing often leads to cutaneous deformities with loss of digits, scarring of the eyelids, nose, lips, scalp, and occasionally blindness due to corneal scarring. Protoporphyria characteristically causes burning pain and erythema with oedema; blistering is absent. Diagnosis is based on finding excess formed porphyrins in blood and excreta. Sunlight exposure should be avoided as much as possible until the porphyrin abnormality is corrected, e.g. by phlebotomy to cause iron depletion in porphyria cutanea tarda, or by liver or haematopoietic stem-cell transplantation in some (rare) cases.

Introduction

The haem biosynthetic pathway holds great fascination for biochemists who marvel at the evolution of ancient enzymes which interact to bring about the formation of the pigments of life, haemoglobin, the cytochromes, chlorophyll, and the cobalamins (vitamin B_{12}). It is unfortunate that, because of complexities in their chemical structure and nomenclature, the important diseases associated with their disturbed haem metabolism are perceived as obscure. These considerations apply particularly to the acute porphyrias which are rare but distressing syndromes that mimic other acute illnesses but for which recognition may be critical for the patient's survival; too often the diagnosis is not established until permanent disability (or even death) supervenes.

The porphyrias are caused by disturbances in the multistep pathway for the formation of haem, a pigment essential for oxygen transfer and the energy-yielding reactions of electron transport.

The formation of haem is tightly regulated so that acquired or hereditary defects of any of its component reactions lead to the overproduction of haem precursors. Potentially photoactive macrocyclic compounds and toxic precursors of pyrroles thus accumulate. Most of the human porphyria syndromes result from uncommon genetically determined deficiencies of unitary enzymes of the haem biosynthetic pathway, but certain toxins including lead, iron, and hydrocarbons influence the pathway and cause porphyria in susceptible individuals. Similarly the metabolism of endogenous molecules, including steroid hormones, and xenobiotics, such as alcohol and many therapeutic drugs, may disturb the delicate equilibrium that is achieved in asymptomatic patients with latent porphyria. Thus gene–environment interactions in previously fit individuals may precipitate sporadic attacks of acute porphyria.

Classification: types of porphyria

The porphyrias are disorders of metabolism characterized by overproduction of the precursors of haem synthesized principally in the liver and bone marrow. About 15 per cent of *de novo* haem biosynthesis occurs in the liver and about 80 per cent in the erythroid marrow. Hepatic synthesis of haem is subject to rapid and wide fluctuations but haem biosynthesis in the erythropoietic bone marrow is, under most circumstances, constitutive and stable. However, haem synthesis may be increased either as the erythron expands and proliferates to meet the demands of blood loss or haemolysis, or in response to ineffective erythropoiesis.

Until now the porphyrias have been classified into the hepatic and erythropoietic types depending on the principal location at which overproduction of haem precursors occurs. For clinical purposes, however, an operational definition of the porphyric syndromes is more usefully presented as the acute and the nonacute porphyrias. The acute porphyrias cause life-threatening neurovisceral manifestations typically precipitated by environmental factors that occur sporadically. The nonacute porphyrias are characterized by photosensitivity syndromes resulting from the overproduction of macrocyclic porphyrins which cause light-induced skin injury. Several of the acute porphyrias may also be associated with the overproduction of porphyrin intermediates and so may be accompanied at times by long-term photosensitivity which is often exacerbated during the acute attacks. In all instances it is the overproduction of haem precursors that characterizes the condition biochemically and this is the principal means by which a diagnosis can be made of the underlying enzymatic defect during the acute attack. Tables 12.5.1, 12.5.2, and 12.5.3 set out the individual defects that characterize the clinical porphyrias and summarize the clinical features of these hereditary syndromes.

Table 12.5.1 The porphyria syndromes

Hereditary porphyria
Acute porphyrias:
Acute intermittent porphyria
Variegate porphyria[a]
Hereditary coproporphyria[a]
Doss porphyria—aminolaevulinate dehydratase deficiency
Non-acute porphyrias:
Congenital erythropoietic porphyria—Gunther's disease
Protoporphyria
Porphyria cutanea tarda[b]—sporadic or familial
Hepatoerythropoietic porphyria[c]
Acquired porphyria
Hexachlorobenzene porphyria
Lead poisoning (plumboporphyria)
Hereditary tyrosinaemia

[a] Acute syndromes also accompanied by long-term skin photosensitivity.

[b] Porphyria cutanea tarda is not a simple monogenic disorder; it is almost always provoked by environmental agents such as hepatitis C, oestrogens, iron excess, or alcohol.

c Homozygous uroporphyrinogen III decarboxylase deficiency.

Formation of haem

Haem biosynthesis is catalysed by eight enzymes and is coordinated between mitochondrial and cytoplasmic compartments in the cell (Fig. 12.5.1). The first committed precursor, 5-aminolaevulinate, is formed in the mitochondria from glycine and the Krebs cycle intermediate succinyl CoA by one or other of the two isozymes of 5-aminolaevulinate synthetase. Precursor 5-aminolaevulinate is then exported to the cytoplasm where it undergoes condensation to form the monopyrrole porphobilinogen, four molecules of which are then condensed to yield the macrocyclic tetrapyrrole uroporphyrinogen III. This reaction is brought about by porphobilinogen deaminase and uroporphyrinogen III synthetase acting coordinately to reverse the orientation of one porphobilinogen molecule to yield the uroporphyrinogen III isoform that is the sole precursor of biological haem. Porphyrins of the I series do not serve as biological intermediates in the formation of protoporphyrin IX or haem.

The cytoplasmic enzyme uroporphyrinogen III decarboxylase decarboxylates the four acetate substituent side chains to yield coproporphyrinogen III, which is then reimported into the mitochondrion for further oxidative decarboxylation. Coproporphyrinogen III oxidase modifies the two propionate side chains to vinyl groups yielding protoporphyrinogen IX, the penultimate precursor of haem. Protoporphyrinogen oxidase removes six hydrogen atoms to yield protoporphyrin IX, which is the substrate for the final step in haem biosynthesis. The insertion of ferrous ions into the porphyrin macrocycle to form ferroprotohaem (haem) is catalysed by the mitochondrial enzyme ferrochelatase.

Haem serves as a key prosthetic group in haem proteins, including cytochromes, myoglobin, and haemoglobin, by which it fulfils its essential biological roles as a transporter of oxygen and electrons in the respiratory chain and in the metabolism of xenobiotics. The two isozymes (constitutive erythroid and the inducible hepatic isozyme) of 5-aminolaevulinate synthetase catalyse the rate-limiting step of haem biosynthesis. Pyridoxal 5-phosphate (derived from vitamin B_6) is an essential cofactor for 5-aminolaevulinate synthetase isozymes. Deficiency of pyridoxine or interference with its metabolism leads to sideroblastic anaemia.

The hepatic isozyme maps to the autosome chromosome 3 but the erythroid isozyme of 5-aminolaevulinate synthetase (ALAS-2) maps to the X chromosome. These enzymes are subject to differential regulation principally involving transcriptional control in the liver and translational and post-translational control mechanisms

Table 12.5.2 Main biochemical abnormalities in the porphyrias

Disorder	Enzyme defect	Biochemical abnormality
Acute intermittent porphyria	Porphobilinogen deaminase	Increased urinary porphobilinogen and 5-aminolaevulinate
Variegate porphyria	Protoporphyinogen IX oxidase	Increased urine 5-aminolaevulinate and porphobilinogen (especially acute attacks)
		Increased stool coproporphyrin III and protoporphyrin
Hereditary coproporphyria	Coproporphyinogen III oxidase	Increased urine 5-aminolaevulinate and porphobilinogen (especially acute attacks)
		Increased stool coproporphyrin III more than protoporphyrin
Doss porphyria	Aminolaevulinate dehydratase	Increased urinary 5-aminolaevulinate
		Faecal porphyrins normal
Porphyria cutanea tarda	Uroporphyrinogen III decarboxylase[a]	Increased urine uroporphyrin I and III
		Increased faecal hepatacarboxylic porphyrin and isocoproporphyrin
Congenital erythropoietic porphyria	Uroporphyrinogen III synthase	Increased urine, plasma, and red cell uroporphyrin I and coproporphyrin I Normal 5-aminolaevulinate and porphobilinogen
		Increased faecal coproporphyrin I
Protoporphyria	Ferrochelatase	Increased protoporphyrin in stool and red cells
Hexachlorabenzene porphyria	Uroporphyrinogen III decarboxylase	Increased urinary uroporphyrin I and III Hepatocarboxylic and other acetic acid substituents
Hereditary tyrosinaemia I	Aminolaevulinate dehydratase[b] (acquired deficiency)	Increased urinary 5-aminolaevulinate and succinylacetone (toxic metabolite)
Lead poisoning	Aminolaevulinate dehydratase, Ferrochelatase ± impaired iron delivery from transferrin	Increased urinary 5-aminolaevulinate raised red-cell protoporphyrin and zinc protoporphyrin

[a] Homozygous deficiency also responsible for hepatoerythropoietic porphyria.
[b] Inborn deficiency of fumarylacetoacetate hydrolase leads to excess formation of the 5-aminolaevulinate hydratase inhibitor, succinyl acetone (4,6-dioxoheptanoate).
Reference ranges: Urine—total porphyrins 20 to 320 nmol/l; 5-aminolaevulinate < 52 μmol/l (urine: creatinine porphobilinogen ratio < 1.5); porphobilinogen < 10.7 μmol/l.
Faeces—total porphyrins 10 to 200 nmol/g dry weight.
Red cell—total porphyrins 0.4 to 1.7 μmol/litre.
Laboratory ranges supplied by Porphyria Service, Department of Medical Biochemistry, University Hospital of Wales NHS Trust, Heath Park, Cardiff CF4 4XW (Professor G.H. Elder).

in the erythroid cell by the end product haem; they ultimately regulate the activity of the whole biosynthetic pathway. Expression of the gene encoding ALAS-1 is rate-limiting for the formation of haem and is increased in response to a key regulator of mitochondrial biogenesis that stimulates activity of the Krebs cycle, the transcription factor peroxisome proliferator-activated receptor coactivator 1α (PGC-1α).

Haem is an essential prosthetic group for many oxidative enzymes as well as transcription factors that regulate circadian activities; haem binds reversibly to a nuclear receptor (Rev-erbα),

Table 12.5.3 Principal manifestations of the porphyrias

Acute intermittent porphyria	Acute neurovisceral attacks
Variegate porphyria	Acute neurovisceral attacks
	Skin photosensitivity with scarring, hairiness, and pigment changes
Hereditary coproporphyria	Acute neurovisceral attacks, blistering skin lesions, photosensitivity
Doss porphyria	Acute neurovisceral attacks, susceptibility to lead exposure
Porphyria cutanea tarda	Blistering skin lesions on light exposure, pigment changes, atrophy and scarring— also may be associated with manifestations of iron storage disease
Congenital erythropoietic porphyria	Haemolytic anaemia, hypersplenism, porphyrinuria, extreme photosensitivity with skin ulceration and injury; adult- or late-onset reported
Hepatoerythropoietic porphyria	Resembles congenital erythropoietic porphyria: blisters, photosensitive skin with scar formation, haemolysis, red urine
Protoporphyria	Photosensitivity; early-onset, characterized by burning pain, oedema—scarring rare
	Occasional cholestatic liver disease, protoporphyrin gallstones—fulminant or subfulminant hepatic failure complicated by neurovisceral syndrome, especially in perioperative state
Hexachlorobenzene porphyria	Resembles sporadic porphyria cutanea tarda
Lead poisoining	Neurovisceral manifestations with signs of disordered red-cell haemoglobinization
Hereditary tyrosinaemia I	Toxic neurovisceral disease

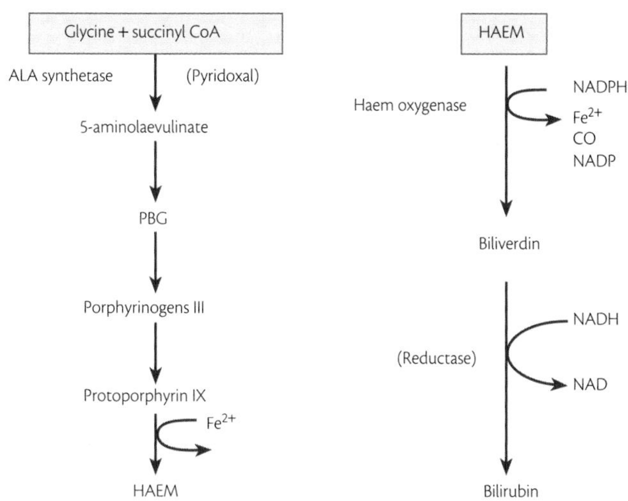

Fig. 12.5.1 Main pathways for haem biosynthesis and degradation in humans.

which is a crucial regulator of the core clock functions in biological rhythms. Haem suppresses the action of Rev-erbα on expression of proteins involved in maintenance of glucose homeostasis and gluconeogenesis. A molecular understanding of these recently discovered interactions holds much promise for elucidating how acute attacks of porphyria are induced by starvation, sepsis, endogenous hormonal factors, and xenobiotics.

The second enzyme of the haem biosynthetic pathway, 5-aminolaevulinate dehydratase, is a multimeric enzyme with reactive sulphydryl groups that are particularly sensitive to the toxic effects of heavy metals, especially lead, so that 5-aminolaevulinate dehydratase activity is a sensitive measure of environmental and industrial toxicity. Moreover, 5-aminolaevulinate dehydratase is inhibited competitively by the metabolite succinylacetone, concentrations of which rise to inhibitory levels in patients who have the defect of aromatic amino acid degradation tyrosinaemia type I. Patients with tyrosinaemia type I and lead poisoning have neurovisceral manifestations that resemble the acute porphyrias, and it appears likely that overproduction of aminolaevulinate, as a result of arrest at the 5-aminolaevulinate dehydratase reaction, contributes to this effect.

In living cells most of the macrocyclic precursors of the haem biosynthetic pathway are present as their reduced porphyrinogen precursors which are not photoreactive. However, when these tetrapyrroles (uroporphyrinogen, coproporphyrinogen, and protoporphyrinogen) are produced in excess, they diffuse into plasma and tissues where they react with ambient oxygen to form their parent porphyrins, which are spectacularly fluorescent. The double-bond resonance structure of these macrocyclic compounds promotes the formation of singlet oxygen by the transfer of absorbed energy to ground-state oxygen through light activation. It appears that generation of singlet oxygen brings about the photodermatoses associated with the porphyrias; these are characterized by photosensitization of the skin and tissues exposed to light in a broad region of the spectrum including the visible range (350–430 nm). Porphyrias associated with overproduction of formed macrocyclic haem precursors are thus associated with photosensitivity, and the particular skin reactions that develop differ between the particular enzyme defects. This may be explained principally by the degree of hydrophobicity of the overproduced porphyrins and their solubility in cellular membranes.

The first tetrapyrrole that serves as an immediate precursor to haem is uroporphyrinogen III, formation of which requires coordinated action of the two cytoplasmic enzymes uroporphyrinogen I synthase (porphobilinogen deaminase) and uroporphyrinogen III cosynthase. In the absence of adequate cosynthase activity, there is a marked overproduction of porphyrins of the I series, which do not form biologically active ferroprotohaem. Deficiency of uroporphyrinogen III cosynthase leads to the very rare but disabling syndrome of Gunther's disease (congenital erythropoietic porphyria). This disorder is characterized by extreme photosensitivity, haemolysis, and the passage of pink urine containing abundant porphyrins of the I isoform. Persistently high concentrations of these toxic molecules in body fluids leads to staining of the teeth and bones and extreme photosensitive damage, often with cruel and painful skin disfigurement and hair loss.

Porphyria cutanea tarda is caused by deficiency of uroporphyrinogen decarboxylase, defects of which involve complex interactions between heredity and environmental factors. The enzyme activity is markedly decreased in the presence of excess tissue iron and, although rare familial cases of porphyria cutanea tarda occur, most patients have a sporadic disease that is provoked by exposure to environmental toxins such as alcohol, oestrogens, hydrocarbons, iron (often associated with mutations in the haemochromatosis gene *HFE*), and hepatitis C. At the time of writing, the pathogenic relationship between these external factors and the manifestations of uroporphyrinogen decarboxylase deficiency is unclear.

The final step in the haem biosynthetic pathway involves insertion of ferrous iron into the protoporphyrin nucleus generated enzymatically from protoporphyrinogen IX by protoporphyrinogen IX oxidase. This last step occurs in the mitochondrion. Ferrochelatase depends on the iron–transferrin cycle for the delivery of iron from plasma transferrin. In the bone marrow, when the iron supply is deficient, freely available zinc may be preferentially converted to zinc protoporphyrin rather than ferroprotohaem thus offering a convenient means to monitor iron-deficient erythropoiesis. Similarly, industrial lead exposure, which inhibits both iron delivery and the activity of the sulphydryl enzyme ferrochelatase, causes accumulation of zinc protoporphyrin and free protoporphyrin in erythroid precursors and reticulocytes. Deficiency of ferrochelatase leads to the accumulation of free protoporphyrin in liver tissue, plasma, and the skin where it induces marked photosensitivity. The accumulation of excess protoporphyrin in red-cell precursors leads to the characteristic fluorocytes (young red cells containing excess free protoporphyrin) that are the easily recognized hallmark of patients with burning photosensitivity caused by protoporphyria.

The highly regulated control mechanism of haem biosynthesis ensures that the free concentrations of the toxic intermediates involved in the pathway are kept low unless there is a metabolic arrest at one of the biosynthetic reactions; under these circumstances an overproduction of the intermediate compounds occurs which can be used for diagnosis. This overproduction predisposes to the development of the particular clinical porphyric syndrome. A knowledge of the enzymatic steps and of the differential solubility of the haem precursors facilitates appropriate diagnostic testing for the precise identification of suspected porphyria. In principle, overproduction of the early precursors such as aminolaevulinic acid is

Table 12.5.4 Solubility and routes of excretion of haem precursors

	Plasma	Urine	Faeces
5-Aminolaevulinate	++	+++	–
Porphobilinogen	++	+++	–
Uroporphyrins I and III	+	++	+
Coproporphyrins I and III	+	+	+++
Protoporphyrin IX	+	–	+++

a common feature of those syndromes associated with neurovisceral manifestations or acute attacks of porphyria. Aminolaevulinate, in particular, represents a common biochemical marker of such attacks and those syndromes that mimic the porphyrias, such as hereditary tyrosinaemia type I and lead poisoning. In patients with cutaneous photosensitivity, overproduction of the formed porphyrin macrocycles can also be detected in plasma, urine, and faeces in which they are distributed according to their aqueous solubility (Table 12.5.4).

The profile of molecules that are overproduced in a given syndrome may be predicted from the level at which the enzymatic arrest occurs, as flux through the pathway is stimulated by diminished negative feedback. In those porphyrias where the principal site of production appears to be in the liver, including the acute porphyrias and porphyria cutanea tarda, fluctuations through the biosynthetic pathway as a result of regulatory effects from environmental or endogenous factors can occur very rapidly; indeed minute-to-minute oscillations in biosynthetic haem fluxes have been recorded in the liver. Thus in starvation and on challenge with xenobiotic reagents (which place a demand for the production of haem to meet the needs for new cytochrome formation), as well as with endogenous hormonal changes, enhanced flux through the pathway leads to toxic overproduction of 5-aminolaevulinic acid. By the same token, rapid repression of the haem biosynthetic pathway in the liver can be induced by the administration of exogenous haem, a useful agent in the control of acute attacks and which rapidly corrects the disturbed metabolism (see below).

Haem formation in the erythron is more rapid than that in the liver but is not subject to sudden oscillations in synthetic rates. Nonetheless in patients with erythropoietic porphyrias, such as congenital porphyria, enhanced rates of red-cell destruction when hypersplenism supervenes or in response to light exposure greatly exacerbate the overproduction of porphyrin intermediates and aggravate photosensitivity due to increased porphyrin release. Short-term experiments indicate that exogenous haem may partially repress the endogenous haem biosynthetic pathway in erythroid tissue but this has not proved to be useful for long-term relief in the erythropoietic porphyrias. Blood transfusion to suppress erythropoiesis or definitive replacement of bone marrow by transplantation has, however, proved to be successful in controlling the devastating manifestations of congenital erythropoietic porphyria.

Pathogenesis

The individual porphyria syndromes are described briefly below but the main manifestations (neurovisceral or phototoxic) remain the subject of further clinical research.

Acute neurovisceral attacks

These attacks occur in four of the porphyrias indicated in Tables 12.5.1 to 12.5.3. In all but one, Doss' porphyria (aminolaevulinate dehydratase deficiency), the inheritance is as an autosomal dominant trait. 5-Aminolaevulinate dehydratase deficiency is inherited as an extremely rare recessive condition. Clinical expression is characterized by acute, life-threatening attacks of neuropathy that include abdominal pain, psychiatric symptoms, and signs of sympathetic and hypothalamic autonomic overactivity, sometimes accompanied by convulsions and motor and sensory deficits. The syndrome is characteristically precipitated by drugs that induce hepatic haem formation and are metabolized by the hepatic cytochrome P-450 system. Neuropathological examination shows axonal degeneration and central chromatolysis in anterior horn cells and in the brain. Electromyography may reveal denervation compatible with a primary axonal neuropathy of peripheral nerves.

Although this acute porphyria is associated with lone overproduction of 5-aminolaevulinic acid, common to all those associated with acute manifestations, a toxic effect of this precursor is not the only potential mechanism of injury. The structure of aminolaevulinate is analogous to the inhibitory neurotransmitters γ-aminobutyric acid and L-glutamate. It seems likely that 5-aminolaevulinate may interfere with the action of the γ-aminobutyric acidergic system, the best evidence for which appears to be its ability to inhibit melatonin production in the rat pineal gland *in vivo*, as has been described in patients with recurrent acute porphyric attacks. It has been further postulated that under the conditions of the acute attack there may be a deficiency of essential haem proteins, such as the cytochrome P-450 isozymes in the liver, with further disturbances in secondary metabolism; other possibilities include a decrease in the activity of hepatic tryptophan dioxygenase, leading to increased formation of 5-hydroxytryptamine (serotonin).

At present there is no clear resolution between combined or individual effects of acute porphyria on the production of neurotoxic pseudotransmitters (aminolaevulinate) or secondary local deficiency of haem. However, early unpublished but apparently beneficial results of liver transplantation in patients with disabling recurrent attacks of acute intermittent porphyria indicate that the principal cause of the acute syndrome is the hepatic overproduction of toxic haem precursors. In any event, there is convincing evidence of abnormal neurotransmitter function and increased serotonin production, as well as direct interference of γ-aminobutyric acid receptors by toxic concentrations of 5-aminolaevulinate. Supplying exogenous haem during the acute attack, however, would be expected to correct both arms of this disturbed metabolism, which may account for the beneficial biochemical and clinical effects observed with its use. The recent development of a mouse model of porphyrinogen deaminase deficiency showing sensitivity to barbiturates serves as an authentic model of the biochemical and neuropathological manifestations of acute porphyria and may clarify much about the pathogenesis of this disturbing clinical syndrome. Detailed observations of the effects of hepatic transplantation in acute human porphyrias are also eagerly awaited.

Photosensitivity

Porphyrins absorb light maximally in the Soret region (400–420 nm) and in the visible wavelength region (between 500 and 600 nm); they re-emit this light energy at lower wavelengths to give pink, orange, or red fluorescence. This fluorescence is associated with the photodynamic effects and excitation to form triplet states; in the presence of oxygen in biological tissues, transfer of electronic energy leads to the generation of reactive oxygen species, including singlet oxygen, leading to complement activation and cutaneous toxicity. Careful studies examining the photoactive spectrum of skin from patients with various porphyrias has confirmed a cause-and-effect relationship between irradiance within the absorbing wavelength range of the given porphyrin and the development of weal-and-flare and other cutaneous phototoxic responses.

Distinct porphyric syndromes are associated with the accumulation of a specifically formed macrocyclic porphyrin, each with its particular solubility properties in plasma and in cell membranes. In porphyria cutanea tarda, skin biopsies show subepidermal bullas and electron microscopy reveals vacuoles in the cells of the superficial dermal epithelium. In this disease, as in protoporphyria, the endothelium of the dermal capillary is thickened and the vessels are surrounded by complement and mucopolysaccharide deposits. In protoporphyria, an adequate oxygen supply has been shown to be critical for the development of experimental phototoxicity *in vivo*. Singlet oxygen and other radicals may lead to lipid peroxidation and cross-linking of membrane proteins with activation of late complement components. In the more severe disease, congenital erythropoietic porphyria, egress of uroporphyrin I from circulating erythrocytes, which may be destroyed within capillaries, leads to gross accumulation of porphyrin in dermal tissue and juxtaposed epithelium. Exposure to light is known to promote photohaemolysis, indicating that light of the visible wavelength can penetrate the skin sufficiently to induce porphyrin photoactivation *in situ*.

Induction of acute porphyric attacks

Acute attacks of porphyria may be life-threatening illnesses that occur in genetically predisposed individuals who usually remain asymptomatic. The acute episodes develop on exposure to environmental or endogenous factors that place a demand for hepatic haem biosynthesis; this leads to the overproduction of porphyrin intermediates and pyrrole precursors. The most frequent precipitating factors are changes in reproductive steroid hormones either due to natural hormone cycles or the administration of exogenous gonadal steroids. Starvation, including that associated with surgical procedures and anaesthesia, intercurrent infections, and many xenobiotics, including alcohol as well as prescription drugs, over-the-counter agents, and chemicals present in health foods can precipitate acute porphyria.

Tables 12.5.5 and 12.5.6 list drugs that have been classified as unsafe in patients with porphyria either because they have been shown to be porphyrinogenic in animals or *in vitro* studies, or have been associated with acute attacks in patients with porphyria. The table is taken from the British National Formulary published by the British Medical Association and the Royal Pharmaceutical Society of Great Britain. It is pointed out in this publication that slight changes in the chemical structure can lead to marked differences in the ability of the drug to induce attacks of porphyria. A more complete list of drugs is provided in a review by Anderson *et al.* (2001) (see 'Further reading').

Acute attacks of porphyria occur in the four conditions known as the hepatic porphyrias and particularly occur for the first time in latent carriers who are aged between 15 and 40 years. Attacks have been recorded in children before puberty but are extremely rare and usually occur during febrile illnesses precipitated by the use of porphyrinogenic cough medicines. Although the porphyrias occur in a latent state in men with a frequency that is equal to that in women, women who have acute porphyria outnumber men by at least 2 to 1. The recent description of Rev-erbα, a haem sensor involved in the coordination of metabolic pathways and circadian rhythms, as well as PGC-1α, a transcriptional coactivator involved in the regulation of ALAS-1 expression, offers the hope that a better understanding of the mechanism by which environmental influences trigger acute porphyria in susceptible individuals will be forthcoming. Genetic variation in these pathways also may go some way to explain the immense variation that individuals show in their susceptibility to the attacks.

Table 12.5.5 Drug classes unsafe in acute porphyrias (some class members may be used)

Amphetamines
Anabolic steroids
Antidepressants (tricyclic and monoamine oxidase inhibitors)
Antihistamines
Barbiturates
Benzodiazepines
Cephalosporins
Steroid contraceptives
Diuretics
Ergot derivatives
Gold salts
Hormone replacement therapy
Progestagens
Sulphonamides
Sulphonylureas

For individually unsafe drugs see Table 12.5.6.
From the British National Formulary (2001).
Published by the British Medical Association and Royal Pharmaceutical Society of Great Britain.

Clinical features of acute porphyria

The clinical manifestations of an acute attack are very diverse and the condition may be indistinguishable from many other disorders. The common neurovisceral symptoms of acute porphyric attacks are listed in Table 12.5.7 and, of these, abdominal pain is the most common presenting symptom. The pain itself may be difficult to identify since it is usually constant but poorly localized and usually unassociated with tenderness. There may be an associated colicky component and later ileus with abdominal distension which may mimic a surgical emergency. Constipation is a characteristic symptom but diarrhoea with increased borborygmi can also occur. The patient is usually markedly distressed and tachycardia is the rule.

Development of pain in the limbs is a frequent feature, particularly in the upper thighs and also in other somatic muscles of the chest, lumbar region, shoulders, and neck. Ultimately, muscle weakness and respiratory paralysis may occur. The patient becomes restless

Table 12.5.6 Individual drugs unsafe in acute porphyria

Alcohol	Erythromycin	Nifedipine
Aluminium-containg antacids	Ethamsylate	Nitrofurantoin
Aminoglutethimide	Ethionamide	Orphenadrine
Amiodarone	Ethosuximide	Oxybutynin
Azopropazone	Etomidate	Oxycodone
Baclofen	Fenfluramine	Oxymetazoline
Bromocriptine	Flucloxacillin	Oxytetracycline
Busulphan	Flupenthixol	Pentazocine
Captopril	Griseofulvin	Phenoxybenzamine
Carbamazepine	Halothane	Phenylbutazone
Carisoprodol	Hydralazine	Phenytoin
Chloral hydrate	Hyoscine	Piroxicam
Chlorambucil	Isometheptene mucate	Prilocaine
Chloramphenicol	Isoniazid	Pyrazinamide
Chloroform	Ketoconazole	Ranitidine
Clonidine	Lignocaine	Rifabutin
Cocaine	Lisinopril[a]	Rifampicin
Colistin	Loxapine	Simvastatin
Cyclophosphamide	Mebeverine	Sulphinpyrazone
Cycloserine	Mefenamic acid	Sulpiride
Cyclosporin	Meprobamate	Tamoxifen
Danazol	Methotrexate	Theophylline
Dapsone	Methyldopa	Thioridazine
Dexfenfluramine	Metoclopramide	Tinidazole
Dextropropoxyphene	Metyrapone	Triclofos
Diclofenac	Miconazole	Trimethoprim
Doxycycline	Mifepristone	Valproate
Enconazole	Minoxidil	Verapamil
Enflurane	Nalidixic acid	Zuclopenthixol

From the British National Formulary (2001).
Published by the British Medical Association and Royal Pharmaceutical Society of Great Britain.
[a] In previous editions. This author has associated the agent with induction of porphyria.
The following drugs are thought to be safe in acute porphyrias:
Antihistamines: cetirizine, chlorpheniramine, cyclizine.
Diuretics: acetazolamide, amiloride, bumetanide, cyclopenthiazide, triamterene.
Ergot derivatives: oxytocin is probably safe.
Sulphonylureas: glipizide.
Analgesics: morphine, diamorphine, codeine, dihydrocodeine, fentanyl, and pethidine are safe.
Tranquillizers: chlorpromazine, haloperidol.
Local anaesthetics: bupivacaine, lignocaine can be used with caution.
Antimicrobials: rifamycins have been used without ill effect in some patients.

or frankly disturbed or deluded as in a toxic confusional state. The inability of attending medical personnel to identify the cause of the pain and the distress associated with it often leads to alienation and an exaggeration of the patient's complaints which may be difficult to diagnose; often a suggestion of hysterical conversion syndrome or worse, malingering, is made by attending staff. Hypertension, sweating, and tremor together with tachycardia indicate marked sympathetic overactivity, and cardiac arrhythmias may ensue. In about 10 per cent of severe attacks grand mal seizures develop, treatment of which may prolong the attack since many anticonvulsants are highly porphyrinogenic. With sustained attacks there may be signs of a peripheral neuropathy that is related to axonal degeneration, principally affecting motor nerves. Peripheral neuropathy in its early stages may not affect the limb and tendon reflexes but with time these will be decreased or absent. In prolonged porphyric attacks, an ascending muscle weakness rapidly affecting the respiratory muscles and diaphragm and with bulbar paralysis may lead to ventilatory failure and death, if lifesaving cardiorespiratory resuscitation and intensive care measures are delayed.

Table 12.5.7 Clinical manifestations of acute porphyria

Abdominal pain
Vomiting
Constipation
Limb, head, neck, and chest pain
Muscle weakness
Sensory loss
Hypertension
Tachycardia
Convulsions
Respiratory paralysis
Fever
Psychiatric symptoms

In a full-blown attack, mental symptoms including anxiety, sleeplessness, and depression are often prominent; the terrifying nature of the illness only aggravates the patient's distress. If the porphyric attack is sustained as a result of failed diagnosis or inadequate management, progressive alienation, visual and auditory hallucinations, and frank paranoia with homicidal outbursts may occur. Such disturbances are difficult to contain within the environment of the busy acute hospital. Although seizures may be a presenting sign of the acute attack, they often occur in association with fulminant hyponatraemia resulting from the inappropriate secretion of antidiuretic hormone and other rapid disturbances of sodium metabolism, including excess renal excretion. Treatment of hyponatraemia due to this cause in the acute attack poses special difficulties (see below). The use of large volumes of hypotonic dextrose will aggravate the hyponatraemia—and seizures—and may induce fatal cerebral herniation due to severe brain oedema.

Diagnosis of the acute attack is suspected on the basis of the past history, including photosensitivity or the intermittent discolouration of urine. The passage of frank wine-coloured or permanganate-coloured urine is unusual but if present indicates a full-blown established attack. The family history is often informative, with a history of abdominal pain in first-degree family members, with or without photosensitivity. Confirmation of an acute attack of porphyria requires the demonstration of increased porphyrin precursors in the urine. Most commonly, increased excretion of the monopyrrole, porphobilinogen, is accompanied by increased excretion of urinary 5-aminolaevulinate. However, porphobilinogen excretion is not increased in the rare aminolaevulinate dehydratase deficiency or in the pseudoporphyria of lead poisoning.

Acute attacks of porphyria appear to be more common in women as a result of changes in sex steroids, and many women who have periodic attacks do so in the 1 or 2 days before the onset of menstrual bleeding; as the menopause approaches, the pattern may worsen, but with the onset of oligomenorrhoea or amenorrhoea, severe attacks of porphyria usually cease. Sometimes, acute attacks lasting a day or two may have their onset in the midmenstrual period around the time of ovulation. Many mild attacks of porphyria resolve spontaneously within a few days, either as a result of withdrawal of the precipitating factor or because of natural hormonal rhythms. Prolonged attacks are usually the consequence of multiple factors and delays in the institution of definitive therapy. The ensuing neurological injury, accompanied in severe attacks by bulbar and respiratory paralysis, may lead to prolonged or permanent disability. Experience shows that in many such cases inappropriate drugs have been given to counter the early manifestations of the condition, e.g. analgesics, psychotropic drugs, and anticonvulsants. Thus the initiating medical interventions ultimately prove to be critical determinants of outcome where the diagnosis is not suspected or, if known, has been perilously ignored.

Outcome

An early series showed that during the first acute attack of porphyria half the patients died. However, perhaps as a result of better hospital facilities to deal with severe or adverse outcomes, the mortality and effects of the disease in patients with acute attacks have improved. Reports from a single centre reported that about three-quarters of patients with acute intermittent porphyria or variegate porphyria were able to lead normal lives after an acute attack. Recurrent attacks of pain occurred only in a minority during a period of prolonged follow-up; these recurrent attacks were most likely to occur in the first 3 years.

The development of national centres for the treatment of porphyria, the early detection of genetic predisposition in at-risk first-degree relatives, and the dramatic reduction in prescriptions of porphyrinogenic drugs, such as barbiturates and sulphonamides, together with better treatment of acute attacks can undoubtedly contribute to improved outcome. Nonetheless, acute porphyria remains life-threatening, and deaths or marked disability due to prolonged, mismanaged, or undiagnosed attacks are all too frequent. Rapidly recurrent attacks of porphyria may be associated with severe motor neuropathy and sustained hypertension; postural hypotension may result from autonomic neuropathy. In severe cases, cranial nerve palsies occur, typically affecting the facial nerve and the vagus nerve. Ischaemia of the occipital cortex during acute attacks has been associated, in several instances, with failed recognition of colours or of human faces (prosopagnosia) and cortical blindness.

Although it appears that progestogens are principally responsible for cyclical or periodic attacks in women and are more porphyrinogenic than oestrogens, pregnancy itself is not invariably associated with adverse outcomes in women at risk from acute attacks. Seizures and hypertension due to acute porphyria may be erroneously attributed to eclampsia. However, drugs that provoke attacks, such as metoclopramide, may be used mistakenly to control gastrointestinal symptoms in pregnancy and thus place the woman and her unborn infant at risk.

Individual porphyrias

Acute porphyrias

These are, in a descending order of frequency: acute intermittent porphyria, variegate porphyria, hereditary coproporphyria, and Doss' porphyria (aminolaevulinate dehydratase deficiency). The first three of these disorders occur in at-risk heterozygotes for a single mutant allele in the cognate gene as autosomal dominant traits; 5-aminolaevulinate dehydratase deficiency is inherited as a very rare autosomal recessive trait.

The overall frequency of heterozygosity for acute porphyrias is estimated to be 1 in 10 000 of the population, of whom only 1 in 5 to 1 in 10 will develop an acute attack. In certain populations (in South Africa and in the Lapps of Northern Sweden) the frequency rises to 1 in 1000 of the population. In South Africa, a high gene frequency results from the founder effects of the migration of a Dutch settler in the 17th century. Variegate porphyria has thus spread to all ethnic groups within the South African population, molecular analysis of which confirms the presence of a single dominant mutant allele of the protoporphyrinogen IX oxidase gene.

In the 2000s very rare homozygous forms of porphyria, where the presence of two mutant alleles of the causative gene are generally responsible for severe clinical disease, have been recognized. In most instances, the condition is not truly homozygous since those individuals affected prove to be compound heterozygotes for two mutant alleles of the cognate gene rather than true homozygotes for the many discrete but rare mutations that occur in porphyria but which would only be expected to occur in consanguineous pedigrees.

Acute intermittent porphyria

This, the most frequent of the acute porphyrias, is caused by mutations in the porphobilinogen deaminase gene that maps to human chromosome 11q23 in which well over 200 mutations have been identified. Several widespread mutations have been identified in certain populations but most are reported in only one or two pedigrees.

Two isozymes of the human porphobilinogen deaminase enzyme occur in the tissues: an erythroid mRNA variant and a nonerythroid transcript that encodes 17 additional amino acid residues in its N-terminus leading to synthesis of a housekeeping ubiquitous isozyme and an erythroid-specific isozyme. Most mutations cause a decrease in the abundance as well as the activity of the porphobilinogen deaminase enzyme in all tissues. A small proportion of mutations associated with lack of the detectable protein product from the mutant allele are associated with reduction of the housekeeping isozyme but normal enzymatic activity of the erythroid-specific isozyme. Thus, in such patients, hepatic porphobilinogen deaminase activity may be reduced to approximately half normal values while the activity of the easily accessed red-cell enzyme is within the normal range.

A few mutations lead to the synthesis of a catalytically impaired but stable porphobilinogen deaminase protein from the cognate mutant allele, but these are a minority. Molecular analysis of the porphobilinogen deaminase gene in patients with acute intermittent porphyria has been very valuable in establishing diagnosis of latent heterozygotes at risk in the affected family, for the provision of appropriate counselling, and for the introduction of preventative strategies (see below).

Acute intermittent porphyria is characterized solely by acute porphyric attacks and cutaneous photosensitivity does not occur. In most instances the patients do not notice any change in their urine, but when the urine is allowed to stand the increased excretion of pyrroles leads to the formation of coloured oxidation products of porphobilinogen (loosely called porphobilin) which may lead to obvious discoloration (Fig. 12.5.2). During the increased excretion of porphyrin precursors water-soluble porphyrins, formed as a result of nonenzymatic photochemical reactions, induce a pink discolouration. During severe acute attacks copious excretion of pyrrole precursors, including porphobilin, may occasionally give the urine a striking appearance resembling blackcurrant juice or strong solutions of potassium permanganate.

The incidence and severity of acute attacks in acute intermittent porphyria and variegate porphyria are generally greater than in hereditary coproporphyria. Various estimates indicate between 1 in 10 to 1 in 5 of heterozygotes experience acute attacks of porphyria during their lifetime. However, increasing use of molecular diagnostic methods for screening at-risk families, institution of appropriate avoidance, and the careful dissemination of information to family members and their medical advisers will further reduce the likelihood of disease in latent gene carriers. Latent carriers of acute intermittent porphyria have a high frequency of hypertension and, although this should be treated, the potential for inducing attacks is increased by the uninformed prescription of antihypertensive drugs. A proportion of patients appear to have depression and other chronic mental symptoms and at least one survey has reported an increased prevalence of acute intermittent porphyria in patients attending long-stay psychiatric facilities, which again puts them at risk from the ill-considered use of porphyrinogenic neuroleptic and other psychoactive drugs.

Variegate porphyria

Variegate porphyria is particularly frequent among white South African people and other ethnic groups within that country. The condition is associated with typical acute attacks of porphyria as well as skin manifestations (the van Rooten skin). Acute attacks of porphyria occur very much as in acute intermittent porphyria. In a series of patients, more than one-half presented with skin lesions alone, one-fifth had acute neurovisceral disease, and a similar proportion had acute attacks as well as cutaneous disease.

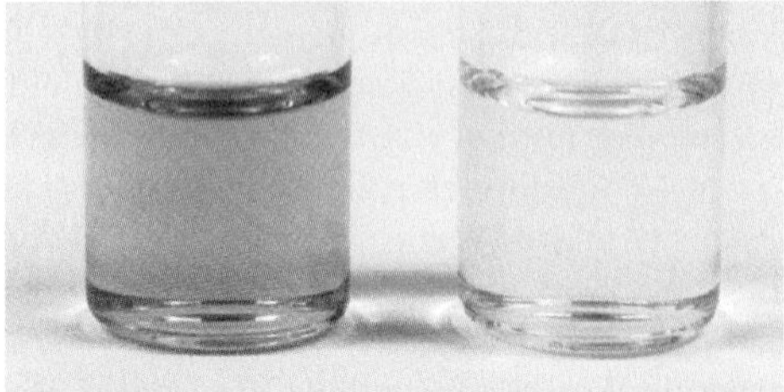

Fig. 12.5.2 Urine from a patient with acute intermittent porphyria around the time of an acute attack (left); control urine (right). A positive reaction with Ehrlich's diazo reagent is shown in the patient's urine following the addition of 50 μl urine to 1 ml of 2 per cent acidic dimethyl benzaldehyde. Subsequent tests showed that the pink diazo adduct was insoluble in chloroform and other organic solvents indicating the presence of excess porphobilinogen. (Urobilinogen in excess may give a positive reaction with the diazo reagent but the product is readily extracted into organic solvents.)

Cutaneous photosensitivity resembles that seen in porphyria cutanea tarda and hereditary coproporphyria (see below) with fragility, milia, hyperpigmentation, and hairiness of light-exposed skin. During acute sunlight exposure, vesicles and even large bullas may form. Microscopic examination of the affected skin shows deposits of immunoglobulin and hyaline material (that stains positively with periodic acid–Schiff reagent) in the dermal capillaries with proliferation of the basal lamina. As with porphyria cutanea tarda, ingestion of reproductive steroid, e.g. the oral contraceptive pill, may induce the cutaneous manifestations of variegate porphyria in otherwise latent heterozygotes.

A few severely affected patients with variegate porphyria have inherited mutations of the protoporphyrinogen oxidase gene (that maps to chromosome 1q22–1q23) from each parent, leading to homozygous 'dominant' variegate porphyria. These individuals present in childhood with a severe phenotype associated with marked photosensitivity, convulsions, and developmental delay; they have several skeletal abnormalities including medially deviated and shortened fifth digits. Developmental retardation is prominent, but surprisingly such patients appear to have few if any attacks of acute porphyria.

Hereditary coproporphyria

This condition is an infrequent and often mild form of acute porphyria which may be associated with cutaneous manifestations. It is due to mutations in the coproporphyrinogen III oxidase gene that maps to chromosome 3q12 and is transmitted as an autosomal dominant trait of low penetrance. The condition usually presents with acute attacks of abdominal pain, as with the other acute porphyrias, and about 30 per cent of patients develop cutaneous photosensitivity. As with some other porphyrias, several children presenting with marked photosensitivity in childhood have been shown to have inherited a mutant allele of the coproporphyrinogen III oxidase gene from each parent giving rise to so-called homozygous dominant hereditary coproporphyria. Particular mutations in the gene are usually restricted to individually infected pedigrees. As with the other acute porphyrias, molecular analysis of the coproporphyrinogen III oxidase gene may be of value in identifying at-risk heterozygotes for genetic counselling and provision of appropriate advice about the prevention and management of symptomatic disease.

5-Aminolaevulinate dehydratase deficiency (Doss' porphyria)

Only a few affected homozygotes for this condition have been identified. Molecular analysis of the cognate gene has revealed the presence of compound heterozygosity and homozygosity for point mutations in the gene which maps to chromosome 9q34. As with the porphobilinogen deaminase gene, there are two promoter regions and alternative noncoding exons that allow for the synthesis of housekeeping and erythroid-specific transcripts. Less than 10 cases of this porphyria have been reported but it seems likely from the individual case histories of those identified that the disease will be under-recognized as the cause of acute abdominal crises usually presenting shortly after puberty and associated with neurological symptoms, including respiratory paralysis. The condition resembles acute lead poisoning. The urine contains an excess of 5-aminolaevulinate but the excretion of porphobilinogen and tetrapyrrolic haem precursors is normal. Heterozygotes for aminolaevulinate dehydratase deficiency have been reported in at least one lead worker in whom peripheral neuropathy was ascribed to simple lead poisoning, but it may have resulted from the susceptibility of the residual 5-aminolaevulinate dehydratase to inhibition by environmental lead.

Cutaneous porphyrias

Congenital erythropoietic porphyria is a classic but very rare syndrome now known to have an astonishing range of presentation from severe haemolytic anaemia *in utero* or severe photosensitivity presenting soon after birth (with excess porphyrins staining the teeth and urine) to mild late-onset forms presenting with skin lesions in adult life. Most patients have a mild to severe haemolysis with increased reticulocytosis, circulating normoblasts, decreased serum haptoglobin, and increased unconjugated bilirubin concentrations. Inclusion bodies are often seen in marrow, erythroid cells, and circulating normoblasts. Splenomegaly develops in childhood, thereby causing pancytopenia as a result of hypersplenism; this accelerates the haemolysis and leads to compensatory erythropoiesis in the bone marrow. Under these circumstances, splenectomy may help to control the condition.

The classic skin manifestations are of severe blistering lesions on sunlight-exposed skin, particularly of the hands and face, with the formation of vesicles and bullas that may become infected. There are pigmentary changes with greatly increased skin fragility. Healing of the lesions with or without consequential infection often leads to cutaneous deformities with loss of digits, scarring of the eyelids, nose, lips, scalp, and occasionally blindness due to corneal scarring. Examination of the teeth shows erythrodontia and deformities, and exposure to ultraviolet light may reveal striking dental fluorescence. The condition is associated with osteoporosis and resorption of long bones as a result of gross expansion of the erythroid bone marrow.

Mutations in the uroporphyrinogen III synthase gene that maps to chromosome 10q25.3–q26.3 have been shown to be responsible for this disease and thus may assist in the prenatal diagnosis of mothers harbouring an at-risk pregnancy and who have previously given birth to an affected infant. Constitutive activation of the haem biosynthetic pathway in erythroid cells leads to persistent overproduction of uroporphyrinogen I and coproporphyrinogen I as by-products of the defective synthesis of uroporphyrinogen III, the sole precursor of protoporphyrin IX and haem. These reduced and colourless metabolites become oxidized to the fluorescent tissue and urinary porphyrins associated with the passage of pink urine that characterizes this often devastating disease.

Congenital erythropoietic porphyria

Several infants and children with congenital erythropoietic porphyria have been successfully treated by haematopoietic stem-cell transplantation and this remains a convincing option for treatment of this very severe and otherwise life-shortening inborn error of haem metabolism.

Porphyria cutanea tarda

This disease is the most common of the cutaneous porphyrias and, unlike other hepatic porphyrias, is never associated with acute porphyric crises. The disease is characterized by skin blistering which is related to sunlight exposure. It occurs in several forms. Porphyria cutanea tarda may result from environmental exposure to dioxin or to hexachlorobenzene, particularly after industrial accidents such as that which occurred in Turkey in the 1960s. Occasional cases have been reported after exposure to other halogenated phenols, but under these circumstances it appears simply to be an environmental toxic syndrome. Toxic cutaneous porphyria appears to be separate from the sporadic porphyria cutanea tarda that is precipitated by other specific environmental factors: increased hepatic storage iron, excess ethanol consumption, administration of oestrogens, hepatitis C virus infection, human immunodeficiency virus infection, and, possibly, nutritional deficiencies including antioxidants such as vitamin C.

Most individuals who develop sporadic porphyria cutanea tarda prove to have increased iron stores in association with the presence of one or more mutant alleles for the *HFE* gene that also predispose to the development of hereditary adult haemochromatosis. In addition, many patients with sporadic porphyria cutanea tarda consume excess alcohol and smoke. There is a clear association between porphyria cutanea tarda and renal impairment in which the development of the disease can be explained by the presence of iron overload (as a result of defective iron utilization with or without routine iron supplementation, particularly in patients on haemodialysis) and failure to excrete excess plasma porphyrins that do not readily diffuse through the peritoneal cavity or haemodialysis membranes. In sporadic porphyria cutanea tarda there is a partial deficiency of uroporphyrinogen III decarboxylase activity in the liver and no family history of the condition. The sequencing of the human uroporphyrinogen decarboxylase gene that maps to human chromosome 1p34 has not provided any evidence of mutations to account for the tissue-specific enzyme deficiency, and no isoforms of the enzyme have yet been identified. At the time of writing the molecular pathogenesis of sporadic porphyria cutanea tarda is unknown, but it is also clear that iron and other environmental influences inactivate hepatic uroporphyrinogen decarboxylase. The relationship between regulators of iron homeostasis and the demand for haem biosynthesis in the hepatocytes of affected individuals is not understood, but it appears likely from studies in experimental animals that genetic variation in the expression and activity of cytochrome isozymes such as P-450 IA2 may be critical for disease expression. Irreversible inhibition of hepatic uroporphyrinogen decarboxylase may also explain the occurrence of toxic porphyria cutanea tarda after exposure to halogenated hydrocarbons, metabolites of which cause experimental uroporphyria in animals.

Less than one-quarter of patients who have porphyria cutanea tarda show a familial susceptibility to the condition. In these cases, mutations occur in one allele of the human uroporphyrinogen decarboxylase gene leading to catalytic deficiency of the enzyme in all cells, including erythrocytes. In most instances the genetic defect leads to partial reduction of the enzyme protein encoded by the mutant allele. Studies of pedigrees affected by familial porphyria cutanea tarda indicate that expressivity of the trait is very low; less than 10 per cent of heterozygotes develop clinical disease. Conversely, a very few patients present with a syndrome that closely resembles congenital erythropoietic porphyria with marked blistering skin lesions, excess hair growth, and cutaneous scarring in association with the excretion of pink or red urine. These individuals represent a homozygous form of uroporphyrinogen decarboxylase deficiency, termed hepatoerythropoietic porphyria, associated with a variety of mutations in the uroporphyrinogen III decarboxylase gene.

In hepatoerythropoietic porphyria, the activity of uroporphyrinogen decarboxylase is markedly deficient, although residual activity

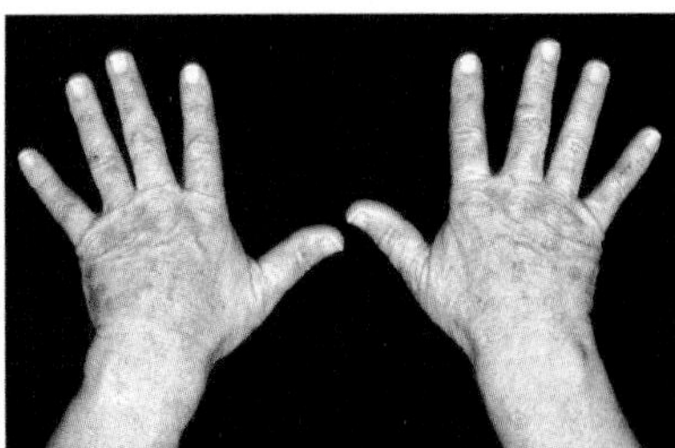

Fig. 12.5.3 Porphyria cutanea tarda in a 60-year-old heterozygote for the *HFE* C282Y mutation. This man, a taxi driver, had noticed irritation after exposure of his hands to light transmitted through the windscreen. He had noticed fragility and blistering combined with pigmentary changes typical of this disorder. After treatment by controlled phlebotomy his skin complaint has regressed.

remains to preserve essential haem biosynthesis in the erythron and liver. Most patients with hepatoerythropoietic porphyria ultimately develop splenomegaly with accelerated haemolysis closely resembling congenital erythropoietic porphyria. Molecular analysis of the human uroporphyrinogen decarboxylase gene may assist the prenatal diagnosis of at-risk pregnancies in women who have already given birth to an affected infant.

The clinical features of porphyria cutanea tarda of whatever form are very characteristic and are confined to light-exposed skin (Fig. 12.5.3). Usually, the only signs are of erosions resulting from minor trauma in skin with increased fragility as a result of light exposure, typically on the dorsum of the hands. Other changes include the development of large subepidermal bullae after exposure to light, which may burst leaving ulcerated lesions that are slow to heal. Increased, often accompanied by areas of decreased, pigmentation is a common feature combined with increased hair growth, particularly on the face.

Patients with porphyria cutanea tarda do not always notice the photosensitivity and rarely experience marked pain unless exposed to brilliant sunlight. Occasionally there is evidence of dermal injury and loss of nails, damage to the conjunctivae, and hair loss. Careful examination of the affected areas shows small depigmented cutaneous scars and the formation of milia. If bacterial infection occurs and there is repeated exposure to sunlight, then severe and permanent scarring may result. Typically, porphyria cutanea tarda occurs in middle-aged men with a history of alcohol use and in women after institution of oestrogen replacement therapy; in young persons, infection with hepatitis C or the immunodeficiency virus may precipitate the disease expression. Frank signs of hepatomegaly or iron overload are rare in porphyria cutanea tarda but have been noted; as with adult haemochromatosis, there is a significantly increased frequency of hepatocellular carcinoma.

Occasionally patients with porphyria cutanea tarda may notice an increase in urine excretion of formed porphyrins which, especially after concentration overnight, may resemble the colour of tea or cola. The stool and urine contain large quantities of coproporphyrins and uroporphyrins that fluoresce intensely on exposure to long-wavelength ultraviolet light when placed in a suitable vessel for its transmission (namely silica rather than standard glass). Similarly, examination of liver biopsy specimens under ultraviolet light reveals bright red/orange fluorescence; microscopic examination may also show coincidental hepatitis with or without excess deposits of stainable tissue iron reflecting the increased iron storage of this disease. In sporadic porphyria cutanea tarda, increased storage iron is reflected by the modest elevations of serum ferritin that often occur in association with the presence of one or more copies of the C282Y allele of the *HFE* gene that maps to human chromosome 6 and which is associated with adult haemochromatosis.

Treatment

Sunlight exposure should be avoided as much as possible until the porphyrin abnormality is corrected. Care is needed to protect fragile skin from mechanical injury and from infection; sunblock creams may also be useful until the metabolic disturbance is controlled.

Patients with porphyria cutanea tarda should moderate or stop their intake of alcohol and avoid the use of iron tonics and sex hormones, especially oestrogens. Screening should be undertaken for chronic infection with human immunodeficiency virus and hepatitis viruses, especially hepatitis C. Management should include imaging or biopsy of the liver if serum liver-related tests are abnormal as well as measurement of α-fetoprotein, since there is a risk of hepatocellular carcinoma in this disease.

Most patients with porphyria cutanea tarda respond to iron depletion by phlebotomy, and initial iron status should be determined by measuring serum ferritin concentrations. Weekly or fortnightly removal of 500 ml of blood will usually correct the abnormal urine and plasma porphyrin profile within a few months but maintenance phlebotomy will be required, usually amounting to the removal of 2 to 4 units of blood at intervals each year. Successful therapy reduces the urinary excretion of porphyrins to normal. Patients with porphyria complicating renal failure should be treated with recombinant human erythropoietin and depleted of iron by gentle phlebotomy or parenteral desferrioxamine, if necessary.

The cutaneous manifestations of porphyria cutanea tarda respond rapidly to low-dose chloroquine treatment, which should be considered in patients with persistent symptoms or at the outset before iron storage has been fully corrected. This action of chloroquine was discovered empirically but the agent forms complexes with uroporphyrin deposits and promotes their external cellular disposal. Chloroquine promotes excretion of uroporphyrin from the liver and induces marked but transient porphyrinuria. Although chloroquine usually provides rapid relief from the cutaneous disease and photosensitivity, it does not correct the underlying metabolic defect in the liver; its long-term use is not recommended unless the other provocative factors in porphyria cutanea tarda have been removed. The usual effective dose of chloroquine is 100 to 200 mg given once or twice weekly; larger doses are associated with marked hepatic toxicity in porphyria cutanea tarda. The drug is reported to have no therapeutic effect on other photosensitive porphyrias.

(Erythropoietic) protoporphyria

Protoporphyria is caused by the overproduction of the immediate precursor of haem, protoporphyrin IX, principally in the bone marrow. Protoporphyria causes an unusual cutaneous photosensitivity syndrome that presents in infancy. Protoporphyria is also a neglected cause of fatal hepatobiliary disease in about 5 per cent of those affected.

Recent studies indicate that protoporphyria is inherited as a recessive condition. Inheritance of mutations in the coding region of the ferrochelatase gene that partially inactivate the enzyme are coinherited in the *trans* isomer with a low-expression allele that occurs at polymorphic frequency in the population. Parent-to-offspring transmission of protoporphyria occurs in less than 10 per cent of cases but in all instances of the disease there is a marked deficiency of the enzyme ferrochelatase (less than 50 per cent of control values). The asymptomatic carrier parent only shows mild ferrochelatase deficiency. The gene for human ferrochelatase maps to chromosome 18q.

Protoporphyria characteristically presents with severe burning pain and cutaneous irritation on exposure to visible light and is usually obvious in infancy or early childhood. Erythema and diffuse oedema may follow marked light exposure but vesicles, blistering, and altered skin fragility are most unusual. After several years, increased pigmentation and thickening of the skin (lichenification) occur, especially over the knuckles. A typical feature is of shallow scarring in the malar regions of the cheeks and at the angle of the lips, where scarring is termed ragades. Overt scarring is unusual. There are no changes in urine colour. Protoporphyria is often the subject of delayed diagnosis because of the marked disparity between the severity of the symptoms and the development of physical signs in the skin.

The cutaneous pathology results from photoactivation of red-cell and plasma-derived protoporphyrin IX in skin capillaries (Figs. 12.5.4 and 12.5.5). Protoporphyrin IX is a hydrophobic molecule that dissolves in cell membranes; it has a photoactivation spectrum in the Soret region with subsidiary activation by green and yellow light. Photoinjury is associated with complement activation and release of vasoactive factors; there is intracellular epidermal oedema accompanied by acute inflammatory changes and extravasated red cells. Deposits of hyaline material are found in superficial capillaries with thickening of the basement membranes. A supply of oxygenated blood appears to be essential for the development of photosensitive damage in protoporphyria.

Mild hypochromic microcytic changes with mild anaemia are usually the only manifestations of disturbed haem biosynthesis and iron metabolism in the bone marrow, although examination of the marrow may reveal occasional sideroblasts with intramitochondrial iron deposits. Haemolysis is usually clinically insignificant until severe cholestatic hepatic disease occurs when splenomegaly and hypersplenism aggravate haemolysis. The photosensitivity worsens under these circumstances and there is upper abdominal pain with splenic enlargement, jaundice, and extreme photosensitivity as concentrations of free protoporphyrin in the plasma rise (Fig. 12.5.5). A vicious cycle of decompensation is established with either fulminant hepatic failure associated with cholestasis due to protoporphyrin deposits within biliary radicals, or the development of cirrhosis. Without treatment, the prognosis is dismal and hepatic transplantation is required (see below).

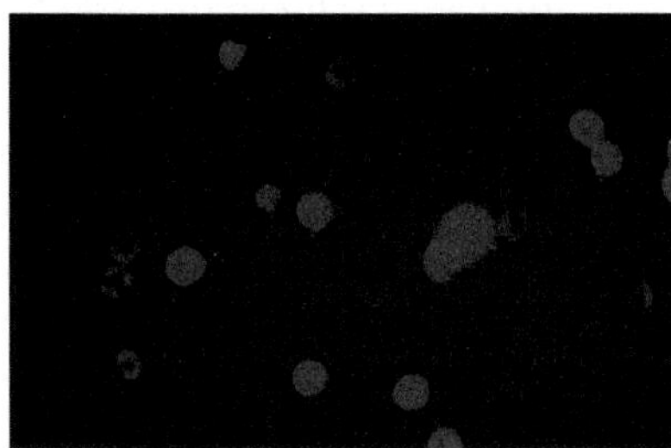

Fig. 12.5.4 Fluorescence microscopy of an unstained blood film from a patient with erythropoietic protoporphyria. Note the fluorescence of increased free protoporphyrin within individual young erythrocytes and reticulocytes.

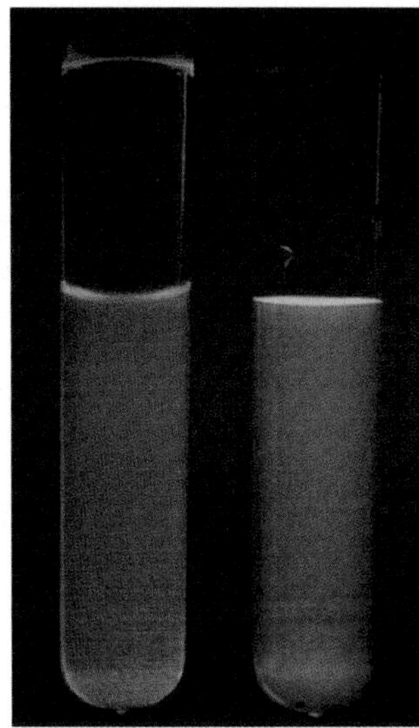

Fig. 12.5.5 Examination of human plasma under long-wave ultraviolet light. Plasma on the left was obtained from a patient with protoporphyrin hepatopathy and greatly increased photosensitivity, and is compared with plasma obtained from a healthy subject on the right. Note the bright red fluorescence due to the presence of high concentrations of free protoporphyrin. Maximum fluorescence was obtained by exposure to visible light in the violet and green–yellow spectral regions, corresponding to the absorbance bands of protoporphyrin.

Protoporphyric hepatic disease

Protoporphyria is normally associated with trivial abnormalities of serum liver-related tests but in a small proportion of patients micronodular cirrhosis with pigment deposition occurs. Examination of the liver under polarized light shows birefringent crystals with a characteristic Maltese-cross appearance and examination under long-wave ultraviolet light reveals bright fluorescence. Gallstones containing precipitated protoporphyrin occur frequently in protoporphyria but cholestasis results principally from intracellular and canalicular precipitation of protoporphyrin.

The principal source of protoporphyrin in protoporphyria is the erythron and although under emergency conditions hepatic transplantation may be effective recurrence of protoporphyrin deposition with injury to the hepatic graft has been reported. The occurrence of this phenomenon, however, is not a contraindication to the use of hepatic transplantation when the illness requires it. Deteriorating hepatic disease is heralded by generalized abdominal pain, splenic enlargement, worsening jaundice, and haemolysis. Interruption of the enterohepatic circulation of protoporphyrin with charcoal or polymeric cationic resins, such as cholestyramine, may arrest the early downhill course by binding protoporphyrin or promoting hepatic bile acid secretion. However, once established, hepatic decompensation and accelerating photosensitivity is rapid.

Surgical management

Severe protoporphyrin hepatotoxicity is an indication for liver transplantation, preferably carried out by an experienced surgical team with the assistance of an informed anaesthetist and expert physicians in attendance. Consideration should be given to the simultaneous removal of the enlarged spleen at the time of the transplantation; there is evidence that splenectomy may reduced the haemolytic component of end-stage protoporphyria.

In some patients with end-stage liver disease due to protoporphyria, a bizarre neurological syndrome has been identified. In the perioperative period, axonal neuropathies requiring mechanical ventilation and cranial nerve palsies have been reported. Under these circumstances, coproporphyrin and uroporphyrins appear in the urine and may account for a blistering photosensitivity in end-stage protoporphyric liver disease.

Operative treatment in patients with protoporphyria can be very dangerous as a result of phototoxic injury to visceral tissues and mucous membranes exposed to brilliant vertical lighting in the operating theatre. Surgical lights are best attenuated by the use of filters that reduce spectral power output below 530 nm; such precautions should be used throughout the perioperative period to reduce overall phototoxicity in the clinical environment. Theoretically, the definitive therapy of protoporphyria will require restoration of erythroid cell ferrochelatase activity in bone marrow. There is a single report of successful marrow transplantation in protoporphyria with coincidental myeloid leukaemia. This procedure cured the symptomatic protoporphyria. In future, either bone marrow transplantation or erythroid progenitor gene therapy will be used to correct this disease in patients with life-threatening liver sequelae. Ancillary treatment by blood transfusion or red cell exchange transfusion will reduce the immediate source of plasma and red-cell protoporphyrin, and in the immediate preoperative period plasmapheresis may also reduce phototoxicity. Neurological complications of fulminant protoporphyria may necessitate prolonged ventilatory support in the postoperative period.

Treatment of photosensitivity

Photosensitivity is managed by avoiding excessive light exposure, remembering that visible light of exciting green and violet wavelengths traverses ordinary window glass. Effective sunscreen preparations may assist management, especially in young children at risk. For many years β-carotene has been given to patients with protoporphyria. β-Carotene may absorb light energy at the appropriate wavelengths and also serve as a free-radical quenching agent. The preparation Lumitene (Hoffmann-La Roche) at a dosage of 120 to 180 mg/day is normally used. This causes orange staining of the skin due to carotenaemia but is otherwise well tolerated. It may improve tolerance to sunlight when plasma carotene concentrations between 10 and 15 μmol/litre are achieved. Increasing melanin formation in the epidermis by narrow-band phototherapy appears to improve light-induced symptoms in patients with protoporphyria. Recently, administration of a depôt preparation of afamelanotide, an α-melanocyte-stimulating hormone analogue, to five patients with protoporphyria, whose tolerance of a standardized source of high-radiance xenon light improved progressively over 120 days, suggests that this agent may usefully ameliorate photosensitivity in the disorder.

Treatment of an acute porphyric attack

It is essential to establish that the symptoms complained of are caused by an acute attack of porphyria. Of key importance is the careful laboratory analysis of urine and blood early in the course of the illness. This demonstrates elevated concentrations of porphyrins and haem precursors typified by elevated urinary 5-aminolaevulinate and porphobilinogen, which should be high in an attack of acute porphyria. The urine sample should be freshly taken from the patient and protected from light before analysis to avoid nonenzymatic conversion of the porphyrin precursors to porphyrins and hence misdiagnosis.

Immediate management of an acute attack of porphyria

An immediate and fastidious review of avoidable factors that would precipitate or aggravate an attack is mandatory. The precipitating factors are usually drugs, alcohol, exogenous or endogenous hormonal changes, fasting (including that due to dieting), or recent surgical procedures. More than 100 drugs may induce attacks of porphyria. Particular care should be taken to exclude agents that are obtained over the counter as tonics or herbal remedies. Tolerance of alcohol varies greatly in patients with porphyria, many of whom appear to tolerate modest amounts of alcohol. Alcohol is, however, best avoided. At the same time it is wise not to implicate alcohol in an acute attack, unless other causes have been excluded.

There is emerging evidence that cigarette smoking, which induces enzymes of the haem-rich cytochrome P_{450} system, is prevalent in patients who have frequent acute attacks of porphyria. The author recommends that persuasive advice to stop smoking is given whenever possible.

Abdominal pain and distress, together with anxiety, require prompt treatment; opiates which are safe in porphyria may be useful, although they often exacerbate constipation. Opiates may be combined with phenothiazine tranquillizers such as chlorpromazine, which may usefully potentiate their action.

Since starvation induces attacks of porphyria and haem biosynthesis may be suppressed by the ingestion of carbohydrate, it is advised that patients with minor attacks should eat regular meals containing carbohydrate in a complex form such as starch for its slow release. One-half to two-thirds of the energy intake should be derived from ingested carbohydrate. The management of an acute attack should involve repeated monitoring for the development of hyponatraemia, which may be very severe as a result of inappropriate secretion of antidiuretic hormone. In the past, intravenous glucose or fructose solutions have been advocated as a means to suppress haem biosynthesis in the liver. Great caution is needed in the use of these agents either as 5 or 20 per cent solutions since they exacerbate hyponatraemia and may cause fatal cerebral oedema. In the author's view, if the patient is sufficiently unwell not to be able to control the attack with oral carbohydrate-rich food, parenteral preparations of haem such as haem arginate, rather than glucose or other sugar solutions, should be administered.

Haem therapy

Haem arginate is administered by a short intravenous infusion in porphyric crises of sufficient severity to merit hospital admission or those associated with limiting pain or metabolic disturbance. Haem arginate (Normosang) supplied by Orphan Europe (see below) is provided as a stable 25 mg/ml concentrate and should be administered at a dosage of 3 mg/kg body weight once daily for up to 4 days to a maximum dose of 250 mg in 100 ml physiological saline infused through a large antebrachial vein over at least 30 min. Haem arginate, like all preparations of haem, tends to polymerize and is unstable; thus the administration should be completed within 1 h after diluting the concentrate. The shelf-life of the concentrate is about 2 years. In the United States of America, haematin is supplied by Abbott Laboratories and appears to be a comparable preparation for suppressing hepatic haem synthesis and correcting the metabolic disturbance of the acute attack. Haem arginate and a preparation of haem albumin are apparently somewhat more stable than haematin, which tends to produce phlebitis or interfere with the action of coagulant proteins.

Recovery from an acute attack depends on the degree of damage to the nervous system and may occur within 1 or 2 days if haem therapy is introduced at the outset. Cast-iron proof of clinical benefit of haem treatment is lacking, but there is sufficient evidence for the beneficial use of therapy for it to be licensed in 19 countries, including the United Kingdom. Haem arginate therapy has a rapid effect on the excretion of aminolaevulinate and porphobilinogen in acute porphyria, and retrospective studies suggest that the outcome of this treatment is better than that in patients previously documented before the use of the agent. Moreover, the results of a double-blind study comparing placebo and haem therapy showed a trend in favour of haem arginate in terms of duration of hospital stay and the requirement for pain relief, but the differences did not quite reach statistical significance in the limited study of 12 patients. On the balance of probabilities, however, the evidence for a beneficial effect of haem arginate therapy, particularly at the onset of a porphyric attack, is very strong.

Haem therapy should be used in any patient with significant hyponatraemia, incipient neuropathy, seizures, or bulbar paralysis, and in any patient with severe symptoms particularly of abdominal pain. It must be recognized that patients with established neuropathy may take many months or even years to recover from an attack and, if it is to be effective, haem therapy should be introduced sufficiently early to halt the progress of the attack. Where haem therapy is not available, parenteral carbohydrate loading is the only alternative treatment for an acute attack; 2 litres of a 20 per cent weight per volume glucose solution is recommended over a 24-h period administered through a central venous catheter. There are risks from giving such therapy as outlined above and in the author's opinion the treatment has been superseded by the introduction of stable preparations of haem. Hypersensitivity reactions to haem arginate are rare and the drug has been used during attacks in pregnant women without injury to either the mother or the child. Haem contains 10 per cent by weight of iron and the maximum daily dose of haem arginate would contain only 23 mg elemental iron; the development of iron storage disease is unlikely, except in very rare instances where an acutely ill patient receives numerous infusions of haematin over prolonged periods.

Occasionally patients, usually women, are seen in whom repeated acute attacks occur irrespective of the use of one or two courses of haem arginate. The reason for this is unknown but it is possible that haem arginate therapy induces tachyphylaxis as a result of exaggerated oscillation of haem catabolism by the induction of haem oxygenase in the liver. For this reason tin protoporphyrin, an inhibitor of haem oxygenase, has been considered. This agent is only available in specialist centres and, because it contains toxic heavy metal and itself may induce photosensitivity, is currently not recommended for routine use. Recently, the combination of recurrent life-threatening porphyric attacks and poor venous access for administration of therapeutic haem preparations has led to the use of liver transplantation in a few young women with this disease. Early (unpublished) reports indicate that this approach may, under exceptional circumstances, be successful. Scrupulous attention to removing all definable risk factors, including smoking, is clearly necessary before such measures are considered.

Young women with cyclical porphyric attacks may benefit temporarily from hormonal intervention by the use of gonadotropin-releasing hormone analogues such as goserelin or buserelin. These agents inhibit androgen, oestrogen, and progestogen production and, as a result, they induce menopausal-like symptoms and depression, as well as rapid decreases in trabecular bone density. Doses sufficient to suppress luteinizing and follicle-stimulating hormone concentrations in serum are required. Prolonged use for more than a few months is not recommended, but buserelin may be used intranasally and may be more convenient. To avoid the worst aspects of hypogonadism in women, low-dose oestrogen therapy under appropriate gynaecological supervision may be coadministered, once cyclical porphyric attacks have come under control. Hypertension is frequent in porphyric attacks and may be very severe as a result of sympathetic overactivity; during the attack, sinus tachycardia is frequent. β-Blockers are effective in the control of the hypertension and labetalol and propranolol are safe; they also relieve the sinus tachycardia.

Hyponatraemia may be very severe and in acute porphyria progresses on a daily basis during the course of the acute attack in most patients. Its management is critical and the rapid onset of severe hyponatraemia clearly contributes to the confusion and other mental symptoms associated with a porphyric attack. Prompt treatment by careful adjustment of fluid balance and fluid restriction is needed. In the presence of hyponatraemia great care should be exercised with the use of intravenous solutions whose prescription should be reviewed frequently. The temptation to place a patient with abdominal pain on a surgical ward and administer a dilute solution of glucose is very great in current hospital practice. In the porphyric attack such management may contribute to death as a result of cerebral oedema or the complications of rapid-onset hyponatraemia. Where hyponatraemia progresses rapidly despite fluid restriction, once the diagnosis of inappropriate secretion of antidiuretic hormone is confirmed by determining urine and plasma osmolalities, hypertonic saline solutions or fluid restriction may be required for its correction.

Grand mal seizures in acute porphyric attacks pose a particular problem for management; they are often precipitated by the hyponatraemia that frequently complicates an acute attack. Clearly appropriate management of the electrolytic abnormality (with the potential for life-threatening cerebral oedema) is an essential element of treatment. Status epilepticus poses special difficulties but has been treated successfully with parenteral diazepam or the related benzodiazepine, temazepam. Carbamazepine, lorazepam, and midazolam are probably (but not definitely) safe in acute porphyria. Clonazepam or valproate have been used for seizure prevention; the generally outmoded therapy of bromide may also have a role. Acetazolamide, which has been used as a minor agent in seizure prophylaxis, has been used safely in acute porphyria but many first-line drugs such as carbamazepine, sodium valproate, phenytoin, and chloral hydrate have been classified as unsafe or are frankly porphyrinogenic. Primidone and phenobarbitone are absolutely forbidden.

Further problems arise in the management of acutely disturbed patients who are not responsive to the safe phenothiazine chlorpromazine. Thioridazine is categorized as unsafe but parenteral haloperidol has been used with good effect in a few patients with uncontrollable or life-threatening manic aggression and paranoid disturbance. In all instances, prescription of any agent to a patient who has had or is having an acute porphyric crisis must involve consultation with a reliable pharmacopoeia with individual drugs categorized for safety.

The ability of most drugs to initiate attacks of porphyria appears in many instances to be related to their effects on the induction of haem biosynthesis in the liver and specifically for the formation of the relevant P-450 xenobiotic-metabolizing isoforms. One key isoform involved in the induction of porphyria is inhibited, at least *in vitro*, by the H_2-antagonist cimetidine. It has been reported that cimetidine at 400 to 800 mg daily is sufficient to inhibit induction of this P-450 isozyme in adult humans. Cimetidine has been administered with occasional success as a means to inhibit or control spontaneous porphyric crises and as a last resort it might be considered in patients with life-threatening and otherwise uncontrollable disease.

There is particular difficulty in young or middle-aged women with cyclical premenstrual attacks. Treatment with high-dose gonadotropins continued for 1 to 2 years is likely to abort the attacks, but given alone will cause distressing symptoms of hypogonadism with depression and osteoporosis. The worst symptoms of hypogonadism can be overcome by the use of low-dose oestrogen replacement, e.g. with oestrogen patches which have a significantly lower risk of provoking an attack of porphyria than progestogen-only hormone preparations. Clearly there is a risk of unopposed oestrogen therapy in patients with an intact endometrium and monitoring for the effects in those receiving oestrogen will be needed.

Acute perimenstrual attacks can be controlled by the prompt administration of haem arginate for 1 to 2 days at the predicted time of susceptibility. Although tachyphylaxis has not been recorded, there may be difficulties in withdrawing the haem arginate because of its effect on inducing haem oxygenase and hence amplifying the potential oscillations of haem biosynthesis in the liver once the haem arginate is withdrawn. The potential for iron overload developing as a result of haem arginate is most unlikely due to its low content of iron at the doses recommended. Some authors have suggested the use of the haem oxygenase inhibitor tin protoporphyrin as an adjunct to the use of haem arginate. Although this may induce a more prolonged biochemical remission of the abnormalities of an acute porphyric attack, it does not induce a more rapid depression of the biochemical abnormality. Experience with tin protoporphyrin where tachyphylaxis of haem arginate is suspected has been favourable in a few patients, but the drug itself induces photosensitivity. Tin is also potentially toxic as a heavy metal of which only limited excretion occurs. At present the use of tin protoporphyrin or its cogener, zinc deuteroporphyrin must remain speculative and more experience is necessary before these agents can be recommended for safe use in the long-term management of patients with recurrent porphyric crises. The role of liver transplantation and, ultimately, corrective gene therapy directed to the liver in acute porphyrias await fuller evaluation in animal models of these diseases and in the few porphyric recipients of hepatic allografts so far recorded.

Sources of information and addresses

British National Formulary, British Medical Association, Tavistock Square, London WC1H 9JP.

United Kingdom and Royal Pharmaceutical Society of Great Britain, 1 Lambeth High Street, London SE1 7JN.

The United Kingdom Drug Information Pharmacists Group website: www.ukdipg.org.uk

Haem arginate (Normosang) is manufactured by Leiras Medica, PO Box 415, SF 20101, Turku, Finland, supplied in the United Kingdom by Orphan Europe (UK) Ltd, 32 Bell Street, Henley-on-Thames, Oxon RG9 2BH. Telephone: 44-(0)1491-414333; Fax: 44-(0)1491-414443; email: info.uk@orphan-europe.com

Patient associations

The British Porphyria Association, 14 Mollison Rise, Gravesend, Kent DA12 4QJ UK. Telephone: 44-(0)1474-350390.

The American Porphyria and Canadian Porphyria Foundations may also be accessed by the internet websites.

Additional information with emphasis on the molecular genetics of individual porphyrias may be found on the Online Mendelian Inheritance in Man (OMIM) website at www.ncbi.nlm.gov/omim

Warning jewellery: it is often valuable in patients with acute porphyrias for them to have a wrist bracelet or neck pendant that provides information about diagnosis in medical emergencies. Details in the United Kingdom can be obtained from The MedicAlert Foundation, 12 Bridge Wharf, 156 Caledonian Road, London N1 9UU. Telephone: 44-(0)207-8333034.

Further reading

Ajioka RS, Phillips JD, Kushner JP (2006). Biosynthesis of heme in mammals. *Biochim Biophys Acta*, **1763**, 723–36.

Anderson KE, *et al.* (1990). A gonadotrophin releasing hormone analogue prevents cyclical attacks of porphyria. *Arch Int Med*, **150**, 1469–74.

Anderson KE, *et al.* (2004). Disorders of heme biosynthesis: X-linked sideroblastic anemia and the porphyrias. In: Scriver CR, *et al.* (eds) *The metabolic and molecular bases of inherited disease*, 8th edition, vol II, pp. 2991–3062. McGraw-Hill, New York. www.ommbid.com. [This is a most comprehensive and up-to-date account of the human biosynthetic pathway in relation to the porphyrias, a large section within a four-volume treatise on inborn errors of metabolism.]

Anderson KE, *et al.* (2005). Recommendations for the diagnosis and treatment of the acute porphyrias. *Ann Int Med*, **142**, 439–50.

Bylesjö I, Wikberg A, Andersson C (2009). Clinical aspects of acute intermittent porphyria in northern Sweden: a population-based study. *Scandanavian Journal of Clinical and Laboratory Investigation* **69**, 612–8.

Collins P, Ferguson J (1995). Narrow-band UVB (TL-01) phototherapy: an effective preventative treatment for the photdermatoses. *British Journal of Dermatology*, **132**, 956–63.

Cox TM (2007). The porphyrias. In: Lomas D (ed) *Horizons in medicine*, vol **19**, pp. 67–83. Royal College of Physicians, London.

Elder GH, Smith SG, Smyth SJ (1990). Laboratory investigation of the porphyrias. *Ann Clin Biochem*, **27**, 395–412.

Elder GH, Hift RJ, Meissner PN (1997). The acute porphyrias. *Lancet*, **349**, 1613–17.

Gorchein A (1997). Drug treatment in acute porphyrias. *Br J Clin Pharmacol*, **44**, 427–34.

Handshin C, *et al.* (2005). Nutritional regulation of hepatic heme synthesis and porphyria through PGC-1α. *Cell*, **122**, 505–15.

Harms J, *et al.* (2009). An α-melanocyte-stimulating hormone analogue in erythropoietic protoporphyria. *New England Journal of Medicine*, **360**, 306–7.

Holme SA, *et al.* (2006) Erythropoietic protoporphyria in the U.K.: clinical features and effect on quality of life. *British Journal of Dermatology*, **155**, 574–81.

Innala E, *et al* .(2010) Evaluation of gonadotropin-releasing hormone agonist treatment for prevention of menstrual-related attacks in acute porphyria. *Acta Obstetrica Gynecol. Scandanvica*, **89**, 95–100.

Kauppinen R, Mustajoki P (1992). Prognosis of acute porphyrias: occurrence of acute attacks, precipitating factors, and associated diseases. *Medicine (Baltimore)*, **71**, 1–13.

Kauppinen R (2005). Porphyrias. *Lancet*, **365**, 241–52.

Mustajoki P, Nordmann Y (1993). Early administration of heme arginate for acute porphyric attacks. *Arch Int Med*, **153**, 2004–8.

Pischik E, Kauppinen R (2009). Neurological manifestations of acute intermittent porphyria. *Cellular and Molecular Biology (Noisy-le-grand)*, **55**, 72–83.

Poh-Fitzpatrick MB (1985). Porphyrin-sensitized cutaneous photosensitivity: pathogenesis and treatment. *Clin Dermatol*, **3**, 41–82.

Schmid R (1998). The porphyrias. *Semin Liver Dis*, **18**, 1–101. [An accessible and comprehensive review of the molecular genetics, biochemistry, clinical features, and treatment of human porphyria.]

Shaw PH, *et al.* (2001). Treatment of congenital erythropoietic porphyria in children by allogeneic stem cell transplantation: a case report and review of the literature. *Bone Marrow Transplantation*, **27**, 101–5.

Soonawalla ZF, *et al.* (2004). Liver transplantation as a cure for acute intermittent porphyria. *Lancet*, **363**, 705–6.

Sylantiev C, *et al.* (2005). Acute neuropathy mimicking porphyria induced by aminolevulinic acid during photodynamic therapy. *Muscle and Nerve*, **31**, 390–3.

Yin L, *et al.* (2007). Rev-erbα, a heme sensor that coordinates metabolic and circadian pathways. *Science*, **318**, 1786–9.

12.6

Lipid and lipoprotein disorders

P.N. Durrington

Essentials

Lipid physiology

Lipids are a heterogeneous group of substances that are distinguished by their low solubility in water and their high solubility in nonpolar (organic) solvents. They are essential as energy stores and respiratory substrates, as structural components of cells, as vitamins, as hormones, for the protection of internal organs, for heat conservation, for digestion, and for lactation.

The main forms of lipid are (1) triglycerides—formed by the esterification of glycerol with fatty acids; provide the body's principal energy store (a 70-kg man contains some 15 kg of stored triglycerides, representing 135 000 kcal of energy); (2) phospholipids—these have at least one fatty acyl group esterified to an alcohol and one phosphate group linked both to the alcohol and to another organic compound; essential components of cell membranes; (3) cholesterol—an essential component of cell membranes; a precursor for the synthesis of steroid hormones, vitamin D, and bile acids.

Lipoproteins—these are macromolecular complexes of lipid and protein: their principal function is to transport lipids through the vascular and extravascular body fluids, and they are also found as components of milk. Their protein components include apolipoproteins and enzymes.

Transport of lipids from the gut to the liver and tissues—this occurs as follows: (1) the products of fat digestion are esterified in the enterocyte, combined with apolipoprotein (apo) B_{48}, and secreted into the lymph (chyle) as chylomicrons; (2) after entry into the blood circulation chylomicrons that have acquired apoC-II (from high-density lipoprotein, HDL) activate lipoprotein lipase, which releases triglycerides to be taken up locally in tissues expressing this lipase; (3) with removal of triglycerides the circulating chylomicrons become smaller and relatively richer in cholesterol and protein; (4) these chylomicron remnants are largely removed from the circulation by the liver, mainly via the 'remnant receptor'.

Transport of lipids and cholesterol from the liver to the tissues—this is important in the fasting state and mainly occurs as follows: (1) the liver secretes a triglyceride-rich lipoprotein known as very low-density lipoprotein (VLDL); (2) these are processed in a similar manner to chylomicrons, with acquisition of apolipoproteins and removal of triglycerides by lipoprotein lipase; but also (3) free cholesterol within VLDL is esterified by a mechanism that involves transfer to high density lipoprotein (HDL) and back to VLDL; and (4) most VLDL is converted to smaller low-density lipoprotein (LDL) particles through the intermediary of intermediate density lipoprotein (IDL); (5) LDL particles deliver cholesterol to the tissues.

'Reverse cholesterol transport'—cholesterol is exported by the gut and liver in quantities which greatly exceed its peripheral catabolism; it gets back from the tissues to the liver via HDL.

Disorders produced by raised concentrations of lipoproteins

The exponential relationship between cholesterol and cardiovascular mortality and morbidity depends on the LDL present. However, except at particularly high levels the risk conferred by LDL is determined by whether or not it is combined with other risk factors (smoking, hypertension, diabetes etc.). Hence cholesterol levels must generally be viewed in the context of an individual's overall risk.

Cardiovascular morbidity and mortality—depending on the LDL cholesterol and its involvement in atherogenesis, there is an exponential relationship between serum cholesterol and the incidence of coronary heart disease within populations. However, the risk conferred by a particular level of cholesterol depends on whether or not it is combined with other risk factors (smoking, hypertension, diabetes, etc.), hence no cholesterol level can be specified which demands a particular therapeutic response: it must always be viewed in the context of an individual's overall cardiovascular risk.

Acute pancreatitis—increase in triglyceride-rich lipoproteins without any increase in LDL is only a modest risk factor for atheroma, but there is an increased likelihood of acute pancreatitis in all types of severe hypertriglyceridaemia.

Particular lipid and lipoprotein disorders

Polygenic hypercholesterolaemia—most hypercholesterolaemia (cholesterol >5 mmol/litre, i.e. 200 mg/dl]) is not due to a single cause, but to some combination of dietary fat, obesity, and individual susceptibility to develop hypercholesterolaemia in the presence of acquired factors such as obesity or a diet high in saturated fat due to overproduction of VLDL by the liver for unknown reasons.

Monogenic familial hypercholesterolaemia—this is dominantly inherited, leads to serum cholesterol concentrations of typically 9 to 11 mmol/litre (350–450 mg/dl), and is due to mutations in the LDL receptor gene. Heterozygotes often have tendon xanthomata, xanthelasmata, corneal arcus at a young age, and premature coronary disease.

Hypercholesterolaemia combined with hypertriglyceridaemia—primary hyperlipoproteinaemia of this type is most commonly due to a polygenic tendency exacerbated by acquired nutritional factors, such as obesity. A rare, severe phenotype can also be caused by decreased clearance of chylomicron remnants and IDL (collectively β-VLDL) at the hepatic 'remnant' (apoE) receptor, when striate palmar xanthomata and tuberoeruptive xanthomata are often seen. Cardiovascular risk is greater for any given level of cholesterol when the serum triglyceride concentration is also elevated.

Severe hypertriglyceridaemia—severe hypertriglyceridaemia ensues when increased hepatic VLDL production, for example due to alcohol excess or diabetes, is associated with decreased triglyceride clearance. Familial lipoprotein lipase deficiency is a rare cause. Eruptive xanthomata are characteristic. Acute pancreatitis may occur when serum triglyceride levels exceed 20 to 30 mmol/litre (2000–3000 mg/dl).

Secondary hyperlipoproteinaemias—these can be caused by diabetes mellitus, obesity, hypothyroidism, chronic kidney disease, drugs, and liver disease.

Management of hyperlipoproteinaemia

Decision to treat—this is not based simply on any particular lipid or lipoprotein value, but on an assessment of individual risk. It is generally agreed that dietary advice to reduce obesity by a decrease in dietary energy intake and to decrease saturated fat consumption is appropriate for all people with LDL cholesterol >2.0 mmol/litre (80 mg/dl), which includes most adults living in the developed world.

Drug treatment—this is justified generally in established atherosclerotic cardiovascular disease, familial hypercholesterolaemia and other severe, monogenic hyperlipoproteinaemias and in diabetes (certainly after the age or forty years and sometimes younger). In other patients cardiovascular risk high enough to warrant statin treatment, (often defined as >20% over 10 years), can be calculated for an individual patient by reference to standard algorithms or charts. The first-line therapy in all forms of hypercholesterolaemia, except that associated with triglyceride levels above 11 mmol/litre (1000 mg/dl), are the statin drugs (3-hydroxy-3-methylglutaryl CoA reductase inhibitors). These should generally be initiated if LDL cholesterol is more than 2.0 mmol/litre (80 mg/dl), with the aim to decrease LDL cholesterol to below this value or by 30%, whichever is the lowest. Other drugs used to reduce cholesterol include bile acid sequestrating agents and ezetimibe (a cholesterol absorption inhibitor). Fibrate drugs are first-line therapy in patients whose hypercholesterolaemia is combined with marked hypertriglyceridaemia, with nicotinic acid (niacin) also used for this indication.

Lipid physiology

Triglycerides (triacylglycerols)

These are formed by the esterification of glycerol with fatty acids, which have a hydrocarbon group attached to a carboxyl group. Generally the hydrocarbon moiety is in the form of a long chain. Naturally occurring fatty acids usually have even numbers of carbon atoms, most of them linked by single bonds, but some contain double bonds. Those with double bonds are termed unsaturated, whereas those with only single bonds are the saturated fatty acids. Fatty acids with one double bond are termed monounsaturated and those with more are termed polyunsaturated. Each double bond creates the possibility of two stereoisomers according to whether the hydrogen atoms of the –CH=CH– are both on the same side of the double bond (*cis*) or on opposite sides (*trans*). Naturally occurring fatty acids are mostly *cis* isomers. *Trans* isomers are, however, present in the milk of ruminants such as the cow and in margarines.

Triglycerides in adipose tissue provide our principal energy store. The body of a 70-kg man contains some 15 kg of stored triglycerides, representing 135 000 kcal (560 kJ) of energy, which would permit survival during total starvation for up to 3 months (compare this with the 225 g of stored glycogen, representing only 900 kcal (3800 J)). Obesity represents an excess of stored fat, and it is unfortunate for those wishing to slim that considerable and very prolonged dietary energy restriction is necessary to lose weight, given the large amount of energy stored in fat. Each gram of triglyceride produces 9 cal (38 J) of energy, whereas the same mass of carbohydrate or protein only produces 4 cal (17 J), and the latter are more difficult to store because they require an aqueous environment. Thus a muscle or liver cell can only store a minimal amount of glycogen whereas the adipocyte contains a droplet of hydrophobic triglyceride surrounded by only a tiny rim of cytoplasm and about 85% of the cell is triglyceride. Thus each gram of adipose tissue yields almost 8 cal (33 J) of energy, whereas tissues containing cells packed to capacity with glycogen would not even approach a yield of 1 cal (4.2 J) for each gram.

For other organs to utilize the energy in adipose tissue the stored triglyceride must first be hydrolysed to its constituent glycerol and nonesterified fatty acids, a process known as lipolysis. This is accomplished by adipose tissue lipase, an intracellular enzyme which is inhibited by insulin. This enzyme is not to be confused with lipoprotein lipase, an extracellular enzyme located on the vascular endothelium of fat and muscle and which is activated by insulin (see below).

The products of lipolysis are released into the circulation and nonesterified fatty acids bind to albumin. The normally circulating concentration of nonesterified fatty acids is 300 to 800 μmol/litre (8–23 mg/dl), but this falls when insulin is secreted following a meal and rises in starvation when insulin secretion is low. The importance of these fatty acids as a system for transporting lipid energy should not be underestimated, even at low concentrations, since their half-life in the circulation is only 2 to 3 min and their turnover is thus 100 to 200 g/day, and even more in starvation or uncontrolled diabetes.

Nonesterified fatty acids can be oxidized to acetyl CoA by some tissues, such as muscle and liver, and then entered into the Krebs (tricarboxylic acid) cycle. Other tissues, which in the fed state rely on glucose as an oxidative substrate, cannot directly utilize nonesterified fatty acids. During starvation these tissues are supplied with water-soluble ketone bodies (acetone, acetoacetate, β-hydroxybutyrate), which the liver produces by partial oxidation (β-oxidation) of nonesterified fatty acids transported to it from adipose tissue. These ketone bodies, which can readily be entered into the Krebs cycle by tissues lacking the ability to oxidize fatty acids, constitute the second system for the transport of lipid energy. They are vital for survival when dietary energy is at a premium, but are also the cause of diabetic ketoacidosis when insulin production is insufficient to suppress the flux of nonesterified fatty acids from adipose tissue, so that the production of ketone bodies takes place at a faster rate than they can be respired. The amount of insulin required to decrease blood glucose increases in the presence of high levels of circulating nonesterified fatty acids. The higher flux of nonesterified fatty acids out of adipose tissue in diabetes thus contributes to insulin resistance. In the case of type 2 diabetes a high rate of release of nonesterified fatty acids may have predated the development of hyperglycaemia by many years because obesity, which is a common antecedent of this type of diabetes, is itself associated with an increased flux of nonesterified fatty acids through the circulation and with insulin resistance.

Phospholipids

These have at least one fatty acyl group esterified to an alcohol and one phosphate group linked both to the alcohol and to another organic compound. The glycerolipids have glycerol as the alcohol. Examples of these are phosphatidylcholine (lecithin) and lysophosphatidylcholine (lysolecithin). Another abundant class of phospholipids is the sphingolipids, such as sphingomyelin. Phospholipids are essential components of cell membranes and, because of the great diversity of physical properties permitted by their structure, are responsible for much of the variation in membrane structure.

Cholesterol

Cholesterol is also an essential component of cell membranes where it allows the phospholipid molecules to pack more closely thus increasing membrane rigidity. It is also a precursor for the synthesis of steroid hormones, vitamin D, and bile acids. It is present in arterial fatty streaks and in atheromatous plaques (see below).

Cholesterol is an alcohol and may be unesterified as free cholesterol or esterified with a fatty acyl group (Fig. 12.6.1).

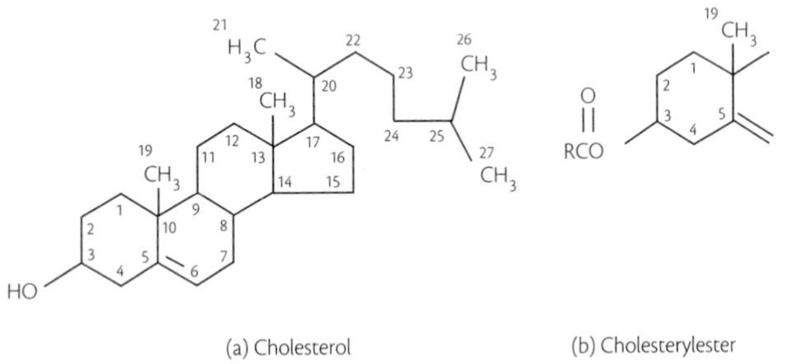

(a) Cholesterol (b) Cholesterylester

Fig. 12.6.1 The structure of free cholesterol and cholesteryl ester.

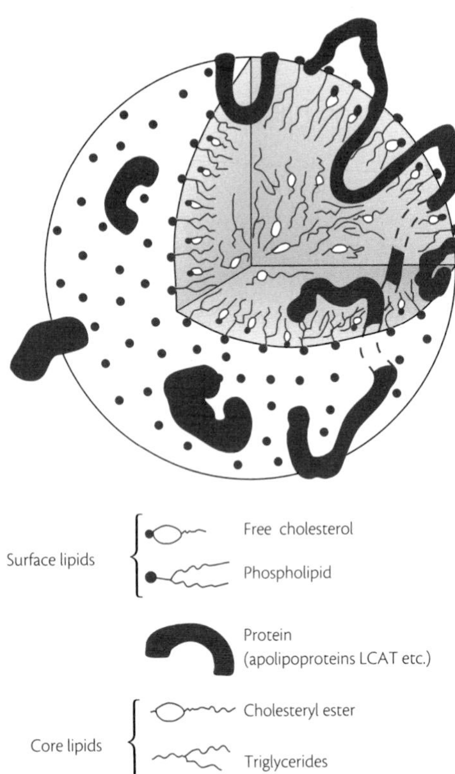

Fig. 12.6.2 Lipoprotein structure. The most hydrophobic lipids (triglycerides, cholesteryl esters) form a central droplet-like core that is surrounded by more polar lipids (phospholipids, free cholesterol) at the water interface. Apolipoproteins are anchored by their more hydrophobic regions, with their more polar regions often exposed to the surface.
(From Durrington (2007) with permission.)

Lipoprotein physiology

Lipoprotein structure

The general structure of lipoprotein molecules is globular (Fig. 12.6.2). The physicochemical considerations, which govern the arrangement of their constituents, are similar to those involved in the formation of mixed micelles in the lumen of the intestine. Thus, within the outer part of the lipoprotein are found the more polar lipids, namely the phospholipids and free cholesterol, with their charged groups pointing out towards the water molecules. In physical terms, however, the role of bile salts, which are also in the outer layer in the mixed micelle, is assumed by proteins, so that the surface structure of a lipoprotein resembles the outer half of a cell membrane. Within the core of the lipoprotein particle are the more hydrophobic lipids, the esterified cholesterol, and triglycerides. These form a central droplet to which are anchored, by their hydrophobic regions, the surface-coating molecules, phospholipids, free cholesterol, and proteins. The exception to this general structure is the newly formed or nascent high-density lipoprotein (HDL), which lacks the central lipid droplet and appears to exist as a disc-like bilayer consisting largely of phospholipids and proteins.

The protein components of lipoproteins are the apolipoproteins, a group of proteins of immense structural diversity, some of which have a largely structural role and others of which are important metabolic regulators. In addition, enzymes are found as components of lipoproteins. One example is lecithin:cholesterol acyltransferase (LCAT) which is located on HDLs that are also its site of action.

Lipid transport from liver and gut to peripheral tissues

The products of fat digestion (fatty acids, monoglycerides, lysolecithin, and free cholesterol) enter the enterocytes from the mixed micelles. They are re-esterified in the smooth endoplasmic reticulum of these cells. Long-chain fatty acids (those with more than 14 carbon atoms) are esterified with monoglycerides to form triglycerides and with lysolecithin to form lecithin. Free cholesterol is esterified by the enzyme acyl CoA:cholesterol *O*-acyltransferase.

The triglycerides, phospholipids, and cholesteryl esters are then combined with an apolipoprotein, known as apoB-48, in the enterocyte. The lipoproteins thus formed are secreted into the lymph (chyle) as chylomicrons. These are large (diameter >75 nm, density <950 g/litre) and are rich in triglycerides but contain only relatively small amounts of protein (Fig. 12.6.3). They travel through the lacteals to join lymph from other parts of the body and enter the blood circulation via the thoracic duct. In addition to cholesterol absorbed from the diet, the chylomicrons may also receive cholesterol that has been newly synthesized in the gut or transferred from other lipoproteins present in the lymph and plasma. The newly secreted or nascent chylomicrons receive C apolipoproteins from HDL, which in that respect appears to act as a circulating reservoir since later in the course of the metabolism of the chylomicron

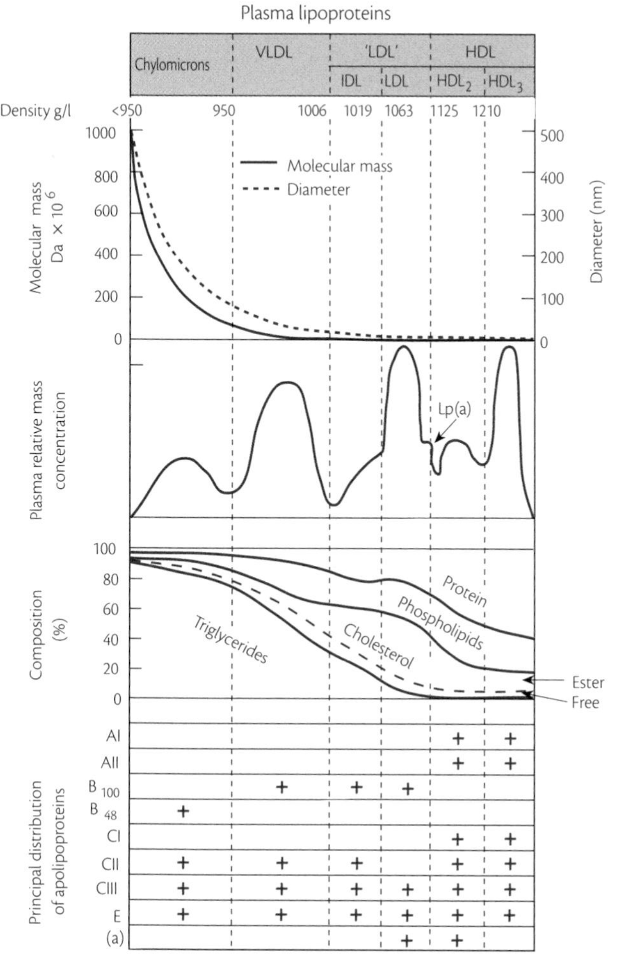

Fig. 12.6.3 The spectrum of plasma lipoprotein particles according to their hydrated density, molecular mass, molecular diameter, relative concentration, lipid composition, and apolipoprotein composition.
(From Durrington (2007) with permission.)

the C apolipoproteins are transferred back to the HDL pool. The chylomicrons also receive apolipoprotein E (apoE), although the manner in which they do so is unclear. Unlike other apolipoproteins, which are synthesized either in the liver or the gut or both, apoE is exceptional in that it is synthesized (and perhaps secreted) by a large number of tissues: liver, brain, spleen, kidney, lungs, and adrenal gland.

Once the chylomicron has acquired the apolipoprotein apoC-II it is capable of activating lipoprotein lipase (Fig. 12.6.4a). This enzyme is located on the vascular endothelium of tissues with a high requirement for triglycerides, such as skeletal and cardiac muscle (for energy), adipose tissue (for storage), and lactating mammary gland (for milk). Lipoprotein lipase releases triglycerides from the core of the chylomicron by hydrolysing them to fatty acids and glycerol, which are taken up by the tissues locally. In this way the circulating chylomicron becomes progressively smaller. Its triglyceride content decreases and it becomes relatively richer in cholesterol and protein. As the core shrinks, its surface materials (phospholipids, free cholesterol, C apolipoproteins) become too crowded and they are transferred to HDL. The cholesteryl ester-enriched, triglyceride-depleted product of chylomicron metabolism is known as the chylomicron remnant. The apoB-48, present from the time of assembly, remains tightly anchored to the core throughout. The apoE also remains and regions of its structure are exposed, permitting chylomicron remnant catabolism via the 'remnant receptor' of the liver and also the low-density lipoprotein (LDL) receptors, which can be expressed by virtually every cell in the body including the liver. The 'remnant receptor' involves the LDL receptor-related protein, LRP, which in addition to its binding site for apoB also has receptor sites for other proteins. ApoE is inhibited from binding to its receptors earlier in the metabolism of chylomicrons because its receptor-binding domain is blocked by the apolipoprotein, apoC-III. Remnants are largely removed from the circulation by the liver. Although the clearance of these particles by the LDL receptor is theoretically possible, this route is not likely to contribute greatly to remnant uptake in the adult since the binding of remnant particles to LRP is enhanced by a trapping mechanism involving heparan sulphate in the space of Disse, whereas elsewhere the remnant particles must compete for binding to the LDL receptor with LDL, the particle concentration of which is much higher than that of the chylomicron remnants (even more so in the tissue fluid than in the plasma). Also the LDL receptor is rapidly down-regulated by the lysosomal release of free cholesterol into the cell, which follows the entry of lipoprotein–receptor complexes into the cell, whereas expression of the remnant clearance pathway is unaffected by entry of cholesterol into the liver.

The liver itself secretes a triglyceride-rich lipoprotein known as very low density lipoprotein (VLDL) which allows the supply of triglycerides to tissues in the fasting state as well as postprandially. VLDL particles are somewhat smaller than the chylomicrons (diameter 30–75 nm, density <1006 g/litre). Once secreted they undergo exactly the same sequence of changes as chylomicrons, i.e. the acquisition of apolipoproteins and the progressive removal of triglycerides from their core by the enzyme lipoprotein lipase. However, some additional transformations are involved in their metabolism in the human. The human liver, unlike the human gut and the liver of other animal species such as the rat, does not esterify cholesterol before its secretion. Most of the cholesterol released from the liver each day into the circulation is thus

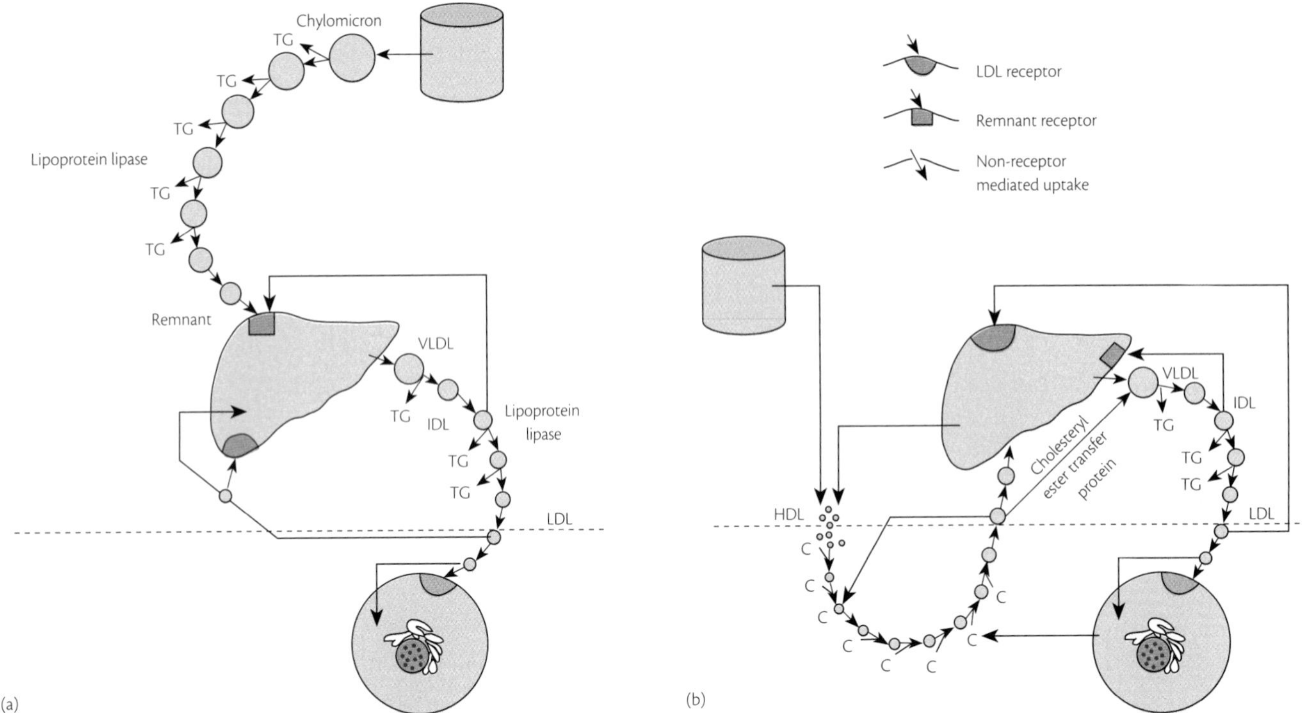

Fig. 12.6.4 Metabolism of (a) triglyceride-rich lipoproteins secreted by the gut and liver, and (b) hepatic triglyceride-rich lipoproteins and lipoproteins transporting cholesterol to and from the tissues.

secreted in the VLDL as free cholesterol, and it undergoes esterification in the circulation. Free cholesterol is transferred to HDL along a concentration gradient. There it is esterified by the action of lecithin:cholesterol acyltransferase, which esterifies the hydroxyl group in the 3-position of cholesterol to a fatty acyl group. This it selectively removes from the 2-position of lecithin to give lysolecithin. The fatty acyl group in this position is generally unsaturated and the cholesteryl esters thus formed are frequently cholesteryl oleate or cholesteryl linoleate.

Esterified cholesterol on HDL is transferred back to VLDL. This cannot take place by simple diffusion, because cholesteryl ester is intensely hydrophobic and because the concentration gradient is unfavourable. A special plasma protein, cholesteryl ester transfer protein (CETP) or lipid transfer protein, transports cholesteryl ester from HDL to VLDL. It does this in exchange for triglycerides in VLDL and thus also contributes to the removal of core triglycerides from VLDL. The principal mechanism for the removal of triglycerides from VLDL is, however, lipolysis catalysed by lipoprotein lipase.

Another major difference between VLDL and chylomicrons is that the apoB produced by the human liver is not apoB-48 but is almost entirely apoB-100. As in the case of chylomicrons, the quantum of apoB packaged in the VLDL remains tightly associated with the particle until its final catabolism; its amount does not vary after secretion. Each molecule of VLDL contains one molecule of apoB-100. The apoB-100 produced in the liver contains the protein sequence necessary to bind to the LDL receptors, whereas that produced by the gut, although derived from the same gene, does not; a process of 'gene editing', which stops the ribosome translating the messenger RNA before the receptor-binding sequence, leads to an apoB with 48% of the molecular mass of that from the liver. Microsomal triglyceride transfer protein is essential for the process by which both apoB-48 and apoB-100 are packaged with triglyceride in the enterocyte and hepatocyte to form chylomicrons or VLDL, respectively; this is defective in abetalipoproteinaemia (see below).

The circulating VLDL particles become progressively smaller as their core is removed by lipolysis and surface materials are transferred to HDL. In humans most of the VLDL is normally converted to smaller LDL particles through the intermediary of a lipoprotein known as intermediate-density lipoprotein (IDL). This has a density of 1006 to 1019 g/litre and contains apoE. In this latter respect it is similar to chylomicron remnants. In some species, such as the rat, it is largely removed by the hepatic receptors, and LDL formation is thus bypassed. The enzyme hepatic lipase may be important in the conversion of IDL to LDL.

In humans, LDL particles, which are relatively enriched in cholesterol but are small enough (diameter 18–25 nm, density 1019–1063 g/litre) to cross the vascular endothelium and enter the tissue fluid, serve to deliver cholesterol to the tissues. Their concentration in the extracellular fluid is probably about 10% of that in the plasma. Cells require cholesterol for membrane repair and growth and, in the case of specialized tissues such as the adrenal gland, gonads, and skin, as a precursor for the syntheses of steroid hormones and vitamin D. LDL is able to enter cells by two routes making a major contribution to its catabolism: one which is regulated according to the cholesterol requirement of each individual cell and one which appears to depend almost entirely on the extracellular concentrations of LDL.

The first of these two routes is by the LDL receptor, a cell-surface receptor which specifically binds lipoproteins that contain apoB-100 or apoE. As mentioned previously, the receptor, although capable of binding apoE-containing lipoproteins, in practice binds mainly to the apoB-100-containing lipoproteins, of which LDL is the most widely distributed. After binding, the LDL–receptor complex is internalized and undergoes intracellular lysosomal degradation. The apoB moiety is hydrolysed to its constituent amino acids, and the cholesteryl ester is hydrolysed to free cholesterol. The release of this free cholesterol is the signal which regulates the cellular cholesterol content by three coordinated reactions. First the enzyme which is rate-limiting for cholesterol biosynthesis (3-hydroxy-3-methylglutaryl-CoA reductase) is repressed, thus effectively centralizing cholesterol biosynthesis to organs such as the liver and gut. Second, the synthesis of the LDL receptor itself is suppressed. Third, acyl CoA:cholesterol *O*-acyltransferase is activated so that any cholesterol that is surplus to immediate requirements can be converted to cholesteryl ester, which because of its hydrophobic nature forms into droplets within the cytoplasm and is thus conveniently stored. The effect of the lysosomal release of free cholesterol on the expression of the LDL receptor contrasts with its effect on the hepatic remnant receptor, which is not subject to any similar down-regulatory process. Free cholesterol released by lysosomal digestion of cholesteryl ester-rich, apoE-containing lipoproteins entering the hepatocyte via LRP does not influence LRP expression, but it will, nevertheless, down-regulate the hepatic LDL receptors. Defective uptake of LDL by the LDL receptor is the basis of familial hypercholesterolaemia (see below).

The other quantitatively important mechanism by which LDL cholesterol may enter cells is by a non-receptor-mediated pathway; LDL binds to cell membranes at sites other than the LDL receptors and some of it passes through the membrane by pinocytosis. The absence of a receptor means that the 'binding' is of low affinity and thus, at low concentrations, LDL entry by this route may have little significance. However, unlike receptor-mediated entry, non-receptor-mediated LDL uptake is not saturable, but continues to increase with increasing extracellular LDL concentrations. When LDL levels are relatively high, entry of cholesterol into the cells by this route may thus assume greater quantitative importance than that via the LDL receptor, which will be both saturated and down-regulated. This appears to be the situation in the typical adult consuming a high-fat diet whose LDL cholesterol is high compared with most animals and in whom only about one-third of LDL is catabolized by receptors and two-thirds by non-receptor-mediated pathways. In hypercholesterolaemia, an even greater proportion of LDL is catabolized via the non-receptor pathway (four-fifths in patients heterozygous for familial hypercholesterolaemia, virtually all in homozygotes; see below).

LDL may also be removed from the circulation by receptors other than the classic LDL receptor. These are probably responsible for the catabolism of only relatively minor amounts of LDL, but two groups of receptors present on the macrophage have excited considerable interest because they are pertinent to atherogenesis. They are the β-VLDL receptor, a modified LDL receptor that allows the uptake of the β-migrating VLDL in patients with type III hyperlipoproteinaemia (see below), and the scavenger or oxidized LDL receptors that permit the uptake of modified LDL by macrophages. Uptake by these receptors is so rapid that foam cells resembling those in arterial fatty streaks and atheromatous lesions are formed *in vitro*. On the other hand, uptake of unmodified LDL by macrophages via the LDL receptor is too slow to allow foam cells to be formed. Modifications of LDL, which may occur *in vivo* and allow macrophage scavenger receptor uptake, are thus of potential relevance to atherogenesis; these are oxidation and glycation (see below).

Lipoprotein(a)

The protein moiety of lipoprotein(a) (Lp(a)), like that of LDL, contains apoB-100, but in addition apolipoprotein(a) (apo(a)) is also present disulphide linked to the apoB-100. The exact location of Lp(a) in the LDL and HDL2 (see below) varies from individual to individual, as does its serum concentration. It may be undetectable in some people or present at concentrations equalling those of LDL in others. Apo(a) contains amino acid sequences homologous to plasminogen. Part of its plasminogen-like protein sequence (the kringle 4 domain) is repeated many times. The number of these repeats, which is determined at a genetic locus adjacent to the plasminogen gene, determines the molecular mass of apo(a), and individuals expressing polymorphisms with fewer kringle 4 repeats have the highest serum concentrations of Lp(a). Lp(a) is associated with the risk of coronary heart disease in individuals of European origin, particularly when serum cholesterol levels are also raised and when there is a family history of premature coronary heart disease. Lp(a) does not give rise to fibrinolytic activity because of amino acid differences in the region of its structure resembling the active site of plasminogen. It has been proposed that it may interfere with thrombolysis. Furthermore, because Lp(a) binds to many different cells and connective tissue matrices, it is retained in the arterial wall longer than LDL and is thus more likely to be oxidized and taken up by macrophages, leading to atheroma (see below).

Transport of cholesterol from tissues back to liver

Cholesterol is exported by the gut and liver in quantities which greatly exceed its peripheral catabolism (largely conversion to steroid hormones and sebum). Therefore, except when the requirement for membrane synthesis is high, e.g. during growth or active tissue repair, the greater part of the cholesterol transported to the tissues (if it is not to accumulate there) must be returned to the liver for elimination in the bile, as bile acids and faecal sterols, or for reassembly into lipoproteins. The return of cholesterol from the tissues to the liver is termed 'reverse cholesterol transport'. It is less well understood than the pathways by which cholesterol reaches the tissues but it may well be critical in the development of atheroma. HDL has many features that make it very likely that it is directly involved in the reverse transport process.

The precursors of plasma HDL (nascent HDL) are disc-shaped bilayers composed largely of protein and phospholipid secreted by the gut and liver (Fig. 12.6.4b). These are small enough to cross the renal glomerulus where they are catabolized in the proximal convoluted tubule. To survive in the circulation the newly secreted HDL must rapidly expand in size through the formation of a central core of cholesteryl ester. It acquires this in two stages. First it receives unesterified cholesterol which leaves cells through a channel called the ATP binding cassette A1 (ABCA1). Most of this cholesterol comes from the liver, but excess tissue cholesterol, e.g. that accumulating in macrophages, can also be acquired by HDL through ABCA1. Homozygosity or compound heterozygosity for mutations in the *ABCA1* gene causes analphalipoproteinaemia (Tangier disease, see below) in which nascent HDL disappears rapidly from the circulation due to renal catabolism before it can acquire cholesterol.

The newly acquired unesterified cholesterol enters the surface layer of the HDL molecule with its more hydrophilic hydroxyl group oriented outwards. The enzyme lecithin:cholesterol acyltransferase

(LCAT) located within HDL then esterifies this hydroxyl group (Fig. 12.6.1) with a long-chain fatty acid, usually oleate or linoleate from the Sn2 position of lecithin (phosphatidylcholine). The resulting strongly hydrophobic cholesteryl ester then moves away from the surface where it was in contact with water to enter the central droplet-like core of the HDL molecule which thus becomes globular. In familial LCAT deficiency HDL acquires unesterified cholesterol, but its core cannot develop and, as in Tangier disease, it is rapidly catabolized by the kidney. Unlike Tangier disease, however, proteinuria and renal impairment ensue associated with presence of cholesterol laden macrophages in the glomeruli (see below)

Components of HDL are also derived from surplus surface material (phospholipids, free cholesterol, and apolipoproteins) from triglyceride-rich lipoproteins released as their triglyceride core shrinks as a consequence of lipolysis. ApoA-I and apoA-II, the major apolipoproteins of HDL, and apoE have been identified in nascent HDL. Other apolipoproteins and the bulk of its lipid are acquired as it circulates through the vascular and other extracellular fluids. In this respect the transformation of HDL from its lipid-depleted precursor to a relatively lipid rich molecule is the inverse of that undergone by other lipoproteins following their secretion.

Even the mature HDL particle is small compared to other lipoproteins (diameter 5–12 nm, density 1063–1210 g/litre) and easily crosses the vascular endothelium, so that its concentration in the tissue fluids is much closer to its intravascular concentration than is the case for LDL. Because the serum HDL cholesterol concentration is only about one-quarter that of LDL, it is often wrongly assumed that its particle concentration is lower. In fact, the particle concentrations of HDL and LDL in human plasma are often similar, and in the tissue fluids there are several times as many HDL molecules as those of other lipoproteins unless the capillary endothelium is fenestrated. Generally, therefore, cells are in contact with higher concentrations of HDL molecules than of any other lipoprotein. This probably accounts for the presence on HDL of the enzyme paraoxonase 1, which appears to remove oxidized lipids that might otherwise damage outer cell membrane proteins or the apoB of LDL.

Cholesteryl ester can leave mature HDL by at least two mechanisms. In the circulation it can be transferred from HDL to VLDL and larger LDL particles in exchange for triglyceride by CETP. When circulating VLDL levels are high there is increased CETP activity leading to low HDL cholesterol levels. On the other hand, in familial CETP deficiency almost all serum cholesterol may be HDL cholesterol. By transferring cholesteryl ester to VLDL, which is itself the precursor for LDL, CETP could be seen as proatherogenic. On the other hand, because much of the LDL is cleared by the liver, CETP could be viewed as contributing to reverse cholesterol transport.

The other mechanism by which HDL can dispose of its cholesteryl ester is via the hepatic scavenger receptor B1. This receptor mechanism can remove cholesteryl ester from HDL during its passage through the liver without catabolizing the whole HDL particle. It thus contributes directly to the reverse cholesterol transport function of HDL.

It is incorrect to regard HDL as a single homogeneous species, since it is known to be a mixture of particles differing in size, in lipid and apolipoprotein composition, and in function. Two main species can be resolved by ultracentrifugation, the less dense of which is designated HDL2 (density 1063–1125 g/litre) and the more dense HDL3 (density 1125–1210 g/litre). HDL3 may be converted to HDL2 by the acquisition of cholesterol, HDL3 thus being a precursor of HDL2. Whereas antisera to apoA-I precipitate virtually all of the HDL, antisera to apoA-II do not, suggesting that some molecules of HDL contain apoA-I and apoA-II, whereas others contain only apoA-I. The apoA-I-only HDL molecules, which predominate in HDL2, may arise from different metabolic channels than do the apoA-I/A-II particles. HDL containing apoE may also have a different metabolic fate, e.g. in the fetus and in the central nervous system it, rather than LDL, may constitute the major system delivering cholesterol to the tissues. Furthermore, HDL may contain other molecular species with overlapping density ranges, such as Lp(a); it is thus a highly diverse lipoprotein class.

Disorders produced by raised concentrations of lipoproteins

The incidence of coronary heart disease varies greatly in different parts of the world. Those countries with a northern European culture (and in particular diet) have the highest rates and China, Japan, and rural Africa the lowest. Mediterranean countries are intermediate. There are, of course, many differences between these countries, but the variable that relates most closely to coronary heart disease is the median serum cholesterol of the middle-aged male population. It is of considerable interest that in a country such as Japan, where the average serum cholesterol is low, other coronary risk factors do not seem to operate. Thus in Japan coronary

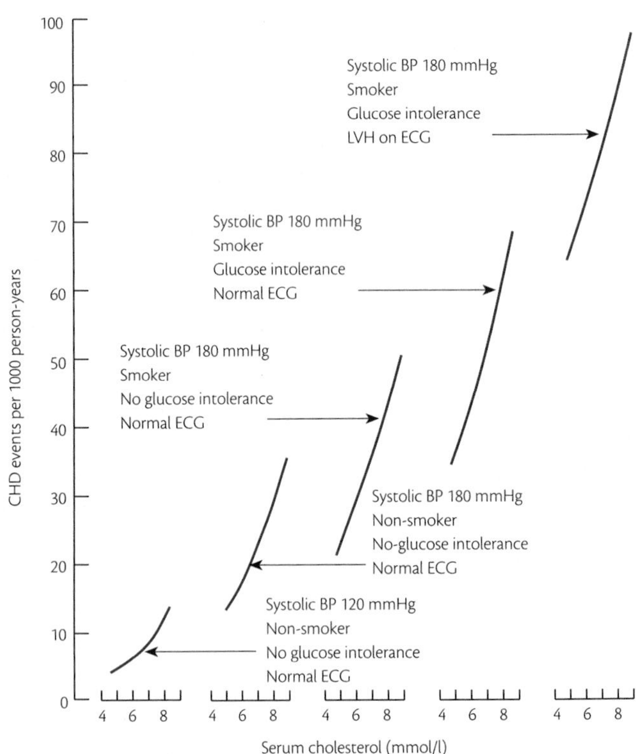

Fig. 12.6.5 The probability of 50-year-old men developing coronary heart disease each year as a function of serum cholesterol concentration, in the absence and in the presence of increasing numbers of risk factors.

(Data from Kannel WB, et al. (1973). *The Framingham Study. An epidemiological investigation of cardiovascular disease. Section 28: the probability of developing certain cardiovascular diseases in eight years at specific values of some characteristics*. Publication 74-618, US Department of Health Education and Welfare. Government Printing Office, Washington DC.)

heart disease is comparatively uncommon, even in cigarette smokers and people with diabetes and hypertension.

Within populations there is an exponential relationship between serum cholesterol and the incidence of coronary heart disease (Fig. 12.6.5). This depends on the LDL cholesterol which comprises some 70 to 80% of the total cholesterol in men and a little less in women. The greater part of the residual cholesterol in serum is on HDL, and the concentration of this HDL cholesterol is inversely related to the likelihood of developing coronary heart disease.

In populations in which death from coronary heart disease is common, fatty streaks are evident in the arteries, such as the aorta, of men dying in their late teens of causes unrelated to cardiovascular disease. This was noted in American casualties of the Korean and Vietnam wars. The fatty streak is the precursor of atheroma (see Section 16). The epidemiological and histopathological evidence implicating LDL in atherogenesis seems overwhelming. Yet in tissue culture, LDL uptake by macrophages or smooth muscle cells proved disappointingly slow and foam cells were not formed. Subsequently it was found that the macrophage has receptors that will allow the rapid uptake of LDL to form foam cells if the LDL has undergone some chemical modification. Several types of macrophage receptors, including scavenger receptors and the oxidized LDL receptors, are now known to be responsible for the uptake of modified LDL. It is likely that the chemical modification leading to LDL uptake in human atherogenesis is oxidation of the polyunsaturated fatty acyl groups of phospholipids of LDL that have crossed the arterial endothelium to enter the subintimal space. The lipid peroxides so formed break down to lysophospholipids and aldehydes, which directly damage the apoB of the LDL which then binds to the scavenger and oxidized LDL receptors. The same substances are directly cytotoxic and may further damage the overlying arterial endothelium, increasing its permeability. The oxidized LDL itself and the release of the cytokines it stimulates are chemotactic to blood monocytes (from which arterial-wall macrophages are derived) and may thus recruit more inflammatory cells into the lesion. HDL may protect LDL against oxidative modification by a process which involves paraoxonase 1, which is tightly bound to HDL. In addition to uptake of LDL through scavenger and oxidized LDL receptors, macrophages phagocytose aggregated LDL to become foam cells and take up LDL–antibody complexes via Fc (immunoglobulin crystallizable fragment) receptors. Glycated LDL is also rapidly taken up by macrophages. Other lipoproteins can be taken up to form foam cells. In particular, the β-VLDL (a mixture of chylomicron remnants and IDL), which accumulates in the circulation in type III hyperlipoproteinaemias (see below), is rapidly taken up by macrophages.

Triglyceride-rich lipoproteins can also be taken up by macrophages by phagocytosis to form foam cells, but these are not located in the arterial wall, perhaps because these large particles cannot cross the vascular endothelium unless it is fenestrated. Thus, in extreme hypertriglyceridaemia lipid-engorged macrophages are present in the mononuclear phagocyte system and may be observed, e.g. on bone marrow biopsy. They are also the cause of the hepatosplenomegaly associated with extreme hypertriglyceridaemia. When hypertriglyceridaemia occurs in association with elevated levels of LDL cholesterol, it increases the likelihood of atheroma developing still further, perhaps because this combination is associated with low serum HDL cholesterol, perhaps because of an increase in circulating IDL and delayed clearance of chylomicron remnants, perhaps because it is associated with smaller LDL particles that are more readily oxidized, or perhaps because there are associated increases in the coagulability of blood due to increased plasma fibrinogen levels and factor VII activity. When, however, triglyceride-rich lipoproteins are increased without any increase in LDL, as in familial lipoprotein lipase deficiency (see below), there appears to be only a modest risk of atheroma. There is, however, an increased likelihood of acute pancreatitis in all types of severe hypertriglyceridaemia, both primary and secondary, particularly when serum triglyceride levels exceed 20 to 30 mmol/litre (2000–3000 mg/dl). The cause of this is not known for certain, but may be attributed to the release of fatty acids by lipolysis *in situ* due to pancreatic lipase.

Normal serum lipid concentrations

Whereas the average serum concentrations of most substances, e.g. sodium or fasting glucose, are much the same in all parts of the world, cholesterol displays considerable variation. In the United Kingdom the median serum cholesterol for a middle-aged man is 5.8 mmol/litre and deaths from coronary heart disease are around 40% of total mortality at this age. In China the average for men of middle age used to be 2 mmol/litre or less, and coronary heart disease accounted for less than 5% of their deaths. Unfortunately serum cholesterol, particularly in Chinese cities, is rising and with it the incidence of coronary heart disease.

Conventionally, the normal range for a variable in a particular population is chosen to include values between the 2.5th and 97.5th percentiles, or sometimes the 1st and 99th percentiles, on the assumption that 19 out of 20 of the population, or 49 out of 50 of the population, respectively, are normal. To be rational, the implication in a medical context must also be that those people in the normal range are healthy. In the case of cholesterol, which is clearly linked to coronary heart disease, the healthy range would be more representative if it included values from societies in which coronary heart disease is uncommon, such as China or Japan. This led the National Institutes of Health in the United States of America and the European Atherosclerosis Society to define healthy limits for serum cholesterol based on the risk of coronary heart disease. Thus the optimal serum cholesterol was considered to be 5.0 mmol/litre (200 mg/dl) or less. The equivalent LDL cholesterol would be 3 mmol/litre (120 mg/dl). More recently it has become clear that LDL cholesterol continues to operate as a risk factor for coronary disease even at these levels, and truly healthy levels are likely to be less than 2 mmol/litre (80 mg/dl). However, the risk conferred by a particular level of cholesterol frequently depends on whether it is combined with other risk factors (Fig. 12.6.5). This is why there can be no single cholesterol level that demands a particular therapeutic response; the cholesterol value must always be viewed in the context of an individual's overall cardiovascular risk (see below).

Until recently 2.3 mmol/litre (200 mg/dl) was regarded as an upper limit of normality for fasting serum triglycerides. This is close to the 90th percentile for men and the 95th percentile for women. More recently, with the recognition that triglyceride levels contribute to coronary heart disease risk, an upper limit of 1.7 mmol/litre (150 mg/dl) has been proposed, e.g. in the definition of metabolic syndrome (Table 12.6.1). In the definition of metabolic syndrome, HDL cholesterol concentrations of not more than 1.0 mmol/litre (<40 mg/dl) for men and less than 1.3 mmol/litre (50 mg/dl) for women are used to denote low HDL.

Table 12.6.1 Components of the metabolic syndrome

Metabolic syndrome is present if three or more of the following are present[a]		
1.	Waist circumference	≥102 cm (≥40 ins) in men
		≥88 cm (≥35 ins) in women
2.	Fasting triglyceride	≥1.7 mmol/litre (≥150 mg/dl)
3.	HDL cholesterol	≤1.0 mmol/litre (≤40 mg/dl) in men
		≤1.3 mmol/litre (≤50 mg/dl) in women
4.	Blood pressure	≥130/≥85 mmHg
		Or on drug treatment for hypertension
5.	Fasting glucose	≥5.6 mmol/litre (≥100 mg/dl)
		Or known diabetes

[a]American Heart Association/National Heart, Lung, and Blood Institute criteria. The International Diabetes Federation makes central obesity an essential component and has specific ethnic cut-off points for waist circumference. Certain European definitions still employ 6.1 mmol/litre (110 mg/dl) as the lower limit for fasting glucose.

(From Grundy SM (2006). Does the metabolic syndrome exist? *Diabet Care*, **29**, 1689–92. Reprinted with permission from The American Diabetes Association.)

The Fredrickson/WHO classification

The concentration of four classes of serum lipoproteins when elevated can be regarded as pathological. These are chylomicrons, VLDL, LDL, and β-VLDL. The hyperlipoproteinaemias can be classified according to which of them is increased (Table 12.6.2).

The Fredrickson/WHO classification causes great confusion, largely because it is difficult to remember and is frequently wrongly regarded as a diagnostic classification when it is simply a way of reporting which of the serum lipoproteins is elevated. It is usually sufficient to remember that when cholesterol alone is elevated there is a type IIa hyperlipoproteinaemia (OMIM# 144000). When both cholesterol and triglycerides are elevated the hyperlipoproteinaemia is generally type IIb, but occasionally it is type V (OMIM# 144650)—the serum will look milky if it is—and rarely type III (OMIM# 107741). Type I (OMIM# 238600) is extraordinarily rare. An isolated increase in fasting serum triglycerides almost invariably signifies type IV hyperlipoproteinaemia (OMIM# 144600).

In addition to measuring cholesterol and triglyceride levels, all hospital laboratories should measure HDL cholesterol in patients whose overall cardiovascular risk is being critically assessed when treatment of their hyperlipoproteinaemia with drugs is under consideration. Particularly in women, an elevated level of cholesterol may result from a relatively high HDL cholesterol concentration

Table 12.6.2 The Fredrickson/WHO classification of hyperlipoproteinaemia

Type	Lipoprotein increased	Lipids increased
I	Chylomicrons	Triglycerides
IIa	LDL	Cholesterol
IIb	LDL and VLDL	Cholesterol and triglycerides
III	β-VLDL (=IDL+chylomicron remnants)	Cholesterol and triglycerides
IV	VLDL	Triglycerides
V	Chylomicrons and VLDL	Cholesterol and triglycerides

β-VLDL, β-migrating very low density lipoprotein; IDL, intermediate-density lipoprotein; LDL, low-density lipoprotein; VLDL, very low density lipoprotein.

and thus not signify any increased risk of coronary heart disease. High serum HDL cholesterol does not have a Fredrickson/WHO class but as evidence suggests it is associated with longevity it cannot be regarded as hyperlipoproteinaemia in the pathological sense. It is low HDL cholesterol which is associated with an increased cardiovascular risk, particularly if total serum cholesterol and triglycerides are also elevated.

Primary hyperlipoproteinaemias

Primary hyperlipoproteinaemias in which there is hypercholesterolaemia (type IIa)

Serum cholesterol levels exceeding 5 mmol/litre (200 mg/dl) are common in adults in the United Kingdom and much of Europe, the United States of America, Australia, and New Zealand. In the United Kingdom, for example, 80% of middle-aged people have levels exceeding this, and the proportion in the United States of America is at least 50%. Most of this hypercholesterolaemia does not represent the effect of any single cause but is due to some combination of dietary fat, obesity, and individual susceptibility to develop hypercholesterolaemia. This susceptibility is partly genetic, probably involving more than one gene, and this common type of hypercholesterolaemia is usually referred to as polygenic hypercholesterolaemia. At the very top end of the cholesterol distribution are to be found individuals who have the less common monogenic condition, familial hypercholesterolaemia.

Familial hypercholesterolaemia

Heterozygous familial hypercholesterolaemia

Familial hypercholesterolaemia (OMIM#143890) is dominantly inherited. The heterozygous form of the condition affects about 1 in 500 people in the United Kingdom and the United States of America making it one of the most common genetic disorders in these countries. In some populations, such as the Lebanese Christians, the Afrikaner and Cape Coloured peoples of South Africa, and French Canadians, it is considerably more common. This is because such people have descended from a relatively small number of early settlers, a few of whom by chance had familial hypercholesterolaemia. This is known as a founder effect. In yet other populations, such as Africans who have not intermingled with Europeans, familial hypercholesterolaemia appears to be rare.

Typically, the serum cholesterol in adult heterozygotes is 9 to 11 mmol/litre (350–450 mg/dl). The condition is expressed regardless of diet or age, and elevated cholesterol levels are present throughout childhood. The lipoprotein phenotype is usually IIa, but occasionally there is a moderate increase in fasting serum triglycerides to produce a IIb pattern. There is a tendency for HDL cholesterol to be at the lower end of the range, particularly if triglycerides are elevated.

The clinical hallmark of familial hypercholesterolaemia is the presence of tendon xanthomas. These appear in heterozygotes from the age of 20 onwards. The most common sites for tendon xanthomas are in the tendons overlying the knuckles and in the Achilles tendons. It is also common to find subperiosteal xanthomas on the upper tibia where the patellar tendon inserts. The skin overlying tendon xanthomas is of normal colour and they do not appear yellow. The cholesteryl ester deposits are deep within the tendons. Tendon xanthomas feel hard because they are fibrotic. Indeed, it is not uncommon for those in the Achilles tendons to become inflamed from time to time, sometimes presenting as chronic Achilles tenosynovitis. More generalized tendinitis may follow rapid therapeutic reduction in serum cholesterol levels. Tendon xanthomas occur in only two disorders apart from familial hypercholesterolaemia, and these are so rare as not to pose any diagnostic difficulty. They are cerebrotendinous xanthomatosis, in which plasma cholestanol is elevated and deposited in tendons, and phytosterolaemia (β-sitosterolaemia), in which there is abnormal intestinal absorption of plant sterols, which are then deposited in tendons.

Corneal arcus is also a frequent occurrence in familial hypercholesterolaemia. When it occurs in adolescence or early adulthood it is more likely to be associated with familial hypercholesterolaemia than corneal arcus occurring in middle age or later. It is, however, not uncommon to encounter patients with familial hypercholesterolaemia who have florid tendon xanthomas but no arcus. It is thus not a very valuable physical sign. Palpebral xanthelasmas, although occurring with greater frequency and at a younger age in familial hypercholesterolaemia, affect only a minority of heterozygotes. Xanthelasmas are not specific for any particular type of hypercholesterolaemia and occur in polygenic hypercholesterolaemia, pregnancy, primary biliary cirrhosis, and hypothyroidism. They are also common in middle-aged women, often overweight, with no very marked increase in serum cholesterol, if any. They may run in families apparently independently of hypercholesterolaemia.

Identifying those heterozygous for familial hypercholesterolaemia as early as possible is important because of their risk of coronary heart disease. If untreated, over half of affected men die before the age of 60 years. It is not uncommon for men to have their first myocardial infarction or develop angina in their thirties and occasionally even earlier. Some 15% of women with familial hypercholesterolaemia die of coronary heart disease before the age of 60 years and the majority have symptomatic coronary disease by that age. Perhaps as many as 10% of women have some evidence of cardiac ischaemia before their menopause. However, whereas it is exceptional for a man with familial hypercholesterolaemia to live to 70 without symptomatic coronary heart disease, almost a quarter of women do so. This largely explains why a family history of premature coronary heart disease is absent in as many as one-quarter of patients discovered to have familial hypercholesterolaemia on screening, or in men who are discovered to have familial hypercholesterolaemia when they present with a heart attack in early life; the condition has been inherited from their mother who has herself not yet developed coronary symptoms. Most people with familial hypercholesterolaemia are not overweight and do not have risk factors for coronary heart disease other than hypercholesterolaemia and a family history of the premature disease. Those without a family history of premature coronary heart disease (*c*.25%) will be missed in screening programmes for risk factors for coronary heart disease in which cholesterol is only measured selectively.

Those patients with familial hypercholesterolaemia who develop coronary heart disease particularly early often come from families in which the affected members have all tended to develop coronary heart disease early. This may be because other genetic factors in the family predispose to coronary heart disease. Thus low serum HDL cholesterol and increased fasting triglycerides are associated with a worse prognosis. Serum Lp (a) is increased in familial hypercholesterolaemia and any familial tendency to run a high level of Lp(a) is exacerbated in those members who also have familial hypercholesterolaemia. The apoE-4 genotype (see below) is also associated with more aggressive atheroma in familial hypercholesterolaemia. A knowledge of the average age at which affected members of a family developed coronary heart disease may be helpful in planning how actively to treat boys and young adult women.

There is an increased risk of atheroma in other parts of the arterial tree in heterozygous familial hypercholesterolaemia, but this is strikingly less so than in the coronary arteries. Some heterozygotes have aortic systolic cardiac murmurs due to deposits of atheroma in the aortic root, sometimes involving the aortic cusps (supravalvar aortic stenosis).

Homozygous familial hypercholesterolaemia

Most cases of homozygous familial hypercholesterolaemia occur in societies in which consanguineous marriages and heterozygous familial hypercholesterolaemia are frequent. The chance of marriage between unrelated heterozygotes meeting by chance in countries such as the United Kingdom or the United States of America is 1 in 250 000 (500^2), and each of their children would have a 1 in 4 chance of being homozygotes. Assuming no adverse effect on the survival of the conceptus, an incidence of homozygous familial hypercholesterolaemia of 1 in 10^6 births would be predicted—a rare disorder.

Clinically, homozygous familial hypercholesterolaemia is characterized by the development of cutaneous xanthomas in childhood. These may be present in the first year of life or may not develop until late childhood. They are typically orange-yellow, subcutaneous, planar xanthomas occurring on the buttocks, antecubital fossae, and the hands, frequently in the webs between the fingers. Tuberose subcutaneous xanthomas on the knees, elbows, and knuckles are also a feature. Serum cholesterol is typically greater than 15 mmol/litre (600 mg/dl). Myocardial infarction and angina frequently occur in childhood, sometimes even in infancy. Atheromatous deposits at the aortic root, invariably present by puberty, are so marked as to produce significant aortic stenosis, which contributes to the risk of sudden death. Death before the age of 30, and often considerably younger, was the rule before the advent of plasmapheresis and similar techniques for the extracorporeal removal of LDL (see below).

Polyarthritis, predominantly affecting the ankles, knees, wrists, and proximal interphalangeal joints, is common in homozygotes for familial hypercholesterolaemia.

Metabolic defect in familial hypercholesterolaemia

In familial hypercholesterolaemia there is decreased catabolism of LDL so that it remains for longer in the circulation. Normally the plasma half-life of LDL is 2.5 to 3 days, whereas in familial hypercholesterolaemia heterozygotes it is 4.5 to 5 days and even longer in homozygotes. The molecular defect which causes this has been elucidated following the discovery of the LDL receptor (see above) by Goldstein and Brown. The gene encoding the LDL receptor protein is located on chromosome 19. Heterozygotes express only about half the LDL receptors of a normal person. Homozygotes have between none and 25% of normal receptor activity. The mutations in the LDL receptor gene produce either receptors with no binding activity (receptor negative because the receptor is not synthesized, is not transported to the cell surface, or, if it gets there, cannot be internalized after binding to LDL) or receptors that allow some LDL to be bound and to enter the cell, but this occurs only slowly because the binding site is abnormal (receptor defective). Almost 1000 mutations have been described and more may exist.

In populations with a founder gene, far fewer mutations are associated with familial hypercholesterolaemia. For example, three mutations account for 90% of familial hypercholesterolaemia in Afrikaners. In societies such as the United Kingdom and the United States of America, however, the most frequent of these mutations is likely to occur in no more than 3 to 4% of patients with familial hypercholesterolaemia. This poses a difficulty in developing a DNA test for this condition in most countries. It also means that true homozygotes are only likely to occur in populations with a small number of mutations or where intermarriage is common. Otherwise most clinically diagnosed homozygotes will actually be compound heterozygotes. However, some of the heterogeneity of the severity of the clinical syndrome of homozygous familial hypercholesterolaemia relates to the nature of the two LDL mutations present. Thus, the worst prognosis is associated with inheritance of two receptor-negative mutations and the best is with two receptor-defective mutations. The type of receptor mutation in heterozygotes is also probably of some importance but here it is blurred against a background of other acquired or genetic factors, which can find expression over a much longer time than in homozygotes.

A small proportion (3%) of patients who have the same clinical features as heterozygotes for familial hypercholesterolaemia do not have an LDL receptor defect but a mutation of apoB in which glutamine is substituted for arginine at amino acid residue 3500, which is part of the LDL receptor binding domain. This disorder has been termed familial defective apoB-100, and probably has a frequency of 1 in 500 to 1 in 600 in the United Kingdom and the United States of America. Only a minority of affected individuals have tendon xanthomas and typically the serum cholesterol associated with it is around 8.0 mmol/litre (310 mg/dl), which is less than in most heterozygotes for familial hypercholesterolaemia. Mutations of *PCSK9* also account for some cases of heterozygous familial hypercholesterolaemia. This gene encodes proprotein convertase subtilisin-like kexin type 9, which is involved in LDL receptor degradation. Rarely a syndrome resembling homozygous familial hypercholesterolaemia can arise due to autosomal recessive inheritance (OMIM# 603813). Most cases have originated from Sardinia and the gene involved is *ARH*.

Common or polygenic hypercholesterolaemia

When a diagnosis of familial hypercholesterolaemia can be made, either because hypercholesterolaemia is present in childhood or an adult has the clinical features of the syndrome, a reasonably accurate estimate of clinical risk can be made and appropriate therapy given. In the United Kingdom, however, familial hypercholesterolaemia probably accounts for no more than 3% of men dying of coronary heart disease before the age of 60. There is overlap between the range of LDL cholesterol levels encountered in familial hypercholesterolaemia and those due to the more common polygenic hypercholesterolaemia. Epidemiological studies have not included sufficient numbers of people with particularly high cholesterol levels to be certain, but it is probable that the risk in familial hypercholesterolaemia is greater than in polygenic hypercholesterolaemia. This may be because in the familial condition the hypercholesterolaemia has been present since birth, whereas polygenic hypercholesterolaemia is frequently not fully developed until the fourth to sixth decade. Furthermore familial hypercholesterolaemia, unlike many other types of hypercholesterolaemia, is associated with increased serum concentrations of Lp(a).

Table 12.6.3 Estimates of the proportion of men in the United Kingdom dying before the age of 60 years from coronary heart disease according to their serum cholesterol and whether they have the familial hypercholesterolaemia clinical syndrome

Serum LDL cholesterol (mmol/litre)	Risk of death before the age of 60[a] (per 1000)	Percentage of UK male population with these cholesterol levels	Percentage of UK male population dying before the age of 60 from CHD with these cholesterol levels
<3	25	20	0.50
3–4	34	35	1.19
4–5	43	30	1.29
5–6	55	10	0.55
6–7	74	4	0.30
>7	130	1	0.13
Heterozygous FH	500	0.2	0.1
Total			4.1

CHD, coronary heart disease; FH, familial hypercholesterolaemia; LDL, low-density lipoprotein.

[a]Death up to 60 years of age in men is chosen because of limited data about cholesterol in older age groups and in women and about morbidity. The combined CHD death and nonfatal symptomatic CHD rate is probably two to three times that of CHD death.

Sources: www.statistics.gov.uk/downloads/theme-health/DL2_32/DH2_No32_2005.pdf (accessed 29 January 2007); Slack J (1969). *Lancet*, **ii**, 1380–2; *Health survey for England 2003* (2004). The Stationery Office, London; Anderson KM, *et al.* (1991). *Circulation*, **83**, 356–62.

Estimates of how much different levels of LDL cholesterol contribute to the overall cumulative male mortality from coronary heart disease by the age of 60 years are given in Table 12.6.3. Most of such premature deaths come from the middle part of the cholesterol distribution and it has therefore been argued that if a significant reduction in the incidence of coronary heart disease is to be achieved in countries such as the United Kingdom, efforts to lower cholesterol cannot simply be confined to those individuals whose plasma cholesterols lie at the upper end of the distribution. Nevertheless, because the number of people in the middle range is so large (the vast majority of whom are not at increased risk of premature coronary heart disease) a different strategy must be applied to reducing their cholesterol from that applied to those in the upper part of the cholesterol distribution. This is the 'low-risk' or 'population' strategy that aims to lower serum cholesterol by public health measures aimed at encouraging the adoption of a lower-fat diet and avoidance of obesity. Some patients from the middle range of serum cholesterol are, however, at much greater individual risk from their cholesterol level than the majority because they have other risk factors for coronary heart disease which combine to increase their susceptibility. Probably the most potent of these is that the individual already has coronary heart disease.

In middle-aged survivors of myocardial infarction, serum cholesterol is an important indicator of cardiac prognosis (Fig. 12.6.6a), ranking after left ventricular function but ahead of most of the other risk factors for coronary heart disease. Lipoproteins are also the most important risk factors for occlusion of coronary artery bypass grafts after the initial postoperative period. In people who have not yet developed coronary heart disease, the effect of risk factors such as cigarette smoking, hypertension, and diabetes

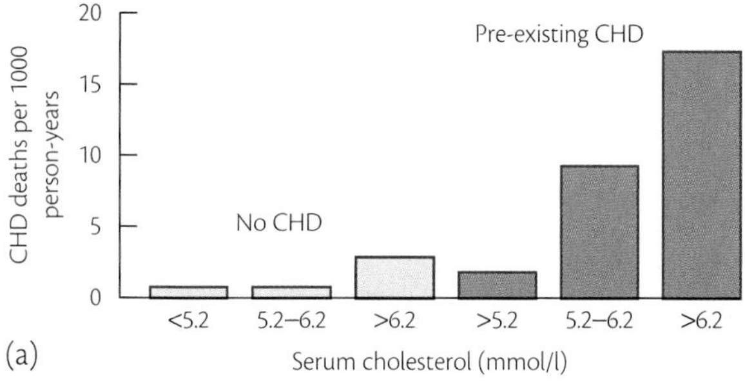

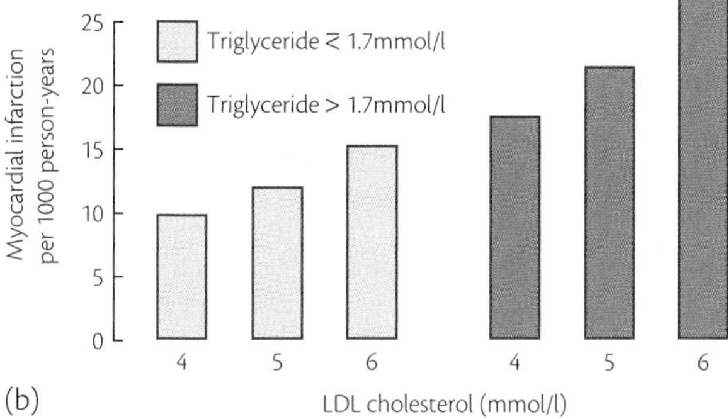

Fig. 12.6.6 (a) The risk of subsequent fatal myocardial infarction in survivors of myocardial infarction according to their serum cholesterol concentration. (b) The likelihood of myocardial infarction occurring in the next 6 years in 60-year-old men according to their LDL cholesterol and triglyceride levels adjusted for variation in serum HDL cholesterol. Calculated using the multiple logistic function from the Prospective Cardiovascular Munster Study using the Spirit 6 calculator.

(Source: (a) Data from Pekkanan J, *et al.* (1990). Ten-year mortality from cardiovascular disease in relation to cholesterol level among men with and without pre-existing cardiovascular disease. *N Engl J Med*, **322**, 1700–7; (b) from Assman G, Schulte H (1992). Relation of HDL-cholesterol and triglycerides to atherosclerotic coronary artery disease (the PROCAM experience). *Am J Cardiol*, **70**, 733–7.)

synergizes with the risk from any given level of cholesterol (Fig. 12.6.5). A family history of coronary heart disease at an early age in a first-degree relative also increases the likelihood of coronary heart disease, and part of this effect is independent of other risk factors for coronary heart disease. The combination of all these factors with a relatively modestly increased serum cholesterol level can increase individual risk substantially to a level where clinical intervention is as justified as it is with more marked elevations in serum cholesterol. This is the 'high-risk' or clinical approach to prevention of coronary heart disease.

Metabolic defect in polygenic hypercholesterolaemia

In polygenic hypercholesterolaemia there is overproduction of VLDL by the liver. If this is rapidly converted to LDL there is no increase in serum triglyceride levels. Otherwise both VLDL and LDL are raised (combined hyperlipidaemia). The build-up of LDL cholesterol in most patients is not due to any defect in the LDL receptor. Obesity and a high-fat diet (particularly saturated fat) are probably the major reasons for the enormous differences in the prevalence of polygenic hypercholesterolaemia in different parts of the world. Undoubtedly, however, individual responses to diet vary greatly and there is a complex interplay between dietetic and genetic factors in the genesis of polygenic hypercholesterolaemia. The rise in cholesterol with age, which occurs in both men and women until the climacteric, seems less evident in societies where the cholesterol level is, for nutritional reasons, lower. There is an impression that dietary modification aimed at lowering cholesterol in middle age in societies where serum cholesterol is high does not reduce it to the extent that might be anticipated from populations habitually consuming such a diet. Whether this is simply a matter of noncompliance with diet or represents some imprinted change in metabolism caused by a high-fat diet in early life is, at present, uncertain.

Primary hyperlipoproteinaemias in which there is hypercholesterolaemia combined with hypertriglyceridaemia

Type III hyperlipoproteinaemia

Type III hyperlipoproteinaemia has several synonyms: broad beta disease, floating beta disease, dysbetalipoproteinaemia, and remnant removal disease. It is rare, probably occurring in fewer than 1 in 5000 people. Type III hyperlipoproteinaemia has the distinction of being the first clinical syndrome associated with hyperlipoproteinaemia to be described (by Addison and Gull in 1851).

Type III hyperlipoproteinaemia is due to the presence in the circulation of increased amounts of chylomicron remnants and IDL, often collectively termed β-VLDL. This is the result of decreased clearance of these lipoproteins at the hepatic 'remnant' (or apoE) receptor. There is an increase in both the serum cholesterol and fasting triglyceride concentrations. Typical levels are 7 to 12 mmol/litre (270–470 mg/dl) for cholesterol and 5 to 20 mmol/litre (450–1800 mg/dl) for triglycerides. Often the concentrations of cholesterol and triglycerides are similar and this may be a clue that a patient has type III hyperlipoproteinaemia. Occasionally the condition is associated with marked hypertriglyceridaemia due to overwhelming chylomicronaemia.

Xanthomas are present in more than half of the patients who have the type III lipoprotein phenotype. Characteristic of the condition are striate palmar xanthomas and tuberoeruptive xanthomas. Striate palmar xanthomas may simply be an orange-yellow discolouration within the creases of the skin of the palms of the hands. They may, however, be more florid and appear as raised, seed-like lesions (sometimes even larger) in the skin creases of the palms, fingers, and flexor surfaces of the wrists. Tuberoeruptive xanthomas are raised yellow lesions, usually on the elbows and knees. They may be nodular or cauliflower-like, often surrounded by smaller satellites. Sometimes they may be found over other tuberosities, such as the heels and dorsum of the interphalangeal joints of the fingers. They resolve entirely with successful treatment of the hyperlipidaemia.

Type III hyperlipoproteinaemia is rare in women before the menopause, perhaps because hepatic uptake of remnant particles is enhanced by oestrogen. It is also rare in childhood but has a definite incidence in men by early adulthood. Type III hyperlipoproteinaemia is generally an autosomal recessive condition with variable penetrance. In all cases there appears to be a mutation or polymorphism of the *APOE* gene, which impairs the receptor binding of apoE. The most frequent is a polymorphism, called apoE2, in which cysteine is substituted for arginine at position 158 of the amino acid sequence. At least 90% of patients with type III hyperlipoproteinaemia are homozygous for apoE2. More often than not, however, apoE2 homozygosity, which is present in around 1% of the population, does not itself impose such a severe strain on lipoprotein metabolism that hyperlipoproteinaemia develops; its combination with some other disorder, leading to overproduction of VLDL or some additional catabolic defect, is required. This explains the association of type III hyperlipoproteinaemia with diabetes and hypothyroidism. More often, however, the additional stimulus to hyperlipoproteinaemia is obesity or the coinheritance of a polygenic tendency to hypertriglyceridaemia. Rarer mutations of apoE have been described that cause the type III phenotype either as an autosomal recessive or, if the mutation involves the receptor-binding domain of apoE (amino acids 124–150), as an autosomal dominant.

Type III hyperlipoproteinaemia undoubtedly causes accelerated atherosclerosis in the coronary, femoral, and tibial arteries. Intermittent claudication occurs at least as frequently as coronary heart disease and the incidence of the latter is about the same as that in familial hypercholesterolaemia. It is notable that in familial hypercholesterolaemia peripheral arterial disease is uncommon relative to coronary heart disease, indicating that the leg arteries are much more susceptible to the larger lipoprotein particles in type III hyperlipoproteinaemia.

In the presence of typical xanthomas, the diagnosis of type III hyperlipoproteinaemia is not difficult. When these are absent the diagnosis must be made in the laboratory. Type IIb or V hyperlipoproteinaemia can give similar serum lipid levels. However, genotyping, available in many specialized centres, can identify apoE2 homozygosity and this, in the presence of hyperlipidaemia, makes type III virtually certain. When there is a rare apoE mutation other than apoE2 homozygosity the only way to confirm the diagnosis is to send plasma to a centre that can provide ultracentrifugation to identify the cholesterol-rich VLDL (β-VLDL) typical of type III hyperlipoproteinaemia. It is also important when apoE2 homozygosity is absent to exclude paraproteinaemia, which can produce both hyperlipoproteinaemia and hypolipoproteinaemia and can mimic typical type III hyperlipoproteinaemia.

Type IIB hyperlipoproteinaemia

The common lipoprotein phenotype associated with a combined increase in serum cholesterol and triglycerides is IIb. In most people with this, in whom it is primary, the cause is probably best regarded as a polygenic tendency exacerbated by acquired nutritional factors, such as obesity. A few patients will have tendon xanthomas, indicating familial hypercholesterolaemia (see above), but the great majority will not. Cardiovascular risk is greater for any given level of cholesterol when the serum triglyceride concentration is also elevated (Fig. 12.6.6b). Often the HDL level is low, which further compounds the risk. In addition, patients with hypertriglyceridaemia frequently have increased levels of a cholesterol-depleted small, dense LDL that contributes little to the total serum cholesterol concentration but which is susceptible to oxidation and to which increasing attention is being paid because it may be highly atherogenic. Some authorities also believe that there is a specific syndrome in which there is a combined increase in serum cholesterol and triglycerides and a greatly increased coronary risk. They term this familial combined hyperlipidaemia. In this, multiple lipoprotein phenotypes occur in different family members: some IIa, some IIb, some IV, or occasionally even V. It is more than probable that what is being observed is the genetic tendency for hypercholesterolaemia and hypertriglyceridaemia running in the same family to combine in some members and not in others, and that when this occurs in a family susceptible to coronary disease a particularly high premature mortality ensues. However, until the arguments about whether familial combined hyperlipidaemia is a distinct genetic entity are resolved, for practical purposes hypertriglyceridaemia (especially when HDL cholesterol is low) should be considered as an additional factor increasing the risk of hypercholesterolaemia. When these abnormalities are combined with a family history of premature coronary heart disease, there is a greatly increased risk of cardiovascular disease unless the condition is detected and treated.

Primary hyperlipidaemias in which hypertriglyceridaemia predominates

Severe hypertriglyceridaemia (types I and V)

Diagnosis and underlying mechanism

In any circumstance in which the serum triglycerides exceed 11 mmol/litre (1000 mg/dl) chylomicrons in addition to VLDL will be major contributors to the hyperlipidaemia, even when the patient is fasting. This is because in the circulation both chylomicrons and VLDL compete for the same clearance mechanism (lipoprotein lipase). The lipoprotein phenotype is usually type V. This severe hypertriglyceridaemia generally ensues when an increase in hepatic VLDL production, either familial or secondary to, e.g. obesity, diabetes, alcohol, or oestrogen administration, is associated with decreased triglyceride clearance, which again may be genetic or acquired, e.g. hypothyroidism, β-blockade, or diabetes mellitus (diabetes can cause both an overproduction of VLDL and decreased lipoprotein lipase activity). With the clearance mechanism already overloaded with VLDL, the postprandial elevation in serum triglyceride concentrations when chylomicrons enter the circulation may be astronomic and they may spend days rather than hours in the circulation. The plasma takes on the appearance of milk and triglycerides may exceed 100 mmol/litre (9000 mg/dl). Thus a patient who might otherwise have a fasting serum triglyceride level of 5 mmol/litre can, with the injudicious use of alcohol or the development of intercurrent diabetes, achieve extraordinarily high serum triglyceride levels. Overall the frequency of severe hypertriglyceridaemia (>11 mmol/litre (1000 mg/dl)) is probably no more than 1 in 1000 in adults and less in children.

Rarely, severe hypertriglyceridaemia is caused by familial lipoprotein lipase deficiency, a genetic deficiency in lipoprotein lipase activity. This is inherited as an autosomal recessive trait. Usually it is due to mutation in the lipoprotein lipase gene leading to defective function or production, but occasionally it is due to a genetic deficiency of apoC-II, the activator of lipoprotein lipase. In familial lipoprotein lipase deficiency, severe hypertriglyceridaemia may be encountered in childhood. Occasionally in children and young adults presenting for the first time it produces type I hyperlipoproteinaemia in which only serum chylomicron levels are elevated. It is not known why the VLDL is not also raised, but with advancing age the increase in both VLDL and chylomicrons, which might be expected if lipoprotein lipase is ineffective, becomes the rule.

Severe hypertriglyceridaemia leading to pancreatitis also occurs in younger people with insulin resistance due to abnormalities of fat distribution. These include partial lipodystrophies such as Dunnigan–Kobberling syndrome (OMIM#151660 and 608600) (loss of subcutaneous adipose tissue from below the neck, acanthosis nigricans, severe insulin resistance, diabetes, polycystic ovaries, androgenization, steatohepatitis), acquired partial lipodystrophy (loss of subcutaneous adipose tissue from thighs upwards, diabetes, type 2 mesangiocapillary glomerulonephritis, C3 complement deficiency), acquired generalized lipodystrophy (general loss of subcutaneous adipose tissue, autoimmunity, steatohepatitis, acanthosis nigricans, insulin-resistant diabetes, lytic bone lesions), and familial generalized lipodystrophy (absent adipose tissue from birth, acanthosis nigricans, diabetes, steatohepatitis, polycystic ovaries). At the other end of the spectrum severe hypertriglyceridaemia frequently accompanies inherited obesity syndromes such as Alström's syndrome (generalized obesity, diabetes, steatohepatitis, cardiac anomalies, retinitis pigmentosa, sensorineural deafness).

Physical signs in severe hypertriglyceridaemia

Tuberoeruptive xanthomas are characteristic of extreme hypertriglyceridaemia. These appear as yellow papules on the extensor surfaces of the arms and legs, buttocks, and back. Often there is hepatosplenomegaly. Liver imaging shows the liver to be fatty, and bone marrow biopsy may reveal macrophages engorged with lipid droplets (foam cells). Because the triglyceride-rich lipoprotein may interfere with the determination of transaminases, giving spuriously high values, liver disease, in particular alcoholic liver disease, may be difficult to exclude, other than by the prompt resolution of the syndrome when a low-fat diet is instituted. Other features include lipaemia retinalis (pallor of the optic fundus, with both the retinal veins and arteries appearing white).

Complications of severe hypertriglyceridaemia

Atheroma is not a prominent complication of familial lipoprotein lipase deficiency, but it does complicate severe hypertriglyceridaemia in which there is residual lipoprotein lipase activity. It is difficult to make a precise estimate of the risk from the hyperlipidaemia *per se* because it is so frequently associated with insulin resistance or frank diabetes, which are themselves risk factors for atherosclerosis. If these are included as part of the syndrome, both coronary heart disease and peripheral arterial disease are common. The explanation for the only modest risk of atheroma in patients lacking lipoprotein lipase is not understood but it may be because the incidence of diabetes is not increased in familial lipoprotein lipase deficiency. Fibrinogen and factor VII activity are not increased, and it is also notable that the conversion of VLDL and chylomicrons to the atherogenic LDL and remnant lipoproteins, respectively, is impaired in the absence of lipoprotein lipase.

Although atheroma may not be directly due to the high levels of triglyceride-rich lipoproteins, other complications are; acute pancreatitis may occur when serum triglyceride levels exceed 20 to 30 mmol/litre (2000–3000 mg/dl) (see above). The presentation of acute pancreatitis is similar to that from other causes. However, the diagnosis may not be confirmed by detecting increased serum amylase activity because falsely low values may be encountered due to interference by triglyceride-rich lipoproteins in the laboratory method. All laboratories should inspect plasma or serum samples for milkiness before reporting normal or only moderately raised serum amylase activity in patients with severe abdominal pain. Clinicians may otherwise wrongly exclude the diagnosis of acute pancreatitis in favour, for example, of perforated peptic ulcer. Some patients do not develop acute pancreatitis even when serum triglyceride levels exceed 100 mmol/litre (9000 mg/dl). Others who are more susceptible experience recurring acute episodes. Generally the pain subsides within a few hours or days of commencing nasogastric aspiration and intravenous fluids with nothing taken by mouth. Occasionally, if such treatment is delayed, pancreatic pseudocysts or abscesses may develop. Recurrent abdominal pain, not typical of pancreatitis, sometimes occurs in patients prone to marked hypertriglyceridaemia; it may mimic irritable bowel syndrome. Severe abdominal pain may also sometimes be the result of splenic infarction.

Pseudohyponatraemia is another consequence of extreme hypertriglyceridaemia, which may lead to serious misdiagnosis if the artefact is unrecognized. Spuriously low serum sodium values are reported because much of the volume of the serum aliquot on which the sodium measurement is made is occupied by lipoproteins rather than water. When the serum triglycerides exceed 40 to 50 mmol/litre (3500–4500 mg/dl) the concentration of sodium in the aqueous phase (and thus the serum osmolality) may be normal while spurious serum sodium levels of 120 to 130 mmol/litre are being reported. The hazard is that these will be misinterpreted by the clinician and a patient already seriously ill with pancreatitis, or occasionally uncontrolled diabetes, will be made worse by restricting fluid intake or the infusion of hypertonic saline.

Focal neurological syndromes such as hemiparesis, memory loss, and loss of mental concentration may complicate extreme hypertriglyceridaemia, perhaps because of ischaemia due to sluggish microcirculation caused by the high concentrations of chylomicrons in the blood. Uniocular visual loss due to occlusion of the retinal microcirculation may likewise complicate hypertriglyceridaemia and is an indication for rapid institution of lipid-lowering therapy and, possibly, antiplatelet agents. Paraesthesiae, especially in the feet, may also be an occasional feature, even in the absence of diabetes. Sicca syndrome and polyarthritis have also been described, but undoubtedly the commonest articular association is gout (see below).

Moderate hypertriglyceridaemia (type IV)

Raised fasting serum triglyceride levels in the range 1.7 to 10.0 mmol/litre (150–900 mg/dl) in the absence of a cholesterol level exceeding 5.0 mmol/litre (200 mg/dl) are occasionally discovered. Diabetes and excess ingestion of alcohol are important causes. Sometimes marked hypertriglyceridaemia is present in a fit, nonobese person with none of these factors. Family studies may then reveal similar increases in relatives, when the condition is called familial as opposed to sporadic hypertriglyceridaemia. Epidemiological studies show a univariate association between plasma triglyceride concentration and the risk of coronary heart disease, but there is little evidence that triglycerides are directly causal. Hypertriglyceridaemia is associated with low levels of HDL, glucose intolerance, and an increased level of cholesterol-depleted, small, dense LDL. The presence of the latter may not be evident from the cholesterol level. Such patients are likely to benefit from statin therapy if they have diabetes, cardiovascular disease, or a risk of cardiovascular disease exceeding 20% over the next 10 years. Those not yet diabetic have a greatly increased risk of developing diabetes mellitus over the next few years particularly if they already have impaired fasting glucose or impaired glucose tolerance. The criteria for the diagnosis of metabolic syndrome are shown in Table 12.6.1.

Hypertriglyceridaemia increases the risk of any associated increase in serum cholesterol (Fig. 12.6.6b) but present evidence would not favour its specific treatment, e.g. with fibrate drugs, as a means of primary prevention of coronary heart disease. Occasionally triglyceride concentrations of 5 mmol/litre (450 mg/dl) or less must receive specific treatment if they occur in patients prone to periodic exacerbations of more severe hypertriglyceridaemia associated with acute pancreatitis. Generally, levels exceeding 10 mmol/litre justify therapy, but for lower levels individual judgement should apply.

Nonalcoholic steatohepatitis

Many patients with dyslipidaemia, particularly if there is an element of hypertriglyceridaemia, will have abnormal serum liver function tests. Most cases in which the transaminases are elevated will be due to nonalcoholic steatohepatitis (also called nonalcoholic fatty liver disease). It is important, however, to exclude other causes such as alcohol, chronic viral hepatitis, haemochromatosis, and autoimmune liver disease. Abdominal ultrasonography will confirm the fatty liver and is essential, if alkaline phosphatase is raised, for seeking biliary obstruction. When alkaline phosphatase is raised, smooth muscle and antimitochondrial antibodies should also be requested to exclude primary biliary cirrhosis. Occasionally liver biopsy is necessary to exclude a primary cause of liver disease. When the diagnosis of nonalcoholic steatohepatitis can be established with reasonable certainty it is not usually a contraindication to statin therapy. Spontaneous fluctuations in transaminase levels in patients with nonalcoholic steatohepatitis can lead to the unnecessary discontinuation of statin therapy. In randomized, placebo-controlled trials of statins, significant liver dysfunction attributable to active treatment was uncommon.

Secondary hyperlipoproteinaemias

Secondary hyperlipoproteinaemias are those which are caused by another primary disorder (Table 12.6.4). When a disease that has hyperlipidaemia as a complication occurs in an individual who has a primary hyperlipoproteinaemia, the two frequently combine to produce marked hyperlipoproteinaemia. This means that in societies in which polygenic hyperlipoproteinaemia is prevalent, secondary hyperlipoproteinaemia will have most impact. The best-known example of this is diabetes mellitus; in Japan it is infrequently complicated by coronary heart disease, whereas in the United Kingdom and the United States of America coronary heart disease is the most common cause of premature death in both type 1 and type 2 diabetes.

Table 12.6.4 The more common causes of secondary hyperlipoproteinaemia

Endocrine/metabolic	Diabetes mellitus and metabolic syndrome
	Thyroid disease
	Pregnancy
	Hyperuricaemia
Nutritional	Obesity
	Alcohol excess
	Anorexia nervosa
Renal disease	Nephrotic syndrome
	Chronic renal failure
Drugs	β-Adrenoreceptor blockers
	Thiazide diuretics
	Steroid hormones
	Microsomal enzyme-inducing agents
	Retinoic acid derivatives
	HIV protease inhibitors
Hepatic disease	Cholestasis
	Hepatocellular dysfunction
	Cholelithiasis
Immunoglobulin excess	Paraproteinaemia

Diabetes mellitus

The dominant hyperlipidaemia in diabetes is hypertriglyceridaemia. This is more likely to be associated with hypercholesterolaemia and with decreased HDL cholesterol in type 2 diabetes. Despite this, the risks of coronary heart disease and peripheral arterial disease are increased in both types 1 and 2 diabetes. This may be because in both disorders the hypertriglyceridaemia results not only simply in an increase in VLDL, but also from an increase in IDL and a small triglyceride-rich, cholesterol-depleted LDL particle. Since neither of these may contribute greatly to an increase in lipids, the term dyslipoproteinaemia is particularly aptly applied in diabetes. Although lipoprotein abnormalities may be less frequent in type 1 diabetes than in type 2, the risk of coronary heart disease in type 1 is more often compounded by the presence of proteinuria. In diabetes uncomplicated by proteinuria, the risk of coronary heart disease is about two to three times that of nondiabetic people of a similar age (Fig. 12.6.5). Proteinuria increases the risk by as much as 40 times. This may stem partly from hypertension and an exacerbation of the dyslipoproteinaemia, both of which may reflect the development of proteinuria. However, the increase in risk is greater than can be explained in this way (see Chapter 12.11) and may result because the proteinuria reflects a generalized increase in the permeability of arterial endothelium, enhancing the entry of macromolecules into the subintima and thus accelerating atherogenesis (see above).

The increased blood glucose in diabetes mellitus results from insulin resistance, insulin deficiency, or both. Insulin resistance may be present in nondiabetic, usually obese people who are still able to secrete sufficient insulin to maintain control of blood glucose, but in such people there is often hypertriglyceridaemia with low HDL cholesterol, hypertension, and increased risk of coronary heart disease. This syndrome is now referred to as the metabolic syndrome (Table 12.6.1). Clearly it has features in common with familial combined hyperlipidaemia and also with diabetes. Indeed, a proportion of people with metabolic syndrome ultimately develop diabetes, sometimes not until after they have already developed coronary heart disease. This may explain in part why glycaemic control in diabetes seems to have little impact in preventing its atheromatous complications.

Diabetic women, particularly those with type 2 disease, tend to have a distribution of adipose tissue resembling that of obese men, being mostly around the abdomen and waist rather than the more female pattern which involves the buttocks and thighs, but leaves the waist relatively small. The relative protection from coronary heart disease which most women have, even those with familial hypercholesterolaemia, is largely lost by diabetic women, and it has been suggested that this may result from this androgenization. Many women with a similar body habitus but who have not yet developed diabetes are insulin resistant and have other features of metabolic syndrome, which predisposes them to premature cardiovascular disease.

Other secondary hyperlipoproteinaemias

Obesity

Obesity is a potent cause of hyperlipidaemia and has most impact in people with glucose intolerance. In its own right, obesity predominantly causes hypertriglyceridaemia, but there is no form of primary hyperlipidaemia that it will not exacerbate. It therefore frequently accompanies hypercholesterolaemia as well as hypertriglyceridaemia. Alcoholic beverages, particularly wine and beer, are energy rich and may be a cause of obesity. Alcohol itself also induces hypertriglyceridaemia. Weight loss is generally associated with decreases in serum cholesterol and triglyceride levels. Anorexia nervosa is paradoxical in that it may be associated with quite marked elevations of serum cholesterol.

Thyroid failure

In hypothyroidism, serum LDL cholesterol and, less frequently, serum triglycerides are raised. Levels of HDL tend to be increased. There is decreased receptor-mediated LDL catabolism and lipoprotein lipase activity may be decreased. Hypothyroidism should always be considered in the diagnosis of hyperlipidaemia, and it is particularly important to exclude it when marked hyperlipidaemia occurs in women and in diabetic patients.

Renal disease

Renal disease is becoming an important cause of secondary hyperlipidaemia in clinical practice because improvements in long-term renal management are now exposing coronary heart disease as the major cause of premature death in many renal disorders. In nephrotic syndrome the major lipoprotein disorder is a rise in serum LDL cholesterol. In chronic renal failure hypertriglyceridaemia is produced by an increase in both VLDL and in LDL triglycerides. Haemodialysis, chronic ambulatory peritoneal dialysis, and high-energy diets exacerbate the hyperlipidaemia. Following renal transplantation many of the lipoprotein abnormalities resolve if good renal function is established, but corticosteroid therapy, weight gain, antihypertensive therapy, and perhaps cyclosporin treatment mean that even then hyperlipidaemia persists in about one-quarter of patients. Lp (a) is markedly elevated in renal disease, even after transplantation.

Drugs

Drugs are a common cause of hyperlipidaemia. β-Adrenergic antagonists without intrinsic sympathetic activity raise triglycerides and lower HDL cholesterol. Thiazide diuretics tend to increase both cholesterol and triglycerides. These effects may be relatively small in people whose serum lipids are not elevated at the outset, but in patients with hypertriglyceridaemia or with diabetes they may be substantial. Oestrogens tend to raise serum triglycerides, but will often lower LDL cholesterol after the menopause. They also raise serum HDL. Androgens and anabolic steroids have the opposite effect, decreasing triglycerides, raising LDL cholesterol, and lowering HDL. They may contribute to premature cardiac death in athletes unwise enough to use them in training. Glucocorticoids increase serum LDL cholesterol and triglycerides and often HDL cholesterol. Retinoic acid derivatives used in the management of skin disorders cause hypertriglyceridaemia. Phenytoin and phenobarbitone raise serum HDL cholesterol. Protease inhibitors used to treat human immunodeficiency virus infection are associated with hypertriglyceridaemia and occasionally with a lipodystrophy in which subcutaneous fat is lost from the face and limbs and collects in the trunk and between the scapulae and back of the neck as a hump.

Liver disease

Cholestatic liver diseases, such as primary biliary cirrhosis, produce hypercholesterolaemia. This is not due to an increase in apoB-containing LDL, but to an abnormal lipoprotein designated lipoprotein X produced largely as the result of reflux of biliary phospholipids into the circulation. Xanthelasmas are common in biliary obstruction and other xanthomas occasionally develop. In the later phase of chronic biliary obstruction, when secondary biliary cirrhosis and hepatocellular disease sets in, hepatic lipid biosynthesis plummets and the hyperlipidaemia of biliary obstruction resolves. Hepatocellular diseases may be associated with moderate hypertriglyceridaemia, probably because of impaired hepatic lipoprotein clearance. Concentrations of HDL are markedly decreased and lecithin:cholesterol acyltransferase activity is low. Some authorities believe that this defect in cholesterol esterification contributes to the complications of liver failure.

Hyperuricaemia

Hyperuricaemia is present in as many as half the men with hypertriglyceridaemia. It may lead to gout, particularly if such patients are receiving diuretic therapy. The association of hypertriglyceridaemia and hyperuricaemia appears to be more common than can be entirely explained by the coincidence of common aetiological factors such as obesity and high alcohol consumption. Yet they are not causally related because specifically lowering one does not usually decrease the other. They must, therefore, have some unknown antecedent in common.

Management of hyperlipoproteinaemia

Clinical trials have established beyond all doubt that reduction of LDL cholesterol decreases both coronary morbidity and mortality and can prolong survival. The risk of coronary heart disease ascribable to a particular LDL cholesterol level varies widely in different individuals, however, depending on the presence of other risk factors for coronary heart disease. Thus a LDL cholesterol value of 4.0 mmol/litre (160 mg/dl) in a 50-year-old woman with a HDL cholesterol level of 1.9 mmol/litre (75 mg/dl) who does not smoke and is neither hypertensive nor diabetic will carry a risk of a coronary event of 1 in 40 over the next 10 years, whereas the same LDL cholesterol level in a man of similar age with a HDL cholesterol value of 0.9 mmol/litre (35 mg/dl) and who is hypertensive, smokes, and has diabetes will carry a risk of 1 in 3 over the same time interval. His likelihood of benefit from a given reduction in LDL cholesterol will thus be much greater than hers, although both have the same concentration of LDL cholesterol. The coronary risk attaching to the LDL cholesterol level in individual patients could, were it known with reasonable accuracy, thus guide the clinician in deciding how rigorously treatment should be given. Below a certain level of risk, treatment may be more trouble than it is worth for the patient's lifestyle, presence of mind, or pocket. For a state health care system there will also be a level of risk below which the cost of cholesterol lowering may jeopardize the financing of other areas of clinical practice.

Another consideration, as with any therapeutic intervention, is that there may be side effects of treatment which should limit it to those patients whose risk of the disease it is intended to prevent (in this case primarily coronary heart disease) is substantially higher than the potential risk of serious side effects. Dietary management is generally viewed as safe, and meta-analyses of dietary trials show no increase in noncardiac mortality. Until recently cholesterol-lowering drugs were often viewed with suspicion. Since 1994, however, results from clinical trials of statins have established that these drugs are safe with adequate medical supervision for the duration of the trials. The same trials also showed that statin therapy decreases stroke risk, which might not have been anticipated from the epidemiological relationship between LDL cholesterol and the incidence of cerebral infarction, which is weaker than that with coronary heart disease. The overall statin effect was to decrease the likelihood of a cardiovascular event (coronary or stroke) by 21% for each 1 mmol/litre (39 mg/dl) statin-induced decrease in LDL cholesterol. This was regardless of the absolute risk of cardiovascular disease, of whether there had been a previous cardiovascular event, of age, or of the presence of other risk factors including type 1 or 2 diabetes, smoking, hypertension, low HDL cholesterol, or raised triglycerides. The lowest average annual coronary risk of participants in these trials was 1% (1 event per 100 people per year) and the highest 4.5%. The relative reduction in risk was similar regardless of the absolute level of risk, so a greater number of coronary events was prevented when the risk was highest. Other cholesterol-lowering drug therapies such as fibrates, bile acid sequestrating agents, and nicotinic acid decrease coronary risk, but their safety and the magnitude of their overall benefit is not as clear as with statins, partly because design and analysis of clinical trials were better in the more recent statin trials.

The essential point to grasp is that the decision to treat hyperlipidaemia is not based simply on any particular lipid or lipoprotein value but on an assessment of individual risk. It is sensible to select for treatment those patients with a high overall probability of dying prematurely of cardiovascular disease. If the balance of risk suggests that they are not, they will be exposed to any possible ill-effects of such treatment with no likelihood of benefit. The identification of patients with established atherosclerotic cardiovascular disease, diabetes, familial hypercholesterolaemia, or with more modest increases in serum cholesterol combined with multiple risk factors, including an unfavourable family history (Figs. 12.6.5 and 12.6.6a,b) allows the targeting of cholesterol-lowering management to high-risk individuals who can benefit most. Charts that can assist in the assessment of coronary risk are to be found in section 15.16.1 of the Joint British Societies' Guidelines.

Dietary management

It is generally agreed that dietary advice should be given to people whose LDL cholesterol exceeds a concentration of 2.0 mmol/litre (80 mg/dl). In a country such as the United Kingdom, however, more than two-thirds of men and women between the ages of 18 and 69 years have LDL cholesterol concentrations exceeding this value. Thus, except in the case of the patients considered to be at high coronary risk, individual dietetic supervision beyond the provision of a diet sheet is not reasonable. It is particularly important to remember that cigarette smoking is a greater cause of ill-health than are minor elevations of serum cholesterol, and advice to stop smoking should be reiterated whenever a medical consultation occurs.

Table 12.6.5 Dietary fatty acids and their sources

Type	Fatty acid	Source
Saturated	Myristic, palmitic, stearic	Pork, beef, sheep fat, dairy products
Monounsaturated	Oleic	Olive oil, rapeseed oil
Polyunsaturated	Linoleic	Sunflower, safflower, corn, soybean oil
	Eicosapentaenoic, docosahexaenoic	Fish oil

All can contribute to obesity. Saturated fats lead to raised cholesterol and triglyceride levels. Oleic acid and linoleic acid decrease LDL cholesterol and often triglycerides. Oleic acid is widely distributed in foods rich in saturated fats, but these sources are not helpful in a diet designed to decrease saturated fat intake. Fish oil decreases triglycerides, but does not decrease LDL cholesterol.

The principal aims of a cholesterol-lowering diet are to reduce obesity by a decrease in dietary energy intake and to decrease saturated fat consumption. Fat is a major source of dietary energy and the reduction in its intake should be the main objective of any weight-reducing diet. In the nonobese, dietary advice should focus on decreasing saturated fat to below 10% of dietary energy intake and substituting it with a mixture of unrefined carbohydrate and monounsaturated and polyunsaturated fats (Table 12.6.5). Polyunsaturated fats in the form of linoleic acid (corn oil, sunflower oil) should not be the only fats to replace saturated fat because it is not certain that in large amounts they do not have harmful long-term effects. In patients with established coronary disease there is increasing interest in the long-chain ω– 3 fatty acids such as those found in fish oil (Table 12.6.5) which are more unsaturated and reduce sudden cardiac death, probably by suppressing ventricular arrhythmias. Eating fatty fish twice a week is thus recommended. Increasingly, too, oils rich in monounsaturated oleic acid such as olive oil, present in the diet of Mediterranean people since time immemorial, are being encouraged by nutritionists as substitutes for saturated fat. Rapeseed oil, which is much cheaper, contains almost as much oleic acid as olive oil. Dietary cholesterol itself, although featuring prominently on food labels, usually has a smaller effect on serum cholesterol concentrations than saturated fat. Decreasing its absorption with foods enriched in plant sterol or stanol esters has a small hypocholesterolaemic effect, as also does mucilaginous fibre in fruit, vegetables, and oats. Avoiding coffee is probably pointless. Some authorities believe that the epidemiological evidence indicating that alcohol is protective against coronary heart disease is strong enough to justify encouraging moderate indulgence (red wine finds particular favour, in view of the lower risk of coronary heart disease in southern as opposed to northern Europe). However, alcoholic beverages in excess can lead to obesity, hypertension, atrial fibrillation, and exacerbation of hypertriglyceridaemia (see above), and a trial of abstinence should be considered in the patient with hyperlipidaemia suspected of overindulgence.

These dietary aims do not need to be modified for the treatment of moderate hypertriglyceridaemia and are also suitable for the management of diabetes. Carbohydrate-restricted diets are no longer in general use for either of these purposes. In patients with severe hypertriglyceridaemia it is necessary to limit the production of chylomicrons and so any fat in the diet must be avoided. Often a 25- to 30-g low-fat diet (in which, if the patient is not obese, carbohydrate is substituted to maintain dietary energy intake) can be employed, but occasionally even lower fat intakes must be achieved. Lipid-lowering drugs are frequently ineffective in patients with severe hypertriglyceridaemia, whereas dietary treatment can be particularly effective. Referral to a specialized centre with experienced dietetic services is often desirable.

Drug therapy of hyperlipidaemia

The indication for drug therapy is not the failure of serum cholesterol concentration to decrease below some arbitrary level despite dietary treatment in all patients. There are people with serum cholesterol concentrations as high as 8 mmol/litre (310 mg/dl) whose risk of coronary heart disease is not sufficiently high to justify the use of lipid-lowering drugs. However, when cardiovascular risk is high statin treatment should generally be initiated if the LDL cholesterol is persistently above 2 mmol/litre (80 mg/dl) and the aim of treatment should be to decrease LDL cholesterol to less than 2.0 mmol/litre (<80 mg/dl) or by 30%, whichever is the lowest. Whether dietary management should be instituted at the same time as lipid-lowering drug therapy or before in order to establish whether it alone will suffice is determined by the degree of risk and the degree to which the serum cholesterol is elevated. Dietary management does not typically decrease serum cholesterol by more than 0.5 mmol/litre (20 mg/dl). Certainly in patients with established coronary heart disease, statin treatment should be introduced without delay. High-risk categories are discussed in the subsections below.

Patients with established coronary heart disease or other significant atherosclerotic disease

Secondary prevention trials of cholesterol lowering using statin drugs provide strong evidence of prolonged survival due to a decrease in coronary events and strokes. Coronary angiography also provides evidence of regression of atheroma with lipid-lowering therapy. Lipid-lowering drugs are therefore indicated in patients with coronary heart disease (including those who have undergone coronary surgery or angioplasty) and with cerebral arteriosclerosis or with peripheral arterial, aortic, or significant carotid atherosclerosis.

Familial hypercholesterolaemia and type III hyperlipoproteinaemia

The high risk of coronary heart disease and the known metabolic defects in these conditions justify the use of lipid-lowering drug therapy. Familial hypercholesterolaemia should, if possible, be detected in childhood or early adulthood, and the age at which statin therapy should be commenced has therefore to be considered. Generally in boys a statin should be prescribed by the age of 20 years. Some authorities advocate even earlier use of statins and this should certainly be considered if the family history of coronary disease is particularly adverse. Pregnancy should be avoided in woman receiving statin treatment. Should they plan to conceive, the statin should be discontinued 3 months before conception is attempted and not recommenced until breast feeding is complete. Few women aged less than 30 years would justify statin treatment on the basis of their immediate cardiovascular risk. However, to wait until a woman with familial hypercholesterolaemia has completed her family before beginning statin treatment could often delay it until she is in her forties, which is too late. Thus the age at which statin treatment should be commenced should be negotiated with the patient after she has been fully informed. Often she will decide to begin treatment around the age of 20 in the knowledge that when she discontinues treatment to have a baby she can look back at several years of treatment and we do know from surrogate measures, such as arterial ultrasonography, that carotid intima-media thickening is evident in both boys and girls who have inherited familial hypercholesterolaemia before the age of 20 and that it can be ameliorated by statin treatment.

Patients with type III hyperlipoproteinaemia are generally encountered in adulthood and treatment should be initiated with a statin drug in all save the minority who respond to dietary management alone. It should not be assumed that dietary control is adequate if any degree of hypertriglyceridaemia persists because this generally indicates that significant β-VLDL is still present in the circulation. Type III is also very responsive to fibrate drugs, which with adequate monitoring for myositis may be combined with statin treatment.

Multiple risk factors

The risk of coronary heart disease in some patients with additional adverse factors, whose serum cholesterol remains elevated despite diet, justifies the use of lipid-lowering drugs. Just how high the risk needs to be and how it can be determined with any degree of exactitude is a persisting problem for the clinician. Most national and international recommendations for primary prevention of coronary heart disease provide a means of assessing an individual patient's risk to assist in the clinical decision as to when to introduce lipid-lowering medication and increasingly when to treat mild hypertension. The National Cholesterol Education Program recommends a scoring system to determine the 10-year risk of myocardial infarction. The Joint European Guidelines include a chart to estimate the 10-year risk of fatal cardiovascular disease (coronary or stroke death). In the Joint British Societies' Guidelines a chart is provided (section 15.16.1) to assess risk of cardiovascular disease (myocardial infarction, new angina, stroke, or transient ischaemic attack) over the next 10 years. The charts are to be found in the British National Formulary and a computer program is also available (http://www.bhsoc.org/Cardiovascular_Risk_Charts_and_Calculators.stm). In the United Kingdom, the National Institute for Health and Clinical Excellence recommends the use of statin treatment when the cardiovascular risk estimated using the charts or computer program is 20% or more over the next 10 years. It is always important to seek evidence of existing coronary heart disease since, if present, this clarifies the decision to start lipid-lowering therapy and justifies investigation in its own right.

Diabetes mellitus

Statin treatment decreases cardiovascular disease risk in both type 1 and type 2 diabetes regardless of whether there is preexisting atherosclerotic disease or microvascular complications. Furthermore, the relative decrease in cardiovascular risk of 21% for each 1 mmol/litre (39 mg/dl) reduction in LDL cholesterol is the same in patients with diabetes as in those without. It is also clearly the case that this benefit extends down to LDL cholesterol levels of 2 mmol/litre or less. There has been much discussion about whether in primary prevention there are patients with diabetes whose cardiovascular risk does not justify statin treatment. By the age of 40 years typically in both type 1 and type 2 diabetes cardiovascular risk is likely to exceed 20% over 10 years or indeed to be equivalent to that of a nondiabetic of similar age who has already experienced a cardiovascular event. Thus all diabetic patients should be offered statin treatment from the age of 40 onwards. Before that statin treatment also should be considered in those at greatest future risk because of the presence of nephropathy, retinopathy, hypertension, or particularly marked hyperlipidaemia. Clearly clinical judgement is important in this age group and female patients will require similar advice about avoiding pregnancy to that given to women with familial hypercholesterolaemia. The target of statin therapy should be a LDL cholesterol of less than 2 mmol/litre (80 mg/dl). When triglyceride levels are raised the laboratory may be unable to report LDL cholesterol levels. In these circumstances a total serum cholesterol target of less than 4 mmol/litre (160 mg/dl) or non-HDL cholesterol target of 2.8 mmol/litre (110 mg/dl) may be substituted. Consideration should also be given as to whether to add a triglyceride-lowering drug, particularly in secondary prevention.

Markedly elevated cholesterol with no other risk factors and no clearly identifiable genetic syndrome

The American National Cholesterol Education Program Adult Treatment Panel III recommends drug treatment when serum LDL cholesterol is 4.9 mmol/litre (190 mg/dl) or over with an option to treat at 4.1 mmol/litre (160 mg/dl) or over regardless of estimated cardiovascular risk.

The purpose of this recommendation is to ensure that people with familial hypercholesterolaemia who have not developed tendon xanthomas are not denied treatment and because risk estimation may underestimate risk at higher LDL concentrations. For similar reasons the Joint British Societies recommend drug treatment regardless of estimated risk when the total serum cholesterol to HDL cholesterol ratio exceeds 6.

Lipid-modifying drugs

No major therapeutic decision, such as the introduction of a particularly restrictive diet or of lipid-modifying drug therapy, should be taken as the result of a single cholesterol determination because this will be influenced both by biological and by laboratory variation. A laboratory result for cholesterol concentration is generally within ±10% of the true mean value, but may occasionally fluctuate more widely. Increasingly, portable or 'on-site' cholesterol analysers are being used in an attempt to make cholesterol measurement as immediate for the clinician as that of blood pressure. This has some advantages, but it must be remembered that such tests may be more expensive than those performed in the laboratory, they are generally less accurate unless performed by someone who is trained and regularly uses the instrument, and the calibration may differ from that employed in hospital laboratories.

Nonfasting cholesterol concentrations are satisfactory for the management of patients responding to simple dietary measures, but for those in whom drug therapy is under consideration two fasting determinations of cholesterol, triglycerides, and HDL cholesterol are generally necessary (serum cholesterol and HDL cholesterol concentrations are not affected by meals, but serum triglyceride levels are). Knowledge of the HDL and triglyceride levels is essential at this stage because abnormal values for these would be an additional factor in favour of lipid-lowering drug therapy and because their concentration may influence the choice of drug. Fasting blood glucose and serum creatinine and transaminases should also be measured, and urine should be tested for protein. Serum thyroxine should be measured if there is any suspicion of hypothyroidism.

The first-line therapy in all forms of hypercholesterolaemia, except that associated with triglyceride levels exceeding 11 mmol/litre (1000 mg/dl), are the statin drugs (3-hydroxy-3-methylglutaryl CoA reductase inhibitors) atorvastatin, fluvastatin, lovastatin, pravastatin, rosuvastatin, and simvastatin. These agents are often effective, even in marked hypercholesterolaemia, as monotherapy. They also have a triglyceride-lowering effect that tends to be related to the extent to which they lower cholesterol but which is generally less than that of a fibrate drug. Evidence that statins decrease cardiovascular events is provided by 14 large trials using atorvastatin, lovastatin, pravastatin, and simvastatin. Their use in combination with fibrate drugs requires strict clinical supervision because there is an increased risk that myositis may ensue. There is a small incidence of this occurring spontaneously in patients on statins, and creatine kinase levels should be monitored. Cyclosporin, macrolide antibiotics such as erythromycin, and antifungal agents also increase the risk of myositis, as does untreated hypothyroidism. Statins may be particularly valuable in patients with renal disease in whom fibrates are contraindicated and in whom bile acid sequestrating agents may exacerbate hypertriglyceridaemia; these latter agents are particularly poorly tolerated in patients already receiving multiple drug regimes. The cholesterol absorption inhibitor ezetimibe lowers LDL cholesterol by reducing the absorption of dietary cholesterol and more importantly the reabsorption of the cholesterol exported into the intestine in bile. Its combination with statins has so far proved safe and it allows many with high pretreatment levels of LDL or who are intolerant of larger statin doses to reach target. So far there are no randomized trials with clinical endpoints to support its efficacy or long-term safety. It may be used in patients with renal disease.

Bile acid sequestrating agents can be used in the treatment of hypercholesterolaemia in the absence of hypertriglyceridaemia, which they may exacerbate. A dose (two sachets) is best taken well soaked in fruit juice before breakfast. In larger, more frequent doses these agents often cause nausea, heartburn, and constipation. Generally for this reason they have been increasingly relegated to the sidelines since the introduction of statins, although recently a tablet form has become available. In children and women of childbearing potential who have heterozygous familial hypercholesterolaemia it is often better to wait until it is safe to commence statin treatment (which is better tolerated) rather than to alienate the patient from the clinic with unpalatable treatment earlier. If bile acid sequestrating agents are prescribed, folate and vitamin D supplementation should be considered, particularly in women who may become pregnant.

In patients whose hypercholesterolaemia is combined with more marked hypertriglyceridaemia, the fibrate drugs (bezafibrate, ciprofibrate, fenofibrate, gemfibrozil) are first-line therapy. They are also often highly effective in type III hyperlipoproteinaemia and useful in primary type V hyperlipoproteinaemia and in the dyslipoproteinaemia of diabetes mellitus. Fibrates are less effective in lowering LDL cholesterol than are statins. Most of their cholesterol-lowering effect is due to a decrease in VLDL cholesterol. They do, however, decrease small dense LDL levels. This is not readily evident from routine laboratory tests because it is unaccompanied by any substantial reduction in cholesterol. In some particularly high-risk patients with combined hyperlipidaemia, statin therapy may be added to fibrate therapy in order to satisfactorily lower LDL cholesterol. The fibrate drugs raise HDL cholesterol by more than many statins.

They must be avoided in patients with disturbed hepatic or renal function. They potentiate anticoagulants. The mode of action of fibrate drugs, which diminish serum triglyceride levels by stimulating lipoprotein lipase and decreasing circulating non-esterified fatty acids, involves stimulation of the nuclear peroxisome proliferator-activated receptor α.

Nicotinic acid (niacin) can be used to lower serum cholesterol and triglyceride levels and raise HDL. The effective dose is usually associated with unpleasant flushing. This can be minimized with long-acting preparations and if aspirin is taken before the nicotinic acid. There are also many other side effects, and liver function must be monitored. Nicotinic acid has not found great therapeutic favour outside the United States of America until its recent availability combined with laropiprant, a prostaglandin D2 receptor blocking agent which ameliorates nicotinic acid-induced flushing. Unlike other lipid-lowering drugs, it is effective in lowering serum Lp(a). Pharmacological preparations of fish oil have triglyceride-lowering properties in daily doses of several millilitres, but do not lower LDL cholesterol and may even exacerbate diabetic hyperlipidaemia. Preparations which concentrate the $\omega - 3$ long-chain fatty acids eicosapentaenoic and docosahexaenoic acid (Table 12.6.5) may have greater therapeutic potential. They improve survival after myocardial infarction in doses that have little effect on serum triglycerides, and may relate to a decreased likelihood of ventricular arrhythmias. $\omega - 3$ fatty acids can be given in renal disease, do not interact adversely with statins, and offer an alternative to fibrates in the treatment of moderate hypertriglyceridaemia.

In patients with type 2 diabetes or impaired fasting glucose (or impaired glucose tolerance) use of metformin should also be considered. The agent both lowers triglycerides and can delay the onset of more severe glycaemia.

Non-pharmacological lipid-lowering treatment

In addition to pharmacological agents and diet, extracorporeal removal of LDL is available in many centres for severe hypercholesterolaemia, usually homozygous familial hypercholesterolaemia in which it improves survival. Plasmapheresis or LDL apheresis, using systems that absorb LDL, are the two methods employed. Plasmapheresis and most methods of LDL apheresis also lower serumLp(a). They must be repeated every 2 to 4 weeks. Occasionally patients with homozygous familial hypercholesterolaemia have also been treated with liver transplantation to provide an organ with normally functioning LDL receptors. Partial ileal bypass surgery has been used to treat heterozygous familial hypercholesterolaemia (it is ineffective in homozygotes), but with the advent of more effective lipid-lowering drugs this is now very rarely necessary. In some patients with severe hypertriglyceridaemia, successful treatment with pancreaticobiliary diversion has been reported.

Hypolipoproteinaemia

Hypolipoproteinaemia is an increasing clinical problem because more cases are being discovered as a result of population screening for high cholesterol. People who have had a low serum cholesterol level all their lives do not seem to be at any disadvantage unless the decrease is profound, as in abetalipoproteinaemia. Indeed, their relative freedom from cardiovascular disease may lead to longevity. When the condition is discovered for the first time it is often difficult, however, to be sure that the low cholesterol is not due to an acquired disease, such as malignancy (e.g. colonic or prostatic neoplasms, leukaemia, reticulosis, or myeloma) or malabsorption (e.g. due to a short bowel, blind-loop syndrome, coeliac disease, pancreatic exocrine insufficiency, or giardiasis).

Some people with serum cholesterol levels around 1.0 to 3.5 mmol/litre (40–140 mg/dl) will have heterozygous familial hypobetalipoproteinaemia (OMIM# 605019) an autosomal dominant condition in which truncated apoB mutations have been described. The condition is benign. However, homozygous hypoapobetalipoproteinaemia and another condition, abetalipoproteinaemia (OMIM#200100) (inherited as an autosomal recessive), which produce more profound hypocholesterolaemia, are associated with retinitis pigmentosa, unusually shaped erythrocytes (acanthocytes), a syndrome resembling Friedreich's ataxia (preventable with administration fat-soluble vitamins), steatorrhoea (which can create diagnostic confusion with other causes of malabsorption leading to secondary hypocholesterolaemia), and fatty liver. Mutation of the *MTTP* gene rather than of the *APOB* gene is associated with abetalipoproteinaemia.

Analphalipoproteinaemia (Tangier disease, OMIM# 205400) is a very rare autosomal recessive disorder due to mutations of *ABCAI* with virtually absent HDL, reduced LDL cholesterol, and cholesteryl ester deposition throughout the body, leading to hepatosplenomegaly and in some cases enlarged orange-yellow tonsils and adenoids, lymph node enlargement, bone marrow infiltration (thrombocytopenia), orange-brown spots on the rectal mucosa, and neuropathy. Heterozygotes for this condition are at increased risk of premature coronary artery disease. Another condition associated with profoundly low HDL levels is familial lecithin:cholesterol acyltransferase deficiency (OMIM# 245900). More than 80% of serum cholesterol is unesterified and corneal opacities, proteinuria, and renal failure ensue. A less severe form of this disorder (fish-eye disease, OMOM 136120) has been described. In another disorder combined deficiency of apoA-I and apoC-III, due to a rearrangement of DNA affecting the transcription of both their genes which are clustered together on chromosome 11, leads to markedly decreased serum HDL levels, accelerated atherosclerosis, and corneal opacities. Some authorities believe that a much more common genetic HDL deficiency is the cause of HDL cholesterol levels in the lower 10% of the frequency distribution. Evidence for this contention is incomplete.

Further reading

Anderson KM, *et al.* (1991). An updated coronary risk profile. A statement for health professionals. *Circulation*, **83**, 356–62.

Arca M, *et al.* (2002). Autosomal recessive hypercholesterolaemia in Sardinia, Italy and mutations in ARH: a clinical and molecular genetic analysis. *Lancet*, **359**, 841–7.

Armitage J (2007). The safety of statins in clinical practice. *Lancet*, **370**, 1781–90.

Assmann G, von Eckardstein A, Brewer HB (2001). Familial analphalipoproteinemia: Tangier disease. In: Scriver CR, *et al.* (eds) *The metabolic and molecular bases of inherited disease*, 8th edition, pp. 2937–60. McGraw-Hill, New York.

Baigent C, *et al.* (2005). Efficacy and safety of cholesterol-lowering treatment: prospective meta-analysis of data from 90,056 participants in 14 randomised trials of statins. *Lancet*, **366**, 1267–78.

Ballantyne CM, *et al.* (2003). Risk for myopathy with statin therapy in high-risk patients. *Arch Intern Med*, **163**, 553–64.

Barter PJ, *et al.* (2006). Apo B versus cholesterol to estimate cardiovascular risk and to guide therapy: report of the Thirty Person/Ten Country Panel. *J Intern Med*, **259**, 247–58.

Bhatnagar D, Soran H, Durrington PN (2008). Hypercholesterolaemia and its management. *BMJ*, **337**, a993.

Brewer HB Jr, *et al.* (2004). Regulation of plasma high-density lipoprotein levels by the ABCA1 transporter and the emerging role of high-density lipoprotein in the treatment of cardiovascular disease. *Arterioscler Thromb Vasc Biol*, **24**, 1755–60.

British Hypertension Society (2009). *Proposed Joint British Societies cardiovascular disease new risk assessment charts.* http://www.bhsoc.org/Cardiovascular_Risk_Prediction_Chart.stm

British National Formulary 52 (2006). BMJ Publishing Group and Royal Pharmaceutical Society of Great Britain, London.

Cannon CP, *et al.* (2006). Meta-analysis of cardiovascular outcomes trials comparing intensive versus moderate statin therapy. *J Am Coll Cardiol*, **48**, 438–45.

Cholesterol Treatment Trialists (2008). Benefits of reducing LDL cholesterol among 18,686 patients with diabetes: meta-analysis of 14 randomised trials of a statin versus control. *Lancet*, **371**, 117–25.

Davies MJ, Woolf N (1993). Atherosclerosis: what is it and why does it occur?. *Br Heart J*, **69** Suppl, S3–11.

DeMott K, *et al.* (2008). Clinical guidelines and evidence review for familial hypercholesterolaemia: the identification and management of adults and children with familial hypercholesterolaemia: London: National Collaborating Centre for Primary Care and Royal College of General Practitioners.

Durrington PN (2003). Dyslipidaemia. *Lancet*, **362**, 717–31.

Durrington PN (2007). *Hyperlipidaemia. Diagnosis and management*, 3rd edition. Hodder Arnold, London.

Durrington PN, Charlton-Menys V (2006). Diabetic dyslipidaemia. In: Barnett AH (ed) *Diabetes. Best practice and research compendium*, pp. 157–67. Elsevier, London.

Expert Panel on Detection, Evaluation and Treatment of High Blood Cholesterol in Adults (1993). Summary of the second report of the National Cholesterol Education Program (NCEP) Expert Panel on detection, evaluation and treatment of high blood cholesterol in Adults (Adult Treatment Panel II). *JAMA*, **269**, 3015–23.

Garg A (2004). Acquired and inherited lipodystrophies. *N Engl J Med*, **350**, 1220–34.

Goldstein JL, Hobbs HH, Brown MS (2001). Familial hypercholesterolaemia. In: Scriver CR, *et al.* (eds) *The metabolic and molecular bases of inherited disease*, 8th edition, pp. 2863–913. McGraw-Hill, New York.

Graham I, *et al.* (2007).European guidelines on cardiovascular disease prevention in clinical practice. Fourth Joint Task Force of European Society of Cardiology and other Societies on Cardiovascular Disease Prevention in Clinical Practice (constituted by representatives of eight societies and by invited experts) *Eur Heart J*, **28**, 2375–414.

Grundy SM, *et al.* for the Co-ordinating Committee of the National Cholesterol Education Program (2004). Implications of recent clinical trials for the National Cholesterol Education Program Adult Treatment Panel III Guidelines. *Circulation*, **110**, 227–39.

Hadfield SG, Humphries SE (2005). Implementation of cascade testing for the detection of familial hypercholesterolaemia. *Curr Opin Lipidol*, **16**, 428–33.

Havel RJ, Kane JP (2001). Introduction: structure and metabolism of plasma lipoproteins. In: Scriver CR, *et al.* (eds) *The metabolic and molecular bases of inherited disease*, 8th edition, pp. 2705–16. McGraw-Hill, New York.

Hokanson JE, Austin MA (1996). Plasma triglyceride level is a risk factor for cardiovascular disease independent of high-density lipoprotein cholesterol level: a meta-analysis of population-based prospective studies. *J Cardiovasc Risk*, **3**, 213–19.

Kane JP, Havel RJ (2001). Disorders of the biogenesis and secretion of lipoproteins containing the B apolipoproteins. In: Scriver CR, *et al.* (eds) *The metabolic and molecular bases of inherited disease*, 8th edition, pp. 2717–52. McGraw-Hill, New York.

Laing SP, *et al.* (2003). Mortality from cerebrovascular disease in a cohort of 23 000 patients with insulin-treated diabetes. *Stroke*, **34**, 418–21.

Laing SP, *et al.* (2003). Mortality from heart disease in a cohort of 23,000 patients with insulin-treated diabetes. *Diabetologia*, **46**, 760–5.

Law MR, Wald NJ, Rudnicka AR (2003). Quantifying effect of statins on low density lipoprotein cholesterol, ischaemic heart disease, and stroke: systematic review and meta-analysis. *BMJ*, **326**, 1423–7.

Mahley RW, Rall SC (2001). Type III hyperlipoproteinemia (dysbetalipoproteinemia): the role of apolipoprotein E in normal and abnormal lipoprotein metabolism. In: Scriver CR, *et al.* (eds) *The metabolic and molecular bases of inherited disease*, 8th edition, pp. 2835–62. McGraw-Hill, New York.

McAvoy NC, *et al.* (2006). Non-alcoholic fatty liver: natural history, pathogenesis and treatment. *Br J Diabetes Vasc Dis*, **6**, 251–60.

Miller JP (1999). Liver disease. In: Betteridge DJ, Illingworth DR, Shepherd J (eds) *Lipoproteins in health and disease*, pp. 985–1009. Arnold, London.

National Institute for Health and Clinical Excellence (2006). *Statins for the prevention of cardiovascular events in patients at increased risk of developing cardiovascular disease or those with established cardiovascular disease. Technology appraisal 94.* NICE, London. www.nice.org.uk/page.aspx?0=TA094 [accessed 22 January 2007].

Naukkarinen J, Ehnholm C, Peltonen L (2006). Genetics of familial combined hyperlipidemia. *Curr Opin Lipidol*, **17**, 285–90.

Pekkanen J, *et al.* (1990). Ten-year mortality from cardiovascular disease in relation to cholesterol level among men with and without pre-existing cardiovascular disease. *N Engl J Med*, **322**, 1700–7.

Robins SJ, Bloomfield HE (2006). Fibric acid derivatives in cardiovascular disease prevention: results from the large clinical trials. *Curr Opin Lipidol*, **17**, 431–9.

Santamarina-Fojo S, *et al.* (2001). Lecithin cholesterol acyltransferase deficiency and fish eye disease. In: Scriver CR, *et al.* (eds) *The metabolic and molecular bases of inherited disease*, 8th edition, pp. 2817–33. McGraw-Hill, New York.

Short CD, Durrington PN (1999). Renal disorders. In: Betteridge DJ, Illingworth DR, Shepherd J (eds) *Lipoproteins in health and disease*, pp. 943–66. Arnold, London.

Thompson GR (2003). LDL apheresis. *Atherosclerosis*, **167**, 1–13.

Whiteley L, *et al.* (2005). Should diabetes be considered a coronary heart disease risk equivalent? Results from 25 years of follow-up in the Renfrew and Paisley survey. *Diabetes Care*, **28**, 1588–93.

Wiegman A, *et al.* (2004). Efficacy and safety of statin therapy in children with familial hypercholesterolemia: a randomised controlled trial. *JAMA*, **292**, 331–7.

Wood DA, *et al.* (2005). JBS2: Joint British Societies' guidelines on prevention of cardiovascular disease in clinical practice. *Heart*, **91** Suppl V, v1–52.

12.7

Trace metal disorders

Contents

12.7.1 Hereditary haemochromatosis *1673*
William J.H. Griffiths and Timothy M. Cox

12.7.2 Inherited diseases of copper metabolism: Wilson's disease and Menkes' disease *1688*
Michael L. Schilsky and Pramod K. Mistry

12.7.1 Hereditary haemochromatosis

William J.H. Griffiths and Timothy M. Cox

Essentials

Haemochromatosis is an hereditary disorder generally caused by inappropriate absorption of iron by the small intestine which leads to iron deposition in the viscera, endocrine organs, and other sites, causing structural injury and impaired function. The most common form is classical adult haemochromatosis, but juvenile and neonatal forms are recognized, and several other genetic syndromes associated with iron storage have been identified; these may rarely involve specific tissues selectively, such as the lens of the eye or basal ganglia of the brain, or a characteristic range of tissues including the liver, heart, and endocrine system. Early-onset (juvenile) haemochromatosis has a predilection for the heart, pituitary gonadotrophs and the pancreatic islet—thus myocardial disease (which may be fatal if untreated), hypogonadism and diabetes mellitus are prominent features. Prompt diagnosis and depletion of tissue iron by chelating agents—and venesection where possible—may be life-saving.

Classical adult haemochromatosis

Aetiology and pathogenesis—the condition is inherited as a recessive trait and due to mutations in the MHC class I-related *HFE* gene that appear to affect the function of key intestinal iron transport proteins such as divalent metal transporter 1 (DMT 1) and ferroportin, also reducing liver production of hepcidin that normally inhibits iron export from enterocytes and macrophages via its interaction with ferroportin (a similar phenotype can be produced by mutation in other genes involved in iron metabolism). The mutant allele, designated *C282Y* of *HFE*, is carried by about 1 in 10 individuals of European ancestry, hence about 1 in 400 are homozygotes or compound heterozygotes with biochemical abnormalities of iron storage that may lead to full-blown clinical haemochromatosis.

Clinical features—expression of disease may range from slight abnormality of blood parameters that reflect iron metabolism to the established clinical syndrome of cutaneous pigmentation (generalized slate-grey or localized bronzed coloration), cardiomyopathy, endocrine failure (especially diabetes mellitus and hypogonadism), arthritis (most typically affecting the second and third metacarpophalangeal joints of the hands and feet), and pigment cirrhosis.

Diagnosis—this can be usually established by demonstrating abnormalities of iron metabolism, with fasting serum transferrin iron saturation above 55% and elevated serum ferritin concentration. Molecular analysis of the *HFE* gene for homozygosity for the *C282Y* allele may be very useful in patients of European ancestry. Liver biopsy with histochemical determination (and preferably chemical quantification) of tissue iron content is required if there is doubt as to the diagnosis.

Management—since it is the toxicity of iron that is responsible for the manifestations of all forms of haemochromatosis, treatment is directed to the removal of iron at the earliest possible stage by phlebotomy, typically (in an adult) of 500 ml of blood each week until the serum ferritin concentration is reduced to within the low normal range and, if possible, there is a mild iron-deficiency anaemia, after which the frequency of phlebotomy is reduced. Patients with severe clinical manifestations, e.g. life-threatening cardiac arrhythmias, or who are incapable of withstanding frequent phlebotomy, require chelation therapy with the parenteral agent, desferrioxamine. End organ failure, e.g. diabetes mellitus, hypogonadism, may need treatment. Patients with cirrhosis should undergo 6-monthly surveillance by ultrasonography and serum α-fetoprotein (AFP) estimation for early detection of hepatocellular carcinoma.

Prognosis—the main causes of death in untreated patients are hepatocellular failure and carcinoma of the liver, with cardiomyopathy and diabetes also contributing. Life expectancy is probably improved by removing iron and maintaining normal iron homeostasis, and most patients feel better on iron-depletion therapy.

Family members—the diagnosis of haemochromatosis in an individual has immediate implications for first-degree relatives. Those in whom HLA typing or molecular analysis of the *HFE* or non-*HFE* iron overload genes indicates a genetic predisposition to the disease require re-evaluation by clinical and biochemical testing at intervals of not more than 5 years.

Identification of mutations in the genes encoding haemojuvelin and hepcidin, which predispose to severe iron loading, also permit genetic testing and presymptomatic diagnosis of juvenile haemochromatosis before irreversible organ injury occurs in first-degree family members at risk. Predictive genetic testing is not available for neonatal haemochromatosis.

Pathological storage of iron

The body contains about 4 g of iron, 3 g of which is complexed with haem to form haemoglobin, myoglobin, and the cytochromes. The nonhaem storage compartment, which consists of ferritin and its proteolytic degradation product haemosiderin, represents up to 0.5 g of elemental iron in adult women and slightly more than 1 g in adult men. Excess storage of body iron (iron overload) is associated with an increase in hepatic iron concentrations and of the surrogate biomarker, serum ferritin. Minimal iron storage occurs when more than 1.5 g of total body iron is present. This is reflected in a hepatic iron concentration of approximately 30 μmol/g of tissue with a serum ferritin level of usually less than 250 μg/litre. Moderate iron storage disease is reflected by a serum ferritin of approximately 500 μg/litre. Under these circumstances, the hepatic iron concentration rises to 100 μmol/g. Severe iron storage disease (>5 g of storage iron) is shown by a hepatic iron concentration of over 200 μmol/g liver tissue, with a serum ferritin level of at least 750 μg/litre. Under these circumstances, tissue injury with impaired function is almost invariably present.

Clinical subtypes of haemochromatosis

Adult haemochromatosis

The familiar form of haemochromatosis is the classical adult type, which typically presents in middle age and is usually expressed in men. The disorder is inherited as a recessive trait and is due to mutations in a gene, *HFE*, that maps to the short arm of chromosome 6 in close apposition to the HLA class I loci of the human major histocompatibility complex (MHC). Expression of iron storage disease in individuals carrying mutations in the *HFE* gene is very variable and is influenced by several environmental and sexual factors, as well as emerging genetic modifiers. Mutant alleles of the *HFE* gene that predispose to adult-type haemochromatosis are widespread and frequent in populations of northern European origin. There is evidence from haplotype analysis that a single mutation arose on an ancestral chromosome 6 and spread throughout this population, probably as a result of the migration of the Vikings from Scandinavia. The disease occurs throughout the world as a result of intermarriage but is at its highest frequency in France, Germany, Great Britain, Ireland, Northern Italy, Scandinavia, Spain, and Eastern Europe as far as European Russia. Colonization has led to its appearance in all populations of the United States and in Australasia, and for the same reason hereditary adult-type haemochromatosis also occurs in South America.

Classical adult-type haemochromatosis is a slowly progressive disease affecting the liver, endocrine system, heart, and joints; it is often only diagnosed when irreversible tissue injury has occurred. The condition predisposes to the development of primary carcinomas of the liver. A rare genetic form of adult haemochromatosis occurs in patients homozygous for mutations in the transferrin receptor 2 (*TFR2*). This form has mainly been described in southern Europeans and is termed type 3 haemochromatosis using the OMIM classification (see Table 12.7.1.1). The phenotype resembles *HFE*-related haemochromatosis (type 1) although generally more severe and presenting at a younger age. The TFR2 protein is mainly expressed in the liver and has a lower affinity for iron uptake than the ubiquitous transferrin receptor. Within the small intestine its specific localization to the crypts has previously suggested a programming role interacting with *HFE* in a signalling pathway for body iron status.

Identification of the protein responsible for iron transport across the basolateral surface of enterocytes provided a candidate for a recently recognized atypical form of haemochromatosis. The iron exporter in question has been termed ferroportin and appears to also control iron release from hepatocytes and, importantly, macrophages. Single missense mutations in the ferroportin gene are associated with a specific dominantly inherited phenotype. Haemochromatosis due to heterozygous ferroportin mutations has been coined ferroportin disease and also referred to as type 4 haemochromatosis. The disorder is typified by a raised ferritin level with normal or low transferrin saturation and a tendency for anaemia with poor venesection tolerance. Not restricted to white people, the condition is recognized in Asians and a unique and common polymorphism (Q248H) in Southern African populations may contribute to the indigenous iron overload observed.

Iron loading occurs predominantly within the reticuloendothelial system with splenic uptake visible on MRI. On liver microscopy, Kupffer cells are iron-laden with relative sparing of hepatocytes.

Table 12.7.1.1 Inherited disorders of iron storage

Disorder	OMIM no.	Locus	Gene/protein
Atransferrinaemia	209300	3q21	transferrin
Acaeruloplasminaemia	604290	3q23–q25	caeruloplasmin
Haemochromatosis (HFE 1) (adult)	235200	6p21.3	HFE
Haemochromatosis (HFE 2) (juvenile)	602390	1q	unknown
Haemochromatosis (HFE 3) (adult)	604250	7q22	transferrin receptor 2
Haemochromatosis (HFE 4) (adult, dominant)	606069	2q32	ferroportin
Haemochromatosis (neonatal)	231100	unknown	unknown†

† Autosomal recessively inherited in only a few families.

Ferroportin mutations appear to trap iron within macrophages and it has been proposed that the reduced availability of plasma iron either directly or via an ensuing anaemia drives increased intestinal absorption. As well as the phenotype described above, where spillover of iron into hepatocytes is minimal and disease course benign, a second phenotype, less commonly observed, is characterized by an elevated transferrin saturation, hepatic parenchymal iron deposition, and liver disease.

Juvenile haemochromatosis

Since the identification of adult iron storage disease by several European physicians during the 19th century, a similar disease has been recognized in children and young adults who may develop iron storage disease of a more severe character, now designated juvenile haemochromatosis. This is defined as iron storage disease occurring before the age of 35 years. It evolves rapidly, typically affects the heart and endocrine system, and causes infantilism and hypogonadism, as well as life-threatening cardiac arrhythmias. Juvenile haemochromatosis is inherited as a very rare recessive trait in which there is an increased frequency of consanguinity among the parents of affected subjects. Juvenile haemochromatosis resembles the severe iron storage disease associated with the iron-loading anaemias, such as β-thalassaemia. Juvenile haemochromatosis affects males and females equally—an observation that reflects the overwhelming nature of the iron homeostatic defect. Iron overload develops before the modifying effects of menstruation and dietary factors supervene.

Recently, the genetic basis of juvenile haemochromatosis has been elucidated and revealed key proteins involved in iron metabolism. Most cases have been associated with mutations in the *HJV* gene on chromosome 1q, encoding the protein haemojuvelin; the homozygous mutation *G320V* accounts for approximately 50% of *HJV*-associated or type 2A haemochromatosis. Haemojuvelin is expressed predominantly by hepatocytes but also in cardiac and endocrine tissues; its precise role is obscure. The common mutations abrogate expression at the cell surface where haemojuvelin may act as a coreceptor for bone morphogenetic protein as part of an intracellular signalling mechanism. A smaller number of cases are explained by mutations in the *HAMP* gene on chromosome 19 which codes for the peptide hepcidin. In mice with disruption of murine *HAMP*, or its promoter sequence, hepatic iron loading occurs. Conversely, overexpression of murine *HAMP* results in anaemia in keeping with hepcidin suppressing intestinal iron absorption. Indeed, *HAMP* overexpression overrides the effect of the *C282Y* mutation on dietary iron uptake and prevents haemochromatosis in HFE-deficient mice. This finding supports the more severe phenotype observed in this form of juvenile disease (type 2B) compared with *HFE*-related haemochromatosis. Hepcidin is thought to play a central role in iron homeostasis and current models are premised on hepcidin acting as a putative iron-regulatory hormone with effects on end organs, including the intestine and the monocyte/macrophage system.

Neonatal haemochromatosis

Neonatal haemochromatosis is a newly identified syndrome of uncertain cause, characterized by congenital cirrhosis or fulminant hepatitis associated with the widespread deposition of iron in hepatic and extrahepatic tissues. Approximately 100 cases of neonatal haemochromatosis have been reported. Neonatal haemochromatosis occurs in the context of maternal disease (including viral infection) and in the presence of maternal antinuclear factor, as a complication of metabolic disease in the fetus, and sporadically or recurrently, without overt cause, in siblings, including maternal half-siblings. This latter observation indicates that conception by the use of sperm donors in women who have had a previously affected infant should not be recommended. Although infants with neonatal haemochromatosis die of liver disease shortly after birth, there are many instances where survival is associated with a complete recovery and thereafter normal growth and development with no signs of abnormal iron metabolism. Recently, it has been shown that the outcome of pregnancies at risk for neonatal haemochromatosis is improved by treatment of the mother with high-dose intravenous infusions of pooled human immunoglobulin, thereby suggesting the operation of a humoral factor. However, the involvement of genetic determinants, possibly of paternal origin, in an alloimmune response has not been excluded. In other pedigrees, although neonatal haemochromatosis appears to have a clear hereditary basis, no predictive genetic test is yet available to inform the outcome of at-risk pregnancies for this devastating disease.

Prevalence and epidemiology

Juvenile and neonatal haemochromatosis are rare disorders that occur sporadically, but hereditary adult haemochromatosis is widely disseminated and of global importance. Removal of toxic iron by repeated venesection improves the outcome for adult haemochromatosis. If this treatment is instituted before irreversible tissue injury occurs, venesection may restore health and a normal life expectancy. For these reasons, there has been much discussion about the early recognition of iron storage disease by the introduction of population-based screening programmes, using genetic testing or phenotypic biochemical screening methods, that can be applied to communities at risk.

In European populations, about 1 in 10 individuals carries one copy of an allele of the *HFE* gene that predisposes to iron storage disease, and between 1 in 100 and 1 in 400 persons in these populations are homozygotes or compound heterozygotes with biochemical abnormalities of iron storage that may lead to full-blown clinical haemochromatosis. Thus, the mutant allele, designated *C282Y* of *HFE*, which is the principal determinant of iron storage disease, occurs at polymorphic frequency and is one of the most common genetic abnormalities leading to an autosomal recessive disease in populations of northern European origin. In European patients with iron storage disease due to hereditary haemochromatosis, the frequency of homozygosity for the *C282Y HFE* allele ranges from about 35% in southern Italy to more than 90% in the British Isles, including Ireland. In Australia, homozygosity for *C282Y* occurs in almost 100% of patients with hereditary haemochromatosis. However, as discussed later, although useful for diagnosis, homozygosity for the *C282Y* mutation of *HFE* is not tantamount to a diagnosis of established iron storage disease nor, therefore, of clinical haemochromatosis.

Clinical expression of haemochromatosis is highly dependent on age and it is very rare for there to be detectable disease in adults below the age of 20 years. As clinical disease is much more common in men than women, it is likely to reflect environmental factors and the modification of disease expression due to blood loss associated with menstruation and the investment in pregnancies, as well as the comparatively reduced dietary complement of iron in women. Other environmental factors, particularly the consumption of alcohol, appear to interact with predisposing genetic factors to induce the clinical expression of iron storage disease in *C282Y* homozygotes. Most patients with the disease develop symptoms at, or above, the age of 40 years. However, studies of iron metabolism by biochemical measurements or tissue biopsy may reveal early evidence of iron storage in the long presymptomatic phase of this condition. With greater awareness of the diverse clinical manifestations of adult type hereditary haemochromatosis, detection on the basis of early symptoms, for example arthritis or endocrine disease, may be possible. Thus, although the mutations that predispose to the development of haemochromatosis as a clinical entity are frequent in populations of European ancestry, there is a marked disparity in populations in which *C282Y* homozygosity is prevalent and the frequency with which symptomatic haemochromatosis is diagnosed.

Phenotypic expression of disease

For epidemiological purposes, since there is no internationally agreed case definition of haemochromatosis, caution is needed in interpreting claims that haemochromatosis is the most common inherited disorder affecting European peoples. Phenotypic expression of the disease may range from the established clinical syndrome (which includes cutaneous pigmentation, cardiomyopathy, endocrine failure—especially diabetes mellitus and hypogonadism, arthritis, and pigment cirrhosis) to a slight abnormality of blood parameters that reflect iron metabolism—elevated serum transferrin iron saturation and serum ferritin measurements. Such studies that are available to determine the penetrance and expressivity of the haemochromatosis gene have provided widely varying results in different populations. In Australia, where the mean intake of iron in the diet appears to be much greater than in the average European population today, most middle-aged male *C282Y* homozygotes appear to express at least one clinical manifestation of iron storage disease. Similarly, a study of homozygous relatives (principally siblings) within pedigrees known to have haemochromatosis suggest that about one-half of the men over 40 years of age, and about 1 in 6 of the women over 50 years of age, have at least one haemochromatosis-related clinical disorder. This latter survey, conducted in the United States, suggests that an important proportion of homozygous relatives of patients with established haemochromatosis, especially men, have conditions such as cirrhosis and arthropathy, as well as abnormalities of serum liver-related tests that are not detected by spontaneous clinical referral.

Many reports of disease expression in haemochromatosis may, however, be questioned because of the prevalence of co-segregating genes within affected pedigrees, as well as early household environmental factors common to siblings that may predispose to disease expression. Studies in mice support this explanation, since it has been shown that several independent genetic determinants control the extent of iron loading observed in mouse models of iron storage disease generated by targeted disruption of the murine homologue of the *HFE* gene. In contrast, surveys conducted in outbred populations, for example in Jersey, show a great disparity between the predicted frequency of homozygosity for *C282Y* and the number of recorded cases with the disease attending local hospitals. These latter studies may reflect the widely suspected inability of clinicians to diagnose haemochromatosis, and an inability to bring together the unitary clinical manifestations of the disease into a unifying diagnostic category. However, widely differing degrees of disease penetrance almost certainly account for the apparent shortfall of diagnosed cases in populations at risk.

At present, no clear data in large unbiased population surveys are available to assess disease penetrance and the modifying effects of lifestyle factors such as alcohol, nutrition, and diet, as well as pregnancy and menstruation, that are likely to influence the effects and rate of iron storage in human *C282Y* homozygotes. Mortality figures show that death is rarely attributed to hereditary haemochromatosis in populations at risk. This fact contrasts starkly with the well-established known complications of the full clinical syndrome, in which early death results from cirrhosis of the liver, hepatocellular carcinoma, endocrine failure, or cardiac complications.

A contemporary study that examined the frequency of the most common symptoms of haemochromatosis in *C282Y* homozygotes, *C282Y/H63D* compound heterozygotes, and persons who are wild-type at these loci has been reported from California. In more than 41 000 individuals attending a health appraisal clinic, no evidence of an increased frequency of symptoms was identified in those genetically predisposed to iron storage disease. The only significant clinical history identified in the at-risk group was that of hepatitis or prior liver complaints. Only one of the 152 identified *C282Y* homozygotes had signs and symptoms of adult haemochromatosis. This provocative report, indicating a very low clinical penetrance (less than 1%) of the haemochromatosis genotype in an unusual group of adults over the age of 26 years, raises important questions about the introduction of mass population screening for this potentially treatable iron storage disease by genetic or even biochemical methods. However, the high prevalence of impotence, joint symptoms, chronic fatigue, and other complaints such as cardiac arrhythmias in the study group as a whole, raises disturbing questions about the valid application of this report to other populations. It is perhaps not surprising that in a group where, on average, more than 40% complained of a general limitation of their health and/or joint symptoms, and in which more than 35% of the male participants scored positively on symptom enquiry about impotence, a significant contribution from predisposing haemochromatosis alleles could not be identified. Nonetheless, this large study raises key questions about the utility of screening for adult haemochromatosis as a genetic disease.

Before screening for haemochromatosis is introduced, there is clearly a need for other population surveys to be carried out in which the morbidity and mortality of individuals with the wild-type genotype, as well as those harbouring disease alleles, are investigated. More recent investigations to determine the effects of iron storage in *C282Y* homozygotes have been reported in a comprehensive study of about 30 000 individuals aged between 40 and 69 years from Melbourne, Australia. Of 203 subjects found to be homozygous for the *C282Y* allele, 'iron-overload-related disease' occurred in 28% of the men and 1.2% of the women. Longitudinal studies have shown that iron overload in *C282Y* homozygotes is not always progressive and indeed may recede in some cases. In the Melbourne study, follow-up for an average of 11.4 years showed that the hazard ratio for death from any cause was 1.04 (confidence limits 0.67–1.62) in *C282Y* homozygotes compared with subjects who did not harbour any copy of this mutant *HFE* allele. Not all individuals with mild iron loading require treatment and this clearly has implications for the introduction of mass population screening programmes for *HFE*-related haemochromatosis.

Pathophysiology and pathogenesis

Young patients with haemochromatosis absorb an increased amount of dietary iron in their upper intestine compared with normal control subjects. In established iron storage disease, iron absorption continues at a rate that is inappropriate for the level of iron stores, as reflected by serum ferritin and tissue iron determinations.

In the absence of an effective excretory pathway, the increased absorption of iron by the intestine leads to a progressive accumulation of the metal in the parenchymal cells of the liver, heart, endocrine glands, and specialized type B synoviocytes. Excess iron accumulates in the pancreas where it is found in both acinar and endocrine cells of the islet, although there is a particular predisposition in the early phases of iron loading to the islet β-cell. Iron also accumulates to toxic levels in the gonadotrophs of the anterior pituitary gland, leading to hypogonadotrophic hypogonadism. Iron may accumulate in the adrenal gland, where it is concentrated particularly in those cells that secrete aldosterone, in the zona glomerulosa. Iron accumulates in the cardiac myocytes and conducting tissue of the heart, in the chief cells of the parathyroid, and in parenchymal cells throughout the body. The consequences of toxic iron storage include diabetes mellitus, cirrhosis of the liver, cardiomyopathy with or without conduction defects, hypogonadism, arthritis with chondrocalcinosis, adrenocortical deficiency, and, rarely, hypoparathyroidism. Evidence for the intrinsic toxicity of iron in haemochromatosis is provided by the regression of the pathological changes following measures taken to reduce iron, for example the use of iron chelators and removal of body iron by venesection. Venesection stimulates the mobilization and removal of iron from the storage compartment by increasing the demand for red cell production in the bone marrow.

Mechanism of iron toxicity

High concentrations of iron salts are toxic to cultured cells. The administration of iron chelates to experimental animals has induced diabetes with iron loading in the liver and pancreas, as well as the generation of (renal) carcinomas. Injections of iron salts induce local sarcomas in experimental animals, with evidence of species susceptibility. In humans, sarcomas or carcinomas have arisen, albeit rarely, at sites of therapeutic injections of iron, and it is possible that the complications of silicosis and asbestos exposure result from the complement of iron associated with these particulates. A wealth of indirect but corroborative evidence indicates that the primary effect of excess free iron is to promote the formation of oxygen free radicals, which mediate the damage to cells and tissues that is observed in iron storage disease. In established haemochromatosis, the iron-binding capacity of plasma transferrin may be exceeded, so that a proportion of the iron present in the blood remains reactive as a low-molecular-weight species only loosely attached to plasma proteins. Nontransferrin iron in human plasma stimulates the peroxidation of unsaturated lipids and can form reactive complexes that react with DNA, thus suggesting a mechanism for genome toxicity and carcinogenesis related to iron overload. Iron is highly electroreactive, and coupling of the Fenton and Haber–Weiss reactions leads to the formation of hydroxyl radicals as a result of the catalytic interactions between superoxide and ferric ions. Tissues with significant iron storage show peroxidative injury in membrane lipid fractions.

The lysosomal compartment appears to be particularly susceptible to iron-mediated damage, since iron in the form of ferritin and its degradation product haemosiderin accumulates within lysosomes to form the particulate ferrugineous granules known as siderosomes. In haemochromatosis, there is an increased activity of lysosomal enzymes with biochemical evidence of increased lysosomal fragility indicating disruption of the integrity of the lysosomal membrane by iron. These changes revert to normal when the tissue iron is removed by venesection or by the use of specific iron chelators. It seems likely that the electrochemical reactivity of iron, and its particular propensity to accelerate the formation of oxygen free radicals, mediate its injurious effects on cell membranes, and on the nuclear genome, leading to cancerous change. However, despite great advances in the understanding of free-radical chemistry, the cause-and-effect relationship between iron storage and tissue injury is difficult to prove unequivocally. Nonetheless, much experimental evidence points to the development of iron-mediated peroxidative injury of cellular membranes including the lysosome, as well as iron-mediated genotoxicity. Whatever their physiochemical basis might be, common mechanisms of iron toxicity clearly exist, since the pathological and clinical manifestations of all iron storage syndromes, including secondary haemochromatosis associated with blood transfusion and the iron-loading anaemias, are almost identical.

Pathology of iron storage

Heavy deposits of iron in the tissues are associated with fibrosis and cell loss. Simple inspection reveals an overt rust-like discolouration of the liver, spleen, pancreas, heart, and lymph nodes. The liver is usually enlarged and haemosiderin is found in all cell types with the formation of fibrous septa and hyperplastic nodules. These nodules, which may be the forerunners of adenomas and hepatocellular carcinomas, contain little stainable iron, unlike the adjacent parenchyma.

The dominant site of iron deposition during the early phases is within hepatocytes, but soon iron loading may be observed in all

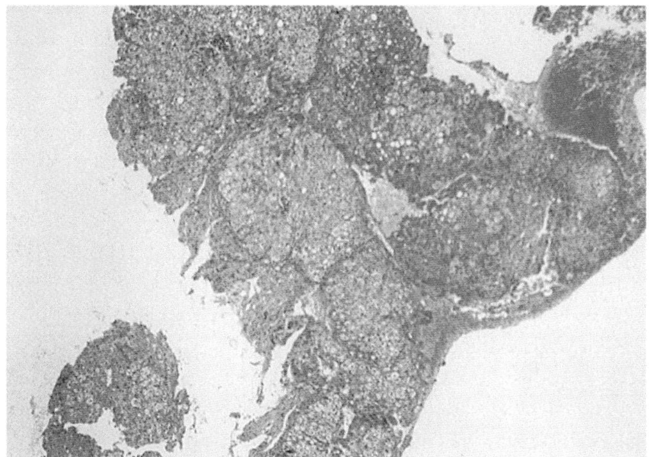

Fig. 12.7.1.1 Low-power needle-biopsy appearance of liver specimen stained with haematoxylin and eosin from a 67-year-old man with adult haemochromatosis due to homozygosity for the *C282Y* mutation. Note the large hyperplastic nodules and fibrosis.

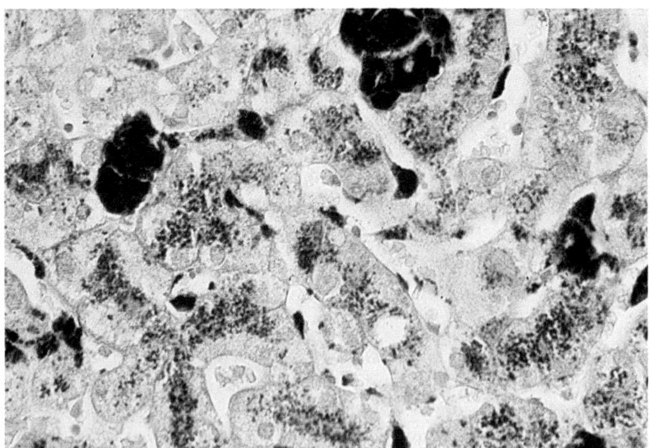

Fig. 12.7.1.2 High-power micrograph of the liver biopsy specimen shown in Fig. 12.7.1.1 stained with Perls' reagent. Note the extensive deposits of ferric iron in all cell types including Kupffer cells, cells lining small biliary radicles, and in a punctate distribution within parenchymal hepatocytes. Liver cells are hyperplastic.

cell types, including the lining cells of biliary canaliculi, Kupffer cells, and stellate cells (see Figs. 12.7.1.1 and 12.7.1.2).

Similarly, in the pancreas there is fibrosis and iron deposition in the acini, ducts, and islets of Langerhans. Staining with Perls' reagent reveals marked haemosiderin deposition in the exocrine and endocrine glands, including many cell types in the testes. Haemosiderin is also markedly increased in the chief cells of the parathyroid, the anterior pituitary, the zona glomerulosa of the adrenal, and the thyroid.

In the joints, there is loss of the intra-articular space with chondrocalcinosis and deposits of haemosiderin in the synovium. Electron microscopy shows selective deposits of ferritin and haemosiderin within type B synoviocytes. Radiological examination of the joints shows collapse of articular surfaces, subchondral cyst formation, and prominent formation of periarticular osteophytes. In the heart, pericardial constriction with fibrosis may occasionally be observed, but the principal abnormality is seen in the myocardium with degeneration and vacuolation of cardiac myocytes and intermyocyte fibrosis that involves conducting tissue in the septa. Surviving myocytes show eosinophilic degeneration and evidence of hypertrophy. Microscopical examination shows that, in established cases of haemochromatosis, all tissues except the choroid plexus are affected by the iron storage process. In the past, it was considered that transfusional and other types of secondary iron storage disease predominantly affected the cells of the mononuclear macrophage system, such as the Kupffer cells of the liver, rather than the parenchymal cells. Iron deposits in the macrophage system may be less damaging than in other cell types, but it is difficult at present to relate evidence of iron-mediated injury to its cellular distribution. Progressive tissue injury follows the long-term cumulative toxicity of iron storage and its consequential effects on organ structure and cellular function. A striking, but unexplained, feature of iron storage disease in the liver and other tissues is the absence of overt necrosis. Careful study of the cellular effects of iron storage on apoptotic mechanisms in diseased tissues is clearly warranted.

Quantitative aspects of iron storage disease

Chemical determination of tissue iron content yields useful information about the severity of iron loading in haemochromatosis, and may also provide a means to judge local responses to iron-depletion therapy, such as venesection. In normal individuals, the total concentrations of liver iron do not exceed 0.15% by dry weight, but in established haemochromatosis the value is usually 1% or more. In severely affected patients with untreated hereditary haemochromatosis or secondary haemochromatosis the amount of iron may exceed 5% of the dry weight of tissue. The overall burden of body iron in patients with haemochromatosis is usually in excess of 5 g in hereditary disease, a figure that rises with age. Estimates indicate that the total burden in patients with advanced haemochromatosis can be as much as 40 to 60 g, most of this accumulating in the liver. The pancreas and other organs such as the lymph, thyroid, pituitary, and salivary glands typically show an increase of more than 10 times the normal iron content.

Nature of the metabolic defect

In established haemochromatosis, where the burden of iron may increase body iron stores by at least 10-fold, measurements usually show that iron absorption is within the normal range. Studies in young patients with rapidly progressive disease show a markedly increased absorption of iron, and all the evidence points to an increase in iron absorption to 2 to 3 mg daily throughout the lifetime of patients with haemochromatosis. After depletion therapy, the rate of recovery of iron stores is greatly enhanced for many years in patients with haemochromatosis, reflecting a persistent homeostatic abnormality in the retention of dietary iron. The daily absorption of between 2 and 4 mg of iron over a period of 30 to 40 years accounts for the degree of iron loading that occurs at presentation in patients with haemochromatosis, and compares with the normal absorption of 0.8 to 1.0 mg in men and in women, up to 2 mg daily. In effect, the abnormal absorption of iron represents a disturbed regulation of the final common pathway for the acquisition of iron from the environment by the small intestinal mucosa.

Iron absorption in hereditary haemochromatosis

A report, describing the transplantation of intestine and liver from an *HFE C282Y* homozygote into a recipient without haemochromatosis, has provided evidence that the small intestine is a key site of expression of the hereditary defect in adult haemochromatosis. The transplantation was associated with early iron overloading in the recipient, together with raised serum transferrin iron saturations—a phenomenon not observed in recipients of hepatic allografts obtained from donors later found to be homozygous for the haemochromatosis gene. Studies *in vitro* and *in vivo* have suggested that there is a qualitative abnormality of the uptake and transfer of iron from the intestinal lumen in patients with hereditary haemochromatosis, although until recently the nature of this abnormality was unclear.

Recently, genetic studies of mutant strains of mice with abnormalities of iron metabolism have shed light on the iron-absorption mechanism. The identification of a single gene encoding the divalent metal transporter protein, DMT1, which is expressed in the upper small intestine and cells of the erythron, provides a molecular understanding of the iron deficiency and the microcytic anaemia that occurs in the *mk/mk* mouse strain. A single point mutation in the *DMT1* gene interferes with the uptake of ferrous iron, since it disrupts the cognate transmembrane carrier protein mainly expressed in the mucosa of the proximal small intestine, at the site of iron absorption, and in the erythroid precursor cells. Since *in vitro* studies of the expressed protein DMT1 show that it serves only as a carrier of divalent cations, and that interference with this pathway is sufficient to induce iron deficiency in a mammalian species, ferrous iron uptake is probably the main pathway by which inorganic iron is acquired by the intestine. Human *DMT1* maps to the long arm of chromosome 12 and encodes a 12-membrane-spanning protein that is expressed in the apical membrane of the upper intestine and in the apical membrane of differentiated human CaCo-2 cells of small intestinal phenotype. DMT1 is also expressed in developing erythroid cells in which it is responsible for the intracellular delivery of iron derived from transferrin for haemoglobin synthesis.

The discovery of DMT 1 immediately indicated a possible role for this important protein in human haemochromatosis. Overexpression of *DMT1* mRNA has been identified in the intestinal mucosa of patients homozygous for the *C282Y* mutation with hereditary haemochromatosis, as well as in mice with iron storage disease due to targeted disruption of the *HFE* gene. At the same time, studies in experimental animals have identified a cytochrome-containing ferrireductase that is also localized to the intestinal brush-border membrane; this reductase has been cloned from murine intestine and its human homologue has been identified. Expression of mucosal ferrireductase is specific to the apical microvillous membrane of mammalian intestinal mucosa and appears to be induced in response to nutritional iron deficiency. Mucosal ferrireductase reduces ferric irons derived from the diet in the lumen for delivery to the DMT1 carrier protein, the final divalent pathway for inorganic iron uptake by intestinal mucosa. The mRNA species encoding murine *DMT1* exist in two isoforms, one of which contains an iron-response element in its 3′ region, which would allow for the post-transcriptional regulation of protein expression controlled by intracellular iron status. A similar translational control of transferrin receptor expression has been described with the 3′ iron-response element in the mRNA encoding the human transferrin receptor. Since the isoform of DMT1 containing the iron-response element is preferentially expressed in the duodenum, it seems likely that changes in intracellular iron status regulate the expression of this carrier protein in iron deficiency and haemochromatosis. Studies in *HFE* knockout mice indicate that the functional expression of the DMT1 protein is enhanced in the murine model of haemochromatosis, leading to increased iron uptake across the brush-border membrane of iron presented in the ferrous form. The action of rate-limiting ferrireductases at the brush-border membrane functionally coupled to DMT1 activity appears to explain the enhanced isotopic uptake of ferric iron in this model of haemochromatosis.

At present, our molecular understanding of transepithelial iron uptake in haemochromatosis and in health is somewhat rudimentary. After initial uptake, the enhanced transfer of iron across the mucosal epithelium in haemochromatosis and iron deficiency is mediated by as yet unknown iron-binding proteins. Delivery of the iron to the systemic circulation is mediated by the regulated downstream coexpression of the membrane protein ferroportin. It seems likely that, in hereditary haemochromatosis and physiological iron deficiency, post-transcriptional control of carrier proteins responsible for the uptake and transfer of iron occurs in the absorptive epithelium on the tips of the intestinal villi. Thus, homeostatic mechanisms in the proximal intestine operate to bring about the coordinated transfer of iron presented in the intestinal lumen specifically to meet body requirements. Proteins, including hephaestin, encoded on the X chromosome, which is mutated in the sex-linked anaemic mouse *sla*, also mediates the transfer of iron across the intestinal mucosa.

The signal for regulating the absorptive activity of the ferrous ion transport pathway is not known. However, it seems likely that interactions between the wild-type HFE protein and transferrin receptors, including the newly described transferrin receptor 2 isoform that may be expressed in intestinal crypts, in some way instruct the developing epithelial cells within the intestinal crypt about body iron requirements. Although functional interactions of HFE molecules with the identified components of the absorptive pathway have yet to be clarified, the HFE protein probably influences iron status in intestinal stem cells within the crypt. By these means, the expression of key transport proteins such as DMT1 and ferroportin may be imprinted, thus influencing their subsequent functional activity during ascent up the villus.

At present, however, much more experimental work will be required to further our understanding of the signalling pathways by which the body iron status regulates the avidity of the proximal small intestine for nutritional iron presented within the lumen. Recently, the putative antimicrobial peptide hepcidin has been the subject of investigation. It is proposed that hepcidin is a negative stimulator of intestinal iron absorption and that hepatic synthesis increases in response to iron overload and inflammation but decreases in the iron-deficient state. Hepcidin appears to a key mediator of iron homeostasis, although exactly how the molecular machinery of intestinal iron absorption responds to changes in the concentration of plasma hepcidin remains to be defined.

A variable, but often substantial, component of dietary iron is present in the organic form as haem. A full molecular understanding of the uptake and transfer pathways for the absorption of iron complexes to the porphyrias is also needed. Whole-body studies show that the absorption of the radiolabelled iron moiety of haemoglobin is enhanced in patients with adult type haemochromatosis. Early studies in dogs have shown that, in the presence of proteolytic digestion products of globin, the haem complex is taken up intact by mucosal epithelial cells; free iron is then released by the action of intracellular haem oxygenases. The contribution of haemoglobin, myoglobin, and cytochromes to the iron overload in patients with haemochromatosis has not been quantified, but iron complexed to haem may well represent an important component of the total burden of body iron in symptomatic haemochromatosis. Recent identification of a putative transporter of haem iron on the brush border of mammalian duodenum is a key advance. Haem carrier protein 1 (HCP1) is up-regulated in response to iron deficiency and hypoxia, but its contribution to the dysregulated absorption of iron in hereditary haemochromatosis is unclear.

Genetics and molecular biology of haemochromatosis

The principal determinant of adult haemochromatosis has long been known to be tightly linked to the human MHC loci on the short arm of chromosome 6. In 1996, mutations in the HLA class

I-linked haemochromatosis gene, *HFE*, were shown to predispose to the adult form of the disease. The most common mutation in the nonclassical MHC class I HFE protein affects a key cysteine residue, which contributes to the formation of the conserved α-3 helix that interacts cotranslationally with the β_2-microglobulin protein. This association is required for the cell-surface expression of all class I MHC molecules. Most patients with haemochromatosis are thus homozygous for a cysteine to tyrosine mutation at codon 282 (*C282Y*) of the nascent HFE protein. An increased frequency of this mutation, in association with the more common *H63D* missense mutation, also occurs in adult haemochromatosis (see Fig. 12.7.1.3). A minor variant, affecting the same region in the α_1 helix, *S65C*, is also occasionally associated with the *C282Y* allele in compound heterozygotes with adult iron storage disease.

These missense mutations in HFE occur at a much lower frequency in control populations without iron overload. Apart from reducing cell-surface expression of the mutant C282Y polypeptide, and thus the abundance of this protein within a population of cytoplasmic vesicles, a functional explanation for the qualitative abnormality of iron metabolism that characterizes haemochromatosis is not available. Recent unsubstantiated experiments have indicated the coexpression of HFE with transferrin receptor isoforms within a vesicular intracellular compartment. Structural studies have provided a molecular basis for this interaction based on the expression of truncated soluble HFE and transferrin receptor protein *in vitro*, combined with elegant structural studies using X-ray diffraction. Recently, a novel isoform of the transferrin receptor, transferrin receptor 2, has been identified in intestinal crypt cells where it may colocalize with the HFE protein within intracellular vesicles. Since rare cases of adult haemochromatosis have been reported with nonsense and inactivating (null) mutations in the transferrin receptor 2 gene (*TFR2*), it seems likely that the HFE protein participates in the regulation of iron delivery to cells through the transferrin ligand. HFE may affect the delivery of transferrin-bound iron by way of the transferrin receptor, or, also plausibly, by the transferrin receptor 2 isoform in intestinal crypt cells, thereby influencing their subsequent absorptive behaviour.

The recently identified peptide hepcidin has become the focus of attention as the potential circulatory signal for body iron status with a key role in the disturbed iron homeostasis of hereditary haemochromatosis. Rather than the expected compensatory increase, hepcidin expression is paradoxically decreased and unresponsive in haemochromatosis caused by mutations in *HFE*, *TFR2*, and *HJV*. The proteins encoded by these genes are predominantly synthesized within the liver. Given that these types of haemochromatosis are qualitatively similar and differ mainly in severity, it has been argued that these observations point to a common pathway in hepatocytes which signals hepcidin production downstream. In support of this argument, the distribution of tissue iron in HFE-related haemochromatosis can be altered after inducing experimental overexpression of hepcidin.

Many recent studies suggest that hepcidin production in hepatocytes is linked to a haemojuvelin-dependent signalling pathway which is responsive to plasma iron saturations. Recent studies also suggest an effector function of hepcidin, whereby direct interaction with ferroportin at the cell surface results in its internalization and degradation with consequent reduced export of iron from macrophages and enterocytes. Ferroportin mutations appear either to abrogate cell surface expression of the encoded protein or interfere with the ability of membraneous ferroportin to bind hepcidin; differential effects on cellular iron export correlate with what appear to be the two discrete phenotypes observed in type 4 haemochromatosis. Serum hepcidin concentrations appear to be increased in ferroportin iron overload as opposed to other forms of haemochromatosis.

In summary, a reduction in circulating hepcidin as a consequence of haemochromatosis gene defects, or directly as a result of *HAMP* gene mutations, appears to enhance plasma iron and subsequent tissue loading; it has been proposed that attenuated

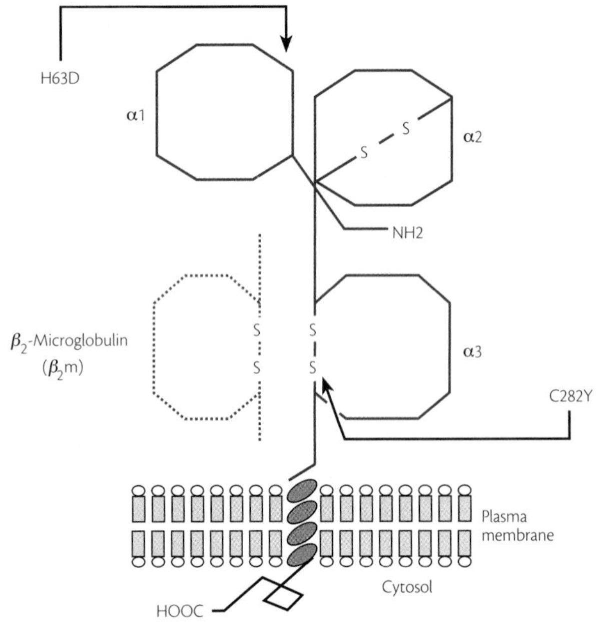

Fig. 12.7.1.3 Diagram of nonclassical MHC class I-like HFE molecule shown in juxtaposition with the β_2-microglobulin. The location of the two frequent amino acid substitutions (*C282Y* and *H63D*) that predispose to the development of adult haemochromatosis is indicated by the arrows.

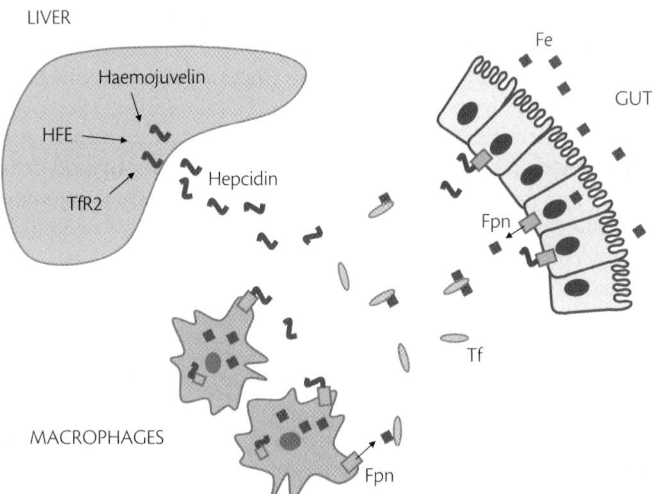

Fig. 12.7.1.4 Molecular regulation of iron homeostasis. This is maintained by hepcidin, a peptide released by hepatocytes into the circulation under stimulatory control of a common pathway involving HFE, hemojuvelin, and transferrin receptor 2. Hepcidin normally inhibits iron export from enterocytes and macrophages via its interaction with ferroportin. Mutations in haemochromatosis genes reduce hepcidin expression and allow excess iron to enter the plasma compartment and bind to transferrin with consequent tissue iron loading.

inhibition of macrophage and enterocyte ferroportin activity is responsible for this effect. An action of hepcidin as an effector molecule after hepatic signalling is central to several current models of iron homeostasis (see Fig. 12.7.1.4).

Clinical features

Adult haemochromatosis

The clinical features of adult haemochromatosis include skin pigmentation. The pigment may be manifest as a generalized slate-grey coloration, due principally to melanin, or localized bronzed pigmentation particularly of the lower limbs, associated with iron deposits in adnexal dermal structures, as well as melanin. Histological examination of the skin reveals increased melanocyte activity in conjunction with iron deposits, particularly in cutaneous sweat and apocrine glands. Increased skin pigmentation is a common, but not invariable, manifestation of haemochromatosis. It increases as the disease progresses and may be a late manifestation of the condition. Absence of pigmentation should consequently never be regarded as a contraindication to the diagnosis of iron storage disease.

Iron storage disease invariably affects the liver, which is usually enlarged and may be cirrhotic, but portal hypertension and splenomegaly are rare end-stage features of haemochromatosis. The enlarged liver, even in the absence of cirrhosis, may contain single or multifocal hepatocellular carcinomas. Hypogonadism is often present and is typically preceded by a long history of fatigue, sexual asthenia, and impotence, as well as premature menopause and loss of libido in women. In men, there is gynaecomastia, circumoral vertical skin wrinkling, and loss of body hair; the genitalia show premature atrophy.

Many patients with haemochromatosis suffer from arthritis at an early phase in the illness and this may indeed be the sole manifestation of the condition for many years. The arthritis typically affects the second and third metacarpophalangeal joints of the hands and feet (Fig. 12.7.1.5). These joints show painful swelling without obvious inflammatory changes. Distal interphalangeal joint disease is also recorded and is usually considered to be typical of osteoarthritis. Many joints, including the wrist, elbow, shoulder, and knee, may be affected and the changes in these joints are typically associated with chondrocalcinosis that is detected radiologically. The affected joints show loss of joint space, subchondral cysts, and, especially in the digits, prominent osteophyte formation (Fig. 12.7.1.6). Recent studies show that premature and disabling arthritis in the hip and other large joints is a characteristic feature of haemochromatosis.

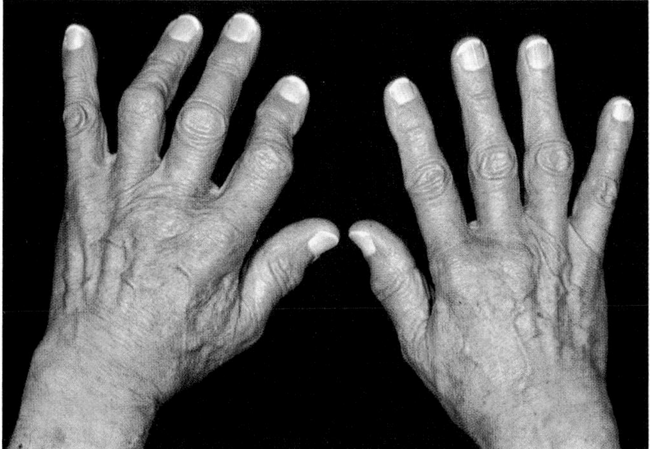

Fig. 12.7.1.5 Arthropathy in a man with adult haemochromatosis forced to stop manual work because of painful arthritis, especially in the second and third metacarpophalangeal joints. Note the increased skin pigmentation.

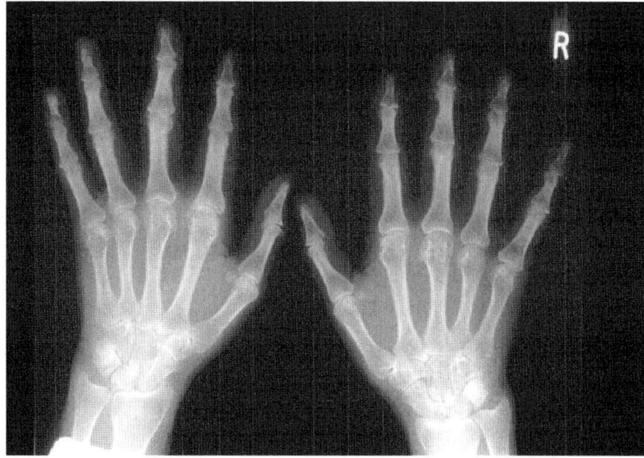

Fig. 12.7.1.6 Radiograph of hands in a 51-year-old woman with haemochromatotic arthropathy of the hands for many years. Note the loss of joint space, especially in metacarpophalangeal joints with subchondral cyst formation and osteophyte growth. Chondrocalcinosis is present in the ulnar fibrocartilage at the wrist.

The symptoms of haemochromatosis are notoriously nonspecific and slow in their progression. Fatigue is often reported and may be a manifestation of hypogonadism and the onset of diabetes mellitus. Atrial fibrillation may be an early manifestation of cardiomyopathy. Later, paroxysmal arrhythmias and cardiac failure supervene, leading to shortness of breath and fatigue. Occasional patients with haemochromatosis present with isolated features, such as abnormal liver-related tests detected during a routine examination for health insurance, or with arthralgia and signs of arthropathy in association with either diabetes, impaired libido, or sexual failure. Cardiomyopathy with heart failure or isolated arrhythmias is an unusual lone presentation of the disease.

The differential diagnosis of haemochromatosis is very wide, but the presence of diabetes with abnormal liver function or hepatomegaly, or an association with endocrine failure or arthropathy, should prompt consideration of iron storage disease. Likewise, the presence of seronegative polyarthropathy with pigmentation, hepatomegaly, or any of the associated endocrinological changes should initiate immediate testing for evidence of haemochromatosis.

In young patients with hypogonadism or cardiomyopathy, iron storage disease should be considered. Juvenile haemochromatosis is often neglected by endocrinologists investigating young patients for infantilism or hypogonadotrophic hypogonadism. The condition may be responsible for cases of undiagnosed seronegative polyarthropathy. Haemochromatosis should be considered in any patient with signs and symptoms of chronic liver disease, including those with sustained mild elevation of serum transaminase activities, particularly since the liver is affected early in the course of the iron overload.

In fully established cases, skin pigmentation which may be either of a grey colour, as a result of increased melanin, or, especially on the shins, a yellow-brown bronze colour. Pigmentation in association with diabetes with or without arthropathy and hepatomegaly almost always signifies established iron storage disease.

Diagnosis

It is critically important to make a diagnosis of haemochromatosis at the earliest opportunity. There is strong evidence that if treatment to remove iron before established structural injury occurs, then tissue function and symptoms improve. Several surveys indicate that removal of iron from patients diagnosed in the precirrhotic phase of adult haemochromatosis is associated with a normal or near-normal life expectancy.

Laboratory investigations

In adult haemochromatosis, the diagnosis can be usually established by demonstrating abnormalities of iron metabolism (fasting serum transferrin saturation with iron greater than 55%) together with a measurement of serum ferritin concentration that provides evidence of increased iron stores. In most, but not all, untreated patients with pathological iron storage disease due to haemochromatosis, the serum concentration of ferritin is elevated. Molecular analysis of the *HFE* gene for homozygosity for the common (*C282Y*) predisposing allele to the development of adult haemochromatosis may be very useful in patients of European ancestry. There is an increased frequency of compound heterozygotes for the *C282Y/H63D* or, more rarely, *C282Y/S65C* genotypes in patients with evidence of iron storage disease. For patients with elevated ferritin but normal or low transferrin saturation, ferroportin disease should be considered.

Given the genetic variants that are now recognized as causes of haemochromatosis, it is clear that if any doubt exists as to the diagnosis, or molecular analysis of the *HFE* gene or of non-*HFE* iron overload genes fails to identify known pathogenic mutations, then tissue diagnosis is indicated. This is usually carried out by liver biopsy with histochemical determination, and preferably chemical quantification, of tissue iron content. Although a liver biopsy is associated with small but definable risks, it does offer a key opportunity for the evaluation of liver structure and of the injury consequent upon iron deposition. The finding of cirrhotic change carries with it a worse prognosis. Cirrhotic change is also a major predictor of the occurrence of hepatocellular carcinoma, which occurs rarely in noncirrhotic subjects with iron storage disease (Fig. 12.7.1.7). For *C282Y* homozygotes, liver biopsy may be reserved for those at risk of significant liver fibrosis. When serum aminotransferase values are normal, hepatomegaly is absent and the serum ferritin is below 1000 μg/litre, the risk of significant fibrosis is negligible. This validated tool applies also to asymptomatic individuals identified through family screening or routine blood testing.

Serum iron-saturation determinations, and particularly serum ferritin concentrations, may signify conditions other than iron storage disease. Serum ferritin is elevated in inflammatory states, in certain malignancies such as Hodgkin's disease and in any condition associated with significant necrosis of parenchymal liver cells. Under these circumstances liver biopsy is recommended, since it is most likely to provide a definitive diagnosis of iron storage disease. Sometimes, however, liver biopsy is not possible, either because the patient will not consent to it, or because of the presence of ascites and a bleeding disorder, especially thrombocytopenia. Under these circumstances, MRI of the liver can demonstrate iron storage if moderate or severe. A reduced signal on T2-weighted imaging correlates with significant iron deposition and a crude assessment of hepatic iron concentration is possible with dedicated data manipulation.

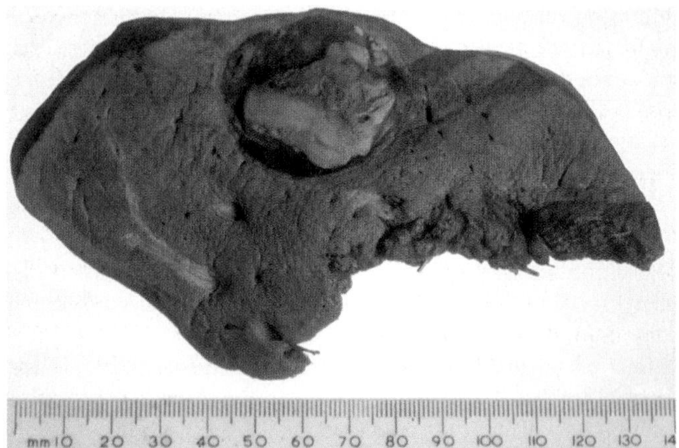

Fig. 12.7.1.7 Adult haemochromatosis. Section of liver lobe after surgical resection to remove a primary hepatocellular carcinoma arising in an iron-loaded but, unusually, noncirrhotic liver in this disorder. The patient, aged 62 years, had been partially treated by venesection but recently noticed increasing lethargy. A raised serum α-fetoprotein concentration led to the diagnosis. Moderate histochemical evidence of iron storage was found in the nonmalignant tissue excised at surgery.

If a liver biopsy is not possible and MRI of the liver does not reveal increased ferromagnetic signals indicative of iron storage, there are two further options: measurement of urinary iron excretion after parenteral administration of desferrioxamine, and, where the patient will tolerate it, quantitative phlebotomy. Injection of 500 mg of desferrioxamine intramuscularly in a patient with iron overload will usually induce the daily excretion of more than 2 mg of iron as the ferrioxamine complex in the urine. Ferrioxamine excretion may be increased in patients with haemolytic anaemia but, when elevated, is generally indicative of iron storage disease. Weekly phlebotomy of 500 ml will remove approximately 225 mg of iron, and thus provides a means of estimating the amount of iron removed from the storage compartment when undertaken to induce a mild hypochromic anaemia of approximately 10.5 to 11.0 g of haemoglobin/dl or a serum ferritin concentration of less than 30 μg/litre. Iron overload exists when the estimated iron removed by this method exceeds 1.5 g. Unfortunately, quantitative phlebotomy is cumbersome and may not be possible in patients with severe liver disease associated with hypoalbuminaemia.

Diagnosis in family members

The diagnosis of haemochromatosis, whether it be of the adult or juvenile form, has immediate implications for that individual's first-degree relatives. All forms of haemochromatosis have a strong hereditary basis and even some forms of neonatal haemochromatosis may, in some families, be inherited as an autosomal recessive trait. A dominant transmission pattern has been established in the case of type 4 haemochromatosis.

Although the penetrance and expressivity of homozygosity for the various alleles that predispose to haemochromatosis is not yet established, the risks of the disease in first-degree family members is sufficiently high to warrant systematic study. Clearly, the implications for asymptomatic or undiagnosed relatives of the index case are potentially very large. Hence, considerable care and sensitivity are needed in the means of informing them about the condition through the identified index case. In large families there may be formidable difficulties, so that the help of genetic counselling services, as well as formal assistance from physicians practised in medical genetics, may be needed. There can be little doubt, however, that at-risk relatives should be offered the opportunity for further diagnostic and clinical evaluation in relation to iron storage disease. The condition is readily susceptible to iron-depletion therapy in its early stages. Moreover, there may be additional considerations for patients who wish to make reproductive choices and who will need to be reassured that appropriate testing can be carried out on their future offspring.

In HFE haemochromatosis, molecular analysis of the *HFE* gene (and, formerly, the tightly linked class I HLA class typing) may assist in assessing the risk of disease, particularly in asymptomatic siblings. Phenotypic screening, however, is useful at the level of clinical evaluation for evidence of liver disease, hypogonadism, arthritis, pigmentation, and diabetes. Determining the biochemical phenotype first involves assay of the serum parameters of disordered iron metabolism. Since the serum parameters may be abnormal before iron-mediated tissue injury has occurred, liver biopsy should be considered particularly if the serum ferritin is greater than 1000 µg/ml or the serum transaminases are raised.

In first-degree relatives, in whom HLA typing or molecular analysis of the *HFE* or non-*HFE* iron overload genes indicates a genetic predisposition to the disease, periodic re-evaluation is needed by clinical and biochemical testing at intervals of not more than 5 years. In members of families affected by haemochromatosis due to mutations in the *HFE* or non-*HFE* iron overload gene who were not found to carry the predisposing mutations and whose ferritin and iron parameters are normal, liver biopsy is not mandatory and the risk of the development of significant iron storage disease in less than 5 or 10 years is extremely low. In patients with no known pregenetic disposition and normal tissue biopsy findings, further follow-up screening is not indicated.

From the foregoing it can be seen that there is an urgent need to characterize the genotype–phenotype relationship in both *HFE* and non-*HFE* haemochromatosis. Unfortunately, no genetic locus has yet been identified for neonatal haemochromatosis, although this is a subject of continuing research. In at-risk pregnancies, neonatal haemochromatosis may be occasionally recognized by MRI during the third trimester, which may show increased iron signals in the fetal liver. After birth, biopsy of the oral mucosa on the gums or inner lip may reveal histological evidence of iron storage in minor salivary glands of affected infants.

Environmental cofactors and disease expression

Many patients with adult haemochromatosis give a history of excessive current or prior alcohol consumption. In the past, physicians have been tempted to attribute evidence of excess tissue iron in these individuals solely to the consumption of alcohol. In practice, however, it appears that those individuals who have biopsy-proven evidence of hepatic iron storage usually prove to carry two predisposing alleles of the *HFE* gene and therefore have true haemochromatosis. Although no clear predictors for the expressio n of disease in first-degree relatives at risk are available, disease expression is reduced in women of reproductive age. Most practising clinicians consider that age and alcohol consumption are the main identifiable environmental factors that contribute to disease expression in predisposed homozygotes. Other comorbid factors, including heritable factors, that may influence the expression of *HFE* mutations in homozygous subjects, include the presence of adult coeliac disease. There are few data that define the relationship between haemochromatosis and coeliac disease, but subclinical coeliac disease may ameliorate the long-standing effects of iron loading in *C282Y* homozygotes. Cosegregation of haemochromatosis and coeliac disease has not hitherto been reported. Recently, discriminatory polymorphisms in genes which modulate oxidative stress and other fibrogenic cytokine responses have been postulated as influencing expression of haemochromatosis in *C282Y* homozygotes.

The identification, since *HFE*, of several genes associated with haemochromatosis has provided some insight into the phenotypic variation of primary iron overload. The phenotype of type 4 haemochromatosis certainly appears distinct. It is now apparent, however, that individuals with juvenile mutations may present later and with milder disease than described historically for juvenile haemochromatosis patients. Those with *TFR2* mutations have occasionally presented young with a severe iron overload phenotype more reminiscent of juvenile haemochromatosis. Iron overload with varying severity has been accounted for by compound heterozygous forms of *HFE* and juvenile mutations, termed digenic inheritance. Moreover, *C282Y* homozygotes with the most severe iron overload may carry an additional juvenile mutation to account for increased disease expression. The classical haemochromatosis phenotypes overlap and combinations of genetic alteration contribute to a spectrum of disease.

Treatment

Since it is the toxicity of iron that is responsible for the manifestations of all forms of haemochromatosis, treatment is directed to the removal of iron at the earliest possible stage.

Venesection

In adult and juvenile haemochromatosis, the preferred method of treatment is iron depletion by means of phlebotomy. This is best instituted by the removal of approximately 500 ml of venous blood each week by needle puncture of peripheral veins in the antecubital fossa. In young patients, it may be possible to increase the frequency of venesection to twice per week after several once-weekly procedures. In elderly patients and those with hypoalbuminaemia as well as end-organ failure and heart disease, the frequency of venesection should be commuted to within the rate tolerated. Coincidental inflammatory disease may impede the erythropoietin-mediated drive to haemopoiesis, and, particularly in the early phases of treatment, mild haemorrhagic anaemia may ensure. Thus, adjustments need to be made according to the early responses to venesection therapy, and regular monitoring of the haemoglobin concentration or haematocrit is advisable.

Difficulties may arise in delivering this deceptively simple treatment as a result of poor organization of health service provision and of unavailability of suitable health care personnel to carry out the venesection procedure. Venesection should not be carried out by naive or incompetent medical and nursing staff. Every practical effort should be made to ensure that the procedure is convenient for the patient, who is often a young or middle-aged person in full-time employment, and who may find regular access to the treatment centre problematic. In cold weather, or in patients with poor circulation or inconspicuous superficial venous access, the use of local anaesthetics such as lidocaine cream or even local diffusable preparations of glyceryl trinitrate, applied 30 to 60 min before the venesection procedure, may greatly improve venous access. Likewise, the simple technique of immersing the arm in warm water to improve peripheral blood flow may be critical for establishing confidence in treatment staff. Since patients with haemochromatosis usually harbour a large burden of iron, requiring repeated phlebotomy over a period of several years, every effort should be made to preserve the integrity of their peripheral veins. In the authors' view, the use of a local anaesthetic is usually unwarranted since it involves further tissue invasion in the region of the antecubital fossa with needles. Moreover, repeated injections of the irritant fluid often lead to sclerosis around the venous access site. Where blood transfusion services can assume some, if not all, responsibility for the phlebotomy of haemochromatosis patients, the inconvenience of hospital-based services can be circumvented and blood supplies can be enhanced safely.

Duration of venesection therapy

One 500 ml unit of peripheral blood contains approximately 225 mg of elemental iron. Thus most patients with established haemochromatosis will require weekly phlebotomy for a period of 2 to 3 years. The objective of this treatment is to restore serum ferritin concentrations to within the low normal range and, if possible, to induce a mild iron-deficiency anaemia of approximately 11.5 g haemoglobin/dl. Having thus achieved a satisfactory depletion of body iron stores, interval maintenance phlebotomy, carried out according to ferritin measurements, four to six times per year is usually sufficient to maintain normal iron stores with a serum ferritin concentration less than 100 μg/litre. Some authorities suggest that serum ferritin values below 30 μg/litre should ideally be achieved. In patients with juvenile haemochromatosis, who have a higher than normal intestinal iron absorption, more frequent phlebotomy may be needed to maintain a healthy iron balance.

Iron chelation therapy

Alternative methods of iron removal are needed for patients with severe clinical manifestations of haemochromatosis, such as life-threatening cardiac arrhythmias and those with severe liver disease and hypoalbuminaemia, who are incapable of withstanding frequent phlebotomy. The preferred alternative involves chelation therapy with the parenteral agent desferrioxamine. As indicated in Chapter 22.5.4, the subcutaneous administration of desferrioxamine brings about the removal of a maximum of 20 to 25 mg of iron daily and is thus generally less efficient than vigorous weekly phlebotomy. However, desferrioxamine may gain access to cellular pools of iron that are important in the pathogenesis of tissue injury in established iron storage disease, and therefore may offer particular benefit in patients critically ill with arrhythmias due to haemochromatotic cardiomyopathy. Although the nature of this so-called 'chelatable iron pool' is unknown, there is strong circumstantial evidence that its depletion by means of intravenous desferrioxamine treatment may reverse the life-threatening consequences of terminal iron storage disease in patients with haemochromatosis. Moreover, the removal of 140 mg of chelatable iron per week represents about two-thirds of the amount that can be removed by weekly phlebotomy. A biological advantage may also be gained by therapeutic access to a reactive, low molecular weight, chelatable fraction responsible for the injurious effects of cellular iron overload.

Parenteral desferrioxamine may be given intravenously for life-threatening cardiac disease, as described in Chapter 22.5.4, or, in the nonemergent situation, by subcutaneous infusion using portable infusion pumps for 12 to 14 h, five or six times per week. It must be stressed, however, that chelation therapy is not the preferred option for the treatment of established haemochromatosis and should be restricted to those patients unable to tolerate phlebotomy as a result of anaemia or hypoalbuminaemia, or in whom life-threatening cardiomyopathy or liver disease is present. Newer oral iron chelators with promising safety profiles are in development and are becoming established for secondary iron overload. Their use in hereditary haemochromatosis awaits exploration but represent a promising alternative to venesection.

General measures

Attention should be given in patients with haemochromatosis to the diagnosis and treatment of end-organ failure. This particularly applies to the management of diabetes mellitus by diet and insulin where necessary, as well as hormone replacement therapy for hypogonadism (see Chapter 13.8.2). In men, intramuscular depot injections of testosterone enantate (250 mg every 2–3 weeks) are recommended to improve libido and inhibit the development of premature osteoporosis. Similarly, conventional sex hormone replacement therapy should be used in women with premature gonadal failure as a result of haemochromatosis. Cardiac failure in patients with haemochromatosis due to cardiomyopathy and hepatic failure consequential upon pigmentary cirrhosis should be treated by standard methods. Organ transplantation may be used successfully, but correction of systemic iron overload should be undertaken as soon as practicable to restore normal function in all organ systems. Rarely, end-organ hormone deficiencies result from thyroid infiltration and parathyroid and adrenocortical disease. These deficiencies should be vigorously sought for in the clinical evaluation of the patient at presentation. The appearance of lethargy, faintness due to postural hypotension, or symptomatic hypocalcaemia demands immediate investigation and institution of appropriate replacement therapy. Patients with cirrhosis should undergo 6 monthly surveillance by ultrasound examination and α-fetoprotein estimation for early detection of hepatocellular carcinoma.

Prognosis

The main causes of death in untreated patients with haemochromatosis are hepatocellular failure, primary carcinoma of the liver (including hepatocellular carcinoma), and, rarely, cholangiocarcinomas. Cardiac failure due to haemochromatotic cardiomyopathy and untreated diabetes also contribute to death. Although not categorically proven, evidence from retrospective surveys suggest that life expectancy is improved by removing iron from patients with haemochromatosis of whatever cause and the subsequent maintenance of normal iron homeostasis. Most patients experience an improvement in well-being on iron-depletion therapy and, during its early phases, there is evidence that hypogonadotrophic hypogonadism may improve with this therapy. Similarly, the manifestations of cardiomyopathy with intractable cardiac failure or tachyarrhythmias can improve after the removal of iron.

The cirrhosis of haemochromatosis appears not to be reversible, although the earlier precirrhotic manifestations of hepatic disease improve greatly on the removal of iron with an apparent restoration of normal life expectancy. Indeed, there is mounting evidence that hepatic fibrosis, short of cirrhosis, can reverse following iron depletion. In all patients, there is at least a twofold increase in the survival rate at 5 years from the point of diagnosis with the introduction of phlebotomy. In patients studied during the 1950s and 1960s, the 5-year survival rate improved from 18% to more than 65% in all haemochromatosis subjects treated.

In patients diagnosed with haemochromatosis but without cirrhosis, iron-depletion therapy is associated with a near normal or normal life expectancy compared with a sex- and age-matched control cohort derived from the same population. It is notable, however, that the indolent nature of this storage disorder and the long-term survival of patients who are affected by it has, so far, rendered long-term controlled studies of the effects of phlebotomy on eventual outcome almost impossible to achieve. However, a wealth of evidence, based on the understanding of the pathogenesis and documented responses to iron depletion in individual patient cohorts, indicates that early removal of iron is highly desirable—indeed, it may be decisive in determining a good outcome from all forms of human iron storage disease, including all subtypes of hereditary haemochromatosis so far established.

Hepatocellular carcinoma occurs mostly in patients with iron storage disease who have established cirrhosis and the risk appears to persist despite removal of iron. Although hepatocellular carcinoma and cholangiocarcinoma have been reported in noncirrhotic patients with haemochromatosis, these are rare phenomena. Systematic ultrasound surveillance is vital if liver cancer is to be detected at a stage where potentially curative treatment can be offered. Since all the evidence suggests that patients with haemochromatosis are more likely to have diabetes mellitus and other manifestations of the disease, every encouragement should be given to the prompt diagnosis of the condition and early institution of iron-depletion therapy.

Increasingly, it has been recognized that the arthropathy of haemochromatosis can be disabling, whether or not it is associated simply with joint pain (arthralgia) or progressive and noninflammatory joint destruction. The disease is associated with a loss of cartilage and, in many large joints, chondrocalcinosis. Although the response of the arthropathy to iron-depletion therapy is controversial, the weight of observation indicates that, once established, the arthropathy of haemochromatosis progresses independently of body iron status and of iron-depletion treatment. It seems intrinsically likely that effective removal of excess body iron stores before the development of joint symptoms will prevent their onset and progression. However, at present only cross-sectional data are available to support this contention.

In summary, observations in adult haemochromatosis suggest that once the disease is established in association with cirrhosis or diabetes mellitus, it diminishes life expectancy. The prognosis for cardiomyopathy in juvenile haemochromatosis is very poor but it may be improved by early diagnosis and the early institution of vigorous iron-depletion therapy. In several cases, the outcome has been improved by allogeneic cardiac transplantation. In adult patients with established pigment cirrhosis, hepatic transplantation has been undertaken and, provided the other systemic manifestations of haemochromatosis have been adequately treated, the procedure is associated with a good overall prognosis.

Prevention and control

The importance of early recognition and the institution of iron-depletion therapy in all forms of haemochromatosis cannot be overemphasized. Molecular analysis of the *HFE* gene or HLA class I haplotype screening, together with biochemical characterization using serum transferrin iron saturation estimations and serum ferritin concentrations, has the power to assist greatly in the detection of presymptomatic first-degree relatives of patients with haemochromatosis.

In relation to whole populations in which mutations in the *HFE* gene are frequent, the health implications based on mass screening remain contentious. Superficially, adult hereditary haemochromatosis due to mutations in the *HFE* gene appears to be an ideal condition for DNA-based mass population screening. The condition is attributable to a single gene, and a single mutation of diagnostic significance is prevalent (gene frequency 5–10%). Disease-related mutations in *HFE* (especially *C282Y*) are easily tested for by means of techniques based on the polymerase chain reaction. At the same time, HFE-mediated haemochromatosis has a long incubation period without symptoms, and all the evidence suggests that the institution of treatment for presymptomatic disease is cheap, simple, and effective.

On the other hand, genetic identification of at-risk individuals is associated with problems of stigmatization, increased anxiety, and potential life insurance weighting, all of which are familiar aspects in well-rehearsed debates about genetic testing in the general population. These aspects must be considered, together with the age-related penetrance of the homozygous state for *HFE C282Y* variants and, as yet, unknown combined genetic and environmental influences on disease expression. Uncertainty as to the significance of these factors has held back the introduction of mass population screening by DNA-based methods. In light of the present state of knowledge, it is clear that homozygosity for the *C282Y* allele of *HFE* cannot be considered to be tantamount to a diagnosis of hereditary haemochromatosis.

More information is needed from outbred populations, rather than from homozygotes identified as a result of screening family members of index cases having full-blown clinical disease. Family studies provide a false measure of disease expressivity, presumably as a result of shared environments and of the cosegregation of potential disease-modifying genes within defined pedigrees. Finally, it must be emphasized that difficulties also occur for the evaluation of the burden of haemochromatosis in the population at large. Although there are definitions of iron storage disease that reflect the abnormal biochemical genotype, the manifestations of the clinical disease are variable and protean. Moreover, as pointed out earlier, no internationally agreed case definition of haemochromatosis exists, which creates additional difficulties for the introduction of public health measures and appropriate policy review of nationwide screening procedures.

Future directions

Although startling progress has been made in the discovery of many components that serve to regulate iron homeostasis in humans, more information is needed before a full molecular understanding of the mechanisms of iron homeostasis can be achieved. The genetic basis of some neonatal and further variant forms of adult haemochromatosis has yet to be fully explored. The downstream effects of HFE and haemojuvelin require ongoing study and the concept of hepcidin as the principal controlling factor in iron homeostasis needs confirmation. An even more challenging task will be the identification of the environmental cofactors that determine the expression of iron storage disease in genetically predisposed individuals. Alcohol is a long-standing candidate, but the mechanism by which it leads to increased delivery of toxic iron to the tissues is, at present, poorly understood. Recognizing genetic modifiers of disease expression may, in future, inform natural history and treatment decisions in asymptomatic individuals at risk from iron storage disease. Greater understanding of these issues and of penetrance in particular populations will determine local screening practices for disease prevention.

Newly identified iron storage diseases

By general agreement, the term haemochromatosis is used to describe systemic syndromes of pathological iron storage that affect many tissues and disturb the function of diverse organ systems. Conversely, several distinct clinical syndromes of local iron toxicity have been identified, especially in the eye and brain. Although these syndromes are individually rare, they are important because they are potentially accessible to measures that reduce cellular free iron (e.g. metal chelation, mentioned above), and because they demonstrate the central importance of metabolic iron in selected tissues. A fuller understanding of these disorders, and the cognate cell metabolic pathways they affect, may well shed light on ill-understood aspects of tissue iron physiology. Additional information is available by reference to the Online Mendelian Inheritance in Man (OMIM) website at http://www.ncbi.nlm.nih.gov/omim.

Hereditary hyperferritinaemia cataract syndrome (OMIM 600886)

The sole clinical manifestation of this condition is of congenital bilateral ferrugineous nuclear cataracts due to the disposition of excess ferritin light chain polypeptide in the ocular lenses. The serum ferritin concentrations are moderately elevated but no evidence of systemic iron storage is found. The disorder is caused by mutations in the 5′ noncoding iron-response element of the ferritin light-chain gene that leads to unregulated translational overexpression of ferritin light chains. These polypeptides accumulate in the lenses and disturb their tissue organization and refractile properties. The hyperferritinaemia cataract syndrome is, as expected for an overexpression disease, inherited as a dominant trait. Measurement of serum ferritin concentrations may identify at-risk family members. The gene encoding ferritin light chain polypeptide maps to chromosome 19q3.3-qter.

Adult-onset basal ganglia disease (OMIM 606159)

A single pedigree has been identified with a dominantly inherited disorder showing features of late-onset extrapyramidal dysfunction resembling parkinsonism or Huntington's disease. Imaging and autopsy studies revealed cavitation of the basal ganglia with deposition of iron and ferritin protein in adjacent tissue, especially in the putamen and the globus pallidus. The macroscopic appearances showed widespread reddish discolouration of affected tissues. This disorder was mapped to chromosome 19q13.3 and a single mutation, a point insertion of a single adenine at nucleotide 461, was identified in exon 4 of the ferritin light-chain gene. The mutation is predicted to disrupt the C-terminal sequence of the ferritin light-chain molecule and disturb the iron-binding core of the hetero or homomeric protein. Serum ferritin concentrations were found to be abnormally low in affected heterozygotes. Although this disorder has so far only been identified in a single large pedigree, it further illustrates the importance of ferritin in tissue iron metabolism and, especially, in selective regions of the brain. This disorder has been termed a 'neuroferritinopathy' and may be the first of several diseases affecting cellular iron pathways in iron-rich brain tissue.

Acaeruloplasminaemia with iron deposition (haemosiderosis) in basal ganglia (OMIM 277900)

This disorder is associated with mild systemic iron deposition and deficiency of the plasma copper-binding protein, caeruloplasmin. Caeruloplasmin has long been known to possess ferroxidase activity and the ability to enhance the mobilization and delivery of iron to and from macrophages and hepatocytes. It promotes iron loading of intact ferritin micelles. Acaeruloplasminaemia, due to mutations in the gene encoding caeruloplasmin on chromosome 3q21–24, is an autosomal recessive trait. The deficiency is associated with diabetes mellitus, dementia, and extrapyramidal features including parkinsonism, with choreoathetosis as well as cerebellar ataxia. MRI shows altered signals in the basal ganglia, and retinal degeneration may be apparent by fundoscopy. Excess systemic iron is demonstrable by examination of liver tissue and the serum ferritin concentration is moderately elevated; however, low serum iron transferrin saturations with hypochromic microcytic anaemia, reminiscent of copper deficiency, are usually present.

Infusions of plasma or purified caeruloplasmin may correct the systemic abnormalities of iron metabolism, but probably do not influence the dementia or the other neurological deficits, at least once these are established. The role of caeruloplasmin replacement or indeed parenteral chelation therapy with desferrioxamine or trientine, especially in the early evolution of the neurological syndrome, has not yet been established. The interplay between copper and iron metabolism is well illustrated by this severely disabling illness. Acaeruloplasminaemia illustrates the particular sensitivity of the basal ganglia to disturbances of iron metabolism. In this context, it is notable that caeruloplasmin expression is abundant in glia in the brain microvasculature juxtaposed to the pigment-containing dopaminergic neurones of the substantia nigra and inner layer of the retina.

Hallervorden–Spatz disease: pantothenate kinase-associated neurodegeneration (OMIM 234200)

This disease has been familiar to neurologists and neuropathologists since its original description by two, now discredited, German neuroscientists of the Nazi period. The clinical features indicate basal ganglia disease and dementia with retinal degeneration leading to optic atrophy. The disorder often presents with club foot deformity in children and adolescents; extrapyramidal rigidity preceded by choreoathetosis usually follows rapidly. Dementia, optic atrophy, and generalized seizures occur in the latter stages, and death usually ensues by the age of 30 years. Although late-onset forms of the disease are known, a striking feature is the presence of iron pigment in the basal ganglia and substantia nigra, now easily recognized by MRI. The heredofamilial nature of this syndrome has been known since its first description. Hallervorden–Spatz disease is now known to be an autosomal recessive trait due to mutations in the pantothenate kinase 2 (*PANK2*) gene that maps to chromosome 20p13.

Pantothenate kinase 2 is abundant in the retina and target regions of the brain and regulates the formation of coenzyme A. Deficiency of pantothenate kinase 2 would deplete sensitive neural tissues with a high metabolic rate of coenzyme A; the defect may also lead to a consequential accumulation of cysteine, which normally condenses with the enzyme product, phosphopantothenate. In the presence of high concentrations of free iron, excess cysteine may accelerate the formation of cytotoxic oxygen free radicals. For some years, cysteine accumulation has been independently observed in the iron-rich nigrostriatal regions of the brain affected by this disorder. Identification of *PANK2* mutations offers the hope of improved diagnosis of this neurodegenerative disorder, and, more importantly, the prospect of specific therapy using supplementation to enhance local coenzyme A activity and phosphopantothenate concentrations in affected neural tissue.

Further practical information

Many patients' associations and societies exist to serve the needs of patients in their respective countries. In the United Kingdom, useful information can be obtained from The Haemochromatosis Society, Hollybush House, Hadley Green Road, Barnet, EN5 5PR. Fax: 44 (0) 208 449 1363; Email: info@haemochromatosis.org.uk.

The society's website (http://www.haemochromatosis.org.uk) includes links to similar societies in other parts of the world.

Further reading

Adams PC, Speechley M, Kertesz, AE (1991). Long-term survival analysis in hereditary haemochromatosis. *Gastroenterology*, **101**, 368–72.

Adams PC, *et al.* (2005). Hemochromatosis and iron-overload screening in a racially diverse population. *N Engl J Med*, **352**, 1769–78.

Adams PC, Barton JC. (2007). Haemochromatosis. *Lancet*, **370**, 1855–60.

Adams P, *et al.* (2009). Screening for iron overload: Lessons from the HEmochromatosis and IRon Overload Screening (HEIRS) Study. *Canadian Journal of Gastroenterology*, **23**, 769–72.

Allen KJ, *et al.* (2008). Iron-overload-related disease in *HFE* hereditary hemochromatosis. *N Engl J Med*, **358**, 221–30.

Andersen RV, *et al.* (2004). Hemochromatosis mutations in the general population: iron overload progression rate. *Blood*, **103**, 2914–19.

Babitt JL, *et al.* (2006). Bone morphogenetic protein signaling by hemojuvelin regulates hepcidin expression. *Nat Genet*, **38**, 531–39.

Beutler E, *et al.* (2002). Penetrance of 845G→A (C282Y). *HFE* hereditary haemochromatosis mutation in the USA. *Lancet*, **359**, 211–18.

Bomford A, Williams R (1976). Long-term results of venesection therapy in idiopathic haemochromatosis. *Q J Med (N S)*, **45**, 611–23.

Brissot P, *et al.* (2008). Current approach to hemochromatosis. *Blood Rev*, **22**, 195–210.

Bulaj ZJ, *et al.* (2000). Disease-related conditions in relatives of patients with hemochromatosis. *N Engl J Med*, **343**, 1529–35.

Burke W, *et al.* (1998). Hereditary hemochromatosis. Gene discovery and its implications for population-based screening. *JAMA*, **280**, 172–78.

Camaschella C, *et al.* (2000). The gene TfR2 is mutated in a new type of haemochromatosis mapping to 7q22. *Nat Genet*, **25**, 14–15.

Camaschella C, Poggiali E (2009). Rare types of genetic hemochromatosis. *Acta Haematologica*, **122**, 140–5.

De Gobbi M, *et al.* (2002). Natural history of juvenile haemochromatosis. *Br J Haematol*, **117**, 973–99.

Falize L, *et al.* (2006). Reversibility of hepatic fibrosis in treated genetic hemochromatosis: a study of 36 cases. *Hepatology*, **44**, 472–7.

Fargion S, *et al.* (1992). Survival and prognostic factors in 212 Italian patients with genetic haemochromatosis. *Hepatology*, **15**, 655–59.

Fargion S, *et al.* (2001). Tumor necrosis factor alpha promoter polymorphisms influence the phenotypic expression of hereditary hemochromatosis. *Blood*, **97**, 3707–12.

Feder JN, *et al.* (1996). A novel MHC class I-like gene is mutated in patients with haemochromatosis. *Nat Genet*, **13**, 399–408.

Finch SC, Finch CA (1955). Idiopathic hemochromatosis, an iron storage disease. Iron metabolism in hemochromatosis. *Medicine (Baltimore)*, **34**, 381–430.

Fleming ME, *et al.* (1999). Mechanism of increased iron absorption in murine model of hereditary haemochromatosis: increased duodenal expression of the iron transporter, DMT-1. *Proc Natl Acad Sci U S A*, **96**, 3143–48.

Fleming RE, Bacon BR (2005). Iron homeostasis. *N Engl J Med*, **352**, 1741–44.

Gao J, *et al.* (2009). Interaction of the hereditary hemochromatosis protein HFE with transferrin receptor 2 is required for transferrin-induced hepcidin expression. *Cell Metabolism*, **9**, 217–27.

Griffiths WJ (2007). Review article: the genetic basis of haemochromatosis. *Aliment Pharmacol Ther*, **26**, 331–42.

Kellerher T, *et al.* (2004). Increased DMT1 but not IREG1 or HFE mRNA following iron depletion therapy in hereditary haemochromatosis. *Gut*, **53**, 1174–9.

Kelly AL, *et al.* (1998). Hereditary juvenile haemochromatosis: a genetically heterogenous life-threatening iron storage disease. *Q J Med*, **91**, 607–18.

Kelly AL, *et al.* (2001). Classification and genetic features of neonatal haemochromatosis: a study of twenty-seven affected pedigrees and molecular analysis of genes implicated in iron metabolism. *J Med Genet*, **38**, 599–10.

Le Gac G, *et al.* (2004). The recently identified type 2A juvenile haemochromatosis gene (HJV), a second candidate modifier of the C282Y homozygous phenotype. *Hum Mol Genet*, **13**, 1913–18.

Lee PL, Beutler E (2009). Regulation of hepcidin and iron-overload disease. *Annual Reviews in Pathology*, **4**, 489–515.

McCance RA, Widdowson EM (1937). Absorption and excretion of iron. *Lancet*, **233**, 680–4.

McKie AT, *et al.* (2000). A novel duodenal iron-regulated transporter, IREG1, implicated in baso-lateral transfer of iron to the circulation. *Mol Cell*, **5**, 299–309.

McKie AT, *et al.* (2001). An iron-regulated ferric reductase associated with the absorption of dietary iron. *Science*, **291**, 1755–9.

Merryweather-Clarke AT, *et al.* (1998). The effect of HFE mutations on serum ferritin and transferrin saturation in the Jersey population. *Br J Haematol*, **101**, 369–73.

Merryweather-Clarke AT, *et al.* (2003). Digenic inheritance of mutations in HAMP and HFE results in different types of haemochromatosis. *Hum Mol Genet*, **12**, 2241–7.

Meynard D, *et al.* (2009). Lack of the bone morphogenetic protein BMP6 induces massive iron overload. *Nature Genetics*, **41**, 478–81.

Montosi G, *et al.* (2001). Autosomal-dominant hemochromatosis is associated with a mutation in the ferroportin (SLC11A3) gene. *J Clin Invest*, **108**, 619–23.

Nemeth E, *et al.* (2004). Hepcidin regulates cellular iron efflux by binding to ferroportin and inducing its internalization. *Science*, **306**, 2090–3.

Nicolas G, *et al.* (2003). Constitutive hepcidin expression prevents iron overload in a mouse model of hemochromatosis. *Nat Genet*, **34**, 97–101.

Niederau C, *et al.* (1996). Long-term survival in patients with hereditary haemochromatosis. *Gastroenterology*, **110**, 1107–19.

Olynyk JK, *et al.* (2004). Evolution of untreated hereditary hemochromatosis in the Busselton population: a 17-year study. *Mayo Clin Proc*, **79**, 309–13.

Papanikolaou G, *et al.* (2004) Mutations in HFE2 cause iron overload in chromosome 1q-linked juvenile hemochromatosis. *Nat Genet*, **36**, 77–82.

Roetto A, *et al.* (1999). Juvenile hemochromatosis locus maps to chromosome 1q. *Am J Hum Genet*, **64**, 1388–93.

Roetto A, *et al.* (2003). Mutant antimicrobial peptide hepcidin is associated with severe juvenile hemochromatosis. *Nat Genet*, **33**, 21–2.

Sheldon JH (1935). *Haemochromatosis*. London: Oxford University Press.

Simon M, Bourel M, Genetet B (1977). Idiopathic hemochromatosis: demonstration of recessive transmission and early detection by family HLA typing. *N Engl J Med*, **297**, 1017–21.

Wallace DF, et al. (2009). Combined deletion of Hfe and transferrin receptor 2 in mice leads to marked dysregulation of hepcidin and iron overload. *Hepatology*, **50**, 1992–2000.

Whitington PF, Kelly S (2008). Outcome of pregnancies at risk for neonatal hemochromatosis is improved by treatment with high-dose intravenous immunoglobulin. *Pediatrics*, **121**, e1615–21.

Zoller H, Cox TM (2005). Hemochromatosis: genetic testing and clinical practice. *Clin Gastroenterol Hepatol*, **3**, 945–58.

Zoller H, *et al.* (2005). Primary iron overload with inappropriate hepcidin expression in V162del ferroportin disease. *Hepatology*, **42**, 466–72.

12.7.2 Inherited diseases of copper metabolism: Wilson's disease and Menkes' disease

Michael L. Schilsky and Pramod K. Mistry

Essentials

Copper is an essential metal that is an important cofactor for many proteins and enzymes. Two related genetic defects in copper transport have been described.

Wilson's disease

An uncommon disorder (1 in 30 000) caused by autosomal recessive loss of function mutations in a metal-transporting P-type ATPase (*ATP7B*) that result in defective copper excretion into bile and hence copper toxicity. Typical presentation is in the second and third decade of life with liver disease (ranging from asymptomatic hepatomegaly to fulminant hepatic failure) or neuropsychiatric disorder (dystonia, dysarthria, Parkinsonian tremor, psychiatric). Kayser–Fleischer corneal rings may be seen. No single biochemical test or clinical finding is sufficient for establishing the diagnosis, but typical findings include low serum ceruloplasmin, high urinary copper excretion, and elevated liver copper content. Treatment is with copper chelating agents and zinc. Liver transplantation is required for fulminant hepatic failure and decompensated liver disease unresponsive to medical therapy.

Menkes' disease

A rare disorder (1 in 300 000) caused by X-linked loss of function mutations in a P-type ATPase homologous to ATP7B (*ATP7A*) that result in defective copper transport across intestine, placenta and brain and hence cellular copper deficiency. Clinical presentation is in infancy with facial dimorphism, connective tissue disorder, hypopigmentation, abnormal hair, seizures and failure to thrive, usually followed by death by age 3 years. Treatment, which is only effective when presymptomatic diagnosis is made in a sibling after florid presentation in a previous affected sibling, is with intravenous copper histidine.

Introduction

Copper is an essential metal that is an important cofactor for many proteins and copper-containing enzymes involved in cellular respiration, antioxidant defence, pigment production, neurotransmitter formation, connective tissue synthesis, and iron homeostasis. Therefore in states of impaired copper homeostasis resulting in copper excess or copper deficiency, tissue injury and organ dysfunction ensue. The average diet provides substantial amounts of copper, typically between 2 and 5mg/day, most of which is eventually excreted in the bile. Copper is absorbed by enterocytes mainly in the duodenum and proximal small intestine and transported in the portal circulation bound to albumin and histidine to the liver where it is avidly removed from the circulation. The liver utilizes some copper for metabolic needs, synthesizes and secretes the copper containing the protein ceruloplasmin and excretes excess copper into the bile (see Fig. 12.7.2.1).

Wilson's disease (OMIM 277900)

Wilson's disease (hepatolenticular degeneration) was first described in 1912 by Kinnear Wilson as progressive lenticular degeneration, a familial, lethal neurological disease accompanied by chronic liver disease leading to cirrhosis. Over the next few decades, the role of copper in the pathogenesis of Wilson's disease was established, and the pattern of inheritance was determined to be autosomal recessive. In 1993 the gene defect in Wilson's disease was identified. The *ATP7B* gene encodes a metal-transporting P-type ATPase, which is expressed mainly in hepatocytes and functions in the transmembrane transport of copper. The absent or reduced function of ATP7B protein leads to impaired excretion of excess copper into the bile, leading to copper accumulation and toxicity. Eventually copper is released into the bloodstream and deposited in extrahepatic tissues. Failure to incorporate copper into ceruloplasmin is an additional consequence of the loss of functional ATP7B protein. Ceruloplasmin devoid of copper, apoceruloplasmin, has a short half-life, which causes decreased plasma levels found in most patients with Wilson's disease (see Fig. 12.7.2.1).

Wilson's disease occurs worldwide with an average incidence of approximately 30 per million. The carrier frequency is approximately 1 in 90. There is protean phenotypic presentation comprising various combinations of liver disease, progressive neurological disorder, and psychiatric disorder. Presentation with liver disease occurs more frequently in children and younger adult patients than in older adults. Overt liver disease is the most common presenting feature in childhood with the age of presentation between 10 and 13 years. In contrast, neurological disease occurs as the initial presenting feature in adults, usually in the third or fourth

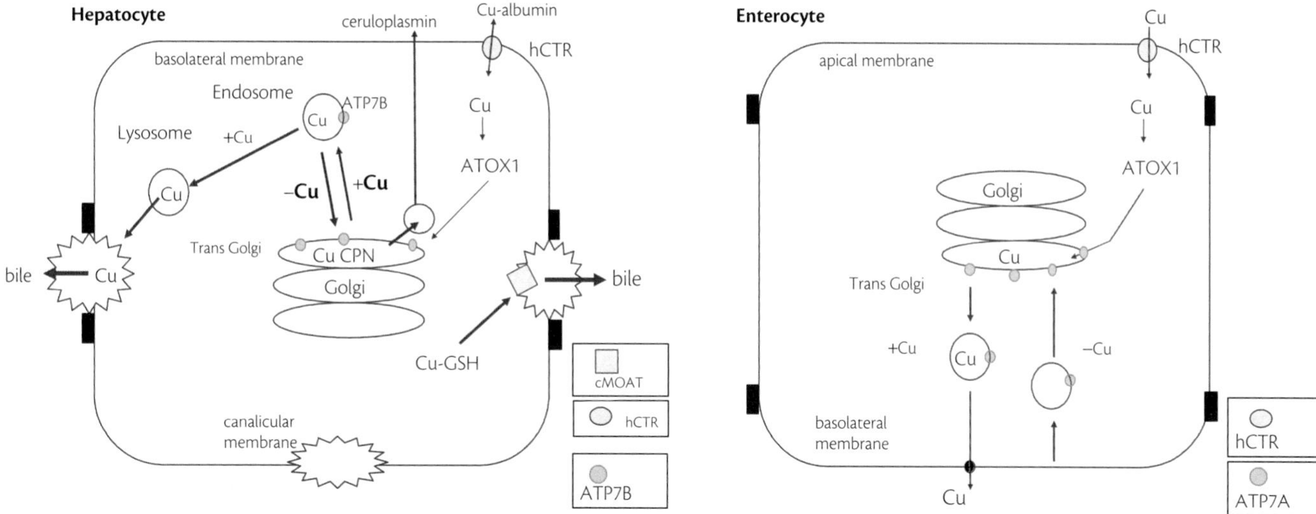

Fig. 12.7.2.1 Cellular copper trafficking in the hepatocyte and enterocyte depicting the contrasting metabolic defects in Wilson's disease and Menkes' disease. ATP7B is the major copper transporter in the hepatocyte, and ATP7A fulfils this role in the enterocyte. Copper gains access to both cell types via copper transporter 1, hCTR, and is delivered by the copper chaperone ATOX1 to ATP7B and APT7A, respectively, residing in the trans-Golgi network. Increasing cell copper content is associated with trafficking of ATP7B towards the apical canalicular membrane and copper excretion in bile in the hepatocyte. In contrast, in the enterocyte, increasing copper leads to net absorption of copper via the basolateral surface. While ATP7B expression is relatively restricted to hepatocytes and a few other cell types, ATP7A expression is more ubiquitous except that it is not expressed in the liver. In the other cells that express ATP7A, the basolateral presence of ATP7A when copper is abundant, and this protein's copper transport activity, result in the cellular excretion of excess copper. In the kidney, ATP7A and ATP7B are active in copper reabsorption or excretion from the body.

decade of life. This sequence reflects the natural history of primary hepatic involvement followed by neurological and other extrahepatic organ dysfunction. Symptoms at any age are frequently nonspecific and there is considerable overlap between distinct hepatic and neurological presentations frequently cited in the literature.

Wilson's disease was uniformly fatal until treatments were developed half a century ago, when it became one of the first liver diseases for which effective pharmacological treatment was identified. The first chelating agent introduced in 1951 for the treatment of Wilson's disease was British Anti-Lewisite (BAL or dimercaptopropanol). The identification and testing of an orally administered chelator, D-penicillamine, by John Walsh in 1956 revolutionized the treatment of this disorder. Other treatment modalities have since been introduced, including the use of zinc salts to block enteral copper absorption, tetrathiomolybdate to chelate copper and block enteral absorption, and orthotopic liver transplant, which may be life-saving and curative for this disorder since the primary site of the metabolic disorder is the liver.

Clinical features

Over the years diagnostic advances have enabled a more systematic evaluation of individuals suspected to have Wilson's disease before they develop neurological symptoms. These include the recognition of corneal Kayser–Fleischer rings (see Fig. 12.7.2.2), reduced serum ceruloplasmin of most patients, and the ability to measure copper concentration in percutaneous liver biopsy specimens. More recently, molecular diagnostic studies have made it feasible to identify presymptomatic individuals by analysing the *ATP7B* gene. Since *de novo* genetic diagnosis is currently expensive and not universally available (and sometimes inconclusive), a combination of clinical findings and biochemical testing is usually necessary to establish the diagnosis of Wilson's disease.

A patient presenting with liver disease aged between 5 and 40 years with decreased serum ceruloplasmin and detectable Kayser–Fleischer rings represents the classic form of Wilson's disease. However, about one-half of patients presenting with liver disease do not possess two of these three criteria and pose a challenge in trying to establish the diagnosis. Moreover, as with other liver diseases, patients may not come to medical attention when their clinical disease is comparatively mild.

Spectrum of disease

The diversity of liver disease encountered in patients with Wilson's disease is summarized in Table 12.7.2.1.

Wilson's disease should be considered in the differential diagnosis of patients with unexplained liver disease and when neurological and/or psychiatric symptoms occur concurrently with liver disease. Liver involvement can range from asymptomatic, with only biochemical abnormalities, to fulminant hepatic failure. Children may be entirely asymptomatic, with hepatomegaly or abnormal serum aminotransferases found only incidentally. Some patients may have a brief clinical illness resembling an acute viral hepatitis, and others may present with features indistinguishable from autoimmune hepatitis. Some may present with only biochemical abnormalities or histological findings of steatosis on liver biopsy

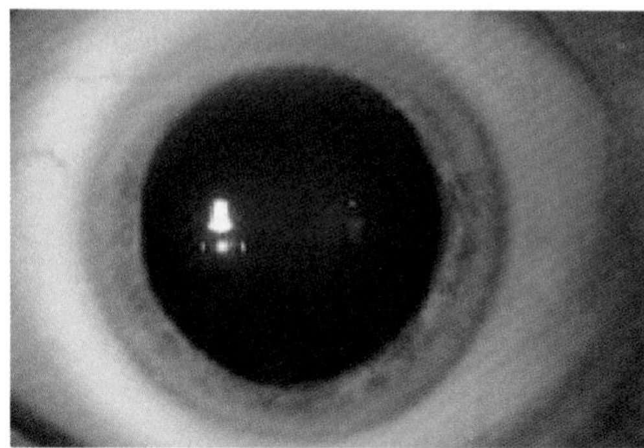

Fig. 12.7.2.2 Florid Kayser–Fleischer rings in a patient with Wilson's disease. (Courtesy of Dr Susan Hall Forster, Yale School of Medicine.)

Table 12.7.2.1 Clinical patterns of hepatic, neurological and psychiatric disease in patients with Wilson's disease

Hepatic	Asymptomatic hepatomegaly
	Isolated splenomegaly
	Persistently elevated serum aminotransferase activity (AST, ALT)
	Fatty liver
	Acute hepatitis
	Resembling autoimmune hepatitis
	Cirrhosis—compensated or decompensated
	Fulminant hepatic failure
Neurological	Movement disorders (tremor, involuntary movements)
	Drooling, dysarthria
	Rigid dystonia
	Pseudobulbar palsy
	Dysautonomia
	Migraine headaches
	Insomnia
	Seizures
Psychiatric	Depression
	Neurotic behaviours
	Personality changes
	Psychosis
Other systems	Renal abnormalities: aminoaciduria and nephrolithiasis
	Skeletal abnormalities: premature osteoporosis and arthritis
	Cardiomyopathy, dysrhythmias
	Pancreatitis
	Hypoparathyroidism
	Menstrual irregularities; infertility, repeated miscarriages

and many others with signs of chronic liver disease and evidence of compensated or decompensated cirrhosis. Patients may present with isolated splenomegaly due to clinically unapparent cirrhosis and portal hypertension. Wilson's disease may also present as fulminant hepatic failure with an associated Coombs' negative haemolytic anaemia and acute renal failure. Some patients have transient episodes of jaundice, due to haemolysis. Low-grade haemolysis may be associated with Wilson's disease when liver disease is not clinically evident.

Neurological manifestations of Wilson's disease typically present later than the liver disease, most often in the third decade of life. However, earlier subtle findings may appear in paediatric patients, including changes in behaviour, deterioration in school work or the inability to perform activities requiring good hand–eye coordination. Patient may exhibit small handwriting as in Parkinson's disease (micrographia). Other common findings in those presenting with neurological disease include tremor, lack of motor coordination, drooling, dysarthria, dystonia, and spasticity. Because of pseudobulbar palsy, transfer dysphagia may also occur, with a risk of aspiration if severe. Dysautonomia may be present. Migraine headaches and insomnia may be reported, but seizures are infrequent. Along with behavioural changes, other psychiatric manifestations include depression, anxiety, and even frank psychosis. Many individuals with neurological or psychiatric manifestations may have cirrhosis, but frequently they are not symptomatic from their liver disease.

Age

Even when presymptomatic siblings are excluded, the age at which Wilson's disease may present is both younger and older than generally appreciated, though the majority present between the ages of 5 and 35 years. Wilson's disease is increasingly diagnosed in children younger than 5 years old, with atypical findings in children under 2 years old that include cirrhosis in a 3 year old and fulminant hepatic failure in a 5 year old. The oldest patients diagnosed with Wilson's disease were in their early seventies.

Eye manifestations

Kayser–Fleischer rings represent deposition of copper in the Descemet's membrane of the cornea (see Fig. 12.7.2.2). When they are visible by direct inspection, they appear as a band of golden-brownish pigment near the limbus. A slit-lamp examination by an experienced observer is required to identify Kayser–Fleischer rings in most patients. Rarely, they may be found in patients with chronic cholestatic diseases and in children with neonatal cholestasis; however, these disorders can usually be distinguished from Wilson's disease on clinical grounds. Kayser–Fleischer rings are present in approximately 95% of patients with a neurological presentation but in only approximately 40 to 50% of patients with predominant hepatic disease at the time of diagnosis.

Sunflower cataracts, also found by slit lamp examination, represent deposits of copper in the lens. These typically do not obstruct vision, and—along with Kayser–Fleischer rings—will gradually disappear with effective medical treatment or following liver transplant. Reappearance of either of these ophthalmological findings in a medically treated patient in whom these had previously disappeared suggests non-compliance with therapy.

Diagnostic testing

A diagnosis of Wilson's disease should be considered in any patient with unexplained liver disease, especially if associated with neurological and psychiatric disease; patients with fulminant liver failure, especially if haemolysis is present; and first-degree relatives of affected patients. No single biochemical test or clinical finding is sufficient to establish the diagnosis. A combination of clinical and biochemical evaluation is necessary to make the diagnosis.

Biochemical liver tests

Serum aminotransferase activities are generally abnormal in Wilson's disease except at a very early age. In many individuals, the degree of elevation of aminotransferase activity may be mild and does not reflect the severity of the liver disease.

Ceruloplasmin

Ceruloplasmin is a 132-kDa protein synthesized mainly in the liver and is also an acute phase reactant. The vast majority of ceruloplasmin is secreted into the circulation from hepatocytes as a copper-carrying protein containing six copper atoms per molecule (holoceruloplasmin), and the remainder as the protein lacking copper (apoceruloplasmin). Ceruloplasmin is the major carrier for copper in the blood, accounting for 90% of the circulating copper in normal individuals. It is also a ferroxidase and a nitric oxide oxidase, so it influences nitric oxide homeostasis. Levels of serum ceruloplasmin may be measured enzymatically by their copper-dependent oxidase activity towards these substrates, or by antibody-dependent assays. Results generally are regarded as equivalent, but it should be noted that immunological assays routinely in clinical use may overestimate ceruloplasmin concentrations since they do not discriminate between apoceruloplasmin and holoceruloplasmin.

A serum ceruloplasmin level of less than 200 mg/L (<20 mg/dl) is considered consistent with Wilson's disease, and diagnostic if associated with Kayser–Fleischer rings. Low ceruloplasmin levels are found in approximately 95% of Wilson's disease patients. Serum ceruloplasmin alone as a screening test for Wilson's disease in patients referred with liver disease has a low positive predictive value (approximately 6%). Moreover, a low ceruloplasmin level is found in 20% of healthy heterozygote carriers of Wilson's disease, and in other disorders including protein-losing states, poor hepatocellular synthetic function, and aceruloplasminemia.

Serum copper

Although a disease of copper overload, the total serum copper in Wilson's disease is usually decreased in proportion to the decreased ceruloplasmin in the circulation. In patients with severe liver injury, serum copper may be within the normal range despite a decreased serum ceruloplasmin level. In the setting of acute fulminant hepatic failure due to Wilson's disease, levels of serum copper may be markedly elevated due to the sudden release of the metal from tissue stores. Normal or elevated serum copper levels in the face of decreased levels of ceruloplasmin indicate an increase in circulating free or non-ceruloplasmin-bound copper.

Urinary copper excretion

The amount of copper excreted in the urine in a 24-h period, which reflects the amount of nonceruloplasmin copper in circulation, may be helpful for diagnosing Wilson's disease and for monitoring treatment. Basal measurements can provide useful diagnostic information so long as copper does not contaminate the collection apparatus (this is less problematic with current plastic disposables) and the urine collection is complete. Basal 24-h urinary excretion of copper in Wilson's disease is typically more than 100 µg (1.6 µmoles) in symptomatic patients, but a level above 40 µg (>0.6 µmoles) may indicate Wilson's disease and requires further investigation.

Liver copper concentration

Liver copper content of more than 250 µg/g dry weight provides critical diagnostic information and should be obtained in cases where the diagnosis is not straightforward and in younger patients. In untreated patients, normal hepatic copper content (<40–50 µg/g dry weight) almost always excludes a diagnosis of Wilson's disease. Further diagnostic testing is indicated for patients with intermediate copper concentrations (70–250 µg/g dry weight) especially if there is active liver disease or other symptoms of Wilson's disease. The major problem with hepatic parenchymal copper concentration is that in the later stages of Wilson's disease distribution of copper within the liver is often inhomogeneous. In extreme cases, nodules lacking histochemically detectable copper are found next to cirrhotic nodules with abundant copper.

Liver biopsy findings

The earliest histological abnormalities in the liver include microvesicular and macrovesicular steatosis, glycogenated nuclei, and focal hepatocellular necrosis. The liver biopsy may show classic histological features of autoimmune hepatitis. With progressive parenchymal damage, fibrosis and subsequently cirrhosis develops and is frequently found in most patients by the second decade of life. Cirrhosis is usually macronodular, although occasionally micronodular. In the setting of fulminant hepatic failure, there is marked hepatocellular degeneration, hepatocytes apoptosis, and parenchymal collapse, typically on the background of cirrhosis.

Detection of copper in hepatocytes by orcein or rhodanine staining is highly variable. Electron microscopy reveals characteristic mitochondrial abnormalities in hepatocytes in the early phase of the disease (when steatosis is evident).

Neurological findings and radiological imaging of the brain

Neurological disease may manifest with parkinsonian features of dystonia, hypertonia, and rigidity, with tremors and dysarthria. Muscle spasms, which can lead to contractures, dysarthria, dysphonia, and dysphagia can be incapacitating. At this stage of the disease, MRI or CT of the brain may detect structural abnormalities in the basal ganglia. Most frequently found are increased density on CT and hyperintensity on T2 MRI in the region of the basal ganglia.

Genetic studies

ATP7B mutation analysis can be difficult because of the multiplicity of mutations, the occurrence of mutations in noncoding sequence and the large size of the gene that spans around 80 kb. Pedigree analysis using haplotypes of polymorphisms flanking the Wilson's disease gene can be used but it is being replaced by methods relying on high throughput sequencing. Therefore, direct mutation analysis is becoming increasingly feasible. Most patients are compound heterozygotes. Currently over 300 mutations of *ATP7B* have been identified (see the HUGO database at http://www.medgen.med.ualberta.ca/database.html for the updated catalogue).

Mutation analysis is an especially valuable diagnostic strategy for certain well defined populations harbouring prevalent *ATP7B* mutations. Populations with a single predominant mutation include those of Iceland, Japan, Korea, Sardinia, Spain and the Canary Islands, and Taiwan. Certain populations in eastern Europe also show predominance of the H1069Q mutation, accounting for nearly 40% of disease alleles. Genotype–phenotype correlation is not perfect as in most other inherited metabolic diseases of the liver, indicating an important role for modifier genes and environmental factors in the determination of ultimate phenotypic characteristics. However, a large multinational study and a meta-analysis suggest that homozygosity for H1069Q mutation is associated with neurological presentation in adults. The H1060Q Wilson ATPase resides in a highly conserved sequence in the cytoplasmic loop, SEHPL, and appears to result in defective trafficking of the mutant protein.

Diagnostic considerations in specific target populations

Liver diseases which mimic Wilson's disease

Patients with Wilson's disease, especially younger ones, may have clinical features and histological findings on liver biopsy indistinguishable from autoimmune hepatitis. All children with apparent autoimmune hepatitis and any adult patient with the presumptive diagnosis of autoimmune hepatitis failing to respond appropriately to corticosteroids must be evaluated for Wilson's disease. Hepatic steatosis in Wilson's disease is rarely as severe as in non-alcoholic fatty liver disease. Nevertheless occasional patients with Wilson's disease closely resemble non-alcoholic fatty liver disease or may have both diseases.

Fulminant liver failure

A high level of clinical suspicion is essential for the diagnosis as simple indices of laboratory findings do not reliably distinguish patients with fulminant hepatic failure from those with acute liver failure due to viral infection or drug toxicity. Most patients with the fulminant hepatic failure presentation of Wilson's disease have a characteristic pattern of clinical findings:

- Coombs' negative haemolytic anaemia with features of acute intravascular haemolysis
- coagulopathy unresponsive to parenteral vitamin k administration
- rapid progression to renal failure
- relatively modest rises in serum aminotransferases (typically <<2000 IU/litre) from the beginning of clinical illness
- normal or markedly subnormal serum alkaline phosphatase (typically <40 IU/litre)
- female to male ratio of 2:1.

Serum ceruloplasmin is usually decreased, but the predictive value of this test in the setting of acute liver failure is poor. Serum copper and 24-h urinary excretion of copper are greatly elevated. The serum copper is usually greater than 200 µg/dl (31.5 µmol/litre). Kayser–Fleischer rings may be identified to support the diagnosis of Wilson's disease but may be absent in 50% of these patients. Expeditious diagnosis is critically important since, without timely liver transplantation, death is almost inevitable.

Family screening

First-degree relatives of any patient newly diagnosed with Wilson's disease must be screened. Assessment should include serum copper, ceruloplasmin, liver function tests, slit-lamp examination of the eyes for Kayser–Fleischer rings, and basal 24-hour urinary copper. Individuals without Kayser–Fleischer rings who have subnormal ceruloplasmin and abnormal liver tests undergo liver biopsy to confirm the diagnosis. Molecular analysis of the *ATP7B* gene is increasingly available and may be used as primary screening tool, especially for family screening once the proband is identified. Treatment should be initiated for all individuals over 3 years old identified as patients by family screening.

Treatment

In general, the approach to treatment is dependent upon whether there is active disease or symptoms, whether neurological or hepatic, or whether the patient is identified prior to the onset of clinical symptoms. This distinction helps in determining the choice of therapy and the dosages of medications utilized. The recommended initial treatment of symptomatic patients or those with active disease is with chelating agents. The largest treatment experience worldwide is with penicillamine; however, there is now more frequent consideration of trientine for primary therapy. Combination therapy, in which zinc is utilized in conjunction with a chelating agent (temporally separated), has a theoretical basis in both blocking copper uptake and eliminating excess copper. Studies of the use of tetrathiomolybdate as an alternative chelating agent for the initial treatment of neurological Wilson's disease suggest that this drug may be useful as initial therapy for patients presenting with neurological symptoms (see Table 12.7.2.2).

Once the disease symptoms or biochemical abnormalities have stabilized, typically in 2 to 6 months after the initiation of therapy, a reduced dosage of chelators or zinc therapy can be used for maintenance treatment. Patients presenting without symptoms may be

Table 12.7.2.2 Pharmacological treatments of Wilson's disease

Drug/dose	Mode of action	Neurological deterioration	Side effects	Comments
Penicillamine 750–1500 mg in 2 or 3 divided doses; requires supplemental pyridoxine	General chelator Induces cupruria	10–20% during the initial phase of treatment	Fever, rash, proteinuria, Lupus-like reaction Aplastic anaemia Leukopenia Thrombocytopenia Nephrotic syndrome Degenerative changes in skin; Elastosis perforans serpiginosa Serous retinitis Hepatotoxicity	Reduce dose for surgery to promote wound healing and during pregnancy to reduce teratogenicity
Trientine 750–1500 mg in 2 or 3 divided doses	General chelator Induces cupruria	10–15% during the initial phase of treatment	Gastritis; Aplastic anaemia rare Sideroblastic anaemia	Reduce dose for surgery to promote wound healing and during pregnancy
Zinc 75–150 mg in 3 divided doses	Metallothionein inducer Blocks intestinal absorption of copper	Can occur during the initial phase of treatment	Gastritis; biochemical pancreatitis; Zinc accumulation; Possible changes in immune function	No dosage reduction for surgery or pregnancy
Tetrathio-molybdate 120 mg in 6 divided doses (with meals and apart from meals)	Chelator Blocks copper absorption	Reports of rare neurological deterioration during the initial treatment	Anaemia; neutropenia Hepatotoxicity	Experimental in the United States and Canada

treated with either maintenance dosages of a chelating agent or with zinc from the outset. Failure to comply with lifelong therapy has led to recurrent symptoms and liver failure, the latter requiring liver transplant for survival. Monitoring of therapy includes monitoring for compliance as well as for potential treatment induced side effects.

Liver transplantation

Liver transplantation is the only effective option for those with Wilson's disease who present with fulminant hepatic failure and is indicated for all Wilson's disease patients with decompensated liver disease unresponsive to medical therapy. In fulminant liver failure due to Wilson's disease, interventions to rapidly reduce elevated free circulating copper may reduce secondary organ injury while the patient awaits a suitable organ donor. Liver transplantation corrects the hepatic metabolic defects of Wilson's disease and may reverse extrahepatic copper disposition. Living donor liver transplantation has been successfully performed for Wilson's disease, including the use of donor livers from heterozygote carriers for Wilson's disease. One year survival following liver transplantation ranges from 79 to 87%, and those who survive this early period continue to survive long term. Less definite indications for liver transplantation exist for patients with respect to severe neurological disease. A liver transplant is not recommended as the primary treatment for neurological Wilson's disease since the liver disease is stabilized by medical therapy in most of these individuals and outcomes with a liver transplant in the setting of advanced neurological disease are not always beneficial.

Menkes' disease (OMIM 309400)

Menkes' disease is an X-linked recessive neurodegenerative disorder presenting in infancy due to mutations in the *ATP7A* gene, which encodes a p-type ATPase homologous to *ATP7B*. The pathology and disease manifestations reflect decreased activities of enzymes that require copper as a cofactor, such as dopamine-β-hydroxylase, cytochrome *c* oxidase, and lysyl oxidase. Affected infants appear healthy at birth but by the age of approximately 2 months develop hypotonia, seizures, and failure to thrive, usually followed by death by 3 years of age from endstage neurodegenerative disease. Treatment with daily injections of copper histidine may improve the outcome if started presymptomatically soon after birth. Thus this type of pre-emptive treatment is only amenable when presymptomatic diagnosis is made in a sibling after florid presentation in a previous affected sibling. However, newborn screening is not routinely available, and early detection is difficult because clinical abnormalities in affected newborns are absent or subtle. Furthermore, the usual biochemical markers, low serum copper and ceruloplasmin, are unreliable in the neonatal period. Molecular diagnosis can be potentially performed, but its use is hindered by the large size of *ATP7A* (150 kb) and diversity of mutation types including large deletions and chromosomal rearrangements. Recently, a promising test for neonatal diagnosis of Menkes' disease has been developed involving the measurement of serum neurotransmitter levels. Dopamine-β-hydroxylase converts dopamine to noradrenaline and these transmitters in turn can be further metabolized to dihydroxyphenylacetic acid to dihydroxyphenylglycol, respectively. Therefore, in Menkes' disease, deficiency of dopamine-β-hydroxylase leads to a high ratio of dopamine to norepinephrine as well as of dihydroxyphenylacetic acid to dihydroxyphenylglycol. These characteristic abnormalities can be used to identify presymptomatic disease, allowing pre-emptive therapy with copper histidine, and resulting in marked improvement of clinical outcomes. Occipital Horn syndrome is a milder allelic variant of Menkes' disease.

Further reading

Culotta VC, Gitlin JD (2007). *Disorders of copper transport.* In: Valle, D, *et al.* (eds) *The online metabolic and molecular bases of inherited disease (OMMBID)*, Part 14, Chapter 126. McGraw-Hill, New York (http://www.ommbid.com/).

de Bie P, *et al.* (2007). Molecular pathogenesis of Wilson and Menkes disease: correlation of mutations with molecular defects and disease phenotypes. *J Med Genet*, **44**(11), 673–88.

Emre S, *et al.* (2001). Orthotopic liver transplantation for Wilson's disease: a single-center experience. *Transplantation*, **72**, 1232–6.

Ferenci P, *et al.* (2007). Late-onset Wilson's disease. *Gastroenterology*, **132**(4), 1294–8.

Kaler SG, *et al.* (2008). Neonatal diagnosis and treatment of Menkes disease. *N Engl J Med*, **358**, 605–614.

Menkes JH (1999). Menkes disease and Wilson disease: two sides of the same copper coin. Part I: Menkes disease. *Europ J Paediatr Neurol*, **3**, 147–58.

Merle U, *et al.* (2007). Clinical presentation, diagnosis and long-term outcome of Wilson's disease: a cohort study. *Gut*, **56**(1), 115–20.

Payne AS, Kelly EJ, Gitlin JD (1998). Functional expression of the Wilson disease protein reveals mislocalization and impaired copper-dependent trafficking of the common H1069Q mutation. *Proc Natl Acad Sci U S A*, **95**, 10854–9.

Roberts EA, Schilsky ML, American Association for Study of Liver Diseases (2008). Diagnosis and treatment of Wilson disease: an update. *Hepatology*, **47**(6), 2089–111.

Stapelbroek JM, *et al.* (2004). The H1069Q mutation in ATP7B is associated with late and neurologic presentation in Wilson disease: results of a meta-analysis. *J Hepatol*, **41**(5), 758–763.

12.8

Lysosomal disease

P.B. Deegan and Timothy M. Cox

Essentials

Lysosomal function and classification of diseases

The lysosome is an intracellular organelle which recycles biological macromolecules derived either endogenously, from digestion of cellular components (autophagy), or from the breakdown of material that has been incorporated from outside the cell by, for example, phagocytosis.

Lysosomal diseases may be classified according to the nature of the primary storage molecules (biochemical classification) or according to the defective molecular cell physiology (functional classification). Biochemical classification readily identifies: (1) sphingolipidoses, (2) mucopolysaccharidoses, (3) glycoproteinoses, (4) glycogenosis -with or without lysosomal debris derived from subcellular organelles-due to impaired autophagy and (5) others or miscellaneous conditions with multiple classes of storage material. Functional classification describes (1) deficiency of a specific acid hydrolase activity, (2) deficiency of an activator protein, (3) deficiency of a lysosomal membrane protein or transporter, (4) abnormal post-translational modification of lysosomal proteins, and (5) abnormal biogenesis of lysosomes. A combination of two classification systems may allow the best description of the pathological basis of particular conditions.

General aspects of lysosomal diseases

At least 70 single-gene defects are responsible for inborn errors of lysosomal function: these are most often caused by deficiency of specific acid hydrolases, but mutations occur in protein activators necessary for their action, or in membrane proteins that transport the substrates for, or products of, lysosomal digestion. About one in 5000 live-born infants have a lysosomal disorder, with Gaucher disease and Fabry disease (both glycosphingolipidoses) probably the most frequent.

Lysosomal diseases occur at all ages and are clinically diverse; they differ greatly in their rate of progression and represent a large burden of illness in the population. The range of manifestations includes organomegaly, disturbed function of visceral organs, skeletal effects and neurological features.

A detailed family history, including careful analysis of the extended pedigree, is of critical importance. Simple histochemical stains of existing biopsy material and examination of urine metabolites, including lipids and oligosaccharides, may point to the diagnosis. Specific enzymatic assays on leucocytes or cultured fibroblasts are often definitive but may be supported by molecular analysis of genes encoding proteins destined for the lysosome.

There is no specific or curative treatment for most lysosomal disorders: supportive and palliative measures are nonetheless of great benefit. However, proteins can be delivered directly to lysosomes from the extracellular fluid phase by means of specific glycoprotein receptors, hence recombinant DNA technology which with protein engineering allows large-scale manufacture and post-translational modification of human proteins for targeting to this intracellular compartment. This technology has led to the development of enzyme-replacement therapy for several lysosomal diseases. The success of such treatment is predicated on characterization of single-gene defects responsible for lysosomal disorders and the discovery of lectin-like ligands and their receptors, by which nascent lysosomal proteins are specifically delivered to the organelle during biogenesis. Orally active agents are in development for at least one important class of lysosomal disorders, the sphingolipidoses; these treatments, based on small molecules, may allow access to the brain - which is often affected.

Particular lysosomal diseases

Gaucher disease—one of the most common lysosomal diseases; autosomal recessive; usually caused by catalytic deficiency of acid glucocerebrosidase. Characteristic manifestations of the most frequent form—'adult non-neuronopathic' (type I)—include (1) pancytopenia, with bleeding due to thrombocytopenia; (2) splenic enlargement; and (3) bone pain with osteoporosis and episodic avascular necrosis. Diagnosis is based on white-cell acid β-glucosidase activity; biopsy material may show characteristic multinucleate storage cells with striated cytoplasm on Leishmann staining. Enzyme-replacement therapy (imiglucerase) is extremely expensive but corrects cytopenia, reduces hepatosplenomegaly and the frequency of episodic bone infarction and improves quality of life.

Fabry disease—an X-linked disorder caused by deficiency of α-galactosidase A that leads to the accumulation of globotriaosylceramide (Gb3). Typically manifest in early childhood with lancinating pain and background burning sensations in the extremities,

Fabry disease rivals Gaucher disease in frequency. Other features include diarrhoea, lack of peripheral sweating, impotence, high-tone deafness, angiokeratomas (small, raised, red, vascular lesions, particularly around the buttocks and genital region), chronic kidney disease (progressing to renal failure), cardiac hypertrophy and stroke. Affected male hemizygotes are diagnosed by finding excess glycolipid in urine or plasma supported by finding deficient α-galactosidase A activity in white cells or cultured skin fibroblasts; molecular analysis of the α-galactosidase A gene is usually needed for identifying heterozygote females. Enzyme replacement with recombinant human α-galactosidase A is very costly but improves neuropathic pain and cardiac hypertrophy and may stabilize renal function particularly if given before proteinuria becomes florid.

Other diseases discussed in this chapter include (1) the mucopolysaccharidoses, (2) Pompe disease (glycogen storage disease type II), (3) Niemann-Pick disease, (4) Danon disease, and (5) diseases more recently attributed to lysosomal defects.

Lysosomal function

Since their discovery more than 50 years ago by the Nobel prizewinner Christian de Duve, lysosomes and their associated endosomal structures have been a focus of research into molecular cell biology. Lysosomes are an integral part of the intracellular digestive system: they acquire complex macromolecules for breakdown and recycling by three main pathways: (1) receptor-mediated endocy-tosis; (2) engulfment and fusion (phagocytosis); and (3) autophagy, a variant of which, crinophagy, represents the fusion of lysosomes with secretory granules to degrade their unused contents. Greater understanding of lysosomal function has arisen from biochemical definition of cellular macromolecules that accumulate when the organelle is affected by hereditary diseases and from exploration of the ebb and flow of substrates and products as they traverse the lysosomal compartment.

Endocytosis and membrane flow

Receptor-mediated endocytosis occurs by means of clathrin-coated pits, a process by which molecules are delivered after internalization to a peripheral, and later to a perinuclear endosomal compartment, 'the endolysosome'. The endolysosome undergoes maturation to form a lysosome after the loss of certain membrane components and further acidification. Some molecules acquired by receptor-mediated endocytosis (for example, apolipoprotein B in low-density lipoproteins) are specifically retrieved and ultimately returned to the cell surface having despatched their cargo to the lysosome. Other molecules that are not retrieved are ultimately degraded by fusion with mature lysosomes and enzymatic hydrolysis (for example, the epidermal growth factor receptor system). The endosomal system also mediates the traffic of nascent acid hydrolases from the trans-Golgi network to the lysosome, employing a specific mannose 6-phosphate receptor targeting system. Plasma membrane proteins bound for degradation in the lysosomal system are incorporated into membrane-bound vesicles within the endosomal lumen and thus enter the lysosome upon fusion. In contrast, structural or transporter proteins bound for incorporation into the lysosomal membrane remain within the limiting membrane of the endosome and form part of the lysosomal membrane on fusion.

Phagocytosis

Lysosomes are also involved in a specialized process for the degradation of exogenous particulates and proteins, including microbes and effete cells such as erythrocytes and neutrophils. Although this engulfment and fusion process involving phagolysosomes is distributed throughout nature, it is particularly active in macrophages and dendritic cells. A specialized phagolysosome variant occurs in osteoclasts that are derived from myeloid cells of mononuclear phagocyte origin. The osteoclastic resorptive vacuole serves as a large exteriorized lysosomal compartment which is independently acidified for the process of bone resorption. In macrophages, cell-surface components on bacteria and yeast, as well as exogenous cells, are recognized and bound by specific receptors on the plasma membrane. The phagocytes engulf foreign material to form large vesicles in which acidification and proteolysis, as well as the secretion of degradative molecules (including reactive oxygen and nitrogen species), is initiated. The phagolysosome fuses with lysosomes and further acidification occurs, so that the acid hydrolases are activated to bring about the breakdown of the ingested material.

Autophagy

Autophagy occurs within cells: microautophagy describes the degradation of cytosolic components trapped during invagination of endosomes and lysosomes; macroautophagy describes the engulfment of relatively large volumes, including organelles. In a constant process of membrane fusion and flow, the endoplasmic reticulum, ribosomes, mitochondria, peroxisomes and other lysosomes, and particulate material such as macromolecular complexes of glycogen, are engulfed by autophagic vacuoles. Formation of these vacuoles is initiated when a flattened cisterna composed of membrane encircles cytoplasm to form a double-layered vesicle; acidified late endosomes and lysosomes fuse with the nascent vacuoles to form an autolysosome: after continued acidification, the complement of lysosomal hydrolases effects breakdown of the inner membrane and digestion of the vacuolar contents. After digestion is completed, the autolysosome acquires an electron-dense—and often autofluorescent—core known as a residual body. When lysosomal function is impeded, the breakdown of endogenous macromolecules is impaired; this, together with a failure to breakdown exogenous macromolecular substrates, results in a characteristic pattern of pathological storage of the biological residue. Disturbed autophagy is a spectacular feature in Pompe and Danon diseases but probably contributes to the pathogenesis of many, if not all, lysosomal diseases.

Autophagy—and crinophagy—retrieve the basic building blocks of cellular components and proceed hand-in-hand with *de novo* synthesis and the renewal of intracellular compartments throughout life; the process is stimulated under conditions of starvation and disuse—for example, in immobilized muscles or during involution of the anterior pituitary gland after pregnancy. When starvation is prolonged, macroautophagy slows down in favour of the lysosomal uptake of a class of large cellular proteins harbouring particular amino acid sequences which are recognized by receptors that mediate import into the organelle. The intrinsic and highly glycosylated lysosomal membrane protein, LAMP2, is implicated in the uptake of such cytosolic proteins: LAMP2 is mutated in the X-linked disorder Danon disease in which liver, as well as cardiac and skeletal muscle, show prominent vacuoles engorged with glycogen and other debris, including remnants of cellular organelles.

Degradation and recycling of complex macromolecules

At least 40 lysosomal hydrolases have been described, including proteases, glycosidases, sulphatases, phosphatases, and lipases. These enzymes require an acidic pH for optimal function, which in the lysosome is maintained at a pH of 4 to 5.5 by an ATP-dependent proton transporter. The lysosomal membrane and the acidic pH optimum of the hydrolases protect the remainder of the cell, at neutral pH, from indiscriminate autodigestion. Activator proteins are required for several lysosomal enzymes: saposin C is required for the in vivo catalytic function of glucocerebrosidase, deficiency of which causes Gaucher disease—a Gaucher disease-like phenotype has been observed in the rare individuals with saposin C deficiency. Targeting of hydrolases to the lysosomal compartment is achieved in most cases by post-translational modification of the carbohydrate moiety of these glycoproteins, with the addition of a phosphate group on the sixth carbon of mannose residues. This mediates binding to the MPR on the inner membrane of the trans-Golgi network; the complex is incorporated into a clathrin-coated vesicle and trafficked to the lysosome through the endo-somal pathway.

Transporter proteins of the lysosomal membrane are less well characterized than the acid hydrolases. Transporters are required to export the products of lysosomal digestion, amino acids, monosaccharides, nucleosides, and ions, for re-use in cellular metabolism. Most transporters are uncharacterized, although those for cystine and sialic acid are better understood as a result of study of the deficiency syndromes cystinosis and Salla disease, and the subsequent identification of genes encoding the transport proteins cystinosin and sialin. Recent research has identified mucolipin as a channel for monovalent cations; impaired function of which causes mucolipidosis IV. The protein CLN3, deficiency of which results in juvenile Batten disease, is implicated in the egress of arginine.

Antigen presentation

Proteases of lysosomal origin, particularly the cysteine proteinases or cathepsins, are responsible for the cleavage of endocytosed protein antigens to generate peptide fragments. In antigen-presenting cells, where abundant expression of several of these proteases is necessary, peptide fragments of the cognate antigens are presented in association with major histocompatibility complex (MHC) class II molecules as a key step in the pathway that orchestrates the adaptive immune response. In mouse models of autoimmunity, deficiency of acid proteases—such as cathepsins B and S, generated experimentally by gene disruption technology—can ameliorate many of the disease manifestations.

Definition

Lysosomal diseases result from inherited defects in lysosomal hydrolases and the mechanisms for delivering them to the organelle; lysosomal enzyme activators and cofactors; lysosomal membrane proteins; and carrier systems for the transport of the substrates and products of lysosomal digestion between the organelle and the cytoplasm. Most of the enzymatic defects are restricted to the activity of a single hydrolase but defects of activators and cofactors, as well as proteins involved in the processing of nascent lysosomal enzymes for organellar delivery, can lead to generalized defects of lysosome function.

Classification

Lysosomal disorders may be classified according to the nature of the primary storage compounds (biochemical classification) or according to the nature of the physiological defect (functional classification). A combination of two classification systems may allow a clearer description of the pathological basis of the condition.

As the clinical manifestations for the 70 or more diseases associated with inborn errors of lysosomal function are very diverse, the reader is referred to specialized literature for further information (see Further reading).

Biochemical classification

Sphingolipidoses

Sphingolipids are amphiphilic compounds with a lipophilic moiety based on the amino-alcohol sphingosine (usually linked to a long-chain fatty acid to form ceramide) and a polar hydrophilic mono- or oligosaccharide chain. Sphingolipids are found in all plasma membranes and concentrated in lipid rafts: the lipophilic moiety is anchored in the outer leaflet of the lipid bilayer and the carbohydrate element extends into the extracellular space. Sphingolipids mediate diverse cellular functions and serve as specific receptors and cell-recognition markers. Ultimately they are delivered to the lysosomal compartment in the course of membrane turnover in endocytosis and phagocytosis. Deacylated forms of the sphingolipids (glucosylsphingosine, a 'psychosine', is the deacylated form of glucosylceramide) are water soluble and hence freely diffusible. Exploration of the roles of such lysolipids and other small water-soluble lipid molecules, such as sphingosine 1-phosphate and ceramide, and their metabolites in signal transduction and other cellular processes, is an expanding field of research and holds promise for a more comprehensive understanding of the molecular pathogenesis of sphingolipid diseases.

Mucopolysaccharidoses

Mucopolysaccharides, or glycosaminoglycans (GAGs), are complex linear polysaccharides, composed of repeating units of polar disaccharides which are strongly negatively charged under physiological conditions. When associated with a linear core protein, the GAGs form even larger three-dimensional complexes, known as proteoglycans. By virtue of their negative charge and extended structure, proteoglycans attract water molecules and have important gel-like properties. Proteoglycans are essential components of ground substance in intercellular spaces and connective tissue, including cartilage, vitreous humour, and synovial fluid. Lysosomal degradation of the carbohydrate moieties requires the participation of several glycosidases orchestrated in series.

Glycoproteinoses

Glycoproteins are proteins to which one or more oligosaccharide chains are attached covalently. The carbohydrate moiety is often branched and complex, mediating specific recognition by cell surface receptors. As with the glycosaminoglycans, lysosomal degradation of the carbohydrate element requires the ordered participation of several glycosidases operating in sequence. Deficiency of one glycosidase, in effect, blocks the subsequent release of sugars in the reaction series, thus causing accumulation of oligosaccharides and other complex glycan molecules.

Glycogenosis (Pompe disease)

Deficiency of α1, 4-glucosidase, acid maltase, causes intra- and extra-lysosomal accumulation of glycogen in muscle and other tissues. This storage molecule is common to conditions of impaired autophagy (e.g. Danon disease) and confirms the role of the lysosome in constitutive remodelling of glycogen deposits.

Multiple classes of storage material

Several lysosomal hydrolases are not specific to one substrate: β-galactosidase deficiency, for example, leads to accumulation of a glycophingolipid (GM1 ganglioside) and glycosaminoglycans (kera-tan sulphate and β-galactosyl oligosaccharides). This deficiency is responsible for a range of phenotypes, extending from a predominantly neurodegenerative disease, GM1 gangliosidosis, and the largely skeletal disorder of Morquio β—a mucopolysaccharidosis.

All eukaryotic sulphatases, including the eight sulphatases destined for the mammalian lysosome—where they desulphate glycosaminoglycans, glycolipids, and glycopeptides—require the conversion of a conserved cysteine residue to formylglycine for their activation. Genetic defects in the enzyme, sulphatase modifying factor (SUMF1), which mediates this conversion in the endoplasmic reticulum, leads to Austin disease (multiple sulphatase deficiency)—a condition which usually resembles late-infantile metachromatic leucodystrophy but with prominent clinical and biochemical features of a complex mucopolysaccharidosis as well as icthyosis, due to an accompanying deficiency of steroid sulphatase.

Deficiency in the precursor of the small sphingolipid activator proteins (SAPs) leads to loss of activity of the cognate hydrolases, whose activity depends on interaction with the activators saposins A to D. Depending on the selectivity of the defect, a distinct disease complex, characterized by accumulation of a broad panel of glycosphingolipids, occurs when these proteins are deficient.

A genetically and biochemically distinct activator, GM2 activator protein, interacts crucially to form a ternary complex with hex-osaminidase A and its specific natural substrate in the lysosome, GM2 ganglioside. Deficiency of this activator protein gives rise to a phenocopy of the severe neurodegenerative disorder, Tay-Sachs disease but characteristically the activity of the hexosaminidase when determined with the usual fluorogenic substrates is unimpaired. A similar phenomenon occurs in the disorders due to saposin deficiencies and may render correct diagnosis difficult for the unwary.

Most acid hydrolases are glycoproteins that are specifically targeted to the lysosomal system through interaction between a mannose-phosphate moiety and membrane mannose-phosphate receptors. Failure to generate the mannose-phosphate signal gives rise to widespread mistargeting of hydrolases and intralysosomal deficiency of the respective activities with consequent accumulation of many substrates (I-cell disease); characteristically, body fluids, including plasma, have increased activities of many lysosomal hydrolases and although the disease shares many features of a mucopolysaccharidosis, the urine is usually free of glycosaminoglycans.

Miscellaneous

Please see Table 12.8.1 for details.

Functional classification

Classification based on the nature of the defect in cell biological terms is particularly relevant in relation to potential therapeutic approaches. Examples of the type of defects listed here are given in the 'Biochemical classification' section and throughout the text:

- deficiency of a specific acid hydrolase activity;
- deficiency of an activator protein;
- deficiency of a lysosomal membrane protein or transporter;
- abnormal post-translational modification of lysosomal proteins;
- abnormal lysosomal biogenesis.

Pathophysiology

Lysosomal storage of primary substrates

In the initial period of discovery of lysosomal diseases, limited availability of investigative tools influenced how the conditions were viewed. Pathological examination and microscopy showed not only organ enlargement but intracellular 'storage' bodies of remarkable appearance. Biochemical characterization of storage compounds guided research into discovery of enzyme activities and gene products. This led to a somewhat simplistic view of the pathogenesis of lysosomal storage diseases as being related to the expansion of cells and organs containing relatively inert 'storage' material. In most cases, the contribution of storage material to organ enlargement is quantitatively very small and the widespread effects of lysosomal diseases on cell-cell interactions with paracrine, inflammatory, and immunological consequences, remain unsolved. Latterly the pathogenesis of lysosomal diseases in relation to secondary metabolites and their specific roles in signalling and cell biology is receiving attention; investigations are also underway into the effects of storage on membrane flow and trafficking within the cell.

Although the amount of storage material that accumulates within lysosomes in the lysosomal diseases is several hundred- or thousandfold greater than normal, the absolute amount of material may amount to only a few grams, even in an enlarged viscus such as the spleen, which may exceed 5 kg in some disorders. For example, the presence of a few grams of the sphingolipid, sphingomyelin, in Niemann-Pick disease, is associated with massive visceral enlargement with accompanying inflammatory, ischaemic, and other destructive changes due to the presence of storage cells. Similarly, marked pathological injury occurs: in the viscera and bone marrow spaces of patients with Gaucher disease; in the heart and skeletal muscles of patients with α-glucosidase deficiency (with glycogen accumulation in the sarcoplasm of striated and cardiac myocytes); in the kidney and heart of patients with Fabry disease; and affecting neurons throughout the nervous system of patients with ceroid neuronal lipofucsinosis, Tay-Sachs disease, and GM1 gangliosidosis.

Table 12.8.1

Sphingolipidoses

Cer: ceramide, GlcCer: glucosylceramide, Gb3: globotriaosylceramide, gangliosides GM1 and GM2, SM: sphingomyelin

Disease	Synonym	OMIM	Locus gene	Gene product	Storage material
Farber	Lipogranulomatosis	228000	8p22 ASAH	Acid ceramidase	Cer
Fabry	Anderson-Fabry	301500	Xq22 GLA	α-Galactosidase A	Gb3
Gaucher	G lucosylceram idosis	606463 230900 231000 230800	1q21 GBA	Glucocerebrosidase	GlcCer
GM1 gangliosidosis		230500 230600	3p21 GLB1	β-Galactosidase	GM1
Tay-Sachs	GM2-gangliosidosis B	272800	15q23 HEXA	β-Hexosaminidase α-subunit	GM2
Sandhoff	GM2-gangliosidosis O	268800	5q13 HEXB	β-Hexosaminidase β-subunit	GM2
Tay-Sachs AB variant	GM2 gangliosidosis AB	272750	5q32 GM2A	GM2 activator protein	GM2
Krabbe	Globoid cell leucodystrophy	245200	14q31 GALC	β-Galactosylceramidase	GalCer
Metachromatic leucodystrophy	Arylsulphatase A deficiency	250100	22q13 ARSA	Arylsulphatase A	Sulphatide
Prosaposin deficiency		176801	10q22 PSAP	Prosaposin	Multiple lipids
Saposin B deficiency	Metachromatic leucodystrophy variant	249900	10q22 PSAP	Saposin B	Sulphatide
Saposin C deficiency	Gaucher variant	610539	10q22 PSAP	Saposin C	GlcCer
Niemann-Pick types AandB		257200 607616	11p15 SPMPD1	Acid sphingomyelinase	SM
Other lipidoses	**Synonym**	**OMIM**	**Locus**	**Gene product**	**Storage material**
Niemann-Pick type C1		257220	18q11 NPC1	NPC1	Cholesterol,GSL
Niemann-Pick type C2		607625	14q24 NPC2	NPC2	Cholesterol,GSL
Wolman	Cholesteryl ester storage disease	278000	10q23.2 LI PA	Acid lipase	Cholesterol-ester

Mucopolysaccharidoses (MPS)

DS: dermatan sulphate, HS: heparan sulphate, KS: keratan sulphate, CS: chrondoitin sulphate, HA: hyaluronan

Disease	Synonym	OMIM	Locus	Gene product	Storage
MPS1	Hurler Hurler/Scheie Scheie	607015 (MPS 1H) 607015 (MPS 1HS) 607016 (MPS 1S)	4p16 IDUA	α-Iduronidase	DS, HS
MPS II	Hunter	309900	Xq28 IDS	Iduronate sulphatase	DS, HS
MPS IIIA	Sanfilippo A	52900	17q25 SGS	Heparan N-sulphatase	HS
MPS IIIB	Sanfilippo B	252910	17q21 NAGLU	N-Acetyl glucosaminidase	HS
MPS IIIC	Sanfilippo C	252930	8p11 TMEM76 HGSNAT	α-Glucosaminide acetyl-CoA transferase	HS HS
MPS IIID	Sanfilippo D	252940	12q14 GNS	N-acetylglucosamine 6-sulphatase	HS
MPS IVA	Morquio A	253000	16q24 GALNS	Galactosamine 6-sulphatase	KS,CS
MPS IVB	Morquio B	253010	3p21 GLB1	Acid β-galactosidase	KS
MPS VI	Maroteaux-Lamy	253200	5q12 ARSB	Arylsulphatase B N-Acetyl galactosamine 4-sulphatase	DS
MPS VII	Sly	253220	7q21 GUSB	Glucuronidase	DS, HS, CS
MPS IX	Haluronidase Deficiency	601492	3p21 HYL1	Hyaluronidase 1	HA

Glycogen storage disease

Disease	Synonym	OMIM	Locus	Gene product	Storage
Pompe	Glycogen storage Disease type II	232300	17q25 GAA	α-Glucosidase	Glycogen

Multiple substrate storage due to single gene defects

Disease	Synonym	OMIM	Locus	Gene product	Storage product
Multiple sulphatase deficiency	Austin disease	272200	3p26 SUMF1	Formyl-glycine generating enzyme	Sulphatide,Mucopolysaccharides
Galactosialidosis		256540	20q13 PPCA	Protective protein Cathepsin A	GSL, Polysaccharides
Mucolipidosis Type II	I-cell disease	252500	12q23 GNPTAB	UDP-GlcNac Phospho transferase α/β unit	Multiple lipids & oligosaccharides

(Continued)

Table 12.8.1 *(Cont'd)*

Multiple substrate storage due to single gene defects					
Disease	**Synonym**	**OMIM**	**Locus**	**Gene product**	**Storage product**
Mucolipidosis Type IIIa	Classic pseudo-Hurler polydystrophy	252600	12q23 GNPTAB	UDP-G1cNac Phosphotransferase α/β unit	see above
Mucolipidosis Type III	Pseudo-Hurler polydystrophy	352605	16p GNPTG	UDP-G1cNac Phosphotransferase γ-subunit	see above
Mucolipidosis Type IV		252650	19p13 MCOLN1	Mucolipin-1 cation channel	see above
Glycoproteinoses					
Disease	**Synonym**	**OMIM**	**Locus**	**Gene product**	**Storage product**
Aspartylglucosaminuria		208400	4q32 AGA	Glycosyl-asparaginase	Aspartyl-glucosamine
Fucosidosis		230000	1p34 FUCA	α-Fucosidase	Oligosaccha rides
α-Mannosidosis		248500	19q12 MAN2B1	α-Mannosidase	Oligosaccha rides
β-Mannosidosis		248510	4q22 MANBA	β-Mannosidase	Oligosaccha rides
Sialidosis	Sialidase deficiency Mucolipidosis type 1	256550	6p21 NEU1	α-Sialidase Neuraminidase	Oligosaccha rides
Schindler	NAGA deficiency Kanzaki disease	609242 609241	22q13 NAGA	α-N-Acetyl galactosaminidase	Oligosaccha rides
Lysosomal transport defects					
Disease	**Synonym**	**OMIM**	**Locus**	**Gene product**	**Storage product**
Cystinosis		219800 219900 219750	17p13 CTNS	Cystinosin (cystin transport)	Cystine
Methylmalonic-Aciduria	Vitamin B12 lysosomal release defect	277380	unknown	Vitamin B12 carrier (Cb1F)	Vitamin B12
Salla	Sialuria	604322	6q14 SLC17A5	Sialin (sialic acid transport)	Sialic acid
Lysosomal protease defect					
Disease	**Synonym**	**OMIM**	**Locus**	**Gene product**	**Storage**
Pycnodystostosis		265800	1q21 CTSK	Cathepsin K	Collagen fibrils (osteoclasts)
Autophagy defects (with glycogenosis)					
Disease	**Synonym**	**OMIM**	**Locus**	**Gene product**	**Storage Product**
Danon	PseudoglycogenosisII	300257	Xq24 LAMP2	LAMP2	Vacuoles
X-linked myopathy		310440	Xq28 XMEA	XMEA	Vacuole
Vacuolar myopathy	Muscular dystrophy With vacuoles	601846	19p13 MDRV	MDRV	Vacuoles

Autophagy defects

Disease	Synonym	OMIM	Locus	Gene product	Storage Product
Autophagic vacuolar myopathy		609500	unknown	unknown	Vacuoles

Neuronal Ceroid Lipofuscinosis (NCL)
SAPs: sphingolipid activator proteins, SCMAS: subunit c mitochondrial ATP synthase

Disease	Synonym	OMIM	Locus	Gene product	Storage Product
CLN1	Haltia-Santavuori	256730	1p32 CLN1	PPT1 palmitoyl protein thioesterase 1	SAPs
CLN2	Jansky-Bielchowsky	204500	11p15 CLN2	TPP1 tripeptidyl peptidase 1	SCMAS
CLN3	Spielmeyer-Sjögren Batten	204200	16p12 CLN3	CLN3	SCMAS
CLN4A	Kufs	204300	unknown	unknown	SCMAS
CLN4B	Parry disease	162350	unknown	unknown	SAPs
CLN5	vLINCL Finnish	256731	13q22 CLN5	CLN5	SCMAS
CLN6	Lake-Cavanagh	601780	15q21 CLN6	CLN6	SCMAS
CLN7	vLINCL Turkish	610951	unknown	unknown	SCMAS
CLN8	Northern epilepsy	600143	8p32 CLN8	CLN8	SCMAS
CLN9	Variant Batten Disease	609055	unknown	regulator of dihydroceramide synthase	SCMAS
CLN10	Congenital NCL	610127	11p15 CTSD	Cathepsin D	SAPs

Disorders in extended lysosomal apparatus (melanosomes, lamellar bodies)

Disease	Synonym	OMIM	Locus	Gene product	Storage Product
Chediak-Higashi		214500	1q42 LYST	LYST	Enlarged vacuoles Melanosomes
MYOV	Griscelli type 1	214450	15q21 MYO5A	Myosin 5A	Melanin granules
RAB27A	Griscelli type 2	603868	15q21 RAB27A	RAB27A	Melanin granules
Melanophilin	Griscelli type 3	609227	2q37 MLPH	Melanophilin	Melanin granules
HPS-1	Hermansky Pudlak type 1	604982	10q23 HPS-1	HPS-1	Multiple vacuoles
HPS-2	Hermansky-Pudlak type 2	608233	5q14 AP3B1	AP3 β-subunit	See above
HPS-3	Hermansky-Pudlak type 3	606118	3q24 HPS-3	HPS-3	See above

(Continued)

Table 12.8.1 *(Cont'd)*

Disorders in extended lysosomal apparatus (melanosomes, lamellar bodies)					
Disease	**Synonym**	**OMIM**	**Locus**	**Gene product**	**Storage Product**
HPS-4	Hermansky-Pudlak type 4	606682	22q11 HPS-4	HPS-4	See above
HPS-5	Hermansky-Pudlak type 5	607521	11p15	HPS-5	See above
			HPS-5	HPS-6	See above
HPS-6	Hermansky-Pudlak type 6	607522	10q24 HPS-6		
HPS-7	Hermansky-Pudlak type 7	607145	6p22 DTNB1	Dysbindin	See above
HPS-8	Hermansky-Pudlak type 8	609762	19q13 BLOC1S3	BLOC1S3	See above
Surfactant metabolism dysfunction-4	SMPD3	610921	16p13 ABCA3	ABCA3	Alveolar proteins
Congenital and lamellar Ichthyosis	Harlequin fetus	242500 601277	2q34 ABCA12	ABCA12	Abnormal keratin

Secondary metabolites and their effects

Although there often appears to be an anatomical relationship between the extent of lysosomal storage and the development of overt disease in a particular organ, at present, there is little mechanistic understanding of this relationship in molecular terms. Sphingolipids participate in cell-recognition events and receptor biology; sphingolipid metabolites (the deacylated lysosphingolipids) also function as signalling molecules in apoptotic and proliferative responses. However, in two striking instances (Gaucher and Krabbe disease, due to acid β-glucocerebrosidase and β-galactocerebrosidase deficiencies, respectively), multinucleated macrophages resembling the pathognomonic Gaucher or globoid cell can be induced *in vitro* by the water-soluble molecules glucosylpsychosine and galactosylpsychosine, which are overproduced in these diseases. At pathophysiological concentrations in culture, psychosines and related glycolipids inhibit cytokinesis—and are thus implicated in the cellular pathways that are responsible for a key feature of the disease. Psycho sines interact with G-protein-coupled receptors (TCAG 8) on the plasma membrane of human monocytic-lineage cells. Recently, another deacylated glycosphingolipid, lyso-globotriaosylceramide (lyso-GB3) has been identified in the plasma of patients with Fabry disease; lyso-GB3 has powerful effects on smooth muscle and endothelial proliferation and is thus implicated in the devastating systemic vascular manifestations that characterize Fabry disease. These findings may signify new approaches to the understanding of several lysosomal disorders associated with cell loss due to apoptosis and fibro-inflammatory responses; since lysolipids diffuse readily from their site of formation, different approaches to their treatment other than targeted enzyme replacement, may be appropriate.

Cellular effects

The cellular reaction associated with lysosomal storage is often restricted and stereotypical. In neural tissue, several pathological hallmarks such as meganeurite formate and ectopic dendritogenesis, accompany the accumulation of a wide assortment of storage compounds. It appears that lysosomal storage gives rise to a generalized defect in the complex traffic flow mediated by the endosomal system with effects on autophagy, signal propagation at the synapse, axonal transport, myelin formation, and arborization of dendrites. Lipid rafts, detergent-resistant islands within the plasma membrane, contain high local concentrations of gangliosides and play an important role in many cell signalling events. Disordered lateral movement and recycling of raft components, as part of a general or specific endosomal 'traffic jam', may have profound effects on cell signalling, as well as recycling processes mediated by autophagy.

Tissue and organ malfunction

In a scientific era which offers powerful analytical techniques to explore complex functional networks that lead to tissue pathology, the lysosomal diseases represent a promising field for investigation using large-scale, high-throughput methods to investigate altered protein and gene expression in the context of cell signalling responses. An early application of this work has been the use of authentic experimental models of some of the more severe storage diseases generated by gene knockout technology; these models facilitate research on otherwise inaccessible tissues such as the brain during the development of the storage phenotype. Gene-expression profiling experiments conducted during periods of neuronal cell death have shown upregulation of genes related to the inflammatory process in the nervous system of mice that serve as a model of GM_2 gangliosidosis. The activation of local microglia is shown by the signature of upregulated macrophage expression markers and lymphocyte chemoattractants, as well as genes encoding antigen-presenting MHC class II molecules. Since GM_2 gangliosidosis in mice is mitigated by bone marrow transplantation, which supplies a population of genetically competent immune cells (and which is accompanied by the use of powerful immunosup-pressant agents), it seems probable that the altered immunity accompanying bone marrow transplantation may itself modify the clinical expression of lysosomal storage diseases affecting the brain—such an effect may be independent of the storage material.

Several indirect studies have indicated the release of inflammatory cytokines in at least one lysosomal storage disease (Gaucher disease), which may explain the metabolic and plasma protein abnormalities associated with a sustained inflammatory response that characterizes the clinical syndrome. Hypertrophy and fibrosis characterize the organ responses in many lysosomal diseases. Whether the response is mediated at a cellular, paracrine, or endocrine level remains unclear. In Fabry disease, lyso-Gb3, is a promising candidate for an elusive, endocrine-like factor in the cardiac and vascular aspects of this condition.

The clinical presentation of malfunctioning organs in lysosomal storage disorders generally resembles the pathological outcomes of hypertrophy, fibrosis, and organ failure observed in other chronic conditions. Neurological syndromes vary with the anatomical site of greatest injury and with the relative involvement of grey or white matter (neuronopathic or myelination defects).

Clinical presentation

Natural course and severity range

All lysosomal diseases disturb the catabolism of complex molecules in numerous tissues and their manifestations are usually progressive and permanent; they show no relationship to food intake and are generally independent of intercurrent illness. The rate of deterioration depends in part on the degree of residual activity of the deficient enzyme or process; subtotal deficiencies present early in childhood with rapid evolution of disease. Partial deficiencies emerge more slowly and often present in later childhood or adult life. The disease may be insidious, as in the indolent splenomegaly of adults with Gaucher disease, the renal impairment of Fabry disease, or the muscle weakness of adult-onset Pompe disease. Acute episodes may punctuate this process, giving rise to a step-wise impairment of function, such as occurs with the avascular necrosis that typically affects the epiphyses of the long bones in Niemann-Pick disease type B or Gaucher disease.

Organomegaly and disturbed visceral function

Those disorders that affect metabolically active organs, such as the liver and kidney, often cause functional impairment, including the manifestations of liver failure, portal hypertension, and, in the case of the kidney, rickets, metabolic acidosis, for example as a consequence of the Fanconi syndrome in cystinosis. Cardiac involvement leads to hypertrophy, diastolic malfunction, conduction and rhythm disturbances, as well as thickening of the valves. Respiratory manifestations of the mucopolysaccharidoses are usually first evident as a result of narrowing of large airways but restricted ventilation due to skeletal disease often supervenes. Splenomegaly, complicated by marked functional hypersplenism, is characteristic of untreated Gaucher disease.

Skeletal manifestations

In several of the mucopolysaccharidoses, skeletal effects predominate and are particularly cruel. Severe growth retardation, joint stiffness, and atlantoaxial instability impair the quality and duration of life. In Gaucher disease, diverse osseous manifestations include marrow infiltration, osteoporosis, lytic lesions, pathological fractures, and occasional plasmacytoma or frank myelomatosis.

Neurologic features

Lysosomal diseases are a prominent cause of progressive neurological and mental deterioration in patients whose disease starts during adolescence up to mature adult life, and should always be considered in the diagnostic examination.

Ataxia is a feature of GM1 and GM2 gangliosidoses, and a flaccid paraparesis in young children might suggest metachromatic leucodystrophy; widespread white-matter disease in association with frontal dementia and spastic paraparesis is a characteristic presentation of juvenile and adult forms of metachromatic leucodystrophy and Krabbe disease. In both disorders, polyneuropathy and pyramidal signs are superimposed. Early-onset leucodystrophy is caused by metachromatic leucodystrophy, multiple sulphatase deficiency, and Krabbe disease—Krabbe disease is a rare but important diagnostic entity in this group since the disease may be mitigated by allogeneic marrow transplantation in early life. Lysosomal diseases with prominent neurological manifestations are often associated with progressive mental deterioration, with or without the onset of spasticity, myoclonic seizures, and optic atrophy. Extrapyramidal signs including parkinsonism, athetoid movements, and dystonia are frequent in this group of disorders.

Corneal opacities suggest cystinosis, I-cell disease, mucopolysaccharidoses, mannosidosis, Fabry disease, and galactosialidosis, as well as one form of Gaucher disease with neuronopathic features (the D409H type IIIc variant). Perifoveal pallor with the appearance of pigmentation in the macula (the 'cherry-red spot' in white persons) is a hallmark of Tay-Sachs disease and other gangliosidoses affecting infants and young adults. Specific syndromes are described in later sections.

Diagnosis

Clinical suspicion and family history

Even in the critically ill, it is essential, where possible, to establish the definitive diagnosis where a lysosomal disease is suspected, for several reasons: (1) specific treatment may be available; (2) these disorders are inherited either as X-linked or as autosomal recessive traits, and have important consequences for reproductive choice in other family members; and (3) the diagnosis may clarify unexplained symptoms in at-risk relatives. Increasingly, enzyme replacement therapy, bone marrow transplantation, or even oral substrate-reduction and enzyme enhancement therapies may be available. Furthermore, several disorders respond well to supportive measures including renal transplantation and hepatic transplantation. Finally, a great deal of expertise and practical support is available from specialist groups.

Charitable associations now exist in many countries for members to share their experiences and provide advice and counselling. Above all, invaluable information about available medical services for specific conditions can be obtained through patient organizations. The World Wide Web provides a useful entry into this often untapped resource where important information for patients, their doctors, and other relevant healthcare personnel, is to be found.

The key to making the diagnosis is enthusiastic suspicion and dogged persistence. In most circumstances, once suspected, the lysosomal disease can be identified with relative ease by referral to a specialized regional reference laboratory for the diagnosis of metabolic disorders; senior laboratory staff will usually advise about the handling of appropriate tissue material for diagnostic studies.

In the first instance, simple histochemical stains of existing biopsy material and examination of urine metabolites, including lipids and oligosaccharides, may narrow down the diagnosis. More commonly, specific enzymatic assays are used—generally carried out on leucocytes isolated from fresh heparinized blood samples, or on fibroblasts cultured from small biopsy specimens of skin; the latter are particularly valuable since, once established, fibroblast cultures can be stored indefinitely for repeated and definitive study.

Fabry disease, Niemann-Pick disease type B and C, as well as Gaucher disease, have often come to light in young or adult patients with particular syndromic presentations. Apart from paediatricians, general physicians, haematologists, nephrologists, neurologists, gastroenterologists and hepatologists, dermatologists, and even orthopaedic surgeons may be the first to evaluate the patient—all of whom should be able to identify the condition by following diagnostic pathways appropriate to their specialty. In any event, the diagnosis of lysosomal storage diseases is rarely difficult, provided the expertise of trusted laboratory services is available for the conduct of biochemical assays, diagnostic DNA studies, and wide-ranging histopathological examination. The value of good communications between laboratory staff and clinical investigators, to whom these patients are referred, cannot be overestimated.

A detailed family history, taking care to investigate the extended pedigree, is of critical importance. The differential diagnosis narrows substantially if there is evidence of X-linked inheritance characteristic of Fabry disease, MPS II (Hunter), or Danon disease. At-risk family members will be identified, often living with pre-symptomatic or undiagnosed disease. Tracing family members is best carried out sensitively in cooperation with professional genetic counselling services and with the general oversight of patient representative organizations. The high frequency of several mutant alleles of the *HEXA* gene responsible for Tay-Sachs disease in Ashkenazi Jews has led to greatly enhanced awareness of the disorder in this population, with successful international programmes for carrier detection. The birth of infants affected by Tay-Sachs disease is now exceptional in Jews but attenuated, late-onset forms of the disease occur in several populations.

Radiology

Ultrasonography, magnetic resonance imaging (MRI), and computed X-ray tomography (CT) may reveal visceral enlargement and infiltration, for example Niemann-Pick disease, mucopolysaccharidoses, and Gaucher disease. Skeletal radiographs may reveal bone expansion in vertebrae and in the phalangeal and long bones, sometimes associated with infarction and collapse, particularly in

Niemann-Pick disease type B and Gaucher disease. Echocardiography may reveal thickening and calcification of the cardiac valves (particularly of the aortic ring), infiltration of cardiac muscle causing ventricular hypertrophy in Pompe disease, Fabry disease, mucopolysaccharidoses I, IV, and VI, and, often strikingly, in Danon disease.

Neuroradiology is of value—particularly in patients with mucopolysaccharidoses, and in Morquio syndrome as well as MPS syndromes I, II, and VI where instability of the atlantoaxial joint may cause fatal subluxation in relation to diseased connective tissue surrounding the dens. MRI of the cervical spine in MPS is critical in judging the need for joint stabilization by posterior fusion. Similarly, investigations of the lower spine may determine the cause of progressive spinal deformity due to lumbar kyphosis, and assist in the evaluation of the need for surgery. MRI of the brain is invaluable in the assessment of dementing illnesses: cortical and/or white-matter disease may be delineated. MRI is often critical for diagnosing the striking white-matter changes that occur in patients with Krabbe disease, multiple sulphatase deficiency, and metachromatic leucodystrophy (Fig. 12.8.1).

Extensive white-matter lesions and eventual cerebral atrophy characterize the advanced stage of the neurological aspects of Fabry disease (Fig. 12.8.2).

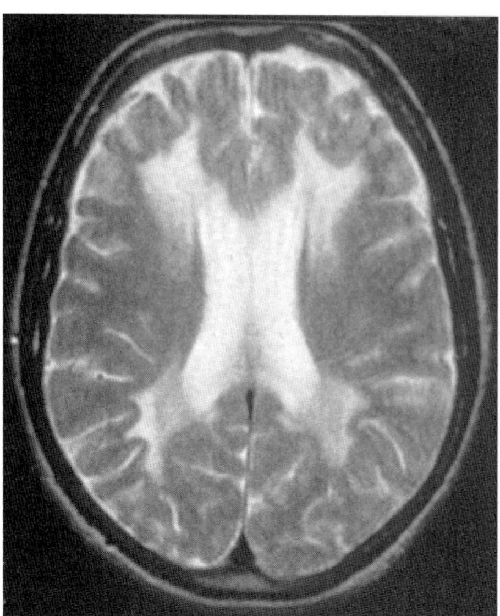

Fig. 12.8.2 Extensive white-matter lesions and eventual cerebral atrophy characterize the advanced stage of the neurological aspects of Fabry disease; ectopic calcification within the basal ganglia, cerebral cortex, and cerebellum is thought to locate to the media of small penetrating arteries. This 62-year-old patient with Fabry disease died of a dementing illness having suffered multiple stroke-like events, 15 years after a successful renal transplant.

Pathology

Although lysosomal defects occur in all tissues, the principal focus of each disease is observed in those tissues with the most rapid turnover of the parent macromolecule whose degradation is impaired. For example, in Gaucher disease, the turnover of parent glycolipids appears to be greatest in the mononuclear phagocytes.

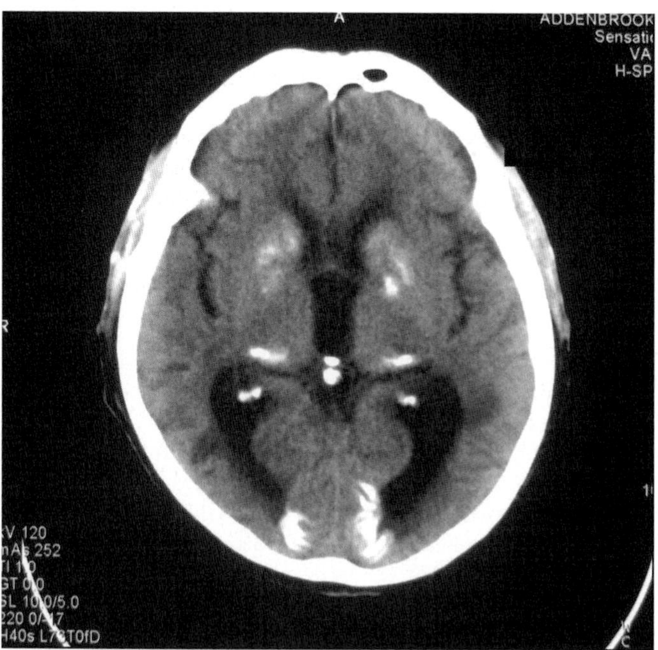

Fig. 12.8.1 Magnetic resonance imaging of the brain of a young woman with adult-onset metachromatic leucodystrophy. Notice the high signal intensity especially in the frontal white matter and periventricular regions. This patient presented with bizarre behaviour due to a frontal-type dementia; there are no neurological signs or symptoms. Short-term memory loss and lack of planning and higher executive functions are prominent features of her illness.

Here the accumulation of glycolipids derived from the breakdown of membranes present in the formed blood elements occurs; with mild or moderate impairment of the responsible enzyme, glucocer-ebrosidase, the pathology is restricted to the macrophage-containing tissues of the liver, spleen, bone marrow, and, occasionally, the lung. When inherited defects further impair the activity of glucocerebrosidase, additional pathology is seen in the nervous system where the source of accumulating glycolipid is principally endogenous neural sphingolipids.

Microscopic pathology shows storage within dilated vesicular spaces, which represent diseased lysosomes. Sphingolipids, being amphipathic molecules, tend to accumulate in whorls known as 'membranous cytoplasmic bodies' where they assume a lamellar structure within lysosomal spaces. Paracrystalline and crystalline material in distended lysosomes may also be seen under electron microscopy, for example in the accumulation of the charged glycolipid, sulphatide, that occurs in metachromatic leucodystrophy (arylsulphatase A deficiency). With more water-soluble substrates, granular material accumulates within the vesicular spaces. These spaces represent distended and often fused lysosomes, filled for example with undegraded glycogen macromolecular complexes in acid maltase deficiency (Pompe disease).

As emphasized earlier, the pathological manifestations of the lysosomal diseases are diverse. They may range from enlargement of viscera with infiltration by abnormal macrophages containing storage material (foam cells of Niemann-Pick disease or Gaucher's cells) to bone infarction, neuronophagia, vacuolation of renal tubular cells, and diverse tissue infiltrates. Inclusion bodies may be observed in metachromatic-stained cells of the urine deposit or in circulating neutrophils and lymphocytes (Maroteaux-Lamy disease); staining with a periodic acid-Schiff reagent may reveal diastase-resistant glycolipid storage in the kidney and other organs in Fabry disease and other glycosphingolipidoses. The presence of metachromatic storage material in nervous tissue, including

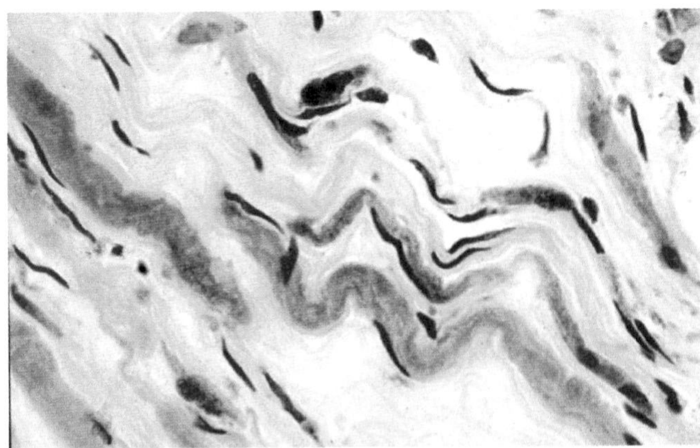

Fig. 12.8.3 Sural nerve biopsy stained with toluidine blue from the patient shown in Fig. 12.8.1 with metachromatic leucodystrophy. Note the brown-staining granular material within Schwann cells and perineurial macrophages typical of this disorder due to the deposition of the glycolipid sulphatide. (Courtesy of Dr. J. Xuereb, Addenbrooke's Hospital.)

peripheral nerves, is characteristic of the sphingolipidosis, metachromatic leucodystrophy (Fig. 12.8.3).

Ultrastructural examination is often diagnostic for lysosomal diseases: membrane-bound vesicles containing storage material that may show a crystalline or concentric appearance, or, in the case of glycogen in Pompe disease, vacuoles with a granular appearance. The appearance of concentric arrays of material, strongly suggest a sphingolipidosis. Amorphous material accumulates within the lysosomal vacuoles in the mucopolysaccharidoses and glycoproteinoses. The secondary effects of lysosomal hypertrophy include increased staining for tartrate-resistant acid phosphatase and other lysosomal markers, including intrinsic lysosomal membrane proteins, for example LAMP1.

Diagnostic biochemistry

For most of the lysosomal storage diseases, the suspected diagnosis can be confirmed by biochemical studies. Storage compounds can, as in the case of the glycoproteinoses and mucopolysacchaidoses, be detected in the urine. Initial colorimetric screening methods may confirm the presence of elevated concentrations of glycosaminoglycans but are not specific; chromatographic separation of individual glycoconjugates will assist further. More often, the diagnosis is established by confirming reduced or absent activity of an acid hydrolase. Specialized laboratories carry out panels of these assays depending on the clinical details provided by the clinician. Most assay systems are based on the cleavage of synthetic fluorescent analogues of the natural substrate in question. Accurate clinical information greatly assists the laboratory in deciding which enzyme activity, of many, to assay. The usual sample is a peripheral blood leucocyte preparation made from whole blood, although fibroblast cultures obtained from skin biopsies or biopsy specimens of other tissues may be required.

The biochemistry laboratory has a further role in determining the presence and concentration of markers of disease activity or response to treatment. Such biomarkers play an increasing role in clinical management, pharmaceutical development, and research. Markers in clinical practice include the chitinase, chitotriosidase, and the chemokine, CCL 18/PARC, as markers of the presence and extent of tissue infiltration by the eponymous cell in Gaucher disease.

Molecular diagnosis

Molecular analysis of genes encoding lysosomal enzymes may often support the enzymatic diagnosis, and may, on occasion, provide a rough prediction about the behaviour of the disease. DNA-based studies are of particular value for future prenatal diagnosis in a particular pedigree, and for the diagnosis of carrier status in at-risk females for heterozygosity in the X-linked diseases such as Hunter, Danon, and Fabry diseases. Lately, there has been a strong and justified trend in favour of specific enzymatic and genetic diagnoses, rather than for diagnoses based on the examination of biopsy material by light microscopy with or without the additional use of special histochemical stains. Ultrastructural examination of biopsy material may be of particular value in recognizing the type of disorder but is rarely crucial for a specific diagnosis. Hitherto, histochemical and histopathological methods have led to diagnostic inaccuracies, but it must be admitted that many cases of lysosomal disease—particularly as they affect adults—have in the past come to light as a result of bone marrow examinations, liver and muscle biopsies, and other procedures carried out in an attempt to arrive at a diagnosis in an otherwise puzzling condition.

Treatment

Lysosomal diseases have been the focus of several prominent therapeutic discoveries. The cooperation of informed patient groups, applied medical research funded by government organizations, and the commercial interest of medium-sized pharmaceutical companies has been promoted by recently introduced Orphan Drug legislation. This legislation has facilitated the early exclusive licensing of products for rare diseases—and has greatly enhanced corporate pharmaceutical investment. Orphan diseases are variously defined as those affecting fewer than one in 2000 of the population (Europe) or fewer than 200 000 individuals (United States); each lysosomal disease is, in effect, an ultra-orphan disorder, that is a disease affecting fewer than one in 50 000 individuals. Despite attracting great attention as a result of the high individual costs of treatment, the total national burden of treatments for these diseases in countries with developed healthcare systems is low (in England, the costs of specific treatments for lysosomal diseases amounts to about 0.1 per cent of the health budget).

At present, about a dozen recombinant human enzyme preparations are in use or in late clinical investigation. Indeed, several companies are expanding interest in this rarefied field, with additional recombinant proteins (including biosimilar molecules), small-molecule products—and even gene therapy—in robust competitive development. The orphan drug industry has drawn encouragement from the commercial success of recombinant human products such as human insulin, erythropoietin and other haematopoietic growth factors, and therapeutic antibodies and interferons. These are top-selling agents which have brought handsome rewards for the biotechnology companies prepared to invest heavily in medical sciences—and whose manufacturing patents have sometimes been defended with almost brutal vigour. At the time of writing, Genzyme Therapeutics, the United States-based company first involved in the development of targeted enzyme replacement therapy, imiglucerase (Cerezyme) for Gaucher disease, is providing treatment to about 5000 patients in more than 90 countries. The company, now the third largest biotechnology company in the world, reports revenues of about $4 billion, of which in 2007 nearly 30 per cent was attributed to Cerezyme; over the same period, the revenue from their enzyme product for Fabry disease was $424 million. Commercial success on an international scale has enabled Genzyme to invest in treatments for increasingly challenging disorders, including Pompe disease (the first inborn disorder to be recognized as a lysosomal defect by colleagues of de Duve). This fatal condition is associated with glycogen deposition in cardiac and skeletal muscle and requires the delivery of the therapeutic protein Myozyme (recombinant human acid alpha-glucosidase (maltase)) to a large bulk of diseased tissue, to which it is targeted by surface expression of mannose 6-phosphate residues.

The challenge here is met by the administration of gram quantities of the modified pure recombinant protein for adult patients at each infusion.

As described here, many of the 70 or so known human lysosomal disorders are disabling and distressing conditions that cause pain and disability in infants, children, and adults of all ages, and for which, until recently, no definitive treatments have been available. To enhance the availability of treatment for these diseases, compassionate programmes that grant access to patients disadvantaged by living in countries with undeveloped healthcare systems have been put in place. In 2007, Genzyme made global product donations of $110 million—such initiatives often appear to stimulate local investment in infrastructural services for diagnosis and treatment. The arrival of at least five additional pharmaceutical companies (Actelion, Amicus, Biomarin, Protalix, Shire Human Genetic Therapies) committed to obtaining a commercially realistic portion of this unique global market in ultra-orphan agents has introduced a powerful element of competition to the field and the fascination of continued research to develop improved products based on better understanding of lysosomal diseases—as well as the means to access niche markets during periods of unprecedented change in healthcare provision.

The magnification of interest that has accompanied successful medical research into this area has been a model of utility and progress: fundamentally it continues to provide for many patients and their families the hope that, at last, definitive relief is forthcoming.

Supportive and palliative

For most of the lysosomal disorders, no specific or curative treatment is available and, as a consequence, the psychological and social burdens are pervasive. As discussed earlier, the organ response to the metabolic defect is often stereotypical and similar to that seen in other diseases. Thus treatment is limited to those supportive and palliative measures shared with other chronic diseases. Occasionally, organ transplantation is required to deal with heart, liver, or kidney failure. Orthopaedic surgical techniques, such as joint replacement surgery and stabilization of kyphosis using Harrington rods, are frequently required and beneficial. Patients with obstructive hydro-cephalus benefit from the placement of shunts for cerebrospinal fluid. Middle ear effusions and glue ear are also treated conventionally with grommets. Physiotherapy for restricted joint movement and muscle weakness is valuable. Mobility aids and ventilatory support add to the range of expensive and invasive measures required in the absence of definitive treatment.

Augmentation of deficient activity

Early experiments by Elizabeth Neufeld and colleagues using fibroblasts in which glycosaminoglycans accumulate due to mucopolysaccharidoses such as Hurler disease (autosomal recessive) and Hunter syndrome (X-linked), showed that the rate of degradation—rather than the rates of synthesis or secretion—of ^{35}S sulphate-labelled substrate, is severely disrupted. When (as a result, initially, of a laboratory error), fibroblasts obtained from these genetically distinct storage disorders were co-cultured, the pathological accumulation of glycosaminoglycans in lysosomes was prevented. The biosynthetic labelling technique was also used to show that degradation of the substrates was restored to normal in these co-culture experiments. Further investigation of this phenomenon by the Neufeld group demonstrated that each of the fibroblast cultures elaborated and delivered a specific corrective factor to the medium, which ultimately proved to be a high-molecular-weight form of the hydrolases that were specifically lacking in fibroblasts from each disease. These corrective factors were identified in several comparable experiments using fibroblasts derived from other mucopolysaccharidoses and also several different classes of lysosomal disease; when taken up from the medium the factors restore the impaired intracellular degradation of cognate substrates. Thus functional correction of the biochemical defects permitted an early classification of distinct complementation groups among the mucopolysaccharidosis syndromes—often before the individual enzymatic defects had been characterized.

Specific receptor pathways for the biosynthesis and uptake of nascent lysosomal proteins during the course of organelle biogenesis have been identified: the secretion-recapture process is usually brought about by the so-called 'recognition marker', man-nose 6-phosphate. This terminal sugar is generated by a specific mechanism involving two post-translational modifying enzymes during the biosynthesis of soluble glycoproteins destined for the lysosomal matrix. Receptors, serving as intracellular lectins for mannose 6-phosphate ligands are densely expressed on pre-lysosomal membranes and mediate uptake of suitably labelled nascent proteins into the developing organelle. However, this trafficking process is not foolproof and 10 to 20 per cent of newly-formed soluble lysosomal proteins are misdirected to the plasma membrane from which they are released; by the same token, an appreciable population of cation-independent mannose 6-phosphate receptors is expressed on the plasmalemma. The 'leakiness' of this targeting system represents a default pathway for lysosomal protein secretion and recapture—as well as mutual complementation between different cells and tissues.

Functional complementation of lysosomal storage disorders by supplying particular molecular isoforms of the enzymes that are deficient in individual diseases provides a scientific justification for enzyme replacement treatment. Successful application of enzyme-replacement is dependent on an understanding of glycoprotein chemistry, receptor-mediated endocytosis, and the molecular cell biology of lysosomal biogenesis: identification of the secretion and recapture mechanism has provided further practical underpinning.

The mannose 6-phosphate pathway is not the only mechanism for delivering proteins to the lysosome: indeed the first successful enzyme replacement therapy for Gaucher disease employs human glucocerebrosidase that is modified specifically to reveal terminal unphosphorylated mannose residues that greatly enhance delivery of the therapeutic protein to cells of the macrophage lineage that are the principal focus the disease. Characterization of lysosomal recognition markers occurred at a time when other cell-surface glycoprotein recognition systems were being identified: the asialoglycoprotein receptor, the first mammalian lectin identified by Ashwell and Morell can mediate the uptake of modified plasma proteins by parenchymal liver cells *in vivo*. Recent studies show that in some cells, for example in the inner ear and brain, as well as lymphocytes (but not fibroblasts or macrophages), delivery of nascent acid glucocerebrosidase to lysosomes is dependent on a unique tissue-specific chaperone function supplied by a lysosomal membrane protein (LIMP2). Mutations in the human *LIMP2* gene appear to account for some atypical cases of Gaucher disease with neurological manifestations (including myotonic epilepsy), kidney disease, and perplexing enzymology when examined in peripheral blood cells and cultured skin fibroblasts; in these patients glucocerebrosidase deficiency is found in fibroblasts but not leucocytes.

Haematopoietic stem cell transplantation

Cellular complementation, by providing a source of wild-type enzyme delivered from allogeneic bone marrow transplantation, has also had spectacular successes in several lysosomal disorders. In Gaucher disease, where the pathogenic cell is of haematopoietic origin, bone marrow transplantation was effective in the past. Successful engraftment led to full correction of the biochemical defect and reversal of most of the visceral and haematological effects of the condition that had not already progressed irrevocably. Now that a safer treatment in the form of enzyme replacement is available, bone marrow transplantation, with its attendant risks, is very rarely indicated. In diseases due to deficiency of soluble hydrolases, donor cells that repopulate the microglia (the brain equivalent of tissue macrophages) may participate in the secretion-recapture mechanism; and in this form of cell-replacement therapy would be expected to provide a source of enzyme to vicinal cells. Haematopoietic stem cell transplantation has been successful, when administered at an early stage, in several of the neurodegenerative lysosomal storage disorders, such as Hurler disease (MPS I), and Krabbe disease.

Enzyme replacement therapy

The whole field of the lysosomal diseases is attracting much attention as a promising area of clinical research and pharmaceutical investment. The earlier definition of Orphan diseases as 'those in which treatments offer little or no financial incentive for commercial development' has been abandoned: these rare diseases are now conveniently defined as 'those which individually affect fewer than 0.05 per cent of the population'.

Discovery of mechanism by which lysosomal proteins are delivered to the nascent organelle have gone hand-in-hand with the hope of treatment based on the targeting of therapeutic enzymes to diseased tissues. Nonetheless the first commercial preparation of glucocerebrosidase (alglucerase, Ceredase) was not licensed until 1991 and 1994 by the FDA and EMEA, respectively, after decades of painstaking research. This preparation was purified from placentae and the glycan structure was modified enzymatically to reveal terminal mannose groups that bind the mannose receptor on cells of macrophage origin. Alglucerase mitigated many features of the Gaucher disease when given parenterally. The therapeutic and commercial success of algucerase, albeit at the height of the human immunodeficiency virus (HIV) epidemic related to use of natural human coagulation factor VIII in haemophiliacs, and iatrogenic Creutzfeldt-Jakob disease, as well as potential difficulties in maintaining the supply of suitable placentae, stimulated the demand for a recombinant preparation (imiglucerase, Cerezyme, licensed in 1994 and 1998) and the later expansion of the concept to include diseases that would be targeted using the more general lysosomal recognition marker, mannose 6-phosphate. Since 2001, recombinant protein therapies have also become available for Fabry disease, MPS I, MPS II, Maroteaux-Lamy disease (MPS VI), Pompe disease, and alpha-mannosidosis. Universal availability of these treatments is limited by their exorbitant financial cost (licensed doses cost upwards of $200 000 per annum for an average adult) and by the requirement for a sophisticated healthcare infrastructure to support the delivery and monitoring of the therapy.

Thus, even imiglucerase (Cerezyme) the lead product, which has been available for over 15 years and whose efficacy is clear, is available to fewer than 20 per cent of patients globally for whom it is indicated. The mature therapeutic position of the newer enzyme products will emerge given time; but it must be recognized that the conditions for which they are designed are heterogeneous and, it appears, generally more intractable than Gaucher disease.

Pharmacological chaperone therapy

This strategy is based on the ability of small molecules to bind to key regions of mutant proteins that are misfolded and thus prematurely degraded in the endoplasmic reticulum and Golgi network. Aberrant protein folding is increasingly recognized as a frequent molecular mechanism in inherited diseases and leads to an operational deficiency of protein function at the normal cellular point of action as a result of disrupted co-translational processing. Pharmacological chaperones are molecules which bind to the active site of mutant lysosomal enzymes and thus assist delivery to the site of action in the correct compartment. In the case of lysosomal enzymes, the chaperone molecule often proves to be a weak inhibitor of the target from which it is ultimately proposed to dissociate on reaching the destination within the acidic environment of the organelle. Pyrimethamine, a licensed antimicrobial has chaperone-like effects in cells harbouring some HEXA mutations from Tay-Sachs patients; this drug is currently undergoing clinical trials.

Several iminosugars correct the misfolding of mutant lysosomal glucocerebrosidases in experimental cell systems, including cultured fibroblasts obtained from Gaucher patients: one of these, isofagomine, is currently undergoing clinical evaluation by the Amicus company in Gaucher disease. Clinical trials are also underway with another iminosugar (1-deoxygalactonojirimycin) in patients with Fabry disease in whom *in vitro* studies indicate the potential for functional enhancement of several mutant α-galactosidase variants which occur in this disorder. Although the use of pharmacological chaperones is an attractive concept for the oral treatment of lysosomal diseases—and in some cases the molecules may penetrate injured tissue across the blood-brain barrier—hitherto no small molecule has been reported to show clinical efficacy in any putative misfolding disease, including the misfolded cystic fibrosis transmembrane regulator (CFTR). Suitable models of these diseases in which to test the strategy are hard to identify and in the authors' view, there are other formidable barriers in the translation of preclinical experiments in cultured cells to the successful use of chaperones in human patients, not least of which is the need to obtain sufficiently high concentrations of the chaperone molecules specifically to restore adequate lysosomal function at the relevant sites without inducing toxicity. However, the late entry of chaperones onto the competitive stage subtended by lysosomal diseases is to be welcomed—for the limelight will linger only on those actors seen in context to have useful parts to play.

Restriction of substrate flux

For many years the accumulation of storage material within lysosomes has been considered to be the precipitating factor for the development of tissue injury and the inflammatory response that accompanies the lysosomal storage disorders. By analogy with the development of atherosclerosis due to impaired catabolism of cholesterol bound to low-density lipoproteins, it is principally a failure of degradation or export from the lysosome that leads to the pathological storage. Thus, like the statins which inhibit the first committed step in the biosynthesis of cholesterol, the concept of depleting the supply of macromolecular substrate to prevent the accumulation of injurious material has been developed experimentally and brought to clinical trial in the sphingolipid disorders. Two classes of inhibitor are prominent in therapeutic studies: iminosugars derived from naturally-occurring compounds (acting principally as sugar mimetics) and synthetic morpholino compounds, which act as analogues of the ceramide moiety of sphingolipids.

Of leading developmental interest has been the discovery that certain iminosugars related to deoxynojirimycin selectively inhibit the ceramide-specific UDP-glucosyltransferase reaction as the first committed step in the biosynthesis of glycosphingolipids. Experimental studies in cultured cells with pathological storage of glycolipids in lysosomes showed regression of the intralysosomal material after exposure to low concentrations of these natural product derivatives.

In the absence of a living model of Gaucher disease at the time, demonstration of reduced storage and delayed symptom onset in murine models of debilitating human glycosphingolipidoses such as Tay-Sachs disease and Sandhoff disease provided preclinical data to support clinical trials in Gaucher disease. N-butyldeoxynojirimycin, a particular analogue of these iminosugars, had previously been used in clinical trials in an attempt to inhibit the replication of HIV, as a result of its related inhibitory activity towards α-glucosidases; in these trials, such drugs appear to be relatively non-toxic in large doses. With these data in mind, studies were undertaken to investigate the concept of substrate depletion as a treatment for established glycosphingolipidoses. Evidence of disease regression was obtained in an open-labelled trial of N-butyldeoxynojirimycin in patients with Gaucher disease, as shown by the reduction in visceral enlargement, enzymatic markers of Gaucher disease activity (plasma chitotriosidase activity), and a slow improvement in haematological parameters. In Gaucher disease, it was anticipated that the beneficial effects of substrate depletion would be indirect, since they would result from the decrease in the delivery to the macrophage system of glycoli-pid substrates on the membrane of blood cells. In any event, since the iminosugars are small molecules with the potential to penetrate the blood-brain barrier, the possibility of their use (either as a monotherapy or as a synergistic treatment with enzyme therapy) for neuronopathic Gaucher disease has been raised, as well as for the treatment of the otherwise intractable glycosphingolipidoses that cause severe neurological disease.

No effective treatment is currently available for Tay-Sachs disease, Sandhoff disease, and GM1 gangliosidosis, and the juvenile and late-onset variants are thus potential targets for substrate depletion with inhibitory small molecules. Substrate depletion therapy depends upon the presence of residual enzymatic activity in the lysosomes. Disturbances of the dynamic equilibrium in the supply and handling of macromolecular lysosomal substrates occur, but most, if not all, patients with glycosphingolipid disorders express residual enzymatic function. Clinical trials have taken place not only in Gaucher disease but in Niemann-Pick-disease type C. This latter disorder is itself associated with a secondary accumulation of toxic glycolipids within neuronal lysosomes.

The iminosugars appear to be relatively well tolerated apart from causing diarrhoea, probably as a result of impaired biosynthesis of intestinal disaccharidases as a subsidiary effect on oligosaccharide processing. Indeed, experience shows that they are usually well tolerated once appropriate dietary restrictions are introduced. However, several cases of peripheral neuropathy have been reported in long-term studies of patients with Gaucher disease. The sugars are absorbed after oral ingestion and offer the hope of a therapy to arrest the progression of several severe neurological sphingolipidoses that are otherwise beyond therapeutic correction.

At present, the outcome of the clinical trials based on promising animal experiments with several iminosugars and the morpholino inhibitors of glycolipid biosynthesis derivatives is urgently awaited. Early clinical results indicate that the morpholino compound, GENZ 112638, a ceramide analogue with a highly selective inhibitory action on glycolipid biosynthesis, has strong salutary effects in non-neuronopathic Gaucher disease. GENZ 112638 so far appears to have an acceptable side-effect profile but clearly long-term studies will be needed to determine the efficacy and safety profile of this oral drug if it is to become an acceptable alternative to enzyme therapy. Substrate reduction therapy may, however, have wider applications in the treatment of certain sphingolipidoses, including late-onset Tay-Sachs disease, GM1 gangliosidosis, and Niemann-Pick disease type C, which affect the brain and for which no other therapy is currently available. Several agents have been found to be effective in animal models of glycosphingolipidoses—an action which is dependent on their capacity to enter brain tissue and in this respect, successors to N-butyldeoxynojirimycin are actively undergoing preclinical study.

Examples of lysosomal disorders

Gaucher disease

This disorder may occur at any age and is the most frequent of the lysosomal storage diseases. The condition is usually due to a catalytic deficiency of glucocerebrosidase, although rare cases of deficiency of its cognate sphingolipid activator protein (SAP-C) may cause a severe disorder intermediate between Gaucher disease and metachromatic leucodystrophy. Numerous mutations responsible for the enzymatic deficiency have been identified in the human glucocerebrosidase gene and the reader is referred to the specialist literature for those genotype/phenotype correlations that broadly apply to this protean disorder.

Rarely, infants are born with an almost complete lack of glucocerebrosidase activity: they die within a few days of birth or are stillborn due to skeletal deformities and/or dehydration as a result of loss of skin integrity (collodion babies). Infantile Gaucher disease (classified as type II disease) is a rare condition that is associated with death in the first 2 years of life: there is neuronopathic disease with bulbar palsy, opisthotonus, and minor visceral enlargement. This disease is invariably fatal and does not respond to either systemic or intrathecal enzyme replacement therapy. While neurological disease may occur in children, adolescents, and young adults with Gaucher disease, it is less severe than in the infantile variant. In such patients the disease is associated with supranuclear gaze palsies, ataxia, nerve deafness, myoclonus, and, occasionally, seizures. The neurological condition usually deteriorates slowly but is exacerbated if splenectomy is performed for the accompanying splenomegaly and associated pancytopenia.

Where possible, and with vigorous enzyme therapy, splenectomy is best avoided—partial splenectomy may be carried out to ameliorate pressure effects and life-threatening thrombocytopenia. Subacute neuronopathic disease is not always fatal and often improves with combined bone marrow transplantation and enzyme replacement therapy. Affected children may show striking visceromegaly, with the associated gaze palsies often playing a small part in the clinical presentation. Although juvenile subacute neuronopathic Gaucher disease (type III) occurs sporadically in all populations, there is a small isolate in Northern Sweden where all individuals are homozygous for a single point mutation in the glucocerebrosidase gene *(L444P)* that has arisen by descent from a common ancestor.

The most frequent form of Gaucher disease is the so-called 'adult non-neuronopathic form' (type I). This disease is found in all populations, but is over-represented in Jews of Ashkenazi origin. Although the condition does not commonly affect the nervous system, visceral and skeletal manifestations are prominent. Rare patients develop extrapyramidal disease resembling parkinsonism in middle life; the response to dopaminergic agents is often disappointing and the disorder may progress rapidly. This complication may reflect the emerging but ill-understood relationship between mutant glucocerebrosidase alleles and Parkinson disease in several populations. The pathognomic abnormality is the presence of large storage cells, which are activated macrophages (Gaucher cells), typically found in the splenic sinusoids. The Gaucher cells (Figs. 12.8.4 and 12.8.5) replace the Kupffer cells of the liver, alveolar macrophages of the lung and in the bone marrow.

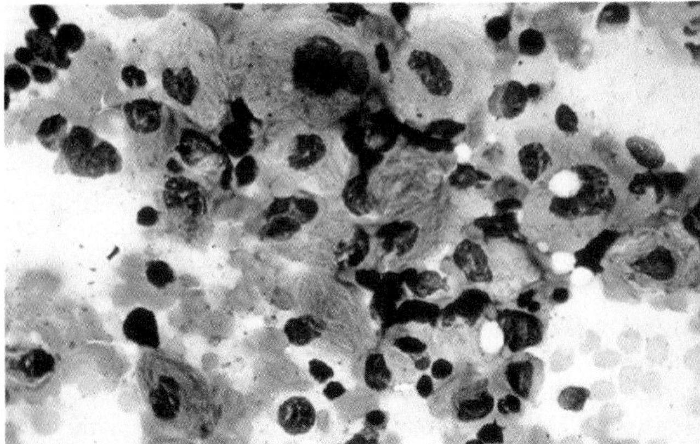

Fig. 12.8.4 Light micrograph of a Leishmann-stained bone marrow biopsy obtained from a 23-year-old man with type 1 Gaucher disease. Note that the large, pale-blue staining Gaucher cells with striated cytoplasm replace the Kupffer cells of the liver, alveolar macrophages of the lung, and of the bone marrow.

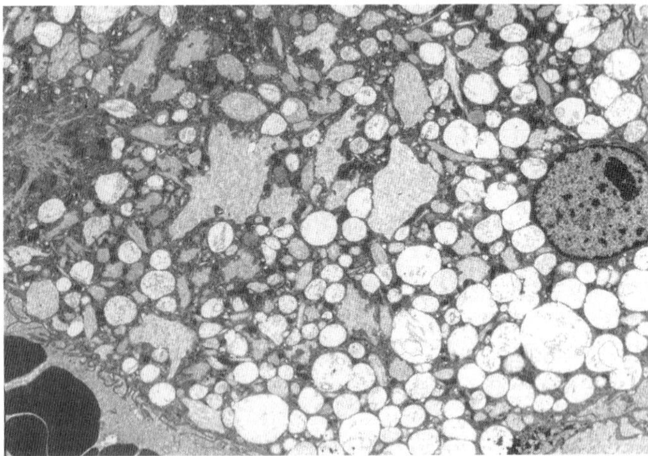

Fig. 12.8.5 Electron micrograph showing the cytoplasm of a Gaucher cell in the spleen of a 56-year-old man removed because of life-threatening thrombocytopenia and pain due to a recent splenic infarct. Note the vesicular spaces filled with fibrillary glycolipid storage material.

Characteristically, Gaucher disease presents with pancytopenia, with bleeding due to thrombocytopenia and splenic enlargement. Acutely painful episodes also occur in the bones, particularly during growth; these episodes are followed by avascular necrosis of the bone with consequential effects on the integrity of large joints, including the hip, knee, and shoulder (Fig. 12.8.6). The increased frequency of infarction events is an important aspect of Gaucher disease that, as yet, has not been explained. Bone necrosis remains an aspect of the condition that often persists despite enzyme therapy and presents a significant challenge for clinical research. In the era before enzyme replacement therapy, splenectomy was often carried out during childhood to relieve the pressure effects of the enlarged

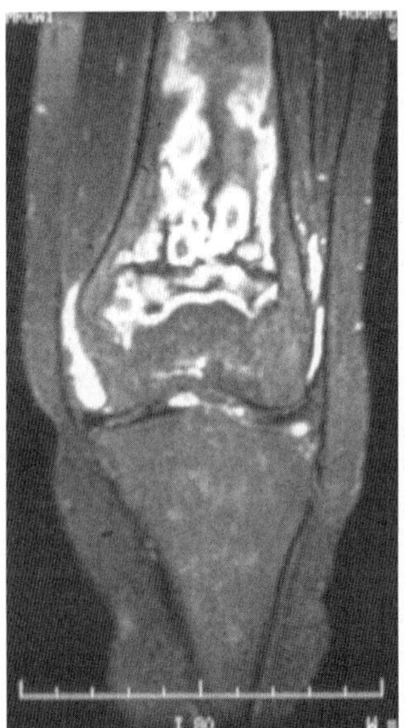

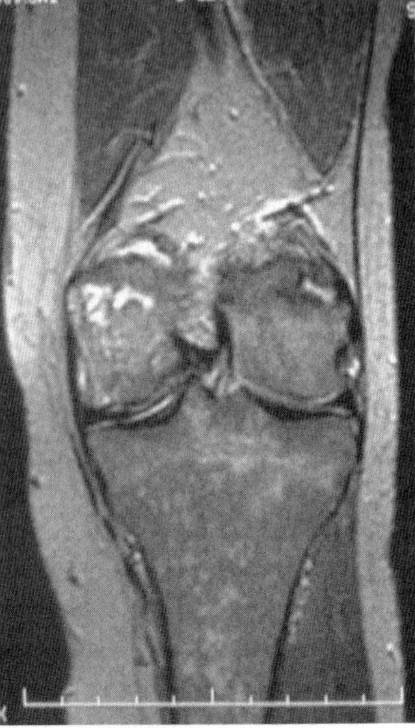

Fig. 12.8.6 T1 (left)- and T2 (right)-weighted magnetic resonance images obtained from the lower femur and upper tibia of a 30-year-old woman with non-neuronopathic Gaucher disease experiencing pain due to acute avascular necrosis of bone. Note the geographical areas of increased signal intensity on the T_2-weighted image due to increased tissue water representing oedema surrounding the necrotic tissue.
(Courtesy of Professor D. Lomas, Addenbrooke's Hospital.)

organ and to ameliorate the effects of accompanying cytopenias. Although there appears to be an association between splenectomy and the development of severe bone disease, it is unclear as to whether this is directly due to the effects of the splenectomy or the consequential manifestations of disease severity. Nonetheless, splenectomy is best avoided where at all possible. Splenectomy in Gaucher disease carries a greatly enhanced risk of overwhelming infection; this includes infection with protozoa, such as babesia and malaria, as well as capsulated bacteria, for example *Streptococcus pneumoniae*, *Haemophilus influenzae*, and *Neisseria meningitidis.*

Gaucher disease is a truly multisystem disorder, which is accompanied by many ill-understood plasma and metabolic abnormalities. These include a polyclonal immunoglobulin response that may progress to monoclonal gammopathy, amyloidosis, or even frank myeloma. Low-density lipoprotein and high-density lipoprotein cholesterol fractions are abnormal in the plasma. Some lysosomal enzymes are elevated, including tartrate-resistant acid phosphatase, hexosaminidase, and a human chitinase, chitotriosidase. Chitotriosidase has proved to be very useful for monitoring Gaucher disease activity in response to treatment, and may reflect the severity of the disease. The enzyme is elevated sometimes several hundredfold above normal in untreated Gaucher disease.

Gaucher disease may rarely be associated with pulmonary infiltrates, including reticulonodular opacities, restrictive lung defects, and various abnormalities of the pulmonary circulation causing pulmonary hypertension. The hepatopulmonary syndrome, accompanied by platypnoea and associated with severe scarring liver disease or cirrhosis and portal venous hypertension, has also been reported in severely affected adults. In addition to the effects of avascular necrosis, the osseous manifestations of Gaucher disease are very diverse and include the presence of expanded bone lesions (Fig. 12.8.7) with surrounding cortical thinning related to Gaucher cell infiltrates within the bone marrow ('Gauchomas'). Diffuse osteoporosis accompanied by pathological fractures may also compound the skeletal manifestations of Gaucher disease.

Kyphoscoliosis due to crush fractures and avascular necrosis of vertebrae are common in untreated adults, particularly in postmenopausal women.

In its untreated state, Gaucher disease is a miserable condition leading to progressive skeletal deformity, pancytopenia, and visceral enlargement with failing organ function punctuated by painful visceral bone crises. The mean age of death in a single large series reported from Pittsburgh, Pennsylvania, was 60 years during the pretreatment era, but this does not take into account the poor quality of life of most affected individuals. Some homozy-gotes for 'mild' missense mutations in the glucocerebrosidase gene (especially the widespread mutation, N370S) may escape detection and remain asymptomatic throughout a long adult life. Detailed investigation reveals only a mild thrombocytopenia and trivial splenomegaly in some cases. However, monoclonal gammopa-thy is frequently present after the age of 45 years. It is uncertain as to what extent the presence of such mutations in the population at large (homozygosity for N370S occurs in about one in 960 Ashkenazi Jews) contributes to the development of β-cell lymphoproliferative disorders, such as B-cell lymphoma and myeloma, in this at-risk group.

The diagnosis of Gaucher disease is based on white-cell acid β-glucosidase activity, which may be accompanied by the elevation of one or more related marker enzymes such as chitotriosidase or tartrate-resistant acid phosphatase in the serum. Spleen tissue, liver

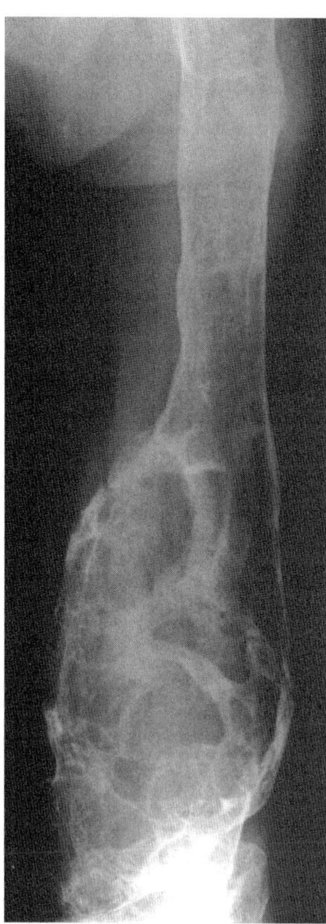

Fig. 12.8.7 Expanded lytic lesion at the distal end of the femur in a 44-year-old woman with severe Gaucher disease complicated by osteoporosis, avascular necrosis, and, as shown, expanded lytic lesions in long bones leading to local infiltration of the marrow space by Gaucher tissue.

biopsy material, or bone marrow aspirates may show the characteristic oligonucleate storage cells demonstrating striated cytoplasm on Leishmann staining (see Fig. 12.8.4), but which appear as pink sheets in tissue sections stained with haematoxylin and eosin. Molecular analysis of the glucocerebrosidase gene may identify widespread mutant glucocerebrosidase alleles that cause this disease and may assist in the diagnosis and investigation of family members at risk for this recessive disorder.

Treatment

Until recently, the treatment for Gaucher disease was palliative. Bone marrow transplantation has been undertaken in a few infants and children with rapidly progressive disease, including those with the subacute neuronopathic form type III. When successful, this may correct most of the systemic manifestations of the condition and restore growth. Some observers believe that it may arrest further neurological deterioration. However, bone marrow transplantation is no longer in routine use because of the accompanying severe risk resulting from the procedures and constraints in the supply of donors, especially MHC-matched, first-degree relatives.

Enzyme replacement therapy was introduced during the early 1990s in the form of a natural product extracted from the human placenta, alglucerase (Ceredase). A recombinant glycoform, imi-glucerase (Cerezyme), is now available that, like alglucerase, is modified to reveal terminal mannose residues. The recombinant protein is supplied as a lyophilized powder which is reconstituted for intravenous infusion; the preparation is given at variable frequencies, from three times a week to once every 2 weeks, and infused over approximately 60 min. Modification of the sugar residues on this protein facilitates targeting to mannose receptors on macrophages, in which it complements the enzyme deficiency of the pathological storage cells. After a few weeks of enzyme administration, most patients show an improvement in the blood parameters of disease activity and a reduction of the chronic inflammatory response that accompanies Gaucher disease: the platelet count rises; and there is a correction of the hypersplenic blood picture, with a reduction in hepatosplenomegaly and an improvement in the asthenia that complicates Gaucher disease. Quality-of-life measures also show clear improvement.

Controversy remains as to the appropriate dose of imiglucerase; however, most authorities agree that the administration of the enzyme should be lifelong. There are several schools of thought as to whether enzyme therapy should be administered at a high dose to start with, perhaps then reducing as evidence of disease regression becomes clear, or whether a more variable but lower dose be given and altered according to response. Disease activity is assessed by objective parameters, including visceral enlargement, and by determination of surrogate biomarkers such as chitotriosidase and blood counts. At present, there is no agreed protocol for therapy in adults with Gaucher disease; but by analogy with other chronic disorders, the application of simple defined therapeutic goals with close monitoring of individual patients has much to recommend it. Achievement of key goals and amelioration of disease-associated parameters is more rapid when high-dose enzyme therapy is administered. In patients with the subacute neuronopathic form of the condition, international guidelines suggest that a dose of at least 120 units of enzyme per kg bodyweight per month is necessary to secure disease regression.

Although it would not be expected that enzyme replacement therapy would improve the neuronopathic aspects of Gaucher disease, there is evidence that useful clinical improvement may be induced by enzyme replacement therapy and the drug is specifically licensed for this indication. Enzyme replacement therapy for Gaucher disease is very expensive and the doses recommended range from below 10 to at least 120 IU/kg per month. Thus for an adult, this may cost as much as £200 000 per year, so placing demands on healthcare provision for a single rare patient in the long term.

In response to these pressures and to the inconvenience of parenteral administration, there have been initiatives to develop alternative methods to treat the condition, including the use of an oral agent that inhibits the formation of the substrate delivered to macrophages. When taken for several months, miglustat (Zavesca; N-butyldeoxynojirimycin) appears to reduce the content of gangliosides in circulating white cells, and has salutary effects on key laboratory and clinical parameters of Gaucher disease activity. In relation to treatment with iminosugars, short-duration unwanted effects (including diarrhoea due to inhibition of intestinal disaccharidases) are frequent, although they usually respond well to dietary adjustments. Zavesca is licensed in the United States and Europe by the Actelion company for use in mild to moderate type I Gaucher disease, albeit with certain restrictions. The occurrence of peripheral neuropathy after long-term administration in a few patients with non-neuronopathic Gaucher disease may restrict the indications for its use. The results of a trial to determine whether or not Zavesca is inferior to maintenance therapy with Cerezyme in patients with type 1 Gaucher disease after stable control of their disease who then switch to the oral agent are awaited and should clarify its mature therapeutic position.

Further orally-active compounds are in advanced clinical development, including the substrate-reducing agent and ceramide analogue developed by Genzyme (GENZ 112638). Isofagomine, a compound supplied by Amicus as AT2101 is under clinical investigation as a pharmacological chaperone aimed at improving the folding and stability of mutant glucocerebrosidases in Gaucher disease and thus increasing delivery of active enzyme to the lysosome, but preliminary results at going to press have been disappointing. In addition to these agents, at least two 'biosimilar' preparations of mannose-terminated recombinant human glu-cocerebrosidase are in late-phase clinical trials (one, manufactured by Shire Human Genetic Therapies using selective gene activation in a human fibrosarcoma cell line, and another recombinant product engineered for expression in carrot cell cultures by the biotechnology company, Protalix).

Enzyme replacement therapy, although very expensive, is a successful treatment for Gaucher disease, and, since most patients do express the protein antigen endogenously, hypersensitivity and immune reactions are very rare. Apart from the inconvenience of periodic intravenous infusions, treatment is well tolerated and many patients in Europe and the United Kingdom choose to take their treatment as self-administered infusions at home. Treatment for Gaucher disease should include appropriate immunization and antimicrobial prophylaxis in the fortunately diminishing number of patients who have undergone splenectomy. Osteoporosis may be an indication for bisphosphonate drugs. Patients may require joint-replacement surgery to ameliorate the effects of bone infarction crises and, in rare instances, liver transplantation for end-stage liver disease. All surgical procedures carry a risk of haemorrhage in the face of thrombocytopenia or blood coagulation factor abnormalities. It is thus critically important to engage expert assistance from a haematologist in planning surgical interventions. Bone marrow transplantation probably does not have a role today, except in rare circumstances. Evidence of metabolic bone disease complicating the disorder should be always sought and osteoporosis should be treated promptly with enzyme replacement therapy, with the additional consideration of orally active or parenteral bisphosphonates. Where present, a deficiency of 25-hydroxyvitamin D should probably be treated with appropriate supplements; some patients develop deficiency of vitamin B_{12} and this should be sought for and treated promptly. On account of the increased risk of infection due to intrinsic chemotactic and phagocytic defects as well as splenectomy, patients with Gaucher disease undergoing surgery or with systemic infection should be promptly treated—preferably with parenteral antimicrobial agents.

Fabry disease

This disease is an X-linked disorder, unlike many of the lysosomal diseases, apart from Danon and Hunter disease (MPS II). A notable feature of Fabry disease, unlike MPS II, is the presence of clinical signs and symptoms in most heterozygous female carriers of the condition. Although these manifestations are usually less severe and of later onset than in affected hemizygous males, florid and life-shortening clinical disease has often been observed (and ignored) in affected women. Deficiency of α-galactosidase A causes the accumulation of ceramidetrihexoside (otherwise known as globotriaosylceramide), which principally derives from the breakdown of lipids present in senescent red cells.

The most characteristic symptoms of the disease are the onset in early childhood of lancinating pain with background burning sensations in the extremities that are made worse by exercise and exposure to extremes of temperature. These attacks can be very disabling and represent neuropathic pain, which is notoriously difficult to control. The acroparasthesias are frequently attributed to Raynaud phenomenon but this relationship is unclear. Nonetheless, many of the symptoms of Fabry disease can be explained by neuropathy affecting autonomic nervous tone. Patients with Fabry disease have disturbing gastrointestinal symptoms, characterized by diarrhoea shortly after eating; attacks of abdominal pain associated with unexplained fever also occur. The abdominal symptoms may also be related to autonomic neuropathy.

Most men with established disease notice a striking absence of peripheral sweating, and are frequently impotent. High-toneloss of hearing is also a common feature of Fabry disease; it appears to reflect selective injury to cochlear neurons. Affected male hemizygotes have small, raised, red vascular skin lesions (angiokeratomas) particularly around the buttocks and genital region. These lesions are often detected in limited areas of affected heterozygous females and reflect X-chromosome inactivation patterns in the skin.

With increasing age, impaired capillary circulation and progressive tubular, interstitial, and glomerular disease in the kidney leads to proteinuria and renal failure. Many patients require renal support, including haemodialysis, peritoneal dialysis, or kidney transplantation. Cardiac hypertrophy, especially of the left ventricle, occurs with conduction defects leading to a shortened PR interval and a prolonged QRS complex—later accompanied by tachyarrhythmias and complete heart block. Left ventricular hypertrophy may be associated with hypertension and cardiac embolic disease; disease of capillaries and medium-sized vessels in the brain is associated with unusual microvascular changes, particularly in the posterior cerebral circulation, and also causes stroke.

Stroke and renal failure are the most common causes of death in patients with Fabry disease; in men, death occurs at a median age of 48 to 49 years, with a greatly reduced quality of life during the antecedent symptomatic period. Life expectancy in affected heterozygous women is also shortened. Sometimes the lancinating acroparasthesias are sufficient to cause severe depression and even suicide. Disease expression in many carrier females, who may rarely develop renal failure, is often accompanied by angiokeratomas restricted to certain dermatomes on careful examination and asymptomatic corneal opacification with whorl-like cataracts on slit-lamp examination.

Diagnosis is made by demonstrating the abnormal glycolipid in urine or plasma, as well as by assay of α-galactosidase A in tears, plasma, white cells, or other tissue material. Molecular analysis of the α-galactosidase A gene on the long arm of the X chromosome is worthwhile because it allows the unambiguous detection of female heterozygotes and may thus be useful during the reproductive period, particularly for antenatal diagnosis. Despite the presence of active disease, ceramidetrihexoside concentrations and α-galactosidase A assays are often within normal limits in affected female heterozygotes.

Hitherto, the treatment for Fabry disease has been palliative, involving the use of anticonvulsants (including gabapentin) for the acroparasthesiae and neuropathic pain. Gastrointestinal symptoms sometimes respond to antimotility agents or to pancreatic enzyme supplements but these agents have not been subjected to control trials. Renal failure is managed by dialysis or by renal transplantation; occasionally, cardiac transplantation has been required for cardiomyopathy; pacemakers and antiarrhythmic drugs may also be needed. There is a rare cardiac variant in this disease, which appears to be predominantly manifested by restrictive cardiomyopathy in elderly patients with appreciable residual α-galactosidase activity.

Recently, enzyme replacement using recombinant human α-galactosidase A has been developed as a more definitive treatment. To date, two preparations—which may differ slightly in their post-translational glycosylation status for delivery to endothelial, epithelial, and other cells that represent the pathological focus of this disease—have been licensed: agalsidase-alfa (Replagal—not approved in the United States) and agalsidase-beta (Fabrazyme). Administration of these preparations to male hemizygotes has improved lipid accumulation in the plasma and in renal biopsy samples from male hemizygotes with this disease. Both products have also been shown in double-blind, placebo-controlled trials to improve clinical endpoints of the disease, including neuropathic pain, stabilization of renal function, and ventricular mass, as well as conduction defects that represent infiltrative cardiomyopathy. Substantial reversal of established organ malfunction has been less easily achieved with enzyme treatment for Fabry disease. Unlike Gaucher disease, targeting to the affected cells and tissues in Fabry disease probably results from receptor-mediated uptake of protein molecules harbouring the common lysosomal recognition marker, mannose-6 phosphate. In one remarkable instance, therapy with galactose infusions appears to have mitigated this condition by stabilizing the nascent mutant enzyme, thereby enhancing residual α-galactosidase A activity with slow clearance of cardiac glycolipid storage. Clinical trials of the putative pharmacological chaperone, 1-deoxyglactonojirimycin, which is predicted to stabilize certain residual α-galactosidase A variants in Fabry disease and by preventing misfolding, increase their delivery to the lysosome, are in progress.

Mucopolysaccharidoses

These disorders are caused by a deficiency of lysosomal hydrolases that catalyse the cleavage of complex glycosaminoglycans—macromolecular components of connective tissues including joints, bones, heart, and major arteries. Clinical manifestations of each of these disorders reflect an individual enzymatic deficiency and the resulting accumulation of mucopolysaccharide derivatives, of which dermatan, keratan, chondroitin, and heparan sulphates are the principal components. In general, the accumulation of the complex substrates that are normally linked to proteins to form proteoglycans is associated with visceral enlargement, as well as bony abnormalities, joint stiffness, corneal clouding, and short stature; the accumulation of heparan sulphate may particularly be associated with the development of brain disease, including thickening of the leptomeninges. Thus hydrocephalus is an often-neglected factor in cerebral impairment that may also be attributed to lysosomal storage affecting neurons of the brain and peripheral ganglia—as well as the retina.

Clinical features and pathology

Typically, these disorders are associated with coarse facial features, bone shortening, and skeletal abnormalities, as well as disturbances of dentition, the gums, and middle ear. Abnormalities of the tracheobronchial cartilages and upper airways may be associated with respiratory infections and obstructive lung disease. In the heart, the coronary arteries and valves may be infiltrated by glycosaminoglycans, leading to nodular thickening of aortic and mitral valves with clinical evidence of valvular malfunction. In some cases, accumulation of glycosaminoglycan occurs in the coronary arteries, which may be occluded. Similar changes may occur in peripheral arteries—particularly those supplying the viscera. In the eye, the basal layers of the cornea show swelling, cytoplasmic vacuolization, and storage granules leading to opacification. Scleral thickening may impinge upon the optic nerve.

Excess urinary excretion of glycosaminoglycan products, including dermatan sulphate and heparan sulphate, characteristically occur in the mucopolysaccharidoses. This abnormality should immediately prompt further investigations by enzymatic and genetic studies in blood leucocytes and/or fibroblasts obtained from cultured skin-biopsy samples. The inheritance pattern of the mucopolysaccharidoses is typical of autosomal recessive traits—with the exception of Hunter disease (MPS II, which is due to iduronate sulphatase deficiency) that maps to the X chromosome and, unlike Fabry disease, is expressed predominantly in boys and men. Female heterozygotes for Hunter disease only very rarely show evidence of neurological impairment or connective tissue abnormalities.

Treatment of the mucopolysaccharidoses

Palliative treatment is a very important aspect of the management of these diseases, and should include the provision of multidisciplinary support for children and young adults with the accompanying developmental disabilities. Sustained provision for the long-term management of the condition in affected families is desirable.

Surgical procedures

Corneal transplantation may be required to improve vision where retinal degeneration is not dominant. Carpel tunnel syndrome with compression neuropathy of the median nerve is very common in the mucopolysaccharidoses and, when indicated, surgical treatment is often beneficial. Particular care is required in patients with mucopolysaccharidoses such as Hurler syndrome when surgical procedures under general anaesthetic are required for relief of hydrocephalus, myringotomy, hernia repair, relief of airways obstruction due to laryngeal disease, and corrective spinal or joint surgery. Infiltration of the soft tissues of the upper and lower airways, as well as the heart and cervical spine (which may include subluxation of the atlanto-occipital joint) is associated with high perioperative mortality. Complications thus arise with the administration of a general anaesthetic beyond that of difficulties with endotracheal intubation. In particular, a tracheostomy may be required to avoid life-threatening complications of intubation. An extensive preoperative examination should be conducted when an anaesthetic is required for any procedure, particularly to assess the stability of the atlantoaxial joint, the airway, and the presence of coronary artery disease (that may predispose to perioperative myocardial infarction).

Specific treatment

Bone marrow transplantation using HLA-identical sibling and HLA-matched non-sibling donors has been extensively investigated in the mucopolysaccharidoses. Long-term clinical trials have confirmed the beneficial effects of successful transplantation with reversal of hepatosplenomegaly and obstructive airways disease. In some cases there is improved longevity, with a possible reduction also in the incidence of secondary hydrocephalus. However, at present, transplantation does not cure the condition and is unable to reverse established brain injury and most of the crippling skeletal manifestations of the mucopolysaccharidoses. If it is to be considered, bone marrow transplantation should thus be carried out early in the course of these diseases. The therapeutic position of bone marrow and cord-blood derived stem cell therapy is most clearly established for Hurler disease (the more severe variant of MPS I).

Enzyme replacement therapy has long been under investigation in MPS I (Hurler syndrome, Hurler-Scheie syndrome, and Scheie syndrome), which was one of the first of such disorders to be subjected to intensive laboratory study. In clinical trials, recombinant human α-L-iduronidase, now licensed as laronidase (Aldurazyme) given by weekly infusion intravenously, after 1 year clearly showed a reduction in lysosomal storage: liver volume decreased; there was an improved rate of growth as well as improvement in the range of joint movements at sites characteristic of connective tissue infiltration in this condition. With a reduction in the storage material in the upper airways, there was also an improvement in episodes of hypoventilation during sleep. After a few weeks of enzyme treatment, urinary glycosaminoglycans abnormalities were corrected. Although many patients developed serum antibodies, only transient immune reactions, including urticaria, occurred during the infusions. In patients with this disease, the first to be shown by experiments with fibroblasts *in vitro* to be corrected by enzymatic complementation, treatment with a recombinant human product reduces lysosomal storage and ameliorates several of the important clinical manifestations. Enzyme replacement therapies have received market authorization for patients suffering from MPS II (Hunter syndrome with iduronate sulphatase deficiency) and MPS VI (Maroteaux-Lamy disease due to arylsulphatase B deficiency) following successful clinical trials. Favourable responses to enzyme replacement therapy have also been reported in animal models of related disorders, including the cone-head mouse that represents a faithful model of MPS VII (Sly disease), due to deficiency of acid β-glucuronidase.

Although enzyme therapy is in an emerging phase of application in the mucopolysaccharidoses, there has been a remarkable response from the pharmaceutical industry for the therapeutic development of enzyme replacement therapy for lysosomal diseases. With the present state of knowledge, bone marrow transplantation seems to be ineffective for many patients with MPS; if it is to be restricted to use before the development of mental decline, the risks associated with the procedure and the need for matched donors to provide competent marrow cells limit its acceptability. Questions still arise of how clinical benefits and an improved quality of life can be best assessed. However, encouraging results showing an improved quality of life, mobility, nutrition, and educational achievements have already been documented in several MPS disorders in response to enzyme therapy—even where pre-existing developmental effects and mental retardation are established. The combined effects of marrow transplantation and enzyme replacement have yet to be systematically evaluated in clinical trials for evidence of therapeutic synergy.

Pompe disease

Glycogen storage disease type II, due to acid maltase deficiency, otherwise known as Pompe disease, is an autosomal recessive disorder of glycogen metabolism caused by deficient activity of lysosomal acid maltase—α-glucosidase. The disease occurs in many countries and ethnic groups. The prevalence of this disorder is one in about 150 000 and males and females are affected equally.

Acid maltase deficiency was the first of the lysosomal storage diseases to be so characterized by H.-G. Hers, a colleague of de Duve.

Pompe first reported infants with massive cardiac hypertrophy and skeletal weakness with hypotonia, enlargement of the tongue and liver—and a uniformly fatal outcome. Acid maltase releases glucose units from the carbohydrate storage macromolecule, glycogen, as well as from the disaccharide, maltose. The enzyme is profoundly deficient in infants with Pompe disease and partial deficiencies in the enzyme, detectable in all cells, are responsible for later onset forms in children, adolescents, and adults. No clear correlation between the degree of enzyme deficiency and the severity of disease is possible. Pathological accumulation of glycogen within vacuolar lysosomal spaces occurs in skeletal muscles and, on occasion, other tissues but it is noteworthy that in certain muscles, microscopic examination may be normal or show only trivial abnormalities— especially in patients with late-onset disease. Hence, the diagnosis of late-onset Pompe disease may be difficult and routine muscle biopsies may not identify all those affected. The combined use of muscle biopsy with, biochemical assays and molecular analysis of the acid glucosidase gene (at least for the common IVS1 mutation) should be considered in patients with unclassified myopathy. Acid maltase is normally responsible for constitutive autophagy and molecular remodelling of intracytoplasmic glycogen; when deficient, abnormal glycogen accumulates within the lysosomal vacuole and elsewhere in the cell. In pathways not yet completely understood, this pathological accumulation is associated with tissue injury but large cytoplasmic collections of autophagic debris appear to disrupt the contractile apparatus. Since glycogen is a storage molecule abundant in muscle cells, it is these cells that are the principal focus of acid maltase deficiency.

Patients with infantile onset of symptoms have predominantly skeletal muscle disease, hypertrophic cardiomyopathy, or mac-roglossia; in the absence of cardiac failure, hepatomegaly is not a feature of Pompe disease. Onset of disease in children and adults with weakness and poor athletic performance is associated with delayed achievement of developmental motor milestones. Ultimately the clinical appearance is dominated by proximal muscle weakness with lordosis of the spine; patients adopt the Gower manoeuvre in rising from the squatting position. Late-onset forms observed in adults usually present as a progressive proximal myopathy with the variable addition of diaphragmatic and respiratory muscle paralysis leading to respiratory failure but the rate of progression is unpredictable. The onset of symptoms varies between the age of 10 and 60 years. In most patients there is a history of longstanding proximal weakness with involvement of the truncal muscles and weakness in the hips in advance of the upper limb girdle. Poor physical strength and failure in gymnastic activities may be the clue. In children and adolescents the condition may be misdiagnosed as a late-onset muscular dystrophy or even polymyositis—leading to inappropriate treatment. Ultimately the progressive proximal weakness is apparent, associated with respiratory failure: the latter is pressaged by fatigue, breathlessness on exertion and sleepiness due to marked ventilatory failure—carbon dioxide retention causes morning headaches. Occasionally dysphagia for solids may result from weakness of voluntary pharyngeal muscle that initiate swallowing.

Myozyme (alglucosidase alpha) has been developed as a mannose 6-phosphate-containing recombinant human acid α-glucosidase (rhGAA) for the treatment of patients of any age with Pompe disease (GSD-II). Enzyme replacement therapy is administered to restore enzymatic activity, deplete accumulated glycogen, and prevent its further accumulation to allow repair of damaged myocytes. In the very severe infantile form of the condition, where survival beyond 1 year of age is unusual, treatment with Myozyme has been associated with prolonged survival. In a trial of rhGAA in infants aged 6 months or younger, all were alive at 18 months but only 2 per cent of the historical cohort group survived to this age. Most patients treated with rhGAA had normal growth and significant motor development during the treatment period. In another report, two severely affected patients (wheelchair- and ventilator-dependent) remained stable during an 8-year period of enzyme therapy and in a third, moderately affected patient, muscle strength improved markedly and the ability to walk was regained.

In some instances the outcome has been disappointing and, in general, better outcomes are seen with early treatment and in patients who do not develop antibody responses to the recombinant protein. Taken as a whole, the efficacy of enzyme replacement therapy for acid maltase deficiency emphasizes the need for prompt clinical recognition and diagnosis—especially in infants and young children.

Several studies have confirmed the therapeutic efficacy of rhGAA in patients suffering from attenuated forms of Pompe disease. In the present authors' experience with adult patients suffering from acid maltase deficiency, improvements in skeletal and respiratory muscle function are seen in the first year of treatment, with stability maintained thereafter. It is unclear if, once lost, diaphragmatic function can be regained; we contend that restricting treatment to those with severely weak and wasted limbs and respiratory failure due to diaphragmatic paralysis will greatly under-estimate its capacity to improve life quality or restore the function of injured muscles.

Even with specific treatment, the role of physical therapy, respiratory assessment and support, nutritional care, and measures aimed at general rehabilitation remain crucial for functional outcome and improved quality of life.

Niemann-Pick diseases

Niemann-Pick disease types A and B are, respectively, neuronopathic and non-neuronopathic variants of acid sphingomyelinase deficiency, a sphingolipid disorder leading to the accumulation of sphingomyelin. Niemann-Pick disease resembles many of the manifestations of Gaucher disease with a characteristic secondary storage cell which is also a macrophage. The Niemann-Pick cell has a foamy appearance rather than the characteristic striated cytoplasm of the Gaucher cell. In Niemann-Pick disease, there is prominent infiltration of the lungs as well as the marrow cavity. At present, no specific treatments are available apart from the prompt treatment of pulmonary infection and the management of the consequences of skeletal infiltrates and episodes of avascular necrosis. Some patients, including those previously misdiagnosed as having

Gaucher disease, may have undergone splenectomy to relieve pressure symptoms or the haematological effects of hypersplenism.

Niemann-Pick disease type A is associated with disabling neuronopathic features and dementia. At the present time no specific therapy for it exists. Niemann-Pick disease type B may occur in adults who have only trivial splenomegaly and minor pulmonary infiltrates that are only exacerbated at times of intercurrent pneumonic infection; they are at risk from osseous disease related to marrow infiltration, as with Gaucher disease. Since this disease is primarily a disorder of macrophages, it should be susceptible to enzymatic complementation using the mannose receptor. At the time of writing, clinical research to develop macrophage-targeted, recombinant, human acid sphingomyelinase is well advanced. Unfortunately, no pharmaceutical inhibitors are available for substrate reduction therapy for the neuronopathic manifestations of Niemann-Pick disease type A, since the biosynthesis of sphingomyelin is not regulated by the uridine diphosphate-glucosylceramide synthase reaction.

Niemann-Pick disease type C (NPC) may present with jaundice in infants or children, but the initial hepatitic illness usually resolves. Later evidence of neuronopathic disease occurs, with ataxia, seizures (vertical), supranuclear gaze palsy, and progressive diffuse cortical injury. NPC is not due to a primary defect of acid sphingomyelinase but to mutations in two distinct lysosomal proteins, NPC1 and NPC2 that when mutated, reflect subtypes of the disease. Although the function of the NPC1 and NPC2 proteins is not fully understood, they are implicated in the intracel-lular transport of cholesterol and cholesterol esters to and from the lysosomal compartment. NPC is also associated with the appearance of foam cells in the macrophages; the Kupffer cells of the liver may be enlarged and a cholesterol trafficking defect is apparent in most cells.

Thus the NPC defect, though not manifest in the skin, may be detected in skin and fibroblasts after culture and exposure to low-density lipoprotein-cholesterol: in NPC, cholesterol is taken up and accumulates in intracellular droplets that stain positively with the fluorescent dye filipin. Within the brain, NPC causes neuronophagia and the accumulation of gangliosides and other complex sphingolipid storage products that may induce neuronal injury. There is a strong perception among treating physicians and patients of clinical benefit with an iminosugar in arresting progression of the neurological disease in some patients. Clinical trials using *N*-butyldeoxynojirimycin in patients with NPC have followed the delayed onset and increased survival of mice homozygous for a spontaneous mutation in the *NPC1* gene that serves as an authentic model, recapitulating many features of the human disease. This research, recently presented to licensing authorities, has led to marketing approval of N-butyldeoxynojirimycin (miglustat, Zavesca) suppplied by the Actelion Company. After appraisal by the European Medicines Evaluation Agency, miglustat received market authorization for treatment of Niemann–Pick C disease in 2009.

NPC is an intractable condition associated with progressive neurological disease in childhood and early adult life. Biological deterioration progresses inexorably and death usually occurs in the third or fourth decade. The use of statins and other agents that interfere with cholesterol metabolism has not been effective in arresting the course of this cruel illness.

Danon disease

In 1981 two cases of cardiomyopathy in male infants with skeletal myopathy and mental retardation were reported by Danon and colleagues. The skeletal pathology suggested type II glycogenosis but no deficiency of acid maltase activity was present. Defects in LAMP2, a major lysosomal membrane protein, have subsequently been identified in Danon disease due to mutations in the gene encoding LAMP2, located on the X-chromosome. In affected males, the clinical features include a dramatic hypertrophic cardiomyopathy, a mild skeletal myopathy, and mild to moderate learning difficulties. The cardiomyopathy is particularly prone to give rise to malignant ventricular arrhythmias. Before the introduction of implanted defibrillation devices the median age of death of classically affected hemizygotes was about 20 years. A milder pheno-type, apparently restricted to the heart, is seen in heterozygous women. Recently, mutations in the *LAMP2* gene have been found at a surprisingly high frequency (6 per cent) in men with unexplained severe hypertrophic cardiomyopathy. LAMP2 is a highly glycosylated integral membrane protein of the lysosome with a role in mediating fusion of the autophagic vacuole with the lysosome. Deficiency leads to accumulation of vacuoles containing autophagic debris, including mitochondria and granular deposits of glycogen. Apart from supportive measures, no specific treatment is currently available, although a few hemizygous male patients have been successfully treated by cardiac transplantation.

Diseases recently attributed to lysosomal dysfunction

The characterization of lysosomal defects in several ill-understood disorders with diverse clinical manifestations continues to reveal much about the role of the lysosome in cellular functions of significance in medicine and molecular physiology. Several recently studied lysosomal diseases in this category are briefly described here.

Neuronal ceroid lipofuscinoses

The neuronal ceroid lipofuscinoses (CLN) represent the most common group of progressive brain diseases that affect children and young adults; 10 independent genetic groups have so far been identified. Childhood forms of these disorders are inherited as recessive traits and result in a progressive dementia combined with epilepsy, blindness, and an early death. The most familiar form of these diseases was previously known in English-speaking countries as Batten disease. Pathological studies show the characteristic accumulation of an autofluorescent storage material within neurons and lysosomes in other cells; this material consists of several oxidized and ubiquitinated proteins The storage of this material occurs preferentially in lysosomes of the nervous system and is associated with progressive neuronal death leading to a marked atrophy of the brain; cerebral atrophy is particularly obvious in the early-onset forms of the neuronal lipofuscinoses. Although this complex of neurodegenerative conditions associated with lipofuscin pigments has long been recognized, the diseases were previously thought to represent disorders of other organelles. Mitochondria were implicated because degraded fragments of mitochondrial cytochrome C polypeptide were found to be one of the prominent storage molecules in neuronal tissue from patients with Batten disease. Latterly, advances in molecular genetics have allowed the identification of defective genes and their protein products in several distinct clinical phenotypes.

Typical clinical forms of the neuronal ceroid lipofuscinoses include late infantile and juvenile neurodegenerative disorders; at least 10 genetic loci, which encode proteins implicated in different aspects of lysosomal metabolism, have been assigned to distinct CLN phenotypes. Neuronal ceroid lipofuscinosis type I (CLN1) is due to mutations in a gene encoding palmitoyl: protein thioeste-rase 1. CLN2 is due to defects in the gene encoding tripeptidyl-peptidase. CLN3 is the most frequent form and is due to deficiency of a lysosomal arginine transporter. To date, two lysosomal proteins of membrane location, CLN4 and CLN5, have also been identified. CLN7 is related to deficiency of a lysosomal membrane transporter of unknown function. CLN8 is due to defects in the gene encoding human cathepsin D. No specific therapy for Batten disease yet exists, but the discovery of the basis of the condition and the genes involved allows for prenatal and postnatal diagnosis in affected pedigrees by molecular analysis of the implicated cognate genes. In most instances, neuronal ceroid lipofuscinoses represents defects in elements of intralysosomal protein catabolism, indicating that the turnover of the cognate proteinsis very high in cortical neurons. Very recent *in vitro* studies have suggested that the use of the thiol agent, cysteamine, which is used with benefit in patients with cystinosis, may activate residual palmitoyl-protein phytoesterase activity in patients with CLN1.

The realization that the CLN indeed represent inherited disorders of lysosomal protein metabolism is very recent but the discovery clearly has important consequences for better understanding the pathology of this family of cruel neurodegenerative disorders and for developing better diagnostic tools (especially for prenatal application) as well as innovative treatments.

Papillon-Lefèvre syndrome

This is an unusual syndrome resulting in periodontal disease with tooth loss and palmoplantar keratosis. Papillon-Lefèvre syndrome is associated with a selective deficiency of cathepsin C activity within the specific granules of neutrophilic polymorphonuclear leucocytes. It appears that the enzyme deficiency leads to the failure of bacterial clearance in the gums, thereby causing destructive periodontitis and tooth loss. The corresponding role of cathepsin C within the dermal epithelium is not known, but a failure of cathepsin C activity reproducibly leads to epithelial abnormalities and thickening of the skin, particularly on the soles of the feet. Papillon-Lefèvre syndrome is inherited as an autosomal recessive trait and several mutations have been identified within the gene encoding the cathepsin C polypeptide. Some patients with disabling skin manifestations have obtained benefit by the use of retin-oids. These agents are, however, unlikely to improve early-onset destructive periodontal disease.

The importance of the Papillon-Lefèvre syndrome rests not only on the identification of lysosomal cathepsin C as an important component of immune defences against bacteria that specifically invade the privileged periodontal site, but also on the involvement of this enzyme in the normal turnover of keratinized skin. The molecular characterization of this disorder illustrates the protean manifestations of lysosomal defects and of the ubiquitous importance of lysosomes in the destruction and recycling of exogenous microbial, as well as endogenous cellular components.

Defects of organellar assembly: Chediak-Higashi and Hermansky-Pudlak syndromes

These rare disorders are inherited as autosomal recessive traits. Both cause oculocutaneous albinism in association with abnormal platelet granules and melanosomes in the skin and eyes. Chediak-Higashi syndrome predisposes to microbial infection and there are giant lysosomal granules in peripheral blood granulocytes; ceroid storage occurs in the nervous system and lungs. Although very rare, Hermansky-Pudlak syndrome occurs at a high frequency in the Swiss Alps and the Puerto-Rican population where it is the most common single-gene defect. Hermansky-Pudlak syndrome causes a mild bleeding diathesis and platelet dense bodies are absent. Granulomatous colitis occurs and pulmonary changes lead to interstitial lung fibrosis; unexplained cardiomyopathy has been reported.

The Hermansky-Pudlak syndrome is caused by mutations in the β-3A adaptin gene which is associated with altered trafficking of lysosomal proteins in melanosomes, lysosomes, and platelet-dense granules leading to storage pool deficiency. The gene maps to chromosome 10q. Chediak-Higashi syndrome has a clinical pheno-type with a complex set of immune defects affecting natural killer cells and neutrophic leucocytes. Recurrent cutaneous and systemic pyogenic infections occur with defective neutrophil and monocyte migration; natural killer-cell cytotoxicity is absent. Neutrophils, melanocytes, neurons, muscle cells, and Schwann cells show giant inclusion bodies. Neurodegeneration is a prominent feature of the disease in young adults, but death often results from a rapidly progressive lymphoproliferative disorder. Chediak-Higashi syndrome is caused by mutations in the lysosomal trafficking regulator gene located on chromosome 1q44. There are clear similarities between Hermansky-Pudlak syndrome and Chediak-Higashi syndrome, and further functional studies of their respective cognate proteins should reveal important information about the synthesis and assembly of lysosomes and related organelles.

Further reading

Key website addresses

Scriver CR, *et al.* (2004). *Metabolic and Molecular Bases of Inherited Disease*, 8th edn. Part 16: Lysosomal disorders, Chapters 134–54. McGraw-Hill, New York. http://www.ommbid.com. [This is the definitive reference work in English; it is now available in a readily accessible and, for its size, frequently updated, online format.]

Online mendelian inheritance in man: http://www.ncbi.nlm.nih.gov [This database is a comprehensive catalogue of human genes and genetic disorders authored and edited by the late Dr. Victor McKusick and his colleagues at Johns Hopkins University and elsewhere, and developed for the World Wide Web by the National Centre for Biotechnology Information (NCBI). The database contains textual information and references. It also provides numerous links to MEDLINE and sequence records in the Entrez system, and links to additional related resources at NCBI and elsewhere.]

Books

Saftig P (ed) (2005). *Lysosomes.* Springer Science, New York.

Barranger JA and Cabrera-Salazar MA (eds) (2007). *Lysosomal Storage Disorders.* Springer Science, New York.

Nyhan WL, Barshop BA, Ozand PT (eds), 2005). *Atlas of Metabolic Diseases*, 2nd edn. Hodder Education, London

Journal articles

Aerts JM, *et al.* (2008). Biomarkers for lysosomal storage disorders: identification and application as exemplified by chitotriosidase in Gaucher disease. *Acta Paediatrica* **97**(Supplement 457), 7–14.

Barton NW, *et al.* (1991). Replacement therapy for inherited enzyme deficiency macrophage-targeted glucocerebrosidase for Gaucher's disease. *New Engand Journal of Medicine* **324**, 1464–70.

Cox TM, *et al.* (2003). The role of the iminosugar N-butyldeoxynojirimycin (miglustat) in management of type 1 (non-neuronopathic) Gaucher disease. *Journal of Inherited Metabolic Disease* **26**, 513–26.

Cox TM, *et al.* (2008). Management of non-neuronopathic Gaucher disease with special reference to pregnancy, splenectomy, bisphosphonate therapy, use of biomarkers and bone disease monitoring. *Journal of Inherited Metabolic Disease* **31**, 319–36.

Eng CM, *et al.* (2001). Safety and efficacy of recombinant human alpha-galactosidase A-replacement therapy in Fabry's disease. *New England Journal of Medicine* **345**, 9–16.

Eng CM, *et al.* (2007). Fabry disease: baseline medical characteristics of a cohort of 1765 males and females in the Fabry Registry. *Journal of Inherited Metabolic Disease* **30**, 184–92.

Fratantoni JC, *et al.* (1969).The defect in Hurler and Hunter syndromes. II. Deficiency of specific factors involved in mucopolysaccharide degradation. *Proceedings of the National Academy of Sciences (USA)* **6**, 360–6.

Kishnani PS, *et al.* (2007) Recombinant human acid [alpha] -glucosidase: major clinical benefits in infantile-onset Pompe's disease. *Neurology* **68**, 99–109.

Laforet P, *et al.* (2008). Neuromuscular Disorders 2008 (18) 832;T.O.4).

Maegawa GH *et al.* (2006). The natural history of juvenile or subacute GM2 gangliosidosis: 21 new cases and literature review of 134 previously reported. *Pediatrics* **118**, e1550–62. [Erratum: Pediatrics (2007) 120,936].

Maegawa GH, *et al.* (2007). Pyrimethamine as a potential pharmacological chaperone for late-onset forms of GM2 gangliosidosis. *Journal of Biological Chemistry* **282**, 9150–61.

McEachern KA, *et al.* (2007). A specific and potent inhibitor of glucosylceramide synthase for substrate inhibition therapy of Gaucher disease. *Molecular Genetics and Metabolism* **91**, 259–67.

Meikle PJ, *et al.* (1999). Prevalence of lysosomal storage disorders. *Journal of the American Medical Association* **281**, 249–54.

Neudorfer GM, *et al.* (2005). Late-onset Tay-Sachs disease: phenotypic characterization and genotypic correlations in 21 affected patients. *Genetic Medicine* **7**, 119–23.

Pellegrini N, *et al.* (2005). Respiratory and limb muscle weakness in adults with Pompe disease. *European Respiratory Journal* **26**, 1024–31.

Robertson PL, Maas M, Goldblatt J (2007). Semiquantitative assessment of skeletal response to enzyme replacement therapy for Gaucher's disease using the bone marrow burden score. *American Journal of Roentgenology* **188**, 1521–8.

Saftig P, *et al.* (2001). Disease model: LAMP-2 enlightens Danon disease. *Trends in Molecular Medicine* **7**, 37–9.

Schiffmann R, *et al.* (2001). Enzyme replacement therapy in Fabry disease: a randomized controlled trial. *Journal of the American Medical Association* **285**, 2743–9.

van Capelle CI, *et al.* (2008). Eight years experience with enzyme replacement therapy in two children and one adult with Pompe disease. *Neuromuscular Disorders* **18**, 447–52.

Van den Hout HM, *et al.* (2003). The natural course of infantile Pompe's disease: 20 original cases compared with 133 cases from the Literature. *Pediatrics* **112**, 332–40.

Von Figura K (1991). Molecular recognition and targeting of lysosomal proteins. *Current Opinion in Cell Biology* **3**, 642–6.

Weinreb NJ, *et al.* (2002). Effectiveness of enzyme replacement therapy in 1028 patients with type 1 Gaucher disease after 2 to 5 years of treatment: a report from the Gaucher Registry. *American Journal of Medicine* **113**, 112–19.

Winkel LP, *et al.* (2004). Enzyme replacement therapy in late-onset Pompe's disease: a three-year follow-up. *Annals of Neurology* **55**, 495–502.

12.9

Disorders of peroxisomal metabolism in adults

Anthony S. Wierzbicki

Essentials

The peroxisome is a specialized organelle which employs molecular oxygen in the oxidation of complex organic molecules including lipids. Enzymatic pathways for the metabolism of fatty acids, including very long-chain fatty acids (VLCFA) enable this organelle to carry out β-oxidation in partnership with mitochondria. A peroxisomal pathway for isoprenoid lipids derived from chlorophyll, such as phytanic acid, utilizes α-oxidation, but a default mechanism involving ω-oxidation may also metabolize phytanic acid and its derivatives.

The biochemical manifestations, molecular pathology, and diverse clinical features of many peroxisomal disorders have now been clarified, offering the promise of prompt diagnosis, better management and useful means to provide appropriate genetic counselling for affected families. At the same time, specific treatments including rigorous dietary interventions and plasmapheresis to remove undegraded toxic metabolites offer credible hope of improvement and prevention of disease in affected individuals.

Inborn errors of peroxisomal metabolism usually present in infancy and childhood, but some disorders typically become manifest later in life and in adults, in whom the progress is often slow.

Particular adult peroxisomal disorders

X-linked adrenoleukodystrophy (X-ALD)—due to mutation in the gene for an ATP-binding cassette (ABC) protein of unknown function and characterized by accumulation of unbranched saturated VLCFAs, particularly hexacosanoate (C26), in the cholesterol esters of brain white matter, adrenal cortex and certain sphingolipids of the brain. The disease has multiple phenotypes: it may present in adolescence with slowly progressive stiffness, clumsiness, weakness, weight loss, and skin pigmentation typical of Addison's disease; it may present in adults with primarily psychiatric manifestations. Most cases develop increasing handicap; management is palliative and supportive in most instances.

Adult Refsum's disease—due in most cases to mutation in the gene for phytanoyl CoA-hydroxylase (PhyH) such that patients are unable to detoxify phytanic acid by α-oxidation and have greatly elevated levels of this in their plasma. Usually presents in late childhood with progressive deterioration of night vision, the occurrence of progressive retinitis pigmentosa, and anosmia; late features include deafness, ataxia, polyneuropathy, ichthyosis and cardiac arrhythmias. Treatment is by restriction of dietary phytanic acid, with or without its elimination by plasmapheresis or apheresis.

Neuropsychiatric adult peroxisomal disorders

Historical perspective

The likely first description of X-linked adrenoleukodystrophy (X-ALD; OMIM 300100) was in 1910 when a 6-year-old child developed abnormal eye movements, apathy, and mental deterioration. His gait then deteriorated and skin darkening was noted prior to his death a few months later. Examination of the brain by Schilder showed central demyelination, perivascular lymphocytes, foam cells, and gliosis which he termed encephalitis periaxalis diffusa. Other cases he later described are likely due to other leukodystrophies. Adrenoleukodystrophy was defined in 1970, with its characteristic adrenal changes of excess very long chain fatty acids (VLCFAs) and cholesterol esters present in cell inclusion bodies. These VLCFAs were later identified as pathognomic and identifiable in plasma samples and the primary defect was identified as an inability to metabolize them. The gene was mapped to Xq18 and identified as a member of the ATP-binding cassette (ABC) transporter family. X-ALD was localized to the peroxisome. Subsequently, mouse models have been developed which show similar clinical features to human disease.

Aetiology

Adrenoleukodystrophy is characterized by the accumulation of unbranched saturated VLCFAs with a chain length of 24 to 30 carbons, particularly hexacosanoate (C26), in the cholesterol esters of brain white matter, in the adrenal cortex, and in certain sphingolipids of the brain. The disorder shows X-linked inheritance with expression in female heterozygotes. The disruptive effects of the accumulation of VLCFAs, especially hexacosanoic acid (C26:0), on cell membrane structure and function may explain the neurological manifestations seen in adrenoleukodystrophy patients. VLCFAs cause alterations in membrane fluidity and affect cortisol secretion from cultured cells of adrenal cortical origin. In addition, albumin has only one C26 binding site compared with more than six for shorter fatty acids, so limiting its efficacy as a reverse transport protein for excess VLCFAs.

Clinical features

X-ALD is heterogeneous. Seven phenotypes occur in males and five are recognized in females (see Table 12.9.1). Childhood cerebral adrenoleukodystrophy presents between the ages of 5 and 10 years with emotional lability, hyperactivity/withdrawal, and mental deterioration, mimicking attention deficit disorder which evolves to parietal lobe dysfunction with apraxia, astereognosis, and later dementia. MRI shows a characteristic pattern of symmetric involvement of the posterior parieto-occipital white matter in 85% of patients, frontal involvement in 10%, and an asymmetric pattern in the rest.

The adolescent form is adenomyeloneuropathy which presents with slowly progressive stiffness, clumsiness, weakness, weight loss, and skin pigmentation typical of Addison's disease. Autonomic function including micturition and erectile function are affected later. Somatosensory, auditory, and brainstem evoked potential are abnormal with some cases of abnormal visual and peripheral nerve conduction abnormalities. Brain MRI scans are abnormal in 50% of men and 80% of women, usually affecting corticospinal tracts with later parenchymal changes. Depression and emotional lability are common. Adult cerebral adrenoleukodystrophy is a variant of adenomyeloneuropathy occurring after age 20 without spinal cord symptoms. The primary signs are psychiatric with a presentation of psychotic mania and may include schizophrenia or dementia.

Some cases show a pure initial addisonian picture with no neurological involvement; all are autoantibody negative. The onset of Addison's disease is usually in childhood but the neurological changes follow in 20 to 30 years. Subtle hyperreflexia or impaired vibration sense and subtle MRI or neurophysiological signs may be detected earlier in these cases.

In female adrenoleukodystrophy heterozygotes, adrenal cortical insufficiency rarely develops, although isolated mineralocorticoid insufficiency may occur. Furthermore, adrenoleukodystrophy heterozygotes are predisposed to hypoaldosteronism related to the use of nonsteroidal anti-inflammatory agents (NSAIDs). A subclinical decrease in glucocorticoid reserve, as measured by synthetic ovine corticotropin-releasing hormone testing, may be present in most of these women. Aldosterone levels should be included in ACTH stimulation testing done to detect adrenal insufficiency in affected women. NSAIDs should be considered a risk factor for the development of hypoaldosteronism in women who are heterozygous for adrenoleukodystrophy.

Rare presentations include olivopontocerebellar atrophy which has been described as X-ALD ataxia in Japanese. Other uncommon presentations include unilateral masses which can mimic brain tumours and cases of spontaneous remission of neurological symptoms.

Women who are X-ALD heterozygotes usually present with adenomyeloneuropathy at age 30 to 40. Subtle signs are often detected prior to presentation but eventually the full picture occurs, with late-onset dementia.

Neuropathology

There are two distinct forms of neuropathology associated with X-ALD. Pure adrenomyeloneuropathy is a distal axonic neuropathy while the cerebral forms are associated with inflammation. In cerebral X-ALD, brain pathology is often grossly normal though

Table 12.9.1 Psychiatric signs and inborn errors of metabolism in adolescents and adults

Disorder	Confusion	Mental retardation	Behavioural disturbance	Catatonia	Visual hallucination	Psychosis	Depression
Urea cycle defect	+	+/−	+	+	+	+	+
Homocysteine disorders	+	+	+	+	+	+/−	+
Porphyria	+		+	+		+/−	+/−
Wilson's disease		+/−	+			+/−	+
CTX		+	+	+		+	
MLD			+			+	
GM_2 gangliosidosis			+	+	+	+	+
Mannosidoses	+	+	+		+	+	
X-ALD			+			+	+
Nonketotic hyperglycinemia		+	+				
Monoamine oxidase A deficiency		+	+				
Creatine transporter deficiency		+	+				
Succinic semi-aldehyde dehydrogenase deficiency		+	+				
Niemann–Pick C			+	+	+	+	+

CTX, cerebrotendinous xanthomatosis; MLD, metachromatic leukodystrophy; X-ALD, X-linked adrenoleukodystrophy.

Reproduced from Sedel F *et al.* (2007a). Psychiatric manifestations revealing inborn errors of metabolism in adolescents and adults. *J Inherit Metab Dis*, **30**, 631–41, with permission.

with signs of cerebral atherosclerosis. Grey matter is unaffected but white matter disease occurs in a rostrocaudal direction with demyelination prominent in the parieto-occipital cortex and the cerebellum. The detailed pathology shows oligodendroglial cell loss, astrocytosis, and a perivascular inflammatory infiltrate. In the noncerebral form, demyelination is seen in the corticospinal tracts with no obvious inflammation and only mild gliosis and occasional macrophages. In the adrenal cortex, cells are filled with lamellar deposits of cholesterol esters with primary cortical atrophy and no evidence of inflammation or antibodies, with milder changes in the adrenomyeloneuropathy form. In men with X-ALD, the testes show Leydig cell alterations, again with lamellar deposits. It has been estimated that at least 10% of males with Addison's disease (adrenocortical failure) have X-linked adrenomyeloneuropathy or unrecognized X-ALD.

Metabolism of VLCFAs

VLCFAs are derived from the diet and endogenous synthesis with between 20 and 80% derived from synthesis, depending on the study. The synthetic pathway occurs in brain microsomes with repeated additions of malonyl-CoA units to palmitic (C16:0) or stearic (C18:0) acid precursors. There are probably separate pathways for C20: 0 and C22:0 (behenic) fatty acids with the C22:0 pathway also elongating C22:1 (erucic) acid. Degradation of VLCFAs occurs by β-oxidation within peroxisomes after activation by specific acyl-CoA ligases which are chain length specific, so that a very long chain-CoA synthetase exists. In actuality, there are multiple very long chain-CoA synthetases with differing tissue and organelle specificities, all of which contain AMP-binding domains and a long chain synthetase domain. Both very long chain-CoA synthetases and microsomal fatty acid transfer protein-1 have very long chain-CoA synthetase activity but may function differently in the synthesis and degradation of VLCFAs.

The X-ALD protein and its homologues

The X-ALD gene was mapped to a region of the X-chromosome close to the glucose-6-phosphate dehydrogenase gene. The gene was established to code for an ABC protein of still unknown function but likely to involve the translocation of a variety of substrates across extra and intracellular membranes, including lipids, sterols, and drugs. The ABCD1 protein (adrenoleukodystrophy protein) maps to Xq28 and is mutated in X-ALD.

ABCD1 is a member of the ABC transporter superfamily. It expresses a half transporter which is located in the peroxisome. The gene has an open reading frame of 2235 bases which encodes a 745-amino acid protein with 38.5% amino acid identity and 78.9% similarity to another peroxisomal protein (ABCD3).

Mutations in *ABCD1* result in X-ALD in animal models, with elevated VLCFAs. *ABCD1* is one of four related peroxisomal transporters that are found in the human genome, the others being *ABCD2* (adrenoleukodystrophy related protein) (OMIM 601081), *ABCD3* (peroxisomal membrane protein 70) (OMIM 170995), and *ABCD4* (P70R/PMP69) (OMIM 603214). The adrenoleukodystrophy protein and the adrenoleukodystrophy-related protein are expressed on oligodendroglia, while the adrenoleukodystrophy-related protein and peroxisomal membrane protein 70 are found in neurons of the central nervous system. These genes are highly conserved in evolution, and two homologous genes are present in the yeast genome, *PXA1* and *PXA2*, which also transport long chain fatty acids. The 80-kDa protein encoded by this gene is absent in patients with X-ALD, in whom X-ALD mRNA was undetectable. Most of the *ABCD1* mutations (>450) in X-ALD are point mutations, but large deletions have been described. There is no correlation between genotype and phenotype. In 15 to 20% of obligate female heterozygotes, false-negative results occur for plasma VLCFAs. Mutation analysis is the only reliable method for the identification of heterozygotes.

Overexpression of the adrenoleukodystrophy protein and its homologue, the adrenoleukodystrophy-related protein (ABCD2), can restore the impaired peroxisomal β-oxidation in the fibroblasts of adrenoleukodystrophy patients. However, it seems that functional replacement of the adrenoleukodystrophy protein by adrenoleukodystrophy-related protein is not due to stabilization of the mutated adrenoleukodystrophy protein. Similarly, the adrenoleukodystrophy-related protein and peroxisomal membrane protein 70 could restore the peroxisomal β-oxidation defect in the liver of adrenoleukodystrophy protein-deficient mice by stimulating *Aldr* and *Pmp70* gene expression through a dietary treatment with the peroxisome proliferator fenofibrate. These results suggested that a correction of the biochemical defect in adrenoleukodystrophy might be possible by drug-induced overexpression or ectopic expression of the adrenoleukodystrophy-related gene. The adrenoleukodystrophy protein transporter may facilitate the interaction between peroxisomes and mitochondria, the two sites within the cells where β-oxidation of VLCFAs occurs.

Epidemiology

Screening and diagnostic records suggest that the prevalence is a minimum of 1 in 22 500 to 62 000. In contrast, the use of the Hardy–Weinberg approach and genetic frequency data suggests a combined male to female frequency of 1 in 18 000 similar to phenylketonuria (1 in 12 000).

Differential diagnosis

The differential diagnosis of neuropsychiatric abnormalities is shown in Table 12.9.2. X-ALD can mimic attention deficit disorder, multiple sclerosis, organic dementias, and psychoses among neurological diseases and Addison's disease and hypogonadism among endocrine disorders (see Table 12.9.2). The critical clinical differential element is the finding of abnormal ACTH levels and skin pigmentation with neurological signs, however subtle.

Clinical investigation

Clinical biochemistry

The primary abnormality in X-ALD is an accumulation of VLCFAs (>C22) which occur in myelin. C26:0 can account for up to 5% of brain cerebrosides and sulphatides. In X-ALD, both saturated and unsaturated forms of C26:0 (cerotic) and C24:0 (lignoceric) acids accumulate with reductions in C24:1(n − 9) (nervonic) acid. Normally shorter fatty acids accumulate in brain cholesterol esters, but in X-ALD, by contrast, these are mostly C26:0 and are enriched in myelin and in areas of demyelination. Similarly, C26:0 accumulates in white matter phosphatidylcholine phospholipids, C24:0 and C24:1 in gangliosides. Erythrocytes, plasma, and cultured fibroblasts all contain a 2 to 10-fold excess of VLCFAs. The diagnostic test relies on measurement of C26:0 levels and the ratios of

Table 12.9.2 Differential diagnosis of X-ALD

Presentation	Differential diagnosis
Childhood neurological with normal endocrinology	Hyperactivity; attention deficit disorder
	Epilepsy/seizures
	Brain tumour
	Metachromatic/globoid leukodystrophy
	Postencephalitic syndromes,: e.g. subacute sclerosing panencephalitis
	Myelinoclastic diffuse sclerosis
Childhood neurological with hypoadrenalism	Addison's disease with posthypoglycaemic damage
	X-linked glycerol kinase deficiency
	Central pontine myelinolysis
	Glucocorticoid deficiency with achalasia
Hypoadrenalism	Secondary causes of hypoadrenalism
Adrenomyeloneuropathy	Multiple sclerosis
	Familial or other spastic parapereses
	Spinocerebellar/olivopontocerebellar degeneration
	Cervical spondylosis
	Spinal cord tumour, e.g. ependymoma
Adult cerebral	Schizophrenia
	Depression
	Epilepsy/ organic psychosis
	Alzheimer's disease or other dementias
	Brain tumour
Heterozygote with symptoms	Multiple sclerosis
	Chronic spinal disease
	Spinal cord tumour
	Cervical spondylosis

C26 to C22:0 (docosahexaenoic acid) and C26:0 to C24:0 (tetracosanoic acid).

Results can be confirmed by fibroblast studies or by the use of sequencing techniques. Highly elevated VLCFA levels are also found in peroxisomal biogenesis disorders but these show a different clinical presentation to X-ALD or transiently with ketogenic diets for seizures. False negative results may occur in patients consuming excess C22:1; ω – 9 (erucic acid; Lorenzo's oil) which is found in mustard and rapeseed oils. A few affected males (0.1%) have borderline normal C26:0 levels and 15% of obligate female carriers have normal results. Effective mutation detection in these families is therefore fundamental to the unambiguous determination of genetic status. Of particular concern are female members of kinships with segregating X-ALD mutations, because normal levels of VLCFA do not guarantee a lack of carrier status. Prenatal diagnosis is possible from cultured amniocytes or chorionic villus cells.

Radiology

An MRI scan often reveals biochemical changes before the development of clinical symptoms. Eighty per cent of childhood cerebral adrenoleukodystrophy patients have symmetric periventricular white matter changes in the posterior parietal and occipital lobes with a dorsocaudal progression with time. Contrast studies show up areas of active demyelination, inflammation with breakdown of the blood–brain barrier and gliosis. Proton spectroscopy using *N*-acetyl aspartate shows up neuronal loss, while choline compound studies assaying phosphocholine and glycerophosphocholine indicate membrane turnover and demyelination, and myo-inositol compounds seem to be indices of gliosis. The presence of lactate indicates the anaerobic metabolism of the inflammatory cell infiltrate. In the adrenomyeloneuropathy brain, MRIs may be normal in 50% of men and 80% of women but diffuse spinal cord atrophy is present.

Endocrinology

Overt hypoadrenalism occurs in 40% of patients with childhood cerebral adrenoleukodystrophy and 80% have a deficient cortisol response on Synacthen testing. In childhood disease 80% show abnormal adrenal stimulation test results, while in adrenomyeloneuropathy between 30% and 50% show normal responses. Clinical Addison's disease is found in 1% of female heterozygotes. In adrenoleukodystrophy heterozygotes, adrenal cortical insufficiency rarely develops, although hypoaldosteronism may occur, especially if NSAIDs are being used. ACTH levels are increased in male patients. Levels of follicle-stimulating hormone (FSH) or luteinizing hormone (LH) are increased in 50% to 70% of patients with adrenomyeloneuropathy, while testosterone levels are reduced in 20% with low normal levels of dehydroepiandrosterone sulphate.

Neurophysiology

Hearing is normal but brainstem auditory evoked potentials are abnormal in 95% of adrenomyeloneuropathy patients and 42% of heterozygote patients. Abnormalities in visual evoked potentials are also found as latencies and are increased in 20% of men with adrenomyeloneuropathy but in more than 70% with childhood cerebral disease. Electroretinograms are normal. Subtle demyelination and axonal loss patterns of nerve conduction are found in 90% of men and 67% of women with adrenomyeloneuropathy, usually affecting the legs more than the arms. Neuropsychological tests can show up deficits in parieto-occipital function affecting visuospatial parameters and auditory processing, while frontal lobe lesions affect executive functions, emotions, problem solving, and anticipatory processing.

Treatment

The progressive nature of X-ALD means that comprehensive family and professional management support services are required. Leukodystrophies are associated with progressive learning difficulties, psychiatric disturbance, and increasing disability. Painful muscle spasms are common and should be managed with diazepam, baclofen, or gabapentin. Bulbar muscle function may be lost with disease progression, thus requiring special attention to feeding to reduce the risk of aspiration pneumonia.

Dietary therapy was based on the restriction of the intake of C26:0 to less than 15% of normal intake, but early trials showed no effect of this on levels of VLCFA levels. Addition of oleic acid normalized VLCFA levels in fibroblasts and oral glyceryl trioleate reduced VLCFA levels by 50% with an improvement in nerve conduction measures. A 4:1 combination of glyceryl trioleate and trierucate (Lorenzo's oil) normalized VLCFA levels within 1 month and prompted mass use of this intervention. No evidence of a clinically relevant benefit from dietary treatment with Lorenzo's oil has been seen in many studies of patients with neurological involvement and X-ALD, and asymptomatic thrombocytopenia was noted in 30% of patients. The fatty acid composition of the plasma and liver, but not that of the brain, improves with this therapy, suggesting that little erucic acid crossed the blood–brain barrier. Thus, dietary supplementation with Lorenzo's oil is of limited value in correcting the accumulation of saturated VLCFAs in the brain of patients with established neurological adrenoleukodystrophy.

In a study of 89 asymptomatic boys with X-ALD who had normal MRI scans, Lorenzo's oil and moderate fat restriction were prescribed for 6.9±2.7 years. Plasma fatty acids and clinical status were followed as measures of outcome. Twenty-four per cent developed MRI abnormalities and 11% developed neurological and MRI abnormalities. The trial concluded that the reduction of C26:0 by Lorenzo's oil was associated with a reduced risk of developing MRI abnormalities. Lorenzo's oil therapy is indicated in asymptomatic boys with X-ALD who have normal brain MRI scans. Experience with other adrenoleukodystrophy patients indicated that total fat intake in excess of 30 to 35% of total calories may counteract or nullify the C26:0-reducing effect of Lorenzo's oil.

Patients who develop progressive MRI abnormalities should be considered for haematopoietic stem cell transplantation, but the 5-year mortality is 38% and survival is increased by 8 months on average. Results in 283 boys with X-ALD who received haematopoietic cell bone marrow transplantation showed that the estimated 5-year survival was 66%. The leading cause of death was disease progression. Donor-derived engraftment occurred in 86% of patients. Demyelination involved parietal–occipital lobes in 90%, leading to visual and auditory processing deficits in many boys. Bone marrow transplantation must be considered very early, even in a child without symptoms but with signs of demyelination on MRI, if a suitable donor is available. There are few data on the usefulness of bone marrow transplantation in adrenomyeloneuropathy.

Adrenal function must be monitored since 80% of asymptomatic patients with adrenoleukodystrophy develop evidence of adrenal insufficiency and adrenal hormone replacement therapy should be provided when indicated by laboratory findings.

Given the inflammation associated with X-ALD, a number of immunosuppressive regimes have been investigated. Studies of cyclophosphamide, immunoglobulin, and interferon-β have been unsuccessful.

Prognosis

The prognosis in X-ALD depends on the presentation. As yet, there are no methods of determining which type of disease will result from a given mutation as genotype–phenotype correlation is poor. Once leukodystrophy begins, the prognosis is poor as progression is inevitable.

Future developments

Other potential therapeutic approaches to X-ALD include the use of lipid-lowering drugs. Lowering cholesterol activates human ABCD2 in cultured cells. In mice, a sterol regulatory element exists in the ABCD2 promoter and overlaps sites for liver X receptor/retinoid X receptor heterodimers. Adipose ABCD2 is induced by SREBP1c, whereas hepatic ABCD2 expression is down-regulated by concurrent activation of liver X receptor-α and SREBP1c. Hepatic ABCD2 expression in liver X receptor-α/β mice is inducible to levels vastly exceeding wild type.

Statins (3-HMG-CoA reductase inhibitors) are capable of normalizing VLCFA levels in primary skin fibroblasts derived from X-ALD patients. They block the induction of proinflammatory cytokines through effects on rho kinase. Twelve patients with X-ALD were treated with lovastatin for up to 12 months. Levels of C26:0 declined from pretreatment values and stabilized at various levels during a period of observation of up to 12 months, which does not correlate with the type of adrenoleukodystrophy gene mutation. In six patients, erythrocyte C26:0 levels fell by 50%. All patients with adrenomyeloneuropathy remained neurologically stable. However, follow-up trials have been unsuccessful.

The PPAR-α agonist-mediated induction of *ABCD2* expression seems to be indirect and possibly mediated by the sterol-responsive element-binding protein 2 in mice, but there are no published human studies of fibrate therapy. Sodium 4-phenylbutyrate reduces VLCFA levels through its effects on peroxisomal function and increases adrenoleukodystrophy-related protein levels. However human studies have failed to show consistent beneficial effects.

Omega oxidation is an alternative oxidation route for VLCFAs. These fatty acids are substrates for the ω-oxidation system in human liver microsomes and are converted into ω-hydroxy fatty acids and further oxidized to dicarboxylic acids via cytochrome P450-mediated reactions. The high sensitivity towards the specific P450 inhibitor 17-octadecynoic acid suggested that ω-hydroxylation of VLCFAs is catalysed by the CYP4A/F subfamilies, particularly CYP4F2 and CYP4F3B, and that therapies capable of increasing ω-oxidation may have the potential to reduce the progression of the disease. Recently gene therapy has been attempted for X-ALD using lentivirus transformation of white cells and 9-14% of cells showed reconstitution of ABC-D1 expression over 24 months.

Neuro-ophthalmic adult peroxisomal disorders

Introduction

Though survival is improving for peroxisomal biogenesis disorders and more subtle defects are now diagnosed, most still present in the neonatal period or in infancy. This is also true for most single enzyme peroxisomal deficiencies. Only one group of disorders presents later, with the onset of symptoms often in early teenage years but, due to delays in diagnosis, many are not identified until they reach adulthood. In contrast to the neuropsychiatric or endocrine presentation associated with adrenoleukodystrophy, these peroxisomal disorders present as central and peripheral neuropathies—a neuro-ophthalmic picture. They are often termed Refsum's disease though, given the multiple underlying genetic defects, it would be better to refer to them as Refsum's syndrome.

The syndrome comprises three genetic disorders: phytanoyl-CoA hydroxylase deficiency (classical adult Refsum's disease), atypical rhizomelic chondrodysplasia punctata type 1, and the newly described α-methyl-acylCoA racemase deficiency.

Historical perspective

Adult Refsum's disease (OMIM 266510), also called heredopathia atactica polyneuritiformis, is a hereditary sensory motor neuropathy type IV. It was first described in 1947, but only recognized as a syndrome by Refsum in 1962. He described a constellation of signs comprised of retinitis pigmentosa, anosmia, deafness, ataxia, and polyneuropathy allied with raised levels of protein in the cerebrospinal fluid. The biochemical defect was identified in 1963 when phytanic acid was noted in the plasma of affected patients and defective α-oxidation was later suggested as the cause of adult Refsum's disease. This disease was thought to be unifactorial with admittedly some rare aberrant complementation studies until 1995 when, after the localization of the gene for phytanoyl-CoA hydroxylase, up to 50% of cases in one series were shown not to be linked to chromosome 10 but to chromosome 6. Eventually the novel defect was identified as a variant of rhizomelic chondrodysplasia punctata type 1 and caused by mutations in peroxin 7. In parallel with this discovery three patients were described in 1997 with a phenotype of sensory neuropathy and a subtle bile acid disorder but whose families included siblings with a Refsum's-like syndrome which was identified as due to a deficiency in α-methylacyl-CoA racemase.

Clinical features

In contrast to Zellweger's syndrome (OMIM 214100), neonatal adrenoleukodystrophy (OMIM 202370), infantile Refsum's's disease (OMIM 266500), and rhizomelic chondrodysplasia (OMIM 601757), adult Refsum's disease usually presents in late childhood with progressive deterioration of night vision, the occurrence of progressive retinitis pigmentosa and anosmia (see Fig. 12.9.1). Anosmia, contrary to early reports, is a constant feature of adult Refsum's disease. After 10 to 15 years, deafness, ataxia, polyneuropathy, ichthyosis, and cardiac arrhythmias can occur. Short metacarpals or metatarsals are found in about one-third of patients. Rare findings include psychiatric disturbance and proteinuria. Premature death may result from cardiac arrhythmias.

α-Methylacyl-CoA racemase (OMIM 604489) presents with adult-onset sensorimotor neuropathy. It may be accompanied by retinitis pigmentosa, visual field restriction and loss of acuity, axonal sensorimotor neuropathy, and myopathy-like adult Refsum's disease. Other features described have included primary hypogonadism, hypothyroidism, spastic paraparesis, epileptic seizures, and mild developmental delay. More severe childhood-onset cases have shown a phenotype of defects in bile acid synthesis allied with fat-soluble vitamin deficiencies, coagulopathy, and cholestatic liver disease and a resemblance to a Niemann–Pick type C phenotype.

Differential diagnosis

The differential diagnoses of the neuropathic disorders and relevant signs and investigations are shown in Tables 12.9.3 and 12.9.4. With classical adult Refsum's disease, the differential diagnosis includes the various genetic retinitis pigmentosa syndromes if neurological signs are subtle and other rare neurological disorders (Table 12.9.5).

Aetiology

Phytanic acid (3*R*,*S*,7*R*,11*R*,15-tetramethylhexadecanoic acid) is an isoprenoid lipid derived from the phytol side chain of chlorophylls by bacterial degradation in ruminants, invertebrates, or pelagic fish (see Fig. 12.9.2). Phytol can be oxidized to an unsaturated fatty acid, phytenic acid, and this is saturated to phytanic acid by a pathway involving fatty aldehyde dehydrogenase 10 (FALDH-10) in microsomes. The significance of this pathway in humans is unclear though high phytanic acid levels have been described in some patients deficient in FALDH-10 with Sjögren–Larsson syndrome. Most phytanic acid is ingested from the adipose tissue and muscle of herbivores or pelagic fish. The average human daily dietary intake of phytanic acid in Western societies is between 50 and 100 mg, of which about 50% is absorbed and metabolized.

Phytanic acid is transported in plasma bound to very low density lipoprotein and later low density lipoprotein, with its

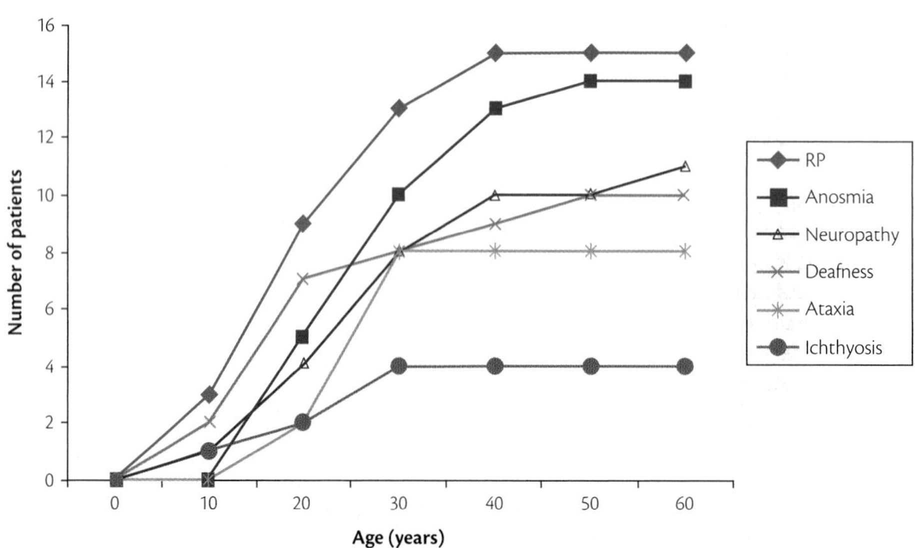

Fig. 12.9.1 Cumulative incidence of clinical features on presentation of 15 patients with Refsum's's disease. RP, retinitis pigmentosa.
(From Wierzbicki AS, *et al.* (2002). Refsum's disease: a peroxisomal disorder affecting phytanic acid alpha-oxidation. *J Neurochem*, 80, 727–35, with permission.)

Table 12.9.3 Differential diagnosis of treatable adult neuropathies caused by inborn errors of metabolism

Disease	Onset	Neurology	Signs	Chemistry	Treatment	Screening
Fabry's disease	10–20	Small fibre Sensory	Stroke; cardiomyopathy; renal	Low α-galactocerebrosidase	ERT	WBC α-Gal
Serine deficiency	10–20	Axonal	Growth delay; ichthyosis	Low CSF/plasma serine	Serine	Plasma amino acids
Cerebrotendinous xanthomatosis	10–40	Axonal, Demyelination, Sensorimotor	Mental retardation; ataxia, spastic paraperesis. Tendon xanthomata	Cholestanol	Chenodeoxycholate	Cholestanol
Adult Refsum's disease/ syndrome	10–50	Demyelination Sensorimotor	Retinitis pigmentosa, ataxia, anosmia	Phytanic acid	Low phytanic acid diet	Phytanic acid
Porphyrias	10–50	All	Neuropsychiatric Dermatological	PBG and δALA	Various	PBG and δALA
Wilson's disease	15–50	Axonal Demyelination Sensorimotor	Movement disorder	Copper/Caeruloplasmin	Chelation	Copper/ caeruloplasmin

CSF, cerebrospinal fluid; δALA, δ-aminolaevulanic acid; PBG, porphobilinogen.
Reproduced from Sebel F et al (2007) Peripheral neuropathy and inborn errors of metabolism in adults. *J Inherit Metab Dis*, **30**, 642–53, with permission.

elimination allied to reverse cholesterol transport (high density lipoprotein). Phytanic acid is preferentially taken up by the liver and may account for up to 50% of the free fatty acid pool in hepatocytes. This pool is labile and can be acutely mobilized by stress, infection, or starvation, resulting in rapid phytanic acid release. Plasma phytanic acid concentrations are less than 10% of the levels found in adipose tissue and neurons, which accumulate phytanic acid because of its hydrophobicity. The elimination half-life of total body phytanic acid is usually between 1 and 2 years.

Most fatty acids are metabolized by the β-oxidation pathways in peroxisomes and mitochondria. Phytanic acid cannot be metabolized by this route owing to the presence of a β-methyl group.

Table 12.9.4 Differential diagnosis of other adult neuropathies caused by inborn errors of metabolism.

Disease	Age of onset	Neuropathy	Signs	Chemistry	Treatment	Screening
Mitochondrial myopathy	15–50	All	Retinitis pigmentosa, epilepsy, ataxia	CSF/plasma lactate	None	Lactate, muscle biopsy
Metachromatic leukodystrophy	15–50	Demyelination Sensorimotor	Psychiatry, ataxia	Aryl-sulphatase A	None/Bone marrow transplant	Aryl-sulphatase A
Krabbe's disease	15–50	Demyelination Sensorimotor	Spastic paraparesis	WBC galacto-cerebrosidase	None/Bone marrow transplant	WBC galacto-cerebrosidase
GM_2 gangliosidosis	15–50	All	Psychiatry; ataxia,	Hexosaminidase	None	WBC hexosaminidase
AMACR	10–50	Demyelination Sensorimotor	Retinitis pigmentosa, ataxia, anosmia, IQ	Pristanic acid, D/ THCA	Low PA diet	Pristanic acid
Abetalipoproteinaemia	5–20	Axonal, Sensory, Sensorimotor	Ataxia, movement disorder, retinitis pigmentosa, acanthocytes	Low cholesterol, Low apolipoprotein B, vitamins A and E	Vitamins A and E	Apolipoprotein B
Vitamin E deficiency	10–20	Axonal, Demyelination Sensorimotor	Ataxia, movement disorder, retinitis pigmentosa, acanthocytes	Vitamin E	Vitamin E	Vitamin E
Homocysteine metabolism (CblC)	15–50	Axonal, motor neuron disease Sensorimotor	Psychiatric, stroke, leukoencephalopathy; Macrocytosis	Homocysteine; methylmalonic acid	Folate, vitamins B_{12} and B_6, betaine	Homocysteine
X-ALD	15–50	Axonal, demyelination Sensorimotor	Neuropsychiatric leukoencephalopathy; adrenal failure	Very long chain fatty acids	?Lorenzo's oil	Very long chain fatty acids

AMACR, α-methylacyl-CoA racemase; WBC, white blood cell.
Reproduced from Sedel F, *et al.* (2007). Peripheral neuropathy and inborn errors of metabolism in adults. *J Inherit Metab Dis*, **30**, 642–53, with permission.

Table 12.9.5 Differential diagnosis of retinitis with neurological signs

Presentation	OMIM	Neurological and other signs
Abetalipoproteinaemia	200100	Ataxia, movement disorder, retinitis pigmentosa, acanthocytes
Vitamin E deficiency	600415	
Ornithine aminotransferase deficiency	258870	Gyrate atrophy
		Myopathy
Usher's syndrome Ia	276900	Congenital deafness, ataxia
Usher's syndromes II	276901	Moderate progressive deafness
Bardet–Biedl–Moon syndrome	209900	Polydactyly
		Truncal obesity
		Hypogonadism
		Short stature
		Mental retardation
Kearns–Sayre syndrome	530000	Ophthalmoplegia
		Cardiomyopathy
Ceroid lipofuscinosis (Batten's disease)	204300	Seizures
		Dyskinesia
		Dementia
X-linked macular degeneration	304020	Ataxia
		Myoclonic encephalopathy

Instead, phytanic acid is metabolized either by α-oxidation to pristanic acid, or by ω-oxidation from the other end of the molecule. Using radiolabelled [^{14}C]-phytanic acid as a substrate, an enzyme activity responsible for the α-oxidation of phytanic acid in cell lysates was described in 1967. This activity was eventually localized within peroxisomes and, after 30 years, the pathway responsible for α-oxidation has been clarified.

Alpha oxidation of phytanic acid

Most phytanic acid metabolism occurs in the liver and kidney by α-oxidation, though skin fibroblasts are used for clinical diagnostic purposes. Phytanic acid from plasma enters the peroxisome in association with the sterol carrier protein-2 (SCP-2) and is metabolized by a four-step initial α-oxidation pathway. Unusually, it appears this pathway can metabolize two stereoisomers of its substrate equally well. One carbon atom is then removed from the latter in a lyase reaction to give pristanal and formyl-CoA. Pristanal is then oxidized to pristanic acid which is thio-esterified using CoA to give a racemic mixture. The action of a α-methylacyl-CoA racemase converts the (2*R*)-epimer to the (2*S*)-epimer. Further degradation of (2*S*)-pristanic acid by the stereospecific β-oxidation pathway then occurs, with the release of propionyl and acetyl-CoA units. Further β-oxidation reactions (including epimerization) are required to generate the dimethylundecanoic and dimethylnonanoic and methyl-heptanoic acid derivatives, which are finally exported for mitochondrial β-oxidation.

Molecular genetics

The defect in adult Refsum's disease was soon identified as being due to the lack of an α-oxidase. It took 30 years for the enzyme responsible, phytanoyl CoA-hydroxylase, to be identified. Two groups identified the gene for phytanoyl CoA-hydroxylase simultaneously in 1997. The phytanoyl CoA-hydroxylase gene includes nine exons and codes for a 338 amino acid protein including the 30 amino acid signal domain, which is cleaved on entry into the peroxisome. Like all the peroxisomal targeting sequence type 2 proteins, phytanoyl CoA-hydroxylase is transported into the peroxisomes by the protein transporter peroxin 7. Deficiency in this transporter is responsible for rhizomelic chondrodysplasia punctata type 1. Phytanoyl CoA-hydroxylase is an iron (II) and 2-oxoglutarate-dependent oxygenase, with little overall sequence similarity to other human oxygenases. Numerous point and splice mutations in phytanoyl CoA-hydroxylase have now been described in adult Refsum's disease patients, many of which affect 2-oxoglutarate conversion. Significantly, all cause complete inactivation of the protein; no partial function mutations have yet been identified.

Genetic mapping studies have shown that in most cases, but not all, classical adult Refsum's disease maps to chromosome 10. The locus for the second form of adult Refsum's disease, comprising about 10% of cases, was localized to chromosome 6q22–24 and biochemical studies of fibroblasts from patients with adult Refsum's disease established that these patients have subtle deficiencies of peroxisomal targeting sequence type-2 dependent enzyme functions (plasmalogen synthesis) consistent with mild variants of rhizomelic chondrodysplasia punctata, though they lack any clinical signs specific to childhood-onset rhizomelic chondrodysplasia punctata. Ironically, one of the original patients described with adult Refsum's disease turned out to have the rhizomelic chondrodysplasia punctata variant. A limited number of mutations have been described that cause Refsum's–rhizomelic chondrodysplasia punctata and it is unclear why these mutations should preferentially lead to mislocalization of phytanoyl CoA-hydroxylase in contrast to other peroxin 7 imported proteins. A third locus for adult Refsum's disease has recently been described on chromosome 20p11.21-q12 in a consanguineous family but the causative gene remains to be identified.

Disordered ω-oxidation

Patients with adult Refsum's disease are unable to detoxify phytanic acid by α-oxidation, and so the ω-oxidation pathway is the only metabolic pathway available for its degradation. This pathway produces 3-methyladipic acid as the final metabolite, which is excreted in the urine. Thus, 3-methyladipic acid concentrations can be used as an index of the molar activity of the ω-oxidation pathway. After ingestion of a test load of phytanic acid, 3-methyladipic acid is detected in the urine of healthy controls and adult Refsum's disease heterozygotes showing that ω-oxidation plays a significant role in postprandial metabolism of phytanic acid in humans.

The activity of the ω-oxidation pathway is approximately doubled in patients with adult Refsum's disease, but this microsomal pathway has considerable reserve capacity. The balance of intake of phytanic acid and its ω-oxidation is likely to determine long-term concentrations of the lipid. Patients with adult Refsum's disease often clinically relapse during episodes of illness or drastic weight loss. Fasting induces ketosis and lipolysis and acute mobilization of phytanic acid in hepatocyte and adipocyte fatty acid pools. This process can induce a release of 5000 mg (*c.*15 mmol) per day of phytanic acid (50 times normal). In experimental ketosis, following acute starvation, phytanic acid doubled in 29 h in patients with adult Refsum's disease and a 80% rise was seen in urinary 3-methyladipic acid levels, indicating that ω-oxidation was buffering part of this rise. Phytanic acid concentrations can exceed the capacity of the residual α- and ω-oxidation pathways. Excess phytanic acid is excreted by low-affinity pathways. Phytanic acid can be glucuronidated and it can also be lost nonspecifically in the urine as nephropathy is a feature of adult Refsum's disease.

The enzymology of the ω-oxidation pathway in adult Refsum's disease has been clarified and occurs through the microsomal cytochrome P450 (CYP) 4A system as well as the peroxisome. The capacity of the ω-oxidation pathway has been measured by the excretion of 2,6-dimethyloctanedioic acid (the C10 ω-2-methyl thioester derivative of phytanic acid) at 30 mg phytanic acid (89 μmol) per day. However, other studies measuring 3-methyladipic acid excretion showed a far lower capacity of 6.9 mg (20.4 μmol) per day. These differences in activity may reflect the metabolic fates of the respective markers. Both 2,6-dimethyloctanedioic acid and 3-hexanedioic acid are products of the initial steps of ω-oxidation and may be dependent on carnitine ester formation for activation and further metabolism. The initial steps of ω-oxidation appear to have a greater capacity than that of the whole pathway when measured by the final product 3-methyladipic acid.

Molecular toxicology of Refsum's syndrome

The exact mechanism of the toxicity of phytanic acid to neuronal, cardiac, and bone tissue is gradually being clarified. Some studies indicated that phytanic acid is directly toxic to ciliary ganglion cells and induces calcium-driven apoptosis in Purkinje cells. Structural homology between phytanic acid and vitamin A, vitamin E, geranyl-pyrophosphate, and farnesyl pyrophosphate has been noted and it has been suggested that phytanic acid may have a role in the regulation of isoprenoid metabolism and protein prenylation. More recent studies have focused on the role of phytanic acid as a direct toxin to mitochondria and it has been found that phytanic acid has a rotenone-like action in uncoupling complex I in the oxidative phosphorylation chain in the mitochondrial inner membrane, with subsequent likely production of reactive oxygen species. This metabolic toxicity may explain why neuronal or allied retinal pigment tissues rich in mitochondria are the prime tissues affected in adult Refsum's disease.

The molecular toxicology of pristanic acid is unknown, although it is likely that the mild ophthalmic features seen in some cases may relate to phytanic acid toxicity as for phytanoyl CoA-hydroxylase deficiency. Although both di- and trihydroxycholestanoic acids levels are elevated in α-methylacyl-CoA racemase, there is no phenotype of itching associated with this disorder. The cause of the sensory neuropathy in α-methylacyl-CoA racemase still remains to be determined.

Epidemiology

Neuropathic adult peroxisomal disorders are rare, with a prevalence of 1 in 10^6 in Europe and, for unexplained reasons, 10-fold less in the United States of America. As with all recessive conditions, they are more common in cultures or localities with strong founder effects where consanguineous marriages are frequent. The classical Refsum's phenotype is usually found in genetic ophthalmic services where it may represent 1% of retinitis pigmentosa cases. No surveys have been performed on the incidence of α-methylacyl-CoA racemase among patients with neuropathy.

Clinical investigation

The key investigations in the case of suspected neuropathic adult Refsum's disease are the measurement of phytanic acid (for adult Refsum's disease) and pristanic acid (for suspected α-methylacyl-CoA racemase). These are diagnostic.

For clinical staging purposes, electroretinograms are often performed but often show flat responses characteristic of well-established retinitis pigmentosa. Visual fields should be assessed regularly as functional diplopia is a long-term complication of adult Refsum's disease. Slit-lamp examination for cataracts is also indicated, as these can be treated. Ideally, retinal photography should be performed so that the extent of retinitis pigmentosa and its progression can be monitored on a long term basis. Anosmia can be detected by screening using the standard four-bottle smell test, but is best quantified by more extensive profiles, e.g. the University of Pennsylvania smell identification test. Auditory function should be assessed by auditory evoked potentials and hearing tests and monitored every 5 years. Peripheral neuropathy should be investigated by peripheral nerve conduction studies for somatosensory potentials and electromyography. A nonspecific demyelination pattern is typical of adult Refsum's disease. Osteo- or chondrodysplasia is best identified by a radiological survey of hands and feet for short metatarsals and knee radiology for signs of current or previous chondrodysplasia.

Subtler signs that may accompany these definitive tests include an electrolyte profile showing mild hypokalaemia and a Fanconi-like aminoaciduria which can occur in adult Refsum's disease. Liver function tests should be performed. If bilirubin is raised or α-methylacyl-CoA racemase is suspected, a detailed bile acid profile should be performed by mass spectrometric methods. As the differential diagnoses include vitamin deficiencies, vitamin A and E levels should be measured to exclude retinol-deficiency retinopathy and tocopherol-deficient ataxia. Vitamin B_{12} and folate determinates are used to exclude cobalamin/folate deficient neuropathy.

To differentiate phytanoyl-CoA hydroxylase from peroxin 7 adult Refsum's disease, it is necessary to measure plasma VLCFAs and plasmalogens. However, often the deficiencies are subtle and these investigations may appear normal. For a definitive diagnosis, a skin biopsy should be taken, fibroblasts grown, and detailed enzyme and immunofluorescence profiles examined in a specialist peroxisomal laboratory.

Criteria for diagnosis

The pathognomic finding in adult Refsum's disease is greatly elevated phytanic acid concentrations in the plasma (>200 μmol/litre; normal <30 μmol/litre), in contrast to other peroxisomal disorders where levels are usually lower and other metabolic abnormalities are also present. Unlike in rhizomelic chondrodysplasia punctata or the peroxisomal biogenesis disorders, no intellectual defects are seen, bone abnormalities are mild (if present at all), and there is no defect in plasmalogen synthesis. In infantile Refsum's disease, which is a mild clinical variant of the peroxisomal biogenesis disorder encompassing Zellweger's disease as its most severe form, numerous subtle peroxisomal defects are present and the condition presents from birth.

In α-methylacyl-CoA racemase neuropathy, the pathognomic findings are raised levels of pristanic acid (>100 μmol/litre) allied with increases in di- and trihydroxycholestanoic acids.

A secondary elevation of phytanic acid may be seen, but levels are usually between 50 and 100 μmol/litre.

Treatment

Long-term prospects for the treatment of adult Refsum's disease (or at least for some forms) are good as it is one of the few inherited disorders of metabolism with an exogenous precipitating cause. The disease is treated symptomatically by restriction of phytanic acid intake in the diet or its elimination by plasmapheresis or apheresis. These regimes reduce plasma phytanic acid levels by between 50 and 70%, to values typically around 100 to 300 μmol/litre, and can eliminate phytanic acid completely from fat stores in some patients. Treatment successfully resolves symptoms of ichthyosis, sensory neuropathy, and ataxia in approximately that order. However, it has uncertain effects on the progression of retinitis pigmentosa, anosmia, or deafness although it seems to stabilize these signs.

Prognosis

The prognosis in adult Refsum's disease depends on the degree to which phytanic acid concentrations are decreased. In untreated disease, presentation is with progressive weakness and neuropathy usually following an acute infective illness which leads to anorexia and acute hepatic phytanic acid release exacerbating the condition. Concentrations of phytanic acid in the plasma usually exceed 1000 μmol/litre. Left untreated, cardiomyopathy and sudden death can occur. If phytanic acid levels are reduced by plasmapheresis and by adequate parenteral nutrition, and then a low phytanic acid diet is followed, prognosis is good. Any myopathy usually resolves within 2 to 3 weeks, though acute visual and auditory deterioration may be irrecoverable. In long-term cases patients are blind, deaf, and anosmic, have extensive peripheral myopathy, and are often wheelchair bound.

In acute adult Refsum's disease, once phytanic acid levels fall to less than 500 μmol/litre, ichthyosis resolves followed by improvement in myopathy and neuropathy. If phytanic acid levels can be restored to normal values, then it is likely that ophthalmological changes will be minimal or slow, but sudden step-like deteriorations can occur. The principal long-term disability is increasing loss of visual field with subsequent diplopia and progressive cataract formation. Auditory function generally remains good unless phytanic acid levels are substantially raised, in which case audiological deterioration occurs with the need for cochlear implants. Although acute myopathy resolves, patients may have muscle spasms or contractures which may be either related to the adult Refsum's disease or secondary to the osteodystrophy. Splints and the surgical correction of osteopathy may be required.

Other issues

Adult Refsum's disease is a potentially treatable cause of retinitis pigmentosa or neuropathy. The average delay to diagnosis is 12 years and a simple biochemical screening test exists for these disorders. Given that earlier implementation of dietary restriction of phytanic acid would likely arrest the disease process before retinitis is established, screening for phytanic and pristanic acidaemias should be considered as an important investigation in retinitis pigmentosa or peripheral neuropathy.

Future developments

The causes of neuropathic adult peroxisomal disorders are incompletely delineated. Cases of pristanic acidaemia with an adult Refsum's disease phenotype exist for which no cause has yet been found. Similarly, all cases of adult Refsum's disease currently described are null-function variants, so the phenotype associated with low partial function has not been identified. It may be entirely normal, but it is possible that some cases of retinal dystrophy or peripheral neuropathy may actually be caused by mild phytanoyl-CoA hydroxylase mutations. No cases of deficiency of phytanic acid lyase have been described although, given the gene location overlapping the biotinidase locus on 3p25, a complex phenotype of adult Refsum's disease neuropathy and ichthyosis with biotinidase-deficiency induced hypotonia, ataxia, hearing loss, optic atrophy, skin rash, alopecia, and organic aciduria might be expected. Alternatively, this combination may be lethal. A number of lyase enzymes with peroxisomal targeting signal motifs remain to be placed on the α-oxidation pathway and these may be associated with neuropathy or retinitis pigmentosa syndromes.

Reduction of dietary phytanic acid is already successful in ameliorating some symptoms but newer, more efficacious, therapies are still required to fully reverse the progression of this disease. The signalling pathways which regulate α-oxidation in humans are unclear. In rodents, the retinoid X receptor β and peroxisomal proliferator activating receptor α pathways control α-oxidation and thus fibrate (PPAR-α agonist) therapy increases activity, but this does not seem to be true in humans. As ω-oxidation is capable of large increases in activity and is principally mediated through cytochrome P450 enzymes, it forms a good candidate for therapeutic interventions to induce enzyme activity and reduce phytanic acid levels in Refsum's disease. However, at the present time, no drug therapy trials of compounds capable of modulating either the α- or the ω-oxidation pathways have been conducted in humans.

Further information

Adult Refsum's Disease Website: information for patients, carers and clinicians: http://refsumdisease.org

United Leukodystrophy Foundation Website: http://www.ulf.org

X-linked Adrenoleukodystrophy Data base: http://www.X-ald.nl

Further reading

Aubourg P, *et al.* (1993). A two-year trial of oleic and erucic acids ('Lorenzo's oil') as treatment for adrenomyeloneuropathy. *N Engl J Med*, **329**, 745–52. [Original randomized control trial of Lorenzo's oil in X-ALD.]

Brown PJ, et al. (1993). Diet and Refsum's disease. The determination of phytanic acid and phytol in certain foods and application of this knowledge to the choice of suitable convenience foods for patients with Refsum's disease. *J Hum Nutr Diet*, **6**, 295–05. [Diet for Refsum's disease.]

Brown FR III, *et al.* (1983). Myelin membrane from adrenoleukodystrophy brain white matter—isolation and physical/chemical properties. *J Neurochem*, **41**, 341–8. [Finding increased very long chain fatty acids in myelin in X-ALD.]

Budka H, Sluga E, Heiss WD (1976). Spastic paraplegia associated with Addison's disease: adult variant of adrenoleukodystrophy. *J Neurol*, **213**, 237–50. [Description of adenomyeloneuropathy variant of X-ALD.]

Cartier N, *et al.* (2009). Hematopoietic stem cell gene therapy with a lentiviral vector in X-linked adrenoleukodystrophy. *Science*, **326**, 818–23. [Gene therapy for X-ALD.]

Eichler F, *et al.* (2007). Magnetic resonance imaging detection of lesion progression in adult patients with X-linked adrenoleukodystrophy. *Arch Neurol*, **64**, 659–64. [MRI of X-ALD.]

Ferdinandusse S, *et al.* (2000). Mutations in the gene encoding peroxisomal alpha-methylacyl-CoA racemase cause adult-onset sensory motor neuropathy. *Nat Genet*, **24**, 188–91. [Description of the genetic defect in α-methyl-acylCoA racemase deficiency.]

Fiskerstrand T, *et al.*(2009). A novel Refsum-like disorder that maps to chromosome 20. *Neurology*, **72**, 20–7. [Description of the third locus for adult Refsum disease.]

Goldman JM, *et al.* (1985). Screening of patients with retinitis pigmentosa for heredopathia atactica polyneuritiformis (Refsum's disease). *Br Med J (Clin Res Ed)*, **290**, 1109–10. [Screening for adult Refsum's disease in retinitis pigmentosa patients.]

Griffin JW, *et al.* (1977). Adrenomyeloneuropathy: a probable variant of adrenoleukodystrophy. *Neurology*, **27**, 1107–3 [Description of adrenomyeloneuropathy in X-ALD.]

Haberfeld W, Spieler F (1910). Zur diffusen Hirn-Rueckmarksclerose im Kindesalter. *Dtch Z Nervenh*, **40**, 436–63. [Original description of X-ALD.]

Hirsch D, Stahl A, Lodish AF (1998). A family of fatty acid transporters conserved from mycobacterium to man. *Proc Natl Acad Sci USA*, **95**, 8625–29. [Review of X-ALD related ABC transporters.]

Jansen GA, *et al.* (1997). Refsum disease is caused by mutations in the phytanoyl-CoA hydroxylase gene. *Nat Genet*, **17**, 190–93. [Description of genetic defect in adult Refsum's disease.]

Jansen GA, Waterham HR, Wanders RJ (2004). Molecular basis of Refsum disease: sequence variations in phytanoyl-CoA hydroxylase (PHYH) and the PTS2 receptor (PEX7). *Hum Mutat*, **23**, 209–18. [Mutation spectrum in adult Refsum's disease.]

Kemp S, *et al.* (2001). ABCD1 mutations and the X-linked adrenoleukodystrophy mutation database: role in diagnosis and clinical correlations. *Hum Mutat*, **18**, 499–515. [Mutation spectrum in X-ALD.]

Kishimoto Y, *et al.* (1980). Adrenoleukodystrophy: evidence that abnormal very long chain fatty acids of brain cholesterol esters are of exogenous origin. *Biochem Biophys Res Commun*, **96**, 69–76. [Possibility of diet therapy in X-ALD.]

Komen JC, Wanders RJ (2006). Identification of the cytochrome P450 enzymes responsible for the omega-hydroxylation of phytanic acid. *FEBS Lett*, **580**, 3794–98. [Identification of the ω-oxidation pathway.]

Kumar AJ, *et al.* (1995). MR findings in adult-onset adrenoleukodystrophy. *Am J Neuroradiol*, **16**, 1227–37. [MRI findings in X-ALD.]

Mahmood A, *et al.* (2007). Survival analysis of haematopoietic cell transplantation for childhood cerebral X-linked adrenoleukodystrophy: a comparison study. *Lancet Neurol*, **6**, 687–92. [Outcomes of bone marrow transplantation in X-ALD.]

Mihalik SJ, *et al.* (1997). Identification of PAHX, a Refsum's disease gene. *Nat Genet*, **17**, 185–89. [Description of gene defect in adult Refsum's disease.]

Moser AB, *et al.* (1999). Plasma very long chain fatty acids in 3000 peroxisome disease patients and 29,000 controls. *Ann Neurol*, **45**, 100–10. [Screening for peroxisomal disorders and X-ALD.]

Moser HW, *et al.* (1987). The adrenoleukodsytrophies. *Crit Rev Neurobiol*, **3**, 29–88. [Clinical survey of X-ALD.]

Moser HW, *et al.* (1991). Clinical aspects of adrenoleukodystrophy and adrenomyeloneuropathy. *Dev Neurosci*, **13**, 254–61. [Signs in X-ALD heterozygotes.]

Moser HW, *et al.* (2005). Follow-up of 89 asymptomatic patients with adrenoleukodystrophy treated with Lorenzo's oil. *Arch Neurol*, **62**, 1073–80. [Long-term outcomes with Lorenzo's oil.]

Moser HW, Mahmood A, Raymond GV (2007). X-linked adrenoleukodystrophy. *Nat Clin Pract Neurol*, **3**, 140–51. [Use of bone marrow transplant in X-ALD.]

Mosser J, *et al.* (1993). Putative X-linked adrenoleukodystrophy gene shares unexpected homology with ABC transporters. *Nature*, **361**, 726–30. [Description of X-ALD gene as an ABC transporter.]

Mukherji M, *et al.* (2001). Structure-function analysis of phytanoyl-CoA 2-hydroxylase mutations causing Refsum's's disease. *Hum Mol Genet*, **10**, 1971–82. [Structure function correlation for phytanoyl-CoA hydroxylase.]

Mukherji M, *et al.* (2003). The chemical biology of branched-chain lipid metabolism. *Prog Lipid Res*, **42**, 359–76. [Review of the α-oxidation pathway.]

National Center for Biotechnology Information. *Online Mendelian Inheritance in Man (OMIM) database*. http://www.ncbi.nlm.nih.gov/omim/

Odone A, Odone M (1989). Lorenzo's oil. A new treatment for adrenoleukodystrophy. *J Pediatr Neurosci*, **5**, 55–60. [Original description of Lorenzo's oil.]

Powers JM, Schaumburg HH (1974). Adrenoleukodystrophy (sex-linked Schilder's disease). A pathogenetic hypothesis based on ultrastructural lesions in adrenal cortex, peripheral nerves and testis. *Am J Path*, **76**, 481–91. [A hypothesis for X-ALD.]

Prescott AG, Lloyd MD (2000). The iron(II), 2-oxoacid-dependent dioxygenases and their role in metabolism. *Nat Prod Rep*, **17**, 367–83. [Review of the role of oxygenases.]

Purdue PE, *et al.* (1999). Rhizomelic chondrodysplasia punctata, a peroxisomal biogenesis disorder caused by defects in Pex7p, a peroxisomal protein import receptor: a minireview. *Neurochem Res*, **24**, 581–86. [Review of rhizomelic chondrodysplasia punctata.]

Refsum's S (1946). Heredopathia atactica polyneuritiformis. *Acta Psychiatr Scand*, **38** Suppl, 9–15. [Original clinical description of adult Refsum's disease.]

Rizzo WB, *et al.* (1986). Adrenoleukodystrophy: oleic acid lowers fibroblast saturated C22-C26 fatty acids. *Neurology*, **36**, 357–61. [Exogenous fatty acids can affect C22:C26 ratios.]

Schilder P (1924). Die Encephalitis periaxalis diffusa. *Arch Psychiatr Nervenkr*, **71**, 327–35. [Original description of full spectrum X-ALD.]

Schonfeld P, Reiser G (2006). Rotenone-like action of the branched-chain phytanic acid induces oxidative stress in mitochondria. *J Biol Chem*, **281**, 7136–42. [Neurotoxicology of phytanic acid.]

Sedel F, *et al.* (2007a). Psychiatric manifestations revealing inborn errors of metabolism in adolescents and adults. *J Inherit Metab Dis*, **30**, 631–41. [Review of psychiatric presentations of inborn errors of metabolism.]

Sedel F, *et al.* (2007b). Peripheral neuropathy and inborn errors of metabolism in adults. *J Inherit Metab Dis*, **30**, 642–53. [Review of neuropathy presentations of inborn errors of metabolism.]

Singh I, *et al.* (1984). Adrenoleukodystrophy; impaired oxidation of very long chain fatty acids in white blood cells, cultured skin fibroblasts and amniocytes. *Pediatr Res*, **18**, 286–90. [Description of very long chain fatty acid oxidation defect in X-ALD.]

Steinberg D, *et al.* (1967). Refsum's disease: nature of the enzyme defect. *Science*, **156**, 1740–42. [Description of the enzyme defect in adult Refsum's disease.]

van den Brink DM, *et al.* (2003). Identification of PEX7 as the second gene involved in Refsum's disease. *Am J Hum Genet*, **72**, 471–77. [Identification of variant rhizomelic chondrodysplasia punctata as adult Refsum's disease phenocopy.]

Wierzbicki AS, *et al.* (2002). Refsum's disease: a peroxisomal disorder affecting phytanic acid alpha-oxidation. *J Neurochem*, **80**, 727–35. [Review of adult Refsum's disease.]

Wierzbicki AS, *et al.* (2003). Metabolism of phytanic acid and 3-methyl-adipic acid excretion in patients with adult Refsum's disease. *J Lipid Res*, **44**, 1481–88. [Clinical significance of ω-oxidation in adult Refsum's disease.]

12.10

Hereditary disorders of oxalate metabolism—the primary hyperoxalurias

Christopher J. Danpure and Dawn S. Milliner

Essentials

Oxalate is an end-product of metabolism with no known useful biological function in humans. Anything that increases the body burden of oxalate, or elevates the concentration of oxalate in the urine, increases the risk of calcium oxalate deposition in the kidney and/or urinary tract, resulting in nephrocalcinosis and/or urinary stones.

Hyperoxaluria can be due to excessive dietary intake, enhanced gut absorption (e.g. after small intestinal resection or bypass), ill-defined multifactorial disease (as in idiopathic calcium oxalate urinary stone disease, see Chapter 21.14), or—less commonly—as a consequence of a number of inherited monogenic disorders, only two of which have been well characterized.

Primary hyperoxaluria type 1 (PH1, alanine:glyoxylate aminotransferase deficiency) and type 2 (PH2, glyoxylate/hydroxypyruvate reductase deficiency)

Clinical features and diagnosis—presentation is with symptoms or findings related to urolithiasis, usually in childhood but sometimes in adult life. Recurring stone formation is characteristic, and with progressive loss of kidney function (reaching endstage renal failure at median 30 years) a rising plasma oxalate level leads to deposition of calcium oxalate in many organs (systemic oxalosis), manifesting as painful, nonhealing skin ulcers, fracturing osteodystrophy, refractory anemia, complete heart block, and heart failure due to oxalate cardiomyopathy. Variability of clinical expression is marked, with some patients reaching end-stage renal failure in early childhood, while others retain renal function into late adulthood. Diagnosis is by DNA analysis of peripheral blood samples, or by enzyme assay of percutaneous liver biopsy tissue. Prenatal diagnosis can be accomplished in the first trimester by DNA analysis of chorionic villus samples.

Management—this initially involves (1) maintenance of high fluid intake; (2) medications to inhibit calcium oxalate crystallization—pharmacological doses of pyridoxine (vitamin B_6) are useful in some patients; and (3) urological procedures as required. Management of endstage renal failure is difficult: (1) haemodialysis and peritoneal dialysis are not capable of preventing progression of systemic oxalosis; (2) kidney transplantation alone is problematic in PH1—patients who respond fully to pyridoxine (with normalization or near normalization of urine oxalate) can do well, but otherwise the new kidney is at significant risk from oxalate deposition, particularly if there is delayed graft function; (3) combined liver and kidney transplantation—the treatment of choice in patients with PH1 who do not respond well to pyridoxine and are approaching endstage renal failure.

Introduction

Oxalate, hyperoxaluria, and oxalosis

Oxalate is an end product of metabolism with no known useful biological function in humans. In fact, oxalate can be distinctly detrimental to complex life forms because of the low solubility of its calcium salt. The solubility product of calcium oxalate is readily exceeded in urine, resulting in its crystallization and aggregation into calculi. Under physiological conditions oxalate, especially calcium oxalate, is only poorly absorbed from the gut, so only a minority of the body's oxalate is supplied directly by the diet. Most is derived by endogenous synthesis from dietary, mostly carbohydrate, precursors.

Most oxalate in the body is removed by urinary excretion. A small proportion appears to be excreted into the gut, but the physiological importance of intestinal elimination, especially in the presence of normal renal function, is unclear. The predominant role of the kidney in oxalate removal makes it the prime target for calcium oxalate deposition (see below). In normal adults, plasma oxalate levels are 1 to 3 μmol/litre and urinary excretion is less than 450 μmol/24 h. In healthy children, the 24 h oxalate excretion and random urine oxalate/creatinine ratios vary according to age. However, when normalized for body surface area, urinary excretion rates for children 2 years or older are similar to those of adults (i.e. <450 μmol/1.73 m^2 per 24 h).

Anything that increases the body's burden of oxalate, or elevates the concentration of oxalate in the urine, increases the risk of calcium oxalate deposition in the kidney and/or urinary tract. Environmental causes include excessive dietary intake of oxalate (particularly when combined with low calcium intake) and extended periods of dehydration. Intake of oxalate precursors, such as intravenous ascorbic acid, in patients receiving parenteral nutrition, or accidental ingestion of ethylene glycol are occasionally responsible. Enhanced gut absorption of oxalate is often encountered in patients with gastrointestinal disease or after bowel resection or bypass (but with intact colons), and can be seen in patients receiving medications that alter fat absorption, such as tetrahydrolipstatin (orlistat).

Hyperoxaluria is a well-recognized risk factor in the common condition of idiopathic calcium oxalate kidney stone disease. Although its causes in such patients remain unclear, they are almost certainly multifactorial in nature, with both environmental and genetic components. The number of different genetic causes of hyperoxaluria is unknown. Well-characterized monogenic causes of hyperoxaluria are rare, but can be severe; the best studied are primary hyperoxaluria type 1 and type 2.

Historical perspectives

The condition now recognized as primary hyperoxaluria was first identified by Lepoutre in 1925. However, it was another quarter of a century before it was described in detail, and it was not until 1957 that it was recognized as a metabolic disorder. The next great leap forward came in 1968 when Williams and Smith realized that primary hyperoxaluria was at least two disorders, now known as primary hyperoxaluria type 1 and type 2 (PH1 and PH2). The basic enzyme defect in PH2 was recognized at the time, but the basic defect in PH1 did not emerge until 1986. Since then, advances in understanding of the primary hyperoxalurias have been rapid, offending genes having been cloned and numerous mutations identified.

Treatments have evolved in parallel with our increased understanding of the aetiology and pathophysiology of the condition. Until 20 years ago the outlook for primary hyperoxaluria patients was bleak. However, in the past two decades, life expectancy for most patients has improved markedly following the introduction of more rational medical and surgical treatments. In the latter case, enzyme replacement therapy by liver transplantation stands out. Many primary hyperoxaluria patients are alive today who would not be were it not for liver transplantation. Our increased understanding, especially of enzyme genotype–phenotype relationships, has led to the exciting prospect of new, possibly mutation-specific, pharmacological treatments in the not too distant future.

Aetiology, genetics, pathogenesis, and pathology

The primary hyperoxalurias are a group of disorders of which only two, PH1 (OMIM 259900) and PH2 (OMIM 260000), are well characterized. Both types are simple autosomal recessive disorders of glyoxylate metabolism that result in marked increases in the metabolic production of oxalate and the inappropriate deposition of insoluble calcium oxalate in the kidney and urinary tract. Despite these apparent similarities, the molecular bases of these two disorders are completely different. PH1 is caused by a deficiency of the liver-specific peroxisomal enzyme alanine–glyoxylate aminotransferase (AGT, EC 2.6.1.44), whereas PH2 is caused by a deficiency of the more widely distributed cytosolic and mitochondrial enzyme glyoxylate/hydroxypyruvate reductase (GRHPR, EC 1.1.1.26/79). Like all aminotransferases, AGT requires a metabolite of vitamin B_6, pyridoxal phosphate, as cofactor. GRHPR does not require a cofactor.

AGT normally catalyses the conversion of the intermediary metabolite glyoxylate to glycine, but its absence in PH1 allows glyoxylate to be oxidized to oxalate and reduced to glycolate instead (Fig. 12.10.1). GRHPR normally catalyses the reduction of

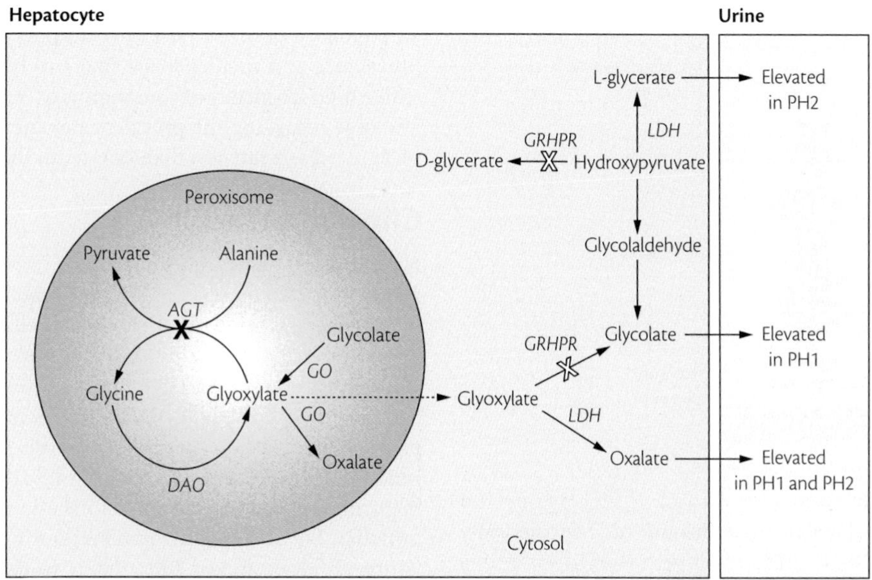

Fig. 12.10.1 Main pathways of glyoxylate metabolism in human liver cells. The black 'X' indicates the location of the enzyme defect in primary hyperoxaluria type 1 and the white 'X' indicates the enzyme defects in PH2. The peroxisomal membrane is likely to be permeable to most or all of the metabolites shown. However, only the peroxisomal efflux of glyoxylate (dotted line) is shown to highlight the relationship between AGT deficiency and the concomitant hyperoxaluria and hyperglycolicaciduria characteristic of primary hyperoxaluria type 1. AGT, alanine–glyoxylate aminotransferase; GO, glycolate oxidase; DAO, D-amino acid oxidase; GRHPR, glyoxylate/hydroxypyruvate reductase; LDH, lactate dehydrogenase; PH1, primary hyperoxaluria type 1; PH2, primary hyperoxaluria type 2.

glyoxylate to glycolate as well as the reduction of hydroxypyruvate to D-glycerate. However, its deficiency in PH2 allows glyoxylate to be oxidized to oxalate and hydroxypyruvate to be reduced to L-glycerate (Fig. 12.10.1). Oxalate cannot be further metabolized and can only be removed from the body by renal and, to a lesser degree, gastrointestinal excretion. Although glycolate and L-glycerate can be further metabolized, their increased rate of synthesis in PH1 and PH2, respectively, exceeds their ability to be removed metabolically. Therefore, large amounts of these metabolites are also removed by renal excretion. Concomitant hyperoxaluria and hyperglycolicaciduria used to be considered pathognomonic of PH1, and concomitant hyperoxaluria and hyper-L-glyceric aciduria pathognomonic of PH2. However, up to one-quarter of PH1 patients do not exhibit hyperglycolicaciduria, and some PH2 patients do not have hyper-L-glyeric aciduria.

PH1, in particular, is heterogeneous at the level of molecular phenotype. Three major enzymic categories are recognized: (1) absence of both AGT catalytic activity and AGT immunoreactive protein; (2) absence of AGT catalytic activity but the presence of AGT immunoreactive protein; (3) presence of both AGT catalytic activity and AGT immunoreactive protein. Surprisingly for a recessive disease, many patients in the last category can have AGT activity similar to that found in asymptomatic heterozygotes (Fig. 12.10.2). In most of the latter patients, disease is caused by an unparalleled protein trafficking defect in which AGT is mistargeted from its normal location in the peroxisomes to the mitochondria. Although mistargeted AGT is still enzymically active, it is unable to fulfil its metabolic function (i.e. glyoxylate transamination) properly when located in the mitochondria.

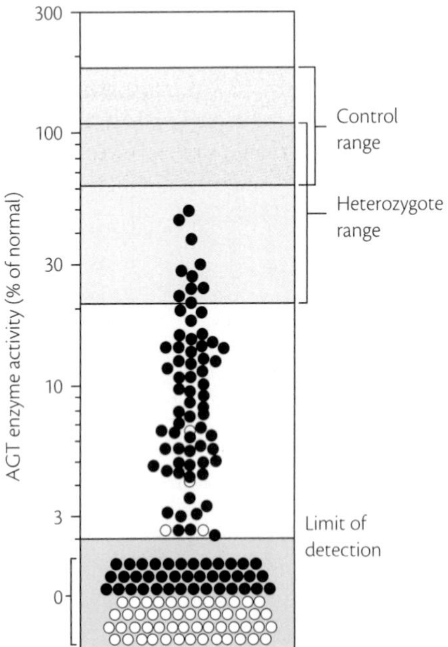

Fig. 12.10.2 Hepatic alanine–glyoxylate aminotransferase (AGT) heterogeneity in patients with primary hyperoxaluria type 1. AGT enzyme activity, expressed as a percentage of the mean normal control value, is shown for 162 patients. Almost all patients with significant AGT enzyme activity express the peroxisome-to-mitochondrion mis-targeting phenotype. Black circles, biopsies with detectable levels of immunoreactive AGT protein; white circles, biopsies with undetectable levels of immunoreactive AGT protein.

AGT is encoded by the *AGXT* gene, which contains 11 exons, spanning approximately 10 kb on chromosome 2q37.3. GRHPR is encoded by the *GRHPR* gene, which contains nine exons and spans approximately 9 kb in the pericentromeric region of chromosome 9. At least 150 mutations and polymorphisms have been identified at the *AGXT* locus, the three most common of which are described in Table 12.10.1. Rather fewer mutations have been found at the *GRHPR* locus. Many mutations in *AGXT*, including some of the most common, segregate and functionally interact with a very common polymorphism that results in a Pro11Leu amino acid replacement. The X-ray crystal structures of both AGT (Fig. 12.10.3) and GRHPR have been determined, enabling the effects of many of the missense mutations and, in the case of AGT, their interactions with the Pro11Leu polymorphism to be rationalized.

The most common mutation found in PH1, with an allelic frequency of 30 to 40%, leads to a Gly170Arg amino acid replacement. This mutation, together with a very common Pro11Leu polymorphism, is responsible for AGT peroxisome-to-mitochondrion mistargeting. The Pro11Leu polymorphism generates a functionally weak N-terminal mitochondrial targeting sequence, the efficiency of which is enhanced by the additional presence of the Gly170Arg mutation. Interestingly, the Gly170Arg mutation on its own is predicted to be without any untoward consequences.

The outcome of AGT or GRHPR deficiency, in PH1 or PH2 respectively, is increased synthesis and urinary excretion of oxalate. In most, but not all, patients hyperoxaluria is accompanied by hyperglycolicaciduria (in PH1) and hyper-L-glyceric aciduria (in PH2). Although glycolate and L-glycerate are useful in the differential diagnosis of PH1 and PH2 (see below), they themselves appear to cause no ill effects. All the pathological sequelae of the primary hyperoxalurias are associated with the increased synthesis and excretion of oxalate.

Epidemiology

The primary hyperoxalurias are rare disorders. In Europe, PH1 has an estimated prevalence of 1.0 to 2.9 per million people and an incidence of 0.12 to 0.15 per million per year. However, both prevalence and incidence are likely to be greater in populations with a high frequency of consanguinity. Although there are no data available regarding the prevalence or incidence of PH2, cases are recognized at a rate less than one-tenth that of PH1.

Clinical features

High concentrations of oxalate in the urine result in the formation of calcium oxalate crystals in renal tubules. The crystals are then endocytosed by renal tubule epithelial cells and migrate to the renal interstitium. There, the crystals incite an inflammatory, giant-cell reaction that results in renal injury, ultimately leading to interstitial fibrosis. Widespread calcium oxalate deposition in the renal parenchyma is termed nephrocalcinosis and is usually visible on renal imaging studies. Aggregation of calcium oxalate crystals in the urinary space leads to stone formation (nephrolithiasis or urolithiasis). For reasons that remain poorly understood, infants and young children appear more likely to develop nephrocalcinosis, although it can occur at any age. Stones in the absence of nephrocalcinosis are more characteristic in older children and adults.

Although marked hyperoxaluria is present from early infancy, the age at which symptoms develop is highly variable, ranging from

Table 12.10.1 The three most common mutations and polymorphisms found in alanine–glyoxylate aminotransferase

Polymorphism/ mutation	**Description**	**Allelic frequency[a]**		**Notes**
		PH1 patients (%)	**Normal population (%)**	
Polymorphisms				
Pro11Leu[b]	Substitution of proline by leucine at residue 11	*c*.50	15–20	These three polymorphic variations define the minor *AGXT* allele
Intron 1 duplication	A 74bp partial duplication of intron 1	*c*.50	15–20	
Ile340Met	Substitution of isoleucine by methionine at residue 340	*c*.50	15–20	
Mutations				
Gly170Arg[b]	Substitution of glycine by arginine at residue 170	30–40		Segregates with the minor *AGXT* allele
33–34*insC*	Insertion of a single base (C) leading to a shift in the reading frame	*c*.12		
Ile244Thr	Substitution of isoleucine by threonine at residue 244	6–9[c]		Segregates with the minor *AGXT* allele

[a] In European and North American populations.
[b] Pro11Leu and Gly170Arg synergistically interact to misdirect AGT from its normal location in hepatocyte peroxisomes to mitochondria.
PH1, primary hyperoxaluria type 1.
[c] Ile244Thr has a much higher frequency in some North African and Spanish populations.

a few months to well into adulthood. In most patients, symptoms or findings related to urolithiasis (pain, haematuria, stone passage) are evident in early childhood. Recurring stone formation is characteristic, often requiring multiple stone-removal procedures. Over time, the damaging effects of calcium oxalate deposition in the kidney, episodes of transient obstruction due to stones, and injury related to stone-removal procedures or infection result in irreversible loss of renal function. Endstage renal failure can occur at any age, from infancy to the sixth decade of life, with a median of approximately 30 years (Fig. 12.10.4).

In a minority of patients, the first clinical manifestation of primary hyperoxaluria is renal failure. Symptoms of uraemia prompt patients to seek medical attention. On evaluation, nephrocalcinosis and/or bilateral renal stones are usually found. Occasionally, the diagnosis is made on renal biopsy in a patient in whom primary hyperoxaluria was not considered on clinical grounds. A severe infantile form of PH1 results in irreversible renal failure during the first year or two of life, presenting as failure to thrive.

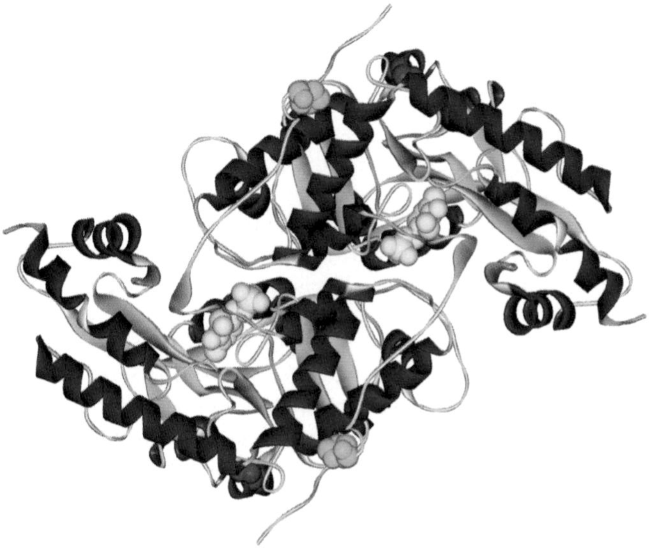

Fig. 12.10.3 Crystal structure of the human alanine–glyoxylate aminotransferase dimer. The carbon backbone is coloured as follows: red, α-helix; cyan, β-sheet; grey, random coil. Specific amino acids are coloured as follows: green, Pro11; blue, Gly170; yellow, pyridoxal phosphate attached to Lys209.

When renal function falls below a GFR of about 30 to 35 ml/min per 1.73 m^2, the kidney is unable to excrete the excess oxalate produced by the liver and the plasma oxalate concentration begins to rise abruptly. When the calcium oxalate concentration in plasma exceeds saturation, it is deposited in many organs and tissues (systemic oxalosis) resulting in progressively severe multisystem disease. Painful, nonhealing ulcers of the skin, fracturing osteodystrophy, refractory anaemia, complete heart block, and heart failure due to oxalate cardiomyopathy are features of systemic oxalosis. Without prompt and definitive management, death ensues.

Although there are no clinical features that can reliably differentiate PH1 from PH2 in an individual patient, PH2 is characterized by slightly lower oxalate excretion rates, fewer stone episodes, and better preservation of renal function than PH1.

Differential diagnosis

PH1 or PH2 should be considered in any child with urinary tract stones or nephrocalcinosis and in adults with recurrent calcium oxalate stones, especially if the clinical history extends back into childhood. Impaired renal function in a patient with calcium urolithiasis or nephrocalcinosis, or in a sibling, should also suggest the diagnosis. A presumptive diagnosis of PH1 or PH2 can often be made on the basis of 24 h urinary oxalate, glycolate, and L-glycerate excretion. Due to highly age-dependent normal ranges in young children, random urine oxalate/creatinine ratios are best regarded as an initial screen. If the ratio appears elevated, a timed (12–24 h) urine collection should be obtained for more reliable diagnostic information. It should be kept in mind that urinary oxalate excretion can be misleadingly low in patients with advanced renal failure, and concomitant hyperglycolicaciduria (in PH1) or hyper-L-glycericaciduria (in PH2) are not always present. Plasma levels of oxalate, glycolate, and glycerate are rarely of diagnostic benefit in patients whose renal function is well maintained, though can be valuable in those with renal failure.

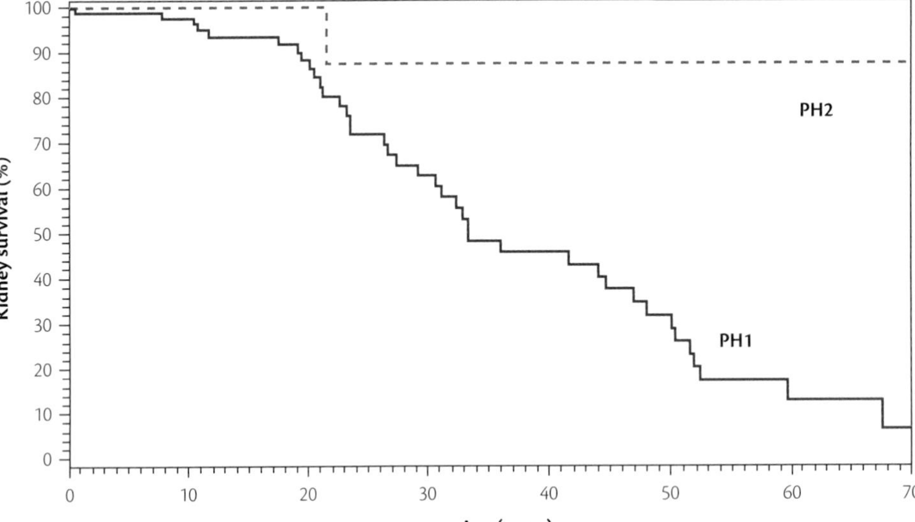

Fig. 12.10.4 Actuarial analysis of kidney survival in primary hyperoxaluria type 1 (solid line, n = 94) and PH2 (dotted line, n = 10) patients enrolled in the International Primary Hyperoxaluria Registry. By 34 years of age, half of the patients with primary hyperoxaluria type 1 developed end-stage renal failure. Better preservation of renal function is seen in patients with PH2.

Definitive diagnosis requires confirmation of homozygosity or compound heterozygosity for known mutations of AGT or GRHPR, or the determination of either AGT (for PH1) or GRHPR (for PH2) enzyme activity on a percutaneous needle biopsy of the liver. Although AGT expression is limited to hepatocytes, GRHPR is expressed in other tissues as well. This allows the possibility that the activity of GRHPR in peripheral blood leucocytes might be able to be used for PH2 diagnosis. For both AGT and GRHPR the assays of enzyme activity can be supported by the measurement of AGT and GRHPR immunoreactivity by western blotting. AGT peroxisome-to-mitochondrion mistargeting in PH1 can be confirmed by immunoelectron microscopy, but this is rarely needed nowadays. The identification of over 150 mutations in PH1 allows the possibility of diagnosis by DNA analysis in suitable families. It has been estimated that, even in the absence of family history, screening possible European or North American PH1 patients for the three most common mutations (Table 12.10.1) would be able to diagnose PH1 with an efficiency of 34%. When coupled with family and linkage analysis studies the success rate is greatly improved. Increasingly, more comprehensive gene sequencing is also being used, leading to improved diagnostic efficiency.

Prenatal diagnosis

Until the early 1990s, PH1 was diagnosed prenatally by measuring AGT enzyme activity and immunoreactivity in fetal liver biopsies in the second trimester. However, this approach has now been superseded by DNA (mutation or linkage) analysis of material obtained from chorionic villus samples in the first trimester. In suitable families this method can be used for both types of primary hyperoxaluria.

Treatment

There are a number of different levels at which treatment for PH1 and PH2 can be addressed, depending on the position of the defect being targeted along the pathophysiological pathway (Fig. 12.10.5). Those treatments addressing the distal stages of the pathway (e.g. stones or renal failure) are suitable for both types of primary hyperoxaluria. On the other hand, those addressing proximal stages (e.g. enzyme dysfunction) are more likely to be disease-specific.

Patients with primary hyperoxaluria who have adequate renal function should maintain high oral fluid intake in order to keep oxalate in the urine as dilute as possible. A suitable target level is 2 litres/m^2 body surface area. In infants and young children placement of a feeding or gastrostomy tube may be needed to assure sufficient intake. Reduction in calcium oxalate crystal formation can be accomplished by lowering the urine oxalate concentration and by the use of medication. Citrates, either as sodium citrate (0.1–0.15 g/kg per day) or equivalent doses of either sodium/potassium citrate or effervescent anhydrous sodium acid phosphate reduce the degree of calcium oxalate saturation in the urine. Neutral phosphates (providing 20–30 mg/kg per day of elemental phosphorus in divided doses) increase the excretion of pyrophosphate ions, which inhibit heterogeneous calcium oxalate crystal nucleation, seeded growth, and aggregation. This medication also reduces calcium absorption. Magnesium supplements (e.g. magnesium oxide 200 mg/day in adult patients) also inhibit crystal growth and aggregation. The doses used should be sufficient to produce a material increase in the urinary excretion of either phosphate or magnesium. Phosphate and magnesium should be avoided if there is renal insufficiency.

In about one-third of PH1 patients pharmacological doses (5–8 mg/kg per day) of pyridoxine (vitamin B_6) cause a significant reduction in urinary oxalate levels and improvement in clinical condition. Although it is well known that pyridoxal phosphate, a metabolite of pyridoxine, is the cofactor for AGT, the metabolic basis of pyridoxine responsiveness is unclear. Recent studies have shown that most pyridoxine-responsive PH1 patients carry one or two copies of the AGT mistargeting mutant allele containing the Gly170Arg mutation and Pro11Leu polymorphism. Pyridoxal phosphate is not required for the activity of GRHPR. Thus, pyridoxine would be expected to be ineffective in PH2 patients, as has been confirmed in clinical studies.

Obstructive uropathy requires prompt stent placement or percutaneous nephrostomy to relieve the obstruction. Ureteroscopic basket retrieval, nephroscopic lithotomy, endoscopic lithotripsy

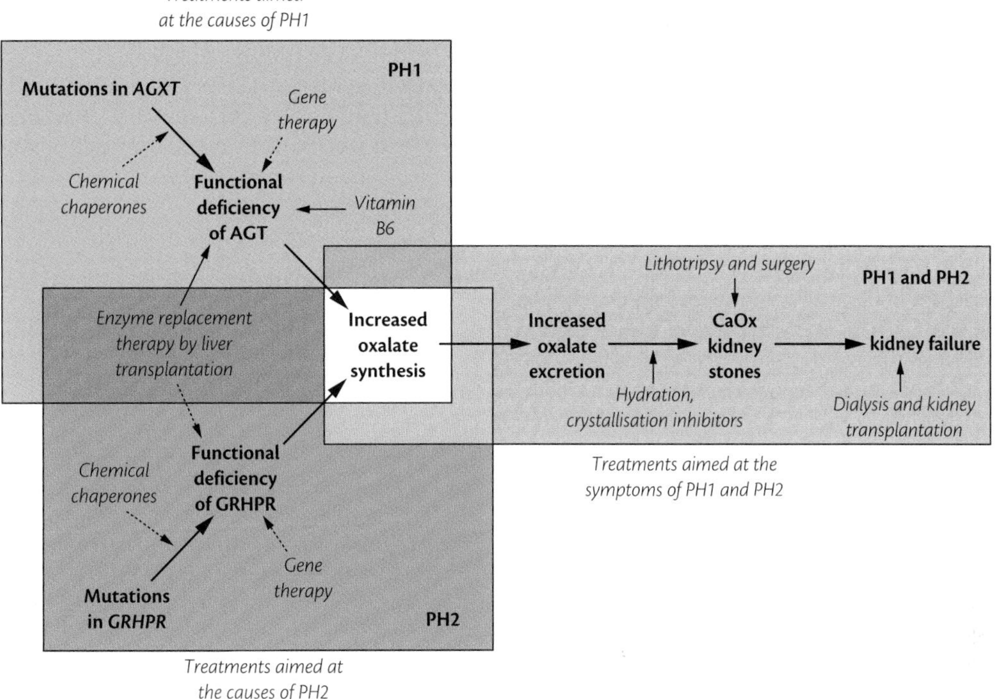

Fig. 12.10.5 Current and future approaches to the treatment of primary hyperoxaluria types 1 and 2. Current treatments (solid arrows) and potential treatments (dashed arrows) are superimposed on the molecular aetiological and pathophysiological pathways in primary hyperoxaluria types 1 and 2. Treatments aimed at the pathways on the left tend to be directed at the causes of disease and are usually specific for either type 1 or type 2 primary hyperoxaluria. The treatments for the pathway on the right are aimed at the clinically observable symptoms and are likely to be common to types 1 and 2. CaOx, calcium oxalate; AGT, alanine–glyoxylate aminotransferase; GRHPR, glyoxylate/hydroxypyruvate reductase.

with ultrasonic, electrohydraulic, and laser techniques, as well as extracorporeal shockwave lithotripsy can be used to deal with stones. Open lithotomy for large calculi should now rarely be needed. Stone debris may require either external drainage via a nephrostomy or internal drainage via a stent. However, stents and other foreign bodies in the urinary tract rapidly become encrusted with calcium oxalate deposits. The kidneys should be kept as free from stones as possible; close follow-up is essential with regular radiological and/or ultrasonographic assessment.

Management of endstage renal failure poses particular challenges in patients with primary hyperoxaluria. The high rate of oxalate synthesis exceeds the rate of its removal by either conventional haemodialysis or peritoneal dialysis. The condition of patients with renal failure invariably worsens as calcium oxalate is deposited throughout the body (systemic oxalosis). Transplantation in the treatment of primary hyperoxaluria can be divided into two categories: kidney transplantation and liver transplantation. It is essential to realize that the aims of, and rationale behind, these procedures are completely different. Whereas kidney transplantation aims to resolve the uraemic consequences of kidney failure and to reduce plasma oxalate concentrations to levels that fall below the supersaturation threshold for calcium oxalate, liver transplantation is a rather specialized form of enzyme replacement therapy.

Kidney transplantation can provide temporary benefit, although 'temporary' in this context can mean years, or sometimes decades, particularly for pyridoxine-responsive PH1 patients and patients with PH2. The problem with kidney transplantation is that it does not address the basic cause of the disease. Although the transplanted kidney can provide efficient excretion of oxalate and keep plasma oxalate concentrations at levels low enough to minimize or avoid systemic calcium oxalate deposition, it has no effect on the underlying enzyme deficiency. Frequently, the transplanted kidney accumulates insoluble calcium oxalate as before. Indeed, the newly transplanted kidney is in a very vulnerable position, especially for patients who have been on haemodialysis for long periods. Not only does it have to deal with the increased synthetic load of oxalate resulting from the enzyme deficiency, it also has to deal with all the oxalate accumulated throughout the body following deteriorating or nonexistent renal function.

AGT is more or less liver-specific and, although GRHPR is more widely distributed, its activity in the liver greatly exceeds that in other tissues. Therefore, liver transplantation has the potential to replace all, or almost all, the body's requirement for AGT and, to a lesser extent, GRHPR. Unlike kidney transplantation, liver transplantation is a form of enzyme replacement therapy. Several hundred liver transplantations, often combined with kidney transplantation, have been carried out worldwide for PH1. At the time of writing, no such procedures have been carried out for PH2. Experience has shown that liver transplantation is able to achieve a metabolic cure for PH1, although it may take many years for the urinary excretion of oxalate to be normalized. This is especially the case if patients have spent many years with poor renal function or on haemodialysis, during which time the corporeal load of calcium oxalate has built up, particularly in the bones.

It has been suggested that PH1 patients who are either unresponsive or only partially responsive to pyridoxine should progress straight from approaching endstage renal failure (GFR <30 ml/min per 1.73m^2) to combined liver and kidney transplantation. PH1 patients who respond fully to pyridoxine, with normalization or near normalization of urine oxalate while on treatment and patients with PH2, can do well with kidney transplantation alone. The approach to transplantation may vary depending on individual patient factors.

Initiation of maintenance dialysis or transplantation should be accomplished as soon as the plasma oxalate concentration begins to exceed the solubility threshold for calcium oxalate. This occurs in most patients at a GFR of 20 to 25 ml/min per 1.73 m^2, though can occur earlier in some patients. The purpose of early initiation of renal replacement therapy is to minimize systemic oxalosis and reduce the risk of calcium oxalate deposits in the grafted kidney. If dialysis is needed, the time should be kept to a minimum before transplantation is performed. Vigorous dialysis, required daily in most patients, is needed. The plasma oxalate concentration and urine oxalate excretion rate should be followed sequentially before and after operation in these patients until normal. Elimination of tissue oxalate stores can take up to 3 years following successful transplantation. Careful management of the hyperoxaluria throughout this time is essential to avoid damage to the renal allograft. Pre-emptive liver transplantation before the glomerular filtration rate has decreased to 30 ml/min per 1.73 m^2 is an option if the disease is diagnosed early and is following an aggressive course. The risks of the transplant procedure, the added years of immunosuppression, and the difficulty in accurate prediction of rate of loss of renal function in PH patients must be balanced against the benefit. Heterotopic auxiliary liver transplantation is theoretically unsound, since the remaining native liver would continue to make large amounts of oxalate.

Other forms of primary hyperoxaluria

There are other forms of primary hyperoxaluria in addition to PH1 and PH2. They are indeterminate in number and poorly characterized. Although sometimes grouped under the heading 'primary hyperoxaluria type 3', this is misleading and unhelpful. Case studies have been published of individuals with elevated urinary oxalate of presumed metabolic origin, but who have normal AGT and GRHPR activities. At least one publication reported an individual with hyperoxaluria and hyperglycolicaciduria, yet who still had normal AGT. Potential explanations of the basic defects in these non-PH1, non-PH2 patients have included dysfunction of other metabolic enzymes involved indirectly in oxalate synthesis, abnormalities in enteric oxalate absorption, and defects in renal oxalate excretion. However, no conclusive proof has been forthcoming for any of these possibilities.

Likely future developments

Just as the discovery of AGT deficiency in PH1 heralded the introduction of enzyme replacement therapy by liver transplantation 20 years ago, so recent discoveries on the functional relationships between mutations and enzyme dysfunction will lead to the design of pharmacological countermeasures. Mutation-specific chemical chaperones have definite potential as future treatments patients with PH1 or type 2 who have missense mutations in AGT or GRHPR.

Gene therapy for primary hyperoxaluria was forecast more than 15 years ago. Unfortunately, the general lack of suitable vectors that are both safe and able to deliver high enough levels of AGT or GRHPR to their sites of action has resulted in almost no progress in this direction. However, recent studies using hepatocyte transplantation in an AGT knockout mouse model, in which the hepatocytes were made to express AGT by retroviral transduction, might indicate a way forward.

Further reading

Am J Nephrol, **25**, 263–310 and Urol Res, **33**, 315–407. [23 articles dealing with various experimental aspects of primary hyperoxaluria and calcium oxalate kidney stones presented at the 7th International Workshop on Primary Hyperoxaluria held in October 2004 at the Mayo Clinic, Rochester, Minnesota.]

Barratt TM, Danpure CJ (1999). Hyperoxaluria. In: Barratt TM, Avner ED, Harmon WE (eds) *Paediatric nephrology*, 4th edition, pp. 609–24. [Review with emphasis on paediatric patients.]

Booth MP, *et al.* (2006). Structural basis of substrate specificity in human glyoxylate reductase/hydroxypyruvate reductase. *J Mol Biol*, **360**, 178–89. [First reported crystal structure of human GRHPR.]

Cochat P (1999). Primary hyperoxaluria type 1. *Kidney Int*, **55**, 2533–47. [Contains a good discussion of transplantation.]

Coulter-Mackie MB, Rumsby G (2004). Genetic heterogeneity in primary hyperoxaluria type 1: impact on diagnosis. *Mol Genet Metab*, **83**, 38–46. [Comprehensive list of mutations and polymorphisms in PH1.]

Cramer SD, *et al.* (1999). The gene encoding hydroxypyruvate reductase (GRHPR) is mutated in patients with primary hyperoxaluria type II. *Hum Mol Genet*, **8**, 2063–9. [First cloning of human GRHPR cDNA and discovery of first mutations in GRHPR in PH2.]

Danpure CJ (2001). Primary hyperoxaluria. In: Scriver CR, *et al.* (eds). *The metabolic and molecular basis of inherited disease*, 8th edition, vol. II, pp. 3323–67. McGraw-Hill, New York. [Comprehensive review.]

Danpure CJ (2009). Oxalate and primary hyperoxaluria. In: O'Brien PJ, Bruce WR (eds). *Endogenous toxins: targets for disease treatment and prevention*. **11**, 269–290. Wiley [Review of PH in the context of oxalate toxicity.]

Danpure CJ, Jennings PR (1986). Peroxisomal alanine:glyoxylate aminotransferase deficiency in primary hyperoxaluria type I. *FEBS Lett*, **201**, 20–4. [First report of the basic enzyme deficiency in PH1.]

Danpure CJ, Rumsby G (1996). Strategies for the prenatal diagnosis of primary hyperoxaluria type 1. *Prenat Diagn*, **16**, 587–98. [Review of different approaches to the prenatal diagnosis of PH1.]

Danpure CJ, *et al.* (1989). An enzyme trafficking defect in two patients with primary hyperoxaluria type 1: peroxisomal alanine:glyoxylate aminotransferase re-routed to mitochondria. *J Cell Biol*, **108**, 1345–52. [First report of AGT protein trafficking defect in PH1.]

Hoppe B, Beck BB, Milliner DS (2009). The primary hyperoxalurias. *Kidney Int*, **75**, 1264–71. [Up to date review of the clinical aspects of PH.]

Lumb MJ, Birdsey GM, Danpure CJ (2003). Correction of an enzyme trafficking defect in hereditary kidney stone disease in vitro. *Biochem J*, **374**, 79–87. [Correction in vitro of AGT trafficking defect by protein stabilization.]

Lumb MJ, Danpure CJ (2000). Functional synergism between the most common polymorphism in human alanine:glyoxylate aminotransferase and four of the most common disease-causing mutations. *J Biol Chem*, **275**, 36415–22. [Demonstration of mutation-polymorphism interaction in AGT in PH1.]

Monico CG, Milliner DS (2001). Combined liver-kidney and kidney-alone transplantation in primary hyperoxaluria. *Liver Transpl*, **7**, 954–63. [Discussion of the relative merits of liver-kidney and kidney transplantation.]

Monico CG, Rossetti S, Olson JB, Milliner DS (2005). Pyridoxine effect in type I primary hyperoxaluria is associated with the most common mutant allele. *Kidney Int*, **67**, 1704–9. [Report of the relationship between pyridoxine responsiveness in primary hyperoxaluria type 1 patients and the AGT mistargeting mutation Gly170Arg.].

National Center for Biotechnology Information. *Online Mendelian Inheritance in Man (OMIN)*. Main web page: http://www.ncbi.nlm.nih.gov/entrez/query.fcgi?db=OMIM; Primary hyperoxaluria type 1 web page: http://www.ncbi.nlm.nih.gov/entrez/dispomim.cgi?id=259900; Primary hyperoxaluria type 2 web page: http://www.ncbi.nlm.nih.gov/entrez/dispomim.cgi?id=260000.

Purdue PE, Takada Y, Danpure CJ (1990). Identification of mutations associated with peroxisome-to-mitochondrion mistargeting of alanine:glyoxylate aminotransferase in PH1. *J Cell Biol*, **111**, 2341–51. [Identification of first mutations in AGT in PH1.]

Purdue PE, *et al.* (1991). Characterization and chromosomal mapping of a genomic clone encoding human alanine: glyoxylate aminotransferase. *Genomics*, **10**, 34–42. [First cloning of human AGT genomic DNA and identification of intron–exon boundaries.]

Rumsby G, Cregeen D (1999). Identification and expression of a cDNA for human hydroxypyruvate/glyoxylate reductase. *Biochim Biophys Acta*, **1446**, 383–8. [First cloning of human GRHPR cDNA.]

Salido EC, *et al.* (2006). Alanine-glyoxylate aminotransferase-deficient mice, a model for primary hyperoxaluria that responds to adenoviral gene transfer. *Proc Natl Acad Sci USA*, **103**, 18249–54. [Retrovial gene therapy in a mouse AGT knockout model.]

Santana A, *et al.* (2003). Primary hyperoxaluria type 1 in the Canary Islands: a conformational disease due to I244T mutation in the P11L-containing alanine:glyoxylate aminotransferase. *Proc Natl Acad Sci USA*, **100**, 7277–82. [Correction in vitro of mutation-induced AGT aggregation.]

Takada Y, *et al.* (1990). Human peroxisomal L-alanine:glyoxylate aminotransferase. Evolutionary loss of a mitochondrial targeting signal by point mutation of the initiation codon. *Biochem J*, **268**, 517–20. [First cloning of the human AGT cDNA.]

Watts RW, *et al.* (1987). Successful treatment of primary hyperoxaluria type 1 by combined hepatic and renal transplantation. *Lancet*, **2**, 474–5. [First successful hepatorenal transplantation in PH1.]

Williams HE, Smith LH Jr (1968). L-glyceric aciduria. A new genetic variant of primary hyperoxaluria. *N Engl J Med*, **278**, 233–8. [First report of the basic enzyme deficiency in PH2.]

Zhang X, *et al.* (2003). Crystal structure of alanine:glyoxylate aminotransferase and the relationship between genotype and enzymatic phenotype in primary hyperoxaluria type 1. *J Mol Biol*, **331**, 643–52. [First reported crystal structure of human AGT.]

12.11

Disturbances of acid–base homeostasis

R.D. Cohen and H.F. Woods

Essentials

Acid–base physiology and terminology

Despite a daily load of protons, derived mainly from metabolism, the hydrogen ion concentration of arterial blood in health is tightly maintained within a slightly alkaline range (pH 7.36–7.42); concentrations of intracellular hydrogen ions are also controlled. Failure adequately to excrete or neutralize protons causes acidic conditions to prevail (decreased pH): undue intake of base, uncompensated loss of protons—or the substrates from which they are derived—induces an alkaline milieu (raised pH).

The term acidosis refers to the pathological reduction of pH, also to the circumstance when pH would have been decreased were it not for the occurrence of compensatory mechanisms; an equivalent but reciprocal definition applies to alkalosis.

In health, the principal source of protons is CO_2, which originates from aerobic metabolism, is volatile and thus eliminated readily by the lungs. Lesser contributions come from urea synthesis and the generation of lactate and other organic anions such as 3-hydroxybutyrate and acetoacetate, which are eliminated by metabolism in the liver, kidneys and other tissues. Less than 1% of the proton burden is derived from the breakdown of sulphur- and phosphorus-containing molecules; these are ultimately converted to non-volatile sulphuric and phosphoric acids, which are excreted exclusively by the kidneys.

The body has limited capacity to offset rapid changes in pH by using extracellular and intracellular buffers, which are chiefly proteins (e.g. haemoglobin) or bicarbonate and phosphate ions. Acid–base buffering allows decompensation to be avoided transiently, but the proton burden must in the end be eliminated.

When the primary acid–base disorder is related to abnormal CO_2 elimination, it is termed 'respiratory'. All other primary disturbances of acid production or elimination are 'metabolic'. Primary processes are to be distinguished from those that are compensatory, which are termed 'secondary', e.g. secondary respiratory alkalosis as a compensatory mechanism for primary metabolic acidosis.

Clinical aspects of acid–base disturbances

Disturbances of acid–base balance have major effects on the body, including respiration, consciousness, cardiac function (acidosis decreases cardiac contractility and alkalosis has a small opposite effect, with both conditions predisposing to cardiac arrhythmia), renal function, and drug metabolism (Moviat, 2008). Potassium homeostasis is critically affected, with hypokalaemia a usual association of metabolic alkalosis and hyperkalaemia of metabolic acidosis.

Primary acid–base syndromes—these include: (1) respiratory acidosis due to respiratory failure; (2) metabolic acidosis due to diabetic ketoacidosis, lactic acidosis from multiple causes, renal acidosis, and poisoning by agents such as salicylate and methanol; (3) respiratory alkalosis due to hyperventilation; and (4) metabolic alkalosis due to the use of potassium-losing diuretics and persistent severe vomiting.

Arterial blood gas analysis—clinical evaluation cannot determine arterial pH, $Paco_2$, and bicarbonate concentration. Sampling of arterial blood is required. Blood gas analysers measure pH and Pco_2 directly, and calculate plasma bicarbonate. They also generally provide at least two other derived acid–base variables that are attempts to provide a measurement independent of respiratory disturbance and thus indicative of any underlying pure metabolic disturbance: (1) standard bicarbonate, which represents what the plasma bicarbonate would be if the blood had the normal $Paco_2$ of 5.33 kPa (40 mmHg) rather than its actual value; and (2) base excess or deficit, which is the amount of alkali in mmol needed to restore the pH of 1 litre of the patient's blood *in vitro* to normal (pH 7.4) at a Pco_2 of 5.33 kPa. An acid–base diagram is recommended for interpreting the results. Plasma urea, creatinine, sodium, potassium, and chloride, and—when appropriate—lactate, ketoacid, and salicylate concentrations are useful.

Anion gap—the sum of the concentrations of plasma cations (Na^+ and K–) normally exceeds that of the anions (Cl^- and HCO_3^-). This so-called anion gap (range 10–18 mmol/litre) is usually attributable to the net negative charge on plasma proteins, phosphate, sulphate, and organic acids. Metabolic acidoses may have a high or normal anion gap. Those with a high anion gap are due to the ingestion or endogenous generation of acids, usually organic, whose anions are not routinely measured in plasma. Calculation of the anion gap is therefore valuable for diagnosis of metabolic acidosis, but the regre ttable practice of omitting chloride estimations frequently prevents its application.

Management—the mainstay of treatment of acid–base disorders is to eliminate the cause, with restoration of acid–base balance occurring in due course as physiological control mechanisms are able to compensate. It may occasionally be necessary to restore or partly restore normal acid–base status directly, but some interventions of this kind, e.g. infusion of bicarbonate solutions in metabolic acidosis, remain controversial.

Acid–base homeostasis

In resting humans, arterial blood pH (pHa) is normally maintained between 7.36 and 7.42 by controlling the arterial partial pressure of CO_2 ($Pa\text{CO}_2$) and plasma bicarbonate (HCO_3^-) between the limits 4.7 to 5.8 kPa and 24 to 30 mmol/litre, respectively. Intracellular pH is also controlled, but varies substantially between organs within the range 6.3 to 7.4, depending on the prevailing physiological or pathological circumstances. Some intracellular organelles are particularly acid, notably lysosomes. There is a substantial daily burden of hydrogen ions (protons) derived principally from metabolism (Table 12.11.1), and disordered neutralization or elimination of this burden shifts pH in the acid direction. Inappropriate loss of protons or proton-generating substrates, or excessive input of alkali, shifts pH in the alkaline direction.

Extra- and intracellular buffers, notably haemoglobin, other proteins, bicarbonate, and phosphate, play a transient role in countering acute pH changes, but normally the acid burdens listed in Table 12.11.1 are ultimately eliminated quantitatively or neutralized. These burdens have been grouped into three classes according to their mode of disposal. CO_2 derived from cellular respiration is much the largest potential generator of protons, the burden in the resting subject being an order of magnitude greater than that resulting from lactic and other organic acid production as well as from urea synthesis. Protons derived from the metabolism of sulphur- and phosphorus-containing compounds constitute the smallest source and represent a burden that is around 1% that derived from CO_2. Disposal of CO_2 is dependent on adequate respiratory function. The metabolism of sulphur-containing amino acids in the diet eventually results in the production of so-called 'fixed acids', namely sulphuric acid and phosphoric acid, which may originate from many sources. Neither of these acids is volatile and they are thus excreted by the kidney.

The organic acids listed in Table 12.11.1 have pK values much below that of blood pH. They are therefore present in the blood as acid anions, rather than as the undissociated acids. The equivalent amount of hydrogen ions, generated at the site of production of these acids, titrate with local tissue and blood bicarbonate, and with other buffers. The organic acid anions (lactate, 3-hydroxybutyrate, acetoacetate, and fatty acids) are nonvolatile but, unlike the fixed acids, may be eliminated by metabolism. Figure 12.11.1 shows an example of the important principle that when these organic acid anions are metabolized to electroneutral products (e.g. glucose, or CO_2 and water) protons are consumed and the bicarbonate consumed at their site of production is regenerated. Protons from organic acids can also be eliminated in the urine, but normally this is a much slower process than the metabolic route. Particularly in the case of the ketone bodies, for which the renal threshold is relatively low, substantial amounts can be lost in the urine when their plasma concentration is elevated. Although in maximally acidified urine (pH 4.5) about half of the urinary ketone bodies are in the form of the undissociated acid, the remaining free anion moiety represents loss of potential alkali, since it eludes metabolism to bicarbonate.

Despite the large quantitative differences in the burden due to the three classes of acid shown in Fig. 12.11.1, their correct elimination is, in a sense, equally important, for no class is able substantially to be disposed of by a route normally used to eliminate another class. Normally, the rates of production and elimination of each class of acid are matched in a long-term steady state. The homeostasis of

Table 12.11.1 Production and elimination of hydrogen ions

Class	Daily production (mol)	Source	Excreted by lungs	Metabolic removal possible	Normal main organs of elimination
I CO_2	15	Tissue	Yes	Very minor	Lungs
II Organic acids and urea synthesis					
Lactate	1.2	Many tissues	No	Yes	Liver (50–70%), kidneys
Ketoacids[a]	0.6	Liver	No	Yes	Most tissues, urine
Free fatty acids	0.7	Adipose tissue	No	Yes	Most tissues
H^+ generated during urea synthesis	1.1[b]	Liver	No	Yes	Liver and other tissues
III Fixed acids					
Sulphuric		Dietary sulphur-containing amino acids	No	No	
	} 0.1				} Urinary excretion
Phosphoric		Organic phosphate metabolism	No	No	

The daily production rates for the organic acids are calculated from data in resting 70-kg men after an overnight fast, and are proportioned up to 24 h.

[a] Because of food ingestion during the daytime, the values for the ketoacids (3-hydroxybutyric and acetoacetic) may be overestimates.

[b] On a 100 g protein diet.

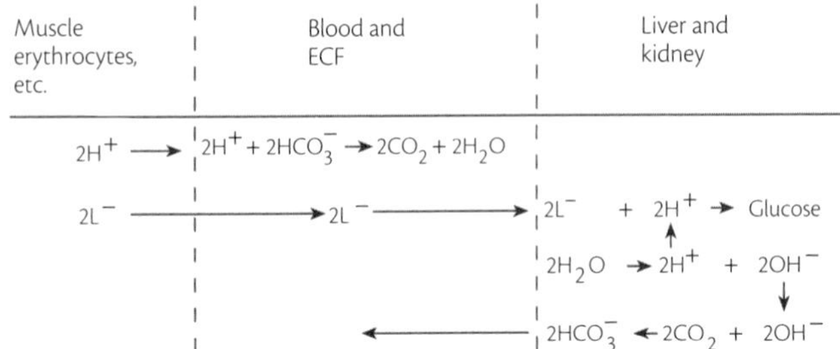

Fig. 12.11.1 A scheme, using L-lactate conversion to glucose as an example, showing how conversion of the anion of an organic acid of low pK to an electroneutral substance consumes H^+ and regenerates HCO_3^-.

arterial blood pH thus provided is given quantitative expression in the Henderson–Hasselbalch equation:

$$pHa = 6.1 + \log_{10}\{[HCO_3^-]_a/(0.225 \times Paco_2)\}$$

The constancy of arterial plasma bicarbonate concentration ($[HCO_3^-]_a$) is maintained by the removal of class I and II acids and by proton generation during ureagenesis (see below) and that of *Paco*$_2$ by the lungs, thereby fixing pHa within a narrow range.

Roles of the kidneys and liver in acid–base homeostasis

The interplay of these organs in acid–base homeostasis has been a matter of controversy. The authors' view is that the contribution of the kidneys is not entirely what it has appeared to be, and that the role of the liver requires emphasis. Classical descriptions are based on the kidneys as the principal controllers of $[HCO_3^-]$. Yet, as may be seen in Table 12.11.1, the liver is responsible for the major part of lactate disposal and consequent bicarbonate regeneration as well as the generation of keto acids, with the opposite acid–base consequence. There is, however, evidence that both these hepatic functions are normally controlled in an attempt to preserve acid–base homeostasis. Thus at normal concentrations of blood lactate, deviations in the acid direction enhance hepatic lactate disposal. As will be seen in the case of lactate, the homeostasis may be lost at higher concentrations of lactate. Ketogenesis is itself suppressed by increasing acidosis.

Urea production is another important feature of hepatic metabolism. The production of each molecule of urea (ultimately from NH_4^+ and CO_2) is accompanied by the generation of two protons. Ureagenesis is therefore a potential acidifying mechanism. Most of the protons produced in ureagenesis are neutralized by the bicarbonate generated during the oxidation of the carbon skeleton of amino acids, but normally there is a slight excess of protons produced, which have to be eliminated by the kidneys. Urea synthesis and accompanying proton production are negatively regulated by acidosis, which constitutes another acid–base regulatory system intrinsic to the liver.

The renal tubules secrete protons and those not involved in the process of bicarbonate reabsorption are buffered by urinary phosphate. Under normal conditions, about 30 mmol/day of protons are excreted in this way. Classically, urinary ammonia (NH_3) is regarded as another buffer for hydrogen ions, which are therefore removed as NH_4^+. Normally, the excretion of hydrogen ions in the supposed NH_4^+ buffer amounts to about 70 mmol/day, but may increase to 500 mmol/day under severe acidifying stress in maximally acidified urine. It is, however, not possible to reconcile this view with the physicochemical fact that the NH_3/NH_4^+ equilibrium is almost entirely in the form of NH_4^+ at the time of generation from glutamine and is therefore not available for buffering further protons. A more plausible explanation of the role of the kidneys is that the increase in NH_4^+excretion during acidosis serves to divert nitrogen from hepatic urea synthesis and consequent proton production, thus countering the acidosis.

These considerations provide a background to the interpretation of many acid–base syndromes described below.

Acid–base disorders

Definitions

The terminology of acid–base disturbances has always been confused. The terms acidaemia and alkalaemia simply indicate that pHa is lower or higher than the normal range. Here we use the term acidosis to encompass both the situation where pHa is low and also that in which, although pHa is normal, it would have been lowered if compensatory mechanisms had not occurred; an equivalent definition applies to alkalosis. When the primary disturbance is related to abnormal CO_2 elimination, the disturbance is referred to as 'respiratory'. All other primary disturbances, that is those related to disturbances of class II or III acid production or removal, are referred to as 'metabolic' or 'nonrespiratory'. The term 'primary' is used to distinguish these processes from those which are compensatory in nature. Thus primary metabolic acidosis (lowering $[HCO_3^-]_a$) is compensated for by hyperventilation, which decreases *Paco*$_2$. Respiratory acidosis (elevation of *Paco*$_2$) is compensated for by metabolic events that result in an elevation of $[HCO_3^-]_a$.

Diagnosis of acid–base disturbances

Since the clinical manifestations of acid–base disturbances, described later, are frequently nonspecific and may not be apparent until the disturbance is quite severe, laboratory investigation, though a method has been published for converting venous values to arterial values (Toftegaard *et al.*, 2009), is indispensable. Measurement of pHa, *Paco*$_2$, and $[HCO_3^-]_a$ on arterial blood is the primary investigation. Estimation of plasma urea, creatinine, sodium, potassium, and chloride, and, when appropriate, lactate, keto acids, and salicylate provides further important information. Adrogué *et al.* (2009) present a common-sense and practical critique of the many proposed schemes for diagnosis of acid-base disorders.

Measurement of pHa and Paco$_2$: Paco$_2$ acid–base diagram

Blood gas analysers measure pH and *Paco*$_2$ and calculate plasma bicarbonate from the Henderson–Hasselbalch equation. Interpretation of results is best achieved by the use of an acid–base diagram that has pHa and *Paco*$_2$as its axes. Diagrams that use $[HCO_3^-]_a$ on one of the axes are less suitable, since $[HCO_3^-]_a$ is calculated from pHa and *Paco*$_2$ and is not only subject to compounding errors in those measurements, but is affected by some poorly understood variations in pK_a in the Henderson–Hasselbalch equation in blood from severely ill patients.

The acid–base diagram in Fig. 12.11.2 has bands drawn to show the ranges of data expected in uncomplicated acid–base disorders. It not only aids the diagnosis of acid–base disorders, but, in addition, the course of an individual patient's disturbance and the response to treatment can be followed by serial plotting of data. The shaded

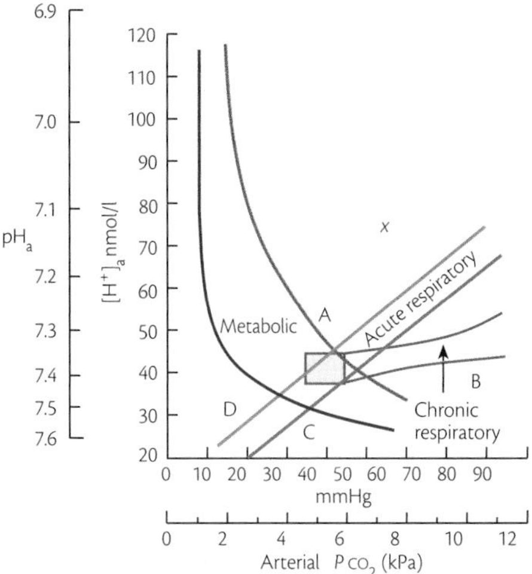

Fig. 12.11.2 A practical acid–base diagram. The band marked 'acute respiratory' is the 95% confidence range of values obtained in normal individuals voluntarily hyperventilating or breathing air/CO_2 mixtures for short periods. After a few days of CO_2 retention, an increase in plasma HCO_3^- produces substantial or complete compensation for the respiratory acidosis; the band in chronic respiratory acidosis is therefore different from the acute response, the presence of the extra HCO_3^- decreasing the fall in pHa expected for a given rise in $Paco_2$.

rectangle represents the approximate limits of pHa and $Paco_2$ in normal individuals. Thus a patient with uncomplicated metabolic acidosis will have values lying in the band marked 'metabolic' in the region above and to the left of the normal zone; the metabolic band is the envelope of measurements of pHa and $Paco_2$ in patients with uncomplicated metabolic acidosis and alkalosis. The metabolic band is rather restricted on the alkalotic side, below and to the right of the normal zone. This is because compensation by hypoventilation for metabolic alkalosis is often poor; hypoxia may limit the degree of hypoventilation and metabolic alkaloses may be associated with intracellular acidosis, which could stimulate the respiratory centre. Marked hypocapnia is, however, occasionally seen in metabolic alkalosis.

In some patients pHa and $Paco_2$ measurements will not fall within any of the defined bands in Fig. 12.11.2. Such patients have a mixture of acid–base disorders. Thus a patient whose pHa and $Paco_2$ are represented by the point marked 'x' on the figure has mixed respiratory and metabolic acidosis, e.g. a patient with uraemic acidosis and an exacerbation of chronic bronchitis with respiratory failure. Values of pHa and $Paco_2$ lying in sectors A and C result from a combination of two primary acid–base conditions; in sectors B and D one of the two disturbances might be compensatory for the other.

Acid–base analytical equipment usually also provides at least two additional derived acid–base variables—the standard bicarbonate and the base excess or deficit. The standard bicarbonate represents what the plasma bicarbonate would be if the blood had the normal $Paco_2$ of 5.33 kPa (40 mmHg) rather than its actual value. Standard bicarbonate was introduced in an attempt to provide a measurement which was independent of respiratory disturbance and thus indicative of the underlying pure metabolic disturbance. Base deficit represents the amount of alkali in mmol needed to restore the pH of 1 litre of the patient's blood *in vitro* to normal (pH 7.4) at a Pco_2 of 5.33 kPa, and might, at first sight, be considered a quantitative measure of metabolic acidosis. Unfortunately, the titration curve of blood *in vitro* is different from that of blood circulating *in vivo*, since in the latter situation the interstitial and intracellular fluids also interact in the titration and may gain or lose bicarbonate from it; in addition, their buffering capacity differs from that of blood. These considerations detract from the usefulness of base excess or deficit as a guide either to diagnosis or therapy.

Further difficulties arise from ambiguities in the interpretation of base excess or deficit. Thus a patient with chronic respiratory acidosis will have a high standard bicarbonate and a base excess due to the compensatory increase of plasma bicarbonate. It could be said, therefore, that this patient has simultaneously a respiratory acidosis and a metabolic alkalosis, as a base excess indicates the latter. This way of regarding the situation seems to us confusing and is incompatible with the definitions of acidosis and alkalosis we have given, which are intended to indicate the direction of the primary disturbance.

Use of the anion gap

In measurements of plasma electrolytes, the sum of the cations ($Na^+ + K^+$) normally exceeds that of the anions ($Cl^- + HCO_3^-$) by about 14 mmol/litre (reference range 10–18mmol/litre). This difference is known as the anion gap and in health is attributable largely to the net negative charge on plasma proteins, but also to phosphate, sulphate, and several organic acids. Calculation of the anion gap is of great value in the differential diagnosis of metabolic acidosis, but the (regrettably increasingly common) practice of omitting chloride estimation from sets of plasma electrolytes frequently deprives the clinician of this important diagnostic tool.

Metabolic acidoses may be divided broadly into those with a high anion gap and those with a normal anion gap. Metabolic acidoses with a high anion gap are due to the ingestion or endogenous generation of acids, usually organic, whose anions are not measured in routine sets of plasma electrolytes. Plasma bicarbonate is titrated by these acids and therefore decreases; the anion gap is thus widened by the presence of these unmeasured anions. The most frequent organic acids concerned are lactic acid and keto acids. In uremic acidosis the anion gap seldom exceeds 28 mmol/litre, but considerably higher values may be found in severe lactic acidosis and ketoacidosis. It should be noted that there are causes of raised anion gap other than metabolic acidosis, e.g. therapy with sodium salts of relatively strong acids (e.g. lactate, acetate) and high-dose sodium carbenicillin treatment.

Metabolic acidoses with a normal anion gap are due to the direct loss of bicarbonate from the body, either through the gut or fistulae or through the kidney, or, rarely, as a result of the ingestion or infusion of acid or acidifying substances. When bicarbonate is lost more chloride is retained by the renal tubules; thus low plasma bicarbonate is accompanied by hyperchloraemia and the anion gap remains unchanged.

Caution should be exercised in interpreting the anion gap in the presence of substantial paraproteinaemia, because of the uncertain charge on the abnormal protein. Hypoalbuminaemia may lead to underestimation of the true anion gap, since the anion gap is largely due to the negative charge of albumin.

Causes of acid–base disturbance

Table 12.11.2 classifies those conditions associated with high anion gap metabolic acidosis by the principal organic acid involved. Often a mixture of acids is involved but, where possible, the predominant acid has been shown in italics.

Table 12.11.2 High anion gap metabolic acidoses

Condition	Associated plasma anions[a]
Predominant ketoacidosis	
Diabetic ketoacidosis	*3-hydroxybutyrate*, acetoacetate, lactate
Starvation ketoacidosis	*3-hydroxybutyrate*, acetoacetate
Alcoholic ketoacidosis	*3-hydroxybutyrate*, acetoacetate, lactate
Ketotic hypoglycaemia of childhood	*3-hydroxybutyrate*, acetoacetate, lactate
Predominant lactic acidosis	
Type A lactic acidosis	
Exercise	Lactate
Postepileptic	Lactate
Shock (traumatic, haemorrhagic, cardiogenic, septic)	Lactate
Severe hypoxia, including acute pulmonary oedema	Lactate
Type B lactic acidosis	
Biguanide-associated (phenformin, metformin, buformin)	Lactate
Ethanol-associated	Lactate
Following recovery from diabetic ketoacidosis	Lactate
Fructose, sorbitol, or xylitol infusion	Lactate
Severe falciparum malaria	Lactate
Fulminant hepatic necrosis, severe liver disease	Lactate
Leukaemia and reticuloses	Lactate
Paracetamol poisoning	Lactate
Associated with sodium nitroprusside therapy	Lactate
Thiamine deficiency, acute beriberi	Lactate
D(−)-lactic acidosis (short gut syndromes, jejunoileal bypass, *Lactobacillus* ingestion)	D(−)-lactate
Type 1 glycogenosis (hepatic glucose 6-phosphatase deficiency)	Lactate
Hepatic fructose-1,6-bisphosphatase deficiency	Lactate
Associated with mitochondrial myopathies and encephalomyopathies	Lactate
Treatment with nucleoside reverse transcriptase inhibitors	
Inherited syndromes, e.g. MELAS	
Inherited or acquired single or multiple carboxylase deficiencies	*Lactate*, other organic acid anions
Conditions with mixed or ill-defined source of acidosis	
Uraemic acidosis	Phosphate, sulphate, etc.
Salicylate poisoning (acidotic phase)	Salicylate, ketoacids, lactate
Methanol poisoning	Formate, lactate
Ethylene glycol poisoning	Lactate, glycolate, oxalate
Paraldehyde poisoning	Unknown
Reye's syndrome	Lactate (principally)
Jamaican vomiting sickness	Unknown
Numerous inherited organic acidurias	Various
Toluene toxicity	Benzoate, hippurate

[a] The predominant anion is shown in italics.
Except when otherwise stated, lactate refers to the L(+)-isomer.
MELAS, mitochondrial encephalopathy, lactic acidosis, and stroke-like episodes.

Normal anion gap metabolic acidoses are shown in Box 12.11.1, classified according to whether they are due to gut or renal bicarbonate loss, or to ingestion or infusion of acidifying agents.

Metabolic alkalosis is due either to the ingestion or infusion of excessive alkali in circumstances when it cannot be excreted (e.g. poor renal function), or to the secretion of urine that is inappropriate both in its acidity and in its NH_4^+ content (Box 12.11.2). Most of the causes of the latter occurrence are related to the complex events in potassium and chloride deficiency and are dealt with later, as is the pathogenesis of the metabolic alkalosis of acute hepatic failure.

In Box 12.11.3 the causes of respiratory acidosis are classified according to the level of the problem, namely, the lungs and airways, the neuromuscular and mechanical aspects of respiration, and the central nervous system.

Except in the case of deliberate or inadvertent external hyperventilation, respiratory alkalosis is always due to some form of stimulus to the respiratory centre, as classified in Box 12.11.4.

The effects of acid–base disturbances

These are widespread and we limit ourselves here to a brief description of those with known clinical consequences.

Respiratory effects

Both metabolic acidosis and acute respiratory acidosis induced by breathing high $P\text{CO}_2$ gas mixtures result in hyperventilation. Deep, sighing respiration (Kussmaul breathing) is a familiar sign of metabolic acidosis. pH control of ventilation is determined by the pH perceived by the carotid and aortic body chemoreceptors and by receptors in the medulla that appear to monitor the pH of brain extracellular fluid. In the steady state, brain extracellular fluid pH is closely similar to that of cerebrospinal fluid. Sudden development of metabolic acidosis, resulting in low pHa and arterial bicarbonate, induces hyperventilation by stimulating the carotid body and aortic chemoreceptors and $P\text{aCO}_2$ is thus lowered. However, the first effect on brain extracellular fluid pH is to raise it. This is because brain extracellular fluid $P\text{CO}_2$ is lowered since CO_2 is rapidly equilibrated across the blood–brain barrier. However, it takes many hours for the brain extracellular fluid bicarbonate to fall in response to the lowering of plasma bicarbonate because movement of bicarbonate across the barrier is much slower than that of CO_2. The temporary alkalinization of brain extracellular fluid somewhat offsets the extra ventilatory drive from the carotid and aortic chemoreceptors, so the hyperventilatory

Box 12.11.1 Metabolic acidoses with normal ion gap

Gastrointestinal bicarbonate loss

- Diarrhoea
- Pancreatic fistula
- Ureteroenterostomy

Renal causes

Renal tubular acidosis type 1 (gradient type)

- Primary

Transient infantile type
Permanent (childhood or adult)

- Secondary

Hypergammaglobulinaemia, amphotericin B therapy, autoimmune states
Vitamin D intoxication, hyperthyroidism, carnitine palmitoyl transferase I deficiency

Renal tubular acidosis type 2 (bicarbonate wastage)

- Primary

Isolated, idiopathic Fanconi's syndrome

- Secondary

Hyperthyroidism, vitamin D deficiency, outdated tetracycline, uraemia (occasionally), myeloma, Sjögren's syndrome, heavy metal poisoning
Hereditary disorders: cystinosis, Wilson's disease, fructose intolerance, galactosaemia, Lowe's syndrome
Treatment with carbonic anhydrase inhibitors

Renal tubular acidosis Type 4

- Hypoaldosteronism, aldosterone insensitivity, hyporeninaemia, diabetes mellitus, pyelonephritis, pseudohypoaldosteronism (types I and II), nonsteroidal anti-inflammatory agents, angiotensin converting enzyme inhibitors
- Moderate renal insufficiency

Ingestion or infusion of acidifying agents

- Ammonium chloride, arginine hydrochloride, hydrochloric acid, intravenous feeding with solutions containing excess basic amino acids
- Rapid intravenous hydration (dilutional acidosis)

compensatory response takes some hours to reach its maximum. Though clinical circumstances usually prevent the observation of this sequence of events, the opposite—persistence of hyperventilation after restoration of normal pH during therapy of metabolic acidosis—is commonly seen and may last for more than 24 h.

In chronic respiratory failure, with high $Paco_2$, direct depression of the respiratory centre occurs; the respiratory response to increments of $Paco_2$ is progressively lost and ventilation becomes increasingly dependent on hypoxic drive. Alkalosis also may depress respiration and increases the difficulties of weaning artificially ventilated patients from the respirator.

Box 12.11.2 Causes of metabolic alkalosis

- Ingestion or infusion of alkali in excess of excretion

Milk-alkali syndrome
Alkaline overshoot during therapy of lactic acidosis or diabetic ketoacidosis

- Inappropriate loss of acid (gastric or renal routes)

Pyloric stenosis, self-induced persistent vomiting
Potassium depletion other than in renal tubular acidosis or laxative abuse
Chloride depletion

Hyperaldosteronism (primary or secondary)

- Contraction alkalosis

Rapid diuresis
Other causes of mild extracellular fluid depletion

- Failure of ureagenesis
- Fulminant hepatic failure

Cardiovascular effects

Acidosis decreases cardiac contractility (negative inotropism) and alkalosis has smaller but opposite effects. Acidosis and alkalosis both predispose to cardiac arrhythmias. The negative inotropic effects are particularly related to changes in myocardial intracellular pH and are experimentally found to be rather greater in acute respiratory than in acute metabolic acidosis. In the rat, progressive metabolic acidosis reduces cardiac output as a result of bradycardia and negative inotropy; there is consequent hypotension and decreased renal and hepatic blood flow. This sequence of events may provide a model for the circulatory collapse that often occurs

Box 12.11.3 Causes of respiratory acidosis

- Structural and mechanical pulmonary disease

Chronic obstructive pulmonary disease
Severe asthma
Large airway obstruction

- Neuromuscular and mechanical problems

Acute ascending polyneuritis (Guillain–Barré syndrome)
Poliomyelitis
Acute porphyria
Myasthenia gravis
Motor neurone disease
Muscular dystrophies
Traumatic flail chest
Ankylosing spondylitis
Severe kyphoscoliosis
Gross obesity, sleep apnoea syndromes
Muscle relaxant drugs

- Respiratory centre disorders

Organic disease affecting the respiratory centre
Respiratory depressant drugs
Respiratory arrest

Box 12.11.4 Causes of respiratory alkalosis

- Spontaneous or psychogenic hyperventilation
- Reflex hyperventilation (e.g. pulmonary embolism)

Other stimuli to respiratory centre

- Via chemoreceptors:

  Low inspired oxygen concentration (e.g. high altitude)
  Alveolocapillary diffusion block (e.g. fibrosing alveolitis)
  Right-to-left shunt
  Carbon monoxide poisoning

- Via drugs or metabolites:

  Salicylate poisoning
  Acute liver failure, chronic liver disease
  Persistent hyperventilation after recovery from metabolic acidosis
  Local lesion affecting respiratory centre

- Overventilation during anaesthesia or assisted ventilation

in patients after some hours of metabolic acidosis not originally attributable to shock. Mild-to-moderate metabolic acidosis has not often been associated with negative inotropic effects in the intact animal; this appears to be due to the protective effects of catecholamine release, which is increased in acidosis. In more severe acidosis, this protection breaks down. Patients receiving β-blockers may be more susceptible to the negative inotropic effects of acidosis.

Cerebral arterioles are very sensitive to the pH of brain extracellular fluid; they dilate when this falls and constrict when the pH rises. The cerebrovascular resistance is thus subject to the same type of phased responses to acid–base disturbances as described above for ventilation. Dilatation is also the response of most systemic arterioles to acidosis, although this response may be modified by catecholamine effects. The peripheral veins, however, constrict in acidosis, resulting in a shift of blood from the peripheral capacitance vessels to the central circulation. This effect has been shown to have important clinical consequences during treatment (see below) (Celloto, 2008).

Effects on the endocrine system

Chronic metabolic acidosis decreases growth hormone secretion and the response of insulin-like growth factor 1 (IGF-1) secretion to growth hormone. The sensitivity of parathyroid hormone secretion to changes in plasma calcium is reduced, as is the activation of vitamin D. In view of this it is perhaps surprising that both acute metabolic and respiratory alkalosis also lower plasma parathyroid hormone concentrations (in dogs). Insulin-mediated glucose metabolism is also decreased. Plasma thyroxine and triiodothyronine levels are decreased and plasma thyroid-stimulating hormone is elevated.

Effects on intermediary carbohydrate metabolism

In all tissues in which observations have been made, glycolysis is inhibited by acidosis and stimulated by alkalosis because of the effect of intracellular pH on phosphofructokinase, a rate-limiting enzyme of glycolysis. Respiratory alkalosis might therefore be expected to raise blood lactate, but this effect is usually small, probably due to removal of lactate by the liver. However, in the presence of severe liver disease, gross elevation of blood lactate may be seen in association with respiratory alkalosis, and the increased production of protons with lactate may partially compensate for the alkalosis.

Animal studies have shown that hepatic gluconeogenesis from lactate is inhibited by acidosis because of an effect on the metabolic step between pyruvate and oxaloacetate. This phenomenon may override the stimulatory effect on hepatic lactate disposal described earlier, and may be responsible for perpetuating and worsening lactic acidosis.

Effects on nitrogen balance

Chronic acidosis produces negative nitrogen balance, mainly due to accelerated proteolysis by the enzyme caspase-3 in skeletal muscle. There is also increased expression of the genes coding for ubiquitin and proteasome subunits. Ubiquitin is a small protein that binds fragments of actin and myosin and targets them for internalization into proteosomes, organelles which further degrade the protein into small peptides. Treatment with alkali reverses this process. Metabolic acidosis leads to the development of insulin resistance, including blunting of the protein-anabolic effect of insulin on skeletal muscle. This effect may be partly mediated by stimulation of branched chain keto-acid dehydrogenase, thus depleting the tissue of leucine, isoleucine, and valine.

Effects on blood oxygen uptake and delivery to the tissues

One of the factors determining the uptake of oxygen by blood during passage through the lungs, and the subsequent delivery of oxygen to the tissues, is the position of the blood-oxygen dissociation curve with respect to the abscissa (Po_2). Right shifts of this curve improve the unloading of oxygen in the tissues, but under some circumstances may impair oxygen uptake in the lungs. Left shifts have the opposite effect. The position of the curve is determined by three haemoglobin ligands, namely hydrogen ions, CO_2, and 2,3-bisphosphoglycerate. Increases in any of these shift the curve to the right. Changes in intraerythrocytic pH and Pco_2 are often rapid, but those of 2,3-bisphosphoglycerate are much slower. In chronic acidosis, the synthesis of 2,3-bisphosphoglycerate is inhibited and marked reductions in the erythrocyte content of this metabolite may occur, with opposite effects in alkalosis. These changes are, however, slow in comparison with the immediate effects of changes in pH and Pco_2 (the Bohr effect).

The effect of these differences in time scale on oxygen delivery gives rise to a characteristic sequence of events during the development and treatment of acute metabolic acidosis. Initially, the acute acidosis causes a right shift of the curve, and thus improved oxygen release to the tissues. After several hours erythrocyte 2,3-bisphosphoglycerate falls, thus restoring the position of the curve towards normal. If the patient is now rapidly treated with alkali, the Bohr effect results in rapid shift to a position to the left of normal because of the low level of 2,3-bisphosphoglycerate. The resulting sudden deterioration of oxygen release may have adverse clinical effects unless the consequences of left shift are ameliorated by other factors, such as an increase in tissue blood flow. It may be many hours or days before erythrocyte 2,3-bisphosphoglycerate concentration is restored to normal.

Effects on the nervous system

Severe acidosis is frequently associated with impairment of consciousness, varying from mild drowsiness to coma. This effect is not closely related to systemic pH, and the mechanism is poorly understood. The effects on the respiratory and cardiovascular centres have been discussed above. The excitability of neural and muscular tissues is increased by alkalosis and diminished by acidosis. Tetany is a common feature of respiratory alkalosis, and may also be seen when chronic metabolic acidosis is corrected in patients with hypocalcaemia, a sequence of events that may occur in chronic renal failure. Epileptic attacks in susceptible individuals may be precipitated by alkalosis and suppressed by acidosis.

Effects on potassium homeostasis

Acute acidosis results in a shift of potassium out of the intracellular compartment into the extracellular fluid. Hyperkalaemia is thus often seen in the acidosis of renal failure, untreated diabetic ketoacidosis, and in acute respiratory failure. Its mechanism is not entirely clear, factors other than extracellular pH being implicated. Alkali therapy in such patients causes a shift of potassium back into cells. As substantial amounts of potassium may be lost in the urine during the period of hyperkalaemia, overall depletion of body potassium occurs; thus alkali therapy may result in a rapid fall of plasma potassium to dangerous levels. This is a well-known hazard in the treatment of diabetic ketoacidosis and is even more dangerous in types 1 and 2 renal tubular acidosis, in which plasma potassium is frequently low in the presence of acidosis (see also under 'Treatment' below).

Chronic metabolic alkalosis is also frequently accompanied by potassium depletion, which results from distal tubular potassium secretion uninhibited by competition with hydrogen ions for secretion.

Effects on the kidney

The kidney is a major organ of acid–base regulation and many of its responses are therefore geared to acid–base homeostasis. Proton secretion is a principal function of tubular cells and in the proximal tubule is a crucial part of the mechanism for the apparent reabsorption of the large quantities of bicarbonate filtered at the glomerulus. In the cortical and medullary collecting tubules, where the main acidification of the urine takes place, the α-intercalated cell is equipped with an H^+ ATPase residing in the apical (luminal) membrane and a band 3 general anion exchanger in the basolateral membrane. The β-intercalated cell has the opposite polarity in respect of the H^+ ATPase and the anion exchanger. In acidotic conditions β-intercalated cells are converted into α-cells, a process mediated by the extracellular protein hensin. Under acid conditions, protons and bicarbonate are generated by carbonic anhydrase within these intercalated cells. The protons are secreted into the lumen, where they titrate the phosphate buffer or convert any bicarbonate still present into CO_2 and water; the bicarbonate is transported by the anion exchanger in the opposite direction into the bloodstream. Under alkaline conditions the maximum urinary pH which can be achieved is about 8.0, whereas in acid conditions the minimum urinary pH attainable is in the range 4.5 to 5.3.

As indicated earlier, there is a large increase in renal NH_4^+ production and excretion in the urine in acidosis. The NH_4^+ ions are derived from glutamine by the action of glutaminase in the proximal tubule; they are mainly secreted by pH-dependent nonionic diffusion into the collecting tubule lumen, where the blood–lumen pH gradient is the greatest in acidosis. Chronic acidosis results in an increased expression of the proximal tubule glutamine transporter and of glutaminase and phosphoenolpyruvate carboxykinase. The latter enzyme is rate-limiting for gluconeogenesis, and an increase in renal gluconeogenesis is thought to play a crucial role in the high rate of NH_4^+ production. A reinterpretation of the role of increased NH_4^+ excretion in acidosis has been discussed above.

Effects on the distribution of metabolites and drugs

Many weak acids and bases are distributed between body compartments by the simple physicochemical process of pH-dependent nonionic diffusion, which is based on movement of the non-dissociated hydrophobic moiety across the lipid membranes separating compartments, quite independently of any transporter. The pH differences between the compartments will determine the relative concentrations in the two spaces at equilibrium. Weak acids accumulate in the more alkaline compartment and weak alkalis in the more acid compartment. Examples of physiological metabolites distributed by this mechanism include NH_3/NH_4^+ (weak base) and urobilinogen (weak acid). The distribution between blood and cerebrospinal fluid of NH_4^+ and other amines present in advanced liver disease is partly determined in this way. Examples of drugs exhibiting this behaviour are salicylates and phenobarbitone (weak acids); use of their pH-dependent distribution is made in the treatment of poisoning with these drugs by forced alkaline diuresis.

Effects on bone

Bone acts as a buffer in chronic metabolic acidosis. The leaching out of bone calcium carbonate and the exchange of extracellular phosphate for carbonate within the apatite crystal result in the neutralization of protons. Metabolic acidosis also inhibits osteoblast function. These mechanisms cause a negative calcium balance in chronic metabolic acidosis, and in chronic uraemic acidotic subjects it has been shown that calcium balance can be restored by treatment with sodium bicarbonate. Although chronic metabolic acidosis in rats results in osteoporosis, renal tubular acidosis and the acidosis associated with ureterosigmoidostomy may lead to osteomalacia, which can be corrected by alkali therapy alone.

Effects on inflammatory cytokines

In animals with experimental septic shock, metabolic acidosis results in greater increases in blood levels of inflammatory cytokines such as tumour necrosis factor-α (TNFα) and interleukins 6 and 10, than seen in nonacidotic animals.

Effects on leucocytes

Severe acidosis is often associated with marked leucocytosis, unrelated to the presence of infection. Blood leucocyte counts of up to 60×10^9/litre have been recorded in lactic acidosis, and high values are also common in diabetic ketoacidosis. This phenomenon may be partly a specific reaction to acidosis and not merely a general manifestation of stress, dehydration or infection.

Major acid–base syndromes

Lactic acidosis

In normal resting individuals, venous blood lactate concentration is in the range 0.6 to 1.0 mmol/litre. In extreme exercise this may rise to 20 mmol/litre or more. Lactate is the end product of anaerobic glycolysis. Its production by many tissues, even at rest, is accompanied by equal amounts of protons, since its pK is low (3.8) and the undissociated acid is therefore present only in minute amounts. These protons react with blood and tissue bicarbonate to form CO_2 and water, but the lost bicarbonate is quantitatively restored when the lactate is converted to glucose (see Fig. 12.11.1), mainly in the liver, or oxidized in many tissues to CO_2 and water. When lactate is produced at a rate which exceeds the disposal rate, the regeneration of bicarbonate is incomplete and acidosis results. The pathological mechanisms leading to lactic acidosis are therefore excess production, defective disposal, or commonly, a mixture of both. As the acidosis develops, hepatic disposal of lactate by gluconeogenesis may become further inhibited (see above), leading to a cycle which provides a model for the often fulminating course of lactic acidosis.

Clinically, lactic acidosis falls into two main categories. In type A lactic acidosis, much the more common, there is clinical evidence of shock, poor tissue perfusion, or hypoxia. Though increased peripheral glycolysis is an important contributor, associated poor hepatic and renal perfusion limit the lactate disposal mechanisms. Indeed in circulatory failure, the liver and kidneys may produce lactate rather than dispose of it. In type B lactic acidosis there is no evidence, at the outset, of circulatory insufficiency or hypoxia, although after many hours of increasing acidosis these may supervene. The original diagnosis and cause of acidosis may be obscured if the patient does not present until this late stage. Type A lactic acidosis is a frequent manifestation of haemorrhagic, septic, cardiogenic, or traumatic shock and there is a direct relationship between the concentration of blood lactate and poor prognosis. The causes of type B lactic acidosis (Table 12.11.2) are varied and some of the mechanisms will be described below.

The initial clinical presentation in type B lactic acidosis is fairly uniform and consists of hyperventilation or dyspnoea, drowsiness or coma, vomiting, and abdominal pain, in approximately that order of frequency. The condition usually develops over a few hours, but may be more chronic, e.g. in the mitochondrial myopathies. Although by definition there is initially no clinical evidence of poor tissue perfusion or hypoxia, patients with severe type B lactic acidosis commonly become shocked after a few hours.

The diagnosis of lactic acidosis is based on the clinical circumstances, including the presence of a known aetiological factor, the presence of a high anion gap acidosis, and the measurement of blood lactate, for which automated apparatus is now widely available.

Biguanide-induced lactic acidosis

The biguanide class of oral hypoglycaemic agents has widespread metabolic effects, including inhibition of gluconeogenesis and the monocarboxylate transporter responsible for the movement of lactate ions across cell membranes, and stimulation of glycolysis. This lactic acidosis is of the type B variety although, as indicated above, circulatory insufficiency may eventually supervene. Lactic acidosis caused by phenformin and buformin had a mortality rate of about 50%, but these biguanides are no longer used. Metformin is widely used, however, and the incidence of lactic acidosis with this drug is less than one-tenth of that with phenformin. Since metformin is almost entirely excreted in the urine, lactic acidosis may be largely avoided by taking care not to prescribe it in patients with even mild degrees of renal insufficiency or conditions such as uncontrolled heart failure, which might be expected to diminish renal function. Attempts have been made to show that the risk of lactic acidosis in diabetics taking metformin is no greater than in diabetics not receiving the drug. There have, however, been serious criticisms of those studies. It is now clear that metformin is indeed a cause of lactic acidosis, principally in the presence of poor renal function.

Postictal lactic acidosis

The violent muscular contractions during convulsions may produce severe lactic acidosis in the same way as vigorous exercise. The finding of lactic acidosis in these circumstances occasionally gives rise to confusion, but may be distinguished from other causes of lactic acidosis by the rapid decline of blood lactate after the cessation of convulsions, with a half-life of approximately 20 min.

Lactic acidosis in liver disease

Although impaired disposal of an administered lactate load is readily demonstrable in chronic liver disease, clinical lactic acidosis is uncommon. However, in the later stages of fulminant hepatic necrosis it may be an important part of the clinical picture. Acid–base disturbances in the earlier stages are discussed below.

Lactic acidosis in severe falciparum malaria

Lactic acidosis is a common feature of severe malaria due to *Plasmodium falciparum*, particularly in children, where it is a strong predictor of poor prognosis. Although shock may be a factor, the lactic acidosis is frequently of the type B variety and is attributable to many factors, including production of lactate by the parasite itself, occlusion of the microcirculation by parasites, the direct effects of high circulating levels of certain cytokines, notably TNF, inhibition of gluconeogenesis from lactate because of decreased hepatic blood flow, and overproduction of lactate during the convulsions that are a common feature of cerebral malaria. Hypoglycaemia in severe malaria may be linked with lactic acidosis; it may be a manifestation of decreased gluconeogenesis or of insulin release during quinine therapy. Acidosis appears to increase the attachment of infected erythrocytes to capillary walls, perhaps thus worsening the capillary blockage seen in the cerebral circulation and other sites. It may also inhibit the uptake of antimalarial drugs into erythrocytes. It should be noted that lactic acidosis by no means wholly accounts for the acidosis of severe malaria, ketoacids also playing a major role.

Lactic acidosis associated with treatment with nucleoside reverse transcriptase inhibitors

There have been reports of lactic acidosis, which may be severe, associated with AIDS therapy with nucleoside reverse transcriptase inhibitors. Two mechanisms have been described: riboflavin deficiency and a mitochondrial disorder (with myopathy associated with the characteristic ragged red fibres seen in inherited mitochondrial myopathies). In the former type, the lactic acidosis rapidly responds to the administration of riboflavin.

Ethanol- and methanol-induced lactic acidosis

Ingestion of ethanol after a period of fasting is a well-known cause of hypoglycaemia, which may be severe. The phenomenon is due to the inhibition of gluconeogenesis, which is the sole source of endogenous glucose output when glycogen stores have been depleted. The defect in gluconeogenesis may result in moderate lactic acidosis because ethanol diverts some of the NAD^+ needed for the oxidation of lactate to pyruvate, the first step in lactate disposal, for its own oxidation (catalysed by alcohol dehydrogenase). Following the withdrawal of ethanol, the administration of glucose, and re-feeding, the condition is normally self-limiting.

In methanol poisoning the main contributor to the acidosis is formic acid, but lactic acidosis also plays a part because of inhibition of gluconeogenesis by similar mechanisms to those in ethanol-induced lactic acidosis.

Lactic acidosis in Reye's syndrome

Reye's syndrome is described elsewhere (see Chapter 12.2.1) and is mentioned here to note that the metabolic acidosis component is principally lactic acidosis, the degree of which corresponds with the stage of coma, blood NH_3 only correlating with coma level in the early stages.

Salicylate and ethylene glycol poisoning

See Chapter 9.2.

D(−) lactic acidosis

In all the lactic acidoses described above the stereoisomer involved is L(+)-lactate, the end product of mammalian glycolysis. However, a few cases have been described in which the acidosis has been due to D(−)-lactate. There is a very minor pathway of D(−)-lactate production in mammalian tissues, but in D(−) lactic acidosis the D(−)-lactate arises as a product of glycolysis in bacteria in the gut, and all cases have been associated with short gut or jejunal–ileal bypass syndromes or the therapeutic ingestion of large quantities of *Lactobacillus acidophilus*. The lactic acidosis may be severe and is often associated with disturbances of consciousness; it is presumably due to the absorption of large quantities of D(−)-lactate from the gut, since it may be treated by appropriate oral antibiotics. In healthy individuals, infused D(−)-lactate is cleared at approximately 70% of the rate for L(+)-lactate, but by the nonspecific 2-hydroxybutyrate dehydrogenase rather than L(+)-lactate dehydrogenase. The main problem in diagnosing D(−)-lactate acidosis is that D(−)-lactate is not detectable by the routine blood lactate assay, which employs the enzyme L(+)-lactate dehydrogenase. If the condition is suspected because of unexplained high anion gap metabolic acidosis in a patient with a predisposing condition, then D(−)-lactate should be assayed either by gas chromatography or using a bacterial D(−)-lactate dehydrogenase.

Diabetic ketoacidosis

The pathogenesis and clinical features of diabetic ketoacidosis are described elsewhere (Chapter 13.11.1). Only the acid–base disturbance is discussed here. Though the acidosis is conventionally regarded as being due mainly to the overproduction of keto-acids by the liver, recent evidence has suggested that the protons are wholly or partly derived from other tissues, although the liver is, of course, the source of keto acid anions. Hepatic gluconeogenesis, a major source of the hyperglycaemia of diabetic ketoacidosis, proceeds at increased rates in spite of potential inhibition by systemic acidosis. This is because, unlike in acidoses of other origins, hepatic intracellular pH does not fall in diabetic ketoacidosis because of mechanisms discussed elsewhere.

Diabetic ketoacidosis has usually been regarded as a typical high anion gap metabolic acidosis in which extracellular bicarbonate has simply been titrated by the keto acids. If this were the case, the fall in plasma bicarbonate should roughly equal the rise in anion gap and the plasma concentration of keto acids. However, Adrogué and colleagues have shown that, whereas in some cases this is true, the situation is frequently more complex. Patients who present in ketoacidosis with relatively well-preserved renal function tend to have an increase in anion gap that is much less than the decrease in bicarbonate. This is due to the loss of large quantities of keto acid anions in the urine, with concomitant tubular reabsorption of chloride to maintain electroneutrality. Hyperchloraemia develops and, together with the urinary loss of keto acids, results in a relatively small elevation of the anion gap compared with the bicarbonate deficit. In contrast, patients who have relatively poor renal function on presentation, e.g. because of dehydration, have much smaller urinary losses of keto acids and present with a more classical high anion gap metabolic acidosis.

The total blood ketone body concentration in the well-controlled diabetic is about 0.1 mmol/litre. In diabetic ketoacidosis the concentration is often more than 10 mmol/litre and can rise as high as 30 mmol/litre. Some of the most severe acidoses seen in clinical practice occur in diabetic ketoacidosis, occasionally with pHa values as low as 6.8; urinary pH reaches its minimum possible value (4.5–5.3). At the lower of these values about half the urinary keto acids are undissociated, and some protons are lost in this way. Severe depletion of erythrocyte 2,3-bisphosphoglycerate occurs, leading to left shift of the oxygen dissociation curve, especially during treatment, and with potentially adverse consequences (see below).

In 5 to 10% of patients with diabetic ketoacidosis there is an accompanying element of lactic acidosis, with blood lactate more than 5 mmol/litre. Lactic acidosis occurs particularly when the patient is shocked, but there are rare instances of lactic acidosis supervening when treatment of the initial ketoacidosis is well advanced. There are also occasional ketotic diabetics in whom the blood lactate is low. This effect is readily reproducible in experimental animals and is thought to be related to increased hepatic disposal of lactate and suppression of peripheral glycolysis by the acidosis.

Acidosis of renal failure

Metabolic acidosis of varying degree is a classical feature of acute and chronic renal failure. It has traditionally been attributed to failure of the kidneys to excrete protons derived from fixed acids—the class III acids of Table 12.11.1. In chronic renal failure the remaining functional nephrons are usually able to lower the urinary pH to the normal minimum. However, failure of proximal tubular bicarbonate reabsorption may occasionally occur and lead to a bicarbonate leak, as in type 2 renal tubular acidosis (see Chapter 21.15); in this case urinary pH does not fall to its minimum until the filtered load of bicarbonate has been substantially reduced by the fall in plasma bicarbonate. In some conditions, e.g. chronic pyelonephritis and chronic obstructive uropathy, the renal medulla is particularly affected and acidification of the urine may be impaired. Nevertheless, the usually normal acidification in chronic renal failure means that the phosphate buffers in the tubular lumen are titrated by protons to the same extent as is possible in normal kidneys. However, the excretion of NH_4^+ ions is lower than normal in chronic renal failure because of the loss of glutaminase-containing proximal tubules, and reduced renal blood flow decreases the supply of glutamine. The conventional explanation of the acidosis of renal failure has been that the diminished supply of NH_3 from the glutaminase reaction lowers the ability of the luminal contents to buffer secreted protons, with the result that the minimum urinary pH is attained with fewer protons in the NH_3/NH_4^+ buffering system, and thus fewer protons are disposed of in the urine.

However, as indicated above, the NH_3/NH_4^+ buffering system is already virtually entirely in the protonated form (i.e. NH_4^+) at the time of its generation in the glutaminase reaction, so this system has no remaining capacity to act as a urinary buffer, either in health or in renal failure. An alternative explanation is therefore required for the acidosis of renal failure. Atkinson and Camien have suggested that in chronic renal failure the nitrogen which would, in health, be excreted as NH_4^+ ions in the urine is effectively diverted to the liver, where it is converted to urea with accompanying generation of protons (see above). The acidosis of renal failure is therefore due to relative overproduction of urea, rather than to failure of excretion of protons in the urine as NH_4^+ ions.

The anion gap in uraemic acidosis seldom exceeds 28 to 30 mmol/litre. The elevation is due to the accumulation of a relatively small quantity of several acid anions, including phosphate, sulphate, citrate, and other less well-characterized contributions. When there is an element of proximal bicarbonate wastage the anion gap may not be grossly raised; chloride may be reabsorbed instead of bicarbonate, leading to moderate hyperchloraemia.

The renal tubular acidoses, which are tubular disorders not initially accompanied by glomerular failure, are discussed in Chapter 21.15.

Metabolic alkaloses associated with potassium and chloride deficiency

The most common cause of metabolic alkalosis is that associated with the use of potassium-losing diuretics. Pyloric stenosis and Bartter's and Gitelman's syndromes provide further examples of a complex aetiology. Chloride deficiency, indicated by low plasma chloride, may be due to a direct action of the diuretics, to loss from the gastrointestinal tract—as in pyloric stenosis—or to potassium deficiency itself, which has been shown experimentally to impair renal retention of chloride.

Normally, most renal sodium reabsorption takes place in the proximal tubule, and it has to be accompanied by a readily reabsorbable anion to maintain electroneutrality. The most readily reabsorbable anion is chloride, and if the filtered load of chloride is low because of hypochloraemia, some of the sodium which normally would have been reabsorbed proximally passes to the distal segment of the nephron. Here, sodium is reabsorbed by exchange with cations, principally potassium and protons, rather than accompanied by an anion. Since priority over acid–base regulation is accorded to the demands of extracellular volume control, the sodium reabsorption thus dictated causes further loss of potassium and protons into the urine, when the homeostatic response would have been to retain these latter ions. This accounts for the observation that the urine in these circumstances is acid when it should be alkaline (paradoxical aciduria) and contains substantial quantities of potassium. Potassium loss in the urine is the principal cause of potassium depletion in pyloric stenosis, not loss in the vomit. The hypokalaemia is exacerbated by the fact that extracellular fluid volume is depleted in both diuretic therapy and in pyloric stenosis, leading to activation of the renin–angiotensin–aldosterone system, with further potassium loss. These considerations have important implications for therapy (see below).

An important cause of hypokalaemic hypochloraemic alkalosis is deliberate overuse by patients of diuretics, notably furosemide, for reasons that may be related to psychological disturbances of body image. Many of these patients are secretive about their use of diuretics; measurement of plasma furosemide is one way of diagnosing this dangerous condition. It should be noted that even use of diuretics in the normal way may produce metabolic alkalosis.

Acid–base disturbances in fulminant hepatic failure

The most frequent acid–base disturbance in the earlier stages of fulminant hepatic failure is respiratory alkalosis, presumably due to the stimulatory effects of NH_4^+ and other amines on the respiratory centre. Metabolic alkalosis is also frequent, probably due to the failure of ureagenesis and its accompanying proton generation, but in some cases could be contributed to by potassium deficiency. Whatever the mechanism of the alkalosis, blood lactate concentration is frequently elevated, even in the absence of circulatory insufficiency. This phenomenon has been attributed to stimulation of peripheral glycolysis by alkalosis and to impairment of hepatic lactate disposal. Lactic acidosis may be a major feature in the later stages when the circulation is compromised, but is also occasionally seen in the very early stages. This early lactic acidosis is observed in paracetamol poisoning, a common cause of fulminant hepatic failure; it is associated with hypoglycaemia and may be largely related to a direct effect of paracetamol metabolites on hepatic gluconeogenesis from lactate. However, mild hypotension and dehydration may also contribute.

Principles of treatment of acid–base disorders

The mainstay of treatment of acid–base disorders is to eliminate the cause of the disorder, the acid–base control mechanisms then restoring the normal situation in due course. However, it may occasionally be necessary to make a direct attempt to restore or partly restore normal acid–base status.

The treatment of respiratory acidosis is discussed in Chapter 18.3.

Acute metabolic acidosis

The advantages of treatment, especially with sodium bicarbonate, are still highly controversial. Randomized controlled trials have not resolved these issues completely, largely because of the great variation of the physiological state of patients on presentation and the difficulty in establishing adequately sized and matching groups for trial purposes. Here we attempt to distinguish between conditions in which there is a consensus as to the best therapeutic approach and those in which there is less agreement. This is not an ideal approach, but is unavoidable at present.

The potential advantages of treating severe acidosis directly are improvement in cardiac performance, reduced risk of cardiac arrhythmia, redistribution of the blood volume away from the central circulation, correction of hyperkalaemia, and restoration of hepatic lactate disposal. Disadvantages lie in adverse effects on the oxygen dissociation curve, circulatory overload, especially if isotonic solutions have to be used, alkaline 'overshoot' when the acidosis is due to organic acids such as lactic acid and ketone bodies, and, allegedly, if bicarbonate is used, paradoxical intracellular acidification.

Paradoxical intracellular acidification is a concept arising from the observation that when sodium bicarbonate is infused, a significant rise in $Paco_2$ is observed because of the titration of bicarbonate by protons. Since there is an expectation that CO_2 will diffuse into cells much more rapidly than bicarbonate is translocated, it would be expected that intracellular pH would fall at the same time as pHa rises; since many of the adverse effects of acidosis are directly related to effects on intracellular pH, this would be undesirable. A related observation is that in circulatory insufficiency, Pco_2 may be much greater in mixed venous blood than in arterial blood, where it is often normal. On occasion, bicarbonate therapy may exaggerate this difference and it has been inferred that bicarbonate must be acidifying the intracellular compartment by the mechanisms outlined above. However, considerations of the mechanisms responsible for the mixed venous hypercapnia suggest that only if arterial Pco_2 is raised after passage of the blood through the lungs is bicarbonate therapy likely to cause intracellular acidification. Whether $Paco_2$ is indeed elevated by intravenous bicarbonate therapy is dependent on numerous factors, including cardiac output, ventilation, the pulmonary dead space to total volume ratio, and, in particular, the rate of administration of bicarbonate.

Paradoxical intracellular acidification can indeed be demonstrated in closed systems, such as platelets, in which the CO_2 is not removed, and has been the reason for the development of alternative therapies such as an equimolar mixture of sodium bicarbonate and carbonate ('carbicarb'), for which the rise in $Paco_2$ during administration is substantially attenuated. However, it is difficult to demonstrate such an effect *in vivo*, when CO_2 is removed by the lungs, and in experimental animals either no change or actual elevation in intracellular pH in heart, liver, and skeletal muscle may be observed during bicarbonate administration, despite elevation of mixed venous Pco_2. In any case, if doubts remain concerning this issue, the problem may be avoided by the simple expedient of administering bicarbonate slowly. Hindman has made useful calculations of the rates of bicarbonate administration that avoid rises in $Paco_2$ under a range of circumstances.

The situations in which sodium bicarbonate therapy is generally agreed to be advantageous are as follows:

- Metabolic acidosis in severe renal failure. In acute renal failure, sodium bicarbonate treatment may correct hyperkalaemia by shifting potassium into the intracellular compartment. It may also relieve distressing hyperventilation and make time for definitive renal support therapy to be introduced. If the patient is already fluid-overloaded the bicarbonate may be administered as a hypertonic solution (e.g. 8.4%; 1000 mmol/litre). If the patient is dehydrated then the isotonic solution (1.4%; 163 mmol/litre) may be given. During haemofiltration for acute renal failure in the presence of lactic acidosis, there is little doubt that the use of bicarbonate rather than lactate-containing replacement fluid is preferable because of failure of metabolism of lactate to bicarbonate in this situation (see below). In chronically uraemic patients, the use of oral bicarbonate to treat the acidosis may improve well-being, nitrogen balance, and the osteomalacic component of renal osteodystrophy.
- Acidosis of severe diarrhoea. It has been shown, in the specific instance of cholera, where circulatory insufficiency and loss of alkali are prominent factors, that treatment with bicarbonate is superior to that with sodium chloride solutions. These patients have severe peripheral venoconstriction, displacing their blood volume towards the lungs. The administration of saline solutions may thus induce pulmonary oedema before the volume deficit has been replaced. Sodium bicarbonate appears to relieve the peripheral venoconstriction and full replacement is therefore less hazardous.
- Renal tubular acidosis, both chronic and exacerbations. This subject is discussed elsewhere (Chapter 21.15), but it is necessary to re-emphasize here that in types 1 and 2 renal tubular acidosis, where hypokalaemia is a prominent feature, it is mandatory to deal with the hypokalaemia either before or at least simultaneously with the acidosis. Treatment of the acidosis first will result in a further fall in plasma potassium, by driving potassium into the cells, with potentially fatal consequences.

It is in the treatment of lactic acidosis, particularly type A, and in diabetic ketoacidosis that the uncertainty of the value of bicarbonate therapy principally lies. In animal models of lactic acidosis, treatment with bicarbonate has been shown to produce less favourable or no better haemodynamic and metabolic results than with sodium chloride. Interestingly, in an acute model of haemorrhagic shock there was little difference between bicarbonate and saline therapies; in these experiments there had been no time for erythrocyte 2,3-bisphosphoglycerate to fall. In contrast, in a model of diabetic ketoacidosis, developing over 48 h, in which 2,3-bisphosphoglycerate was now virtually undetectable, treatment with bicarbonate produced a fall in blood pressure and evidence of tissue hypoxia, despite intracellular alkalinization. This suggests that acute acidoses of more than a few hours' duration may become increasingly susceptible to the adverse effects of bicarbonate. In a small prospective randomized trial of bicarbonate compared with saline in critically ill patients with lactic acidosis due to shock there was no advantage of one therapy over the other, but this trial was not exempt from the general difficulties in mounting such trials.

The following practical guidance is therefore empirical, and largely based on current practice rather than formal trials.

Lactic acidosis

Of paramount importance in type A lactic acidosis is the correction of hypovolaemic, cardiogenic, and other factors which are the primary cause of the condition. Such correction will promote aerobic metabolism and promote intracellular metabolism of lactate, with consequent regeneration of bicarbonate (Fig. 12.11.1). Whether the administration of exogenous bicarbonate can hasten this process or confer other benefits is uncertain. In short-duration lactic acidosis there may be less concern about effects on oxygen dissociation related to 2,3-bisphosphoglycerate levels, but it should be remembered that unless therapy directed at the primary cause has improved the circulation, alkalinization itself may produce an unfavourable effect on oxygen release from haemoglobin. Nevertheless, the possibility of bicarbonate helping in some circumstances cannot be ruled out. If it is given, this should be relatively slowly and as the isotonic solution, unless there is a circulatory overload problem, and only in amounts sufficient to raise pHa to a relatively 'safe' level. In the special case of the acidosis of cardiac arrest, the previous priority given to bicarbonate administration has disappeared because of lack of evidence of efficacy and the risk of alkaline overshoot when the high levels of lactate are metabolized on restoration of cardiac output. Hypertonic sodium bicarbonate is only now recommended as a secondary treatment after prolonged arrest. In type B lactic acidosis due to biguanides it has been conventional to use bicarbonate therapy at least to bring pHa to 7.2 to 7.4 over several hours, and survival has been linked to the achievement of that goal. However, an alternative interpretation of the data is that those patients in whom acid–base status was restored to normal would have achieved this without the aid of bicarbonate, or with the use of saline instead. Other therapies for type B lactic acidoses of different causes are discussed below.

Diabetic ketoacidosis

It is generally accepted that provided pHa is not below 7.0, bicarbonate treatment is not indicated. Rehydration and insulin therapy result in improved renal function, a fall in ketone-body production and an increase in ketone-body metabolism, all of which contribute to correction of the acidosis. When pHa is below 7.0 many give just sufficient bicarbonate (isotonic) to bring pHa just above 7.0, with careful attention to changes in plasma potassium. There is, however, no evidence that this regimen is better than rehydration (with saline), insulin, and potassium replacement alone, and there are data showing that such therapy delays falls in ketone body levels and lactate (if raised). The delayed fall in lactate is consistent with tissue hypoxia related to low erythrocyte 2,3-bisphosphoglycerate, as discussed above. It is therefore common practice not to give bicarbonate, even at low pHa levels. If bicarbonate is given then it must be isotonic (1.4%, 163 mmol/litre); to give hypertonic bicarbonate would merely exacerbate the already present hyperosmolality. The amount required seldom exceeds 0.5 to 1 litre.

The amount of alkali therapy, if given, should be determined by an iterative process of administration of a relatively small amount (e.g. 80 mmol), followed by reassessment of the clinical state, pHa, and $Paco_2$, with the aid of serial plots on the acid–base diagram in Fig. 12.11.2, before repeating the cycle.

Alkalinizing agents other than bicarbonate have been considered. Sodium lactate has the disadvantage that it has to be metabolized to neutral products plus bicarbonate before it has an alkalinizing effect (Fig. 12.11.1) and if lactate metabolism is impaired, as in shock and hypoxia in particular, it has no effect. Lactate is not a buffer in its own right at pH values encountered in health or disease. The mixture of bicarbonate and carbonate referred to above has not been shown to have clinical advantages and is less effective than saline in animal models of diabetic ketoacidosis. THAM [tris(hydroxymethyl)aminomethane] buffer has the theoretical advantage of producing intracellular as well as extracellular alkalinization, but is seldom used because of unwanted effects. Sodium dichloroacetate increases lactate disposal via oxidation by activation of pyruvate dehydrogenase, and markedly lowers blood lactate in critically ill patients with lactic acidosis. However, in a multicentre trial it did not improve survival over that in a saline control group, possibly because of the severity of the associated pathologies and the diverse clinical state of the patients. However, it is of proven value in the treatment of some congenital lactic acidoses. Thiamine produces dramatic resolution of the severe lactic acidosis sometimes seen in beriberi. Riboflavin has produced similar results in lactic acidosis associated with nucleoside reverse transcriptase inhibitor therapy.

Treatment of metabolic alkalosis

The first imperative is to identify the primary cause and if possible eliminate it. Where potassium-losing diuretics are responsible they can be replaced by potassium-sparing preparations. In the most common form of chronic metabolic alkalosis, namely that associated with potassium and chloride deficiency, the primary therapies are potassium and chloride replacement. It has been shown that the potassium deficiency and alkalosis cannot be fully corrected unless there is also replenishment of chloride. Potassium supplements, whether oral or intravenous, should therefore be in the form of potassium chloride or contain other sources of chloride. It is also necessary to deal with any element of extracellular fluid volume contraction to switch off the drive to the renin–aldosterone system. It is seldom necessary to resort to administration of acid.

Further reading

Adrogué HJ, *et al.* (1982). Plasma acid-base patterns in diabetic ketoacidosis. *N Engl J Med*, **307**, 1603–10.

Adrogué HJ, *et al.* (2009). Assessing acid-base disorders. *Kidney International*, **76**, 1239–47.

Alberti KGMM, *et al.* (1972). 2,3-bisphosphoglycerate and tissue oxygenation in uncontrolled diabetes mellitus. *Lancet*, **3**, 391–5.

Atkinson DE, Camien MN (1982). The role of urea synthesis in the removal of metabolic bicarbonate and the regulation of blood pH. *Curr Top Cell Regul*, **21**, 261–302.

Beech JS, *et al.* (1989). Gluconeogenesis and the protection of hepatic intracellular pH during diabetic ketoacidosis in rats. *Biochem J*, **263**, 737–44.

Bellingham A, Detter JC, Lenfant C (1971). Regulatory mechanisms of hemoglobin oxygen affinity in acidosis and alkalosis. *J Clin Invest*, **50**, 700–6.

Bruijstens LA, *et al.* (2008). Reality of severe metformin induced acidosis in the absence of chronic renal impairment. *Neth J Med*, **66**, 185–90.

Celloto AC, *et al.* (2008). Effects of acid-base imbalance on vascular reactivity. *Braz J Med Biol Res*, **41**, 439–45.

Chariot P, *et al.* (1999). Zidovudine-induced mitochondrial disorder with massive steatosis, myopathy, lactic acidosis, and mitochondrial myopathy. *J Hepatol*, **30**, 156–60.

Cohen RD (1990). The metabolic background to acid-base homeostasis and some of its disorders. In: Cohen RD, *et al.* (eds). *The metabolic and molecular basis of acquired disease*, pp. 962–1001. Ballière Tindall, London.

Cohen RD (1991). Roles of the liver and kidney in acid-base regulation and its disorders. *Br J Anaesth*, **67**, 154–64.

Cohen RD (1994). Lactic acidosis—new perspectives on origins and treatment. *Diabetes Rev*, **2**, 86–97.

Cohen RD, Woods HF (1976). *Clinical and biochemical aspects of lactic acidosis.* Blackwell, Oxford.

Cohen RD, Woods HF (1983). Lactic acidosis revisited. *Diabetes*, **32**, 181–91.

Cohen RD, Woods HF (1999). Metformin and lactic acidosis. *Diabet Care*, **22**, 1010.

Cooper DJ, *et al.* (1990). Bicarbonate does not improve hemodynamics in critically ill patients who have lactic acidosis. *Ann Intern Med*, **112**, 492–8.

Dickson RP, Luks AM, (2009). Toluene toxicity as a cause of elevated anion gap metabolic acidosis. *Respir Care*, **54**, 1115–17.

Di Grande A, *et al.* (2008). Metformin-induced lactic acidosis in a type 2 diabetic patient with acute renal failure. *Clin Ter*, **159**, 87–9.

Doberer D, *et al.* (2009). A critique of Stewart's approach: the chemical mechanism of dilutional acidosis. *Intensive Care Med*, **35**, 2173–80.

Emmett M, Narins RG (1977). Clinical use of the anion gap. *Medicine (Baltimore)*, **56**, 38–54.

Goldsmith DJA, Forni LG, Hilton PJ (1997). Bicarbonate therapy and intracellular acidosis. *Clin Sci*, **93**, 593–8.

Hale PJ, Crase J, Nattrass M (1984). Metabolic effects of bicarbonate in the treatment of diabetic ketoacidosis. *Br Med J*, **289**, 1035–8.

Hilton PJ, *et al.* (1998). Bicarbonate-based haemofiltration in the management of acute renal failure with lactic acidosis. *Q J Med*, **91**, 279–83.

Hindman BJ (1990). Sodium bicarbonate in the treatment of subtypes of acute lactic acidosis: physiologic considerations. *Anesthesiology*, **72**, 1064–76.

Hood VL, Tannen RL (1998). Protection of acid-base balance by pH regulation of acid production. *N Engl J Med*, **339**, 819–26.

Kassirer JP, *et al.* (1965). The critical role of chloride in the correction of hypokalaemic alkalosis in man. *Am J Med*, **209**, 655–8.

Kellum JA, Song M, Almasri E (2006) Hyperchloremic acidosis increases circulatory inflammatory molecules in experimental sepsis. *Chest*, **130**, 962–7.

Krishna S, *et al.* (1994). Lactic acidosis and hypoglycaemia in children with severe malaria: pathophysiological and prognostic significance. *Trans R Soc Trop Med Hyg*, **88**, 67–73.

Lopez I, *et al.* (2003). Direct suppressive effect of acute metabolic and respiratory alkalosis on parathyroid hormone secretion in the dog. *J Bone Miner Res*, **18**, 1478–85.

Luzatti R, *et al.* (1999). Riboflavine and severe lactic acidosis. *Lancet*, **353**, 901–2.

Mitch WE (2006). Metabolic and clinical consequences of metabolic acidosis. *J Nephrol*, **19** Suppl 9, 570–5.

Mitchell JH, Wildenthal K, Johnson RL (1972). The effects of acid-base disturbances on cardiovascular and pulmonary function. *Kidney Int*, **1**, 375–89.

Moviat M, *et al.* (2008). Contribution of various metabolites to the "unmeasured" anions in critically ill patients with metabolic acidosis. *Crit Care Med*, **36**, 752–8.

Narins RG, *et al.* (1995). Anion gap. In: Aneff AI, De Fronzo RA (eds) *Fluid, electrolyte and acid-base disorders*, 2nd edition, pp. 111–14. Churchill Livingstone, New York.

Oh MS, *et al.* (1979). D-lactic acidosis in a man with the short bowel syndrome. *N Engl J Med*, **301**, 249–52.

Orringer CE, *et al.* (1977). Natural history of lactic acidosis after grand mal seizures. *N Engl J Med*, **297**, 796–9.

Quintard H, Hubert S, Ichai C, (2007). [What is the contribution of Stewart's concept in acid-base disorders analysis?]. *Ann Fr Anesth Reanim*, **26**, 423–33.

Record CO, *et al.* (1975). Acid-base and metabolic disturbances in fulminant hepatic failure. *Gut*, **16**, 144–9.

Schwarz GJ, *et al.* (2002). Acid incubation reverses the polarity of intercalated cell transporters, an effect mediated by hensin. *J Clin Invest*, **109**, 89–99.

Stacpoole PW, *et al.* (1999). Treatment of congenital lactic acidosis with dichloroacetate. *Arch Dis Child*, **77**, 535–41.

Toftegaard M, Rees SE, Andreassen S, (2009). Evaluation of a method for converting venous values of acid-base and oxygenation status to arterial values. *Emerg Med J*, **26**, 268–272.

Tonsgard JH, Huttenlocher PR, Thisted RA (1982). Lactic acidaemia in Reye's syndrome. *Pediatrics*, **69**, 64–9.

Weil MH, *et al.* (1986). Difference in acid-base state between venous and arterial blood during cardiopulmonary resuscitation. *N Engl J Med*, **315**, 153–6.

Yee AH, Rabinstein AA. (2010). Neurologic presentations of acid-base imbalance, electrolyte abnormalities, and endocrine emergencies. *Neurol Clin* , **28**, 1–16.

12.12

The acute phase response, amyloidoses and familial Mediterranean fever

Contents

12.12.1 The acute phase response and C-reactive protein *1752*
M.B. Pepys

12.12.2 Hereditary periodic fever syndromes *1760*
Helen J. Lachmann and Philip N. Hawkins

12.12.3 Amyloidosis *1766*
M.B. Pepys and Philip N. Hawkins

12.12.1 The acute phase response and C-reactive protein

M.B. Pepys

Essentials

The acute phase response—trauma, tissue necrosis, infection, inflammation, and malignant neoplasia induce a complex series of nonspecific systemic, physiological, and metabolic responses including fever, leucocytosis, catabolism of muscle proteins, greatly increased *de novo* synthesis and secretion of a number of 'acute phase' plasma proteins, and decreased synthesis of albumin, transthyretin, and high- and low-density lipoproteins. The altered plasma protein concentration profile is called the acute phase response. All endothermic animals mount a similar response, suggesting that it may have survival value, and increased availability of proteinase inhibitors, complement, clotting, and transport proteins presumably enhances host resistance, minimizes tissue injury, and promotes regeneration and repair.

Acute phase proteins—these are mostly synthesized by hepatocytes, in which transcription is controlled by cytokines including interleukin 1, interleukin 6, and tumour necrosis factor. The circulating concentrations of complement proteins and clotting factors increase by up to 50 to 100%; some of the proteinase inhibitors and α_1-acid glycoprotein can increase three- to fivefold; but C-reactive protein and serum amyloid A protein (an apolipoprotein of high-density lipoprotein particles) are unique in that their concentrations can change by more than 1000-fold.

C-reactive protein (CRP)—this consists of five identical, nonglycosylated, noncovalently-associated polypeptide subunits. It binds to substances which contain phosphocholine, including phospholipids, some plasma lipoproteins, and the plasma membranes of damaged cells, also to small nuclear ribonucleoprotein particles when these are exposed in dead or damaged cells. By activating the classical complement pathway after binding to ligand it can trigger the inflammatory, opsonizing, and complex-solubilizing activities of the complement system, perhaps thereby protecting against infection with organisms that express phosphocholine (e.g. pneumococci and *Haemophilus influenzae*) and aiding in recognition and 'scavenging' of cellular debris.

Clinical features—(1) determination of CRP in serum or plasma is the most useful marker of the acute phase response in most inflammatory and tissue damaging conditions. It is a stable analyte, easy to measure, and has proven value in monitoring therapeutic responses. (2) Acute phase proteins may be harmful in some circumstances. Sustained increased production of serum amyloid A protein can lead to the deposition of AA-type, reactive systemic amyloid, a serious and usually fatal condition that can complicate chronic infective and inflammatory diseases. CRP, through its capacity to activate complement, can exacerbate ischaemic (and possibly also other forms) of tissue damage.

Introduction

The principal plasma proteins that change in concentration in the acute phase response are listed in Table 12.12.1.1. C-reactive protein (CRP) has particular clinical utility as a robust and easily measured systemic marker for monitoring the extent, activity and response to therapy in many inflammatory and tissue damaging conditions.

C-reactive protein (CRP)

CRP was the first protein to be discovered that behaves as an acute phase reactant, and was named for its calcium-dependent interaction

Table 12.12.1.1 Plasma proteins in the acute phase response

Protein	Increased	Decreased
Proteinase inhibitors	α_1-antitrypsin	Inter α-antitrypsin
	α_1-antichymotrypsin	
Coagulation proteins	Fibrinogen	
	Prothrombin	
	Factor VIII	
	Plasminogen	
Complement proteins	Cls	Properdin
	C2, B	
	C3,C4,C5	
	C56	
	C1INH	
Transport proteins	Haptoglobin	
	Haemopexin	
	Caeruloplasmin	
Miscellaneous	C-reactive protein	Albumin
	Serum amyloid A protein	Transthyretin (prealbumin)
	Fibronectin	High density lipoprotein
	α1-acid glycoprotein	Low density lipoprotein
	Gc globulin	

with the somatic C-polysaccharide of pneumococci, in which CRP recognizes phosphocholine residues. CRP also binds to other substances that contain phosphocholine, including phospholipids, some plasma lipoproteins, and the plasma membranes of damaged, but not intact cells. In addition, CRP binds specifically to small nuclear ribonucleoprotein particles when these are exposed in dead or damaged cells.

Ligand-bound CRP activates the classical complement pathway via C1, and can trigger the inflammatory, opsonizing, and complex-solubilizing activities of the complement system. A significant biological function of CRP may thus be to recognize and scavenge cellular debris, promoting its safe clearance and helping to maintain tolerance to potential autoantigens. CRP may also protect against infection with pneumococci and *Haemophilus influenzae*, organisms that can express phosphocholine, and may thus contribute to innate immunity. On the other hand, CRP can also have tissue-damaging effects, e.g. complement activation by CRP exacerbates ischaemic injury. However, no structural polymorphism of CRP has been observed nor has any case of CRP deficiency been described, so the functions of human CRP are not yet known for certain.

The CRP molecule consists of five identical, nonglycosylated, noncovalently-associated polypeptide subunits, each of mass 23 027 Da and containing 206 amino acid residues. The subunits have a flattened β-sheet jellyroll fold with a single intrachain disulphide bond, and are arranged in an annular configuration with cyclic pentameric symmetry. There is a single calcium-dependent ligand-binding site on the medial aspect of each subunit, all located on the same planar face of the molecule. A distinct but closely related plasma protein, serum amyloid P component, which is not an acute phase protein in humans, has a very similar molecular structure with the same fold, characteristic of the lectin-fold superfamily. plasma CRP and serum amyloid P component belong to the pentraxin family, which has been highly conserved in evolution.

Serum concentration of CRP

Circulating CRP is produced by the hepatocytes where its synthesis is under transcriptional regulation by the pro-inflammatory cytokines, especially IL 6. CRP is a trace protein in apparently normal healthy individuals, the median value in adults being 0.8 mg/litre, with an interquartile range of 0.3 to 1.7 mg/litre. Ninety per cent of apparently healthy subjects have levels of less than 3 mg/litre and 99 per cent have levels less than 10 mg/litre. Serum CRP concentrations are lower in healthy newborns, but reach adult values within a few days. Normal values in the indigenous Japanese population are substantially lower than in white Caucasians. Serial studies of normal subjects and of monozygotic and dizygotic twins show that each individual's baseline CRP value is rather constant and is substantially genetically determined. Baseline CRP is strongly correlated with body mass index, especially abdominal obesity, and is also higher in smokers, hypertensive subjects, diabetics, those who take little or no exercise, and individuals from the lower socioeconomic classes. Occasional higher values of CRP seen in ostensibly healthy people almost certainly reflect intercurrent subclinical pathology. In large surveys of the unscreened general population there is a trend towards higher values with increasing age, with the median value rising to about 2 mg/litre, and this likely reflects the higher incidence of many different pathological processes with age.

Serum CRP concentration rises rapidly in the acute phase response and can exceed 300 mg/litre by 48 h after a severe stimulus such as myocardial infarction, acute systemic bacterial infection, major trauma, or surgery. With uncomplicated resolution of injury or effective treatment of infection the circulating CRP concentration generally falls equally rapidly.

The speed of change and incremental range of CRP concentrations are exceptional among all the acute phase proteins, apart from serum amyloid A, which behaves in a similar fashion. The half-life of CRP in the circulation is 19 h and is constant in all conditions, regardless of the presence of an acute phase response or its cause. In contrast to other acute phase proteins, such as clotting factors, complement proteins, transport proteins, and proteinase inhibitors, CRP does not undergo significant local sequestration or consumption, fragmentation, or complex formation. This means that, unlike most of the other acute phase reactants, the single major determinant of the circulating concentration of CRP is its rate of synthesis. Since this in turn is dependent on the intensity of the acute phase stimulus, the serum CRP level usually closely reflects the extent and activity of disease. These properties underlie the value in clinical practice of precise measurement of the serum CRP concentration. Drug or other treatments do not affect CRP production unless they also affect the disease process that is responsible for the induction of CRP synthesis. The only exception is combined ciclosporin and steroid treatment given after renal transplantation. This suppresses the CRP response to renal allograft rejection, though not that provoked by infection. The only physical condition that seriously interferes with the capacity to interpret CRP levels is severe hepatocellular impairment, since plasma CRP is made exclusively in the liver.

Clinical measurement of serum C-reactive protein concentration

Conditions associated with marked elevation of serum CRP

Most tissue-damaging processes, infections, inflammatory diseases of unknown aetiology, and malignant neoplasms are associated with a major acute phase response of CRP. CRP production is exquisitely sensitive to all these pathologies and is thus a nonspecific response to disease. It can never, on its own, be used as a diagnostic test. However, if the CRP result is interpreted in the light of full clinical information about the patient it can provide exceptionally useful information for clinical management. Thus in nearly all the conditions listed in Box 12.12.1.1 the CRP level reflects quite precisely the extent and activity of disease. With deterioration the CRP level rises, whereas with spontaneous or therapeutically induced remission the CRP level falls, and it thereby supplies an objective index of progress that is rarely available in any other way.

Infection

Most forms of systemic microbial infection are associated with high levels of serum CRP and, although the peak values attained in different patients cover a wide range, serial assays in individual subjects usually show an excellent correlation between the serum plasma CRP concentration and the severity of disease and its response to treatment. Acute systemic Gram-positive and Gram-negative bacterial infections are among the most potent stimuli for CRP production. Systemic fungal infections occurring in immunodeficient hosts are also associated with high CRP values, whereas the levels in chronic bacterial infections such as tuberculosis and leprosy are usually rather lower, though nevertheless still markedly raised. Uncomplicated viral infections, particularly meningitis, may induce only a very modest response or none at all. Clinical rhinovirus infection (common cold) and influenza are associated with minor CRP elevation in a proportion of individuals, though this may reflect secondary bacterial infection. However, systemic cytomegalovirus or herpes simplex infection of immunosuppressed patients does cause a major CRP response. Little is known about the CRP response to metazoan parasitic infestation in otherwise healthy subjects but malaria, especially *Plasmodium falciparum* infection, is associated with high CRP values, as are *Pneumocystis* spp. and *Toxoplasma* spp. infections in immunodeficient patients.

Minor or localized low-grade infection may not stimulate CRP production greatly, but the major CRP response in acute, serious bacterial infection is almost invariable and is present at all ages from premature neonates to older people. It also occurs in patients who are immunosuppressed or immunocompromised, whether by a primary disease such as leukaemia, lymphoma, or other malignancy, by AIDS, or by treatment with cytotoxic drugs, corticosteroids, or irradiation. This is of particular importance in the very young, in older people, in compromised hosts, and in any other patient in whom the usual clinical signs and symptoms of infection, including fever and neutrophil leucocytosis, may be masked or lacking (Figs. 12.12.1.1 and 12.12.1.2). Furthermore, at the onset of bacterial infection, especially in patients who are otherwise well following elective surgery or myocardial infarction, the CRP response frequently precedes clinical symptoms, including fever, by up to 24 to 48 h.

Once infection is diagnosed or suspected and antimicrobial treatment has been commenced, frequent monitoring of the serum CRP concentration provides an objective means of assessing the response, which is often not otherwise available. Effective therapy is associated with a rapid, exponential fall in CRP level, with a half-life of about 24 h, and occurrence of this pattern is an encouraging prognostic sign (Fig. 12.12.1.2). Normalization of the CRP usually corresponds to clinical cure of the infection and may thus be used to determine the necessary duration of antimicrobial therapy. On the other hand, especially in neutropenic or immunodeficient patients, persistent elevation of CRP at the end of a course of antibiotics often presages relapse or recurrence of infection.

When bacterial infection is complicated by abscess formation or for any other reason is less readily eradicated by antimicrobial drugs, the serum CRP concentration may remain elevated or may fall linearly rather than exponentially during treatment. Such a pattern should raise questions regarding the dosage of the drugs, the sensitivity of the organism, and/or stimulate a diagnostic search both for localized pus and for other underlying, noninfective pathology such as malignancy. Indeed, in the absence of one of the chronic idiopathic inflammatory conditions which are known to be associated with high CRP levels (see below), the persistence of a raised serum CRP concentration is usually a grave prognostic sign indicating the presence of either uncontrolled infection and/or other serious pathology likely to cause death. However, with alteration in

Box 12.12.1.1 Conditions associated with major elevation of serum CRP concentration

Infections

Allergic complications of infection
- rheumatic fever
- erythema nodosum leprosum

Inflammatory disease
- rheumatoid arthritis
- juvenile chronic (rheumatoid) arthritis
- ankylosing spondylitis
- psoriatic arthritis
- systemic vasculitis
- polymyalgia rheumatica
- Reiter's disease
- Crohn's disease
- familial Mediterranean fever

Necrosis
- myocardial infarction
- tumour embolization
- acute pancreatitis

Trauma
- surgery
- burns
- fractures

Malignant neoplasia
- lymphoma, Hodgkin's disease,
- carcinoma, sarcoma

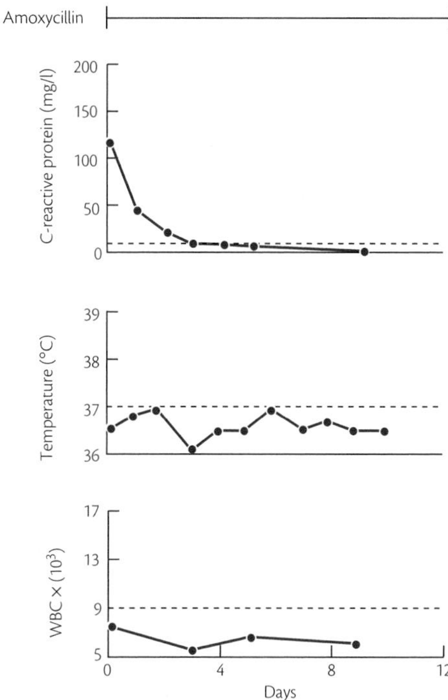

Fig. 12.12.1.1 A 69-year-old diabetic man was admitted with a 3-day history of confusion, cough, and incontinence of urine. There was clinical and radiological evidence of a left-sided pneumonia and although both the temperature and white cell count remained normal, the CRP was high (119 mg/litre), confirming the suspicion of infection. Following treatment with amoxicillin, 250 mg the times daily, the CRP level fell rapidly, in a characteristic exponential manner, and he made a speedy recovery with return of continence and improved mental state.

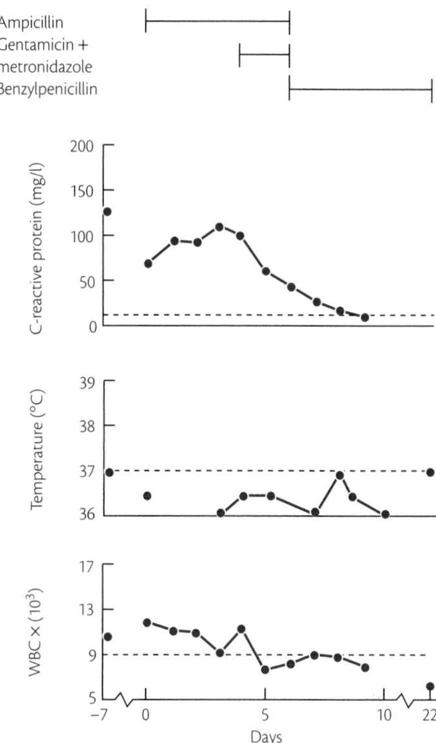

Fig. 12.12.1.2 An 86-year-old woman had been refusing food and drink for 6 weeks. She was dehydrated, but rehydration in hospital failed to improve hermental state. She was paranoid and refused nursing and medical care. Paraphrenia was diagnosed and deterioration continued. A CRP of 130 mg/litre and a white cell count of 13.5 × 10⁹/litre were then found. Chest radiograph, normal on admission, now showed a cavitating lesion from which 150 ml of pus were aspirated. Intravenous ampicillin reduced neither the CRP nor the white cell count, prompting a change of therapy to gentamicin and metronidazole. *Streptococcus equinus* was finally identified in the pus and treatment was changed to benzylpenicillin alone. The CRP then fell exponentially but rather slowly. The patient's clinical and mental state gradually improved and she was eventually discharged.

antimicrobial drug regimen or the evacuation of pus or elimination of other pathology, the rapid fall in CRP that may then be observed is an encouraging objective sign of clinical improvement.

These considerations apply at all ages and regardless of intercurrent pathology, with the exception of severe hepatocellular impairment. In view of the very small amount of serum required for the assay and the speed and precision of automated CRP immunoassays, it is apparent that routine monitoring of serum CRP makes a valuable contribution to the recognition and management of infectious diseases. Situations in which these applications have been well documented are listed in Box 12.12.1.2.

Meningitis is of particular interest in view of its potential severity and the importance of rapid diagnosis and appropriate treatment. Bacterial meningitis is associated with much higher serum CRP levels at presentation than cases of aseptic or proven viral meningitis. The latter frequently have CRP concentrations within the normal range or which are only very slightly raised, unless they develop secondary bacterial infective complications, whereas patients with tuberculous meningitis have intermediate values. Appropriate therapy for either bacterial or tuberculous meningitis causes the CRP level to fall, and this can be used to monitor objectively the response to treatment.

Baseline CRP values are much lower at birth and for the first few days than in older children or adults. Also, neonatal infections progress much more rapidly and can have a fatal outcome before the CRP response has produced concentrations detectable in routine assays. It is therefore essential to use highly sensitive methods capable of detecting and precisely measuring CRP in the range 0.05 to 5.0 mg/litre, otherwise the critical initial acute phase response to infection will be missed.

Inflammatory disease

Most of the chronic inflammatory diseases of unknown aetiology (Box 12.12.1.1), with some notable exceptions described below, are associated with high CRP values when they are active. Serial measurements of CRP in individuals with any of these diseases generally reflect the extent and activity of their condition as determined by clinical examination and other laboratory tests. Rheumatoid arthritis is the most common and important disease in this group and the correlation between CRP values in individual patients and the extent and activity of arthritis is very well established. Importantly, there are appreciable differences between the CRP levels attained in different subjects with apparently similar severity of arthritis, but in each case the CRP value always reflects current disease activity. Furthermore, CRP values precisely predict future progression of bone erosion and joint damage. Left unchecked, high CRP levels are inevitably followed by progressive erosive disease, whereas treatments that lower CRP retard or arrest this process.

In some of the inflammatory disorders, e.g. systemic vasculitis or Crohn's disease (Fig. 12.12.1.3), unlike rheumatoid arthritis, the pathology is relatively inaccessible to direct examination, and serum CRP measurement provides the best available, objective index of

Box 12.12.1.2 Applications of serum CRP measurement in infectious disease

- Bacteraemia and septicaemia in children and adults
- Bacteraemia and septicaemia in neonates
- Bacterial and other infections in immunosuppressed patients
- Deep fungal infections
- Meningitis: viral < TB < bacterial
- Bacterial infections after major elective surgery or other invasive procedures
- Infective relapse after abdominal surgery for sepsis
- Peritonitis in patients on chronic ambulatory peritoneal dialysis
- Acute appendicitis (differential diagnosis)
- Evaluation of antibiotic therapy for female pelvic infection
- Laryngotracheitis/pharyngitis/epiglottitis in children
- Chorioamnionitis after premature rupture of membranes
- Disseminated versus localized gonococcal infection
- Infection precipitating sickle cell crisis

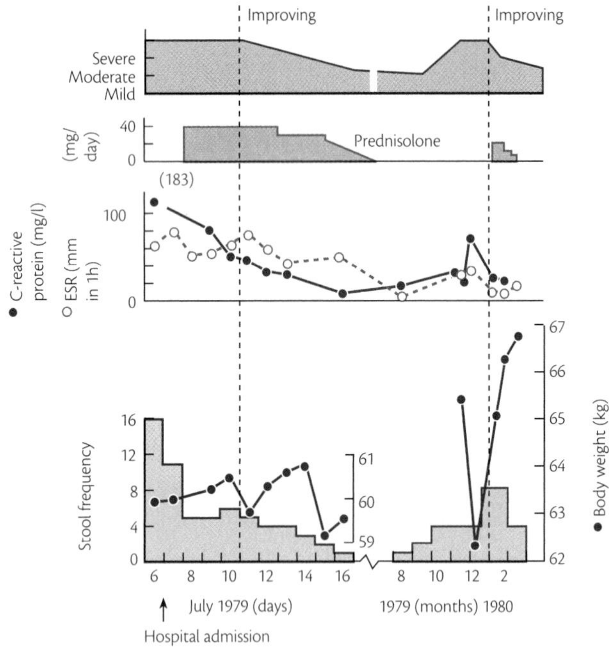

Fig. 12.12.1.3 A 26-year-old man with pancolonic Crohn's disease. He was admitted with severe exacerbation; temperature 38°C; pulse 110 beats/min; 16 stools per day; haematocrit 41.5 per cent, leucocytes 13.8×10^9/litre. Rectal mucosa severely inflamed with histiocytic granulomas on biopsy. Rapid improvement occurred with oral and rectal prednisolone, ampicillin, and metronidazole, with complete clinical and histological remission on day 11. Relapse 5 months later responded promptly to a short course of oral and rectal prednisolone. CRP and ESR were both high during the initial exacerbation. The rapid response to treatment was paralleled by a prompt fall in CRP, whereas the ESR responded more slowly. Despite clinical remission and a normal ESR, the CRP remained slightly elevated, suggesting persistent low-grade inflammatory activity, and it rose further during a subsequent relapse when the ESR did not change. (From Fagan A, *et al.* (1982). Serum levels of C-reactive protein in Crohn's disease and ulcerative colitis. *Eur J Clin Invest*, **12**, 351–9, with permission.)

disease activity. Furthermore, the presence or absence of a CRP response can distinguish between symptoms or organ dysfunction that are due to currently active inflammation and those that are the consequence of fibrosis and scarring from previous episodes. This can be very important when treatments include steroids and other powerful and potentially hazardous immunosuppressive, anti-inflammatory, and cytotoxic drugs. It permits precise titration of dosages and may help to avoid excessive or unnecessary use.

Induction of clinical remission and control of the underlying disease process is associated with prompt normalization of the CRP. However, CRP also becomes abnormal with intercurrent infection, a common complication of some of these disorders and their treatments, and this serves to focus diagnostic attention often before the infection has become too severe or even before it is clinically evident. Monitoring the CRP response to antimicrobial therapy can then help to confirm the diagnosis and the efficacy of therapy. Persistent elevation of the CRP after eradication of infection may indicate relapse of the underlying inflammatory disease, requiring additional anti-inflammatory treatment.

Necrosis

Myocardial infarction is invariably associated with a major CRP response, as is elective embolization leading to necrosis of tumours in the liver and elsewhere. The peak level of CRP occurs about 50 h after the onset of pain in myocardial infarction patients who do not undergo revascularization, and may be earlier and smaller following effective early revascularization. CRP production usually correlates in magnitude, though not in timing, with the peak serum level of the specific myocardial markers creatine kinase MB and troponin. In patients who recover uneventfully, the CRP falls rapidly towards normal in the usual exponential fashion. However, complications such as persistent cardiac dysfunction, further infarction, aneurysm formation, intercurrent infection, thromboembolism, or postinfarction syndrome are associated with either persistently raised CRP levels or secondary elevation after the initial decrease. Myocardial rupture is seen only in patients with high peak CRP values (>200 mg/litre) and the peak CRP concentration after acute myocardial infarction is inversely correlated with overall outcome, including survival, in the short, medium, and long term.

Stable angina and invasive investigation, such as coronary arteriography, do not stimulate CRP production, whereas some other causes of chest pain, such as pulmonary embolism, pleurisy, or pericarditis, are usually associated with raised CRP levels. Routine assays of CRP after infarction or in patients with chest pain may thus assist in diagnosis and in the recognition and management of complications, including iatrogenic infection associated with invasive cardiovascular monitoring.

Serum CRP levels closely reflect the severity and progress of acute pancreatitis, providing a better guide to intra-abdominal events than other markers such as leucocyte counts, erythrocyte sedimentation rate (ESR), temperature, and the plasma concentrations of antiproteinase. A CRP concentration greater than 100 mg/litre at the end of the first week of illness is associated with a more prolonged subsequent course and a higher risk of the development of a pancreatic collection. Serial CRP measurements can therefore guide the use of appropriate imaging techniques and help to confirm resolution before discharge from hospital.

Trauma

The CRP concentration always rises after significant trauma, surgery, or burns, peaking after about 2 days and then falling towards normal with recovery and healing. Infections or other tissue-damaging complications alter this normal pattern of CRP response and the failure of the CRP to continue falling, or the appearance of a second peak, may precede clinical evidence of intercurrent infection by 1 to 2 days.

Malignancy

Most malignant tumours, especially when they are extensive and metastatic, induce an acute phase response. This is particularly so with those neoplasms that cause systemic symptoms such as fever and weight loss, e.g. Hodgkin's disease (stage B) and renal carcinoma, but raised CRP levels are seen with many others. In some studies, notably of prostatic carcinoma and bladder carcinoma, the CRP level at presentation has been found to correlate with the overall tumour load and also with the prognosis, being higher for a given mass of tumour in those patients who subsequently fare worse. The CRP may also correlate better with progress and regression of tumour than other, more specific tumour markers. However, given the nonspecific nature of the acute phase response and the limited number of studies performed so far, a definite role for CRP measurement in the management of cancer patients, other than in cases of intercurrent infection, has not yet been established.

Allograft rejection

In the era before routine immunosuppression with combined ciclosporin and steroid treatment, rejection episodes following renal allografting were generally associated with increased production of CRP. However, such treatment almost completely suppresses the CRP response in this situation. In contrast, the acute phase response of serum amyloid A is unaffected and, importantly, intercurrent infection still stimulates high levels of both CRP and serum amyloid A.

Conditions associated with minor elevation of serum CRP

Despite unequivocal evidence of active inflammation and/or tissue damage, the conditions listed in Box 12.12.1.3 are usually associated with only minor elevations of the serum CRP concentration, and in many cases it may even remain normal in the face of severe disease. The contrasts between systemic lupus erythematosus (SLE) and rheumatoid and other arthritic conditions shown in Box 12.12.1.1, and between ulcerative colitis and Crohn's disease, are very striking. However, intercurrent microbial infection provokes a major CRP response in all the conditions shown in Box 12.12.1.3, and this is of great value in diagnosis and management, especially in SLE and leukaemia. The basis of the apparently selective failure of the acute phase response of CRP (which is also shown by serum amyloid A) is not known, but presumably involves defect(s) in the pathways that mediate the acute phase response to autologous inflammation and tissue damage.

Pyrexia is common in SLE and may be caused by microbial infection or by activity of the lupus itself. Both SLE and its treatment predispose to infection, and steroids and immunosuppressives can mask the usual symptoms and signs of infection. Furthermore, infection can trigger exacerbations of SLE. This is a serious clinical situation and infection remains one of the most common causes of death in patients with SLE. CRP values of 60 mg/litre or more are very rare in SLE in the absence of infection, whereas levels below 60 mg/litre are seen in patients with documented infection only when it is rather mild and often localized, e.g. to the skin or lower urinary tract. Differential diagnosis and management of fever in SLE are thus considerably improved by the measurement of serum CRP concentration (Fig. 12.12.1.4).

The reason why leukaemia patients fail to mount more than a modest CRP response, even during induction therapy when there is massive death of leukaemia cells, is not known. However, they do respond to infection. Since all febrile episodes in leukaemia must initially be treated as infective, the main value of CRP monitoring is to determine the response to therapy and assist in decisions about its duration. Acute or chronic graft-vs-host disease

Box 12.12.1.3 Conditions associated with minor elevation of serum CRP concentration

- Systemic lupus erythematosus
- Scleroderma
- Dermatomyositis
- Ulcerative colitis
- Leukaemia
- Graft-versus-host disease

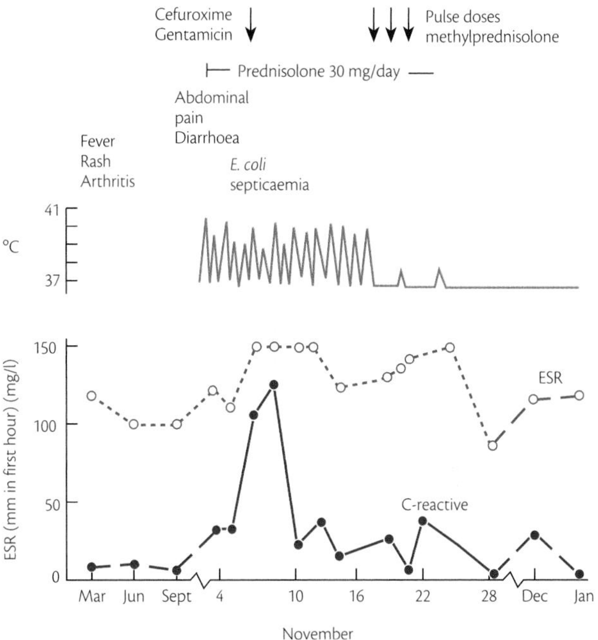

Fig. 12.12.1.4 A 12-year-old girl with a 3-year history of SLE; recurrent febrile episodes, polyarthritis, cutaneous vasculitis, and episodes of asymptomatic bacteriuria. Intermittent treatment was with prednisolone, azathioprine, and plasma exchange. Serum CRP was only marginally elevated throughout but erythrocyte sedimentation rate was persistently raised. Fever recurred with diarrhoea and abdominal pain. All microbial cultures were negative except for growth of *Escherichia coli* from the urine. Despite oral cefalexin and prednisolone her condition deteriorated, with severe neutropenia, probably due to azathioprine. CRP rose from 36 to 101 mg/litre and then 137 mg/litre, and at this stage her blood culture grew *Escherichia coli*. Intravenous antibiotics were given and the serum CRP level fell rapidly, but there was little clinical improvement. Active SLE appeared then to be the sole cause of the fever and this was confirmed by the development of a diffuse vasculitic rash and polyarthritis. Three pulse doses of methylprednisolone were given intravenously on successive days and produced a dramatic improvement in her clinical state with resolution of the fever. This case illustrates: (1) the differential response of CRP to fever resulting from activity of SLE alone and fever due to bacterial infection; (2) the rapid response of CRP both to the onset and to the effective treatment of serious bacterial infection; and (3) the failure of ESR measurements to provide any useful information in this complex and rapidly evolving clinical situation.

(From Pepys MB, Langham JG, de Beer FC (1982). C-reactive protein in systemic lupus erythematosus. *Clin Rheum Dis*, **8**, 91–103, with permission.)

after bone marrow transplantation is usually associated with only a modest CRP response, if any. However, the immunosuppressive treatments used to prevent bone marrow rejection and to control graft-vs-host disease render the patients susceptible to intercurrent infections, often with unusual microorganisms, and these are always associated with high levels of CRP. CRP monitoring therefore plays a valuable role in management in the post-transplant period.

Interpretation of clinical serum CRP measurements

The CRP response is not specific and CRP measurements on their own can therefore never be diagnostic of any particular condition, nor should they be used in isolation for any other clinical purpose. The CRP value can only be interpreted in the light of all other available clinical and laboratory information. Provided this is done it can make a most useful contribution to overall assessment of the patient and determination of the best management.

Routine CRP measurement

The applications fall into three main categories:

- Screening for organic disease
- Monitoring of extent and activity of disease:
  - infection
  - inflammation
  - malignancy
  - necrosis
- Detection and management of intercurrent infection

Screening for organic disease

CRP production is a very sensitive response to organic disease. A normal CRP therefore eliminates many possible types of pathology and is a reassuring finding. Those serious conditions that stimulate CRP production only weakly, if at all, e.g. SLE, ulcerative colitis, and leukaemia, are all readily recognized by clinical examination and other simple tests such as blood counts, rectal biopsy, and serology. The presence of a raised CRP is unequivocal evidence of active pathology, though this may not necessarily be the cause of the complaint for which the patient presented. Such a finding, in the absence of other obvious abnormality, warrants a repeat CRP assay after a few days when a trivial cause such as an upper respiratory tract infection will have resolved. Further investigation of a persistently raised CRP level will then depend on the severity of the complaint and other clinical findings.

Monitoring extent and activity of disease

Once the diagnosis is established, in those diseases which cause major elevation of the CRP, serial measurements reflect activity and response to treatment and can be used for monitoring. However, they can only be interpreted provided other possible intercurrent causes of an acute phase response, particularly infections, are excluded.

Detection and management of intercurrent infection

Production of CRP is a very sensitive response to most forms of infection and a raised level is thus a useful guide to the possible presence of infection in otherwise normal subjects or individuals with a primary condition that predisposes to infection. In disorders that themselves elevate the CRP concentration, the decision as to whether infection is present or not must depend on clinical examination and other laboratory tests; the role of CRP testing is then to demonstrate rapidly and objectively whether there is a response to whatever treatment is used. Effective antimicrobial therapy of infection is always associated with a prompt fall in the CRP, whereas persistent CRP elevation indicates continuing infection and/or activity of the underlying disease. There is no other objective test that yields this sort of information so accurately. Changes in the results of clinical examinations and tests of organ function usually lag hours or days behind the CRP response.

CRP and body temperature

The acute phase response, which is best measured clinically by quantification of the serum CRP, is part of the systemic response of the body to disease. Monitoring of this same response by measurement of body temperature is an integral part of the physical examination and of patient management. CRP production is triggered by the same cytokines that cause fever, and the serum CRP concentration therefore may be considered in part to be a biochemical measurement of the body temperature. However, the CRP response is not susceptible to the many vagaries of thermoregulation itself and routine clinical measurement of body temperature. The precise numerical value of the CRP concentration and its changes over time reflect much more accurately than the temperature the intensity of the underlying stimulus. Furthermore, there is often a CRP response in the absence of fever, especially in neonates and older people, though also at any age in many chronic inflammatory conditions, and a case therefore exists for the inclusion of a regular serum CRP chart together with the standard temperature chart in appropriate patients.

CRP or ESR?

The only other comparable nonspecific index of the presence of disease that is routinely measured is the ESR. The ESR reflects, in part, the intensity of the acute phase response, especially that of fibrinogen and the α-globulins, but is also largely determined by the concentration of immunoglobulins, which are not acute phase reactants. These proteins all have half-lives of days to weeks. The rate of change of the ESR is thus very much slower than that of the CRP level, and it rarely reflects precisely the clinical status of the patient at the actual time of testing. ESR is also dependent on the number and morphology of the red cells, which bear no relationship to the acute phase response. Finally, there is a significant diurnal variation in ESR, depending on food intake, which is not seen in the CRP. The ESR is therefore of limited use as an objective index of disease activity on which management decisions can be based. The dynamic range of the ESR is also much less than that of CRP and the precision and reproducibility of ESR measurement is poor compared to the robust immunoassays available for CRP. Thus, in all clinical situations that have been carefully evaluated, ranging from acute bacterial infections to the chronic remittent inflammatory diseases, such as Crohn's disease, rheumatoid arthritis and other inflammatory arthropathies, and systemic vasculitis in its various forms, frequent prospective measurements of CRP reflect disease activity very much more closely than measurements of the ESR. However, the ESR remains a useful screening test for the detection of paraproteinaemias, especially multiple myeloma, which do not necessarily provoke an acute phase response.

CRP and cardiovascular disease

The 1994 report of a prognostic association between increased CRP and serum amyloid A values and outcome in severe unstable angina, and the discovery of a significant predictive association between baseline CRP values in the general population and future coronary events, triggered an avalanche of work in this field. These observations have become increasingly controversial, but forthcoming publications of very large-scale observational and genetic epidemiological studies should resolve the major issues. The key questions are whether the measurement of baseline CRP concentration provides information useful for the assessment and management of cardiovascular disease risk, and whether CRP itself contributes to the pathogenesis of atherosclerosis, atherothrombosis, and/or ischaemic tissue injury.

The possible involvement of CRP in atherogenesis was first suggested by the binding of CRP to low density lipoprotein and the presence of CRP in atherosclerotic lesions. In recent years an extraordinarily wide range of proinflammatory and cell-activating effects have been claimed for CRP, based on *in vitro* studies with various cell types. Unfortunately, nearly all this work has been done with commercial CRP preparations produced in recombinant bacteria, and none of the positive observations have been reproducible with authentic pure human CRP isolated from human source material. The amazing range of potent proinflammatory and cell-activating properties ascribed to CRP is not consistent with the fact that neither the administration of vast doses of pure human CRP in normal healthy animals nor the 1000-fold natural acute phase response of CRP in patients are associated with any such effects. In experimental animal models of atherosclerosis CRP either has no effect on atherogenesis *in vivo* or is atheroprotective. Human epidemiological studies of atherosclerosis burden have had varying results, but overall provide no compelling evidence for an association with CRP values.

Baseline CRP values are significantly associated with all the known risk factors and pathogenetic mechanisms for coronary heart disease events, and about 70 per cent of the variance in baseline CRP is ascribable to these factors. Although CRP concentration is thus not independently associated with cardiovascular disease risk, a statistically significant association remains even after maximal adjustment. However, the level of association is markedly less than was originally reported and is comparable with the association with cardiovascular disease risk of other nonspecific systemic markers of inflammation, such as low plasma albumin, raised white cell count, ESR, and serum amyloid A. Despite persisting controversy, most studies show that CRP measurement adds no useful information to risk assessment by the major established risk scores, such as Framingham. Also, since statins lower risk when administered at any level of low-density cholesterol and in all subgroups of the population, regardless of intercurrent disease or additional risk factors, there is no justification for the use of CRP measurement to select patients for statin treatment. Indeed, measuring the exquisitely nonspecific CRP in this context, without comprehensive review of a patient with a raised value, risks missing other important pathology.

The unfortunate conflation of association with causality triggered much speculation about whether CRP is a pathogenetic factor for cardiovascular disease events. However, mendelian randomization genetic epidemiological studies looking at hereditary polymorphisms associated with higher or lower baseline CRP values all show no association with cardiovascular disease risk. This negative outcome is entirely consistent with the negative *in vivo* animal studies of CRP and atherogenesis. In contrast, experimental animal studies robustly show that human CRP can exacerbate pre-existing ischaemic injury and that this can be blocked by experimental drugs that inhibit CRP function. Future testing of such compounds in patients will reveal whether this mechanism is clinically relevant.

Serum amyloid A protein

Serum amyloid A, an apolipoprotein of high-density lipoprotein particles, is a marked acute phase reactant, its concentration rising from normal levels of about 2 mg/litre by as much as 1000-fold. It is essential to monitor and control serum amyloid A levels in patients with reactive systemic, AA type amyloidosis (see Chapter 12.12.3). The other indication for routine serum amyloid A measurement is in renal allograft recipients, in whom the serum amyloid A response is the most sensitive marker of rejection episodes, despite suppression of the CRP response by immunosuppression with ciclosporin and steroids.

Further reading

Boralessa H, *et al.* (1986). C-reactive protein in patients undergoing cardiac surgery. *Anaesthesia*, **41**, 11–15.

Casas JP *et al.* (2008). C-reactive protein and coronary heart disease: a critical review. *J Intern Med*, **264**, 295–314.

Elliott P *et al.* (2009). Genetic Loci associated with C-reactive protein levels and risk of coronary heart disease. *JAMA*, **302**, 37–48.

Emerging Risk Factors Collaboration (2009). C-reactive protein concentration and risk of coronary heart disease, stroke and mortality: an individual participant meta analysis. *Lancet*, **375** (9709),132–140.

Fagan EA *et al.* (1982). Serum levels of C-reactive protein in Crohn's disease and ulcerative colitis. *Eur J Clin Invest*, **12**, 351–60.

Griselli M *et al.* (1999). C-reactive protein and complement are important mediators of tissue damage in acute myocardial infarction. *J Exp Med*, **190**, 1733–9.

Hartmann A *et al.* (1997). Serum amyloid A protein is a clinically useful indicator of acute renal allograft rejection. *Nephrol Dial Transplant*, **12**, 161–6.

Kushner I, Rzewnicki D, Samols D (2006). What does minor elevation of C-reactive protein signify? *Am J Med*, **119**, 166, e117–28.

Liuzzo G *et al.* (1994). The prognostic value of C-reactive protein and serum amyloid A protein in severe unstable angina. *N Engl J Med*, **331**, 417–24.

Lowe GDO, Pepys MB (2006). C-reactive protein and cardiovascular disease: weighing the evidence. *Curr Atheroscler Rep*, **8**, 421–8.

Pepys MB (2005). CRP or not CRP? That is the question. *Arterioscler Thromb Vasc Biol*, **25**, 1091–4.

Pepys MB, Hirschfield GM (2003). C-reactive protein: a critical update. *J Clin Invest*, **111**, 1805–12.

Pepys MB, Lanham JG, de Beer FC (1982). C-reactive protein in systemic lupus erythematosus. *Clin Rheum Dis*, **8**, 91–103.

Pepys MB *et al.* (2005). Proinflammatory effects of bacterial recombinant human C-reactive protein are caused by contamination with bacterial products, not by C-reactive protein itself. *Circ Res*, **97**, e97–103.

Pepys MB *et al.* (2006). Targeting C-reactive protein for the treatment of cardiovascular disease. *Nature*, **440**, 1217–21.

Ridker PM *et al.* (1997). Inflammation, aspirin, and the risk of cardiovascular disease in apparently healthy men. *N Engl J Med*, **336**, 973–9.

Starke ID *et al.* (1984). Serum C-reactive protein levels in the management of infection in acute leukaemia. *Eur J Cancer*, **20**, 319–25.

van Leeuwen MA *et al.* (1997). Individual relationship between progression of radiological damage and the acute phase response in early rheumatoid arthritis. Towards development of a decision support system. *J Rheumatol*, **24**, 20–7.

Wasunna A *et al.* (1990). C-reactive protein and bacterial infection in preterm infants. *Eur J Pediatr*, **149**, 424–7.

12.12.2 Hereditary periodic fever syndromes

Helen J. Lachmann and Philip N. Hawkins

Essentials

The hereditary periodic fever syndromes are autoinflammatory diseases that mostly present in childhood and are characterized by recurrent, self-limiting, seemingly unprovoked episodes of fever and systemic inflammation that occur in the absence of autoantibody production or identifiable infection.

Disorders include (1) familial Mediterranean fever (FMF), due to mutation in the gene encoding pyrin; (2) tumour necrosis factor (TNF) receptor associated periodic syndrome (TRAPS), due to mutation in a gene for a TNF receptor; (3) Mevalonate kinase deficiency and period fever (MKD), caused by mutations in the mevalonate kinase gene; and (4) the cryopyrin associated periodic syndromes (CAPS), which include (a) familial cold urticarial syndrome, (b) Muckle–Wells syndrome, and (c) chronic infantile neurological, cutaneous and articular syndrome. Understanding of the molecular pathogenesis of these disorders provides unique insights into the regulation of innate immunity and inflammation.

Diagnosis—this relies on recognition of suggestive clinical features (e.g. fever with peritonitis and/or pleurisy, arthralgia/arthritis) that are almost always accompanied by a substantial acute phase response, and is supported by genetic testing. With the exception of FMF, which is prevalent in certain geographic areas, hereditary periodic fever syndromes are rare and easily overlooked in the differential diagnosis of recurrent fevers.

Clinical features and management—attacks can be mild to debilitating and short to prolonged, whilst their most feared complication is AA amyloidosis. Effective therapies are available for some syndromes, e.g. (1) FMF—daily prophylactic colchicine prevents clinical attacks and susceptibility to AA amyloidosis; (2) CAPS—daily treatment with anakinra (recombinant IL-1 receptor antagonist) produces rapid and often complete clinical and serological remission; (3) TRAPS—anti-TNF therapy with etanercept is useful in some patients.

Introduction

The hereditary periodic fever syndromes are a group of multisystem disorders characterized by fluctuating or irregularly recurring episodes of fever and systemic inflammation, notably affecting the joints, eyes, skin, and serosal surfaces. They include familial Mediterranean fever (FMF), tumour necrosis factor receptor-associated periodic syndrome (TRAPS), Mevalonate kinase deficiency and periodic fever (previously known as the hyper-IgD and periodic fever syndrome (HIDS)), and the cryopyrin-associated periodic syndromes (CAPS). The latter are a spectrum of three hitherto apparently distinct disorders of increasing severity: familial cold urticarial syndrome (now known as familial cold autoinflammatory syndrome; FCAS), Muckle–Wells syndrome (MWS), and chronic infantile neurological, cutaneous, and articular syndrome (CINCA). The latter is also known in the United States of America as neonatal-onset multisystem inflammatory disorder (NOMID).

Although many symptoms of these disorders are shared, there are clear distinctions in the pattern of their inheritance, the duration and frequency of attacks, and their overall clinical picture (Table 12.12.2.1). With the exception of CINCA, these diseases are usually compatible with normal life expectancy, though with the ever-looming grave threat of AA amyloidosis. Recent insights into their molecular pathogenesis have led to enhanced diagnosis through DNA analysis and the development of rational therapies, and have shed important new light on regulation of the innate immune system.

Historical perspective

Although the hereditary periodic fever syndromes have only been identified as such during the last few decades, there are various ancient references to them, particularly FMF. Perhaps the earliest extant clinical description is found in William Heberden's 1802 *Commentaries on History and Care of Disease*: 'Pains which are regularly intermittent, the fits of which return periodically as those of an ague; such as I have known in the bowels, stomach, breast, loins, arms and hips, though it be but seldom that such parts suffer in such a manner'.

Familial Mediterranean fever (FMF)

Genetics

FMF is predominantly inherited in a recessive manner. The gene associated with FMF, *MEFV*, which encodes a protein called pyrin, was identified through positional cloning in 1997. *MEFV* is expressed in polymorphonuclear leucocytes and monocytes, and expression is up-regulated in response to inflammatory activators such as interferon-γ and tumour necrosis factor-α (TNFα). The more than 40 *MEFV* mutations that are associated with FMF encode either single amino acid substitutions or deletions. The mutations that cause FMF are mostly in exon 10, but also occur elsewhere, particularly in exons 1, 3, 5, and 9. Mutations in each of the two *MEFV* alleles can be identified in most patients with FMF, whereas most individuals with a single mutated allele remain healthy carriers. While it is inherently likely that different mutations will affect the function of a protein to differing extents, several findings suggest that the methionine residue at position 694 is especially important. Four different pathogenic exon 10 mutations involving Met694 have been identified, and individuals homozygous for Met694Val tend to have particularly severe disease. Simple heterozygous deletion of this residue, which is likely to produce especially marked structural disruption, is associated with autosomal dominant FMF of variable penetrance. More extensive disruption of a single *MEFV* allele by one or more mutations may account for other rare reports of dominant FMF. Much more commonly, FMF affecting more than one generation of a family is pseudodominantly inherited, reflecting consanguinity or a high local prevalence of the heterozygous carrier state.

One particular pyrin variant, *E148Q* encoded in exon 2, is extremely frequent in Asian populations, with an allele frequency of 10 to 20%, and occurs in other populations at a much lower frequency. Although pyrin *E148Q* can cause typical FMF when coupled with various exon 10 mutations, homozygosity for *E148Q* alone is thought not to be associated with disease in the vast majority

Table 12.12.2.1 Features of inherited periodic fever syndromes

Periodic fever syndrome	Gene	OMIM	Mode of inheritance	Predominant population	Usual age at onset	Potential precipitants of attacks	Distinctive clinical features	Typical duration of attacks	Typical frequency of attacks	Characteristic laboratory abnormalities	Treatment
FMF	*MEFV* Chromosome 16	608107	Autosomal recessive (dominant in rare families)	Eastern Mediterranean	Childhood/ early adulthood	Usually none Occasionally menstruation, fasting, stress, or trauma	Short severe attacks Colchicine-responsive Erysipelas-like erythema	1–3 days	Variable	Marked acute phase response during attacks	Colchicine
TRAPS	*TNFRSF1A* Chromosome 12	142680	Autosomal dominant (can be *de novo*)	Northern European, but reported in many ethnic groups	Childhood/ early adulthood	Usually none	Prolonged symptoms	More than a week (may be very prolonged)	Variable (may be continuous)	Marked acute phase response during attacks Low levels of soluble TNFR1 when well	Etanercept, anti IL-1therapies High-dose corticosteroids
MKD	*MVK* Chromosome 12	260920	Autosomal recessive	Northern European	Infancy	Immunizations	Diarrhoea and lymphadenopathy.	3–7 days	1–2 monthly	Elevated IgD and IgA, acute phase response, and mevalonate aciduria during attacks	Anti-TNF and anti-IL-1 therapies
FCAS	*NLRP3* Chromosome 1	611762	Autosomal dominant	Northern European	Childhood	Exposure to cold environment	Cold-induced fever, arthralgia, rash, and conjunctivitis	24–48 h	Depends on environmental factors	Acute phase response during attacks; to a lesser extent when well	Cold avoidance Anti-IL-1 therapies
MWS	*NLRP3* Chromosome 1	191900	Autosomal dominant,	Northern European	Neonatal/ infancy	Marked diurnal variation Cold environment, but less marked than in FCAS	Urticarial rash Conjunctivitis Sensorineural deafness	Continuous (often worse in the evenings)	Often daily	Varying but marked acute phase response most of the time	Anti-IL-1 therapies
CINCA/ NOMID	*NLRP3* Chromosome 1	607115	Sporadic	Northern European	Infancy	None	Urticarial rash Aseptic meningitis Deforming arthropathy Sensorineural deafness Mental retardation	Continuous	Continuous	Varying but marked acute phase response most of the time	Anti-IL-1 therapies
PAPA	*PSTPIP1 (CD2BP1)* Chromosome 15	604416	Autosomal dominant	Northern European (only three families reported)	Childhood	None	Pyogenic arthritis, pyoderma gangrenosum, and cystic acne	Intermittent attacks with migratory arthritis	Variable (may be continuous)	Acute phase response during attacks	Anti-TNF therapy
Blau's syndrome	*NOD2 (CARD15)* Chromosome 16	605956 186580	Autosomal dominant	None	Childhood	None	Granulomatous polyarthritis, iritis, and dermatitis	Continuous	Continuous	Sustained modest acute phase response	Corticosteroids

CINCA/NOMID, chronic infantile neurological, cutaneous, and articular syndrome/neonatal-onset multisystem inflammatory disorder; FCAS, familial cold autoinflammatory syndrome; FMF, familial Mediterranean fever; HIDS, hyper-IgD periodic fever syndrome; IL-1, interleukin 1; MWS, Muckle–Wells syndrome; PAPA, pyogenic arthritis, pyoderma gangrenosum, and acne syndrome; TNF, tumour necrosis factor; TNFR1, tumour necrosis factor receptor 1; TRAPS, tumour necrosis factor receptor-associated periodic syndrome.

of cases. There is, however, a suggestion that the presence of pyrin *E148Q* might intensify non-FMF types of inflammation.

Pathology

The structure and function of pyrin have not yet been characterized in detail, although subtle abnormalities of leucocyte function have been reported in FMF. The putative 781 amino acid protein has sequence homologies with a number of proteins of apparently disparate function and cellular localization. Recent work suggests that pyrin is not primarily a nuclear protein, but interacts via its N-terminal death domain with microtubules and the actin cytoskeleton, consistent with a role in directed cell migration and by the C-terminal domain to active IL-1 beta and NF- κ B; other proteins that have homology with pyrin's N-terminal sequence are now classified generically to have a pyrin domain.

Members of the death-domain superfamily play important roles in the assembly and activation of apoptotic and inflammatory complexes through homotypic protein-protein interactions. Proteins with pyrin domains are involved in inflammation, apoptosis, and NF-κB signalling and have been implicated in pathways in CAPS as well. It is thought that *MEFV* mutations associated with FMF may disrupt an interaction between pyrin domains that normally exerts a stabilizing, down-regulating effect on neutrophil activation.

Epidemiology

Familial Mediterranean fever occurs worldwide, though predominantly in populations arising from the eastern Mediterranean basin, particularly non-Ashkenazi Jews, Armenians, Turks, and Levantine Arabs. The prevalence of FMF has been estimated to be 1 in 250 to 1 in 500 among non-Ashkenazi Jews and 1 in 1000 in the Turkish population. The carrier frequency is as high as 1 in 5 among Armenian, Turkish, and North African Jewish populations, fuelling speculation that the FMF trait may have conferred survival benefit, possibly through enhanced resistance to microbial infection mediated by up-regulation of the innate inflammatory response. Males and females are equally affected. FMF usually presents in childhood, in 60% before the age of 10 years and in 90% by 20 years.

Clinical features

Attacks of FMF occur irregularly at variable frequencies and may be precipitated by physical and emotional stress, menstruation, and diet. The onset is rapid and symptoms resolve spontaneously within 6 to 72 h. Fever with peritonitis and/or pleurisy are the hallmark features, but occur with widely varying intensity from very mild to severely incapacitating. The clinical picture may mimic an acute surgical abdomen with ileus and vomiting, and 40% of patients undergo laparoscopy before the diagnosis is made. Pleuritic attacks occur in 40% of patients, characteristically unilaterally, either alone or in association with peritonitis. Pericarditis is rare and cardiac tamponade extremely rare. Headache with meningism is reported, but generally the nervous system is not involved in attacks. Orchitis occurs in less than 5% of males, most commonly in early childhood, when it can be confused with torsion of the testis. Transient arthralgia in lower-limb joints is not infrequent in acute attacks, and usually subsides within 2 to 4 days; chronic arthritis is rare, but can be destructive. A characteristic erysipelas-like erythematous rash occurs in 20% of patients (Fig. 12.12.2.1), usually on the lower extremities. Myalgia can be part of the constitutional upset during acute attacks, but up to one-fifth of patients complain of persistent muscle pain on exertion, usually affecting the calves. The rare but distinct syndrome of protracted febrile myalgia presents as severe pain, mainly affecting the lower limbs or abdominal musculature; symptoms may persist for weeks and be accompanied by a vasculitic rash, but usually respond to corticosteroids.

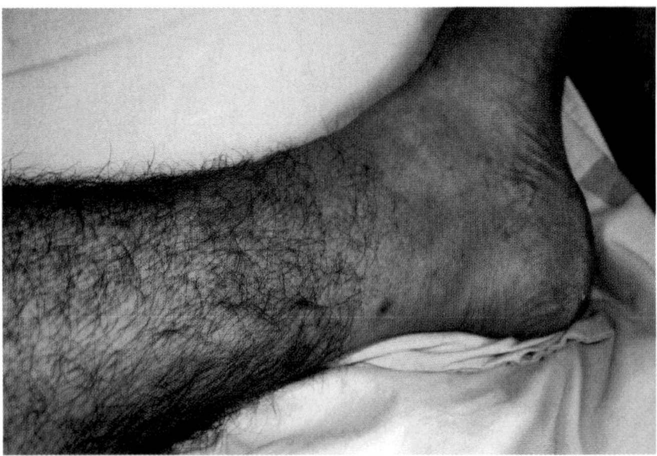

Fig. 12.12.2.1 Typical erythematous erysipelas-like rash in a man with familial Mediterranean fever.

Clinical investigation

Acute attacks are accompanied by a number of laboratory abnormalities including neutrophilia, raised erythrocyte sedimentation rate (ESR) and a dramatic acute phase response. Investigations may be required to exclude other potential causes of symptoms but, in general, imaging by radiography, ultrasonography, or echocardiography during acute attacks is unrewarding.

The results of genetic testing must be interpreted with care, since some individuals with paired pathogenic *MEFV* mutations remain completely healthy, and others with apparent carrier status develop classical FMF. Furthermore, *MEFV* spans 10 exons, and most diagnostic laboratories offer only limited screening. However, in the absence of a mutation in exon 10, a diagnosis of FMF is unlikely.

Treatment

Supportive treatment, including analgesia, may be required in acute attacks, but the mainstay of therapy in FMF is prophylaxis with colchicine, a serendipitous discovery made by Goldfinger in 1972. Continuous treatment with colchicine 1 to 2 mg daily prevents or substantially reduces the symptoms of FMF in at least 95% of cases. Colchicine binds to tubulin and evidently modulates neutrophil function in a presumably rather specific and certainly very beneficial manner in patients with variant forms of pyrin. Recent data also suggest that colchicine may also suppress the effect of N-terminal cleaved pyrin in enhancing NF- κ B activation in FMF.

Long-term use of colchicine is advisable in every patient with FMF and mandatory in those with AA amyloidosis. Although colchicine is extremely toxic in overdose, the small regular doses required for the treatment of FMF are generally very well tolerated, but may cause diarrhoea that sometimes responds to a lactose-free diet. Despite concerns about antimitotic potential, colchicine does not appear to cause infertility or birth defects, even when used throughout pregnancy. The concentration of colchicine in breast milk is sufficiently low to permit breastfeeding. Initiating or increasing the dose of colchicine does not usually ameliorate acute attacks.

Very few patients are genuinely resistant to colchicine; there have been reports of benefit in such patients following treatment with etanercept or recombinant human interleukin 1 (IL-1) receptor antagonist (anakinra).

TNF receptor-associated periodic syndrome (TRAPS)

Genetics

TRAPS is an autosomal dominant disease associated with mutations in the 10-exon tumour necrosis factor receptor superfamily 1A gene (*TNFRSF1A*) on chromosome 12p13. A disproportionate number of the 50 or so associated mutations disrupt the coding of the first and second cysteine residues of the extracellular domains.

Pathology

TNF is a key mediator in the inflammatory response, with several activities including increased expression of adhesion molecules, induction of cytokine secretion and activation of leucocytes. TNF receptor 1 (TNFR1) is a member of the death-domain superfamily and comprises an extracellular region containing four cysteine-rich domains, a transmembrane domain, and an intracellular death domain. Binding of TNF results in trimerization of the receptor and activation of NF-κB, with downstream induction of inflammation or apoptosis. Under normal circumstances TNF signalling is terminated by cleavage of the extracellular domain; this results in the release of soluble TNFR1 into the plasma, competitively inhibiting the binding of circulating TNF to cell-surface receptors.

The mechanisms by which heterozygous *TRFRSF1A* mutations cause TRAPS are still unclear, and may well vary according to the specific mutation.

Epidemiology

TRAPS was first described in 1982, somewhat tongue-in-cheek, as 'familial Hibernian fever', reflecting a preponderance of patients from Ireland and Scotland in early reports. It is now clear that TRAPS occurs in many populations, including white, Jewish, Arab, and Central American populations, but the disease is rare and we are aware of fewer than 100 patients in the United Kingdom. Males and females are affected equally and the median age at presentation is 4 years. Most mutations are associated with high penetrance, but two variants that can be associated with TRAPS (*P46L* and *R92Q*) are present in approximately 1% of healthy chromosomes, and are thus variously regarded as low-penetrance mutations or polymorphisms.

Clinical features

Attacks of TRAPS are far less distinct than in FMF, sometimes lasting many weeks, and almost one-third of patients have fairly continuous symptoms. Approximately one-half of patients have no clear family history; many of these have the *P46L* or *R92Q* variants, which tend to be associated with milder disease and older age at presentation. Symptoms are rather variable: more than 95% of patients experience fever and 80% complain of arthralgia or myalgia; abdominal pain occurs in 70%, and a faint but sometimes quite diffuse erythematous rash occurs in 60%. Other features include pleuritic pain, lymphadenopathy, conjunctivitis, and periorbital oedema. There are also reports of central nervous system manifestations resembling multiple sclerosis.

Clinical investigation

Symptoms are almost universally accompanied by a very marked acute phase response. The plasma concentration of soluble TNFR1 can be abnormally low in patients whose mutations are associated with decreased receptor shedding, though only when their disease is quiescent. Genetic testing is pivotal in establishing the diagnosis.

Treatment

Despite high hopes for anti-TNF biological agents, the treatment of TRAPS has proved disappointing in many patients. Acute attacks can be suppressed with corticosteroids, but prolonged treatment may be required at potentially harmful doses. Anti-TNF therapy in the form of etanercept, though interestingly not infliximab, has proved useful in some patients, although the response may decline over time. There are case reports suggesting that IL-1 blockade can also be effective in TRAPS.

Mevalonate kinase deficiency (MKD)

Genetics

MKD (also known as HIDS) is an autosomal recessive disease caused by mutations in the mevalonate kinase gene (*MVK*) on the long arm of chromosome 12. To date, 58 MKD-associated mutations have been described, spanning exons 2 to 11, the most common of which encode *MVK* variants *V377I* and *I268T*. The gene carriage rate in the population of the Netherlands, in which MKD is most prevalent, is 1 in 350.

Pathology

The *MVK* mutations associated with MKD result in 85 to 95% deficiency in mevalonate kinase activity. This enzyme is involved in cholesterol, farnesyl, and isoprenoid biosynthesis. It is not yet known how mevalonate kinase deficiency causes recurrent inflammation, although there is speculation that reduced protein isoprenylation causes defective lymphocyte apoptosis. Other mutations in *MVK* result in even greater reduction in enzyme activity, and cause the much more severe disease known as mevalonic aciduria.

Epidemiology

MKD is most prevalent in the Netherlands, where it was first described as HIDS in 1984. It has subsequently been reported in other populations, including Arabs and South-East Asians, though is least rare among northern European whites. The disease usually presents in the first year of life and occurs equally in both sexes. There are only about 200 patients with HIDS on the Dutch disease registry, and only some dozens recognized in the United Kingdom.

Clinical features

Symptoms are episodic and are often well circumscribed. Attacks are irregular, usually last 4 to 6 days, and can be provoked by vaccination, minor trauma, surgery, or stress. Fever, cervical lymphadenopathy, and abdominal pain with vomiting and diarrhoea are typical. Other common symptoms include headache, arthralgia, large joint arthritis, erythematous macules and papules, and aphthous ulcers. The disease typically ameliorates in early adult life and older patients may remain free of symptoms for years.

Clinical investigation

A diagnosis of HIDS is supported by a high serum IgD concentration (>100 IU/ml) although, particularly in very young patients, this value may occasionally be normal. The serum IgA concentration is also elevated in 80% of patients, and is more routinely available. Clinical attacks are accompanied by an acute phase response, leucocytosis, and the presence of melvalonic acid in the urine. A mutation in both alleles of *MVK* can be identified in most patients, more than 80% of whom have the most common *V337I* variant.

Treatment

Treatment remains largely supportive, including nonsteroidal anti-inflammatory drugs. Colchicine and thalidomide have been pursued with no convincing effect, though there have been some preliminary reports of responses to etanercept and anakinra. A recent study indicated a degree of benefit from treatment with simvastatin, an inhibitor of 3-hydroxy-3-methylglutaryl coenzyme A (HMG-CoA) reductase.

Cryopyrin-associated periodic syndromes (CAPS)

Genetics

CAPS comprises a spectrum of disease associated with mutations in the gene *NLRP3/CIAS1* on chromosome 1q44 that encodes the death-domain protein variously known as NLRP3 (previously NALP3) and cryopyrin. Dominant inheritance is evident in about 75% of patients with Muckle–Wells syndrome (MWS) and familial cold autoinflammatory syndrome (FCAS), whereas chronic infantile neurological, cutaneous, and articular syndrome (CINCA), the most severe phenotype, is usually due to *de novo* mutation. More than 60 single amino acid substitutions have been reported; all but three of which are in exon 3. The relationship between mutation and clinical phenotype can differ markedly between individuals, even within a family.

Pathology

NLRP3 is expressed in peripheral blood leucocytes and chondrocytes, and encodes a pyrin-like protein that contains a pyrin domain, a nucleotide-binding site domain, and a leucine-rich repeat motif. Following recognition and binding, via its leucine-rich repeat, of an intracellular pathogen-associated molecular pattern, NLRP3 associates with other members of the death-domain superfamily to form a multimeric cytosolic assembly, the inflammasome. This results in activation of caspase 1, which processes pro-IL-1 to produce the active cytokine; it also up-regulates NF-κB expression, resulting in increased IL-1 gene expression. IL-1 is a major proinflammatory cytokine involved in mediating local and systemic responses to infection and tissue injury. The remarkable response to IL-1 receptor blockade in CAPS confirms that the clinical features are substantially mediated by IL-1.

Epidemiology

So far, most reported patients have European ancestry, but CAPS probably occurs worldwide. Onset of disease is almost always in early infancy, and there is no sex bias.

Clinical features

FCAS was first described in 1940 as recurrent episodes of cold-induced fever, arthralgia, conjunctivitis, and rash. MWS was described in 1962 as a much more persistent urticaria-like rash, conjunctivitis, arthralgia, and fever, complicated by progressive sensorineural deafness and a high risk of AA amyloidosis (Fig. 12.12.2.2). CINCA was described as a sporadic severe inflammatory disorder that presents in the neonatal period with involvement of many organs including the skin, skeletal system, and central nervous system. Bony overgrowth and premature ossification may occur, particularly in the skull and knees, and chronic aseptic meningitis can result in severe developmental delay, optic atrophy, and deafness. It is now evident that FCAS, MWS, and CINCA represent a spectrum of a single disease entity.

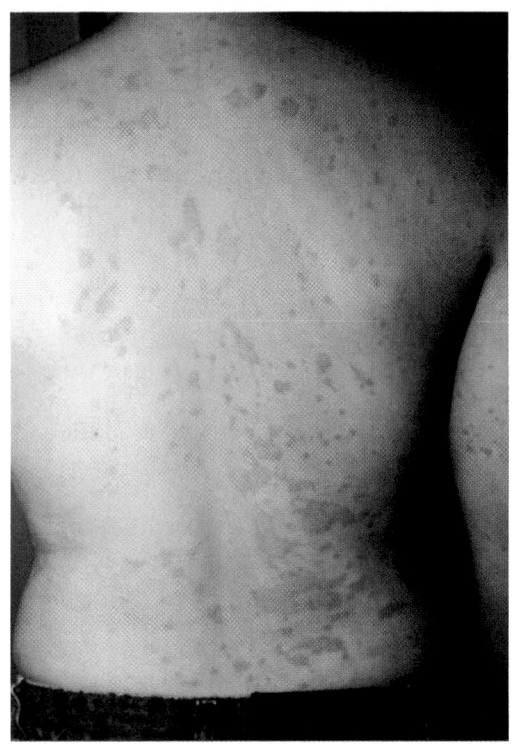

Fig. 12.12.2.2 Urticarial rash of Muckle–Wells syndrome. These lesions, accompanied by conjunctivitis, arthralgia, and fever, appeared daily in the early evenings prior to treatment with anakinra.

Clinical investigation

There is usually an acute phase response, and often leucocytosis and thrombocytosis that can vary substantially between measurements, and may not at times be present in some patients at the milder end of the disease spectrum, i.e. with FCAS and mild MWS. Audiometric evidence of sensorineural hearing loss should be sought, and characteristic bony abnormalities may be radiologically evident in CINCA. Features consistent with chronic meningitis may be evident on fundoscopy and MRI. A mutation in *NLRP3* can be readily identified in most patients with FCAS and MWS, though curiously not in about half of those with CINCA.

Treatment

Daily treatment with anakinra produces rapid and often complete clinical and serological remission of CAPS. Various new IL-1 inhibitors have also proved to be very effective in trials. There is hope that early treatment with anti IL-1 therapies may prevent neurological and skeletal abnormalities.

Table 12.12.2.2 Differential diagnosis of inherited periodic fever syndromes

Abdominal pain and fever	Thoracic pain and fever	Arthritis and fever	Fever, rash, and myalgia	Nonhereditary periodic fever syndromes
Acute surgical abdomen	Myocardial infarction	Septic arthritis	Viral illness	PFAPA (periodic fever, aphthous stomatitis, pharyngitis, and adenopathy)
Acute cholecystitis	Pneumonia/pleurisy	Juvenile inflammatory arthritis	Systemic lupus erythematosus	
Pyelonephritis	Acute pericarditis	Rheumatic fever	Cellulitis/erysipelas	
Pelvic inflammatory disease	Pulmonary embolism	Lyme disease	Behçet's disease	
Endometriosis		Palindromic arthritis	Cyclic neutropenia	
Mesenteric adenitis		Crystalline arthritis (gout) and calcium pyrophosphate dihydrate crystal deposition disease	Malignancy	
Systemic vasculitis				
Hereditary or acquired angioedema (not associated with fever)				

Other hereditary periodic fever syndromes

Pyogenic arthritis, pyoderma gangrenosum, and acne (PAPA) syndrome

This exceptionally rare autosomal dominant disease is caused by mutations in *PTSTPIP*, the gene encoding CD2 binding protein 1. The underlying pathogenesis remains poorly understood, although there is evidence that CD2 binding protein 1 interacts with the pyrin pathway. It is characterized by severe acne and recurrent sterile arthritis that typically occur after minor trauma. Early reports suggest that therapy with anakinra may be effective.

Blau syndrome

This was first described in 1985 as an autosomal dominant syndrome of sarcoid-like granulomatous infiltration of the joints (causing camptodactyly), eyes, skin, and sometimes viscera. It is caused by missense mutations in *NOD2/CARD15*, which is another member of the death-domain superfamily. *NOD2* mutations have also been implicated in familial Crohn's disease. Treatment is with corticosteroids.

Differential diagnosis of the hereditary periodic fever syndromes

These diseases have a broad differential diagnosis, particularly at first presentation, that is influenced by age and encompasses a vast spectrum of infectious, immune and neoplastic disorders (Table 12.12.2.2). Conversely, symptoms such as fever, arthralgia, and rashes in a patient known to have a hereditary periodic fever syndrome may also result from an alternative intercurrent disorder.

Prognosis

Although CINCA/NOMID can be sufficiently severe to cause death within the first few decades, life expectancy among most patients with inherited periodic fever syndromes is relatively good, and excellent in those for whom there is now effective therapy. The most serious and life-threatening complication of these diseases generally is AA amyloidosis.

AA amyloidosis

This usually presents with proteinuric kidney dysfunction. AA amyloid fibrils are derived from the circulating acute phase protein serum amyloid A protein (SAA), which is synthesized by hepatocytes under the transcriptional regulation of IL-1, IL-6, and TNFα. The terminology is either serum amyloid A protein or SAA. The circulating concentration of SAA in health is less than approximately 3 mg/litre, but this can rise by up to 1000-fold in the presence of inflammation. In chronic inflammatory diseases generally, AA amyloidosis occurs in up to 5% of patients after a median duration of about 20 years, but is much more frequent among patients with untreated inherited periodic fever syndromes. This may reflect their lifelong nature and their capacity to stimulate remarkably high plasma concentrations of SAA, even when they seem clinically quiescent. Before the widespread introduction of colchicine prophylaxis, up to 60% of patients with FMF died of amyloidosis, and even recently it was reported in 13% of a large Turkish series. The incidence of AA amyloidosis in TRAPS and MWS is approximately 25%, but is less than 5% in MDK, perhaps because the disease often ameliorates in early adulthood.

The natural course of AA amyloidosis is renal failure and early death, but this can be prevented by treatment of the underlying inflammatory disorder that substantially suppresses the production of serum amyloid A. Indeed, treatment such as colchicine in FMF and anakinra in CAPS can halt further deposition of AA amyloid, facilitate gradual regression of existing deposits, and lead to preservation or even improvement in renal function. Regular long-term measurement of serum amyloid A is vital in patients with AA amyloidosis.

Likely future developments

The recent elucidation of the pathogenesis of these diseases has led to major advances in their treatment, most notably in CAPS. It is likely that continued studies will shed further light on aspects of the innate immune system and inflammation generally, and on strategies for the treatment of TRAPS and MKD in particular. The clinical significance of low penetrance mutations and polymorphisms in the genes associated with inherited periodic fever syndromes will be sought. CAPS provides a powerful model of IL-1-driven disease, and a uniquely informative test bed for the early-phase development of novel IL-1 inhibitors that may have applications in many common inflammatory disorders, ranging from gout and rheumatoid arthritis to sepsis.

Further reading

Aganna E, *et al.* (2003). Heterogeneity among patients with tumor necrosis factor receptor-associated periodic syndrome phenotypes. *Arthritis Rheum*, **48**, 2632–44. [Case series and review of TRAPS.]

Ben-Chetrit E, Levy M (2003). Reproductive system in familial Mediterranean fever: an overview. *Ann Rheum Dis*, **62**, 916–9. [Review from an experienced group of the effect of FMF and its treatment on fertility and pregnancy outcomes.]

Chae JJ, Aksentijevich, Kastner DL (2009). Advances in the understanding of familial mediterranean fever and possibilities for targeted therapy. *Br J Haematol*, **146**, 467–78 (Review of the current understanding of the pathogenesis of FMF and the role of pyrin).

Goldbach-Mansky R, *et al.* (2006). Neonatal-onset multisystem inflammatory disease responsive to interleukin-1beta inhibition. *N Engl J Med*, **355**, 581–92. [First description of the use of anakinra in children with NOMID.]

Houten SM, *et al.* (2005). Caspase recruitment domain 15 mutations and rheumatic diseases. *Curr Opin Rheumatol*, **17**, 579–85. [Review including Blau syndrome and early-onset sarcoidosis.]

Lachmann HJ, *et al.* (2006). Clinical and subclinical inflammation in patients with familial Mediterranean fever and in heterozygous carriers of MEFV mutations. *Rheumatology*, **45**, 746–50. [First demonstration of a heterozygote phenotype in FMF with up-regulated inflammatory activity.]

Lachmann HJ, *et al.* (2007). Natural history and outcome in systemic AA amyloidosis. *N Engl J Med*, **356**, 2361–71. [Description of the presentation and outcome in a large series of patients with AA amyloidosis, demonstrating the importance of reducing long-term inflammation and serum amyloid A production.]

Leslie KS, *et al.* (2006). Phenotype, genotype, and sustained response to anakinra in 22 patients with autoinflammatory disease associated with CIAS-1/NALP3 mutations. *Arch Dermatol*, **142**, 1591–7. [Large case series of patients with an excellent response to anakinra.]

Niel E, Scherrmann JM (2006). Colchicine today. *Joint Bone Spine*, **73**, 672–78. [Up-to-date review of colchicine.]

Onen F (2006). Familial Mediterranean fever. *Rheumatol Int*, **26**, 489–96. [Clinical review of FMF.]

Schneiders MS, *et al.* (2005). Manipulation of isoprenoid biosynthesis as a possible therapeutic option in mevalonate kinase deficiency. *Arthritis Rheum*, **54**, 2306–13. [Evidence that failure of isoprenylation contributes to the inflammatory phenotype in HIDS.]

Ting JP, Kastner DL, Hoffman HM (2006). CATERPILLERs, pyrin and hereditary immunological disorders. *Nat Rev Immunol*, **6**, 183–95. [Review of the molecular pathogenesis of the hereditary fever syndromes.]

Tschopp J, Martinon F, Burns K (2003). NALPs: a novel protein family involved in inflammation. *Nat Rev Mol Cell Biol*, **4**, 95–104. [Review of the inflammasome and related pathways.]

12.12.3 Amyloidosis

M.B. Pepys and Philip N. Hawkins

Essentials

Amyloidosis is the clinical condition caused by extracellular deposition of amyloid in the tissues. Amyloid deposits are composed of amyloid fibrils, abnormal insoluble protein fibres formed by misfolding of their normally soluble precursors. About 25 different proteins can form clinically or pathologically significant amyloid fibrils in vivo as a result of either acquired or hereditary abnormalities. Small, focal, clinically silent amyloid deposits in the brain, heart, seminal vesicles, and joints are a universal accompaniment of ageing. However, clinically important amyloid deposits usually accumulate progressively, disrupting the structure and function of affected tissues and lead inexorably to organ failure and death. No treatment yet exists which can specifically clear amyloid deposits, but intervention which reduces the availability of the amyloid fibril precursor proteins may lead to amyloid regression with clinical benefit.

Pathology—amyloid fibrils of all types are similar: straight, rigid, and non branching; of indeterminate length and 10–15 nm in diameter; and with their subunit proteins arranged in a stack of twisted antiparallel β-pleated sheets. The fibrils bind Congo red dye producing pathognomonic green birefringence when viewed in polarized light, and the protein type can be identified by immunostaining or proteomic analysis. Amyloid deposits always contain a non fibrillar plasma glycoprotein, amyloid P component, the universal presence of which is the basis for use of radioisotope-labelled serum amyloid P component as a diagnostic tracer.

Clinicopathological correlation—amyloid may be deposited in any tissue of the body, including blood vessels walls and connective tissue matrix; clinical manifestations are correspondingly diverse. Although there are some typical clinical presentations related to fibril type, there are many forms of amyloidosis in which there is little or no concordance between the fibril protein, or the genotype of its precursor, and the clinical phenotype. Identification of the amyloid fibril protein is always essential for appropriate clinical management.

Specific types of amyloidosis

Reactive systemic (AA) amyloidosis—fibrils composed of AA protein derived from the acute phase protein, serum amyloid A protein (SAA). Occurs as a complication of any chronic inflammatory disorders (e.g. rheumatoid arthritis) or infections in which SAA concentrations are persistently increased. Most commonly presents with proteinuria and/or organomegaly, e.g. hepatosplenomegaly: nephrotic syndrome may develop before progression to endstage renal failure. Treatment is directed towards the underlying condition, aiming to reduce SAA values to normal.

Monoclonal immunoglobulin light chain (AL) amyloidosis—fibrils consists of all or part of the variable (VL) domain of monoclonal immunoglobulin light chains. May complicate any B-cell dyscrasia but most cases are associated with otherwise 'benign' monoclonal gammopathy. Highly variable idiotypic disease but characteristic presentations include involvement of the heart (restrictive cardiomyopathy), kidneys (proteinuria, renal failure), gut (motility disorders, malabsorption), tongue (macroglossia), and nerves (painful sensory polyneuropathy). Treatment is cytotoxic chemotherapy aimed at elimination or suppression of the causative B-cell clone, as for myeloma.

Hereditary systemic amyloidoses—include familial amyloid polyneuropathy, which is caused by mutations in the gene for the plasma protein transthyretin and characterized by progressive peripheral and autonomic neuropathy and varying degrees of visceral involvement.

Clinical amyloidosis

It is useful for diagnosis, management, and the development of new treatments to distinguish clearly between amyloidosis, in which extracellular amyloid deposits are the unequivocal cause of tissue damage and disease, and other diseases in which amyloid deposits of unknown pathogenic significance are present in the tissues. In systemic amyloidosis, in which amyloid can accumulate in the viscera, blood vessels, and connective tissue throughout the body (except within the brain substance itself), the deposits definitely cause the clinical disease. By contrast, amyloid deposits in the brain and cerebral blood vessels are a central part of the pathology of Alzheimer's disease, the fourth most common cause of death in the Western world, and amyloid is present in the islets of Langerhans of the pancreas in all patients with type 2 diabetes; however, the extent to which these local amyloid deposits are responsible for disease, if at all, is uncertain.

Systemic amyloidosis is responsible for about 1 in 1000 of all deaths in developed countries, and is a serious and important disease because it is often difficult to diagnose, it is usually fatal, and its management is complex and costly. Most systemic amyloidosis is a complication of other underlying primary conditions, which include monoclonal gammopathies of all types, chronic inflammatory disorders, and dialysis for endstage renal failure. Hereditary amyloidosis is very rare, except in a few geographic foci, but its diversity is remarkable. It is important because of its poor prognosis, the complexity of clinical management, the difficult genetic issues involved, and its considerable value as a model for understanding the pathogenesis of amyloid deposition.

Although there are some correlations between fibril protein type and clinical manifestations, there are also many forms of acquired and hereditary amyloidosis in which there is little or no concordance between the fibril protein, or the genotype of its precursor, and the clinical phenotype (Tables 12.12.3.1 and 12.12.3.2). There are evidently genetic and/or environmental factors, distinct from the amyloid fibril protein itself, that determine whether, when, and where clinically significant amyloid deposits form. The nature of these important determinants of amyloidogenesis is obscure. Furthermore, the mechanisms by which amyloid deposition causes disease are poorly understood. While a heavy amyloid load is invariably a bad sign, there may be a poor correlation between the local amount of amyloid and the level of organ dysfunction. Active deposition of new amyloid is often associated with accelerated deterioration compared with stable, long-standing deposits. Nascent or newly formed amyloid fibrils generated *in vitro* are also cytotoxic to cultured cells, whereas aged or *ex vivo* fibrils are generally inert, but it is not known if or how this relates to effects *in vivo*. In most forms of systemic amyloidosis there is overwhelming evidence that tissue damage and resultant disease are caused by the physical presence and accumulation of amyloid deposits, and not by cytotoxicity of the amyloidogenic proteins or their prefibrillar aggregates.

Table 12.12.3.1 Acquired amyloidosis syndromes

Clinical syndrome	Fibril protein
Systemic AL amyloidosis, associated with immunocyte dyscrasia, myeloma, monoclonal gammopathy, occult dyscrasia	AL derived from monoclonal immunoglobulin light chains
Local nodular AL amyloidosis (skin, respiratory tract, urogenital tract, etc.) associated with focal immunocyte dyscrasia	AL derived from monoclonal immunoglobulin light chains
Reactive systemic AA amyloidosis, associated with chronic active diseases	AA derived from SAA
Senile systemic amyloidosis	Transthyretin derived from plasma transthyretin
Sporadic cerebral amyloid angiopathy	Aβ derived from APP
Haemodialysis-associated amyloidosis; localized to osteoarticular tissues or systemic	β_2-microglobulin derived from high plasma levels
Primary localized cutaneous amyloid (macular, papular)	? Keratin-derived
Ocular amyloid (cornea, conjunctiva)	Not known
Orbital amyloid	AL or AH derived from monoclonal Ig

Abbreviations: AL, monoclonal immunoglobulin light chain; AA, amyloid A; SAA, serum amyloid A protein; APP, amyloid precursor protein; AH, monoclonal immunoglobulin heavy chain fragment; Ig, immunoglobulin.

Reactive systemic (AA) amyloidosis

Associated conditions

AA amyloidosis occurs in association with chronic inflammatory disorders, chronic local or systemic microbial infections, and, occasionally, malignant neoplasms. In western Europe and the United States of America the most frequent predisposing conditions are idiopathic rheumatic diseases (Table 12.12.3.3). Amyloidosis complicates up to 10% of cases of rheumatoid arthritis and juvenile inflammatory arthritis, although, for reasons that are not clear, the incidence is lower in the United States than in Europe. Amyloidosis is exceptionally rare in systemic lupus erythematosus, related connective tissue diseases, and in ulcerative colitis, by contrast with Crohn's disease; probably because in lupus and ulcerative colitis there is a blunted acute phase response of serum amyloid A protein, the precursor of AA amyloid fibrils. Tuberculosis and leprosy are important causes of AA amyloidosis, particularly where these infections are endemic. Chronic osteomyelitis, bronchiectasis, chronically infected burns, and decubitus ulcers, as well as the chronic pyelonephritis of paraplegic patients, are other well-recognized associations (see Table 12.12.3.3). Hodgkin's disease and renal carcinoma, which often cause fever, other systemic symptoms, and a major acute phase response, are the malignancies most commonly associated with systemic AA amyloidosis.

Clinical features

AA amyloid involves the viscera, but may be widely distributed without causing clinical symptoms. More than 90% of patients

Table 12.12.3.2 Hereditary amyloidosis syndromes

Clinical syndrome	Fibril protein
Predominant peripheral nerve involvement, familial amyloid polyneuropathy. Autosomal dominant	Transthyretin variants (commonly Met30, over 80 described)
	A-I N-terminal fragment of variant Arg26
Predominant cranial nerve involvement with lattice corneal dystrophy. Autosomal dominant	Gelsolin, fragment of variants Asn187 or Tyr187
Oculoleptomeningeal amyloidosis. Autosomal dominant	Transthyretin variants
Non-neuropathic, prominent visceral involvement (Ostertag-type). Autosomal dominant	Apolipoprotein A-I N-terminal fragment of variants
	Lysozyme variants
	Fibrinogen α–chain variants
Predominant cardiac involvement, no clinical neuropathy. Autosomal dominant	Transthyretin variants
Hereditary cerebral haemorrhage with amyloidosis (cerebral amyloid angiopathy). Autosomal dominant:	
Icelandic type (major asymptomatic systemic amyloid also present)	Cystatin C, fragment of variant Glu68
Dutch type	Aβ derived from APP variant Gln693
Familial Mediterranean fever, prominent renal involvement. Autosomal recessive	AA derived from SAA
Muckle–Well's syndrome and other heridiatry periodic fevers. Autosomal recessive (see Chapter 12.12.2)	AA derived from SAA
Cutaneous deposits (bullous, papular, pustulodermal)	Not known

Amino acids: Met, methionine; Arg, arginine; Asn, asparagine; Tyr, tyrosine; Glu, glutamic acid; Gln, glutamine.
Abbreviations: Aβ, amyloid β APP, amyloid precursor protein; SAA, serum amyloid A protein.

Table 12.12.3.3 Conditions associated with reactive systemic amyloid A amyloidosis

Chronic inflammatory disorders
Rheumatoid arthritis
Juvenile inflammatory arthritis
Ankylosing spondylitis
Psoriasis and psoriatic arthropathy
Reiter's syndrome
Adult Still's disease
Behçet's syndrome
Crohn's disease
Chronic microbial infections
Leprosy
Tuberculosis
Bronchiectasis
Decubitus ulcers
Chronic pyelonephritis in paraplegics
Osteomyelitis
Whipple's disease
Malignant neoplasms
Hodgkin's disease
Renal carcinoma
Carcinomas of gut, lung, urogenital tract
Basal cell carcinoma
Hairy cell leukaemia

present with nonselective proteinuria resulting from glomerular deposition, and nephrotic syndrome may develop before progression to endstage renal failure. Haematuria, isolated tubular defects, nephrogenic diabetes insipidus, and diffuse renal calcification rarely occur. Kidney size is usually normal, but may be enlarged, or, in advanced cases, reduced. End-stage chronic renal failure is the cause of death in 40 to 60% of cases, but acute renal failure may be precipitated by hypotension and/or salt and water depletion following surgery, excessive use of diuretics, or intercurrent infec tion, and may be associated with renal vein thrombosis. The second most common presentation is with organ enlargement, such as hepatosplenomegaly or thyroid goitre, with or without overt renal abnormality, but in any case amyloid deposits are almost always widespread at the time of presentation. Involvement of the heart and gastrointestinal tract is frequent, but rarely causes functional impairment.

AA amyloidosis may become clinically evident early in the course of associated disease, but the incidence increases with the duration of the primary condition. The mean duration of chronic rheumatic diseases, such as rheumatoid arthritis, ankylosing spondylitis, or juvenile rheumatoid arthritis, before amyloid is diagnosed is 12 to 14 years, although they can present much sooner. For most patients the prognosis is closely related to the degree of renal involvement and the effectiveness of treatment for the underlying inflammatory condition. In the presence of persistent uncontrolled inflammation, 50% of patients with AA amyloidosis die within 5 years of diagnosis; however, if the acute phase response can be consistently suppressed proteinuria can cease, renal function can be retained, and the prognosis is much better. The availability of chronic haemodialysis and transplantation prevents early death from uraemia *per se*, but amyloid deposition in extrarenal tissues may be responsible for a less favourable prognosis than for some other causes of endstage renal failure.

Amyloidosis associated with immunocyte dyscrasia: monoclonal immunoglobulin light chain (AL) amyloidosis

Associated conditions

Monoclonal immunoglobulin light chain (AL) amyloidosis may complicate almost any dyscrasia of cells of the B-lymphocyte lineage, including multiple myeloma, malignant lymphomas, and macroglobulinaemia, but most cases are associated with otherwise benign monoclonal gammopathy. Amyloidosis occurs in up to 15% of cases of myeloma, in a lower proportion of other malignant B-cell disorders, and probably in fewer than 5% of patients with a benign monoclonal gammopathies, which are, of course, much more common than myeloma. In some cases, deposition of AL amyloid may be the only evidence of the B-cell dyscrasia.

A monoclonal paraprotein or free light chains can be detected in the serum or urine of about 90% of patients with AL amyloidosis, while in the remaining 10% of cases detection of immunoglobulin gene rearrangement in the bone marrow or peripheral blood sometimes confirms a monoclonal gammopathy. The paraprotein may also appear after presentation and diagnosis of the amyloidosis, and subnormal levels of some or all serum immunoglobulins, or increased numbers of marrow plasma cells, may provide less direct clues to the underlying aetiology. Until recently it has been the practice to diagnose apparently primary cases of amyloidosis, with no previous predisposing inflammatory condition or family history of amyloidosis, as AL type by exclusion. However, it has now been recognized that autosomal dominant hereditary non-neuropathic amyloidosis, particularly that caused by variant fibrinogen α-chain, may be poorly penetrant and of late onset, so there may be no family history. The coincident occurrence of a monoclonal gammopathy may then be gravely misleading, and it is essential to exclude by genotyping all known amyloidogenic mutations, and to seek positive immunohistochemical or biochemical identification of the amyloid fibril protein in all cases.

Clinical features

AL amyloidosis occurs equally in men and women, usually over the age of 50 years, but occasionally in young adults. It has a lifetime incidence (and is the cause of death) of between 0.5 and 1 in 1000 individuals in the United Kingdom. The clinical manifestations are protean, as virtually any tissue other than the brain may be directly involved. Uraemia, heart failure, or other effects of amyloidosis usually cause death within a year of diagnosis, unless the underlying B-cell clone is effectively suppressed.

The heart is affected in 90% of patients with AL amyloidosis. In 30% of these, restrictive cardiomyopathy is the presenting feature and in up to 50% of these patients it is fatal. Other cardiac presentations include arrhythmias and angina. Measurement of circulating brain natriuretic peptide provides a sensitive index of cardiac dysfunction in cardiac AL amyloidosis, and often shows rapid improvement when there is a clonal response to cytotoxic chemotherapy. This suggests that the amyloidogenic light chains may themselves have intrinsic cardiotoxicity, in addition to their deposition as amyloid fibrils. Renal AL amyloidosis has the same manifestations as renal AA amyloidosis, but the prognosis is worse. Gut involvement may cause disturbances of motility (often secondary to autonomic neuropathy), malabsorption, perforation, haemorrhage, or obstruction. Macroglossia occurs rarely, but is almost pathognomonic. Hyposplenism sometimes occurs in both AA and AL amyloidosis. Painful sensory polyneuropathy, with early loss of pain and temperature sensation, followed later by motor deficits, is seen in 10 to 20% of cases, and carpal tunnel syndrome in 20%. Autonomic neuropathy leading to orthostatic hypotension, impotence, and gastrointestinal disturbances may occur alone or together with the peripheral neuropathy, and has a very poor prognosis. Skin involvement takes the form of papules, nodules, and plaques, usually on the face and upper trunk, and involvement of dermal blood vessels results in purpura, occurring either spontaneously or after minimal trauma, and is very common. Articular amyloid is rare, but may mimic acute polyarticular rheumatoid arthritis, or it may present as asymmetrical arthritis affecting the hip or shoulder. Infiltration of the glenohumeral joint and surrounding soft tissues occasionally produces the characteristic 'shoulder pad' sign. A rare but serious manifestation of AL amyloidosis is an acquired bleeding diathesis that may be associated with deficiency of factor X, and sometimes also factor IX, or with increased fibrinolysis. It does not occur in AA amyloidosis, although in both AL and AA disease there may be serious bleeding in the absence of any identifiable coagulation factor deficiency.

Senile amyloidosis

Some amyloid is seen in all autopsies on individuals over 80 years of age, but it is not known whether this contributes to the ageing process or whether it is an epiphenomenon that becomes clinically important only when it is extensive.

Senile systemic (cardiac) amyloidosis

Up to 25% of older people have microscopic, clinically silent systemic deposits of transthyretin amyloid involving the walls of the heart and blood vessels, smooth and striated muscle, fat tissue, renal papillae, and alveolar walls. By contrast with most other forms of systemic amyloidosis (including hereditary transthyretin amyloid caused by point mutations in the transthyretin gene), the spleen and renal glomeruli are rarely affected. The brain is not involved. Occasionally, more extensive deposits in the heart, affecting the ventricles and atria and situated in the interstitium and vessel walls, cause significant impairment of cardiac function and may be fatal. The transthyretin involved is usually of the normal wild type, but cases with transthyretin variants have been described that may be hereditary. The isoleucine 122 variant, which occurs in about 1.3 million African Americans, including about 13 000 individuals homozygous for this polymorphism, is associated with a greatly increased risk of senile cardiac amyloidosis, suggesting that this condition may be substantially underdiagnosed; cases of congestive cardiac failure in older people presumably being assumed to reflect coronary artery disease.

Senile focal amyloidosis

Microscopic and clinically silent amyloid deposits of different fibril types, localized to particular tissues, are very commonly present in older people. Deposits of β-protein (see below) as amyloid in cerebral blood vessels and intracerebral plaques seen in normal older brains may or may not have been the harbinger of Alzheimer's disease had the patient survived long enough. Amyloid deposits composed of apolipoprotein A-I are present in most osteoarthritic joints at surgery or autopsy, usually in close association with calcium pyrophosphate deposits, and affect the articular cartilage and joint capsule. However, the significance of this age-associated articular amyloid, the amount of which is correlated with neither the presence nor clinical severity of osteoarthritis, is not known. The corpora amylacea of the prostate are composed of β_2-microglobulin amyloid fibrils. Amyloid in the seminal vesicles is derived from semenogelin I, an exocrine secretory product of the vesicle cells. Isolated deposits of cardiac atrial amyloid consist of atrial natriuretic peptide. The focal amyloid deposits commonly present in atheromatous plaques of older subjects are of two types: containing fibrils either composed of medin, a fragment of lactadherin, or the N-terminal fragment of apolipoprotein A-I.

Table 12.12.3.4 Cerebral amyloidosis

Age-related amyloid angiopathy with or without intracerebral deposits
Hereditary amyloid angiopathy of meningeal and cortical vessels associated with cerebral haemorrhage: Icelandic type Dutch type
Hereditary amyloid angiopathy affecting the entire central nervous system
Alzheimer's disease: sporadic, familial, or associated with Down's syndrome
Cerebral amyloid associated with prion disease: Sporadic spongiform encephalopathy, Creutzfeldt–Jacob disease, variant Creutzfeldt–Jakob disease Familial prion disease, familial Creutzfeldt–Jacob disease, GSS syndrome atypical familial prion disease
Familial oculoleptomeningeal amyloidosis

Cerebral amyloid

The brain is a very common and important site of amyloid deposition (Table 12.12.3.4), although, possibly because of the blood–brain barrier, there are never any deposits in the cerebral parenchyma itself in any form of acquired systemic visceral amyloidosis. However, cerebrovascular transthyretin amyloid may occur in familial amyloid polyneuropathy resulting from the most common transthyretin variant (methionine for valine at residue 30), and oculoleptomeningeal amyloidosis is caused by other very rare transthyretin variants. The common and major forms of brain amyloid are confined to the brain and cerebral blood vessels, with the single exception of cystatin C amyloid in hereditary cerebral haemorrhage with amyloidosis, Icelandic type, in which there are major, though clinically silent, systemic deposits.

Alzheimer's disease

By far the most frequent and important type of amyloid in the brain is that related to Alzheimer's disease, which is the most common cause of dementia and affects more than 3 million individuals in the United States of America and a corresponding proportion of other Western populations. It is generally a disease of older people, and its prevalence is therefore increasing. The clinical differential diagnosis of senile dementia and the positive identification of Alzheimer's disease are difficult and often of limited precision in life. However, intracerebral and cerebrovascular amyloid deposits are hallmarks of the neuropathological diagnosis.

The amyloid fibrils are composed of β-protein (Aβ), a 39- to 43-residue cleavage product of the large amyloid precursor protein. The vast majority of cases of Alzheimer's disease are sporadic, but there are also families with an autosomal dominant pattern of inheritance and usually early onset. In about 20 families there are causative mutations in the *APP* gene for amyloid precursor protein on chromosome 21, and most other kindreds have mutations in the genes for presenilin 1 (chromosome 14) and presenilin 2 (chromosome 1). All these mutations are associated with increased production from amyloid precursor protein of Aβ1–42, the most amyloidogenic form of Aβ. Since all individuals with Down's syndrome (trisomy 21) develop Alzheimer's disease if they survive into their forties, there is evidently a close link between amyloid precursor protein, Aβ overproduction, Aβ amyloidosis, and the pathogenesis of Alzheimer's disease. However, it remains unclear whether or how Aβ *per se*, or the amyloid fibrils that it forms, contribute to the neuronal loss that underlies the dementia.

Synthetic Aβ fibrils formed *in vitro* are markedly cytotoxic, and cause the death of cultured cells by apoptosis and necrosis. Although it is not clear to what extent these findings reflect phenomena that may be responsible for neurodegeneration *in vivo*, there is increasing evidence, from both transgenic mouse models of Alzheimer's disease and *in vivo* intracerebral injection of different molecular conformations of Aβ, that small oligomeric prefibrillar aggregates of Aβ are associated with and cause cognitive dysfunction. There is controversy about the correlation between the severity of dementia in Alzheimer's disease and the extent of amyloid angiopathy and plaques. Nevertheless, the fact that patients with Alzheimer's disease caused by amyloid precursor protein and presenilin mutations have exactly the same neuropathology as sporadic cases, including tangles, argues strongly that the amyloid precursor protein and Aβ pathway can be of primary pathogenetic significance.

In addition to the Aβ deposits in the brains of patients with Alzheimer's disease and Down's syndrome, there are also extensive 'amorphous' deposits throughout the brain. These do not stain with Congo red, and are detectable only by immunohistochemical staining. Their significance is unknown. They apparently precede the appearance of histochemically identifiable amyloid, but are not necessarily the precursor of it because they are present in areas such as the cerebellum in which Aβ is never seen. The nonfibrillar, nonamyloid protein apolipoprotein E is demonstrable in many amyloid deposits, including those of Alzheimer's disease. The *APOE4* gene (chromosome 19), encoding one of the three isoforms of this apolipoprotein, is strongly associated with a predisposition to develop Alzheimer's disease and with increased amounts of amyloid in the brain, but the underlying mechanisms are unknown.

Another neuropathological feature of Alzheimer's disease, and some other neurodegenerative conditions, is the neurofibrillary tangle located intracellularly within neuronal cell bodies and processes. These tangles have a characteristic ultrastructural morphology of paired helical filaments, and are composed of an abnormally phosphorylated form of the normal neurofilament protein, tau. They bind Congo red and then give the pathognomonic green birefringence of amyloid when viewed in polarized light. Although their electronmicroscopic ultrastructure is completely different from that of amyloid fibrils, the most recent review of amyloid nomenclature includes them as amyloid.

Senile cerebral amyloidosis and amyloid (congophilic cerebral) angiopathy

Up to 60% of the brains of nondemented older individuals contain Aβ in the cerebral blood vessels, and there may also be focal intracerebral Aβ plaques. These deposits are usually clinically silent and may or may not have been harbingers of Alzheimer's disease, had the patients survived long enough. Sometimes the amyloid angiopathy is more extensive, and is increasingly recognized as an important cause of cerebral haemorrhage and stroke, to be distinguished from atherosclerotic cerebrovascular disease.

Hereditary cerebral haemorrhage with amyloidosis: hereditary cerebral amyloid angiopathy

Icelandic type **(OMIM#604312)**

Cerebrovascular amyloid deposits composed of a fragment of a genetic variant of cystatin C are responsible for recurrent major cerebral haemorrhages starting in early adult life in members of families originating in western Iceland. There is autosomal dominant inheritance and appreciable, but clinically silent, amyloid deposits are present in the spleen, lymph nodes, and skin. There is no extravascular amyloid in the brain, and the neurological deficits, often including dementia, of surviving patients are compatible with their cerebrovascular pathology.

Dutch type (OMIM#605714)

In families originating from a small region on the coast of the Netherlands the autosomal dominant inheritance of a genetic variant of Aβ, which is deposited as cerebrovascular amyloid, results in recurrent normotensive cerebral haemorrhages starting in middle age. There are also amorphous Aβ deposits in the brain and early senile plaques, without congophilic amyloid cores. Multi-infarct dementia occurs in survivors, but some patients become demented in the absence of stroke. Amyloid outside the brain has not been reported.

Cerebral amyloid associated with prion disease

The neuropathology of a group of progressive, invariably fatal spongiform encephalopathies sometimes, but certainly not always, includes intracerebral amyloid plaques. These diseases are transmissible and in some cases hereditary. The sporadic and familial Creutzfeldt–Jacob disease, the familial Gerstmann–Sträussler–Scheinker syndrome, and kuru are caused by prions (PrP^{Sc}), conformational isoforms of the normal physiological cellular prion protein (PrP^{C}). The human diseases are closely related to the animal diseases scrapie of sheep and goats, transmissible encephalopathy of mink, elk, and male deer, and bovine spongiform encephalopathy. Variant Creutzfeldt–Jacob disease is apparently the result of transmission of bovine spongiform encephalopathy to humans.

The significance of amyloid *per se* in these disorders is not clear because it is not always histologically detectable, and in some disorders is not seen, e.g. fatal familial insomnia and bovine spongiform encephalopathy (which is apparently a result of the transmission of ovine scrapie to cattle). When scrapie or its human counterparts are transmitted to experimental animals by inoculation of affected brain tissue, the development of intracerebral amyloid depends on the strain of infectious agent and the genetic background of the recipient. Even when amyloid is present in the brain it is not seen elsewhere, e.g. in the spleen, although the latter is a rich source of the infective agent. However, when the infective agent is exhaustively and highly purified from brain or spleen it forms typical congophilic amyloid fibrils composed of the proteinase-resistant subunit PrP^{Sc}, and when amyloid deposits are present in affected brains they immunostain with antiprion antibodies.

The amyloid fibril protein is thus directly related to the cause of the encephalopathy, but histologically demonstrable amyloid deposition is evidently not necessary for the expression of disease. Indeed, recent work in transgenic and knockout mouse strains clearly demonstrates both that prion amyloid deposition is not a necessary condition for the development of transmissible spongiform encephalopathy, and that expression of the normal cellular isoform, PrP^{C}, is absolutely required. Neuronal damage may perhaps be caused by a cytotoxic interaction between prefibrillar PrP^{Sc} aggregates and the normal PrP^{C}, or indeed by other mechanisms entirely. This is a different situation from the extracerebral amyloidosis, and from cystatin C and nonhereditary cerebral amyloid angiopathies, in which amyloid deposition is invariably present when there is clinical disease, and is unequivocally the cause of tissue damage.

Hereditary systemic amyloidosis

Familial amyloid polyneuropathy (hereditary transthyretin amyloidosis) (OMIM*176300)

Familial amyloid polyneuropathy is an autosomal dominant syndrome with onset at any time from the second decade onwards. It is characterized by progressive peripheral and autonomic neuropathy and varying degrees of visceral involvement especially affecting the vitreous of the eye, the heart, kidneys, thyroid, and adrenals. There are usually amyloid deposits throughout the body involving the walls of blood vessels and the connective tissue matrix; the pathology is due to these deposits. Apart from major foci in Portugal, Japan, and Sweden, familial amyloid polyneuropathy has been reported in most populations throughout the world. There is considerable variation in the age of onset, rate of progression, and involvement of different systems; although within families the pattern is usually quite consistent. There is remorseless progression and the disorder is invariably fatal. Death results from the effects and complications of peripheral and/or autonomic neuropathy, or from cardiac or renal failure.

Familial amyloid polyneuropathy is caused by mutations in the gene for the plasma protein transthyretin (formerly known as prealbumin). The most frequent of these causes a methionine for valine substitution at position 30 in the mature protein, but more than 80 amyloidogenic mutations have been described. There is often little correlation between the underlying mutation and the clinical phenotype, which is evidently determined by other genetic and possibly also environmental factors, although in a few cases certain mutations are uniquely associated with particularly aggressive or relatively organ-limited disease. The amyloidogenic transthyretin mutations are not always penetrant, and asymptomatic methionine-30 homozygotes over the age of 60 years have been reported. Rare kindreds with the apolipoprotein A-I arginine 26 variant, which usually causes nonneuropathic amyloidosis, may present with prominent peripheral neuropathy resembling transthyretin familial amyloid polyneuropathy (OMIM*107680).

Familial amyloid polyneuropathy with predominant cranial neuropathy (OMIM*137350)

Originally described in Finland, but now reported in other populations, this autosomal dominant hereditary amyloidosis presents in adult life with cranial neuropathy, lattice corneal dystrophy, and distal peripheral neuropathy. There may be skin, renal, and cardiac manifestations and microscopic amyloid deposits are widely distributed in connective tissue and blood vessel walls; life expectancy approaches normal. The amyloid fibrils are derived from variants of the actin-modulating protein gelsolin, encoded by point mutations. Individuals homozygous for these mutations have severe renal amyloidosis in addition to the usual neuropathy.

Nonneuropathic systemic amyloidosis (OMIM#105200)

In this rare autosomal dominant syndrome of major systemic amyloidosis without clinical evidence of neuropathy, the patterns of organ involvement and overall clinical phenotype vary between families. The kidneys are often the most severely affected organ, leading to hypertension and renal failure, but the heart, spleen, liver, bowel, connective tissue, and exocrine glands may all be involved. Following clinical presentation there is inexorable progression to death or organ failure requiring transplantation. Clinical presentation is usually in early adulthood, although in a few kindreds it may be as late as the sixth decade. The amyloid proteins so far identified are genetic variants of apolipoprotein A-I and A-II, lysozyme, and the fibrinogen α-chain.

Cardiac amyloidosis

Cardiac amyloidosis without overt involvement of other viscera or neuropathy, progressing inexorably to death, is associated with certain transthyretin gene mutations and is inherited in an autosomal dominant manner with variable penetrance (see Table 12.12.3.2). By far the most common variant is transthyretin iseoleucine 122, which occurs in 4% of African Americans and frequently causes cardiac amyloidosis from the sixth decade onwards.

Familial Mediterranean fever (OMIM#249100)

Familial Mediterranean fever is an autosomal recessive autoinflammatory disorder caused by mutations in the gene *MEFV* on chromosome 16 that encodes a neutrophil-specific protein of unknown function called pyrin or marenostrin (see Chapter 12.12.2). The disease is characterized by recurrent episodes of fever, abdominal pain, pleurisy, or arthritis, and predominantly occurs in non-Ashkenazi Jews, Armenians, Anatolian Turks, and Levantine Arabs. Among Sephardi Jews of North African origin, and in the other populations (except Armenians and, to a lesser extent, Ashkenazi Jews), untreated familial Mediterranean fever is eventually complicated in a high proportion of cases by typical systemic AA amyloidosis. Furthermore, some patients with familial Mediterranean fever present with AA amyloidosis before they have experienced any symptoms, and this is consistent with the recent finding that a substantial acute phase plasma protein response is frequently present, even in asymptomatic individuals. The variable incidence of amyloidosis in patients with familial Mediterranean fever from different populations is not wholly explained by their specific pyrin gene mutations, and is another illustration of the unknown genetic determinants of clinical amyloidosis.

Haemodialysis-associated amyloidosis

Almost all patients with endstage renal failure who are maintained on haemodialysis for more than 5 years develop amyloid deposits composed of β_2-microglobulin. These deposits are predominantly osteoarticular and are associated with carpal tunnel syndrome, large-joint pain and stiffness, soft-tissue masses, bone cysts, and pathological fractures. Renal tubular amyloid concretions may also form. The serious clinical problems associated with β_2-microglobulin amyloidosis constitute the major cause of morbidity in patients on long-term dialysis. Furthermore, in some patients more extensive deposition occurs, most commonly in the spleen but also in other organs, and a few cases of death associated with systemic β_2-microglobulin amyloid have been reported. The β_2-microglobulin is derived from the high plasma concentrations that develop in renal insufficiency and are not cleared by dialysis. This type of amyloidosis also occurs in patients on continuous ambulatory peritoneal dialysis, and has even been reported in a few patients with chronic renal failure who have never been dialysed. Improved clearance of β_2-microglobulin by current dialysis membranes and procedures encouragingly seems to be reducing the incidence of this form of amyloidosis.

Endocrine amyloid

Many tumours of APUD cells that produce peptide hormones have amyloid deposits in their stroma. These are probably composed of the hormone peptides; in the case of medullary carcinoma of the thyroid the fibril subunits are derived from procalcitonin. In insulinomas the amyloid fibril protein is a novel peptide first identified in that site and subsequently shown to be the fibril protein in the amyloid of the islets of Langerhans seen in type 2 (maturity onset) diabetes. This peptide is called islet amyloid polypeptide, or amylin, and shows appreciable homology with calcitonin gene-related peptide. Amyloid of this type is an almost universal feature of the pancreatic islets in type 2 diabetes, and becomes more extensive with increasing duration and severity of the disease. Although the amyloid itself is probably not initially responsible for the metabolic defect in this form of diabetes, it is likely that progressive amyloid deposition, leading to islet destruction, subsequently does contribute to the pathogenesis. The possible hormonal or other role of islet amyloid polypeptide itself, which is produced by the islet β-cells, is also not yet clear.

Rare localized amyloidosis syndromes

Amyloid deposits localized to the skin occur in both acquired and hereditary forms of amyloidosis. Primary localized cutaneous amyloidosis presents in adult life as macular or papular lesions, the fibrils of which may be derived from keratin. Hereditary cutaneous amyloid lesions are rare, of unknown fibril type, and are sometimes associated with other, nonamyloid, multisystem disorders. Amyloid deposits in the eye cause local problems in the cornea (corneal lattice dystrophy) or conjunctiva, while orbital amyloid presents as mass lesions that can disrupt eye movement and the structure of the orbit. In one such case the fibril protein has been identified as a fragment of IgG heavy chain. Lactoferrin and keratoepithelin have been identified as the amyloid fibril proteins in different cases of corneal amyloidosis.

Localized foci of AL amyloid can occur anywhere in the body in the absence of systemic AL amyloidosis, the most common sites being the skin, upper airways and respiratory tract, and the urogenital tract. They may be associated with a local plasmacytoma or B-cell lymphoma producing a monoclonal immunoglobulin, but often the cells, which must be present to produce the amyloidogenic protein, are scattered inconspicuously in the affected tissue. The clinical problems caused by these space-occupying amyloidomas are usually cured by surgical resection, but this is not always possible.

Amyloid fibrils

Regardless of their very diverse protein subunits, amyloid fibrils of different types are remarkably similar: straight, rigid, nonbranching, of indeterminate length, and 10 to 15 nm in diameter. They are insoluble in physiological solutions, relatively resistant to proteolysis, and bind Congo red dye, producing pathognomonic green birefringence when viewed in polarized light. Electron microscopy reveals that each fibril consists of two or more protofilaments, the precise number varying with the fibril type. The X-ray diffraction patterns of all the different *ex vivo* amyloid fibrils, and of synthetic fibrils formed *in vitro*, that have been studied demonstrate the presence of a common core structure within the filaments: the subunit proteins are arranged in a stack of twisted antiparallel β-pleated sheets lying with their long axes perpendicular to the long axis of the fibril.

Recent observations have shown that many different proteins, including molecules totally unrelated to amyloidosis *in vivo*, can be refolded after denaturation *in vitro* to form typical, stable, congophilic cross-fibrils. Although it is not clear why only the 26 known amyloidogenic proteins adopt the amyloid fold and persist as fibrils *in vivo*, a major unifying theme that is currently emerging is that, in all cases studied, the precursors are relatively destabilized. Even under physiological or other conditions they may encounter *in vivo*, they adopt partly unfolded states that involve the loss of tertiary or higher-order structure. These readily aggregate, with retention of β-sheet secondary structure, into protofilaments and fibrils. Once the process has started, seeding may also play an important facilitating role, so that amyloid deposition may progress exponentially as expansion of the amyloid template captures further precursor molecules.

Amyloid fibril proteins and their precursors

Immunoglobulin light chain

AL proteins are derived from the N-terminal region of monoclonal immunoglobulin light chains and consist of all or part of the variable domain. Intact light chains may occasionally be found, and the molecular weight therefore varies between about 8 and 30 kDa. The light chain of the monoclonal paraprotein is either identical to, or clearly the precursor of, AL isolated from the amyloid deposits.

AL is more commonly derived from λ chains than from κ chains, despite the fact that κ chains predominate among both normal immunoglobulins and the paraprotein products of immunocyte dyscrasias. A new λ-chain subgroup, λ_{VI}, was initially identified as an AL protein in two cases of immunocyte dyscrasia-associated amyloidosis, before it had been recognized in any other form, and it has subsequently been observed in many more cases of AL amyloidosis. Furthermore, there is increasing evidence from sequence analysis of Bence Jones proteins of both κ and λ type from patients with AL amyloidosis, and of AL proteins themselves, that these polypeptides contain unique amino acid replacements or insertions compared with nonamyloid monoclonal light chains. In some cases these changes involve the replacement of hydrophilic framework residues by hydrophobic residues, changes likely to promote aggregation and insolubilization; in others the monoclonal light chains from amyloid patients have been directly demonstrated to have decreased solubility and a greater propensity for precipitation than control nonamyloid proteins. The inherent amyloidogenicity of particular monoclonal light chains has been elegantly confirmed in an *in vivo* model in which isolated Bence Jones proteins were injected into mice. Animals receiving light chains from AL amyloid patients developed typical amyloid deposits composed of the human protein, whereas animals receiving light chains from myeloma patients without amyloid did not.

Amyloid A (AA)

The AA protein is a single nonglycosylated polypeptide chain usually of mass 8000 Da and containing 76 residues corresponding to the N-terminal portion of the 104-residue serum amyloid A protein (SAA). Smaller and larger AA fragments, even some whole SAA molecules, have also been reported in AA fibrils. SAA is an apolipoprotein of high density lipoprotein particles, and is the polymorphic product of a set of genes located on the short arm of chromosome 11. It is highly conserved in evolution and is a major acute phase reactant in all species in which it has been studied. Most of the SAA in plasma is produced by hepatocytes, in which the synthesis is under transcriptional regulation by cytokines (especially interleukin 1, interleukin 6, and tumour necrosis factor) acting via NF-κB-like transcription factors, and possibly others. After secretion it is rapidly associated with high density lipoproteins, from which it displaces apolipoprotein A-I. The circulating concentration can rise from normal levels of up to 3 mg/litre to over 1000 mg/litre within 24 to 48 h of an acute stimulus, and with ongoing chronic inflammation the level may remain persistently high. Certain isoforms of SAA, the products of different genes, are predominantly synthesized elsewhere in the body by macrophages, adipocytes, and certain other cells. Although they also associate with high density lipoproteins, their acute phase synthesis is stimulated differently and they presumably have different functions. There is also a closely related family of high density lipoprotein trace apoproteins that are not acute phase reactants; they have been designated constitutive SAAs, although they do not form amyloid.

The precursor of amyloid fibril AA protein is circulating SAA, from which amyloid fibril AA protein is derived by proteolytic cleavage. Such cleavage can be produced by macrophages and by a variety of proteinases, but since further cleavage of AA is readily demonstrable *in vitro* it is not clear why the AA peptide persists in amyloid. Furthermore, it is not known whether the process of AA fibril generation involves cleavage of SAA before and/or after aggregation of monomers. Persistent overproduction of SAA causing sustained high circulating levels is a necessary condition for deposition of AA amyloid, but it is not known why only some individuals in this state develop amyloidosis. In mice, only one of the three major isoforms of SAA is the precursor of AA in amyloid fibrils. Human SAA isoforms are more complex, but homozygosity for particular types seems to favour amyloidogenesis, although there may also be ethnic differences.

The normal functions of SAA are not known, although modulating effects on reverse cholesterol transport and on lipid function in the microenvironment of inflammatory foci have been proposed. A protein, homologous with SAA, produced by rabbit fibroblasts has been reported to act as an autocrine stimulator of collagenase production *in vitro*. Other reports of potent cell-regulatory functions of isolated denatured delipidated SAA have yet to be confirmed in physiological preparations of SAA-rich high density lipoproteins. Regardless of its physiological role, the behaviour of SAA as an exquisitely sensitive acute phase protein with an enormous dynamic range makes it an extremely valuable empirical clinical marker. It can be used objectively to monitor the extent and activity of infective, inflammatory, necrotic, and neoplastic disease. Furthermore, routine monitoring of SAA should be an integral part of the management of all patients with AA amyloidosis or disorders predisposing to it, as control of the primary inflammatory process in order to reduce SAA production is essential if amyloidosis is to be halted, enabled to regress, or prevented. Automated immunoassay systems for SAA are available that meet a World Health Organization international reference standard.

Transthyretin

Transthyretin, formerly known as prealbumin, is a normal nonglycosylated plasma protein with a relative molecular mass of 55 044 Da. It is composed of four identical noncovalently associated subunits, each of 127 amino acids. It is produced by hepatocytes and the choroid plexus, and is a significant negative acute phase protein. Each tetrameric molecule is able to bind a single thyroxine or triodothyronine molecule and up to 15% of circulating thyroid hormone is transported in this way. Transthyretin also forms a 1:1 molecular complex with retinol-binding protein, which transports vitamin A.

Transthyretin is encoded by a single-copy gene, but is appreciably polymorphic and more than 90 different point mutations encoding single residue substitutions have been identified. Normal wild type transthyretin is an inherently amyloidogenic protein that forms the fibrils in senile systemic amyloidosis. *In vitro* exposure to reduced pH is sufficient to generate transthyretin amyloid fibrils from the pure protein. Most of the variant forms of transthyretin have been associated with hereditary amyloidosis, and show decreased stability *in vitro* compared with the wild type. Transgenic mice expressing variant human transthyretin with a methionine 30 substitution sometimes develop systemic amyloid deposits, though unfortunately not in the peripheral nerves, even when the transgene is expressed in the choroid plexus and transthyretin amyloid is deposited in the meninges and choroid plexus. This is another example of the important unknown factors, other than the presence of an amyloidogenic protein itself, that determine where and when clinical amyloidosis develops.

Individuals heterozygous for transthyretin mutations have a mixture of wild type and variant transthyretin monomers in their circulating transthyretin, and if they develop amyloidosis both forms are often present, although the variant may predominate in the amyloid fibrils. Although cleavage fragments of transthyretin are commonly present, intact transthyretin subunits are also found and fibrillogenesis does not depend on an initial proteolytic step.

Amyloid beta (Aβ)

The fibril protein in the intracerebral and cerebrovascular amyloid of Alzheimer's disease, Down's syndrome, and hereditary amyloid angiopathy of the Dutch type is a 39- to 43-residue sequence derived by proteolysis from a precursor protein of high molecular weight, the amyloid precursor protein (APP), encoded on the long arm of chromosome 21. Several isoforms of APP are generated by alternative splicing of transcripts from the 19-exon gene, yielding three major forms: APP695, APP751, and APP770. These are each single-chain, multidomain glycoproteins with the 47 residues of the C-terminal lying within the cytoplasm, a 25-residue membrane-spanning region, and the rest of the molecule lying extracellularly. APP751 and APP770 contain a 56-residue Kunitz-type serine proteinase inhibitor domain encoded by exon 7.

Following glycosylation and membrane insertion APPs are cleaved extracellularly, close to the transmembrane sequence, by so-called APP secretase activity. This releases, in the case of APP751 and APP770, a molecule known as proteinase nexin II, which avidly binds factor XIa, trypsin, and chymotrypsin, as well as epidermal growth factor-binding protein and the γ subunit of nerve growth factor. The predominant species of mRNA found in the brain encodes APP695, which lacks the proteinase inhibitor domain, while mRNA for APP751 is the most abundant in other tissues. Despite this, 85% of secreted APP in the brain is proteinase nexin II. Interestingly, APP secreted by a glial cell line is substantially glycosylated with chondroitin sulphate glycosaminoglycan chains. APP also undergoes high-affinity interactions with heparan sulphate. These observations suggest that APP may have important functions in cell adhesion, cell migration, and modulation of growth-factor activities. APP proteinase nexin II is present in and released by platelets, and probably functions in the clotting cascade.

The amyloidogenic peptide Aβ, encoded by parts of exons 16 and 17, corresponds to the part of the APP sequence that extends from within the cell membrane into the extracellular space. Secretase cleavage of APP to release the soluble form cannot therefore generate intact Aβ itself, or larger fragments containing it. However, there is an alternative processing pathway for APP, in which it is taken up whole by lysosomes and cleaved to yield fragments that do contain the whole Aβ sequence. Furthermore, APP cleaved at the N-terminus of Aβ, and soluble Aβ itself, are normally produced by cell lines and by mixed brain cells in culture, and are present in the cerebrospinal fluid. However, the source of the Aβ in the intracerebral amorphous deposits, and that which aggregates as amyloid fibrils in the brain and cerebral blood vessels, is still not known. The 42-residue form of Aβ (Aβ1–42) is markedly the most amyloidogenic, and all the mutations in the APP and presenilin genes that are associated with hereditary Alzheimer's disease result in increased production of this amyloid. Increased availability of the precursor is thus responsible for amyloidogenesis, but the pathogenesis of neuronal damage and dementia remain unclear.

Cystatin C

Cystatin C (formerly called γ-trace) is an inhibitor of cysteine proteinases, including cathepsin B, H, and L. It is encoded by a gene on chromosome 20 and consists of a single nonglycosylated polypeptide chain of 120 residues. It is present in all major human biological fluids at concentrations compatible with a significant physiological role in proteinase inhibition. The normal concentration in cerebrospinal fluid is 6.5 mg/litre (range 2.7–13.7), but is much lower (2.7 mg/litre, range 1.0–4.7) in patients with the Icelandic type of hereditary cerebral amyloid angiopathy, in whom fragments of the glutamine 68 genetic variant of cystatin C form the amyloid fibrils. This reduced concentration is diagnostically useful, and is evident even in presymptomatic carriers of the cystatin C gene mutation.

The point mutation that causes the disease encodes a glutamine for leucine substitution in the mature protein, and the amyloid fibril protein consists of the C-terminal 110 residues of the variant. This N-terminally truncated form is not detectable in the cerebrospinal fluid of affected patients, suggesting that cleavage takes place either in close proximity to fibril deposition or after the fibrils have formed. The variant cystatin C is less stable than the wild type and readily forms fibrils *in vitro*. It is not known whether cerebral haemorrhage in cystatin C amyloidosis is caused simply by the damaging effects of vascular amyloid deposition, or whether deficiency in inhibitory capacity for cysteine proteinases also plays a part.

Gelsolin

Gelsolin is a widely distributed 90 kDa cytoplasmic protein that binds actin monomers, nucleates actin filament growth, and severs actin filaments. Alternative transcriptional initiation and message processing from a single gene on chromosome 9 are responsible for the synthesis of a secreted form of gelsolin (93 kDa), which circulates in the plasma at a concentration of about 200 mg/litre. Its function in the blood is not known, but may be related to the clearance of actin filaments released by dying cells. In the Finnish type of hereditary amyloidosis the amyloid fibril protein is a 71-residue fragment of variant gelsolin, with asparagine substituted for aspartic acid at position 15 (corresponding to residue 187 of the mature molecule), and the same mutation has been discovered in affected kindreds from different ethnic backgrounds. In one Danish family with the same phenotype there is a different mutation at the same nucleotide, predicting a tyrosine for aspartic acid substitution at residue 187. Synthetic and recombinant peptides that include the asparagine for aspartic acid substitution at residue 187 are less soluble than the wild type sequence and readily form amyloid fibrils *in vitro*.

Apolipoprotein A-I and A-II

Apolipoprotein A-I is the most abundant apolipoprotein among the high density lipoprotein particles, and participates in their central function of reverse cholesterol transport from the periphery to the liver. Apolipoprotein A-I variants are extremely rare, and may be phenotypically silent or may affect lipid metabolism. However, 15 different variants of apolipoprotein A-I, including single- and multiple-residue substitutions and deletions, have been associated with amyloidosis. These are inherited in an autosomal dominant manner and are usually highly penetrant, but there are marked variations in the age and manner of presentation, even within the same family and in different kindreds with the same mutation.

The amyloid fibril protein consists, in all cases studied, of the first 90 or so N-terminal residues, even when the causative variant residue(s) are more distal. Wild type apolipoprotein A-I is also amyloidogenic, forming the deposits associated with atheromatous plaques in older people; the various amyloidogenic mutations presumably encode sequence changes that render apolipoprotein A-I less stable and/or more liable to cleavage that yields the fibrillogenic N-terminal fragment. Predominantly renal amyloidosis has also been described in a handful of families in association with several different mutations in a normal stop codon in the gene for apolipoprotein A-II, which results in a peptide extension from residue 78.

Lysozyme

Lysozyme is the classic bacteriolytic enzyme of external secretions, discovered by Fleming in 1922. It is also present at high concentration within articular cartilage and in the granules of polymorphs, and is the major secreted product of macrophages. Lysozymes are present in most organisms in which they have been sought, although their physiological role is not always clear. The complete structures of hen egg-white and human lysozymes are known to atomic resolution, and their catalytic mechanism, epitopes, folding, and other aspects of their structure–function relationship have been analysed exhaustively. This contrasts with the absence of detailed three-dimensional structural information on any other amyloid fibril protein or its precursor, except transthyretin and β_2-microglobulin.

Lysozyme, unlike transthyretin and β_2-microglobulin, is not inherently amyloidogenic, and is therefore a valuable model for the investigation of amyloid fibrillogenesis. There is only one copy of the lysozyme gene in the human genome, and no disease is associated with lysozyme other than amyloidosis. The first mutations identified to cause amyloidosis were substitution of threonine for isoleucine at residue 56 in one family, and histidine for aspartic acid at residue 67 in another. These dramatic changes in residues that are extremely conserved throughout the lysozyme and related α-lactalbumin protein families destabilize the native fold, so that the variants readily adopt partly unfolded states, even under physiological conditions, and spontaneously aggregate *in vitro*, and evidently also *in vivo*, into amyloid fibrils. Several further amyloidogenic variants of lysozyme have recently been described.

Islet amyloid polypeptide

Islet amyloid polypeptide (amylin; IAPP) is a 37-residue molecule encoded by a gene on chromosome 12 and with 46% sequence homology to the neuropeptide calcitonin gene-related peptide. Islet amyloid polypeptide is produced in the β-cells of the pancreatic islets of Langerhans, and is stored in and released from their secretory granules together with insulin. It has been reported to modulate insulin release and to induce peripheral insulin resistance, vasodilatation, and lowering of plasma calcium, but neither its physiological role nor its contribution to diabetes are yet known.

The amyloidogenicity of islet amyloid polypeptide depends on the amino acid sequence between residues 20 and 29, as shown by *in vitro* fibrillogenesis with synthetic peptides. The synthetic decapeptide IAPP20–29, and even the hexapeptide IAPP25–29, form amyloid-like fibrils *in vitro*, whereas other islet amyloid polypeptide fragments do not. There is also a correlation between conservation of this sequence and deposition of the amyloid in the islets of diabetic animals of different species. However, the role of the amyloid in diabetogenesis remains to be established. In the degu, a South American rodent, spontaneous diabetes is associated with islet amyloid composed of insulin, and xenogeneic insulin can also form amyloid in humans at the site of repeated therapeutic insulin injections.

β_2-Microglobulin

β_2-Microglobulin is a nonglycosylated, nonpolymorphic, single-chain protein of 99 residues, with a single intrachain disulphide bridge and a relative molecular mass of 11 815, encoded by a single gene on chromosome 15. It becomes noncovalently associated with the heavy chain of major histocompatibility class I antigens, and is required for transport and expression of the major histocompatibility complex (MHC) at the cell surface. Amino acid sequence homology places β_2-microglobulin in the superfamily that includes immunoglobulins, T-cell receptor α- and β-chains, Thy-1 (CD90), MHC class I and II molecules, secretory component, etc. Its three-dimensional structure is a typical β-barrel with two antiparallel pleated sheets comprising three and four strands, respectively, and closely resembles an immunoglobulin domain.

β_2-Microglobulin is produced by lymphoid and a variety of other cells, in which it stabilizes the structure and function of MHC class I antigens at the cell surface. When these complexes are shed by cleavage of the heavy chain at the cell surface, free β_2-microglobulin is released. The circulating concentration of β_2-microglobulin is 1 to 2 mg/litre and the protein is rapidly cleared by glomerular filtration and then catabolized in the proximal renal tubule. Impairment of renal function is associated with retention of β_2-microglobulin and increased circulating levels because there is no other site for its catabolism. Daily production of β_2-microglobulin is about 200 mg, and in patients in endstage renal failure on haemodialysis, plasma β_2-microglobulin levels rise to and remain at levels of about 40 to 70 mg/litre. Isolated unaltered β_2-microglobulin can form amyloid-like fibrils itself *in vitro*, and most studies of *ex vivo* β_2-microglobulin fibrils show the whole intact molecule to be the major subunit, although fragments and altered forms of β_2-microglobulin have also been reported.

Glycosaminoglycans

Amyloidotic organs contain more glycosaminoglycans than normal tissues, and at least some of this is a tightly bound integral part of the amyloid fibrils. These fibril-associated glycosaminoglycans are heparan sulphate and dermatan sulphate in all forms of amyloid that have been investigated. Fibrils isolated by water extraction and separated from other tissue components contain 1 to 2% by weight glycosaminoglycan, none of which is covalently associated with the fibril protein. Interestingly, in systemic AA and AL amyloidosis, the only forms in which this has been studied so far, there is markedly restricted heterogeneity of the glycosaminoglycan chains, suggesting that particular subclasses of heparan and dermatan sulphates are involved. Immunohistochemical studies demonstrate the presence of proteoglycan core proteins in all amyloid deposits, and that these are closely related to fibrils at the ultrastructural level. However, in isolated fibril preparations much of the glycosaminoglycan material is free carbohydrate chains, and it is not yet clear whether this represents aberrant glycosaminoglycan metabolism related to amyloidosis or is just an artefact of postmortem degradation of core protein.

The significance of glycosaminoglycans in amyloid remains unclear, but their universal presence, intimate relationship with the fibrils, and restricted heterogeneity all suggest that they may be important. Glycosaminoglycans are known to participate in the organization of some normal structural proteins into fibrils and they may have comparable fibrillogenic effects on certain amyloid fibril precursor proteins. Furthermore, the glycosaminoglycans on amyloid fibrils may be ligands to which serum amyloid P component, another universal constituent of amyloid deposits, binds.

Amyloid P component and serum amyloid P component

Amyloid deposits in all different forms of the disease, both in humans and in animals, contain the nonfibrillar glycoprotein amyloid P component. Amyloid P component is identical to and derived from the normal circulating plasma protein, serum amyloid P component, a member of the pentraxin protein family that includes C-reactive protein. Human serum amyloid P component is secreted only by hepatocytes, is a trace constituent of plasma (women: mean 24 mg/litre, range 8–55, men: mean 32 mg/litre, range 12–50), and is not an acute phase reactant. Nevertheless, apart from the fibrils themselves, amyloid P component is always by far the most abundant protein in all amyloid deposits.

Serum amyloid P component consists of five identical noncovalently associated subunits, each with a molecular mass of 25 462 Da, arranged in a pentameric disc-like ring. The tertiary fold of the subunit is dominated by antiparallel β-sheets, forming a flattened β-barrel with jellyroll topology and a core of hydrophobic side chains. This is the lectin fold, shared with a variety of other animal, plant, and bacterial carbohydrate-binding proteins (lectins). Serum amyloid P component is a calcium-dependent ligand-binding protein; its best-defined specificity is for the 4,6-cyclic pyruvate acetal of β-D-galactose, but it also binds avidly and specifically to DNA, chromatin, glycosaminoglycans (particularly heparan and dermatan sulphates), and to all known types of amyloid fibrils. The latter interaction is responsible for the unique specific accumulation of serum amyloid P component in amyloid deposits. Aggregated, but not native, serum amyloid P component also binds specifically to C4-binding protein and fibronectin from plasma, although serum amyloid P component is not complexed with any other protein in the circulation. In addition to being a plasma protein, human serum amyloid P component is also a normal constituent of certain extracellular matrix structures. It is covalently associated with collagen and/or other matrix components in the lamina rara interna of the human glomerular basement membrane, and is present on the microfibrillar mantle of elastin fibres throughout the body.

Although no deficiency of serum amyloid P component has been described, and it has been stably conserved in evolution, its physiological function remains unclear. There is a single copy of its gene on chromosome 1, no polymorphism of the amino acid sequence, and the single biantennary oligosaccharide chain attached to asparagine at residue 32 is the most invariant glycan of any known glycoprotein. Studies of serum amyloid P component knockout mice have shown that serum amyloid P component is involved in host resistance to some infections, and contributes to the pathogenesis of others, but these animals are otherwise healthy and have a normal lifespan.

The serum amyloid P component molecule is highly resistant to proteolysis and, although not itself a proteinase inhibitor, its binding to amyloid fibrils *in vitro* protects them against proteolysis. Once bound to amyloid fibrils *in vivo*, serum amyloid P component persists for very prolonged periods and is not catabolized at all, by contrast with its rapid clearance from the plasma (half-life 24 h) and prompt catabolism in the liver. These observations suggest that serum amyloid P component may contribute to the persistence of amyloid deposits *in vivo*; serum amyloid P component knockout mice show retarded and reduced induction of experimental AA amyloidosis, confirming that serum amyloid P component is significantly involved in the pathogenesis of amyloidosis.

Other proteins in amyloid deposits

A number of plasma proteins, other than the fibril proteins themselves and serum amyloid P component, have been detected immunohistochemically in some amyloid deposits. These include α_1-antichymotrypsin, some complement components, apolipoprotein E, and various proteins of the extracellular matrix and basement membrane. None of these is as universal, abundant, or selective as serum amyloid P component, and their role, if any, in the pathogenesis or effects of amyloid deposition is not known.

Diagnosis and monitoring of amyloidosis

Introduction

Until recently, amyloidosis was an exclusively histological diagnosis, and green birefringence of deposits stained with Congo red and viewed in polarized light remains the gold standard. Furthermore, immunohistochemical staining of amyloid-containing tissue is the simplest method for identifying the type of amyloid fibril present. However, biopsies provide extremely small samples and therefore can never provide information on the extent, localization, progression, or regression of amyloid deposits. A major advance in clinical amyloidosis has been the development of radiolabelled serum amyloid P component as a specific tracer for amyloid. Combined scintigraphic imaging and metabolic analysis using labelled serum amyloid P component have provided a wealth of new information on the natural history of many different forms of amyloid and their response to treatment.

Histochemical diagnosis of amyloidosis

Biopsy

Amyloid may be an incidental finding on biopsy of the kidneys, liver, heart, bowel, peripheral nerves, lymph nodes, skin, thyroid, or bone marrow. When amyloidosis is suspected clinically, biopsy of the rectum or subcutaneous fat is the least invasive. Amyloid is present at these sites in more than 90% of cases of systemic AA or AL amyloidosis. Alternatively, a clinically affected tissue may be biopsied directly.

Congo red and other histochemical stains

Many cotton dyes, fluorochromes, and metachromatic stains have been used, but Congo red staining, and its resultant green birefringence when viewed with high-intensity polarized light, is the pathognomonic histochemical test for amyloidosis. The stain is unstable and must be freshly prepared every 2 months or less in alkaline alcoholic solution. It is critical to have a section thickness of 5 to 10 μm and include in every staining run a positive control tissue containing modest amounts of amyloid.

Immunohistochemistry

Although many amyloid fibril proteins can be identified immunohistochemically, the demonstration of amyloidogenic proteins in tissues does not, on its own, establish the presence of amyloid. Congo red staining and green birefringence are always required, and immunostaining may then enable the amyloid to be classified. Antibodies to serum amyloid A protein are commercially available and always stain AA deposits, similarly with anti-β_2-microglobulin antisera and haemodialysis-associated amyloid. In AL amyloid the deposits are stainable with standard antisera to κ or λ immunoglobulin light chains in only about one-half of cases, probably because the light-chain fragment in the fibrils is usually the N-terminal variable domain, which is largely unique for each monoclonal protein. Immunohistochemical staining of transthyretin, Aβ, and prion protein amyloid may require pretreatment of sections with formic acid or alkaline guanidine, or deglycosylation.

Electron microscopy

Amyloid fibrils cannot always be convincingly identified ultrastructurally, and electron microscopy alone is not sufficient to confirm the diagnosis of amyloidosis.

Problems of histological diagnosis

The tissue sample must be adequate (e.g. the inclusion of submucosal vessels in a rectal biopsy specimen), and failure to find amyloid does not exclude the diagnosis. The unavoidable sampling problem means that biopsy cannot reveal the extent or distribution of amyloid. Experience with Congo red staining is required if clinically important false negative and false positive results are to be avoided. Immunohistochemical staining requires positive and negative controls, including demonstration of the specificity of staining by absorption of positive antisera with isolated pure antigens. The recent development of powerful proteomic analysis methods applicable to histological sections suggests that, in specialist centres, direct identification of all amyloid fibril proteins may soon be possible on microscopic tissue samples.

Nonhistological investigations

Two-dimensional echocardiography showing small, concentrically hypertrophied ventricles, generally impaired contraction, dilated atria, homogeneously echogenic valves, and 'sparkling' echodensity of ventricular walls is virtually diagnostic of cardiac amyloidosis. However, clinically significant restrictive diastolic impairment may be difficult to detect, even by comprehensive Doppler echocardiography and other functional studies. Cardiac magnetic resonance imaging appearances are also characteristic in amyloidosis and coupled with late gadolinium enhancement can be diagnostic.

In cases of known or suspected hereditary amyloidosis, the gene defect must be characterized. If amyloidotic tissue is available the fibril protein may be known and the corresponding gene can then be studied, but if no tissue containing amyloid is available, screening of the genes for known amyloidogenic proteins must be undertaken.

Biochemical and immunochemical tests exist for screening the plasma for amyloidogenic variant protein products of mutant genes, e.g. for transthyretin and apolipoprotein A-I variants, but molecular genetic analysis of DNA is easier to perform and is the most direct approach. However, regardless of the DNA results, it is desirable, if possible, directly to identify the respective protein in the amyloid.

Serum amyloid P component as a specific tracer in amyloidosis

The universal presence in amyloid deposits of amyloid P component, derived from circulating serum amyloid P component, is the basis for the use of radioisotope-labelled serum amyloid P component as a diagnostic tracer in amyloidosis. No localization or retention of labelled serum amyloid P component occurs in healthy subjects or in patients with diseases other than amyloidosis (Fig. 12.12.3.1a). Radioiodinated serum amyloid P component has a short half-life (24 h) in the plasma and is rapidly catabolized, with complete excretion of the iodinated breakdown products in the urine. However, in patients with systemic or localized extracerebral amyloidosis, the tracer rapidly and specifically localizes to the deposits, in proportion to the quantity of amyloid present, and persists there without breakdown or modification (Fig. 12.12.3.1b, c). Highly purified serum amyloid P component, isolated from donor plasma according to pharmaceutical current good manufacturing practice, is oxidatively iodinated under conditions that preserve its function intact. The medium-energy, short half-life, pure γ-emitter ^{123}I is used for scintigraphic imaging, and the long half-life isotope ^{125}I is used for metabolic studies. The dose of radioactivity administered (<4 mSv) is well within accepted safety limits and more than 10 000 studies have been completed without any adverse effects. In addition to high-resolution scintigraphs, the uptake of tracer into various organs can be precisely quantified and, together with highly reproducible metabolic data on the plasma clearance and whole-body retention of activity, the progression or regression of amyloid can be monitored serially and quantitatively.

Important observations regarding amyloid include the following: the different distribution of amyloid in different forms of the disease; amyloid in anatomical sites not available for biopsy (adrenals, spleen); major systemic deposits of forms of amyloid previously thought to be organ-limited; a poor correlation between the quantity of amyloid present in a given organ and the level of organ dysfunction; a nonhomogeneous distribution of amyloid within individual organs; and evidence for rapid progression and sometimes regression of amyloid deposits with different rates in different organs (Fig. 12.12.3.2). Examples of major regression of amyloidosis, when it has been possible to reduce or eliminate the supply of fibril precursor, are very encouraging. Studies with labelled serum amyloid P component thus make a valuable contribution to the diagnosis and management of patients with systemic amyloidosis, and in the United Kingdom these are routinely available for all known or suspected cases of amyloidosis in the

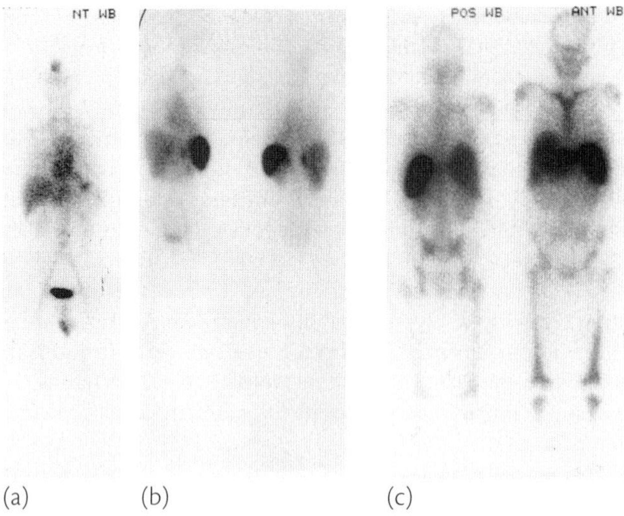

Fig. 12.12.3.1 Whole-body scintigraphs 24 h after intravenous injection of ^{123}I-labelled human serum amyloid P component. (a) Anterior view of a normal control subject showing the distribution of residual tracer in the blood pool and radioactive breakdown products in urine in the bladder; note the absence of localization or retention of tracer anywhere in the body. (b) Posterior (left) and anterior (right) views of a patient with juvenile chronic arthritis complicated by AA amyloidosis. There is uptake of tracer in the spleen, kidneys, and adrenal glands, a typical distribution of AA amyloid in which the spleen is involved in 100% of cases, kidneys in 75%, and adrenals in 40%. Note the reduced blood pool and bladder signal compared with (a). This patient, whose amyloid was diagnosed by renal biopsy 15 years before when nephrotic syndrome developed, and who was then treated with chlorambucil, had been in complete remission for 10 years during which there had been no acute phase response. At the time of this scan there was no biochemical abnormality in blood or urine, despite the very appreciable amyloid deposits, illustrating the discordance between the presence of amyloid and clinical effects. (c) Posterior (left) and anterior (right) views of a patient with monoclonal gammopathy complicated by extensive AL amyloidosis. There is uptake and retention of tracer in the liver, spleen, kidneys, bone marrow, and soft tissues around the shoulder. This scintigraphic pattern of amyloid distribution is pathognomonic for AL amyloidosis; bone-marrow uptake has not been seen in any other type. Note the complete absence of blood pool or bladder signal resulting from complete uptake of the tracer dose into the substantial amyloid deposits.

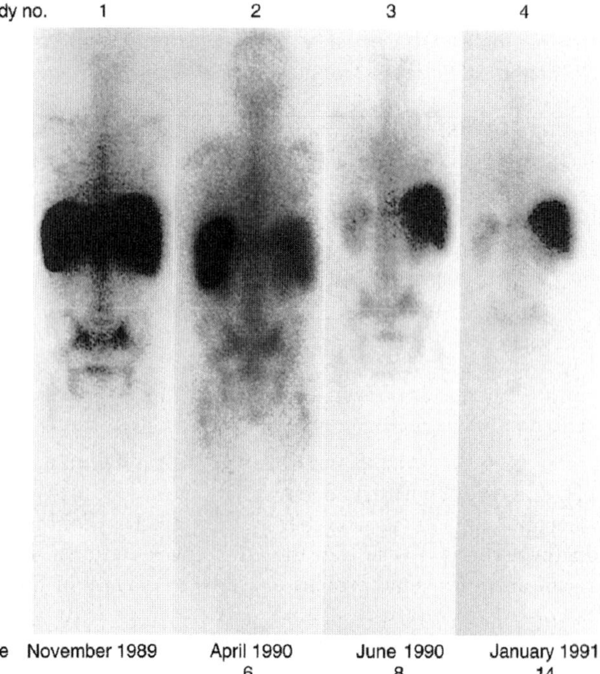

Fig. 12.12.3.2 Serial posterior whole-body ^{123}I-serum amyloid P component scintigraphs of a man with AL amyloidosis complicating benign monoclonal gammopathy. At presentation (scan 1) there was uptake in the spleen, liver, and bone marrow, obscuring any possible renal signal. Chemotherapy was given before scan 2, which shows increased spleen uptake, reduced liver uptake, and some renal uptake, but no change in total amyloid load determined by measurements of the clearance and retention of the tracer (not shown). Subsequently, he had recurrent splenic infarctions and splenectomy was performed. Thereafter (scan 3) there was increased tracer uptake in the liver, although a notably lower total amyloid load. Six months later (scan 4) liver and kidney uptake, plasma clearance, and whole body retention of tracer were all reduced, indicating regression of amyloid. He was clinically much improved and remained well.

National Health Service National Amyloidosis Centre at the Royal Free Hospital, London.

Management of amyloidosis

Although no treatments yet exist that specifically promote the mobilization of amyloid, there have been substantial recent advances in the management of systemic amyloidosis, in particular active measures to support failing organ function while attempts are made to reduce the supply of the amyloid fibril precursor protein. Serial serum amyloid P component scintigraphy in more than 2000 patients with various forms of amyloid has shown that control of the primary disease process, or removal of the source of the amyloidogenic precursor, often results in regression of existing deposits and recovery or preservation of organ function. This strongly supports aggressive intervention, and relatively toxic drug regimes or other radical approaches can be justified by the poor prognosis. Such an approach, leading to reduced morbidity and improved survival, was the basis for the establishment of the National Health Service National Amyloid Centre. However, clinical improvement in amyloidosis is often delayed long after the underlying disorder has remitted, reflecting the very gradual regression of the deposits that is now recognized to occur in most patients. Continuing production of the amyloid precursor protein should be monitored as closely as possible in the long term, to determine the requirement for and intensity of treatment for the underlying primary condition. In AA amyloidosis this involves frequent estimation of the plasma SAA level, and in AL amyloidosis it requires monitoring of the serum free light-chain concentration or other markers of the underlying monoclonal plasma-cell proliferation.

The treatment of AA amyloidosis ranges from potent anti-inflammatory and immunosuppressive drugs in patients with rheumatoid arthritis, to lifelong prophylactic colchicine in familial Mediterranean fever, and surgery in conditions such as refractory osteomyelitis and the tumours of Castleman's disease. The biological cytokine-inhibiting agents antitumour necrosis factor and recombinant interleukin 1 receptor antagonist can induce rapid and complete remission of inflammatory activity in many patients with rheumatoid or juvenile idiopathic arthritis, and those with inherited periodic fever syndromes.

Treatment of AL amyloidosis is based on that for myeloma, although the plasma-cell dyscrasias in AL amyloidosis are often very subtle. Prolonged low-intensity cytotoxic regimes, such as oral melphalan and prednisolone, are beneficial in about 20% of patients.

More dose-intensive chemotherapy regimes, such as oral melphalan and dexamethasone, and thalidomide-based regimes, notably oral cyclophosphamide, thalidomide and dexamethasone, are associated with responses in more than 50% of patients, along with manageable toxicity. High-dose chemotherapy with autologous peripheral blood stem-cell transplantation may be associated with even higher response rates, although procedural mortality is high in individuals with multiple amyloidotic organ involvement, especially patients with autonomic neuropathy, severe cardiac amyloidosis, or a history of gastrointestinal bleeding, and in those aged over about 60 years.

The disabling arthralgia of β_2-microglobulin amyloidosis may partially respond to nonsteroidal anti-inflammatory drugs or corticosteroids, but even the most severe symptoms usually rapidly vanish following renal transplantation. The basis for this remarkable clinical response is unclear, since although transplantation rapidly restores normal β_2-microglobulin metabolism, regression of β_2-microglobulin amyloid may not be evident for many years.

Hepatic transplantation is effective in familial amyloid polyneuropathy associated with transthyretin gene mutations, since the variant amyloidogenic protein is produced mainly in the liver. Outcome has proved best among younger patients with the methionine-30 substitution, though even in this group the peripheral neuropathy usually only stabilizes. Unfortunately, paradoxical progression of established cardiac amyloidosis with wild type transthyretin has been observed in many older patients, particularly those with nonmethionine-30 substitutions. Important questions therefore remain about the selection of patients and timing of the procedure but, so far, early intervention seems advisable. On a similar basis, hepatic transplantation has also been successfully undertaken in some patients with hereditary fibrinogen α-chain and apolipoprotein A-I amyloidosis.

Supportive therapy remains critical in systemic amyloidosis, with the potential for delaying target organ failure, maintaining quality of life, and prolonging survival while the underlying process can be treated. Rigorous control of hypertension is vital in renal amyloidosis. Surgical resection of amyloidotic tissue is occasionally beneficial but, in general, a conservative approach to surgery, anaesthesia, and other invasive procedures is advisable. Should any such procedure be undertaken, meticulous attention to blood pressure and fluid balance is essential. Amyloidotic tissues may heal poorly and are liable to bleed. Diuretics and vasoactive drugs should be used cautiously in cardiac amyloidosis because they can reduce cardiac output substantially. Dysrhythmias may respond to conventional pharmacological therapy or to pacing. Replacement of vital organ function, notably dialysis, may be necessary, and cardiac, renal, and liver transplant procedures have a role in selected cases.

Finally, a number of different therapies aimed specifically at inhibiting the formation of amyloid fibrils or promoting fibril regression are currently under development, and some are already being evaluated clinically. The latter include approaches directed at precursor protein production, glycosaminoglycans, serum amyloid P component, preventing aberrant protein folding, and various kinds of immunotherapy, offering hope that amyloidosis may become more readily treatable.

Further reading

Booth DR, *et al.* (1997). Instability, unfolding and aggregation of human lysozyme variants underlying amyloid fibrillogenesis. *Nature*, **385**, 787–93.

Drüeke TB (1998). Dialysis-related amyloidosis. *Nephrol Dial Transplant*, **13** Suppl 1, 58–64.

Gertz MA, Merlini G, Treon SP (2004). Amyloidosis and Waldenstrom's macroglobulinemia. *Hematology Am Soc Hematol Educ Program*, 257–82.

Hardy J (1997). Amyloid, the presenilins and Alzheimer's disease. *Trends Neurosci*, **20**, 154–9.

Hawkins PN (2002). Serum amyloid P component scintigraphy for diagnosis and monitoring amyloidosis. *Curr Opin Nephrol Hypertens*, **11**, 649–55.

Hawkins PN, Lavender JP, Pepys MB (1990). Evaluation of systemic amyloidosis by scintigraphy with ^{123}I-labeled serum amyloid P component. *N Engl J Med*, **323**, 508–13.

Kyle RA, Gertz MA (1995). Primary systemic amyloidosis: clinical and laboratory features in 474 cases. *Semin Hematol*, **32**, 45–9.

Lachmann HJ, *et al.* (2002). Misdiagnosis of hereditary amyloidosis as AL (primary) amyloidosis. *N Engl J Med*, **346**, 1786–91.

Lachmann HJ, *et al.* (2003). Outcome in systemic AL amyloidosis in relation to changes in concentration of circulating free immunoglobulin light chains following chemotherapy. *Br J Haematol*, **122**, 78–84.

Lachmann HJ, *et al.* (2007). Natural history and outcome in systemic AA amyloidosis. *N Engl J Med*, **356**, 2361–2371.

Pepys MB (2006). Amyloidosis. *Annu Rev Med*, **57**, 223–41.

Westermark P *et al.* (2007). A primer of amyloid nomenclature. *Amyloid*, **14**, 179–83.

12.13

α_1-Antitrypsin deficiency and the serpinopathies

David A. Lomas

Essentials

α_1-Antitrypsin is an acute phase glycoprotein synthesized by the liver that functions as an inhibitor of a range of proteolytic enzymes, most importantly neutrophil elastase. Severe plasma deficiency of α_1-antitrypsin results from homozygocity for the Z allele, which causes the protein to undergo a conformational transition and form ordered polymers that are retained within hepatocytes as PAS-positive inclusions.

Clinical features—(1) Liver—all adults with the Z allele of α_1-antitrypsin have slowly progressive hepatic damage that is often subclinical and only evident as a minor degree of portal fibrosis, but up to 50% of Z homozygotes present with clinically evident cirrhosis and occasionally with hepatocellular carcinoma. (2) Lung—patients with Z α_1-antitrypsin deficiency develop panlobular emphysema that tends to affect the bases rather than the apices of the lungs and is greatly exacerbated by smoking; cor pulmonale and polycythaemia are late features.

Diagnosis and management—severe genetic deficiency of α_1-antitrypsin is readily diagnosed by low plasma levels and the virtual absence of the α_1-band on protein electrophoresis. Patients should be very strongly advised to abstain from smoking, and to avoid agents that cause hepatic injury (such as excessive alcohol and obesity). Treatment otherwise involves conventional trials of bronchodilators and inhaled corticosteroids, pulmonary rehabilitation and—where appropriate—assessment for long-term oxygen therapy and lung transplantation. α_1-Antitrypsin replacement therapy is widely used in North America, but its value is uncertain.

Other serpinopathies—the polymerization that underlies α_1-antitrypsin deficiency is found in other members of the serine protease inhibitor (or serpin) superfamily to cause diseases as diverse as thrombosis (antithrombin), angioedema (C1 inhibitor), and dementia (neuroserpin).

Introduction

α_1-Antitrypsin deficiency was first described by Carl-Bertil Laurell and Sten Eriksson in 1963 when they reported five individuals in whom there was a deficiency of the α_1 band on serum protein electrophoresis. Three of the individuals had emphysema and one had a family history of emphysema. α_1-Antitrypsin is a 394 amino acid, 52-kDa acute phase glycoprotein synthesized by the liver and macrophages and by intestinal and bronchial epithelial cells. It is present in the plasma at a concentration of between 0.9 and 1.8 g/litre and functions as an inhibitor of a range of proteolytic enzymes of which the most important is neutrophil elastase. α_1-Antitrypsin deficiency results from point mutations that cause the protein to misfold and be retained within hepatocytes which in turn causes liver disease. The lack of circulating α_1-antitrypsin causes uncontrolled tissue digestion within the lung and hence emphysema.

Genetics and pathogenesis of disease

Genetics

α_1-Antitrypsin is subject to genetic variation resulting from mutations in the 12.2-kb, 7-exon *SERPINA1* gene on the long arm of chromosome 14 (14q32.1) (OMIM 107400). Over 100 allelic variants have been reported and classified using the PI (protease inhibitor) nomenclature that assesses α_1-antitrypsin mobility in isoelectric focusing analysis. Normal α_1-antitrypsin migrates in the middle (M) and variants are designated A (anodal) to L if they migrate faster than M, and N to Z if they migrate more slowly. Many of these variants have been sequenced at the DNA level and shown to result from point mutations in the α_1-antitrypsin gene (Table 12.13.1). For example, the Z allele results from the substitution of a positively charged lysine for a negative glutamic acid at position 342. The S allele results from the substitution of a neutral

Table 12.13.1 Some alleles of *SERPINA1*. The letter denotes the migration on isoelectric focusing (PI) and the name denotes the origin of the mutation

	Mutation
Normal alleles	
M1	Val213Ala
M2	Arg101His
M3	Glu376Asp
$X_{christchurch}$	Glu363Lys
Deficiency alleles	
F	Arg223Cys
I	Arg39Cys
Mheerlen	Pro369Leu
Mmalton	Phe52del or Phe51del
Mmineral springs	Gly67Glu
Mprocida	Leu41Pro
Plowell	Asp256Val
S	Glu264Val
Siiyama	Ser53Phe
Z	Glu342Lys
Null alleles	
QObellingham	Lys217X
QObolton	Pro362X
QOgranite falls	Tyr160X
QOhongkong-1	Leu318 deletion of 2 bp and premature stop codon at 334
QOludwigshafen	Ile92Asn
Dysfunctional alleles	
Pittsburgh*	Met358Arg

* Antithrombin activity that results in a bleeding diathesis.

valine for a glutamic acid at position 264. Point mutations are inherited by simple mendelian trait; the normal genotype is designated PI MM or PI M, a heterozygote for the Z gene is PI MZ, and a homozygote is PI ZZ or PI Z. α_1-Antitrypsin alleles are codominantly expressed, with each allele contributing to the plasma level of protein. Therefore each of the deficiency alleles results in a characteristic decrease in the plasma concentration of α_1-antitrypsin; the S variant forms 60% of the normal M concentration and the Z variant 10 to 15%. Null alleles produce no α_1-antitrypsin. Thus combinations of alleles have predictable effects, the MZ heterozygote has an α_1-antitrypsin plasma level of 60% (50% from the normal M allele and 10% from the Z allele), the MS heterozygote 80% and the SZ heterozygote 40%. Very rarely point mutations can result in dysfunctional α_1-antitrypsin that no longer inhibits neutrophil elastase or which can inhibit other serine proteases. The most striking example is the Pittsburgh mutant (Met358Arg) which converted α_1-antitrypsin into an inhibitor of thrombin, thereby causing a fatal bleeding diathesis.

The molecular basis of α_1-antitrypsin deficiency

Liver disease

α_1-Antitrypsin functions by presenting its reactive-centre methionine residue on an exposed loop of the molecule such that it forms an ideal substrate for the enzyme neutrophil elastase (Fig. 12.13.1). The conformational transition that ensues results in the formation of a stable complex that inhibits the enzyme and allows it to be eliminated from sites of inflammation. The Z mutation (Glu342Lys) results in normal translation of the gene, but 85% of the Z α_1-antitrypsin is retained within the endoplasmic reticulum with only 10 to 15% entering the circulation. The Z mutation distorts the relationship between the loop and the A β-pleated sheet that forms the major feature of the molecule. The consequent perturbation in structure allows the reactive-centre loop of one α_1-molecule to lock into the A sheet of a second to form a dimer which then extends to form chains of loop-sheet polymers (Fig. 12.13.1). The formation of these polymers is temperature and concentration dependent and is localized to the endoplasmic reticulum of the hepatocyte (Fig. 12.13.2). These chains of polymers become interwoven to form the insoluble aggregates that are the hallmark of α_1-antitrypsin liver disease. The process of intrahepatic polymerization also underlies the severe plasma deficiency of the rare Siiyama (Ser53Phe) and Mmalton (deletion of residue 52) deficiency alleles and the mild plasma deficiency of the S (Glu264Val) and I (Arg39Cys) variants. There is a strong genotype–phenotype correlation that can be explained by the molecular instability caused by the mutation and in particular the rate at which the mutant forms polymers. Those mutants that cause the most rapid polymerization cause the most retention of α_1-antitrypsin within the liver. This in turn correlates with the greatest risk of liver damage and cirrhosis, and the most severe plasma deficiency. Misfolded Z α_1-antitrypsin within hepatocytes is cleared by the proteosome but the ordered polymers are not detected by the unfolded protein response and are handled by less well understood pathways including autophagy.

Lung disease

The development of emphysema associated with α_1-antitrypsin deficiency is greatly accelerated by tobacco smoking. Emphysema results from uncontrolled enzymatic activity within the lung with those individuals with plasma α_1-antitrypsin levels of $<40\%$ of normal being most at risk. This is compounded by a fivefold reduction in association rate kinetics with neutrophil elastase caused by the Z mutation and the polymerization of secreted Z α_1-antitrypsin within the airways and alveoli. The formation of polymers inactivates α_1-antitrypsin (thereby further reducing the protein available to inhibit neutrophil elastase) and the polymers themselves may drive some of the excessive inflammation that characterizes this condition.

Epidemiology

Two point mutations have been shown to explain the vast majority of cases of α_1-antitrypsin deficiency. The Z allele causes the most severe plasma deficiency and is most prevalent in southern Scandinavia and the north-western European seaboard where 4% of the population are MZ heterozygotes and 1 in 1700 are PI Z homozygotes. The gene frequency of the Z allele reduces towards the south and east of Europe. In contrast, the S allele causes only mild plasma deficiency and is most common in southern Europe where up to 28% of the population

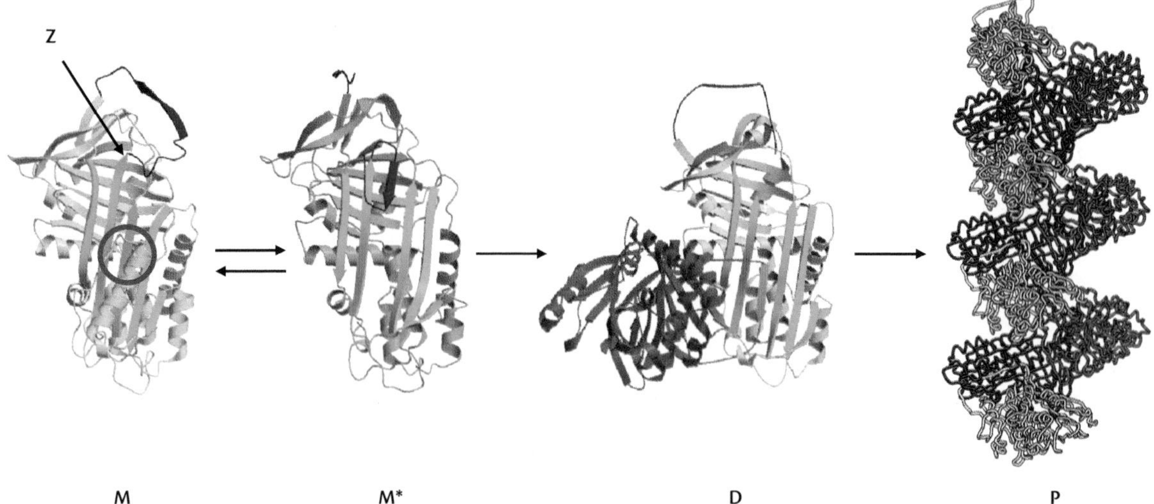

Fig. 12.13.1 Mutant Z α_1-antitrypsin is retained within hepatocytes as polymers. The structure of α_1-antitrypsin is centred on β-sheet A (green) and the mobile reactive centre loop (red). Polymer formation results from the Z variant of α_1-antitrypsin (Glu342Lys at P_{17}; arrowed) or mutations in the shutter domain (blue circle) that open β-sheet A to favour partial loop insertion and the formation of an unstable intermediate (M*). The patent β-sheet A can either accept the loop of another molecule to form a dimer (D) which then extends into polymers (P). The individual molecules of α_1-antitrypsin within the polymer are coloured red, yellow and blue. (From Gooptu, B., Hazes, B., Chang, W.-S.W., Dafforn, T.R., Carrell, R.W., Read, R. & Lomas, D.A. (2000). Inactive conformation of the serpin a1-antichymotrypsin indicates two stage insertion of the reactive loop; implications for inhibitory function and conformational disease. *Proc. Natl. Acad. Sci* (USA), **97**, 67–72. with permission.)

are MS heterozygotes. The S allele becomes less frequent as one moves north-east. The frequencies of the Z allele in the United States of America are similar to the lowest frequencies in Europe but the S allele is more common than in northern Europeans. α_1-Antitrypsin deficiency is infrequent in Asian, African, and Middle Eastern populations. It is also rare in Japan, but when present it is usually due to the Siiyama mutation (Ser53Phe). In the genetically isolated island of Sardinia the commonest cause of severe α_1-antitrypsin deficiency is the Mmalton mutation (deletion of residue 52).

The Z allele is believed to have arisen from a single origin 66 generations or 2000 years ago. The high frequency in southern Scandinavia suggests that the mutation arose in the Viking population. The date of origin implies that the allele arose when the Vikings populated mid/northern Europe and before their migration to Scandinavia. It is likely that the Z allele of α_1-antitrypsin was then distributed across northern Europe by the Viking raiders between 800 and 1100 AD, and then to the United States and the rest of the world during migration over the past 200 years. The S allele appears to have arisen in the north of the Iberian peninsula, but the date of origin is uncertain. This mutation was similarly introduced into North America by mass migration.

Clinical features

α_1-Antitrypsin deficiency and liver disease

The accumulation of abnormal protein starts *in utero* and is characterized by diastase-resistant, periodic acid–Schiff (PAS) positive inclusions of α_1-antitrypsin in the periportal cells (Fig. 12.13.2).

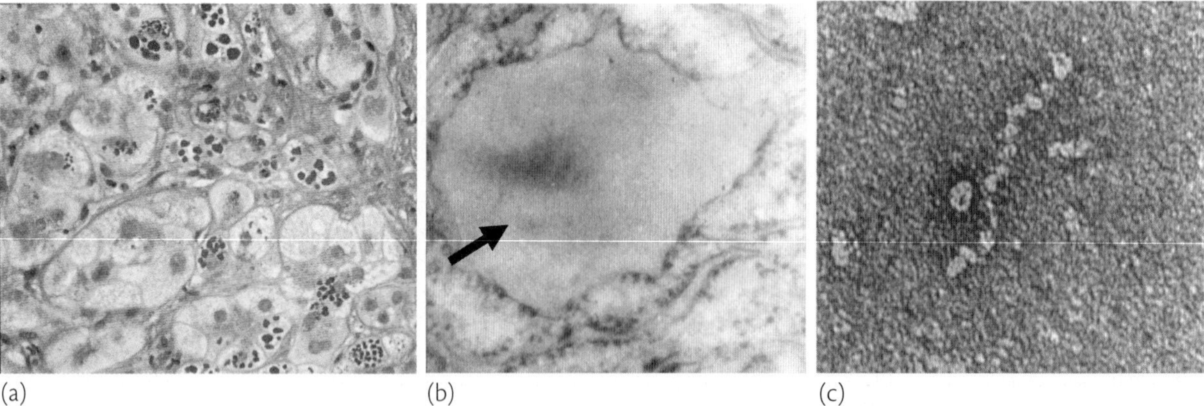

Fig. 12.13.2 Z α_1-antitrypsin is retained within hepatocytes as intracellular inclusions. These inclusions are PAS positive and diastase resistant (a) and are associated with neonatal hepatitis and hepatocellular carcinoma (b). Electron micrograph of an hepatocyte from the liver of a patient with Z α_1-antitrypsin deficiency shows the accumulation of α_1-antitrypsin within the rough endoplasmic reticulum (arrow). These inclusions are composed of chains of α_1-antitrypsin polymers (c).
((b) and (c) reproduced from (i) Lomas, D.A., Evans, D.L., Finch, J.T. & Carrell, R.W. (1992). The mechanism of Z a 1-antitrypsin accumulation in the liver. *Nature*, **357**, 605–607. (ii) Lomas, D.A., Finch, J.T., Seyama, K., Nukiwa, T. & Carrell, R.W. (1993). a_1-antitrypsin Siiyama (Ser^{53}→Phe); further evidence for intracellular loop-sheet polymerisation. *J. Biol. Chem.*, **268**, 15333–15335, with permission.)

Seventy-three per cent of Z α_1-antitrypsin homozygote infants have a raised serum alanine aminotransferase in the first year of life but in only 15% of people is it still abnormal by 12 years of age. Similarly serum bilirubin is raised in 11% of PI Z infants in the first 2–4 months but falls to normal by 6 months of age. One in 10 infants develops cholestatic jaundice and 6% develop clinical evidence of liver disease without jaundice. These symptoms usually resolve by the second year of life but approximately 15% of patients with cholestatic jaundice progress to juvenile cirrhosis. The overall risk of death from liver disease in PI Z children during childhood is 2 to 3%, with boys being at more risk than girls. All adults with the Z allele of α_1-antitrypsin have slowly progressive hepatic damage that is often subclinical and only evident as a minor degree of portal fibrosis. However, up to 50% of Z α_1-antitrypsin homozygotes present with clinically evident cirrhosis and occasionally with hepatocellular carcinoma.

α_1-Antitrypsin deficiency and emphysema

Patients with emphysema related to α_1-antitrypsin deficiency usually present with increasing dyspnoea with cor pulmonale and polycythaemia occurring late in the course of the disease. Emphysema associated with Z α_1-antitrypsin deficiency differs from 'usual chronic obstructive pulmonary disease (COPD)' with normal levels of M α_1-antitrypsin in that it affects predominantly the bases rather than the apices of the lungs, it is associated with panlobular rather than centrilobular disease, and it results from the expression of different genes when assessed by microarray analysis. However in many cases the distribution of disease is indistinguishable from 'usual COPD'. High-resolution CT scans are the most accurate method of assessing the distribution of panlobular emphysema and for monitoring the progress of the pulmonary disease, although this currently has little value outside clinical trials. Lung function tests are typical for emphysema with a reduced FEV_1/FVC ratio (forced expiratory volume in 1 s/forced vital capacity) and FEV_1, gas trapping (raised residual volume/total lung capacity ratio), and a low gas-transfer factor. As in many individuals with COPD, partial reversibility of airflow obstruction (as defined by an increase of 12% and 200 ml in FEV_1) is common in individuals with COPD secondary to α_1-antitrypsin deficiency. The most important factor in the development and progression of emphysema in α_1-antitrypsin deficiency is tobacco smoking.

Other conditions associated with α_1-antitrypsin deficiency

α_1-Antitrypsin deficiency is associated with an increased prevalence of asthma, panniculitis, Wegener's granulomatosis and possibly pancreatitis, gallstones, bronchiectasis, and intracranial and intra-abdominal aneurysms. There appears to be a reduced risk of cerebrovascular disease.

Clinical investigation

The severe genetic deficiency of α_1-antitrypsin is readily diagnosed by low plasma levels and the virtual absence of the α_1-band on protein electrophoresis. As α_1-antitrypsin is an acute phase protein, most laboratories will report levels with another acute-phase reactant, such as α_1-antitchymotrypsin, which allows the clinician to assess the likelihood of deficiency in the context of the inflammatory response. The acute phase response raises the plasma level of α_1-antitrypsin, but the plasma level of the PI Z homozygote can never reach the normal range. The deficiency variant is then assigned a PI phenotype according to the migration of the protein on an isoelectric focusing gel. The mutation underlying the deficiency can be determined by sequencing the *SERPINA1* gene. Commercial kits permit detection of the Z and S alleles but will not detect null or other rare alleles.

Treatment

The treatment of α_1-antitrypsin deficiency depends largely on the avoidance of stimuli causing repeated pulmonary inflammation—primarily smoking. Patients with α_1-antitrypsin deficiency-related emphysema should receive conventional therapy with trials of bronchodilators and inhaled corticosteroids, pulmonary rehabilitation and, where appropriate, assessment for long-term oxygen therapy and lung transplantation. The role of lung volume-reduction surgery in this group is unclear as the disease is basal rather than apical and resections of this region are technically more difficult. Mixed results have been reported in uncontrolled trials.

The lung disease results from a deficiency in the antielastase screen. This may be rectified biochemically by intravenous infusions of α_1-antitrypsin. Registry data suggest that individuals with α_1-antitrypsin deficiency and an FEV_1 of 35 to 49% predicted may derive benefit from replacement therapy. The only controlled trial showed a nonsignificant trend towards reduced progression of emphysema in individuals receiving intravenous α_1-antitrypsin. α_1-Antitrypsin replacement therapy is not currently available in many European countries, including the United Kingdom, but it is widely used in North America.

All *Z* homozygotes have some liver damage and, as such, would be wise to avoid alcohol abuse and obesity. PI Z homozygotes should be monitored for the persistence of hyperbilirubinaemia as this, along with deteriorating results of coagulation studies, indicates the need for liver transplantation. Parents with a child with severe Z α_1-antitrypsin liver disease may require genetic counselling. The likelihood of similar severe liver damage in a subsequent Z homozygote sibling is approximately 20%.

The uncommon α_1-antitrypsin deficiency-associated panniculitis usually responds to dapsone, 100 to 150 mg daily, for 2 to 4 weeks, but occasionally it necessitates the administration of intravenous α_1-antitrypsin replacement therapy.

Prognosis

Estimates of the annual rate of decline in FEV_1 range from 41 to 109 ml in individuals with α_1-antitrypsin deficiency although one study reported a rate of decline of 316 ml/year in current smokers. The fastest rate of decline is in current smokers (and to a lesser extent ex-smokers), men, individuals aged 30–44 years, those with FEV_1 values between 35 and 79% predicted and those with a bronchodilator response. Respiratory failure accounts for 50 to 72% of deaths in individuals with α_1-antitrypsin deficiency with the second most common cause of death being liver cirrhosis (10–13%). Most children avoid significant liver damage in childhood but are still at risk of disease in adult life. The factors that predict progressive liver disease are unclear but males and the obese appear to be most at risk. The only significant cohort study has followed 184 individuals with α_1-antitrypsin deficiency (127 PI Z, 2 PI Z–, 54 PI SZ, and

1 PI S–) from birth to 26 years of age. One PI SZ and 5 PI Z children died in early childhood (2 of liver disease and 2 of other causes but were found to have histological signs of cirrhosis or fibrosis at post-mortem) and 12% and 6% of PI Z subjects had abnormal liver function tests at 18 and 26 years respectively but no clinical evidence of liver disease. All the 26-year-olds had normal lung function (including the 17% of individuals who were current or ex-smokers).

A logical follow-on from the association of α_1-antitrypsin antitrypsin deficiency with emphysema is an assessment of the risk of COPD in heterozygotes who carry an abnormal Z allele and a normal M allele. These individuals have plasma α_1-antitrypsin levels that are approximately 60% of normal. A population-based study demonstrated that PI MZ heterozygotes do not have a clearly increased risk of lung damage. However if groups of patients are collected who already have COPD, then the prevalence of PI MZ individuals appears to be elevated. In addition, a longitudinal study has demonstrated that among COPD patients, the PI MZ heterozygotes have a more rapid decline in lung function. These data suggest that either all PI MZ individuals are at slightly increased risk for the development of COPD, or that a subset of the PI MZ subjects are at substantially increased risk of pulmonary damage if they smoke.

Other 'serpinopathies'

α_1-Antitrypsin is the archetypal member of a superfamily of proteins termed the serine protease inhibitors, or serpins, that have closely related structures and functions. These inhibitors control various inflammatory cascades, including coagulation (antithrombin), complement activation (C1-inhibitor), and fibrinolysis (α_2-antiplasmin). Pathological processes that underlie the deficiency of one member may account for deficiency of others. Indeed the process of polymer formation has also been reported in deficiency-mutants of antithrombin, C1-inhibitor, α_1-antichymotrypsin, and heparin co-factor II. These polymers are inactive as proteinase inhibitors and so predispose the individual to thrombosis (antithrombin) and angio-oedema (C1-inhibitor). The plasma deficiency that results from the polymerization of mutants of α_1-antichymotrypsin has been associated with COPD in some (but not all) association studies, but the plasma deficiency of heparin cofactor II has yet to be associated with a clinical phenotype. Perhaps the most striking serpinopathy results from the polymerization of mutants of a neuron-specific serpin, neuroserpin, to cause the novel inclusion-body dementia known as familial encephalopathy with neuroserpin inclusion bodies (FENIB; OMIM 604218). This is inherited as an autosomal dominant trait with the inclusions of neuroserpin in the brain being PAS-positive and diastase-resistant, identical to those of Z α_1-antitrypsin in the liver. The five mutations that have been described show a striking inverse correlation between the rate that the protein forms polymers and the age of onset/severity of the dementia.

New and emerging treatments

Other treatments at earlier stages of development include gene therapy, the administration of retinoic acid and chemical chaperones. Vectors carrying the α_1-antitrypsin gene have been targeted to liver, lung, and muscle in animals. There is good expression of α_1-antitrypsin but further data is required to assess whether this can be achieved in humans. In particular it is important to determine the length of time of protein expression and whether the levels of α_1-antitrypsin in the epithelial lining fluid of the lung are sufficient to prevent ongoing proteolytic damage. Chemical chaperones are effective in stabilizing Z α_1-antitrypsin *in vitro* and increasing secretion from cell lines and in mouse models of disease, but have not been effective *in vivo*. Similarly, although the effects of retinoic acid on alveolar regeneration in the rat look promising they have yet to be demonstrated in patients with emphysema. Perhaps more promising is the exploitation of our understanding of the pathogenesis of α_1-antitrypsin deficiency to develop small molecules to block polymerization and so treat the associated liver and lung disease.

Further reading

Davis RL, *et al.* (2002). Association between conformational mutations in neuroserpin and onset and severity of dementia. *Lancet*, **359**, 2242–7. [Description of families with mutations in the serpin, neuroserpin, that form polymers *in vivo* and an inclusion-body dementia.]

Eriksson S, Carlson J, Velez R (1986). Risk of cirrhosis and primary liver cancer in alpha$_1$-antitrypsin deficiency. *N Engl J Med*, **314**, 736–9. [Post-mortem study demonstrating a high prevalence of liver disease in adults with PiZ α_1-antitrypsin deficiency.]

Laurell C-B, Eriksson S (1963). The electrophoretic α_1-globulin pattern of serum in α_1-antitrypsin deficiency. *Scand J Clin Lab Invest*, **15**: 132–40. [The first report of α_1-antitrypsin deficiency in five individuals of whom three had emphysema and one had a family history of emphysema.]

Gooptu, B., Lomas, D.A. (2009). Conformational pathology of the serpins - themes, variations and therapeutic strategies. *Ann. Rev. Biochem*, **78**, 147–176.]

Lomas DA (2006). The selective advantage of α_1-antitrypsin deficiency. *Am J Resp Crit Care Med*, **173**, 1072–7. [Discussion of the reason for the high prevalence of the Z allele of α_1-antitrypsin in the white population.]

Mahadeva R, *et al.* (2005). Polymers of Z α_1-antitrypsin co-localise with neutrophils in emphysematous alveoli and are chemotactic *in vivo*. *Am J Pathol*, **166**, 377–86. [Demonstration that polymers co-localise with neutrophils in lungs from individuals with α_1-antitrypsin deficiency and that they are chemotactic when instilled into the lungs of mice.]

Owen MC, *et al.* (1983). Mutation of antitrypsin to antithrombin. α_1-antitrypsin Pittsburgh (358 Met to Arg), a fatal bleeding disorder. *N Engl J Med*, **309**, 694–8 [Description of a point mutation in α_1-antitrypsin that converted it to an inhibitor of thrombin and so caused an episodic bleeding disorder in a 14 year-old-boy.]

Piitulainen E, Eriksson S (1999). Decline in FEV$_1$ related to smoking status in individuals with severe alpha$_1$-antitrypsin deficiency. *Eur Resp J*, **13**, 247–51. [Report of rate of decline in lung function of 608 patients followed for 1–31 years. Current smokers have an accelerated rate of decline in lung function but ex-smokers have the same rate as non-smokers. The values are likely to be more representative than other reports as many subjects were ascertained from screening and family studies.]

Piitulainen E, *et al.* (2005). Alpha$_1$-antitrypsin deficiency in 26-year-old subjects: lung, liver, and protease/protease inhibitor studies. *Chest*, **128**, 2076–81. [Report on the follow up of individuals with α_1-antitrypsin deficiency from birth to 26 years. This is the only long-term prospective study of patients with α_1-antitrypsin deficiency and therefore the only study that is free from selection bias.]

Stoller JK, Aboussouan LS (2005). Alpha-1-antitrypsin deficiency. *Lancet*, *365*, 2225–36 [A review of the pathophysiology, clinical features and management of α_1-antitrypsin deficiency.]

Sveger T (1976). Liver disease in alpha$_1$-antitrypsin deficiency detected by screening of 200,000 infants. *N Engl J Med*, **294**, 1316–21. [Prospective study of liver disease in 120 Pi Z, 48 Pi SZ, two PI Z-and one Pi S-infants in the first 6 months of life.]

Index

Note: Numbers in italic refer to tables and/or illustrations separate from the text.

Species names for animals, plants, fungi and insects are listed by their Latin names, followed by their common name where appropriate.

abacavir
  HIV/AIDS 636, *638*
  mode of action *444*
abatacept, rheumatoid arthritis 3598, *3599*, 3600
abdomen, infections, anaerobic 751
abdominal actinomycoses 853
abdominal aortic aneurysm 2963
  definition 2963
  detection before rupture 2964, *2964*
  epidemiology 2963
  management
    endovascular repair 2965
    medical 2965
    surgery 2965
  rupture 2964, *3120*
abdominal migraine 2207
abdominal pain 2207
  acute abdomen 2207
  functional 2387
  lower abdomen 2207
  management 2387
  upper abdomen 2207
abetalipoproteinaemia
  differential diagnosis *1725*
  haematological changes 4559
Abiotrophia spp. *962*
ABO system 4562, *4563*
  compatibility *290*
  incompatibility 4458
abscess
  cerebral *4780*, 4780
  diverticular 2392
  epidural 700, *702*
  filarial 1156
  intracranial 5013
  liver, pyogenic 2543, *2543*
  postinjection 833
  spleen 4338
absolute effect size 51
absolute risk reduction 51, *51*
absorption enhancers 4732
absorption 1455, 2326
  drug interactions 1470
  mechanisms of 2327
  rate of 1455
    coadministered drugs 1456
    first-pass metabolism 1456
    food 1456
    gastrointestinal motility 1455
    malabsorption 1456
  sites of 2327
absorptive capacity 2326
acaeruloplasminaemia *1674*
  with iron deposition 1686
Acanthamoeba 1036, *1042, 1043*
  amoebic keratitis 1043
acanthocytes *4195*
acanthocytosis 4452, 4468
  with neurological disease and normal lipoproteins 4560
Acanthoparyphium tyosenense 1220
Acanthophis spp. (death adder) 1329
  antivenom *1340*
acanthosis nigricans 4719, *385, 4719*
  insulin resistance 1996
acatalasia *1552*
accidents
  drowning *see* drowning
  work-related 1389, *1389*
acclimatization
  heat 1394
  high altitude 1402
    blood 1403
    circulation 1403
    extreme altitudes 1404
    fluid balance 1403
    ventilation 1403
accountability 60
ACE inhibitors 2624
  adverse effects, in pregnancy *2188*
  ascites 2489
  in breast milk *2101*
  dilated cardiomyopathy 2776
  drug interactions *3968*
  effects on renin-angiotensin-aldosterone system 3843
  focal segmental glomerulosclerosis 3984
  heart failure 2722, *2722*
  hypertension 2042, *3050*, 3052
  hypertensive emergencies *3079*
  poisoning 1280
  systemic sclerosis 3675
  teratogenicity *1468*
  transposition of great arteries 2863
  vibration injury 1435
acebutalol, in breast milk *1469*
acetaldehyde 2475
acetaminophen *see* paracetamol
acetazolamide
  adverse effects, renal toxicity *3860*
  epilepsy 4821
  mountain sickness 1404
  vertigo *4861*
acetohexamide, hepatotoxicity *2529, 2532*
acetone poisoning 1306
acetylation, genetic variability 1473
acetylcholinesterase
  endplate deficiency 5183
  in sarcoidosis 3409
achalasia 2294, *2295*
Achilles tendinitis *3248*
Achilles tendinopathy *5382*
achlorhydria 2247, 2320
achondrogenesis *3721*
  mutations in *3757*
achondroplasia *3721*, 3758
achondroplasia-like dwarfism 3758
Achromobacter spp. *962*
aciclovir
  adverse effects *455*
  gingivostomatitis 2263
  herpes labialis 2264
  herpes zoster 493
  HSV 487
  mode of action *444*
  pregnancy *2172*
  prophylactic *440*
  in renal failure *4185*
  renal toxicity *3860*
  resistance 488
  varicella zoster 492
α_1-acid glycoprotein *1753*
acid lipase deficiency *1553*
acid maltase deficiency 5215
  see also Pompe's disease
Acidaminococcus spp. *962*
acid-base disorders
  causes 1741, *1742–4*
  clinical aspects 1738
  CNS complications 5155
  definitions 1740
  diagnosis 1740
    anion gap 1741
    pHa and $Paco_2$ *1740, 1741*
  effects of 1742
    blood oxygen uptake/delivery 1744
    bone 1745
    cardiovascular 1743
    distribution of metabolites and drugs 1745
    endocrine 1744
    inflammatory cytokines 1745
    intermediary carbohydrate metabolism 1744
    kidney 1745
    leucocytes 1745
    nervous system 1745
    nitrogen balance 1744
    potassium homeostasis 1745
    respiratory 1742
  lactic acidosis *see* lactic acidosis
  treatment 1748
acid-base homeostasis 1739, *1739–40, 3189, 3197, 3197–8*
  CKD 3908
  disturbances of *see* acid-base disorders
  hepatocellular failure 2497
    management 2503
  physiology/terminology 1738
  poisoned patients 1277, *3197*
  potassium homeostasis *3833*
  renal regulation of 3813
  role of kidneys and liver 1740
  strong ion approach 3198
acidosis
  CKD 3916
  and hyperkalaemia 3844
  metabolic *3198*
    acute renal trauma 3890
  respiratory 3197, *3198*
Acidovorax (Pseudomonas) spp. *962*
acids
  carcinogenesis *1380*
  poisoning 1306
Acinetobacter iwoffii 3436
Acinetobacter spp. *962*
acne arthralgia 3706
acne 4678, *4679–80*
  conglobata 4682
  cosmetic 4681
  drug-induced 4681
  dysmorphophobia 4681
  excorié 4681
  fulminans 4682
  Gram-negative folliculitis 4681
  infantile 4681
  occupational 1382
  in pregnancy 2149
  pyoderma faciale 4682
  SAPHO syndrome 4682
aconite 68

aconitine 1363, 1370
Aconitum napellus (monkshood/aconite) *1363*
acoustic neuroma 366
ACP Journal Club 23
acrivastine 3282
acrocyanosis 4687
acrodermatitis chronica atrophicans 863
acrogeria *3776*
acromegaly 1806
  amenorrhoea 1907
  clinical features 1807, *1807*
    myopathy 5217
  diagnosis 1807
  pregnancy 2140
  treatment 1807
acromesomelic chondrodysplasia, mutations in *3757*
acrylamide
  CNS effects *1386*
  peripheral nervous system effects *1387*, 5087
ACST-1 trial 36
ACTH stimulation test 1883
ACTH 1800, 1812
  Cushing's disease 1813
  deficiency 1882, 1812
  ectopic ACTH syndrome 3522
  ectopic secretion 1872, *1872, 2062, 2063*
    treatment 1880
  measurement 1803
  morning plasma 1875, *1875*
  Nelson's syndrome 1813
  reference values *5441*
actin 131, 179
actinic prurigo 4669, *4669*
Actinobacillus actinomycetemcomitans 2260
Actinobacillus spp. *962*
Actinobaculum spp. *962*
actinolite 3498
Actinomadura spp. *962*
Actinomyces actinomycetemcomitans 859
Actinomyces georgiae 851
Actinomyces gerencseriae 850–1
Actinomyces israelii 850–1, 1042
Actinomyces meyeri 851
Actinomyces naeslundi 851
Actinomyces neuii 851
Actinomyces odontolyticus 851
Actinomyces spp. *962*
  osteomyelitis *3789*
Actinomyces viscosus 851, 2257, 2260
Actinomycetes spp., diseases caused by 855
actinomycin D, hepatotoxicity *2536*
actinomycoses 850
  aetiology 851
  clinical features 852
    abdominal actinomycoses 853
    actinomycotic endocarditis 854
    bone infections 854
    central nervous system infections 853
    cervicofacial actinomycoses 852, *852–3*
    cutaneous actinomycoses 854
    thoracic actinomycoses 853, *853*
  definition 850
  diagnosis 854
    laboratory 854
    radiography 854
  epidemiology 855
  pathogenesis and pathology 851
    histopathology 851, *852*
    synergistic polymicrobial infection 851, *852*
  prognosis 855
  treatment 854
action potentials 161
  cardiac 2603, 2610
activated partial thromboplastin time 4502
activated protein C 416
  recombinant human 417
activator protein-1, 154
activin 1795
activities of daily living 5406
Actractaspididae 1327
acupressure 67
acupuncture 65, 67
  description 67
  efficacy 67
  mode of action 67
  safety 67
acute abdomen 2232, 2207
  assessment 2232
  causes *2233*, 2234
    acute appendicitis 2234
    diverticulitis 2235
    intestinal obstruction 2234
    perforated viscus 2234
  examination 2233
  history 2233, *2233*
  investigations 2234, *2235*
  management, principles of 2232
  medical causes 2236
  medical ward 2235
    acute pseudo-obstruction (adynamic ileus) 2235
    chronic liver disease 2236
    iatrogenic 2236
    immunosuppressed patients 2236
    older patients 2236
    peritoneal dialysis 2236
  pain 2233
  presentation 5474
acute coronary syndromes 2630, *2879, 2880, 2914*
  clinical presentation and definition 2913, *2914*
  ECG 2643, 2653
    role of 2653
    triage 2653
  management 2911
  non-ST-elevation
    coronary artery bypass surgery 2924
    integrated approach 2922, *2923–4*
    management 2917
    risk stratification 2922
  outcome 2914, *2915*
  plaque erosion 2879
  plaque rupture 2880
  presentation 5458
  risk characterization 2916, *2916*
  vulnerable plaque 2880, *2881*
  see also angina; myocardial infarction
acute erythroid leukaemias 4226
acute fatty liver of pregnancy 2105, 2127
  clinical features *2130*
  differential diagnosis *2131*
  laboratory variables *2130*
acute interstitial nephritis 3901, 4002
  aetiology 4002, *4003*
    drugs 4002
    immune-mediated disease 4004
    infections 4002
  clinical features 4005
  clinical investigation 4005
  differential diagnosis 4005
  epidemiology 4005
  historical perspective 4002
  pathogenesis 4004
  pathology 4004, *4005*
  prognosis 4006
  treatment 4006
acute interstitial pneumonia 3369, *3369*
acute lung injury *see* acute respiratory distress syndrome
acute lymphoblastic leukaemia 4215, 4229
  B-lineage 4215
    Bcr-abl 4215
    E2A fusion genes 4216
    MLL fusion genes 4216
    MYC 4217
    Tel-aml 1, 4216
  management 4230
    leukaemogenesis and novel therapies 4231
    sensitivity/resistance to chemotherapy 4232
  presentation and diagnosis 4229
  prognostic factors 4230
  T-lineage 4217
    activation of tyrosine kinases, RAS and PI3K signalling 4218
    dysregulated expression of oncogenic transcription factors 4217
    NOTCH1 mutations 4217
  therapeutic targets 4232
acute lymphocytic leukaemia, translocations *341*
acute lymphoid leukaemia 4213
acute megakaryoblastic leukaemia 4226
acute monoblastic leukaemia 4226
acute monocytic leukaemia 4226
acute myeloblastic leukaemia
  with maturation 4226
  minimally differentiated 4226
  without maturation 4226
acute myeloid leukaemia 4218, 4233, 4224
  activation of tyrosine kinase and RAS signalling pathways 4219
  AML1-ETO 4218
  CBFβ-MYH11, 4219
  children 4212
  diagnosis 4234
  epidemiology and causation 4234, *4234*
  infection 4238
  molecular biology
    MLL fusion genes 4219
    NPM mutations 4219
    PML-RARα fusion 4218
  with multilineage dysplasia 4226
  not otherwise categorized *4223, 4225, 4226*
  prognostic factors 4234, *4234*
  recurrent genetic abnormalities 4225
  supportive care 4237
    blood products 4238
    chemotherapy-induced pancytopenia 4238
    initiation of therapy 4237
  therapy-related 4226
    alkylating agents 4350
    topoisomerase II inhibitors 4226
  translocations *341*
  treatment 4234, *4235*
    bone marrow transplantation 4237
    chemotherapy 4235
    definition of remmission 4235
    maintenance therapy 4236
    older patients 4236
    outcomes 4235
    relapse 4236
    targeted 4236
acute myelomonocytic leukaemia 4226
acute phase proteins *1753*
  rheumatic fever 2801
acute phase response 1752
acute promyelocytic leukaemia 4239
  complications 4239
  supportive care 4239
  treatment 4239
acute respiratory distress syndrome (ARDS) 3132, 3141
  causes *3141*
  definition 3141, *3141*
  epidemiology 3142
  incidence 3142
  investigations 3142, *3143*
  management 3143, *3143*
    fluids 3144
    lung protection 3144
    mechanical ventilation 3144
    nonventilatory adjuncts 3145
    nutrition 3143
  morbidity and mortality 3142
  pathophysiology 3142
acylcarnitine, analysis 1563
adalimumab 158
  pregnancy *2158*
  psoriasis 4615
  rheumatoid arthritis 3598, *3599*
ADAMS proteinases 3552
Adams-Oliver syndrome 2595
ADAMTS proteinases 3548
ADAMTS13, 2178
  deficiency *see* thrombotic thrombocytopenic purpura
adapalene, acne *4680*
adaptation 13, 1464
  and adverse drug reactions 1464
adaptive immunity 224, 152
  alcoholic liver disease 2476
  antigen specificity 225
    antigen recognition by T cells 225, *226*
  diversity 227
    B-cell receptors and antibody 228
    immunoglobulins *228*
    MHC molecules 229
    T-cell receptors 227, *228*
  down-regulation of immune response 232

T-cell tolerance 232
future developments 234
immunological memory 229
generation and maintenance of memory 232
naive state 229, *229*
priming of immune response 230, *230*
T-cell effector functions 230
uses of 233
diagnostics 233
prophylaxis 233
therapy 233
Addenbrooke's Sedation Score *3155*
Addison's disease *1871*, 1880, *1881*
aetiology 1880, *1881*
clinical features
hypercalcaemia *3745*
myopathy 5217
pregnancy 2143
Addisonian crisis 5481
adenine phosphoribosyl transferase deficiency *4101*
adenine 138
adenocarcinoma
and DIC *4543*, 4543
oesophagus *2299*, 2301
small intestine 2222, *2222*, 2338
adenoidal facies 3171
adenomyeloneuropathy 1720
adenosine deaminase deficiency 1632
treatment 1632
adenosine triphosphate (ATP) 129
adenosine, cardiac arrhythmias 2700, *2701*
adenosyl-homocysteinase/ S-adenosyl-homocysteine hydrolase deficiency *1566*
adenoviruses *474*, 477
enteric 538
adenylosuccinase deficiency 1631
adhesive capsulitis *3248*
adiponectin 1790, 2135
adipose tissue lipase 1653
aditory input 4788
ADMA *2598*
adolescents
contraception 1263
growth *1954*
suicide attempts 5295
adrenal cortex
development *1788*
disorders of 1869, *1871*
Cushing's syndrome 1869, 1871, *384*, *1871*
glucocorticoid deficiency 1870, *1871*, 1880
mineralocorticoid deficiency 1870, *1871*, *1889*
mineralocorticoid excess 1870, *1871*, 1884
drug-induced 2068
steroid biosynthesis *1871*
adrenal gland
disorders of 1869, 2066
adrenal cortex 1869
congenital adrenal hyperplasia 1891
haematological changes 4559
in pregnancy 2143
steroidogenesis *1892*
adrenal hyperplasia, congenital *1871*, 1891
clinical presentation 1891, *1893*
genetics 1894, *1894*
21-hydroxylase deficiency 1891
17α-hydroxylase deficiency 1898
11β-hydroxylase deficiency 1899
3β-hydroxysteroid dehydrogenase deficiency 1898
lipoid adrenal hyperplasia 1898
longer-term outcome 1896, *1896*
adult stature and medical management 1896
reproductive function 1897
management in infancy and childhood 1892
medical 1892
surgical 1893, *1894*
neonatal screening 1896
P450 oxidoreductase deficiency 1899
pregnancy 2143
prenatal diagnosis/ treatment 1895, *1895*
sexual development disorders 1969
adrenal hypoplasia, congenital *1871*
adrenal insufficiency 1889
CNS complications 5153
drug-induced 2068
adrenal tumours
adenoma 1872
carcinoma 1872
prognosis 1878
incidentalomas 1890
adrenalectomy 1878
adrenaline 3129
anaphylaxis 3111
intramuscular 3112
intravenous 3112
metabolic effects *1481*
peptic ulcer disease 2312
reference values *5441*
self-injectable 3113
adrenergic receptors 3129
adrenocorticotrophic hormone *see* ACTH
adrenoleucodystrophy *1552*, 4961, 5104
pseudo-neonatal *1552*
X-linked *1552*, 1881
adrenoleukodystrophy protein 1721
adrenomyeloneuropathy 1720
adriamycin, adverse effects *400*
Adson's manoeuvre 3558
adult T-cell leukaemia/ lymphoma 651, 4333
advance directives 19
advanced glycation endproducts 2033
advanced life support 3097, *3099*, *3100*
nonshockable rhythms 3100, *3102*
reversible causes of arrest 3101
shockable rhythms 3099, *3101*
Advenella spp. *962*
adventitia 4484
adverse drug reactions 1449, 1464
allergic 1465–6
classification 1465, 4724
dose-related 1465
cutaneous 4724
causality 4729, *4729*
clinical patterns 4725
maculopapular eruption/toxic erythema 4726
type I 4726, *4727*
type II 4726, *4727*
type III 4726
type IV 4726
delayed effects causing 1467
drugs in breast milk 1468, *1469*, *2188*, *2189*
due to adaptation 1464
incidence 1464
long-term effects causing 1467
adaptive changes 1467
rebound phenomena 1467
pharmacovigilance 46, 1469
prevention 1469
reproductive effects 1467
teratogenesis *see* teratogenesis
type B 4724, *4725*
see also individual drugs
adynamic ileus 2235
Aedes aegypti 575
Aedes scutellaris 559
Aedes spp. *1226*
Aedes vigilax 559
Aerococcus spp. *962*
Aeromonas hydrophila 734, 807, 1326
Aeromonas spp. *962*
aerosol toxicity 3456
acute pneumonitis 3457
acute tracheobronchitis 3457
acute upper airway 3456
treatment 3457
aerospace medicine 1408
clinical aspects 1414
infectious disease spread 1415
jet lag 1414, *1414*
newly emerging infectious disease 1415
passenger fitness to fly 1415
traveller's thrombosis 1414
physics of flight environment 1409, *1409*
atmospheric pressure 1409, *1410*
atmospheric temperature 1409
atmospheric zone 1409
cosmic radiation 1410
physiology of flight 1410
altitude-induced decompression illness 1413, *1413*
hypoxia 1410, *1411–12*
mechanical effects of pressure change 1413, *1413*
oxygen equipment and pressure cabins 1412, *1413*
Afipia spp. *962*
aflatoxin 309, *338*, 1014
Africa
corruption in 116, *116*
demographic entrapment 82
scale of 117
types of 116
disentrapment 116, *118*
population policy 118
African tick-bite fever *912*
afterload 2622, *2623*
and ventricular volume 2624
agammaglobulinaemia
autosomal recessive *238*
X-linked *238*, 244
Agamomermis spp. *1176*
age
acute pancreatitis mortality 2562
and cancer susceptibility 303
maternal, in pregnancy 2086
and osteoarthritis 3630
ageing 13
haematological changes 4560
hypogonadism 1920
age-related macular degeneration 5252
aggrecan 3548
Aggregatibacter (Actinobacillus) actinomycetemcomitans 852
agitation, management 3156
agraphia 4790
Agrobacterium spp. *962*
Ahlback's disease *3804*
Aicardi-Goutières syndrome 5111
air pollution
indoor 3314
outdoor 3314
air travel 466
DVT prevention *3008*
heart failure 2721
see also jet lag; travel medicine
air-crescent sign *3213*
airflow limitation 3470, *3471*
airway hyper-responsiveness 3285, *3285–6*
COPD 3315
tests of 3292
exercise testing 3292
inhaled histamine/ methacholine 3293
airway inflammation 3286
airway remodelling 3285
airway resistance 3190
airway 3173, 3100
acute respiratory failure 3136, *3136–7*
anaphylaxis 3111
clearance 3360
critical illness 3116, *3116*
design 3173, *3174*
dynamic compression 3177, *3177*
management 5516
poisoned patients 1276
protection of 3172
smooth muscle 3178
see also individual parts
airways disease 2635, *3183*
COPD *3319–20*
HIV-related 3252
small airways 3321, *3321–2*
upper airways, cystic fibrosis 3361
see also asthma; chronic obstructive pulmonary disease
airways obstruction 3254
causes *3255*, 3256
aspiration 3256, *3257*
infections 3258, *3258*
laryngeal dysfunction 3260
oedema 3257
tracheal abnormalities 3259
tracheal compression 3259, *3259*
tracheal stenosis 3259, *3259*
tumours 3258, *3259*
definition 3254
diagnosis 3254
differential diagnosis 3296
examination 3255
history 3254
lung function tests 3255, *3255–6*
ajmaline, adverse effects, hepatotoxicity *2529*, *2532–3*
Al Khumra haemorrhagic fever virus *566*, 574

Alagille's syndrome 2538, 2580
pulmonary valve stenosis 2848
renal involvement 4102
alanine transaminase, reference values *5436*
albendazole
ascariasis 1170
cystic hydatid disease 1187
cysticercosis 1198
filariasis 1158
giardiasis *1113*
gnathostomiasis 1184
hookworm 1166
intestinal flukes 1221
isosporiasis 1115
strongyloidiasis 1164
trichuriasis 1176
Albers-Schönberg disease *see* osteopetrosis
albinism
oculocutaneous
type I 4663
type II 4663
partial, immunodeficiency with *238*
Albright's hereditary osteodystrophy *1530*, 1798
albumin *1753*
intravenous infusion 2489
microalbuminuria 3867
pregnancy *2126*
reference values *5435, 5444*, 5447
urinary excretion *3867*
Albustix 3865
Alcaligenes spp. *962*
alclometasone dipropionate 4731
alcohol abuse 5271
brief interventions 5352
extended 5355
identification of drinkers 5353, *5354*
implementation 5355
simple 5353
definitions 5351
binge drinking 5352
hazardous/harmful drinking 5351
history 5260, *5261*
oesophageal symptoms *2297*
possible dependence 5355
prevalence 5352
suicide attempts 5295
see also alcohol dependence
alcohol consumption, heart failure 2720
alcohol dehydrogenase, mutations 13
alcohol dependence 5341
aetiology 5343
diagnosis 5342, *5342*
epidemiology 5342
pathology 5343
cancer 5344
cardiovascular 5343
endocrinological 5344, *5345*
gastrointestinal 5343
injury 5344
liver 5343, *5344*
neurological 5344
pulmonary 5344
pregnancy complications 5346
treatment 5346
alcohol withdrawal 5346, *5347*, 5503
pharmacotherapy 5348
alcohol
and acute pancreatitis 2558
and blood pressure 1519
and cancer 305
CNS effects 5155
and coronary heart disease 2891
drowning accidents 1398
haematological effects 4557
and hypertension 3030, 3048
and hypoglycaemia 2056
intoxidation 5369
and peptic ulcer disease 2308
in pregnancy 2090
fetal alcohol syndrome *1468*, 2090, 5146
reference values *5435*
teratogenicity *1468*, 2090
alcohol-associated pseudo-Cushing's syndrome 1872
alcoholic hepatitis
clinical features 2477
treatment 2478
corticosteroids 2478
alcoholic ketoacidosis *1742*
alcoholic liver disease 2474
clinical features 2477
alcoholic fatty liver 2477
alcoholic hepatitis 2477
cirrhosis 2477
diagnosis 2477
epidemiology 2476
hormonal abnormalities *2066*
pathogenesis 2475
adaptive immune system 2476
ethanol metabolism *2475–6, 2210*
innate immune system 2476
recurrence post-transplantation 2512
susceptibility 2476
treatment 2478
abstinence 2478, *2478*
alcoholic cirrhosis 2479
alcoholic hepatitis 2478
transplantation 2479, 2507
alcoholic myopathy 5156, 5218
alcoholic neuropathy 5089, 5156
aldolase deficiency 4472
aldosterone antagonists, heart failure 2723
aldosterone 1870
action of *1791, 3815*
biosynthesis defects 1889
in Conn's syndrome 3063
ectopic secretion 2065
potassium excretion *3833*
potassium homeostasis *3833*
reference values *5441*, 5447
signalling pathways *1797*
aldosteronism *1871*
glucocorticoid-remediable 3071, *3073*
glucocorticoid-suppressible 1887, *1887*
primary *see* Conn's syndrome
alefacept, psoriasis 4615
alemtuzumab 292, *294, 376*
post-transplantation *3954*
alendronate
adverse effects, oesophagitis *2294*
hyperparathyroidism 1859
osteoporosis *3799*
Paget's disease 3744
Alenquer virus *581*
Alexander technique *66*
Alexander's disease 5105
alexia 4790
alfentanil 3155, *3155*
Alfuy virus *566*
algid malaria 1064
treatment 1080
alginates, in renal failure 4176
alglucosidase alfa 1715
Alishewanella spp. *962*
Alistipes spp. *962*
alkali poisoning 1307
alkaline phosphatase 3727, *3729*
CKD-MBD *3922*
pregnancy *2126*
reference values *5436*
children *5438*
alkalosis
metabolic *3198*
respiratory 3197, *3198*
alkaptonuria 1586, *1566*, 3720, *3721*, 3754
clinical features *3731, 3755*
diagnosis 1587
treatment and outcome 1587
alkylating agents 398
carcinogenesis *338*
resistance *399*
alleles, segregation 136
allelic affinity 138
allelic heterogeneity 138
allergen immunotherapy 265, 3282
asthma 3299
allergens 260
drugs 263
food 262, *263*
hymenoptera venom 263
latex 264
allergic bronchopulmonary aspergillosis 3295, 3346
allergic bronchopulmonary mycosis 3430, *3430*
allergic rhinitis 261, 3277
aetiology 3278
clinical diagnosis 3279, *3280*
environmental factors 3278
occupational rhinitis 3278
perennial allergic rhinitis 3278
seasonal allergic rhinitis 3278, *3278*
epidemiology 3278
examination 3280
genetic influences 3278
historical perspective 3277
history 3279, *3280*
investigations 3280
skin prick tests 3280, *3281*
pathogenesis 3279, *3279*
treatment 3281, *3281*
allergen avoidance 3281
allergen immunotherapy 3282
pharmacotherapy 3281
allergy 258, 15
aetiology 258–9
see also allergens
and asthma 3286
clinical features 261
allergic rhinitis 261
angio-oedema 219, 262
asthma 261
conjunctivitis 261
eczema 261
nonallergic rhinitis 261
urticaria 261
development 259, *259*
diagnosis 265
differential diagnosis 264
food *see* food allergy
health economics 265
historical aspects 259
investigations 264
challenge tests 264
intradermal tests 264
specific IgE 264
tryptase 264
non-IgE mediated reactions 259
pathogenesis 258–9
prevalence 259
atopy 259
clinical 259
sensitization as predictor 259
prevention 258, 261
treatment 258, 265, *265*
allergen avoidance 265
anti-IgE 265
immunotherapy 265
pharmacotherapy 265
type I (allergic) hypersensitivity reactions 233, 259, *259*
uncertainties 266
see also anaphylaxis
Alligator mississippiensis 1325
Alligator mississippiensis 1325
alligators 1325
allodynia 5412
allografts *281*
rejection 280–1, *282*
Alloiococcus spp. *962*
allopurinol
adverse effects 1624–5
hepatotoxicity *2529, 2532, 2535*
renal toxicity *3860*
calcium stone prevention *4130*
drug interactions *3968*
gout 1624, 3643
Lesch-Nyhan syndrome 1629
allorecognition 283
costimulation 283
direct 283, *285*
indirect 283, *285*
pathways of 283
T-cells in 283
almitrine bismethylate, chronic respiratory failure 3474
almotriptan, migraine *4917–18*
aloe vera 4736
aloe, drug interactions *69*
alopecia areata 4702, *4703*
alopecia, scarring 4703
Alpers' syndrome 5103
Alpers-Huttenlocher syndrome *5223*
α-blockers
hypertension 3052
hypertensive emergencies *3079*
in renal failure 4179
α-fetoprotein, neural tube defects 5136
alphaviruses 557, *558*
arthritis and rash 557
neuroinvasive disease 560
see also individual viruses
Alphitobius diaperinus 1236
Alport's syndrome 4098
antiglomerular basement membrane disease in 3999
genetic counselling and treatment 4099

pathogenesis 4098
symptoms 4098
Alström's syndrome *1530*, 1664
Alternaria spp. *3436*
alternobaric vertigo 1419
altitude-induced decompression illness 1413, *1413*
altitude-related illness 2171
acclimatization 1402
blood 1403
circulation 1403
extreme altitudes 1404
fluid balance 1403
ventilation 1403
cerebral oedema 1402, 1405
cough 1407
high-altitude environment 1402, *1402–3*
hypobaric hypoxia 1403
mountain sickness
acute 1402, 1404, *1404*
chronic (Monge's disease) 1402, 1408
peripheral oedema 1407
pre-existing medical conditions 1407
pulmonary hypertension 1408
pulmonary oedema 1402, *1405*, *1405–6*
retinal haemorrhage 1407, *1407*
aluminium phosphide poisoning 1301
aluminium
and cancer *1380*
CKD-MBD *3922*
poisoning 1296
antidote *1274*
hypercalcaemia *3745*
skeletal effects 3768
reference values *5445*
alveolar haemorrhage 3396, *3397*
autoimmune rheumatic disorders *3390*
SLE 3392
alveolar hypoventilation 4267
alveolar interdependence 3179
alveolar rhabdomyosarcoma, translocations *341*
alveolar ventilation *3469*
improving 3474
alveoli 3173
design 3173, *3174*
drug reactions 3463, *3463*
capillary leakage 3463
inflammation/fibrosis 3464, *3464–5*
pulmonary eosinophilia 3465
alveolitis, extrinsic allergic 3296
Alzheimer's disease 187, 1770, 4798, 5100
clinical features 4800
definition 4798, *4799*
epidemiology and risk factors 4798
genetics 148, *143*
investigations 4800, *4800*, *4801*
management and prognosis 4802
pathology 4799, *4799*
pathophysiology 4800, *4800*
Amanita muscaria (fly agaric) *1366–7*
Amanita pantherina (panther cap) *1368*
Amanita phalloides (death cap) *1368*
Amanita virosa (destroying angel) *1369*
amantadine
influenza virus 480
mode of action *444*
Parkinson's disease 4886
amatoxins *1367*, 1368, *1369*
amaurosis fugax 5239
Amblyomma americanum 915
Amblyomma cajennense 904, *1228*
Amblyomma hebraeum 904, *1228*
amblyopia, tobacco-alcohol 5157
AMD *1939*, 3100
amegakaryocytic thrombocytopenic purpura 4515
amenorrhoea 1901, 1905, *1905*
idiopathic hypothalamic 1907, *1907*
weight-loss related 1906
see also female athlete triad
amephetamines, poisoning 1280
amikacin
mycobacterial disease 835
nocardiosis 857
Pseudomonas aeruginosa 737
in renal failure *4185*
serum levels *5449*
spectrum of activity *446*
amiloride
ascites 2487
heart failure *2722*
amilsulpride 5266
amineptine, adverse effects, hepatotoxicity *2534*
amino acidaemias 5109
amino acids
analysis 1563, *1563*
daily intake *1480*
metabolism 1485, *1486*, 2442
regulation of gene expression *1482*
renal tubular reabsorption 3872
stores *1480*
amino aciduria 4140, 4146, *4148*
see also individual conditions
4-aminobiphenyl *1380*
aminoglutethimide
adverse effects, hepatotoxicity *2532*, *2533*
Cushing's syndrome 1880
ectopic ACTH secretion 2064
reproductive effects *1917*
aminoglycosides
adverse effects *455*
drug interactions *3968*
mode of action *443*
nephrotoxicity *3860*, 3897
pregnancy *2172*
5-aminolaevulinate 1640
aminolaevulinate dehydratase deficiency 1640, 1643–4
aminophylline
COPD 3334
see also theophylline
4-aminopyrine, vertigo *4861*
aminorex, thromboembolism 3465
5-aminosalicylates
Crohn's disease 2366
ulcerative colitis 2378
5-aminosalicylic acid nephritis 4011, *4008*, *4012*
clinical features 4011, *4012*
diagnosis and treatment 4012
pathogenesis and pathology 4011
aminosidine, leishmaniasis *1138*
amiodaquine, adverse effects, hepatotoxicity *2529*
amiodarone *2701*
adverse effects, hepatotoxicity *2535*
in breast milk *2189*
drug interactions *1471*
heart failure 2724
induction of thyrotoxicosis 1843, 2067
in renal failure *4179*
thyroiditis 1843
2-amionadipic aciduria *1566*
amisulpiride *5337*
schizophrenia *5325*
amitriptyline
adverse effects *5313*
hepatotoxicity *2529*, *2532–3*
diabetic neuropathy 2039
migraine prevention *4916*
serum levels *5449*
amlodipine
hypertensive emergencies *3079*
Raynaud's phenomenon *3671*
ammonia
metabolism 2442
poisoning 1307
reference values *5435*
children *5438*
amniotic fluid embolism 2122
amodiaquine 1075
amoebae, free-living 1036, 1042
amoebiasis 1035–6, *1385*
clinical features 1037
cutaneous and genital amoebiasis 1040
hepatic amoebiasis 1038, *1039–40*
invasive intestinal amoebiasis 1037
epidemiology 1036
laboratory diagnosis 1040, *1040*
management 1041
chemotherapy 1041
supportive and surgical 1041
pathology 1037, *1037*
prevention 1042
prognosis 1041
amoebic infections 1035
amoebic keratitis 1043
amoebicides, reproductive effects *1917*
amoeboma 1037–8
amosite 3498
amotivational states 4794
amoxicillin/clavulanate *706*
adverse effects, hepatotoxicity *2533*, 2535
animal-related injuries 1326
bacterial overgrowth *2334*
cellulitis, mastitis and pyomyositis *699*
H. influenzae 762
impetigo *697*
melioidosis *771*
pelvic inflammatory disease *1260*
septic bursitis/arthritis *700*
spectrum of activity *446*
amoxicillin
actinomycoses 854
in breast milk *1469*
cellulitis, mastitis and pyomyositis *699*
H. influenzae 762
H. pylori 2312, *2313*
impetigo *697*
infective endocarditis *2817*, 2817
Lyme borreliosis *864*
pharmacokinetics *449*
pneumococcal pneumonia 687
pneumonia *3238*
in renal failure *4185*
septic bursitis/arthritis *700*
spectrum of activity *446*
typhoid carriers *742*
typhoid fever *742*
urinary tract infection *4114*
amphetamine, serum levels *5449*
amphetamines 5384
adverse effects, hepatotoxicity *2529*
contraindication in porphyria 1641, 5484
amphibians, poisonous 1343, *1344*
amphotericin B
adverse effects *455*
coccidioidomycosis 1022
cryptococcosis 1020
disseminated candidosis 1013
fungal infections 1015
leishmaniasis *1138*
oral candidiasis 2269
paracoccidioidomycosis 1028
Penicillium marneffei 1034
in renal failure *4185*
renal toxicity *3860*
ampicillin *706*
bacteraemia *703*
cellulitis, mastitis and pyomyositis *699*
chlamydial infections *943*
endocarditis *704*
epidural abscess *702*
infective endocarditis *2817–18*
listeriosis 898
nocardiosis 857
osteomyelitis *701*
pharmacokinetics *449*
pneumonia *702*
postantibiotic effect *451*
spectrum of activity *446*
toxic shock syndrome *697*
typhoid carriers *742*
urinary tract infection *702*
amplicons 342
amplitype polymarker DNA 5371
amprenavir, mode of action *444*
amrinone 3130
Amycolatopsis spp. *962*
amylase, reference values *5436*, 5447
amylin 1992
amyloid A 1773
amyloid fibrils 1772
proteins and precursors 1773
amyloid A 1773
amyloid β 1774
amyloid P component 1776
apolipoprotein A-I/A-II 1775
cystatin C 1774
gelsolin 1774
glycosaminoglycans 1775
immunoglobulin light chain 1773
islet amyloid polypeptide 1775
lysozyme 1775
β_2-microglobulin 1775
transthyretin 1779
amyloid neuropathy 5064
amyloid P component 1776–7, *1778*
amyloid β 1774
amyloidosis 1766, 3707

cardiac 1772, 2785
cerebral 1770, *1770*
Alzheimer's disease 1770
hereditary cerebral amyloid angiopathy 1770
prion disease 1771
senile 1770
clinical 1767, *1767–8*
diagnosis and monitoring 1776
histochemistry 1776
nonhistological investigations 1777
dialysis patients 3942
endocrine 1772
haemodialysis-associated 1772, 3942
hepatic involvement 2545
hereditary systemic 1771
familial amyloid polyneuropathy 1771
nonneuropathic 1771
immunoglobulin light-chain 4056
late gadolinium enhancement 2676
leprosy 4089
localized syndromes 1772
malabsorption 2221, *2221*
management 1778
monoclonal immunoglobulin light chain 1768
neuropathy 5086
primary 4353
aetiology and epidemiology 4353
clinical features 4353, *4354*
diagnosis 4354, *4354*
laboratory findings 4354
prognosis 4354
treatment 4354
pulmonary 3451
reactive systemic 1767
associated conditions 1767, *1768*
clinical features 1767
renal involvement 4075
and rheumatoid arthritis 3589
senile 1769
focal 1769
systemic (cardiac) 1769
amyotrophic lateral sclerosis 5070, 5124, *384*, 5172
clinical features 5070
clinical variants 5071
differential diagnosis and investigation 5071
giving diagnosis 5072
pathology 5070
prognosis 5071
treatment 5072
anabolic steroids 5383, *5384*
adverse effects, hepatotoxicity *2533*
contraindication in porphyria 1641
anaemia 4374
acquired pernicious 4408
adaptation to 4375, *4375*
cardiovascular changes 4377
erythropoietin 4376
pulmonary function 4377
red cells 4376, *4376*
tissue perfusion 4377
aplastic *see* aplastic anaemia
autoimmune haemolytic *276, 385*
bartonellosis *937*
cancer-associated 383, *4548, 4549*
causes 4377, *4378*
blood loss 4379
cobalamin deficiency 4382
defective proliferation of red-cell precursors 4378, *4378*
defective red-cell maturation 4378
folate deficiency 4383
haemolytic 4379, *4379*
infection 4383
malabsorption 4384
of chronic disorders 4400
CKD 3923
epidemiology and clinical significance 3924
management 3924
pathogenesis 3923, *3924*
clinical assessment 4380
clinical effects 4377
congenital dyserythropoietic 4449
consequences 4382
defective maturation of red cells 4445
definition 4375, *4382, 4382*
developing countries 4382, 4383
dialysis patients 3941
exercise-induced 5381
haematological investigation 4380, *4380*
haemolytic *see* haemolytic anaemia
and heart failure 2726
inherited 4384, *4384*
iron deficiency 4382
pregnancy 2174
malaria 1063, *1065, 1067*
treatment 1079
management 4381
megaloblastic *see* megaloblastic anaemia
microangiopathic haemolytic *385*, 4459, *4459*
normochromic, normocytic 4400, *4400*
management 4401
pernicious *see* pernicious anaemia
pregnancy 2173
aplastic 2177
haemolytic 2177
iron deficiency 2174
vitamin B12 and folate deficiency 2174
prevalence 4375, 4382, *4382*
prevention 4385
refractory 4259
with excess blasts 4260
with ringed sideroblasts 4259
sideroblastic 4446
SLE 3659
vitamin deficiency 4418
and world health 4381
anaerobic bacteria 748
antibiotic resistance *753*
clinical spectrum 751
definition 749
diagnosis 752
epidemiology 749
history 748
human commensal flora 749, *750*
pathogenesis 750
taxonomy 749, *749*
treatment 752
Anaerobiospirillum spp. *962*
Anaerococcus spp. *962*
Anaeroglobus spp. *962*
Anaerorhabdus spp. *962*
anaesthesia
and anaphylaxis 3108
renal failure 4184
anaesthetics, topical 4736
anakinra 157
rheumatoid arthritis 3598, *3599*, 3600
anal sphincter, anatomy 2202
analgesia
critical illness 3153
hazards of 3154, *3155*
analgesic ladder 5413, *5421*
analgesic nephropathy 4008, *4008, 4010*
analgesics
antagonists 3156
critical illness 3155, *3155*
neuropathic pain 5414, *5414*
nociceptive pain 5413, *5413*
in renal failure 4182, *4182*
analphalipoproteinaemia 1657, 1671
anaphylactic shock
malignant 5465
see also anaphylaxis
anaphylactoid reactions 1466
anaphylatoxins 286
anaphylaxis 3106, 262, *262, 3107*
aetiology 3107, *3108*
allergist/immunologist referral 3113
anaesthesia-related 3108
clinical features 3109, *3110*
cardiovascular manifestations 3110
cutaneous and general reactions 3110, *3110*
gastrointestinal manifestations 3110
neurological manifestations 3110
respiratory manifestations 3110
continuing treatment 3113
definition 3107, *3107*
differential diagnosis 3110
drug-induced 3108
epidemiology 3109
exercise-induced 3109
fatal 3109
food-induced 3108
future developments 3114
grading *3108*
hospital admissions *260*, 3109
hymenoptera stings 1350, 3108
idiopathic 3109
immediate treatment 3111, *3111*
adrenaline 3111
fluid replacement 3112
oxygen and airway patency 3111
investigations 3111
IgE skin testing, *in vitro* testing and challenge testing 3111
mast cell tryptase and histamine 3111
latex-induced 3108
observation 3112
pathophysiology 3109
mast cell/basophil inflammatory mediators 3109
mediator actions 3109
prevention 3113
drug and allergen avoidance 3114
education 3113
long-term desensitization (immunotherapy) 3113
pretreatment 3113
skin testing and short-term desensitization 3113
second-line treatments 3112
summation 3109
treatment 258
see also allergy
Anaplasma phagocytophilum 914, 863, 903, 916
anaplasmosis 903, 914
bacteriology, taxonomy and genomics 914, *915*
human granulocytic 916, *917–18*
anaplastic large T/null-cell lymphoma 4328, 4332
anastrozole, breast cancer *1937*
Anatrichosoma spp. *1176*
ANCA-associated vasculitis *3855*, 4032, 4036–7, 4631
aetiology and genetics 4034
areas of uncertainty 4043
clinical features 4036, *4037*
differential diagnosis *4039, 4033*, 4039, *4042*
epidemiology 4036, *4036*
historical perspective 4034
investigation 4038, *4039*
pathogenesis and pathology 4034, *4035*
prognosis 4042, *4042*
quality of life 4042
treatment 4040
adverse events 4041
induction therapy 4040
maintenance therapy 4040
refractory disease 4041
renal transplantation 4041
see also individual syndromes
ancrod *4540*
Ancylostoma braziliense 1166
Ancylostoma caninum 1163, *1176*
gastroenteritis 1166
Ancylostoma duodenale 1163, 1165
Ancylostoma malayanum *1176*
Andersen syndrome 166, *1598*, 1602
Anderson-Fabry disease *see* Fabry's disease
Andes virus *581*
andioendothelioma, vasculitis 5162
androgen insensitivity syndrome *1917, 1966, 1971*
androgen receptor defects *1917*
androgen replacement 1921
testosterone preparations 1921
androgens
actions of *1915, 1966*
biosynthesis *1965*
defects in 1970
deficiency *1915*
maternal excess 1969
resistance to 1971
Andrographis paniculata 68
andromedotoxins 1364
Anemonia sulcata 1347
anencephaly 5136
antenatal screening *102*
aneuploidy 341
aneurysm
abdominal aortic 2963
Behçet's disease *3685*
endovascular repair 2965
syphilitic 2827

Angelman's syndrome 139, *139*, 145
  hypopigmentation 4663
angiitis
  cutaneous leucocytoclastic *3650*
  isolated CNS *3650*
angina 2629, *2630*, *2886*, *2887*
  atypical 2631
  causes *2903*
  clinical evaluation 2904
  diabetes mellitus 2043
  diagnosis 2904, *2905*
  and heart failure 2725
  investigation 2905, *2905*
  Ludwig's 2258
  management 2902, *2903*
    coronary artery bypass surgery 2943
  Prinzmetal's 2631
  prognosis *2904*
  referral 2903, *2903*
  refractory 2910
  risk assessment 2906
    biomarkers 2907
    clinical indicators 2907
    invasive testing 2907
    noninvasive 2907
    risk scores 2907
  treatment 2907, *2908*
    antianginal drugs 2908
    lifestyle modification 2908
    revascularization 2909, *2910*
    secondary prevention 2907
  unstable *2915*
    ECG 2653
    hypertension 3081
    management 2917
  walk-through angina 2629
angiodysplasia, GI bleeding 2241
angiogenesis 355, *2601*, *2602*
angiogenic switch 397
angiography
  cerebral 4770
  digital subtraction 3880
  renal *3874*, 3880, *3880*
angiokeratoma corporis diffusum *see* Fabry's disease
angiomatosis
  bacillary 927, 930
    diagnosis *931*
    treatment 933
angiomyolipoma 2521
angio-oedema 218, *262*, *4591*, *4652*, *4653*
  airways obstruction 3257
  allergic (IgE-mediated) 262
  allergy 219
  hereditary 262
angiopoietin 2595
angiosarcoma 4694
  liver 2519, *2519*
angiostrongyliasis *see* parastrongyliasis
angiotensin converting enzyme (ACE) 2600
angiotensin II receptor antagonists 2042
  dilated cardiomyopathy 2776
  effects on renin-angiotensin-aldosterone system 3843
  heart failure *2722*, 2723
  hypertension *3050*, 3052
  Raynaud's phenomenon *3671*
angiotensin II 2623, *4482*
angiotensin-converting enzyme, reference values *5436*
angular cheilitis 2268, *2268*
anhydrotic ectodermal dysplasia with immunodeficiency *238*
animal-related injuries 1324–5
  clinical features 1326
  epidemiology 1325
  prevention 1326
  treatment 1326
anion gap 1741, 3190
anisakiasis 1168, 1170
  clinical features 1170, *1171*
  diagnosis 1171
  epidemiology and control 1170
  life cycle 1170
  treatment 1171
anisochromia *4195*
anistreplase, pulmonary embolism 3016
ankle
  pain *3557*
  rheumatoid arthritis 3588
ankylosing spondylitis 3509, 3603, 3607
  clinical features *3605*, 3607
  diagnosis 3608, *3608*
  epidemiology 3607
  extra-articular involvement 3609
  immunopathology and pathogenesis 3607
  laboratory and radiological features 3608, *3609*
  neurological complications 5160
  ocular involvement 5242, *5243*
  physical examination 3608
  prognosis 3610
  pulmonary involvement 3393
  treatment 3610
Anncaliia algerae *1116*
Anncaliia connori *1116*
Anncaliia vesicularum *1116*
anogenital warts 602, *602*
  clinical features 602, *602–3*
  diagnosis and management 603
  epidemiology 602
anomalous pulmonary venous drainage
  partial 2860
  total 2859
anomia 4789
Anopheles arabiensis 1053
Anopheles funestus 1053
Anopheles gambiae 1053
Anopheles quadriannulatus 1053
Anopheles spp. 1053, *1226*
  blood feeding and host preference 1053
  breeding habitat 1054
  distribution and density 1054, *1054*
  genetics and insecticide resistance 1055, *1055*
  immunity to malaria 1055
  vectorial capacity and transmissibility 1054
anorchia 1973
anorectal disease, benign 2241
anorexia nervosa 5319
  haematological changes 4559
  hormonal abnormalities 2066, *2066*
  management 5323
anorexia
  male *1917*
  palliative care 5427
anorgasmia 1942, 1947
anosmia 5033
anovulation 1904
anoxic brain damage 5151
anserine bursitis *3248*, *3557*
ant stings 1349
antabuse syndrome 1370
antacids, in renal failure 4176
antenatal screening 101, *102*
anterior abdominal wall defects 2397
  exomphalos 2397
  gastroschisis 2398
anterior pituitary gland
  adenohypophysis 1800
  anatomy and embryology 1800
  disorders of 1799
    clinical features 1802
    craniopharyngioma 1815
    hypophysitis 1816
    hypopituitarism 1814
    neuro-ophthalmological evaluation 1804
    pituitary adenoma 1814
    pituitary apoplexy 1815
    pituitary carcinoma 1814
    pituitary function testing 1803
    radiological assessment 1804
    Rathke's cleft cysts 1817
  hormone-producing cells *1801*
  hormones 1805
    see also individual hormones
  neurohypophysis 1800
  physiology 1802
  radiotherapy 1805
  surgery 1805
anthophyllite 3498
anthracyclines 399
anthraquinone glycosides *1362*
anthrax 783, 1442
  aetiology and genetics 784
  clinical features 785
    cutaneous anthrax 785, *786*
    gastrointestinal anthrax 786, *786*
    inhalation anthrax 787, *787*
    meningeal anthrax 787
  diagnosis 787
  epidemiology 784
  history 783
  pathogenesis and pathology 784
  prevention 785
  prognosis 788
  treatment 787
Anti Thrombotic Trialists' Collaborative Group 38
antiandrogens, skin disorders 4739
antianginal drugs 2908
  β-blockers 2908
  calcium antagonists 2909
  nitrates 2909
  potassium channel openers 2909
  in renal failure 4180
antianxiety drugs 5336
  benzodiazepines *see* benzodiazepines
  in renal failure 4181
antiarrhythmics 2700, *2700–1*, *4179*
  class I, II, III, IV 2700, *2701*
  in renal failure 4178
  STEMI 2933
  see also individual drugs
antibacterial drugs *see* antimicrobials
antibiotics
  acute pancreatitis 2565
  adverse effects
    colitis 2429
    diarrhoea 431
  bronchiectasis 3350, *3351*
  COPD 3337, 3342
  Crohn's disease 2366
  failed therapy 456
  gastrointestinal infections 2432
  malaria 1077
  mode of action 443, *443*
  NNT *52*
  osteomyelitis 3793
  poisoning 1280
  in pregnancy 2171, *2172*
  prophylactic 452
  Pseudomonas aeruginosa 737
  Raynaud's phenomenon *3671*
  resistance 447, *447–8*
    altered target site 448
    enzymatic inactivation 448
    impermeability 448
    metabolic bypass 448
    surveillance of 448
  sepsis 417
  typhoid fever 742, *742*
antibody deficiency 235, 244
  autosomal recessive with B lymphopenia 245
  cancer medicine *376*
    diseases associated with *238*
  clinical features *245*
  drugs causing *244*
  normal serum immunoglobulins *238*, 247
  outcome 248
  physiological 246
  supplementary management 248
  thymoma 247
  transient of infancy *238*
  treatment 248
antibody-dependent enhancement 576
anti-C1 inhibitor antibodies 221
anti-C1q antibodies 221
anti-CCP antibodies 3568
anticholinergics, COPD 3334, *3335*
anticholinesterases, snake bite 1343
α_1-antichymotrypsin *1753*
anticoagulants
  acute coronary syndromes 2919
  COPD 3343
  dilated cardiomyopathy 2776
  haemodialysis 3935
  heart failure 2724
  new 3022, *3022*
  poisoning, antidote *1274*
  pregnancy *2160*
  pulmonary arterial hypertension 2987
  in renal failure 4180
  STEMI 2932
  stroke 4941
  see also individual drugs
anticoagulation cascade 416
anticoagulation
  atrial fibrillation 3021
  perioperative management 3021, *3022*
  therapeutic 3018
  venous thromboembolism 3018
anticonvulsants 4819
  adverse effects
    osteomalacia 3740
    reproductive *1917*

behavioural teratology 2189
breastfeeding 4823
choice of 4819, *4819*
diabetic neuropathy 2039
drug monitoring 4822, *4823*
enzyme induction 4822
folate deficiency 4413
mechanisms of action 4820, *4820*
poisoning 1280
pregnancy 4822
teratogenicity 2147, 2187
see also individual drugs
antidepressants 5330, *5331*
contraindication in porphyria 1641, *5484*
monoamine oxidase inhibitors 5332
neuropathic pain 5414, *5414*
poisoning 1281
post-traumatic stress disorder 5290
in renal failure 4181
serotonin reuptake inhibitors 5331
tricyclics *see* tricyclic antidepressants
antidiarrhoeal drugs 2433, *2433*
antidiuretic hormone
action of 3815, *3815*
excess *384*
reference values *5441*
antidotes *1274*, 1278
anti-dsDNA antibodies, SLE 3654, *3654*, 3660
antiemetics
palliative care 5424, *5423–4*
in renal failure 4182
antiendomysial antibody 2339
antifibrinolytic drugs, in renal failure 4181
antifungals
mode of action 444
skin disorders
oral 4739
topical 4735
see also individual drugs
antigen receptors 4313, *4313*
antigenic variation 411
antigen-presenting cells 379
antigens, human cancer 375
antiglomerular basement membrane disease 3995
aetiology and pathogenesis 3996
anti-GBM antibodies and T-cell-mediated immune response 3996
disease associations 3996
environmental factors 3996
genetic predisposition 3996
Goodpasture antigen 3996
in Alport's syndrome 3999
clinical features 3997, *3998*
pulmonary 3997, *3997*
renal 3997
clinical investigation 3998, *3998*
differential diagnosis 3998
epidemiology *3997*
historical perspectives 3995
pathology 3996, *3997*
prognosis 3999, *4000*
treatment 3998, *3999*
see also Goodpasture's syndrome
antihistamines
allergic rhinitis 3281
anaphylaxis 3112
contraindication in porphyria 1641, *5484*
poisoning *1274*, 1282
in renal failure 4181
topical 4735
antihypertensive agents 3049, *3050*
α-blockers 3052
behavioural teratology 2190
β-blockers 3051
in breast milk *2101*
calcium antagonists 3051
centrally acting sympatholytics 3052
CKD 3915, *3915*
diuretics 3050
in pregnancy *2099*
in renal failure 4178
renin-angiotensin system blockers 3051
vasodilators 3052
anti-inflammatory agents
ARDS 3145
bronchiectasis 3351
cystic fibrosis 3360
anti-inflammatory cascade 415
anti-La antibodies, Sjögren's syndrome 3660
antileukotrienes, asthma 3304
anti-lymphocyte globulin, post-transplantation *3954*
antimalarials 1073, *1074*
adverse effects, ocular 5251, *5251*
4-aminoquinolines 1075
8-aminoquinolines 1076
antibiotics 1077
arylaminoalcohols 1074
bisquinolines 1075
folate-synthesis inhibitors 1076
hydroxynaphthoquinones 1077
peroxides 1076
poisoning 1282
skin disorders 4739
see also individual drugs
antimetabolites 398
anti-Mi-2 antibodies 3696
antimicrobials 441
adverse drug reactions 455, *454–6*
bactericidal vs. bacteriostatic agents 453
combined therapy 445, *446–7*
dose selection 452
duration of treatment 453
guidelines and formularies *457*, 458
minimum inhibitory concentration *452*
mode of action 443, *443–4*
pharmacodynamics 450, *450–2*
pharmacokinetics 449
bioavailability 449, *449*
distribution 449, *450*
excretion 450
metabolism 450
principles of use *451*, *452–3*, *453*
in renal failure *4185*
spectrum of activity 444
susceptibility testing 445, *445–6*
see also antibiotics; antifungals; antivirals
antimuscarinics, intravenous 3309
antimycobacterial agents, pregnancy *2172*
antineuronal antibodies 5167, *5167–8*
antineuronal nuclear antibodies (ANNA-1) 3523
antinuclear antibodies *3568*, 3568–9
autoimmune rheumatic disease *3651*
antinuclear cytoplasmic antibodies *see* ANCAs
antiobesity drugs 1533, 2010
antioncogenes *see* tumour suppressor genes
antioxidants
ARDS 3145
dietary supplements 1503
protective function 1511
Raynaud's phenomenon *3671*
skin preparations 4732
antiparasitic agents
mode of action 444
pregnancy *2172*
see also individual drugs
antiphospholipid antibodies, SLE 3655, 3660
antiphospholipid antibody nephropathy 4050
antiphospholipid syndrome 3568, *3650*, 3658, 4543
cardiac involvement 2783
cognitive impairment 5281
pregnancy 2154, *2157*, *2159*
management 2160, *2160*
antiplasmin 4497
antiplatelet agents
acute coronary syndromes 2917
coronary bypass 2945
drug interactions *1471*
heart failure 2724
peptic ulcer disease 2313
in renal failure 4180
stroke 4941
antipruritics 4732
calamine 4732
camphor 4733
menthol 4733
antipsychotics 5335
adverse effects 5335, *5336–7*
atypical 3156, *5266*, *5337*
drug interactions 5336
indications and use 5335
poisoning 1283
in renal failure 4181
reproductive effects *1917*
antiretroviral therapy 636
entry inhibitors 636
integrase inhibitors 637
non-nucleoside reverse transcriptase inhibitors 636
nucleoside analogues 636, *638*
protease inhibitors 636
anti-Ro antibodies, Sjögren's syndrome 3660
antisense nucleotides *1939*
antisense therapy 4322
antiseptics 4734
benzoyl peroxide 4734
cetrimide 4734
chlorhexidine 4734
poisoning 1316
povidone-iodine 4735
triclosan 4735
antisignal recognition particle antibodies 3696
antispasmodics, in renal failure 4176
antisynthetase autoantibodies 3696
antisynthetase syndrome 3695–6
antithrombin III 2601, *4196*
deficiency 4529
laboratory tests *4522*
antithrombin 416, *4490*, 4494
deficiency *2118*
antithymocyte globulin 3482
systemic sclerosis *3677*
anti-thymocyte globulin, post-transplantation *3954*
antithyroid drugs 1840, *1841*
adverse effects, in pregnancy *2188*
α_1-antitrypsin *1753*
COPD 3323, *3323*
reference values *5444*
α_1-antitrypsin deficiency 1780, 2539, 4650
clinical features 1782
clinical investigation 1783
epidemiology 1781
genetics *139*, 1780
molecular basis 1781, *1782*
prognosis 1783
treatment 1783
emerging 1784
anti-TNF agents 401
ankylosing spondylitis 3610
nephrotoxicity 4053
rheumatoid arthritis 3598, *3598*
antituberculous drugs 825, *825*
children *825*
interactions with antiretroviral drugs 827
toxicity 825
antitussives, COPD 3337
antivenom 1339
contraindications 1340
dose *1340*, 1341
indications 1339
Australia 1339
Europe 1339
USA and Canada 1339
prediction of reactions 1340
reactions to 1341
response to 1341
selection/administration 1340, *1340–1*
antivirals
mode of action 444, *444*
skin disorders 4739
see also individual drugs
anti-Xa inhibitors, acute coronary syndromes 2921
Antley-Bixler syndrome 1899
ants, and hygiene 1236
anuria 3852
anus, imperforate 2403
anxiety 5308
diagnosis and clinical features 5310, *5311*
epidemiology 5309, *5309*
history taking 5259, *5260*
impact 5309
pathophysiology 5310
somatic presentation 5301
somatized *5260*, *5261*
symptoms *5261*
treatment *5313*, *5312*
aorta, hypertensive changes 3035
aortic aneurysm
abdominal, rupture *3120*
back pain 3574
GI involvement 2422
screening *106*
aortic coarctation 2856, *2844*, 3061, *3062*
follow-up 2857, *2858*
investigations 2856, *2857*

pregnancy 2112
presentation 2856
repair 2857
aortic disease, echocardiography 2668, *2669*
aortic dissection 2631, *3120*
blood pressure management 3082
clinical features *2632*
presentation 5459
thoracic 2953
aortic regurgitation 2737, 2750
causes 2750, *2751*
differential diagnosis 2753
echocardiography 2664
investigations 2752
cardiac catheterization 2753
chest radiograph 2752, *2752*
ECG 2752
echocardiography 2752, *2752–3*
management 2753
medical 2753
surgical 2753
pathophysiology and complications 2751
physical examination 2751
pregnancy 2113
symptoms 2751
syphilis 2827, *2827*
aortic root abscess *793*
aortic root dilatation, pregnancy 2112, *2112*
aortic stenosis 2736, 2746
causes 2746
differential diagnosis 2749
echocardiography 2663, *2664*
familial supravalvar 2836, *2836*
investigations 2748
cardiac catheterization/ angiography *2684*, 2749
chest radiograph 2748
ECG 2748
echocardiography 2748, *2749*
management 2750
medical 2750
surgical 2750
pathophysiology and complications 2747
coronary circulation 2747
left ventricular response 2747
percutaneous treatment 2942
physical examination 2747
pregnancy 2113
supravalvar 2851
symptoms 2747
aortic valve vegetation *793*
aortic valve
bicuspid *2844*, 2851
in pregnancy 2113
mixed disease 2754
see also various diseases of
aorto-enteric fistula 2585
aortopathy
pregnancy 2112
aortic coarctation 2112
dilated aortic root 2112, *2112*
aortopulmonary window 2858
APACHE II score 2561, *2562*, 3158
apatite-associated syndromes 3638, 3647
acute calcific periarthritis 3647, *3647*
and osteoarthritis 3647
APC gene 349, *363*
Apert's syndrome *3721*
mutations in *3757*
Apeu virus *581*
apex, tapping 2739
aphasia 4743, 4789
atypical 4790
Broca's 4789
comprehension 4789
conduction 4790
fluency and paraphasic errors 4789
global 4790
repetition 4789
Wernicke's 4790
aphthous stomatitis 2269
aetiology 2269, *2270–1*
clinical features 2271
herpetiform ulcers *2271*, 2272
major aphthous ulcers *2271*, 2272
minor aphthous ulcers *2270*, 2271
course and prognosis 2272
diagnosis *2271*, 2272
pathology 2271
treatment 2272
Apis cerania (honey bee) 1349
Apis dorsata (honey bee) 1349
Apis mellifera (honey bee) 1349
aplastic anaemia 4287, 4212
acquired 4288, *4289*
aetiology and incidence *4289*, 4289
clinical features *4291*, 4290
clinical investigation 4291, *4292*
definition 4288
differential diagnosis 4290
pathogenesis 4289
treatment and prognosis *4292*, *4294*, *4295*
bone marrow failure 4287, *4289*
classification and definition 4288
congenital 4294, *4291*
dyskeratosis congenita 4295
Shwachman-Diamond syndrome 4296
see also Fanconi's anaemia
pregnancy 2177
pure red-cell aplasia 4784
apocrine gland disorders 4676
bromhidrosis 4677
chromhidrosis 4677
Fox-Fordyce disease 4676
hidradenitis suppurativa 4676
trimethylaminuria 4677
Apoi virus *566*
apolipoprotein A-I/A-II 1775
Apophallus donicus *1222*
apoptosis 177, 336
activation of 179
bystander 596
caspases *see* caspases
and cell stress 183
DNA damage response 183
heat shock response 183
stress-activated kinase response 183
unfolded protein response 183
death-signalling receptors 179, *180*
and disease 186
cardiovascular disease 187
central nervous system degeneration 187
immunity 186
infective disorders 186
tumour biology 187, *187*
gene mutations 351, *352*
mitochondrial signals coupled to 180, *181–2*
recognition by macrophages 185, *185*
SLE 3655
structural changes 177, *178*
apoptotic cells, role in autoimmunity 269
appendicitis
acute 2234
amoebic 1038
nutritional causes 1522
in pregnancy 2132
apraxia 4793
APRIL 156
aquaporins 1791, 2602
arabinoside, adverse effects, hepatotoxicity *2532*
arachnodactyly
congenital contractural *3721*
Marfan's syndrome 3752
Arcanobacterium spp. *962*
archaebacteria 127
archexin *1939*
Arcobacter spp. *962*
arcus juvenilis 3730
Arcyophora spp. 1236
Arcyophora spp. 1236
ARDS *see* acute respiratory distress syndrome
Ardystil syndrome 3458
Areca catechu 1374
arenaviruses 588, 1442
aetiology and genetics 588
areas of uncertainty 595
clinical features 591
diagnosis/differential diagnosis 594, *594*
epidemiology 589
future developments 595
management 590, *590*
pathogenesis/pathology 588
postexposure prophylaxis 590
prevention 590
treatment 594
vaccines 591
see also individual viruses
Argasidae (soft ticks) *1228*
argatroban, haemodialysis 3935
Argentine haemorrhagic fever *see* South American haemorrhagic fever
argininaemia *1566*
arginine hydrochloride 1565
arginine, reference values 5447
argininosuccinic aciduria *1566*
Argyll-Robertson pupil 5034
argyria 1382
aripiprazole 5266
Aristolochia 68
aristolochic acid nephropathy *see* Chinese herb nephropathy
Arizona hinshawii 1240
arm ischaemia 2963
Armillifer agkistrodontis 1238
Armillifer armillatus 1237–8
Armillifer spp. 1237–8, *1238–9*
Arnold-Chiari malformation 3260
Aroa virus *566*
aromatase deficiency *1917*
placental 1969
aromatase inhibitors, breast cancer *1937*
aromatherapy *66*
aromatic amines *308*, *338*, *1380*
aromatic L-amino acid decarboxylase deficiency *1566*, 1588
arrhythmias *see* cardiac arrhythmias
arrhythmogenic right ventricular cardiomyopathy 2715, 2765, 2778, 2850
causes 2778
clinical features 2779
definition 2778
investigations 2779, *2780*
ECG 2779, *2780*
echocardiography 2779
endomyocardial biopsy 2780
exercise testing 2779
MRI 2780, *2781*
management 2780
pathology and pathophysiology 2779
arrhythmogenic right ventricular dysplasia *2840*
arsenic
and cancer *307–8*, *338*, *1380*
poisoning 1297
antidote *1274*
peripheral nervous system effects *1387*, 5087
reference values *5445*
arsenicals, hepatotoxicity *1385*, *2536*
arsine poisoning 1307
arsphenamine, adverse effects, hepatotoxicity *2532*
artemether *1074*, 1076, *1078*
artemisinin 1076
suppositories 1076
arterial blood gases 3189, *3195*, *5514*, *5515*
acid-base balance 3197, *3197–8*
acute respiratory failure 3134, *3134*
anatomical shunt 3196
COPD 3329, *3330*
haemoglobin-oxygen dissociation curve 3195, *3196*
pulmonary embolism 3014
respiratory acidosis/alkalosis 3197
respiratory failure 3196
ventilation-perfusion mismatching 3196, *3196*
arterial cannulation 5511, *5512*
arterial disease 2953
cholesterol embolism 2966
oral contraceptives 2193, *2194*
peripheral *see* peripheral arterial disease
Takayasu's arteritis *see* Takayasu's arteritis
thoracic aortic dissection 2953
arterial occlusive disease 4935
arterial oxygen saturation *see* SaO2
arterial oxygen tension 3468, *3468*
arterial pressure 3125
mean *2621*, 3125
regulation of 2622
baroreceptors 2620, 2623
blood volume 2623
natriuretic peptides 2623
renin-angiotensin system 2623
arterial wall 2874, *2875*
adventitia 2874

intima 2874
media 2874
arteries 2594
hypertensive changes 3035
arteriography, pulmonary/bronchial 3205, *3205*
arteriovenous fistulae 4688
artesunate 1076, *1078*
arthritis
brucellar *791*, 793
chlamydial 945
Chlamydia pneumoniae 948
and coeliac disease 3615
cricoarytenoid 3509
filarial 1157
gouty 1623, *1623*
and hypogammaglobulinaemia 958, *958*
and inflammatory bowel disease 3603, 3613
juvenile chronic *see* juvenile chronic arthritis
meningococcal 718
immune complex-mediated 718
patterns of *3556*
psoriatic *see* psoriatic arthritis
pyogenic 3617
reactive 3622, *3605*
rheumatic fever 2800
rheumatoid *see* rheumatoid arthritis
septic 698, *700*
Arthrobacter spp. *962*
arthrochalasis 3777
arthrography 3564
arthrogryposis multiplex congenita *166*
arthropathies
collagenous colitis 3615
crystal-related 3637
intestinal bypass surgery 3615
arthropods
allergic reactions 1235
bites 1226
accidental 1229
infestations 1229
nonvenomous 1225
see also individual species
artificial nutrition support 1535
complications 1539
enteral feeding 1539
parenteral feeding 1541
cost-effectiveness 1544
disease-specific/therapeutic feeds *1544*
estimating nutrition requirements 1538
ethical issues 1542
indications 1537, *1537*
long-term 1542
nutrition support team 1544
perioperative 1544
special situations 1542
critical illness 1542, *1543*
gastrointestinal disease 1543, *1544*
liver disease 1543
renal disease 1543
artificial sweeteners, and bladder cancer 328
Artyfechinostomum mehrai 1220
asbestos *308*, 320, *338*, *1380*, *3185*
benign pleural disease 3487, 3491, 3498
clinical features 3499, *3499–500*
pathogenesis 3498, *3499*
mesothelioma 3535
asbestosis 3414, *3420*, *3420*
aetiology and pathology 3420, *3421*
clinical features 3421, *3421–2*
differential diagnosis 3422
prevention and management 3422
risk in nonoccupationally exposed population 3422
ascariasis 1168
clinical features 1169, *1170*
diagnosis 1170, *1170*
epidemiology and control 1169
life cycle 1168, *1169*
treatment 1170
Ascaris lumbricoides 1168
and acute pancreatitis 2560
Ascaris suum 1176
ascites 2482
aetiology 2483
causes *2484*
clinical features 2484, *2485*
complications 2490, *2490*
hepatorenal syndrome 2490
hypercatabolic state 2490
paraumbilical hernia 2490
pleural effusion 2490
respiratory difficulties 2490
spontaneous bacterial peritonitis 2490, *2490–1*
drug prescribing 2492
epidemiology 2483
hepatocellular failure 2496
diagnosis 2500
laboratory diagnosis 2484
ascitic fluid 2485, *2486*, *2488*
paracentesis 2485
pancreatic 2566
pathogenesis 2483
prognosis 2489
refractory 2489
treatment 2486, *2487*
ACE inhibitors 2489
bed rest 2486
dietary salt restriction 2486
diuretics 2487, *2488*
intravenous albumin infusion 2489
therapeutic paracentesis 2488, *2488*
water restriction 2486
ascitic amylase 2485
ascitic fluid
culture 2486
cytology 2486
investigations 2485
microscopy 2486
protein concentration 2485, *2486*
volume 2486
ascorbic acid *see* vitamin C
ASK-1, 184
Askanazy cells 1835
asparaginase, adverse effects, hepatotoxicity *2534*
aspartate transaminase
reference values *5436*
children *5438*
aspartylglucosaminuria 1698, 5122
aspergillosis 1014
allergic bronchopulmonary 3295, 3346
diseases associated with *1014*
HIV-related 3251
Aspergillus clavatus 3436
Aspergillus flavus 306, 309, 1014
Aspergillus fumigatus 1014, *3436*
HIV-associated infection *3247*
Aspergillus niger 1014
Aspergillus spp. *3436*
Aspergillus terreus 1014
Aspergillus versicolor 3436
asphyxiants 3457
asphyxiating thoracic dystrophy 3510
aspiration 3256, *3257*
in pregnancy 2123
aspirin
acute coronary syndromes 2917
adverse effects
hepatotoxicity *2529*, *2535*
oesophagitis *2294*
peptic ulceration 2307
in pregnancy *2188*
and asthma 3288
drug cross-reactions *3289*
in breast milk *1469*
cancer pain 394
clinical trials *40*
drug interactions *1471*
limb ischaemia 2962
migraine *4917*
stroke prevention 30
see also salicylates
assassin bug 1229
asterixis 2495, *2496*, 3890
asthenozoospermia 1922
asthma *3120*, 3283, *3285*
acute exacerbations 3284, *3302*, *3306*, *3307*, *3309*
management 3308, *3308*
allergic 261
bronchoscopy *3223*, 3224
clinical features 3283, 3290
breathlessness *2633*
cough-variant 3291
diagnosis 3283, 3291
airflow limitation 3291, *3292*
tests of airway hyper-responsiveness 3292
differential diagnosis 3296, *3327*
difficult 3305, *3305*
drug-induced 3461, *3461–2*
with eosinophilic pneumonia 3430
food intolerance 2254
and heart failure 2725
imaging 3295
management 3283
action plan *3298*
allergen avoidance 3298
drug treatments 3299
immunotherapy 3299
objectives 3297, *3297*
patient education 3298
stepped approach 3284, 3304
treatment selection 3298
morbidity *3316*
occupational *see* occupational asthma
pathophysiology 3285
airway hyper-responsiveness 3285, *3285–6*
airway inflammation 3286
pregnancy 2123
presentation 5468
prevalence 3289
prognosis 3290
signs 3291
symptoms 3291
triggers 3283, 3286
atopy and allergy 3286
drugs 3287
occupation 3287, *3288*
respiratory virus infections 3287
astroviruses 539
diarrhoea 2427
epidemiology 540
replication 539
structure and classification 539
asystole 2694
ataxia telangiectasia 255, 302, *238*, 307, *360*, 368, *4908*, 5099
genetics *139*
and leukaemia 332
ataxia-like syndrome *238*
ataxias 4902
autosomal recessive 4907, *4908*
with defective DNA repair 4907
with oculomotor apraxia 4908
see also individual conditions
cerebellar 4904
acute/subacute onset 4905, *4905*
autosomal dominant 4908, *4909*
chronic progressive course 4905
developmental disorders 4904, *4904*
episodic course 4905
vascular disorders 4905
cerebellar symptoms 4903
eye movements 4904
gait and posture 4903
limb ataxia 4904
muscle tone 4904
speech 4903
tremor 4904
differential diagnosis *4903*
episodic
type 1, 162, 166
type 2, 162, 166
familial episodic 5115
Friedreich's *see* Friedreich's ataxia
gait disturbance 4902
hereditary 5114
idiopathic degenerative late-onset 4909
progressive metabolic 4906
degenerative 4907
spinocerebellar
autosomal dominant 5115, *5116*
type 6, 162, 166
symptoms 4902
ataxia-telangiectasia 1845, 4692
atazanavir
HIV/AIDS 636, *638*
mode of action *444*
toxicity *640*
atelectasis, rounded 3487, *3499*, *3500*
Atelopsus spp. 1346
atelosteogenesis, mutations in *3757*
atenolol *2701*
in breast milk *1469*, *2101*
hypertensive emergencies *3079*
ATG *290*, 292
atherectomy 2938, *2938*
directional coronary 2938, *2939*
rotational ablation 2938, *2938*
Atherix spp. *1226*
atherogenesis 2875, *2876*
atheroma 2418, 2875

atherogenesis 2875, *2876*
atheroprotection 2877
cellular senescence 2877
evolution of 2877, *2878*
calcification 2878
cell death in plaque 2878
disease progression and positive remodelling 2879
extracellular matrix 2877, *2879*
neovascularization 2878
smooth muscle cells 2877
in hypertension 3035
leucocyte recruitment 2876
atheromatous renovascular disease 4078
clinical features 4079
epidemiology 4079
future developments 4080
investigation 4079
prognosis 4080
treatment 4079, *4080*
atherosclerosis *2875*, 3035
aorta and large arteries 3035
biology and pathology 2873
C. pneumoniae 948
post-transplant 3963, *3963*
resistance vessels 3035
see also atheroma
atherosclerotic ulcer 2958, *2958*
athetosis *4890*
ATM kinase 344, *346*
atmospheric pressure 1409, *1410*
atmospheric temperature 1409
atmospheric zone 1409
atoms 1429
atopic eczema, pregnancy 2153
atopic eruption of pregnancy 2151, *2150–1*
Atopobium spp. *962*
atopy 259, 3278
and asthma 3286
and COPD 3315
atorvastatin 1670
atovaquone *1074*, 1077
babesiosis 1090
prophylactic 1086
toxoplasmosis *1096*
ATP binding cassette A1, 1657
ATP synthase deficiency 1572
Atractaspididae 1333
Atractaspis aterrima (burrowing asp) *1328*
Atractaspis microlepidota 1327
atransferrinaemia *1674*
atrial extrasystoles 2702, *2703*
atrial fibrillation 2641, 2689, 2703
anticoagulation 3021
clinical features 2703, *2703*
diagnosis 2704, *2704*
echocardiography 2666, *2666*
and heart failure 2725
management 2704
mechanisms 2703
and mitral stenosis 2738
paroxysmal 2704
permanent 2705
persistent 2705, *2705*
pre-excited 2709, *2710*
prevention of thrombo-embolism 2704, *2705*
atrial flutter 2706, *2706, 2714*
atrial hypertrophy, ECG 2650, *2650–1*
atrial natriuretic factor 2609
atrial septal defects 2851, *2851, 2851*
clinical signs 2852
coronary sinus defect 2853
indications for closure 2853
investigations 2853
ostium secondum 2648, 2852
patent foramen ovale 2851
pregnancy 2113
and pulmonary vascular disease 2852
sinus venosus 2853
atrial septostomy 2988
atrioventricular block 2692
aetiology 2692, *2693*
asystole 2694
first-degree 2693, *2693*
ECG *2648*
second-degree 2693
type I (Wenckebach) *2693*
type II (Mobitz) *2693*
third-degree 2694, *2694*
atrioventricular nodal re-entry tachycardia 2707
clinical features 2707
management 2707
mechanism 2707, *2707–8*
atrioventricular node 2619, *2619*
atrioventricular re-entry tachycardia 2708, *2708–9*
atrioventricular septal defect 2855, *2856*
atrophie blanche *4690*
atropine *1274*
anaphylaxis 3112
poisoning 1361
snake bite 1343
ATT trial *40*
attention 4788, *4789*
Auchmeromyia luteola *1226, 1233*
Aura virus *558*
auramine manufacture *1380*
Aureobasidium pullulans 3436
aureomycin, adverse effects, hepatotoxicity *2534*
Aurora kinases 343
auscultation, chest 3187
Austin's disease 1697, 1698, 5105
Austin-Flint murmur 2752
Austroleptis spp. *1226*
autoantibodies
antinuclear *see* ANCAs
polymyositis/dermatomyositis 3695, *3696*
rheumatoid arthritis 3584
SLE 3654, *3654*, 3660
systemic sclerosis 3670, *3670*
autoantigens
acquisition of adjuvant properties 275, *276*
expression in target tissue 277
autogenic training *66*
autografts *281*
autohaemolysis *4196*
autoimmune disease 267
aetiology 267–8
environmental factors 270
genetic factors 268
amplification 275
autoantigen expression in target tissues 277
disease-specific autoantigens 275
clinical features 277
complement deficiency 218, 222
epidemiology 268
nonsustained 267
pathogenesis 267, 270
central and peripheral tolerance 270
effector mechanisms 275
immune response to self antigens 271, *272–4*
and pericarditis 2791
prognosis 277
rheumatic 3649
systemic 267, *277*
tissue-specific 267
treatment 278
see also individual disorders
autoimmune haemolytic anaemia *276, 385*, 4454, *4455*
autoimmune hepatitis *276*, 3560
aetiology 2460
associated conditions *2461*, 2462
clinical manifestations 2461, *2461*
diagostic criteria 2461
differential diagnosis 2461
epidemiology 2461
histology 2460, *2461*
immunopathogenesis 2460, *2461*
investigations 2461
natural history 2462
subtypes 2462, *2462*
treatment 2462
autoimmune hypoglycaemia 2056
autoimmune insulin syndrome 2056
autoimmune limbic encephalitis 5175, *5176*
autoimmune lymphoproliferative syndrome *238*
autoimmune polyendocrine syndrome type I 269
autoimmune polyendocrinopathy, candidiasis, ectodermal dysplasia syndrome (APCED) *238*
autoimmune rheumatoid disease pulmonary involvement 3387, *3389*
clinically significant disease 3394
disease detection 3393
prognosis and when to treat 3394
treatment 3394
see also individual conditions
autoinflammatory syndromes 3708, *238, 3709–10*
autonomic failure 5059, *5063–4*
chronic 5059, *5062*
drugs 5066
investigations *5062*
see also individual conditions
autonomic nervous system diseases *5056–7*, 5055
classification 5056, *5057–9*
clinical features 5056, *5060–1*
investigations 5059, *5062*
management 5059, *5063*
see also individual disorders
autonomic nervous system
diurnal variation 2626
heart 2625
autonomy 17
definition of 17
respect for 20
autophagic vacuolar myopathy 1698
autophagy 1703, 178
defects in 1698
autosomal dominant polycystic kidney disease 4095
diagnosis 4095, *4096*
genetic counselling 4097
pathogenesis 4097
symptoms 4096
treatment 4097
urinary tract infection 4117
autosomal recessive disorders 138, *139*
autosomal recessive polycystic kidney disease 4097
Avalon virus *581*
avascular necrosis, post-transplant 3964
axillary nerve neuropathy 5081
Ayurvedic medicine 67
Azadirachta indica 1374
azathioprine
adverse effects 3955, *3955*
hepatotoxicity *2532, 2533, 2536*
renal toxicity *3860*
aphthous ulcers 2272
Behçet's disease 3687
carcinogenesis *307*
Crohn's disease 2366
lupus nephritis 4047, 4049
polymyositis/dermatomyositis 3697
post-transplantation 291, *290, 2511, 3482*
primary biliary cirrhosis *2467*
renal transplantation *3954*
rheumatoid arthritis *3595*
sarcoidosis *3411*
skin disorders 4737
Still's disease 3706
azithromycin *707*
babesiosis 1090
bartonellosis 939
chancroid 764
chlamydial infections *943*
gonorrhoea 726
leptospirosis 878
Lyme borreliosis *864*
mycobacterial disease 835
mycoplasmal infections *960*
pelvic inflammatory disease *1260*
pertussis *766*
pneumonia *3238*
in renal failure *4185*
rickettsioses 914
S. pyogenes 675
syphilis 894
toxoplasmosis *1096*
typhoid fever *742*
azo dyes, carcinogenesis *338*
azoles 1015
azoospermia 1385, 1922
obstructive 1924
Azospirillum spp. *962*
azothioprine, pregnancy *2158*
aztreonam
pneumonia *3238, 3245*
Pseudomonas aeruginosa 737

B cells
antibodies *244*
antigen recognition 227, *227*
combined T/B cell deficiency *238*
diagnostics 233

lymphopenia 245
malignancies *244*
naive *229*, 229
priming and functions 231, *231*
rheumatoid arthritis 3584
SCID *251*
SLE 3654, *3654*
therapy 233
tolerance 233
B lymphocyte stimulator protein 156
Babanki virus *558*
Babesia divergens 1089
Babesia microti 863, 1089
babesiosis 1089
clinical features 1089
diagnosis 1089, *1090*
epidemiology 1089
pathogenesis 1089
treatment and prevention 1090
bacille Calmette-Guérin *see* BCG
Bacillus anthracis 783
Bacillus spp. *962*
Bacillus subtilis *3436*
back pain 3571
causes *1257*
diagnosis 3249, *1257*
investigations 3264
management 3245
medical causes 3573
nonspecific pain 3574
sciatica/neurological deficits 3269
surgical emergencies 3572
mechanical *3557*
neurological signs 3574
occupational 1383
physical examination *3573*, 3573
pregnancy 2146
red flag signs 3573
sciatica 3574
surgical emergencies 3574
underlying medical causes 3573
backward failure 3128
baclofen
adverse effects, hepatotoxicity *2529*, *2532*
vertigo *4861*
Bacon, Francis 9
bacteraemia *421*, 927
anaerobic 751
bartonella 927, 930
diagnosis *931*
nosocomial 431
occult 761
Pseudomonas aeruginosa 736
staphylococcal 702, *703*
coagulase-negative 704
streptococcal 674, *674*
bacteria, anaerobic 748
bacterial endocarditis 2871, *2871*
bacterial infections
and cancer 306
haematological changes 4550–1, *4551*
immunocompromised patients 249
immunosuppressed patients 3958
intracranial 4780
liver involvement 2541, *2543*
ocular 5245, *5245*
pregnancy 2169
renal involvement 4071, 4073
skin 4673
bacterial killing defects 252
bacteriuria
asymptomatic 4108
treatment 4112
maternal, antenatal screening *102*
Bacteroides fragilis, antibiotic sensitivity *446*
Bacteroides spp. *962*, 1257
antibiotic resistance *753*
Bacteroides ureolyticus *852*
Bagaza virus *566*
bagiliximab, lymphoma *4320*
Balamuthia mandrillaris 1043, *1044*
Balamuthia 1036, 1042
balantidiasis 1111, *1114*, *1114*
historical perspective 1112
Balint's syndrome 4791
Balkan nephropathy 327, *4008*, *4015*, *4015*
clinical features 4016
diagnosis and treatment 4016
pathogenesis 4015
environmental factors 4015
genetic factors 4015
pathology 4016
balloon angioplasty 2936, *2936–7*
Balneatrix spp. *962*
balsalazide, ulcerative colitis 2378, *2380*
Baltic myoclonus 5103
bamboo spine 3509, *3610*
Bangui virus *581*
Bannayan-Riley-Ruvalcaba syndrome 5099
Bannwarth's syndrome 861
Banzi virus *566*
Barakat's syndrome *1855*
barbiturates
in breast milk *2189*
contraindication in porphyria 1641, *5484*
drug interactions *3968*
folate deficiency 4413
poisoning *1274*, 1283
Bardet-Biedl syndrome *148*, *140*, *1530*, *1917*, 5142
renal involvement 4102
Bardet-Biedl-Moon syndrome, differential diagnosis *1722*
bariatric surgery 1534, 2010
baritosis 3424
barium studies
colorectal cancer *2225*
diverticular disease *2391*
gastro-oesophageal reflux disease 2289
small intestine 2219
ulcerative colitis *2376*
Barker-Hales hypothesis 2004
Barmah Forest virus *558*, 559
baroreceptors 2623
barotrauma
diving 1418, 1419
Barrett's oesophagus 2407, 2291
aetiopathogenesis 2292
definition and nomenclature 2291
management 2292, *2292*
see also oesophageal cancer
barrier creams 1382
Barth syndrome *1566*, 1572
Barthel Scale 5406
bartholinitis
chlamydial 943
mycoplasmal infections *956*
Bartlett, Elisha 10
Bartonella alsatica *928*
Bartonella bacilliformis 934, 1227, *928*, *934–5*
Bartonella birtlesii *928*
Bartonella bovis *928*
Bartonella capreoli *928*
Bartonella chomelii *928*
Bartonella clarridgeiae *928*
Bartonella doshiae *928*
Bartonella elizabethae *928*
Bartonella grahamii *928*
Bartonella henselae 634, 1326
stellar retinitis *930*
Bartonella koehlerae *928*
Bartonella peromysci *928*
Bartonella phoceensis *928*
Bartonella quintana 860, 872, *928*, 1231
infective endocarditis 2816
Bartonella rattimassiliensis *928*
Bartonella schoenbuchensis *928*
Bartonella spp. 926, *962*
aetiology and genetics 927, *927*
bacillary angiomatosis 930
bacillary peliosis 930
cat-scratch disease 929
clinical features 928
bacteraemia and endocarditis 930
trench fever 929
diagnosis 927, *930*, *931*
direct 931, *931–2*
indirect 932, *933*
specimen collection 930
encephalopathy and neuroretinitis 929, *930*
epidemiology 928
history 927
osteomyelitis *931*
pathogenesis/pathology 927
prevention 927
treatment 927, 932
see also bartonellosis
Bartonella talpae *928*
Bartonella taylorii *928*
Bartonella tribocorum *928*
Bartonella vinsonii *928*
Bartonella washoensis *928*
bartonellosis 934
aetiology 934, *935*
clinical features *938*, *936*, *937–8*
diagnosis 938
epidemiology 934, *935–6*
geographical distribution *936*
laboratory features 938
pathogenesis 935, *937*
prevention 939
prognosis 938
treatment 938
Bartter's syndrome *165*, 166, *3073*, *3838*
nephrocalcinosis *4128*
pregnancy 2143
type I (*NKCC2* mutations) 3838, *4145*
type II (*ROMK* mutations) 3838, *4145*
type III (*CLCNKB* mutations) 3839, *4145*
type IV 3839, *4145*
basal cell carcinoma 4708, *4708*
basal cell naevus syndrome *see* Gorlin's syndrome
basal ganglia 4874
anatomy
functional 4874
gross 4874, *4874*
disease, adult-onset 1686
function/dysfunction 4877
hyperdirect pathway and oscillations 4876
pathways 4875, *4875*
rate model of function 4876, *4876*
basal transcription factors 1803
base excess *5515*
basic life support 3097
basic reproductive number 1243
basidiobolus 1008
basiliximab 292, 3482
post-transplantation *3954*
basophilic stippling *4195*
basophils *4196*, 4311
inflammatory mediators 3109
Bassen-Kornzweig disease 1497, 5113
Bateson, William 362, 1550
Batten's disease 1717
differential diagnosis *1722*
variant 1698
Batu cave virus *566*
Bax protein *181*
Bayesian theory, clinical trials 45
Baylisascaris procyonis *1176*
Bayou virus *581*
Bay 11-7082 1939
Bazin's disease 4674
B-cell prolymphocytic leukaemia 4227
B-cell receptors 174
diversity 228, *228*
BCG vaccine 830
Bcl-2 proteins *182*
BCNU, adverse effects *400*
Beal's syndrome 3752, 3778
Bean syndrome 2585
Bebaru virus *558*
Becker muscular dystrophy 5129, 5195
cardiac involvement *2788*, *2840*
carriers 5195
diagnosis 5195, *5196*
genetic counselling *5197*
management 5197
prognosis 5196, *5196*
Becker's disease 164
Becker's sign 2751
Beckwith-Wiedemann syndrome 1957, *2766*
beclometasone diproprionate, asthma 3300
beclomethasone, COPD 3334
bedbugs 1225, *1227*, *1228*
bee stings 1349
renal toxicity 4092
beetle stings 1351, *1351*
behavioural change 4793
behavioural problems 5263
alcohol and drug states 5266
calming the situation 5264
Emergency Department facilities 5264
inpatient units 5264
staff behaviour 5264
care following tranquillization 5266
emergency medication 5265, *5265*
atypical antipsychotics 3156, 5266
major tranquillizers 5265
minor tranquillizers 5265
evaluation 5263, *5264*

legal rights and duties 5266
psychosis 5266
see also cognitive disorders
behavioural teratology 2189
behavioural therapy, obesity 1533
Behçet's disease 2586, 3649
aetiology and genetics 3684
cardiac involvement 2785
clinical features 3685, *3685*
cardiac 3687
gastrointestinal 3686
mucocutaneous 3685, *3685*
musculoskeletal 3686
neurological 3686
ocular 3686, *5241, 5241*
oral 2272, *3685*
vascular 3686, *3688*
diagnosis 3687, *3687*
differential diagnosis 3687
epidemiology 3685
investigations 3687
management 3687
neurological complications 5163
pathogenesis/pathology 3684
pregnancy 2162
prognosis 3688
pulmonary involvement 3401
skin involvement 4722
treatment 5163
Behr's syndrome *4908*
bejel *see* syphilis, endemic
Bell's palsy 5036
pregnancy 2146
belladonna alkaloids 1361, *1362*
Bence Jones proteinuria 4346
bendrofluazide, in breast milk *1469*
bendroflumethiazide, heart failure *2722*
bends 3802
benorylate, adverse effects, hepatotoxicity *2529*
benoxaprofen, adverse effects, hepatotoxicity *2529, 2533*
benzbromarone, gout 1625, 3644
benzene
carcinogenesis *308, 1380*
poisoning 1307
γ-benzene hexachloride, scabies 1230
benzidine *1380*
benznidazole, Chagas' disease 1132
benzodiazepines 5336
adverse effects, in pregnancy *2188*
breastfeeding *2189*
contraindication in porphyria 1641
poisoning *1274*, 1283
antidote *1274, 5505*
benzoic acid 4733
benzoyl peroxide 4734
3,4-benzpyrene *338*
benzyl alcohol poisoning 1308
benzylpenicillin
diphtheria 668
meningitis 719, *719*
relapsing fevers 872
in renal failure *4185*
S. moniliformis 859
Bergeyella spp. *962*
beriberi 1491
Bernard, Claude, *Introduction to the Study of Experimental Medicine* 11
Bernard-Soulier syndrome, laboratory tests *4504*
Bertiella mucronata 1190
Bertiella studeri 1190
berylliosis 3423, *3424*
beryllium
carcinogenesis *308*
and sarcoidosis 3404
best interests 17
composite theories 18
desire-fulfilment theories 18
mental state theories 17
objective list theories 18
β-agonists 2618
adverse effects, in pregnancy *2188*
COPD 3334
NNT *52*
β_2-agonists
asthma 3301, *3302*
COPD *3335*
long-acting 3302
performance enhancement 5384
poisoning 1284
β-blockers 2618
acute coronary syndromes 2917
adverse effects, in pregnancy *2188*
angina 2908
and asthma 3287
in breast milk *2189*
dilated cardiomyopathy 2776
and exercise testing 2661
heart failure *2722*, 2723
hypertension 2042, *3050*, 3051
hypertensive emergencies *3079*
performance enhancement 5385
poisoning 1284
antidote *1274*
in pregnancy *2099, 2188*
in renal failure 4178
see also individual drugs
beta-lactams
adverse effects *455*
acute interstitial nephritis 4005
endocarditis *704*
infective endocarditis 2811
pregnancy *2171*
Pseudomonas aeruginosa 737
urinary tract infection *4113*
betahistine dihydrochloride, vertigo *4861*
betamethasone dipropionate 4731
betamethasone valerate *2151*, 4731
betamethasone, SLE 2156
betel chewer's cancer 312
bevacizumab *376*, 401, *1939*
cost-effectiveness ratio *53*
bezafibrate 1670
BH3-only proteins 181
BH4 deficiency *1566*
Bhanja virus *581*, 587
biallelic mismatch repair *2406*
bias *33*, 33–4
minimization of 37
bicalutamide, reproductive effects *1917*
bicarbonate dialysis *3933*
bicarbonate wasting 3964
bicarbonate *5515*
duodenal secretion 2306
performance enhancement 5385
plasma/serum *3837*
reference values *5435*
children *5438*
Bichat, Xavier 10
bicipital tendinitis *3248*
biclonal gammopathies 4346
bicycle ergometry 2659
Bifidobacterium matruchotii 851
Bifidobacterium spp. *962*
bifonazole, fungal infections 1015
bile acid sequestrating agents 1670
in renal failure 4177
bile ducts
extrahepatic, cancer 316
malignant obstruction, ERCP 2218
vanishing bile duct syndrome 2470
bile pigment gallstones 2550
bile salts
absorption 2229
malabsorption *2328*
metabolism *2440*, 2441
bile
composition 2548
formation 2440, *2440*
'limey' 2552
physiological functions *2440*
bilharzia *see* schistosomiasis
biliary atresia 2579
classification 2579
differential diagnosis 2580
extrahepatic 2580
imaging 2580
intrahepatic 2580
laboratory investigations 2580
symptoms and signs 2579, *2580*
treatment and prognosis 2580
biliary cirrhosis, primary 2464
aetiology 2464
clinical features 2466
hepatic granuloma 2520
clinical investigation 2466
diagnostic criteria 2466
differential diagnosis 2466
epidemiology 2465
future developments 2468
genetics 2464
historical perspective 2464
pathogenesis 2464, *2465*
pathology 2465, *2465*
prognosis 2467
recurrence post-transplantation 2512
treatment 2466, *2467*
immunosuppressive agents 2467
liver transplantation 2467, 2507
biliary cystadenoma 2521
biliary secretions 2227
biliary strictures 2554
malignant 2554, *2554–5*
biliary tract 2435
anatomy 2436, *2547, 2547*
congenital disorders 2579
biliary atresia 2579
Caroli's disease 2554, *2580–1, 2581*
fibropolycystic disease 2580
in cystic fibrosis 3354
diseases 2546
cholestasis *see* cholestasis
imaging 2548, *2548*
infections 2554
investigation 2547
laboratory investigations 2547
symptoms and signs 2547
bilirubin 14
metabolism 2441, *2441*
physiology 2444, *2445*
reference values *5435*
children *5438*
biliverdin 14, 2445
Bilophila spp. *962*
bioavailability 1451, *1455, 1456*
antimicrobials 449, *449*
biogenic amines *1791*
biomarkers 45
acute coronary syndromes 2916
angina 2907
cardiomyopathy 2775
coronary heart disease 2892
biomedical publications, annual flow *23*
biopsy
bone *see* bone biopsy
bronchial 3220
liver, Wilson's disease 1691
lung *see* lung biopsy
mediastinal masses 3540
muscle *see* muscle biopsy
pleural 3225, 3491
renal *see* renal biopsy
sentinel node 386
skin *see* skin biopsy
biopterin metabolism defects 1583, *1585*
clinical presentation 1584
diagnosis 1585
treatment and outcome 1585
bioterrorism 1440
biological weapons 1441, *1441*
clinical features 1443
decontamination 1444
differential diagnosis 1443
dissemination of bioweapons 1442
epidemiological investigation 1444
epidemiology 1442, *1442*
future developments 1445
history 1441
infectious/contagious diseases 1442
isolation and quarantine 1444
legal and ethical aspects 1445
postexposure prophylaxis 1444
prevention 1443
public education and risk communication 1444
surveillance and early detection 1443
toxins 1442
uncertainty and controversy 1445
biotin 1494
requirements 1494
biotinidase deficiency *1566*, 1578
aetiology/pathophysiology *1577*, 1578
clinical presentation 1578, *1578*
diagnosis 1578
treatment and outcome 1578
bipolar disorder 5325
birds, poisonous 1344, *1344*
birth asphyxia/trauma, child mortality *75*
birthmarks 4692
angiokeratoma corporis diffusum *see* Fabry's disease
blue rubber bleb naevus syndrome 4692
cutis marmorata 4692

Klippel-Trenaunay syndrome 4692
Maffucci's syndrome 4692
port-wine stain 4692
Birt-Hogg-Dube syndrome *363*, 368, 371, 3500
renal carcinoma in 4166
bisacodyl *5426*
bis-chloromethyl ether, carcinogenesis *308*
bismuth chelate, poisoning 1284
bismuth salts, peptic ulcer disease 2311, *2313*
bismuth subsalicylate *2433*
bisoprolol, heart failure *2722*
bisphosphonates 383
adverse effects 1857
osteoporosis *3799*, 3800
Paget's disease 3744
bites
animal 5499
arthropod 1226
human 5369
bithionol, paragonimiasis 1219
Bitis arietans (puff adder) 1328
antivenom *1340*
Bitis rhinoceros (rhinoceros viper) *1238*
bivalirudin, acute coronary syndromes 2920
BK virus 600, 605
black cohosh 68
drug interactions *69*
toxicity 68
Black Creek Canal virus *581*
black piedra 1004
blackflies 1227
blackheads 1382
bladder cancer 327, 4163
aetiology
artificial sweeteners 328
medicines 328
occupational 327
parasitic infection 328
smoking 328
genetic changes 4163
incidence *301*
risk factors 4163, *4163*
staging and grading 4163, *4164*
high-risk superficial 4164
low-risk noninvasive 4163
metastatic transitional cell carcinoma 4165
muscle invasion 4164, *4165*
transitional cell carcinoma of kidney or ureter 4165
bladder
abnormal emptying 4116
cancer 4162
care of in poisoned patients 1278
painful bladder syndrome 4111
Blalock-Taussig shunt 2865, *2865*
Blarina brevicauda (North American short-tailed shrew) 1327
Blastocystis hominis 1118
aetiology and biology *1112, 1114*, 1118, *1119*
clinical features and treatment 1118
diagnosis 1118
epidemiology 1118
pathogenicity 1119
Blastomyces dermatitidis 1011
HIV-associated infection *3247*
pneumonia 3237
Blastomyces spp., osteomyelitis *3789*
blastomycosis *1009*, 1011
clinical features 1012
epidemiology 1011
Blatta orientalis (common cockroach) 1236
Blattella germanica (German cockroach) 1236
Blau syndrome *1761*, 1765
bleach, poisoning by 1317
bleeding diatheses 5244
bleeding tendency 4498
acquired haemophilia 4506
clinical assessment 4499
clinical examination 4500
mucosa 4501
musculoskeletal system 4501
skin 4500
splenomegaly 4501
critically ill patients 4505
disseminated intravascular coagulation 4505
drug-induced bleeding 4503
history 4499
investigations 4503, *4504*
massive transfusion 4505
neonate 4506
surgical bleeding 4505
thrombocytopenia 4505
von Willebrand disease 4505
acquired 4506
bleeding time *4196*, 4503
acute renal trauma 3894, *3894*
bleeding
treatment 4506
acute bleeding 4506
nonacute bleeding 4506
bleomycin 398
adverse effects *400*
hepatotoxicity *2534*
lymphoma *4320, 4320*
malignant pleural effusion 391
skin disorders 4738
blepharospasm 4892, *4893*
Blighia sapida (Ackee fruit) *1363*
blindness 5252
blisters, drug poisoning 1274
bloating 2386
blockbuster drugs 61
Blomstrand's chondrodysplasia *1855, 1865, 3721*, 3729
mutations in *3757*
blood coagulation *see* coagulation
blood count 4194, 4502
SLE 3661
blood disorders 4191
approach to 4191
blood workup 4191
clinical features, oral 2284, *2284*
hepatic involvement 2541
history 4191
physical examination 4191
pregnancy 2173
anaemia 2173
haemoglobinopathies 2173–4
haemostasis 2173, 2177
see also individual conditions
blood doping 5385
blood film 4194, *4195*
blood gases *5437*
blood group systems 4562, *4563*
ABO 4562, *4563*
compatibility *290*
incompatibility 4458
antibody detection 4563
Rh 4562
incompatibility 4457
blood pressure
CKD 3913
clinical trials 43, *43*
and coronary heart disease 2888, *2891*
measurement 3041, *3041*
ambulatory blood pressure 3041, *3042*
home blood pressure 3042
monitors 3041, *3041*
pregnancy 2088
and sleep 3030, 3048
see also hypertension
blood substitutes 4570
blood transfusion 4561
autoantibodies 4564
autologous 4570
compatibility testing 4564
complications 4566, *4566*
acute intravascular haemolytic reactions 4566
allergic reactions 4567
delayed extravascular haemolytic reactions 4567
febrile nonhaemolytic reactions 4567
graft-vs-host disease 4568
septic reactions 4567
transfusion-related acute lung injury 4568
cytomegalovirus-safe 4570
disease transmission 4568, *4569*
irradiation 4570
leucoreduction 4569
liver disorders 2541
massive 4535, 4515
plasma, cryoprecipitate and plasma derivatives 4565
platelets 4565
red blood cells 4564, *4564*
see also blood group systems
blood vessels 2593
adventitia 2594, 2602
in cyanosis 2846
disorders of 4683
arterial and peripheral ischaemic disorders 4686
cutaneous manifestations 4684, *4684*
lymphatic disorders 4694
pressure ulcers 4688
telangiectasis 4690, *4690*
vascular birthmarks 4692
vascular tumours 4693
venous disorders 4688
endothelium 2594, *2594*
integrated responses of 2593
intima 2594
media 2594
pathophysiology 2594
wall 4481, *4481*
adventitia 4484
endothelial cells 4481
extracellular matrix 4483, *3550, 4483–4*
role in coagulation 4495, *4496*
smooth muscle cells *see* vascular smooth muscle cells
see also vascular
blood volume *2620, 2623, 4196*, 4198
blood
cerebrospinal fluid 4750
constituents of 4194, *4194*
transfusion, granulocytes 4566
Bloom's syndrome 302, *341, 360, 368, 4668*
and leukaemia 332
Blount's disease *3804*
blubber finger 958
blue rubber bleb naevus syndrome 4692
bocavirus *474*, 481
BODE index *3331*
body dysmorphic disorder 5302
body lice 1231
body mass index *1528*, 1537
as predictor of endstage renal disease *3917*
Boerhaave's syndrome 2303
Bohr effect 1744
Bolivian haemorrhagic fever *see* South American haemorrhagic fever
bombesin 2319
Bombus spp. (bumble bee) 1349
bone age 1953
bone biopsy
bone disease 3733
osteomalacia 3738
bone cells 3722, *3722*
see also individual cell types
bone density
changes in *3562*
familial high *3721*
increased 3759
bone disease
deformity and short stature 3729
diagnosis 3729, *3734*
dialysis patients 3942
ectopic calcification 3762, *3763*
chondrocalcinosis 3764
dystrophic 3764
in hyperphosphataemia 3764
with hypocalcaemia 3764
idiopathic soft-tissue 3764
in inherited hypophosphataemia 3764
metastatic 3764
without bone formation 3762
ectopic ossification 3720, 3762, *3763*, 3764
acquired 3764
after neurological injury 3764
inherited 3765
posttraumatic 3764
history 3729
hyperparathyroidism *see* hyperparathyroidism
intestinal failure-associated 1542
investigations 3731
biochemistry 3731, *3731*
bone biopsy 3733
radiology 3733
metabolic 3719, *3721*
osteoporosis *see* osteoporosis
Paget's *see* Paget's disease of bone
physical signs 3730
presentation 3719
skeletal dysplasia 1956, 3720
see also musculoskeletal disease; and individual conditions
bone formation *3550*, 3723

bone infections
actinomycotic 854
anaerobic 752
Pseudomonas aeruginosa 737
tuberculosis 820
bone marrow failure 4401
bone marrow transplantation
adenosine deaminase deficiency 1632
aplastic anaemia *4295*, 4288
complications, haemorrhagic cystitis 605
leukaemia 4237
mucopolysaccharidoses 1712
multiple myeloma 4349
bone marrow
activity and distribution 4192
anatomy 4200, *4200–2*
erythropoiesis 4369
examination 4191
in malaria 1062
bone mass 3725
see also osteoporosis
bone mineral density, osteoporosis 3798
bone mineralization 3727
bone morphogenetic proteins 158, 3720
bone pain 3730
bone resorption 3724
bone tumours 320
incidence *321*
metastatic 381
bone turnover
markers of 3799
measurement of 3729, *3729*
bone 3549, 3719
acidosis 1745
collagen 3548, *3548, 3725–6*
cortical 3721
cysts 3713
modelling 3719
noncollagen proteins 3726
physiology 3720
structure 3721
trabecular 3721
borage, drug interactions *69*
Bordeaux mixture *3436*
Bordetella pertussis 764
aetiology, genetics, pathogenesis and pathology 765
clinical features 765
clinical investigation 766
diagnosis 766
differential diagnosis 766
epidemiology 765
history 765
morbidity 765
mortality 765
prevention 765
prognosis 767
treatment 766, *766*
vaccine adverse events 767, 767
Bordetella spp. *962*
Bornholm disease 530, 3185
Borrelia afzelii 861
Borrelia burgdorferi 860–1, 2763
osteomyelitis *3789*
Borrelia crocidurae 867
Borrelia duttonii 866
Borrelia garinii 861
Borrelia hermsii 867
Borrelia hispanica 867
Borrelia parkeri 867
Borrelia recurrentis *866*, 866–7, 1231
Borrelia spp. *962*
Borrelia turicatae 867
bortezomib
adverse effects, neuropathy 5088
multiple myeloma 4350
Bosea spp. *962*
bosentan, pulmonary arterial hypertension 2988
bosutinib 4254
Bothrops (Bothriopsis) bilineatus, antivenom *1340*
Bothrops asper, antivenom *1340*
Bothrops atrox, antivenom *1340*
Bothrops jararaca, antivenom *1340*
Bothrops marajoensis 1335
Bothrops spp. (lancehead vipers) *1239*, 1329
botox 804, 1442
botrocetin *4540*
botulism 803, 804
definition 804
diagnosis 805
history 805
infant 806
occurrence 804
pathogenesis 805
physical examination 805
toxin 804, 1442
treatment 806
wound 806
Bouboui virus *566*
Bouchard's nodes 3632
bourgeons conjunctifs 3385
Bourneville's disease *see* tuberous sclerosis
boutonnière deformity 3587
Bowditch phenomenon 2624
bowel-associated dermatosis-arthritis syndrome 4634
Bowen's disease *4675*, 4707
bowstring sign 3588
bracheobronchiomegaly 3260
brachial plexopathy, postirradiation 5079
brachial plexus neuropathy 5079
Brachylaima cribbi *1223–4*
Brachyspira spp. *962*
brachytherapy 2940
Bracycephalus spp. 1346
Bradley, Andrew 190
bradycardias 2688, 2691
aetiology and mechanisms 2691
atrioventricular block *see* atrioventricular block
management 2691, *2691*
acute 2691
pacemaker therapy 2694
neurogenic syncope 2692
presentation 5459
sick sinus syndrome 2639, *2688, 2692, 2692–3*
and syncope *2638*, 2639
Bradyrhizobium spp. *962*
brain death 4847, 4848
actions 4849
children 4848
diagnosis 4848
testing for 4848
brain imaging 5274
brain natriuretic peptide *2635*
reference values *5441*
brain tumours 328, *328*
cognitive impairment 5276
metastatic 390
brain
basal ganglia 4874
cerebellum 4872
cognitive domains 4788
effects of malnutrition 1510
hypertensive damage 3036
cerebral infarction 3036
cognitive function 3037
encephalopathy 3037
intracerebral haemorrhage 3036
imaging
cerebral angiography 4770
computed tomography 4769
contrast enhancement 4770
MRI 4769, *4770*
myelography 4771
see also individual modalities
in malaria *see* cerebral malaria
motor area 4787
relapsing fever *869*
sensory inputs 4787
auditory 4788
somatosensory 4787
vision 4787
thalamus 4877
brainstem auditory-evoked potentials 4757
brainstem death 3161
concept of 3161
diagnosis 3162, *3162*
non-organ donors 3163
patient management 3161, *3162*
potential organ donors 3163
brainstem encephalitis 5171
brainstem glioma 4779
brainstem syndromes 4929
diencephalic 4929, 5274
investigations and treatment 4932
medullary 4932, *4932*
midbrain 4930, *4930*
pontine 4930
pseudobulbar palsy 4932
tectal deafness 4930
thalamic 4930
thalamic stroke syndrome 4930
branchio-oto-renal syndrome 4102
BRCA1/2 genes 302, 358, 361, *363*, 364, 1930
breast cancer 1928, 323
anthropometric factors 1929
clinical approach 1930
clinical assessment 1928
diagnosis *1930–1*, 1931
dietary factors 1929
disease burden 1928
epidemiology 1928
familial 1929, *1930*
female reproductive hormones in 1929
future developments 1938, *1939*
genetic predisposition 364
genome association 141, *361*
hereditary 1929
histopathology 1931
ductal carcinoma *in situ* 1931, *1932*
invasive carcinoma 1932, *1932*
predictive markers 1933, *1933*
and hormone replacement therapy 50
HRT effects 2197
incidence *301*, *323*
migrants vs residents *302*
management 1928
monitoring 1931
radiotherapy 1934, *1936*
surgery 1933, *1934*
surveillance 1931
systemic therapy 1935, *1937*
biological therapy 1935
chemotherapy 1935
endocrine therapy 1935
metastatic 1937, *1938*
mortality *323*
pregnancy 2183
prevention 1929
screening 105, *106, 1930, 1930*
staging 1931
breast disease, benign 1940
congenital abnormalities 1940
cystic change 1941
diabetic mastopathy 1941
fat necrosis 1941
fibroadenoma 1940, *1940*
fibromatosis 1941
hamartoma 1941
inflammation 1941
macrocysts 1941
male breast 1942
mastalgia 1941
nipple/areola complex 1941, *1941*
phylloides tumours 1941
breast mice 1940, *1940*
breastfeeding, drugs and 1468, *1469*, 2188, *2189*, 4823
breath tests
bacterial overgrowth 2333
carbon dioxide *2227*
glucose-hydrogen *2230*
hydrogen *2227*
lactose-hydrogen *2228*
urea *2230*
breathing *see* respiration; respiratory
breathlessness 2628, *2632, 2632, 3182, 3183*
causes *3183*
conditions causing *2633*
airways disease 2635
hypertrophic cardiomyopathy 2781
left ventricular failure 2633
pulmonary embolism 2635
lung cancer 3519
modified Borg scale *3326*
modified MRC dyspnoea scale *3326*
New York Heart Association classification *2633*
palliative care 5425, *5426*
prediction of heart failure *2634*
pregnancy 2088
with preserved left ventricular function 2636
Brescia-Cimino fistula 3939
bretylium, in renal failure *4179*
Brevibacterium spp. *962*
Brevundimonas spp. *962*
Brill-Zinsser disease 912
Briquet's syndrome 5301
Bristol Activities of Daily Living Scale (BADLS) 5406
British National Formulary 1451
'brittle' diabetes 2018
Broca's aphasia 4789
bromhidrosis 4677
bromide, reference values *5445*

bromocriptine
adverse effects,
hepatotoxicity *2529*, *2532*
in breast milk *1469*
prolactinoma 1811
in pregnancy 2140
bronchi 3175, *3176*
radiographic view 3207
bronchial adenoma 3532
bronchial carcinoid 3532
bronchial thermoplasty *3223*, 3224
bronchiectasis 3345
aetiology and pathogenesis 3346, *3346–7*
developmental defects 3346
excessive immune response 3347
immune deficiency 3347
mechanical obstruction 3348
mucociliary clearance disorders 3347
postinfective 3348
toxic insult 3348
associated conditions 3348
autoimmune rheumatic disorders *3390*, 3391
complications 3351
definition 3345
epidemiology 3345
examination 3348
future developments 3352
history 3348
idiopathic 3348
imaging 3215, *3215*
investigation and diagnosis 3348
cause of disease 3349, *3350*
disease state 3349, *3349*
radiological imaging 3348, *3349*
management 3350, *3350–1*
anti-inflammatory therapy 3351
antibiotics 3350
bronchodilators 3351
monitoring response 3351
surgery 3351
pathology 3346
microscopic features 3346
prognosis 3352
systemic sclerosis *3672*
bronchioles 3175, *3176*
terminal 3178, *3179*
bronchiolitis obliterans syndrome *3483*
bronchiolitis obliterans *1599*, *3379*, 3383
autoimmune rheumatic disorders *3390*, 3391
clinical features 3383
differential diagnosis 3384
histopathology 3383, *3383*
investigations 3383
imaging 3383, *3384*
lung function tests 3384
and rheumatoid arthritis 3588
treatment 3384
bronchiolitis 3321, *3321*, *3368*
follicular 3386
obstructive 3312
viral aetiology *474*
bronchitis
chronic 3312, *3318*, *3320*
morbidity *3316*
bronchoalveolar lavage 3220, *3221*
diffuse parenchymal lung disease 3373
organizing pneumonia 3385
pulmonary fibrosis 3378
bronchoconstriction 3170
bronchodilatation 3170
bronchodilators
acute asthma 3308
in breast milk *2189*
bronchiectasis 3351
COPD 3334, *3335–6*, 3342
cystic fibrosis 3360
inhaled 3308
intravenous 3308
in renal failure 4181
bronchogenic cysts *3542*, 3543
bronchography, complications 3466
bronchoscopy 3216–17
contraindications 3217
diagnostic role 3222
diffuse lung disease 3222
lung cancer 3222
respiratory infection 3223
disinfection 3218
equipment 3218
indications 3217, *3217*
lung cancer 3524
patient preparation 3218, *3218*
procedure 3219, *3219*
techniques and sampling 3220
bronchial biopsies 3220
bronchial brushings 3220
bronchial washings 3220
bronchoalveolar lavage 3220, *3221*
endobronchial ultrasound 3221, *3221*
fine needle aspiration 3220
fluorescence bronchoscopy 3222
lung biopsy 3220
magnetic navigation 3221, *3222*
therapeutic role 3223
asthma *3223*, 3224
emphysema 3223, *3223*
lung cancer 3223
bronchovascular bundle 2974
broom
drug interactions *69*
toxicity 68
Brown-Séquard syndrome 4743
Brown-Violetto-van Laere syndrome 5073
Brucella abortus 789
renal toxicity *4086*
Brucella canis 789
Brucella melitensis 789
Brucella spp. *962*
infective endocarditis *2812*
osteomyelitis *791*, *793*, *3789*
Brucella suis 789
brucellosis 789
aetiological agent 789
clinical features 790, *790*
diagnosis 793
epidemiology 789
localizations 790, *791–3*
mode of transmission 789
pathogenesis 789
prevention 794
treatment 794
Brugada syndrome 2612, 2715
sudden unexplained death during sleep 3840
Brugia malayi 1153–5
renal toxicity 4088
Brugia spp. *1176*
Brugia timori 1153–5
Brugmansia suaveolens (angel's trumpet) *1362*
Bruton's agammaglobulinaemia tyrosine kinase (BTK) 244
bryostatin *11939*
bubonic plague *see Yersinia pestis*
buccal drug administration 1452
Buchner, Eduard 11
Budd-Chiari syndrome 2483
liver transplantation 2508
pregnancy 2130
budesonide
asthma 3300
COPD 3334
primary biliary cirrhosis *2467*
Buerger's disease 2960, 4687
Bukalasa bat virus *566*
bulimia nervosa 5319
management 5323
bullae *4591*
Bulleidia spp. *962*
bullosis diabeticorum 2048
bullous emphysema 3343
bullous pemphigoid *4603*, 4606, *4606*
bumetanide, heart failure *2722*
bundle branch block 2650
left 2650, *2651*, 2657
right 2651, *2652*
bundle of His *see* His bundle
Bungarus caeruleus (common krait) 1328
antivenom *1340*
Bunina bodies 5070
Bunostomum trigonocephalum *1176*
Bunyamwera virus 580, *581*
Bunyaviridae 579
Hantavirus 582
Nairovirus *581*, 585
Orthobunyavirus 580
Phlebovirus *581*, 586
viral taxonomy and vectors 580, *581–2*
see also individual viruses
buprenorphine 1290
palliative care 5423
buprioprion, adverse effects *5313*
Burkholderia cepacia, cystic fibrosis 3356
Burkholderia mallei 771
Burkholderia pseudomallei 768
osteomyelitis *3789*
renal toxicity *4086*
Burkitt's lymphoma 300
endemic ('African') 502, 505, 1082
sporadic 505
translocations *341*
Burkitt's lymphoma/leukaemia 4227
burns
electrical 1425
lightning injuries 1424
nutrition support 1542, *1543*
radiation 1431
burr cells *4195*
bursitis
anserine *3248*, *3557*
olecranon *3248*, 3588
prepatellar *3248*
septic 698, *700*
trochanteric *3248*
Buruli ulcer 833, 848
aetiology 848
clinical features 849
disseminated disease 849
localized disease 849, *849*
differential diagnosis 849
epidemiology and transmission 848
laboratory diagnosis 850
pathogenesis 849
pathology 849
prevention and control 850
socioeconomic impact 850
treatment 850
buspirone 5338
Bussuquara virus *566*
busulfan 398
adverse effects,
hepatotoxicity *2533*, *2536*
busulphan, carcinogenesis *307*
butcher's warts *4675*
butoconazole, candidiasis 1258
butterburr, migraine prevention *4916*
butterfly stings 1351
Buttiauxella spp. *962*
Butvrivibrio spp. *962*
butyrophenones, poisoning 1283
Bwamba virus *581*, 587
bystander apoptosis 596

C1 esterase inhibitor, reference values *5444*
C1 inhibitor *216*, *1753*
antibodies 221
deficiency 218, *254*
C1q, deficiency *254*
C1r, deficiency *254*
C1s *1753*
deficiency *254*
C2, *1753*
deficiency *254*
C3 *224*, *1753*
deficiency *254*
unregulated activation 219, *220*
C3 nephritic factor 221
C3a 286
C3b 286
C4 *224*, *1753*
deficiency *254*
C4b 286
C4-binding protein *216*
C5, deficiency *254*
C 56, *1753*
C5a 286
C6, deficiency *254*
C7, deficiency *254*
C8, deficiency *254*
C9, deficiency *254*
CA125, reference values *5442*
CA19–9, reference values *5442*
Cabassou virus *558*
cabergoline
prolactinoma 1811
in pregnancy 2140
Cabot's rings *4195*
Cacipacore virus *566*
caclizumab 292
CADASIL 5110
cadmium
carcinogenesis *308*, *338*
poisoning 1297, *3739*, 4018
skeletal effects 3769
reference values *5445*
reproductive effects *1917*
caeruloplasmin *1753*
reference values *5444*

caffeine
in breast milk *1469*
orthostatic hypotension *5063*
performance enhancement 5385
in pregnancy 2090
caftazidime, pneumonia *3238*
Caisson disease 3802
calamine 4732
calcidiol
CKD-MBD *3922*
deficiency 3918, *3918*
calcific arteriolopathy 4721
calcific periarthritis 3647, *3647*
calcific tendinitis *3248*
calcification 3564
ectopic, of renal disease 3714
calcineurin inhibitors
adverse effects 3955, *3955*
effects on renin-angiotensin-aldosterone system 3843
post-transplantation *290,* 291, 3482, *3954*
psoriasis 4614
calcinosis cutis 3694
calcinosis 3564
calciotropic hormones, ectopic secretion 2061
calciphylaxis *4686*, 4687
calcipotriol 4733
calcitonin gene-related peptide 1803, 2320
calcitonin
calcium balance 3728
ectopic secretion 2065
hypercalcaemia 1857
Paget's disease 3744
reference values *5442*
calcitriol, CKD-MBD *3922*
calcium antagonists
acute coronary syndromes 2917
angina 2909
contraindication in porphyria *5484*
and exercise testing 2661
heart failure 2724
hypertension 2042, *3050*, 3051
hypertensive emergencies *3079*
mode of action 1461
poisoning 1285
antidote *1274*
pulmonary arterial hypertension 2987
Raynaud's phenomenon *3671*
in renal failure 4180
STEMI 2933
see also individual drugs
calcium balance 3727, *3727*
calcitonin 3728
parathyroid hormone 3728
parathyroid-hormone-related protein 3729
vitamin D 3728, *3728*
calcium channel blockers *see* calcium antagonists
calcium channels 160
calcium gluconate, drug interactions *1471*
calcium oxalate *1362*
stones *4124*
calcium phosphate
stones *4124*, 4129
calcium pyrophosphate deposition disease 3633
calcium sodium edetate 1462
calcium
CKD-MBD *3922*
dietary reference values *1502*
homeostasis 1852, *1852–3*, 1854
hyperkalaemia *3891*
malabsorption 3890
osteoporosis 3800
reference intake *1524*
reference values *5435*, *5446*
children *5438*
requirements in pregnancy 2083
serum, control of 3921, *3922*
stones 4126
genetics and environment *4126*, *4128*
pathology/pathogenesis 4126, *4129–30*
prevention 4124
urinary *3837*
calcium-sensing receptor abnormalities 1866
caliciviruses 538
diarrhoea 2427
epidemiology 540
immune response 539
replication 538
structure and classification 538, *539*
California encephalitis 580, *581*
Callilepsis laureola (impila) poisoning 4092
Calliphora spp. *1233*
Calliphoridae (Congo floor maggot) *1226*, *1233*
Calloselasma rhodostoma (Malayan pit viper) 1329, *1335*
antivenom *1340*
calnexin 129
Calotropis spp. 1373
Calovo virus *581*
calprotectin 2230
faecal 2375
calreticulin 129
calsequestrin 2607
Calyptra eustrigata 1236
Calyptra eustrigata 1236
cAMP response element binding proteins *see* CREBs
Campbell de Morgan spots 4691
camphor 4733
campomelic dysplasia *3721*
mutations in *3757*
Campylobacter gracilis *852*
Campylobacter jejuni 801, 2247
Campylobacter spp. 727, *733*, *962*
clinical features 734
epidemiology 733
laboratory diagnosis 734
pathogenesis 733
treatment 734
Camurati-Engelmann disease 175, *3721*, *3759*, *3759*
Canale-Smith syndrome 186
Canavan's disease *1566*, 1580, 5107
cancer antigens 372, 375
cancer/testis 375
differentiation 376
overexpressed 377
unique 377
viral 377
cancer cachexia syndrome 382
cancer 299, 333, 380
causes 302
avoidable 304
alcohol 305
diet 309
drugs 307
immunosuppression 307
infection 306
interacting factors 311
ionizing radiation 305
occupation 307
physical inactivity 311
pollution 308
reproduction and hormone secretion 310
tobacco 304, *304–5*
ultraviolet radiation 306
biological factors
age 303
delay between cause and effect 303
gender 303
genetic susceptibility 302
chance 304
diagnosis, histopathological 383
emergency situations 389
carcinomatous 'meningitis' 390
cerebral metastasis 390
pericardial effusion 391
pleural effusion 391
spinal cord/cauda equina compression 389, *389*
epidemiology 299
site of origin 312
genetic alterations 340
genetic counselling 369
identification of at-risk families 370
risk assessment 369
genetic predisposition 358, 364
breast cancer 364
clinical management 370
colon cancer 364, *364*
identification and management 369
lifestyle changes 370
melanoma 365
ovarian cancer 365
pancreatic cancer 365
prevention strategies 370
prostate cancer 365
response to treatment 370
upper GI cancer 365
genetic testing 370
haematological changes 4548, *4549*
anaemia 383, *4548*, *4549*
chemotherapy-induced changes 4550
haemophagocytic syndrome 4550
platelets and blood coagulation 4548, *4549–50*
polycythaemia 4548
white-cell abnormalities 4550
HIV-related 3251
human antigens 375
immune adjuvants 372
immune surveillance 374, *374*
immune tolerance 373
immunity 372
incidence
between communities 300, *301*
changes in migrant groups 301, *302*
changes with time 301
inherited 358
clinical features 358
historical aspects 359
management 358
mechanisms *358*, *360*
association studies 362
linkage analysis 362
phenotypic features 362
rare syndromes 365, *365*
investigation 383
malignant phenotype 336, *336*
management 388, *388*
antibodies *376*
chemotherapy *388*, 397
immunotherapy 372, 377
radiotherapy *388*, 401
surgery 388
metastatic 337, 354
fron unknown primary site 392, *392*
staging 386
mortality rate *76*, *311*
nutrition-related 1521, *1521*
occupational 307, *308*, 1379
bladder 327
lung 318
post-transplant 3962, *3962*
predisposition genes 361
risks associated with 362, *363*
pregnancy 2181
breast cancer 2183
cervical cancer 2183
colon cancer 2184
gestational trophoblastic disease 2182
leukaemia 2184
lymphoma 2184
melanoma 2184
ovarian cancer 2183
thyroid cancer 2184
preventability 300
renal involvement 4076, *4072*
direct 4076
immune reactions 4077
metabolic effects 4076
remote effects 4076
treatment effects 4078
screening 105, 370
staging 386, *387*
distant metastases 386
lymph node spread 386
notation 387, *388*
surgical 387
supportive care 393
long-term consequences of treatment 394
pain management 394
psychological support 393
symptoms and signs 381
anaemia 383
fever 382
hypercalcaemia 383
pain 381
paraneoplastic syndromes 383
tumour mass 382
weight loss 382
two-hit hypothesis 335, *335*
vaccines 376, *376*
viral carcinogenesis 355, 653, *653*
HPV *306*, *357*, *601*, 604, *3962*
mechanisms 654
treatment and prevention 654
viral treatments 654
see also individual cancer sites
cancer/testis (CT) antigens 375
cancrum oris (noma) 2269

candesartan
heart failure *2722*
migraine prevention *4916*
Candida albicans 1256, *1258*, *3436*
infective oesophagitis *2293*
Candida glabrata 1258
candida intertrigo 1003
Candida spp. 801
endophthalmitis *438*
osteomyelitis *3789*
pregnancy *2171*
candidiasis
mucocutaneous without endocrinopathy *238*
oesophageal 629
oral (thrush) *1000*, 1002, 2267
aetiology 2267
clinical features 2267, *2268*
differential diagnosis 2268
HIV/AIDS *626*, *2266*
pathology 2267
treatment 2269
superficial 998, 1002
aetiology 1002
chronic 1003
clinical features 1003
epidemiology 1003
laboratory diagnosis 1004
predisposing factors *1003*
treatment 1004
systemic *1009*, 1012, *1012*
aetiology 1012
clinical features 1013
epidemiology 1013
laboratory diagnosis 1013
treatment 1013
vulvovaginal 1256, 1258
Candiru virus *581*
cannabis
poisoning 1285
reproductive effects *1917*
canthariasis 1225, *1235*, 1235
Capecchi, Mario 191
capecitabine, breast cancer *1937*
Capillaria hepatica 1168, 1171
Capillaria philippinensis 2357, *2357*
capillariasis 1168, 1171, 1240
hepatic 1171, *1172*
intestinal 1171, *1171*
capillaries 2594
capillary leakage syndrome 588
Caplan's syndrome 3391, 3416
Capnocytophaga canimorsus 1326
Capnocytophaga spp. *852*, *962*, *2260*
capnography, acute respiratory failure 3136
capsaicin
diabetic neuropathy 2040
neuropathic pain 5415
Capsicum spp. 1373
captopril
adverse effects
hepatotoxicity *2529*, *2532–3*
oesophagitis *2294*
renal toxicity *3860*
heart failure *2722*
hypertensive emergencies *3079*
Caraparu virus *581*
carate *see* pinta
carbamate insecticide poisoning *1274*, 1302
antidote *1274*
carbamazepine 5334
adverse effects 5334
hepatotoxicity *2529*, *2532–3*, *2535*
in breast milk *1469*, *2189*
diabetic neuropathy 2039
dose levels *4823*
drug interactions *1471*, *3968*, *5334*
epilepsy 4820
indications and use 5334
metastatic brain tumours 390
poisoning 1280
serum levels *5449*
teratogenicity *1468*, 2148, *2187*, *4823*
vertigo *4861*
carbamylation 3871
carbapenem, pneumonia *3238*
carbenicillin, adverse effects, hepatotoxicity *2529*
carbimazole 1840
adverse effects, hepatotoxicity *2529*, *2532–3*
in breast milk *1469*, *2189*
carbocisteine 3337
carbohydrate intolerance syndrome 2348, *2348*
lactose intolerance 2348
sucrase-isomaltase deficiency 2350
trehalase deficiency 2350
carbohydrate metabolism, disorders of 1596
acidosis 1744
galactose, pentose and pyruvate metabolism 1610
glycogen storage diseases 1596
inborn errors of fructose metabolism 1604
carbohydrate-response element binding protein (ChREBP) *1482*
carbohydrates
absorption 2228, *2228*
daily intake *1480*
digestion 2347, *2348*
luminal phase 2347
mucosal phase 2347
links with fats 1484
metabolism *1480*, 1481, 2441, *2441*
diabetes mellitus type 1 2000
insulin effects 1994, *1995*
postabsorptive state 1481
postprandial 1482
in pregnancy 2081
requirements 1539
stores *1480*
carbon dioxide breath test *2227*
carbon dioxide
narcosis 3507
poisoning 1308
carbon disulphide
poisoning 1308
CNS effects *1386*
peripheral nervous system effects *1387*
carbon monoxide
poisoning 1308
antidote *1274*
CNS effects 1379
peripheral nervous system effects *1387*
uptake 3189, 3194, *3194–5*
carbon tetrachloride, hepatotoxicity *1385*
carbonic anhydrase II deficiency 3761
carboplatin
breast cancer *1937*
lung cancer 3529–30
carboxyhaemoglobin, drug overdose *5505*
carboxyhaemoglobinaemia 4444
carbuncles 697, *698*
carbutamide, adverse effects, hepatotoxicity *2529*
carcinoembryonic antigen, reference values *5442*
carcinogenesis 337, *337*, 1467
and apoptosis 187, *187*
cancer stem cell hypothesis 340, *340–1*
cellular transformation 338
initiators and promotors 338
monoclonal theory *338–40*, 339
multistep pathway 361
mutation *338*
origin of cancer cells 339
carcinogens *338*
alcohol 305
asbestos *308*, 320
chemotherapeutic agents 307, *307*
ingestion of 309
polycyclic hydrocarbons 338, *307–8*
tobacco 304, *304–5*
carcinoid syndrome 2322
biochemistry 2323, *2323*
bronchial 3532
clinical features 2323
intestinal 2222
investigations 2323, *2324*
prognosis 2324
treatment 2324
carcinoma erysipeloides 4695, *4695*
carcinomatous meningitis 390
cardiac action potential 2603, *2603*, *2610*, *2612*
membrane potential 2610
ion channels 2610
origin of 2610
phase 0 *2610*, *2612*
phase 1 *2612*, *2614*
phase 2 2613
phase 3 2614
phase 4 2614
regional variation in 2614, *2615*
see also myocytes, cardiac
cardiac allograft vasculopathy 2731, *2731*
cardiac arrest 3097
advanced life support 3097, 3099
audit and research 3104
basic life support 3097
chain of survival *3098*
CPR 3097–8
decision-making 3104
defibrillation 3101
DNAR order 3097
electrophysiological assessment 3104
epidemiology 3098
future developments 3105
historical perspective 3097
postresuscitation care 3097, 3102
airway and breathing 3103
cerebral perfusion 3103
circulation 3103
disability and exposure 3103
seizure control 3103
temperature control 3103
therapeutic hypothermia 3104
presentation 5453, *5453*
prevention 3098
prognosis 3104
cardiac arrhythmias 2688, *3120*
bradycardias *see* bradycardias
definition 2690
ECG 2647
exercise testing 2661
genetic syndromes 2690, 2714
hypertension-induced 3036
investigation 2690
ambulatory ECG 2690
ECG 2690, *2690*
electrophysiological studies 2691, *2691*
poisoned patients 1277
pregnancy 2114
symptoms 2690
tachycardias *see* tachycardias
cardiac catheterization/angiography 2678
cardiac flow/output 2681
complications 2687, *2687*
coronary artery anatomy/function 2685
indications 2679
aortic regurgitation 2753
cardiac myxoma 2832
congenital heart disease 2679
congestive heart failure 2679
coronary artery disease 2679
dilated cardiomyopathy 2776
hypertrophic cardiomyopathy 2770
mitral regurgitation 2745
mitral stenosis *2684*, 2740
pericardial disease 2679, *2679*
pulmonary vascular disease 2680
valvular heart disease 2679
intracardiac pressures 2681, *2681*
intracardiac shunts 2683
left heart 2680
left ventricular dysfunction 2685, *2685*
patient preparation 2680
pregnancy 2109
quantitative 2683
right heart 2680
pulmonary arterial hypertension 2986
valvular regurgitation 2684
valvular stenosis 2684, *2684*
vascular access 2680
vascular resistance 2683, *2684*
cardiac cycle 2619, *2619*
mechanical events 2620, *2620*
cardiac flow 2681
cardiac function 2622
afterload 2622, *2623*
Frank-Starling relationship 2622, *2622*
preload 2622, *2622*
cardiac glycosides 1363, *1363*, *1364*
in renal failure 4177
cardiac muscle channelopathies 163
cardiac output 2621, 2681, 3126
angiographic output 2682
dye dilution 2682, *2682*
oximetry 2681, *2682*
pregnancy 2076, *2076*
thermodilution 2682

cardiac pacemaker *see* sinoatrial node
cardiac pacing *see* pacing
cardiac repair 201
cardiac reserve 2626
cardiac sarcoidosis 2763
cardiac stem cells 200
cardiac syncope *2637–8*, 2639, 4816
  bradycardia *2638*, 2639
  structural cardiovascular disease *2638*, 2639
  tachycardia *2638*, 2639
cardiac tamponade 2790, *2792*, *3120*
  causes 2792
  clinical features 2793
  differential diagnosis 2793
  investigations 2793, *2793–4*
  management 2793
  pathophysiology 2792
  presentation 5465
cardiac transplantation 2729
  complications 2730
    cardiac allograft vasculopathy 2731, *2731*
    hyperlipidaemia 2731
    renal dysfunction 2731
  donor-recipient matching 2730
  heart failure 2727
  immunosuppression 2730, *2730*
    see also transplantation immunology
  outcome 2730, *2731*
  recipient selection 2730, *2730*
cardiac tumours 2830
  benign 2832
  metastatic 2832
  myxoma 2830
    clinical features 2831
    investigations 2831, *2831*
    pathology 2830
    treatment and prognosis 2832
  pericardial 2796
cardial malformations, antenatal screening *102*
Cardiobacterium hominis 859
Cardiobacterium spp. *962*
cardiogenic shock 3122, 3127
cardiomegaly, bartonellosis *937*
cardiomyopathy 2764
  arrhythmogenic right ventricular *see* arrhythmogenic right ventricular cardiomyopathy
  dilated *see* dilated cardiomyopathy
  hypertrophic *see* hypertrophic cardiomyopathy
  pregnancy 2110
    peripartum 2110, *2111*
  restrictive *see* restrictive cardiomyopathy
cardiopulmonary resuscitation
  cardiac arrest 3097–8
  drowning *1400*
  mechanism of action 3098, *3100*
  renal failure patients 4180
  risks to rescuer 3098
  starting 3098, *3099*
cardiorespiratory collapse *3120*
  presentation 5454, *5455–6*
cardiotoxins, plant-derived *1362*, 1363
cardiovascular disease
  anoxic brain damage 5151
  C-reactive protein 1758
  dialysis patients 3941
  fetal and postnatal effects 2900, *2900*
  hepatic involvement 2538
  HRT 2196, *2197*
  mortality rate 75, *76*
  occupational 1383
  and polycystic ovary syndrome 1910
  polycythaemias 4267
  rabies 547, *549*
  risk factors 76
  role of apoptosis in 187
  and syncope *2638*
  syphilis *see* syphilis, cardiovascular
cardiovascular function, poisoned patients 1276
cardiovascular homeostasis 3123
  arterial pressure and vascular circuit 3125
  cardiac output, oxygen delivery and oxygen consumption 3126
  ventricular pump function 3123
cardiovascular system 2591
  acidosis 1743
  diphtheria complications 667
  effects of malnutrition 1510
  pregnancy 2075, 2088, 2093, *2094*, 2121
    blood pressure 2088
    fluid balance 2076
    increased cardiac output 2076, *2076*
    mechanism of changes 2076
    oedema 2088
    palpitations 2088
  respiratory disease 3187
  in SLE 2783, *2783–4*, 3659
  structure and function 2593
    blood vessels and endothelium 2593
    clinical physiology 2168
    myocytes and action potential 2603
cardioversion 2700, 5512
carditis
  Lyme borreliosis 862
  rheumatic fever 2800
care, rationing of 58
caretaker genes 342, 361
Carey Island virus *566*
caries *see* dental caries
carmustine
  adverse effects
    carcinogenesis *307*
    hepatotoxicity *2529*
  lymphoma *4320*
Carnett's sign 2206
Carney complex 1845, 1985, 2830
Carney's syndrome, and Cushing's syndrome 1872, *1872*
carnitine palmitoyltransferase deficiency 5216
carnitine 1563
  deficiency 5216
Caroli's disease 2554, *2580–1*, *2581*
β-carotene 1488
  reference values *5443*
    children *5438*
carotenoids 1488
  and cancer risk 310
carotid endarterectomy 4941
carotid sinus hypersensitivity 2638
carotid sinus syncope 4816
carp bile, renal toxicity 4092
carpal tunnel syndrome 1383, *3557*, *3587*, 5082, *5082*
  pregnancy 2089, 2146
Carrión's disease *see* bartonellosis
cartilage 3547, *3548*
  age-related changes *3550*
  disorders of 3713
Carukia barnesi 1347
Carvajal-Huerta syndrome 2778
carvedilol, heart failure *2722*
cascara, drug interactions *69*
case series 50, *50*
case-control studies 49, *49*
case-finding 90
caspase 1, 158
caspases 178, *178*
  and cell-cycle proteins 179
  DNA damage/repair 179
  inhibitors of activation 184
  role in apoptosis 185
  substrates 179
caspofungin
  fungal infections 1016–17
  in renal failure *4185*
CAST trial *40*
Castellani's paint 1016
Castleman's disease 499, *3542*, 3543
  HIV-associated 499
  IL-6 in 158
catamenial pneumothorax 3503
cataplexy 4826, 4831
  differential diagnosis 4817
cataracts *168*, 5252
  diabetes mellitus 2036
catecholaminergic polymorphic ventricular tachycardia 2715
catecholamines
  biochemistry 3066, *3066*
  potassium homeostasis *3833*
  reference values *5441*
β-catenin *1939*
caterpillar stings 1351
Catha edulis (khat leaf), nephrotoxicity *4093*
cathartics 1279
cathepsin B 3552
cathepsin G, COPD *3323*
cathepsin K 3551
cathepsin L 3552
cathepsins 178, 209
Catonella spp. *962*
Catostomus commersoni 1215
catroxobin *4540*
cat-scratch disease 927
  clinical features 929
  diagnosis *931*
  treatment 932
Catu virus *581*
cauda equina syndrome 389, 3574
causalgia 4688
caustic ingestion 2303
caveolae 2595
cavitating pulmonary lesions 3213, *3213*
CCR5 211
CCR7 *209*
CCS2-COMMIT trial *40*
CD11c *209*
CD123 *209*
CD133 2595
CD134 *287*
CD137 *287*
CD14 208, 211
CD15 253
CD152 *284*, *287*
CD15–3, reference values *5442*
CD154 *284*, *287*
CD16 209
CD18 253
CD1a *209*
CD25, antibodies *290*
CD27 *287*
CD273 *287*
CD274 *287*
CD279 *287*
CD28 *186*, *284*, *287*
CD3, SCID *251*
CD34 2595
CD4 157
  antigen presentation 226
    MCH class II 226
  functions of 231
  idiopathic lymphopenia *238*
  SCID *251*
  SLE *3656*
CD40 *209*, *245*, 284, *287*
CD40 ligand deficiency *see* hyper-IgM syndrome
CD55 221
CD56 209
CD59 *216*, 221
  deficiency *254*
CD62P *see* P-selectin
CD68 208
CD70 *287*
CD8 157, 210
  antigen presentation 225
    binding to MHC class I 225
    peptide transport 225
    proteasome 225
    T-cell receptor recognition 226
  functions of 230
  SCID *251*
CD80 *208*, *209*, *284*, *287*
CD86 *208*, *209*, *287*
Cedecea spp. *962*
cefalexin *706*
  adverse effects, hepatotoxicity *2532*
  cellulitis, mastitis and pyomyositis *699*
  impetigo *697*
  pharmacokinetics *449*
  septic bursitis/arthritis *700*
  urinary tract infection *4114*
cefazolin *706*
  bacteraemia *703*
  endocarditis *704*
  epidural abscess *702*
  osteomyelitis *701*
  pneumonia *702*, *3238*
  septic bursitis/arthritis *700*
  toxic shock syndrome *697*
  urinary tract infection *702*
cefepime
  pneumonia *3238*, *3245*
  Pseudomonas aeruginosa 737
cefixime
  pharmacokinetics *449*
  in renal failure *4185*
  typhoid fever *742*
cefotaxime
  animal-related injuries 1326
  H. influenzae 762
  leptospirosis 878
  Lyme borreliosis *864*
  meningitis 719, *719*
  nocardiosis 857
  pelvic inflammatory disease *1260*
  pneumococcal pneumonia 687

  pneumonia *3238*
  postantibiotic effect *451*
  in renal failure *4185*
  spectrum of activity *446*
  yersiniosis 777
cefoxitin
  anaerobic infections *753*
  pelvic inflammatory disease *1260*
cefradine, in renal failure *4185*
ceftazidime
  melioidosis *771*
  pneumonia *3245*
  Pseudomonas aeruginosa 737
  in renal failure *4185*
  spectrum of activity *446*
ceftriaxone
  chancroid 764
  chlamydial infections *943*
  gonorrhoea 726
  H. influenzae 762
  infective endocarditis *2817*
  leptospirosis 878
  Lyme borreliosis *864*
  meningitis 719, *719*
  pelvic inflammatory disease *1260*
  pneumococcal pneumonia 687
  pneumonia *3238*
  in renal failure *4185*
  syphilis 894
  typhoid fever *742*
ceftriazone, yersiniosis 777
cefuroxime axetil
  Lyme borreliosis *864*
  pharmacokinetics *449*
cefuroxime
  pneumonia *3238*
  spectrum of activity *446*
celecoxib
  ankylosing spondylitis 3611
  and asthma *3289*
  rheumatoid arthritis *3594*
cell cycle checkpoints
  and cancer 344
  DNA damage 343
  G1/S 345, *345–6*
  G2/M 346
  spindle 343
cell death 177
  activation-induced 186
  gene mutations 351
  see also apoptosis
cell growth 2601
cell stress responses 183
cell surface receptors 169
cell-mediated immunity
  impaired 235, 248
    categories of 249
    causes of *249*
    clinical phenotype 249
cells 127
  cytoskeleton 131
  dynamics of 131
  endocytosis 131
  lipid bilayers 128
  membrane proteins 128
  organelles 128
    endoplasmic reticulum 129
    Golgi apparatus 130
    lysosomes 130
    mitochondria 129
    nucleus 127–8
    peroxisomes 129
  vesicles *128*
cellular adhesion 2601
cellular transformation 338
cellulitis 4673, 4695
  H. influenzae 760
  and lymphoedema 3088
  staphylococcal 696, *697*
  streptococcal 673, *673*
  treatment *3091*
Cellulomonas spp. *962*
Cellusimicrobium spp. *962*
Centipeda spp. *962*
centipede bites 1356, *1356*
central core disease 164
central nervous system
  acquired metabolic disorders 5150
  cystic fibrosis 3363
  degeneration 187
  development of 5135
  developmental abnormalities 5134
    cerebral palsies 5146
    complex 5143
    cortical development disorders 5139, *5140*
    diagnosis and genetic counselling 5148
    extrinsically caused 5145
    migration disorders 5139, *5140*
    neural tube defects 5135, *5136*
    regionalization disorders 5138
    sacral agenesis 5138
    syringomyelia 5138
  disorders
    demyelinating 4948
    in pregnancy 2146
    see also individual conditions
  electrophysiology 4752
  infections 4976
    actinomycotic 853
    anaerobic 751
    bacterial 4976
    intracranial abscess 5013
    neurosyphilis/neuro-AIDS 5015
    prion diseases 5023
    tick-borne encephalitis 572, *566, 573*
    viral 4998
    see also individual infections
  occupational disorders 1386, *1386*
  superficial siderosis 5157
  tuberculosis 820
central pontine myelinolysis 4960, 5154
central sleep apnoea 3261, 3273, *3273*
  apparent 3275
  overnight ventilation 3275
central vein cannulation 5510
Centrocestus armatus 1222
Centrocestus caninus 1222
Centrocestus cuspidatus 1222
Centrocestus formosanus 1222
Centrocestus kurokawai 1222
Centrocestus longus 1222
centromere 138
  fission 147
Centruroides (Sculpturatus) exilicauda (Arizona bark scorpion) *1352*
Centruroides spp. 1351
cephalexin
  adverse effects, hepatotoxicity *2535*
  bacterial overgrowth *2334*
cephalocele 5136
cephalosporins
  adverse effects, hepatotoxicity *2533*
  contraindication in porphyria 1641
  mode of action *443*
  pharmacokinetics *449*
Cephalosporium spp. *3436*
Ceratopogonidae (biting midges) *1226*
Cerbera odollam 1373, *1373*
cercarial dermatitis 1202, 1205
cercopithecine herpesvirus 1 483, 500
cerebellar aplasia/hypoplasia 5142, *5142*
cerebellar ataxia, malaria 1068
cerebellar degeneration *384*
  alcoholic 5156
  paraneoplastic 5169, *5171*
cerebellum 4872
  anatomy
    functional 4872
    gross 4872
  cryoarchitecture 4872, *4872*
  function/dysfunction 4873
  pontocerebellum 4873, *4873*
  spinocerebellum 4872
  vestibulocerebellum 4872
Cerebera odollam (suicide tree) *1373*
cerebral abscess *4780*, 4780
cerebral amyloidosis 1770, *1770*
  Alzheimer's disease 1770
  hereditary cerebral amyloid angiopathy 1770
  prion disease 1771
  senile 1770
cerebral angiography 4770
cerebral arteriovenous malformations 4944
cerebral circulation 4935, *4935*
  circle of Willis *4935*
cerebral demyelination 3822
cerebral herniation *3149*
cerebral infarction *see* stroke
cerebral ischaemia
  investigations 4937
  see also individual ischaemic conditions
cerebral malaria *1061*, 1062, 1065, *1066–7*
  treatment 1077
cerebral oedema
  altitude-related 1402, 1405
  brain defences 3820, *3820*
  hepatocellular failure 2497
    management 2503
cerebral palsies 5146
  aetiology 5147
  brain imaging *5144*, 5147
  classification 5146
  epidemiology 5147
cerebral perfusion pressure 3148
cerebral perfusion 3103
cerebral tumours
  intrinsic *4777*, 4777
  secondary *4779*, *4779*
cerebral vasculitis 5161, *5161*
cerebral venous sinus thrombosis *4774*, 4775
cerebral venous thrombosis, pregnancy 2147
cerebrospinal fluid 4750
  analysis 4975
  blood 4750
  drainage, intracranial hypertension *3150*
  glucose 4752
  immunoglobulins 4752
  lactate 4752
  leucocytes and cytology 4750, *4751*
  low volume headache 4925, *4925*
  microbiological and serological reactions 4752
  multiple sclerosis 4957
  opening pressure 4750
  pigment 4751
  pressure 4974
  protein 4752
  raised volume headache 4926
  reference values *5447*
cerebrotendinous xanthomatosis 5110
  differential diagnosis *1725*
  psychiatric signs *1720*
cerebrovascular disease
  arterial occlusive disease 4935
  imaging *4771*, 4771
  magnetic brain stimulation 4784
  pregnancy 2145
  stroke *see* stroke
cerebrovascular syncope *2638*, 2639
ceruloplasmin 1690
cervical cancer 324, *601, 603, 604*
  epidemiology 604
  incidence *301, 324*
    migrants vs residents *302*
  pregnancy 2183
  prevention and control 604
  screening *106*
  vaccines 604
cervical cap *26*
cervicitis
  chlamydial 943, *944*
  mycoplasmal infections *956*
cervicofacial actinomycoses 852, *852–3*
cervicogenic headache 4926
cervix, strawberry 1257
cestodes *see* tapeworms
cetirizine 3282
  anaphylaxis 3113
cetrimide 4734
cetuximab *376*, 401
  cost-effectiveness ratio *53*
c-fms 4201
Chadwick, Edwin 11
Chagas' disease 1127
  aetiology 1128, *1128, 1129*
  clinical features *1130, 1131*,1133
  epidemiology 1129
  future research 1129
  gut peptides 2322
  laboratory diagnosis 1132
  myocarditis 2763
  pathogenesis/pathology 1130, *1130, 1131*
  prevention and control 1133
  treatment 1132
Chagres virus *581*
chain of survival *3098*
challenge tests 3111
  foods 2254
chamomile, drug interactions *69*
chancre, trypanosomal *1122*, 1122
chancroid 764, 1243
  aetiology 763
  clinical features 763
  epidemiology 763
  and HIV 764
  laboratory diagnosis 763
  pathology/pathogenesis 763
  prevention and control 764

treatment 764
Changuinola virus 556
channelopathies 162, 5218
cardiac muscle 163
cognitive impairment 5281
cystic fibrosis *see* cystic fibrosis
kidney 165
Bartter's syndrome 165
Liddle's syndrome 165
nephrogenic diabetes insipidus 165
nephrolithiasis 165
pseudohypoaldosteronism type 1, 165
neuronal 162
benign familial neonatal convulsions 162
Charcot-Marie-Tooth disease 136, 143, 148, 163
episodic ataxia type 1 162
episodic ataxia type 2 162
familial hemiplegic migraine 162
generalized epilepsy with febrile seizures 162
spinocerebellar ataxia type 6 162
startle disease (hyperekplexia) 162
nonsyndromic deafness 168
periodic paralyses 5218
skeletal muscle 163
malignant hyperthermia and central core disease 164
myasthenia gravis 163
myotonia 164
periodic paralyses 164
slow-channel syndrome 163
chaparrall 68
chaperones 1254
charcoal, activated 1278
multiple-dose 1279
Charcot's arthropathy 1990, 2046, 3712
Charcot-Bouchard aneurysm 3036
Charcot-Marie-Tooth disease 136, *148, 148, 163, 166, 5093, 5093*
Chase-Aurbach test 1864
chasteberry, drug interactions *69*
Chediak-Higashi syndrome *238*, 1698, 1717, 4309
hypopigmentation 4663
Cheilospirura spp. *1176*
cheiroarthropathy 2047
chelates, in renal failure 4176
chelating agents 1462
chelation therapy *66*
chemoembolization, transarterial 2517
chemokines 212
chemotaxis 209
chemotherapy 397, *388, 397*
adjuvant 397
adverse effects 399, *400*
oesophageal problems 2303
antimicrobial 441
classes 398
hormonal abnormalities *2066*
neoadjuvant 397
resistance 399, *399*
targeted 400
see also individual drugs and classes
chenodeoxycholic acid 2548
adverse effects, hepatotoxicity *2529*
cherry angioma 4691
cherry-red spot-myoclonus epilepsy syndrome 5102
chest aspiration 5517, *5518*
chest decompression 5517
chest drain 5517
chest pain *2629, 2628–9, 3185,* 3185
acute coronary syndromes 2630
angina pectoris 2629
aortic dissection 2631
at rest 2629
atypical angina 2631
coronary spasm 2631
differential diagnosis *2630*
noncardiac 2296
peptic stricture 2291
pericarditis 2631
Prinzmetal's angina 2631
syndrome X 2631
chest wall disease 3214, *3214*
and chronic respiratory failure 3470
chest wall, in pregnancy 2121
chest X-ray 3200
acute respiratory failure 3135
aortic dissection 2955, *2955*
aortic regurgitation 2752, *2752*
aortic stenosis 2748
ARDS *3143*
Chagas' disease *1131*
COPD 3331, *3331*
cystic fibrosis *3356*
diffuse parenchymal lung disease 3371
dilated cardiomyopathy 2775
disease signs 3209
cavitating pulmonary lesions 3213, *3213*
increased transradiancy of hemithorax 3211, *3212*
multiple pulmonary nodules 3213, *3214*
pulmonary collapse 3209, *3210–11*
pulmonary consolidation 3209, *3210*
pulmonary nodule/mass 3212, *3212*
specific 3214
hypertrophic cardiomyopathy 2770
infections 421
interpretation 3208
lung cancer *3518–21*
mediastinal mass *3542*
melioidosis *769*
mitral regurgitation 2744, *2744*
mitral stenosis 2739, *2740*
pleural effusion *3489–90*
pleural empyema *3495*
Pneumocystis jirovecii 1030, *627–8, 1030*
pneumonia 3236, *3233–4*
pneumothorax *3501*
pregnancy 2088, 2109
pulmonary arterial hypertension *2984*
pulmonary embolism 3013, *3014*
pulmonary fibrosis 3377
pulmonary oedema 2998, *2998*
high-altitude *1406*
radiographic anatomy 3206, *3206*
diaphragm and thoracic cage 3207
hilar structures 3207
lateral view *3206*, 3207
mediastinum 3206, *3206*
pulmonary fissues, vessels and bronchi 3207
renal disease 3873
standard views 3201
technical considerations 3200
Cheyne-Stokes breathing 3186
Chiari malformations 5142
chickenpox *489*
chiggers *see* scrub typhus
Chikungunya virus 557, *558*
chilblains 4687
child mortality
causes 74, *75*
measures to reduce 77
children
chronic granulomatous disease 2526
Cushing's syndrome 1874
endocarditis 2811
glomerulonephritis 3979
growth 1951
hereditary bulbar palsy 5073
HIV/AIDS 641
hypertension 3056
immunizations 77, 467
lactase restriction 2349
magnetic brain stimulation 4784
multiple sclerosis 4956
obesity *1529*
poisoning 1273
reference values *5438*
screening 105
suicide attempts 5295
tuberculosis *825*
ulcerative colitis 2382
chimeric F-box protein *1939*
Chinese herb nephropathy 4012, *3860, 4008, 4084*
clinical features 4013
diagnosis and treatment 4013
pathogenesis and pathology 4012, *4013*
Chinese herbs
hepatotoxicity *2529*
renal toxicity *3860*, 4084
Chinese restaurant syndrome 2254
chirality 1462
Chironex fleckeri (box jellyfish) 1347
chiropractic *66*
Chiropsalmus quadrigatus 1347
Chiropsalmus quadrumanus 1347
Chlamydia abortus 940, 948
Chlamydia felis 948
Chlamydia pneumoniae 940, 947
arthritis 948
atherosclerosis 948
epidemiology 948
pharyngitis 3227
pneumonia 3231, 3235
respiratory disease 947
treatment *3238*
Chlamydia psittaci 940, 948
clinical features 948
infective endocarditis 2816
pneumonia 3231
treatment *3238*
Chlamydia spp. *962*
eye infection 5246
pregnancy 2169
Chlamydia trachomatis 939, *940*
pregnancy 2169
see also chlamydial infections
chlamydial infections 939, *186, 1246, 1247*
classification 940
diagnosis 940
culture and staining 948
enzyme immunoassay 949
nucleic acid amplification 949
serological tests 949
genital tract 939
growth cycle, serovars and protein profile 940
immune response 949
immunocompromised patients 945
incidence *1247*
laboratory diagnosis *947*, 948
neonatal 945, *945*
pathogenesis 949
screening *106*
trachoma 939, 941
treatment 940, *943*, 949
see also individual infections
Chlamydophila psittaci, community-acquired pneumonia *453*
Chlamydophila spp. *962*
chloasma 2149, *2150*
chloracne 1382
chloral hydrate, contraindication in porphyria *5484*
α-chloralose poisoning 1302
chlorambucil 398
adverse effects, hepatotoxicity *2532, 2533*
carcinogenesis *307*
contraindication in porphyria *5484*
lymphoma *4320*
membranous nephropathy 3987
pregnancy *2158*
primary biliary cirrhosis *2467*
chloramphenicol
adverse effects, hepatotoxicity *2532*
anthrax 787
bacterial overgrowth *2334*
bartonellosis 938
H. influenzae 762
listeriosis 898
meningitis 719, *719*
mode of action *443*
prognosis 923
relapsing fevers 872
in renal failure *4185*
rickettsioses 914
S. moniliformis 859
scrub typhus 921
tularaemia 782
typhoid fever *742*
chlorate poisoning 1303
chlordane, CNS effects *1386*
chlordecone
CNS effects *1386*
reproductive effects 1385
chlordiazepoxide 3156
adverse effects, hepatotoxicity *2532–3*
chlorhexidine 4734
chloride channels, drugs acting on 1461
chloride deficiency, metabolic alkalosis 1748
chloride
dietary reference values *1502*

plasma/serum *3837*
reference values *5435*, *5446*
children *5438*
urinary *3837*
chlorinated hydrocarbons, hepatotoxicity *1385*
chlorinated naphthalenes, hepatotoxicity *1385*
chlorine poisoning 1309
chlornaphazine, carcinogenesis *307*, 328
4-chloro-*ortho*-toluidine *1380*
chloroform, adverse effects, hepatotoxicity *2529*
chloromethane, hepatotoxicity *1385*
chloromethyl methyl ether *308*, *1380*
chlorophenoxy herbicide poisoning 1303, *1303*
Chlorophyllum molybdites 1370
chloroquine *1074*, 1075
poisoning 1282
pregnancy *2158*
prophylactic *1086*, 1087
rheumatoid arthritis *3595*
chlorozotocin, adverse effects, hepatotoxicity *2529*, *2532*
chlorproguanil-dapsone 1076
chlorpromazine 5265
adverse effects, hepatotoxicity *2532*, *2533*, *2535*
schizophrenia *5325*
chlorpropamide 2014
adverse effects, hepatotoxicity *2529*, *2532–3*, *2535*
chlorthalidone
adverse effects, hepatotoxicity *2533*
calcium stone prevention *4130*
cholangiocarcinoma 2517
diagnosis 2518
epidemiology and aetiology 2518
pathogenesis 2518
pathology 2518
treatment and prognosis 2518
cholangitis 2551
bacterial 2554
sclerosing 2555, *2555*
liver transplantation 2507
recurrence post-transplantation 2511
cholecalciferol 1495
cholecystectomy, postcholecystectomy synromes 2553
cholecystitis
acute 2551
aetiology 2551
complications 2551
differential diagnosis 2551
laboratory investigations 2551
symptoms and signs 2551
treatment 2551
chronic 2552
cholecystokinin 2318
choledochal cyst 2582, *2582*
choledocholithiasis 2552
clinical features 2552
differential diagnosis 2553, *2553*
imaging 2553, *2553*
laboratory investigations 2553
treatment 2553
cholelithiasis, pregnancy 2130, *2131*
cholera 754
aetiology, genetics and pathophysiology 754
clinical assessment *758*
clinical features 757, *757*
diagnosis 757
differential diagnosis 757
epidemiology 755
geographical distribution *756*
history 754
mortality *121*
prevention 756, *757*
prognosis 758
treatment 757, *758*
vaccines 468, *466*, 756
cholestasis 2449, 2501
drug-induced *2533*, 2450, 2533
intrahepatic *2447*
benign recurrent 2450
drug-induced 2536, *2537*
of pregnancy 2126, *2150*, 2450
differential diagnosis *2131*
neonatal 2449
see also jaundice
cholesterol 1654, *1654*, 2548
crystals 3648
gallstones 2549
pregnancy *2126*
raised
mortality *88*
treatment 1670
reference values *5435*, *5444*
regulation of gene expression *1482*
reverse transport 1657
cholesterol embolism *2966*, 2966–8
cholesteryl ester transfer protein 1657
cholic acid 2548
^{14}C-cholylglycine breath test 2333
chondrocalcinosis 3564, 3727, 3764
familial *3721*
chondrocytes 3548
age-related changes *3550*
chondrodysplasia punctata, mutations in *3757*
chondrodysplasia punctatum rhizomelia *1552*
chondrodysplasia
Blomstrand's 3729, *1855*, *1865*, *3721*
clinical features *3731*
Jansen's metaphyseal 1862, *1855*, *3721*, *3729*
chondroectodermal dysplasia *see* Ellis-van Creveld syndrome
chondroitin sulphate, osteoarthritis 3635
chondrosarcoma 320
chorea 4887, *4890*, *4894*, 4894
hemiballism 4896
Huntington's disease *see* Huntington's disease
pregnancy 2144
Sydenham's 2801, 4895
treatment 2804
chorea-acanthocytosis 5113
chorioamniotis, mycoplasmal infections *956*
choriocarcinoma 2145
choriomeningitis, lymphocytic *see* lymphocytic choriomeningitis
chromium 1498, *1498*
carcinogenesis *308*, *1380*
poisoning 1298
reference values *5445*
Chromobacterium spp. *962*
chromoblastomycosis 999, 1005
aetiology 1005
clinical features 1006, *1006*, *1018*
diagnosis 1006
epidemiology 1006
pathogenesis 1006
treatment 1007
chromogranin A, reference values *5442*
chromogranin B 1789
reference values *5442*
chromogranin-derived peptides 2320
chromogranins 1977
chromosomal instability 343
chromosomal translocations 341, 344
complex 344
simple 344
chromosome aberrations 145
numerical 145
triploidies and tetraploidies 145
trisomies and monosomies 145
structural 145
centromere fission 145, 138, 147
complex rearrangements 146
deletions and duplications 145
heterochromatin variants 147
insertions 146
inversions 146
isochromosomes 147
mosaicism 147
reciprocal translocations 146
ring chromosomes 146
Robertsonian translocations 146
chromosome fragility syndromes 368
see also individual syndromes
chromosomes 138
autosomal 138
centromere 138
marker 145
sex 138
telomere 138
chronic actinic dermatitis *4670*, 4671
chronic eosinophilic leukaemia 4228
chronic fatigue syndrome 5304, 532, 1388
aetiology 5305
biological factors 5305
psychological factors 5305
social and iatrogenic factors 5306
clinical features 5306
clinical investigation 5307
diagnostic criteria 5307, *5307*
differential diagnosis 5306, *5306*
epidemiology 5306
historical perspective 5305
prevention 5306
prognosis 5307
treatment 5307
chronic granulomatous disease *238*, *2250*, *4308*
of childhood 2526
chronic idiopathic axonal polyneuropathy 5094
chronic infantile neurological, cutaneous and articular syndrome *see* CINCA
chronic inflammatory demyelinating polyradiculoneuropathy 5090
chronic lymphocytic leukaemia 4220, 4331, *244*, 4227, 4240
aetiology and genetics 4241
areas of uncertainty 4245
clinical features 4242
clinical investigation 4242, *4243*
diagnostic criteria 4243
differential diagnosis 4242, *4243*
epidemiology 4242
future developments 4246
historical perspective 4240
pathogenesis/pathology 4241
prevention 4242
prognosis 4245
renal involvement 4063
staging 4243
treatment 4244
complications 4245
quality of life 4245
relapse/refractory disease 4244
second malignancies 4245
chronic mucocutaneous candidiasis *2250*
chronic myelogenous leukaemia 4227
translocations *342*
chronic myeloid leukaemia 4247, *4220*, *4248*
aetiology 4248
clinical features and diagnosis 4248, *4249*
epidemiology 4247
management 4251, *4252*, *4254–5*
molecular biology 4249, *4250*
natural history 4248, *4248–9*
prognostic factors 4251, *4251*
translocations *341*
chronic myelomonocytic leukaemia 4228
chronic neutrophilic leukaemia 4228
chronic obstructive pulmonary disease (COPD) 3311, *3120*
aetiology 3311, 3313
air pollution 3314
atopy and airways hyper-responsiveness 3315
chronic bronchopulmonary infection 3314
diet 3315
environmental factors 3313
occupation 3314
prenatal factors 3315
socioeconomic factors 3315
tobacco smoke 3313, *3314*
chest X-ray 3214, *3215*
clinical features 3311
airflow limitation 3470, *3471*
clinical history 3326
smoking and occupation 3327
definition 3311
differential diagnosis 3327, *3327*
epidemiology 3315
exacerbations 3325, 3341
assessment of severity 3341, *3342*
oxygen therapy 3342
examination 3327
cardiovascular 3327
chest 3327
general inspection 3327
and gender 3315
genetic factors 3315
imaging 3331
investigation 3312
arterial blood gases 3014, 3329
BODE index 3300
carbon monoxide transfer 3329
exercise testing 1587

flow volume loops 3329
lung volumes 3329
peak expiratory flow 3329, *3324, 3329*
respiratory function and exercise capacity 3328, *3328*
respiratory muscle function 1726
reversibility testing 3328, *3329*
sleep studies 5062
spirometry 3328, *3328*
management 3312, 3334
antibiotics 3337
antitussives 3337
bronchodilators 3334, *3335–6*
corticosteroids 3337
drug delivery devices 3336
home nebulizer therapy 3336
mucolytics 3337
oxygen therapy 3338, *3473*
pulmonary rehabilitation 3339, *3339–40*
surgery 3343
vaccines 3337
vasodilators 3337
ventilatory support 3339
morbidity 3316, *3316*
mortality 3317, *76, 3317*
natural history 3317, *3318*
pathogenesis 3322, *3322*
inflammatory cells/ mediators 3322, *3322*
oxidative stress 3323
protease/antiprotease imbalance 3323
pathology 3311, *3318, 3319*
bronchiolitis/small airways disease 3321, *3321*
chronic bronchitis 3318, *3320*
emphysema 3319
pulmonary vasculature 3321
small airways disease 3321, *3321–2*
pathophysiology 3311, 3323
airflow limitation and hyper-inflation 3324, *3324–5*
gas exchange abnormalities 3324
impaired respiratory muscle function 3325
mucus hypersecretion and ciliary dysfunction 3324
pulmonary hypertension 3325
prevalence 3315, *3316*
prevention 3312, 3333
smoking cessation 3333, *3333*
prognosis 3317
risk factors *3313*
surgery in 3341
symptoms 3326, *3326*
systemic effects 3325, *3325*
chronic pulmonary disease 832
chronotropism, positive 2618
Chryseobacterium spp. *962*
Chrysomya bezziana *1233*, 1234
Chrysops spp. (mangrove fly) 1150
Chrysops spp. *1226*
chrysotile *see* asbestosis
Churg-Strauss syndrome 3397, *3430, 3650, 4033*
aetiology and pathogenesis 3397
cardiac involvement *2783*, 3397
central nervous system 3398
clinical presentation 3397, *3399*
gastrointestinal involvement 3398
GI tract involvement 2422
investigation 3398
imaging *3409, 3399*
musculoskeletal system 3398
pregnancy 2162
pulmonary involvement *3396, 3398*
asthma 3306
eosinophilic pneumonia 3295
renal disease 3398, 4038
skin lesions 3397
treatment 3402
Chuvash polycythaemia 4268
Chvostek's sign 2327, 3731
chylomicrons 1655
chylothorax 3486, 3495
aetiology 3495, *3497*
clinical features 3496
diagnosis 3496, *3497*
pathophysiology 3495
treatment 3496
chylous reflux 4696
chyluria 1156, *1157*, 4089
ciclosporin
adverse effects 3955, *3955*
hepatotoxicity *2533*
nephrotoxicity 4053
aplastic anaemia *4295*, 4288
carcinogenesis *307*
focal segmental glomerulosclerosis 3984
lupus nephritis 4049
membranous nephropathy 3987
minimal-change nephropathy 3982
post-transplantation 291, 3482, *290, 2511, 2730, 3954*
pregnancy *2158*
primary biliary cirrhosis *2467*
psoriasis 4615
psoriatic arthritis 3613
rheumatoid arthritis *3595*
skin disorders 4737
systemic sclerosis *3677*
therapeutic drug monitoring *1475*, 1476
ulcerative colitis 2379
cicutoxin 1362
cidofovir, adenovirus 477
ciftriaxone, mycobacterial disease 835
ciguatera toxin 1346
ciliary dysfunction 3324
ciliary dyskinesia 3347
cilostazol, limb ischaemia 2962
cimetidine
adverse effects, hepatotoxicity *2532*
drug interactions *1471*, 2311
peptic ulcer disease 2311
reproductive effects *1917*
Cimex lectularius (bedbug) 1227, *1228*
cinacalcet 1853
hyperparathyroidism 1859
CINCA 1764, *1761, 3709*
cinchonism 1282
ciprofibrate 1670
ciprofloxacin *707*
adverse effects, hepatotoxicity *2529*
anthrax 787
bacterial overgrowth *2334*
bartonellosis 938
in breast milk *1469*
brucellosis 794
chancroid 764
cyclosporiasis 1107
drug interactions *1471*
endocarditis *704*
gonorrhoea 726
mycobacterial disease 835
mycoplasmal infections *960*
nocardiosis 857
P. multocida 779
pharmacokinetics *449*
pneumonia *3245*
postantibiotic effect *451*
Pseudomonas aeruginosa 737
Q fever 926
in renal failure *4185*
septic bursitis/arthritis *700*
spectrum of activity *446*
tularaemia 782
typhoid carriers *742*
typhoid fever *742*
urinary tract infection *4113*
yersiniosis 777
circadian rhythms
disorders of 4835
advanced sleep phase syndrome 4836
delayed sleep phase syndrome 4835
shift-work sleep disorder 4836
drug interactions with 1463
melatonin 2071
circinate balanitis *3625*
circulatory failure, acute pancreatitis 2564
circulatory support, critical illness 3122, *3117*, 3117
cirrhosis 2482
ascites *see* ascites
clinical features 2477
lung disease 2538
drug-induced 2536, *2536*
epidemiology 2483
reproductive effects *1917*
treatment 2479
cisplatin 398
adverse effects *400*
hepatotoxicity *2532, 2534*
renal *3860*
lung cancer 3529–30
lymphoma *4320*
mesothelioma 3537
resistance *399*
citalopram
adverse effects *5313*
poisoning 1281
citrin deficiency *1566*
Citrobacter spp. *962*
citrullinaemia *1566*
Citrullus colocynthus 1372
CKD *see* renal disease, chronic
c-kit 4201
Cladophialophora carrionii 1005
Cladotanytarsus lewisi 1236
clarithromycin *707*
H. pylori 2312, *2313*
legionnaire's disease 902
leprosy 846
Lyme borreliosis *864*
mycobacterial disease 835, *835*
mycoplasmal infections *960*
pertussis *766*
pneumococcal pneumonia 687
pneumonia *3238*
in renal failure *4185*
rickettsioses 914
S. pyogenes 675
toxoplasmosis *1096*
clavulanic acid, actinomycoses 854
clear cell sarcoma, translocations *341*
clearance 1454
cleidocranial dysostosis, mutations in *3757*
cleidocranial dysplasia 3759
Cleistanthus collinus 1374
clindamycin colitis 801
clindamycin *706*
acne *4680*
adverse effects, hepatotoxicity *2529, 2532*
anaerobic infections *753*
babesiosis 1090
bacterial vaginosis 1257
cellulitis, mastitis and pyomyositis *699*
chlamydial infections *943*
gas gangrene 808
impetigo *697*
mode of action *443*
mycoplasmal infections *960*
P. multocida 779
pelvic inflammatory disease *1260*
Pneumocystic jirovecii 1031
pneumonia *3238*
in renal failure *4185*
S. pyogenes 675
scalded skin syndrome 696
septic bursitis/arthritis *700*
skin disorders 4739
spectrum of activity *446*
toxic shock syndrome *697*
toxoplasmosis *1096*
clinical effectiveness 51
absolute effect size 51
comparative 52
heterogeneous patient populations 52
see also clinical trials
clinical evaluation of medicines 48
methodology 49
clinical oncology 372
clinical pharmacology 1449
adverse drug reactions 1449, 1464
drug interactions 1449, *1470, 1471*
effectiveness 1450
efficacy 1450
efficiency 1450
formularies 1451
WHO Model List of Essential Drugs 1451
medicines management 1451
prescribing 1449
principles 1451, *1452*
pharmaceutics 1451
pharmacodynamics 1459
pharmacokinetics 1454
therapeutic process 1462
risk-benefit ratio 1450
therapeutic index 1450
clinical questions 23, *24*
clinical trials 45
advanced technology 46
biomarkers 45
case-control studies 49, *49*
comparisons between treatment options 46
controlled observational studies 49

design of 45
developing countries 47
effect size 32, *32*
ethical issues 47
expectations 31
historical controlled *4603*, 49
and individual patient treatment 28
large-scale 31
placebo effects 47
presentation of results 46
randomized controlled *see* randomized controlled trials
stroke prevention 30
surrogate endpoints 45
clobazam, epilepsy 4821
clobetasol propionate *2151*
clobetasol *4734*
clobetasone butyrate *2151*
clodronate
hypercalcaemia 1854
hyperparathyroidism 1859
clofazimine
leprosy *845*, 845
pigmentation *845*
pregnancy *2172*
clofibrate, adverse effects, hepatotoxicity *2529*
clomacetin, adverse effects, hepatotoxicity *2529*
clomethiazole 5337
poisoning 1285
clomipramine, cataplexy *4833*
clonazepam
dose levels *4823*
epilepsy 4821
serum levels *5449*
sleep disturbance *4833*
clonidine 3156
hypertension 3052
opioid withdrawal *5347*
orthostatic hypotension *5063*
in pregnancy *2099*
clonorchiasis 1212
clinical features 1213
diagnosis 1214, *1214*
epidemiology and control 1212
pathology 1213, *1213*
treatment 1214
Clonorchis sinensis 307, *315, 1212, 1213*
life cycle 1212, *1213*
clopidogrel 2314
acute coronary syndromes 2918
drug interactions *1471*
stroke prevention 30
Clostridium botulinum 803, 804
Clostridium difficile 800
aetiology, pathogenesis and pathology 801
areas of controversy
antibiotic selection 802
diagnostic testing 802
infection control 802
strain identification 802
treatment 802
clinical features 801
diagnosis 801
diarrhoea 431
differential diagnosis 801
epidemiology 801
future developments 803
history 800
NAP1 strain 801
prevention 801
toxin 802
treatment 802
Clostridium fallax 806
Clostridium histolyticum 804, 806
Clostridium novyi 806–7, 804
Clostridium perfringens 800–1, 804, 807
food poisoning 804, 808
gastrointestinal infections 804, 808
Clostridium septicum 804, 806
Clostridium sordellii 804, 806–7
Clostridium spp. *962*
osteomyelitis *3789*
toxins 807
clotrimazole
candidiasis 1258
fungal infections 1015
Clouston's syndrome *4599*, 4600
cloxacillin, adverse effects, hepatotoxicity *2532*
clozapine *5337*
schizophrenia *5325*
clubbing *see* digital clubbing
cluster headache 4918, *4918–20*
clusterin *216*
c-myc 183
CNS *see* central nervous system
coagulase-negative staphylococci 704
bacteraemia 704
endocarditis 705
peritoneal dialysis-associated peritonitis 708
therapy *705*
coagulation cascade *414, 415, 4504, 4519–20*
coagulation disorders
acquired 4531, *4533*
coumarin over-anticoagulation 4534, *4536*
DIC *see* disseminated intravascular coagulation
haemodilution and massive transfusion 4535
heparin and heparin-like anticoagulants 4539
hyperfibrinolysis 4539
immunoglobulin-mediated factor deficiency 4537
liver disease *4537*, 4535
plasma-cell dyscrasias 4539, *4540*
prohaemorrhagic 4534
prothrombotic 4542
treatment of 4532, *4533*
venom-induced *4540*
in cyanosis 2846
dialysis patients 3941
genetic 4518
ADAMTS13 deficiency 4527
factor V/factor VIII deficiency 4527
factor XI deficiency 4527
factor XIII and fibrinogen deficiency 4528
haemophilia 4518
tissue factor and common pathway deficiencies 4527
von Willebrand disease *see* von Willebrand disease
coagulation factors 4489, *4490–1*
cofactors 4492
concentrates 4533
deficiency, immunoglobulin-mediated 4537
non-vitamin K dependent 4491
vitamin K-dependent 4489, 4534
see also individual factors
coagulation inhibitors 4494–5, *4496*
coagulation pathways 4494, *4494*
tissue factor cells 4495, *4495*
coagulation 2601, 4489
in cancer 4548, *4549–50*
in pregnancy 2078
coagulopathy
dilutional 4505
meningococcal septicaemia *717*
coal tar *1380*, 4733
psoriasis 4614
coal/coke production, and cancer *1380*
coal-worker's pneumoconiosis 3414–15
aetiology and pathology 3415, *3415–16*
clinical features 3416, *3417*
prevention and management 3417
co-amoxiclav
P. multocida 779
in renal failure *4185*
coarctation of aorta *see* aortic coarctation
cobalamin E defect 1594
cobalamin G defect 1594
cobalamin 1493, *4403, 4404*
absorption 2229, *4404, 4405*
acquired disorders of metabolism 4417
biochemistry 4403, *4403–4*
deficiency 4382, 1494
causes 4411
diagnosis 4415
dietary 4412
neuropathy 5089
in pregnancy 2174
treatment 4416
dietary reference values *1502*
homocysteine metabolism 1494
inborn errors of metabolism 4417
malabsorption *2328, 2332*
nutrition 4404
reference intake *1524*
reference values *5443*
requirements 1494
serum *4196*
transport 4405, *4405*
cobalt 1498, *1498*
carcinogenesis *1380*
extrinsic allergic alveolitis *3436*
poisoning 1298
reference values *5445*
cocaine abuse 5364
clinical and pathological aspects 5365
cocaine 5384
adverse effects, hepatotoxicity *2529*
poisoning 1285
reproductive effects *1917*
serum levels *5449*
Coccidioides immitis 1020
HIV-associated infection *3247*
osteomyelitis *3789*
pneumonia 3237
Coccidioides posadasii 1020
coccidioidomycosis 1020, *1009*
clinical presentation 1021
central nervous system involvement 1022, *1022*
chronic pulmonary coccidioidomycosis 1021
coccidioma formation 1021
disseminated coccidioidomycoses *1021–2*, 1022
osteoarticular disease 1022, *1022*
pneumonia 1021
diagnosis 1021
pathogenesis 1021
persons at risk 1021
pregnancy 2124
treatment 1022, *1022*
Cochliomyia hominivorax *1233*, 1234
Cochliomyia macelleria *1233*
Cochrane Collaboration 24
Cochrane Controlled Trials Register (CCTR) 24
Cochrane Database Systematic Reviews 24
Cochrane, Archie 37
Cockayne's syndrome *4668, 4908, 5099*
Cockcroft-Gault equation 3847, 3869
cockroaches, and hygiene 1236
codanthrusate *5426*
codeine
in breast milk *2189*
diarrhoea *2433*
co-dydramol, cancer pain 394
coeliac axis compression 2420
coeliac disease 2335, *2220, 2221, 2253, 2336*
aetiology 2336
and arthralgia 3711
and arthritis 3615
clinical features 2337, *2337*
neuropathy 5088
oral 2279
osteomalacia 3739
diagnosis 2340
serological tests 2329
differential diagnosis 2338, *2339*
epidemiology 2337
extraintestinal manifestations 2338
future developments 2341
haematological abnormalities 2339
hepatic involvement 2540
historical perspective 2336
hormonal abnormalities *2066*
IgA deficiency 2339
intestinal complications 2338
enteropathy-associated T cell lymphoma 2338
small-bowel adenocarcinoma 2338
ulcerative jejunitis 2338
investigations
antibody tests 2339
biochemistry 2339
HLA DQ typing 2340
radiology 2339
wireless capsule enteroscopy 2340
moulage phenomenon *2221*
neurological complications 5164
pathology 2338
persistent 2341
pregnancy 2132
prognosis 2341, *2341*

refractory 2338
screening 2341
selective IgA deficiency 2249
treatment 2340, *2340–1*
see also malabsorption
coenzyme Q10, migraine prevention *4916*
coeur en sabot 2864
coevolution 14
Cogan's syndrome 5162
ocular involvement 5243
cognition 4746
cognitive assessment 5274
cognitive behavioural therapy *5330*, 5340
pain relief 5415
post-traumatic stress disorder 5290
cognitive disorders
acute *5270*, 5269–70
alcohol and substance abuse 5271, *5272*
delirium 5270–1, *5271*
investigation 5271, *5272*
management 5272
psychiatric disorder 5271
chronic 5269, *5272*, *5273*
dementia 5272, *5273*
focal cognitive disorders 5273
investigation 5274
cognitive and behavioural change 5269
conditions giving rise to 5276, *5276*
extracerebral disorders 5279
neurological disorders 5276
in hypertension 3037
organic comorbidity 5275, *5275*
organic mood disorder 5276
organic personality disorder 5276
organic psychotic disorder 5275
reversible vs irreversible 5270
specific vs generalized 5270
vs psychiatric disorders 5270
see also psychiatric disorders
Cohen syndrome *1530*
coital insufficiency *1917*
colchicine 1364, *1362*, *1365*
adverse effects, hepatotoxicity *2532*
Behçet's disease 3687
drug interactions *3968*
gout 1624, 3643
primary biliary cirrhosis *2467*
Colchicum autumnale (autumn crocus) *1365*
Colchicum autumnale (meadow saffron), nephrotoxicity *4093*
cold agglutinin syndrome 4455
cold agglutinin titre *4196*
cold injury 4687
cold sore *see* herpes labialis
cold-related illness 1395
falling core temperature 1394
frostbite 1395, 1397
hypothermia 1394–5
nonfreezing cold injury 1395–6
thermoregulation 1395
Coley, William 372
colistin, bacterial overgrowth *2334*
colitis
amoebic with dysentery 1037
antibiotic-associated 2429
collagenous 2584
cystica profunda 2586
fulminant 1039
lymphocytic 1063
microscopic 2584
presentation 5472, *5472*
colitiviruses 555
Colorado tick fever 555
Eyach 556
collagen disorders
GI tract 2417
intestinal effects 2421
collagen propeptides *3729*
collagen 3548, *3548*, 3725, *3725–6*
collagenase inhibitors, osteoarthritis 3636
collagenous colitis 2584
arthropathies in 3615
collecting duct (of kidney) 3814, *3815*
acid-base homeostasis 4133, *4135*
Colles' fracture 3796–7
Collinsella spp. *962*
collodion babies 1709
colloid cyst *4778*, 4778
colon
anatomy 2201, 2224
atresia 2402
bacterial flora *2330*
diverticular disease 1521
function of 2203
pathology 2224
see also individual conditions
pseudo-obstruction 2235, 2589
radiology 2224
salt and water absorption *2208*
colonic diverticula *see* diverticular disease
colonic irrigation *66*
colonoscopy 2210
cleaning and disinfection 2210
contraindications 2212
cost-effectiveness 2214
equipment 2210
indications 2213
GI bleeding 2242
limitations 2212
medication 2211
patient preparation 2211
risks 2212
total 2212
ulcerative colitis 2375
colony-stimulating factors 2601
Colorado tick fever 555
colorectal adenoma-carcinoma sequence 361, *362*
colorectal cancer 2225, *2225*, 2405, 2410
bleeding 2241
epidemiology 2410, *2410*
genetic predisposition 364, *364*
hereditary nonpolyposis *2406*
HRT effects 2197
incidence *301*, 2410, *2410*
migrants vs residents *302*
mortality 2410
nutrition-related 1521, *1521*
pregnancy 2184
risk factors 2410
screening *106*
Colostethus spp. 1346
Colubridae 1327, 1333
coma
adverse effects *3154*
assessment and examination 4844
continuation of care 4847
definition 4842, *4843*
Glasgow Coma Score 1281, *5488*
history 4843
investigation 4845, *4846*
value of 4846
neurological examination 4844, *4845*
Oxfordshire Community Stroke Subclassification System *5488*
presentation 5486
prognosis 4846
Comamonas spp. *962*
combined oral contraceptive pill *1265*
comfrey 68
common peroneal nerve neuropathy 5085
common variable immuno-deficiency *238*, 244, 2246
clinical features 2247, *2247*
small intestine 2247
stomach 2247
definition 2246
management 2249
communication 109
disease prevention 109
health information 109
comparative genomic hybridization, array-based 136
compartment syndrome 5382
snake bite 1328
competence 18
lack of 18
complement proteins *1753*
complement system *211*, 213, *215*, *288*
acquired complement deficiency 220
in autoimmune disease 222
activation 213–14
alternative pathway 214
classical pathway 214
MBL pathway 215
terminal pathway 215
autoantibodies to 221
anti-C1q antibodies 221
antiC1 inhibitor antibodies 221
C3 nephritic factor 221
biology 208, *216*
defects 712
defensins 209, 211
deficiency *254*
in disease *211*, 213, 216
autoimmune disease 218
haemolytic anaemia 222
infectious diseases 217, 223
inherited deficiency 217
paroxysmal nocturnal haemoglobinuria 221
mannose-binding lectin 211
measurement of complement 214, 223
diagnosis of disease 223
methods 224
monitoring of disease 223
pentraxins 212
reference values *5444*
regulation *208*, 213, 216
abnormalities 218
acquired 221
SLE 3655
viral subversion of *223*
complementary and alternative medicine *65*, 66, *66*
definition 65
heart failure 2721
popularity of 65, 67
prevalence 66
skin disorders 4736
types of 65
see also individual modalities
complex regional pain syndrome 4688
compliance 1453
assessment of 1454
doctor's behaviour 1453
illness 1453
improvement of 1454
patient's behaviour 1453
prescribing regimen 1453
composite theories 18
comprehension 4789
computed tomography (CT) 3200
acute pancreatitis 2561, *2562*
acute respiratory failure 3135
angina 2906, *2907*
ankylosing spondylitis 3609
ARDS *3143*
bronchiectasis *3349*
bronchiolitis obliterans *3384*
cardiac 2671, *2676*, 2676
clinical uses 2676
chest 3201, *3202*
anatomy of mediastinum 3208, *3209*
Conn's syndrome *3064*
COPD 3332, *3332*
Cushing's disease *1877–8*
diffuse parenchymal lung disease 3372, *3372*
epilepsy 4818
high-resolution 3203, *3203*
infective endocarditis *2810*
lung cancer 3524, *3520–2*
mediastinal mass *3542*
mesothelioma *3535*
neurological disorders
historical perspective 4769
stroke *4771*, *4772*
transient ischaemic attacks *4773*
organizing pneumonia *3385*
pancreatic tumours 2576
Parkinson's disease 4882
pleural effusion 3490, *3490*
pleural empyema *3493*
pneumothorax *3503*
pregnancy 2109
pulmonary arterial hypertension *2984*
pulmonary fibrosis 3377, *3377–8*
renal disease *3874*, 3877, *3877*
renal parenchyma 3878
rheumatic disorders 3565
sarcoidosis *3407*
small intestine 2220
solitary fibrous tumour of pleura *3535*
spiral (helical) 3202, *3202*
pulmonary embolism 3011, *3012*
systemic sclerosis *3390*
urinary tract obstruction 4154, *4155*
Wegener's granulomatosis *3400*
condoms *1265*

condyloma acuminata 605
cone shell envenoming 1348, *1348–9*
cone-nose bugs 1228
confidentiality 20
confusion
  definition 4842
  management 3156
  presentation 5486
congenital anomalies, child mortality *75*
congenital dyserythropoietic anaemia 4449
congenital heart disease 2834, 2842
  arrhythmogenic right ventricular cardiomyopathy 2715
  arterial disorders 2856
  atrial septal defects 2851, *2851*
  Brugada syndrome 2611, 2715
  cardiac catheterization/angiography 2679
  catecholaminergic polymorphic ventricular tachycardia 2715
  classification 2842, *2844*, 2844
    atrial arrangement 2844, *2845*
    sequential segmental analysis 2844, *2844*
  connective tissue disorders 2834, 2837
  cor triatatrium *2844*, 2850
  cyanosis 2845, *2845*
  Ebstein's anomaly *2844*, 2849
  echocardiography 2667
  Eisenmenger's syndrome 2851, 2683, *2844*, 2847
  Fallot's tetralogy 2851
  hypertrophic cardiomyopathy 2715
  hypoplastic left heart syndrome 2870
  infundibular stenosis *2844*, 2849
  long QT syndrome 2714, *2714*
  MRI 2676
  pregnancy and contraception 2113, *2871*
  pulmonary valve stenosis 2848
  pulmonary venous anomalies 2859
  short QT syndrome 2715
  syndromic 2834–5
  systemic venous anomalies 2859, *2859*
  transposition complexes 2860, *2861*
  ventricular septal defects 2851, 2853
  see also individual conditions
congestive heart failure
  cardiac catheterization/angiography 2679
  hepatic involvement 2538
conidiobolus 1008, *1008*
Conium maculatum (hemlock) *1363*
conivaptan *1824*
conjunctival haemorrhage, infective endocarditis *2809*
conjunctivitis
  allergic 261
  meningococcal 719
  viral 531
Conn's syndrome 1884, 3062
  aetiology and pathology 3062
  clinical features 3063
    myopathy 5217
  diagnosis 1885, *1885*
  differential diagnosis 1885, *1886*, 3063
  drug-induced 2068
  epidemiology 3062
  history 3062
  investigations 3063
    aldosterone 3063
    aldosterone/renin ratio 3063
    electrolytes 3063
    fludrocortisone suppression 3064
    functional lateralization 3064, *3065*
    genetic testing 3064
    renin 3063
    scanning 3064, *3064*
  prognosis 3066
  treatment 3065
connective tissue disorders 4691
  cardiac involvement 2834, 2837
  hepatic involvement 2544
  vasculitis associated with 4631
  see also individual conditions
connective tissue tumours 321
  incidence *321*
connective tissue 3547
  breakdown 3551, *3551*
connexins 2608
consciousness 4746, *4842*, 4842
consent 18
  competence 18
consequentialism 20
constipation 1522, *2209*, 2209
  abdominal pain 2237
  causes *2208*
  chronic 5302
  functional 2386
  palliative care 5426, *5426*
contact dermatitis 4618
  allergic 4620, *4621*
    scalp 4702
  irritant 4618, *4619*
  occupational 1381
continuous positive airway pressure (CPAP) 3140, 5514
Contracaecum spp. *1176*
contraception 1262
  contraindications *1265*
  effectiveness 1263
  eligibility criteria 1267
  emergency *26*
  heart disease patients 2115
  ideal contraceptive *1262*
  methods 1263
  and STIs 1263
  young people 1263
contraceptive implants *1267*
contrast media
  allergy to 3015
  nephrotoxicity 3898
  ultrasound 3877
Conus geographus 1348
conversion disorder 5302
convulsants, plant-derived 1362, *1362*
convulsions
  benign familial neonatal/infantile 162, 5101
  poisoned patients 1277
COPD *see* chronic obstructive pulmonary disease
co-phenotrope, opioid withdrawal *5347*
copper sulphate poisoning 4094
copper 1498, *1498*
  dietary reference values *1502*
  excretion 1691
  liver content 1691
  poisoning 1298
    antidote *1274*
  reference values *5445–6*
  serum levels 1691
coproporphyria, hereditary 1637, *1637*, 1644
coproporphyrin 1640
  reference values *5446*
co-proxamol, cancer pain 394
copy number variation 142, *143*
cor pulmonale, imaging 3333
cor triatriatum 2850, *2844*, 2997
Cordylobia anthropophaga 1233, 1234
Cordylobia rodhaini 1233
Corfou virus *581*
Cori cycle *1480*
Cori's disease 1598, *1598*
  differential diagnosis *1600*
Cori-Forbes disease 5216
corneal arcus 1661
coronary angioplasty 2948
coronary arteries
  anomalies 2858
  imaging 2895
coronary arteriography/angiography 2685, *2686*
coronary artery bypass surgery 2942, 2924, 2948
  complications 2944
  historical perspectives 2942
  indications 2943, *2943*
    angina pectoris 2943
    non-STEMI 2943
    STEMI 2943
  outcomes 2942, 2944
  and percutaneous intervention 2945, *2945*
  procedure 2943
  secondary prevention 2945
  STEMI 2929
coronary artery disease
  cardiac catheterization/angiography 2679, 2685
  cold working conditions 2951
  CT angiography 2677, *2677–8*
  driving 2949
  exercise testing 2949
  HIV/AIDS 2824
  hot working conditions 2951
  implanted devices 2951
  late gadolinium enhancement 2675, *2675*
  MRI 2676
  rehabilitation 2948
  retirement and end of life 2951
  risk evaluation 2948
  seafarers 2951
  and stress 2949
  toxic exposure 2950
  travel 2950
coronary calcification, CT 2676, *2677*
coronary heart disease 2873, 2881
  acute coronary syndromes 2630, *2879, 2880*
  angina pectoris *see* angina pectoris
  atherosclerosis *see* atherosclerosis
  biomarkers 2892, *2895*
  definition of 2884
  diabetes mellitus 2043
  ethnicity 2888
  fetal origins hypothesis 2898
    fetal nutrition 2898
  future developments 2896
  genetic influences 2894
  genome association 141
  historical perspective 2882, *2883*
  life before 2946
  life course influences 2894
  life and work *2947*, 2947, *2947*
  morbidity 2884, *2885*
  mortality 2885, *2885*
  myocardial infarction
    see myocardial infarction
  nutrition-related 1517, *1518*
    age-adjusted risk *1518*
    promoters *1518*
    protectors *1518*
  older patients 2886
  prevention 2895
    population-based strategies 2895
  psychosocial factors 2885, *2887*
  risk factors 1669, *2875, 2876, 2888, 2893*
    alcohol 2891
    blood pressure 2888
    combined 2892, *2893*
    diet and lipids 2889
    lack of exercise 2892
    obesity and diabetes 2892
    smoking 2888
  screening 2894, *2895*
  social class gradient 2885, *2886*
  women 2886
coronary ostial stenosis 2827, *2827*
coronary sinus defect 2853
  ostium primum 2853
coronary spasm 2631, 2655
coronaviruses *474*, 476
  SARS-like 659
Coronella austriaca (smooth snake) 1327
corpus callosum, agenesis 5143, *5144*
Corrigan's pulse 2751
corruption 116
cortical dysgenesis, nonlissencephalic 5141
cortical microdysgenesis/dysplasia 5141, *5142*
corticobasal degeneration 4807
corticobasal ganglionic degeneration 4887
corticosteroids
  adverse effects 3954, *3954*
    inhaled corticosteroids 3300–1
    ocular 5251
    oesophagitis *2294*
    in pregnancy *2188*
    reproductive *1917*
  alcoholic hepatitis 2478
  allergic rhinitis 3282
  anaphylaxis 3112
  aplastic anaemia 4288
  ARDS 3141
  asthma 3299, *3300*
    acute 3306
    inhaled 3300
    oral 3300
  in breast milk *2189*
  COPD 3337, 3343
  Crohn's disease 2366
  cystic fibrosis 3360

focal segmental glomerulosclerosis 3984
H. influenzae 762
herpes zoster 493
intracranial hypertension *3150*
lymphoma *4320*
membranous nephropathy 3987
meningitis 720
multiple myeloma 4350
osteoarthritis 3635
polymyositis/dermatomyositis 3697
post-transplantation 290, *290, 2730*, 3482
psoriasis 4614
in renal failure 4181
rheumatic fever 2804
rheumatoid arthritis 3597
sarcoidosis 3410
skin disorders
oral 4737
topical 4733, *4734*
topical *2151*
potency 4731
tuberculosis 828
vertigo *4861*
corticotrophs *1801*
corticotropin-releasing factor (CRF), ectopic production 1872
corticotropin-releasing factor test 1876
Cortinarius rubellus (speciossimus) *1369–70*
cortisol binding globulin 1790
cortisol 1790
actions *1791*
metabolic effects *1481*
midnight plasma/salivary 1875
reference values *5441*, *5446*
signalling pathways *1797*
urinary free 1874
cortisone, uses *3798*
Corvisart, J.N. 10
Corynebacterium diphtheria *see* diphtheria
Corynebacterium matruchotii *851*
Corynebacterium spp. *962*
osteomyelitis *3789*
coryza, viral aetiology *474*
cosmic radiation 1410
doses 1410
health risks 1410
protection against 1410
costameres 2606, *2607*
Costeff optic atrophy *1566*, 1572
Costeff's syndrome *4908*
cost-effectiveness analysis 53, 55
criticisms of 56
costochondritis 3712
costs
healthcare 61–2
minimization of 53
opportunity 53
cost-utility analysis 53, *53*
cotrimoxazole
adverse effects, hepatotoxicity *2529*, *2532*
infective endocarditis 2811
co-trimoxazole
adverse effects, hepatotoxicity *2533*
adverse reactions 1031
animal-related injuries 1326
bartonellosis 938
cyclosporiasis 1107
drug interactions *3968*
isosporiasis 1115
listeriosis 898
Madura foot 1005
measles *523*
nocardiosis 857
paracoccidioidomycosis 1028
Pneumocystic jirovecii 1031
prophylactic *440*
in renal failure *4185*
spectrum of activity *446*
toxoplasmosis *1096*
typhoid carriers *742*
typhoid fever *742*
Cotylurus japonicus *1223*
cough headache 4921
cough syncope 4816
cough 3183, *3184*
altitude-related 1407
causes *3184*
drug-induced 3463
lung cancer 3518
mechanism 3170
coumarin-induced skin necrosis *4544*, 4544
coumarin-induced venous limb gangrene 4544
coumarins
adverse effects, hepatotoxicity *2529*
overanticoagulation 4534, *4536*
counselling 5340
Cowbone Ridge virus *566*
Cowden's disease 1845, *352, 2406*
Cowden's syndrome 358, *360*, 367
and breast cancer *1930*
cowpox 512, *512*
cows' milk protein enteropathy 263, 2253
COX inhibitors
and asthma *3289*
rheumatoid arthritis *3594*
COX-1 inhibitors 2307
COX-2 inhibitors 2307
Coxiella burnetii 923, *924*
infective endocarditis *2812*, 2816
pneumonia 3231
community-acquired *453*
treatment *3238*
see also Q fever
Coxiella spp. *962*
coxsackievirus
clinical features *529*
exanthema 531, *531*
hand-foot-and-mouth disease 531, *531*
herpangina 531, *531*
C-peptide 1992
CPR *see* cardiopulmonary resuscitation
CR1, *216*
crab yaws *882*
crackles 3187
cranberry 68
drug interactions *69*
urinary tract infection 4114
cranial irradiation 3530
cranial nerve disorders 5033
facial nerve 5036
glossopharyngeal nerve 5037
hypoglossal nerve 5038
olfactory nerve 5033
palsies 2039
pupillary abnormalities 5034
spinal accessory nerve 5038
third, fourth and sixth cranial nerves 5034
trigeminal nerve 5035
vagus nerve 5037
cranial nerves, diagnosis of brainstem death 3162
craniopharyngioma 1815
imaging 4779
morbidity and mortality 1816
presentation 1815
treatment 1816
Crasydactylus punctatus 1235
crbamoylphosphate synthetase I deficiency *1566*
C-reactive protein 1752, *1753*
acute pancreatitis 2557, *2563*
and body temperature 1758
cardiovascular disease 1758
clinical measurement 1754
interpretation 1758
routine 1758
elevation 1754, *1754*
allograft rejection 1757
infection 1754, *1755–6*
inflammatory disease 1755, *1756*
malignancy 1757
minor 1757, *1757*
necrosis 1756
trauma 1756
reference values *5444*
serum concentration 1753
creams 4731
creatine kinase
marathon runners 5380, *5380*
reference values *5436*
children *5438*
creatine transporter deficiency, psychiatric signs *1720*
creatine, performance enhancement 5384
creatinine clearance 3868, *3869*
prediction of 3869
Cockcroft-Gault equation 3847, 3869
MDRD equation 3870, *3870*
reference values, children *5438*
creatinine
measurement *3847*
reference values *5435*, *5446*
children *5438*
urine:plasma ratio *3896*
CREBs 1788
crepitations 3187
CREST syndrome *see* systemic sclerosis
Creutzfeldt-Jakob disease 1771
iatrogenic 5027, *5027*
sporadic 5025, *5025–6*
clinical features 5031
diagnosis 5031
variant *5028*, 5028, *5028*
clinical features *5031*
cognitive impairment 5278
diagnosis *5030*
cricoarytenoid arthritis 3509
cricothyroidotomy 5516
needle 5516, *5517*
surgical 5516, *5517*
Crigler-Najjar syndrome 2441, 2448
Crimean-Congo haemorrhagic fever *581–2*, 585, *585*
crinophagy 1703
critical illness
acute respiratory failure 3132
airway and breathing 3116, *3116*
cardiorespiratory collapse *3120*
circulatory support 3122, *3117*, 3117
clinical approach 3115
communication 3121
discontinuing treatment 3158
fluid therapy 3118
haemodynamic monitoring *3127*
hepatic involvement 2545, *2545*
patient discomfort *3154*
polyneuropathy 5087, 5152
psychological disturbances 3154
raised intracranial pressure 3147
recognition of 3115, *3116*
sedation and analgesia 3153
underlying condition 3121
venous access 3117, *3118–119*
ventilation 3116
volume overload 3121
see also individual illnesses
crocidolite 3498
crocodiles 1325
Crocodilus niloticus (Nile crocodile) 1325
Crocodilus niloticus 1325
Crocodilus porosus (saltwater crocodile) 1325
Crocodilus porosus 1325
Crohn's disease 2361, 2222
aetiology 2361
environmental factors 2361
genetics 2362
areas of controversy 2369
clinical features 2363
extraintestinal manifestations 2363
hepatic granuloma 2523
signs 2363
symptoms 2363
colorectal 2225
complications 2368
neurological 5163
diagnostic criteria 2365
differential diagnosis 2364, *2364*
epidemiology 2362
future developments 2369
genetics *143*
genome association 141
heredity, fertility and pregnancy 2369
history 2361
IL-6 in 157
investigations 2364, *2365*
orofacial granulomatosis 2278
pathology, *2365*, 2362,
history *2363*
prognosis 2369
radiology *2223*
skin involvement 4722
surgery 2367
treatment 2365
5-aminosalicylates 2366
antibiotics 2366
biological therapies 2367
corticosteroids 2366
diet and nutrition 2366
immunosuppressants 2366
smoking cessation 2365
Cronkhite-Canada syndrome 2222
Croptostroma corticale *3436*

Crosby capsule 2336
crotalase *4540*
Crotalus adamanteus, antivenom *1340*
Crotalus atrox, antivenom *1340*
Crotalus durissus cascavella (South American tropical rattlesnake) *1332*
Crotalus oreganus, antivenom *1340*
Crotalus spp. (rattlesnakes) 1329
Crotalus viridis, antivenom *1340*
Croton tiglium 1372
croup, viral aetiology *474*
Crouzon's syndrome, mutations in *3757*
cryoglobulinaemia
  arthralgia 3708
  essential mixed *3650*
  hepatic involvement 2545
  hepatitis C virus 3858
  pulmonary involvement *3396*
  renal involvement 4061, *4062*
cryoglobulinaemic vasculitis *4033*, 4629
  aetiology, pathogenesis and pathology 4629
  clinical features 4630, *4630*
  clinical investigation 4630
  treatment 4042, 4630
cryoprecipitate 4533, 4565
cryopyrin-associated periodic syndromes *1761*, 1764
cryotherapy 4737
Cryptelytrops (Trimeresurus) albolabris (Southeast Asian white-lipped green viper) *1332*
cryptic determinants 271, *272–3*
Cryptobacterium spp. *962*
cryptococcosis 1018, *1009*
  aetiology and epidemiology 1018
  clinical features 1019, *1019*
  diagnosis 1019
  treatment 1020
Cryptococcus albidus *3436*
Cryptococcus neoformans 1018
  HIV patients 5019, *3247, 5020*
Cryptocotyle lingua *1222*
cryptorchidism 1923, *1917*, 1972
cryptosporidiosis 1098
  age and sex distribution 1100
  clinical features
    immunocompetent patients 1101
    immunocompromised patients 1101
  control of transmission 1104
  diagnosis 1103, *1102–4*
  differential diagnosis 1102
  epidemiology 1098
  foodborne transmission 1100
  frequency of occurrence 1100
  human-to-humantransmission 1099
  infectivity 1103
  laboratory investigations 1101
  nosocomial transmission 1100
  pathology 1100
  resistance and disinfection 1103
  temporal distribution 1100
  treatment 1102
  waterborne transmission 1099
  zoonotic transmission 1099
Cryptosporidium parvum 1098
  malabsorption *2357*
Cryptosporidium spp. 1098
  biology 1098, *1099*
  molecular biology 1098
crysotile 3498
crystal-related arthropathies 3637
  apatite-associated syndromes 3638, 3647
  crystal deposition and clearance 3638, *3639*
  diversity and terminology 3638, *3638*
  gout *see* gout
  inflammation and tissue damage 3639
  pyrophosphate arthropathy 3564, 3637, 3644
crystaluria 3867
CT angiography, renal disease 3878, *3878*
CT *see* computed tomography
CT urography 3878
Ctenocephalides felis (cat flea) *1232*
Ctenocephalides felis 907
Ctenopharyngodon idellus (grass carp) 1347
Culex spp. *1226*
Culicidae (mosquitoes) *1226*
Culicoides spp. *1226*
Culiseta spp. *1226*
Cullen's sign 2563
Cupriavidus spp. *962*
CURB-65 score 3231, 3240
CURE trial *40*
Cushing's disease 1813, 1871
  vs ectopic ACTH secretion *2063*
Cushing's syndrome 1869, 1871, *384, 1871*
  amenorrhoea 1907
  causes *1872*
    ACTH-dependent 1871
      Cushing's disease 1871
      ectopic ACTH syndrome 1872
      ectopic production of CRF 1872
    ACTH-independent 1872
      aberrant receptor expression 1872
      adrenal adenoma/carcinoma 1872, 1874
      alcohol-associated pseudo-Cushing's syndrome 1872
      Carney's syndrome 1872
      McCune-Albright syndrome 1872
  in children 1874
  clinical features 1873, *1872–3*
    myopathy 5217
  CNS complications 5153
  cognitive impairment 5280
  cyclical 1874
  definition 1871
  drug-induced 2068
  investigation 1874
    diagnostic tests 1874, *1874*
    differential diagnostic tests 1875, *1875*
  pregnancy 1874, 2141
  prognosis 1878
  reproductive effects *1917*
  treatment 1878
    adrenal causes 1878
    ectopic ACTH syndrome 1880
    medical 1880, *1880*
    pituitary-dependent disease 1878, *1879*
cutaneous actinomycoses 854
cutaneous larva migrans 1166, *1167*
Cuterebra spp. *1233*
Cuterebridae *1233*
cutis laxa 4586
cutis marmorata 4692
cutting balloon 2938
cyanide poisoning 1309
  antidote *1274*
cyanogenic glycosides *1362*, 1365
cyanosis 2845, *2845*
  complications *2845*, 2846
  disorders of coagulation and blood vessels 2846
  pregnancy 2114
  respiratory disease 3186
  secondary erythrocytosis 2845, *2846*
  venesection *2846*
cyclandelate, vibration injury 1435
cyclin-dependent kinases 345, *345*
cyclizine *5423*
Cyclodontostomum purvisi *1176*
cyclooxygenase (COX) 2307
cyclophosphamide 398
  adverse effects *400*
    hepatotoxicity *2529, 2536*
    aplastic anaemia 4288
  Behçet's disease 3687
  breast cancer *1937*
  carcinogenesis *307*, 328
  contraindication in porphyria *5484*
  lung cancer 3530
  lupus nephritis 4047–8
  lymphoma *4320*, 4320
  membranous nephropathy 3987
  polymyositis/dermatomyositis 3697
  pregnancy *2158*
  sarcoidosis *3411*
  skin disorders 4737
  SLE 3662
  systemic sclerosis *3677*
cyclophyllidian tapeworms 1188, *1189*
  life cycle *1190–1*
cyclopropane, adverse effects, hepatotoxicity *2529*
cycloserine, pregnancy *2172*
Cyclospora cayetanensis 1105
Cyclospora spp. 1105
cyclosporiasis 1105
  clinical features 1105
  diagnosis 1105, *1107–8*
  epidemiology 1105
  life cycle 1105, *1106–7*
  pathology 1107, *1108*
  prevention 1107
  treatment 1107
cyproterone acetate
  polycystic ovary syndrome 1910
  reproductive effects *1917*
  skin disorders 4739
γ-cystathionase deficiency *1566*
cystathioninuria 1594
cystatin C 1774, 3871
cysteine proteinases, COPD *3323*
cystic fibrosis transmembrane regulator (CFTR) 133, 3347, 3353
cystic fibrosis 139, 167, *168*, 3353
  antenatal screening *102*
  and bronchiectasis 3350
  care team 3363
  central nervous system 3363
  definition 3353
  diabetes mellitus 3362
  diagnosis 3356
    genotype 3357
    nasal electrical potential difference 3357
    sweat testing 3357, *3358*
  epidemiology 3355
    genotype 3355
    phenotype 3355, *3355*
    survival 3355, *3357*
  future prospects 3364
  gastrointestinal management 3361
    distal intestinal obstruction syndrome 3361
    nutrition 3361
    pancreatic insufficiency 3361
  genetics *139, 3354,* 3354
  hepatic involvement 2539
  infection issues 3359
    cross-infection 3359
  kidneys 3363
  liver disease 3362
  lung transplantation 3363, *3363, 3478*
  microbiology 3355
    B. cepacia complex 3356
    H. influenzae 3356
    P. aeruginosa 3356
    S. aureus 3355
  osteoporosis 3363
  pathogenesis 3354
    biliary tract 3354
    gut 3354
    heterozygote advantage 3355
    pancreas 3354
    respiratory tract 3354
    sweat ducts 3354
  presenting feature 3356, *3357*
  reproductive effects *1917*, 3362
  respiratory complications 3361
    haemoptysis 3361
    pneumothorax 3361
    upper airway disease 3361
  respiratory failure 3363
  respiratory management 3359
    airway clearance 3360
    altered mucus properties 3360
    anti-inflammatory therapy 3360
    antibiotics 3359
    bronchodilators 3360
    oxygen therapy 3360
  screening 3358
  skin and joints 3363
  terminal care 3363
cystic hydatid disease 1185
  aetiology 1185
  clinical features 1186, *1186–7*
  diagnosis 1186, *1187*
  epidemiology 1186, *1186*
  pathogenesis 1186
  prevention and control 1188
  treatment 1187
cystic hygroma 4696
cysticercosis 1193
  aetiology 1194, *1194*
  clinical features 1195, *1195*
  diagnosis
    immunological tests 1198

neuroimaging 1197, *1197*
parasitological 1198
epidemiology 1194
future developments 1199
pathogenesis 1194
pathology 1195, *1196–7*
prevention and control 1199
prognosis 1199
treatment 1198
cystine
reference values *5446*
stones *4124*, 4130
cystinosis 1698, *1551, 1552, 3730, 3739, 4148, 4149*
renal involvement 4101
cystinuria 4147, *1551, 4128, 4148*
nephrolithiasis *4101*
cystitis 4107, *4107*
drug-induced 4111
interstitial 4111
radiation-induced 4111
treatment 4112, *4113–114*
cysts *4591*
bone 3713
bronchogenic *3542*, 3543
choledochal 2582, *2582*
colloid *4778*, 4778
dermoid 3541
epidermoid 4706
mediastinal 3543
pericardial 3543
pilar 4706
popliteal *3557*
spleen 4339
thymus 3541
cytarabine 398
adverse effects, hepatotoxicity *2529, 2533*
lymphoma *4320*
cytochrome *b* deficiency *2766*
cytochrome P450
genetic variability *see* pharmacogenomics
isoforms *1458*
cytogenetics 135
cytokine receptors 3279
cytokine storm 596
cytokine superfamilies 398
cytokines 152, 212, *212, 1791*
acidosis 1745
chemokines 212
classification 153, *153*
interferons 213
measurement in biological fluids 159
mode of action 155
post-translational regulation 155
proinflammatory 2601
receptor interactions *253*
rheumatoid arthritis 3585, *3586–7*
SLE 3656, *3656*
superfamilies 155, *156*
interleukin-1, 156
TNF 155
synthesis, expression and regulation 154, *154*
T-cell function regulators 157
as therapeutic targets 158
transcriptional/post-transcriptional regulation 154
cytomegalovirus retinitis 5248, *5248*
cytomegalovirus 483, *484*, 494
aetiology 494
and cancer 496
clinical features 494
congenital 495, *244*, 5146
epidemiology 494
historical background 494
HIV patients 5020
immunosuppressed patients 495, *3956, 3958*
treatment 496
infective oesophagitis *2293*
laboratory diagnosis 496
pathogenesis 494
pathology 496
and peptic ulcer disease 2308
pregnancy 497, *2167*, 2167
prevention and control 497
renal involvement 4073
treatment 496
see also individual conditions
cytopenia
refractory
with multilineage dysplasia 4259
with multilineage dysplasia and ringed sideroblasts 4260
cytosine arabinoside, carcinomatous 'meningitis' 391
cytosine 138
adverse effects, hepatotoxicity *2532*
cytoskeleton 131
cytotoxic drugs
drug interactions *1471*
reproductive effects *1917*
secondary immunodeficiency *244*
cytotoxic T cells 186, 287
cytotoxins
fungal 1368, *1367, 1369*
plant-derived 1364, *1367*

D-2-hydroxyglutaric aciduria 1579, *1566, 1580*
Daboia (Vipera) palaestinae, antivenom *1340*
Daboia russelii 1328
antivenom *1340*
Daboia siamensis (Eastern Russell's viper) *1331*
antivenom *1340*
dacarbazine
adverse effects, hepatotoxicity *2529, 2536*
lymphoma *4320*, 4320
daclizumab 3482
lymphoma *4320*
post-transplantation *3954*
dactylitis *881*
Dakar bat virus *566*
dalbavancin *706*
bacteraemia *703*
cellulitis, mastitis and pyomyositis *699*
dalteparin, pregnancy 2118
danazol
adverse effects
hepatotoxicity *2533*
hirsutism 2068
teratogenicity *2187*
Dandy-Walker malformation *5142*, 5143
Danon's disease 1716, 1698
autophagy 1703
dantrolene
adverse effects, hepatotoxicity *2529*
amphetamine/ecstasy poisoning 1280
dapsone
adverse effects, hepatotoxicity *2529, 2535*
leprosy *845*
Madura foot 1005
poisoning 1286
pregnancy *2172*
skin disorders 4739
spider bites 1355
toxoplasmosis *1096*
daptomycin *707*
bacteraemia *703*
cellulitis, mastitis and pyomyositis *699*
endocarditis *704*
epidural abscess *702*
mode of action *443*
toxic shock syndrome *697*
Darier's disease 4596
photoaggravation *4670*
darmbrand 808
darunavir
HIV/AIDS *638*
toxicity *640*
Darwin, Charles 13
dasatinib 400
leukaemias 4253
data entry, remote 46
Database of Abstracts of Reviews of Effectiveness (DARE) 24
DaTSCAN, Parkinson's disease 4882, *4885*
daunorubicin, adverse effects *400*
D-dimer
deep venous thrombosis 3004
in pregnancy 2119
pulmonary embolism 3010
reference values 5444
DDS syndrome 845
DDT 1150
CNS effects *1386*
peripheral nervous system effects *1387*
de Musset's sign 2751
de Quervain's disease 1383
De Quervain's tenosynovitis *3248, 3557*
De Quervain's thyroiditis 1843
deafness *168*
neonatal screening *104*
nonsyndromic 168
Paget's disease of bone 3742
death
causes of 5363
cocaine abuse 5364
medical care related 5363
sudden death syndrome 5364, *5365*
sudden infant death 5363
sudden unexpected nocturnal death 5364
duties at 5360, *5361*
brain death 5362
confirming and documenting 5361
death certification 5362
excluding foul play 5362
reporting to legal authorities 5362–3
time of death 5362
Debaryomyces hansenii 3436
debrancher enzyme deficiency 5216
decay accelerating factor *216*
decompression illness
altitude-induced 1413, *1413*
diving-related 1420, *1420*
Decticus verrucivorus 1229
deep venous thrombosis 3003, 4688
clinical features 3003
complications 3004
detection of 3004
diagnostic strategy *3005*, 3004
differential diagnosis 3003
incidence and pathology 3003
investigation 3004
pregnancy 2116
presentation 5462, *5463–4*
prevention *3006, 3004, 3007–8*
spinal cord injuries 5051
treatment *3008*, 3004
defence against disease 15
defensins 209, 211
deferasirox 4397
deferiprone 4397
defibrillation 3101
factors affecting success 3101
electrode position 3101
pads versus paddles 3102
shock energy and waveforms 3102, *3103*
transthoracic impedance 3101, *3102*
safety 3102
dehydroemetine, amoebiasis 1041
delavirdine
HIV/AIDS 636
mode of action *444*
Delftia spp. *962*
delirium tremens 1464, 5155
delirium 5263, *5270, 5271*
alcohol and substance abuse 5271, *5272*
causes *5264*
clinical features *4789, 5264*
definition 4842
differential diagnosis 4798
investigation 5271, *5272*
management 3156, 5272
older patients 5389, 5402, 5406
causes 5403
clinical challenges 5403
definition 5403, *5403*
management 5403
precipitating factors *5272*
and psychiatric disorder 5271
risk factors *5271*
Demansia atra (whip snake) *1238*
demeclocycline, renal toxicity *3860*
dementia 4795, *384*, 4790, 5100, 5272, 5407
alcoholic 5156
Alzheimer's disease *see* Alzheimer's disease
causes *4796, 5273*
classification *4796–8*
clinical features *5273*
differential diagnosis 4797
and driving 5402
frontotemporal 4802, 5100
Lewy body 4803, *4805*, 4886, 5100
subcortical 4807
treatable causes 4807
vascular 4806
Demodex folliculorum 4672, 4675
demographic entrapment 82
scale of 117
types of 116, *116*

demographic risk 89
demyelinating disorders 4948
  central pontine myelinolysis 4960
  inflammation, neurodegeneration and remyelination 4951
  isolated 4952
  leucodystrophies 4960
  multiple sclerosis *see* multiple sclerosis
  neurobiology 4950
  pathophysiology 4950
  recovery of function 4950, *4951*
  see also individual disorders
dendritic cells 209, *288*
  myeloid 208, *209*
  plasmacytoid 208, *209*
Dendrobates histrionicus (poison frog) *1344*
dengue fever 575
  aetiology 575
  clinical features 576
    classic dengue fever 576, *577*
    dengue haemorrhagic fever 577, *577–8*
    renal toxicity *4086*
  differential diagnosis 578
  epidemiology 575
  global distribution *576*
  laboratory diagnosis 578
  management 578
  outcome 579
  pathogenesis 576
  prevention 579
dengue virus *566*
Dent's disease *165,* 166, *3721, 3739, 4135, 4149*
  nephrolithiasis *4101, 4128*
dental caries 1522, 2257
  aetiology 2257
  clinical features 2258, *2259*
  course and prognosis 2259
  differential diagnosis 2259
  pathology 2258
  treatment 2259
dentatorubral-pallidoluysian atrophy 5115
dentinogenesis imperfecta 3730, 3747
Denver shunts 2489
Denys-Drash syndrome 1970
deodorants, poisoning by 1317
dependency syndrome 3088
depolarization 161
depression 4163
  diagnosis and clinical features 5310, *5311*
  and dysthymia 5311, *5311*
  epidemiology 5309, *5309*
  history taking 5259, *5260*
  impact 5309
  older people 5407
  palliative care 5426
  pathophysiology 5310
  recognition of 5262, *5262*
  somatic presentation 5301
  somatized 5261, *5261*
  symptoms *5261*
  treatment *5312, 5313*
Dermabacter spp. *962*
Dermacentor andersoni 1228
Dermacentor marginatus 1228
Dermacentor silvarum 1228
Dermacentor variabilis 1228
Dermacoccus spp. *962*
dermatitis herpetiformis *4603,* 4608, *4609*
  coeliac disease 2338
dermatitis
  contact *see* contact dermatitis
  exfoliative *385*
  infective 650, *652*
  see also eczema
Dermatobia hominis 1233–4
dermatofibroma 4706
dermatological vehicles 4731
  additives 4732
    absorption enhancers 4732
    antioxidants 4732
    emulsifiers 4732
    preservatives 4732
  choice of 4732
  creams 4731
  gels 4732
  lotions 4732
  ointments 4731
dermatomyositis *see* polymyositis/dermatomyositis
Dermatophagoides spp. *see* house dust mites
Dermatophilus spp. *962*
dermatophytoses 998–9
  aetiology 999
  clinical features 1000
    dry type infections of soles and palms 1000
    HIV and immunocompromised patients 1001
    onychomycosis 1000
    tinea capitis 1000
    tinea corporis 1000
    tinea cruris 1000
    tinea imbricata 1001
    tinea pedis 1000
  epidemiology 999
  laboratory diagnosis 1001
  treatment 1001
dermatotoxins, plant-derived *1362,* 1365, *1365–6*
Dermestes peruvianus 1236
dermis
  failure of 4586
  structure 4584
dermographism, in pregnancy 2153
dermoid cysts 3541
desferrioxamine 1462
  aluminium poisoning 1296
  haemochromatosis 1684, 4397
desflurane, adverse effects, hepatotoxicity *2529*
desipramine
  adverse effects *5313*
    hepatotoxicity *2529, 2532*
desire-fulfilment theories 18
desloratidine 3282
Desmodontinae (vampire bats) 1327
desmopressin 4534
  diabetes insipidus 1823
  orthostatic hypotension *5063*
  structure 1819
desmosomes 2608, *4594, 4604*
desquamative interstitial pneumonia 3368, *3368*
Desulfomicrobium spp. *962*
Desulfomonas spp. *962*
Desulfovibrio spp. *962*
detergents
  effects on skin 1382
  poisoning by 1317
developed countries, priority setting 58
developing countries
  clinical trials 47
  priority setting 58
Devic's disease 4953
devil's claw 68
dexamethasone suppression test *5449*
  high-dose 1876
  low-dose 1875
  overnight 1875
dexamethasone
  congenital adrenal hyperplasia 1893
  meningitis 4989
  metastatic brain tumours 390
  SLE 2156
dexamfetamine, narcolepsy *4833*
dexmedetomidine 3156
dextroproxyphene, adverse effects, hepatotoxicity *2533*
Di George syndrome *2250*
diabetes insipidus 1819, 1821, 3852
  causes *1822*
  central 3830
  cranial 1822, *1822, 3829*
    treatment *1822,* 1823
  differential diagnosis 1821
  nephrogenic 165, 166, *1822,* 1823, *3829,* 3830
    treatment 1823
  in potential organ donors *3162, 3164*
  pregnancy 1874
  primary polydipsia 1823, 3828
  water deprivation test *1822*
diabetes mellitus 1666, 1987
  aetiology 1998
    autoimmune 1999
    enterovirus 531
    environmental factors 1999
    genetic 1998
  annual review *2022*
  'brittle' 2018
  cardiac involvement 2786
  care structures 2021
  classification *1998*
  cognitive impairment 5280
  complications 1989
    autonomic failure 5065
    chronic 2030
    CNS 5153
    metabolic 1988, 2024
      hyperosmolar nonketotic state (HONK) 1989, 2027
      hypoglycaemia 1989, 2028
      ketoacidosis *see* diabetic ketoacidosis
      lactic acidosis 2028
  and coronary heart disease 2892
  cystic fibrosis 3362
  diagnosis 1990, *1990*
  education 2021
  employment, driving and insurance 2021
  flatbush 2008
  genome association 141
  gestational 2007
    and polycystic ovary syndrome 1909
  glycaemic control 2020
    blood glucose monitoring 2020
    during infections 2023
    HbA1c and fructosamine 2020
    monitoring schedules 2020
    urinary glucose and ketones 2020
haematological changes 4559
infections 2021
intercurrent illness *2023*
malnutrition-related 2007
management 1988, 2008
  diet and lifestyle 2008, *2009*
    antiobesity drugs and bariatric surgery 2010
    dietary composition 2009
    optimization of meal patterns 2009
    physical activity 2010
    smoking 2010
    total energy intake 2009
  insulin 2010
  oral hypoglycaemic agents 2014
  statins 1669
  treatment targets *2006*
  type 1 diabetes 2017
  type 2 diabetes 2019
maturity-onset diabetes of the young (MODY) 1988, *2005, 2007*
metabolic basis 1992
  insulin 1992
  islets of Langerhans 1992
mitochondrial 2008
monogenic 1988, 2005
mortality rate *76*
neonatal 2006
oesophageal symptoms *2297*
in pancreatic disease 2007
poor control 2018
pregnancy 2133
  aetiology and genetics 2135
  classification 2134, *2134*
  diagnosis 2136, *2136*
  effect of 2137
  epidemiology 2134
  fetal assessment 2138
  gestational 2133
  historical perspective 2134
  pathogenesis/pathology 2135
  postpartum considerations 2138
  pregestational 2133
  risk factors *2135*
  screening 2135
  timing/mode of delivery 2138, *2138*
  treatment 2137, *2137*
screening 1991, *1991*
skin involvement 4717
  acanthosis nigricans and insulin resistance 4719, *4719*
  diabetic dermopathy 4717
  diabetic neuropathy 4719
  granuma annulare 4717, *4718*
  infection 4718
  necrobiosis lipoidica 4718, *4718*
stem cell therapy 202
surgery 2023
type 1 *276,* 1987, 1997
  clinical features 2002, *2002*
  epidemiology and demographic features 1997
  experimental treatments 2018
  fulminant 2008
  management 2017

metabolic disturbance 2000
carbohydrate metabolism 2000
fat metabolism 2000
natural history 2000, *2001*
poor glycaemic control *2018*
prognosis 2002
protein metabolism 2000
counter-regulatory hormones 2000
type 2 1520, *1520*, 1987, 2003
aetiology 2003
β-cell failure 2004
environmental factors 2004
genetic factors 2003
clinical features *2002*, 2005
epidemiology and demographic features 2003
fetal and postnatal effects 2899, *2899*
management 2019
metabolic disturbances 2005
natural history 2004
and polycystic ovary syndrome 1910
prognosis 2005
risk factors 2004
diabetic bullae 4719
diabetic dermatopathy 4717
diabetic dermopathy 2048
diabetic hand syndrome 2047
diabetic ketoacidosis *1742*, 1747, 2003, 2024
abdominal pain 2236
causes 2024
clinical features 2025
complications 2026, *2027*
investigations and diagnosis 2025, *2025*
management 2025
fluid replacement 2025
insulin replacement 2026
potassium replacement 2026
subsequent 2027
pathophysiology *2023*, 2024
presentation 5477
treatment 1750
diabetic nephropathy *1989, 2022*, 4021
areas of uncertainty 4031
characteristics 3857, *3858*
clinical features 4027
blood pressure 4028
glomerular filtration rate 4028
urinary albumin excretion rate 4027
clinical investigation 4028, *4028*
diagnostic criteria 4029, *4029*
differential diagnosis 4028
epidemiology 4025, *4025–6*
genetics 4024
historical perspective 4022, *4022*
blood pressure 4022
fetal programming 4023
growth factors 4023
haemodynamic factors 4022, *4023*
mechanical and structural factors 4023
pathology/pathogenesis 4024, *4024*
prevention 4025
blood pressure control 4026
glycaemic control *4026*
prognosis 4030, *4030*
treatment 4029
glycaemic control and blood pressure 4029
diabetic neuropathy 1989, *2022*, 2036, 4719, 5085
clinical syndromes 2036, *2036*
acute mononeuropathies 2038
autonomic neuropathy 2037
cranial nerve palsies 2039
diabetic amyotrophy 2038
diffuse small fibre neuropathy 2037
diffuse symmetrical polyneuropathy 2036
insulin neuritis 2039
pressure palsies 2039
diagnosis 2039
treatment 2039
diabetic retinopathy *2022*, 2032, 5235, 5252
advanced 2034
aetiology and pathogenesis 2033
background 2033
clinical findings 5236, *5236–7*
epidemiology 2033
eye examination 2034, *2035*
incidence 5236
maculopathy 2034
management 2035, *5237*
specific treatments 2035
pathology 5236, *5236*
preproliferative 2034
prognosis 5236
progression 5236
proliferative 2034
risk factors 5236
screening 5237, *106, 5237*
stages of 2033, *2033*
symptoms 2034
diagnostic accuracy *24*
diagnostic test results 25, *25–6*
Dialister spp. *962*
dialyser reactions 3941
dialysis bone disease 3768
dialysis osteodystrophy 5218
dialysis 3932
poisoned patients 1279
and pregnancy 2107
see also haemodialysis; peritoneal dialysis
diamorphine *3155*
diaphragm, contraceptive *26*
diaphragm
disorders of 3511
aetiology 3511, *3511*
in pregnancy 2121
radiographic view 3207
investigations 3512
pathophysiology 3511
symptoms and signs 3512
treatment 3512
diaphyseal aclasis 3759
diarrhoea 536, *2208*
acidosis 1749
antibiotic-associated 431
functional 2387
and gut peptides 2322
hypokalaemia 3836
immunocompromised patients 249
inflammatory 2428
bacteria 2429
diagnosis 2431
parasites 2429
noninflammatory 2426, *2427*
bacteria 2426
chronic 2428
diagnosis 2431
viruses 2427
in renal failure 4176
small bowel resection 2355
travellers' 2428
prevention/management 468, *468*
diarrhoeal disease
child mortality *75*
interventions 77
mortality *121*
diastolic function, cardiac catheterization/angiography 2685
diastolic pressure *2621*
diastrophic dysplasia *3721*
mutations in *3757*
diazepam 3156, *5423, 5265*
adverse effects, hepatotoxicity *2529, 2532, 2535*
amphetamine/ecstasy poisoning 1280
contraindication in porphyria *5484*
diazoxide
adverse effects, hirsutism 2068
hypertensive emergencies *3080*
1:2,5:6-dibenzpyrene *338*
1,2-dibromo-3-chloropropane, reproductive effects 1385
DIC *see* disseminated intravascular coagulation
dicarboxylic aminoaciduria *4148*
Dichelobacter spp. *962*
diclazuril, isosporiasis 1115
diclofenac
adverse effects, hepatotoxicity *2532*
ankylosing spondylitis 3610
and asthma *3289*
rheumatoid arthritis *3594*
dicloxacillin *706*
cellulitis, mastitis and pyomyositis *699*
impetigo *697*
septic bursitis/arthritis *700*
dicrocoeliasis 1215, *1216*
Dicrocoelium dendriticum 1212, *1213*, 1215, *1216*, 1238
dicylomine, opioid withdrawal *5347*
didanosine
HIV/AIDS *638*
mode of action *444*
dideoxyinosine, adverse effects, hepatotoxicity *2529*
diencephalic syndromes 4929, 5274
Dientamoeba fragilis 1036, 1042
diet
and cancer 309
fibre 310
ingestion of preformed carcinogens 309
meat and fat 309
overnutrition 309
retinoids and carotenoids 310
and COPD 3315
coronary heart disease risk 2889
Crohn's disease 2366
diabetes mellitus 2008, *2009*
dietary composition 2009
optimization of meal patterns 2009
total energy intake 2009
dialysis patients 3940
gastrointestinal infections 2432
hypertension 3048
macrobiotic 65
obesity treatment 1532
post-renal transplant 3967
potassium in *3842*
ulcerative colitis 2380
dietary change 1520, 1523
dietary reference values *1502*, 1503, *1523* 1523,
diethylcarbamazine, filariasis 1158
diethylene glycol
metabolism *1311*
poisoning 1310
antidote *1274*
diethylenetriaminepentaacetic acid (DTPA) 3881
diethylstilboestrol, teratogenicity *1468*
Dietzia spp. *962*
diffuse alveolar haemorrhage 3427
diffuse idiopathic skeletal hyperostosis (DISH) *see* Forestier's disease
diffuse parenchymal lung disease 3365, *3367*
bronchiolitis obliterans 3382
classification 3366
clinical examination 3370
clinical history 3370
clinical issues 3373
criteria for biopsy 3374
integrated diagnosis 3373
management principles 3373
cryptogenic organizing pneumonia 3382
definition 3366
diagnostic approach 3370, *3370*
blood tests 3372
bronchoalveolar lavage 3373
chest X-ray 3371
high-resolution CT 3372, *3372*
lung biopsy 3373
lung function tests 3371
differential diagnosis *3367*
idiopathic interstitial pneumonias *3367*, 3365–6
idiopathic pulmonary fibrosis 3375
diflunisal
adverse effects, hepatotoxicity *2532, 2533*
and asthma *3289*
rheumatoid arthritis *3594*
digenic inheritance 139, 140
DiGeorge syndrome 235, *238*, 252
cardiac involvement 2837
and hypoparathyroidism *1855*, 1864
DiGeorge/velocardiofacial syndrome *148*, 145
digital clubbing *385*
cirrhosis *2499*
cyanosis 2846
interstitial lung disease 3388
lung cancer 3523
Digitalis purpurea (foxglove) *1364*
digitalis
poisoning 1286
antidote *1274*
reproductive effects *1917*
digoxin
in breast milk *1469, 2189*
cardiac arrhythmias 2700, *2701*

dilated cardiomyopathy 2776
drug interactions *1471*
and exercise testing 2661
heart failure 2724
poisoning, antidotes *5505*
in renal failure *4179*
serum levels *5449*
therapeutic drug monitoring 1475, *1475*
thyrotoxicosis 1840
dihydroergotamine
migraine *4918*
orthostatic hypotension *5063*
dihydrofolate reductase inhibitors 4413
dihydropyrimidine dehydrogenase deficiency 1634
dihydrotestosterone
actions *1791*
signalling pathways *1797*
2,8-dihydroxyadeninuria 1630
dilated cardiomyopathy 2765, 2773
arrhythmias in 2774
causes 2773, *2773*
definition 2773
history 2774
investigations 2775
cardiac biomarkers 2775
cardiac catheterization 2776
chest radiography 2775
ECG 2775
echocardiography 2775, *2775–6*
electrophysiological testing 2776
exercise testing 2775
MRI 2776
late gadolinium enhancement 2676
management 2776
nonpharmacological 2777
pharmacological 2776
and mitral regurgitation 2743
and myocarditis 2760
pathology and pathophysiology 2774
physical examination 2774
pregnancy 2111
prognosis 2774
X-linked *2788*
diloxanide, amoebiasis 1041
diltiazem
adverse effects, hepatotoxicity *2532*, *2535*
in breast milk *1469*
Raynaud's phenomenon *3671*
in renal failure *4179*
dimercaprol *1274*, 1462
dimercaptosuccinic acid (DMSA) 3880
dimethylaminoazobenzene *338*
dimethylnitrosamine *338*
dimorphism 999
dinitrophenol, hepatotoxicity *1385*
Dinobdella ferox 1238
Dioctophyma renale 1176
Diorchitrema formosanum 1222
Diorchitrema pseudocirratum 1222
Dioscorea quartiniana (yam), nephrotoxicity *4093*
diphenoxylate *2433*
diphenyl methane diisocyanate *3436*
diphosphoglycerate mutase deficiency 4472
diphtheria 664
clinical features 666
anterior nasal 666
cutaneous 666
malignant 666, *666–7*
tonsillar (faucial) 666, *666*
tracheolaryngeal 666, *666*
ulceration *667*
clinical investigation 668
complications 667
cardiovascular 667
neurological 667, *668*
diagnosis 668
differential diagnosis 668
epidemiology 665
history 664
immunization *91*
pathogenesis 665
prevention 669
treatment 668
vaccines *466*, 669
diphtheritic neuropathy 5091
diphyllobothriasis 1199, *1200*
Diphyllobothrium latum 1200
Diphyllobothrium nihonkaiense 1200
Diphyllobothrium pacificum 1200
Diphyllobothrium yonagoense 1200
diplopia 4973, 5034
Diploscapter coronata 1176
Dipylidium caninum 1190, 1193
dipyridamole, stroke prevention 30
Dirofilaria immitis 1176
renal toxicity 4088
Dirofilaria repens 1176
Dirofilaria tenuis 1176
Dirofilaria ursi 1176
disability-adjusted life years *74*, 1506
disaccharidase deficiency 2347
carbohydrate intolerance syndrome 2348
treatment 2350
disasters 1436, *1437*
earthquakes 1438
floods 121, 1440
human 82
definition 119
divisiveness of 122
famines 120, *121–2*
natural-social distinction 120
policy intervention 121
hurricanes 1439
postdisaster relief 1440
predisaster measures 1438
volcanic eruptions 1439
discoid lupus erythematosus 2278
discontinuing treatment 3158
basic care provision 3160
decision not to escalate 3160
do not resuscitate orders 3160
making the decision 3159
family's input 3159
medical team's input 3159
patient's input 3159
means of withdrawal 3159
outcomes of medical treatment 3158
patients without hope 3158
Disease Control Priorities Project 76
lowering child mortality *77*, *78*
disease control, priority setting 76
disease genetics 148
see also individual diseases
disease modelling, stem cells 202
disease prevention 109
disease, major causes of 74
disease-modifying anti-rheumatic drugs *see* DMARDS
disequilibrium syndrome *4904*
dishwashing liquids, poisoning by 1317
disinfectants, poisoning by 1317
disomy, uniparental 139
disopyramide *2701*
adverse effects, hepatotoxicity *2532*, *2533*
in renal failure *4179*
disorders 1740
Dispholidus typus (boomslang) 1327
disseminated intravascular coagulation 4535, 4505, 4513, 5506
acute haemolysis 4537
adenocarcinoma-associated *4543*, 4543
causes *4537*, *4514*
diagnosis and treatment 4536
immunological disorders 4537
infection 4537
malaria 1080
meningitis 720
neonate 4545
obstetrical complications 4357
pathogenesis *4538*
pregnancy 2178
trauma and shock 4536
vascular anomalies 4537
disseminated tuberculosis 820
distal intestinal obstruction syndrome 3361
distal tubule (of kidney) 3814, *3815*
nephrolithiasis *4101*
renal tubular acidosis
with hyperkalaemia 4137
with hypokalaemia 4137
distribution 1456
antimicrobials 449, *450*
protein binding 1456
tissue 1457
distributive shock 3122, 3128
disulfiram 5348
adverse effects, hepatotoxicity *2529*
diterpene esters *1362*
dithranol 4733
psoriasis 4614
diuretics
ascites 2487, *2488*
contraindication in porphyria 1641
COPD 3343
dilated cardiomyopathy 2776
drug interactions *1471*, *3968*
heart failure 2721, *2722*
hypertension 2042, *3050*
hypertensive emergencies *3079*
hypokalaemia 3835
intracranial hypertension *3150*
mode of action 1461
osmotic 1462
performance enhancement 5385
poisoning 1286
potassium-sparing 3844
in renal failure 4177, *4178*
diverticular disease 1521, 2224, *2224*, 2235, 2389
aetiology 2389
clinical features 2390
complicated 2391
abscess 2392
acute diverculitis 2391, *2392*
colonic fistulas 2393
faecal peritonitis 2393
haemorrhage 2393
intestinal obstruction 2393
perforation 2392, *2393*
epidemiology 2389
GI bleeding 2241
investigations *2235*
jejunal 2221
pathogenesis 2390, *2390*
pathology 2390
uncomplicated 2391, *2391*
diving medicine 1416, *1417*
ascent 1419
barotrauma 1419
decompression illness 1420, *1420*
hypoxia 1419
isobaric decompression 1421
barotrauma 1418
bottom of dive 1418
high-pressure nervous syndrome 1419
hypercapnia 1419
inert gas narcosis 1418
oxygen toxicity 1419, *1419*
descent 1418
fitness to dive 1421
immersion effects 1417, *1418*
limitations to diving 1417, *1417–18*
problems after dive 1421
dizziness 4860, *4861*
management 4863, *4861–5*
djenkol beal poisoning 4092
DMARDS
ankylosing spondylitis 3610
psoriatic arthritis 3613
rheumatoid arthritis *3595*
clinical trials 3596
DNA damage checkpoint 343
DNA identikit 5371
DNA profiling 5370
HLA *DQ*α 5371
mitochondrial DNA 5371
polymerase chain reaction 5371
population frequency of DNA patterns 5371
variable number of tandem repeats 5370
DNA repair defects *238*, 255, 5099
DNA strand break pathways 343
DNA 138, 127
complementary (cDNA) 136
damage checkpoint 187
damage response 183
damage/repair 179
mismatch 344
nucleotide excision 343
nucleotides 138
repetitive elements 141
secondary structures 142
transcription 127
DNA-ligase IV deficiency *238*
DNAR *see* do not attempt resuscitation order
do not attempt resuscitation order 3097, 3159
Dobrava virus *581*
dobutamine 3130
docetaxel, breast cancer *1937*
docobalt edetate *1274*
doctors
health advertising to 109
preventive responsibilities 90

docusate *5426*
dog bites 1325
dolichostenomelia 3778
Dolichovespula spp. 1350
Dolosicoccus spp. *962*
Dolosigranulum spp. *962*
domperidone *5423*
donovanosis 745
  aetiology 746
  clinical features 746, *746*
  diagnosis 746
  pathogenesis 746
  treatment 746, *747*
dopamine agonists
  acromegaly 1807
  prolactinoma 1811
dopamine β-hydroxylase deficiency *1566*, 1589, 5065
dopamine 3129
dopexamine 3130
Doppler echocardiography 2663, *2664*
  heart failure 2719
doripenem, pneumonia *3238*, *3245*
Doss porphyria 1643–4, 1637, 1637, 1640
dosulepin, migraine prevention *4916*
DOT therapy, tuberculosis 811, 826
double outlet right ventricle 2866
Down's syndrome 145, *148*,
  antenatal screening *98*, 101, *102*
  cardiac involvement 2835
  and leukaemia 332
doxazosin
  hypertensive emergencies *3079*
  in pregnancy *2099*
doxepin, adverse effects *5313*
doxorubicin 399
  adverse effects *400*
  breast cancer *1937*
  lung cancer 3530
  lymphoma *4320*
  resistance *399*
doxycycline *706*
  acne *4680*
  adverse effects, oesophagitis *2294*
  animal-related injuries 1326
  anthrax 787
  bacterial overgrowth *2334*
  brucellosis 794
  cellulitis, mastitis and pyomyositis *699*
  chlamydial infections *943*
  impetigo *697*
  infective endocarditis *2818*
  leptospirosis 878
  Lyme borreliosis *864–5*
  melioidosis *771*
  mycoplasmal infections *960*
  pelvic inflammatory disease *1260*
  pneumonia *3238*
  prophylactic *1086*, 1087
  Q fever 926
  in renal failure *4185*
  rickettsioses 914
  septic bursitis/arthritis *700*
  syphilis 894
  tularaemia 782
2,3-DPG deficiency 4268
D-penicillamine *1274*, 1462
  adverse effects
    hepatotoxicity *2532*, *2533*
    renal toxicity *3860*
  pregnancy *2158*
  primary biliary cirrhosis *2467*
  rheumatoid arthritis *3595*
  Wilson's disease *1692*
dracunculiasis *see* guinea worm disease
Dressler's syndrome 2791
driving
  coronary artery disease 2949
  diabetes mellitus 2021
  epilepsy 4823
  obstructive sleep apnoea 3273
  older patients 5390, 5402
    dementia 5402
    risk ascertainment 5402
  spinal cord injuries 5053
drop attacks, differential diagnosis 4817
drotrecogin alfa 417
droughts 121
drowning 1397
  causes 1399, *1399*
  clinical features 1399
  definition 1397
  epidemiology 1397
    alcohol 1398
    ethnicity 1398
  mortality/morbidity 1397
  pathophysiology 1398
    hypothermia 1398
  prevention 1401, *1401*
  prognostic indicators 1399
    cardiovascular status 1399
    neurological status 1400
  treatment 1400
    hospital 1400
    immediate 1400, *1400*
drug action, modification of 1463
drug allergy 263
drug clearance, in pregnancy 2190, *2190*
drug dependence 5341, *5350*
  aetiology 5343
  epidemiology 5342
  opioids
    pathology 5345
    withdrawal *5347*, 5347–8
  pain management 5349, *5349*
  pregnancy complications 5346
  stimulants
    pathology 5344, *5345*
    withdrawal 5347–8
  suicide attempts 5295
  treatment 5346
drug development 63
drug discovery 202, *203*
drug formulations 1451
  combinations 1453
  inhaled 1452
  modified-release 1451
  subcutaneous, intramuscular and local injections 1452
  sublingual, buccal and rectal 1452
  transdermal 1452
drug interactions 1449, 1470, *1471*, 5266
  pharmaceutical 1470
  pharmacodynamic *1471*, 1472
  pharmacokinetic 1470, *1471*
    absorption 1470
    excretion 1472
    induction of metabolism 1471
    inhibition of metabolism 1471
    protein-binding displacement 1470
  physiochemical *1471*
  phytotherapy *69*
  renal transplant patients 3967
  see also individual drugs
drug metabolism 1457, *1458*
  antimicrobials 450
  induction of 1471
  inhibition of 1471
  pharmacogenetic variation *see* pharmacogenetics
  and renal function 4174
drug overdose 5503
  antidotes *5505*
  clinical features *5504*
  laboratory data *5505*
  treatment *5505*
  see also poisoning
drug protein binding, pregnancy 2190
drug-disease interactions 1463
drug-induced acute pancreatitis 2558
drug-induced anaphylaxis 3108
drug-induced endocrine manifestations 2059, 2067
drug-induced nephropathies 4008
drug-receptor interactions 1459
  altered effects of endogenous ligands 1460
    increased endogenous release 1460
    inhibition of endogenous metabolism 1461
    inhibition of endogenous reuptake 1460
    prevention of endogenous release/synthesis 1460
  inhibition of ion movements 1461
  long-term effects 1460
  receptor subtypes 1460
  second messengers 1460
drugs
  clinical evaluation 48
  clinical trials *see* clinical trials
  cost of 62
  economic evaluation 53
  evaluation and efficacy 48
  global access 63
  innovation in 60
    incentives 61
  long-term therapy 1464
  onset and duration of effects 1463
  personalized prescribing 46, 61, 1474
  pharmacological actions 1463
  provision 54
  short-term effects 1462
  see also clinical pharmacology; healthcare provision
dry eye 5234
Dubin-Johnson syndrome 2450
Duchenne muscular dystrophy 5129, 5195
  cardiac involvement *2840*, *2788*
  carriers 5195
  and chronic respiratory failure 3471, *3472*
  diagnosis 5195, *5196*
  genetic counselling *5197*
  management 5197
  prognosis 5196, *5196*
duck-billed platypus, envenoming 1327
Duffy blood group system 4563
Dugbe virus *581*
duloxetine 5331, *5331*
  adverse effects *5313*
  diabetic neuropathy 2039
Dunnigan-Kobberling syndrome 1664
duodenum
  bicarbonate secretion 2306
  obstruction 2399
Dupuytren's contracture *3248*
dural sinus thrombosis 4973
Dürck's granulomas 1062
Duroziez's sign 2751
Duvenhage virus 554
DVT *see* deep venous thrombosis
dwarfism, proportionate 3759
dynamic mutations 142
dynein 131
dynorphin 2319
dysarthria 4743, 4903
dysautonomia
  acute/subacute 5062
  Wilson's disease 1690
dysbaric osteonecrosis 1421, 3802
dysentery
  with amoebic colitis 1037
  mortality *121*
dysexecutive syndrome 4793
Dysgonomonas spp. *962*
dyskeratosis congenita 4295
dyslexia 4790
dyslipidaemia
  diabetes mellitus 2041, *2041*
  management 2041
  risks of 2041
dysmorphophobia 4681
dyspareunia 1942, *1947*
dyspepsia 2206
  peptic ulcer disease 2309
dysphagia 2205
  management 2298
dyspnoea *see* breathlessness
dystonia 4887, 4889
  aetiology 4890, *4891*
  blepharospasm and oromandibular 4892, *4893*
  classification 4889, *4891*
  definition 4889
  dopa-responsive 4887, 4891
  generalized idiopathic torsion 4887
  idiopathic (torsion) 4890
  paroxysmal 4894
  spasmodic 4894
  spasmodic torticollis 4891, *4892*
  writer's cramp 4892, *4893*
dystrophia myotonica *244*
  cardiac involvement *2840*
dystrophin 2606, *2607*

Eagle effect 673
Eale's disease 5163
Early Breast Cancer Trialists' Collaborative Group 38
earthquakes 1438, *1439*
Eastern equine encephalitis *558*, 560
eating disorders 5317
  atypical 5302
  classification and diagnosis 5317, *5318*
  clinical features 5318
  development and course 5319
  epidemiology 5320

management 5323
medical complications 5321, *5322*
neurobiological findings 5321
pathogenesis 5320, *5321*
genetic factors 5320
prevention 5323
see also individual disorders
Ebola virus *see* filoviruses
EBP50, 133
ebrotidine, adverse effects, hepatotoxicity *2529*
Ebstein's anomaly *2844*, 2849
associated abnormalities 2849
clinical presentation 2849
investigations 2850, *2850*
physical signs 2849
treatment 2850
e-cadherin 355
ecarin *4540*
eccrine gland disorders 4677
hyperhidrosis 4677, *4677*
hypohidrosis/anhidrosis 4678
miliaria 4678
ECG 2643
acute coronary syndromes 2643, 2653, *2914*, 2915
role of 2653
triage 2653
acute respiratory failure 3135
ambulatory 2690
aortic dissection 2955
aortic regurgitation 2752
aortic stenosis 2748
arrhythmogenic right ventricular cardiomyopathy 2779, *2780*
atrial hypertrophy 2650, *2650–1*
atrioventricular block *2648*
axis 2647, *2647*
cardiac arrhythmias 2690, *2690*
coronary heart disease 2895
dilated cardiomyopathy 2775
errors in interpretation 2657
exercise testing 2644, 2657
cardiovascular response 2657, *2658*
conduction of test 2659
as diagnostic tool 2660
exercise protocols 2659, *2659*
interpretation of 2660
and medication 2661
problems of 2660
prognostic value 2660, *2661*
risks of 2660
special groups 2661
technical issues 2661
when to stop 2660
heart disease, pregnancy 2109
heart failure 2718, *2719*
heart rate 2646
heart rhythm 2647
hemiblocks 2650
bundle branch block 2650
left anterior 2650
left posterior 2650
history 2644
hyperkalaemia *3891*
hypertrophic cardiomyopathy 2769
left ventricular hypertrophy 2649, *2649*
mitral regurgitation 2744
mitral stenosis 2739
palpitation 2641
pericardial effusion *2793*
pulmonary arterial hypertension 2985, *2986*
pulmonary embolism 3013, *3013*
resting 12-lead 2643–4
chest leads 2646, *2646*
interpretation 2646, *2647*
lead nomenclature 2645
limb leads 2645, *2645*
rheumatic fever *2801*
right ventricular hypertrophy 2649
syncope 2640
torsades de pointes 2713, *2713*
ventricular pre-excitation 2651
Mahaim-type 2652
short PR-type 2652
Wolff-Parkinson-White syndrome 2648, *2651, 2652*
ventricular tachycardia 2710, *2710*
waveform 2644, *2645*
P wave 2644, 2648
PR interval 2648
QRS complex 2645, 2648
QT interval 2649
ST segment 2649
T wave 2645, 2649
U wave 2649
see also individual conditions
ECG-gated SPECT 2673, *2674*
Echinochasmus fujianeusius 1220
Echinochasmus japonicus 1220
Echinochasmus perfoliatus 1220
Echinochasmus recurvatum 1220
Echinococcus granulosus, cystic hydatid disease 1185
Echinostoma cinetorchis 1220
Echinostoma echinatum 1220
Echinostoma hortense 1220
Echinostoma ilocanum 1220
Echinostoma macrorchis 1220
Echinostoma malayanum 1220
Echinostoma melis 1220
Echinostoma revolutum 1220
echinostomiasis 1221, *1221*
Echis leucogaster, antivenom *1340*
Echis ocellatus (carpet viper) 1328, *1332*
antivenom *1340*
Echis pyramidum, antivenom *1340*
echocardiography
2D (cross-sectional) 2662, *2663*
3D 2670, *2670*
acute respiratory failure 3135
aortic regurgitation 2752, *2752–3*
aortic stenosis 2748, *2749*
arrhythmogenic right ventricular cardiomyopathy 2779
cardiac myxoma 2831, *2831*
dilated cardiomyopathy 2775, *2775–6*
Doppler 2663, *2664*
heart failure 2719
history 2662
HIV/AIDS 2825
hypertrophic cardiomyopathy 2770, *2770*
infective endocarditis 2812, *2813*
intracardiac 2669, *2670*
M-mode 2663, *2663*
mitral regurgitation 2744, *2744–5*
mitral stenosis 2739, *2740*
pericardial effusion *2793*
portable 2670, *2670*
pregnancy 2109
pulmonary arterial hypertension 2985
pulmonary embolism 3014
pulmonary fibrosis 3379
stress 2669, *2670*
angina 2906
transoesophageal 2667, *2667*
aortic disease 2668, *2669*
endocarditis 2668, *2669*
patient selection 2668, *2668*
thromboembolism 2669, *2669*
valvular heart disease 2668
transthoracic 2663
abnormal left ventricular function 2666, *2666*
atrial fibrillation 2666, *2666*
congenital heart disease 2667
infective endocarditis 2667
left ventricular hypertrophy 2666
pericardial disease 2667, *2667*
post-stroke/embolism 2666, *2667*
pulmonary embolism 2667
valvular heart disease 2663
echovirus, clinical features *529*
eclampsia *2095*, 2100, 2128
differential diagnosis *2131*
ecological footprint 75, 83, 84
econazole, fungal infections 1015
economic evaluation 53
cost minimization 53
cost-effectiveness analysis 53
cost-utility analysis 53, *53*
opportunity cost 53
economics of health 74
health care 82
reducing child mortality *78*
screening 100
ecstasy
adverse effects, hepatotoxicity *2529*
poisoning *1274*, 1280
clinical features 1280
management 1280
Ectobius lapponicus 1236
ectodermal dysplasia/skin fragility syndrome 4600
ectodermal dysplasias 4600
hidrotic 4600
hypohidrotic 4601
keratosis, ichthyosis, deafness syndrome 4600
ectoparasites 4675
ectopia lentis *3779–80*
ectopic ACTH syndrome 1872, *1872*, 3522
treatment 1880
eculizumab 221
paroxysmal nocturnal haemoglobinuria 4301–2, *4302*
eczema herpeticum 485
eczema 4618
asteatotic 4624, *4624*
atopic 261, 4621
clinical features 4621, *4622*
definitions 4621
incidence, prevalence and natural history 4621
pathogenesis 4622
treatment 4623, *4623*
classification 4618, *4619*
contact *see* contact dermatitis
dyshidrotic (pompholyx) 4624
photoaggravation *4670*
scalp 4702
seborrhoeic 4624
UV-induced (photodermatitis) 4625
varicose 4624
eczematous reactions, drug-induced 4728
Edge Hill virus *566*
edrophonium, snake bite 1343
education, diabetes mellitus 2021
Edwards' syndrome 145, *148*
Edwardsiella spp. *962*
Edwardsiella tarda 1240
EEG *see* electroencephalography
efalizumab, psoriasis 4163
efavirenz
HIV/AIDS 636, *638*
mode of action *444*
toxicity *640*
effectiveness of drugs 1450
efficacy of drugs 1450
efficiency of drugs 1450
eflornithine
adverse reactions *1125*
trypanosomiasis 1126, *1124–5*
egg allergy 263
Eggerthella spp. *962*
Ehlers-Danlos syndrome 2840, *3721*, 3752, 3771–2, 4586
aortic dissection 2955
classification *3753*
clinical features *3773–5*
clinical genetics 3772
autosomal dominant types 3772
autosomal recessive types 3772
mutations *3757*
X-linked type 3774
diagnostic criteria *3775*
investigations 3774
molecular pathology 3777, *3777–8*
types of
arthrochalasis 3777
classical 3774
hypermobile 3774
kyphoscoliosis 3777
vascular 3775, *3776*
Ehrlich, Paul 372
Ehrlichia chaffeensis 903, *962*
Ehrilichia spp. *962*
Ehrlichia ewingii 903, 915
ehrlichioses 903, 914
bacteriology, taxonomy and genomics 914, *915*
E. ewingii granulocytic 915
monocytic 915
Eikenella corrodens *852*, 859
Eikenella spp. *962*
Eisenmenger's syndrome 2683, *2844*, 2847, 2851
clinical findings 2842
investigations 2847, *2847*
lung transplantation *3478*
outcome and complications 2848, *2848*
pregnancy and contraception 2848
treatment 2848
ejaculation, retrograde *1917*

Ekböm's syndrome *see* restless legs syndrome
Elapidae 1328, 1333
antivenom *1340*
elastance, left ventricular 3125
elastase 209
elastic compression stockings 2118
elbow
pain *3557*
rheumatoid arthritis 3588
elder abuse 5408
elderly patients *see* older patients
electroacupuncture 67
electrocardiogram *see* ECG
electroconvulsive therapy 5315
electrocution 1422
burns 1425
cardiovascular consequences 1425
epidemiology 1423
mechanisms of 1423
neurological and muscular consequences 1425
presentation 1424
psychological consequences 1425
treatment 1425
electroencephalography 4753
abnormal EEG 4775
epilepsy 4817
indications 4753
method *4753, 4754*
normal EEG 4754
electrolyte disorders, post-transplant 3964
electrolytes
CKD 3908
Conn's syndrome 3063
gastrointestinal fluids *1538*
hepatocellular failure 2497
management 2503
malaria 1079
poisoned patients 1277
requirements 1538, *1538*
electromyography 4759
clinical correlations *4762, 4760, 4760–1, 4763*
indications 4758
measurements 4759, *4759*
method 4759
polymyositis/dermatomyositis 3697
electronic patient records 46
Electrophorus electricus (electric eel) 1325
Electrophorus electricus 1325
electroretinography 4757
elephantiasis 1156, *1156*
nonfilarial *see* podoconiosis
eletriptan, migraine *4917–18*
elimination diets 2254
Elizabethkingia spp. *962*
elliptocytes *4195*
elliptocytosis *4464*, 4466
hereditary 4452
hereditary spherocytic 4452
Ellis-van Creveld syndrome 2837
mutations in *3757*
Ellsworth-Howard test 1864
elretinate, adverse effects, hepatotoxicity *2529*
elvitegravir, HIV/AIDS *638*
EMBASE 24
embolism
amniotic fluid 2122
arterial 2418
cholesterol 2966
pulmonary *see* pulmonary embolism
embryonic stem cells 189
Emery-Dreifuss muscular dystrophy 5129, *5199, 5200–1*
reproductive effects *1917*
emesis, poisoning 1279
Emmonsia crescens 1012
Emmonsia parva 1012
emollients 1382, *4732*
Empedobacter spp. *962*
emphysema 3177, *3312, 3319, 3321*
α_1-antitrypsin deficiency 1781, 1783
bullous 3343
centriacinar 3320
morbidity *3316*
periacinar 3320
treatment, bronchoscopy 3223, *3223*
emphysematous pyelonephritis 4120, *4120*
employment, diabetes mellitus 2021
empyema, pneumococcal 688
emtricitabine
HIV/AIDS *638*
mode of action *444*
emulsifiers 4732
emulsifying ointment 4736
enalapril
adverse effects, hepatotoxicity *2529*
heart failure *2722*
encapsulating peritoneal sclerosis 3947
encephalitis 5002
autoimmune limbic 5175, *5176*
brainstem 5171
California 580, *581*
clinical features 4984
Eastern equine *558*, 560
enterovirus 530
granulomatous amoebic 1044, *1044*
herpes simplex 486, 4999, 5002–3
HSV 486
Japanese 565, *568, 5002, 5004, 5005–6*
limbic 5171, *5172*
measles-related 521
mumps 514
Murray Valley *566*, 572
Nipah virus 5002, *5004, 5006*
Bangladesh and India 526
relapse and late onset 526
Powassan *566*, 574
presentation 5497
St Louis 565, *566*, 569
tick-borne 572, *566, 573, 5002*
varicella 490
Venezuelan equine *558*, 560
viral *4781*, 4781
West Nile virus *566*, 569, *570*, 5002, 5004
Western equine *558*, 561
Encephalitozoon cuniculi 1115, *1116*
Encephalitozoon hellem 1116
Encephalitozoon intestinalis 1116
encephalization 4747
encephalomyelitis, acute disseminated 4952
encephalopathy 2501
cognitive impairment 5278
hepatic 2494
clinical features 2495, *2495–6*
diagnosis 2499
management 2502, *2502*
hypertensive 3037, 3079
hyponatraemic 3821
hypoxia in 3821, *3822*
risk factors 3821
treatment 3821, *3824*
endobronchial ultrasound 3221, *3221*
endocarditis
actinomycotic 854
bacterial 2871, *2871*
bartonella 927, 930
diagnosis *931*
treatment 933
brucellar *793*
candida 1013
echocardiography
transoesophageal 2668, *2669*
transthoracic 2667
HIV/AIDS *2822*, 2823
infective 2806
Liebman-Sachs 2738
pneumococcal 691
staphylococcal 702, *703–4*
coagulase-negative 705
endocrine disease 1797, *1797–8*
anaemia in 4401
CKD 3909
cognitive impairment 5279
drug-induced 2059, 2067
adrenal cortex 2068
gonads 2068
gynaecomastia 2068
parathyroid 2069
posterior pituitary 2069
prolactin 2068
thyroid 2067
hepatic involvement 2541
polycythaemia 4268
pregnancy 2140
adrenal 2143
parathyroid disorders 2143
pituitary disorders 2140, *2141*
thyroid disorders 2141, *2142*
skin involvement 4559
endocrine system
acidosis 1744
endocrine gland development 1788, *1801*
in pregnancy 2078
endocytosis 1695, 131
end-of-life (terminal) care 19, *5427, 5428–9*
heart failure 2729
mercy killing 19
endogenous repair 202
Endolimax nana 1042
endolysosomes 1695
endometrial cancer 324
incidence *301*
migrants vs residents *302*
and polycystic ovary syndrome 1909
endometriosis 2587
endophthalmitis, *Candida* spp. *438*
endoplasmic reticulum 129
endoscopic mucosal resection 2217
endoscopic retrograde cholangiopancreatography (ERCP) 2217, 2227
acute pancreatitis 2564
benign strictures 2218
gallstones 2218
gastric outlet obstruction 2218
malignant bile duct obstruction 2218
pancreatic tumours 2576
pancreatitis 2218
endoscopic sphincterotomy 2550
endoscopic ultrasound, pancreatic tumours 2576
endoscopy units 2215
endoscopy 2214
development 2215
diagnostic 2215
disinfection 2215
gastro-oesophageal reflux disease 2289
hazards and complications 2218
infection risk 2215
malabsorption 2329
oesophagus 2287
pancreas and biliary tree 2217
small bowel (enteroscopy) 2216
video capsule 2216
therapeutic 2216
assisted nutrition 2217
endoscopic mucosal resection 2217
endoscopic ultrasound 2217
gastrointestinal bleeding 2216
laser therapy 2217
malignant gastro-oesophageal strictures 2216
oesophageal stricture 2216
polyps and mucosal cancers 2217
removal of foreign objects 2217
see also endoscopic
endostatin *1939*
endothelial cells 4481, *4482*
anticoagulant properties 4482, *4482*
procoagulant properties 4482, *4482–3*
receptors 4483, *4483*
role in coagulation 4495, *4496*
vascular tone 4482
endothelial progenitor cells 2595
endothelial-leucocyte adhesion molecule 1 (ELAM-1) *see* E-selectin
endothelin receptor antagonists, pulmonary arterial hypertension 2988
endothelin 2320, *2599, 4482*
endothelium, blood vessels *see* vascular endothelium
endotoxic shock 210
endotoxin 2476, 2598
endotracheal intubation 3136, *5516, 5516*
complications *3137*
indications *3136*
end-systolic elastance 3125
energy balance, regulation of *1531*
energy requirements 1538
in pregnancy 2080, *2081*
enflurane, adverse effects, hepatotoxicity *2529*
enfuvirtide
HIV/AIDS 636, *638*
toxicity *640*
enkephalins 2319

enoxaparin, pregnancy 2118, *2120*
Entamoeba chattoni 1042
Entamoeba coli 1042
Entamoeba dispar 1036, 1042
Entamoeba gingivalis 1042
Entamoeba hartmanni 1042
Entamoeba histolytica 1035–6
  biology and pathogenicity 1036
  see also amoebiasis
Entamoeba moshkovskii 1042
Entebbe bat virus *566*
enteral nutrition 2217
  access devices *1540*
  complications 1539
  indications for *1537*
enteric fever 2432
enteritis necroticans 808
enteritis
  measles-related 520, *522*
  postradiation 2223
Enterobacter spp. *962*
Enterobacteriaceae 728
  community-acquired pneumonia *453*
  treatment *3238, 3245*
enterobiasis 1168, 1172
  clinical features 1172, *1172*
  diagnosis 1173, *1173*
  epidemiology and control 1172
  life cycle 1172, *1172*
  treatment 1173
Enterobius vermicularis 1168, 1172
enterococci 678
  antibiotic sensitivity and treatment 678
  infections caused by 678
Enterococcus avium 678
Enterococcus casseliflavus 678
Enterococcus durans 678
Enterococcus faecalis 678
  antibiotic sensitivity *446*
Enterococcus faecium 678
Enterococcus spp. *962*
  infective endocarditis *2812*, 2815
  osteomyelitis *3789*
Enterocytozoon bieneusi 1115, *1116*
  malabsorption *2357*
enteroglucagon 2319
  inhibition *2320*
enteropathy, tropical 2358
enteropathy-associated T-cell lymphoma 2338, 2344
  clinical features 2345
    pathology 2345, *2345*
  genetics 2346
  immunophenotype 2346, *2346*
  precursor lesions 2346
  prognosis 2347
enterovirus 71, 5002
  clinical features 5004
enteroviruses *474*, 476, 527
  clinical features 529, *529*
    see also individual viruses and conditions
  epidemiology 532
  laboratory diagnosis 532
    genome detection 532
    serology 532
    virus isolation 532
  neonatal infections 530
  pathogenesis 529
  pregnancy *2171*
  prevention 533
  viruses 527, *528*
enthesitis *3605*, 3607
entry inhibitors 636
  toxicity *640*
envenoming
  animals 1327
  mammals 1327
environmental change 91
environmental diseases 1393
  aerospace medicine 1408
  bioterrorism 1440
  cold 1395
  disasters 1436
  diving medicine 1416
  drowning 1397
  heat 1393
  high altitude 2171
  lightning and electrical injuries 1422
  noise 1432
  podoconiosis 1426
  radiation 1429
  vibration 1434
environmental disruption 74
environmental factors
  autoimmunity 270
  obesity 1529
environmental overload 81
environmental stress 81
enzastaurin *1939*
enzyme replacement therapy 1708
  Fabry's disease 1712
  Gaucher's disease 1709
  mucopolysaccharidoses 1712
enzymes
  activation 1461
  inhibition 1461
eosinophilia 4356
  diseases associated with 4357
    allergic and immunological disorders 4357
    endocrine diseases 4358
    gastrointestinal diseases 4357
    HIV and retroviral infections 4357
    infectious diseases 4357
    myeloproliferative and neoplastic diseases 4357
    pulmonary syndromes 4357, *4358*
    rheumatological diseases 4358
    skin and subcutaneous diseases 4357
  pulmonary 3465
  tropical 3429
eosinophilic fasciitis 4646
eosinophilic gastroenteritis 2221
eosinophilic oesophagitis 2293, *2293*
eosinophilic pneumonia 3295, 3428
  acute 3429
  with asthma 3430
  chronic 3429
  diagnosis 3429
  treatment 3429
eosinophils 152, *288, 4196, 4311*
  infants and children *4197*
ephedra, drug interactions *69*
ephedrine 5384
  orthostatic hypotension *5063*
ephelides 4706
epicondylitis 1383, *3557*
epidemics, tracing of 13
epidermal growth factor receptor 400
epidermal growth factor 348
epidermis
  failure of 4586
  structure 4584, *4593, 4594*
    basement membrane zone 4593
    desmosomes 4594
    gap junctions 4594
    hemidesmosomes 4593
    keratins 4594
epidermodysplasia verruciformis 605, *4675*
epidermoid cyst 4706
epidermolysis bullosa acquisita *4603*, 4608, *4608*
epidermolysis bullosa 4594, *4595*
  diagnosis and management 4596
  dystrophic 4596
  genetics *4595*
  hemidesmosomal 4596
  junctional 4595
    Herlitz 4595
    non-Herlitz 4596
  simplex 4594, *4595*
    Dowling-Meara 4595
    Loebner 4595
    Weber-Cockayne 4595
Epidermophyton floccosum 1000
epididymis *1914*
epididymitis
  chlamydial 942
  mycoplasmal infections *956*, 957
epidural abscess 700, *702*
epidural anaesthesia 3156
epigenetics 353, *354*
epiglottitis *3258*
  H. influenzae 760, 761
epilepsia partialis continua 4899
epilepsy 4810
  causes 4815
    alcohol 4816
    cerebrovascular disease 4815
    dementia 4816
    genetic 4815
    idiopathic focal epilepsies 4815
    idiopathic generalized epilepsies 4815
    infection 4815
    malformations of cortical development 4815
    metabolic disorders 4816
    multiple sclerosis 4816
    trauma 4815
    tumour 4815
  childhood/juvenile absence 5102
  classification 4811, *4812*
  clinical features 4812
    generalized seizures 4813, *4814*
    partial seizures 4812
  cognitive impairment 5277, *5278*
  definitions 4811
  differential diagnosis 4816
    drop attacks 4817
    hyperventilation 4817
    migraine 4817
    narcolepsy and cataplexy 4817
    parasomnias 4817
    psychogenic nonepileptic seizures 4817
    syncope 4816
    transient ischaemic attacks 4816
  driving 4823
  epidemiology 4811
  generalized
    with febrile seizures 5101
    with febrile seizures and absence 5101
  genetics 5101
  gestational 2148
  investigations 4817
    CT 4818
    EEG 4817
    MRI 4818, *4818*
    PET 4819, *4819*
    SPECT 4819
  juvenile myoclonic 166, 5101
  malaria chemoprophylaxis 1087
  myoclonic 4899
  myoclonic with ragged red fibres (MERFF) *2766*, 5102
  nocturnal frontal lobe 166
  northern 1698
  pathophysiology 4811
  precipitants 4816
  pregnancy 2147
  prognosis 4825, *4825*
  progressive myoclonus 5102
  psychiatric aspects 4825
  pyridoxal-phosphate-dependent *1566*, 1590
  pyridoxine-dependent *1566*
  specialist nurses and GP's role 4825
  sudden death 4824
  syndromes 4814
  temporal lobe, reproductive effects *1917*
  treatment
    pharmacological *see* anticonvulsants
    surgery 4824
epileptic encephalopathy 5103
epinephrine *see* adrenaline
EpiPen 1350
epipodophyllotoxins, carcinogenesis *307*
epirubicin, breast cancer *1937*
episcleritis, meningococcal 718, *719*
epistasis 140, 4500
  hypertension 3040
Episthmium caninum *1220*
eplerenone, heart failure 2723
Epstein-Barr virus *246, 484,* 501
  and cancer 187
    B-cell tumours 502
    endemic ('African') Burkitt's lymphoma 505
    gastric carcinoma 507
    hairy leukoplakia 507
    Hodgkin's lymphoma 506
    nasopharyngeal 312, 506
    NK-cell lymphoma 507
    salivary gland lymphoepithelioma 507
    smooth-muscle tumours 507
    sporadic Burkitt's lymphoma 505
    T-cell lymphoma 507
  chronic active 505
  epidemiology 502, *503*
  immunosuppressed patients 506, *3957, 3958*
  infectious cycle 502
  infectious mononucleosis 501–2
  oncoproteins *356*
  virus-coded proteins 502

X-linked lymphoproliferative disease 504
Epworth Sleepiness Scale *3268*
Erb's palsy 2138, 5080
ERCP *see* endoscopic retrograde cholangiopancreatography
Erdheim-Chester disease 2587
erectile dysfunction 1927, *1942*
ergocalciferol 1495
ergot alkaloids, contraindication in porphyria 1641, *5484*
ergotamine, migraine *4917–18*
erionite, mesothelioma 3535
Eristalis spp. 1232
Eristalis tenax *1233*
erlotinib 400, *1939*
lung cancer 3529
ertapenem, in renal failure *4185*
erucism 1351
Erwinia spp. *962*
erysipelas 673, *673*
Erysipelothrix spp. *962*
erythem migrans 4652
erythema ab igne 4686
erythema annulare centrifugum 4651, *4651*
erythema gyratum repens 4652
erythema infectiosum 608
erythema marginatum 2801
erythema migrans 861, *862*, 4652
erythema multiforme 2277, *4727*, 4728, *4729*, 4739
aetiology 2277
clinical features 2277, *2277*
course and prognosis 2278
differential diagnosis 2277
HSV 486
pathology 2277
photoaggravation *4670*
treatment 2277
erythema nodosum 4648, *4650*
Behçet's disease *3685*
erythema
annular 4651
migratory *385*
erythrocyte sedimentation rate 1758, 3230, 4198
erythrocytes *see* red cells
erythrocytosis *385*
secondary 2845, *2846*
erythroderma 4740
erythroid precursors 4368
erythroid production, perturbations in 4371
erythroid progenitors 4368
erythrokeratoderma variabilis *168*, 4599
erythromelalgia 4688
erythromycin *707*
acne *4680*
adverse effects, hepatotoxicity *2529*, *2532–3*
animal-related injuries 1326
anthrax 787
bacillary angiomatosis 933
bartonellosis 938
cellulitis, mastitis and pyomyositis *699*
chancroid 764
chlamydial infections *943*
diphtheria 668
drug interactions *1471*
legionnaire's disease 902
listeriosis 898
Lyme borreliosis *864*
mycoplasmal infections 959, *960*
peliosis hepatis 933
pertussis *766*
pharmacokinetics *449*
pneumococcal pneumonia 687
pneumonia *3238*
postantibiotic effect *451*
Raynaud's phenomenon *3671*
relapsing fevers 872
in renal failure *4185*
S. moniliformis 859
S. pyogenes 675
septic bursitis/arthritis *700*
skin disorders 4738
spectrum of activity *446*
syphilis 894
erythropoiesis 4204, *4205*, *4265*, *4368*
bone marrow 4369
erythroid compartment 4368
and iron balance 4387, *4387*
iron deficiency 4394
negative regulation 4204
ontogeny 4369
regulation of 4370
yolk sac 4369
erythropoietic porphyria, congenital 1637, 1645
erythropoietin 1403, *4201*, *4370*
acquired/congenital defects 4371
hypoxia-inducible regulation *4205*
orthostatic hypotension *5063*
performance enhancement 5385
signalling, acquired/congenital defects 4371
Escherichia coli 727, 729, 1256
antibiotic sensitivity *446*
enteroaggregative 730
enterohaemorrhagic 730
enteroinvasive 730
enteropathic 729
enterotoxigenic 730
osteomyelitis *3789*
urinary tract infection 2104
Escherichia spp. *962*
E-selectin 2601
esmolol
hypertensive emergencies *3080*
in renal failure *4179*
essential hypertension *see* hypertension
essential thrombocythaemia 4282
aetiology and pathogenesis 4282
clinical features 4283
diagnostic criteria *4284*, 4284
epidemiology 4283
future directions 4286
laboratory evaluation 4283
pathobiology 4283
prognosis 4282
risk assessment 4284
treatment 4284, *4286*
esthiomene *946*
etanercept
pregnancy *2158*
psoriasis 4615
rheumatoid arthritis 3598, *3599*
Still's disease 3706
ethambutol
adverse effects, ocular 5251
mycobacterial disease *835*
pregnancy *2172*
in renal failure *4185*
toxicity 826
tuberculosis *825*
dose *826*
ethanol
and hyperuricaemia 1626
lactic acidosis 1746
metabolism 2475, *2475*
poisoning 1287, *1287*
reproductive effects *1917*
ethical issues
artificial nutrition support 1542
clinical trials 47
ethics 16
autonomy 17
best interests 17
confidentiality 20
consent 18
end of life 19
ethionamide, pregnancy *2172*
ethnicity
drowning accidents 1398
and osteoarthritis 3630
ethnopharmacology 47
ethosuximide
dose levels *4823*
epilepsy 4821
serum levels *5449*
ethyl ether, adverse effects, hepatotoxicity *2529*
ethylene glycol poisoning 1310, *1742*, 4094
antidote *1274*
clinical features *1311*
ethylene oxide *1380*
ethylmalonic encephalopathy *1566*, 1581
aetiology/pathophysiology 1581
clinical presentation 1582, *1582*
diagnosis 1582
treatment and outcome 1582
etidronate
hypercalcaemia 1857
osteoporosis *3799*
Paget's disease 3744
etodolac
and asthma *3289*
rheumatoid arthritis *3594*
etoposide *338*, 399
lung cancer 3530
lymphoma *4320*
resistance *399*
etoricoxib
ankylosing spondylitis 3611
rheumatoid arthritis *3594*
etravirine, HIV/AIDS 636, *638*
eubacteria 127
Eubacterium spp. *962*
euglobulin lysis time *4196*
eukaryotes 127, *129*
Eunectes murinus 1325
Eunectes murinus 1325
European Medicines Evaluation Agency (EMEA) 199
Eurotium spp. *3436*
Eurytrema pancreaticum *1213*
Eustrongylides spp. *1176*
evening primrose oil, Raynaud's phenomenon *3671*
Everglades virus *558*
everolimus, transplantation 292, *2730*
Evidence Based Mental Health 23
Evidence-Based Medicine 23
evidence-based medicine
application of 27
clinical questions 23, *24*
definition of 28
diagnostic test results 25, *25–6*
finding answers 24
history 23
need for 23
point of care 22
treatment studies 25, *26*
evoked potentials 4755
brainstem auditory-evoked potentials 4757
electroretinography 4757
indications 4756
motor-evoked potentials *4758*, 4758
near-field and far-field responses 4756
somatosensory-evoked potentials *4757*, 4757
visual-evoked potentials *4756*, 4756
evolutionary aetiology 14, 15
evolutionary biology 12
application of 13
levels of selection 13
natural selection and adaptation 13
research implications 15
teaching implications 15
utility of 15
Ewing's sarcoma 389
translocations *341*
Ewing's tumour of bone 320
Ewingella spp. *962*
exanthem subitum 497
exanthema
coxsackievirus 531, *531*
echovirus 531, *531*
excitation-contraction coupling 2615
excitotoxicity 187
excretion 1459
active tubular secretion 1459
antimicrobials 450
drug interactions 1472
glomerular filtration 1459
passive tubular reabsorption 1459
exemestane, breast cancer *1937*
exercise ECG testing 2644, 2657
angina 2905
cardiovascular response 2657, *2658*
conduction of test 2659
as diagnostic tool 2660
exercise protocols 2659, *2659*
bicycle ergometry 2659
Bruce protocol 2659
interpretation of 2660
and medication 2661
problems of 2660
prognostic value 2660, *2661*
risks of 2660
special groups 2661
technical issues 2661
when to stop 2660
exercise testing 3190, 3199
asthma 3292
COPD 3330
coronary artery disease 2949
pregnancy 2109
pulmonary arterial hypertension 2985
exercise training, COPD 3340
exercise
cardiac response to 2626

training effects 2627
in diabetes mellitus 2010
in heart failure 2721
and hyperkalaemia 3844
hypertension *3047*, 3048
in obesity 1533
potassium homeostasis *3833*
in pregnancy 2090
see also sports medicine
exercise-induced anaphylaxis 3109
exertional headache 4921
exfoliative dermatitis 4740
Exiguobacterium spp. *962*
exomphalos 2397
exons 138
exotoxins, producers of 734
Expanded Program on Immunization 463, *463*
expedition medicine *see* travel medicine
expert opinion 50
expert witnesses 5360, *5361*
expiration, flow-volume curves 3193, *3193*
exposure-prone procedures 1381
extracellular matrix 4483, *3550, 4483–4*
extracorporeal circulation 4515
extracorporeal gas exchange 1360
extracorporeal membrane oxygenation 1401
meningitis 721
extracorporeal shock-wave lithotripsy 2550
extractable nuclear antigens 3568
extrapulmonary restriction 3392
extrapulmonary tuberculosis 810, *818*
bone and joint 820
central nervous system 820
genitourinary 819
lymphatic 819
miliary and disseminated 820
pleural 818
sites of *818*
tuberculous meningitis 819
extrasystoles
atrial 2702, *2703*
junctional 2703
ventricular 2703, *2703*
extrinsic allergic alveolitis 3296, 3434
aetiology 3435, *3436*
clinical features 3441
clinical investigation 3443
diagnostic criteria 3445
environmental exposure 3444
hypersensitivity 3444, *3445*
pulmonary 3443, *3444*
differential diagnosis 3442, *3443*
epidemiology 3440
incidence 3440
prevalence 3440
historical perspective 3434
management 3445
pathogenesis 3438
coeliac disease 3440
immune mechanisms 3438, *3438–9*
smoking 3440
pathology 3435
prevention 3441
prognosis 3445
extrinsic crystals 3648
Eyach virus 556
eye disorders 5234
age-related macular degeneration 5252
cataracts *see* cataracts
diabetes mellitus *see* diabetic retinopathy
dry eye 5234
glaucoma 5252
hypertension *see* hypertensive retinopathy
inherited diseases 5250, *5250*
ischaemia 5240
loss of vision 5234, *5235*
ocular vascular occlusion 5239
red eye 5234, *5234*
trachoma *see* trachoma
trauma 5252
see also under individual conditions
eye movements 4858
nystagmus 4859, *4859*
saccades 4860
smooth pursuit 4860
eye position 4859
eye 5233
examination 5235
fluorescein angiography 5235
ophthalmoscope 5235, *5235*
moths and beetles frequenting 1236
pupil *see* pupil; pupillary
retina *see* retina; retinal
signs of poisoning 1275
visual fields 5235
ezetimibe, adverse effects, hepatotoxicity *2529*
ezrin 133

fabric conditioners, poisoning by 1317
Fabry's disease 1694, 1696, 1698, 1709, 1969, 4099, 4693
cardiac involvement 2789, *2840*
corneal opacity 1704
diagnosis 1704
differential diagnosis *1725*
treatment 1712
facial nerve disorders 5036
facial palsy *see* Bell's palsy
facies latrodectismica, spider bites 1355, *1355*
Facklamia spp. *962*
factitious disorder 5303
factor D, deficiency *254*
factor H *216*
deficiency 219, *220, 254*
factor I *216*
deficiency 219, *220, 254*
factor II *see* prothrombin
factor IX 4490
inhibitors 4539
laboratory tests *4504, 4522*
factor IXa 4495, *4495*
factor V Leiden *2118*, 4530
factor V 4492, *4492*
deficiency 4527
inhibitors 4539
laboratory tests *4504, 4522*
factor VII 4490
inhibitors 4539
laboratory tests *4504, 4522*
factor VIII inhibitors, acquired 2179
factor VIII *1753*, 4492, *4493*
deficiency 4527
inhibitor, acquired *4535*, 4538
laboratory tests *4504, 4522*
factor X 4490
inhibitors 4539
laboratory tests *4504, 4522*
factor Xa 4495, *4495*
factor XI 4491
deficiency 2179, 4527
inhibitors 4539
laboratory tests *4504, 4522*
factor XII *4490*, 4491
factor XIII *4490*, 4492
deficiency 4528
inhibitors 4539
laboratory tests *4504, 4522*
faecal elastase, reference values *5446*
faecal fat 2328
faecal incontinence 5389, 5399
aetiology 5400
conditions affecting *5400*
evaluation 5400
treatment 5400
faecal output 2226
faecal peritonitis 2234, 2393
faecal reference values 5447
Fallot's tetralogy 2851, *2864*
with absent pulmonary valve 2865
associations 2864
clinical course and management 2864
palliated history 2865, *2865*
pregnancy 2114
radical repair 2865, *2866*
falls clinic 5395
falls 5389, 5394
aetiology 5394
assessment 5394
investigations 5395
management 5395
prevention 5394
prognosis 5395
famciclovir
herpes zoster 493
HSV 487
mode of action *444*
pregnancy *2172*
varicella zoster 492
familial adenomatous polyposis 315, 358, *2406*
familial amyloid polyneuropathy 1771, 5092
with predominant cranial neuropathy 1771
familial cold autoinflammatory syndrome *238, 1761*, 1764, *3709*
familial expansile osteolysis *3721*, 3744
familial haemophagocytic lymphohistiocytosis *238*
familial hypercholesterolemia, genetics *139*
familial hyperphosphataemic tumoral calcinosis *3721*
familial hypocalciuric hypercalcaemia *3745*
familial juvenile hyperuricaemic nephropathy 1626
familial Mediterranean fever *238*, 1760, *1761*, 1772, *3708, 3709–10*
clinical features 1762, *1762*
clinical investigation 1762
epidemiology 1762
genetics 1760
pathology 1762
treatment 1762
familial papillary renal cell carcinoma 368
familial polyposis coli, genes associated with *363*
familial risk 89
familial supravalvar aortic stenosis 2836, *2836*
famines 120, *122*
excess mortality *121*
famotidine, peptic ulcer disease 2311
Fanconi syndrome 3872
causes *1627*
clinical features, osteomalacia *3737, 3739*
Fanconi's anaemia 302, *360*, 369, 4294
clinical features 4294
genetics, incidence and epidemiology *4291*, 4294
laboratory diagnosis 4295
and leukaemia 332
molecular biology 4295
treatment and prognosis 4295
Fanconi's syndrome
renal 4135, 4140, 4147
causes *4149*
Fanconi-Bickel syndrome *1598*, 1602, *4149*
differential diagnosis *1600*
Fannia canicularis 1233
Farber's disease 1698
farmer's lung *see* extrinsic allergic alveolitis
Fas ligand 186
Fas 169, 186
fascia adherens 2608
fasciitis *421*
Fasciola gigantica 1213
Fasciola hepatica 1212, *1213*, 1238
fascioliasis 1212, 1214
clinical features 1215
diagnosis 1215
epidemiology and control 1215
life cycle 1214
pathology 1215
treatment 1215
fasciolopsiasis *1221*, 1222
Fasciolopsis buski 1221
fascioscapulohumeral muscular dystrophy 5130, *5199, 5200*
fasciotomy, snake bite 1328
fat necrosis of breast 1941
fatal infectious mononucleosis 504
fatigue 2628, 2632
palliative care 5427
in pregnancy 2088
fats *see* lipids
fatty acids
dietary *1668*
nonesterified 1484, 1653
oxidation 1485, *1485*
regulation of gene expression *1482*
fatty liver
clinical features 2477
pathogenesis 2475
fatty streaks 1659
Faxio-Londe disease 5073
Fcγ-receptors, polymorphism 713
febrile pneumonitis *436*
febrile seizures 162
felbamate
adverse effects, hepatotoxicity *2529*
epilepsy 4822

Felty's syndrome 4307
hepatic involvement 2544
and rheumatoid arthritis 3589
female athlete triad 5376, *5376–7*
history 5376
incidence and aetiology 5376, *5376*
investigation and management 5377, *5377–8*
pathophysiology 5376, *5377*
skeletal effects 5377
femfibrozil 1670
femoral nerve neuropathy 5084
femoral vein cannulation 5510, *5511*
fenbrufen, adverse effects, hepatotoxicity *2532*
fenofibrate 1670
adverse effects, hepatotoxicity *2529*
fenoprofen
and asthma *3289*
rheumatoid arthritis *3594*
fenoterol
asthma 3302
COPD *3335*
fentanyl 3155, *3155*
palliative care 5422
feprazon, adverse effects, hepatotoxicity *2532*
ferpexide, adverse effects, hepatotoxicity *2529*
ferritin 4389
reference values *5435*, *5444*
fertility *see* infertility
fetal alcohol syndrome *1468*, 2090, 5146
fetal programming 2083
fetal switch 4201
α-fetoprotein, reference values *5442*
fetus
adverse drug reactions 1468, 2187
effects of maternal diabetes 2138
growth and adult disease 2899
thyroid function 2142
fever of unknown origin 423
causes 423, *424–5*
common diseases 426
diagnostic spectrum 423
subpopulations 423
characteristics of 426
definition 423, *424*
drug-induced 426
factious 426
habitual hyperthermia 426
imaging techniques 426
immunocompromised host 435, *435*
prognosis 427
selective testing 427
therapeutic trials 427
watchful waiting 427
fever
acute pancreatitis 2564
cancer 382
dialysis patients 3941
feverfew, migraine prevention *4916*
fexofenadine 3282
fibrates 1670
fibreoptic bronchoscopy 3135
fibrillary glomerulonephropathies 4060
fibrillin 1 mutations, Marfan's syndrome 2838, *3779*, *3781*
fibrinectin *1753*
fibrinogen titre *4196*
fibrinogen *1753*, *4490*, *4494*, 4494, *4503*
deficiency 4528
laboratory tests *4522*, *4504*
plasma *4196*
pregnancy *2126*
reference values *5444*
fibrinolysis 416, 2601
meningitis 721
myocardial infarction *38*, 40, *42*
venous thromboembolism 3020
fibrinolytic system 4496, *4496–7*
Fibrinolytic Therapy Trialists' Collaborative Group 38
fibroadenoma of breast 1940, *1940*
fibroblast growth factor 2601
fibrodysplasia ossificans progressiva 3713, *3721*, 3765
clinical features *3731*, 3765, *3765–6*
differential diagnosis 3765
management 3766
pathophysiology 3765
fibrogenesis imperfecta ossium 3769
clinical features *3731*
fibroma, cardiac 2832
fibromatosis of breast 1941
fibropolycystic disease 2580
choledochal cyst 2582, *2582*
congenital hepatic fibrosis 2581
microhamartomas 2582
polycystic liver disease 2581, *2581*
fibrosing alveolitis
cryptogenic 3375
and rheumatoid arthritis 3588
systemic sclerosis 3673, *3673*
fibrous dysplasia 3720, *3721*, *3761*, *3762*
clinical features *3731*
monostotic 3762
polyostotic 3762
fibrous erionite pneumoconiosis 3423
Fick principle 2681, *2682*
fifth disease 608
filarial nephropathy 4088
clinical features 4088
management 4089
pathogenesis 4088
pathology 4088
filariasis 3085
cutaneous 1145
lymphatic 1153, *1154*
aetiology 1154
clinical features 1155, *1156–7*
diagnosis 1157
epidemiology and transmission 1155
Global Programme to Eliminate Lymphatic Filariasis 1158
mosquito vectors *1154*, 1155
pathogenesis 1155
treatment 1159
renal involvement 4075
see also individual conditions
Filifactor spp. *962*
Filler formula 3871
Filodes fulvidorsalis 1236
filoviruses 595, 1442
aetiology and genetics 596
areas of uncertainty 599
clinical features 598, *598–9*
diagnosis/differential diagnosis 599, *599*
epidemiology 597
future developments 600
pathogenesis/pathology 596
prevention 597
prognosis 599
treatment 599
finasteride
NNT *52*
skin disorders 4739
fine needle aspiration
bronchial 3220
thyroid cancer 1847
Finegoldia spp. *962*
fingers
boutonnière deformity 3587
clubbing *see* digital clubbing
dactylitis *3606*
swan-neck deformity 3587
fire smoke 3457
first-pass metabolism 1456
Fischoederius elongatus *1223*
fish allergy 263
fish odour syndrome 4677
fish oils
in pregnancy 2090
Raynaud's phenomenon *3671*
fish poisoning 1346
carp gallbladder 1347
diagnosis and treatment 1347
gastrointestinal and neurotoxic syndromes 1346
prevention 1346
fish stings 1325, *1344*, *1344–5*
clinical features 1345
epidemiology 1344, *1345*
incidence 1344
prevention 1345
treatment 1345
venom composition 1345
Fisher's syndrome 5034, 5037, 5090
fitness factors 411
FitzHugh-Curtis syndrome 944, *945*, 1260
flail chest 3510
flatbush diabetes 2008
flavin adenine dinucleotide 1487–8
flaviviruses 564
mosquito-borne 564–5
taxonomy *566*
tick-transmitted 565
see also individual viruses
Flavobacterium spp. *962*
flavoproteins 1490
flea-borne spotted fever 907
fleas 1225, *1232*, 1232
flecainide *2701*
adverse effects, hepatotoxicity *2532*
in renal failure *4179*
fleroxacin, typhoid fever *742*
Flexispira spp. *962*
Flexner, Abraham 11
flexor hallucis longus tendonitis *5382*
flies
blood-sucking 1226, *1226*
and hygiene 1236
FLIP protein 184
floods 121, 1440
flow-volume curves 3192, *3193*
expiration 3193, *3193*
inspiration 3193, *3193*
Flt-3, 4201
flucloxacillin *706*
adverse effects, hepatotoxicity *2533*
bacteraemia *703*, *705*
endocarditis *704–5*
epidural abscess *702*
infective endocarditis *2817*, *2818*
osteomyelitis *701*
pharmacokinetics *449*
pneumonia *702*, *3238*
Raynaud's phenomenon *3671*
in renal failure *4185*
septic bursitis/arthritis *700*
spectrum of activity *446*
toxic shock syndrome *697*
urinary tract infection *702*
fluconazole
adverse effects, hepatotoxicity *2529*
in breast milk *1469*
candidiasis 1258
coccidioidomycosis 1022
cryptococcosis 1020
dermatophytoses 1002
disseminated candidosis 1013
drug interactions *1471*
oral candidiasis 2269
prophylactic *440*
in renal failure *4185*
flucytosine
fungal infections 1016–17
in renal failure *4185*
fludarabine 398
lymphoma *4320*
fludrocortisone suppression test 3064
fludrocortisone
congenital adrenal hyperplasia 1893
orthostatic hypotension *5063*
fluid balance
high altitude 1403
malaria 1079
pregnancy 2076
fluid replacement
acute renal trauma 3892
anaphylaxis 3112
critical illness 3118
diabetic ketoacidosis 2025
fluid restriction, heart failure 2720
fluid, requirements 1538, *1538*
flukes 1212
intestinal 1219
liver 1212
lung 1216
schistosomiasis 1202
flumazenil *1274*, 3156, 5265
hepatic encephalopathy 2502
flunarizine, migraine prevention *4916*
fluorescein angiography 5235
fluorescence bronchoscopy 3222
Fluorobacter spp. *962*
fluoroquinolone, pneumonia *3238*
fluorosis 3767
5-fluorouracil 398, 4736
adverse effects *400*
breast cancer *1937*
resistance *399*
fluoxetine
adverse effects *5313*
hyperprolactinaemia 2068
cataplexy *4833*
poisoning 1281
Raynaud's phenomenon *3671*

flupentixol decanoate, schizophrenia *5325*
fluphenazine decanoate, schizophrenia *5325*
fluphenazine
  adverse effects, hepatotoxicity *2529, 2532*
  diabetic neuropathy 2039
flurandrolone *2151*
flurazepam, adverse effects, hepatotoxicity *2529, 2532–3*
flurbiprofen
  adverse effects, hepatotoxicity *2532*
  and asthma *3289*
  rheumatoid arthritis *3594*
fluroxene, adverse effects, hepatotoxicity *2529*
flutamide
  adverse effects, hepatotoxicity *2529*
  polycystic ovary syndrome 1910
  reproductive effects *1917*
fluticasone propionate *2151*
fluticasone
  asthma 3300
  COPD 3334
fluvastatin 1670
fluvoxamine
  adverse effects *5313*
  poisoning 1281
focal cognitive disorders 5273
focal nodular hyperplasia 2520, *2521*
fodrin 179
foetor hepaticus 2497
fogo selvagem *1227*
folate synthesis inhibitors 1076
folic acid (folate) 1492, *4404*, 4405
  absorption 4406
  acquired disorders of metabolism 4417
  biochemistry 4405, *4405–6*
  and coronary heart disease 2890
  deficiency 4382, 1488, 1493, *4408*, 4412
    blood disorders 4413
    diagnosis 4415–16
    drug-induced 4413
    excess urinary loss 4413
    increased utilization 4412
    inflammatory diseases 4413
    malabsorption 4412
    malignant disease 4413
    metabolic 4413
    nutritional 4412
    pregnancy 2174, 4412
    prematurity 4413
    treatment 4416
  dietary reference values *1502*
  homocysteine metabolism 1494
  inborn errors of metabolism 4417
  nutrition 4406
  in pregnancy 2089, 2148
  red cell *4196*
  reference intake *1524*
  reference values *5443*
  requirements 1493
  serum *4196*
  transport 4407
folinic acid-responsive seizures *1566*, 1589
follicle-stimulating hormone (FSH) 1790, 1799, 1808, 1903
  deficiency 1809
  insensitivity *1917*
  measurement 1803
  menstrual cycle 1904
  reference values *5441*
follicular bronchiolitis 3386
follicular lymphoma, translocations *341*
folliculitis 696, *697*, 4673
folliculogenesis 1902
fomepizole *1274*
fondaparinux 3022
  acute coronary syndromes 2921
Fonsecaea compactum 1006
Fonsecaea pedrosoi 1005
Fontan circulation, pregnancy 2114
food allergy 262, *263*, 2251
  aetiology 2252
  classification *2252*
  clinical features 2252, *2252*
    gut-related symptoms 2252
  coeliac disease *see* coeliac disease
  cows' milk 263, 2253
  definition 2252
  diagnosis 2254
    elimination diets and challenge tests 2254
    skin tests and radioallergosorbent tests 2254
    unproven tests 2255
  eggs 263
  fish/shellfish 263
  kiwi fruit 263
  nuts 263
  oral allergy syndrome 263
  prevalence 2252
  remote symptoms 2253
  treatment 2255
    alternative therapies 2255
    dietary management 2255
    immunotherapy 2255
    sodium cromoglicate 2255
  ulcerative colitis 2373
food cravings in pregnancy 2083
food industry, advertising to patient 110
food intolerance 2252
  asthma 2254
  behavioural problems in children 2254
  Chinese restaurant syndrome 2254
  irritable bowel syndrome *see* irritable bowel syndrome
  lactose intolerance 2254
  migraine and headache 2254
  psychological distress in adults 2254
  urticaria 2254
  see also food allergy
food poisoning 2427
  bacterial 727
  C. perfringens 804, 808
    aetiology 809
    occurrence and clinical findings 808
  fish 1346
  prevention 734
food, and drug absorption 1456
food-borne illness 696
food-induced anaphylaxis 3108
foot ulcers 4690, *4690*
foot/feet
  diabetic *2022*, 2045, *2045*
    Charcot's arthropathy 2046
    ulceration 2046
  pain *3557*
  rheumatoid arthritis *3557*
foot-and-mouth disease 531
Forbes' disease 1598, *1598, 2766*
  differential diagnosis *1600*
forced expiration 3192
forced expiratory volume 3192
  asthma 3292
  COPD 3470
forced vital capacity 3192
foreign bodies, gastrointestinal, removal 2217
forensic medicine 5359, *5360*
  access to information 5370
  causes of death 5363
    cocaine abuse 5364
    medical care related 5363
    sudden death syndrome 5364, *5365*
    sudden infant death 5363
    sudden unexpected nocturnal death 5364
  courts 5359
  DNA profiling 5370
    HLA *DQα* 5371
    mitochondrial DNA 5371
    polymerase chain reaction 5371
    population frequency of DNA patterns 5371
    variable number of tandem repeats 5370
  duties at death 5360, *5361*
  expert witnesses 5360, *5361*
  intoxication 5369
  violence 5366
    describing wounds 5368, *5368*
    human bites 5369
    legal context of wounding 5368
    medical notes 5367, *5368*
    photographs of injury 5369
    sexual assaults 5366
forest plot 51
Forestier's disease 3607, 3713, 3768
fork stalling and template switching 145
formaldehyde poisoning 1311
formoterol, COPD *3335*
formularies 1451
fosamprenavir, HIV/AIDS 636, *638*
foscarnet
  cytomegalovirus 496
  mode of action *444*
  in renal failure *4185*
Fos-Jun transcription complex 1803
Fox-Fordyce disease 4676
fractures 3730
  osteoporosis 3796–7
    prevention of *3799*
  Paget's disease 3742
fragile X syndrome *148, 1530, 1917*
fragile X tremor/ataxia syndrome 5115
frailty 5389–90
  clinical definition of 5391
  complexity of 5390, *5391–2*
  and disease presentation 5392
  patient management 5392, *5393*
framboesia *see* yaws
frameshift mutations 138
Francisella spp. *962*
Francisella tularensis 780, 1442
  aetiology and genetics 780
  clinical features 780, *780–1*
  diagnosis 782
  differential diagnosis 781, *782*
  epidemiology 780
  history 780
  pathogenesis and pathology 780
  prevention 780
  prognosis 782
  treatment 782
Frank-Starling relationship 2622, *2622, 3123, 3124*
Frasier's syndrome 1970
freckles 4706
free fatty acids *1739*
Freiberg's disease *3804*
fresh-frozen plasma 4532
Friedlander's pneumonia 3235
Friedreich's ataxia 1497, 142, *148, 1552, 1917, 2766*, 4907, *4908*, 5114
  cardiac involvement *2840*
FRISC-II trial 2921
frontal lobe syndromes 5273
frontotemporal dementia 4802, 5100
  clinical features 4803
  definition 4802
  diagnosis 4803, *4804*
  epidemiology 4802
  management and prognosis 4803
  pathology and genetics 4802
frostbite 1395, 1397
frovatriptan, migraine *4917–18*
fructosaemia 1605
  diagnosis 1607, *1607*
  metabolic defect 1606
  pathology and molecular genetics 1606, *1606*
  prognosis 1608
  treatment 1608, *1608*
fructosamine 2020
fructose diphosphatase deficiency 1608
  description 1608
  diagnosis 1609
  metabolic defect 1608
  treatment 1609
fructose intolerance, hereditary *4149*
fructose
  hereditary intolerance 1605
  malabsorption 1605
  metabolism 1604, *1604*
    inborn errors of 1604
fructosuria, essential (benign) 1605
frusemide *see* furosemide
fucisidosis *1553*
fucosidosis 1698
Fukuyama's syndrome 5142
Fuller's earth pneumoconiosis 3423
fulminant type 1 diabetes 2008
fulvestrant, breast cancer *1937*
fumaric acid esters, psoriasis 4615
fumarylacetoacetase deficiency 1586
functional bowel disorders 2384
  abdominal pain 2387
  bloating 2386
  constipation 2386
  definition 2384, *2385*
  diarrhoea 2387

see also irritable bowel syndrome
functional residual capacity 3174, 3190
functional somatic syndromes 3557
fungal infections 998
diagnosis 998
HIV-related 648
immunocompromised patients 249
immunosuppressed patients 3959
infective endocarditis 2816
liver involvement 2542
management 1015
azoles 1015
deep infections 1016
polyenes 1015
superficial infections 1016
nail 4699, *4699–700*
ocular 5246, *5247*
opportunistic 1012
scalp 4702
skin 4675
subcutaneous 999, 1004
superficial 998–9
systemic 999, *1008, 1009*
urinary tract 4116
see also individual infections
fungal poisoning 1361, 4093
aetiology 1366
classification 1366, *1367*
cytotoxins *1367,* 1368, *1369*
diagnosis 1366
epidemiology 1366
essentials 1365
gastrointestinal irritants 1366, *1367*
hallucinogens 1368, *1368*
neurotoxins 1367, *1367*
prevention 1366
rhabdomyolysis 1370
fungicides, reproductive effects *1917*
furazolidone
giardiasis *1113*
H. pylori 2312
furosemide
adverse effects
hepatotoxicity *2529*
renal toxicity *3860*
ascites 2487
heart failure *2722*
intracranial hypertension *3150*
furuncles 697, *698*
furunculosis 4673
Fusarium spp. *3436*
fusidic acid
adverse effects, hepatotoxicity *2529*
impetigo *697*
mode of action *443*
in renal failure *4185*
S. pyogenes 675
Fusobacterium nucleatum 2261
Fusobacterium spp. *962, 852*

G protein-coupled receptors 169, *171, 1792, 1792, 1794–5*
genetic defects *1798*
GABA metabolism defects 1592, *1592*
GABA transaminase deficiency *1566,* 1592
gabapentin
diabetic neuropathy 2039
dose levels *4823*
epilepsy 4821
migraine prevention *4916*
neuropathic pain 5415
poisoning 1281
Gadgets Gully virus *566*
gain-of-function mutations 138, 361
galactokinase deficiency (galactose diabetes) 1611
galactosaemia 1612, *3739, 4149*
clinical and pathological features 1612
diagnosis 1613
genetic studies 1613
neonatal screening 102
prognosis 1614
treatment 1613
galactose 1-phosphate uridylyltransferase deficiency *see* galactosaemia
galactose diabetes 2349
galactose metabolism 1611, *1611*
inborn errors 1610
galactosialidosis 1698
corneal opacity 1704
galanin 2320
gallbladder disease, investigations *2235*
gallbladder
cancer 316
diseases *see* cholecystitis; gallstones
gangrene 2551
gallium nitrate, hypercalcaemia 1857
galloping consumption 816
gallstones
and acute pancreatitis 2558
bile pigment 2550
cholesterol 2549
dissolution/disruption 2550
contact 2550
endoscopic sphincterotomy 2550
extracorporeal shock-wave lithotripsy 2550
oral bile acid therapy 2550
patient selection and results 2550
side effects and toxicity 2551
ERCP 2218
formation *2549,* 2549
natural history 2550
nutritional causes 1522
small bowel resection 2355
treatment 2550
γ-globulin, pregnancy *2126*
γ-hydroxybutyrate, poisoning 1287
Gambierdiscus toxicus 1346
ganciclovir
adenovirus 477
cytomegalovirus 496
mode of action *444*
prophylactic *440*
in renal failure *4185*
ganglioneuroblastoma 3543
ganglioneuroma 3543
gangliosidoses 5117
GM1, 5117
GM2, 5120
psychiatric signs *1720*
gangosa *882*
gangrene, wet of foot 4719
Ganjam virus *581*
gap junctions 2608, *2611,* 2619, 4594
Gardener's syndrome 2222
Gardner syndrome 1845
Gardnerella spp. *962*
Gardnerella vaginalis 1256–7, 2169
Garissa virus *566, 581, 661*
garlic 68
drug interactions *69*
Garrod, Archibald 136, 1550, 1560
Garrod's knuckle pads 2047, *2047*
gas exchange 3173
in pregnancy 2121
gas gangrene 804, 806
aetiology 806
of bowel *see* necrotizine enterocolitis
definition 806
diagnosis 807
history 807
physical examination 807
prevention 808
spontaneous 807
toxins 807
treatment 807
gases, toxicity 3456
acute pneumonitis 3457
acute tracheobronchitis 3457
acute upper airway 3456
fire smoke 3457
treatment 3457
Gasterophilus spp. *1233*
gastrectomy, and cobalamin deficiency 4411
gastric acid 2306
gastric aspiration/lavage 1279
gastric banding 1534
gastric bypass 1534
gastric cancer 2405
endoscopy 2217
and Epstein-Barr virus 507
gastric emptying 2229
gastric hypersecretion 2355
gastric inhibitory polypeptide, inhibition *2320*
gastric outlet obstruction, ERCP 2218
gastric pathology 2320, *2321*
gastric polyps 2217
gastric secretion 2227
gastric ulcer, detection of 2215
gastrin 2317
elevation *1978*
inhibition *2320*
reference values *5442*
gastrinoma 1979
treatment 1981
Gastrodiscoides hominis 1223
gastroenteritis
abdominal pain 2237
eosinophilic 2221
viral 536, *537,* 539
adenovirus 538
astrovirus 539
calicivirus 538
clinical features 539
diagnosis 539, *539*
enterovirus 532
outbreak control 541
rotaviruses 536
treatment 539
vaccines 540
gastrointestinal bleeding 2237, *3120, 4555, 4556*
acute lower GI tract 2240
aetiology 2240, *2241*
clinical features 2241
epidemiology 2240
presentation 5471
treatment 2241
acute upper GI tract 2237
aetiology and pathogenesis 2237, *2238*
clinical features 2238, *2238*
differential diagnosis 2238
epidemiology 2238
investigations 2238
presentation 5470, *5470–1*
prevention 2238
Rockall score *2239*
definition 2237
future developments 2242
investigation 2242
colonoscopy 2242
radiology 2242
obscure 2242
prognosis 2240
therapeutic endoscopy 2216
treatment 2239, *2239,* 2242
surgery 2242
gastrointestinal bypass surgery 2540
gastrointestinal cancer syndromes *2406*
gastrointestinal cancers 2405
colorectal *see* colorectal cancer
oesophageal *see* oesophageal cancer
stomach *see* gastric cancer
gastrointestinal disease
Behçet's disease 3686
gut peptides 2320
diarrhoea 2322
intestinal resection 2321
intestinal tumours 2322
malabsorption 2321, *2321*
neuropathic disease 2322, *2322*
haematological changes 4555
hepatic involvement 2539
immune-mediated 2246
primary immuno-deficiency 2246, *2250*
secondary immuno-deficiency 2250
immunocompromised host 431, *439*
and immunodeficiency 2251
infections, anaerobic 751
investigation 2210
colonoscopy and flexible sigmoidoscopy 2210
gastrointestinal function 2226
radiology 2219
upper gastrointestinal endoscopy 2214
malaria 1063
mesenteric ischaemia 2417, *2418*
acute 2419
chronic 2420
compression of coeliac axis 2420
compression of mesenteric vessels 2417
intestinal reperfusion injury 2420
intraluminal occlusion 2417
intrinsic vascular pathology 2418, *2418*
ischaemic colitis 2420, *2420*
nonocclusive 2419, *2419*
nutrition support 1543
occupational 1384

pregnancy 2132
acute appendicitis 2132
coeliac disease 2132
gastro-oesophageal reflux 2132
inflammatory bowel disease 2132
rabies 547
symptomatology 2205
abdominal pain 2207
altered bowel habit 2208
dyspepsia 2206
heartburn 2206
irritable bowel 2207
nausea 2206
oesophageal 2205–6
vomiting 2206
systemic sclerosis 3676, *3676*
vascular and collagen disorders 2417
see also various parts
gastrointestinal fluids, electrolyte composition *1538*
gastrointestinal function 2202
absorption 2202, 2228
bile salts 2229
carbohydrates 2228, *2228*
fat 2229
vitamin B12, 2229
digestive secretions 2202, 2227
biliary 2227
gastric 2227
intestinal 2228
pancreatic 2228
integrity and barrier functions 2230
infection 2230, *2230*
mucosal damage 2230
investigations 2226
breath tests *2227*
faecal output 2226
nutritional assessment 2226
transit time 2229
gastric emptying 2229
intestinal 2229
oesophageal function 2229
gastrointestinal hormones 2316, *2317*
bombesin 2319
cholecystokinin 2318
chromogranin-derived peptides 2320
elevated *1978*
enteroglucagon 2319
gastrin 2317
ghrelin 2319
glucagon-like peptide 1, 2319
glucagon-like peptide 2, 2319
glucose-dependent insulinotropic peptide 2318
motilin 2319
neuropeptide Y 2319
neurotensin 2320
obestatin 2319
opioids 2319
oxyntomodulin 2319
peptide tyrosine tyrosine 2319
secretin 2318
somatostatin 2320, *2320*
tachykinins 2320
vasoactive intestinal peptide 2318, *2318*
gastrointestinal infections 2424
clinical syndromes 2426
antibiotic-associated colitis 2429
food poisoning 2427
inflammatory diarrhoea 2428
invasive infections 2430
noninflammatory diarrhoea 2426, 2428
travellers' diarrhoea 2428
Clostridium perfringens 804, 808
complications *2425*
diagnosis 2430, *2431*
differential diagnosis 2431
management 2432, *2433*
antibiotics 2432
antidiarroeal agents 2433, *2433*
diet 2432
rehydration 2432
pathophysiology 2425
host factors 2425
microbial factors 2425
prevention 2433
gastrointestinal irritants
fungal 1366, *1367*
plant-derived *1362*, 1365
gastrointestinal lymphoma 2342, *2342*
enteropathy-associated T-cell lymphoma 2338, *2344, 2345–6*
immunoproliferative small intestinal disease 2344
MALT lymphoma 2343
gastrointestinal motility 1455, *1456*
gastrointestinal symptoms, exercise-induced 5380
gastrointestinal tract
anatomy 2201, *2202*
epithelial layer 2202
neuromusculature 2202
commensal flora 749, 2425
congenital abnormalities 2395
anterior abdominal wall defects 2397
atresia/stenosis of small intestine 2398, *2399*
colonic atresia 2402
duplication 2399
embryology 2395
Hirschsprung's disease 2402, *2403*
histology 2396
imperforate anus 2403
Meckel's diverticulum 2401
meconium ileus 2401
oesophageal atresia 2396, *2397*
pyloric stenosis 2398
short intestine 2402
small-intestinal lymphangiectasia 2400
small-intestinal malrotation 2400
tracheo-oesophageal fistula 2396, *2397*
in cystic fibrosis 3354
duplication 2399
effects of malnutrition 1510
function 2246
gut-associated lymphoid tissue 2245, *2245*
immune function 2202–3, 2425
local responses 2246
systemic responses 2246
systemic tolerance 2246
intramural bleeding 2423
neural control 2203, *2203*
disturbances of 2204
intrinsic nervous system 2203
migrating motor complex 2203
peristaltic reflex 2203, *2203*
in pregnancy 2077, 2089
radiology 2219
colon 2224
small intestine 2219
salt and water absorption *2208*
in SLE 3659
see also various parts
gastro-oesophageal reflux disease 2288, *2288, 2289*
aetiology 2288
barium swallow and meal 2289
complications 2288, 2291
cystic fibrosis 3362
definition 2288
diagnosis 2289
endoscopy 2289
history 2289
function tests 2289, *2289*
management 2290
acid suppression 2291
antireflux surgery 2291
endoscopic procedures 2291
motility stimulants 2291
nondrug measures and antacids 2290
tailoring/titration of therapy *2289*, 2290
post-transplantation 3484
pregnancy 2089, 2132
symptoms 2288
gastroschisis 2398
gastrostomy
endoscopically placed *1541*
percutaneous endoscopically placed *1540*
radiologically placed *1540*
GATA1, acquired/congenital defects 4371
GATA3, 157
gatekeeper genes 342, 361
gatifloxacin *707*
pharmacokinetics/pharmacodynamics *452*
pneumonia *3245*
Pseudomonas aeruginosa 737
typhoid fever *742*
Gaucher's disease *1553*, 1698, 1694, 1696, *3721*, 3757, 5120
cardiac involvement 2789
clinical features 1710, 1709, 1711
diagnosis 1704, 1706
neuronopathic 5102
pathology 1710
skeletal involvement 1711–3
splenomegaly 1703
treatment 63, 1709, 1555
GAWK peptide 1977, 2320
gaze-holding 4859
Gc globulin *1753*
G-CSF 153, 158, 397, 4201, 4207
management of neutropenia 4308
gefitinib 400, *1939*
lung cancer 3529
gelling phenomenon 3632
gels 4732
gelsemine 1363
gelsolin 179, 1774
gemcitabine
breast cancer *1937*
cost-effectiveness ratio *53*
hepatocellular carcinoma 2517
lung cancer 3529
Gemella morbillorum, infective endocarditis 2815
Gemella spp. *962*
gemfibrozil
adverse effects, hepatotoxicity *2529*
drug interactions *1471*
gemtuzumab ozogamicin *376*
gender (sex) assignment 1966
gender attribution 1966
gender dysphoria 1966
gender identity 1966
gender roles 1966
gender
and cancer susceptibility 303
and COPD 3315
and osteoarthritis 3630
gene amplification 342, *342, 344, 345*
gene expression, differential 132
gene replacement 1555
gene silencing 342
post-transcriptional 133
gene splicing 138, 132
generalized anxiety disorder 5316
genes 138
genetic (locus) heterogeneity 138
genetic analysis 137
genetic counselling
cancer 369
central nervous system abnormalities 5148
genetic damage, repair of 342
genetic disease
cardiac involvement 2834
renal involvement 4095
genetic instability 342
genetic susceptibility, cancer 302
genetic variation 140
repetitive DNA elements 141
single nucleotide polymorphisms (SNPs) 140
genetics
disease 148
autoimmune 268
endocrine 1797, *1797–8*
inherited cancers 358
obesity 1529, *1530*
genital amoebiasis 1040
genital filariasis 1156, *1157*
genital herpes 486, *486*, 1247
genital ulcers, Behçet's disease *3685*
genitourinary tract
commensal flora 750
disease, occupational 1384
infections
anaerobic 752
candidosis 1014
chlamydial 939, *942, 944*
and infertility 1924
mycoplasmal infections 951, 955, *955–6*
see also individual infections
genitourinary tuberculosis 819
genome association studies 141
genome sequencing 148
genomic analysis 148, 137
genomic disorders 143
chromosome aberrations 145
structural 145
low-copy repeats 144
marker chromosomes 145

molecular mechanisms 143
new mutation rates 144
genomic imprinting 139
genomics 135
websites 141
gentamicin
animal-related injuries 1326
chlamydial infections *943*
endocarditis *704–5*
infective endocarditis *2817*, *2817–18*
listeriosis 898
nephrotoxicity 3897
pelvic inflammatory disease *1260*
pneumonia *3238*
postantibiotic effect *451*
Pseudomonas aeruginosa 737
in renal failure *4185*
serum levels *5449*
spectrum of activity *446*
therapeutic drug monitoring *1475*, 1476
tularaemia 782
vertigo *4861*
yersiniosis *777*
Genzyme 63
Geotrichum candidum 1012
Geriatric Depression Scale (GDS) 5406
germander, hepatotoxicity *2529*
germ-cell tumours 386, 3541
malignant 3542
Germiston virus *581*
Gerstmann-Sträussler-Scheinker syndrome 1771
gestational diabetes 2007, 2133
dermoid cysts 3541
and polycystic ovary syndrome 1909
preconception care 2136
see also diabetes mellitus, pregnancy
gestational trophoblastic disease 2182
Getah virus *558*
Ghon complex 815
ghrelin 2319
actions *1791*
GI *see* gastrointestinal
giant cell arteritis *3650*, *4033*, 4632, *5163*
anaemia 4401
cardiac involvement 2785
GI tract involvement 2422
headache 4926
neurological complications 5163
ocular involvement 5241, *5242*
pulmonary involvement *3396*, 3401
treatment 5163
giant cell myocarditis 2763
Giardia lamblia 2247, *2248*
malabsorption *2357*
giardiasis 1111–12
aetiology 1112
clinical features 1113
epidemiology 1113
historical perspective 1112
immunocompromised host 431
laboratory diagnosis 1113
pathogenesis/pathology 1112, *1112*
prevention 1113
treatment 1113, *1113*
Gibbium psylloides 1236
gibbus 820
gigantism 1958
Gilbert's syndrome 2447–8
Gillespie's syndrome *4904*
ginger, drug interactions *69*
gingival bleeding 4500
gingival/periodontal disease 2259
aetiology 2259, *2260*
classification *2260*
clinical features *2260*, 2261
course and prognosis 2261
differential diagnosis 2261
pathology 2261
treatment 2261
gingivitis
acute (necrotizing) ulcerative 2261
aetiology 2261
clinical features 2262, *2262*
course and prognosis 2262
diagnosis 2262
pathology 2262
treatment 2262
and leukaemia *2285*
gingivostomatitis
primary herpetic 485, *485*, 2262
aetiology 2262
clinical features 2262
course and prognosis 2263
diagnosis 2263
pathology 2262
treatment 2263
Ginkgo biloba 68
ginseng, drug interactions *69*
GISSI trial 36
Gitelman's syndrome 1499, 3073, 3837–8, *3838*, 4144
glafenine, adverse effects, hepatotoxicity *2529*
glanders 771
Glanzmann's disease, laboratory tests *4504*
Glasgow Coma Score 1281, *4965*, *5488*
drowning 1400
glaucoma 5252
glibenclamide 2014
adverse effects, hepatotoxicity *2532*, *2533*, *2535*
pregnancy 2137
glimepiride 2014
glioma
brainstem 4779
pregnancy 2147
gliquidone 2014
Glisson's capsule 2435
global access to medicines 62
Global Alliance for Vaccination and Immunization (GAVI) 60
global disease burden *88*
global risk factors *87*
Globicatella spp. *962*
globoid cell leukodystrophy *see* Krabbe's disease
globotriaosylceramide 1712
globozoospermia *1917*
globus hystericus 2205
glomerular disease, tropical 4083, *4083*
glomerular filtration rate *5449*, 3812, 3863
estimation of *3847*, 3868
carbamylation 3871
creatinine clearance 3868, *3869*
cystatin C 3871
isotopic methods 3871
radiological methods 3871
reference values *5435*
glomerular filtration 1459
glomerulonephritis
acute 4073
with C3 deposition 3989
children 3979
classification 3979, *3980*
complement in *222*
familial primary 4100
filarial 1157
infection-associated 4071
leprosy 4089
management 3979
mesangiocapillary 3991
proliferative 3988
rapidly progressive 3855
causes *3856*
clinical presentation 3856, *3856*
rheumatoid arthritis 4053
sickle cell disease 4070
SLE 3658, *3659*
systemic sclerosis 3676
glomerulosclerosis, focal segmental 3979, 3982
aetiology *3982*
clinical presentation 3983
adults 3984
children 3983
pathogenesis 3983
pathology 3983, *3983*
primary (idiopathic) 3983
prognosis 3984
secondary 3982
treatment 3984
glomerulus 3811, *3811*
function 3811
structure 3811
glomus tumour 4693
Glossina morsitans (tsetse fly) 1121, *1121*, *1226*
Glossina spp. *1226*
glossitis 2284, *2284–5*
glossopharyngeal nerve disorders 5037
Gloydius himilayanus 1327
glucagon stimulation test 1804
glucagon 1993, *2443*
actions *1791*
anaphylaxis 3112
β-blocker poisoning *1274*, 1284
elevation *1978*
inhibition *2320*
metabolic effects *1481*
reference values *5442*
glucagon-like peptides 1993, 2319
glucagonoma 1980
treatment 1981
glucocorticoids 1870
deficiency *see* hypoadrenalism
excess *see* Cushing's syndrome
and osteoporosis 3801
replacement therapy 1884
resistance to *1871*, 1888
glucosamine, osteoarthritis 3635
glucose tolerance test 1804, *1991*, 1991
glucose transporter 1 deficiency syndrome 5103
glucose transporters 3813
glucose
blood monitoring 2020
cerebrospinal fluid 4752
hyperkalaemia *3891*
impaired fasting glucose 1991–2
impaired glucose tolerance 1991
reference values *5435*, *5446–7*
children *5438*
regulation of fatty acid oxidation 1485, *1485*
regulation of gene expression *1482*
renal tubular reabsorption 3872
urinary 2020
glucose-6-phosphatase deficiency *see* von Gierke's disease
glucose-6-phosphate dehydrogenase deficiency *1031*, *4082*, *4453*, 4473, *4454*
biochemistry and pathophysiology 4476
clinical features 4474
acute haemolytic anaemia 4474, *4474–5*
chronic nonspherocytic haemolytic anaemia 4476, *4476*
favism 4475, *4475*
neonatal jaundice 4475
definition 4474
drugs causing haemolysis *4459*
epidemiology 4474
genetics 4474
laboratory diagnosis 4476
management 4477
molecular basis 4477, *4477–8*
glucose-6-phosphate isomerase deficiency 4471
glucose-dependent insulinotropic peptide 2318
glucose-fatty acid cycle 1485, *1485*
glucose-hydrogen breath test *2230*
glucose-lowering drugs
insulin *see* insulin
oral hypoglycaemic agents 2014
α-glucosidase inhibitors 2017
glucuronidation, genetic variability 1473
glutamine, and immune system 5378
γ-glutamyl transferase
reference values *5436*
children *5438*
glutaric aciduria type I *1566*, 1575
aetiology/pathophysiology 1575, *1575*
clinical presentation 1575, *1576*
diagnosis 1576
treatment and outcome 1577
glutathione reductase deficiency 4471
gluten-induced enteropathy 4412
glycated haemoglobin 2020
reference values *5435*
glyceryl trinitrate 2629, 3130
hypertensive emergencies *3080*
glycine *N*-methyltransferase deficiency *1566*, 1594
glycinuria *4148*
glycogen storage diseases 1596, *1597–8*, 1698
future developments 1602
hepatic 1597
diagnosis 1600, *1600*
treatment 1601
type I (von Gierke) 1597, *1598–9*

type III (Cori/Forbes) 1598, *1600*
type VI (Hers) 1599
type IX 1599
historical perspective 1596
incidence 1597
skeletal muscle 1601
diagnosis 1602
treatment 1602
type II (Pompe) *see* Pompe's disease
type V (McArdle) 1601
type VII (Tarui) 1601
type IV 5109
glycogen synthase deficiency 1602
glycogenosis
type I 1630
type II *1553*
glycoprotein hormones *1791*
glycoprotein Ia-IIa 4485
glycoprotein Ib-IX-V 4484
glycoprotein IIb-IIIa inhibitors, acute coronary syndromes 2918, *2919*
glycoprotein IIb-IIIa 4485
glycoprotein IV 4485
glycoprotein VI-Fc receptor α-chain complex 4485
glycoproteinoses 1697, *1553*, 1698
Glycorrhiza glabrata (liquorice), nephrotoxicity *4093*
glycosaminoglycans 1775, *4482*
glycosphingolipidoses 1697
glycosuria 3865, 4140–1
renal 4141
renal glucose handling 4141
glyphosate-containing herbicide poisoning 1303
glypressin, orthostatic hypotension *5063*
GM1 gangliosidosis 1698
GM2 activator protein 1697
GM-CSF 158, *212*, 4201, 4207
gnathostomiasis 1182
aetiology and genetics 1182
clinical features 1182, *1183*
differential diagnosis 1183
epidemiology 1182
genetics 1182
histopathology 1182
investigations 1183
pathogenesis 1182
pathology 1182
prevention 1182
prognosis 1184
treatment 1184
goblet cells 3177
goitre 1498, *1826*, *1831*, *1831*
causes *1832*
endemic 1831
grading of *1831*
sporadic 1832
toxic multinodular 1838
treatment 1842
gold neuropathy 4052
gold salts
adverse effects
hepatotoxicity *2532–3*, *2535*
renal toxicity *3860*
contraindication in porphyria 1641
pregnancy *2158*
rheumatoid arthritis *3595*
gold, reference values *5445*
gold-induced thrombocytopenia 4512
golfer's elbow *3557*
Golgi apparatus 130
gonadal dysfunction, cognitive impairment 5281
gonadal dysgenesis 1969
gonadotrohin-releasing hormone (GnRH) 1790, 1903, 1914
insensitivity to *1917*
gonadotrophs *1801*
adenoma 1809
gonadotropin-releasing hormone analogues 1961
gonadotropins
excess *384*
folliculogenesis 1903
gonads
disorders of 2066
drug-induced 2068
Gongylonema pulchrum 1176
gonorrhoea 722, 1243, *1245*, 1259
complications 724
diagnosis 724
epidemiology 722, *723*
incidence *1245*
men 724
pathogenesis 723
pregnancy 2170
risk factors 1244
treatment 726
women 723
complications 723
signs and symptoms 723
see also Neisseria gonorrhoeae
good manufacturing practice 199
Goodpasture's syndrome 437, 3426
anaemia 4558
clinical features 3426
treatment and prognosis 3426
see also antiglomerular basement membrane disease
Gordon's syndrome 1889, 3073, 3844
Gordonia spp. *962*
Gorham's syndrome 3496
Gorlin's syndrome 172, 358, *360*, 367
goserelin, breast cancer *1937*
Gottron's sign 3694, *3694*
gout 1622, 3637, 3639
causes *1621*
classification 3640, *3641*
primary 3641
secondary *3640*, 3641
clinical features 3639
acute attacks 3639
hyperuricaemia 3639
intercritical periods 3640
tophi 3640, *3640*
clinical investigation *3641*, 3642
differential diagnosis 3642
genetics *1622*
and heart failure 2726
post-transplant 3964
and renal disease 3641
chronic urate nephropathy 3642
urolithiasis 3641
renal failure 4183
tophaceous 1623
treatment 1624, *1624*, 3643
gouty arthritis 1623, *1623*
Gradenigo's syndrome 5034–5
graft-vs-host disease 2510
haematopoietic stem cell transplantation 4576, *4576–7*
transfusion-associated 4568
Graham-Steell murmur 2753
Granulicatella spp. *962*
granulocyte colony-stimulating factor *see* G-CSF
granulocyte-macrophage colony stimulating factor *see* GM-CSF
granulocytes 209
transfusion 4566
granulocytosis *385*
granuloma annulare 4717, *4718*
granulomatous disorders, and hypercalcaemia 1861
Graphium spp. *3436*
Graves' disease *276*
clinical features 1839
pathology 1839
pregnancy 1842, *2142*
surgery 1841
treatment 1840
see also Thyrotoxicosis
Graves' ophthalmopathy 5249, *5249*
differential diagnosis 5249
Graves' ophthalmoplegia 5217
gravity, and lung function 3180
green accounting 84
green fluorescent protein 131
green tea 68
greenhouse gases 83
grey hepatization 684
Grey Turner's sign 2563
grief 5284
clinical features 5285
normal grief 5285, *5286*
pathological grief 5285, *5286*
differential diagnosis 5287
epidemiology 5285
mortality 5285
prevention 5288
prognosis 5287
psychiatric comorbidity 5285
treatment 5287
cognitive/behavioural therapies 5287
pharmacological 5287
psychotherapies 5287
self-help 5287
Grifola fondosa 3436
Grimontia spp. *962*
Griscelli syndrome 1698, *238*
griseofulvin
adverse effects, hepatotoxicity *2532*, *2533*
dermatophytoses 1002
fungal infections 1016
Grönblad-Strandberg syndrome *see* pseudoxanthoma elasticum
gross domestic product (GDP)
health care spending as share of *113*
health effects on 74
growth disorders 1951
causes *1951*
excessive growth 1948, 1957
causes 1957
constitutional 1957
familial tall stature 1957
pituitary gigantism 1958
precocious sexual maturation 1957
treatment 1958
growth failure 1948, *3729*, *3730*
chronic disease 1955
constitutional delay 1952
familial short stature 1952
growth hormone deficiency 1956
idiopathic short stature 1952
juvenile hypothyroidism 1955
Laron's syndrome 1957
Prader-Willi syndrome 1956
psychosocial short stature 1955
skeletal dysplasia 1956
Turner's syndrome 1955
growth standards 1951
simple errors 1951
small for gestational age 1952
growth factor receptors *348*
growth factors 334, *334–5*
growth hormone (GH) 1799, 1804–5
actions *1791*
deficiency 1799, 1806, *1806*
primary 1957
secondary 1956
ectopic secretion 2065
excess, acromegaly 1806
inhibition *2320*
measurement 1803
metabolic effects *1481*
reference values(GH) 5441
growth hormone receptor antagonists, acromegaly 1807
growth hormone releasing hormone (GHRH), ectopic secretion 2065
growth plate 3548, *3549*
growth 1948
adolescence 1951
childhood 1951
infancy 1951
normal 1948, *1953–4*
Guaitará fever *see* bartonellosis
Guama virus *581*
guanine 138
guanosine triphosphate cyclohydrolase deficiency 1585, 4887, 4891
clinical presentation 1585
diagnosis 1586
treatment and outcome 1586
Guaroa virus *581*
Guillain-Barré syndrome *384*, 805, 5089
epidemic *276*
presentation 5492
guinea worm disease (dracunculiasis) 1160
aetiology 1160, *1161*
clinical features 1161, *1162*
control and eradication 1162
diagnosis 1162
epidemiology 1161
geographical distribution 1161, *1161*
patient management 1162
Gunther's disease 1638
gut-associated lymphoid tissue (GALT) 2245, *2245*
intraepithelial lymphocytes 2245
lamina propria lymphocytes 2246
Peyer's patches 2202, *2245*
secretory immunoglobulins 2246
Gymnophalloides seoi 1223
gynaecomastia 1385
drug-induced 2068
lung cancer 3523
nonendocrine conditions associated with 2066, *2067*

gyrate atrophy of choroid and retina *1566*
gyromitrin *1367*, 1370

HAART therapy 3252
IRIS syndrome 640
see also antiretroviral therapy
Habershon's jaundice 2541
HACEK organisms, infective endocarditis *2812*, 2816
haem arginate 1648
haem, biosynthesis 1637, *1639*
Haemagogus spp. *1226*
haemangioma
cardiac 2832
infantile 4693
intestinal 2585
liver 2520, *2520*
synovial 3713
Haemaphysalis concinna 1228
Haemaphysalis spinigera 1228
Haemaphysalis turturis 1228
haematemesis 2238, 2309
haematite lung 3424
haematocrit, infants and children *4197*
haematological disease *see* blood disorders
haematological values
adults *4196*
infants and children *4197*
haematopoietic growth factor transfusion 4570
haematopoietic stem cell transplantation
autologous, indications for 4578
conditioning 4575, *4575*
donors 4575
graft-vs-host disease 4576, *4576–7*
immune reconstitution and infections 4577, *4577*
indications *4573*, 4578
lysosomal storage diseases 1697
multiple myeloma 4348
relapse 4578
Haematopota spp. *1226*
haematuria 3865
asymptomatic microscopic 3849
causes 3849, *3850*
management 3850
benign familial 4099
loin pain-haematuria syndrome 3853
macroscopic 3852
causes *3851*
with proteinuria 3849
sickle cell disease 4070
haemochezia 2238
haemochromatosis 1673
adult 1673–4, *1674*
clinical features 1681, *1681–2*
cardiac involvement 2787, *2840*
clinical features 1681
diagnosis 1682
family members 1682
laboratory investigations 1682, *1682*
environmental cofactors 1683
epidemiology 1675
future directions 1685
genetics and molecular biology 1679, *1680*
iron absorption 1678
iron storage 1677, *1677–8*
pathological 1674
iron toxicity 1677
juvenile 1675
neonatal *1674*, 1675
pathophysiology/ pathogenesis 1677
phenotypic expression 1676
prevalence 1675
prevention and control 1685
prognosis 1684
reproductive effects *1917*
secondary 4395, *4395*
treatment 1683
iron chelation therapy 1684, 4396
venesection 1683
haemodiafiltration 3935, *3935–6*
haemodialysis 3930
acute renal trauma 3893
adequacy of 3936
duration and frequency 3937, *3937*
incremental dialysis 3937
quotidian dialysis 3937
target *Kt/V* 3937
urea kinetic modelling 3936, *3937*
urea reduction ratio 3936, *3936*
complications 3940
amyloidosis 1772, 3942
anaemia 3941
bone disease 3942
cardiovascular disease 3941
coagulation problems 3941
dialyser reactions 3941
disequilibration 3940
fevers 3941
hypotension 3941
development of 3931
adequacy 3931
changing demographics 3932
expanding services 3931, *3931–2*
impact of conservative management 3932
impact of transplantation 3932
pioneers 3931
drug elimination 4175
future of 3942
hyperkalaemia *3891*
outcomes 3942
patient management 3938
diet and nutrition 3940
dry weight 3938
hyperlipidaemia 3940
hypertension 3939
infection control 3940
initiation of dialysis 3938
monitoring dialysis delivery 3938
predialysis care 3938, *3938*
prescribing dialysis 3938
technical aspects 3932
anticoagulation 3935
control of ultrafiltration 3934, *3935*
dialysis 3932
dialysis machine 3934
dialysis water and fluids 3933, *3933–4*
extracorporeal circuit 3934, *3934*
membranes and dialysers 3932, *3933*
techniques 3935
conventional haemodialysis 3935
haemodiafiltration 3935, *3935–6*
haemofiltration 3935
high-flux haemodialysis 3935
vascular access 3939
permanent 3939
recirculation 3940
temporary 3939
vs. peritoneal dialysis 3944
haemodilution 4515, 4535
haemodynamic homeostasis 3126, *3127*
haemofiltration 3935
acute renal trauma 3893
drug elimination 4175
haemoglobin A2, *4196*
haemoglobin Alc 4445
haemoglobin Bart's hydrops syndrome 4433, *4433*
haemoglobin H disease 4434
haemoglobin H 2176
haemoglobin Pb 4445
haemoglobin S *see* sickling haemoglobinopathies
haemoglobin SC disease 4441
haemoglobin variants 4437, *4437*
abnormal oxygen binding 4442
haemolysis due to 4441
nomenclature 4437
sickling disorders 4437, *4437*
haemoglobin 4195, *4196*
fetal, in adult life 4445
function 4422
genetic control 4423, *4423–4*
glycated 2020
glycosylated 4445
high-affinity 4267
infants and children *4197*
nephrotoxicity 3899
plasma *4196*
structure 4422, *4445*
synthesis 4424, *4424*
variants, in pregnancy 2176
haemoglobin F *4196*
haemoglobinopathies 4420
classification 4424, *4424*
pregnancy 2173–4
screening *2175*
thalassaemias 2176
variant haemoglobins and sickle cell syndromes 2176
skeletal involvement 3767
thalassaemias 4424
unstable haemoglobin disorders 4442, *4442*
see also haemoglobin variants
haemoglobin-oxygen dissociation curve 3195, *3196*, *3468*
haemoglobinuria 3853
malaria *1068*
march 4460
paroxysmal cold 4456
paroxysmal nocturnal 4298, 221, 4212
haemolysis
chemicals causing *4459*
hepatic involvement 2541
intravascular, malaria *1068*
thermal 4460
venom-induced 4460
haemolytic anaemia 4450, *4451*
acquired 4454
immune haemolytic anaemias 4454, *4455*
nonimmune haemolytic anaemias 4458, *4458–9*
alloimmune 4456
complement system in 222
congenital 4446
red cell enzyme disorders 4452, *4453–4*
red cell membrane disorders 4451
drug-induced 4456
pregnancy 2177
haemolytic disease of newborn 4457
antenatal screening *102*
haemolytic uraemic syndrome 4065, 3862, 4459, 4513
diagnosis 4066
diarrhoeal 4066
histopathology 4066
nondiarrhoeal 4067
drug-related 4068
familial 4067
HIV related 4068
idiopathic 4067
malignancy related 4068
post-renal transplantation 4067
pregnancy related 4068
treatment 4068
pathogenesis 4066, *4066*
Haemonchus contortus 1176
haemoperfusion, poisoned patients 1279
haemopexin *1753*
haemophagocytic lymphohistiocytosis 4362, *4362–3*, 4364
management 4365
haemophagocytic syndrome 4514, 4550
haemophilia A, pregnancy 2179
haemophilia B, pregnancy 2179
haemophilia 4518
antenatal screening *102*
arthralgia 3708
gene transfer 4524
treatment 4522
complications of 4523
Haemophilus aphrophilus 762, 859
Haemophilus ducreyi 764
Haemophilus influenzae 759
antibiotic resistance 761
antibiotic sensitivity *446*
clinical features 761
noncapsulate 761
type b 761, *761*
community-acquired pneumonia *453*
cystic fibrosis 3356
description 759
epidemiology 760
nonapsulate/ nonwerotypeable 760
type b 760
HIV-associated infection *3247*
immunization *90–1*
laboratory diagnosis 762
pathogenicity 410, 760
pneumonia 760, 3231, *3232*, 3234
prevention and control 762
treatment 762, *3238*
Haemophilus parainfluenzae 762
Haemophilus paraphrophilus 762

Haemophilus segnis 762
Haemophilus spp. *962*
osteomyelitis *3789*
haemopoiesis 4199
fetal liver 4369
phylogeny and ontogeny 4200
spleen 4335
haemopoietic growth factors 4207
haemopoietic stem cell disorders 4199
multilineage involvement 4209, *4210*
haemopoietic stem cell transplantation 4571, *197*, *4573*
histocompatibility 4573
haemopoietic stem cells 4573
plasticity 4575
sources of 4574
bone marrow 4574
peripheral blood 4574
umbilical cord blood 4574
haemoptysis 2848, *3184*
cystic fibrosis 3361
lung cancer 3518
haemorrhage
leptospirosis 875
peptic ulcer disease 2309
haemorrhagic diathesis 2496
diagnosis 2500
management 2504
haemosiderin 1677
haemosiderosis 1686
idiopathic pulmonary 4558
haemostasis 4480
assessment of 4502
coagulation pathways 4494, *4494*
coagulation proteins 4489, *4490–1*
fibrinolytic system 4496, *4496–7*
newborns 4541
platelets in 4508
screening assays *4533*, *4535*
haemostatic defects
pregnancy 2173, *2177*
acquired factor VIII inhibitors 2179
factor XI deficiency 2179
haemophilias 2179
thrombocytopenia 2177, *2177*
von Willebrand's disease 2179
snake bite 1332, *1331*, *1333*
haemothorax 3486, 3497
iatrogenic 3498, *3498*
nontraumatic 3498
traumatic 3497
Hafnia spp. *962*
Hailey-Hailey disease 4596
hair
disorders of 4701
alopecia areata 4702, *4703*
eczema 4702
fungal scalp disease 4702
liver disease 4720
scalp psoriasis 4701, *4702*
scarring alopecia 4703
systemic disease 4703
greying 4662
in pregnancy 2078, 2149
hairy cell leukaemia 4227
hairy leukoplakia 507
oral *2266*
halitosis 2285
Hallervorden-Spatz disease 1686
hallucinations
around sleep 4831
visual 4857
hallucinogens
fungal 1368, *1368*
plant-derived 1362, *1362*
haloperidol decanoate, schizophrenia *5325*
haloperidol 3156, *5265*, *5423*
adverse effects, hepatotoxicity *2532*, *2533*
schizophrenia *5325*
halothane
adverse effects, hepatotoxicity *2529*
hepatotoxicity *1385*
Haltia-Santavuori disease 1698
hamartin 367
hamartoma
of breast 1941
cardiac 2832
Hamman-Rich syndrome 3369, 3375
hand, foot and mouth disease 531, *531*, 2264
hand-arm vibration syndrome 1387
handedness 4787
hands
diabetic hand syndrome 2047
mechanic's 3694, *3694*
osteoarthritis *3632*, 3633
pain *3248*
rheumatoid arthritis 3587, *3588*
Hand-Schüller-Christian disease 3446
Hansen's disease *see* leprosy
Hantaan virus *581*
hantavirus *581*, 582
clinical features
acute interstitial nephritis 3859, 3901
pneumonia *3238*
renal toxicity *4086*
haemorrhagic fever with renal syndrome 582, *583*
pulmonary syndrome 584, *584*
renal involvement 4073
Haplorchis microchis 1222
Haplorchis pleurophocerca 1222
Haplorchis pumilio 1222
Haplorchis taichui 1222
Haplorchis vanissimus 1222
Haplorchis yokogawai 1222
HapMap project 149, 362
haptoglobin, serum *4196*
haptoglobins *1753*
reference values *5444*
harlequin fetus 1698, 4598
Harmonia axyridis 1236
Hartnup's disease 1490, *4147*, *4148*
harvest mites 1229
Harvey, William 10, 12
Hashimoto's thyroiditis 1834–5, 1847
Haverhill fever 858
aetiology 858
clinical features 859
hawthorn 68
drug interactions *69*
hay fever *see* allergic rhinitis
Hazara virus *581*
hazard ratio 52
head and neck, infections, anaerobic 751
head injuries 4963
cognitive impairment 5277, *5277*
complications 4966
chronic subdural haematoma 4967
cognitive symptoms 4966
epilepsy 4967
hydrocephalus 4967
infection 4966
intracranial haematoma 4966, *4966*
deteriorating conscious level 4964, *4965*
early management 4964
epidemiology 4963
follow-up 4966, *4967*
golden hour 4964, *4964*
primary and secondary 4963
severity 4964
head lice 1231, *1231*
headache 4911
causes *4912*
chronic daily 4923, *4923*
new onset 4924, *4924*
cluster 4918, *4918–20*
CSF volume
low 4925, *4925*
raised 4926
differential diagnosis *4920*
hypertension 3040
medication overuse 4924
migraine *see* migraine
pregnancy 2089, 2146
primary syndromes 4912, *4912–14*
cough headache 4921
exertional headache 4921
hypnic headache 4922
sex headache 4921
stabbing headache 4921
thunderclap headache 4922
secondary *4912*, 4913, *4915*
cervicogenic 4926
food intolerance 2254
giant cell arteritis 4926
post-traumatic 4926
SUNCT/SUNA 4921
tension-type 4917
health advertising 109
to patients 109
food industry 110
health care providers 110
medical devices 110
pharmaceutical companies 109
to physicians 109
USA 110
rest of world 110
Health and Safety at Work etc. Act (1974), 1377, 1389
health anxiety 5301
health care costs 82
components of *114*, 112–13
consequences 115
cost-control policies 114, *114*
as policy issue 112
reasons for interest 112
health care spending
explanations of 113
as share of GDP *113*
health education 110
health information 109
health, economic benefits 74
health-adjusted life years (HALYs) 55
healthcare provision 54
health maximization vs health equity 58
innovation 60
reasonableness in 57
accountability 57
societal investment 61
spending 61–2
see also medicines
hearing disorders 4865
clinical examination 4867, *4867*
investigations 4867, *4867–8*
management 4868
pathophysiology 4866, *4866–7*
tinnitus 4869
heart disease
amyloid 2785
autoimmune rheumatic disorders 2783, *2783–4*
antiphospholipid syndrome 2783
polymyositis and dermatomyositis 2784
rheumatoid arthritis 2784
seronegative arthropathies 2784
systemic lupus erythematosus 2783
systemic sclerosis 2783
clinical investigation 2643
catheterization and angiography 2678
ECG 2643
echocardiography 2662
imaging techniques 2671
clinical presentation 2628
chest pain, breathlessness and fatigue 2628
syncope and palpitations 2636
clinical trials 43, *43*
congenital *see* congenital heart disease
endocrine disorders 2786
diabetes 2786
hyperthyroidism 2786
hypothyroidism 2787
haematological changes 4560
HIV/AIDS 2822, *2822*
assessment 2825
cardiac tumours 2823
coronary artery disease 2824
endocardial disease 2823
heart muscle 2823
pericardium 2822
pulmonary hypertension 2823, *2824*
right ventricular dysfunction 2823, *2824*
sudden death 2824
inherited metabolic disorders 2787
haemochromatosis 2787
lysosomal diseases 2787
leptospirosis 876
malaria 1063
myocarditis *276*, 2758
myopathies *see* cardiomyopathy
neuromuscular disorders 2787, *2788*
pregnancy 2108
antenatal care 2110
aortopathy 2112, *2112*
arrhythmias 2115
cardiac surgery 2110
cardiomyopathy 2110, *2111*
congenital 2113, *2871*, *2871*
contraception 2115
investigations 2109

ischaemic heart disease 2111
labour and delivery 2110
management 2110
prepregnancy assessment 2109
prosthetic valves 2114, *2114*
pulmonary hypertension 2112
risk stratification 2109, *2110*
small left-to-right shunts 2113
valvular lesions 2113
relapsing fever *869*
sarcoid 2786, *2786*
vasculitides 2784
Behçet's disease 2785
giant cell arteritis 2785
Kawasaki's disease 2785
microscopic polyangiitis 2785
polyarteritis nodosa 2785
Takayasu's arteritis 2784, *2784*
Wegener's granulomatosis *2783*, 2785
see also individual conditions
heart failure 2618, 2717
acute 2719
aetiology 2719, *2720*
clinical features 2717
communication with patient/carer 2728, *2728*
comorbidity 2725
anaemia 2726
angina 2725
asthma/chronic airways disease 2725
atrial fibrillation 2725
gout 2726
renal dysfunction 2725
diabetes mellitus 2044
diagnosis 2718, *2718–19*
Doppler echocardiography 2719
ECG 2718, *2719*
disease monitoring 2728, *2728*
end of life issues 2729
management 2717, 2720
drug therapy 2721
drugs to avoid 2725
implantable cardioverter defibrillator 2727
implantable pacemakers 2726, *2726*
left ventricular assist devices 2727
lifestyle measures 2720
noninvasive ventilation 2728
revascularization 2727
transplantation 2727
ultrafiltration 2728
valve replacement/repair 2727
nonsystolic 2726
Paget's disease 3742
prognosis 2719, *2720*
rheumatic fever 2804
heart murmurs
Austin-Flint 2752
Graham-Steell 2753
heart muscle disease in HIV/AIDS 2823, *2822, 2824*
heart rate 2624, 2646
heart sounds 2620
heart transplantation *see* cardiac transplantation
heart
blood flow 2625
cardiac cycle 2619, *2619*
clinical physiology 2168
exercise response 2626
training effects 2627
hypertensive damage 3035, *3036*
cardiac arrhythmias 3036
myocardial ischaemia 3036
regression of left ventricular hypertrophy 3036
innervation 2625
autonomic efferent 2626
isomerism *2845*
myocardial mechanics 2621, *2622*
in respiratory disease 3187
univentricular 2868
see also cardiac; myocardial
heartburn 2206
heart-lung transplantation, pulmonary arterial hypertension 2988
heat shock proteins 183
heat stroke 5379
presentation 5507
prevention *5380*
heat-related illness 1393
acclimatization 1394
drug-induced 1395
heat exhaustion 1394
heat stroke 1394
susceptibility to 1394
thermoregulation 1393
heavy-chain diseases 4353
Heberden's nodes 3632
Hedgehog pathway 169, *172, 351, 352*
hedonism 17
Heimlich manoeuvre 3256, *3257*
Heinz bodies *4195*
Helcococcus spp. *962*
Helicobacter heilmannii, and peptic ulcer disease 2308
Helicobacter pylori 306, 314, 2227, 2230
and peptic ulcer disease 2237, *2306, 2307*
treatment 2312
urea breath test *2230*
see also peptic ulcer disease
Helicobacter spp. *962*
HELLP syndrome 2096, 2128, 2178, 3862
clinical features *2129–30*
complications *2129*
differential diagnosis *2131*
laboratory variables *2130*
helmet cells *4195*
helminthic infections
HIV-related 648
ocular 5247
see also individual species
Heloderma suspectum (Gila monster) *1343*
hemiballism 4896
hemicrania continua 4922
hemidesosomes 4593
hemifacial spasm 4899, 5037
Hemiscorpius lepturus 1352
hemispheric dominance 4787
hemithorax
increased transradiency 3211, *3212*
opacification of 3211
hemlock 1363, *1363*
Henderson-Paterson molluscum bodies 658
Hendra virus 525
Henoch-Schönlein purpura *222, 3650, 4033, 4629*
GI tract involvement 2422
pregnancy 2162
pulmonary involvement *3396*
renal involvement 3974, *3974*, 4037
treatment 3976, 4041
heparan sulphate 2601
heparin cofactor II *4196*
heparin
acute coronary syndromes 2919
adverse effects, in pregnancy *2188*
in breast milk *2189*
complications of treatment 3019
effects on renin-angiotensin-aldosterone system 3843
haemodialysis 3935
low molecular weight *see* low molecular weight heparin
pregnancy 2108, 2117
in renal failure 4180
venous thromboembolism 3018
heparin-induced thrombocytopenia *4542*, 4512, 4542
hepatic adenoma 2520, *2521–2*
hepatic amoebiasis 1038, *1039*
complications 1039, *1040*
differential diagnosis 1039, *1040*
hepatic artery aneurysm 2586
hepatic coma 5151
hepatic encephalopathy 2494
chronic 5152
clinical features 2495, *2495–6*
diagnosis 2499
management 2502, *2502*
acute illness 2502
chronic illness 2502
hepatic epithelioid haemangioendothelioma 2520
hepatic granulomas 2523
aetiology 2513, 2517
clinical presentation 2517
infectious causes 2517
hepatitis C 2525
histoplasmosis 2518
HIV/AIDS 2518
leprosy 2518
Q fever 2518
schistosomiasis 2518
tuberculosis 2518
investigation and management 2520
noninfective causes 2519
chronic granulomatous disease of childhood 2526
Crohn's disease 2523
drugs and chemicals 2526, *2526*
hepatic granulomatous disease 2526
neoplasia 2526
primary biliary cirrhosis 2520
sarcoidosis 2519
pathogenesis 2513
hepatic stellate cells 2439
hepatitides 4524
hepatitis A *611*, 610, 2452
features of 2453
vaccines *466*, 468
hepatitis B *611*, 610, 612, 2452
antenatal screening *102*
and cancer *306*
chronic 613, *2456, 2457*
grading *2457*
treatment 2457
features of 2453
genome organization 612, *612*
HIV coinfection 635
host immune response and pathogenesis 613
immunization *91*
nephropathy 4074
pregnancy 2168
recurrence post-transplantation 2511
renal toxicity 3858, *4086*
vaccines *466*, 468
viral replication 612, *613*
hepatitis D 610, *611*, 614, 2452
chronic 2459
features of 2454
host immune response and pathogenesis 614
hepatitis E *611*, 614, 2452
features of 2454
hepatitis G 615
hepatitis *611, 482, 1609, 2452, 2453*
acute cholestatic, drug-induced *2532*, 2532
alcoholic
clinical features 2477
treatment 2478
autoimmune 3560, *276*
aetiology 2460
associated conditions *2461*, 2462
clinical manifestations 2461, *2461*
diagostic criteria 2461
differential diagnosis 2461
epidemiology 2461
histology 2460, *2461*
immunopathogenesis 2460, *2461*
investigations 2461
liver transplantation 2507
natural history 2462
recurrence post-transplantation 2511
subtypes 2462, *2462*
treatment 2462
clinical associations
arthralgia 3711
Q fever 925
clinical examination 2454
clinical outcome 2453
differential diagnosis 2454
drug-induced *2529, 2528, 2531*
granulomatous, drug-induced 2535, *2535*
laboratory investigations 2454, *2455–6*
liver transplantation 2459, 2463, 2507
management 2455
nonalcoholic steatotic, drug-induced 2535
occupational *1385*
in pregnancy 2130, *2131*
prevention 2456
prognosis 2463
see also various types
hepatitis C 615, *611*, 2452
aetiology and genetics 616
areas of uncertainty 619
and cancer *306*
chronic 2458, *2459*
treatment 2459
clinical features 617
acute infection 617, *618*
chronic infection 617

hepatic granuloma 2525
renal toxicity *4086*
cryoglobulinaemia 3858
diagnosis 618
pretreatment evaluation 619
RNA testing 618
serology 618
epidemiology 617
features of 2454
future developments 619
historical perspective 616
HIV coinfection 635
nephropathy 4075
pathogenesis/pathology 616
postexposure prophylaxis 617
pregnancy 2169
prevention 617, 2459
prognosis 618
recurrence post-transplantation 2511
treatment 619
hepatoblastoma 2517
hepatocellular carcinoma 2513
aetiology and prevention 2513
clinical presentation 2514
epidemiology 2513
fibrolamellar 2517
investigations 2514, *2515*
liver biopsy 2515, *2516*
liver imaging 2515, *2516*
serum markers 2514
surveillance 2516
pathogenesis 2514
prognosis 2517
treatment 2516
ablative therapies 2517
chemotherapy 2517
liver transplantation 2507, 2516
surgical resection 2516
transarterial chemoembolization 2517
hepatocellular failure 2493
acute 2494
aetiology 2494
course and prognosis 2500
management 2503
aetiology 2494
chronic 2494
aetiology 2495
course and prognosis 2501
clinical features 2495, *2495*
abnormal protein metabolism 2499
acid-base and electrolyte changes 2497
ascites 2496
cardiovascular changes 2497
cerebral oedema and raised intracranial pressure 2497
endocrine changes 2499, *2499*
fatigue 2499
foetor hepaticus 2497
haemorrhagic diathesis 2496
hepatocellular jaundice 2496
hepatopulmonary syndrome 2498
hepatorenal syndrome 2497
hypoglycaemia 2497
portopulmonary hypertension 2498
skin changes 2498, *2498–9*
susceptibility to infection 2497
course and prognosis 2500
diagnosis 2499
ascites 2500
haaemorrhagic diathesis 2500
hepatocellular jaundice 2500
fulminant 2494
course of *2505*
management 2503
future developments 2504
hepatic encephalopathy 2494
clinical features 2495, *2495–6*
diagnosis 2499
management 2502, *2502*
management 2501
pathology 2500
prevention 2495
hepatocyte growth factor 355
hepatocytes *2438*
hepatoerythropoietic porphyria 1637
hepatopathy
congestive 2585
ischaemic 2586
hepatopulmonary syndrome 2498, 3472
management 2504
hepatorenal syndrome 2490, 2497, 3902
management 2504
hepatotoxicity, drug-induced, diferential diagnosis *2131*
hepatotoxins
occupational *1385*
plant-derived *1362*, 1365
hepcidin 4388
HER2, 1933
herbalism 65
Herbaspirillum spp. *962*
Herbert's pits 941
hereditary bulbar palsy of infancy and childhood 5073
hereditary cerebral amyloid angiopathy 1770
hereditary endotheliopathy with retinopathy, nephropathy, and stroke 5110
hereditary hyperferritinaemia cataract syndrome 1686
hereditary nonpolyposis colorectal cancer (HNPCC) syndrome 315, *363*
hereditary periodic fever syndromes 1760
cryopyrin-associated 1764
differential diagnosis 1765, *1765*
familial Mediterranean fever 1760, 3708, *238*, *3709–10*
future developments 1765
hyper-IgD syndrome 1763
prognosis 1765
TRAPS 1763
hereditary spastic paraplegia 5074, 5125, *5125–6*
Hermansky-Pudlak syndrome 1717, 1698
hypopigmentation 4663
hermaphroditism 1967
hernia
hiatus *see* hiatus hernia
paraumbilical 2490
heroin, renal toxicity *3860*
herpangina 2264
coxsackievirus 531, *531*
herpes gestationis 2150, *2152*, 2152
herpes gladiatorum 485
herpes labialis 2263
aetiology 2263
clinical features 2263, *2263*
course and prognosis 2264
diagnosis 2264
pathology 2263
treatment 2264
herpes simplex encephalitis 486, 5002
clinical features 5003, *5004*
herpes simplex virus 482–3
aetiology 484
clinical features 484
cutaneous infectons 485, *489*
encephalitis 486
genital herpes 486, *486*
gingivostomatitis 485, *485*, 2262
immunosuppressed patients 487
keratitis *485*, 486
meningitis 487
neonatal infection and pregnancy 487
congenital 5146
epidemiology 484
genital *see* genital herpes
historical background 483
immunosuppressed patients 3957
infective oesophagitis *2293*
laboratory diagnosis 487
pathogenesis 484
pathology 487
pregnancy 2168
prevention and control 488
treatment 487
type 1 *484*
type 2 *484*
herpes zoster 490, *490–1*
abdominal pain 2236
autonomic 491
motor 491
ophthalmic 490, *491*, 5036
oral 2264, *2264*
pregnancy 2168
treatment 493
varicelliformis *492*
herpesvirus infections, childhood, severe *238*
herpesviruses 482, *483*, *484*
see also individual viruses
herpetic whitlow 485
Hers' disease *1598*, 1599
differential diagnosis *1600*
heterochromatin variants 147
heterologous immunity 289
heterophyasis 1223, *1223*
Heterophyes heterophyes 1222
Heterophyes katsuradai 1222
Heterophyes nocens 1222
Heterophyopsis continua 1222
heteroplasmy 140, 5222
transmission of 5222
heterotopia 5141
heterozygosity 138
hexachlorobenzene, porphyria *1637*
hexamethylene diisocyanate *3436*
hexokinase deficiency 4471
hexosaminidase deficiency 5073
hiatus hernia
rolling or para-oesophageal 2301
sliding 2301
hidradenitis suppurativa 4676
hierarchy of evidence 22
high density lipoprotein (HDL) 1656, *1753*
reference values *5444*
Highlands J virus *558*
high-molecular weight kininogen 4493
high-pressure nervous syndrome 1419
Hill, Bradford 23
Himasthia muehlensi 1220
hip
arthritis *3557*
osteoarthritis *3629*, *3633*
pain *3248*
rheumatoid arthritis 3588
Hippoboscidae *1226*
Hippocrates 9, *10*, 27
Hirschsprung's disease 140, 2402
clinical features 2402
diagnosis 2402, *2403*
gut peptides 2322
management 2403
hirsutism 1902
causes 1911, *1911*
investigation and diagnosis 1912, *1912*
management 1912
polycystic ovary syndrome 1910
hirudin 1357
acute coronary syndromes 2920
in renal failure 4180
His bundle 2609, 2619
histamine challenge 3293
histamine 3111
histamine$_2$-antagonists
in breast milk *2189*
in renal failure 4176
histamine-like syndrome 1346
histidinuria *4148*
histiocytoses 4361, *4361*
aetiology and epidemiology 4361
classification 4362
clinical features 4363
management 4365
Histoplasma capsulatum
HIV-associated infection *3247*
pneumonia 3237
Histoplasma spp., osteomyelitis *3789*
histoplasmosis 1009
African 1011, *1009*, *1011*
classic/small-form 1009, *1009*
aetiology 1009
clinical features 1010, *1010–11*
epidemiology 1009
and hepatic granuloma 2518
HIV encephalopathy 631
HIV/AIDS 620, *244*, 432
aetiology 2264
antenatal screening *102*
cellular biology 620, 623
HIV receptors and cellular tropism 624
viral replication cycle 623, *623–4*
child mortality *75*
children 641
clinical associations
bacillary angiomatosis 634
chancroid 764
cytomegalovirus 495, *495*
hepatitis B virus 635
hepatitis C virus 635
musculoskeletal disease 3712
mycoplasmal infections 958
Pseudomonas aeruginosa 737
syphilis 895
tropical disease 647

clinical features 621, 625, 2265
  advanced disease 647
  developing world 646
  early infection 626, *626*, 646
  gastrointestinal 2250, *2251*
  liver damage 2518, 2544
  nonprogression 627
  ocular 5247, *5248*
  primary infection 625, *625*
  symptomatic disease 626, *626*, 646, 647
cobalamin deficiency 4411
cognitive impairment 5278
complications 627, *637*
  bacterial pneumonia 628, 3248
  dermatological 634, 1001
  gastrointestinal 629
  haematological 634
  HIV-associated nephropathy 3858, 635, *4086*, 4090
  immune restoration syndromes 3252
  Mycobacterium avium complex 629
  nervous system 630, 1020
  ocular 631
  oesophageal candidiasis 629
  Pneumocystis jirovecii pneumonia 627, *627–8*
  respiratory disease *3247–8*, 3246
  risk factors 3247
  tuberculosis 628, 647, 3250
counselling and testing *649*
developing world 644
diagnosis 621, 625
  developing world 648
differential diagosis 2267
epidemiology 622, *622*
  developing world 645
genetics *143*
heart disease 2822, *2822*, 2823
  assessment 2825
  cardiac tumours 2823
  endocardial disease 2823
  heart muscle 2823
  pericardium 2822
  pulmonary hypertension 2823, *2824*
  right ventricular dysfunction 2823, *2824*
  sudden death 2824
hormonal abnormalities *2066*
immunosuppressed patients 3957
interactions with STIs 1248, *1248*
management 621, *447*, 635
  antiretroviral therapy 636
  developing world *649*, 649
  drug resistance 639
  drug toxicity/interactions 639, *640*
  patient adherence 638
  salvage therapy 639
mortality rate *76*
neoplasms *306*, 632
  Kaposi's sarcoma 307, *322*, *632*, *633*, *3247*, *3251*, *3251*
  lung cancer 3252
  lymphoma 506, 633, 3251
neurological complications 5017
  clinical approach 5017
  opportunistic infections 5018, *5017–20*
  opportunistic tumours 5021
neuropathy 631, 5022, *5023*, 5091
opportunistic infections *642*, 641
oral 2264, *2265*, *2267*
pathology 2264
pregnancy 2166
prevention 621, 642
  blood products 643, 646
  developing world 645, 649
  injecting drug use 643, 646
  mother-to-child transmission 643, *646*, 646
  occupational exposure 643
  sexual transmission 642, 645
prognosis 621
renal involvement 4074
reproductive effects *1917*
role of apoptosis in 187
screening 621
staging 648, *648*
and syphilis 2828
transmission 620
vaccines 643
viral encephalitis *4781*, 4781
see also immunocompromised host
HIV-associated nephropathy 3858, 635, *4086*, 4090
HIV-dementia complex 5021, *5022*
HLA DQα 5371
HLA-B27 *3604*, *3605*
HMG co-A reductase, adverse effects, hepatotoxicity *2529*
Hodgkin's lymphoma 329, 506, 4322
  age distribution *329*
  clinical features 4323
    multiorgan involvement *3408*
  hepatic involvement 2541
  incidence and epidemiology 4323, *4323*
  pathology 4323, *4323*
  Pel-Ebstein fever 382
  prognostic factors 4324
  renal involvement 4063
  treatment *4320*
    complications 4325
    primary *4321*, 4324
    relapse 4325
Hoek formula 3871
Holdemania spp. *962*
Holmes-Adie syndrome 5034
holocarboxylase synthetase deficiency *1566*, 1579
holoprosencephaly 5138, *5139*
Holt-Oram syndrome 2837, *2837*
homeopathy 65, 68
  description 68
  efficacy 68
  mode of action 68
  safety 4398
homocysteine disorders, psychiatric signs *1720*
homocysteine
  and coronary heart disease 2890
  metabolism 1494
homocystinuria 1593, 3720, *1566*, *1593*, *3721*, 3754
  cardiac involvement *2840*
  clinical features 1593, *3731*, 3754
  diagnosis 1593
  pathophysiology 3754
  treatment and outcome 1593
homosexuality 1250–1
homovanillic acid
  reference values *5441*, *5446*
    children *5438*
homozygosity 138
hookworm 1163, 1165
  clinical features 1165
  diagnosis 1165
  epidemiology 1165
  haematological changes 4553
  immune modulation 1166
  nonhuman 1163, 1166
    A. caninum-associated gastroenteritis 1166
    cutaneous larva migrans 1166, *1167*
    Oesophagostomum spp. 1167, *1167*
    Trichostrongylus spp. 1167
  pathogenesis and life cycle 1165
  treatment, prevention and control 1166, *1166*
Hoover's sign 3327
hops, drug interactions *69*
hormone binding proteins 1790
hormone replacement therapy 307, 2196
  adverse effects/risks 2197
    breast cancer 2197
  benefits 2196
    cardiovascular disease 2196, *2197*
    colorectal cancer 2197
    osteoporosis 2196
    vasomotor symptoms 2196
  and breast cancer development 50, 307
  contraindication in porphyria 1641
  osteoporosis *3799*, 3800
  STEMI 2932
  therapeutic regimens 2197, *2198*
hormone response element 1788
hormone-directed cancer therapy 399
hormones 1787
  actions 1791, *1791*
  anterior pituitary gland 1805
  control of production 1789, *1789*
  development of endocrine glands 1788, *1788*
  ectopic secretion 2059–60
    ACTH secretion 2062, *2063*
    aldosterone 2065
    calciotropic hormones 2061
    calcitonin 2065
    chemical structure 2060
    definition 2060
    GHRH and GH 2065
    hCG secretion 2064, *2064*
    human placental lactogen 2065
    insulin-like growth factors 2064
    pathogenesis 2061
    prevalence 2060
    prolactin 2065
    renin 2065
    syndrome of inappropriate antidiuresis 2062, *2062*
    treatment 2061
  functions of 1790, *1791*
  gastrointestinal 2316, *2317*
    bombesin 2319
    cholecystokinin 2318
    chromogranin-derived peptides 2320
    enteroglucagon 2319
    gastrin 2317
    ghrelin 2319
    glucagon-like peptide 1, 2319
    glucagon-like peptide 2, 2319
    glucose-dependent insulinotropic peptide 2318
    motilin 2319
    neuropeptide Y 2319
    neurotensin 2320
    obestatin 2319
    opioids 2319
    oxyntomodulin 2319
    peptide tyrosine tyrosine 2319
    secretin 2318
    somatostatin 2320, *2320*
    tachykinins 2320
    vasoactive intestinal peptide 2318, *2318*
  and intermediary metabolism *1481*
  nature of 1788
  nonendocrine diseases 2059, 2066, *2066–7*
    adrenal 2066
    calcium 2067
    gonads 2066
    gynaecomastia 2066
    hypothalamopituitary function 2066
    thyroid 2066
  reference values *5441*
  synthesis, processing and secretion 1788, *1788*
  see also individual hormones
Horner's syndrome 5034
  lung cancer 3519
hornet stings 1349
  renal toxicity 4092
horse chestnut 68
  drug interactions *69*
hot tub dermatitis 736
house dust mites, allergic rhinitis 3278
household products, poisoning by 1316
Howell-Jolly bodies *4195*
HPV *see* human papillomavirus
HRT *see* hormone replacement therapy
HSV *see* herpes simplex virus
HTLV *see* human T-lymphotrophic virus
HTLV-associated infective dermatitis 652, *652*
HTLV-associated myelopathy 651
Hugues-Stovin syndrome 2785
human bocavirus 660
human chorionic gonadotrophin (hCG)
  ectopic secretion 2064, *2064*
  reference values *5441–2*
Human Genome Project 15, 138, 149, 359, 362
human genome 138, 136
  sequencing 136
human growth hormone, performance enhancement 5383
human herpesvirus 1 *see* herpes simplex virus
human herpesvirus 2 *see* herpes simplex virus
human herpesvirus 3 *see* varicella zoster virus
human herpesvirus *4484*
  and cancer *306*

human herpesvirus 5484
human herpesvirus 6 484, 497
  immunosuppressed patients 498
  pregnancy 2171
human herpesvirus 7 483, 484, 498
human herpesvirus 8 483, 484, 498
  aetiology 499
  and cancer 306
  clinical features 499
  epidemiology 499
  laboratory diagnosis 499
  pathogenesis 499
  pathology 499
  prevention and control 500
  treatment 499
human metapneumovirus 474, 479
human papillomavirus 600–1, 601, 1247
  clinical associations 601–2
    anogenital wards 602
    cancer 306, 357, 601, 604, 3962
    cervical cancer 601, 603, 604
    epidermodysplasia verruciformis 605
    respiratory papillomatosis 603
  immunosuppressed patients 3957
  open reading frames 601
  pregnancy 2171
  skin 4675
human parechovirus 660
human placental lactogen, ectopic secretion 2065
human polyomavirus 600, 605
  clinical associations 605
    bone marrow transplant-associated haemorrhagic cystitis 605
    progressive multifocal leukoencephalopathy 606, 606
    renal transplant-associated nephropathy 605, 606
    tumours 607
  immunosuppressed patients 3957
human T-cell leukaemia virus type 1306
human T-lymphotrophic virus 187
human T-lymphotropic virus 650
  diagnosis 651
  epidemiology 650
  future developments 653
  historical perspective 650
  HTLV-1 651, 651
  HTLV-2 651, 653
  pathogenesis 650
  prevention 651
HUMARA gene 4210
humectants 4732, 4732
Humicola fuscoatra 3436
humidifier lung 3435
humoral immune response 287
Hunter's syndrome 1553, 3756
  cardiac involvement 2840
Huntington's disease 4807, 142, 148, 4894, 5106
  aetiology 4894
  diagnosis 4895
  genetic testing 4895
  symptoms 4895
  treatment 4895
Huntington's disease-like syndromes 5112
Huntington's disease-like 2, 5114
Huriez disease 4600
Hurler syndrome 1698, 1553, 2766, 3756
Hurler-Scheie synddrome 1698
hurricanes 1439
Hürthle cell carcinoma 1846
Hürthle cells 1835
Hyalomma spp. 1228
hyaluronan 3550, 3551
hyaluronic acid, osteoarthritis 3635
hyaluronidase deficiency 1698
hycanthone, adverse effects, hepatotoxicity 2529
hydralazine
  adverse effects, hepatotoxicity 2529, 2532–3, 2535
  heart failure 2724
  hypertension 3052
  hypertensive emergencies 3080
hydranencephaly 5145
hydrocephalus 5145, 5145
  communicating 4781
  imaging 4778, 4781
  normal-pressure 4807
hydrochlorothiazide, calcium stone prevention 4130
hydrocortisone 17-butyrate 2151
hydrocortisone acetate 4731
hydrocortisone 2151, 4731
  aphthous ulcers 2272
  congenital adrenal hyperplasia 1892
  hypoadrenalism 1884
hydrogen breath test 2227
hydrogen fluoride/hydrofluoric acid poisoning 1312
hydrogen ions 5515
hydrogen sulphide poisoning 1312
  antidote 1274
hydromorphone, palliative care 5423
hydronephrosis, in pregnancy 2105
Hydrophis semperi 1327
hydroureter, acute 2105
Hydrous piceus 1229
hydroxocobalamin 1274
β-hydroxy-β-methylbutyrate 5385
hydroxyapatite 3719
hydroxycarbamide, adverse effects, hepatotoxicity 2529
hydroxychloroquine
  pregnancy 2158
  rheumatoid arthritis 3595
  sarcoidosis 3411
  Sjögren's syndrome 3691
hydroxyindole acetic acid, reference values 5446
21-hydroxylase deficiency 1891
17α-hydroxylase deficiency 1898
4-hydroxyphenylpyruvate dioxygenase deficiency 1586
17-hydroxyprogesterone, reference values 5441
hydroxyproline 3729, 3733
3β-hydroxysteroid dehydrogenase deficiency 1898
11β-hydroxysteroid dehydrogenase type 2, abnormalities of 1887, 1888
5-hydroxytryptamine, metabolism 2323
hydroxyurea 398
  skin disorders 4738
hygiene hypothesis 3279
hygiene, insects and 1236
Hymenolepsis diminuta 1190
Hymenolepsis nana 1189, 1190, 1192
hymenoptera stings 1349, 1349, 3108
  clinical features 1350
  epidemiology 1349
  prevention 1349
  treatment 1350
hymenoptera venom allergy 263
hyoscine 5423
hyoscyamine, poisoning 1361
hyperaldosteronism, primary see Conn's syndrome
hyperammonaemia 1568
hyperamylasaemia 2559, 2559
hyperandrogenism in women
  androgen production 1911
  androgen-dependent hair growth 1911
  polycystic ovary syndrome see polycystic ovary syndrome
hyperbaric oxygen, gas gangrene 808
hyperbilirubinaemia
  conjugated 2447, 2447
  unconjugated 2446–7
    familial 2447
  see also jaundice
hypercalcaemia 384, 1851, 1854, 2067, 3730, 3733, 3745
  cancer 383, 3522
  causes 1856, 3745
  CKD 3922
  clinical features 1854, 1856
  CNS complications 5154
  diseases causing 1851, 1857
    endocrine causes 1862
    granulomatous disorders 1861
    hyperparathyroidism 1857, 1858
    malignancy 1861
  drug-induced 1862
  familial benign 1855, 1862
  familial hypocalciuric 3745, 4145
  genetics 1855
  investigations 1854, 1857
  management 1856
  paraneoplastic 2061
  post-transplant 3964
  presentation 5481
  renal effects 4019
hypercalciuria
  hypocalcaemic 4128
  idiopathic 4127, 4130
    nephrolithiasis 4101
hypercapnia 1419, 3469, 3469
  scoliosis 3507
hypercatabolic state 2490
hypercholesterolaemia 1660
  common/polygenic 1662, 1662–3
    metabolic defect 1663
  familial 1660
    drug therapy 1669
    heterozygous 1660
    homozygous 1661
    metabolic defect 1661
  nephrotic syndrome 3980
hypercoagulable disease 4529
  antithrombin III deficiency 4529
  factor V Leiden and prothrombin 20210 mutation 4530
  proteins C and S deficiency 4530
  vitamin K epoxide reductase complex, subunit 1 4530
hyperekplexia 166, 162, 4900
hyperemesis gravidarum 2089, 2126
  differential diagnosis 2131
  hormonal abnormalities 2066
hypereosinophilic syndromes 3431, 4359
  aetiology 4359
  clinical features 4359
  definition 4359
  diagnosis 4360
  treatment 4360
hyperfibrinolysis 4506
hypergammaglobulinemia, sarcoidosis 3409
hyperglycaemia
  and complications of diabetes 2030
  stress-induced 2043
  tissue damage 2031
    abnormal microvascular blood flow 2032
    glycation of proteins/macromolecules 2032
    overactivity of polyol pathway 2032
    protein kinase C activation 2032
  type 1 diabetes 2031, 2031
  type 2 diabetes 2031, 2032
  see also diabetes mellitus
hyperglycinaemia
  nonketotic 1591, 1566, 1591
    psychiatric signs 1720
hyperhidrosis 4677, 4677, 5068
hyper-IgD syndrome 238, 1761, 1763
  clinical features 1763
  clinical investigation 1764
  epidemiology 1763
  genetics 1763
  pathology 1763
  treatment 1764
hyper-IgE syndrome 238, 256
hyper-IgM syndrome 238, 245, 2250
  X-linked 238
hyperimmunoglobulin D syndrome 3709
hyperinflation 3324, 3324–5
hyperinsulinaemia, congenital 167, 168
hyperinsulinism 2052
  chemical pathology 2053
  diagnosis 2053
  insulinoma 2052
  treatment 2054
hyperkalaemia 3832, 3840
  causes 3840, 3841
    abnormal external potassium balance 3842
    abnormal internal potassium balance 3844
    acidosis 3844
    acute renal trauma 3890, 3891
    exercise 3844
    mineralocorticoid deficiency 3842
    renal transport abnormalities 3843
  clinical features 3840
    periodic paralysis 164, 166, 3844, 5219
  CNS complications 5155
  distal tubule renal acidosis 4137
  drug overdose 5505
  post-transplant 3964

presentation 5479
treatment 3840, *3891*
hyperkalaemic periodic paralysis 164, 166, 3844
hyperleucocytosis 4237
hyperlipidaemia
and arthralgia 3711
dialysis patients 3940
drug therapy 1669
post-transplant 2731
hyperlipoproteinaemia 1652, *1658, 1658*
and acute pancreatitis 2559
Fredrickson/WHO classification 1660, *1660*
genetics *139*
management 1653, 1667
dietary 1668, *1668*
primary 1660
with hypercholesterolaemia *see* hypercholesterolaemia
with hypertriglyceridaemia 1664
type IIB 1664
type III 1663, 1669
secondary 1666, *1666*
diabetes mellitus 1666
drug-induced 1667
hyperuricaemia 1667
liver disease 1667
obesity 1667
renal disease 1667
thyroid failure 1667
hyperlysinaemia *1566*, 1575
hypermagnesaemia, CNS complications 5155
hypernatraemia 3818, 3826
clinical features 3827
CNS complications 5154
diagnosis 3827, *3827*
pathogenesis 3826, *3826*
treatment 3827, *3828*
hyperornithinaemia 1577
hyperornithinaemia-hyperammonaemia-homocitrullinuria (HHH) syndrome *1566*, 1568
hyperosmolar nonketotic state (HONK) 2027
hyperoxaluria 4127, *4128*
dietary 4127
enteric 4127
nephrolithiasis *4101*
primary 4128
renal effects 4018
hyperoxalurias 1730
aetiology and genetics 1731, *1731–3*
clinical features 1732, *1734*
differential diagnosis 1733
epidemiology 1732
future developments 1736
historical perspectives 1731
pathogenesis/pathology 1731, *1731–3*
prenatal diagnosis 1734
treatment 1734, *1735*
type 1 *1551–2*, 1730
type 2, 1730
hyperparathyroidism 1857
and acute pancreatitis 2559
clinical features
bone disease *3731*
calcium stones 4127
hypercalcaemia *3745*
myopathy 5218
familial isolated 1860
familial primary 1860
management 3923
neonatal *1855*, 1862, *3721*
primary 1857, *1859*
secondary 3745, 3920
prophylaxis *3923*
severe neonatal *4145*
sporadic *1855*
uraemic 1859
hyperparathyroidism–jaw tumour syndrome *1855*, 1860–1
hyperphosphataemia
acute renal trauma 3890
CKD 3918
hyperphosphataemic familial tumoral calcinosis 4143, *4143*
hyperpigmentation *see* pigmentation disorders
hyperpipecolic acidaemia *1552*
hyperpolarizing factor 2599
hyperprolactinaemia 1907
in men 1916
in polycystic ovary syndrome 1909
hyperprolinaemia type II *1566*, 1590
hypersensitivity reactions *4725*
delayed-type 287
type I (anaphylaxis) 233, 259, *259,* 1466, *4725*, 4726
type II (cytotoxic) 233, 1466, *4725*, 4726
type III (immune-complex) 233, 1466, *4725*, 4726
type IV (cell-mediated) 233, 1466, *4725*, 4726
hypersomnia 4830, *4830*
hypersplenism 4337, 4515
hypertension 3023
accelerated-phase 3900
assessment 3040
cardiovascular risk reduction 3055
chronic pulmonary thromboembolic 3017
clinical presentation 3040
epistaxis 3040
headache 3040
male impotence 3040
nocturia 3040
target organ symptoms 3040
definitions of 3024
development of 3031
endothelium 3032
large arteries 3032
natriuretic peptides 3034
oxidative stress 3032
renal factors 3031
renin-angiotensin-aldosterone system 3032, *3033*
small arteries 3031
sympathetic nervous system 3033, *3034*
diabetes mellitus 2041
causes 2042
impact of 2042
management 2042
treatment targets 2042
diagnostic thresholds *3041*
dialysis patients 3939
early origins 3031
epidemiology 3025
cardiovascular morbidity and mortality 3026, *3027–8*
global prevalence 3025, *3026*
lifetime risk 3025, *3026*
systolic blood pressure as main risk factor 3026, *3028*
essential *see* essential hypertension
fetal and postnatal effects 2900, *2900*
genetics 3029, *3029*
intracranial 4972
see also intracranial pressure, raised
malignant 3076, *3076*
clinical features 3077
complications 3077, *3077–8*
epidemiology 3076
investigation 3077
management 3078, *3079–80*
presentation 5465
prognosis 3079, *3081*
management 3046
follow-up 3055
initial *3041–2,* 3046, *3046–7*
lifestyle advice 3047, *3047–8*
pharmacological 3049, *3050*
treatment strategy 3053, *3053–4*
treatment targets 3047
withdrawal of therapy 3055
masked 3042
Mendelian disorders causing 3071, *3071*
genetic defects 3073, *3073*
glucocorticoid-remediable aldosteronism 3071, *3072*
Gordon's syndrome 3073
Liddle's syndrome 3073
syndrome of apparent mineralocorticoid excess 3072
metabolic syndrome 3034
mineralocorticoid, differential diagnosis 1884, *1885*
mortality rate *76*
nutrition-related 1519
pathogenesis and pathophysiology 3027
environment and lifestyle 3028
genetic factors 3028, *3029*
physical examination 3041
blood pressure measurement 3041, *3041*
fundal examination 3042, *3042–4*
poisoned patients 1277
post-transplant 3963, *3963*
pregnancy 2093
causes and terminology 2094, *2094*
eclampsia 2100
long-term sequelae 2101
pre-eclampsia *see* pre-eclampsia
pre-existing 2100
puerperium 2101, *2101*
secondary 2101
treatment 2100
resistant 3054, *3054*
routine examination 3044, *3045*
cardiovascular disease risk 3045
secondary 3057, *3060*
age-related prevalence 3058, *3059*
clinical approach 3059
coarctation of aorta 3061
Conn's syndrome 3062
endocrine causes 3070
phaeochromocytoma 3066
renal hypertension 3059
renovascular hypertension 3059
specialist referral 3055, *3055*
specific patient groups 3055
subtypes 3024, *3024–5*
target organ damage 3034
brain 3036
evolution of 3037, *3038*
eye 3037
heart 3035
kidney 3037
vascular structural changes and atherosclerosis 3035
white coat (office) 3042
hypertensive emergencies 3074, *3075*
acute coronary syndromes 3081
encephalopathy 3037, 3079
left ventricular failure 3079
malignant hypertension 3076, *3076*
pathophysiology 3075, *3076*
hypertensive phenotype 3034
hypertensive retinopathy *3042–3, 3077*, 3077, *5238*
grading *5238*
histopathology 5238
retinal changes 5238
hyperthecosis 1911
hyperthermia
habitual 426
malignant 164, 1474, 5220
poisoned patients 1277
treatment 3103
hyperthyroidism
cardiac involvement 2786
drug-induced 2067
pregnancy 2141
hypertriglyceridaemia 1664
moderate (type IV) 1665
nonalcoholic steatohepatitis 1666
severe (types I and V) 1664
complications 1665
physical signs 1665
hypertrophic cardiomyopathy 2715, 2764–5
causes 2766, *2766*
clinical approach to individual symptoms 2772
arrhythmia 2772
chest pain 2772
dyspnoea 2781
clinical features *2771*
definition 2765
diagnosis 2767, *2768*
history 2768
investigations 2769
cardiac catheterization 2770
chest radiography 2770
ECG 2769
echocardiography 2770, *2770*
electrophysiological studies 2771
exercise testing 2770
management 2771
alcohol septal ablation 2771
pacing 2772
pharmacological 2771
screening and follow-up 2771
surgical 2771
pathology 2766, *2767*
pathophysiology 2766

diastolic dysfunction 2766
myocardial ischaemia 2767
systolic function and dynamic outflow-tract obstruction 2767
physical examination 2768
pregnancy 2111
prevention of sudden death 2772
risk stratification 2772, *2772*
prognosis 2769
hypertrophic pulmonary osteoarthropathy 3523, *3523*, 3714
hyperuricaemia 1622, *1624*, 3639
asymptomatic 1625
causes *1621*
ethanol in 1626
and hyperlipidaemia 1667
renal effects 4019, 4183
treatment 1624
see also gout
hyperuricosuria 4128
renal effects 4019
hyperventilation syndrome *2633*
hyperventilation 3296
differential diagnosis 4817
hyperviscosity *2846*
hypnic headache 4922
hypnosis 3153
hypnotherapy *66*, 5291
hypnotics 3155
antagonists 3156
in renal failure 4181
hypoadrenalism 1870, *1871*, 1880
aetiology *1881*
clinical features 1882, *1882*
laboratory investigations 1883, *1883*
primary 1880
Addison's disease 1880, *1881*
congenital adrenal hyperplasia 1880
secondary 1882
treatment 1884
hypoaldosteronism, hyporeninaemic 1889, 3842
hypobaric hypoxia 1403, 4266
hypocalcaemia 1851, 1862, 3733
autosomal dominant *4145*
causes 1852, *1860*, 1863
acute renal trauma 3890
calcium-sensing receptor anomalies *1853*, 1866
hypoparathyroidism 1863
pseudohypoparathyroidism 1866, *1867*
clinical features 1862, *1863*
CNS complications 5154
familial hypocalciuric *3721*
genetics *1855*
investigations 1862
management 1863
hypocalcaemic hypercalciuria *1855*
hypocalciuria 3733
hypochondriasis 5301
hypochondroplasia *3721*
mutations in *3757*
hypochromia *4195*
hypocitraturia 4128
hypocretin 4826
Hypoderaeum conoideum *1220*
Hypoderma spp. *1233*
hypogammaglobulinaemia
and arthralgia 3710
and arthritis 958, *958*
transient of infancy 247
hypogammaglobulinaemic sprue 2248
hypoglossal nerve disorders 5038
hypoglycaemia *384*, 2049, 2028
accidental 2056
alcohol-induced 2056
autoimmune 2056
causes 2049, *2050*
classification 2050
clinical features 2028
CNS complications 5153
definition 2050
diagnosis/detection 2029
confirmation 2052
drug overdose *5505*
endocrine 2057
factitious 2056
felonious 2056
hepatocellular failure 2497
management 2504
hyperinsulinism 2052
inborn errors of metabolism 2057
intractable recurrent 2030
investigation 2051, *2052*
malaria 1064–5, 1080
malnutrition 1513
non-islet-cell tumour 2054
and organ failure 2057
physiological considerations 2050
postprandial syndrome 2055
presentation 2051, 5477
prevention and treatment 2029, *2030*
reactive 2055
alcohol-induced 2055
sequelae 2029
symptoms 2029
awareness of 2029
treatment
asymptomatic patients 2051
emergency 2051
stuporose/comatose patients 2051
unawareness 2049
hypoglycaemic agents, poisoning 1288
hypogonadism 1913, *1916*, *4908*
aetiology 1916, *1917*
clinical investigation 1920
diagnosis 1916
hypergonadotropic *1960*
specific conditions 1919
treatment 1920
androgen replacement 1921
hypohidrosis/anhidrosis 4678
hypohidrotic ectodermal dysplasia *4599*
hypokalaemia 3831, 3834, 3873
causes 3834, *3835*
diarrhoea 3836
diuretics 3835
familial periodic paralysis 3840
mineralocorticoid excess 3837
renal tubular abnormalities 3837
sporadic periodic paralysis 3840
sudden unexplained death during sleep 3840
thyrotoxic periodic paralysis 3839, *3839*
ureteric diversion into colon 3839
vomiting 3836
clinical features 3834
periodic paralysis *3839*, 3840, 5219
CNS complications 5155
and Cushing's disease 1876
diagnosis 3836, *3837*
distal tubule renal acidosis 4137
drug overdose *5505*
management 3834
presentation 5480
renal effects 4018
hypolipoproteinaemia 1671
hypomagnesaemia 1499, 1852
autosomal dominant renal with hypocalciuria *4145*, 4146
CNS complications 5155
familial
with hypercalciuria and nephrocalcinosis *4128*, *4145*, *4146*
with secondary hypocalcaemia *4145*, 4146
gestational 2143
post-transplant 3964
hypomelanosis of Ito 147
hypomyelination and congenital cataract 5107
hyponatraemia 3817, 3819, 3873
acute porphyria 1649
clinical features 3820
hyponatraemic encephalopathy 3821
CNS complications 5154
complications, cerebral demyelination 3822
DDAVP withdrawal 3824
diagnosis 3821, *3823*
elderly patients 3826
exercise-associated 3823
exercise-induced 5381, *5381*
malaria 1064
pathogenesis 3820, *3820*
cerebral oedema 3820
post-transplant 3964
postoperative 3823
presentation 5480
syndrome of inappropriate diuresis 3825, *3825*
treatment 3821, *3824*
hypoparathyroidism 1863, 3745
acquired 1864
associations *1855*, 1864
Blomstrand's disease *1855*, 1865
complex congenital syndromes *1855*
deafness and renal anomalies *1855*, 1864
DiGeorge syndrome *1855*, 1864
Kearns-Sayre syndrome *1855*, 1865
Kenney-Caffey syndrome *1855*, 1865
MELAS syndrome *1855*, 1865
mitochondrial disorders 1865
polyglandular autoimmune syndrome *1855*
Sanjad-Sakati syndrome *1855*, 1865
clinical features *1866*, *3731*
inherited 1864
isolated *1855*, 1864
neonatal 1864
polyglandular autoimmune 1865, *1865*
hypophosphataemia
post-transplant 3964
X-linked *3721*, *3737*, *3739*, 3739
hypophosphataemic rickets 3739, *3737*, *3739*
hypophosphatasia 3720, *3721*, 3755
clinical features *3731*, 3755, *3756*
and hypercalcaemia *3745*
management 3756
pathophysiology 3755
hypophysitis 1816
hypopigmentation *see* pigmentation disorders
hypopituitarism 1814
causes *1814*
in men *1917*
myopathy 5217
postpartum 2141
hypoplastic left heart syndrome 2870
hypoprothrombinaemia 4539
hyporeninaemia *1871*
hyporeninaemic hypoaldosteronism 1889
hypospadias 1972
hypotension
dialysis patients 3941
malaria 1080
poisoned patients 1276
snake bite 1352
hypothalamic syndrome 1825
hypothalamic/pituitary dysfunction 1906, 2066
hyperprolactinaemia 1907
idiopathic hypothalamic amenorrhoea 1907, *1907*
weight-loss related amenorrhoea 1906
hypothalamic-pituitary tumours 1916
hypothalamic-pituitary-ovarian axis 1903, *1903*
hypothalamic-pituitary-testicular axis *1914*
assessment 1920
hypothalamic-pituitary-thyroid axis *1801*
hypothermia 1395–6
and acute pancreatitis 2559
causes 1396
drowning 1398
intracranial hypertension *3150*
malnutrition 1513
poisoned patients 1277
presentation 5508
therapeutic 3104
and thrombocytopenia 4515
hypothyroidism 1826, 1833
aetiology 1833, *1834*
cardiac involvement 2787
clinical features 1834, *1835*
myopathy 5217
drug-induced 2068
epidemiology 1833
hyperlipidaemia 1667
juvenile 1955
laboratory diagnosis *1835*, 1835
neonatal screening *104*
pathogenesis 1833
pathology 1835
pregnancy 1837, 2142
prognosis 1836
screening 107, *1837*
treatment 1836
uncertainties 1837, *1837*

hypotonia-cystinuria
syndrome *4148*
hypouricaemia
causes *1627*
congenital renal 1627
hypoventilation
sleep-induced 3261, 3273
overnight ventilation 3275
hypovolaemia, malaria 1064
hypovolaemic shock 3122, 3127
hypoxaemia 3468, *3468*
nocturnal 3469
hypoxia
diving 1419
flight-induced 1410, *1411–12*
hepatic involvement 2538
hypobaric 1403, 4266
Hypsizigus marmoreus *3436*

ibandronate
osteoporosis *3799*
Paget's disease 3744
ibfenac, adverse effects,
hepatotoxicity *2532*
ibritumomab tiuxetan *376*
ibuprofen
adverse effects,
hepatotoxicity *2532*
and asthma *3289*
cystic fibrosis 3360
migraine *4917*
opioid withdrawal *5347*
rheumatoid arthritis *3594*
ICAM-1, 2601
I-cell disease 1698
corneal opacity 1704
ichthammol 4733
ichthyoses *385*, 4596
bullous ichthyosiform
erythroderma 4597
congenital/lamellar 1698
harlequin 4598
ichthyosis bullosa of
Siemens 4597
ichthyosis vulgaris, autosomal
dominant 4596
lamellar 4597
Netherton's syndrome 4597
nonbullous ichthyosiform
erythroderma 4597
Sjögren-Larsson syndrome 1724,
4597
X-linked recessive 4597
ICOS *287*
idiopathic thrombocytopenia *276*
idiopathic thrombocytopenic
purpura 4510
ifosfamide 398
adverse effects *400*
lymphoma *4320*
toxicity *3739*
Ignavigranum spp. *962*
Iguape virus *566*
Ilesha virus *581*
ileum, bacterial flora *2330*
Ilheus virus *566*
iliopsoas bursitis *3248*
iliotibial band friction syndrome *5382*
imaging
thoracic 3200
see also different modalities and conditions
imatinib mesylate *1939*
leukaemias 4251, *4252*
resistance 4252, *4252*
imatinib 400
cost-effectiveness ratio *53*
uses *3798*
Imerslund's disease 4411
imidazoles, contraindication in
porphyria *5484*
imiglucerase 1709
iminoglycinuria *4148*
imipenem/cilastin, anaerobic
infections *753*
imipenem
nocardiosis 857
P. aeruginosa *737*
P. multocida *779*
pneumonia *3238*, *3245*
postantibiotic effect *451*
imipramine
adverse effects *5313*
hepatotoxicity *2529*, *2532–3*
diabetic neuropathy 2039
imiquimod 4736
anogenital warts 603
immersion effects 1417, *1418*
immotile cilia syndrome *1917*
immune adjuvants 372
immune dysregulation, polyendocrinopathy, enteropathy,
X-linked (IPEX) *238*, 269, 293
immune function, disorders of
homeostasis *238*
immune privilege 271
immune reconstitution
inflammatory syndrome
(IRIS) 640, 827, 3252, 5023
immune rejection, stem cells 201
immune response 1510
against self antigens 271
down-regulation 232
B-cell tolerance 233
failure of regulation 233
regulatory mechanisms 233
T-cell tolerance 232
humoral 287
memory 232
central 232
effector 232, *232*
priming 230, *230*
immune surveillance,
cancer 374, *374*
immune system 207, 372
adaptive immunity 224
apoptosis in 186
complement *see* complement system
effects of malnutrition 1510
innate 207
in pregnancy 2077
immune thrombocytopenic purpura,
pregnancy 2178
immune tolerance, cancer 373
immunization 460, *90*, *90*
childhood 77, 467
heart failure patients 2721
immunology 460
influenza virus 481, *90–1*
leprosy 847
measles *91*, *517*, *523*
meningitis 4981
mumps *91*, 515
pretravel *466*
programmes
aims of 462
delivery of 463
evaluation 463, *464*
routine programme *91*
rubella 563
travellers 467
tuberculosis 830
vaccine antigens 461, *461–2*
vaccine delivery 462
WHO Expanded Program on
Immunization 463, *463*
see also vaccines
immunocompromised host 235, 2246
antibody deficiency 235, 244
bronchiectasis 3347
chlamydial infections 945
classification 236, *237*, 432, *432*
primary immuno-
deficiency *238*, 432
secondary
immunodeficiency *244*
common variable
immunodeficiency *238*, 2246
dermatophytoses 1001
diagnosis *246*
immunodeficiency with partial
albinism *238*
impaired cell-mediated
immunity 235, 248
infection *237*, 237, 431
acute gastrointestinal
syndromes 439, *439*
acute neurological syn-
dromes 437, *437–8*
clinical syndromes 433
duration of immuno-
suppression 434, *434*
fever *see* fever of unknown
origin
fungal 249
history 433
investigations 434
mycoplasmal 958
physical examination 433, *434*
prevention 440, *440*
pulmonary infiltrates 436, *436*
relation to underlying
condition 432, *433*
speed of progression 434
underlying disease 434
phagocyte deficiency 236, *238*, 252
see also HIV/AIDS;
immunosuppression
immunodominance 271
immunoglobulin A
nephropathy 3971
aetiology 3971
clinical associations 3974
clinical features 3973
acute renal injury 3974
asymptomatic haematuria/
proteinuria 3974
chronic renal failure 3974
Henoch-Schönlein purpura
nephritis 3974, *3974*
IgAN 3973, *3974*
macroscopic haematuria 3974
nephrotic syndrome 3974
clinical investigation 3975
diagnostic criteria 3975
differential diagnosis 3974
epidemiology 3973
genetics 3972
pathogenesis 3972
pathology 3972
immune deposits 3972, *3972–3*
light microscopy 3972, *3973*
prognosis 3976, *3976*
treatment 3975, *3975*
immunoglobulin A *228*
deficiency *238*, 247
coeliac disease 2339
reference values *5440*, *5444*
immunoglobulin D, M *228*
immunoglobulin E *228*
angio-oedema 262
antibodies 265
antibody test 3293
reference values *5444*
skin testing 3111
immunoglobulin G *228*
reference values *5440*, *5444*
subclass deficiency *238*, 247
immunoglobulin light
chain 1773
immunoglobulin light-chain
amyloidosis
clinical presentation 4056
definition and
epidemiology 4056, *4057*
diagnosis 4056
renal involvement 4056
treatment 4057
immunoglobulin M
nephropathy 3989
immunoglobulin M, reference
values *5440*, *5444*
immunoglobulin replacement
therapy 246, 248
adverse effects 248
dosage *248*
immunoglobulins
class switching 245
diversity *228*
increased loss of *244*
intravenous
lupus nephritis 4049
pregnancy *2158*
immunological memory 288
heterologous immunity 289
homeostatic proliferation 290
sensitization 289
immunological tolerance 292, *293*
immunology, transplantation *see*
transplantation immunology
immunonutrition 1503
immunoproliferative small intestinal
disease 2344
immunoreceptor tyrosine activation
motifs *see* ITAMs
immunoreceptor tyrosine-based
inhibitory motifs *see* ITIMS
immunoregulation, abnormal 271
immunosuppressants *244*
carcinogenesis *307*
Crohn's disease 2366
lupus nephritis 4047–8, *4048*
post-transplantation 280, *290*
primary biliary cirrhosis 2467
skin disorders 4737
SLE 3662
targets of *291*
immunosuppression
acute abdomen 2236
adverse effects 3954–5
opportunistic infection 433
opportunistic infections 3956,
3956–7
and cancer 307, 506
cardiac transplantation 2730,
2730

HSV infection 487
liver transplantation 2510, *2511*
lung transplantation 3481
in pregnancy 2077
renal transplantation 3953, *3954*
immunotactoid glomerulopathy 4060, *4061*
immunotherapy
allergen 265, 3282
anaphylaxis 3113
asthma 3299
cancer 372, 377
antigen-presenting cells 379
antigens 378
T cells/T-cell modulation 378
food allergy 2255
leukaemias 4253, *4254*
impetigo 4673
staphylococcal 696, *697*
streptococcal 673
implantable cardioverter-defibrillators 2701, *2702*
heart failure 2727
implied contract 20
impotence, hypertension 3040
in vitro fertilization 1926
inborn errors of metabolism 1549
animal genetic models 1557
carbohydrate metabolism 1596
fructose 1604
galactose, pentose and pyruvate 1610
glycogen storage diseases 1596
carrier identification 1556
clinical features 1549
diagnosis 1553, *1554*
genetic basis 1549
heterogeneity in 1552
hypoglycaemia 2057
inherited 1550, *1551*
and IVF 1557
lysosomal storage diseases 1552
mitochondrial 1551
pathogenesis 1549
prenatal diagnosis 1556
protein-dependent 1559, *1566*
aetiology and genetics 1561
diagnostic work-up 1561
emergency treatment 1564, *1564*
epidemiology 1561
future developments 1565
historical perspective 1560
monitoring of treatment 1565
pathogenesis and pathology 1561
prevention 1561
treatment 1563, *1564*
see also individual defects
screening for 1556
treatment 1553, *1554*
see also individual diseases
incidentaloma 108
adrenal 1890
incontinence
faecal 5389
urinary 5389, 5397
incontinentia pigmenti 4660
incremental cost-effectiveness ratio (ICER) 53, *53*
incretin mimetics 2017
incretin 1993
indapamide, calcium stone prevention *4130*
indels 138
Indian Hedgehog 3549, *3549*
indinavir
HIV/AIDS 636, *638*
mode of action *444*
renal toxicity *3860*
toxicity *640*
indometacin
adverse effects
hepatotoxicity *2532*
in pregnancy *2188*
and asthma *3289*
gout 1624
orthostatic hypotension *5063*
rheumatoid arthritis *3594*
Industrial Injuries Advisory Council 1378
Inermicapsifer madagascariensis *1190*
inert gas dilution method 3191
inert gas narcosis 1418
infant botulism 806
infantile myopathy and lactic acidosis *5223*
infants
growth 1951
hereditary bulbar palsy 5073
small for gestational age 1952
see also children
infections 1510
apoptosis in response to 186
areas of uncertainty 418
bacterial *see* bacterial infections
biliary tract 2554
bacterial cholangitis 2554
infestations 2554
and cancer 306, *306*
central nervous system 4976
actinomycotic 853
anaerobic 751
bacterial 4976
intracranial abscess 5013
neurosyphilis/neuro-AIDS 5015
prion diseases 5023
tick-borne encephalitis 572, *566*, *573*
viral 4998
clinical approach 420
clinical examination 421
clinical features and diagnosis 416
complement deficiency 217, 223
MBL deficiency 217
Neisseria 217
pyogenic infection 217
congenital 5146
diabetes mellitus 2021
differential diagnosis 417
epidemiology 416
fungal *see* fungal infections
gastrointestinal 2424
clinical syndromes 2426
complications *2425*
diagnosis 2430, *2431*
differential diagnosis 2431
management 2432, *2433*
pathophysiology 2425
prevention 2433
haematological changes 4550
history 421, *422*
immune response 1510
immunodeficiency-associated 237, *237*
inflammatory response 1510
intracranial *4780*, 4780
investigations 417, 421
second phase 422
life-threatening situations 420, *421*
liver involvement 2541, *2542*
management prediagnosis 421
occupational risk 1381
opportunistic 3956, *3956–7*
parasitic *see* parasitic infections
pathophysiology 414
anti-inflammatory cascade 415
anticoagulation cascade 416
coagulation cascade 415
inflammatory cascade 414, *414*
pleural *see* pleural empyema
pregnancy 2165
antimicrobial agents 2171, *2172*
bacterial 2169
protozoal 2170
viral 2166
see also individual infections
prognosis 418
renal involvement 4071
skin 4672
bacterial 4673
ectoparasites 4675
fungal 4675
tuberculosis 4674, *4674*
viral 4675
see also individual infections
therapeutic trials 422
viral *see* viral infections
infectious diseases
cardiac involvement 2797
acute rheumatic fever 2797
HIV/AIDS 2822
infective endocarditis 2806
syphilis 2826
newly emerging 1415
renal involvement 3858
general systemic syndromes 3859
nephrotoxicity 3859
spread by air travel 1415
infectious mononucleosis 501–2
clinical course 503
complications 503
differential diagnosis 503
laboratory diagnosis 504
pathogenesis 504
signs 503, *504*
symptoms 502, *503*
treatment 504
see also Epstein-Barr virus
infective endocarditis 2806
in children 2811
clinical features 2808
bacteraemia 2808
circulating immune complexes 2808, 2809–11, *2813*
prosthetic valve 2810
systemic or pulmonary emboli 2808
tissue destruction 2808
diagnosis 2811
criteria for 2813, *2814*
echocardiography 2812
laboratory methods 2811, *2814*
epidemiology 2807
historical background 2807
intravenous drug users 2811
microbiology 2814
pathogenesis 2807
prevention and prophylaxis *2818–19*, 2819
renal involvement 4072, *4072*
right-sided 2811
surgery 2820
treatment 2816, *2816–18*
inferior caval vein anomalies 2859, *2860*
inferior petrosal sinus sampling, Cushing's disease 1876, *1876*
inferior vena cava occlusion 3016
infertility 2086
and cancer treatment 394
cirrhosis and ascites 2492
Crohn's disease 2369
idiopathic *1917*
immunological *1917*
male 1913, 1922
aetiology 1922
azoospermia/oligozoospermia 1922
asthenozoospermia 1922
chromosomal disorders 1923
clinical features 1924
counselling 1927
diagnosis 1924
history 1924
laboratory investigation *1917*, 1925
target tissue defects 1923
coital disorders 1924
cryptorchidism 1923
excurrent duct obstruction 1924
genital tract infections 1924
sperm autoimmunity 1924
testicular tumours 1923
varicocele 1924
teratozoospermia 1922
treatment *1917*, 1925
Y-chromosome microdeletions 1923
mycoplasmal infections and *956*
polycystic ovary syndrome 1909
premature (primary) ovarian failure 1906
infestations 1225, 1229
canthariasis 1225, *1235*
fleas 1225, *1232*
lice 1230, *1230*
myiasis 1225, *1232*, *1233*
scabies 1225, *1229*, *1229–30*
tungosis 1232
inflammation, cytokine targeting 158
inflammatory bowel disease *276*, 2225
and arthritis 3603, 3613
common variable immunodeficiency 2248
GI bleeding 2241
haematological changes 4556
hepatic involvement 2539, *2540*
ocular involvement 5244
pregnancy 2132
selective IgA deficiency 2249
small intestine 2222
see also Crohn's disease; ulcerative colitis
inflammatory cascade 414, *414*
inflammatory mediators, anaphylaxis 3109
inflammatory response 1510
infliximab 158

Crohn's disease 2367
pregnancy *2158*
psoriasis 4615
rheumatoid arthritis 3598, *3599*
sarcoidosis *3411*
Still's disease 3706
ulcerative colitis 2371
influenza virus *474*, 479
antiviral therapy 480
clinical features 480
epidemiology 479
immunity 480
immunization *90–1*, 481
pathogenesis 480
pregnancy 2124
vaccines *466*, 481, 762
Informant Questionnaire on Cognitive Decline in the Elderly (IQCODE) 5406
information overload 22–3
infundibular stenosis *2844*, 2849
inhalation testing 3293
inhaled drugs 1452
inheritance 138
digenic 139, 140
Mendelian 138
mitochondrial 140
monogenic *139*, 139
nonmendelian 138
triallelic 140
inhibin A 1903
inhibin B 1903
inhibin 1795
inhibitor of caspase-activated DNase (ICAD) 179
inhibitors of apoptosis proteins (IAPs) 184
injuries
child mortality *75*
mortality rate *76*
Inkoo virus 580, *581*
innate immunity 152, 207
alcoholic liver disease 2476
cell types 208, *208*, *288*
cytokines 152, 212, *212*
chemokines 212
interferons 213
defects in *238*, 255
lymphoid cells 209
natural killer (NK) cells 209
NKT cells 210
myeloid cell lineage 208
dendritic cells 209, *209*
granulocytes 209
mast cells 209
monocytes/macrophages 208
receptors 210
natural killer receptors 211, *211*
Toll-like receptors 210, *210*
soluble factors 211
complement 211
in transplant rejection 285, *288*
inositol, vibration injury 1435
inotropes 3130
heart failure 2724, *2725*
see also individual drugs
inotropism, positive 2618
Inquilinus spp. *962*
insect stings 1324, 1349
beetles 1351, *1351*
butterflies and moths 1351, *1351*
hymenoptera 1349, *1349*
insects, and hygiene 1236
insomnia 4829, *4830*
inspiration, flow-volume curves 3193, *3193*
inspissated bile syndrome 2580
insulin analogues 2012
insulin C-peptide, reference values *5441*
insulin neuritis 2039
insulin receptor 1993, *1994*
autoantibodies 2056
defects in 1994
postreceptor mechanisms 1994
turnover 1994
insulin resistance 1995
causes of 1995
inherited 1995
obesity 1995
metabolic and clinical features 1996
insulin therapy 2010
adverse effects 2012
diabetic ketoacidosis 2026
dosage 2013
inhaled insulin 2013
injections 2013
insulin analogues 2012
manufacture 2010
preparations 2011
time course of *2011*
pumps 2014
continuous intraperitoneal infusion 2014
continuous subcutaneous infusion 2014
regimens 2012, 2017
starting 2018
types of insulin 2013
insulin tolerance test 1803
insulin 1790, *1992*, *2443*
absorption 2011
actions *1791*, *1795*
allergy 2013
biosynthesis 1992
hyperkalaemia *3891*
and hypoglycaemia 2057
inhibition *2320*
manufacture 2010
metabolic actions *1481*, 1994
carbohydrate metabolism 1994, *1995*
lipid metabolism 1995
measurements of 1995
protein metabolism 1995
pregnancy 2137
reference values *5441*
regulation of gene expression *1482*
secretion 1992
carbohydrate-induced 1485
ectopic 2054
glucose-stimulated 1992
normal pattern 1993
skin reactions to 4719
uses *3798*
insulin-like growth factor binding proteins 1790
insulin-like growth factors
and cancer 311
ectopic secretion 2064
metabolic effects *1481*
reference values *5441*
insulinoma 1979, 2052
insulinopathies 1992
insulitis 1999
insurance, diabetes mellitus 2021
integrase inhibitors 637
intention-to-treat analysis 34
intercalated disc *2611*
interferons 152, 213
cancer therapy 401
interferon-α
hepatitis C 619
lymphoma *4320*
pancreatic neuroendocrine tumours 1982
interferon-β *212*
interferon-γ 209, *212*
interleukin-1 antagonists, osteoarthritis 3636
interleukin-1 receptor associated kinase deficiency *238*
interleukin-1, 156, 2598
interleukin-10, 152, 158
interleukin-12, *212*
interleukin-15, 152
interleukin-18, 152, 157
interleukin-1α 156, *212*
interleukin-1β 156, *212*
interleukin-2, *212*
hepatotoxicity *2533*
receptor blockers 3482
interleukin-3, 4201
interleukin-33, 157
interleukin-4, *212*
interleukin-5, 209, 4201
interleukin-6 152, 157, *212*, 4201
interleukin-8 *209*, *212*
intermediate density lipoprotein (IDL) 1657
intermittent positive pressure ventilation, asthma 3309
internal jugular vein cannulation 5510, *5511*
International Agency for Research on Cancer (IARC) 1379
International HapMap Project 140
International Union of Immunological Societies (IUIS) 236
intersex 1967
interstitial nephritis, infection-associated 4073
interstitial pneumonias, idiopathic 3365–6
acute 3369, *3369*
desquamative 3368, *3368*
lymphocytic 3369, *3369*
nomenclature *3367*
nonspecific 3369, *3369–70*
respiratory bronchiolitis-interstitial lung disease 3368, *3368*
intestinal amoebiasis 1037
amoebic colitis with dysentery 1037
intestinal failure
bone disease 1542
complications 2585
liver disease 1542, *1542*
intestinal flukes 1219
diagnosis 1220
prevention 1221
treatment 1221
intestinal lymphangiectasia 2221, *2251*, 2251
intestinal obstruction 2234
investigations *2235*
intestinal pseudo-obstruction 2589, *2589*
acute colonic 2589
intestinal reperfusion injury 2420
intestinal resection, and gut peptides 2321
intestinal secretions 2228
intestinal transit 2229
intestinal transplantation 1542
intestine
cystic disorders 2586
colitis cystica profunda 2586
pneumatosis cystoides intestinalis 2586
ulcers of 2588
vascular disorders
angiodysplasia 2241
aorto-enteric fistula 2585
haemangioma 2585
spontaneous intramural haemorrhage 2585
see also colon; rectum; small intestine
intracardiac pressures *2621*
cardiac catheterization/angiography 2681, *2681*
intracardiac shunts 2683
intracellular signalling *see* signal transduction
intracerebral haemorrhage 4944
amyloid 4944
causes 4944, *4944*
cavernous malformations 4945
cerebral arteriovenous malformations 4944
diagnosis 4945
hypertensive 3036, *4944*, *4945*
treatment 4945
intracranial abscess 5013
aetiology 5013
clinical features 5014
diagnosis 5014, *5014*
management 5014
microbiology 5013
pathology 5013
prognosis 5015
intracranial haematoma 4966, *4966*
intracranial haemorrhage, imaging 4772, *4774*
intracranial hypertension 4972
aetiology 4973
clinical features 4972
drug-induced 4974
incidence 4972
investigations 4974
management 4975
pathogenesis 4974
prognosis 4975
intracranial infections *4780*, 4780
intracranial pressure
monitoring 3150
Monro-Kellie doctrine 3147
normal 3147
pathophysiology 3147, *3148*
raised 3147
diagnosis 3149
hepatocellular failure 2497, 2503
imaging 3149
lumbar puncture 3150
reasons to treat 3148, *3149*
symptoms 3149
treatment 3150, *3150–1*
signs 3149
temporal patterns of change 3148, *3148–9*
intracranial tumours 4967

aetiology 4968, *4969*
clinical features 4968
diagnosis 4970
epidemiology 4968
imaging *4776*, *4776*, 4782
pathogenesis 4968
pathology 4970, *4970*
prognosis 4971
treatment 4970
intraluminal occlusion 2417
intramural haematoma, spontaneous 2958
intramuscular drug administration 1452
intrapleural space 3175
intrauterine device, copper *1267*
heart disease patients 2115
intrauterine growth retardation, Lesch-Nyhan syndrome *1628*
intravenous urography 3873, *3874*
urinary tract obstruction 4153
intrinsic factor
congenital deficiency 4411
structural abnormality 4411
introns 138
invasive monitoring 5510
Iodamoeba bütchlii 1042
iodapamide, adverse effects, hepatotoxicity *2529*
iodine 1498, *1498*
in breast milk *2189*
dietary reference values *1502*
goitre 1832
in pregnancy 2090
radio-iodine 1841
reference intake *1524*, 1848
requirements in pregnancy 2082
iodoquinol, amoebiasis 1041
ion channels 160
action potentials 161
autoantibodies to *166*
channelopathies 162
disease-associated genes 166
gating 161
and intracellular signalling 169
macroscopic currents 161
open probability 160
single-channel current 160
structure 160
synaptic potentials 161
threshold potential 161
ionizing radiation 1429
acute radiation syndrome 1430
and cancer 305, *308*, *1380*
bone tumours 320
clinical investigations 1431
haematopoietic syndrome 1431
health effects 1430
mechanism of harm 1429
reproductive effects *1917*
tissue reactions 1430
treatment 1431
burns 1431
gastrointestinal syndrome 1431
iopanoic acid, adverse effects, hepatotoxicity *2529*
ioscarboxacid, poisoning 1282
ipecacuanha, syrup of 1279
IPEX syndrome 1999
ipratropium bromide
allergic rhinitis 3282
COPD *3335*
iprindole, adverse effects, hepatotoxicity *2532*
iproniazid, adverse effects, hepatotoxicity *2529*
iridodonesis 3730
iridology 65, *66*
irinotecan, sensitivity *1472*
iron chelation therapy 1684
iron deficiency anaemia *4401*
pregnancy 2174
iron deficiency 4390
causes 4390
clinical and laboratory features 4392
diagnosis 4392
investigations and management 4392
iron metabolism, disorders of 4390
iron overload, hormonal abnormalities 2066
iron storage diseases
acaeruloplasminaemia with iron deposition 1686
adult-onset basal ganglia disease 1686
cardiac involvement 4398
haemochromatosis *see* haemochromatosis
Hallervorden-Spatz disease 1686
hereditary hyperferritinaemia cataract syndrome 1686
pathophysiology/ pathogenesis 1677, *1677–8*
quantitative aspects 1678
secondary 4395, *4395*
clinical features 4396
diagnosis 4396
in pregnancy 4398
prognosis and outcome 4339
treatment 4396
iron supplements 2174, 4393
administration 4394
adverse effects 4394
oesophagitis *2294*
parenteral preparations 4393
prophylactic in pregnancy 4393
iron 1510
absorption 4388
haemochromatosis 1678
body status 4387, *4387*, 4389
dietary reference values *1502*
homeostasis 4386
loss of 4391
blood loss 4391
intestinal parasites 4391
malabsorption 4390
malnutrition 1513
metabolism 4386
pathological storage of 1674
poisoning 1288
antidote *1274*, *5505*
clinical features 1288
mechanisms of 1288
reference intake *1524*
reference values *5435*, *5445–6*
requirements in pregnancy 2082, 2174
serum *4196*
storage 1677, *1677–8*
diseases of 4395
storate 4386
toxicity 1677
transport 4386
irritable bowel syndrome 2384, 1522, 2207, 2224, 2253
clinical features 2385
examination 2385
history 2385
definition 2384
pathophysiology 2385
diet 2385
neuromuscular dysfunction 2385
psychiatric disease 2385
visceral hypersensitivity 2385
recognition 2385
Isaac's syndrome 5281
isaxonine, adverse effects, hepatotoxicity *2529*
ischaemia
arm 2963
leg 2960
acute 2960
chronic 2961
critical 2960
investigation 2961, *2961*
management *2962*, 2961–2
mesenteric 2417, *2235*, *2418*, *2963*
myocardial 2767
small intestine 2223
ischaemic colitis 2420, *2420*
ischaemic heart disease
fetal and postnatal effects 2899, *2899*
mortality rate *76*
pregnancy 2111
ischaemic myopathy 5218
ischemic lactate test *5449*
Iselin's disease *3804*
ISIS trial 36, *1939*, 3521
ISIS-2 trial 34, *35*, *38*, *39–40*
ISIS-4 trial 42
islet amyloid polypeptide 1775
islet-cell stimulating antibodies 2056
islets of Langerhans 1992
isobaric decompression 1421
isochromosomes 147
isoconazole, fungal infections 1015
isoflurane, adverse effects, hepatotoxicity *2529*
isografts *281*
isoniazid
adverse effects
hepatotoxicity *2529*, *2535*
neuropathy 5088
shoulder-hand syndrome 3714
in breast milk *1469*
chemoprophylaxis 828
drug interactions *1471*
hepatotoxicity 829
mycobacterial disease 835
poisoning 1289
prophylactic *440*
in renal failure *4185*
tuberculosis *825*
dose *826*
isoprenaline, asthma 3302
isopropanol poisoning 1312
isopropyl alcohol, and cancer *1380*
isosorbide dinitrate, NNT *52*
Isospora belli 2357
isosporiasis 1111, *1114*, *1115*
historical perspective 1112
isotretinoin
acne *4680*
adverse effects, hepatotoxicity *2532*
teratogenicity *1468*
isovaleric aciduria *1566*, 1570
aetiology/pathophysiology 1570, *1570*
clinical presentation 1570
diagnosis 1571, *1562–3*
treatment and outcome 1571
isoxazoles 1367, *1367–8*
Israel Turkey meningoencephalitis virus *566*
itai-itai disease 1297, 1384
ITAMs 174
Itaqui virus *581*
ITIMS 211
Ito cells *2438*
itraconazole
coccidioidomycosis 1022
dermatophytoses 1002
fungal infections 1015, 1017
oral candidiasis 2269
paracoccidioidomycosis 1028
Penicillium marneffei 1034
prophylactic *440*
in renal failure *4185*
ivabridine, angina 2909
ivermectin
filariasis 1158
onchocerciasis 1149
scabies 1230
strongyloidiasis 1164
trichuriasis 1176
Ixodes hexagonus 1229
Ixodes pacificus 1228
Ixodes persulcatus 1228
Ixodes ricinus 1228
Ixodes scapularis 1089, *1228*
Ixodes ticks *861*
Lyme borreliosis 860
Ixodidae (hard ticks) *1228*

Jaccoud's arthropathy
Sjögren's syndrome 3689, *3690*
SLE 3657, *3658*
Jackson-Weiss syndrome, mutations in *3757*
JAK3, 158
Jak-Stat pathways 155, *1793*, 1794, *1796*, 4201
Jamaican vomiting disease 1363
Jamaican vomiting sickness *1742*
Jamestown Canyon virus 580, *581*
Janeway lesions, infective endocarditis *2809*
Janibacter spp. *962*
Jansen's metaphyseal chondrodysplasia *1855*, 1862, *3721*, *3729*
hypercalcaemia *3745*
mutations in *3757*
Jansky-Bielchowsky disease 1698
Janus kinases 1794, *1796*, 4371
Japanese B encephalitis virus 565, *568*, 5002
clinical features 5004, *5005–6*
pregnancy *2171*
vaccines *466*
jararhagin *4540*
jargon aphasia 4789
Jarisch-Herxheimer reaction 860, 868, *869*, 871
leptospirosis 878
relapsing fever 868, *869*, 871
syphilis 895, 2828
treatment 873
Jatropha curcas 1374
jaundice 2444

clinical examination 2446
Habershon's 2541
hepatocellular 2496
diagnosis 2500
history 2446
in malaria 1065, *1067*
management 2446, *2446*
neonatal 2449
postoperative 2450
in pregnancy 2129
see also cholestasis
JC virus 600, 605
HIV patients 5019, *5021*
jejunoileal obstruction 2399, *2399*
jejunostomy *1540*
jejunum, bacterial flora *2330*
jellyfish envenoming 1347, *1347*
clinical features 1347
epidemiology 1347
prevention 1347
treatment 1348
Jervall-Lange-Nielsen syndrome 163, 166
jet lag 466, *1414*, 1414
melatonin 2071
Jeune's disease 3510
JNK 158
Jod-Basedow phenomenon 1832, 1843
Johnsonella spp. *962*
joint infection
anaerobic 752
Pseudomonas aeruginosa 737
tuberculosis 820
joints 3547
in Behçet's disease *3685*
hypermobility 3774
lavage 3635
prevention of destruction 3553
rheumatoid arthritis 3583, *3583–4*
synovium 3550
josamycin, rickettsioses 914
Joubert's syndrome *4904*, 5142–3
judgement 59
Jugra virus *566*
jugular venous pulse 2620
junctional extrasystoles 2703
Juquitiba virus *581*
Jutiapa virus *566*
juvenile chronic arthritis
ocular involvement 5243
renal involvement 4053
juvenile myelomonocytic leukaemia 4228
juvenile myoclonic epilepsy 166, 5101
juvenile nephronophthisis 4100
juvenile polyposis *2406*, *363*
juvenile xanthogranuloma 4362
management 4365
juxtaglomerular apparatus 3814, *3815*

Kadam virus *566*
Kallmann's syndrome 1907, *1917*, 1919
delayed/absent puberty 1961
renal involvement 4102
Kanzaki's disease 1698, 5122
kaolin pneumoconiosis 3423
Kaposi's sarcoma 307, 322, 499, 632, *633*, *2251*, 3247, 3251, *3251*, 4693, 4697
incidence *301*
oral *2267*
post-transplant 3962
Kaposi's sarcoma-associated herpesvirus *see* human herpesvirus 8
Kaposi-Stemmer sign 3087, *3088*
Karshi virus *566*
Kartagener's syndrome *1917*, 3279, 3349
karyolysis 178
Kashin-Beck disease 1500
Kasokero virus *581*
Katayama fever 1205, *1205*
Kaufman, Matt 190
kava 68
drug interactions *69*
toxicity 68
Kawasaki disease *3650*, 3698, 4632
aetiology and genetics 3699
clinical features 3701, *3700–1*
cardiac 2785
ocular 5244
pulmonary *3396*
diagnosis 3702, *3702*
differential diagnosis 3701
epidemiology *3699*, 3700
future developments 3703
historical perspective 3699
investigations *3701*, 3702
long-term management *3700*, 3703
pathogenesis/pathology 3699
prevention 3700
prognosis 3703, *3703*
risk stratification *3700*
treatment 3702
Kayser-Fleischer rings *1689*, 1690
Kearns-Sayre syndrome *1552*, *5223*
differential diagnosis *1722*
and hypoparathyroidism *1855*, 1865
kebuzone, adverse effects, hepatotoxicity *2532*
Kedougou virus *566*
Kell blood group system 4563
keloids *1008*
Kemerovo virus 556
Kennedy's syndrome *1917*, 1923, 5073
Kenney-Caffey syndrome *1855*, 1865
keratinocytes 199
keratins 4594
keratitis 833
HSV *485*, 486
Pseudomonas aeruginosa 737
keratoacanthoma 4710
keratoderma blennorrhagica 3625, *3625*
keratodermas 4598, *4598–9*
diffuse palmoplantar 4599
focal 4599
syndromic 4600
keratolytics 4733
propylene glycol 4733
salicylic acid and benzoic acid 4733
urea 4733
keratosis, ichthyosis, deafness syndrome 4600
keraunoparalysis 1424
kernicterus 2445
Kerstersia spp. *962*
Keshan disease 1500
ketanserin, Raynaud's phenomenon *3671*
Keterah virus *581*
ketoacidoses
alcoholic *1742*
diabetic *see* diabetic ketoacidosis
starvation *1742*
ketoacids *1739*
ketoconazole
adverse effects *455*
gynaecomastia 2068
hepatotoxicity *2529*, *2533*
ARDS 3145
Cushing's syndrome 1880
ectopic ACTH secretion 2064
fungal infections 1015
leishmaniasis *1138*
paracoccidioidomycosis 1028
reproductive effects *1917*
ketone bodies 1653
ketones, urinary 2020
ketoprofen
and asthma *3289*
cancer pain 394
rheumatoid arthritis *3594*
ketoralac, and asthma *3289*
KI virus 660
Kidd blood group system 4563
kidney 3809
acidosis 1745
adverse drug effects *3860*
blood supply 3809
channelopathies 165
cystic fibrosis 3363
distal tubule/collecting duct 3814, *3815*
effects of malnutrition 1510
glomerulus 3811, *3811*
interstitium 3816
juxtaglomerular apparatus 3814, *3815*
loop of Henle 3809, *3813*, *3814*
nephron 3809, *3810*
in pregnancy 2077, 2103
proximal convuluted tubule 3812
water handling 3818
see also renal
Kienböck's disease *3804*
killer-cell immunoglobulin-like receptors (KIR) 211
kinases 132
kinesin 131
kinesiology, applied *66*
Kingella kingae, osteomyelitis *3789*
Kingella spp. *962*
Kinyoun staining 822
kisspeptin 1790, 1920
kiwi fruit allergy 263
Klebsiella oxytoca 801
Klebsiella pneumoniae, pneumonia 3235
Klebsiella spp. *962*
antibiotic sensitivity *446*
Kleine-Levin syndrome 4833
Klinefelter's syndrome *1917*, 1919, 1923, 1957, 1967
Klippel-Trenaunay syndrome 3085, 4692
Klumpke's paralysis 5080
Kluyvera spp. *962*
knee
osteoarthritis *3629*, *3634*
pain *3248*
rheumatoid arthritis 3588
Kniest's dysplasia *3721*
mutations in *3757*
knockout transgenics 136
Knudson's two-hit hypothesis 361
Koch, Robert 811, 821
Kocuria spp. *962*
Koebner phenomenon 3611, 3705, 4612
Köhler's disease *3804*
koilonychia 4700
Kokobera virus *566*
konzo 5074
Koplik's spots *520*, 2264
Koutango virus *566*
Krabbe's disease 1555, 1698, 1969, 4960, 5105
differential diagnosis *1725*
neurological features 1703
kraits 1335
Krukenberg's tumour 2409
Kufs's disease 1698
Kugelberg-Welander disease 5072
Kunjin virus *566*, 572
Kupffer cells *2438*, 2439
Kurthia spp. *962*
kuru 1771, 5029, *5029*
Kussmaul breathing 3186
Kussmaul's sign 2795
Kviem-Siltzbach agent 3409
kwashiorkor 1507
Kyasanur Forest disease virus *566*, 574
kyphoscoliosis 3470
Ehlers-Danlos syndrome 3777
and respiratory disease 3187
kyphosis 3508, 3730
Kytococcus spp. *962*
Kyzylagach virus *558*

L-2-hydroxyglutaric aciduria *1566*, 1580, *1581*
La Crosse virus 580, *581*
labetalol
in breast milk *1469*, *2101*
hypertensive emergencies *3080*
in pregnancy *2099*
laboratory tests, effects of pregnancy *2126*
laboratory values 5431
biochemistry in diagnosis/management 5433
limitations 5433
normal range 5434
reference intervals 5434
lactate dehydrogenase, reference values *5436*
lactate *1739*
cerebrospinal fluid 4752
reference values *5435*, *5447*
children *5438*
lactation 2091
drugs in breast milk, antihypertensive agents *2101*
lactic acidosis *1742*, 1745, 2028
biguanide-induced 1746
ethanol/methanol-induced 1746
falciparum malaria 1746
D(-)lactic acidosis 1747
in liver disease 1746
nucleoside reverse transcriptase inhibitors 1746
postictal 1746
Reye's syndrome 1747
treatment 1749
Lactobacillus acidophilus 1747, 2257

Lactobacillus casei 2257
Lactobacillus spp. *962*
Lactococcus spp. *962*
lactose intolerance 2254, *2348, 2349*
congenital 2348
diagnosis 2350
lactase deficiency
of prematurity 2349
secondary 2350
lactase restriction 2349
lactose tolerance test 2228
lactose
digestion of 13
malabsorption *2328*
lactose-hydrogen breath test *2228*
lactotrophs *1801*
lactulose *5426*
lacunar syndromes 4940
Ladd's bands 2400
Laennec, R.T.H. 10
Lafora's body disease 5102
Lagos bat virus 554
Laguna Negra virus *581*
Lake-Cavanagh disease 1698
Lambert-Eaton myasthenic syndrome *166, 385*, 3523, 5166, 5173, 5182
clinical features 5182
diagnosis 5182
epidemiology 5182
pathogenesis 5182
prognosis 5182
treatment 5182
Lambl's excrescences 2832
lamins 179
lamivudine
HIV/AIDS 636, *638*
mode of action *444*
lamotrigine
dose levels *4823*
epilepsy 4821
poisoning 1281
serum levels *5449*
teratogenicity *2187*
Lance-Adams syndrome 4899
Langerhans' cell histiocytosis 4362, 4713
clinical features 4363
bone 4363, *4364*
bone marrow and blood 4364
central nervous system 4364
diabetes insipidus 4363
ears 4363
gut 4364
liver 4363
lungs 3447, *3447*, 4363
lymph nodes 4364
skin 4363
management 4365
language disorders 4789
lanolin 4736
lanreotide, acromegaly 1807
lansoprazole, peptic ulcer disease 2311
lapatinib *1939*
large granular lymphocyte leukaemia 4227
large granular lymphocytosis 4308
Laron's syndrome 1957
Larrea tridentate (chapparal), nephrotoxicity *4093*
Larsson formula 3871
larva migrans
cutaneous 1166, *1167*
ocular 1174
visceral 1173
laryngeal cancer 317
incidence *301, 317*
migrants vs residents *302*
laryngeal mask airway 5516, *5517*
larynx 3171, *3172*
communication and neuromuscular function 3172
dynamic control of lung volume 3172, *3172*
protection of airway 3172
recurrent laryngeal nerve paralysis 3172
laser photocoagulation 2035
Lassa fever
clinical features 591, *591–2*
diagnosis/differential diagnosis 594
epidemiology 589
pregnancy *2171*
treatment 594
late gadolinium enhancement 2675
coronary artery disease 2675, *2675*
dilated cardiomyopathy 2676
inflammatory/infiltrative heart disease 2676
lateral cutaneous nerve of thigh, neuropathy 5084
lateral geniculate nucleus lesions 4856
latex allergy 264, 2253, 3108
lathyrism 5074
Lathyrus sativus 1374
Laticauda colubrina (sea krait) *1330*
Latrodectus curassaviensis 1354
Latrodectus hasselti (Australian redback spider) *1354*
Laurence-Moon syndrome *1530, 1917*
Lautropia spp. *962*
lavatory cleaners, poisoning by 1317
lavender, drug interactions *69*
laxatives
abuse 3837
in breast milk *2189*
palliative care *5426*
in renal failure 4177
L-dopa, orthostatic hypotension *5063*
Le Veen shunts 2489
lead poisoning 1299, 1384, 4017
antidote *1274*
clinical features 1299, 4017
CNS effects *1386*
diagnosis and treatment 4017
management 1300
mechanisms of toxicity 1299
medical surveillance 1300
pathogenesis/pathology 4017
peripheral nervous system effects *1387*, 5087
porphyria *1637*
skeletal effects 3768
toxicokinetics 1299
lead
reference values *5445–6*
reproductive effects *1917*
leadership 58
learning disability 5279
Leber's hereditary optic neuropathy *1552*, 4855, *5223*
Leblond, Charles 195
Lebombo virus 556
Lechiguanas virus *581*
lecithin 1654
lecithin:cholesterol acyltransferase (LCAT) 1657
lecithin-cholesterol acyl transferase (LCAT) deficiency 4099
Leclercia spp. *962*
lectins *1362*, 1364
leeches 1357
aquatic 1357
clinical features of intrusion 1358
land 1357
prevention of intrusion 1357
treatment 1358
leflunomide
pregnancy *2158*
rheumatoid arthritis *3595*
sarcoidosis *3411*
left atrium
ball thrombus 2997
dilatation 2738
myxoma 2997
left ventricular dysfunction
cardiac catheterization/ angiography 2685, *2685*
echocardiography 2666, *2666*
HIV/AIDS *2822*
and mitral regurgitation 2742
and mitral stenosis 2739
left ventricular end-systolic pressure-volume relationship 3125
left ventricular failure 2633
hypertensive 3079
left ventricular hypertrophy
ECG 2649, *2649–50*
echocardiography 2666
left ventricular outflow tract obstruction 2851
left ventricular pressure-volume loop 3124, *3124*
left-to-right shunt *2844*
leg ischaemia 2960
acute 2960
chronic 2961
critical 2960
investigation 2961, *2961*
management *2962*, 2961–2
leg movements
restless legs syndrome 5078
of sleep 4835
leg ulcers 4689, *4689*
Legg-Calvé-Perthes disease *3804*
Legionella bozemanii 899
Legionella longeachae 899
Legionella micdadei 899
Legionella pneumophila 899
Legionella spp. *962*
pneumonia 900, *902*, 3235
community-acquired *453*
treatment *3238*
legionellosis *see* legionnaires' disease
legionnaires' disease 899, 3235
aetiology 899
areas of uncertainty 902
clinical features 900, *901*
legionella pneumonia 900, *902*
Pontiac fever 900
epidemiology 899
future developments 902
history 899
laboratory diagnosis 900
pathology 899
prevention 900
prognosis 902
treatment 902
Leifsonia spp. *962*
Leigh's syndrome *1552*, 1617, *5223*
leiomyomatosis, hereditary *363*, 368
Leiperia cincinnalis 1240
Leishmania aethiopica 1135
Leishmania amazonensis 1135
Leishmania brasiliensis 1135
Leishmania chagasi 1135
Leishmania donovani 1135
Leishmania guyanensis 1135
Leishmania infantum 1135
Leishmania major 1135
Leishmania Mexicana 1135
Leishmania panamensis 1135
Leishmania peruviana 1135
Leishmania tropica 1135
leishmaniasis 1134
aetiology 1135, *1135*
cutaneous 1135
American mucosal leishmaniasis 1137, *1137, 1138*
clinical features *1136, 1137*
diffuse *1137*, 1137
laboratory findings 1138
leishmaniasis recidivans *1137*, 1137
treatment *1138*, 1138
haematological changes 4553
HIV-related 634, 648
prevention and control 1141
visceral 1140
clinical features *1140*, 1140
economic impact 1141
epidemiology 1139
and HIV infection 1140
laboratory diagnosis 1141
pathogenesis/pathology 1139
post-kala-azar *1140*, 1140
treatment 1141
Leloir pathway 1611
Lemierre syndrome 3229
Leminorella spp. *962*
lenalidomide, multiple myeloma 4350
lentigines-associated syndromes 4706
Lentinus edodes 3436
Leoconostoc spp. *962*
LEOPARD syndrome *2766*, 2835
lepidopterism 1351
lepirudin 3022
leprechaunism 1995
leprosy 836
aetiology 836
areas of uncertainty 847
bacterial load 838
clinical features 836, 839
anaesthesia 839
borderline lepromatous leprosy 840
borderline leprosy 840, *840*
borderline tuberculoid leprosy 840, *840*
early lesions 839
hepatic granuloma 2518
lepromatous leprosy 840, *841–2*
neuritis *844*, 846–7
peripheral neuropathy 839, *839*

renal involvement 4089
skin 839
tuberculoid leprosy 840
diagnosis 836, 844
slit skin smears 844
differential diagnosis 844
nerves 844
skin *844*, 844
epidemiology 837
eye disease in 842
further research 848
and HIV 837
Lucio's 841
nerve damage 838
pathogenesis 837
patient education 846
and pregnancy 847
prevention 847
of disability 846
vaccines 847
prognosis 847
reactions 838, 842
type 1 (reversal) 842, *842–3*
type 2 (ENL) 843, *843*, 846
rehabilitation 847
Ridley-Jopling classification 837, *838*
risk factors 837
spectrum 837
transmission 837
treatment 836, 845
chemotherapy *845*, 845
management of reactions 846
new reactions 846
vaccines 847
variant forms 841
women 847
leptin *1531*, 1790, 2135
actions *1791*
deficiency 1530, *1530*
metabolic effects *1481*
and obesity *1531*
Leptospira biflexa 874
Leptospira borgpetersenii 874
Leptospira icterohaemorrhagica, renal toxicity *4086*
Leptospira inadai 874
Leptospira interrogans 874
renal toxicity 4089
Leptospira kirshneri 874
Leptospira noguchii 874
Leptospira santarosai 874
Leptospira spp. *962*
Leptospira weilii 874
leptospirosis 874, *1240, 1385*
aetiology 874
clinical features 876, *876*
anicteric leptospirosis 876
icteric leptospirosis (Weil's disease) 877, *877*
renal disease 3901, 4089
diagnosis 877
epidemiology 874
liver involvement 2542
nephrotoxicity 3859
pathology and pathogenesis 875
eye 876
haemorrhage 875
heart 876
kidney 875
liver 875
lungs 875
meningitis 875
striated muscle 875
prevention 878
prognosis 878
treatment 878, *878*
Leptotrichia buccalis 852
Leptotrichia spp. *962*, 2261
lergotrile, adverse effects, hepatotoxicity *2529*
Leriche's syndrome 2961
Lesch-Nyhan syndrome 1627, 4418
clinical features *1628*, 1629
clinical genetics 1630
growth patterns *1628*
haematological changes 4559
intrauterine growth retardation *1628*
nephrolithiasis *4101*
treatment 1629
Leser-Trélat sign 4705
letrozole, breast cancer *1937*
Letterer-Siwe disease 3446
leucocyte adhesion deficiencies *238*, 253, 4304, 4309
leucocyte count 4197, *4196*
differential 4197, *4196*
infants and children *4197*
leucocyte esterase, urinary 3865
leucocyte immunoglobulin-like receptors (LILR) 211
leucocytes 4303
abnormalities in cancer 4550
acidosis 1745
depletion 293
extravasation *289*
migration defects 253
recruitment 286
see also various types
leucocytotoxic testing 2255
leucodystrophies 4960, 5103
adult-onset 4960
autosomal dominant 5111
childhood-onset 4960
classic dysmyelinative 5104
globoid cell *see* Krabbe's disease
hypomyelinative 5106
metachromatic 1698, 4961, 5104
leucoencephalopathy
with ataxia, hypodontia and hypomyelination 5107
with childhood onset 5111
hereditary diffuse with spheroids 5111
megalencephalic with subcortical cysts 5108
progressive cavitatory 5109
secondary inherited 5109
vaculoating 5107
leuconychia, cirrhosis 2498, *2498*
leucoreduction 4569
leucovorin, toxoplasmosis *1096*
leu-enkephalin 2319
leukaemia cutis 4713
leukaemias 331
acute 4223, *4224–5*
precursor lymphoid cell neoplasms 4223
arthralgia 3708
chronic *4223, 4222*, 4226
mature B-cell neoplasms 4227
mature T-cell and natural killer cell neoplasms 4227
of myeloid origin 4227
classification 4221
WHO 4222, *4222–3*, 4228
incidence *331*
molecular genetic changes 4214, *4220*
ocular involvement 5244, *5244*
pregnancy 2184
renal involvement 4063, *4063*
see also individual types
leukocytoclastic vasculitis 5162
leukoplakia 2274
aetiology 2274
clinical features 2274
pathology 2274
course and prognosis 2275
differential diagnosis 2274
treatment 2274
leuprorelin, breast cancer *1937*
levamisole, adverse effects, hepatotoxicity *2529*
levetiracetam
dose levels *4823*
epilepsy 4822
poisoning 1281
levodopa, hepatotoxicity *2529*
levofloxacin *707*
pelvic inflammatory disease *1260*
pharmacokinetics/ pharmacodynamics *452*
pneumonia *3245*
septic bursitis/arthritis *700*
levomepromazine *5423*
levonorgestrel, contraception *1267*
levosimendan, heart failure 2725
levothyroxine, in breast milk *1469*
Lewy body dementia 4803, *4805*, 4886, 5100
Leydig cells 1914
Lhermitte-Duclos disease 367
lice *see* louse infestation
lichen planopilaris 4703
lichen planus 4616, *4616–17*
actinic, photoaggravation *4670*
liver disease 4720
oral 2273
aetiology 2273
clinical features 2273, *2273*
course and prognosis 2274
differential diagnosis 2274
pathology 2273
treatment 2274
lichen sclerosus 1256
lichen simplex 1256
lichenoid reactions, drug-induced 4728
Liddle's syndrome 166, 165, 1887, 3073, 3873
lidocaine (lignocaine) *2701*
contraindication in porphyria *5484*
neuropathic pain 5415
in renal failure *4179*
Liebman-Sachs endocarditis 2738
life expectancy 73
by geographic region *74*
changes in 73
trends 73
life 4748
lifestyle changes, cancer 370
Li-Fraumeni syndrome 320–1, 358, *360*, 367
and breast cancer *1930*
ligaments 3551
lightning injury 1422
cardiovascular and pulmonary consequences 1423
epidemiology 1423
eye, ear and explosive injuries 1424
keraunoparalysis and burns 1424
mechanisms of 1423
neurological consequences 1424
presentation 1423
psychological consequences 1425
treatment 1425
Lignac's disease *3739*
likelihood ratio *99*
lily of the valley, drug intractions *69*
limber neck 804
limb-girdle muscular dystrophies 5130, *5131–2, 5201, 5204*
cardiac involvement *2788*
clinical approach *5201*, 5201
dominant *5201*
investigations 5204, *5205*
management 5206
recessive *5192*
limbic encephalitis *384*, 5171, *5172*
LIMIT-2 trial 42
Limnatis nilotica 1238
lindane poisoning 1304
linear IgA disease *4603*, 4607, *4608*
in pregnancy 2153
linezolid *707*
bacteraemia *703, 705*
cellulitis, mastitis and pyomyositis *699*
endocarditis *704–5*
epidural abscess *702*
impetigo *697*
mode of action *443*
osteomyelitis *701*
P. multocida 779
pneumonia *702, 3238, 3245*
in renal failure *4185*
septic bursitis/arthritis *700*
spectrum of activity *446*
toxic shock syndrome *697*
urinary tract infection *702*
Linguatula serrata 1237
Linguatula spp. 1237
clinical features 1237
linitis plastica 2215
linkage analysis 362
lip, cancer 312
lipid bilayers 128
membrane proteins *132*
lipid disorders 1652
lipid peroxidation 2475, *2476*
lipid rafts 285
lipid transport 1655
lipid-modifying drugs 1670
lipids
absorption 2229
and coronary heart disease 2889
cholesterol and LDL cholesterol 2889
genes and environment 2890, *2891*
HDL cholesterol and apolipoproteins 2890
daily intake *1480*
links with carbohydrates 1484
metabolism 1483, *1484, 2442, 2442*
circulating fats 1483
diabetes mellitus type 1, 2000
dietary fat 1484
disorders of 5216
insulin effects 1995

nonesterified fatty acids and energy transport 1484
in pregnancy 2081
physiology 1652–3
requirements 1539
serum concentrations 1659, *1660*
stores *1480*
lipodermatosclerosis *3089*
lipodystrophies 1995
lipodystrophy
partial 3993, *3994*
total *2766*
lipoedema 3088, *3090*
lipogranulomatosis 1698
lipohypertrophy 2011, 2013
lipoid (lipid) pneumonia 3452
endogenous 3454
exogenous 3453
aetiology 3453
clinical features 3453, *3453*
prevention and treatment 3453
post-bronchography 3466
lipoid adrenal hyperplasia 1898
Liponyssoides sanguineus 909
lipopolysaccharide 154
lipoprotein lipase 1656, *1656*, 2602
lipoprotein(a) 1657
lipoproteins *1655*
disorders of 1652
metabolism 2442, *2442*
physiology 1654
raised concentrations *see* hyperlipoproteinaemia
reference values *5444*
structure 1654, *1654*
Lipoptena cervi (deer fly) *1227*
Lipoptena cervi 1226, *1226–7*, 1236
lipotoxicity 2004
liquorice root
drug interactions *69*
toxicity 68
Lisbon Declaration *5360*
lisinopril
adverse effects, hepatotoxicity *2529*
heart failure *2722*
migraine prevention *4916*
lissencephaly 5140
cobblestone 5140
Listeria spp. *962*
immunosuppressed patients 3959
pregnancy 2169
Listeria grayi 898
Listeria innocua 898
Listeria ivanovii 898
Listeria monocytogenes 896, 898
Listeria seeligeri 898
Listeria welshimeri 898
listeriosis 896
aetiology and genetics 896
areas of uncertainty 898
clinical features 897
diagnostic criteria 898
differential diagnosis 897
epidemiology 897
food industry 898
future developments 898
history 896
pathogenesis/pathology 896
prevention 897
prognosis 898
treatment 898
lithium 5333
adverse effects 5333, *5334*
in breast milk *1469, 2189*
drug interactions *1471*, 5334
indications and use 5333
and iodine uptake 2068
poisoning 1289, 4013
clinical features 4014
diagnosis and treatment 4014
pathogenesis and pathology 4013
in renal failure 4181
serum levels *5449*
teratogenicity *1468, 2187*
therapeutic drug monitoring 1475, *1475*
thyrotoxicosis 1840
toxicity *3745*, 5334
renal *3860*
livedo reticularis *2967, 3659*, 4633, *4633, 4686*
livedoid vasculopathy 4633, *4634*
liver biopsy
hepatocellular carcinoma 2515
Wilson's disease 1691
liver cancer 315
incidence *301, 316*
migrants vs residents *302*
liver disease
alcoholic *see* alcoholic liver disease
α_1-antitrypsin deficiency 1781–2, *1782*
chronic
acute abdomen 2236
in pregnancy 2126
congenital hepatic fibrosis 2581
cystic fibrosis 3362
drug-induced 2527, *2528–9*
folate deficiency 4414
haematological changes 4555, *4557, 4557*
hyperlipidaemia 1667
immunocompromised patients 3961
intestinal failure-associated 1542, *1542*
lactic acidosis 1746
leptospirosis 875
malaria 1063
nutrition support 1543
and osteomalacia 3739
polycystic 2581, *2581*
pregnancy 2125, *2126*
abnormal liver blood tests *2131*
acute fatty liver 2105, 2127
Budd-Chiari syndrome 2130
cholelithiasis 2130
chronic liver disease 2131
clinical features/laboratory variables *2130*
effects of pregnancy on laboratory tests *2126*
HELLP syndrome 2096, 2128, 3862
hyperemesis gravidarum *see* hyperemesis gravidarum
hypertension-associated 2128, *2129*
intrahepatic cholestasis of pregnancy 2126
jaundice 2129
liver tumour 2131
post-liver transplantation 2132
variceal haemorrhage 2131
viral hepatitis 2130, *2131*
skin involvement 4719
hair, nail and collagen changes 4720
lichen planus 4720
pigmentary changes 4719
porphyria cutanea tarda 4720
pruritus 4719
vascular changes 4720
ulcerative colitis 2378
liver enzymes, coeliac disease 2338
liver failure 5151
acid-base disorders 1748
acute hepatic coma 5151
and immunodeficiency *244*
liver transplantation 2507
presentation 5472, *5473*
Wilson's disease 1692
liver flap 2495, *2496*, 3890
liver flukes 1212, *1213*
liver function tests, SLE 3661
liver transplantation 2505
assessment and waiting period 2506
future of 2512
immune suppression 2510, *2511*
indications 2506, *2506*
alcoholic liver disease 2479, 2507
autoimmune hepatitis 2507
Budd-Chiari syndrome 2508
hepatobiliary malignancy 2507
hepatocellular carcinoma 2516
inborn errors of metabolism 1555
liver failure 2507
metabolic/genetic disease 2508
nonalcoholic steatohepatitis 2507
primary biliary cirrhosis 2467, 2507
primary sclerosing cholangitis 2507
viral hepatitis 2459, 2463, 2507
Wilson's disease 1693
post-transplant course 2509
acute rejection and graft-vs-host disease 2510
anastomotic complications 2509
chronic rejection 2510
malignancy 2510
osteodystrophy 2510
renal failure and cardiovascular disease 2510
sepsis 2509
pregnancy after 2132
procedure 2508
anaesthesia 2509
donor organ 2508
surgery 2508
recurrent disease 2511
alcoholic liver disease 2512
autoimmune hepatitis 2511
hepatitis B 2511
hepatitis C 2511
primary biliary cirrhosis 2512
primary sclerosing cholangitis 2511
liver tumours 2512
benign 2520
angiomyolipoma 2521
biliary cystadenoma 2521
focal nodular hyperplasia 2520, *2521*
haemangioma 2520, *2520*
hepatic adenoma 2520, *2521–2*
lymphangioma 2521
mesenchymal hamartoma 2521
cholangiocarcinoma 2517
drug-induced *2536*, 2536
hepatoblastoma 2517
hepatocellular carcinoma *see* hepatocellular carcinoma
in pregnancy 2131
secondary 2522
vascular 2519
angiosarcoma 2519, *2519*
hepatic epithelioid haemangioendothelioma 2520
liver 2435
cellular elements 2438
endothelial lining cells 2438
hepatic stellate cells 2439
Kupffer cells 2439
pit cells 2439
effects of malnutrition 1510
functional anatomy 2437
biliary canaliculi 2437, *2438*
sinusoids 2437, *2438*
structural organization 2437, *2437*
metabolic processes 2440
amino acid and ammonia metabolism 2442
bile salt metabolism 2441
bilirubin metabolism 2441, *2441*
carbohydrate metabolism 2441, *2441*
lipid and lipoprotein metabolism 2442, *2442*
protein synthesis 2442
morphological anatomy 2435
lobes 2435, *2436*
lymphatics 2436
nerve supply 2437
vascular 2436, *2436*
physiological processes 2439
bile formation 2440, *2440*
blood flow 2439
sinusoidal perfusion 2439
pregnancy 2077
spontaneous rupture 2128
regeneration 2501
tumours, metastatic 386
vascular disorders 2585
congestive hepatopathy 2585
hepatic artery aneurysm 2586
ischaemic hepatopathy 2586
portal vein thrombosis 2586
see also biliary tract
Living Planet Index 83
lizards, venomous 1343, *1343*
loa loa 1145
see also loiasis
loading doses 1455
Lobo's disease 1008, *1008*
Lobocraspis griseifulva 1236
Lobocraspis griseifulva 1236
locked-in syndrome 4843, *4844*, 4931
LOD score 362
Loeys-Dietz syndrome 2839, *2839, 3721*, 3752, 3776
see also Marfan's syndrome
Löffler's syndrome 3429
Löfgren's syndrome 3404, 3407
loiasis 1150
clinical features 1151, *1152*

renal toxicity *4086*, 4088
epidemiology 1151, *1151*
laboratory diagnosis 1152
parasitology 1150
prevention 1152
treatment 1152
loin pain haematuria syndrome 5303
loin pain 3853
loin pain-haematuria syndrome 3853
lomefloxacin *707*
lomustine
carcinogenesis *307*
lymphoma *4320*
Lone Star tick 915
long QT syndrome 163, 166, 2611, 2713
acute management 2713
aetiology 2713, *2713*
congenital 2714, *2714*
ECG characteristics 2713, *2713*
Lonomia obliqua 1351
loop of Henle 3809, *3813, 3814*
loperamide 2433, *2433*
lopinavir
HIV/AIDS 636
toxicity *640*
lopinvir, HIV/AIDS *638*
loratadine 3282
lorazepam 3156
lordoscoliosis, osteogenesis imperfecta *3747*
Lorenzo's oil 1723, 1882
losartan
gout 3644
Raynaud's phenomenon *3671*
loss-of-function mutations 138, 361
lotions 4732
Louis, Pierre 10
Louis-Bar syndrome 4692
louping ill virus *566*, 574
louse infestation 1230, *1230*
body lice 1231
head lice 1231, *1231*
pubic lice 1231, *1231*
louse-borne relapsing fever 866
clinical features 870, *870–1*
epidemiology 867
prevention 873
treatment 872
lovastatin 1670
low back pain *see* back pain
low birth weight, child mortality *75*
low density lipoprotein (LDL) *1656–7*, 1659, *1753*
extracorporeal removal 1671
reference values *5444*
low molecular weight heparin
acute coronary syndromes 2919, *2920*
pregnancy 2117–18, *2120*
in renal failure 4180
venous thromboembolism 3019
low-copy repeats 138, 144
fork stalling and template switching 145
microdeletion and microduplication syndromes 144
nonallelic homologous recombination 144
nonhomologous end joining 145
recombination hot spots 144
Lowe's syndrome *3739, 4149*
Lown-Ganong-Levine syndrome 2652, 2709
loxapine, adverse effects, hepatotoxicity *2529*
Loxosceles laeta (South American recluse spider) *1353*
LRP5, 3722
Lucilia spp. *1233*
Lucio's leprosy 841
Ludwig's angina 2258
lumbar puncture 4749, *5514, 5518*
complications 4750
contraindications 4749
meningitis 4984, *4985*
raised intracranial pressure 3150
lumbosacral radiculopathy, postirradiation 5073
lumefantrine *1074*, 1075
lung biopsy 3206, 3217, 3220
diffuse parenchymal lung disease 3373
lung cancer 3525
percutaneous 3225, *3225*
percutaneous needle 3526
pulmonary fibrosis 3379
transbronchial 3525
transoesophageal 3525
lung cancer 318, 3456
aetiology 3515
occupation 318, *3516, 3516*
pollution 319, 3516
radon 320
smoking 299, 3515
biology 3517
clinical features 3518, *3518–19*
extrapulmonary, intrathoracic 3519
extrathoracic metastatic 3520, *3521–2*
intrapulmonary 3518, *3519–21*
diagnosis, bronchoscopy 3222
epidemiology 3515
general management 3531
genetics 3517
geographical differences 320
HIV-related 3252
incidence *301, 318*
migrants vs residents *302*
investigations 3524, *3525*
biopsy 3525
bronchoscopy 3524
CT 3524
lung function tests 3526
PET 3526
radiological assessment 3524
sputum cytology 3524
thoracoscopy 3526
metastatic 387, 1932
survival *3534*
mortality *318, 3515*
non-small cell, staging *388*
paramalignant syndromes 3521
endocrine/metabolic manifestations 3521
finger clubbing and hypertrophic pulmonary osteo-arthropathy 3523, *3523*
neuromyopathies 3523
pathology 3516
adenocarcinoma 3517
bronchioloalveolar carcinoma 3517
large-cell carcinoma 3517
small-cell anaplastic carcinoma 3517
squamous (epidermoid) carcinoma 3516
prevention 3531
prognosis 3527, *3530, 3530*
screening 3531
staging *3525, 3527, 3527*
systemic sclerosis *3672*
treatment 3527
bronchoscopy 3223
chemotherapy 3529–30
duration of 3531
intensity of 3531
non-small-cell lung cancer 3527
radiotherapy 3528, 3530
small-cell lung cancer 3530
surgery *3525*, 3527, *3528*, 3530
lung disease *see* pulmonary disease
lung flukes 1216
lung function tests 3189
acute respiratory failure 3135
airway resistance 3190
airways obstruction 3255, *3255–6*
bronchiolitis obliterans 3384
carbon monoxide uptake 3194, *3194–5*
diffuse pulmonary lung disease 3371
dynamic 3178
exercise testing 3190, 3199
forced expiration 3192
forced expiratory volume 3192
forced vital capacity 3192
functional residual capacity 3174, 3190
interpretation of 3194
lung cancer 3526
lung elasticity 3190, *3191*
lung volume 3191
normal vs abnormal 3195, *3195*
occupational asthma 3293, *3294*
organizing pneumonia 3385
peak expiratory flow rate 3192
pulmonary arterial hypertension 2985
pulmonary fibrosis 3378
reference values 3194
respiratory muscles 3193
sarcoidosis 3409
ventilation 3190
lung function, and gravity 3180
lung injury, acute 3132
lung transplantation 3476
complications 3483
airway-related 3484, *3484–5*
gastro-oesophageal reflux 3484
malignancy 3484
donor selection 3477
donor/recipient matching 3478
immunosuppression 3481
antiproliferative agents 3482
calcineurin inhibitors 3482
corticosteroids 3482
induction agents 3482
indications
bronchiectasis 3351
COPD 3344
cystic fibrosis 3363, *3363, 3478*
Eisenmenger's syndrome *3478*
pulmonary fibrosis 3381, *3478*
pulmonary hypertension *3478*
long-term monitoring 3482
outcome 3484
postoperative care 3480
early extubation 3480
early mobilization 3480
fluid restriction and diuresis 3480
nutrition 3480
prevention of infection 3480, *3481*
recipient selection 3477, *3478*
rejection 3483
acute 3483
chronic 3483, *3483*
hyperacute (antibody-mediated) 3483
surgery 3478, *3479*
transplant process 3477
lung volume 3174
abnormalities of *3191–2*, 3192
COPD 3329
dynamic control of 3172, *3172*
measurement of 3191
inert gas dilution 3191
whole-body plethysmography 3192
in pregnancy 2121
reduction surgery 3343
lung
elastic properties 3174, *3190, 3191*
functional residual capacity 3174
functional unit 3179
gas exchange in 3173
infections, anaerobic 751
lymphocytic infiltrations 3431
mechanical instability 3179
residual volume 3174
surface tension 3179
surfactant 3142, *3180, 3180*
thoracic cavity 3174
total lung capacity 3174
vital capacity 3174
lupus anticoagulant 4554
lupus erythematosus
cutaneous 4634
acute 4636
aetiology and pathogenesis 4634
chronic 4635, *4636–8*
classification 4635, *4635*
clinical investigation 4638
differential diagnosis 4637
nonspecific signs 4636, *4639*
pathology 4635
in pregnancy 2153
prognosis 4639
subacute 4635, *4638*
treatment 4639, *4639*
discoid 2278, 4703
photoaggravation *4670*
systemic *see* systemic lupus erythematosus
lupus nephritis 4045
antiphospholipid antibody nephropathy 4050
clinical presentation 4045
diagnosis 4046, *4046–7*
long-term outcome 4050
pathogenesis 4045
prognostic factors 4054
treatment 4046
immunosuppressants 4047–8, *4048*
plasma exchange 4049
lupus pernio *3407*
lupus vulgaris *4674*
lupus, with glomerulonephritis *143*

lusitropism, positive 2618
luteinizing hormone (LH) 1790, 1799, 1808, 1903, 1914
deficiency 1809
insensitivity *1917*
measurement 1803
menstrual cycle 1904
in polycyclic ovary syndrome 1908
reference values *5441*
Lutembacher's syndrome 2852
Luteococcus spp. *962*
Lutzomyia spp. *1226*
Lutzomyia verrucarum 935
LY450139, *1939*
Lycoperdon spp. *3436*
Lyell's syndrome 4586
Lyme borreliosis 860
clinical features 861
acrodermatitis chronica atrophicans 863
carditis 862
erythema migrans 861, *862*
neurological disease 863
rheumatological disease 863
coinfection 863
epidemiology 861
Eurasian *862*
laboratory diagnosis 863
neuropathy 5091
North American *862*
prevention 864
reinfections 863
treatment 864, *864–5*
Lyme carditis 2763
Lyme disease, pregnancy *2171*
lymecycline, acne *4680*
lymph cysts, traumatic 4696
lymph nodes 4312, *4312*
lymphadenectomy, penile cancer 4173
lymphadenitis 833
filarial 1156
lymphadenopathy 3542, 4314
evaluation 4315
biopsy 4315
genetic studies 4316
immunohistochemistry and flow cytometry 4316
lymphangiectasia, intestinal 2221, 2251, *2251*, 2400, 4696
lymphangiogenesis 4694
lymphangiography, complications 3466
lymphangioleiomyomatosis 3447, *3448*
lymphangioma 2521, *4687, 4695, 4696*
acquired 4696
lymphangiosarcoma 4696
lymphangitis 4695
filarial 1156
lymphatic disorders 4694
lymphatic drainage, manual 3090
lymphatic oedema 2994, 2997
lymphatic tuberculosis 819
lymphocytes *4196*, 4312
development, block in *242*
infants and children *4197*
intraepithelial 2245
lamina propria 2246
localization 230
ontogeny 4313, *4314*
see also B cells; T cells
lymphocytic choriomeningitis
clinical features 592
epidemiology 589
transplantation-associated 592
treatment 595
lymphocytic colitis 2376
lymphocytic hypophysitis 2141
lymphocytic interstitial pneumonitis 3432
autoimmune rheumatic disorders *3390*
lymphocytosis 4314
large granular 4308
lymphoedema 1156, *1855, 4694, 4694*
cobblestone papillomatosis *3088*
facial 3091
filarial 4695
genital 3091
primary 3085
secondary 3085
see also oedema
lymphogranuloma venereum 946, 1247
clinical features 946, *946*
diagnosis 947, *947*
epidemiology 946
treatment 947
lymphohistiocytosis, familial haemophagocytic *238*
lymphoid cells 209
natural killer (NK) cells 209
NKT cells 210
lymphoma 3432, 4317
anaplastic large T/null-cell 4332
angiocentric 3401, 3433
arthralgia 3708
B-cell 4328
high-grade 3433
low-grade 3433
Burkitt's 300, 502
translocations *341*
clinical features
hypercalcaemia *3745*
ocular 5244
cutaneous 4333, 4712
diagnosis 4318, *4319*
diffuse large B-cell 4328, *4334*
evaluation 4318, *4319*
follicular 4326, *4327*, 4329
gastrointestinal 2342
genetics 4320, *4320*
herpetic stomatitis 431, 439
HIV-related 631, 3251
Hodgkin's *see* Hodgkin's lymphoma
immunology 4319, *4319*
lymphoblastic of B-cell/T-cell origin 4328
MALT 4334
mantle-cell 4328, *4328*
misdiagnosis 383, *386*
NK-cell 507
non-Hodgkin's *see* non-Hodgkin's lymphoma
pathobiology 4319
pregnancy 2184
presenting symptoms 4318
renal involvement 4063, *4063*
small intestine 2222, *2222*
small lymphocytic *4328*, 4328
staging *4319*
T-cell 507
enteropathy-associated 2338
peripheral *4328*, 4328
thymus 3541
thyroid 1850
treatment *3433, 4320, 4321, 4322*
lymphoma-like disorders 4333
lymphomatoid
granulomatosis 3401, 3433
vasculitis 5162
lymphopenia, SLE 3659
lymphoproliferative disorders 4314, *4315*
lymphadenopathy 4314
lymphocytosis 4314
post-transplant 3962, *3962*
lymphoscintigraphy 3089, *3090*
lymphotoxin 156
lymphuria 1156, *1157*
Lynch's syndrome 344, 361, 364
Lyon hypothesis 1568
Lyophyllum aggregatum *3436*
lysergic acid diethylamide (LSD), poisoning 1289
lysine intolerance *1566*
lysine, reference values *5446*
lysinuric protein intolerance 4147, *4148*
lysoglobotriaosylceramide 1969
lysolecithin 1654
lysophosphatidylcholine 1654
lysosomal diseases *1552, 1553*, 1694, *3720, 3756, 5117, 5118*
classification 1696
functional 1696
glycoproteinoses 1697
glycosphingolipidoses 1697
mucopolysaccharidoses *see* mucopolysaccharidoses
multiple defects 1697
clinical presentation 1703
natural course and severity 1703
neurological features 1704
organomegaly 1703
skeletal manifestations 1704
diagnosis 1703
biochemical 1706
clinical suspicion and family history 1704
molecular 1706
pathology 1705, 1706
radiology 1704
pathophysiology 1697
cellular dysfunction 1697
primary substrate storage 1696
secondary metabolites 1969
tissue and organ malfunction 1703
treatment 1706
augmentation of deficient activity 1707
enzyme replacement therapy 1708
haematopoietic stem cell transplantation 1708
pharmacological chaperones 1708
restriction of substrate flux 1705
supportive and palliative care 1709
see also various types and individual diseases
lysosomal function 1694, 1695
antigen presentation 1696
autophagy 1703
endocytosis and membrane flow 1695
phagocytosis 1695
lysosomal hydrolases 1696
lysosomal protease defects 1698
lysosomal transport defects 1698
lysosomes 130
lysozyme 1775
lyssaviruses 554
African 554
Australian bat *554*, 554
European bat 554
see also rabies

macrobiotic diet 65
macrocephaly 5139
macrochimerism 292
macrocysts of breast 1941
macrocytosis *4195*
macrolides
adverse effects *455*
cystic fibrosis 3360
mode of action *443*
pregnancy *2172*
macromolecular crowding 127
macronutrients 1479
gene regulation of metabolism *1482*
regulation of flux 1479, *1480–1*
macrophage infectivity potentiator (mip) protein 899
macrophages 152, *208, 288*
recognition of apoptotic cells 185, *185*
macular degeneration
genome association 141
X-linked, differential diagnosis *1722*
macules *4591*
maculopapular eruption 4726
maculopathy, diabetic 2034
Madrid virus *581*
Madura foot 999, 1004
aetiology 1004
causes *1005*
clinical features 1005, *1005*
epidemiology 1004
laboratory diagnosis 1005
treatment 1005
Madura madurellae, osteomyelitis *3789*
Maffucci's syndrome 4692
Magendie, François 11, *11*
magenta manufacture *1380*
MAGE-related genes 375
magic mushrooms 1368, *1368*
MAGIC trial 42
magnesium hydroxide *5426*
magnesium *1498*, 1499
CKD-MBD *3922*
dietary reference values *1502*
intravenous 3308
in myocardial infarction 42, *42*
physiological control 4143
plasma/serum *3837*
reference values *5435, 5446*
urinary *3837*
magnesium-handling disorders 4140, *4143, 4144–5*
magnetic brain stimulation 4782
central motor conduction time 4783
cerebrovascular disease 4784
children 4784

degenerative neurological diseases 4784
magnetic stimulators 4782
motor neuron disease 4784
movement disorders 4784
multiple sclerosis *4784*, 4783
neurosurgical monitoring 4785
physiology 4782
safety of 4783
spinal cord lesions 4784
magnetic resonance angiography, renal disease 3880
magnetic resonance imaging (MRI)
Alzheimer's disease *4804*
ankylosing spondylitis 3609, *3609*
aortic dissection *2956*
arrhythmogenic right ventricular cardiomyopathy 2780, *2781*
cardiac 2671, 2674
clinical uses 2674, *2675*
chest 3200, *3203, 3204*
Crohn's disease *2223*
Cushing's disease *1877–8*
dilated cardiomyopathy 2776
epilepsy 4818, *4818*
lymphoedema 3089
multiple sclerosis 4956
neurological disorders
historical perspective *4770*, 4769
stroke *4772*
transient ischaemic attack *4774*
osteomyelitis *3792*
pancreatic tumours 2576
Parkinson's disease 4882
pleural effusion 3490
polymyositis/ dermatomyositis 3697, *3697*
pregnancy 2109
pulmonary embolism 3012, *3013*
pyogenic arthritis *3619*
renal disease 3878, *3874, 3879*
nephrogenic systemic fibrosis 3879
rheumatic disorders 3565
sarcoidosis *3408*
small intestine 2220
magnetic resonance urography, urinary tract obstruction 4154
magnetic resonance venography, renal disease 3880
Maguari virus *581*
Mahaim-type ventricular pre-excitation 2652, 2709
major histocompatibility complex
class I
deficiency *238*, 252
II 229, 225–6
class II, autoimmune disease 268
diversity 229
mal de Meleda *4599*
malabsorption 2326, 2220, 2321
amyloidosis 2221, *2221*
causes *2328*
coeliac disease *see* coeliac disease
diagnosis 2327
differential diagnosis 2327, *2328*
disaccharidase deficiency 2347
and drug absorption 1456
examination 2327
gastrointestinal lymphoma 2342
history 2327
investigation 2328
coeliac disease testing 2329
endoscopy and small bowel histology 2329
function tests 2328
microbiology 2329
radiology 2329
osteomalacia 3739
response to treatment 2329
small bowel resection 2354
small-bowel bacterial overgrowth 2330
tropical syndromes 2357
Whipple's disease *see* Whipple's disease
Maladera matrida 1235
malakoplakia 2589, 4120
malaria 1045
acquired resistance 1060, *1060*
child mortality *75*
clinical features 1046, 1064
anaemia 1063, *1065, 1067*
falciparum malaria 1064, *1065*
malnutrition 1061
nephrotoxicity 3859, 4084
congenital/neonatal 1070
diagnosis 1047, 1071
differential diagnosis 1071, *1071*
epidemiology 1046, 1055
changing face of 1057
spatial limits 1055, *1056*
varied intensity of transmission 1056
haematological changes 4552, *4552*
HIV-related 648, 1061
immunity and innate resistance 1046, 1059
immunological complications 1081
endemic Burkitt's lymphoma 1082
quartan malarial nephrosis 1081
tropical splenomegaly syndrome 1081
laboratory diagnosis 1072–3
microscopy 1072, *1072*
rapid malarial antigen detection 1073
serological techniques 1073
in monkeys 1069
morbidity 1059
mortality *121*, 1059
mosquito vector *see Anopheles* spp.
organ pathology 1062
bone marrow 1062
brain *1061*, 1062, 1065
gastrointestinal tract 1063
heart 1063
kidney 1063
liver 1063
lung 1063
placenta 1063
retina 1062
spleen 1063
parasite *see Plasmodium* spp.
pathology 1046, *1061, 1061–2*
pathophysiology 1046, 1063
acute renal failure 1064
anaemia and thrombocytopenia 1063
cerebral malaria 1063
hypoglycaemia 1064
hyponatraemia 1064
hypovolaemia and shock 1064
pulmonary oedema 1064
in pregnancy 1058, 1070
pregnancy 2171
presentation 5495
prevention 1047, 1082
access to medicines 1084
indoor residual house spraying 1084
insecticide-treated nets 1083
intermittent preventive treatment 1084
reducing vector abundance 1084
repellents 1084
in travellers *468, 1086, 1085, 1086*
vaccines 1085
prognosis 1081
public health burden 1057, *1058*
renal involvement 4075
transmission 1045
blood transfusion 1070
needlestick 1070
nosocomial 1070
treatment 1047, 1073
chemotherapy 1073, *1074*
falciparum malaria *1074*, 1077, *1078*
in pregnancy 1080
malarial glomerulopathy 4084
clinical features 4085
management 4086
pathogenesis 4085
pathology 4085
malarial psychosis 1068
Malassezia globosa 998
Malassezia spp. 1002
malathion, louse infestation 1231
male reproductive disorders 1913
aetiology *1917*
classification *1917*
hypogonadism 1913, 1916
infertility 1913, 1922
aetiology 1922
diagnosis 1924
treatment 1925
malignant hypertension 3076, *3076*
malignant hyperthermia 164, 1474
malignant melanoma *see* melanoma
malingering 5303
Mallory-Weiss tears 2238, *2238*, 2302
malnutrition 1505, 1515
aetiology 1509
antioxidant protection 1511
classification 1505, *1507*
clinical presentation 1508
clinical syndromes 1507, *1507*
and diabetes mellitus 2007
diarrhoea 1513
effects of
body function 1509
body structure 1509
facility-based care 1512, *1512*
phases of treatment *1506*, 1512, *1512*
resuscitation 1513
general care 1514
identification 1508
management *1506*, 1513
maternal 2080, *2081*
measles-related 522
mortality *1506*
natural history 1508
oedema 1511, *1512*
pathophysiology 1509
prevention 1505, 1508
recovery syndrome 1514
reductive adaptation 1509
functional and metabolic cost 1510
replacing lost weight 1514
screening 1508, *1536*
severe acute 1505, 1507
small bowel resection 2355
specific nutrient deficiencies 1511
see also nutrition
Malpolon monspessulanus (Montpellier snake) 1336
MALT lymphoma 4334
gastric 2343, *2343–4*
immunoproliferative small intestinal disease 2344
Malthus, Thomas 81
Mammomonogamus (Syngamus) laryngeus 1176, 1238
management 58–9
Mandl's disease *3804*
manganese *1498*, 1499
CNS effects *1386*
reference values *5445*
mania, older people 5407
mannitol, intracranial hypertension *3150*
mannose 6-phosphate pathway 1707
mannose-binding lectin 211, 214–15
defects 713
deficiency 217
mannosidoses *1553*, 1698
corneal opacity 1704
psychiatric signs *1720*
Mansonella (Dipetalonema) perstans 1227
Mansonella ozzardi 1227
Mansonella spp. 1145
see also mansonellosis
mansonellosis 1152
clinical features 1152
diagnosis 1152
epidemiology 1152
treatment 1153
Mansonia spp. *1226*
mantle-cell lymphoma *4328*, 4331
Mantoux test 821
MAP kinases 183
maple syrup urine disease *1566*, 1569, *1570*
diagnosis 1569
presentation 1569, *1570*
treatment and outcome 1570
marasmus 1507
maraviroc
HIV/AIDS 637, *638*
toxicity *640*
marble bone disease *see* osteopetrosis
Marburg virus *see* filoviruses
march haemoglobinuria 4460
Marchiafava Bignami syndrome 1615, 5156
Marfan's syndrome 139, 1957, 2736, *3721*, 3749, 3771, 3778
aortic dissection 2954, *2954*
aortic root dilatation 2112, *2112*
clinical features *3731, 3750–1*, 3751, 3778, *3780*, 3782
cardiac involvement 2837, *2838, 3781*
ectopia lentis *3779–80*

iridodonesis 3730, *5250, 5251*
pneumothorax 3500
scoliosis 3507
clinical management 2839
diagnosis 2838, *3751, 3778, 3779, 3784*
genetic counselling 3752
genetics 3779, *3779*
fibrillin 1 mutations 2838, *3779, 3781*
transforming growth factor β 3780, *3782*
pathophysiology 3750
prognosis 3782
treatment 3752, 3780
marine invertebrates, envenoming 1347
Cnidarians 1347, *1347*
cone shells and octopuses 1348, *1348–9*
starfish and sea urchins 1348, *1348*
Marinesco-Sjögren syndrome *4908*
Marituba virus *581*
marker chromosomes 145
Maroteaux-Lamy disease 1698
diagnosis 1706
Marrara syndrome 1237
Marshall Critical Illness Scoring System *2562*
Martorell's syndrome *see* Takayasu's arteritis
Martorell's ulcer 4633
mass communication 108
massage 65
Massilia spp. *962*
Masson bodies 3385
mast cell tryptase 3111
mast cells 209
inflammatory mediators 3109
mast-cell tryptase, reference values *5444*
mastitis 698
mastocytosis, malabsorption 2221
Mathevotaenia symmetrica 1190
matrix Gla protein 3726
matrix metalloproteinases *3550*, 3551, *3552, 4484*
COPD *3323*
matter 4748
maximin rule 56
Mayaro virus *558*, 560
MBD *see* mineral and bone disorder
McArdle's disease 1601, *1598*, 5215
McArdle's sign 5040
McCullogh, Ernest 195
McCune-Albright syndrome 1798, *1855*, 1985, 4143
and Cushing's syndrome 1872, *1872*
hyperpigmentation 4660, *4660*
McLeod's syndrome 5114
Meaban virus *566*
mean arterial pressure *2621*, 3125
mean cell haemoglobin concentration *4196*
infants and children *4197*
mean cell haemoglobin *4196*
infants and children *4197*
mean cell volume *4196*
infants and children *4197*
measles 515
child mortality *75*
clinical features 519, *520*
oral 2264
prodrome 519, *520*
rash 519, *521–2*
complications 520
diagnosis 523
elimination/eradication 524
epidemiology 516, *516*
immunization *91, 517, 523*
pathogenesis and immune response 517, *518–19*
at-risk groups 519, *519*
persistent infection 522
popular beliefs 517
prevention 523
treatment 523
virus and antigens 517, *518*
mebendazole
adverse effects, hepatotoxicity *2529*
ascariasis 1170
cystic hydatid disease 1188
mansonellosis 1153
trichuriasis 1176
mechanic's hands 3694, *3694*
mechanical circulatory support 2729, 2732
mechanical ventilation
acute respiratory failure *3138*, 3139, *3140*
complications *3140*
high frequency 3144
indications *3136*
lung protection 3144
modes of *3138*, 3139
pregnancy 2124
prone positioning 3144
weaning from 3140
mechlorethamine, lymphoma *4320*
Meckel's diverticulum 2401
Meckel-Gruber syndrome 5142
meclofenamate, and asthma *3289*
meconium ileus 2401
mecysteine 3337
median nerve neuropathy 5081, *5082*
mediastinal masses 3539
anatomy 3539, *3539–40*
anterior 3541
germ-cell tumours 3541
thymus 3541
thyroid masses 3542
clinical features 3540, *3541*
investigations 3540
biopsy 3540
radiological assessment 3540
middle 3542
lymphadenopathy 3542
mediastinal cysts 3543
posterior 3543
mediastinum
chest X-ray 3206, *3206*
CT imaging 3208, *3209*
drug reactions 3466
medical ethics *see* ethics
medical screening *see* screening
Medic-Alert bracelet 1350
MedicAlert 3113
medically unexplained symptoms *1388*, 5296, *5297*
aetiology and pathophysiology 5298, *5298*
clinical features 5298
definition and terminology 5296
differential diagnosis 5299
epidemiology 5298
historical perspective 5297
management 5299, *5299–300*
patient assessment 5299
prevention 5298
prognosis 5300
specific syndromes 5300, *5301*
syndromes 5297, *5297*
medicines management 1451
medicines *see* drugs
Mediterranean spotted fever *912*
medium chain acyl CoA ehydrogenase deficiency, neonatal screening *104*
MEDLINE 24, 50
medroxyprogesterone acetate *1263*
medullary syndromes 4932, *4932*
medullary thyroid carcinoma 1984
clinical features 1985
Mee's lines 1297, 4701
mefenamic acid
and asthma *3289*
poisoning 1290
mefenanic acid, contraindication in porphyria *5484*
mefloquine 1075
prophylactic *1086*, 1087
megacolon, Chagas' disease 1133
megakaryocytes, progenitors in disease 4207
megakaroycytopoiesis 4206, 4281
circulating platelets 4207
thrombopoietin 4206
megaloblastic anaemia 4402
acquired 4418
acquired disturbances of cobalamin or folate metabolism 4417
biochemical analysis *4406*, 4407
clinical features and causes 4407, *4407–8*
congenital 4418
inborn errors of metabolism 4417
laboratory investigation 4414, *4414–15*
pregnancy 2174
skin involvement 4558
treatment 4416
Megalopyge spp. 1351
megaoesophagus, Chagas' disease 1132
Megasalia spp. *1233*
Megasphaera spp. *962*
mega-trials 35
megestrol acetate, breast cancer *1937*
meglitinides 2014
adverse effects 2015
efficacy and potency 2011
indications and contraindications 2015
mode of action 2011
pharmacokinetics 2015
meglumine antimoniate, leishmaniasis *1138, 1139*
Meigs' syndrome 2483, 3085
melaena 2238, *2238*, 2309
melan-A 376
melanin, synthesis *4657*
melanocytic naevi (moles)
acquired 4706, *4707*
congenital 4707
melanocytosis 4660
melanoma 321, *4710, 4711*
aetiology and genetics 4710
clinical features 4711, *4711*
clinical investigation 4712
differential diagnosis 4712
epidemiology 4711
genes associated with *363*
genetic predisposition 365
incidence *301, 322*
pathogenesis/pathology 4710
pregnancy 2184
prevention 4711
prognosis 4712
treatment 4712
see also skin cancer
melarsoprol
adverse reactions *1125*
trypanosomiasis 1124, *1124–5*
MELAS syndrome *1552, 1855*, 1865, *2766, 5223*
melasma 2149, *2150*, 4658
melatonin 2071
circadian rhythms 2071
pharmaceutical use 2071
photoperiodism 2071
melioidosis 768
clinical features 768, *769*
clinical investigation 769, *770*
diagnosis 768
differential diagnosis 768
epidemiology and aetiology 768
future developments 771
genetics and pathogenesis 768
management 770, *771*
prevention 768
prognosis and outcome 770
Melkersson-Rosenthal syndrome 2278
Meloidogyne (Heterodera) spp. *1176*
Melophagus ovinus 1226
melorheostosis 3714
meloxicam
ankylosing spondylitis 3610
rheumatoid arthritis *3594*
melphalan *338*, 398
carcinogenesis *307*
membrane attack complex 215
membrane cofactor protein *216*
membrane receptors, signalling by 1791, *1791, 1793*
membranes, biological 132, *132*
biological, fluid mosaic model 132
membranous cytoplasmic bodies 1706
membranous nephropathy 3985, 4077
aetiology 3985, *3986*
clinical presentation 3986
with crescentic glomerulonephritis 3987
renal vein thrombosis 3987
pathogenesis 3986
pathology 3986, *3986*
prognosis 3988
treatment 3987–8
untreated, clinical evolution 3987
memory 4791
episodic *4789*, 4792, *4792*
semantic 4792
working 4791
MEN *see* multiple endocrine neoplasia
men, reproductive system, occupational disease 1385
Menangle virus 526

Mendel, Gregor 136
Mendelian inheritance 138
penetrance, expressivity and age of onset 139
Menière's disease *4863*
meningioma, pregnancy 2147
meningitis 709
bacterial 4976
aetiology 4977, *4978*
clinical features 4982
clinical investigations 4984
community-acquired 4982, *4983*
differential diagnosis 4984
emergency management 4986, *4987–9*
epidemiology 4981
genetics 4978, *4978*
pathogenesis 4978
pathology 4980, *4980*
post-traumatic 4984
prevention 4981
prognosis 4991
recurrent 4986
shunt infections 4984
carcinomatous 390
clinical features 709
clinical presentations 715, *715*
arthritis 718
immune complex-induced 718
cutaneous vasculitis and episcleritis 718, *718–19*
distinct meningitis
and persistent shock 718
without persistent shock 715
meningococcaemia 718, *718*
ocular infections 719
pericarditis 718
persistent septic shock 716, *716–17*
pneumonia 719
cryptococcal, HIV-related 630, 1020
diagnosis 709
enterovirus 530
epidemiology 710
age distribution 711
carriage 712
developing countries 711, *712*
genetic diversity 711
industrialized countries 710
nasopharyngeal colonization 712
preceding infections 711
reservoirs of infection 712
season 711
sub-Sarahan Africa 711, *712*
H. influenzae 760, *761*
handling of clinical specimens 710
HSV 487
invasive infection 713, *713–14*
bacteraemic phase 713
rash 713, *714–15*
leptospirosis 875
Mollaret's 5003
mumps 514
pneumococcal 689
predisposing factors 712, *712*
complement system defects 713
Fcγ-receptor polymorphisms 713
lack of protective antibodies 712
mannose-binding lectin defects 713
presentation 5496
prevention 710, 721
chemoprophylaxis 4982, *4989*
immunization 4981
prognosis 709
sequelae 721
treatment 710, 719
antibiotics 719
initial hospital evaluation 719
prehospital antibiotics 719
supportive 720
tuberculous 819, 4991
viral 5002
clinical features 5002
meningocele 5137
meningococcaemia *421*
meningococcal disease, vaccines *91*, 468, *466*, *721*
meningococcal septicaemia 716, 4740
coagulopathy 717, *717*
inhibited fibrinolysis 717
laboratory findings 717
pathophysiology 716, *717*
proinflammatory and anti-inflammatory mediators 717
subarachnoid space 717
thrombus formation 717
meningoencephalitis
Israel Turkey *566*
trypanosomal *1122*, 1122
zoster 491
Meningonema peruzzii 1176
Menkes' kinky hair disease 1688, 1693, *3721*, 5103
menorrhagia 4500
menstrual cycle 1904, *1904*
Mental Capacity Act 19 2005, 3159
mental disorders
older patients 5406
delirium 5406
dementia 5407
depression 5407
mania/hypomania 5407
neurosis and personality disorders 5408
paranoid disorders 5407
Mental Health Act (2007) 3159
mental state theories 17
menthol 4733
mepacrine, adverse effects, hepatotoxicity *2529*
meperidine *see* pethidine
mercaptoacetyltriglycine (MAG3) 3881
6-mercaptopurine
Crohn's disease 2366
hepatotoxicity *2534*, 2535
mercury
reference values *5445*
reproductive effects *1917*
mercury poisoning 1300
antidote *1274*
CNS effects *1386*
peripheral nervous system effects *1387*, 5087
renal effects 1384
mercy killing 19
MERFF *2766*, 5102, *5223*
Mermis nigrescens 1176
meropenem
pneumonia *3238*, *3245*
Pseudomonas aeruginosa 737
in renal failure *4185*
Merulius lacrymans 3436
mesalazine
Crohn's disease 2366
ulcerative colitis 2378, *2380*
mesangiocapillary glomerulonephritis 3991, *3992*
clinical features 3994
epidemiology 3994
pathogenesis 3992
association with partial lipodystrophy 3993, *3994*
complement activation 3992
complement system 3992, *3993*
prognosis 3994
treatment 3994
mesenchymal hamartoma 2521
mesenteric ischaemia 2417, *2418*, 2963
acute 2419
chronic 2420
compression of coeliac axis 2420
compression of mesenteric vessels 2417
intestinal reperfusion injury 2420
intraluminal occlusion 2417
intrinsic vascular pathology 2418, *2418*
investigations *2235*
ischaemic colitis 2420, *2420*
nonocclusive 2419, *2419*
Mesocestoides lineatus 1190
mesocestoidiasis 1240
Mesorhizobium spp. *962*
mesothelioma 320, 3535
aetiology 3535
clinical features and diagnosis 3536
pathology 3535, *3535–6*
prognosis 3536
treatment 3536
chemotherapy 3537
multimodal 3537
pain control 3536
pleurodesis 3536, *3536*
radiotherapy 3536
messenger RNA 127
MET equivalents *2659*
meta-analysis 31, 37, 46, 51
reliability of 38
small trials 40
metabolic acidosis *3198*
acute renal trauma 3890
drug overdose *5505*
malaria 1067, *1068*, 1080
presentation 5479
treatment 1748
metabolic alkalosis *3198*
potassium and chloride deficiency 1748
treatment 1750
metabolic deficiencies *244*
metabolic syndrome 1520, *1520*, 1622, *1660*, 1997, *1997*, 2631, 2892
hypertension 3034
reproductive effects *1917*
metabolism *see* drug metabolism
metachromatic leucodystrophy 1698, 4961, 5104
diagnosis 1704
differential diagnosis *1725*
psychiatric signs *1720*
Metagonimus minutus 1222
Metagonimus miyatai 1222
Metagonimus takahashii 1222
Metagonimus yokogawai 1222, *1223*, 1223
metahexamide, adverse effects, hepatotoxicity *2529*, *2532*
metal fume fever 3457
metaldehyde poisoning 1304
metalloids, and cancer 1380
metals
and cancer 1380
poisoning 1296
see also individual metals
metanephrine, reference values *5441*
metaphyseal chondrodysplasia *3721*
mutations in *3757*
metastases, cancer 354
Metastrongylus elongatus 1176
met-enkephalin 2319
metformin 2015
pregnancy 2137
methacholine, and airway reactivity 3293
methadone
palliative care 5423
serum levels *5449*
methaemoglobin *4196*
methaemoglobinaemia 1310, 4268, 4443
antidote *1274*
genetic 4443
with haemolytic anaemia 4444
methanol
lactic acidosis 1746
metabolism *1313*
poisoning *1274*, 1313, *1742*
antidote *1274*
CNS effects *1386*
methenamine hippurate, urinary tract infection 4114
methicillin-resistant *S. aureus see* MRSA
methimazole 1840
adverse effects, hepatotoxicity *2529*, *2532–3*
methionine adenosyltransferase deficiency 1594
methionine adenosyltransferase I deficiency *1566*
methionine synthase deficiency *1566*, 1594
methionine synthase reductase deficiency *1566*, 1594
methocarbamol, opioid withdrawal *5347*
methotrexate 398
adverse effects *400*
hepatotoxicity *2534*, *2536*
renal toxicity *3860*
carcinomatous 'meningitis' 391
Crohn's disease 2367
lupus nephritis 4049
lymphoma *4320*
polymyositis/dermatomyositis 3697
pregnancy *2158*
primary biliary cirrhosis *2467*
psoriasis 4614
psoriatic arthritis 3613
resistance *399*

  rheumatoid arthritis *3595*
  sarcoidosis 3410, *3411*
  skin disorders 4738
  systemic sclerosis *3677*
  teratogenicity *1468*
methoxsalen, adverse effects, hepatotoxicity *2529*
methoxyflurane, adverse effects, hepatotoxicity *2529*
methoxypsoralen, carcinogenesis *307*
3-methoxytyramine, reference values *5441*
methyl bromide poisoning 1304
methyl chloride, hepatotoxicity *1385*
methyl mercury, CNS effects *1386*
methyl methacrylate *3436*
methyl *n*-butane ketone, peripheral nervous system effects *1387*
2-methyl-3-hydroxybutyryl-CoA dehydrogenase deficiency *1566*, 1573
  aetiology/pathology 1573
  clinical presentation 1573
  diagnosis 1573
  treatment and outcome 1573
α-methylacyl-CoA racemase 1724
  differential diagnosis *1725*
methylation, genetic variability 1474
3-methylcrotonyl aciduria, type I *1566*
3-methylcrotonylglycinuria *1566*, *1570*, *1571*
  clinical presentation 1571
  diagnosis 1571
  treatment and outcome 1572
methyldiphosphonate (MDP) 3882
methyldopa
  adverse effects, hepatotoxicity *2529*, *2532*, *2535*
  in breast milk *2101*, *2189*
  hypertension 3052
  in pregnancy *2099*
4,4'-methylene bis(2-chloraniline), hepatotoxicity *1385*
methylene chloride poisoning 1313
methylene dianiline, hepatotoxicity *1385*
methylene tetrahydrofolate reductase deficiency 1594
5,10-methylene-tetrahydrofolate reductase deficiency *1566*
3-methylglutaconic aciduria 1572
  type I, IV *1566*, 1572–3
  type II (Barth syndrome) *1566*, 1572
  type III (Costeff optic atrophy) *1566*, 1572
methylhistamine, reference values *5446*
methylmalonic aciduria *1566*, 1574
  aetiology/pathophysiology 1574
  clinical presentation 1574
  diagnosis 1575
  treatment and outcome 1575
methylmalonicaciduria 1698
Methylobacterium spp. *962*
methylphenidate
  adverse effects, hepatotoxicity *2529*
  narcolepsy *4833*
  orthostatic hypotension *5063*
methylprednisolone acetate *4734*
methylprednisolone
  COPD *3335*
  lymphoma *4320*
methylthioninium chloride *1274*
methylxanthines
  asthma 3303, *3303*
  chronic respiratory failure 3474
  COPD 3334, *3335*
methysergide, migraine prevention *4916*
metoclopramide *5423*
  adverse effects, hyperprolactinaemia 2068
  contraindication in porphyria *5484*
  drug interactions *1471*
  orthostatic hypotension *5063*
  poisoning 1289
metolazone, heart failure *2722*
metoprolol
  adverse effects, hepatotoxicity *2529*
  in renal failure *4179*
metorchiasis 1215
Metorchis conjunctus 1212, *1213*, 1215
metronidazole
  amoebiasis 1041
  anaerobic infections *753*
  animal-related injuries 1326
  bacterial overgrowth *2334*
  bacterial vaginosis 1257
  in breast milk *2189*
  C. difficile 801–2
  contraindication in porphyria *5484*
  drug interactions *1471*
  giardiasis *1113*
  gingivitis 2262
  H. pylori 2312, *2313*
  mode of action *443*
  pelvic inflammatory disease *1260*
  pharmacokinetics *449*
  in renal failure *4185*
  skin disorders 4739
  trichomoniasis 1257
metyrapone test 1876
metyrapone
  Cushing's syndrome 1880
  ectopic ACTH secretion 2063
mexiletine
  adverse effects
    hepatotoxicity *2532*
    oesophagitis *2294*
mexilitine, in renal failure *4179*
MI *see* myocardial infarction
mianserin, adverse effects, hepatotoxicity *2532*
mica pneumoconiosis 3423
miconazole
  candidiasis 1258
  fungal infections 1015
microangiopathic haemolytic anaemia *385*, 4459, *4459*
microangiopathy, thrombotic 4544, 4076
Microbacterium spp. *962*
microcephaly 5139
Micrococcus spp. *962*
microcytosis *4195*
microdeletions 144
microduplications 144
β_2-microglobulin 1775
  reference values *5444*, *5446*
micrographia, Wilson's disease 1690
Micronema deletrix *1176*
micronutrients *see* trace elements; vitamins
microorganisms 409
  adaptation to environment 411
  antigenic variation 411
  future challenges 412
  genomes 412
  nosocomial infections 429
  pathogenicity 410
  virulence vs fitness factors 411
microRNA 133, *184*
  as oncogenes 353, *354*
microsatellite instability 344
microsatellite sequences *344*
microsatellites 5371
microscopic polyangiitis *222*, 3401, *3650*, *4033*
  cardiac involvement 2785
  investigation, imaging *3399*, *3409*
  pulmonary involvement *3396*, 3401, *3409*
microsporidiosis 1111, 1115
  aetiology and genetics 1115
  clinical features 1116, *1116*
  epidemiology 1115
  historical perspective 1112
  laboratory diagnosis 1117
  pathogenesis/pathology 1115, *1115–16*
  prevention 1116
  treatment and prognosis 1117
Microsporidium africanum *1116*
Microsporidium ceylonensis *1116*
Microsporum audouinii 1000
Microsporum canis 999
Microsporum ferrugineum 1000
Microsporum gypseum *1000*
Microsporum soudanense 1000
microthrombosis 2418
microtubules 131
microvascular occlusion 4685, *4686*
Micrurus corallinus (painted coral snake) *1330*
micturition syncope 4816
micturition 3852
  anuria 3852
  frequency 3852
  nocturia 3852
  oliguria 3852
  polyuria 3852
midazolam 3156
midbrain syndromes 4930, *4930*
Middleburg virus *558*
midges 1227
midodrine, orthostatic hypotension *5063*
mifepristone, ectopic ACTH secretion 2064
miglustat 1709
Migraine Disability Assessment Score (MIDAS) *4915*
migraine 4915
  abdominal 2207
  causes, food intolerance 2254
  chronic 4923
    prevention 4924
  clinical features 4915
  diagnostic criteria *4915*
  differential diagnosis 4817
  familial hemiplegic 162
  frequent 4915
  investigations, PET *4914*
  management 4916
    acute 4917, *4917–18*
    nonpharmacological 4916
  pathophysiology *4913*
  pregnancy 2146
  prevention 4916, *4916*
  vestibular *4865*
  see also headache
milia 4706
miliaria 4678
miliary tuberculosis 820
milk-alkali syndrome 1862, *3745*
milkmaid's grip 2801
Mill, John Stuart, *On Liberty* 17
Millennium Development Goals 60, 76
Miller-Dieker syndrome 5140
millipede bites 1356, *1357*
milrinone 3130
Milroy's disease 3085
miltefosine, leishmaniasis *1138*
Mimivirus 661
mind 4746
  biology of 4747
  function 4747
  ontogeny 4747
  phylogeny 4747
mind-brain problem 4747
mineral and bone disorder 3917
  biochemical abnormalities 3920, *3922*
  pathogenesis 3918
    1,25-dihydroxy vitamin D deficiency 3918, *3918*
    phosphate excess 3918
  secondary hyperparathyroidism 3920
  symptoms and signs 3919, *3920–1*
  see also individual conditions
mineral oils *1380*
mineralocorticoid hypertension, differential diagnosis 1884, *1885*
mineralocorticoid receptor, mutations in 1888
mineralocorticoids
  deficiency 1870, *1871*, 1889, *1889*, 3842
    adrenal insufficiency 1889
    defects in aldosterone biosynthesis 1889
    hyporeninaemic hypoaldosteronism 1889
    pseudohypoaldosteronism *1871*, 1889
  excess 1870, *1871*, 1884, 3837
    apparent 1887, *1888*, 3837
    Conn's syndrome 1884
    single gene defects 1886, *1886*
  replacement therapy 1884
minerals
  replacement of 1462
  requirements 1539
minimal-change nephropathy 3979–80, 4077
  aetiology and pathogenesis 3980
  clinical features in adults 3982
  clinical features in children 3980
    clinical presentation 3981
    diagnosis 3981
    in glomerular disease *3980*, 3981
    long-term outcome 3981
    treatment 3981
  pathology 3980, *3981*
Minimata disease 1346

Mini-Mental State Examination (MMSE) 5406
minisatellite repeat mapping 5371
minisatellites 141
minocycline *706*
  acne *4680*
  adverse effects, hepatotoxicity *2529*
  bacterial overgrowth *2334*
  cellulitis, mastitis and pyomyositis *699*
  impetigo *697*
  leprosy 846
  nocardiosis 857
  septic bursitis/arthritis *700*
minoxidil 4739
  adverse effects, hirsutism 2068
  contraindication in porphyria *5484*
  hypertension 3053
miosis 5034
MIP-1α *212*
MIP-1β *212*
Mirizzi's syndrome 2552
mirtazapine, adverse effects *5313*
mismatch repair 361
mismatch 14
misoprostol
  peptic ulcer disease 2311
  teratogenicity *1468*
missense mutations 138, 341
mistletoe
  drug intractions *69*
  hepatotoxicity *2529*
mithramycin
  adverse effects, hepatotoxicity *2529*
  hypercalcaemia 1857
mitochondria 129
  permeability transition pore *182*
mitochondrial diabetes 2008
mitochondrial diseases 1551, *1552*, 5117
  clinical features *1551*
mitochondrial DNA 5371
mitochondrial encephalomyopathies 5221
  genetics 5222, *5222*
  respiratory chain disorders 5223
mitochondrial inheritance 140
mitochondrial myopathy *2766*
  differential diagnosis *1725*
mitochondrial neurogastrointestinal encephalomyopathy *5223*
mitogen-activated protein kinase 348
mitomycin C, adverse effects, hepatotoxicity *2536*, *2534*
mitomycin, adverse effects, hepatotoxicity *2532*
mitosis 340
mitotane, Cushing's syndrome 1880
mitoxantrone, lymphoma *4320*
mitral regurgitation 2736, 2742
  causes 2742, *2742*
    dilated cardiomyopathy 2743
    ischaemic 2742
    mitral valve prolapse 2742
  differential diagnosis 2745
  echocardiography 2665, *2665*
  investigations 2744
    cardiac catheterization 2745
    chest radiograph 2744, *2744*
    ECG 2744
    echocardiography 2744, *2744–5*
  management 2745
    medical 2745
    surgical 2745
  pathophysiology and complications 2743
    afterload 2743
    left atrium 2743
    regurgitant orifice and jet 2743
    right heart 2743
  percutaneous treatment 2942
  physical examination 2743
  pregnancy 2113
  symptoms 2743
mitral stenosis 2736, 2738
  causes 2738
  congenital *2844*
  differential diagnosis 2740
  echocardiography 2665, *2665*
  investigations 2739
    cardiac catheterization/angiography *2684*, 2740
    chest radiography 2739, *2740*
    ECG 2739
    echocardiography 2739, *2740*
  juvenile 2800
  management 2740
    medical 2741
    surgical 2741, *2741*
  pathophysiology and complications 2738
    atrial fibrillation 2738
    left atrial dilatation 2738
    left ventricular dysfunction 2739
    pulmonary hypertension 2739
    right heart disease 2739
  percutaneous treatment 2941, *2941*
  physical examination 2739
  pregnancy 2113
  symptoms 2739
mitral valve prolapse 2742
mitral valve 2738
  anatomy and function 2738
  cleft 2855
  congenital anomalies 2851
  mixed disease 2746, *2747*
  parachute 2851
  see also various diseases of
mitrazapine *5331*
Mitsuokelia spp. *962*
mixed connective tissue disease
  neurological complications 5160, *5161*
  oesophageal symptoms *2297*
  pulmonary involvement 3393
  renal involvement 4054
mixed gonadal dysgenesis *1917*
mizolastine 3282
M-line 2605
MMR vaccine 563
Mobiluncus spp. *962*, 1257
moclobemide 5333
  poisoning 1282
modafinil, narcolepsy *4833*
modified-release formulations 1451
Modoc virus *566*
Moellerella spp. *962*
Mogibacterium spp. *962*
moisturizers 4732, *4732*
Mokola virus 554
molecular genetics 135
molecular mimicry 273, *273*
  mechanisms of 273
Mollaret's meningitis 5003
molluscum contagiosum 657
  aetiology 657
  clinical features 657, *658*
  diagnosis 658, *658*
  differential diagnosis 658
  epidemiology 657
  prevention 659
  treatment 658
molybdenum *1498*, 1499
mometasone furoate *2151*, *4734*
Mondor's disease 1941
Monge's disease 1402, 1408
monkeypox 511
  clinical features *511*
monoamine metabolism disorders 1587, *1588*
  aromatic L-amino acid decarboxylase deficiency 1588
  dopamine β-hydroxylase deficiency 1589
  folinic acid-responsive seizures 1562
  tyrosine hydroxylase deficiency 1587
monoamine oxidase A deficiency, psychiatric signs *1720*
monoamine oxidase inhibitors 5332
  adverse effects 5333
  drug interactions *1471*, 5333
  indications and use 5332
  poisoning 1282
monoamine oxidase *4482*
monoclonal antibodies 158, 401
  leukaemia classification *4223*
  leukaemia therapy 4233
  rheumatoid arthritis 3598, *3598*
monoclonal gammopathy of undetermined significance 4344, *4344–6*
  differential diagnosis 4346
  pathophysiology 4345
  prognosis and treatment 4346
monoclonal Ig deposition disease 4059
  clinical presentation 4059
  definition and epidemiology 4059
  diagnosis 4059, *4060*
  non-Randall-type 4060
  treatment 4059
monoclonal immunoglobulin light chain amyloidosis 1768
monoclonal theory of cancer 339, *338–40*
monocyte derived chemokine 3279
monocytes 152, *208*, *4196*, *4310*
  infants and children *4197*
monocytopenia 4311
monocytosis 4310, *4310*
monogenic inheritance 138, 139
Monomorium pharaonis (Pharaoh's ants) 1236
mononeuropathies, pregnancy 2146
Monongahela virus *581*
monosodium glutamate 2254
monosomy 145
Monro-Kellie doctrine 3147
Montana myotis leukoencephalitis virus *566*
mood disorders
  depression *see* depression
  organic causes 5276
mood stabilizers 5333
  see also individual drugs
MOPP regimen 397
  carcinogenesis *307*
moral hazard 113
Moraxella catarrhalis
  HIV-associated infection *3247*
  pneumonia 3231
  treatment *3238*
Moraxella spp. *962*
Morelia amethistina 1325
Morganella spp. *962*
morning glory syndrome 4852
morning sickness, and thyroid dysfunction 2066
morphine 3155, *3155*
  in breast milk *1469*
  cancer pain 394
  palliative care *5423*
morphoea
  generalized *3667*
  plaque *3667*
Morquio's syndrome *1553*, 1698, *3756*, *3757*
  cardiac involvement *2840*
  diagnosis 1704
mortality *32*
  adult 75
  cancer-related *311*
    see also individual types
  child 74
    causes *75*
  drowning 1397
  famines *121*
  major causes of 74
  poisoning 1273
  women *87*
Morton's neuroma *3248*
Morvan's syndrome 5176, 5281
Moryella spp. *962*
mosaicism 139, 147
moth stings 1351, *1351*
motilin 2319
  inhibition *2320*
motion sickness 466
motor input 4787
motor neuron diseases 5069, 5123, 5172
  amyotrophic lateral sclerosis 5070, 5172
  classification *5071*
  lower 5072, *5124*
    hereditary bulbar palsy of infancy and childhood 5073
    hexoaminidase deficiency 5073
    monomelic, focal and segmental 5073
    multifocal motor neuropathy with conduction block 5074
    postirradiation lumbosacral radiculopathy 5073
    postpolio syndrome 5073
    proximal childhood spinal muscular atrophy 5072
    X-linked recessive bulbospinal neuronopathy 5073
  magnetic brain stimulation 4784
  upper 5074
    hereditary spastic paraplegia 5074
    konzo 5074
    lathyrism 5074
    primary lateral sclerosis 5074
motor-evoked potentials *4758*, 4758
Mouchet's disease *3804*

Mounier-Kuhn syndrome 3260, 3346
mountain sickness
acute 1402, *1404*
chronic (Monge's disease) 1402, 1408
mouth 2257
acute (necrotizing) ulcerative gingivitis 2261
aphthous stomatitis 2269
bacterial infections 2269
benign soft tissue conditions 2279
blood disorders 2284, *2284*
bony neoplasms 2283
bullous lesions 2275
pemphigus vulgaris 2275
cancer 312, 2280
aetiology 2280, *2280*
clinical features 2280, *2280*
course and prognosis 2281
differential diagnosis 2280
pathology 2280
treatment 2281
cysts 2283
dental caries 2257
dermatological conditions 2273
discoid lupus erythematosus 2278
erythema multiforme 2277
leukoplakia 2274
lichen planus 2273, *2273*
mucous membrane pemphigoid 2276
developmental lesions 2283
fungal infections 2267
gastrointestinal conditions 2278
coeliac disease 2279
Crohn's disease and orofacial granulomatosis 2278
ulcerative colitis 2279
gingival/periodontal disease 2259
osteodystrophies 2283
ulcers 2269, *2270*
aphthous *see* aphthous stomatitis
Behçet's disease 2272, *3685*
viral infections 2262
HIV/AIDS 2264
movement disorders 4889, *4890*
athetosis *4890*
chorea 4887, *4890, 4894, 4894*
pregnancy 2144
drug-induced 4900, *4900*
dystonia *see* dystonia
hyperekplexia 162, 166, 4900
magnetic brain stimulation 4784
myoclonus *4890*, 4898, *4898*
neurodegenerative 5111
Parkinson's disease *see* Parkinson's disease
in pregnancy 2148
psychogenic 4900
restless legs syndrome *see* restless legs syndrome
sleep-related 4817
stiff person syndrome 4900, *276*, 5174
tics 4897, *4890, 4897*
tremor 4896, *4890, 4896*
movicol *5426*
Mowat-Wilson syndrome 5143
moxibustion 67
moxifloxacin *707*
anaerobic infections *753*
mycoplasmal infections *960*
pharmacokinetics/pharmacodynamics *452*
Pseudomonas aeruginosa 737
in renal failure *4185*
moxonidine, hypertension 3052
M-proteins 4343, *4344*
MRI *see* magnetic resonance imaging
MRSA 693, 695
community-associated (CA-MRSA) 693, 695
health care-associated 694
osteomyelitis *3789*
mTOR inhibitors, post-transplantation *290*, 292, 3482
Mucambo virus *558*
Muckle-Wells syndrome 157, *238, 1761, 1764, 3709*
mucociliary carpet 3169
mucocutaneous candidiasis, chronic without endocrinopathy *238*
mucolipidoses 1698, *1553*, 5122
mucolytics, COPD 3337
mucopolysaccharidoses *1551, 1553*, 1696, 1698, 1712, *3721, 3731, 3739*, 3756
clinical features 1712, *3731*
corneal opacity 1704
diagnosis 1704
Hunter's syndrome 1698, 3756
Hurler syndrome 1698, *2766*, 3756
Morquio's syndrome 1698, *3756, 3757*
pathology 1712
treatment 1712
bone marrow transplantation 1712
surgical 1712
Mucor stolonifer 3436
mucormycosis 1014
clinical features, renal disease 4090, *4091*
invasive *438*
mucous membrane pemphigoid 2276, *4603*, 4606
aetiology 2276, 4607
clinical features 2276, *2276, 4603, 4607, 4607*
course and prognosis 2277
differential diagnosis 2277
pathology 2276, 4607
treatment 2277, 4607
mucus hypersecretion 3315, 3324
Muehrcke's bands 4701
Muir-Torre syndrome 365, *363*, 4710
Mullis, Kary 12
multicentric reticulohistiocytosis 3707
multifocal motor neuropathy 5074, 5090
multiple carboxylase deficiency 1577, *1577*
multiple chemical sensitivity 1388
multiple endocrine neoplasia *1855*, 1982
ocular involvement 5250
type I (MEN1) *360, 366, 358–9, 1855, 1860, 1982, 3721*
clinical features and classification 1982, *1982*
genetics 1983
pancreatic neuroendocrine tumours 1983
parathyroid hyperplasia/adenoma 1983
pituitary adenoma 1983
screening and management 1983
type II (MEN2) *358–9, 360, 366, 1855, 1860, 1984, 3721*
clinical features and classification 1984, *1984*
genetics 1985
screening and management 1985
type IIA (MEN2A) 1984, 3745
type IIB (MEN2B) 1984, *1984*
multiple epiphyseal dysplasia *3721*
mutations in *3757*
multiple myeloma 330, *3739*, 4346
biological aspects 4347
clinical manifestations 4347
diagnosis 4348
epidemiology and aetiology 4347
history 4346
laboratory findings 4347
organ involvement 4347
neurological 4348
renal 4347
prognosis 4348
smouldering 4345
supportive care 4350
anaemia 4351
emotional support 4351
hypercalcaemia 4351
hyperviscosity 4351
infection 4351
neurological 4351
renal failure 4351
skeletal complications 4350
treatment 4348
allogeneic bone marrow transplantation 4349
autologous stem cell transplantation 4348
chemotherapy 4349
maintenance therapy 4349
variant forms 4351
extramedullary plasmacytoma 4352
nonsecretory myeloma 4351
plasma-cell leukaemia 4351
POEMS syndrome 4351
solitary plasmacytoma of bone 4352
multiple regional pain syndromes, investigations 3564, *3570*
multiple sclerosis *276*, 4954
aetiology 4954, *4954*
childhood 4956
clinical course and prognosis 4956
cognitive impairment 5279
differential diagnosis 4957
imaging *4775*, 4775
laboratory investigations 4956
cerebrospinal fluid 4957
electrophysiology 4956
MRI 4956
magnetic brain stimulation *4783*, 4784
ocular involvement 5243
pregnancy 2148
symptoms 4954
treatment 4958
neuroprotection 4960
multiple sulphatase deficiency 1698, 1697, 5105
multiple-system atrophy 4886
multiplex ligation-dependent probe amplification 148
multisystem atrophy 2639, 3260, 3270
mumps 513
aetiology and genetics 513, *514*
clinical features 513
fetus and infant 515
meningitis and encephalitis 514
orchitis 514
parotitis 513
epidemiology and pathogenesis 513
historical perspective 513
immunization *91*, 515
laboratory diagnosis 515
treatment 515
Munchausen's syndrome 5303
mupirocin
herpes labialis 2264
impetigo *697*
S. pyogenes 675
skin disorders 4738
murine typhus 910
clinical features 910
epidemiology 910
treatment 914
muromonab, post-transplantation *3954*
Murphy's sign 2551
Murray Valley encephalitis virus *566*, 572
Murutucu virus *581*
Musca domestica 1233
Musca sorbens 1236
muscarine 1367, *1367*
Muscidae *1233*
Muscina stabulans (stable fly) 1232, *1233*
Muscina stabulans 1232, *1233*
muscle biopsy, polymyositis/dermatomyositis 3697
muscle cramps, pregnancy 2145
muscle disorders 5185, *5188*
channelopathies *see* channelopathies
clinical history 5188
investigation 3569, *3569*
investigations *5187*, 5189, *5190*
metabolic and endocrine 5212
mitochondrial encephalomyopathies 5221
muscular dystrophy *see* muscular dystrophies
myopathies 163
myotonia 164, 5207
physical examination 5189
see also myopathies
muscle soreness 5379
muscle
anatomy 5185, *5186*
contraction, sliding filament theory 5186, *5186–7*
effects of malnutrition 1510
energy production 5188
motor unit 5187, *5187–8*
muscular dystrophies 5129, 5190
classfication 5191, *5192*
congenital 5131, *5192, 5193*
classification 5193, *5202*
diagnosis 5194
differential diagnosis 5193

genetic counselling 5195
prognosis and management 5194
diagnosis 5192, *5192, 5196*
dystrophin deficiency 5195
management 5192
pathophysiology 5192, *5192*
see also various types
musculocutaneous nerve neuropathy 5081
musculoskeletal disorders
and acute respiratory failure *3134*
Behçet's disease 3686
cystic fibrosis 3363
leptospirosis 875
Lyme borreliosis 863
mycoplasmal 951, 957
occupational 1382
affecting occupation 1383
clinical investigations and management 1383
low back pain 1383
occupations associated with 1383
upper limbs 1382
post-transplant 3964
in pregnancy 2089
rheumatic *see* rheumatic disorders; and individual conditions
SLE 3657, *3658*
systemic sclerosis 3676
musculoskeletal pain, diffuse 3758
mushroom poisoning *see* fungal poisoning
mustard gas *308, 1380*
mutagenesis, directed 191
mutation rates 144
mutations 138, *338*
apoptosis and cell death pathways 351
cancer-causing 341, *341*
dynamic 142
frameshift 138
gain-of-function 138, 361
loss-of-function 138, 361
missense 138, 341
silent 138
MutTH syndrome 359
myasthenia gravis 163, *166, 276, 5173, 5178, 5179*
anti-MuSK 5181
clinical features 5179, *5180*
thyroid disease 5217
diagnosis 5180
differential diagnosis 5180
early onset seropositive 5181
epidemiology 5178
haematological changes 4559
late-onset 5181
natural course 5180
ocular 5181
oesophageal symptoms *2297*
pathogenesis 5178
pregnancy 2145
in pregnancy 5181
presentation 5493
prognosis 5181
seronegative 5181
treatment 5180
myasthenic crisis 5181
myasthenic syndromes, congenital 5182
endplate acetylcholinesterase deficiency 5183
postsynaptic 5183
presynaptic 5183
myc oncogene 349
mycetism 999
mycetoma *see* Madura foot
Mycobacterial Growth Indicator Tube (MGIT) 823
mycobacterial infections
environmental 831
Buruli ulcer 833
chronic pulmonary disease 832
disseminated 834, *834*
ecology and epidemiology 832
keratitis 833
lymphadenitis 833
postinjection abscess 833
surgical innoculation 834
swimming pool/fish tank granuloma 833
treatment 835, *835*
immunosuppressed patients 3958
Mendelian susceptibility to *238*, 254
renal involvement 4075
see also individual species
Mycobacterium abscessus 832
Mycobacterium africanum 812
Mycobacterium avium avium 832
Mycobacterium avium complex, HIV-associated infection *3247*
Mycobacterium avium intracellulare 821, *832*, 835, 3419
Mycobacterium avium, bronchiectasis 3349
Mycobacterium bovis 812
Mycobacterium chelonei 832, 4674
Mycobacterium fortuitum 832, 4674
Mycobacterium gordonae 832
Mycobacterium haemophilum 832
Mycobacterium kansasii 3419
Mycobacterium leprae 813
biological characteristics 836
genome 836
immune response to 837
in vivo cultivation 836
renal toxicity *4086*, 4089
see also leprosy
Mycobacterium malmoense 832
Mycobacterium marinum 832
swimming pool/fish tank granuloma 833, *833*
Mycobacterium scrofulaceum 832
Mycobacterium simiae 832
Mycobacterium spp. *962, 3436*
Mycobacterium szulgai 832
Mycobacterium terrae 832
Mycobacterium tuberculosis 812, 2170
HIV-associated infection *3247*
malabsorption *2357*
osteomyelitis *3789*
pneumonia 3237
renal toxicity *4086*, 4089
see also tuberculosis
Mycobacterium ulcerans 832, 4674
Buruli ulcer 848
Mycobacterium xenopi 832
Mycograb 1017
mycophenolate mofetil
adverse effects 3955, *3955*
lupus nephritis 4047, 4049
minimal-change nephropathy 3982
post-transplantation *290*, 291, *2511*, 3482, *3954*
pregnancy *2158*
primary biliary cirrhosis *2467*
SLE 3662
systemic sclerosis *3677*
Mycoplasma amphoriforme 952, *952*
Mycoplasma buccale 952
Mycoplasma faucium 952
Mycoplasma fermentans 952, *952–3*
Mycoplasma genitalium 1259, *952–3*
Mycoplasma hominis 952, *951–2*, 957, 1259, 1256–7, 2169
pregnancy *2171*
Mycoplasma hyorhinis 952
Mycoplasma lipophilum 952
Mycoplasma orale 952, *952*
Mycoplasma penetrans 952
Mycoplasma pirium 952
Mycoplasma pneumoniae 950, 952, 952, *953*
chronic respiratory disease 954
clinical features 953
epidemiology 954
extrapulmonary manifestations 954, *954*
immunopathology 954, *955*
laboratory diagnosis 959
pharyngitis 3227
pneumonia 3231, *3232*, 3234
treatment 959, *3238*
Mycoplasma pulmonis 951
Mycoplasma salivarium 952
Mycoplasma spermatophilum 952
Mycoplasma spp. *962*
mycoplasmal infections 950, *951*
genitourinary *951, 955, 956*
history 952
immunodeficiency states 958
laboratory diagnosis 959
genitourinary and other infections 959, *959*
M. pneumoniae 959
musculoskeletal 951, 957
neonate 957
occurrence *952, 953*
in pregnancy 957
prevention 960
respiratory 950, 952
treatment 959, *960*
genitourinary infections 960
M. pneumoniae infections 959
wounds 958
mycoses *see* fungal infections
mycosis fungoides 4333, 4712
mycotoxicosis 999
mydriasis, belladonna alkaloids 1362, *1362*
myelination 4950
myelitis 5172
transverse 4953
myelodysplasia 4212, 4256
classification 4259, *4260*
5q-syndrome 4260
refractory anaemia 4259
refractory anaemia with excess blasts 4260
refractory anaemia with ringed sideroblasts 4259
refractory cytopenias with multilineage dysplasia 4259
refractory cytopenias with multilineage dysplasia and ringed sideroblasts 4260
clinical features 4258
definition 4257
differential diagnosis 4259
further research 4263
laboratory diagnosis 4258, *4258*
pathogenesis and pathophysiology 4257
prognosis *4262*, 4263
treatment 4261
myelofibrosis, idiopathic 4274, *4275*
aetiology 4275, *4275, 4277*
clinical features 4276
complications 4278, *4279*
course and prognosis 4277
laboratory studies 4276, *4276–7*
treatment 4278
myeloma 4342
renal involvement 3857, *3858*, 4058
myelomatosis *244*
myelomeningocele 5137
myelopathy *384*
HIV-related 631
myeloperoxidase deficiency 4309
myelopoiesis *4202*, 4206
suppression of phagocyte production 4206
myeloproliferative disorders 4211, *4211*
pregnancy 2180
myiasis 1225, *1232, 1233*
dermal 1234, *1234*
ophthalmic 1234
wound 1234, *1235*
myoadenylate deaminase deficiency 1631, 5216
myocardial contractility
control of 2617
and inotropic state 2624, *2624*
mechanical events 2620, *2620*
see also cardiac action potential; myocytes, cardiac
myocardial infarction 2630, *2886, 3120*
breathlessness *2633*
diabetes mellitus 2043, *2043*
diagnosis 2654
atrial infarction 2655
coronary artery spasm 2655
right ventricular infarction 2654, *2656*
septal ischaemia vs posterior infarction 2655
and hypertension 3081
location of *2653*
and mitral regurgitation 2742
non-STEMI 2643
coronary bypass 2943
ECG 2653–4
and pericarditis 2791
risk stratification *2631*
STEMI *see* STEMI
stress-induced hyperglycaemia 2043
TIMI risk score *2631*
treatment
fibrinolysis *38*, 40, *42*
magnesium infusion 42, *42*
myocardial ischaemia 2767
hypertension-induced 3036
myocardial perfusion imaging 2671
angina 2906, *2906*
clinical uses

    coronary artery disease 2672, *2673*
    left ventricular volume/function 2673
  practical considerations 2672
  principles 2671, *2672*
  stress testing 2672
myocardial perfusion, MRI 2676
myocardial viability, MRI 2674
myocarditis *276*, 2758
  aetiology and pathogenesis *2759*, 2759
  clinical features 2758
  future developments 2764
  and idiopathic dilated cardiomyopathy 2760
  late gadolinium enhancement 2676
  peripartum, specific forms 2762
  specific forms 2762, *2763*
    cardiac sarcoidosis 2763
    Chagas' disease 2763
    giant cell 2763
    Lyme carditis 2763
    postviral and nonspecific lymphocytic 2761, *2761–2*
  and ventricular tachycardia 2761
myoclonus 4898, *4890, 4898*
  benign essential 4898
  epilepsia partialis continua 4899
  focal 4899
  hemifacial spasm 4899
  Lance-Adams syndrome 4899
  myoclonic epilepsy 4899
  progressive myoclonic encephalopathies 4899
  spinal 4899
myocytes, cardiac 2603
  connections between 2607, *2611*
  contractile apparatus 2605
    intermediate filaments 2606
    thick filaments 2605, *2606*
    thin filaments 2605, *2606*
  excitation-contraction coupling 2615
  functional anatomy 2603–4, *2604–6*
  myofibrillar contraction 2615, *2616–17*
  plasma membrane *2608*
  plasma membrane currents *2613*
  subtypes 2609
  termination of contraction 2616
myoglobin, nephrotoxicity 3898, *3898*
myoglobinuria 5220, *5220*
myopathies 3730, *5214*
  alcoholic 5156, 5218
  autophagic vacuolar 1698
  drug-induced 5218, *5219*
  endocrine 5216
  inherited 5129
  mitochondrial *2766*
    differential diagnosis *1725*
  nutritional 5218
  post-transplant 3964
  primary metabolic 5214, *5214*
  toxic 5218
  vacuolar 1698
  X-linked 1698
myopathy, ischaemic 5218
myopericarditis, enterovirus 530
myophosphorylase deficiency *see* McArdle's disease
myosin, motor proteins 131
myosin-binding protein-C 2606
myositis ossificans 3713
myotonia congenita 5219
myotonia *164*, 5207, *5208*
  classification 5209, *5209*
myotonic dystrophies 5130
  cardiac involvement *2788*
  oesophageal symptoms *2297*
  pregnancy 2145
  reproductive effects *1917*
  type 1 *5209, 5210–11*
  type 2, 5212
Myrmecia spp. (Australia bull ants) 1350
Myroides spp. *962*
myxoedema coma *1837*
myxoedema 1834
  CNS complications 5153
  neuropathy 5086
myxoid liposarcoma, translocations *341*
myxoma
  cardiac 2830
  left atrial 2997

Na+, Ca2+ exchanger 2617
Na+,K+-ATPase 2617
nabumetone
  and asthma *3289*
  rheumatoid arthritis *3594*
N-acetylaspartic aciduria (Canavan's disease) *1566*, 1580
  aetiology/pathology 1580
  clinical presentation 1580, *1581*
  diagnosis 1581
  treatment and outcome 1581
N-acetylcysteine *1274*, 1293
  dosing regimens *1293*
  uses *3798*
N-acetylglutamate synthetase deficiency *1566*
NADH-coenzyme Q reductase deficiency *2766*
NADPH oxidase 209
Naegleria fowleri 1043
Naegleria 1036, 1042
naevus flammeus 4692
nafcillin *706*
NAGA deficiency 1698
nail disorders 4698
  Beau's lines 4700
  clubbing 4700, *4700–1*
  colour changes 4700, *4701*
  fungal infection (onychomycosis) 4699, *4699–700*
  koilonychia (spooning) 4700
  liver disease 4720
  Mee's lines 4701
  Muehrcke's bands 4701
  nail anatomy *4699*
  nail fold vessels 4700
  polymyositis/dermatomyositis 3694, *3695*
  psoriasis 4612, *4612*, 4698
  splinter haemorrhages 4700
  Terry's nail 4700
  thyroid disease 4700
  uraemic half and half nail 4701
  white, cirrhosis 2498, *2498*
nail-patella syndrome 4099
Nairobi eye 1351
Nairobi sheep disease *581*
Nairovirus 581, 585
  Crimean-Congo haemorrhagic fever *581–2*, 585, *585*
Naja haje (Egyptian cobra) *1239*
Naja kaouthia, antivenom *1340*
Naja naja (Sri Lankan cobra) *1329*
  antivenom *1340*
Naja nigricollis (spitting cobra) *1334–5*
Naja spp. (spitting cobras) 1328
Nakalanga syndrome 1149
nalidixic acid
  adverse effects, hepatotoxicity *2532*
  in breast milk *1469*
  pharmacokinetics *449*
naloxone *1274*, 3156
  drug interactions *1471*
Nam Dinh virus 661
Naonphyetus salmincola 1223
2-naphthylamine *338*, 1379, *1380*
Naples virus *581*, 586
naproxen
  adverse effects, hepatotoxicity *2532, 2533*
  and asthma *3289*
  cancer pain 394
  migraine *4917*
  rheumatoid arthritis *3594*
Naranjal virus *566*
naratriptan, migraine *4917–18*
narcolepsy *3269*, 4828, *4827, 4830, 4831*
  clinical features 4826
  diagnosis 4832
  differential diagnosis 4817, *4827*
  HLA association 4826
  hypocretin 4826
  pathogenesis 4832
  pathophysiology 4827, *4827*
  secondary 4832
  subtypes *4833*
  symptomatic 4827
  treatment 4828, *4828, 4832, 4833*
nasal cancer 317
nasal congestion 3229
nasogastric tubes 1539, *1540*
nasojejunal tubes *1540*
nasopharyngeal cancer 312
  differential diagnosis 507
  and Epstein-Barr virus 312, 506
  incidence *301, 313*
  laboratory diagnosis 507
  pathogenesis 507
  symptoms and signs 506
  treatment 507
natamycin, fungal infections 1015
nateglinide 2014
National Health Service, priority setting 58
National Institute for Health and Clinical Excellence (NICE) 47, 58–9
  Citizen's Council 58–9
National Institute of Neurological Diseases and Stroke (NINDS) 30
National Institutes of Health stroke scale *5489*
natriuretic peptides 2623
  and hypertension 3034
Natrix natrix helvetica (British grass snake) 1327
natural anticancer drugs 399
natural contraception *26*
natural killer (NK) cell leukaemia, aggressive 4227
natural killer (NK) cell lymphoma 507
natural killer (NK) cells 152, *208–9, 286, 288*
  SCID *251*
natural killer receptors 211
natural killer T (NKT) cells 208, 210
natural selection 13
  levels of 13
nausea 2206
  in palliative care *5423–4*, 5424
  pregnancy 2089
Naxos disease 2778, *4599*
N-carbamyl-β-aminoaciduria 1634
Ndumu *558*
nebivolol, heart failure *2722*
nebulin 2606
Necator americanus 1163, 1165
Necator suillus 1176
neck
  pain 3278
    investigation 3227
    management 3254
    whiplash-associated *3575*
  rheumatoid arthritis 3588
necrobiosis lipoidica 4718, *4718*
necrobiosis 2047, *2047*
necrosis 178
necrotizing enterocolitis 804, 808
  aetiology 808
  definition 808
  history and physical examination 808
  treatment and prevention 808
necrotizing fasciitis 673
necrotizing myelopathy 5172
nedocromil sodium, asthma 3304
nefazodone, adverse effects *5313*
Neisseria gonorrhoeae 722, 1259, 2170
  antibiotic sensitivity *446*
  antimicrobial resistance 725
    chromosomally mediated 725
    plasmid-mediated 725
    susceptibility testing 726
  laboratory detection 724
  molecular detection 725
  osteomyelitis *3789*
Neisseria meningitidis 709–10, *711*
  antibiotic sensitivity *446*
  and complement deficiency 217
  pneumonia 3231
  visualization of 710
Neisseria spp. *962*
nelfinavir
  HIV/AIDS *638*
  mode of action *444*
  toxicity *640*
Nelson's syndrome 1813, *1878, 1879*
nematodes 1145
  cutaneous filariasis 1145
  gnathostomiasis 1182
  guinea worm disease 1160
  lymphatic filariasis 1153
  parastrongyliasis 1179
  strongyloidiasis and hookworm 1163
Neodiplostomum seoulensis 1223
neologisms 4789

Neomys anomalus (southern water shrew) 1327
Neomys fodiens (northern water shrew) 1327
neonatal infection
 S. agalactiae 676
 S. pyogenes 674
neonatal-onset multisystem inflammatory disorder *see* NOMID
neonate
 benign familial convulsions 162
 bleeding tendency 4506
 chlamydial infection 945, *945*
 cholestasis 2449
 cytomegalovirus 495
 diabetes 2006
 DIC 4545
 enterovirus 530
 haemochromatosis *1674*, 1675
 HSV infection 487
 hyperparathyroidism *1855*, 1862, *3721*
 hypoparathyroidism 1864
 jaundice 2449
 lupus syndromes 2157
 mycoplasmal infections 957
 screening *101, 104*, 162
 thyroid function 2142
 vitamin K deficiency 4534
neostigmine
 snake bite 1343
 uses *3798*
Neotrombicula autumnalis 1229
nephritis
 acute interstitial 4002, 3901
 chronic tubulointerstitial 4006
 infective endocarditis 2809
 interstitial, infection-associated 4073
nephroblastoma *see* Wilms' tumour
nephrocalcinosis 4126, 4129
 disorders of *4128*
 X-linked hypercalciuric *165*, 166, *3721, 3739*
nephrogenic fibrosing dermopathy 4721
nephrogenic systemic fibrosis 3879
nephrolithiasis 165, *4124*
 genetic disorders with 4100, *4101*
 ultrasound 3876
 X-linked *3721*
 see also urolithiasis; and different stone types
nephron 3809, *3810*
nephrotic syndrome *244*, 3854
 causes *3855*
 clinical features 3854, *3854*
  hypercholesterolaemia 3980
  rapidly progressive glomerulonephritis 3855
  thromboembolic disease 3980
 congenital of Finnish type 4099
 definition 3854, *3854*
 minimal-change *see* minimal-change nephropathy
 sickle cell disease 4070
nephrotoxins 3897, *3897*
 chemical 4094
 endogenous 3898
 exogenous 3897
 plant-derived *1362*, 1365, 4092, *4093*
Nepuyo virus *581*
Nerium oleander (oleander) *1364*
nerve agents
 poisoning *1274*
  antidote *1274*
nerve conduction studies 4762
 clinical correlations 5
 demyelinating neuropathy *4766, 4767*
 focal nerve lesions *4764*, 4765
 motor disorders 4767
 motor nerves *4763*, 4762
 neuromuscular transmission disorders 4768
 peripheral neuropathy *4765*, 4766, *4766*
 sensory nerves 4762
nerve deafness *1855*
nerve palsies, obstetric 2145
nerves
 to serratus anterior, neuropathy 5079
 tumour infiltration 382
nervous system
 acidosis 1745
 diphtheria complications 667, *668*
nervous tissue, stem cells 200
Netherton's syndrome 4597
netilmicin, spectrum of activity *446*
nettle 68
 drug intractions *69*
neural tube defects 5135, *5136*
 aetiology 5136
  folic acid deficiency 1493
 cranial abnormalities 5136
 epidemiology 5135
 management 5138
 prenatal diagnosis 5136, *5137*
 spinal abnormalities 5137
neuralgia, postherpetic 492
neuralgic amyotrophy 5079
neuritis, in leprosy 847, *844*
neuroacanthocytosis 4887
neuroblastoma 3543
neurocanthocytosis 5113
neurocutaneous syndromes 5097
 see also individual diseases
neurodegenerative diseases 5096
 dementia syndromes *see* dementia
 DNA repair defects 5099
 epilepsy *see* epilepsy
 hereditary ataxias 5114
 hereditary neuropathies 5127
 hereditary spastic paraplegia 5074, *5125, 5125–6*
 inherited myopathies 5129
 leucodystrophies *see* leucodystrophies
 lysosomal 5117
 mitochondrial 5117
 motor neuron diseases *see* motor neuron diseases
 movement disorders 5111
 neurocutaneous syndromes 5097
neurofibromatosis
 ocular involvement 5250
 type 1 358, *360*, 366, 5098
  pregnancy 2147
 type 2 *360*, 366, 5098
neuroglycopenia 2049
neurological disorders 4743
 Behçet's disease 3686
 history 4743
 imaging 4768
  congenital anomalies and paediatric 4782
  see also individual conditions
 immunocompromised patients 3961, *3961*
 infection 437, *437*
 investigation 4744
 Lyme borreliosis 863
 management 4745
 occupational 1386
  chemical exposure 1386, *1386–7*
  physical factors 1387
 pregnancy 2144
  central nervous system 2146
  cerebrovascular disorders 2145
  malignancies 2145
  movement disorders 2144
  muscle disorders 2145
  myasthenia gravis 2145
  myotonic dystrophy 2145
  nerves and nerve roots 2146
  obstetric nerve palsies 2145
  thiamine deficiency 2144
 rabies 468
 SLE 3659
 systemic disease 5158
  organ-specific autoimmune disease 5163
  rheumatoid arthritis 5160
  sarcoidosis 5163
  seronegative arthritides 5160
  systemic lupus erythematosus 5158, *5159*
  vasculitis 5160, *5161*
 vasculitis 5160
  clinical features 5160
  complicating nonvasculitis systemic disorders 5162
  complicating systemic vasculitides 5161
  diagnosis and management 5161, *5161*
  treatment 5162
neurological examination 4744
neurological repair 201
neurological signs of poisoning 1274
 abnormal movements 1275
 lateralizing signs 1274
 loss of ocular reflexes 1275
 ocular signs 1275
 pupillary changes 1275
 pyramidal tract 1274
 visual impairment 1275
neuromuscular disorders
 oesophageal symptoms *2297*
 and respiratory failure
  acute *3134*
  chronic 3470
neuromuscular junction 162
 disorders of 5177
  congenital myasthenic syndromes 5182
  Lambert-Eaton myasthenic syndrome *see* Lambert-Eaton myasthenic syndrome
  myasthenia gravis *see* myasthenia gravis
  neuromyotonia *166*, 5174, 5183
neuromuscular transmission 5177, *5178*
neuromyelitis optica 4953
neuromyotonia 5174, 5183
 acquired *166*
neuronal ceroid lipofuscinoses 1698, 1717, 5102, 5123
 congenital 1698
 variant late infantile
  Finnish 1698
  Turkish 1698
neuron-specific enolase, reference values *5442*
neuro-ophthalmological pathways *1802*
neuropathic pain *5412*
 treatment 5414, *5414*
neuropathies *see* peripheral neuropathies
neuropeptide Y 2319
neurophysiology 5275
neuroprotective agents 4941
 multiple sclerosis 4960
neuropsychiatry *see* cognitive disorders
neurosis, older patients 5408
neurosyphilis 5016
 clinical features 888, *5016, 5017*
 cognitive impairment 5278
 diagnosis 893, *5016, 5017*
 differential diagnosis 892
 treatment 5017
neurotensin 2320
 reference values *5442*
neurotoxins
 fungal 1367, *1367*
 plant-derived 1361, *1362*
neurotransmitter diseases 1587, *1587*
neutriceuticals, migraine prevention *4916*
neutropenia 252, *4306, 4306*
 acquired 4307
  drugs and toxins 4307
  nutritional deficiencies 4307
  postinfectious 4307
 autoimmune 4307
 congenital 4306
 cyclic 4307
 evaluation 4308
 hypersplenism/ sequestration 4306
 management 4308
  G-CSF 4308
neutrophil elastase, COPD *3323*
neutrophilia 4304, *4305*
 acquired 4305
  drugs 4305
  infection 4305
  myeloproliferative disorders 4305
  primary haematological conditions 4305
 evaluation of 4306
 hereditary 4304
neutrophilic dermatoses 3706, *3707*, 4634
neutrophils 152, *288, 4196*, 4304
 disorders of function 4308
  Chediak-Higashi syndrome 4309
  chronic granulomatous disease 4308
  leucocyte adhesion deficiency 4309
  myeloperoxidase deficiency 4309
  specific granule deficiency 4310

  infants and children *4197*
  maturation 4304
  morphology 4304
nevirapine
  adverse effects, hepatotoxicity *2529*
  HIV/AIDS 636, *638*
  mode of action *444*
  toxicity *640*
Newton, Isaac 11
NF-κB essential modulator (NEMO) 245
NF-κB 154, 158
Ngari virus 661
n-hexane poisoning 1311
  CNS effects *1386*
  peripheral nervous system effects *1387*
niacin 1489–90
  adverse effects, hepatotoxicity *2529*
  clinical use 1491
  deficiency anaemia 4419
  dietary reference values *1502*
  drug interactions *1471*
  hypercholesterolaemia 1670
  requirements 1491
nicardipine, hypertensive emergencies *3079–80*
nickel *1498*, 1500
  carcinogenesis *308, 338, 1380*
  poisoning 1301
niclofalan, paragonimiasis 1219
niclosamide
  intestinal flukes 1221
  Taenia saginata 1191
nicotinamide adenine dinucleotide (NAD) 1487–8
nicotinamide *see* niacin
nicotinic acid *see* niacin
Niemann-Pick disease 1696, 1698, 1713, 5121
  diagnosis 1704, 1706
  psychiatric signs *1720*
nifedipine
  adverse effects, hepatotoxicity *2529, 2532–3*
  in breast milk *2101*
  hypertensive emergencies *3079*
  in pregnancy *2099*
  Raynaud's phenomenon *3671*
  vibration injury 1435
nifurtimox
  adverse reactions *1125*
  Chagas' disease 1132
  trypanosomiasis *1124–5*, 1126
Nijmegen breakage syndrome *238, 255, 345, 346*
Nikolsky sign 2276
nilotinib, leukaemias 4253
nimesulide, adverse effects, hepatotoxicity *2529, 2533*
Nipah virus encephalitis 5002
Nipah virus 525
  bat as host 526
  clinical features 525, *5004, 5006*
  encephalitis 5002
    Bangladesh and India 526
    relapse and late-onset 526
  epidemiology 525
  laboratory investigations 525, *526*
  pathology/pathogenesis 526, *526*
  treatment 525
nipple, benign disease 1941, *1941*
nitazoxanide
  bacterial overgrowth *2334*
  fascioliasis 1215
  giardiasis *1113*
nitisinone 1555, 3711
nitrate poisoning 1290
nitrates
  acute coronary syndromes 2917
  angina 2909
  heart failure 2724
  Raynaud's phenomenon *3671*
  in renal failure 4180
nitric oxide synthase *2597*
nitric oxide 2597, *2597, 3130, 4482*
  ARDS 3141
  pathophysiology 2598
  physiology 2597
nitrites
  poisoning 1313
  urinary 3865
nitrobenzene, hepatotoxicity *1385*
nitrofurantoin
  adverse effects
    hepatotoxicity *2532, 2533, 2535*
    neuropathy 5088
  in breast milk *1469*
  in renal failure *4185*
  reproductive effects *1917*
  urinary tract infection *4113–14*
nitrogen balance *1538*
  acidosis 1744
nitrogen dioxide
  poisoning 1314
  toxicity *3443*
nitrogen intake *1538*
nitrogen mustard *338*
nitrosamines, carcinogenesis *338*
nitrosoalbumin 2600
nitrosocysteine 2600
nitrosoglutathione 2600
nitrosohaemoglobin 2600
nitrosurea *338*
nizatidine, peptic ulcer disease 2311
NK4, *1939*
Nocardia asteroides 856
Nocardia brasiliensis 856
Nocardia farcinica 856
Nocardia otidiscaviarum 856
Nocardia spp. *962*
  immunosuppressed patients 3959
  osteomyelitis *3789*
  treatment *3238*
Nocardia transvalensis 856
Nocardiopsis spp. *962*
nocardiosis 856
  clinical features 856
    disseminated nocardiosis 857
    nocardia mycetoma 856
    primary cutaneous nocardiosis 856, *856*
    pulmonary nocardiosis 856
  epidemiology 856
  laboratory diagnosis 857
  pathogenesis 856
  treatment 857
nociceptive pain 5411, *5412*
  treatment 5413, *5413*
nocturia 3852
  hypertension 3040
nocturnal enuresis, sickle cell disease 4070
NOD-like receptors 398
nodular lymphoid hyperplasia 2247, *2249*
nodular vasculitis 4650
nodules *4591*
noise-induced hearing loss 1432
  clinical features 1433, *1433*
  diagnosis 1433
  exposure 1433
  management, prevention and surveillance 1433
NOMID *238, 1761*
nomifensine, adverse effects, hepatotoxicity *2529, 2533, 2535*
nonalcoholic fatty liver disease *see* steatohepatitis, nonalcoholic
nonallelic homologous recombination 144
noncommunicable diseases
  mortality rate *75, 76*
  prevention and treatment *78*
nonfreezing cold injury 1395–6
nongranulomatous jejunoileitis 2249
non-Hodgkin's lymphoma *244*, 307, 330, 4326
  aetiology 4326, *4327*
  HIV-associated 633
  incidence *301, 330, 4326*
    migrants vs residents *302*
  International Prognostic Index 4327, *4328*
  REAL/WHO classification *4321, 4324, 4326*
  renal involvement 4063
  treatment *4320*
nonhomologous end joining 145
noninvasive ventilation 3139
  contraindications *3140*
  limitations of *3141*
  nasal positive-pressure 3474
non-islet-cell tumour 2054
  chemical pathology 2054
  diagnosis 2054
  ectopic insulin secretion 2054
  treatment 2054
non-nucleoside reverse transcriptase inhibitors 636
  toxicity *640*
nonsense mediated decay 138
non-STEMI 2643
  coronary bypass 2943
  ECG 2653–4
non-steroidal anti-inflammatory drugs *see* NSAIDs
Noonan's syndrome *2766*
  aortic dissection 2955
  cardiac involvement 2835, *2835*
  pulmonary valve stenosis 2848
Noonan-Leopard syndrome *1917*
noradrenaline 3129
  reference values *5441*
norepinephrine *see* noradrenaline
norfloxacin, bacterial overgrowth *2334*
normetanephrine, reference values *5441*
noroviruses, diarrhoea 2427
northern epilepsy 1698
nortriptyline
  adverse effects *5313*
  migraine prevention *4916*
nose 3169
  anterior nares 3169
  secretory function and sensory innervation 3170
  turbinates 3169
  vascular supply 3169, *3170*
nosocomial infections 428
  antibiotic-associated diarrhoea 431
  bacteraemia 431
  definitions 428
  future developments 431
  hospital infection control 429
  host factors 428
  intravascular devices 430
  microorganisms 429
  pneumonia *430*, 430, 3243
    aetiology 3243, *3243*
    clinical features 3244
    epidemiology 3243
    laboratory diagnosis 3244
    outcome 3245
    pathogenesis 3244, *3244*
    prevention 3245
    treatment 3245, *3245*
  prosthetic devices 430
  respiratory viruses 481
  scale and costs 428, *428*
  surgical wounds 429
  urinary tract 429
Notch pathway 170, 176, 2596
notecarin *4540*
Notechis scutatus (tiger snake) 1329
  antivenom *1340*
Notonecta glauca 1229
NSAIDs
  adverse effects
    diverticular disease 2390
    nephrotoxicity *3860*, 4005, 4011, 4053
    oesophagitis *2294*
  ankylosing spondylitis 3610
  and asthma 3288, *3289*
  breast cancer *1939*
  cancer pain 394
  drug interactions *1471, 3968*
  effects on renin-angiotensin-aldosterone system 3843
  gout 3643
  osteoarthritis 3634
  peptic ulcer disease 2306–7
    prevention 2313, *2313*
  poisoning 1290
  rheumatoid arthritis *3594*
    clinical trials 3595
  SLE 2156
  Still's disease 3706
Ntaya virus *566*
nuclear imaging
  cardiac 2671
  pulmonary arterial hypertension *2985*
  renal disease 3880, *3880*
    dynamic 3881
    static 3880
  small intestine 2220
    Crohn's disease *2223*
  see also individual modalities
nuclear pores 129
nuclear proteins 349
nuclear receptors, signalling by 1794, *1797*
nucleoside analogues 636, *638*
  toxicity *640*
nucleoside reverse transcriptase inhibitors
  toxicity *640*
    neuropathy 5088
nucleotide instability 343
nucleotides 138

excision repair 343
nucleus 127–8
number needed to harm (NNH) 1450
number needed to treat (NNT) *52*, 52, 1450
nut allergy 263
nutcracker oesophagus 2296, *2296*
nutrition
acute renal trauma 3893
ARDS 3143
artificial *see* artificial nutrition support
CKD 3916
Crohn's disease 2366
cystic fibrosis 3361
dialysis patients 3940
dietary change 1520, 1523
dietary reference values *1502*, 1503
economic and technical development 1515, *1516*
immunonutrition 1503
macronutrient metabolism 1479
malnutrition 1505
micronutrient supplements 1503
overnutrition 1516
pregnancy 2079
developing world 2080, *2081*
energy requirements 2080, *2081*
fetal programming 2083
food cravings 2083
foods to avoid 2083
metabolic changes 2081
weight gain 2080, *2080*
small bowel resection 2356
vitamins and trace elements 1487
nutritional deficiencies *244*
nutritional screening 1535
nutritional status 1535
assessment of 2226
nutritional supplements, in heart failure 2721
nutritional support
acute pancreatitis 2565
COPD 3340
nutrition-related diseases 1516
cancer 1521, *1521*
constipation and irritable bowel syndrome 1522
coronary heart disease 1517, *1518*
age-adjusted risk *1518*
promoters *1518*
protectors *1518*
dental caries 1522
diabetes mellitus and metabolic syndrome 1520, *1520*
diverticular disease 1521
epidemiological methods 1516
hypertension and stroke 1519
obesity *see* obesity
osteoporosis 1522
Nyando virus *581*, 587
Nycticebus coucang (slow loris) 1327
NY-ESO-1, 376
nystagmus 4859, *4859*
nystatin, fungal infections 1015

O'nyong-nyong virus *558*, 560
obesity syndromes 1529, *1530*
obesity 1527, 1517, 1667
acute pancreatitis mortality 2562
aetiology 1528
environmental factors 1529
genetic factors 1529, *1530–1*
programming and epigenetics 1530
causes 1527
in children *1529*
classification *1528*
clinical history 1530
and coronary heart disease 2892
definition 1527, *1528*
examination 1530
genome association 141
hepatic involvement 2540
history-taking *1532*
and hypertension 3030
insulin resistance 1995
investigation 1530, *1532*
management 1527, 2008
medical complications *1528*
and osteoarthritis 3630
in polycyclic ovary syndrome 1908, 1911
prevalence 1528
reproductive effects *1917*
and respiratory failure 3472
treatment 1532
bariatric surgery 1534, 2010
behavioural therapy 1533
diet 1532
drug therapy 1533, 2010
exercise 1533
weight loss 1532
obesity-hypoventilation syndrome 1527, 3472
obestatin 2319
obidoxime *1274*
objective list theories 18
observational studies 49
before-and-after studies 50
case-control studies 49, *49*
historical controlled 49, *49*
obsessive-compulsive disorder 5316, 5326
obstructive nephropathy 4151
causes 4152, *4152*
clinical approach 4153
incidence 4152
lower urinary tract
acute 4155
chronic 4157
upper urinary tract
acute 4153, *4155*
chronic 4155, *4156–7*
obstructive shock 3122, 3128
obstructive sleep apnoea 3261, 3263
aetiology 3263, *3264*
anatomical causes 3264, *3265*
neuromuscular function 3264
definition 3263
diagnosis 3268
differential diagnosis 3269
driving regulations 3273
epidemiology 3271
immediate consequences 3265, *3266–7*
prognosis and long-term complications 3272, *3272–3*
reproductive effects *1917*
symptoms and presentation 3268, *3268–9*
treatment 3270, *3270–2*
obturator nerve neuropathy 5084
occipital lobe 4856
cortical blindness 4856
occlusive vasculopathies 4629, 4633
occupational asthma 3287, *3288*
diagnosis 3293
immunological tests 3293
inhalation testing 3293, *3295*
lung function tests 3293, *3294*
management 3299
specific causes 3295
occupational cancers 307, *308*, 1379
background 1379
bladder 327
causes 1379, *1380*
diagnosis 1379
industrial processes 1381
infections 1381
lung cancer 318, 3516, *3516*
see also individual agents
occupational diseases 1376
assessment of workforce/workplace 1378
evaluation 1378
remedial action 1379
cancer *see* occupational cancers
cardiovascular system 1383
compensation 1378
COPD 3314
definition and scope 1377
gastrointestinal tract 1384
genitourinary system 1384
haemopoietic system 1384
historical aspects 1377
individual proof system 1378
musculoskeletal disorders 1382
affecting occupation 1383
clinical investigations and management 1383
low back pain 1383
occupations associated with 1383
upper limbs 1382
neurological 1386
chemical exposure 1386, *1386–7*
physical factors 1387
prevention 1378
psychological aspects 1387
medically unexplained symptoms *1387*, 1388
occupational stress 1387, *1387*
reproductive system 1385
female 1385
male 1385
respiratory 1387
skin 1381
contact dermatitis 1381
employers'/employees' attitudes to 1381
nondermatitic dermatoses 1382
protection against 1381
see also environmental diseases
occupational health services 1377
occupational rhinitis 3278
occupational safety 1388
advice and assistance 1392
audit and review 1390
competence 1391
management 1390
monitoring performance 1390
planning 1390
policy 1390
safety management and culture 1391
sensible risk 1391, *1391*
size of problem 1390
work-related road risk 1391
Ochrobactrum spp. *962*
ochronosis 3711
octopus envenoming 1348, *1348–9*
octreotide
acromegaly 1807
carcinoid syndrome 2324
hepatocellular carcinoma 2517
pancreatic neuroendocrine tumours 1981
ocular larva migrans 1174
ocular myasthenia 5181
oculocephalic reflex, loss of 1275
oculocerebrorenal syndrome *3739*
oculocutaneous albinism
type I 4663
type II 4663
oculomycosis 1015
oculopharyngeal muscular dystrophy 5206
oculovestibular reflex, loss of 1275
odds ratio 49, 52
odynophagia 2206
Oeciacus hirundinis 1227
oedema 3083
aetiology 3085, *3086*
primary lymphoedema 3085
secondary lymphoedema 3085
clinical features 3087, *3088*
cellulitis 3088
clinical investigation 3088
colour Doppler duplex ultrasound 3089
gene testing 3089
lymphoscintigraphy 3089, *3090*
MRI 3089
diagnosis *3088*
differential diagnosis 3087–8
'armchair' legs 3088
lipoedema 3088, *3090*
'venous' oedema 3088
epidemiology 3087
facial lymphoedema 3091
genital lymphoedema 3091
history 3087
idiopathic, of women 3093
clinical features 3093
definition and diagnosis 3093
management 3094
pathophysiology 3094
malnutrition 1511, *1512*
nephrotic syndrome *3854*
pathophysiology 3083, *3084*
pregnancy 2088
prevention 3087
treatment 3090
drug therapy 3091
physical therapy 3090
prevention of infection 3091, *3091*
surgery 3091
upper airway 3257
allergic 3257
angio-oedema 3257
smoke inhalation 3258
oenanthotoxin 1362
Oerskovia spp. *962*
oesophageal atresia 2396, *2397*
clinical features 2396
diagnosis 2397
management 2397
oesophageal cancer 313, 2405, 2406
clinical features 2407, *2407*
incidence *301*, *314*, 2406

migrants vs residents *302*
management 2407
palliative 2407
surgery 2406
predisposing factors 2406
oesophageal columnar metaplasia *see* Barrett's oesophagus
oesophageal disease
symptoms 2205
dysphagia 2205
heartburn 2206
pain 2206
oesophageal diverticula 2302
oesophageal function 2229
oesophageal performation, iatrogenic 2303
oesophageal rupture 2303
oesophageal spasm 2295
oesophageal stricture
endoscopy
benign strictures 2216
malignant strictures 2216
oesophageal transit 2288
oesophageal varices 2238, *2238*
therapeutic endoscopy 2216
uncontrolled haemorrhage 2240
oesophagitis 2206, 2292
eosinophilic 2293, *2293*
GI bleeding *2238*
infective 2292, *2293*
medication-induced 2293, *2294*
oesophagogas-troduodenoscopy 2287
Oesophagostomum spp. 1167, *1167*
oesophagus
anatomy 2201
abnormalities of 2301
Barrett's oesophagus 2291
gastro-oesophageal reflux disease 2288
investigation 2287
management 2298
motor disorders 2294, 2297
neoplasms 2298, *2299, 2301*
peptic stricture 2291
extrinsic compression 2302
function of 2202
radiology 2287
trauma 2302
oestradiol 1903
actions *1791*
17-β-oestradiol, reference values *5441*
oestradiol, signalling pathways *1797*
Oestridae *1233*
oestrogens
deficiency 3630
insensitivity *1917*
reproductive effects *1917*
role in men 1915
Oestrus ovis *1233*, 1234
ofloxacin *707*
brucellosis 794
leprosy 846
mycoplasmal infections *960*
pelvic inflammatory disease *1260*
in renal failure *4185*
typhoid fever *742*
Ohm's law 161, 2683
ointments 4731
OKT3 *290*, 292
adverse effects 3955
olanzapine 5266, *5337*
schizophrenia *5325*
older patients 5389
abuse of 5408
acute abdomen 2236
assessment 5406
coronary heart disease 2886
driving 5390, 5402
ECG exercise testing 2661
faecal incontinence 5389, 5399
falls 5389, 5394
frailty 5389–90
hyponatraemia 3826
mental disorders 5406
delirium 5389, 5402, 5406
dementia 5407
depression 5407
mania/hypomania 5407
neurosis and personality disorders 5408
paranoid disorders 5407
prescribing for 5390, 5401
pressure sores 5389, 5395
suicide attempts 5295
surgery 5390, 5396
urinary incontinence 5389, 5397
oleander poisoning, antidote *1274*
olecranon bursitis *3248*, 3588
olfaction 3170
olfactory nerve disorders 5033
Oligella spp. *962*
oligodendrocytes 4950
oligodendroglioma *4778*, 4778
oligomenorrhoea 1905, *1905*
oligospermia 1385
oligozoospermia 1922
oliguria 3852, 3886
snake bite 1352
olsalazine, ulcerative colitis 2378, *2380*
Olsenella spp. *962*
omega-3 fatty acids, in pregnancy 2090
Omenn's syndrome *238*, 250
omeprazole
adverse effects, hepatotoxicity *2529*
peptic ulcer disease 2240, 2311
Omsk haemorrhagic fever virus *566*, 574
Onchocerca spp. *1176*
Onchocerca volvulus 1227
renal toxicity *4086*, 4088
see also onchocerciasis
onchocerciasis *1146*, 1145–6
clinical features 1147
eye damage 1147, *1148*, 5252
skin disease 1148, *1148–9*
diagnosis 1149
epidemiology 1146
parasitology 1146, *1147*
prevention and control 1150
treatment 1149
oncogenes 335, 342, 346, 361
cytoplasmic protein tyrosine kinases 348, *348*
microRNA 353, *354*
nuclear proteins 349
receptor protein tyrosine kinases 347, *347*
oncogenic hypophosphataemic osteomalacia 4142
oncology
clinical 372
see also cancer
oncostatin M 3552
ondansetron *5423*
ontogeny 4747
Onychocola canadensis 1002
onychomycosis 1000, *4699*, *4699–700*
oogonia 1902
open reading frames, human papillomavirus *601*
Ophionyssus natricis 1240
ophthalmia, venom 1334, *1335*, 1353
ophthalmopathy
thyroid-associated *1839*
treatment *1841*
ophthalmoplegia
chronic progressive *1552*
chronic progressive external *5223*
ophthalmoscopy 5235, *5235*
opiates *see* opioids
opioids
in breast milk *1469, 2189*
cancer pain 394
critical illness 3155, *3155*
dependence 5345
diabetic neuropathy 2039
drug interactions *1471*
palliative care 5422, *5422–3*
poisoning *1274*, 1290
antidote *1274*, *5505*
reproductive effects *1917*
withdrawal 5347, *5347*
Opisthorchis felineus *1213*, 1214
Opisthorchis guayaquilaris *1213*
Opisthorchis viverrini 307, 315, 1212, *1213*, 1214
opisthotonos 795, *796, 798*
opportunistic infections 3956, *3956–7*
opsoclonus-myoclonus 5171
opsonization 208
optic atrophy 4854, *4852, 4854*
optic chiasma, disorders of 4856
optic disc anomalies 4852
colobomas 4852
morning glory syndrome 4852
myelinated nerve fibres 4852
papilloedema 4853, *4853*
swelling 4852
tilting 4852
optic nerve
drusen 4852
dysplasia 4852
glioma 358
hypoplasia 4852
occlusion of vessels supplying 5240
tumours 4855
gliomas 4855
meningiomas 4855
optic neuritis 4854, *384, 4855, 4952*
optic neuropathies
heredofamilial 4853, 4855
arteritis 4853
ischaemic, nonarteritic 3043, 4853
nutritional and toxic 4855
optic pits 4852
optic radiations 4856
optic tract lesions 4856
oral allergy syndrome 263
oral anticoagulants, in renal failure 4180
oral cavity, commensal flora 749
oral contraceptives *1265, 2191, 2192*
adverse effects, hepatotoxicity *2536*
benefits 2191
in breast milk *1469, 2189*
contraindication in porphyria 1641, *5484*
disadvantages 2192
circulatory disease 2192, *2193–4*
tumours 2192, *2192*
heart disease patients 2115
prescribing 2194, *2195*
oral glucose tolerance test *5449*
oral hypoglycaemic agents 2014
α-glucosidase inhibitors 2017
incretin mimetics 2017
meglitinides 2014
metformin 2015
in pregnancy 2137
sulphonylureas 2014
thiazolidinediones 2016
Oran virus *581*
orbitofrontal syndrome 4794
orbiviruses 556
Changuinola 556
Kemerovo 556
Lebombo 556
Orungo 556
orchidectomy *1917*
orchitis *1917*
mumps 514
orellanine 1369, *1367, 1370*
orf 655
aetiology 655
clinical features 655, *656*
diagnosis 656
differential diagnosis 656, *656*
epidemiology 655
immunopathology 655
treatment 657
organ donors 3161, 3163
acceptability 3163, *3163*
clinical management 3163
cardiovascular problems 3163, *3164*
coagulation abnormalities 3164
endocrine problems *3162*, 3164
respiratory problems 3164
temperature control 3164
donor operation 3164
organ system profiles *5436*
organic acidaemias 5109
organic acids, analysis 1563
organic acidurias
clinical chemical indices *1563*
presentation *1562*
organic dusts, toxic syndrome *3443*
organic solvents, CNS effects *1386*
organizing pneumonia *3379, 3383*, 3384
autoimmune rheumatic disorders 3390, *3390*
clinical features 3385
differential diagnosis 3386
histopathology 3384, *3385*
investigations 3385
bronchoalveolar lavage 3385
imaging 3385, *3385*
lung function tests 3385
prognosis 3386
treatment 3386
organophosphate poisoning *1274*, 1304
antidote *1274*

CNS effects *1386*
peripheral nervous system effects *1387*, 5087
organotin compounds, CNS effects *1386*
orgasmic disorders in women 1947
Oriboca virus *581*
Orientia spp. *962*
Orientia tsutsugamushi 903, *919*, 919
oritavancin *706*
bacteraemia *703*
cellulitis, mastitis and pyomyositis *699*
orlistat, in renal failure 4182
ornidazole, giardiasis *1113*
ornithine aminotransferase, differential diagnosis *1722*
ornithine carbamoyltransferase deficiency *1566*
ornithine, reference values *5446*
Ornithodoros spp. *1228*
Ornithorhynchus anatinus (duck-billed platypus) 1327
orofacial granulomatosis 2278
aetiology 3, 2278
clinical features 2278, *2278*
management 2279
oromandibular dystonia 4892, *4893*
oropharyngeal cancer 605
Oropouche virus 582, *581, 583*
oroticaciduria 1633, 4418
Oroya fever *see* bartonellosis
orphan diseases 1706
orphan receptors 1794
orphenadrine, poisoning *1274*
Orthobunyavirus 580, *581*
Bunyamwera virus 580
California encephalitis, Inkoo, Jamestown Canyon, La Crosse, Tahyna and snowshoe hare viruses 580
Oropouche virus 582
Orthoperus spp. 1236
orthopnoea 3507
orthostatic hypotension 2638, *2638*
drugs causing *2639*
treatment *5063*
ortho-toluidine *1380*
Orungo virus 556
os trigonum *5382*
oseltamivir
influenza virus 480
mode of action *444*
pneumonia *3238, 3245*
Osgood Schlatter disease *3804, 5382*
Osler's nodes, infective endocarditis *2809*
Osler-Weber-Rendu disease 2586, 4691
osmolality
potassium homeostasis *3833*
reference values *5435, 5446*
osmoreceptors 1790
osmotic agents, intracranial hypertension *3150*
osmotic diuretics 1462
Ossa virus *581*
osseous heteroplasia
progressive *3721*
clinical features *3731*
osteitis deformans *see* Paget's disease of bone
osteitis fibrosa 3919, *3920*
osteoarthritis 3628, 3564
aetiology 3628
clinical features 3628, *3632*, 3632
definition 3629, *3629*
epidemiology/risk factors 3630, *3630*
age, sex and race 3630
biomechanical factors 3631
genetics 3630
obesity 3630
oestrogen deficiency 3630
reactive oxygen species 3631
hip *3629*
investigations 3633, *3633–4*
knee *3629*
management 3628
pathogenesis 3628, 3631
pathology 3631
protective factors 3631
treatment 3633, *3634*
aids and appliances 3635
analgesics 3634
corticosteroids 3635
exercise and psychosocial support 3633
hyaluronic acid 3635
joint lavage 3635
NSAIDs 3634
surgery 3635
weight loss 3633
osteoarthropathy, hypertrophic pulmonary *385*
osteoblasts 3548, *3719, 3722, 3723*
osteocalcin 3550, *3726, 3729*
CKD-MBD *3922*
osteochondritis dissecans 3803
osteochondrosis 3803
classification *3804*
clinical features 3804
diagnosis 3804
epidemiology 3804
future developments 3804
pathophysiology 3804
treatment 3804
osteoclast differentiation factor 3550
osteoclasts 3548, *3719, 3722, 3724*
osteocytes 3550, 3719, 3722
osteodystrophies
mouth 2283
post-liver transplantation 2510
renal *1858*, 3737
osteogenesis imperfecta 3719, *3721*, 3730, 3745
biochemistry 3748
cardiac involvement *2840*
classification *3746*
clinical features 3746, *3731, 3747–8*
diagnosis 3748
genetic counselling 3748
management 3749
mutations in *3757*
pathophysiology 3746
prenatal diagnosis 3749
prognosis 3749
osteogenic sarcoma 320
osteolysis, familial expansile *3721*, 3744
osteomalacia *384*, 3719, 3734, *3735*
anticonvulsant 3740
autosomal dominant hypophosphataemic *3721*
biochemical changes *3736*
causes *3735*, 3736
CKD 3917, 3919
clinical features *3731*, 3736
myopathy 5218
diagnosis 3738
histology *3735*
investigations 3737
biochemistry *3736*, 3737
bone biopsy 3738
radiology 3737, *3737*
and malabsorption 3739
nutritional 3738
oncogenic 2061
oncogenic hypo-phosphataemic 4142
pathophysiology 3734
and renal disease 3739, *3739*
treatment 3738
osteomyelitis 3788, *699, 701*
acute 3788
treatment 3793
aetiology 3617, *3788, 3789–90*
Bartonella 931
Brucella *791, 793, 3789*
chronic 3788
treatment 3793
clinical features 3791, *3792*
diagnosis 3793
differential diagnosis 3791
epidemiology *4269*
future developments 3794
historical perspective 3788
investigations 3791
occupational aspects 3794
pathogenesis/pathophysiology 3788, *3789–90*
prevention and control 3791
prognosis 3794
psychosocial aspects 3794
quality of life 3794
treatment 3793
adjunctive 3794
antibiotics 3793
surgery 3793
osteonecrosis 3802
clinical features 3803
dysbaric 1421, 3802
epidemiology 3803
genetic factors 3802
imaging 3803
pathophysiology 3802, *3803*
treatment 3803
vascular interruption 3802
osteonectin 3550, 3726
osteopathy 65
osteopenia
CKD 3919
diabetic 2048
osteoperiostitis *881*
osteopetrosis *168*, 3720, *3721*, 3760
clinical features *3731, 3760–1*
mild 3760
severe 3760
osteopontin 3726
osteoporosis circumscripta *3742*
osteoporosis pseudoglioma syndrome, clinical features *3731*
osteoporosis 3796, 1522
bone mineral density 3798
clinical features 3797, *3731, 3797*
cystic fibrosis 3363
diagnosis 3798
bone turnover markers 3799
radiology 3799
epidemiology 3796
glucocorticoid-induced 3801
HRT 2196
non-pharmacological interventions 3800
pathogenesis 3797, *3797*
pathophysiology 3797, *3798*
post-transplant 3964
pseudoglioma *3721*
in rheumatoid arthritis 3589
risk factors 3798, *3798*
treatment 3799
compliance and persistence 3800
duration of therapy 3800
positioning of 3799
rate of commencement 3800
see also individual drugs
osteoprotegerin 156, 3550, 3724
osterix 3722
Ostertagia spp. *1176*
ostium primum defect 2853
ostium secondum defect 2648, 2852
otitis externa, *Pseudomonas aeruginosa* 736
otitis media
chlamydial 945
pneumococcal 690
otomycosis 1015
ovarian cancer 325
genetic predisposition 365
incidence *325*
migrants vs residents *302*
pregnancy 2183
ovarian failure *1960*
ovarian hyperstimulation syndrome 2087
ovary
development *1788*, 1902
disorders of 1904
folliculogenesis 1902
organogenesis and follicle formation 1902, *1902*
overdistension syndrome 2105
overlap syndromes 3268, 3270
overnutrition 309, 1516
overpopulation 74
overtraining syndrome 5378
aetiology 5378
clinical features 5379
pathophysiology 5378
prevention 5379
treatment 5379
overuse injuries 5382, *5382*
overweight
classification *1528*
see also obesity
ovulation disorders 1904
amenorrhoea 1905, *1905*
anovulation 1904
hypothalamic/pituitary dysfunction 1906
management 1905, *1905*
oligomenorrhoea 1905, *1905*
polycystic ovary syndrome 1907
polycystic ovary syndrome (PCOS) *1871*, 1907, *1908*
premature (primary) ovarian failure 1905
ovulation induction 1910, *1910*
Owen, Robert 1377
oxacillin *706*
adverse effects, hepatotoxicity *2529, 2535*
bacteraemia *703, 705*
endocarditis *704–5*

epidural abscess *702*
osteomyelitis *701*
pneumonia *702, 3238*
septic bursitis/arthritis *700*
urinary tract infection *702*
oxalate crystals 3648
oxalate 1730
reference values *5446*
oxalic acid *1362*
oxalosis 1730
oxamniquine, schistosomiasis 1210
oxandrolone 1962
oxaprozin
adverse effects, hepatotoxicity *2529*
and asthma *3289*
oxazolidinone, adverse effects *455*
oxcarbazepine
dose levels *4823*
epilepsy 4822
Oxfordshire Community Stroke Subclassification System *5488*
oxicillin, toxic shock syndrome *697*
oxidation, genetic variability 1472, *1473–4*
oxidative stress 1633, *2475, 2476*
COPD 3323
and hypertension 3032
oximes *1274*, 1305
oximetry 2681, *2682*
oxitropium bromide, COPD *3335*
2-oxoadipic aciduria *1566*
oxycodone
contraindication in porphyria *5484*
palliative care 5423
oxygen consumption 3126
oxygen delivery systems *3138*
fixed performance 3138
variable performance 3139
oxygen delivery 3126, 3470, *3470*
acidosis 1744
oxygen equipment 1412, *1413*
see also ventilation
oxygen therapy
acute asthma 3308
acute respiratory failure 3138, *3138*
air travel 3339
ambulatory 3339
anaphylaxis 3111
chronic respiratory failure 3473, *3473*
COPD 3338, 3342
critical illness 3116
cystic fibrosis 3360
pulmonary arterial hypertension 2987
oxygen uptake, acidosis 1744
oxygen
hyperbaric, gas gangrene 808
toxicity 1419, *1419*
oxymetholone
aplastic anaemia 4288
carcinogenesis *307*
oxyntomodulin 1535, 2319
oxyphenbutazone, adverse effects, hepatotoxicity *2532, 2535*
oxytetracycline, acne *4680*
oxytocin 1824
actions *1791*
structure 1819
Oxyuranus scutellatus canni (Papua New Guinean taipan) *1330*
Oxyuranus scutellatus, antivenom *1340*

P wave 2644, 2648
p38MAPK 158
P450 oxidoreductase deficiency 1899
p53 gene product 349
pacemakers *see* pacing
pachyonychia 4599, *4599*
pacing 2694
complications 2695, *2696*
follow-up 2696
hypertrophic cardiomyopathy 2772
mode selection 2695, *2695*
permanent 2695
heart failure 2726, *2726*
principles of 2694, *2694*
temporary 5512, *5512*
external (transcutaneous) 5512
failure of *5514*
transvenous 5513, *5513–14*
ventricular, temporary 2694
packed cell volume 4195, *4191, 4196*
infants and children *4197*
paclitaxel 401
breast cancer *1937*
cost-effectiveness ratio *53*
lung cancer 3529
$Paco_2$, 1740, 3469
Paeccilomyces spp. *3436*
Paederus crebripunctatus (vesicating beetle) *1351*
Paenibacillus spp. *962*
Paget's disease (of bone) 320, *3719, 3721, 3741, 3741*
clinical features *3731*, 3742
deafness and nerve compression 3742
heart failure 3742
oral 2283
pain, deformity and fracture 3742
diagnosis 3743
sarcoma 3743, *3743*
incidence 3741, *3741*
investigations 3742
biochemistry 3742
radiology 3742, *3742–3*
juvenile *3721*, 3744
clinical features *3731*
oesophageal symptoms *2297*
pathophysiology 3741, 3743
medical 3743
treatment, surgical 3744
Paget's disease (of nipple) 4713
pain ladder 5413, *5421*
pain 5409
cancer-related 381
bone infiltration 381
management 394
nerve infiltration 382
visceral pain 382
history 5412
mechanisms and syndromes 5412, *5412*
in palliative care 5420, *5421–3*
recording of 5413
resistant pain 5415
sensation and transmission 5411
treatment 5413, *5413*
mixed pain 5415
neuropathic pain 5414, *5414*
nociceptive pain 5413, *5413*
types and descriptors *5421*
visceral 382
Paine's syndrome *4904*
painters, cancer in *1380*
palivizumab, respiratory syncytial virus 478
palliative care 5419
emergencies 5427, *5427*
end-of-life care 5427, *5428–9*
future developments 5429
heart failure 2729
history 5419
models of *5420*
symptom management 5420, *5420–1*
anorexia 5427
breathlessness 5425, *5426*
constipation 5426, *5426*
depression 5426
fatigue 5427
nausea and vomiting 5424, *5423–5*
pain 5420, *5421–3*
Pallister-Killian syndrome 147
palmar erythema, cirrhosis 2498, *2498*
palpation, chest 3187
palpitation 2641
history 2641
atrial fibrillation 2641
paroxysmal supraventricular tachycardia 2641
premature beats 2641
sinus tachycardia 2641
ventricular tachycardia 2641
investigation 2641
ambulatory monitoring 2641
ECG 2641
electrophysiological 2641
management 2641
palpitations, pregnancy 2088
pamidronate
adverse effects, renal toxicity *3860*
hypercalcaemia 1857
osteogenesis imperfecta 3749
Paget's disease 3744
p-aminosalicylic acid, adverse effects, hepatotoxicity *2529, 2532*
PAMPS 207, 210, 410
panbronchiolitis, diffuse 3387
Pancoast syndrome 382
Pancoast tumour 3519, 3524
pancreas 2435, 2442
agenesis 2582
annular 2573, 2582
congenital disorders 2582
agenesis 2582
annular pancreas 2582
hereditary pancreatitis 2582
pancreas divisum 2582, *2582*
in cystic fibrosis 3354
development and congenital anomalies 2442
developmental anomalies 2573
diseases 2557
see also pancreatitis
divisum 2573, *2582, 2582*
endocrine 2443, *2443*
exocrine 2442
islets of Langerhans 1992
development *1788*
structure and function 2442
pancreatic disease 1976
diabetes mellitus in 2007
multiple endocrine neoplasia 1982
pancreatic duct stricture 2559
benign 2559
tumours 2559
pancreatic enzyme deficiencies 2573
pancreatic hormones, potassium homeostasis *3833*
pancreatic insufficiency, cystic fibrosis 3361
pancreatic lipase inhibitors 1533
pancreatic neuroendocrine tumours 1977
aetiology and genetics 1977
definition 1977
gastrinoma 1979
glucagonoma 1980
imaging 1978, *1978–9*
immunohistochemical markers 1977
insulinoma 1979
MEN1, 1983
natural history 1979
PPoma 1981
serum markers 1977, *1978*
somatostatinoma 1980
treatment 1981
surgical 1981
symptomatic 1981
VIPoma 1979
pancreatic polypeptide *2443*
elevation *1978*
inhibition *2320*
reference values *5442*
tumours secreting 1981
pancreatic pseudocyst 2566
pancreatic secretions 2228
pancreatic stem cells 200
pancreatic tumours 2574, 317
aetiology and genetics 2574
clinical features 2575
clinical investigation 2575
diagnosis and staging 2575
differential diagnosis 2575
future developments 2578
genetic predisposition 365
histopathology 2577
incidence, migrants vs residents *302*
pathogenesis/pathology 2574
prevention 2575
prognosis 2578
treatment 2577
tumour markers 2577
pancreatin 4177
pancreatitis *3120*
acute 2557
aetiology 2558, *2558*
clinical features 2560
clinical progress and outcome 2563
complications 2566
diagnosis 2561
differential diagnosis 2561, *2561*
disease severity 2561, *2561*
epidemiology 2557
hereditary 2559
iatrogenic 2559
management 2564, *2564*

organ failure scoring 2562, *2562–3*
pathology 2560
surgical intervention 2565, *2565*
traumatic 2559, *2559*
aetiology, enterovirus 531
autoimmune 2560
bile duct obstruction 2555
chronic 2567
aetiology 2567, *2568*
clinical features 2568
complications 2572, *2572*
genetics *143*
incidence 2568
investigation/diagnosis 2569, *2569–71*
management 2571, *2572*
pathophysiology 2568
ERCP 2218, 2564
hereditary 2559, 2573, 2582
investigations *2235*
ocular involvement 5244
pancreolauryl test 2228, 2328
panda sign *4685*
Pangonia spp. *1226*
panitumumab *376*, 401
Panner's disease *3804*
panniculitis *385, 3707*, 4648, *4649*
cold 4651, *4651*
lobular 4650
sclerosing *4649*
septal 4648
see also α_1-antitrypsin deficiency
Pannonibacter spp. *962*
pannus *941*
panophthalmitis, meningococcal 719
Panstrongylus megistus (triatomine bug) *1128*, 1228
Pantoea spp. *962*
Panton-Valentine leukocidin 694, 4673
pantoprazole, peptic ulcer disease 2311
pantothenate kinase-associated neurodegeneration 1686, 5113
pantothenic acid 1491
deficiency anaemia 4419
requirements 1491
PaO_2 3467
PAPA *1761*, 1765
papaverine, adverse effects, hepatotoxicity *2529*
papillary fibroelastoma 2832
papillary muscle rupture 2742
papillary necrosis 4119
papilloedema 4973
Papillon-Lefèvre syndrome 1717, *4599*, 4600
papules *4591*
papulonecrotic tuberculid *4674*
papulosquamous disease 4610
psoriasis *see* psoriasis
Parabacteroides spp. *962*
Paracapillaria philippinensis 1168, 1171
paracentesis
diagnostic 2485
therapeutic 2488, *2488*
benefits 2488
colloid replacement 2488
contraindications 2489
practical aspects 2488
paracetamol
adverse effects, hepatotoxicity *2529*
and asthma *3289*
in breast milk *2189*
cancer pain 394
metabolism *1291*
migraine *4917*
mountain sickness 1404
poisoning 1272, *1291, 1292, 3860*
antidote *1274, 1293, 1292–3, 5505*
clinical features 1291
management of severe liver damage 1293
mechanisms of toxicity 1291
prediction of liver damage 1292, *1293*
prognostic factors 1292
risk factors 1291
serum levels *5449*
SLE 2156
Parachlamydia spp. *962*
Paracoccidioides brasiliensis 1023
paracoccidioidomycosis 1023
aetiology 1023
host-fungus interaction 1024, *1025*
mycology 1024, *1024*
pathogenesis 1024
pathology 1024
virulence 1024
clinical features 1025, *1025*
acute form (juvenile type) 1025, *1026*
chronic form 1026, *1026–7*
definition 1023
diagnosis 1027
histopathology 1027
immunological tests 1027
microbiological 1027
ecology 1023
epidemiology 1023
history 1023
prognosis 1028
treatment 1028
Paracoccus spp. *962*
paraesthesia 5078
paraffin oil (kerosene) poisoning 1314
parafibromin 1861
Parafossarulus manchouricus 1212
paragonimiasis 1216
aetiology and life cycle 1216, *1216–17*
clinical features 1217
extrapulmonary paragonimiasis 1217
pulmonary paragonimiasis 1217, *1217*
clinical investigation 1218, *1218–19*
differential diagnosis 1218
epidemiology 1217
pathogenesis and pathology 1217
prevention and control 1219
prognosis 1219
treatment 1219
Paragonimus africanus 1216
Paragonimus heterotremus 1216
Paragonimus kellicotti 1216
Paragonimus mexicanus 1216
Paragonimus skrjabini 1216
Paragonimus uterobilateralis 1216
Paragonimus westermani 1216
parainfluenza virus *474*, 478
paraldehyde poisoning *1742*
paramyotonia congenita 5219
paraneoplastic syndromes 383, *384*
neurological 5166, *3515, 3519*
amyotrophic lateral sclerosis 5172
brainstem encephalitis 5171
cerebellar degeneration 5169, *5171*
diagnosis *5168, 5168, 5169*
limbic encephalitis 5171, *5172*
myelitis 5172
necrotizing myelopathy 5172
neuromuscular junction and muscle 5173, *5173*
opsoclonus-myoclonus 5171
pathogenesis 5169
peripheral nerves *5173*, 5173
sensory neuronopathy 5172, *5173*
tumours associated with 5168
visual loss 5172
treatment 5169, *5170*
paranoid disorders, older people 5407
paraplegia, hereditary spastic 5074
paraproteinaemias 4342, *4344*
paraquat poisoning 1305, *1306*
parasitic infections 2430
and acute pancreatitis 2560
and cancer 307
bladder cancer 328
diarrhoea 2429
haematological changes 4552
immunosuppressed patients 3959
parasomnias 4834, *4834*
deep non-REM sleep 4834
differential diagnosis 4817
REM sleep 4835
sleep-wake transition 4834
parastrongyliasis 1179
Parastrongylus cantonensis 1179
aetiology 1179
clinical features 1180, *1180*
diagnosis 1180
epidemiology 1179
pathology 1180
treatment, prognosis and control 1180
Parastrongylus costaricensis 1179–80
parathyroid carcinoma *1855*
parathyroid glands 1851
and bone disease 3744
molecular mechanisms 3744
calcium homeostasis 1852, *1852–3*, 1854
disorders of
aetiology and genetics 1854, *1855*
drug-induced 2069
haematological changes 4559
hypercalcaemia 1851, 1854
hypocalcaemia 1851, 1862
ocular involvement 5249
in pregnancy 2143
historical perspective 1852, *1853*
hyperplasia/adenoma 1983, 1985
tumour-like growth 3923
parathyroid hormone
actions *1791*
calcium/phosphorus balance 3728
CKD-MBD *3922*
reference values *5441*
parathyroid hormone-related protein 383, 3720
calcium balance 3729
parathyroidectomy 1859, 3923
parathyroid-hormone peptides, osteoporosis 3800
paratrachoma 945
paratyphoid fever 745
paraumbilical hernia 2490
Paré, Ambroise 23
parenchyma, COPD *3319*
parenteral nutrition
access devices *1540*
complications 1541, 2585
indications for *1537*
parietal lobe syndromes 5274
Parinaud's oculoglandular syndrome 929
Parkinson's disease 4879, 187, 5112
cognitive impairment 5279
dementia 4807
diagnosis 4882
confirmation of 4882, *4885*
epidemiology, incidence and prevalence 4880
genetics *143, 4881, 4881*
management 4884
anticholinergics 4886
dopamine agonists 4885
monoamine oxidase-B inhibitors 4885
surgery 4886
nonmotor symptom complex 4882, *4883*
pathophysiology 4881, *4882–3*
risk factors 4880, *4881*
stem cell therapy 201
symptoms and signs 4881, *4884*
parkinsonism, drug-induced 4886
paromomycin, amoebiasis 1041
paronychia 1003, 1382
parosmia 5033
parotitis, epidemic *see* mumps
paroxetine
adverse effects *5313*
poisoning 1281
paroxysmal cold haemoglobinuria 4456
paroxysmal hemicrania 4920
paroxysmal nocturnal haemoglobinuria 221, 4212, 4298
complications *4301*, 4300
definition 4299
epidemiology *4299*, 4299
laboratory investigations and diagnosis *4299, 4300*, 4300
pathophysiology 4299
bone marrow failure *4301*, 4300
haemolysis 4299
thrombosis 4300
treatment *4302*, 4301
paroxysmal supraventricular tachycardia 2641
Parry's disease 1698
parthenolide *1939*
partial thromboplastin time *4196*
Parvimonas spp. *962*
parvovirus B19 607, *607*
aetiology 607
clinical features 608, *609*
diagnosis 609

epidemiology 608
pathogenesis/pathology 608, *608*
pregnancy 2166, *2167*
prevention 609
treatment 609
Pasqualini's syndrome *1917*
passenger lymphocyte haemolysis 4457
Pasteurella multocida 777, 1326
aetiology and genetics 778
clinical features 778, *778*
clinical investigation 779
differential diagnosis 779
epidemiology 778
history 778
pathogenesis and pathology 778
prevention 778
prognosis 779
treatment 779, *779*
Pasteurella spp. *962*
Patau's syndrome 145
patellar tendinopathy *5382*
patellofemoral joint syndrome *5382*
patello-femoral syndrome *3248*
patent arterial duct 2858
patent ductus arteriosus, pregnancy 2113
patent foramen ovale 2851
pathergy phenomenon, Behçet's disease *3685–6*
pathogen-associated molecular patterns *see* PAMPS
pathogens
coevolution 14
vulnerability to 14, *14*
patient education, COPD 3340, *3340*
patients 3
electronic records 46
health advertising to 109
food industry 110
health care providers 110
medical devices 110
pharmaceutical companies 109
Pauli's reagent *3436*
Paxillus syndrome 1370
pCO_2, *5515*
peak expiratory flow rate 3192
airways obstruction 3256, *3256*
asthma *3292*
COPD *3324*, 3329, *3329*
Pearson's syndrome 1572, *5223*
pectus carinatum 3510
Marfan's syndrome *3750*
pectus excavatum 3509
Marfan's syndrome *3750*
Pediculus humanus 912, *1230, 1230*
Pediococcus spp. *962*
Peel, Robert 1377
pefloxacin *706*
leprosy 846
Pelagia noctiluca 1347
Pelamis platurus 1327
Pel-Ebstein fever 382
peliosis hepatis 927, 930
diagnosis *931*
drug-induced 2535
treatment 933
Pelizaeus-Merzbacher disease 4962, 5106
Pelizaeus-Merzbacher-like disease 5107
pellagra 1490
Pelodera (Rhabditis) strongyloides 1176
pelvic inflammatory disease *944, 944–5*, 1259
aetiology 1259
chlamydial *944–5*
clinical features 1260
complications 1261
diagnosis 1260
differential diagnosis 1260
mycoplasmal infections *956*, 957
prevention 1261
treatment 1261
Pemberton's sign 1833
pemetrexed, mesothelioma 3537
pemoline, adverse effects, hepatotoxicity *2529*
pemphigoid gestationis 2150, 2152, *2152, 4603*
pemphigoid, photoaggravation *4670*
pemphigus foliaceus *1227*, 4603, *4603*
pemphigus vulgaris *276*, 2275, 4602, *4603–4*
aetiology 2275, 4602
clinical features 2275, *2275, 4603, 4603, 4605*
course and prognosis 2276
differential diagnosis *2275*, 2276
pathology 2275, 4602
in pregnancy 2153
treatment 2276, 4603
pemphigus
paraneoplastic *4603*, 4605
photoaggravation *4670*
pemphogoid gestationis *4603*
Pendred's syndrome 4134
penicillamine neuropathy 4052
penicillin G
Lyme borreliosis *864*
pneumonia *3238*
syphilis 894
penicillin V, in renal failure *4185*
penicillin *3798, 706*
adverse effects, hepatotoxicity *2533, 2535*
bacteraemia *703*
bartonellosis 938
cellulitis, mastitis and pyomyositis *699*
diphtheria 668
endocarditis *704*
epidural abscess *702*
gas gangrene 807
impetigo *697*
in breast milk *2189*
infective endocarditis *2817*, 2817
mode of action *443*
osteomyelitis *701*
pharmacokinetics *449*
pneumococcal pneumonia 687
pneumonia *702*
rheumatic fever 2803
S. moniliformis 859
septic bursitis/arthritis *700*
spectrum of activity *446*
Spirillum minus 860
toxic shock syndrome *697*
urinary tract infection *702*
Penicillium camembertii 3436
Penicillium casei 3436
Penicillium chrysogenum/cyclopium 3436
Penicillium citrinum 3436
Penicillium frequentens 3436
Penicillium marneffei 999, 1032
aetiology 1032
clinical features 1032, *1033*
diagnosis 1034, *1034*
natural history 1032
treatment 1034
Penicillium nalgiovense 3436
Penicillium verucosum 3436
penile cancer 326, 4172
diagnosis and staging 4172
treatment 4173
penile deformity 1943
pennyroyal 68
hepatotoxicity *2529*
pentamidine
adverse reactions *1125*
leishmaniasis *1138*
Pneumocystic jirovecii 1031
trypanosomiasis 1124, *1124–5*
pentastomiasis 1237
aetiology 1237
diagnosis 1240
prevention 1240
treatment 1240
Pentastomida 1237, *1238*
pentazocine, contraindication in porphyria *5484*
pentostatin, lymphoma *4320*
pentosuria 1610, 1614
pentoxifylline, sarcoidosis *3411*
pentraxins 212
peperacillin/ticarcillin, pneumonia *3245*
peperaquine 1075
pepsin 2306
peptic stricture 2291
peptic ulcer disease 2237, 2305
aetiology, pathogenesis and pathology 2306
duodenal bicarbonate secretion 2306
gastric acid and pepsis 2306
tobacco, alcohol and stress 2308
ulcerogenic drugs 2307
areas of uncertainty 2314
clinical features 2309
dyspepsia 2309
haemorrhage 2309, *2309*
obstruction 2310
perforation 2309
clinical investigation 2310, *2310*
complications 2314
differential diagnosis 2310
epidemiology 2308
Forrest classification 2310
prevention 2312
antiplatelet drug-associated ulcer 2313
NSAID-associated ulcer 2313, *2313*
treatment 2311
acute symptoms and complications 2311
bleeding 2311, *2312*
H. pylori infections 2312, *2313*
peptide hormones *1791*
peptide tyrosine tyrosine 2319
Peptococcus spp. *962*
Peptoniphilus spp. *962*
Peptostreptococcus spp. *962*
perceptual disorders 4790
percussion, chest 3187
percutaneous coronary intervention 2935
atherectomy 2938, *2938*
balloon angioplasty 2936, *2936–7*
brachytherapy 2940
closure of cardiac defects 2942
complications 2940, *2940*
abrupt closure and distal embolization *2939*, 2940
restenosis 2940
stent thrombosis 2940
cutting balloon 2938
economic considerations 2941
indications 2936
outcomes 2941
angina 2941
myocardial infarction 2941
unstable angina 2941
STEMI 2927
stents 2937
thrombectomy 2939
valvular disease 2941
aortic stenosis 2942
mitral regurgitation 2942
mitral stenosis 2941, *2941*
pulmonary stenosis 2942
percutaneous needle biopsy, lung 3526
perfloxacin, typhoid fever *742*
perforated viscus 2234
investigations *2235*
performance enhancing drugs 5383
anabolic-androgenic steroids 5383, *5384*
β_2-agonists 5384
creatine 5384
human growth hormone 5383
stimulants 5384
pergolide, prolactinoma 1811
pergomide, adverse effects, hepatotoxicity *2529*
perianal infection, streptococcal 672
pericardial clot 2795
pericardial constriction 2790
pericardial cysts 3543
pericardial disease 2790
anatomy and physiology 2790
cardiac catheterization/angiography 2679, *2679*
congenital 2796
echocardiography 2667, *2667*
post-surgery complications 2795
tight pericardium 2796
see also individual conditions
pericardial effusion 2790–1, *2792–3*
HIV/AIDS 2822, *2822*
malignant 391
pericardial tamponade *see* cardiac tamponade
pericardial tumours 2796
pericardiocentesis 5513
pericarditis 2631, 2790–1
causes 2791
autoimmune disease 2791
irradiation 2791
myocardial infarction 2791
clinical features 2791
constrictive 2794
clinical features 2794
differential diagnosis 2795
hepatic involvement 2538
investigations 2795
loculated 2997

management 2795
pathophysiology 2794, *2795*
infective 2791
meningococcal 718
pneumococcal 691
streptococcal 674, *675*
restrictive 2796
systemic sclerosis 3674
pericytes *2596*, 2594–5
roles of *2596*
perifosine *1939*
perihepatitis 1260
perinephric abscess 4119
perinosis 4687
periodic paralyses 5218
hyperkalaemic 166, 164, 3844, 5219
hypokalaemic *3839*, 5219
familial 3840
sporadic 3840
periodontal disease *see* gingival/periodontal disease
peripartum cardiomyopathy 2110, *2111*
peripartum myocarditis 2762
peripheral arterial disease 2959
abdominal aortic aneurysm 2963
aetiology and epidemiology 2959, *2960*
ischaemia of arm 2963
leg ischaemia 2960
acute 2960
chronic 2961
critical 2960
investigation 2961, *2961*
management 2961–2, *2962*
mesenteric ischaemia *see* mesenteric ischaemia
peripheral nervous system
electrophysiology 4752
physiology 5077
structure 5077
peripheral neuropathies *384*, *5076–7*, *5173*, *5173*
clinical categories 5078
deficiency 5088
alcoholic neuropathy 5089, 5156
cobalamin deficiency 5089
coeliac disease 5088
pyridoxine deficiency 5089
Strachan's syndrome 5089
thiamine deficiency 5088
vitamin E deficiency 5089
diagnosis and investigation 5079
genetic 5092
Charcot-Marie-Tooth disease 5093, *5093*
chronic idiopathic axonal polyneuropathy 5094
congenital hypomyelinating neuropathy 5093
distal hereditary motor neuropathies 5094
familial amyloid polyneuropathy 5092
hereditary neuropathy with liability to pressure palsies 5093
hereditary sensory and autonomic neuro-pathies 5094, *5094*
porphyria 5092
Refsum's disease *see* Refsum's disease
hereditary 5127, *5127*
inflammatory and postinfective 5089
chronic inflammatory demyelinating poly-radiculoneuropathy 5090
Fisher's syndrome 5090
Guillain-Barré syndrome 5089
leprosy 839, *839*
multifocal motor neuropathy 5090
metabolic and endocrine disorders
acromegaly 5087
amyloidosis 5086
critical illness polyneuropathy 5087
diabetes *see* diabetic neuropathy
myxoedema 5086
uraemia 5086
neoplastic/paraneoplastic 5092
nerves affected
axillary nerve 5081
brachial plexus 5079
common peroneal nerve 5085
femoral nerve 5084
lateral cutaneous nerve of thigh 5084
median nerve 5081, *5082*
musculocutaneous nerve 5081
nerve to serratus anterior 5079
obturator nerve 5084
phrenic nerve 5079
radial nerve 5080
sciatic nerve 5084
sural nerve 5085
tibial nerve 5084
ulnar nerve 5082
occupational 1386, *1387*
paraprotein-associated 5090
diphtheritic neuropathy 5091
HIV infection 631, 5091
Lyme borreliosis 5091
sarcoid neuropathy 5091
symptomatology 5078
toxic 5087
vasculitis 5092
peripheral oedema, altitude related 1407
peripheral vascular disease 2044
Periplaneta americana (American cockroach) 1236
perisinusoidal fibrosis, drug-induced 2535
peristaltic reflex 2203, *2203*
peritoneal cancer 320
peritoneal dialysis 3943
complications 3946
acute abdomen 2236
encapsulating peritoneal sclerosis 3947
exit-site infection 3947, *3947*
mechanical failure 3947
peritonitis 3946
ultrafiltration failure 3947
drug elimination 4175
historical perspective 3944
peritoneal access 3945
predictors of survival 3944
principles of 3945
solute clearance 3945
ultrafiltration 3945, *3946*
quality monitoring 3945
solute clearance 3945
ultrafiltration 3946
uses of
acute renal trauma 3893, 3944
chronic kidney disease 3944
vs. haemodialysis 3944, *3944*
peritoneal disorders 2587, *2587*
peritonitis
faecal 2234, 2393
peritoneal dialysis-associated 708, 3946
pneumococcal 691
spontaneous bacterial 2490, *2490–1*
prophylaxis 2491
risk factors 2490, *2491*
treatment 2491, *2492*
permethrin, NNT *52*
pernicious anaemia
achlorhydria 2320, *2321*
acquired 4408
aetiology 4408
clinical features 4409
cardiovascular disease 4410, *4410*
malignancy 4410
neural tube defects 4409
neurological complications 4409
stroke 4410
definition 4408
juvenile 4411
pathology 4409
selective IgA deficiency 2249
peroxisomal diseases 1719, *1552*
future developments 1723
neuro-ophthalmic *see* Refsum's disease
neuropsychiatric *see* X-linked adrenoleukodystrophy
prognosis 1723
treatment 1722
peroxisome proliferator activated receptors (PPARs) *1483*
peroxisomes 129
peroxynitrite 2598
persistent mullerian duct syndrome *1917*
personal protection equipment 1390
skin exposure 1381
personality change 4793
personality disorders *5327*, 5327
older patients 5408
organic causes 5276, *5276*
personalized medicine 149, 46, 61, 1474
pertussis, immunization *91*
pes planus, Marfan's syndrome *3750*
pesticides
poisoning 1301
see also individual pesticides
reproductive effects *1917*
PET *see* positron emission tomography
petechiae *4591*
pethidine 3155, *3155*
in breast milk *1469*
petrol poisoning 1314
Peutz-Jeghers syndrome *302*, *363*, *365*, *1845*, 2222, *2406*
and breast cancer *1930*
Peyer's patches 2202, *2343*, *2245*, 2425
Peyronie's disease 1942–3
Pezizia domiciliana 3436
Pfeiffer's bacillus *see Haemophilus influenzae*
Pfeiffer's syndrome, mutations in *3757*
pH *5515*
of urine 3865
pHa 1740
PHA665752, *1939*
phacomatoses *see* neurocutaneous syndromes
Phaeoanellomyces werneckii 1004
phaeochromocytoma 358, 3066
aetiology and pathology 3066, *3066–7*
clinical features 1985, 3067
clinical investigation 3067
CNS complications 5152
cognitive impairment 5280
epidemiology 3067
localisation 3068, *3069*
malignant 3070
pregnancy 2184
prognosis 3070
treatment 3069
Phagicola spp. *1222*
phagocytes 236, *238*, 252
deficiency
bacterial killing defects 252
neutropenia 252
leucocyte migration defects 253
suppression of production 4206
phagocytosis 177, 208, 1695
spleen 4335
phakomatoses
renal involvement 4100
see also individual disorders
Phalen's sign 3558
Phaneropsulus bonnei 1223
Phaneropsulus spinicirrus 1223
pharmaceutical companies, advertising to patients 109
pharmaceutical industry 60
pharmaceutics 1451
adverse drug reactions 1465
compliance and concordance 1453
drug formulations 1451
systemic availability 1451
pharmacodynamics 1459
adverse drug reactions 1465
antimicrobials 450, *450–2*
defects in 1474
malignant hyperthermia 1474
porphyria 1474
red cell enzymes 1474
vitamin D-resistant rick-ets 1474
warfarin sensitivity 1474
drug-receptor interactions 1459–60
enzyme activation/direct enzymatic activity 1461
enzyme inhibition 1461
inhibition of ion movements 1461
second messengers 1460
stereoisomerism 1462
pharmacogenetics 46, *1472*, 1472
pharmacodynamic defects 1474
pharmacokinetic variability 1472, *1472*
pharmacogenomics 46, 1474

pharmacokinetics 1454
absorption and systemic availability 1455
adverse drug reactions 1465
antimicrobials 449, *449*
clearance 1454
distribution 1456
excretion 1459
genetic variability 1472, *1472*
acetylation 1473
glucuronidation 1473
methylation 1474
oxidation 1472, *1473–4*
suxamethonium hydrolysis 1474
loading doses 1455
metabolism 1457, *1458*
nonlinear 1459, *1460*
plasma half-life 1454, *1455*
in renal impairment 4175
repeated dosing 1454
volume of distribution 1454
pharmacological chaperones 1708
pharmacovigilance 46, 1469
pharyngeal cancer 312
pharyngitis/tonsillitis 3227
clinical presentation 3227
Lemierre syndrome 3229
recurrent attacks 3229
streptococcal 672, *672*
throat swabs, rapid tests and clinical algorithms 3228
treatment 3228
choice of antibiotic 3229
patients with rheumatic fever 3229
prevention of complications 3228
symptoms 3228, *3228*
viral aetiology *474*
pharynx 3170
anatomical divisions 3170
lymphoid tissue 3171
muscles of 3170, *3171*
phenacetamide, adverse effects, hepatotoxicity *2529*
phenacetin, carcinogenesis *307*, 328
phenelzine
adverse effects, hepatotoxicity *2529*
poisoning 1282
phenindione, adverse effects, hepatotoxicity *2532*
pheniprazine, adverse effects, hepatotoxicity *2529*
phenobarbital
adverse effects
hepatotoxicity *2532, 2533*
shoulder-hand syndrome 3714
in breast milk *1469, 2189*
dose levels *4823*
epilepsy 4821
serum levels *5449*
teratogenicity 4822
phenocopies 364
phenol poisoning 1314
phenopyrazone, adverse effects, hepatotoxicity *2532*
phenothiazines
poisoning 1283
antidote *5505*
phenotype 138
phenotypic risk 89
phenoxybenzamine, hypertensive emergencies *3079*
phenoxymethyl penicillin, gingivitis 2262
phenoxypropazine, adverse effects, hepatotoxicity *2529*
phentolamine, hypertensive emergencies *3080*
phenylbutazone, adverse effects, hepatotoxicity *2532, 2533, 2535*
phenylephrine 3129
orthostatic hypotension *5063*
phenylketonuria 1560, *1566*, 1582
aetiology/pathophysiology 1582, *1582*
clinical presentation 1583
diagnosis 1583
maternal 1583, *1585*
neonatal screening 162, *104*, 1583
Guthrie test 1561
treatment and outcome 1583, *1584*
phenytoin
adverse effects
adrenal function tests 2068
adrenal insufficiency 2068
hepatotoxicity *2529, 2532–3*
hirsutism 2068
neuropathy 5088
oesophagitis *2294*
in pregnancy *2188*
renal toxicity *3860*
in breast milk *1469, 2189*
diabetic neuropathy 2039
dose levels *4823*
drug interactions *1471, 3968*
epilepsy 4821
metastatic brain tumours 390
poisoning 1275, 1280
serum levels *5449*
teratogenicity *1468, 2187, 4822*
therapeutic drug monitoring 1475, *1475*
phethenylate, adverse effects, hepatotoxicity *2529*
Phialophora verrucosa 1006
Philadelphia chromosome 146, 341
Philodryas olfersii 1327
Philometra spp. *1176*
phlebectasia 4691
Phlebotomidae (sand flies) *1226*
Phlebotomus spp. *1226*
Phlebovirus 581, 586
Rift Valley fever virus 586, *587*
sandfly fever, Naples and Sicilian viruses 586
Phnom Penh bat virus *566*
phobias 5316
Phocanema spp. *1176*
Phoneutria nigriventer (Brazilian armed spider) *1354*
phoratoxin 1364
Phoridae (scuttle flies) *1233*
phosgene poisoning 1315
phosphatases 132
phosphate deficiency rickets 3740
phosphate
CKD-MBD *3922*
physiological control 4141, *4142–3*
reference values *5435, 5446*
children *5438*
in renal failure 4183
renal tubular reabsorption 3872
phosphate-handling disorders 4140–1
decreased phosphate excretion 4143
increased phosphate excretion 4142, *4143*
inherited *4143*, 4142–3
sporadic/acquired 4142
phosphatidylcholine 1654
phosphatidylinositol-3-OH kinases 352
phosphine poisoning 1315
phosphodiesterase inhibitors 3130
drug interactions *1471*
pulmonary arterial hypertension 2988
in renal failure 4177
phosphofructokinase deficiency 4472, *5215*, 5216
3-phosphoglycerate dehydrogenase deficiency *1566, 1591, 1592*
phosphoglycerate kinase deficiency 4472
phospholipidosis, drug-induced 2535
phospholipids 1654
amphipathic 127
phosphoproteins 3726
phosphoribosyl pyrophosphate synthetase superactivity 1630
phosphoric acid *1739*
phosphorus balance 3727, *3727*
parathyroid hormone 3728
phosphorus *1498*, 1500
dietary reference values *1502*
phosphorylation, reversible 132
photoaggravated conditions *4670*, 4671
Photobacterium spp. *962*
photochemotherapy, psoriasis 4614
photodermatitis 4625
photodermatoses 4667, *4668*
clinical features 4668
DNA repair-deficient
diagosis 4668
treatment 4668
idiopathic 4668
actinic prurigo 4669
actinic prurigo 4669, *4669*
chronic actinic dermatitis *4670*, 4671
polymorphic light eruption 4665, 4669
solar urticaria 4670, *4671*
photodynamic therapy 4737
photographing injuries 5369
Photorhabdus spp. *962*
photosensitivity 4665, *4666*
DNA repair-deficient photodermatoses 4667
drug-induced 4667, *4667*
effects of sunlight 4665
erythema 4665
immune suppression 4666
photoageing and photocarcinogenesis 4666
pigmentation 4665
idiopathic photodermatoses 4668
porphyria 1640, *4666, 4667*
phototherapy 4736
broadband 4736
narrowband 4736
psoralen and UVA (PUVA) 4736
psoriasis 4614
phrenic nerve neuropathy 5079
phthalic anhydride *3436*
phthisis 811
see also tuberculosis
phycomycosis 1014
phylloides tumour 1941
phylogeny 4747
Physalia spp. (Portuguese man-o'-war) 1347
Physaloptera caucasica 1176
physiotherapy, COPD 3343
phytanic acid 1725
α oxidation 1726
phytomenadione *1274*
phytotherapy 65, 67
description 67
drug interactions *69*
efficacy 68
mode of action 67
safety 68
Pick's disease *see* frontotemporal dementia
Pickwickian syndrome 1527
picnodysostosis *3721*
piebaldism 4662
piedra
black 1004
white 1004
Pierce, Barry 190
pig bel 808
pigmentation disorders 4656
hyperpigmentation 4657, *4658*
chemical and drug-induced 4658, *4659*
dermal melanocytosis 4660
endocrine causes 4657
incontinentia pigmenti 4660
McCune-Albright syndrome 4660, *4660*
melasma 4658
post-inflammatory 4660, *4661*
urticaria pigmentosa 4659, *4659*
hypopigmentation 4661, *4661*
Chédiak-Higashi syndrome 4663
depigmentation/greying of hair 4662
endocrine causes 4662
Hermansky-Pudlak syndrome 4663
oculocutaneous albinism type I 4663
oculocutaneous albinism type II 4663
piebaldism 4662
Prader-Willi and Angelman syndromes 4663
vitiligo 4661, *4661*
Waardenburg's syndrome 4662
liver disease 4719
normal skin pigmentation 4656
renal disease 4720
UV radiation-induced (tanning) 4657, *4657*
pilar cyst 4706
pimozide
adverse effects, hyperprolactinaemia 2068
schizophrenia *5325*
pindolol, orthostatic hypotension *5063*

pine tar 4733
pineal gland 2070
pathology 2070
photoperiodism 2071
structure 2070
pinta 879, 882
clinical features 882, *883–4*
diagnosis 883
prevention/control 884
treatment 883
pioglitazone, adverse effects, hepatotoxicity 2531
Piophila casei 1232, *1233*
Piophilidae *1233*
piperacillin, *Pseudomonas aeruginosa* 737
piperacillin/tazobactam, anaerobic infections *753*
piperacillin/ticarcillin, pneumonia *3238*
piperadeine-6-carboxylate dehydrogenase deficiency 1590
piperazine, adverse effects, hepatotoxicity *2529*
piroxicam
adverse effects, hepatotoxicity *2532*, *2533*
and asthma *3289*
rheumatoid arthritis *3594*
piroxicates, adverse effects, hepatotoxicity *2529*
pirprofen, adverse effects, hepatotoxicity *2534*
pit cells *2438*, 2439
Pitohui dichrous (hooded pitohui) *1344*
Pitt-Hopkins syndrome 5143
pituitary adenoma 1814
pituitary apoplexy 1815, 5482
pituitary carcinoma 1814
pituitary deficiency 4559
pituitary disorders, cognitive impairment 5280
pituitary function testing 1803
basal tests 1803
ACTH 1803
FSH/LH 1803
GH 1803
prolactin 1803
THS 1803
dynamic tests 1803
glucagon stimulation test 1804
insulin tolerance test 1803
oral glucose tolerance test 1804
short Synacthen test 1804
pituitary gigantism 1958
pituitary gland *1801*
adenoma 1983
anterior *see* anterior pituitary gland
development *1788*
disorders of, in pregnancy 2140
posterior *see* posterior pituitary gland
in pregnancy 2078
pituitary tumours *4779*, 4778
pityriasis rosea 4617
pityriasis versicolor 998, 1002
aetiology 1002
clinical features 1002
epidemiology 1002
laboratory diagnosis 1002
treatment 1002
Pixuna *558*
pizotifen, migraine prevention *4916*
placebo effects 47
placenta
in malaria 1063
role of 2901
Plagiorchis harinasutai 1223
Plagiorchis javensis 1223
Plagiorchis muris 1223
Plagiorchis philippinensis 1223
plague *see Yersinia pestis*
plainopsia 4857
planetary overload 82
Planorbis spp. 1346
plant toxins 1361
cardiotoxins *1362*, 1363
aconitine 1363, 1370
cardiac glycosides 1363, *1363, 1364*
cytotoxins *1362*, 1364
colchicine 1364, *1365*
cyanogenic glycosides *1362*, 1365
lectins *1362*, 1364
ricin *1362*, 1364
dermatotoxins 1365, *1362, 1365–6*
epidemiology 1361
gastrointestinal irritants *1362*, 1365
hepatotoxins *1362*, 1365
Indian poisonous plants 1371, *1371*
Areca catechu 1374
Azadirachta indica 1374
Calotropis spp. 1373
Capsicum spp. 1373, *1373*
Cerbera odollam 1373, *1373*
Citrullus colocynthus 1372
Cleistanthus collinus 1374
Croton tiglium 1372
Jatropha curcas 1374
Lathyrus sativus 1374
Podophyllum spp. 1372
Ricinus communis 1371, *1372*
Semecarpus anacardium 1372
nephrotoxins *4093*, *1362*, 1365, 4092
neurotoxins 1361, *1362*
belladonna alkaloids 1361
convulsants 1362, *1362*
hallucinogens 1362, *1362*
nicotine effects 1361, 1363
plantar fasciitis *3248*, *5382*
plaque, atheromatous
calcification 2878
cell death in 2878
erosion 2879
rupture 2880
vulnerable 2880, *2881*
see also atherosclerosis
plaque, dental *962*
plaques (skin) *4591*
plasma cell dyscrasias, renal involvement 4055, *4056*
plasma exchange, lupus nephritis 4049
plasma half-life 1454, *1455*
plasma oncotic pressure 2994
plasma viscosity *4196*
plasma volume *4196–7*
plasma
fresh-frozen 4532
transfusion 4565
plasma-cell leukaemia 4351
plasmacytoma
extramedullary 4352
solitary, of bone 4352
plasmapheresis, meningitis 721
plasminogen activator inhibitor 1, 2601, 4497
plasminogen *1753*, *4196*, 4497, *4497*
Plasmodium falciparum 1048, *1052–3*, 4084
renal toxicity *4086*
Plasmodium knowlesi 1048, *1052*, *1069*, *1069*
treatment 1081
Plasmodium malariae 1048, *1052*, 1069, 4084
renal toxicity *4086*
treatment 1081
Plasmodium ovale 1048, *1052*, 1069, 4084
treatment 1081
Plasmodium spp. 1048
development in erythrocyte 1050, *1052–3*
development in mosquito 1048, *1050–1*
development of oocyst into sporozoites 1048, *1050*
exo/pre-erythrocytic (liver) stages 1049
genomic organization 1048, *1048*
life cycle 1048, *1049*
movement 1048, *1051*
sexual development 1052
see also malaria
Plasmodium vivax 1048, *1052–3*, 1068, 4084
treatment 1081
plateau principle 1454
platelet count 4197, *4196*
platelet disorders 4507
adhesion/aggregation 4517
decreased production 4514
acquired 4514
congenital 4514
distribution and sequestration 4515
function 4516
acquired 4517
congenital 4516
immune-mediated 4510
increased destruction 4510
nonimmune 4513
number 4508
procoagulant activity 4517
secretion 4517
thrombocytopenia *see* thrombocytopenia
platelet factor *44196*
platelet-derived growth factor 2601
platelets 2600, 4484
activated 4486, *4486*
calcium metabolism 4487
cAMP pathway 4488
coagulant activity 4487
cytoskeletal reorganization 4487, *4488*
phospholipid metabolism 4486
role in coagulation 4495, *4496*
secretion 4488, *4489*
soluble agonists 4488
adhesion 4484, *4485*
glycoprotein Ia-IIa 4485
glycoprotein Ib-IX-V 4484
glycoprotein IIb-IIIa 4485
glycoprotein IV 4485
glycoprotein VI-Fc receptor α-chain complex 4485
aggregation 4489
cancer 4548, *4549–50*
circulating 4207
function analysis 4503
in haemostasis 4508
surface structures 4508
transfusion 4565
platinum neuropathy 5088
pleiotropy 140
Pleistophora ronneafiei 1116
Plesiomonas shigelloides 1240
Plesiomonas spp. *962*
pleura 3175
drug reactions 3466, *3466*
pleural biopsy 3225
pleural cancer 320
pleural disease *3214*, 3214, 3486
autoimmune rheumatic disorders *3390*, 3391, 3393
benign asbestos-induced 3487, 3491, 3498
systemic sclerosis *3672*
see also individual conditions
pleural effusion *3183*, *3489*, *3486–7*
aetiology 3487, *3488*
benign asbestos-related 3487, 3491
in cirrhosis 2490
diagnosis 3489, *3490*
drug-induced *3488*
exudative 3488
formation of 3487
investigations 3487
biopsy 3491
imaging 3490, *3490–1*
malignant 391
physiological consequences 3487
pneumococcal 688
pulmonary embolism 3491
recurrent 3538
rheumatoid arthritis 3491
SLE 3491
transudative 3488
treatment *see* pleurodesis
tuberculous 3486, 3494
pleural empyema 3491
aetiology 3492, *3493*
bacteriology 3491, *3492*
clinical features 3492, *3494–5*
management 3493, *3495*
pathogenesis 3492, *3494*
prognosis 3491, *3493*
pleural fluid
analysis 3488
cytology 3488
normal physiology 3487
see also pleural effusion
pleural plaques, asbestos-related 3499, *3499*
pleural rub *3185*, 3187
pleural thickening, asbestos-related 3499
pleural tuberculosis 818
pleural tumours 3534
benign 3534
solitary fibrous tumour 3534, *3535*
malignant 3535
mesothelioma 3535
metastatic 3537, *3537*
clinical features 3537
diagnosis 3537

management 3537
pleuritic pain 3185, *3185*
pleurodesis
mechanism of 3538
mesothelioma 3536, *3536*
talc toxicity 3538
technical aspects 3538
pleurodynia, epidemic *see* Bornholm disease
pleuropneumonia-like organisms 952
Pleurotus osteatus/ergngi 3436
pluripotent stem cells *4202,* 4203, *4205*
pneumatosis cystoides intestinalis 2586
pneumococcal infections 677, 679, 680
antibiotic resistance 681
epidemiology 681
mechanisms of 683
carriage, transmission and serotypes 681
clinical features 686
endocarditis and pericarditis 691
meningitis 689
otitis media 690
peritonitis 691
pleural effusion/empyema 688
pneumonia 686, *687–8*
septicaemia 691
diagnosis 685, *685*
epidemiology 680
history 680
immunity 683
incidence 680, *681–2*
pathogenesis 683
prevention 684
red hepatization *684*
risk factors 681, *682*
pneumococcus, immunization *91*
pneumoconioses 3414
asbestosis 3414, 3420
berylliosis 3423, *3424*
coal-worker's 3414–15
fibrous erionite 3423
Fuller's earth 3423
kaolin 3423
mica 3423
silicosis 3417
talc 3423
Pneumocystis jirovecii 1028, *235, 249, 627, 627–8*
aetiology 1029
areas of uncertainty 1031
clinical presentation 1029
definition 1028, 1030
arterial blood gases/oximetry 1030
bronchoscopy 1030
computed tomography 1030, *1030*
empirical therapy 1031
induced sputum 1030
molecular detection tests 1031
HIV-associated infection *3247*
immunocompromised patients 3959
investigations, chest radiograph 1030, *1030*
pathogenesis 1029
pathology 1029, *1029*
persons at risk 1029
pneumonia 3237
prophylaxis 1031
treatment 1031
pneumocystis pneumonia 3249, *3249*
clinical features 3249
microbiologial diagnosis 3250
prevention 3250
respiratory failure 3250
treatment 3250
pneumonia *3120,* 3231
aetiology 3231, *3232*
breathlessness *2633*
clinical features 3233, *3233*
abdominal pain 2236
anaerobic bacteria 3234, *3234*
C. pneumoniae 3235
Gram-negative bacilli 3235
H. influenzae 3234
Legionella 3235
liver disease 2538
M. pneumoniae 3234
S. aureus 3235
viruses 3236
coccidioidomycosis, pregnancy 2124
community-acquired
aetiology *453*
pregnancy 2123
controversies 3241
antibiotic selection 3241, *3242*
microbial aetiology 3241
pneumococcal vaccine 3242
CURB-65 score 3231, 3240
eosinophilic 3295, 3428
epidemiology 3232, *3232*
haematological changes 4558
HIV-related 3248
idiopathic interstitial 3365–6
acute 3369, *3369*
desquamative 3368, *3368*
lymphocytic 3369, *3369*
nonspecific 3369, *3369–70*
respiratory bronchiolitis-interstitial lung disease 3368, *3368*
laboratory diagnosis 3236, *3236*
chest X-ray 3236
microbial aetiology 3237
legionella 900, *902*
lipoid (lipid) 3452
measles-related 520, *522*
meningococcal 719
nosocomial 3243
organizing *3379, 3383,* 3384
pathogenesis 3232, *3233*
pneumococcal 686, *687–8*
Pneumocystis jirovecii see Pneumocystis jirovecii
pregnancy 2123
presentation 5469
prevention/control 3240, *3241*
prognosis 3240, *3240*
Q fever 924, *925*
staphylococcal 701, *702*
treatment 3237
antibiotics 3237, *3238–9*
failure to respond 3239
monitoring response 3239
timing 3239
varicella, pregnancy 2123
viral aetiology *474*
pneumonitis
acute 3457
cytomegalovirus 496
lymphocytic interstitial 3432
autoimmune rheumatic disease *3390*
measles-related 522
radiation 3458
varicella 489
ventilation 3435
pneumothorax *3212,* 3175, *3183,* 3487, 3500
aetiology 3500, 3502
air travel after 3502
breathlessness *2633*
catamenial 3503
clinical features 3500, *3502, 3503*
cystic fibrosis 3361
diagnosis 3501, *3501*
iatrogenic 3503
incidence 3500
pathophysiology 3500
prevention of recurrence 3502
prognosis 3502
secondary 3487, 3502
spontaneous 3500
systemic sclerosis *3672*
tension 3116, *3120,* 3487, 3501
presentation 5467
traumatic 3503
treatment 3501–2
pO_2 *5515*
podoconiosis 1426, 3087
aetiology 1426
clinical features 1427, *1427–8*
clinical investigation 1427
differential diagnosis 1427, *1428*
ecology 1426, *1427*
economic burden and social stigma 1428
epidemiology 1426
future developments 1428
genetics 1426
history 1426
pathogenesis 1426
pathology 1426
prevention 1426
prognosis 1428
treatment 1428
podophyllin, anogenital warts 603
podophyllotoxin, anogenital warts 603
Podophyllum spp. 1372
podophyllum 4736
POEMS syndrome 3710, 4064, 4351
poikilocytes *4195*
point of care 22
point-of-care testing 5433
poisoning
children 1273
diagnosis 1273
circumstances under which found 1274
circumstantial evidence 1274
feature clusters 1274, *1274*
neurological signs 1274
suicide notes 1274
drugs and chemicals 1271
epidemiology 1272
fish 1346
fungal 1361
history 1273
hospital admissions 1272
investigations 1275, *1275*
management 1276
antidotes *1274,* 1278
immediate 1276
increasing elimination 1279
reducing absorption 1278
mortality 1273
ocular signs 5251
plants 1361
self-harm 1272
see also insect stings; snake bites; spider bites
Poland's syndrome 1940
polaxamers 1425
polidocanol, peptic ulcer disease 2312
polio 5002
clinical features 529, *529–30, 5003,* 5003
eradication and surveillance 534, *534–5*
vaccines *91, 466, 533,* 533
poliovirus 527, *528*
Polistes spp. (paper wasp) 1350
politics 58–9
pollution
and cancer 308
lung cancer 319, 3516
polyarteritis nodosa *222, 3650, 4033, 4632*
cardiac involvement *2783,* 2785
cutaneous 4632, *4632*
GI tract involvement 2422
hepatic involvement 2544
ocular involvement 5243
pulmonary involvement *3396*
renal involvement 4038
treatment 4042
polychlorinated biphenyls, hepatotoxicity *1385*
polychondritis, relapsing 3260
ocular involvement 5243
polycyclic aromatic hydrocarbons *307–8,* 338, 1379
polycystic ovary syndrome (PCOS) *1871,* 1907, *1908*
definition 1907
diagnostic criteria 1907, *1908*
endocrine features 1908
long-term consequences 1909
cardiovascular risk 1910
endometrial carcinoma 1909
gestational diabetes 1909
type 2 diabetes 1910
management 1910, *1910*
metabolic abnormalities 1909, *1909*
reproductive consequences 1909
polycystic renal disease 1626
autosomal dominant 4095
autosomal recessive 4097
polycythaemia vera 4269, *4269*
biological and molecular aspects 4269
clinical features 4270
diagnostic criteria 4272
epidemiology 4269
laboratory evaluation 4271
pathobiology 4270
polycythaemias 4264
absolute 4266
approach to 4272, *4272*
cancer-associated 4548
Chuvash 4268
classification *4265*
erythropoiesis 4265
management 4273
primary 4268

familial/congenital 4268
prognosis 4274
relative 4265
scoliosis 3507
secondary
appropriate erythropoeitin secretion 4266
inappropriate erythropoietin secretion 4268
prolyl hydroxylase mutations 4268
tumour-associated 4268
polydipsia, primary 1823, 3828
vs diabetes insipidus 3828
polyenes 1015
polymerase chain reaction 710, 5371
amoebiasis 1041
polymicrogyria 5141
polymorphic eruption of pregnancy 2151, *2152*
polymorphic light eruption 4665, 4669
polymyalgia rheumatica 3679
aetiology 3680
anaemia 4401
clinical features 3680–1
diagnosis and classification 3682, *3681–2*
differential diagnosis 3682, *3683*
epidemiology 3680, *3681*
hepatic involvement 2544
historical perspective 3680
investigations 3682
pathology and immunology 3680
prognosis 3683
relationship to temporal arteritis 3680
treatment 3682
polymyositis/dermatomyositis *277, 385, 3650,* 3692, *3693,* 5174
autoantibodies 3695, *3696*
myositis-associated 3696
myositis-specific 3695
clinical features 3693
antisynthetase syndrome 3695
cardiac 2784, *2784,* 3695
dermatomyositis 3694, *3694*
gastrointestinal 3695
malignancy 3695
ocular involvement 5244
polymyositis 3693
pulmonary 3389, *3390,* 3695
cutaneous 4640
aetiology and genetics 4640
clinical features 4640, *4640–2*
clinical investigation 4641
diagnostic criteria 4641
differential diagnosis 4640
pathogenesis and pathology 4640
prognosis 4642
treatment 4642
diagnosis 3696
electromyography 3697
MRI 3697, *3697*
muscle biopsy 3697
skin biopsy 3697
differential diagnosis 3697, *3698*
epidemiology 3693
future developments 3698
historical perspective 3693
oesophageal symptoms *2297*
pathology and pathophysiology 3693
photoaggravation *4670*
prevalence *3650*
prognosis 3698
treatment 3697
polyneuritis, acute inflammatory *see* Guillain-Barré syndrome
polyneuropathy, diffuse symmetrical 2036
aetiology 2036
epidemiology and natural history 2037
symptoms and signs 2037, *2038*
polyomavirus 481
KI virus 660
renal involvement 4073
WU virus 660
polyposis coli 302
polyps
colorectal 2225, *2225*
gastric 2217
rectal 2213
polyuria 3852
polyuria-polydipsia syndromes *see* diabetes insipidus; polydipsia
Pompe's disease *1598,* 1601, 1697, 1715, 3187
autophagy 1695
diagnosis 1706
treatment 1715
Pongola virus *581*
Pontiac fever 900
pontine syndromes 4930
basal (locked-in syndrome) 4931
midpontine 4931, *4931*
superior 4931, *4931*
popliteal cyst *3557*
population genetics 13
population growth 80
contribution to environmental disruption 74
planetary overload 82
subsistence crises 82
porencephaly 5144, *5144*
Porocephalus crotali 1240
porphobilinogen 1640
reference values *5446*
porphyria cutanea tarda *385,* 1637, 1637–8, 1645, *1646,* 4720
treatment 1646
porphyrias 1474, 1636
abdominal pain 2237
acquired 1637
acute 1637, 1636, 1641, 1643
clinical features 1641
induction of attacks 1641, 1641–2
outcome 1643
presentation 5483, *5484*
treatment 1648
acute intermittent 1637, 1637, 1643, *1644*
acute neurovisceral attacks 1640
biochemical abnormalities 1637
classification 1637, *1637*
congenital erythropoietic 1637, *1637,* 1645
contraindicated drugs 1641, 1642
cutaneous 1645
differential diagnosis *1725*
Doss 1637, 1637, 1640, 1643–4
haem formation *1637, 1639,* 1640
hepatoerythropoietic 1637
hereditary coproporphyria 1637, 1637, 1644
hexachlorobenzene 1637, 1637
lead poisoning 1637, 1637
neuropathy 5092
nonacute 1636, 1637
pathogenesis 1640
photosensitivity 1640, 1648
protoporphyria 1637, *1637–8,* 1646, *1647*
psychiatric signs *1720*
variegate 1637, *1637,* 1644
porphyrins, reference values *5446*
Porphyromonas gingivalis 2260–1
Porphyromonas spp. *962*
portal vein thrombosis 2586
portopulmonary hypertension
hepatocellular failure 2498
management 2504
port-wine stain 4692
posaconazole
coccidioidomycosis 1022
fungal infections 1015
positive end-expiratory pressure (PEEP) 3139, 3144
positron emission tomography (PET)
cardiac 2671, 2673
comparison with other techniques 2673
principles 2673
chest 3200, *3204, 3205*
epilepsy 4819, *4819*
lung cancer *3522,* 3526
pancreatic tumours 2576
Parkinson's disease 4882
renal disease 3882
postabortal fever, mycoplasmal infections *956,* 957
postcode prescribing 54
posterior fossa tumour 4778
posterior pituitary gland 1819
anatomy 1819, *1820*
drug-induced disorders 2069
postnatal depression 2091
postpartum fever, mycoplasmal infections *956,* 957
postpolio syndrome 5073
postpolypectomy syndrome 2212
postprandial syndrome 2055
reactive hypoglycaemia 2055
post-thrombotic syndrome 4688
post-traumatic headache 4926
post-traumatic stress disorder 5289
clinical features 5289
differential diagnosis 5289
epidemiology 5289
prognosis 5291
treatment 5289, *5290*
crisis intervention 5290
pharmacological 5290
psychological 5290
postural tachycardia syndrome 5067, *5068*
Potamotrygon hystrix 1345
Potamotrygon spp. *1345*
potassium channel openers
acute coronary syndromes 2917
angina 2909
potassium channels 160–1
drugs acting on 1461
potassium chloride, adverse effects, oesophagitis *2294*
potassium citrate, calcium stone prevention *4130*
potassium deficiency, metabolic alkalosis 1748
potassium excretion, factors modifying *3833*
potassium homeostasis 3832
acidosis 1745
disorders of 3831
hyperkalaemia 3832, 3840
hypokalaemia 3831, 3834
external balance 3833
internal balance 3832, *3833*
potassium magnesium citrate, calcium stone prevention *4130*
potassium perchlorate, thyrotoxicosis 1840
potassium replacement, diabetic ketoacidosis 2026
potassium
and blood pressure 1519
dietary intake *3833*
dietary reference values *1502*
in foodstuffs *3842*
plasma, acute renal trauma 3892
reference values *5435, 5446*
children *5438*
serum concentration *3833*
total body *3833*
urinary *3837*
Potiskum virus *566*
Potocki-Lupski syndrome 145, *148*
Potocki-Shaffer syndrome 145
Pott, Percival 1379
Pott's disease 810, 820, 3508
povidone-iodine 4735
adverse effects, hepatotoxicity *2529*
Powassan encephalitis *566,* 574
power-frequency electric/magnetic fields 1432
poxviruses 508
biology 509, *509–10*
classification 508, *509*
expression vectors 511
genome sequences 511
pathogenesis 509, *510–11*
see also individual viruses
PR interval 2648
short 2652
practolol, oculomucocutaneous syndrome 3466
Prader-Willi syndrome *145, 148, 1530, 1917*
growth failure in 1956
hypopigmentation 4663
prajmaline, adverse effects, hepatotoxicity *2532*
pralidoxime *1274*
pramlintide 1535
pravastatin 1670
hepatocellular carcinoma 2517
praziquantel
clonorchiasis 1214
cysticercosis 1198
intestinal flukes 1221
paragonimiasis 1219
schistosomiasis 1210
Taenia saginata 1191
prazosin
hypertensive emergencies *3079*
in pregnancy *2099*
precordial thump 3100, *3101*

precursor B-lymphoblastic
leukaemia 4223
precursor lymphoid cell
neoplasms 4223
precursor T-lymphoblastic
leukaemia 4224
prednisolone
anaphylaxis 3113
aphthous ulcers 2272
asthma 3300
in breast milk *1469*
polymyalgia rheumatica 3682
post-transplantation *2511*, *3954*
primary biliary cirrhosis *2467*
sarcoidosis *3411*
SLE 2156
temporal arteritis 3683
prednisone
asthma 3300
COPD *3335*
lymphoma *4320*
sarcoidosis *3411*
pre-eclampsia 2094, 2123, 2128,
3862
aetiology and pathogenesis 2095,
2095
antenatal screening *102*
and CKD 3912
clinical features 2095, *2096*,
2129–30
complications *2129*
convulsions 2099
critical care 2099
definition and diagnosis 2096,
2097
differential diagnosis *2131*
laboratory variables *2130*
management 2098, *2099*
prevention 2098, *2098*
prophylaxis 2090
risk factors 2097, *2098*
superimposed 2097
preencephalopathy 2501
pre-excitation syndromes 2689
atrial fibrillation 2709, *2710*
ventricular 2651, 2709
see also Wolff-Parkinson-White
syndrome
prefrontal syndromes 4793
pregabalin
epilepsy 4822
neuropathic pain 5415
pregnancy
acute fatty liver 2105
adrenal disorders, Cushing's
syndrome 1874
alcohol dependence 5346
antenatal care, heart disease 2110
antenatal screening 2087
anticonvulsants 4822
autoimmune rheumatic
disorders 2154
antiphospholipid
syndrome 2154, 2157
rheumatoid arthritis 2154,
2161
systemic lupus
erythematosus 2154–5
behavioural habits 2090
alcohol 2090
caffeine 2090
exercise 2090
tobacco 2090
travel 2090
blood disorders 2173
anaemia 2173
haemoglobinopathies 2173–4
haemostasis 2173, 2177
cancer 2181
breast cancer 2183
cervical cancer 2183
colon cancer 2184
gestational trophoblastic
disease 2182
leukaemia 2184
lymphoma 2184
melanoma 2184
ovarian cancer 2183
thyroid cancer 2184
cardiac clinical features 2109
cardiovascular changes 2108
cholestasis 2126, 2150, *2150*, 2450
differential diagnosis *2131*
congenital heart disease 2871, *2871*
complex 2113
Crohn's disease 2369
cytomegalovirus 497
D-dimer testing 3015
depression in 5314
diabetes mellitus 2133
aetiology and genetics 2135
classification 2134, *2134*
diagnosis 2136, *2136*
effect of 2137
epidemiology 2134
fetal assessment 2138
gestational 2133
historical perspective 2134
pathogenesis/pathology 2135
postpartum
considerations 2138
pregestational 2133
risk factors *2135*
screening 2135
timing/mode of delivery 2138,
2138
treatment 2137, *2137*
diagnosis 2087
dietary modification 2089
folic acid 2089
iodine and thyroxine 2090
multivitamins 2089
sea food, fish oils and
omega-3 fatty acids 2090
drug dependence 5346, *5346*
eclampsia *2095*, 2100, 2128
Eisenmenger's syndrome 2848
endocrine disease 2140
adrenal 2143
parathyroid 2143
pituitary 2140, *2141*
thyroid 2141, *2142*
factors influencing
outcome 2086
infertility and multiple
pregnancies 2086
maternal age 2086
maternal weight 2086
past medical history 2086, *2086*
viral infections 2086
folate deficiency 2174, 4412
gastrointestinal disease 2132
acute appendicitis 2132
coeliac disease 2132
gastro-oesophageal reflux 2132
inflammatory bowel
disease 2132
gestational diabetes 2007
and polycystic ovary
syndrome 1909
heart disease 2108
antenatal care 2110
aortopathy 2112, *2112*
arrhythmias 2115
cardiac surgery 2110
cardiomyopathy 2110, *2111*
congenital 2113, *2871*, 2871
contraception 2115
investigations 2109
ischaemic heart disease 2111
labour and delivery 2110
management 2110
prepregnancy assessment 2109
prosthetic valves 2114, *2114*
pulmonary hypertension 2112
risk stratification 2109, *2110*
small left-to-right shunts 2113
valvular lesions 2113
HELLP syndrome 2096, 3862
HSV infection 487
hypertension 2093
causes and terminology 2094,
2094
long-term sequelae 2101
pre-existing 2100
puerperium 2101, *2101*
secondary 2101, *2101*
treatment 2100
infections 2165
antimicrobial agents 2171, *2172*
bacterial 2169
protozoal 2170
viral 2166
see also individual infections
iron storage diseases 4398
liver disease 2125, *2126*
abnormal liver blood
tests *2131*
acute fatty liver 2127
Budd-Chiari syndrome 2130
cholelithiasis 2130
chronic liver disease 2131
clinical features/laboratory
variables *2130*
effects of pregnancy on
laboratory tests *2126*
HELLP syndrome 2096, 2128,
3862
hyperemesis gravidarum *see*
hyperemesis gravidarum
hypertension-associated 2128,
2129
intrahepatic cholestasis of
pregnancy 2126
jaundice 2129
liver tumour 2131
post-liver transplantation 2132
variceal haemorrhage 2131
viral hepatitis 2130, *2131*
malaria 1058, 1070
treatment 1080
maternal nutrition 2901
medical management 2085
myasthenia gravis 5181
mycoplasmal infections in 957
neurological disorders 2144
central nervous system 2146
cerebrovascular disorders 2145
malignancies 2145
movement disorders 2144
muscle disorders 2145
myasthenia gravis 2145
myotonic dystrophy 2145
nerves and nerve roots 2146
obstetric nerve palsies 2145
thiamine deficiency 2144
nutrition 2079
developing world 2080, *2081*
energy requirements 2080, *2081*
fetal programming 2083
food cravings 2083
foods to avoid 2083
metabolic changes 2081
weight gain 2080, *2080*
physiological changes 2075
cardiovascular 2075, *2093*, *2094*
coagulation 2078
endocrine 2078
gastrointestinal system 2077
immune system 2077
kidney 2077, 2103
liver 2077
respiratory system 2077
skin and hair 2078
post-delivery 2091
future maternal health 2091,
2091
lactation 2091
postnatal depression 2091
pre-eclampsia *see* pre-eclampsia
preparation for 2075
prescribing in 2186
behavioural teratology 2189
drug effects on fetus 2187
drugs and breastfeeding 2188,
2189
effects of pregnancy on
drugs 2190, *2190*
first trimester 2187
later pregnancy 2188, *2188*
therapeutic drug
monitoring 2190
see also teratogenesis
pseudoxanthoma elasticum 3786
renal disease 2103, 3861, *3861*
acute renal failure 2104, *2105*
hydroureter, hydronephrosis
and overdistension
syndrome 2105
management 2106
pre-existing 2106
renal transplant patients 2107
rupture of urinary tract 2106
urinary tract infection 2104
women on dialysis 2107
renal transplant patients 3968
respiratory changes 2121, *2122*
cardiovascular 2121
chest wall and diaphragm 2121
lung volumes 2121
ventilation and gas
exchange 2121
respiratory diseases 2121
amniotic fluid embolism 2122
aspiration 2123
asthma 2123
mechanical ventilation 2124
pneumonia 2123
pre-eclampsia 2123
pregnancy-associated
rhinitis 2122
pulmonary oedema 2123
venous air embolism 2122
venous
thromboembolism 2122
rubella 562

vaccination 564
scleroderma 2162
skin disorders 2149
atopic eczema 2153
autoimmune dermatoses 2153
cutaneous infections 2150
hair changes 2149
pigmentary changes and lesions 2149, *2150*
pilosebaceous changes 2149
pregnancy dermatoses 2150, *2150*
psoriasis 2153
striae gravidarum 2150
vascular changes and lesions 2149, *2150*
SLE 3663
symptoms and signs 2088
cardiovascular system 2088
fatigue 2088
gastrointestinal system 2089
musculoskeletal 2089
neurological 2089
respiratory system 2088
skin 2089
thrombosis 2116
antithrombotic therapy 2117
causes *2118*
diagnosis 2119
risk factors 2117, *2117*
thromboprophylaxis 2118, *2119*
thyroid disease
cancer 1849
hypothyroidism 1837
thyrotoxicosis 1842
thyroid function 1830
travel 469, 2090
treatment 2120, *2120*
ulcerative colitis 2382
urinary tract infection 4118
varicella infection 490
vasculitides 2162
venous thromboembolism 2116, 2122
diagnosis 2119
risk factors 2117, *2117*
treatment 2120, *2120*, 3021
prehypertension 3031
prekallikrein *4490*, 4491
preload 2622, *2622*
premature (primary) ovarian failure 1905
chromosomal/genetic 1906
fertility 1906
iatrogenic 1906
idiopathic 1906
treatment 1906
premature beats 2641
Premolis semirufa 1352
prenatal diagnosis
central nervous system abnormalities 5149
hyperoxalurias 1734
inborn errors of metabolism 1556
osteogenesis imperfecta 3749
prenatal factors, COPD 3315
preotact, osteoporosis *3799*
prepatellar bursitis *3248*
prescribing 1449
older patients 5390, 5401
compliance 5401
drug efficacy 5401
prevention of unwanted drug effects 5401
personalized 46, 61, 149, 1474
preservatives 4732
pressure cabins 1412, *1413*
pressure change, mechanical effects 1413, *1413*
pressure palsies 2039
pressure sores 5049, 5389, 5395
clinical features 5396
prevention 5395
treatment 5396
types of 5395
pressure ulcers 4688
preterm labour, mycoplasmal infections *956*, 957
pretest probabilities *24*
prevention paradox 88
preventive medicine 81
at-risk population 89
demographic risk 89
familial risk 89
phenotypic risk 89
public and individual interventions 89
registration, screening and case-finding 90
changing behaviour 90
doctors' responsibilities 90
environmental change 91
global risk factors *87*
immunization 90, *90*
implementation 92
cultural constraints 92, *93*
programme effectiveness 93
time constraints 93, *93*
prevention paradox 88
primary prevention 89
prophylaxis 91
risk identification/reduction 87, *87*
risk modification 90
risk paradox 88, *88*
screening *see* screening
secondary prevention 89
strategic choices 89
see also public health
Prevotella intermedia 2261
Prevotella spp. *962*, 1257
priapism 1944, *1944–5*
treatment *1945*
primapterinuria dehydratase *1566*
primaquine *1074*, 1076
poisoning 1283
primary biliary cirrhosis *see* biliary cirrhosis, primary
primary lateral sclerosis 5074
primary prevention 89
primary sclerosing cholangitis *see* sclerosing cholangitis, primary
primidone
in breast milk *1469*
serum levels *5449*
Prinzmetal's angina 2631
prion diseases 1771, 5023, *5025*, 5101
aetiology and genetics 5024
Creutzfeldt-Jakob disease *see* Creutzfeldt-Jakob disease
diagnosis 5030, *5030*
hereditary 5026, *5028*
historical perspective 5024, *5024*
investigations *5031*, 5031, *5032*
kuru 1771, *5029*, 5029
pathogenesis/pathology 5024
priority setting 58
judgement, politics and management 59
qualifications and consequences 59
Probarbus jullienii 1347
probenecid
adverse effects, hepatotoxicity *2532*
drug interactions *1471*
gout 1625, 3644
probiotics, urinary tract infection 4115
problem solving therapy 5340
procainamide *2701*
adverse effects, hepatotoxicity *2532*, *2535*
in renal failure *4179*
procarbazine
adverse effects, hepatotoxicity *2529*, *2535*
lymphoma *4320*, 4320
procedures 5510
airway and respiratory 5514
arterial blood gases *see* arterial blood gases
arterial cannulation 5510
cardiac 5512
central vein cannulation 5510
invasive monitoring 5510
Procerovum calderoni 1222
Procerovum varium 1222
prochlorperazine *5423*
adverse effects, hepatotoxicity *2532*, *2533*
procollagen 1 peptide, reference values *5441*
procollagen type 3, reference values *5441*
proctitis 2378
progestagens, contraindication in porphyria 1641
progesterone
actions *1791*
reference values *5441*
signalling pathways *1797*
progestins, reproductive effects *1917*
progestogen-only pill *1265*
progestogens, breast cancer *1937*
prognosis *24*
progressive familial intrahepatic cholestasis, genetics *139*
progressive multifocal leukoencephalopathy 606, *606*, 5011
HIV-related 631
progressive osseous heteroplasia 3767, *3767*
progressive rubella panencephalitis 5012
progressive supranuclear palsy 4807, 4886
proguanil *1074*
prophylactic 1086–7, *1086*
prokaryotes 127
prolactin 1799, 1809
actions *1791*
in CKD 3909
deficiency 1810
drug-induced secretion 2068
ectopic secretion 2065
hyperprolactinaemia *1810*
measurement 1803
reference values *5441*
prolactinoma 1810
investigations 1810
pregnancy 2140
presentation 1810
treatment 1811
treatment withdrawal 1812
proliferative glomerulonephritis 3988, *3989*
endocapillary 3989
idiopathic diffuse 3991
mesiangial 3989
nonstreptococcal 3990, *3991*
poststreptococcal 3990, *3990*
prolyl hydroxylase mutations 4268
prolymphocytic leukaemia
B-cell 4227
T-cell 4227
promazine, adverse effects, hepatotoxicity *2532*
pro-opiomelanocortin 1530, *1521*, *1531*, *2062*
see also ACTH
propafenone *2701*
adverse effects, hepatotoxicity *2532*
in renal failure *4179*
properdin *216*, *1753*
deficiency *254*
prophylaxis 91
Propionibacterium acnes 3706, 4672
Propionibacterium propionicum 850–1, *851*
Propionibacterium spp. *852*, *962*
propionic aciduria *1566*, 1573
aetiology/pathophysiology 1573
clinical presentation 1573, *1574*
diagnosis 1574
treatment and outcome 1574
Propionimicrobium spp. *962*
propofol 3156
propoxyphene, adverse effects, hepatotoxicity *2532*
propranolol
migraine prevention *4916*
orthostatic hypotension *5063*
in renal failure *4179*
propylene glycol 4733
poisoning 1315
propylthiouracil 1840
adverse effects, hepatotoxicity *2529*, *2532*
in breast milk *1469*, *2189*
proquazone, adverse effects, hepatotoxicity *2532*
prosaposin deficiency 1698
prosopagnosia 4791, 4857
Prospect Hill virus *581*
prostacyclin *4482*
prostaglandin G2, *4482*
prostaglandin H2, *4482*
prostaglandins, vibration injury 1435
prostanoids 2599–600
pulmonary arterial hypertension 2987
prostate cancer 325, 4162, 4167
age distribution *326*
diagnosis, staging and grading 4168, *4169*
genetic changes 4168
genetic predisposition 365
genome association 141
incidence *301*
migrants vs residents *302*
risk factors 4168
screening 105, 4168

treatment 4169
locally advanced disease 4169
metastatic disease 4170
radical radiotherapy 4169
radical surgery 4169, *4170*
prostate specific antigen (PSA) 105, 325, 376, 4168
reference values *5442*
prostate specific membrane antigen (PSMA) 376
prostatitis 4115, *4115*
acute bacterial 4115
chlamydial 942
chronic bacterial 4115
chronic prostatitis/chronic pelvic pain syndrome 4115
mycoplasmal infections *956*, 957
treatment 4116
prosthetic heart valves
echocardiography 2666
endocarditis 2810
pregnancy 2114, *2114*
Prosthodendrium molenkampi 1223
protamine, in renal failure 4180
protease inhibitors 636
toxicity *640*
proteases 179
see also caspases
proteasome 225
protein binding 1456
drug interactions 1470
protein catabolic ratio *3937*
protein kinase C 2032
protein kinases 179
see also caspases
protein Z 4492
protein Z-dependent protease inhibitor 4494
protein C 2601, *4196*, 4490
deficiency *2118*, 4530
laboratory tests *4522*
protein S 2601, *4196*, 4492
deficiency *2118*, 4530
laboratory tests *4522*
proteinase 3, COPD *3323*
proteinases *3551*
protein-calorie malnutrition, and immunodeficiency *244*
protein-losing enteropathy *244*, 2588, *2588*
proteins
cerebrospinal fluid 4752
daily intake *1480*
deficiency anaemia 4419
dietary, restriction of 3916
metabolism 1485, *1486*
diabetes mellitus type 1, 2000
insulin effects 1995
in pregnancy 2082
reference values *5435*, *5446–7*
children *5438*
renal handling 3813
requirements 1538, *1538*, *1564*
stores *1480*
synthesis 2442
proteinuria 3863
detection 3848
management 3849, *3849*
measurement of 3867, *3867*
with microscopic haematuria 3849
reduction of 3915
renal tubular 3868
screening 3848, *3848*
selectivity of 3868
spill-over 3868
proteoglycans 3548, 3727
age-related changes *3550*
proteome 132
Proteus mirabilis, antibiotic sensitivity *446*
Proteus spp. *962*
prothrombin G20210A *2118*
prothrombin time *4196*, 4502
prothrombin 20210 4530
prothrombin *1753*, *4522*, 4490
laboratory tests *4504*
Protobothrops flavoviridis (habu) 1329
proton pump inhibitors
adverse effects, acute interstitial nephritis 4005
peptic ulcer disease 2311, *2313*
in renal failure 4176
proto-oncogenes 335, 346, 361
protoporphyria, erythropoietic 1637, *1637–8*, 1646, *1647*
hepatic disease 1647
surgical management 1647
protoporphyrin IX 1640
protozoal infections 1035
amoebic 1035
liver involvement 2543
malaria *see* malaria
ocular 5247, *5247*
pregnancy 2170
protriptyline, adverse effects *5313*
protrusio acetabuli, Marfan's syndrome *3750*
Providencia spp. *962*
provocation-neutralization testing 2255
proxies 19
proximal tubule (of kidney) 3812
acid-base homeostasis 4134, *4134*
amino acid handling 4146
functions 3812
protein handling 3813
sodium and water reabsorption 3812
renal acidosis 4135
cell biology and genetics 4135
clinical and biochemical features 4135
structure 3812, *3813*
pruritus
liver disease 4719
of pregnancy 2150, *2150*
uraemic 4720
without rash 4723
Prussian blue *1274*
P-selectin 282, 2601
Pseudallescheria boydii, osteomyelitis *3789*
Pseudechis textilis, antivenom *1340*
pseudoachondroplasia *3721*, 3759
mutations in *3757*
pseudoallergic reactions 1466
pseudobulbar palsy 4932
pseudocholinesterase, reference values *5436*
pseudochylothorax 3486, *3497*, 3497
pseudocowpox 512
pseudodementia 4797
pseudogout 3644
treatment 3647
pseudohermaphroditism
female 1968
congenital adrenal hyperplasia 1969
maternal androgen excess 1969
male 1969
androgen biosynthesis defects 1970
androgen resistance 1971
gonadal dysgenesis 1969
pseudo-Hurler polydystrophy 1698
pseudohyperkalaemia 3841
pseudohypoaldosteronism *1871*, 1889
and hyperkalaemia 3844
type 1, 165, 3073
type 2 *see* Gordon's syndrome
pseudohypoparathyroidism *1855*, 1866, *3721*, 4143, *4143*
clinical features *1866*, *3731*
pseudomembranous colitis 800
Pseudomonas aeruginosa 735
antibiotic sensitivity *446*
antimicrobial therapy 737
bacteraemia 736, *736*
bone and joint infection 737
colonization 735
cystic fibrosis 3356
ear infection 736
environmental 735
eye infection 737
genetics and pathogenesis 735
HIV-associated infection 737, *3247*
osteomyelitis *3789*
pneumonia 3235, *3245*
prevention 738
pulmonary infection 736
skin and soft tissue infection 736
treatment *3238*
urinary tract 736
Pseudomonas fluorescens 3436
Pseudomonas spp. *962*
Pseudonaja spp. (brown snakes) 1329
Pseudonocardia spp. *962*
pseudopseudohypo-parathyroidism *4143*
Pseudoramibacter spp. *962*
pseudoxanthoma elasticum 3771, 3782
cardiac involvement *2840*
clinical features 3782, *3784*
cardiovascular 3783
cutaneous 3782, *3783*
ophthalmic 3783, *3784*
clinical genetics 3782
diagnosis 3784
differential diagnosis 3785
molecular genetics 3785, *3785*
pathology 3785
pregnancy 3786
prognosis 3786
treatment 3785
pseudo-Zellweger syndrome *1552*
Psilocybe semilanceata (magic mushrooms) *1368*
psilocybin *1367*
psoralens, phototoxic *1362*
psoriasis 1382, 4610
clinical features *4607*, *4610*, *4611*, 4611
comorbid diseases 4612
erythroderma 4611
flexural psoriasis 4611
generalized pustural psoriasis 4611
guttate psoriasis 4611
Koebner phenomenon 4612
metabolic syndrome 4612
nails 4612, *4612*
psoriatic arthritis 4612
scalp 4612, *4612*
sebopsoriasis 4611
histology 4613, *4613*
management 4613
biological agents 4615
phototherapy 4614
systemic therapies 4614
topical therapies 4614
neurological complications 5160
pathogenesis 4613
photoaggravation *4670*
pregnancy 2153
psychosocial aspects 4613
scalp 4701, *4702*
psoriatic arthritis 3603, *3611*, *4612*, *4613*
clinical features 3611, *3611*
definition 3611
diagnosis 3612
epidemiology 3611
laboratory and radiological features 3612, *3612*
pathogenesis 3611
prognosis 3613
treatment 3613
psychiatric disorders 5271
anxiety and depression 4163
chronic fatigue syndrome 5304
and delirium 5271
eating disorders 5317
grief, stress and post-traumatic stress disorder 5284
medically unexplained symptoms 5296
schizophrenia, bipolar disorder, obsessive-compulsive disorder and personality disorder 5324
suicide 5292
see also cognitive disorders
psychiatric medicine 5257
acute behavioural problems 5263
alcohol and drug states 5266
calming the situation 5264
care following tranquillization 5266
emergency medication 5265, *5265*
evaluation 5263, *5264*
legal rights and duties 5266
psychosis 5266
history taking 5259
screening questions 5259
neuropsychiatry 5268
psychoactive drugs, drug interactions *1471*
Psychodidae *1233*
psychogenic nonepileptic seizures 4817
psychogenic unresponsiveness 4843
psychological disturbances 3154
psychological therapy 5338
definition of 5338
heart failure 2721
iatrogenesis 5339
medical consultation 5338

psychotherapeutic aspects 5338–9
referral 5340
specialist treatments 5339
psychopharmacology 5339
psychotropic drugs *5330*
psychosis 5266
malarial 1068
organic causes 5275
psychosocial intervention, COPD 3340
psychosocial short stature 1955
psychotherapy 5315
psychotropic drugs *5330*
classification *5330*
compliance and concordance 5330
drug overdose 5330
mood stabilizers 5333
pharmacokinetics 5330
withdrawal of 5330, *5330*
Psychrobacter spp. *962*
Pterois volitans (lion fish) *1344*
PTH gene 1854
Pthirus pubis 1230–1, *1231*
puberty 1958
constitutional delay 1952
constitutionally advanced 1957
delayed/absent 1958, 1961
causes and evaluation *1960*, 1961
investigation 1961
treatment 1962
physiological mechanisms 1958
precocious 1958–9
causes and evaluation 1959, *1960*
investigation 1960
treatment 1961
timing of 1959
variants of normal 1959, *1959*
pubic lice 1231, *1231*
public health 90
interventions 91, *92*
screening programs *see* screening
see also preventive medicine
public opinion 58–9
Pubmed 24
puerperal fever
S. agalactiae 676
S. pyogenes 674
puffer fish 1346
pulmonary alveolar microlithiasis 3454
aetiology and genetics 3454
clinical features 3454, *3455*
clinical investigation 3455
epidemiology 3454
pathogenesis and pathology 3454
treatment and prognosis 3455
pulmonary alveolar proteinosis 3448
aetiology, genetics and pathogenesis 3449
clinical features 3449
clinical investigation 3449
diagnostic criteria 3449, *3450*
prognosis 3450
treatment 3450
pulmonary amyloidosis 3451
clinical features 3451
diffuse alveolar-interstitial disease 3451, *3452*
localized laryngotracheobronchial disease 3451
localized parenchymal nodules 3451
treatment and prognosis 3452
pulmonary angiography 3011, *3012*
pulmonary artery flotation catheter 5510, *5511*
pulmonary artery occlusion (wedge) pressure 3127
pulmonary atresia
with ventricular septal defect 2867
clinical findings 2867, *2867*
pulmonary circulation 2974
pulmonary blood flow 2976
gravity-dependent 2976, *2976*
gravity-independent 2977
pulmonary vascular resistanct 2975
pulmonary vasomotor tone 2976
hypoxic pulmonary vasoconstriction 2976
ventilation-perfusion relationships 2977, *2977*
structure 2974, *2975*
pulmonary collapse 3209
left lower lobe 3211, *3211*
left upper lobe 3211, *3211*
right lower lobe 3211, *3211*
right middle lobe 3210, *3210*
right upper lobe 3210, *3210*
pulmonary consolidation 3209, *3210*
pulmonary disease *3183*
and acute respiratory failure *3134*
α_1-antitrypsin deficiency 1781, 1783
autoimmune rheumatic disorders 3387
chronic 832
diffuse
bronchoscopy 3222
chronic 3215
parenchymal 3365
drug-induced 3460
hepatic involvement 2538
immunocompromised patients 3960, *3960*
interstitial 3470
leptospirosis 875
polycythaemias 4266
relapsing fever *870*
systemic sclerosis 3672
pulmonary embolectomy 3017
pulmonary embolism 3004, *3120*, *3183*
breathlessness *2633*, 2635
chronic thromboembolic hypertension 3017
clinical assessment 3009, *3011*
clinical features 3005
signs 3008, *3010*
symptoms 3005, *3009*
diagnosis 3014
allergy to contrast materia 3015
critically ill patients 3015
high probability 3015
impaired renal function 3015
low probability 3015
moderate probability 3015
pregnant women 3015
women of reproductive age 3015
differential diagnosis 3010
echocardiography 2667
incidence 3004
infective endocarditis 2808
investigation 3010
arterial blood gases 3014
chest X-ray 3013, *3014*
D-dimer 3010
ECG 3013, *3013*
echocardiography 3014
MRI 3012, *3013*
pulmonary angiography 3011, *3012*
spiral computed tomography 3011, *3012*
ventilation-perfusion lung scans 3010, *3011*
pleural effusion 3491
predisposing factors 3004, *3009*
pregnancy 2116, 2120
presentation 5462, *5463–4*
and pulmonary oedema 2997
treatment 3016
antithrombosis 3016
resuscitation 3016
pulmonary endarterectomy *2990*
pulmonary eosinophilia 3465
haematological changes 4558
tropical 1157
pulmonary fibrosis 3375
autoimmune rheumatic disorders *3390*
clinical features 3377
diagnosis 3376, *3376*, 3379
blood tests 3378
bronchoalveolar lavage 3378
chest X-ray 3377
echocardiography 3379
high-resolution CT *3377–8*
lung biopsy 3379
lung function tests 3378
epidemiology and aetiology 3375
histology and pathogenesis 3376, *3377*
prognosis 3379, *3379*
routine monitoring 3380
systemic sclerosis *3672*
treatment 3380
acute exacerbations 3381
lung transplantation 3381, *3478*
supportive therapy 3381
pulmonary haemorrhage, breathlessness *2633*
pulmonary haemorrhagic disorders 3425, *3426*
eosinophilic pneumonia 3295, 3428
Goodpasture's syndrome 3426
pulmonary haemosiderosis 3426
pulmonary haemosiderosis
idiopathic 3426
clinical features 3427
treatment and prognosis 3427
pulmonary hypertension 2978
altitude-related 1408
arterial 2978, *2979*
clinical features 2982, *2982*
clinical investigation *2983*, 2983, *2984–6*
differential diagnosis 2983
disease-targeted therapies 2987, *2988*
epidemiology and aetiology 2978
genetics 2979
pathogenesis 2980, *2981–2*
pathology 2980, *2980*
treatment 2987
autoimmune rheumatic disorders *3390*, 3392
chronic thromboembolic 2989
clinical presentation 2990
investigation 2990
pathogenesis 2989
treatment 2990, *2990*
classification 2978, *2979*
COPD 3325
HIV-related 3252
HIV/AIDS *2822*, 2823, *2824*
imaging 3333
lung transplantation *3478*
and mitral stenosis 2739
pregnancy 2112
prognosis 2989
SLE 2157
systemic sclerosis *3672*, 3674
pulmonary infiltrates 436, *436*
pulmonary nocardiosis 856
pulmonary nodules
multiple 3213, *3214*
solitary 3212, *3212*
pulmonary oedema 2992, *3120*, *3183*
acute renal trauma 3890
altitude-related 1402, 1405, *1405–6*, 2997
breathlessness *2633*
cardiogenic 2123
causes *2993*, 2996, *2996*
capillary permeability disorders 2998
heart failure 2996
left atrial myoxoma, ball thrombus of left atrium and cor triatriatum 2997
loculated constrictive pericarditis 2997
neurogenic 2997
pulmonary embolism 2997
pulmonary venous thrombosis 2997
clinical features 2998
diagnosis 2998
chest X-ray 2998, *2998*
expansion 2997
lymphatic 2997
malaria 1064, 1067, *1068*, 1080
mechanisms of 2993
high permeability 2994, *2996*
hydrostatic 2993
lymphatic oedema 2994
reduced plasma oncotic pressure 2994
pathogenesis 2992
oedema accumulation 2995, *2995–6*
reduced interstitial pressure 2995
resolution 2996
postobstructive 2997
pregnancy 2123
presentation 5461
pulmonary function 2999
re-expansion 3504
tocolytic-induced 2123
treatment 3000
unilateral 2998
pulmonary regurgitation 2737, 2756

pulmonary rehabilitation 3339, *3339–40*
pulmonary rheumatoid nodules 3391
pulmonary stenosis 2737, 2756
congenital *2844*
percutaneous treatment 2942
pregnancy 2113
pulmonary tuberculosis 810, *816, 817*
pulmonary valve disease, echocardiography 2665
pulmonary valve stenosis, congenital 2848
pulmonary valve, absent 2865
pulmonary vascular disease 3395, *3396*
and acute respiratory failure *3134*
autoimmune rheumatic disorders *3390,* 3391
cardiac catheterization/angiography 2680
clinical manifestations 3396
diffuse alveolar haemorrhage 3396, *3397*
isolated gas transfer deficit 3396
diagnosis 3401
prognosis 3401
and respiratory failure 3472
treatment 3402
pulmonary vascular resistanct 2975
pulmonary veno-occlusive disease 3401
pulmonary venous thrombosis 2997
pulse oximetry, acute respiratory failure 3135
pulse, Corrigan's 2751
pulsus paradoxus, pericardial tamponade 2794
pumpkin seed, drug intractions *69*
Punta Toro virus *581*
pupil, changes in poisoning 1275
pupillary abnormalities 5034
pure red-cell aplasia 4296
aetiology and pathogenesis 4296, *4296*
clinical investigation *4297*
conditions associated with *4296*
diagnostic criteria 4296
future developments 4297
treatment and prognosis 4297
purine 5'-nucleotidase deficiency 1633
purine metabolism 1619, *1620*
disorders of 1619, 1631
see also individual conditions
purine nucleoside phosphorylase deficiency 1632
Purkinje fibres 2609, 2619
purpura fulminans 4532
neonatal 4545
purpura 4500, *4591,* 4683–4
palpable 4685
simple macular 4684, *4685*
pustuloderma, toxic *4727,* 4728
Puumala virus *581*
pycnodysostosis 1698, 3761
mutations in *3757*
pyelography, urinary tract obstruction 4154
pyelonephritis
acute 4108
treatment 4112
emphysematous 4120, *4120*
mycoplasmal *956,* 958
xanthogranulomatous 4119
Pygidiopsis summa 1222
pyloric stenosis, congenital 2398
pyoderma faciale 4682
pyoderma gangrenosum 4721, *4721*
pyoderma 4673
measles-related 521
streptococcal 673
pyogenic arthritis 3617
aetiology 3617
areas of uncertainty 3620
clinical features 3618
diagnosis 3619
differential diagnosis 3619
epidemiology 3618
future developments 3620
investigations 3619, *3619*
pathogenesis/pathophysiology *3617,* 3618, *3618*
prevention/control 3618
prognosis 3620
treatment 3619
pyogenic arthritis, pyoderma gangrenosum and acne syndrome *see* PAPA
pyogenic granuloma 4693
pregnancy 2149, *2150*
pyogenic infection, and complement deficiency 217
pyogenic liver abscess 2543
pyogenic sterile arthritis, pyoderma gangrenosum and acne *3709*
pyomyositis 698, *699*
pyonephrosis 4119
pyrantel embonate, ascariasis 1170
pyrazinamide
pregnancy *2172*
toxicity 826
tuberculosis *825*
dose *826*
pyrethroid poisoning 1306
pyrethrum *3436*
pyrexia *see* fever
pyridinium compounds *3729*
pyridostigmine, orthostatic hypotension *5063*
pyridoxal-phosphate-dependent epilepsy *1566,* 1590
pyridoxine metabolism isorders 1589, *1589*
pyridoxine 1492
adverse effects, neuropathy 5088
clinical aspects 1492
deficiency
anaemia 4419
neuropathy 5089
dietary reference values *1502*
homocysteine metabolism 1494
reference values *5443*
requirements 1492
pyridoxine-dependent epilepsy 1590, *1566*
pyrimethamine-sulphadiazine
isosporiasis 1115
malaria 1076
toxoplasmosis *1096*
pyrimidine 5'-nucleotidase deficiency 1634, 4471
pyrimidine 5'-nucleotidase superactivity 1634
pyrimidine metabolism disorders 1619, *1633, 1633*
oroticaciduria 1633
pyrophosphate arthropathy 3564, 3637, 3644
classification and associations 3645, *3645*
familial predisposition 3645
metabolic disease 3645, *3645*
osteoarthritis and joint insult 3646
clinical features 3644
acute 3644
chronic 3644
incidental 3645
uncommon presentations 3645
differential diagnosis 3646
investigations and diagnosis 3646, *3646*
treatment 3647
pyropoikilocytosis *4464,* 4466
hereditary 4452, *4452*
pyrrolizidine alkaloids *1362*
pyrrolozidium *338*
pyruvate carboxylase deficiency 1617
clinical features 1617
diagnosis and treatment 1617
genetics 1617
metabolic defect 1617
pyruvate dehydrogenase deficiency 1615
biochemical defect 1615
clinical features and prognosis 1615
diagnosis and treatment 1616
genetics 1616
pyruvate kinase deficiency 4453, 4471
pyruvate metabolism disorders 1610, 1615
hyperoxalurias 1730
Python molurus 1325
Python molurus 1325
Python reticulatus 1325
Python reticulatus 1325
Python sebae 1325
Python sebae 1325
pythons 1325

Q fever 923, *1240, 1385*
chronic 925
clinical features 924
acute Q fever 924
hepatic granuloma 2518
hepatitis 925
liver injury 2542
neurological 925
pneumonia 924, *925*
diagnosis 926
epidemiology 924
history 923
in pregnancy 925
prevention 926
treatment 926
18q- syndrome 5106
5q- syndrome 4260
QRS axis 2647, *2647*
QRS complex 2645, 2648
QT interval 2649
Q-tip test 1256
quality-adjusted life years (QALYs) 53, 55
quartan malarial nephrosis 1081
quetiapine 5266, *5337*
adverse effects, hepatotoxicity *2533*
schizophrenia *5325*
quinacrine, giardiasis *1113*
quinagolide, prolactinoma 1811
Quincke's capillary pulsations 2751
quinidine 1075, *1078, 2701*
adverse effects
hepatotoxicity *2529, 2535*
oesophagitis *2294*
drug interactions *1471*
in renal failure *4179*
quinine
adverse effects *455*
hepatotoxicity *2532, 2535*
babesiosis 1090
malaria 1075, *1078*
poisoning *1274,* 1282
pregnancy *2172*
quinolones
adverse effects *455*
mode of action *443*
pharmacodynamics *452*
pharmacokinetics *449, 452*
quinupristin/dalfopristin *707*
bacteraemia *703*
cellulitis, mastitis and pyomyositis *699*
endocarditis *704*
toxic shock syndrome *697*

Rab 38, 376
rabeprazole, peptic ulcer disease 2311
rabies 541
animal *546,* 546
animal reservoirs *542,* 544, *544*
clinical features 546, *547*
cardiovascular 547, *549*
furious rabies *547, 548, 549*
gastrointestinal 547
nervous system 468
paralytic/dumb rabies 547
prodromal symptoms 546, *547*
respiratory 547
control in animals 551
diagnosis 547
furious rabies 548
laboratory 550, *551*
paralytic/dumb rabies 549
epidemiology *542,* 543, *543*
global distribution *543*
human 543
immunological response 543
to rabies infection 545
to rabies vaccination 545
pathogenesis 545
pathology *550,* 550
presentation 5499
prevention 551
postexposure prophylaxis 552
pre-exposure prophylaxis 551
prognosis 550
transmission *545,* 554
treatment 550
vaccines *466,* 468, 552
see also rhabdoviruses
Rabson-Mendenhall syndrome 1994
RAc 2 deficiency *238,* 253
radial nerve neuropathy 5080
radiation nephropathy 4016
clinical features 4016
diagnosis and treatment 4017
pathogenesis and pathology 4016

radiation pneumonitis 3458
clinical features 3459, *3459*
pathogenesis 3459
treatment 3460
radiation 1429
history 1429
ionizing *see* ionizing radiation
nonionizing 1429, 1431
power-frequency electric/magnetic fields 1432
radio-frequency electromagnetic waves 1432
static magnetic fields 1432
ultraviolet 1431
and pericarditis 2791
risk measurement 1429
radioactivity 1429
radioallergosorbent tests *2251*, 2254
radiofrequency ablation 2702, *2702*, 2711, 3206
radio-frequency electromagnetic waves 1432
radio-iodine
thyroid cancer 1848
thyrotoxicosis 1841
radionuclide imaging
thyroid cancer 1847
urinary tract obstruction 4154
ventilation-perfusion 3200, *3203*, *3204*
radionuclide ventriculography
equilibrium 2673
first pass 2673
radiopharmaceuticals, pancreatic neuroendocrine tumours 1982
radiotherapy *388*, 401
anterior pituitary gland 1805
cancer 403, *403*
breast 1934, *1936*
complications 402
hormonal abnormalities *2066*
lung cancer 3528, 3530
mesothelioma 3536
metastatic brain tumours 390
pancreatic neuroendocrine tumours 1982
radon, and lung cancer 320, *1380*
Raeder's syndrome 5034
Rahnella spp. *962*
Raillietina celebensis *1190*
Raillietina demerariensis *1190*
Raillietiella gehyrae 1240
raloxifene 2198
hyperparathyroidism 1859
osteoporosis *3799*, 3800
Ralstonia spp. *962*
raltegravir
HIV/AIDS *638*
toxicity *640*
raltitrexed, mesothelioma 3537
Ramazzini, *De Morbis Artificium* 1377
ramipril, heart failure *2722*
Ramsay-Hunt syndrome *4908*, 5037
random errors 33, *33*, 35
minimization of 37
randomization 35
randomized controlled trials 22, 27, 49
entry procedures 36
lumping 29
mega-trials 35
meta-analysis 37
proper running of 34
data-dependent emphasis 34, *35*
intention-to-treat analysis 34
lack of bias 34
no foreknowledge of treatment 34
random errors 35
randomization 35
relevance to clinical practice 44
theoretical and practical limitations 28
usefulness of 29
see also individual trials
ranitidine
adverse effects, hepatotoxicity *2532*, *2535*
anaphylaxis 3113
H. pylori *2313*
peptic ulcer disease 2311
RANK 3723, *3723*
Ranke's complex 815
RANKL 156, 3550, 3722, 3724
ranolazine, angina 2909
Raoultella spp. *962*
rapamycin, post-transplantation *2511*
rare diseases, challenges of 62
Ras proteins 348
Rasbo spp. *962*
rasburicase, gout 1624
rashes
drug-induced *4740*
meningitis 713, *714–15*
typhoid *740*
Rasmussen's encephalitis *166*, *276*
rat-bite fever 857
prevention 860
S. moniliformis 858
aetiology 858
clinical features 858
diagnosis 859
differential diagnosis 859
epidemiology 858
prognosis 859
treatment 859
Spirillum minus 859
aetiology 859
clinical features 859
diagnosis 860
differential diagnosis 860
epidemiology 859
prognosis 860
treatment 860
Rathke's cleft, cysts 1817
Rathke's pouch 1800
rationing of care 58
Raynaud's phenomenon *3666*, 3671, 4687
clinical features 3668
autoimmune *3666*
primary *3666*
management *3671*
Sjögren's syndrome 3690
reactive arthritis 3622, *3605*
areas of uncertainty 3627
clinical features 3624
arthritis 3624, *3624*
extra-articular *3623–5*, 3624
preceding illness 3624
definition 3622, *3623*
differential diagnosis 3625, *3625*
epidemiology 3623
historical perspective 3622
laboratory features 3625
immunology 3626
microbiology 3625
radiology 3626
pathogenesis 3623
postinfectious *3623*
psychological issues 3626
quality of life 3626
treatment 3626
reactive nitrogen intermediates 156
reactive oxygen intermediates 156
reactive oxygen species 208
osteoarthritis 3631
reboxetine 5331, *5331*
receiver-operator characteristic (ROC) curve 97, *97–8*
reciprocal translocations 146
rectal cancer 315
incidence *301*
migrants vs residents *302*
screening *106*
rectal drug administration 1452
rectum
anatomy 2201
cancer *see* colorectal cancer
function of 2203
salt and water absorption *2208*
solitary rectal ulcer syndrome 2588
recurrent laryngeal nerve paralysis 3172, 3260
red cell count *4196*
infants and children *4197*
red cell enzymopathies 4468, *4470*
aldolase deficiency 4472
diagnosis 4472–3
diphosphoglycerate mutase deficiency 4472
genetics 4470
glucose-6-phosphate isomerase deficiency 4471
glutathione reductase deficiency 4471
glutathione synthesis enzymes 4471
hexokinase deficiency 4471
high adenosine deaminase activity 4472
phosphofructokinase deficiency 4472
phosphoglycerate kinase deficiency 4472
pyrimidine 5'-nucleotidase deficiency 4471
pyruvate kinase deficiency 4453, 4471
triosephosphate isomerase deficiency 4471
red cell mass *4197*
red cell membrane 4461
composition and function 4461
disorders of *4451*, 4451, 4461
elliptocytosis and pyropoikilocytosis 4466
hereditary spherocytosis 4462
red cells
density *4196*
diameter *4196*
enzyme defects 1474
enzyme disorders 4452, *4453–4*
homeostasis 4372
lifespan *4196*
maturation defects 4561, *4446*
alcohol- and drug-induced 4449
copper deficiency 4449
lead, arsenic or zinc ingestion 4449
metabolism 4469, *4469*
premature destruction 4372
shape disorders 4461, *4462*
transfusion 4564, *4564*
volume *4196*
red clover 68
red eye 5234, *5234*
red hepatization 683, *684*
5α-reductase defects *1917*
Reduvius personatus 1229
Reed-Sternberg cells 4323
re-expansion pulmonary oedema 3504
refeeding syndrome 1539
reference nutrient intakes *1524*
reflex apnoea 3275
reflexology 65
reflux nephropathy 4118, *4118*
Refsum's disease *1552*, 1723
aetiology *1724*, 1724
clinical features 1724
clinical investigation 1727
diagnostic criteria 1727
differential diagnosis 1724, *1725–6*
epidemiology 1727
future developments 1728
historical perspective 1724
molecular genetics 1726
disordered omega-oxidation 1726
molecular toxicology 1727
prognosis 1728
treatment 1728
regenerative medicine 193, 191
cardiac repair 201
diabetes mellitus 202
history *197*
neurological repair 201
requirements 193
see also stem cells
regional anaesthesia 3156
regional pain disorders 3578
regional pain syndrome, chronic 3712
regulatory T cells *see* Tregs
regurgitation, peptic stricture 2291
rehydration therapy *758*, 2432
Reichel's syndrome 3713
Reifenstein's syndrome 1923
Reiter's syndrome 3622
mycoplasmal *956*, 958
neurological complications 5160
ocular involvement 5242
relapsing fevers 866
aetiology 866
clinical features
Jarisch-Herxheimer reaction 868, *869*, 871
louse-borne 870, *870–1*
severe disease 871
spontaneous crisis 871
tick-borne 870
diagnosis 872
differential diagnosis 872
epidemiology
louse-borne 867
tick-borne 867, *868*
history 866, *866–7*
immunopathology 868
laboratory findings 872
louse-borne 866

pathology 869
cerebral haemorrhage *869*
heart *869*
pulmonary *870*
spleen *869*
pathophysiology 868
prevention and control 873
prognosis 872
relapse phenomenon 868
tick-borne 866
treatment 872
Jarisch-Herxheimer reaction 873
supportive 873
relapsing polychondritis, pulmonary involvement 3393
relative risk 49, 52
remifentanil 3155, *3155*
renal acid-base homeostasis 4134
collecting duct 4134, *4135*
proximal tubule 4134, *4134*
renal angiography *3874*
renal arteriography, interventional 3880
renal artery stenosis 3900
nuclear imaging 3881, *3881*
renal biopsy 3864, *3882, 3883*
acute renal trauma 3893
complications 3883
contraindications 3882
indications 3882, *3883*
technique 3883
renal blood flow 3872
renal calcium handling disorders 4124
renal cancer 327, 371, 4162, 4165
diagnosis, staging and grading 4166
familial papillary renal cell carcinoma 368
genetic changes 4166
incidence *301*
paraneoplastic phenomena 4166
prognosis 4167, *4167*
risk factors 4165
treatment 4166
laparoscopic surgery 4167
metastatic disease 4167
open surgery *4166*, 4167
renal carbuncle 4119
renal colic, investigations *2235*
renal cysts and diabetes syndrome 4098
renal disease
acute cortical necrosis 3899
acute kidney injury 3885, 5475
Acute Kidney Injury Network classification 3886, *3887*
assessment 3885, 3888
bleeding time 3894, *3894*
causes 3886, *3887–8*, 3894
clinical features 3890
definition 3886, *3887*
diagnosis 3885, 3887
drug prescribing 3894
epidemiology 3886
fluid requirements 3892
life-threatening complications 3890
management 3885
nutrition 3893
renal biopsy 3893
renal replacement therapy 3892
Risk Injury Failure Loss and Endstage kidney disease (RIFLE) classification 3886, *3887*
sepsis 3894
volume depletion 3892
acute tubular necrosis 3894
asymptomatic 3846
chronic 3850, *3851*, 3863, 3904
causes 3907, *3907–8*
clinical assessment 3911
clinical presentation 3910, *3911*
definition 3905
family history 3912
global overview *3907*
infections 3858
investigations *3914*
lifestyle measures 3916, *3916*
management 3905, 3916
mineral and bone disorder 3917
mortality risk *3906*
palliative care 3905, *3926, 3928*
pathophysiology 3904, 3908
peritoneal dialysis 3944
physical examination 3912, *3913*
prevalence and incidence 3906, *3906*
prevention of progression 3904, 3912
progression of 3909, *3910*
protein restriction 3916
screening for 3847
stages of *3870*
tropical 4084, *4085*
clinical presentation 3846
cystic 1626, *4095, 4096*
autosomal dominant polycystic disease 4095
autosomal recessive polycystic kidney disease 4097
renal cysts and diabetes syndrome 4098
disease associations 3856, *3857*
diabetic nephropathy 3857, *3858*
infectious diseases 3858
myeloma 3857, *3858*
renovascular disease 3857, *3858*
drug-induced *3860*, 3861
nephrotoxicity 3861
obstruction 3861
salt and water depletion 3861
ectopic calcification 3714
glomerular, tropical 4083, *4083*
glomerulonephritic 3900, *3901*
and gout 3641
chronic urate nephropathy 3642
urolithiasis 3641
haematological changes 4554
anaemia 4554
platelets and coagulation 4555
polycythaemia 4555
white cells 4555
and heart failure 2725
hyperlipidaemia 1667
hypertensive 3037
inflammatory conditions 3889, *3889*
investigations 3863
biopsy 3864, *3882, 3883*
GFR *see* glomerular filtration rate
imaging 3864, *3873, 3874*
renal blood flow 3872
tubular function 3864, 3872
urine *see* urine
leptospirosis 875
malaria 1063
nephrotic syndrome *244*, 3854
nutrition support 1543
and osteomalacia 3739, *3739*
polycythaemia 4268
post-transplant 2731
in pregnancy 3861, *3861*
pregnancy 2103, 3861, *3861*
acute renal failure 2104, *2105*
hydroureter, hydronephrosis and overdistension syndrome 2105
management 2106
pre-existing 2106
renal transplant patients 2107
rupture of urinary tract 2106
urinary tract infection 2104
women on dialysis 2107
prerenal failure 3894
prevalence *3847*
renal failure *see* renal failure
screening 3847
drug-induced disease 3848
employment/insurance 3848
families 3848
population and risk group 3847
proteinuria 3848, *3848*
secondary care 3848
skin involvement 4720
calcific arteriolopathy 4721
nephrogenic fibrosing dermopathy 4721
pigmentary changes 4720
uraemic pruritus 4720
SLE 3658, *3659*
stages of *3906*
symptomatic 3850
loin pain 3853
urinary symptoms 3852
systemic sclerosis 3675
tropical 4082
acute renal failure 4083, *4084–5*
CKD 4084, *4085*
glomerular 4083, *4083*
infections 4084, *4086*
toxins 4090
tubulointerstitial 3843
vasculitis 3900, *3901*
renal failure
acidosis 1747
acute 3851
leptospiral 4089
malarial 1064, 1079, 4086
obstetric 2105, *2105*
pregnancy 2104, *2105*
with thrombotic microangiopathy 2104
tropical 4083, *4084–5*
acute pancreatitis 2564
anaemia in 4401
chronic
complications 3925, *3926*
reproductive effects *1917*
sickle cell disease 4070
CNS complications 5152
drug handling 4172
iatrogenic disease 5152
and immunodeficiency *244*
malignant hypertension 3078, *3078*
prescribing in 4176, *4184*
cardiovascular system 4177
central nervous system 4181
endocrine system 4183
gastrointestinal system 4176
immunological products and vaccines 4183
malignant disease and immunosuppression 4183
nutrition 4183
obstetrics, gynaeology and urinary tract 4183
respiratory system 4181
skin 4183
snake bite 1352
symptoms 3912
renal functional capacity *5449*
renal hypertension 3059
renal masses, ultrasound 3876
renal osteodystrophy *1858*
post-transplant 3964
renal replacement therapy 3930
acute renal trauma 3892
preparation for 3925
see also individual modalities
renal stones *see* nephrolithiasis
renal transplantation 3947
allocation of kidneys 3951
complications 3948, 3952, 3963
accelerated atherosclerosis 3963, *3963*
cosmetic 3965
electrolyte disorders 3964
gastrointestinal 3965
haematological 3965
hypertension 3963, *3963*
nephropathy 605, *606*
rejection 3948, *3952, 3953*
surgical 3952, *3952*
immunosuppression 3953, *3954*
adverse effects 3954–5
ischaemia times 3951
kidney donation 3948
deceased donors 3950, *3950*
living donors 3949, *3949*
outcome 3966
chronic allograft nephropathy 3966
de novo glomerulonephritis 3967
graft and patient survival 3966, *3965–7*
recurrence of original disease 3967
patient management
diet 3967
drug interactions 3967, *3968*
follow-up 3968
pregnancy 3968
postoperative management 3951
pregnancy after 2107
prescribing after 4184, *4184*
prognosis 3948
recipient assessment 3950
and skin cancer 4720
supply and demand 3948
surgical technique 3951
technical aspects 3947
ultrasound 3876, *3877*
urinary tract infection 4117
renal tubular acidosis *3739, 4128*, 4133
causes *4136*

clinical presentation *4134,* 4136, *4136*
distal tubule with hyperkalaemia 4137
distal tubule with hypokalaemia 4137
mixed 4138
proximal tubule 4135
diagnosis 4138, *4138*
and hyperkalaemia 3843
management 4139
treatment 1749
renal tubular function 3864, 3872
distal tubule 3873
electrolyte handling disorders 4140
electrolyte imbalances 3873
proximal tubule 3872
amino acids 3872
glucose 3872
phosphate 3872
renal vasculitis 4053
renal vein thrombosis 3900
renal venography 3880
renal-coloboma syndrome 4102
renin
in Conn's syndrome 3063
ectopic secretion 2065
reference values *5441*
renin-angiotensin system 2600, 2623
drugs affecting 4179
renin-angiotensin-aldosterone system
drug effects on 3843
role in hypertension 3032, *3033*
renovascular disease 3857, *3858*
ultrasound 3876
renovascular hypertension 3059, *3061*
diagnosis 3060
mechanism 3060
treatment 3061
repaglinide 2014
repetitive strain injury 1382
reproduction, health effects 15
reproductive system
occupational disease 1385
female 1385
male 1385
reptilase time 4503
residual volume 3174
resistance vessels, hypertensive changes 3035
resistant ovary syndrome 1906
respiration
pattern of 3186
sleep-related disorders 3261
respiratory acidosis 1742, *3197, 3198*
respiratory alkalosis 3197, *3198*
respiratory bronchiolitis-interstitial lung disease 3368, *3368*
respiratory chain disorders 5223
clinical syndromes 5223, *5223*
investigation 5224
management 5226
nonspecific presentations 5224, *5223, 5225*
prognosis 5226
respiratory chain 5221, *5222*
respiratory disease
auscultation 3187
child mortality *75*
Chlamydia pneumoniae 947
clinical investigation 3189
bronchoscopy, thoracoscopy and tissue biopsy 3216
respiratory function tests 3189
thoracic imaging 3200
clinical presentation 3186
cyanosis 3186
exercise 3187
heart and cardiovascular system 3187
impaired cerebral function 3186
skeleton and muscles 3187
skin and subcutaneous tissues 3186
stridor and pattern of breathing 3186
CNS effects 5152
history 3185
investigations 3188, *3188*
malaria 1063
mortality *76, 121*
mycoplasmal infections 950, 952
observation, palpation and percussion 3187
occupational 1387
peptic stricture 2291
rabies 547
SLE 3659
symptoms 3182
breathlessness *see* breathlessness
chest pain 3185, *3185*
cough 3183, *3184*
haemoptysis 2848, *3184,* 3184
systemic sclerosis *3672*
see also individual conditions
respiratory failure 3132, 3196
acute pancreatitis 2564
causes *3134*
chronic 3467
assessment 3472, *3472*
causes 3470, *3471*
treatment 3473
clinical investigations 3134
arterial blood gases 3134, *3134*
blood tests 3135, *3135*
chest radiograph 3135
CT 3135
ECG and echocardiography 3135
fibreoptic bronchoscopy 3135
screening for infection 3135
ultrasound 3135
cystic fibrosis 3363
definition and epidemiology 3133
history and examination 3133, *3134*
management 3136
airway 3136, *3136–7*
mechanical ventilation *3138,* 3139, *3140*
noninvasive ventilation 3139
oxygen therapy 3138, *3138*
presentation 5467
respiratory monitoring 3135
arterial oxygen saturation/pulse oximetry 3135
capnography 3136
indwelling arterial catheter 3135
lung function assessment 3135
type 1, 3133
type 2, 3133
respiratory function tests *see* lung function tests
respiratory papillomatosis 603
respiratory stimulants 3343
respiratory syncytial virus *474,* 477
respiratory system
commensal flora 749
in cystic fibrosis 3354
dead space 3176
distribution of ventilation 3178
mucociliary function 3177
particle deposition 3176
pregnancy 2077, 2088
chest X-ray 2088
dyspnoea 2088
subacute toxic injury 3458
upper 3169
see also various parts
viruses 473, *474*
laboratory diagnosis 475
seasonality 475
transmission 475
see also individual viruses
respiratory tract infection 3227
diagnosis, bronchoscopy 3223
HIV-related 3246
pneumonia *see* pneumonia
upper respiratory tract 3221
nasal congention and rhinorrhoea 3229
pharyngitis/tonsillitis 3227
rhinitis 3227, 3230
sinusitis 3227, 3230
Restan virus *581*
restless legs syndrome 4899, 5078
pregnancy 2145
restrictive cardiomyopathy 2765, 2777
causes 2777
clinical features and investigation 2778, *2778*
definition 2777
management 2778
pathology 2777
resuscitation *5453*
cardiopulmonary *see* cardiopulmonary resuscitation
malnutrition 1513
pulmonary embolism 3016
RET proto-oncogene 1845
retching 2206
reteplase, pulmonary embolism 3016
reticulocyte count 4197, *4196*
infants and children *4197*
retina, in malaria 1062, *1066*
retinal arteriolar embolization 3043
retinal artery occlusion 5239, *5239*
retinal artery
microaneurysms 3043
occlusion 3043, *3044*
retinal haemorrhage, altitude-related 1407, *1407*
retinal neoavascularization 5245
retinal vein occlusion 3043, *3044, 5239, 5240*
retinitis pigmentosa *168,* 140
retinitis
bartonella *931*
cytomegalovirus *495,* 497
HIV-related 631, *632*
differential diagnosis *1722*
varicella zoster 492
retinoblastoma gene 349
retinoblastoma 302, 358, *360,* 361, 365
retinoic acid
actions *1791*
signalling pathways *1797*
retinoids 1485, 1488, 4733
acne *4680*
and cancer risk 310
oral 4737
psoriasis 4615
teratogenicity *1468, 2187*
retinol 1485
retinopathy, hypertensive *3042–3,* 3077, *3077*
retroperitoneal fibrosis 4158, *4158*
aetiology 4158
clinical features 4158
diagnosis 4159, *4159–60*
epidemiology 4158
management 4160, *4161*
pathogenesis 4158
prognosis 4161
secondary 4158, *4158*
retrotransposons 141
retroviruses 346, *651*
Rett's syndrome 138
revascularization 2909, *2910*
acute coronary syndromes 2921
Reye's syndrome *1742,* 5010
lactic acidosis 1747
Rh system 4562
incompatibility 4457
Rhabditis spp. *1176*
rhabdomyolysis 3859
causes 3898, *3898*
fungal poisoning 1370
poisoned patients 1278
presentation 5475
rhabdomyoma, cardiac 2832
Rhabdophis tigrinus (Japanese yamakagashi) 1327
rhabdoviruses 541
transmission *545,* 554
virology *545,* 543
see also rabies
rhabomyolysis 5379
Rhagionidae (snipe flies) *1226*
rheumatic disorders
autoimmune 3649
ANCAs *3651*
clinical features 3651
clinical spectrum 3650, *3650*
definition and epidemiology 3649, *3650*
immunopathogenesis 3651
lung in 3387, *3389*
in pregnancy 2154
see also individual conditions
autoinflammatory 3708
clinical presentation 3554
diagnosis *3555–6,* 3554
drugs producing 3714
examination 3558
focal 3557, *3557*
functional somatic syndromes 3557
gastroenterological and metabolic 3711
haematological 3708
investigations 3558, 3560
arthrography 3564
blood tests 3565, *3566–7*
calcification 3564
CT 3565
erosions 3563, *3563–4*
immunological tests 3567
MRI 3565
osteoarthritis 3564

plain radiography 3562, *3562–3*
scintigraphy 3565, *3565*
specific clinical tests 3569
synoval fluid analysis 3561, *3561–2*
ultrasound 3565
paraneoplastic presentations 3714
prognostic markers 3560, *3561*
signs/symptoms *3556*
systemic 3556
treatment 3558
vasculitides *3650*
rheumatic fever 2797
clinical features 2800, *2800*
acute phase reactants 2801
arthritis 2800
carditis 2800, *2801*
erythema marginatum 2801
fever 2801
poststreptococcal syndromes 2802
subcutaneous nodules 2801
Sydenham's chorea 2801
diagnosis 2802, *2803*
epidemiology 2798, *2798*
pathogenesis 2799, *2799*
host factors 2799
immune response 2800
organism factors 2799
site of infection 2800
and pharyngitis 3229
prevention 2805
prognosis and follow-up 2804
recurrences 2804
treatment 2802
rheumatoid arthritis *277*, 3579, *3650*
aetiology 3579, 3581
environmental factors 3582
genetic factors 3581, *3582*
host factors 3583
clinical course 3589
disease activity 3589
structural damage 3590
clinical features 3579, 3586
ankles and feet 3588
elbows and shoulders 3588
hands and wrists 3587, *3588*
hip 3588
joint distribution 3587
knees 3588
neck 3588
presentation 3586
cutaneous involvement 4647, *4647–8*
definition 3580, *3580*
diagnosis 3579, 3591
differential diagnosis 3591
infection-related polyarthritis 3591
osteoarthritis 3591
polyarthritis of connective tissue disease 3591
spondyloarthropathies 3591
epidemiology 3581, *3581*
extra-articular disease 3588
amyloidosis 3589
cancer 3589
cardiac involvement *2783–4*, 2784, 3589
eye complications *3589*, 5248, *5242*
Felty's syndrome 3589
fibrosing alveolitis 3588
infections 3589
neurological 3589
nodules 3588, *3588*
obliterative bronchiolitis 3588
osteoporosis 3589
serositis 3588
systemic vasculitis 3588
genome association 141
haematological changes 4553
hepatic involvement 2544
historical background 3580
investigations 3591
imaging 3592, *3592*
laboratory tests 3591
management 3579, 3592
aims of 3592
drug therapy 3592, *3594–5*
extra-articular disease 3594
mild disease 3593
moderate/severe disease 3593
nonpharmacological measures 3593
mycoplasmal 957
neurological complications 5160
oesophageal symptoms *2297*
pathogenesis 3579, *3584, 3585*
B cells and autoantibodies 3584
cytokines 3585, *3586–7*
T cells 3585
pathology 3583
extra-articular disease 3584, *3584*
joints 3583, *3583*
pregnancy 2154, 2161
effect of disease on pregnancy 2161
effect of pregnancy on disease 2161
management 2161
prevalence *3650*
prognosis 3579, *3590, 3590*
prognostic factors 3590
remission 3590
pulmonary involvement 3390, *3390*
pleural effusion 3491
renal involvement 4051, *4052*
reproductive effects *1917*
rheumatoid factor 3567, *3568*
rhinitis 3227, 3230
allergic *see* allergic rhinitis
nonallergic 261
pregnancy-associated 2122
rhinopharyngitis mutans *882*
rhinorrhoea 3229
rhinoscleroma 747
aetiology 747
clinical features 3, 747, *747–8*
diagnosis 748
pathogenesis 747
treatment 748
rhinosporidiosis 1015
rhinoviruses *474*, 475
Rhipicephalus sanguineus 1228
Rhodnius prolixus 1228
Rhodococcus equi, HIV-associated infection *3247*
Rhodococcus spp. *962*
rhodopsin 1489
Rhodotorula spp. *3436*
ribavirin
adenovirus 477
hepatitis C 619
human metapneumovirus 479
Lassa fever 594
parainfluenza virus 479
pregnancy *2172*
respiratory syncytial virus 478
riboflavin 1489–90
deficiency anaemia 4419
dietary reference values *1502*
dietary sources 1490
migraine prevention *4916*
reference values *5443*
requirements 1490
ribs
disorders of 3509
congenital abnormalities 3509
see also individual disorders
ricin *1362*, 1364, 1442
Ricinus communis (castor oil plant) *1372*
Ricinus communis 1371
rickets 1488, *1496, 3719, 3734, 3735*
autosomal dominant hypo-phosphataemic 4142, *4143*
autosomal recessive with hypercalciuria 4142, *4143*
autosomal recessive hypo-phosphataemic 4142, *4143*
biochemical changes *3736*
clinical features *3731*
hypophosphataemic *3737*, 3739, *3739*
oncogenic *3721*
phosphate deficiency 3740
tumour-associated 3740
vitamin D dependent *3721*, 3740
vitamin D-resistant 1474, *3739*
X-linked hypo-phosphataemic 4142, *4143*
see also osteomalacia
Rickettsia aeschlimannii 905
Rickettsia africae 905
Rickettsia akari 904, 908
Rickettsia australis 905
Rickettsia bellii 905
Rickettsia canadensis 905
Rickettsia conorii caspia 905
Rickettsia conorii conorii 905
Rickettsia conorii indica 905
Rickettsia conorii israelensis 905
Rickettsia conorii 912
Rickettsia felis 904
Rickettsia heilongjiangensis 905
Rickettsia helvetica 905
Rickettsia honei 905
Rickettsia japonica 905
Rickettsia massiliae 905
Rickettsia parkeri 905
Rickettsia prowazekii 904, 1231
Rickettsia rickettsii 905
Rickettsia sibirica mongolitimonae 905
Rickettsia sibirica sibirica 905
Rickettsia slovaca 905, 911
Rickettsia spp. *962*
ocular involvement 5247
Rickettsia typhi 904
rickettsialpox 908
clinical features 909
epidemiology 908
rickettsioses 903
bacteriology 903
clinical features 903
diagnosis 903
epidemic typhus 911
epidemiology 903
flea-borne spotted fever 907
future developments 918
murine typhus 910
pathophysiology 904
prevention 903, 918
prognosis 903, 914
taxonomy and genomics 904
tick-borne 904, *905*
agents and diseases 907
clinical features 907
epidemiology 904, *907–10*
treatment 903, 914
see also individual conditions
rickety rosary 3736
Rictularia spp. *1176*
Ridley-Jopling classification of leprosy 837, *838*
rifabutin, contraindication in porphyria *5484*
rifampicin *707*
adverse effects
adrenal insufficiency 2068
hepatotoxicity *2532, 2533*
brucellosis 794
contraindication in porphyria *5484*
drug interactions *1471, 3968*
endocarditis *704–5*
H. influenzae 762
hepatotoxicity 825
infective endocarditis *2811, 2817, 2818*
leprosy *845*
listeriosis 898
Madura foot 1005
mode of action *443*
mycobacterial disease *835*
pharmacokinetics *449*
pneumonia *3238, 3245*
poisoning 1280
postantibiotic effect *451*
pregnancy *2172*
Q fever 926
septic bursitis/arthritis *700*
tuberculosis *825*
dose *826*
rifaximin, bacterial overgrowth *2334*
rifecoxib, and asthma *3289*
Rift Valley fever *581*, 586, *587*
renal toxicity *4086*
right ventricle, double outlet 2866
right ventricular anomalies 2850, *2859*
right ventricular dysfunction, HIV/AIDS *2822*, 2823, *2824*
right ventricular hypertrophy, ECG 2649
Riley-Day syndrome 5064
rimantadine
influenza virus 480
mode of action *444*
rimonabant 1533
ring chromosomes 146
ringworm
body 998, 1000
scalp 1000
Rio Bravo virus *566*
Rio Negro *558*
risedronate, osteoporosis *3799*
risk modification 90
risk paradox 88, *88*
risk
familial 89

phenotypic 89
risk-benefit ratio 1450
risperidone 5266, *5337*
adverse effects, hepatotoxicity *2533*
schizophrenia *5325*
risus sardonicus *797*
RITA 3 trial 2921
ritonavir
adverse effects, hepatotoxicity *2529*
HIV/AIDS *638*
mode of action *444*
toxicity *640*
rituximab *244*, *376*, *401*
cost-effectiveness ratio *53*
lupus nephritis 4049
lymphoma *4320*
polymyositis/ dermatomyositis 3697
post-transplantation *3954*
pregnancy *2158*
rheumatoid arthritis 3598, *3599*, 3600
SLE 3662
rivaroxaban 3022
rizatriptan, migraine *4917–18*
RNA 138
see also various types
road traffic accidents, mortality rate *76*
Robertson, Elizabeth 191
Robertsonian translocations 146
Rocio virus *566*, 572
Rockall score *2239*
rodenticides, anticoagulant, poisoning 1302
Romaña's sign *1130*
Romano-Ward syndrome 163, 166
Romanus lesion *3609*
Romberg's sign 5040
rosacea 4691
roseola infantum 497
Roseomonas spp. *962*
rosiglitazone, adverse effects, hepatotoxicity 2531
Ross River virus *558*, 559
rosuvastatin 1670
rotational ablation 2938, *2938*
rotator cuff
rupture *3248*
tendinitis *3248*
rotaviruses 536
classification 537
diarrhoea 2427
epidemiology 540
immune response 538
pathogenesis 538
replication 537
structure 536, *537*
Roth spots, infective endocarditis 2809
Rothia dentocariosa *851*
Rothia spp. *962*
Rothmund-Thomson syndrome *360*, 369
Rotor syndrome 2450
Rous sarcoma virus 346
Royal Farm virus *566*
rubber industry, cancer in *1380*
rubella syndrome, antenatal screening *102*
rubella 561
aetiology 562
congenital *244*, 562, 5146
clinical features 562, *563*
laboratory diagnosis 562
risk to fetus 562
epidemiology 562
immunization *91*
management in pregnancy 562
postnatal 562
pregnancy 2166
prevention 563
progressive panencephalitis 5012
rugger jersey spine 3737
rumination 2207
Ruminococcus spp. *962*
Runx 3549, *3549*
RUNX2, 3722
Russell's viper venom *4540*
Russell-Silver syndrome 1953
ryanodine receptors 2607

S100, reference values *5442*
Sabethes spp. *1226*
Saboya virus *566*
sabre tibia 882
Saccharomonospora viridis *3436*
saccharopinuria *1566*, 1575
Saccharopolyspora rectivirgula 3435, *3436*
sacral agenesis 5138
sacroilliitis, brucella *792*
sage, drug intractions *69*
Sal Vieja virus *566*
salazopyrine
adverse effects, hepatotoxicity *2529*
Still's disease 3706
salbutamol
anaphylaxis 3112
COPD *3335*
hyperkalaemia *3891*
salicylates
adverse effects, hepatotoxicity *2529*
metabolism *1294*
poisoning *1274*, 1293, 2028
clinical features 1294, *1295*
pathophysiology *1295*
rheumatic fever 2804
serum levels *5449*
uses *3798*
salicylic acid 4733
saline diuresis, hypercalcaemia 1857
salivary calculus 2282
salivary glands
diseases of 2281
cancer 312, *313*, 507, 2283
salivary duct obstruction 2282
sialadenitis 2282
xerostomia 2281, *2281*
Salla's disease *1552*, 1698, *3739*
salmeterol, COPD *3335*
Salmonella enteritidis 2429
Salmonella spp. 727, *801*, *962*
clinical features 733
epidemiology 732
immunosuppressed patients 3959
laboratory diagnosis 733
osteomyelitis *3789*
pathogenesis 733
prevention 733
treatment 733
Salmonella typhi, renal toxicity *4086*
salmonellosis 1240
Salmonid virus *558*
salsalate, and asthma *3289*
salt restriction
ascites and cirrhosis 2486
heart failure *2720*
hypertension 3048
salt, and blood pressure 1519, 3030
saltwater aspiration syndrome 1417
Samter's triad 3288
San Perlita virus *566*
sanctity of life 19
sandflies, bartonellosis 935
sandfly fever *581*, 586
Sandhoff's disease 1698
Sanfilippo's disease 1698
sanitizers, poisoning by 1317
Sanjad-Sakati syndrome *1855*, 1865
SaO_2, acute respiratory failure 3135
SAPHO syndrome 3604, 3614, *3614–15*, 4682
saposin B deficiency 1698
saposin C deficiency 1696, 1698
saquinavir
HIV/AIDS 636, *638*
mode of action *444*
toxicity *640*
sarafotoxins 1331
Sarcocystis spp. 1109
sarcocystosis 1109, *1109*
clinical features 1110
diagnosis 1110, *1110*
prevention 1111
treatment 1110
sarcoid nephropathy 4007
clinical features 4007
diagnosis and treatment 4008
sarcoid neuropathy 5091
sarcoid, cardiac involvement 2786, *2786*
sarcoidosis 3403, 5163
aetiology 3404
areas of uncertainty 3412
cardiac 2763
clinical features 3403, 3405, *3405–7*
hepatic involvement 2519, 2539
hypercalcaemia *3745*
lupus pernio *3407*
multiorgan involvement *3408*
ocular 5240
skin 4715, *4716*
complications 3412
differential diagnosis *3406*
epidemiology 3404, *3404*
future developments 3413
hormonal abnormalities *2066*
hypercalcaemia 2067
investigations 3403, 3409
imaging 3409
lung function tests 3409
serum ACE levels 3409
management 3403
pathogenesis 3405
pathology 3408
prevalence *3404*
prognosis 3412
renal involvement 3860
treatment 3410, *3410–11*
corticosteroids 3410
strategy 3412
sarcoma 358
cardiac 2832
in Paget's disease 3743, *3743*
Sarcophaga spp. *1233*
Sarcophagidae *1233*
sarcoplasmic reticulum 2603
calcium channels 160
coupling of plasma membrane to 2607, *2608–10*
sarcoplasmic/endoplasmic reticulum ATPase type 2 *see* SERCA2
SARS-like coronaviruses 659
saruplase, pulmonary embolism 3016
Saumarez Reef virus *566*
saw palmetto 68
scabbard trachea 3260
scabies 1225, 1229
immunocompromised patients 3959
treatment 1230
scalded skin syndrome 696, *696*
scalp
allergic contact dermatitis 4702
eczema 4702
fungal disease 4702
irritant dermatitis 4702
psoriasis 4701, *4702*
seborrhoeic dermatitis 4702
Scardovia spp. *962*
Scarites sulcatus 1235
scarlet fever 672
Schatzki ring 2302, *2302*
Scheie syndrome 1698
cardiac involvement *2840*
Scheuermann's disease *3804*
Schilder's disease 4960
Schilling test 2229, 2328
Schindler's disease 1698, 5122
Schisotosoma mansoni 1203
schistocytes *4195*
Schistosoma haematobium 307, 327, 1202–3
Schistosoma intercalatum 1203
Schistosoma japonicum 315, 1202–3
Schistosoma mansoni, renal toxicity *4086*
Schistosoma mekongi 1203
schistosomal nephropathy 4087, *4088*
schistosomiasis 1202, *1385*
clinical features 1202, 1205
cercarial dermatitis/ swimmer's itch 1205
hepatic granuloma 2518
intestinal schistosomiasis 1206, *1206–8*
nervous system involvement 1208
pulmonary manifestations 1208, *1208*
renal disease 1208, 4087
stage of maturation 1205, *1205*
urinary schistosomiasis *1205*, *1206*, 4121
diagnosis 1202
diagnosis and investigations 1209
direct parasitological methods 1209
immunodiagnosis 1209
indirect methods 1209
ultrasonography 1209
geographical distribution *1203*
haematological changes 4553
parasite life cycle 1203, *1204*
pathophysiology/ pathogenesis 1209
pregnancy *2171*
prevention and control 1202, 1211
prognosis 1202, 1210
renal involvement 4075

transmission and epidemiology 1210, *1211*
treatment 1202, 1210
schizencephaly 5144, *5144*
schizophrenia 5324
  aetiology 5324
  clinical features 5324
  differential diagnosis 5324
  management 5325, *5325*
  prognosis 5325
Schmidt's syndrome 1999
Schober test 3609
Schwachman-Diamond syndrome 2573
schwannomin 366
Sciates sulcatus 1235
sciatic nerve neuropathy 5084
sciatica 3574
  management 3245
science in medicine 9
scimitar syndrome 2860, *2861*
scintigraphy
  adrenal *1878*
  pulmonary arterial hypertension *2985*
  rheumatic disorders 3565, *3565*
scleroderma renal crisis 3900
scleroderma *277*, *3650*, *3666*, *4642*
  clinical features *3667–8*, 3668
    bacterial overgrowth *2332*
    en coup de sabre *3666–7*
    generalized morphoea *3667*
    linear *3666–7*
    plaque morphoea *3667*
    skin lesions 3672
  differential diagnosis *3668*
  epidemiology 3668
  genetics 3666
  localized 4646, *4646–7*
  pathogenesis *3667*
  pregnancy 2162
    effect of disease on pregnancy 2162
    effect of pregnancy on disease 2162
    management 2162
  solvent-induced 1382
  see also systemic sclerosis
sclerosing cholangitis, primary 2468, *2469*
  aetiology 2469
    cellular immune abnormalities 2470
    exposure to bacterial components 2470
    humoral immune abnormalities 2469
    immunogenetic factors 2469
  clinical features 2470
  diagnosis *2469*, 2470, *2471*
  disease associations 2471, *2471*
  natural history and prognosis 2472
  pathological features 2470, *2471*
  small duct 2471
  treatment 2472
sclerosteosis *3721*, 3760
scoliosis 3505, *3506*
  causes *3506*
  hypercapnia 3507
  investigations 3507
  Marfan's syndrome *3750–1*
  pathophysiology 3506
  prognosis 3507
  sleep apnoea 3506
  symptoms and physical signs 3507
  treatment 3508, *3508*
Scolopendra spp. (Thai centipede) *1356*
scombrotoxins 1346
scopolamine, poisoning 1361
Scopulariopsis brevicaulis 1002
scorpion bites 2560
scorpion stings 1351, *1352–3*
  clinical features 1352
  epidemiology 1351
  prevention 1352
  treatment 1353
screening 81, 90–1
  acceptability 100
  adults 105
    cancers 105
  antenatal 101, *102*, 2087
  breast cancer 105, *106*, 1930, *1930*
  children 105
  coeliac disease 2341
  contraindications 94
  coronary heart disease 2894, *2895*
  criteria for 94
  cystic fibrosis 3358
  definition 95
  diabetes mellitus 1991, *1991*
  diabetic retinopathy *106*, 5237, *5237*
  facilities 100
  financial considerations 100
  gestational diabetes 2135, *2135*
  HIV/AIDS 621
  hypothyroidism 107, *1837*
  inborn errors of metabolism 1556
  incidentalomas 108
  indications 94
  lung cancer 3531
  malnutrition 1508, *1536*
  multiple endocrine neoplasia 1983, 1985
  neonatal 104, 101
  non-malignant diseases *106*, 107
  performance *107*
  prostate cancer 105, 4168
  proteinuria 3848, *3848*
  renal disease 3847
    drug-induced 3848
    employment/insurance 3848
    families 3848
    population and risk group 3847
    secondary care 3848
  requirements 95, *100*, *101*
    disorder 95
    natural history 95
    prevalence/incidence 95
    remedy 95
    screening test 95
  risk factors *100*
  STIs 1248
  tautological 95, 107
  terminology 107
  test performance 96, *96*
    detection rate 96, *96*
    detection rate cannot be determined 100
    false-positive rate 96, *96*
    odds of being affected if result positive 96, *98–9*
  Wilson's disease 1692
scrofuloderma *4674*
scrub typhus 919
  aetiology and epidemiology 903, 919, *919–21*
  clinical features 920, *921–2*
  diagnosis 921
  pathology/pathogenesis 920
  prevention and control 923
  treatment 921
scurvy 1488–9, 3767
Scytalidium dimidiatum 1002
Scytalidium hyalinum 1002
scytalidium infections 1002
sea snakes 1335
sea urchin envenoming 1348, *1348*
Seadornaviruses 556
seafoods, in pregnancy 2090
seal finger 958
sebaceous adenoma 4705
sebaceous gland disorders *see* acne
sebaceous hyperplasia 4705
seborrhoeic dermatitis, scalp 4702
seborrhoeic eczema 4624
seborrhoeic keratosis *385*, 4705, *4706*
second messengers 1460
secondary prevention 89
secretin 2318
  inhibition *2320*
Securidacea longepedunculata (violet tree), nephrotoxicity *4093*
sedation
  colonoscopy 2211
  critical illness 3153
  hazards of 3154, *3155*
sedatives, reproductive effects *1917*
sedimentation rate *4196*
Segawa's syndrome *see* guanosine triphosphate cyclohydrolase deficiency
SeHCAT test 2229
seizures
  acute porphyria 1649
  folinic acid-responsive *1566*, 1589
  pyridoxine-dependent 5103
  see also epilepsy
selective IgA deficiency 2249
  aetiology 2249
  clinical features 2249
    gastrointestinal 2249, *2249*
  definition 2249
  management 2249
selective oestrogen receptor modulators (SERMs)
  breast cancer
    prevention 1929
    treatment *1937*
  hyperparathyroidism 1859
selective serotonin reuptake inhibitors 5312
  vertigo *4861*
selegiline
  drug interactions *1471*
  poisoning 1282
Selemonas spp. *962*
selenium *1498*, 1500
  clinical applications 1500
  deficiency syndromes 1500
  dietary reference values *1502*
  optimal intake 1501
  reference values *5445*
  sepsis and critical care 1501
  toxicity 1501
selenocysteine 1500
Selenomonas spp. 2261
self-harm 1274
  suicide notes 1274
Semacarpum anacardium (marking nut) 1372
  nephrotoxicity *4093*
SEN virus 615
senile squalor (Diogenes) syndrome 5408
senna *5426*
sensory input 4787
sensory neuronopathy 5172, *5173*
Seoul virus *581*
Sepik virus *566*
sepsis syndromes *421*
sepsis 3859
  acute renal trauma 3894
  child mortality *75*
  clinical features, jaundice 2450
  post-liver transplantation 2509
  prevention of complications 418
  puerperal 2169
  treatment 417
    antibiotics 417
    drotrecogin alfa 417
    goal-directed resuscitation 417
    mechanical ventilation 418
    recombinant human activated protein C 417
    source control 417
  see also infections
Septata intestinalis 2357
septic arthritis 698, *700*, 3617
septic bursitis 698, *700*
septic shock
  meningitis 716, *716–17*
  presentation 5501
  see also sepsis
septic vasculitis 4631
septicaemia 4545
  H. influenzae 760
  meningococcal *see* meningococcal septicaemia
  pneumococcal 691
septo-optic dysplasia 5145
SERCA2, 2616, 2618
serine deficiency, differential diagnosis *1725*
serine proteases, COPD *3323*
serine proteinases *3551*
serine/threonine kinase 1788
seronegative arthritides, neurological complications 5160
seronegative arthropathies
  cardiac involvement 2784, *2784*
  oesophageal symptoms *2297*
serositis, and rheumatoid arthritis 3588
serotonin antagonists, Raynaud's phenomenon *3671*
serotonin reuptake inhibitors (SSRIs)
  drug interactions *1471*, 5331
  poisoning 1281
serotonin reuptake inhibitors 5331, *5331*
  adverse effects 5331
  indications and use 5331
SERPINA1, alleles of *1781*
serpinopathies 1780
Serratia spp. *962*
  antibiotic sensitivity *446*
sertraline
  adverse effects *5313*
  poisoning 1281
serum amyloid A protein *1753*, 1759

acute pancreatitis 2557
serum-ascites albumin
gradient 2485, *2486*
Sever's disease *3804*
severe combined immunodeficiency
(SCID) 236, *238, 249, 2250*
blood lymphocyte profile *251*
clinical features 249
diagnosis 250
gene therapy 251
immunological and molecular
classification 250
lymphocyte phenotyping *251*
MHC class I deficiency 252
treatment and prognosis 251
sex determination 1966
sex headache 4921
sex hormone binding globulin 1790
sex hormones, and cancer *307*, 310
sex-hormone binding protein,
reference values *5441*
sexual activity, in heart failure 2721
sexual arousal disorders 1946
sexual assaults 5366
sexual aversion disorders 1946
sexual behaviour 1250
age at first heterosexual
intercourse 1250
heterosexual partners 1251
homosexual lifestyles 1250–1
risk reduction strategies 1252
sexual desire disorders 1946
sexual development disorders 1967
assessment 1973
causes *1968*
classification of 1967, *1967–8*
examination 1973
investigations 1973, *1973–4*
management 1974
sex chromosomes 1967
46,XX 1968
46,XY 1969
sexual differentiation 1963
fetal sex development 1963,
1963–6
sexual dysfunction 1942
female 1942, *1945, 1946*
orgasmic disorders 1947
sexual arousal disorders 1946
sexual aversion disorders 1946
sexual desire disorders 1946
sexual pain disorders 1947
male 1942
drug-induced *1943*
erectile dysfunction 1927,
1942, *1942*
penile deformity/Peyronie's
disease 1943
priapism 1944, *1944–5*
rapid (premature)
ejaculation 1945
sexual health promotion 1252
sexual history 1253, *1254*
sexual orientation 1250, 1966
sexual pain disorders 1947, *1947*
sexually transmitted infections
and contraception 1263
developed countries 1244
developing countries 1247
epidemiology 1243
examination 1254
chaperones 1254
extragenital symptoms *1254*
incidence 1243, *1244*
interactions with HIV 1248, *1248*
presenting symptoms *1254*
prevention
primary 1248
secondary 1248
risk factors 1244
screening 1248
sexual behaviour 1250
sexual history 1253
transmission of 1243
travellers 467
vaginal discharge 1256
see also individual conditions
Sezary syndrome 4333
shale oils *1380*
Shaver's disease 3424
shawl sign 3694
shear stress 2598
Sheehan's syndrome
pregnancy 2141
snake bite 1336
sheep bile, renal toxicity 4092
shellfish allergy 263
shellfish poisoning
amnesic 1346
paralytic 1346
Shewanella spp. *962*
Shigella dysenteriae 2429
renal toxicity *4086*
Shigella flexneri 186
Shigella spp. *962*
Shigella 727, 731
clinical features 732
control 732
epidemiology 731
laboratory diagnosis 732
pathogenesis 732
treatment 732
shock
anaphylactic
presentation 5465
see also anaphylaxis
cardiogenic 3122, 3127
distributive 3122, 3128
hypovolaemic 3122, 3127
obstructive 3122, 3128
pathophysiology 3122, 3126
snake bite 1352
Shokwe virus *581*
Shone's syndrome 2851
short intestine, congenital 2402
short QT syndrome 2715
short stature *see* growth disorders
short Synacthen test 1804, *5449*
short-bowel syndrome 2221
shoulder
pain *3248, 3557*
rheumatoid arthritis 3588
Shprintzen-Goldberg syndrome 3778
shrews, envenoming 1328
shrinking lung syndrome 3392
Shulman's syndrome 4646
Shuni virus *581*
shunt nephritis 4072
shunts
anatomical 3196
ascites 2489
peritoneovenous 2489
transjugular intrahepatic
portosystemic (TIPS) 2489
Shwachman-Diamond
syndrome 4296
Shy-Drager syndrome 2639, 3260,
3270
gut peptides 2322
SIADH 3522
sialadenitis 2282
sialic acid storage disorders 5123
sialidosis 1698, 5122
type 1 5102
sialoproteins 3726, *3729*
sibutramine 1533
in renal failure 4182
Sicilian virus *581*, 586
sick building syndrome 1388
sick sinus syndrome 2639, *2688,
2692, 2692–3*
sickle cell crisis 5506
sickle cell disease 3711, 4687
antenatal screening *102*
hepatic involvement 2541
jaundice 2449
pregnancy 2176
renal involvement 4069
clinical syndromes 4070
medullary 4069
reproductive effects *1917*
sickle cells *4195*
sickle retinopathy 5245
sickling haemoglobinopathies 4437,
4437, 5245
clinical features 4438
complications 4438, *4438*
chronic 4439, *4439*
control and management 4440
course and prognosis 4440
distribution 4438
laboratory diagnosis 4440, *4440*
pathogenesis 4437, *4438*
sideroblastic anaemia *4446–7*
acquired idiopathic *4447*, 4448
hereditary 4446, *4447–8*
sideroblasts, ringed 4259–60
siderocytes *4195*
siderosis 3424
CNS 5157
sigmoidoscopy
flexible 2211
ulcerative colitis 2375, *2375*
see also colonoscopy
signal transduction 169, *348*
and autoimmunity 269
cell surface receptors 169
genetic defects *1798*
growth factor receptors *348*
integration 170
ion channel activation 169
nuclear receptors 169
robustness 170
sensitivity 170
spatial resolution 170
T-cell receptors 285, *288*
temporal resolution 170
signalling pathways 170
G-protein coupled-receptors 169,
171
Hedgehog 172
Notch 170, 176
Toll-like receptors 169, 175
transforming growth factor β
superfamily 175
tyrosine kinase-dependent 174
Wnt 169, 171
sildenafil *2598*, 2988
drug interactions *1471*
pulmonary arterial
hypertension 2988
silent mutations 138
silhouette sign *3210*
silica, carcinogenesis *308*
silicon *1498*, 1501
silicosis 1377, 3417
aetiology and pathology 3417,
3418
clinical features 3418, *3419–20*
prevention and
management 3419
silver, reference values *5445*
Simkania spp. *962*
Simulidae (blackflies) *1226*
Simulium spp. *1226*
simvastatin 1670
Sin Nombre virus *581*
Sindbis virus *558*, 559
Sinding-Larsen-Johansson
disease *3804*
single nucleotide polymorphisms
(SNPs) 154, 140
single photon emission computed
tomography *see* SPECT
sinoatrial disease *see* sick sinus
syndrome
sinoatrial node 2604, *2609*, 2619,
2619
sinus arrest *2693*
sinus histiocytosis with massive
lymphadenopathy 4362
clinical features 4364
management 4366
sinus of Valsalva, aneurysm 2858
sinus tachycardia 2641
sinus venosus 2853
sinusitis 3227, 3230
Siphunculina funicola (oriental eye
fly) 1236
Siphunculina funicola 1236
Sipple's syndrome 1984, 3745
sirolimus *1939*
post-transplantation *3954*
transplantation *290*, 292, *2730*
sitagliptin 2017
Sitophilus spp. 1236
situs inversus, atrial *2845*
situs solitus, atrial *2845*
sixth disease 497
Sjögren's syndrome *277, 3650*, 3688
aetiology and pathology 3689
clinical features 3689
systemic 3689, *3690*
diagnosis 3690, *3690–1*
future developments 3692
hepatic involvement 2545
historical perspective 3689
neurological complications 5160
oesophageal symptoms *2297*
prevalence *3650*
prognosis 3691
pulmonary involvement *3390*, 3392
renal involvement 4053
treatment 3691
Sjögren-Larsson syndrome 1724,
4597, 5109
skeletal disorders *see* bone
disease; musculoskeletal
disorders
skeletal dysplasias 1956, 3720, 3757
clinical features 3758
mutations in *3757*
see also individual conditions
skeletal growth 3548
skeletal hyperphosphatasia,
expansile *3721*

skeletal muscle *see* muscle
skin biopsy 4592
  polymyositis/dermatomyositis 3697
skin cancer 322
  aetiology, HPV 605
  incidence *301*
  melanoma *see* melanoma
skin disorders
  adverse drug reactions 4724
  amoebiasis 1040
  distribution 4587, *4588*
  eczema *see* eczema
  examination 4587
  history taking 4587, *4588*
  infections 4672
    bacterial 4673
    ectoparasites 4675
    fungal 4675
    tuberculosis 4674, *4674*
    viral 4675
    see also individual infections
  inherited 4593
    ectodermal dysplasias 4600
    epidermolysis bullosa 4594, *4595*
    ichthyoses 4596
    keratodermas 4598
  investigations 4592
    biopsy 4592
    immunofluorescence tests 4592
    skin scrapings 4592
    Woods light examination 4592
  lesion shape and grouping 4589, *4591*
  management 4731
    antiandrogens 4739
    antifungal agents 4735, 4739
    antimalarial agents 4739
    antimicrobials 4738
    antipruritics 4732
    antiseptics 4734
    antivirals 4739
    biological treatments 4738
    complementary medicines 4736
    compliance and adherence 4731
    corticosteroids 4733, *4734*
    cryotherapy 4737
    immunosuppressants and cytotoxics 4737
    keratolytics 4733
    moisturizers 4732, *4732*
    photodynamic therapy 4737
    phototherapy 4736
    preparations *see* dermatological vehicles
    sunscreens 4735, *4735*
    tars 4733
  morphology 4588, *4588, 4591*
  occupational 1381
    contact dermatitis 1381
    employees' and employers' attitudes to 1381
    nondermatitic dermatoses 1382
    protection against 1381
  onchocerciasis 1148, *1148–9*
  papulosquamous disease 4610
  photosensitivity 4665
  pigmentation 4656
  pregnancy 2149
    atopic eczema 2153
    autoimmune dermatoses 2153
    cutaneous infections 2150
    hair changes 2149
    pigmentary changes and lesions 2149, *2150*
    pilosebaceous changes 2149
    pregnancy dermatoses 2150, *2150*
    psoriasis 2153
    striae gravidarum 2150
    vascular changes and lesions 2149, *2150*
  site of 4588, *4589–90*
  skin failure 4739
  SLE 3658, *3658*
  symmetry 4587
  systemic diseases 4715
    see also relevant diseases
  terminology *4591*
  vesiculobullous disease 4602
  see also individual disorders
skin lesions
  leprosy 839
  poisoned patients 1278
skin prick tests 2254, *3280, 3281*
skin protection 1381
skin tags 4705
skin tumours 4705
  benign 4705
    melanocytic 4706
    nonmelanocytic 4705
  malignant 4708
    melanocytic 4710
    nonmelanocytic 4708
  metastases 4713, *4713*
  premalignant lesions 4707
    Bowen's disease 4707
    solar keratosis 4707
  see also individual tumours
skin 4583, *4584*
  commensal flora 749
  cystic fibrosis 3363
  dermis
    failure of 4586
    structure 4584
  effects of malnutrition 1510
  epidermis
    failure of 4586
    structure 4583–4, *4593, 4594*
  failure of 4586
  functions of 4584, *4585*
  infections, anaerobic 752
  origin of 4583
  pigmentation 4656
  in pregnancy 2078, 2089
  renewal 4584
  in respiratory disease 3186
  structure 4583
    regional variations 4584, *4585*
skullcap 68
Slackia spp. *962*
slapped cheek disease 608
SLE *see* systemic lupus erythematosus
sleep apnoea
  central 3261, *3273, 3273*
  obstructive *see* obstructive sleep apnoea
  reflex 3275
  REM 3274
sleep disorders 4828, *4829*
  assessment 4836, *4836–7*
  hypersomnia 4830, *4830*
  insomnia 4829, *4830*
  narcolepsy *see* narcolepsy
  parasomnias 4834, *4834*
sleep paralysis 4831
sleep studies, COPD 3330
sleep
  at high altitude 1403
  blood pressure during 3030, 3048
  breathing during 3261, *3262*
  disorders of 3261
    obstructive sleep apnoea 3263
  NREM 3261, *3262*
  periodic leg movements 3269
  REM 3261, *3262*
  sudden unexplained death during 3840
slim disease 2357
slow loris, envenoming 1328
slow-channel syndrome 163
Sly's disease 1698
small airways disease 3321, *3321–2*
small intestine
  absorption 2203
    salt and water *2208*
  anatomy 2201, 2220
  atresia/stenosis 2398
    duodenal obstruction 2399
    jejunoileal obstruction 2399, *2399*
  bacterial flora 2330, *2330*
    drugs metabolized by *2331*
  bacterial overgrowth 2330, 2356
    associated clinical conditions 2331, *2332*
    clinical features *2330*, 2331
    diagnosis 2333, *2333*
    endogenous factors preventing *2331*
    management 2334, *2334*
    mechanisms 2331
  cancers 2405
  common variable immunodeficiency 2247
  endoscopy 2216
  function of 2203
  ischaemia 2223
  lesions of *4407*, 4411
  lymphangiectasia 2400
  malrotation 2400
  pathology 2220
    see also individual conditions
  radiology 2219
  resection 2354
    aetiology and prevention 2354, *2355*
    bacterial overgrowth 2356
    future directions 2356
    management 2355
    metabolic consequences 2354
    pathophysiology 2354
    physiology 2354
  tumours of 2222
    adenocarcinoma 2222, *2222*
    carcinoid 2222
    lymphoma 2222, *2222*
smallpox 1442, *510–11*
  clinical features *510–11*
  eradication of 510
  mortality *121*
Smithies, Oliver 191
Smith-Lemli-Opitz syndrome 1572
Smith-Magenis syndrome 145, *148*
smoke inhalation 3258
smoker's keratosis *2285*
smoking cessation, COPD 3333, *3333*
smoking
  and blood pressure 3049
  and cancer 304, *304–5*
    bladder cancer 328
    lung cancer 299, *3515*, 3515
  and COPD 3313, *3314*
  and coronary heart disease 2888
  diabetic patients 2010
  and heart failure 2721
  mortality rate from smoking-related diseases 75
  passive 3314, 3516
  and peptic ulcer disease 2308
  in pregnancy 2090
smooth muscle, tumours 507
smouldering multiple myeloma 4345
snake bites *1324, 1327*, 1327, 4541
  biting apparatus 1329
  classification of snakes 1327
    Atractaspididae 1327, *1328*
    Colubridae 1327, *1327*
    Elapidae 1328, *1329–30*
    Viperidae 1328, *1331–2*
  clinical features 1346, *1334*, 4091
    Atractaspididae 1333
    Colubridae 1333
    Elapidae 1333, *1334–5*
    European vipers 1336
    sea snakes and kraits 1335
    Viperidae 1335, *1335–6*
  distribution 1327
  epidemiology 1328
  immunization 1330
  immunodiagnosis 1337
  incidence/importance 1328, *1332*
  interval between bite and death 1343
  laboratory investigations 1337
  management 1337
    antivenom 1339
    first aid 1337, *1338*
    haemostatic defects 1332
    hospital treatment 1339
    hypotension and shock 1342
    intracompartmental syndrome and fasciotomy 1328
    local envenoming 1342
    local infection 1353
    neurotoxic envenoming 1342
    oliguria and renal failure 1352
    pressure-immobilization 1338, *1338*
    supportive treatment 1342
    venom ophthalmia 1353
  pathophysiology 1331, *1333*
  prevention of bites 1329
snake venom
  properties 1330
    pharmacology 1331
    polypeptide toxins 1331
  renal toxicity 4090, *4091*
Sneathia spp. *962*
sneezing 3170
snowshoe hare virus 580, *581*
sodium benzoate 1565
sodium bicarbonate
  drug interactions *1471*
  hyperkalaemia *3891*
  metabolic acidosis 1749
sodium calcium edetate *1274*
sodium channels 160

sodium cromoglicate
allergic rhinitis 3282
asthma 3304
food allergy 2255
sodium fusidate *706*
bacteraemia *703*
endocarditis *704*
infective endocarditis *2818*
sodium homeostasis disorders 3817
hypernatraemia 3818, 3826
hyponatraemia 3817, 3819
sodium nitrite *1274*
sodium nitroprusside 3130
hypertensive emergencies *3080*
sodium oxybate, narcolepsy *4833*
sodium phenylacetate 1565
sodium potassium citrate, calcium stone prevention *4130*
sodium stibogluconate, leishmaniasis *1138*, *1139*
sodium tetradecyl sulphate, peptic ulcer disease 2312
sodium thiosulphate *1274*
sodium urate nephropathy, chronic 1625
sodium valproate 5334
adverse effects 5335
hepatotoxicity *2529*, *2534*
in breast milk *1469*, *2189*
diabetic neuropathy 2039
dose levels *4823*
drug interactions 5335
epilepsy 4821
indications and use 5335
migraine prevention *4916*
poisoning 1281
serum levels *5449*
teratogenicity *1468*, 2148, *2187*, *4822*
vertigo *4861*
sodium
dietary reference values *1502*
fractional excretion *3896*
reference intake *1524*
reference values *5435*, *5446*
children *5438*
renal reabsorption 3812
urinary *3837*
acute renal trauma 3892
prerenal failure *3896*
sodoku 858–9, 872
sodum oxybate
cataplexy *4833*
narcolepsy *4833*
sleep disturbance *4833*
soft tissue, infections, anaerobic 752
Sokoluk virus *566*
sokosha 858–9
solar keratosis 4707
solar lentigo 4706
solar urticaria 4670, *4671*
Soldado virus *581*
Solenodon (Apotogale) cubanus 1327
Solenodon paradoxus 1327
solenodons, envenoming 1328
Solenopsis spp. (American fire ants) 1350
solid organs, stem cell generation 202
solute diuresis 3830
solvent drag 2327
solvents 1382
somatic cell nuclear transfer 199
somatosensory cortex 4787
somatosensory-evoked potentials *4757*, 4757
somatostatin analogues 1981
somatostatin 1992, *2320*, *2443*
inhibitory actions *2320*
reference values *5442*
somatostatinoma 1980
treatment 1982
somatotrophs *1801*
soots *1380*
sorafenib 401, *1939*
hepatocellular carcinoma 2517
sotalol *2701*
Sotos syndrome 145, 1957
South American haemorrhagic fever *593*
clinical features 593, *593*
diagnosis/differential diagnosis 594
epidemiology 589
treatment 595
South-East Asian ovalocytosis 4467
Southern elephant seal virus *558*
Sox 3549, *3549*
Spaniopsis spp. *1226*
Spanish fly 1351
sparfloxacin *706*
sparganosis 1200, *1200–1*, 1240
spatial neglect 4791
specific granule deficiency 4310
SPECT
ECG-gated 2673, *2674*
epilepsy 4819
spectinomycin, gonorrhoea 726
spectrin 2606, *2607*
Spelotrema brevicaeca 1223
sperm autoimmunity 1924
spermatogenesis 1916
spermicides *26*
spherocytosis *4195*
hereditary 4452, 4462
aetiology and pathogenesis 4462
classification *4463*
clinical features 4462, *4462–3*
complications 4463
diagnosis 4464, *4464–5*
differential diagnosis *4465*, 4465
inheritance 4463
treatment 4465
sphincter of Oddi 2438, *2438*
dyskinesia 2560, *2560*
Sphingobacterium spiritivorum 3436
Sphingobacterium spp. *962*
sphingolipidoses *1553*, 5117
sphingolipids 1654
Sphingomonas spp. *962*
sphingomyelin 1654
spider bites 1325, 1353, *1353–4*
epidemiology 1353
facies latrodectismica 1355, *1355*
necrotic araneism 1354, *1354*, 1355
neurotoxic araneism 1355, *1355*
treatment 1355
spider naevi 4691
cirrhosis 2498, *2498*
pregnancy 2149
Spielmeyer-Sjögren Batten disease 1698
spina bifida occulta 5137
spina bifida 5137
antenatal screening *102*
spinal accessory nerve disorders 5038
spinal cord compression 389, *389*
spinal cord diseases 5039, *5041–2*
aetiology and pathogenesis 5040, *5041*
clinical features 5040, *5042*
clinical investigation 5042
diagnostic criteria 5043
differential diagnosis 5042
treatment and prognosis 5044
spinal cord injuries 5047, 5065, *5065*
epidemiology 5046
functional outcome *5048*
long-term issues 5052
discharge home 5052
driving 5053
emotional problems 5052
employment 5053
fertility 5053
leisure pursuits 5053
medical problems 5053
sexual life 5052
magnetic brain stimulation 4784
management 5046, *5048*
spinal cord injury centre 5048
steroids 5048
surgical vs conservative 5047
presentation 5491
problems in 5048, *5049*
autonomic dysreflexia 5050
bladder disorders 5049
bowel care 5050
deep venous thrombosis 5051
heterotopic ossification 5050
pain and dysaesthesia 5051
pressure sores 5049
respiratory 5049
spasticity and contractures 5050
rehabilitation 5051, *5051*
reproductive effects *1917*
spinal disorders 3505
ankylosing spondylitis *see* ankylosing spondylitis
kyphosis 3508
osteoarthritis *3634*
scoliosis 3505, *3506*
straight-back syndrome 3509
spinal fusion 3508
spinal manipulation 65, 70
spinal muscular atrophy 5123
proximal of childhood 5072
adult-onset form 5073
intermediate form 5072
Kugelberg-Welander disease 5072
Werdnig-Hoffmann disease 5072
spindle checkpoint genes 343
spiramycin, toxoplasmosis *1096*
Spirillum minus 857, 859, 872, 1326
Spirillum spp. *962*
spiritual healing 65
Spirobolus (giant Papua New Guinea millipede) *1357*
Spirocerca lupi 1176
spirometry 3192
airways obstruction 3256, *3256*
COPD 3328, *3328*
spironolactone
adverse effects
gynaecomastia 2068
hepatotoxicity *2532*
ascites 2487
heart failure 2723
polycystic ovary syndrome 1910
reproductive effects *1917*
skin disorders 4739
spleen 4334
abcess 4338
blood flow 4335
cysts 4339
functions 4335, 4339, *4339–40*
blood pool 4336
cell sequestration, phagocytosis and pooling 4335
haemopoiesis 4335
immune function 4336
plasma volume 4336
history 4334
injury 4338
in malaria 1063, 1080
relapsing fever *869*
structure 4334, *4335*
tumours 4338
splenectomy
clinical complications 4341
indications 4340, *4341*
splenic hypoplasia/atrophy 4339
splenic infarction 4339
splenomegaly 4336, 4501, 4515
causes 4337, *4337*
Gaucher's disease 1703
infective endocarditis *2810*
investigation 4336
nontropical idiopathic 4338
storage disease 4338
tropical splenomegaly syndrome 4338
splinter haemorrhage, infective endocarditis *2809*
Spondweni virus *566*
spondylitis, brucellar *792*, 794
spondyloarthritides 3603
clinical features *3605–6*
definitions 3604
diagnosis 3605
differential diagnosis 3606, *3606–7*
epidemiology 3604, *3604–5*
HLA-B27 association *3605*
pathogenesis 3604, *3605*
prevalence *3604*
prognosis 3607
see also individual conditions
spondyloarthritis, undifferentiated 3603, 3610
clinical features 3611
definition 3610
diagnosis 3611
epidemiology 3611
prognosis 3611
treatment 3611
spondyloepiphyseal dysplasia congenita 3759
spondyloepiphyseal dysplasia tarda (X-linked) *3721*, 3758
mutations in *3757*
spondyloepiphyseal dysplasias *3721*, 3758
spondylolisthesis, Marfan's syndrome *3750*
spondylolysis *3248*
Sporobolomyces spp. *3436*
Sporothrix schenckii 1007
osteomyelitis *3789*
sporotrichosis 999, 1007

aetiology 1007
clinical features 1007, *1007*
epidemiology 1007
systemic 1012
treatment 1008
sports medicine 5375
drugs and ergogenic aids 5383
female athlete triad 5376, *5376–7*
fitness to exercise 5381
medical complications 5379
overtraining syndrome 5378
overuse injuries 5382, *5382*
sprue
hypogammaglobulinaemic 2248
tropical 2358–9, 4412
sputum 3177
clearance 3350
lung cancer 3524
squamous cell carcinoma antigen, reference values *5442*
squamous cell carcinoma 4709, *4710*
oesophagus 2300, *2301*
ST elevation myocardial infarction *see* STEMI
St John's wort 68
drug intractions *69*
St Louis encephalitis virus 565, *566*, 569
ST segment 2649
staircase phenomenon 2624
stanazolol, vibration injury 1435
stannosis 3424, *3424*
stanozolol, adverse effects, hepatotoxicity *2533*
Staphyloccus epidermidis 1256
staphylococcal scalded skin syndrome 4740
staphylococci 693
antimicrobial resistance 694
clinical features 695
coagulase-negative 704
epidemiology 694
microbiology 694
molecular genetics 694
pathogenesis 694
prevention 695
regulation and virulence determinants 694
Staphylococcus aureus 801, 807, *852*, 1256
antibiotic sensitivity *446*
CA-MRSA 695
clinical features 695
clinical syndromes 695
bacteraemia 702, *703*
endocarditis 702, *703–4*
epidural abscess 700, *702*
food-borne illness 696
furuncles and carbuncles 697, *698*
impetigo, folliculitis and cellulitis 696, *697*
mastitis 698
osteomyelitis 699, *701*
pneumonia 701, *702, 3232*
pyomyositis 698, *699*
scalded skin syndrome 696, *696*
septic arthritis 698, *700*
septic bursitis 698, *700*
toxic shock syndrome 696, *697*
urinary tract infections 701, *702*
colonization 694
cystic fibrosis 3355
epidemiology 694
health care-associated MRSA 694
HIV-associated infection *3247*
infective endocarditis *2812*, 2815
methicillin-resistant *see* MRSA
osteomyelitis *3789*
pneumonia 3231, 3235
community-acquired *453*
prevention 695
risk factors 695
secular trends and morbidity 695
treatment *3238, 3245*
vancomycin-resistant *see* VRSA
Staphylococcus epidermidis 4672
Staphylococcus lugdunensis 708
Staphylococcus saprophyticus 708, 4672
Staphylococcus spp. *962*
infective endocarditis 2815
osteomyelitis *3789*
staphylokinase, pulmonary embolism 3016
starfish envenoming 1348, *1348*
Stargardt disease, genetics *139*
startle disease (hyperekplexia) 162, 166
starvation ketoacidosis *1742*
static magnetic fields 1432
statins 1670, 2041
adverse effects
hepatotoxicity 2531
renal toxicity *3860*
contraindication in porphyria *5484*
drug interactions *1471, 3968*
heart failure 2724
limb ischaemia 2962
NNT *52*
osteonecrosis 3803
in renal failure 4181
stroke prevention 4942
status epilepticus 4823
acute porphyria 1649
presentation 5490
stavudine
HIV/AIDS *638*
mode of action *444*
steakhouse syndrome 2302
steatocystoma multiplex 4600
steatohepatitis, nonalcoholic *1666*, 2474, *2481*
clinical presentation 2480
epidemiology 2480
investigation 2481
management 2482
liver transplantation 2507
natural history 2480
steatorrhoea 2331
steatosis, drug-induced 2534, *2534*
Steel factor 4201
Steele-Richardson-Olszewski syndrome 4807, 4886
Stellantchasmus amplicaecus 1222
stem cells 193, *336–7*, 4199
barriers to progress 189
and cancer 340, *340–1*
as cellular immunomodulators 202
as cellular vehicles 202
disease modelling and drug discovery 202, *203*
embryonic *see* embryonic stem cells
endogenous repair 202
expansion of numbers 199
cardiac tissue 200
donor cell developmental stage 199
nervous tissue 200
pancreatic tissue 200
function of 4201, *4202*
history 195, *197*
identification of source 199
pluripotent *4202*, 4203, *4205*
progenitors 4201, *4202*
solid organ transplantation 202
sources *194*
target conditions 193, 195
therapeutic applications *196*, 197, *198*
validation of functional recovery 200
overcoming immune rejection 201
reproducibility and scale 201
route/location of delivery 201
survival, engraftment and connectivity 200
STEMI 2643, *2654–5*, 2924
complications 2929
arrhythmias 2930
cardiogenic shock 2929
failure of reperfusion 2929
left ventricular dysfunction and heart failure 2930
left ventricular thrombus 2931
pericarditis 2931
ventricular septal defect, papillary muscle rupture and myocardial rupture 2930
continuing management 2927, *2927*, 2931
coronary artery bypass surgery 2929
percutaneous coronary intervention 2927
thrombolytic treatment 2928
coronary bypass 2943
diagnostic problems
late presentation 2657
left bundle branch block 2657
noninfarct causes of ST segment elevation 2656
pre-excitation 2657
'stuttering' infarction 2656
T wave inversion 2657, *2658*
differential diagnosis 2926
ECG 2653–4
old infarction 2657, *2657*
outcome 2924
pharmacological interventions 2932, *2932*
antiarrhythmics 2933
anticoagulants 2932
calcium antagonists 2933
hormone replacement therapy 2932
prehospital care 2925, 2931
presentation 5456, *5457–8*
secondary prevention 2931
triage and management 2926, *2926*, 2931
Stenotrophomonas spp. *962*
stents 2937, 2948
drug-eluting 2938
metal 2937, *2937–8*
thrombosis 2940
stercoral ulcers 2588
stereoisomerism 1462
sterile pyuria 3866
sterilization (contraceptive) *1265*
heart disease patients 2115
sternum
disorders of 3509
congenital abnormalities 3509
see also individual disorders
steroids, NNT *52*
Stevens, Leroy 189
Stevens-Johnson syndrome 4586, 4728, 4739
Stewart-Treves syndrome 4696
Stickler's syndrome *3721*
mutations in *3757*
Stictodora fuscata 1222
Stictodora lari 1222
stiff person syndrome *276*, 4900, 5174
Still's disease
adult 3705, *3706*
IL-6 in 157
stings 5499
ants 1349
beetle 1351, *1351*
butterfly 1351
caterpillar 1351
fish 1325, 1344, *1344–5*
hymenoptera 1349, *1349*, 1350, 3108
renal toxicity 4092
moth 1351, *1351*
scorpion 1351, *1352–3*
Stokes-Adams attacks 2690, 2694
see also atrioventricular block
stomach cancer 314, 2408
clinical features 2409
diagnosis 2409
incidence *301*, 2408,
migrants vs residents *302*, 315
management 2409, *2409*
mortality *314*
pathology 2409
predisposing factors 2408, 2409
stomach
anatomy 2201
bacterial flora *2330*
common variable immunodeficiency 2247
function of 2203
stomatitis
herpetic *439*
measles-related 520, *522*
stomatocytosis 4467, *4467*
hereditary 4452
Stomolophus nomurai (Chinese jellyfish) 1347
Stomoxys calcitrans *1226, 1233*
stop codons 138
strabismus, phenytoin poisoning 1275
Strachan's syndrome 5089
straight-back syndrome 3509
Stratford virus *566*
streptobacillary rat-bite fever 858
aetiology 858
clinical features 858
Streptobacillus moniliformis 857–8, 1326
Streptobacillus spp. *962*
streptococci 670
classification 671
group A 670
see also Streptococcus pyogenes
group B 670

see also Streptococcus agalactiae
group C 676
group G 676
pyogenic 671
infective endocarditis 2815
viridans, infective endocarditis 2815
Streptococcus adjacens 671
Streptococcus agalactiae 675, 1256
carriage 675
infections caused by 676
in adults 676
neonatal infection 676
puerperal infection 676
laboratory diagnosis 676
pathogenicity, virulence and typing 675
prevention 676
puerperal sepsis 2169
treatment 676
Streptococcus anginosus 677
Streptococcus bovis 677
infective endocarditis *2812*, 2815
Streptococcus constellatus 677
Streptococcus defectivus 671
Streptococcus faecalis 671
Streptococcus faecium 671
Streptococcus intermedius 677
Streptococcus milleri 677
Streptococcus mitis 677
Streptococcus morbillorum, infective endocarditis 2815
Streptococcus mutans 677, 2257
Streptococcus pneumoniae 677, 680
antibiotic sensitivity *446*
community-acquired pneumonia *453*
HIV-associated infection *3247*
infective endocarditis 2815
osteomyelitis *3789*
pneumonia 3231, *3232*
treatment *3238*
Streptococcus pyogenes 671, 807
antibiotic sensitivity *446*
carriage 671
infections caused by 672
bacteraemia 674, *674*
perianal infection 672
pericarditis 674, *675*
pharyngitis 672, *672*
puerperal and neonatal infection 674
scarlet fever 672
skin and soft tissue infections 673, *673*
toxic shock syndrome 674, *674*
vulvovaginitis 673
laboratory investigations 674
management 675
pathogenicity, virulence and typing 671
pneumonia 3231
puerperal sepsis 2169
Streptococcus salivarius 677
Streptococcus sanguis 677, 2257
Streptococcus spp. *962*
infective endocarditis 2815
osteomyelitis *3789*
Streptococcus suis 677, *678*
streptokinase, pulmonary embolism 3016
Streptomyces albus *3436*
Streptomyces somaliensis 1004
Streptomyces spp. *962*
osteomyelitis *3789*
streptomycin
brucellosis 794
Madura foot 1005
in renal failure *4185*
S. moniliformis 859
toxicity 826
tuberculosis *825*
dose *826*
uses *3798*
streptozotocin, adverse effects, hepatotoxicity *2529*, *2532*
stress echocardiography 2669, *2670*
angina 2906
stress testing, myocardial perfusion imaging 2672
stress 5288
and blood pressure 3031
occupational 1387, *1387*
and peptic ulcer disease 2308
stressors 5288
striae gravidarum 2150
stridor 3186–7
lung cancer 3518
stroke prevention, clinical trials 30
stroke work 2621
stroke 3036, 4933
causes *4938*
classification 4938
clinical trials 43, *43*
cognitive impairment 5276
diabetes mellitus 2044
diagnosis 4937, *4939*, *4945*
echocardiography 2666, *2667*
epidemiology 4935
fetal and postnatal effects 2899
and hypertension 3081
imaging *4771*, 4771, *4772*
mortality rate *76*
NIH stroke scale *5489*
nutrition-related 1519
outcome *4939*
pregnancy 2147
presentation 5487
secondary prevention 4941
anticoagulants 4942
antihypertensive drugs 4942
antiplatelet agents 4942
carotid endarterectomy 4941
statins 4942
and SLE 5159
syndromes 4939, *4940*
thrombolysis *5489*
treatment 4940
anticoagulants 4941
antiplatelet agents 4941
neuroprotective agents 4941
stroke units vs general wards 4940
surgical decompression 4941
thrombolysis 4941
Strongyloides fuelleborni 1165
Strongyloides stercoralis 1163, *2357*
immunocompromised host 431
pathogenesis and life cycle 1163
see also strongyloidiasis
strongyloidiasis 1163, 1240
clinical features 1164, *1164*
diagnosis 1164
epidemiology 1163
HIV-associated infection *3247*
immunocompromised patients 3959
treatment and prevention 1164
strontium ranelate, osteoporosis *3799*, 3800
struvite stones *4124*, 4131
stupor 4842
Sturge-Weber syndrome 5099
'stuttering' infarction 2656
subacromial impingement *3248*
subacute sclerosing panencephalitis 5011
measles-related 522
subaortic stenosis *2844*, 2851
subarachnoid haemorrhage 4946
causes 4946, *4946*
diagnosis *4946*, 4947
presentation 5490
treatment 4947
subclavian vein cannulation 5510, *5511*
subcortical dementia 4807
subcutaneous drug administration 1452
subdural empyema *4780*, 4780
subdural haematoma, chronic 4807
sublingual drug administration 1452
submersion injury 1397
subsistence crises 82
substance abuse 5271
substituted judgement 19
succimer *1274*
succinic semialdehyde dehydrogenase deficiency 1592
psychiatric signs *1720*
Succinivibrio spp. *962*
sucralfate, peptic ulcer disease 2311
sucrase-isomaltase deficiency 2350
sudden death in sport 5381, *5381*
cardiac screening 5381
prevention 5382
sudden death syndrome 5364, *5365*
sudden infant death 5363
Sudeck's atrophy 4688
suicidal intent 5293, *5294*
suicide
attempted 5292
alcohol and drug abusers 5295
arrival at hospital 5293
care after 5294
children and adolescents 5295
clinical services 5295
coping resources and supports 5294
elderly patients 5295
medical care 5293
psychosocial assessment 5293, *5294*
risk of repetition 5294, *5295*
mortality rate *76*
risk of 5311
sulbactam *706*
bacteraemia *703*
cellulitis, mastitis and pyomyositis *699*
endocarditis *704*
epidural abscess *702*
osteomyelitis *701*
pneumonia *702*
toxic shock syndrome *697*
urinary tract infection *702*
sulfadiazine, nocardiosis 857
sulfafurazole, nocardiosis 857
sulfamethoxazole, pharmacokinetics *449*
sulfapyridine, skin disorders 4739
sulfasalazine
ankylosing spondylitis 3611
psoriatic arthritis 3613
reproductive effects *1917*
sulfinpyrazone, stroke prevention 30
sulindac
adverse effects, hepatotoxicity *2532*
and asthma *3289*
rheumatoid arthritis *3594*
sulphadiazine
adverse effects, hepatotoxicity *2532*
paracoccidioidomycosis 1028
sulphaemoglobinaemia 4444
sulphasalazine
adverse effects, hepatotoxicity *2535*
pregnancy *2158*
ulcerative colitis 2378, *2380*, *2380*
sulphinpyrazone, gout 1625
sulphonamides
adverse effects
hepatotoxicity *2529*, *2532*, *2535*
renal toxicity *3860*
in breast milk *2189*
contraindication in porphyria 1641, *5484*
mode of action *443*
pregnancy *2172*
uses *3798*
sulphones, adverse effects, hepatotoxicity *2533*
sulphonylureas 2014
adverse effects 2015
contraindication in porphyria 1641
efficacy and potency 2015
and hypoglycaemia 2057
indications and contraindications 2015
mode of action 2014
pharmacokinetics 2015
sulphsalazine, rheumatoid arthritis *3595*
sulphur dioxide poisoning 1315
sulphur *1498*, 1501
sulphuric acid *1739*
carcinogenesis *308*
sulpiride
adverse effects, hyperprolactinaemia 2068
schizophrenia *5325*
sumatriptan
drug interactions *1471*
migraine *4917–18*
summer penile syndrome 1229
sun protection factor 4735, *4735*
SUNCT/SUNA 4921
sunitinib 401, *1939*
sunscreens 4735, *4735*
Supella longipalpa (banded cockroach) 1236
superior mesenteric artery syndrome 2422
superior vena cava, anomalies 2859, *2859–60*
superior vena cavography 3205, *3205–6*
superoxide anion 2598
superoxide 2599–600
supravalval stenosis *2844*

supraventricular tachycardias 2689, 2706
atrioventricular nodal re-entry tachycardia 2707, *2707–8*
atrioventricular re-entry tachycardia 2708, *2708–9*
sural nerve neuropathy 5085
suramin
adverse reactions *1125*
trypanosomiasis 648,*1125*
surfactant metabolism dysfunction 4, 1698
surfactant 3180, *3180*
ARDS 3142, 3180
impaired activity 3180
surgery
abdominal aortic aneurysm 2965
adrenalectomy 1878
anterior pituitary gland 1805
aortic dissection 2957
bariatric 1534, 2010
duodenal switch 1534
gastric banding 1534
gastric bypass 1534
cancer 388
breast 1933, *1934*
lung 3525, *3527–8*, 3530
cardiac, in pregnancy 2110
congenital adrenal hyperplasia 1893, *1894*
in COPD 3341
coronary bypass *see* coronary artery bypass surgery
Crohn's disease 2367
diabetic patients 2023
gastrointestinal bypass 2540
Graves' disease 1841
infective endocarditis 2820
limb ischaemia 2963
neurosurgery, DVT prevention *3007*
oesophageal cancer 2406
older patients 5390, 5396
antibiotic prophylaxis 5397
choice of anaesthetic 5397
postoperative management 5397
preoperative assessment 5396
orthopaedic, DVT prevention *3007*
osteoarthritis 3635
osteomyelitis 3793
pancreatic tumours 2577
parathyroidectomy 1859, 3923
peptic ulcer 2314
thoracic, video-assisted 3224, *3225*
tonsillectomy 3229
ulcerative colitis 2380
sustainability 74
Sutterella spp. *962*
Suttonella spp. *962*
suxamethonium
apnoea *1472*
hydrolysis 1474
swallowing, difficulty in *see* dysphagia
swan-neck deformity 3587
sweat glands
apocrine, disorders of 4676
in cystic fibrosis 3354
eccrine, disorders of 4677
Sweet's syndrome *3707*, 4634, *4634*
swimmer's itch 1202, 1205
swimming pool/fish tank granuloma 833, *833*
Swyer's syndrome 1906, *1967, 1969, 2766*
Sydenham, Thomas 10
Sydenham's chorea 2801, 4895
treatment 2804
syk 158
sympathoadrenal system 2618
sympathomimetics, in renal failure 4180
Symphoromyia spp. *1226*
Synanceja verrucosa 1345
synaptic potentials 161
syncope 2636, 4838
assessment 2639
cardiac *2637*, 2639
bradycardia *2638*, 2639
structural cardiovascular disease *2638*, 2639
tachycardia *2638*, 2639
cerebrovascular *2638*, 2639
clinical features 4839, *4840*
clinical investigations 4840
definition 2636
differential diagnosis 2637, *2637, 4816, 4840, 4840*
epidemiology 4839
history 2640
family history 2640
preceding symptoms 2640
provocative factors 2640
recovery period 2640
syncopal episode 2640
investigation 2640
ambulatory monitoring 2640
ECG 2640
electrophysiological 2640
tilt testing 2638, *2638*, 2640
neurally mediated 2637, *2638, 2692, 5066–7*, 5067
carotid sinus hypersensitivity 2638
situational reflex-mediated syncope 2638
vasovagal syncope 2638
orthostatic hypotension 2638, *2638*
pathogenesis 4838, *4838*
prognosis 2637
psychogenic *2638*, 2639
treatment 2641
treatment and prognosis 4841
syndrome of apparent mineralocorticoid excess 3072
syndrome of inappropriate antidiuresis (SIAD) *1819*, 1823, *2062*, 2062
causes *1824*
treatment 1823
types of *1824*
syndrome of inappropriate diuresis 3825, *3825*
syndrome of inappropriate secretion of antidiuretic hormone *see* SIADH
syndrome X *see* metabolic syndrome
synercid, in renal failure *4185*
synovial (osteo-)chondromatosis 3713
synovial fluid 3551
analysis 3561
crystal identification 3561, *3562*
Gram stain and culture 3561
macroscopic appearance 3561, *3561*
synovial haemangioma 3713
synovial sarcoma, translocations *341*
synovitis, pigmented villonodular 3712
synovium 3550
disorders of 3712
Syphacia spp. *1176*
syphilis 885, *1245, 1246*
aetiology and genetics 886
cardiovascular 2826
clinical features 891
clinical presentation 2826, *2827*
diagnosis 893, 2828, *2828*
differential diagnosis 892
and HIV infection 2828
laboratory investigation 2828
medical treatment 2828
pathogenesis/pathology 2826
surgical treatment 2829, *2829*
clinical features 887
infective oesophagitis *2293*
oral 2269
clinical investigation 892
direct detection 892, *892*
nonspecific tests 892, *893*
serology 892, *893*
specific tests 893
congenital
antenatal screening *102*
clinical features 891, *891*
diagnosis 894
diagnosis 885, 893
differential diagnosis 891
endemic *880*, 882
diagnosis 883
differential diagnosis 883
prevention/control 884
treatment 883
epidemiology 886
future developments 895
gummatous (late benign)
clinical features 890, *891*
diagnosis 893
differential diagnosis 892
history 885
HIV infection 895
incidence *1246*
latent
clinical features 888
diagnosis 893
differential diagnosis 892
lumbar puncture in 895
neurosyphilis *see* neurosyphilis
pathogenesis/pathology 886
pregnancy 2170
prevention 885, 887
primary
clinical features 887, *887–8*
diagnosis 893
differential diagnosis 891
prognosis 895
renal involvement 4075
risk factors 1244
secondary
clinical features 888, *889–90*
diagnosis 893
differential diagnosis 891
tertiary, clinical features 888, *890*
treatment 885, *894, 894*
choice of antibiotics 894
contacts 894
follow up 894
Jarisch-Herxheimer reaction 895
venereal 879
syringomyelia 5138
Syrphidae *1233*
systematic reviews 23, *50, 51*
systemic availability 1451, *1455, 1456*
systemic inflammatory diseases, renal involvement 3859, *3859*
systemic inflammatory response syndrome 416
systemic lupus erythematosus *277, 3650*, 3652, *5158, 5159*
aetiology and pathology 3654, *3654*
apoptosis and complement 3655
B lymphocytes and auto-antibodies 3654, *3654*
cytokines 3653, 3656
histopathology 3656, *3656*
T lymphocytes 3655
classification *3653*
clinical features 3654, 3657
cardiovascular involve-ment 2783, *2783–4*, 3659
constitutional symptoms 3657
cutaneous and mucosal involvement 3658, *3658*
gastrointestinal involvement 3659
GI tract 2421
haematological involvement 3659
musculoskeletal involvement 3657, *3658*
neuropsychiatric involvement 3659
ocular 5243
oesophageal symptoms *2297*
renal involvement 3658, *3659*
respiratory involvement 3659
cognitive impairment 5281
complement deficiency 218, 222
controversies 3663
diagnosis 3653, 3661
differential diagnosis 3660
drug-induced 3714
epidemiology 3656
future prospects 3663
genetics *143*
haematological changes 4553
hepatic involvement 2544
historical perspective 3653
investigations 3653, 3660
autoantibodies *3654*, 3660
disease activity and end-organ damage 3661
management 3653, *3661*, 3661
biologic therapies 3662
drug side effects 3662
immunosuppression 3662
neonatal syndromes 2157
neurological complications 5159
diagnosis 5159
management 5159
occupational and psychological aspects 3663
pregnancy 2154–5, 3663
effect of disease on pregnancy 2155
effect of pregnancy on disease 2155
management 2155, *2156*
prevalence *3650*
prognosis 3653, 3663

pulmonary involvement *3390*, 3392
pleural effusion 3491
renal involvement *see* lupus nephritis
and stroke 5159
systemic sclerosis 3665, *3666*, 3675, 3900
aetiology and genetics 3666, *3667*
autoimmune serology 3670, *3670*
clinical features 3665
cardiac involvement 2783, *2783–4*, 3674
diffuse cutaneous 3669, *3666*, *3669*
GI tract 2421, *2421*
limited cutaneous *3666*, 3669, *3669*
oesophagus *2297*, 2298
overlap syndromes *3666*, 3670
pulmonary involvement 3388, *3390*
sine scleroderma *3666*, 3670
complications 3665
cardiac 3674, *3675*
gastrointestinal 3676, *3676*
macrovascular disease 3671
musculoskeletal 3676
organ-based *3670*, 3671
pulmonary disease 3672
renal disease 3675
respiratory tract *3672*
skin lesions 3672
cutaneous 4642
aetiology and genetics 4642
clinical features 4643, *4643*
CREST syndrome 4643, *4643–4*
diffuse 4644, *4645*
epidemiology 4643
pathogenesis/pathology 4642
future developments 3678
management 3665, *3670*, *3677*
neurological complications 5160
pathogenesis/pathology 3666, *3667*
prevalence *3650*
prognosis 3665, 3677
renal involvement 4050
clinical presentation 4051
diagnosis 4051
pathogenesis 4050
pathology 4051, *4051*
prognosis 4051
treatment 4051
see also Raynaud's phenomenon; scleroderma
systemic vasculitis *see* vasculitides
systolic pressure *2621*

T cells 287
activation 283, *286*
allorecognition 283
antigen recognition 225, *226*
in cancer 378
combined T/B cell deficiency *238*
costimulation molecules *287*
cytokines regulating 157
cytotoxic 186, 287
depletion 293
diagnostics 233
disorders of 235
effector functions 230
CD4+ 231
CD8+ 230
homing 230
proliferation 230
modulation by antibodies 378
naive *229*, 229
natural killer 210
regulatory *see* Tregs
rheumatoid arthritis 3585
SLE 3655
therapy 234
tolerance 232
T wave 2645, 2649
inversion 2657
T53, 358
Tabanidae (horse flies and clegs) *1226*
Tabanus spp. *1226*
taboos 117, *117*
Tacaiuma virus *581*
TACE 158
tachycardia-bradycardia syndrome 2691–2
tachycardias 2688, 2696
antidromic 2708, *2708–9*
atrial 2706, *2706*
atrial fibrillation *see* atrial fibrillation
atrial flutter 2706, *2706*, *2714*
differential diagnosis 2697, *2698*
extrasystoles 2702
atrial 2702, *2703*
junctional 2703
ventricular 2703, *2703*
management 2698
acute 2698, *2699*
antiarrhythmic drugs 2700, *2700–1*
cardioversion 2700
implantable cardioverter-defibrillators 2701, *2702*
radiofrequency ablation 2702, *2702*
surgery 2702
mechanisms 2696, *2696*
automaticity 2696
re-entry 2697, *2697*
triggered activity 2697
narrow-complex 2697, *2698*
orthodromic 2708, *2708–9*
paroxysmal supraventricular 2641
pericardial tamponade 2794
pre-excitation syndromes 2689, 2708
atrial fibrillation 2709, *2710*
ventricular 2651, 2709
see also Wolff-Parkinson-White syndrome
presentation 5460, *5461*
sinus 2641
supraventricular 2689, 2706
atrioventricular nodal re-entry tachycardia 2707, *2707–8*
atrioventricular re-entry tachycardia 2708, *2708–9*
and syncope *2638*, 2639
ventricular *see* ventricular tachycardias
ventricular fibrillation 2690, *2714*, 2714
wide-complex 2697
tachykinins 2320
tacrolimus
adverse effects 3955, *3955*
post-transplantation 3482, *290*, *2730*, *3954*
liver *2511*
pregnancy *2158*
psoriasis 4614
TACTICS trial 2921
tadalafil 2988
Taenia asiatica *1190*, 1192
Taenia saginata 1189, *1190*, 1191
clinical features 1191, *1191*
control 1192
diagnosis 1191, *1191*
epidemiology 1191
geographical distribution 1191
treatment 1191
Taenia solium 1189, *1190*, *1192*, 1192
life cycle *1194*
see also cysticercosis
tafenoquine 1076
Tahyna virus 580, *581*
Takayasu's arteritis 2968, *2969*, *3650*, *4033*, 4633
aetiology and pathology 2969
clinical features 2970, *2970*
cardiac involvement *2783*, 2784
ocular involvement 5244
pulmonary involvement *3396*, 3401
diagnostic criteria 2972
differential diagnosis 2971
epidemiology 2970
historical perspective 2969, *2969*
investigation 2971, *2971*
prognosis 2973
renal involvement 4038, *4039*
treatment 4042
treatment 2972
talc pneumoconiosis 3423
talc *1380*
pleurodesis toxicity 3538
Tamdy virus *581*
Tamm-Horsfall protein 1626, 3866
tamoxifen
adverse effects, hepatotoxicity *2532*, *2533*
breast cancer *1937*
carcinogenesis *307*
clinical trials 39, *41*
hepatocellular carcinoma 2517
tanapox 512, *512*
tandem repeats 138
short (STR) 141
variable number of (VNTR) 141
Tangier disease 1657, 1671
Tannerella spp. *962*
tannic acid, adverse effects, hepatotoxicity *2529*
tanning (of skin) 4657, *4657*
tapeworms 1185
cyclophyllidian 1188
cystic hydatid disease 1185
cysticercosis 1193
diphyllobothriasis 1199
sparganosis 1200, *1200*
see also individual species
tardive dyskinesia 4887
target cells *4195*
target of rapamycin inhibitor *2730*, 2732
Taricha spp. 1346
tars 4733
tartrate-resistant acid phosphatase *3729*
reference values *5442*
Tarui's disease 1601, 4472, *1598*, *5215*, 5216
Tataguine virus *581*, 587
Tatumella spp. *962*
tau protein, reference values *5447*
taxanes 399
neuropathy 5088
taxins 1364
taxol, adverse effects *400*
Tay-Sachs disease 1698, *1553*, 1697, 3757
antenatal screening *102*
macular pigmentation 1704
tazarotene, psoriasis 4614
tazocin, in renal failure *4185*
TBOX 1, 252
T-cell costimulatory molecules 284
T-cell dependent immunity *see* cell-mediated immunity
T-cell lymphoma 507
T-cell prolymphocytic leukaemia 4227
T-cell receptors
diverse 227, *228*
recognition 226
signal transduction 285, *288*
tea tree (melaleuca) oil 4736
tectal deafness 4930
teicoplanin *706*
bacteraemia *703*
endocarditis *704*
infective endocarditis *2818*
mode of action *443*
pneumonia *3238*
in renal failure *4185*
spectrum of activity *446*
toxic shock syndrome *697*
telangiectasia 3672, *4690*, 4690
hereditary haemorrhagic *see* Osler-Rendu-Weber disease
primary 4691
secondary 4690
telavancin *706*
bacteraemia *703*
cellulitis, mastitis and pyomyositis *699*
telithromycin, adverse effects, hepatotoxicity *2529*
Telmatoscopus albipunctatus *1233*
telogen effluvium 4703
telomere 138
telomeric repeats 138
Tembusu virus *566*
temozolomide, cost-effectiveness ratio *53*
temporal arteritis 3679
aetiology 3680
clinical features 3680–1
cardiovascular and large artery 3681
cerebrovascular 3681
ophthalmological 3681
diagnosis and classification *3681–2*, 3682
differential diagnosis 3682, *3683*
epidemiology 3680, *3681*
historical perspective 3680
investigations 3682
pathology and immunology 3680
prognosis 3683
relationship to polymalgia rheumatica 3680
treatment 3682
temporal lobe syndromes 4794, 5274
temporomandibular joint disorders 2285
temsirolimus *1939*

tenascin-X 3772
Tenckhoff catheter 3944
tendinitis
  Achilles *3248*
  bicipital *3248*
  calcific *3248*
  rotator cuff *3248*
tendons 3551
  rupture, post-transplant 3964
  xanthoma 1660
Tenebrio molitor 1236
tennis elbow *3557*
tenofovir
  HIV/AIDS *638*
  mode of action *444*
  toxicity *640*
tenosynovitis 1383
  De Quervain's *3248*, *3557*
  digital flexor *3557*
tenoxicam, rheumatoid arthritis *3594*
Tensaw virus *581*
Tensilon test 1343
tension pneumothorax 3116, *3120*, 3487, 3501
  presentation 5467
tension-type headache 4917
teratocarcinomas 189
teratogenesis *1467*, *1468*, 2186, 2187, *2187*
  drug identification 2186
  prevention 2188
  thalidomide 2186
  see also individual drugs
teratozoospermia 1922
terbinafine
  fungal infections 1002, 1016
  NNT *52*
terbutaline, COPD *3335*
terconazole, candidiasis 1258
teriparatide, osteoporosis *3799*
terpenes *1362*
Terranova spp. *1176*
Terry's nail 4700
testicular agenesis *1917*
testicular cancer 326, 4163, 4171
  age distribution *326*
  histological subtypes 4171, *4171*
  incidence, migrants vs residents *302*
  mortality *327*
  presentation and diagnosis 4171
  risk factors 4171
  staging 4171, *4172*
  treatment 4171, *4172*
testicular failure *1960*
testicular feminization 1923
testicular torsion *1917*
testicular trauma *1917*
testicular tumours *1917*
  infertility 1923
testis 1913, *1914*
  development *1788*
  spermatogenesis 1916
  undescended *1917*, 1923, 1972
  vanishing 1973
testosterone replacement 1921
  older patients 1922
testosterone 1914
  actions *1791*
  physiological actions *1915*
  in polycyclic ovary syndrome 1908
  reference values *5441*
  signalling pathways *1797*
  synthesis *1915*
tetanus 795
  Ablett score *798*
  aetiology and genetics 795
  child mortality *75*
  clinical features 796, *796–8*
  differential diagnosis 798
  epidemiology 796
  history 795
  immunization *91*
  management *797*, 799
  pathogenesis and pathology 795
  presentation 5498
  prevention 796
  severity score *799*
tetrachloroethylene
  extrinsic allergic alveolitis *3436*
  hepatotoxicity *1385*
  poisoning 1316
tetracosactrin, gout 1624
tetracycline(s)
  adverse effects
    oesophagitis *2294*
    in pregnancy *2188*
  anaplasmosis 916
  animal-related injuries 1326
  aphthous ulcers 2272
  bacterial overgrowth *2334*
  chlamydial infections *943*
  gas gangrene 808
  H. influenzae 762
  H. pylori 2312, *2313*
  listeriosis 898
  malignant pleural effusion 391
  mode of action *443*
  mycoplasmal infections 959, *960*
  osteoarthritis 3636
  pharmacokinetics *449*
  pneumonia *3238*
  relapsing fevers 872
  S. moniliformis 859
  scrub typhus 921
  skin disorders 4738
  spectrum of activity *446*
  teratogenicity *1468*
tetracycline
  acne *4680*
  adverse effects, hepatotoxicity *2534*
Tetrameres fissispina *1176*
tetraploidy 145
tetrathio-molybdate, Wilson's disease *1692*
tetrodotoxin 1346, 2611
Th17 cells 157
Th2 cells 157
thalamic stroke syndrome 4930
thalamic syndromes 4930
thalamus 4877
  anatomy
    functional 4878, *4878*
    gross 4877
  cytoarchitecture 4878
  function/dysfunction 4879
thalassaemias 4424, *4425*
  definition and classification 4425, *4425*
  hepatic involvement 2541
  hereditary persistence of fetal haemoglobin 4431
  history 4424
  laboratory diagnosis 4435
  prenatal diagnosis 4436
  prevention 4435
  symptomatic treatment 4436
  thalassaemia intermedia 4434, *4435*
  α-thalassaemias 4431, *4434*
    differential diagnosis 4435
    distribution 4431, *4431*
    genotype-phenotype relationships 4432
    haemoglobin Bart's hydrops syndrome 4433, *4433*
    haemoglobin H disease 4434
    inheritance and molecular pathology 4431, *4432–4*
    intellectual disability 4434
    pathophysiology *4432*, 4433
    pregnancy 2176
  β-thalassaemias 4425
    antenatal screening *102*
    in association with haemoglobin variants 4429, *4430*
    distribution 4425, *4425*
    heterozygous 4429
    jaundice 2449
    major 2177
    minor 2177
    molecular pathology 4426, *4426*
    pathophysiology 4427, *4427*
    pregnancy 2176
    severe homozygous/compound heterozygous forms *4425*, 4427, *4428–9*
  $\delta\beta$-thalassaemias *4425*, 4431
  $\varepsilon\gamma\delta\beta$-thalassaemias 4431
thalidomide
  Behçet's disease 3687
  leprosy 846
  multiple myeloma 4350
  neuropathy 5088
  pregnancy *2172*
  sarcoidosis *3411*
  skin disorders 4738
  teratogenicity *1468*, 2186
thallium
  poisoning
    antidote *1274*
    peripheral nervous system effects *1387*, 5087
  reference values *5445*
thanatophoric dysplasia *3721*
  mutations in *3757*
Thaumetopoea processionea 1351
theatre sign 3632
Thelazia californiensis *1176*
Thelazia callipaeda *1176*
Thelotornis capensis 1327
Thelotornis kirtlandii (tree snake) 1327
T-helper cells 157
theophylline
  adverse effects *3336*
    oesophagitis *2294*
  asthma 3303
  COPD 3334
  drug interactions *1471*
  factors affecting plasma concentration *3337*
  mechanisms of action *3336*
  poisoning 1295
  serum levels *5449*
  therapeutic drug monitoring *1475*, 1476
therapeutic drug monitoring 1475
  ciclosporin *1475*, 1476
  digoxin 1475, *1475*
  gentamicin *1475*, 1476
  lithium 1475, *1475*
  phenytoin 1475, *1475*
  pregnancy 2190
  theophylline *1475*, 1476
therapeutic index 1450
therapeutic process 1462
therapeutic window 1455
Thermoactinomyces sacchari 3435, *3436*
Thermoactinomyces vulgaris 3435, *3436*
thermoregulation
  cold 1395
  heat 1393
Thevetia peruviana (yellow oleander) *1364*
thiamine 1488, 1491
  clinical aspects 1491
  deficiency 2144
    anaemia 4419
    neuropathy 5088
  dietary reference values *1502*
  reference values 5434
  requirements 1492
    in pregnancy 2082
thiazide diuretics
  hypertension 3050
  toxicity *3745*
thiazolidinediones 2016
Thibault, George 28
thin membrane nephropathy 3977
  aetiology, genetics and pathogenesis 3977
  clinical features 3978
  definition 3977
  differential diagnosis 3978
  pathology 3977, *3978*
  prognosis 3978
thiobendazole, adverse effects, hepatotoxicity *2533*
thioguanine, adverse effects, hepatotoxicity *2536*
thiopentone 3156
thiopurine, sensitivity *1472*
thioridazine
  adverse effects, hepatotoxicity *2532*
  poisoning *1274*
  schizophrenia *5325*
thioridizine, adverse effects, hepatotoxicity *2533*
thiotepa
  carcinogenesis *307*
  carcinomatous 'meningitis' 391
thiouracil, adverse effects, hepatotoxicity *2532*, *2533*
Thomsen's disease 164
Thomson, Jamie 191
thoracic actinomycoses 853, *853*
thoracic aortic dissection 2953
  aetiology 2954, *2954*, *2958*, 2958
    penetrating atherosclerotic ulcer 2958, *2958*
    spontaneous intramural haematoma 2958, *2958*
  classification 2954, *2954*
  clinical features 2955
  follow-up and prognosis 2957
  investigation 2955, *2956*
    blood tests 2955
    chest X-ray 2955, *2955*
    ECG 2955

imaging 2956, *2956–7*
management 2956
emergency 2956
surgery 2957
pathogenesis 2953, *2954*
thoracic cage, radiographic view 3207
thoracic cavity 3174
thoracic outlet syndromes 5080
thoracoplasty 3510, *3510*
thoracoscopy 3217, 3224
contraindications 3224
equipment 3224
indications 3224
lung cancer 3526
mesothelioma *3536*
patient preparation 3224
procedure 3224
sterilization 3224
therapeutic role 3224
video-assisted thoracic surgery 3224, *3225*
threadworms *see* enterobiasis
threonine proteinases 3551
thrombectomy 2939
distal protection 2939, *2939*
thrombin inhibitors 4539
acute coronary syndromes 2920
thrombin time *4196*, 4503
thrombin-activatable fibrinolytic inhibitor 4498
thromboangiitis obliterans 2960, 4687
thrombocythaemia 4515, *4516*
thrombocytopenia 4505, 4508
alcohol-induced 4515
alloimmune 2178, *4510*, 4512
autoimmune 4510
classification 4508, *4509*
destructive 4513
drug-induced 4512
gestational 2177
heparin-induced 4512, *4542*, 4542
history and physical examination 4509
idiopathic *276*
laboratory evaluation 4509
laboratory tests *4504*
liver disease 4506
malaria 1063
pregnancy 2177, *2177*
renal disease 4505
secondary immune 4511
sepsis and infection 4514
thrombocytosis 4280, *385*, 4515
essential thrombocythaemia 4282
normal megakaryocytopoiesis 4281
pathophysiology and classification 4281, 4282
secondary 4516
thromboembolic disease, nephrotic syndrome 3980
thromboembolism
drug-induced 3465
echocardiography 2669, *2669*
prevention of 2704, *2705*
β-thromboglobulin *4196*
thrombolysis
pulmonary embolism 3016
stroke 4941
thrombomodulin *4482*, *4490*, *4493*
thrombophilia
ocular involvement 5245
screening for 2117
thrombophlebitis
Behçet's disease *3685*
superficial 4689
thrombopoiesis 4508
thrombopoietin 4201, 4206
recombinant human 4207
thromboprophylaxis, pregnancy 2118, *2119*
thrombosis 4480
macrovascular 4542
mesenteric 2417
microvascular 4543
traveller's 1414
thrombotic microangiopathy 4076, 4544
thrombotic thrombocytopenic purpura 3862, 4460, 4513, 4527
classification *4513*
pregnancy 2178
thrush *1000*, 1002
thunderclap headache 4922
thymic aplasia *see* DiGeorge syndrome
thymic tolerance induction, incomplete 269
thymine 138
thymocyte associated and released chemokine 3279
thymoma 3541
with antibody deficiency *238*, 247
thymus
cysts 3541
lymphoma 3541
thyroglobulin, reference values *5442*
thyroid acropachy 1839, *1839*
thyroid cancer 1845, 328
follicular epithelial tumours 1845, *1846*
incidence *329*
lymphoma 1850
medullary carcinoma *1846*, 1849, *1849*
familial 366
nonepithelial tumours *1846*
pregnancy 2184
secondary tumours *1846*
cancer *see* thyroid cancer
causes 1831, *1831*
cognitive impairment 5280
destructive thyroiditis 1843
drug-induced 2067
goitre 1498, 1826, 1831
Graves' ophthalmopathy 5249, *5249*
haematological changes 4559
hyperthyroidism 2067
hypothyroidism 1826, 1833
and myasthenia 5217
neurological complications 5164
in pregnancy 2141, *2142*
hyperthyroidism 2141
hypothyroidism 2142
postpartum 2142
thyroid nodules 2142
skin involvement 4723
thyrotoxicosis 1826, 1837
thyroid failure 1667
thyroid follicular epithelial
tumours 1845, *1846*
aetiology 1845
anaplastic carcinoma 1848
clinical features 1846
diagnosis 1847
epidemiology 1846
follow-up 1848
pathology 1846, *1847*
in pregnancy 1849
prevention 1849
prognosis 1848, *1849*
treatment 1848
thyroid gland 1826
anatomy and histology 1827, *1827*
development *1788*, 1827
function 1830, 1830
non-thyroidal illness 1830
pregnancy 1830
regulation 1829
medullary carcinoma 1984
in pregnancy 2078
structure 1827
thyroid hormone
actions *1791*, 1829, *1829*
metabolism 1828, *1829*
resistance syndrome 1843
synthesis and secretion 1827, *1828*
transport 1828, *1828*
thyroid masses 3542
thyroid ophthalmopathy 5217
thyroid peroxisomal antibodies, reference values *5444*
thyroid replacement therapy 1848
thyroid stimulating hormone 1800, 1813
abnormal concentrations *1830*
deficiency 1813
excess, and follicular epithelial tumours 1845, *1846*
hypothyroidism 1836
inhibition *2320*
measurement 1803
thyrotropinoma 1813
thyroid storm *1842*
thyroid-binding globulin, reference values *5441*
thyroiditis 1843
acute 1843
atrophic 1834
Hashimoto's 1834–5, 1847
silent 1843
subacute (de Quervain's) 1843
thyroid-stimulating hormone
reference values *5441*
children *5438*
thyrotoxic crisis 5482
thyrotoxic periodic paralysis 3839, *3839*, 5217
thyrotoxicosis 1826, 1837
aetiology 1837, *1838*
amiodarone-induced 1843
areas of uncertainty 1842
clinical features 1838, *1838*
hypercalcaemia *3745*
myopathy 5216
ophthalmopathy *1839*
thyroid acropachy 1839, *1839*
CNS complications 5153
epidemiology 1837
and hypercalcaemia 1862
laboratory diagnosis 1839
pathogenesis 1837
pathology 1839
pregnancy 1842
prognosis 1842
reproductive effects *1917*
treatment 1840
thyrotrophs *1801*
thyrotropinoma 1813
diagnosis 1813
treatment 1813
thyroxine binding globulin 1790
thyroxine
in CKD 3909
levels in pregnancy 2090
poisoning 1296
uses *3798*
tiabendazole, adverse effects, hepatotoxicity *2532*
tiagabine
dose levels *4823*
epilepsy 4822
poisoning 1281
tibial nerve neuropathy 5084
tibolone 2198
ticarcillin, *Pseudomonas aeruginosa* 737
tick bites 1325, 1356
clinical features 1356
epidemiology 1356
taxonomy 1356
treatment 1356
tick-borne encephalitis *566*, 572, *573*, *5002*
vaccines *466*
tick-borne haemorrhagic fever 574
tick-borne relapsing fever 866
clinical features 870
epidemiology 867, *868*
prevention 873
treatment 872
tick-borne rickettsioses 904
tick-borne viruses 555
coltiviruses 555
orbiviruses 556
prevention 556
seadornaviruses 556
ticks 1225, *1228*, 1228
ticlopidine
acute coronary syndromes 2918
adverse effects, hepatotoxicity *2532*
stroke prevention 30
tics *4890*, 4897, *4897*
Gilles de la Tourette's syndrome 4897
Tietze's syndrome 3712
tigecycline *706*
cellulitis, mastitis and pyomyositis *699*
Till, James 195
tilt testing 2638, *2638*, 2640
tiludronate, Paget's disease 3744
time-varying elastance 3125, *3125*
TIMI 3B trial 2921
TIMPS 355, 3552
tinea capitis 998, 1000
tinea corporis 998, 1000
tinea cruris 1000
tinea imbricata 1001, *1001*
tinea nigra 1004
tinea pedis 998, 1000
tinea versicolor *see* pityriasis versicolor
Tinel's sign 3558
tinidazole
amoebiasis 1041
bacterial vaginosis 1257
giardiasis *1113*
trichomoniasis 1257
tinnitus 4869
tioconazole, fungal infections 1015

Tioman virus 526
tiotropium, COPD *3335*
tipranavir
 HIV/AIDS *638*
 mode of action *444*
 toxicity *640*
Tissierella spp. *962*
tissue distribution 1457
tissue factor pathway inhibitor
  protein 416, *4482, 4490,* 4494
tissue factor *4482, 4490, 4493*
 in microparticles 4496
tissue growth factor β 152, *212*
tissue necrosis 210
tissue plasminogen activator *4482,*
  4497
 pulmonary embolism 3016
tissue transglutaminase 2329, 2339
tissue-specific element 1788
titin 2606
Tityus serrulatus (South American
  scorpion) *1352*
TNF *see* tumour necrosis factor
TNF-receptor associated periodic
  syndrome *3709*
TNM staging system 387, *388*
tobacco use *see* smoking
tobacco-alcohol amblyopia 5157
tobramycin
 Pseudomonas aeruginosa 737
 spectrum of activity *446*
tocainide, adverse effects,
  hepatotoxicity *2535*
tocolytics, and pulmonary
  oedema 2123
tocopherols 1497
tokelau 1001, *1001*
tolazoline, vibration injury 1435
tolbutamide 2014
 adverse effects, hepato-
  toxicity *2532, 2533, 2535*
tolerance 1464
 metabolic 1464
 physiological 1464
 withdrawal 1464
tolfenamic acid, migraine *4917*
Toll-like receptors 152, 210, *210,* 398
 in autoimmunity 275
 in graft rejection 281
 TLR3, 211
 TLR4, 211
 TLR5, 211
 TLR9, 211
tolmetin, and asthma *3289*
tolnaftate 4735
Tolosa-Hunt syndrome 5034
toluene diamine,
  hepatotoxicity *1385*
toluene diisocyanate *3436*
toluene poisoning 1316
 CNS effects *1386*
tolvaptan *1824*
tongue
 cancer 312
 geographical *2285*
 glossitis 2284, *2284–5*
 see also mouth
tonsillectomy 3229
tonsillitis *see* pharyngitis/tonsillitis
tophaceous gout 3640, *3640*
topiramate
 dose levels *4823*
 epilepsy 4821
 migraine prevention *4916*
 poisoning 1281
 vertigo *4861*
torasemide, heart failure *2722*
Torpedo spp. 1325
Torpedo spp. 1325
torsades de pointes 2713
 acute management 2713
 aetiology 2713
 ECG characteristics 2713, *2713*
torticollis, spasmodic 4891, *4892*
Toscana virus *581,* 661
tositumomab, lymphoma *4320*
tositumomab-131, *376*
Tospovirus 581
total iron-binding capacity *4196*
total lung capacity 3174
 reduced *3192*
total parenteral nutrition
 and bone disease 3767
 hepatic involvement 2540, *2540*
 and hypercalcaemia *3745*
Tourette's syndrome 4897
Touton giant cells 4706
toxalbumins 1364
toxic epidermal necrolysis 4728, 4739
 SCORTEN system *4728*
toxic erythema 4726
toxic metabolite hypothesis 1561
toxic neuropathy 5087
toxic shock syndrome *421*
 staphylococcal 696, *697*
 streptococcal 674, *674*
toxins 2425
 amatoxins 1368, *1367, 1369*
 andromedotoxins 1364
 bioterrorism 1442
 botulinum 804, 1442
 cardiotoxins *1362,* 1363
 cicutoxin 1362
 ciguatera 1346
 Clostridium spp. 802, 807
 exotoxins 734
 gas gangrene 807
 oenanthotoxin 1362
 phoratoxin 1364
 sarafotoxins 1331
 scombrotoxins 1346
 tetrodotoxin 1346, 2611
 uraemic 3909
toxocariasis 1168, *1173, 1173*
 ocular larva migrans 1174
 visceral larva migrans 1173
Toxoplasma gondii 1091
 HIV-associated infection *3247*
 immunocompromised
  patients 3960
 see also toxoplasmosis
toxoplasmosis 1090
 aetiology 1091, *1091*
 areas of uncertainty 1097
 cerebral, HIV-related 630, *630*
 clinical features 1093
  congenital toxoplasmosis 1094
  immunocompetent
   patients 1093
  immunocompromised
   patients 1094
  ocular toxoplasmosis 1093
 congenital 5146
 epidemiology 1092, *1093–4*
 haematological changes 4552
 historical perspective 1091
 HIV patients 5017, *5017–20*
 pathogenesis 1092
 pathology 1092
 pregnancy *2167,* 2170, *2170*
 prevention 1093
 treatment 1095, *1096*
  choroidoretinitis 1095
  immunocompetent
   patients 1095, *1096*
  immunocompromised
   patients 1095
  maternal and fetal
   infection 1095
TP53 gene 349
Trabulsiella spp. *962*
trace elements 137, 1488
 dietary reference values *1502*
 in pregnancy 2082
 properties *1498*
 requirements 1539
 supplements 1503
 see also individual elements
trace metal disorders 1673
 haemochromatosis 1673
 Menkes' disease 1688
 Wilson's disease 1688
trachea 3175
 scabbard 3260
tracheal compression 3259, *3259*
tracheal intubation 3100
tracheal stenosis 3259, *3259*
tracheobronchial disease
 gases/aerosols 3457
 Sjögren's syndrome 3392
tracheobronchopathia
  osteochondroplastica 3260
tracheomalacia 3259
tracheo-oesophageal fistula 2396,
  2397
 clinical features 2396
 diagnosis 2397
 management 2397
tracheostomy 3136
 complications *3137*
 decannulation *3141*
 management in non-ICU
  setting 3137
 types of *3137*
*Trachipleistophora
  anthropophthera 1116*
Trachipleistophora hominis 1116
trachoma 939, 941, 5252
 clinical features 941, *941–2*
 diagnosis 942
 epidemiology 941
 treatment 942, *943*
traction lesions 5079
tramadol
 contraindication in
  porphyria *5484*
 drug interactions *1471*
trandolapril, heart failure *2722*
tranquillizers 5265, *5265*
 major 5265
 minor 5265
 patient care 5266
transcobolamine II deficiency *244*
transcription factors 154, 349
 retinoblastoma gene 349
 TP53 gene and p53 gene
  product 349
transcription 127
transferrin saturation, reference
  values *5435*
transferrin *4196*
 congenital deficiency 4394
β_1-transferrin, reference values *5444*
transforming growth factor β 175,
  2601
 Marfan's syndrome 3780, *3782*
transforming growth factor 1795,
  1796
transfusion-related acute lung
  injury 4568
transgenics 351
transient ischaemic attacks
 causes *4938*
 diagnosis 4936
 differential diagnosis 4816, 4937,
  4937
 imaging *4772–4*
 prognostic implications 4937
 types of 4936
transitions, genetic 135
translation 127
transoesophageal
  echocardiography 2667, *2667*
 aortic disease 2668, *2669*
 endocarditis 2668, *2669*
 patient selection 2668, *2668*
 thromboembolism 2669, *2669*
 valvular heart disease 2668
transparency 60
transplantation immunology 280
 ABO compatibility *290*
 chronic graft dysfunction *283*
 clinical perspective 280
 effector mechanisms 285
 immune response to transplanted
  tissue 280
 immunological memory 288
 immunosuppression 280, *290*
 rejection 280–1, *282*
  acute *283*
  hyperacute *283*
  innate immune system in 285,
   288
  role of graft in *284*
 T-cell allorecognition and
  activation 283
 terminology *281*
 tolerance 292, *293*
transplantation
 heart *see* cardiac transplantation
 kidney *see* renal transplantation
 lung *see* lung transplantation
transposition of great arteries 2860,
  2861
 arterial switch operation 2862
 congenitally corrected 2862, *2863*
  pregnancy 2114
 Mustard/Senning
  operations 2861, *2862*
 palliative surgery 2862
 pregnancy 2113
 Rastelli operation 2862, *2863*
trans-sulphuration defects 1592,
  1593
transthoracic
  echocardiography 2663
 abnormal left ventricular
  function 2666, *2666*
 atrial fibrillation 2666, *2666*
 congenital heart disease 2667
 infective endocarditis 2667
 left ventricular hypertrophy 2666
 pericardial disease 2667, *2667*
 post-stroke/embolism 2666, *2667*
 pulmonary embolism 2667
 valvular heart disease 2663